5/31/89 [illegible] III MD

217 428 5889

CANCER

Principles & Practice of Oncology

EDITED BY

Vincent T. DeVita, Jr., M.D.

Physician-in-Chief
Benno C. Schmidt Chair in Clinical Oncology
Memorial Sloan-Kettering Cancer Center
Professor of Medicine
Cornell University Medical College
Visiting Physician
The Rockefeller University Hospital
New York, New York

Samuel Hellman, M.D.

Dean and A. N. Pritzker Professor
Biological Sciences Division
and Pritzker School of Medicine
Vice President for the Medical Center
The University of Chicago
Chicago, Illinois

Steven A. Rosenberg, M.D., Ph.D.

Chief of Surgery
National Cancer Institute
Professor of Surgery
Uniformed Services University of the
Health Sciences School of Medicine
Bethesda, Maryland

161 Contributors

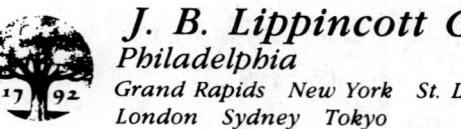

J. B. Lippincott Company
Philadelphia
Grand Rapids New York St. Louis San Fra
London Sydney Tokyo

CNCER

Prciples & Practice of ncology

3rd Edition

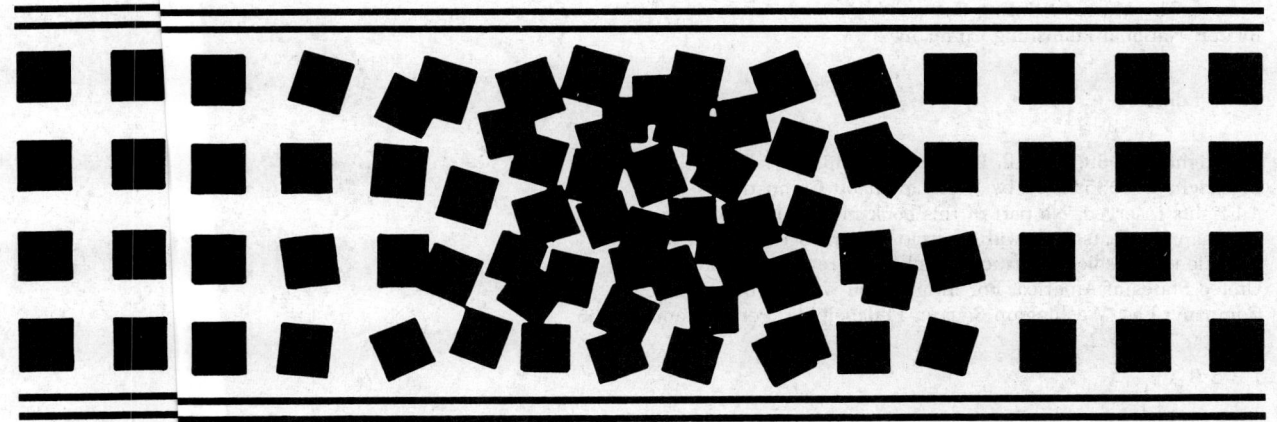

Sponsoring Editor: Richard Winters
Project Editor: Virginia Barishek
Indexer: Alexandra Weir Nickerson
Design Coordinator: Ellen C. Dawson
Production Manager: Carol A. Florence
Production Supervisor: Charlene Squibb
Production Assistant: Pamela Milcos
Compositor: Digitype, Inc.
Printer: The Murray Printing Company
Binder: National Publishing Company

Third Edition

1 3 5 6 4 2

Library of Congress Cataloging-in-Publication Data

Cancer : principles and practice of oncology.

Also issues in 2 v.
Includes bibliographies and index.
1. Cancer. 2. Oncology. I. DeVita, Vincent T. II. Hellman, Samuel. III. Rosenberg, Steven A. [DNLM: 1. Neoplasms. QZ 200 C21537]
RC261.C274 1989 616.99′4 89-2389
ISBN 0-397-50840-9 (1-vol. ed.)
ISBN 0-397-50843-3 (2-vol. ed. : set)

The authors and publisher have exerted every effort to ensure that drug selection and dosage set forth in this text are in accord with current recommendations and practice at the time of publication. However, in view of ongoing research, changes in government regulations, and the constant flow of information relating to drug therapy and drug reactions, the reader is urged to check the package insert for each drug for any change in indications and dosage and for added warnings and precautions. This is particularly important when the recommended agent is a new or infrequently employed drug.

Dedicated to

Mary Kay

Rusty

Alice

Contributors

Daniel A. Albert, M.D.
David G. Cogan Professor of Ophthalmology
Harvard Medical School
Surgeon in Ophthalmology
Director
David G. Cogan Eye Pathology Laboratory
Massachusetts Eye and Ear Infirmary
Boston, Massachusetts

Tom Anderson, M.D.
Professor of Medicine
Chief
Division of Hematology/Oncology
Medical College of Wisconsin
Milwaukee County Medical Complex
Milwaukee, Wisconsin

Karen H. Antman, M.D.
Associate Professor of Medicine
Harvard Medical School
Assistant Physician
Dana Farber Cancer Institute
Boston, Massachusetts

Ehud Arbit, M.D.
Associate Professor of Surgery
Cornell University Medical College
Attending Surgeon and Associate Member
Memorial Sloan-Kettering Cancer Center
New York, New York

Alan R. Baker, M.D.
Senior Investigator
Surgery Branch
National Cancer Institute
Bethesda, Maryland

Charles M. Balch, M.D.
Professor of Surgery
Head
Division of Surgery
University of Texas
M. D. Anderson Cancer Center
Houston, Texas

J. Andrew Billings, M.D.
Assistant Clinical Professor
Harvard Medical School
Assistant Physician
Massachusetts General Hospital
Boston, Massachusetts

Richard S. Bockman, M.D., Ph.D.
Associate Professor of Medicine
Endocrinology Division
Cornell University Medical College
Associate Attending
The Hospital for Special Surgery and New York Hospital
New York, New York

David G. Bragg, M.D.
Professor and Chairman
Department of Radiology
University of Utah School of Medicine
Senior Consultant
Veterans Administration Hospital
Salt Lake City, Utah

Murray F. Brennan, M.D., M.Ch., F.R.A.C.S.
Professor of Surgery
Cornell University Medical College
Alfred P. Sloan Professor and Chairman
Department of Surgery
Memorial Sloan-Kettering Cancer Center
New York, New York

Samuel Broder, M.D.
Director
National Cancer Institute
Bethesda, Maryland

Paul A. Bunn, Jr., M.D.
Director
University of Colorado Cancer Center
Head
Division of Medical Oncology
Professor of Medicine
University of Colorado
Health Sciences Center
University Hospital
Denver, Colorado

J. Robert Cassady, M.D.
Head
Department of Radiation Oncology
University of Arizona
Health Sciences Center
Tucson, Arizona

Nicholas J. Cassisi, D.D.S., M.D.
Professor and Chief
Division of Otolaryngology
Department of Surgery
University of Florida
Shands Hospital
Gainesville, Florida

Bruce A. Chabner, M.D.
Director
Division of Cancer Treatment
National Cancer Institute
Bethesda, Maryland

Alfred E. Chang, M.D.
Associate Professor of Surgery
Chief
Division of Surgical Oncology
University of Michigan Medical Center
Ann Arbor, Michigan

Richard Chang, M.D.
Assistant Professor of Radiology
Georgetown University
Washington, D.C.
Staff Radiologist
Diagnostic Radiology Department
National Institutes of Health
Bethesda, Maryland

Grace Christ, M.A., A.C.S.W.
Director
Program Planning and Project Pending
Department of Social Work
Memorial Hospital
New York, New York

John R. Clark, M.D.
Instructor in Medicine
Harvard Medical School
Clinical Associate in Medicine
Dana Farber Cancer Institute
Boston, Massachusetts

Alfred M. Cohen, M.D.
Associate Professor of Surgery
Cornell University Medical College
Chief
Colorectal Service
Department of Surgery
Memorial Sloan-Kettering Cancer Center
New York, New York

C. Norman Coleman, M.D.
Alvan T. and Viola D. Fuller American Cancer Society Professor
Harvard Medical School
Chairman
Joint Center for Radiation Therapy
Boston, Massachusetts

E. David Crawford, M.D.
Professor and Chairman
Division of Urology
University of Colorado
Health Sciences Center
Denver, Colorado

Joseph W. Cullen, M.D.
Deputy Director
Division of Cancer Prevention and Control
National Cancer Institute
Bethesda, Maryland

Michael Dean, Ph.D.
Program Resources Inc.
NCI–Frederick Cancer Research Facility
Frederick, Maryland

Albert B. Deisseroth, M.D., Ph.D.
Anderson Professor of Cancer Treatment and Research
Chairman
Department of Hematology
University of Texas
M.D. Anderson Cancer Center
Houston, Texas

Thomas F. Delaney, M.D.
Senior Investigator
Radiation Oncology Branch
National Cancer Institute
Bethesda, Maryland

Joel A. DeLisa, M.D.
Professor and Chairman
Department of Rehabilitation Medicine
U.M.D.N.J.–New Jersey Medical School
Medical Director and Chief Medical Officer
Kessler Institute for Rehabilitation
West Orange, New Jersey

Susan S. Devesa, Ph.D.
Epidemiology and Biostatistics Program
Division of Cancer Etiology
National Cancer Institute
Bethesda, Maryland

Sarah A. Donaldson, M.D.
Professor
Department of Radiation Oncology
Stanford University School of Medicine
Stanford University Hospital
Stanford, California

John L. Doppman, M.D.
Chief of Radiology
National Institutes of Health
Professor of Radiology
Georgetown University Medical School
Bethesda, Maryland

Patricia L. Duffey, B.S.N., R.N.
Chemotherapy Research Nurse
Biologic Response Modifier Program
Division of Cancer Treatment
National Cancer Institute
Bethesda, Maryland

John D. Earle, M.D.
Chairman
Division of Radiation Therapy
William H. Donner Professor of Oncology
Mayo Medical School
Rochester, Minnesota

Lawrence H. Einhorn, M.D.
Distinguished Professor of Medicine
Indiana University Medical Center
Department of Medicine
Distinguished Professor of Medicine
University Hospital
Indianapolis, Indiana

William R. Fair, M.D.
Chief
Urology Service
Memorial Sloan-Kettering Cancer Center
Professor of Surgery
Cornell University Medical College
New York Hospital
New York, New York

Geoffrey Falkson, M.B.Ch.B., M.Med.(Int.), M.D.
Professor and Head
Department of Medical Oncology
University of Pretoria
Pretoria, Republic of South Africa

Philip J. Fialkow, M.D.
Professor and Chairman
Department of Medicine
University of Washington
Physician-in-Chief
University Hospital
Seattle, Washington

Kathleen M. Foley, M.D.
Associate Professor of Neurology and Pharmacology
Cornell University Medical College
Chief
Pain Service
Department of Neurology
Attending Neurologist
Memorial Sloan-Kettering Cancer Center
New York, New York

Joseph F. Fraumeni, Jr., M.D.
Associate Director for Epidemiology and Biostatistics
National Cancer Institute
Bethesda, Maryland

Michael A. Friedman, M.D.
National Cancer Institute
Bethesda, Maryland

R. J. Michael Fry, M.D.
Head
Cancer Biology Section
Biology Division
Oak Ridge National Laboratory
Oak Ridge, Tennessee

Zvi Fuks, M.D.
Chairman
Department of Radiation Oncology
Memorial Sloan-Kettering Cancer Center
New York, New York

Lynn H. Gerber, M.D.
Associate Professor of Medicine
George Washington University
Washington, D.C.
Chief
Department of Rehabilitation Medicine
Warren Grant Magnuson Clinical Center
National Institutes of Health
Bethesda, Maryland

Roy Geronemus, M.D.
Assistant Professor of Dermatology
New York University Medical Center
New York, New York

Eli J. Glatstein, M.D.
Professor of Radiology
Uniformed Services University of Health Science
Chief
Radiation Oncology Branch
National Cancer Institute
Bethesda, Maryland

Richard J. Gralla, M.D.
Associate Professor of Medicine
Cornell University Medical College
Head
Section of Thoracic Surgery
Memorial Sloan-Kettering Cancer Center
New York, New York

Peter Greenwald, M.D., Dr.P.H.
Director
Division of Cancer Prevention and Control
National Cancer Institute
Bethesda, Maryland

Thomas W. Griffin, M.D.
Professor of Radiation Oncology
Chairman
Department of Radiation Oncology
Director
University Cancer Center
University of Washington
School of Medicine
Seattle, Washington

Jerome E. Groopman, M.D.
Associate Professor of Medicine
Harvard Medical School
Chief
Division of Hematology/Oncology
New England Deaconess Hospital
Boston, Massachusetts

Leonard L. Gunderson, M.D., M.S.
Professor of Oncology
Mayo Medical School
Consultant in Radiation Oncology
Mayo Clinic
Rochester, Minnesota

Philip H. Gutin, M.D.
Associate Professor
Departments of Neurological Surgery and Radiation Oncology
School of Medicine
University of California
San Francisco, California

H. Ric Harnsberger, M.D.
Associate Professor
ENT/Neuroradiology
University of Utah Medical Center
Cottonwood Hospital
Salt Lake City, Utah

Jay R. Harris, M.D.
Associate Professor
Harvard Medical School
Clinical/Educational Director
Joint Center for Radiation Therapy
Boston, Massachusetts

Daniel M. Hays, M.D.
Professor of Surgery and Pediatrics
University of Southern California
School of Medicine
Attending Physician and Surgeon
Departments of Surgery and Pediatrics
Children's Hospital of Los Angeles
Los Angeles, California

I. Craig Henderson, M.D.
Associate Professor of Medicine
Harvard Medical School
Medical Coordinator
Breast Evaluation Center
Dana Farber Cancer Center
Boston, Massachusetts

Alan D. Hillel, M.D.
Assistant Professor
Department of Otolaryngology/Head and Neck Surgery
University of Washington
Chief
Otolaryngology/Head and Neck Surgery
Veterans Administration Medical Center
Seattle, Washington

Jimmie C. Holland, M.D.
Professor
Department of Psychiatry
Cornell University Medical College
Chief
Psychiatry Service
Memorial Sloan-Kettering Cancer Center
New York, New York

Robert N. Hoover, M.D., Sc.D.
Chief
Environmental Epidemiology Branch
National Cancer Institute
Bethesda, Maryland

Marc E. Horowitz, M.D.
Senior Investigator
Pediatric Branch
National Cancer Institute
Clinical Center
National Institutes of Health
Bethesda, Maryland

William J. Hoskins, M.D.
Associate Professor of Obstetrics and Gynecology
Cornell University Medical College
Associate Chief
Gynecology Service
Memorial Sloan-Kettering Cancer Center
New York, New York

Alan N. Houghton, M.D.
Head
Laboratory of Solid Tumor Immunology
Cornell University Medical College
Head
Melanoma/Sarcoma Section
Department of Medical Oncology
Memorial Sloan-Kettering Cancer Center
New York, New York

Peter M. Howley, M.D.
Chief
Laboratory of Tumor Virus Biology
National Cancer Institute
Bethesda, Maryland

Susan M. Hubbard, R.N.
Associate Director
International Cancer Information Center
National Cancer Institute
Bethesda, Maryland

Daniel C. Ihde, M.D.
Professor of Medicine
Uniformed Services University of the Health Sciences
Head
Clinical Investigations Section
NCI–Navy Medical Oncology Branch
Naval Hospital
Bethesda, Maryland

Elaine S. Jaffe, M.D.
Chief
Hematopathology Section
Deputy Chief
Laboratory of Pathology
National Cancer Institute
Bethesda, Maryland

Robert T. Jensen, M.D.
Senior Investigator
Digestive Diseases Branch
National Institute of Diabetes, Digestive, and Kidney Diseases
National Institutes of Health
Bethesda, Maryland

David Kelsen, M.D.
Associate Professor of Medicine
Cornell University Medical College
Head
Gastrointestinal Section
Division of Medical Oncology
Memorial Sloan-Kettering Cancer Center
New York, New York

Nancy E. Kemeny, M.D.
Associate Professor of Clinical Medicine
Cornell University Medical College
Associate Attending
Memorial Sloan-Kettering Cancer Center
New York, New York

Leo J. Kinlen, M.B., B.S., D.Phil., F.R.C.P.
Director
CRC Cancer Epidemiology Unit
University of Edinburgh
Edinburgh, Scotland

David W. Kinne, M.D.
Associate Professor of Surgery
Cornell University Medical College
Chief
Breast Service
Attending Surgeon
Memorial Sloan-Kettering Cancer Center
New York, New York

Timothy Kinsella, M.D.
Professor and Chairman
Department of Human Oncology
University of Wisconsin School of Medicine
Deputy Director
University of Wisconsin Clinical Cancer Center
University of Wisconsin Hospital and Clinics
Madison, Wisconsin

Libby L. Klein, M.S.W., A.C.S.W.
Social Work Researcher
Memorial Sloan-Kettering Cancer Center
New York, New York

Larry E. Kun, M.D.
Chairman
Department of Radiation Oncology
St. Jude Children's Research Hospital
Professor
Departments of Radiology and Pediatrics
Director
Division of Radiation Oncology
University of Tennessee
Memphis, Tennessee

Marguerite S. Lederberg, M.D.
Clinical Associate Professor of Psychiatry
Cornell University Medical Center
Associate Attending Psychiatrist
Memorial Sloan-Kettering Cancer Center
New York, New York

Lawrence P. Leichman, M.D.
Associate Professor of Medicine
University of Southern California
Associate Director for Medical Oncology
Los Angeles County Hospital
University of Southern California Medical Center
Los Angeles, California

Victor A. Levin, M.D.
Professor and Chairman
Department of Neuro-Oncology
University of Texas
M. D. Anderson Cancer Center
Houston, Texas

Allen S. Lichter, M.D.
Professor and Chairman
University of Michigan Medical School
University of Michigan Hospital
Ann Arbor, Michigan

W. Marston Linehan, M.D.
Head
Urologic Oncology Section
Surgery Branch
National Cancer Institute
Assistant Professor of Surgery
Uniformed Services University of the Health Sciences
School of Medicine
Bethesda, Maryland

Michael P. Link, M.D.
Associate Professor of Pediatrics
Stanford University School of Medicine
Staff Hematologist/Oncologist
Children's Hospital at Stanford
Stanford, California

Lance A. Liotta, M.D., Ph.D.
Chief
Laboratory of Pathology
National Cancer Institute
Bethesda, Maryland

Patrick J. Loehrer, M.D.
Associate Professor of Medicine
Section of Hematology-Oncology
Indiana University School of Medicine
Indiana University Hospital
Indianapolis, Indiana

Dan L. Longo, M.D.
Biological Response Modifiers Program
Division of Cancer Treatment
National Cancer Institute
Bethesda, Maryland

Matthew Loscalzo, A.C.S.W.
Assistant Director
Department of Social Work/Educational Coordinator
Memorial Sloan-Kettering Cancer Center
New York, New York

Michael T. Lotze, M.D.
Assistant Professor
Uniformed Services University of the Health Sciences
Senior Investigator
Surgery Branch
National Cancer Institute
Bethesda, Maryland

Bert L. Lum, Pharm.D.
Associate Professor
University of the Pacific
Stockton, California
Research Associate
Department of Oncology
Palo Alto Veterans Administration Medical Center
Palo Alto, California

John S. Macdonald, M.D.
Professor of Medicine
Director
Division of Hematology and Oncology
Lucille Markey Cancer Center
University of Kentucky Medical Center
Lexington, Kentucky

Martin M. Malawer, M.D.
Associate Professor of Orthopedic Surgery and Child Development
Children's Hospital National Medical Center and George Washington University School of Medicine
The Washington Hospital Center
Washington, D.C.

Mary Jane Massie, M.D.
Associate Professor of Clinical Psychiatry
Cornell University Medical College
Associate Attending Psychiatrist
Psychiatry Service
Department of Neurology
Memorial Sloan-Kettering Cancer Center
New York, New York

Peter Mauch, M.D.
Associate Professor
Department of Radiation Therapy
Harvard Medical School
Boston, Massachusetts

Rosalie Raps Melnick, Ph.D., M.B.A.
Clinical Assistant Professor
Department of Rehabilitation Medicine
University of Washington
Associate Chief of Staff/Education
Seattle Veterans Administration Medical Center
Seattle, Washington

Joel D. Meyers, M.D.
Professor of Medicine
University of Washington
School of Medicine
Head
Program in Infectious Diseases
Fred Hutchinson Cancer Research Center
Seattle, Washington

Anthony B. Miller, M.B., F.R.C.P.
Professor
Department of Preventive Medicine and Biostatistics
Faculty of Medicine
University of Toronto
Toronto, Ontario, Canada

Donald L. Miller, M.D.
Associate Professor of Radiology
Georgetown University School of Medicine
Associate Professor of Radiology
Uniformed Services University of the Health Sciences
School of Medicine
Director of Vascular/Interventional Radiology
Diagnostic Radiology Department
National Institutes of Health
Bethesda, Maryland

Robert M. Miller, Ph.D.
Clinical Assistant Professor
Speech and Hearing Sciences, Otolaryngology, and Rehabilitation Medicine
University of Washington
Chief
Audiology and Speech Pathology Service
Seattle Veterans Administration Medical Center
Seattle, Washington

Rodney R. Million, M.D.
Professor and Chairman
Department of Radiation Oncology
University of Florida
Shands Hospital
Gainesville, Florida

John D. Minna, M.D.
Professor of Medicine
Uniformed Services University of the Health Sciences
Chief
NCI–Navy Medical Oncology Branch
Naval Hospital
Bethesda, Maryland

James B. Mitchell, Ph.D.
Deputy Chief
Radiation Oncology Branch
National Cancer Institute
Bethesda, Maryland

Drogo K. Montague, M.D.
Director
Center for Sexual Function
Head
Section of Urodynamics and Prosthetic Surgery
Department of Urology
Cleveland Clinic Foundation
Cleveland, Ohio

John J. Mulvihill, M.D.
Chief
Clinical Genetics Section
Clinical Epidemiology Branch
National Cancer Institute
Director
Interinstitute Medical Genetics Program
Warren Grant Magnuson Clinical Center
National Institutes of Health
Bethesda, Maryland

Charles E. Myers, M.D.
Chief
Medicine Branch and Clinical Pharmacology Branch
Clinical Center
National Institutes of Health
Bethesda, Maryland

Jeffrey A. Norton, M.D.
Head
Surgical Metabolism Section
Surgery Branch
National Cancer Institute
Bethesda, Maryland

James R. Oleson, M.D., Ph.D.
Associate Professor
Division of Radiation Oncology
Duke University Medical Center
Durham, North Carolina

Stanley E. Order, M.D., Sc.D.
Willard and Lillian Hackerman Professor of Radiation Oncology
The Johns Hopkins Medical Institution
School of Medicine
Director
Radiation Oncology
The Johns Hopkins Hospital
Baltimore, Maryland

Morag Park, Ph.D.
Ludwig Institute for Cancer Research
BRI–Basic Research Program
NCI–Frederick Cancer Research Facility
Frederick, Maryland

Harvey Pass, M.D.
Head
Thoracic Oncology Section
Senior Investigator
Surgery Branch
National Cancer Institute
Bethesda, Maryland

Jennifer A. K. Patterson, M.D.
Assistant Professor
Department of Dermatology
New York University Medical Center
Director of Inpatient and Consultative Services
Department of Dermatology
Bellevue Hospital Center
New York, New York

Carlos A. Perez, M.D.
Director
Radiation Oncology Center
Mallinckrodt Institute of Radiology
Washington University Medical Center
St. Louis, Missouri

Lester J. Peters, M.D.
Professor and Head
Division of Radiotherapy
John G. and Marie Stella Kenedy Chair
University of Texas
M. D. Anderson Hospital Cancer Center
Houston, Texas

Theodore L. Phillips, M.D.
Professor and Chairman
Department of Radiation Oncology
University of California
Attending Physician
Long/Moffitt Hospital
San Francisco, California

Henry C. Pitot, M.D., Ph.D.
Professor of Oncology and Pathology
The Medical School
University of Wisconsin
Pathologist
University Hospitals
Madison, Wisconsin

Philip A. Pizzo, M.D.
Chief of Pediatrics
Head
Infectious Disease Section
National Cancer Institute
Clinical Center
National Institutes of Health
Bethesda, Maryland

David G. Poplack, M.D.
Head
Leukemia Section
Pediatric Branch
National Cancer Institute
Bethesda, Maryland

Abram Recht, M.D.
Assistant Professor
Joint Center for Radiation Therapy
Department of Radiation Therapy
Harvard Medical School
Radiation Therapist
Beth Israel Hospital
Assistant Physician
Dana Farber Cancer Institute
Boston, Massachusetts

Jerome P. Richie, M.D.
Elliott Carr Cutler Professor of
Urological Surgery
Chairman
Harvard Program in Urology
Chief of Urology
Brigham and Women's Hospital
Boston, Massachusetts

E. Chester Ridgway, M.D.
Professor of Medicine
Head
Division of Endocrinology
University of Colorado Health Sciences Center
Denver, Colorado

Anita B. Roberts, Ph.D.
Senior Scientist
Laboratory of Chemoprevention
National Cancer Institute
Bethesda, Maryland

J. C. Rosenberg, M.D., Ph.D.
Professor of Surgery
Wayne State University
Chief of Surgery
Hutzel Hospital
Detroit, Michigan

Jack A. Roth, M.D.
Johnson Professor and Chairman
Department of Thoracic Surgery
Professor of Tumor Biology
M.D. Anderson Cancer Center
Houston, Texas

Janet D. Rowley, M.D.
Professor
Department of Medicine
University of Chicago School of Medicine
Chicago, Illinois

Angelo Russo, M.D., Ph.D.
Head
Experimental Phototherapy
Radiation Oncology Branch
National Institutes of Health
Bethesda, Maryland

Jose Alain Sahel, M.D., Ph.D.
Professor of Ophthalmology
University of Strasbourg
Clinique Ophtalmologique
Centre Hospitalier Regional
Strasbourg, France

Sydney E. Salmon, M.D.
Professor
Internal Medicine
Director
Arizona Cancer Center
University of Arizona College of Medicine
Tucson, Arizona

Wendy S. Schain, Ed.D.
Adjunct Clinical Professor
Georgetown University Medical School
Kensington, Maryland

Claudia A. Seipp, R.N., O.C.N.
Oncology Nurse Clinician
Surgery Branch
National Cancer Institute
Bethesda, Maryland

Brenda Shank, M.D., Ph.D.
Associate Professor of Radiation Oncology in Medicine
Cornell University Medical Center
Associate Member
Memorial Sloan-Kettering Cancer Center
Associate Attending Radiation Oncologist
Memorial Hospital
New York, New York

Glenn E. Sheline, Ph.D., M.D.
Professor of Radiation Oncology
University of California School of Medicine
University of California Hospitals
San Francisco, California

Richard J. Sherins, M.D.
Director
Division of Andrology
Genetics and I.V.F. Institute
Fairfax, Virginia

Moshe Shike, M.D.
Associate Professor of Clinical Medicine
Cornell University Medical College
Associate Attending Physician
Department of Medicine
Memorial Sloan-Kettering Cancer Center
New York, New York

William U. Shipley, M.D.
Associate Professor of Radiation Therapy
Harvard Medical School
Radiation Therapist
Department of Radiation Medicine
Massachusetts General Hospital
Associate Director
Massachusetts General Hospital Cancer Center
Boston, Massachusetts

Edward H. Shortliffe, M.D., Ph.D.
Associate Professor of Medicine and of Computer Science
Stanford University School of Medicine
Attending Physician
Stanford University Medical Center
Stanford, California

Leslie R. Shover, Ph.D.
Head
Section of Psychosexual Disorders
The Center for Sexual Function
The Cleveland Clinic Foundation
Cleveland, Ohio

Richard M. Simon, Ph.D.
Chief
Biometric Branch
National Cancer Institute
Bethesda, Maryland

William F. Sindelar, M.D., Ph.D.
Senior Investigator
Surgery Branch
National Cancer Institute
Bethesda, Maryland

Jack W. Singer, M.D.
Professor of Medicine
University of Washington
Chief of Medical Oncology
Verterans Administration Medical Center
Seattle, Washington

Stephen T. Sonis, D.M.D., D.M.Sc.
Associate Professor of Oral Medicine
Harvard School of Dental Medicine
Chief
Dental Service
Brigham and Women's Hospital
Boston, Massachusetts

Michael B. Sporn, M.D.
Chief
Laboratory of Chemoprevention
National Cancer Institute
Bethesda, Maryland

Glenn Steele, Jr., M.D., Ph.D.
The William McDermott Professor of Surgery
Harvard Medical School
Chairman
Department of Surgery
New England Deaconess Hospital
Boston, Massachusetts

William G. Stetler-Stevenson, M.D., Ph.D.
Senior Staff Fellow
Laboratory of Pathology
National Institutes of Health
Bethesda, Maryland

Rainer Storb, M.D.
Professor of Medicine
University of Washington School of Medicine
Head
Program in Transplant Biology
Fred Hutchinson Cancer Research Center
Seattle, Washington

Diane E. Stover, M.D.
Associate Professor of Medicine
Cornell University Medical College
Chief of Pulmonary Service
Associate Attending Physician
Memorial Sloan-Kettering Cancer Center
New York, New York

Paul H. Sugarbaker, M.D.
Director of Surgical Oncology
Winship Cancer Center
Emory University School of Medicine
Atlanta, Georgia

Ian F. Tannock, M.D., Ph.D.
Associate Professor of Medicine and Medical Biophysics
University of Toronto
Staff Physician/Senior Scientist
Princess Margaret Hospital and Ontario Cancer Institute
Toronto, Ontario, Canada

William M. Thompson, M.D.
Professor and Chairman
Department of Radiology
University of Minnesota
Chairman
Department of Radiology
University of Minnesota Hospital and Clinic
Minneapolis, Minnesota

Frank M. Torti, M.D.
Associate Professor of Medicine
Stanford University
Chief
Oncology Section
Veterans Administration Medical Center
Palo Alto, California

Margaret A. Tucker, M.D.
Chief
Family Studies Section
Environmental Epidemiology Branch
Division of Cancer Etiology
National Cancer Institute
Bethesda, Maryland

John E. Ultmann, M.D.
Professor of Medicine
Director
Cancer Research Center
Division of Biological Science
University of Chicago
Pritzker School of Medicine
Attending Physician
The University of Chicago Hospitals
Chicago, Illinois

George F. Vande Woude, Ph.D.
Director
BRI–Basic Research Program
NCI–Frederick Cancer Research Facility
Frederick, Maryland

Susan Vande Woude, D.V.M.
Post Doctoral Fellow
Division of Comparative Medicine
The Johns Hopkins University
Baltimore, Maryland

Ralph Wallerstein, Jr., M.D.
Assistant Clinical Professor of Medicine
University of California
San Francisco, California

Harold J. Wanebo, M.D.
Professor of Surgery
Director of Surgical Oncology
Brown University
Chief
Department of Surgery
Roger Williams General Hospital
Providence, Rhode Island

Raymond P. Warrell, Jr., M.D.
Assistant Professor of Medicine
Cornell University Medical College
Associate Member
Memorial Sloan-Kettering Cancer Center
New York, New York

Lois L. Weinstein, A.C.S.W.
Department of Social Work
Memorial Sloan-Kettering Cancer Center
New York, New York

Peter H. Wiernik, M.D.
Gutman Professor and Chairman
Department of Oncology
Montefiore Medical Center
Head
Division of Medical Oncology
Albert Einstein College of Medicine
Associate Professor for Clinical Research
Albert Einstein Cancer Center
Bronx, New York

Stephen D. Williams, M.D.
Professor of Medicine
Indiana University
Chief
Hematology-Oncology
Indianapolis Veterans Administration Medical Center
Indianapolis, Indiana

Richard E. Wilson, M.D.
Professor of Surgery
Harvard Medical School
Chief
Surgical Oncology
Brigham and Women's Hospital
Dana Farber Cancer Institute
Boston, Massachusetts

Donald C. Wright, M.D.
Clinical Neurosurgery Section
Surgical Neurology Branch
National Institutes of Neurological and Communicative Disorders and Stroke
Clinical Center
National Institutes of Health
Bethesda, Maryland

Alan Yagoda, M.D.
Instructor in Medicine
Cornell University Medical College
New York, New York
Assistant Clinical Professor of Medicine
Yale University School of Medicine
New Haven, Connecticut
Attending Physician
Memorial Sloan-Kettering Cancer Center
New York, New York

Joachim Yahalom, M.D.
Assistant Professor
Cornell University Medical Center
Assistant Attending
Department of Radiation Oncology
Memorial Sloan-Kettering Cancer Center
New York, New York

Robert C. Young, M.D.
Associate Director
Centers and Community Oncology Program
National Cancer Institute
Bethesda, Maryland

Preface

Early diagnosis and prompt treatment with carefully integrated, multimodal management continues to provide cancer patients with the best chance of surviving the disease. The integrated, multimodal approach to the treatment of cancer, with a balanced view of how the majority of cancer patients are managed today, was the *raison d'etre* of the first edition of *Cancer: Principles and Practice of Oncology* in 1982 and remains a hallmark of the third edition.

Dramatic changes in cancer research and the management of cancer patients have resulted in a sense of urgency to put the freshest information in the hands of practicing physicians. This sense of urgency has necessitated the timely production of this edition. The first section, "Principles of Oncology," has once again been entirely revised to reflect the rapid accumulation of new information about the etiology and development of cancer at the molecular level. It reflects the need of physicians to have at their disposal a succinct yet comprehensive discussion of the scientific basis of the cancer process. More information has been added on useful aspects of the technology of the molecular biology of cancer and the metastatic process. In addition, the discussions of the increasingly beneficial approaches to cancer prevention have been amplified.

With each passing year, more patients with cancer are curable and treatments are associated with less morbidity than in the past. The second portion of the book, "Practice of Oncology," has been extensively revised to reflect this continued integration of local and systemic treatments and the growing sophistication of multimodality treatments. Since the second edition of this book, new treatments have been developed for the more common visceral tumors. The newest information on the results of these clinical trials is included, where appropriate, as is the latest information on the increasingly widespread benefits of the use of biologics (such as colony-stimulating factors and various lymphokines). The complications of cancer and its treatment, and presentations on approaches to treatments under development, are the main features of the final portion of the book. We have continued to emphasize the need for practicality. The information presented in each chapter is both fresh and usable.

Thus, *Cancer: Principles and Practice of Oncology* continues to be a book for both oncologists and physicians of other specialties whose practices include a significant number of cancer patients. By retaining freshness and practicality without sacrificing comprehensiveness, we have attempted to place at the fingertips of the physician all the necessary data to manage cancer patients within a single book. The pace of discovery in the medical sciences makes this task an increasingly difficult challenge with each edition. We hope that a comprehensive text like *Cancer: Principles and Practice of Oncology* is useful to physicians and their patients.

Vincent T. DeVita, Jr., M.D.,
Samuel Hellman, M.D.
Steven A. Rosenberg, M.D., Ph.D.

Acknowledgments

The editors are especially grateful to those whose excellent help and unflagging enthusiasm contributed to this book.

Alice Rosenberg assumed responsibility for the overall compilation of the contributions to this book and for many of the organizational details involved in its assembly.

Rhanda Steele and Susan Hubbard contributed to the preparation and compilation of many of the manuscripts.

Richard Winters provided valuable editorial assistance in the preparation of the second and third editions.

Stuart Freeman, Editor, Oncology Program, J. B. Lippincott Company, has worked closely with the editors from the book's inception in 1978 through the completion of all three editions. His valuable advice and continuing encouragement have contributed greatly to the preparation of all three.

Contents

CANCER

Principles & Practice of Oncology

PART 1 *Principles of Oncology*

IAN F. TANNOCK

CHAPTER 1 Principles of Cell Proliferation: Cell Kinetics

Human tumors have a wide range of growth rates. The introduction of tritiated thymidine and autoradiography in the 1950s allowed the growth of selected human tumors to be analyzed in terms of properties of the constituent cells, and later applications of flow cytometry have allowed more rapid and automated analysis of cell kinetics. These data may provide useful prognostic information, and the ability of flow cytometry to detect aneuploid cell populations makes it an important aid in tumor diagnosis. Many anticancer drugs are selective for proliferating cells, and most drugs, as well as ionizing radiation, vary in their activity around the cell cycle. Tissues containing rapidly proliferating cells such as the bone marrow or intestinal mucosa are frequently dose-limiting in cancer chemotherapy, and an understanding of their cell kinetics provides a basis for the scheduling of anticancer drugs. This chapter describes principles of cell kinetics and uses of flow cytometry, with emphasis on those properties that may have direct application to the diagnosis, prognosis, and treatment of human cancer.

GROWTH OF HUMAN TUMORS

TUMOR DOUBLING TIMES

Determination of the rate of growth of tumors is limited to sites that are accessible to measurement, and most growth curves have been derived from measurements of pulmonary metastases in serial chest radiographs. Steel[1] has reviewed published data on the growth of 780 human tumors in patients who were not receiving treatment. Many of the investigators made only two or three measurements on each tumor, but in a small number of studies, multiple serial estimates of tumor volume were available. Many of these serial measurements could be fitted by a straight line when tumor volume (on a logarithmic scale) was plotted against time (on a linear scale); that is, the growth curve was exponential (Fig. 1-1). Exponential growth implies that the tumor takes a constant time to double its volume, and representative values of volume doubling time (T_D) for different types of human tumor are shown in Table 1-1.

The following general conclusions can be drawn from the available data on tumor growth rate:

1. Lung metastases derived from many of the more common solid tumors in humans have mean values of T_D in the range of 2 to 3 months. There is, however, a wide range of growth rates among tumors of the same histologic type and tissue of origin.
2. Tumors that are responsive to anticancer drugs (*e.g.*, lymphomas, testicular cancer, and tumors in children) usually grow more rapidly than do less responsive tumors.
3. Lung metastases from tumors of the colon and breast tend to grow more rapidly than do the primary tumors from which they are seeded.

PRECLINICAL GROWTH OF HUMAN TUMORS

The smallest tumor that is likely to be detected by physical or radiologic examination will have a diameter of about 1 cm

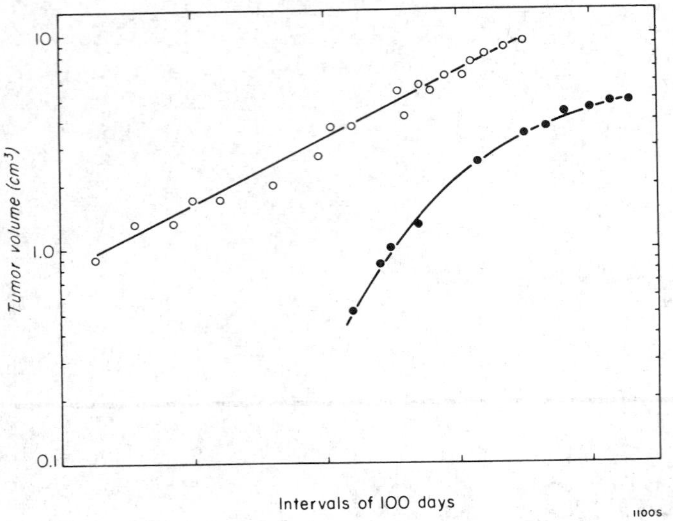

FIG. 1-1. Growth curve for pulmonary metastases from cancer of the breast *(open symbols)* and cancer of the rectum *(closed symbols)*. The breast cancer metastasis grew exponentially with a volume doubling time of 3 months, but the rectal cancer metastasis showed decreasing growth rate with increasing size. (Hill RP, Bush RS-Unpublished data)

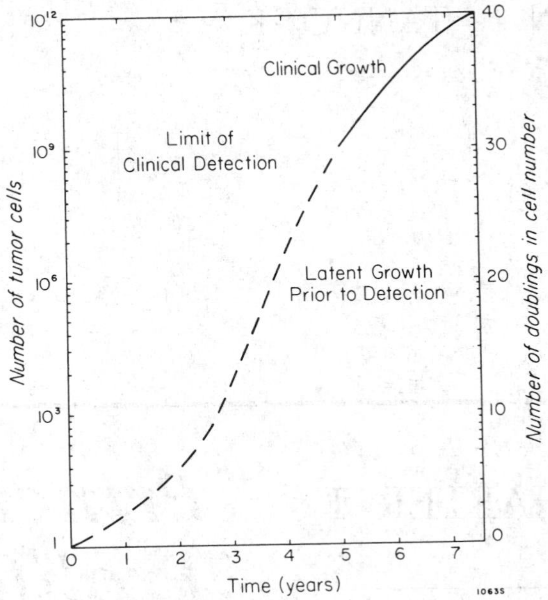

FIG. 1-2. Hypothetical growth curve for a human tumor. Note that the tumor grows for 5 years before attaining a size of ~1 g (~10^9 cells), when it can first be clinically detected. Thereafter, despite some slowing of growth, it attains a lethal mass of ~1 kg (~10^{12} cells) in a further 2.5 years.

and may contain 10^8 to 10^9 tumor cells, depending on the contribution of stroma and other elements to tumor bulk. Such a tumor will have undergone about 30 doublings in cell number if it is clonally derived from a single transformed cell (Fig. 1-2). Growth from a tumor of 1 g (the minimum size detectable) to a potentially lethal mass of 1 kg requires only 10 further doublings of cell number. Thus, the period of tumor growth that is clinically evident represents a rather short period in the total life history of a tumor. There is ample opportunity for seeding of metastases before detection of a primary tumor.

TABLE 1-1. Representative Values of Volume Doubling Time for Different Types of Human Tumors

Tumor Type	*Number of Tumors*	*Volume Doubling Time in Weeks (geometric mean value)*
Primary lung cancer		
Adenocarcinoma	64	21
Squamous-cell carcinoma	85	12
Anaplastic carcinoma	55	11
Breast cancer		
Primary	17	14
Lung metastases	44	11
Soft-tissue metastases	66	3
Colorectal cancer		
Primary	19	90
Lung metastases	56	14
Lymphoma		
Lymph node lesions	27	4
Lung metastases of:		
Carcinoma of testis	80	4
Childhood tumors	47	4
Adult sarcomas	58	7

Reproduced from Tannock and Hill[2] with permission, and adapted from data reviewed by Steel.[1]

If human tumors grew exponentially from inception to death of the host (or to institution of some form of treatment), the time of origin of the malignancy could be estimated by extrapolating growth curves back to a single cell. If this is done for growth of the lung metastasis of the human breast cancer that is shown in Figure 1-1 (with the assumption that a tumor of volume 1 cm^3 contains 10^9 cells), the latency period from a single cell origin of the metastasis would be about 7.5 years.

Although the latency period of slowly growing human tumors is long, some tumors show decelerating growth with time (Fig. 1-1), so the above example may overestimate the latency period. Deceleration of growth is commonly observed for transplantable tumors in animals and probably results in part from decreasing tumor vascularity and cellular nutrition leading to slowing of cell proliferation and increasing cell death.[3] Many human tumors also develop necrosis and are subject to the same processes, so that more rapid growth of small, well-vascularized preclinical tumors seems likely. Mathematical models have been used to fit tumor growth curves that show deceleration of growth, such as the Gompertz equation, but clinical data are insufficient to define a precise model.

Shackney and co-workers[4] have estimated the period of preclinical growth of some human tumors. They studied groups of patients in whom a proportion of tumors were cured by treatment and assumed that tumor recurrence in the remainder was due to proliferation from a small number of residual tumor cells. The time of appearance of recurrent nodules in the chest wall after mastectomy for breast cancer suggested that tumor growth was more rapid during the preclinical phase. In contrast, rapidly progressive tumors such as Burkitt's lymphoma and Wilms' tumor appeared to have grown exponentially at a fairly constant rate.

It is possible that there is a period of slow growth following initiation of some tumors because of the requirement for stimulation of a blood supply[5] and the possibility that the tumor has to escape immunologic and other host defense mechanisms. This effect is observed after transplantation of some tumors in animals, but there are no data for human tumors that allow one to judge the validity of this concept.

Analysis of tumor growth in terms of the proliferation and death of constituent cells will be explored in the following sections.

CELL KINETICS OF HUMAN TUMORS

BASIC CONCEPTS

Must of the available information about cell kinetics of human tumors and normal tissues has been derived from studies using ^{3}H-thymidine and autoradiography. More recently these techniques have been largely superseded by techniques based on flow cytometry, but many of the principles of experimental design are similar.

When ^{3}H-thymidine is injected into animals (including humans), it is incorporated into the DNA that is being synthesized while the remainder is rapidly broken down and excreted as tritiated water. Labeled cells can be recognized in autoradiographs that are prepared by covering tissue sections with photographic emulsion followed by prolonged exposure in the dark (Fig. 1-3); the short range of β-particles released from tritium (mean range ~0.5 μm) exposes only the film immediately overlying the cell nucleus and leads to good resolution of labeled and unlabeled cells.

FIG. 1-3. Autoradiograph of a tumor section. Labeled cells that have taken up ^{3}H-thymidine may be recognized by grains in the photographic emulsion immediately overlying the cell nucleus.

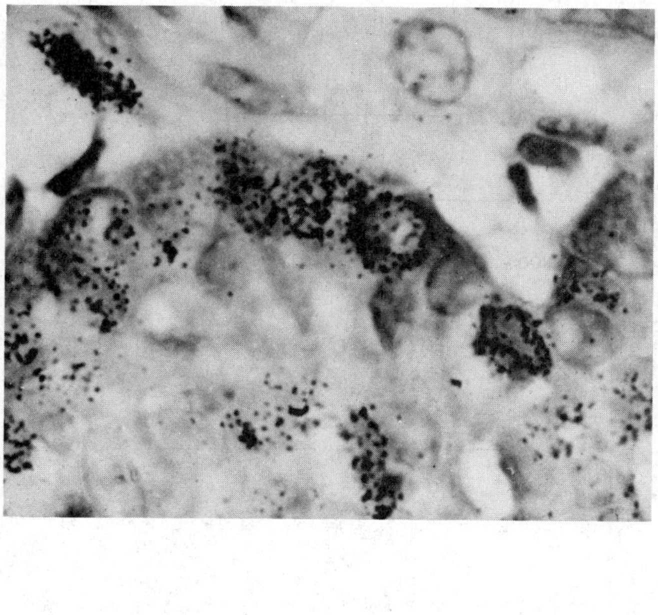

Classification of the cell cycle into discrete phases followed the demonstration that DNA synthesis took place during a defined time interval, rather than continuously during interphase.[6] The intervals between mitosis (M) and DNA synthesis (S) were termed the G_1 and G_2 phase (G = gap), thus providing the familiar terminology of Figure 1-4.

In normal renewal tissues such as the bone marrow, small intestine, and skin, cells lose their ability to proliferate as they undergo differentiation, and the production of new cells by mitosis is matched by loss of differentiated cells from the population. Mendelsohn[7] showed that many cells in tumors may also be nonproliferative, and there is evidence that both differentiation and poor nutrition may cause cells to become quiescent. The term growth fraction was applied to the proportion of cells that were in cycle; because most anticancer drugs have greater activity for cycling cells, tumors with high values of growth fraction might be expected to be most responsive to chemotherapy.

The presence of necrosis or pyknotic cells is evidence for cell death in tumors, and the rate of cell death or loss from human tumors can be a high proportion of the rate of cell production.[8] Because of nonproliferating cells and cell loss, the volume doubling time of human tumors is (fortunately) much longer than the mean cell cycle time of the constituent cells. Many tumors may be thought of as analogous to renewal tissues, with only a slight imbalance between production and loss of cells which leads to tumor growth; indeed, tumors have been described as "caricatures" of normal tissue renewal.[9]

The analogy between tumors and renewal tissues may be extended to include the concept of stem cells. In normal renewal populations, there is evidence for the existence of a small population of stem cells whose progeny can proliferate and differentiate to repopulate the tissue. The following evidence suggests that in many tumors there may be only a small subpopulation (also referred to as stem cells) that has the capacity for indefinite proliferation.

1. Tissue-specific differentiation occurs in many human tumors, suggesting the retention of properties of renewal tissues. Studies of thymidine labeling in some animal tumors have shown that differentiated cells (which cannot form tumors on transplantation) are

FIG. 1-4. Model of a tumor cell population. The tumor contains proliferating cells (referred to as the growth fraction) and nonproliferating cells. The latter population may include cells that have lost the ability to proliferate (*e.g.*, by differentiation) or cells that can revert to proliferation if factors such as cellular nutrition improve. Most tumors contain a high rate of cell death or loss from the tumor.

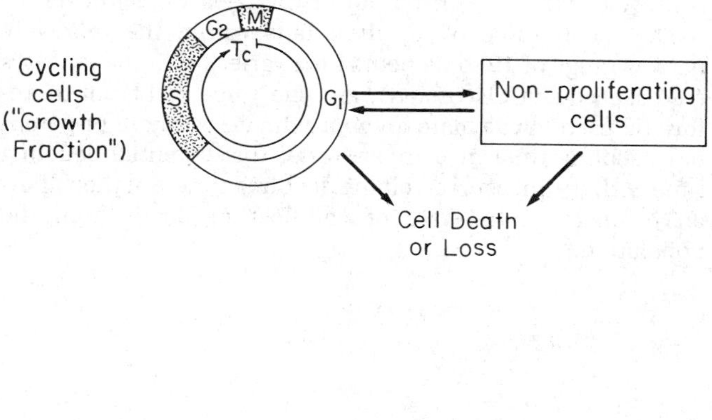

derived from undifferentiated cells that have the ability to generate tumors when implanted into new hosts.[10]

2. The ability to control some human tumors by tolerated doses of radiation is consistent with the radiobiological properties of constituent cells only if one assumes that the target cell population (*i.e.*, stem cells) is much smaller than the total number of cells in the tumor.[11]
3. Growth of colonies from human tumor cells in culture occurs from only a small proportion (usually < 0.1%) of the population.[12,13] Although this property may reflect the imperfect nature of the tissue culture environment, cells from some tumors may be separated by physical means into those with colony-forming potential (*i.e.*, putative stem cells) and those with markers of differentiation.[14]

It is important to distinguish between the proliferative state of a cell and its proliferative potential. There is evidence that pluripotential stem cells in the bone marrow have low frequency of cell division in the absence of stress;[15] in contrast, myeloblasts and myelocytes proliferate rapidly but are not stem cells. Similarly, the proliferative state of a tumor cell gives no information about its ability to produce large numbers of progeny, or its "stemness." Commonly used techniques involving thymidine autoradiography or flow cytometry give information about the proliferative status of the entire cell population. Recognition of cells with large proliferative potential requires an assay of colony formation, and special techniques are required to examine the proliferation kinetics of colony-forming tumor cells.

TRITIATED THYMIDINE AND AUTORADIOGRAPHY

The proportion of cells that is labeled following a short (usually 1 hr) exposure to ^{3}H-thymidine has been termed the labeling index (LI). The LI is often determined by incubation of tissue biopsies with ^{3}H-thymidine in vitro. Provided that the isotope is available to all of the cells, LI represents the proportion of cells in DNA synthesis at the time of ^{3}H-thymidine exposure. LI is thus a measure of the rate of cell production and is related to the duration of DNA synthesis (T_s) and potential doubling time (T) of a tumor population by the formula

$$LI = \lambda \frac{T_s}{T} \qquad (1)$$

Here λ is a factor that is typically about 0.8.[1] The potential doubling time (T) is the doubling time that the tumor would have in the absence of cell loss; it would be equal to mean cell cycle time (T_c) only if all of the cells were in cycle.

The mean value of T_s often falls within the relatively narrow range of 12 to 24 hours for a variety of human tumors (see subsequent discussion), and the value of LI can therefore be used to calculate an approximate estimate of potential doubling time. A comparison of this potential doubling time with the measured volume doubling time can then allow an estimate of the rate of cell loss or death from the population.[8]

Estimation of the duration of individual phases of the cell cycle requires more complex techniques, such as the percent labeled mitoses (PLM) method. The technique requires a single injection of ^{3}H-thymidine followed by the preparation of autoradiographs from sections of serial biopsies; for this reason it is now rarely used in humans, but historically it has provided the most detailed information about the kinetics of selected human tumors.

Percent labeled mitoses curves are generated by plotting the percentage of mitotic cells that are labeled in autoradiographs as a function of time after administration of ^{3}H-thymidine. Under idealized conditions in which there is no variation in the duration of cell cycle phases, the cohort of labeled cells that were initially in S-phase generates successive waves of labeled mitoses as it passes around the cell cycle (Figs. 1-5A and B). These waves of labeled mitoses are of width T_s (*i.e.*, the "width" of the labeled cohort), and of periodicity T_c. In practice, the PLM curve becomes damped because of variability in the duration of cell cycle phases (Fig. 1-5C) but can be analyzed by computer methods to obtain an approximate distribution of cell cycle phase times.

The growth fraction may be estimated from the value of LI

FIG. 1-5. The percent labeled mitoses (PLM) technique. After administration of ^{3}H-thymidine, the cohort of labeled cells moves around the cycle as shown in **A**. Under the idealized conditions in which individual phase times do not vary, the percentage of labeled mitoses varies with time as shown in **B**. Here points a, b, c, d, and e on the curve are derived from the corresponding cycle diagrams of panel A. **C** depicts an experimental curve, derived by Shirakawa *et al*[16] for human melanoma. Damping occurs because of variability in cell cycle phase times, but the PLM curve can be analyzed by computer methods to give a distribution of cell cycle times (and of individual phase duration) for the tumor.

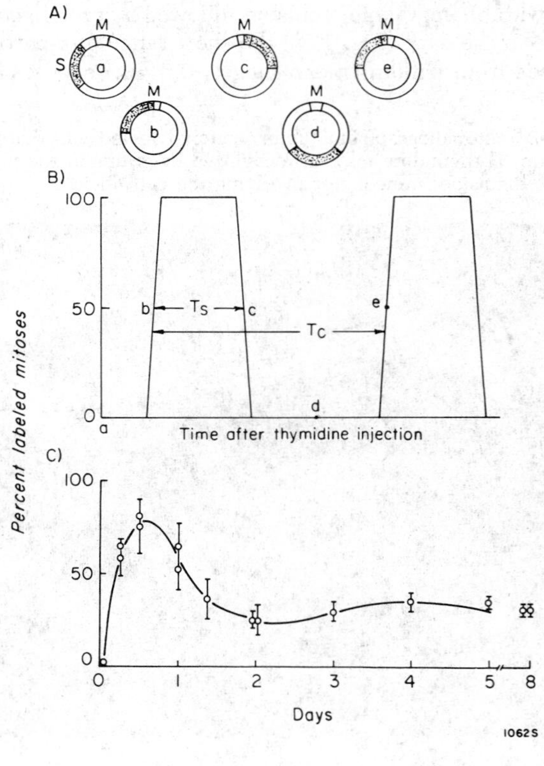

and the distribution of cell cycle phase times. Information about the phase distributions of cycling cells allows calculation of the proportion of proliferating cells that are in S-phase. Since the measured LI is the proportion of total cells in S-phase, the ratio of measured LI to the estimated S-phase fraction of cycling cells is a measure of growth fraction. An alternative method of estimating growth fraction is through determination of the proportion of cells that contain enzymes (*e.g.*, DNA-dependent DNA polymerase) that appear to be induced only in cycling cells.[17] Estimates of growth fraction should be regarded as approximate since techniques are not available to distinguish nonproliferating cells from those with cycle times longer than the mean.

FLOW CYTOMETRY

Techniques using ^{3}H-thymidine have the advantage of preserving tissue geometry, but they are labor-intensive and slow. Newer techniques based on flow cytometry have the major advantages of speed and automation.

The principal features of flow cytometry are the production of a suspension of single cells, their staining with a fluorescent dye, and the derivation of a distribution of fluorescence intensity. The latter is achieved by passing the cells in single file through a laser beam which excites the fluorescence, as shown in Figure 1-6.
An electric charge may be applied to cells of different fluorescence intensity, so that they can be separated in an electrostatic field, allowing their further chemical or biological characterization. This is known as fluorescence-activated cell sorting. Flow cytometry may be used to study a wide variety of cellular properties, depending only on the availability of appropriate fluorescent probes.

For most studies of cell kinetics, fluorescent dyes are used (*e.g.*, acridine orange or propidium iodide) whose binding is proportional to DNA content. The fluorescence intensity thus allows derivation of the distribution of DNA content among the cells of the population (Fig. 1-7). Computer methods are used to estimate the proportion of cells in the G_1, S, and G_2/M phases of the cell cycle from the DNA distribution. Estimates of the proportion of S-phase cells by flow cytometry tend to be slightly higher than estimates of LI determined using ^{3}H-thymidine and autoradiography. By comparison with normal diploid cells as a standard, the flow cytometer also allows detection of aneuploid cells.

Recent innovations have allowed more complex analysis of cell cycle parameters by flow cytometry. Many of these methods have utilized "labeling" of cells by nonradioactive

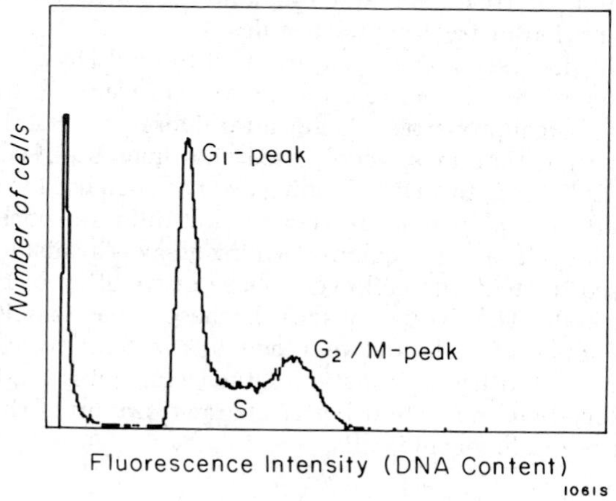

FIG. 1-7. A DNA histogram produced by flow cytometry. Cells of a human bladder cancer cell line were labeled with acridine orange. The peak at the origin represents cellular debris. The DNA distribution may be analyzed by computer methods to estimate the proportion of cells in G_1, S, and G_2/M phases of the cell cycle.

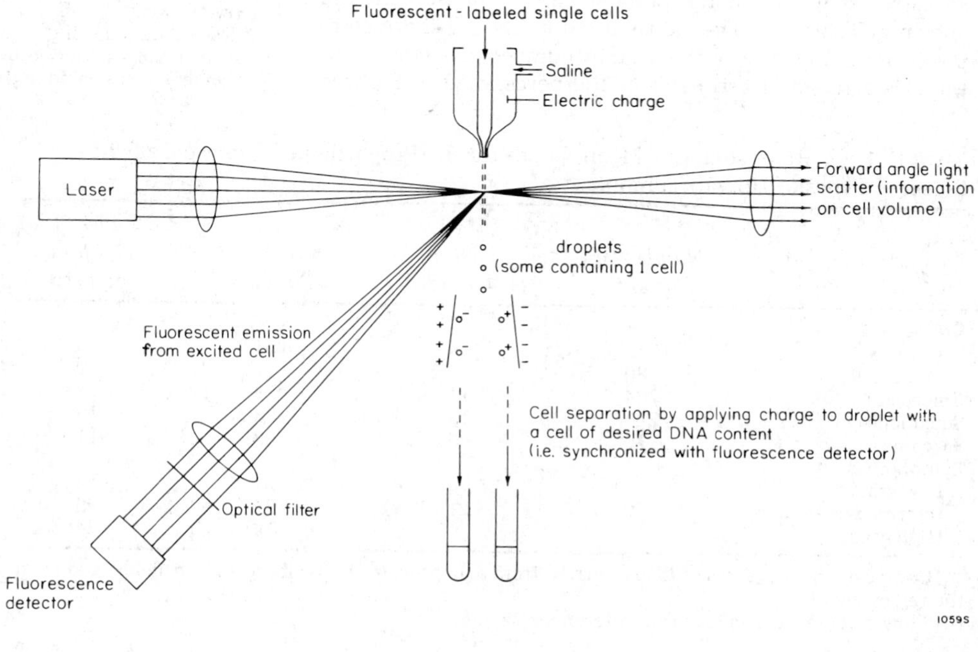

FIG. 1-6. The principal features of a flow cytometer. Single cells are labeled with a fluorescent probe and are directed in single file through a laser beam. Analysis of forward angle light scatter can be used to estimate cell volume. Fluorescence emission from the excited cell then provides a distribution of fluorescence intensity. Electric charge that is related to fluorescence intensity can also be applied to droplets containing single cells, allowing their separation in an electrostatic field. This process is known as fluorescence-activated cell sorting.

bromodeoxyuridine (BrdUrd), which, like thymidine, is taken up into S-phase cells of the cycle.[18] BrdUrd that is incorporated into DNA may then be detected by flow cytometry, using a fluorescent labeled monoclonal antibody directed against incorporated BrdUrd. A recent application of the BrdUrd method allows estimation of T_s and potential doubling time from a single biopsy.[19] The biopsy is usually taken about 3 hours after i.v. administration of BrdUrd, and two-parameter flow cytometry then allows recognition of the movement of the BrdUrd tagged cells (recognized by the fluorescent monoclonal antibody) through S-phase (defined by their DNA content using propidium iodide or a similar stain). The method is currently being used to determine the potential doubling time of selected human tumors before initiation of treatment and might find application in the optimization of treatment schedules.

Most fluorescent dyes that are used to bind DNA require fixation of the cells or are cytotoxic, thus preventing study of the biological properties of cells after fluorescence-activated cell sorting. The most widely used vital fluorescent stain is Hoechst 33342; this DNA-binding dye has been used to study properties of cells that are separated at different phases of the cell cycle and, if a colony-forming assay is available, can be used to study the cell cycle phase distribution of clonogenic cells. The dye is not ideal because it has toxicity for some types of cells and may add to the toxicity of cells treated with drugs or radiation. Other vital stains are being developed and may allow better characterization of the cell kinetics of clonogenic cells.

KINETIC PROPERTIES OF HUMAN TUMORS

The proportion of tumor cells undergoing DNA synthesis, as measured by thymidine labeling index or from DNA histograms generated by flow cytometry, gives a relatively simple measure of the overall rate of cell proliferation. Data are available for most types of human malignancy, and representative estimates of the percentage of S-phase cells are shown in Table 1-2. The values listed in Table 1-2 are composite means derived from a large number of studies, and there is a range of estimates of the percentage of S-phase cells for each type of tumor. In general, there is a correlation between the proportion of S-phase cells with increasing tumor grade and with aneuploidy.

The data in Table 1-2 indicate that many solid tumors in humans contain at most 10% cells that are in DNA synthesis, although higher proportions of S-phase cells are found in some rapidly growing tumors such as high-grade lymphomas. Proliferating cells in normal bone marrow and intestinal crypts have values of labeling index in the ranges of 30% to 70% and 12% to 18%, respectively. Thus, tumors do not have a higher proportion of S-phase cells than some normal tissues.

Published information about the duration of the cell cycle and its constituent phases in human tumors has been derived mainly from percent labeled mitoses experiments, and some of these data are summarized in Table 1-3. Recently, flow cytometry after administration of BrdUrd has allowed rapid estimation of the duration of DNA synthesis for several types of human tumor. These studies suggest that the mean duration of DNA synthesis is usually in the range of 12 to 24

TABLE 1-3. Estimates of Mean Duration of DNA Synthesis (T_s) and Cycle Time (T_c) Obtained for Selected Human Tumors

	Mean T_s (h)		*Mean T_c (days)*
Tumor Type	*By FCM**	*By PLM†*	*By PLM†*
Melanoma	9	21	2.5
Breast		21	2.5
Squamous cell of head and neck	12	20	2.5
Lung	26	20	4.5
Colon and rectum	25	17	3.0
Lymphomas	16	12	2.0
Acute leukemias	11	22	2.5

*Unpublished data of Wilson GD et al (personal communication) obtained by in vivo administration of BrdUrd followed by flow cytometry (FCM).

†Data obtained using the percent labeled mitoses method (PLM). Includes results reviewed by Steel[1] and Tannock.[29] Mean values of T_c have been estimated to the nearest ½ day.

TABLE 1-2. Representative Mean Values for the Proportion of S-Phase Cells in Selected Types of Human Tumors

Tumor Type	*Number of Patients*	*LI* (%) (using ³H-thymidine)*	*Number of Patients*	*S-Phase† (%) (by flow cytometry)*
Breast				
Primary	1075	4	151	8
Metastatic	80	9	12	10
Colorectal	284	11	53	18
Squamous cell	244	13	73	19
Sarcomas	70	5	68	11
Lymphomas				
Low grade			127	4
Intermediate grade	79	21	179	9
High grade			74	24

*Composite mean values of LI are derived from data provided by Wolberg and Ansfield[20] and from the review by Meyer.[21]

†Flow cytometric data are from references 22–28.

hours, with mean cell cycle times of 2 to 4 days. The latter estimates must be regarded as approximate because the available techniques are not sufficiently sensitive to distinguish between nonproliferating cells and those with longer cycle times. The mean cycle time of cells within human tumors (typically 2–4 days) is much shorter than the mean volume doubling time of the tumors (typically 2–3 months for common solid tumors). Two factors contribute to this difference: a high proportion of nonproliferating cells and a high rate of cell death.

Estimates of growth fraction obtained by comparing the measured proportion of S-phase cells (by flow cytometry or labeling index) with that predicted from the phase distribution of cycling cells are often consistent with values of growth fraction of the order of 20% to 30%. Tumor cells may be out of cycle because of differentiation or because of limited access to nutrients. There is marked heterogeneity in patterns of thymidine labeling within solid tumors, and the rate of cellular proliferation has been found to decrease rapidly with increasing distance from capillaries in both animal and human tumors.[30,31] This effect may lead to large errors in estimates of LI that are obtained from small biopsies. The observation may also be relevant to therapy in that it defines a population of poorly nourished cells that is known to be resistant to radiation because of hypoxia, and that may be resistant to chemotherapy because of limited drug access and a low rate of cellular proliferation.

The observation of necrosis and pyknotic cells in human tumors is evidence for cell death, and cells may also be lost from the tumor by shedding (*e.g.*, into the bowel) or through blood vessels and lymphatics. Steel[8] has estimated the rate of cell loss in various human tumors by comparing their potential doubling time (see Equation 1), which is the expected doubling time of the tumor in the absence of cell loss, with measured volume doubling times. The rate of cell loss is frequently found to be 80% or more of the rate of cell production. This observation supports the concept that tumors may be regarded as analogues of cell renewal tissues, but where the normal balance between cell production and loss is modified in favor of a slight excess of cell production.

DIAGNOSIS AND PROGNOSIS

FLOW CYTOMETRY AS A DIAGNOSTIC TOOL

Flow cytometry is being used increasingly as an aid in cancer diagnosis and histologic classification. Useful information can be obtained from DNA histograms and from using an increasing array of monoclonal antibodies to detect surface markers or cytoplasmic determinants of cells.

About 70% of all tumors have cells with abnormal DNA content.[32] DNA-specific staining of effusions or tissue biopsies, followed by flow cytometry, can detect a small proportion of aneuploid tumor cells mixed with normal diploid cells. This technique has been used to study the urine of patients who are suspected of having bladder cancer, and in one large study was shown to have a sensitivity of 80%, superior to that of conventional cytology.[33] The technique has also been studied as an alternative to cervical and vaginal cytology; it has the potential advantages of automation and objectivity, but the presence of inflammatory cells and cellular debris and clumps, resulting from imperfect methods for dissociation of tissue into single cells, may complicate the analysis. Future improvements in techniques for cellular dissociation, and simultaneous measurement of DNA content and cellular size by forward-angle light scatter, may allow increased use of flow cytometry in the diagnosis of solid tumors.

Dispersion of cells is not a problem in the study of lymphoma and leukemia, and flow cytometry is used increasingly in their diagnosis and classification. Subtypes of human leukemia and lymphoma may be differentiated by using fluorescence-labeled monoclonal antibodies directed against a variety of cellular antigens, including T-cell antigens, surface or cytoplasmic immunoglobulins, and common acute lymphocytic leukemia antigen (CALLA), among others. These methods not only are useful as a guide to classification but also may influence treatment, since different subtypes of leukemia are optimally treated with different drugs. Similar techniques may provide diagnostic information in the acquired immune deficiency syndrome (AIDS). The ratio of T-helper to T-suppressor cells can be measured by flow cytometry as the ratio of lymphoid cells expressing the T_4 or T_8 antigens, and in healthy individuals is usually in the range of 1.7 to 2.0. In patients with AIDS, the ratio is less than 1.0, although it may also be slightly decreased in homosexual men who are not infected with the AIDS virus.

It is sometimes difficult to diagnose B-cell lymphomas, as compared to reactive hyperplasia, by histologic criteria. B-cells express immunoglobulins on their cell surface, and differential diagnosis can be achieved by using a flow cytometric technique that detects an excess of cells expressing either κ or λ light chains with the aid of fluorescent monoclonal antibodies.[34] The ratio of κ- to λ-expressing cells is normally close to 1.0, and an excess of either cell type indicates clonal proliferation of one type of cell and implies the presence of lymphoma.

An increasing number of monoclonal antibodies are becoming available that react with antigenic determinants that have some degree of specificity for various types of malignant cells. Flow cytometry may allow the detection of a small subpopulation of cells that carry such determinants among a much larger population of normal cells, and it is likely to be used increasingly in cancer diagnosis.

PROGNOSIS

Before the availability of flow cytometry, a number of studies had attempted to correlate values of pretreatment labeling index of human tumors (measured usually by in vitro incubation with ^{3}H-thymidine) and prognosis. Some investigators reported improved prognosis with lower values of labeling index, but others reported the opposite. The probable reason for this discrepancy is that patients with tumors having a lower labeling index were likely to have slowly progressive disease but, because most drugs are more active against proliferating cells, were also less likely to respond to chemotherapy. The technique is time consuming, and most studies were based on small samples of patients with various stages of disease and other prognostic factors.

The ability of flow cytometry to provide rapid, automated analysis of large numbers of cells has prompted a reexamination of the relevance of cell kinetic parameters to prognosis. It is now possible to perform flow cytometry studies using cells dissociated from paraffin-embedded sections.[35] Series of patients who have received uniform treatment in clinical trials and for whom complete clinical follow-up is available can thus be studied retrospectively using archival material obtained from pathology departments. This powerful approach is being applied to large groups of patients with several types of tumors.

Two properties of DNA histograms may be correlated with prognosis: ploidy as measured by the DNA index (the mean DNA content of G_1-cells in the tumor as compared to a DNA index of 1 for normal diploid G_1 cells); and the percentage of S-phase cells. Data from some larger studies are summarized in Table 1-4, and for most (but not all) tumor types, aneuploidy is associated with higher grade and poorer prognosis. In ovarian cancer, for example, aneuploidy was the most critical determinant of prognosis when analyzed with other potential prognostic factors by multivariate analysis.[36] Aneuploid tumors also tended to have a higher proportion of S-phase cells, but in general the correlation of prognosis with S-phase proportion was weak.

Flow cytometry may also provide useful information about hormone receptors in malignant cells. The presence of high estrogen and progestin receptor levels in breast cancer is known to be associated with a more favorable prognosis and is strongly predictive of response to hormonal therapy. Hormone receptors in cells may be detected by flow cytometry with the aid of fluorescence-labeled hormones that recognize the receptors. When perfected, this technique will have the advantage of speed and automation and will allow assessment of heterogeneity of receptor content among the cells of the population, rather than just the average value that is obtained by conventional methods. This information may be of additional prognostic value and might also guide the more appropriate use of hormones in cancer treatment.

TABLE 1-4. Prognostic Significance of Cellular DNA Content in Selected Human Tumors

Tumor Type	*Survival Advantage for Diploid Tumors*
Breast*	+
Ovary*	+
Cervix	+
Endometrium	+
Prostate	+
Bladder	+
Kidney	+
Lung	+
Colon	+
Melanoma	−
Brain tumors	−
ALL	−
AML	+
Myeloma*	+
Lymphomas	±

From data reviewed in Friedlander, et al[36] and Cornelisse, et al.[37]
*Ploidy has been shown to be an independent prognostic variable in postmenopausal breast cancer, ovarian cancer, and myeloma.

CELL KINETICS AND TREATMENT

CYCLE-DEPENDENCE OF THERAPY

Rapidly growing tumors tend to be most sensitive to chemotherapy. Also, damage to normal tissues at short intervals after chemotherapy or wide-field radiation is most often observed in organs such as the bone marrow or the intestine, which are renewal tissues known to contain rapidly proliferating cells. These observations suggest that rapidly proliferating cells may be more susceptible to therapy and have led to several studies of the relationship between cytotoxicity and proliferative rate.

When mammalian cells are cultured, they show a period of exponential growth when all cells are proliferating, followed by slowing of growth as cells become crowded and consume available nutrients. The culture reaches a maximum size in plateau phase, when cell proliferation is very slow (Fig. 1-8A). The effects of a given treatment on rapidly and slowly proliferating cells may therefore be studied by assessing colony formation in new cultures following treatment of cells in exponential and plateau phase. Frequently this type of experiment leads to survival curves similar to those in Figure 1-8B, which show that rapidly proliferating cells are more sensitive to the drug. This technique and others (*e.g.*, the spleen colony assay[38]) have demonstrated that some drugs (*e.g.*, methotrexate, cytarabine, and vinca alkaloids) exert lethal effects only against proliferating cells. Others, including anthracyclines and most alkylating agents, have some activity against slowly proliferating cells but are considerably more toxic to rapidly proliferating cells.[29] Only for a few drugs, including cisplatin, nitrosoureas, and bleomycin, is there little or no selectivity, and this may be cell-line dependent.

Most drugs and ionizing radiation vary in their lethal effects at different phases of the cell cycle. This phenomenon has been studied either by synchronizing cells in a given cell cycle phase[39] or by sorting cells at different phases of the cycle immediately before or after treatment, followed by a cloning assay to assess their viability. Cells may be separated in different phases of the cell cycle by using fluorescence-activated cell sorting, although this technique is currently limited because available nontoxic fluorescent stains for DNA may influence the cytotoxicity of anticancer drugs or radiation.[40] An alternative method, centrifugal elutriation, separates cells on the basis of size in a continuous flow centrifuge and has been useful in obtaining information about treatment effects during the cell cycle. These methods have demonstrated that many drugs exert their maximum lethal effects when cells are synthesizing DNA (Fig. 1-9); this is true for most of the antimetabolites and for anthracyclines. Vinblastine and vincristine also exert their cytotoxic action in the S-phase, although cells may arrest and die when they subsequently attempt to pass through mitosis. For ionizing radiation and many alkylating agents, the pattern of toxicity

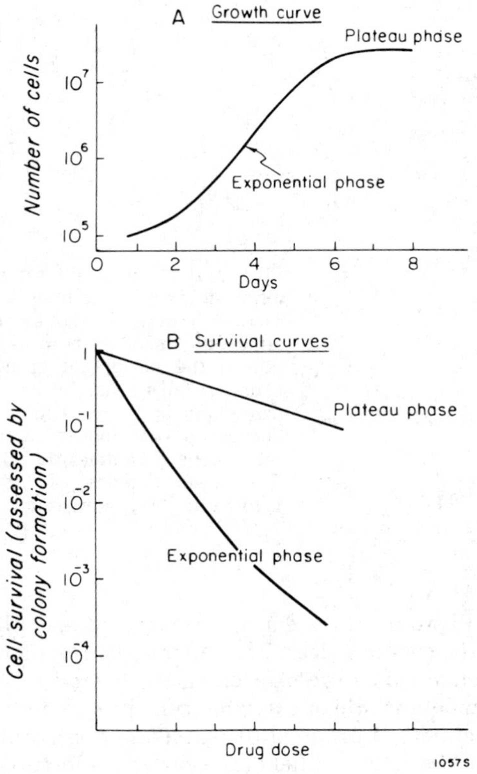

FIG. 1-8. **A.** Cells in tissue culture show a period of rapid proliferation and exponential growth, followed by slowing of growth and a plateau phase as nutrients are depleted and cell concentration increases. **B.** The effect of drugs against slowly and rapidly proliferating cells can be assessed by treatment of cell cultures in exponential and plateau phase. Cells are then replated to assess survival by colony formation. Most drugs show greater toxicity for rapidly proliferating cells in exponential growth phase, as in the example shown.

FIG. 1-9. The position in the cell cycle at which anticancer drugs and radiation most often exert their maximum lethal toxicity. Drugs and radiation may also act to delay progression around the cycle (*e.g.*, vinblastine and vincristine induce mitotic arrest).

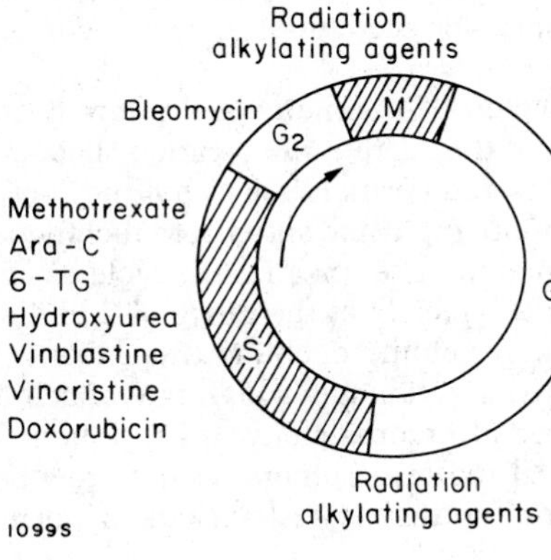

is more complex with two periods of maximum activity, one for cells near the G_1/S transition and one for G_2-phase or mitotic cells.

SCHEDULING OF CHEMOTHERAPY

Because most drugs have varying toxicity for cells in different phases of the cell cycle, immediately after treatment a high proportion of surviving cells will be partially synchronized in a resistant phase. Several investigators have proposed that drug treatment might be scheduled at intervals that allow the synchronized surviving tumor cells to progress to a drug-sensitive phase of the cell cycle, or, conversely, such that cells in critical normal tissues are again in a drug-resistant phase. In practice, the wide heterogeneity of cell cycle parameters among individual cells and of drug distribution makes this difficult to achieve.

It has been demonstrated that therapeutic outcome is markedly dependent on scheduling interval for drug treatment of experimental tumors,[41] but it has been difficult to predict the optimum scheduling interval from knowledge of cell cycle kinetics.[29] It is probable that the interval between injection of cycle-specific drugs within a given course of chemotherapy could have a strong influence on therapeutic outcome in humans, but, at present, any improvements in scheduling are likely to be achieved by empirical means.

Knowledge of the cell population kinetics in critical normal tissues is important in understanding the basis for scheduling of successive courses of chemotherapy. Scheduling is based on a need for recovery between courses of critical normal tissues, most frequently the bone marrow or intestinal mucosa. A schematic illustration of cell proliferation in the bone marrow is shown in Figure 1-10. Pluripotential stem cells normally have a low rate of cell proliferation and are therefore protected from toxicity of cycle-dependent drugs. In contrast, rapidly proliferating granulocyte precursors (myeloblasts, promyelocytes, and myelocytes) are depleted by chemotherapy; this leads to a delayed fall in granulocyte count, since more mature nonproliferating precursors such as metamyelocytes and bands continue to differentiate into mature granulocytes within the first few days after drug treatment. Thereafter, the granulocyte count falls rapidly to a nadir, usually reached at 10 to 14 days after treatment. For some drugs (*e.g.*, vinblastine), the nadir occurs earlier, and there is evidence that many other drugs delay the process of maturation.

Drugs also exert toxic effects against proliferating red cell precursors and megakaryocytes, but the granulocyte count is most susceptible to chemotherapy because mature cells have a short lifespan. When the granulocyte count falls, feedback mechanisms induce stem cells to cycle, leading to recovery that for most drugs is complete within 3 to 4 weeks. This provides the basis for the usual interval between courses of chemotherapy; reinitiation of chemotherapy at earlier intervals may expose stem cells to drugs when they are cycling and cause permanent damage to bone marrow.

The delayed fall in granulocyte count has allowed the development of schedules in which cycle-active drugs are given on days 1 and 8 of a 4-week cycle. This strategy has been used in regimens such as mechlorethamine, vincristine, pro-

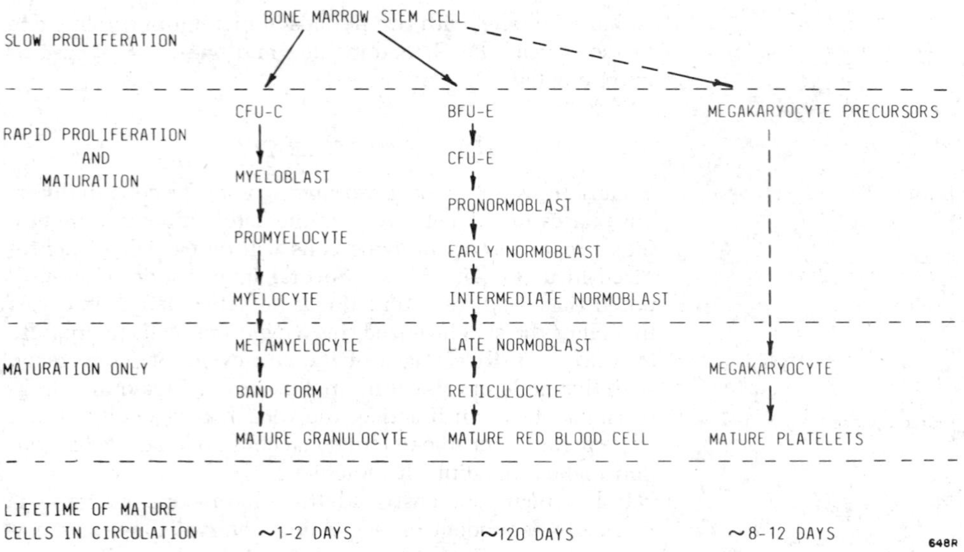

FIG. 1-10. Cell proliferation and differentiation in the bone marrow. Toxicity of drugs for rapidly proliferating precursors leads to a delayed fall in the peripheral granulocyte count. A fall in platelet or erythrocyte count is observed more rarely because of the longer lifetime of these cells. (Tannock IF, Hill RP: The Basic Science of Oncology. Elmsford, NY, Pergamon Press, 1987)

carbazine, and prednisone (MOPP) for Hodgkin's disease and cyclophosphamide, methotrexate, and 5-fluorouracil (CMF) for breast cancer. The second injection of drugs at 1 week after the first is tolerated because the bone marrow stem cells have not yet been stimulated to proliferate, since the second treatment precedes the fall in peripheral granulocyte count.

Some drugs, including melphalan, nitrosoureas, and mitomycin C, cause more prolonged myelosuppression. These drugs show little selectivity for cycling cells and may therefore be expected to damage stem cells. Evidence for damage to stem cells is shown by the decreased ability of murine stem cells to repopulate the marrow following serial treatment with BCNU or melphalan, as compared to treatment with cyclophosphamide, doxorubicin, or 5-fluorouracil.[42,43] These results agree with the clinical experience that cumulative myelosuppression is more common after treatment with BCNU or melphalan.

SCHEDULING OF RADIOTHERAPY

It has been found empirically that radiation treatment may be both effective and tolerated when delivered as a course of small dose fractions (usually 200 cGy or less) over several weeks. Several processes take place between fractions, including repair of sublethal damage, repopulation of surviving cells, redistribution of surviving cells to more radiosensitive phases of the cell cycle, and, in tumors, improvement in cellular oxygenation. Repair and repopulation between fractions are the major processes that allow normal tissues to tolerate protracted fractionated radiation with acceptable levels of damage.

Scheduling of radiotherapy has developed empirically, and most patients are treated daily from Monday to Friday. It is known from animal models that the interval between radiation doses may influence the outcome of therapy, and there has been recent interest in attempting to modify radiation fractionation in an attempt to improve therapeutic index. Tumor cell proliferation during fractionated radiotherapy may limit the overall success of treatment; hence, there may be therapeutic gain from shortening the overall treatment time for tumors in which surviving cells proliferate rapidly during treatment,[44] provided that dose-limiting normal tissues within the radiation field are slowly proliferating. Several investigators are attempting to measure pretreatment cell cycle parameters, particularly the potential doubling time of constituent cells, using BrdUrd incorporation and flow cytometry. Tumors with rapid proliferation are then treated using accelerated fractionation in which three or more doses are delivered each day, whereas slowly proliferating tumors are treated by conventional fractionation schedules. Data are not yet available to judge the benefits of this approach, but it represents an attempt to improve the outcome of radiotherapy that is based on sound scientific principles.

CONCLUSION

Human tumors often grow exponentially during a period of clinical observation, and typical volume doubling times for common solid tumors are in the range of 2 to 3 months. Tumors have a long period of preclinical growth, offering ample opportunity for seeding of metastases before clinical detection.

Methods based on ^{3}H-thymidine and autoradiography have provided much of the current information about cell kinetics of human tumors and normal tissues, but they are now being supplanted by more rapid and automated techniques employing flow cytometry. The mean cell cycle time of many human tumors is typically in the range of 2 to 4 days, much shorter than their volume doubling time; this is consistent with a low growth fraction and a high rate of cell loss. There is a large degree of heterogeneity in cell kinetic properties within individual tumors. Tumors do not grow because the rate of cell proliferation is faster than in normal tissues;

rather, they grow because the rate of cell production exceeds the rate of cell death.

About 70% of all tumors have abnormal DNA content, and flow cytometry can aid diagnosis by detecting a small proportion of aneuploid tumor cells mixed with normal diploid cells. With the aid of fluorescence-labeled monoclonal antibodies, flow cytometry is used increasingly to characterize the phenotype of malignant cells, especially in the classification of lymphomas and leukemias. DNA histograms have also been generated from paraffin-embedded sections of a variety of tumors, and for many human tumors aneuploidy is associated with poor prognosis.

Most anticancer drugs show greater toxicity for rapidly proliferating cells, and drugs and radiation have variable activity around the cell cycle. It is unlikely that these effects can be used to increase therapeutic index through synchronization of cells because of heterogeneity in cell cycle parameters and drug distribution. The greater sensitivity of rapidly proliferating cells suggests an explanation for the greater responsiveness of rapidly growing tumors to chemotherapy and allows an understanding of the fall and recovery of the granulocyte count following drug treatment. Proliferation of tumor cells during a course of fractionated radiation therapy may limit the success of treatment, and it may be possible to develop accelerated fractionation schedules for tumors with rapid cell proliferation following evaluation of their cycle kinetics by flow cytometry.

REFERENCES

1. Steel GG: Growth Kinetics of Tumours: Cell Population Kinetics in Relation to the Growth and Treatment of Cancer. Oxford, Clarendon Press, 1977
2. Tannock IF, Hill RP: The Basic Science of Oncology. Elmsford, NY, Pergamon Press, 1987
3. Tannock IF: Biology of tumor growth. Hosp Pract [Off] 18:81, 1983
4. Shackney SE, McCormack GW, Cuchural GJ Jr: Growth rate patterns of solid tumors and their relation to responsiveness to therapy. An analytical review. Ann Intern Med 89:107, 1978
5. Folkman J: Tumor angiogenesis: A possible control point in tumor growth. Ann Intern Med 82:96, 1975
6. Howard A, Pelc SR: Nuclear incorporation of P^{32} as demonstrated by autoradiographs. J Exp Cell Res 2:178, 1951
7. Mendelsohn ML: The growth fraction: A new concept applied to tumours. Science 132:1496, 1960
8. Steel GG: Cell loss as a factor in the growth rate of human tumours. Eur J Cancer Clin Oncol 3:381, 1967
9. Pierce GB, Shikes R, Fink LM: Cancer: A Problem of Developmental Biology. Englewood Cliffs, NJ, Prentice-Hall, 1978
10. Pierce GB, Wallace C: Differentiation of malignant to benign cells. Cancer Res 31:127, 1971
11. Bush RS, Hill RP: Biological discussion augmenting radiation effects and model systems. Laryngoscope 85:1119, 1975
12. Hamburger AW, Salmon SE: Primary bioassay of human myeloma stem cells. J Clin Invest 60:846, 1977
13. Courtenay VD, Selby PJ, Smith IE, et al: Growth of human tumour cell colonies from biopsies using two soft-agar techniques. Br J Cancer 38:77, 1978
14. MacKillop WJ, Stewart SS, Buick RN: Density/volume analysis in the study of cellular heterogeneity in human ovarian carcinoma. Br J Cancer 45:812, 1982
15. Fauser AA, Messner HA: Proliferative state of human pluripotent hemopoietic progenitors (CFU-GEMM) in normal individuals and under regenerative conditions after bone marrow transplantation. Blood 54:1197, 1979.
16. Shirakawa S, Luce JK, Tannock I, et al: Cell proliferation in human melanoma. J Clin Invest 49:1188, 1970
17. Nelson JRS, Schiffer LM: Autoradiographic detection of DNA polymerase containing nuclei in sarcoma 180 ascites cells. Cell Tissue Kinet 6:45, 1973
18. Gray JW (ed): Monoclonal antibodies against bromodeoxyuridine. Cytometry 6:499, 1985
19. Begg AC, McNally NJ, Schrieve DC, et al: A method to measure the duration of DNA synthesis and the potential doubling time from a single sample. Cytometry 6:620, 1985
20. Wolberg WH, Ansfield FJ: The relation of thymidine labeling index in human tumors *in vitro* to the effectivness of 5-fluorouracil chemotherapy. Cancer Res 81:448, 1971
21. Meyer JS: Cell kinetic measurements of human tumors. Hum Pathol 13:874, 1982
22. Frankfurt OS, Greco WR, Slocum HK, et al: Proliferative characteristics of primary and metastatic human solid tumors by DNA flow cytometry. Cytometry 5:629, 1984
23. Johnson TS, Williamson KD, Cramer MM, et al: Flow cytometric analysis of head and neck carcinoma DNA index and S-fraction from paraffin-embedded sections: Comparison with malignancy grading. Cytometry 6:461, 1985
24. McDivitt RW, Stone KR, Craig RB, et al: A comparison of human breast cancer cell kinetics measured by flow cytometry and thymidine labeling. Lab Invest 52:287, 1985
25. Srigley J, Barlogie B, Butler JJ, et al: Heterogeneity of non-Hodgkin's lymphoma probed by nucleic acid cytometry. Blood 65:1090, 1985
26. Christensson B, Tribukait B, Linder I-L, et al: Cell proliferation and DNA content in non-Hodgkin's lymphoma: Flow cytometry in relation to lymphoma classification. Cancer 58:1295, 1986
27. Juneja SK, Cooper IA, Hodgson GS, et al: DNA ploidy patterns and cytokinetics of non-Hodgkin's lymphoma. J Clin Pathol 39:98, 1986
28. Kallioniemi O-P, Hietanen T, Mattila J, et al: Aneuploid DNA content and high S-phase fraction of tumor cells are related to poor prognosis in patients with primary breast cancer. Eur J Cancer Clin Oncol 23:277, 1987
29. Tannock I: Cell kinetics and chemotherapy: A critical review. Cancer Treat Rep 62:1117, 1978
30. Tannock IF: The relation between cell proliferation and the vascular system in a transplanted murine mammary tumour. Br J Cancer 22:258, 1968
31. Moore JV, Hasleton PS, Buckley CH: Tumour cords in 52 human bronchial and cervical squamous cell carcinomas: Inferences for their cellular kinetics and radiobiology. Br J Cancer 51:407, 1985
32. Barlogie B, Raber MN, Schumann J, et al: Flow cytometry in clinical cancer research. Cancer Res 43:3982, 1983
33. Badalament RA, Kimmel M, Gay H, et al: The sensitivity of flow cytometry compared with conventional cytology in the detection of superficial bladder carcinoma. Cancer 59:2078, 1987
34. Ault KA: Detection of small numbers of monoclonal B lymphocytes in the blood of patients with lymphoma. N Engl J Med 300:1401, 1979
35. Hedley DW, Friedlander ML, Taylor IW, et al: Method for analysis of cellular DNA content of paraffin embedded pathological material using flow cytometry. J Histochem Cytochem 31:1333, 1983
36. Friedlander ML, Hedley DW, Taylor IW: Clinical and biological significance of aneuploidy in human tumours. J Clin Pathol 37:961, 1984
37. Cornelisse CJ, Van de Velde CJH, Caspers RJC, et al: DNA ploidy and survival in breast cancer patients. Cytometry 8:225, 1987
38. Till JE, McCulloch EA: A direct measurement of the radiation sensitivity of normal mouse bone marrow cells. Radiat Res 14:213, 1961
38. Nias AH, Fox M: Synchronization of mammalian cells with respect to the mitotic cycle. Cell Tissue Kinet 4:375, 1971
40. Pallavicini MG, Lalande ME, Miller RG, et al: Cell cycle distribution of chronically hypoxic cells and determination of the clonogenic potential of cells accumulated in G_2 and M phases after irradiation of a solid tumor *in vivo*. Cancer Res 39:1891, 1979
41. Skipper HE, Schabel FM Jr, Wilcox WS: Experimental evaluation of potential anticancer agents. XXI. Scheduling of arabinosylcytosine to take advantage of its S-phase specificity against leukemic cells. Cancer Chemother Rep 54:125, 1967
42. Trainor KJ, Seshadri RS, Morley AA: Residual marrow injury following cytotoxic drugs.Leuk Res 3:205, 1979
43. Botnick LE, Hannon EC, Vigneulle R, et al: Differential effects of cytotoxic agents on hematopoietic progenitors. Cancer Res 41:2338, 1981
44. Denekamp J: Cell kinetics and radiation biology. Int J Radiat Biol 49:357, 1986

MICHAEL DEAN

GEORGE F. VANDE WOUDE

CHAPTER 2 *Principles of Molecular Cell Biology of Cancer: Introduction to Methods in Molecular Biology*

For a major portion of this century and as recently as 1979, there was considerable controversy over whether viruses cause cancer or whether environmental insults to normal cell genes can initiate the cancer process.[1] Only during the past 4 years have we learned, as a result of extraordinary advances in biotechnology, that both viruses and genetic mutations can mediate neoplastic disease by similar mechanisms. Diverse basic research disciplines, woven together by technological breakthroughs in molecular biology and genetic engineering, have provided new concepts of the molecular basis of neoplastic disease. Absolute measurements in molecular biology and genetic engineering technologies have provided us with our first descriptions of the molecular elements responsible for triggering the events that lead to cancer. The terms DNA sequence, hybridization, molecular cloning, linkage analyses, and pulsed-field gel electrophoresis are part of a growing armamentarium of techniques used to identify, isolate, and characterize the molecular elements that have been implicated in normal and abnormal biological processes in human and animal cells (see Appendix.)

The recent achievements promise important applications of this new information for clinical diagnostics in human diseases and cancer, and for this purpose it is important to understand the technology and how it is used. Certainly, if specific cellular genes are shown to be associated with specific tumor types, like c-*myc* in Burkitt's lymphoma,[2] or c-*abl* in chronic myelogenous leukemia,[3–5] then the molecular biology tools become unambiguous diagnostic reagents. In cancer, we may be relating molecular alterations to types of proliferative growth, and it may be only the temporary lack of technical sophistication that prevents correlation of genetic and molecular changes with benign and preneoplastic (*e.g.*, hyperplasia, metaplasia, dysplasia, anaplasia) or malignant neoplastic cellular changes. The rapidly emerging biotechnology requires familiarization with the specialized terminology of molecular biology, including the key terms mentioned above. It is necessary to introduce the names of molecular structures and techniques used in molecular biology, molecular genetics, and genetic engineering.

GENE EXPRESSION: TRANSCRIPTION TRANSLATION

The flow of information in eukaryotic cells is from DNA to RNA, a process termed RNA transcription, and from RNA into protein, a process termed translation (Fig. 2-1). The

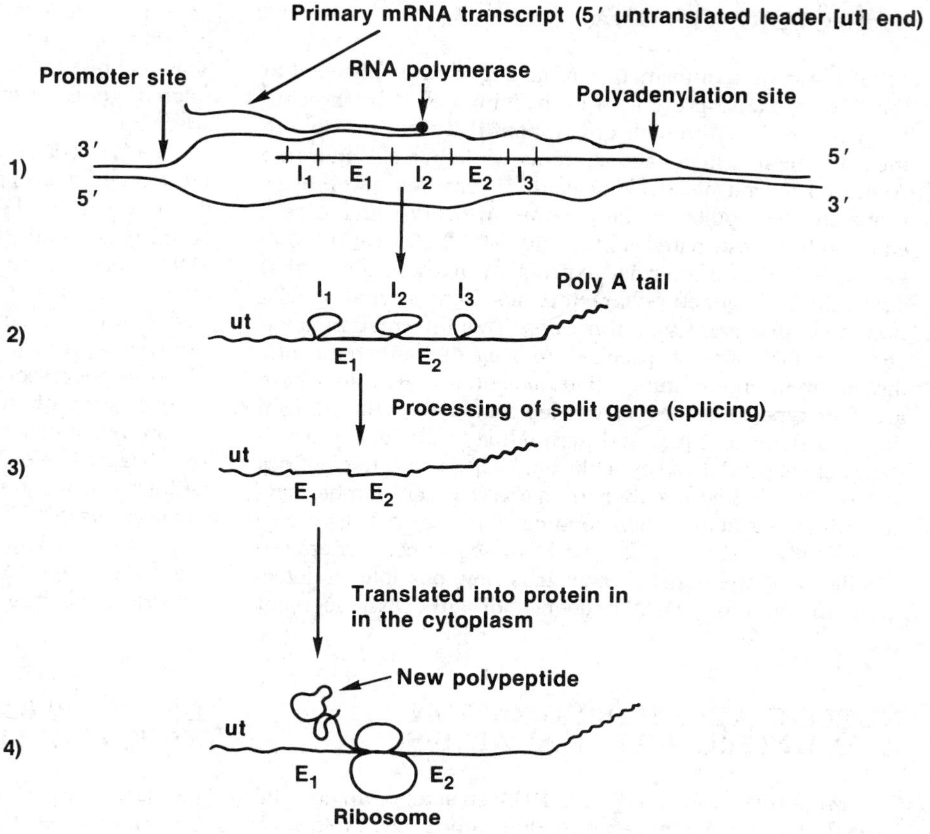

FIG. 2-1. Gene transcription and translation. Messenger RNA synthesis by polymerase II is initiated from a site in the gene called a promoter, and RNA is transcribed from the complementary (nonsense) DNA strand of the structural (protein coding) gene. Thus the 5′ (upstream) end of the RNA is transcribed from a DNA sequence in the 3′ to 5′ orientation (line 1). The first portion usually lacks structural (protein coding) information and is referred to as untranslated (ut) leader. The newly transcribed structural information is interrupted by intervening sequences (introns, I_1 to I_3), which are processed (spliced) from the transcript to leave only structural coding exons (E_1 and E_2) (lines 2 and 3). The transcribed messenger RNA (mRNA) is terminated by the addition of approximately 200 adenine nucleotide bases. The process is called polyadenylation, and the sequence is referred to as the poly A tail. The mRNA is transported to the cytoplasm, where it is translated or decoded into protein. This occurs in cytoplasmic structures called polyribosomes, and the decoding is performed by transfer RNA (tRNA) molecules that recognize the specific nucleotide codon information and provide the appropriate amino acid for linking to the growing polypeptide chain.[93]

enzyme RNA polymerase copies or transcribes genes that encode proteins into RNA[6,7] using monomeric nucleotides similar to, but with subtle differences from, the four nucleotides present in DNA. These monomeric nucleotides are called ribonucleotide bases. The RNA copy of the DNA is referred to as messenger RNA (mRNA) (see Fig. 2-1). Genes that are transcribed into mRNA are translated into the cytoplasm into proteins by a translation system that deciphers the amino acid sequence encoded in the mRNA transcript.[8] RNA synthesis is initiated from a promoter region in the DNA[6,7,9,10] (see Fig. 2-1), and the primary RNA transcript consists of a series of coding and noncoding regions (termed exons and introns, respectively). During processing, introns are removed (spliced out) from the primary transcript and adenylic acid residues added to one end in a process termed polyadenylation. The mature mRNA is then transported to the cytoplasm and subsequently translated into protein on structures termed polyribosomes. The first portion of mRNA usually does not code for a protein sequence and is referred to as untranslated leader. The coding region of the mRNA is dictated by a series of triplets of nucleotide bases called codons, each specifying an amino acid in the translated protein. Thus, the precise order of nucleotides in the DNA sequence determines the precise order of amino acids in a protein chain. The order of the amino acids in a protein chain is responsible for the three-dimensional structure of the protein and its biochemical activity.

The advances in modern biology are paced by the advances in technology which allow the measurements of the various processes, beginning with DNA and its structure and ending with the protein product, its structure and function. Techniques have been developed that allow analysis at each step in the process of information flow from DNA to protein (see Fig. 2-1). For example, the technique first developed by E. Southern and referred to as Southern analysis[11] provides a means for examining DNA structural elements of a single gene in the presence of all the other genes of a eukaryotic organism. Somewhat later, a technique was developed to identify specific mRNA species (transcripts) in the presence of all RNA transcripts expressed within a single cell type.[12] Even though this technique was developed on the west coast of the United States, it has been termed Northern analysis by its founders. Likewise, a technique that detects a single protein species from among all the proteins expressed in a specific cell or tissue has been termed Western blot analysis by its founders.[13] In this chapter we describe the structure and function of DNA and the methods in current use that allow the determination of its primary structure and organization. This will ultimately lead to physical mapping and sequencing of the entire human genome. In the following chapter describing gene regulation, we discuss the methods used for its study and for analysis of the protein products translated from RNA. The descriptions of the methods are coordinated with the presentation of molecular biology of the process.

STRUCTURE OF DNA

All of the genetic information of an organism is encoded in the DNA genome present in each living cell.[14] In the cell, DNA is condensed into chromatin, but if it were possible to measure the length of each DNA molecule in a chromosome from end to end, it could measure 10 cm long. Moreover, there are two copies of the genome in every somatic cell, each with an estimated complexity of 50,000 to 100,000 genes. It is the differential expression of these genes that determines all genetic characteristics from animal speciation to cellular and tissue functions. This information is encoded in DNA by the precise ordering of four chemically distinct monomeric units called nucleotides, of which there are two types: purine bases (deoxyadenylic acid [A] and deoxyguanylic acid [G]) and pyrimidine bases (deoxythymidylic acid [T] and deoxycytidylic acid [C]). These nucleotides or bases are linked together in chains that can number several billion per mammalian genome (Fig. 2-2).[14] The precise order of nucleotides, called the DNA sequence, confers the specificity of the genetic code. It is now possible to determine the absolute DNA sequence of any DNA segment (Fig. 2-3).[15,16]

NUCLEIC ACID HYBRIDIZATION AND HETERODUPLEX ANALYSIS

The properties associated with DNA structure provide the basis for modern genetic engineering technology. First, each DNA molecule consists of two strands (each somatic cell is diploid and therefore possesses four strands) paired together in what is referred to as the Watson-Crick double helix[17] (see Fig. 2-2). Each nucleotide has polarity, and this direction in each DNA strand is indicated by a 5′ to 3′ notation. Note also that each strand is complementary to the other in the double helix and they run in opposite directions. In the complementary strands, the *A* nucleotide pairs with *T*, whereas *G* always pairs with *C* (called base pairs).[14] The chemical bonds responsible for base pairing and holding the complementary strands together are weak, and in vitro the two strands can be denatured (separated or melted apart) by temperatures of 70 to 80°C or by alkaline pH conditions. Likewise, the precise order of base pairing between the two strands allows the strands to reanneal at low temperatures in neutral solution because the energy of each base pair is reinforced by that of its neighbors.[18-21] As few as 15 base pairs are sufficient for two strands to anneal.[22-24] The length of the strands can influence annealing efficiency markedly, and very long strands can actually interfere with the process.

The ability to denature or separate the two strands and to allow them to reanneal is the basic principle in the nucleic acid hybridization technique (see Appendix). Annealing can occur between DNA sequences in which fewer than 75% of the bases are complementary (homologous), and the strands will still form base pairs or hybridize.[18] Thus, a DNA sequence from a human gene such as the globin gene, under defined annealing conditions, can form a hybrid with the globin DNA sequences in mouse genomic DNA because the latter share partial homology with the human sequence. If one of the sequences is first isotopically labeled, then the hybridized sequences can be visualized on autoradiographs. This technique has permitted us to identify the presence of related genes, such as oncogenes, in cells of different species.

We can visualize individual hybrid DNA molecules in the electron microscope (Fig. 2-4). The homologous stretches of sequences in two DNA molecules can be compared and measured in a technique known as heteroduplex analysis. The DNA molecules to be compared are mixed, denatured into single strands, and allowed to form hybrids (double strands) under nondenaturing, annealing conditions.[25] The molecules are then spread on a surface of water, picked up onto an electron microscope grid, and shadowed with metal to allow identification of the DNA single- and complementary double-stranded structures of individual molecules in an electron beam. The example shown is a heteroduplex between a cellular oncogene (c-*ras*^{H}, see Chap. 4) and its viral homologue (v-*ras*^{H}).[26] The regions of DNA sequence homology are observed as double-stranded, whereas nonhomologous regions are single-stranded, as revealed by the relative thicknesses of the strands.

DNA DUPLICATION AND NICK TRANSLATION

The DNA molecule is duplicated in vivo by a DNA polymerase enzyme[27,28] that copies the template or parental strand by linking together the individual nucleotides as they base pair with the template DNA (see Fig. 2-2). The new DNA molecules, each consisting of parental strand and a newly synthesized strand, are partitioned to each new daughter cell during cell division.

The DNA polymerase enzyme is used extensively in vitro in the laboratory to copy a DNA sequence that has been treated with the enzyme deoxyribonuclease (DNase) under conditions that cause nicks in single-stranded DNA. The DNA polymerase begins at the nick and replaces (in the 5′ to 3′ direction) the nucleotides in the nicked strand. When isotopically labeled nucleotides (usually ^{32}P or ^{3}H isotopes) are included in the reaction, the DNA becomes uniformly labeled.[29,30] This reaction is referred to as nick translation (see Appendix). The isotopically labeled DNA sequence can then be used as a probe to detect, by hybridization, its homologous sequence in other DNA fragments. In this manner, a labeled DNA sequence such as a fragment of the globin gene will hybridize only to the unique globin gene copy among the more than 50,000 genes in the DNA molecule of a mammal and is the molecular biologist's tool for finding the proverbial needle in a haystack.

A variation of this technique known as *random priming* uses a randomly generated set of six base-pair oligonucleotides as primers to generate labeled DNA of very high specific activity.[31] A related technique, called the polymerase chain reaction (PCR), uses specific primers to copy and amplify a specific DNA sequence.[32] PCR technology has been used to amplify and then detect or clone selected regions of mammalian DNA.[33] It is possible by this technique

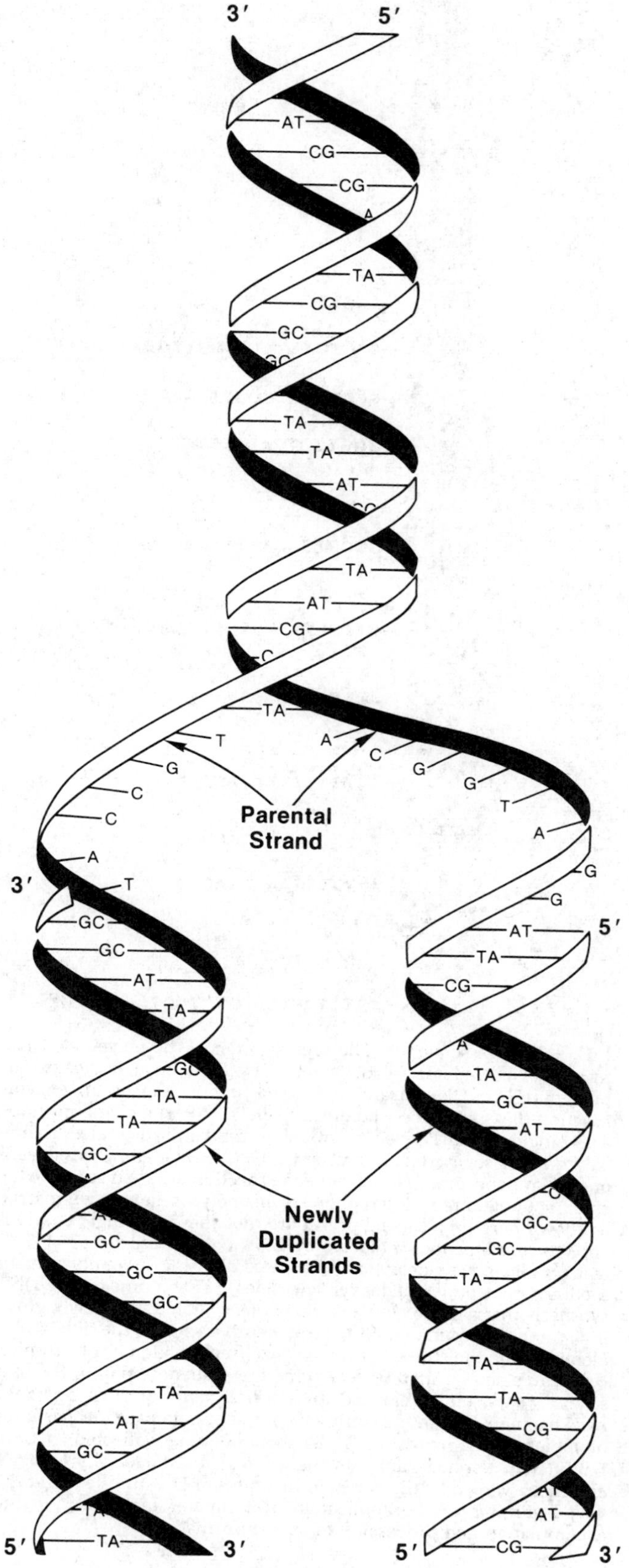

FIG. 2-2. Structure of DNA. The precise order of monomeric deoxyribonucleic acids (adenylic [A], thymidylic [T], guanylic [G], and cytodylic [C] acids) in the DNA molecule encodes all the genetic information for each organism. The DNA molecule consists of two strands in opposite polarity as determined by the orientation of the monomer nucleotide bases and indicated by a 5′ to 3′ notation. The two strands of opposite polarity are held together by weak bonds between pairs of nucleotide bases. Note that A always pairs with T and G with C. When DNA is duplicated by DNA polymerase, the newly synthesized strand is formed by linking the appropriate base pairs as directed by the template of the parental strand.

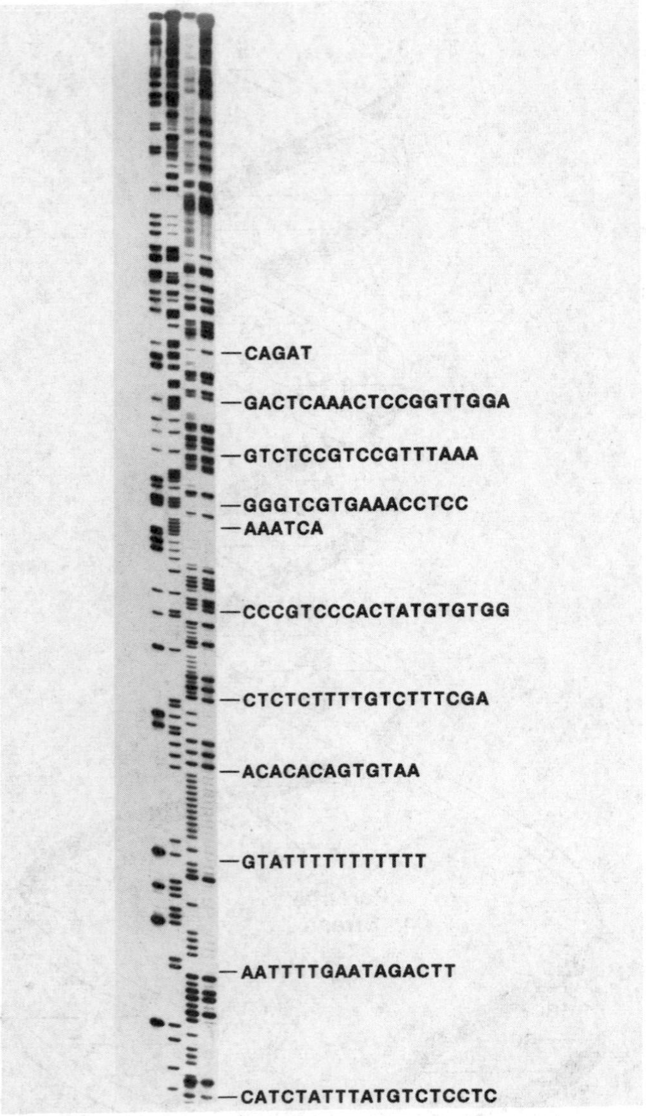

FIG. 2-3. DNA sequence. The precise order of the nucleotide bases in a DNA strand can be determined by DNA sequencing. In one procedure,[15] a DNA strand is labeled at one end by an enzyme reaction that can place isotopically labeled ^{32}P in a single position. The single-strand labeled fragment is randomly degraded chemically in four separate reactions at C, T+C, A+G, and G residues,[15] and the random fragments from each reaction are then subjected to size fractionation by electrophoresis in a polyacrylamide gel matrix, as shown here. In a second procedure, not shown, a single strand is copied from a primer molecule by DNA polymerase (see Fig. 2-1) using radioactive nucleotide bases and limiting amounts of four modified nucleotides (dideoxynucleotides).[16] Each time during DNA synthesis that a dideoxynucleotide is incorporated, the newly growing strand is terminated. Since the incorporation of the dideoxynucleotides into the strand is random, size fractionation by electrophoresis can again be used to determine the sequence. Within the past several years, more than 2.8 million base pairs of DNA sequence have been entered into a common computer data bank for purposes of molecular comparisons. DNA sequences are collected in GenBank (Bolt, Beranek, and Newman, Inc., Cambridge, MA) under a contract awarded by the National Institutes of Health. We are at the very beginning of the application of computer technology in the accumulation and processing of such information.

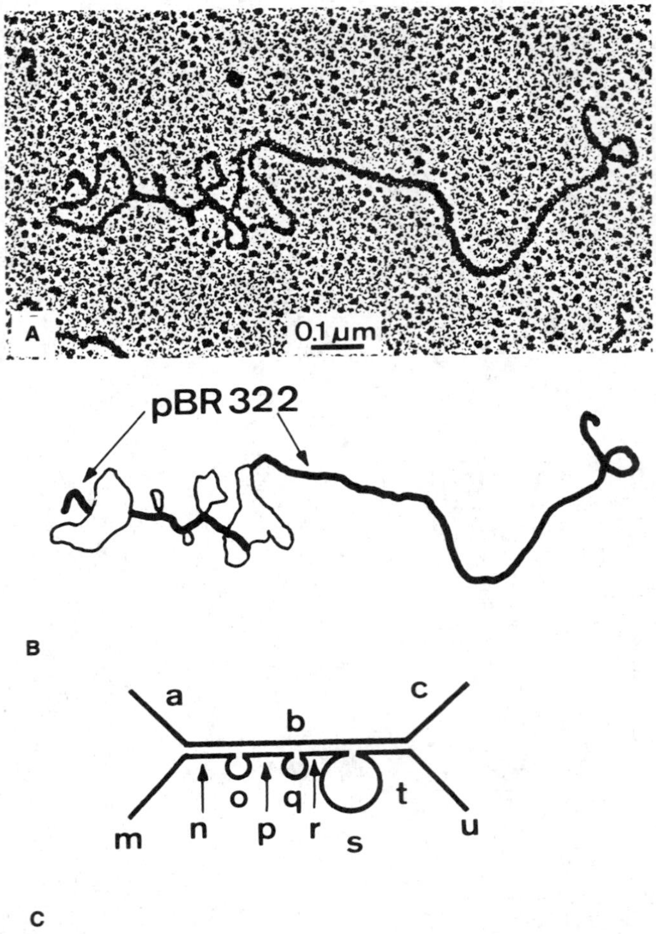

FIG. 2-4. Heteroduplex analysis. Two molecularly cloned DNA molecules containing, respectively, the human cellular oncogene locus of *ras*^{H} and the viral oncogene locus of *ras*^{H}, were mixed, denatured, and allowed to anneal. The DNA molecules were spread, treated for visualization in the electron microscope,[26] and examined for heteroduplex hybrid molecules. This technique allows individual DNA molecules to be visualized and identifies regions of homology (double-stranded) and nonhomology (single-stranded). In this example, the homologous region represents the human cellular oncogene *ras*^{H} locus in a double-stranded hybrid with the viral *ras*^{H} gene. The magnification is approximately ×100,000. Note that because v-*ras*^{H} is a cDNA copy of the *ras*^{H} gene, the regions o, q, and s, which are introns in c-*ras*,^{H} are deleted in v-*ras*.^{H}

to determine point mutations or DNA rearrangements in very small samples of material.

DNA RESTRICTION ENZYMES

The precise order of nucleotides in the DNA molecules is the basis for the genetic code. If it were possible to reproducibly fragment genomic DNA by cutting at specific nucleotide sequences and to fractionate the fragments by size, we could identify by hybridization (using a radioactive probe prepared as described above) those DNA fragments in the total array of fragments that contain a unique gene.

Restriction Enzyme	Site
*Hind*III	5′ A↓AGCTT 3′ / 3′ TTCGA↑A 5′
*Bam*HI	5′ G↓GATCC 3′ / 3′ CCTAG↑G 5′
*Eco*RI	5′ G↓AATTC 3′ / 3′ CTTAA↑G 5′
*Kpn*I	5′ GGTAC↓C 3′ / 3′ C↑CATGG 5′
*Taq*I	5′ T↓CGA 3′ / 3′ AGC↑T 5′
*Not*I	5′ GC↓GGCCGC 3′ / 3′ CGCCGG↑CG 5′
*Sfi*I	5′ GGCCN↓NNNNGGCC 3′ / 3′ CCGGNNNN↑NCCGG 5′

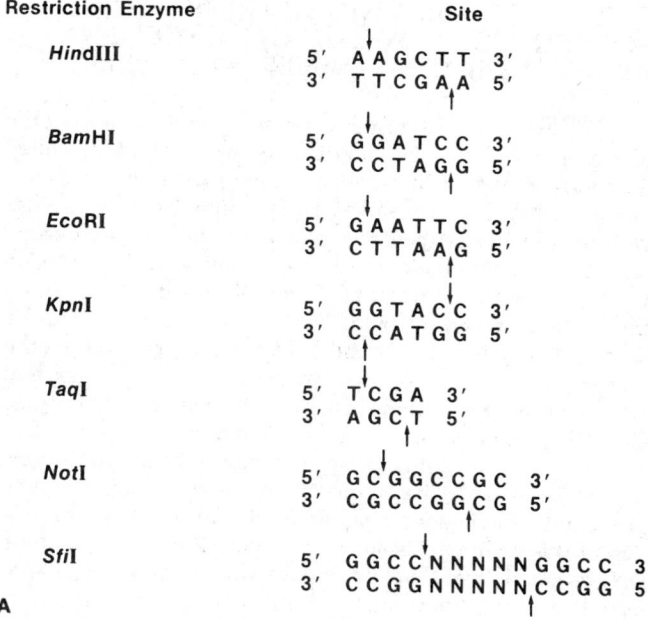

A

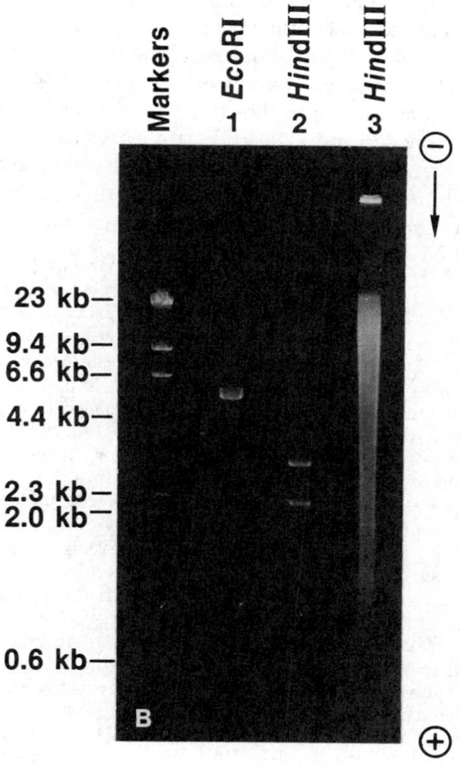

B

FIG. 2-5. **A.** Restriction enzyme recognition sites. The six-base nucleotide sequence recognition sites[35] in double-stranded DNA for *Hind*III, *Bam*HI, *Eco*RI, and *Kpn*I are underlined. The orientation 5′ to 3′ is important because with these enzymes the double-strand enzyme cleavage is staggered, leaving a four-base 5′ single-strand overhang (*Hind*III, *Bam*HI, and *Eco*RI) or a four-base 3′ overhang (*Kpn*I). Three additional recognition sites for the enzymes *Taq*I, *Not*I, and *Sfi*I are shown. These enzymes will cleave double-stranded DNA everywhere in the molecule that the recognition sequence appears. The overhang allows recombinant DNA gene splicing in the presence of DNA ligase to occur between a heterogeneous population of similarly digested DNA fragments. **B.** Fractionation of restriction fragments by electrophoresis. One microgram of purified polyoma virus DNA is digested with *Eco*RI (lane 1) or *Hind*III (lane 2) and subjected to agarose gel electrophoresis. Ten micrograms of human placental DNA is digested with *Hind*III (lane 3) and likewise subjected to electrophoresis. After being stained with ethidium bromide, the resolved DNA fragments can be visualized by long-wave UV light in the gel. The extreme left lane shows DNA fragments of known size. kb, kilobase pairs in length.

One of the most important contributions to the study of DNA was the identification of enzymes, known as restriction enzymes, that cut double-stranded DNA at specific nucleotide sequence recognition sites.[34] Several hundred restriction enzymes that recognize more than 150 specific nucleotide sequences in double-stranded DNA have been identified. The recognition sites of several restriction enzymes are shown in Figure 2-5A. These enzymes are produced in bacteria and are part of an elaborate restriction/modification system that protects the bacteria from invasion by foreign DNA.[34–38] Such sites, present in the genome of the bacterial host cell, are protected by a modification enzyme that methylates one of the nucleotide bases in the restriction enzyme recognition site and thereby protects the host DNA from being cleaved.[38] Foreign DNA entering the cell is not modified and is subject to digestion by the restriction enzyme. In vitro, these enzymes provide powerful tools for dissecting DNA genetic information and are fundamental to the principles of recombinant DNA technology.[39]

Most of the restriction enzymes that have been identified, many of which are commercially available, recognize either six, five, or four nucleotide base pairs of DNA sequence.[34] In a DNA molecule of random nucleotide base sequences, a six-base recognition sequence would be expected to occur once in every 4096 base pairs (*i.e.,* once in 4^6 base pairs). In human DNA, which is approximately 3×10^9 base pairs in length, a six-base recognition restriction enzyme would be expected to cut the DNA into several million fragments, whereas the DNA genome of a small DNA tumor virus (*e.g.,* 5300 base pairs in length) would be cut only a few times by the same enzyme. Examples of each are shown in Figure 2-5B. It is possible to fractionate the digested DNA fragments according to size in an agarose gel matrix by electrophoresis. The mobilities of the DNA fragments in this matrix are approximately proportional to the log of their length in base pairs.[40] The DNA fragments can be visualized with ultraviolet light after staining with the fluorescing dye ethidium bromide.[41] Thus, in the example shown in Figure 2-4B, polyoma virus DNA is 5292 base pairs in length,[42] and the *Hind*III recognition sequence AAGCTT occurs twice in the molecule. Therefore, digestion with the *Hind*III enzyme yields two fragments, 3030 and 2262 base pairs in length. By comparison, the genomic DNA from human cells is cut several million times by the same enzyme and appears as a smear when resolved by gel electrophoresis and visualized by ethidium bromide staining (Fig. 2-5B).

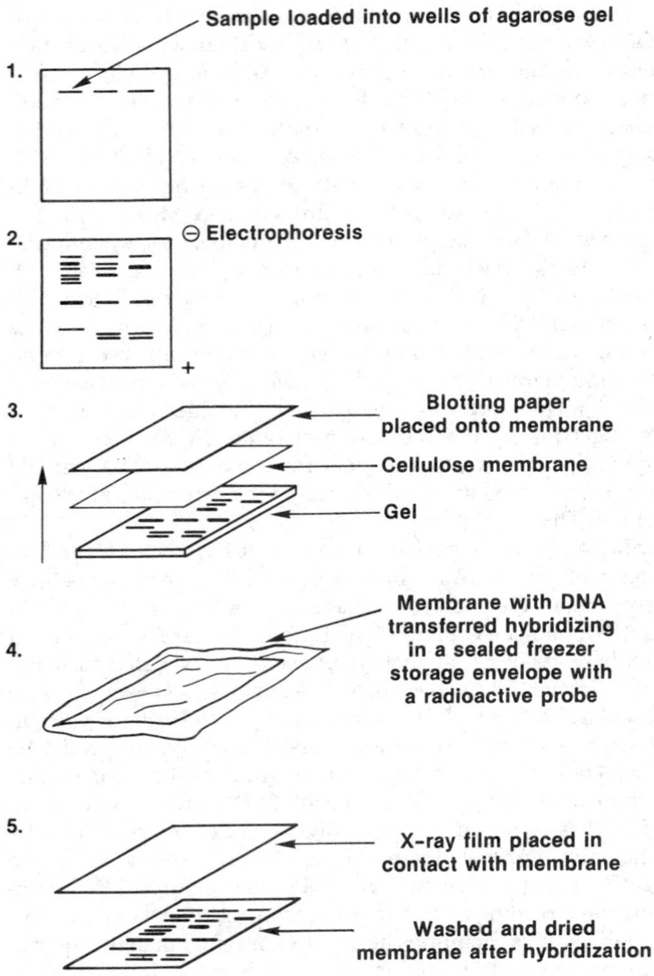

Schematic of Steps in the Southern Transfer Analysis

A

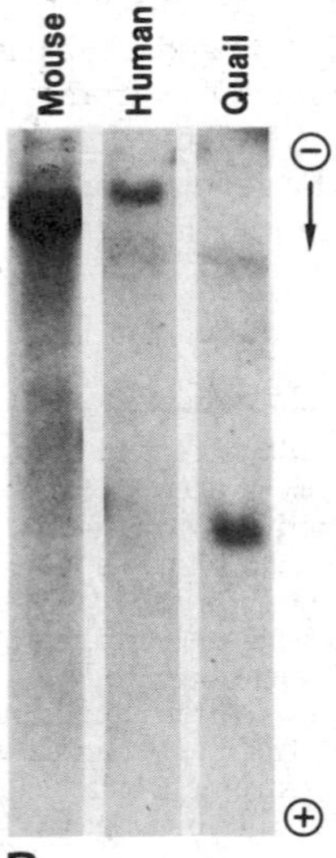

B

DETECTION OF UNIQUE GENE SEQUENCES IN TOTAL GENOMIC DNA BY SOUTHERN TRANSFER ANALYSIS

Any one of the 50,000 or more genes present in the genome of mammalian DNA can be detected by a technique called Southern transfer analysis,[43] in which restriction-enzyme–cleaved DNA that is resolved in one dimension by agarose gel electrophoresis (see Fig. 2-5B) is denatured and transferred to a membrane that traps the resolved single-stranded DNA (Fig. 2-6A). When this target DNA is immobilized on the membrane, an isotopically labeled DNA probe can be used to hybridize to the bound DNA pattern. By exposing the membrane to x-ray film, we can detect a gene that occurs only once in the genome, such as the *mos* oncogene (see Chap. 3), and determine its location in relation to restriction sites (Fig. 2-6B). Using these relatively simple procedures, we can develop restriction enzyme maps of a specific genetic locus in the total genome of a mammalian cell. One application of this technique is shown in Figure 2-6B. The genomic DNA isolated from chicken, mouse, and human cells is subjected to Southern transfer analysis using an isotopically labeled mouse *mos* oncogene probe.[43] The mouse probe detects the homologous sequences in mouse DNA as well as the related nucleotide sequences of the *mos* gene in human and chicken genomic DNA. This result shows that *mos* gene sequences are conserved between all three animal species. Similarly, thousands of probes have been used to detect genomic sequences in the DNA of both viruses and living organisms. A variation of the Southern blot technique is the Northern blot. In this method RNA is run on denaturing gels, blotted to membranes, and hybridized to radioactive probes. This method allows the size and abundance of specific RNA

FIG. 2-6. **A**. Schematic of steps in the Southern transfer analysis.[42] *1*. A 20 cm × 20 cm 0.5% to 1.0% agarose gel, 3 mm or 4 mm thick, is formed in a conventional gel electrophoresis apparatus. 2. Restriction-enzyme-digested DNA samples are loaded into preformed wells, and the gel is subjected to an electrophoretic field to fractionate the restricted DNA fragments. 3. For blotting, the gel is placed in a tray on top of absorbent paper wetted with buffer, and a cut-to-size wetted membrane is placed atop the gel and is sandwiched with dry absorbent paper to draw (blot) the resolved DNA fragments onto the DNA-trapping membrane. *4*. After the DNA is fixed to the membrane and nonspecific binding sites are blocked with a special medium, the membrane is sealed in a plastic envelope along with a suitable isotopically labeled probe and placed under hybridization conditions, usually overnight. 5. The excess isotopic label is washed off and the membrane exposed to x-ray film for 12 hours or more. The film is subsequently developed to reveal hybridizing fragments. **B**. Southern transfer analysis detection of the *mos* oncogene in mouse, quail, and human cellular genomic DNA. Twenty micrograms each of mouse BALB/c DNA digested with *Eco*RI, human placental DNA digested with *Hind*III, and quail QT6 cell line DNA digested with *Bam*HI were subjected to electrophoresis in an agarose gel. The electrophoretically resolved DNA in the gel was then transferred to a cellulose nitrate membrane by the procedure of Southern analysis,[42] and a mouse *mos*-specific isotopically labeled probe[94] was hybridized to the DNA blotted onto the membrane. After hybridization, the membrane was exposed to x-ray film for 12 hours to detect the radioactive fragments containing nucleotide sequences homologous to *mos*. Here we use a radioactive probe to detect the hybrid; a similar hybrid was visualized in the heteroduplex analysis shown in Figure 2-3.

species to be determined. The Western blot involves the electrophoresis and transfer of proteins, which are subsequently detected by antibodies.

PULSED-FIELD GEL ELECTROPHORESIS

The traditional Southern blot technique is useful for a wide variety of applications in the analysis of DNA but suffers from the limitation that fragments larger than 20 kb are poorly resolved on conventional agarose gels. Recent variations of this technique have been described that use alterations in the electrical field applied to the DNA and result in increased resolution of large DNA fragments. Although there are several variations of this method, they all use pulses of current[44] instead of a constant field to increase resolution, hence the name pulsed-field gel electrophoresis (PFGE). Variations of this method involve applying current at different angles to the gel and are referred to as orthogonal field agarose gel electrophoresis (OFAGE).[45]

During conventional electrophoresis, as depicted in Figure 2-5, large DNA fragments run together through the gel. In one version of PFGE, not only are pulses of current applied to the gel, but also the polarity of the field is biased to favor DNA mobility in one direction. This technique is referred to as field-inversion gel electrophoresis (FIGE).[46] This presumably causes large DNA fragments to be oriented in the gel. The size range in which fragments resolve by this method depends on the placement of the electrodes in the gel box and the duration of the pulses, but the separation of fragments as large as 7 million base pairs has been reported.[47] This technique has been made possible by the discovery of restriction enzymes that contain 8 bp recognition sequences (see Fig. 2-5A) (*i.e.,* 4^8 or once in every 65,536 base pairs; yielding ~45,000 fragments per human genome or ~2000–3000 per chromosome). These enzymes generate large DNA fragments 50 to 500 kb long that can be analyzed by PGFE.

With the power to resolve large fragments of DNA, researchers have been able to tackle problems that were previously impossible. The *Escherichia coli* genome is approximately 10 million pairs long, a size too large to map by conventional gel electrophoresis. A complete physical map of the *E. coli* genome was recently reported[48] and will allow the structure of the genome and the organization of its genes to be known in greater detail. The maps of other bacterial genomes, yeast chromosomes, and eventually mammalian chromosomes can now be constructed by PFGE techniques. An example of one application of this technique is shown in Figure 2-7. DNA from a human cell line containing a DNA rearrangement in the *met* oncogene[49,50] is digested with the enzyme Sfi I and subjected to FIGE. The DNA fragments are transferred to and immobilized on a membrane by slight modifications of the conventional procedure described in Figure 2-6. Isotopically labeled DNA probes are again used to detect the sequence homologue on a DNA fragment. In the example shown (see Fig. 2-7) a novel 350-kb DNA fragment is depicted in an Sfi I DNA fragment carrying the rearranged oncogene locus. The normal (allele) fragment, also present in this cell, is revealed on a ~150-kb Sfi I fragment. The oncogene activation event resulted from a DNA rearrangement and generated the new Sfi fragment. By subjecting normal DNA to limited (partial) digestion with these rare cutting enzymes, maps of larger segments of DNA can be generated and used for linking two or more markers, thereby generating a physical restriction map.[51] The size markers often used in these analyses represent the chromosomes of *Saccharomyces cerevisiae.*

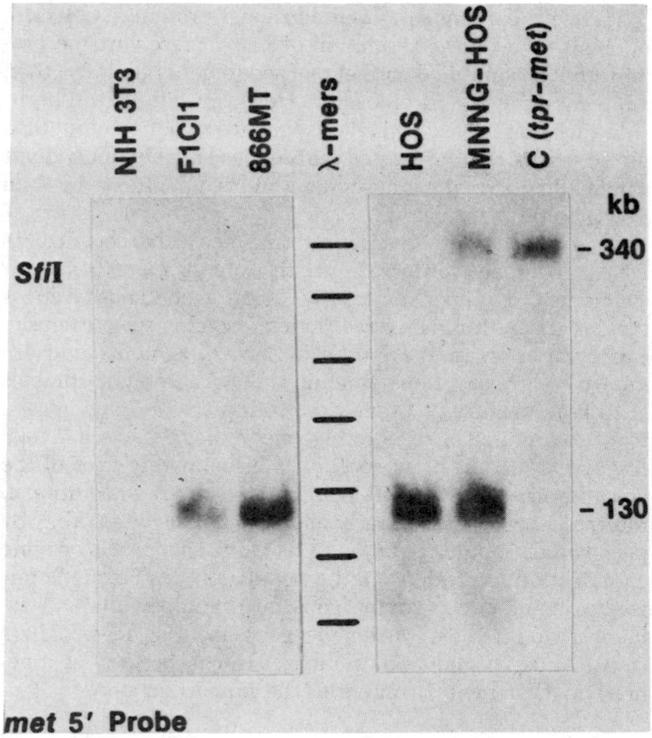

FIG. 2-7. DNA fragments separated by pulsed-field gel electrophoresis. DNA from several human cell lines was digested with the enzyme Sfi I, separated by the pulsed-field technique and Southern blotted. The filter was hybridized with a probe from the *met* oncogene. The appearance of a rearranged allele of the *met* gene can be observed in the DNA from the MNNG-HOS line, a chemically transformed human cell. Note the separation of the fragments between 120 and 340 kb.

RESTRICTION FRAGMENT LENGTH POLYMORPHISMS: DNA-BASED GENETIC MARKERS

In the last few years we have seen dramatic advances in our understanding of several human diseases, including muscular dystrophy, cystic fibrosis, retinoblastoma, and colon and small lung cell cancers. These breakthroughs have been made possible by dramatic developments in the field of human genetics. Genetic analysis of an organism requires the identification of genetic markers that reveal the inherited differences between individuals. Early human genetic markers included ABO blood groups, isozymes, and HLA antigens.[52–54] Progress in linking these markers together was hampered by their small number compared to the size of the human genome.

The development of two-dimensional protein gel electrophoresis allowed the resolution of many more variable proteins, but this method cannot be used to generate more than a few markers per chromosome. However, because all heritable variation is based on DNA sequence variation, a method for detecting DNA sequence differences between individuals would allow virtually any segment of the genome to be used as a genetic marker.

As we have seen, restriction enzymes can recognize in DNA the precise order of specific four to eight base pair segments of a sequence (see Fig. 2-5A). Genetic differences that create or eliminate a restriction enzyme recognition site cause variation in the length of DNA fragments and are known as restriction fragment length polymorphisms (RFLPs).[55] Figure 2-8 shows an example of a unique probe from the long arm of chromosome 7 that detects a 7.5-kb fragment with the enzyme *Taq*I. Approximately 50% of the chromosomes in the white population contain an additional, internal *Taq*I site, creating an additional allele of 4.0 kb.[56] By performing Southern blot analysis using this probe/enzyme combination, individuals in the population can be characterized as being either homozygous for the upper allele (1,1), heterozygous (1,2), or homozygous for the lower allele (2,2). Thus fragments of cloned DNA can be used as a genetic marker for this region of the human genome.

These differences in sequence (between two alleles) occur at a frequency of an estimated 1 per 200 to 500 base pairs[57] and are responsible for the genetic differences between any two individuals. RFLPs can be characterized by both the degree to which they are useful in genetic analysis and their chromosomal location. The frequency of a polymorphism is determined by typing a large number of unrelated individuals and determining the frequency of each allele. For example, if a two allele polymorphism is analyzed in 50 individuals (100 chromosomes) and 60 copies of allele 1 and 40 copies of allele 2 are detected, the frequency is 0.60/0.40. The heterozygosity of an RFLP is related to the frequency and is a measure of the percentage of individuals who are heterozygotes. The polymorphism information content (PIC) is a measure of the percentage of families in which both parents are heterozygous for a given polymorphism.[55]

Probes that detect RFLPs can be mapped to chromosomes by both physical and genetic methods. The physical methods include somatic cell hybridization[58] and in situ hybridization.[59] Briefly, a gene can be assigned to a chromosome by following its segregation in a panel of interspecies hybrids segregating human chromosomes (*i.e.*, human X hamster hybrids). The technique of in situ hybridization is performed by hybridizing an isotopically labeled DNA fragment directly to mitotic phase chromosomes. After the probe is annealed,

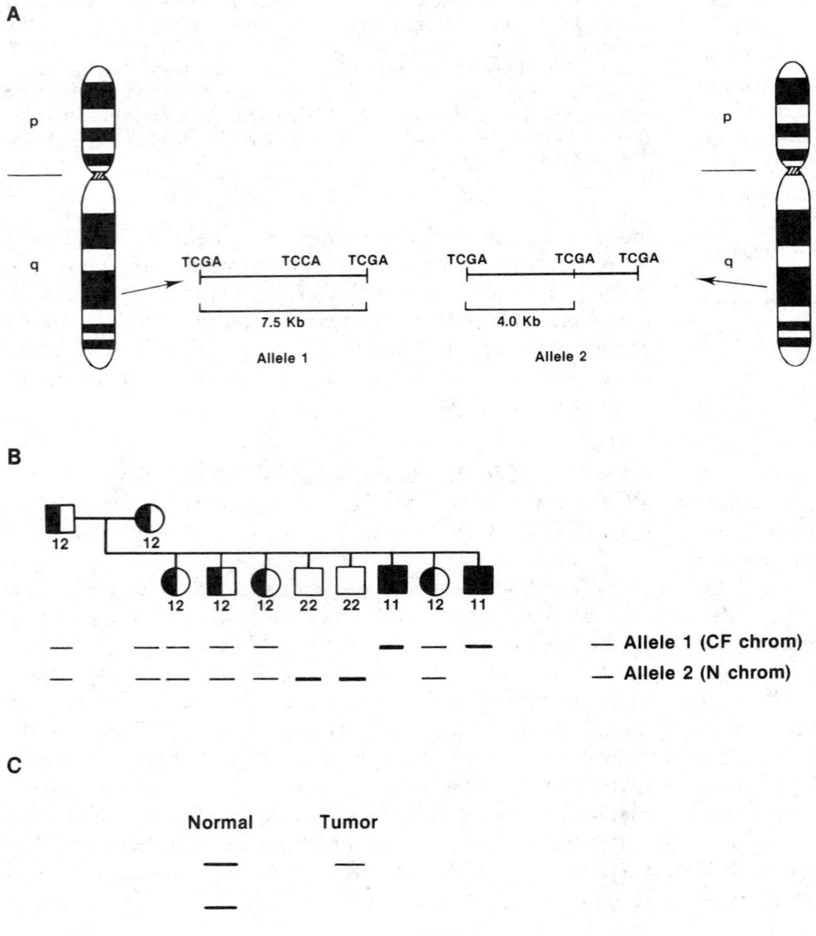

FIG. 2-8. Use of a DNA-based genetic marker. **A**. An example of an RFLP. A diagram of human chromosome 7 shows the position of the *met* proto-oncogene at 7q31.[95] The sequence TCGA is the recognition sequence of the *Taq*I restriction enzyme, which generates a 7.5-kb fragment. **B**. Use of an RFLP in genetic diagnosis. The *met* gene is tightly linked to the cystic fibrosis (CF) gene,[56] and therefore they are almost always inherited together. In this family, allele 1 is on the CF chromosome and the affected children (*filled symbols*) have a 1,1 genotype. Individuals with a 1,2 genotype are unaffected carriers and 2,2 children are unaffected noncarriers. **C**. RFLP detection of DNA deletion in a tumor. This hypothetical example shows how the deletion of all or part of a chromosome can be detected by comparing tumor and normal DNA from the same patient.

a photographic emulsion is applied, the sample is exposed, and, after developing, the grains are counted over the chromosomes. This technique allows the gene to be assigned not only to a chromosome but also, when combined with chromosome banding techniques, to a band or region on a chromosome (Fig. 2-9). A more precise method for positioning an RFLP is by linking it physically or genetically to another polymorphism. This requires the RFLPs to be typed in the same group of pedigrees. The most efficient families for linking RFLPs have been determined to be three generation families with large sibships.[60] Two RFLPs that are near each other on a chromosome will be inherited together in a family in a meiotic recombination dependent fashion. The genetic distance between two markers is determined by the recombination frequency, the percentage of meioses in which a recombination is detected between two markers. If the recombination is observed in one of 100 meiosis (a frequency of 1%), a genetic distance of 1 centimorgan (cM) occurs between the two markers. In the human genome this is approximately equivalent to one million base pairs in physical distance; for example, ~20 markers spaced 5 cM apart could provide a genetic *linkage map* of a human chromosome (~2.0 /10^8 base pairs).[61]

LINKAGE ANALYSIS

A major use of RFLPs is in the analysis of families that segregate a human disease. DNA from individuals in the pedigree is analyzed by Southern blot using DNA probes that detect RFLPs. The inheritance of the alleles of the genetic marker is correlated with the inheritance of the disease. The data are statistically analyzed by calculating the odds that the association between the marker and the disease occurred by chance. This information is used to calculate a LOD score (the log of the odds), and a LOD score of three (odds of 1000 to 1) is taken as formal proof of linkage.[62] An example of linkage is displayed in Figure 2-8B. RFLP markers that we discovered in the *met* proto-oncogene locus on human chromosome 7 were used by White and co-workers[56] to analyze pedigrees segregating the recessive genetic disease cystic fibrosis. In the first families that could be scored for the inheritance of the marker, there was a perfect correlation between the marker and the disease, generating a LOD score of 8.0. The odds that this situation could occur by chance is greater than 100,000,000 to 1, providing conclusive evidence that the gene responsible for cystic fibrosis lies next to the *met* gene on the long arm of human chromosome 7. These genetic markers were also found to be useful in carrier detection and prenatal diagnosis of families affected by this disease.[63]

FIG. 2-9. In situ DNA hybridization to a human chromosome. A histogram of human chromosome 7 is displayed showing the results of an in situ hybridization experiment using the *met* oncogene as a probe. In this experiment a radioactive fragment of the gene was hybridized to spreads of human chromosomes. After washing and applying a photographic emulsion, the grains depicting hybridization are recorded. A representation of the number of grains and their location is depicted here, demonstrating that the *met* gene lies on chromosome 7q31.1–31.3.

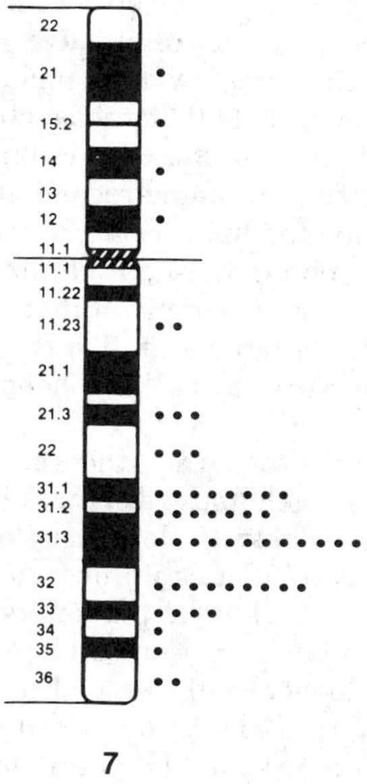

CHROMOSOMAL ALTERATIONS IN HUMAN TUMORS

Several human tumor types have been described that contain deletions of specific chromosomal regions. These were first detected by analyzing the karyotypes of the tumor cells in cases such as retinoblastoma[64,65] and Wilms' tumor.[66] More recently, nonrandom deletions have been described for secondary acute nonlymphocytic leukemia, colon, kidney, and lung cancers.[67–70] RFLP markers are a particularly powerful tool for this type of analysis. To analyze tumor samples with RFLPs, samples of the tumor DNA (as free as possible of normal tissue) are compared to DNA obtained from normal tissue or cells from the same patient. The DNA is analyzed with probes that identify polymorphisms. If the normal DNA is heterozygous and the tumor DNA homozygous, this demonstrates that one copy of that gene or chromosomal region has been deleted in the tumor (see Fig. 2-8C). This type of analysis has recently been applied to the analysis of breast tumors, renal cell cancer (see also Chap. 3), lung cancer, and colon cancer. This technique is particularly powerful for analyzing tumors that contain deletions too small to be detected by karyotypic analyses, or for solid tumors in which reliable karyotypic analyses are hard to perform.

CHARACTERIZING THE HUMAN GENOME

Recently much attention has been given to the suggestion that the complete DNA sequence of the human genome be determined, a project that can be described as biology's equivalent to the moon landing. Although few doubt that much valuable information is to be gained from the complete characterization of human genetic material, many worry that such a project would take research money away from other, more productive endeavors.[71] In fact, the idea should be thought of as a series of projects, each with very real promise of benefits to medical research. For example, if a specific genetic locus is identified by RFLP analysis to be linked to a disease, then careful characterization of this locus (*i.e.*, physical mapping and sequence analyses) would serve to assist in the identification of the responsible genetic element. The rest of this chapter will detail the stages and techniques involved characterizing the human genome.

MOLECULAR CLONING

Modern molecular biology is dependent on the technology of molecular cloning—the isolation and propagation of defined DNA fragments. In addition to cutting DNA with restriction enzymes, we also can reseal the cut ends using enzymes called DNA ligases.[72] The combination of restriction and ligation enzymes has provided the basis for recombinant DNA technology.[39] For example, the genome of polyoma virus is a circular double-stranded DNA molecule (see Fig. 2-5B) that is 5292 base pairs in length[42] and contains a single *Bam*HI recognition site (see Fig. 2-5A).[42] Cutting this DNA molecule with *Bam*HI yields a linear fragment. With DNA ligase, the two ends of the linearized, double-stranded DNA can be resealed (covalently linked), and some percentage of the molecules return to the original configuration. However, head-to-head or head-to-tail joining also may occur. The simplest condition for ligation is one in which a single cut has been made in a circular DNA molecule. Obviously, the more unique ends that are introduced into the reaction, the more complex the ligation products become.[39,72]

In bacteria, DNA plasmids carrying drug resistance genes have been used as vectors for cloning DNA fragments. Plasmids are small, circular DNA molecules that replicate as an episome (autonomously from the chromosome). DNA fragments can be inserted into a plasmid vector and thus can replicate with the plasmid. The most commonly used vector for molecular cloning, pBR322,[39,73,74] is a plasmid that replicates episomally in *E. coli*. It consists essentially of three regions that control different genetic functions (Fig. 2-10). One region, the origin of replication (*ori*) where DNA synthesis originates, allows the plasmid to replicate as an episome in *E. coli*. This plasmid also contains two genes (Tet^r and Amp^r) that, when expressed, confer to strains of *E. coli* harboring the plasmid, resistances to the drugs tetracycline and ampicillin, respectively. If a DNA segment is introduced into one of the drug resistance genes, then the gene is rendered inactive and the *E. coli* cell harboring the plasmid becomes sensitive to the drug. In this way, plasmids that contain molecularly cloned fragments can be identified. The procedures for hybridization with bacterial colonies[75] or lambda phage vectors[76] are analogous to the Southern transfer procedure described earlier. DNA from *E. coli* colonies growing on agar in a Petri dish is transferred to a membrane, and a single colony or a single virus plaque in hundreds of thousands can be identified and isolated. DNA from this plasmid or virus vector may contain a single molecularly cloned DNA fragment from the original population of more than one million fragments present in the animal genome. The plasmid or lambda phage vectors are generally amplified in *E. coli* so that each cell contains many copies of the molecularly cloned fragment.[39] From 1 liter of bacterial culture, 100 μg to 1 mg of purified vector DNA can be recovered. In the example shown in Figure 2-10, the plasmid DNA containing the polyoma viral genome inserted in the pBR322 *Bam*HI site is purified from the transformed *E. coli* cells and subjected to digestion with *Bam*HI to release the polyoma DNA insert from the vector. Here, the insert is recovered after subjecting the digested DNA to gel electrophoresis.[77,78] The desired fragment, isolated and purified in large quantities, can be characterized by DNA sequencing for the determination of absolute genetic information (see Fig. 2-3). *E. coli* host/vector systems have been the most widely applied for molecular cloning, but other cloning vector systems, such as those using mammalian viruses, are also used.[79]

Although well suited for the cloning of small DNA fragments, plasmids are not very suitable for the cloning of DNA fragments larger than 10 kb. Derivatives of the bacteriophage lambda have been developed that allow DNA molecules of up to 20 kb to be cloned (Fig. 2-11). By removing genes that are not essential for the replication of lambda, vectors have been designed to accommodate foreign DNA. By combining the recombinant DNA with the enzymes and proteins required to package lambda DNA into virus particles, recombinant viruses are generated. If the collection of DNA fragments inserted into phage is representative of the entire genome (*i.e.*, at least one or more copies of every region) the collection of lambda phage particles generated is termed a genomic library.[80] Because the packaging of lambda phage is very efficient and the clones can be stably stored, this method is in wide use in molecular biology laboratories.

Researchers have continued to develop vectors that can clone fragments larger than ~20 kb. One such vector (called a cosmid) is a hybrid vector[81] with part plasmid and part phage functions; it contains the phage sequences for packaging DNA into lambda phage particles, but once inside the bacterial cell it replicates using plasmid functions. The advantage of cosmids is that they can be used to clone up to 50 kb of DNA. This allows representative genomic libraries to be constructed that are fewer in number than lambda phage genomic libraries. Both lambda phage and cosmid libraries are useful for "chromosome walking" studies, that is, one end of an insert from one recombinant can serve as probe for rescreening the libraries for purposes of obtaining recombinants that contain adjacent chromosomal DNA sequences.[82] Clearly, more genetic information is spanned when cosmid libraries are used. Large segments of the mouse and human MHC locus have been isolated in this manner.[83]

The recent impetus to narrow the gap between genetic methods of analyzing genomes (distances in the millions of base pairs) and the molecular level has led researchers to develop cloning vectors that can propagate DNA fragments larger than 100 kb. A technique that offers great promise is the generation of minichromosomes in yeast.[84] Analysis of the structural components of yeast chromosomes has allowed researchers to identify and isolate yeast DNA sequences with centromeric and telomeric functions. By add-

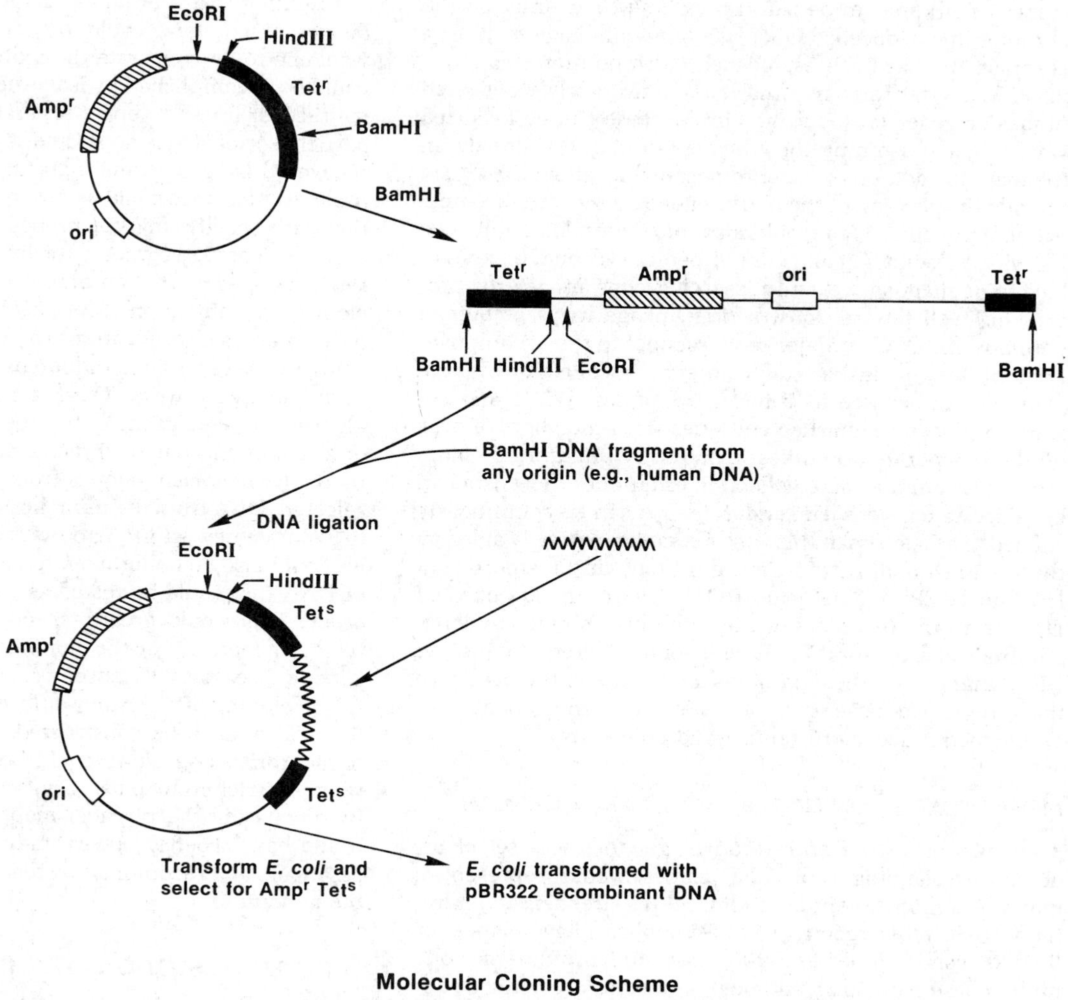

FIG. 2-10. Molecular cloning scheme. The circular plasmid pBR322 is digested with *Bam*HI restriction enzyme (see Fig. 2-4A) at its single recognition site, which resides in the tetracycline (Tet) gene to yield a linear fragment (*e.g.*, see pBR322, Fig. 2-9, lane 3). This linearized plasmid is mixed with *Bam*HI-digested DNA from any source (*e.g.*, polyoma DNA as in Fig. 2-9, lane 1) and the mixed sample is ligated (see Fig. 2-9, lane 4). A certain fraction of the molecules obtained will have the recombinant structure as shown. The plasmid molecules are transformed into *E. coli* and cells harboring the plasmids are selected by their resistance to the unaltered ampicillin resistance gene. Ampicillin-resistant colonies are tested for resistance to tetracycline; any that are sensitive to tetracycline (Tet) could have new DNA fragments cloned into the *Bam*HI site. Plasmid DNA is prepared from these cells and tested for the presence of the desired insert.

ing these sequences to large fragments of human DNA, large segments of the human chromosomes can be replicated in yeast cells as chromosomes. Recently DNA molecules larger than 125 kb have been successfully cloned into yeast cells.[84] Naturally occurring yeast chromosomes are several million base pairs in length, so there is sufficient reason to believe that recombinant chromosomes of this size can also be generated. This could greatly facilitate human genome analyses by providing a system where genetic markers can be linked to physical restriction maps.

THE HUMAN GENETIC LINKAGE MAP

The first step toward sequencing the human genome is to generate a road map of spaced genetic markers for each chromosome by developing a genetic linkage map.[85] Just as RFLPs are shown to be linked to a gene for a genetic disease, recombination frequencies can be used to link two RFLPs to each other and thereby address whether they are near each other on the same chromosome. By studying the inheritance of RFLPs in the same families, the genetic distance between pairs of markers can be determined and their order on the chromosome deduced.[60] Once a complete linkage map for a chromosome has been established (with no more than 10–20 cM between any two markers), any newly discovered probes or genes on the same chromosome can be localized simply by determining their linkage to markers already on the map. In addition to the chromosomal location, these data provide the position of the marker gene on the chromosome. A human genetic map would also allow any human disease for which a suitable collection of pedigrees could be assembled to be mapped. Several research groups are already progressing well toward constructing linkage maps of human chromosomes.[60,61] A major tool essential to the accomplishment of this goal is the establishment of a collection of large pedigrees to be used as reference families. White and coworkers[60] have established cell lines from members of over 60 three-generation families with 6 to 12 children. By mapping RFLPs in the same collection of families, new data can be added to previous data and the maps can be continuously refined. The success of this venture has been greatly aided by the establishment of the Centre d'Etude du Polymorphism Humain (CEPH). The goal of CEPH is to provide purified DNA from the members of the reference families to collaborating investigators. Each collaborator agrees to analyze RFLP markers in these families and combine the data with the genetic data base, the result being that the genome can be mapped much more rapidly and efficiently.

MOLECULAR CLONING OF THE HUMAN GENOME

The isolation of the entire human genome as a set of ordered, overlapping molecular clones would represent a major accomplishment for biological researchers. At a minimum, this would require 150,000 lambda phage clones, or 60,000 cosmid clones or 3,000 yeast minichromosomes one million base pairs long. Although strategies are being developed to directly link phage or cosmid clones, the task would be much more straightforward with minichromosomes.

Assuming that a library of large minichromosomes could be generated, how could they be ordered? One strategy would be to first separate the individual chromosomes. This could be accomplished by isolating chromosomes in somatic hybrid cell lines[86,87] or by separating them by size using a particle sorter. Once separated, each chromosome could be recovered by generating 1 to 200 minichromosomes. The minichromosomes could be ordered by using DNA hybridization with specific marker probes to detect clones that contain overlapping segments, or by using the DNA probes already mapped on that chromosome to identify and order the clones. A combination of the two approaches would probably have to be used to fill in all the gaps.

An ordered set of one million base pair fragments would be useful in many ways. Once a region of the genome was identified as containing either the gene for a genetic disease or a region associated with chromosomal abnormalities in a particular neoplasm, clones from that region could be easily selected. DNA from the minichromosome could then be used to generate new RFLP markers for that region. Further studies could also be undertaken to identify genes in this stretch of DNA that could be tested as candidate genes for the disorder. This would greatly speed up the process known as reverse genetics[88]; or the cloning of a gene responsible for a genetic disease by its chromosomal location.

The cloning of a chromosome would also allow a complete physical map to be constructed, that is, probes from each minichromosome clone could be used to generate a long-range restriction map using pulse-field gel electrophoresis.[51] By comparing the physical map with the genetic map, we would have a better understanding of the relation between base pairs and recombination distance for specific regions of the genome.

FURTHER DISSECTION OF THE GENOME

To analyze specific regions of the genome in greater detail, the yeast minichromosome DNA fragments could be sub-

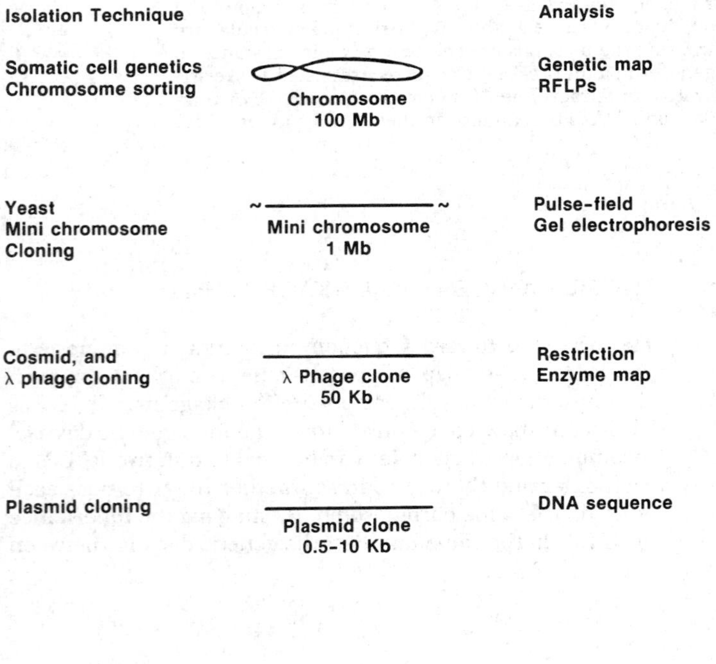

FIG. 2-11. Cloning and analyzing the human genome. A comparison of techniques for capturing portions of genetic information and the types of analyses that they make possible. Somatic cell hybrids and fluorescence-activated cell sorting allow whole chromosomes (50–200 mb) to be isolated.[96] These techniques assist in the construction of genetic lineage maps of chromosomes. Chromosomes can be broken down into 0.1 to 1.0 mb fragments by cloning into yeast minichromosomes.[84] These fragments can be used to generate a physical map using PFGE.[44,45] Minichromosomes can be subdivided by cloning into cosmid and phage vectors,[80,81] and these subclones can then be characterized by conventional restriction curve mapping. Finally, fragments for the phage clones can be inserted into plasmid vectors and the nucleotide sequence determined.

cloned into either cosmid or phage vectors. Restriction mapping and hybridization could be used to order the subcloned DNA by generating a series of overlapping DNA clones spanning the entire minichromosome. The DNA subclones could then be used to generate a detailed restriction map of the region. Having cloned a portion of a gene, a researcher could select the appropriate subclones likely to contain the rest of the gene. This would allow the entire gene and its control sequences to be rapidly characterized.

Once fully automated DNA sequencing procedures are developed,[89,90] the entire genome could be efficiently sequenced. The sequence would allow us to learn a great deal about the organization of the human genome. Gene families would become greatly expanded, allowing researchers to rapidly select new genes that might be of biological and medical importance.

POLYMERASE CHAIN REACTION

A technique has been developed that allows direct analysis of a segment of DNA that is uniquely present in the genome of a single cell in the presence of hundreds of thousands of cells.[32,91,92] This technology is based on a process referred to as the polymerase chain reaction (PCR), and the sensitivity is made possible because the DNA sequence of interest is specifically amplified several hundred thousand times. The PCR can be automated and, because of its extraordinary sensitivity, will have a significant impact in clinical diagnostics. One of the most important applications will be in genetic screening[32] and in detection of minimal residual cells in patients after cancer treatment.[91,92]

AUTOMATION OF MOLECULAR GENETICS

A crucial requirement to determine the sequence of the three billion base pairs of the human genome is the development of machines that automate repetitive tasks. Moreover, it will be necessary to dedicate powerful computers to store the information and to generate the relevant software to process it. Machines have been constructed that extract DNA from cells, synthesize small DNA fragments or oligonucleotides, and determine the DNA sequence of DNA fragments. Cloning and sequencing projects now routinely require the use of oligonucleotides. Oligonucleotides can be used as probes for Southern analysis or for screening genetic libraries; they also can be used to generate specific mutations in the sequence of cloned genes for identifying important sequence elements by altering their function in vitro and in vivo. The first machines able to automatically perform DNA sequence analysis of fragments more than five hundred bases in length are now commercially available. In the near future, then, DNA sequencing will not be the rate-limiting step, but genetic and physical mapping still represent major obstacles. Obviously, the enormous volume of data now being generated by genetic studies and DNA sequencing projects requires the use of increasingly powerful computers and innovative software. More emphasis is being placed on the development of software that predicts molecular structure and facilitates drug design. In 1987, the National Cancer Institute established the first supercomputer facility dedicated totally to biomedical research.

CONCLUSION

The techniques of molecular biology are responsible for many major advances in the biological sciences, especially in genetics, biology, and medicine. By using genetic analyses to identify disease genes, and molecular cloning to determine the structure of genes, complex biological problems can begin to be unraveled. Such advances as the identification of oncogenes and the cloning of the muscular dystrophy and retinoblastoma genes are examples of the power of this approach. There is no doubt that the continued application of molecular methods to biological problems will lead to a greater understanding of normal cellular functions and the mechanisms of abnormal cellular responses.

Research was sponsored by the National Cancer Institute, Department of Health and Human Services, under Contract No. N01-CO-74101 with Bionetics Research, Inc. The contents of this chapter do not necessarily reflect the views or policies of the Department of Health and Human Services, nor does mention of trade names, commercial products, or organizations imply endorsement by the U.S. government.

GLOSSARY OF TERMS USED IN MOLECULAR BIOLOGY AND ONCOGENE RESEARCH

Acute transforming retroviruses: Viruses that have acquired sequences from the host genome that give them the property of causing rapid tumor formation in animals or morphologic transformation in cells in culture. The acquired sequences are termed viral oncogenes.

Antisense: The noncoding strand of the DNA within the RNA-coding region of the gene. It is complementary to the "sense" strand and is used as a template for RNA synthesis.

CAT: Chloramphenicol acetyl transferase, a prokaryotic enzyme that is used in a reporter gene assay to measure protein synthesis in vitro.

cDNA libraries: A collection of clones representative of the mRNA of a given cell type that is formed using the enzyme reverse transcriptase.

Centimorgan (cM): A unit of genetic distance. A centimorgan is equivalent to a meiotic recombination frequency of 1%. In the human genome with approximately 3×10^6 base pairs and 3000 cM, 1 cM is roughly equal to one million base pairs.

cis-acting DNA elements: DNA segments that serve as binding sites for transcriptional activators or repressors; a nondiffusible control element.

Coding sequence: That part of the genome or mRNA that is translated into protein.

Conditional expression: Gene expression that occurs only in response to certain stimuli or specific conditions.

Consensus sequence: A characteristic nucleotide sequence that is identified with a gene regulation function.

Constitutive expression: A gene that is expressed at the same level for most of the cell cycle.

Cosmid: A cloning vector designed to carry large fragments of DNA. The vector contains sequences of lambda bacteriophage that allow the DNA to be packaged as a phage particle. Once inside the bacterium, the cosmid replicates as a plasmid. Cosmid vectors can be used to clone fragments as large as 50 kb.

DNA sequence: The precise order of the four nucleotides, adenine [*A*], guanine [*G*], cytosine [*C*], thymidine [*T*], as they are linked together to form the DNA chain. This DNA sequence encodes the genetic information of an organism.

DNA transfection: The transfer of DNA into cells in culture. The foreign DNA can associate with the host chromosome and be expressed as an identifiable phenotype.

DNase footprinting: A technique that allows the determination of the specific DNA sequence in the binding sites of a DNA binding protein or protein complex.

Enhancers: DNA elements of varying length that can be located upstream or downstream from a gene in either polarity and enhance gene transcription.

Exon: Gene sequences that are retained in fully mature mRNA. Most often they contain protein coding information.

Gene transcription: Synthesis of an RNA molecule by polymerization of nucleotides complementary to a DNA template. This RNA molecule is a precursor of mRNA and represents a faithful complementary copy of the DNA sequence from which it was transcribed. A specific sequence in front of the gene (promoter) acts to identify the initiation site for transcription. In RNA, uridine *(U)* occupies positions that thymidine *(T)* occupies in DNA.

Genomic Library: A collection of clones containing genomic DNA fragments. The library should contain enough clones so that every region of the genome is represented at least once.

Heteroduplex: A double-stranded DNA molecule formed by hybridization of complementary single strands derived from two different sources. Only stretches of homologous or complementary DNA sequences can form double-stranded regions, whereas noncomplementary DNA stretches remain as single strands and are visible as such in the electron microscope.

Hybridization: The annealing or base pairing of two single-stranded DNA or RNA molecules that are homologous or complementary.

Inducible: Capable of being "turned on" in a specific situation; that is, the β-lactamase gene of *E. coli* is "induced" under conditions of low glucose and high galactose concentrations.

Initiation codon: The ribonucleotides "AUG" that translate into the amino acid methionine; is always the first amino acid codon of every mRNA.

Insertional mutagenesis: The process of interrupting the structure —either regulatory elements or protein coding information—of a gene by insertion of foreign genetic information.

Intron: Noncoding DNA sequences that interrupt the coding portions of a gene (exons); it is excised in the fully processed mRNA.

Linkage map: A set of closely spaced genetic markers, generally RFLPs, that have been mapped to the same chromosome. If the linkage map covers the entire chromosome, any gene responsible for an inherited disease can in theory be located.

Linker scanning: A method of in vitro mutagenesis wherein restriction enzyme cleavage sites are inserted at different positions along the gene so that sequences 5′ and 3′ to the insertions are not altered. Gene function is then assayed to identify functional domains.

Long terminal repeat: A repetitive element of the integrated provirus that is generated during viral DNA synthesis and contains the transcription control elements that regulate virus expression.

Messenger RNA: An RNA molecule that represents a faithful copy of the amino acid–coding sequences of a gene. Noncoding sequences (introns) have been removed. With few exceptions, mRNA possesses a stretch of about 200 adenine bases (poly A tail) attached to its 3′ end; this tail is not encoded by DNA.

Minichromosome: A large fragment of DNA that can replicate in yeast cells. Minichromosomes are constructed by adding yeast centromere and telomere sequences onto foreign DNA fragments. Human DNA fragments as large as 125 kb have been cloned in yeast, and it may be possible to clone one million base pair or longer segments.

Mobility Shift: An assay that allows identification of extracts that contain specific DNA binding proteins.

Molecular cloning: The insertion of a foreign DNA segment of finite length into a vector that replicates in a specific host. The host-vector systems are defined by the NIH "Guidelines for Research Involving Recombinant DNA Molecules" (Federal Register 47:38050–38068, 1982).

Nick translation: A method that replaces nucleotides in double-stranded DNA with the same but isotopically labeled nucleotides after treatment with DNase I and repair with DNA polymerase. Both strands are labeled by this technique.

Null mutations: Mutations that eliminate or inactivate a gene from the genome of an organism.

Polyadenylation: The addition of a stretch of approximately 200 riboadenylic acid residues to the end of an RNA *pol*II transcript.

Primer extension: An assay that utilizes mRNA and a complementary oligonucleotide primer to synthesize a DNA antisense copy of the mRNA. It is used to determine mRNA 5′ structure.

Promoter: A DNA sequence that signals RNA polymerase to initiate transcription.

Pulsed-field gel electrophoresis (PFGE): A modification of agarose gel electrophoresis of DNA in which fragments several megabases can be resolved. The technique uses pulses of current in either the reverse direction or at angles to the gel to accomplish the increased resolution.

Recombinant DNA: A DNA molecule constructed by joining a fragment of DNA from a different source to a vector, such as a circular bacterial plasmid. The vector is opened at a specific site, a given DNA fragment from another source is inserted, and the circle is closed again. The recombinant DNA is amplified in a host cell that can replicate the vector.

Reporter gene: A gene whose activity can be easily assayed; it is used as a marker of gene expression in transcription or translation systems, or both.

Restriction enzymes: Enzymes made by certain strains of bacteria to protect themselves against invading foreign DNA (*e.g.*, bacteriophage DNA). These enzymes cut DNA at specific recognition sites.

Restriction fragment length polymorphism (RFLP): A variation between individuals in the size of fragments produced by restriction enzyme digestion. The variation is inherited and can be used as a genetic marker in linkage analysis.

Retrovirus: A plus-stranded RNA genome virus that is reverse transcribed into DNA during infection and replication. The DNA copy integrates into the host chromosomal DNA. This DNA template, called a provirus, is transcribed into virion RNA and produces translatable mRNA that codes for virion or oncogene protein products.

Reverse genetics: The use of information on the chromosomal location of a genetic disease gene to clone the gene itself. In some instances chromosomal abnormalities have provided the essential clues, and in other cases genetic linkage data have been used to localize the gene.

Reverse transcriptase: An enzyme produced by retroviruses that makes complementary DNA (cDNA) copies of RNA. The process is called reverse transcription.

S1 nuclease protection analysis: An assay designed to elucidate mRNA structure; it utilizes RNA–DNA hybridization conditions and single-strand specific S1 nuclease enzyme to digest nonannealed RNA or DNA species.

Site-directed mutagenesis: Used to introduce a specific mutation at a specific site in a DNA sequence using DNA techniques.

Southern analysis: A technique for detecting specific sequences in

DNA. A DNA sample is digested with restriction enzymes. The restriction fragments are fractionated by size on agarose gels, transferred to a nitrocellulose membrane, and subjected to hybridization using an isotopically labeled nucleic acid probe.

Subtraction cloning: Use of serial RNA–DNA hybridization reactions with removal of annealed species to enrich for transcripts unique to a particular cell type.

trans-acting factors: Diffusible products that act to regulate transcription at specific sites along the DNA strand.

Transgenic mouse: A mouse generated by the introduction of a recombinant DNA molecule at the one-cell embryo stage. The founder mouse is shown to contain the recombinant DNA molecule by, for example, examining DNA extracted from a segment of the tail, and new strains are developed if the founder mouse is able to transmit the acquired gene in a mendelian fashion.

Tyrosine kinases: Protein enzymes that have specificity for phosphorylating tyrosine residues on target proteins.

Upstream elements: DNA sequences upstream from the RNA start site of a gene that are involved in regulating its expression.

REFERENCES

1. Temin HM: Viral oncogenes. Cold Spring Harbor Symp Quant Biol 44:1, 1979
2. Leder P, Battey J, Lenoir G, et al: Translocations among antibody genes in human cancer. Science 222:765, 1983
3. Groffen J, Stephenson JR, Heisterkamp N, et al: Philadelphia chromosomal breakpoints are clustered within a limited region, *bcr,* on chromosome 22. Cell 36:93, 1984
4. Canaani E, Steiner-Saltz D, Aghai E, et al: Altered transcription of an oncogene in chronic myeloid leukaemia. Lancet 1:593, 1984
5. Collins SJ, Kubonishi I, Miyoshi I, et al: Altered transcription of the c-*abl* oncogene in K-562 and other chronic myelogenous leukemia cells. Science 225:72, 1984
6. Roeder R: Eukaryotic nuclear RNA polymerases. In Losick R, Chamberlin M (eds): RNA Polymerases, pp 285–329. Cold Spring Harbor, NY, Cold Spring Harbor Laboratory, 1986.
7. Corden J, Wasylyk B, Buchwalder A, et al: Expression of cloned genes in new environment. Science 209:1406, 1980
8. Watson JD: Molecular Biology of the Gene, 3rd ed. Menlo Park, NJ, Benjamin/Cummings, 1976
9. Darnell JE Jr: Variety in the level of gene control in eukaryotic cells. Nature 297:365, 1982
10. Ziff E, Evans RM: Coincidence of the promoter and capped 5′ terminus of RNA from the adenovirus 2 major late transcription unit. Cell 15:1463, 1978
11. Southern EM: Detection of specific sequences among DNA fragments separated by gel electrophoresis. J Mol Biol 98:503, 1975
12. Alwine JC, Kemp DJ, Stark GR: Method for detection of specific RNAs in agarose gels by transfer to diazobenzyloxymethyl-paper and hybridization with DNA probes. Proc Natl Acad Sci USA 74:5350, 1977
13. Towbin H, Staehelin T, Gordon J: Proc Natl Acad Sci USA 76:4350, 1986
14. Lewin B: Genes, 3rd ed. New York, John Wiley & Sons, 1987
15. Maxam AM, Gilbert W: A new method for sequencing DNA. Proc Natl Acad Sci USA 74:560, 1977
16. Sanger F, Nicklen S, Coulson AR: DNA sequencing with chain-terminating inhibitors. Proc Natl Acad Sci USA 74:5463, 1977
17. Watson JD, Crick FHC: Molecular structure of nucleic acid. A structure for deoxyribose nucleic acid. Nature 171:737, 1953
18. Bonner TI, Brenner DJ, Beufeld BR, et al: Reduction in the rate of DNA reassociation by sequence divergence. J Mol Biol 81:123, 1973
19. Casey J, Davidson N: Rates of formation and thermal stabilities of RNA:DNA and DNA:DNA duplexes at high concentrations of formamide. Nucleic Acids Res 4:1539, 1977
20. Hutton JR: Renaturation kinetics and thermal stability of DNA in aqueous solutions of formamide and urea. Nucleic Acids Res 4:3537, 1977
21. McConaughy BL, Laird CD, McCarthy BJ: Nucleic acid reassociation in formamide. Biochemistry 8:3289, 1969
22. Suggs, SV, Wallace RB, Hirose T, et al: Use of synthetic oligonucleotides as hybridization probes: Isolation of cloned cDNA sequences for human b2-microglobulin. Proc Natl Acad Sci USA 78:6613, 1981
23. Wallace RB, Shaffer J, Murphy RF, etal: Hybridization of synthetic oligodeoxyribonucleotides to FX174DNA: The effect of single base pair mismatch. Nucleic Acids Res 6:3543, 1979
24. Wallace RB, Johnson MJ, Hirose T, et al: The use of synthetic oligonucleotides as hybridization probes: II. Hybridization of oligonucleotides of mixed sequence to rabbit b-globin DNA. Nucleic Acids Res. 9:879, 1981
25. Tiemeir DC, Tilghman SM, Polsky FI, et al: A comparison of two cloned mouse b-globin genes and their surrounding and intervening sequences. Cell 14:237, 1978
26. Lowy DR, Gonda MA, Furth ME, et al: The human genes homologous to P21 ras viral oncogenes. In Scolnick EM, Levine AJ (eds): Tumor Viruses and Differentiation, p 435. New York, Alan R. Liss, 1983
27. Richardson CC: Enzymes in DNA metabolism. Annu Rev Biochem 38:795, 1969
28. Kornberg A: Aspects of DNA replication. Cold Spring Harbor Symp Quant Biol 43:1, 1980
29. Rigby PWJ, Dieckmann M, Rhodes C, et al: Labeling deoxyribonucleic acid to high specific activity in vitro by nick translation with DNA polymerase I. J Mol Biol 113:237, 1977
30. Maniatis T, Jeffrey A, Kleid DG: Nucleotide sequence of the rightward operator of phagel. Proc Natl Acad Sci USA 72:1184, 1975
31. Feinberg AP, Vogelstein B: A technique for radiolabelling DNA restriction endonuclease fragments to high specific activity. Ann Biochem 132:6, 1983
32. Saiki RK, Scharf S, Faloona KB, et al: Enzymatic amplication of *β*-globin genomic sequences and restriction site analysis for diagnosis of sickle cell anemia. Science 230:1350, 1985
33. Scharf SJ, Horn GT, Erlich HA: Direct cloning and sequence analysis of enzymatically amplified genomic sequences. Science 233:1076, 1986
34. Roberts R: Restriction and modification enzymes and their recognition sequences. Nucleic Acid Res 10:117, 1982
35. Linn S, Arber W: Host specificity of DNA produced by *Escherichia coli.* X. In vitro restriction of phage fd replicative form. Proc Natl Acad Sci USA 59:1300, 1968
36. Smith HO, Wilcox KW: A restriction enzyme from Hemophilus influenzae. I. Purification and general properties. J Mol Biol 51:379, 1970
37. Kelly TJ Jr, Smith HO: A restriction enzyme from Hemophilus influenzae. II. Base sequence of the recognition site. J Mol Biol 51:393, 1970
38. Roberts RJ: Restriction and modification enzymes and their recognition sequences. Nucleic Acids Res 9:75, 1981
39. Maniatis T, Fritsch, EF, Sambrook J: Molecular Cloning: A Laboratory Manual. Cold Spring Harbor Laboratory, Cold Spring Harbor, NY, 1982
40. Helling RB, Goodman HM, Boyer HW: Analysis of endonuclease RvEcoRI fragments of DNA from lambdoid bacteriophages and other viruses by agarose-gel electrophoresis. J Virol 14:1235, 1974
41. Sharp PA, Sugden B, Sambrook J: Detection of two restriction endonuclease activities in Haemophilus parainfluenzae using analytical agarose-ethidium bromide electrophoresis. Biochemistry 12:3055, 1973
42. Soeda E, Arrand JR, Smolar N, et al: Coding potential and regulatory signals of the polyoma virus genome. Nature 283:445, 1980
43. Southen EM: Detection of specific sequences among DNA fragments separated by gel electrophoresis. J Mol Biol 98:503, 1975
44. Schwartz DC, Cantor CR: Separation of yeast chromosome-sized DNAs by pulsed field gradient gel electrophoresis. Cell 37:67, 1984
45. Carle GF, Olson MV: Separation of chromosomal DNA molecules from yeast by ortiogonalified alternation gel electrophoresis Nucleic Acids Res 12:14, 1984
46. Chu C, Vollrath D, Davis RW: Separation of large DNA molecules by contour-clamped homogenous electric fields. Science 234:1582, 1986
47. Vollrath D, Davis RW: Resolution of DNA molecules greater than 5 megabases by contour-clamped homogeneous electric fields. Nucleic Acids Res 15:7865, 1987
48. Smith CL, Econome JG, Schutt A, et al: A physical map of the *Escherichia coli* K12 genome. Science 236:1448, 1987
49. Park M, Dean M, Cooper CS, et al: Mechanism of *met* oncogene activation. Cell 45:895, 1986
50. Dean M, Park M, Vande Woude GF: Characterization of the rearranged *tpr-met* oncogene breakpoint. Mol Cell Biol 7:921, 1987
51. Lawrance SK, Smith CL, Srivastava R, et al: Megabase-scale mapping of the HLA gene complex by pulsed field gel electrophoresis. Science 235:1387, 1987
52. Race R, Sadnger R: Blood Groups in Man, 6th ed, p 610. Oxford, Blackwell, 1975
53. Thomas G, Bodmer W, Bodmer J: Karlin S, Nevo E (eds): The HLA system as a model for studying the interaction between selection, migration and linkage. In Population Genetics and Ecology, p 465. New York, Academic Press, 1976
54. Ploegh HL, Orr HT, Strominger JL: Major histocompatibility antigens: The human (HLA-A, -B, -C) and murine (H-LK,-D) class I molecules. Cell 24:287, 1981
55. Botstein D, White R, Skolnick M, et al: Construction of a genetic linkage map in man using restriction fragment length polymorphisms. Am J Hum Genet 32:314, 1980.
56. White R, Woodward S, Leppert M, et al: A closely linked genetic marker for cystic fibrosis. Nature 318:45, 1985
57. White RL, Barker D, Holm T, et al: Approaches to linkage analysis in the human. In Caskey CT, White RL (eds): Banbury Report 14: Recombinant DNA Applications to Human Disease. Cold Spring Harbor, NY, Cold Spring Harbor Laboratory, 1983.
58. O'Brien SJ, Nash WG: Genetic mapping in mammals: Chromosome map of domestic cat. Science 216:257, 1982
59. Harper ME, Saunders GF: Localization of single copy DNA sequences on G-banded human chromosomes by in situ hybridization. Chromosoma 83:431, 1981
60. White R, Leppert M, Bishop DT, et al: Construction of linkage maps with DNA markers for human chromosomes. Nature 101:5, 1985
61. Donis-Keller H, Green P, Helms C, et al: A genetic linkage map of the human genome. Cell 51:319, 1987
62. Morton NE: Sequential tests for the detection of linkage. Am J Hum Genet 7:277, 1955
63. Dean M, O'Connell P, Leppert M, et al: Three additional DNA polymorphisms in the *met* gene and D7S8 locus: Use in prenatal diagnosis of cystic fibrosis. J Pediatr 111:490, 1987

64. Knudson AG, Hethcote HW, Brown BW: Mutation and childhood cancer: A probabilistic model for the incidence of retinoblastoma. Proc Natl Acad Sci USA 72:5116, 1975
65. Francke U: Specific chromosome changes in the human heritable tumors retinoblastoma and nephroblastoma. In Rowley JD, Ultmann JE (eds): Chromosomes and Cancer. Bristol-Myers Symposia Series vol 5, p 99. New York, Academic Press, 1983
66. Cavenee WK, Dryja TP, Phillips RA, et al: Expression of recessive alleles by chromosomal mechanisms in retinoblastoma. Nature 305:779, 1983
67. Bodmer WF, Bailey CJ, Bodmer J, et al: Localization of the gene for familial adenomatous polyposis on chromosome 5. Nature 328: 614, 1987
68. Solomon E, Voss R, Hall V, et al: Chromosome 5 allele loss in human colorectal carcinomas. Nature 328:616, 1987
69. Zbar B, Brauch H, Talmadge C, et al: Loss of alleles of loci on the short arm of chromosome 3 in renal cell carcinoma. Nature 327:721, 1987
70. Rowley JD, Golomb HM, Vardiman JW: Nonrandom chromosome abnormalities in acute leukemia and dysmyelopoietic syndromes in patients with previously treated malignant disease. Blood 58:759, 1981
71. Roberts L: Human genome: Questions of cost. Science 237:1411, 1987
72. Dugaiczyk A, Boyer HW, Goodman HM: Ligation of EcoRI endonuclease-generated DNA fragments into linear and circular structures. J Mol Biol 96:171, 1975
73. Bolivar F, Backman K: Plasmids of *Escherichia coli* as cloning vectors. Methods Enzymol 68:245, 1979
74. Bernard HU, Helinski DR: Bacterial plasmid cloning vehicles. In Setlow JK, Hollaender A (eds): Genetic Engineering, vol 2, p 133. New York, Plenum Press, 1980
75. Grunstein M, Hogness D: Colony hybridization: A method for the isolation of cloned DNAs that contain a specific gene. Proc Natl Acad Sci USA 72:3961, 1975
76. Benton WD, Davis RW: Screen λgt recombinant clones by hybridization to single plagues in situ. Science 196:180, 1977
77. Wu R, Jay E, Roychoudburg R: Nucleotide sequence analysis of DNA. Methods Cancer Res 12:87, 1976
78. Smith HO, Bernstiel ML: A simple method for DNA restriction site mapping. Nucleic Acids Res 3:2387, 1976
79. Gluzman Y: Eukaryotic Viral Vectors. Cold Spring Harbor, NY, Cold Spring Harbor Laboratory, 1982
80. Maniatis T, Hardison RC, Lacy E, et al: The isolation of structural genes from libraries of eucaryotic DNA. Cell 15:687, 1978
81. Saito I, Stark GR: Charomids: Cosmid vectors for efficient cloning and mapping of large or small restriction fragments. Proc Natl Acad Sci USA 83:8664, 1986
82. Watson JD, Tooze J, Kurtz DT: Recombinant DNA: A Short Course. New York, Scientific American Books, 1983
83. Steinmetz M, Moor KW, Frelinger JA, et al: A pseudogene homologous to mouse transplantation antigens: Transplantation antigens are encoded by light exons that correlate with protein domains. Cell 25:683, 1981
84. Steinmetz M, Winoto A, Minard K, et al: Clusters of genes encoding mouse transplantation antigens. Cell 28:489, 1982
85. Burke DT, Carle GF, Olson MV: Cloning of large segments of exogenous DNA into yeast by means of artificial chromosome vectors. Science 236:806, 1987
86. Moore EE, Jones C, Kao FT, et al: Synteny between glycineamide ribonucleotide synthetase and superoxide dismutase soluble. Am J Hum Genet 29:389, 1977
87. Kunkel LM, Tantravahi U, Eisenhard M, et al: Regional localization on the human X of DNA segments cloned from flow sorted chromosomes. Nucleic Acids Res 10:1557, 1982
88. Orkin SH: Reverse genetics and human disease. Cell 47:845, 1986
89. Smith LM, Sanders JZ, Kaiser RJ, etal: Fluorescence detection in automated DNA sequence analysis. Nature 321:674, 1986
90. Prober JM, Trainor GL, Dam RJ, et al: A system for rapid DNA sequencing with fluorescent chain-terminating dideoxynucleotides. Science 238:336, 1987
91. Lee M-S, Chang K-S, Cabanillas F, et al: Detection of minimal residual cells carrying the t(14;18) by DNA sequence amplification. Science 237:175, 1987
92. Crescenzi M, Seta M, Herzig GP, et al: Thermophilic polymerase chain amplification of t(14/18) breakpoints and the detection of minimal residual disease. Proc Natl Acad Sci USA (in press)
93. Watson JD, Tooze J: The DNA Story. San Francisco, WH Freeman, 1981
94. Blair DG, Oskarsson M, Wood TG, et al: Activation of the transforming potential of a normal cell sequence: A molecular model for oncogenesis. Science 212:941, 1981
95. Dean M, Park M, Le Beau MM, et al: The human *met* oncogene is related to the tyrosine kinase oncogenes. Nature 318:385, 1985
96. Gray JW, Dean PN, Fuscoe JC, et al: High-speed chromosome sorting. Science 238:323, 1987

SUSAN VANDE WOUDE

GEORGE F. VANDE WOUDE

CHAPTER 3 *Principles of Molecular Cell Biology of Cancer: General Aspects of Gene Regulation*

The human genome contains 50,000 to 100,000 genes encoded in its DNA sequence. Each codes for a specific product, either an RNA or a protein, which has a unique function in cellular metabolism. Whether the individual cell is a neuron or hepatocyte, its genetic information is essentially the same. How each cell determines its phenotype and maintains its cellular function throughout its life is a marvelous, albeit complex, achievement.

Genomic DNA is contained in chromosomes as described in a previous chapter. Were it possible to stretch out a DNA molecule, a human chromosome would measure several centimeters in length; in the cell nucleus it is highly coiled in an exquisitely ordered structure to facilitate regulated expression. A myriad of complex protein-nucleotide interactions occur in the process of gene expression that ultimately results in specific protein synthesis. Initially, DNA is copied into RNA in a process called transcription, and the RNA is then used as a template for protein synthesis in a process called translation. The host of events that occur during these processes is discussed in greater detail in the following sections. As will be seen, while some of the particular enzymes and proteins that regulate the actual processes are being characterized, much is yet to be discovered about genes, their control elements, and the protein complexes which control this process. Gene expression, the molecular basis for cell division, specialization, and differentiation, is a vast topic; current molecular biological techniques have just begun to reveal the mechanisms of the detailed cellular processes leading to phenotypic expression. The elucidation of these processes has enormous implications not only for understanding normal cell function, but also for unraveling mechanisms in cell dysfunction.

TRANSCRIPTION

In eukaryotes, the enzyme RNA polymerase II (RNA *pol*II) copies (transcribes) genes (DNA sequences) into messenger RNA (mRNA)[1,2] using monomeric nucleotides similar to the four bases used in DNA. The bases in RNA differ from that of DNA by a single substitution of an alcohol group for a hydrogen at the 2′ position of the ribose backbone (hence ribonucleic acid versus *deoxy*ribonucleic acid). Also note that uracil (U) replaces thymidine (T) as one of the four basic subunits of RNA structure. RNA polymerase begins transcription at a promoter initiation site that lies "upstream" of the DNA coding sequence,[1,2] the part of the gene which, once transcribed into RNA, forms a template for protein synthesis.

Many eukaryotic promoter regions have been shown to contain characteristic (consensus) nucleic acid sequences. With many genes these regions consist of a TATA box located 25 to 30 nucleotides upstream of the mRNA start site,[3-8] and one or more sites designated as "upstream elements" which lie 20 to 70 bp further upstream.[9] The upstream elements often contain GC rich regions[3,4,10,11] and the sequence CCAAT.[12] The promoter region is responsible for directing the correct initiation point of mRNA transcription; the upstream elements influence frequency of transcription initiation.[3,9,13] Transcription initiation in these regions is mediated or influenced by protein factors in addition to RNA *pol*II that are required as coactivators of initiation. Before transcription initiation, the appropriate regions of DNA must be exposed so that RNA polymerase and transcription activation protein complexes can begin RNA synthesis.[14]

DNA sequences called enhancers are involved in the regulation of transcription. Enhancers are specific DNA sequences that may be 50 to 200 nucleotides in length and are often repeated several times. They are found hundreds to thousands of bases (1000 nucleotides is referred to as a kilobase or kb) on either side (upstream or downstream) of the DNA coding sequence (Fig. 3-1A). These are recognition sequences or targets for DNA binding proteins that participate in enhancing (or suppressing) transcription.[9,13] Enhancers were first identified as control elements of viral transcription and are often constitutively turned on (positively regulated) in host cells to provide the virus access to cell expression systems. In contrast, cellular gene enhancers can be strictly conditional and limit expression to specific cell types. For example, the IgG enhancers only function in lymphoid cells.[15,16] The recognition sequences encoded in the DNA are called cis acting while the factors that bind to these sites act in trans.[17] Thus, gene expression, or transcription, is regulated by cis recognition elements and trans acting factors.

The DNA molecule is double-stranded; one strand is called the sense strand and contains the encoded protein information. The nucleotide sequence is linked via a phosphate backbone in a 5′ to 3′ direction while the other, complementary DNA strand, contains antisense information and its nucleotide sequence is 3′ to 5′ in orientation (see Chapter 2). The RNA transcript is transcribed 5′ to 3′ from the antisense DNA strand. The initial 5′ portion of the RNA transcript usually does not encode amino acid sequence information and consequently is known as untranslated (UT) leader. The next segment of the newly synthesized RNA contains coding (exon) and noncoding (intron) information.[18] Most eukaryotic gene primary transcripts contain one or more introns, and during mRNA maturation these introns are removed by processing or splicing to yield the mature mRNA molecule (Fig. 3-1B). The functions of introns are not completely understood,[18] and in most cases, they represent a much greater portion of the genetic locus than the actual coding sequences.

With few exceptions, the protein coding region is followed by noncoding sequences which are referred to as the 3′ untranslated region (U). The end of the RNA is terminated by posttranscriptional modification called polyadenylation. A polymer of adenylic (A) ribonucleotides (poly A tail) approximately 200 bp long[19] is added in response to a cis-acting polyadenylation signal and a specific polyadenylation site usually 20 bases downstream from this signal. Thus, characteristic sequences are identified at the point in mRNA where polyadenylation begins, yet there is not a DNA template for the poly A tail[20,21] (see Fig. 3-1).

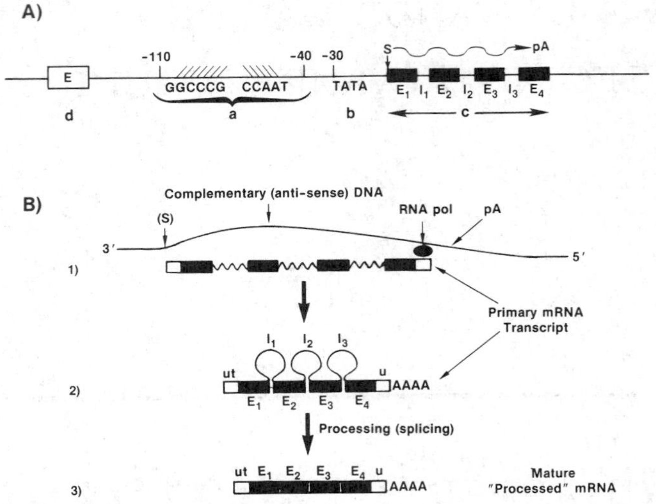

FIG. 3-1. **A**. Diagram of important elements of a eukaryotic transcription unit. *(a)* Upstream elements important for control of transcription initiation. Found 40 to 110 nucleotides upstream from the mRNA start site S, these regions variously contain GC rich and/or CCAAT sequences.[3,9,13] *(b)* The RNA *pol*I binding region or promoter located 30 bp upstream from the mRNA start site and consisting of the sequence TATA. *(c)* The DNA region actually copied into its complementary RNA sequence. S represents the beginning of the untranslated leaders; black (E_1, E_2, E_3, E_4) signifies exons or regions corresponding to amino acid sequences in the corresponding protein product while the introns (I_1, I_2, I_3) represent nonprotein coding regions which are spliced out during mRNA processing. pA signifies the end of the mRNA sequence where polyadenylation occurs. A polyadenylation signal is encoded in the DNA. *(d)* Enhancers are required in cis for efficient transcription to occur from eukaryotic promoters. They can be located hundreds or thousands of bases upstream or downstream or in the DNA coding sequence.[9,13,15,16] **B**. Eukaryotic messenger RNA transcription. mRNA synthesis by polymerase II is initiated from the promoter site described in the text and in **A**. RNA is transcribed from the complementary DNA strand of the structural (protein coding) region of the gene. Thus, the 5′ end of the RNA is transcribed from the upstream DNA sequence in the 3′ to 5′ direction (line 1). Supercoiled DNA must be unwound during this process. For clarity, only the complementary antisense DNA strand is shown. The first portion of the mRNA strand is designated the untranslated (ut) leader as the immediate 5′ end of the message usually lacks protein coding information. The newly transcribed mRNA (primary transcript) structural coding information (exons, E_1, E_2, E_3, and E_4) is interrupted by several noncoding regions (introns, I_1, I_2, and I_3), which are processed (spliced) out to form the mature mRNA (lines 2 and 3). The 3′ end also often contains untranslatable information (U). Both the 5′ and 3′ untranslated regions have been implicated in regulating translational efficiency and mRNA stability. The mRNA is terminated by addition of approximately 200 adenine nucleotide bases by the process of polyadenylation.[19] The mature transcript (line 3) is transported to and translated in the cytoplasm.

CHARACTERIZATION OF SPECIFIC mRNA SPECIES

Central to the study of gene transcription is the ability to isolate mRNA species from the cellular milieu. This process is complicated by the fact that mRNA represents only 1% to 2% of total cellular RNA and because destructive RNases are prevalent in the environment.[22] The other major cellular RNA species are transfer RNA (tRNA), which plays a key role in amino acid polymerization during protein synthesis, and ribosomal RNA (rRNA), which makes up the nucleotide structure of cytoplasmic ribosomes, the structures on which protein translation occurs. mRNA extraction is performed with great care to avoid contamination with RNases, and the unique feature of a poly A tail is used to selectively enrich for the mRNA fraction. Under appropriate salt conditions poly A sequences will anneal (hybridize) to an oligo dT-cellulose column (a polymer of deoxythymidine), while other RNA species and contaminating protein or DNA species are washed through (Fig. 3-2A). The mRNA can then be eluted from the column by lowering the salt concentration and collecting fractions.[23,24]

S1 NUCLEASE PROTECTION AND NORTHERN ANALYSIS

Specific mRNA transcripts from cells can be identified by several methods. One method, S1 nuclease protection analysis, utilizes hybridization (base pairing) between mRNA and a specific DNA probe. An isotopically labeled DNA fragment complementary to the specific RNA in question is denatured and mixed with total or poly A-enriched RNA. Conditions are then provided that favor RNA-DNA hybridization. A DNase S1 nuclease reaction is performed that digests all single-stranded RNA and DNA present in the reaction, but not the DNA-RNA hybrids.[25,26] These complexes are then analyzed or resolved by polyacrylamide gel electrophoresis (Fig. 3-3).[25,26] This technique is extremely sensitive because RNA/DNA annealing conditions are very selective. Therefore, genes that are expressed at very low levels can be identified in the presence of very large quantities of "other" RNA because of the sensitivity of single-stranded molecules to S1 nuclease.[27] Recently, procedures have been developed that allow radioisotopically labeled RNA probes with high specific activity to be generated using specific prokaryotic promoter systems. Assays that utilize RNA/RNA hybridization conditions and RNA nuclease enzymes that digest single- but not double-stranded RNA molecules can then be performed.[28]

Perhaps the most widely used technique for detecting mRNA transcripts is a method analogous to the DNA Southern blot analysis (see Chap. 2) and is known as Northern analysis.[29] In this technique, total RNA or poly-A enriched RNA is extracted as described above and subjected to electrophoresis on a gel matrix where it is resolved based on size. The RNA can then be transferred and covalently linked to a membrane filter.[29] Specific mRNA species can then be identified by hybridization with isotopically labeled probes. Northern analyses can reveal quantitative and qualitative information on steady state RNA transcripts and have been useful for identification of amplified gene expression (*e.g.*, c-*myc* in promyelocytic cells, HL60, see Chap. 4) or hybrid RNA transcripts in rearranged genomic loci (*e.g.*, the novel 8.0 kb *bcr-abl* hybrid transcript expressed in chronic myelogenous leukemia that arises from the Philadelphia chromosome 9;22 translocation between *bcr* and *abl*).[30,31]

FIG. 3-2. mRNA isolation and cDNA cloning. **A**. In order to isolate mRNA from total RNA, the latter is applied to an oligo dt-cellulose column under high salt conditions. Non-poly A sequences wash through as poly A sequences greater than 20 nucleotides can anneal. When a low salt buffer is applied to the column, the bound mRNA will elute off. **B**. To make a cDNA library, the mRNA isolated as described in **A** is incubated with free deoxynucleotides and other cofactors and the enzyme reverse transcriptase (RT) (usually isolated from avian myeloblastosis virus) is added to copy the RNA sequence into DNA. The single-strand DNA copy made from the RNA template ends with a hairpin loop and a 3′ double-strand DNA region remains (line 1). The DNA copy of the RNA template is isolated; DNA polymerase is added to complete synthesis of the second DNA strand (line 2). S1 nuclease is then utilized to hydrolyze the single-strand loop (line 3) and the resultant complementary DNAs (cDNAs) are cloned using protocols similar to those discussed in Chapter 2 (line 4).

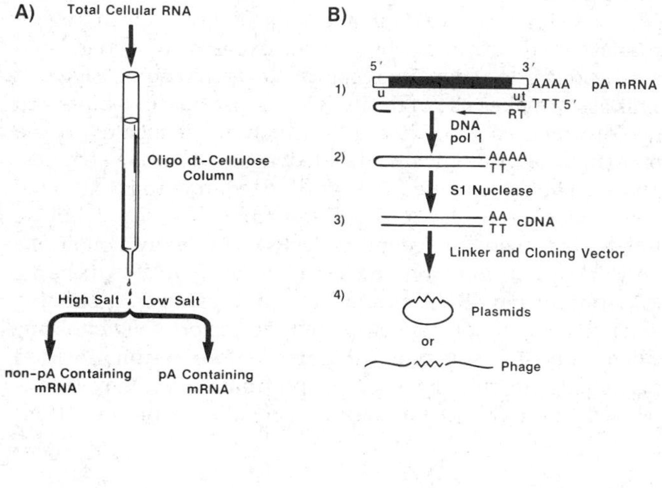

DETERMINING THE STRUCTURE OF THE mRNA

S1 nuclease protection analysis (see Fig. 3-3) is also useful for identifying RNA transcript structure. For example, if a genomic DNA fragment that overlaps an exon/intron junction is used as probe (*i.e.*, the labeled end is in an exon), hybridization with its homologous RNA will contain a single-stranded region which will be degraded by S1 nuclease. For example, if the -N-N-N- portion of the DNA fragment in Figure 3-3 is intron sequence, this region is processed out of the RNA and the S1 nuclease would truncate the probe corresponding to the exon/intron splice junction, thereby approximating its position in the DNA sequence.[32]

A procedure called primer extension is used to identify the 5′ end of an RNA transcript. In this technique, a complementary antisense oligonucleotide primer of finite length (~2–50 bases) which has been isotopically labeled (*e.g.*, at its 5′ end) is hybridized with its homologous mRNA. Reverse transcriptase, a retroviral enzyme that promotes DNA synthesis from RNA precursors, is then used to generate a copy of the mRNA toward its 5′ end. The product is analyzed by gel electrophoresis for size estimation. It is also possible from this reaction to directly determine the DNA sequence from

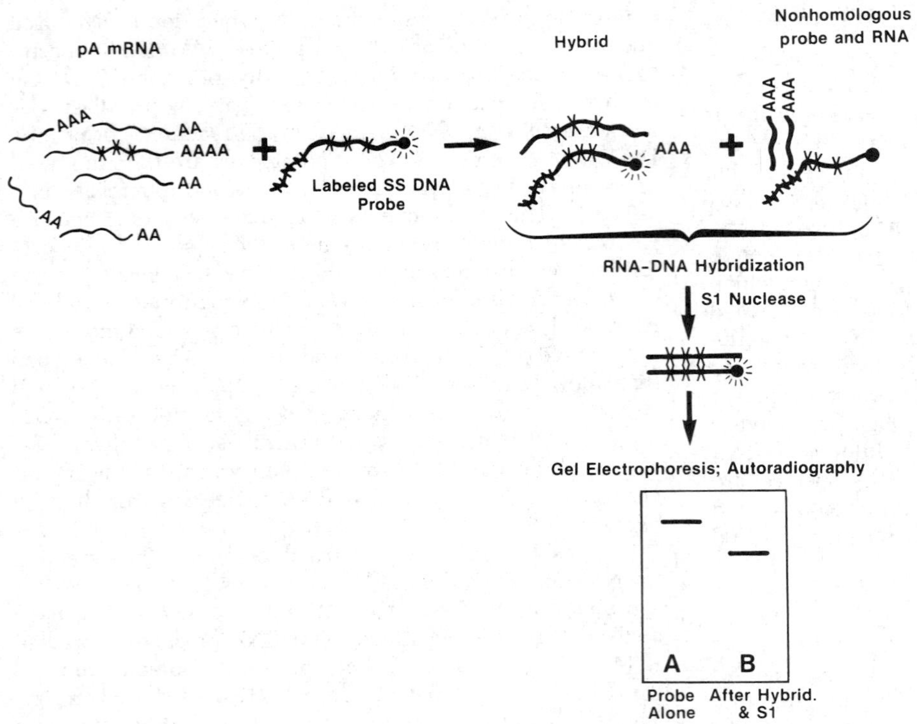

FIG. 3-3. S1 nuclease analysis. S1 nuclease is used to demonstrate that a specific transcript is present in a population of mRNAs. A radioactively labeled single-stranded DNA probe is denatured and mixed with the mRNAs. Buffer and temperature conditions favoring RNA-DNA annealing are provided. S1 nuclease is added, which degrades all single-strand DNA and RNA in the mixture; only the double-strand RNA/DNA product is resistant to digestion. The product is analyzed by gel electrophoresis and autoradiography for size and abundance.

which the RNA was synthesized. This information can be used to localize the transcription initiation site in genomic DNA.[33,34]

COMPLEMENTARY DNA (cDNA) CLONING AND SUBTRACTION CLONING

Techniques to isolate and characterize mRNA provide an important tool for study of gene transcription. Expression of mRNA in various tissues can be identified, quantified, and further studied. In addition, mRNA extraction techniques allow use of a powerful technique called cDNA cloning. mRNAs are isolated from a specific tissue type using oligo dT-cellulose chromatography or a similar method. Reverse transcriptase is used to generate single-stranded DNA copies from the mRNA molecules (see Fig. 3-2B). DNA polymerase is then used to generate double-stranded DNA fragments which can be cloned into conventional prokaryotic vectors as described in Chapter 2 to yield cDNA libraries.[23] cDNA libraries differ from genomic libraries by being limited to only the transcribed portion of genes and therefore are greatly reduced in sequence complexity. These libraries are useful in providing amplified copies of specific sequences; for example, a cDNA library from bone marrow RBC precursors will contain many copies of globin cDNA, whereas this gene occurs only once in a genomic library.

cDNA libraries prepared in a similar manner have been extremely useful for identifying transcripts that are differentially regulated in related cell types in the so-called subtraction cloning technique. For example, to identify novel transcripts specifically expressed in mitogenically stimulated cells compared to resting cells, single-stranded cDNA prepared from the former is annealed with an excess of RNA prepared from the latter. RNA-DNA hybrids representing sequences common to both cell types are removed by chromatographic procedures. After repeating the cycle several times, the remaining noncomplementary single-strand cDNA is recovered. A library is generated from this enriched cDNA fraction and can be screened with isotopically labeled total RNA from each cell type to identify the novel transcripts.[35,36] Obviously, this technique or variation of it can be used to identify transcripts specific for transformed versus normal cell types as well as differentiation specific gene transcripts.

RUN ON, IN VITRO, AND GENE TRANSFER TRANSCRIPTION ASSAYS

Run on transcription is a technique used to study whether a gene is being transcribed in a specific cell type, or in kinetic studies, to determine whether its expression is regulated during differentiation in response to a mitogenic signal.[37] This assay makes use of in situ RNA transcription factors and nuclei prepared from test cells which are incubated in the presence of isotopically labeled ribonucleotide triphosphates. The radioactive RNA synthesized in vitro is extracted and annealed to DNA fragments fixed to nitrocellulose filters that span the genomic locus. The assay conditions only favor continuation and completion of RNA synthesis; initiation of new RNA strands and processing (*i.e.*, splicing and polyadenylation) of completed transcripts will not occur. Thus, only the transcripts initiated before nuclei isolation participate (or run on) in vitro, and from these analyses it is possible to define the kinetics of regulation of gene transcription within a cell cycle and approximate the size of the transcription locus. RNA transcription usually proceeds beyond pA signals, but thus far transcription termination has not been shown to be independent of polyadenylation.[38]

RNA synthesis initiation and characterization of promoters can be studied in vitro (in vitro transcription) by the addition of a DNA substrate to enriched cellular factors containing RNA polymerase and labeled ribonucleotide triphosphates.[37,40–42] The DNA substrate is cleaved by several restriction enzymes downstream from a putative transcription start site, and the size of the RNA products synthesized from the DNA template allows mapping of promoter regions.[25,41–43]

DNA-mediated gene transfer in tissue culture is used to assay gene expression. Under appropriate conditions, recombinant DNA constructs containing a promoter and an appropriate reporter gene can be transferred (transfected) into cells, and expression can be measured by reporter gene activity.[44–47] Analysis of mRNA or a reporter gene product produced by intact cells can be used to reveal cis-acting promoter elements. A sensitive reporter assay has been developed in which a prokaryotic enzyme, chloramphenicol acetyl transferase (CAT), is used as a marker of gene expression.[48] This gene is responsible for inducing chloramphenicol resistance in strains of bacteria. It inactivates chloramphenicol by forming monoacetylated and diacetylated derivatives[49] using acetyl coA as a substrate. If the CAT gene is linked to a eukaryotic transcription control element and these constructs are transfected into mammalian or eukaryotic cells, cell extracts can be readily assayed for CAT activity as a measure of gene expression (Fig. 3-4). Different transcription control elements can reveal quantitative differences in CAT activity and serve to identify tissue-specific enhancers. Mutations introduced into the transcription control element which alter relative CAT activity can identify the responsible cis DNA sequences.

TRANSLATION

The mature processed mRNA (with spliced out introns and a poly A tail) is transported to the cytoplasm where it is prepared as a substrate for protein synthesis. The 5′ sequences of mRNA are methylated or capped[50] during mRNA processing or maturation; this may serve as a protective mechanism by making the mRNA resistant to certain ribonucleases, or may serve a function in ribosomal recognition or transport of the molecule from the nucleus.[51,52] Protein synthesis occurs in the cytosol on large protein-RNA structures known as ribosomes.[53–55] Eukaryotic ribosomes consist of two unequal subunits; they bind mRNA molecules in the presence of appropriate factors and tRNA and direct amino acid polymerization into protein molecules. The mechanism for transport of mRNA from nucleus to cytoplasm and subsequent initiation of ribosomal binding is a complex process where structural features of the mRNA (*e.g.*, 5′ and 3′ untranslated regions) may play a role.[51,55]

In order for mRNA to be translated into the specific protein for which it encodes, interactions between translation initiation enzymes, cofactors, amino acid charged tRNA, and ribosomes must take place. The protein coding information of mRNA, the series of codons or triplet nucleotides, serve as recognition sites for aminoacyl tRNA (genetic code, Table 3-1). The first amino acid codon of every mRNA is methionine. It is required in all cells for the initiation of translation and therefore AUG is called the initiation codon. Subsequent triplets of nucleotides encode for one of the 20 amino acids found in eukaryotic proteins. The decoding occurs on the surface of the ribosome via the complementary pairing of a specific tRNA, charged with its specific amino acid, to its respective codon. The ribosome translocates from 5′ to 3′ in an energy-dependent reaction and at each codon the respective charged tRNA contributes its amino acid covalently to a growing peptide chain. Many ribosomes spaced at finite intervals can participate in translation of the same mRNA simultaneously; these structures with multiple growing protein chains are referred to as polyribosomes.[30,54,56,57] The codons UAA, UAG, and UGA are translation termination signals that cause the dissociation of ribosomes from the mRNA and the cessation of the protein synthesis reaction. The protein is released from the ribosome and further processed, transported to its site of action, incorporated into cellular structure, or used as is. Examples of post-translational modifications that can occur and are most often required for biological activity include glycosylation (addition of one or more sugar moieties), phosphorylation (addition of a phosphate group), proteolytic cleavage (*e.g.*, cleavage of proinsulin into C peptide and insulin), or subunit binding (*e.g.*, oligomeric structures such as the adult hemoglobin molecule, which consists of independently synthesized α and β subunits.)[58]

As with transcription, translation can be carried out in vitro in a cell-free extract. Two such systems commonly employed are attained from rabbit reticulocytes[58–60] and wheat germ extract.[58,61,62] Translational activity is studied by uses of radioactively labeled amino acids which are incorporated into protein end products. Gel electrophoresis is then used to separate the synthesized polypeptide; two-dimensional separation can be achieved by subjecting the sample to isoelectric focusing using a pH gradient in the second dimension.[63] Autoradiography then allows visualization of the protein. If antibodies against the protein under study are

FIG. 3-4. CAT assay for analysis of gene expression in cells. **A**. Constructs are developed using cloning techniques that link an appropriate promoter or enhancer, or both, to the chloramphenicol acetylase gene (CAT). **B**. Tissue culture cells are transfected with the genomic construct. **C**. After an appropriate amount of time, cell extracts containing the CAT protein are mixed with radiolabeled chloramphenicol and acetyl CoA. **D**. Mixtures from **C** are spotted on thin layer silica gels. The separation of chloramphenicol (cm), 1-acetate cm, 3-acetate cm, and 1,3 diacetate cm are rapidly separated by this method of chromatography. Autoradiography subsequently allows visualization of the end products and allows calculation of enzymatic activity and ultimately the level of gene expression.

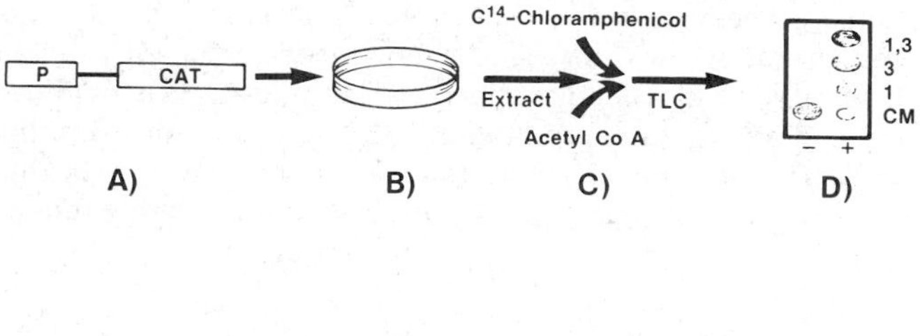

TABLE 3-1. The Genetic Code*

First Position in Codon	Second Position in Codon U	C	A	G	Third Position in Codon (3′ end)
U	Phe	Ser	Tyr	Cys	U
	Phe	Ser	Tyr	Cys	C
	Leu	Ser	Ter	Ter	A
	Leu	Ser	Ter	Trp	G
C	Leu	Pro	His	Arg	U
	Leu	Pro	His	Arg	C
	Leu	Pro	Gln	Arg	A
	Leu	Pro	Gln	Arg	G
A	Ile	Thr	Asn	Ser	U
	Ile	Thr	Asn	Ser	C
	Ile	Thr	Lys	Arg	A
	Met	Thr	Lys	Arg	G
G	Val	Ala	Asp	Gly	U
	Val	Ala	Asp	Gly	C
	Val	Ala	Glu	Gly	A
	Val	Ala	Glu	Gly	G

*The three RNA nucleotide bases coding for amino acid codons are given in first, second, and third positions in the 5′ to 3′ notation. For example, the codon 5′ AUG 3′ on mRNA specifies methionine, whereas CUC specifies leucine. UAA, UAG, and UGA are translational termination signals. AUG codes for methionine and is the first amino acid or initiation signal of every protein, but also codes for internal methionines. Uridine (U), cytidine (C), adenine (A), and guanine (G) are nucleotide bases. Alanine (Ala), arginine (Arg), asparagine (Asn), aspartic (Asp), cysteine (Cys), glutamic (Glu), glutamine (Gln), glycine (Gly), histidine (His), isoleucine (Ilc), leucine (Leu), lysine (Lys), methionine (Met), phenylalanine (Phe), proline (Pro), serine (Ser), threonine (Thr), tyrosine (Tyr), tryptophan (Trp), and valine (Val) are amino acids.

available, immunoprecipitation can be used as an identification method.[64] Tryptic digestion[65–67] and amino acid sequencing[68] are alternative methods of protein analysis and used for comparing one product to another as in a fingerprint (see Chap. 2).

Independent or simultaneous transcription and translation can be performed in *Xenopus laevis* oocytes. These cells have two advantages for use as expression systems; they are extremely large (approximately 1.2 mm in diameter) and contain large stores of gene transcription and mRNA translation machinery. DNA or mRNA can be introduced into the prepared oocyte by microinjection techniques, and protein or RNA end products are assayed as described above.[34,69]

Specific polypeptides and proteins can be detected in cells in culture by in vivo amino acid labeling procedures, followed by immunoprecipitation, gel analysis, and autoradiography as described above. Steady-state levels of polypeptides can be measured by Western blot analysis,[70] in which proteins from either cells or tissues solubilized in ionic detergents are subject to polyacrylamide gel electrophoresis, which fractionates them based on size. The fractionated cell proteins are then transferred to nitrocellulose or nylon membrane,[71] and, following incubation with appropriate antibodies, individual polypeptide bands recognized by the antibody can be visualized by either isotopic or nonisotopic enzymatic labeling procedures.[71]

OVERVIEW

Now that the processes of transcription and translation have been outlined, it may be helpful to discuss the processing of an expressed gene from start to finish to illustrate some of the aforementioned points (Fig. 3-5). We describe insulin because its synthesis has been fairly well characterized. Insulin is a 5700-dalton protein comprising an A and B chain connected by two disulfide bonds between cysteine residues on each polypeptide.[72] It is synthesized primarily in the beta cells of the islets of Langerhans of the pancreas. Secretion of insulin appears to be mediated by glucose[72,73] and other soluble factors such as amino acids, catecholamines, glucagon, and hormones;[73,74] it is likely that these metabolites play a role both as transcriptional inducers and by increasing post-transcriptional levels of insulin.[75–79]

The human insulin gene is located on chromosome 11 in the terminal band of the short arm (parathyroid hormone, β-globin, and LDH-A genes are also located in this region) and occupies 1.5 kb of the DNA.[80] It contains two introns, an untranslated leader and a noncoding 3′ untranslated region.[81,82] As mentioned, glucose is a positive regulator for insulin RNA transcription in the islet cells and increases in cAMP levels seem to correspond to induction of insulin gene expression.[79,83,84] Rising cAMP levels are also induced in islet cells under the influence of glucagon-like peptide with concurrent rise in insulin mRNA transcripts. Thus, insulin gene expression seems to be regulated via cellular second messengers. mRNA stability seems to be increased in high glucose conditions[83] and, as will be discussed later, translational processing is also accelerated in the presence of high concentrations of glucose. An enhancer region of the rat insulin gene has been mapped to flanking sequences 5′ of the coding region approximately 330 bp upstream from the transcription start site and extends approximately 130 bp toward the gene. The sequence in this region is highly reiter-

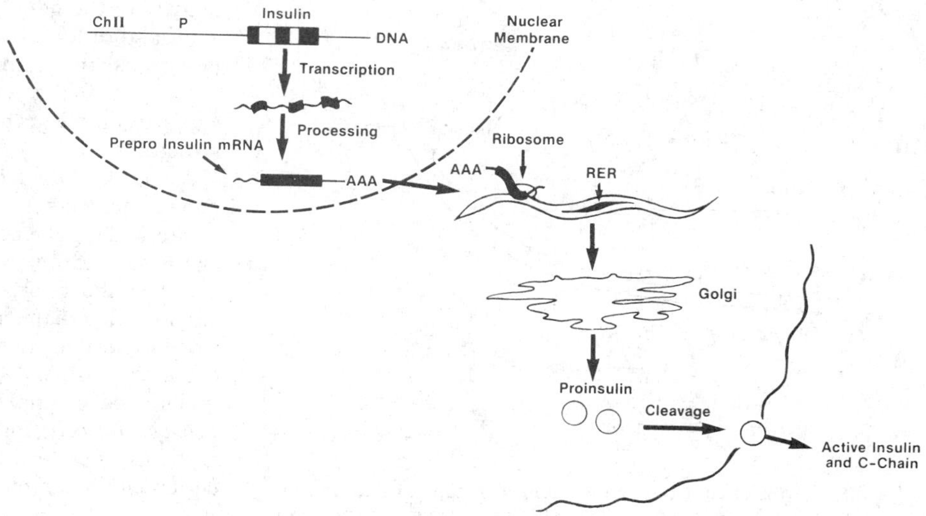

FIG. 3-5. Synthesis of insulin occurs within the β cells of the pancreas. Glucose and other positive regulators likely act through a second messenger intermediate to induce mRNA synthesis. mRNA transcription and processing occur within the nucleus; the initial preproinsulin mRNA is transported through the nuclear membrane to the ribosomes and rough endoplasmic reticulum (RER). The initial translation product (preproinsulin) is 11,500 daltons; a 23 amino acid sequence at the amino terminal end aids transport through the RER, and then is cleaved off. This results in proinsulin, which is subsequently transported to the Golgi apparatus, where it is packaged into vesicles with zinc. While transversing toward the cell membrane, the C peptide is cleaved from the molecule to form mature insulin. The vesicles are released into the pancreatic ducts by emicytosis, an energy-dependent process. ChII, chromosome 11; AAA, poly A tail.

ated and most likely contains several binding sites for various trans-acting factors.[85] A negative regulatory element has also been mapped upstream of the rat insulin gene that seems to suppress enhancer activity.[86]

Once gene activation occurs, the mRNA transcript is synthesized and processed by intron splicing, capping, and polyadenylation. The 600 nucleotide mature transcript is transported from the nucleus to the ribosomes where its initial translation product is an 11,500-dalton protein called preproinsulin. The 23-amino acid sequence at the amino terminus of this polypeptide (a signal peptide) facilitates transport of the molecule through the initial part of the cell secretory apparatus (the endoplasmic reticulum) where it is cleaved to the proinsulin molecule.[72,87] Human proinsulin differs from mature insulin by the presence of an additional 35 amino acid residue referred to as the C chain. This polypeptide links the carboxy terminus of the B chain to the amino terminus of the A chain; it is this form of the molecule that is packaged into secretory granules within the β cell.[72,87]

Recent experimental evidence indicates that at least in vitro, glucose can enhance transcription by stimulating rate of initiation of transcription, increasing elongation rate of the polypeptide (*i.e.*, speeding up synthesis postinitiation of translation), and can increase the rate of transfer of newly synthesized preproinsulin into secretory membranes.[88]

The secretory granules previously alluded to are formed at the Golgi apparatus by pinocytosis. They contain a dense core of insulin within a membranous sac;[89] zinc is also present, most likely in a complex with the insulin molecules, and high concentrations of calcium are also present in the vesicle.[90] The granules move toward the cell membrane via movements of the β cell microtubule microfilament system. As they traverse the cell, the C chain of proinsulin is cleaved from the A and B chains to produce mature insulin molecules. This reaction involves proteolytic cleavage by tryptic and carboxypeptidase enzymes and may be dependent on pH changes occurring within the vesicle.[91-93] The rate of conversion can also be increased in the presence of glucose.[94] Once at the plasma membrane, fusion of the granules with the β cell membrane occurs and mature insulin is released into the extracellular space.[90] This process, called emicytosis, is an energy dependent process that also requires calcium (see Fig. 3-5).[95] Thus, it is clear that at every level from initiation or induction of gene transcription through release of the biologically active protein product, there are mechanisms that can stoichiometrically influence the amount of gene product expressed.

CONTROL OF GENE EXPRESSION

The preceding sections have described mechanisms of transcription and translation and current techniques being used to elucidate rate and molecular details of these processes for various eukaryotic genes. It is apparent at this point that the production of proteins which alternately determined phenotype and function of a cell can be regulated at many levels. Outlined below are possible sites where various molecular mechanisms could halt or turn on specific gene expression (Fig. 3-6).

REGULATION OF RNA TRANSCRIPTION

This level of gene control is probably the most widely studied by molecular biologists, yet detailed mechanisms of gene regulation at this level remain to be elucidated. Within a specific cell type, certain genes are "switched on" while others are "switched off" and thus inaccessible to the cell's transcriptional machinery. The resultant combination of gene products are responsible for the cell's phenotype (or necessary for expression of the appropriate phenotype). Addition of methyl groups to nucleotide residues, a process termed DNA methylation, is one mechanism that has been proposed as a regulator of gene expression.[51,96] Nuclease

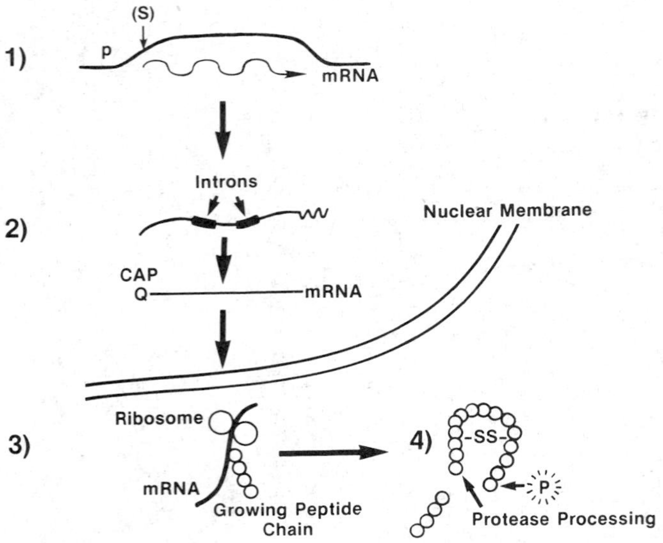

FIG. 3-6. Levels of control of gene expression can exist at *(1)* transcription of DNA into mRNA; *(2)* mRNA processing and transport; *(3)* protein synthesis; and *(4)* post-translational modification and transport. P, phosphorylation; -SS-, disulfide link; CAP Q, mRNA cap site.

sensitive sites have been mapped in chromatin in important transcription control elements[97] implicating chromosomal unwinding and uncovering of DNA as a possible gene control mechanism. How and when the switching on and off of genes occurs, how the activity of genes may be altered in diseased states and aging, and what outside mechanisms can alter cell behavior via changes in gene regulation are key questions currently being addressed. Considering nature's frugality, it is likely that this level of gene control is the major mechanism for cell diversity.

REGULATION OF mRNA PROCESSING

This level of gene control considers polyadenylation, capping, intron splicing, and transport of mRNA to the ribosome as processes that could alter levels of gene expression. Other factors that regulate mRNA stability may play a role in determining mRNA half-life and utility and thus could conceivably alter levels of transcription products.

REGULATION OF TRANSLATION

Translational initiation and amino acid sequence elongation rate are two areas that can affect product synthesis. In addition, activation of specific ribosome particles may also play a role in rate of protein synthesis.[99,100]

POST-TRANSLATIONAL MODIFICATIONS

Proteins often require cleavage, molecular alterations, or transport before activation. It is evident in some cases that the rate of these processes can be altered to satisfy the changing needs of the cell, tissue, organ, or body. Insulin, for example, can be processed from proinsulin at a faster rate in the presence of high serum glucose as previously discussed. The most common forms of modification are glycosylation and phosphorylation.[58] The latter modification is a major activity of the gene products that regulate cell growth, division, and differentiation.[101] There are many other types of post-translational modification such as fatty acid acylation and N-terminal glycine myristylation[102] that can apparently serve to direct proteins to the cell membrane and surface structures.

As can be inferred from the above discussion, eukaryotic gene expression is complex to dissect and investigate, and it is likely that gene control exists in multiple levels of protein synthesis and involves complex feedback mechanisms. Because of the relative simplicity of prokaryotes, which are single-celled, haploid, and have no nucleus, the best understood molecular models of gene control have been defined in these organisms. A brief discussion of the simplest and best understood example of gene induction, the lac operon of *Escherichia coli,* follows in order to illustrate some fundamental principles that most likely underlie gene expression control in eukaryotes as well.

The Lac Operon

The bacteria *E. coli* will use glucose as its energy source when it is available. If, however, the disaccharide lactose is presented in lieu of glucose, it too can be utilized via hydrolysis into its constituents, glucose and galactose. This requires production of the enzyme β-galactosidase, which is normally present in minute quantities within the cell. The gene is "induced" or turned on by interaction of lactose with the lac repressor protein. Normally the repressor binds to a specific nucleotide sequence in the operator region of the β-galactosidase gene, thereby blocking its promoter; the repressor has a second binding site for lactose. The lactose-repressor complex is sterically unable to continue to bind the operator, thus the bacterial RNA polymerase can now bind the β-galactosidase promoter and initiate gene transcription (Fig. 3-7A).[103]

Furthermore, high levels of glucose in the presence of lactose has been shown to inhibit β-galactosidase expression. The mechanism for this control operates through the action of cyclic AMP (cAMP). As glucose levels fall, cAMP concentrations rise within the bacterium; cAMP molecules then associate with a bacterial protein called cap that catalyzes RNA polymerase binding to the promoter site of β-galactosidase, thus stimulating its expression (Fig. 3-7B).[104] This simple example of gene control conveys the following points which are relevant to eukaryotic systems:

Certain genes are constitutive, that is, they are produced at constant levels throughout the routine processes of the cell. The constitutively produced proteins generally provide the housekeeping functions of the cell. Other genes are inducible or conditional, that is, the level of their expression can be altered in response to outside stimuli. An example would be the induction of a cascade of host functions in response to a growth factor binding to its receptor. Platelet-derived growth factor (PDGF) and its receptor, a member of the tyrosine

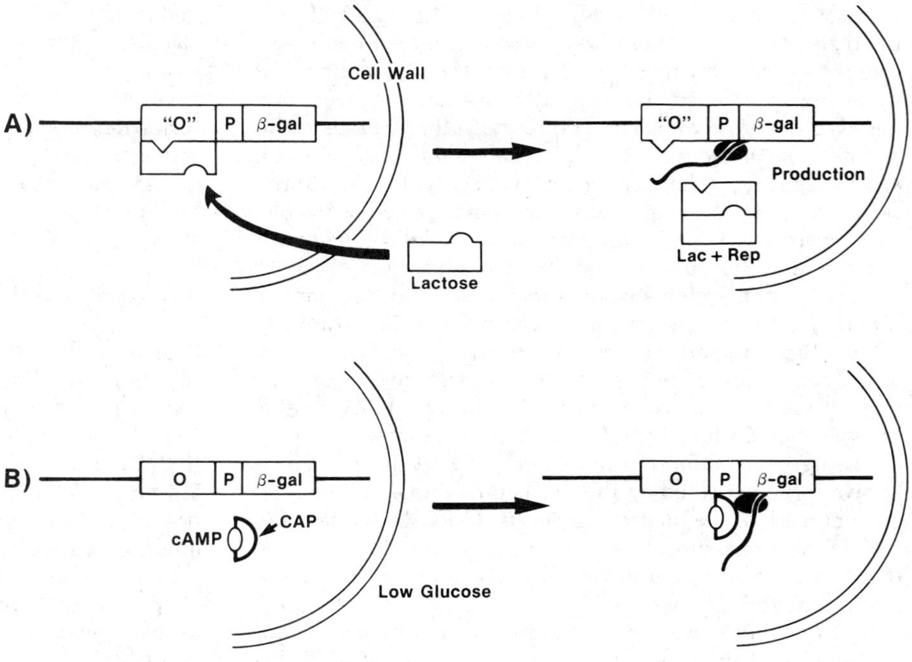

FIG. 3-7. Control of β-galactosidase gene expression of *E. coli*. **A**. A repressor binds to the operator-promoter region of the *E. coli* genome that prevents RNA transcription. Lactose present at high concentration can diffuse through the cell wall, bind a second site on the repressor, and open up the transcription start site for mRNA synthesis. **B**. Cyclic AMP (cAMP) overcomes the catabolite repression exerted over the β-galactosidase gene by high concentrations of glucose. cAMP binds a soluble binding protein (CAP, for catabolite gene activator protein) which subsequently assists the binding of RNA polymerase to the operator-promoter site. cAMP levels are normally inverse of those of glucose in situ. O, operator; p, promoter; β-gal, β-galactosidase gene.

kinase family of growth factor receptors, are examples. PDGF interacts with receptors and induces a cascade of host functions.[105] This occurs via ligand binding with subsequent phosphorylation of specific tyrosine residues on target substrates.

As mentioned earlier, two types of genetic elements are generally identified in control of expression. Cis elements are those DNA segments which serve as binding sites for transcriptional activators or repressors and repress or facilitate transcription. Thus, the operator and promoter regions of the lac operon, and upstream elements, promoters, and enhancers of eukaryotic genes are cis elements. Note that these factors are nondiffusible. Trans elements are diffusible substances which can bind to DNA (at a cis-sequence) and exert control over transcription. Examples in the lac operon model are lactose and cAMP-CAP. Thus, trans elements can activate at multiple sites in the genome.

Some DNA-protein interactions serve to enhance expression and others repress expression. This generalization can be applied to eukaryotic gene expression in many instances, as in the control of DNA expression by the glucocorticoid hormones in eukaryotes.

GLUCOCORTICOID-INDUCED GENE EXPRESSION

It has long been noted that glucocorticoid hormones exert a wide variety of activities such as growth and differentiation of certain eukaryotic cells. It is well accepted that the mechanism for such actions involves diffusion of the hormone into the cytosol with subsequent binding to a soluble receptor (Fig. 3-8). This hormone receptor complex then activates gene expression through a less well-understood mechanism which involves DNA binding at an enhancer sequence. Two human glucocorticoid receptors (HGR) have been fairly well characterized at the molecular level. They consist of chains of 777 (α) and 742 (β) amino acids that have several functional domains as determined by mutant construction. One area of importance is the steroid binding area; surprisingly, deletion of this domain results in constitutive expression of genes induced by the HGR-glucocorticoid complex,[107] indicating that induction may be associated with the removal of a repressor. A second functional domain is responsible for DNA binding and trans-activation of susceptible genes. This domain is a central cysteine-rich region of protein and has sequence homology to several other DNA binding proteins, including the thyroid hormone receptor or the v-*erb*A onco-

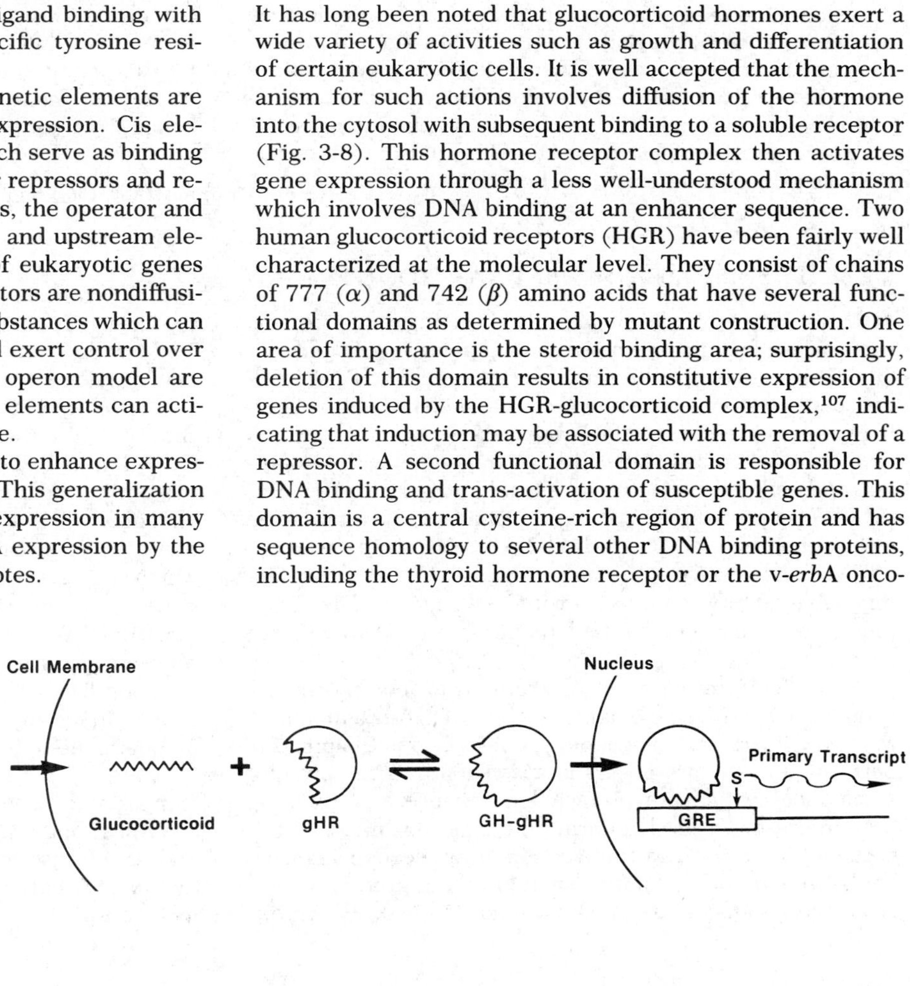

FIG. 3-8. Glucocorticoid binds a soluble cell receptor (*gHR*) upon entering a mammalian cell. This GH-gHR complex then can bind DNA at an enhancer sequence that results in mRNA transcription.

gene of avian erythroblastosis virus. An immunologic domain also exists that seems to play a minor role in enhancement of gene activity.[108] In light of these domains, the following mechanism for steroid activation has been proposed: the steroid molecule enters the cell and binds HGR, and because of the induced conformational change can now bind a specific enhancer sequence and induce transcription.[107] Because the major activation function seems to colocalize with the DNA binding domain, DNA GHR complex binding may be sufficient to induce transcription. Other gene activation systems studied map these two functions to different domains, suggesting that interaction at a third site is sometimes required for trans-activation (see Fig. 3-8).[109] Thus, eukaryotic gene expression, although more complex than in prokaryotes, relies on similar protein-DNA binding complexes (receptor-ligand) which alter gene expression.

The tyrosine amino transferase gene of liver cells is known to be activated by the glucocorticoid-GHR complex; current work in the mouse suggests its GH-GHR binding site lies 2.5 kb upstream of its transcription initiation site, and that binding of the activator causes local alterations in chromatin structure.[110]

One technique used to study functional domains of proteins is that of in vitro mutagenesis. In the case of GHR this was accomplished by linker scanning. Amino acid codons containing restriction enzyme *Bam*HI sites are inserted in such a way that the reading frame for the protein is not disturbed but the amino acid sequence at the site of the insertion is altered. The insertion sites are generated by partial digestion of previously constructed fragments with a frequent cutting restriction enzyme(s). These manipulations result in a series of DNA mutations along the different domains of the plasmid. The constructs are then assayed for various activities to determine the effects of disrupting the DNA sequence in different locations.[109]

MOBILITY SHIFT ASSAYS AND DNASE FOOTPRINTING

Methods commonly used to identify cis-acting sequences and trans-acting factors are known as DNA footprinting and mobility shift assays.[111] In the latter assay, candidate DNA binding sequences (cis elements) are used to identify trans binding proteins present in soluble nuclear-derived cell fractions by mixing isotopically labeled DNA fragments with the protein fraction and subjecting the sample to gel electrophoresis.[112] The protein-DNA complex significantly retards the electrophoretic mobility of the DNA fragment. In this manner, specific-cell types can be screened for trans-acting factors. DNA affinity columns prepared with specific DNA fragments are subsequently used to purify the DNA binding protein.[113]

DNase footprinting methods are used to identify the sequences in the specific binding region of DNA fragments.[114] Maxam-Gilbert DNA sequencing as described in Chapter 2 is performed in the presence and absence of binding protein. Nucleotides which are protected by an overlying binding protein are not degraded during the digestion phase of the sequencing assay. Thus, comparison of two sequencing gels, one with and one without protection by the protein, allows sequence specific analysis of the binding region.[114] An oligonucleotide can then be synthesized with the sequence derived from the footprinting assay and used in mobility shift assays as confirmation of both having identified the appropriate DNA sequence and its protein. More rigorous characterization of the binding sequence is made by site-directed mutagenesis. Search of the DNA sequence in the gene sequence data base can reveal other genes that possess possible binding sites.

TRANSCRIPTIONAL FACTORS

One area currently under intense investigation that may implicate gene dysfunction as a mechanism for oncogenesis is that of transcriptional factors; several have been characterized. For example, Spl has been isolated from HeLa cells, initially as a factor required for optimal function of the Simian virus 40 (SV40) early promoter.[115–117] Subsequently, it has been shown to enhance transcription 10- to 50-fold via binding to a GC-rich sequence.[118] Viral promoters that are responsive to Spl binding besides SV40 include the herpes simplex virus immediate early promoters[119] and the human immunodeficiency virus (HIV) long terminal repeat promoter.[118] Cellular responsive promoters include human metallothionein genes and the mouse dehydrofolate reductase gene.[118] How such a transcription factor operates at the molecular level is not yet understood. Because tandem repeats exist within binding sequences, each with varying affinities to induce transcription, and because multiple transcriptional factors must interact to initiate mRNA transcription, a complex interaction involving DNA-protein binding must occur. Appropriate conformational changes must take place to enhance RNA *pol*II binding initiation and transcription.[118]

jun ONCOGENE, GCN-4 AND AP-1

GCN-4 is a transcriptional control element in yeast that enhances expression of coregulated genes involved in amino acid biosynthesis.[120,121] Its optimal DNA binding sequence is the nearly palindromic oligonucleotide ATGACTCAT.[122] The *jun* oncogene of avian sarcoma virus[121,123] has no specific sequence homology to other oncogenes or to the tyrosine-specific protein kinases,[123,124] but recently it has been shown that it has considerable sequence homology with GCN-4 in its carboxy terminal region.[124] A chimeric protein containing the amino terminus of GCN-4 and the carboxy terminus of the *jun* oncogene can induce amino acid biosynthesis in yeast cells in the absence of functional GCN-4, which suggests that the two genes have functional as well as structural homology.[125] A human transcriptional factor, Apl, binds to DNA sequences homologous to GCN-4 binding sites, further suggesting *jun* is derived from a normal cellular transcription factor.[125] Apl binds to promoter regions of phorbol diester inducible genes (human collagenase, stromelysin, metalothione II, SV40).[126] Phorbol diesters are potent tumor promoters[127–129] and may exert their effect by altering gene expression.[126] The analogies between GCN-4, *jun* oncogene, and Apl strongly suggest that one mechanism of oncogenesis may be a transcriptional element gone awry; since such factors undoubtedly play a major role in cellular function and metabolism.[130,131]

DNA REARRANGEMENT AS A MECHANISM OF GENE CONTROL

DNA recombination plays a role in diversity of antibody variable regions. Before B cell differentiation, the coding region of the heavy and light chain of the immunoglobulin gene are dispersed throughout multiple sites on the chromosome.[132,133] For example, the promoter region of an unrearranged immunoglobulin gene is located approximately 300 kb upstream from the 3′ end of the gene in the germ line configuration. A complex rearrangement event occurs during B cell maturation that draws the various DNA segments of the gene into proximity to form a final transcription unit of 3 kb.[132] The joining sequences in these events are hot spots for imprecise alignment; the resultant reading frame therefore can exhibit enormous diversity in DNA sequence and explains the millions of unique antibody idiotypes produced in a single individual.[132,133]

This example illustrates how genomic rearrangement may be important as a control of gene expression and how such DNA breakage, repair, and mutation may serve as a normal process in certain cellular functions. It has been known for years that chromosomal rearrangements and translocations may also be a common mechanism in neoplastic transformation. For example, translocation of material from chromosome 9 to 22 has long been used as a marker for chronic myelogenous leukemia (the Philadelphia chromosome).[134] It is now known that this rearrangement results in adjoining of two specific genomic regions: breakpoint cluster region (*bcr* of chromosome 9) and the Abelson proto-oncogene (*abl* of chromosome 22).[135,136] The fusion of these genes allows expression of a novel 8.5 kb mRNA[30,31] that encodes for a 210,000 dalton chimeric protein.[137] This protein is a nonintegral tyrosine kinase that may play a role in signal transduction;[138] how it acts to produce a cancer phenotype is not well understood. A more thorough discussion of the phenomenon of genetic rearrangement allowing novel RNA transcripts and protein production which results in neoplasia can be found in Chapter 4.

GENE TRANSFER METHODS IN VITRO AND IN VIVO

GENE TRANSFER/TRANSFECTION

As described earlier, genes and their transcription control elements are now routinely studied by gene transfer methods. These assays are usually performed as transient expression assays, that is, within 48 hours after transfection the cells are disrupted and RNA is extracted and analyzed for quality and quantity of the product that is expressed from the DNA recombinant. In contrast, there has been wide usage of gene transfer technology, where the introduced genes become stably associated with the genetic information of the cell and their influence on the cell phenotype can be monitored in tissue culture. DNA can be introduced into cells by DNA transfection,microinjection,[139] electroporation,[140,141] and the use of specific viral vectors,[142] and have provided biologists with important systems not only for identifying essential regions in promoter transcription control elements but also for studying the properties and phenotype of a gene product. This technique has been especially important for identifying transforming oncogenes. The DNA transfection assay was actually developed to study and identify the transforming regions of DNA tumor viruses. The assay consists of introducing the DNA to be tested onto recipient nontransformed cell monolayers (described in more detail in Chap. 3). Transformation of cells by DNA is assayed by the appearance of focal areas of morphologically altered cells and by use of less labor intensive modification of the assay in which these cells are injected into nude mice and assayed for tumorigenicity.[143] The major limitations of this assay is that it does not reveal how expression of a specific gene influences normal cell growth and differentiation in the developing embryo and in adult animals. These questions are now being addressed by generating transgenic animals.

TRANSGENIC ANIMALS

The term transgenic was coined to define organisms that carry genetic material that has been introduced into the germ line. The inserted genetic information or transgene can be a segment of genomic DNA from a homologous or a heterologous species or even from viruses complete with its normal regulatory sequences and coding information. Most often, however, genes are introduced into the germ line of these animals using regulatory sequences which direct expression to specific cells or tissue types. Many genes have been introduced into the mouse germ line by direct microinjection into the male pronucleus of a fertilized egg. The egg is then reimplanted into a foster mother to allow normal development.[144] In a fraction of the injected embryos, the recombinant DNA becomes inserted into the germ line at a single chromosomal locus. Most often the newly acquired genetic is transmitted to progeny in mendelian fashion.

Despite the recombinant DNA being arbitrarily localized in the genome, in most cases it is subjected to normal gene regulation.[145] Thus, many new mouse strains have been generated with novel phenotypes that can be traced to the newly inserted genetic information and its expression in specific cells or organs. There have been many examples of the use of tissue-specific upstream regulatory sequences to drive novel structural genetic information. In a number of cases, these promoters have been used to express transforming viral genes and oncogenes in selected tissue types. Regulatory control regions from the elastase[146] or insulin genes have been used to direct SV40 T antigen expression to the pancreas. In these cases, tumors arise in the appropriate target cells. Using the regulatory sequence of a lens crystalline gene, SV40 T antigen expression was confined to the lens of the eye and it was shown that these animals developed heritable lens tumors.[147] Ectopic or increased expression of oncogenes in transgenic animals frequently generates phenotypes that can aid in understanding gene function. A *mos* oncogene transgene expressed at high levels during postnatal eye development caused alterations in lens fiber epithelial cell differentiation (Fig. 3-9). The earliest effect observed because of this ectopic expression was altered polarity in the elongation of lens fiber epithelial cells.[148]

The use of the transgenic mouse provides an exceptional system for studying protocols for gene therapy and several different genetic defects have been corrected using this pro-

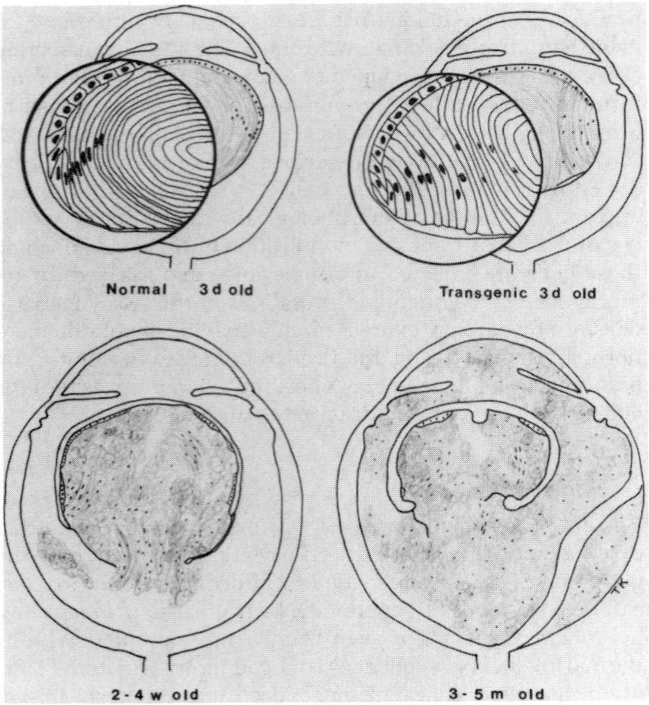

FIG. 3-9. Schematic drawing to summarize histologic findings on lenses of transgenic *mos* mice. In the normal mouse, lens fibers are formed by differentiation of epithelial cells at the equator. Nuclei of concentrically elongating cells form the bow configuration. Abnormality of the transgenic lens becomes apparent on the third postnatal day. The basal ends of the fiber cells extend only a short distance from the equator. The capsule in this area becomes thickened. The posterior capsule is not formed beyond this zone. By 2 to 4 weeks, the attenuated posterior capsule ruptures and lens fiber cells escape into the vitreal cavity. Lens fiber cells become globular in shape. Epithelial cells remain present and newly formed fiber cells are occasionally recognizable. By 3 to 5 months, the anterior capsule becomes very thick and the whole eye cavity, including anterior chamber and subretinal space, fills with globular lens cells.

cedure. For example, a strain of dwarf mice which is defective in growth hormone production was partially corrected by the introduction of a rat growth hormone transgene.[149] Likewise, immune defects have been corrected in mutant animals,[50–152] and most recently, a mutant strain of mice deficient in β-globin synthesis was corrected by introducing β-globin as a transgene. Although this technology raises ethical questions about performing gene therapy in humans, the mouse serves well as an experimental model system for determining the conduct of such procedures. Perhaps the greatest potential of the transgenic system lies in the possibility of introducing mutations into the normal genes of the animal and substituting modifications or mutant genes which will mimic human disease. This is clearly one of the most exciting areas in biology and can provide experimental systems which currently do not exist for studying treatment and therapy modalities for human diseases.

CONCLUSION

It is evident that much is to be learned about specific details of control of gene expression in eukaryotes; it is also being noted with increasing frequency the role that oncogenes play in altering normal cellular activity. For instance, oncogenes may in function resemble cell receptors which conditionally regulate expression of inducible genes, but become constitutively exprssed by the altered oncogene form. Alternatively, mutation of a cis element would alter gene expression and cause subsequent aberrant growth. The rearrangement in a cis regulatory region of the first exon of c-*myc* in Burkitt's lymphoma is an example.[153] Because it is likely that normal gene control relies on a precise sequence of events occurring in a cascade response and often a subsequent diminution reaction, alteration of one important control element could have devastating effects on cell metabolism and growth. It has also been noted that suppressor cancer genes may exist; disruption of the function of these genes can be correlated with the appearance of a neoplastic phenotype.[154] In the ongoing studies of gene expression, it is certain that the current explosion of information will reveal the molecular mechanisms for normal as well as neoplastic processes.

Research sponsored by the National Cancer Institute, Department of Health and Human Services, under Contract No. NO1-CO-74101 with Bionetics Research, Inc. The contents of this chapter do not necessarily reflect the views or policies of the Department of Health and Human Services, nor does mention of trade names, commercial products, or organizations imply endorsement by the U.S. government.

REFERENCES

1. Roeder R: Eukaryotic nuclear RNA polymerases. In Losick R, Chamberlin M (eds): RNA Polymerases, pp 285–329. Cold Spring Harbor, NY, Cold Spring Harbor Laboratory, 1976
2. Corden J, Wasylyk B, Buchwalder A, et al: Expression of cloned genes in new environment. Science 209:1406–1414, 1980
3. Breathnach R, Chambon P: Organization and expression of eukaryotic split genes encoding for proteins. Annu Rev Biochem 50:349–383, 1981
4. Shenk T: Transcriptional control regions: Nucleotide sequence requirements for initiation by RNA polymerase II and III. Curr Top Microbiol Immunol 93:25–40, 1981
5. Benoist C, Chambon P: *In vivo* sequence requirements of the SV40 early promoter region. Nature 290:304–310, 1981
6. Myers RM, Rio DC, Robbins AK, et al: SV40 gene expression is modulated by the cooperative banding of T antigen to DNA. Cell 25:373–384, 1981
7. McKnight SL: Functional relationships between transcriptional control signals of the thymidine kinase gene of herpes simplex virus. Cell 31:355–366, 1982
8. McKnight SL, Kingsbury R: Transcriptional control signals of a eukaryote protein coding gene. Science 217:316–324, 1982
9. Sassone-Corsi P, Borrelli E: Transcriptional regulation by *trans*-acting factors. Trends Genet 2:215–219, 1986
10. Lebowitz P, Ghosh PK: Initiation and regulation of simian virus 40 early transcription *in vitro*. J Virol 41:449–461, 1982
11. Everett R, Baty D, Chambon P: The repeated GC rich motifs upstream from the TATA box are important elements of the SV40 early promoter. Nucleic Acids Res 11:2447–2464, 1983
12. Efstratiadis A, Posakony JW, Maniatis T, et al: The structure and evolution of the human β-globin gene family. Cell 21:653–668, 1980
13. Maniatis T, Goodbourn S, Fisher JA: Regulation of inducible and tissue-specific gene expression. Science 236:1237–1244, 1987
14. Lewin B: RNA polymerase-promoter interactions control initiations. In Genes, Vol 3, p 183. New York, John Wiley & Sons, 1987
15. Voss S, Schlokat U, Gruss P: The role of enhancers in the regulation of cell-type-specific transcriptional control. Trends Biol Sci 11:287–289, 1986
16. Gluzman Y, Shenk T: Current Communications in Molecular Biology: Enhancers and Eukaryotic Gene Expression. Cold Spring Harbor, NY, Cold Spring Harbor Laboratory, 1983
17. Lewin B: The panoply of operons: The lactose paradigm and others. In Genes, Vol 3, p 219. New York, John Wiley & Sons, 1987
18. Gilbert W: Why genes in pieces? Nature 271:501, 1978
19. Adesnik M, Darnell JE: Biogenesis and characterization of histone messenger RNA in HeLa cells. J Mol Biol 67:397–406, 1972

20. Proudfoot NY, Brownlee GG: 3′ non-coding region sequences in eukaryotic messenger RNA. Nature 263:211–214, 1976
21. Fitzgerald M, Shenk T: The sequence 5′ AAUAAA-3′ forms part of the recognition site for polyadenylation of late SV40 mRNAs. Cell 24:251–260, 1981
22. Clemens MJ: Purification of eukaryotic messenger RNA. In Hames BD, Higgins SJ (eds): Transcription and Translation: A Practical Approach, p 211. Oxford, IRC Press, 1984
23. Maniatis T, Fritsch EF, Sambrook J: Molecular Cloning: A Laboratory Manual. Cold Spring Harbor, NY, Cold Spring Harbor Laboratory, 1982
24. Aviv H, Leder P: Purification of biologically active globin messenger RNA by chromatography on oligothymidylic acid cellulose. Proc Natl Acad Sci USA 69:1408–1412, 1972
25. Berk AJ, Sharp PA: Sizing and mapping of early adenovirus mRNAs by gel electrophoresis of S1 endonuclease-digested hybrids. Cell 12:721–732, 1977
26. Favaloro J, Treisman R, Kamen R: Transcriptional maps of polyoma virus-specific RNA: Analysis by two-dimensional nuclease S1 gel mapping. Methods Enzymol 65:718–749, 1980
27. Propst F, Vande Woude G: Expression of c-mos proto-oncogene transcripts in mouse tissues. Nature 315:516–518, 1985
28. Melton DA, Krieg PA, Rebagliati T, et al: Efficient *in vitro* synthsis of biologically active RNA and RNA hybridization probes from plasmids containing a bacteriophage SP6 promoter. Nucleic Acids Res 12:7035–7056, 1984
29. Alwine JC, Kemp DJ, Stark GR: Method for detection of specific RNAs in agarose gels by transfer to diazobenzyloxymethyl paper and hybridization with DNA probes. Proc Natl Acad Sci USA 74:5340–5354, 1977
30. Shtivelman E, Lifshitz B, Gale RP, et al: Fused transcript of *abl* and *bcr* genes in chronic myelogenous leukemia. Nature 315:550–554, 1986
31. Grosveld G, Verwoerd T, Van Agthoven T, et al: The chronic myelocytic cell line k562 contains a breakpoint in *bcr* and produces a chimeric *bcr*/c-*abl* transcript. Mol Cell Biol 6:607–616, 1986
32. Berk AJ, Sharp PA: Sizing and mapping of early adenovirus mRNAs by gel electrophoresis of S1-endonuclease-digested hybrids. Cell 12:721–732, 1977
33. Davies RW: DNA sequencing. In Rickwood D, Hames BD, eds. Gel Electrophoresis of Nucleic Acids: A Practical Approach, pp 117–172. Oxford, IRL Press, 1982
34. Coleman A: Expression of exogenous DNA in *Xenopus* oocytes. In Hames BD, Higgins SJ (eds): Transcription and Translation: A Practical Approach, pp 49–69. Washington, DC, IRL Press, 1984.
35. Alt FW, Kellems RE, Bertino JR, et al: Selective multiplication of dihydrofolate reductase genes in methotrexate resistant variants of cultured murine cells. J Biol Chem 253:1357–1361, 1978
36. Alt FW, Enea V, Bothwell ALM, et al: Probes for specific mRNAs by subtractive hybridization: anomalous expression of immunoglobulin genes. In Axel R, Maniatis T, Fox CF (eds): Eukaryotic Gene Regulation, pp 407–419. New York, New York Academic Press, 1979
37. Greenberg ME, Ziff EB: Stimulation of 3T3 cells induces transcription of the c-*fos* proto-oncogene. Nature 311:433–438, 1984
38. McGeady ML, Wood TG, Maizel JV, et al: Sequence upstream to the mouse c-*mos* oncogene may function as a transcription termination signal. DNA 5:289–298, 1986
39. Dignam JD, Lebovitz RM, Roeder RG: Accurate transcription initiation by RNA polymerase II in a soluble extract from isolated mammalian nuclei, Nucleic Acids Res 11:1475, 1983
40. Manley JL: Analysis of the expression of genes encoding animal mRNA by *in vitro* techniques. Prog Nucleic Acids Res Mol Biol 30:196–242, 1983
41. McMaster GK, Carmichael GC: Analysis of single- and double-stranded nucleic acids on polyacrylamide and agarose gels by using glyoxal and acridine orange. Proc Natl Acad Sci USA 74:4835–4838, 1977
42. Manley JL: Transcription of eukaryotic genes in a whole cell extract. In Hames BD, Higgins SJ (eds): Transcription and Translation: A Practical Approach, p 74. Oxford, IRL Press, 1984
43. Manley JL: Transcription of eukaryotic genes in a whole cell extract. In Hames BD, Higgins SJ (eds): Transcription and Translation: A Practical Approach, p 79. Oxford, IRL Press, 1984
44. Wigler M, Pellicer A, Silverstein S, et al: DNA-mediated transfer of the adenine phosphoribosyltransferase locus into mammalian cells. Proc Natl Acad Sci USA 76:1373–1376, 1979
45. Lewis WH, Srinivasan PR, Stokoe N, et al: Parameters governing the transfer of genes for thymidine kinase and dihydrofolate reductase into mouse cells using metaphase chromosomes or DNA. Somatic Cell Mol Genet 6:333–347, 1980
46. Graham FL, Bacchetti S, McKinnon R: Transformation of mammalian cells with DNA using the calcium technique. In Baserga R, Croce C, Rovera G (eds): Introduction of Macromolecules into Viable Mammalian Cells. The Wistar Symposium Series 1, pp 3–25. New York, Alan R. Liss, 1980
47. Spandidos DA, Wilkie NM: Expression of exogenous DNA in mammalian cells. In Hames BD, Higgins SJ (eds): Transcription and Translation: A Practical Approach, pp 1–48. Oxford, IRL Press, 1984
48. Gorman C, Moffat L, Howard B: Recombinant genomes which express chloramphenicol acetyltransferase in mammalian cells. Mol Cell Biol 2:1044–1051, 1982
49. Shaw W: The enzymatic acetylation of chloramphenicol by extracts of R factor resistant *Escherichia coli*. J Biol Chem 242:687–693, 1975
50. Bannerjee AK: 5′-terminal cap structure in eukaryotic messenger ribonucleic acids. Microbiol Rev 44:175–205, 1980
51. Lewin B: Gene Expression-2, Eucaryotic Chromosomes, p 677. New York, John Wiley & Sons, 1980
52. Furiuchi Y, LaFiandra A, Shatkin AF: 5′-terminal structure and mRNA stability. Nature 266:235–239, 1977
53. Lewin B: The ribosome translation factory. In Genes, Vol 3, p 144. New York, John Wiley & Sons, 1987
54. Nomura M, Tissieres A, Lengyel P: Ribosomes. Cold Spring Harbor, NY, Cold Spring Harbor Laboratory, 1974
55. Watson JD, Tooze J: The DNA story. San Francisco, WH Freeman, 1981
56. Lewin B: The messenger RNA template. Genes, Vol 2, p 151. New York, John Wiley & Sons, 1985
57. Wittman HG: Architecture of prokaryotic ribosomes. Annu Rev Biochem 52:35–65, 1983
58. Clemens MJ: Translation of eukaryotic messenger RNA in cell-free extracts. In Hames BD, Higgins SJ (eds): Transcription and Translation: A Practical Approach, pp 231–270. Oxford, IRL Press, 1984
59. McDowell M, Joklik WK, Villa-Komaroff L, et al: Translation of reovirus messenger RNAs synthesized *in vitro* into reovirus polypeptides by several mammalian cell-free extracts. Proc Natl Acad Sci USA 69:2649–2653, 1972
60. Pelham HRB, Jackson RJ: An efficient mRNA dependent translation system from rabbit reticulocyte lysates. Eur J Biochem 67:247–256, 1976
61. Olliver CL, Grobler-Rabie A, Boyd CD: *In vitro* translation of messenger RNA in a wheat germ extract cell-free system. In Walker JM (ed): Methods in Molecular Biology, Vol 2, pp 137–144. Clifton, NJ, Humana Press, 1984
62. Roberts BE, Paterson BM: Efficient translation of tobacco mosaic virus RNA and rabbit globin 9S RNA in a cell free system from commercial wheat germ. Proc Natl Acad Sci USA 70:2330–2334, 1973
63. Sinclair J, Rickwood D: Two-dimensional gel electrophoresis. In Hames BD, Rickwood D (eds): Gel Electrophoresis of Proteins: A Practical Approach. Washington, DC, IRL Press, 1981
64. Kessler SW: Use of a protein A bearing staphylococci for the immunoprecipitation and isolation of antigens from cells. Methods Enzymol 73:441–459, 1981
65. Dobos P, Kerr IM, Martin M: Synthesis of capsid and noncapsid viral proteins in response to encephalomyocarditis virus ribonucleic acid in animal cell-free systems. J Virol 8:491, 1971
66. Heywood SM, Rourke AW: Cell free synthesis of myosin. Methods Enzymol 30:699, 1974
67. Woodward WR, Wilairat P, Herbert E: Preparation of reticulocyte aminoacyl-tRNA and the assay of codon recognition properties of isoacceptor tRNA's in a reticulocyte cell-free system. Methods Enzymol 30:740, 1974
68. Devillers-Thiery A, Kindt T, Scheele G, et al: Homology in amino-terminal sequence of precursors to pancreatic secretory proteins. Proc Natl Acad Sci USA 72:5016, 1975
69. Richter JD, Lorenz LJ, Crawford DR, et al: The control of translation by RNA binding proteins in *xenopus laevis* oocytes. In Matthews MB (ed): Translational Control, Current Communications in Molecular Biology, pp 144–149. Cold Spring Harbor, NY, Cold Spring Harbor Laboratory, 1986
70. Towbin H, Staehelin T, Gordon J: Electrophoretic transfer of proteins from polyacrylamide gels to nitrocellulose sheets: Procedure and some applications. Proc Natl Acad Sci USA 76:4350–4354, 1979
71. Bers G, Garfin D: Protein and nucleic acid blotting and immunobiochemical detection. Bio Tech 3:276–288, 1985
72. Smith EL, Hill RL, Lehman JR, et al: Principles of Biochemistry: Mammalian Biochemistry, pp 474–497. McGraw Hill, New York, 1983
73. Cooperstein SJ, Watkins D: The Islets of Langerhans: Biochemistry, Physiology and Pathology. New York, Academic Press, 1981
74. Drucker DJ, Philippe J, Mojsov S, et al: Glucagon-like peptide I stimulates insulin gene expression and increases cyclic AMP levels in a rat islet cell line. Proc Natl Acad Sci USA 84:3434–3438, 1987
75. Permutt MA, Kipnis DM: Insulin biosynthesis: On the mechanism of glucose stimulation. J Biol Chem 247:1194–1199, 1972
76. Itch N, Okamoto H: Translational control of proinsulin synthesis by glucose. Nature 283:100–102, 1980
77. Brunstead J, Chan SJ: Direct effect of glucose on the prepoinsulin mRNA level in isolated pancreatic islets. Biochem Biophys Methods 106:1383–1389, 1982
78. Giddings SJ, Chirgwin J, Permutt MA: Effects of glucose on proinsulin messenger RNA in rats *in vivo*. Diabetes 31:624–629, 1982
79. Welsh M, Chirgwin J, Permutt MA: Effects of D-glucose, L-leucine and 2 ketoisocaproate on insulin messenger-RNA levels in mouse pancreatic islets. Diabetes 35:228–231, 1986
79. Lebo RV, Cheung MC, Bruce BD, et al: Mapping parathyroid hormone, β-globin, insulin, and LDH-A genes within the human chromosome 11 short arm by spot blotting sorted chromosomes. Hum Genet 69:316–320, 1985
80. Rotwein P, Naylor SL, Chirgwin JM: Human insulin-related DNA sequences map to chromosomes 2 and 11. Somatic Cell Mol Genet 12:625–631, 1986
81. Lewin B: The organization of interrupted genes. In Genes, Vol 2, p 312. New York, John Wiley & Sons, 1985
82. Lomedico P, Rosenthal N, Efstratiadis A, et al: The structure and evolution of the two nonallelic rat preproinsulin genes. Cell 18:545–558, 1979
83. Welsh M, Nielsen DA, Mackrell AJ, et al: Control of insulin gene expression in pancreatic β-cells and in an insulin-producing cell line, R1N-5F cells. J Biol Chem 260:13590–13594, 1985
84. Ashcroft SJH: Metabolic controls of insulin secretion. In Cooperstein SJ, Watkins D (eds): Islets of Langerhans, pp 117–148. Academic Press, New York, 1981
85. Ohlsson H, Edlund T: Sequence specific interactions of nuclear factors with the insulin gene enhancer. Cell 45:35–44, 1986

86. Laimins L, Holmgren-Konig M, Khoury G, et al: Transcriptional "silencer" element in rat repetitive sequencers associated with the rat insulin 1 gene locus. Proc Natl Acad Sci USA 83:3151–3155, 1986
87. Pemutt MA: Biosynthesis of insulin. In Copperstein SJ, Watkind D (eds): Islets of Langerhans, pp 75–95. New York, Academic Press, 1981
88. Welsh M, Scherberg N, Gilmore R, et al: Translational control of insulin biosynthesis. Biochem J 235:459–467, 1986
89. Howell SL, Lacy PE: In Memoirs of the Society for Endocrinology: Subcellular Organization and Function in Endocrine Tissues. London, Cambridge University Press, 19:469–480, 1970
90. McDaniel ML, Lacy PE: Interactions in cell organelles in insulin secretin. In Cooperstein SJ, Watkins D (eds): Islets of Langerhans, pp 97–115. New York, Academic Press, 1981
91. Docherty K, Steiner DF: Post-translational proteolysis in polypeptide hormone biosynthesis. Annu Rev Physiol 44:625–638, 1982
92. Docherty K, Carrol R, Steiner DF: Conversion of proinsulin to insulin, involvement of a 31,500 molecular weight thiol protease. Proc Natl Acad Sci USA 79:4613–4617, 1982
93. Orci L, Ravazzola M, Amherdt M, et al: Conversion of proinsulin to insulin occurs coordinately with acidification of maturing secretory vesicles. J Cell Biol 103:2273–2281, 1986
94. Bajas JS (ed): Insulin and metabolism, pp 24–28. New York, Excerpta Medica, 1977
95. Grodsky GM: A threshold distribution hypothesis for packet storage of insulin. Diabetes 21:584–593, 1972
96. Rugin R, Riggs AD: DNA methylation and gene function. Science 210:604–610, 1980
97. Groudine M, Weintraub H: Propagation of globin DNAse-1 hypersensitive sites in absence of factors required for induction: A possible mechanism for determination. Cell 30:131–139, 1982
98. Nelson EM, Winkler MM: Regulation of mRNA entry into polysomes. J Biol Chem 262:11501–11506, 1987
99. Hershey JWR, Duncan R, Matthews M: Introduction: Mechanisms of translational control. In Matthews MD (ed): Translational Control, Current Communications in Molecular Biology, pp 1–19. Cold Spring Harbor, NY, Cold Spring Harbor Laboratory, 1986
100. Brown D: Gene expression in eukaryotes. Science 211:667–674, 1981
101. Hunter T: A thousand and one protein kinases. Cell 50:823–829, 1987
102. Towler DA, Gordon JI, Adams SP, et al: The biology and enzymology of eukaryotic protein acylation. Annu Rev Biochem (in press)
103. Jacob F, Monod J: Genetic regulatory mechanisms in the synthesis of proteins. J Mol Biol 3:318–356, 1961
104. Pastan I, Pearlman R: Cyclic AMP in bacteria. Science 169:339–344, 1969
105. Stiles CD, Capone GT, Scher CD, et al: Dual control of cell growth by somatomedins and platelet-derived growth factor. Proc Natl Acad Sci USA 76:1279, 1979
106. Hollenberg SM, Weinberger C, Ong E, et al: Primary structure and expression of a functional human glucocorticoid receptor cDNA. Nature 318:635–641, 1985
107. Hollenberg SM, Giguere V, Segui P, et al: Colocalization of DNA binding and transcriptional activation functions in the human glucocorticoid receptor. Cell 49:39–46, 1987
108. Giguere V, Hollenberg, SM, Rosenfeld MG, et al: Functional domains of the human glucocorticoid receptor. Cell 46:645–652, 1986
109. Keegan L, Gill G, Ptashne M: Separation of DNA binding from the transcription-activating function of a eukaryotic regulatory protein. Science 231:699–704, 1986
110. Jantzen HM, Strahle U, Gloss B, et al: Cooperativity of glucocorticoid response elements located far upstream of the tyrosine aminotransferase gene. Cell 49:29–38, 1987
111. Garner MM, Revzin A: A gell electrophoresis method for quantifying the binding of proteins to specific DNA regions: Application to components of the *Escherichia coli* lactose operon regulatory system. Nucleic Acids Res 9:3047–3060, 1981
112. Garner MM, Revzin A: The use of gel electrophoresis to detect and study nucleic acid-protein interactions. Trends Biol Sci 11:395–396, 1986
113. Kadonaga JT, Tijian R: Affinity purification of sequence specific DNA binding proteins. Proc Natl Acad Sci USA 83:5589–5893, 1986
114. Galas DJ, Schmitz A: DNAse foot printing: A simple method for the detection of protein-DNA binding specificity. Nucleic Acids Res 5:3157–3170, 1978
115. Short NJ: Are some controlling factors more equal than others? Nature 326:740–741, 1987
116. Briggs MR, Kadonaga JT, Bell SP, et al: Purification and biochemical characterizatin of the promoter-specific transcription factor, Sp1. Science 234:47–52, 1986
117. Dynan WS, Tijian R: Control of eukaryotic messenger RNA synthesis by sequence specific DNA-binding proteins. Nature 316:774–777, 1985
118. Kadonaga JT, Jones KA, Tjian R: Promoter-specific activation of RNA polymerase II transcription by Sp1. Trends Genet 2:20–23, 1986
119. Jones KA, Tjian R: Sp1 binds to promoter sequences and activates herpes simplex virus immediate-early gene transcription *in vitro*. Nature 317:179–182, 1985
120. Hope IA, Struhl K: GCN4 protein, synthesized *in vitro*, binds to HIS3 regulatory sequences: Implications for the general control of amino acid biosynthetic genes in yeast. Cell 43:177–188, 1985
121. Arndt K, Fink G: GCN4 protein, a positive transcription factor in yeast, binds general control promoters to all 5′ TGACTC 3′ sequences. Proc Natl Acad Sci USA 83:8516–8520, 1986
122. Hill DE, Hope IA, Macke JP, et al: Saturation mutagenesis of the yeast *his3* regulatory site: Requirements for transcriptional induction and for binding by GCN4 activator protein. Science 234:451–457, 1986
123. Maki Y, Bos TJ, Davis C, et al: Avian sarcoma virus 17 carries the *jun* oncogene. Proc Natl Acad Sci USA 84:2848–2852, 1987
124. Vogt PK, Bos TJ, Doolittle RF: Homology between the DNA-binding domain of the GCN4 regulatory protein of yeast and the carboxyterminal region of a protein coded for by the oncogene *jun*. Proc Natl Acad Sci USA 84:3316–3319, 1987
125. Struhl K: The DNA-binding domains of the jun oncoprotein and the yeast GCN4 transcriptional activator protein are functionally homologous. Cell 50:841–846, 1987
126. Angel P, Imagawa M, Chiu R, et al: Phorbol ester-inducible genes contain a common *cis* element recognized by a TPA-medulated *trans*-acting factor. Cell 49:729–739, 1987
127. Weinstein IB, Lee LS, Fisher PB, et al: Action of phorbol esters in cell culture: Mimicry of transformation, altered differentiation and effects on cell membrane. J Supramol Struct 12:195–208, 1979
128. Blumberg PM: In vitro studies on the mode of action of the phorbol esters, potent tumor promoters. CRC Crit Rev Toxicol 9:153–197, 1981
129. Slaga TJ: Cellular and molecular mechanisms of tumor promotion. Cancer Surv 2:595–612, 1983
130. Bohmann D, Bos TJ, Admon A, et al: Human proto-oncogene *c-jun* encodes a DNA binding protein with structural and functional properties of transcription factor AP-1. Science 238:1386–1392, 1987
131. Varmus HE: Oncogenes and transcriptional control. Science 238:1337–1339, 1987
132. Tonegawa S: Somatic generation of antibody diversity. Nature 302:575–581, 1983
133. Nossal GJV: Current concepts in immunology: The basic components of the immune system. N Engl J Med 316:1320–1325, 1987
134. Rowley JD: Ph′-positive leukaemia including chronic myelogenous leukaemia. Clin Haematol 9:54, 1980
135. Collins SJ, Kubonishi I, Miyoshi I, et al: Altered transcription of the c-*abl* oncogene in K-562 and other chronic myelogenous leukemia cells. Science 225:72, 1984
136. Gale RP, Canaani E: An 8-kilobase *abl* RNA transcript in chronic myelogenous leukemia. Proc Natl Acad Sci USA 81:5648–5652, 1984
137. Konopka JB, Watanabe SM, Witte ON: An alteration of the human c-*abl* protein in K562 leukemia cells unmasks associated tyrosine kinase activity. Cell 37:1035, 1984
138. Konopka JB, Witte ON: Detection of c-*abl* tyrosine kinase activity *in vitro* permits direct comparison of normal and altered *abl* gene products. Mol Cell Biol 5:3116, 1985
139. Mulcahy LS, Smith MR, Stacey DW: Requirement for *ras* proto-oncogene function during serum-stimulated growth in NIH 3T3 cells. Nature 313:241–243, 1985
140. Chu G, Hayakawa H, Berg P: Electroporation for the efficient transfection of mammalian cells with DNA. Nucleic Acids Res 15:1311–1325, 1987
141. Toneguzzo F, Keating A: Stable expression of selectable genes introduced into human hematopoietic stem cells by electric field-mediated DNA transfer. Proc Natl Acad Sci USA 83:3496–2499, 1986
142. Gluzman Y: Eukaryotic Viral Vectors. Cold Spring Harbor, NY, Cold Spring Harbor Laboratory, 1982
143. Blair DG, Cooper CS, Oskarsson MK, et al: New method for detecting cellular transforming genes. Science 218:1122–1125, 1982
144. Gordon JW, Scangos GA, Plotkin DJ, et al: Genetic transformation of mouse embryos by microinjection of purified DNA. Proc Natl Acad Sci USA 77:7380–7384, 1980
145. Palmiter RD, Brinster RL: Germ-line transformation of mice. Annu Rev Genet 20:465–499, 1986
146. Ornitz DM, Palmiter RD, Messing A, et al: Elastase 1 promoter directs expression of human growth hormone and SV40 T-antigen genes to pancreatic acinar cells in transgenic mice. Cold Spring Harbor Symp Quant Biol 50:399–409, 1985
147. Mahon KA, Chepelinsky AB, Khillan JS, et al: Oncogenesis of the lens in transgenic mice. Science 235:1622, 1987
148. Khillan JS, Oskarsson MK, Propst F, et al: Defects in lens fiber differentiation are linked to c-*mos* overexpression in transgenic mice. Genes Dev 1:1327–1335, 1987
149. Hammer RE, Palmiter RD, Brinster RL: Partial correction of murine hereditary disorder by germ-line incorporation of a new gene. Nature 311:65–67, 1987
150. LeMeur M, Gerlinger P, Benoist C, et al: Correcting an immune-response deficiency by creating Eα gene transgenic mice. Nature 316:38–42, 1985
151. Pinkert CA, Widera G, Cowing C, et al: Tissue-specific, inducible and functional expression of the Eα^d MHC class II gene in transgenic mice. EMBO J 4:2225–2230, 1985
152. Yamamura K, Kikutani H, Folsom V, et al: Functional expression of microinjected Eα^d gene in C57BL/6 transgenic mice. Nature 316:67–69, 1985
153. Cesarman E, Dalla-Favera R, Bentley D, et al: Mutations in the first exon are associated with altered transcription of c-*myc* in Burkitt lymphoma. Science 238:1272, 1987
154. Klein G: The approaching era of the tumor suppressor genes. Science 238:1539–1545, 1987
155. Park M, Dean M, Cooper CS, et al: Mechanism of *met* oncogene activation. Cell 45:895–904, 1986

MORAG PARK

GEORGE F. VANDE WOUDE

CHAPTER 4 *Principles of Molecular Cell Biology of Cancer: Oncogenes*

During the past several years we have witnessed extraordinary advances in our understanding of the mechanisms of oncogenesis. This understanding has come about primarily through a synthesis of what were until recently separate cancer research disciplines. The application of the techniques of molecular biology led to the discovery of, in tumor virology, the transforming genes of tumor viruses[1]; in cytogenetics, the genes activated at the breakpoints of nonrandom chromosomal translocations of lymphomas and leukemias[2]; in cell biology, the correlation between growth factors or growth factor receptors and certain transforming genes[3]; and the existence of transforming genes which are activated in vivo and in vitro by direct acting chemical carcinogens.[4] These transforming genes are collectively called oncogenes and their study has elucidated the process of cellular transformation and may ultimately reveal the intricate processes by which cells communicate, grow, divide, and differentiate.

The preceding two chapters describe the advances in technologies that researchers are using to unravel the mysteries of genome order and gene regulation. They provide a useful introduction to this chapter because the genes and their products described herein appear to regulate, at some level, the biological processes of cell division and differentiation. The emerging description of how these biological processes are regulated has far-reaching implications.

All biological systems must faithfully duplicate genetic information and partition it equally among progeny, whether the process is somatic or germ cell division in higher organisms or virus replication in host cells (*i.e.*, amplification and packaging of viral genomes into virions) (Fig. 4-1). These processes are not perfect; errors (mutations) do occur. Such mutations can alter normal physiologic processes, and, indeed, the frequency of chromosomal abnormalities in cancer cells[5] is almost certainly the result of interference with the normal regulation of DNA duplication and chromosome partitioning.

In this chapter we describe oncogenes and their normally functioning cellular counterparts termed proto-oncogenes. Proto-oncogene products are important regulators of biological processes. They are localized in different cell compartments, are expressed at different stages of the cell cycle, and appear to be involved in the cascade of events that serve to maintain the ordered procession through the cell cycle (Fig. 4-2). The cell cycle is regulated by external mitogens (growth factors, peptide and steroid hormones, and lymphokines [Fig. 4-3]) which bind to their specific cell receptors (for example, the insulin, platelet-derived growth factor and epidermal growth factors bind to members of the tyrosine kinase family of growth factor receptors, as shown in Fig. 4-2B.) This activates a process termed signal transduction whereby specific signals are transmitted throughout the cell to the nucleus. The process is also mediated by nonintegral membrane associated proteins belonging to the tyrosine kinase and *ras* gene families (Figs. 4-2C and 4-2D). Signals

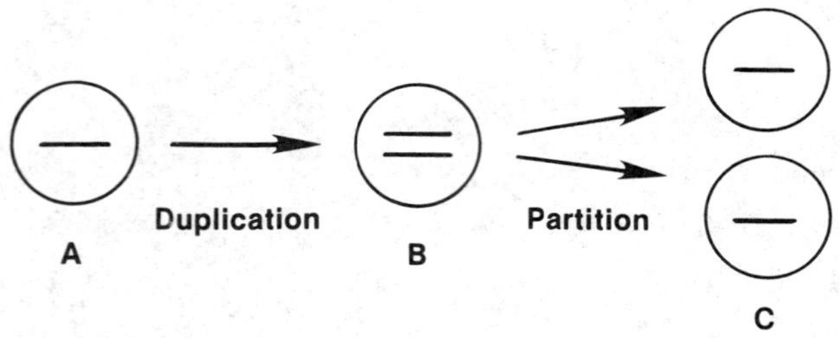

FIG. 4-1. Schematic representation of the process of duplication of genetic information and its partitioning to progeny cells.

generated by mitogenic stimulation can lead to the expression of specific genes coding for proteins localized to the nucleus (Figs. 4-2E and 4-3). Certain members of the oncogene nuclear protein products have been shown to be trans-activators of specific RNA transcripts.

Mutations that alter levels of gene expression or alter the form of the gene products in this pathway have been shown to activate their oncogenic potential (Table 4-1). Indeed, the discovery and study of oncogenes has provided the common link between, for example, a growth factor gene–like platelet derived growth factor (PDGF) and nuclear protein proto-oncogenes, c-*fos* and c-*myc* (see Fig. 4-2).[6,7] In the cancer cell, this ordered procession (see Fig. 4-2) is partially lost when more than one of these pathway members (see Fig. 4-3) are activated as oncogenes. For example, instead of maintaining conditional regulation at a specific stage in the cell cycle, the oncogene may provide a constitutive signal that perhaps initiates a cascade of subordinate functions out of sync with the normal events.

The term proto-oncogene is misleading because it wrongly implies that these genes latently reside in the genome for the sole purpose of expressing the neoplastic phenotype, when in fact they are essential to the normal biological processes such as cell division. The risk of errors (*e.g.*, chromosomal translocations) which activate their oncogenic potential suggests that numerous safeguards preventing facile activation of oncogenes must exist in the animal genome. The presence of these safeguards is certainly related to the multiple

FIG. 4-2. Stimulation of quiescent murine fibroblasts to enter the G1 phase of growth by addition of platelet-derived growth factor (PDGF) or fibroblast growth factor (FGF). A transient increase in the expression of both c-*fos* and c-*myc* follows PDGF or FGF stimulation or treatment of cells with phorbol ester TPA plus a calcium ionophore. Cells rendered competent require epidermal growth factor and insulin-like growth factors to progress through DNA synthesis and the cell cycle.

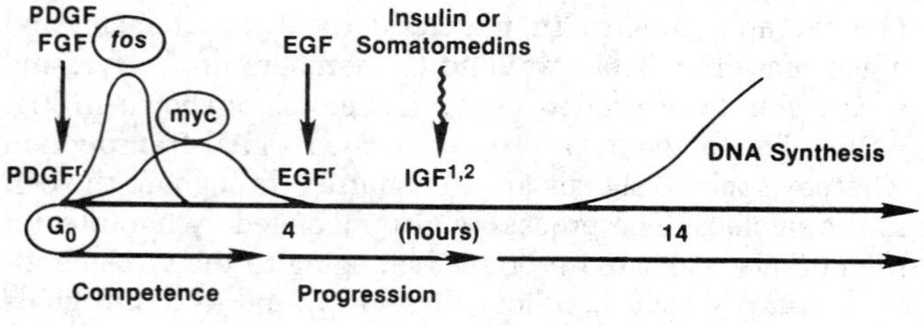

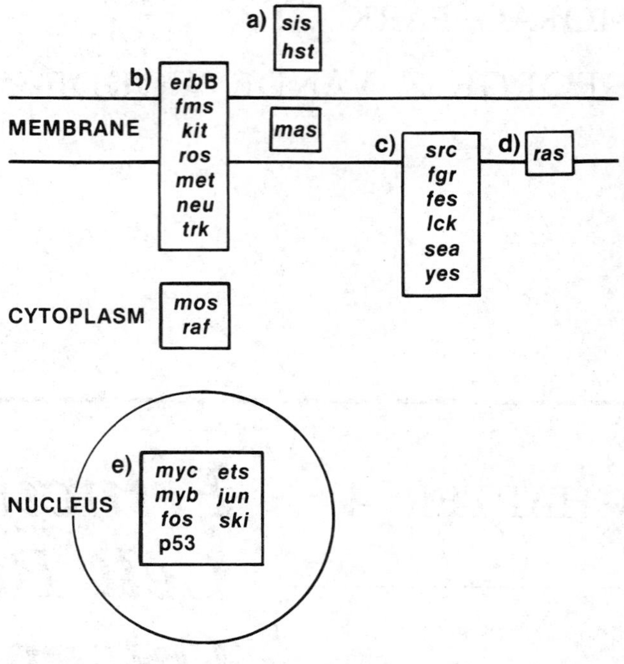

FIG. 4-3. Schematic presentation of the cellular compartments where oncogene or proto-oncogene products are localized. The growth factors (external mitogenic signals) *(a)*, transmembrane tyrosine kinase growth factor receptor membranes *(b)*, nonintegral membrane associated proteins of the *src* gene family *(c)*, and *ras* gene family *(d)* plus oncogenes localized in the nucleus *(e)*.

events (multiple genetic alterations or oncogene activation events occurring in a single cell)[2] believed to occur prior to the onset of neoplastic transformation and tumor progression.

IDENTIFICATION OF ONCOGENES

For a major portion of this century, there was considerable controversy over whether viruses or environmental insults to normal cell genes cause cancer.[8–13] The first oncogenes were identified in studies of cancer-causing retroviruses. An important step in the retrovirus infection cycle is the stable integration of the provirus into the host chromosome.[14,15] By determining the DNA sequence of the integrated retrovirus provirus, researchers learned that these proviruses resemble transposons, or movable genetic elements, which have been studied widely in prokaryotes and lower eukaryotes.[16] These genetic elements move to alternate positions in the chromosomes of a cell. They were first characterized[17] and subsequently studied because of their ability to alter or modify expression of the genetic loci into which they insert.[18] Studies showed that provirus insertion also modifies expression of the region of the host chromosome into which it inserts; when the locus is a proto-oncogene, the provirus insertion can result in tumorigenesis.[19,20] Oncogenes have been isolated also in DNA tumor viruses and in various tumor cells associated with chromosomal breakpoints.

TABLE 4-1. Oncogenes: Source and Properties

Reference	RNA Tumor Virus	Oncogene	Alternative Method of Identification	Species of Origin	Source	Properties
src Family						*Proto-oncogene*
Tyrosine Kinases: Integral Membrane						characteristic of growth factor receptors
351	Susan McDonough feline sarcoma virus	v-*fms*		Cat	Sarcoma	From CSF-1 receptor
351	Avian erythroblastosis virus	v-*erb*B		Chicken	Sarcoma/ erythroblastosis	From EGF-receptor
352	HZ4 feline sarcoma virus	v-*kit*		Cat	Sarcoma	
351	UR2 avian sarcoma virus	v-*ros*		Chicken	Sarcoma	
57		*neu*	DNA transfection	Rat	Neuroblastoma	
60		*met*	DNA transfection	Human	MNNG-treated human osteocarcinoma cell line	
61		*trk*	DNA transfection	Human	Colon carcinoma	
Tyrosine Kinases: Membrane Associated						
351	Rous sarcoma virus	v-*src*		Chicken	Sarcoma	
351	Yamaguchi-79 sarcoma virus	v-*yes*		Chicken	Sarcoma	
351	Gardner-Rasheed feline sarcoma virus	v-*fqr*		Cat	Sarcoma	
351	Fujinami sarcoma virus	v-*fps*		Chicken	Sarcoma	
351	Snyder-Theilen feline sarcoma virus	v-*fes*		Cat	Sarcoma	
351	Abelson murine leukemia virus	v-*abl*		Mouse	Leukemia	
351	Hardy Zuckerman 2 feline sarcoma virus	v-*abl*		Cat	Sarcoma	
Serine/Threonine Kinases						
351	Moloney murine sarcoma virus	v-*mos*		Mouse	Sarcoma	
351	3611 murine sarcoma virus	*raf*		Mouse	Sarcoma	
Growth Factor Families						
353	Simian sarcoma virus	v-*sis*		Woolly monkey	Glioma/ fibrosarcoma	B chain PDGF
87		*int*-2	Proviral insertion	Mouse	Mammary carcinoma	Member of FGF family
63		KS3	DNA transfection	Human	Kaposi's sarcoma	Member of FGF family
62		*hst*	DNA transfection	Human	Stomach carcinoma	Member of FGF family
ras Family						
42	Harvey murine sarcoma virus	v-H-*ras*		Rat	Erythroleukemia	GTP binding/ GTPase
43	Kirsten murine sarcoma virus	v-K-*ras*		Rat	Sarcoma	GTP binding/GTPase
47		N-*ras*	DNA transfection	Human DNA	Various	GTP binding/GTPase
Nuclear protein family						
351	Myelocyto-matosis-29 virus	v-*myc*		Chicken	Carcinoma myelocytomtosis	Binds DNA
175		N-*myc*	Gene amplification	Human	Neuroblastoma	?

(continued)

TABLE 4-1. Oncogenes: Source and Properties *(Continued)*

Reference	*RNA Tumor Virus*	*Oncogene*	*Alternative Method of Identification*	*Species of Origin*	*Source*	*Properties*
Nuclear protein family (continued)						
324		L-*myc*	Gene amplification	Human	Small cell lung carcinoma	?
117	Avian myeloblastosis virus	v-*myb*		Chicken	Myeloblastosis	Binds DNA
351	FBJ murine sarcoma virus	v-*fos*		Mouse	Osteosarcoma	Binds DNA
351	Sloan-Kettering avian sarcoma virus	v-*ski*		Chicken	Carcinoma	?
278		v-*jun*		Chicken		Binds DNA
194		P53		Mouse/human	Expressed at high levels in transformed cells	Binds SV40 large T/and adenovirus E1B
Others						
351	Reticulo-endotheliosis virus, strain T	v-*rel*		Turkey	Lymphatic leukemia	
351	E26 avian leukemia virus	v-*ets*		Chicken		
351	Avian erythroblastosis virus	v-*erb*A		Chicken	Erythroblastosis	Derived from steroid receptor for triiodothyronine
33		*mas*	DNA transfection	Human	Mammary carcinoma	Transmembrane protein
118		*int*-1	Proviral insertion	Mouse	Mammary carcinoma	

RETROVIRUSES AND ONCOGENES

Acute transforming retroviruses have been isolated from many avian and mammalian sources and can be divided into two classes based on the latency period between infection and the appearance of a tumor. Leukemia or leukosis viruses[16] produce leukemia or lymphoma in animals after long latent periods (more than 3 months). Acute transforming retroviruses can produce tumors in newborn animals in less than 2 weeks; this characteristic led early investigators to believe that they had identified agents responsible for neoplastic transformation. The difference between the latent periods for disease caused by these two virus classes can be traced to differences in their genetic content. The acute transforming retroviruses possess nucleic acid sequences acquired (transduced) from the genetic information of the host cell, and these gene sequences are responsible for the rapid transforming activity (Fig. 4-4). These host-derived genes are called viral oncogenes (v-*onc*), and many have been identified in acute transforming retroviruses (see Table 4-1). In contrast, the leukemia retroviruses do not contain transduced host oncogenes (see Fig. 4-4). The long latent period for disease caused by these retroviruses is partially the result of the low probability that proviruses will integrate into or adjacent to a host cellular oncogene. The integration activates oncogene expression in the same way as does an acute transforming retrovirus.

Because retroviruses can integrate at many loci in the host chromosome, their insertions can interrupt various normal genetic functions. Provirus insertion can cause mutations by interrupting coding sequences or regulatory elements. Expression of adjacent host genes also can be activated or elevated because of enhancer activity (see Chap. 3) of the viral transcription control element or long terminal repeat (LTR) (Fig. 4-5). When integration occurs in a proto-oncogene locus, elevated or unregulated expression of this gene can result in tumor formation. Figure 4-5 shows several models for retroviral activation of oncogene expression and presents a model for provirus acquisition or transduction of a cellular oncogene. There is little question that oncogenes are acquired by retroviruses from the normal genome of the cell.[16]

FIG. 4-4. Schematic representation of the general structure of leukemia retroviral and acute transforming retroviral genomes.

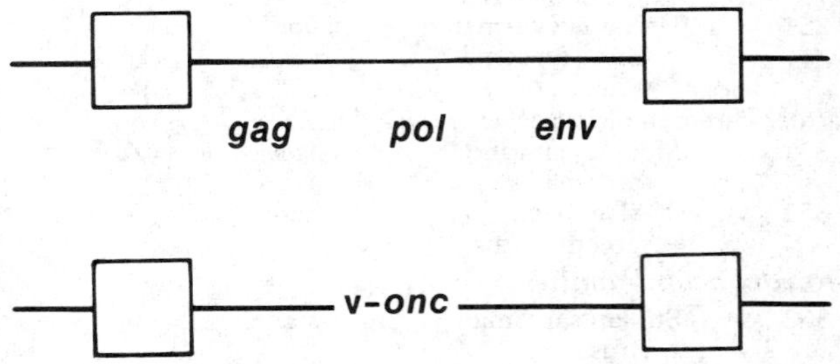

In the first model (Fig. 4-5, line I), a retrovirus provirus integrates adjacent to a cellular oncogene. In the second model, the transformation/transduction model (Fig. 4-5,

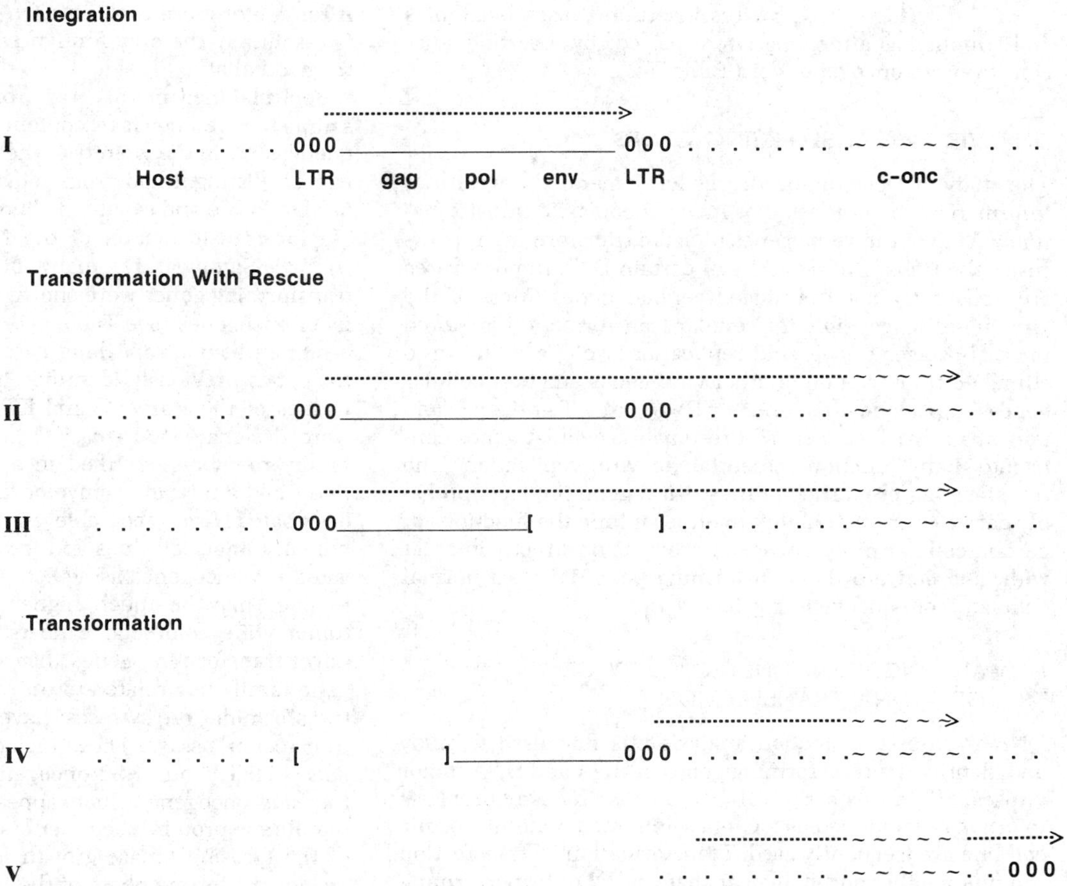

FIG. 4-5. Oncogene activation by provirus insertion. The retrovirus provirus inserts randomly into host chromosomal DNA. If integration occurs adjacent to a cellular oncogene (c-*onc*) and if sufficient levels of RNA are expressed, transformation is possible (lines II and III). However, most LTR-mediated provirus transcripts occur between the LTR elements (line II), and few transcripts proceed into the c-*onc* locus. A DNA rearrangement that results in the loss of the downstream LTR (line III) allows transcription into the c-*onc* locus. With either model the elevated or unregulated LTR-promoted c-*onc* transcription can result in transformation if the c-*onc* portion of the transcript is in the proper configuration to be translated into protein. Neither arrangement (line II or III) may permit transcription of a translatable c-*onc* mRNA, but both could result in transduction of the c-*onc* into a retroviral genome. The viral portion of the transcript can provide the necessary sequences for the entire fused viral c-*onc* transcript to be packaged into virions. As part of the viral genome, the transcript is subject to an enormous increase in genetic rearrangements, and events that generate efficient expression of a c-*onc* transforming product (now as v-*onc*) can result in the generation of an acute transforming retrovirus. The transduced c-*onc* becomes the transforming element or v-*onc* (see Table 4-1). Transformation by provirus insertion is observed more frequently, as shown in lines IV and V with either upstream or downstream insertions.

line II), provirus expression extends beyond the downstream LTR into the cellular oncogene locus. However, most of the transcripts terminate within this LTR element, and it is unlikely that this level of expression would lead to transformation. In the third model (Figure 4-5, line III), the downstream LTR sequences of the provirus have been lost and now proviral transcripts originating in the upstream LTR proceed through into the oncogene locus. This rearrangement can result in a high level of expression of the cellular oncogene and could lead to transformation. These models illustrate the mechanism by which cellular oncogenes can be transduced by retroviruses; c-*onc*-containing transcripts (Fig. 4-5, lines II and III) can be encapsidated into virions and acquired as part of the viral genome. The event is extremely rare.

The transformation models (Fig. 4-5, lines IV and V) show that activation of expression can occur with an LTR either upstream or downstream to the oncogene.[19–22] The activations are, in large part, the result of the transcription enhancer effect which causes unregulated expression of the oncogene from its own promoter (see Chap. 3).

Many novel oncogenes have been discovered on the basis

of the knowledge that provirus insertion causes leukemias and lymphomas after long latent periods by inserting adjacent to proto-oncogene loci (Table 4-2).

DNA VIRUS TRANSFORMING GENES

The study of DNA tumor viruses has generated a wealth of information about genes that induce neoplastic transformation.[23] Unlike the v-*onc* genes of acute transforming retroviruses, the transforming genes of certain DNA tumor viruses are apparently not transduced cellular genes. Most of the viral genes responsible for cellular transformation, required for early stages of the viral replication cycle, are known to stimulate transcription of other viral genes and host cellular genes (*e.g.,* adenovirus E1A,[24,25] SV40 large T antigen,[26] and polyoma large T antigen.)[27] Presumably, cellular genes contribute many functions essential for viral replication. The transforming properties of these viral gene products probably derive from their ability to either mimic the functions of certain cellular proto-oncogene products or directly interact with, and activate the transforming potential of, a normal cellular proto-oncogene product.

HUMAN ONCOGENES DETECTED BY GENE TRANSFER/DNA TRANSFECTION

DNA transfer/transfection analysis was first used to study and identify the transforming genes of RNA and DNA tumor viruses.[28,29] In this assay, NIH/3T3 cells (mouse fibroblasts in origin) maintained as a contact-inhibited nontumorigenic cell line are frequently used. Transformation by transfection is monitored by morphological changes[30,31] or by performing tumorigenesis assays in nude mice[32,33] (Fig. 4-6A and B). Genomic DNA from mouse and human chemically induced or naturally occurring tumor cell lines were shown to give rise to foci of morphologically altered cells when transfected onto nontransformed mouse cell monolayers.[34,35] DNA from the newly transformed mouse cells can be extracted and cycled again onto nontransformed mouse cell monolayers. After two or more cycles of DNA transfection, the oncogene is essentially the only foreign DNA detectable in the transformed cells.

Foci obtained in this way from human tumor cell DNA samples were shown to contain human repetitive DNA sequences[36,37] in the vicinity of the oncogene. These sequences can be distinguished from mouse sequences[38] and can be used to locate and isolate the human DNA segment responsible for transformation of the NIH/3T3 cells (see Fig. 4-6).[39–41] Significantly, many of the transfectable human transforming genes were shown to be related to the *ras* family of oncogenes (see Table 4-1). The transforming genes of a human bladder and lung carcinoma were homologous to *ras* genes previously identified in acute transforming retroviruses of the Harvey[42] and Kirsten[43] sarcoma viruses and were designated c-H-*ras*[44–46] and c-K-*ras*.[44–46] A *ras* gene family member identified in a human neuroblastoma cell line[47] and a human promyelocytic leukemia cell line[48] were designated N-*ras* (see Table 4-1).[49–51] Approximately 15% of human tumor cell lines and fresh tumor biopsies have activated *ras* oncogenes as detected by this assay,[52–54] and this number may be much higher in certain specific human tumors like colorectal cancers.[55,56] A growing number of novel transforming genes that are not members of the *ras* gene family nor related to the viral oncogenes of the acute transforming retroviruses have been identified by DNA transfection assays. These include the *neu*,[57–59] *met*,[60] *trk*,[61] *mas*,[33] HST,[62] and KS3 oncogenes.[63] With the exception of the *mas* oncogene which appears to be a unique integral membrane protein, the other oncogenes are either members of the tyrosine kinase growth factor receptor family (*neu*, *met*, or *trk*) or members of the fibroblast growth factor family (FGF), (HST, KS3).

ONCOGENES IDENTIFIED BY CHROMOSOME ABNORMALITIES

Oncogenes have been associated with the nonrandom chromosomal abnormalities identified by cytogeneticists. Micro-

TABLE 4-2. Cellular Genes Activated by Insertional Mutagenesis

Gene	*Virus*	*Disease*	*Animal*	*Reference*
c-myc	ALV, CSV, REV	Bursal lymphoma	Chicken	310,311
	MLV	T cell lymphoma	Mouse	
	FeLV	T cell lymphoma	Cat	312
c-*erb*B	ALV	Erythroleukemia	Chicken	116
c-*myb*	MLV	Lymphosarcoma	Mouse	313
c-H-*ras*	MAV	Nephroblastoma	Chicken	314
c-*mos*	IAP	Plasmacytoma cell line	Mouse	315
IL-2	GaLV	T cell lymphoma cell line	Ape	124
IL-3	IAP	Myelomonocytic leukemia	Mouse	125
int-1	MMTV	Mammary carcinoma	Mouse	118
int-2	MMTV	Mammary carcinoma	Mouse	87
Pim-1	M-MLV	T-cell lymphoma	Mouse	316
tck(1skT)	M-MLV	Thymoma cell line	Mouse	317
pvt(mis-1)	M-MLV	T or B cell lymphoma	Mouse/rat	318,319
Mlvi-1	M-MLV	T cell lymphoma	Rat	320
Mlvi-2	M-MLV	T cell lymphoma	Rat	320
Mlvi-3	M-MLV	T cell lymphoma	Rat	320
Evi-1	MCF-MLV	Myeloid lymphoma	Mouse	321
Evi-2	MCF-MLV	Myeloid lymphoma	Mouse	322

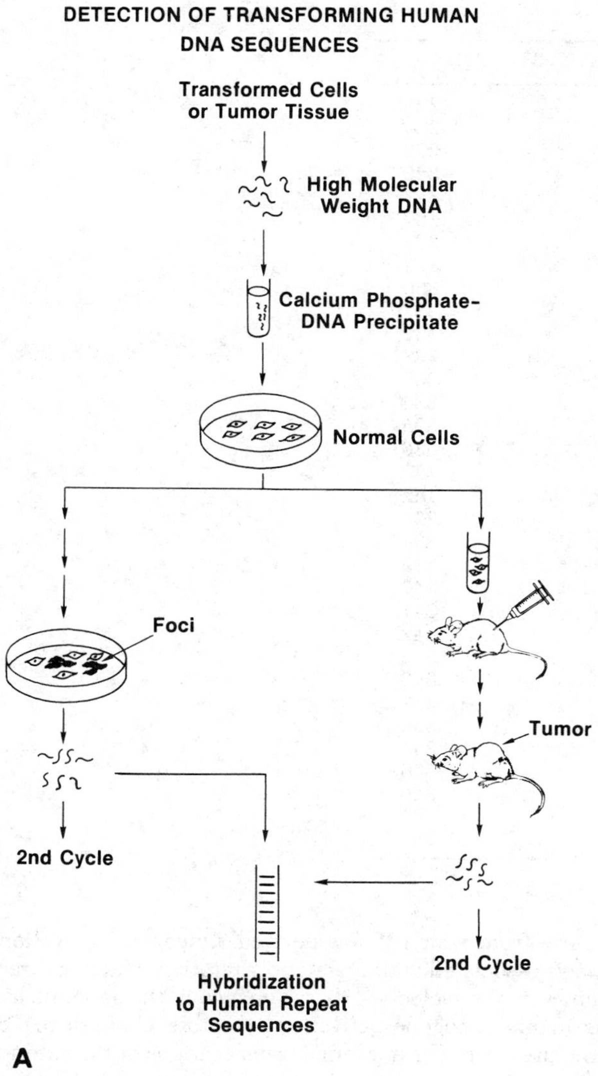

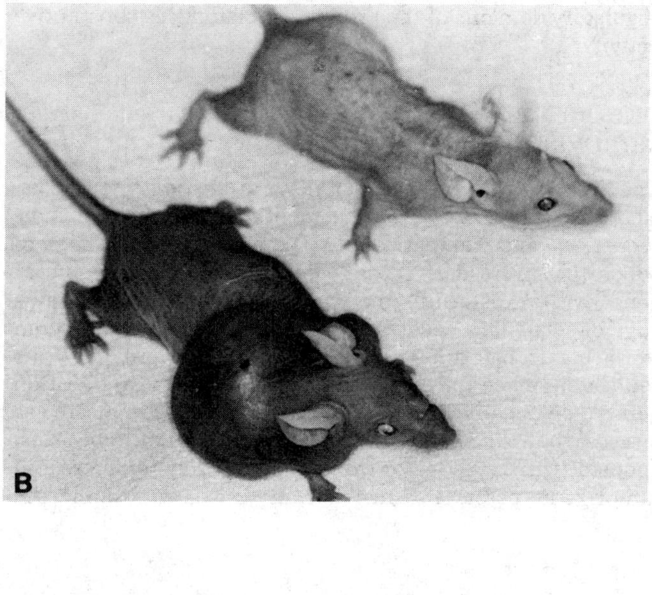

scopic structural changes of chromosomes, such as nonrandom chromosomal translocations and homogeneously staining regions (HSR), are associated with mammalian and human tumors.[64–67] This association was the basis for speculation that the chromosome abnormalities were activating oncogenes by mechanisms similar to provirus activation in animal model systems.[65,66] The chromosomal localization of cellular proto-oncogenes determined by in situ hybridization (Table 4-3) revealed proto-oncogenes at or near chromosomal translocation breakpoints.[67,68] Nonrandom chromosomal translocations are consistently associated with some types of leukemias and myelodysplasias.[69,70] In many cases the DNA breakpoints involved in the translocation have been isolated. Oncogenes have been identified at translocation breakpoints in Burkitt's lymphoma (c-*myc*)[71] and chronic myelogenous leukemia *(bcr-abl)*.[72] Possible oncogenic loci have been identified by isolating the DNA segments associated with the translocation breakpoints in adult B cell lymphomas, follicular lymphomas, and diffuse histiocytic leukemias (*bcl*I and *bcl*II.)[73,74]

Other oncogenes have been identified in chromosomal abnormalities associated with amplification of specific DNA segments. In human neuroblastomas, up to a 700-fold amplification of a sequence with limited homology to c-*myc*, termed N-*myc*, has been found in homogeneously staining regions of the tumor cells.[75,76]

The loss of DNA from certain regions of chromosomes, thought to unmask recessive mutations present in the remaining allele and often referred to as recessive oncogenes, have been associated with several tumors, especially childhood tumors such as retinoblastoma and Wilms'.[77–79] These chromosomal abnormalities involve deletions of various lengths in portions of chromosomes in different patients; however, analysis of the chromosomes reveals common deleted regions. Patients with retinoblastoma have deletions in chromosome 13 band ql4[80] and patients with Wilms' tumor have deletions in chromosome 11 band p13.[81] Recently, a candidate retinoblastoma gene was isolated[82,83] but its function in normal or tumor cells is not yet known.

GROWTH FACTORS AND GROWTH FACTOR RECEPTORS THAT ARE ONCOGENES

The discovery that certain oncogenes (v-*sis* and v-*erb*B) were homologs of a growth factor PDGF[84,85] and growth factor receptor (epidermal growth factor receptor [EGFR])[86] pro-

FIG. 4-6. **A**. DNA transfection. The DNA transfection schemes show the calcium phosphate-dependent protocols used for detecting transforming genes in transformed cells and tumors. The DNA from either primary foci or tumors is recycled in the transfection assay to facilitate the loss of extraneous nontransforming sequences that are carried with the transforming gene in the first transfection. After several cycles, the major portion of the foreign DNA in the focus or tumor is responsible for the transforming activity and can be isolated by conventional recombinant DNA technology. **B**. Nude mouse tumor assay. Both animals received subcutaneous injections of 3×10^6 NIH 3T3 cells that had been transfected 4 days earlier with either normal human DNA or DNA from a pancreatic-carcinoma–derived cell line. Tumor appearance was first noted 6 weeks after the cells had been injected.

TABLE 4-3. Chromosomal Location of Oncogenes

Chromosome	*Location*	*Proto-Oncogene*	*Reference*
1	1p36	*fgr*	323
1	1p32	L-*myc*	324
1	1p11-13	N-*ras*	325
1	1q22-qter	*ski*	326
1	1q32	*trk*	327
2	2p23-24	N-*myc*	157
2	2p11-12	*rel*	328
3	3p25	*raf*	329
5	5q34	*fms*	330
6	6p21	*pim*-1	331
6	6q21-22	*ros*	332
6	6q22-24	*myb*	333
6	6q24-27	*mas*	332
7	7p11-13	*erb*B	334
7	7q31	*met*	335
8	8q22	*mos*	336
8	8q24	*myc*	127
9	9q34.1	*abl*	142
11	11p14.1	H-*ras*	337
11	11q13	*int*-2	338
11	11q23-24	*ets*-1	339
12	12p12.1	K-*ras*	340
12	12pter-q14	*int*-1	341
14	14q21-31	*fos*	342
15	15q26.1	*fes*	333
17	17p23	p53	343
17	17q12-22	*neu*	59
17	17q21-22	*erb*A	334
18	18q21.3	*yes*	344
20	20q12-13	src	345
21	21q22	*ets*-2	346
22	22q11	*bcr*	72
22	22q13.1	*sis*	347

vided a direct link with genes responsible for regulating cell division and differentiation, but raised the question whether other members of these families have oncogenic potential. The list has recently expanded to include other growth factors such as members of the fibroblast growth factor family (HST,[62] *int*-2[87] and KS3[63]) a known hematopoietic growth factor receptor (colony-stimulating factor [CSF-1], v-*fms*,[88] and v-*erb*A, the receptor for a thyroid hormone.[89,90] Several oncogenes have been identified that resemble tyrosine kinase growth factor receptor family members (*neu*,[57] *met*,[60] and *trk*[61]), but no candidate ligands are yet known for their products. The increasing number of correlations between oncogenes and growth factors raises the interesting consideration that many growth factors and cell receptors can, under the appropriate circumstances, behave as oncogenes. In the past, oncogenes were identified by a few methods and assays. As their normal functions are revealed, new and better approaches will be developed for their identification; already, it is becoming more common to identify possible oncogenes from structural analyses of genes (Fig. 4-7).

MECHANISMS OF ONCOGENE ACTIVATION

Mechanisms of oncogene activation are best studied by directly comparing the activated oncogene with the proto-oncogene from which it was derived. Oncogene activation is always associated with a genetic alteration which can range from a single nucleotide (base) change in the genomic locus (as in *ras* oncogene activation) to gross changes in DNA structure (as in chromosomal translocations or the extensive changes observed in transduced viral oncogenes).[91,92] In general, however, the changes that activate proto-oncogenes result from an unregulated increase or unscheduled expression of the normal product, or from mutations or deletions in regulatory domains of the protein which induces constitutive activity.

ONCOGENES IN ACUTE TRANSFORMING RETROVIRUSES

The acute transforming retroviruses are, in many respects, laboratory curiosities, but the identification of their v-*onc* sequences and comparison to the proto-oncogenes from which they were derived have provided a unique source of genes with transforming potential and fundamental knowledge of sequences necessary for their activation. Most often the acute transforming retroviruses are impaired in virus replication since they lack a full complement of replication genes (see Fig. 4-4). However, because they are replicated as viruses, they are subject to a very high mutation rate. This, coupled with investigator-mediated selection for increased tumorigenic potential, can result in viruses with numerous

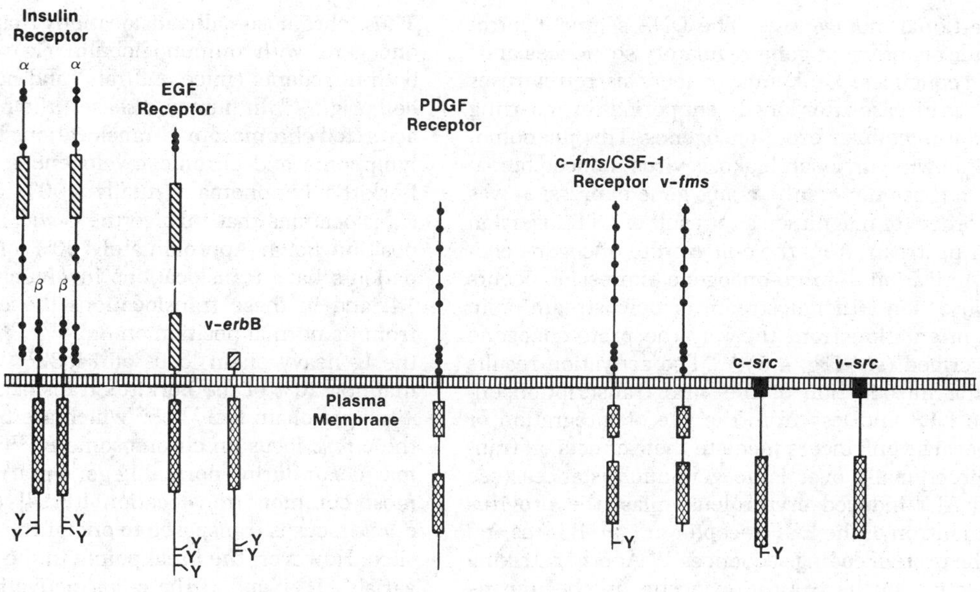

FIG. 4-7. Schematic comparison of structural features of cell surface receptors and tyrosine kinase oncogene products. Regions of high cysteine concentration are shown as hatched boxes and single cysteine residues are filled circles. The tyrosine kinase domain is represented as cross-hatched boxes and the position of carboxy terminal tyrosine residues is shown as Y. The deletions that activate v-*erb*B, v-*fms*, and v-*src* are illustrated. EGF, epidermal growth factor; PDGF, platelet derived growth factor; CSF-1, mononuclear phagocyte colony stimulating factor.

changes in v-*onc* sequences when compared with the proto-oncogene. Thus, mutations can be identified that increase tumorigenic potential. Such mutations include multiple point mutations, deleted upstream or downstream exons, and transcriptional and posttranscriptional regulatory elements. For example, a 3′ noncoding region sequence that normally inhibits c-*fos* expression posttranscriptionally allows v-*fos* to be produced at high levels.[93,94] Many v-*onc* genes are expressed as fusion gene products with viral genes (*gag* and *env*) and at high levels under constitutive control of the retroviral LTR.[95] *gag*- or *env-onc* fusion products may serve to contribute to transforming potential by misdirecting an oncogene product to an improper cellular location. Moreover, the target cell specificity of the retrovirus can result in the expression of the oncogene in an inappropriate cell type. For instance, the presence of *gag* sequences is required for v-*abl* transformation of lymphoid cells.[96] The v-*ras* genes contain point mutations in the same position as in activated c-*ras* genes in human tumors,[97] whereas the v-*src* gene in Rous sarcoma virus contains both point mutations and a C-terminal deletion.[98] The latter deletion has been shown to be essential for activating the *src* proto-oncogene.

The products of the cellular and viral *src* genes possess intrinsic protein tyrosine kinase activity.[99] The tyrosine residue deleted in the v-*src* product (tyr 527)[100,101] may be required for down-regulating the intrinsic *src* kinase activity.[100,102] Other nonintegral tyrosine kinase genes in the *src* family (*yes, fgr, fps, fms*) also have tyrosine residues in their C-terminal amino acid sequences[99] and activated *yes, fgr,* and *fms* oncogenes lack the C-terminal region containing a tyrosine codon thought to be equivalent in function to the tyrosine 527 in c-*src*.[88,103–106] However, the v-*erb* oncogene, a modified form of the EGF receptor of avian erythroblastosis virus (AEV), in addition to having a C-terminal deletion, has a deletion in its N-terminal ligand-binding domain[107] and is presumed to function as a constitutively activated growth factor receptor.[99,108,109] Thus, as with other members of the *src* family, the truncation of the C terminus may activate the gene. However, a hybrid protein expressed from the EGF receptor locus activated by the insertion of ALV contains the appropriate C-terminal amino acids and, in this case, the deletion of the ligand-binding domain is sufficient for activation.[110] Similarly, the v-*kit* oncogene (see Table 4-1) has both N-terminal and C-terminal deletions and is derived from an oncogene related to the PDGF receptor.[111] However, two oncogenes identified by the DNA transfection assay, *met*[112,113] and *trk*[61] (see Table 4-1), also putative tyrosine kinase receptor genes, appear to be activated by a DNA rearrangement that eliminates the putative ligand-binding domain and substitutes protein domains derived from other genes; this rearrangement may be essential for efficient transformation.[61,113]

ONCOGENE ACTIVATION BY INSERTIONAL MUTAGENESIS

Insertional mutagenesis is an alteration resulting from the insertion of foreign DNA sequences into a defined genetic locus. Provirus insertion or transposition of a movable genetic element that interrupts host genomic sequences are forms of insertional mutagenesis. The DNA segment introduced can alter or interrupt gene regulatory sequences and/or structural sequences. Leukemia or leukosis retroviruses cause neoplastic disease after long latent periods by inserting into or adjacent to cellular proto-oncogenes. This phenomenon was first shown with avian leukosis virus-induced bursal lymphomas. In these tumors the c-*myc* gene expression was elevated two orders of magnitude as a result of LTR insertion adjacent to or upstream from the c-*myc* proto-oncogene coding locus.[114] Activation of proto-oncogene expression occurs by provirus insertion either upstream or downstream or in the opposite orientation from the way the proto-oncogene locus is transcribed (see Fig. 4-5).[115] The activation results more from the introduction of the viral transcription enhancer in the LTR and less from the site of integration or orientation because enhancers mediate their effects on transcription bidirectionally over large genomic distances (see Chap. 3). In ALV-induced erythroleukemias, the provirus inserts into an intron of the EGF receptor or c-*erb*B locus and decapitates the protein coding sequences.[116] Another striking example of activation by truncation occurs in the murine leukemia virus-induced myeloid tumors. In these tumors the provirus insertion occurs in the N-terminal coding domain of the c-*myb* locus.[117]

Leukemia retroviruses can cause many different types of tumors by virtue of the cell types they infect, the genes they integrate adjacent to (and the genes' relevance to the growth properties of that particular cell type), and the influence of the cell-type on the transcriptional enhancement of the LTR. Studies analyzing these variables have identified many oncogenes (see Table 4-2). Specific examples are *int*-1 and *int*-2, which are activated in mouse mammary tumors by provirus insertion.[87,118] Sometimes proviruses are found adjacent to both *int*-1 and *int*-2 in the same tumor.[119] Many times the protein coding domain of oncogenes activated by insertional mutagenesis remain unaltered and in these instances, activation presumably occurs as a result of inappropriate levels of gene expression. *int*-1 and *int*-2 genes are normally only transiently expressed during embryogenesis[120,121] but integration of mouse mammary tumor virus provirus into mammary epithelial cells results in low levels of expression. Although the exact mechanism is unknown, expression of *int*-1 and *int*-2 appears to be required for the development of mammary tumors. Similarly, hematopoietic cell lines that grow in the absence of growth factors have been induced to make their own growth factors as a consequence of proviral insertions adjacent to lymphokine genes IL-2 and IL-3.[122,123] Other studies have shown that when IL-2 or IL-3 genes are introduced by recombinant DNA techniques into retrovirus vectors, the viruses generated render factor-dependent cell lines factor-independent and tumorigenic[124,125] through an autocrine stimulation mechanism.

ONCOGENE ACTIVATION BY CHROMOSOMAL (DNA) REARRANGEMENTS

Nonrandom chromosomal translocations in leukemias and lymphomas of human and animal origin provide some of the most compelling indirect evidence for implicating oncogenes in the formation and progression of neoplastic disease. Thus, chromosomal translocations that juxtapose the c-*myc* oncogene with immunoglobulin (Ig) sequences are found both in rodents (mice and rats) and humans in tumors of B cell origin.[126] In human diseases, the most extensively characterized chromosomal translocations have been in Burkitt's lymphoma and chronic myelogenous leukemia (CML). In Burkitt's lymphoma virtually 100% of the patients have translocations that involve the c-*myc* locus on chromosome position 8q24. Approximately 80% of Burkitt's lymphoma patients have translocations involving chromosomes 8 and 14, and in these translocations the c-*myc* locus is moved from its normal position on 8q24[127,128] to a position distal to the Ig heavy chain locus at 14q32[129] (Table 4-4). The remaining 20% of the Burkitt's translocations involve the κ or λ Ig light chain loci,[130–132] which are translocated distally to the c-*myc* locus on chromosome 8.[131,133] The translocations may occur during normal Ig gene rearrangement, and in the most common translocation [t8:14] (see Table 4-4), the c-*myc* locus is transposed to one of the Ig heavy chain switch sites. However, the breakpoints in the c-*myc* locus are quite variable.[134] None of the c-*myc* activations can be explained by a single model, although the rearranged c-*myc* gene appears to be expressed constitutively and several mechanisms have been proposed to account for this. First, translocation events appear to alter the first exon of the c-*myc* locus where cis-acting transcription regulatory sequences reside.[135–138] Quite strikingly, even when the translocation breakpoint is quite distant from the first exon, mutations are found in the same first exon cis-acting sequences.[138–140] In some instances, the translocation of the immunoglobulin enhancer cis-acting sequences into the vicinity of c-*myc* has been proposed as a transcriptional activation mechanism for c-*myc* expression.[139–141]

At least 95% of patients with CML possess a typical Philadelphia chromosome resulting from the translocation between chromosome 9 and 22 (9;22) (q34;q11).[167] In this translocation, the c-*abl* proto-oncogene (see Table 4-1) is translocated from chromosome 9 band q34 to chromosome 22 at band q11.[142,143] The breakpoints that occur in chromosome 22q11 are clustered within a 5-kb genomic region, and this region has been referred to as the breakpoint cluster region *(bcr)*. In contrast, the breakpoints in the c-*abl* locus on chromosome 9q34 differ considerably from patient to patient with estimated differences of greater than 100 kb. In spite of this, a transcription unit in the *bcr* locus[144] provides the promoter and 5′ end sequences that result in a fused 8.5-kb *bcr-abl* hybrid mRNA[145,146] encoding a novel fusion protein of 210 kilodaltons (kd)[147] (see Table 4-4). Thus, in this disease, DNA rearrangements in the *bcr* locus, the expression of the novel 8.5-kb *bcr-abl* mRNA, and the detection of the novel 210-kd *bcr-abl* protein are all diagnostic for the Philadelphia positive CML.[148] It is not understood how this rearrangement contributes to CML. The normal c-*abl* product is a member of the tyrosine kinase family and may be involved in signal transduction,[56] and it is possible that the *bcr* locus which appears to be expressed in many cell types provides a mechanism for expressing the *abl* tyrosine kinase gene in an unregulated fashion analogous to immunoglobulin rearrangement that results in an enhanced level of c-*myc* expression in Burkitt's lymphoma. However, the *bcr* locus

TABLE 4-4. Chromosomal Translocations in Human Malignancies

Gene Locus	*Human Neoplasm*	*Percentage of Tumors with Translocation or Gene Rearrangement*	*Chromosome Translocation*	*Reference*
c-*myc*	Burkitt's lymphoma	80	t(8;14)(q24;q32)	348
		15	t(8;22)(q34;q11)	349
		5	t(2;8)(q11;q24)	141
bcr-abl	Chronic myelogenous leukemia	90–95	t(9;22)(q34;q11)	144
	Acute lymphocytic leukemia	10–15	t(9;22)(q34;q11)	350
bcl-1	Chronic lymphocytic leukemia of B cell type	10–20	t(11;14)(q13;q32)	73
bcl-2	Follicular lymphoma	85–95	t(14;18)(q32;q21)	74

provides N-terminal sequences to the c-*abl* product; this could either alter protein function or direct the tyrosine kinase to a different cellular location.[149] The acute transforming retroviruses possessing the v-*abl* oncogene have been shown to render hematopoietic cells growth factor independent after infection.[150] Thus, the *bcr-abl* rearrangement may stimulate proliferation of certain hematopoietic cells and prevent terminal differentiation. The *bcr-abl* rearrangement may serve as a paradigm for how other tyrosine kinase gene family members, such as the tropomyosin-*trk* or *tpr-met* oncogenes, are activated.

Homogeneously staining chromosomal regions and double minute chromosomes are karyotypes frequently found in tumor cells and tumor cell lines. These atypical chromosome characteristics represent multiple (amplified) copies of a single gene-containing DNA segment, and cellular oncogenes have been found in multiple copies in cells showing this karyotype.[151,152] Even in the absence of these microscopic chromosomal changes, studies using nucleic acid hybridization have shown that cellular oncogenes can be amplified.[151] Gene amplification has been best characterized in studies on the development of cell resistance to cytotoxic drugs[153]; the mechanism of DNA amplification is poorly understood. However, during a single cell cycle, DNA replication must occur repeatedly in a segment of DNA 200 to 2000 kb in size.[154]

Several cellular oncogenes have been found amplified in human tumors (Table 4-5). The c-*myc* proto-oncogene locus is shown to be amplified in a promyelocytic leukemia both in the primary tumor as well as in the cell line HL-60 derived from the tumor.[155,156] Other oncogenes like c-*erb*B (EGFR), *neu* (HER-2), and c-*myc* family members have been shown to be amplified in specific tumor types (see Table 4-5) and presence of multiple copies have been associated with poor prognosis. Thus, the presence of multiple copies of N-*myc* (which was first identified as an amplified gene in human neuroblastoma[157]) has been shown to correlate with advanced stages of disease.[158] The presence of multiple copies of *myc* gene family members in small cell lung carcinoma is also associated with more malignant progression of the disease.[159] Thus the *myc* family members appear to be associated with the progression of neuroblastomas and small cell lung carcinomas, whereas the c-*erbB* or EGFR gene has been found amplified in glioblastomas and squamous carcinomas.[160,161] The human homolog of the *neu* gene, HER-2, is closely related to the EGF receptor or c-*erb*B gene and is often found amplified in adenocarcinomas and breast tumors.[162] Also, human mammary tumors that have amplified copies of the HER-2 gene are more advanced, are hormone-independent, and have a poor prognosis.[163,164] Tumors with amplified copies of oncogenes express high levels of the oncogene RNA, a finding consistent with experiments showing that overexpression of some of the oncogenes like c-*erb*B and *neu* in NIH/3T3 cells results in morphological transformation.[165,166]

ONCOGENE ACTIVATION BY POINT MUTATIONS

The c-H-*ras* oncogene isolated from a human bladder carcinoma cell line was the first oncogene shown to be activated in a human tumor cell line. This gene was activated by a single point mutation that resulted in a change from a glycine to a valine codon in the 12th amino acid position.[167–169] The *ras* oncogene has been identified in many animal and

TABLE 4-5. Cellular Oncogenes Amplified in Human Tumors

Tumor	*Oncogene*	*Amplification*	*Reference*
Small-cell lung cancer	c-*myc*	up to 80×	159
	N-*myc*	up to 50×	158
	L-*myc*	up to 20×	324
Neuroblastomas	N-*myc*	up to 250×	152
Glioblastomas	c-*erb*B(EGFR)	up to 50×	153
Mammary carcinoma	c-*erb*B2(HER2)	up to 30×	163,164

human tumor samples[54,96] (see Fig. 4-7). *ras* oncogenes in tumors have been shown to be activated by mutations in the 12th, 13th and the 59th to 61st codons.[96] In addition, studies have shown that mutations created in vitro by site-directed mutagenesis in codons 63, 116, and 119 can also activate *ras* as a transforming gene.[96] Although it is not completely clear how these point mutations or codon changes result in the *ras* protein activation. The normal gene product binds guanidine nucleotides and possesses GTPase activity[170] whereas mutant *ras* oncogene products have greatly reduced GTPase activity, suggesting that this dysfunction may be a factor.

Several studies have shown that *ras* genes are the target of chemical carcinogens in animal tumor model systems. Certain carcinogens cause G to T base transversions or G to A base transitions that are often observed in activated *ras* genes.[171,172] Thus, topical application of the carcinogen dimethylbenzanthracene (DMBA) followed by treatment with tumor promoters, results in benign skin papillomas that contain activated c-H-*ras* genes.[173] In addition, studies using a mammary carcinoma model system showed that treatment of newborn rats with a single dose of nitrosomethylurea (NMU) results in the development of mammary carcinomas 2 to 3 months after animals reach sexual maturity. Eighty-five percent of these tumors contain an activated c-H-*ras* oncogene with the same G to A base transition in the 12th *ras* codon.[174,175] In both of these animal model systems, the *ras* gene participates in a multistep process of carcinogenesis. In the latter case, c-H-*ras* activation must occur as an initiation step since NMU is only active for a few minutes after injection. Thus, although the *ras* gene is the target of the genotoxic chemical carcinogen, expression of the transformed phenotype requires additional steroid dependent promoter activity. Other studies show that *ras* activation can also play a role in tumor progression.[176] With the exception of the *neu* gene in rodents, the *ras* family represent the only known oncogenes thus far that can be activated by a single point mutation. This may explain the predominance of *ras* gene mutations found in animal and human cancers.

ONCOGENE/PROTO-ONCOGENE ACTIVITY

The products of oncogenes presumably display at least a subset of the activities of the proto-oncogene product. Therefore, the functional properties of the proto-oncogene product must be characterized in order to understand the role of an oncogene in tumorigenesis. As was mentioned earlier, proto-oncogenes appear to function in the biological processes of cell division and differentiation (see Figs. 4-2 and 4-3). Because these genes have been conserved in the evolutionary process, they have closely related counterparts in multicellular organisms. Thus, these biological processes can be studied in animal model systems and in genetically well-characterized organisms. Transgenic mouse strains have been developed in which oncogene transgenes have been introduced into the germline so that their in vivo roles in tumorigenesis can be studied. Other techniques are being applied as well and some of these techniques are discussed below.

EVOLUTIONARY CONSERVATION OF PROTO-ONCOGENES

The conservation of proto-oncogenes in different animal species can be studied with the use of nucleic acid hybridization techniques (see Chap. 2). The DNA sequences of certain proto-oncogenes are more highly conserved between species than the DNA sequences of others, a measure that must be related to their function. Some proto-oncogenes have been found in all multicellular organisms studied, indicating that their products have essential biological roles.[177] Of special interest are the proto-oncogene homologs found in organisms that are well suited for classic genetic studies, such as yeast or *Drosophila*. In these organisms, the phenotypic influence of mutated proto-oncogene homologs on cell division or differentiation and embryological development can be tested, and genes can be identified that suppress the mutant phenotype, thereby revealing other members of the biochemical pathway. The nucleotide sequences of most of the oncogenes listed in Table 4-1 have been determined, and in many cases, both their RNA and protein products have been characterized. They have also been compared to the nucleotide or predicted amino acid sequences of the host proto-oncogene from which they were derived and to the proto-oncogene homologs in other species, especially in humans. For instance, recently the *int*-1 oncogene was shown to be a developmentally regulated gene of *Drosophila*.[178] Studies of *ras* genes in yeast are increasing our understanding of what is apparently a highly conserved biochemical pathway of signal transduction.[179–187]

COOPERATING ONCOGENE ASSAY

Oncogenes can be divided into two complementation groups based on their activities in DNA transfection assays performed in rat embryo fibroblast cells (REF cells). Transforming genes of certain DNA tumor viruses display different biological activities in REF cells. REF cells normally undergo a finite number of passages in culture before they become senescent. One class of genes, adenovirus (Ad) E1A and polyoma (Py) large T antigen genes, rescue REF cells from senescence. Thus, the expression of the products of these two DNA tumor virus genes allows cells to be continuously maintained in culture (immortalized). A second class of genes, Ad E1B and Py middle T antigen genes, cause morphological transformation of the rescued cells and render them tumorigenic in nude mice.[188–190] Many of the oncogenes display one or the other of these phenotypes and can be assigned to two complementation groups. For example, foci of transformed cells appear when REF cells are transfected with both v-H-*ras* and v-*myc* oncogenes.[52,53,190,191] Moreover, members from one complementation group, whether a viral gene or an oncogene, can act synergistically with members of the second complementation group. Members of the oncogene group that rescues cells from senescence have products that are localized to the nucleus,[190–194] whereas the genes that morphologically transform the immortalized REF cells are membrane associated and contain members of the *ras* gene family and Py middle T antigen.[52,53,195]

NIH/3T3 cells are similar to REF cells immortalized by a member of the first complementation group. NIH/3T3 cells have been particularly useful for identifying genes that morphologically transform cells in DNA transfection assays. Many of the oncogenes are in the same complementation groups as genes from DNA tumor viruses, suggesting that they may transform cells through similar pathways. For example, the Ad E1A and Py large T antigen gene products bind DNA as shown for some oncogene products located in the nucleus (see Table 4-1) and the DNA tumor virus early genes have been shown to transactivate expression of cellular genes.[26,192] These viral genes are expressed early during DNA tumor virus replication before the onset of viral DNA synthesis. Thus these similarities indicate that the early virus genes may be to virus replication what c-*myc* is to cell cycle regulation and cell division (see Fig. 4-3). Another interesting correlation has been made among members of the second complementation group. The gene for Py middle T antigen is a membrane-associated phosphoprotein that forms a complex with the c-*src* protein.[196] In the complex, the kinase activity of the c-*src* protein is elevated to levels similar to those of the activated v-*src* product.[53,99,197] Considering the extraordinary differences between these biological systems, that is, between genes that function early during adenovirus or polyomavirus infection and cellular proto-oncogenes, it is striking that they can elicit similar phenotypes. The findings suggest that there are similar gene product requirements for the replication of cells and viruses.

ONCOGENES AND TRANSGENIC MICE

Transgenic mice provide a new and powerful model system for studying the role of oncogenes in tumor development. In this system the expression of foreign genes (transgenes) can be assessed in animals capable of producing normal physiologic responses. As described in Chapter 3, transgenes are introduced into the germ line of mice by microinjection of recombinant DNA molecules into the male pronucleus of fertilized eggs.[198] In this manner, oncogenes under transcriptional regulation of different promoter elements have been studied in transgenic mice.[198–201] A striking finding is that neoplasia or hyperplasia occurs only in clonal populations in specific tissues. For example, mice carrying a c-*myc* gene coupled with a mouse mammary tumor virus (MMTV) steroid-responsive LTR promoter develop mammary tumors and occasional B cell lymphomas[199] even though *myc* is expressed at high levels in other tissues. Similarly, mice carrying the v-H-*ras* gene with the same MMTV LTR promoter develop salivary gland tumors, mammary tumors, and display hyperplasia of the Harderian gland.[202] Long latent periods of 6 to 14 months are required for tumor development in mice bearing the MMTV LTR *myc* transgene, which clearly indicates that additional changes are required for tumor development.[203] The synergistic action of two oncogenes in vivo has also been tested by crossing the transgenic mouse strain containing the MMTV LTR *ras* gene with the strain possessing the MMTV LTR *myc* transgene.[202] Transgenic animals carrying both *myc* and *ras* have a higher incidence of tumors (*e.g.*, B cell malignancies were 10-fold higher) with a shorter latent period than found in mouse strains carrying either oncogene alone.[202] However, the tumors, were clonal, and most of the cells expressed both oncogenes without expressing a transformed phenotype.

The best evidence indicating that c-*myc*-Ig gene rearrangements act as an initiating event in B cell tumors (discussed earlier in Oncogene Activation by Chromosomal Rearrangements and Translocations) was obtained by generating transgenic mice containing a c-*myc* gene regulated by a lymphoid-specific heavy chain Ig enhancer.[204] The lymphoid cells of these animals expressed high levels of the *myc* gene regulated by the IgH enhancer and the animals developed lymphoid tumors. However, these tumors were rare and clonal, indicating that additional events are necessary to promote tumorigenesis. These experiments demonstrated, however, that this specific gene rearrangement predisposes the animal to B cell tumors and is indirect evidence supporting the role of similar Ig-c-*myc* rearrangements in Burkitt's lymphoma in mouse B cell tumors.

These studies fully support the model that tumorigenesis is the result of multiple events in the same cell. One possible explanation for the low incidence of neoplasia in the *myc*-Ig transgenic mice is that the oncogene may not have been expressed at a critical stage of development or differentiation. It also indicates that oncogenes, as transgenes, are not necessarily dominant transforming genes. It is possible, therefore, that they may require the concomitant loss or alteration of expression of the resident normal gene, which would occur at low frequency, for example, by somatic recombination events as has been described for the retinoblastoma gene.[79] These early transgenic mice experiments demonstrate the power of the technique for addressing specific questions in tumor development and progression.

PROPERTIES OF ONCOGENES/PROTO-ONCOGENES AND THEIR PRODUCTS

GROWTH FACTORS

Growth factors provide the mitogenic signal mediated through their respective receptors that results in the proliferation and/or differentiation of cells.[205,206] In tissue culture, they must be supplied to stimulate proliferation of cell growth and are essential for the propagation of normal, nontransformed cells in culture.[207] However, transformed cells show partial or complete relaxation of requirements for growth factors. Factor dependence is also abrogated by infecting cells with specific acute transforming retroviruses.[208] Thus, viral oncogene products can override factor dependency by perhaps mimicking the action of ligands, their receptors,[209] or some intermediate in the ordered procession of events that follows mitogenic stimulation.

The first correlation of an oncogene with a growth factor was revealed by computer-assisted comparisons showing that the amino acid sequence of the v-*sis* oncogene was highly related to the beta chain of PDGF.[209–211] PDGF is an important serum mitogen required for mesenchymal cell growth in culture.[212] Connective tissue tumors such as sarcomas and glioblastomas express the c-*sis* proto-oncogene, whereas their counterparts in normal tissue do not.[212] Presumably, the sarcoma and glial tumor cells synthesize the mitogen to which they respond. Many oncogenes have been shown to be identical to, or related to, polypeptide growth factors. *int*-2, activated by MMTV proviral insertion in mouse mammary carcinomas,[213,214] the KS3 oncogene identified in gene transfer experiments in genomic DNA from a Kaposi's sarcoma,[63] and HST, a transforming gene identified in a human stomach cancer by DNA transfection[62,215] are all members of the basic or acidic fibroblast growth factor family.[216] The human KS3 and HST oncogenes are identical, but distinct from the closely related mouse *int*-2 gene. *int*-2 expression is most abundant in primitive mouse endodermal cells. Its low level of expression activated by proviral insertion in mouse mammary tumors may serve, in an autocrine fashion, to stimulate inappropriate cell proliferation. The fibroblast growth factors exhibit angiogenic properties and are related polypeptide mitogens[217] apparently recognizing different cell-type receptors.

Tumor cells often express transforming growth factors and two, referred to as TGF-α and TGF-β are expressed by rodent cells transformed with acute transforming retroviruses.[218] TGF-α binds to the EGF receptor, and TGF-β binds to a unique cell receptor.[219] TGF-α is normally synthesized only during embryogenesis.[220] It is believed that the transforming growth factors function in an autocrine fashion to stimulate cell proliferation.[221]

TYROSINE PROTEIN KINASES

The tyrosine protein kinases can be subdivided into at least three families. The first is the transmembrane protein tyrosine kinase family to which the growth factor receptors belong. In addition to being homologous in a tyrosine-specific protein kinase domain, these receptor-related molecules traverse the membrane once and have extracellular ligand-binding domains (see Fig. 4-7). It was early shown that the v-*erb*B oncogene product (see Table 4-1) is a truncated version of the EGF receptor.[222-224] More recently, the v-*fms* oncogene has been shown to be the activated form of the macrophage colony-stimulating factor receptor (CSF-1).[88] Other members of the tyrosine kinase growth factor receptor family are the *ros,*[225] *kit,*[111] *met,*[113] *trk,*[61] and *neu*[57,60] oncogenes (see Table 4-1 and Fig. 4-7). Both N-terminal and C-terminal rearrangements appear to activate the transforming potential of these transmembrane receptor tyrosine kinase family members. These alterations may remove down-modulating domains of the protein and result in the constitutive activation of what is normally a conditionally regulated enzyme activity.

The second family consists of a large number of nonintegral membrane-associated protein tyrosine kinases. The protein product of v-*src,* the prototype of this family, is associated with the plasma membrane but does not traverse the membrane. Other members of this family are *fes, abl, fgr,* and *yes* (see Table 4-1). All of these proto-oncogene products are homologous in the tyrosine kinase domains and each seems to have a myristylated N-terminal glycine residue.[226] The tyrosine kinase domain, as in the growth factor receptor tyrosine kinase family, is responsible for catalyzing the transfer of phosphate groups from ATP to tyrosine residues during autophosphorylation or transphosphorylation of target molecules. Tyrosine phosphorylation may regulate cell shape with cell growth[227] but it is a rare activity in normal cells and accounts for only a fraction of total protein phosphorylation.[228] Several cellular cytoskeletal proteins are known to be targets of *src* protein tyrosine kinase phosphorylation. Thus, v-*src* transforming activity may result from unregulated tyrosine phosphorylation of target molecules present in certain cell lineages.[227] Similarly, although the c-*abl* proto-oncogene is expressed in many tissues, it only appears to transform cells of the hematopoietic lineage,[229] suggesting that a special target or substrate may be present in these cell lineages.

The members of this subfamily appear to be expressed at high levels and in specific cell types. Thus, the *src* proto-oncogene product is expressed at low levels in most vertebrate cells but at high levels in platelets and certain neural cell types.[230,231] A similar expression pattern for c-*src* also is observed in *Drosophila* where the highest levels are detected in the eye and brain.[232] These findings suggest that *src* is coupled to a signal transduction system from a cell surface receptor or ion channel specific for neurons.

The third and least understood members of this subtype of proto-oncogenes are the members of the serine kinase family. Certain domains of the proteins of the *raf* and *mos* (see Table 4-1) are somewhat homologous to those of *src* kinase family members, but there is evidence that the phosphorylation specificity of these members is for serine and threonine.[233,234] Curiously, no tyrosine kinase genes have been identified in yeast although many proteins with serine/threonine kinase have. Studies of cell division cycle mutants (cdc) have shown that the serine/threonine kinases are required for movement through the specific point in the yeast cell cycle.[235,236] Several other protein kinase genes have been identified in yeast and some of these genes have also been found in mammals.[237-239] Strikingly, one of the genes isolated from humans complements a mutation in the homologous gene from the yeast strain *Schizosaccharomyces pombe* indicating that its function is highly conserved during evolution.[237] The study of the serine/threonine kinases in yeast may provide a model for understanding how the serine/threonine kinase genes, such as *mos* and *raf,* function in mammalian cells. Recently, the *mos* gene has been shown to be expressed in male and female germ cells in vertebrates during postmeiotic cell maturation, suggesting that *mos* gene product may be involved in reductive division.[240-242]

THE *RAS* FAMILY OF ONCOGENES AND PROTO-ONCOGENES

The *ras* gene family members are found in human cancers more often than any other oncogene[54] and therefore are among the most intensively studied oncogenes. These investigations have focused primarily on understanding the normal proto-oncogene function and comparing it to the oncogene product activated by point mutations. Because the *ras* gene is highly conserved,[177] members of this family have been studied in mammals, chickens,[243] fruit flies *(Drosophila melanogaster),*[177] slime molds,[244] and yeast.[245,246] Even in yeast, *ras* is significantly (65%) homologous with the *ras* family members found in humans.

In the mammalian genome, three *ras* gene family members designated c-H-*ras,* c-K-*ras,* and N-*ras* have been characterized (see Table 4-1). The three proto-oncogenes all encode a protein of 21,000 daltons (p21)[247] and are very homologous in amino acid sequence differing primarily at their C termini. The *ras* protein has been shown to bind guanine nucleotides and to possess GTPase activity.[248,249] As with certain members of the *src* kinase family, p21 *ras* is associated with the cytoplasmic surface of the plasma membrane and is a nonintegral membrane-associated product.[250,251] The amino acid sequence of the *ras* gene product is somewhat homologous to α subunit of G proteins that are also involved in guanidine nucleotide binding and signal transduction.[252] The G proteins are effectors of adenylcyclase[253] and include stimulatory G_S and inhibitory G_I effectors. Members of the G protein family also include transducin, a regulator of retinal rod cyclic GMP, phosphodieserase,[254] and cytoskeletal proteins such as tubulin.[255] G proteins are functionally regulated by the binding of guanidine nucleotides after receiving signals from receptors. The regulatory effect is mediated in the GTP-bound state but is transient because of intrinsic G protein GTPase activity. The biochemical activities of p21 *ras* are similar to G proteins; p21 *ras* exists in an equilibrium between an active conformation with bound GTP and an inactive conformation when the GTP is hydrolyzed (Fig. 4-8). Presumably, a receptor-mediated signal results in exchange of GDP for GTP, converting p21 from an inactive to an active form[256,258] and allowing it to interact as an effector with target molecules (see Fig. 4-8).[50] A decrease in the GTPase activity observed in the activated *ras* oncogene product is believed to be responsible for its transforming activity.[259] Thus, the binding of GTP with the diminished capacity to hydrolyze it would maintain the protein in a constitutively active state, thus sending a continuous signal to the cell along the mitogenic pathway. The mechanism by which the normal p21 product (expressed from the normal allele) and its intrinsic GTPase activity influence the signal transduction properties of the activated oncogene product is not yet understood.

The identification of *ras* genes in yeast has made it possible to study *ras* functions by classical and molecular genetics.[260,261] In *Saccharo-myces cerevisiae,* there are two *ras* genes that are 65% homologous in the N-terminal catalytic domains to mammalian p21 *ras.* [260] The *ras* genes in yeast are necessary for the survival of the organism. In experiments in which yeast *ras* genes were replaced with the human *ras* gene,[262] the yeast survived, demonstrating that the functional activity of *ras* in yeast has been conserved in evolution. In addition, the yeast *ras* gene mutated at the corresponding codon (along with certain other modifications), which activates the mammalian *ras* gene, transforms mouse NIH/3T3 cells.[245,260] These findings are the basis of the remarkable conclusion that the normal activity of p21 must be coupled to its transforming activity. Yeast *ras* genes also bind GTP and have an intrinsic GTPase activity[263,264]; however, in yeast the genes appear to regulate cyclic AMP levels through adenylcyclase,[265,266] and suppressor mutations that rescue *ras*-defective strains of yeast have been shown to map to components of the adenylcyclase pathway.[265,266] In contrast, the *ras* gene in other organisms does not appear to function through adenylcyclase[244,267] and in mammals and higher vertebrates it is probably involved in the second messenger pathways. Its function and its activity in these higher organisms are unknown.

NUCLEAR ONCOGENE/PROTO-ONCOGENE PROTEINS

The nuclear proteins encoded by proto-oncogenes and oncogenes are believed to be directly involved in the regulation of gene expression that leads to cell proliferation, division, and differentiation. Many of these nuclear proteins appear to be able to bind DNA; however, none are as homologous to each other as are the members of the *src* protein kinase or *ras*

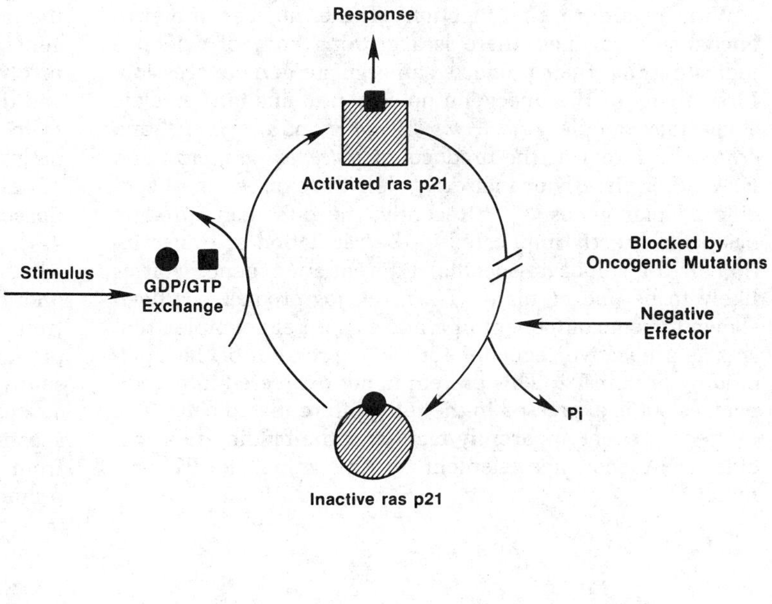

FIG. 4-8. Model for regulation of the *ras* p21 product. The alternating relaxed and activated states of the protein are shown. These are at least in part controlled by the rate of GTP hydrolysis by the intrinsic *ras* GTPase. GTP is diagrammatically represented as the filled small square and GDP as the filled small circle. The putative stimulus that positively regulates and an effector that negatively regulates the activity of p21 *ras* are shown.

gene families, although there are several *myc*-related genes (c-*myc*, N-*myc*, and L-*myc*).[268] Several have been shown to be participate in the same complementation group of the cooperative oncogene assay or have been shown to be transcriptionally activated by mitogenic stimulation (*e.g.*, *myc*, *fos*, Fig. 4-3).[269] Thus, when quiescent serum-starved (growth-arrested) murine fibroblasts are stimulated with serum or growth factors, the cells immediately enter G_1, and there is a transient increase in the level of c-*myc* and c-*fos*. The induction varies from a peak at 30 minutes for c-*fos*[269-271] to 2 hours for c-*myc*[272] (see Fig. 4-3). p53 RNA expression is also stimulated, but at a much later time; it peaks 18 to 24 hours poststimulation.[273] The induction of the expression of these nuclear protein–encoding proto-oncogenes is observed with either PDGF or fetal calf serum,[271] but the cells only become competent for DNA replication. If PDGF is removed, the cells remain competent, and apparently the expression of a family of genes referred to as competence genes (which includes *fos* and *myc*) has already occurred.[274,275] EGF and insulin-like growth factors are required for cells to progress through G_1 and enter S phase[276] (see Fig. 4-3). These studies suggest that the transient expression of nuclear protein–encoding oncogenes is required for cells to traverse specific points in the cell cycle. The expression of *fos* and *myc* in this system greatly precedes the onset of DNA synthesis and probably is not directly involved in DNA replication. In the cooperative oncogene assay the early genes of DNA tumor viruses are in the same complementation group as *myc*. These early viral genes are not directly involved in viral DNA replication but rather are involved with the transactivation of other viral and host cell genes.

Expression of c-*myb* and c-*myc* decreases dramatically during terminal differentiation, indirect evidence that they play a role in cell proliferation.[277-280] It is also postulated that constitutive expression of c-*myc* prevents differentiation and promotes cell division.[281] Since the expression of these genes appears to occur at specific points in the cell cycle, their expression may either promote proliferation or promote differentiation by being specifically expressed, as shown for c-*fos* where expression is observed during promonocyte differentiation and macrophage proliferation.[282]

With regard to the function of the nuclear protein–encoding oncogenes, there is a growing body of evidence indicating that their products can regulate gene expression. First, many of the oncogene nuclear proteins bind nucleic acids (for example, *myc*,[282] *fos*,[284] *myb*,[285] p53,[194] *jun*,[286] and *erb*A).[287] Moreover, the products of *myc*, *fos*, *jun*, *erb*A and E1A either directly or indirectly alter the expression of specific cellular genes.[288,289] Recently, the c-*fos* gene product has been directly implicated in the regulation of transcription of an adipocyte-specific differentiation gene.[290] It is likely to be one of many. Thus, the *fos* product has been shown to be a component of a nuclear protein complex that acts as a negative regulator for the expression of the lipid-binding protein P2. This protein is not expressed in preadipocytes but is expressed in the fully differentiated cells. The *fos* gene product apparently facilitates the binding to a specific DNA sequence element in the adipocyte P2 promoter.[290]

Perhaps the most dramatic evidence demonstrating the role of nuclear protein–encoding oncogenes as trans-acting factors comes from the studies of the v-*jun* oncogene.[291] DNA sequence analysis revealed that the C terminus of the v-*jun* protein was homologous to the C terminus of the transcriptional activator protein GCN4 from yeast *Saccharomyces cerevisiae*.[292] Furthermore, a chimeric GCN4 gene sequence containing the DNA-binding domain of v-*jun* rescued yeast strains that lacked the GCN4 gene (*null mutations*).[286] The consensus DNA-binding sequence for the yeast GCN4 gene is the same as the mammalian transcription factor AP1. This led to the demonstration that the v-*jun* oncogene clearly is the viral homolog of the normal AP1 transcription factor gene.[293] The AP1 product interacts not only with phorbol ester-inducible promoter elements, but with the enhancer elements found in many viral and cellular transcription control sequences. This finding suggests that the unregulated or ectopic expression of a normal transcription regulator protein contributes to tumor development. Moreover, and most importantly, researchers should be able to identify genes regulated by AP1 or c-*jun* that directly affect growth and expression of a neoplastic phenotype.

A different role has been proposed for the nuclear protein oncogene v-*erb*A, which was first shown to be related to a receptor for steroid hormones[294] and was subsequently identified as a nuclear receptor for thyroid hormones, triiodothyronine, and thyroxin.[295,296] v-*erb*A by itself does not appear to express transforming potential, but its presence potentiates the transforming potential of v-*erb*B by specifically interrupting differentiation of erythryoblasts.[297] The thyroid hormone receptor T3 is known to both positively and negatively regulate the expression of many genes.[298] v-*erb*A arrests expression of genes that play an important role in erythroid differentiation, the anion transporter,[299] and δ aminolevulinic (Ala S),[300] a key enzyme in hemin synthesis. Because of mutations in the v-*erb*A gene, it does not bind T3 or T4 and is therefore ligand independent. As with other nuclear protein–encoding oncogenes, its product probably acts constitutively to either up- or down-regulate expression of target genes, apparently interrupting the regulation of genes that are essential for erythroblast differentiation.

Beginning with mitogenic growth factors and ending with the nuclear proteins encoded by oncogenes and proto-oncogenes, we have described a component of pathways that are involved in the control and regulation of cell proliferation and differentiation and that have been identified primarily from the study of oncogenes. There are, however, additional pathways, the so-called second messages, that are also important in signal transduction. One example is the phospholipase C-mediated cleavage of phosphoinositol[301] (see Fig. 4-9). In this pathway diacylglycerol (DAG) is generated, which activates C kinase and mediates production of phosphorylated inositols.[301] The latter mobilizes calcium stores from the endoplasmic reticulum, increases the cytoplasm pH, and stimulates calcium-dependent protein kinase, resulting in the phosphorylation of specific protein substrates.[302] Protein C kinase also phosphorylates numerous substrates and its implication in mitogenic response stems from its activity as a receptor for phorbol ester tumor promoters.[302]

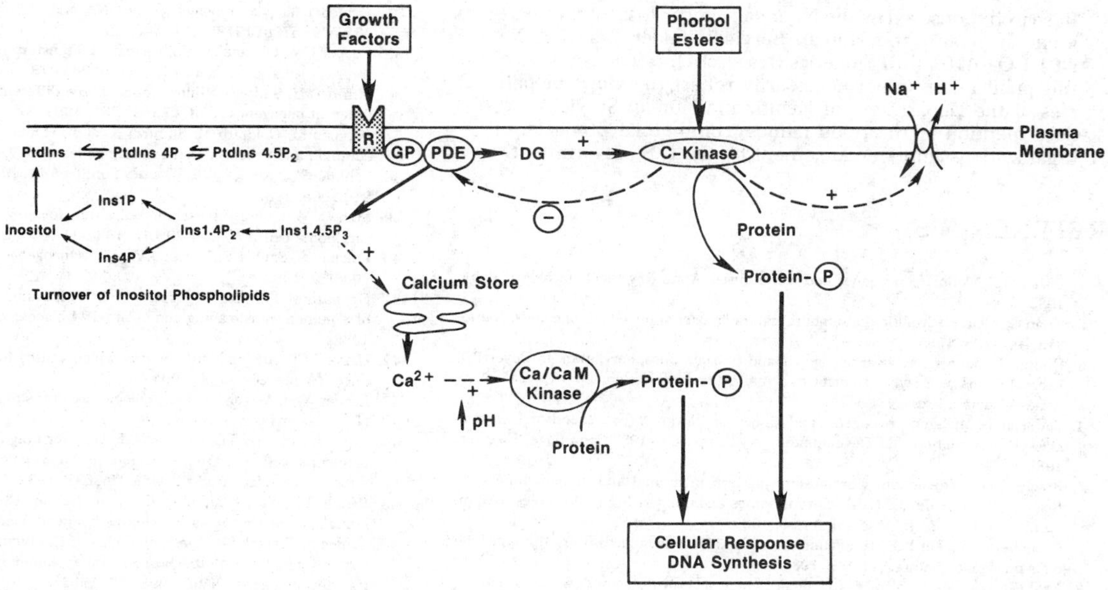

FIG. 4-9. Role of diacylglycerol (DG) and inositol lipid hydrolysis in the control of DNA synthesis. Some growth factors acting on specific receptors (R) uses a GTP-binding protein (GP) to stimulate a phosphodiesterase (PDE) which cleaves phosphatidylinositol (4,5-biphosphate) (Ptd Ins $4,5P_2$) to diacylglycerol (DG) and inositol 1,4,5-triphosphate (Ins $1,45P_3$). Diacylglycerol has several functions, including the stimulation of the same c-kinase that can be activated by phorbol esters with the subsequent activation of an Na^+-H^+ exchanger. Ins $1,4,5P_3$ acts to mobilize intracellular calcium, which results in stimulation of a calmodulin kinase (CaM).
#cf

FUTURE CONSIDERATIONS

Much of our understanding of proto-oncogene function will come from studies using classic and molecular genetics in organisms such as yeast and *Drosophila* since they are well-characterized genetically and can be easily manipulated. However, clearly the new emerging technology for performing studies in molecular genetics directly in higher mammals has enormous promise, as is already evidence for mouse transgenic technology. There is currently a great effort to generate techniques that will produce null mutations in genes of higher organisms,[303,304] which will open new vistas for experimentation.

Numerous techniques already exist in molecular biology to alter the structure of gene products and to express the gene products at very high levels, first in prokaryotic vector systems and more recently in insect and higher eukaryotes, using mammalian viral vector systems. With these techniques, oncogene protein structure and biochemical function can be studied and the three-dimensional structure determined. These studies are the basis for both elucidating the interaction of the protein with its substrate and designing drugs that can perhaps specifically target the activated oncogene product. The three-dimensional protein crystal structure for the *ras* oncogene has recently been described[305] and there is a great effort to determine the three-dimensional structure of other proto-oncogenes products.

We have not described the class of molecules that are referred to as suppressor genes or antioncogenes.[306] The genetic evidence is compelling that such genes exist, but at present it is not understood how these genes function.

Clinical applications of this new information and technology are beginning to emerge. New diagnostic techniques such as the polymerase chain reaction (see Chap. 2) will provide new methods for determining genetic alterations and identifying mutations. For example, with the polymerase chain reaction, which is already automated, it has been possible to identify the breakpoints in the DNA in follicular lymphomas.[307,308] The sensitivity of this technique will allow the detection of one lymphoma cell in the presence of a million normal cells. The procedure is superb for identifying subclinical presence of leukemia cells in patients and for determining the effectiveness of protocols designed to purge malignant cells from bone marrow. It also enables researchers to rapidly sequence chromosomal breakpoints at the DNA level.[308] It will markedly improve the detection of minimal residual disease and improve the ability to assess the stage of cancer in patients and evaluate therapy. We can expect that this is just one of many of the innovations that will have profound impact on the practice of medicine. History demonstrates that improved diagnostic procedures ultimately result in improved therapies. The ability to identify oncogenes associated with a specific tumor type should provide a remarkable way to diagnose disease and improve treatment.[309]

Research sponsored by the National Cancer Institute, Department of Health and Human Services, under Contract No. N01-CO-74101 with Bionetics Research, Inc. The contents of this publication do not necessarily reflect the views or policies of the Department of Health and Human Services, nor does mention of the trade names, commercial products, or organizations imply endorsement by the U.S. government.

REFERENCES

1. Bishop JM: Cellular oncogenes and retroviruses. Annu Rev Biochem 52:301–354, 1983
2. Klein G, Klein E: Evolution of tumours and the impact of molecular oncology. Nature 315:190–195, 1985
3. Hunter T, Cooper JA: Viral oncogenes and tyrosine phosphorylation. In Boyer PD, Krebs EG (eds): Enzyme Control by Protein Phosphorylation, pp 191–246. New York, Academic Press, 1986
4. Barbacid M: Mutagens, oncogenes and cancer. In Stewart A (ed): Trends in Genetics: DNA Differentiation and Development, vol 2, pp 188–192. Cambridge, Elsevier, 1986
5. Rowley JD: Introduction: Chromosome pattern in animal and human tumors. In Rowley JD, Ultmann JE (eds): Chromosomes and Cancer: From Molecules to Man, pp 57–60. New York, Academic Press, 1983
6. Greenberg ME, Ziff EB: Stimulation of mouse 3T3 cells induces transcription of the *c-fos* oncogene. Nature 311:433, 1984
7. Leof EB, Wharton W, Van Wyk JJ, et al: Epidermal growth factor (EGF) and somatomedin C regulate G1 progression in competent BALB/c-3T3 cells. Exp Cell Res 141:107, 1982
8. Temin HM: On the origin of genes for neoplasia: G.H.A. Clowes Memorial Lecture. Cancer Res 34:2835, 1974
9. Cairns J: Mutation selection and the natural history of cancer. Nature 255:197, 1975
10. Cairns J: The origin of human cancers. Nature 289:353, 1981
11. Klein G: The role of gene dosage and genetic transpositions in carcinogenesis. Nature 294:313, 1981
12. Rous P: A sarcoma of the fowl transmissible by an agent separable from the tumor cells. J Exp Med 13:397, 1911
13. Gross L: Oncogenic Viruses. New York, Pergamon Press, 1970
14. Temin HM: Origin of retroviruses from cellular moveable genetic elements. Cell 21:599, 1980
15. Temin HM: Structure, variation and synthesis of retrovirus long terminal repeat. Cell 27:1, 1981
16. Weiss R, Teich N, Varmus H, et al: RNA Tumor Viruses. Cold Spring Harbor, NY, Cold Spring Harbor Laboratory, 1982
17. McClintock B: Chromosome organization and genic expression. Cold Spring Harbor Symp Quant Biol 16:13–47, 1952
18. Campbell A: Some general questions about movable elements and their implications. Cold Spring Harbor Symp Quant Biol 45:1–9, 1981
19. Hayward WS, Neel BG, Astrin SM: Activation of a cellular *onc* gene by promoter insertion in ALV-induced lymphoid leukosis. Nature 290:475–479, 1982
20. Blair DG, Oskarsson M, Wood TG, et al: Activation of the transforming potential of a normal cell sequence: A molecular model for oncogenesis. Science 212:941–943, 1981
21. Wood TG, McGeady ML, Blair DG, et al: Long terminal repeat enhancement of v-*mos* transforming activity: Identification of essential regions. J Virol 46:726–736, 1983
22. Payne GS, Bishop JM, Varmus HE: Multiple arrangements of viral DNA and an activated host oncogene in bursal lymphomas. Nature 295:209–214, 1982
23. Tooze J: Molecular biology of tumor viruses. In DNA tumor viruses, 3rd ed. Cold Spring Harbor, NY, Cold Spring Harbor Laboratory, 1980
24. Berk AJ, Lee F, Harrison T, et al: A pre-early adenovirus 5 gene product regulates synthesis of early viral messenger RNAs. Cell 17:935, 1979
25. Jones N, Shenk T: An adenovirus type 5 early gene function regulates expression of other early viral genes. Proc Natl Acad Sci USA 76:3665, 1979
26. Rigby PWJ, Lane DP: Structure and function of simian virus 40 large T-antigen. In Klein G (ed): Viral Oncology, vol 3, pp 31–57. New York, Raven Press, 1983
27. Green MR, Treisman R, Maniatis T: Transcriptional activation of cloned human B-globin genes by viral immediate-early gene products. Cell 35:137, 1983
28. Hill M, Hillova J: Virus recovery in chicken cells tested with Rous sarcoma cell DNA. Nature 237:35, 1972
29. Graham FL, Van Der Eb AJ: A new technique for the assay of infectivity of human adenovirus 5DNA. Virology 52:456, 1973
30. Weinberg RA: Use of transfection to analyze genetic information and malignant transformation. Biochem Biophys Acta 651:25, 1981
31. Cooper GM, Okenquist S, Silverman L: Transforming activity of DNA of chemically transformed and normal cells. Nature 284:418, 1980
32. Blair DG, Cooper CS, Oskarsson MK, et al: New method for detecting cellular transforming genes. Science 218:1122, 1982
33. Fasano O, Birnbaum D, Edlund L, et al: New human transforming genes detected by a tumorigenicity assay. Mol Cell Biol 4:1695, 1984
34. Shih C, Shilo BZ, Goldfarb MP, et al: Passage of phenotypes of chemically transformed cells via transfection of DNA and chromatin. Proc Natl Acad Sci USA 76:5714–5718, 1979
35. Cooper GM, Okenquist S, Silverman L: Transforming activity of DNA of chemically transformed and normal cells. Nature 284:418–421, 1980
36. Murray MJ, Shilo BZ, Shih C, et al: Three different human tumor cell lines contain different oncogenes. Cell 25:355–361, 1981
37. Perucho M, Goldfarb M, Shimizu K, et al: Human tumor-derived cell lines contain common and different transforming genes. Cell 27:467–476, 1981
38. Schmid CW, Jelinek WR: The *alu* family of dispersed repetitive sequences. Science 216:1065, 1982
39. Shih C, Weinberg RA: Isolation of a transforming sequence from a human bladder carcinoma cell line. Cell 29:161, 1982
40. Pulciani S, Santos E, Lauver AV, et al: Oncogenes in solid human tumours. Nature 300:539, 1982
41. Goldfarb M, Shimizu K, Perucho M, et al: Isolation and preliminary characterization of a human transforming gene from T24 bladder carcinoma cells. Nature 296:404, 1982
42. Harvey TT: An unidentified virus which causes the rapid production of tumors in mice. Nature 204:1104, 1964
43. Kirsten WH, Meyer LA: Morphologic responses to a murine erythroblastosis virus. J Natl Cancer Inst 39:311, 1967
44. Der CJ, Krontiris TG, Cooper GM: Transforming genes of human bladder and lung carcinoma cell lines are homologous to the *ras* genes of Harvey and Kirsten sarcoma viruses. Proc Natl Acad Sci USA 79:3637, 1982
45. Parada LF, Tabin CJ, Shih C, et al: Human EJ bladder carcinoma oncogene is homologue of Harvey sarcoma virus *ras* gene. Nature 297:474, 1982
46. Santos E, Tronick SR, Aaronson SA, et al: T24 human bladder carcinoma oncogene is an activated form of the normal human homologue of BALB- and Harvey -MSV transforming gene. Nature 298:343, 1982
47. Perucho M, Goldfarb M, Shimizu K, et al: Human tumor–derived cell lines contain common and different transforming genes. Cell 27:467, 1981
48. Murray MJ, Shilo B-Z, Shih C, et al: Three different human tumor cell lines contain different oncogenes. Cell 25:355, 1981
49. Hall A, Marshall CJ, Spurr NK, et al: Identification of the transforming gene in two human sarcoma cell lines as a new member of the *ras* gene family located on chromosome 1. Nature 303:396, 1983
50. Murray MJ, Cunningham JM, Parada LF, et al: The HL-60 transforming sequence: A *ras* oncogene coexisting with altered *myc* genes in hematopoietic tumors. Cell 33:749, 1983
51. Shimizu K, Birnbaum D, Ruley MA, et al: Structure of the Ki-*ras* gene of the human lung carcinoma cell line Calu-1. Nature 304:497, 1983
52. Marshall C: Human oncogenes. In Weiss R, Teich N, Varmus H et al (eds): RNA Tumor Viruses, 2nd ed, pp 487–565. Cold Spring Harbor, NY, Cold Spring Harbor Laboratory, 1984
53. Varmus HE: The molecular genetics of cellular oncogenes. Annu Rev Genet 18:553, 1984
54. Barbacid M: *ras* genes. Annu Rev Biochem 56:779, 1987
55. Forrester K, Almoguera C, Han K, et al: Detection of high incidence of K-*ras* oncogenes during human colon tumorigenesis. Nature 327:298, 1987
56. Bos JL, Fearon ER, Hamilton SR, et al: Prevalence of *ras* gene mutations in human colorectal cancers. Nature 327:293, 1987
57. Bargmann CI, Hung M-C, Weinberg RA: Multiple independent activations of the *neu* oncogene by a point mutation altering the transmembrane domain of p185. Cell 45:649, 1986
58. Yamamoto T, Ikawa S, Akiyama T: Similarity of protein encoded by the human c-*erb*-B-2 gene to epidermal growth factor receptor. Nature 319:230, 1986
59. Coussens L, Yang-Feng TL, Liao Y, et al: Tyrosine kinase receptor with extensive homology to EGF receptor shares chromosomal location with *neu* oncogene. Science 230:1132, 1985
60. Cooper CS, Park M, Blair DG, et al: Molecular cloning of a new transforming gene from a chemically transformed human cell line. Nature 311:29, 1984
61. Martin-Zanca D, Hughes SH, Barbacid M: A human oncogene formed by the fusion of truncated tropomyosin and protein tyrosine kinase sequences. Nature 319:743, 1986
62. Yoshida T, Miyagawa K, Odagiri H, et al: Genomic sequence of *hst*, a transforming gene encoding a protein homologous to fibroblast growth factors and the *int*-2-encoded protein. Proc Natl Acad Sci USA 84:7305, 1987
63. Bovi PD, Curatola AM, Kern FG: An oncogene isolated by transfection of Kaposi's sarcoma DNA encodes a growth factor that is a member of the FGF family. Cell 50:729, 1987
64. Yunis JJ: The chromosomal basis of human neoplasia. Science 221:227–236, 1983
65. Klein G: The role of gene dosage and genetic transpositions in carcinogenesis. Nature 294:313–318, 1981
66. Klein G: Specific chromosomal translocations and the genesis of B-cell-derived tumors in mice and men. Cell 32:311–315, 1983
67. Rowley J: Human oncogene locations and chromosome aberrations. Nature 301:290–291, 1983
68. Yunis JJ, Soreng AL, Bowe AE: Fragile sites are targets of diverse mutagens and carcinogens. Oncogene 1:59, 1987
69. Mitelman F: Catalogue of Chromosome Aberrations in Cancer, 2nd ed. New York, Alan R. Liss, 1985

70. Rowley JD, Testa JR: Chromosome abnormalities in malignant hematologic diseases. Adv Cancer Res 36:103, 1982
71. Croce CM, Nowell PC: Molecular basis of human B cell neoplasia. Blood 65:1, 1985
72. Heisterkamp N, Stephenson JR, Groffen J, et al: Localization of the *c-abl* oncogene adjacent to a translocation break point in chronic myelocytic leukemia. Nature 306:239, 1983
73. Tsujimoto Y, Jorge Y, Onorato-Showe L, et al: Molecular cloning of the chromosomal breakpoint of B-cell lymphomas and leukemias with the t(11;14) chromosome translocation. Science 224:1403, 1984
74. Tsujimoto Y, Finger LR, Yunis J, et al: Cloning of the chromosome breakpoint of neoplastic B cells with the t(14;18) chromosome translocation. Science 226:1097, 1984
75. Kohl NE, Kanda N, Schreck RR, et al: Transposition and amplification of oncogene-related sequences in human neuroblastomas. Cell 35:359–367, 1983
76. Schwab M, Alitalo K, Klempnauer K-H, et al: Amplified DNA with limited homology to *myc* cellular oncogene is shared by human neuroblastoma cell lines and a neuroblastoma tumor. Nature 305:245–248, 1983
77. Vogel F: Genetics of retinoblastoma. Hum Genet 52:1, 1979
78. Benedict WF, Murphree AL, Banerjee A, et al: Patient with 13 chromosome deletion: Evidence that the retinoblastoma gene is a recessive cancer gene. Science 219:973, 1983
79. Cavenee WK, Dryja TP, Phillips RA, et al: Expression of recessive alleles by chromosomal mechanisms in retinoblastoma. Nature 305:779, 1983
80. Sparkes RS: Cytogenetics of retinoblastoma. Cancer Surv 3:479, 1984
81. Van-Heyningen V, Boyd PA, Searwright A, et al: Molecular analysis of chromosome 11 deletions in aniridia-Wilms' tumor syndrome. Proc Natl Acad Sci USA 82:8592, 1985
82. Friend SH, Bernards R, Rogel S, et al: A human DNA segment with properties of the gene that predisposes to retinoblastoma and osteosarcoma. Nature 323:643, 1986
83. Lee W-H, Bookstein R, Hong F, et al: Human susceptibility gene: Cloning, identification and sequence. Science 235:1394, 1987
84. Waterfield MD, Scaqrce GT, Whittle N, et al: Platelet-derived growth factor is structurally related to the putative transforming protein p28^{sis} of simian sarcoma virus. Nature 304:35–39, 1983
85. Doolittle RF, Hunkapiller MW, Hood LE, et al: Simian sarcoma virus *onc* gene, v-*sis*, is derived from the gene (or genes) encoding a platelet-derived growth factor. Science 221:275–277, 1983
86. Downward J, Yarden Y, Mayes E, et al: Close similarity of epidermal growth factor receptor and v-*erb*-B oncogene protein sequences. Nature 307:521–527, 1984
87. Peters G, Brookes S, Smith R, et al: Tumorigenesis by mouse mammary tumor virus: Evidence for a common region for provirus integration in mammary tumors. Cell 33:369, 1983
88. Sherr CJ, Rettenmier CW, Sacca R, et al: The c-*fms* proto-oncogene product is related to the receptor for the mononuclear phagocyte growth factor, CSF-1. Cell 41:665, 1985
89. Sap J, Munoz A, Damm K, et al: The v-*erb*A protein is a high affinity receptor for thyroid hormone. Nature 324:635, 1986
90. Weinberger C, Thompson C, Ong E, et al: The C-v-*erb*A gene encodes a thyroid hormone receptor. Nature 324:641, 1986
91. Bishop JM: The molecular genetics of cancer. Science 235:305–311, 1987
92. Coffin JM, Tsichlis PN, Barker CS, et al: Variation in avian retrovirus genomes. Ann NY Acad Sci 354:410, 1980
93. Curran T, Miller Ad, Zokas L, et al: Viral and cellular *fos* proteins: A comparative analysis. Cell 36:259, 1984
94. Meijlink F, Curran T, Miller AD, et al: Removal of a 67-base-pair sequence in the noncoding region of proto-oncogene *fos* converts it to a transforming gene. Proc Natl Acad Sci USA 82:4987, 1985
95. Bishop JM: Cellular oncogenes and retroviruses. Annu Rev Biochem 52:301, 1983
96. Levinson AD: Normal and activated *ras* oncogenes and their encoded products. Trends Genet 2:81, 1986
97. Prywes R, Foulkes JG, Rosenberg N, et al: Sequences of the A-MuLV protein needed for fibroblast and lymphoid cell transformation. Cell 34:569, 1983
98. Takeya T, Hanafusa H: Structure and sequence of the cellular gene homologous to the RSV *src* gene and the mechanism for generating the transforming virus. Cell 32:881, 1983
99. Hunter T, Cooper JA: Epidermal growth factor induces rapid tyrosine phosphorylation of proteins in A431 human tumor cells. Cell 24:741, 1981
100. Courtneidge SA: Activation of the pp60c-*src* kinase by middle T antigen binding or by dephosphorylation. EMBO J 4:1471, 1985
101. Cooper JA, Gould KL, Cartwright CA, et al: Tyr527 is phosphorylated in pp60c-*src*: Implications for regulation. Science 231:1431, 1986
102. Cooper JA, King CS: Dephosphorylation or antibody binding to the carboxy terminus stimulates pp60c-*src*. Mol Cell Biol 6:4467, 1986
103. Kawakami T, Pennington CY, Robbins KC: Isolation and oncogenic potential of a novel human *src*-like gene. Mol Cell Biol 6:4195, 1986
104. Sukegawa J, Semba K, Yamanashi Y, et al: Characterization of cDNA clones for the human c-*yes* gene. Mol Cell Biol 7:41, 1987
105. Browning PJ, Bunn HF, Cline A, et al: "Replacement" of COOH-terminal truncation of v-*fms* with c-*fms* sequences markedly reduces transformation potential. Proc Natl Acad Sci USA 83:7800, 1986
106. Coussens L, Van Beveren C, Smith D, et al: Structural alteration of viral homologue of receptor proto-oncogene *fms* at carboxyl terminus. Nature 320:277, 1986
107. Downward J, Yarden Y, Mayes E, et al: Close similarity of epidermal growth factor receptor and v-*erb*-B oncogene protein sequences. Nature 307:521, 1984
108. Downward J, Parker P, Waterfield MD: Autophosphorylation sites on the epidermal growth factor receptor. Nature 311:483, 1984
109. Schlessinger J: Allosteric regulation of the epidermal growth factor receptor kinase. J Cell Biol 103:2067, 1986
110. Gould KL, Woodgett JR, Cooper JA, et al: Protein kinase C phosphorylates pp60c-*src* at a novel site. Cell 42:849, 1985
111. Yarden Y, Kuang WJ, Yang-Feng T, et al: Human proto-oncogene c-*kit*: A new cell surface receptor tyrosine kinase for an unidentified ligand. EMBO J 6:3341, 1987
112. Park M, Dean M, Cooper CS, et al: Mechanism of *met* oncogene activation. Cell 45:895, 1986
113. Park M, Dean M, Kaul K, et al: Sequence of *met* proto-oncogene cDNA has features characteristic of the tyrosine kinase family of growth factor receptors. Proc Natl Acad Sci USA, 84:6379, 1987
114. Hayward WS, Neel BG, Astrin SM: Activation of the cellular *onc* gene by promoter insertion in ALV-induced lymphoid leukosis. Nature 290:475, 1981
115. Payne GS, Bishop JM, Varmus HE: Multiple arrangements of viral DNA and an activated hos oncogene in bursal lymphomas. Nature 295:209, 1982
116. Nilsen TW, Maroney PA, Goodwin RG, et al: c-*erb*B activation in ALV-induced erythroblastosis: Novel RNA processing and promoter insertion result in expression of an amino-truncated EGF receptor. Cell 41:719, 1985
117. Klempnauer K-H, Ramsay G, Bishop JM: The product of the retroviral transforming gene v-*myb* is a truncated version of the protein encoded by the cellular oncogene c-*myb*. Cell 33:345, 1983
118. Nusse R, Varmus HE: Many tumors induced by the mouse mammary tumor virus contain a provirus integrated in the same region of the host genome. Cell 31:99, 1982
119. Peters G, Lee AE, Dickson C: Concerted activation of two potential proto-oncogenes in carcinomas induced by mouse mammary tumor virus. Nature 320:628, 1986
120. Jakobovits A, Shackleford GM, Varmus HE, et al: Two proto-oncogenes implicated in mammary carcinogenesis, *int*-1 and *int*-2, are independently regulated during mouse development. Proc Natl Acad Sci USA 83:7806, 1986
121. Wilkinson DG, Bailes JA, McMahon AP: Expression of the proto-oncogene *int*-1 is restricted to specific neural cells in the developing mouse embryo. Cell 50:79, 1987
122. Metcalf D, Begley CG, Nicola NA, et al: Quantitative responsiveness of murine hemopoietic population *in vitro* and *in vivo* to recombinant multi-CSF (IL-3). Exp Hematol 15:288, 1987
123. Hapel AJ, Vande Woude GF, Campbell HD, et al: Generation of an autocrine leukemia using a retroviral expression vector carrying the interleukin-3 gene. Lymphokine Res 5:249, 1986
124. Chen SJ, Holbrook NJ, Mitchell KF, et al: A viral long terminal repeat in the interleukin 2 gene of a cell line that constitutively produces interleukin 2. Proc Natl Acad Sci USA 82:7284, 1985
125. Ymer S, Tucker QJ, Sanderson CJ, et al: Constitutive synthesis of interleukin-3 by leukaemia cell line WEH1-3B is due to retroviral insertion near the gene. Nature 317:255, 1985
126. Klein G, Klein E: *Myc*/Ig juxtaposition by chromosomal translocations: some new insights, puzzles and paradoxes. Immunol Today 6:208–215, 1985
127. Neel BG, Jhanwar SC, Chaganti RSK, et al: Two human c-*onc* genes are located on the long arm of chromosome 8. Proc Natl Acad Sci USA 79:7842, 1982
128. Dalla-Favera R, Franchini G, Martinotti S, et al: Chromosomal assignment of the human homologues of feline sarcoma virus and avian myeloblastosis virus *onc* genes. Proc Natl Acad Sci USA 79:4714, 1982
129. Kirsch IR, Morton CC, Nakahara K, et al: Human immunoglobulin heavy chain genes map to a region of translocations in malignant B lymphocytes. Science 216:301, 1982
130. Erikson J, Martins J, Croce CM: Assignment of the genes for human K immunoglobulin chains to chromosome 22. Nature 294:173, 1981
131. Erikson J, Nishikura K, Ar-Rushdi A, et al: Translocation of an immunoglobulin J locus to a region 3′ of an unrearranged c-*myc* oncogene enhances c-*myc* transcription. Proc Natl Acad Sci USA 80:7581, 1983
132. McBride OW, Hieter PA, Hollis GF, et al: Chromosomal location of human kappa and lambda immunoglobulin light chain constant region genes. J Exp Med 155:1480, 1982
133. De La Chapelle A, Lenoir G, Boué J, et al: Lambda Ig constant region genes are translocated to chromosome 8 in Burkitt's lymphoma with t(8;22). Nucleic Acids Res 11:1133, 1983
134. Croce CM, Nowell PC: Molecular basis of human B cell neoplasia. Blood 65:1, 1985
135. Piechacyzk M, Yang J-Q, Blanchard J-M, et al: Posttranscriptional mechanisms are responsible for accumulation of truncated c-*myc* RNAs in murine plasma cell tumors. Cell 42:589, 1985
136. Rabbitts PH, Watson JV, Lamond A, et al: Metabolism of c-*myc* gene products: c-*myc* mRNA and protein expression in the cell cycle. EMBO J 4:2009, 1985
137. Remmers EF, Yang J-Q, Marcu KB: A negative transcriptional control element located upstream of the murine c-*myc* gene. EMBO J 5:899, 1986
138. Cesarman E, Dalla-Favera R, Bentley D, et al: Mutations in the first exon are associated with altered transcription of c-*myc* in Burkitt lymphoma. Science 238:1272, 1987
139. Leder P, Battey J, Lenoir G, et al: Translocations among antibody genes in human cancer. Science 222:765, 1983
140. Taub R, Moulding C, Battey J, et al: Activation and somatic mutation of the translocated c-*myc* gene in Burkitt lymphoma cells. Cell 36:339, 1984

141. Croce CM, Thierfelder W, Erickson J, et al: Transcriptional activation of an unrearranged and untranslocated c-*myc* oncogene by translocation of a C K locus in Burkitt lymphoma cells. Proc Natl Acad Sci USA 80:6922, 1983
142. Heisterkamp N, Groffen J, Stephenson JR, et al: Chromosomal localization of human cellular homologues of two viral oncogenes. Nature 299:747, 1982
143. De Klein A, Van Kessel AG, Grosveld G, et al: A cellular oncogene is translocated to the Philadelphia chromosome in chronic myelocytic leukaemia. Nature 300:765, 1982
144. Groffen J, Stephenson JR, Heisterkamp N, et al: Philadelphia chromosomal breakpoints are clustered within a limited region, *bcr*, on chromosome 22. Cell 36:93, 1984
145. Canaani E, Steiner-Saltz D, Aghai E, et al: Altered transcription of an oncogene in chronic myeloid leukaemia. Lancet 1:593, 1984
146. Collins SJ, Kubonishi I, Miyoshi I, et al: Altered transcription of the c-*abl* oncogene in K-562 and other chronic myelogenous leukemia cells. Science 225:72, 1984
147. Konopka, JB, Watanabe SM, Witte ON: An alteration of the human c-*abl* protein in K562 leukemia cells unmasks associated tyrosine kinase activity. Cell 37:1035, 1984
148. Witte ON: Functions of the *abl* oncogene. Cancer Surv 5:183, 1986
149. Konopka JB, Witte ON: Detection of c-*abl* tyrosine kinase activity *in vitro* permits direct comparison of normal and altered *abl* gene products. Mol Cell Biol 5:3116, 1985
150. Pierce JH, Di Fiore PP, Aaronson SA, et al: Neoplastic transformation of mast cells by Abelson-MuLV: Abrogation of IL-3 dependence by a nonautocrine mechanism. Cell 41:685, 1985
151. Alitalo K, Schwab M, Lin CC, et al: Homogeneously staining chromosomal regions contain amplified copies of an abundantly expressed cellular oncogene (c-*myc*) in malignant neuroendocrine cells from a human colon carcinoma. Proc Natl Acad Sci USA 80:1707, 1983
152. Schwab M, Alitalo K, Klempnauer K-H, et al: Amplified DNA with limited homology to *myc* cellular oncogene is shared by human neuroblastoma cell lines and a neuroblastoma tumour. Nature 305:245, 1983
153. Schimke RT: Gene amplification in cultured animal cells. Cell 37:705, 1984
154. Shilo Y, Shipley J, Brodeur GM, et al: Differential amplification, assembly, and relocation of multiple DNA sequences in human neuroblastomas and neuroblastoma cell lines. Proc Natl Acad Sci USA 82:3761, 1985
155. Collins S, Groudine M: Amplification of endogenous *myc*-related DNA sequences in a human myeloid leukaemia cell line. Nature 298:679, 1982
156. Dalla Favera R, Wong-Staal F, Gallo RC: *onc* gene amplification in promyelocytic leukaemia cell line HL-60 and primary leukaemic cells of the same patient. Nature 299:61, 1982
157. Schwab M, Varmus HE, Bishop JM: Chromosome localization in normal cells and neuroblastomas of a gene related to c-*myc*. Nature 308:288, 1984
158. Brodeur GM, Seeger RC, Schwab M, et al: Amplification of N-*myc* in untreated human neuroblastomas correlates with advanced disease stage. Science 224:1121, 1984
159. Little CD, Nau MM, Carney DN, et al: Amplification and expression of the c-*myc* oncogene in human lung cell lines. Nature 306:194, 1983
160. Libermann TA, Nusbaum HR, Razon N, et al: Amplification, enhanced expression and possible rearrangement of EGF receptor gene in primary human brain tumours of glial origin. Nature 313:144, 1985
161. Yamamoto T, Kamat N, Kawano H, et al: High incidence of amplification of the epidermal growth factor receptor gene in human squamous carcinoma cell lines. Cancer Res 46:414, 1986
162. Yokota J, Terada M, Toyoshima K, et al: Amplification of the c-*erb*B-2 oncogene in human adenocarcinomas *in vitro*. Lancet 1:765, 1986
163. Zhou D, Battifora H, Yokota J, et al: Association of multiple copies of the c-*erb*B-2 oncogene with spread of breast cancer. Cancer Res 47:6123, 1987
164. King CR, Kraus MH, Aaronson SA: Amplification of a novel v-*erb*B-related gene in a human mammary carcinoma. Science 229:974, 1985
165. Hudziak RM, Schlessinger J, Ullrich A: Increased expression of the putative growth factor receptor p185 HER2 causes transformation and tumorigenesis of NIH 3T3 cells. Proc Natl Acad Sci USA 84:7159, 1987
166. Di Fiore PP, Pierce JH, Kraus MH, et al: *erb*B-2 is a potent oncogene when overexpressed in NIH/3T3 cells. Science 237:178, 1987
167. Reddy EP, Smith MJ, Srinivasan A: Nucleotide sequence of Abelson murine leukemia virus genome: Structural similarity of its transforming gene product to other *onc* gene products with tyrosine-specific kinase activity. Proc Natl Acad Sci USA 80:3623, 1983
168. Tabin CJ, Bradley SM, Bargmann CI, et al: Mechanism of action of a human oncogene. Nature 300:143, 1982
169. Taparowsky E, Shimizu K, Goldfarb M, et al: Structure and activation of the human N-*ras* gene. Cell 34:581, 1983
170. Shih TY, Weeks MO: Oncogenes and cancer: p21 *ras* genes. Cancer Invest 2:109, 1984
171. Eadie JS, Conrad M, Toorchen D, et al: Mechanism of mutagenesis by 06-methylguanine. Nature 308:201, 1984
172. Loechler EL, Green CL, Essignmann JM: In vivo mutagenesis by 06-methylguanine built into a unique site in a viral genome. Proc Natl Acad Sci USA 81:6271, 1984
173. Balmain A, Pragnell IB: Mouse skin carcinomas induced in vivo by chemical carcinogens have a transforming Harvey-*ras* oncogene. Nature 303:72, 1983
174. Sukumar S, Notario V, Martin-Zanca D, et al: Induction of mammary carcinomas in rats by nitroso-methylurea involves malignant activation of H-*ras*-1 locus by single point mutations. Nature 306:658, 1983
175. Zarbl H, Sukumar S, Arthur AV, et al: Direct mutagenesis of Ha-ras-1 oncogenes by N-nitroso-N-methylurea during initiation of mammary carcinogenesis in rats. Nature 315:382, 1985
176. Vousden KH, Marshall CJ: Three different activated *ras* genes in mouse tumours; evidence for oncogene activation during progression of a mouse lymphoma. EMBO J 3:913, 1984
177. Shilo B-Z, Weinberg RA: DNA sequences homologous to vertebrate oncogenes are conserved in Drosophila melanogaster. Proc Natl Acad Sci USA 78:6789, 1981
178. Rijsewijk F, Schuermann M, Wagenaar E, et al: The drosophila homolog of the mouse mammary oncogene int-1 is identical to the segment polarity gene wingless. Cell 50:649–657, 1987
179. Kataoko T, Powers S, Cameron S, et al: Functional homology of mammalian and yeast *ras* genes. Cell 40:19, 1985
180. Defeo-Jones D, Tatchell K, Robinson LC, et al: Mammalian and yeast *ras* gene products: Biological function in their heterologous systems. Science 228:179, 1985
181. Tatchell K, Chaleff DT, Defeo-Jones D, et al: Requirement of either of a pair of *ras*-related genes of Saccharomyces cerevisiae for spore viability. Nature 309:523, 1984
182. Kataoka T, Powers S, McGill C, et al: Genetic analysis of yeast RAS1 and RAS2 genes. Cell 37:437, 1984
183. Tamanoi F, Walsh M, Kataoka T, et al: A product of yeast RAS2 gene is a guanine nucleotide binding protein. Proc Natl Acad Sci USA 81:6924, 1984
184. Temeles GL, Gibbs JB: Yeast and mammalian *ras* proteins have conserved biochemical properties. Nature 313:700, 1985
185. Broek D, Samiy N, Fasano O, et al: Differential activation of yeast adenylate cyclase by wild-type and mutant *ras* proteins. Cell 41:763, 1985
186. Toda T, Uno I, Ishikawa T, et al: In yeast, *ras* proteins are controlling elements of adenylate cyclase. Cell 40:27, 1985
187. Beckner SK, Hattori S, Shih TY: The *ras* oncogene product p21 is not a regulatory component of adenylate cyclase. Nature 317:71, 1985
188. Shiro K, Shimojo H, Swaada Y, et al: Incomplete transformation of rat cells by a small fragment of adenovirus 12 DNA. Virology 95:127, 1979
189. Houweling A, Van Den Elsen PJ, Van Der Eb AJ: Partial transformation of primary rat cells by the left-most 4-5 D fragment of adenovirus 5 DNA. Virology 105:537, 1980
190. Van Den Elsen P, De Pater S, Houweling A, et al: The relationship between region E1a and E1b of human adenoviruses in cell transformation. Gene 18:175, 1982
191. Ruley HE: Adenovirus early region 1A enables viral and cellular transforming primary cells in culture. Nature 304:602, 1982
192. Parada LF, Land H, Weinbert RA, et al: Cooperation between gene encoding P53 tumour antigen and *ras* in cellular transformation. Nature 312:648, 1984
193. Eliyahu D, Raz A, Gruss P, et al: Participation of p53 cellular tumor antigen in transformation of normal embryonic cells. Nature 312:647, 1984
194. Yancopoulos GD, Nisen PD, Tesfaye A, et al: N-*myc* can cooperate with *ras* to transform normal cells in culture. Proc Natl Acad Sci USA 82:5455, 1985
195. Land H, Parada LF, Weinbert RA: Cellular oncogenes and multistep carcinogenesis. Science 222:771–778, 1983
196. Courtneidge SA, Smith AE: Polyoma virus transforming protein associates with the product of the c-*src* cellular gene. Nature 303:435, 1983
197. Bolen JP, Thiele CJ, Israel MA, et al: Enhancement of cellular *src* gene product associated tyrosyl kinase activity following polyoma virus infection and transformation. Cell 38:767, 1984
198. Brinster RL, Chen HV, Trumbauer ME, et al: Factors effecting the efficiency of introducing foreign DNA into mice by microinjecting eggs. Proc Natl Acad Sci USA 82:4438, 1985
199. Stewart TA, Pattengale PK, Leder P: Spontaneous mammary adenocarcinomas in transgenic mice that carry and express MTV/*myc* fusion genes. Cell 38:627, 1984
200. Hanahan D: Heritable formation of pancreatic B cell tumours in transgenic mice expressing recombinant insulin/simian virus 40 oncogenes. Nature 315:115, 1985
201. Messing A, Chen H-Y, Palmiter RD, et al: Peripheral neuropathies, hepatocellular carcinomas and islet cell adenomas in transgenic mice. Nature 316:461, 1985
202. Sinn E, Muller W, Pattengale P, et al: Coexpression of MMTV/v-Ha-*ras* and MMTV/c-*myc* genes in transgenic mice: Synergistic action of oncogenes in vivo. Cell 49:465, 1987
203. Leder A, Pattengale PK, Kuo A, et al: Consequences of widespread deregulation of the c-*myc* gene in transgenic mice: Multiple neoplasms and normal development. Cell 45: 485, 1986
204. Adams JM, Harris AW, Pinkert CA, et al: The c-*myc* oncogene driven by immunoglobin enhancers induces lymphoid malignancy in transgenic mice. Nature 318:533, 1985
205. Robb RJ: Interleukin 2: The molecule and its function. Immunol Today 5:203, 1984
206. Tushinski RJ, Oliver IT, Guilbert LJ, et al: Survival of mononuclear phagocytes depends on a lineage-specific growth factor that the differentiated cells selectively destroy. Cell 28:71, 1982
207. Hamilton JA, Stanley ER, Burgess AW, et al: Stimulation of macrophage plasminogen activator activity by colony-stimulating factors. J Cell Physiol 103:435, 1980
208. Weissman BE, Aaronson SA: Balb and Kirsten murine sarcoma viruses alter growth and differentiation of EGF-dependent Balb/c mouse epidermal keratinocyte lines. Cell 32:599, 1983
209. Doolittle RF, Hunkapiller MW, Hood LE, et al: Simian sarcoma virus *onc* gene, v-*sis*, is derived from the gene (or genes) encoding a platelet-derived growth factor. Science 221:275, 1983
210. Chiu I-M, Reddy EP, Givol D, et al: Nucleotide sequence analysis identifies the human c-*sis* proto-oncogene as a structural gene for platelet-derived growth factor. Cell 37:123, 1984

211. Waterfield MD, Scrace GT, Whittle N, et al: Platelet-derived growth factor is structurally related to the putative transforming protein p28 *sis* of simian sarcoma virus. Nature 304:35, 1983
212. Ross R, Glomset J, Kariya B, et al: A platelet-dependent serum factor that stimulates the proliferation of arterial smooth muscle cells in vitro. Proc Natl Acad Sci USA 71:1207, 1974
213. Dickson C, Smith R, Brookes S, et al: Tumorigenesis by mouse mammary tumor virus: Proviral activation of a cellular gene in the common integration region *int*-2. Cell 37:529, 1984
214. Dickson C, Peters G: Potential oncogene product related to growth factors. Nature 326:833, 1987
215. Taira M, Yoshida T, Miyagawa K, et al: cDNA sequence of human transforming gene *hst* and identification of the coding sequence required for transforming activity. Proc Natl Acad Sci USA 84:2980, 1987
216. Abraham JA, Mergia A, Whang JL, et al: Nucleotide sequence of a bovine clone encoding the angiogenic protein, basic fibroblast growth factor. Science 233:545, 1986
217. Esch F, Baird A, Ling N, et al: Primary structure of bovine pituitary basic fibroblast growth factor (FGF) and comparison with the amino-terminal sequence of bovine brain acidic FGF. Proc Natl Acad Sci USA 82:6507, 1985
218. Delarco JE, Todaro GJ: Growth factors from murine sarcoma virus-transformed cells. Proc Natl Acad Sci USA 75:4001, 1978
219. Roberts AB, Sporn MB: Growth factors and transformation. Cancer Surv 5:405, 1986
220. Twardzik DR, Todaro GJ, Marquardt H, et al: Transformation induced by abelson murine leukemia virus involves production of a polypeptide growth factor. Science 216:894, 1982
221. Kaplan PL, Ozanne B: Cellular responsiveness to growth factors correlates with a cell's ability to express the transformed phenotype. Cell 33:931, 1983
222. Weber W, Gill GN, Spiess J: Production of an epidermal growth factor receptor-related protein. Science 224:294, 1984
223. Merlino GT, Xu Y-H, Ishii S, et al: Amplification and enhanced expression of the epidermal growth factor receptor gene in A431 human carcinoma cells. Science 224:417, 1984
224. Ullrich A, Coussens L, Hayflick JS, et al: Human epidermal growth factor receptor cDNA sequence and aberrant expression of the amplified gene in A431 epidermoid carcinoma cells. Nature 309:418, 1984
225. Ebina Y, Ellis L, Jarnagin K, et al: The human insulin receptor cDNA: The structural basis for hormone-activated transmembrane signalling. Cell 40:747, 1985
226. Hunter T, Cooper JA: Protein-tyrosine kinases. Annu Rev Biochem 54:897–930, 1985
227. Cooper JA, Bowen-Pope DF, Raines E, et al: Similar effects of platelet-derived growth factor and epidermal growth factor on the phosphorylation of tyrosine in cellular proteins. Cell 31:263, 1982
228. Sefton BM, Hunter T, Beemon K, et al: Evidence that the phosphorylation of tyrosine is essential for cellular transformation by Rous sarcoma virus. Cell 20:807, 1980
229. Whitlock CA, Witte ON: The complexity of virus-cell interactions in Abelson virus infection of lymphoid and other hematopoietic cells. In Dixon FJ (ed): Advances in Immunology, vol 37, pp 73–98. New York, Academic Press, 1985
230. Spector DH, Smith K, Padgett T, et al: Uninfected avian cells contain RNA related to the transforming gene of avian sarcoma viruses. Cell 13:371, 1978
231. Brugge JS, Cotton PC, Queral AE, et al: Neurones express high levels of a structurally modified, activated form of pp60c-*src*. Nature 316:554, 1985
232. Simon MA, Drees B, Kornberg T, et al: The nucleotide sequence and tissue-specific expression of Drosophila c-*src*. Cell 42:831, 1985
233. Moelling K, Pfaff E, Beug H, et al: DNA-binding activity is associated with purified *myb* proteins from AMB and E26 viruses and is temperature-sensitive for E26 *ts* mutants. Cell 40:983, 1985
234. Maxwell SA, Arlinghaus RB: Serine kinase activity associated with Moloney murine sarcoma virus-124-encoded p37^{mos}. Virology 143:321, 1985
235. Reed SI, Hadwiger JA, Lorincz AT: Protein kinase activity associated with the product of the yeast cell cycle gene CDC28. Proc Natl Acad Sci USA 82:4055, 1985
236. Simanis V, Nurse PM: The cell cycle control gene *cdc*2+ of yeast encodes a protein kinase potentially regulated by phosphorylation. Cell 45:261, 1986
237. Lee MG, Nurse P: Complementation used to clone a human homologue of the fission yeast cell cycle control gene *cdc*2. Nature 327:31, 1987
238. Hanks SK: Homology probing: Identification of cDNA clones encoding members of the protein-serine kinase family. Proc Natl Acad Sci USA 84:388, 1987
239. Draetta G, Brizuela L, Potashkin J, et al: Identification of p34 and p13, human homologs of the cell cycle regulators of fission yeast encoded by *cdc*2+ and *suc*1+. Cell 50:319, 1987
240. Propst F, Rosenberg MP, Iyer A, et al: c-*mos* proto-oncogene RNA transcripts in mouse tissues: Structural features, developmental regulation and localization in specific cell types. Mol Cell Biol 7:1629–1637, 1987
241. Propst F, Rosenberg MP, Oskarsson MK, et al: Genetic analysis and developmental regulation of testis-specific RNA expression of *Mos, Abl*, actin and *Hox-1.4*. Oncogene 2:227–233, 1988
242. Keshet E, Rosenberg M, Mercer JA, et al: Developmental regulation of ovarian-specific *mos* expression. Oncogene 2:235–240, 1988
243. Westaway D, Papkoff J, Moscovici C, et al: Identification of a provirally activated c-Ha-*ras* oncogene in an avian nephroblastoma via a novel procedure: cDNA cloning of a chimaeric viral-host transcript. EMBO J 5:301, 1986
244. Reymond CD, Gomer RH, Mehdy MC, et al: Developmental regulation of a Dictyostelium gene encoding a protein homologous to mammalian *ras* protein. Cell 39:141, 1984
245. Defeo-Jones D, Skolnick E, Koller R, et al: *ras*-related gene sequences identified and isolated from *Saccharomyces cerevisiae*. Nature 306:707, 1983
246. Powers S, Kataoka T, Fasano O, et al: Genes in *S. cerevisiae* encoding proteins with domains homologous to the mammalian *ras* proteins. Cell 36:607, 1984
247. Shih TY, Weeks MO, Young HA, et al: Identification of a sarcoma virus-coded phosphoprotein in nonproducer cells transformed by Kirsten or Harvey murine sarcoma virus. Virology 96:64, 1979
248. Gibbs JB, Sigal IS, Poe M, et al: Intrinsic GTPase activity distinguishes normal and oncogenic *ras* p21 molecules. Proc Natl Acad Sci USA 81:5704, 1984
249. McGrath JP, Capon DJ, Goeddel DV, et al: Comparative biochemical properties of normal and activated human *ras* p21 protein. Nature 310:644, 1984
250. Willingham MC, Pastan I, Shih TY, et al: Localization of the *src* gene product of the Harvey strain of MSV to plasma membrane of transformed cells by electron microscopic immunocytochemistry. Cell 19:1005, 1980
251. Shih TY, Weeks MO: Oncogenes and cancer: The p21 *ras* genes. Cancer Invest 2:109, 1984
252. Hurley JB, Simon MI, Teplow DB, et al: Homologies between signal transducing G proteins and *ras* gene products. Science 226:860, 1984
253. Gilman AG: G proteins and dual control of adenylate cyclase. Cell 36:577, 1984
254. Stryer L: Cyclic GMP cascade of vision. Annu Rev Neurosci 9:87, 1986
255. Hughes SM: Are guanine nucleotide binding proteins a distinct class of regulatory proteins? FEBS Lett 164:1, 1983
256. McCormick F, Clark BFC, La Cour TFM, et al: A model for the tertiary structure of p21, the product of the *ras* oncogene. Science 228:96, 1985
257. Clanton DJ, Hattori S, Shih TY: Mutations of the *ras* gene product p21 that abolish guanine nucleotide binding. Proc Natl Acad Sci USA 83:5076, 1986
258. Willumsen BM, Christensen A, Hubbert NL, et al: The p21 *ras* C-terminus is required for transformation and membrane association. Nature 310:583, 1984
259. Seeburg PH, Colby WW, Capon DJ, et al: Biological properties of human c-Ha-*ras*1 genes mutated at codon 12. Nature 312:71, 1984
260. Kataoko T, Powers S, Cameron S, et al: Functional homology of mammalian and yeast *ras* genes. Cell 40:19, 1985
261. Defeo-Jones D, Tatchell K, Robinsin LC, et al: Mammalian and yeast *ras* gene products: Biological function in their heterologous systems. Science 228:179, 1985
262. Kataoka T, Powers S, McGill, C, et al: Genetic analysis of yeast RAS1 and RAS2 genes. Cell 37:437, 1984
263. Tamanoi F, Walsh M, Kataoka T, et al: A product of yeast RAS2 gene is a guanine nucleotide binding protein. Proc Natl Acad Sci USA 81:6924, 1984
264. Temeles GL, Gibbs JB: Yeast and mammalian *ras* proteins have conserved biochemical properties. Nature 313:700, 1985
265. Broek D, Samiy N, Fasano O, et al: Differential activation of yeast adenylate cyclase by wild-type and mutant *ras* proteins. Cell 41:763, 1985
266. Toda T, Uno I, Ishikawa T, et al: In yeast, *ras* proteins are controlling elements of adenylate cyclase. Cell 40:27, 1985
267. Beckner SK, Hattori S, Shih TY: The *ras* oncogene product p21 is not a regulatory component of adenylate cyclase. Nature 317:71, 1985
268. Kohl NE, Kanda N, Schreck RR, et al: Transposition and amplification of oncogene-related sequences in human neuroblastomas. Cell 35:359, 1983
269. Greenberg ME, Ziff EB: Stimulation of mouse 3T3 cells induces transcription of the c-*fos* oncogene. Nature 311:433, 1984
270. Kruijer W, Cooper JA, Hunter T, et al: Platelet-derived growth factor induces rapid but transient expression of the c-*fos* gene and protein. Nature 312: 711, 1984
271. Moller R, Bravo R, Burckhardt J, et al: Induction of c-*fos* gene and protein by growth factors precedes activation of c-*myc*. Nature 312:716, 1984
272. Thompson CB, Challoner PB, Neiman PE, et al: Expression of the c-*myb* proto-oncogene during cellular proliferation. Nature 319:374, 1986
273. Reich NC, Levine AJ: Growth regulation of a cellular tumour antigen, p53, in non-transformed cells. Nature 308:199, 1984
274. Leof EB, Wharton W, Van Wyck JJ, et al: Epidermal growth factor (EGF) and somatomedin C regulate G1 progression in competent BALB/c-3T3 cells. Exp Cell Res 141:107, 1982
275. Curran T, Morgan JI: Superinduction of the c-*fos* by nerve growth factor in the presence of peripherally active benzodiazeprines. Science 229:1265, 1985
276. Stiles CD, Capone GT, Scher CD, et al: Dual control of cell growth by somatomedins and platelet-derived growth factor. Proc Natl Acad Sci USA 76:1279, 1979
277. Eisenman RN, Thompson CB: Oncogenes with potential nuclear function: myc, myb, and fos. Cancer Surv 5:309–327, 1986
278. Westin EH, Gallo RC, Arya SK, et al: Differential expression of the *amv* gene in human hematopoietic cells. Proc Natl Acad Sci USA 79:2194, 1982
279. Campisi J, Gray HE, Parchee AB, et al: Cell-cycle control of c-*myc* but not c-*ras* expression is lost following chemical transformation. Cell 36:241, 1984
280. Torelli G, Selleri L, Donelli A, et al: Activation of c-*myb* expression by phytohemagglutinin stimulation in normal human T lymphocytes. Mol Cell Biol 5:2874, 1985
281. Prochowkni EV, Kukowska J: Deregulated expression of c-*myc* by murine erythroleukemia cells prevents differentiation. Nature 32:848, 1986
282. Mitchell RL, Zokas L, Schreiber RD, et al: Rapid induction of the expression of proto-oncogene *fos* during human monocytic differentiation. Cell 40:209, 1985
283. Donner P, Greiser-Wilke I, Moelling K: Nuclear localization and DNA binding of

the transforming gene product of avian myelocytomatosis virus. Nature 296:262, 1982

284. Sambucetti L, Curran T: The *fos* protein complex is associated with DNA in isolated nuclei and binds to DNA cellulose. Science 234:1417, 1986
285. Moelling K, Pfaff E, Beug H, et al: DNA-binding activity is associated with purified *myb* proteins from AMV and E26 viruses and is temperature-sensitive for E26 *ts* mutants. Cell 40:983, 1985
286. Struhl K: The DNA-binding domains of the *jun* oncoprotein and the yeast GCN4 transcriptional activator protein are functionally homologous. Cell 50:841, 1987
287. McLeod K, Baxter J: Chromatin receptors for thyroid hormones. J Biol Chem 251:7380, 1976
288. Kingston RE, Baldwin AS, Sharp PA: Transcription control by oncogenes. Cell 41:3, 1985
289. Kaddurah-Daouk R, Greene JM, Baldwin AS Jr, et al: Activation and repression of mammalian gene expression by the c-*myc* protein. Genes Dev 1:347, 1987
290. Distel RJ, Ro H-S, Rosen BS, et al: Nucleoprotein complexes that regulate gene expression in adipocyte differentiation: Direct participation of c-*fos*. Cell 49:835, 1987
291. Maki Y, Bos TJ, Davis C, et al: Avian sarcoma virus 17 carries the *jun* oncogene. Proc Natl Acad Sci USA 84:2848, 1987
292. Vogt PK, Bos TJ, Doolittle RF: Homology between the DNA-binding domain of the GCN4 regulatory protein of yeast and the carboxyl-terminal region of a protein coded for by the oncogene *jun*. Proc Natl Acad Sci USA 84:3316, 1987
293. Bohmann D, Bos TJ, Admin A, et al: Human proto-oncogene c-*jun* encodes a DNA binding protein with structural and functional properties of transcription factor AP-1. Science 238:1386, 1987
294. Weinberger C, Hollenberg SM, Rosenfeld MG, et al: Domain structure of the human glucocorticoid receptor and its relationship to the v-*erb*A oncogene product. Nature 318:670, 1985
295. SAP J, Munoz A, Damm K, et al: The v-*erb* A protein is a high affinity receptor for thyroid hormone. Nature 324:635, 1986
296. Weinberger C, Thompson C, Ong E, et al: The C-v-*erb*A gene encodes a thyroid hormone receptor. Nature 324:641, 1986
297. Frykberg L, Palmieri S, Beng H, et al: Transforming capacities of avian erythroblastosis virus mutants deleted in the V-*erb*A or *erb*B oncogenes. Cell 32:227, 1983
298. Oppenheimer JH, Samuels HH (eds): Molecular Basis of Thyroid Hormone Action. New York Academic Press, 1983
299. Woods CM, Boyer B, Vogt PK, et al: Asychronous expression of the anion transporter and the peripheral components of the membrane skeleton in AZV- and S13-transformed cells. J Cell Biol 103:1789, 1986
300. Zenke M, Kahn P, Disela C, et al: v-*erb*A specifically suppresses transcription of the avian erythrocyte anion transporter (band 3) gene. Cell 52:107–119, 1988
301. Nishizuka Y: Studies and perspectives of protein kinase C. Science 233:305, 1986
302. Berridge MJ: Inositol triphosphate and diacylglycerol: Two interacting second messengers. Annu Rev Biochem 56:159, 1987
303. Smithies O, Gregg RG, Boggs SS, et al: Insertion of DNA sequences into the human chromosome β-globin locus by homologous recombination. Nature 317:230–234, 1985
304. Thomas KR, Folger KR, Capecchi MR: High frequency targeting of genes to specific sites in the mammalian genome. Cell 44:419–428, 1986
305. De Vos AM, Tong L, Milburn MV, et al: Three-dimensional structure of an oncogene protein: Catalytic domain of human c-H-*ras* p21. Science 239:888–893, 1988
306. Klein G: The approaching era of the tumor suppressor genes. Science 238:1539–1545, 1987
307. Lee M-S, Chang K-S, Cabanillas F, et al: Detection of minimal residual cells carrying the t(14;18) by DNA sequence amplification. Science 237:175–178, 1987
308. Crescenzi M, Seto M, Herzig GP, et al: Thermophilic polymerase chain amplification of t(14;18) breakpoints and the detection of minimal residual disease. Proc Natl Acad Sci USA (in press)
309. Miser JS, Kinsella TJ, Triche TJ, et al: Treatment of peripheral neuroepithelioma in children and young adults. J Clin Oncol 5:1752–1758, 1987
310. Hayward WS, Neel BG, Astrin SM: Activation of a cellular *onc* gene by promoter insertion in ALV-induced lymphoid leukosis. Nature 290:475, 1981
311. Payne GS, Bishop JM, Varmus HE: Multiple arrangements of viral DNA and an activated host oncogene in bursal lymphomas. Nature 295:209, 1982
312. Neil JC, Hughes D, McFarlane R, Wilkie NM: Transduction and rearrangement of the *myc* gene by feline leukaemia virus in naturally occurring T-cell leukaemias. Nature 308:814, 1984
313. Schen-Ong GLC, Morse HC III, Potter M, et al: Two modes of c-*myb* activation in virus-induced mouse myeloid tumors. Mol Cell Biol 6:380, 1986
314. Silver J, Kozak C: Common proviral integration region on mouse chromosome in lymphomas and myelogenous leukemias induced by Friend murine leukemia virus. J Virol 57:526, 1986
315. Canaani E, Dreazen O, Klar A, et al: Activation of the c-*mos* oncogene in a mouse plasmacytoma by insertion of an endogenous intracisternal A-particle genome. Proc Natl Acad Sci USA 80:7118, 1983
316. Voronova AF, Sefton BM: Expression of a new tyrosine protein kinase is stimulated by retrovirus promoter insertion. Nature 319:682, 1986
317. Marth JD, Peet R, Krebs EG, et al: A lymphocyte-specific protein-tyrosine kinase gene is rearranged and overexpressed in the murine T cell lymphoma LSTRA. Cell 43:393, 1985
318. Tsichlis PN, Strauss PG, Hu LF: A common region for proviral DNA integration in MoMuLV-induced rat thymic lymphomas. Nature 302:445, 1983
319. Villeneuve L, Rassart E, Jolicoeur P, et al: Proviral integration site *Mis*-1 in rat thymomas corresponds to the *pvt*-1 translocation breakpoint in murine plasmacytomas. Mol Cell Biol 6:1834, 1986
320. Cuypers HT, Selten G, Quint W, et al: Murine leukemia virus-induced T-cell lymphomagenesis: Integration of proviruses in a distinct chromosomal region. Cell 37:141, 1984
321. Mucenski ML, Taylor BA, Ihle JN, et al: Identification of a common ecotropic viral integration site, *Evi*-1, in the DNA of AKXD murine myeloid tumors. Mol Cell Biol 8:301, 1988
322. Buchberg AM, Bedigian HG, Taylor BA, et al: Localization of Evi-2 to Chromosome 11: Linkage to other proto-oncogene and growth factor loci using interspecific backcross mice. Oncogene Res (in press)
323. Nishizawa M, Semba K, Yoshida MC, et al: Structure, expression and chromosomal location of the human c-*fgr* gene. Mol Cell Biol 76:511, 1986
324. Nau MM, Brooks BJ, Battey J, et al: L-*myc*, a new *myc*-related gene amplified and expressed in human small lung cancer. Nature 318:69, 1985
325. Rabin M, Watson M, Barker PE, et al: N-*ras* transforming gene maps to region p11-p13 on chromosome 1 by *in situ* hybridization. Cytogenet Cell Genet 38:70, 1984
326. Rowley JD: Biological implications of consistent chromosome rearrangements in leukemia and lymphoma. Cancer Res 44:3159, 1984
327. Barbacid M: Personal communication
328. Brownell E, Kozak CA, Fowle JR, et al: Comparative genetic mapping of cellular *rel* sequences in man, mouse, and the domestic cat. Am J Hum Genet 39:194, 1986
329. Bonner T, O'Brien SJ, Nash WG, et al: The human homologous of *raf* (*mil*) oncogene are located on human chromosomes 3 and 4. Science 223:71, 1984
330. Roussel MF, Sherr CJ, Barker PE, et al: Molecular cloning of the c-*fms* locus and its assignment to human chromosome 5. J Virol 48:770, 1983
331. Nagarajan L, Louis E, Twsujimoto Y, et al: Localization of the human *pim* oncogene (PIM) to a region of chromosome 6 involved in translocations in acute leukemias. Proc Natl Acad Sci USA 83:2556, 1986
332. Rabin M, Birnbaum D, Young D, et al: Human *ros*1 and *mas* 1 oncogenes located in regions of chromosome 6 associated with tumor-specific rearrangements. Oncogene Res 1:169, 1987
333. Harper ME, Franchini G, Love J, et al: Chromosomal sublocalization of human c-*myb* and c-*fes* cellular *onc* genes. Nature 304:169, 1983
334. Spurr NK, Solomon E, Jansson M, et al: Chromosomal localization of the human homologues to the oncogenes v-*erb*A and B. EMBO J 3:159, 1984
335. Park M, Testa JR, Blair DG, et al: Two rearranged *met* alleles in MMNG-HOS cells reveal the orientation of *met* on chromosome 7 to other markers tightly linked to the cystic fibrosis locus. Proc Natl Acad Sci USA (in press)
336. Caubet J-F, Mathieu-Mahul D, Berhneim A, et al: Human proto-oncogene c-*mos* maps to 8q11. EMBO J 4:2245, 1985
337. De Martinville B, Giacalone J, Shih C, et al: Oncogene from human EJ bladder carcinoma is located on the short arm of chromosome 11. Science 219:498, 1983
338. Horn TM, Huebner K, Croce C, et al: Chromosomal locations of members of a family of novel endogenous human retroviral genomes. J Virol 58:955, 1986
339. Detaisne C, Gegonne A, Stehelin D, et al: Chromosomal localization of the human proto-oncogene c-*ets*. Nature 310:581, 1984
340. McBride OW, Swan DC, Tronick SR, et al: Regional chromosomal location of N-*ras*, K-*ras*-1, K-*ras*-2 and *myb* oncogenes in human cells. Nucleic Acid Res 11:8221, 1983
341. Van't Veer LJ, Van Kessel AG, Van Heerikhuizen H, et al: Molecular cloning and chromosomal assignment of the human homolog of *int*-1, a mouse gene implicated in mammary tumorigenesis. Mol Cell Biol 4:2532, 1984
342. Barker PE, Rabin M, Watson M, et al: Human c-*fos* oncogene mapped within chromosomal region 14q21-q31. Proc Natl Acad Sci USA 81:5826, 1984
343. McBride OW, Merry D, Givol D: The gene for human p53 cellular tumor antigen is located on chromosome 17 short arm (17p13). Proc Natl Acad Sci USA 83:130, 1986
344. Semba K, Yamanashi Y, Nishikawa M, et al: Location of the c-*yes* gene on the human chromosome and its expression in various tissues. Science 227:1038, 1985
345. Sakaguchi AY, Naylor SL, Shows TB: A sequence homologous to Rous sarcoma virus v-*src* is on human chromosome 20. Prog Nucleic Acid Res Mol Biol 29:279, 1983
346. Watson DK, Sacchi N, McWilliams-Smith MJ, et al: The avian and mammalian *ets* genes: Molecular characterization, chromosome mapping and implication in human leukemia. Anticancer Res 6:631–636, 1986
347. Dalla Favera R, Gallo RC, Giallongo A, et al: Chromosomal localization of the human homolog (c-*sis*) of the simian sarcoma virus *onc* gene. Science 218:686, 1982
348. Erikson J, Finan J, Nowell PC, et al: Translocation of immunoglobuin VH genes in Burkitt lymphoma. Proc Natl Acad Sci USA 79:5611, 1982
349. Lenoir GM, Preud'Homme JL, Bernheim A, et al: Correlation between immunoglobin light chain expression and variant translocation in Burkitt's lymphoma. Nature 298:474, 1982
350. Sandberg A, Kohno S, Wake N, et al: Chromosome and causation of human cancer and leukemia: XLII. Cancer Genet Cytogenet 2:145, 1980
351. Vande Woude GF, Gilden RV: Principles of cancer biology: The molecular biology of cancer. In DeVita VT Jr, Hellman S, Rosenberg SA (eds): Cancer: Principles and Practices of Oncology, vol 2, pp 23–47. Philadelphia, JB Lippincott, 1985
352. Besmer P, Murphy JE, George PC, et al: A new acute transforming feline retrovirus and relationship of its oncogene v-*kit* with the protein kinase gene family. Nature 320:415, 1986
353. Robbins KC, Devare SG, Reddy EP, et al: *In vivo* identification of the transforming gene product of simian sarcoma virus. Science 218:1131, 1982

ANITA B. ROBERTS
MICHAEL B. SPORN

CHAPTER 5 Principles of Molecular Cell Biology of Cancer: Growth Factors Related to Transformation

This chapter reviews the role of peptide growth factors and their receptors in the control of cell differentiation and proliferation. Study of peptide growth factors and their role in malignant transformation is important because it is likely that control of the expression of growth factors eventually will lead to new modalities of cancer prevention or therapy.

In the broadest sense, this approach to prevention or therapy rests on the assumption that cancer is a disease of abnormal cell differentiation, in some cases of arrested cell differentiation.[1–3] Fundamental to this approach are the concepts that neoplasms are caricatures of normal processes of tissue development and renewal[1] and that the malregulated expression of developmentally relevant cellular genes appears to underlie all cancers.[2] It is becoming increasingly clear that many critical developmental phenomena in both normal and malignant tissues are mediated by peptide growth factors and that study of these agents is now of major significance in cancer biology.[4–6]

To understand the role of peptide growth factors in either the genesis of cancer or its prevention and reversal, one must first consider the oncogene concept. Bishop has summarized this concept as follows:[7]

> It now appears likely that normal cells bear the seeds of their own destruction in the form of cancer genes, whose anomalous activities mediate tumorigenesis. The term, cancer genes, is a convenience, of course, and is viewed by some as a misnomer: the loci in question may be physiologically essential constituents of the cell's genetic apparatus that become pathogenic only when their structure or control is disturbed by oncogenic agents.

Mintz and Fleischman have suggested that "the gene at issue [may be] any of the numerous "banal" or ordinary genes involved in cell growth and differentiation, rather than special or exotic cancer genes.[2] They have emphasized that

> there may be numerous "mundane" genes . . . in normal cells that might cause neoplastic conversion if they were made to function at levels above normal; genes of this sort might promote the growth and proliferation of initially normal stem cells beyond the usual period, thereby "locking" them into the stem-cell mode and making them unresponsive toward stimuli (*e.g.*, specific inducers) to differentiate.

Very recent work has shown that the expression of several different oncogenes within a cell may be needed to achieve tumorigenicity[8,9]; these molecular findings fit very well with classical concepts of initiation-promotion and multistage carcinogenesis.[10] With the above as background, the significance of the peptides growth factors that control cell proliferation and differentiation becomes much clearer because recent discoveries have shown that oncogenes can control expression of certain peptide growth factors and their receptors and can alter their signaling pathways. In a broader sense, it can be considered that the genes for all peptide growth factors, their receptors, and intermediates in their signaling pathways have oncogenic potential.[11] In this chapter we will describe some fundamental properties of peptide growth factors and their receptors before discussing their relationships to oncogenes.

NATURE OF PEPTIDE GROWTH FACTORS AND THEIR RECEPTORS

The term growth factor is difficult to define because there is no consensus as to what properties allow a substance to be considered a growth factor.[12] In general parlance, growth factors are not the typical macronutrients and micronutrients that are well defined in biochemistry textbooks but rather are an ill-defined set of polypeptides that can modulate cell function and exert specific and potent growth regulatory action on target cells. In contrast to micronutrients that act within the cell, growth factors are secreted by cells and interact with specific, membrane-bound glycoprotein receptors that function as transducers of the signal generated by these effector substances. Growth factors are among the most potent known biological substances involved in control of cellular physiology; in many cell culture systems they are active at concentrations as low as 10^{-12}M, and amounts as small as a few picograms (one picogram is one millionth of a microgram) can induce a highly specific biological response. The specificity of the response is believed to reside in the membrane-bound receptor for the growth factor rather than in the growth factor itself. Several different although structurally related polypeptides may bind to the same receptor; for example, insulin and insulin-like growth factors (IGFs) may bind to either the insulin receptor or to IGF receptors.[13,14] The role of the polypeptide growth factor in binding to the receptor is to trigger the receptor to express its program; as Roth has succinctly expressed it, "The receptor has the message."[15]

Receptors for growth factors may be viewed as similar to allosteric enzymes that are in an inactive state until their ligands bind. This binding then triggers the functional activity of the receptor and its intrinsic enzymatic activity. Many of the important receptors for growth factors are now known to have growth factor-dependent tyrosine kinase activity.[6] While many of the polypeptide growth factors are relatively small (5000–25,000 molecular weight), highly stable molecules, typical receptors are much larger (150,000–350,000 molecular weight) and are much less stable, particularly when isolated. For example, during a typical isolation procedure, many growth factors can be subjected to very harsh conditions such as exposure to strong acid, organic solvents such as ethanol, propanol, or acetonitrile, or high temperatures without loss of biological activity. In contrast, receptor molecules, which are integral components of the cell membrane, will often be irreversibly inactivated by such rigorous treatment, and much gentler conditions are required for their isolation in a physiologically active state. Consequently, because it has been much more difficult to purify receptors than growth factors, knowledge of the molecular properties of receptors is at present much more limited. However, new chemical methods of purification involving affinity chromatography, monoclonal antibodies, and nonionic detergents used to solubilize receptors have recently allowed the purification of the receptors for many of the polypeptide growth factors. Although certain receptors are known to have specific enzymatic activities (such as tyrosine kinase activity),[6,16] very little is known about the mechanism whereby the signal from the receptor is transduced into a specific biological response within the cell itself. Since both the effector and its receptor are often internalized after the binding of the effector, it is possible that the only role of the effector is to translocate the receptor (or a fragment of the receptor) to another compartment of the cell, where its intrinsic enzymatic activity may be manifested.

It is now beginning to be appreciated that most growth factors are multifunctional and can act on a broad range of target cells.[17] Thus not only can they stimulate cell proliferation, but also, under appropriate conditions, they can inhibit cell proliferation or have effects on cell function unrelated to proliferation. Indeed, a specific polypeptide growth factor that may be a potent mitogenic agent in one cellular context may have an entirely different function in another. For example, epidermal growth factor (EGF), a potent mitogen for fibroblasts throughout the body, has recently been identified in the central nervous system of both immature and adult rats, where it has been suggested that it functions as a neurotransmitter substance in the brain.[18] Many other small polypeptides of the gut, which in some contexts may have growth factor activity, likewise may be functioning in the brain as neurotransmitter substances.[19] In a similar vein, transforming growth factor-beta (TGF-beta), which acts synergistically with EGF to enhance mitogenesis of a rat kidney fibroblast cell line (NRK cell line) when grown in soft agar, acts antagonistically to EGF and thus is an antimitogenic agent for the human lung cancer cell line A-549 when it is grown in soft agar.[20]

Another important concept is that the action of any growth factor is not an intrinsic property of that individual peptide but rather a property of a set of conditions that are operant on a cell at a particular time.[17] That set of conditions includes not only the various growth factors to which the cell is exposed but also the extracellular environment of the cell. Thus, in a defined rat fibroblastic cell line (FR3T3, *myc* transfected), TGF-beta synergizes with one growth factor, platelet-derived growth factor (PDGF), to promote anchorage-independent growth but antagonizes the mitogenic effects of a second growth factor (EGF) and suppresses anchorage-independent growth.[20] Moreover, while TGF-beta may be mitogenic for cells growing under anchorage-independent conditions (in soft agar culture), it may be antimitogenic for the same cells (with the same set of added growth factors) growing under anchorage-dependent conditions (in monolayer cultures on a plastic surface).[20] It is difficult, therefore, to be rigid about defining the action of any particular polypeptide growth factor. Rather what appears to have happened during evolution is that polypeptide effectors and their corresponding receptors, which have exquisitely high affinity and specificity for each other and are classic "lock and key" signaling systems, have been used for many different purposes in many different cells throughout the body. Under some circumstances the signal generated by the effector-receptor complex may be mitogenic, whereas under other circumstances the signal may be antimitogenic; the signal may also be used in yet other circumstances for purposes that have nothing to do with the control of the cell cycle.[17]

With an understanding of the multifunctionality of growth factors comes the realization that the names of most growth factors are misnomers. Growth factors have traditionally been named within the context of their original discovery, which may have little to do with their ultimate physiologic role or even with their total tissue distribution. For example, EGF clearly is a highly potent agent for stimulating growth and multiplication of fibroblastic cells, as well as epidermal and other epithelial cells.[21,22] In some situations, EGF can also be a potent antimitogenic agent, as is the case with the A431 human vulvar squamous carcinoma cell line.[23] In another example, polypeptides very similar in structure (perhaps identical) to PDGF have recently been found in cells other than platelets, such as endothelial cells, vascular smooth muscle cells, and many different types of tumor cells.[24] Yet another growth factor that is misnamed is TGF-beta (originally discovered in a phenotypic transformation assay in cell culture), which has been found in high concentration in platelets and would appear to have a physiologic role in promotion of wound healing.[25] It is apparent that the descriptive value of the names of polypeptide growth factors is no greater than the descriptive value of the names of the investigators who discovered them.

AUTOCRINE SECRETION OF GROWTH FACTORS AND CANCER

Autocrine secretion (Fig. 5-1) is an important new concept that is emerging as a unifying theme in studies of the role of polypeptide growth factors in malignancy.[26–28] It has been known for many years that malignant cells in culture require fewer exogenous growth factors for optimal growth and multiplication than do their normal counterparts.[29,30] One explanation is that malignant cells are relatively independent of exogenous growth factors because they are capable of endogenous synthesis of their own growth factors. In 1978, De Larco and Todaro[31] suggested that the endogenous production of polypeptide growth factors, which act on their producer cells via functional external receptors, could be responsible for the malignant transformation of cells. To the extent that a cell is dependent on an exogenous supply of growth factors, provided by endocrine secretion (via the blood) or paracrine secretion (from an adjacent cell), its growth can be controlled by regulating that supply. However, if a cell acquires the ability to produce its own growth factors and has the functional receptors for them (this process has been called autocrine secretion),[26–28] it then is under less-stringent external growth control and has a selective growth advantage over neighboring cells, which are still subject to external regulation.

FIG. 5-1. Diagrammatic representation of endocrine, paracrine, and autocrine secretion. Peptide growth factors are shown in latent form within the cell. The thickened, semicircular regions of the cell membrane represent receptor sites.[26]

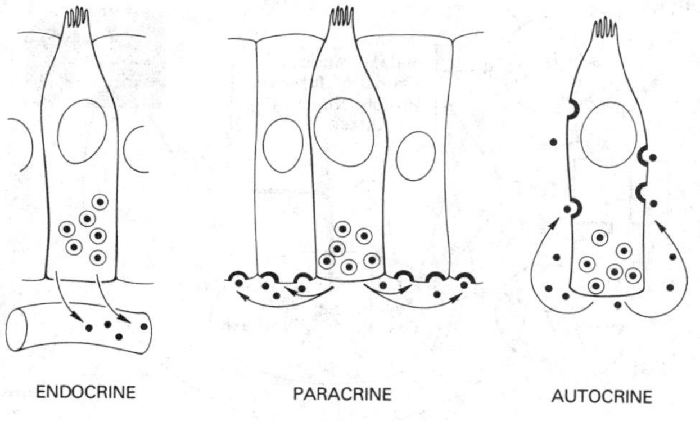

Autocrine action of growth factors in cancer cells was first shown in rat and mouse cells transformed by Moloney and Kirsten sarcoma viruses.[31] When grown in culture, these tumor cells were found to release polypeptides resembling EGF (originally called "sarcoma growth factor") into the extracellular medium. These polypeptides had the important property of causing reversible, phenotypic transformation (anchorage-independent growth in soft agar) of non-neoplastic indicator cells, and this transformation assay has been used as a primary method for screening and purifying the entire set of "transforming growth factors."[32] It soon became apparent that the EGF-like peptides released by the virally transformed cells were not the same as EGF itself, although their mechanism of action was mediated by binding to the EGF receptor. These EGF-like peptides have subsequently been called type-alpha transforming growth factors (TGF-alpha); their entire amino acid sequences have been determined and their genes cloned from both human and rodent sources. A wide variety of tumor cells, of both human and rodent origin, are now known to synthesize and release TGF-alpha, and it is believed that the autocrine action of this polypeptide growth factor plays an important role in the malignant behavior of these cells.[33]

Other polypeptide growth factors known to have an autocrine action are PDGF[34] and bombesin, the small tetradecapeptide secreted by human small cell lung cancer cells (SCLC).[35] The data on the autocrine action of PDGF are particularly impressive. Several human osteosarcoma and glioma cell lines are known to produce PDGF-like substances that are believed to mediate their abnormal growth. Antisera to PDGF have been shown to block the growth of rodent tumor cells transformed by simian sarcoma virus; these data strongly suggest that the synthesis of PDGF-like molecules is one of the primary factors responsible for the malignant behavior of the transformed cells.[36] Likewise, as illustrated in Figure 5-2, antibodies to bombesin inhibit both the in vitro clonal growth of SCLC cells and the growth of xenografts of these cells in nude mice, suggesting that they have interfered with an essential autocrine pathway responsible for the uncontrolled growth of the tumor cells.[35]

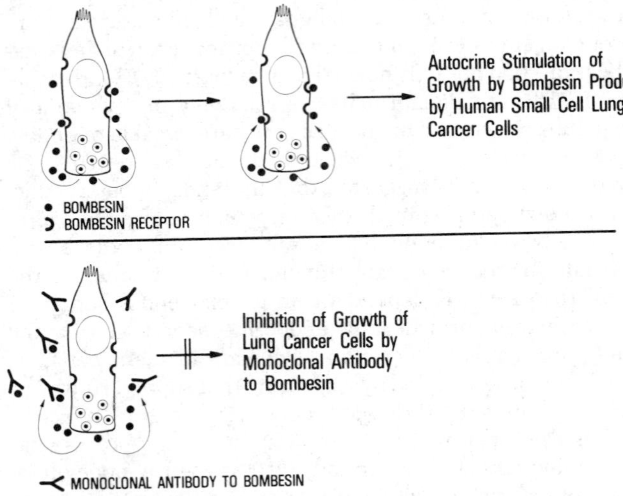

FIG. 5-2. Inhibition of growth of human small cell lung cancer cells by monoclonal antibodies to bombesin.[140]

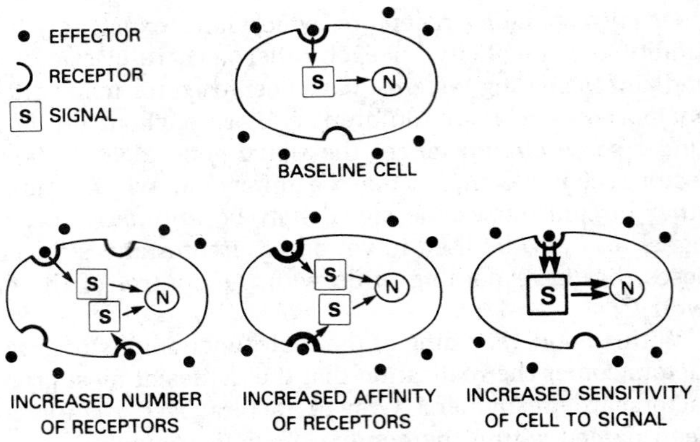

FIG. 5-3. Mechanisms for increasing receptivity of a cell to a peptide growth factor.

Although we have discussed the importance of autocrine secretion and action of growth factors on the cancer cell, it should not be assumed that autocrine phenomena pertain only to tumor cells. During growth and tissue injury of vascular endothelium and vascular smooth muscle, there is substantial autocrine secretion of PDGF-like molecules.[37] It is likely that embryonic, rapidly growing, or injured tissues are all capable of autocrine secretion of growth factors and that this is an entirely normal physiologic response. The pathologic aspect of autocrine secretion in the cancer cell should be viewed as the continuous inappropriate expression of the polypeptide growth factors or the constant hypersensitivity of the cancer cell to its own growth factors, by mechanisms that will be discussed later.

Although it is apparent that the autocrine concept can be the basis of the uncontrolled growth of tumor cells, paracrine action of tumor growth factors on cellular components of tumor stroma also clearly plays a role in development of the malignancy.[38,39] Thus, for example, fibroblast growth factor (FGF) stimulates the growth of endothelial cells, in that way promoting neovascularization of the tumor,[40] and TGF-beta stimulates fibroblasts to elaborate connective tissue.[25] Such indirect effects of growth factors on tumor growth will be discussed in greater detail later.

Although the original autocrine hypothesis stressed the production of growth factors by tumor cells, it is now clear that the tumor cell may also achieve the same type of autonomy by modification of the synthesis of receptors for growth factors or by alteration of the postreceptor signaling pathway for a particular growth factor rather than by a direct increase in the synthesis and release of the growth factor itself.[27] Thus, as shown in Figure 5-3 (left), increased receptiveness to stimulation by a peptide growth factor may result from either an increased number of receptors on the surface of a cell or an increased affinity of the receptors for the peptide (Fig. 5-3, middle). Either or both of these mechanisms have been shown to be operative in human squamous cell carcinomas of the head and neck or vulva that have been grown in cell culture. These cells have either extremely high numbers of receptors for EGF[41] or receptors with unusually high affinity for EGF.[42] A third subset of increased sensitivity (Fig. 5-3, right) is the possibility that the availability, number, or affinity of effector or receptor molecules is not altered in a cancer cell but that it becomes more sensitive to the signal generated by the effector-receptor complex (*i.e.*, that there is greater amplification of the signal generated by a peptide growth factor occupying a specific receptor). Signaling cascades are known to involve such intermediates as ion transport channels, phosphoinositol metabolites, protein kinase C, and ribosomal S6 kinase; in addition, activation of nuclear expression of the *myc* and *fos* proto-oncogenes follows mitogenic stimulation of cells (Fig. 5-4). The sequence of events that link the membrane tyrosine kinase activity, the cytoplasmic signals, and the nuclear signals is not yet understood. However, the overlap between activation of these signals by growth factors and by oncogenes suggests that

FIG. 5-4. Diagrammatic representation of intermediates thought to function in intracellular signalling pathways of growth factors. Indicated are cytoplasmic and nuclear elements known to become activated or elevated in concentration following binding of mitogenic peptides to receptors that have tyrosine kinase activity; the sequence of events is not known. In contrast, a growth inhibitor like TGF-beta appears to signal through distinct pathways; treatment of mitogenically stimulated cells with TGF-beta blocks DNA synthesis without interfering with any of the signals generated by the mitogenic growth factors.[25,115,182]

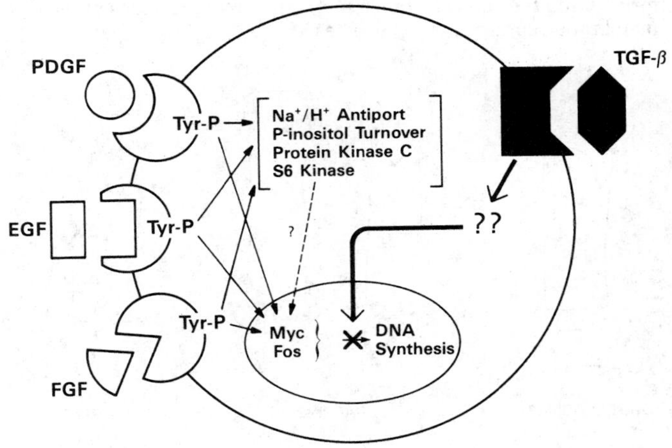

increased sensitivity to signals might result from background oncogene activity; we have already noted that peptide growth factors and oncogene expression may generate similar signals, for example, tyrosine kinase activity. In this way, one can understand how the activities of certain peptide growth factors and oncogenes are permissive for each other.

NEGATIVE GROWTH FACTORS: A REVISED AUTOCRINE HYPOTHESIS

A significant recent finding is that the signaling pathway activated by an autocrine polypeptide may evoke a negative growth response rather than a positive one. The best example of such a negative growth factor is TGF-beta, which has been shown to be a bifunctional regulator of cell growth.[20,25] Interestingly, the signaling pathways of TGF-beta and perhaps of other negative growth regulators appear to be distinct from those of mitogenic peptides whose receptors have intrinsic tyrosine kinase activity; thus, as shown in Figure 5-4, TGF-beta blocks DNA synthesis in cells treated simultaneously with such mitogens without impairing any of the signals they generate.[25] The discovery of the identity of TGF-beta with a growth inhibitor produced by monkey kidney cells demonstrates the existence of negative autocrine pathways, since the monkey kidney cells that produce TGF-beta have receptors for it and respond with an inhibition of cell growth.[43,44] The concept of a cell producing its own growth inhibitory substances is old, but it lacked experimental support until this demonstration of the identity of a growth inhibitor with a homogeneous polypeptide of known amino acid sequence.

Based on these new findings, we have recently suggested that the autocrine hypothesis be extended to include the concept that malignant transformation may be the result not only of excessive production, expression, and action of positive autocrine growth factors, but also of the failure of cells to synthesize, express, or respond to specific negative growth factors that the cells ordinarily release to control their own growth.[27] This loss of negative growth control might be the result of a biochemical lesion in the growth inhibitor, a failure of cells to effectively process and release the inhibitor, a loss or defect of the receptors or the postreceptor signaling pathway for the negative effector, or the failure of cells to activate the release negative growth factor. Examples of two of these mechanisms can be found in the response of transformed cells to TGF-beta. As an example of failure of cells to activate a released negative effector, human lung carcinoma cells (A549) are unable to activate the latent, biologically inactive, TGF-beta that they secrete; however, their growth is inhibited by exogenous active TGF-beta, demonstrating that the receptors and signaling pathways are still functional.[45] An example of alterations in signaling pathways, which have made transformed cells refractory to inhibition by TGF-beta, is found in hepatocytes transformed in vitro by aflatoxin; these cells no longer respond to TGF-beta even though the parental cells, from which they were derived, are exquisitely sensitive to inhibition by TGF-beta.[46] Finally, as an example of cells that have escaped from negative growth control by loss of receptors for TGF-beta, a human squamous cell carcinoma, SCC-25, is not inhibited by TGF-beta and has no detectable cell surface receptors for the factor; in contrast, the growth of normal human prokeratinocytes, which do have TGF-beta receptors, is strongly inhibited by the peptide.[47]

RELATIONSHIPS BETWEEN GROWTH FACTORS AND ONCOGENES

During the past 7 years, two fields of scientific investigation, which had previously been unrelated to each other, have merged into a single domain. As recently as 1980, it was not generally appreciated that there is any significant relationship between polypeptide growth factors and oncogenes. A series of major scientific discoveries has altered this belief, so that it is now almost impossible to discuss the topic of growth factors without immediate reference to oncogenes; conversely, any contemporary review of oncogenes must consider the role of growth factors in their ultimate phenotypic expression. One way to conceptualize the role of oncogenes in causation of cancer is to state that oncogenes confer growth factor autonomy on cells. In this conceptual framework, autocrine secretion and action of growth factors play a central role. The interplay of oncogenes and growth factors occurs at every level: the growth factor itself, the receptor for the growth factor, and the pathways whereby the signal generated by the binding of the growth factor to its receptor is transmitted to the nucleus of the cell. These relationships, some of which will be described in detail, are summarized in Figure 5-5.

The first significant linking of growth factor research and oncogene research came in 1981 when Cohen, Erikson, Hunter, and colleagues[48–50] showed that there is a common enzymatic mechanism shared by the receptor for EGF and the transforming protein, pp60^{src}, encoded by the Rous sarcoma virus oncogene, *src*. In this case, it was found that two apparently unrelated phenomena—namely, a biochemical mechanism whereby a receptor for a growth factor causes a signal to be transduced across the plasma membrane of the cell and a biochemical mechanism whereby the unique transforming protein of an oncogenic virus exerts its effects—were one and the same, that is, a mechanism to initiate enzymatic activity with the capacity to phosphorylate a variety of target proteins on tyrosine residues. Subsequently, it has been found that several other important growth factor receptors, including those for insulin,[51] insulin-like growth factor I (IGF-I),[52] and PDGF[53] are also tyrosine kinases (*i.e.*, they induce phosphorylation of tyrosine residues on target proteins). Moreover, it is now known that the gene products of numerous oncogenes other than *src*, including the *fps, yes, ros, abl,* and *fes* genes, are also tyrosine kinases.[6,16]

In 1983, a second major discovery linking growth factors and oncogenes was announced independently by two research groups. They found that the simian sarcoma virus (*sis*) oncogene codes for the production of a polypeptide that has striking sequence homology with the B chain of PDGF.[54,55] Further studies have confirmed the importance of this work, and it is now known that the N-terminal 109 amino acid residues of the B chain of PDGF are almost identical with the sequence of the transforming protein produced by simian sarcoma virus.[56]

A third important discovery linking growth factors and oncogenes was the 1984 report of major sequence homology

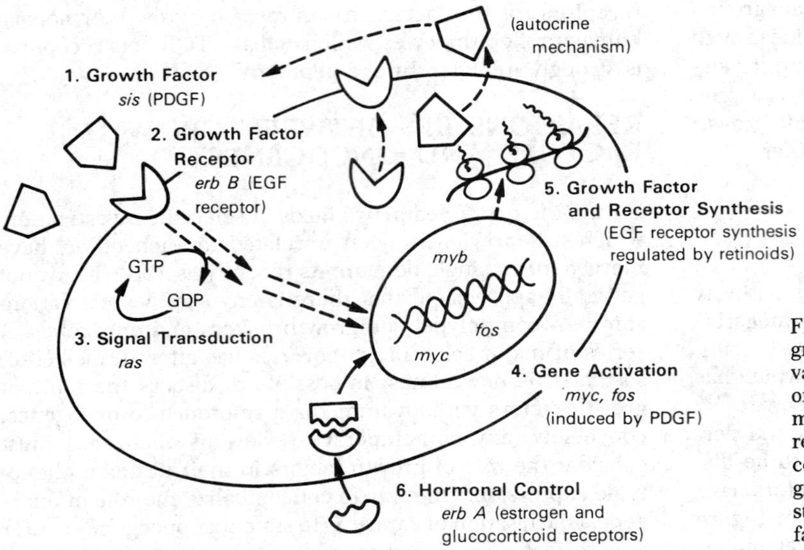

FIG. 5-5. Hierarchic levels of interaction between growth factors and oncogenes. Many oncogenes activate biochemical pathways that facilitate expression of peptide growth factors in an autocrine loop; intermediates include the growth factors (process 1), their receptors (process 2), and signalling pathways (processes 3 and 4). Also shown are mechanisms whereby growth-regulatory molecules such as retinoids and steroids interact with oncogenes and peptide growth factors (processes 5 and 6).

between the receptor for EGF and the viral *erbB* oncogene.[57,58] In this case, the viral oncogene codes for a protein that strikingly resembles the transmembrane and cytoplasmic (tyrosine kinase) domains of the EGF receptor. The protein encoded by *erb*B lacks the portion of the EGF receptor believed to be responsible for the extracellular binding of the ligand, EGF, to the receptor itself. This virally coded "truncated receptor" is believed to be able to generate a mitogenic signal, even in the absence of its natural ligand. It is as if the truncation of the receptor has short-circuited the normal physiologic mechanism for controlling its activity, and the truncated receptor is now permanently turned on, even though no EGF may be present.

A fourth major advance was the demonstration that a specific growth factor, PDGF, can control the expression of specific oncogenes, *myc* and *fos*.[59–61] *Myc* and *fos* both code for nuclear proteins that are believed to have some critical function, as yet unknown, in control of the cell cycle.[62] In particular, the expression of *myc* in turn appears to make a cell more sensitive to the effects of other growth factors, such as EGF.[63] It had been known for some time from the work of Stiles and colleagues[64] that PDGF exerts a permissive action for other growth factors such as EGF or IGF-I. The terms competence and progression have been used to describe this phenomenon, implying that PDGF induces a state of competence in the cell, so that it can respond to a mitogen such as EGF or IGF-I and progress through the cell cycle. The discovery that the action of two oncogenes, *myc* and *fos*, are involved in this process, is yet another example of intimate relationships between growth factors and oncogenes.

These four discoveries have had an overwhelming impact on growth factor and oncogene research. They have made clear that it is no longer possible to separate the two fields conceptually and that the most likely path for future advances will be elucidation of the various mechanisms whereby growth factors control the expression of oncogenes, and oncogenes in turn control the expression of growth factors.

PROPERTIES OF SPECIFIC GROWTH FACTORS: RELEVANCE TO CANCER

Specific, well-defined polypeptide growth factors play a prominent role in control of cellular proliferation, cellular differentiation, and cellular function.[5,6,12,16] A tumor is a complex tissue composed not only of the tumor cells themselves but also of the stromal elements, including inflammatory cells, fibroblasts, and endothelial cells.[38,39] Therefore, consideration of the roles that these growth factors play in carcinogenesis must take into account which specific cell types are secreting a particular growth factor and which specific cells types can respond to the growth factor. In some instances, stimulation of the proliferation of tumor cells by growth factors may be a direct result of autocrine action of these peptides on the tumor cells; however, in other cases it may be indirect via paracrine stimulation of the supporting stromal elements, as evidenced by increased elaboration of connective tissue and increased neovascularization, or by suppression of immune surveillance. Table 5-1 provides a selected listing of several of the most thoroughly characterized of these peptides that have been demonstrated to play a role in cellular transformation. It is not meant to be comprehensive because peptides such as colony stimulating factors, interleukins, and interferons, which principally control the function of cells of haematopoietic lineages, will not be considered in this chapter. Categorization of polypeptide growth factors into families is based on their chemical structure; receptor and antibody cross-reactivity also may be found within families of growth factors. A brief discussion of each family of growth factors and its mechanistic link to carcinogenesis follows.

TABLE 5-1. Polypeptide Growth Factors Related to Transformation

Growth Factor	Source	Target Tissue	Biological Activity	Molecular Weight (daltons): Growth Factor	Molecular Weight (daltons): Membrane Receptor	Human Chromosomal Location: Growth Factor	Human Chromosomal Location: Receptor	References (cloning)
Insulin Family								
Insulin	β-Islet cells of pancreas	Liver, adipose, muscle	Supports growth, modulates metabolism of lipids, amino acids, and sugars	5,800	350,000	11	19	(171,172)
IGF-1 and IGF-II	Human plasma	Liver, adipose, muscle, cartilage, fibroblasts	Insulin-like metabolic effects; mitogens; stimulate incorporation of sulfate into cartilage proteoglycans	I:7,600 II:7,500	I:350,000 II:250,000	12 11	15 ?	(173,174) (175,176)
EGF Family								
EGF	Mouse submaxilary gland, human urine	Epidermal cells, fibroblasts, epithelial cells	Mitogen, promotes keratinization, inhibits gastric acid secretion	6,200	180,000	4	7	(86,87)
TGF-alpha	Transformed cells	Identical to EGF	Identical to EGF	5,500	180,000	2	7	(178)
PDGF Family								
Dimers of A and B chains	α-Granules platelets	Fibroblasts, smooth muscle cells, glial	Supports growth of various mesenchymal cells, chemotactic agent	28,000–35,000	200,000	A: 7 B: 22	5 5	(107) (54,55)
TGF-beta Family								
TGF-beta 1 and 2	α-Granules platelets	All cell types	Often inhibits growth, augments matrix accumulation, chemotactic	25,000	500,000	1: 19 2: ?	? ?	(179) (180*)
MIS	Testis	Müllerian duct	Inhibits growth of cells derived from the Müllerian duct	54,000	?	?	?	(121)
FGF Family								
aFGF bFGF	Brain Pituitary	All cell types	Mitogenic for cells of mesodermal and neuroectodermal origin	17,000 17,000	125,000 145,000	5 4	? ?	(134) (133)

(continued)

TABLE 5-1. Polypeptide Growth Factors Related to Transformation *(Continued)*

Growth Factor	*Source*	*Target Tissue*	*Biological Activity*	*Molecular Weight (daltons)*		*Human Chromosomal Location*		*References (cloning)*
				Growth Factor	*Membrane Receptor*	*Growth Factor*	*Receptor*	
Bombesin/GRP								
Bombesin	Frog skin	Many epithelial and mesenchymal cells	Mitogenic for gastrointestinal, respiratory tract, and 3T3 cells	1,400	?	?	?	(181*)
GRP	Porcine gut			2,700	?	?	?	(139*)

*Reference to amino acid sequence.

INSULIN FAMILY

Several polypeptide growth factors belong to the insulin family, including, in addition to insulin, the insulin-like growth factors IGF-I and IGF-II, nerve growth factor (NGF), and relaxin.[65-68] Human somatomedin C has been shown to be identical with IGF-I.[69] Of these five peptides, all except relaxin have been implicated in carcinogenesis. Insulin and the IGFs have similar biologic activities (generally stimulating growth and cellular metabolism) and a high degree of structural relatedness, including conservation of all three disulfide bonds.[70] The insulin and IGF-I receptors have a similar subunit structure, and the two ligands show a limited degree of receptor cross-reactivity.[13,14] Each receptor has associated with it tyrosine kinase activity that when activated leads to phosphorylation of various cellular proteins including autophosphorylation of the beta subunits of the receptors for both of these peptides (the ligand binding sites are on the alpha subunits). In contrast, the IGF-II receptor has a distinct structure and no associated tyrosine kinase activity[13,14,71]; it cannot bind insulin, even with low affinity. However, treatment of responsive cells with insulin increases expression of IGF-II receptors. Thus the action of these three growth factors on cells is highly cooperative, given the receptor cross-reactivity and the inducibility of the IGF-II receptor by insulin.

There is now substantial evidence suggesting an involvement of IGF-II in a variety of embryonal neoplasms. Wilms' tumor (nephroblastoma), rhabdomyosarcoma, and hepatoblastoma all express significantly elevated levels of IGF-II mRNA relative to nonmalignant adult tissues.[72,73] The level of expression in the tumors is similar to that found in fetal tissues, consistent with the observations that IGF-II plays an important role in embryonic development.[74,75] The IGF-II gene has been localized to chromosome 11p, and loss of heterozygosity for 11p markers has been demonstrated in all three of these tumors that express elevated levels of IGF-II mRNA.[72,73] A human fibrosarcoma cell line that secretes IGF-II has also been described.[76] Whether IGF-II may contribute to the growth of any of these tumors is not known; however, it is to be expected that constitutive synthesis of a mitogenic peptide could provide a cell with significant growth advantage. Exogenous IGF-II can also act as a transforming growth factor in that it can induce phenotypic transformation of untransformed Balb/c cells as measured by their growth as colonies of cells in soft agar medium.[77]

Insulin is permissive for the actions of several polypeptide growth factors on cells in addition to IGF-II.[78,79] Also, both insulin and IGF-I receptors have tyrosine kinase activity that has specific features in common with the tyrosine kinase coded by the Rous sarcoma virus *src* oncogene.[51,52] Thus, in chick heart mesenchymal cells, insulin and EGF, which also stimulates tyrosine kinase activity, synergize to stimulate growth at the same level found in cells infected with Rous sarcoma virus.[80-82]

NGF, a structural homologue of proinsulin, binds to a unique receptor. Although its effects on growth of sympathetic neurons are well understood, the role of its increased secretion by a variety of tumor cells including melanoma, fibrosarcoma, and glioblastoma cells is not currently known.[67]

EPIDERMAL GROWTH FACTOR FAMILY

In addition to EGF (also called urogastrone), this family comprises the TGF-alphas[33,83-85] and possibly other less well-characterized peptides including putative EGF-like molecules encoded in the large messenger RNA transcript for EGF.[86,87] Two protein products of members of the poxvirus family, vaccinia virus protein[88] and a protein encoded by the Shope fibroma virus[89] also have significant homology to EGF and TGF-alpha in their amino acid sequences. Although the various members of this growth factor family share only limited amino acid sequence homology, the positions of all three disulfide bonds are conserved, as was found to be the case in the insulin family of growth factors.

With regard to the EGF family, there has thus far been identified only a single receptor species, the well-characterized EGF receptor, which binds all members of the family with nearly equal affinities[33,88-91]; thus, the infectivity of vaccinia virus can be blocked by pretreatment of the cells with EGF.[92] Like the insulin and IGF-I receptors, this receptor also has intrinsic tyrosine kinase activity that is activated by binding of its ligand; this kinase again has specific features in common with the tyrosine kinase domain of the *src* family of oncogenes.[48-50] All members of the family of tyrosine kinase associated oncogenes, including *src, fes, fps, fgr, abl*, and *erbB*, have in common a region of 250 amino acids which comprise the protein kinase domain. Moreover, the *erbB* oncogene of avian erythroblastosis virus has been shown to specifically represent the transmembrane portions and tyrosine kinase domains of the EGF receptor.[57,93–94] In the case of v-*erbB*, the extracellular ligand binding domain is missing from the receptor, leading to constitutive activation of the receptor in the absence of ligand binding.

Different types of human tumor cells overexpress the EGF receptor; these include glioblastomas and several squamous epidermoid carcinomas, of which the A431 cell line is representative.[41,95,96] In brain tumors of glial origin and in A431 cells there is amplification and rearrangement of the gene encoding the EGF receptor.[97] It is not known whether this plays a role in the development of the malignancy. However, a characteristic feature of human glioblastomas is an increase in the number of copies of chromosome 7, often with rearrangements[98]; since the EGF receptor maps to the short arm of chromosome 7, a relationship between effects on the EGF receptor and the malignant phenotype might be expected.[97]

Both EGF and TGF-alpha usually stimulate proliferation of target cells, and overexpression of either of these peptides has, in certain instances, been correlated with transformation. TGF-alpha was named on the basis of its ability to induce phenotypic transformation of non-neoplastic fibroblasts,[85] and EGF can potentiate the viral and chemical transformation of cultured cells.[99–101] Certain retrovirus-transformed cells and human tumor cell lines synthesize TGF-alpha, whereas their untransformed counterparts do not.[83,85,102] In addition, higher molecular weight peptides related to TGF-alpha are secreted in the urine of patients with tumors but not of controls.[103] However, the original concept that TGF-alpha secretion would be restricted to tumor cells has been disproved; TGF-alpha is secreted by normal bovine anterior pituitary cells in culture,[104,105] and transcriptional activity of TGF-alpha is high in the early mouse embryo.[106]

PLATELET-DERIVED GROWTH FACTOR FAMILY

This family of growth factors appears to be restricted to three homodimeric and heterodimeric combinations (AA,AB,BB) of the A and B chains of PDGF, each of which can cross-react with the same PDGF receptor, and each of which appears to have similar activity in stimulating growth of responsive cells.[24,107] The B chain of PDGF is 96% homologous with the putative transforming protein (p28^{sis}) of simian sarcoma virus (SSV),[54,55] and many different lines of evidence show that transformation induced by SSV is mediated by a PDGF-like growth factor.[24,36] To date, the PDGF B chain homodimer is the only growth factor for which there has been identified a corresponding oncogene product. The genes for both the B and the A chains of PDGF are expressed in tumor cells, principally glioma and osteosarcoma cell lines, although some tumor cells express exclusively A chain or B chain transcripts.[107] As with TGF-alpha, elevated urinary levels of proteins antigenically related to PDGF have been associated with some cancer patients.[108] However, secretion of PDGF is not unique to cancer cells; many normal cells also express these transcripts. Thus, activated macrophages express PDGF B chain transcripts, whereas rat skeletal myoblasts and arterial smooth muscle cells express only PDGF A chain transcripts.[109] Interestingly, a different splicing pattern of the A chain RNA has been found in glioma cells, which may lead to preferential secretion of A chain homodimers with markedly enhanced mitogenic activity.[110,111]

Like the other growth factor receptors described thus far, the PDGF receptor also has associated tyrosine kinase activity.[53,112,113] However, in contrast to the receptors for the insulin, EGF, and TGF-beta families of growth factors, which are more or less ubiquitous, PDGF receptor expression is highest in connective tissue cells, vascular smooth muscle cells, and glial cells; it is never found associated with epithelial or endothelial cells.[112] Nonetheless, PDGF secretion by tumor cells is not restricted to PDGF-responsive cells such as glioblastoma and sarcoma cells; certain bladder carcinoma cells, erythroleukemic cells, and leukemia cells, which do not display PDGF receptors, also secrete PDGF-like peptides.[24] This suggests either that secretion of PDGF by these cells is irrelevant to their transformation or that it may support tumor growth indirectly by acting on responsive connective tissue cells in the tumor stroma, as will be discussed in greater detail later.

TRANSFORMING GROWTH FACTOR-BETA FAMILY

The largest growth factor family is that of peptides structurally related to TGF-beta in terms of the homologous positioning of seven to nine cysteine residues, and recent discoveries suggest that yet more family members may be found.[25,114,115] Like PDGF, TGF-beta can exist in both homodimeric and heterodimeric combinations of TGF-beta 1 and 2 chains,[114] and the biologic activity of the dimers is identical in most systems studied[114,116] with only a few exceptions.[117] Other members of the family include the mammalian inhibins[118] and activins,[119,120] mullerian inhibitory substance (MIS),[121] and the predicted products of a pattern gene in *Drosophila* (decapentaplegic gene complex, DPP-C)[122] and of an amphibian gene, Vg1, expressed in oocytes.[123] Thus far, only TGF-beta 1 and 2 and MIS have been implicated in carcinogenesis.

The biologic activities of the TGF-betas are extremely diverse[25,115]; however, unlike the previously described growth factors, TGF-betas often inhibit cell growth and block the action of peptides belonging to the insulin, EGF, and PDGF families. TGF-beta is thought to play an important role in maintaining quiescence in adult tissues, being turned off during specific bursts of growth such as in the pubescent mammary gland[124] or in the regenerating liver.[125] Many of its effects are probably mediated through specific effects on elaboration of extracellular matrix proteins.[25,115]

TGF-beta 1 and 2 react with a unique cell membrane receptor[116,126] that is not yet well characterized like those of the insulin, EGF, and PDGF families, all of which have been cloned and sequenced. However, data suggest that it does not have an associated tyrosine kinase activity[127,128] and therefore probably signals through different intracellular pathways. The TGF-beta receptor is expressed on nearly all cell types, and transformed cells that overexpress the receptor have not been found.[45] Rather, control of TGF-beta activity probably is at the level of activation of the biologically inactive, latent, secreted form of TGF-beta.[45] Many tumors cells exhibit high levels of TGF-beta mRNA,[129] and most tumor cell lines secrete TGF-beta; however, these tumor cells are often refractory to growth control by the TGF-beta they secrete. For example, in human A549 lung carcinoma cells it has been shown that the uncontrolled growth of the cells results from their inability to activate the latent TGF-beta they secrete; growth of the cells is strongly inhibited by activated TGF-beta.[45] Other malignant cells seem to have escaped from the growth-inhibitory actions of TGF-beta by other mechanisms, since they are no longer responsive to active TGF-beta, in contrast to their untransformed counterparts that are inhibited by TGF-beta.[46,47] For these reasons, it has been suggested that TGF-beta secreted by tumor cells may support their growth indirectly by stimulating formation of tumor stroma.[115]

Another member of the TGF-beta family, MIS, a testicular product that causes regression of the mullerian ducts (the anlage of the female reproductive system) in the male embryo,[121] has been found to be inhibitory to the growth of epithelial ovarian carcinomas derived from these tissues.[130,131] Neoplastic progression of the serosal surface of the ovary in the adult recapitulates the development of the embryonic mullerian ducts. This finding suggests that MIS, as well as other yet undiscovered embryonic inhibitors, may herald a new therapeutic approach to tumors derived from their corresponding target tissues.[130]

FIBROBLAST GROWTH FACTOR FAMILY

Basic and acidic fibroblast growth factor (bFGF; aFGF) are two closely related single-chain peptides of approximately 16 kDa that act principally to stimulate mitogenesis in cells of mesodermal and neuroectodermal origin.[40,132] They are probably the most potent known stimulators of the growth of endothelial cells and as such have been postulated to play a role in neovascularization in vivo. Since the cloning and sequencing of the FGFs,[133,134] it has become apparent that many peptides of different cellular origin and ostensibly different biological activities are actually identical to the FGFs.[135] bFGF is synthesized by a wide variety of both normal and transformed cells, including chondrosarcoma, melanoma, rhabdomyosarcoma, hepatoma, retinoblastoma, and osteosarcoma; synthesis of aFGF appears to be more restricted but is also found in both normal and transformed cells. FGFs have high affinity for heparin, a property that has aided significantly in the purification of these peptides.[132] Evidence also suggests that FGF secreted from cells may be integrally associated with extracellular matrix, possibly complexed to heparan sulfate.[136] Both FGFs bind to the same receptors, glycosylated species of 125 and 145 kDa, although there is some evidence for preferential binding of aFGF and bFGF, respectively.[137] These receptors, like those for other mitogenic peptides such as insulin, EGF, and PDGF, are linked to tyrosine kinase activity.[138]

Although direct evidence is lacking, it seems clear that FGF will play a role in tumorigenesis. It is secreted by a wide variety of tumor cells, is a potent mitogen for many cell types of mesenchymal origin, and can stimulate angiogenesis. It may have autocrine effects on proliferation of tumor cells, as well as paracrine effects by stimulation of the neovascularization of the tumor.[40,135,136]

BOMBESIN/GASTRIN-RELEASING PEPTIDE

Bombesin is a tetradecapeptide purified initially from frog skin; it is homologous to the mammalian peptide gastrin-releasing peptide (GRP) that contains 27 amino acids[35,139]; both bind to the same receptor and elicit identical biological activities, including mitogenesis. There is clear evidence that these very small peptides play a pivotal role in control of the growth of human SCLCs.[35] These tumors have long been known to secrete a variety of regulatory peptides, including GRP. The central role of this peptide in autocrine control of tumor growth has been demonstrated by the finding that specific blocking monoclonal antibodies to GRP block both the clonal growth of SCLC in vitro and the growth of SCLC xenografts in vivo (see Fig. 5-2).[140] As in previous examples, it has been postulated that the role of GRP in SCLC reflects its possible role in fetal lung development. This is the first direct evidence that blocking of the autocrine action of a tumor cell mitogen might be useful therapeutically and suggests that peptide antagonists and antibodies that bind to growth factor receptors might be equally useful.

COOPERATIVE INTERACTIONS OF GROWTH FACTORS RELEVANT TO TRANSFORMATION

DIRECT FUNCTIONAL INTERACTIONS OF POLYPEPTIDE GROWTH FACTORS

Many polypeptide growth factors belonging to different structural families are functionally interactive.[141] Thus three distinct peptides—TGF-beta, a peptide related to EGF/TGF-alpha, and PDGF—all found in human platelets, cooperate in inducing phenotypic transformation of nonneoplastic fibroblasts.[142] The transformation response depends on the concentration of each of the three growth factors, and the aberrant expression of any one of them will predispose to transformation.[142] Conversely, as shown by the ability of monoclonal antibodies to bombesin/GRP to block growth of SCLC cells[140] and of monoclonal antibodies to the EGF receptor to block anchorage independent growth of fibroblastic indicator cells induced by the combined actions of EGF and TGF-beta,[143] blocking of one of the obligatory growth factors in a set is sufficient to block the response. Not only are many biological responses the result of the action of a set of growth factors, but also the direction of the response is determined by the particular set of growth factors acting on the cells, not by any intrinsic activity of the individual peptides. Thus, in fibroblasts transfected with a *myc* oncogene, it has been demonstrated that TGF-beta inhibits the formation of colonies of the cells in the presence of EGF but stimulates the formation of colonies of the cells in the presence of PDGF.[20] Finally, there is evidence that functionally interactive growth factors can alter either receptor number or receptor affinity for other members of the set. This inter-receptor communication represents another mechanism for regulation of cellular response patterns.[14,141] Thus TGF-beta can induce the synthesis of cellular receptors for EGF and increase the sensitivity of the cellular response to EGF,[144] and insulin can increase cellular binding of IGF-II.[14] These examples of the obligatory nature of direct cooperative interactions between growth factors suggest possible therapeutic applications.

INDIRECT INTERACTIONS OF GROWTH FACTORS

In addition to cooperative interactions of several growth factors on a particular target cell, the complex nature of tumor tissue suggests that indirect cooperative interactions of several growth factors, each acting on different target cells found within the tumor, can have significant consequences for tumor growth; nontumor target cells include inflammatory cells, fibroblasts, and endothelial cells, all components of tumor stroma.[38,39] Suppression by growth factors of immune surveillance and enhancement of connective tissue and neovascularization can all stimulate tumorigenesis. In this regard, TGF-beta, which is secreted by many tumor cells, has been shown to inhibit growth and expression of differentiated function by all lymphocytic cells, including T-cells,[145] B-cells,[146] cytotoxic killer cells,[147] and lymphokine activated killer cells[148]; to activate fibroblasts to synthesize connective tissue proteins, including type I collagen, fibronectin, and proteoglycans[25,115]; and to stimulate angiogenesis in vivo.[149] Moreover, PDGF and FGF both stimulate proliferation of fibroblasts,[24] while FGF is thought to be the principal endothelial cell mitogen.[136]

The importance of angiogenesis on tumor growth should not be underestimated. It has been known for a long time that tumors implanted into perfused tissues in which mechanisms of neovascularization have degenerated will remain viable but static until reimplanted into an environment in which the tumor can become vascularized.[150] Although FGF is the principal endothelial cell mitogen,[136] TGF-beta has also been shown to stimulate angiogenesis in vivo.[149] Another peptide, angiogenin, isolated from medium conditioned by a human adenocarcinoma cell line, is active in two models of angiogenesis, the chick embryo chorioallantoic membrane assay and the rabbit corneal pocket assay,[151-153] but whether it plays a role in tumor angiogenesis is not known.[154] Control of angiogenesis has been suggested as an alternative therapeutic approach to control of tumor growth.[155,156]

It has been proposed that excessive stimulation of connective tissue by growth factors secreted by tumor cells could contribute to desmoplasia, an increase in connective tissue formation in the immediate vicinity of tumor cells, found most often in malignancies such as melanoma, colorectal carcinoma, and scirrhous carcinoma of the breast.[157] Effects of both TGF-beta[25,115] and PDGF[24] on connective tissue suggest that action of these two growth factors may be found to be associated with desmoplasia. In addition to effects of growth factors, connective tissue proteins themselves may contribute to regulation of tumor cell growth. Thus both collagen fragments and fibronectin are chemotactic for mesenchymal cells,[158] and fibronectin has been shown to stimulate both proliferation and differentiation of certain mesenchymal cells.[159,160] Polymers, too, such as heparin secreted by mast cells, have been suggested to further stimulate neovascularization of tumors.[161]

Yet another aspect of indirect effects of growth factors on tumor growth is their ability to stimulate the migration of different cell types toward a tumor and then activate those cells to produce yet other growth factors. For example, both TGF-beta and PDGF, secreted by tumor cells that themselves might not be responsive to the factors, have chemotactic activity for monocytes, fibroblasts, and smooth muscle cells.[24,25] Both TGF-beta and PDGF, at somewhat higher concentrations, then activate monocytes to secrete other mitogens such as interleukin-1 beta,[162] which acts on fibroblasts. Yet another mechanism for perpetuating growth factor action in tumor stroma is the secretion of growth factors by activated inflammatory cells; thus activated macrophages have been shown to secrete both PDGF and TGF-beta,[163,164] and activated T-lymphocytes also secrete TGF-beta.[145]

In summary, it is clear that growth factors can act at many different levels to modulate carcinogenesis and that understanding of their roles in this process involves consideration of their actions not only on the tumor cells but also on stromal elements of the tumor. Moreover, to understand the complex role of growth factors in this process, it is necessary to consider not only growth factor secretion by the tumor cells but also growth factor secretion by other cell types in the tumor mass.

INHIBITION OF THE ACTION OF POSITIVE GROWTH FACTORS AS A THERAPEUTIC APPROACH TO CANCER

The hope that it will eventually be possible to control growth factor synthesis and expression has given a new rationale to approaching cancer therapy. The autocrine hypothesis provides a conceptual framework for designing new therapeutic agents.[27] One direct new approach to therapy would be to control autocrine growth factor pathways by preventing interactions of the effector polypeptide with its receptor. This could be accomplished in three ways: action of the growth factor could be blocked by use of specific antibodies to the growth factor which bind to its active site; binding of the growth factor to its receptor could be blocked by antibodies to the receptor; or an extracellular antagonist of a presumed autocrine polypeptide, which would compete for receptor binding (but not be functionally active upon binding), could be used. The first approach has recently been accomplished in an experimental model by using monoclonal antibodies to the tetradecapeptide bombesin, which is produced and released by most human small cell lung cancer cells (oat cell cancers). As discussed earlier in this chapter, these highly malignant cells have functional receptors for this peptide and release it in large quantities.[35] Monoclonal antibodies raised against bombesin not only inhibit the binding of bombesin to its receptor but also markedly inhibit both the growth of lung cancer cells in vitro and their ability to form tumors in nude mice (see Fig. 5-2).[140] As an example of the second approach, monoclonal antibodies raised to the EGF receptors of the human epidermoid carcinoma cell line, A431, compete with EGF for receptor binding, and both block the proliferation of the cells in culture and inhibit A431 tumor growth in nude mice.[165] It is clear that these types of experiments provide a paradigm for other growth factors that are presumed to act by an autocrine mechanism and that antibodies against either growth factors or growth factor receptors could potentially prove to be therapeutically useful.

The other approach, that of developing growth factor antagonists, is still untested, but the cloned genes, which are available for many growth factors, should be amenable to methods of in vitro site-directed mutagenesis. In this way, specific amino acid substitutions can be made at any locus in a growth factor molecule. Such mutated growth factors can then be screened for potential antagonist activity. The potential usefulness of such an approach has been demonstrated in several instances with human insulin, where it has been shown that a mutational substitution of a single amino acid in a critical location can convert an agonist to an antagonist. (In these cases the mutations occurred naturally, and the patients with such mutations had clinical diabetes.[166–167]) Thus, although this has not yet been done successfully with other growth factors, recombinant DNA technology has made this a practical laboratory problem.

ENHANCEMENT OF THE ACTION OF NEGATIVE GROWTH FACTORS FOR PREVENTION OF CANCER

In the previous section, we have discussed the possible use of antagonists of positive growth factors as a means to arrest the growth of cancer cells. The discovery of negative autocrine growth factors now opens up a new approach to the cancer problem, particularly for the prevention of cancer. Thus, we would propose that any drug or biological response modifier that could potentially increase the activity of a negative growth factor could represent a practical approach to the prevention of cancer, particularly since preneoplastic cells are more sensitive to the action of negative autocrine factors than their malignant counterparts. One important advance in this regard is the recent demonstration that the estradiol antagonist tamoxifen markedly increases the secretion of TGF-beta in estrogen-sensitive human MCF-7 breast carcinoma cells[168]; this increase in TGF-beta has been linked to a suppression of growth in these cells. These studies demonstrate that increasing the activity of a negative autocrine factor by use of an estrogen analogue is one possible mechanism that can be exploited for control of epithelial cell growth; they are of obvious relevance to animal experiments that have shown that tamoxifen can prevent experimental mammary cancer in rats[169] or to the potential clinical use of tamoxifen to prevent breast cancer in women at high risk.[170]

REFERENCES

1. Pierce GB, Shikes R, Fink LM: Cancer: A Problem of Developmental Biology. Englewood Cliffs, NJ, Prentice-Hall, 1978
2. Mintz BH, Fleischman RA: Teratocarcinomas and other neoplasms as developmental defects in gene expression. Adv Cancer Res 34:211–278, 1981
3. Sachs L: Control of normal cell differentiation and the phenotypic reversion of malignancy in myeloid leukemia. Nature 274:535–539, 1978
4. Sporn MB, Roberts AB: Peptide growth factors and inflammation, tissue repair, and cancer. J Clin Invest 78:329–332, 1986
5. Goustin AS, Leof EB, Shipley GD, et al: Growth factors and cancer. Cancer Res 46:1015–1029, 1986
6. Heldin CH, Westermark B: Growth factors: Mechanism of action and relation to oncogenes. Cell 37:9–20, 1984
7. Bishop JM: Retroviruses and cancer genes. Adv Cancer Res 37:1–32, 1982
8. Land H, Parada LF, Weinberg RA: Tumorigenic conversion of primary embryo fibroblasts requires at least two cooperating oncogenes. Nature 304:596–602, 1983
9. Ruley HE: Adenovirus early region 1A enables viral and cellular transforming genes to transform primary cells in culture. Nature 304:602–606, 1983
10. Land H, Parada LF, Weinberg RA: Cellular oncogenes and multistep carcinogenesis. Science 222:771–778, 1983
11. Roberts AB, Sporn MB: Growth factors and transformation. Cancer Surv 5:405–412, 1986
12. James R, Bradshaw RA: Polypeptide growth factors. Annu Rev Biochem 53:259–292, 1984
13. Rechler MM, Nissley SP: The nature and regulation of the receptors for insulin-like growth factors. Annu Rev Physiol 47:425–442, 1985
14. Czech MP: New perspectives on the mechanisms of insulin action. Recent Prog Hormone Res 40:347–377, 1984
15. Roth J: Insulin binding to its receptor: Is the receptor more important that the hormone? Diabetes Care 4:27–32, 1981
16. Kris RM, Libermann TA, Avivi A, et al: Growth factors, growth-factor receptors and oncogenes. Biotechnol: 1:135–140, 1985
17. Sporn MB, Roberts AB: Peptide growth factors are multifunctional. Nature 332:217–219, 1988
18. Fallon JH, Seroogy KB, Loughlin SE, et al: Epidermal growth factor immunoreactive material in the central nervous system: Location and development. Science 224:1107–1109, 1984
19. Dockray GJ: Evolutionary relationships of the gut hormones. Fed Proc 38:2295–2301, 1979
20. Roberts AB, Anzano MA, Wakefield LM, et al: Type Beta transforming growth factor: A bifunctional regulator of cellular growth. Proc Natl Acad Sci USA 82:119–123, 1985
21. Carpenter G, Cohen S: Epidermal growth factor. Annu Rev Biochem 48:193–216, 1979
22. Hollenberg MD: Epidermal growth factor-urogastrone, a polypeptide acquiring hormonal status. Vitam Horm 37:69–110, 1979
23. Gill GN, Lazar CS: Increased phosphotyrosine content and inhibition of proliferation in EGF-treated A431 cells. Nature 293:305–307, 1981
24. Ross R, Raines EW, Bowen-Pope DF: The biology of platelet-derived growth factor. Cell 46:155–169, 1986
25. Sporn MB, Roberts AB, Wakefield LM, et al: Some recent advances in the chemistry and biology of transforming growth factor-beta. J Cell Biol 105:1039–1045, 1987
26. Sporn MB, Todaro GJ: Autocrine secretion and malignant transformation of cells. New Engl J Med 308:878–880, 1980
27. Sporn MB, Roberts AB: Autocrine growth factors and cancer. Nature 313:747–751, 1985
28. Sporn MB, Roberts AB: Autocrine, paracrine and endocrine mechanisms of growth control. Cancer Surv 4:627–632, 1985
29. Temin HM: Studies on carcinogenesis by avian sarcoma viruses VI. Differential multiplication of uninfected and of converted cells in response to insulin. J Cell Physiol 69:377–384, 1967
30. Holley RW: Control of growth of mammalian cells in cell culture. Nature 258:487–490, 1975
31. De Larco JE, Todaro GJ: Growth factors from murine sarcoma virus-transformed cells. Proc Natl Acad Sci USA 75:4001–4005, 1978
32. Roberts AB, Sporn MB: Transforming growth factors. Cancer Surv 4:683–705, 1985
33. Todaro GJ, Lee DC, Webb NR, et al: Rat type-alpha transforming growth factor: Structure and possible function as a membrane receptor. Cancer Cells 3:51–58, 1985
34. Williams LT: The *sis* gene and PDGF. Cancer Surv 5:233–241, 1986
35. Cuttitta F, Carney DN, Mulshine J, et al: Autocrine growth factors in human small cell lung cancer. Cancer Surv 4:707–727, 1985
36. Johnsson A, Betsholtz C, Heldin C-H, et al: Antibodies against platelet-derived growth factor inhibit acute transformation by simian sarcoma virus. Nature 317:438–442, 1985
37. Seifert RA, Schwartz SM, Bowen-Pope DF: Developmentally regulated production of platelet derived growth factor-like molecules. Nature 311:669–671, 1984
38. Dvorak HF: Tumors: Wounds that do not heal. New Engl J Med 315:1650–1659, 1986
39. Haddow A: Molecular repair, wound healing, and carcinogenesis: Tumor production a possible overhealing? Adv Cancer Res 16:181–234, 1972
40. Gospodarowicz D, Neufeld G, Schweigerer L: Molecular and biological characterization of fibroblast growth factor: An angiogenic factor which also controls the proliferation and differentiation of mesoderm and neuroectoderm derived cells. Cell Differ 19:1–17, 1986
41. Cowley G, Smith J, Gusterson B, et al: The EGF receptor is expressed at high levels on squamous cell carcinomas. Cancer Cells 1:5–10, 1984
42. Kawamoto T, Sato JD, Le A, et al: Growth stimulation of A431 cells by epidermal growth factor: Identification of high-affinity receptors for epidermal growth factor by an anti-receptor monoclonal antibody. Proc Natl Acad Sci USA 80:1337–1341, 1983
43. Holley RW: Control of animal cell proliferation. J Supramolec Struct 13:191–197, 1980
44. Tucker RF, Shipley GD, Moses HL, et al: Growth inhibitor from BSC-1 cells closely related to those isolated from tumor cells. Science 226:705–707, 1984
45. Wakefield LM, Smith DM, Masui T, et al: Distribution and modulation of the cellular receptor for transforming growth factor-beta. J Cell Biol 105:965–975, 1987
46. McMahon JB, Richards WL, del Campo AA, et al: Differential effects of transforming growth factor-beta on proliferation of normal and malignant rat liver epithelial cells in culture. Cancer Res 46:4665–4671, 1986
47. Shipley GD, Pittelkow MR, Wille JJ Jr, et al: Reversible inhibition of normal human prokeratinocyte proliferation by type beta transforming growth factor-growth inhibitor in serum-free medium. Cancer Res 46:2068–2071, 1986

48. Chinkers M, Cohen S: Purified EGF receptor-kinase interacts specifically with antibodies to Rous sarcoma virus transforming protein. Nature 290:516–519, 1981
49. Erikson E, Shealy DJ, Erikson RL: Evidence that viral transforming gene products and epidermal growth factor stimulate phosphorylation of the same cellular protein with similar specificity. J Biol Chem 256:11381–11384, 1981
50. Cooper JA, Hunter T: Similarities and differences between the effects of epidermal growth factor and Rous sarcoma virus. J Cell Biol 91:878–883, 1981
51. Kasuga M, Fujita-Yamaguchi Y, Blithe M, et al: Characterization of the insulin receptor kinase purified from human placental membranes. J Biol Chem 258:10973–10980, 1983
52. Rubin JB, Shia MA, Pilch PR: Stimulation of tyrosine-specific phosphorylation in vitro by insulinlike growth factor I. Nature 305:438–440, 1983
53. Heldin C-H, Ek B, Ronnstrand L: Characterization of the receptor for platelet-derived growth factor on human fibroblasts. J Biol Chem 258:10054–10061, 1983
54. Doolittle RF, Hunkapiller MW, Hood LE, et al: Simian sarcoma virus onc gene, *v-sis*, is derived from the gene (genes) encoding a platelet-derived growth factor. Science 221:275–277, 1983
55. Waterfield MD, Scrace GT, Whittle N, et al: Platelet-derived growth factor is structurally related to the putative transforming protein p28^{sis} of simian sarcoma virus. Nature 304:35–39, 1983
56. Johnsson A, Heldin C-H, Wasteson A, et al: The *c-sis* gene encodes a precursor of the B chain of platelet-derived growth factor. EMBO J 3:921–928, 1984
57. Downward J, Yarden Y, Mayes E, et al: Close similarity of epidermal growth factor receptor and v-*erb*-B oncogene protein sequences. Nature 307:521–528, 1984
58. Martin GS: The *erb*B gene and the EGF receptor. Cancer Surv 5:199–219, 1986
59. Kelly K, Cochran BH, Stiles CD, et al: Cell-specific regulation of the c-myc gene by lymphocyte mitogens and platelet-derived growth factor. Cell 35:603–610, 1983
60. Greenberg ME, Ziff EB: Stimulation of 3T3 cells induces transcription of the *c-fos* proto-oncogene. Nature 311:433–438, 1984
61. Curran T, Bravo R, Muller R: Transient induction of *c-fos* and *c-myc* is an immediate consequence of growth factor stimulation. Cancer Surv 4:655–681, 1985
62. Eisenman RN, Thompson CB: Oncogenes with potential nuclear function: *myc, myb* and *fos*. Cancer Surv 5:309–327, 1986
63. Stern DL, Roberts AB, Roche NS, et al. Differential responsiveness of *myc*- and *ras*-transfected cells to growth factors: Selective stimulation of *myc*-transfected cells by EGF. Mol Cell Biol 6:870–877, 1986
64. Stiles CD, Capone GT, Scher CD, et al: Dual control of cell growth by somatomedins and platelet-derived growth factor. Proc Natl Acad Sci USA 76:1279–1283, 1979
65. Humbel RE, Bosshard HR, Zahn H: Chemistry of Insulin. In Greep RO, Astwood EB (eds): Handbook of Physiology, vol 1, pp 311–332. Washington, DC, American Physiological Society, 1972
66. Zapf J, Froesch ER, Humbel RE: The insulin-like growth factors (IGF) of human serum: Chemical and biological characterization and aspects of their possible physiological role. Curr Top Cell Regul 19:257–309, 1981
67. Bradshaw RA: Nerve growth factor. Annu Rev Biochem 47:191–216, 1978
68. Schwage C, Steinetz B, Weiss G, et al: Relaxin. Recent Prog Horm Res 34:123–211, 1978
69. Svoboda ME, Van Wyk JJ, Klapper DG, et al: Purification of somatomedin-C from human plasma: Chemical and biological properties, partial sequence analysis and relationship to other somatomedins. Biochemistry 19:790–797, 1980
70. Blundell TL, Bedarker S, Humbel RE: Teritary structures, receptor binding, and antigenicity of insulin-like growth factors. Fed Proc 42:2592–2597, 1983
71. Morgan DO, Edman JC, Standring DN, et al: Insulin-like growth factor II receptor as a multifunctional binding protein. Nature 329:301–397, 1987
72. Reeve AE, Eccles MR, Wilkins RJ, et al: Expression of insulin-like growth factor-II transcripts in Wilms' tumour. Nature 317:258–260, 1985
73. Scott J, Cowell J, Robertson ME, et al: Insulin-like growth factor-II gene expression in Wilms' tumour and embryonic tissue. Nature 317:260–262, 1985
74. Adams SO, Nissley SP, Handwerger S, et al: Developmental patterns of insulin-like growth factor-I and -II synthesis and regulation in rat fibroblasts. Nature 302:150–153, 1983
75. Han VKM, D'Ercole AJ, Lund PK: Cellular localization of somatomedin (insulin-like growth factor) messenger RNA in the human fetus. Science 236:193–197, 1987
76. Todaro GJ, De Larco JE, Marquardt H, et al: Polypeptide growth factors produced by tumor cells and virus-transformed cells: A possible growth advantage for the producer cells. Cold Spring Harbor Conferences on Cell Proliferation. 6:113–127, 1979
77. Massagué J, Kelly B, Mottola C: Stimulation by insulin-like growth factors is required for cellular transformation by type beta transforming growth factor. J Biol Chem 260:4551–4554, 1985
78. Oppenheimer CL, Pessin JE, Massague J, et al: Insulin action rapidly modulates the apparent affinity of the insulin-like growth factor II receptor. J Biol Chem 258:4824–4830, 1983
79. Rozengurt E: Early signals in the mitogenic response. Science 234:161–166, 1986
80. Carpenter G: The biochemistry and physiology of the receptor-kinase for epidermal growth factor. Mol Cell Endocrinol 31:1–19, 1983
81. Balk SD, Shiu RPC, LaFleur MM, et al: Epidermal growth factor and insulin cause normal chicken heart mesenchymal cells to proliferate like their Rous sarcoma virus-infected counterparts. Proc Natl Acad Sci USA 79:1154–1157, 1982
82. Soderquist AM, Carpenter G: Developments in the mechanism of growth factor action: Activation of protein kinase by epidermal growth factor. Fed Proc 42:2615–2620, 1983
83. Todaro GJ, Fryling C, De Larco JE: Transforming growth factors (TGFs) produced by certain human tumor cells: Polypeptides that interact with epidermal growth factor (EGF) receptors. Proc Natl Acad Sci USA 77:5258–5262, 1980
84. Marquardt H, Hunkapiller MW, Hood LE, et al: Transforming growth factors produced by retrovirus-transformed rodent fibroblasts and human melanoma cells: Amino acid sequence hormology with epidermal growth factor. Proc Natl Acad Sci USA 80:4684–4688, 1983
85. Roberts AB, Frolik CA, Anzano MA, et al: Transforming growth factors from neoplastic and non-neoplastic tissues. Fed Proc 42:2621–2626, 1983
86. Gray A, Dull TJ, Ullrich A: Nucleotide sequence of epidermal growth factor cDNA predicts a 128,000-molecular weight protein precursor. Nature 303:722–725, 1983
87. Scott J, Urdea M, Quiroga M, et al: Structure of a mouse submaxillary messenger RNA encoding epidermal growth factor and seven related proteins. Science 221:236–240, 1983
88. Blomquist MC, Hunt LT, Barker WC: Vaccinia virus 19-kilodalton protein: Relationship to several mammalian proteins, including two growth factors. Proc Natl Acad Sci USA 81:7363–7367, 1984
89. Chang W, Upton C, Hu S-L, et al: The genome of Shope fibroma virus, a tumorigenic poxvirus, contains a growth factor gene with sequence similarity to those encoding epidermal growth factor and transforming growth factor alpha. Mol Cell Biol 7:535–540, 1987
90. Marquardt H, Hunkapiller MW, Hood LE, et al: Rat transforming growth factor type I: Structure and relation to epidermal growth factor. Science 223:1079–1082, 1984
91. Stroobant P, Rice AP, Gullick WJ, et al: Purification and characterization of vaccinia virus growth factor. Cell 42:383–393, 1985
92. Eppstein DA, Marsh YV, Schreiber AB, et al: Epidermal growth factor receptor occupancy inhibits vaccinia virus infection. Nature 318:663–665, 1985
93. Privalsky ML, Ralston R, Bishop JM: The membrane glycoprotein encoded by the retroviral oncogene v-*erb*-B is structurally related to tyrosine-specific protein kinases. Proc Natl Acad Sci USA 81:704–707, 1984
94. Ullrich A, Coussens L, Hayflick J, et al: Human epidermal growth factor receptor cDNA sequence and aberrent expression of the amplified gene in A431 epidermoid carcinoma cells. Nature 309:418–425, 1984
95. Libermann TA, Rason N, Bartal AD, et al: Expression of epidermal growth factor receptors in human brain tumors. Cancer Res 44:753–760, 1984
96. Thompson DM, Gill GN: The EGF receptor: Structure, regulation and potential role in malignancy. Cancer Surv 4:767–788, 1985
97. Libermann TA, Nusbaum HR, Rason N, et al: Amplification enchances expression and possible rearrangement of the EGF receptor gene in primary human brain tumors of glial origin. Nature 313:144–147, 1985
98. Mark J, Westermark B, Ponten J, et al: Banding patterns in human glioma cell lines. Heredity (Edinburgh) 87:243–260, 1977
99. Fisher PB, Mufson A, Weinstein IB, et al: Epidermal growth factor, like tumor promoters, enhances viral and radiation-induced cell transformation. Carcinogenesis 2:183–187, 1981
100. Harrison J, Auersperg N: Epidermal growth factor enhances viral transformation of granulosa cells. Science 213:218–219, 1981
101. Rose SP, Stahn R, Passovoy DS, et al: Epidermal growth factor enhancement of skin tumor induction in mice. Experientia 32:913–915, 1976
102. De Larco JE, Preston YA, Todaro GJ: Properties of a sarcoma-growth-factor-like peptide from cells transformed by a temperature-sensitive sarcoma virus. J Cell Physiol 109:143–152, 1981
103. Twardzik DR, Sherwin SA, Ranchalis J, et al: Transforming growth factors in the urine of normal, pregnant, and tumor-bearing humans. JNCI 69:793–798, 1982
104. Samsoondar J, Kobrin MS, Kudlow JE: Alpha-transforming growth factor secreted by untransformed bovine anterior pituitary cells in culture. J Biol Chem 261:14408–14413, 1986
105. Kobrin MS, Samsoondar J, Kudlow JE: Alpha-transforming growth factor secreted by untransformed bovine anterior pituitary cells in culture. J Biol Chem 261:14414–14419, 1986
106. Lee D, Rochford R, Todaro GJ, et al: Development expression of rat transforming growth factor-alpha RNA. Mol Cell Biol 5:3644–3646, 1985
107. Betsholtz C, Johnsson A, Heldin C-H, et al: cDNA sequence and chromosomal localization of human platelet-derived growth factor A-chain and its expression in tumor cell lines. Nature 320:695–699, 1986
108. Niman HL, Thompson AMH, Yu A, et al: Anti-peptide antibodies detect oncogene-related proteins in urine. Proc Natl Acad Sci USA 82:7924–7928, 1985
109. Sejersen T, Betsholtz C, Sjolund M, et al: Rat skeletal myoblast and arterial smooth muscle cells express the gene for the A chain but not the gene for the B chain *(c-sis)* of platelet-derived growth factor (PDGF) and produce a PDGF-like protein. Proc Natl Acad Sci USA 83:6844–6848, 1986
110. Tong BD, Auer DE, Jaye M, et al: cDNA clones reveal differences between human glial and endothelial cell platelet-derived growth factor A-chains. Nature 328:619–621, 1987
111. Collins T, Bonthron DT, Orkin SH: Alternative RNA splicing affects function of encoded platelet-derived growth factor A chain. Nature 328:621–623, 1987
112. Bowen-Pope DF, Ross R: The platelet-derived growth factor receptor. In Birnbaumer L, O'Malley BW (eds): Peptide Hormones. Methods in Enzymology, vol 109, pp 69–101. New York, Academic Press, 1985
113. Yarden Y, Escobedo JA, Kuang WJ, et al: Structure of the receptor for platelet-derived growth factor helps define a family of closely related growth factor receptors. Nature 323:226–232, 1986
114. Cheifetz S, Weatherbee JA, Tsang ML-S, et al: The transforming growth factor-beta

system, a complex pattern of cross-reactive ligands and receptors. Cell 48:409–415, 1987

115. Roberts AB, Flanders KC, Kondaiah P, et al: Transforming growth factor beta: Biochemistry and roles in embryogenesis, tissue repair and remodeling, and carcinogenesis. Recent Prog Horm Res 144:157–197, 1988
116. Segarini PR, Roberts AB, Rosen DM, et al: Membrane binding characterization of two forms of transforming growth factor-beta. J Biol Chem (in press)
117. Ohta M, Greenberger JS, Anklesaria P, et al: Two forms of transforming growth factor-beta distinguished by multipotential haematopoietic progenitor cells. Nature 329:539–541, 1987
118. Mason AJ, Hayflick JS, Ling N, et al: Complementary DNA sequences of ovarian follicular fluid inhibin show precursor structure and homology with transforming growth factor-beta. Nature 318:659–663, 1985
119. Vale W, Rivier J, Vaughan J, et al: Purificiation and characterization of an FSH releasing protein from porcine ovarian follicular fluid. Nature 321:776–779, 1986
120. Ling N, Ying S-Y, Ueno N, et al: Pituitary FSH is released by a heterodimer of the beta-subunits from the two forms of inhibin. Nature 321:779–782, 1986
121. Cate RL, Mattaliano RJ, Hession C, et al: Isolation of the bovine and human genes for müllerian inhibiting substance and expression of the human gene in animal cells. Cell 45:685–698, 1986
122. Padgett RW, St Johnston RD, Gelbart WM: A transcript from a *Drosophila* pattern gene predicts a protein homologous to the transforming growth factor-beta family. Nature 325:81–84, 1987
123. Weeks DL, Melton DA: A maternal messenger RNA localized to the vegetal hemisphere in Xenopus eggs codes for a growth factor related to TGF-beta. Cell 51:861–867, 1987
124. Silberstein GB, Daniel CW: Reversible inhibition of mammary gland growth by transforming growth factor-beta. Science 237:291–293, 1987
125. Fausto N, Mead JE, Braun L, et al: Protooncogene expression and growth factors during liver regeneration. Symp Fundam Cancer Res 39:69–86, 1987
126. Cheifetz S, Like B, Massague J: Cellular distribution of type I and type II receptors for transforming growth factor-beta. J Biol Chem 261:9972–9978, 1986
127. Fanger BO, Wakefield LM, Sporn MB: Structure and properties of the cellular receptor for transforming growth factor type beta. Biochemistry 25:3083–3091, 1986
128. Libby J, Martinez R, Weber MJ: Tyrosine phosphorylation in cells treated with transforming growth factor-beta. J Cell Pysiol 129:159–166, 1986
129. Derynck R, Goeddel DV, Ullrich A, et al: Synthesis of messenger RNAs for transforming growth factors alpha and beta and the epidermal growth factor receptor by human tumors. Cancer Res 47:707–712, 1987
130. Donahoe PK, Fuller Jr, AF, Scully RE, et al: Mullerian inhibiting substance inhibits growth of a human ovarian cancer in nude mice. Ann Surg 194:472–480, 1981
131. Fuller Jr AF, Krane IM, Budzik GP, et al: Mullerian inhibiting substance reduction of colony growth of human gynecologic cancers in a stem cell assay. Gynecol Oncol 22:135–148, 1985
132. Baird A, Esch F, Mormede P, et al: Molecular characterization of fibroblast growth factor: Distribution and biological activities in various tissues. Recent Prog Horm Res 42:143–205, 1986
133. Abraham JA, Mergia A, Whang JL, et al: Nucleotide sequence of a bovine clone encoding the angiogenic protein, basic fibroblast growth factor. Science 233:545–548, 1986
134. Jaye M, Howk R, Burgess W, et al: Human endothelial cell growth factor: cloning, nucleotide sequence, and chromosome localization. Science 233:541–545, 1986
135. Gospodarowicz D: Fibroblast growth factor: Structural and biological properties. Nucl Med Biol 14:421–434, 1987
136. Gospodarowicz D, Ferrara N, Schweigerer L, et al: Structural characterization and biological functions of fibroblast growth factor. Endocr Rev 8:1–20, 1987
137. Neufeld G, Gospodarowicz D: Basic and acidic fibroblast growth factor interact with the same cell surface receptor. J Biol Chem 261:5631–5637, 1986
138. Huang SS, Huang JS: Association of bovine brain-derived growth factor receptor with protein tyrosine kinase activity. J Biol Chem 261:9568–9571, 1986
139. McDonald TJ, Jornvall H, Vagne M, et al: Characterization of a gastrin releasing peptide from porcine non-antral gastric tissue. Biochem Biophys Commun 90:227–233, 1979
140. Cuttitta F, Carney DN, Mulshine J, et al: Bombesin-like peptides can function as autocrine growth factors in human small cell lung cancer. Nature 316:823–826, 1985
141. Zachary I, Rozengurt E: Modulation of the epidermal growth factor receptor by mitogenic ligands: Effects of bombesin and role of protein kinase C. Cancer Surv 4:729–765, 1985
142. Assoian RK, Grotendorst GR, Miller DM, et al: Three growth factors from human platelets coordinating phenotypic transformation. Nature 309:804–806, 1984
143. Carpenter G, Stoscheck CM, Preston YA, et al: Antibodies to the epidermal growth factor receptor block the biological activities of sarcoma growth factor. Proc Natl Acad Sci USA 80:5627–5630, 1983
144. Assoian RK, Frolik CA, Roberts AB, et al: Transforming growth factor-beta controls receptor levels for epidermal growth factor in NRK-fibroblasts. Cell 36:35–41, 1984
145. Kehrl JH, Wakefield LM, Roberts AB, et al: Production of transforming growth factor beta by human T lymphocytes and its potential role in the regulation of T cell growth. J Exp Med 163:1037–1050, 1986
146. Kehrl JH, Roberts AB, Wakefield LM, et al: Transforming growth factor beta is an important immunomodulatory protein for human B lymphocytes. J Immunol 137:3855–3860, 1986
147. Rook AH, Kehrl JH, Wakefield LM, et al: Effects of transforming growth factor beta on the functions of natural killer cells: Depressed cytolytic activity and blunting of interferon responsiveness. J Immunol 136:3916–3920, 1986
148. Mulé JJ, Schwarz SL, Roberts AB, et al: Transforming growth factor-beta inhibits the *in vitro* generation of lymphokine-activated killer cells and cytotoxic T cells. Cancer Immunol Immunother 26:95–100, 1988
149. Roberts AB, Sporn MB, Assoian RK, et al: Transforming growth factor type beta: Rapid induction of fibrosis and angiogenesis *in vivo* and stimulation of collagen formation *in vitro*. Proc Natl Acad Sci USA 83:4167–4171, 1986
150. Folkman J: Toward an understanding of angiogenesis: Search and discovery. Perspect Biol Med 29:10–36, 1985
151. Fett JW, Strydom DJ, Lobb RR, et al: Isolation and characterization of angiogenin, and angiogenic protein from human carcinoma cells. Biochemistry 24:5480–5486, 1985
152. Strydom DJ, Fett JW, Lobb RR, et al: Amino acid sequence of human tumor derived angiogenin. Biochemistry 24:5486–5494, 1985
153. Kurachi K, Davie EW, Strydom DJ, et al: Sequence of cDNA and gene for angiogenin, a human angiogenesis factor. Biochemistry 24:5494–5499, 1985
154. Weiner HL, Weiner LH, Swain JL: Tissue distribution and developmental expression of the messenger RNA encoding angiogenin. Science 237:280–282, 1987
155. Folkman, J: Tumor angiogenesis. Adv Cancer Res 43:175–203, 1985
156. Folkman J: How is blood vessel growth regulated in normal and neoplastic tissue? G.H.A. Clowes Memorial Award Lecture. Cancer Res 46:467–473, 1986
157. Liotta LA, Rao CN, Barsky SH: Tumor invasion and the extracellular matrix. Lab Invest 49:636–649, 1983
158. Yamada KM: Cell surface interactions with extracellular materials. Annu Rev Biochem 52:761–799, 1983
159. Hynes RD: Molecular biology of fibronectin. Annu Rev Cell Biol 1:67–90, 1985
160. Ignotz RA, Massague J: Transforming growth factor-beta stimulates the expression of fibronectin and collagen and their incorporation into the extracellular matrix. J Biol Chem 261:4337–4345, 1986
161. Folkman J: Regulation of angiogenesis: A new function of heparin. Biochem Pharmacol 34:905–909, 1985
162. Wahl SM, Hunt DA, Wong HL, et al: Transforming growth factor beta is a potent immunosuppressive agent which inhibits interleukin 1-dependent lymphocyte proliferation. Immunol 140:3026–3032, 1988
163. Assoian RK, Fleurdelys BF, Stevenson HC, et al: Expression and secretion of type Beta transforming growth factor by activated human macrophages. Proc Natl Acad Sci USA 84:6020–6024, 1987
164. Shimokado K, Raines EW, Madtes DK, et al: A significant part of macrophage-derived growth factor consists of at least two forms of PDGF. Cell 43:277–286, 1985
165. Hamui H, Tomoyuki K, Sato JD, et al: Growth inhibition of human tumor cells in athymic mice by anti-epidermal growth factor receptor monoclonal antibodies. Cancer Res 44:1002–1007, 1984
166. Tager H, Given B, Baldwin D, et al: A structurally abnormal insulin causing human diabetes. Nature 281:122–125, 1979
167. Haneda M, Chan SJ, Kwok CM, et al: Studies on mutant human insulin genes: Identification and sequence analysis of a gene encoding Ser^{B24} insulin. Proc Natl Acad Sci USA 80:6366–6370, 1983
168. Knabbe C, Lippman ME, Wakefield LM, et al: Evidence that transforming growth factor-beta is a hormonally regulated negative growth factor in human breast cancer cells. Cell 48:417–428, 1987
169. McCormick DL, Moon RC: Retinoid-tamoxifen interaction in mammary cancer chemoprevention. Carcinogenesis 7:193–196, 1986
170. Carbone P: In Jordan VC (ed): Estrogen/Antiestrogen Action and Breast Cancer Therapy, p 492. Madison, WI, University of Wisconsin Press, 1986
171. Bell GI, Pictet RL, Rutter WJ, et al: Sequence of the human insulin gene. Nature 284:26–32, 1980
172. Ullrich A, Dull TJ, Gray A, et al: Genetic variation in the human insulin gene. Science 209:612–615, 1980
173. Jansen M, van Schaik FMA, Ricken AT, et al: Sequence of cDNA encoding human insulin-like growth factor I precursor. Nature 306:609–611, 1983
174. Ullrich A, Berman CH, Dull TJ, et al: Isolation of the human insulin-like growth factor I gene using a single synthetic DNA probe. EMBO J 3:361–364, 1984
175. Bell GI, Merryweather JP, Sanchez-Pescador R, et al: Sequence of a cDNA encoding human preproinsulin-like growth factor II. Nature 310:775–777, 1984
176. Dull TJ, Gray A, Hayflick JS, et al: Insulin-like growth factor II precursor gene organization in relation to insulin gene family. Nature 310:777–781, 1984
177. Ullrich A, Gray A, Berman C, et al: Human beta-nerve growth factor gene sequence highly homologous to that of mouse. Nature 303:821–825, 1983
178. Derynck R, Roberts AB, Winkler ME, et al: Human transforming growth factor-alpha: Precursor structure and expression in E. coli. Cell 38:287–297, 1984
179. Derynck R, Jarrett JA, Chen EY, et al: Human transforming growth factor-beta complementary DNA sequence and expression in normal and transformed cells. Nature 316:701–705, 1985
180. Marquardt H, Lioubin MN, Ikeda T: Complete amino acid sequence of human transforming growth factor type beta2. J Biol Chem 262:12127–12131, 1987
181. Anastasi A, Erspamer V, Bucci M: Isolation and structure of bombesin and alytesin, two analogous active peptides from the skin of the European amphibians *Bombina* and *Alytes*. Experientia 27:166–167, 1971
182. Chambard J-C, Pouysségur J: TGF-β inhibits growth factor-induced DNA synthesis in hamster fibroblasts without affecting the early mitogenic events. J Cell Physiol 135:101–107, 1988

JANET D. ROWLEY

CHAPTER 6 *Principles of Molecular Cell Biology of Cancer: Chromosomal Abnormalities*

The close association of specific chromosome abnormalities with particular types of human cancer has been established by a number of investigators in the past decade. A few of the genes involved in consistent chromosome rearrangements, notably translocations, have already been identified, and it is likely that most of the genes affected by these aberrations will be identified within the next decade. Moreover, for several of the rearrangements, some of the changes in gene structure and function have been defined. Therefore, some general principles that may be applicable to all chromosome rearrangements in human malignant disease are beginning to emerge.

Much of the detailed information on the relevant chromosome rearrangements is contained in a number of recent reviews,[1–6] and only a general summary will be presented here. Mitelman has published three editions of his "Catalogue of Chromosome Aberrations in Cancer."[1,7,8] The proportions of abnormal karyotypes listed in the Catalogues according to type of neoplasia are shown in Figure 6-1. Although carcinomas account for the greatest proportion of malignant disease, they represent only about 15% of the karyotypic data; most of the available information concerns leukemia and lymphoma. Only data obtained in untreated patients will be considered here.

From the beginning of the cytogenetic analysis of human malignant disease, it has been clear that virtually all solid tumors, including the non-Hodgkin's lymphomas, have an abnormal karyotype and that some of these abnormalities are limited to a given tumor.[2–6] With regard to the leukemias, it appeared from studies in the 1960s and early 1970s that only about 50% had an abnormal karyotype.[3–5] With improved culture techniques and with the development of processing methods that resulted in longer chromosomes with a larger number of more clearly defined bands, Yunis and associates have provided evidence that a karyotypic abnormality can be detected in virtually all leukemias as well.[6] Some malignant diseases, such as Hodgkin's disease or multiple myeloma, continue to show a high frequency of normal karyotypes. These diseases are characterized by malignant cells with a low mitotic index, and therefore it is likely that the dividing cells studied do not represent the malignant cells. The discussion will be restricted to clonal abnormali-

At the Human Gene Mapping 9 (HGM9) meeting in Paris in September 1987, it was decided to identify human genes with capital letters in italics. This change is reflected herein; other chapters may use the formerly accepted convention of lower-cased letters in italics.

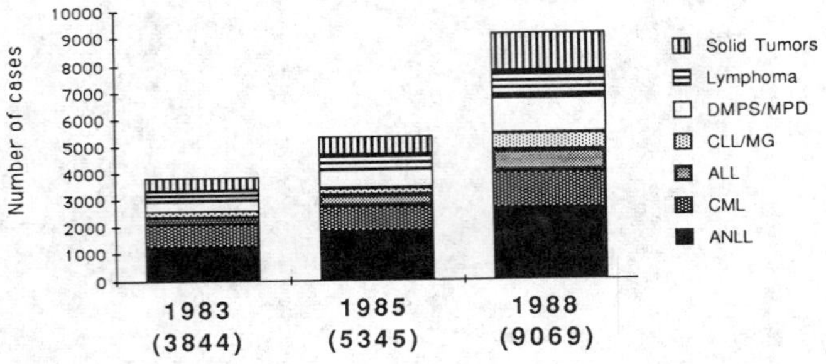

FIG. 6-1. Proportion of abnormal karyotypes by disease type in Mitelman's three catalogs of chromosome aberrations in cancer. The number in parentheses below the date is the total number of abnormal karyotypes in each edition. Patients with CML and only a t(9;22) are not included.

ties, which are defined as at least two cells with the same extra chromosome or structural rearrangement (identified with banding) or three cells with the same missing chromosome.[9] As can be seen from Table 6-1, with the exception of the t(9;22) the chromosome abnormalities in the myeloid leukemias differ from those in the lymphoid leukemias and lymphomas. Molecular analysis of the 9;22 translocation junction has revealed that the break in No. 22 may be different in myeloid and lymphoid leukemia.

Different chromosome changes have been observed in neoplastic cells, and these often occur in combination. This leads to great difficulty in trying to identify precisely the unique abnormalities in a particular cancer. The simplest change is either a gain or a loss of a whole chromosome. Common structural alterations are *translocations,* with involve the exchange of material between two or more chromosomes, and *deletions,* which involve loss of DNA from a chromosome and thus from the affected cell (Fig. 6-2). In chromosome *inversions* a single chromosome is broken in two places, and the central portion is inverted and rejoined to the ends of the chromosome.

A number of international meetings over the last 25 years have led to the establishment of a universally accepted system for chromosome nomenclature; that standard nomenclature will be used here. Each chromosome band is numbered.[10] The total chromosome number is followed by the sex chromosomes, and gains and losses of whole chromosomes are identified by a + or − before the chromosome number. A gain or loss of part of a chromosome is identified by a + or − after the chromosome number; *p* and *q* represent the short and long arm, respectively. Translocations are indicated by *t*; the chromosomes involved are noted in the first set of brackets and the breakpoints in the second set of brackets. Other abnormalities will be defined when they are first described.

TABLE 6-1. Common Chromosome Changes in Leukemia

Type	*Gains*	*Losses*	*Rearrangements*
	Myeloid Leukemia		
CML			
Chronic phase			t(9;22)(q34;q11)
Blast crisis	+8, +Ph^1	Rare; −7	t(9;22), i(17q)
ANLL			
AML (M2)	+8	−7; less −5	t(8;21)(q22;q22)
APL (M3)			t(15;17)(q22;q11−12)
AMMoL (M4) (abn. eosinophils)	+8 +22	−7	inv(16)(p13q22) t(16;16), del(16q)
AMoL (M5)			t(9;11)(p22;q23), t(11q), del (11q)
M2/M4 (incr. basophils)			t(6;9)(p23;q34)
M4 (incr. platelets)			t(3;3)(q21;q26), inv(3)
	Lymphoid Leukemia		
CLL			
B-cell	+12		14q+ (q32)
T-cell			t(8;14)(q24;q11) inv(14)(q11q32)
ALL			
Early B-precursor*			t(4;11)(q21;q23)
Common	+21, +6	Rare	t(9;22), del (6q)(q15−q21), near haploid
pre-B			t(1;19)(q23;p13)
B-cell			t(8;14)(q24;q32) t(2;8)(p12;q24) t(8;22)(q24;q11)
Early T-precursor			t(9p), del(9p) (p21−22)
T-cell			t(11;14)(p13;q11), t(8;14)(q24;q11) inv(14)(q11q32)

*CALLA+.

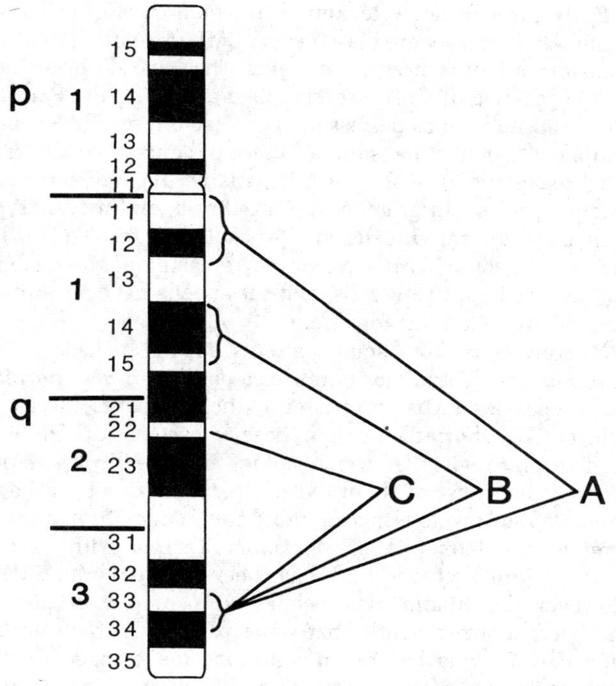

FIG. 6-2. Examples of various deletions of chromosome No. 5. The types are based on the amount of chromosome material missing from the deleted compared with the normal No. 5. Type A is the most extreme example and type C is the least extreme example. The brackets indicate the limits of uncertainty where the band containing the breakpoint has been defined by different staining techniques.

To be relevant to the malignant disease, chromosomes for analysis must be obtained from the tumor cells. Thus, for leukemia, bone marrow cells processed directly or after 1- to 3-day culture are used[11]; lymph nodes or solid tumors are minced to yield a single cell suspension that can be harvested immediately or cultured for a short period of time. The cells are exposed to a hypotonic solution, fixed, and stained according to a variety of protocols.[12]

MYELOID LEUKEMIAS

CHRONIC MYELOID LEUKEMIA

The subtype of leukemia termed *chronic myeloid leukemia* (CML) is important because the first consistent chromosome abnormality in any malignant disease was identified in CML. The abnormality is the Philadelphia or Ph^1 chromosome,[13] which was shown with banding to involve No. 22 (22q−). The correct chromosome defect was shown to be a translocation involving Nos. 9 and 22; this was the first consistent translocation specifically associated with any human or animal disease (Fig. 6-3).[14] The reciprocal nature of the translocation was established only recently, when the Abelson proto-oncogene, *ABL*, normally on No. 9, was identified on the Ph^1 chromosome.[15] Other studies with fluorescent markers or chromosome polymorphisms have shown that, in a particular patient, the same No. 9 and No. 22 are involved in each cell. The karyotypes of many Ph^1+ patients with CML have been examined with banding techniques by a number of investigators; in a recent review of 1129 Ph^1

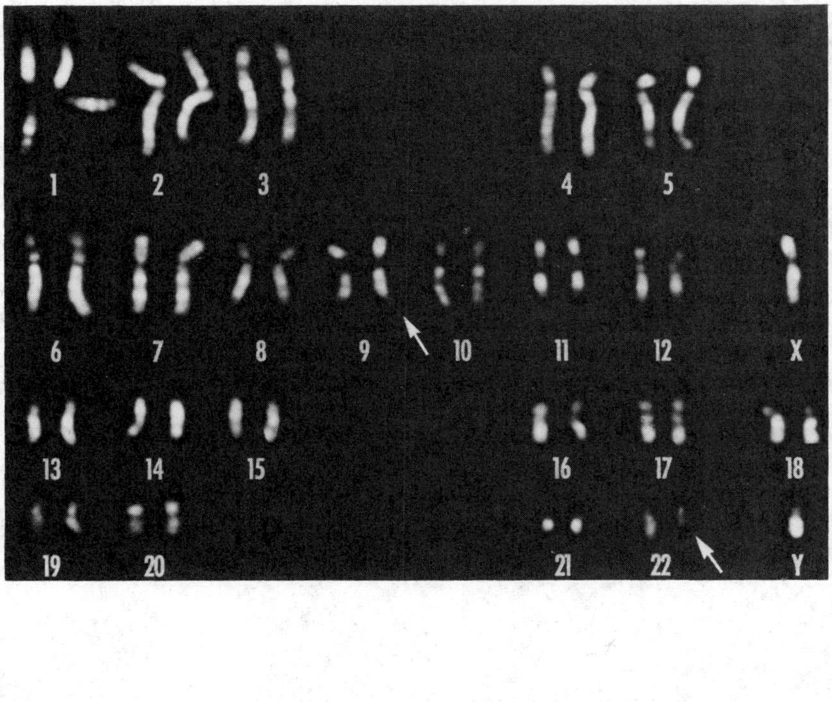

FIG. 6-3. Karyotype of a metaphase cell from a bone marrow aspirate obtained from an untreated male with chronic myeloid leukemia illustrating the t(9;22)(q34;q11). The Philadelphia chromosome (Ph^1) is the chromosome on the right in pair 22 (↑). The material missing from the long arm of this chromosome (22q−) is translocated to the long arm of chromosome 9 (9q+) (↑), and is the additional pale band that is not present on the normal chromosome 9. Chromosomes were treated with trypsin and stained with Giemsa.

patients, the 9;22 translocation was identified in 1036 (92%).[4] Variant translocations have been discovered, however, in addition to the typical t(9;22). Until very recently, these were thought to be of two kinds: one appeared to be a simple translocation involving No. 22 and some chromosome other than No. 9 (about 4%), and the other was a complex translocation involving three or more different chromosomes, two of which were No. 9 and No. 22 (about 4%). Recent data clearly demonstrate that No. 9 is affected in the simple as well as the complex translocations, and that its involvement had been overlooked.[16] Virtually all chromosomes have been involved in these variant translocations, but No. 17 is affected more often then are other chromosomes. The genetic consequences of the standard t(9;22) or the complex translocation involving at least three chromosomes is to move the *ABL* proto-oncogene on No. 9 next to a gene on No. 22, called *BCR*, whose function is currently unknown. (Fig. 6-4)

When patients with CML enter the terminal acute phase, about 10% to 20% appear to retain the 46, Ph^1+ cell line unchanged, whereas most patients show additional chromosome abnormalities, resulting in cells with modal chromosome numbers of 47 to 50.[4] During the acute phase of CML, different abnormal chromosomes occur singly or in combination in a distinctly nonrandom pattern. In patients who have only a single new chromosome change, this most commonly involves a second Ph^1, an isochromosome for the long arm of No. 17 [i(17q)], or a +8, in descending order of frequency. Chromosome loss occurs only rarely; that most often seen is −7, which occurs in 3% of patients.[4]

FIG. 6-4. Diagrammatic representation of chromosome translocation that produces the 9q+ and 22q− (Ph^1) chromosomes. One proto-oncogene, *ABL*, is moved to No. 22 adjacent to a gene of unknown function called *BCR*; the break in No. 22 is distal to the IG lambda locus, which is not involved in the translocation. The *SIS* proto-oncogene is moved to the 9q+ chromosome. It is located some distance from the breakpoint on No. 22 and there is no evidence that it is altered as the result of the translocation.

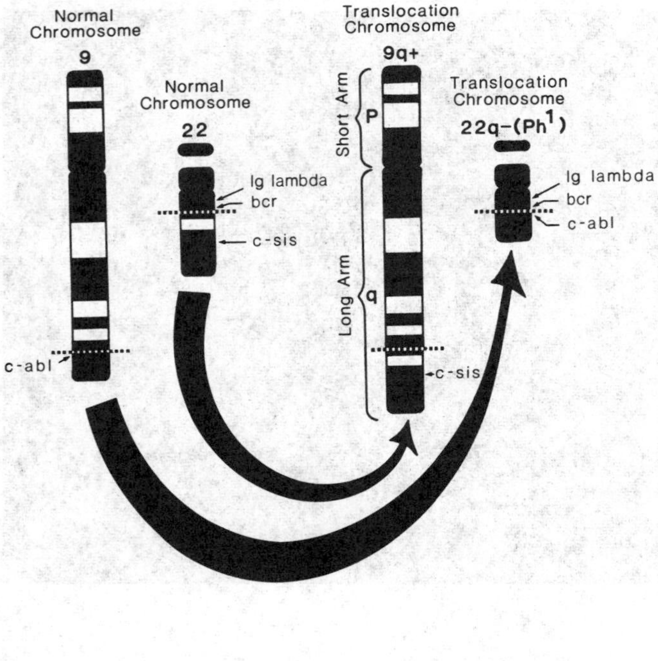

Early cases of acute leukemia in which the Ph^1 chromosome was present were classified as CML presenting in blast transformation; at present, patients who have no prior history suggestive of CML are classified as having Ph^1+ acute leukemia. In fact, as discussed in the section on Ph^1+ acute lymphocytic leukemia, some of these patients have a different breakpoint in *BCR*. In CML patients, the Ph^1 chromosome is present in granulocytic, erythroid, and megakaryocytic cells, in some B-cells, and probably in a few T-cells. In blast crisis, some blasts have intracytoplasmic IgM, which is characteristic of pre-B-cells, and these cells have an immunoglobulin gene rearrangement.[17]

Marrow cells from some patients appear to lack a Ph^1 chromosome. The majority of these patients have a normal karyotype. Somewhat surprisingly, these patients survive a substantially shorter time than those whose cells are Ph^1+.[18] Our recent review of the histology of 25 Ph^1− patients showed that most of them did not have CML but did have some type of myelodysplasia, most commonly chronic myelomonocytic leukemia or refractory anemia with excess blasts.[19] Similar observations have been reported by others.[20] However, the situation has become more complex because it has been shown recently that some patients with clinically typical CML who lack a Ph^1 chromosome cytogenetically have evidence of the insertion of *ABL* sequences into the *BCR* gene.[21,22] Thus it can be proposed that the sine qua non of CML is the juxtaposition of *BCR* and *ABL*.

ACUTE NONLYMPHOCYTIC LEUKEMIA DE NOVO

With initial banding analysis, clonal chromosome abnormalities were detected in about 50% of patients with acute nonlymphocytic leukemia (ANLL). This percentage has increased with improved banding and culture techniques; many laboratories currently are finding that at least 80% of patients have an abnormal karyotype. The most frequent abnormalities are a gain of No. 8 and loss of No. 7, changes that are seen in most subtypes of ANLL.[3-6,23] Specific rearrangements are closely associated with a particular subtype of ANLL as defined by the French–American–British Cooperative Group (FAB classification).[24] The chromosome abnormalities associated with each subtype are diagrammed in Figure 6-5.

The 8;21 Translocation in ANLL

A translocation between chromosomes 8 and 21 [t(8;21)(q22;q22)] was first identified in 1973.[25] The frequency with which this translocation is detected varies from one laboratory to another; it accounted for 25 (10%) of the 249 abnormal cases reviewed by Rowley and Testa [4] and 12% of the abnormal karyotypes reviewed at the Fourth International Workshop on Chromosomes in Leukemia.[23] The t(8;21) is the most frequent abnormality in children with ANLL, being reported in 10 (17%) of 60 karyotypically abnormal cases.[4] The abnormality initially appeared to be restricted to patients with a diagnosis of M2 (acute myeloblastic leukemia with maturation) according the FAB classification. However, 7% of t(8;21) patients analyzed at the Fourth Workshop had a diagnosis of M4.[23]

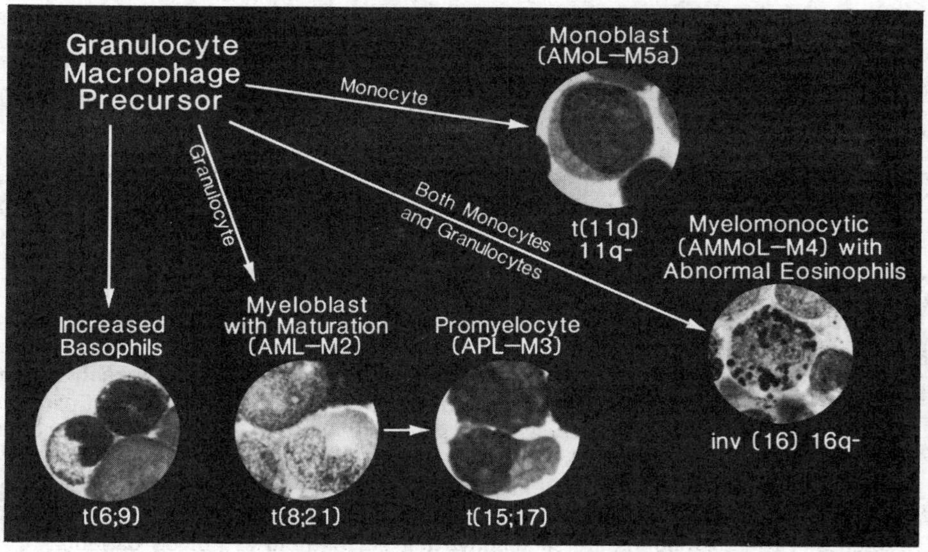

FIG. 6-5. Relationship of the subtypes of ANLL, and particular chromosome abnormality associated with each subtype. Photomicrographs illustrate the special features of the leukemic bone marrow cells obtained from untreated patients; the particular chromosome rearrangements associated with that type of leukemia are listed under the photomicrograph.

The 8;21 translocation is of interest for three other reasons. First, chromosomes 8 and 21 can participate in three-way rearrangements similar to those involving chromosomes 9 and 22 in CML. Second, the t(8;21) is often accompanied by the loss of a sex chromosome; among the cases reviewed at the Fourth Workshop, 28 (85%) of 33 males were −Y and 8 (67%) of 12 females were −X.[23] This association is particularly noteworthy because sex chromosome abnormalities are otherwise rarely observed in ANLL. Third, this translocation has never been reported as a constitutional abnormality or observed in other malignant diseases (Rowley JD: Unpublished observations).

The 15;17 Translocation in Acute Promyelocytic Leukemia

A structural rearrangement involving chromosomes 15 and 17 in acute promyelocytic leukemia was first recognized in 1977.[26] Of the 61 patients whose cases were analyzed at the Fourth Workshop, 43 (70%) had a t(15;17) (q22;q11−12), 3 had other abnormalities, and only 15 (25%) patients had a normal karyotype.[23] This rearrangement is unique to APL. In our recent review, all 44 patients with APL had a t(15;17).[3]

The 6;9 Translocation in ANLL with Increased Basophils

A translocation involving chromosomes 6 and 9 [t(6;9) (p23;q34)] was first described in two patients in 1976, but no common features were detected.[9] Slides from 9 patients with this translocation were recently reviewed; 8 of the 9 patients had an increase in basophils in the bone marrow ranging from 1.5% to 12% (normal value, 0.2%). Similar increases were noted in only 3% of other ANLL de novo patients.[27] Because the marrow in all biopsy specimens was hypercellular, this represents a marked increase in the total basophil count. The basophils appeared to be morphologically normal. Of the 9 patients, 5 were classified as having M2, 3 as having M4, and 1 as having M1. The breakpoint in No. 9 is in the same band as the t(9;22) in CML, and a marked increase in basophils is a regular feature of Ph¹+ CML. However, molecular analysis has shown that the breakpoint in chromosome 9 is distal to the *ABL* gene.[28]

Structural Alterations of 11q in Acute Monocytic Leukemia

The close association of translocations, or less often deletions, of the long arm of No. 11 (11q) and acute monoblastic leukemia (M5) was first observed by Berger et al.[29] Abnormalities of 11q occurred most frequently in children with monoblastic leukemia (type *a*) (6 of 8); adults with monoblastic leukemia had the next highest incidence (5 of 16). The incidence in monocytic leukemia type *b* was low (1 of 3 children and 0 of 7 adults). At the Fourth Workshop, 33 patients had some structural rearrangement involving 11q; 21 (63.6%) of the 33 were classified as having M5, 5 as having M4, and 3 as having M2.[23] Of the 21 patients with M5, 15 had the monoblastic type, 3 had the monocytic type, and the slides of 3 could not be subclassified. Five of the patients were less than 1 year old, and 7 others were less than 20 years old. When all patients with M5 leukemia were considered, about 22% had an aberration involving 11q.

Aberrations of 11q differ from the t(8;22) and t(15;17) in two ways. First, the breakpoint in 11q involves band 11q23−24 in about two thirds of patients, but it can also occur in 11q13−14. Second, although translocations are more common (21 of 33 Fourth Workshop patients), 11 patients appeared to have what was identified as a terminal deletion of 11q. Although the other chromosome involved in the translocation is variable, a t(9;11)(p22;q23) is common.[30]

Structural Alterations in No. 16 in Acute Myelomonocytic Leukemia with Abnormal Eosinophils

Another clinical-cytogenetic association recently identified involves myelomonocytic (M4) leukemia with abnormal eosinophils. Arthur and Bloomfield described 5 cases of M2 or M4 in which the bone marrow contained an excess of eosinophils (8%–54%); all 5 patients had a deleted No. 16 [del(16)(q22)].[31] Our group has reported on a related entity, first in 18 patients and then in a larger series of 33 patients.[32] Most of these patients had M4 leukemia with eosinophils that showed unique morphological changes [M4Eo], including large and irregular basophilic granules; one third lacked increased eosinophils because the marrow contained fewer than 5% eosinophils. Twenty-seven patients had an inversion of No. 16, inv(16)(p13q22), and six had a t(16;16)(p13;q22). The strong correlation between abnormal eosinophils and structural rearrangements of No. 16 was confirmed at the Fourth Workshop.[23] In fact, the morphological features of the eosinophils are so specific that our pathologists can accurately predict which patients will have either an inv(16) or a t(16;16) by examining the bone marrow aspirate. It appears that this relatively common (25% of our AMMoL patients have this aberration) but subtle chromosome aberration was undetected in the past, in part because of poor morphology. This chromosome abnormality has clinical implications as well. Among 32 treated patients, 78% achieved a complete remission, compared with 36% of 58 other AMMoL patients. The median survival time was more than 65 weeks for patients with an abnormal No. 16, compared with 29 weeks for those with a normal No. 16.[32] These data confirm an observation reported by Keating that an increase in marrow eosinophils is a good prognostic sign.[33] In fact, at the Fourth Workshop it was clearly shown that the type rather than the presence of a chromosome abnormality has prognostic importance (Table 6-2). Thus, although the projected median survival for all patients was 8 months, those with a t(8;21) had the longest median survival (13 months), while those with abnormalities of chromosomes 5 and 7, t(15;17), or hyperdiploidy had the shortest survivals (3 to 4 months.)

ANLL AND MYELODYSPLASTIC SYNDROME ASSOCIATED WITH TREATMENT

A distinctive disorder of bone marrow morphology and function that terminates in myelodysplastic syndrome (MDS) or in ANLL has been recognized as a late complication of cytotoxic therapy used in the treatment of both malignant and nonmalignant diseases.[34] Characteristic nonrandom chromosome abnormalities are commonly observed in bone marrow cells of patients with t-MDS/t-ANLL. These abnormalities differ in their type and frequency from those noted in ANLL developing de novo. We reported previously that part or all of chromosome Nos. 5 and/or 7 was lost in cells from 23 (86%) of 26 t-MDS/t-ANLL patients.[35] More recently 61 of 63 patients were found to have an abnormal karyotype, and 55 of these had an abnormality of one or both chromosomes 5 and 7.[35] These observations have been confirmed by others.[36,37] After analyzing data in 17 patients with a deletion of the long arm of No. 5 we were able to identify a region, 5q23 to 5q32, that was consistently missing in every patient. In contrast, only about 16% of patients with ANLL de novo have a similar abnormality of chromosome No. 5 or No. 7 or both.[38] Moreover, the latter patients frequently have had significant occupational exposure to potential environmental carcinogens, such as chemicals, solvents, or pesticides.[39,40] Furthermore, one seldom finds the specific rearrangements in t-ANLL that are closely associated with the distinct morphological subsets of ANLL de novo, such as t(8;21), t(15;17), or inv(16).

A number of growth factors or growth factor receptors have been mapped to the region 5q23–32 that is consistently deleted; whether any of them play a role in mutagen-associated leukemia is unknown.[41]

TABLE 6-2. Correlation of Karyotype and Survival of 660 Patients with ANLL de novo*

Karyotype	*Number of Patients*	*Complete Remission: Median Duration, Months (% of patients)†*	*Median Survival, Months‡*
Normal	307	13 (45)	10
−5 or 5q−	29	4 (28)	4
−7 or 7q−	28	25+ (21)	3
Abn. 5 and 7	21	Too few	3
t(15;17)	43	10 (40)	3
t(8;21)	44	10 (77)	13
llq abn.	29	6 (21)	8
+8	36	8 (22)	6
+21	12	19+ (67)	10
46 abnormal	67	13 (31)	5
>46 chromosomes	31	12 (16)	4
<46 chromosomes	13	6 (46)	5

*Data from Fourth Workshop on Chromosomes in Leukemia. Cancer Genet Cytogenet 11:249–360, 1984.
†Percentage of patients with each karyotype who achieved a complete remission.
‡Difference in survival is significant (p = 0.0002).

MALIGNANT DISEASES AFFECTING LYMPHOCYTES

The chromosome abnormalities in lymphoid disorders, especially in the non-Hodgkin's lymphomas, have been reviewed in considerable detail.[4,42–45] This section reviews the consistent translocations seen in Burkitt's lymphoma and in some cases of B-cell ALL, the other aberrations in ALL, and aberrations in some T-cell disorders.

LYMPHOMA

In 1972, Manolov and Manolova discovered that cells of Burkitt's lymphomas had an additional band at the end of the long arm of the one chromosome No. 14 (14q+).[46] Zech and co-workers in 1976 first observed that the end of the one No. 8 was consistently absent, and they suggested that the missing part of No. 8 was translocated to No. 14 [t(8;14)(q24;q32)].[47] The t(8;14) has also been observed in nonendemic Burkitt's tumors from America, Europe, and Japan that are Epstein-Barr virus negative; thus, it is a highly characteristic chromosome anomaly in Burkitt's tumors. This translocation has also been observed in other lymphomas, particularly those of the diffuse large cell type. Two other, related translocations were later identified in Burkitt's tumors. All three translocations involved No. 8 with a break in the same band, 8q24. One variant translocation involved chromosome No. 2 with a break in the short arm [t(2;8)(p12;q24)], and the other involved No. 22 with a break in the long arm in the band (22qll) that is affected in CML. All three translocations have been identified in patients with B-cell ALL.

The data on Burkitt's lymphoma indicate that No. 8 is the consistently involved chromosome. When the karyotypic aberrations seen in lymphoid disease are considered as a whole, a break in No. 14 at q32, with translocation of material from elsewhere to the broken No. 14, is the single most common change. The only other recurring translocation, t(14;18)(q32;q21), is in fact the most common translocation in lymphoma (Fig. 6-6). This was first identified by Fukuhara and co-workers in 6 of 9 patients with poorly differentiated lymphocytic lymphoma,[48] now called "malignant lymphoma, follicular, predominantly small cleaved cell" (FSC) in the International Classification System.[49] This finding was confirmed by many others.[42–45] The correlation between karyotype and histologic type in 260 cases reviewed at the Fifth International Workshop on Chromosomes in Leukemia and Lymphoma is summarized in Figure 6-7.[45] Fifteen percent of the 260 workshop patients had a normal karyotype. The karyotypic pattern varies greatly among the different subgroups. The t(14;18) is common in follicular lymphomas, whereas the t(8;14) is common in small noncleaved cell lymphoma.

What are the implications of the t(14;18) in tumors with a large cell or diffuse morphology? Analysis of the karyotypic pattern in these tumors shows that certain additional chromosome changes, especially a gain of No. 7 or a deletion of the long arm of No. 6 [(del)6q], appear to correlate with a more malignant phenotype (see Fig. 6-6).[43,44] The translocation junction has been cloned and a gene on No. 18 called

FIG. 6-6. R-banding karyotype of a cell in the leukemic phase illustrating the many complex changes that can occur. There is an extra X and No. 20 and loss of the Y chromosome. Note the deletion of 1q (*left*), 1p (*center*), 2q, 5q (*left*), 6q, 8q, 11q (*right*), and 18q; addition to 4q, 5p (*right*), 10q, 11q (*left*), 13p, and both 14q's; a gain of the abnormal No. 7 (7q+); and four unknown markers (M1 to M4). The 1q− chromosome originates from a translocation with 5p [t(1;5)(q11;p15), and the 1p− chromosome could result from a translocation with No. 17 [t(1;17)(q?21;p?13). The two 14q+ chromosomes result from a 14q translocation with 8q and 18q, [t(8;14)(q24;q32) and [t(14;18)(q32;q21), respectively. The 5q− and the 6q− chromosome each could have an interstitial deletion of the long arm, [del(5)(q13q31)] and [del(6)(q21q23)]. The 11q− chromosome has lost the whole long arm. M4 could be a ring chromosome.

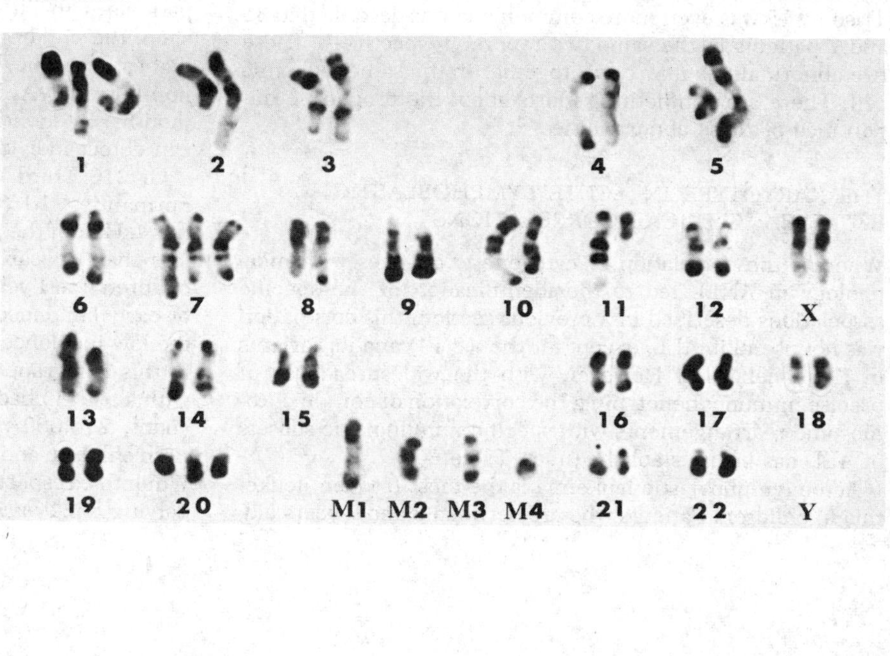

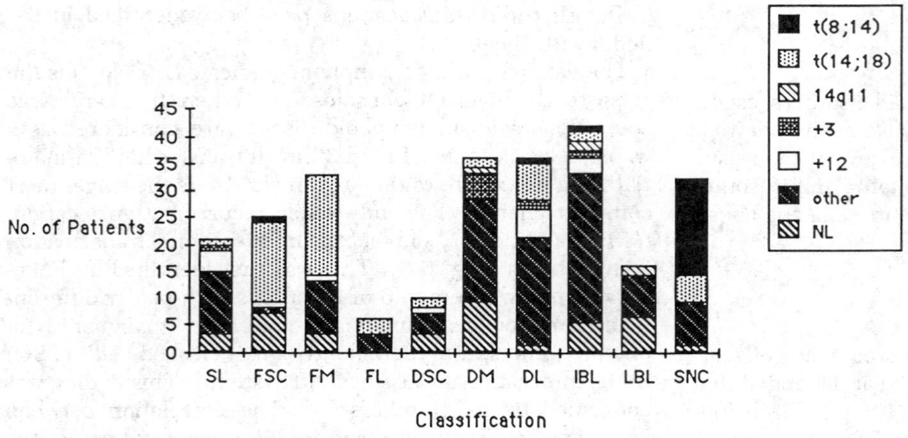

FIG. 6-7. Histogram showing the most common chromosome changes identified in 260 lymphomas studied before treatment and reviewed at the Fifth International Workshop on Chromosomes in Leukemia/Lymphoma; each tumor was classified according to the Working Formulation.

BCL2 (the second B-cell leukemia gene) has been identified.[50] Breakpoints cluster in at least two sites on the gene; the major cluster is in the 3′ untranslated region of the second exon. In the lymphoma cells, the expression of the normal gene is suppressed and an abnormal chimeric *BCL2–IGH* messenger RNA (mRNA) is expressed. This leads to inappropriate expression of a structurally normal protein whose function is unknown.[51]

THE KARYOTYPE IN CHRONIC LYMPHOCYTIC LEUKEMIA

Chronic lymphocytic leukemia (CLL) is the most common leukemia in the United States and Europe, accounting for about 30% of all leukemias. It is considered to be a monoclonal neoplastic proliferation of small lymphocytes which are of B-cell origin in 95% of cases. The early studies of the cytogenetic pattern in CLL showed a normal karyotype in most samples. As better culture and banding methods have been applied to these studies, nonrandom clonal abnormalities have been detected. These include translocations involving 14q32 and trisomy for chromosome 12.[1,52–55] In two reports, translocations of 14q were observed in 17 of 87 patients and in 5 of 16 patients with abnormal karyotypes.[8,54] Trisomy 12 was even more common and was described in 33 and 7 patients in the same two reports, respectively. These two abnormalities may occur together in the same leukemic cell. There are conflicting reports about the prognostic importance of these abnormalities.[53–55]

THE KARYOTYPE IN ACUTE LYMPHOBLASTIC LEUKEMIA: CLINICAL CORRELATIONS

Whereas the correlation of cytogenetic changes with morphology in ANLL led to the identification of the specific associations described in a previous section, this correlation was not useful in ALL, except for the t(8;14) and its variants in L3, B-cell ALL. However, with the widespread use of precise immunophenotyping, the correlation of certain chromosome rearrangements with specific immunologic subsets of ALL has been established (see Table 6-1).

Acute lymphoblastic leukemia is the most frequent leukemia in children. Patients who are between 3 and 7 years old, who have a white blood cell (WBC) count of less than 10,000/mm³, and whose leukemic cells have non-T, non-B surface markers have the best prognosis. For many years metaphase chromosomes from ALL patients had poor morphology with indistinct bands, making an accurate analysis difficult, and there have been fewer reports of chromosome patterns in ALL than in ANLL. Recent improvements permit correlation of the karyotype with other recognized prognostic factors. It was rigorously demonstrated for the first time at the Third International Workshop on Chromosomes in Leukemia that the karyotype is an important independent prognostic factor in ALL.[56] Of 330 patients whose cases were reviewed at the Third Workshop, 112 appeared to have a normal karyotype; the largest group (39 patients) with a well-defined abnormality had a Ph¹ chromosome. Eighteen patients had a t(4;11), 16 had a t(8;14), and 15 had an abnormality of No. 14 not involving chromosome 8. Other patients with abnormalities were classified by the modal chromosome number.

The Ph¹ chromosome is the most frequent rearrangement, accounting for 17.3% of cases of adult ALL. At the cytogenetic level, the breakpoints appear identical to those in CML; recent molecular analysis indicates that the breakpoint in the *BCR* gene on No. 22 may be more proximal in some patients with Ph¹+ ALL than in CML. At the Third Workshop, the children with a Ph¹ chromosome had the second highest median leukocyte count (75,000/mm³), all had non-B, non-T ALL, and their median survival was only 15 months. By identifying this chromosomal abnormality, one can detect individuals who have a poor prognosis.

Of 216 Third Workshop patients with chromosomal abnormalities, 18 (8.3%) had a t(4;11)(q21;q23) rearrangement. Half of the patients were children, most of whom were less than 1 year old; and the median age of the affected children was 1 year. The association of t(4;11) with neonatal or early childhood ALL is particularly interesting in view of the low incidence of ALL in this age group; acute leukemias in this age group are usually of the myeloid type. Children with a t(4;11) had very high leukocyte counts (median WBC count, 214,000/mm³), which is a poor prognostic factor. Both children and adults had a short median survival—9 and 7 months, respectively. Only patients with abnormalities involving 8q24 or 14q32 had shorter survivals.

Although the morphology of some cells with a t(4;11) often appears lymphoid, other features are more suggestive of monocytic leukemia. A t(4;11) cell line showed rearranged heavy and light chain (κ) genes, although cells lacked cytoplasmic immunoglobulin and thus were probably in a very early stage of B-cell differentiation.[57] However, when cells were cultured with the phorbol ester TPA, a monocytic-like phenotype was induced. Thus these cells appear to be very early precursor cells that have dual lineage capabilities.

Another recurring chromosome abnormality is the t(1;19) (q21;p13), which has been identified in about 25% of patients with a pre-B phenotype, that is, they have cytoplasmic immunoglobulin and are classified as CALLA+.[58–60]

The leukemic cells of some patients with ALL are characterized by a gain of many chromosomes and fewer structural abnormalities.[61–62] Chromosome numbers usually range from 50 to 60, and a few patients have up to 65 chromosomes. Although identical karyotypes are unusual, certain additional chromosomes are commonly seen. Among 31 Third Workshop patients with hyperdiploidy (14% of patients with abnormalities), +21, +6, +18, +14, +4, and +10 in decreasing frequency were seen in 10% to 33%.[56] It is interesting that some of these chromosomes, particularly Nos. 10, 18 and 21, were also seen as additional chromosomes in patients with near-haploidy, with chromosome numbers of 26 to 36 (median, 28). The median age of the 22 children with this abnormality was 3 years, and that of all 31 patients was 5 years, less than that of patients with other abnormalities. The WBC count was low (median, 6,000/mm^3). Thus, these patients have all of the previously recognized factors, including age between 3 and 7 years, low WBC count, and non-T, non-B markers, that indicate a good prognosis. In a follow-up study of the Third Workshop patients, the complete remission rate for children was 95%, with a median remission duration that will be greater than 5 years. The median survival of the children with hyperdiploidy is longer than for those with a normal karyotype; for adults, the medial survival for the two groups is comparable. Chromosome losses were less frequent and involved No. 9, 7, 13, 20, or 8 in that order. The three translocations seen in B-cell ALL were described under Burkitt's lymphoma. With regard to karyotype and age, patients with a deletion of 6q and a modal chromosome number greater than 50 were younger, and those with a Ph^1 chromosome or a 14q+ were older than patients with other abnormalities. In summary, the highest remission rates were in patients with a normal karyotype and a modal number greater than 50; the lowest were seen in patients with a Ph^1 chromosome, a 14q+ chromosome, a t(8;14), and a t(4;11).[63]

T-CELL DISORDERS

Although fewer leukemias of T-cell origin have been studied, a distinct pattern of nonrandom karyotypic abnormalities is emerging. Rearrangements involving the proximal bands of chromosome 14 (14q11–q13) are relatively common. Those involving two regions of chromosome 7 (7q35-q36 and 7p15) also occur in T-cell malignancies but have been observed in nonmalignant T-cell disorders as well; breaks involving these regions are very rare in other malignant diseases. One recurring rearrangement in T-cell neoplasia, particularly CLL, is a paracentric inversion of chromosome 14 with a proximal breakpoint at q11 and a distal breakpoint at q32.[64,65] A closely related rearrangement, t(14;14)(q11;q32), is seen in T-cell neoplasia [64,66] and in phytohemagglutinin-stimulated T-lymphocytes from patients with ataxia-telangiectasia (A-T) as well as in the leukemic cells of A-T patients in whom this disease evolved.[66,67] A number of reports from Japan have described the frequent occurrence of 14q11 breaks in adult T-cell leukemia–lymphoma patients [68,69]; fewer such patients have been described in Western countries, and 14q11 breaks are much less common.[70,71] Williams et al have described a t(11;14)(p13;q13) in the leukemic cells of 4 of 16 patients with T-cell acute lymphoblastic leukemia.[60] Thus, in some of these T-cell diseases, breaks occur in either 14q11 or 14q32, or in both bands in the same patient. In B-cell disorders, however, breaks occur essentially only in 14q32, and they rarely involve 14q11.[54] The data confirm the observation made some time ago that the proximal region of chromosome 14 is important in T-cell neoplasia.[66] More detailed analysis of rearrangements of 7q in T-cell disorders has revealed that a few patients have breaks at 7q32 to 7q36, the location of the β chain for the T-cell receptor.[64,72]

KARYOTYPES OF CANCERS AND OF BENIGN TUMORS

Whereas the karyotype of the leukemic cells has been determined in thousands of patients with either acute or chronic myeloid leukemia, the karyotype has been defined from fewer than 100 samples of any specific cancer. Several reasons account for this discrepancy. First, it is difficult to obtain successful chromosome preparations from solid tumors because of extensive fibrosis or necrosis. Second, until recently, many investigators questioned the relevance of the chromosome changes in malignant cells, and therefore this area of research, was not pursued. Third, the karyotypes of the tumor cells frequently show high modal numbers, often 60 to 90 chromosomes, with many bizarre marker chromosomes, and it is very difficult to distinguish the primary change from changes related to secondary evolution with progression of the malignant phenotype. Those changes that appear to be consistent are summarized in Table 6-3.

TUMORS ORIGINATING IN EMBRYONIC CELLS

Tumors originating in embryonic cells are of particular interest to the cytogeneticist because some of them occur in patients who have specific *constitutional* chromosome abnormalities. In all preceding sections, the karyotypic changes were somatic mutations in malignant cells and were not present in other unaffected cells. In contrast, some patients at risk of developing retinoblastoma have a variable deletion of chromosome 13 that always includes 13q14, whereas other patients with a deletion of No. 11 (band 11p13) are at risk of developing Wilms' tumor. In general, these deletions also are associated with various phenotypic abnormalities (for review, see refs. 2 and 73). Relatively few

TABLE 6-3. Recurring Chromosome Abnormalities in Solid Tumors

Involving embryonic cells	
Neuroblastoma	Deletion of No. 1 (p32–p36)
Ewing's sarcoma/peripheral neuroepithelioma	t(11;22)(q24;q12)
Wilms' tumor	Deletion of No. 11 (p13)* Trisomy 1q
Retinoblastoma	Deletion of No. 13 (q14)* Trisomy lq
Testicular tumors	i(12p)
Adult cancers	
Malignant melanoma	Deletion of No. 1 (p11–p22)
Small cell lung carcinoma	Deletion of No. 3 (p14–p23)
Renal carcinoma	Deletion of No. 3 (p14–p21)
Liposarcoma	t(12;16)(q13;p11)
Synovial sarcoma	t(X;18)(p11.2;q11.2)
Rhabdomyosarcoma (alveolar)	t(2;13)(q37;q14)
Benign tumors	
Pleomorphic adenomas	t(3;8)(p21;q12); t(9;12)(p13–22; q13–15)
Meningioma	Loss of No. 22 or deletion (q11)
Lipoma	t(3;12)(q27–q28;q13–q14)

*Observed as a constitutional abnormality as well as in some tumors.

tumors have been analyzed, and deletions of No. 13 or much less often, of No. 11 have been observed in tumor cells from some retinoblastomas or Wilms' tumors, respectively. The most common change that we have observed in Wilms' tumors is trisomy for the long arm of No. 1 (+1q).[74]

Both Wilms' tumors and retinoblastomas have two patterns of inheritance, one as an autosomal dominant and one as a sporadic mutation. The age at tumor detection as well as other observations led Knudsen to propose the two-mutation hypothesis.[75] According to this hypothesis, in patients who inherit the predisposing gene, only one other change is needed for transformation of retinal cells to tumor cells, and in these individuals multiple tumors are diagnosed at a very early age. In sporadic cases, two independent mutations must affect the same cell for transformation to occur; since this event is relatively uncommon, the tumors are unifocal and develop at an older age. Based on the consistent loss of chromosome band, 13q14, this band was thought to be the locus for the retinoblastoma or *RB* gene. Studies confirming that No. 13 was the critical chromosome included the discovery that tumor cells frequently homozygous for DNA markers on chromosome 13 were heterozygous in cells of nontumor tissue from the same patient.[76] Using probes cloned from 13q14, Dryja et al discovered that copies of one of the probes had been deleted from both chromosomes in one of 20 tumors; DNA probes from this region detected mRNA in a retinal cell line that was absent in some retinoblastomas.[77] By making a DNA copy of the mRNA, they identified deletions or mutations in about 30% of retinoblastoma tumors or cell lines.[78] Others have identified mRNA abnormalities in each of six retinoblastomas.[79] Thus, we now have the tools to identify the complete *RB* gene, to understand its function in normal cells, and then to determine why its abnormal function or its absence leads to malignant transformation of these cells. The current assumption is that the *RB* gene, and the genes that will be identified in the deleted chromosome segments in other tumor cells, function as tumor suppressors or "anti-oncogenes." Presumably these genes inhibit the function of genes stimulating cell proliferation, and their loss allows the growth-promoting genes to function without modulation.[80]

Recurring chromosome abnormalities limited to the malignant cells have also been observed in other childhood tumors. For example, a deletion of some of the long arm of chromosome 1 (1p−) has been noted in neuroblastomas.[81] Neuroblastomas are also of interest because of their proclivity to undergo gene amplification, which is manifested chromosomally as hundreds or thousands of small discrete pieces of chromosomes called *double minutes,* or long unbanded regions on chromosomes called *homogeneously staining regions,* or HSR.[82] In some cell lines, these have been shown to represent amplification of *NMYC*.[83] Amplification of *NMYC* has also been identified in tumor samples; it is highly correlated with advanced stage (III and IV) and with poor survival.[84]

CANCER IN ADULTS

Although karyotypes have been determined for a number of individual tumors, it has been difficult to establish a consistent pattern comparable to that described earlier for ANLL, for reasons already discussed. Loss of chromosomal material may be an important factor in some of the more common tumors in adults, including lung cancer and colon cancer. A deletion of the long arm of No. 1 has been observed in malignant melanoma[85]; the deleted region may be larger than that noted in neuroblastoma. A deletion of the short arm of No. 3 (p14–p23) has been described by Whang-Peng et al[86] in small cell lung carcinoma, and a somewhat different deletion (3p14-p21) has been described in renal cancer.[87,88] Examination of various different types of lung cancers, including small cell, squamous cell, and adenocarcinoma, has revealed the development of homozygosity for DNA markers that are located near 3p21.[89,90] Using the strategies developed for retinoblastoma, a number of laboratories are trying to identify the critical gene within the deletion. Atkin and Baker have noted an isochromosome for the short arm of No. 12 [i(12p)] in testicular tumors.[91]

CHROMOSOME TRANSLOCATIONS IN SARCOMAS

Soft tissue (mesenchymal) tumors are relatively rare, accounting for less than 1% of all human neoplasms. They are very heterogeneous, and may present diagnostic problems. Recently, cytogenetic and molecular analysis of these tumors in their malignant (sarcoma) and benign forms has yielded important clues to the hitherto unsuspected relationship of some of these rare neoplasms and has aided in classifying some of the undifferentiated forms of these tumors. Moreover, the fact that the benign and malignant forms have related karyotypic changes provides an important resource for identifying the additional genetic changes that occur in the malignant compared with the benign form.

Although chromosome translocations have not been a

prominent cytogenetic feature of solid tumors, a number of them have been identified in certain specific tumors, especially sarcomas. One example is the 11;22 translocation [t(11;22)(q24;q12)] in Ewing's sarcoma,[92-93] which has been detected in more than 90% of these tumors. The identity of the genes involved in this translocation has not been established. Cytogeneticists and oncologists were both surprised when it was reported that peripheral neuroepithelial tumors also had the 11;22 translocation.[94] In fact, the neuronal phenotype of Ewing's sarcoma and neuroepithelioma is the same. The similarity is substantiated by molecular analysis: Ewing's sarcoma and neuroepithelioma have identical levels of proto-ocogene expression which differ from those in neuroblastoma.[95] Amplification of *NMYC* is limited to neuroblastoma. Treatment of neuroepithelial tumors had been disappointing; however, use of therapy for Ewing's sarcoma resulted in a remarkable improvement in response.

Recurring translocations have recently been described in both liposarcoma and synovial sarcoma.[2,96-98] Sandberg and his colleagues have described a t(12;16)(q13;p11) only in the myxoid subgroup of liposarcomas; other abnormalities, including ring chromosome, appeared to be more frequent in well-differentiated sarcomas.[97] The chromosome abnormality in synovial sarcoma [t(X;18)(p11.2;q11.2)] is of interest because it is the first one involving a sex chromosome. This abnormality does not appear to be restricted to a particular histologic pattern.[98]

BENIGN TUMORS

Although much of the discussion in this chapter implies that chromosome aberrations are equivalent to a malignant phenotype, there are a number of exceptions. In the myeloproliferative disorders, patients with clonal chromosome abnormalities in marrow cells have been observed for up to 12 to 15 years without undergoing leukemic transformation.[4,5] Several benign tumors have clonal abnormalities, of which the meningiomas described by Mark et al[99] and by Zankl and Zang[100] have been studied most extensively. Each group has noted either the loss of all of No. 22 or, less commonly, a deletion of the long arm with a break in 22q11. This information led Gusella and his colleagues to examine various neuronal tumors with DNA markers; they discovered the loss of heterozygosity for chromosome 22 probes in acoustic neuromas.[101] Mark et al examined parotid gland tumors and noted a translocation [t(3;8)(p25;q21)] in many of them.[102] Cytogenetic analyses of uterine leiomyomas have only recently been reported; however, it appears that breaks in 14q22–24 and in 12q14–15 are not uncommon.[103,104] An identical translocation, t(12;14)(q14–15;q23–24) was found as the only abnormality in 4 of 34 leiomyomas.[104]

Of special interest with regard to the sarcomas is that many benign neoplasms affect the same cell type. Thus, of 26 lipomas karyotyped, 70% had consistent chromosome rearrangements; 13 of them had a reciprocal translocation involving 12q13–14, the same breakpoint noted in liposarcomas. It may be significant that this region of No. 12 is involved in lipomas–liposarcomas, leiomyomas, and mixed salivary gland tumors.

MOLECULAR ANALYSIS OF CONSISTENT CHROMOSOME ABNORMALITIES, PARTICULARLY TRANSLOCATIONS

HOW AND WHEN CONSISTENT TRANSLOCATIONS OCCUR.

We do not know how consistent structural rearrangements occur, but there are at least two possibilities.[105] The rearrangements may be random, but selection may act to eliminate the vast majority that do not provide the cell with a proliferative advantage. Alternatively, certain changes may occur preferentially and thus may be the ones we see. Some tantalizing data show an association of chromosome rearrangements in tumor cells from patients with fragile sites affecting one of the chromosome bands broken in the tumor cells.[106-108] However, much more research is required to clarify the role of fragile sites as a predisposing factor to malignant transformation.

Croce[109] has proposed that many of the chromosome rearrangements in B- and T-cell tumors involve sequences used in the normal recombination of the V-D-J segments of the immunoglobulin and T-cell receptor genes. The presence of heptamer and nanomer sequences in the nonimmunoglobulin gene at the site of the translocation, namely *MYC* and *BCL2* has been reported. We have no indication at present that the genes involved in the translocations in myeloid leukemias undergo similar DNA rearrangements.

An equally important question is, when in the multistage process of malignant transformation of a particular cell do translocations or other chromosome aberrations occur? Some chromosome changes occur as part of the further evolution of the malignant phenotype (*e.g.*, blast crisis of CML) and they are therefore relatively late events. But what about the occurrence of the t(9;22) in CML, for example? Does the Ph^1 occur in a single normal cell that becomes the progenitor of the leukemic clone, or is there expansion of a clone, possibly a leukemic one, in which a translocation occurs in one of these already abnormal cells? Fialkow et al [110] have presented detailed evidence supporting the latter proposal.

Adams et al[111] have constructed transgenic mice whose cells all have a vector containing the *MYC/IgH* junction from a murine plasmacytoma. All cells contain this construct; however, the B-cell tumors that occurred in every animal were clonal, indicating that one or more additional charges occurred in one cell, resulting in clonality.

CHROMOSOME LOCATION OF PROTO-ONCOGENES

One of the most surprising revelations in the recent past has involved the cellular oncogenes and their chromosome location. Much of the excitement derives from the observation that many proto-oncogenes are located in the bands that are involved in consistent translocations (Fig. 6-8).[105,111-116] The evidence in Burkitt's lymphoma and in CML clearly points the way for future research in this area. The gene for the proto-oncogene *MYC* (the cellular homologue of the avian myelocytomatosis virus) is on chromosome 8(q24). The immunoglobulin genes (heavy chain, and κ and λ light chain genes) are located at the breakpoints on the three chromo-

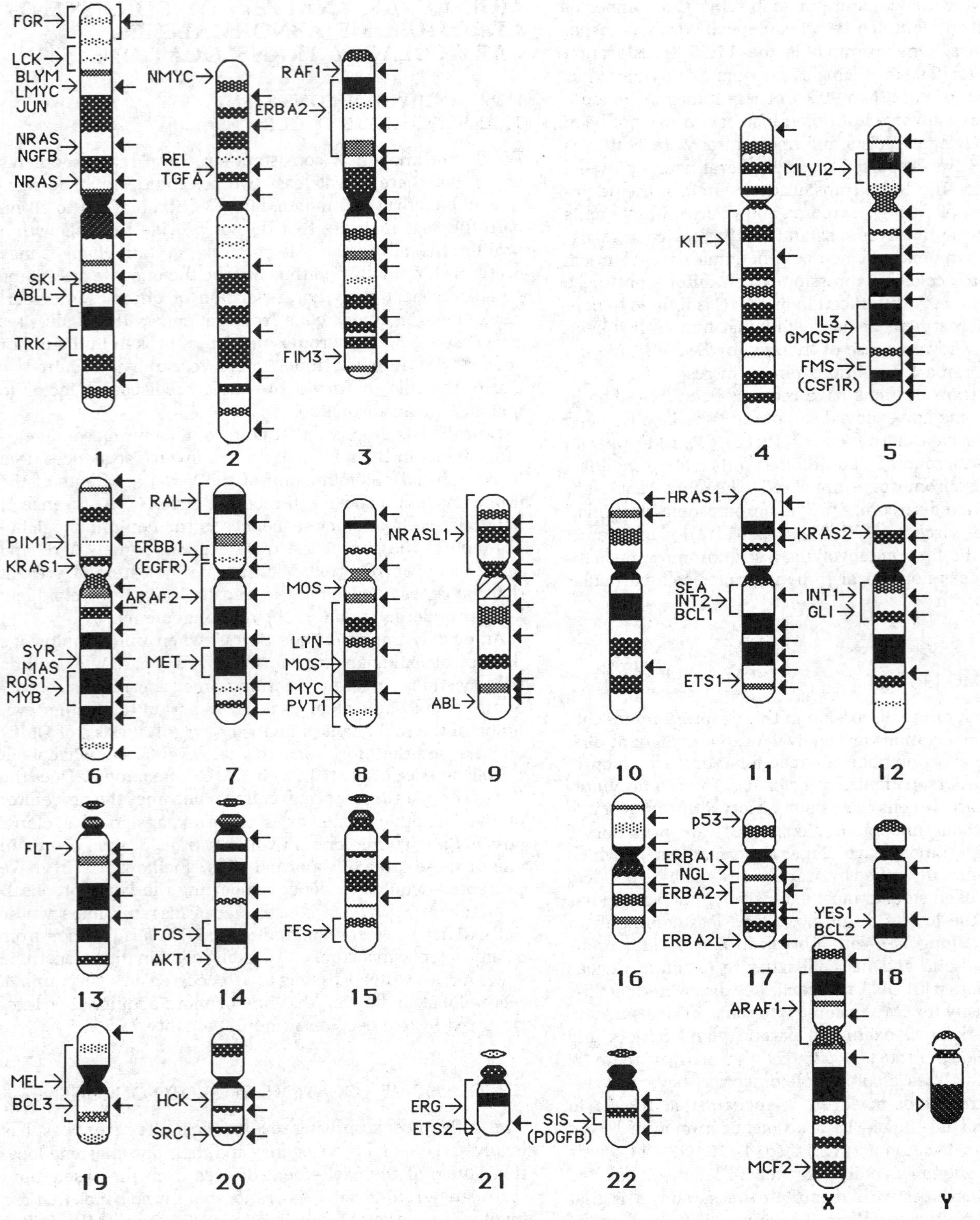

FIG. 6-8. Map of the chromosome location of proto-oncogenes or of genes with transforming properties and the breakpoints observed in recurring chromosome abnormalities in human leukemia, lymphoma, and solid tumors. The proto-oncogenes and their locations are placed to the left of the appropriate chromosome band (*arrow*) or region (indicated by a bracket). The breakpoints in recurring translocations, inversions, deletions, and so forth are indicated with an arrow to the right of the affected chromosome band. The location of the cancer specific breakpoints are based on the Human Gene Mapping 9 report.[5]

somes, other than No. 8, that are involved in the translocations in Burkitt's lymphoma: 14q23, 2p12, and 22q11 respectively. These translocations result in the aberrant juxtaposition of *MYC* and one of the immunoglobulin genes; this in turn leads to abnormal regulation of *MYC* expression, although the precise nature of the derangement is not presently understood.[113,115] Comparable chromosome translocations and gene rearrangements have been observed in mouse plasmacytomas.[116]

An analogous chromosome abnormality has been defined recently in T-cell leukemia. In this translocation the breakpoint also involves *MYC* at 8q24, but the other gene is the α chain for the T-cell receptor (*TCRA*) which is located at 14q11.[117,118] In SKW3, we and others have shown that the break in *MYC* is 3′ of the third exon and *MYC* remains on chromosome 8; in *TCRA* the break is just 5′ of a Jα segment (JαD).[119,120] This translocation is similar to these involving the immunoglobulin light chain genes in which *MYC* also remains on No. 8. The *TCRA* gene is also involved with translocations affecting 14q32 and the heavy chain gene in the inv(14).[121]

Investigators are now in the process of unraveling the mystery of the Ph[1] translocation in CML and ALL. In the t(9;22) in CML and ALL, the Abelson proto-oncogene (*ABL*) is translocated to the Ph[1] chromosome.[15] This was an important observation, because *ABL* was the first gene known to be on No. 9 that was shown to translocate to No. 22, thus establishing that the translocation was reciprocal. The *ABL* gene was first identified because of its homology with the viral oncogene that had been isolated from a mouse pre-B-cell leukemia. The breakpoint junction in CML was cloned and the site on the Ph[1] was called *bcr*, for breakpoint cluster region,[122] since the majority of breaks cluster in a small, 5.8-kilobase (kb) region. In contrast, the breaks on No. 9 occur over an incredible distance of more than 200 kb. We have used pulse field gel electophoresis (PFGE) to great advantage in the study of the *ABL* proto-oncogene. Southern blotting with standard gel electrophoresis leads to separation of DNA fragments in the size range of 2 to about 25 kb. Since the *ABL* gene is larger than 200 kb, mapping it in 10- to 20-kb pieces is a formidable task. In contrast, by using PFGE one can separate fragments more than 1,000 kb in size, and this technique is also very effective in the 100-to 600-kb range. A normal chromosome band contains roughly 3000 to 5000 kb, and thus several very large, overlapping fragments could contain a single band. Using many probes for *ABL* provided by various investigators, Westbrook, Rubin and co-workers have constructed a map of the normal *ABL* gene.[123] This is a complex gene that normally uses one of two alternative beginnings, exon Ia or Ib. During transcription, either of these can be spliced at the same point on the remainder of the gene, which is called the common splice acceptor site, or exon II. One of their first discoveries was that the type Ib exon mapped more than 200 kb upstream from exon II. As a result, a very large segment of the RNA transcript is removed or spliced out to form the mature mRNA. This is a remarkable feat, not identified before in biologic systems. The breakpoints in the chromosomes of various CML patients and cell lines occur in many locations upstream (5′) of exon II. However, the same size (8.5 kb) mRNA is found in all CML patients; this occurs because the *bcr* exons are spliced to *ABL* exon II, resulting in a chimeric mRNA that is translated into a chimeric protein (p210 BCR-ABL).[124,125]

With regard to Ph[1]+ ALL, it has always been an enigma why the typical Ph[1] translocation is seen in ALL and in fact is the most common translocation in adults with ALL.[56] One relatively trivial explanation would be that the patients really had CML in lymphoid blast crisis with an undiagnosed chronic phase, and this may occur in some patients. However, analysis of DNA from some Ph[1]+ ALL cells indicates that the breakpoint in the *BCR* gene on No. 22 differs from that in CML. In one study, the majority of adult patients (13 of 17) appeared to have the *BCR* rearrangement seen in CML, whereas it was not found in any of 7 children, who presumably had a more 5′ breakpoint in the *BCR* gene.[126]

Data from our laboratory as well as others indicate that the breakpoints on No. 22 are more than 50 kb proximal to the CML break but are still within the *BCR* gene.[127] The breakpoints on No. 9 are similar to those in CML. In our studies, 4 of 6 Ph[1]+ (*bcr*-negative) ALL patients have a rearrangement of *BCR* detected on PFGE. Several investigators have shown that these Ph[1]+ ALL patients have an abnormal-sized chimeric *BCR-ABL* mRNA (7.0–7.4 kb) and *ABL* protein (p185 BCR-ABL).[128,129] It should be possible to use several DNA probes from the *BCR* gene and PFGE to distinguish the CML from the ALL breakpoint. In the future, we will understand the role of the *BCR* and *ABL* proteins in normal cells and that of the two different chimeric *BCR-ABL* proteins in CML and in ALL. Thus, the genetic analysis of what appeared to be a simple chromosome change, namely, the 9;22 translocation, has revealed unexpected complexity. An understanding of the altered function of the ABL protein will probably be central to the development of more specific and more effective forms of therapy.

Remarkable progress is being made in the molecular genetic analysis of solid tumors. In addition to the amplification of *NMYC* in neuroblastoma, Slamon and co-workers have recently reported that amplification of the *HER2/neu* gene in breast tumor tissue occurred in 40% of patients with positive axillary lymph nodes. This gene amplification showed a more significant correlation with survival than did the extent of lymph node involvement.[130] Bodmer et al reported that the gene for familial polyposis coli (FPC) was very closely linked to a DNA marker on the long arm of chromosome 5 near 5q21-q22.[131] The same group found that at least 20% of patients with sporadic colorectal cancers showed loss of heterozygosity for a very polymorphic DNA probe on 5q.[132] These observations, based initially on the identification of an interstitial deletion of chromosome 5 (bands 5q15–q22)[133] in a patient with FPC, will permit cloning of the involved gene using strategies already described for retinoblastoma. As noted earlier, the observation by Whang-Peng et al[86] of a deletion of the short arm of chromosome 3 in small cell lung cancer provided the essential clue to examining these tumors for loss of heterozygosity for DNA markers on 3p.[89,90]

It is interesting to speculate that the difference in frequency of carcinomas compared with leukemia, lymphoma or sarcoma may be related to the difference in size of the target DNA. The latter tumors are associated with relatively specific chromosome rearrangements (translocations or inversions) that lead to the abnormal juxtaposition of two specific genes. Although the breakpoints may show some variability on the DNA level, they must bring together the critical functional elements of the two genes. The identity of the two genes is determined by the cell type within which the rearrangement occurs. These factors lead to the relatively low probability that the critical genetic rearrangement will occur in the appropriate cell type. In contrast, if the preliminary data on the more common cancers (*e.g.*, lung cancer and colon cancer) are confirmed, than a different genetic or cytogenetic mechanism, or both, would be involved in malignant transformation. In these cancers, homozygous chromosome deletion or gene inactivation appears to be a prominent feature, presumably leading to loss of genes that regulate or inhibit cell proliferation. The extent of the detectable deletions is quite variable, the only requirement being that both alleles of the critical gene must be deleted or inactivated. Thus any two chromosome breaks that lead to loss of the critical gene in the appropriate cell type would provide one step in the multistep process of transformation. It is too simplistic to relate the incidence of various neoplasias only to the precision of the DNA changes required, namely, specific translocations versus variable size deletions, but future research may confirm that this difference is a contributing factor.

SPECIFICITY OF CHROMOSOME REARRANGEMENTS

The evidence presented in this chapter clearly demonstrates the remarkable specificity of certain chromosome rearrangements for particular subtypes of tumors, especially leukemia or lymphoma. The mechanisms by which this specificity is achieved are unknown; however, a number of investigators have shown that certain proteins required for promotion of gene expression are synthesized in a very cell-type–specific manner.[134] These proteins are only present in the appropriate cell type, and therefore the particular gene is activated only in that cell type. The chromosome rearrangements affecting *MYC* in B-cell and T-cell tumors strongly support the interpretation that the specificity resides in the gene that is uniquely active in a particular cell type. Thus the immunoglobulin genes are highly regulated in B-cells and they can therefore serve as the switch or activator mechanism for *MYC* in B-cells; on the other hand, *TCRA* is an active gene in T-cells with a strong enhancer/promotor and it clearly is an activator for *MYC* in T-cells. A reasonable paradigm is that translocations bring together in an inappropriate manner a growth factor or growth factor receptor gene (the proto-oncogene in the examples defined to date) adjacent to an active cell specific gene. It should be emphasized that many of the proto-oncogenes were identified in viruses that cause tumors. However, these genes have not been conserved through evolution from yeast and *Drosophila* to the chicken, mouse, and man to cause cancer! Where we have any insight into the function of these genes in normal cells, they are growth factors or growth factor receptors. It is not unexpected that the genes which a virus might coopt if it developed into a tumor-producing virus would be genes that control proliferation, genes that, under viral regulation, would function abnormally with regard to cell growth. Further support for the concept that oncogenes are growth factors gone wrong is provided by studies performed at the Hall Institute in Melbourne. Investigators inserted the cloned gene for granulocyte–macrophage colony-stimulating factor into a viral vector, transfected mouse myeloid cells with this gene, and injected the cells into mice which developed leukemia.[135] The term "oncogene" is too short and easy for it to be discarded, but it really refers to respectable genes for growth factors or their receptors.

As has been described in this chapter, analysis of various tumors for alterations in proto-oncogenes has revealed that a number are abnormal as a result of translocations, amplification, or mutations. In some situations the relationship of the change in the proto-oncogene to the multistage process of malignant transformation is unclear.[114] Such ambiguity is not a problem with chromosome translocations; the evidence is overwhelming that the t(8;14) in Burkitt's lymphoma and the t(9;22) in CML are an integral component of the cascade of events leading to the transformation of a normal to a malignant cell. The ever-increasing number of translocations reviewed in this chapter provide a potential gold mine for identifying new genes that are unequivocally related to the malignant phenotype of the affected cell. The challenge is to isolate these translocation breakpoint junctions, to identify the genes that are located at these breakpoints, and then to determine the change in gene function that occurs as a consequence of the translocation. The ultimate measure of success, however, will be in the application of these new insights to the development of new, more effective treatments for cancer. In the future, each particular subtype of tumor will be treated in a uniquely defined way that is most appropriate for the specific genetic defect present in that tumor. This should lead to a new era of cancer therapy that is both more effective and less toxic.

GLOSSARY OF CYTOGENETIC TERMINOLOGY

centromere The constriction along the length of the chromosome that is the site of the spindle fiber attachment. The position of the centromere determines whether chromosomes are metacentric (X-shaped, *e.g.*, chromosomes 1, 3, 16, 19, 20) or acrocentric (inverted V-shaped, *e.g.*, chromosomes 13-15, 21, 22, Y). During mitosis the two exact copies of the DNA in each chromosome are separated by shortening of the spindle fibers attached to opposite sides of the dividing cell.

clone In the cytogenetic sense, defined as two cells with the same additional or structurally rearranged chromosome or three cells with loss of the same chromosome.

deletion A segment of a chromosome is missing as the result of two breaks and loss of the intervening piece (see Fig. 6-2).

diploid Normal chromosome number and composition of chromosomes.

haploid Only half the normal complement (*i.e.*, 23 chromosomes).

hyperdiploid Additional chromosomes; therefore the modal number is 47 or greater.

hypodiploid Loss of chromosomes; modal number is 45 or less.

inversion Two breaks occur in the same chromosome with rotation of the intervening segment. If both breaks are on the same side of the centromere, it is called a *paracentric inversion*. If the breaks are on opposite sides it is called a *pericentric inversion*.

isochromosome A chromosome consisting of identical copies of one chromosome arm with loss of the other arm. Thus an isochromosome for the long arm of No. 17 [i(17q)] contains two copies of the long arm (separated by the centromere) with loss of the short arm of the chromosome.

karyotype Arrangement of chromosomes from a particular cell according to a well-established system such that the largest chromosomes are first and the smallest ones are last (see Fig.6-3). Normal female karyotype is 46,XX; normal male karyotype is 46,XY. Karyotype symbols: p = short arm, q = long arm, t = translocation, del = deletion, inv = inversion, i = isochromosome. A + before the chromosome indicates a gain of a whole chromosome (*e.g.*, +8); a + after the chromosome indicates gain of part of the chromosome (*e.g.*, 14q+ denotes added material at the end of the long arm of No. 14). A − before the chromosome indicates a loss of a whole chromosome (*e.g.*, −7); a − after the chromosome indicates loss of part of the chromosome (*e.g.*, 5q− denotes loss of part of the long arm of No. 5). A ? indicates uncertainty about the identity of the chromosome or band listed just after the ?.

translocation A break in at least two chromosomes with exchange of material. In a reciprocal translocation there is no obvious loss of chromosomal material (see Fig. 6-4).

REFERENCES

1. Mitelman F: Catalog of Chromosome Aberrations in Cancer. New York, Alan R Liss, 1988
2. Heim S, Mitelman F: Cancer Cytogenetics. New York, Alan R Liss, 1987
3. Rowley JD: Chromosome abnormalities in leukemia. J Clin Oncol 6:194–202, 1988
4. Rowley JD, Testa JR: Chromosome abnormalities in malignant hematologic diseases. Adv Cancer Res 36:103–148, 1982
5. Bloomfield CD, Trent JM, van den Berghe H: Report of the Committee on Structural Chromosome Changes in Neoplasia. Human Gene Mapping 9. (1987) Cytogenet Cell Genet 46:344–366, 1987
6. Yunis JJ: The chromosomal basis of human neoplasia. Science 221:227–236, 1983
7. Mitelman F: Catalogue of chromosome aberrations in cancer. Cytogenet Cell Genet 36:1–515, 1983
8. Mitelman F: Catalog of chromosome aberrations in cancer. In Sandberg AA (ed): Progress and Topics in Cytogenetics, Vol 5. New York, Alan R Liss, 1985
9. Rowley JD, Potter D: Chromosomal banding patterns in acute nonlymphocytic leukemia. Blood 47:705–721, 1976
10. ISCN: An international system for human cytogenetic nomenclature: High resolution banding. Cytogenet Cell Genet 31:1–23, 1981
11. Testa JR, Rowley JD: Chromosomes in leukemia and lymphoma with special emphasis on methodology. In Catovsky D (ed): The Leukemic Cell, pp 184-202. Edinburgh, Churchill-Livingstone, 1981
12. First International Workshop in Solid Tumors. Cancer Genet Cytogenet 19:3–197, 1986
13. Nowell PC, Hungerford DA: A minute chromosome in human granulocytic leukemia. Science 132:1497, 1960
14. Rowley JD: A new consistent chromosomal abnormality in chronic myelogenous leukemia. Nature 243: 290–293, 1973
15. de Klein A, van Kessel AG, Grosveld G et al: A cellular oncogene is translocated to the Philadelphia chromosome in chronic myelocytic leukemia. Nature 300:765–767, 1982
16. de Klein, Hagemeijer A: Cytogenetic and molecular analysis of the Ph[1] translocation in chronic myeloid leukemia. Cancer Surveys 3:515–529, 1984
17. Bakhshi A, Minowada J, Arnold A et al: Lymphoid blast crises of chronic myelogenous leukemia represent stages in the development of B-cell precursors N Engl J Med 309:826–831, 1983
18. Whang-Peng J, Canellos GP, Carbone PP et al: Clinical implications of cytogenetic variants in chronic myelocytic leukemia (CML). Blood 32:755–766, 1968
19. Pugh WC, Pearson M, Vardiman JW et al: Philadelphia chromosome-negative chronic myelogenous leukaemia: A morphologic reassessment, Br J Haematol 60:457–467, 1985
20. Travis LB, Pierre RV, DeWald GW: Ph[1]-negative chronic granulocytic leukemia: A nonentity. Am J Clin Pathol 85:186–193. 1986
21. Morris CM, Reeve AE, Fitzgerald PH et al: Genomic diversity correlates with clinical variation in Ph[1]-negative chronic myeloid leukemia. Nature 320:281–283, 1986
22. Bartram CR: Molecular genetic analyses of chronic myelocytic leukemia. In Huhn D, Hellriegel P, Niederle N (eds): Chronic Myelocytic Leukemia and Interferon. New York, Springer-Verlag (in press)
23. Fourth International Workshop on Chromosomes in Leukemia. Cancer Genet Cytogenet 11:249–360, 1984
24. Bennett JM, Catovsky D, Daniel M-T et al: Proposals for the classification of the acute leukemias: French–American–British (FAB) Cooperative Group. BR J Haematol 33: 451–458, 1976
25. Rowley JD: Identification of a translocation with quinacrine fluorescence in a patient with acute leukemia. Ann Genet (Paris) 16:109–112, 1973
26. Rowley JD: Golomb HM, Vardiman J et al: Further evidence for a non-random chromosomal abnormality in acute promyelocytic leukemia. Int J Cancer 20:869–872, 1977
27. Pearson MG, Vardiman JW, Le Beau MM et al: A new cytogenetic subset of acute non-lymphocytic leukemia: t(6;9) associated with bone marrow basophilia. Am J Hematol 18:393-403, 1985
28. Westbrook CA, LeBeau MM, Diaz MO et al: Chromosomal localization and characterization of *c-abl* in the t(6;9) of acute nonlymphocytic leukemia. Proc Natl Acad Sci USA 82:8742–8746, 1985
29. Berger R, Bernheim A, Sigaux F et al: Acute monocytic leukemia chromosome studies. Leuk Res 6:17–26, 1982
30. Hagemeijer A, Hahlen K, Sizoo W et al: Translocation (9;11)(p21;q23) in three cases of acute monoblastic leukemia. Cancer Genet Cytogenet 5:95–105, 1982
31. Arthur DC, Bloomfield CD: Partial deletion of the long arm of chromosome 16 and bone marrow eosinophilia in acute nonlymphocytic leukemia: A new association. Blood 61:994–998, 1983
32. Larson RA, Williams SF, Le Beau MM et al: Acute myelomonocytic leukemia with abnormal eosinophils and inv(16) or t(16;16) has a favorable prognosis. Blood 68:1242–1249, 1986
33. Keating MJ: Early identification of potentially cured patients with acute myelogenous leukemia: A recent challenge. In Bloomfield CD (ed): Adult Leukemias I, pp 237–263. Boston, Martinus Nijhoff, 1982
34. Le Beau MM, Albain KS, Larson RA et al: Clinical and cytogenetic correlations in 63 patients with therapy-related myelodysplastic syndromes and acute nonlymphocytic leukemia: Further evidence for characteristic abnormalities of chromosomes No. 5 and 7. J Clin Oncol 4:325–345, 1986
35. Rowley JD, Golomb HM, Vardiman JW: Nonrandom chromosome abnormalities in acute leukemia and dysmyelopoietic syndromes in patients with previously treated malignant disease. Blood 58:759–767, 1981
36. Arthur DC, Bloomfield CD: Banded chromosome analysis in patients with treatment-associated acute non-lymphocytic leukemia. Cancer Genet Cytogenet 12:189–199, 1984
37. Pedersen-Bjergaad J, Philip P, Pederson NT et al: Acute nonlymphocytic leukemia, preleukemia, and acute myeloproliferative syndrome secondary to treatment of other malignant diseases. Cancer 54:452-462, 1984
38. Larson RA, Le Beau MM, Vardiman JW et al: The predictive value of initial cytogenetic studies in 148 adults with acute nonlymphocytic leukemia. Cancer Genet Cytogenet 10:219–236, 1983
39. Mitelman F, Nilsson PG, Brandt C et al: Chromosome pattern, occupation and clinical features in patients with acute nonlymphocytic leukemia. Cancer Genet Cytogenet 4:187–214, 1981
40. Golomb HM, Alimena G., Rowley JD et al: Correlation of occupation and karyotype in adults with acute nonlymphocytic leukemia. Blood 60:404–411, 1982
41. Le Beau MM, Pettenati MJ, Lemons RS et al: Assignment of the *GM-CSF, CSF*-1, and *FMS* genes to human chromosome 5 provides evidence for linkage of a family of genes regulating hematopoiesis and for their involvement in the deletion (5q) in myeloid disorders. In: Molecular Biology of Homo Sapiens. Cold Spring Harbor Symp Quant Biol 51:899–909, 1986
42. Bloomfield CD, Arthur DC, Frizzera G et al: Nonrandom chromosome abnormalities in lymphoma. Cancer Res 43:2975–2984, 1983
43. Koduru PRK, Filippa DA, Richardson ME et al: Cytogenetic and histologic correlations in malignant lymphomas. Blood 69:97–102, 1987
44. Yunis JJ, Frizzera G, Oken MM et al: Multiple recurrent genomic defects in follicular lymphoma: A possible model for cancer. N Engl J Med 316:79–84, 1987
45. Fifth International Workshop on Chromosomes in Leukemia-Lymphoma: Correlation of chromosome abnormalities with histologic and immunologic characteristics in

non-Hodgkin's lymphoma and adult T-cell leukemia–lymphoma. Blood 70:1554–1564, 1987
46. Manolov G, Manolova Y: Marker band in one chromosome 14 from Burkitt lymphomas. Nature 237:33–34, 1972
47. Zech L, Haglund U, Nilsson K et al: Characteristic chromosomal abnormalities in biopsies and lymphoid-cell lines from patients with Burkitt and non-Burkitt lymphomas. Int J Cancer 17:47–56, 1976
48. Fukuhara S, Rowley JD, Variakojis D et al: Chromosome abnormalities in poorly differentiated lymphocytic lymphoma. Cancer Res 39:3119–3128, 1979
49. Working formulation for clinical usage: National Cancer Institute sponsored study of classification of non-Hodgkin's lymphomas. Cancer 49:2112–2135, 1982
50. Tsujimoto Y, Finger LR, Yunis JJ et al: Cloning of the chromosome breakpoint of neoplastic B cells with the t(14;18) chromosome translocation. Science 226:1098–1099, 1984
51. Cleary ML, Sklar J.: Cloning and structural analysis of cDNA's for *bcl*-2 and a hybrid bcl-2/immunoglobulin transcript resulting from the t(14;18) translocation. Cell 47:19–28, 1986
52. Gahrton G, Robert K-H, Fribert K et al: Nonrandom chromosomal aberrations in chronic lymphocytic leukemia revealed by polyclonal B-cell mitogen stimulation. Blood 56:640-647, 1980
53. Han T, Ozer H, Sadamori N et al: Prognostic importance of cytogenetic abnormalities in patients with chronic lymphocytic leukemia. N Engl J Med 310:288–292, 1984
54. Bird ML, Ueshima Y, Rowley JD et al: Chromosome abnormalities in B-cell chronic lymphocytic leukemia and their clinical correlations. Leukemia (in press)
55. Robert K-H, Gahrton G, Friberg K et al: Extra chromosome 12 and prognosis in chronic lymphocytic leukemia. Scand J Haematol 28:163–168, 1982
56. Third International Workshop on Chromosomes in Leukemia. Cancer Genet Cytogenet 4:95–142, 1981
57. Stong RC, Korsmeyer SJ, Parkin JL et al: Human acute leukemia cell line with the t(4;11) chromosomal rearrangement exhibits B-lineage and monocytic characteristics. Blood 67:391–397, 1986
58. Michael PM, Levin MD, Garson OM et al: Translocation 1;19: A new cytogenetic abnormality in acute lymphocytic leukemia. Cancer Genet Cytogenet 12:333–341, 1984
59. Carroll AJ, Crist WM, Parmley RT et al: Pre-B cell leukemia associated with chromosome translocation 1;19. Blood 63:721–724, 1984
60. Williams DL, Look AT, Melvin SL et al: New chromosomal translocations correlate with specific immunophenotypes of childhood acute lymphoblastic leukemia. Cell 36:101–109, 1984
61. Secker-Walker LM, Swansbury GJ, Hardisty RM et al: Cytogenetics of acute lymphoblastic leukemia in children as a factor in the prediction of long-term survival. Br J Haematol 52:389–399, 1982
62. Williams DL, Tsiatis A, Brodeur GMG et al: Prognostic importance of chromosome number in 136 untreated children with acute lymphoblastic leukemia. Blood 60:864–871, 1982
63. Bloomfield CD, Goldman AI, Alimena G et al: Chromosomal abnormalities identify high-risk and low-risk patients with acute lymphoblastic leukemia. Blood 67:415–420, 1986
64. Ueshima Y, Rowley JD, Variakojis D et al: Cytogenetic studies on patients with chronic T cell leukemia/lymphoma. Blood 63:1028–1038, 1984
65. Zech L, Gahrton G. Hammarstrom L et al: Inversion of chromosome 14 marks human T-cell chronic lymphocytic leukemia. Nature 308:858–860, 1984
66. Kaiser-McCaw B, Hecht F, Harnden DG et al: Somatic rearrangement of chromosome 14 in human lymphocytes. Proc Natl Acad Sci USA 72:2071–2075, 1975
67. Aurias A: Analyse cytogenetique de 21 cas d'ataxie-telangiectase. J Genet Hum 29:235–247, 1981
68. Miyamoto K, Tomita N, Ishii A et al: Chromosome abnormalities of leukemia cells in adult patients with T-cell leukemia. JNCI 73:353–362, 1984
69. Sadamori N, Nishino K, Kusano M et al: Significance of chromosome 14 anomaly at band q11 in Japanese patients with adult T-cell leukemia. Cancer 58:2244–2250, 1986
70. Rowley JD, Haren JM, Wong-Staal F et al: Chromosome pattern in cells from patients positive for human T-cell leukemia virus. In Gallo RC, Essex ME, Gross L (eds): Human T-Cell Leukemia-Lymphoma Viruses; pp 85-89. Cold Spring Harbor, NY, Cold Spring Harbor Laboratory 1984
71. Whang-Peng J, Bunn PA, Knutsen T et al: Cytogenetic studies in human T-cell lymphoma virus (HTLV)-positive leukemia–lymphoma in the United States. JNCI 74:357–369, 1985
72. Raimondi SC, Pui C-H, Behm FG et al: 7q32–q36 translocations in childhood T cell leukemia: Cytogenetic evidence for involvement of the T cell receptor β-chain gene. Blood 69: 131–134, 1987
73. Francke U: Specific chromosome changes in the human heritable tumors retinoblastoma and nephroblastoma. In Rowley JD, Ultmann JE (eds): Chromosomes and Cancer. Bristol–Myers Symposia Series, Vol 5, pp 99–115, New York, Academic Press 1983
74. Kondo K, Chilcote RR, Maurer HS et al: Chromosome abnormalities in tumor cells from patients with sporadic Wilms' tumor. Cancer Res 44:5376–5281, 1984
75. Knudson AG: Mutation and cancer: Statistical study of retinoblastoma. Proc Natl Acad Sci USA 68:800–823, 1971
76. Cavenee WK, Dryja TP, Philllips RA et al: Expression of recessive alleles by chromosomal mechanisms in retinoblastoma. Nature 305:779–784, 1983
77. Dryja TP, Cavenee WK, White R et al: Homozygosity of chromosome 13 in retinoblastoma. N Engl J Med 310:550–553, 1984
78. Friend SH, Bernards R, Rogelj S et al: A human DNA segment with properties of the gene that predisposes to retinoblastoma. Nature 323:643–646, 1986
79. Lee W-H Bookstein R, Hong F et al: Human retinoblastoma susceptibility gene: Cloning, identification, and sequence. Science 235:1394–1399, 1987
80. Murphree AL, Benedict WF: Retinoblastoma: Clues to human oncogenesis. Science 219:1028–1033, 1984
81. Brodeur GM, Green AA, Hayes FA et al: Cytogenetic features of human neuroblastomas and cell lines. Cancer Res 41:4678–4686, 1981
82. Biedler JL, Spengler BA: Metaphase chromosome anomaly: Association with drug resistance and cell-specific products. Science 191:185–187, 1976
83. Schwab M, Alitalo K, Klempnauer K-H et al: Amplified DNA with limited homology to myc cellular oncogene is shared by human neuroblastoma cell lines and a neuroblastoma tumour. Nature 305:245–248, 1983
84. Brodeur GM, Seeger RL, Schwab M: Amplification of N-myc in untreated neuroblastoma correlates with advanced disease stage. Science 224:1121–1124, 1984
85. Balaban G, Herlyn M, Guerry D et al: Cytogenetics of human malignant melanoma and pre-malignant lesions. Cancer Genet Cytogenet 3:243–250, 1981
86. Whang-Peng J, Bunn PA Jr, Kao-Shan CS et al: A nonrandom chromosomal abnormality, del 3p(14-23), in human small cell lung cancer (SCLC). Cancer Genet Cytogenet 6:119–134, 1982
87. Yoshida MA, Ohyashiki K, Ochi K et al: Rearrangement of chromosome 3 in renal cell carcinoma. Cancer Genet Cytogenet 19:351–354, 1986
88. Szucs S, Muller-Brechlin R, DeRiese W, et al: Deletion 3p: The only chromosome loss in a primary renal cell carcinoma. Cancer Genet Cytogenet 26:369–373, 1987
89. Naylor SL, Johnson BE, Minna JD et al: Loss of heterozygosity of chromosome 3p markers in small cell lung cancer. Nature 329:451–454, 1987
90. Kok K, Osinga J, Carritt B et al: Deletion of a DNA sequence at the chromosomal region 3p21 in all major types of lung cancer. Nature 330:578–581, 1987
91. Atkin NB, Baker MC: Specific chromosome change, i(12p), in testicular tumours? Lancet 2:1349, 1982
92. Aurias A, Rimbaut C, Buffe D et al: Chromosomal translocation in Ewing's sarcoma. N Engl J Med 309:496, 1983
93. Turc-Carel C, Philip I, Berger M-P et al: Chromosomal translocation in Ewing's sarcoma. N Engl J Med 309:497–498, 1983
94. Whang-Peng J, Triche TJ, Knutsen T et al: Chromosome translocation in peripheral neuroepithelioma. N Engl J Med 311:584-585, 1984
95. Israel MA, Helman LJ, Miser J: Patterns of proto-oncogene expression: A novel approach to the development of tumor markers. In DeVita VT Jr, Hellman S, Rosenberg SA (eds): Important Advances in Oncology 1987. Philadelphia, JB Lippincott, 1987
96. Dal Cin P, Sandberg AA: Chromosome changes in soft tissue tumors: Benign and malignant. Cancer Invest (in press)
97. Turc-Carel C, Limon J, Dal Cin P et al: Cytogenetic studies of adipose tissue tumors: II. Recurrent reciprocal translocation t(12;16)(q13;p11) in myxoid liposarcomas. Cancer Genet Cytogenet 23: 291–299, 1986
98. Turc-Carel C, Dal Cin P, Limon J et al: Involvement of chromosome X in primary cytogenetic changes in human neoplasia: Nonrandom translocation in synovial sarcoma. Proc Natl Acad Sci USA 84:1981–1985, 1987
99. Mark J, Mitelman F, Levan G: On the specificity of the G abnormality in human meningiomas studied by the fluorescence technique. Acta Pathol Microbiol Immunol Scand [A] 80:812–820, 1972
100. Zankl H, Zang KD: Marker chromosome 20q– does not arise only in bone marrow disorders. Cancer Genet Cytogenet 3:85–87, 1981
101. Seizinger BR, Martuza RL, Gusella JF: Loss of genes on chromosomes 22 in tumorigenesis of human acoustic neuroma. Nature 322:644–647, 1986
102. Mark J, Dahlenfors R, Ekedahl C et al: Cytogenetics of the human mixed salivary gland tumor. Hereditas 99:115–129, 1983
103. Turc-Carel C, Dal Cin P, Boghasian L et al: Consistent breakpoints in region 14q22–q24 in uterine leiomyoma. Cancer Genet Cytogenet 32:25–31, 1988
104. Heim S, Nilbert M, Vanni R et al: A specific translocation, t(12;14)(q14–15;q23–24) characterizes a subgroup of uterine leiomyomas. Cancer Genet Cytogenet 32:13–17, 1988
105. Rowley JD: The biological implications of consistent chromosome rearrangements. Cancer Res 44:3159–3165, 1984
106. Sutherland GR, Hecht F: Fragile Sites on Human Chromosomes. New York, Oxford University Press, 1985
107. Yunis JJ, Soreng AL: Constitutive fragile sites and cancer. Science 226:1199–1204, 1984
108. Le Beau MM: Chromosomal fragile sites and cancer-specific rearrangements. Blood 67:849–858, 1986
109. ar-Rushdi A, Nishikura K, Erickson J: Differential expression of the translocated and the untranslocated c-myc oncogene in Burkitt lymphoma. Science 222:390–393, 1983
110. Fialkow PJ, Singer JW: Tracing development and cell lineages in human hemopoietic neoplasia. In: Weissman IL (ed): Leukemia: Dahlem Konferenzen, pp 203–222. Berlin; Springer-Verlag, 1985
111. Adams JM, Harris AW, Pinkert CA et al: The c-myc oncogene driven by immunoglobulin enhancers induces lymphoid malignancy in transgenic mice. Nature 318:533–538, 1985
112. Bishop JM: The molecular genetics of cancer. Science 235:305–311, 1987
113. Klein G, Klein E: Conditioned tumorigenicity of activated oncogenes. Cancer Res 46:3211–3224, 1986

114. Duesberg PH: Retroviruses as carcinogens and pathogens: Expectations and reality. Cancer Res 47:1199–1220, 1987
115. Leder P, Battey J, Lenoir G et al: Translocations among antibody genes in human cancer. Science 222:765–771, 1983
116. Klein G: Specific chromosomal translocations and the genesis of B-cell derived tumors in mice and men. Cell 32:311–315, 1983
117. Croce CM, Isobe M, Palumbo A et al: Gene for α-chain of human T-cell receptor: Location on chromosome 14 region involved in T-cell neoplasms. Science 227:1044–1047, 1985
118. Caccia N, Bruns GA, Kirsch IR et al: T cell receptor α-chain genes are located on chromosome 14 at 14q11–14q12 in humans. J Exp Med 161:1255–1260, 1985
119. Shima EA, Le Beau MM, McKeithan TW et al: Gene encoding the α chain of the T-cell receptor is moved immediately downstream of c-*myc* in a chromosomal 8;14 translocation in a cell line from a human T-cell leukemia. Proc Natl Acad Sci USA 83:3439–3443, 1986
120. Mathieu-Mahul D, Caubet JF, Bernheim A: Molecular cloning of a DNA fragment from human chromosome 14(14q11) involved in T cell malignancies. EMBO J 4:3427–3433, 1985
121. Baer R, Chen K-C, Smith SD et al: Fusion of an immunoglobulin variable gene and a T cell receptor constant gene in the chromosome 14 inversion associated with T cell tumors. Cell 44:705–713, 1985
122. Groffen J, Stevenson JR, Heisterkamp N et al: Philadelphia chromosomal breakpoints are clustered within a limited region, bcr, on chromosome 22. Cell 36:93–99, 1984
123. Westbrook CA, Rubin CM, Carrino JJ et al: Long-range mapping of the Philadelphia chromosome by pulsed-field gel electrophoresis. Blood 71:697–702, 1988
124. Konopka JB, Watanabe SM, Witte ON: An alteration of the human c-abl protein in K562 leukemia cells unmasks associate tyrosine kinase activity. Cell 37:1035–1042, 1984
125. Shtivelman E, Lifshitz B, Robert P et al: Fused transcript of abl and bcr genes in chronic myelogenous leukemia. Nature 315:550–554, 1985
126. de Klein A, Hagemeijer A, Bartram CR et al: Rearrangement and translocation of the c-*abl* oncogene in Philadelphia positive acute lymphoblastic leukemia. Blood 68:1369–1375, 1986
127. Rubin CM, Carrino JJ, Dickler MN et al: Heterogeneity of genomic fusion of *BCR* and *ABL* in Philadelphia chromosome–positive acute lymphoblastic leukemia. Proc Natl Acad Sci USA 85:2795–2799, 1988
128. Clark SS, McLaughlin J, Crist WM et al: Unique forms of the abl tyrosine kinase distinguish Ph¹-positive CML from Ph¹-positive ALL. Science 235:85–88, 1987
129. Chan LC, Karhi KK, Rayter SI et al: A novel *abl* protein expressed in Philadelphia chromosome positive acute lymphoblastic leukemia. Nature 325:635–637, 1987
130. Slamon DJ, Clark GM, Wong SG et al: Human breast cancer: Correlation of relapse and survival with amplification of the HER-2/*neu* oncogene. Science 235:177–182, 1987
131. Bodmer WF, Bailey CJ, Bodmer J et al: Localization of the gene for familial adenomatous polyposis on chromosome 5. Nature 328:614–616, 1987
132. Solomon E, Voss R, Hall V et al: Chromosome 5 allele loss in human colorectal carcinoma. Nature 328:616–619, 1987
133. Herrera L, Kakati S, Gibas L et al: Gardner syndrome in a man with an interstitial deletion of 5q. Am J Med Genet 25:473–476, 1986
134. Nomiyama H, Fromental C, Xiao JH et al: Cell-specific activity of the constituent elements of the simian virus 40 enhancer. Proc Natl Acad Sci USA 84:7881–7885, 1987
135. Lang RA, Metcalf D, Gough NM et al: Expression of a hemapoietic growth factor cDNA in a factor-dependent cell line results in autonomous growth and tumorigenicity. Cell 43:531–542, 1985

LANCE A. LIOTTA
WILLIAM G. STETLER-STEVENSON

CHAPTER 7 *Principles of Molecular Cell Biology of Cancer: Cancer Metastasis*

CLINICAL SIGNIFICANCE OF INVASION AND METASTASES

Tumor invasion and metastasis is the major cause of treatment failure in cancer patients. Approximately 30% of patients with newly diagnosed solid tumors (excluding skin cancers other than melanoma) already have clinically detectable metastases. Of those 70% of cancer patients who are clinically free of metastases, approximately half can be cured by local tumor therapy alone. The remaining patients have clinically occult micrometastases that ultimately become manifest. Thus, 60% of patients have microscopic or clinically evident metastases at the time of primary tumor treatment. Most patients have multiple metastases. The formation of metastatic colonies is a continuous process that begins early in the growth of the primary tumor and increases with time.[2–9] A few large identifiable metastases in a given organ are frequently accompanied by a greater number of micrometastases that were seeded more recently. The size and age variation in metastases, their dispersed anatomical location, and their heterogeneous composition hinder surgical removal and limit the effective concentration of anticancer drugs that can be delivered to the metastatic colonies.[1–4] The patient with metastatic disease dies of the direct anatomical compromise caused by the metastases or of complications associated with antimetastatic therapy.

Tumors of comparable size can have widely divergent metastatic potential, depending on their intrinsic aggressiveness and histologic type.[3–5] For many common epithelial tumors, tumor cell dissemination begins soon after primary tumor vascularization. It has been calculated that the majority of metastases from breast carcinomas are initiated when the primary tumor is less than 0.125 cm^3;[6–8] this is in accord with experimental studies.[9] Indeed, Fidler and Hart have shown that the subpopulation of highly metastatic tumor cells preexists at a very early stage in the development of the heterogeneous primary tumor.[4] These highly aggressive cells may be selected out because they have a higher probability of successfully producing a metastatic colony compared with other subpopulations of primary tumor cells.

HETEROGENEITY OF THE METASTATIC PHENOTYPE

In the last 10 years the biologic heterogeneity of neoplasms has become widely recognized. At the time of diagnosis, most neoplasms consist of different populations of cells with diverse biologic characteristics (Fig. 7-1). Subpopulations differ in immunogenicity, growth rates, karyotype, pigment production, hormone production, receptor content, and susceptibility to cytotoxic drugs. Fidler and Hart have emphasized that neoplasms can be heterogeneous in their propensity to invade and metastasize, and that the aggressive

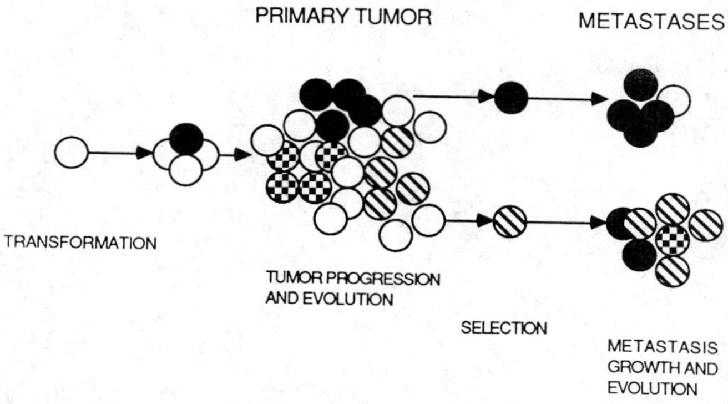

FIG. 7-1. Tumor cell heterogeneity. Clinically detectable tumors comprise a variety of subpopulations of tumor cells with diverse biologic characteristics. These subpopulations differ in growth rate, karyotype, immunogenicity, production of hormones or pigments, cell surface receptors, cytotoxic drug susceptibility, and so forth. The generation of cellular diversity within a tumor is attributed to genetic instability, either inherent in malignant cells or acquired during tumor growth. Selective pressures such as the events of the metastatic cascade or chemotherapeutic treatment result in survival of minor subpopulations of cells that preexisted in the primary neoplasm.

subpopulation may be selected out in the formation of metastasis. The first experimental proof of metastatic heterogeneity was provided by Fidler and Kripke in 1977.[10] Working with the murine B16 melanoma, the investigators used a modified fluctuation assay developed by Luria and Delbruck.[11] They discovered that preexisting subpopulations growing in the same tumor exhibit heterogeneous metastatic potential.

The process of metastasis is not random. Instead, it is a cascade of linked sequential steps that must be traversed by tumor cells if a metastasis is to develop. Each step involves multiple tumor–host interactions. A metastatic tumor cell, in order to be successful, must leave the primary tumor and invade local host tissue. It must then enter the circulation, survive in the circulation, arrest at the distant vascular bed, extravasate into the organ interstitium and parenchyma, and multiply to initiate a metastatic colony. Interruption of the metastatic cascade at any of these steps can prevent the production of clinically symptomatic metastasis. A large foundation of experimental work suggests that during each stage of the process of metastasis the rules of survival of the fittest tumor cells apply. Metastasis thus is the end result of a highly selective competition favoring the survival of a minor subpopulation of metastatic cells that preexist within the primary neoplasm.

TABLE 7-1. Tumor-Host Interactions During the Metastatic Cascade

Metastatic Cascade Event	*Potential Mechanisms*
1. Tumor initiation	Carcinogenic insult, oncogene activation or derepression, chromosome rearrangement
2. Promotion and progression	Karyotypic, genetic, and epigenetic instability; gene amplification; promotion-associated genes and hormones
3. Uncontrolled proliferation	Autocrine growth factors or their receptors, receptors for host hormones such as estrogen
4. Angiogenesis	Multiple angiogenesis factors including known growth factors
5. Invasion of local tissues, blood and lymphatic vessels	Serum chemoattractants, autocrine motility factors, attachment receptors, degradative enzymes
6. Circulating tumor cell arrest and extravasation	Tumor cell homotypic or heterotypic aggregation
a. adherence to endothelium	Tumor cell interaction with fibrin, platelets, and clotting factors; adhesion to RGD-type receptors
b. retraction of endothelium	Platelet factors, tumor cell factors
c. adhesion to basement membrane	Laminin receptor, thrombospondin receptor
d. dissolution of basement membrane	Degradative proteases, type IV collagenase, heparanase, cathepsins
e. locomotion	Autocrine motility factors, chemotaxis factors
7. Colony formation at secondary site	Receptors for local tissue growth factors, angiogenesis factors
8. Evasion of host defenses and resistance to therapy	Resistance to killing by host macrophages, natural killer cells, and activated T-cells; failure to express, or blocking of, tumor-specific antigens; amplification of drug resistance genes

THE METASTATIC CASCADE

A metastatic colony is the end result of a complicated series of tumor–host interactions (Table 7-1), (Fig. 7-2A). Primary tumor initiation and progression is followed by the transition from in situ to locally invasive cancer, which is accompanied by angiogenesis (Fig. 7-2B).[3,4,12] Newly formed tumor vessels are often defective and easily invaded by tumor cells within the primary mass.[9,13] At the invasion front tumor cells also invade preestablished host blood vessels. Tumor cells are discharged into the venous drainage in single-cell form and in clumps. For rapidly growing tumors 1 cm in size, millions of tumor cells can be shed into the circulation every day.[9] Fortunately for the patient, only a very small percentage ($<0.01\%$) of circulating tumor cells initiate metastatic colonies.[3] Tumors generally lack a well-formed lymphatic network.[14] Therefore, communication of tumor cells with lymphatic channels occurs only at the tumor periphery and not within the tumor mass. Tumor cells entering the lymphatic drainage are carried to regional lymph nodes where they arrest in the large lymphatics of the subcapsular sinus. Within 10 to 60 minutes after initial arrest in the lymph node, a significant fraction of the tumor cells detach and enter the efferent lymphatics. These tumor cells eventually end up in the regional or systemic venous drainage owing to the existence of numerous lymphatic–hematogenous communications. Thus, the regional lymph node does not function as a true mechanical barrier to tumor

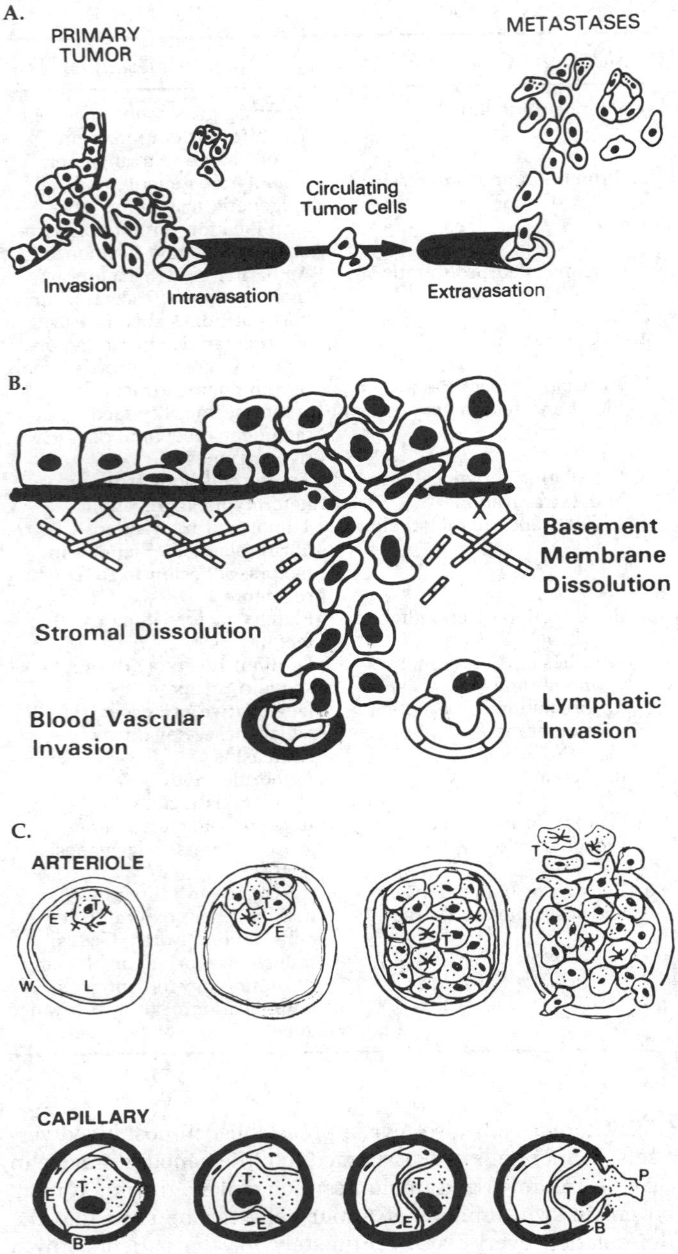

FIG. 7-2. **A**. Overview of the metastatic cascade. Tumor cells invade at the primary tumor site and enter the interstitial stroma, gaining access to blood vessels for further dissemination. Tumor cells invade the vascular wall and are dislodged into the circulation both as single cells and in tumor cell clusters. Circulating tumor cells arrest in the precapillary venules of the target organ by adherence or mechanical trapping. They must then exit the circulation by disrupting the endothelial basement membrane to initiate a metastatic colony. **B**. Early events of the metastatic cascade. The progression from in situ to invasive carcinoma is accompanied by dissolution of the basement membrane (*black line*), penetration of tumor cells into the surrounding stroma, and disruption of the interstitial stroma. Expansion of the primary tumor is accompanied by angiogenesis. Once in the stroma, the tumor cells may invade these newly formed vessels, as well as preexisting host vessels and lymphatics, allowing tumor cell dissemination from the primary tumor site. To enter the bloodstream the tumor cells must penetrate the continuous endothelial basement membrane. This is not the case for lymphatics, which lack a basement membrane. **C**. Late events of the metastatic cascade. Approximately 90% of the circulating tumor cells leave the circulation at the venule or capillary level (lower sequence from left to right). Tumor cells (*T*) arrest by adherence to the luminal surface of endothelial cells. This stimulates retraction of the endothelial cells to expose the underlying basement membrane (*B*). Tumor cells adhere to the basement membrane via cell surface matrix receptors. The retracted endothelial cells migrate over the tumor cell, separating it from the circulation. Over a period of 8 to 24 hours, the tumor cell degrades the basement membrane using a variety of proteases, including type IV collagen–degrading metalloproteinases. The tumor cell then protrudes a pseudopodia (*P*) through the zone of basement membrane lysis; this is followed by migration of the whole tumor cell. Approximately 10% of circulating tumor cells exit at the level of the artery (upper sequence from left to right). Tumor cells (*T*) complexed with fibrin and platelets attach to the artery luminal (*L*) surface. Endothelial cells (*E*) encase the proliferating tumor cell colony, which expands and fills the lumen. Once the lumen is filled (2–4 weeks), individual tumor cells invade the arterial wall (*W*) and exit the circulation.

dissemination. Lymphatic and hematogenous dissemination occur in parallel.

CIRCULATING TUMOR CELL ARREST AND EXTRAVASATION

Circulating tumor cells use a variety of means to arrest in the vessels of the target organ where they will initiate metastatic colonies (Fig. 7-2C). Approximately 80% of the circulating tumor cells are in single-cell form and attach directly to the intact endothelial surface, or to preexisting regions of exposed subendothelial basement membrane. Clumps of circulating tumor cells or tumor cells aggregated with host leukocytes, fibrin, or platelets can directly embolize in the precapillary venules by mechanical impaction (Fig. 7-3A). Tumor cells in single-cell or clump form adhere to the endothelial luminal surface of arterioles. The fate and time course of the arrested tumor cells differ depending on the mechanism and location of lodgement. Tumor cells adherent to the surface of venule or capillary endothelium rapidly (within 1–4 hours) induce the active retraction of the endothelial cells (Figs. 7-3B and C).[3,15–17] The tumor cell then attaches avidly to the exposed basement membrane. Once the tumor cells have attached, the adjacent endothelial cells extend over the tumor cell and separate it from the bloodstream (Figs. 7-3D and E). Tumor cells located between the

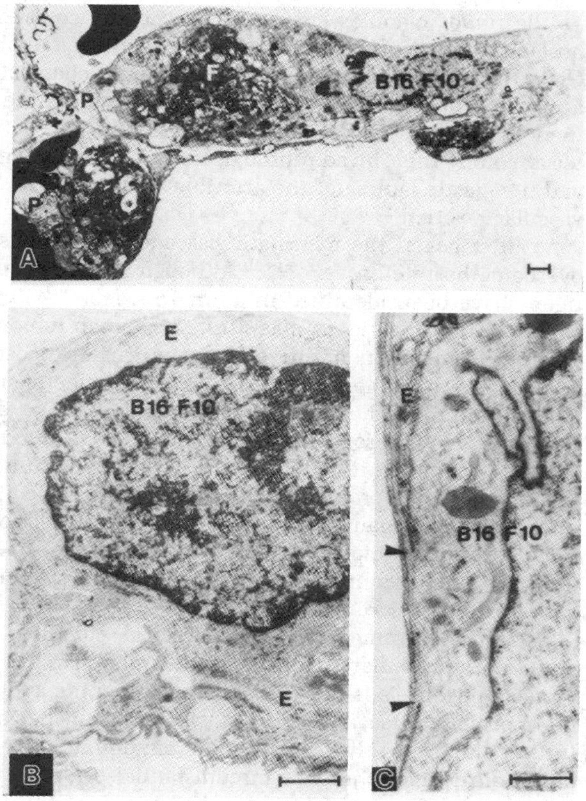

FIG. 7-3. **A.** A B16-F10 tumor cell in a lung capillary 3 hours after IV inoculation. Nonpolymerized fibrin (*F*) and platelets (*P*) are adherent to the tumor cell. (Scale bar: 1 μm; magnification ×4250) **B.** At 6 hours after IV inoculation, the endothelium (*E*) adjacent to the attached tumor cell is still intact. A narrow slit can be observed between the tumor cell and the endothelium. (Scale bar: 1 μm; magnification ×12,800) **C.** A tumor cell in a capillary 12 hours after IV inoculation. Over a small surface area, the tumor cell is tightly adherent to the basement membrane (*arrowheads*). *E* = endothelium. (Scale bar: 1 μm; magnification ×12,800) **D.** Tumor cell in a lung capillary 12 hours after inoculation. The tumor cell is adherent to the basement membrane (*BM*) over a large surface area. An endothelial cell (*E*) has detached from the basement membrane (*arrow*) and moved over the tumor cell, separating it from the fibrin (*F*) deposit. *M* = melanosomes. (Scale bar: 1 μm; magnification ×9600). **E.** A group of tumor cells completely surrounded by an endothelial covering (*E*) in the lumen of an arteriole, 2 weeks after inoculation of tumor cells. (Scale bar: 10 μm; magnification ×1060) **F.** A portion of a tumor colony in an arteriole 2 weeks after IV inoculation. A tumor cell pseudopodium traverses a focal defect of the elastica interna basement (*EI*). *M* = melanosomes. (Scale bar: 1 μm; magnification ×9600)

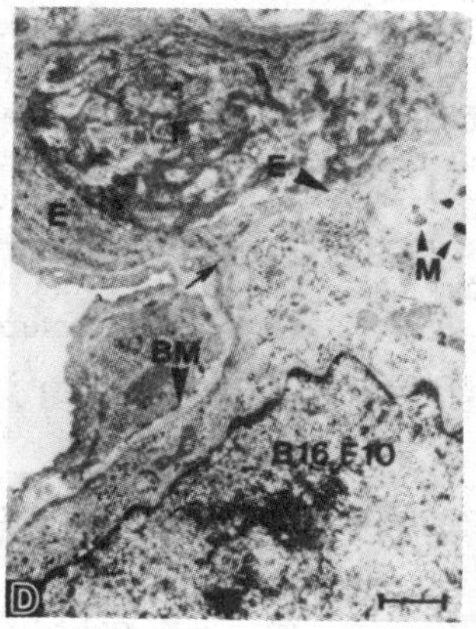

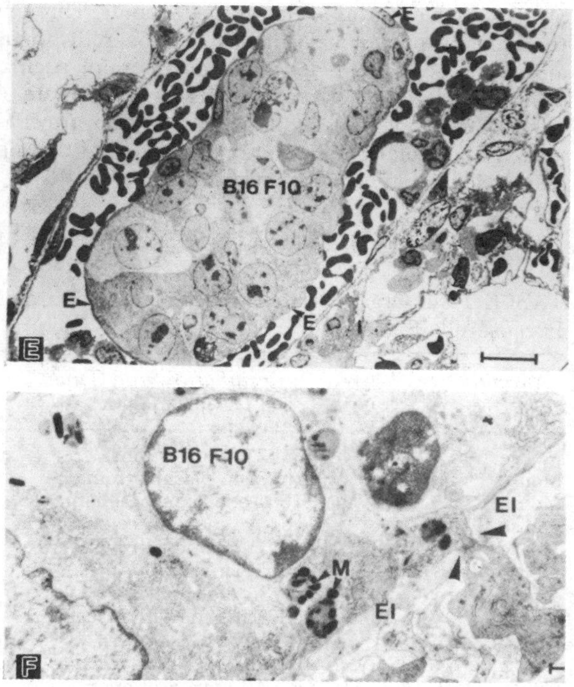

endothelium and the basement membrane are held up in this location for 8 to 24 hours. Local dissolution of the basement membrane then occurs in association with a tumor cell pseudopodium traversing the basement membrane (Fig. 7-3F). This step is soon followed by complete extravasation of the tumor cell and quite often reestablishment of blood flow in the breached vessel.[15] Tumor cells arrested in the arterial tree can remain in this location for 2 to 3 weeks. Endothelial retraction does not occur after arterial arrest. Intra-arterial tumor cells can actually proliferate and expand as colonies.

As the tumor colonies enlarge, they become covered by a host endothelial surface that lacks a basement membrane. Once the tumor colony fills the arteriole, mechanical damage to the endothelium occurs, and this exposes the basement membrane. Tumor cells at the periphery of the intraarterial colony then invade through the basement membrane and the elastic lamina of the arteriole wall to gain an extravascular position.[15]

At all stages of the metastatic cascade, tumor cells must overcome host defenses.[3–5,18,20] Although tumor-specific antigens have been identified in animal models, it is unclear whether similar antigens play a role in human tumors, and whether recognition of these antigens can be boosted by adjuvant immunotherapy.[18,19] The limited effectiveness of adjuvant immunotherapy for metastases may be due to tumor antigen heterogeneity, tumor antigen shedding, or absence of tumor cell immunogenicity. "Nonspecific" host defenses such as macrophages and natural killer cells may be more effective against heterogeneous tumor cell populations.[20] In animal models these effector cells play an important role in the elimination of circulating tumor cells and destruction of micrometastases.[20]

Extravasated tumor cells proliferate as colonies but require a new vascular supply to grow larger than 0.5 mm.[13] Thus angiogenesis is necessary at the beginning and end of the metastatic cascade. A metastasis can itself metastasize, further amplifying the level of tumor dissemination. Numerous clinical reports provide circumstantial evidence for the existence of dormant metastases.[1,3] Up to one third of the mortality from breast cancer, for instance, occurs more than 5 years after removal of the primary tumor. Three potential mechanisms of tumor dormancy have been distinguished in animal models.[3]: (1) immunologic restraint such that the tumor population death rate equals its growth rate, (2) constitutive dependency of tumor cells on host growth factors, and (3) avascularity, which limits the size of the metastasis due to deficiency in nutrient diffusion.

DISTRIBUTION OF METASTASES BY TARGET ORGAN

The distribution of metastases varies widely, depending on the histologic type and anatomical location of the primary tumor. The most frequent organ location of distant metastasis in many types of cancer appears to be the first capillary bed encountered by the circulating cells. Examples include sarcomas metastasizing to lung, lung cancer metastasizing to brain, and colorectal tumor disseminating to liver.

However, many metastatic sites cannot be predicted from anatomical considerations alone and can be considered examples of organ tropism. For example, clear cell carcinoma of the kidney often metastasizes to bone and thyroid, breast carcinoma to ovaries, and ocular melanoma to the liver.

An increasing number of animal tumor models show preference for metastasizing to one or more distant sites. In many cases, target organ preference in these models cannot be explained based on anatomical considerations. Organ preference of metastatic colonization can be observed in some animal tumors that have not undergone purposeful selection (Table 7-2). In other models, organ selectivity has been experimentally amplified by sequential in vivo passage through the target organ (Table 7-3).

A number of investigators have implanted organ grafts into ectopic sites. The transplanted organ grafts were used as target sites for tumor cell hematogenous colonization. Hart and Fidler[4] observed that intravenously injected B16-F10 melanoma cells colonized the native lung as well as subcutaneous lung grafts. In order to colonize the ectopic site, the tumor cells must have left the first capillary arrest site in the lungs and traveled to the ectopic site. In control mice, ectopic kidney grafts were not colonized by circulating B16-F10 tumor cells, indicating a clear organ selectivity for lung but not kidney.

Theoretical mechanisms for organ tropism include the following[3,17]: (1) Tumor cells disseminate equally in all organs, but preferentially grow only in specific organs. Pref-

TABLE 7-2. Organ Preference of Metastatic Colonization in Animal Tumors Not Purposefully Selected*

Animal Species	*Designation and Type of Tumor*	*Common Colonization Site(s)*
Mouse	X5563 plasmacytoma	Spleen
Mouse	Kobayashi plasmacytoma	Bone
Mouse	C198 reticuloendothelioma	Liver > lung, spleen
Mouse	Type A reticulum cell sarcoma	Liver > spleen
Mouse	RAW117 large cell lymphoma	Liver > other sites
Mouse	B16 melanoma	Lung > other sites
Mouse	K-1735 melanoma	Lung
Mouse	M-5076 monocytic sarcoma	Liver > ovary > other sites
Rat	R39 sarcoma	Kidney, adrenal
Rat	Flexner-Jobling carcinoma	Kidney, adrenal
Guinea pig	Line 10 hepatocarcinoma	Liver, lymph node
Chicken	HV-transformed lymphoma	Liver
Rabbit	VX_2 carcinoma	Liver, lung

* Modified from Nicolson GL: Organ specificity of tumor metastasis: Role of preferential adhesion, invasion and growth of malignant cells at specific secondary sites. Cancer Metastasis Rev 7:143, 1988.

TABLE 7-3. Organ Preference of Metastases in Some Selected Human and Animal Tumor Models*

Tumor System Subline	*Lung*	*Liver*	*Brain*	*Ovary*	*Spleen*	*Lymph Node*
Murine B16 melanoma (IV or IC)						
B16-F10	++++	±	−	+	±	±
B16-B15b	+++	−	+++	−	−	±
B16-013	++	−	−	+++	−	±
Murine RAW117 large cell lymphoma (IV or IC)						
RAW117-L17	+++	++++	−	−	++	−
Murine Lewis lung carcinoma (IM, IC, or IS)						
HL	++++	−	−	−	−	+
HH	±	++++	±	±	−	+
Chicken MD lymphoma (IV)						
AL-2	−	++++	−	±	−	−
AL-3	−	+	−	+++	−	−
Human A375 melanoma (IV in nude mice)						
A375-SM	++	−	−	−	−	+
A375-L	+	++	−	−	−	−
Human PC-3 prostatic carcinoma (IV in athymic mice)						
PC-3-125-IN	++++	−	−	−	−	−
PC-3-1-LN	++++	+	−	+	±	+++
Human KM12 colon carcinoma (IS or ICM in nude mice)						
KM20C	+	+++	−	−	−	+
KM23C	+	+++	−	−	−	++
Human MeWo melanoma (IV in nude mice)						
MeWo	+	−	−	−	−	−
MeWo-70-W	++	−	++	+	−	−

* Modified from Nicolson GL: Organ specificity of tumor metastasis: Role of preferential adhesion, invasion and growth of malignant cells at specific secondary sites. Cancer Metastasis Rev Cancer Metastasis Rev 7:143, 1988.

Metastases: − = none, ± = sometimes, + = few, ++ = moderate, +++ = many, ++++ = large numbers and heavy tumor burden. IS = intra-splenic, IC = intra-cardia. ICM = intraceum.

erential growth may be induced by local growth factors or hormones present in the target organ for metastasis. (2) Circulating tumor cells may adhere preferentially to the endothelial luminal surface only in the target organ. This hypothesis predicts organ-specific endothelial determinants. (3) Circulating tumor cells may respond to soluble factors diffusing locally out of the target organ. Such factors could act in a chemotactic fashion to attract the tumor cells to extravasate. They could also cause the circulating tumor cells to aggregate and therefore embolize in the target organ. Research with animal models indicates that all of these mechanisms play a role to various degrees, depending on the tumor model system (Table 7-4).[3,17]

BASEMENT MEMBRANE DISRUPTION DURING TRANSITION FROM IN SITU TO INVASIVE TUMORS

The mammalian organism is composed of a series of tissue compartments separated from each other by two types of extracellular matrix: basement membranes and interstitial stroma.[5] The matrix determines tissue architecture, has important biologic functions, and is a mechanical barrier to invasion. During the transition from in situ to invasive carcinoma, tumor cells penetrate the epithelial basement membrane and enter the underlying interstitial stroma. Once the tumor cells enter the stroma they gain access to lymphatics and blood vessels for further dissemination (see Fig. 7-2B). Fibrosarcomas and angiosarcomas, developing from stromal cells, invade surrounding muscle basement membrane and destroy myocytes. Tumor cells must cross basement membranes to invade peripheral nerves and most types of organ parenchyma. During intravasation or extravasation, tumor cells of any histologic origin must penetrate the subendothelial basement membrane.[3,5] In the distant organ where metastatic colonies are initiated, extravasated tumor cells must migrate through the perivascular interstitial stroma before tumor colony growth occurs in the organ parenchyma. Therefore, tumor cell interaction with the extracellular matrix occurs at multiple stages in the metastatic cascade.

General and widespread changes occur in the organization, distribution, and amount of the epithelial basement membrane during the transition from benign to invasive carcinoma.[21,22] The human breast is illustrative. Benign proliferative disorders of the breast such as fibrocystic disease, sclerosing adenosis, intraductal hyperplasia, fibroadenoma, and intraductal papilloma are all characterized by disorganization of the normal epithelial stromal architecture. Extreme forms can mimic the appearance of invasive carcinoma. However, no matter how extensive the architectural disorganization, these benign disorders are always characterized by a continuous basement membrane separating the epithelium from the stroma.[21] In contrast, invasive ductal carcinoma, invasive lobular carcinoma, and tubular carcinoma consistently possess a defective extracellular basement membrane with zones of basement membrane loss around the invading tumor cells in the stroma.[21] The base-

TABLE 7-4. Evidence for Some Tumor Cell and Host Properties Important in Organ Preference of Blood-borne Metastases*

	Properties Associated with Blood-borne Metastases to Specific Sites								
Tumor System	*Increased Primary Invasion†*	*Increased Entry into Blood*	*Increased Homotypic Adhesion*	*Increased Heterotypic Adhesion‡*	*Increased Attachment to Organ Endothelial Cells*	*Increased Attachment to Organ BM§*	*Increased Invasion of Target Organ*	*Increased Organ Growth Properties‖*	*Decreased Sensitivity to Host Responses¶*
MuB16 melanoma	Yes	Yes	Yes	Yes	Yes	Yes	Yes	Yes	Yes
Mu RAW117 large cell lymphoma	No	No	No	No	Yes	No	Yes	Yes	Yes
Mu L5178Y T-lymphoma (ESb)	Yes	Yes	No	Yes	Yes	Yes	Yes	Yes	Yes
My 3LL lung carcinoma	Yes	Yes	ND**	Yes	Yes	No	Yes	ND	Yes
Rat 13762NF mammary carcinoma	Yes	Yes	Yes	No	Yes	Yes	Yes	Yes	Yes
Rat RMS 9-4 rhabdomyosarcoma	No	Yes	ND	ND	Yes	Yes	ND	No	No

* Modified from Nicolson GL: Organ specificity of tumor metastasis: Role of preferential adhesion, invasion and growth of malignant cells at specific secondary sites. Cancer Metastasis Rev 7:143, 1988.
† Invasion measured at a SC or IM site.
‡ Adhesion measured with syngeneic or nonsyngeneic platelets, lymphocytes, or other blood cells.
§ Attachment measured to organ-derived subendothelial matrix.
‖ Growth stimulation measured with organ-derived soluble factors.
¶ Sensitivity measured as cytolysis or cytostasis by syngeneic host macrophages, lymphocytes, or natural killer cells.
** ND = not determined.

ment membrane is also markedly defective adjacent to tumor cells in lymph node and organ metastases. In some focal regions of well-differentiated carcinoma, partial basement membrane formation can be identified. These findings are directly applicable to diagnostic problems in surgical pathology such as the differentiation of tangential sections of in situ lesions from true invasion, or the differentiation of severe adenosis from invasive carcinoma. Loss of basement membranes in human rectal carcinomas significantly correlates with an increased incidence of metastasis and a poor 5-year survival.[22]

THREE-STEP THEORY OF INVASION

A three-step hypothesis has been proposed to describe the sequence of biochemical events during tumor cell invasion of the extracellular matrix.[5] The first step is tumor cell attachment to the matrix. This attachment may be mediated through specific glycoproteins such as laminin and fibronectin and through tumor cell plasma membrane receptors. Following attachment, the tumor cell secretes hydrolytic enzymes (or induces host cells to secrete enzymes) that can locally degrade the matrix (including degradation of the attachment glycoproteins). Matrix lysis most likely takes place in a highly localized region close to the tumor cell surface where the amount of active enzyme outbalances the natural protease inhibitors present in the serum and in the matrix itself. In contrast to the invasive tumor cell, when a normal cell or benign tumor cell attaches to the matrix it may respond by shifting into a resting or differentiated state. The third step is tumor cell locomotion into the region of the matrix modified by proteolysis. The direction of the locomotion may be influenced by host-derived chemotactic factors and tumor cell–derived motility factors. The chemotactic factors derived from serum, organ parenchyma, or the matrix itself[3,17] may influence the organ specificity of metastasis. Continued invasion of the matrix may take place by cyclic repetition of these three steps.

LAMININ RECEPTORS

Cell surface receptors for the basement membrane glycoprotein laminin mediate adhesion of tumor cells to the basement membrane prior to invasion.[23,24] Laminin as visualized by rotary shadowing electron microscopy has a distinctive cruciform shape with three short arms (35 nm) and one long arm (75 nm) (Fig. 7-4).[25] All arms have globular end regions. The specialized structure of the laminin molecule may contribute to its multiple biologic functions. Laminin plays a role in cell attachment, cell spreading, mitogenesis, neurite outgrowth, morphogenesis, and cell movement. Many types of neoplastic cells contain high affinity (nM Kd) cell surface binding sites (laminin receptors) for laminin.[23] The molecular weight of the isolated receptor is 65 kDa.[7] The laminin receptor binds to the B chain (short arm) region of the laminin molecule.[26] Laminin receptors may be altered in number or degree of occupancy in human carcinomas. This may be the indirect result of defective basement membrane organization in the carcinomas. Breast carcinoma and colon carcinoma tissue contains a higher number of exposed (unoccupied) receptors than benign lesions. The laminin receptors of normal epithelium may be polarized at the basal surface and occupied by laminin in the basement membrane. In contrast, the laminin receptors on invading carcinoma cells are amplified and may be distributed over the entire surface of the cell (Fig. 7-5). The laminin receptor can be shown experimentally to play a role in hematogenous metastasis.[27] Treating tumor cells with the receptor-binding fragment of laminin at very low concentrations markedly inhibits or abolishes lung metastasis from hematogenously introduced tumor cells. The mechanism of action involves blocking the adhesion of circulating tumor cells to the subendothelial basement membrane.

RGD RECOGNITION RECEPTORS

A family of cell surface glycoproteins termed *integrins* has been identified whose members bind with low affinity to a

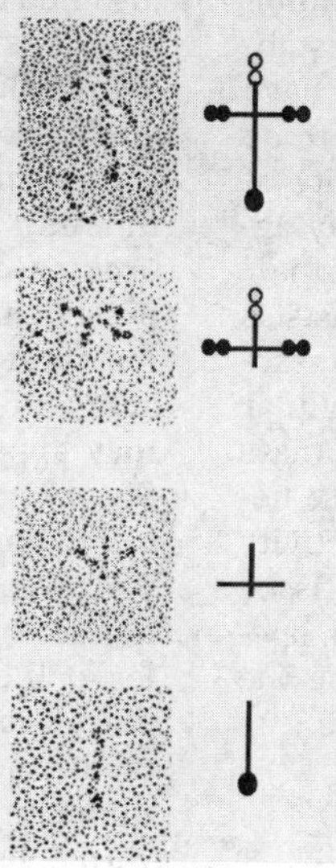

Molecule or fragment	Structural features	Biologic functions
Whole laminin	-short arms 35nm -long arms 76nm -rich in alpha-D-mannopyranosyl residues	Promotes cell attachment, spreading, migration, growth morphogenesis, and metastases
Short arm domain	-globular ends rich in alpha-D-galactosyl end groups. -arms may be composed of more than one type of chain	-globular ends bind to type IV collagen, and sulfatides -promotes cell attachment and spreading
Rod shaped intersection of short arms	-disulfide bonded "knot" -relatively protease resistant -contains mannose terminated oligosaccharide units	-contains laminin receptor binding domain -inhibits cell attachment and metastases
Long arm	-may contain alpha helix structure -protease labile	-binds heparin sulfate proteoglycan -promotes neurite outgrowth

FIG. 7-4. Laminin functional domains. Laminin is a cross-shaped glycoprotein with three short arms and one long arm, all terminating in globular end regions. Electron micrographs of an individual whole laminin molecule or purified fragments are shown; associated structural features and biologic functions are noted.

variety of adhesion proteins including fibronectin, von Willebrand factor, fibrin, vitronectin, type I collagen, and thrombospondin.[28] The integrins are a complex of alpha (140 kDa) and beta (95 kDa) subunit proteins. The functions of several of the integrins are inhibited by peptides related to the Arg-Gly-Asp (RGD) sequence of fibronectin. RGD sequences present on a wide variety of proteins may serve as the recognition site for binding of the integrins. It is likely that specific ligand sequences adjacent to the RGD site may confer preferential recognition of one type of adhesion protein by certain members of the integrin family.[30] Integrin proteins are thought to align adhesion proteins such as fibronectin on the cell surface with cytoskeletal components such as talin and actin, thus altering cell shape.[31] Integrin-type proteins may play an adhesive role in platelet–tumor cell interactions, binding of lymphoid cells to endothelium, and the interaction of circulating tumor cells with endothelial surfaces, fibrin, von Willebrand factor, or thrombospondin. In keeping with this concept, it has been reported that co-injection of tumor cells with large quantities of RGD peptides will inhibit metastasis formation in animal models.[32] The RGD peptides may interfere with the adhesion of tumor cells to the endothelial surface, which may be mediated directly or indirectly through integrin proteins.

PROTEINASES AND TUMOR CELL INVASION

In vitro studies have shown that tumor cell invasion is not a passive process in response to pressure from excessive cellular proliferation alone but rather is an active process requiring protein synthesis and extracellular proteolysis. Inhibitors of metalloproteinases or protein synthesis, but not of DNA synthesis, block tumor cell invasion into the matrix.[33–35] As outlined earlier, various tissue compartments are separated from each other by interstitial stroma and/or a basement membrane. During the process of invasion, tumor cells must traverse these barriers to cross tissue boundaries. Therefore, it has been suggested that invasive tumor cells secrete matrix-degrading enzymes with activities directed against the major components of these barriers, namely collagens type I, IV, and V, fibronectin, and proteoglycans.[35–38]

Many investigators have explored the possible involvement of proteinases in tumor cell invasion and have proposed a role for a variety of matrix-degrading en-

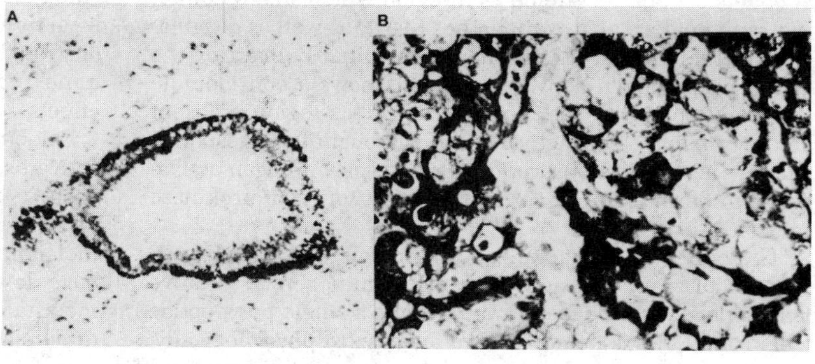

FIG. 7-5. Immunohistochemistry of laminin receptor distribution. **A.** Normal endometrial gland stained with anti-laminin receptor antibodies. These cells show clear polarization, with the majority of the laminin receptor staining in the basal portion of the cells adjacent to the basement membrane. **B.** Endometrial adenocarcinoma cells stained with anti-laminin receptor antibodies. These cells show an increased staining intensity and lack of polarization when compared with the normal endometrial gland.

zymes.[35,37,39–41] These include enzymes from three of the four major categories of proteinases—serine proteinases, neutral metalloproteinases, and cysteine proteinases. Some of these enzymes have been identified and have well-established substrates in the extracellular matrix. Others have ill-defined substrates or substrates that are not known to be localized in the extracellular matrix. The heterogeneity of solid tumors with respect to both the mixture of highly aggressive tumor cells with those of low metastatic potential[4] and the admixture of inflammatory cells and fibroblasts is well documented.[3] The variety of enzymatic activities associated with tumor cell invasion is in part due to this cellular heterogeneity. Homogenates or extracts of a tumor mass may not accurately reflect tumor cell protease activity because of stromal cell or inflammatory cell protease activity or because of the release of protease inhibitors during tissue processing. Recently developed molecular probes for specific proteases now offer a means for directly studying the expression of these enzymes by individual tumor cells.

SERINE PROTEINASES

There is considerable experimental evidence documenting increased plasminogen activator and plasmin activity in virally transformed and malignant cells.[36,37] These studies are traced to early observations of the ability of cancer tissue explants to dissolve the plasma clots on which they were grown. Renewed interest in plasminogen activators followed the demonstration that cell transformation by a variety of oncogenic viruses induced a drastic increase in the extracellular release of plasminogen activators. Tumor promoters such as phorbol esters may further potentiate this increase in virally transformed cells.[42,43]

Plasminogen activators exist in at least two forms [36–38,41]: urokinase-type plasminogen activator, so called because it was originally discovered in human urine, and tissue-type plasminogen activator. Tissue-type plasminogen activator is somewhat larger than urokinase and was originally purified from tissue extracts. These forms of plasminogen activators are independent gene products, as has been demonstrated with amino acid sequence analysis and confirmed by cDNA cloning and nucleotide sequencing. In vitro, both enzymes are secreted as single polypeptide, proenzyme forms that are converted to active, disulfide-bonded forms by cleavage at a single proteolytic site. Although the A chains of these forms differ considerably in size, they share structurally conserved regions that are similar to other serine proteinases.[36–38] The A chains contain a cysteine-rich region which shows homology with epidermal growth factor (EGF), as well as coagulation factors IX and X. The amino-terminal domain of the tissue plasminogen activator A chain shows a considerable degree of homology with fibronectin.[37] This region is absent in the urokinase-type activator and is thought to be responsible for the efficient absorption of tissue plasminogen activator onto fibrin clots, an ability that most forms of urokinase lack.

The only well-characterized physiologic substrate known for the plasminogen activators is plasminogen.[36,38] Native plasminogen is produced in the liver as a single polypeptide chain of 92,000 daltons.[44,45] Two forms exist physiologically, and both forms are activated by plasminogen activators to yield the active protease plasmin. Plasmin consists of two disulfide bonded polypeptide chains and its proteolytic specificity is similar to that of trypsin.

Investigators from a number of laboratories have shown by analysis of tumor extracts that plasminogen activator activity is associated with a variety of human and animal tumors.[36,37,41,46–48] Most commonly, this activity is of the urokinase type, although tissue-type plasminogen activator is present in extracts of some tumors. These results must be interpreted cautiously, however, since tissue plasminogen activator is present in endothelial cells and its concentration may appear falsely elevated in highly vascularized tumors. Short-term organ cultures and cell cultures of neoplastic cell origin have been reported to produce urokinase alone, tissue plasminogen activator alone, or both forms, as well as a nondetermined type of plasminogen activator. In other studies, cell cultures of neoplastic tissue have been found to lack plasminogen activator when analyzed immediately after establishment of the cell culture. In still other cell lines plasminogen activator activity, although initially present, is lost with subsequent cell passages.[46,47]

Experiments with several tumor cell lines have indicated that matrix glycoproteins are susceptible to plasmin-mediated proteolytic degradation.[36–38,41,49,50] These lines include human rhabdomyosarcoma cells, human fibrosarcoma cell lines, hamster fibrosarcoma cells, and murine melanoma cell lines. Depending on the cell line, the matrix-degrading activity may or may not become independent of plasminogen conversion to plasmin at high cell density. Human rhabdomyosarcoma cells required the presence of plasminogen at all cell densities in order to effect matrix degradation. For the fibrosarcoma cells and murine melanoma cells, matrix degradation became independent of exogenous plasminogen at high cell densities.[51] This suggests that an additional, as yet unidentified proteolytic activity may be involved in matrix degradation at high cell densities. Metastatic mouse sarcoma cells show laminin-degrading activity that is mostly plasminogen dependent. However, most of the plasminogen-independent laminin degrading activity is removed by inhibitors of metalloproteinases.[38,52]

Studies with the human epidermoid cell line HEP-3 have provided some of the best evidence for the role of plasminogen activators in tumor invasion.[53] Antibodies that specifically inhibit human urokinase activity, but do not cross-react with chicken urokinase, significantly reduced or prevented pulmonary metastases from HEP-3 tumors transplanted onto chick embryo chorioallantoic membranes without reducing local tumor growth. Appropriate immunologic controls demonstrated that this effect was due to inhibition of the human tumor urokinase activity and not secondary immunologic effects.

Evidence for a positive correlation between plasminogen activator activity and tumor invasiveness remains unclear. A positive correlation between plasminogen activator activity and metastatic potential has been established for the murine melanoma cell line B16.[54] Low metastatic cell lines (B16F1) have low plasminogen activator activity, whereas highly metastatic cell lines (B16F10) show high levels in primary tumors and even higher levels in the pulmonary metastases from these primary tumors. The correlation of plasminogen activator activity with metastatic potential has also been observed in the rat mammary adenocarcinoma model.[55] However, in human tumors the situation is not clear-cut. Although there may be some correlation with invasion, plasminogen activator levels certainly do not show a correlation with the metastatic capacity of human tumors when assayed by protein methods. This possibly is a result of a general protease activity that destroys this activity, low levels of active enzyme, or rapid "physiologic" protein turnover of plasminogen activator. A recent report demonstrated a significant (sixfold) elevation of urokinase mRNA levels in human primary lung and breast carcinomas when compared with levels in nonmalignant tissues.[56] Furthermore, a significant correlation between urokinase mRNA levels in lung carcinomas and the presence of regional lymph node metastasis was found. These results need to be confirmed by further studies, but it appears that important prognostic information may be obtained from such investigations. As the investigators suggest, urokinase mRNA content may help identify patients at risk for recurrence or early metastasis. These patients could then be selected for adjuvant therapy.

Metalloproteinases

Tumor cell invasion requires crossing tissue compartment barriers such as basement membranes and interstitial connective tissues. Both of these barriers have various collagen types that compose the structural scaffolding upon which other matrix components such as fibronectin, laminin, and proteoglycans are assembled. In this section we shall consider the metalloenzymes that may be involved in tumor invasion and metastasis.

Tumor-derived collagenases that degrade interstitial collagen types I, II, and III have been purified and characterized by a number of laboratories. The properties of these enzymes are similar to those of the classic collagenase first described by Gross and co-workers.[57] The cDNA for human fibroblast interstitial collagenase has recently been cloned and sequenced.[58,59] The collagenases are calcium- and zinc-dependent metalloproteinases that function at neutral pH. These enzymes produce a single cleavage across all three alpha chains of the native type I collagen molecule, resulting in characteristic fragments corresponding to a cleavage site located 75% of the distance from the amino terminus of the full length substrate. Interstitial collagenase activity has been reported in a number of human tumors and has been correlated with the aggressiveness of human bladder carcinomas.[60,61] Immunohistochemical studies suggest that the tumor cells themselves do not secrete type I collagenase, but instead directly stimulate fibroblast secretion of this enzyme.[60]

Basement membrane collagens types IV and V differ markedly from the interstitial collagenases (types I, II, and III) both in structure and in proteolytic susceptibility. These basement membrane collagens are not susceptible to proteolytic attack by the interstitital collagenases described above. Ultrastructural studies of tumor cell extravasation and invasion demonstrated local dissolution of basement membrane materials and suggested that tumor cells produce a distinct collagenolytic enzyme to degrade basement membranes. In support of this concept, highly metastatic tumor cells, endothelial cells, and polymorphonuclear leukocytes have been found to produce a type IV collagen-specific metalloproteinase.[62] Unique metalloproteinases that degrade type V collagen have also been described.

Type IV collagen–specific metalloproteinase, type IV collagenase, was first identified and purified from a metastatic murine tumor cell line.[63] Type IV collagenase is a neutral metalloproteinase with a *p*H optimum of 7.6 and is not inhibited by serine protease inhibitors or cysteine protease inhibitors. The enzyme has an apparent molecular weight of approximately 70,000 daltons and generates characteristic cleavage products from native type IV collagen (Fig. 7-6). Human type IV collagenases with similar characteristics have been isolated from fibrosarcoma and melanoma cell lines.[62–65]

Type IV collagenolytic activity correlates with metastatic activity in murine tumor models.[66–68] Highly aggressive human tumors, such as carcinomas, melanomas, hepatomas, fibrosarcomas, and reticulum cell sarcomas, all have elevated levels of type IV collagenase when compared with benign control cells.[66–68] Anti-type IV collagenase antibodies react with invading colon and breast cancer cells as well as lymph node metastases of primary breast cancers on immunohistochemical staining.[21] Furthermore, a quantitative relationship between type IV collagenase activity and in vitro invasion of tumor cells through isolated human amnion membrane has been observed. The penetration of human tumor cells can be inhibited in this assay by metalloproteinase inhibitors.[34] These results suggest that type IV collagenase activity may serve as a useful marker of the invasive capacity and possibly the metastatic potential of some human tumors.

Studies have shown a possible linkage between augmented type IV collagenase activity and the genetic induction of a metastatic phenotype.[68–70] Plasmids containing various Harvey-*ras* oncogene constructs or cellular proto-oncogene constructs were used to transfect NIH-3T3 cells. A series of transfectants were identified that were nontumorigenic, tumorigenic but nonmetastatic, and tumorigenic, metastatic. This observation allows the tumorigenic and metastatic phenotypes to be separated out for further study. A series of NIH-3T3 cell transfectants that exhibited metastatic capacity in vivo all secreted high levels of type IV collagenase. Spontaneously transformed NIH-3T3 cells that were tumorigenic but not metastatic as well as parental NIH-3T3 cells both produced only very low levels of type IV collagenase. Thus, type IV collagenase may be one of a number of possible metastasis-associated gene products.

A new metalloproteinase activity secreted by phorbol ester–stimulated synovial fibroblasts has been characterized.[71] This enzyme, referred to as stromelysin, is secreted as a 51,000-dalton proenzyme and is capable of degrading a variety of extracellular matrix proteins, including fibronectin, laminin, elastin, IgG, and proteoglycans.[71,72] The enzyme has been cloned from rabbit and human sources, and the amino acid sequences as determined with cDNA sequencing show homology with the rat protein transin, which is a secreted protease.[72,73] This is of interest because the rat

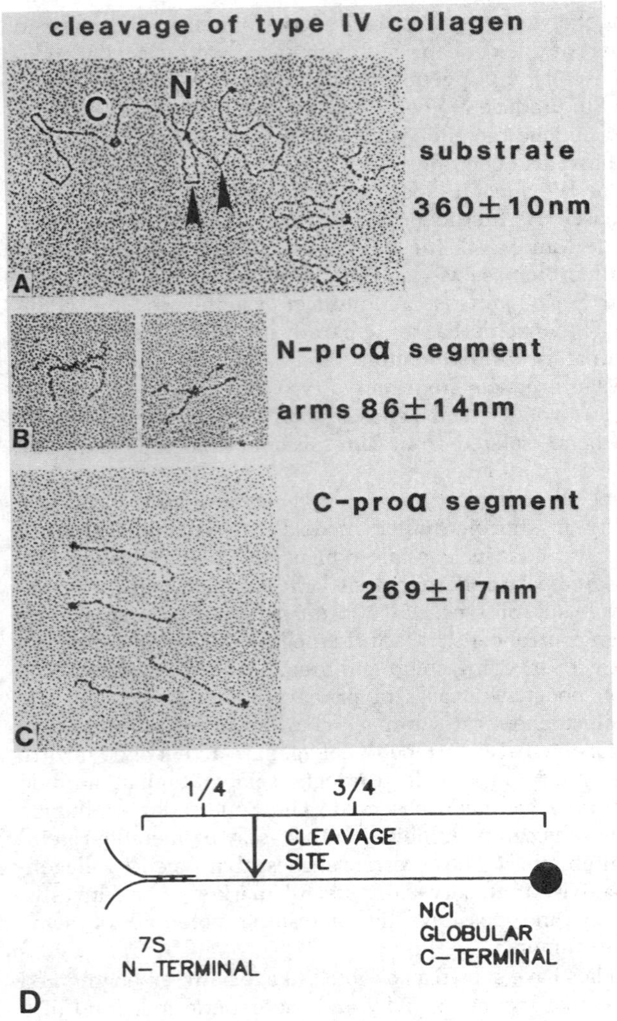

FIG. 7-6. Electron micrographs of type IV collagen fragments cleaved by tumor cell-derived type IV collagenolytic metalloproteinase (*CIV*). **Panel A.** Type IV basement membrane collagen molecules (pro-alpha chains) spontaneously link together to form a network with two to four molecules combining at the N-terminus (*N*) and two molecules combining at the globular C-terminus (*C*). Purified tumor cell-derived CIV cleaves the type IV collagen substrate at a location one-fourth the distance from the N-terminus (*arrow*), producing a small cleavage product (**panel B**) and a large C-terminal fragment (**panel C**). **Panel D.** Schematic representation of type IV collagen molecule showing the cleavage site of type IV collagenase.

transin gene is greatly increased in experimentally induced rat carcinomas.[74] In cell lines of fibroblast origin, stromelysin and interstitial collagenase show similar rates of secretion and coordinate gene regulation in response to phorbol ester treatments.[73] Induction was blocked by cycloheximide, which suggests that the signal transduction pathway is indirect and requires new protein synthesis. However, phorbol ester treatment failed to induce stromelysin synthesis in normal human keratinocytes, endothelial cells, or human tumor cell lines, such as melanoma, fibrosarcoma, and *ras*-transformed bronchial epithelial cells.[72] Thus, the possible role of this enzyme in tumor cell invasion awaits further elucidation.

Cysteine Proteinases and Endoglycosidases

As with the other proteases described in this section, there is an accumulating body of correlative evidence that suggests a role for the cysteine protease cathepsin B in tumor cell invasion and metastasis.[39,40] Cathepsin B is a lysosomal acid hydrolase with a broad range of endopeptidase activity against substrates that include myosin, actin, proteoglycans, fibronectin, laminin, and nonhelical portions of type IV collagen.

Cathepsin B activity has been found in association with the plasma membrane fraction of tumor cells, and in the conditioned media from tumor cell cultures.[39] The tumor cell cathepsin B activity isolated from a variety of human tumors appears to be a different enzyme from the lysosomal protease of normal cells, based on *p*H stability profiles. Studies using the murine melanoma cell line B16 have shown a correlation of cathepsin B activity with potential for metastatic colony formation in the mouse lung. Cathepsin B activity in extracts of human tumors has shown a positive correlation with malignant behavior of these tumors.[39,40]

Studies have also focused on enzymatic activities that degrade the proteoglycan components of the extracellular matrix barriers. Nicolson and colleagues have characterized an endoglycosidase activity produced by murine melanoma cells that releases heparan sulfate chains from matrix proteoglycans.[75,76] This heparanase activity correlated with the metastatic potential of the melanoma subline, that is, highly metastatic cells produced greater levels of endoglycosidase activity than cells of low metastatic potential. A similar heparanase activity has been demonstrated in human melanoma cells, and variants of these human cell lines with high metastatic potential produced significantly higher heparanase activities than parental cells of low metastatic potential.[77]

Thus, the increased expression of a variety of enzyme activities, some capable of degrading specific extracellular matrix components (collagenase, heparanase), have been correlated with the invasive or metastatic potential of many different malignant tumor cell types. The malignant cell apparently produces a spectrum of matrix-degrading enzyme activities that varies with cell type, tumor preparation, and cell culture conditions. This finding led investigators to begin dissecting these concerted enzyme activities by using protease-specific inhibitors and activators.[78,79] Results of such studies have suggested the presence of proteolytic activation cascades, such as plasminogen activator–plasmin–collagenase, which may account for the spectrum of enzyme activities associated with malignant cell types. Regulation of proteolysis may occur at many levels, including tumor cell–host cell interactions and protease inhibitors produced by the host or by the tumor cells themselves. Expression of matrix-degrading enzymes is by no means tumor-cell specific. The actively invading tumor cells may merely respond to different regulatory signals than their noninvasive counterparts.

TUMOR CELL MOTILITY FACTORS

Cell motility is necessary for tumor cells to traverse many stages in the complex cascade of invasion. Such stages could include the detachment and subsequent infiltration of cells from the primary tumor into adjacent tissue, the migration of cells through the vascular wall into the circulation (intravasation), and the extravasation of cells to a secondary site. The movement of cells through biologic barriers such as the endothelial basement membranes of the vasculature may well occur by means of chemotactic mechanisms. Indeed, studies on in vitro chemotaxis of some tumor cells indicate that a variety of compounds such as complement-derived materials, collagen peptides, formyl peptides, and certain connective tissue components can act as chemoattractants.[10,80,81] Although these agents may contribute to the directional aspects of a motile response, they are not sufficient to initiate the intrinsic locomotion of tumor cells. The availability of soluble attractants to the tumor cell is greatly dependent on the host, even when the production of attractants is the result of tumor cell–host tissue interaction. At best, it seems that the cell would have access to such motility stimuli at sporadic and irregular intervals. Such conditions are unfavorable to a sustained migration of highly invasive cells. With these considerations in mind, and stimulated by studies of Anzano et al[82] demonstrating autocrine growth factors for transformed cells, the possibility that such cells could elaborate autocrine motility factors was investigated. The action of these substances might, in part, explain both the markedly invasive character and the metastatic property of malignant neoplastic cells. Thus, under the influence of such an autocrine material, a tumor cell might move out into the surrounding host tissue and also exert a "recruiting" effect on adjacent tumor cells in the presence of an attractant gradient. Conceivably, such factors might also attract fibroblastic cells of the host, resulting in the phenomenon of desmoplasia, characteristic of invasive tumors.

It was found that the human melanoma cell line A2058 and human breast carcinoma cells produce in culture a material that markedly stimulates their own motility.[83–85] These cells respond in a dose-dependent manner to various concentrations of conditioned medium obtained by incubating confluent cells in serum-free medium, an indication that the motility factor is derived from the cell. Motility was measured by the modified Boyden chamber procedure. This assay and "checkerboard" analysis,[83] revealed that the conditioned medium factor has both chemotactic (directional) and chemokinetic (randomly motile) properties. The transducer system activated by autocrine motility factor (AMF) involves phospholipase C and phospholipase A_2 (Fig. 7-7).[84]

Early events in migration may involve pseudopodia protrusion.[85] During the course of invasion, the same tumor cell must interact with a variety of extracellular matrix proteins as it traverses each tissue barrier. For example, the tumor cell encounters laminin and type IV collagen when it penetrates the basement membrane, and type I collagen and fibronectin when it crosses the interstitial stroma. It has recently been shown that cells express specific cell surface receptors that recognize extracellular matrix proteins as decribed above. The first example of such a receptor is the laminin receptor, which binds to laminin with a nanomolar affinity. Laminin receptors have been shown to be augmented in actively invading tumor cells, and may play an important role in tumor cell interaction with the basement membrane. Arg–Gly–Asp (RGD) recognition receptors are another class of cell surface proteins that bind extracellular matrix proteins, which in turn contain the protein sequence

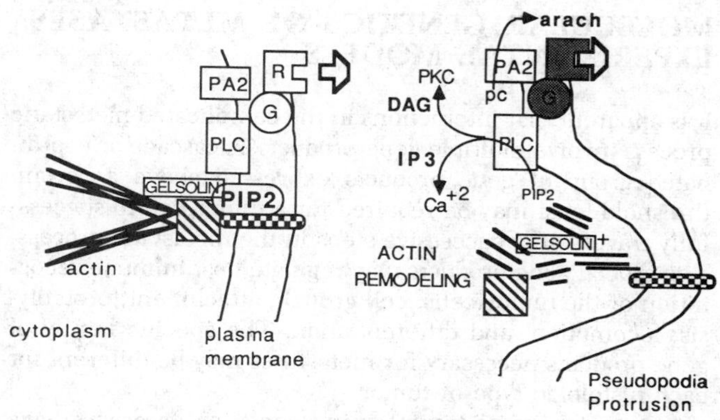

FIG. 7-7. Hypothetical role of membrane lipids in tumor cell motility induced by cytokines such as AMF. Rapid cytoskeleton remodeling may be regulated in part by receptor mediated pathways through guanyl nucleotide–binding proteins (*G*) coupled to phospholipase C (*PLC*) and phospholipase A_2 (*PA2*). Phospholipase C mediates the hydrolysis of phosphatidylinositol 4,5-bisphosphate (*PIP2*), one of the inositol lipids in the plasma membrane. PIP2 strongly inhibits the actin filament–severing properties of gelsolin, a calcium-dependent actin binding protein. PIP2 is cleaved by PLC to form diacylglycerol (*DG*) and insositol 1,4,5-triphosphate (*IP3*). DG stimulates protein kinase C (*PKC*). IP3 induces a rapid release of calcium (*Ca^{2+}*) from intracellular stores. The turnover of PIP2 and the increase in local calcium availability could both contribute to an increase in actin depolymerization via gelsolin. Furthermore, PIP2 is known to form a complex with the cytoplasmic domain of transmembrane proteins such as glycophorin, which in turn facilitates binding of membrane skeletal proteins such as protein 4.1, which promotes associations between actin and spectrin. Turnover of PIP2 could therefore uncouple the tethering of the cytoskeleton to the plasma membrane. Phospholipase A_2 cleaves membrane phosphatidylcholine (*pc*) to generate arachidonic acid (*arach*). Arachidonic acid and its metabolites contribute to lipid methylation events that alter membrane fluidity. Such a combination of events may affect pseudopodial protrusion.

Arg–Gly–Asp.[28] Such proteins include fibronectin, collagen type I, and vitronectin. The process of cell migration undoubtedly requires a series of adhesion and detachment steps resulting in traction and propulsion. Studies using AMF-stimulated motility as the model system have revealed an important function of pseudopodia protrusion in this process. AMF stimulates motility on a variety of different substrates. Therefore, its action is independent of the mechanism of attachment. Furthermore, AMF induces the rapid protrusion of pseudopodia in both a time- and dose-dependent manner.[83] Isolation of the induced pseudopodia reveals that they are highly enriched in their content of laminin and fibronectin matrix receptors. Since cell pseudopodia formation is known to be a prominent feature of actively motile cells, we can now set forth a working hypothesis to explain the early events in cell motility. Cytokines such as AMF that stimulate intrinsic motility may induce exploratory pseudopodia prior to cell translocation. Such pseudopodia may express augmented levels of matrix receptors (and possibly proteinases). The protruding pseudopodia may serve multiple functions, including (1) acting as "sense organs" to interact with the extracellular matrix proteins and thereby locate directional cues, (2) providing propulsive traction for locomotion, and (3) inducing local matrix proteolysis to assist in the penetration of the matrix.[86,87]

MOLECULAR GENETICS OF METASTASES: EXPERIMENTAL MODELS

It is apparent that interactions in the complicated metastatic process involve multiple gene products. A cascade or coordinated group of gene products expressed above a certain threshold level may be required for a tumor cell to successfully traverse the successive steps in the metastatic process. The crucial gene products may regulate host immune recognition of the tumor cells, cell growth, attachment, proteolysis, locomotion, and differentiation. The specific family of gene products necessary for metastases may be different for each histologic type of tumor.

A growing list of transforming genes or *oncogenes* have been identified that may be involved in the genetic alterations leading to tumor growth, invasion, and metastasis.[88–91] Following introduction into suitable recipient cells, oncogenes confer anchorage-independent colony growth in soft agar, and in many cases, tumorigenicity in animal hosts. Cancer cells must, of course, be tumorigenic in order to grow as a metastatic colony. However, not all tumorigenic cells are necessarily invasive and metastatic. This is because the metastatic phenotype is independent from the tumorigenic phenotype. Most of the past work on oncogene function has emphasized mechanisms related to alteration of growth control. Investigators studying oncogene-transformed cells rarely tested these cells for the ability to produce metastases in animal models.

It is now recognized that some oncogene classes can induce the complete metastatic phenotype in the appropriate recipient cell.[69,92–101] An important example is the H-*ras* oncogene. Transfection of members of the *ras* family oncogene into rat or mouse embryo–derived fibroblasts[69,92,95,100] will lead to full expression of the metastatic phenotype. The mechanism of metastasis induction by *ras* is not related to changes in sensitivity to killing by immune cells. Metastasis induction by *ras* is associated with a cascade of gene expression that elevates the intrinsic aggressiveness of the tumor cells.

Thorgeirsson et al[92] were the first to report the metastatic propensity of murine cells transformed with human tumor genomic DNA. Mouse embryo–derived fibroblasts (NIH-3T3 cells) transfected with AML or bladder cancer tumor DNA produced numerous metastases when injected into immunodeficient nude mice. When the resulting metastatic clones were examined, they were found to have acquired exogenous activated *ras* oncogene sequences. To test whether the *ras* oncogene itself or associated genomic DNA was responsible for the metastatic induction, cloned, defined *ras* oncogenes were transferred into NIH-3T3 cells. The resulting *ras*-transformed cells were fully metastatic but had not become resistant to natural killer cell or macrophage lysis. *ras*-Transfected cells also produce metastases in a nonmammalian system, the chick embryo, as reported by Bondy et al.[93]

Muschel et al.[69,99] transformed NIH-3T3 cells with the viral H-*ras* oncogene or the H-*ras* oncogene from the T24 human bladder carcinoma cell line and isolated multiple independent clones. All of the clones are metastatic following injection into nude mice. Egan et al[95] confirmed these results and found that the number of lung metastases produced was proportional to the level of the *ras* oncogene–encoded P21 protein in each transformant. The rare metastatic variants isolated from cells with barely detectable H-*ras* were found to have high levels of *ras* expression caused by rearrangement or amplification at the DNA level. Egan et al[95] also used a steroid-responsive promoter to show the importance of *ras* oncogene transcript dose on metastasis production. The level of *ras* expression in these experimental models correlates directly with metastatic potential. The H-*ras* oncogene is distinguished from its normal cellular counterpart by one or more point mutations.[89] In the viral and T24 *ras,* the mutation is at the position coding for the 12th amino acid. Transfection of the normal proto-oncogene lacking the mutation will not cause transformation. However, Chang et al[90] demonstrated that the *ras* proto-oncogene joined to a viral promoter and transcriptional enhancer would cause elevated production of the normal P21 protein and could transform NIH-3T3 cells. The cells transformed with elevated levels of the normal *ras* (encoding normal P21 protein) produced tumors at a rate comparable to cells transformed with the mutated *ras.*[90] However, when the same cells were tested for metastatic propensity, the cells transformed by the mutated *ras* were much more efficient in the production of metastases[69,95] than were cells transformed by normal *ras.* Nevertheless, very high levels of the normal P21 could also lead to metastasis production.[95] Taken together, all the results are consistent with a dominant role for *ras*-encoded protein dose in the induction of metastases. Very low levels of the mutated P21 protein will result in poorly metastatic tumors, and moderate to high levels of the mutated P21 protein will result in highly metastatic tumors. In contrast, low or moderate levels of normal P21 will result in tumors and very high levels of P21 will produce metastatic tumors.

The use of NIH-3T3 cells in experimental models of metastasis induction by oncogenes has been criticized because these cells are aneuploid and have a high rate of spontaneous transformation.[94] It was conceivable that *ras* oncogene induction of metastases might require cellular or genetic properties present only in NIH-3T3 cells. Therefore, Muschel et al[69] and Pozzatti et al[100] tested the metastatic propensity of *ras*-transfected diploid primary cells. Muschel et al[69] found that rat skin cells, rat muscle cells, and Chinese hamster lung fibroblasts were induced to become metastatic by transfection of *ras* linked to an enhancer, using a construct of Spandidos and Wilkie. Pozzatti et al[100] examined a series of diploid rat embryo cell clones that had been transformed by H-*ras* alone or H-*ras* linked to an SV-40 enhancer cotransfected with a dominant selectible marker (pRSVneo). These clones were all highly metastatic after intravenous, subcutaneous, or intramuscular injection into nude mice. Thus, the ability of the H-*ras* oncogene to induce metastases is not limited to NIH-3T3 cells but occurs even after transformation of certain diploid primary cells.

The *ras* oncogene can also amplify the metastatic potential in certain poorly metastatic or nonmetastatic established tumor cell lines that were not originally transformed by H-*ras*. Vousden et al[96] transfected H-*ras* into a highly tumorigenic cell line derived from a murine mammary carcinoma.

Although the parent cell line was very weakly metastatic, the subclones transfected with *ras* were all highly metastatic. Multiple clones were isolated from the resulting lung metastases, and most retained the metastatic phenotype. One of the clones was no longer metastatic; it was found to have lost the introduced *ras* oncogene. Collard et al[98] obtained similar results when mutated *ras* oncogenes were inserted into T-lymphoma cells. The lymphoma cells became invasive and metastatic in proportion to the level of H-*ras*–specific mRNA. Kerbel et al[97] had similar results with SP1, a cell line isolated from a nonmetastatic murine mammary carcinoma. Metastatic primary tumors were produced by all clones that incorporated the mutated but not the normal *ras*.

The ability of the H-*ras* oncogene to induce metastases is dependent on the cell type. Transfection of H-*ras* into C127 murine cells will result in highly tumorigenic cells that fail to form metastases after intravenous or subcutaneous injection into nude mice. The carcinogen *N*-nitrosomethylurea will induce skin papillomas and mammary tumors in appropriate strains of mice.[101,102] The vast majority of the induced tumors have an activated *ras* oncogene[102] but are nonmetastatic. Only 10% of DMBA tumors will produce metastases. These results lead to the conclusion that activation of the H-*ras* oncogene is not sufficient to induce metastases in certain cultured cell types or spontaneous tumors. The *ras* oncogene may fail to induce metastases in a particular cell because that cell lacks an appropriate cooperation factor. On the other hand, the resistant cell may possess a means of suppressing the ability of *ras* to induce metastases. The adenovirus 2 E1A is an example of a gene that can suppress metastases caused by H-*ras*. Pozzatti et al[100] showed that cotransfection of E1A with *ras* results in nonmetastatic tumors. The mechanism of inhibition may involve the 12S E1A transcript (Pozzatti, personal communication) and is not related to histocompatibility antigen changes or increased sensitivity to immune cell killing. The results lead us to predict the existence of normal genes that function to suppress the metastatic cascade induced by certain oncogenes such as *ras*.[103]

The mechanism by which the H-*ras* oncogene can induce metastases in the appropriate cell recipient is unknown. It must involve the activation of a multigene cascade since the H-*ras*–transformed cells acquire a large number of new functional properties, including increased adhesiveness, changes in cell surface carbohydrates associated with metastases,[104] motility, and ability to invade tissue barriers.[83,92,104–106] One potential explanation is that H-*ras* transfection leads to genetic or karyotypic instability with the resulting selection of metastatic variants.[91] A second possible mechanism could involve the selected integration of H-*ras* into a specific location in the genome next to metastases-associated genes. Both of these explanations seem unlikely, based on the data obtained so far. Diploid rat embryo fibroblasts transfected with H-*ras* become metastatic as soon as enough cells (four passages) can be grown to inject into nude mice. The resulting metastatic clones do not contain any consistent gross karyotypic alteration and indeed may remain fully diploid.[100] All of the transfectant clones expressing the activated P21 protein are metastatic,[69,95,100] implying that induction of metastases is not a rare event as would be expected if there were a requirement for *ras* to be integrated into a specific site. The explanation we are left with is that the *ras* P21 protein alters some general pathway in the cell and that this pathway is involved in the metastatic cascade. A likely candidate pathway is the G protein–mediated transducer systems involved in phosphatidylinositol-4,5-bisphosphate and catabolites thereof, as well as the arachidonic acid pathways mediated through phospholipase A_2 (see Fig. 7-4).[83,106,107]

H-*ras* is not the only oncogene that can induce metastatic potential in 3T3 cells. Egan et al[107] recently reported that certain transforming oncogenes encoding protein kinases (*mos, raf, src, fes,* and *fms*) but not nuclear oncogenes such as *myc* or p53 induced 3T3 cells to produce lung metastases after intravenous injection. Whether or not these oncogenes will induce the spontaneous metastatic phenotype in diploid primary cells is unknown. Transformation of cells by *src, fes,* and *fms* may be mediated through a *ras*-dependent mechanism, as Smith et al[108] have shown that transformation by these oncogenes is blocked by antibodies to *ras*-encoded P21. Oncogenes have been found to have multifactorial effects on a variety of general cell pathways.[109,110]

Regardless of the mechanism by which oncogene transfection induces metastases in animal systems, it constitutes a revolutionary model system for studying the biochemical mechanisms of metastases. For example, specific classes of collagenase[70,92] and motility-stimulating cytokines[83] have been shown to be biochemically linked to the induction of metastases by the H-*ras* oncogene. With appropriate combinations of H-*ras* oncogenes with viral enhancers or other oncogenes such as E1A, diploid cells will become either fully tumorigenic but non metastatic or poorly metastatic, or fully metastatic. The metastatic clones are very aggressive, producing more than 200 metastases in the lungs of nude mice after intravenous injection of only 5×10^4 cells. A wide variety of organs are the site of spontaneous metastases produced from primary tumors arising from subcutaneous or intramuscular injection of transfected cells. Virtually unlimited numbers of clones of metastatic or nonmetastatic tumor cells can be produced using transfection methods. The transfection model system has a number of advantages compared to previous metastases models, which were the result of multiple selection steps applied to heterogeneous transplantable tumors.[3,4]

ONCOGENE EXPRESSION CORRELATION WITH HUMAN TUMOR METASTATIC AGGRESSIVENESS

Proto-oncogenes may be activated and may contribute to neoplastic transformation and progression to the metastatic phenotype.[88–90,102,104–114] Activation can occur by multiple pathways, including (1) amplification of the number of copies of the oncogene in the genome of tumor cells, (2) mutation within the coding sequence of the oncogene, (3) chromosomal breaks and translocation with subsequent enhanced expression of the oncogene-encoded protein, and (4) insertion of a retroviral promoter near the proto-oncogene. Yokota et al[115] studied proto-oncogene alteration in 72 samples of tumor tissue and corresponding normal tissue from the same patient. Alterations were frequently found in c-*myc*, c-*ras*, and c-*myb*. No oncogene alterations were observed in the normal tissue. Oncogene alterations may merely be a hallmark of the genetic instability of tumors. On the other hand, if proto-oncogene alterations play an actual functional role in malignant behavior, they might provide a survival advantage and be selected out in the expanding tumor cell population. This could result in increased expression of relevant oncogene products in more aggressive tumors with a higher propensity to metastasize. In fact, oncogene expression does correlate with metastatic behavior in certain classes of human tumors studied to date. However, a different class of oncogene appears to be important for each histologic type of tumor.

Amplification of the *HER-2/neu* oncogene has been correlated with metastases in human breast carcinoma. The *HER-2/neu (neu)* oncogene is a member of the *erb*-B–like oncogene family, and is related to, but distinct from, the gene encoding the epidermal growth factor receptor. Slamon et al[112] studied alterations in the gene in 189 primary human breast cancer specimens and found that *neu* was amplified in 30% of the tumors. Amplification was a significant predictor of overall survival, time to relapse, estrogen receptor status, size of primary tumor, and number of axillary lymph nodes positive for metastasis. Van de Vijver et al[114] detected amplification of *neu* in 16 of 95 human breast tumor samples; the amplification was accompanied by overexpression in the tumors from which intact RNA could be isolated. No correlation was found in this study between *neu* amplification and estrogen receptor content, patient age, or clinical stage of disease.

Increased expression of the H-*ras* oncogene has also been correlated with lymph node metastases in human breast carcinoma. Agnantis et al[116] found a significant elevation of H-*ras* transcripts in malignant compared with normal breast tissue, with a higher mean value of expression in cases with lymph node metastases. Horan-Hand et al[117] immunologically assayed the H-*ras* P21 protein in samples of human breast carcinoma and colon carcinoma. Enhanced expression was documented in 66% of breast and 100% of colon carcinomas compared to normal counterparts, with levels in breast carcinoma ranging from 18.4 to 51.7 pg P21/μg protein. Clair et al[118] extended this finding to report a correlation of breast carcinoma P21 expression with advanced-disease stage and positive axillary lymph node metastasis. Lundy et al[119] reported a positive correlation between H-*ras* P21 protein levels and lymph node metastasis, but not between H-*ras* P21 levels and patient age or estrogen receptor status.

N-*myc* amplification is associated with rapid progression of neuroblastomas. Seeger et al[120] studied 89 patients with untreated primary neuroblastoma to determine the relation between the number of copies of the N-*myc* oncogene and survival without disease progression. Analysis of progression-free survival in all patients revealed that amplification of N-*myc* was associated with the worst prognosis. The estimated progression-free survival at 18 months was 70%, 30%, and 5% for patients whose tumors had one, three to ten, or more than ten N-*myc* copies, respectively. It is unclear whether or not the poor survival in patients with amplified N-*myc* is due to an increased number of metastases. However, amplified N-*myc* is prevalent in Stage 4 neuroblastomas[121] with distant metastases from hematogenous or lymphatic dissemination. The mechanism by which N-*myc* augments tumor aggressiveness is unknown. Experimental animal studies to date have not shown a significant role for N-*myc* transfection (N-*myc* alone or in combination with H-*ras*[69,107]) in the induction of the metastatic phenotype. However, these experiments have not been conducted with neural cell lines. In patients whose neuroblastoma tumor cells can be grown in vitro as a cell line, there is a very high association with amplified N-*myc* and poor prognosis. Thus, it is conceivable that N-*myc* amplification somehow facilitates the independent growth of neuroblastoma cells in a harsh environment. This would favor the growth of metastatic colonies in distant organ sites. Neuroblastoma cells without N-*myc* amplification may have a greater requirement for cooperating local host factors that support growth.

Tumors other than neuroblastoma have not shown as strong a correlation between N-*myc* amplification and clinical prognosis or extent of metastasis. In contrast to *neu* amplification and H-*ras* overexpression, C-*myc* or N-*myc* oncogene amplification was not correlated with human breast cancer stage of disease, hormonal receptor status, or axillary lymph node metastasis.[111,112] C-*myc* and N-*myc* are amplified in small cell lung cancers and gastrointestinal malignancies, but the level of amplification has not been shown to correlate with metastasis.[122,123] Thus, if oncogenes are indeed important in human tumor progression, the effect of any given oncogene may depend on the genetic background of the host cell.

NEW STRATEGIES FOR METASTASIS DIAGNOSIS AND THERAPY

The elucidation of biochemical and genetic mechanisms that play a role in cancer metastasis (see Table 7-1) has led to new strategies for cancer diagnosis and therapy. Normal host parenchymal cells do not invade and metastasize. Thus, the biochemical changes that are expressed in the malignant phenotype may be a target for strategies that are more selective for the tumor cells than are conventional cytotoxic agents.

The most immediate application of these basic research findings is in the area of tumor diagnosis and prognosis. The clinical aggressiveness of an individual tumor could be more accurately predicted by the measurement of genes or gene products functionally associated with the phenotype of invasion and metastases. These include oncogenes such as *ras*, *myc*, *neu*, newly discovered genes that may be associated with suppression of the metastatic phenotype,[103] and genes that encode receptors, proteinases, and motility factors associated with invasion. The average levels of such metastasis markers could be measured in a sample of the tumor tissue. On the other hand, antibodies or genetic probes for the markers could be applied to a histologic section of the tumor to study the tumor cell population distribution of the marker. In this manner, the proportion of tumor cells reacting with the marker could be used as an index of the aggressive tumor subpopulation. Application of antibodies to metastases-associated antigens by the surgical pathologist may provide increased accuracy in the identification of micrometastases in lymph nodes. Furthermore, immunohistochemical applications are not limited to tumor-associated antigens. Host antigens may also be altered in the vicinity of the tumor. This is the case for host basement membranes which are locally fragmented or lost in the area of tumor cell invasion. Loss of basement membrane antigens has already proved useful in the detection of breast cancer microinvasion and in the grading and staging of colorectal tumors.[21,22]

Some of the proteins associated with invasion and metastasis are secreted by the tumor cell. Examples are degradative enzymes such as type IV collagenase and heparanase, or hormone-like proteins such as tumor autocrine motility factors and growth factors. Following secretion by the tumor cell, the proteins (whole or as fragments), may accumulate in the blood or urine of the patient. Measurement of the level of the proteins by sensitive immunoassay procedures may be a means to (1) detect the existence of occult metastases, (2) estimate the body burden of metastatic disease, and (3) detect local tumor recurrence. Furthermore, in the case of bladder cancer, the level of the marker in the urine may reflect the invasive stage of the transitional cell carcinoma.

Tumor cell proteins functionally associated with the metastatic phenotype may be quantitatively augmented in tumor cells composing the metastatic foci. Systemically administered antibodies or synthetic ligands that bind to the tumor cell proteins may preferentially accumulate in the metastatic foci, compared with other body sites. This could be of use in the radioscintigraphic detection of clinically occult metastases. Furthermore, if the antibody or ligand is coupled to a toxic agent, it may selectively kill the tumor cells in the metastatic foci.

An increased understanding of the mechanisms of tumor cell invasion may lead to the development of pharmacologic agents or strategies that block tumor cell invasion. In theory, blocking any of the necessary steps for invasion listed in Table 7-1 could prevent tumor cell invasion. Tumor angiogenesis may depend on mechanisms similar to cancer invasion, including proteolysis. Consequently, an anti-invasion agent may also block tumor angiogenesis. Chronic systemic treatment or local administration with an anti-invasion agent may be clinically useful in the following settings: (1) preventing the transition from in situ to invasive cancer in high-risk patients, (2) reducing local tumor recurrence and invasion following surgical removal of primary tumors, and (3) inhibiting metastasis formation by circulating tumor cells disseminated by inoperable primary tumors, metastases, or released during surgical manipulation of the primary tumor.

The ultimate goal of metastasis prevention would be the selective eradication of established metastases, perhaps by targeting toxic agents to the metastatic foci. However, actual killing of the tumor cells in the metastatic foci may not be necessary to prevent the usual clinical outcome of metastatic disease. Inhibition of metastatic growth by chronic treatment regimens may achieve the same end. This is a hopeful area for therapy strategies because it has been found that common cellular pathways may be deranged by genetic events, such as increased *ras* expression, in such a way as to increase both the growth and invasion of tumor cells. An example of a common pathway is the inositol phosphate cascade operating through phospholipase C. This pathway may be altered by a number of oncogenes. Agents that normalize this pathway in tumor cells may act to suppress both growth and invasion.

REFERENCES

1. Sugarbaker EV: Patterns of metastasis in human malignancies. Cancer Biol Rev 2:235, 1981
2. Weiss L, Gilbert HA: Bone Metastases. Boston, GK Hall, 1981
3. Schirrmacher V: Cancer metastasis: Experimental approaches, theoretical concepts, and impacts for treatment strategies. Adv Cancer Res 43:1, 1985
4. Fidler IJ, Hart IR: Biologic diversity in metastatic neoplasms: Origins and implications. Science 217:998, 1982
5. Liotta LA: Tumor invasion and metastases: role of the extracellular matrix. Rhoads Memorial Award Lecture. Cancer Res 46:1, 1986
6. Tubiana M, Chauvel P, Renaud A et al: Vitresse de croissance et histoire naturelle du cancer du sein. Bull Cancer 62:341, 1975
7. Koscielny S, Tubiana M, Valleron A-J: A simulation model of the natural history of human breast cancer. Br J Cancer 52:515, 1985
8. Bauer W, Igot J-P, Le Gal Y: Chronologie du cancer mammaire utilisant un modele de croissance de Gompertz. Ann Anat Pathol (Paris) 25:39, 1980
9. Liotta LA, Kleinerman J, Saidel GM: Quantitative relationships of intravascular tumor cells, tumor vessels, and pulmonary metastases following tumor implantation. Cancer Res 34:997, 1974
10. Fidler IJ, Kripke ML: Metastasis results from pre-existing variant cells within a malignant tumor. Science 197:893, 1977
11. Luria SE, Delbruck M: Mutations of bacteria from virus sensitivity to virus resistance. Genetics 28:491, 1945
12. Furcht LT: Editorial: Critical factors controlling angiogenesis: Cell products, cell matrix, and growth factors. Lab Invest 55:505, 1986
13. Folkman J: Tumor angiogenesis. Adv Cancer Res 43:175, 1985
14. Gullino PM, Grantham F: The vascular space of growing tumors. Cancer Res 24:1727, 1964
15. Lapis K, Paku S, Liotta LA: Endothelialization of embolised tumor cells during metastasis formation. Clin Exp Metastasis 6:73, 1988
16. Wallace AC, Chew E, Jones DS: The arrest and extravasation of cancer cells in the lung. In Weiss L, Gilbert HA (eds): Pulmonary Metastasis, p 26. Boston, GK Hall, 1978
17. Nicolson GL, Dulski K, Basson C et al: Preferential organ attachment and invasion in vitro by B16 melanoma cells selected for differing metastatic colonization and invasive properties. Invasion Metastasis 5:144, 1985
18. Frost P, Kerbel RS: Immunology of metastasis: Can the immune response cope with disseminated tumor? Metastasis Rev 2:239, 1983
19. Old LJ: Cancer immunology: The search for specificity. Cancer Res 41:361, 1981
20. Hanna N, Fidler IJ: Relationship between metastatic potential and resistance to natural killer cell mediated cytotoxicity in three murine tumor systems. JNCI 66:1183, 1981
21. Barsky SH, Siegal GP, Jannotta F et al: Loss of basement membrane components by invasive tumors but not their benign counterparts. Lab Invest 49:140, 1983
22. Forester SJ, Talbot IC, Critshley DR: Laminin and fibronectin in rectal adenocarcinoma: Relationship to tumor grade stage and metastasis. Br J Cancer 50:51, 1984
23. Wewer UM, Liotta LA, Jaye M et al: Altered levels of laminin receptor mRNA in various human carcinoma cells that have different abilities to bind laminin. Proc Natl Acad Sci USA 83:7137, 1986
24. Rao CN, Margulies M, Tralka S et al: Isolation of a subunit of laminin and its role in molecular structure and tumor cell attachment. J Biol Chem 257:9740, 1982
25. Engel J, Odermatt E, Engel A et al: Shapes, domain organization and flexibility of laminin and fibronectin: Two multifunctional proteins of the ECM. Mol Biol 150:97, 1981
26. Wewer UM, Taraboletti G, Sobel ME et al: Laminin receptor: Role in tumor cell migration. Cancer Res 47:5691, 1987
27. Barsky SH, Rao CN, Williams JE et al: Laminin molecular domains which alter metastasis in a murine model. J Clin Invest 74:843, 1984
28. Hynes RO: Integrins: A family of cell surface receptors. Cell 48:549, 1987
29. Ruoslahti E, Pierschbacher MD: Arg-Gly-Asp: A versatile cell recognition signal. Cell 44:517, 1986
30. Yamada KM, Kennedy DW: Dualistic nature of adhesive protein function: Fibronectin and its biologically active peptide fragments can autoinhibit fibronectin function. J Cell Biol 99:29, 1984
31. Horwitz A, Duggan C et al: Binding of fibronectin receptors to talin. Nature 320:531, 1986
32. Humphries MJ, Olden K, Yamada KM: A synthetic peptide from fibronectin inhibits experimental metastasis of murine melanoma cells. Science 233:467, 1986
33. Thorgeirsson UP, Turpeenniemi-Hujanen T, Neckers LM et al: Protein synthesis but

not DNA synthesis is required for tumor cell invasion *in vitro*. Invasion Metastasis 4:73, 1984

34. Thorgeirsson UP, Liotta LA, Kalebic T et al: Effect of natural protease inhibitors and a chemoattractant or tumor cell invasion *in vitro*. JNCI 69:1049, 1982
35. Liotta LA, Thorgeirsson UP, Garbisa S: Role of collagenases in tumor cell invasion. Cancer Metastasis Rev 1:277, 1982
36. Goldfarb RH: Plasminogen activators. Ann Rep Med Chem 18:257, 1983
37. Dano K, Andreasen PA, Grondahl-Hansen J et al: Plasminogen activators, tissue degradation, and cancer. Adv Cancer Res 44:139, 1985
38. Goldfarb RH, Liotta LA: Proteolytic enzymes in cancer invasion and metastasis. Semin Thromb Hemost 12:294, 1986
39. Sloane BF, Rozhin J, Ryan RE et al: Cathepsin B-like cysteine proteinases and metastases. In Honn KV, Powers WE, Sloan BF (eds): Mechanisms of Cancer Metastasis: Potential Therapeutic Implications, p. 377. Boston, Martinus Nijhoff, 1986
40. Sloane BF, Honn KV: Cysteine proteinases and metastasis. Cancer Metastasis Rev 3:249, 1984
41. Markus G: Plasminogen activators in malignant growth. In Davidson JF (ed): Progress in Fibrinolysis, p 587. Edinburgh, Churchill Livingstone, 1983
42. Goldfarb RH, Quigley JP: Purification of plasminogen activator from Rous sarcoma virus transformed chick embryo fibroblasts treated with the tumor promoter phorbol 12-myristate 13-acetate. Biochemistry 19:5463, 1980
43. Goldfarb RH, Quigley JP: Synergistic effect of tumor virus transformation and tumor promoter treatment on the production of plasminogen activator by chick embryo fibroblasts. Cancer Res 38:4601, 1978
44. Lijnen HR, Collen D: Interaction of plasminogen activation and inhibitors with plasminogen and fibrin. Semin Thromb Hemost 8:2, 1982
45. Castellino FJ, Powell SR: Human plasminogen. Methods Enzymol 80:365, 1981
46. Cajot J-F, Sordat B, Kruithof EKO et al: Human primary colon carcinomas xenografted into nude mice: I. Characterization of plasminogen activators expressed by primary tumors and their xenografts. JNCI 77:703, 1986
47. Markus G, Camiolo SM, Kohga S et al: Plasminogen activator secretion of human tumors in short-term organ culture, including a comparison of primary and metabolic tumors. Cancer Res 43:5517, 1983
48. Markus G: The role of hemostasis and fibrinolysis in the metastatic spread of cancer. Semin Thromb Hemost 10:61, 1984
49. Jones PA, DeClerck YA: Extracellular matrix destruction by invasive tumor cells. Cancer Metastasis Rev 1:289, 1982
50. Kramer RH, Bensch KG, Wang J: Invasion of reconstituted basement membrane matrix by metastatic human tumor cells. Cancer Res 46:1980, 1986
51. Bogenman E, Jones PA: Role of plasminogen in matrix degradation by neoplastic cells. JNCI 71:1177, 1983
52. Liotta LA, Goldfarb RH, Brundage R et al: Effect of plasminogen activator (urokinase), plasmin, and thrombin on glycoprotein and collagenous components of basement membrane. Cancer Res 41:4629, 1981
53. Ossowski L, Reich E: Antibodies to plasminogen activator inhibit tumor metastasis. Cell 35:611, 1983
54. Wang BS, McLouglin GA, Richie JP et al: Correlation of the production of plasminogen activator with tumor metastasis in B16 mouse melanoma cell lines. Cancer Res 40:288, 1980
55. Carlsen SA, Ramshaw JA, Warrington RC: Involvement of plasminogen activator production in a rat model. Cancer Res 44:3012, 1984
56. Sappino A-P, Busso N, Belin D et al: Increase of urokinase type plasminogen activator gene expression in human lung and breast carcinomas. Cancer Res 47:4043, 1987
57. Gross J, Nagai Y: Specific degradation of the collagen molecule by tadpole collagenolytic enzyme. Proc Natl Acad Sci USA 54:1197, 1965
58. Goldberg GI, Wilhelm SM, Kronberger A et al: Human fibroblast collagenase: Complete primary structure and homology to an oncogene transformation-induced rat protein. J Biol Chem 261:6600, 1986
59. Fini ME, Plucinska IM, Mayer AS et al: A gene for rabbit synovial cell collagenase: Member of a family of metalloproteinases that degrade the connective tissue matrix. Biochemistry 26:6156, 1987
60. Huang C-C, Blitzer A, Abramson M: Collagenase in human head and neck tumors and rat tumors and fibroblasts in monolayer cultures. Ann Otol Rhinol Laryngol 95:158, 1986
61. Wirl G, Frich J: Collagenase: A marker enzyme in human bladder cancer. Urol Res 7:103, 1979
62. Liotta LA, Rao CN: Role of the extracellular matrix in cancer. Ann NY Acad Sci 460:333, 1985
63. Liotta LA, Abe S, Robey PG et al: Preferential digestion of basement membrane collagen by an enzyme derived from a metastatic murine tumor. Proc Natl Acad Sci USA 76:2268, 1979
64. Salo T, Liotta LA, Tryggvason K: Purification and characterization of a murine basement membrane collagen-degrading enzyme secreted by metastatic tumor cells. J Biol Chem 258:3058, 1983
65. Liotta LA, Rao CN, Barsky SH: Tumor invasion and the extracellular matrix. Lab Invest 49:636, 1983
66. Liotta LA, Tryggvason K, Garbisa S et al: Metastatic potential correlates with enzymatic degradation of basement membrane collagen. Nature 284:67, 1980
67. Nakatsukasa H: Type IV collagen-degrading enzyme activity in hepatocellular carcinoma. Acta Med Okayama 40:83, 1986
68. Turpeenniemi-Hujanen T, Thorgeirsson UP, Hart IR et al: Expression of collagenase IV (basement membrane collagenase) activity in murine tumor cell hybrids that differ in metastatic potential. JNCI 75:99, 1985
69. Muschel R, Williams JE, Lowy DR et al: Harvey *ras* induction of metastatic potential depends upon oncogene activation and type of recipient cell. Am J Pathol 121:1, 1985
70. Garbisa S, Pozzatti R, Muschel RJ et al: Secretion of type IV collagenolytic protease and metastatic phenotype: Induction by transfection with c-Ha-ras but not c-Ha-ras plus Ad2-Ela. Cancer Res 47:1523, 1987
71. Chin JR, Murphy G, Werb Z: Stromelysin, a connective tissue-degrading metalloendopeptidase secreted by stimulated rabbit synovial fibroblasts in parallel with collagenase. J Biol Chem 260:12367, 1985
72. Wilhelm SM, Collier IE, Kronberger A et al: Human skin fibroblast stromelysin: Structure, glycosylation, substrate specificity, and differential expression in normal and tumorigenic cells. Proc Natl Acad Sci USA 84:6725, 1987
73. Frisch SM, Clark EJ, Werb Z: Coordinate regulation of stromelysin and collagenase genes determined with cDNA probes. Proc Natl Acad Sci USA 84:2600, 1987
74. Matrisian LM, Leroy P, Ruhlmann C et al: Isolation of the oncogene and epidermal growth factor-induced transin gene: Complex control in rat fibroblasts. Mol Cell Biol 6:1679, 1986
75. Nakajima M, Irimura T, Di Ferrante D et al: Heparan sulfate degradation: Relation to tumor invasive and metastatic properties of mouse B16 melanoma sublines. Science 220:611, 1983
76. Nakajima M, Irimura T, Di Ferrante N et al: Metastatic melanoma cell heparanase characterization of heparan sulfate degradation fragments produced by B16 melanoma endoglucuronidase. J Biol Chem 259:2283, 1984
77. Nakajima M, Irimura T, Nicolson GL: Tumor metastasis-associated heparanase (heparan sulfate endoglycosidase) activity in human melanoma cells. Cancer Lett 31:277, 1986
78. Mignatti P, Robbins E, Rifkin DB: Tumor invasion through the human amniotic membrane: Requirement for a proteinase cascade. Cell 47:487, 1986
79. Persky B, Ostrowski LE, Pagast P et al: Inhibition of proteolytic enzymes in the *in vitro* amnion model for basement membrane invasion. Cancer Res 16:4129, 1986
80. Lam WC, Delikatny JE, Orr FW et al: The chemotactic response of tumor cells: A model for cancer metastasis. Am J Pathol 104:69, 1981
81. McCarthy JB, Basara ML, Palm SL, et al: Stimulation of haptotaxis and migration of tumor cells by serum spreading factor. Cancer Metastasis Rev 4:125, 1985
82. Anzano MA, Roberts AB, Smith JM et al: Sarcoma growth factors from conditioned media of virally transformed cells composed of both type α and type β growth factors. Proc Natl Acad Sci USA 80:6264, 1983
83. Liotta LA, Mandler R, Murano G et al: Tumor cell autocrine motility factor: Tumor cell autocrine motility factor. Proc Natl Acad Sci USA 83:3302, 1986
84. Stracke ML, Guirguis R, Liotta LA et al: Pertussis toxin inhibits stimulated motility independently of the adenylate cyclase pathway in human melanoma cells. Biochem Biophys Res Commun 146:339, 1987
85. Guirguis R, Margulies IMK, Taraboletti G et al: Cytokine-induced pseudopodial protrusion is coupled to tumor cell migration. Nature 329:261, 1987
86. Bokoch GM, Gilman AG: Inhibition of receptor-mediated release of arachidonic acid by pertussis toxin. Cell 39:301, 1984
87. Smith CD, Cox CC, Snyderman R: Receptor-coupled activation of phosphoinositide-specific phospholipase C by an N protein. Science 232:97, 1986
88. Weinberg RA: Oncogenes of spontaneous and chemically induced tumors. Adv Cancer Res 36:149, 1982
89. Hunter T: Oncogenes and proto-oncogenes: How do they differ? JNCI 73:773, 1984
90. Chang EH, Furth ME, Scolnick EM et al: Tumorigenic transformation of mammalian cells induced by a normal human gene homologous to the oncogene of Harvey murine sarcoma virus. Proc Natl Acad Sci USA 78:3328, 1981
91. Nicolson GL: Tumor cell instability, diversification, and progression to the metastatic phenotype: From oncogene to oncofetal expression. Cancer Res 47:1473, 1987
92. Thorgeirsson UP, Turpeenniemi-Hujanen T, Williams JE et al: NIH/3T3 cells transfected with human tumor DNA containing activated ras oncogenes express the metastatic phenotype in nude mice. Mol Cell Biol 5:259, 1985
93. Bondy GP, Wilson S, Chambers AF: Experimental metastatic ability of H-ras transformed NIH-3T3 cells. Cancer Res 45:6005, 1985
94. Greig RG, Koestler TP, Trainer DL et al: Tumorigenic and metastatic properties of "normal" and ras-transfected NIH/3T3 cells. Proc Natl Acad Sci USA 82:3698, 1985
95. Egan SE, McClarty GA, Jarolim L et al: Expression of H-ras correlates with metastatic potential: Evidence for direct regulation of the metastatic phenotype in 10T1/2 and NIH 3T3 cells. Mol Cell Biol 7:830, 1987
96. Vousden KH, Eccles SA, Purvies H et al: Enhanced spontaneous metastasis of mouse carcinoma cells transfected with an activated c-Ha-ras-1 gene. Int J Cancer 37:425, 1986
97. Kerbel RS, Waghorne C, Man MS et al: Alteration of the tumorigenic and metastatic properties of neoplastic cells is associated with the process of calcium phosphate-mediated DNA transfection. Proc Natl Acad Sci USA 84:1263, 1987
98. Collard JG, Schijven JF, Roos E: Invasive and metastatic potential induced by ras-transfection into mouse BW5147 T-lymphoma cells. Cancer Res 47:754, 1987
99. Muschel RJ, Nakahara K, Chu EW et al: Karyotypic analysis of diploid or near diploid metastatic Harvey ras transformed rat embryo fibroblasts. Cancer Res 46:4104, 1986
100. Pozzatti R, Muschel R, Williams J et al: Primary rat embryo cells transformed by one or two oncogenes show different metastatic potentials. Science 232:223, 1986
101. Gullino PM, Pettigrew NM, Grantharn FH: N-nitrosomethylurea as a mammary gland carcinoma in rats. JNCI 54:401, 1975
102. Sukumar S, Notairo V, Martin-Zanca et al: Induction of mammary carcinomas in rats by NMU involves malignant activation of Ha-ras-1 locus by a single point mutation. Nature 306:658, 1983

103. Steeg PS, Bevilacqua G, Kopper L et al: Evidence for a novel gene associated with low tumor metastatic potential. JNCI 80:200, 1988
104. Dennis JW, Laferte S, Waghorne C et al: 1-6 branching of Asn-linked oligosaccharides is directly associated with metastasis. Science 236:582, 1987
105. Stryer L, Bourne HR: G proteins: A family of signal transducers. Annu Rev Cell Biol 2:391, 1986
106. Fleischman LF, Chahwala SB, Cantley L: Ras-transformed cells: Altered levels of phosphatidylinositol-4,5-bisphosphate and catabolites. Science 231:407, 1986
107. Egan SE, Wright JA, Jarolim L et al: Transformation by oncogenes encoding protein kinases induces the metastatic phenotype. Science 238:202, 1987
108. Smith MR, DeGudicibus SJ, Stacey DW: Requirement for c-ras proteins during viral oncogene transformation. Nature 320:540, 1986
109. Jaggi R, Salmons B, Muellener D et al: The v-mos and H-ras oncogene expression represses glucocorticoid hormone-dependent transcription from the mouse mammary tumor virus LTR. EMBO J 5:2609, 1986
110. Rabin MS, Doherty PJ, Gottesman MM: The tumor promoter phorbol 12-myristate 13-acetate induces a program of altered gene expression similar to that induced by platelet-derived growth factor and transforming oncogenes. Proc Natl Acad Sci USA 83:357, 1986
111. Cline MJ, Battifora H, Yokota J: Proto-oncogene abnormalities in human breast cancer: Correlations with anatomic features and clinical course of disease. J Clin Oncol 5:999, 1987
112. Slamon DJ, Clark GM, Wong SG et al: Human breast cancer: Correlation of relapse and survival with amplification of the HER-2/neu oncogene. Science 235:177, 1987
113. Kolata G: Oncogenes give breast cancer prognosis. Science 235:160, 1987
114. van de Vijver M, van de Bersselaar R, Devilee P et al: Amplification of the neu (c-erbB-2) oncogene in human mammary tumors is relatively frequent and is often accompanied by amplification of the linked c-erbA oncogene. Mol Cell Biol 7:2019, 1987
115. Yokota J, Tsunetsugu-Yokota Y, Battifora H et al: Alterations of myc, myb, and ras^{ha} proto-oncogenes in cancers are frequent and show clinical correlation. Science 231:261, 1986
116. Agnantis NJ, Parissi P, Anagnostakis D et al: Comparative study of Harvey-ras oncogene expression with conventional clinicopathologic parameters of breast cancer. Oncology 43:36, 1986
117. Horan Hand P, Vilasi V, Thor A et al: Quantitation of Harvey ras p21 enhanced expression in human breast and colon carcinomas. JNCI 79:59, 1987
118. Clair T, Miller WR, Cho-Chung YS: Prognostic significance of the expression of a ras protein with a molecular weight of 21,000 by human breast cancer. Cancer Res 47:5290, 1987
119. Lundy J, Grimson R, Mishriki Y et al: Elevated ras oncogene expression correlates with lymph node metastases in breast cancer patients. J Clin Oncol 4:1321, 1986
120. Seeger RC, Brodeur GM, Sather H et al: Association of multiple copies of the N-myc oncogene with rapid progression of neuroblastomas. N Engl J Med 313:1111, 1985
121. Brodeur GM, Seeger RC, Schwab M et al: Amplification of N-myc in untreated human neuroblastomas correlates with advanced disease stage. Science 224:1121, 1984
122. Nau MM, Brooks BJ, Carney DN et al: Human small-cell lung cancers show amplification and expression of the N-myc gene. Proc Natl Acad Sci USA 83:1092, 1986
123. Tsuboi K, Hirayoshi K, Takeuchi K et al: Expression of the c-myc gene in human gastrointestinal malignancies. Biochem Biophys Res Commun 146:699, 1987

HENRY C. PITOT

CHAPTER 8 *Principles of Carcinogenesis: Chemical*

The first source of our knowledge of chemical carcinogenesis was clinical observations in humans. In 1775, Percival Pott, an eminent English physician and surgeon, described the occurrence of cancer of the scrotum in a number of his male patients.[1] The common history of these patients was employment as chimney sweeps when they were young. On the basis of this observation, Dr. Pott, with remarkable insight, concluded that the childhood occupation of these men was directly and causally related to their malignant disease, and that the soot was the causative agent. Strangely enough, Pott did not suggest avoiding the soot as a means of prevention, although his report in 1775 apparently inspired the Danish Chimney Sweepers' Guild to rule 3 years later that its members should bathe daily. It was not until more than a century later that Butlin[2] reported the relative rarity of scrotal cancer in chimney sweeps on the European continent compared with those in England. It appeared that the lower incidence of the disease was the result of frequent bathing and protective clothing.

The lesson from Pott's report took a long time to be learned. One hundred years after its publication, the high incidence of skin cancer among certain German workers finally was traced to their exposure to coal tar, the chief constituent of the chimney sweeps' soot. However, it took another 40 years before the disease was reproduced experimentally, and even today, more than two centuries after Pott's original scientific report on the association of soot and smoke products with the later development of cancer, many of us still disregard the obvious hazards of the carcinogenic products resulting from the combustion of tobacco in cigarettes and of many of the organic fuels of our industrialized world.

Polycyclic hydrocarbons, soots, and tars, however, were not the only chemicals in the human environment exhibiting a causal relationship with specific human cancers. The chemical dye industry developed and flourished during the last half of the 19th century in Europe. Before World War I, Germany provided more than 80% of the world's supply of aniline, its derivatives, and related aromatic amines, the bases for the synthesis of most dyes used at that time. In 1895 Rehn described the occurrence of bladder cancer in several workers in the aniline dye industry.[3] Other epidemiologic studies incriminated several related aromatic amines, especially naphthylamines and benzidine, as carcinogenic for humans. Although the exact chemical dye responsible for the bladder cancers in workers was not identified in Rehn's report, the distinctly different chemical nature of the crude soots and tars implicated by Pott and Butlin compared with the relatively pure, synthetic aromatic amines used in the dye industry suggested that chemicals of diverse structure were capable of causing cancer in the human. Unfortunately, it took almost another 50 years before experimental proof of the exact nature of the carcinogenic aniline dyes was obtained.[4]

The term *carcinogen* generally has been used by oncologists to indicate an agent that causes cancer. Today such a simplistic definition is not sufficient. We have proposed the following definition to include most instances of agents that are carcinogens.

> A *carcinogen* is an agent whose administration to previously untreated animals leads to a statistically significant increased incidence of neoplasms of one or more histogenetic types as compared with the incidences in appropriate untreated animals, whether the control animals have low or high spontaneous incidences of the neoplasms in question.

This definition includes the induction of neoplasms that are not usually observed, the earlier induction of neoplasms that are usually observed, and the induction of more neoplasms than are usually found. Although it would be important to distinguish between agents that induce neoplasms by direct action on the cells that become neoplastic and those that produce neoplasia by indirect actions in the animal as a whole, at present it is seldom possible to do so. Some agents, such as immune suppressants, can increase the incidence of neoplasms in tissues previously exposed to carcinogens by indirect effects on the host. Agents acting through such effects should not be termed carcinogens.

CHEMICAL CARCINOGENESIS

One hundred forty years after Pott's report of the association of soot from the combustion of coal with skin cancer of the scrotum, an experimental basis for Pott's clinical observation was reported. In 1915, the Japanese pathologists Yamagiwa and Ichikawa reported the first production of skin tumors in animals by the application of coal tar to the skin.[5] These investigators repeatedly applied crude coal tar to the ears of rabbits for a number of months, finally producing both benign and, later, malignant epidermal neoplasms. Later studies demonstrated that the skin of mice was also susceptible to the carcinogenic action of such organic tars. During the next 15 years, extensive attempts were made to determine the nature of the material in the crude tars that caused malignancy. In 1925, Kennaway reported the production of carcinogenic tars by pyrolysis of simple organic compounds comprising only carbon and hydrogen.[6] In the early 1930s, several such polycyclic hydrocarbons were isolated from active crude tar fractions. In 1930, the first synthetic carcinogenic compound was made.[7] This compound, dibenz*[a,h]*anthracene (1,2,5,6-dibenzanthracene), was tested for carcinogenic activity by being painted on the skin of mice and was found to be a potent carcinogen. The isolation from coal tar and synthesis of the carcinogen, benzo*[a]*pyrene (3,4-benzpyrene) was achieved in 1932. Polycyclic hydrocarbons vary in their carcinogenic potencies; for example, the isomer of dibenz*[a,h]*anthracene, dibenz*[a,c]*anthracene (1,2,3,4-dibenzanthracene), has very little carcinogenic activity. Structures of some polycyclic hydrocarbons are noted in Figure 8-1.

In 1935, Sasaki and Yoshida extended the field of chemical carcinogenesis by demonstrating that the feeding of the azo dye, *o*-aminoazotoluene, to rats resulted in the development of liver tumors.[8] Kinosita later demonstrated that 4-dimethylaminoazobenzene in the diet also caused neoplasms

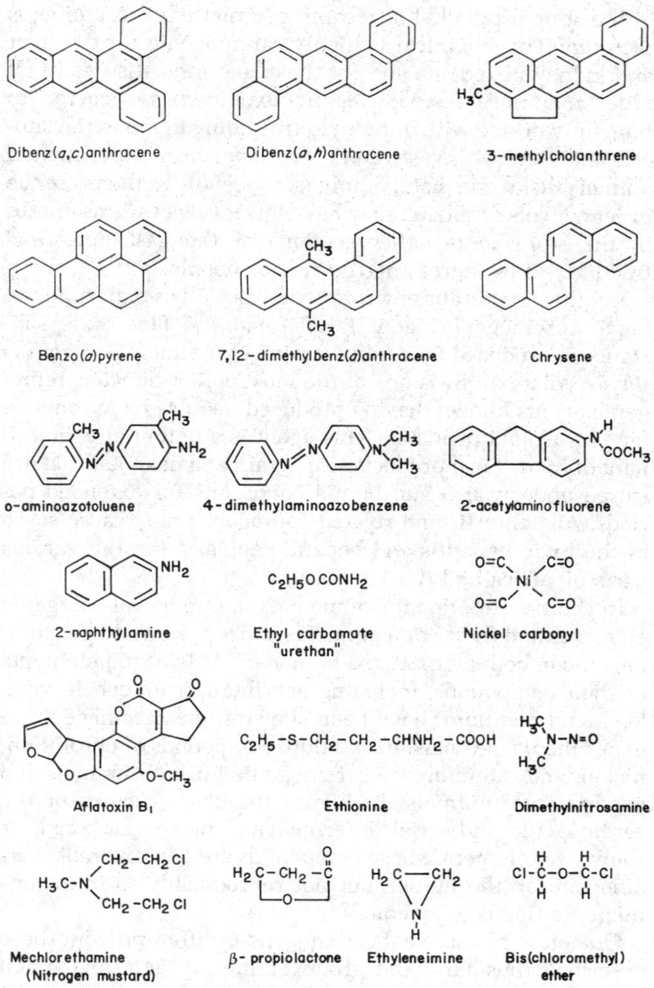

FIG. 8-1. Chemical structures of representative chemical carcinogens. (Adapted from Pitot HC: Fundamentals of Oncology, 3rd ed. New York, Marcel Dekker, 1986)

in the liver.[9] A number of analogues of this compound were also prepared. An interesting correlation arising from these later studies was that the amino group of carcinogenic dyes usually had at least one methyl substituent, although *o*-aminoazotoluene does not. Unlike the polycyclic hydrocarbons, the azo dyes generally did not act at the site of first contact of the compound with the organism, but rather in a remote area, namely, the liver. Painting of the skin with most azo dyes resulted in few or no tumors, and the ingestion of polycyclic hydrocarbons generally resulted in no hepatomas except in neonates.

2-Acetylaminofluorene, first synthesized as an insecticide but fortunately never used for that purpose, is a model laboratory chemical carcinogen. The best known representative of aromatic amines, carcinogenic for the urinary bladder in humans, is 2-napthylamine, although benzidine and related dyes are equally carcinogenic (see below). The nitrosamines are a class of compounds many members of which are effective chemical carcinogens and of potential importance in the genesis of neoplasia in humans. In Figure 8-1 the structure of the simplest dialkyl nitrosamine, dimethylnitrosamine, is pictured. This chemical is highly carcinogenic for the liver and kidney in rodents and for these and other tissues in all other mammals tested. Hepatic toxicity has occurred in humans working with dimethylnitrosamine in industrial situations.[10] Several investigators have shown in experimental animals that some dietary amines, especially in the presence of high levels of nitrite, may have low levels of nitrosamines in the stomach or other sections of the gastrointestinal tract,[11-13] thus increasing the risk of neoplasia.[14]

Another important environmental as well as experimental hepatocarcinogenic agent is aflatoxin B_1. This toxic substance is produced by certain strains of the mold *Aspergillus flavus.* Aflatoxin B_1 is one of the most potent hepatocarcinogenic agents known, having produced neoplasms in rodents, fish, birds, and primates. This agent is a potential contaminant of many farm products (*e.g.*, grain and peanuts) that are stored under warm and humid conditions for extended periods. Aflatoxin B_1 and related compounds may cause some of the toxic hepatitis and hepatic neoplasia seen in various parts of Africa and the Far East.[15]

In addition to organic compounds, a number of inorganic elements and their compounds have been shown to be carcinogenic in both animals and humans.[16] At least ten elements or their compounds, including beryllium, iron, cobalt, zinc, lead, and platinum, have been shown to be carcinogenic in experimental animals. In addition, compounds of chromium, nickel, and cadmium are carcinogenic for both humans and experimental animals. In Figure 8-1 the structure of the carcinogenic industrial intermediate, nickel carbonyl, is shown. An element whose compounds are demonstrably carcinogenic in the human but not reproducibly so in experimental animals is arsenic.[17]

One class of chemical carcinogens is different from those described thus far—the group of inert plastic and metal films that cause sarcomas at the implantation site, usually subcutaneous, in some rodents.[18] Rats and mice are highly susceptible to this form of carcinogenesis, but guinea pigs appear to be resistant.[19] The carcinogenic properties of the implant are largely dependent on its physical characteristics and surface area. Multiple perforations, pulverization, or roughening of the surface of the implant markedly reduce the incidence of neoplasms.[20]

The chemical nature of the implant is not the critical factor in its ability to transform normal cells to neoplastic cells. Studies by Brand and associates[18] have shown that DNA synthesis occurs in the film-attached cell population throughout the preneoplastic phase and that preneoplastic cells may be identified well before neoplasms develop.[21] These studies may have significance in human neoplasia in view of the recent report that orthopaedic implant materials may induce the same phenomenon in rats.[22]

METABOLISM OF CHEMICAL CARCINOGENS IN RELATION TO CARCINOGENESIS

Although the discovery that polycyclic hydrocarbons and other compounds could induce cancer gave hope that the complete understanding of the nature of neoplasia might follow, we still appear to be far from such an understanding. The principal excretory metabolites of polycyclic hydrocarbons were hydroxylated derivatives, which usually had little or no carcinogenic activity. Similarly, hydroxylation in vivo of the rings of the aromatic amine carcinogens, such as 2-acetylaminofluorene (AAF) and 4-dimethylaminoazobenzene (DAB), usually resulted in a complete loss of activity and facilitated the further metabolism and excretion of the parent compounds.

As is evident from Figure 8-1, the different classes of chemical carcinogens do not have common structural features. The complexity of the various chemicals that can induce cancer posed a striking dilemma in attempts to understand the mechanisms of action of these agents. The beginning of our present-day understanding of the solution to this dilemma was reported in 1947 by the Millers, who first demonstrated that, during the process of hepatocarcinogenesis, carcinogenic azo dyes became covalently bound to proteins of the liver but not to proteins of the resulting neoplasms.[23] The initial studies of the Millers led them to propose that the binding of carcinogens to proteins might lead to the loss or deletion of critical proteins for growth control. At the time this hypothesis was proposed, in 1947, the molecular concept of the gene was in its infancy.

As an extension of this work, Elizabeth Miller[24] demonstrated the covalent binding of benzo*[a]*pyrene or its metabolite(s) to proteins in the skin of mice treated with the hydrocarbon. This finding strongly suggested that an important step in the induction of cancer by chemicals was the covalent interaction of some form of the chemical with proteins and other macromolecules. Because the parent compound in all cases studied could not bind directly with macromolecules, it was concluded that the interaction of chemicals with macromolecules was the result of the metabolic action of the cell. In 1960 the Millers and Cramer[25] reported that 2-acetylaminofluorene was metabolized not only by ring hydroxylation, but also by hydroxylation of the nitrogen of the acetylamino group. They isolated *N*-hydroxy-2-acetylaminofluorene (Fig. 8-2) and, in subsequent investigations, found this compound to be more carcinogenic that the parent compound, 2-acetylaminofluorene. *N*-hydroxy-2-acetylaminofluorene also induced neoplasms not found following administration of the parent compound, such as subcutaneous sarcomas at the site of injection. Further, in animals (such as the guinea pig) that convert little of the 2-acetylaminofluorene to its *N*-hydroxy derivative in vivo, cancer of the liver was not produced by feeding the parent compound. These studies strongly supported the suggestion that, at least for 2-acetylaminofluorene, the parent compound was not the direct carcinogen, but rather that certain metabolic derivative(s) were the active components in the induction of neoplasia. These studies led to the finding of the activation of carcinogens by means of their metabolism by cellular enzymes.[26]

The Millers continued their investigations of the metabolism of *N*-hydroxy-2-acetylaminofluorene and demonstrated that the *N*-hydroxy group could be esterified to yield a highly reactive compound that can react nonenzymatically with nucleophilic sites on proteins and nucleic acids and with specific amino acids and nucleosides. These results led to a

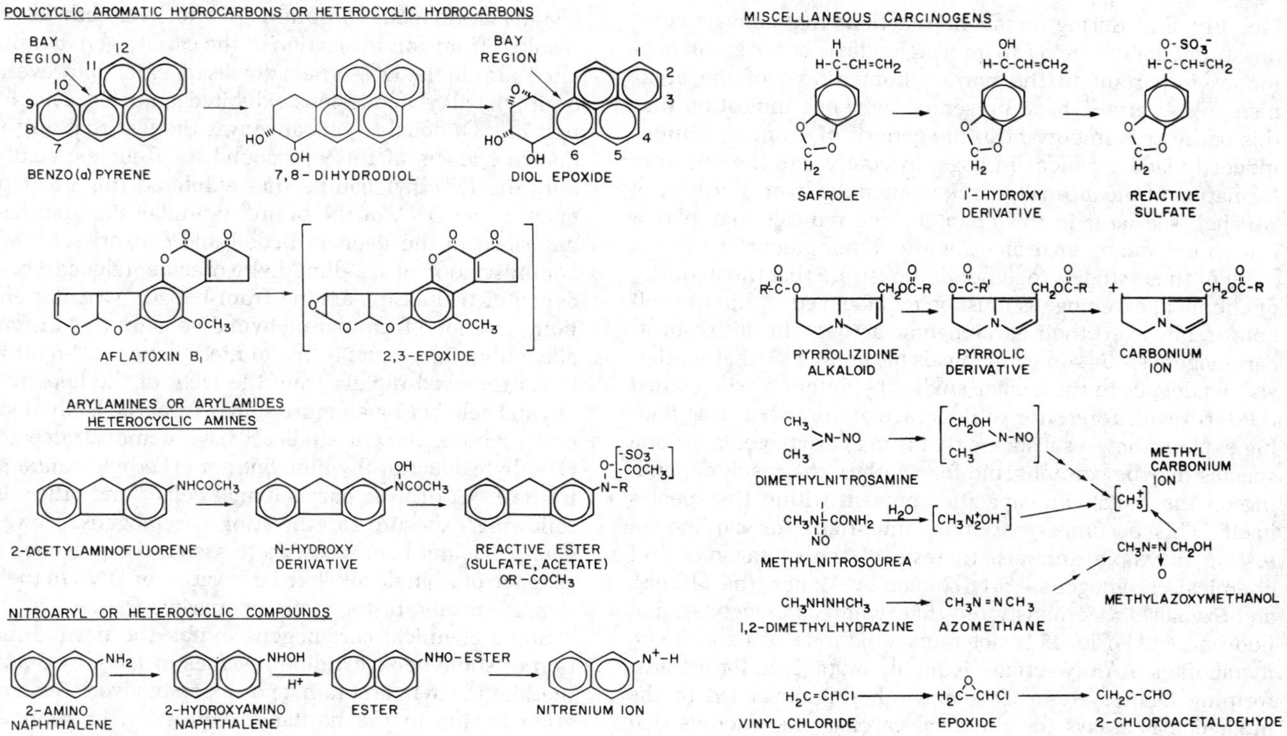

FIG. 8-2. Structures of representative procarcinogens, proximate and ultimate forms of chemical carcinogens. (Adapted from Pitot HC: Fundamentals of Oncology, 3rd ed. New York, Marcel Dekker, 1986)

solution of the dilemma of the variety of structurally unrelated chemical carcinogens. They proposed that chemical carcinogens are, or are converted by metabolism into, electrophilic reactants (chemicals with electron-deficient sites) that exert their biologic effects by covalent interaction with cellular macromolecules. The critical target most probably is DNA.[27]

After the demonstration by the Millers of the critical significance of electrophilic metabolites in chemical carcinogenesis, a number of "proximate" and "ultimate" forms, especially those of aromatic amines, were described (see Fig. 8-2). The ultimate form of the carcinogen, that is, the form that actually interacts with cellular constituents to cause the neoplastic transformation, is the final product shown in most of the pathways in Figure 8-2. However, the carcinogenic polycyclic hydrocarbons still posed a problem. As early as 1950, Boyland[28] had proposed the formation of epoxide intermediates in the metabolism of these chemicals. Later investigations showed that epoxides of polycyclic hydrocarbons could react with nucleic acids and proteins in the absence of any metabolizing system. In 1974, Sims and associates[29] proposed that a diol epoxide of benzo*[a]*pyrene was the ultimate form of this carcinogen. Subsequent studies by a number of investigators[30,31] have demonstrated that the structure of this ultimate form is (+)-*anti*-benzo*[a]*pyrene-7,8-dihydro-9,10-epoxide (see Fig. 8-2).

One of the interesting ramifications of these findings is the importance of oxidation of the carbons of the "bay region" of potentially carcinogenic polycyclic hydrocarbons. Figure 8-2 shows the bay region of benzo*[a]*pyrene. Levin and associates[32] as well as others[31] have proposed that epoxidation of a dihydro, angular benzo ring that forms part of a bay region of a polycyclic hydrocarbon is the most likely ultimate carcinogenic form of the hydrocarbon. The bay region is the sterically hindered region formed by the angular benzo ring. Although the bay region concept has not been tested with all known carcinogenic polycyclic hydrocarbons, it appears to be generally applicable thus far.

In addition to the electrophilic intermediates comprising the structures of the ultimate forms of chemical carcinogens, recent evidence also indicates that free radical derivatives of chemical carcinogens may be produced both metabolically and nonenzymatically during their metabolism.[33] Free radicals carry no charge but do possess a single unpaired electron, making the radical extremely reactive. That such forms may be important in the induction of neoplastic transformation by chemicals comes from two lines of evidence. Various molecules that inhibit the formation of free radicals, many of which are termed antioxidants, can inhibit the carcinogenic action of many chemical carcinogens.[34] Although there is no doubt that free radical intermediates are sometimes formed during the metabolism of chemical carcinogens, only recently have relatively specific metabolic reactions of certain chemical carcinogens, particularly polycyclic hydrocarbons, been shown to proceed through free radical intermediates. Marnett[35] has described the co-oxygenation of polyunsaturated fatty acids with polycyclic aromatic hydrocarbons, leading to the formation of the ultimate diol epoxide form (see Fig. 8-2) during metabolic reactions that convert polyunsaturated fatty acids to prostaglandins, a series of hormones important in the normal homeostasis of the organism. Wise et al[36] have presented evidence indicating that this pathway is important in the genesis of aromatic amine-induced bladder cancer in dogs, in contrast to the enzymic formation of the ultimate carcinogen in the liver. Further, as we shall see later in this chapter, free radicals may play a role in enhancing or promoting the development of cancer.

All of these studies together demonstrate that the majority of chemical carcinogens must be metabolized within the cell before they exert their carcinogenic activity. In this respect, carcinogenesis by some chemicals becomes a "lethal synthesis" analogous to the earlier studies by Peters,[37] who coined the term with reference to fluoroacetate. Further, this finding explains how a substance that is not carcinogenic for one species may be carcinogenic for another, the result depending on the metabolic capacities present within the species itself. This becomes extremely important for carcinogen testing in whole animals. In tests of the mutagenicity of chemical carcinogens, early studies by Maher, the Millers, and Szybalski[38] demonstrated that, whereas 2-acetylaminofluorene (AAF) itself is not mutagenic, one of its ultimate metabolites, AAF-*N*-sulfate, is highly mutagenic for a transforming DNA system. This and other findings led to the mutagenesis assays for chemical carcinogens, such as that developed by Ames and colleagues,[39] which involves the in vitro metabolism of suspected carcinogens by liver microsomal preparations in the presence of a highly mutable strain of bacteria (see below).

Not all chemical carcinogens require intracellular metabolism to become ultimate carcinogens. Examples are the direct alkylating agents β-propiolactone, nitrogen mustard, ethyleneimine, and bis(chloromethyl)ether (see Fig. 8-1), the latter having been shown to be carcinogenic for humans (see below).

One important aspect of chemical carcinogenesis is the nature of the critical molecular interactions between ultimate carcinogens and those components of the cell whose reactions with the carcinogen lead to the neoplastic change. Metabolic studies with labeled carcinogens have investigated the loss of radioactivity from protein, RNA, and DNA and have shown in several instances that adducts are lost almost entirely from the former two components but are retained to a greater or lesser extent in the DNA of cells.[40] These findings have led to the postulation that an interaction critical for the neoplastic transformation occurs between the ultimate form of the carcinogen and DNA. However, not all of the molecular interactions between the ultimate form of a chemical carcinogen and DNA share in the causation of the neoplastic transformation. Goth and Rajewsky[41] emphasized the importance of such an understanding by demonstrating that the presence of *persistent* DNA–carcinogen adducts appeared to be related directly to the susceptibility of a tissue to cancer development. These investigators administered the carcinogen, ethylnitrosourea, to newborn rats and compared the quantitative and qualitative aspects of the ethylation of DNA in a tissue showing no carcinogenic effects of this ethylating agent, the liver, with one in which cancer subsequently developed, the brain. In the liver, ethylated DNA resulted from administration of the carcinogen, but the alkylated sites in the DNA gradually disappeared; however, in the brain, the alkylated lesions exhibited a much greater biologic half-life. Of equal significance was the fact that, of the then known adducts of this compound with nucleic acid, it was only the O^6-ethylguanine that exhibited this great persistence in the DNA of the brain. A similar situation has been described in the liver by Bedell and co-workers,[42] wherein administration of 1,2-dimethylhydrazine induced a high incidence of neoplasms arising from hepatic vascular endothelium, but none from parenchymal cells. In this instance the alkylation that occurs is that of methylation. O^6-methylguanine is removed rapidly from the DNA of the hepatic parenchymal cell, but much more slowly from the DNA of vascular endothelium. Recent studies[43] have demonstrated that the O^4-ethyl adduct of thymine but not O^6-ethylguanine persists in the DNA of liver parenchymal cells[44] and other tissues[45] following exposure to ethylating carcinogens. However, to date it has not been possible to assign the presence or persistence of a single alkylated derivative of DNA to the formation of specific histogenetic neoplasms.[45]

Some chemical carcinogens inhibit the normal methylation of some deoxycytidine residues in DNA by *S*-adenosylmethionine in liver, brain, and spleen in vivo.[46] Such methylation results in the heritable expression or repression of specific genes in eukaryotic cells. The inhibition of this process appears to occur by several mechanisms, including formation of covalent adducts (see above), single-strand breaks in the DNA, and the direct inactivation of the enzyme, DNA-*S*-adenosylmethionine methyltransferase, which is responsible for normal methylation.[46] Thus the inhibition of DNA methylation by chemical carcinogens is another potential pathway by which these agents may induce the neoplastic transformation.

A potential application of our knowledge of the presence and persistence of covalent adducts of carcinogenic chemicals in macromolecules is the determination of the amounts of such adducts in human tissues.[47] Immunoassays including the enzyme-linked immunosorbent assay (ELISA)[48] and the radioimmunoassay (RIA)[49] allow the determination of individual specific chemical adducts of DNA with a very high degree of sensitivity and specificity. In addition, a technique of ^{32}P-postlabeling analysis of DNA[50] allows an even greater degree of sensitivity (detection of a single adduct in 10^7–10^8 nucleotides) but without the same specificity as the immunoassays. (For details of the immunoassay method, the reader is referred to Volume 92 of the series *Methods in Enzymology*.[51]) These techniques are indispensable to the new field of "molecular epidemiology."[52] Recent studies have indicated that such techniques can be utilized to detect polycyclic hydrocarbon adducts in DNA of smokers and individuals exposed to high levels of smoke and soot in their work.[52,53] In addition, a marked increase in the form of the aromatic amine carcinogen, 4-aminobiphenyl, covalently bound to hemoglobin in the serum has been reported by use of techniques of gas chromatography and mass spectrometry.[54] Because of DNA excision repair (see below) the levels of DNA adducts found in humans probably represent steady-state levels rather than peak levels, which may be seen shortly after a single exposure. However, these techniques can be used to monitor the risk of individuals exposed to potential environmental carcinogens, allowing the institution of preventive measures to reduce such risk.

The methods by which alkylated lesions in DNA are removed include a number of processes collectively termed DNA repair. Although it is beyond the scope of this chapter to consider the various pathways of DNA repair,[55,56] many features of the processes of DNA repair are important for the process of carcinogenesis. Substantial experimental evidence has demonstrated the existence of chemical damage to DNA after the administration of chemical carcinogens, even at very low doses.[57] Further, there is some evidence that such damage appears to persist, at least in some experimental systems such as murine hepatocarcinogenesis.[58] Although there is some evidence that carcinogenic chemicals and radiation activate some form of "error-prone" mechanism of DNA repair or replication,[59] other evidence suggests that the persistence of unrepaired DNA damage, including DNA-chemical adducts (see above), may be the cause of mutation, resulting in initiation of the affected cell.[60,61] For example, the *N*-(guan-8-yl)-2-acetylaminofluorene adducts formed in DNA from 2-acetylaminofluorene are repaired rather rapidly with a half-life of 7 days. However, the 3-(guan-N^2-yl)-acetylaminofluorene and *N*-(guan-8-yl)-2-aminofluorene adducts in DNA are not repaired and thus remain in the cellular genome.[62] The administration of some carcinogens such as dimethylnitrosamine actually stimulates the repair of O^6 alkylation guanines in DNA by such carcinogens given chronically.[63] Perhaps the strongest evidence that faulty DNA repair may lead to carcinogenesis is seen in the high incidence of skin cancer in patients with the autosomal recessive disease, xeroderma pigmentosum.[64] Persons with this condition have a markedly lowered ability to repair damage to DNA caused by ultraviolet light and by certain carcinogenic chemicals. The mechanism for the increased incidence of skin cancer seen in these patients is not known, but several theories have been proposed, including the mismatching of bases in DNA during the process of replicating an unrepaired, damaged DNA template. Sirover and Lobe[65] have suggested that inorganic metallic carcinogens may be carcinogenic by increasing the infidelity of DNA synthesis. With both of these mechanisms, an increase in mutation frequency as well as carcinogenesis would be expected.

Knowledge of both the metabolism of chemical carcinogens and the effects of the reactions of products formed by these metabolic pathways has led to a better understanding not only of the process of chemical carcinogenesis, but also of the relation of the neoplastic transformation by chemicals to the mutagenicity of the same agents. We now know that the vast majority of chemical carcinogens either are themselves mutagens or may be converted in the cell to active mutagens. This fact, coupled with the potential importance of faulty DNA repair associated with an increased incidence of neoplasia in certain genetic conditions, strongly supports the suggestion that chemical carcinogens may exert their effects as both mutagens and carcinogens by direct interaction of their ultimate forms with cellular DNA.

NATURAL HISTORY OF CHEMICAL CARCINOGENESIS: STAGES OF INITIATION, PROMOTION, AND PROGRESSION

One of the ubiquitous characteristics of the natural history of the development of a neoplasm in vivo is the extended time period between the initial application of a carcinogen—be it physical, chemical, or biologic—and the appearance of a neoplasm. Since there is now substantial evidence that neoplasms result from the alteration of a single cell whose progeny develop into the neoplastic lesion which then becomes clinically evident,[66] the latent period preceding cancer development may be simply the result of the continued growth of such clones until one or more are large enough to be called cancer. Foulds proposed such a concept but suggested that changes were continually occurring in this process, which he termed the progression of neoplasia.[67] However, an alternative explanation of this latent period of the development of neoplasia became apparent from studies conducted some four decades ago[68–70] and more recently.[71,72] These studies, carried out principally with mouse epidermis in vivo, suggested that the latent period during epidermal carcinogenesis of the skin of the mouse consisted of at least two stages, now termed *initiation* and *promotion* (Fig. 8-3).

Both Foulds' concept of progression[67] and the concepts of initiation and promotion were developed from model systems in animals, mammary carcinogenesis and epidermal carcinogenesis respectively in the mouse. Today, however, it is apparent that the multistage characteristic of carcinogenesis is not unique to these experimental systems but occurs with the process of carcinogenesis in a number of tissues in

FIG. 8-3. Natural history of neoplastic development, beginning with the initiated cell resulting from administration of an initiating agent with subsequent promotion to a visible lesion, followed by progression of this tumor to metastatic cancer. Euploidy and aneuploidy refer to the karyotypes of the cells during the various stages of neoplastic development. Euploidy indicates a normal complement of chromosomes; aneuploidy denotes abnormalities in the number or structure of one or more chromosomes. (Adapted from Pitot HC: Fundamentals of Oncology, 3rd ed. New York, Marcel Dekker, 1986)

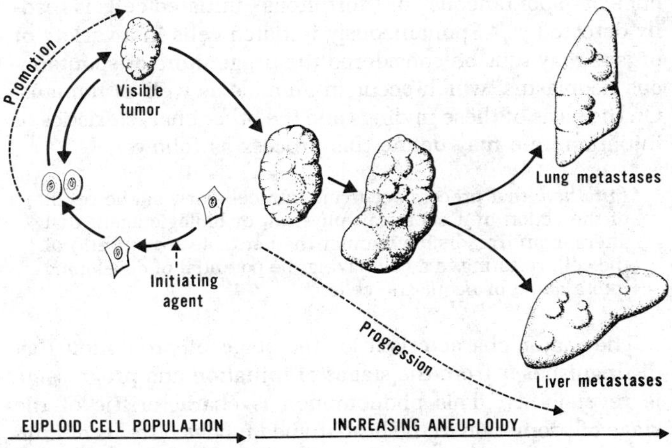

TABLE 8-1. Morphologic and Biologic Characteristics of the Stages of Initiation, Promotion, and Progression in Hepatocarcinogenesis in the Rat*

Initiation	*Promotion*	*Progression*
Irreversible with constant "stem cell" potential; initiated "stem cell" not morphologically identifiable	Reversible	Irreversible Measurable and/or morphologically discernible alteration in cell genome's structure
Efficacy sensitive to xenobiotic and other chemical factors	Promoted cell population existence dependent on continued administration of the promoting agent	
Spontaneous (fortuitous) occurrence of initiated cells can be quantified	Efficacy sensitive to dietary and hormonal factors	Growth of altered cells sensitive to environmental factors during early phase
Requires cell division for "fixation"		
Dose-response does not exhibit a readily measurable threshold	Dose-response exhibits measurable threshold and maximal effect dependent on dose of initiating agent	Benign and/or malignant neoplasms characteristically seen
Relative effect of initiators depends on quantitation of focal lesions following defined period of promotion	Relative effectiveness of promoters depends on time and dose rate to reach maximal effect and on dose rate	"Progressor" agents act to advance promoted cells into this stage but may not be initiating agents

* Adapted from Pitot HC et al: Multistage carcinogenesis: The phenomenon underlying the theories. In Iverson OH (ed): Theories of Carcinogenesis, p. 159. Washington, DC, Hemisphere Publishing, 1987.

several species, including the human.[73] On the basis of such experimental findings, predominantly in the most intensively studied multistage carcinogenesis model systems (those of the skin of the mouse[72] and the liver of the rat[74]), three stages have been characterized (Table 8-1). The irreversibility and "memory" characteristics of the process of initiation are well characterized.[71,75] Evidence of the additivity of initiation comes from numerous investigations of the linearity of the dose-response to carcinogenic agents that initiate cells.[76] As yet it has not been possible to identify unequivocally single initiated cells, but the early clonal progeny of an initiated cell may be recognized in several model multistage carcinogenesis systems, notably that of rat hepatocarcinogenesis.[77] Furthermore, in this system the presence of "spontaneous" or "fortuitous" initiated cells is readily detected.[78,79] Spontaneously initiated cells in a variety of organs may thus be considered the progenitors of spontaneous neoplasms, which occur in animals as well as humans. On the basis of these findings and the other characteristics of initiation, one may define this process as follows:

> *Initiation:* that process occurring intracellularly as the result of the action of a chemical, physical, or biologic agent that alters in an irreversible manner the heritable structure(s) of the cell, resulting in a cell having the potential of developing into a clone of neoplastic cells.

The major characteristic of the stage of promotion that distinguishes it from the stages of initiation and progression is reversibility. This phenomenon is characteristic of the stage of promotion in the best-studied model systems of multistage carcinogenesis in the rodent[80,81] and in human neoplasia as well.[82] Furthermore, at least in multistage hepatocarcinogenesis in the rat, preneoplastic cells in the stage of promotion that develop from initiated cells are actually dependent on the presence of the promoting agent for their existence in that tissue.[81] Promoting agents by definition cannot initiate but may promote cells that have been initiated by fortuitous events such as background radiation, dietary contaminants, environmental "toxins," and other factors. The existence of fortuitously initiated cells has been discussed above. Therefore, promoting agents are carcinogenic in that they may promote such spontaneously initiated cells to neoplasia. Agents capable of initiation, promotion, and progression to cancer are termed *complete carcinogens,* but even these, at sufficiently low doses, only initiate cells without subsequent promotion. Under these circumstances, such complete carcinogens may act as "pure" initiating agents or *incomplete carcinogens.* Some carcinogenic agents, such as urethan, can induce neoplasms in some internal tissues but not in the skin. However, after systemic urethan administration, subsequent treatment of the skin with croton oil results in the appearance of papillomas and carcinomas of the skin.[83] On the basis of these data, urethan was termed an incomplete carcinogen or pure initiating agent for the skin, although this compound is a complete carcinogen for the lung and the liver.

Studies in cell culture[84,85] have demonstrated that initiating agents are most effective at certain stages of the cell cycle, usually at the beginning of DNA synthesis. Further, the ability of a carcinogenic agent to initiate cells may depend on the capacity of the cell to metabolize the agent to its ultimate carcinogenic form. Several studies[86–88] have indicated the importance of one or several rounds of cell division in the presence of the initiating agent in vivo or in vitro for a cell to become initiated. Further, it is possible to inhibit the process of carcinogenesis with agents that have been termed anticarcinogens or to stimulate the process of initiation with agents that have been termed cocarcinogens. Both types of agents usually act during the production of the ultimate form of the carcinogen, although other mechanisms for such processes have also been described.[89,90] On the other hand, tumor promotion may be modulated by various environmental factors, including diet, age, hormonal balance, and sex. Therefore, on the basis of the characteristics of tumor promotion, one may define the process as follows:

> *Promotion:* that stage in the natural history of neoplastic development which, if existent, is characterized by (1) the reversible expansion of the initiated cell population and (2) the reversible alteration of genetic expression.

Boutwell[71] was among the first to propose that promoting agents exert their effects by altering the expression of genetic information within the cell. Since this stage is reversible, these effects of promoting agents during the stage are also reversible. As indicated previously, major characteristics of the process of initiation involve its dose dependency, with the absence of any readily measurable threshold or no-effect dose level and the presence of a maximal effective dose short of lethal cellular toxicity. The existence of a threshold can be predicted from the reversibility characteristic of promotion, whereas a maximal response to the promoting agent, after a single dose of an initiating agent, would be expected if the promoting agent lacked initiating activity. Furthermore, the maximal yield of promoted neoplasms or preneoplastic foci would reflect the number of cells initiated by exposure to the initiating agent.

The diversity of promoting agents can be seen in the structures depicted in Figure 8-4. Several of these compounds act as promoting agents in various tissues and show a relatively high degree of tissue specificity. For example, saccharin is an effective promoting agent in bladder carcinogenesis but not in hepatocarcinogenesis, while phenobarbital, although an effective promoting agent in the liver, was totally ineffective as a promoter for bladder carcinogenesis.[92] Not only estrogens but other hormones have been shown to serve as effective promoting agents in vivo.[93] Not shown in Figure 8-4 is the foreign body or plastic film carcinogenesis discussed previously. Experimental studies[94,95] have indicated that such foreign bodies can act as promoting agents, probably promoting initiated cells already present in normal tissue. Further, Topping and Nettesheim[96] have presented evidence that asbestos acts as a promoting agent in experimental tracheal carcinogenesis. This finding correlates well with the known epidemiologic phenomenon of the marked enhancement of bronchogenic carcinoma in humans exposed to asbestos who are smokers as compared with smokers who were not exposed to abestos (see below).

The reversibility of the stage of tumor promotion makes it an obvious target for some form of regulation of the development of neoplasia in vivo. Paramount among such approaches is that of active chemoprevention by dietary, chemical, or other related mechanisms.[97] Although not all agents

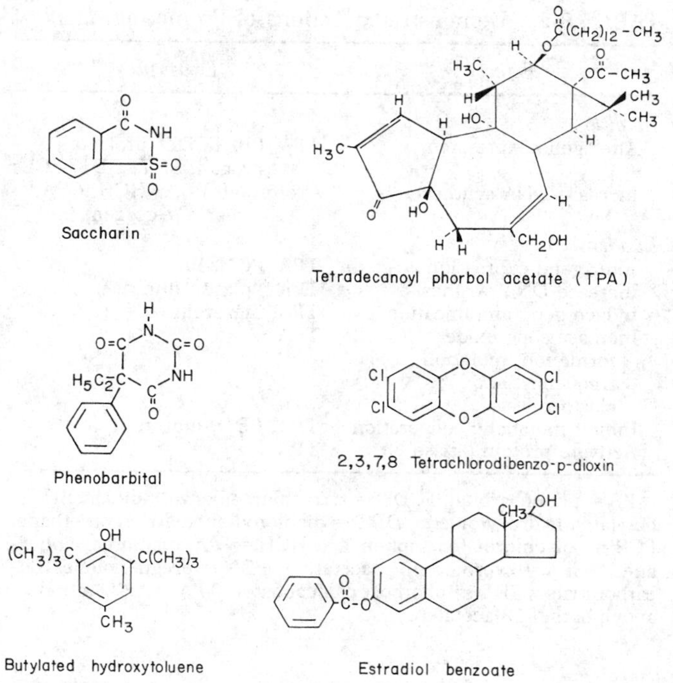

FIG. 8-4. Chemical structures of several promoting agents active in carcinogenesis in several tissues and species. (Adapted from Pitot HC: Fundamentals of Oncology, 3rd ed. New York, Marcel Dekker, 1986)

that have been utilized in such studies specifically inhibit neoplastic development at the stage of promotion, those that have been utilized for potential chemoprevention of cancer in humans, including derivatives of vitamins A, C, and E and selenium, appear to act predominantly at the stage of promotion.[98] This approach is consonant with our knowledge of the importance of promoting agents in the human environment associated with the development of cancer in people (see below).

Our knowledge of the mechanism of action of tumor promotion is still relatively unclear. Unlike the activity of initiating agents, there is little evidence of a major direct role for the metabolism of promoting agents in their mechanism of action. However, various promoting agents do exhibit a variety of actions in vivo and in vitro. Some of these are listed in Table 8-2. In addition to their effects in altering the genetic expression, many tumor-promoting agents have been shown to be mitogenic, at least to certain cell populations. Croton oil, when applied to mouse skin, causes a rapid increase in DNA synthesis in most basal skin cells.[99] Several promoters of hepatocarcinogenesis have been shown to enhance DNA synthesis in early progeny of initiated cells selectively compared with the remaining hepatocytes.[100] Many studies have shown that cell replication is required to "fix" the step of initiation of chemical carcinogenesis, but that such fixation in itself is not sufficient to assure the continuance of the process of promotion and ultimate tumor formation.[91]

Tumor promoters also alter gene expression and increase DNA synthesis in vitro. Several of the phorbol ester promot-

TABLE 8-2. Demonstrated Actions of Promoting Agents

Effect	*Examples*
In vivo	
Alter gene expression	TPA, PB, TCDD, prolactin, estrogen, BHT, DDT, PCBs
Increase DNA synthesis	Croton oil, PB, α-HCH, CPA, saccharin, estrogen
In vitro	
Alter gene expression	TPA, PCN, PB
Increase DNA synthesis	TPA, "plastic film" (?)
Induce gene amplification	TPA, mezerein
Increase superoxide formation, mutation frequency, and clastogenesis	TPA
Inhibit metabolic cooperation	TPA, PDD, mezerein
Activate protein kinase C	TPA

PB = phenobarbital, TCDD = tetrachlorodibenzo-*p*-dioxin, BHT = butylated hydroxytoluene, DDT = dichlorodiphenyltrichloroethane, PCB = polychlorinated biphenyl, α-HCH = α-hexachlorocyclohexane, CPA = cyproterone acetate, PCN = pregnenolone-16α-carbonitrile, PDD = phorbol didecanoate, TPA = 12-*O*-tetradecanoylphorbol-13-acetate.

ing agents can stimulate the amplification of specific genes within cultured cells.[101,102] Direct effects of tumor promoters on the genome of the cell have not, generally, been considered as a major mechanism of their effects in neoplastic development. However, several studies in vitro[103,104] have demonstrated an indirect effect of 12-*O*-tetradecanoylphorbol-13-acetate (TPA) in the presence of leukocytes, resulting in the formation of DNA strand breaks, chromosomal abnormalities, and structural modification of bases in DNA.[105] Such changes may be the result of action of reactive oxygen metabolites, especially superoxide radicals. Evidence of the importance of such radicals can also be found from the inhibition of tumor promotion by antioxidants, which eliminate the accumulation of oxygen metabolites.[106] Recently, however, Fischer and her associates have reported experiments suggesting that such indirect effects of TPA are not essential for tumor promotion in mouse skin.[107] Another possible mechanism of action of tumor promoters studied extensively by Trosko and his co-workers[108] is the inhibition of intercellular communication (metabolic cooperation) between cells in culture. Although such a phenomenon has not been shown to be a ubiquitous characteristic of promoting agents,[109] a relationship between reactive oxygen species and the inhibition of intercellular communication by promoting agents has been described.[110]

One of the most recent exciting findings in relation to the action of TPA is the demonstration of specific cellular membrane receptors for this tumor promoter in many cells[111] and its identity with the enzyme, protein kinase C.[112,113] This enzyme has been shown to respond to an endogenous ligand, diacylglycerol, and to have multiple effects on a variety of cellular substrates.[113] Several cDNAs for the mRNA of the protein kinase C have been isolated, providing evidence that this important receptor-enzyme consists of a multigene family compatible with its ubiquitous nature and function.[114,115] However, the relationship of this enzyme to promoting agents other than TPA, if any, remains to be elucidated in the mechanisms of promoting agents.

The stage of progression in the natural history of neoplastic development (see Fig. 8-2) has not yet been clearly defined; however, on the basis of the known action of initiating and promoting agents, irreversible benign and/or malignant neoplasms are characteristic of this stage of neoplastic development. Progression has been defined as that stage of carcinogenesis exhibiting measurable (by recombinant DNA technology or related methods) and/or morphological karyotypic changes in the structure of the cell genome.[116] Furthermore, the karyotypic changes seen in this stage are a reflection of karyotypic instability, which in turn can lead to a variety of other changes characteristically seen in malignant neoplasms, including a less differentiated morphology, increased growth rate, invasion and metastases, gene amplification, and chromosomal translocations and related abnormalities leading to alterations in gene expression. The stage of progression has been identified in both epidermal carcinogenesis in the mouse[117] and in multistage hepatocarcinogenesis in the rat.[118] Although complete carcinogens effectively advance cells through the entire natural history of neoplastic development, agents that act primarily in the final stage of carcinogenesis exist, as evidenced by the effect of benzoyl peroxide in multistage epidermal carcinogenesis in the mouse.[119] Theoretically, such agents should be capable of inducing major genetic changes as defined above for the entrance of a cell into the stage of progression. Protocols exemplified by the initiation–promotion–initiation format[120] have been described both in the mouse skin[121] and rat liver.[122] In the latter case, morphological evidence for the existence of a transition between the stages of promotion and progression is seen with the appearance of "foci within foci." The initial focus results from the clonal expansion of initiated cells, whereas the focus of cells developing within a promoted clone appears to represent further genetic alterations induced by the administration of a second initiating agent during the stage of promotion. Such foci within foci are probably the direct precursors of malignant neoplasms.[123] Furthermore, in multistage epidermal carcinogenesis in the mouse, Aldaz et al have described a systematic study of the karyotypic evolution of mouse skin papillomas to carcinomas, in concert with the stage of progression as defined above.[124]

From the characteristics (see Table 8-1) and definitions of the three stages of neoplastic development, it is obvious that two stages, initiation and progression, appear to involve changes in the structure of the genome of the cell. Initiation probably is the result of multiple point mutations and related subtle genomic alterations, whereas progression results from more major genetic abnormalities, including chromosomal translocation, karyotypic instability, deletions, and so forth. While it is entirely possible that a complete carcinogen, especially at high doses, may directly convert a normal cell to one in the stage of progression, it is likely that most examples of human carcinogenesis do exhibit the reversible stage of promotion (see below). In the concept of the natural history of the development of neoplasia as described here (see Fig. 8-2), there is a clear analogy between the two genetic alterations of initiation and progression and the two-hit theory of Knudson[125] developed from studies of neoplasms in the human that exhibit a clear Mendelian pattern of inheritance.

TARGETS OF CHEMICAL CARCINOGENS

Although the interaction and reaction of chemical carcinogens with DNA appear to be the principal mechanisms for their carcinogenic effects, the probability that such mutational events would occur at one or more specific genetic sites has long been considered. With the demonstration that specific oncogenic viruses, especially retroviruses, contain within their genome genes directly concerned with the oncogenic process, studies in both experimental and human systems have been directed toward investigating the structures and expression of cellular oncogenes (proto-oncogenes) in neoplastic cells as well as normal cells treated with chemical carcinogens.

There is now considerable evidence[126] that a number of proto-oncogenes are expressed at higher levels in many human neoplasms than in their normal tissues of origin. The mechanisms for such increased expression or "activation" have been studied and include genetic mechanisms ranging from base mutations or deletions in sequences to altered expression resulting from enhanced transcription, gene amplification, or changes in gene methylation. Therefore, the mechanism involved in proto-oncogene "activation" may be mutational, transcriptional, or both. Since it is difficult to monitor transcriptional activation during the early stages of neoplastic development, a number of studies have been directed toward determining whether mutational activation of proto-oncogenes occurs during this period. Quintanilla et al[127] have demonstrated that more than 90% of tumors, benign and malignant, exhibit specific mutations in the Harvey-*ras* proto-oncogene that are related directly to the structural changes in DNA induced by the chemical carcinogen used for initiation. This type of activation was also demonstrated in both adenomas and carcinomas of livers of mice given chemical carcinogens as well as the control animals that received no such agents. While the mutations in control animals were limited to a single codon, those seen in this gene in the livers of mice given chemical carcinogens were found in other codons as well.[128] A more extensive investigation with different chemical carcinogens by Wiseman et al[129] showed quite clearly the correlation between specific mutations at the 61st codon and the chemical agent utilized to induce the neoplasms. In a more direct test of the role of mutationally activated oncogenes in multistage epidermal carcinogenesis in the mouse, Brown et al[130] demonstrated that introduction of viral Harvey-*ras* genes into epidermal cells in vivo resulted in papillomas and carcinomas when the animals were subsequently treated with TPA, but no lesions occurred in the absence of the promoting agent. Similar correlative studies have been done in the rat mammary gland[131] and liver,[132] but only on examination of resultant carcinomas. These studies suggest that mutational activation of a specific proto-oncogene may be involved in initiation or promotion of carcinogenesis in these systems.

Because it is much more difficult to investigate the early stages of carcinogenesis in humans, most investigations on proto-oncogene activation have been carried out on lesions in the stage of progression. Transcriptional activation of the Harvey-*ras* proto-oncogene has been described in human gastric carcinoma,[133] prostatic cancer,[134] and pulmonary and pleural neoplasms,[135] the results suggesting that increased progression of the tumor was related to increased expression of the gene. In colorectal tumors this proto-oncogene was expressed at higher levels in primary than in metastatic tumors.[136] Increased expression of the *myc* proto-oncogene in human carcinomas of the uterine cervix was correlated with a higher incidence of early relapse,[137] while in an extensive study Yokota and his associates[138] demonstrated that amplification of this proto-oncogene occurred in advanced, widespread neoplasms as well as in aggressive primary tumors. Thus, studies in the human suggest an important role for proto-oncogene activation in the stage of progression, and it remains to be determined whether mutational activation of proto-oncogenes during initiation represents the major carcinogen-DNA target that initiates the entire process of chemical carcinogenesis in general.

PROMOTING AGENTS IN THE HUMAN ENVIRONMENT

On the basis of our knowledge of the epidemiology of human neoplasia and the demonstrated promoting action of various agents in the human environment, it is likely that the appearance of cancer in humans is related to the stages of tumor promotion and progression more than to the stage of initiation. Some promoting agents that are a significant part

TABLE 8-3. Promoting Agents in the Human Environment and Neoplasms Associated with Prolonged Contact with Those Agents*

Agent	*Resultant Neoplasm*
Dietary fat	Mammary adenocarcinoma
High caloric intake	Increased cancer incidence in general
Cigarette smoke	Bronchogenic carcinoma (esophageal and bladder cancer)
Asbestos	Bronchogenic carcinoma and mesothelioma
Halogenated hydrocarbons (TCDD, PCBs)	Liver cancer†
Phorbol esters	Esophageal cancer
Saccharin	Bladder cancer
Phenobarbital	Liver cancer†
Prolactin	Mammary adenocarcinoma†
Synthetic estrogens	Liver adenomas
Alcoholic beverages	Oral cancer, liver, and esophageal cancer

* Adapted from Pitot HC: The natural history of neoplastic development: The relation of experimental models to human cancer. Cancer 49:1206, 1982.

† Promotion demonstrated in experimental animals but not in humans as yet.

of the human environment[139] are listed in Table 8-3. Although not all of these agents have been shown by epidemiologic studies to be important factors in human cancer, a number clearly are, and others well may be. Doll and Peto[140] reviewed the importance of caloric intake and dietary fat in the genesis of human cancer. In addition, experimental evidence has clearly indicated that dietary fats, especially unsaturated fatty acids, may act as promoting agents in experimental mammary carcinogenesis and possibly in several other histogenetic types of neoplasms.[141] Cigarette smoke is a complete carcinogen but contains many promoting agents, and epidemiologic evidence argues strongly that tumor promotion is an important, if not the major, factor in the final development of pulmonary cancer in humans as a result of smoking.[142] Asbestos fibers have been shown to be promoting agents in experimental systems,[96] and their effects in humans may be explained on the basis of their action as a promoter for both bronchogenic carcinoma and mesothelioma.[143] Although there are numerous controversies over the relation of artificial sweeteners to human bladder cancer and of dioxins in insecticides to human neoplasia, there is ample experimental evidence that both of these agents are potent promoters for bladder and liver cancers in experimental systems.[139] As Berenblum[93] has suggested, all endogenous hormones may be considered to be promoting agents, and the action of synthetic estrogens in inducing liver cell adenomas in humans as well as in rodents argues strongly for a major promoting role of these compounds.[144] Finally, substantial epidemiologic evidence indicates that alcoholic beverages promote esophageal, gastric, and hepatic cancer in humans, although relatively little evidence has been uncovered to demonstrate their promoting action in animals.[145]

CHEMICAL CARCINOGENESIS IN HUMANS

Knowledge of carcinogenesis in humans as a result of the action of specific chemicals has come largely from epidemiologic and statistical investigations on both large and small groups of humans. However, epidemiologic studies can only identify factors that are different between two populations and that are sufficiently important in the etiology of the condition under study to play a determining role under the conditions of exposure. Further, on the basis of epidemiologic studies alone, it is extremely difficult to determine whether a specific chemical is carcinogenic for the human. The reasons for this include the extended lag period between exposure and clinical occurrence of the neoplasm, the high background incidence in the general population, and the relatively imprecise knowledge of the nature of the exposure in most instances. Only under exceptional circumstances is it possible to identify carcinogenic agents solely from epidemiologic studies when the incidence of a cancer induced by an agent is less than 50% greater than the occurrence of that kind of cancer in the total human population. Thus, many negative epidemiologic studies must be considered as inconclusive for indicating the risk factor of relatively weak carcinogens for inducing neoplastic disease in humans.

Because epidemiologic studies in themselves are often insufficient to establish the carcinogenicity of an agent for humans, other techniques involving studies in lower forms of life have been used to complement or, in some cases, supplant existing epidemiologic observations. Later in this chapter we shall consider such methodologies, but at this point our discussion will be restricted to a consideration of epidemiologic data in the determination of the carcinogenicity of agents for humans. One of the pioneer agencies in the establishment of the carcinogenic risk of chemicals for humans has been the International Agency for Research on Cancer (IARC). In a supplement to their monograph series,[146] the IARC has categorized the degrees of evidence of carcinogenicity from studies in humans. Their categorization is as follows:

1. *Sufficient evidence* of carcinogenicity indicates that there is a causal relation between the agent and human cancer.
2. *Limited evidence* of carcinogenicity indicates that a causal interpretation is credible but that alternative explanations, such as chance, bias, or confounding of the data, could not be excluded completely.
3. *Inadequate evidence* indicates that one of three conditions prevailed: (a) there were few pertinent data; (b) the available studies, although showing evidence of association, did not exclude chance, bias, or confounding of the findings; (c) studies were available that did not show evidence of carcinogenicity.

It is evident that epidemiologic studies have many limitations in determining etiologic factors in human cancer. On the other hand, one can never prove that an agent is truly carcinogenic for humans unless epidemiologic evidence in support of such a thesis is forthcoming.

CARCINOGENIC CHEMICAL AGENTS ASSOCIATED WITH LIFE-STYLE

Table 8-4 lists a number of agents, conditions, or processes in our life-styles that are causally related to the development of specific neoplasms in humans on the basis of epidemiologic studies. The carcinogenicity of alcoholic beverages for humans is related almost entirely to their action in association with another known carcinogenic agent. The combination of excessive alcohol ingestion and cigarette smoking markedly increases the risk in men and women of oral and laryngeal cancer, compared with the effect of either of these agents alone or in their absence.[147,148] Cancer of the liver is associated with excessive alcohol consumption,[149] and recent data by Ohnishi and co-workers[150] suggest that habitual alcoholic intake can promote the development of hepatocellular carcinoma in patients infected with the hepatitis B virus, a known oncogenic virus for the human liver. Several recent studies have also indicated an important association between alcohol consumption, even at moderate levels, and a significantly increased risk of breast cancer in women.[151–153] Although some alcoholic beverages contain known chemical carcinogens, including nitrosamines,[154] and different alcoholic beverages may have slightly different influences on the incidence of certain types of human cancer,[155] most evidence suggests that the principal effect is caused by alcohol

TABLE 8-4. Chemical Agents Associated with Life-Style and Posing a Carcinogenic Risk to Humans on the Basis of Epidemiologic Studies

Chemical, Physiologic Condition, or Process	*Associated Neoplasm*	*Evidence for Carcinogenicity**
Alcoholic beverages	Esophagus, liver, oropharynx, larynx	Sufficient
Aflatoxins	Liver	Limited
Betel chewing	Mouth	Sufficient
Dietary factors (fat, protein, calories)	Breast, colon, endometrium, gallbladder	Sufficient
Reproductive history:		
Late age at first pregnancy	Breast	Sufficient
Zero or low parity	Ovary	Sufficient
Sexual promiscuity	Cervix uteri	Sufficient
Tobacco smoking	Mouth, pharynx, larynx, lung, esophagus, bladder	Sufficient

* This terminology refers to the IARC categorization and is based on the findings reviewed in the IARC monographs[146] and the review by Doll and Peto.[140]

itself and is largely independent of the form in which it is drunk.[140]

Epidemiologic studies have shown that the geographic regions in which there is extensive contamination of foodstuffs by aflatoxin (see Fig. 8-1 and 8-2) are also the areas where the incidence of human liver cancer is relatively high.[15] Several studies have shown a direct association between the aflatoxin content of food and the frequency of hepatomas in the population. In parts of Africa and East Asia where aflatoxin is found in the diet, levels of 100 to 1000 parts per billion in individual foodstuffs are not unusual. Thus, unlike most other environmental carcinogenic agents for humans, the dose of aflatoxin to which those humans are exposed greatly exceeds that known to produce cancer in experimental animals. Although other mold toxins, such as sterigmatocystin, have been suggested as additional etiologic factors in human liver cancer, their role in this disease has not been proved.

Another example of the induction of cancer in humans by naturally occurring dietary contaminants is that described in several provinces of the People's Republic of China. In these locales, there is a positive correlation between the extremely high incidence of esophageal carcinoma and the consumption of pickled and otherwise moldy foodstuffs,[156] which may contain nitrosamines.[157]

A general association of diet and human cancer incidence has been demonstrated. Doll and Peto[140] have outlined a number of the hypothetical or demonstrable ways in which diet may alter the incidence of human cancer, including carcinogen ingestion (*e.g.*, aflatoxin B_1 and alcoholic beverages). Although food additives, pesticide contaminants, and dietary nitrites are potentially important because of their effects on human carcinogenesis, there is no evidence for a significant role of these factors in human cancer. A major factor in the relation of diet to the incidence of human cancer is caloric intake. There is substantial epidemiologic evidence that the incidence of various human cancers is increased in overweight people.[158] Ample experimental evidence supports such a concept.[159] Thus, although one is unwilling to accept the suggestion that 40% of human cancer is directly related to diet, there is increasing evidence that diet and related factors play a major role in the incidence of human cancer. However, this role is quite complex and, in all likelihood, does not result from the direct conversion of normal to neoplastic cells by dietary constituents, but rather stems from an alteration in the development of cells within the organism that have the potential for cancerous growth, that is, by tumor promotion.

The fact that certain types of reproductive and sexual behavior alter the incidence of human cancer has been known since the time of Ramazzini (see below). Doll and Peto[140] pointed out that pregnancy and childbirth seem to play a significant role in the prevention of cancers of the endometrium, ovary, and breast; all of these conditions are less common in women who have borne children at an early age than in women who have had no children. This relation is most striking in respect to the incidence of breast cancer: parous women become progressively less likely to develop this cancer as the age at the time of the first pregnancy decreases.[160] However, early menarche, late first full-term pregnancy, and late menopause generally have been accepted as the three major factors that increase the risk of breast cancer in the human.[161]

Perhaps the most common single, direct, chemical cause of human cancer is tobacco smoking. Doll and Peto[140] have estimated, from epidemiologic data, that 85% to 90% of the lung cancer cases in the United States annually are the direct result of tobacco smoking. If one adds to this the number of cancers of the bladder and gastrointestinal tract that can be attributed to tobacco smoking, about 30% of all cancer deaths in the United States result from this habit. If all deaths from neoplasms causally related to tobacco smoking are removed from the statistics, there is essentially no annual increase in the overall age-adjusted cancer death rate in men and a continual decreasing cancer death rate in women. Thus, tobacco smoke represents the major known cause of human cancer in our society, and it is the only known factor causing a continual increase in the overall age-adjusted cancer death rate of Americans.

CARCINOGENIC AGENTS ASSOCIATED WITH OCCUPATIONS

In 1713, Bernardino Ramazzini published *De Morbis Artificum [Diseases of Workers]*, which was translated in 1964 by Wright. In this text Ramazzini described the high incidence of mammary cancer in nuns and attributed it to their celibate life. Scrotal cancer in one-time chimney sweeps, described by Pott, was another example of occupational cancer. During the 19th century, several reports of the association of specific cancers in the mining, smelting, dye, and lubricating processes industries were published. Unfortunately, in many instances little was done for many years to protect the workers, a neglect from which we are not entirely free today (Table 8-5).

The association of occupational exposure to asbestos and the subsequent development of bronchogenic carcinoma and mesothelioma has been well established. However, in virtually all of the studies undertaken in this field, the highest incidence of bronchogenic carcinoma was found in those persons exposed to asbestos who also had a history of cigarette smoking. One study of 17,800 asbestos insulation workers in the United States and Canada indicated that the risk of bronchogenic carcinoma in nonsmokers who had been exposed to asbestos was very much lower than in smokers; this suggests the probable requirement for multiple environmental agents in the production of lung cancer in persons exposed to asbestos. On the other hand, there have been several documented cases of people developing mesotheliomas many years after an extremely short exposure to asbestos.[163] Further evidence in support of the direct carcinogenic effect of asbestos is the fact that mesotheliomas can be induced in rodents by appropriate exposure to this material.[164] However, although other fibrous materials such as fiberglass have been shown to be carcinogenic in rodents,[165] there is essentially no evidence to date that fiberglass causes human cancer. Although the mechanism of asbestos induction of cancer is not yet known, the demonstration that the type and size of fiber are important for the carcinogenicity of

TABLE 8-5. Chemical Agents Associated with Occupations and Posing a Carcinogenic Risk to Humans on the Basis of Epidemiologic Studies

Chemical, Process, or Industry	*Associated Neoplasm*	*Evidence for Carcinogenicity**
Acrylonitrite	Lung, colon, prostate	Limited
Arsenic	Lung	Sufficient
Asbestos	Lung, mesothelioma, gastrointestinal tract (?)	Sufficient
Manufacture of auramine	Bladder	Limited
Aromatic amines (aminobiphenyl, benzidine, 2-naphthylamine, 4-nitrobiphenyl)	Bladder	Sufficient
Benzene	Leukemia	Sufficient
Beryllium and its compounds	Lung	Limited
Bis(chloromethyl)ether	Lung	Sufficient
Boot and shoe manufacture and repair	Nasal carcinoma	Sufficient
Cadmium and its compounds	Lung, prostate (?)	Limited
Chromium and some of its compounds	Lung	Sufficient
Furniture manufacture (hardwood)	Nasal carcinoma	Sufficient
Hematite mining (underground)	Lung	Sufficient
Isopropyl alcohol manufacture	Cancer of paranasal sinuses	Sufficient
Nickel refining	Lung, nasal sinuses	Sufficient
Occupational exposure to phenoxyacetic acids and herbicides	Soft tissue sarcoma	Limited
Rubber industry (certain occupations)	Leukemia, bladder	Sufficient
Soots, tars, and oils	Skin, lung, bladder, gastrointestinal tract	Sufficient
Vinyl chloride	Liver (angiosarcoma)	Sufficient

* This terminology refers to the IARC categorization and is based on the findings reviewed in the IARC monographs[146] and the review by Doll and Peto.[140]

this material indicates that its carcinogenic action may be similar to that of the plastic film carcinogenesis discussed earlier in this chapter.

Aromatic amines, especially those used in the dye industry, have long been known to be potential risks for cancer, especially bladder cancer, in humans. Although the severity of the risk to workers in the dye industry varied with the exposure, 100% of the workers who distilled 2-naphthylamine developed bladder cancer.[166] Not until 1938 was verification of the carcinogenicity of these compounds, especially 2-naphthylamine, obtained in experimental animals. Exposure, usually prolonged, to another organic chemical, benzene, has now been linked by epidemiologic studies to the induction of leukemia in persons exposed in an occupational setting.[167]

A review by the IARC in 1975 reported 43 cases of angiosarcoma in ten different countries. All of the patients had a history of working with vinyl chloride. Hepatic angiosarcoma is an extremely rare neoplasm in humans, and the incidence seen in this group is therefore far from what might be expected in the general population. Although the low incidence of these neoplasms suggests that vinyl chloride is a relatively weak carcinogen, the rarity of hepatic angiosarcoma in the general population strongly supports a causal relationship between exposure to the organic monomer and the induction of this mesenchymal neoplasm.

The United States government has sponsored publications that suggest that occupational causes of neoplasia in humans may be responsible for as much as 20% of total cancer mortality, but Doll and Peto[140] have presented compelling arguments that such is not the case. Their review of the currently available statistical and epidemiologic evidence indicates that only about 4% of all cancer deaths in the United States can be attributed to occupational causes. The increasingly strict governmental regulation of actual and potential industrial health hazards promises to decrease this figure to even lower levels in the future.

CARCINOGENIC AGENTS ASSOCIATED WITH MEDICAL THERAPY AND DIAGNOSIS

In modern times, the dictum of Hippocrates that above all a physician should do no harm to his patient has been modified to a consideration of the benefit to the patient in relation to the risk of the procedure or therapy involved. Many times in the past the risk to the patient was unknown or unsuspected, and only later did the risk factor become evident. A good example of such unsuspected risk was the administration of diethylstilbesterol to pregnant women to avert a threatened abortion. The benefit of such a procedure is obvious, but the risk did not become obvious until many years later, when a small percentage of the female offspring of mothers treated with this estrogenic analogue during gestation developed vaginal carcinomas, usually shortly after puberty (Table 8-6).[168] Further evidence of the carcinogenicity of some synthetic estrogen preparations has been obtained as a result of the demonstrated association of liver cell adenomas with the prolonged use of oral contraceptives that contain synthetic steroidal estrogens.[169] In postmenopausal women, the use of estrogens to prevent a variety of symptoms has been clearly documented as associated with an increased risk of endometrial carcinoma, ranging from eightfold to 16-fold.[169]

Although there is no doubt of the association of lung

TABLE 8-6. Chemical Agents Associated with Medical Diagnosis and Treatment That Pose a Carcinogenic Risk to Humans on the Basis of Epidemiologic Studies

Chemical or Drug	*Associated Neoplasm*	*Evidence for Carcinogenicity**
Alkylating agents (cyclophosphamide, melphalan)	Bladder, leukemia	Sufficient
Inorganic arsenicals	Skin, liver	Sufficient
Azathioprine (immunosuppressive drugs)	Lymphoma, reticulum cell sarcoma, skin, Kaposi's sarcoma (?)	Sufficient
Chlornaphazine	Bladder	Sufficient
Chloramphenicol	Leukemia	Limited
Diethylstilbesterol	Vagina (clear cell carcinoma)	Sufficient
Estrogens:		
Premenopausal	Liver cell adenoma	Sufficient
Postmenopausal	Endometrium	Limited
Methoxypsoralen with UV light	Skin	Sufficient
Oxymetholone	Liver	Limited
Phenacetin	Renal pelvis (carcinoma)	Sufficient
Phenytoin (diphenylhydantoin)	Lymphoma, neuroblastoma	Limited
Thorotrast	Liver (angiosarcoma)	Sufficient

* This terminology refers to the IARC categorization and is based on the findings reviewed in the IARC monographs[146] and the review by Doll and Peto.[140]

cancer with chronic exposure to arsenic in industrial situations, arsenic compounds were widely used in the treatment of various diseases in the early 20th century. Organic arsenicals were used to treat syphilis, and there is some evidence of their association with skin cancer in people receiving such treatment for prolonged periods. The association of skin cancer as well as liver cancer with the chronic administration of Fowler's solution has now been well documented.[170] This medicament, in the form of a solution of 1% potassium arsenite in aqueous alcohol, was used to treat dermatitis, arthritis, and other conditions, including chronic leukemia. Since the material was often administered for years, some patients received many grams of arsenic during their period of treatment.

A number of agents known to damage DNA have been used in the diagnosis and treatment of various diseases, especially neoplasia. Alkylating agents are used primarily for the treatment of malignant neoplasms, and a number, including melphalan and cyclophosphamide (Cytoxan), have been causally associated with the induction of carcinoma of the bladder, especially in children receiving intensive therapy for acute leukemia. In addition, the induction of acute nonlymphocytic leukemia in adults receiving such chemotherapy, especially for Hodgkin's disease, has been reported.[171] Methoxypsoralen, which interacts with DNA, has been used in combination with ultraviolet light in the treatment of psoriasis. Definite evidence of the induction of squamous cell carcinoma of the skin by this regimen has been presented.[172]

Of the drugs that have been used in the chemical immunosuppression of patients in preparation for transplantation of organs and tissues from one person to another, azathioprine has been associated with an increased incidence of neoplasia. Although this drug and others used during clinical immunosuppression interact with DNA, it is not clear whether such compounds are actually carcinogenic or act by suppressing the natural resistance of the host. Since the predominant neoplasms appearing in such immunosuppressed patients are those derived from the immune system, it is reasonable to suggest that a major mechanism for the induction of neoplasia in immunosuppressed patients is the loss of host resistance to neoplastic cells already present but normally prevented from expressing their neoplastic potential by immune mechanisms of the host. The recent outbreak of acquired immune deficiency syndrome (AIDS) has further substantiated the role of immunodeficiency in cancer development by the finding of a significant increase in lymphomas and Kaposi's sarcoma in such patients.[173]

The association of leukemia with administration of the antibiotic chloramphenicol may be related to its depressive action on the bone marrow.[171] The association of carcinoma of the renal pelvis with excessive abuse of the analgesic phenacetin is now well known, but the association of lymphomas with the chronic administration of phenytoin for the control of epilepsy is not so well documented.[171] Phenytoin induces lymphoid reactions that are at times difficult to distinguish from neoplasia, but there is limited evidence of its causal association with lymphoma, although the risk is probably much less than the benefit to the epileptic patient. Some forms of medical therapy and diagnosis do present significant carcinogenic risks to the patient, but the total number of cancer cases resulting from such actions is extremely small compared with the incidence of cancer in general in the human population.[174]

PREVENTION OF CHEMICAL CARCINOGENESIS: TESTING OF CHEMICALS FOR CARCINOGENIC ACTIVITY

The prevention of cancer development by active intervention in the natural history of carcinogenesis in the stages of initiation or promotion is a potential reality. Alternatively, cancer may be prevented by eliminating causative agents in the environment. Thus, the identification of chemicals that pose a carcinogenic risk to humans has received major attention in the last two decades. A number of methods have been devised for the bioassay of carcinogenic agents found in the environment. The principal standard for these tests is the induction of neoplasia in experimental animals. Although these studies are tedious and expensive, at present they are the best and most reliable procedures available. However, the mere production of a neoplasm in an experimental animal provides no information about the molecular and biologic processes that precede the appearance of the neoplasm. The induction of neoplasia in animals at a statistically higher level than in controls has been considered indicative of carcinogenicity of the agent under study; however, modern concepts of the natural history of neoplastic development, that is, initiation and promotion, require that this simplistic evaluation of the data be reconsidered.

Although whole-animal bioassay procedures are the basis for determining the potential risk of a chemical for inducing cancer in humans, it became clear some time ago that the testing of all potentially dangerous chemicals by whole-animal bioassays would be physically and financially impossible. Thus, in the last two decades, considerable effort has been directed toward devising "screening" bioassays that may indicate which chemicals can be potentially dangerous and should be selected for whole-animal bioassay. A summary of these short-term tests for carcinogenicity and mutagenicity is given in Table 8-7. The reader is referred to the discussion by Pitot[175] for detailed references to Table 8-7.

One of the most popular screening methods for potential carcinogenicity is the Ames test. Since most carcinogenic chemicals are mutagenic per se or are metabolized in vivo to mutagenic compounds, the Ames assay, which depends on the induced mutation of one or more highly mutable bacterial strains, is a reasonable screening procedure for carcinogenicity. An outline of the Ames test as it is commonly used at present is shown in Figure 8-5. The specifics of the test are given in the legend. If the test agent or its metabolite is mutagenic, a mutation converting the histidine gene back to its normal structure will allow the bacteria to synthesize histidine again de novo, resulting in visible growth of revertant colonies on the Petri dish.

In a study of 300 compounds of known carcinogenic potential, McCann and Ames[176] found that only about 10% of the compounds tested produced false-negative tests. A similar or greater percentage of such false-negative tests occurs

TABLE 8-7. Short-Term "Screening" Assays for Carcinogenicity and Mutagenicity*

Test	*End Point*
Prokaryote mutagenesis in vitro (*e.g.*, Ames test)	Back or forward mutations in specific bacterial strains (with added liver homogenate)
Host-mediated prokaryote mutagenesis in vivo	Back or forward mutations in specific bacterial strains
Dominant lethal assay	Death of fertilized egg in mammalian implanted spectra
Sperm abnormality induction	Microscopically abnormal sperm
Mutagenesis in cultured cells	Scoring of dominant or linked mutations
Mutations in *Neurospora*	Scoring of mutations
Mitotic recombination in yeast alleles to homozygous state	Conversion of heterozygous to homozygous state
Drosophila	Recessive lethal test
Induced chromosomal aberrations	Visible alterations in karyotype
Micronucleus test	Appearance of micronuclei in bone marrow cells in vivo
Sister chromatids differentially exchanged	Visible exchange of labeled sister chromatids
DNA repair in vivo or in vitro	Unscheduled DNA synthesis or DNA strand breaks
Fidelity of DNA polymerases in vitro	Altered fidelity of DNA synthesis in cell-free system

* Adapted from Pitot HC: Relationships of bioassay data on chemicals to their toxic and carcinogenic risk for humans. J Environ Pathol Toxicol 3:431, 1980.

with virtually all of the "screening" bioassay tests that are used. Thus, no single screening procedure is necessarily definitive in identifying a compound that should be subjected to a whole-animal bioassay. In fact, prokaryotic mutagenicity tests have been shown to miss (score negative) from 10%[176] to 23%[177] of known or suspected carcinogenic agents tested.

As indicated in Table 8-7, many of the tests involve the determination of mutations as an end point. Other tests involve the demonstration of DNA repair or changes in the structure of chromosomes of cells in culture. Not shown in Table 8-7 is the use of cell transformation in culture as a method for identifying chemicals that can cause the malignant transformation or a related phenomenon in cells grown in culture. Although this test has the advantage of relative rapidity, not all cells transformed in culture exhibit biologic neoplasia when transplanted in vivo. Further, although human tissues in culture may be used directly as test agents for mutagenesis, certain metabolic activation reactions that must take place for many compounds to be effective as carcinogens do not occur to an appreciable extent in many tissues cultured in vitro. In these cases, some supplementary activating system, such as a feeder layer, is necessary.

Although short-term screening assays for carcinogens and mutagens are relatively convenient and inexpensive, the final proof of carcinogenicity of an agent is its ability to induce neoplasms in mammals. Thus, whole-animal bioassay procedures remain the standard for judging whether an agent is carcinogenic. Many attempts at estimating the risk of environmental agents to humans are based on extrapolations from whole-animal bioassay data to the situation in humans.

Whole-animal bioassay systems, however, are not without problems. One of the most difficult variables found in whole-animal bioassay systems is the "spontaneous" tumor incidence of control animal populations. Neoplasms may appear in test animals, but unless the incidence of such tumors exceeds the spontaneous incidence of neoplasms by a statistically significant margin, the incidence of tumors may be considered as false positive. Most animal tests use 50 control and 50 treated animals. Even when controls have a 0% incidence, at least 10% of the 50 treated animals must exhibit tumors to ensure that the result is statistically significant.[178] By increasing the number of controls, this percentage may be decreased, but even at a tenfold higher number of control animals with 0% incidence, at least a 4% incidence of tumors in the treated animals would be required for statistical significance. Thus it is apparent that the sensitivity of the animal bioassay is markedly limited by statistical considerations.

In addition to the problem of sensitivity of whole-animal bioassays, a number of other problems have arisen, especially in the interpretation of the data obtained. At present it is generally considered, and rather strictly adhered to by regulatory agencies, that chemical carcinogens exert their effects through mechanisms that do not allow the determination of no-effect or threshold levels. This concept is based largely on the extrapolation of data from whole-animal bioassays to very low doses at which no measurements can be obtained by the usual assay procedures. Gehring and Blau[179] discussed various factors related to this problem; a variety of mechanisms tend to invalidate the concept of a no-effect level for various chemicals. Further, promoting agents both theoretically and in practice exhibit no-effect levels, as discussed earlier in this chapter. As Fears and associates[180] have pointed out, false-positive results are much less likely to occur at tissue sites with low spontaneous tumor rates. In fact, even the appearance of a very low

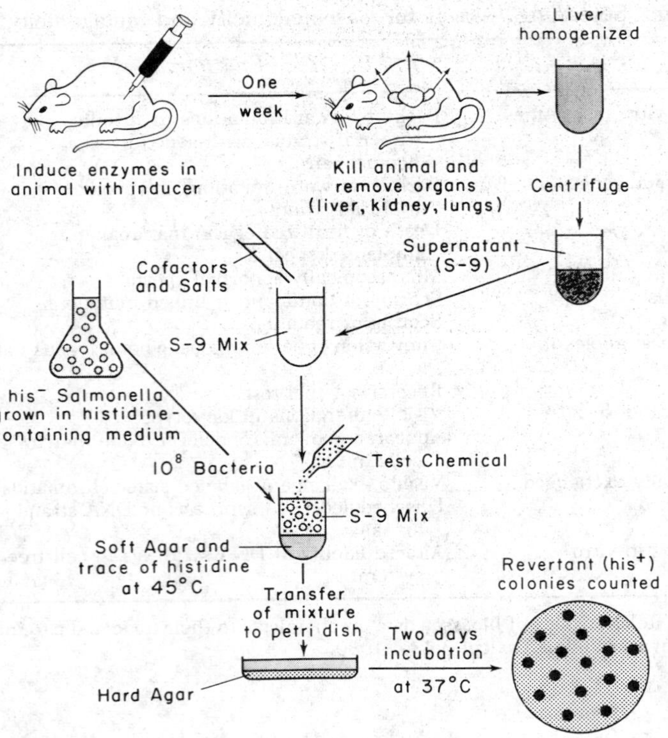

FIG. 8-5. The *Salmonella* (Ames) test to detect mutagenic activity by chemicals requiring metabolic activation. After intraperitoneal drug injection (usually for 1 week) to induce enzyme activity, the liver (and other organs, if desired) of the rodent are removed and homogenized and the mixture is centrifuged. The supernatant (S-9) may be stored frozen, or immediately combined with other biochemicals that promote activation (cofactors and salts). The S-9 mix, the test chemical, and about 10^8 salmonellae unable to synthesize histidine (his$^-$) are added to a test tube containing soft agar with a trace of histidine. The trace of histidine is necessary to allow the his$^-$ salmonellae to go through at least one or two rounds of replication, allowing "fixation" of any mutations that occur. This entire mixture is then transferred to a Petri dish containing hard agar and incubated for 2 days. If the activated chemical is mutagenic, histidine biosynthesis resumes in the mutated bacterium, and the growth of revertant colonies is later visible on the dish.

incidence of neoplasms at a site that seldom, if ever, exhibits spontaneous tumor formation is considered much more significant in the interpretation of the test results than is a barely statistically significant increase in tumor incidence at a tissue site with a high spontaneous tumor rate. Most bioassays are carried out in at least two different species of rodent, usually rats and mice. A major problem has been in the interpretation of the induction of hepatomas in mice by an agent with no other evidence of carcinogenic effect in either species. Although the whole-animal bioassay, when distinctly positive and exhibiting a reproducible dose-response, is the standard for extrapolation of such data to risk in humans, many, if not most, positive whole-animal bioassays must have other data to support findings of carcinogenicity if an extrapolation to humans is to be meaningful.

Another consideration in the establishment and interpretation of whole-animal bioassays is our increased understanding of the natural history of neoplastic development.[59] The bioassay most commonly used in determining the carcinogenicity of chemicals is the induction of neoplasms in any tissue of the test animals by chronic administration of the test compound for most of the animal's life span. This test does not distinguish complete carcinogens from promoting agents because the latter may promote cells initiated by incidental environmental factors, such as dietary contaminants, background radiation, and spontaneous mutations. Despite the fact that promoting agents are quite different from complete carcinogens and initiating agents (see Table 8-1), regulatory legislation does not yet distinguish among these types of agents.

CONCLUSIONS

Because we live in an environment permeated with chemicals whose number and diversity increase every year, it is important that we know and understand the mechanisms by which chemicals can induce the neoplastic transformation. Identification of such chemicals and their classification as incomplete or complete carcinogens, promoting agents, or the new class of "progressor" agents is essential for a rational approach to the prevention of chemical carcinogenesis in humans. Although it is the responsibility of all persons to limit their exposure to known cancer-causing chemicals, such as those that occur in cigarette smoke, alcoholic beverages, or in the form of excess calories, the prevention of cancer in the general population ultimately will remain the responsibility of society as a whole through research, education, and, where necessary, regulatory legislation.

REFERENCES

1. Pott P: Chirurgical Observations Relative to the Cataract, the Polypus of the Nose, the Cancer of the Scrotum, the Different Kinds of Ruptures, and the Mortification of the Toes and Feet. London, Hawkes, Clarke and Collins, 1775
2. Butlin HT: Cancer of the scrotum in chimney-sweeps and others: II. Why foreign sweeps do not suffer from scrotal cancer. Br Med J 2:1, 1892
3. Rehn L: Blasengeschwülste bei Fuchsin-Arbeitern. Arch Klin Chir 50:588, 1895
4. Hueper WC, Wiley FH, Wolfe HD: Experimental production of bladder tumors in dogs by administration of beta-naphthylamine. J Indust Hyg Toxicol 20:46, 1938
5. Yamagiwa K, Ichikawa K: Experimentelle Studie Über die Pathogenese der Epithelialgeschwülste. Mitteilungen Med Facultat Kaiserl Univ Tokyo 15:295, 1915
6. Kennaway EL: Experiments on cancer-producing substances. Br Med J 2:1, 1925
7. Kennaway EL, Hieger I: Carcinogenic substances and their fluorescence spectra. Br Med J 1:1044, 1930
8. Sasaki T, Yoshida T: Experimentelle Erzeugung des Lebercarcinoms durch Fütterung mit o-Amidoazotoluol. Virchows Arch Pathol Anat 295:175, 1935
9. Kinosita R: Researches on the cancerogenesis of the various chemical substances. Gann 30:423, 1936
10. Coulston F, Olajos EJ: Toxicology of *N*-nitroso compounds. Ecotoxicol Environ Safety 6:89, 1982
11. Magee PN, Swann PF: Nitroso compounds. Br Med Bull 25:240, 1969
12. Lijinsky W: Nitrosamines and nitrosamides in the etiology of gastrointestinal cancer. Cancer 40:2446, 1977
13. Matsukura N, Kawachi T, Sasajima K et al: Induction of liver tumors in rats by sodium nitrite and methylguanidine. Z Krebsforsch 90:87, 1977
14. Bartsch H, Montesano R: Relevance of nitrosamines to human cancer. Carcinogenesis 5:1381, 1984
15. Shank RC: Epidemiology of aflatoxin carcinogenesis. In Kraybill HFE, Mehlman MA (eds): Environmental Cancer, p 291. New York, John Wiley & Sons, 1977
16. Martell AE: Chemistry of carcinogenic metals. Environ Health Perspect 40:207, 1981
17. Landrigan PJ: Arsenic: State of the art. Am J Ind Med 2:5, 1981
18. Brand KG, Buoen LC, Johnson KH et al: Etiological factors, stages, and the role of the foreign body in foreign body tumorigenesis: A review. Cancer Res 35:279, 1975
19. Stinson NE: The tissue reaction induced in rats and guinea pigs by polymethylacrylate (acrylic) and stainless steel. Br J Exp Pathol 45:21, 1946
20. Ferguson DJ: Cellular attachment to implanted foreign bodies in relation to tumorigenesis. Cancer Res 37:4367, 1977

21. Thomassen MJ, Buoen LC, Brand I et al: Foreign-body tumorigenesis in mice: DNA synthesis in surface-attached cells during preneoplasia. JNCI 61:359, 1978
22. Memoli VA, Urban RM, Alroy J et al: Malignant neoplasms associated with orthopedic implant materials in rats. J Orthop Res 4:346, 1986
23. Miller EC, Miller JA: The presence and significance of bound amino azo dyes in the livers of rats fed *p*-dimethylaminoazobenzene. Cancer Res 7:468, 1947
24. Miller EC: Studies on the formation of protein-bound derivatives of 3,4-benzopyrene in the epidermal fraction of mouse skin. Cancer Res 11:100, 1951
25. Miller JA, Cramer JW, Miller EC: The N- and ring-hydroxylation of 2-acetylaminofluorene during carcinogenesis in the rat. Cancer Res 20:950, 1960
26. Miller JA: Carcinogenesis by chemicals: An overview. Cancer Res 30:559, 1970
27. Miller EC: Some current perspectives on chemical carcinogenesis in humans and experimental animals: Presidential Address. Cancer Res 38:1479, 1978
28. Boyland E: The biological significance of metabolism of polycyclic compounds. Biochem Soc Symp 5:40, 1950
29. Sims P, Grover PL, Swaisland A et al: Metabolic activation of benzo(a)pyrene proceeds by a diol-epoxide. Nature 252:326, 1974
30. Harvey RG: Activated metabolites of carcinogenic hydrocarbons. Acc Chem Res 14:218, 1981
31. Conney AH: Induction of microsomal enzymes by foreign chemicals and carcinogenesis by polycyclic aromatic hydrocarbons: GHA Clowes Memorial Lecture. Cancer Res 42:4875, 1982
32. Levin W, Thakker DR, Wood AW et al: Evidence that benzo(*a*)anthracene 3,4-diol-1,2-epoxide is an ultimate carcinogen on mouse skin. Cancer Res 38:1705, 1978
33. Nagata C, Kodama M, Ioki Y et al: Free radicals produced from chemical carcinogens and their significance in carcinogenesis. In Floyd RA (ed): Free Radicals and Cancer, p 1. New York, Marcel Dekker, 1982
34. Kahl R: Synthetic antioxidants: Biochemical actions and interference with radiation, toxic compounds, chemical mutagens and chemical carcinogens. Toxicology 33:185, 1984
35. Marnett LJ: Peroxyl free radicals: Potential mediators of tumor initiation and promotion. Carcinogenesis 8:1365, 1987
36. Wise RW, Zenser TV, Kadlubar FF et al: Metabolic activation of carcinogenic aromatic amines by dog bladder and kidney prostaglandin H synthase. Cancer Res 44:1893, 1984
37. Peters RA: Mechanism of the toxicity of the active constituent of *Dichapetalum cymosum* and related compounds. Adv Enzymol 18:113, 1957
38. Maher VM, Miller EC, Miller JA et al: Mutations and decreases in density of transforming DNA produced by derivatives of the carcinogens 2-acetylaminofluorene and N-methyl-4-aminoazobenzene. Mol Pharmacol 4:1, 1968
39. Ames BN, Durston WE, Yamasaki E et al: Carcinogens are mutagens: A simple test system combining liver homogenates for activation and bacteria for detection. Proc Natl Acad Sci USA 70:2281, 1973
40. Bresnick E, Eastman A: Alkylation of mammalian cell DNA, persistence of adducts, and relationship to carcinogenesis. Drug Metab Rev 13:189, 1982
41. Goth R, Rajewsky MF: Persistence of O^6-ethylguanine in rat-brain DNA: Correlation with nervous system-specific carcinogenesis by ethylnitrosourea. Proc Natl Acad Sci USA 71:639, 1974
42. Bedell MA, Lewis JG, Billings KC et al: Cell specificity in hepatocarcinogenesis: Preferential accumulation of O^6-methylguanine in target cell DNA during continuous exposure of rats to 1,2-dimethylhydrazine. Cancer Res 42:3079, 1982
43. Swenberg JA, Dyroff MC, Bedell MA et al: O^4-Ethyldeoxythymidine, but not O^6-ethyldeoxyguanosine, accumulates in hepatocyte DNA of rats exposed continuously to diethylnitrosamine. Proc Natl Acad Sci USA 81:1692, 1984
44. Müller R, Rajewsky MF: Enzymatic removal of O^6-ethylguanine *versus* stability of O^4-ethylthymine in the DNA of rat tissues exposed to the carcinogen ethylnitrosourea: Possible interference of guanine-O^6 alkylation with 5-cytosine methylation in the DNA of replicating target cells. Z Naturforsch [C] 38:1023, 1983
45. Singer B: *In vivo* formation and persistence of modified nucleosides resulting from alkylating agents. Environ Health Perspect 62:41, 1985
46. Riggs AD, Jones PA: 5-Methylcytosine, gene regulation, and cancer. Adv Cancer Res 40:1, 1983
47. Farmer PB, Neumann H-G, Henschler D: Estimation of exposure of man to substances reacting covalently with macromolecules. Arch Toxicol 60:251, 1987
48. Oellerich M: Enzyme-immunoassay: A review. J Clin Chem Clin Biochem 22:895, 1984
49. Yalow RS: Radioimmunoassay: A probe for the fine structure of biologic systems. Science 200:1236, 1978
50. Gupta RC, Reddy MV, Randerath K: ^{32}P-postlabeling analysis of non-radioactive aromatic carcinogen-DNA adducts. Carcinogenesis 3:1081, 1982
51. Langone JJ, Van Vunakis H (eds): Methods in Enzymology, Vol 92, Immunochemical Techniques, Part E, Monoclonal Antibodies and General Immunoassay Methods. New York, Academic Press, 1983
52. Perera FP, Weinstein IB: Molecular epidemiology and carcinogen-DNA adduct detection: New approaches to studies of human cancer causation. J Chronic Dis 35:581, 1982
53. Harris CC, Vahakangas K, Newman MJ et al: Detection of benzo[*a*]pyrene diol epoxide-DNA adducts in peripheral blood lymphocytes and antibodies to the adducts in serum from coke oven workers. Proc Natl Acad Sci USA 82:6672, 1985
54. Bryant MS, Skipper PL, Tannenbaum SR et al: Hemoglobin adducts of 4-aminobiphenyl in smokers and nonsmokers. Cancer Res 47:602, 1987
55. Brash DE, Hart RW: DNA damage and repair in vivo. J Environ Pathol Toxicol 2:79, 1978
56. Teebor GW, Frenkel K: The initiation of DNA excision-repair. Adv Cancer Res 38:23, 1983
57. Brambilla G, Carlo P, Finollo R et al: Viscometric detection of liver DNA fragmentation in rats treated with minimal doses of chemical carcinogens. Cancer Res 43:202, 1983
58. Stout DL, Becker FF: Progressive DNA damage in hepatic nodules during 2-acetylaminofluorene carcinogenesis. Cancer Res 40:1269, 1980
59. Sarasin A, Bourre F, Benoit A: Error-prone replication of ultraviolet-irradiated simian virus 40 in carcinogen-treated monkey kidney cells. Biochimie 64:815, 1982
60. Wintersberger U: Chemical carcinogenesis: The price for DNA repair? Naturwissenschaften 69:107, 1982
61. Stewart BW: Generation and persistence of carcinogen-induced repair intermediates in rat liver DNA in vivo. Cancer Res 41:3238, 1981
62. Neumann H-G: Role of extent and persistence of DNA modifications in chemical carcinogenesis by aromatic amines: Recent results. Cancer Res 84:77, 1983
63. Yarosh DB: The role of O^6-methylguanine-DNA methyltransferase in cell survival, mutagenesis and carcinogenesis. Mutat Res 145:1, 1985
64. Hanawalt PC, Sarasin A: Cancer-prone hereditary diseases with DNA processing abnormalities. Trends Genet 2:124-129, 1900
65. Sirover MA, Lobe LA: Infidelity of DNA synthesis in vitro: Screening for potential metal mutagens or carcinogens. Science 194:1434, 1976.
66. Fialkow PJ: Clonal origin of human tumors. Biochim Biophys Acta 458:283, 1976
67. Foulds L: Neoplastic Development. Academic Press, New York, 1969
68. Rous P, Kidd JG: Conditional neoplasms and subthreshold neoplastic states. J Exp Med 73:365, 1941
69. Mottram JC: A developing factor in experimental blastogenesis. J Pathol Bacteriol 56:181, 1944
70. Berenblum I, Shubik P: The role of croton oil applications associated with a single painting of a carcinogen in tumor induction of the mouse's skin. Br J Cancer 1:379, 1947
71. Boutwell RK: Some biological aspects of skin carcinogenesis. Prog Exp Tumor Res 4:207, 1964
72. Slaga TJ: Overview of tumor promotion in animals. Environ Health Perspect 50:3, 1983
73. Pitot HC, Beer D, Hendrich S: Multistage carcinogenesis: The phenomenon underlying the theories. In Iversen OH (ed): Theories of Carcinogenesis, p 159. Washington, DC, Hemisphere Publishing, 1987
74. Goldsworthy TL, Hanigan MH, Pitot HC: Models of hepatocarcinogenesis in the rat: Contrasts and comparisons. CRC Crit Rev Toxicol 17:61, 1986
75. Pitot HC: Drugs as promoters of carcinogenesis. In Estabrook RW, Lindenlaub E (eds): The Induction of Drug Metabolism, p 471. New York, Schattauer Verlag, 1979
76. Port R, Schmähl D, Wahrendorf J: Some examples of dose-response studies in chemical carcinogenesis. Oncology 33:66, 1976
77. Weinberg WC, Berkwits L, Iannaccone PM: The clonal nature of carcinogen-induced altered foci of gamma-glutamyl transpeptidase expression in rat liver. Carcinogenesis 8:565, 1987
78. Schulte-Hermann R, Timmermann-Trosiener I, Schuppler J: Promotion of spontaneous preneoplastic cells in rat liver as a possible explanation of tumor production by nonmutagenic compounds. Cancer Res 43:839, 1983
79. Popp JA, Scortichini BH, Garvey LK: Quantitative evaluation of hepatic foci of cellular alteration occurring spontaneously in Fischer-344 rats. Fundam Appl Toxicol 5:314, 1985
80. Stenbäck F: Tumor persistence and regression in skin carcinogenesis. Z Krebsforsch 91:249, 1978
81. Hendrich S, Glauert HP, Pitot HC: The phenotypic stability of altered hepatic foci: Effects of withdrawal and subsequent readministration of phenobarbital. Carcinogenesis 7:2041, 1986
82. Bühler H, Pirovino M, Akovbiantz A et al: Regression of liver cell adenoma: A follow-up study of three consecutive patients after discontinuation of oral contraceptive use. Gastroenterology 82:775, 1982
83. Berenblum I, Haran-Ghera A: A quantitative study of the systemic initiating action of urethane (ethyl carbamate) in mouse skin carcinogenesis. Br J Cancer 11:77, 1957
84. Grisham JW, Greenberg DS, Kaufman DG et al: Cycle-related toxicity and transformation in 10T1/2 cells treated with N-methyl-N′-nitro-N-nitrosoguanidine. Proc Natl Acad Sci USA 77:4813, 1980
85. McCormick PJ, Bertram JS: Differential cell cycle phase specificity for neoplastic transformation and mutation to ouabain resistance induced by N-methyl-N′-nitro-N-nitrosoguanidine in synchronized C3H10T1/2 C18 cells. Proc Natl Acad Sci USA 79:4342, 1982
86. Columbano A, Rajalakshmi S, Sarma DSR: Requirement of cell proliferation for the initiation of liver carcinogenesis as assayed by three different procedures. Cancer Res 41:2079, 1981
87. Berwald Y, Sachs L: In vitro transformation of normal cells to tumor cells by carcinogenic hydrocarbons. JNCI 35:641, 1965
88. Kakunaga T: The role of cell division in the malignant transformation of mouse cells treated with 3-methylcholanthrene. Cancer Res 35:1637, 1975
89. Lakowicz JR, Englund F, Hidmark A: Particle-enhanced membrane uptake of a polynuclear aromatic hydrocarbon: A possible role in cocarcinogenesis. JNCI 61:1155, 1978
90. Hozumi M, Ogawa M, Sugimura T et al: Inhibition of tumorigenesis in mouse skin by leupeptin, a protease inhibitor from *Actinomycetes*. Cancer Res 32:1725, 1972
91. Boutwell RK: The function and mechanism of promoters of carcinogenesis. Crit Rev Toxicol 2:419, 1974

92. Nakanishi K, Fukushima S, Hagiwara A et al: Organ-specific promoting effects of phenobarbital sodium and sodium saccharin in the induction of liver and urinary bladder tumors in male F344 rats. JNCI 68:497, 1982
93. Berenblum I: Established principles and unresolved problems in carcinogenesis JNCI 60:723, 1978
94. Brand KG, Buoen LC, Johnson KH et al: Etiological factors, stages, and the role of the foreign body in foreign body tumorigenesis: A review. Cancer Res 35:279, 1975
95. Ryan WL, Stenback F, Curtis GL: Tumor promotion by foreign bodies (IUD). Cancer Lett 13:299, 1981
96. Topping DC, Nettesheim P: Two-stage carcinogenesis studies with asbestos in Fischer 344 rats. JNCI 65:627, 1980
97. Wattenberg LW: Chemoprevention of cancer. Cancer Res 45:1, 1985
98. Bertram JS, Kolonel LN, Meyskens FL Jr: Rationale and strategies for chemoprevention of cancer in humans. Cancer Res 47:3012, 1987
99. Frankfurt OS, Raitcheva E: Fast onset of DNA synthesis stimulated by tumor promoter in mouse epidermis at the initiation stage of carcinogenesis. JNCI 51:1861, 1973
100. Schulte-Hermann R, Schuppler J, Timmermann-Trosiener I et al: The role of growth of normal and preneoplastic cell populations for tumor promotion in rat liver. Environ Health Perspect 50:185, 1983
101. Varshavsky A: Phorbol ester dramatically increases incidence of methotrexate-resistant mouse cells: Possible mechanisms and relevance to tumor promotion. Cell 25:561, 1981
102. Hayashi K, Fujiki H, Sugimura T: Effects of tumor promoters on the frequency of metallothionein I gene amplification in cells exposed to cadmium. Cancer Res 43:5433, 1983
103. Birnboim HC: DNA strand breakage in human leukocytes exposed to a tumor promoter, phorbol myristate acetate. Science 215:1247, 1982
104. Emerit I, Cerutti PA: Tumor promoter phorbol 12-myristate 13-acetate induces a clastogenic factor in human lymphocytes. Proc Natl Acad Sci USA 79:7509, 1982
105. Frenkel K, Chrzan K, Troll W et al: Radiation-like modification of bases in DNA exposed to tumor promoter-activated polymorphonuclear leukocytes. Cancer Res 46:5533, 1986
106. Ito N, Hirose M: The role of antioxidants in chemical carcinogenesis. Jpn J Cancer Res 78:1011, 1987
107. Fischer SM, Baldwin JK, Jasheway DW et al: Possible dissociation of the phorbol ester–induced oxidant response and tumor promotion in the F_1 offspring of SSIN × C57BL/6J mice. Carcinogenesis 8:1521, 1987
108. Loch-Caruso R, Trosko JE: Inhibited intercellular communication as a mechanistic link between teratogenesis and carcinogenesis. CRC Crit Rev Toxicol 16:157, 1985
109. Kinsella AR: Elimination of metabolic co-operation and the induction of sister chromatid exchanges are not properties common to all promoting or co-carcinogenic agents. Carcinogenesis 3:499, 1982
110. Ruch RJ, Klaunig JE: Antioxidant prevention of tumor promoter-induced inhibition of mouse hepatocyte intercellular communication. Cancer Lett 33:137, 1986
111. Leach KL, James ML, Blumberg PM: Characterization of a specific phorbol ester aporeceptor in mouse brain cytosol. Proc Natl Acad Sci USA 80:4208, 1983
112. Ashendel CL: The phorbol ester receptor: A phospholipid-regulated protein kinase. Biochim Biophys Acta 822:219, 1985
113. Nishizuka Y: Studies and perspectives of protein kinase C. Science 233:305, 1986
114. Housey GM, O'Brian CA, Johnson MD et al: Isolation of cDNA clones encoding protein kinase C: Evidence for a protein kinase C-related gene family. Proc Natl Acad Sci USA 84:1065, 1987
115. Knopf JL, Lee M-H, Sultzman LA et al: Cloning and expression of multiple protein kinase C cDNAs. Cell 46:491, 1986
116. Pitot HC: Fundamentals of Oncology, 3rd ed. New York, Marcel Dekker, 1986
117. Weinstein IB, Gattoni-Celli S, Kirschmeier P et al: Multistage carcinogenesis involves multiple genes and multiple mechanisms. J Cell Physiol Suppl 3:127, 1984
118. Schulte-Hermann R: Tumor promotion in the liver. Arch Toxicol 57:147, 1985
119. O'Connell JF, Klein-Szanto AJP, DiGiovanni DM et al: Enhanced malignant progression of mouse skin tumors by the free-radical generator benzoyl peroxide. Cancer Res 46:2863, 1986
120. Potter VR: A new protocol and its rationale for the study of initiation and promotion of carcinogenesis in rat liver. Carcinogenesis 2:1375, 1981
121. Hennings H, Spangler EF, Shores R et al: Malignant conversion and metastasis of mouse skin tumors: A comparison of SENCAR and CD-1 mice. Environ Health Perspect 68:69, 1986
122. Scherer E, Feringa AW, Emmelot P: Initiation-promotion-initiation: Induction of neoplastic foci within islands of precancerous liver cells in the rat. In Börzsönyi M, Lapis K, Day NE et al: (eds): Models, Mechanisms and Etiology of Tumor Promotion, p 57. Lyon, International Agency for Research on Cancer, IARC Scientific Publications, 1984
123. Scherer E: Neoplastic progression in experimental hepatocarcinogenesis. Biochim Biophys Acta 738:219, 1984
124. Aldaz CM, Conti CJ, Klein-Szanto AJP et al: Progressive dysplasia and neuploidy are hallmarks of mouse skin papillomas: Relevance to malignancy. Proc Natl Acad Sci USA 84:2029, 1987
125. Knudson AG Jr: Hereditary cancer, oncogenes, and antioncogenes. Cancer Res 45:1437, 1985
126. Pitot HC: Oncogenes and human neoplasia. Clin Lab Med 6:167, 1986
127. Quintanilla M, Brown K, Ramsden M et al: Carcinogen-specific mutation and amplification of Ha-*ras* during mouse skin carcinogenesis. Nature 322:78, 1986
128. Reynolds SH, Stowers SJ, Patterson RM et al: Activated oncogenes in B6C3F1 mouse liver tumors: Implications for risk assessment. Science 237:1309, 1987
129. Wiseman RW, Stowers SJ, Miller EC et al: Activating mutations of the c-Ha-*ras* protooncogene in chemically induced hepatomas of the male B6C3 F_1 mouse. Proc Natl Acad Sci USA 83:5825, 1986
130. Brown K, Qunitanilla M, Ramsden M et al: v-*ras* genes from Harvey and BALB murine sarcoma viruses can act as initiators of two-stage mouse skin carcinogenesis. Cell 46:445, 1986
131. Zarbl H, Sukumar S, Arthur AV et al: Direct mutagenesis of Ha-*ras*-1 oncogenes by *N*-nitroso-*N*-methylurea during initiation of mammary carcinogenesis in rats. Nature 315:382, 1985
132. McMahon G, Davis E, Wogan GN: Characterization of c-Ki-*ras* oncogene alleles by direct sequencing of enzymatically amplified DNA from carcinogen-induced tumors. Proc Natl Acad Sci USA 84:4974, 1987
133. Tahara E, Yasui W, Taniyama K et al: Ha-*ras* oncogene product in human gastric carcinoma: Correlation with invasiveness, metastasis or prognosis. Jpn J Cancer Res 77:517, 1986
134. Viola MV, Fromowitz F, Oravez S et al: Expression of *ras* oncogene p21 in prostate cancer. N Engl J Med 314:133, 1986
135. Lee I, Gould VE, Radosevich JA et al: Immunohistochemical evaluation of *ras* oncogene expression in pulmonary and pleural neoplasms. Virchows Arch [Cell Pathol] 53:146, 1987
136. Gallick GE, Kurzrock R, Kloetzer WS et al: Expression of $p21^{ras}$ in fresh primary and metastatic human colorectal tumors. Proc Natl Acad Sci USA 82:1795, 1985
137. Riou G, Le MG, Le Doussal V et al: c-*myc*- protooncogene expression and prognosis in early carcinoma of the uterine cervix. Lancet 1:761, 1987
138. Yokota J, Tsunetsugu-Yokota Y, Battifora H et al: Alterations of *myc*, *myb*, and ras^{Ha} proto-oncogenes in cancers are frequent and show clinical correlation. Science 231:261, 1986
139. Pitot HC: The natural history of neoplastic development: The relation of experimental models to human cancer. Cancer 49:1206, 1982
140. Doll R, Peto R: The Causes of Cancer. New York, Oxford University Press, 1981
141. Carroll KK, Hopkins GJ: Dietary polyunsaturated fat versus saturated fat in relation to mammary carcinogenesis. Lipids 14:155, 1979
142. Hammond EC: Tobacco. In Fraumeni JF Jr (ed): Persons at High Risk of Cancer: An Approach to Cancer Etiology and Control, p 13. New York, Academic Press, 1975
143. Nicholson WJ: Cancer following occupational exposure to asbestos and vinyl chloride. Cancer 39:1792, 1977
144. Ishak KG: Hepatic lesions caused by anabolic and contraceptive steroids. Semin Liver Dis 1:116, 1981
145. Lieber CS, Seitz HK, Garro AJ et al: Alcohol-related diseases and carcinogenesis. Cancer Res 39:2863, 1979
146. Chemicals, Industrial Processes and Industries Associated with Cancer in Humans. IARC Monogr Eval Carcinog Risk Chem Hum [Suppl] 4, 1982
147. Bross IDJ, Coombs J: Early onset of oral cancer among women who drink and smoke. Oncology 33:136, 1976
148. Herity B, Moriarty M, Daly L et al: The role of tobacco and alcohol in the aetiology of lung and larynx cancer. Br J Cancer 46:961, 1982
149. Tuyns AJ: Epidemiology of alcohol and cancer. Cancer Res 39:2840, 1979
150. Ohnishi K, Iida S, Iwama S et al: The effect of chronic habitual alcohol intake on the development of liver cirrhosis and hepatocellular carcinoma: Relation to hepatitis B surface antigen carriage. Cancer 49:672, 1982
151. O'Connell DL, Hulka BS, Chambless LE et al: Cigarette smoking, alcohol consumption, and breast cancer risk. JNCI 78:229, 1987
152. Harvey EB, Schairer C, Brinton LA et al: Alcohol consumption and breast cancer. JNCI 78:657, 1987
153. Willett WC, Stampfer MJ, Colditz GA et al: Moderate alcohol consumption and the risk of breast cancer. N Engl J Med 316:1174, 1987
154. Tuyns AJ, Griciute LL: Carcinogenic substances in alcoholic beverages. In Davis W, Harrap KR, Stathopoulos G (eds): Human Cancer: Its Characterization and Treatment, p 130. Amsterdam, Excerpta Medica, 1980
155. Tuyns AJ, Pequignot G, Abbatucci JS: Oesophageal cancer and alcohol consumption: Importance of type of beverage. Int J Cancer 23:443, 1979
156. Yang CS: Research on esophageal cancer in China: A review. Cancer Res 40:2633, 1980
157. Singer GM, Chuan J, Roman J et al: Nitrosamines and nitrosamine precursors in foods from Linxian, China, a high incidence area for esophageal cancer. Carcinogenesis 7:733, 1986
158. Garfinkel L: Overweight and cancer. Ann Intern Med 103:1034, 1985
159. Birt DF: Fat and calorie effects on carcinogenesis at sites other than the mammary gland. Am J Clin Nutr 45:203, 1987
160. McMahon B, Cole P, Brown J: Etiology of human breast cancer: A review. JNCI 50:21, 1973
161. Pike MC, Krailo MD, Henderson BE et al: "Hormonal" risk factors, "breast tissue age" and the age-incidence of breast cancer. Nature 303:767, 1983
162. Hammond EC, Selikoff IJ: Relation of cigarette smoking to risk of death of asbestos-associated disease among insulation workers in the United States. IARC Sci Publ 8:312, 1973

163. Chen WJ, Karle Mottet N: Malignant mesothelioma with minimal asbestos exposure. Hum Pathol 9:253, 1978
164. Pigott GH, Gaskell BA, Ishmael J: Effects of long term inhalation of alumina fibres in rats. Br J Exp Pathol 62:323, 1981
165. Stanton MF, Layard M, Tegeris A et al: Carcinogenicity of fibrous glass: Pleural response in the rat in relation to fiber dimension. JNCI 58:587, 1977
166. Connolly JG, White EP: Malignant cells in the urine of men exposed to beta-naphthylamine. Can Med Assoc J 100:879, 1969
167. Rinsky RA, Young RJ, Smith AB: Leukemia in benzene workers. Am J Indust Med 2:217, 1981
168. Herbst AL: Clear cell adenocarcinoma and the current status of DES-exposed females. Cancer 48:484, 1981
169. Huggins GR, Zucker PK: Oral contraceptives and neoplasia: 1987 update. Fertil Steril 47:733, 1987
170. Pershagen G: The carcinogenicity of arsenic. Environ Health Perspect 40:93, 1981
171. Hoover R, Fraumeni JF Jr: Drug-induced cancer. Cancer 47:1071, 1981
172. Stern RS, Thibodeau LA, Kleinerman RA: Risk of cutaneous carcinoma in patients treated with oral methoxsalen photochemotherapy for psoriasis. N Engl J Med 300:809, 1979
173. Volberding PA: Kaposi's sarcoma, B-cell lymphoma and other AIDS-associated tumours. Clin Immunol Allergy 6:569, 1986
174. Schmähl D: Iatrogenic carcinogenesis. J Cancer Res Clin Oncol 99:71, 1981
175. Pitot HC: Relationships of bioassay data on chemicals to their toxic and carcinogenic risk for humans. J Environ Pathol Toxicol 3:431, 1980
176. McCann J, Ames BN: Detection of carcinogens as mutagens in the *Salmonella*/microsome test: Assay of 300 chemicals. Discussion. Proc Natl Acad Sci USA 73:950, 1976
177. Rinkus SJ, Legator MS: Chemical characterization of 465 known or suspected carcinogens and their correlation with mutagenic activity in the *Salmonella typhimurium* system. Cancer Res 39:3289, 1979
178. Sontag JM: Aspects in carcinogen bioassay. In Hiatt H, Watson J, Winsten J (eds): Origins of Human Cancer, Book C, p 1327. Cold Spring Harbor, New York, Cold Spring Harbor Laboratory, 1977
179. Gehring PJ, Blau GE: Mechanisms of carcinogenesis: Dose response. J Environ Pathol Toxicol 1:163, 1977
180. Fears TR, Tarone RE, Chu KC: False-positive and false-negative rates for carcinogenicity screens. Cancer Res 37:1941, 1977

R. J. MICHAEL FRY

CHAPTER 9 *Principles of Carcinogenesis: Physical*

This chapter discusses the induction of cancer by three types of physical agents: ionizing radiation, ultraviolet radiation, and foreign bodies and fibers. Studies of cancer induction by these agents have two aims: first, the estimate of risk of cancer following exposure, and second, the elucidation of mechanisms of cancer induction. Studies with different agents can help identify features that are independent of the type of carcinogen and those that are agent-specific.

IONIZING RADIATION

Studies of the carcinogenic action of ionizing radiations have been carried out in humans,[1-12] experimental animals,[4,13-17] and in vitro cell systems.[18-21] The ability to determine or calculate absorbed doses of radiation and the knowledge of the effects at the molecular, chromosomal, cellular, tissue, and whole-body levels make ionizing radiation a remarkable tool for investigating the quantitative aspects and mechanisms of cancer induction.

Ionizing radiations have the characteristic of localized release of sufficient energy to break strong chemical bonds. The many types or qualities of radiation usually are divided into electromagnetic radiation, such as x-rays and γ-rays, and particulate radiation, including electrons, protons, neutrons, alpha particles, and heavy ions. Radiation can interact with biologic targets both directly and indirectly. Ionization of the atoms of the target may be caused directly, whereas in the so-called indirect effect radiation interacts with other molecules or atoms in the cell, especially water, producing free radicals that reach critical targets by diffusion. The rate at which energy is deposited is characteristic of the type of radiation and is called the linear energy transfer (LET). LET indicates an average rate of energy deposition at the micron level.

Exposure to sufficient doses of ionizing radiation may result in cancer induction. The susceptibility of tissue varies markedly, but all tissues appear to be at risk,[13,22] although not necessarily in relation to natural incidence. Because we all are exposed to radiation from natural and other sources, the issue of the dose-response relationships and risk estimates is important.

Humans have evolved in a radiation environment, but changes in that environment over time are not known precisely. The latest estimate by the National Council on Radiation Protection Measurements (NCRP) of the average annual effective dose equivalent from all sources in the U.S. population is about 3.6 milli-Sievert* (360 mrem).[23] About 82% of the total dose is from natural sources comprising cosmic rays, radionuclides, terrestrial γ-rays, and radon daughters (Fig. 9-1). About 40% of the total annual dose is considered to be due to radon daughters but with large individual variations. Most soils and rocks contain widely varying concentrations of uranium-238 and radium-226. The decay of radium-226 leads to release of radon into the surrounding water or air. The home is the major source of exposure to radon for the general population. Radon (radon-222) and

* Sievert (Sv) is the unit of dose equivalent in International Standard units. $Sv = 1\ J \cdot kg^{-1} = 100$ rem.

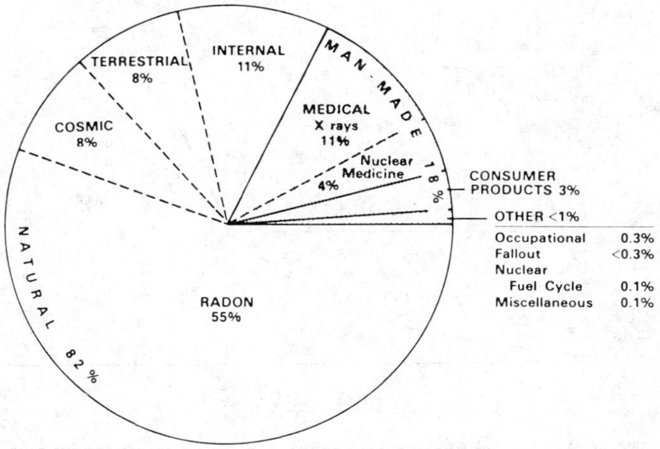

FIG. 9-1. Estimated contribution of various radiation sources to the total average effective dose equivalent in the U.S. population. The estimates of some of the contributing sources, for example, radon, have uncertainties on the order of a factor of two or three. (NCRP Report 93: Ionizing Radiation Exposure of the Population of the United States. Bethesda, MD, NCRP, 1987)

thoron (radon-220) emanate from the ground and building materials, disperse in the air, and decay into short-lived daughters or progeny that are isotopes of polonium, lead, and bismuth. The radon and thoron daughters attach to aerosol particles, and the alpha emitters are deposited with the particles in the tracheobronchial tree.[24,25] The concern is the risk of lung cancer from the high-LET radiation from the decay daughters such as polonium-218 and polonium-214.[24–26]

The potential exposure to radon varies markedly in different parts of the country, depending on geological features. An important variable is the level of thoron daughters, which is not measured separately in most assessments of populations exposure. It has been suggested that thoron can be a significant contributor to the lung dose,[27] but less by a factor of 3 than the exposure due to the progeny of radon-222.[25]

There is as yet no complete survey of indoor radon levels in the United States. Based on the uranium content of rock and soil, locations that have a potential for high indoor radon levels have been mapped and are widespread over the country. Obviously, houses built on reclaimed lands that have been mined and that have ores or soils near the surface may have significant radon levels. But houses in areas with no association of phosphate or uranium mining have also been found with radon at levels that remedial action is considered prudent, for example, in parts of the states of New York, New Jersey, and Pennsylvania.

The estimates of risk of excess lung cancer caused by exposure to radon are shown in Table 9-1. The estimates are based on epidemiologic studies of miners of uranium and of other underground miners.[2,24,25,27] The risk estimates vary with the assumptions made and the models used.

Current epidemiologic studies should establish whether or not living in homes in districts with high radon levels does, in fact, increase the risk of lung cancer. As is the case with some other lung carcinogens, smoking is an important cofactor. It is estimated that smokers exposed to radon have

TABLE 9-1. Estimates of Excess Lifetime Risk of Lung Cancer Mortality as a Result of Lifetime Exposure to Radon Daughters

Report, Year (Reference)	*Risk Estimate (deaths from lung cancer/ 10^6 person WLM)**
UNSCEAR, 1982 (27)	200–450
National Research Council (BEIR III) 1980 (2)	730
NCRP Report 77, 1984 (24)	130
National Research Council (BEIR IV), 1987 (25)	350

* Working level month (WLM): A unit of exposure to air concentrations of potential alpha energy released from radon daughters. One working level month is defined as the exposure to an average of 1 working level (a unit of air concentration of potential alpha energy released from radon and its daughters which has the energy release of 1.3×10^5 MeV/liter of air or 2.08×10^{-5} J/m^3) for a working month of 170 hours or 3.5×10^{-3} Jh/m^3.[24] Measurements of radon in homes are expressed in terms of picocuries (pCi) of radon per liter of air. Approximately 4 pCi/liter of radon equals 0.02 WL, and if 12 hours per day is spent in the home, the occupants would be exposed to about 0.5 WLM over a period of a year.

ten times the risk of lung cancer than nonsmokers similarly exposed.

It is estimated that 8% to 12% of houses across the nation may have annual average radon levels greater than 4 pCi/liter of air, which is considered by the Environmental Protection Agency to be the level at which remedial measures should be considered. A number of different remedial measures are being used, all based on two main principles: (1) stopping the entry of or diverting radon from the house, and (2) removing radon by increasing the rate of ventilation, especially in the basement. For smokers the best advice is to give up smoking. The evidence for an interaction between smoking and irradiation from alpha emitters and the associated increased risk of lung cancer is sufficient to be a warning.

Medical procedures contribute about 15% of the total annual effective dose equivalent, but again, individual doses vary markedly. About 250 million medical radiologic examinations are performed annually in the United States, and the average bone marrow dose has been estimated to be about 1 mSv (100 mrem).[23] With increasing use of techniques that provide more information and involve midplane doses of 1 to 3 rad,[28,29] the average dose may rise.

IONIZING RADIATION AND CANCER

HISTORICAL PERSPECTIVE

A causal relation between the exposure to radiation and cancer was suspected within 6 years of the discovery of roentgen rays.[30] Causal relations between carcinogenic agents and cancer in humans, even if suspected, usually take a long time to establish, mainly because of the long latent period between exposure and the appearance of the cancer.

The cancer that was observed first was skin cancer, not unusual in the early days of radiation, although the dose required to induce cancer of skin is in the hundreds of rads.

An association between radiation and leukemia was suspected some years later.[31] The information about radiation-induced leukemogenesis in humans[2,32–34] and animals is now extensive,[35–40] partly because the latent period for leukemia is shorter than that for solid cancers.

The induction of cancer in humans by radionuclides was suspected first by Martland in radium dial painters in 1931.[41] Osteosarcomas were detected first; later, carcinomas of the mastoid and nasal sinuses were seen.[42] Full accounts have been published of the early radiation workers[43] and of the early studies of radiation-induced cancer in humans and experimental animals.[44]

An increase in our understanding of the risks associated with radiation exposure and the effectiveness of protection[45,46] is underlined by the fact that the maximum permissible lifetime dose for radiation workers has been decreased by a factor of about 10 from 1936, when the level was about 2400 R. The basis of the past, current, and future protection standards has been reviewed recently,[47] and future trends have been outlined.[48] The major factors that influence the estimates of risk are listed in Table 9-2.

PHYSICAL FACTORS

RADIATION QUALITY

X-rays give rise to electrons that are energetic but that have a small mass and are sparsely ionizing. In contrast, alpha particles, with a greater mass and slower velocity, are densely ionizing. Exposures to equal doses of these different radiations do not have the same biologic effect. The relative biologic effectiveness (RBE)† of the high-LET radiations, such as alpha particles and neutrons, is greater than that of the low-LET radiations, such as x-rays and γ- rays. The induction of cancer is no exception. Experimental data suggest that the dose-response relationships are of the forms shown schematically in Figure 9-2. The initial linear slope of the dose-response curve for induction of tumors by high-LET radiation is markedly steeper than that for cobalt-60 γ-rays. The curve for low-LET radiation is initially linear but curves upward as the dose-squared (D^2) component of the response becomes

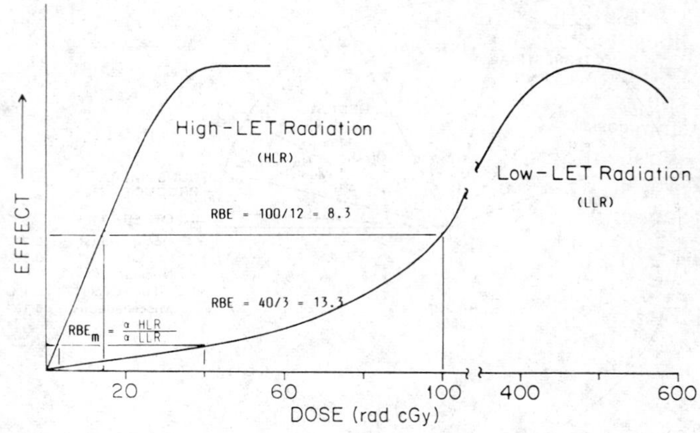

FIG. 9-2. Dose-response relationships for cancer induction by high- and low-LET radiation. Note inverse relationship of RBE to dose and the maximum RBE (RBE_m).

predominant. The curves for both high- and low-LET radiation bend over but at very different dose levels. It is suggested that the response curves bend over because cell killing reduces the probability of a cancer. However, especially in the case of high-LET radiation, other factors contribute to the complex shape.

RBE values, which are used to describe quantitatively the differences in effectiveness between different types of radiation, vary with dose, dose rate, fractionation, and the tissue involved. As can be seen from Figure 9-2, the RBE increases with decrease in dose down to dose levels at which both curves become linear and the RBE becomes maximum (RBE_m). RBE_m values derived from experimental animal studies are used in the selection of quality factors (Q) for the determination of dose equivalents for different types of radiation because there are no human data for radiations such as neutrons. In 1985 the International Commission on Radiological Protection recommended increasing the Q for neutrons from 10 to 20.[49]

DOSE AND DOSE RESPONSES

The ability to measure the absorbed dose of radiation is a great advantage to both the clinician and the experimenter. However, organ dose becomes a less useful measurement in experimental studies, especially with high-LET radiation at very low doses, because few of the cells will be traversed by particles. The measurement of interest is the absorbed energy in the cell traversed, which is not indicated by the absorbed dose in the tissue. Similarly, at the dimensions of interest in relation to targets (at the micrometer or nanometer level), mean absorbed dose and dose–rate become inappropriate. Another example of the problem is the high dose that is localized in tissue at the sites of deposition of energy from alpha emitters in either the lung or bone. In the case of high-LET particles, both fluence and track structure become essential to the understanding of the relationship of energy deposition and biologic effects. The reader is referred to expert reviews for details of the current concepts of dose and microdosimetry.[50–53]

† A ratio of the absorbed dose of a reference radiation, conventionally x-rays but in practice often γ rays, to the absorbed dose of a test radiation to produce the same level of biological effect.

TABLE 9-2. Factors that Influence the Estimate of Risk for Radiation-Induced Cancer

Physical	*Biological*	*Analytical*
Radiation quality	Genetic factors	Choice of:
Dose	Age	Models for dose response
Dose rate	Sex	Projection models
Fractionation	Radionuclide	Absolute risk
	Metabolism	Relative risk

Three dose-response relationships — linear, quadratic, and linear-quadratic (LQ) — usually are considered relevant, and estimates based on these models have been compared. The aim of protection standards has been well served by the simplest approach, the linear, no-threshold model, but its simplicity ignores the biology. However, the understanding of the dose deposition of radiation and the mechanism of carcinogenesis is not adequate for formulating precise dose-response models. There is not a single form of dose response for carcinogenesis, and the differences reflect differences in the mechanisms. End points, such as chromosomal aberrations that may be associated intimately with carcinogenesis,[54–56] can be described by a linear-quadratic model,[57–59] but radiation-induced cancer involves many factors.[17,60,61] Factors involved in the probability of a cancer being induced include whether or not (1) the targets required for malignant transformation are hit, (2) the transformation events are repaired, (3) the initiated cell survives, and (4) the expression of the initiated cell occurs.

Molecular studies suggest that at least two gene loci on different chromosomes are involved in transformation which is indicative of a large target.[62] A large target is consistent with mechanisms involving chromosome breaks and translocation.[5]

Dose-response curves for incidence of cancer as a function of dose reflect expression as well as initiation. Carcinogenesis usually is considered multistage although there is no obvious requirement for further direct effects on the target cell after initiation, since single exposures to radiation can induce cancer. On the other hand, events involving host factors that in turn alter tissue environment, such as cell–cell interactions,[63] or systemic factors such as hormone levels, or immune capability play an important role and must be considered.[17,60] Models of dose responses should take into account the time-dependent changes in both initiation and expression.[17]

DOSE RATE AND FRACTIONATION

Reductions in dose rate reduce the carcinogenic effect of low-LET radiation both in animals and in in vitro cell systems.[64–67] The reduction may be marked but varies among tumor types, presumably because the mechanisms of carcinogenesis also vary. Reductions in effect are predicted by models of carcinogenesis that involve interaction of lesions or that allow for repair. With low dose rates, the number of tracks per cell does not change, but the probability of interactions between two tracks is diminished. Similarly, with a spatial relationship of two tracks suitable for interaction but separated in time, repair may occur and abrogate interaction. Time is biologically important, and extending the time over which exposure occurs influences a number of responses. With sufficiently low dose rates or low doses, no interactions should occur, and the response will be single track in form and described by $E = \tilde{\alpha}D$, where D = dose and $\tilde{\alpha}$ is an empirically determined coefficient.

Experimental data for many high dose rate, low-LET radiation-induced tumors can be fitted by a linear-quadratic dose-response model. Such a dose response suggests that the slope of the responses to low dose rates and multiple small fractions will be equivalent to the linear component of the linear-quadratic response. It can be seen from Figure 9-3 that experimental data for two tumors with markedly different dose responses (note the differences in the dose scales) support the basis of the linear-quadratic model. When the dose per fraction is within the dose range over which the linear component of the linear-quadratic response is predominant, the dose response is linear and the slope is equivalent to that after low dose exposures.[68]

Fractionation of doses can take many forms. The simplest, splitting the dose into two fractions (a technique used widely to study repair), reduces the carcinogenic effect in skin.[68,69] On the other hand, suitably spaced multiple fractions at a certain dose level greatly increase the probability that thymic lymphoma will develop. The effects of fractionation on in vitro malignant transformation appear to depend on the choice of dose per fraction.[70–72]

Protraction of exposures over a long period may reduce the effect both because of the reduced dose rate and because, with age, the susceptibility decreases. An exception to the sparing effect of protraction is the apparent requirement for protracted exposures to induce myeloproliferative disease in dogs.[40] It is not known whether protraction allows exposure to the high total doses required without death from marrow damage or whether repeated radiation-induced lesions ensure expression of leukemia.

It has not been possible to establish unequivocally that lowering dose rates reduces the carcinogenic effect in

FIG. 9-3. **A.** Incidence of lung cancer in BALB/c mice as a function of dose after single high dose-rate exposures to γ-rays (●—●), and after 2 × 1 Gy (△), 4 × 0.5 Gy (▲), 20 × 0.1 Gy (■) fractions. Low dose-rate exposures (○—○) are also shown. **B.** Incidence of breast cancer after single high dose–rate exposures to γ rays (●—●) and after 5 × 0.05 Gy (◇) and 25 × 0.01 Gy (□). The low dose-rate data are indicated (○—○). Note that the dose scales vary by a factor of 8. (Adapted from Ullrich RL et al: Radiation carcinogenesis: Time-dose relationships. Radiat Res 111:179–184, 1987)

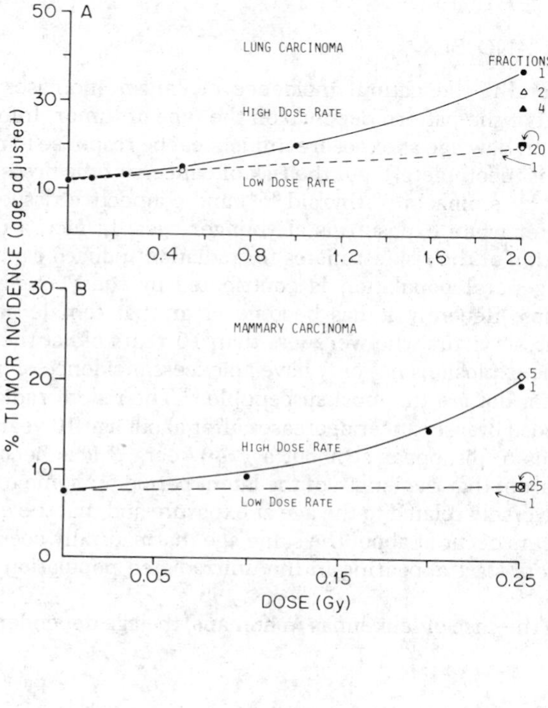

humans, but unless our current understanding of the biophysics and biology of induction of DNA lesions and repair is very wrong, it must be so.

In contrast, not only is the effect of high-LET irradiation not reduced by lowering the dose rate, but, in the case of induction of mammary tumors in mice[73] and malignant transformation in vitro,[74] low dose rate exposures appear to be more effective than single acute exposures.

GENETIC FACTORS

The strain-dependent differences in both natural and radiation-induced incidences of cancer in mice attest to the importance of inherited factors. Evidence has suggested that retroviruses are involved, but it is not clear that the distribution of oncogenes is strain and species dependent. Inherited susceptibility may also be related to host factors that influence expression rather than initiation.

The cells of patients with several human genetic diseases have been shown to be hypersensitive to killing in vitro by ionizing radiation.[75–78] It has been found that cells from individuals with hereditary cutaneous melanoma and familial dysplastic nevus syndrome (FDNS) have an increased sensitivity for induction of chromatid aberrations in G_2.[79] Of particular interest is the finding of the increased sensitivity before clinical expression of the FDNS trait in individuals with FDNS who have increased susceptibility for radiation-induced cancer. The risk of cancer also is elevated in some genetic conditions, for example, ataxia-telangiectasia,[80] but no clear-cut association with an increased susceptibility to induction of cancer by radiation has been established. An important and as yet unanswered question is whether the heterozygotic state of any of the genetic disorders carries an increased risk.

Second cancers in patients treated with radiation for cancer in childhood have a distinct pattern that is related to the type of primary tumor, which suggests a genetically determined susceptibility.

AGE AND SEX

Generally, the natural incidence of cancer increases with age, but the pattern depends on the type of tumor. Information on how age at exposure influences the response to radiation is incomplete,[81] but the risk of cancers of the breast,[10,82] lung,[3,10] stomach,[3,10] thyroid,[83,84] and connective tissues[85] is greater when exposure is at younger ages. In fact, a major fraction of the risk estimates for radiation-induced cancer in the general population is contributed by the younger age groups. Recently it has become clear that female atomic bomb survivors who were less than 10 years old at the time of the explosions not only have an excess incidence of breast cancer but are the most susceptible.[82] The risk of radiation-induced breast cancer decreases after about age 10 years and seems to disappear at about age 40 years.[10] It is becoming apparent that the length of the latent period for some tumors is inversely related to the age at exposure and that the excess cancers occur at about the same age that naturally occurring tumors start appearing in the unirradiated population (Fig. 9-4).[86]

In the case of leukemias in humans, the age dependency of susceptibility is more complex.[87] The risk of leukemia was greater in 50-year-old patients with ankylosing spondylitis than in patients less than 25 years old.[87] In the atomic bomb survivors, the risk of acute leukemias was high in those exposed at a young age, less in those exposed at age 20 to 50 years, and again high in those older than 50 years at the time of the explosion.[3,10]

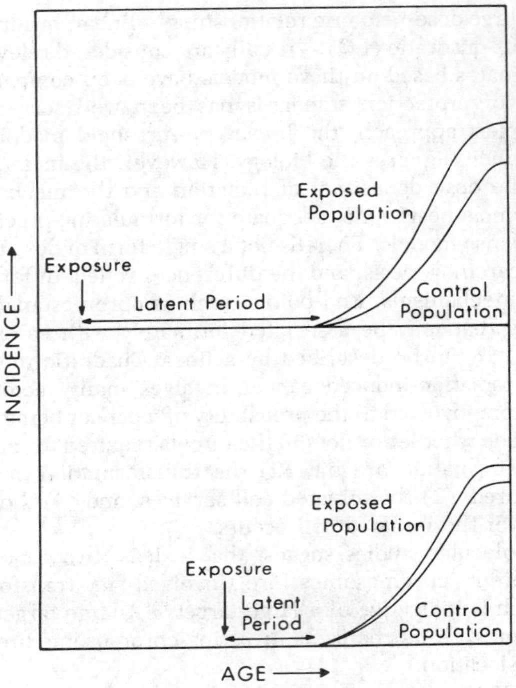

FIG. 9-4. Illustration of inverse relationship of length of latent period with age at exposure found for some cancers, particularly breast cancer. Note greater susceptibility for cancer induction with exposures at a young age compared with exposure at older ages.

Solid cancers induced by radiation tend not to appear until the age at which the naturally occurring cancer is seen. Therefore, the latent period will be longer when exposure is early in life. This suggests that age-dependent host factors are most important and that the expression of cells initiated in the young is suppressed until the necessary host changes occur. If cancer is a multistage process, then the age dependency of the effect of radiation will depend on whether the early or late stages are the most affected. If the number of cells that have gone through some of the multiple stages of the cancer process increases with age and if radiation acts at a late stage, then the absolute effect would increase with age at exposure.[88] The finding for ankylosing spondylitis is consistent with this idea.

The question of the risk of cancer induction when the exposure is prenatal is still in dispute, although the use of ultrasonography has made it clinically irrelevant.

The risk of radiation-induced cancer is estimated to be 30% to 50% greater in women than men.[1] The difference can be accounted for by sex-specific tumors, particularly those in the breast, which appears to be a susceptible tissue. Thyroid cancer after radiation exposure may also occur with higher frequency in women than in men.[83] On the other hand, male atomic bomb survivors appear to have been at greater risk of leukemia than female survivors.

PROJECTION MODELS

Estimates of risk are expressed either in absolute or relative terms. The absolute risk is the added risk caused by irradiation and is expressed as the number of radiation-related cancers in an exposed population per unit time per unit dose (1 cancer/10^6 persons/year/rad). When such risk estimates are used, the number of years of excess risk should be provided. For persons of similar ages at exposure, absolute risk = $a + bd$, where a is the risk of the specific cancer in the control population, b is the excess risk per rad, and d is the dose in rad. The relative risk is the ratio between the risk in the irradiated population and the risk in the nonirradiated population, and is expressed as a multiple of the natural risk. Such a model assumes that the risk resulting from radiation is determined by the natural incidence and that radiation acts in a multiplicative manner.

The models are illustrated in Figure 9-5. It is apparent that neither model applies to all radiation-induced cancers and that the models are simplistic but useful. The importance of projection models is indicated by the fact that the major source of data for radiation risk estimates is the atomic bomb survivors and that more than 60% of the survivors are still alive. To estimate radiation risks for the U.S. population from such data, projections both in time and across populations must be made.

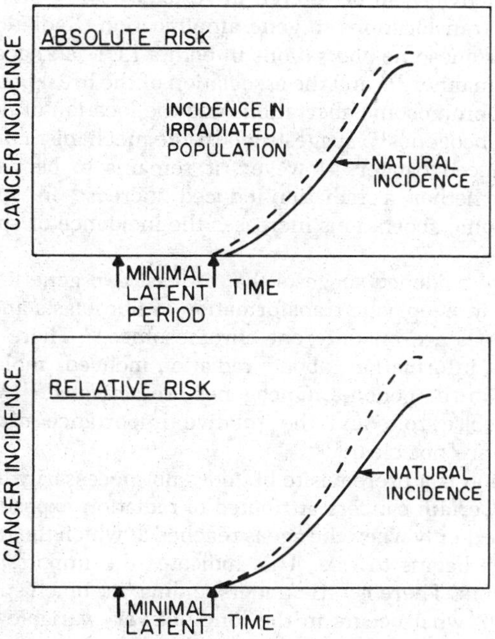

FIG. 9-5. Absolute and relative risk models used in the estimation and projection of risks. The time between exposure to radiation and the time that the specific cancers appear in excess of the natural incidence is indicated, but for some tumors the length of the latent period is age-dependent.

RISK ESTIMATES

Sensible protection standards depend on reliable risk estimates. Despite the breadth of available information, some of the steps in risk estimation still depend on judgment, for example, the choice of a dose-response model and Q values for high-LET radiation. Improvement in the risk estimates will come, as data accumulate and insights develop, from further understanding of mechanisms.

Risk estimates for the induction of cancer by low-LET radiation are based on the human experience. The atomic bomb survivors are the major source of data for high dose-rate whole-body exposure. The doses at Hiroshima and Nagasaki have been reassessed, a major undertaking that is now coming to completion. The new doses indicate that the neutron component was much less than originally thought. The neutron doses are now so low that direct estimates of the effectiveness of neutrons will at best be difficult and at worst impossible to make. The organ doses, except for some surface tissues such as the breast, have not changed markedly. It is likely that any changes in risk estimates will result from the increasing cancer mortality data as the population of atomic bomb survival ages. More than 57,000 of the 91,228 persons in the current Life Span Study are still alive.[11] Almost 7,000 died of cancer between 1950 and 1985. It is estimated that the excess of cancer deaths due to radiation in this population is about 8%.

The estimate of excess risk of radiation-induced leukemia based on the new dosimetry (DS86) and the mortality data for the years 1950 to 1985 is 2.91 per 10^4 person-year Gray (PYGy), compared to 1.75 per 10^4 PYGy with the previous dosimetry (T65D).[11] These estimates are averaged over six categories of sex and age at time of exposure and assume an RBE of 10. The estimates of excess cancer rates for various organs, based on mortality data for 1950 to 1982 and assuming T65D doses, are shown in Figure 9-6.[10]

Risk estimates based on data from all relevant sources were reported in 1985.[8,89] However, the new risk estimates are expected in 1988 when the United Nations Scientific Committee on Effects of Atomic Radiation (UNSCEAR) and the National Academy of Sciences (Biological Effects of Ionizing Radiation V) complete their current deliberations. Not only must the new DS86 dosimetry and updated data from Hiroshima and Nagasaki and other studies be taken into account, but also RBE values, dose-response relationships, and projection models. In the case of the latter, it has become increasingly clear that relative risk is the appropriate model for most solid cancers.[2,90] Not surprisingly, incidence rates are higher and are the appropriate index for tumor induction in organs such as the thyroid.

The recent accidents at Chernobyl in the Soviet Union, Juarez, Mexico, and Goiania, Brazil add impetus to improving estimates of risk.

RADIOLOGIC RISKS

More than 90% of the annual dose received from man-made radiation sources is from medical diagnostic procedures.[23] The differences in the reported organ doses are great and depend on the type of examination and on the techniques; UNSCEAR has reported that doses range from 0.01 to 5 rad

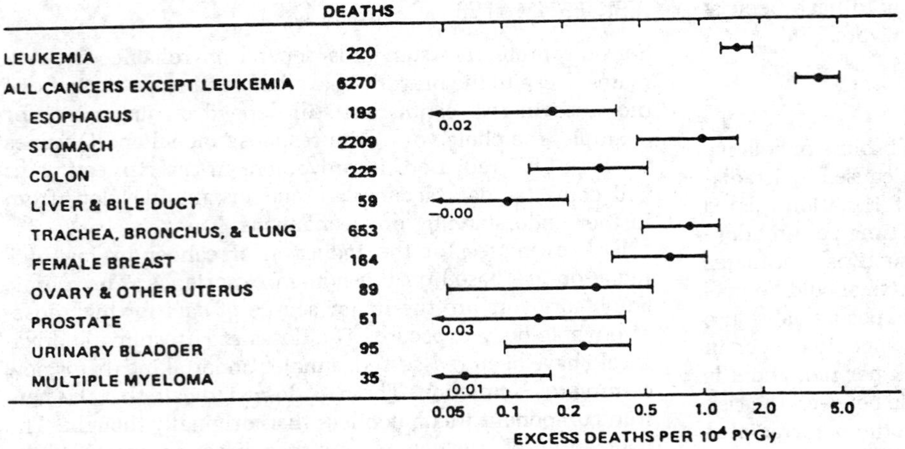

FIG. 9-6. The maximum likelihood estimates and 90% confidence limits for average absolute excess risk of radiation-induced cancer mortality at selected sites in atomic bomb survivors. The estimates are derived from a linear model adjusted for city (Hiroshima or Nagasaki), sex, age at time of exposure, and time since exposure, and are expressed in person-years per Gray (PYGy) (Preston DL et al: Studies of the mortality of A-bomb survivors: 8. Cancer Mortality, 1950–1982. Radiat Res 111:151–178, 1987)

(0.1–50 mGy).[91] The benefit of well-selected procedures is clear, but approaches to reduce exposures make sense.[92] About 250 million diagnostic x-ray examinations are carried out each year, and there has been concern about the risk from routine examinations or methods that result in the accumulation of high doses.[92] There are no direct estimates of cancer induction at very low doses, and the estimates of risk are a matter of judgment. Based on reported radiologic procedures, Harwood and Yaffe estimated the total risk of cancer induction from a diagnostic examination as about $1:10^6$ per year, and small in comparison to the benefit.[93] They exempted barium enema examinations and positive mode mammography from this estimate because of the higher dose with the barium enema examination and the suspected susceptibility of the breast to radiation in positive mode mammography. Evans et al[94] concluded from a study of 75,000 patients that 1% of all cases of leukemia and 0.7% of all cases of breast cancer might be attributed to diagnostic radiography. These figures are probably overestimates. The majority of radiologic examinations are performed on patients who are older than 40 years, and the cancers that the authors considered radiation-induced occurred late in life.

The question of the use of routine x-ray mammography has focused attention on the balance of risk and benefit. In the late 1970s there was concern that the risk of annual mammography in women aged 35 to 49 years might be greater than the benefit. The doses involved in mammography have been reduced since then, and it also has been shown that the risk of radiation-induced breast cancer decreases markedly with age.[82]

Risk estimates of breast cancer have been based on a linear no-threshold dose-response relationship, but this has been questioned recently.[95] If the dose response is, in fact, curvilinear, radiation risk estimates may be adjusted downward. In any case, the current practice of selecting patients for mammography based on age and family history is appropriate.

The use of ultrasonography has made the issue of the risk of exposure in utero of more academic than practical interest. Cancer occurs as a secondary effect of radiation therapy both for benign[7,9,12,96–103] and malignant disease.[5,6,12,104,105] Leukemia is more frequent after chemotherapy than after radiation therapy.[106,107] There are marked differences in susceptibility between organs. For many sites the risk of radiation-induced cancer decreases with age. Conversely, the risk is highest in childhood. Brain tumors have been reported recently in children exposed to 1 Gy.[103] In the case of skin treated with x-rays, subsequent exposure to sunlight[97] or PUVA[108] increases the risk of skin cancer.

The use of magnetic resonance imaging (MRI) has increased and in the future may result in a reduction in the use of diagnostic x-rays. There have been no extensive studies of possible late effects of MRI, but risk of cancer seems unlikely.

MECHANISM OF RADIATION CARCINOGENESIS

A major attraction to the idea that activation of cellular oncogenes is central to initiation of malignant transformation is that it provides a paradigm for explaining a common pathway of effects of very different agents.[109,110]

Gene activity can be altered in various ways, from chromosome translocations to gene amplification. Radiation induces chromosome aberrations in both a LET- and dose-dependent manner,[111] and the association of the breakpoints of specific chromosome aberrations and the location of human cellular oncogenes[112] suggests a possible mechanism of radiation-induced cancer. However, it remains to be demonstrated whether a radiation-induced increase in specific chromosome aberrations increases the incidence of specific cancers.

Current evidence suggests that at least two gene loci are involved in neoplastic transformation of fibroblasts and that these genes are on different chromosomes.[62] There is increasing information about radiation-induced molecular changes in the genome. Oncogenes are activated,[113,114] but their precise role and the relative importance of other changes are not clear.[115]

Initiation is a prerequisite but does not necessarily lead to cancer. Certain cancers attributed to radiation exposure become overt only when the age is reached at which the natural incidence begins to rise. This indicates the importance of host factors. There is little understanding but much speculation about what occurs in the long but very variable latent periods. In some tissues, potential cancer cells may lie dormant for years. In other tissues, cancer may involve a multistep process that includes further mutations and selection. Clearly, different factors are involved in the mechanisms of different types of cancer, especially in the expression stages. In certain tumors, secondary or host factors are the most important determining factors.

ULTRAVIOLET RADIATION CARCINOGENESIS

Skin cancer is by far the most common cancer among whites in the United States. About 400,000 cases of basal cell or squamous cell carcinoma occur each year.[116] Basal cell carcinomas are four times more frequent than squamous cell carcinomas in men; the same ratio in women is 6 : 1.[116] Both types of cancer are found more frequently in men than in women and about 70 times more frequently in whites than in blacks.[116] The cancers usually occur on areas exposed to sunlight, and at higher rates in southern latitudes of the United States. The incidence, mainly of basal cell carcinoma, is increasing, but fortunately the cure rate is above 95%. The marked increase in the incidence of melanoma in developed nations is of greater concern because of the higher mortality rate than in nonmelanoma skin cancer.[117] The evidence for a causal relationship between ultraviolet radiation (UVR) and melanoma is not as watertight as that for nonmelanoma skin cancer but is compelling.[118,119]

Depletion of stratospheric ozone has been a matter of concern for almost 20 years. First, it was feared that supersonic airplanes would inject nitrogen oxides into the stratosphere, resulting in depletion of ozone.[120–122] More recently, the increasing level of chlorofluorocarbons has been suspected as a possible cause of the decrease of ozone in the stratosphere.[123–124] Measurements by the Total Ozone Spectrometer on Nimbus 7 during spring in the Antarctic indicate that the ozone levels have fallen as much as 4%,[125,126] and a "hole" in the ozone layer has appeared. The possibility of a more global reduction has renewed the concern that an increase in skin cancer may result. A recent study of the National Aeronautical and Space Agency concluded that ozone levels have fallen 1% to 3% in the latitudes from Florida to Canada.

The stratospheric ozone layer acts as a highly effective absorbing layer that prevents the most biologically effective wavelengths of UVR, especially UVB (280–320 nm), from reaching humans. Any increase in UVB fluences on Earth would increase the probability of skin cancer. A 1% decrease in stratospheric ozone could result in about a 2% increase in the amount of UVB reaching Earth. It has been estimated that each 1% decrease in ozone might cause about a 4% increase in nonmelanoma cancer. An important question is whether or not the incidence of melanoma would be increased. Scotto et al[127] suggest that there will likely be an increase in the more southern latitudes, and that the increase in melanoma may appear earlier than the predicted increase in nonmelanoma skin cancer. Such a suggestion depends on the validity of the causal relationship between melanoma and UVR. A correlation between the incidence of melanoma and sunspot activity has been claimed,[128] but the study did not take into account the length of the latent period for melanoma induction. The stratospheric changes caused by cyclic changes in sunspot activity are complex and a number of factors, perhaps relevant to skin cancer, vary; for example, galactic cosmic rays can change ozone levels.

Perhaps some comfort may be taken from the report that no increase of UVB was detected between 1974 and 1985 at the various monitoring stations that span the United States from North Dakota to Florida.[127] This finding suggests that ozone depletion may not be as global as feared, or that the attenuation of UVB radiation is more complex than was previously thought. The effect of current levels of chlorofluorocarbons on stratospheric ozone will not be detected for some years. Only time and accurate surveillance will reveal the long-term trend.

HISTORIC PERSPECTIVE

Astute clinical observations were the first stage in understanding the relationship of sunlight to skin cancer in men involved in maritime and outdoor occupations. The association of exposure to greater intensities of sunlight and skin cancer strengthened the evidence that sunlight was a major etiologic factor.[129]

In 1928, it was demonstrated that UVR induced skin cancer in experimental animals[130]; later, the carcinogenic effect was found to be restricted to wavelengths shorter than 320 nm.[131]

MECHANISMS OF UVR CARCINOGENESIS

The evidence that the induction of skin cancer by UVR results in UVR-induced DNA damage is considerable. For example, (1) the action spectra for neoplastic transformation[132] and anchorage-independent growth[133] are similar to those for the induction of cyclobutane pyrimidine dimers; (2) enzymatic photoreactivation of UVR-induced pyrimidine dimers suppresses the induction of in vitro transformation of human fibroblasts,[134] the induction of thyroid neoplasia in fish,[135] and induction of sarcomas in the corneas of opossums[136]; and (3) the cells of patients with Xeroderma pigmentosum, who have a marked susceptibility to melanoma and nonmelanoma skin cancer, lack the ability to repair UVR-induced DNA damage.[137] Although cyclobutane pyrimidine dimers appear to be the pertinent molecular lesion for UVR-induced cancer, the role of other photoproducts, such as pyrimidine-pyrimidine (6-4) photoproduct, may be important.

In humans and experimental animals, protracted or multiple exposures with high total fluences of UVR usually are required to produce carcinomas of the skin. The question is whether the later exposures influence the expression of the changes initiated by the early exposures, and if so, how? It can be seen from Figure 9-7 that the dose–response curve for the experimental induction of skin cancer has an apparent threshold, but that threshold can be altered by treatment with the promoter tissue plasminogen activator (TPA). These results suggest that UVR initiates many cells that do not develop into cancer. There is now a renewed interest in the role of immune surveillance that might explain the apparent suppression of initiated cells.[138,139] It is suggested that

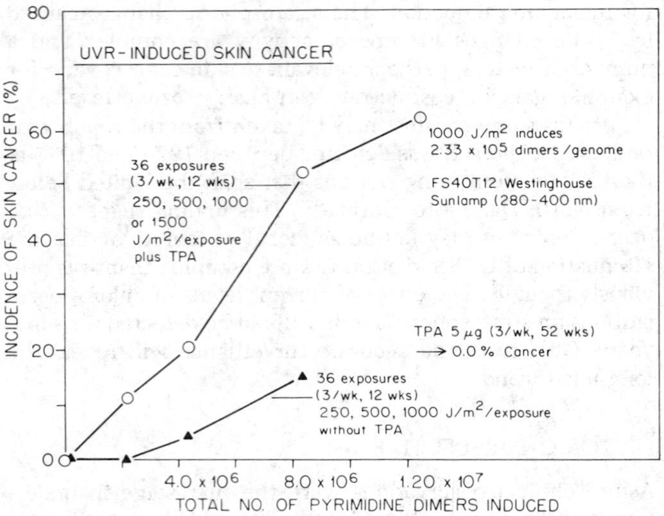

FIG. 9-7. Incidence of squamous cell carcinoma as a function of the number of cyclobutane pyrimidine dimers induced by exposure to UVR (280–400 nm) (▲—▲), and exposure to UVR followed by treatment with 5 μg TPA for 1 year after the end of the UVR regimen (O—O).

UVR affects Langerhans' cells, which are antigen-presenting cells in the epidermis and the most superficial sentinel of the immune system. These effects result in the development of suppressor T-lymphocytes that interfere with the rejection of the tumors.[138]

People are protected from the sequelae of UVR-induced damage by two distinct types of mechanisms. First, pigment, hair, and skin thickness all reduce the absorbed dose. In people of Celtic background, pigmentation is not distributed evenly in the skin, and skin cancer is common. Second, human cells repair UVR-induced DNA damage with great fidelity. This capability is reduced markedly in patients with xeroderma pigmentosum.[137]

XERODERMA PIGMENTOSUM

Xeroderma pigmentosum is a ubiquitous autosomal recessive disease with a frequency of about 1:250,000 in the United States and Europe but reportedly higher in countries such as Egypt and Japan.[140–142] The disease was first described by Hebra and Kaposi 120 years ago.[143] Homozygotes occur more frequently in families of consanguineous marriages, and males and females are equally affected.[140] The disease is characterized by a hypersensitivity to sunlight associated with a marked susceptibility to skin cancer, including melanoma, except in Japan.[141] Almost 50% of patients with xeroderma pigmentosum in the United States, Europe, and Japan also have neurologic abnormalities, but few have all the lesions that are characteristic of the de Sanctis–Cacchione syndrome.[141] Various ocular lesions such as cloudiness of the cornea, pigmentation, and telangiectasia of the conjunctiva have been considered part of the syndrome since the entity was first recognized.[140,141] The description of the early cases concentrated on the degenerative and pigmentation changes as well as telangiectasia,[143,144] and it was not until 1932 that de Sanctis and Cacchione reported the associated neurologic abnormalities.[145] Both the genetic aspects and the possible role of sunlight in xeroderma pigmentosum were noted by Hebra and Kaposi.[143] As early as 1929, it was suggested that the xeroderma pigmentosum trait might be an essential characteristic of persons who developed skin cancer.[146] The parents of patients with xeroderma pigmentosum are heterozygotes and clinically normal.[141] There has been no consistent evidence that the cells of persons heterozygous for the syndrome were significantly defective in DNA repair. However, although it has been suggested that heterozygotes are at a higher risk for skin cancer,[147] the evidence indicates that the gene for xeroderma pigmentosum must be in the homozygous state to result in the clinical syndrome.

In 1968 Cleaver described the finding of defective excision repair of UVR-induced damage in fibroblasts cultured from the skin of xeroderma pigmentosum patients.[148] Thus began the exciting search for a causal relation between a specific DNA lesion and cancer.

No longer is xeroderma pigmentosum thought to be a disease involving a single defect in DNA repair; rather, there is a complex interrelationship of different repair systems, their genetics, and enzymology. The studies of fusing cells from different xeroderma pigmentosum patients with normal cells have revealed the genetic heterogeneity in the syndrome.[149–151] Seven complementation groups (A to G) have been identified that are deficient in excision repair, which implies the involvement of seven genes. An eighth group, known as variant, shows no CNS abnormalities or the characteristic sensitivity to sunlight.[152–154] However, the cells are more susceptible to UVR-induced mutation than are normal cells.[155]

The important molecular defect of cells of the xeroderma pigmentosum variant is reflected in the interruption of replication forks during semiconservative DNA synthesis after exposure to UVR. An examination of the comparative survival of UV-irradiated cells and the clinical conditions in the eight groups indicated that the occurrence of neurologic abnormalities correlates with the severity of the repair defect.[137] A normal karyotype and normal frequency of sister chromatid exchanges are the usual findings in xeroderma pigmentosum cells,[137,156] although abnormalities have been reported in cells from patients of the complementation groups C and D.[157] However, after exposure to UVR or certain chemical carcinogens, both chromosome aberrations and sister chromatid exchanges are increased more than in similarly exposed normal cells.[158–161]

A new form of xeroderma pigmentosum has been reported recently.[162] A family that demonstrated an apparent dominant inheritance of a DNA repair defect with skin cancer also had two members with defective DNA repair but free of cancers. This family is just one more demonstration that a causal relation between defective DNA repair and cancer is far from clear-cut.

FOREIGN BODY CARCINOGENESIS

NONFIBER FOREIGN BODIES

The introduction of foreign material that is not biodegradable usually stimulates a connective tissue or mesothelial reaction. The characteristics of the reaction depend on the final site of the foreign body. In the case of scars and tissue reactions around schistosomal eggs or tubercular lesions, the foreign body reactions have some probability of neoplastic change. Because the reaction frequently involves connective tissues, sarcomas of various types are the tumors that usually arise, but carcinomas also have been found in relation to foreign bodies. The incidental observation that Bakelite disks[163] and cellophane[164] caused sarcomas opened up an area of research with many facets, reviewed by Bischoff and Bryson[165] and Brand.[166]

Central to sarcomagenesis are the size and shape of the implants: the same materials in a powdered or porous form lose most of their tumorigenicity.[165,166] Within limits, the greater the surface area, the greater is the probability of tumors.[166] The chemical nature of the implants is not a predominant determinant of the development of the capsules and tumors because pure carbon disks produce sarcomas. Perforations, even without a reduction in surface area, reduce the incidence of sarcoma. However, the tumor incidence and latency are influenced by the physicochemical properties of the implants; latency is especially influenced by the smoothness and durability of the surface of the implant.[165,166]

The susceptibility to this form of carcinogenesis is species- and strain-dependent but age-independent.[165–167] Foreign body sarcomas are rare in humans but can be induced easily in some rodents. The events that occur from insertion of disks to the development of sarcomas have been fully documented, but the precise mechanism of neoplastic change is unknown.[168] Because chromosome abnormalities are a consistent finding,[168] the application of the new techniques of molecular biology and chromosome analysis should be rewarding.

When a ^{90}Sr-^{90}Y source is incorporated into laminated mylar disks, the radiation advances the time of appearance and increases the incidence of sarcomas in rats.[169] This type of experiment is an in vivo version of the currently popular in vitro radiation transformation experiments.

FIBER CARCINOGENESIS

Tobacco smoke remains the most important cause of lung cancer, but asbestos exposures account for 4000 to 6000 lung cancers and about 2000 cases of mesothelioma per year in the United States[170] and a comparable number of cancers in Great Britain.[171] Fortunately, in the future the number of cases should decrease because industrial and environmental exposures have been markedly reduced.

Although asbestos has dominated the research in fiber carcinogenesis because of its importance as an industrial and environmental carcinogen,[170,172–173] other types of fibers have biologic effects and have been classified by Leineweber into (1) man-made vitreous fibers, (2) synthetic crystalline fibers, and (3) natural mineral fibers.[174] The group of natural mineral fibers includes zeolites, the cause of a high incidence of cancer in parts of Turkey.[175] Omenn et al provide a detailed classification of fibers, some of which have replaced asbestos.[176] The concern is whether or not fibers that differ chemically from asbestos but are physically similar to it will prove carcinogenic. Reliable bioassays are needed in order to predict and prevent potential risks of the newer fibers.

ASBESTOS

A group of hydrated silicates have a fibrous crystalline structure known commercially as asbestos. There are two major classes of asbestos: the amphiboles, which include crocidolite, and the serpentines, which include chrysotile, the most widely used form of asbestos in the United States.

Because the tissue response to fibers is a fibrous reaction, there is the risk of neoplastic change, and the carcinogenic properties of at least one member of all three classes of fibers listed in the preceding paragraph have been shown. It is thought that chrysotile is less likely to cause pleural mesotheliomas than other asbestiform fibers, and it is not correlated with peritoneal mesothelioma.[176]

Physical characteristics such as length and diameter are more important determinants of carcinogenicity than is the chemical composition.[176–178] Studies have indicated that fibers that are carcinogenic tend to be longer than about 8 μm and less than 1.50 μm in diameter.[178]

Asbestos workers have an increased risk of developing mesothelioma and cancer at a number of sites, especially the lung.[170] Mesothelioma is pathognomonic of fiber carcinogenesis, particularly asbestos.[170,176] These tumors arise from the mesothelial surfaces of the pleura and peritoneum and have a pleomorphic histologic appearance. The tumors spread over the pleural and peritoneal surfaces, do not invade the underlying tissues deeply, but do metastasize.

Large numbers of people have been exposed to asbestos industrially or environmentally. Whether the widespread contamination by small amounts of fibers poses a hazard remains to be determined. It is still not known how the risk of mesothelioma is related to the amount of exposure and the different types of asbestos fiber, but the amount and the route of exposure appear to influence the site at which mesothelioma occurs. The importance of the type of exposure in relation to the occupation is illustrated by the finding that most mesotheliomas were pleural in shipyard workers but were peritoneal in asbestos factory workers. Lung cancer is the most common tumor caused by asbestos. The observed rate of lung cancer in asbestos insulation workers was four times that expected.[170] Chrysotile, amosite, anthophyllite, and crocidolite fibers have been implicated. A multiplicative effect of exposure to tobacco increases the risk of lung cancer in asbestos workers four to five times that of the nonsmoker.[179]

The latent period appears to correlate positively with the level of exposure and negatively with the age at first exposure. There is uncertainty about the appropriate models for risk estimates. It has been assumed that the dose responses for both mesotheliomas and lung cancer are linear. An absolute risk model is appropriate for mesothelioma. Death rates for mesothelioma in asbestos workers with protracted exposures appear to be proportional to the third or fourth power of the time from first exposure "irrespective of age, site, fiber type or dust level."[180] In the case of lung cancer a relative risk model is considered more appropriate.

Although the mechanism of induction of cancer by fibers remains a mystery, some progress has been made. It has been shown that asbestos and glass fibers are phagocytized by cells in culture and accumulate in the perinuclear region of the cytoplasm. Cells appear to selectively phagocytose the longer fibers, with the shorter fibers accumulating on the cell surface.[181] The cellular effects, from cell killing to transformation, depend on the fibers taken up by the cells.[182] In Syrian hamster embryo cells in culture, asbestos fibers induce a dose-dependent increase in micronuclei and chromosome aberrations.[182] Both chromosome aberrations and malignant transformation are induced by decreasing the length of the fibers.[182] This and other evidence suggests a correlation between the induction of chromosome aberrations and malignant transformation.[183-185] Aneuploidy is a consistent finding,[183] as it is in the early stages of other types of tumors. In experiments using the C3H 10T1/2 established cell lines, asbestos fibers were found to be cytotoxic in a dose-dependent manner but were ineffective for the induction of malignant transformation.[186] However, the combined treatment with asbestos fibers and γ radiation had a greater than additive effect on the induction of oncogenic transformation.[186]

This chapter has been authored by a contractor of the U.S. government under contract No. DE-AC05-840R21400. Accordingly, the U.S. government retains a nonexclusive, royalty-free license to publish or reproduce the published form of the contribution, or allow others to do so, for U.S. government purposes.

Research was sponsored by the Office of Health and Environmental Research, U.S. Department of Energy, under contract DE-AC05-840R21400 with the Martin Marietta Energy Systems, Inc.

It is a pleasure to acknowledge the valuable help of Mrs. F. Young.

REFERENCES

1. United Nations Scientific Committee on Effects of Atomic Radiation: Sources and Effects of Ionizing Radiation. 1977 Report to the General Assembly with Annexes, New York, United Nations, 1977
2. National Research Council, Committee on the Biological Effects of Ionizing Radiation (BEIR): The Effects on Populations of Exposure to Low Levels of Ionizing Radiation. Washington, DC, National Academy Press, 1980
3. Wakabayashi T, Kato H, Ikeda T et al: Studies of the mortality of A-bomb survivors: Part III. Incidence of cancer in 1959–78, based on the tumor registry, Nagasaki. Radiat Res 93:112–146, 1983
4. Boice JD Jr, Fraumeni JF Jr (eds): Radiation Carcinogenesis: Epidemiology and Biological Significance. New York, Raven Press, 1984
5. Kohn HI, Fry RJM: Radiation Carcinogenesis. N Engl J Med 310:504–511, 1984
6. Boice JD Jr, Day WE, Andersen A et al: Second cancers following radiation treatment for cervical cancer: An international collaboration among cancer registries. JNCI 74:955–975, 1985
7. Darby SC, Nakashima E, Kato H: A parallel analysis of cancer mortality among atomic bomb survivors and patients with ankylosing spondylitis given x-ray therapy. JNCI 75:1–21, 1985
8. Rall JE, Beebe GW, Hoel DG et al. Report of the National Institutes of Health Ad Hoc Working Group to Develop Radioepidemiological Tables. DHHS publication No. (NIH) 85-2748. Washington, DC, U.S. Government Printing Office, 1985
9. Darby SC, Doll R, Gill SK et al: Long-term mortality after a single treatment course with x-rays in patients treated for ankylosing spondylitis. Br J Cancer 55:179–190, 1987
10. Preston DL, Kato H, Kopecky KJ et al: Studies of the mortality of A-bomb survivors: 8. Cancer mortality, 1950–1982. Radiat Res 111:151–178, 1987
11. Preston DL, Pierce DA: The effects of changes in dosimetry on cancer mortality risk estimates in the atomic bomb survivors. RERF TR 9-87. Hiroshima, Radiation Effects Research Foundation, 1987
12. Boice JD Jr: Carcinogenesis: A synopsis of human experience with external exposure in medicine. JNCI (in press)
13. Storer JB: Radiation carcinogenesis. In Becker FF (ed): Cancer: A Comprehensive Treatise, 2nd ed, vol 1, pp 629–659. New York, Plenum Press, 1982
14. Broerse JJ, Hennen LA, Van Zwieten MJ: Radiation carcinogenesis in experimental animals and its implications for radiation protection. Int J Radiat Biol 48:167–187, 1985
15. Burns FJ, Upton AC, Silini G: Radiation Carcinogenesis and DNA Alterations. NATO ASI Series. New York, Plenum Press, 1986
16. Upton AC, Albert RE, Burns FJ et al: (eds): Radiation Carcinogenesis. New York, Elsevier, 1986
17. Fry RJM, Storer JB: External radiation carcinogenesis. Adv Radiat Biol 13:31–89, 1987
18. Borek C: In vitro transformation. Adv Cancer Res 37:159–231, 1982
19. Hall EJ, Hei TK: Oncogenic transformation of cells in culture: Pragmatic comparisons of oncogenicity, cellular and molecular mechanisms. Int J Radiat Oncol Biol Phys 12:1909–1921, 1986
20. Little JB: The radiobiology of in vitro neoplastic transformation. In Burns FJ, Upton AC, Silini G (eds): Radiation Carcinogenesis and DNA Alterations, pp 163–184. NATO ASI Series. New York, Plenum Press, 1986
21. Hill CK, Han A, Elkind MM: Promotion, dose rate, and repair processes in radiation-induced neoplastic transformation. Radiat Res 109:347–351, 1987
22. Beebe GW: Assessment of health risks from exposure to ionizing radiation. In Prentice RL, Whittemore AS (eds): Environmental Epidemiology: Risk Assessment, pp 3–21. Philadelphia, SIAM, 1982
23. National Council on Radiation Protection and Measurements (NCRP): Ionizing Radiation Exposure of the Population of the United States. NCRP Report No 93. Bethesda, MD, NCRP, 1987
24. National Council on Radiation Protection and Measurements (NCRP): Exposures from the Uranium Series with Emphasis on Radon and its Daughters. NCRP Report No. 77. Bethesda, MD, NCRP, 1984
25. National Research Council: Biological Effects of Ionizing Radiation (BEIR): Health Risks of Radon and Other Internally Deposited Alpha Emitters. Washington, DC, National Academy Press, 1987
26. Harley N, Samet JM, Cross FT et al: Contribution of radon and radon daughters to respiratory cancer. Environ Health Perspect 70:17–21, 1986
27. United Nations Scientific Committee on Effects of Atomic Radiation (UNSCEAR): Ionizing Radiation: Sources and Biological Effects. Report to the General Assembly with Annexes, 1987
28. Schlein B, Tucker TT, Johnson DW: The mean active bone marrow dose to the adult population of the United States from diagnostic radiology. Health Phys 34:587–601, 1978
29. McCullough EC, Payne JT: Patient dosage in computed tomography. Radiology 129:457–463, 1978
30. Frieben A: Demonstration lines cancroids des rechten Handruckens, das sich nach langdauernder Einwirkung von Röntgenstrahlen entwichelt hatte. Fortschr Geb Röntgenstr 6:106, 1902
31. von Jagic N, Scwarz G, von Siebenrock L: Blutbefunde bei Röntgenologon. Berl Klin Wochenschr 48:1220–1222, 1911
32. Ishimaru M, Ishimaru T, Mikami M et al: Incidence of leukemia in a fixed cohort of atomic bomb survivors and controls: Hiroshima and Nagasaki, October 1950–December 1978. RERF TR-13-81. Hiroshima, Radiation Effects Research Foundation, 1982
33. Brodsky JB, Lidell R, Groer PG et al: Temporal analysis of a dose-response relationship: Leukemia mortality in atomic bomb survivors. RERF TR 5-82. Hiroshima, Radiation Effects Research Foundation, 1983
34. Boice JD Jr, Blettner M, Kleinerman RA et al: Radiation dose and leukemia risk in patients treated for cancer of the cervix. JNCI 79:1295–1311, 1987
35. Upton AC, Randolph ML, Conklin JW: Late effects of fast neutrons and gamma rays in mice as influenced by the dose rate of irradiation: Induction of neoplasia. Radiat Res 41:467–491, 1970
36. Kaplan HS: Interaction between radiation and viruses in the induction of murine thymic lymphomas and lymphatic leukemias. In Duplan JF (ed): Radiation-Induced Leukemogenesis and Related Viruses, pp 1–18. Amsterdam, North Holland, 1977
37. Ullrich RL, Storer JB: Influence of gamma radiation on the development of neoplastic disease in mice: I. Reticular tissue tumors. Radiat Res 80:303–316, 1979
38. Mole RH: Radiation-induced myeloid leukemia in the mouse: Experimental observations and *in vivo* implications for hypotheses about the basis of carcinogenesis. Leuk Res 7:859–865, 1986
39. Ullrich RL, Preston RJ: Myeloid leukemia in male RFM mice following irradiation with fission spectrum neutrons or gamma rays. Radiat Res 109:165–170, 1987
40. Tolle DV, Fritz TE, Seed TM et al: Leukemia induction in beagles exposed continuously to ^{60}Co gamma irradiation: Hematology. In Baum SJ, Ledney GD, Thierfelder S (eds): Experimental Hematology Today 1982, pp 241–249. Basel, S Karger, 1982
41. Martland HS: The occurrence of malignancy in radioactive persons: A general review of data gathered in the study of the radium dial painters with special reference to the occurrence of osteogenic sarcoma and the interrelationship of certain blood diseases. Am J Cancer 15:2435–2516, 1931
42. Rowland RE, Stehney AF, Lucas HF Jr: Dose-response relationships for female radium-dial workers. Radiat Res 76:368–383, 1978
43. Grigg ERN: The Trail of the Invisible Light. Springfield, IL, Charles C Thomas, 1965
44. Upton AC: Physical carcinogenesis: Radiation—history and sources. In Becker FF (ed): Cancer: A Comprehensive Treatise, 2nd ed, pp 551–567. New York, Plenum Press, 1982
45. Stone RS: Maximum permissible exposure standards. In: Protection in Diagnostic Radiology. New Brunswick, Rutgers University Press, 1959

46. Sinclair WK: Radiation Protection: The NCRP Guidelines and some considerations for the future. Yale J Biol Med 54:471–484, 1981
47. Sinclair WK: Risk, research and radiation protection. Radiat Res 112:191–216, 1987
48. National Council on Radiation Protection and Measurements (NCRP): Recommendations on limits for exposure to ionizing radiation. NCRP Report 91. Bethesda, Md, NCRP, 1987
49. International Commission on Radiological Protection (ICRP): Statement from Paris meeting of the ICRP. Phys Med Biol 30:863, 1985
50. Kellerer AM, Rossi HH: A generalized formulation of dual radiation action. Radiat Res 75:471–488, 1978
51. Kellerer AM, Rossi HH: Biophysical aspects of radiation carcinogenesis. In Becker FF (ed): Cancer: A Comprehensive Treatise, 2nd ed, pp 569–616. New York, Plenum Press, 1982
52. Goodhead DT: An assessment of the role of microdosimetry in radiobiology. Radiat Res 91:45–76, 1982
53. Bond VP, Varma MN: A stochastic, weighted hit size theory of cellular biological action. In Booze J, Ebert HG (eds): Radiation Protection: Proceedings of the 8th Symposium on Microdosimetry, pp 423–438, July 1982, Luxemburg 1983
54. Dalla-Favera R, Martinotti S, Gallo RC et al: Translocation and rearrangements of the c-myc oncogene locus in human undifferentiated B-cell lymphomas. Science 219:963–967, 1983
55. Klein G: Chromosomal translocations and the genesis of B-cell-derived tumors in mice and men. Cell 32:311–315, 1983
56. Rowley JD: Biological implications of consistent chromosome rearrangements in leukemia and lymphoma. Cancer Res 44:3159–3168, 1984
57. Sax K: Chromosome aberrations induced by x-rays. Genetics 23:494–516, 1938
58. Lea DE: Actions of Radiations on Living Cells, 2nd ed. Cambridge, University Press, 1955
59. Lloyd DC, Purrott RJ, Dolphin GW et al: The relationship between chromosome aberrations and low-LET radiation dose to human lymphocytes. Int J Radiat Biol 28:75–90, 1975
60. Upton AC: Radiobiological effects of low doses: Implications for radiological protection. Radiat Res 71:51–74, 1977
61. Little JB: Influence of noncarcinogenic secondary factors on radiation carcinogenesis. Radiat Res 87:240–250, 1981
62. Land H, Parada LF, Weinberg RA: Tumorigenic conversion of primary embryo fibroblasts require at least two cooperating oncogenes. Nature 304:596–602, 1983
63. Terzaghi-Howe M: Inhibition of carcinogen-altered rat tracheal epithelial cell proliferation by normal epithelial cells *in vivo*. Carcinogenesis 8:145–150, 1987
64. Upton AC, Randolph ML, Conklin JW: Late effects of fast neutrons and gamma-rays in mice influenced by the dose rate of irradiation: Induction of neoplasia. Radiat Res 41:467–491, 1970
65. Ullrich RL, Storer JB: Influence of gamma radiation on the development of neoplastic disease in mice: III. Dose-rate effects. Radiat Res 80:325–342, 1979
66. Han A, Hill CK, Elkind MM: Repair of cell killing and neoplastic transformation at reduced dose rates of ^{60}Co gamma rays. Cancer Res 40:3328–3332, 1980
67. National Council on Radiation Protection and Measurements (NCRP): Influence of Dose and Its Distribution in Time and Dose-Response Relationships for Low-LET Radiations. NCRP Report No 64. Washington, DC, NCRP, 1980
68. Ullrich RL, Jernigan MC, Satterfield LC et al: Radiation carcinogenesis: Time-dose relationships. Radiat Res 111:179–184, 1987
69. Burns FJ, Vanderlaan M: Split-dose recovery for radiation-induced tumors in rat skin. Int J Radiat Biol 32:135–144, 1977
70. Terzaghi M, Little JB: Oncogenic transformation *in vitro* after split-dose X-irradiation. Int J Radiat Biol 29:583–587, 1976
71. Miller R, Hall EJ: X-ray dose fractionation and oncogenic transformation in cultured mouse embryo cells. Nature 272:58–60, 1978
72. Borek C: Neoplastic transformation following split doses of X rays. Br J Radiol 52:845–846, 1979
73. Ullrich RL: Tumor induction in BALB/c mice after fractionated or protracted exposures to fission-spectrum neutrons. Radiat Res 97:587–597, 1984
74. Hill CK, Buonaguro FM, Myers CP et al: Fission-spectrum neutrons at reduced dose rates enhance neoplastic transformation. Nature 298:67–69, 1982
75. Taylor AMR, Harnden DG, Arlett CF et al: Ataxia telangiectasia: A human mutation with abnormal radiation sensitivity. Nature 258:427–429, 1975
76. Arlett CF, Lehmann AR: Human disorders showing increased sensitivity to the induction of genetic damage. Annu Rev Genet 12:95–115, 1978
77. Lewis PD, Carr JB, Arlett CF et al: Increased sensitivity to gamma irradiation of skin fibroblasts in Friedrich's ataxia. Lancet 2:474–475, 1979
78. Smith PJ, Paterson MC, Kraemer KH: *In vitro* radiosensitivity in a patient with dermatomyositis and cancer. Lancet 1:216–217, 1981
79. Sandford KK, Parshad R, Green MH et al: Hypersensitivity to G_2 chromatid radiation damage in familial dysplastic naevus syndrome. Lancet 2:1111–1116, 1987
80. Kersey JH, Spector BD: Immune deficiency disease. In Fraumeni JF Jr (ed): Persons at High Risk of Cancer: An Approach to Cancer Etiology and Control, pp 55–67. New York, Academic Press, 1975
81. Tucker MA, Meadows AJ, Boice JD Jr et al: Cancer risk following treatment of childhood cancer. In Boice JD, Fraumeni JF Jr (eds): Radiation Carcinogenesis: Epidemiology and Biological Significance, pp 211–224. New York, Raven Press, 1984
82. Tokunaga M, Land CE, Yamamoto T et al: Incidence of female breast cancer among atomic bomb survivors, Hiroshima and Nagasaki 1950–80. Radiation Effects Research Foundation Technical Report 15-84. Hiroshima, RERF, 1985
83. Shore RE, Woodard ED, Hempelmann LH: Radiation-induced thyroid cancer. In Boice JD Jr, Fraumeni JF Jr (eds): Radiation Carcinogenesis: Epidemiology and Biological Significance, pp 131–138. New York, Raven Press, 1984
84. Ron E, Modan B: Thyroid and other neoplasms following childhood scalp irradiation. In Boice JD Jr, Fraumeni JF Jr (eds): Radiation Carcinogenesis: Epidemiology and Biological Significance, pp 139–151. New York, Raven Press, 1984
85. Kim JH, Chu FC, Woodard MR et al: Radiation-induced soft-tissue and bone sarcoma. Radiology 129:501–508, 1978
86. Land CE: Temporal distributions of risk for radiation-induced cancers. J Chronic Dis 40(suppl 2):45S–57S, 1987
87. Smith PG, Doll R: Mortality among patients with ankylosing spondylitis after a single treatment course with x-rays. Br Med J 284:449–460, 1982
88. Day NE: Radiation and multistage carcinogenesis. In Boice JD Jr, Fraumeni JF Jr (eds): Radiation Carcinogenesis: Epidemiology and Biological Significance, pp 437–443. New York, Raven Press, 1984
89. Gilbert E: Health effects model for nuclear power plant accident consequence analysis. In Evans JS, Moeller DW, Cooper DW (eds): NUREG/CR-414. Washington, DC, U.S. Government Printing Office, 1985
90. Storer JB, Mitchell TJ, Fry RJM: Extrapolation of the relative risk of radiogenic neoplasms across mouse strains and to man. Radiat Res 114:331–353, 1988
91. United Nations Scientific Committee on the Effects of Atomic Radiation: 1982 Report to the General Assembly with Annexes, United Nations, 1982
92. Fawkes FGR, Davies ER, Evans KT et al: Multicenter trial of four strategies to reduce use of a radiological test. Lancet 1:367–369, 1986
93. Harwood AR, Yaffe M: Cancer in man after diagnostic or therapeutic irradiation. In Penn I (ed): Cancer Surveys, vol 1, pp 703–731. Oxford, Oxford University Press, 1982
94. Evans JS, Wennberg JE, McNeil BJ: The influence of diagnostic radiography on the incidence of breast cancer and leukemia. N Engl J Med 315:810–815, 1986
95. Howe GR: Epidemiology of radiogenic breast cancer. In Boice JD Jr, Fraumeni JF Jr (eds): Radiation Carcinogenesis: Epidemiology and Biological Significance, pp 119–129. New York, Raven Press, 1984
96. Smith PG, Doll R: Mortality among patients with ankylosing spondylitis after a single treatment course with x rays. Br Med J 284:449–460, 1982
97. Shore RE, Albert RE, Reed M et al: Skin cancer incidence among children irradiated for ringworm of the scalp. Radiat Res 100:192–204, 1984
98. Shore RE, Woodard E, Hildreth N et al: Thyroid tumors following thymus irradiation. JNCI 74:1177–1184, 1985
99. Shore RE, Woodard E, Dvoretsky P et al: Breast cancer among women given x-ray therapy for acute post partum mastitis. JNCI 77:689–696, 1986
100. Schneider AB, Shore RE, Freedman E et al: Radiation-induced thyroid and other head and neck tumors: Occurrence of multiple tumors and analysis of risk factors. J Clin Endocrinol Metab 63:107–112, 1986
101. Lineletof B, Eklund G: Incidence of malignant skin tumors in 14,140 patients after Grenz-ray treatment for benign skin disorders. Arch Dermatol 122:1391–1395, 1986
102. van Vloten WA, Hermans J, van Daal WAJ: Radiation-induced skin cancer and radiodermatitis of the head and neck. Cancer 59:411–414, 1987
103. Ron E, Modan B, Boice JD Jr: Mortality following radiotherapy for ringworm of the scalp. Am J Epidermiol 127:713–725, 1988
104. Tucker MA, D'Angio GJ, Boice JD Jr et al: Bone sarcomas linked to radiotherapy and chemotherapy in children. N Engl J Med 317:588–593, 1987
105. Griem ML, Justman J, Weiss L: The neoplastic potential of gastric irradiation: IV. Risk estimates. Am J Clin Oncol 7:675–677, 1984
106. Coleman CN: Secondary neoplasms in patients treated for cancer: Etiology and perspective. Radiat Res 92:188–200, 1982
107. Tucker MA, Meadows AT, Boice JD Jr et al: Leukemia after therapy with alkylating agents for childhood cancers. JNCI 78:459–464, 1987
108. Stern RS, Thibodeau LA, Kleinerman RA et al: Risk of cutaneous carcinoma in patients treated with oral methoxsalen photochemotherapy for psoriasis. N Engl J Med 300:809–813, 1979
109. Weinberg RA: The action of oncogenes in the cytoplasm and nucleus. Science 230:770–776, 1985
110. Klein G, Klein J: Evolution of tumors and the impact of molecular oncology. Nature (London) 315:190–195, 1985
111. Lloyd DC, Purott RJ, Dolphin GW: Chromosome aberrations induced in human lymphocytes by neutron irradiation. Int J Radiat Biol 29:169–182, 1976
112. Le Beau MM, Rowley JD: Chromosomal abnormalities in leukemia and lymphoma: Clinical and biological significance. Adv Hum Genet 15:1–54, 1986
113. Guerrero I, Calzava P, Mayer A et al: A molecular approach to leukemogenesis: Mouse lymphomas contain an activated c-ras oncogene. Proc Natl Acad Sci USA 81:202–205, 1984
114. Sawey MJ, Hood AT, Burns FJ et al: Activation of c-myc and c-K-ras oncogenes in primary rat tumors induced by ionizing radiation. Mol Cell Biol 7:932–935, 1987
115. Borek C, Ong A, Mason H: Distinctive transforming genes in x-ray–transformed mammalian cells. Proc Natl Acad Sci USA 84:794–798, 1987
116. Scotto J, Fraumeni JF Jr: Skin (other than melanoma). In Schottenfeld D, Fraumeni JF Jr (eds): Cancer Epidemiology and Prevention, pp 996–1011. Philadelphia, WB Saunders, 1982
117. Magnus K: Incidence of malignant melanoma of the skin in the five Nordic countries: Significance of solar radiation. Int J Cancer 20:477–485, 1977

118. Fitzpatrick TB, Sober AJ: Sunlight and skin cancer. N Engl J Med 313:818–819, 1985
119. Scotto J, Fears TR: The association of solar ultraviolet and skin melanoma incidence among Caucasians in the United States. Cancer Invest 5:275–283, 1987
120. Carter LJ: The global environment: MIT study looks for danger signals. Science 169:660–662, 1970
121. Johnston H: Reduction of stratospheric ozone by nitrogen oxide catalysts from supersonic transport exhaust. Science 173:517–522, 1971
122. Cutchis P: Stratospheric ozone depletion and solar ultraviolet radiation on earth. Science 184:13, 1974
123. National Research Council: Causes and effects of changes in stratospheric ozone: Update 1983. Washington, DC, National Academy Press, 1984
124. Prather MJ, McElroy MB, Wofsy SC: Reductions in ozone at high concentrations of stratospheric halogens. Nature 312:227–231, 1984
125. Farman JC, Gardiner BG, Shanklin JD: Large losses of total ozone in Antarctica reveal seasonal $C10_x/NO_x$ interaction. Nature 315:207–210, 1985
126. Solomon S, Garcia RR, Rowland FS et al: On the depletion of Antarctic ozone. Nature 321:755–758, 1986
127. Scotto J, Cotton G, Urbach F et al: Science 239:762–764, 1988
128. Houghton A, Munster EW, Viola MV: Increased incidence of malignant melanoma after peaks of sunspot activity. Lancet 1:759–760, 1978
129. Urbach F (ed): The Biologic Effects of Ultraviolet Radiation. Oxford, Pergamon Press, 1969
130. Findlay GH: Ultraviolet light and skin cancer. Lancet 2:1070–1073, 1928
131. Roffo AH: Cancer et soleil carcinomas provogues par l'action du soleil in toto. Bull Assoc Franc Etude Cancer 23:590–592, 1934
132. Doniger J, Jacobson ED, Krell K et al: Ultraviolet light action spectra for neoplastic transformation and lethality of Syrian hamster embryo cells correlate with spectrum for pyrimidine dimer formation in cellular DNA. Proc Natl Acad Sci USA 78:2378–2382, 1981
133. Sutherland BM, Delihas NC, Oliver RP et al: Action spectra for ultraviolet light-induced transformation of human cells to anchorage-independent growth. Cancer Res 41:2211–2214, 1981
134. Sutherland BM, Cimino JS, Delihas N et al: Ultraviolet light-induced transformation of human cells to anchorage-independent growth. Cancer Res 40:1934–1939, 1980
135. Hart RW, Setlow RB, Woodhead AD: Evidence that pyrimidine dimers in DNA can give rise to tumors. Proc Natl Acad Sci USA 75:5574–5578, 1977
136. Ley RD, Applegate LA, Fry RJM et al: UVA/visible light suppression of ultraviolet radiation-induced skin and eye tumors of the marsupial Monodelphis domestica. Photochem Photobiol 47:45S, 1988
137. Cleaver JE: Xeroderma pigmentosum. In Stanbury JB, Wyngaarden JB, Fredrickson DS et al (eds): The Metabolic Basis of Inherited Disease, pp 1227–1248. New York, McGraw-Hill, 1983
138. Kripke ML: Immunologic mechanisms in UV radiation carcinogenesis. Adv Cancer Res 34:69–106, 1981
139. Parrish JA (ed): The effect of ultraviolet radiation on the immune system. Skillman, NJ, Johnson & Johnson, 1983
140. Robbins JH, Kraemer KH, Lutzner MA et al: Xeroderma pigmentosum: An inherited disease with sun sensitivity, multiple cutaneous neoplasms and abnormal repair. Ann Intern Med 80:221–248, 1974
141. Kraemer K, Lee MM, Scotto J: Xeroderma pigmentosum: Cutaneous, ocular and neurological abnormalities in 830 published cases. Arch Dermatol 123:241–250, 1987
142. Hashem N, Bootsma D, Keijzer W et al: Clinical characteristics, DNA repair, and complementation groups in xeroderma pigmentosum patients from Egypt. Cancer Res 40:13–18, 1980
143. Hebra F, Kaposi M: On Diseases of the Skin Including the Exanthemata, vol 3, pp 252–258 (Tay W, trans). London, New Sydenham Society, 1974
144. Taylor RN: A further contribution to the study of xeroderma of Hebra. Trans Am Dermatol Assoc 37:37–46, 1979
145. de Sanctis C, Cacchione A: L'idiozia xerodermica. Riv Sper Freniatr 56:269–292, 1932
146. Haxthausen H, Hausmann N: Die Lichterkrankugen der Haut. Vienna, Urban und Schwartzenberg, 1929
147. Swift M, Chase C: Cancer in families with xeroderma pigmentosum. JNCI 62:1415–1421, 1979
148. Cleaver JE: Defective repair replication of DNA in xeroderma pigmentosum. Nature 218:652–656, 1968
149. deWeerd-Kastelein EA, Keijzer W, Bootsma D: Genetic heterogeneity of xeroderma pigmentosum demonstrated by somatic cell hybridization. Nature 238:80–83, 1972
150. Kraemer KH, Coon HG, Pettiga RA et al: Genetic heterogeneity in xeroderma pigmentosum complementation groups and their relationship to DNA repair rates. Proc Natl Acad Sci USA 72:59–63, 1975
151. Kraemer KH, deWeerd-Kastelein EA, Robbins JH et al: Five complementation groups in xeroderma pigmentosum. Mutat Res 33:327–340, 1975
152. Jung EG: New form of molecular defect in xeroderma pigmentosum. Nature 228:361–362, 1970
153. Burk PG, Lutzner MA, Clarke DD et al: Ultraviolet-stimulated thymidine incorporation in xeroderma pigmentosum lymphocytes. J Lab Clin Med 77:759–767, 1971
154. Cleaver JE: Xeroderma pigmentosum: Variants with normal DNA repair and normal sensitivity to ultraviolet light. J Invest Dermatol 58:124–128, 1972
155. Maher VM, Ouelette LM, Curren RD et al: Frequency of ultraviolet light-induced mutations is higher in xeroderma pigmentosum variant cells. Nature 261:593–595, 1976
156. Wolff S, Bodycote J, Thomas GH et al: Sister chromatid exchange in xeroderma pigmentosum cells that are defective in DNA excision repair or post-replication repair. Genetics 81:349–355, 1975
157. German J, Gilleran TG, Setlow RB et al: Mutant karyotypes in cultures of cells from a man with xeroderma pigmentosum. Ann Genet 16:23–27, 1973
158. Parrington JM, Delhanty JDA, Baden HP: Unscheduled DNA synthesis: UV-induced chromosome aberrations and SV40 transformation in cultured cells from xeroderma pigmentosum. Ann Hum Genet 35:149–160, 1971
159. Huang CC, Benerjee A, Hou Y: Chromosomal instability in cell lines derived from patients with xeroderma pigmentosum. Proc Soc Exp Biol Med 148:1244–1248, 1975
160. deWeerd-Kastelein EA, Keijzer W, Rainaldi G et al: Induction of sister chromatid exchanges in xeroderma pigmentosum cells after exposure to ultraviolet light. Mutat Res 45:253–261, 1977
161. Wolff S, Rodin B, Cleaver JE: Sister chromatid exchanges induced by mutagenic carcinogens in normal and xeroderma pigmentosum cells. Nature 265:347–349, 1977
162. Kraemer KH, Slor H, Andrews A: A new form of xeroderma pigmentosum: Reduced repair without neoplasia (abstr). J Invest Dermatol 80:331, 1983
163. Turner FC: Sarcomas at sites of subcutaneously implanted Bakelite disks in rats. JNCI 2:81–83, 1941
164. Oppenheimer BS, Oppenheimer ET, Stout AP: Sarcomas induced in rats by implanting cellophane. Proc Soc Exp Biol Med 67:33–34, 1948
165. Bischoff F, Bryson G: Carcinogenesis through solid state surfaces. Prog Exp Tumor Res 5:86–133, 1964
166. Brand KG: Cancer associated with asbestosis and schistosomiasis foreign bodies and scars. In Becker FF (ed): Cancer: A Comprehensive Treatise, 2nd ed, vol 1, pp 661–692. New York, Plenum Press, 1982
167. Brand I, Buoen LC, Brand KG: Foreign body tumors of mice: Strain and sex differences in latency and incidence. JNCI 58:1443–1447, 1977
168. Brand KG: Solid state carcinogenesis. In Butterworth BE, Slaga TJ (eds). Nongenotoxic Mechanisms in Carcinogenesis. Banbury Report 25. Cold Spring Harbor, New York, Cold Spring Harbor Laboratory, 1987
169. Brues AM, Auerbach H, DeRoche GM et al: Mechanisms of carcinogenesis. In: Argonne National Laboratory, Biological and Medical Research Division Annual Report, ANL 7535, pp 28–30. Argonne, IL, ANL, 1968
170. Nicholson WJ, Perbep G, Selikoff IJ: Occupational exposure to asbestos: Population at risk and projected mortality. Am J Ind Med 3:259–311, 1987
171. Doll R, Peto J: Effects on health of exposure to asbestos. Health and Sujet Commission Report. London, Her Majesty's Stationery Office, 1985
172. Wagner JC (ed): Biological Effects of Mineral Fibers, vols. I and II. IARC Scientific Publications No 30. Lyon, World Health Organization, 1980
173. Harrington JS: Fiber carcinogenesis: Epidemiologic observations and the Stanton hypothesis. JNCI 67:977–989, 1981
174. Leineweber JP: Dust chemistry and physics: Mineral and vitreous fibers. In Wagner JC (ed): Biological Effects of Mineral Fibers, vol 2, pp 881–900. IARC Scientific Publications No. 30. Lyon, World Health Organization, 1980
175. Baris YI, Sahin AA, Ozesmi M et al: An outbreak of pleural mesothelioma and chronic fibrosing pleurisy in the village of Karan/Urgup in Anatolia. Thorax 33:181–192, 1978
176. Omenn GS, Merchant J, Boatman E et al: Contribution of environmental fibers to respiratory cancer. Environ Health Perspect 70:51–56, 1986
177. Harrington JS, Allison AC, Badami DV: Mineral fibers: Chemical, physicochemical and biological properties. Adv Pharmacol Chemother 17:291–402, 1975
178. Stanton MF, Layara M, Tegeris A et al: Relation of particle dimension to carcinogenicity in amphibole asbestosis and other fibrous minerals. JNCI 67:965–975, 1981
179. Selikoff IJ (ed): Cancer from Occupational Asbestos Exposure. Projections 1965–2030. Disability Compensation for Asbestos-Associated Disease in the United States. New York, Environmental Sciences Laboratory, Mount Sinai School of Medicine of the City University, 1982
180. Peto J, Seidman H, Selikoff IJ: Mesothelioma mortality in asbestos workers: Implications for models of carcinogenesis and risk assessment. Br J Cancer 45:124, 1982
181. Hesterberg TW, Butterich CJ, Oshimura M et al: Role of phagocytosis in Syrian hamster cell transformation and cytogenetic effects induced by asbestos and short and long glass fibers. Cancer Res 46:5795–5802, 1986
182. Hesterberg TW, Barrett JC: Dependence of asbestos and mineral dust-induced transformation of mammalian cells in culture on fiber dimension. Cancer Res 44:2170–2180, 1984
183. Hesterberg TW, Barrett JC: Induction of asbestos fibers of anaphase abnormalities: Mechanism for aneuploidy induction and possibly carcinogenesis. Carcinogenesis 6:473–475, 1985
184. Oshimura M, Hesterberg TW, Tsutsui T et al: Correlation of asbestos-induced cytogenetic effects with cell transformation of Syrian hamster embryo cells in culture. Cancer Res 44:5017–5022, 1984
185. Oshimura M, Hesterberg TW, Barrett JC: An early nonrandom karyotypic change in immortal Syrian hamster cell lines transformed by asbestos: Trisomy of chromosome 11. Cancer Genet Cytogenet 22:225–237, 1986
186. Hei TK, Geard CR, Osmak RS et al: Correlation of in vitro genotoxicity and oncogenicity induced by radiation and asbestos fibres. Br J Cancer 52:591–597, 1985

PETER M. HOWLEY

CHAPTER 10 Principles of Carcinogenesis: Viral

Viral oncology has its foundations in observations made at the turn of the century defining the transmissibility of avian leukemia in Denmark, in 1908, and of an avian sarcoma in chickens, in 1911.[1,2] These important discoveries were not appreciated at the time, and their impact on virology and medicine was not recognized for decades. The work of Peyton Rous,[2] who showed that cell-free extracts from a sarcoma in chickens could induce tumors in injected chickens within a few weeks, even when passed through filters that retained bacteria, was finally recognized and led to a Nobel prize in 1966. Rous's original work demonstrated that the infectious agent was not only capable of inducing tumors, but also imprinted the phenotypic characteristics of the original tumor on the recipient transformed cell. At the time Rous's work was relegated to the ranks of avian curiosities, and its importance was not recognized for several decades.

In the 1930s Richard Shope published a series of papers on cell-free transmission of tumors in rabbits. The first studies involved fibromatous tumors, found in the footpads of wild cottontail rabbits, that could be transmitted by injecting cell-free extracts into either wild or domestic rabbits.[3] Subsequent studies have shown that this virus, now referred to as the Shope fibroma virus, is a pox virus. Additional studies carried out by Shope demonstrated that cutaneous papillomatosis in wild cottontail rabbits could also be transmitted by cell-free extracts. He also observed, as did Peyton Rous, that in a number of cases these benign papillomas would progress spontaneously into squamous cell carcinomas in infected domestic rabbits or in the infected cottontail rabbits.[4,5] In general, however, the field of viral oncology lay stagnant until the early 1950s with the discovery of the murine leukemia viruses by Ludwig Gross[6] and of the mouse polyomavirus by Gross, Stewart, and Eddy.[7,8] At this point in the 1950s many cancer researchers and virologists turned to the field of viral oncology, hoping that the initial observations in mammals could be extended to humans and that a fair proportion of human tumors might also be found to have a viral etiology. The Special Viral Cancer Program at the National Cancer Institute grew out of this intense interest in viral oncology and the speculation that human tumor viruses would be identified.

Many of the most important developments in modern molecular biology, including the discovery of reverse transcriptase, the development of recombinant DNA technology, the discovery of mRNA splicing, and the discovery of oncogenes, derived directly from studies in viral oncology conducted in the 1960s and 1970s. Oncogenes were first recognized as cellular genes that had been acquired by retroviruses through some type of recombinational process that converted them into acute transforming RNA tumor viruses. It is now known that oncogenes participate in many different types of tumors and can be involved at different stages of tumorigenesis and viral oncology. This has contributed significantly to our concepts of nonviral carcinogenesis. It is likely that the direct transforming, oncogene-transducing retroviruses do not play a major causative role in naturally occurring cancers in animals or in humans, but rather represent laboratory-generated recombinants. A list of human viruses with oncogenic properties is given in Table 10-1. This list includes viruses such as the transforming adenoviruses, which are capable of

TABLE 10-1. Human Viruses with Oncogenic Properties

Virus Family	*Type*	*Human Tumor*	*Cofactors*
Adenovirus	Types 2, 5, 12	None	. . .
Hepadnavirus	Hepatitis B (HBV)	Hepatocellular carcinoma	Aflatoxin, alcohol, smoking
Herpesvirus	Epstein-Barr (EBV)	Burkitt's lymphoma	Marlaria
		Immunoblastic lymphoma	Immunodeficiency
		Nasopharyngeal carcinoma	Nitrosamines, HLA genotype
Papillomaviruses	HPV-16, 18, 33, 39	Cervical neoplasia	Smoking, ?HSV
	HPV-5, 8, 17	Skin cancer	Genetic disorders, sunlight
Polyomavirus	BK, JC	?Neural tumors	
		?Insulinomas	
Retroviruses	HTLV-1	Adult T-cell leukemia-lymphoma	Uncertain
	HTLV-2	Hairy cell leukemia	Unknown

transforming normal cells into malignant cells in the laboratory but have not been associated with any known human tumors. The list also includes viruses such as the papillomaviruses that have been etiologically associated with specific human cancers and have been shown to encode transforming viral oncogenes. Finally, Table 10-1 includes viruses such as the hepatitis B virus that have been closely linked with specific human tumors but have not been shown to encode a viral oncogene. This chapter focuses on viruses that have been associated with specific human cancers and considers their biology and pertinent molecular biology. The evidence for the association of each of these viruses with specific types of human neoplasia is presented, and the mechanisms by which these viruses may contribute to malignant transformation are discussed.

Also listed in Table 10-1 are cofactors believed to be important in the carcinogenic processes associated with the different viruses. It is clear that none of these viruses alone is sufficient for the induction of the specific neoplasias with which it has been associated. Rather, the viruses associated with human cancers are thought to be involved at an early step in carcinogenesis. Subsequent cellular events such as somatic mutations are thought to be important at the subsequent multiple steps involved in malignant progression.

HUMAN RETROVIRUSES

The first tumor viruses described were both retroviruses. These were the avian leukemia virus, described by Ellermann and Bang in 1908,[1] and the avian sarcoma virus, described by Peyton Rous in 1911.[2] Among the tumor viruses, the retroviruses have been a primary subject of research by virologists, oncologists, and molecular biologists. In the past two decades studies with the retroviruses have provided us with reverse transcriptase and oncogenes, and retroviruses have recently been engineered into vectors for the effective delivery of DNA to cells for gene therapy. Interest in viruses as infectious tumor agents was spurred by the findings of Ludwig Gross in the 1950s when he described retroviruses that caused tumors in mice.[6,7] In the early 1960s William Jarrett discovered the feline leukemia virus (FeLV), which was capable of inducing leukemia as well as aplasia in cats.[9] Subsequent studies established that the leukemia associated with FeLV could be communicated in the natural setting and was not limited to the laboratory. This provided a major impetus to the search for retroviruses as possible tumor viruses causing leukemia in humans. In the retroviruses associated with animal leukemia in chickens, mice, and cats there is extensive viral replication and the virus particles often can be readily visualized with electron microscopy.[10] The studies of the late 1960s through the 1970s that sought human retroviruses in human blood disorders relied heavily on electron microscopy for evidence of such viruses.

As had been shown in 1970 by the Nobel Prize-winning experiments of Howard Temin and David Baltimore, retroviruses contain enzymes called reverse transcriptase which are involved in transcribing the single-stranded RNA copy of the input viral RNA into DNA.[11,12] This enzymatic activity is associated with retrovirus particles and can be readily assayed from infected cells. Thus, assays for reverse transcriptase activities, which are unique to retroviruses, provided an alternative assay for these viruses that was more sensitive to electron microscopy. The first unequivocal evidence of a human retrovirus, HTLV-1, came almost 70 years after Rous's initial description of the avian sarcoma virus.

HUMAN T-CELL LYMPHADENOTROPIC VIRUS TYPE 1

The first substantiated reports of a human retrovirus were published in 1980 and 1981 by Robert Gallo and his colleagues,[13,14] followed in 1982 by reports by Yoshida and his colleagues in Japan.[15] The viral isolates were from T-cell leukemia in humans. The first isolate from Gallo's laboratory was from a patient with a T-cell leukemia and skin abnormalities similar to those seen in mycosis fungoides or Sézary syndrome. Subsequent analysis of other patients with mycosis fungoides and the Sézary syndrome revealed that only a small proportion of such patients had evidence of HTLV-1. The patient studied by Gallo et al was found to have a form of T-cell leukemia known as adult T-cell leukemia (ATL), which differs from mycosis fungoides. ATL, first described in 1977 by Kiyoshi Takatsuki and colleagues of Kyoto University,[16] is endemic in Kyushu and Shikoku, the southernmost islands of Japan; and it was from a case of ATL that the first Japanese isolate of the human retrovirus initially referred to as the adult T-cell leukemia virus was isolated.[15,17] Subsequent studies established that Gallo's initial isolate of HTLV-1 and the ATL virus were identical,[18,19] and by convention the virus is now referred to as HTLV-1.

ATL is a malignancy of mature T4+ lymphocytes.[20] It is endemic in parts of Japan[21] as well as in the Caribbean and in parts of Africa.[22,23] The tumor resembles mycosis fungoides and Sézary syndrome but is more aggressive than these two syndromes. Median survival from the time of diagnosis is only 3 to 4 months. The disease affects visceral organs as well as the skin, and often induces hypercalcemia. The isolation in Gallo's laboratory of HTLV-1 from a leukemia cell line was a consequence and extension of the basic research performed in that laboratory identifying a T-cell growth factor (now referred to as interleukin-2, or IL-2).[24] IL-2 is released by T-cells following stimulation with phytohemagglutinin (PHA), which stimulates T-cells to proliferate. PHA-activated T-cells not only secrete IL-2 but also develop receptor molecules on their surface for the growth factor molecules. With IL-2 bound to its receptor, the cells begin to divide. The characterization and isolation of IL-2 permitted investigators in Gallo's laboratory to grow the human leukemic cells indefinitely and eventually to identify the first human retrovirus.

After the isolation of HTLV-1, immunologic assays were developed to detect antibodies specific for the viral antigens. Such serologic assays became the basis for subsequent epidemiologic and transmission studies. Studies revealed that the viral infection was more common in endemic areas than were malignancies.[21] Less than 1% of seropositive patients ever develop ATL. A preleukemic disease in the form of a chronic lymphocytosis is often seen before the development of acute leukemia or lymphoma.[25]

Although retroviruses are often referred to as leukemia viruses, the spectrum of diseases with which they are associated is not limited to leukemia. Of the animal viruses, the avian leukemia viruses are also associated with an autoimmune wasting disease and osteoporosis. The feline leukemia viruses can be associated with anemia, aplasia, and immunodeficiency. Certain mouse leukemia viruses can induce paralysis and neuropathies. Similarly, HTLV-1 infection in humans has been associated with diseases other than ATL. HTLV-1 has been associated with an increased susceptibility to opportunistic infections as well as with a degenerative neurologic disease. In West Indian patients this disease is referred to as tropical spastic paraparesis,[26,27] and a similar disease in Japan known as HAM (HTLV-I associated myelopathy).[28] Specific risk factors that may be important in determining the development of leukemia, immunodeficiency, or tropical spastic paraparesis in HTLV-1–infected individuals currently are not known.

HUMAN T-CELL LYMPHADENOTROPIC VIRUS TYPE 2

The second human retrovirus, HTLV-2 was described in a cell line established from a patient with an unusual form of hairy cell leukemia.[29] Morphologically the cells of HTLV-2 resemble those of a hairy cell leukemia; however, they contain markers of a T-cell lineage, whereas most hairy cell leukemia cells contain B-cell markers. Unlike HTLV-1, HTLV-2 has not yet been found to be endemic in any specific population of humans. Its association with hairy cell leukemia is somewhat tenuous, although strengthened recently by several other cases of HTLV-2 seropositive T-cell variants of hairy cell leukemia and the isolation of a second HTLV-2 isolate from such a patient.[30] HTLV-2 is distinct from HTLV-1 but shares considerable nucleic acid homology.[31,32]

HUMAN IMMUNODEFICIENCY VIRUS

The human immunodeficiency viruses, HIV-1 and HIV-2, are human retroviruses of the subclass Lentiviridae.[33] Initially referred to as HTLVs, they are now recognized to be distinct viruses. Like HTLV-1 and HTLV-2, the HIVs also infect T4+ cells; in other respects the viruses are not closely related. HIV-1 and HIV-2 are associated with the acquired immune deficiency syndrome (AIDS) but do not appear to directly cause any specific human tumors. However, patients with AIDS have a high incidence of specific tumors.[34] One of the earliest diagnostic features of AIDs in young homosexual men may be Kaposi's sarcoma, which before the AIDs epidemic was regarded as an extremely rare tumor. Other tumors for which AIDS patients are at high relative risk are non-Hodgkin's lymphomas, anogenital warts, and papillomavirus-associated squamous cell carcinomas. In AIDS patients these tumors likely have a viral etiology. The lymphomas may be largely accounted for by the emergence of cells transformed by the Epstein-Barr virus and progressing to malignancy. It is also possible that HTLV-1 may account for some lymphomas in patients with AIDs. The genital warts and perianal squamous cell carcinomas seen in these patients have been shown to harbor specific human papillomavirus DNA types (see below). A viral etiology for Kaposi's sarcoma has been postulated, but no candidate virus has yet been identified.

THE MECHANISM OF TRANSFORMATION

Only a subset of individuals seropositive for HTLV-1 will develop ATL. The virus is not acquired by casual contact but is transmitted through sexual contact, through transfusion of contaminated blood, and possibly from mother to infant through mother's milk.[35–37] The latency period between acquisition of the virus to development of ATL can vary from a few years to as long as 40 years in patients who are destined to develop the malignancy.

How is HTLV-1 involved in leukemogenesis? Several lines of evidence suggest that the virus's role is quite direct. The first is epidemiologic. Infants born in an endemic area who have been infected have the same likelihood of developing ATL if they remain in the endemic area or if they move to an area of low prevalence. Thus it appears that the virus alone is sufficient to initiate the chain of events leading to malignancy, independent of subsequent environmental factors.

Additional evidence supporting the role of HTLV-1 as an etiologic agent in ATL comes from the molecular biology of the virus. In retrovirus-infected cells the provirus (*i.e.,* the double-stranded DNA copy of the viral RNA genome) becomes integrated into the cellular genome. Within HTLV-1–infected cells, the provirus is also randomly integrated into the host chromosome.[38] In the leukemic cells of an ATL patient, however, the viral sequences are found integrated in the same place in each cell, and the site of integration varies from leukemia to leukemia.[39,40] This indicates that ATL is clonal and is derived from a single cell. It also indicates that the viral infection necessarily precedes the origin of the tumor.

HTLV-1 can transform human umbilical cord blood lymphocytes (T-cells) from normal cells into immortalized precancerous cells.[41,42] The mechanism by which HTLV-1 induces leukemogenesis is different from that of the other chronic leukemia retroviruses such as the avian leukosis virus. The combination of the clonality of the tumor cells and the random nature of the integration sites of the provirus from tumor to tumor indicates that HTLV-1 transforms by a novel mechanism for retroviruses. Prior to the detailed studies of HTLV-1, two mechanisms were known by which a retrovirus could induce malignancy. One mechanism involved the transduction of oncogene directly by the retrovirus. Oncogenes are cellular genes often involved in the regulation of cellular growth. For example, the avian sarcoma virus is capable of inducing tumors in chickens because it has acquired extra nucleic acids from a cellular oncogene called *sarc.* Retroviruses containing an oncogene are themselves defective but give rise to a rapidly developing cancer following infection of the appropriate cell. The tumors that result from infection with a retrovirus containing an oncogene are not necessarily monoclonal. The genetic events leading to the recombinational events between the cellular and viral nucleic acids are rare, and these viruses are of importance to the molecular virologist but are of little consequence to the etiology of naturally occurring cancers in humans or animals.

The slow-acting leukemogenic retroviruses such as the feline leukemia virus (FeLV) and the mouse leukemia virus (MuLV) do not contain oncogenes, and they induce leukemia in a manner similar to the HTLV-1–associated human malignancies, in which only a minority of the infected animals develop leukemia. There is also a long latency period between acquisition of the virus and the formation of tumors. In addition, the tumors are clonal. The difference between the mechanisms of leukemogenesis of these slow-acting leukemogenic retroviruses and of HTLV-1 is that although the provirus integrates randomly into the cellular chromosomes in infected cells, it is found preferentially in the vicinity of proto-oncogenes in the tumors that develop. For the slow-acting leukemogenic viruses to induce malignancy, the provirus must integrate in a region of the host genome in a manner that enables the regulatory sequences of the provirus to interact with the nearby oncogene to promote cellular proliferation. The mechanism by which this occurs is referred to as promoter insertion if the proviral long terminal repeat (LTR) acts as a promoter to initiate transcription of the proto-oncogene, or enhancer insertion if it acts as an enhancer to activate the proto-oncogene. In the case of the avian leukosis virus, the integration of the retrovirus occurs in the vicinity of the c-*myc* oncogene, resulting in the deregulation of its expression.[43]

The HTLV-1 provirus can therefore act at a distance. This suggests that the viral genome encodes a factor that is critical in the early stages of leukemogenesis. HTLV-1 and HTLV-2 belong to a distinct group of retroviruses that have been referred to as transregulating retroviruses. This group also includes the bovine leukemia virus, the biology of which is somewhat similar to that of HTLV-1 and HTLV-2.[44] As shown in Figure 10-1, these viruses differ from the chronic leukemia viruses and the acute leukemia viruses in that they contain additional genomic sequences at the 3′ end of the genome, originally called the X region by Yoshida et al, who first brought attention to it.[45] Subsequent studies from a number of laboratories have indicated that this region encodes transregulatory factors.[46–49] There appear to be several small regulatory proteins encoded by this region.[50] One gene serves as a master key for activating transcription from the viral LTR and is called the TAT gene, for transactivator of transcription. The TAT gene product acts to increase the transcriptional activity of the viral promoter in the LTR.[48,51,52]

In addition the TAT gene product has been shown to activate transcription of some nonviral genes, including the IL-2 gene and IL-2 receptor.[53] Thus it seems possible that one mechanism by which HTLV-1 could induce cellular prolifer-

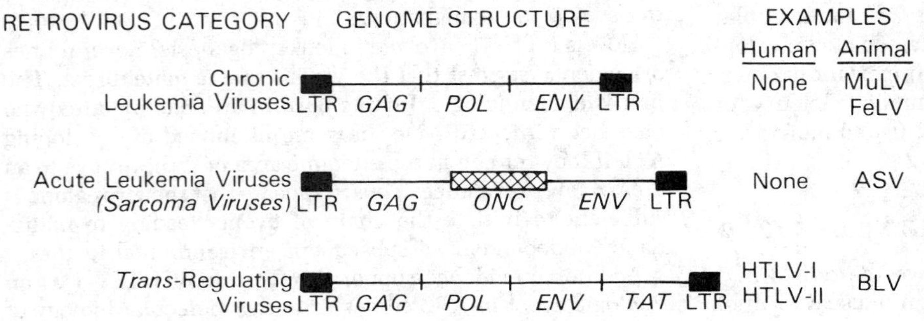

FIG. 10-1. Genomic organization of different types of retroviruses. The prototype retrovirus represented in the figure by the chronic leukemia viruses contains regulatory sequences at each end derived from the long terminal repeat (LTR) elements of the virus as well as coding sequences for the viral proteins *gag, pol,* and *env.* The acute transforming retroviruses are defective viruses. In addition to losing viral gene segments, they have acquired *onc* sequences from the cellular genome. The transregulatory retroviruses contain sequences, 3′ to the *env* gene, that encode regulatory factors. This region has been referred to as the X region and encodes the TAT gene among other regulatory factors.

ation and immortalization could involve the stimulation of both IL-2 and its receptor. The mechanism by which the TAT gene functions is not yet clear. It does not appear to be a direct DNA-binding protein;[54] therefore it does not activate either the viral LTR or the specific cellular genes by direct DNA binding. It most likely acts indirectly by modifying other cellular transcription factors.

HEPATITIS B VIRUS

Hepatitis B virus (HBV) causes hepatitis B infection, a major worldwide public health problem. In endemic parts of the world such as Far East Asia and tropical Africa, approximately 10% of the population are chronic carriers of HBV, and in these areas, chronic active hepatitis and liver cirrhosis associated with HBV infection are the major causes of mortality. Furthermore, HBV has been shown by epidemiologic studies to be of major importance in the etiology of hepatocellular carcinoma (HCC).[55] In China alone, one-half million to one million cases of HCC occur annually.

HBV is a member of a group of animal viruses known as the hepadnaviruses. It is the only member of this group of viruses that has a human reservoir.[56] Other hepadnaviruses include the woodchuck hepatitis virus (WHV), the Beechey ground squirrel hepatitis virus (GSHV), and the Pekin duck hepatitis B virus (DHBV).[57–59] Each of these viruses has a similar structure and each is hepatotropic, leading to persistent viral infections of the liver. Studies of the animal hepatitis viruses have been important in developing our understanding of the molecular biology of the hepadnaviruses. Of the hepadnaviruses, only HBV and WHV have been associated with chronic active hepatitis and HCC.

DISCOVERY

The hepatitis B surface antigen (HBsAg) was discovered in 1963 by Baruch Blumberg and co-workers while studying human serum protein polymorphisms.[60,61] Subsequent studies led to the association of this antigen with acute hepatitis B infection and an intermediate name, hepatitis-associated antigen (HAA), and finally the current name, hepatitis B surface antigen.[62,63] This antigen is the surface or envelope protein of the HBV particle, and its presence in the serum of infected patients remains the most useful marker of active HBV infection.[64] Until recently, HBV had not been successfully grown in tissue culture, and the serum from infected patients became the principal source of viral material for the characterization of the virus.

During an HBV infection, virus particles are present at high titer in the serum: up to 10^5 to 10^9 virions per milliliter are visible by electron microscopy.[65] In addition to the complete virion particles, the serum also contains empty viral envelopes consisting of spherical or filamentous particles 22 nm in diameter.[66] The virion of 42 nm in diameter consists of an envelope and a nucleocapsid containing the double-stranded circular DNA molecule, and the DNA polymerase. This virion particle was first described by Dane[64] and is sometimes referred to as the Dane particle. The outer envelope contains HBsAg, consisting of protein, carbohydrate, and lipid. The capsid carries the hepatitis B core antigen (HBcAg). The outer envelope of the virion with the HBsAg can be removed by treatment with nonionic detergents such as Nonidet P-40, releasing the free core particles (Fig. 10-2). Treatment of the virion core with a strong detergent such as SDS will then release the double-stranded viral DNA. The serum concentrations of the incomplete viral forms usually greatly exceed the concentrations of the complete virions, and concentrations of up to 10^{13} 22-nm spherical particles have been noted in some human sera.[66] The spectrum of viral forms described for HBV is also found in the serum of animals infected with WHV, GSHV, and DHBV.[57–59]

HBV VIRAL DNA

HBV particles contain small circular DNA molecules that are partially double-stranded.[67,68] The DNA consists of a long strand with a constant length of 3220 bases and a short strand that varies in length from 1700 to 2800 bases in different molecules. A map of the HBV DNA genome is shown in Figure 10-3.[69] The virion particles also contain a DNA polymerase activity that is capable of repairing the single-stranded DNA region to make two fully double-stranded molecules, each approximately 3220 bases long.[70] For this reaction, DNA synthesis initiates at the 3′ end of the short strand, which, as noted earlier, is heterogeneous among different DNA molecules. DNA synthesis terminates when it reaches the uniquely located 5′ end of the short strand. The long strand is not a closed molecule but contains a nick at a unique site approximately 300 base pairs from the 5′ end of the short strand.

Recombinant DNA technology has rapidly advanced our understanding of the biology of HBV. The complete genome

FIG. 10-2. HBV forms in the blood of infected humans (*1*), the virion core released by nonionic detergent (*2*), and the viral genome (*3*). (Redrawn from Robinson.[69])

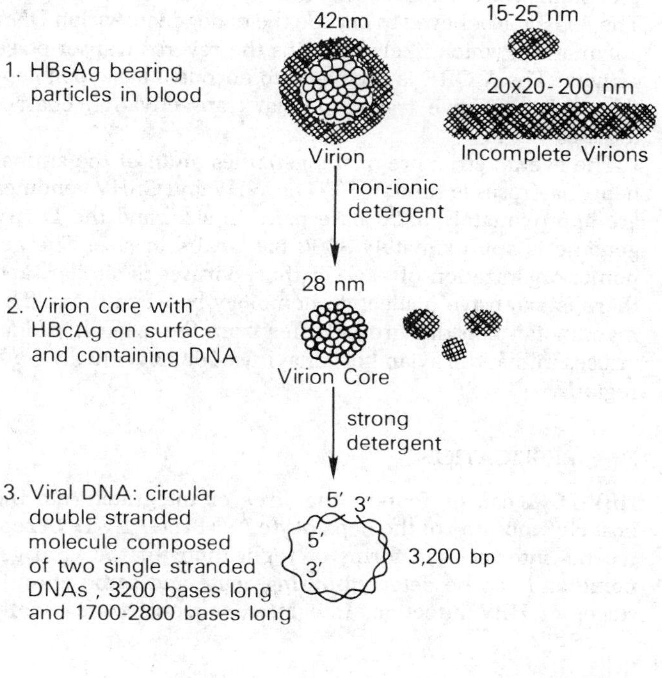

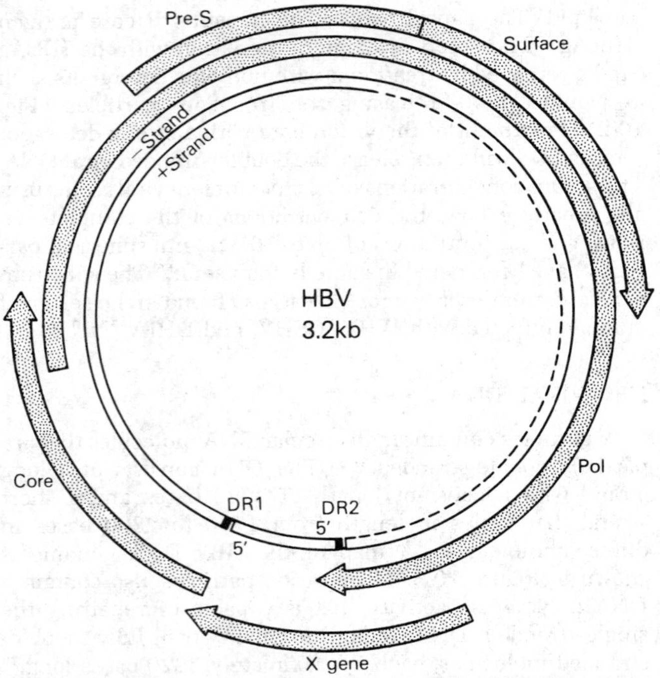

FIG. 10-3. Physical and genetic map of HBV DNA. The arrows surrounding the genome represent the four large open reading frames of the L(−) strand with the genes they encode indicated. The broken line is the S(+) DNA strand. The positions of the 5′ ends of the DNA strands are indicated. The location of the direct repeats (DR1 and DR2) involved in the initiation of DNA replication are also indicated.[72,73]

has been cloned in bacterial cells and the complete nucleotide sequence determined.[71] The viral genome has four open reading frames (ORFs). These ORFs are designated as S and pre-S, C, A, and X.[68,72] S and pre-S represent two contiguous reading frames and code for the HBsAg polypeptides. Region C contains the coding sequences for the core and E antigens. The A ORF is believed to encode the endogenous virion DNA polymerase, which likely contains the reverse transcriptase activity. The X ORF is predicted to encode a basic polypeptide and may have transcriptional transactivation characteristics.

The overall structure of the genomes of all of the animal hepadnaviruses is similar.[72,73] The WHV and GSHV genomes are approximately 3300 base pairs in size, and the DHBV genome is approximately 3000 base pairs in size. The genomic organization of each of these viruses is similar, and there is extensive nucleotide homology between them. The mammalian hepadnaviruses differ from the avian hepadnaviruses in that the avian hepadnaviruses do not contain the X region.[72]

HBV REPLICATION

HBV DNA can be found either free or integrated into the host chromosome of the hepatocyte.[74,75] Free HBV DNA represents intermediate forms of replication for the viral genome and can be detected during acute and some chronic stages of HBV infection. Integrated sequences are usually found during chronic viral infection and in HCC. The replication mechanism for the hepadnaviruses, first discovered by Summers and Mason for DHBV[76] and later confirmed for HBV, is different from that of other DNA viruses.[73] The replication cycle involves a reverse transcription step resembling that of the retroviruses in that a central feature is the use of an RNA copy of the genome as an intermediate in replication. The hepadnaviruses differ from the retroviruses, however, in that the retrovirus virions contain RNA and the intermediate form of replication is integrated DNA. The virions of the hepadnaviruses contain DNA and the intermediate replication form is RNA. It is thought that integration of the hepadnaviral genome is not a necessary intermediate step for viral genome replication. The similarity between the retroviruses and the hepadnaviruses is also reflected in the genomic organization in which all of the genes are necessarily encoded on only one strand. The order of the genes within the retroviruses (*gag, pol,* and *env*) is similar to the order of their counterparts in the hepadnaviruses (core, polymerase, and surface antigen). Other subtle differences in the transcriptional programs utilized to generate the messenger RNAs for these different viruses exist. Of note is that enhancer sequences have been found in both viruses. For the retroviruses, enhancer sequences have been found in the LTRs. For the hepadnavirus, in which no significantly large noncoding region exists, an enhancer element has been found downstream of the S ORF.[77,78] A further similarity between these viruses is the finding that a subset of these viruses encode transcriptional transacting factors. For HTLV-1, described earlier in this chapter, the TAT ORF encodes such a factor. Preliminary evidence from several laboratories indicates that the X gene of the mammalian hepadnaviruses may also encode a factor with transcriptional transactivation functions.

HBV AND HEPATOCELLULAR CARCINOMA

There is considerable evidence of an etiologic involvement of HBV in human HCC. This evidence stems primarily from epidemiologic studies. There is a striking correlation between the worldwide geographic incidence of HCC and the prevalence of HBsAg chronic carriers.[79] Compelling evidence for the role of HBV in HCC comes from the prospective epidemiologic studies performed by Beasley et al in Taiwan and reported in 1981.[55] Those studies revealed that the relative risk for HCC in HBsAg-positive males was 217, compared to the risk in noncarriers. Furthermore, 51% of the deaths in the carriers were caused by cirrhosis of the liver or HCC, compared with only 2% among the control population. Among the noncarriers, 90% had evidence of a prior HBV infection but did not have evidence of HBsAg chronic carrier state. This observation indicated that the high incidence of HCC was clearly related to the carrier state and not to a prior HBV infection per se. The age distribution of HBV infections, which occur at early ages in this Taiwanese population, indicated that the tumors appear after a mean duration of 35 years of HBV infection. Between 60% and 90% of the patients with HCC also had cirrhosis.

These epidemiologic data do not preclude an etiologic role for other factors in HCC, and in fact other factors such as aflatoxin have been recognized as having a role in some cases of liver cancer. However, factors in addition to HBV chronic infection do not need to be implicated in order to explain these striking epidemiologic findings.

HBV infection in humans is not the only hepadnavirus infection associated with HCC in nature. A much higher incidence of hepatoma formation has been observed in woodchucks infected with WHV.[80] Approximately one third of the infected animals held in captivity will develop HCC each year, and no tumors have been observed in noninfected animals. HCC develops in these woodchucks with histologic changes of acute and chronic hepatitis but not in association with cirrhosis.

PAPILLOMAVIRUSES

The viral nature of human warts was first suggested at the turn of the century by Ciuffo, who demonstrated cell-free filtrate transmission.[81] This important group of viruses has remained refractory to standard virologic studies, and no papillomavirus has been successfully propagated in the laboratory in tissue culture. However, advances in basic research through the application of biotechnology have led to a virtual explosion of knowledge concerning the papillomaviruses in the past decade. The molecular cloning of papillomavirus genomic DNA has permitted the generation of sufficient quantities of viral genetic material for systematic investigation of this group of viruses.

BIOLOGY OF HUMAN PAPILLOMAVIRUS INFECTION

The papillomaviruses are widely distributed in nature and infect many higher vertebrate species ranging from birds to man. Although originally classified as papovaviruses because of their icosahedral shape and circular, double-stranded DNA genome, the papillomaviruses are now recognized to be separate from the other papovaviruses such as polyoma and SV40, based on different biologic and genetic characteristics. The papillomaviruses contain a double-stranded circular DNA genome of 8000 base pairs, larger than DNA genome of the polyomaviruses (5000 base pairs), and the virion particles have a correspondingly larger capsid diameter (55 nm versus 40 nm). No papillomavirus has ever been propagated in tissue culture. The development of a permissive cell culture system for papillomavirus replication will be a major step toward elucidating the biology of this virus.

Unlike some other human viruses such as adenoviruses, papillomaviruses cannot be typed by serologic methods because antisera are currently not available that can distinguish among the different HPV types. Consequently, the viruses have been "typed" by DNA hybridization under controlled conditions of stringency.[82] Viruses differing by more than 50% DNA homology when assayed under stringent conditions are considered to be different types. With such methods, a total of 53 types of human papillomavirus have now been categorized, and new types are being recognized on a regular basis. Some of these viruses and the clinical syndromes with which they are associated are listed in Table 10-2.[83–111]

The productive functions of the papillomavirus, including vegetative viral DNA synthesis and the expression of late viral genes, occur only in the fully differentiated squamous epithelial cells of a papilloma. Vegetative viral DNA synthesis has been detected by in situ hybridization techniques only in the squamous epithelial cells of the stratum spinosum and of the granular layer of the epidermis, but not in the basal layer or in the underlying dermal fibroblasts. Viral capsid protein production and virus assembly occur only in the upper stratum spinosum and in the granular layer, where the epithelial cells are terminally differentiated. It is generally believed that the viral genome is present in the epithelial cells of the basal layer and that the expression of specific viral genes in the basal layer and in the lower layers of the epidermis is responsible for cellular proliferation characteristic of a wart. As the cells of the epidermis normally migrate upward through the stratum spinosum into the granular layer, they undergo a program of differentiation. The control of papillomavirus late gene expression is tightly linked to the differentiation state of the squamous epithelial cells.[112] The basis for this transcriptional control is not yet known.

Papillomaviruses are specifically tropic for squamous epithelial cells, and HPV types have specificity for different anatomical sites. HPV-1 has been observed to replicate only in heavily keratinized epithelium such as the palm or the sole, and HPV-16 preferentially replicates in mucosal squamous epithelium. HPV-1 does not replicate in cervical epithelium, and HPV-16 has not been observed in the skin of the hand or foot. Specialized keratinocytes from different anatomical sites may have distinct differentiation patterns, evident from the distinct types of keratin proteins that they synthesize and from the pattern of synthesis of other epithelial specific proteins such as involucrin. The ability of HPV to proliferate at a particular anatomical site may therefore reflect a specific interaction between viral and cellular gene regulatory factors involved in transcription.

HPV GENOMIC ORGANIZATION

All HPV types examined to date have a similar genomic organization. The DNA genomes of each of the HPVs sequenced as well as the other animal papillomaviruses contain approximately 8000 base pairs of genetic information. All of the ORFs that could serve to encode proteins for these viruses are located on only one of the two viral DNA strands. RNA studies have indicated that only one strand, the complementary strand, is transcribed.[113,114]

The HPV genome can be divided into two distinct regions: an "early" region that encodes the viral proteins involved in viral DNA replication, transcription, and cellular transformation, and a "late" region that encodes the viral capsid proteins. This functional division is based on genetic studies carried out with the bovine papillomavirus.[115] The organization of a typical HPV-16 genome is shown in Figure 10-4. The genes located in the early region of the genes are designated as E1, or E2, . . . E7, and the genes located in the late region are designated as L1 and L2. From studies with HPV-1, it is likely that E4 encodes a late gene that is expressed only in productively infected keratinocytes.[116] Thus, although this ORF is located with the early ORFs, its func-

TABLE 10-2. Human Papillomaviruses

*Virus Type**	*Clinical Association†*	*References*
HPV-1	Plantar Warts	83,84
HPV-2	Verruca vulgaris	85
HPV-3	Flat warts	86
HPV-4	Plantar warts	87
HPV-5	Macular lesions in EV	88
HPV-6	Genital warts, laryngeal papillomas	89
HPV-7	Common warts in meat handlers	90, 91
HPV-8	Macular lesions in EV[a]	88, 92
HPV-9	Macular lesions in EV	93
HPV-10	Flat warts	94
HPV-11	Laryngeal papillomas, genital warts	95
HPV-12	Macular lesions in EV	94
HPV-13	Oral focal epithelial hyperplasia	96
HPV-14	Macular lesions in EV	97
HPV-15	Macular lesions in EV	98
HPV-16	Cervical dysplasia, Bowenoid papulosis, cervical carcinoma	99
HPV-17	Macular lesions in EV	98
HPV-18	Cervical dysplasia and carcinoma	100
HPV-19	Macular lesions in EV	98, 101
HPV-20	Macular lesions in EV	98, 101
HPV-21	Macular lesions in EV	98
HPV-22	Macular lesions in EV	98
HPV-23	Macular lesions in EV	98
HPV-24	Macular lesions in EV	98
HPV-25	Macular lesions in EV	101
HPV-26	Flat warts	102
HPV-27	Verruca vulgaris	Zachow et al (unpubl.)
HPV-28	Flat warts	Favre et al (unpubl.)
HPV-29	Verruca vulgaris	Favre et al (unpubl.)
HPV-30	Genital warts, laryngeal carcinoma	103
HPV-31	Cervical dysplasia	104
HPV-32	Oral focal epithelial hyperplasia	105
HPV-33	Genital intraepithelial neoplasia, cervical carcinomas	106
HPV-34	Bowenoid papulosis, Bowen's disease	107
HPV-35	Cervical cancer	108
HPV-36	Macular lesions in EV	109
HPV-37	Keratoacanthoma	110
HPV-38	Detected in malignant melanoma	110
HPV-39	Bowenoid papulosis	111
HPV-42	Vulvar papilloma	111

* HPV types 40, 41, and 43 to 53 have been described at meetings but have not yet appeared in the literature.
† EV = epidermodysplasia verruciformis.

tion may only be important in the vegetative replication of the virus.

In productively infected tissue (*i.e.*, tissues in which viral particles are made, such as a wart), mRNA is transcribed from the early *and* late regions of the genome.[114,117] Nonproductive infection of host cells (as seen in the lower cells of the epithelium in a wart) is accompanied by mRNA transcription from only the early region of the genome.[113] Restriction of genomic expression to only the early region involves regulation of transcription at the level of initiation of RNA synthesis and at the level of transcriptional termination.[112]

The functional analysis of the molecular biology of papillomaviruses has been largely limited to the bovine papillomavirus (BPV-1), which can transform a variety of rodent fibroblast cell lines in tissue culture.[118–120] In these transformed cells, the DNA remains as a stable extrachromosomal plasmid, and this system has served as an excellent model for studying latent infection by papillomavirus.[121] This virus has therefore served as the prototype for unraveling various aspects of the biology of the papillomaviruses over the past decade. Table 10-3 lists the various papillomavirus ORFs and the functions that have been assigned to them in different papillomavirus systems.[122–138] Two independent transforming genes have been mapped to the E5 gene and to the E6 gene of BPV-1 (reviewed in ref. 139). The E2 gene of BPV-1 encodes factors that are involved in the regulation of a conditional transcriptional enhancer located in the viral control region, LCR.[125,128] Mutations in the E2 gene result in decreased transformation efficiency of the BPV-1 and affect DNA replication.[132,133,140] It is believed that this effect may be indirect through the requirement for transcriptional activity of the viral genes that are directly required for transformation (E5 and E6). The E2 genes of other papillomaviruses have also been shown to encode transcriptional regulatory functions.[126,127] In the bovine papillo-

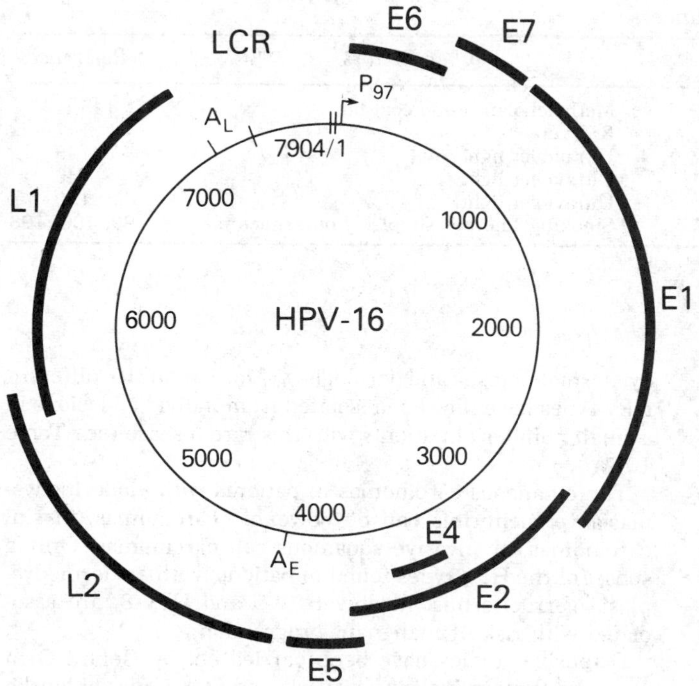

FIG. 10-4. Genomic map of HPV-16 deduced from the DNA sequence. Nucleotide numbers are noted within the circular maps, transcription proceeds clockwise, and the major open reading frames (E1 to E7, L1, and L2) are indicated. The only transcriptional promoter mapped to date for HPV-16 is designated (P_{97}). A_E and A_L represent the putative polyadenylation signals for the early and late transcripts, respectively. The viral long control region (LCR) containing the putative viral transcriptional and replication regulatory elements is noted.

mavirus, the E1 gene is required for extrachromosomal replication.[123,124] The E1 ORF actually encodes at least two genes. The 5′ portion encodes a modulator gene *(mod)* that is required for establishing stable plasmid DNA replication but is not required for transient plasmid DNA replication.[122] The 3′ portion of the E1 ORF encodes a replication function that is required for transient and stable DNA replication.[124] In the BPV system the E7 gene is also required for high copy number DNA plasmid maintenance.[136] No function has yet been found for the E3 ORF of BPV-1. The E8 ORF may also be involved in plasmid replication. The L1 ORF of the papillomaviruses encodes the major caption protein, and the L2 ORF encodes a minor caption protein.[137,138] The L1 and L2 ORFs are expressed only in the terminally differentiated keratinocytes.[112,114]

Although papillomavirus transformation studies have been principally carried out with BPV-1 in which the E5 and E6 ORFs have each been shown to encode independent transforming genes,[139] transformation of rodent cells has also been described for HPV-16[140,141] and for HPV-18.[142] This transforming activity has been localized to the E6/E7 ORFs for HPV-16 and HPV-18.[142,143] In addition HPV-16 has been shown to encode a factor capable of cooperating with the activated *ras* oncogene in the transformation of primary rodent cells.[144] This function has also been mapped to the E7 ORF.[143] A transcriptional regulatory function in addition to that of E2 has been mapped to the E7 ORF of HPV-16.[143] This function is similar to the transcriptional regulatory function of the adenovirus E1a gene in that each of these viral proteins can activate the adenovirus E2 promoter. Analysis of the amino acid structure of the adenovirus E1a gene and the E7 genes of several of the genital papillomaviruses has revealed striking similarities mapping to the conserved domains of 1 and 2 of adenovirus E1a and HPV-16 E7.[143] These domains have been shown to be important for the immortalization of primary cells in the adenovirus E1a gene.

PAPILLOMAVIRUSES IN CANCER

A subgroup of papillomaviruses can induce lesions that may progress to squamous cell carcinomas. These viruses and their associated malignancies are listed in Table 10-4.[145–150] The most extensively studied of these viruses has been the Shope papillomavirus, which infects cottontail rabbits in nature (CRPV). Studies with this virus date to the early 1930s, when Shope identified CRPV as the etiologic agent of cutaneous papillomatosis in rabbits.[151] The Shope system has been extensively studied as a model for papillomavirus-induced carcinogenesis.[145,146] One of the features of carcinogenic progression with the papillomaviruses is the synergy

TABLE 10-3. Papillomavirus Gene Functions

Open Reading Frame	*Function(s) Assigned*	*Virus*	*References*
E1 (5′ portion)	Replication modulator	BPV-1	122
E1 (3′ portion)	Replication	BPV-1	123, 124
E2 (full)	Transcriptional transactivator	BPV-1, HPV-11, HPV-16	125, 126, 127
E2 (3′ portion)	Transcriptional repressor	BPV-1	128
E3	None	. . .	
E4	Cytoplasmic protein in warts	HPV-1	116
E5	Transformation	BPV-1	129–133
E6	Transformation, plasmid copy control	BPV-1	134, 135, 136
E7	Plasmid copy control	BPV-1	136
E8	Possible role in DNA replication	BPV-1	Lusky (unpubl.)
L1	Major capsid protein	BPV-1	137
L2	Minor capsid protein	HPV-1	138

TABLE 10-4. Papillomaviruses and Naturally Occurring Cancers

Papillomaviruses	*Cancers*	*Other Factors*	*References*
CRPV	Skin cancer	Methylcholanthrene coal tar	145, 146
BPV-4	Tongue, esophageal, foregut cancers	Bracken	147
BPV (not typed)	Ocular cancers	Ultraviolet light	148
Ovine papillomavirus	Skin cancer	Ultraviolet light	149
HPV-5, 8 and others	Skin cancer in patients with EV	Ultraviolet light	150
HPV-16, 18, 33	Anogenital cancers, some oral cancers	Smoking,? herpes simplex,? other factors	99, 100, 106

EV = epidermodysplasia verruciformis.

between the virus and carcinogenic external factors (see Table 10-4). In the case of CRPV, carcinomas develop more readily in virally induced papillomas that are painted with coal tar or methylcholanthrene.[152,153] These CRPV-associated carcinomas contain copies of the viral DNA that are transcriptionally active, supporting an active role for these viruses in the cancers that develop.[154,155]

In cattle, BPV-4 has been associated with esophageal papillomatosis and with squamous cell carcinomas of upper alimentary tract.[147,156] Interestingly, however, only those cattle from the highlands of Scotland that are infected with BPV-4 and that also feed on bracken fern, which is known to contain a radiomimetic substance, have a high incidence of squamous cell carcinomas of the esophagus and the foregut.[147] In contrast to the CRPV-associated carcinomas, in which the viral DNA is invariably found, extensive analysis of the squamous cell carcinomas of the upper alimentary tract in cattle infected with BPV-4 has failed to reveal a consistent pattern of viral DNA sequences within the malignant tumors.[157] In the case of these alimentary tract tumors, it is possible that the continued presence of BPV-4 DNA sequences is not required for the maintenance of the carcinogenic stage. However, it is also possible that a different bovine papillomavirus, distinct from BPV-4, may be associated with these carcinomas and that the assays performed to detect the viral DNA sequences have not been sufficiently sensitive.

EPIDERMODYSPLASIA VERRUCIFORMIS

Epidermodysplasia verruciformis is a rare, life-long disease that usually begins in infancy or childhood. The disease is characterized by disseminated polymorphic cutaneous lesions that resemble flat warts, and by reddish macules sometimes referred to as pityriasis-like lesions.[158] Approximately one third of the patients with epidermodysplasia verruciformis develop multiple skin cancers, usually during the third or fourth decade of life. Papillomavirus particles have been detected within the benign lesions but not in the carcinomas. It has been proposed that the disease is linked to a rare, recessive, abnormal allele of an X-linked gene. Patients with epidermodysplasia verruciformis often have impaired cell-mediated immunity, which is believed to play a role in the life-long infection by papillomaviruses. The carcinomas that develop in these patients arise in sun-exposed areas, and ultraviolet radiation is thought to play a cocarcinogenic role with the papillomaviruses in the etiology of these cancers. Epidermodysplasia verruciformis has been intensely studied by dermatologists and virologists. More than 15 different HPV types have now been isolated from individual lesions in a small number of patients with this rare disease (see Table 10-2).

The cutaneous carcinomas in patients with epidermodysplasia verruciformis can be bowenoid carcinomas, in situ carcinomas, or invasive squamous cell carcinomas. Only a subset of the HPV types found in patients with epidermodysplasia verruciformis, notably HPV-5 and HPV-8, are associated with risk of malignant progression.

Extensive studies have been carried out by Gerard Orth from the Pasteur Institute in Paris and Stephonia Jablonska in Warsaw in analyzing the HPVs in cancers from patients with epidermodysplasia verruciformis. They investigated a total of 28 tumors from 14 patients. HPV genomes were found in 27 of the 28 samples. Twenty-one of these contained HPV-5 DNA, five contained HPV-8 DNA, and one contained HPV-14 DNA.[150] HPV-5 has been found in metastatic squamous cell carcinoma lesions in some patients with epidermodysplasia verruciformis.[159,160] Still other investigators have found additional HPVs in carcinomas in epidermodysplasia verruciformis patients. HPV-3 has been found in an in situ vulvar carcinoma of a patient with epidermodysplasia verruciformis,[161] and HPV-17 has been found in a cutaneous epidermodysplasia verruciformis carcinoma by a group of Japanese investigators.[162] Thus the specific association of carcinomas in patients with epidermodysplasia verruciformis is not strictly limited to HPV-5 and HPV-8. Although metastasis is uncommon in the cancers in these patients, the presence of HPV-5 in the two metastatic lymph node lesions examined strengthens the argument for an etiologic role for HPV.[150,159] Further studies have established that the viral genomes are transcriptionally active within these carcinomas.[163]

GENITAL CARCINOMAS

The epidemiology of genital warts follows a pattern characteristic of a venereally transmitted disease, with a high prevalence in populations of women of high promiscuity.[164,165] Two general types of genital wart viral infections are recognized that can be differentiated by their clinical appearance: condylomata acuminata and flat genital warts. It has been known for many years that condylomata acuminata, which can be localized to the penis, the vulva, the perineum, the anus, and rarely the uterine cervix, are caused by papillomaviruses. Particles have been demonstrated by electron microscopy,[166,167] and in 1980 papillomavirus-specific antigens were detected utilizing antisera to a common papillomavirus antigen.[168] HPV-6 was directly cloned from a condyloma acuminatum, and, using its DNA along with that of the closely related HPV-11, zur Hausen and co-workers in West Germany were able to demonstrate HPV DNA in over 90% of the lesions of condyloma acuminatum that have been examined.[169,170] Less frequently other HPV types can be found in condylomata acuminata. Malignant conversion of condylomata acuminata into squamous cell carcinoma is quite uncommon. Buschke and Lowenstein[171] have described a lesion, designated as a giant condyloma, that has characteristics similar to that of a locally invasive squamous cell carcinoma. These tumors have been associated with HPV-6 and HPV-11.[169,172] The majority of cervical carcinomas and other genital tract carcinomas, however, have been negative when examined for HPV-6 and HPV-11.

Compelling evidence linking an HPV infection with cervical carcinoma came from the recognition that the morphological changes previously interpreted as cervical dysplasia on Papanicolaou-stained smears and tissue sections of the cervix were due to a papillomavirus infection.[173-175] The characteristic cell that is diagnostic for a cervical papillomavirus infection is the koilocyte, found in high association in smears with cervical dysplastic changes.[176] Electron microscopy disclosed papillomavirus particles in the koilocytotic cells, proving the papillomavirus etiology.[177,178] Numerous investigators have found papillomavirus-specific capsid antigens and HPV DNA within cervical dysplastic lesions, confirming the viral etiology of cervical dysplasia.

Epidemiologic studies have implicated an infectious agent in the etiology of human cervical carcinoma.[179,180] Venereal transmission of a carcinogenic factor with a long latency has been suggested by such studies. Sexual promiscuity, early age at onset of sexual activity, and poor sexual hygiene are risk factors for cervical carcinoma. There is a correlation between the incidence rates of cervical cancer and penile carcinoma in different geographic areas, although the incidence rates for penile carcinoma are 20-fold lower than those of cervical carcinoma. A similar incidence ratio of cervical carcinoma and penile carcinoma is maintained in areas of high, medium, or low prevalence, suggesting that the etiologic factors for penile and cervical carcinoma may be the same. The "male factor" also appears to implicate a venereally transmitted agent. Monogamous women are at higher risk for cervical carcinoma if their spouses have multiple sexual partners.

The suggestion of possible involvement of an infectious agent in the etiology of cervical carcinoma has prompted many studies evaluating genital pathogens as potential causative agents. Infections by *Trichomonas, Chlamydia,* and bacteria, such as syphilis and gonorrhea, have not been linked to cervical carcinoma. In the late 1960s and early 1970s genital infection by herpes simplex virus (HSV) type 2 was considered a possible etiologic candidate.[181,182] Support for the notion that HSV might be a cancer-associated virus came from studies demonstrating the ability of HSV to transform certain rodent cells in the laboratory in vitro and from serologic studies suggesting a higher frequency of antibodies to HSV-2 in patients with cervical carcinoma. However, subsequent carefully done molecular studies that sought to demonstrate HSV RNA or HSV DNA in cervical cancer tissues could not provide convincing evidence for a role for HSV in cervical cancer.[183] More recently a large prospective epidemiologic study carried out by Vonka et al has failed to support the involvement of HSV-1 or HSV-2 infections in cervical cancer.[184,185]

The association of an HPV with cervical dysplasia (also referred to as cervical intraepithelial neoplasia, CIN) provided impetus for a close examination of cervical cancer for HPV sequences. The natural history linking CIN to carcinoma in situ and to invasive squamous cell carcinoma of the cervix had already been well established.[186-188] Initial experiments from a number of laboratories revealed HPV sequences in occasional cases of cervical carcinoma and anogenital carcinoma, but no consistent pattern of positivity emerged. Using radioactively labeled HPV-11 DNA under conditions of hybridization of low stringency, zur Hausen and his colleagues at Heidelberg examined human cervical carcinoma DNAs for unknown HPV types and were able to identify two new papillomavirus DNAs, HPV-16 and HPV-18, from two cervical cancer tissues.[99,100] Using HPV-16 and HPV-18 DNA as probes they found these DNAs in approximately 70% of all cervical carcinomas examined.[189] The use of low stringency hybridization techniques has led to the identification of approximately a dozen different HPVs now associated with genital tract lesions. HPV-33, HPV-39, and HPV-42 are each associated with a small percentage of cervical carcinomas.[106,111] Thus, specific HPVs are now regularly found in human cervical carcinoma tissues and in other human genital carcinomas, including penile carcinomas, vulvar carcinomas, and perianal carcinomas. The cloning of this set of HPV DNAs has made available DNA probes that permit extensive analysis of specific lesions for a variety of HPV types. It is now recognized, for instance, that bowenoid papulosis of the penis[190,191] is associated with HPV-16. In general, HPV-16, HPV-18, and HPV-33 are found in cases of moderate to severe dysplasia and in invasive cervical carcinomas; and HPV-6, HPV-11, and HPV-31 are found in cases of condyloma acuminatum and in cases of mild cervical dysplasia. Preliminary epidemiologic studies suggest that lesions associated with HPV-16 and HPV-18 may be at higher risk for progression to cervical carcinoma. More extensive epidemiologic studies with proper controls are now under way to establish these associations more firmly and to identify other risk factors.

HPV infections by themselves are not sufficient for carcinogenic progression. Only a small fraction of individuals infected by a specific HPV will eventually develop cervical carcinoma. Thus the genetic information carried by the virus per se is not sufficient for malignant progression. Other factors must be involved in the progression of viral associated lesions to these genital tract cancers and may work synergistically with papillomavirus infections. For example, epidemiologic studies have suggested that smoking is a risk factor for developing cervical carcinoma.[192-194] The tobacco condensate might accumulate in the vaginal fluids bathing the cervix and act as a cofactor with the papillomavirus infection.[195] It has also been postulated that herpes virus infection could act synergistically with specific papillomaviruses to induce human cervical carcinoma.[196] Specific molecular studies to establish cooperativity between these two viruses have not yet been reported in the literature. The striking association of specific HPV types with genital tract carcinomas has been established. RNA and DNA analyses of biopsy specimens has demonstrated a high correlation of viral transcriptional activity with the presence of viral DNA.[197–199]

In addition, over the years several cell lines have been derived from human cervical carcinomas, including the HeLa, SiHa, and Caski cell lines, which have proved useful in studying the HPVs associated with cervical carcinoma. HeLa cells contain approximately ten incomplete copies of HPV-18 genome integrated and the viral DNA is transcriptionally active.[197,200] In the HeLa cell line, the HPV-18 genome is integrated with 50 kilobases of the c-*myc* oncogene on chromosome 8.[201] Integration of the HPV genomes in cervical carcinomas within the vicinity of the c-*myc* locus on chromosome 8 is not a general characteristic of all human cervical carcinomas, however. The SiHa and Caski cell lines contain integrated HPV-16 DNA.[200] The SiHa cell line contains a single copy of HPV-16 and the Caski cell line contains approximately 600 copies of the viral DNA integrated.[200,202] In these cell lines the viral genomes are integrated at other chromosomal sites, indicating that integration is not site specific for the papillomaviruses but apparently can occur at a variety of sites.[201]

Transcriptional analyses of the cervical carcinoma cell lines has shown that a high percentage of these cell lines are positive for HPV transcription and that the E6 and E7 regions of the viral genomes appear to be invariably expressed in the transcriptionally positive lines.[197,200,201] In addition, there is little if any expression of the E2 ORF. In those cell lines in which only a single copy of viral DNA has been integrated, integration appears to be specific for the E1 and E2 ORFs, resulting in disruption of the integrity and expression of the E2 ORF.[197,201] Since the E2 ORF of the human papillomaviruses encodes transcriptional regulatory factors,[126,127] integration resulting in the disruption of the E2 ORF could result in the uncoupling of the control of the HPV promoter in the viral LCR from E2 transregulation. The HPV-16 and HPV-18 control region contains E2-independent enhancer elements that are cell type specific and glucocorticoid responsive.[203,205] Transcription from the LCR promoters leads to expression of the E6 and E7 ORFs, suggesting that expression of the products may be necessary for maintenance of the transformed phenotype. Transformation, immortalization, and transcriptional modulation functions have been mapped to these ORFs in HPV-16 and HPV-18.[140–143]

OTHER HUMAN CANCERS ASSOCIATED WITH PAPILLOMAVIRUSES

The availability of specific HPV DNA probes has allowed investigators to screen a variety of human cancers for HPV sequences. Based on the animal models, it seemed likely that any carcinomas of any squamous epithelium or an epithelium that can undergo squamous metaplasia would be a potential candidate for an HPV association. Studies on oral and upper airway carcinomas have revealed some HPV-positive carcinomas.[103,206,207] HPV DNA has been found in benign oral papillomas,[208–211] and oral focal epithelial hyperplasia has been firmly established as having a papillomavirus etiology.[96,105] In addition, papillomavirus DNA sequences have been found associated with cases of oral leukoplakia.[209,212] HPV-16 sequences have been described in a verrucous carcinoma of the larynx. Recently HPV-11 was found in a squamous cell carcinoma of the lung in a 26-year-old man with a history of laryngotracheobronchial papillomatosis.[213] In this case, HPV-11 DNA was also found within metastatic lesions in the liver and lymph nodes. The viral genome was transcriptionally active, suggesting that expression of the virus may have played an active role in the carcinogenic progression. An association of esophageal carcinomas with HPV has not yet been demonstrated in humans. However there appears to be an excellent candidate for a human cancer that could be associated with an HPV. The esophagus is lined by squamous epithelium, and squamous cell papillomas of the esophagus have been described in humans.[214,215] To date the specific HPVs associated with these papillomas have not been determined, although viral antigens have been detected in several cases.

EPSTEIN-BARR VIRUS

The Epstein-Barr virus (EBV) was the first human tumor virus to be recognized. It was discovered during studies of lymphoma in young children in certain parts of East Africa, which were first described by Dennis Burkitt in 1958.[216] Although this childhood lymphoma had been previously recognized, it had not been clearly defined as a unique entity with characteristic clinical, pathologic, and epidemiologic features. In his early descriptive studies Burkitt suggested that the lymphoma could be due to a virus because its geographic distribution—a belt across equatorial Africa—was similar to that of yellow fever.[216,217] In 1964, Epstein and Barr described virus particles of the herpesvirus family in lymphoblastoid lines cultured from explants of Burkitt's lymphoma.[218,219] The finding of such virus particles in lymphoid lines, however, was not limited to explants of Burkitt's lymphoma tissue since they could also be seen in cell lines established from patients with other malignancies, from patients with infectious mononucleosis, and, occasionally, from normal individuals.

EBV is a double-stranded DNA virus belonging to the herpesvirus family. Other members of the human herpesvirus family include herpes simplex viruses types 1 and 2, varicella zoster virus, cytomegalovirus, and the recently described human B-lymphotropic virus. Morphologically the mature virus is essentially indistinguishable from other members of the herpes family. The viruses are large, 150 to 180 nm in diameter, and contain a large double-stranded DNA genome of approximately 170,000 base pairs. In addition to its central core of genetic material, the virus particle is also composed of a capsid layer made up of capsomeres in an icosahedral shape and an outer lipoprotein envelope. Because of its tropism for lymphoid cells, in vivo and in vitro, EBV is considered a member of the gamma herpesviruses.

Individual members of this group are specific for either B- or T-lymphocytes. EBV and HBLV are the two viruses in this group that cause disease in humans. Other gamma herpesviruses include Marek's disease virus of chickens and two viruses that infect New World monkeys: herpes ateles and herpes saimiri. Our understanding of the biology and clinical importance of HBLV, which was first described in 1986 by investigators at Gallo's laboratory, is still in its infancy.[220,221]

EBV VIRAL GENOME

The EBV viral genome is a double-stranded DNA molecule of approximately 170,000 base pairs.[222] The organization is complex, with regions of repeated DNA sequences and multiple tandem copies (6–12) of a 500-base pair terminal repeat unit at the end of the linear genome. When in one cell nucleus in the latent state, the genome exists in a circular form. Its ability to circularize may involve homologous recombination through the terminal repeated DNA sequences. The EBV genome has now been sequenced in its entirety.[223] The availability of this DNA sequence information has permitted the identification of open reading frames and genes for subsequent genetic and molecular studies.

EBV ANTIGENS

A variety of antigens have been identified in EBV-infected and transformed cells by immunologic methods. The viral capsid antigens and membrane antigens are detected in cells producing EBV particles.[224] The membrane antigens are late antigens; their expression occurs after the onset of vegetative viral DNA synthesis in the life cycle of the virus. The membrane antigens are responsible for eliciting virus-neutralizing antibody.[225] A group of antigens referred to as the EBV-induced early antigens are synthesized early in the virus replication cycle. This group of antigens can be subdivided into diffuse (D) and restricted (R) components based on the distribution of the antigens and the sensitivity of the patterns to fixation.[226] The restricted early antigens are denatured by methanol, whereas the diffuse components are stable. An important complex identified by immunofluorescence procedures is the EBV-induced nuclear antigen (EBNA).[227] This antigen is as an excellent immunologic marker for the presence of the viral DNA because it is expressed in virtually every cell containing the viral genome. EBNA is detected using anticomplement immunofluorescence assays as described by Reedman and Klein in 1973.[227] An additional antigen complex identified in the membranes of EBV-infected cells by lymphocyte cytotoxic assays has been designated LYDMA, for lymphocyte-detected membrane antigen.[228–230] This antigen presumably serves as the target for cytotoxic T-lymphocytes. For the cell biologist and the molecular biologist, the EBNA and LYDMA antigens are the major candidates for transforming proteins because of their expression in transformed cells.

Until recently, the composition and nature of the EBV-induced antigens were unclear because the components of these complexes had not been specifically identified. Monospecific reagents directed against specific constituents of the antigen complex have permitted the definition of specific components. A large amount of data has been generated concerning the EBV proteins over the past few years using monoclonal antibodies.[231,232] The reader is referred to a recent review by Pearson and Luca[233] for a more detailed description of the EBV-determined antigens.

BURKITT'S LYMPHOMA

Burkitt's lymphoma occurs several years after the primary infection with EBV. Studies have indicated that Burkitt's lymphoma is a monoclonal lymphoma,[234] as opposed to infectious mononucleosis, which is a polyclonal disease. African Burkitt's lymphoma is characterized by rapid growth of the tumor at nonlymphoid sites such as the jaw or the retroperitoneum. The tumor is of B-cell origin and is closely related to the small noncleaved cells of normal lymphoid follicles.[235] The biopsy specimens from African Burkitt's lymphoma invariably contain the EBV genome and are positive for EBNA.[236] By contrast, only 15% to 20% of non-African Burkitt's lymphomas contain the EBV genome. EBV has a worldwide distribution and infects most (>90%) individuals by the time they reach adulthood. The clustering of Burkitt's lymphoma in the equatorial belt of East Africa, therefore, remains unexplained. It has been hypothesized that potential alterations of the immune system, possibly due to hyperstimulation by endemic malaria, may play an important role in the outcome of an EBV infection in individuals in this region.[237,238] Individuals from this region have impairment of virus-specific cytotoxic T-cell activity. Normally, it is the T-cell response to EBV infection that limits B-cell proliferation, which is directly stimulated by EBV.[239] It has been postulated that failure of the T-cell immune response to control this proliferation could lead to excessive B-cell proliferation and, as such, provide a suitable background for further mutation, oncogenic transformation, and lymphomogenesis.

Burkitt's lymphomas regularly exhibit abnormalities of the chromosomes that contain the immunoglobulin genes, notably chromosomes 2, 14, and 22. The most common abnormality, observed in more than 90% of Burkitt's lymphomas, is a translocation of the long arm of chromosome 14,[240] which contains the heavy chain immunoglobulin genes, to chromosome 8, which contains the c-*myc* oncogene. Less frequent translocations involve chromosome 2 (κ light chain) and chromosome 22 (λ light chain).[241] These translocations generally involve reciprocal translocations to the distal arm of chromosome 8 (band 824), which contains the c-*myc* proto-oncogene.[242] It is believed that Burkitt's lymphomas exhibit abnormal expression of the c-*myc* oncogene after this translocation, and that the abnormal expression results from proximity of the c-*myc* oncogene to the transcriptional control elements of the immunoglobulin genes.[242,243] Support for this model is provided by the recent experiments of Dalla-Favera et al, who demonstrated tumorigenic conversion of EBV-infected human B-lymphocytes with the introduction of an activated c-*myc* oncogene.[244] This study demonstrates that EBV infection and c-*myc* activation are sufficient for tumorigenic transformation of human B-cells in vitro.

The chromosomal abnormalities noted above are not detected in the peripheral blood lymphocytes of patients with Burkitt's lymphoma, nor are they found in nonmalignant lymphoblastoid cell lines derived from such patients. Thus the translocation appears to be specific for Burkitt's lymphoma and appears to occur at a step following the immortalization by EBV. In 1979 George Klein suggested a scenario for the involvement of EBV in the etiology of African Burkitt's lymphoma.[245] The first step involves the EBV-induced immortalization of B-lymphocytes in a primary infection. The second step involves stimulated proliferation of EBV-positive B-cells. This step is facilitated in the geographic areas where Burkitt's lymphoma is endemic (presumably because of the presence of malaria) through B-cell triggering and the suppression of T-cells involved in the control of the proliferation of EBV-infected cells. This pool of cells thus increases in size as a target cell population for random chromosomal rearrangements. The third and final step is the reciprocal translocation involving a chromosomal locus with an immunoglobulin gene and the c-*myc* gene on chromosome 8. This leads to the deregulation of the c-*myc* gene, the development of the malignant clone, and finally the appearance of a tumor mass.[246] Alternative scenarios have been proposed in which the order of the steps is rearranged such that the B-cell activation by malaria precedes the chromosomal translocation and is followed by EBV infection.[247] Regardless, the components of either of these scenarios account for the geographic distribution of Burkitt's lymphoma, the critical involvement of EBV in lymphomogenesis, and the eventual selection and clonal outgrowth of a population of cells with the critical translocation involving the deregulation of the *myc* gene on chromosome 8.

NASOPHARYNGEAL CARCINOMA

Nasopharyngeal carcinoma has also been linked to EBV (reviewed in ref. 248). Nasopharyngeal carcinoma occurs in adults from ages 20 to 50, although in certain parts of Africa the age distribution extends to children as well. In general, affected males outnumber females in a ratio of 2 : 1, and although worldwide the annual incidence rates are low, some areas in China (especially the southern province) have a high rate of approximately 10 cases per 100,000 population per year. Since the incidence among individuals of Chinese descent remains high irrespective of where they live, a genetic susceptibility has been proposed. For the Cantonese in Singapore, the annual rates of 29 per 100,000 are higher than for other racial groups living in the same locale. A correlation of certain HLA haplotypes has been noted among the Chinese; however, these associations do not hold true for evaluation of nasopharyngeal carcinoma in Tunisia. Environmental factors that have been implicated as risk factors for nasopharyngeal carcinoma include fumes, chemicals, smoke, and ingestion of salt-cured fish.

EBV genomes are found in nearly all biopsies of undifferentiated NPC specimens from all over the world.[249,250] The genome has been demonstrated to exist in the epithelial cells of the tumors.[251] The EBV genome is transcriptionally active within these tumors, and the regions that are transcribed in the biopsies are the same as those expressed in latently infected lymphocytes.[252] These molecular observations are consistent with an active role for EBV in the neoplastic processes involved in nasopharyngeal carcinoma. Patients with nasopharyngeal carcinoma have elevated levels of IgG antibodies to EBV capsid and early antigens. Furthermore, they have serum IgA antibodies to capsid and early antigen, likely reflecting the local production of such antibodies in the nasopharynx. Characteristic chromosomal translocations have been sought in the nasopharyngeal carcinomas but none have yet been identified. Attempts to identify mutated or activated cellular oncogenes thus far have not been successful.

The presence of immunoglobulin markers for EBV (IgA/VCA and IgA/EA) has provided the opportunity for early serologic identification of patients with nasopharyngeal carcinoma. The frequency of IgA antibody to the EBV capsid antigen in 150,000 Chinese studied was 1%. About 20% of the patients with elevated IgA antibodies to VCA had nasopharyngeal carcinoma, however, when biopsied. Thus, early detection using serologic tests can be applied in areas where nasopharyngeal carcinoma is prevalent, possibly leading to early therapeutic intervention.[253]

LYMPHOMA IN IMMUNODEFICIENT INDIVIDUALS

EBV is associated with lymphomas in patients with acquired or congenital immunodeficiencies. These lymphomas can be distinguished from the classic Burkitt's lymphomas in that the tumors are often polyclonal. The tumors also do not demonstrate the characteristic chromosomal abnormalities of Burkitt's lymphoma described earlier. The pathogenesis of these lymphomas involves a deficiency in the effector mechanisms needed to control EBV-transformed cells. The prototypic model for this disease has been the X-linked lymphoproliferative syndrome.[254] Patients with X-linked lymphoproliferative syndrome who develop acute infectious mononucleosis exhibit the usual atypical lymphocytosis and polyclonal elevation of serum immunoglobulins as well as increases in specific antibody to VCA and to EA. During these infections, however, patients with X-linked lymphoproliferative syndrome fail to mount and sustain an anti-EBNA response following acute infection. The unique vulnerability of males with X-linked lymphoproliferative syndrome to EBV infection is most likely due to an inherited immune regulatory defect that results in failure to govern the cytotoxic T-cells and natural killer cells required to cope with EBV.

Patients with iatrogenic immunodeficiencies, such as organ transplant recipients, are at increased risk for lymphomas, and these lymphomas often contain EBV DNA and EBNA. Also, patients with AIDS are at a higher risk for developing polyclonal lymphomas that are associated with EBV.

REFERENCES

1. Ellermann V, Bang O: Experimentelle Leukámie bei Huhnern. Zentralbl Bakteriol Abt [I.] 46:595–609, 1908
2. Rous P: A sarcoma of the fowl transmissible by an agent separable from the tumor cells. J Exp Med 13:397–411, 1911

3. Shope RE: A filtrable virus causing a tumor-like condition in rabbits and its relationship to virus myxomatosum. J Exp Med 56:803–1932
4. Shope RE: Infectious papillomatosis of rabbits. J Exp Med 58:607–629, 1933
5. Rous P, Beard JW: The progression to carcinoma of vinus-induced rabbit papillomas (Shope). J Exp Med 62:523–548, 1935
6. Gross L: Pathogenic properties, and "vertical" transmission of the mouse leukemia agent. Proc Soc Exp Biol Med 78:342–348, 1951
7. Gross L: A filtrable agent, recovered from Akr leukemia extracts, causing salivary gland carcinomas in C3H mice. Proc Soc Exp Biol Med 83:414–421, 1953
8. Stewart SE: Leukemia in mice produced by a filterable agent present in AKR leukemic tissues with notes on a sarcoma produced by the same agent. Anat Rev 117:532, 1953
9. Jarrett WFH, Martin WB, Crighton GW et al: Transmission experiments with leukemia (lymphosarcoma). Nature 202:566–567, 1964
10. Bernard W: The detection and study of tumor viruses with electron microscopy. Cancer Res 20:712–727, 1960
11. Temin HM, Mizutani S: RNA-dependent DNA polymerase in virions of Rous sarcoma virus. Nature 226:1211–1212, 1970
12. Baltimore D: RNA-dependent DNA polymerase in virions of RNA tumor viruses. Nature 276:1209–1211, 1970
13. Poiesz BJ, Ruscetti FW, Gazdar AF, Bunn PA, Minna JD, Gallo RC: Detection and isolation of type C retrovirus particles from fresh and cultured lymphocytes of a patient with cutaneous T-cell lymphoma. Proc Natl Acad Sci USA 77:7415–7419, 1980
14. Poiesz BJ, Ruscetti FW, Reitz MS, Kalyanaraman VS, Gallo RC: Isolation of a new type C retrovirus (HTLV) in primary uncultured cells of a patient with Sezary T-cell leukemia. Nature 294:268–271, 1981
15. Yoshida M, Miyoshi I, Hinuma Y:Isolation and characterization of retrovirus from cell lines of human adult T-cell leukemia and its implication in disease. Proc Natl Acad Sci USA 79:2031–2035, 1982
16. Uchiyama T, Yodoi J, Sagawa K, Takatsuki K, Uchino H: Adult T-cell leukemia: Clinical and hematological features of 16 cases. Blood 50:481–492, 1977
17. Miyoshi I, Kubonishi I, Yoshimoto S et al: Type C virus particles in a cord T-cell line derived by co-cultivating normal human cord leukocytes and human leukaemic T cells. Nature 294:770–771, 1981
18. Watanabe T, Seiki M, Yoshida M: Retrovirus terminology. Science 222:1178, 1983
19. Watanabe T: HTLV type 1 (US isolate) and ATLV (Japanese isolate) are the same species of human retrovirus. Virology 133:238–241, 1984
20. Hattori T, Uchiyama T, Tibana K, Takatsuki K, Uchino H: Surface phenotype of Japanese adult T-cell leukemia cells characterized by monoclonal antibodies. Blood 58:645–647, 1981
21. Hinuma T, Nagata K, Misoka M et al: Adult T cell leukemia: Antigen in an ATL cell line and detection of antibodies of the antigen in human sera. Proc Natl Acad Sci USA 78:6476–7480, 1981
22. Blattner WA, Kalyanaraman VS, Robert-Guroff M et al: The human type C retrovirus, HTLV, in blacks from the Caribbean region, and relationship to adult T cell leukemia/lymphoma. Int J Cancer 30:257–265, 1982
23. Hunsmann G, Schneider J, Schmitt J et al: Detection of serum antibodies to adult T-cell leukemia virus in non-human primates and in people from Africa. Int J Cancer 32:329–332, 1983
24. Morgan DA, Ruscetti FW, Gallo RC: Selective in vitro growth of T-lymphocytes from normal human bone marrows. Science 193:1007, 1976
25. Yamaguchi K, Nishimura H, Kawano K, Jono M, Miyamoto Y, Takatsuki K: A proposal for smoldering adult T-cell leukemia: Diversity in clinical pictures of adult T-cell leukemia. Jpn J Clin Oncol 13:189–200, 1983
26. Gessain A, Barin F, Vemant JC et al: Antibodies to human lymphotropic virus type-1 in patients with tropical spastic paraparesis. Lancet 2:407–410, 1985
27. Bartholomew C, Cleghorn F, Charles W et al: HTLV-1 and tropical spastic paraparesis. Lancet 2:99–100, 1986
28. Osame M, Usuku K, Izumo S et al: HTLV-I associated myelopathy: A new clinical entity. Lancet 1:1031–1032, 1986
29. Kalyanaraman VS, Sarngadharan MG, Robert-Guroff M et al: A new subtype of human T-cell leukemia virus (HTLV-II) associated with a T-cell variant of hairy cell leukemia. Science 218:571–573, 1982
30. Rosenblatt J, Golde JD, Wachsman W et al: A second isolate of HTLV-II associated with atypical hairy-cell leukemia. N Engl J Med 315:372–377, 1986
31. Gelmann EP, Franchini G, Manzari V, Wong-Staal F, Gallo RC: Molecular cloning of a unique human T-cell leukemia virus (HTLV-II). Proc Natl Acad Sci USA 81:993–997, 1984
32. Shaw GM, Gonda MA, Flickinger GH, Hahn BH, Gallo RC, Wong-Staal F: Genomes of evolutionary divergent members of human T-cell leukemia virus family (HTLV-I and HTLV-II) are highly conserved, especially in pX. Proc Natl Acad Sci USA 81:4544–4548, 1984
33. McClure MO, Weiss RA: Human immunodeficiency virus and related viruses. Curr Top AIDS 1:95–117, 1987
34. Pinching A, Weiss RA: AIDS and the spectrum of HTLV-III/LAV infection. Int Rev Exp Pathol 28:1–44, 1986
35. Tajima K, Tominaga S, Suchi T: Epidemiological analysis of the distribution of antibody to adult T-cell leukemia virus. Gann 73:893–901, 1982
36. Kinoshita K, Hino S, Amagasaki T et al: Demonstration of adult T-cell leukemia virus antigen in milk from three sero-positive mothers. Gann 75:103–105, 1984
37. Okochi K, Sato H, Hinuma Y: A retrospective study on transmission of adult T-cell leukemia virus by blood transfusion: Sero-conversion in recipients. Vox Sang 46:245–253, 1983
38. Seika M, Eddy R, Shows TR, Yoshida H: Non-specific integration of the HTLV provirus genome into adult T-cell leukemia cells. Nature 309:640–642, 1984
39. Yoshida M, Seiki M, Yamaguchi K, Takatsuki K: Monoclonal integration of human T-cell leukemia provirus in all primary tumors of adult T-cell leukemia suggests causative role of human T-cell leukemia virus in the disease. Proc Natl Acad Sci USA 81:2534–2537, 1984
40. Wong-Staal F, Hahn B, Manzari V et al: A survey of human leukemias for sequences of a human retrovirus, HTLV. Nature 302:626–628, 1983
41. Yamamoto N, Okada M, Koyanagi Y et al: Transformation of human leukocytes by cocultivation with an adult T-cell leukemia virus producer cell line. Science 217:737–739, 1982
42. Popovic M, Lange-Wantzin G, Sarin PS, Mann D, Gallo RC: Transformation of human umbilical cord blood T-cells by human T-cell leukemia/lymphoma virus. Proc Natl Acad Sci USA 80:502–506, 1983
43. Hayward WS, Neel BG, Astrin SM: Activation of a cellular *onc* gene by promoter insertion in ALV-induced lymphoid leukosis. Nature 290:475–480, 1981
44. Burny A, Buck C, Chantrenne H: Bovine leukemia virus: Molecular biology and epidemiology. In Klein G (ed): Viral Oncology, pp 231–280. New York, Raven Press, 1980
45. Seiki M, Hattori S, Hirayama Y, Yoshida M: Human adult T-cell leukemia virus: Complete nucleotide sequence of provirus genome integrated in leukemia cell DNA. Proc Natl Acad Sci USA 80:3618–3622, 1983
46. Sodroski JG, Rosen CA, Haseltine WA: Trans-acting transcriptional activation of the long terminal repeat of human T lymphotropic viruses in infected cells. Science 225:381–385, 1984
47. Fujisawa J, Seiki M, Kiyokawa T, Yoshida M: Functional activation of long terminal repeat of human T-cell leukemia virus type 1 by transacting factor. Proc Natl Acad Sci USA 82:2277–2281, 1985
48. Febler BK, Paskalis H, Klienman-Ewing C et al: The pX protein of HTLV-I is a transciptional activator of its long terminal repeats. Science 229:675–679, 1985
49. Chen ISY, Slamon DJ, Rosenblatt JD et al: The x gene is essential for HTLV replication. Science 229:54–58, 1985
50. Kiyokawa T, Seiki M, Iwashita S, Imagawa K, Shimizu F, Yoshida M: $p27^{x\text{-}III}$ and $p21^{x\text{-}III}$, proteins encoded by the pX sequence of human T-cell leukemia virus type I. Proc Natl Acad Sci USA 82:8359–8363, 1985
51. Fujisawa J, Seiki M, Sato M, Yoshida M: A transcriptional enhancer sequence of HTLV-1 is responsible for trans-activation mediated by p40 or HTLV-1. EMBO J 5:713–718, 1986
52. Rosen CA, Sodroski JG, Haseltine WA: Location of cis-acting regulatory sequences in the human T-cell leukemia virus type 1 long terminal repeat. Proc Natl Acad Sci USA 82:6502–6506, 1985
53. Greene WC, Leonard WJ, Wano Y et al: Trans-activator gene of HTLV-II induces IL-2 receptor and IL-2 cellular gene expression. Science 232:877–880, 1986
54. Jeang KT, Brady J, Radonovich M, Duvall J, Khoury G: p4-x trans-activation of the HTLV-I LTR promoter. UCLA Symp Mol Cell Biol 67:181–189, 1988
55. Beasley RP, Lin CC, Hwang L et al: Hepatocellular carcinoma and hepatitis B virus: A prospective study of 22,707 men in Taiwan. Lancet 2:1129–1133, 1981
56. Robinson WS, Marion PL, Feitelson M et al: The hepadna virus group: Hepatitis B and related viruses. In Szmuness W, Alter HJ, Maynard JW (eds): Viral Hepatitis — 1981 International Symposium, pp 57–68. Philadelphia, Franklin Institute Press, 1982
57. Summers J, Smolec JM, Snyder R: A virus similar to human hepatitis B virus associated with hepatitis and hepatoma in woodchucks. Proc Natl Acad Sci USA 74:4533–4537, 1978
58. Marion PL, Oshiro L, Regnery DC et al: A virus in Beechey ground squirrels that is related to hepatitis B virus of man. Proc Natl Acad Sci USA 77:2941–2945, 1980
59. Mason WS, Seal G, Summers J: Virus of Pekin ducks with structural and biological relatedness to human hepatitis B virus. J Virol 36:829–836, 1980
60. Blumberg BS, Alter HJ, Visnich S: A "new" antigen in leukemia sera. JAMA 191:541–546, 1965
61. Alter HJ, Blumberg BS: Further studies on a "new" human isoprecipitin system (Australia antigen). Blood 27:297–309, 1966
62. Blumberg BS, Gerstley BJS, Hungerford DA et al: A serum antigen (Australia antigen) in Down's syndrome leukemia and hepatitis. Ann Intern Med 66:924–931, 1967
63. Prince AM: An antigen detected in the blood during the incubation period of serum hepatitis. Proc Natl Acad Sci USA 60:814–821, 1968
64. Dane DS, Cameron CH, Briggs M: Virus-like particles in serum of patients with Australia antigen associated hepatitis. Lancet 2:695–698, 1970
65. Almeida JD: Individual morphological variation seen in Australia antigen positive sera. Am J Dis Child 123:303–309, 1972
66. Kim CY, Tilles JG: Purification and biophysical characterization of hepatitis B antigen. J Clin Invest 52:1176–1186, 1970
67. Summers JA, O'Connell A, Millman I: Genome of hepatitis B virus: Restriction enzyme cleavage and structure of DNA extracted from Dane particles. Proc Natl Acad Sci USA 72:4597–4601, 1975
68. Tiollais P, Pourcel C, Dejean A: The hepatitis B virus. Nature 317:489–495, 1985
69. Robinson WS: Hepatitis B virus. In Fields BN (ed): Virology, pp 1384–1406. New York, Raven Press, 1985
70. Landers TA, Greenberg HB, Robinson WS: Structure of hepatitis B Dane particle DNA and nature of the endogenous DNA polymerase reaction. J Virol 23:368–376, 1977

71. Galibert F, Mandart E, Fitoussi F et al: Nucleotide sequence of hepatitis B virus genome (subtype ayw) cloned in E. coli. Nature 281:646–650, 1979
72. Ganem D, Varmus HE: The molecular biology of hepatitis B virus. Annu Rev Biochem 56:651–693, 1987
73. Seeger C, Ganem D, Varmus HE: Biochemical and genetic evidence for the hepatitis B virus replication strategy. Science 232:477–484, 1986
74. Shafritz DA, Shouval D, Sherman H et al: Integration of hepatitis B virus DNA into the genome of liver cells in chronic liver disease and hepatocellular carcinoma. N Engl J Med 305:1067–1073, 1981
75. Brechot C, Pourcel C, Hadchouel M et al: State of hepatitis B virus DNA in liver diseases. Hematology 2:27–34, 1982
76. Summers J, Mason WS: Replication of the genome of a hepatitis B-like virus by reverse transcription of an RNA intermediate. Cell 29:403–415, 1982
77. Shaul Y, Rutter WJ, Laub O: A human hepatitis B viral enhancer element. EMBO J 4:427–430, 1985
78. Jameel S, Siddiqui A: The human hepatitis B virus enhancer requires transacting cellular factor(s) for activity. Mol Cell Biol 6:710–715, 1986
79. Szmuness W: Hepatocellular carcinoma and the hepatitis B virus: Evidence for a causal association. Prog Med Virol 24:40–69, 1978
80. Popper H, Shih JWK, Gerin JL et al: Woodchuck hepatitis and hepatocellular carcinoma: Correlation of histologic with virologic observations. Hematology 1:91–98, 1981
81. Ciuffo G: Imnfesto positivo con filtrato di verruca volgare. Giorn Ital Mal Venereol 48:12–17, 1907
82. Coggins JR, zur Hausen H: Workshop on papillomaviruses and cancer. Cancer Res 39:545–546, 1979
83. Favre M, Orth G, Croissant O et al: Human papillomavirus DNA: Physical map. Proc Natl Acad Sci USA 72:4810–4814, 1975
84. Gissmann L, zur Hausen H: Human papillomaviruses: Physical mapping and genetic heterogenicity. Proc Natl Acad Sci USA 73:1310–1313, 1976
85. Orth G, Favre M, Croissant O: Characterization of a new type of human papillomavirus that causes skin warts. J Virol 24:108–120, 1977
86. Orth G, Jablonska S, Favre M et al: Characterization of two types of human papillomavirus in lesions of epidermodysplasia verruciformis. Proc Natl Acad Sci USA 75:1537–1541, 1978
87. Gissmann L, Pfister H, zur Hausen H: Human papillomaviruses (HPV): Characterization of four different isolates. Virology 7:569–580, 1977
88. Orth G, Favre M, Breitburd F et al: Epidermodysplasia verruciformis: A model for the role of papillomaviruses in human cancer. Cold Spring Harbor Symp Quant Biol [Conference on Cell Proliferation] 7:259–282, 1980
89. Gissmann L, zur Hausen H: Partial characterization of viral DNA from human genital warts (condylomata acuminata). Int J Cancer 25:605–609, 1980
90. Ostrow RS, Kryzyek R, Pass F et al: Identification of a novel human papillomavirus in cutaneous warts of meat handlers. Virology 108:21–27, 1981
91. Orth G, Jablonska S, Favre M et al: Identification of papillomaviruses in butchers' warts. J Invest Dermatol 76:97–102, 1981
92. Pfister H, Nurnberger F, Gissmann L, zur Hausen H: Characterization of a human papillomavirus from epidermodysplasia verruciformis lesions of a patient from Upper Volta. Int J Cancer 27:645–650, 1981
93. Kremsdorf D, Jablonska S, Favre M, Orth G: Biochemical characterization of two types of human papillomaviruses associated with epidermodysplasia verruciformis. J Virol 43:436–447, 1982
94. Kremsdorf D, Jablonska S, Favre M, Orth G: Human papillomaviruses associated with epidermodysplasia verruciformis: II. Molecular cloning and biochemical characterization of human papillomavirus 3a, 8, 10, and 12 genomes. J Virol 48:340–351, 1983
95. Gissmann L, Diehl V, Schultz-Coulon H, zur Hausen H: Molecular cloning and characterization of human papillomavirus DNA derived from a laryngeal papilloma. J Virol 44:393–400, 1982
96. Pfister H, Hettich I, Runne U et al: Characterization of human papillomavirus type 13 from lesions of focal epithelial hyperplasia Heck. J Virol 47:363–366, 1983
97. Tsumori T, Yutsudo M, Nakano Y et al: Molecular cloning of a new human papillomavirus isolated from epidermodysplasia verruciformis lesions. J Gen Virol 64:967–969, 1983
98. Kremsdorf D, Favre M, Jablonska S et al: Molecular cloning and characterization of the genomes of nine newly recognized papillomavirus types associated with epidermodysplasia verruciformis. J Virol 52:1013–1018, 1984
99. Durst M, Gissmann L, Ikenberg H, zur Hausen H: A papillomavirus DNA from a cervical carcinoma and its prevalence in cancer biopsy samples from different geographic regions. Proc Natl Acad Sci USA 80:3812–3815, 1983
100. Boshart M, Gissmann L, Ikenberg H, Kleinheinz A, Scheurlen W, zur Hausen H: A new type of papillomavirus DNA, its presence in genital cancer biopsies and in cell lines derived from cervical cancer. EMBO J 3:1151–1157, 1984
101. Gassermaier A, Lammel M, Pfister H: Molecular cloning and characterization of the DNAs of human papillomaviruses 19, 20, and 25 from a patient with epidermodysplasia verruciformis. J Virol 52:1019–1023, 1984
102. Ostrow RS, Zachow KR, Thompson O, Faras AJ: Molecular cloning and characterization of a unique type of human papillomavirus from an immune deficient patient. J Invest Dermatol 82:362–366, 1984
103. Kahn T, Schwarz E, zur Hausen H: Molecular cloning and characterization of the DNA of a new human papillomavirus from a laryngeal carcinoma. Int J Cancer 37:61–65, 1986
104. Lorincz AT, Lancaster WD, Temple GF: Cloning and characterization of the DNA of a new human papillomavirus from a woman with dysplasia of the uterine cervix. J Virol 58:225–229, 1986
105. Beaudenon S, Praetorius F, Kremsdorf D et al: A new type of human papillomavirus associated with oral focal epithelial hyperplasia. J Invest Dermatol 88:130–135, 1987
106. Beaudenon S, Kremsdorf D, Croissant O et al: A novel type of human papillomavirus associated with genital neoplasias. Nature 321:246–249, 1986
107. Kawashima M, Jablonska S, Favre M, Obalek S, Croissant O, Orth G: Characterization of a new type of human papillomavirus found in a lesion of Bowen's disease of the skin. J Virol 57:688–692, 1986
108. Lorincz AT, Quinn AP, Lancaster WD, Temple GF: A new type of papillomavirus associated with cancer of the uterine cervix. Virology 159:187–190, 1987
109. Kawashima M, Favre M, Jablonska S, Obalek S, Orth G: Characterization of a new type of human papillomavirus (HPV) related to HPV5 from a case of actinic keratosis. Virology 145:384–389, 1986
110. Scheurlen W, Gissmann L, Gross G, zur Hausen H: Molecular cloning of two new HPV types (HPV37 and HPV38) from a keratoacanthoma and a malignant melanoma. Int J Cancer 37:505–510, 1986
111. Beaudenon S, Kremsdorf D, Obalek S et al: Plurality of genital human papillomaviruses: Characterization of two new types with distinct biological properties. Virology 161:374–384, 1987
112. Baker CC, Howley PM: Differential promoter utilization by the bovine papillomavirus in transformed cells as productively infected wart tissues. EMBO J 6:1027–1035, 1987
113. Heilman CA, Engel L, Lowy DR, Howley PM: Virus-specific transcription in bovine papillomavirus-transformed mouse cells. Virology 119:22–34, 1982
114. Engel LW, Heilman CA, Howley PM: Transcriptional organization of the bovine papillomavirus type 1. J Virol 47:516–528, 1983
115. Lowy DR, Dvoretzky I, Shober R, Law M-F, Engle L, Howley PM: In vitro tumorigenic transformation by a defined subgenomic fragment of bovine papillomavirus DNA. Nature 287:72–74, 1980
116. Doorbar J, Campbell D, Grand RJA et al: Identification of the human papillomavirus type 1a encodes a minor structural protein carrying type-specific antigens. EMBO J 5:355–362, 1986
117. Amtmann E, Sauer G: Bovine papilloma virus transcription: Polyadenylated RNA species and assessment of the direction of transcription. J Virol 43:59–66, 1982
118. Black PH, Hartley JW, Rowe WP, Huebner RJ: Transformation of bovine tissue culture cells by bovine papillomavirus. Nature 199:1016–1018, 1963
119. Thomas M, Boiron M, Tanzer J, Levy JP, Bernard J: In vitro transformation of mice cells by bovine papillomavirus. Nature 202:709–710, 1964
120. Dvoretzky I, Shober R, Lowy DR: Focus assay in mouse cells for bovine papillomavirus. Virology 103:369–375, 1980
121. Law MF, Lowy DR, Dvoretzky I, Howley PM: Mouse cells transformed by bovine papillomavirus contain only extrachromosomal viral DNA sequences. Proc Natl Acad Sci USA 78:2727–2731, 1981
122. Lusky M, Botchan MR: A bovine papillomavirus type 1–encoded modulator function is dispensable for transient viral replication but is required for establishment of the stable plasmid state. J Virol 60:729–742, 1986
123. Sarver N, Rabson MS, Yang Y-C, Bryne JC, Howley PM: Localization and analysis of bovine papillomavirus type 1 transforming functions. J Virol 52:377–388, 1984
124. Lusky M, Botchan MR: Genetic analysis of bovine papillomavirus type-1 trans-acting replication factors. J Virol 53:955–965, 1985
125. Spalholz BA, Yang Y-C, Howley PM: Transactivation of a bovine papillomavirus transcriptional regulatory element by the E2 gene product. Cell 42:183–191, 1985
126. Phelps WC, Howley PM: Transcriptional transactivation by the human papillomavirus E2 gene product. J Virol 61:1630–1638, 1987
127. Hirochika H, Broker TR, Chow LT: Enhancers and trans-acting E2 transcriptional factors of papillomaviruses. J Virol 61:2599–2608, 1987
128. Lambert PF, Spalholz BA, Howley PM: A transcriptional repressor encoded by BPV-1 shares a common carboxy terminal domain with the E2 transactivator. Cell 50:69–78, 1987
129. Yang Y-C, Spalholz BA, Rabson MS, Howley PM: Dissociation of transforming and transactivation functions for bovine papillomavirus type 1. Nature 318:575–577, 1985
130. DiMaio D, Guralski D, Schiller JT: Translation of open reading frame E5 of bovine papillomavirus is required for its transforming activity. Proc Natl Acad Sci USA 83:1797–1801, 1986
131. Schiller J, Vousden K, Vass WC, Lowy DR: The E5 open reading frame of bovine papillomavirus type 1 encodes a transforming gene. J Virol 57:1–6, 1986
132. Groff DE, Lancaster WD: Genetic analysis of the 3′ early region transformation and replication functions of bovine papillomavirus type 1. Virology 150:221–230, 1986
133. Rabson MS, Yee C, Yang Y-C, Howley PM: Analysis of the bovine papillomavirus type 1 3′ early region transformation and plasmid maintenance functions. J Virol 60:626–634, 1986
134. Yang Y-C, Okayama H, Howley PM: Bovine papillomavirus contains multiple transforming genes. Proc Natl Acad Sci USA 82:1030–1034, 1985
135. Schiller JT, Vass WC, Lowy DR: Identification of a second transforming region in bovine papillomavirus DNA. Proc Natl Acad Sci USA 81:7880–7884, 1984
136. Berg LJ, Singh K, Botchan M: Complementation of a bovine papillomavirus low-copy number mutant: Evidence for a temporal requirement of the complementing gene. Mol Cell Biol 6:859–869, 1986
137. Pilacinski WP, Glassman DL, Krzyzek RA et al: Cloning and expression in *Escherichia*

coli of the bovine papillomavirus L1 and L2 open reading frames. Biotechnology 1:356–360, 1984

138. Komly CA, Breitburd F, Croissant O et al: The L2 open reading frame of human papillomavirus type 1a encodes a minor structural protein carrying type-specific antigens. J Virol 60:813–816, 1986
139. Howley PM, Schlegel R: Papillomavirus transformation. In Salzman NP, Howley PM (eds): The Papovaviridae: II. The Papillomaviruses, pp 141–163, New York, Plenum Publishing Corp, 1987
140. DiMaio D: Nonsense mutation in open reading frame E2 of bovine papillomavirus DNA. J Virol 57:475–480, 1986
141. Tsunokawa Y, Takebe N, Kasamatsu T et al: Transforming activity of human papillomavirus type 16 DNA sequences in cervical cancer. Proc Natl Acad Sci USA 83:220–223, 1986
142. Bedell MA, Jones KH, Laimins LA: The E6–E7 region of human papillomavirus type 18 is sufficient for transformation of NIH 3T3 and Rat 1 cells. J Virol 61:3635–3640, 1987
143. Phelps WC, Yee CL, Munger K, Howley PM: The human papillomavirus type 16 E7 gene encodes transactivation and transformation functions similar to adenovirus E1a. Cell 53:539–547, 1988
144. Matlashewski G, Schneider J, Banks L et al: Human papillomavirus type 16 DNA cooperates with activated ras in transforming primary cells. EMBO J 6:1741–1746, 1987
145. Rous P, Beard JW: The progression to carcinoma of virus-induced rabbit papillomas (Shope). J Exp Med 62:523–548, 1935
146. Rous P, Kidd JG, Smith WE: Experiments of the cause of the rabbit carcinomas derived from virus-induced papillomas. J Exp Med 96:159–174, 1953
147. Jarrett WFH, McNeil PE, Grimshaw WIR et al: High incidence area of cattle cancer with a possible interaction between an environmental carcinogen and a papillomavirus. Nature 274:215–217, 1978
148. Ford JN, Jennings PA, Spradbrow PB et al: Evidence for papillomaviruses in ocular lesions in cattle. Res Vet Sci 32:257–259, 1982
149. Vanselow BA, Spradbrow PB, Jackson ARB: Papillomaviruses, papillomas and squamous cell carcinomas in sheep. Vet Rec 110:561–562, 1982
150. Orth G: Epidermodysplasia verruciformis: A model for understanding the oncogenicity of human papillomaviruses. In Evered D, Clark S (eds): Papillomaviruses. Ciba Found Symp 120:157–174, 1986
151. Shope RE: Infectious papillomatosis of rabbits. J Exp Med 58:607–624, 1933
152. Rous P, Kidd JG: The carcinogenic effect of a virus upon tarred skin. Science 83:468–469, 1936
153. Kidd JG, Rous P: Effects of the papillomavirus (Shope) upon tar warts of rabbits. Proc Soc Exp Biol Med 37:518–520, 1937
154. Wettstein FO, Stevens JG: Variable sized free episomes of Shope papilloma virus DNA are present in all non-virus-producing neoplasms and integrated genomes are detected in some. Proc Natl Acad Sci USA 79:790–794, 1982
155. Nasseri M, Wettstein FO: Differences exist between viral transcripts in cottontail rabbit papillomavirus-induced benign and malignant tumors as well as non-virus-producing and virus-producing tumors. J Virol 51:706–712, 1984
156. Jarrett WFH, Murphy J, O'Neil BW et al: Virus-induced papillomas of the alimentary tract of cattle. Int J Cancer 22:323–328, 1978
157. Campo MS, Moar MH, Sartirana ML et al: The presence of bovine papillomavirus type 4 DNA is not required for the progression to, or the maintenance of, the malignant state in cancers of the alimentary canal in cattle. EMBO J 4:1819–1825, 1985
158. Lutzner M: Epidermodysplasia verruciformis: An autosomal recessive disease characterized by viral warts and skin cancer. A model for viral oncogenesis. Bull Cancer 65:169–182, 1978
159. Pass F, Faras AJ: Human papillomavirus DNA in cutaneous primary and metastasized squamous cell carcinomas from patients with epidermodysplasia verruciformis. Proc Natl Acad Sci USA 79:1634–1638, 1982
160. Pfister H, Gassenmaier A, Nurnberger F: HPV-5 DNA in a carcinoma of an epidermodysplasia verruciformis patient infected with various human papillomavirus types. Cancer Res 43:1436–1441, 1983
161. Green M, Brackmann KH, Sanders PR et al: Isolation of a human papillomavirus from a patient with epidermodysplasia verruciformis: Presence of related viral DNA genomes in human urogenital tumors. Proc Natl Acad Sci USA 79:4437–4441, 1982
162. Yutsudo M, Shimakage T, Hakura A: Human papillomavirus type 17 DNA in skin carcinoma tissue of a patient with epidermodysplasia verruciformis. Virology 144:295–298, 1985
163. Yutsudo M, Hakura A: Human papillomavirus type 17 transcripts expressed in skin cancer tissue of a patient with epidermodysplasia verruciformis. Int J Cancer 39:586–589, 1987
164. Underwood PB, Hester LL: Diagnosis and treatment of premalignant lesions of the vulva: A review. Am J Obstet Gynecol 110:849–857, 1971
165. Waugh M: Condylomata acuminata. Br Med J 2:527–528, 1972
166. Dunn AE, Ogilvie MM: Intranuclear virus particles in human genital wart tissue: Observation on the ultrastructure of epidermal layer. J Ultrastruct Res 22:282–295, 1968
167. Oriel JD, Almeida JD: Demonstration of virus particles in human genital warts. Br J Vener Dis 46:37–42, 1970
168. Woodruff JD, Braun L, Cavallieri R et al: Immunological identification of papillomavirus antigen in paraffin-processed condyloma tissues from the female genital tract. Obstet Gynecol 56:727–732, 1980
169. Gissmann L, de Villiers EM, zur Hausen H: Analysis of human genital warts (condylomata acuminata) and other genital tumors for human papillomavirus type 6 DNA. Int J Cancer 29:143–146, 1982
170. Gissmann L, Wolnik L, Ikenberg H, Koldovsky U, Schnurch G, zur Hausen H: Human papillomavirus type 6 and 11 DNA sequences in genital and laryngeal papillomas and in some cervical cancers. Proc Natl Acad Sci USA 80:560–563, 1983
171. Buschke A, Lowenstein L: Über carcinomahnlich condylomata acuminata des penis. Arch Dermatol Syph 163:30–46, 1931
172. Boshart M, zur Hausen H: Human papillomaviruses in Buschke-Lowenstein tumors: Physical state of the DNA and identification of a tandem duplication in the non-coding region of a human papillomavirus 6 subtype. J Virol 58:963–966, 1986
173. Meisels A, Fortin R: Condylomatous lesions of the cervix and vagina: I. Cytologic patterns. Acta Cytol 20:505–509, 1976
174. Purola E, Savia E: Cytology of gynecologic condyloma acuminatum. Acta Cytol 21:26–31, 1977
175. Laverty CR, Russell P, Hillis E et al: The significance of noncondylomatous wart virus infection of the cervical transformation zone. Acta Cytol 22:195–201, 1978
176. Koss LG, Durfee GR: Unusual patterns of squamous epithelium of the uterine cervix: Cytologic and pathologic study of koilocytotic atypia. Ann NY Acad Sci 63:1245–1261, 1956
177. Della Torre G, Pilotti S, dePalo G et al: Viral particles in cervical condylomatous lesions. Tumori 64:549–553, 1978
178. Hills E, Laverty CR: Electron microscopic detection of papilloma virus particles in selected koilocytotic cells in a routine cervical smear. Acta Cytol 23:53–56, 1979
179. Kessler IL: Human cervical cancer as a venereal disease. Cancer Res 36:783–791, 1976
180. zur Hausen H: Human papillomaviruses and their possible role in squamous cell carcinomas. Curr Top Microbiol Immunol 78:1–30, 1977
181. Rawls WE, Tompkins WAF, Figueroa ME et al: Herpes simplex virus type 2: Association with carcinoma of the cervix. Science 161:1255–1256, 1968
182. Nahmias AJ, Josey WE, Naib ZM et al: Antibodies to herpes virus hominis types 1 and 2 in humans: II. Women with cervical cancer. Am J Epidemiol 91:548–552, 1970
183. zur Hausen H: Herpes simplex virus in human genital cancer. Int Rev Exp Pathol 25:307–326, 1983
184. Vonka V, Kanda J, Hirsch I et al: Prospective study on the relationship between cervical neoplasia and herpes simplex type-2 virus: II. Herpes simplex type-2 antibody presence in sera taken at enrollment. Int J Cancer 33:61–66, 1984
185. Vonka V, Kanda J, Jelinek J et al: Prospective study on the relationship between cervical neoplasia and herpes simplex type-2 virus: I. Epidemiologic characteristics. Int J Cancer 33:49–60, 1984
186. Peterson O: Spontaneous course of cervical precancerous conditions. Am J Obstet Gynecol 72:1063–1071, 1956
187. Kinlen LJ, Spriggs AI: Women with positive cervical smears but without surgical intervention: A follow up study. Lancet 2:463–465, 1978
188. Richart RM, Barrow BA: A follow-up study of patients with cervical dysplasia. Am J Obstet Gynecol 105:386–393, 1969
189. Gissmann L, Schwarz E: Persistence and expression of human papillomavirus DNA in genital cancer. In Evered D, Clark S (eds): Papillomaviruses. Ciba Found Symp 120:190–197, 1986
190. Ikenberg H, Gissmann L, Gross G, Grussendorf-Conen E-I, zur Hausen H: Human papillomavirus 16 related DNA in genital Bowen's disease and in bowenoid papulosis. Int J Cancer 32:563–565, 1983
191. Gross G, Hagedorn M, Ikenberg H et al: Bowenoid papulosis: Presence of human papillomavirus (HPV) structural antigens and of HPV-16 related DNA sequences. Arch Dermatol 121:858–863, 1985
192. Clarke EA, Morgan RW, Newman AM: Smoking as a risk factor in cancer of the cervix: Additional evidence from a case control study. Am J Epidemiol 115:59–66, 1982
193. Wigle DT: Smoking and cancer of the cervix: Hypothesis. Am J Epidemiol 111:125–127, 1980
194. Winkelstein W Jr: Smoking and cancer of the uterine cervix. Am J Epidemiol 106:257–259, 1977
195. Hoffmann D, Hecht SS, Haley NJ et al: Tumorigenic agents in tobacco products and their uptake by chewers, smokers and nonsmokers. J Cell Biochem 9C:33, 1985
196. zur Hausen H: Human genital cancer: Synergism between two virus infections or synergism between a virus infection and initiating events. Lancet 2:1370–1372, 1982
197. Schwarz E, Freese UK, Gissmann L, Mayer W, Roggenbuck B, Stemlau A, zur Hausen H: Structure and transcription of human papillomavirus sequences in cervical carcinoma cells. Nature 314:111–114, 1985
198. Smotkin D, Wettstein FO: Transcription of human papillomavirus type 16 early genes in cervical cancer and a cancer derived cell line and identification of the E7 protein. Proc Natl Acad Sci USA 83:4680–4684, 1986
199. Shirasawa H, Tomita Y, Kubota K et al: Transcriptional differences of the human papillomavirus type 16 genome between precancerous lesions and invasive carcinomas. J Virol 62:1022–1027, 1988
200. Yee C, Krishnan-Hewlett I, Baker CC et al: Presence and expression of human papillomavirus sequences in human cervical carcinoma cell lines. Am J Pathol 119:361–366, 1985
201. Durst M, Croce CM, Gissmann L et al: Papillomavirus sequences integrate near cellular oncogenes in some cervical carcinomas. Proc Natl Acad Sci USA 84:1070–1074, 1987

202. Baker CC, Phelps WC, Lindgren V et al: Structural and transcriptional analysis of human papillomavirus type 16 sequences in cervical carcinoma cell lines. J Virol 61:962–971, 1987
203. Theirry F, Heard JM, Dartmann K et al: Characterization of a transcriptional promoter of human papillomavirus 18 and the modulation of its expression by simian virus 40 and adenovirus early antigens. J Virol 61:134–142, 1987
204. Gloss B, Bernard HU, Seedorf K et al: The upstream regulatory region of the human papillomavirus 16 contains an E2 protein-independent enhancer which is specific for cervical carcinoma cells and regulated by glucocorticoid hormones. EMBO J 6:3734–3743, 1987
205. Cripe TP, Haugen TH, Turk OP et al: Transcriptional regulation of the human papillomavirus-16 E6-E7 promoter by a keratinocyte-dependent enhancer, and by viral E2 trans-activator and repressor gene products: Implications for cervical carcinogenesis. EMBO J 6:3745–3753, 1987
206. Loning T, Ikenberg H, Becker J et al: Analysis of oral papillomas leukoplakias, and invasive carcinomas for human papillomavirus type related DNA. J Invest Dermatol 84:417–420, 1985
207. Brandsma JL, Steinberg BM, Abramson AL et al: Presence of human papillomavirus type 16 related sequences in verrucous carcinoma of the larynx. Cancer Res 46:2185–2188, 1986
208. Jenson AB, Lancaster WD, Hartman DP et al: Frequency and distribution of papillomavirus structural antigens cerrucae, multiple papillomas, and condylomata of the oral cavity. Am J Pathol 107:212–218, 1982
209. Lind P, Syrjanen K, Koppang HS et al: Immunoreactivity and human papillomavirus (HPV) on oral precancer and cancer lesions. Scand J Dent Res 94:419–426, 1986
210. de Villiers EM, Neumann C, Le JY, Weidauer H, zur Hausen H: Infection of the oral mucosa with defined types of human papillomaviruses. Med Microbiol Immunol 174:287–294, 1986
211. Naghashfar Z, Sawada E, Kutcher MK et al: Identification of genital tract papillomaviruses HPV-6 and HPV-16 in warts of the oral cavity. J Virol 17:313–324, 1985
212. Syrjanen S, Syrjanen K, Lamberg MA: Detection of human papillomavirus DNA in oral mucosal lesions using in situ DNA hybridization applied on paraffin sections. Oral Surg 62:660–667, 1986
213. Byrne JC, Tsao MS, Fraser RS, Howley PM: Human papillomavirus-11 DNA in patient with chronic laryngotracheobronchial papillomatosis and metastatic squamous-cell carcinoma of the lung. N Engl J Med 317:873–878, 1987
214. Syrjanen K, Pyrhonen S, Aukee S et al: Squamous cell papilloma of the esophagus: A tumor probably caused by human papillomavirus (HPV). Diagn Histopathol 5:291–296, 1982
215. Winkler B, Capo V, Reumann W, Ma A et al: Human papillomavirus infection of the esophagus. Cancer 55:149–155, 1985
216. Burkitt D: A sarcoma involving the jaws in African children. Br. J Surg 46:218–223, 1958
217. Burkitt D: Determining the climatic limitations of a children's cancer common in Africa. Br Med J 2:1019–1023, 1962
218. Epstein MA, Barr YM: Cultivation in vitro of human lymphoblasts from Burkitt's malignant lymphoma. Lancet 1:252–253, 1964
219. Epstein MA, Achong BG, Barr YM: Virus particles in cultured lymphoblasts from Burkitt's lymphoma. Lancet 1:702–703, 1964
220. Salahuddin SK, Ablashi DV, Markham PD et al: Isolation of a new virus, HBLV, in patients with lymphoproliferative disorders. Nature 324:596–601, 1986
221. Josephs SF, Salahuddin SK, Ablashi DV et al: Genomic analysis of the human B-lymphotropic virus (HBLV). Nature 324:601–603, 1986
222. Kieff E, Dambaugh T, Heller M et al: The biology and chemistry of Epstein-Barr virus. J Infect Dis 146:506–517, 1982
223. Baer R, Bankier AT, Biggin MD et al: DNA sequence and expression of B95-8 Epstein Barr virus genome. Nature 310:207–211, 1984
224. Hummel M, Kieff E: Mapping of polypeptides encoded by the Epstein-Barr virus genome in productive infection. Proc Natl Acad Sci USA 79:5698–5702, 1982
225. de Schryver A, Klein G, Henle W et al: Comparison of EBV neutralization tests based on abortive infection or transformation of lymphoid cells and their relation to membrane reactive antibodies (anti-MA). Int J Cancer 13:353–362, 1974
226. Henle G, Henle W, Klein G: Demonstration of two distinct components in the early antigen complex of Epstein-Barr virus-infected cells. Int J Cancer 8:272–282, 1971
227. Reedman BM, Klein G: Cellular localization of an Epstein-Barr virus (EBV) associated complement-fixing antigen in producer and non-producer lymphoblastoid cell lines. Int J Cancer 11:499–520, 1973
228. Rickenson AB, Moss DJ, Pope JH: Long-term T-cell mediated immunity to Epstein-Barr virus in man: II. Components necessary for regression in virus-infected leukocyte cultures. Int J Cancer 23:610–617, 1979
229. Rickenson AB, Wallace LE, Epstein MA: HLA-restricted T-cell recognition of Epstein-Barr virus-infected B cells. Nature 283:865–867, 1980
230. Svedmyr E, Jondal M: Cytotoxic effector cells specific for B cell lines transformed by Epstein-Barr virus are present in patients with infectious mononucleosis. Proc Natl Acad Sci USA 72:1622–1626, 1975
231. Thorley-Lawson DA, Geilinger K: Monoclonal antibodies against the major glycoprotein (gp 350/220) of Epstein-Barr virus neutralize infectivity. Proc Natl Acad Sci USA 77:5307–5311, 1980
232. Pearson GR, Vroman B, Chase B et al: Identification of polypeptide components of the Epstein-Barr virus early antigen complex with monoclonal antibodies. J Virol 47:193–201, 1983
233. Pearson GR, Luka J: Characterization of the virus-determined antigens. In Epstein MA, Achong BG (eds): The Epstein-Barr Virus, pp 47–74. New York, John Wiley & Sons, 1986
234. Fialkow PJ, Klein E, Klein G et al: Immunoglobulin and glucose-6-phosphate dehydrogenase as markers of cellular origin in Burkitt lymphoma. J Exp Med 138:89–101, 1973
235. Mann RB, Bernard CW: Burkitts tumor: Lessons from mice, monkeys, and man. Lancet 2:84, 1979
236. Magrath I: Clinical and pathobiological features of Burkitt's lymphoma and their relevance to treatment. In Levine PH, Ablashi DV, Pearson GR et al: Epstein-Barr Virus and Associated Diseases, pp 631–643. Boston, Martinus Nijhoff, 1985
237. Kafuko GW, Burkitt DP: Burkitt's lymphoma and malaria. Int J Cancer 6:1–9, 1970
238. Morrow RH Jr: Epidemiological evidence for the role of falciparum malaria in the pathogenesis of Burkitt's lymphoma. In Lenoir GM, O'Connor G, Olweny CLM (eds): A Human Cancer Model, IARC Sci Publ 60:177–186, 1985
239. Moss DJ, Burrows SR, Catelino DJ et al: A comparison of Epstein-Barr virus-specific T-cell immunity in malaria-endemic and nonendemic regions of Papua New Guinea. Int J Cancer 31:727–732, 1983
240. Manolov G, Manolova Y: Marker band in one chromosome 14 from Burkitt lymphomas. Nature 237:33–34, 1972
241. Lenoir GM, Taub R: Chromosomal translocations and oncogenes in Burkitt's lymphoma. In Goldman JM (ed): Leukaemia and Lymphoma Research: Vol 2. Genetic Rearrangements in Leukaemia and Lymphoma, pp 152–172. London, Harnden, 1986
242. Leder P, Battey J, Lenoir G et al: Translocations among antibody genes in human cancer. Science 222:765–771, 1983
243. Erikson J, Finan J, Nowell PC, Croce CM: Translocation of immunoglobulin V_H genes in Burkitt's lymphoma. Proc Natl Acad Sci USA 79:5611–5615, 1982
244. Lombardi L, Newcomb EW, Della-Favera R: Pathogenesis of Burkitt's lymphoma: Expression of an activated c-myc oncogene causes the tumorigenic conversion of EBV-infected human B-Lymphocytes. Cell 49:161–170, 1987
245. Klein G: Lymphoma development in mice and human: Diversity of initiation is followed by convergent cytogenetic evolution. Proc Natl Acad Sci USA 76:2442–2446, 1979
246. Klein G, Klein E: Evolution of tumors and the impact of molecular oncology. Nature 315:190, 1985
247. Lenoir GM, Bornkamm GW: Burkitt's lymphoma, a human cancer model for the study of multistep development of cancer: Proposal for a new scenario. Adv Viral Oncol 7:173–206, 1987
248. Henle W, Henle G: Epstein-Barr virus and human malignancies. Adv Viral Oncol 5:201–238, 1985
249. zur Hausen H, Schulte-Holthausen H, Klein G et al: EBV DNA in biopsies of Burkitt tumors and anaplastic carcinomas of the nasopharynx. Nature 228:1056–1058, 1970
250. Andersson-Anvret M, Forsby N, Klein G et al: Relationship between the Epstein-Barr virus and undifferentiated nasopharyngeal carcinoma: Correlated nucleic acid hybridization and histopathological examination. Int J Cancer 20:486–494, 1977
251. Raab-Traub N, Flynn K, Pearson G et al: The differentiated form of nasopharyngeal carcinoma contains Epstein-Barr virus DNA. Int J Cancer 39:25–29, 1987
252. Pagano JS: Epstein-Barr virus transcription in nasopharyngeal carcinoma. J Virol 48:580–590, 1983
253. de The G, Zeng Y: Population screening for EBV markers: Toward improvement of nasopharyngeal carcinoma control. In Epstein MA, Achog BG (eds): The Epstein-Barr Virus, pp 237–248. New York, John Wiley & Sons, 1986
254. Purtilo DT, Sakamoto K, Barnabai V et al: Epstein-Barr virus-induced diseases in boys with the X-linked lymphoproliferative syndrome (XLP): Updates on studies of the registry. Am J Med 73:49–56, 1982

PETER GREENWALD

CHAPTER 11 *Principles of Cancer Prevention: Diet and Nutrition*

Laboratory and epidemiologic research findings of the past several decades have converged to provide strong evidence that dietary factors are major determinants for a large proportion of human cancers. Epidemiologists note wide international variations in the occurrence and prevalence of specific types of cancer. For example, death rates from breast cancer are five times higher in certain Western countries than in less developed countries with very different lifestyles. Migration and time trend data coupled with laboratory results implicate several dietary factors in an increased cancer risk; other dietary factors may reduce cancer risk. Although it is clear that the intake of dietary mutagens and carcinogens or poor dietary practices, including inadequate intake of foods high in important nutrients and fiber or an excessive fat and caloric intake, influence certain types of cancer incidence, the exact mechanisms and nutrient interactions are not understood fully.

The concept of diet as a possible etiologic factor has received momentum from basic carcinogenesis studies and population studies and from the recent substantial increase in commitment to research in this field. Cancer prevention through the identification and elimination of dietary components associated with the development of cancer is not feasible. A more logical preventive strategy is to identify factors that act as inhibitors of carcinogenesis and to increase human exposure to them. Two programs at the National Cancer Institute (NCI) focus on nutrient-related research for cancer prevention: the Chemoprevention Program and the Diet, Nutrition, and Cancer Program. Chemoprevention, a recent area of research emphasis, explores natural and synthetic substances, precisely formulated and measured, that demonstrate the potential to prevent, halt, or reverse carcinogenesis. Particular attention is being directed toward beta-carotene, vitamin A (retinol) and related synthetic retinoids, vitamins C and E, and certain selenium compounds, often in study populations already exposed to cancer-causing agents but before clinical cancer is evident. Many other agents are in preclinical testing. The closely associated Diet, Nutrition, and Cancer Program is looking at less defined macronutrient factors (such as dietary fats or fiber-containing foods) that may affect the risk of cancer development.

The most direct evidence for establishing even a small to moderate causal association for cancer prevention strategies in humans comes from clinical intervention trials. Such trials may provide the only evidence on whether a specific intervention, such as a change in diet, will reduce cancer risk. As data from epidemiologic and carcinogenesis research converged, a sound basis was building for testing hypotheses by initiating human trials. The use of clinical trials to evaluate the efficacy and safety of preventive interventions parallels the earlier work of oncologists who 30 years ago began to set into place a systematic process for clinical testing of new therapies. When the first human cancer prevention trials were begun in the early 1980s, for the most part using specific nutrients thought to have a protective effect, they became the accepted means of proving whether a nutrient or other preventive agent suppresses the carcinogenic process. These studies also began to explore the use of precancerous markers as end points for evaluating the effects of preventive interventions. However, for reasons that will be discussed later in this chapter, clinical trials are not always feasible. When a clinical trial is practical and timely, it should be used. In other instances, we must follow different paths to achieve a scientific consensus on the efficacy and safety of particular interventions for cancer prevention.

This chapter reviews dietary factors associated with the cause and prevention of cancer and addresses the development and potential benefits of diet and cancer research, focusing on the following topics: laboratory studies, epidemiologic studies, specific dietary factors and cancer risk, chemoprevention, prevention research processes, similarities and differences between clinical treatment and prevention trials, an overview of intervention trials completed or in progress, research related to selected diet and cancer hypotheses, the physician's role as a promoter of a healthy diet, and future prospects for cancer prevention research on dietary factors and their impact on carcinogenesis.

OVERVIEW OF DIETARY FACTORS RELATED TO CARCINOGENESIS

Many compounds have been isolated from food sources that can markedly influence the growth and development of cancer in animal models and cell culture systems. These substances represent a structurally diverse group with multiple biologic effects, broad variabilities in efficacy and toxicity, and mechanisms of action as yet not fully elucidated.

Some naturally occurring compounds found to have inhibitory effects on cancer growth are coumarins, phenols, indoles, aromatic isothiocyanates, alkenyl benzenes, methylated flavones, plant sterols, selenium salts, and protease inhibitors. Notable preventive antineoplastic activity also has been demonstrated with pharmacologic amounts of the essential nutrients ascorbic acid (vitamin C), alpha-tocopherol (vitamin E), retinoids (vitamin A and derivatives), and beta-carotene.[1]

Pioneering studies in cancer biology in the early part of the 20th century established that tumors can be chemically induced using coal tar, azo dyes, and polycyclic hydrocarbons. Modifications in study design, particularly the use of oral rather than percutaneous routes of application, led to the observation in 1941 by Kensler that the development of azo dye–induced liver tumors could be retarded by dietary manipulations.[2] Riboflavin (vitamin B_6) was identified as a dietary constituent that expressed a preventive role through enhanced detoxification of the dyes. The macronutrients fiber and fat have been examined for their effect on carcinogenesis in several animal models.[3,4] Restricted caloric intake was found by Tannenbaum and Silverstone to be an important preventive factor in chemical carcinogenesis, with dietary fat tending to augment the carcinogenic process.[5]

A variety of substances have only recently been recognized as major sources of mutagens and carcinogens in the human diet. Large numbers of these substances are synthesized in edible plants, or are produced during the cooking or processing of food, or are used as food additives for preservation or flavor enhancement. Genotoxic, mutagenic, and carcinogenic derivatives, demonstrated in animal models, include dietary phenols, alkaloids and glycoalkaloids, isothiocyanates, alcohol, quinones, and cyclopropenoid fatty acids. Heterocyclic amines isolated from cooked proteins are potent carcinogens. Mycotoxins synthesized by a variety of molds contaminate human food, and several of these toxins are potent carcinogens. Aflatoxin, for example, contaminates grains, peanuts, and other stored foodstuffs and has been shown to be a human carcinogen in animal and epidemiologic studies. Alcohol consumption has been associated with an increased risk of oral, pharyngeal, esophageal, and stomach cancer, especially in smokers. The degree of risk associated with these substances remains largely unknown.[6,7]

Many dietary factors are known to be inhibitors of chemical carcinogenesis. For example, benzyl isothiocyanate (which occurs in cruciferous vegetables) inhibits benzo (*a*)pyrene-induced forestomach neoplasia in mice and induces glutathione *S*-transferase activity in the same system.[8] Several classes of compounds that occur naturally in food, such as phenols and lactones, are active in this system as well. Still others act as inhibitors or suppressors of chemical carcinogenesis in other tumor model systems.[9] Associated with this inhibition of carcinogenesis in some cases are elevated levels of certain enzymes involved in the metabolism of a wide range of carcinogens, including benzo(*a*)pyrene. Elevations in hepatic mixed function oxidase activity and glutathione *S*-transferase activity are postulated as carcinogen detoxification mechanisms that effectively reduce the intracellular concentration of an ultimate carcinogenic species. However, increased activities of these same enzymes also can enhance the conversion of many procarcinogens to the proximate carcinogen structure.[10]

Other types of biologic activities by dietary factors related to chemoprevention of cancer have been reported. Dietary fiber, which inhibits chemically induced cancer of the colon and small intestine in some studies, may enhance carcinogen excretion.[11] Inhibition of carcinogen formation has been demonstrated with ascorbic acid in both humans and experimental animals. For example, oral administration of ascorbic acid with sodium nitrite or nitrate and amines or amides effectively inhibits *N*-nitrosamine generation in the stomach under certain conditions.[12]

Inhibition of mutagenesis through the scavenging of potentially mutagenic free radicals (by alpha-tocopherol) and singlet oxygen (by ascorbic acid or beta-carotenes) is also considered to be a potentially plausible preventive mechanism.[9]

There is some suggestion in the epidemiologic literature of an inverse association between ingestion of vitamin C–containing foods and the development of cancer, particularly cancer of the esophagus[13] and stomach.[14] A possible mechanism for the protective effect of vitamin C is inhibition of nitrosamine formation from secondary and higher amines in combination with nitrite.[12,15] However, vitamin A, beta-carotene, and vitamin C are present together in many fruits and vegetables, and the epidemiologic studies in most cases do not allow clear distinction of the dietary factor responsible for potential benefits. Vitamin E is difficult to study epidemiologically because it is present in a wide variety of foods and can vary greatly with individual foodstuffs. Menkes et al[16] found that serum vitamin E (and serum beta-carotene) levels were lower in persons who later developed squamous cell carcinoma of the lung than in controls, an observation different from that reported by Willett et al.[17] Clinical trials are needed to resolve these differences.

Geographic correlation studies suggest a possible benefit from diets high in selenium.[18,19] Such studies cannot be definitive because of the possibility that an undefined covariable is responsible for the results. Ip has reviewed experimental evidence for a chemopreventive role for certain selenium compounds.[20] Among other minerals, calcium (and vitamin D) was reported to be inversely associated with the development of colorectal cancer in a 19-year prospective study in men.[21] This finding is not entirely consistent with data from international studies but merits testing in clinical trials.

The hypothesis that dietary factors can influence cancer risk, particularly in certain high-risk groups, is supported by both descriptive and analytic epidemiologic research. Taken together, results from epidemiologic and laboratory studies provide a rationale for intensive research into the nature of cancer prevention by nutrient components and their synthetic analogues.

DIETARY FACTORS AND CANCER RISK

VITAMIN A/RETINOIDS/CAROTENOIDS

By far the most extensive and clinically applicable research on dietary factors in carcinogenesis relates to the retinoids. The term *retinoids* generally applies to vitamin A (retinol) and its isomers, derivatives (retinal, retinoic acid), and synthetic analogues. These compounds have been found to directly modify the expression of a neoplastic phenotype, in some cases actually arresting the dedifferentiation of a cell. As discussed in more detail below, retinoids are of special interest for use in clinical prevention because they can exert their antineoplastic activity in cells that are already dedifferentiated or initiated into a malignant state.

Vitamin A (or its derivatives) is essential for proper growth and differentiation of epithelial tissue and bone, reproduction, and vision. In experimental animals, vitamin A deficiency is associated with an increased incidence of several types of cancer and with premalignant changes in some tissues.[22] Except for its role in the visual cycle, the mechanism of action of vitamin A in its numerous physiologic roles has not been fully identified. Beta-carotene is a dietary precursor of vitamin A widely distributed in plants. When cleaved enzymatically in the intestine or liver, one molecule of beta-carotene yields two molecules of retinol.

Lasnitzki,[23] using an organ culture system, discovered that vitamin A was able to suppress abnormal differentiation of prostate gland epithelium induced by treatment with 3-methylcholanthrene (3-MC). Later work established that retinoids could inhibit malignant transformation induced by either 3-MC or radiation in tissue culture systems.[24,25] Transformation was suppressed even when the retinoid was added 1 week after 3-MC. Further, it was shown that following removal of the retinoid from the culture medium, full expression of the malignant phenotype occurred.

Examples also exist of retinoids inducing terminal differentiation from neoplastic to a nonneoplastic phenotype. This has been accomplished with murine F9 teratocarcinoma cells[26] and human promyelocytic leukemia cells,[27] among others. In the human leukemia system, malignant cells are terminally differentiated by retinoic acid to a form with the morphological and biochemical characteristics of a mature granulocyte. The extension of these observations to other cell lines (both established and primary cultures), coupled with the observation that some retinoids are active at nanomolar concentrations, suggests that retinoids have a physiological role in normal hematopoiesis.[28]

The study of retinoid activity has been facilitated by the concerted development of synthetic analogues designed to enhance potency and minimize toxicity. One analogue in particular, 13-*cis*-retinoic acid, has undergone extensive study in several organ-specific animal model systems of chemical carcinogenesis. This compound consistently arrests malignant progression in three different rodent bladder cancer systems.[29] A significant inhibitory effect was seen in Fischer rats even when treatment with 13-*cis*-retinoic acid was delayed for 8 weeks following initiation with *N*-butyl-*N*-(4-hydroxybutyl)nitrosamine.[30] Other retinoid derivatives have similar inhibitory activity in chemically induced model systems of breast cancer and skin cancer.[29,31] Regression of chemically induced tumors and a delay in the appearance of transplanted tumors have been reported for several other synthetic retinoids.[22]

A number of mechanisms have been suggested to account for the interference by retinoids in the progression of carcinogenesis. In mice, retinoids inhibit the activity of ornithine decarboxylase, an enzyme associated with tumor promotion processes.[31] Retinoids also block cell transformation through inhibition of polypeptide transforming factors, such as sarcoma growth factor.[32] Interference with the synthesis of proteins required for neoplastic progression is another possibility.

Carotenoids are also of interest as chemopreventive agents, although there is little laboratory data to confirm that they have any inherent activity independent of their ultimate conversion to retinoids.[33] Specifically, they do not exhibit any serious toxicity, and blood levels of carotenoids are directly related to dietary intake, unlike the retinoids, which are subject to strict homeostatic control. A direct chemopreventive role for beta-carotene has been suggested because of its very efficient ability to deactivate singlet oxygen and trap organic free radicals.[22] The notable inhibitory effects of retinoids observed in the laboratory are also observed in epidemiologic studies. About 20 reports have evaluated cancer incidence and vitamin A or beta-carotene intake. In nine retrospective studies, a significant increase in cancer risk at various sites was associated with diminished vitamin A intake.[34] Risks reported for the groups with low vitamin A intake were about twice those for the high intake groups.

A retrospective Norwegian study found that cancer patients had an increased risk for colon cancer associated with a vitamin A intake lower than that determined for a healthy control group.[35] Similarly, in a Japanese study, patients with gastric metaplasia had lower vitamin A intakes than a healthy control group.[36] Most other retrospective data confirm the inverse association between ingestion of foods containing vitamin A or beta-carotene and relative cancer risk, with risk levels 2 to 2.5 times higher in the low-intake groups than in the high-intake groups.[37]

The interpretation of retrospective epidemiologic studies is complicated by several factors. Dietary recall information usually is incomplete and imprecise. Cancer induction may take many years, and it is uncertain what time period of dietary intake is most relevant to the process. Also, most studies have tended to focus on food groups rather than specific nutrients. For example, foods high in beta-carotene also are high in other nutrients and may be low in fat. The groups under study may come from populations having wide differences in nutrient status, further complicating the estimation of risk associated with one dietary component.

Two large prospective studies that evaluated vitamin A intake and the risk of lung cancer have yielded consistent findings. In a study of 8,278 Norwegian men, Bjelke found an inverse relationship between lung cancer risk and vitamin A intake, [38] an observation that was confirmed in a study update.[39] The same result was found in a 10-year study of more than 250,000 Japanese adults.[40] In a smaller study, lung cancer incidence was inversely correlated with beta-carotene intake in 2,100 American men.[41]

Both retrospective and prospective studies have been conducted correlating serum retinol levels and relative cancer risk. The results have been contradictory.[34,37] This is not surprising, as retinol levels in serum are not directly influenced by dietary intake and vary only slightly among individuals in developed countries where vitamin A deficiencies are unusual.[33] Further, serum retinol levels may not accurately reflect local retinoid concentration in some tissues. It has been suggested that beta-carotene, if not itself an inherently important chemopreventive agent, could be used as a nontoxic means of increasing the quantity of circulating (pre)retinoids.[37]

FAT AND CALORIC INTAKE

Dietary fat is associated with breast, prostate, and colon cancers in population and animal studies, although not all the reported associations are consistent. Tannenbaum[42] and others in the 1940s demonstrated that high-fat diets enhance the occurrence of both spontaneous and chemically induced mammary tumors in mice.[42] Caloric or fat restriction inhibits spontaneous and chemically induced mammary tumors in animal models.[43,44] The reported cumulative tumor incidence in a review of 82 published experiments was, on average, 42% lower in calorie-restricted mice.[45] These studies demonstrate that dietary fat and caloric intake may differentially modify cancer incidence.

In human population studies, comparisons of the fat intake in the diets of various countries indicate that those populations with the highest per capita fat consumption have the highest breast cancer mortality.[46] A fivefold difference is seen between high-risk countries such as Denmark and low-risk countries such as Japan. A strong positive correlation between the intake of dietary fat and breast cancer mortality is seen in data from 39 countries.[47] Similar but weaker correlations were shown for fat intake and cancer of the colon and prostate.

Most case–control studies support an association between fat intake and breast cancer incidence.[48-52] Cohort studies on dietary fat and breast cancer have been less consistent. Notably, Willett et al found no relationship between dietary fat and breast cancer incidence in a cohort of 90,000 nurses.[53] The lack of correlation may be due to the fact that fat intake in this population varied only marginally, from 32% to 44% of total calories. International studies find broader ranges, with some populations reporting intakes as low as 15%.

International correlation studies find an association between colon cancer incidence and the intake of animal fat.[54] However, correlation studies within countries have not supported this association.[55-57] Case–control studies on colon cancer and fat are also inconsistent.[58] Contradictory data suggest that factors other than fat, such as dietary fiber, may influence colon cancer risk. There is some evidence that dietary fiber modifies the promoting effect of dietary fat and colon cancer incidence.[59] In a recent animal study, fiber moderated the effect of a high-fat diet on chemically induced colon tumors. Tumors developed in 63.7% of rats fed high-fat, low-fiber diets but only in 10.9% of rats fed high-fat, high-fiber diets.[60] Several reports indicate that dietary fat can promote chemically induced intestinal tumors in animal models.[61]

The international correlation data on prostate cancer risk support a positive association with fat intake.[58] Two case–control studies found that prostate cancer risk is correlated with diets high in animal fats, cheeses, cream, and eggs.[62,63]

The type of dietary fat implicated in cancer is a current research topic. There is experimental evidence that high-fat diets rich in linoleic acid, found in corn, safflower, sunflower, and other vegetable oils, may act as tumor promoters. Similar diets rich in oleic acid, from olive oil, and eicosapentaenoic acid, in fish oils, do not promote cancer in animals and may be protective. This may explain the low incidence of breast and colon cancer in Eskimos, whose main fat source is fish, and in people in Greece and Spain, whose main fat source is olive oil.[64]

Currently, Americans consume about 36% to 38% of their total daily calories as fat.[65,66] Numerous health experts have recommended that Americans reduce that figure to 30% or less to reduce risks for heart disease, obesity, and cancer.

FIBER

Since the early 1970s, when Burkitt proposed that dietary fiber may reduce the risk of large bowel cancer,[67] numerous epidemiologic and laboratory studies have explored a possible protective role for fiber. A review of results from 40 epidemiologic studies indicated an inverse relationship between total dietary fiber intake and colon cancer incidence in 32 of the 40 studies.[68]

Most international correlation studies using food availability data find that colon cancer mortality or incidence is inversely associated with fiber-rich food intake. Within-country correlational studies are also consistent. The low colon cancer rates in U.S. Mormons and Seventh-Day Adventists and rural Scandinavians, for example, correlate with higher intakes of fiber-rich foods than in the general population.[69,70]

Results from case–control studies generally reflect an inverse or protective association between dietary fiber and the risk of colon cancer. It should be noted that several studies show no association, and a few studies indicate increased risk.[3] However, inconsistent findings may be explained if one considers that dietary fibers from different food sources are heterogeneous mixtures of specific components, including cellulose, hemicellulose, pectin, gums, and lignin, and thus may have varying physiological effects. In addition, fiber components are difficult to quantify accurately in foods.[68]

More information is needed about which specific fiber components are protective. Laboratory results on chemically induced colon cancers in rodents suggest that inhibitory or enhancing effects are related to the type of fiber, the specific carcinogen, and other experimental variables such as route of administration. For example, cellulose inhibited 1,2-dimethylhydrazine-induced tumors in rats, but pectin had no effect.[71] Watanabe et al[72] noted that pectin was protective but alfalfa and bran were ineffective when azoxymethane and methylnitrosourea were administered parenterally. When administered intrarectally, pectin and bran were ineffective, while alfalfa enhanced carcinogenesis. Wheat bran appears to inhibit colon cancer development in animal models more consistently than other fiber sources.[3]

Several mechanisms have been proposed for the inhibitory effect of fiber on colorectal carcinogenesis. Fiber increases fecal bulk, thus reducing fecal mutagen concentrations. Also, enhanced colonic transit time can reduce the period of exposure of colonic mucosa to fecal mutagens. Finally, mutagen formation may be reduced by fiber-induced changes in colonic *p*h or bacterial metabolism.

The mean dietary fiber intake in the U.S. adult population is about 11 g/day.[73] Because of converging evidence that fiber may moderate the effects of fat, and because epidemiologic data consistently show an inverse association of dietary fiber intake with colon cancer, an increase to 20 to 30 g/day of dietary fiber is currently recommended by the NCI.

MUTAGENS AND CARCINOGENS IN FOOD

A variety of carcinogenic and mutagenic substances occur in our diet. The advent of rapid assays for mutagenicity has spurred the identification of many such compounds in food sources. Some of these substances occur naturally in the diet, whereas others result from food additives, preparation and processing procedures, pesticide residues, environmental pollution, and fungal contamination.[6,11]

Naturally occurring carcinogens include tannins, found in herbal teas,[74] hydrazines, found in edible mushrooms,[75] and safrole and related natural alkenyl benzenes, found in flavorings and spices.[76] Naturally occurring flavonoids, widespread in edible plants and fruits, are mutagenic.[77] Fungal contamination of stored food can produce potent carcinogenic mycotoxins such as aflatoxin. In some areas of Africa, aflatoxin contamination of grain is implicated in higher than expected rates of liver cancer.[78,79]

Other notable sources of carcinogens in the human diet are the nitrosamines, derived from the interaction of nitrite with secondary or tertiary amines. Both sodium nitrate and its bacterial reduction product, sodium nitrite, occur naturally in plants, meats, and dairy products. They also are widely used as preservatives in smoked meat and salted fish.[11] The nitrosamines, such as dimethylnitrosamine, are potent carcinogens that generate diverse types of cancer in many animal species. Epidemiologic studies conducted in the United States, England, South America, Iran, Japan, and China demonstrate an association between nitrate and nitrite consumption and the incidence of stomach and esophageal cancer.[58] The formation of nitrosamines in humans following oral administration of nitrite and an appropriate substrate amine has been demonstrated.[80] The generation of nitrosamines, in stored food or in the gut, can be reduced by the presence of ascorbic acid or other antioxidants.[81]

Recent research on pyrolysis products formed during cooking led Sugimura and co-workers to identify a series of mutagenic heterocyclic amines in meat and fish. Rodents fed long-term diets containing mutagenic heterocyclic amines consistently developed multiple tumors in the lung, liver, small and large intestine, and colon. Pyrolysates of tryptophan, glutamic acid, and soybean are carcinogenic.[82] Also found in charbroiled meat are polyaromatic hydrocarbons.[83] As a result of environmental contamination, polyaromatic hydrocarbon levels in the range of parts per billion often occur in plants, meat, fish, and refined fats.[84] Other carcinogenic environmental contaminants in food include the growth promoter diethylstilbestrol, pesticides such as DDT and chlordane, and industrial pollutants such as arsenic, asbestos, heavy metals, and polychlorinated biphenyls.[11]

Most food-derived mutagens and carcinogens that have been studied in detail require metabolic activation to reactive electrophilic species. Some, such as the mutagen caffeine, are believed to act through inhibition of DNA repair processes.[6] In evaluating the risk posed to man from exposure to these chemicals, it is important to consider that chemical carcinogenesis is a multistage process that occurs over a relatively long period of time. Many variables can conceivably impinge on and modulate this process. Individual exposures to dietary carcinogens and mutagens are variable in terms of dose, frequency, and duration. Related factors include modification of metabolic activation and detoxification mechanisms, the presence of other protective or inhibitory substances in the diet, and the impact of other life-style–related factors. Although the carcinogenic risk posed to man by dietary carcinogens and mutagens is uncertain, it is no doubt prudent to avoid mycotoxin-contaminated foods and excessive exposure to nitrosamine sources and to minimize the intake of heterocyclic amines produced during cooking.

ALCOHOL

In the United States, alcohol consumption is widespread and represents a significant component of dietary intake for some persons.[85] Epidemiologic research indicates that high alcohol intake is associated with an increased risk of several types of cancer. Cancer of the esophagus, pharynx, larynx, and mouth is observed with high alcohol use in many correlational and case–control studies.[86,87] These cancers are also associated with smoking. Colorectal cancer is associated with excessive beer drinking in several studies,[58] including a recent prospective report.[88]

Of the approximately 17 cohort and case–control studies on alcohol consumption and breast cancer, all but three showed an increased cancer risk.[89] Two recent cohort studies indicated an increase in breast cancer incidence for even moderate drinkers compared with nondrinkers. Willett et al,[53] using a sample of 90,000 nurses, reported a 60% increase in breast cancer risk in women who had one or more alcoholic drinks per day. In a more representative sample, Schatzkin et al found a 40% to 50% increase in risk among women who consumed three alcoholic drinks per week.[90] These studies are limited by the difficulty of obtaining an accurate history of alcohol intake. In a recent case–control study, increased breast cancer risk associated with alcohol consumption was evident only for women who drank at ages less than 30 years, regardless of current consumption.[91]

Based on an analysis of epidemiologic studies, the International Agency for Research on Cancer considers the evidence sufficient for categorizing alcoholic beverages as carcinogenic. The most compelling studies showed enhanced cancer risk when alcohol is present as a cocarcinogen, for example, in combination with cigarette smoking.[92,93]

A more precise evaluation of epidemiologic research on alcohol consumption is hampered by the fact that the ethanol source is variable. Beer, wine, distilled spirits, and locally prepared beverages contain multiple constituents with potential biologic activity. Although not itself a mutagen, the ethanol in fermented preparations is frequently accompanied by mutagenic constituents.[7] Further, excessive alcohol consumption is often associated with impaired nutritional status, which may also influence cancer risk. Stryker et al[94] reported that an intake of 20 g alcohol per day reduced plasma beta-carotene levels 24% in men and 11% in women. Decreased levels of some micronutrients, especially vitamin A and carotenoids, may be linked to cancer development. Finally, the marked hepatoxicity produced by ethanol may interfere with the successful metabolism and excretion of potentially carcinogenic xenobiotics.

DIETARY INTERVENTION: CLINICAL TRIALS

It is estimated that up to 80% of cancer incidence is associated with life-style and environmental factors and, therefore, theoretically subject to prevention efforts.[93] The compelling evidence accumulated from laboratory and population studies on dietary factors associated with lower risk has provided investigators with strong leads for reducing cancer incidence. The NCI, recognizing the need for confirmatory studies, is sponsoring major clinical research efforts directed toward the chemoprevention of cancer.

The Chemoprevention Program, designed to identify and evaluate the efficacy of discrete, well-defined specific micronutrients, or synthetic analogues, in reducing human cancer, is concerned with questions such as nutrient bioavailability, metabolism, toxicity, and the public health impact of this intervention research. The program depends on the integration of results from epidemiologic and laboratory studies to devise appropriate human intervention trials that test a chemopreventive approach to cancer control. A parallel approach is being used by the Diet, Nutrition, and Cancer Program, which emphasizes the role of macronutrients such as fat and fiber.

The chemoprevention approach to nutrition intervention, defined as the addition of specific micronutrients or synthetic formulations to the diet, has two obvious advantages over the macronutrient approach. First, the biologic effects of chemically defined substances administered in specified dosages are easier to assess than changes associated with the addition or removal of a broadly characterized macronutrient. Second, it usually is much easier to add a dietary supplement than to expect full understanding and compliance with a recommended major dietary change.

RESEARCH STRATEGY

The research and initiation phases of both of the NCI cancer prevention programs follow a prescribed progression of phases designed to systematically and vigorously test a specific proposed intervention strategy. Preclinical investigations select and evaluate candidate substances and determine their efficacy, safety, and pharmacologic parameters in in vitro and in vivo screening systems. Following identification of research leads and method development, controlled intervention trials are used to validate efficacy and safety. Once the value of a preventive intervention has been proved, broad application is targeted to populations at risk or the general population.

In addition to the sequence of cancer control phases within the Chemoprevention Program and the Diet, Nutrition, and Cancer Program at the NCI, "convergence plans," or research flow designs, were developed for assessing the adequacy of pharmacologic, toxicologic, and epidemiologic data. This research flow design, with specified decision and convergence points, is shown for the Chemoprevention Program in Figure 11-1.[95]

If a particular chemoprevention agent or intervention satisfies all of the laboratory and epidemiologic decision points, an evaluation is made as to whether the research data are strong enough to justify intervention in humans. Because of the enormous commitment of resources required for large-scale human intervention trials, studies with the potential for broad public health impact generally have been limited to cancers with the greatest morbidity and mortality. Other studies address populations at very high risk (*e.g.*, asbestos-exposed smokers) or people with precancerous lesions. The research flow designs have been formulated into a series of decision point matrices or stages. Criteria for satisfactory resolutions of the research hypothesis must be met before the research flow is supported for further action. More than 20 human intervention trials sponsored by the NCI Chemoprevention Program are currently in progress. The trials are testing selected chemopreventive agents with

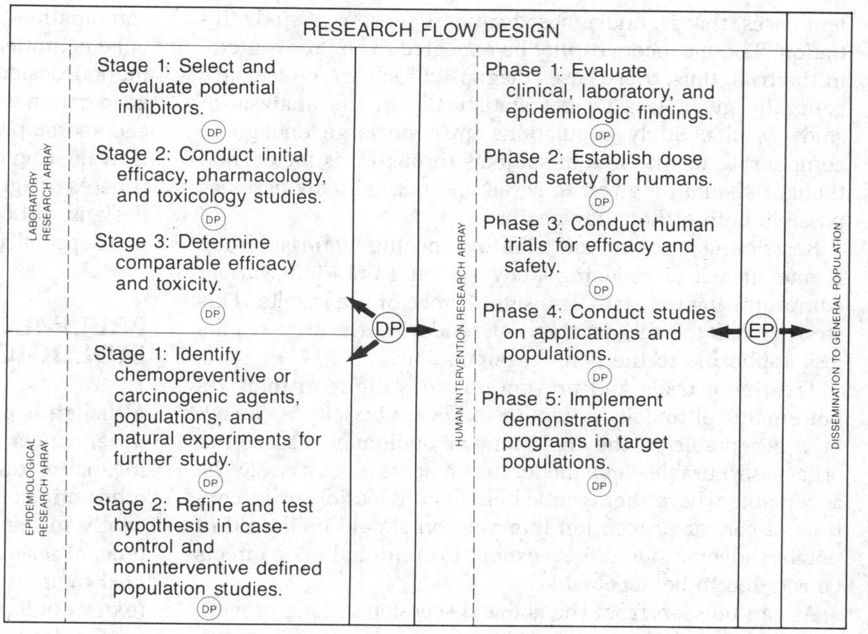

FIG. 11-1. Research flow design of NCI Chemoprevention Program. DP = decision point; EP = evaluation point.

demonstrated potential for inhibiting lung, breast, colon, esophageal, bladder, and skin cancers—some of the most common cancers in humans.

FEATURES OF PREVENTION TRIALS AND TREATMENT TRIALS

Cancer prevention and cancer treatment trials are both designed to evaluate an intervention strategy for efficacy and toxicity in a clinical setting. Features of a sound research design such as randomization, appropriate controls, blinding when feasible, and an appreciation of statistical considerations are important for both types of trials. They differ significantly, however, with respect to study design and evaluation criteria.

Whereas the goal of a cancer treatment trial is to reduce mortality and morbidity, the intent of a prevention trial is to lower the rate of cancer occurrence. The efficacy of a cancer prevention intervention is based on a decrease in cancer incidence in the test population. Alternatively, the trial end point may measure the occurrence or modification of precursor lesions associated with the eventual appearance of malignant disease. Although no precursor markers have yet been identified as reliable indicators of disease incidence, the evaluation of such parameters in a prevention trial can examine human biologic effects in addition to testing whether or not the intervention will lower the cancer occurrence rate.

A prevention trial may also consider the value of an intervention designed to reduce exposure to a cancer-causing substance, such as cigarettes. The goal in this case would be to reduce the amount of smoking in the intervention group.

The study population in a treatment trial consists of cancer patients, whereas a prevention trial may use as test subjects the general population, persons at high risk for cancer or with precancerous lesions, or currently disease-free subjects previously treated for cancer. The principal investigator and the organizational setting influence the choice and recruitment of a test population. Clinicians are more apt to come in contact with persons requiring medical supervision; thus, it may be easier for them to select patients with precancerous lesions or healthy subjects in screening programs or prepaid health plans. Implementation of a prevention trial using a general or specially defined healthy population requires carefully planned recruitment schemes and an organizational framework to support the effort.

The duration of a prevention trial is usually much longer than that of a treatment trial. The choice of study length is not always obvious because it may take several years before any benefit can be expected, and that benefit may build with time.

Due to statistical considerations, the size of the study population in a prevention trial is usually an order of magnitude greater than that in a treatment trial. Even the most common cancers occur only rarely in a random sampling of several thousand people examined over a 5-year period. Adherence (compliance) to an intervention therapy may be difficult to maintain, requiring a larger test population to compensate for "dropouts." A statistical analysis of expected compliance can be used to help estimate the number of subjects required for a given study, and programs designed to maintain a high level of compliance (including counseling and "recapture" of dropouts) can be implemented. Conversely, some subjects may be "drop-ins," particularly in a study lasting several years. Drop-ins are test subjects in the control group who alter their life-style in such a way as to reflect the intervention plan being tested (*e.g.*, by adopting a low-fat diet or by consuming more carrots).

Another problem associated with the choice of a study population in a prevention trial is the occurrence of prevalent cases, that is, undiagnosed cancers present at study initiation. These cancers cannot be expected to be "prevented" in the trial; thus, those cases diagnosed early in the trial are generally given less weight statistically in the analysis of study results. Study populations must be large enough to compensate for the loss of subjects through this factor, and thought should be given to screening out as many cases as possible before the study begins.

Restricting a prevention trial to a specific high-risk group is one means of reducing study size and duration without compromising the statistical significance of the results. This strategy has the disadvantage of rendering the trial results less applicable to the general population.

Treatment trials and prevention trials differ in their requirements of toxicity acceptance. Severe toxicity is considered acceptable in the treatment of malignant disease not otherwise curable, and moderate or acute toxicity may be acceptable where therapeutic benefits are less clear. In contrast, a cancer prevention intervention should be devoid of notable adverse side-effects except for minimal toxic effects considered to be acceptable.

As can be seen from the above discussion, a long prevention trial in a large population has many potential organizational, logistical, and statistical problems. Pilot studies should be conducted for most prevention trials. The variability in study populations, the size and scope of many trials, and the logistics of study implementation and management all can be tested before a full research effort is initiated. The purpose of a pilot study is rarely to measure outcomes, but rather to test for practical problems in study design.

A useful feature of many prevention trial protocols is the inclusion of a "run-in" period—a period of time, before study initiation and subject randomization, when both the intervention and control groups receive placebos. Because dropouts tend to occur early in a trial, the use of a run-in period can eliminate these cases and strengthen the statistical analysis of the results. This may confound the study interpretation because the remaining subjects represent only those achieving good compliance. To the extent allowed by sample size, a run-in also is useful for determining the rate of reported side-effects to be expected in controls.

Beyond administration of a proposed intervention, investigators in some prevention trials will collect baseline biochemical information to strengthen and expand the analysis of trial results. For example, Hennekens[96] collected blood from a large proportion of physicians in a trial designed to test the efficacy of beta-carotene in reducing cancer risk. In addition to the data on cancer incidence, his group now will be able to determine whether benefits accrued for all subjects, or only for those whose initial blood level of beta-carotene was low.

The study design of a treatment trial generally consists of a treatment group versus a placebo group or an alternate treatment group. More complex, factorial designs are often used for preventive intervention trials. A factorial design[97] allows two or more interventions to be evaluated in one trial, with approximately the same number of study subjects (and expense) as would be required to test a single agent (factor). Prevention trials are well suited for factorial designs because most interventions are nontoxic and can be given safely in combination. The number of agents that can be studied at once is limited by the logistics of managing complex experimental designs rather than by statistical considerations. A good rationale should be provided for inclusion of multiple agents in a prevention trial; the largest trial now in progress is evaluating eight groups of agents (including placebo). Estimates of agent interactions are also possible from factorial designs, although the sample size should be increased if this is of special interest.

PRELIMINARY CLINICAL TRIALS: BIOLOGIC MARKER END POINTS

Although a prospective randomized intervention trial with lower cancer incidence as the end point is the most desirable means for testing the efficacy of a chemopreventive agent, other clinical work preceding such a study can add significantly to our knowledge base. For example, for beta-carotene a series of clinical–metabolic studies performed in healthy men examined the effects of short-term dosing for toxicity and pharmacokinetic factors, generating useful data for the design of testing protocols for larger scale chemoprevention trials.[98]

In many cases, retrospective epidemiologic work and laboratory research combine to establish a strong case for the testing of a chemopreventive regimen. An intervention trial with a selected study population is sometimes used to assess not cancer incidence but a change in the nature of precancerous lesions or other biologic markers thought to be associated with the eventual development of malignant disease. This type of study is less costly than a large randomized trial and likely to provide a statistically significant outcome. A small selective study is also useful for initially establishing the biologic activity of a compound in humans when previous work has been conducted exclusively in the laboratory. In addition, the analysis of efficacy, toxicity, and dosage regimens provides important data for the design of larger randomized trials in the future.

The choice of a precursor or precancerous lesion as the end point for a clinical intervention study should be based on the strength of its association with a specific cancer, the ease with which the end point can be quantitatively evaluated, and the prevalence of this lesion in a study population.[99] It should be emphasized that the use of precursor lesions as predictors of future cancer incidence has not been experimentally validated in large-scale clinical trials. This important step must be taken before we can be fully confident of any marker end point in a clinical trial.

Dietary intervention studies in colon cancer have successfully employed protocols using precursor lesions as the clinical end point of interest. For example, the occurrence of rectal polyps in patients with familial polyposis was reduced by the administration of ascorbic acid (vitamin C).[100] Over a period of 3 to 13 months, rectal polyps disappeared or regressed in five of the eight treated patients. A later randomized trial of ascorbic acid intervention in 49 patients confirmed these results.[101]

Also evaluated in a study of colon cancer has been fecal mutagenicity, possibly associated with colon cancer. Fecal extracts contain mutagenic substances, as assessed by the Ames *Salmonella* test.[102] The occurrence and prevalence of such compounds may be influenced by diet, and therefore, the exposure of colonic epithelium to mutagenic substances may be reduced. Supplemental ascorbic acid and alpha-tocopherol (vitamin E) were used by Dion and colleagues[103] to successfully reduce mutagenic substances in 20 healthy subjects.

Other clinical work related to colon cancer concerns the observation that Seventh-Day Adventist vegetarians have a significantly lower incidence of this cancer than the general population. Lipkin and colleagues[104] found that the proliferation of colonic mucosa epithelial cells was markedly less in these vegetarians than in a control group. Further, Lipkin and Newmark[105] found that calcium carbonate supplementation for 2 to 3 months reduced epithelial cell proliferation in persons at high risk for familial colon cancer. Although the association described is of great interest, equally important is the development of a sensitive assay usable in large populations to measure the proliferation of colonic epithelial cells. When validated to predict cancers, such indices may be used in future trials to quantify the effects of a chemopreventive agent.

Retinoids have been tested clinically for their ability to affect the occurrence and regression of precursor lesions associated with lung and oral cancer. A synthetic retinoid, etretinate, was tested for its ability to reduce bronchial squamous cell metaplasia.[106] This work, conducted in a high-risk population (heavy smokers), suggested that the degree of bronchial metaplasia was reduced in treated subjects. In other work, 13-*cis*-retinoic acid, when applied topically, was found to reduce the severity of oral leukoplakia, an epithelial lesion associated with oral cancer.[107] The study examined several dosages (3, 5, or 10 mg/day for 6 months) and provided a particularly detailed enumeration of adverse side-effects. The leukoplakia recurred after cessation of therapy.

Related work on oral cancer used a test for inhibition of genotoxicity as the clinical end point of interest.[108] Betel nut tobacco chewers, persons at high risk of developing oral cancer, were the test population. The occurrence of micronuclei (a genotoxic marker) in exfoliated oral epithelial cells was assessed after treatment with placebo, vitamin A, beta-carotene, or 4,4'-diketo-beta-carotene. Both vitamin A and beta-carotene notably inhibited the occurrence of micronucleated epithelial cells, but 4,4′-diketo-beta-carotene did not. This beta-carotene derivative is not converted to vitamin A in vivo, suggesting that under these conditions, vitamin A is the active moiety, with beta-carotene an equally effective precursor.

These are a few examples of completed clinical intervention studies that used biologic marker end points. They suggest beneficial effects of chemopreventive agents, adding further impetus to this research field. This type of work can contribute to the overall evaluation of the clinical potential of a chemopreventive agent and supplies valuable information regarding biologic activity in humans, toxicity, dose regimens, and candidate target populations. In some cases, important new technologies are developed that provide research tools helpful not only for prevention research but for other types of cancer research as well. However, before marker end points can be used as a substitute for large-scale trials with cancer incidence end points, the markers will have to be validated in the context of clinical trials. This will take many years to accomplish.

INTERVENTION TRIALS IN PROGRESS

At present, more than two dozen large-scale dietary intervention trials are under way. This research is designed to evaluate the influence of a variety of dietary factors and synthetic retinoids on cancer incidence in specifically defined high-risk populations. Each of these studies is a randomized prospective trial ranging in design from simple to complex factorial. Variations in study designs and protocols are illustrated by the trials described below. Aspects of the research methods are highlighted to help those with an interest in developing this type of research trial.

ISOTRETINOIN–BASAL CELL CARCINOMA PREVENTION TRIAL

The synthetic retinoid isotretinoin (13-*cis*-retinoic acid; Accutane) is currently being evaluated in a long-term low-dosage protocol (10 mg/day for 3 years) for its ability to reduce the incidence of basal cell carcinoma. The subject population is a group of 1000 men and women aged 40 to 75 years who have had two or more biopsy-proven basal cell carcinomas during the 5 years before entry into the study. The trial will include a 2-year postintervention follow-up. The objective is to reduce the incidence of new basal cell carcinomas in persons at high risk because of previous basal cell carcinoma. In addition, information will be gathered regarding the toxicity of isotretinoin when taken for long periods at low doses. This randomized, double-blind, multicenter study is being conducted by the NCI with the collaboration of military medical centers, private medical institutions, and Hoffmann-LaRoche, Inc. The simple randomization into two groups (isotretinoin versus placebo) is similar to many therapeutic trials. This trial had a 6-month pilot phase to monitor patient recruitment and enrollment procedures, test data management and study logistics, and evaluate short-term safety and toxicity. Greenberg and colleagues[109] are using a similar design to determine whether beta-carotene influences the recurrence of nonmelanoma skin cancer in patients who have recently had a nonmelanoma skin cancer removed. The trial will involve 2000 subjects. After a 1-month run-in period to improve trial efficacy, subjects receive either 50 mg beta-carotene or a placebo daily.

U.S.–FINLAND LUNG CANCER PREVENTION TRIAL

A large-scale trial, conducted as a collaborative project by the NCI and the National Public Health Institute of Finland, currently is investigating the efficacy of both beta-carotene and alpha-tocopherol (vitamin E) in reducing lung cancer incidence among 28,000 male cigarette smokers. Reduction in the incidence of other cancers also will be evaluated.

This randomized double-blind 6-year intervention study, begun in March 1984, employs a 2×2 factorial design to evaluate four separate treatment groups: placebo (control), beta-carotene (20 mg/day), vitamin E (alpha-tocopherol, 100 mg/day), and beta-carotene in combination with vitamin E.[110] This design allows estimation of effects associated with the individual agents by comparison of vitamin E or beta-carotene with placebo, as well as estimation of any synergistic effects or inhibitory interaction between beta-carotene and vitamin E with regard to cancer incidence.

An 11-month pilot study in one of five participating clinics was used to evaluate recruitment procedures, clinic staff operations, appropriateness of research forms, compliance, usefulness of a run-in period, and side-effects of the study agents before the full research effort was initiated. Incident cancers will be identified through clinical follow-up procedures and by periodic matching of names of study subjects with the Finnish Cancer Registry.

NUTRITION INTERVENTION TRIALS IN LINXIAN, CHINA

The NCI and the Cancer Institute of the Chinese Academy of Medical Sciences are collaborating in the conduct of two randomized, double-blind, 5-year intervention trials in Linxian, China, an area with a particularly high incidence of esophageal cancer. One study, the General Population Trial, which uses a fractional factorial design, will determine the effect of multiple vitamin/mineral combinations on the incidence of esophageal cancer. The test population is composed of 30,000 men and women, ages 40 to 69, divided into eight intervention groups receiving placebos or specified combinations of vitamin A, beta-carotene, zinc, riboflavin, niacin, vitamin C, molybdenum, selenium, and vitamin E at doses one to four times the U.S. recommended daily allowance (RDA).[111] The fractional factorial design is illustrated in Figure 11-2. This statistical technique allows data to be divided into subsets during analysis to examine specific agent effects or interactions of interest. The Linxian design is a half-replication of the full 2^4 factorial, testing only 8 of the possible 16 groups. Ability to test the effect of each main factor under study is retained; however, two-way interactions between factors are confounded with each other.[112] Judicious use of a fractional factorial design can reduce a large factorial study, such as the Linxian trial, to practicable size.

FIG. 11-2. The Linxian esophageal cancer prevention trial is a fractional factorial design based on a 2^4 factorial. The asterisks indicate the eight intervention groups included in a half-replicate of the 2^4 factorial design. Thirty thousand participants, 40 to 69 years old, will receive either a daily placebo or one of the seven vitamin/mineral combinations. Treatment agents are (*A*) vitamin A, beta-carotene, zinc; (*B*) riboflavin, niacin; (*C*) vitamin C, molybdenum; (*D*) selenium, vitamin E.

Intervention Groups

Placebo*	A	B	**AB***
C	**AC***	**BC***	ABC
D	**AD***	**BD***	ABD
CD*	ACD	BCD	**ABCD***

A second study, the Dysplasia Trial, will examine the effect of multiple vitamins/minerals on a high-risk population with severe esophageal dysplasia. In a simple study design, 3400 men and women, ages 40 to 69, will receive either a placebo or a multiple vitamin/mineral supplement at levels one to four times the RDA. Participants will be evaluated for disease progression or regression. In both studies, cancer incidence and mortality will be determined through hospital record pathology slides and radiographic reviews in conjunction with the Linxian Esophageal Cancer Registry.

Before initiation of the full-scale trials, a 6-month pilot study indicated that patient recruitment, compliance, and study logistics were feasible. In addition, nutritional assessment data showed that deficiencies were common and that nutritional status could be improved by low-dose vitamin supplementation.

Of the many other cancer prevention trials in progress, 11 are examining the effects of beta-carotene, alone or in combination with other agents, on cancer incidence. For example, a Boston study[96] of 22,000 healthy male physicians, ages 40 to 84, is evaluating the influence of beta-carotene and aspirin on both total cancer incidence and cardiovascular disease, using a factorial study design (Fig. 11-3).

Grouping beta-carotene intervention research by cancer site, seven studies are directed toward reducing the incidence of lung cancer in smoking and other high-risk groups. In one study, the preventive effect of beta-carotene in combination with vitamin A is being tested in a population at high risk for lung cancer and mesothelioma due to occupational exposure to asbestos. Tin miners at high risk for lung cancer are receiving beta-carotene, retinol, vitamin E, and selenium.

Six intervention studies are investigating the prevention of skin cancer in such high-risk groups as albinos in equatorial Africa and subjects with previous skin cancer and precancerous actinic keratosis. The prevention of colon cancer and

FIG. 11-3. The physicians health study is a 2 × 2 factorial design in which 22,000 healthy physicians receive, on alternate days, either (*A*) beta-carotene and aspirin, (*B*) aspirin and placebo, (*C*) beta-carotene and placebo, or (*D*) placebo only.

Intervention Groups

		Beta-carotene Yes	Beta-carotene No
Aspirin	Yes	A	B
	No	C	D

cervical cancer is the subject of other dietary intervention trials. Five studies on the prevention of colon cancer are testing vitamin C, vitamin E, beta-carotene, or wheat fiber, alone or in combination, in subjects selected on the basis of familial polyposis or adenotomous polyp diagnosis. Women with cervical dysplasia are being treated with *trans*-retinoic acid or folic acid in two separate trials for the prevention of cervical cancer.[34]

THE PHYSICIAN AS AN EFFECTIVE PROMOTER OF HEALTHY DIET

The clinician involved in primary health care has a leading role in counseling patients on life-style as it affects their overall health. Nutritional science, included in many medical school curricula, is a critical part of effective health promotion education. For the best use of the physician's time, patient education might be seen as a cooperative process involving nurses, dietitians, and others.

A number of studies have examined the potential effectiveness of physicians as agents of health-promoting behavior change in their patients.[113-115] There are several reasons why physicians can be effective. Physicians are often good role models. Physicians are also seen as the most authoritative source of medical and health information. About 70% of Americans make at least one visit a year to their doctor, often because they are ill or otherwise amenable to a suggestion about life-style and behavior change. These visits are often excellent "teachable moments" because of the personal relationship and trust that clinicians are able to establish with their patients.

The following guidelines are ways in which physicians can assist their patients to make positive dietary changes:[116]

1. Discuss risk factors and the benefits associated with dietary modification with patients. The personal communication with the patient and individualized counseling based on the patient's history and situation are key to the success of this effort.
2. Assess the patient's current dietary profile. For example, have the patient fill out a diet history. This will reveal problem areas and allow the physician and patient to discuss the patient's dietary habits more concretely and conceive possible ways of making changes.
3. Have the patient choose several changes to work on until the next visit. Small, incremental steps are easier to make than a total modification of the diet.
4. Provide the patient with information materials to assist him or her in behavior change.
5. On subsequent patient visits, review the diet history questionnaire and recommended behavior changes to monitor compliance and encourage progress.

To assist patients in making dietary changes, some simple strategies may be suggested. One of these is a choose more/choose less approach, developed by NCI for use in its cancer prevention materials.[117] This approach does not preclude the use of any food. Rather, it emphasizes a shift away from high-fat, low-fiber foods that may increase cancer risk toward foods low in fat and rich in fiber and nutrients.

Although not all the answers are fully known about diet and its relationship to disease risks, a number of scientific organizations have issued dietary guidelines for the public. These expert groups believe that sufficient data now exist for the public to be informed and that prudent guidelines based on current evidence are likely to lower risks for major chronic diseases, including cancer, and will do no harm.

In 1980, the U.S. Department of Agriculture and the Department of Health and Human Services jointly published "Nutrition and Your Health: Dietary Guidelines for Americans." A slightly edited version was published in 1985. These guidelines were designed to assist healthy adult Americans in improving their nutritional status and overall health.

Most recently, the NCI has developed for the public a compatible set of dietary guidelines (listed below), adding some specificity to aid in interpretation:[118]

1. Reduce fat intake to 30% of calories or less.
2. Increase fiber intake to 20 to 30 g/day, with an upper limit of 35 g/day.
3. Include a variety of vegetables and fruit in the daily diet.
4. Avoid obesity.
5. Consume alcoholic beverages in moderation, if at all.
6. Minimize consumption of salt-cured, salt-pickled, or smoked foods.

The physician can call on numerous other resources to assist in diet counseling. Effective use of information materials and collaboration with nutrition professionals are critical to the patient's successful change. Qualified professionals, including private-practice registered dietitians and nutritionists and health department or extension nutritionists, can do much to support and complement a physician's efforts. Resources for materials include the Food and Nutrition Information Center of the USDA National Agricultural Library; publications of the USDA and USDHHS; and resources from the American Heart Association, American Cancer Society, American Dietetic Association, and Society for Nutrition Education.

FUTURE PROSPECTS FOR CANCER PREVENTION

Approximately 900,000 new cases of cancer are diagnosed in the United States each year, with 450,000 deaths attributed to this disease annually. The NCI has launched an aggressive effort to control cancer by the year 2000 and to reduce the mortality by 50% between 1985 and 2000.[119] Cancer prevention interventions designed to minimize life-style or environmental factors that promote cancer or to maximize exposure to agents that reduce cancer incidence are expected to play a major role in achieving this goal.

The weight of new evidence developed in the second half of this century from laboratory and population studies has focused cancer prevention efforts on two avoidable risks: smoking and dietary factors.[34] The estimated 35% of cancer deaths that may be related to dietary components have stimulated an aggressive effort to explore the roles of diet and nutrition in cancer prevention. Behavior research and nutrition education can contribute much to the success of these prevention efforts and represent major efforts in the prevention programs at the NCI.

The example of retinoids and beta-carotene illustrates how the convergence of basic research and population studies, coupled with developmental research, has led to large prospective clinical intervention trials. The promising clinical work under way with 13-*cis*-retinoic acid emerges from research on the process of carcinogenesis, the development of more active, less toxic retinoid analogues, and epidemiologic research. The specificity of the retinoids in the control of cell function suggests that this group of compounds is a practical tool for the study of several molecular mechanisms of action in cancer prevention. New approaches to the control of cell differentiation are being investigated as a result of the particular interest in the antineoplastic activity of the retinoids. Insights into the expression of oncogenes and modulation of the action of specific peptide growth factors and their membrane-bound receptors have already generated prevention research initiatives.[28]

The identification of human oncogene products and assays for their detection could in the future enable the clinician to screen and intervene before the onset of disease. The development of antisera for the *ras* oncogene product, protein P_{21}, is an example of such a marker under evaluation for the early detection of cancer. The study of tumor suppressor genes that can inhibit the expression of the tumorigenic phenotype is providing evidence, although still fragmentary, of new mechanisms for inhibiting tumor growth potentially more diversified than the oncogenes.[120] Tests such as the micronucleus test[108] for chromosome aberrations may prove useful, when the scoring can be automated, for selecting the most active chemopreventive agents and effective dosages for intervention trials. Further prospects for prevention, although speculative, may be developed with the retroviruses, known to be responsible for animal leukemias and lymphomas and at least one type of human leukemia. It is conceivable that one day there may be an antiviral cancer vaccine available.

In the area of dietary research, all the confounding factors may never be identified; however, this does not preclude testing of specific agents of potential benefit in pilot intervention trials. Thus, literally hundreds of dietary and synthetic agents are under consideration for future study.

Advances in food and agricultural technologies and the development of new dietary synthetic substitutes are contributing to our changing food supply and may have a profound effect on nutritional intake and long-term health effects. Several synthetic fat substitutes such as Simplesse and Olestra are awaiting Food and Drug Administration approval, and if approved, they could have a profound effect on nutritional intake and long-term health effects. Both products are low in calorie and cholesterol content and may appreciably reduce fat intake and chronic disease incidence. Edible plants are now cultivated with specific characteristics that may be nutritionally superior or inferior. This is also true of food production in artificially controlled media such as aquaculture or the rapid multiplication of stock by microculture techniques. Genetic engineering applied to agriculture may revolutionize the production of economically important crops by raising the level of so-called natural pesticides and breeding animals free of genetic or infectious diseases. Obviously, prudence is required in managing the choices of natural and artificial dietary substitutes.

An increasing number of American companies have developed programs aimed at promoting overall health and reducing risk factors for coronary heart disease and cancer. Many major United States employers are participating in cancer education and early detection programs aimed especially at lung, colorectal, breast, and uterine cancers. Diet modification and weight control programs are increasingly found in industry-sponsored wellness programs. In addition, many employers are opting to provide a preventive health care package as part of health insurance benefits, which generally includes a cancer screening schedule that is in accordance with American Cancer Society recommendations. Continued and increased interest in cancer education and prevention in the worksite could contribute greatly to reducing the incidence of certain types of cancer.

The NCI approach to cancer prevention is a rigorous discipline bridging fundamental and applied research that identifies a testable intervention hypothesis by evaluating the scientific evidence, develops intervention methodology, and validates the intervention in clinical trials.

Cancer prevention and control research has intensified in the 1980s, gaining impetus from investigations leading to the recognition that diet and the human nutritional state are linked to the incidence of certain common cancers. To confirm that these correlations directly affect causality, these lines of investigation should be both continued and expanded.

REFERENCES

1. Wattenberg LW: Inhibition of neoplasia by minor dietary constituents. Cancer Res 43:2448–2453, 1983
2. Shimkin MB: Contrary to nature. Washington, DC, Department of Health, Education and Welfare, 1977
3. Pilch SM (ed): Physiological Effects and Health Consequences of Dietary Fiber, pp 118–135. Bethesda, Md, Life Sciences Research Office, FASEB, 1987
4. Ip C, Birt DF, Rogers AE et al (eds): Dietary Fat and Cancer, pp 231–374. New York, Alan R Liss, 1986
5. Tannenbaum A, Silverstone H: Nutrition in relation to cancer. Adv Cancer Res 1:451–501, 1953
6. Ames BN: Dietary carcinogens and anticarcinogens. Science 221:1256–1264, 1983
7. Ames BN, Magaw R, Gold LS: Ranking possible carcinogenic hazards. Science 236:271–280, 1987
8. Sparnins VL, Wattenberg LW: Enhancement of glutathione *S*-transferase activity of the mouse forestomach by inhibitors of benzo(a)pyrene-induced neoplasia of the forestomach. JNCI 66:769–771, 1981
9. Wattenberg, LW: Chemoprevention of cancer. Cancer Res 45:1–8, 1985
10. Miller EC, Miller JA: Biochemical mechanisms of chemical carcinogenesis. In Busch H (ed): The Molecular Biology of Cancer, pp 342–377. New York, Academic Press, 1974
11. Carr BI: Chemical carcinogens and inhibitors of carcinogenesis in the human diet. Cancer 55:218–224, 1985
12. Krytopoulos SA: Ascorbic acid and the formation of *N*-nitroso compounds: possible role of ascorbic acid in cancer prevention. Am J Clin Nutr 45:1344–1350, 1987
13. Mettlin C, Graham S, Priore R et al: Diet and cancer of the esophagus. Nutr Cancer 2:143–147, 1981
14. Haenszel W, Correa P: Developments in the epidemiology of stomach cancer over the past decade. Cancer Res 35:3452–3459, 1975
15. Mirvish SS, Wallcave L, Eagen M et al: Ascorbate-nitrite reaction: Possible means of blocking the formation of carcinogenic N-nitroso compounds. Science 177:65–68, 1972
16. Menkes MS, Comstock GW, Vuilleumier JP et al: Serum beta-carotene, vitamins A and E, selenium and the risk of lung cancer. N Engl J Med 315:1250–1254, 1986

17. Willett W, Polk R, Underwood BA et al: Relation of serum vitamins A and E and carotenoids to the risk of cancer. N Engl J Med 310:430–434, 1984
18. Schrauzer GN, White DA, Schneider CJ: Cancer mortality correlation studies: III. Statistical associations with dietary selenium intakes. Bioinorgan Chem 7:23–31, 1977
19. Shamberger RJ, Tylko SA, Willis CE: Antioxidants and cancer: VI. Selenium and age-adjusted human cancer mortality. Arch Environ Health 31:231–235, 1976
20. Ip C: The chemopreventive role of selenium in carcinogenesis. J Am Coll Toxicol 5:7–20, 1986
21. Garland C, Shekelle RB, Barrett-Conner E et al: Dietary vitamin D and calcium and risk of colorectal cancer: A 19-year prospective study in men. Lancet 1:307–309, 1985
22. Hennekens CH, Mayrent SL, Willet W: Vitamin A, carotenoids, and retinoids. Cancer 58:1837–1841, 1986
23. Lasnitzki I: The influence of a hypervitaminosis on the effect of 20-methylcholanthrene on mouse prostate glands grown *in vitro*. Br J Cancer 9:434–441, 1955
24. Merriman RL, Bertram JS: Reversible inhibition by retinoids of 3-methylcholanthrene-induced neoplastic transformation of C3H/10T-1/2 CL8 cells. Cancer Res 39:1661–1666, 1979
25. Harisiadis L, Miller RC, Hall EJ et al: A vitamin A analogue inhibits radiation-induced oncogenic transformation. Nature 274:486–487, 1978
26. Strickland S, Mahdavi V: The induction of differentiation in teratocarcinoma stem cells by retinoic acid. Cell 15:393–403, 1978
27. Breitman TR, Collins SJ, Keene BR: Terminal differentiation of human promyelocytic leukemia cells in primary culture in response to retinoic acid. Blood 57:1000–1004, 1981
28. Sporn MB, Roberts AB: Role of retinoids in differentiation and carcinogenesis. Cancer Res 43:3034–3040, 1983
29. Sporn MB, Newton DL: Chemoprevention of cancer with retinoids. Fed Proc 38:2528–2534, 1979
30. Becci PJ, Thompson HJ, Grubbs CJ et al: Effect of delay in administration of 13-*cis*-retinoic acid on the inhibition of urinary bladder carcinogenesis in the rat. Cancer Res 39:3141–3144, 1979
31. Boutwell RK: Retinoids and inhibition of ornithine decarboxylase activity. J Am Acad Dermatol 6:796–798, 1982
32. Todaro GJ, DeLarco JE, Sporn MB: Retinoids block phenotypic cell transformation produced by sarcoma growth factor. Nature 276:272–274, 1978
33. Peto R: The marked differences between carotenoids and retinoids: Methodological implications for biochemical epidemiology. Cancer Surveys 2:327–340, 1983
34. Greenwald P, Sondik E, Lynch BS: Diet and chemoprevention in NCI's research strategy to achieve national cancer control objectives. Annu Rev Public Health 7:267–291, 1986
35. Bjelke E: Epidemiologic studies of cancer of the stomach, colon, and rectum, with special emphasis on the role of diet. Scand J Gastroenterol 9:1–53, 1974
36. Nomura A, Yamakawa H, Ishidate T et al: Intestinal metaplasia in Japan: Association with diet. JNCI 68:401–405, 1982
37. Peto R, Doll R, Buckley JD et al: Can dietary beta-carotene materially reduce human cancer rates? Nature 290:201–208, 1981
38. Bjelke E: Dietary vitamin A and human lung cancer. Int J Cancer 15:561–565, 1975
39. Kvale G, Bjelke E, Gart JJ: Dietary habits and lung cancer risk. Int J Cancer 31:397–405, 1983
40. Hirayama T: Diet and cancer. Nutr Cancer 1:67–81, 1979
41. Shekelle RB, Liu S, Raynor WJ Jr et al: Dietary vitamin A and risk of cancer in the Western Electric Study. Lancet 2:1185–1190, 1981
42. Tannenbaum A: The genesis and growth of tumors: III. Effect of a high fat diet. Cancer Res 2:468–475, 1942
43. Tannenbaum A: The dependence of the genesis of induced skin tumors on the caloric intake during different stages of carcinogenesis. Cancer Res 4:673–677, 1944
44. Kritchevsky D, Weber MM, Buck CL et al: Calories, fat and cancer. Lipids 21:272–274, 1986
45. Albanes D: Total calories, body weight, and tumor incidence in mice. Cancer Res 47:1987–1992, 1987a
46. Wynder EL, MacCormick F, Hill P et al: Nutrition and the etiology and prevention of breast cancer. Cancer Detect Prev 1:293–310, 1976
47. Carroll KK, Hopkins GJ: Dietary polyunsaturated fat versus saturated fat in relation to mammary carcinogenesis. Lipids 14:155, 1979
48. Phillips RL: Role of life-style and dietary habits in risk of cancer among Seventh-Day Adventists. Cancer Res 35:3513–3522, 1975
49. Miller AB, Kelly A, Choi NW et al: A study of diet and breast cancer. Am J Epidemiol 107:499–509, 1978
50. Nomura A, Henderson BE, Lee J: Breast cancer and diet among the Japanese in Hawaii. Am J Clin Nutr 31:2020–2025, 1978
51. Lubin JH, Burns PE, Blot HJ et al: Dietary factors and breast cancer risk. Int J Cancer 28:685–689, 1981
52. Papatestas AE, Knittle J, Lesnick G et al: Diet and human carcinogenesis. In: European Organization for Cooperation in Cancer Prevention Studies: Third Annual Symposium Proceedings, Aarhus, Denmark, June 19–21, 1985; p 66
53. Willett WC, Stampfer MJ, Colditz GA et al: Moderate alcohol consumption and the risk of breast cancer. N Engl J Med 316(19):1174–1180, 1987
54. McKeown-Eyssen G, Bright-See E: Dietary factors in colon cancer: International relationships. Nutr Cancer 6:160, 1984
55. Enstrom JE: Colorectal cancer and consumption of beef and fat. Br J Cancer 32:432–439, 1975
56. Bingham SA, William DR, Cole TJ et al: Dietary fiber and regional large-bowel cancer mortality in Britain. Br J Cancer 40:456–463, 1979
57. Kolonel LN, Nomura AMY, Hinds MW et al: Role of diet in cancer incidence in Hawaii. Cancer Res 43:2397s–2402s, 1983
58. Palmer S: Diet, nutrition, and cancer. Prog Food Nutr Sci 9:283–341, 1985
59. Jensen OM, MacLennan R, Wahrendorf J: Diet, bowel function, fecal characteristics, and large bowel cancer in Denmark and Finland. Nutr Cancer 4(1):5–19, 1982
60. Galloway DJ, Owen RW, Jarrett F et al: Experimental colorectal cancer: The relationship of diet and faecal bile acid concentration to tumour induction. Br J Surg 73:233–237, 1986
61. Reddy BS, Cohen LA, McCoy GD et al: Nutrition and its relationship to cancer. Adv Cancer Res 32:237–345, 1980
62. Graham S, Haughey B, Marshall J et al: Diet in the epidemiology of carcinoma of the prostate gland. JNCI 70:687–692, 1983
63. Kolonel LN, Hankin JH, Lee J et al: Nutrient intakes in relation to cancer incidence in Hawaii. Br J Cancer 44:332–339, 1981
64. Kinsella JE: Food components with potential therapeutic benefits: The n-3 polyunsaturated fatty acids of fish oils. Food Technol 40:89–97, 1986
65. USDA: Nationwide food consumption continuous survey of food intake by individuals: Men 19–50 years, 1 day, 1985. Report No 85-3, pp 1–46, November 1986
66. USDA: Nationwide food consumption continuous survey of food intake by individuals: Women 19–50 years and their children 1–5 years, 1 day, 1986. Report No 86-1, pp 1–46, January 1987
67. Burkitt DP: Epidemiology of cancer of the colon and rectum. Cancer 28:3–13, 1971
68. Greenwald P, Lanza E, Eddy GA: Dietary fiber in the reduction of colon cancer risk. J Am Diet Assoc 87(9):1178–1188, 1987
69. Enstrom JE: Cancer mortality among Mormons in California during 1968–75. JNCI 65:1073, 1980
70. Jensen OM: Cancer risk among Danish male Seventh-Day Adventists and other temperance society members. JNCI 70:1011, 1983
71. Freeman HJ, Spiller GA, Kim YS: A double-blind study on the effect of purified cellulose dietary fiber on 1,2-dimethylhydrazine-induced rat colonic neoplasia. Cancer Res 38:2912–2917, 1978
72. Watanabe K, Reddy BS, Weisburger JH et al: Effect of dietary alfalfa, pectin, and wheat bran on azoxymethane- or methylnitrosourea-induced colon carcinogenesis in rats. JNCI 63(1):141–145, 1979
73. Lanza E, Jones DY, Block G et al: Dietary fiber intake in the U.S. population. Am J Clin Nutr 46:790–797, 1987
74. Korpassy B: Tannins as hepatic carcinogens. Prog Exp Tumor Res 2:245–290, 1961
75. Toth B: Mushroom hydrazines: Occurrence, metabolism, carcinogenesis and environmental implications. In Miller EC et al (eds): Naturally Occurring Carcinogens, Mutagens, and Modulators of Carcinogenesis, pp 57–65. Baltimore, University Park Press, 1979
76. Miller JA, Swanson AB, Miller EC: The metabolic activation of safrole and related naturally occurring alkenylbenzenes in relation to carcinogenesis by these agents. In Miller EC et al (eds): Naturally Occurring Carcinogens, Mutagens, and Modulators of Carcinogenesis, pp 111–125. Baltimore, University Park Press, 1979
77. Brown JP: A review of the genetic effects of naturally occurring flavonoids, anthraquinones and related compounds. Mutat Res 75:243–277, 1980
78. Linsell CA, Peers FG: Aflatoxin and liver cell cancer. Trans R Soc Trop Med Hyg 71:471–473, 1977
79. van Rensburg SJ, van der Watt JJ, Purchase IFH et al: Primary liver cancer rate and aflatoxin intake in a high cancer area. S Afr Med J 48:2508a–d, 1974
80. Magee P (ed): Nitrosamines and Human Cancer. Banbury Report 12. Cold Spring Harbor, New York, Cold Spring Harbor Laboratory, 1982
81. Williams GM, Weisburger JH: Chemical carcinogens. In Klassen CD, Amur MO, Doull J (eds): Casarett and Doull's Toxicology: The Basic Science of Poisons, 3rd ed, pp 99–173. New York, Mcmillan, 1986
82. Sugimura T: Carcinogenicity of mutagenic heterocyclic amines formed during the cooking process. Mutat Res 150:33–41, 1985
83. Lijinsky W, Shubik P: Benzo(a)pyrene and other polynuclear hydrocarbons in charcoal-broiled meat. Science 145:53–55, 1964
84. Howard JW, Fazio T: Review of polycyclic aromatic hydrocarbons in foods: Analytical methodology and reported findings of polycyclic aromatic hydrocarbons in foods. J Assoc Off Anal Chem 63:1077–1104, 1980
85. Vitale JJ, Broitman SA, Gottlieb LS: Alcohol and carcinogenesis. In Newell GR, Ellison NM (eds): Nutrition and Cancer: Etiology and Treatment, pp 291–301. New York, Raven Press, 1981
86. Tuyns AJ: Alcohol. In Schottenfeld D, Fraumeni JF Jr (eds): Cancer Epidemiology and Prevention, pp 293–303. Philadelphia, WB Saunders, 1982
87. Rothman KJ: Alcohol. In Fraumeni JF Jr (ed): Persons at High Risk of Cancer: An Approach to Cancer Etiology and Control, pp 139–148. New York, Academic Press, 1975
88. Pollack ES, Nomura AMY, Heilbrun LK et al: Prospective study of alcohol consumption and cancer. N Engl J Med 310(10):617–621, 1984
89. Graham S: Alcohol and breast cancer. N Engl J Med 316(19):1211–1213, 1987
90. Schatzkin A, Jones DY, Hoover RN et al: Alcohol consumption and breast cancer in the epidemiologic follow-up study of the First National Health and Nutrition Examination Survey. N Engl J Med 316(19):1169–1173, 1987

91. Harvey EB, Schairer C, Brinton LA et al: Alcohol consumption and breast cancer. JNCI 78(4):657–661, 1987
92. International Agency for Research on Cancer: Chemicals, Industrial Processes and Industries Associated with Cancer in Humans. IARC Monogr (Suppl) 4, 1982
93. Doll R, Peto R: The causes of cancer: Quantitative estimates of avoidable risks of cancer in the United States today. JNCI 61:1191–1308, 1981
94. Stryker WS, Kaplan LA, Stein EA et al: The relation of diet, cigarette smoking, and alcohol consumption to plasma beta-carotene and alpha-tocopherol levels. Am J Epidemiol 127(2):283–296, 1988
95. Greenwald P, Dewys WD, Carrese LM et al: Chemoprevention program at the National Cancer Institute. In Prasad (ed): Vitamins, Nutrition, and Cancer, pp 282–291. Basel, S Karger, 1984
96. Hennekens CH: Issues in the design and conduct of clinical trials. JNCI 73:1473–1476, 1984
97. Byar DP, Piantadosi S: Factorial designs for randomized clinical trials. Cancer Treat Rep 69:1055-1062, 1985
98. Dimitrov NV, Boone CW, Hay MB et al: Plasma beta-carotene levels: Kinetic patterns during administration of various doses of beta-carotene. J Nutr Growth Cancer 3:227–237, 1986
99. Bruce WR, McKeown-Eyssen G, Ciampi A et al: Strategies for dietary intervention studies in colon cancer. Cancer 47 (suppl):1121–1125, 1981
100. DeCosse JJ, Adams MB, Kuzma JF et al: Effect of ascorbic acid on rectal polyps of patients with familial polyposis. Surgery 78:608–612, 1975
101. Bussey HJR, DeCosse JJ, Deschner EE et al: A randomized trial of ascorbic acid in polyposis coli. Cancer 50:1434–1439, 1982
102. Bruce WR, Varghese AJ, Furrer R et al: A mutagen in human feces. In Hiatt HH, Watson JD, Winsten JA (eds): Origins of Human Cancer, pp 1641–1644. Cold Spring Harbor, New York, Cold Spring Harbor Laboratory, 1977
103. Dion PW, Bright-See EB, Smith CC et al: The effect of dietary ascorbic acid and alpha-tocopherol on fecal mutagenicity. Mutat Res 102:27–37, 1982
104. Lipkin M, Uehara K, Winawer S et al: Seventh-Day Adventist vegetarians have a quiescent proliferative activity in colonic mucosa. Cancer Lett 26:139–144, 1985
105. Lipkin N, Newmark H: Effect of added dietary calcium on colonic epithelial cell proliferation in subjects at high risk for familial colonic cancer. N Engl J Med 313:1381–1384, 1985
106. Gouveia J, Hercend T, Lemaigre G et al: Degree of bronchial metaplasia in heavy smokers and its regression after treatment with a retinoid. Lancet 1:710–712, 1982
107. Shah JP, Strong EW, DeCosse JJ et al: Effect of retinoids on oral leukoplakia. Am J Surg 146:466–470, 1983
108. Stitch HF, Stitch W, Rosin MP et al: Use of the micronucleus test to monitor the effect of vitamin A, beta-carotene and canthaxanthin on the buccal mucosa of betel nut/tobacco chewers. Int J Cancer 34:745–750, 1984
109. Greenberg ER, Baron JA, Beck JR: Carotenoids and cancer prevention. In Saurat (ed): Retinoids: New Trends in Research and Therapy, pp 360–370. Basel, S Karger, 1985
110. Albanes D, Virtamo J, Rautalahti M et al: Pilot study: The U.S.–Finland lung cancer prevention trial. J Nutr Growth Cancer 3:207–214, 1986
111. Li J-Y, Taylor PR, Li G-Y et al: Intervention studies in Linxian, China: An update. J Nutr Growth Cancer 3:199–206, 1986
112. Blot WJ, Li J-Y: Some considerations in the design of a nutrition intervention trial in Linxian, People's Republic of China. Natl Cancer Inst Monogr 69:29–34, 1985
113. Wechsler H, Levine S, Idelson RC et al: The physician's role in health promotion: A survey of primary care practitioners. N Engl J Med 309(2):97–100, 1983
114. Orleans CT: Understanding and promoting smoking cessation: Overview and guidelines for physician intervention. Annu Rev Med 36:51–61, 1985
115. Valente CM, Sobal J, Muncie HL Jr et al: Health promotion: Physicians' beliefs, attitudes, and practices. Am J Prev Med 2(2):82–88, 1986
116. Glanz K: Nutrition education for risk factor reduction and patient education: A review. Prev Med 14:721–752, 1985
117. US Department of Health and Human Services, Public Health Service: Diet, Nutrition and Cancer Prevention: The Good News. NIH publication No 87-2878, 1986
118. Butram RR, Clifford CK, Lanza E: National Cancer Institute dietary guidelines: Rationale. Am J Clin Nutr (in press)
119. US Department of Health and Human Services, Public Health Service, National Institutes of Health: Cancer Control Objectives for the Nation: 1985–2000. NIH (NCI) publication No 86-2880. Washington, DC, US Government Printing Office, 1986
120. Klein G: The approaching era of the tumor suppressor genes. Science 238:1539–1546, 1987

JOSEPH W. CULLEN

CHAPTER 12 *Principles of Cancer Prevention: Tobacco*

Over the past several decades, our understanding of the cancer process has increased substantially; cancer research has generated an impressive knowledge base related to the fundamental biological mechanisms underlying cell growth and regulation and to the management of cancer in its variety of forms. Of particular note has been the gradual accumulation of scientific evidence linking lifestyle to many cancers and therefore the opportunity to develop strategies to modify lifestyles and thereby prevent what was once regarded as the inevitable consequence of aging.

It is estimated that a large majority of cancers are caused or promoted by lifestyle factors that are controllable at the individual or societal level, or both.[1] That human behavior plays a prominent role in our understanding and control of the nation's second leading cause of mortality has led to a national cancer control agenda with a new emphasis on preventing disease and promoting health whenever possible. Risk factors such as diet, radiation (both actinic and ionizing), some occupational and drug exposures, and excessive alcohol consumption have all been implicated in cancer causation. But the most well-documented risk factor is tobacco use, and particularly smoking. Findings from basic laboratory and epidemiological research clearly indicate that if smoking and tobacco use can be reduced in the United States a marked reduction in cancer incidence and mortality is possible. The objectives of this chapter are to review the knowledge base in tobacco carcinogenesis, tobacco use and trends, particularly for cigarette smoking, and opportunities for cancer prevention. The unique and important role that physicians can play in reducing cancer risk by adopting smoking control interventions will also be discussed.

TOBACCO'S CONTRIBUTION TO CANCER ETIOLOGY AND MORTALITY

Knowledge of the link between tobacco use and cancer is not new. In fact, cancer was the first disease to be linked to tobacco use. For more than two centuries scientific evidence has been accumulating on the cancer consequences of tobacco use. From the earliest observations of John Hill,[2] a London physician who in 1761 reported an association between snuff use and cancer of the nose, to recent studies on the effect of environmental tobacco smoke (ETS) in nonsmokers, countless epidemiological, clinical, and experimental studies have conclusively demonstrated that tobacco use significantly increases the risk of developing cancer.

It is obviously not feasible (that is, ethical) to experiment with humans to prove the cause and effect relationship between the use of tobacco and any disease, cancer included. Scientists and public health specialists have relied on preclinical studies and epidemiological evidence to draw such conclusions. In so doing, they have established a rigorous set of criteria which have been outlined and applied in major scientific reviews[3–5] over the past two decades. These criteria are

Consistency of the association: similar observations by multiple investigators in different locations and situations, at different times, and using different methods of study.

Strength of the association: high ratio of disease rate for the population exposed to the suspected risk factor compared to the population not exposed.

Specificity of the association: associations with the exposure exist for the specific or limited set of diseases, and associations with the disease exist for a specific or limited set of exposures.
Temporal relationship of the association: exposure to the suspected etiologic factor precedes the disease.
Coherence of the association: epidemiologic observations are consonant with all else that is known about the disease.

The first Surgeon General's report on *Smoking and Health* in 1964 may be the most conspicuous document to have used these criteria. In that monograph, if these criteria were judged to be satisfied and pathologic and experimental data were supportive, the term "causal" was applied to the association. The designation "major cause" was used when the relative risk for the cancer in tobacco users was high. The term "contributory factor" was used when the body of evidence was less compelling, the relative risk lower, or the ancillary evidence (pathologic and experimental data) not sufficient for a judgment of causality. The term "association" was used when a relationship between tobacco use and a health consequence existed but the data were inadequate for an assessment of the extent of that relationship.

Thousands of studies detail the numerous and severe health consequences of cigarette smoking, and a succession of Surgeons General have reviewed and summarized the health effects associated with smoking.[3,4,6–21] Smoking is responsible for more than 315,000 deaths per year in the United States.[22] This death toll is greater than all other drug and alcohol abuse deaths combined, seven times more than all automobile fatalities per year, and more than all American military fatalities in World War I, World War II, and Vietnam combined.[23]

Cigarette smoking is a major cause of cancers of the lung, larynx, oral cavity, and esophagus, and is a contributory factor for the development of cancers of the bladder, pancreas, and kidney. A link between smoking and stomach cancer and cancer of the uterine cervix has also been noted.[4] Overall, cigarette smoking has been identified as the chief avoidable cause of cancer death in the United States.[4] In 1984, it was responsible for nearly one million years of potential life lost in the United States population.[22] Table 12-1 provides a recent summary of the deaths attributed to tobacco by cancer site.

LUNG CANCER

According to Tso and Gray,[24] the relationship between tobacco smoke and lung cancer in developed countries may be the most researched subject in medical history. In the United States, conclusive evidence of the association between cigarette smoking and lung cancer was first published in 1950. Wynder and Graham,[25] Doll and Hill,[26] and Levin et al,[27] reported a link between smoking and cancer. Yet the first national reviews were not published until 1962 (Report on Smoking of the Royal College of Surgeons[28]) and 1964 (Report of the Advisory Committee to the Surgeon General of the Public Health Service[3]). Both of these reports included epidemiological studies profiling tobacco consumption, composition, and carcinogenicity in animals and humans. The conclusions reached in these assessments and by a large number of comprehensive reviews since that time are impressively uniform and consistent: cigarette smoking causes lung cancer.[4,15,16,20,29]

Some of the epidemiological evidence in the U.S. Surgeon General's Report of 1964 involved 50 retrospective studies and 8 prospective studies that included more than 17 million person years of data.[4] From the prospective studies, lung cancer mortality ratios were concluded to be substantially greater for smokers than for nonsmokers (Table 12-2). As seen from Table 12-3, these mortality ratios are dose dependent. For men who smoke more than 25 cigarettes a day, the risk of death from lung cancer is 25 times that for the nonsmoker.

Whereas smoking alone has serious lung cancer effects, the morbidity is even greater when there is a concomitant exposure to certain environmental or occupational elements. Cigarette smoking and asbestos exposure, for example, together result in a more than additive increase in lung cancer risk.[14,30–35] The same is true for uranium miners who smoke and are exposed to radon daughters.[36,37]

TABLE 12-1. Total Mortality and Smoking-Attributable Mortality (SAM), by Disease, Cancer Site, and Sex—United States, 1984 (Adults ≥ 20 Years Old)

Cancer Site	*Men*		*Women*		*Total*
	Deaths	*SAM*	*Deaths*	*SAM*	*SAM**
Lip, oral cavity, pharynx	5,754	3,958	2,689	1,110	5,068
Esophagus	6,310	3,717	2,345	1,257	4,974
Stomach	8,463	1,455	5,772	1,467	2,922
Pancreas	11,513	3,459	11,634	1,653	5,112
Larynx	2,959	2,385	664	274	2,660
Trachea, lung, bronchus	82,459	65,659	36,227	27,170	92,829
Cervix uteri	0	0	4,562	1,685	1,685
Urinary bladder	6,597	2,447	3,114	853	3,299
Kidney, other urinary	5,424	1,319	3,403	403	1,722

From the Centers for Disease Control: Smoking-attributable mortality and years of potential life lost—United States, 1984. MMWR 30:42, 1987.
* Sums may not equal total because of rounding.

TABLE 12-2. Lung Cancer Mortality Ratios—Prospective Studies

Population	*Size*	*Number of Deaths*	*Cigarette Smokers**
British physicians	34,000 men	441	14.00
	6,194 women	27	5.00
Swedish study	27,000 men	55	7.00
	28,000 women	8	4.50
Japanese study	122,000 men	940	3.76
	143,000 women	304	2.03
ACS 25-state study	358,000 men	2,018	8.53
	483,000 women	439	3.58
U.S. veterans	290,000 men	3,126	11.28
Canadian veterans	78,000 men	331	14.20
ACS 9-state study	188,000 men	448	10.73
California men in nine occupations	68,000 men	368	7.61

From the U.S. Department of Health and Human Services, Office on Smoking and Health: The Health Consequences of Smoking: Cancer. A Report of the Surgeon General, DHHS Pub. No. (PHS) 82–50179, 1982, p 36.

* Ratio of smoker to nonsmoker.

TABLE 12-3. Lung Cancer Mortality Ratios for Men and Women, by Current Number of Cigarettes Smoked per Day—Prospective Studies

Population	*Men*		*Women*	
	Cigarettes Smoked per Day	*Mortality Ratios*	*Cigarettes Smoked per Day*	*Mortality Ratios*
ACS 25-state study	Nonsmoker	1.00	Nonsmoker	1.00
	1–9	4.62	1–9	1.30
	10–19	8.62	10–19	2.40
	20–39	14.69	20–39	4.90
	40+	18.71	40+	7.50
British physicians' study	Nonsmoker	1.00	Nonsmoker	1.00
	1–14	7.80	1–14	1.28
	15–24	12.70	15–24	6.41
	25+	25.10	25+	29.71
Swedish study	Nonsmoker	1.00	Nonsmoker	1.00
	1–7	2.30	1–7	1.80
	8–15	8.80	8–15	11.30
	16+	13.70	16+	
Japanese study: all ages	Nonsmoker	1.00	Nonsmoker	1.0
	1–19	3.49	<20	1.90
	20–39	5.69	20–29	4.20
	40+	6.45		
U.S. veterans study	Nonsmoker	1.00		
	1–9	3.89		
	10–20	9.63		
	21–39	16.70		
	≥40	23.70		
ACS 9-state study	Nonsmoker	1.00		
	1–9	8.00		
	10–20	10.50		
	20+	23.40		
Canadian veterans	Nonsmoker	1.00		
	1–9	9.50		
	10–20	15.80		
	20+	17.30		
California men in nine occupations	Nonsmoker	1.00		
	about ½ pack	3.72		
	about 1 pack	9.05		
	about 1½ packs	9.56		

From the U.S. Department of Health and Human Services, Office on Smoking and Health: The Health Consequences of Smoking: Cancer. A Report of the Surgeon General, DHHS Pub. No. (PHS) 82–50179, 1982, p 38.

Lung cancer is now the leading cause of cancer death for men in the United States.[38] Although breast cancer continues to be the leading cause of cancer death among women, lung cancer is now second in women and in many parts of the United States is the leading cause.[39]

Figure 12-1 presents smoking prevalence in the United States for men and women from 1965 (the year following the first Surgeon General's report on smoking and health) to 1985. Smoking rates for men declined significantly over this period from 51% to 33%.* Smoking rates for women also declined, but not as dramatically, from 31.5% to 28%. In fact, while rates for men had stabilized from the mid 1950s to 1965, rates for women had continued to climb from 24.5% in 1955 to 31.5% in 1965.

Predictably, these divergent smoking profiles have resulted in similar lung cancer rates. As depicted in Figure 12-2, the age-adjusted lung cancer incidence rates for men started to decline in 1983 (for the first time in this century) and continue to decline. Rates for women, on the other hand, continue to increase, and based upon women's smoking prevalence rates since 1955 the rates will continue to incline for some years to come.

Were it not for lung cancer, the overall cancer death rates would actually be decreasing in the United States.[38] As shown in Figure 12-3, there has been a 13% decline in overall mortality rates over the past 35 years for all cancer sites, excluding lung, as compared to a 9% increase in mortality rates for all cancer sites over that same period.

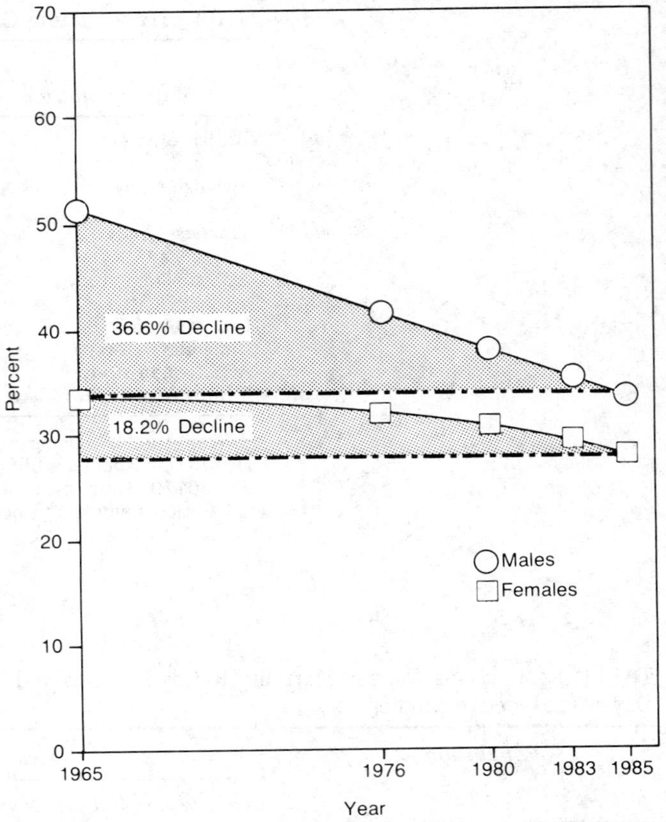

FIG. 12-1. Prevalence of cigarette smoking in the United States. (From the U.S. Department of Health and Human Services, National Center for Health Statistics, National Health Interview Survey)

LARYNGEAL CANCER

Cigarette smoking is the major cause of laryngeal cancer.[4] More than 25 retrospective and 6 major prospective studies have examined the relationship between smoking and cancer of the larynx. Cigarette smokers in the prospective studies have up to 13 times more deaths from laryngeal cancer than nonsmokers, and relative risk ratios for the retrospective studies were consistently above 2.0.[4] Cigar and pipe smokers experience a risk for cancer of the larynx similar to that of cigarette smokers.

The risk of developing laryngeal cancer increases with increased exposure to cigarette smoke; heavy smokers have cancer mortality ratios 20 to 30 times greater than nonsmokers.[4] Furthermore, alcohol can act synergistically with cigarette smoking to increase the risk for cancer of the larynx up to 50% more than the sum of the excess risks posed by either behavior alone.[41]

* In 1986 the Public Health Service's Office of Smoking and Health carried out a telephone survey to study the U.S. adult population's knowledge, attitudes, and practices regarding the use of tobacco. This survey collected data from a national probability sample of 13,031 respondents who were at least 17 years old. The results showed the lowest prevalence of current cigarette smoking among adults ever recorded in the United States: 29.5% for men and 23.8% for women.[40] However, the age group in question is not comparable to the age groups for the samples previously collected through the National Health Interview Surveys (at least 20 years old). In addition, telephone surveys tend to underestimate the number of smokers in the age group surveyed because they often miss low socioeconomic status and minority populations that are at higher risk to smoke.

ORAL CANCER

Cigarette smoking is a major cause of cancers of the oral cavity (including malignant tumors of the lip, tongue, salivary gland, floor of the mouth, mesopharynx, and hypopharynx).[4] A similar risk for oral cancer is posed by pipe and cigar smoking. In studies of U.S. populations, the deaths from oral cancer are from 3 to 14 times greater for smokers than for nonsmokers. This risk is also dose-related. Comparing those who smoke 25 or more cigarettes a day (the standard definition of heavy smokers) to nonsmokers, there is evidence that oral cancer mortality ratios are 5.5 to 33 times greater than in the nonsmoker.

As is true for laryngeal cancer, alcohol synergistically increases the risk of cancer of the oral cavity on a dose-related basis. McLoy and co-workers[42] found that smokers who consumed 7 or more ounces of alcohol per day had a fivefold increase in risk for oral cancer even if they smoked less than half a pack of cigarettes a day. The risk rose to 20-fold for 11 to 20 cigarettes and to 24-fold for more than a pack a day.

ESOPHAGEAL CANCER

Smoking of cigarettes, cigars, and pipes cause carcinoma of the esophagus.[4,22] Death rates for esophageal cancer are up

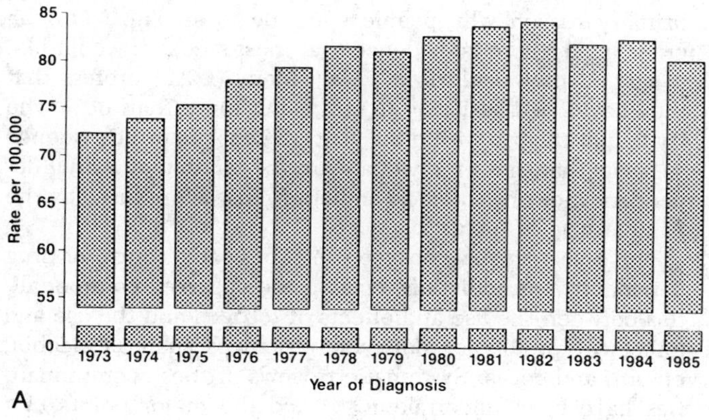

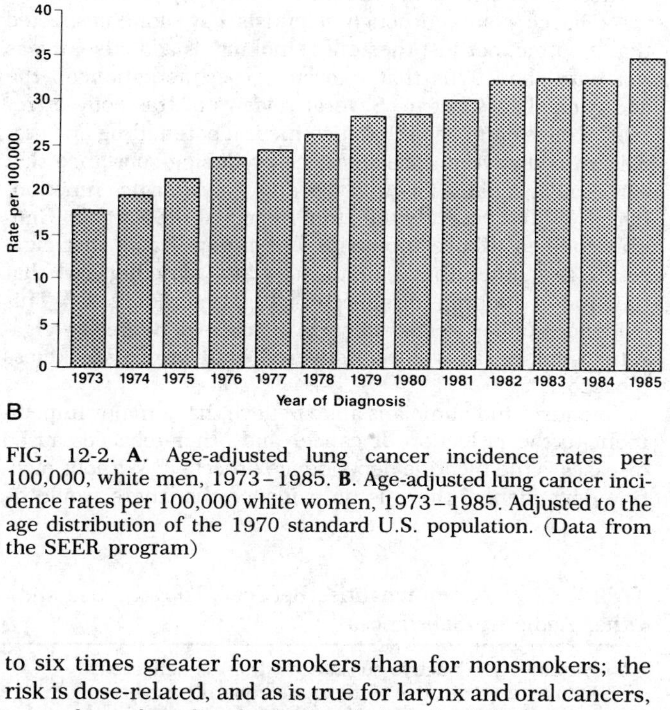

FIG. 12-2. **A**. Age-adjusted lung cancer incidence rates per 100,000, white men, 1973–1985. **B**. Age-adjusted lung cancer incidence rates per 100,000 white women, 1973–1985. Adjusted to the age distribution of the 1970 standard U.S. population. (Data from the SEER program)

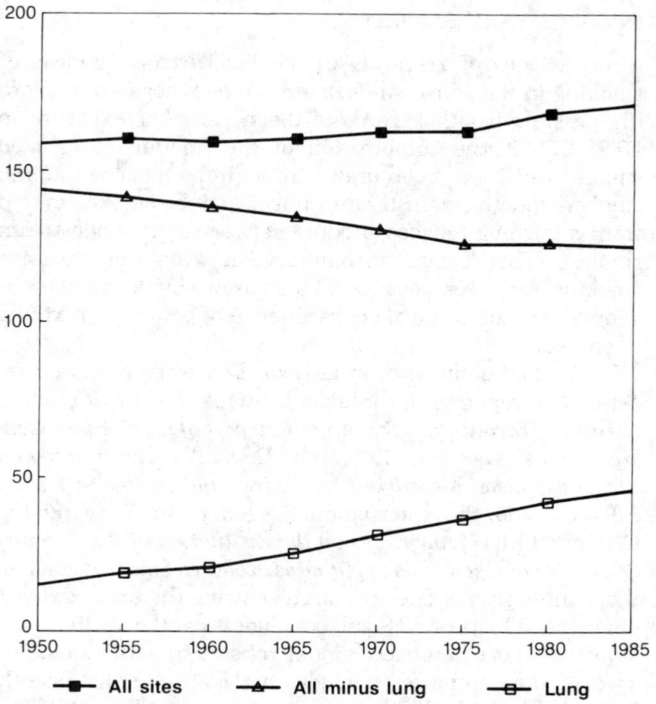

FIG. 12-3. Trends in cancer death rates. (From the National Cancer Institute: Annual Cancer Statistics Review including Cancer Trends: 1950–1985. NIH Pub. No. 88–2789, 1988)

to six times greater for smokers than for nonsmokers; the risk is dose-related, and as is true for larynx and oral cancers, a number of studies have found that alcohol consumption acts synergistically with smoking to increase the risk for developing esophageal cancer.[43–51]

OTHER CANCERS

Cigarette smoking is a contributory factor in the development of bladder, kidney, and pancreatic cancers. An association has also been noted between cigarette smoking and cervical and stomach cancers.[4] The attribution of association noted in the 1982 Surgeon General's report between smoking and cervical cancer continues to be strengthened by recent studies providing positive results.[52–54]

SMOKELESS TOBACCO USE

In the United States, smokeless tobacco consists of chewing tobacco and snuff. Experimental investigations have revealed potent carcinogens in these smokeless tobacco products, including nitrosamines, [55–62] polycyclic aromatic hydrocarbons,[63,64] and radiation emitting polonium.[65] The first evidence of cancer among users of snuff or chewing tobacco appeared in case reports during the early 1940s.[66] The first epidemiologic study of smokeless tobacco was not conducted until the early 1950s.[67]

A comprehensive assessment of the available scientific evidence on the health consequences of using smokeless tobacco is now available as a result of recent reviews by three scientific bodies.[5,68,69] The three reviews are consistent in their conclusions. The scientific evidence is strong that the use of snuff causes cancer in humans, with the strongest evidence of causality for oral cancer. Oral cancer has been shown to occur several times more frequently in snuff dippers than in non–tobacco users, and the excess risk of cancers of the cheek and gum may be nearly 50-fold among long-term snuff users.[70] Some investigations suggest that the use of chewing tobacco may also increase the risk of oral cancer, but the evidence is not as strong and the risks have yet to be quantified.

Evidence for an association between smokeless tobacco use and cancer outside of the oral cavity is sparse. There is suggestive evidence that smokeless tobacco users face increased risks of tumors of the upper aerodigestive tract, but results are currently inconclusive.[5]

INVOLUNTARY SMOKING

After decades of research on the health consequences of smoking in the active smoker, researchers began to explore the possible health hazards to the nonsmoker exposure to ETS. ETS is the combination of the fraction of exhaled smoke after it has been drawn through the tobacco into the smokers mouth (mainstream smoke) and the smoke emitted from a burning tobacco product between puffs (sidestream smoke). The terms "involuntary smoking" or "passive smoking" are used because ETS exposure by nonsmokers is generally an unavoidable consequence of being in proximity to smokers.

The constituents and hazards of ETS were reviewed recently and reported in three publications: *The Health Consequences of Involuntary Smoking: A Report of the Surgeon General*,[21] the National Research Council's *Environmental Tobacco Smoke: Measuring Exposures and Assessing Health Effects*,[71] and the International Agency for Research on Cancer's *IARC Monographs on the Evaluation of the Carcinogenic Risk of Chemicals to Humans: Tobacco Smoke*.[28] Each of these monographs cites research showing the toxic and carcinogenic effects of ETS and concludes that these effects are similar to those of tobacco smoke inhaled by active smokers. Two of these reports conclude that ETS can significantly increase the risk of lung cancer in nonsmokers.[21,71] The third report concludes that nonsmokers exposed to ETS have an increased risk of cancer or are not without risk.[28] Although the magnitude of risk is uncertain, an estimate from epidemiological studies of spousal exposure in various populations in Europe, Asia, and North America places the risk of lung cancer in nonsmokers married to smokers at about 34% higher than it is for nonsmoking spouses of nonsmokers.[71]

Although more complete data on the dose and variability of smoke exposure in the nonsmoking population are needed before an accurate quantitative estimate of the number of ETS-induced lung cancers can be made, many experts believe that a meaningful proportion of the lung cancers that occur in nonsmokers are the result of this risk factor.[21] The National Research Council has estimated that ETS is responsible for 20% or 2,400 of the nonsmoker lung cancer deaths per year, with a range of 10% to 50% or 350 to 6,000 deaths.[71] Such an estimate should and does generate a substantial public health concern. With respect to cancers at sites other than the lung, there are insufficient data to evaluate adequately the role of involuntary smoking.

NICOTINE DEPENDENCE: THE LINK BETWEEN TOBACCO AND TOBACCO-RELATED DISEASES

Although there is a growing body of evidence that lifestyle modification affects cancer incidence, this knowledge has yet to be absorbed fully by the public. For example, there are approximately 50 million Americans who continue to smoke. Why individuals persist in this risk-taking behavior despite the knowledge of the serious cancer and other health consequences of tobacco use is curious. On the one hand, tobacco industry representatives cite personal choice as the primary reason why people continue to smoke.[72] On the other hand, there is evidence that most smokers would like to quit, if they could find a way. Many (60%) profess that they have tried seriously to quit,[73] but more than 80% who try to quit relapse within the year. Recent scientific evidence suggests that these individuals are the victims of a drug dependency, or physiological addiction, that is produced by the habitual use of tobacco.

The assertion that tobacco use is basically a form of drug dependence or addiction rests on the observed commonalities between the use and effects of tobacco and the use and effects of prototype addictive substances such as alcohol, opium, and cocas. Systematic reviews of these commonalities have been undertaken[74-78] and the major points that tobacco and addictive substances have in common are summarized in Table 12-4.

The next major question is, what elements of tobacco are critical in controlling the behavior of the user? The conceptual leap from habitual behavior to drug abuse and addiction can be made only on the basis of evidence that a specific psychoactive drug is critical to the behavior.[5]

Nicotine is one of the naturally occurring constituents of the tobacco plant. Although scientists have long suspected that nicotine, not just the act of smoking, is addictive, it was not until the 1970s that rigorous experimentation on the addiction theory began. Several reviews of this body of research have concluded that nicotine is a potent drug and that it is an addictive and dependence-producing substance that can control behavior and modify physiologic functioning.[5,77,78] Most recently the 1988 Report of the Surgeon General codified this relationship. The report states that cigarettes and other forms of tobacco are addicting and that nicotine is the drug in tobacco that causes addiction.[79] This evidence applies to the effects of nicotine delivered by cigarette smoking as well as delivered orally from smokeless tobacco.

Scientists and clinicians alike believe that a major impediment to the reduction of cancer and other tobacco-caused diseases is the nicotine dependence process.[80] Without nicotine dependence, there is no evidence that there would be

TABLE 12-4. Commonalities Between Tobacco Use and Other Addictive Substances

- A centrally (CNS) active substance (drug) is delivered.
- Discriminate (subjective) effects are centrally mediated.
- The substance (drug) is a reinforcer for animals.
- The patterns of acquisition and maintenance of substance ingestion are orderly.
- The patterns of self-administration of the substance are orderly.
- The patterns of self-administration of the substance vary as a function of the dose that is consumed.
- Tolerance to the behavioral and physiologic effects of the substance develops with repeated use (neuroadaptation).
- Therapeutic effects may be produced by the substance.
- The treatment of addiction resulting from the substance (drug) involves similar strategies.

From the U.S. Department of Health and Human Services. The Health Consequences of Using Smokeless Tobacco: A Report of the Advisory Committee to the Surgeon General, pp 146–147. Bethesda, MD, NIH Publication No. 86-2874, 1986.

widespread and compulsive use of tobacco. Nicotine addiction is truly the bridge between tobacco as an environmental toxin and the multitude of diseases that result from repeated exposure.[81]

The significance of this evidence is demonstrated by the inclusion of a specific category for diseases and deaths caused by "tobacco dependence" in the current (ninth) revision of the International Classification of Diseases[82] and the third edition of the Diagnostic and Statistical Manual of Mental Disorders.[83] Tobacco dependence is defined as follows:

> Continuous use of tobacco for at least a month with either (1) unsuccessful attempts to stop or significantly reduce the amount of tobacco use on a permanent basis, (2) the development of tobacco withdrawal, or (3) the presence of a serious physical disorder (*e.g.*, respiratory or cardiovascular disease) that the individual (or the physician) knows is exacerbated by tobacco use. . . . If the individual with a serious case of one of the tobacco-related physical disorders continues to use tobacco, despite awareness of its harmful effects, a reasonable inference can be made that the individual is tobacco dependent.

Although tobacco dependence is the most common of the addictive disorders, most American physicians are believed to be unaware of either the existence or the importance of this diagnostic category.[84] Appropriate use of this category is particularly important because new pharmacotherapy approaches to deal with tobacco are available and are proving to be successful aids in smoking cessation. The most promising of these approaches is discussed later in this chapter.

OPPORTUNITIES FOR TOBACCO USE PREVENTION AND CESSATION

The evidence is clearly positive that quitting smoking decreases the risk for lung cancer. As is evident in Table 12-5, 15 to 20 years after quitting, the ex-smokers' risk of dying from lung cancer declines to a point where it closely approximates the risk of the nonsmoker.[85,86] The magnitude of the residual risk is largely determined by the cumulative exposure to tobacco prior to smoking cessation, that is, the total amount smoked, the age when smoking began, the degree of inhalation, and the tar level of the products used. Similar benefits of smoking cessation have been demonstrated for laryngeal,[87] esophageal,[88] and oral cavity cancers.[88]

The benefits of quitting cigarette smoking are evident. But in themselves they are not sufficient to get people to quit. A comprehensive public health prevention strategy is needed. In the United States, the message about the health consequences of smoking competes with the tobacco industry's multi-billion dollar campaign annually to convince people to smoke and with smokers' own motivations for smoking. In developing a prevention strategy, one must learn more about smokers themselves: Who are they, and what motivates them to smoke or stop smoking? But much more impor-

TABLE 12-5. Lung Cancer Mortality Ratios in Ex-Cigarette Smokers, by Number of Years Stopped Smoking

Study	*Years Stopped Smoking*	*Mortality Ratio*	
British physicians	1–4	16.00	
	5–9	5.90	
	10–14	5.30	
	15+	2.00	
	Current smokers	14.00	
U.S. veterans*	1–4	18.83	
	5–9	7.73	
	10–14	4.71	
	15–19	4.81	
	20+	2.10	
	Current smokers	11.28	
Japanese men	1–4	4.65	
	5–9	2.50	
	10+	1.35	
	Current smokers	3.76	
		Number of Cigarettes Smoked per Day	
		1–19	20+
ACS 25-state study (men 50–69)	<1	7.20	29.13
	1–4	4.60	12.00
	5–9	1.00	7.20
	10+	0.40	1.06
	Current smokers	6.47	13.67

From the U.S. Department of Health and Human Services, Office on Smoking and Health: The Health Consequences of Smoking: Cancer. A Report of the Surgeon General. DHHS Pub. No. (PHS) 82–50179, 1982, p 46.

* Includes data only for ex-cigarette smokers who stopped for other than physicians' orders.

tantly, there is a need to reduce smoking and tobacco use prevalence by every strategy available that is feasible and effective.

TARGETING HIGH RISK POPULATIONS FOR BEHAVIOR CHANGE

The use of tobacco is an individual decision. As the 1982 Surgeon General's report on smoking and cancer states, "There is no single action an individual can take to reduce the risk of cancer more effectively than quitting smoking, particularly cigarettes."[4] An increasing number of people have heard that message and acted on it. Since the first Surgeon General's report in 1964, approximately 40 million people have quit smoking.[89] Many argue that this immense modification in a society's lifestyle may be the largest sociocultural change in the history of this country. Within this generally positive profile, however, tobacco use in several population groups warrants special surveillance.

First, approximately 50 million American adults, or about one in three,[89] still smoke, and 2 to 3 million young people aged 12 to 17 are currently cigarette smokers.[90]

Second, ethnic minorities are more likely to smoke than whites, and in particular, black men are more likely to smoke than white men (40.6% versus 33.2%, respectively).[89] Lung cancer incidence rates for blacks already exceed those for whites, and these rate differentials are expected to increase substantially over the next decade. Although smoking prevalence is the same in Hispanic men as in white men (albeit 8% less in women),[89] this advantage may be fast disappearing. Recent data suggest that young Hispanics are smoking as much as, if not more than, their white peers.[91]

Third, there is special concern for the heavy smoker, that is, someone who smokes 25 or more cigarettes a day. There are more heavy smokers today than ever before.[89] A heavy smoker is 15 to 25 times more likely to die of lung cancer than a nonsmoker.[4]

Fourth, numerous surveys and studies have shown that smoking is most often initiated during the junior and senior high school years.[89,92,93] This period provides a prime opportunity for cancer prevention, and a number of smoking prevention programs have been oriented toward that age group. Although it appears that smoking is declining among this group,* the level of cigarette use remains alarmingly high, and female high school seniors continue to smoke at higher rates than their male peers.[94]

Fifth, one of the most disturbing trends in tobacco use by young people is the increasing use of smokeless tobacco—snuff and chewing tobacco. Smokeless tobacco users are the fastest growing group of tobacco users, and the pattern of use is steadily shifting from older to younger users. Currently, 16% of males between the ages of 12 and 25—over 12 million people—have used smokeless tobacco in the preceding year; 5% to 8%, or about 6 million, are regular users (at least once a week).[95] Use varies widely across the country. Boyd and co-workers in a recent review reported that less than 7% of sixth-grade boys in New York City but more than 68% of sixth-grade boys in rural Montana were users. Use also varies by ethnic group. Hispanics and whites have comparable use rates, whereas use among Native Americans is higher than among whites, and use among blacks and Asians is lower.[96]

Finally, the problem of tobacco use in all these high-risk populations is influenced by current trends in tobacco advertising and marketing. The tobacco industry is spending more than two billion dollars a year on cigarette advertising and promotion. There are also indications that the cigarette market in the United States has become increasingly segmented in response to the decline in cigarette sales and the proliferation of brands.[97] In order to succeed, manufacturers of new cigarette brands must target specific segments of the market. As a result, marketing campaigns have targeted women, minorities, blue-collar workers, and especially children and adolescents. While representatives of the tobacco and advertising industries maintain that the only purpose and effect of cigarette advertising is to promote brand loyalty and brand switching, many health professionals believe that cigarette advertising perpetuates and increases cigarette consumption. Advertising tobacco products may recruit new smokers, induce former smokers to relapse, make it more difficult for smokers to quit, and increase the level of smokers' consumption by acting as an external cue to smoke.[97]

TOBACCO USE INTERVENTIONS

Intervention research programs designed to develop effective methods of reducing cigarette smoking and other forms of tobacco use have proliferated during the past two decades. The results of these studies have been highlighted in several reviews.[98-105]

Much of the initial behavioral research has focused on gaining an understanding of the factors that influence the development and maintenance of smoking and tobacco use behavior. Smoking and cessation are complex behavioral patterns that proceed through a sequence of stages from initiation of smoking to maintenance of cessation. Psychological, social, and demographic factors are strongly associated with smoking initiation; cessation and maintenance of cessation are affected by a combination of physiological and psychosocial variables.

Considerable progress has been made in developing and testing the effectiveness of a variety of intervention methods or techniques to prevent or control tobacco use. These include approaches to decrease physiological addiction[106] and psychological dependence, strategies aimed at maintenance or relapse,[100,107,108] programs that combine physiological, behavioral, aversive, and maintenance techniques,[109,110] self-help techniques,[111,112] mass media,[113] schools,[114] communities as a whole,[115] and interventions involving physicians and dentists.[116]

* Because national probability sampling for this age category has not been carried out since 1979, except in high school seniors, the data that are available are in question. High school seniors are a self-selected population. They are under-represented by low socioeconomic status and minority populations.

THE PHYSICIAN: AN EFFECTIVE AGENT OF CHANGE

There are a number of reasons physicians can be effective in reducing smoking prevalence. First, physicians are role models for health. Less than 17% smoke, compared with 30% of the general population.[117] Physicians are perceived as the most authoritative source of medical and health information. About 70% of Americans make at least one visit a year to their doctor. Often because they are ill, they may be amenable to a suggestion about lifestyle and behavior change ("the teachable moment"). The personal relationship and trust that clinicians are able to establish with their patients can be used to advantage in counseling patients about cancer prevention habits in general and tobacco use in particular. Some groups, such as smokers, make disproportionately greater use of medical services than other groups, and so there may be more clinical opportunities in which the physician can raise the smoking issue. Table 12-6 illustrates the range of these clinical opportunities.

Many physicians now view health promotion as an important part of their practices. In particular, they consider smoking a serious health hazard and consider it their responsibility to advise their patients to quit.[118] However, recent data indicate that less than 45% of physicians do, in fact, counsel their patients about smoking.[119] Why the disparity between attitude and action? A number of reasons have been cited:[120–122]

1. Lack of time
2. Lack of reimbursement for health promotion counseling
3. Pessimism about their ability to effect behavior change, especially if the patient is there for an unrelated problem
4. Feeling that counseling about lifestyle behaviors, especially if the patient is asymptomatic, is an infringement on the patient's personal freedom
5. Lack of training in health promotion activities and a lack of knowledge about outside health promotion resources
6. Reliance on ineffective health education methods, which then contributes to the sense of pessimism noted earlier

Several of these factors, such as reimbursement and lack of training in health promotion activities, reflect legitimate barriers to effective counseling. Effective ways to eliminate or minimize these barriers must be found to assist physicians in their health promotion efforts. Many of the barriers identified are attitudinal, and a number of studies over the past 20 years belie the belief that physicians are not effective. For example, clinical trial data indicate that even brief advice to the patient from a physician to stop smoking can be effective. A 1979 study by Russell[123] showed that a 1-year quit rate of 5% can be achieved with 1 to 2 minutes of physician counseling supplemented by a four-page brochure and 1- and 12-month telephone follow-up. The seemingly minimal percentage of quitters in this study was achieved with only a very brief intervention by physicians possessing incomplete smoking cessation counseling skills. While the average physician is interested in and accustomed to more successful treatment outcomes than 5%, it is important to note the public health impact of this outcome. Millions of smokers in a decade can be helped to quit, given a success rate of 25 patients per year in the offices of 50,000 physicians (less than 10% of the physicians in the United States). With more commitment and better skills, quit rates could presumably reach much higher levels.

A 1985 study by Goldstein and colleagues[124] also supports the contention that physicians can be effective agents of change. In this study, recently trained family practitioners in Iowa were interviewed about their smoking counseling beliefs, attitudes, and practices. The respondents overwhelmingly expressed strong motivation to counsel their patients who smoked, whether or not they had smoking-related symptoms. They also expressed confidence in their abilities to be effective, particularly if they had received formal training in smoking counseling. Table 12-7 summarizes the attitudes of these physicians[124] and compares them with physicians surveyed in earlier studies.[125]

TABLE 12-6. Clinical Opportunities to Talk About Smoking with Patients

Symptoms
Cough
Sputum production
Shortness of breath
Tests
Electrocardiography
Pulmonary function tests
Total Leukocyte counts
Blood pressure measurements
Hematocrit
Auscultation of heart and lungs
Blood lipid studies
Blood coagulation studies
Serum alpha$_1$-antiprotease determinations
Pregnancy tests
Carboxyhemoglobin determinations
Diagnosis of Disease and Risk Factors
Coronary heart disease
Peripheral vascular disease
Angina pectoris
Hypertension
Emphysema
Chronic bronchitis
Pneumonia
Asthma
Acute bronchitis
Recurrent respiratory infection
Diabetes mellitus
Hypercholesterolemia
Peptic ulcer
Allergy
Drug Prescriptions
Drug and tobacco smoke interactions
Pharmacologic aids to smoking cessation
Nicotine chewing gum

From the National Heart, Lung, and Blood Institute: Clinical Opportunity for Smoking Intervention: A Guide for the Busy Physician. National Heart, Lung, and Blood Institute's Smoking Education Program in cooperation with the American Lung Association and the American Thoracic Society. NIH Publication No. 86–2178, 1986.

TABLE 12-7. Physician Smoking Counseling Studies

	Study Year (%)			
	1978	1981	1984	1985
Respondents who smoke	15		12	2
"Counseling about smoking is important"	85			100
"Quite effective" or "very successful" in counseling	12	3		30
"Physicians have an obligation to counsel"	85	86		99
"I counsel patients whether or not they have a smoking-related illness"	52		89	98
Believed they had influenced patients to stop smoking		14		98

From Goldstein B, et al: Survey of physicians' attitudes and practices in early cancer detection. CA 35:197–213, 1985.

HELPING PATIENTS QUIT SMOKING: A MULTIFACETED APPROACH

A recent consensus conference of smoking intervention researchers reviewed the results from six intervention trials that are testing ways to maximize physician effectiveness in smoking cessation and prevention efforts. The group concluded that physicians can intervene effectively to promote smoking cessation, especially if a specific regimen is followed. The researchers also concluded that an individualized approach to smokers, combined with self-help materials, selected prescriptions of nicotine gum, and follow-up monitoring of a patient's attempt to quit, were more effective than advice alone.[126] Within this consensus, the following program elements, summarized in Table 12-8, were found to be essential in an office-based intervention strategy for physicians.[126]

Conduct Intake and Screening

The physician should determine whether a patient smokes. If the patient does smoke, the physician should assess the smoking history and the patient's motivation to quit. The patient's chart should be flagged, and smoking status should be updated at each subsequent visit.

Recommended Physician Actions

The physician should discuss the hazards of smoking and the benefits of quitting, and should personalize them. A strong recommendation to quit should be given, and if possible, a commitment from the patient to quit by a specific date should be obtained. An individualized quit plan should be outlined, and a pharmacological aid, nicotine gum, should be considered when appropriate. Finally, the physician should assure the patient of support in this effort and state that the office will monitor the patient's progress.

Establish Supportive Office Procedures

The importance of providing an office system that enables a physician-based smoking cessation program to function smoothly and independently of the physician cannot be overstated. Office staff should be involved and their roles should be defined. Office staff activities can include reviewing the quit plan with the patient, reviewing the proper use of nicotine gum, providing self-help materials, assisting with referrals to outside smoking cessation treatments, and scheduling follow-up contacts.

TABLE 12-8. Essential Elements of a Physician-Guided Smoking Cessation Program

Intake and Screening
- Identify smoking status along with vital signs
- Update tobacco use status regularly (6 months and 12 months).
- Obtain basic data on smoking history and readiness to quit (update regularly if possible).

Physicians Actions
- Assess motivation and risk profile.
- Personalize risk of smoking and benefit of quitting.
- Advise to quit.
- Obtain quit commitment (set quit date).
- Triage (quit plan, including nicotine gum).
- Emphasize that progress will be monitored.

Office Staff Actions
- Define office resources.
- Review quit plan.
- Explain nicotine gum use (as necessary).
- Explain self-help materials (review special sections).
- Facilitate referral to outside resources.
- Schedule follow-up contact (link to quit plan).

Follow-up
- Conduct rapid followup of all patients with plan to change.
- Reassess smoking status at next visit.
- Triage and recycle relapsers at next visit.

Office Environment
- Establish smoke-free office (staff and patients)
- Make smoking education materials available.
- Publicize smoking cessation program.

From the U.S. Department of Health and Human Services: Essential Elements of an HMO-Guided Smoking Cessation Program. NCI Prepublication Edition, June 1987.

Establish Follow-up Procedures

The physician or office staff should contact the patient soon after the initial visit to check on progress. At each subsequent visit, the patient's smoking status and progress in quitting should be updated and further assistance provided when necessary. If a patient has relapsed, the doctor or staff should assist in identifying an appropriate treatment plan.

Establish an Appropriate Office Environment

The physician and office staff should reinforce nonsmoking message to patients. The most obvious step is a nonsmoking physician and staff and a smoke-free office. Information on the health effects of smoking and smoking cessation programs should be provided in the office. The fact that the physician provides smoking counseling should be publicized.

Numerous resources are available to help physicians establish and maintain smoking cessation efforts in their offices. These aids cover most aspects of quitting and are available in various formats. Table 12-9 lists some existing resources.

PHARMACOLOGIC AIDS FOR SMOKING CESSATION

Because tobacco use is a form of drug dependence, strategies of treatment used with dependence on other drugs have been applied. The most promising treatment and the first recognized as safe and efficacious by the Food and Drug Administration is nicorette, or nicotine gum. It is used in the same way that methadone substitution is used to treat heroin addiction.[127]

It is important to note that the intended use of the gum is unlike ordinary chewing gum. The manufacturer supplies the product buffered to a pH of 8.0 to 8.4. The nicotine component is meant to be absorbed in the mouth transmucosally, and not in the gut from where the chemically active drug will pass through the liver and lose most of its pharmacologic potency. After a small number of chews (approximately 15), the gum should be "parked" between the cheek and the gums for maximum absorption. The gum's effectiveness in aiding cessation has been demonstrated in several placebo-controlled trials.[128-132] Other studies have also shown that under a wide range of conditions the desire to smoke is reduced, although not eliminated, and withdrawal symptoms are lessened.[133-136] Recent work at the Addiction Research Center of the National Institute on Drug Abuse indicates that nicorette not only meets the criteria of therapeutic efficacy and low toxicity but appears to have a relatively low potential for abuse. It is apparently easier for most people to quit using the gum than to quit tobacco use.[79]

There are caveats regarding the use of nicotine gum, however. First, treatment of tobacco dependence is most efficacious when the gum is used in conjunction with a behavioral intervention. Cigarette smoking, like other forms of drug abuse, is only partially mediated by pharmacologic factors. The gum addresses possible physiological dependence, whereas the behavioral program equips the smoker to deal with psychological hurdles.[106] Second, persons who are most effectively treated with the gum thus far are heavily addicted smokers[137] as measured by the Fagerstrom Tolerance Scale.[128] Finally, it has been suggested that the use of the gum would probably be more efficacious if patient and physician compliance were increased.[138] As few as one third of the patients given a prescription for the gum ever fill it and most patients use the gum for less than the recommended 3 months. It is also important to stress that physicians or their staff instruct the patients in proper use of the gum and provide adequate follow-up of the patient to guarantee com-

TABLE 12-9. Smoking Cessation Resources

Title	*Available from*
Self-Help Manuals	
Clearing the Air—A Guide to Quitting Smoking	Office of Cancer Communications, National Cancer Institute, Bethesda, Maryland 20892
Quit for Good	Office of Cancer Communications, National Cancer Institute, Bethesda, Maryland 20892
Freedom From Smoking in 20 Days	American Lung Association, Local Office
Freedom From Smoking For You and Your Family	American Lung Association, Local Office
The Quitter's Guide—A Seven Day Plan to Help You Stop Smoking	American Cancer Society, Local Office
How to Quit Cigarettes	American Cancer Society, Local Office
Stop Smoking, Stay Trim	American Lung Association, Local Office
Videos	
In Control: A Home Video Freedom From Smoking Program	American Lung Association, Local Office
Why Quit Quiz Video	American Cancer Society, Local Office
Quitting With Nicorette	Minnesota Coalition for a Smoke-Free Society 2000, 2221 University Avenue, S.E., Suite 400, Minneapolis, Minnesota 55414
Motivational Materials	
Fifty Most Often Asked Questions About Smoking and Health and the Answers	American Cancer Society, Local Office
Why Do You Smoke	Office of Cancer Communications, National Cancer Institute, Bethesda, Maryland 20892
Health Hazards Associated With Involuntary Smoking: Cancer Facts	Office of Cancer Communications, National Cancer Institute, Building 31, Room 10A34, Bethesda, Maryland 20892
Second-Hand Smoke: The Fact Series	American Lung Association, Local Office
Physicians/Office Staff Training Guides	
A Physician Talks About Smoking	Office on Smoking and Health, Public Health Service, Rockville, Maryland 20857
Clinical Opportunities for Smoking Intervention—A Guide for the Busy Physician	National Heart, Lung, and Blood Institute in cooperation with the American Lung Association and the American Thoracic Society
The Physicians Guide—How To Help Your Hypertensive Patient Stop Smoking	National High Blood Pressure Education Program, National Heart, Lung, and Blood Institute
Family Physicians' Guide to Smoking Cessation	American Academy of Family Practitioners, 1740 West 92nd Street, Kansas City, Missouri 64114

From the U.S. Department of Health and Human Services: Essential Elements of an HMO-Guided Smoking Cessation Program. NCI Prepublication Edition, June 1987.

pliance and correct usage. When proper instructions are given and compliance is achieved, nicotine gum has a significant effect on short-term cessation and a demonstrable effect on long-term cessation.

PHYSICIAN INTERVENTION OPPORTUNITIES IN THE COMMUNITY

In response to the evidence concerning the health hazards of involuntary smoking, a growing number of states, agencies, and businesses are taking action to restrict smoking in public places. No longer is it solely the smoker's right to smoke if he or she desires. Rather, the nonsmoker has the right to breathe air free of tobacco smoke. As Surgeon General Dr. C. Everett Koop stated in the preface to his report, "The right of smokers to smoke ends where their behavior affects the health and well-being of others."[21]

Physicians have a role to play not only in office practices but also increasingly in the community. As more businesses offer health promotion programs and institute policies to restrict smoking, the need grows for smoking cessation policies and guidelines. Physicians who practice in business and industry can become active in several arenas:[139]

1. They can lay the groundwork for smoking cessation programs by writing articles on smoking in the company newsletter and making presentations to employees and instruction managers.
2. If the company decides to institute a smoking cessation program, the physician can assist in the development of an in-house effort or can assist in selecting a competent professional consultant.
3. They can assist in program implementation through clinical and diagnostic services to screen smoking employees and by advising smokers to participate in smoking cessation programs in the company.
4. They can assist in counseling employees who are either successful (*i.e.*, helping with withdrawal symptoms) or unsuccessful in quitting. They can also prescribe nicotine gum as part of the program.
5. Finally, they can assist in program evaluation and follow-up.

The involvement of physicians in nontraditional roles is also important. These include serving as experts on tobacco control issues to both the lay and medical communities, helping to motivate and mobilize other physicians toward greater involvement, advocating policy and initiatives while sitting on boards of directors for a variety of community organizations, and advocating legislative initiatives while participating in a number of community and state-wide activities.

THE CASE FOR CANCER PREVENTION

The prevention of chronic disease, including cancer, is possible because a modification of lifestyle is possible. A study by Enstrom[140] demonstrates this fact rather dramatically. He showed that the decline in smoking prevalence among California physicians had an important impact on a number of mortality endpoints that included smoking related cancers. Table 12-10 depicts standardized mortality ratios of these physicians compared with other American white men for the periods 1950–1959 and 1970–1979. Reductions in smoking prevalence from 53% in 1950 to about 10% in 1980 resulted in significantly lower death rates from lung cancer. The California physicians' Standard Mortality Ratios (SMR) declined from 62% (already 38% less than the comparison population) in 1950–1959 to 30% in 1970–1979 (70% less than the comparison population). Their SMRs for other smoking-related cancers, ischemic heart disease, and other diseases of the lung and bronchus also declined significantly.

The adoption of risk-reducing behavior patterns is an important element in any effective cancer control strategy. As the first line of authority in health matters, physicians have a critical role to play in a strategy to reduce diseases caused by tobacco use. Helping people to stop smoking and to avoid other forms of tobacco use is one of the greatest challenges facing public health and preventive medicine today. Cancer control authorities recognize that an aggressive, multifaceted strategy to tobacco use prevention and control will be necessary to achieve the National Cancer Institute's mortality reduction goal by the year 2000. An important element of this strategy is the commitment of physicians to actions that will maximize their potential impact as exemplars, authority figures, and interventionists to reduce all tobacco use and cigarette smoking in particular.

TABLE 12-10. Mortality Ratios and Smoking Prevalence

	1950	*1950–1959*	*1970–1979*	*1980*
Standardized mortality rates (%) of California physicians relative to U.S. white men				
Lung cancer		62	30	
Other smoking-related cancers		100	63	
Ischemic heart disease		106	71	
Bronchitis, emphysema, asthma		62	35	
Smoking Prevalence (%)				
California physicians	53			10
U.S. white males	53			38

Enstrom JE: Trends in mortality among California physicians after giving up smoking. Br J Med [Clin Res] 286:1101–1105, 1983.

REFERENCES

1. Doll R, Peto R: The causes of cancer: Quantitative estimates of avoidable risk in cancer in the United States. JNCI 66:1191–1308, 1981
2. Redmond DE: Tobacco and cancer: The first clinical report, 1761. N Engl J Med 282:18–23, 1970
3. US Department of Health, Education, and Welfare, Centers for Disease Control: Smoking and Health: Report of the Advisory Committee to the Surgeon General. PHS Publication No. 1103. Washington, DC, US Government Printing Office, 1964
4. US Department of Health and Human Services, Office on Smoking and Health: The Health Consequences of Smoking: Cancer. A Report of the Surgeon General. Washington, DC, DHHS (PHS) 82–50179, 1982
5. US Department of Health and Human Services, Office on Smoking and Health: The Health Consequences of Using Smokeless Tobacco: A Report of the Advisory Committee to the Surgeon General. Washington, DC, US Government Printing Office, 1986
6. US Department of Health, Education, and Welfare, Public Health Service: The Health Consequences of Smoking: 1967. PHS Publication No. 1696. Washington, DC, US Government Printing Office, 1967
7. US Department of Health, Education, and Welfare, Public Health Service: The Health Consequences of Smoking: 1968. Supplement to the 1967 Public Health Service Review. PHS Publication No. 1696. Washington, DC, US Government Printing Office, 1968
8. US Department of Health, Education, and Welfare, Public Health Service: The Health Consequences of Smoking: 1969. Supplement to the 1967 Public Health Service Review. PHS Publication No. 1696–2. Washington, DC, US Government Printing Office, 1969
9. US Department of Health, Education, and Welfare, Health Services and Mental Health Administration: The Health Consequences of Smoking, A Report to the Surgeon General: 1971. DHEW Publication No. (HSM) 71–7513. Washington, DC, US Government Printing Office, 1972
10. US Department of Health, Education, and Welfare, Health Services and Mental Health Administration: The Health Consequences of Smoking, A Report to the Surgeon General: 1972. DHEW Publication No. (HSM) 71–7516. Washington, DC, US Government Printing Office, 1972
11. US Department of Health, Education, and Welfare, Health Services and Mental Health Administration: The Health Consequences of Smoking: 1973. DHEW Publication No. (HSM) 73–8704. Washington, DC, US Government Printing Office, 1973
12. US Department of Health, Education, and Welfare, Centers for Disease Control: The Health Consequences of Smoking: 1974. DHEW Publication No. (CDC) 74–8704. Washington, DC, US Government Printing Office, 1975
13. US Department of Health, Education, and Welfare, Centers for Disease Control: The Health Consequences of Smoking: 1975. DHEW Publication No. (CDC) 76–8704. Washington, DC, US Government Printing Office, 1976
14. US Department of Health, Education, and Welfare, Public Health Service: Office of the Assistant Secretary for Health, Office on Smoking and Health: The Health Consequences of Smoking: 1977–1978. DHEW Publication No. (PHS) 79–50065. Washington, DC, US Government Printing Office, 1979
15. US Department of Health, Education, and Welfare, Office on Smoking and Health: Smoking and Health: A Report of the Surgeon General. DHEW Publication No. (PHS) 79–50066. Washington, DC, US Government Printing Office, 1979
16. US Department of Health and Human Services, Office on Smoking and Health: The Health Consequences of Smoking for Women: A Report of the Surgeon General. Washington, DC, US Government Printing Office, 1980
17. US Department of Health and Human Services, Office on Smoking and Health: The Health Consequences of Smoking: The Changing Cigarette. A Report of the Surgeon General, 1981. DHHS Publication No. (PHS) 81–50156. Washington, DC, US Government Printing Office, 1981
18. US Department of Health and Human Services, Office on Smoking and Health: The Health Consequences of Smoking: Cardiovascular Disease. A Report of the Surgeon General, 1983. DHHS (PHS) 84–50204. Washington, DC, US Government Printing Office, 1984
19. US Department of Health and Human Services, Office on Smoking and Health: The Health Consequences of Smoking: Chronic Obstructive Lung Disease. A Report of the Surgeon General, 1984. DHHS (PHS) 84–50205. Washington, DC, US Government Printing Office, 1984
20. US Department of Health and Human Services, Office on Smoking and Health: The Health Consequences of Smoking. Cancer and Chronic Lung Disease in the Workplace: A Report of the Surgeon General. Washington, DC, US Government Printing Office, 1985
21. US Department of Health and Human Services, Office on Smoking and Health: The Health Consequences of Involuntary Smoking: A Report of the Surgeon General. Washington, DC, US Government Printing Office, 1986
22. US Department of Health and Human Services, Centers for Disease Control: Smoking-attributable mortality and years of potential life lost. United States, 1984. MMWR 36:693–697, 1987
23. Pollin W: The role of the additive process as a key step in causation of all tobacco-related diseases. JAMA 252:2874–2875, 1984
24. Tso TC, Gray NJ: Personal communication, 1985
25. Wynder EL, Graham EA: Tobacco smoking as a possible etiologic factor in bronchiogenic carcinoma: A study of 684 proved cases. JAMA 143:329–336, 1950
26. Doll R, Hill AB: Smoking and carcinoma of the lung: Preliminary report. Br Med J 2:739–748, 1950
27. Levin ML, Goldstein H, Gerhardt PR: Cancer and tobacco smoking: A preliminary report. JAMA 143:336–338, 1950
28. Royal College of Physicians: Smoking and Health: Summary and Report of the Royal College of Physicians of London on Smoking in Relation to Cancer of the Lung and Other Diseases. New York, Pitman, 1962
29. International Agency for Research on Cancer: IARC Monographs on the Evaluation of the Carcinogenic Risk of Chemicals to Humans: Tobacco Smoking 38:12–20. Geneva, World Health Organization, 1985
30. Berry G, Newhouse ML, Antonis P: Combined effect of asbestos and smoking on mortality from lung cancer and mesothelioma in factory workers. Br J Ind Med 42:12–18, 1985
31. McDonald JC, Liddell FDK, Gibbs GW, et al: Dust exposure and mortality in chrysotile mining, 1910–1975. Br J Ind Med 37:11–24, 1980
32. Liddell FDK, Thomas DC, Gibbs GW, et al: Fibre exposure and mortality from pneumoconiosis, respiratory and abdominal malignancies in chrysotile production in Quebec 1926–1975. Ann Acad Med Singapore (Suppl 2) 13:340–344, 1984
33. Selikoff IJ, Seidman H, Hammond EC: Mortality effects of cigarette smoking among amosite asbestos factory workers. JNCI 65:507–513, 1980
34. Meurman LO, Kiviluoto R, Hakama M: Combined effect of asbestos exposure and tobacco smoking on Finnish anthophyllite miners and millers. Ann NY Acad Sci 330:491–495, 1979
35. Hammond EC, Selikoff IJ, Seidman H: Asbestos exposure, cigarette smoking and death rates. Ann NY Acad Sci 330:473–490, 1979
36. Hornung RW, Samuels S: Survivorship models for lung cancer mortality in uranium mines: Is cumulative dose an appropriate measure of exposure? In Gomez (ed): Radiation Hazards in Mining, pp 363–368. New York, Society of Mining Engineers of the American Institute of Mining, Metallurgical and Petroleum Engineers, 1981
37. Whittemore AS, McMillan A: Lung cancer mortality among US uranium miners: A reappraisal. JNCI 71:489–499, 1983
38. National Cancer Institute: Annual Cancer Statistics Review. NIH Publication No. 87–2789, 1987
39. American Cancer Society: 1987 Cancer Facts and Figures, p 9. New York, American Cancer Society, 1987
40. US Department of Health and Human Services, Centers for Disease Control: Cigarette Smoking in the United States, 1986. MMWR 36:581–585, 1987
41. Flanders WD, Rothman KJ: Interaction of alcohol and tobacco in laryngeal cancer. Am J Epidemiol (in press)
42. McLoy DG, Hecht SS, Wynder EL: The roles of tobacco, alcohol, and diet in the etiology of upper alimentary and respiratory tract cancer. Prev Med 9:622–629, 1980
43. Hirayama T: Prospective studies on cancer epidemiology based on census population in Japan. In Bucalossi P, Veronesi U, Cascinelli N (eds): Cancer Epidemiology, Environmental Factors, Vol 3, pp 26–35. Proceedings of the 11th International Cancer Congress, Florence, Italy, 1974. Amsterdam, Excerpta Medica, 1975
44. Kamionkowski MD, Fleshler B: The role of alcoholic intake in esophageal carcinoma. Am J Med Sci 249:696–700, 1965
45. Kissin B, Kaley MM, Su WH, et al: Head and neck cancer in alcoholics: The relationship to drinking, smoking, and dietary patterns. JAMA 224:1174–1175, 1973
46. Schoenberg BS, Bailar JC III, Fraumeni JF Jr: Certain mortality patterns of esophageal cancer in the United States, 1930–1967. JNCI 46:63–73, 1971
47. Schottenfeld D, Gantt RC, Wynder EL: The role of alcohol and tobacco in multiple primary cancers of the upper digestive system, larynx, and lung: A prospective study. Prev Med 3:277–293, 1974
48. Takano K, Osogoshi K, Kamimura N, et al: [Epidemiology of esophageal cancer—with special reference to the significance of hot food and beverage drinking, smoking, and nutritional deficiency.] Int J Cancer 5:152–156, 1970
49. Williams RR, Horm JW: Association of cancer sites with tobacco and alcohol consumption and socioeconomic status of patients: Interview study from the Third National Cancer Survey. JNCI 58:525–547, 1977
50. Wynder EL, Bross IJ: A study of etiological factors in cancer of the esophagus. Cancer 14:389–413, 1961
51. Wynder EL, Mushinski MH, Spivak JC: Tobacco and alcohol consumption in relation to the development of multiple primary cancers. Cancer 40:1872–1878, 1977
52. Swan S: Smoking and cervical cancer. In Rosenberg MJ (ed): Smoking and Reproductive Health, pp 176–185. Littleton, MA, PSG Publishing, 1987
53. Brinton LA, Schairer C, Haenszel W, et al: Cigarette smoking and invasive cervical cancer. JAMA 255:3265–3269, 1986
54. Baran JA, Byers T, Greenberg ER, et al: Cigarette smoking in women with cancers of the breast and reproductive organs. JNCI 77:677–680, 1986
55. Baumslag N, Keen P, Petering HG: Carcinoma of the maxillary antrum and its relationship to trace and metal content in snuff. Arch Environ Health 23:1–5, 1971
56. Brunnermann KD, Genoble L, Hoffmann D: N-nitrosamines in chewing tobacco: An international comparison. J Agric Food Chem 33:1178–1181, 1985
57. Hoffmann D, Adams JD: Carcinogenic tobacco-specific N-nitrosamines in snuff and in the saliva of snuff dippers. Cancer Res 41:4305–4308, 1981
58. Osterdahl BG, Slorach S: N-nitrosamines in snuff and chewing tobacco on the Swedish market in 1983. Food Addit Contam 1:299–305, 1984
59. Nair J, Ohshima H, Malaveille C, et al: N-nitrosamine compounds (NOC) in saliva and urine of betel quid chewers: studies on occurrence and formation. Carcinogenesis 6:295–303, 1985
60. Hoffmann D, Hecht SS, Ornaf RM, et al: Nitrosonornicotine: Presence in tobacco, formation and carcinogenicity. IARC Sci Publ 14:307–320, 1976

61. Munson JW, Abdine H: Determination of N-nitrosonornicotine in tobacco by gas chromatography/mass spectroscopy. Anal Lett 10:777–786, 1977
62. Adams JD, Brunnemann KD, Hoffman D: Rapid method for the analysis of tobacco-specific N-nitrosamines by gas-liquid chromatography with a thermal energy analyzer. J Chromatogr 256:347–351, 1983
63. Campbell JM, Lindsey AJ: Polycyclic aromatic hydrocarbons in snuff. Chem Ind (Lond) 951, 1957
64. Hoffmann D, Harley NH, Fisenne I, et al: Carcinogenic agents in snuff. JNCI 76:435–437, 1986
65. Harley NH, Cohen BS, Tso TC: Polonium-210: A questionable risk factor in smoking-related carcinogenesis. Banbury Report 3:93–104, 1980
66. Friedell HL, Rosenthal LM: The etiologic role of chewing tobacco in cancer of the mouth. JAMA 116:2130–2135, 1941
67. Moore GE, Bissinger LL, Proehl EC: Tobacco and intraoral cancer. Surg Forum 3:685–688, 1952
68. International Agency for Research on Cancer: Tobacco habits other than smoking: Betel-quid and areca-nut chewing and some related nitrosamines. IARC Monogr Eval Carcinog Risk Chem Hum 37:291, 1985
69. National Institutes of Health: Health implications of smokeless tobacco use. Consensus Development Conference Statement VI 6:1. Bethesda, MD, 1986
70. Winn DM, Blot WJ, Shy CM, et al: Snuff dipping and oral cancer among women in the Southern United States. N Engl J Med 304:745–749, 1981
71. National Research Council, National Academy of Sciences: Environmental Tobacco Smoke: Measuring Exposures and Assessing Health Effects. Washington, DC, National Academy Press, 1986
72. Edwards D: Nicotine: A drug of choice. Sci News 129, 1986
73. US Department of Health and Human Services, National Center for Health Statistics: National Health Interview Survey Smoking Supplement, 1980
74. Jarvik M: The role of nicotine in the smoking habit. In Hunt WA (ed): Learning Mechanisms in Smoking, pp 155–190. Chicago, Aldine, 1970
75. Russell MAH: Cigarette smoking: National history of a dependence disorder. Br J Med Psychol 44:1–16, 1971
76. Jarvik M: Further observations on nicotine as the reinforcing agent in smoking. In Dunn WL (ed): Smoking Behavior: Motives and Incentives, pp 33–49. Washington, DC, Winston, 1973
77. Jaffe JH, Kanzler M: Smoking as an addictive disorder. In Krasnegor NA (ed): Cigarette Smoking as a Dependence Process. NIDA Research Monograph 23, pp 4–23. Washington, DC, US Government Printing Office, 1979
78. Henningfield JE, Griffiths RR, Jasinski DR: Human dependence on tobacco and opioids: Common factors. In Thompson T, Johanson CE (eds): Behavioral Pharmacology of Human Drug Dependence. NIDA Research Monograph. Washington DC, US Government Printing Office, 1981
79. Henningfield JE: Side effects of nicotine dependence. NJ Med 85:108–112, 1988
80. US Department of Health and Human Services, Centers for Disease Control: The Pharmacologic Basis of Tobacco Dependence: A Report of the Surgeon General (in press)
81. Henningfield JE, Nemeth-Costlett R: Nicotine dependence: Interface between tobacco and tobacco-related disease. Chest (in press)
82. World Health Organization: International Classification of Diseases (Ninth Revision). Geneva, World Health Organization, 1978
83. American Psychiatric Association: Diagnostic and Statistical Manual of Mental Disorders, 3rd ed. Washington, DC, American Psychiatric Association, 1979
84. Pollin W, Ravenholt RT: Tobacco addiction and tobacco mortality. JAMA 252:2849–2854, 1984
85. Doll R, Peto R: Mortality in relation to smoking: 20 years' observations on male British doctors. Br Med J 2:1525–1536, 1976
86. Rogot E, Murray JL: Smoking and causes of death among U.S. veterans: 16 years of observation. Public Health Rep 95:213–222, 1980
87. Wynder EL, Stellman SD: Impact of long-term filter cigarette usage on lung and larynx cancer risk: A case-control study. JNCI 62:471–477, 1979
88. Wynder EL, Stellman SD: Comparative epidemiology of tobacco-related cancers. Cancer Res 37:4608–4622, 1977
89. US Department of Health and Human Services, National Center for Health Statistics: National Health Interview Survey, 1985
90. US Department of Health and Human Services, National Institute on Drug Abuse: Drug Abuse Statistics 1985—Population Estimates (based on data from the National Household Survey on Drug Abuse of 1985), November 1986
91. Haynes S: Cigarette smoking among three adolescent Hispanic groups: Results from the Hispanic Health and Nutrition Examination Survey. Presented at the Conference on Tobacco Use Among Blacks and Hispanics, Washington, D.C., March 28–29, 1988
92. Botvin GJ, Eng A, Williams CL: Preventing the onset of cigarette smoking through life skills training. Prev Med 9:135–143, 1983
93. Flay BR, d'Avernas JR, Best JA, et al: Cigarette smoking: Why young people do it and ways of preventing it. In McGrath P, Firestone P (eds): Pediatric and Adolescent Behavioral Medicine, pp 132–183. New York, Springer-Verlag, 1983
94. US Department of Health and Human Services, National Institute on Drug Abuse: Survey of Drug Use Among High School Seniors, 1986
95. US Department of Health and Human Services, National Institute on Drug Abuse: National Household Survey on Drug Abuse, 1985
96. Boyd G, Ary DV, Wirt R, et al: Use of smokeless tobacco among children and adolescents in the United States. Prev Med 16:402–421, 1987
97. Davis R: Current trends in cigarette advertising and marketing. N Engl J Med 316:725–732, 1987
98. Glasgow RE, Bernstein DA: Behavioral treatment of smoking behavior. In Prokop CK, Bradley LA (eds): Medical Psychology: A New Perspective. New York, Academic Press, 1981
99. Glasgow RE, Klesges RC: Smoking intervention programs in the workplace. In US Department of Health and Human Services, The Health Consequences of Smoking: Cancer and Chronic Lung Disease in the Workplace. DHHS Publication No. (PHS) 85–50207. Washington, DC, US Government Printing Office, 1985
100. Lichtenstein E, Brown A: Current trends in the modification of cigarette dependence. In Bellack A, Hersen M, Kazdin AE (eds): International Handbook of Behavior Modification and Therapy, vol 2. New York, Plenum Press, 1983
101. Lichtenstein E, Danaher BG: Modification of smoking behavior: A critical analysis of theory, research, and practice. In Hersen M, Eisler M, Miller PM (eds): Progress in Behavioral Modification. New York, Academic Press, 1976
102. Ockene JK: Changes in cigarette smoking behavior in clinical and community trials. In US Department of Health and Human Services, The Health Consequences of Smoking for Cardiovascular Disease: A Report of the Surgeon General. DHHS Publication No. (PHS) 84–50204. Washington, DC, US Government Printing Office, 1984
103. Pechacek TF: Modification of smoking behavior. In Krasnegor NA (ed): The Behavior Aspects of Smoking, NIDA Research Monograph No. 26. US Department of Health and Human Services, Public Health Service, National Institute on Drug Abuse, DHHS Publication No. (ADM) 79–882, 1979
104. Pechacek TF, Danaher BG: How and why people quit smoking: A cognitive-behavioral analysis. In Kendall PC, Hollen SD (eds): Cognitive-Behavioral Interventions: Theory, Research, and Procedure. New York, Academic Press, 1979
105. US Department of Health and Human Services, Centers for Disease Control: Smoking and health—A national status report: A Report to Congress. DHHS Publication No. (CDC) 87–8396, Rockville, Maryland, 1987
106. Russell MAH: Conceptual framework for nicotine substitution. In Ockene JK (ed): Pharmacologic Treatment of Tobacco Dependence: Proceedings of the World Congress, pp 90–107. Cambridge, MA, Institute for the Study of Smoking Behavior and Policy, Smoking Behavior and Policy Conference Series, 1986
107. Marlatt GA, Gordon JR: Relapse Prevention: Maintenance Strategies in the Treatment of Addiction, New York, Guilford Press, 1985
108. Ockene JK, Broste S, Hymowitz N, et al: For the MRFIT Research Group. Paper presented at Council on Epidemiology, American Heart Association, San Diego, 1983
109. Brown RA, Lichtenstein E, McIntyre KO, et al: The effects of nicotine fading and relapse prevention on smoking cessation. J Consult Clin Psychol 52:307–308, 1984
110. Hall SM, Killen JD: Psychological and pharmacological approaches to smoking relapse prevention. In Grabowski J, Hall SM (eds): Pharmacological Adjuncts in Smoking Cessation. NIDA Research Monograph No. 53, US Department of Health and Human Services, Public Health Service, Alcohol, Drug Abuse and Mental Health Administration, DHHS Publication No. (ADM) 85–1333, 1985
111. Davis AL, Faust R, Ordentilch M: Self-help smoking cessation and maintenance programs: A comparative study with 12-month follow-up by the American Lung Association. Am J Public Health 874:1212–1217, 1984
112. Glasgow RE, Schaeffer L, O'Neil HK: Self-help books and amount of therapist contact in smoking cessation programs. J Consult Clin Psychol 49:659–667, 1981
113. Flay BR: Mass media and smoking cessation. Presented at the International Communication Association Meeting, Chicago, May 1986
114. Snow WH, Gilchrist LD, Schinke SP: A critique of progress in adolescent smoking prevention. Children Youth Serv Rev 7:1–19, 1985
115. Puska P, Koskela K: Community-based strategies to fight smoking: Experiences from the North Karelia Project in Finland. NY State J Med 83:1335–1338, 1983
116. Pederson LL: Compliance with physician advice to quit smoking: A review of the literature. Prev Med 11:71–84, 1982
117. Garfinkel L, Stellman SD: Cigarette smoking among physicians, dentists, and nurses. CA 36:1, 1986
118. Orleans CT: Understanding and promoting smoking cessation: Overview and guidelines for physician intervention. Annu Rev Med 36:51–61, 1985
119. Valente CM, Sobal J, Muncie HL Jr, et al: Health promotion: Physicians' beliefs, attitudes, and practices. Am J Prev Med 2:82–88, 1986
120. Orleans CT, George LK, Houpt JL, et al: Health promotion in primary care: A survey of U.S. family practitioners. Prev Med 14:636–647, 1985
121. Wilson DM, Lindsay-McIntyre E, Best JA, et al: A smoking cessation intervention program for family physicians. Can Med Assoc J 137:613–619, 1987
122. Anda RF, Remington PL, Siento DG, et al: Are physicians advising smokers to quit? A patient's perspective. JAMA 257:14, 1916–1919, 1987
123. Russell MA, Wilson C, Taylor C: The effects of general practitioners' advice against smoking. Br Med J 2:231–235, 1979
124. Goldstein B, Fischer PM, Richards JW, et al: Smoking counseling practices of recently trained family physicians. J Fam Pract 24:195–197, 1987
125. Wechsler H, Levine S, Idelson RK, et al: The physicians's role in health promotion—a survey of primary care practitioners. N Engl J Med 309:97–100, 1983
126. US Department of Health and Human Services, National Cancer Institute: Essential Elements of an HMO-Guided Smoking Cessation Program. Prepublication edition, June 1987
127. Grabowski J, Stitzer ML, Henningfield JE (eds): Behavioral intervention techniques in drug abuse treatment. NIDA Research Monograph Series No. 46. Washington, DC, US Government Printing Office, 1984

128. Fagerstrom K: A comparison of psychological and pharmacological treatment in smoking cessation. J Behav Med 5:343–351, 1982
129. Jarvis MJ, Raw M, Russell MAH, et al: Randomised controlled trial of nicotine chewing-gum. Br Med J 285:337–340, 1982
130. Schneider NG, Jarvik ME, Forsythe AB, et al: Nicotine gum in smoking cessation: A placebo-controlled, double-blind trial. Addict Behav 8:253–261, 1983
131. Hjalmarson AIM: Effect of nicotine chewing gum in smoking cessation: A randomized, placebo-controlled, double-blind study. JAMA 252:2835–2838, 1984
132. Malcolm RE, Sillett RW, Turner JAM, et al: The use of nicotine chewing gum as an aid to stopping smoking. Psychopharmacology (Berlin) 70:295–296, 1980
133. Hughes JR, Hatsukami DK, Pickens RW, et al: Effect of nicotine on the tobacco withdrawal syndrome. Psychopharmacologia 83:82–87, 1984
134. Hughes JR, Hatsukami DK: Short-term effects of nicotine gum. In Grabowski J, Hall SJ (eds): Pharmacological Adjuncts in Smoking Cessation. NIDA Research Monograph No. 53, US Department of Health and Human Services, Public Health Service, Alcohol, Drug Abuse, and Mental Health Administration. DHHS Publication No. (ADM) 85–1333, 1985
135. Schneider NG, Jarvik ME, Forsythe AB: Nicotine versus placebo gum in the alleviation of withdrawal during smoking cessation. Addict Behav 9:149–156, 1984
136. West R, Jarvis MJ, Russell MAH, et al: Effect of nicotine replacement on the cigarette withdrawal syndrome. Br J Addict 79:215–219, 1984
137. Fagerstrom K: Effects of nicotine chewing gum and followup appointment in physician based smoking cessation. Prev Med 13:517–527, 1984
138. Hughes JR: Problems of nicotine gum. In Ockene JK (ed): Pharmacologic Treatment of Tobacco Dependence: Proceedings of the World Congress, pp 141–147. Cambridge MA, Institute for the Study of Smoking Behavior and Policy, Smoking Behavior and Policy Conference Series, 1986
139. Fisher EB, Bishop DB, Mayer JA, et al: The physician's contribution to smoking cessation in the workplace. Chest 93:556–565, 1988
140. Enstrom JE: Health and dietary practices and cancer mortality among California Mormons. In Cairns J, Lyon JL, Skolnick M (eds): Cancer Incidence in Defined Populations, pp 69–92. Cold Spring Harbor, NY, Cold Spring Harbor Laboratory, 1980

Joseph F. Fraumeni, Jr.
Robert N. Hoover
Susan S. Devesa
Leo J. Kinlen

CHAPTER 13 *Epidemiology of Cancer*

Epidemiology is the study of variations in disease frequency among population groups and the factors that influence these variations. Its principal objective is the finding of causes so that, ideally, preventive measures may be applied. By focusing on events that necessarily precede the onset of disease, epidemiology contrasts with clinical medicine in which the primary concern is the diagnosis and treatment of individual patients. In epidemiology, the perennial reference point for individual patients is the population from which they come. This approach encompasses not only unaffected members of the group in question, which may be useful for comparison purposes, but also all affected persons in that population, thereby avoiding the selection factors that can determine the experience of individual clinicians.

Following dramatic improvements in the control of infectious disease during this century, the attention of epidemiologists has increasingly turned toward the study of chronic illnesses. The resulting advances include some of the most important discoveries in the etiology and prevention of cancer. The impact of epidemiology on cancer touches the clinician, experimentalist, policy maker, and even the lay public, whose attention is often drawn to epidemiologic observations and environmental issues by the news media, sometimes in an unbalanced way.

Practicing physicians must often interpret epidemiologic findings for their patients. They have opportunities to use epidemiologic data that will protect high-risk individuals, collaborate in epidemiologic studies, and make clinical observations relevant to etiology. In view of the large volume of current research into the origins of cancer and its prevention, it is increasingly important for the clinical oncologist to understand the principles and methods of epidemiology.

HISTORICAL PERSPECTIVE

Epidemiologic observations in cancer have a long and fascinating history.[1] In 1700, the Italian occupational physician Bernardino Ramazzini noted that breast cancer was more common in nuns than other women, and he suggested the influence of celibacy. In 1775, the British surgeon Percivall Pott reported the first description of occupational carcinogenesis in the form of scrotal cancer among chimney sweeps. In the 18th century there were also reports of cancer risks associated with tobacco, namely snuff taking and nasal cancer by Hill in 1761 and pipe smoking and lip cancer by von Soemmering in 1795. Perhaps the first epidemiologic study of cancer, in any modern sense, was in 1842 by Rigoni-Stern who attempted to quantify the risks of uterine cancer in the city of Verona among nuns and other women and showed that the disease was significantly less common in the former group. Important occupational cancers were also noted in the 19th century: lung cancer (though first described as "mediastinal lymphoma") among the metal miners of Schneeberg and Joachimsthal by Harting and Hesse in 1879, and bladder cancer among aniline dye workers by Rehn in 1895. In 1888 Hutchinson reported the first suggestion of drug-induced cancer with an account of skin cancers in patients treated with an arsenic-containing solution.

These historical observations, and many others that followed,[2,3] illustrate the importance of clinical observations as a source of new discoveries in cancer etiology. They also include an early indication of the long latent interval in human carcinogenesis, for Pott noted that some of the men with scrotal cancer had not worked as chimney sweeps since boyhood. Furthermore, they show how some causes can be detected (and diseases prevented) before specific agents and mechanisms are elucidated by laboratory investigators. Indeed, many decades elapsed before evidence was available to indicate that polycyclic hydrocarbons, radioactive substances, and aromatic amines explained some of the early findings described above.

AIMS OF EPIDEMIOLOGY

It is convenient to stress several key words in the definition of epidemiology, which is the study of the distribution and determinants of disease frequency in human populations.[4] The word "humans" distinguishes the approach from those laboratory disciplines in cancer research that use animals and other test systems in their experiments. The study of "populations" stands in contrast to clinical research, which usually involves investigations at the individual or case series level. The term "frequency" indicates the orientation of epidemiology towards quantifying the occurrence of disease and the risks attributable to various causes. Finally, the phrase "distribution and determinants" points to the two major approaches of epidemiology. In general, descriptive studies examine the distribution of disease frequency in populations that can be useful in generating etiologic hypotheses, while analytical studies test hypotheses by pursuing differences in the personal characteristics or exposures among individuals.

The main contribution of cancer epidemiology is the detection and quantification of the risks associated with specific environmental exposures and host factors. These associations may lead to causal inferences, thus providing the basis for instituting preventive measures. Epidemiologic data support the concept that carcinogenesis is a lengthy multistage process that is affected by a wide variety of factors.[5–7] Some factors appear to act early as initiators, others later as promoters, and still others at both early and late stages. Certain agents act together to accelerate the carcinogenic process, such as the way smoking combines synergistically with asbestos to produce lung cancer or with alcohol to produce oral and esophageal cancers. Furthermore, there is some evidence that the process is retarded by dietary factors, such as certain micronutrients that appear to diminish the risk of various cancer sites including smoking-related lung cancer.

Thus, the aims of epidemiology are to uncover new etiologic leads through peculiarities in the distribution of cancer, quantify the risks associated with different exposures (some of which may be protective), promote insights into the mechanisms of carcinogenesis, and assess the efficacy of preventive measures. While the usual observational methods of epidemiology have succeeded in identifying many causes of cancer, future progress may depend to a considerable degree on innovative strategies that employ laboratory techniques in epidemiologic investigations.

DESCRIPTIVE STUDIES

There is perhaps no disorder that shows a uniform incidence in all human groups. Indeed, cancers are striking in the variations they show according to such factors as age, sex, race, time, socioeconomic class, marital status, and geographic location. Descriptive (or demographic) studies, by revealing the patterns of disease in populations, have provided many clues to cancer etiology. Variations by age, area, and time are often remarkable, even allowing for the fluctuations that might be expected as a result of chance and differences in diagnostic and reporting practices.[6] The descriptive patterns are useful also in monitoring variations and trends that might point to new environmental hazards, in evaluating the effects of cancer prevention, screening, and treatment activities, and in predicting future trends that may help set priorities in various aspects of oncology.[8]

MEASURES OF CANCER FREQUENCY

Descriptive studies measure rates, which are based on three items of information: the number of individuals affected by the disease (numerator), the length of the period covered (time), and the population from which they are derived (denominator). The expression of disease in this manner allows the rates in one population to be compared with the rates in another. Often these rates must be adjusted for such factors as age, race, and social class, which might otherwise spuriously influence the comparison.[9] The rates most often used in cancer epidemiology concern incidence, mortality, and prevalence, with each having its particular uses and limitations. When measures of occurrence are not based on populations at risk, they usually represent proportions, even though sometimes labelled as rates, such as case-fatality rates. Sample calculations of these measures are derived from numbers given in Table 13-1.

The incidence rate provides a direct measure of the probability of developing cancer, and is defined as the

$$\frac{\text{Number of persons developing cancer in a unit of time}}{\text{Total population living at that time}}$$

Most often the unit of time is 1 year, with the mid-year population serving as the denominator. The rates are usually expressed per 100,000 or per million persons. For example, from the data in Table 13-1, the annual occurrence of Hodgkin's disease per 100,000 residents in Connecticut is calculated using the equation on the next page:

TABLE 13-1. Patients with Hodgkin's Disease and Pancreatic Cancer, Connecticut, 1982

Type of Cancer	*Patients Alive at Start of Year**	*New Cases in Year†*	*Deaths in Year‡*
Hodgkin's disease	1151	120	26
Pancreatic cancer	220	326	297

* Prevalence data estimated from data of Feldman AR, et al: The prevalence of cancer. N Engl J Med 315:1394, 1986.

† Incidence data from Connecticut Tumor Registry.

‡ Mortality data from National Center for Health Statistics.

Estimated populations were 3,112,469 on January 1, 1982 for prevalence and 3,126,488 on July 1, 1982 for incidence and mortality.

$$\text{Incidence rate} = \frac{120}{3{,}126{,}488} \times 100{,}000$$
$$= 3.8 \text{ per } 100{,}000 \text{ per year}$$

Incidence rates may be crude (all ages), as in this example, or age-specific. Because of the great dependence of cancer incidence on age, it is much more informative to use age-specific rates. However, when summary figures are necessary to compare rates between population groups with different age distributions, they should be age-adjusted; this is done by multiplying each age-specific rate by the percent of individuals in a standard population (*e.g.*, the 1970 U.S. population) with the same ages, and then summing to produce a single value. For etiologic studies, incidence rates tend to be more informative than mortality rates, because they cover all diagnosed cases (not merely the fatal ones) at a time which is closer to the point of causation. The information on incident cancers is usually more extensive and reliable, with details often available on histologic type and stage.

The mortality or death rate is defined as the

$$\frac{\text{Number of persons dying of cancer in a unit of time}}{\text{Total population living at that time}}$$

From data in Table 13-1, the mortality rate for Hodgkin's disease is computed as follows:

$$\text{Mortality rate} = \frac{26}{3{,}126{,}488} \times 100{,}000$$
$$= 0.8 \text{ per } 100{,}000 \text{ per year}$$

For etiologic research, mortality rates most clearly reflect the occurrence of those cancer sites with the worst prognosis, and are vulnerable to well-known inaccuracies and variations in death-certificate reporting of diagnoses. However, mortality data are often the only statistics available in certain locations and periods, and they have been especially useful for evaluation of long-term trends and geographic variations on a national or international scale. For several cancers with poor survival, mortality rates nearly equal incidence rates. Even with improvements in survival of many cancers, mortality rates help in clarifying incidence trends for certain cancers (*e.g.*, breast and prostate) that may be distorted by heightened efforts at case finding.[6,8] Mortality rates are also very useful in evaluating the impact of advances in cancer prevention and treatment on the general population. The combined analyses of incidence, mortality, and survival statistics that comprise the Surveillance, Epidemiology, and End Results (SEER) Program of the National Cancer Institute (NCI) provide valuable data on the patterns of cancer in the United States.[10]

The case-fatality rate is a measure of the severity or lethality of disease. A proportion rather than a true rate, it is usually expressed as a percentage and defined as the

$$\frac{\text{Number of deaths from cancer}}{\text{Number of persons developing cancer}} \times 100\%$$

From data in Table 13-1, case-fatality rates are estimated as follows:

$$\text{Case fatality (Hodgkin's disease)} = \frac{26}{120} \times 100\% = 21.7\%$$

$$\text{Case fatality (pancreatic cancer)} = \frac{297}{326} \times 100\% = 91.1\%$$

Because the cases and deaths usually refer to the same period of time, this concept is less meaningful in chronic than in acute diseases, and is generally replaced by survival rates that are discussed below.

The prevalence rate is seldom used in etiologic studies of cancer, but provides a useful measure for planning health services by estimating the burden of disease in the population.[11] Also called point prevalence, it is defined as the

$$\frac{\text{Number of persons with cancer at a given point in time}}{\text{Total population living at that time}}$$

From data in Table 13-1, the prevalence of Hodgkin's disease on January 1, 1982 is calculated as follows:

$$\text{Prevalence} = \frac{1{,}115}{3{,}112{,}469} \times 100{,}000 = 37.0 \text{ per } 100{,}000$$

Table 13-2 summarizes the various kinds of rates for Hodgkin's disease and pancreatic cancer. Hodgkin's disease displays lower incidence and mortality rates than pancreatic cancer, but a higher prevalence rate due to its much lower case-fatality rate (or conversely, higher survival rate).

Proportional rates or relative frequencies are used when details of the population that produce a series of cancer cases or deaths are unknown. This may occur in surveys of hospital patients or death certificates, where the proportions of different cancers may be compared with those in the general population for each sex and age group. Proportional mortality ratios are sometimes used in studies of occupational groups.[12] However, since the denominator refers to total deaths rather than the population at risk, the magnitude of the ratio for a particular cancer may be misleading since it also fluctuates according to the number of deaths from other causes. Thus, positive findings emerging from this type of survey should be interpreted cautiously and pursued by more definitive investigation.

CORRELATIONAL STUDIES

Descriptive studies may use the correlational (or ecological) approach, in which the rates of disease in populations are compared with the geographic or temporal distribution of

TABLE 13-2. Measures of Frequency for Hodgkin's Disease and Pancreatic Cancer, Connecticut, 1982*

Measure	*Hodgkin's disease*	*Pancreatic cancer*
Mortality	0.8	9.5
Incidence	3.8	10.4
Prevalence	37.0	7.1

* Crude rates per 100,000 population per year, calculated from data in Table 13-1.

suspected risk factors.[13] The association is often expressed in terms of correlation or regression coefficients. Although a correlational study may be helpful in formulating hypotheses about carcinogenic risks, it falls short of establishing causal relationships. Correlational studies have the advantage of being inexpensive and quick because they often use statistics assembled for other purposes.[13]

The primary weakness of such studies for etiologic research, as with descriptive studies generally, is that they concern populations rather than individuals. Moreover, the exposure measures are usually crude and subject to confounding factors. For example, in early surveys of lung cancer, the temporal increases among men were consistent with the effects of an increasing prevalence of cigarette smoking, but this correlation by itself provided only weak evidence of causation, since other factors such as air pollution and improvements in diagnosis showed a similar pattern. It required analytical studies that pursued these leads to establish the cause-and-effect relationship between smoking and lung cancer. Correlational studies also may provide supporting evidence in evaluating relationships detected by analytical or laboratory studies. This is illustrated by the more recent temporal increases in lung cancer among women, who have lagged about 25 years behind men in their adoption of smoking habits. Another example is the geographic correlation in developing countries between primary liver cancer and intake of foodstuffs contaminated by aflatoxin, a potent hepatocarcinogen in laboratory animals.[6] Nevertheless, while correlational data may provide clues to etiology, one must be careful not to draw a premature or inappropriate conclusion, sometimes referred to as an ecological fallacy.[13]

SOURCES OF DATA

Descriptive studies employ mainly population-based statistics on mortality, incidence, and survival to calculate rates, although clinical series from hospital-based registries or other sources may also provide clues to the etiology and natural history of cancer.

Death Certificates

In many countries, a death certificate is prepared for legal purposes for each person who dies.[14] In addition to a number of demographic variables, the certificate usually includes the underlying and secondary causes of death. Although in 1900 only 11 states in the United States contributed to the national registration system, by 1933 all 48 states were included. Alaska and Hawaii were added in 1959–1960 with their entry into the Union. The National Center for Health Statistics tabulates the deaths annually and calculates rates using population estimates provided by the Census Bureau. The data are also made available on computer magnetic tape for research purposes. A national death registry for the United States was established in 1979. This National Death Index is frequently used to identify persons in epidemiologic studies who have died.

The NCI has examined the national cancer mortality data in several periods. An early tabulation by age, race, sex, and form of cancer included deaths starting in 1930 and continuing through 1955.[15] Geographic variations in cancer mortality at the state level were evaluated for the years 1950–1967.[16] Analyses at the county level for 1950–1969[17] formed the basis for computer-generated color atlases portraying geographic patterns on a small-area scale for whites and nonwhites.[18,19] More recently, cancer mortality was tabulated at the county level by decade from 1950 through 1979.[20] Using data through 1980, maps of cancer mortality were prepared according to state economic area to examine trends in the geographic patterns.[21] Computer graphics have also been used to display national trends by age, race, and sex for 1950–1977.[22] Long-term trends in U.S. cancer mortality and incidence were examined for 1935–1974[23] and more recently for 1947–1984.[24] The geographic and temporal variations of cancer mortality have also been analysed on an international scale.[25]

Despite the value of mortality data for epidemiologic study, reservations are often expressed about the quality of diagnoses reported on death certificates, even though most cancers diagnosed before death are properly recorded on the certificates.[26] However, changes in diagnostic and certification practices as well as in coding rules may produce spurious trends, and it is prudent to consider each observation on its merits. Death certificates are also of great value to epidemiologists in comparing the mortality of a specific group under study with that of the general population. It is important, however, that the death certificates of the study group be coded according to the same rules as for the standard or reference population.

Population-Based Registries

The complete ascertainment of all newly diagnosed cases of cancer in a defined population is a difficult and expensive task. There is no system for gathering incidence data for the entire United States, but such data have been collected for specific areas in different time periods. The longest ongoing population-based resource is the Connecticut Tumor Registry, which has incidence data available from 1935.[27] Several other registries covering states or cities have been in existence for varying time periods.

The NCI has coordinated several periodic surveys of cancer incidence in selected areas of the country. The first survey was in 1937–1939 and the second in 1947–1948,[28] with both covering the same 10 metropolitan areas and referred to as the Ten-Cities Surveys. Information was gathered on cases diagnosed during 1 calendar year in each of the areas, although the specific year varied among the areas. A special survey of cases diagnosed during 1950 was conducted in Iowa to compare cancer incidence patterns among rural and urban residents.[29] The Third National Cancer Survey included cases diagnosed during 1969–1971 in two states and seven cities.[30] Since 1973, the SEER program has included several population-based cancer registries that continuously gather information on cancer incidence, mortality, and survival.[10,31] The SEER registries cover more than 10% of the U.S. population. Although not a probability sample of the entire population, considerable geographic and ethnic variations are represented. It has been possible to evaluate the long-term trends in cancer incidence by focusing on the geographic areas common to the various surveys.[23,24] In other countries a number of cancer reporting systems have been in existence for varying lengths of time, starting with the Danish Cancer Registry in 1942. The International Agency for Research on Cancer has compiled data from many of the registries in five successive volumes of Cancer Incidence in Five Continents. This resource has been immensely valuable for proposing etiologic hypotheses.

In conjunction with the operation of a cancer registry, patients may be followed to ascertain their medical condition and vital status. Such survival data are useful in understanding incidence and mortality trends, and in measuring the dissemination and effect of treatment improvements in the general population. Although not population-based, the End Results Group of the NCI compiled survival data starting in 1950.[32,33] However, since the advent of the SEER program in 1973, it has been possible to continuously monitor population-based survival statistics.[34,35]

Hospital-Based Registries

Although hospital-based cancer registries are valuable for clinical, administrative, and educational purposes, the data have limited use for epidemiologic studies.[36] However, such a registry may be an important component of a population-based cancer reporting system, and provides a means of identifying patients for case-control studies. In addition, a hospital registry may be useful in investigating the natural history of cancer and the risk of developing second primary cancers, and in assembling a clinical series that may provide clues to environmental or genetic factors in cancer etiology.

PATTERNS OF CANCER OCCURRENCE

MAGNITUDE OF THE PROBLEM

In the United States, cancer is second only to heart disease as a cause of death and accounts for 22% of all deaths.[37] Among women aged 35 to 74, it is the leading cause of death. Almost one million newly diagnosed cases of cancer and nearly 500,000 deaths due to cancer are predicted for the United States during 1988 (Table 13-3). Lung cancer is the most common form, accounting for 15% of the cases and 28% of the deaths. Almost as many cases of colorectal cancer occur as lung cancer, but there are more than twice as many deaths from lung cancer. Next most common are cancers of the breast and prostate, so that these four cancers account for 54% and 55% of the total cancer cases and deaths, respectively. The 11 sites shown in Table 13-3 comprise 79% of all cancer cases and 75% of cancer deaths.

TABLE 13-3. Estimated New Cases and Deaths in the United States for Major Forms of Cancer—1988

	Number of Cases	*Number of Deaths*
All sites	985,000	494,000
Lung	152,000	139,000
Colon and rectum	147,000	61,500
Breast	135,900*	42,300
Prostate	99,000	28,000
Urinary tract	68,900	20,000
Uterus	46,900*	10,000
Oral cavity and pharynx	30,200	9,050
Skin	27,300†	7,800‡
Pancreas	27,000	24,500
Leukemia	26,900	18,100
Ovary	19,000	12,000
All other sites	204,900	121,750

From Silverberg E, Lubera JA: Cancer Statistics, 1988. CA 38:5, 1988. Based on incidence data from National Cancer Institute SEER program 1982–1984 and mortality data from the National Center for Health Statistics. All figures are rounded.

* Invasive cancers only; more than 5,000 carcinomas in situ of the breast and 50,000 carcinomas in situ of the cervix are estimated.

† Melanoma only; more than 500,000 nonmelanoma skin cancers are estimated.

‡ Melanoma 5,800; other skin cancers 2,000.

Table 13-4 presents the age-adjusted incidence and mortality rates for 44 forms of cancer among white males and females in the United States for the period 1981–1985. Among males the incidence and mortality rates are highest for lung cancer, followed by prostate and colon cancers, whereas among females the rates are highest for breast cancer, followed by cancers of the lung and colon. However, the differential between incidence and mortality is much less for lung cancer than for the other leading cancers, reflecting well-known survival differences. All cancers show higher rates among men except for those of the breast, gallbladder, and thyroid.

INTERNATIONAL VARIATION

It has been estimated that about 75% to 80% of all cancer in the United States is due to environmental factors.[6] To obtain this estimate, rates for the lowest-risk countries were subtracted from rates prevailing in the United States. It is convenient to regard the lowest risk as the baseline level for "spontaneous" tumors that in theory cannot be prevented.

Table 13-5 shows in rank form the international variation for a number of cancers based on recent statistics from volume 5 of Cancer Incidence in Five Continents.[38] The variation ranges from 155-fold for melanoma to fivefold for leukemia, and is not believed to be greatly affected by differences in diagnostic and reporting practices between countries.[3,6] Although genetic factors may play some role, as in melanoma, which tends to affect fair-skinned populations, the available evidence suggests that the international differences are mainly due to environmental factors. The patterns observed in Table 13-5 are in fact likely to underestimate the true global variation, since some regions with exceptionally high rates of certain cancers are not covered by registries, such as esophageal cancer in parts of China and Iran, liver cancer in parts of Africa and Asia, and urinary tract cancer in areas endemic with schistosomiasis or Balkan nephropathy.[3] Furthermore, the differences would be more pronounced if data were available for certain subtypes of cancer such as Burkitt's lymphoma and Kaposi's sarcoma, or subsites such as the gingival-buccal mucosa which comes in contact with smokeless tobacco and related products.

TABLE 13-4. Average Annual Age-Adjusted Incidence and Mortality Rates per 100,000 Among U.S. Whites by Primary Cancer Site, 1981–1985*

	Incidence (SEER)		*Mortality (U.S.)*	
	Males	*Females*	*Males*	*Females*
All sites	412.1	322.2	211.3	136.2
Lip	3.3	0.3	0.1	0.0
Salivary gland	1.1	0.7	0.3	0.2
Nasopharynx	0.6	0.2	0.4	0.1
Other oral cavity and pharynx	11.9	5.3	4.0	1.4
Esophagus	4.8	1.6	4.6	1.2
Stomach	11.0	4.9	7.1	3.3
Small intestine	1.1	0.8	0.4	0.3
Colon	41.6	32.3	21.2	15.4
Rectum	19.7	12.7	4.1	2.5
Liver	2.8	1.1	2.8	1.3
Gallbladder	0.8	1.6	0.6	1.1
Other biliary	1.6	1.1	1.2	0.9
Pancreas	10.9	8.1	10.1	6.9
Larynx	8.5	1.6	2.5	0.4
Lung and bronchus	82.7	33.8	71.4	24.4
Pleura	1.3	0.2	0.3	0.1
Nasal cavity and sinuses	0.8	0.5	0.3	0.1
Bones and joints	1.0	0.7	0.6	0.3
Soft tissue	2.5	1.7	1.2	1.0
Melanoma of skin	10.7	8.6	3.0	1.7
Other nonepithelial skin	2.5	0.7	1.2	0.3
Breast	0.8	95.7	0.2	27.1
Cervix uteri	—	7.9	—	2.9
Uterus excluding cervix	—	24.2	—	3.7
Ovary	—	14.1	—	8.0
Vagina	—	0.7	—	0.2
Vulva	—	1.6	—	0.3
Prostate	81.3	—	21.4	—
Testis	4.4	—	0.4	—
Penis	0.8	—	0.2	—
Bladder	30.5	7.8	6.4	1.8
Kidney	11.0	4.9	4.7	2.1
Ureter	1.0	0.3	0.2	0.1
Eye and orbit	0.9	0.7	0.1	0.1
Brain and other nervous system	7.5	5.2	5.0	3.5
Thyroid	2.3	5.6	0.3	0.4
Hodgkin's disease	3.5	2.6	1.0	0.6
Non-Hodgkin's lymphoma	14.2	10.2	6.8	4.7
Multiple myeloma	4.5	3.1	3.1	2.1
Acute lymphocytic leukemia	1.6	1.3	0.8	0.5
Chronic lymphocytic leukemia	4.1	2.0	1.7	0.7
Acute myeloid leukemia	3.3	2.2	2.5	1.7
Chronic myeloid leukemia	1.6	0.9	1.0	0.6
Other leukemias	2.6	1.3	2.7	1.6
Miscellaneous	14.8	11.4	15.7	10.8

* Rates age-adjusted based on the 1970 U.S. standard population. Incidence data from the National Cancer Institute SEER program, and national mortality data from the National Center for Health Statistics.

MIGRANT PATTERNS

Further evidence for environmental factors can be found in studies of migrant populations, such as the Japanese who moved to Hawaii and California. After migration, with the adoption of new habits, the risk of various cancers has moved away from the rate prevailing in the country of origin toward that of the new country.[39] Among Japanese migrants, increases in the risk of large bowel cancer were evident within a few decades of migration, whereas changes in breast cancer continue for generations. In contrast to general environmental exposures, lifestyle practices may change slowly among migrants, depending upon the speed and extent of acculturation.

Migrant patterns have been studied by comparing the cancer mortality rates in the U.S. white population by country of birth with the corresponding rates in the country of origin.[40] Figure 13-1 shows the age-adjusted mortality rates for colorectal and stomach cancers.[41] Stomach cancer rates among migrants are generally lower than in the country of

TABLE 13-5. International Variation in Cancer Incidence*

	Ratio (H/L)	High (H) Incidence Area	Rate†	Low (L) Incidence Area	Rate†
Melanoma	155	Australia (Queensland)	30.9	Japan (Osaka)	0.2
Lip	151	Canada (Newfoundland)	15.1	Japan (Osaka)	0.1
Nasopharynx	100	Hong Kong	30.0	U.K. (South Western)	0.3
Prostate	70	U.S. (Atlanta, black)	91.2	China (Tianjin)	1.3
Liver	49	China (Shanghai)	34.4	Canada (Nova Scotia)	0.7
Penis	42	Brazil (Recife)	8.3	Israel (Born Eur. and Am.)	0.2
Oral cavity	34	France (Bas-Rhin)	13.5	India (Poona)	0.4
Cervix uteri (F)	28	Brazil (Recife)	83.2	Israel (non-Jews)	3.0
Esophagus	27	France (Calvados)	29.9	Romania (Urban Cluj)	1.1
Stomach	22	Japan (Nagasaki)	82.0	Kuwait (Kuwaitis)	3.7
Thyroid	22	Hawaii (Chinese)	8.8	Poland (Warsaw City)	0.4
Multiple myeloma	22	U.S. (Alameda, black)	8.8	Phillipines (Rural)	0.4
Kidney	21	Canada (NWT and Yukon)	15.0	India (Poona)	0.7
Corpus uteri (F)	21	U.S. (Bay area, white)	25.7	India (Nagpur)	1.2
Lung	19	U.S. (New Orleans, black)	110.0	India (Madras)	5.8
Colon	19	U.S. (Connecticut, white)	34.1	India (Madras)	1.8
Testis	17	Switzerland (Urban Vaud)	10.0	China (Tianjin)	0.6
Bladder	16	Switzerland (Basel)	27.8	India (Nagpur)	1.7
Lymphosarcoma	12	Switzerland (Basel)	9.2	Japan (Rural Miyagi)	0.8
Pancreas	11	U.S. (Los Angeles, Korean)	16.4	India (Poona)	1.5
Hodgkin's disease	10	Canada (Quebec)	4.8	Japan (Miyagi)	0.5
Brain	9	N.Z. (Polynesian Islanders)	9.7	India (Nagpur)	1.1
Larynx	8	Brazil (Sao Paulo)	17.8	Japan (Rural Miyagi)	2.1
Ovary (F)	8	N.Z. (Polynesian Islanders)	25.8	Kuwait (Kuwaitis)	3.3
Rectum	8	Israel (Born Eur. and Am.)	22.6	Kuwait (Kuwaitis)	3.0
Breast (F)	7	Hawaii (Hawaiian)	93.9	Israel (non-Jews)	14.1
Leukemia	5	Canada (Ontario)	11.6	India (Nagpur)	2.2

From C. Muir and M. Parkin, International Agency for Research on Cancer, based on data abstracted from Muir C, Waterhouse J, Mack T, et al (eds): Cancer Incidence in Five Continents, Vol 5. Lyon, International Agency for Research on Cancer, 1987.

*Among males unless specified as females (F); rates based on less than 10 cases are excluded.

†Average annual rate per 100,000, age-adjusted based on the world standard population; rates generally are for the period 1978–1982.

origin, but higher than among U.S.-born whites. In contrast, colorectal cancer mortality in most countries is lower than in the United States, but the rates among migrants not only approach those of the U.S.-born whites but even exceed them in some instances. Those born in Mexico, however, have retained rates that are about 50% those of native-born white Americans. In addition, colorectal cancer mortality among the foreign-born has not reached U.S. rates as frequently for women as for men. When mortality from other cancers among the U.S. foreign-born is compared with statistics in the countries of origin, the rates for breast, corpus uteri, and prostate cancers are generally more closely aligned with those for U.S. native-born whites. Analytical studies among migrants should provide insights into lifestyle factors in cancer causation.

CANCER MAPS

Although variations within countries are not as great as those seen internationally, the computer-generated mapping of cancer death rates in the United States at the county level for the period 1950–1969 revealed a variety of high-risk areas[18,19] that have led to the investigation of environmental exposures. For example, as shown in Figure 13-2, the elevated rates for lung cancer among men along the eastern seaboard drew attention to the unexpected scale and impact of asbestos exposures in shipyards during World War II.[42] Similarly, a clustering of high-risk areas in Louisiana was traced in part to heavy smoking by the Cajun population.[43] Furthermore, studies of the elevated rates for oral cancer among women in the rural south, shown in Figure 13-3, have pointed to the hazards associated with the practice of snuff dipping.[44] A recent update of the cancer maps through the period 1970–1980 has revealed patterns resembling those in the earlier atlas, but with a tendency toward greater uniformity of rates around the country.[21] Yet some new clustering emerged, including elevated rates of lung and oral cancers among women in Florida and along the Pacific coast that seem related to smoking habits and high rates of non-Hodgkin's lymphoma in central regions that may be associated with agricultural exposure to herbicides.[45] The U.S. cancer maps were soon followed by similar atlases from other countries, the total reaching 15 at last count. Most remarkable are the maps from China that have disclosed dramatic variations in mortality and have stimulated a number of analytical studies in areas with exceptionally high rates.[46] In Scandinavian countries that have national cancer registries, atlases based on incidence data have been useful in identifying high-risk communities, particularly for less lethal tumors (*e.g.*, endometrium) that are not measured well by mortality statistics.

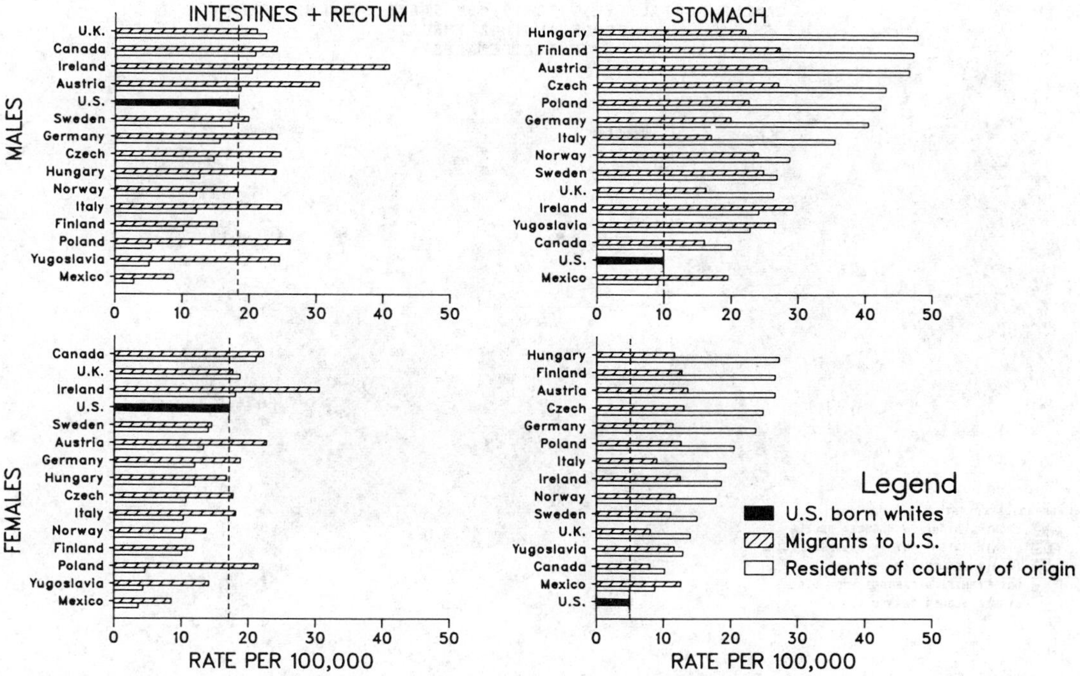

FIG. 13-1. Average annual mortality rates for intestinal and stomach cancers among U.S.-born whites, migrants from selected countries from 1959 to 1961, and residents of the countries of origin, 1960. Rates standardized for age on the 1950 U.S. population. (Data from Lilienfeld AM, Levin ML, Kessler II: Cancer in the United States. Cambridge, MA, Harvard University Press, 1972)

FIG. 13-2. Mapping of lung cancer mortality rates among white males for United States counties, 1950 to 1969. Rates standardized for age on the 1960 U.S. population. (Adapted from Mason TJ, McKay FW, Hoover R, et al: Atlas of Cancer Mortality for U.S. Counties: 1950–1969. DHEW Publication No. [NIH] 75–780. Washington, DC, US Government Printing Office, 1975)

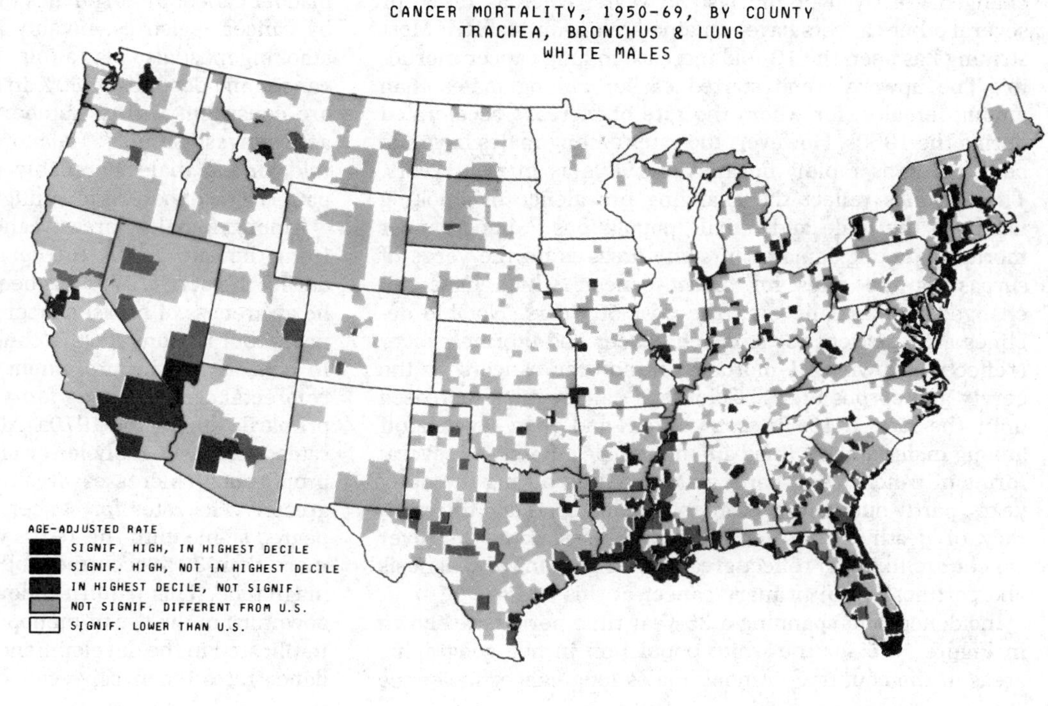

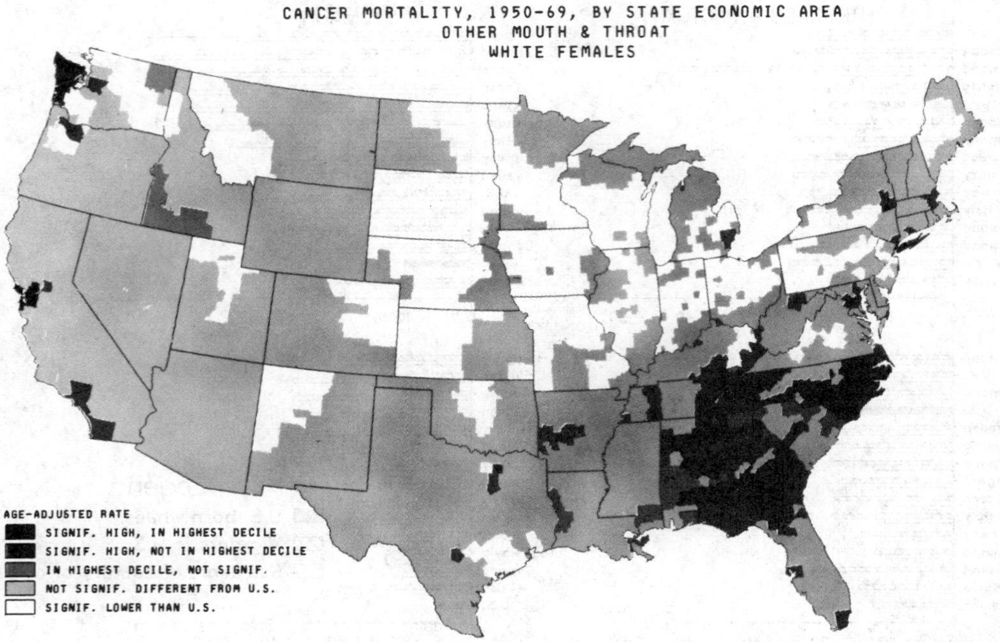

FIG. 13-3. Mapping of oral and pharyngeal cancer mortality rates among white females for United States counties, 1950 to 1969. Rates standardized for age on the 1960 U.S. population. (Adapted from Mason TJ, McKay FW, Hoover R, et al: Atlas of Cancer Mortality for U.S. Counties: 1950–1969. DHEW Publication No. [NIH] 75–780. Washington, DC, US Government Printing Office, 1975)

TIME TRENDS

A major indication of the importance of environmental factors lies in the variation in the mortality and incidence of certain cancers over time. As shown in Figure 13-4, mortality rates for some forms of cancer in the United States have changed greatly over the last 55 years, whereas rates for several other cancers have remained relatively stable.[37] Most striking has been the 10-fold increase in lung cancer mortality. The upward trend started earlier among males than among females, for whom the rate of increase accelerated during the 1960s. However, the rates among males have not been rising as rapidly during the 1980s as in prior years. These trends reflect the changing prevalence of smoking habits in the male and female populations.[47] Lung cancer mortality among females in some areas is on the verge of surpassing the rates for breast cancer, which have not changed substantially over the past 50 years. Notable declines are apparent for stomach cancer and uterine cancer (reflecting downward mortality trends for cancers of the cervix and corpus uteri). Colorectal cancer rates increased until the late 1940s in both sexes, and then leveled off among males and declined among females. Rates for several forms of cancer (*e.g.*, pancreas) increased during the early years, partly due to improvements in diagnosis and the accuracy of death certificates. The decreases noted for liver cancer are likely to reflect greater precision in the diagnosis and certification of primary cancer at this site.

Incidence data spanning a 35-year time period are shown in Figure 13-5 for the white population in five geographic areas of the country.[24] Among males lung cancer incidence increased almost 3% per year to become the most frequent form of cancer, but the decline in the most recent years may reflect a decrease in smoking prevalence. Prostatic cancer incidence increased substantially, particularly since 1970, which must be due at least partly to the improved detection of early-stage or latent carcinomas. Some of the increases in bladder cancer among males may be due to changing criteria by cancer registries, notably for papillomas, but trends in smoking must also play a role. Increases of 60% in colorectal cancer and declines of 69% in stomach cancer among males are consistent with a number of dietary hypotheses under active investigation.[48] Melanoma incidence rose nearly fourfold among males, probably due in part to the changing patterns of exposure to sunlight.[49]

Among females, breast cancer incidence increased 31% from the late 1940s to the mid-1980s. The striking rise during the early 1970s has been attributed to increased public awareness of breast cancer that precipitated earlier diagnoses, but reasons for the continuing increases are unclear. In contrast to the prominent upward trend among males, colorectal cancer among females increased only about 10%, primarily during the 1970s. Although lung cancer incidence rates are considerably lower among females than males, the proportional increases of almost 6% per year have been greater. The rates for cancer of the body of the uterus appeared stable until the 1970s when a substantial increase of more than 30% occurred, followed by decreases of similar magnitude. This pattern follows the upturn and subsequent downturn in the use of menopausal estrogens that have been implicated in the development of endometrial cancer.[50] Incidence rates for invasive cancer of the cervix uteri declined

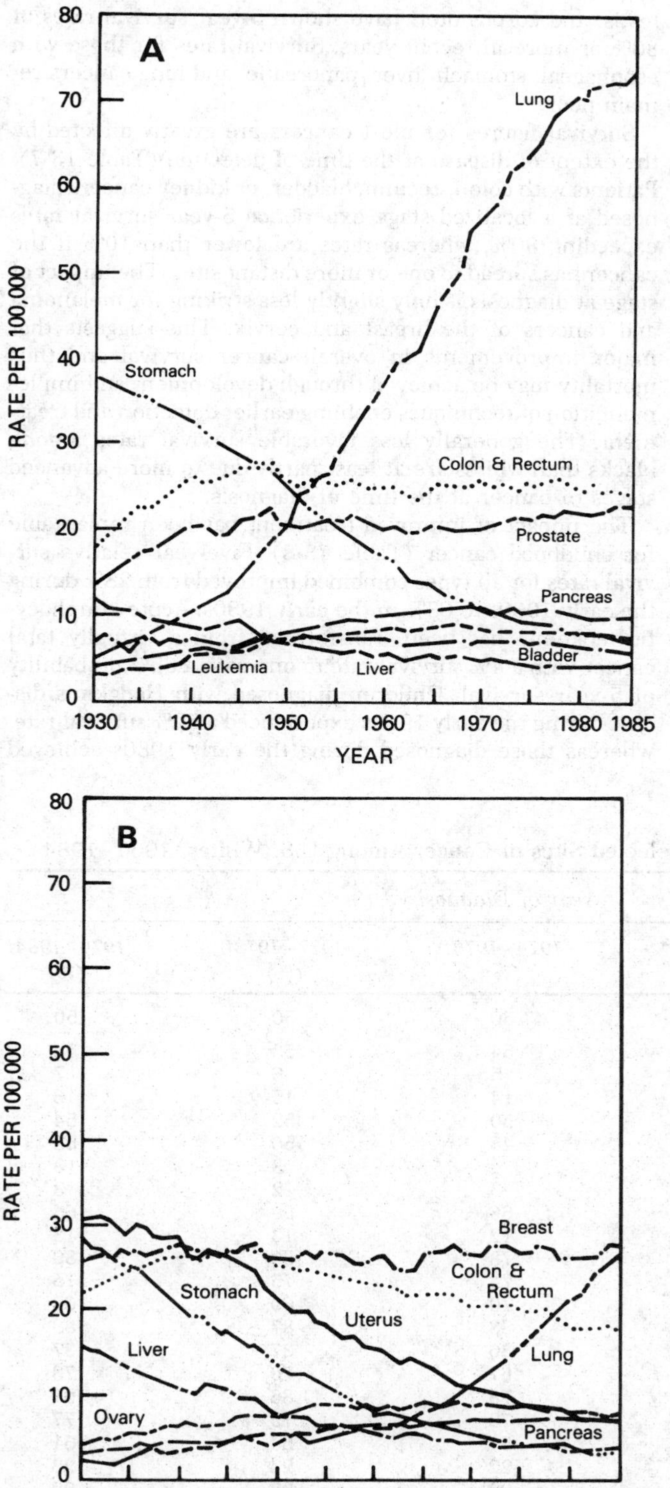

FIG. 13-4. Cancer mortality trends for selected sites in the United States population, 1930 to 1985, among males (**A**) and females (**B**). Rates standardized for age on the 1970 U.S. population. (Data from the National Center for Health Statistics and Bureau of the Census. Modified from Silverberg E, Lubera JA: Cancer Statistics, 1988. CA 38:5, 1988)

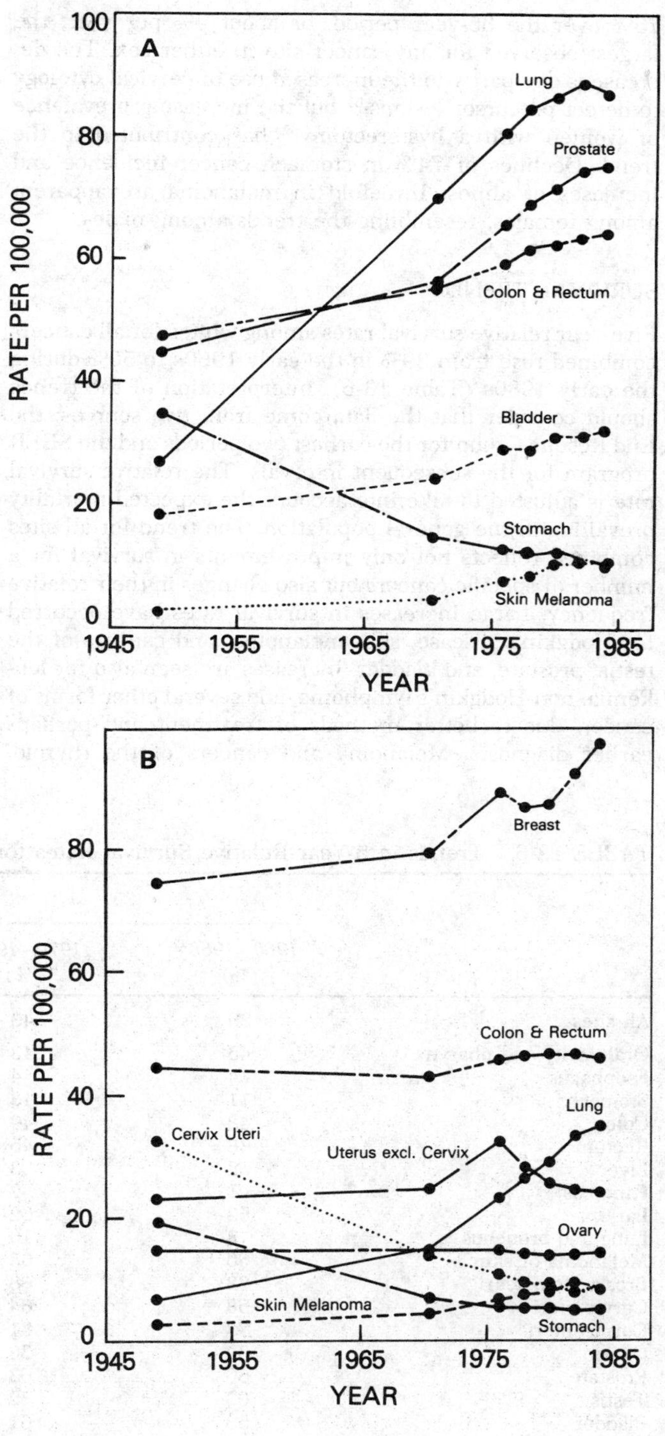

FIG. 13-5. Cancer incidence trends for selected sites in five geographic areas of the United States, 1947 to 1984, among white males (**A**) and white females (**B**). Rates standardized for age on the 1970 U.S. population. (Adapted from Devesa SS, Silverman DT, Young JL Jr, et al: Cancer incidence and mortality trends among whites in the United States, 1947–84. JNCI 79:701, 1987)

75% over the 35-year period, or about 4% per year, the largest observed for any cancer site in either sex. The decrease is due partly to the increased use of cervical cytology to detect precursor lesions,[51] but the increasing prevalence of women with a hysterectomy[52] has contributed to the trend. Declines of 74% in stomach cancer incidence and increases of almost threefold in melanoma are apparent among females, resembling the trends among males.

SURVIVAL TRENDS

Five-year relative survival rates among whites for all cancers combined rose from 39% in the early 1960s to 50% during the early 1980s (Table 13-6). Interpretation of the trends should consider that the data come from two sources: the End Results Group for the earliest two periods and the SEER program for the subsequent intervals. The relative survival rate is adjusted to take into account the expected mortality prevailing in the general population. The trend for all sites combined reflects not only improvements in survival for a number of specific cancers but also changes in their relative frequency. Large increases in survival rates have occurred for Hodgkin's disease, skin melanoma, and cancers of the testis, prostate, and bladder. Increases are seen also for leukemia, non-Hodgkin's lymphoma, and several other forms of cancer, due to better methods of treatment and perhaps earlier diagnosis. Melanoma and cancers of the thyroid, testis, and corpus uteri have shown 5-year survival rates of 80% or more in recent years. Survival rates for those with esophageal, stomach, liver, pancreatic, and lung cancers remain poor.

Survival figures for most cancers are greatly affected by the extent of disease at the time of detection (Table 13-7). Patients with colon, rectum, bladder, or kidney cancers diagnosed at a localized stage experience 5-year survival rates exceeding 80%, whereas rates are lower than 10% if the cancer has spread to one or more distant sites. The impact of stage at diagnosis is only slightly less striking for melanoma and cancers of the breast and cervix. This suggests that major improvements in overall cancer survival and thus mortality may be achieved through development and implementation of techniques enabling earlier detection and treatment. The generally less favorable survival rates among blacks than whites are at least partly due to more advanced stages of cancer at the time of diagnosis.

The impact of improved treatment has been remarkable for childhood cancer (Table 13-8). Five-year relative survival rates for all types combined improved from 28% during the early 1960s to 63% in the early 1980s. Acute lymphocytic leukemia has been transformed from a virtually fatal cancer with a 4% survival rate to one with a 65% probability of 5-year survival. Children diagnosed with Hodgkin's disease during the early 1960s experienced a 52% survival rate, whereas those diagnosed during the early 1980s achieved

TABLE 13-6. Trends in 5-Year Relative Survival Rates for Selected Sites of Cancer Among U.S. Whites, 1960–1984

	Year of Diagnosis				
	*1960–1963** (%)	*1970–1973** (%)	*1974–1976†* (%)	*1977–1978†* (%)	*1979–1984†* (%)
All sites	39	43	50	50	50
Oral cavity and pharynx	45	43	54	53	53
Esophagus	4	4	5	6	7
Stomach	11	13	14	15	16
Colon	43	49	50	52	54
Rectum	38	45	48	50	52
Liver	2	3	4	3	3
Pancreas	1	2	3	2	3
Larynx	53	62	66	69	66
Lung and bronchus	8	10	12	13	13
Melanoma of skin	60	68	78	80	80
Breast (females)	63	68	74	75	75
Cervix uteri	58	64	70	69	67
Corpus uteri	73	81	88	87	83
Ovary	32	36	36	37	37
Prostate	50	63	67	70	73
Testis	63	72	78	86	91
Bladder	53	61	73	75	77
Kidney	37	46	51	50	51
Brain and nervous system	18	20	22	23	23
Thyroid	83	86	92	92	92
Hodgkin's disease	40	67	71	73	74
Non-Hodgkin's lymphoma	31	41	47	48	49
Multiple myeloma	12	19	24	24	24
Leukemia	14	22	34	37	32

From National Cancer Institute: Annual Cancer Statistics Review Including Cancer Trends 1950–1985. Bethesda, MD, 1988.
* Rates based on data from the End Results Group using a series of hospital registries and one population-based registry.
† Rates based on data from the SEER program, with follow-up of patients through 1985.

TABLE 13-7. Five-Year Relative Survival Rates Among U.S. Whites for Selected Sites of Cancer According to Stage at Diagnosis, 1979–1984*

	Localized (%)	*Regional* (%)	*Distant* (%)
Oral cavity and pharynx	77	42	17
Esophagus	15	5	1
Stomach	57	15	2
Colon	87	58	6
Rectum	81	46	3
Pancreas	6	4	1
Larynx	81	53	24
Lung and bronchus	35	14	1
Melanoma of skin	90	52	12
Breast (females)	90	69	18
Cervix uteri	88	52	15
Corpus uteri	91	71	25
Ovary	84	45	20
Prostate	85	74	31
Testis	97	94	61
Bladder	89	45	8
Kidney	83	53	7
Thyroid	99	91	49

From National Cancer Institute: Annual Cancer Statistics Review Including Cancer Trends 1950–1985. Bethesda, MD 1988.
* Rates based on data from the SEER program, with follow-up of patients through 1985.

rates exceeding 90%. For Wilms' tumor, survival rates increased from 33% to 82% over the same period. The improvements in therapy and survival have resulted in dramatic declines in childhood cancer mortality in recent years.[53]

AGE CURVES

The marked rise in cancer incidence with advancing age has suggested in the past that some aspect of the aging process increases susceptibility to cancer, perhaps by impairing immune function. It is now considered, however, that the relationship of many cancers with increasing age mainly reflects the importance of duration of exposure to carcinogens and of long induction periods.[5] The age-specific incidence rates for cancers of individual sites are reproduced in Appendix Tables 13-1 to 13-4. The rates cover the years 1981 to 1985 for the SEER program of the NCI, and are given by sex and race (whites and blacks).

Figure 13-6 shows the age distribution for selected cancers in the white population, with incidence plotted on a semilog scale. Most epithelial cancers are rare under age 30 but then rise progressively with age (*e.g.*, cancers of the colon and rectum, prostate, and bladder), although at the oldest ages a slight downturn in the curve is probably related to underdiagnosis. For cancers of female reproductive sites, the rates appear to reach a plateau or decline at postmenopausal ages, consistent with an influence of endogenous hormones. Only a few nonepithelial cancers rise sharply with age, notably multiple myeloma and chronic lymphocytic leukemia.[5] Deviations from the usual age trend are illustrated by the cancers plotted in Figure 13-6C. Peaks for leukemia and nervous system cancer occur not only at older ages but also in early childhood, suggesting the influence of prenatal factors. The bimodal age curve for Hodgkin's disease has received much attention and there is some evidence suggesting that the young adult peak may result from an infectious agent.[54] Also intriguing is the pattern of testis cancer, with a peak occurrence among young adult men and a rising incidence over time that remains unexplained.[55] The rates for invasive cervical cancer increase sharply with age among young women, but then level off after age 35.

Table 13-9 shows the incidence rates for the major cancers among white children by age group and sex for the period 1981 to 1985. Except for lymphomas and bone tumors, the highest incidence occurs in children under 5 years of age. In general, boys have somewhat higher rates than girls in all three age groups, especially for the lymphomas.

TABLE 13-8. Trends in 5-Year Relative Survival Rates for Selected Forms of Cancer Among U.S. White Children Under 15 Years of Age, 1960–1984

	Year of Diagnosis				
	*1960–1963** (%)	*1970–1973** (%)	*1974–1976†* (%)	*1977–1978†* (%)	*1979–1984†* (%)
All forms	28	45	55	62	63
Acute lymphocytic leukemia	4	34	53	73	65
Acute myeloid leukemia	3	5	16	27	25
Wilms' tumor	33	70	74	80	82
Brain and nervous system	35	45	54	55	56
Neuroblastoma	25	40	48	46	56
Bone	20	30	52	53	48
Hodgkin's disease	52	90	80	82	91
Non-Hodgkin's lymphoma	18	26	43	44	60

From National Cancer Institute: Annual Cancer Statistics Review Including Cancer Trends 1950–1985. Bethesda, MD, 1988.
* Rates based on the End Results Group using a series of hospital registries and one population-based registry.
† Rates based on the SEER program, with follow-up of patients through 1985.

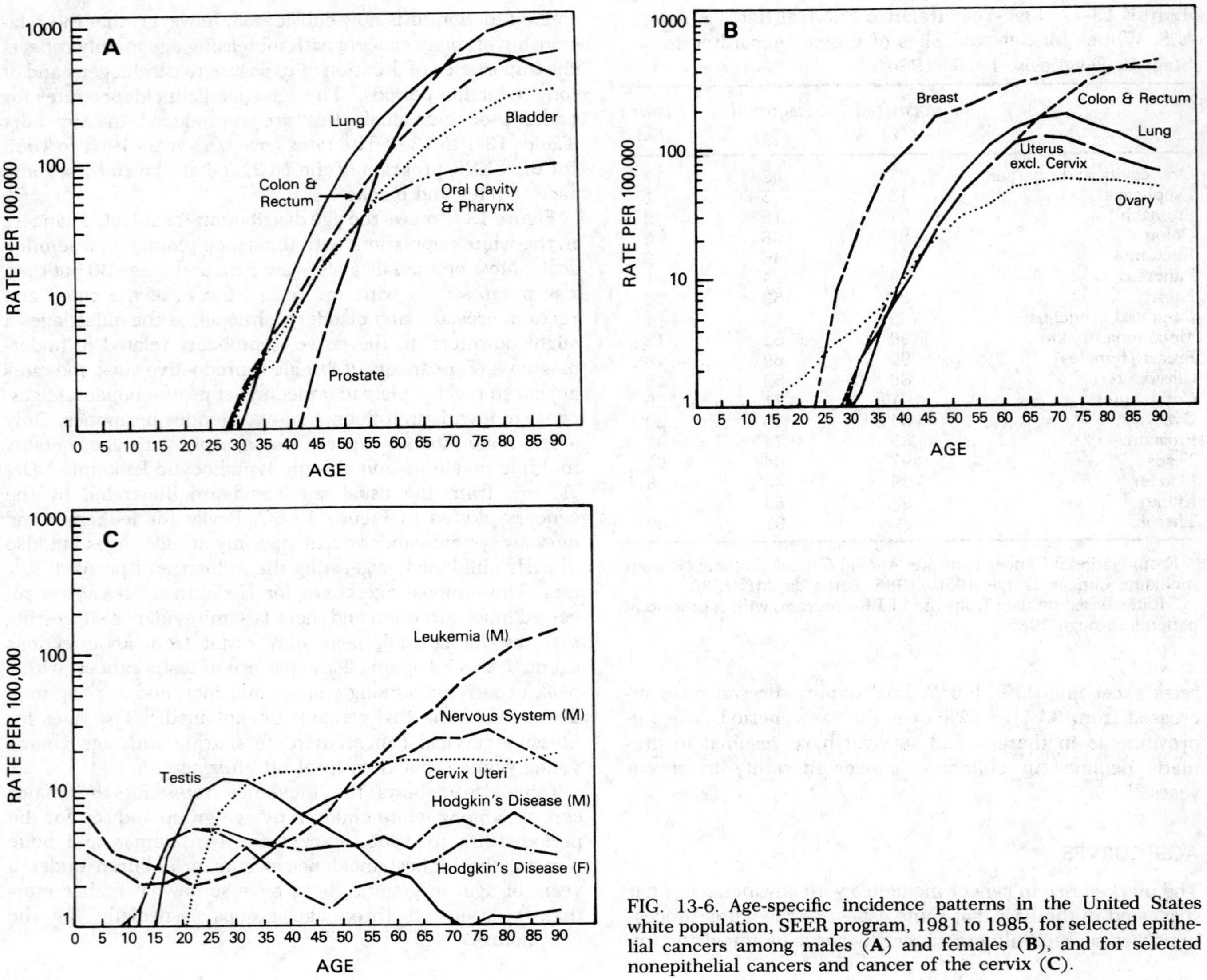

FIG. 13-6. Age-specific incidence patterns in the United States white population, SEER program, 1981 to 1985, for selected epithelial cancers among males (**A**) and females (**B**), and for selected nonepithelial cancers and cancer of the cervix (**C**).

TABLE 13-9. Age-Specific Incidence Rates for Selected Forms of Cancer Among U.S. White Children, 1981–1985*

	Boys			*Girls*		
	0–4	*5–9*	*10–14*	*0–4*	*5–9*	*10–14*
All forms	19.9	11.7	11.8	17.4	9.6	10.7
Leukemia	6.8	3.4	3.0	6.1	3.2	2.3
Brain and central nervous system	3.8	2.8	2.2	2.9	2.6	1.7
Lymphoma	0.8	2.5	3.2	0.3	0.4	1.8
Neuroblastoma	3.3	0.3	0.1	3.0	0.4	0.1
Soft tissue	0.8	0.5	0.6	0.8	0.2	0.6
Wilms' tumor	1.9	0.6	0.2	1.8	0.7	0.1
Bone	0.1	0.7	1.3	0.2	0.7	1.2
Retinoblastoma	1.0	0.1	0.0	1.1	0.1	0.0
All others	2.1	0.9	1.2	2.0	1.4	2.9

* Average annual rates per 100,000 population, based on data from the SEER program.

ETHNIC VARIATION

The SEER program provides data indicating striking racial and ethnic variations in cancer incidence in the United States (Table 13-10). For males, the rates for all cancers combined are highest in blacks, followed by whites and Hawaiians, whereas for females the rates are highest for Hawaiians, followed by whites and blacks. The lowest rates in both sexes are in American Indians. Compared to other groups, whites have especially high rates for melanoma, Hodgkin's disease, non-Hodgkin's lymphoma, leukemia, and cancers of the lip, breast, corpus uteri, ovary, testis, bladder, brain, colon, and rectum. Blacks have elevated rates for multiple myeloma and cancers of the oral cavity, esophagus, colon, pancreas, larynx, lung (males), cervix uteri, and prostate. Hispanics have especially high rates for cervix cancer, and to some extent for cancers of the stomach and biliary tract (females), whereas American Indians have remarkably high rates for cancers of the stomach, biliary tract, cervix, and kidney (females). Chinese experience elevated rates for cancers of the nasopharynx and liver, while Japanese have high rates for stomach cancer and (in males) for cancers of the colon, rectum, and thyroid. Filipinos have high rates for cancers of the thyroid, while Hawaiians show elevated rates for cancers of the lung (notably in females), breast, corpus uteri, stomach, and thyroid. Like migrant populations, the racial and ethnic variations in cancer occurrence within the United States offer special opportunities for studies aimed at clarifying the environmental and host determinants of cancer.

SOCIOECONOMIC PATTERNS

Whereas part of the racial and ethnic variations in rates may reflect genetic influences, many appear strongly influenced by environmental factors, some of which may be associated with socioeconomic status. Data from the Third National Cancer Survey[30] were used to estimate the associations of cancer incidence with median family income and educational achievement as indicated by census tract of residence, and to evaluate the impact of adjustment for socioeconomic disparities on the observed black/white relative risks.[56] Overall, cancer incidence rates among whites were 20% greater in the lowest income group than in the highest, with a continuous gradient in risk (Table 13-11). This pattern varied by primary site, however. Cervix cancer was almost four times as frequent among women in the lowest relative to the highest category, for reasons that are not entirely clear. Rates for esophageal cancer among men varied more than twofold, in line with socioeconomic differences in the use of alcohol and tobacco as well as nutritional status. Striking inverse gradients were also apparent for lung and stomach cancers among males, reflecting smoking and perhaps nutritional patterns. In contrast, positive gradients with income level were apparent for both breast and corpus uteri cancers, which may parallel the distribution of reproductive and menstrual risk factors.

An important question is the extent to which socioeconomic factors account for the black/white differentials in cancer incidence. When adjusted for racial variations in socioeconomic status, the excess risk among blacks is dimin-

TABLE 13-10A. Average Annual Age-Adjusted Incidence Rates per 100,000 for Selected Cancer Sites by Racial and Ethnic Group, 1975–1985, U.S. Males*

	Whites	*Blacks*	*Hispanics*	*American Indians*	*Chinese*	*Japanese*	*Filipinos*	*Hawaiians*
All sites	404.1	490.2	265.5	184.5	292.7	303.6	242.0	398.9
Lip	3.7	0.2	3.3	0.0	0.1	0.1	0.0	0.0
Nasopharynx	0.6	1.0	0.9	0.5	13.9	1.4	2.9	1.5
Other oral cavity and pharynx	11.8	20.5	5.2	1.7	6.2	6.0	6.8	10.1
Esophagus	4.9	18.4	2.9	1.9	6.1	5.6	4.9	15.1
Stomach	11.5	20.5	20.8	26.1	14.5	38.6	9.6	40.4
Colon	40.3	40.7	17.9	8.4	33.6	42.1	24.0	25.8
Rectum	20.0	14.9	11.5	5.0	19.3	23.4	16.9	18.7
Liver	2.7	5.2	4.3	4.5	19.5	7.1	10.2	9.8
Gallbladder	0.8	0.8	1.5	8.9	1.2	1.5	1.2	1.4
Other biliary	1.6	1.2	2.2	2.8	2.2	3.9	2.1	2.5
Pancreas	11.2	16.9	12.4	9.0	8.7	9.9	7.9	10.6
Larynx	8.6	12.3	4.2	1.1	2.9	3.9	2.8	6.5
Lung and bronchus	82.1	119.6	32.2	14.2	61.2	48.4	39.9	108.2
Melanoma of skin	9.8	0.8	1.6	2.2	0.4	1.5	1.2	1.6
Prostate	77.3	122.8	71.5	45.5	32.5	45.7	47.4	59.6
Testis	4.2	0.8	3.0	1.8	1.9	1.3	0.5	2.6
Bladder	30.2	15.1	10.9	3.6	13.9	12.5	6.0	10.6
Kidney	10.3	9.6	8.7	9.2	4.9	6.1	4.6	6.9
Brain and other nervous system	7.3	4.3	4.9	3.1	3.0	3.1	3.4	3.1
Thyroid	2.3	1.4	2.9	2.3	4.5	6.2	6.8	7.4
Hodgkin's disease	3.5	2.7	3.3	0.7	0.8	0.8	1.7	1.4
Non-Hodgkin's lymphoma	13.0	8.5	6.9	4.7	10.2	9.2	9.8	10.9
Multiple myeloma	4.6	10.3	2.8	2.7	2.2	1.7	4.6	5.9
Leukemia	13.8	11.1	7.8	5.5	7.7	6.9	8.8	9.5
All others	27.8	30.7	21.8	18.7	21.3	16.6	18.0	28.6

* Based on data from the SEER program. Data for Hispanics and American Indians are from New Mexico, whereas those for Chinese, Japanese, and Filipinos are from San Francisco and Hawaii. Rates age-adjusted based on the 1970 U.S. standard population.

TABLE 13-10B. Average Annual Age-Adjusted Incidence Rates per 100,000 for Selected Cancer Sites by Racial and Ethnic Group 1975–1985, U.S. Females*

	Whites	*Blacks*	*Hispanics*	*American Indians*	*Chinese*	*Japanese*	*Filipinos*	*Hawaiians*
All sites	316.1	296.6	220.4	168.8	242.2	214.0	202.6	344.1
Lip	0.3	0.1	0.4	0.0	0.0	0.1	0.0	0.0
Nasopharynx	0.3	0.5	0.2	0.0	6.7	0.3	1.6	1.1
Other oral cavity and pharynx	5.2	6.2	1.7	0.6	1.3	2.1	5.3	5.3
Esophagus	1.6	5.0	0.8	0.3	1.2	0.8	1.9	2.2
Stomach	5.1	8.5	10.0	12.3	8.7	19.0	7.2	17.9
Colon	32.3	35.0	16.7	8.1	23.7	25.7	14.9	16.3
Rectum	12.8	10.8	7.6	3.2	10.9	10.9	8.1	8.1
Liver	1.1	1.7	1.9	2.6	4.7	2.4	3.2	2.7
Gallbladder	1.6	1.1	7.1	17.1	1.0	1.7	1.8	1.3
Other biliary	1.1	0.8	1.3	4.4	1.9	2.4	0.7	2.6
Pancreas	7.7	11.5	10.8	4.3	7.8	6.0	4.8	9.2
Larynx	1.5	2.2	0.9	0.0	0.2	0.2	0.7	1.6
Lung and bronchus	29.7	31.2	15.6	4.6	27.6	13.2	17.9	45.8
Melanoma of skin	8.2	0.7	2.2	0.7	0.7	1.0	0.9	1.0
Breast	91.5	76.4	50.9	25.6	58.7	57.1	45.6	104.6
Cervix uteri	8.8	19.7	17.1	20.0	10.5	5.8	10.8	14.5
Uterus excluding cervix	27.1	14.8	11.2	5.2	18.2	17.6	11.0	28.0
Ovary	14.1	9.8	11.3	8.9	10.3	8.5	9.7	13.2
Bladder	7.7	5.5	3.3	0.4	4.0	4.4	3.1	6.0
Kidney	4.7	4.6	4.2	6.2	2.5	2.2	2.2	2.8
Brain and other nervous system	5.1	2.9	2.4	1.8	2.7	2.2	1.3	4.2
Thyroid	5.5	3.5	7.9	6.1	6.9	6.6	17.3	13.7
Hodgkin's disease	2.6	1.2	1.3	0.5	0.8	0.3	1.3	0.9
Non-Hodgkin's lymphoma	9.6	5.7	5.5	4.8	6.5	5.9	7.1	6.6
Multiple myeloma	3.1	6.8	2.8	2.2	1.7	1.3	2.6	5.6
Leukemia	8.0	7.0	6.3	4.5	4.7	5.1	6.4	7.0
All others	20.2	23.6	18.8	24.4	18.1	11.1	15.3	22.2

* Based on data from the SEER program. Data for Hispanics and American Indians are from New Mexico, whereas those for Chinese, Japanese, and Filipinos are from San Francisco and Hawaii. Rates age-adjusted based on the 1970 U.S. standard population.

ished for cancers of the esophagus, stomach, lung, and cervix. Socioeconomic status may also influence cancer survival and mortality patterns by affecting access to diagnosis and treatment.

ANALYTICAL STUDIES

The major contribution of epidemiology has been to test etiologic hypotheses through analytical studies, usually involving cohort or case-control designs. These studies obtain data on suspected risk factors and disease occurrence at the individual instead of at the aggregate (population) level. By using specific methods to select and compare groups of subjects, while controlling for other relevant variables, the risk of disease associated with exposure can be estimated.[4,13,14] In designing these studies, the groups should be sufficiently large and the time intervals between initial exposure and tumor onset sufficiently long to identify the lowest excess risk considered important to detect. Reliable and valid estimates of exposure should be sought, with quantitative measurements to permit dose-response evaluations. Studies must

TABLE 13-11. Relative Risks (RR) for All Cancers and Selected Sites by Socioeconomic Status (SES) and Race, 1969–1971*

	Income Level Among Whites					*Black/White RR*	
	Low	2	3	4	*High*	*SES Unadjusted*	*SES Adjusted†*
All sites (males)	1.20	1.09	1.07	1.02	1.00	1.10	1.0
Esophagus (males)	2.13	1.69	1.34	1.20	1.00	3.05	2.3
Stomach (males)	1.39	1.26	1.16	1.02	1.00	1.48	1.2
Lung (males)	1.65	1.44	1.33	1.18	1.00	1.10	0.9
Breast (females)	0.70	0.73	0.80	0.83	1.00	0.85	0.8
Cervix uteri	3.82	2.69	1.95	1.39	1.00	1.74	1.2
Corpus uteri	0.75	0.83	0.88	0.89	1.00	0.70	0.6

* Data derived from the Third National Cancer Survey, 1969–1971. All relative risks adjusted for age and geographic area.
† Also adjusted for income and education.

be designed to minimize potential sources of bias (*i.e.*, systematic error), and to permit the detection and control of confounding (*i.e.*, the distortion of exposure-disease associations by extraneous variables).

COHORT STUDIES

Cohort studies, also referred to as follow-up studies or prospective studies, identify groups of individuals with and without a particular exposure, follow them over time to determine subsequent health outcomes, and compare their mortality or incidence rates of disease.[4,57] An association is suggested when the rates of disease are different in the exposed than in the unexposed group. These investigations may be based on current exposures and future health outcomes, referred to as a prospective cohort study; but more often they use information on exposures collected in the past, termed a retrospective cohort study. Instead of an unexposed comparison group, general population mortality or incidence rates (specific for age, sex, race, geographic area, and calendar time) are often used to estimate an expected number of events. This method assumes that in the absence of the specific exposure of interest the study group would have the same probability of developing the disease as the general population. The cohort approach is used mainly when it is possible to evaluate high exposures in clearly defined subgroups of the population. It has been especially helpful, for example, in assessing the carcinogenic risk from occupational hazards, smoking, or medical exposures such as radiation and certain drugs.

CASE-CONTROL STUDIES

Case-control studies, also called case-referent studies or retrospective studies, identify persons with a particular disease (cases) and a group of similar persons without the disease (controls), and then collect information on past exposures by interview or other methods.[4,57] If the proportion of cases with a certain exposure is greater than that of the controls, an association may be indicated. The case-control approach is especially well-suited for studying uncommon diseases. Although used primarily to test hypotheses, the approach occasionally has taken the form of an exploratory study when a disease is so poorly understood that hypotheses need to be formulated for subsequent investigation. In general, it is desirable that both cases and controls are selected from the same source, which may be either population-based or hospital-based. However, since factors associated with hospitalization may be over-represented among hospital controls, careful consideration should be given to the diagnostic composition of this group. Bias is minimized by selecting hospital controls with a variety of disorders and excluding conditions related to the exposure in question.[58]

COMPARISON OF METHODS

The case-control and cohort methods have different strengths and weaknesses. Case-control studies provide a more efficient means of studying rare diseases, with fewer individuals needed, a shorter study period, and generally lower costs as compared with the cohort approach. In addition, there are greater opportunities to evaluate more than one risk factor and interactions between them.[59] On the other hand, the case-control approach cannot directly estimate the actual rate associated with a particular exposure, and is subject to recall and other biases that affect the comparability of cases and controls and the precision of past exposure measures.[4] Such studies also are usually limited to evaluating one disease at a time.

The advantages of cohort studies are their capacity to measure directly incidence or mortality rates associated with a particular exposure; to reduce subjective biases by obtaining information before the disease develops; to detect associations between a particular exposure and multiple outcomes; and to evaluate temporal relationships such as latency period and the duration of an effect. However, cohort studies are usually expensive and complex undertakings. They require large numbers of exposed individuals, particularly when uncommon diseases are being investigated, and care in dealing with such problems as persons lost to follow-up or with biased estimates of risk, as produced for example by the healthy worker effect of occupational studies.[4] Moreover, they may not permit as ready an ascertainment of potential confounding factors. To remedy this particular deficiency, case-control studies within defined cohorts, or nested case-control studies, are often initiated.

MEASURES OF ASSOCIATION

For cohort studies, the chief measures of association are based on rates of disease. The relative risk (RR) or risk ratio is the disease rate in the exposed, I_e, divided by the disease rate in the referent (usually nonexposed, I_o) population.[4] As illustrated by Table 13-12, the relative risk from a cohort study is defined as

$$RR = I_e I_o = \frac{a}{n_e} \frac{c}{n_o}$$

This measure gives the relative disease risk between two populations. Thus, an RR of 2.0 would indicate that the exposed group has twice the risk of the unexposed group (*i.e.*, a 100% increase in risk). An important aspect of the calculation is the concept of person-time. Usually individuals are followed for different periods owing to variable times of entry to and exit from observation because of either death or loss to follow-up. In order to accommodate the variable follow-up periods and still preserve the concept of a rate, each person is counted in the denominator only for the interval of time under observation, resulting in measures of person-years or person-months.[4]

An association may also be measured by the risk difference, often referred to as the attributable risk (A_e). This estimate results from the subtraction of the rate among the unexposed from that among the exposed. From Table 13-12, the attributable risk is defined as

$$A_e = I_e - I_o = \frac{a}{n_e} - \frac{c}{n_o}$$

The attributable risk means that if the relationship observed is causal, the difference between the rates of exposed

TABLE 13-12. Measures of Association from a Cohort Study

	Affected Persons (Cases)	*Total Persons (Person-Time)*
Exposed	a	n_e
Not Exposed	c	n_o
Total	a + c	N

Relative risk (RR) $= \frac{a}{n_e} \Big/ \frac{c}{n_o}$

Attributable risk in the exposed $(A_e) = \frac{a}{n_e} - \frac{c}{n_o}$

Attributable risk percent in the exposed $(A_e\%) = \frac{(a/n_e) - (c/n_o)}{a/n_e} = \frac{RR\text{-}1}{RR} \times 100\%$

Population attributable risk $(A_p) = \frac{a+c}{N} - \frac{c}{n_o}$

Population attributable risk percent $(A_p\%) = \frac{(a+c)/N\text{-}(c/n_o)}{(a+c)N} = \frac{RR\text{-}1}{RR + 1/P\text{-}1} \times 100\%$

where P is the proportion of the population that is exposed, or n_e/N

and unexposed groups is the amount of disease attributable to that exposure.[4] When expressed as a percentage of the total disease rate in an exposed group, the attributable risk percent ($A_e\%$) is the proportion of the exposed group's total risk that is due to the exposure.[60]

The measures of relative risk and attributable risk have somewhat different uses. The magnitude of the RR indicates the strength of a relationship between exposure and disease and the likelihood of causality. The A_e is influenced not only by the magnitude of the difference between the exposed and unexposed but also by the rate of disease in the absence of exposure.

The amount of disease attributable to a particular exposure can be estimated not only among the exposed but also in the population as a whole.[60] This measure would thus reflect the amount of disease that would be eliminated in a definable population if the exposure were removed, and is referred to as the population attributable risk (A_p). It is calculated by subtracting the rate among the unexposed from the rate that exists in the total population. Again, from Table 13-12, the population attributable risk is defined as

$$A_p = I_t - I_o = \frac{a+c}{N} - \frac{c}{n_o}$$

Thus, the magnitude of this estimate is influenced by the size of the relative difference in risk between the exposed and unexposed, by the level of the disease among the unexposed, and by the prevalence of the exposure in the population. When the attributable risk is expressed as a proportion of the total disease rate in population, it is called the population attributable risk percent ($A_p\%$) or the etiologic fraction.[61]

These measures are illustrated by a recent cohort study involving 1-year survivors of ovarian cancer from five randomized trials.[62] The incidence rates for acute nonlymphocytic leukemia and preleukemia were evaluated among women treated with no chemotherapy, with cyclophosphamide, and with melphalan. The corresponding rates were 0.18, 3.21, and 11.46 cases per 1000 women per year. Compared to those receiving no chemotherapy, the RR of leukemic conditions was 18 (3.21/0.18) for women given cyclophosphamide and 64 (11.46/0.18) for those given melphalan. The magnitude of these risks suggests that the drugs are causally related to leukemia. However, the risk differences obtained by subtracting rates among the exposed from the unexposed groups were not very great. The A_e associated with cyclophosphamide is about 3 per 1000 per year, and with melphalan about 11 per 1000 per year. Given the life-threatening problems posed by ovarian cancer, these risks should not deter physicians from using therapy whose proven benefit outweighs these risks. Also, when the A_e is not large, one can see how difficult it is for an individual clinician, or even a large group practice, to suspect a leukemia risk related to treatment.

If exposure to all alkylating agents were removed, it would have very little impact on the total leukemia rate in the general population, for relatively few persons are exposed to these drugs. However, in the clinical populations under study, the overall rate of leukemic conditions was 2.29 per 1000 patients per year. As shown in Table 13-13, subtracting the rate among those not treated with chemotherapy (.18 per 1000 per year) from the rate for all patients combined yields a population attributable risk of 2.11 cases per 1000 women per year, or an etiologic fraction of 92% in the clinical populations.

For case-control studies, the enumeration of exposed and unexposed populations is not available, as it is in cohort studies, to directly measure rates (or risks). Fortunately, data from cross-classification tables in a case-control study can be used to calculate reasonable estimates of relative and attributable risks. If the sampling fractions for the cases and the controls are known (*i.e.*, the proportion of all the cases in a defined population that is present in the case series, and the proportion of the same population present in the control series), these can be used to estimate the rates among the exposed and unexposed groups and thus to calculate relative and attributable risks. For most case-control studies, however, sampling fractions are unknown. In this circumstance,

TABLE 13-13. Risks of Leukemia and Preleukemia Associated with Chemotherapy

	Cases	*Person-Years at Risk*	*Rate per 1,000*
Any Chemotherapy	33	4,295	7.68
No Chemotherapy	2	10,983	0.18
Total	35	15,278	2.29

$$\text{Relative risk (RR)} = \frac{33/4{,}279}{2/10{,}983} = \frac{7.68}{0.18} = 42.4$$

$$\text{Attributable risk in the exposed } (A_e) = 33/4{,}279 - 2/10{,}983 = 7.40 \text{ per } 1{,}000$$

$$\text{Attributable risk percent in the exposed } (A_e\%) = \frac{42.4\text{-}1}{42.4} \times 100\% = 98\%$$

$$\text{Population attributable risk } (A_p) = \frac{35}{15{,}278} - \frac{2}{10{,}983} = 2.11 \text{ per } 1{,}000$$

$$\text{Population attributable risk percent } (A_p\%) = \frac{35/15{,}278\text{-}2/10{,}983}{35/15{,}278} \times 100\% = 92\%$$

Adapted from Greene MH, Harris EL, Gershenson DM, et al: Melphalan may be a more potent leukemogen than cyclophosphamide. Ann Intern Med 105:360, 1986.

as shown in Table 13-14, the calculation of relative odds, also termed an odds ratio, usually gives a good approximation of the relative risk.[4] The absolute measures of attributable risk cannot be estimated directly, but algebraic properties of cross-classification tables allow estimations of the attributable risk percent and the etiologic fraction[60] as shown in Table 13-14.

Calculation of these measures is illustrated in Table 13-15, based on a national case-control study of bladder cancer that evaluated the risks associated with smoking.[63] The study estimated a relative risk of 2.2 for cigarette smoking, with 55% of bladder cancer among smokers attributable to their smoking and 43% of bladder cancer in the U.S. population due to smoking. These figures are consistent with the direct estimates of risk from cohort studies.

INTERVENTION STUDIES

Also referred to as experimental studies,[57] controlled intervention trials represent a third strategy of analytical epidemiology that is especially useful for confirming causal relationships suggested by cohort or case-control studies and for directly evaluating the effect of possible preventive measures. This method permits control over extraneous variables and biases that may influence results by the random allocation of subjects to study and control groups. There are no clear guidelines as to when evidence is sufficient to conduct intervention trials, yet when there is a reasonable likelihood of benefit resulting from intervention (as well as any potential for harm), ethical questions may arise. In the field of cancer etiology and prevention, opportunities for inter-

TABLE 13-14. Measures of Association from a Case-Control Study

	Cases	*Controls*
Exposed	a	b
Not exposed	c	d
Total	a + c	b + d

$$\text{Relative odds (R)} = \frac{ad}{bc}$$

$$\text{Attributable risk percent in the exposed } (A_e\%) = \frac{R\text{-}1}{R} \times 100\%$$

$$\text{Population attributable risk percent } (A_p\%) \text{ or etiologic fraction} = \frac{P_o\,(R\text{-}1)}{1 + P_o\,(R\text{-}1)} \times 100\%$$

$$= \frac{(R-1)P_e}{R} \times 100\%$$

where P_o is the exposure rate in the controls, or $\frac{b,}{b+d}$ and P_e is the exposure rate

in the cases, or $\frac{a}{a+c}$

TABLE 13-15. Risks of Bladder Cancer Associated with Cigarette Smoking

	Cases	Controls
Smokers	2324	3581
Nonsmokers	657	2198
Total	2981	5779

$$\text{Relative odds (R)} = \frac{(2324)(2198)}{(657)(3581)} = 2.2$$

$$\text{Attributable risk percent in the exposed } (A_e\%) = \frac{2.2\text{-}1}{2.2} \times 100\% = 55\%$$

$$\text{Population attributable risk percent } (A_p\%) \text{ or etiologic fraction} = \frac{\frac{3581}{5779}(2.2\text{-}1)}{1 + \frac{3581}{5579}(2.2\text{-}1)} \times 100\%$$

$$= 43\%$$

$$\text{Alternatively, } \frac{(2.2\text{-}1)}{2.2} \times \frac{2324}{2981} \times 100\% = 43\%$$

Adapted from Hartge P, Silverman D, Hoover R, et al: Changing cigarette habits and bladder cancer risk: A case-control study. JNCI 78:1119, 1987.

vention have been limited for various reasons, including the long latency periods that may be involved before an effect is seen. However, intervention studies are now gaining emphasis in the evaluation of diet and nutrition, especially the use of various micronutrient supplements that may inhibit late stages of the carcinogenic process. Also underway are hepatitis-B vaccine trials in endemic areas for liver cancer. After intervention the follow-up and analytical procedures to evaluate outcomes resemble those employed for cohort studies.

STRENGTHS AND LIMITS OF EPIDEMIOLOGY

STRENGTHS

In contrast to laboratory studies, epidemiology directly evaluates the experience of human populations and their response to various environmental exposures and host factors (the risk of disease). Thus, the consequences of an exposure can be measured as it actually occurs in the population. Questionable extrapolations from other species are also avoided. Although positive findings from animal studies may indicate a potential human risk, epidemiology offers the only means of quantifying the risk. Furthermore, even when the specific causal agent cannot be clearly identified (*e.g.*, the precise carcinogens in cigarette smoke), sufficient information can be obtained for the disease to be prevented.

LIMITATIONS

However, cancer epidemiology has certain limitations. First, studies are mainly observational, relying on natural occurrences in human populations, and the opportunities for experiment are rare and limited to efforts at prevention. Second, epidemiology can seldom indicate a cause with great specificity, particularly when the exposures are multiple or when surrogate measures of exposure are used (*e.g.*, occupation or area of residence), though laboratory techniques may be helpful in such circumstances. Third, study groups chosen on the basis of one characteristic may be distinctive in another, and it may be difficult to disentangle them even with refined analytical methods. Fourth, it is hard to incriminate an agent when there is relative uniformity of exposure in a given population, which may be the case with some dietary factors (*e.g.*, high fat intake). Finally, evidence of an environmental hazard is usually obtained from high or intermediate levels of exposure. As in animal studies, it is difficult to detect causal relationships when the exposure level is low or the excess risk is small compared to the baseline incidence rate. In such situations, the numbers of subjects needed to provide definite results may be virtually impossible to assemble for the purposes of a single study.

BIOCHEMICAL EPIDEMIOLOGY

The power of certain studies may be increased by incorporating laboratory methods into analytical investigations, so-called biochemical or molecular epidemiology.[64,65] The analysis of biological samples in the laboratory can obviously permit the study of exposure to oncogenic viruses. It may also be possible to detect past exposures to chemical and physical agents and to clarify early preneoplastic events, various host factors, and mechanisms of action. At present the approach is providing new opportunities to evaluate carcinogenic risks associated with dietary factors and with markers of genetic predisposition. In view of rapid experimental advances, biochemical epidemiology represents a challenging multidisciplinary approach that should help to elucidate further the causes of cancer. Such studies are complex undertakings that require careful planning and teamwork, including the collaboration of clinicians.

SOURCES OF CLUES

Since an analytical study is designed to evaluate an association between a disease and an antecedent factor, there must be some prior indication or suspicion of such an association. The lead may come from descriptive or correlational studies or from another analytical study. However, the most fruitful source of etiologic clues has been the alert clinician who has uncovered some of the most striking examples of environmental cancer, starting with Pott's discovery of scrotal cancer among chimney sweeps. Usually the clinician recognizes an excessive number of patients with the same tumor and traces the cluster to a particular cultural, occupational, or iatrogenic exposure.[2] Thus, clinical observations have linked asbestos with mesothelioma, vinyl chloride with hepatic angiosarcoma, furniture-making with nasal adenocarcinoma, radium-dial painting with osteosarcoma, and prenatal exposure to diethylstilbestrol with clear-cell adenocarcinoma of the vagina among the offspring. It was possible for clinicians to detect these associations because they involved tumors that are rare in the general population and they also involved exceptionally high risks. In most instances the associations hardly required epidemiologic study for their confirmation, but only to quantify them. Clinicians have also identified a wide variety of heritable conditions associated with susceptibility to cancer.[66] Opportunities for the practicing physician to make significant etiologic discoveries were highlighted recently at a symposium sponsored by the Princess Takamatsu Cancer fund, entitled "Rare Events as Clues to Cancer Etiology."[67] On the other hand, epidemiologists can identify causes of cancer that may seem less dramatic in relative risks but are very important to public health, such as smoking and asbestos in lung cancer.

Another source of leads has been provided by experimental studies, especially those relating chemicals to tumors in laboratory animals. In the case of mustard gas and 4-aminobiphenyl, for example, carcinogenic risks were found in humans after the substances were shown to induce tumors in animal studies.[2] Whatever the sequence of observations, there is no question that clinical, epidemiologic, and experimental data greatly complement one another in determining the risks and mechanisms involved in carcinogenesis. When all approaches are brought to bear on a particular hypothesis, advances in understanding the carcinogenic process may be extraordinary.

INTERPRETATION OF EPIDEMIOLOGIC STUDIES

SAMPLE SIZE AND POWER

A fundamental aspect of planning or evaluating a study is the number of subjects needed to test an etiologic hypothesis.[13] The power of a study is the likelihood of detecting a postulated level of risk. The larger the sample size, the greater the power to detect a specified risk, and conversely, the smaller the sample size, the weaker the power.

The issues of sample size and power are of great concern when evaluating negative results of epidemiologic studies.[68] Only large studies may confidently exclude low to moderate levels of risk, whereas negative results of a small study should be viewed with caution because they usually lack adequate power.

NONCAUSAL ASSOCIATIONS

When interpreting the results of analytical studies, one must ask whether the associations observed between exposure and disease are the result of bias, confounding, chance, or cause-and-effect. Bias or systematic error is usually the result of imperfections in study design or conduct, and often cannot be corrected in the analysis. Many types of bias have been described,[69] but most can be grouped as biases of selection or information.[58] Selection bias involves systematic differences in exposure between those selected and not selected into the study. For example, a case-control study might include only cases referred to a particular institution or only survivors, so that differences observed might reflect factors influencing referral patterns or survival. A similar bias in a cohort study may result from differences in the loss to follow-up between exposed and unexposed groups. Information bias involves differences in measuring the factor in question between groups, and is best illustrated by recall bias or interviewer bias, both of which may affect the outcome of case-control studies. For example, in studies of childhood cancer, parents of cases might provide more reliable or thorough responses than parents of controls because of the soul-searching they had undergone. Also, interviewers might tend to probe more deeply into past events if a subject is known to be a case rather than a control.

Confounding refers to the effect of an extraneous variable that may account, entirely or partly, for an apparent association between exposure and disease, or may obscure a real association.[13,58] Confounding can usually be evaluated and accommodated during analysis by adjustment procedures, including the stratification of subjects on the suspected variable. To be a confounder, a variable must be related to the exposure and related causally to the disease. For example, cigarette smoking could contribute to an excess of lung cancer among some industrial groups if they smoke more heavily than the average. Conversely, a relationship between oral contraceptives and invasive cervical cancer became apparent only after adjustment was made for interval since last Pap smear, because in this study the frequency of screening was found to be related both to pill use and the development of cervical cancer.[70] Whereas analytical methods can control for known confounders, it cannot do this for unknown confounders, which are free to distort observed risk estimates. The advantage of experimental studies, of course, is that the randomization process tends to ensure that the prevalence of all potential confounders is similar among the randomized groups.

The role of chance is evaluated in epidemiologic studies by the use of significance testing and confidence limits. If a risk estimate is statistically significant at a specified level (*e.g.,* 0.05, or 1 in 20) or if the 95% confidence limits exclude 1.0, chance can be assumed to be an unlikely explanation. It does not of course exclude the operation of a chance event, but only indicates that chance would explain a risk estimate of the observed magnitude or greater only 1 out of 20 times. In studies involving multiple comparisons, some significant associations can be anticipated by the play of chance, and each finding should be considered on its own merits.

DETERMINING CAUSALITY

In interpreting associations found in epidemiologic studies, one is influenced by the magnitude of the risk estimates, their statistical significance (likelihood of being due to chance), and especially the rigor of the study design to avoid methodologic pitfalls. If bias, confounding, and chance are excluded as likely explanations for an association, the issue of causality must be considered through a process of scientific judgment that extends beyond any statement of statistical probability.[13,14,58] During the controversy over cigarette smoking and lung cancer, a set of criteria was formulated to assist the epidemiologist in making causal inferences.[71,72] These criteria provide useful guidelines for determining causality, and refer especially to the strength and specificity of an association, the presence of a dose-response gradient, the consistency and reproducibility of results, biological plausibility and coherence, and an appropriate temporal sequence. It may not be possible to satisfy all the criteria in any particular instance, although evidence that the exposure preceded the disease is obviously crucial.[58] With smaller relative risks, especially when interactions between multiple exposures and susceptibility states seem important, the term risk factors is often used instead of causal agents. The finding of small relative risks should not be readily dismissed as due to chance or bias but explored further by examining possible interactions with other risk factors or susceptible subgroups of the population.

Causal inferences from epidemiology usually develop gradually after taking into account all relevant biological information, including laboratory studies. Although epidemiologic observations can accumulate to the point at which causation is virtually inescapable, strictly speaking it is not possible by these means alone to prove causality. Nevertheless, causation can often be shown to be sufficiently probable to provide a compelling basis for preventive and public health action, and certainly so in the case of cigarette smoking and lung cancer.

CAUSES OF CANCER

This section is intended to provide a brief overview of cancer risk factors, based mainly on evidence from analytical epidemiology, including recent observations relevant to the practicing oncologist. The contributions of epidemiology to cancer etiology and prevention are presented elsewhere in greater detail.[6,7,73,74] Best known is the success of the epidemiologic approach in discovering or confirming a number of lifestyle and other environmental exposures as causes of cancer (Table 13-16).

TOBACCO

Among the carcinogenic hazards identified so far, tobacco smoking is the most important in Western countries and increasingly so in developing countries. Smoking has been firmly linked to cancers not only of the lung but also of the larynx, mouth, pharynx, esophagus, bladder, and pancreas.[75] Recent evidence indicates that smokers are also prone to cancers of the kidney parenchyma[76] and pelvis,[77] cervix,[78] nasal passages,[79] and perhaps stomach cancer[80] and leukemia.[81] The wide variety of neoplasms related to smoking is hardly surprising in view of the large number of chemicals detected in cigarette smoke and delivered to a highly vascular and absorptive organ. In the United States it appears that smoking, especially of cigarettes, accounts for about 40% of all cancer deaths in men and about 20% in women, with lung cancers representing the largest proportion. For smokers of two or more packs per day, the risk of lung cancer is about 20 times that of nonsmokers, and is much greater for squamous and small cell carcinomas than for adenocarcinomas.

Epidemiologic studies have demonstrated the benefits of stopping smoking, with lower risks relative to those of continuing smokers appearing within a few years of quitting.[6,75] This is consistent with evidence that smoking exerts an effect at late as well as early stages of carcinogenesis. The introduction of lower tar levels in cigarettes and of filter tips has also reduced the risk of lung cancer, although not nearly to the extent seen with cessation of smoking.[82] The risks of cigar and pipe smokers resemble those of cigarette smokers for cancers of the oral cavity, larynx, and esophagus, but are lower for lung cancer.

Smokeless tobacco is also of concern, since oral cancer has been linked with snuff dipping, a common practice in rural southern parts of the United States.[44] Under suspicion are the high levels of tobacco-specific nitrosamines that have been detected in snuff and in the saliva of snuff users. In parts of Asia, oral cancer is common in people who use tobacco quids often mixed with betel, lime, and other agents.[83] Overall, these findings have prompted recent public health and legislative measures in the United States aimed at discouraging the use of smokeless tobacco, especially among young people.

Passive smoking has been hotly debated as a risk factor for lung cancer. A review of the available evidence suggests that nonsmoking women married to smokers have experienced an excess risk of the order of 30%.[84] There is little question that passive or involuntary smoking is real, since tobacco smoke constituents and metabolites can be detected in the body fluids of exposed nonsmokers. Moreover, a cause-and-effect relationship with lung cancer is suggested by the replication of findings in different populations, by a dose-response effect with excess risks of about 70% among heavily exposed nonsmokers, by cell type patterns resembling those associated with active smoking, and by the similarity in risk estimates between heavy passive smokers and very light active smokers.

ALCOHOL

Consumption of alcoholic beverages has been shown to potentiate the effects of tobacco smoking on cancers of the mouth, pharynx, esophagus, and larynx, and has been estimated to account for about 3% of all cancer deaths.[85,86] It has been difficult to study the effects of alcohol alone and the

TABLE 13-16. Environmental Causes of Human Cancer

Agent	*Type of Exposure*	*Site of Cancer*
Alcoholic beverages	Drinking	Mouth, pharynx, esophagus, larynx, liver
Alkylating agents (melphalan, cyclophosphamide, chlorambucil, semustine)	Medication	Leukemia
Androgen-anabolic steroids	Medication	Liver
Aromatic amines (benzidine, 2-naphthylamine, 4-aminobiphenyl)	Manufacturing of dyes and other chemicals	Bladder
Arsenic (inorganic)	Mining and smelting of certain ores, pesticide manufacturing and use, medication, drinking water	Lung, skin, liver (angiosarcoma)
Asbestos	Manufacturing and use	Lung, pleura, peritoneum
Benzene	Leather, petroleum, and other industries	Leukemia
Bis(chloromethyl)ether	Manufacturing	Lung (small cell)
Chlornaphazine	Medication	Bladder
Chromium compounds	Manufacturing	Lung
Estrogens	Medication	
Synthetic (DES)		Cervix, vagina (adenocarcinoma)
Conjugated (Premarin)		Endometrium
Steroid contraceptives		Liver (benign)
Immunosuppressants (azathoprine, cyclosporin)	Medication	Non-Hodgkin's lymphoma, skin (squamous carcinoma and melanoma), soft tissue tumors (including Kaposi's sarcoma)
Ionizing radiation	Atomic bomb explosions, treatment and diagnosis, radium dial painting, uranium and metal mining	Most sites
Isopropyl alcohol production	Manufacturing by strong acid process	Nasal sinuses
Leather industry	Manufacturing and repair (boot and shoe)	Nasal sinuses, bladder
Mustard gas	Manufacturing	Lung, larynx, nasal sinuses
Nickel dust	Refining	Lung, nasal sinuses
Parasites	Infection	
Schistosoma haematobium		Bladder (squamous carcinoma)
Clonorchis sinensis		Liver (cholangiocarcinoma)
Phenacetin-containing analgesics	Medication	Renal pelvis
Polycyclic hydrocarbons	Coal carbonization products and some mineral oils	Lung, skin (squamous carcinoma)
Tobacco chews, including betel nut	Snuff dipping and chewing of tobacco, betel, lime	Mouth
Tobacco smoke	Smoking, especially cigarettes	Lung, larynx, mouth, pharynx, esophagus, bladder, pancreas, kidney
Ultraviolet radiation	Sunlight	Skin (including melanoma), lip
Viruses	Infection	
Epstein-Barr virus		Burkitt's lymphoma; nasopharyngeal carcinoma (?)
Hepatitis-B virus		Hepatocellular carcinoma
Human T-lymphotrophic virus, type I		T-cell leukemia/lymphoma
Vinyl chloride	Manufacturing of polyvinyl chloride	Liver (angiosarcoma)
Wood dusts	Furniture manufacturing (hardwood)	Nasal sinuses (adenocarcinoma)

nature of the interaction with smoking because of small numbers in certain categories of exposure (especially drinkers who abstain from smoking). In a large-scale case-control study of oral cancer, the risks shown in Table 13-17 increased with intake of alcohol among nonsmokers, but in combination with smoking the risks multiplied to 35-fold among heavy consumers of both products.[87] Combined exposures were found to account for about three fourths of all oral and pharyngeal cancers. The risks were not uniform for all forms of alcohol, being higher with hard liquor or beer than with wine. For esophageal cancer, the highest recorded risks from alcohol are those associated with the consumption of home-brewed apple brandies in the northwest part of France. For larynx cancer, the alcohol effect is more prominent for tumors occurring in the supraglottic than in the intrinsic segments. Since ethanol is not carcinogenic in laboratory animals, the mechanism by which alcohol acts is not clear, but it may involve nutritional deficiencies that accompany drinking, contaminants such as nitrosamines and hydrocarbons, or increased permeability of mucous membranes to other carcinogens.

Alcohol is an important cause of hepatic cirrhosis, which is sometimes complicated by hepatocellular carcinoma, although alcohol may also have an independent effect on the risk of this cancer. The role of alcohol in other cancers remains uncertain. Rectal cancer in men has shown positive geographic correlations with beer consumption, but the findings from analytical studies have been inconsistent. For example, cohort studies of brewery workers (who receive a free beer allocation) have revealed an excess risk of rectal cancer in Dublin but not in Copenhagen.[88] Recent interest has centered around the possible relationship of alcohol with breast cancer, with a series of prospective studies showing an excess risk and dose-response gradient.[89,90] Further investigation is needed to determine if this relationship is causal, or if indirect, how it is mediated.

OCCUPATIONAL HAZARDS

The study of occupational groups has identified more carcinogens than any other branch of cancer epidemiology and has led to cancer prevention by reducing or eliminating hazardous exposures in the workplace.[91,92] Occupational exposures may account for about 5% of all cancer deaths, while the proportion is higher in certain areas for particular cancers, such as those of the bladder and lung. Most carcinogenic exposures in the workplace were first detected by clinicians, while others were noted initially by epidemiologists as in the case of asbestos (lung cancer), inorganic arsenic (lung cancer), and the leather industry (nasal cancer), or by experimentalists, as in the case of 4-aminobiphenyl.[2] It is noteworthy that all compounds shown to be carcinogenic in humans have been positive in long-term animal testing, except for arsenic and alcohol. This argues for the importance of bioassay programs, but the exceptions remind us that it may not be prudent to rely solely on laboratory work.

Asbestos represents the major occupational carcinogen in many countries due to its induction of lung cancers rather than mesotheliomas. This is true despite the fact that the relative risk for lung cancer is little more than twofold, whereas that for mesotheliomas is well over 100-fold, the reason being that lung cancer is much more common than mesothelioma in people unexposed to asbestos. A multiplicative relationship exists between asbestos exposure and smoking in the development of lung cancer.[93] As shown in Figure 13-7, American shipyard workers (whose exposure to asbestos was heavy during World War II) have experienced a high incidence, but the far greater excess among smokers than nonsmokers indicates a synergism between the risk factors.[42] The risks also vary according to the type of asbestos fiber and are highest for crocidolite, which is now banned in many countries. Much research is in progress on man-made mineral fibers, but as yet there is no clear evidence of a carcinogenic risk to humans.[92]

Many of the occupational cancers listed in Table 13-16 are characterized by high relative risks and specificity of cell type. A challenge facing epidemiologists is to detect hazards with smaller relative risks that may have a greater impact on the public health when the exposure is widespread and the tumor in question is common. This problem is particularly acute for lung cancer because variations in the prevalence and duration of smoking may mask the detection of occupational risks. The discovery of occupational hazards may also have implications beyond the workplace, since they may point to potential risks experienced at a lower level by the general public.

TABLE 13-17. Relative Risks for Oral and Pharyngeal Cancer Associated with Smoking and Drinking

	Number of Alcohol Drinks Per Week				
Smoking Status	*<1*	*1–4*	*5–14*	*15–24*	*30+*
Nonsmoker	1.0	1.3	1.6	1.4	5.8
Former smoker	0.7	2.2	1.4	3.2	6.4
Light smoker	1.7	1.5	2.7	5.4	7.9
Moderate smoker	1.9	2.4	4.4	7.2	23.8
Heavy smoker	7.4	0.7	4.4	20.2	37.7

Adapted from Blot WJ, McLaughlin JK, Winn DM, et al: Smoking and drinking in relation to oral and pharyngeal cancer. Cancer Res 48:3282, 1988.

* Light, moderate, and heavy smokers: 1–19, 20–39, and 40+ cigarettes per day for 20+ years, respectively.

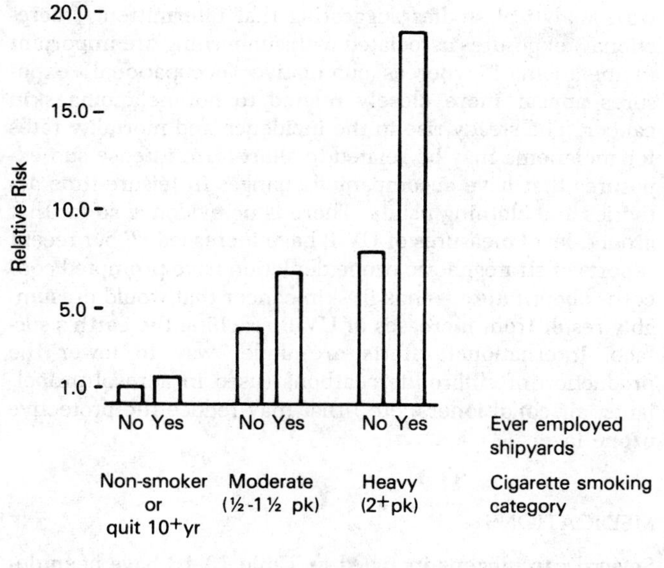

FIG. 13-7. Relative risk of lung cancer according to usual cigarette-smoking category and employment in shipyards during World War II. (Blot WJ, Harrington JM, Toledo A, et al: Lung cancer after employment in shipyards during World War II. N Engl J Med 299:620, 1978)

ENVIRONMENTAL POLLUTION

Pollutants in the urban air have long been suspected in the etiology of lung cancer, with fossil fuel combustion products, especially polycyclic hydrocarbons, being of special concern. The subject has been difficult to study, primarily due to the overpowering effects of smoking, which first became popular in urban areas. Nevertheless, there is suggestive evidence that atmospheric pollution plays a limited role in the causation of lung cancer.[6]

Asbestos bodies and calcified pleural plaques are common in urban populations, but the risks of cancer following non-occupational exposures are uncertain. There are many case reports suggesting that mesotheliomas may result from neighborhood exposures to asbestos industries and from household contact with asbestos dust, perhaps through the laundering of work clothing.[94] A striking example of an environmental carcinogen is the naturally occurring zeolite fiber in parts of Turkey that causes a high mortality from pleural mesothelioma.[95] Another hazard may result from airborne arsenic, because increased mortality rates for lung cancer have been reported in both sexes in the neighborhood of arsenic-emitting smelters that cannot be explained by smoking and occupational exposures.[96]

There is much current interest in the role of indoor air pollution by radon gas and tobacco smoke in lung cancer etiology. In China, the high rates of lung cancer among nonsmoking women have been related to cooking oil vapors generated by wok cooking[97] and to effluents from coal-heating stoves.[98] Also under investigation are contaminants in drinking water, especially since several halogenated organic compounds produced during chlorination are carcinogenic and mutagenic in laboratory tests. A large case-control study of bladder cancer has found a modest excess risk associated with prolonged use of chlorinated surface water,[99] and studies are underway to see if this risk can be confirmed and whether it extends to other cancers. It has been estimated that only about 2% of cancer deaths are due to environmental pollution,[6] but this estimate is based on limited data and may be modified by the results of future research.

IONIZING RADIATION

Along with tobacco smoking, more is known about the carcinogenic effects of ionizing radiation than about any other human carcinogen.[100] This dates from early observations on radiologists to the comprehensive studies among survivors of the atomic bombs in Japan and among patients receiving radiotherapy for ankylosing spondylitis. It is difficult to measure directly the effects of low doses of ionizing radiation, such as x-rays or gamma rays, and extrapolations have to be made from populations exposed to high and moderate doses for medical, occupational, or military reasons. Although a great deal has been learned about the carcinogenic risks of radiation therapy used for many conditions, there is little firm data about risks from the lower doses of diagnostic radiation, except for a 50% increase of leukemia and other childhood cancers associated with prenatal exposures.

It has been estimated that approximately 3% of all cancer deaths may be attributed to radiation,[101] but the upper limit might be twice as high if certain estimates are confirmed about the risks of lung cancer associated with indoor levels of radon emanating mainly from soils containing uranium deposits. Studies of underground miners exposed to relatively high doses of alpha-radiation have shown excess lung cancer risks, even at levels that might be attained through long-term residential exposure in some parts of the United States.[102] More reliable data should come from ongoing case-control studies of lung cancer that involve careful measurements of indoor radon.

Nearly all sites of the body appear vulnerable to the carcinogenic effects of radiation, with the most radiosensitive tissues being the bone marrow, breast, and thyroid.[103] The patterns of risk provide insights into mechanisms of carcinogenesis and guidelines for radiation protection. For example, radiogenic leukemia shows a distinctive wave-like pattern with the excess risk starting 2 to 4 years after exposure, peaking at 6 to 8 years, and declining to normal within 25 years. In contrast, radiogenic carcinomas have a minimal latent period of 5 to 10 years and a temporal distribution that resembles the natural age-specific incidence curve, suggesting the influence of other factors acting at a later stage of carcinogenesis. The advent of large-scale mammography has renewed interest in the breast cancer experience of atomic bomb survivors and women exposed to medical x-rays. Despite a reasonably linear dose-response curve for breast cancer, the radiation effect is most pronounced among young women and is not evident among those who were exposed after age 40. This finding is reassuring for women in midlife who are most likely to undergo periodic screening with mammography.

SOLAR RADIATION

Ultraviolet (UV) radiation from sunlight is the major risk factor for skin cancer, both squamous and basal cell carcinomas and melanoma.[104] The evidence includes the tendency of tumors to arise on sun-exposed sites, the high incidence associated with outdoor activities, and the predisposition of fair-complexioned people who sunburn easily. Exceptionally high risks of skin cancer occur among persons with genetic diseases exacerbated by sunlight (xeroderma pigmentosum and albinism). Furthermore, in experimental animals, repeated doses of UV radiation, particularly in the UV-B spectral range (290 to 320 nm), can induce skin cancer. In addition, about one half of the melanomas appear to arise from dysplastic nevi, a fairly recently described precursor state that should greatly expand opportunities for early detection and treatment.[105]

Since incidence data for nonmelanoma skin cancer are not collected routinely by most population-based cancer registries, special surveys in the United States were conducted in the 1970s as an adjunct to the SEER program together with measures of UV-B radiation at ground level.[106] The gradient with UV-B levels was steepest for squamous cell carcinoma followed by basal cell carcinoma, and was least apparent for melanoma (Figure 13-8). These differences are consistent with analytical studies suggesting that intermittent (recreational) exposures associated with sunburning are important in melanoma,[49] whereas cumulative (occupational) exposures appear more closely related to nonmelanoma skin cancer. The steady rise in the incidence and mortality rates for melanoma may be related to short-term intense sun exposures that have accompanied changes in leisure-time activities and clothing habits. There is no evidence so far that ground-level measures of UV-B have increased,[107] but recent reports of stratospheric ozone depletion have prompted concerns about future trends in skin cancer that would presumably result from increases of UV-B reaching the earth's surface. International efforts are under way to lower the production of chlorofluorocarbons (used in aerosol propellants, air conditioners, etc.) that may reduce the protective ozone layer.

MEDICATIONS

Several carcinogens included in Table 13-16 have been detected by studies of patients exposed to medicinal agents that may account for as much as 2% of all cancers. Some drugs have been withdrawn from clinical practice, whereas others are retained because their benefits are judged to outweigh

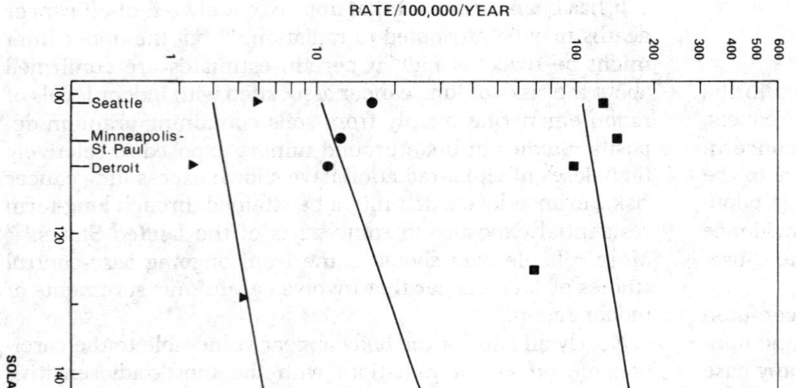

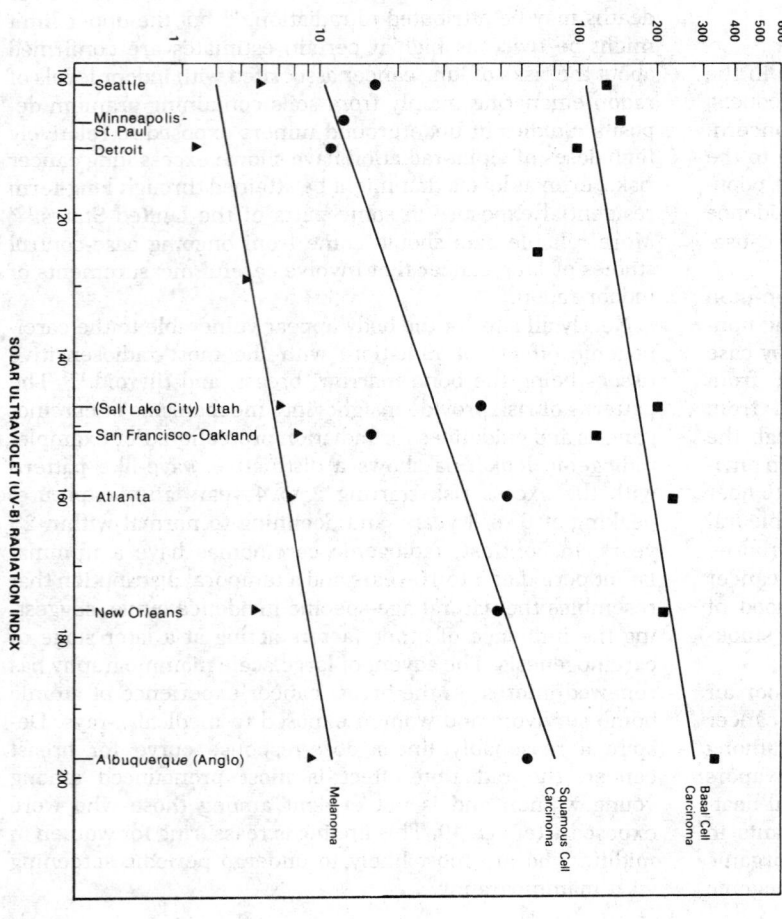

FIG. 13-8. Annual age-adjusted incidence rates for basal and squamous cell carcinomas and melanoma among white females, according to annual UV-B measurements at selected areas of the United States. (Scotto J, Fraumeni JF Jr: Skin (other than melanoma). In Schottenfeld D, Fraumeni JF Jr [eds]: Cancer Epidemiology and Prevention, p 996. Philadelphia, WB Saunders, 1982. Melanoma data are from the SEER program [1973–1976] and nonmelanoma data from a special survey [1977–1978]. Regression lines are based on exponential model.)

their side effects. A major discovery was that synthetic estrogens given during pregnancy produced adenocarcinomas of the vagina and cervix several years later in daughters exposed in utero.[108] This was the first demonstration of transplacental carcinogenesis in humans. Endometrial cancer can result from conjugated estrogens taken for menopausal symptoms, and some studies have suggested an excess of breast cancer in long-term users.[109] Oral contraceptives are still under evaluation, with some studies suggesting an elevated risk of breast cancer when there is early and prolonged use or when there exist predisposing conditions such as familial occurrence or benign breast disease.[110–112] Also, a relationship of pill use to invasive cervical cancer is suggested by recent studies that have controlled carefully for confounding variables such as sexual activity and screening history.[70] It is noteworthy that a reduced risk of endometrial and ovarian cancers has been reported with the combined oral contraceptives, especially following long-term use. The effects of exogenous hormones, along with the relation of female cancers to reproductive and menstrual variables, indicate the importance of investigating endogenous hormones as risk factors.[112,113]

An excess risk of acute nonlymphocytic leukemia has been noted among patients receiving alkylating agents, especially melphalan, cyclophosphamide, and chlorambucil.[62] Thus, the monitoring of carcinogenic risks should be part of randomized therapy trials. For example, when semustine (methyl-CCNU) was evaluated as adjuvant therapy for gastrointestinal cancer, the risks of leukemia and preleukemia were found to be elevated, with a clear dose-response relationship (Table 13-18).[114,115] This finding demonstrates the importance of carefully weighing risks and benefits in designing treatment regimens involving alkylating agents, especially for those cancer patients with a low risk of relapse or for patients with nonmalignant diseases.

Immunosuppressive agents, particularly azathioprine, have been assessed mainly by studies of renal transplant recipients. The risk of non-Hodgkin's lymphoma is very high within a few months of transplantation and remains at about the same level.[116,117] This rapid onset is in marked contrast to the usual behavior of chemical carcinogens and suggests activation of a latent oncogenic virus by immunologic mechanisms. Contrary to the prediction of the "immunosurveillance hypothesis" as first proposed, the increase of other cancers is not generalized but is confined to particular types such as squamous carcinoma of the skin, melanoma, Kaposi's sarcoma, and liver cancer (Table 13-19). Although the risk of post-transplant lymphoma might be influenced by antigenic stimulation by the graft, patients treated with azathioprine for other conditions have shown an approximately 10-fold excess of lymphoma.[117] A predominance of lymphomas has been seen also with primary immunodeficiency disorders such as ataxia-telangiectasia, Wiskott-Aldrich syndrome, and the X-linked lymphoproliferative syndrome.[118] For lymphomas in the latter group as well as in transplant patients, there is evidence of causation by the Epstein-Barr virus (EBV).[119] This finding is consistent with animal experiments, indicating that immunosurveillance primarily operates against viral-induced neoplasms.

VIRUSES

The laboratory discovery of many different oncogenic viruses in animals has long suggested that some human cancers have a similar etiology, but convincing evidence in humans was slow to emerge until recently.[120] The proportion of viral-related cancer in the United States has been roughly estimated at 5%,[6] but one can only speculate about upper bounds as rapid advances in molecular virology are made. However, the estimate must surpass 5% in certain developing countries.

EBV is widely considered the necessary cause of endemic Burkitt's lymphoma and perhaps also nasopharyngeal cancer.[121] In Burkitt's lymphoma, holoendemic malaria appears to enhance the oncogenic effect of EBV and produce uneven distribution and occasional clustering of the lymphoma in Africa. EBV appears involved also in the lymphomas that occur in certain immunodeficiency disorders, perhaps by interacting with immunologic and genetic mechanisms. The relation of EBV to nasopharyngeal cancer has been suggested by the higher antibody levels seen in patients than in controls, and the presence of viral genome in epithelial cells from the tumor. The high rates of this cancer in southern China cannot be attributed to EBV infection alone, and other risk factors such as consumption of salted fish or histocompatibility antigens appear to be involved.

TABLE 13-18. Risk of Leukemic Disorders According to Dose of Semustine

	Cumulative Dosage (mg/m²)				
	0	*1-*	*500-*	*750-*	*1000+*
Number of leukemic disorders	1	3	3	7	5
Number of patients	1,566	714	442	633	278
Relative risk*	1.0	8.7	10.5	18.7	36.9
Five-year cumulative risk (%)†	0.1	0.8	1.2	1.1	2.5

Adapted from Boice JD Jr, Greene MH, Killen JY Jr, et al: Leukemia after adjuvant chemotherapy with semustine (methyl-CCNU)—Evidence of a dose-response effect. N Engl J Med 314:119, 1986.

* The referent category was those who did not receive semustine. Maximum likelihood estimates of relative risk were adjusted for survival times.

† Cumulative probabilities were estimated by the Kaplan-Meier technique (Kaplan EL, Meier P: Nonparametric estimation from incomplete observations. J Am Stat Assoc 53:457, 1958).

TABLE 13-19. Relative Risk of Certain Cancers in Renal Transplant Recipients in Two Major Studies (with Observed Cancers in Parentheses)

Types of Cancer	*United Kingdom-Australasian Study*	*American College of Surgeons Study**
All types†	2.8 (86)	2.8 (136)
Non-Hodgkin's lymphoma	45.9 (42)	26.9 (53)
Primary liver cancer	37.5 (3)	20.0 (4)
Skin melanoma	8.7 (2)	2.5 (5)
Other cancer‡	1.3 (39)	1.7 (74)

Adapted from Kinlen LJ: Immunosuppressive therapy and cancer. Cancer Surv 1:565, 1982.
* Based on unpublished data from Hoover RN and Fraumeni JF Jr.
† Excludes cervix cancer in situ and nonmelanoma skin cancer, although increases in squamous carcinoma of skin have been reported.
‡ Includes excesses of mesenchymal tumors, notably Kaposi's sarcoma.

Hepatitis-B virus (HBV) infection is an important cause of hepatocellular carcinoma, especially in endemic regions of Asia and Africa. The most convincing evidence comes from a cohort study of 22,707 men in Taiwan in which the risk of liver carcinoma was more than 200 times greater among carriers of hepatitis-B surface antigen than among noncarriers (Table 13-20).[122] It is possible that the oncogenic effects of hepatitis-B are enhanced by early-life infection and dietary exposures to aflatoxin.

The high incidence of adult T-cell leukemia in certain areas, such as Japan and the Caribbean, has been linked to infection with the human T-lymphotrophic virus type I (HTLV-I), the first retrovirus to be detected in humans.[123] In endemic areas the virus appears to be transmitted early in life and may also be spread by sexual activity, drug abuse, and blood transfusions.

Another human retrovirus, now called the human immunodeficiency virus (HIV), has been shown to cause the acquired immunodeficiency syndrome (AIDS).[124] Recognized since 1981, AIDS in the United States affects mainly homosexual men, hemophiliacs, and intravenous drug abusers, and predisposes to Kaposi's sarcoma and non-Hodgkin's lymphoma. The much higher incidence of Kaposi's sarcoma among male homosexuals than other high-risk groups with AIDS suggests that an oncogenic agent is superimposed on HIV infection and is also sexually transmitted. The classic or endemic form of Kaposi's sarcoma in Africa and Mediterranean areas has been associated with cytomegalovirus infection in some studies, but the findings in AIDS patients suggest that it is a passenger virus.

The relationship of cervical cancer to multiple sexual partners has long suggested the venereal transmission of an infectious agent. Although herpes simplex virus type 2 has been a candidate agent for some time, the chief suspect at present is the human papillomavirus (HPV). DNA sequences from certain HPV types, notably HPV-16 and HPV-18, have been found in a high percentage of biopsies from invasive cervical cancer.[125] HPV has been isolated also from many vulvar, penile, and anal cancers, as well as from squamous cell skin cancers associated with the genetic syndrome of epidermodysplasia verruciformis.

Investigations of clusters of leukemia or lymphoma in the community have provided no solid clues to etiology, and statistical studies have not detected any general tendency for space-time clustering of these tumors. A viral origin for Hodgkin's disease in young adults has been suggested by its association with certain childhood environments, such as small family size, that would tend to reduce or delay early-life exposures to infections, such as in paralytic poliomyelitis.[54] EBV has been suspected, since antibody levels tend to be higher in cases than controls and an increased risk of Hodgkin's disease has been reported among persons with infectious mononucleosis. However, molecular viral studies have not been supportive and the relationship with EBV may

TABLE 13-20. Deaths from Liver Disease According to Hepatitis-B Surface Antigen (HBsAg) Status on Recruitment into Study

HBsAg Status	*Cause of Death*		*Population at Risk*	*Mortality from Liver Cancer**
	Liver Cancer	*Cirrhosis*		
Positive	40	17	3,454	1158
Negative	1	2	19,253	5
Total	41	19	22,707	181

Adapted from Beasley RP, Hwang L-Y, Lin C-C, et al: Hepatocellular carcinoma and hepatitis-B virus. Lancet 2:1129, 1981.
* Mortality from primary hepatocellular carcinoma per 100,000 during study period.

be indirect. Despite mounting evidence for oncogenic viruses in humans, there is no indication that any form of cancer is contagious.

DIET AND NUTRITION

When viewed in the light of experimental work showing how dietary manipulation can influence the yield of tumors in laboratory animals, the recent growth of interest in dietary causes of human cancer seems not merely logical but overdue. International correlations and migrant studies also suggest that certain aspects of the affluent Western diet contribute to a sizable but uncertain proportion of all cancers. Various hypotheses about causative and protective factors are under intensive study, but the specific dietary components are elusive and the mechanisms of action appear complex. Problems stem from the inherent limitations of nutritional methods such as dietary recall, but progress may come from cohort studies in which specimens have been stored for subsequent biochemical assay and from intervention studies to determine whether certain dietary modifications and nutrient supplements exert a protective effect against cancer.

Dietary fat has been suggested as a risk factor for certain cancers, especially of the breast and large bowel, by the strongly positive correlations that exist between age-adjusted rates in different countries and per capita consumption of fat.[126] However, the results of case-control and cohort studies have not provided strong support for the fat hypothesis.[48,127,128] Furthermore, no positive relationship has been found between the levels of serum cholesterol, which are influenced by fat intake, and subsequent risk of breast or large bowel cancers. The issue is complicated by methodological difficulties in estimating intake of fat and different types of fat, the limited variation in fat consumption within many countries, problems in evaluating dietary habits in early life (which may be especially important for breast cancer), and difficulties in distinguishing fat per se from calories (since fat is more calorigenic than other nutrients). Calories may influence the risk of breast and other reproductive cancers by increasing body weight or size, for obesity is an established risk factor for certain cancers in women, especially cancer of the endometrium.[50] It is possible that obesity elevates the risk of endometrial and breast cancers by increasing the serum levels of circulating estrogens through a conversion from androstenedione in adipose tissue and perhaps also by a lowering of the sex-hormone binding globulin.[112,113]

Evidence is accumulating that a low intake of certain food groups may predispose to cancer, and indeed a lower consumption of green vegetables and fresh fruit has been one of the more consistent findings in dietary studies of cancer. A protective action for fiber was proposed by Burkitt, who was impressed by the low rates of colon cancer in parts of Africa where fiber intake and stool bulk were high. Correlational studies have indicated that fiber intake, especially when measured as nonstarch polysaccharides, tends to be lower in high-incidence regions.[129] Although the results are less consistent, there is some support from case-control studies that fiber protects against colon cancer.[130] However, the subject is complicated by the relatively crude characterization of fiber and by difficulty in separating the effects of micronutrients found in fiber sources such as fruits and vegetables.

Micronutrients may be responsible for the inverse risks associated with the intake of fruits and vegetables. Several epithelial cancers, especially of the lung, show this negative relationship both in case-control studies and some cohort studies employing serologic tests; the effect has been attributed by some workers to beta-carotene.[48,131] More limited evidence suggests that vitamin C may protect against gastric and certain other cancers, perhaps by blocking the endogenous formation of nitrosamines. However, other components of fruits and vegetables have been suggested as protective factors in experimental and epidemiological studies, for example, indole compounds in cruciferous vegetables that may decrease the risk of colon cancer,[132] and allyl sulfide in garlic and onions that may lower the risk of gastric cancer.[80] The effects of vitamin E, selenium, and calcium are also under study. Furthermore, mixed or multiple deficiencies in the diet may be involved in some tumors, especially among populations with high risks of esophageal cancer.[133] Intervention studies are ideally suited to test the micronutrient hypotheses, and the results of several ongoing trials are awaited with interest.

A variety of other dietary factors, including additives and contaminants, have attracted attention. The consumption of aflatoxin, a carcinogenic metabolite of the fungus *Aspergillus flavus*, has been linked to liver cancer by correlation studies and more recently by a case-control study.[134] A relationship between salted foods and stomach cancer has been claimed in some studies,[80] but this has not been consistently observed. The consumption of salted fish containing high concentrations of nitrosamines has been linked to the high rates of nasopharyngeal cancer in Hong Kong and southern China.[135] Coffee intake has been associated with bladder and pancreatic cancers, but this has not been confirmed in many other studies and there is no evidence for a causal relationship. The artificial sweeteners saccharin and cyclamate cause bladder cancer in laboratory animals, but a large case-control study of bladder cancer indicated that the risk in humans at past levels of consumption is very small if present at all.[136] Cooking practices may generate hydrocarbons or other carcinogens in the food at high temperatures, but no relevant epidemiologic data are available.

GENETIC SUSCEPTIBILITY

Although the geographic and ethnic differentials for most cancers appear largely determined by environmental influences, genetic factors may contribute to some high rates (*e.g.*, nasopharyngeal cancer among Chinese and gallbladder cancer among American Indians) as well as some low rates (*e.g.*, testicular cancer and Ewing's sarcoma among blacks in Africa and the United States). Genetic susceptibility is most evident for skin cancer, with geographic and ethnic variations corresponding to the degree of protective skin pigmentation. The apparently limited evidence for genetic factors based on these patterns, however, does not exclude even large variations in individual susceptibility. Furthermore, the relatively small differences in risk between close relatives of patients with cancer and other people for childhood tumors other than retinoblastoma are in fact consistent with large differences in genetic predisposition. The truth of this perhaps surprising statement can be demonstrated mathematically.[137] Only with advances in biochemical and molecular methods, however, does it seem possible to further define the impact of genetic factors or genetic-environmental interactions in cancer etiology.[138] For example, the phenotype associated with the rapid metabolic oxidation of certain drugs appears to influence the risk of smoking-related lung cancer,[139] supporting the long-held suspicion that certain persons have a higher risk of smoking-induced lung cancer than others because of genetic constitution. The claim is sometimes made that the proportion of people who are susceptible to cancer is limited, with variations only in the specific sites affected (Cramer's hypothesis). This notion has been shown to be false[5] and has given way to mutation models and genetic hypotheses[140] that are stimulating further research into the nature of cancer susceptibility genes.

Although only a small fraction of cancer is inherited in a mendelian fashion, over 200 single-gene disorders have been linked to neoplasia.[141] This does not include several constitutional cytogenetic disorders that predispose to cancer, such as Down's syndrome with leukemia, Klinefelter's syndrome with mediastinal teratoma, gonadal dysgenesis with gonadoblastoma, and aniridia with Wilms' tumor.[66] Table 13-21 lists some cancers that occur as an inherited trait (hereditary neoplasms) and Table 13-22 presents those arising as a complication of inherited precursor lesions (preneoplastic states). Included are several syndromes in which sunlight contributes to multiple skin cancers, including the dysplastic nevus syndrome predisposing to melanoma and xeroderma pigmentosum predisposing to a variety of skin cancers. Genetically determined neoplasms tend to occur earlier in life than other cancers of the same anatomic type and often have a multifocal origin. In addition, several common neoplasms such as breast and colon cancers show small familial risks of the order of twofold to threefold, but among subgroups of patients with onset at young ages and bilateral or multifocal origin, the risks may be as high as 20- to 30-fold.[142] Some families show remarkable aggregations of site-specific cancer that appear consistent with autosomal dominant inheritance. However, because cancer is so common, it is sometimes difficult to know whether familial clusters are simply due to chance, especially if different types of cancer are involved.[143] In this circumstance it can be useful to consider the possibility of a familial multiple-cancer syndrome. A distinct pattern is seen, for example, with a familial aggregation involving several childhood and adult cancers, including soft-tissue and bone sarcomas, breast carcinoma, brain tumors, leukemia, and adrenocortical neoplasms (the Li-Fraumeni cancer family syndrome).[144,145] Family members with this syndrome are prone to multiple primary cancers, including radiogenic sarcomas. Currently, molecular studies including DNA probes are attempting to understand the genetic events and biological mechanisms that may be shared by a variety of neoplasms, including breast cancer.[146,147] Thus, by delineating genetic and familial syndromes of cancer, clinicians have been instrumental not only in helping to identify and protect high-risk individuals but also in pointing experimentalists to new research opportunities. A multidisciplinary approach to genetic susceptibility ranging from clinical observations and epidemiology to molecular biology shows promise in identifying carcinogenic mechanisms, and thus may have consequences in cancer prevention that are at least as important as the detection of environmental carcinogens.

Table 13-21. Hereditary Neoplasms

	*Inheritance**	*Features*
Retinoblastoma	AD	Susceptibility to second primary tumors, including osteosarcoma of leg and radiogenic sarcoma of orbit; chromosome deletion (13q14) in some cases
Nevoid basal cell carcinoma	AD	Basal cell cancers of skin increased by UV and ionizing radiation; medulloblastoma, ovarian fibromas, and developmental defects in some cases
Multiple endocrine neoplasia I	AD	Adenomas of anterior pituitary, parathyroid, pancreatic islet cells, thyroid, and adrenal cortex; carcinoid tumors of intestine and bronchus in some cases
Multiple endocrine neoplasia II	AD	Pheochromocytoma and medullary thyroid carcinoma; parathyroid tumors and neurofibromas in some cases
Polyposis coli	AD	Multiple adenomatous polyps and adenocarcinomas of large bowel; some families exhibit osteomas, fibromas, lipomas, and epidermal cysts (Gardner's syndrome)
Dysplastic nevus syndrome	AD	Hereditary melanomas derived from nevi, especially after sun exposure

* AD, autosomal dominant.

TABLE 13-22. Hereditary Preneoplastic Syndromes

	Inheritance*	Neoplasms
Phacomatoses		
Neurofibromatosis	AD	Sarcomatous change in the neurofibromas of 10% of cases; gliomas of brain and optic nerve, acoustic neuromas, meningiomas, and acute leukemia
Tuberous sclerosis	AD	Hamartomatous growths in several organs; brain tumors, chiefly giant-cell astrocytoma, in 1%–3% of patients
von Hippel-Lindau syndrome	AD	Angiomatosis of retina and cerebellum; renal adenocarcinoma, pheochromocytoma, and ependymoma in some cases
Peutz-Jeghers syndrome	AD	Rare malignant change in hamartomatous polyps of gastrointestinal tract; ovarian neoplasms in 5% of female patients
Cowden's multiple hamartoma syndrome	AD	Oral papillomas, cystic mastopathy and breast cancer, thyroid and colonic neoplasms
Genodermatoses		
Xeroderma pigmentosum	AR	Various skin cancers in all patients exposed to sunlight
Albinism	AR	Skin cancers, chiefly squamous, in sun-exposed areas
Epidermodysplasia verruciformis	AR	Skin cancers, chiefly squamous, in multiple warts induced by papillomavirus
Werner's syndrome (adult progeria)	AR	Soft tissue sarcoma, other tumors
Chromosome instability		
Bloom's syndrome	AR	Acute leukemia, non-Hodgkin's lymphoma, other cancers
Fanconi's anemia	AR	Acute myelomonocytic leukemia and squamous carcinoma of mucous membranes; hepatoma reported after androgen-anabolic steroids
Immune deficiency		
Ataxia-telangiectasia	AR	Non-Hodgkin's lymphoma, acute lymphocytic leukemia, stomach cancer, other tumors; heterozygous carriers prone to cancer, especially of the breast
Common variable immunodeficiency	?AR	Non-Hodgkin's lymphoma, stomach cancer
Wiskott-Aldrich syndrome	XR	Non-Hodgkin's lymphoma, acute leukemia
X-linked (Bruton's) agammaglobulinemia	XR	Non-Hodgkin's lymphoma, acute leukemia
X-linked lymphoproliferative syndrome	XR	Non-Hodgkin's lymphoma, plasmacytoma

* AD, autosomal dominant; AR, autosomal recessive; XR, X-linked recessive.

REFERENCES

1. Shimkin MB: Contrary to Nature. National Institutes of Health (NIH) Report 76–720. Washington, DC, US Government Printing Office, 1977
2. Doll R: Pott and the prospects for prevention. Br J Cancer 32:263, 1975
3. Doll R: The epidemiology of cancer. Cancer 45:2475, 1980
4. MacMahon B, Pugh TF: Epidemiology: Principles and Methods. Boston, Little, Brown, 1970
5. Doll R: An epidemiologic perspective of the biology of cancer. Cancer Res 38:3573, 1978
5. Doll R, Peto R: The causes of cancer. JNCI 66:1191, 1981
7. Schottenfeld D, Fraumeni JF Jr (eds): Cancer Epidemiology and Prevention. Philadelphia, WB Saunders, 1982
8. Muir CS, Malhotra A: Changing patterns of cancer incidence in five continents. Gann Monogr Cancer Res 33:3, 1987
9. Hill AB: Principles of Medical Statistics. New York, Oxford University Press, 1966
10. Young JL Jr, Percy CL, Asire AJ (eds): Surveillance, Epidemiology, and End Results: Incidence and Mortality Data, 1973–77. Natl Cancer Inst Monogr 57, 1981
11. Feldman AR, Kessler L, Myers MH, et al: The prevalence of cancer: Estimates based on the Connecticut Tumor Registry. N Engl J Med 315:1394, 1986
12. Decoufle P, Thomas TL, Pickle LW: Comparison of the proportionate mortality ratio and standardized mortality ratio risk measures. Am J Epidemiol 111:263, 1980
13. Kelsey JL, Thompson WD, Evans AS: Methods in Observational Epidemiology. New York, Oxford University Press, 1986
14. Lilienfeld A, Pederson E, Dowd JE: Cancer Epidemiology: Methods of Study. Baltimore, Johns Hopkins Press, 1967

15. Gordon T, Crittenden M, Haenszel W: Cancer mortality trends in the United States, 1930–1955. Natl Cancer Inst Mongr 6:133, 1961
16. Burbank F: Patterns in Cancer Mortality in the United States: 1950–1967. Natl Cancer Inst Mongr 33, 1971
17. Mason TJ, McKay FW: US Cancer Mortality by County: 1950–1969. DHEW Publication No. (NIH)74–615. Washington, DC, US Government Printing Office, 1974
18. Mason TJ, McKay FW, Hoover R, et al: Atlas of Cancer Mortality for US Counties: 1950–1969. DHEW Publication No. (NIH)75–780. Washington, DC, US Government Printing Office, 1975
19. Mason TJ, McKay FW, Hoover R, et al: Atlas of Cancer Mortality among US Nonwhites: 1950–1969. DHEW Publication No. (NIH)76–1204. Washington, DC, US Government Printing Office, 1976
20. Riggan WB, Van Bruggen J, Acquavella JF, et al: US Cancer Mortality Rates and Trends, 1950–1979, Vols 1–3. Publication No. EPA-600/1–83–015a. Washington, DC, US Government Printing Office, 1983
21. Pickle LW, Mason TJ, Howard N, et al: Atlas of US Cancer Mortality Rates and Trends among Whites, 1950–1980. DHHS Publication No. (NIH)87–2900. Washington, DC, US Government Printing Office, 1987
22. McKay FW, Hanson MR, Miller RW: Cancer Mortality in the United States: 1950–1977. Natl Cancer Inst Monogr 59, 1982
23. Devesa SS, Silverman DT: Cancer incidence and mortality trends in the United States: 1935–74. J Natl Cancer Inst 60:545, 1978
24. Devesa SS, Silverman DT, Young JL Jr, et al: Cancer incidence and mortality trends among whites in the United States, 1947–84. JNCI 79:701, 1987
25. Segi M, Aoki K, Kurihara M: World cancer mortality. Gann Monogr Cancer Res 26:121, 1981
26. Percy C, Stanek E III, Gloeckler L: Accuracy of cancer death certificates and its effect on cancer mortality statistics. Am J Public Health 71:242, 1981
27. Heston JF, Kelly JB, Meigs JW, et al (eds): Forty-five Years of Cancer Incidence in Connecticut: 1935–79. Natl Cancer Inst Monogr 70, 1986
28. Dorn HF, Cutler SJ: Morbidity from Cancer in the United States: Parts I and II. Public Health Monogr 56, 1959
29. Haenszel W, Marcus SC, Zimmerer EG: Cancer Morbidity in Urban and Rural Iowa. Public Health Monogr 37, 1956
30. Cutler SJ, Young JL Jr (eds): Third National Cancer Survey: Incidence Data. Natl Cancer Inst Monogr 41, 1975
31. Horm JW, Asire AJ, Young JL Jr, et al (eds): SEER Program. Cancer Incidence and Mortality in the United States, 1973–81. DHHS Publication No. (NIH)85–1837. Bethesda, MD, National Institutes of Health, 1984
32. Axtell LM, Asire AJ, Myers MH: Cancer Patient Survival. Report No. 5. DHEW Publication No. (NIH)77–992. Bethesda, MD, National Institutes of Health, 1976
33. Myers MH, Hankey BF: Cancer Patient Survival Experience. NIH Publication No. (NIH)80–2148. Bethesda, MD, National Institutes of Health, 1980
34. Ries LG, Pollack ES, Young JL Jr: Cancer patient survival: Surveillance, epidemiology, and end results program, 1973–79. JNCI 70:693, 1983
35. Young JL Jr, Ries LG, Pollack ES: Cancer patient survival among ethnic groups in the United States. JNCI 73:341, 1984
36. Newell GR: Hospital- and population-based tumor registries. Cancer Bull 35:283, 1983
37. Silverberg E, Lubera JA: Cancer statistics, 1988. CA 38:5, 1988
38. Muir C, Waterhouse J, Mack T, et al: Cancer Incidence in Five Continents, Vol V. Lyon, International Agency for Research on Cancer, 1987
39. Haenszel W: Migrant studies. In Schottenfeld D, Fraumeni JF Jr (eds): Cancer Epidemiology and Prevention, p 194. Philadelphia, WB Saunders, 1982
40. Lilienfeld AM, Levin ML, Kessler II: Cancer in the United States. Cambridge, MA, Harvard University Press, 1972
41. Ziegler RG, Devesa SS, Fraumeni JF Jr: Epidemiologic patterns of colorectal cancer. In DeVita VT Jr, Hellman S, Rosenberg SA (eds): Important Advances in Oncology 1986, p 209. Philadelphia, JB Lippincott, 1986
42. Blot WJ, Harrington JM, Toledo A, et al: Lung cancer after employment in shipyards during World War II. N Engl J Med 299:620, 1978
43. Pickle LW, Correa P, Fontham E: Recent case-control studies of lung cancer in the United States. In Mizell M, Correa P (eds): Lung Cancer: Causes and Prevention, p 101. Deerfield Beach, FL, Verlag-Chemie International, 1984
44. Winn D, Blot WJ, Shy CM, et al: Snuff dipping and oral cancer among women in the southern United States. N Engl J Med 304:745, 1981
45. Hoar SK, Blair A, Holmes FF, et al: Agricultural herbicide use and risk of lymphoma and soft-tissue sarcoma. JAMA 256:1141, 1986
46. Liu JY, Liu BQ, Li GY, et al: Atlas of cancer mortality in the People's Republic of China: An aid for cancer control and research. Int J Epidemiol 10:127, 1981
47. National Center for Health Statistics: Health: United States, 1985. DHHS Publication No. (PHS)86–1232. Washington, DC, US Government Printing Office, 1985
48. Willett WC, MacMahon B: Diet and cancer—an overview. N Engl J Med 310:633, 697, 1984
49. Elwood JM, Hislop TG: Solar radiation in the etiology of cutaneous malignant melanoma in Caucasians. Natl Cancer Inst Monogr 62:167, 1982
50. Weiss NS: Epidemiology of carcinoma of the endometrium. In Lilienfeld AM (ed): Reviews in Cancer Epidemiology, vol 2, p 46. New York, Elsevier, 1983
51. Cramer DW: Uterine cervix. In Schottenfeld D, Fraumeni JF Jr (eds): Cancer Epidemiology and Prevention, p 881. Philadelphia, WB Saunders, 1982
52. Pokras R, Hufnagel VG: Hysterectomies in the United States, 1965–84. Vital and Health Statistics. Series 13, No. 92. DHHS Publication No. (PHS)88–1753. Washington, DC, US Government Printing Office, 1987
53. Miller RW, McKay FW: Decline in US childhood cancer mortality. JAMA 251:1567, 1984
54. Gutensohn N, Cole P: Epidemiology of Hodgkin's disease. Semin Oncol 7:92, 1980
55. Brown LM, Pottern LM, Hoover RN, et al: Testicular cancer in the United States: Trends in incidence and mortality. Int J Epidemiol 15:164, 1986
56. Devesa SS, Diamond EL: Association of breast cancer and cervical cancer incidences with income and education among whites and blacks. JNCI 65:515, 1980
57. Hutchison GB: The epidemiologic method. In Schottenfeld D, Fraumeni JF Jr (eds): Cancer Epidemiology and Prevention, p 3. Philadelphia, WB Saunders, 1982
58. Rothman KJ: Modern Epidemiology. Boston, Little, Brown, 1986
59. Cole P: The evolving case-control study. J Chronic Dis 32:15, 1979
60. Cole P, MacMahon B: Attributable risk percent in case-control studies. Br J Prev Soc Med 25:242, 1971
61. Miettinen OS: Proportion of disease caused or prevented by a given exposure, trait or intervention. Am J Epidemiol 99:325, 1974
62. Greene MH, Harris EL, Gershenson DM, et al: Melphalan may be a more potent leukemogen than cyclophosphamide. Ann Intern Med 105:360, 1986
63. Hartge P, Silverman D, Hoover R, et al: Changing cigarette habits and bladder cancer risk: A case-control study. JNCI 78:1119, 1987
64. Harris CC (ed): Biochemical and Molecular Epidemiology of Cancer. New York, Alan R. Liss, 1986
65. Perera FP, Weinstein IB: Molecular epidemiology and carcinogen-DNA adduct detection: New approaches to studies of human cancer causation. J Chronic Dis 35:581, 1982
66. Miller RW: Genes, syndromes, and cancer. Pediatr Rev 8:153, 1986
67. Miller RW: Meeting report—Rare events as clues to cancer etiology. Cancer Res 48:3544, 1988
68. Wald NJ, Doll R (eds): Interpretation of Negative Epidemiological Evidence for Carcinogenicity. IARC Scientific Publication No. 65. Lyon, International Agency for Research on Cancer, 1985
69. Sackett DL: Bias in analytic research. J Chronic Dis 32:51, 1979
70. Brinton LA, Huggins GR, Lehman HF, et al: Long-term use of oral contraceptives and risk of invasive cervical cancer. Int J Cancer 38:339, 1986
71. Hill AB: The environment and disease: Association or causation? Proc R Soc Med 58:295, 1965
72. Smoking and Health: Report of the Advisory Committee to the Surgeon General. Public Health Service Publication No. 1103. Washington, DC, US Government Printing Office, 1964
73. Vessey MP, Gray M (eds): Cancer Risks and Prevention. Oxford, Oxford University Press, 1985
74. MacClure KM, MacMahon B: An epidemiologic perspective of environmental carcinogenesis. Epidemiol Rev 2:19, 1980
75. International Agency for Research on Cancer: Tobacco Smoking. IARC Monographs on the Evaluation of the Carcinogenic Risk of Chemicals to Humans, Vol 38. Lyon, International Agency for Research on Cancer, 1986
76. McLaughlin JK, Mandel JS, Blot WJ, et al: A population-based case-control study of renal cell carcinoma. JNCI 72:275, 1984
77. McLaughlin JK, Blot WJ, Mandel JS, et al: Etiology of cancer of the renal pelvis. JNCI 71:287, 1983
78. Brinton LA, Schairer C, Haenszel W, et al: Cigarette smoking and invasive cervical cancer. JAMA 255:3265, 1986
79. Brinton LA, Blot WJ, Becker JA, et al: A case-control study of cancers of the nasal cavity and paranasal sinuses. Am J Epidemiol 119:896, 1984
80. You WC, Blot WJ, Chang YS, et al: Diet and the high risk of stomach cancer in Shandong, China. Cancer Res 48:3518, 1988
81. Kinlen LJ, Rogot E: Leukemia and smoking habits. Br Med J (in press)
82. Lubin JH, Blot WJ, Berino F, et al: Patterns of lung cancer risk according to type of cigarette smoked. Int J Cancer 33:569, 1984
83. International Agency for Research on Cancer: Tobacco Habits Other Than Smoking: Betel-Quid and Areca-Nut Chewing; and Some Related Nitrosamines. IARC Monographs on the Evaluation of the Carcinogenic Risk of Chemicals to Humans, Vol 37. Lyon, International Agency for Research on Cancer, 1985
84. Blot WJ, Fraumeni JF Jr: Passive smoking and lung cancer. JNCI 77:993, 1986
85. Tuyns AJ: Alcohol. In Schottenfeld D, Fraumeni JF Jr (eds): Cancer Epidemiology and Prevention, p 293. Philadelphia, WB Saunders, 1982
86. Rothman KJ: The proportion of cancer attributable to alcohol consumption. Prev Med 9:174, 1980
87. Blot WJ, McLaughlin JK, Winn DM, et al: Smoking and drinking in relation to oral and pharyngeal cancer. Cancer Res 48:3282, 1988
88. Jensen OM: Cancer morbidity and causes of death among Danish brewery workers. Int J Cancer 23:454, 1979
89. Schatzkin A, Jones DY, Hoover RN: Alcohol consumption and breast cancer in the epidemiologic follow-up study of the first National Health and Nutrition Examination Survey. N Engl Med J 316:1169, 1987
90. Willett WC, Stampfer MJ, Colditz GA, et al: Moderate alcohol consumption and the risk of breast cancer. N Engl J Med 316:1174, 1987
91. Decoufle P: Occupation. In Schottenfeld D, Fraumeni JF Jr (eds): Cancer Epidemiology and Prevention, p 318. Philadelphia, WB Saunders, 1982

92. Saracci R: Occupation. In Vessey MP, Gray M (eds): Cancer Risks and Prevention, p 99. Oxford, Oxford University Press, 1985
93. Saracci R: Asbestosis and lung cancer: An analysis of the epidemiological evidence on the asbestos-smoking interaction. Int J Cancer 20:323, 1977
94. Tagnon I, Blot WJ, Stroube RB, et al: Mesothelioma associated with the shipbuilding industry in coastal Virginia. Cancer Res 40:3875, 1980
95. Artvinll M, Baris YI: Malignant mesotheliomas in a small village in the Anatolian region of Turkey: An epidemiologic study. JNCI 63:17, 1979
96. Brown LM, Pottern LM, Blot WJ: Lung cancer in relation to environmental pollutants emitted from industrial sources. Environ Res 34:250, 1984
97. Gao YT, Blot WJ, Zheng W, et al: Lung cancer among Chinese women. Int J Cancer 40:604, 1987
98. Mumford JL, He XZ, Chapman RS, et al: Lung cancer and indoor air pollution in Xuan Wei, China. Science 235:217, 1987
99. Cantor KP, Hoover R, Hartge P, et al: Bladder cancer, drinking water source, and tap water consumption: A case-control study. JNCI 79:1269, 1987
100. Boice JD Jr, Fraumeni JF Jr (eds): Radiation Carcinogenesis: Epidemiology and Biological Significance. Progress in Cancer Research and Therapy, Vol 26. New York, Raven Press, 1984
101. Jablon S, Bailar JC III: The contribution of ionizing radiation to cancer mortality in the United States. Prev Med 9:219, 1980
102. National Research Council, Committee on the Biological Effects of Ionizing Radiations (BEIR) IV: Health Risks of Radon and Other Internally Deposited Alpha-Emitters. Washington, DC, National Academy Press, 1988
103. Boice JD Jr, Land CE: Ionizing radiation. In Schottenfeld D, Fraumeni JF Jr (eds): Cancer Epidemiology and Prevention, p 231. Philadelphia, WB Saunders, 1982
104. Scotto J, Fears TR, Fraumeni JF Jr: Solar radiation. In Schottenfeld D, Fraumeni JF Jr (eds): Cancer Epidemiology and Prevention, p 254. Philadelphia, WB Saunders, 1982
105. Greene MH, Clark WH, Tucker MA, et al: Acquired precursors of cutaneous malignant melanoma: The familial dysplastic nevus syndrome. N Engl J Med 312:91, 1985
106. Scotto J, Fraumeni JF Jr: Skin (other than melanoma). In Schottenfeld D, Fraumeni JF Jr (eds): Cancer Epidemiology and Prevention, p 996. Philadelphia, WB Saunders, 1982
107. Scotto J, Cotton G, Urbach F, et al: Biologically effective ultraviolent radiation: Surface measurements in the United States, 1974 to 1985. Science 239:762, 1988
108. Herbst AL, Cole P, Colton T, et al: Age incidence and risk of diethylstilbestrol-related clear cell carcinoma of the vagina and cervix. Am J Obstet Gynecol 128:43, 1977
109. Brinton LA, Hoover R, Fraumeni JF Jr: Menopausal oestrogens and breast cancer risk: An expanded case-control study. Br J Cancer 54:825, 1986
110. Key TJA, Pike MC: The role of oestrogens and progestogens in the epidemiology and prevention of breast cancer. Eur J Cancer Clin Oncol 24:29, 1988
111. Vessey MP: Exogenous hormones. In Vessey MP, Gray M (eds): Cancer Risks and Prevention, p 166. Oxford, Oxford University Press, 1985
112. Henderson BE, Ross R, Bernstein L: Estrogens as a cause of human cancer. Cancer Res 48:246, 1988
113. Pike MC: Endogenous hormones. In Vessey MP, Gray M (eds): Cancer Risks and Prevention, p 195. Oxford, Oxford University Press, 1985
114. Boice JD Jr, Greene MH, Killen JY Jr, et al: Leukemia and preleukemia after adjuvant treatment of gastrointestinal cancer with semustine (methyl-CCNU). N Engl J Med 309:1079, 1983
115. Boice JD Jr, Greene MH, Killen JY Jr, et al: Leukemia after adjuvant chemotherapy with semustine (methyl-CCNU) — Evidence of a dose-response effect. N Engl J Med 314:119, 1986
116. Hoover R, Fraumeni JF Jr: Risk of cancer in renal-transplant recipients. Lancet 2:55, 1973
117. Kinlen LJ: Immunosuppressive therapy and cancer. Cancer Surv 1:565, 1982
118. Filopovich AH, Spector BD, Kersey J: Immunodeficiency in humans as a risk factor in the development of malignancy. Prev Med 9:252, 1980
119. List AF, Greco FA, Vogler LB: Lymphoproliferative diseases in immunocompromised hosts: The role of the Epstein-Barr virus. J Clin Oncol 5:1673, 1987
120. Evans AS: Viruses. In Schottenfeld D, Fraumeni JF Jr (eds): Cancer Epidemiology and Prevention, p 364. Philadelphia, WB Saunders, 1982
121. Levine PH, Ablashi DV, Nonoyama M, et al (eds): Epstein-Barr Virus and Human Disease. Clifton, NJ, Humana Press, 1987
122. Beasley RP, Hwang LY, Lin CC, et al: Hepatocellular carcinoma and hepatitis B virus: A prospective study of 22,707 men in Taiwan. Lancet 2:1129, 1981
123. Blattner WA: Human retroviruses. In Feigin RD, Cherry JD (eds): Textbook of Pediatric Infectious Diseases, 2nd ed, p 1795. Philadelphia, WB Saunders, 1987
124. Goedert JJ, Blattner WA: The epidemiology and natural history of human immunodeficiency virus. In DeVita VT Jr, Hellman S, Rosenberg SA (eds): AIDS: Etiology, Diagnosis, Treatment and Prevention, 2nd ed. Philadelphia, JB Lippincott, 1988
125. zur Hausen H: Papillomaviruses in human cancer. Cancer 59:1692, 1987
126. Armstrong BK, McMichael AJ, MacLennan R: Diet. In Schottenfeld D, Fraumeni JF Jr (eds): Cancer Epidemiology and Prevention, p 419. Philadelphia, WB Saunders, 1982
127. Graham S: Toward a dietary prevention of cancer. Epidemiol Rev 5:38, 1983
128. Kinlen LJ: Fat and breast cancer. Cancer Surv 6:585, 1987
129. Bingham SA, Williams DRR, Cummings JH: Dietary fibre consumption in Britain: New estimates and their relatin to large bowel cancer mortality. Br J Cancer 52:399, 1985
130. Greenwald P, Lanza E: Role of dietary fiber in the prevention of cancer. In DeVita VT Jr, Hellman S, Rosenberg SA (eds): Important Advances in Oncology, 1986, p 37. Philadelphia, JB Lippincott, 1986
131. Ziegler RG, Mason TJ, Stemhagen A, et al: Carotene intake, vegetables, and the risk of lung cancer among white men in New Jersey. Am J Epidemiol 123:1080, 1986
132. Graham S, Dayal H, Swanson M, et al: Diet in the epidemiology of cancer of the colon and rectum. J Natl Cancer Inst 61:709, 1978
133. Kinlen LJ: Meat and fat consumption and cancer mortality: A study of strict religious orders in Britain. Lancet 1:946, 1982
134. Bulatao-Jayme J, Almero EM, Castro MCA, et al: A case-control dietary study of primary liver cancer risk from aflatoxin exposure. Int J Epidemiol 11:112, 1982
135. Yu MC, Ho JHC, Lai SH, et al: Cantonese-style salted fish as a cause of nasopharyngeal carcinoma: Report of a case-control study in Hong Kong. Cancer Res 46:956, 1986
136. Hoover RN, Strasser PH: Artificial sweeteners and human bladder cancer. Lancet 1:837, 1980
137. Peto J: Genetic predisposition to cancer. Banbury Report 4:203, 1980
138. Chaganti RSK, German JL (eds): Genetics in Clinical Oncology. New York, Oxford University Press, 1985
139. Ayesh R, Idle JR, Ritchie JC, et al: Metabolic oxidation phenotypes as markers for susceptibility to lung cancer. Nature 312:169, 1984
140. Knudson AG: Hereditary cancer, oncogenes, and antioncogenes. Cancer Res 45:1437, 1985
141. Mulvihill JJ: Clinical genetics of pediatric cancer. In Pizzo P, Poplack DP (eds): Principles and Practice of Pediatric Oncology, pp 19–38. Philadelphia, JB Lippincott, 1989
142. Anderson DE: Familial predisposition. In Schottenfeld D, Fraumeni JF Jr (eds): Cancer Epidemiology and Prevention, p 483. Philadelphia, WB Saunders, 1982
143. Mulvihill JJ: Clinical ecogenetics: Cancer in families. N Engl J Med 312:1569, 1985
144. Li FP, Fraumeni JF Jr: Soft-tissue sarcomas, breast cancer, and other neoplasms: A familial syndrome? Ann Intern Med 71:747, 1969
145. Li FP, Fraumeni JF Jr, Mulvihill JJ, et al: A cancer family syndrome in 24 kindreds. Cancer Res (in press)
146. Chang EH, Pirollo KF, Zou ZQ, et al: Oncogenes in radioresistant, noncancerous skin fibroblasts from a cancer-prone family. Science 237:1036, 1987
147. Hansen MF, Cavenee WK: Genetics of cancer predisposition. Cancer Res 47:5518, 1987

APPENDIX TABLE 13-1. Average Annual Age-Specific Cancer Incidence Rates per 100,000 Population by Site, SEER Program, 1981–1985: White Males

	<5	5–9	10–14	15–19	20–24	25–29	30–34	35–39
All sites	19.9	11.7	11.8	21.2	32.3	43.0	61.9	86.3
Oral cavity and pharynx	—	0.0	0.2	0.2	0.6	0.9	2.5	3.2
Digestive system	1.2	0.2	0.1	0.4	1.1	2.1	4.8	10.0
Esophagus	—	—	—	—	—	0.0	0.1	0.2
Stomach	—	—	0.0	0.1	0.1	0.3	0.5	1.3
Small intestine	0.0	0.0	—	—	—	0.1	0.2	0.2
Colon	—	—	0.0	0.3	0.5	0.8	2.1	4.3
Rectum	—	—	—	—	0.1	0.3	0.8	1.6
Anus and anal canal	—	—	—	—	0.0	0.0	0.2	0.3
Liver	0.6	0.0	—	0.0	0.1	0.1	0.2	0.4
Gallbladder	—	—	—	—	0.0	—	0.0	0.1
Other biliary	0.0	—	—	—	0.0	0.1	0.1	0.1
Pancreas	—	—	—	0.0	0.0	0.1	0.4	1.2
Retroperitoneum	0.6	0.2	—	0.0	0.1	0.1	0.2	0.2
Respiratory system	0.4	0.1	—	0.3	0.6	0.6	2.3	8.0
Nasal cavity, sinuses, ear	0.0	0.0	—	0.0	0.0	0.0	0.1	0.3
Larynx	—	—	—	—	0.0	0.1	0.2	0.9
Lung and bronchus	—	—	—	0.2	0.2	0.4	1.8	6.3
Pleura	—	—	—	—	—	—	0.1	0.2
Bones and joints	0.1	0.7	1.3	2.1	1.0	0.7	0.7	0.5
Soft tissue	1.4	0.5	0.6	0.8	1.1	1.4	1.5	2.0
Melanoma of skin	0.1	0.0	0.1	0.9	2.4	4.6	7.9	11.6
Breast	—	—	—	—	—	0.0	0.1	0.1
Male genital system	0.6	0.2	0.2	3.4	9.5	12.6	12.1	9.9
Prostate gland	0.1	—	—	0.0	0.0	—	0.0	0.1
Testis	0.5	0.1	0.2	3.3	9.3	12.5	12.0	9.5
Penis	—	—	—	—	0.0	0.0	0.1	0.2
Urinary system	2.0	0.6	0.2	0.3	0.9	1.3	3.4	7.1
Urinary bladder	0.0	0.0	—	0.3	0.6	0.9	2.4	4.6
Kidney and renal pelvis	1.9	0.6	0.2	0.1	0.2	0.4	0.9	2.4
Ureter	—	—	—	—	—	—	0.1	0.1
Eye and orbit	1.1	0.2	0.1	0.1	0.1	0.2	0.3	0.3
Brain and nervous system	3.8	2.8	2.1	2.2	2.7	2.8	4.3	4.6
Thyroid	0.0	0.0	0.2	0.8	1.1	1.6	2.7	3.2
Other endocrine	1.3	0.2	0.2	0.3	0.3	0.2	0.2	0.4
Hodgkin's disease	—	0.9	1.4	4.3	5.5	5.3	4.4	4.1
Non-Hodgkin's lymphomas	0.8	1.6	1.8	2.1	2.0	2.7	4.0	7.6
Multiple myeloma	—	—	—	—	0.0	0.0	0.2	0.4
Leukemias	6.7	3.5	3.1	2.6	2.1	2.3	2.8	3.9
Lymphocytic leukemia	5.4	3.0	2.1	1.8	0.9	0.7	0.6	0.7
Acute lymphocytic	5.4	3.0	2.1	1.7	0.8	0.6	0.5	0.4
Chronic lymphocytic	—	—	—	—	0.0	0.0	0.0	0.3
Granulocytic leukemia	0.8	0.3	0.7	0.6	0.9	1.5	1.8	2.6
Acute granulocytic	0.4	0.2	0.4	0.4	0.4	0.9	0.9	1.7
Chronic granulocytic	0.2	—	0.1	0.2	0.4	0.5	0.7	0.8
Monocytic leukemia	0.1	—	0.0	0.1	0.1	0.0	0.1	0.1
Acute monocytic	0.1	—	0.0	0.1	0.1	0.0	0.1	0.1
Chronic monocytic	—	—	—	—	—	—	—	—
Other leukemia	0.4	0.2	0.2	0.1	0.2	0.2	0.4	0.5
Ill-defined/unknown	0.5	0.1	0.2	0.3	0.6	0.7	1.2	1.9

From the National Cancer Institute: Annual Cancer Statistics Review Including Cancer Trends 1950–1985. Bethesda, MD, 1988.

APPENDIX TABLE 13-1 *(continued)*

40–44	*45–49*	*50–54*	*55–59*	*60–64*	*65–69*	*70–74*	*75–79*	*80–84*	*85+*
137.5	239.4	436.4	782.7	1233.0	1830.3	2483.1	3101.1	3576.3	3669.4
8.2	17.9	30.9	51.0	63.8	76.4	83.7	80.5	85.9	90.0
22.6	49.3	97.1	180.9	291.2	432.1	598.6	769.6	926.6	1026.9
1.1	2.6	5.5	12.8	18.8	25.0	29.6	32.2	30.8	32.2
3.1	6.2	11.6	21.1	31.1	50.1	67.2	78.5	116.4	141.8
0.8	1.2	1.6	2.6	3.5	4.7	7.1	6.8	7.3	6.0
8.5	18.2	36.7	66.6	118.6	182.7	268.2	368.7	446.2	513.8
3.9	10.0	21.9	41.6	65.0	93.9	120.6	141.5	162.6	151.1
0.4	0.5	0.9	1.9	2.3	2.7	3.0	4.4	4.5	4.3
0.6	1.3	3.1	5.9	9.4	13.1	17.7	21.3	25.6	21.3
0.1	0.1	0.4	0.9	1.8	3.4	5.0	9.5	8.8	13.9
0.4	0.9	1.2	3.0	4.1	7.5	9.4	14.3	18.7	20.3
3.0	7.3	13.1	22.7	33.9	45.1	66.7	86.0	98.7	111.9
0.5	0.6	0.6	0.8	1.1	1.5	1.7	2.3	3.1	4.0
24.2	57.9	124.7	236.3	347.6	483.9	597.6	641.0	610.4	445.0
0.6	0.9	1.1	2.3	2.6	2.9	3.8	4.4	4.3	5.0
2.8	6.8	16.1	27.2	36.2	43.9	44.4	41.9	36.9	25.2
20.2	48.8	106.0	203.3	303.3	428.9	538.8	582.2	557.4	407.5
0.3	1.1	1.3	2.6	4.5	6.7	9.1	11.6	10.2	6.3
0.6	0.4	0.7	1.1	1.7	1.9	2.3	3.5	1.7	1.0
2.3	2.7	3.8	3.9	4.8	5.8	7.6	12.7	11.1	18.9
14.8	17.9	21.2	25.8	29.0	32.7	33.0	36.2	38.3	42.2
0.5	0.6	1.1	2.0	2.2	3.5	4.2	5.5	5.9	6.3
8.6	12.1	31.7	86.6	203.8	393.9	636.2	873.1	1069.6	1154.1
1.3	5.6	26.4	82.1	199.2	388.7	630.4	865.2	1059.4	1138.8
6.8	5.3	4.0	2.6	2.3	1.3	1.0	1.2	1.2	1.3
0.4	1.0	1.2	1.6	1.8	3.1	3.9	5.2	6.4	10.3
14.8	28.9	49.8	87.0	135.1	190.9	248.5	322.5	384.1	394.9
8.6	16.3	31.7	57.4	92.3	138.5	184.1	240.6	301.1	326.1
5.9	12.3	17.1	27.3	37.8	46.4	54.3	67.5	69.6	56.5
0.1	0.2	0.6	1.7	3.3	4.4	6.9	10.0	9.0	6.0
0.7	0.9	1.2	1.4	2.6	2.2	4.1	4.4	5.4	3.7
6.9	8.9	10.7	15.9	19.3	25.0	24.8	28.1	21.8	14.9
3.5	3.7	4.4	4.7	5.2	6.6	5.0	5.7	5.0	6.0
0.4	0.5	0.7	0.6	1.5	1.8	1.3	0.9	1.2	0.3
3.7	3.9	4.0	4.6	3.8	5.8	6.2	5.1	7.1	4.6
11.1	13.7	22.0	27.2	39.9	52.1	65.7	84.4	101.5	88.0
1.5	2.3	4.5	8.8	14.3	20.3	25.2	40.5	43.3	45.8
5.0	7.3	13.1	19.0	30.4	43.1	65.2	89.2	122.4	151.1
1.4	2.3	5.0	8.6	14.0	17.6	28.3	33.8	48.5	67.4
0.4	0.6	0.6	0.8	1.0	1.1	1.9	1.2	4.0	3.3
1.0	1.6	4.2	7.6	12.6	15.7	25.6	31.3	43.1	60.8
2.4	3.4	5.4	7.0	10.5	17.8	24.5	39.0	53.5	60.1
1.4	2.2	3.3	4.2	6.1	10.7	14.8	23.4	29.6	32.5
0.8	1.1	1.6	2.5	3.3	5.5	8.0	12.2	16.8	21.6
0.1	0.3	0.4	0.4	1.0	1.2	0.8	2.4	4.0	3.3
0.1	0.2	0.3	0.2	0.8	1.1	0.6	1.9	3.1	2.3
—	0.0	—	0.0	0.2	0.1	—	0.3	—	0.3
1.1	1.2	2.2	3.0	4.9	6.4	11.5	13.9	16.3	20.3
3.2	6.2	11.7	23.6	34.1	49.5	69.2	91.1	128.5	164.7

APPENDIX TABLE 13-2. Average Annual Age-Specific Cancer Incidence Rates per 100,000 Population by Site, SEER Program, 1981–1985: White Females

	<5	5–9	10–14	15–19	20–24	25–29	30–34	35–39
All sites	17.4	9.6	10.7	19.3	28.5	53.5	91.1	154.7
Oral cavity and pharynx	0.0	0.2	0.2	0.5	0.3	0.7	1.4	2.1
Digestive system	1.0	0.0	0.3	0.3	0.8	1.6	4.0	8.7
Esophagus	—	—	—	—	—	0.0	—	0.0
Stomach	—	—	—	0.1	0.0	0.1	0.4	1.1
Small intestine	—	—	—	0.0	0.1	0.0	0.1	0.3
Colon	—	—	0.1	0.1	0.3	0.6	1.7	3.9
Rectum	—	—	—	0.1	0.2	0.2	0.8	1.7
Anus and anal canal	—	—	—	—	—	0.0	0.1	0.2
Liver	0.5	—	0.2	0.1	0.1	0.3	0.2	0.3
Gallbladder	—	—	—	—	—	—	—	0.1
Other biliary	—	—	—	—	—	0.0	0.1	0.1
Pancreas	0.0	—	—	0.0	0.0	0.1	0.4	0.8
Retroperitoneum	0.4	0.0	0.0	—	0.0	0.1	0.1	0.2
Respiratory system	0.4	0.1	0.1	0.2	0.3	0.8	1.6	5.9
Nasal cavity, sinuses, ear	0.1	0.1	—	0.0	0.0	0.1	0.1	0.3
Larynx	—	—	—	—	0.0	0.1	0.1	0.3
Lung and bronchus	—	—	0.1	0.1	0.2	0.6	1.3	5.3
Pleura	—	—	—	—	0.0	—	0.0	—
Bones and joints	0.2	0.7	1.2	1.1	0.5	0.5	0.4	0.3
Soft tissue	1.6	0.3	0.6	1.0	0.8	0.8	1.1	1.4
Melanoma of skin	0.0	0.1	0.1	1.5	3.5	7.8	11.8	14.1
Breast	—	—	—	0.1	0.9	8.0	26.1	66.0
Female genital system	0.1	0.2	0.7	1.9	4.7	12.3	19.8	28.0
Cervix uteri	0.0	—	—	0.3	2.0	7.6	11.8	14.0
Corpus and uterus, NOS	—	0.0	0.0	0.1	0.1	0.6	2.5	5.9
Ovary	—	0.1	0.6	1.3	1.9	3.3	4.3	7.0
Vagina	0.1	—	—	—	0.2	0.2	0.2	0.2
Vulva	0.0	—	0.0	0.0	0.2	0.2	0.5	0.7
Urinary system	1.9	0.7	0.1	0.3	0.2	0.7	1.3	2.9
Urinary bladder	0.0	0.0	—	0.2	0.1	0.4	0.5	1.5
Kidney and renal pelvis	1.9	0.7	0.1	0.1	0.1	0.3	0.7	1.3
Ureter	—	—	—	—	—	—	0.0	—
Eye and orbit	1.3	0.2	0.1	0.0	0.0	0.2	0.3	0.2
Brain and nervous system	2.9	2.7	1.7	1.7	1.6	2.7	3.0	3.7
Thyroid	—	0.2	0.9	2.6	5.9	8.5	9.3	9.1
Other endocrine	1.0	0.3	0.1	0.1	0.1	0.1	0.2	0.2
Hodgkin's disease	—	0.2	1.4	4.6	5.4	4.9	3.8	2.6
Non-Hodgkin's lymphomas	0.2	0.2	0.4	1.0	1.2	1.7	3.0	3.6
Multiple myeloma	—	—	—	—	—	—	0.1	0.4
Leukemias	6.1	3.3	2.3	2.1	1.6	1.5	2.6	3.0
Lymphocytic leukemia	5.2	2.9	1.5	0.9	0.5	0.3	0.4	0.7
Acute lymphocytic	5.2	2.8	1.5	0.9	0.5	0.3	0.4	0.4
Chronic lymphocytic	—	—	—	—	—	—	0.1	0.3
Granulocytic leukemia	0.5	0.3	0.6	0.9	0.9	1.0	1.7	1.9
Acute granulocytic	0.5	0.2	0.4	0.7	0.5	0.7	1.0	1.3
Chronic granulocytic	0.0	—	0.2	0.2	0.2	0.3	0.4	0.5
Monocytic leukemia	0.2	—	0.1	0.1	0.0	0.1	0.2	0.1
Acute monocytic	0.2	—	0.1	0.1	0.0	0.1	0.1	0.1
Chronic monocytic	—	—	—	—	—	—	—	—
Other leukemia	0.2	0.1	0.1	0.2	0.2	0.1	0.3	0.3
Ill-defined/unknown	0.4	0.1	0.2	0.2	0.2	0.2	0.9	1.8

From the National Cancer Institute: Annual Cancer Statistics Review Including Cancer Trends 1950–1985. Bethesda, MD, 1988.

APPENDIX TABLE 13-2 *(continued)*

40–44	*45–49*	*50–54*	*55–59*	*60–64*	*65–69*	*70–74*	*75–79*	*80–84*	*85+*
247.4	394.4	549.5	761.4	1029.1	1256.6	1475.3	1644.8	1827.9	1876.0
3.3	7.7	11.7	19.6	26.4	30.1	28.1	28.6	27.8	29.5
18.8	39.5	75.3	121.2	185.5	272.7	388.0	524.6	655.2	729.4
0.2	0.6	2.0	4.0	6.5	7.4	8.9	11.1	12.4	13.3
1.5	3.1	5.4	7.6	12.9	17.5	27.8	42.6	54.7	68.1
0.3	1.1	1.4	2.0	2.0	2.8	3.6	4.4	5.8	5.4
8.5	18.3	34.7	57.7	86.7	136.4	193.4	278.7	346.9	390.1
4.0	8.7	16.7	26.2	37.2	50.5	70.8	82.6	97.6	106.0
0.5	0.9	2.0	2.6	3.2	4.0	4.7	4.5	6.7	5.1
0.6	0.5	1.6	2.2	3.1	4.0	6.5	7.9	8.7	10.5
0.4	0.5	1.6	2.3	4.3	6.6	9.7	14.0	19.0	21.8
0.3	0.4	1.5	1.3	3.3	4.3	6.9	9.4	13.7	14.0
2.0	4.4	7.7	13.8	24.2	36.8	52.3	63.5	84.7	88.1
0.2	0.4	0.3	0.6	1.0	0.8	1.1	2.6	1.4	1.2
17.0	37.3	70.5	111.2	153.8	181.2	189.6	159.9	137.6	98.0
0.3	0.5	0.9	0.8	1.8	1.6	1.8	2.5	2.6	1.7
0.8	2.5	3.6	5.1	7.0	8.3	7.3	5.3	3.6	2.5
15.6	33.9	65.7	104.3	144.4	169.6	178.9	150.2	128.7	92.7
0.3	0.1	0.2	0.6	0.5	1.1	1.3	1.6	2.2	0.4
0.3	0.5	0.5	0.5	1.2	1.4	1.5	1.3	2.5	1.7
1.8	1.2	2.1	2.8	3.9	4.5	5.0	5.1	9.3	7.6
14.5	16.7	17.1	18.1	17.7	16.0	18.4	19.3	21.4	22.0
114.5	174.0	201.2	252.0	303.9	344.3	372.0	389.0	400.3	395.0
40.6	65.9	95.1	129.1	184.4	202.7	207.1	190.9	176.9	161.0
14.3	15.0	14.9	16.2	17.2	17.2	17.3	16.8	16.1	19.0
12.1	25.8	47.0	70.9	109.2	123.1	118.9	99.9	82.1	64.1
12.3	21.9	29.3	36.0	49.9	53.2	58.1	55.2	55.6	49.4
0.6	0.8	0.6	1.5	2.2	1.9	2.8	4.0	5.1	5.8
0.8	1.5	2.4	2.6	3.4	5.3	7.7	12.2	15.5	20.1
6.2	11.5	16.6	27.0	43.4	56.6	73.3	89.7	105.3	110.1
2.9	5.9	9.1	14.6	25.6	32.8	46.1	55.1	72.1	82.7
3.4	5.4	7.0	11.5	16.1	21.4	23.4	29.6	28.3	23.0
—	0.1	0.2	0.7	1.0	1.6	2.7	3.4	3.1	2.7
0.6	0.9	0.5	1.7	1.4	2.8	2.5	2.1	2.0	2.1
4.5	4.9	8.8	9.7	13.5	17.0	16.5	16.8	16.1	6.9
9.3	9.4	9.2	8.7	9.3	7.9	9.4	7.0	9.0	6.3
0.3	0.2	0.7	0.7	1.0	0.8	1.3	0.7	0.8	0.3
1.7	1.4	2.0	2.2	2.8	3.1	4.3	4.4	3.9	3.4
6.5	9.6	15.1	22.6	30.1	38.8	53.3	66.0	68.9	66.0
0.7	1.6	3.7	5.2	9.8	14.7	19.2	24.3	29.1	28.5
3.3	5.1	7.5	11.1	15.0	24.1	32.1	41.5	62.3	75.8
0.9	1.3	2.4	3.5	6.3	10.0	14.0	17.7	24.8	32.4
0.6	0.5	0.4	0.3	0.5	0.7	0.6	1.4	1.3	1.7
0.3	0.7	1.9	3.1	5.4	9.2	12.7	15.4	22.0	28.6
1.8	3.1	3.9	5.6	6.5	10.2	14.5	17.7	25.3	28.9
1.0	1.7	2.6	3.8	4.1	6.6	9.2	10.2	14.3	16.1
0.6	1.2	1.2	1.4	1.7	2.5	3.9	5.7	7.6	9.3
0.2	0.2	0.2	0.4	0.4	0.7	0.4	0.8	1.9	2.1
0.1	0.2	0.2	0.3	0.3	0.6	0.4	0.7	1.2	1.0
0.0	—	—	—	0.0	—	—	—	0.5	0.5
0.5	0.5	0.9	1.5	1.9	3.2	3.1	5.4	10.3	12.4
2.8	6.1	11.3	16.9	25.0	36.2	51.6	70.3	94.1	127.2

APPENDIX TABLE 13-3. Average Annual Age-Specific Cancer Incidence Rates per 100,000 Population by Site, SEER Program, 1981–1985: Black Males

	<5	5–9	10–14	15–19	20–24	25–29	30–34	35–39
All sites	10.7	8.4	9.9	14.4	18.3	22.2	43.8	75.5
Oral cavity and pharynx	0.4	0.2	0.7	0.5	0.9	0.7	3.7	8.7
Digestive system	0.2	0.4	0.2	0.2	0.5	2.9	7.9	14.0
Esophagus	—	—	—	—	—	0.2	0.8	1.1
Stomach	—	—	—	—	—	0.2	0.4	3.4
Small intestine	—	—	—	—	—	0.4	—	0.3
Colon	—	—	0.2	0.2	0.2	0.9	2.9	5.6
Rectum	—	—	—	—	—	0.9	1.2	1.1
Anus and anal canal	—	—	—	—	—	—	—	—
Liver	—	0.2	—	—	0.4	0.4	2.1	0.8
Gallbladder	—	—	—	—	—	—	—	—
Other biliary	—	—	—	—	—	—	—	0.3
Pancreas	—	—	—	—	—	—	0.2	1.4
Retroperitoneum	0.2	0.2	—	—	—	—	0.2	—
Respiratory system	0.6	0.6	0.2	—	0.5	1.1	4.1	11.5
Nasal cavity, sinuses, ear	0.2	0.2	—	—	0.2	—	—	—
Larnyx	—	—	—	—	—	—	0.6	1.1
Lung and bronchus	—	—	0.2	—	0.2	0.9	3.1	9.8
Pleura	—	—	—	—	—	0.2	—	—
Bones and joints	0.2	0.4	0.9	2.3	0.4	0.4	0.4	1.4
Soft tissue	0.7	0.2	0.7	0.5	1.1	1.6	2.3	1.4
Melanoma of skin	—	—	—	—	0.2	—	—	0.6
Breast	—	—	—	—	—	—	—	0.3
Male genital system	0.2	—	0.2	0.7	2.0	2.5	1.7	4.2
Prostate gland	—	—	—	—	—	—	—	1.4
Testis	0.2	—	—	0.5	2.0	2.5	1.4	1.7
Penis	—	—	—	—	—	—	0.2	0.3
Urinary system	2.0	1.2	0.4	0.2	0.5	1.4	2.9	3.6
Urinary bladder	—	—	—	0.2	—	0.5	0.6	1.1
Kidney and renal pelvis	2.0	1.2	0.4	—	0.5	0.7	2.3	2.5
Ureter	—	—	—	—	—	—	—	—
Eye and orbit	1.5	0.2	—	—	—	0.2	0.2	0.6
Brain and nervous system	1.7	2.5	1.4	3.1	1.1	0.7	3.1	1.4
Thyroid	—	—	—	0.4	0.4	0.4	0.6	2.2
Other endocrine	0.6	—	—	—	0.2	—	0.6	0.3
Hodgkin's disease	—	0.4	1.1	2.3	4.4	3.0	3.1	3.4
Non-Hodgkin's lymphomas	0.4	0.8	1.4	1.1	2.0	2.7	5.4	6.7
Multiple myeloma	—	—	—	—	—	—	0.6	2.2
Leukemias	2.0	1.6	2.7	2.7	3.0	2.2	2.5	5.6
Lymphocytic leukemia	1.7	1.2	1.8	1.4	—	0.2	—	1.7
Acute lymphocytic	1.7	1.0	1.8	1.4	—	0.2	—	1.1
Chronic lymphocytic	—	—	—	—	—	—	—	0.6
Granulocytic leukemia	0.2	0.4	0.9	1.1	2.3	1.8	2.5	3.4
Acute granulocytic	0.2	0.4	0.7	0.4	1.2	0.9	0.6	1.4
Chronic granulocytic	—	—	0.2	0.7	1.1	0.7	1.9	2.0
Monocytic leukemia	—	—	—	—	—	0.2	—	0.3
Acute monocytic	—	—	—	—	—	0.2	—	—
Chronic monocytic	—	—	—	—	—	—	—	0.3
Other leukemia	0.2	—	—	0.2	0.7	—	—	0.3
Ill-defined/unknown	0.4	—	—	0.2	0.5	0.5	0.4	4.2

From the National Cancer Institute: Annual Cancer Statistics Review Including Cancer Trends 1950–1985. Bethesda, MD, 1988.

APPENDIX TABLE 13-3 *(continued)*

40–44	*45–49*	*50–54*	*55–59*	*60–64*	*65–69*	*70–74*	*75–79*	*80–84*	*85+*
185.0	376.0	689.7	1182.5	1739.3	2315.5	3050.3	3294.1	4068.2	3433.6
24.1	49.6	68.3	95.1	86.2	74.7	65.8	44.8	67.9	39.3
47.9	92.1	182.8	283.7	422.4	533.5	707.1	831.6	1078.3	914.5
12.4	24.1	49.0	65.3	86.2	83.8	75.8	73.5	41.5	39.3
5.8	15.6	32.0	40.0	66.3	93.0	114.9	141.6	222.4	151.5
1.1	2.2	2.8	6.3	4.0	4.6	7.8	7.2	—	5.6
13.2	25.5	42.9	77.0	129.8	178.3	262.1	362.0	456.2	381.5
6.9	8.0	19.8	32.2	48.8	61.0	78.1	82.4	147.0	112.2
—	1.3	1.4	2.4	1.7	3.0	3.3	9.0	3.8	11.2
2.2	2.7	8.0	13.2	18.7	33.5	36.8	19.7	26.4	5.6
0.7	—	0.5	1.5	0.6	3.0	6.7	7.2	11.3	11.2
—	0.9	1.4	2.9	4.0	3.0	10.0	10.8	7.5	11.2
5.5	11.6	25.0	39.5	59.5	66.3	109.3	107.5	154.6	168.3
—	—	—	1.0	1.7	0.8	1.1	1.8	3.8	—
52.6	134.6	253.0	444.5	567.5	707.3	801.9	679.3	667.3	460.1
1.1	1.3	1.4	2.9	1.7	1.5	5.6	7.2	11.3	11.2
9.1	16.1	24.5	43.4	59.0	58.7	59.1	48.4	18.9	33.7
41.7	116.7	226.6	393.4	503.4	644.0	733.9	614.7	629.6	403.9
0.4	0.4	0.5	3.9	2.3	3.0	3.3	7.2	7.5	11.2
0.4	0.4	—	1.5	1.1	—	3.3	1.8	—	—
3.7	4.9	1.4	1.9	5.1	9.1	10.0	7.2	3.8	5.6
—	1.8	0.9	0.5	3.4	3.8	—	3.6	11.3	5.6
—	1.8	1.4	5.4	2.3	1.5	7.8	7.2	15.1	5.6
4.8	13.0	52.8	158.4	389.5	644.0	1032.8	1206.2	1583.5	1408.2
2.6	11.2	51.4	155.0	384.9	638.7	1027.2	1197.2	1576.0	1402.6
0.7	0.4	—	0.5	1.1	—	—	—	—	5.6
1.5	0.9	1.4	1.9	2.8	3.8	4.5	9.0	7.5	—
9.9	21.0	40.5	61.4	83.3	133.4	162.8	179.2	192.3	213.2
4.8	9.4	19.3	30.7	44.2	83.1	99.3	114.7	124.4	157.1
4.8	11.6	19.3	28.8	37.4	45.7	53.5	44.8	56.6	50.5
0.4	—	0.5	0.5	0.6	1.5	5.6	5.4	—	5.6
—	0.4	0.5	—	1.1	0.8	—	—	—	11.2
6.9	6.7	8.5	7.3	15.9	11.4	12.3	9.0	11.3	5.6
2.9	3.1	1.4	4.9	4.0	3.8	3.3	3.6	—	5.6
0.4	1.3	0.9	1.0	2.3	—	—	1.8	—	—
2.9	4.0	0.9	1.5	4.0	3.0	4.5	5.4	3.8	22.4
7.3	8.5	15.5	19.5	27.8	38.9	43.5	43.0	49.0	16.8
3.7	9.8	14.1	29.7	34.6	49.5	49.1	93.2	124.4	50.5
7.7	8.9	11.8	19.0	29.5	38.1	55.8	44.8	101.8	84.2
2.2	2.2	5.7	6.8	11.9	13.7	32.3	30.5	49.0	33.7
0.7	—	0.5	—	—	—	1.1	3.6	7.5	—
1.5	1.3	5.2	6.8	11.3	13.0	30.1	26.9	41.5	33.7
4.4	5.8	3.3	8.8	14.2	17.5	15.6	12.5	37.7	39.3
4.0	1.8	0.9	3.4	6.2	9.9	6.7	9.0	22.6	22.4
0.4	3.1	2.4	4.9	7.4	7.6	5.6	3.6	11.3	16.8
—	—	0.9	1.5	0.6	0.8	—	—	—	5.6
—	—	0.9	1.5	0.6	0.8	—	—	—	5.6
—	—	—	—	—	—	—	—	—	—
1.1	0.9	1.9	1.9	2.8	6.1	7.8	1.8	15.1	5.6
8.0	10.7	31.6	45.8	55.6	59.4	88.1	125.5	150.8	173.9

APPENDIX TABLE 13-4. Average Annual Age-Specific Cancer Incidence Rates per 100,000 Population by Site, SEER Program, 1981–1985: Black Females

	<5	*5–9*	*10–14*	*15–19*	*20–24*	*25–29*	*30–34*	*35–39*
All sites	17.2	7.7	9.3	12.3	17.1	38.5	88.1	154.3
Oral cavity and pharynx	—	—	0.5	0.7	0.5	0.3	1.1	4.1
Digestive system	1.5	—	0.2	0.5	1.0	2.7	4.8	13.9
Esophagus	—	—	—	—	—	—	0.2	1.2
Stomach	—	—	—	—	—	0.6	0.7	1.7
Small intestine	—	—	—	—	0.2	—	—	0.2
Colon	—	—	—	—	0.3	1.1	2.4	7.3
Rectum	—	—	—	—	—	0.8	0.6	1.9
Anus and anal canal	—	—	—	—	—	—	—	0.5
Liver	0.6	—	0.2	0.4	0.3	—	—	0.2
Gallbladder	—	—	—	—	—	—	—	—
Other biliary	—	—	—	0.2	—	—	—	—
Pancreas	—	—	—	—	0.2	0.2	0.7	0.7
Retroperitoneum	1.0	—	—	—	—	—	—	—
Respiratory system	—	—	—	—	0.2	0.5	1.8	6.3
Nasal cavity, sinuses, ear	—	—	—	—	—	0.2	—	—
Larynx	—	—	—	—	—	—	0.2	1.2
Lung and bronchus	—	—	—	—	—	0.2	1.5	5.1
Pleura	—	—	—	—	—	—	0.2	—
Bones and joints	0.4	0.2	0.9	0.7	0.2	0.5	0.6	0.7
Soft tissue	2.1	0.6	0.9	1.4	0.2	0.8	1.3	0.7
Melanoma of skin	—	0.2	—	—	—	—	0.4	0.5
Breast	—	—	—	—	1.5	12.2	39.8	73.0
Female genital system	0.2	0.6	1.1	2.5	6.1	12.1	21.9	32.1
Cervix uteri	—	—	—	0.7	2.6	7.6	14.7	22.1
Corpus and uterus, NOS	—	—	—	—	—	1.1	1.5	3.9
Ovary	—	0.6	1.1	1.4	2.5	2.3	4.4	4.4
Vagina	0.2	—	—	—	0.2	—	0.2	0.2
Vulva	—	—	—	—	—	0.5	0.6	1.5
Urinary system	3.3	1.0	0.5	0.9	0.8	0.5	1.5	1.2
Urinary bladder	—	—	—	0.4	0.2	0.2	0.4	0.7
Kidney and renal pelvis	3.3	1.0	0.5	0.5	0.7	0.3	0.9	0.5
Ureter	—	—	—	—	—	—	—	—
Eye and orbit	1.1	—	—	—	—	—	—	—
Brain and nervous system	2.5	2.8	1.5	0.5	1.0	1.1	1.3	1.2
Thyroid	—	—	0.2	0.5	1.8	2.7	3.9	3.9
Other endocrine	0.4	0.2	—	0.2	0.2	—	—	0.7
Hodgkin's disease	—	0.2	0.9	1.3	0.8	1.4	1.5	2.4
Non-Hodgkin's lymphomas	0.6	0.4	0.2	0.5	1.3	1.3	2.4	2.9
Multiple myeloma	—	—	—	—	—	—	0.7	1.0
Leukemias	4.8	1.4	2.0	1.6	1.5	1.3	2.0	4.4
Lymphocytic leukemia	4.2	0.8	0.5	0.4	—	0.2	0.2	0.2
Acute lymphocytic	4.2	0.8	0.5	0.4	—	0.2	0.2	—
Chronic lymphocytic	—	—	—	—	—	—	—	0.2
Granulocytic leukemia	0.2	0.4	1.1	1.1	1.3	0.8	1.7	2.9
Acute granulocytic	0.2	0.2	0.5	0.5	1.0	0.6	0.7	1.9
Chronic granulocytic	—	0.2	0.2	0.4	0.3	0.2	0.7	0.7
Monocytic leukemia	0.2	—	0.2	0.2	—	0.2	—	—
Acute monocytic	0.2	—	0.2	0.2	—	0.2	—	—
Chronic monocytic	—	—	—	—	—	—	—	—
Other leukemia	0.2	0.2	0.2	—	0.2	0.2	0.2	1.2
Ill-defined/unknown	0.4	—	0.4	0.2	—	0.3	1.5	3.9

From the National Cancer Institute: Annual Cancer Statistics Review Including Cancer Trends 1950–1985. Bethesda, MD, 1988.

APPENDIX TABLE 13-4 *(continued)*

40–44	*45–49*	*50–54*	*55–59*	*60–64*	*65–69*	*70–74*	*75–79*	*80–84*	*85+*
269.9	389.9	514.1	755.0	925.9	1102.4	1378.6	1514.7	1891.1	1695.3
8.8	17.5	21.0	29.5	22.0	16.7	19.7	16.2	12.8	14.6
31.9	60.1	99.1	162.7	230.5	328.5	466.6	523.7	736.8	697.6
3.3	7.8	15.9	17.9	24.4	21.3	19.7	11.5	19.2	14.6
2.3	7.0	7.1	13.7	19.6	34.0	51.1	61.1	108.6	124.4
1.0	1.6	3.2	2.1	3.3	5.8	9.4	4.6	4.3	4.9
13.4	21.7	37.7	72.4	105.7	156.7	229.0	259.6	347.1	309.8
4.9	7.0	13.1	24.6	28.2	46.7	51.9	70.4	80.9	78.1
2.0	1.6	2.8	3.7	4.3	2.9	5.5	1.2	10.6	7.3
—	1.2	2.4	4.2	4.8	6.9	7.9	13.8	4.3	17.1
0.3	0.8	2.0	3.7	2.9	3.5	4.7	11.5	19.2	7.3
—	—	0.8	0.4	2.4	2.9	5.5	5.8	8.5	14.6
4.2	10.1	13.5	18.3	33.5	46.7	77.9	83.1	129.9	112.2
0.7	1.2	0.4	1.2	1.0	0.6	2.4	—	2.1	—
29.3	58.6	85.6	123.2	158.3	159.1	147.9	151.1	134.2	102.4
0.3	1.2	—	0.8	1.4	0.6	1.6	—	6.4	—
2.0	5.0	8.3	7.9	10.5	8.1	6.3	5.8	6.4	—
27.1	52.0	77.3	114.0	146.3	148.7	140.1	144.2	119.3	97.6
—	0.4	—	—	—	1.7	—	1.2	—	2.4
1.0	0.4	0.4	—	1.0	0.6	—	1.2	2.1	2.4
1.6	1.9	2.8	3.3	4.3	6.9	9.4	12.7	10.6	—
—	1.2	1.2	0.8	2.9	3.5	0.8	4.6	—	9.8
114.8	149.0	158.2	209.3	223.8	244.9	307.7	305.7	389.7	302.5
46.0	53.2	75.7	108.2	141.1	155.0	183.3	205.3	215.1	231.7
31.6	29.1	33.3	34.1	34.0	41.5	51.1	56.5	59.6	87.8
7.2	9.3	19.0	38.3	63.1	68.6	77.9	73.9	89.5	85.4
4.9	11.6	17.4	27.1	35.4	35.7	40.1	56.5	38.3	39.0
0.7	1.2	2.0	3.3	3.8	5.8	8.7	5.8	14.9	9.8
1.3	1.2	2.8	2.9	3.3	—	3.9	8.1	2.1	4.9
5.9	8.5	17.4	30.4	34.9	36.9	47.2	63.4	83.1	73.2
1.0	1.2	5.9	15.0	17.7	24.2	26.8	33.5	49.0	56.1
4.6	5.8	9.5	13.3	13.9	12.1	18.9	25.4	29.8	17.1
—	—	—	—	—	—	1.6	1.2	2.1	—
0.7	—	0.4	—	0.5	—	—	—	—	—
2.6	1.2	5.2	4.2	7.7	9.8	7.9	12.7	14.9	—
6.2	7.8	5.2	8.7	5.7	5.8	8.7	1.2	6.4	12.2
—	0.8	0.4	1.2	1.0	2.3	—	—	—	—
1.0	0.4	1.2	1.7	1.4	2.3	2.4	2.3	2.1	—
3.3	8.9	7.5	13.7	18.7	32.3	30.7	36.9	38.3	34.1
3.3	4.7	11.5	13.7	18.2	26.5	44.1	47.3	63.9	46.3
3.3	4.3	6.7	10.8	21.0	21.3	29.9	48.5	42.6	56.1
—	1.2	1.6	3.7	6.2	7.5	11.8	24.2	19.2	19.5
—	0.4	0.8	0.4	0.5	1.7	0.8	—	—	—
—	0.4	0.8	3.3	5.3	5.2	11.0	23.1	17.0	14.6
2.6	2.3	5.2	5.4	10.5	11.5	13.4	16.2	17.0	22.0
2.0	1.6	3.2	2.9	6.7	5.2	4.7	9.2	10.6	12.2
0.7	0.8	2.0	2.5	3.3	4.6	7.9	5.8	6.4	9.8
—	—	—	0.4	1.0	0.6	1.6	—	—	2.4
—	—	—	0.4	1.0	0.6	1.6	—	—	—
—	—	—	—	—	—	—	—	—	—
0.7	0.8	—	1.2	3.3	1.7	3.1	8.1	6.4	12.2
9.8	8.5	14.7	31.6	32.5	50.1	70.0	80.8	138.4	112.2

STEVEN A. ROSENBERG

CHAPTER 14 Principles of Surgical Oncology

Surgery is the oldest treatment for cancer and, until recently, was the only treatment that could cure patients with cancer. The surgical treatment of cancer has changed dramatically over the last several decades. Advances in surgical techniques and a better understanding of the patterns of spread of individual cancers have allowed surgeons to perform successful resections for an increased number of patients. The development of alternate treatment strategies that can control microscopic disease has prompted surgeons to reassess the magnitude of surgery necessary.

The surgeon who treats cancer must be familiar with the natural history of individual cancers and with the principles and potentialities of surgery, radiation therapy, chemotherapy, immunotherapy, and other new treatment modalities.

The surgeon has a central role in the prevention, diagnosis, definitive treatment, palliation, and rehabilitation of the cancer patient. The principles underlying each of these roles of the surgical oncologist are discussed in this chapter.

HISTORICAL PERSPECTIVE

Although the earliest discussions of the surgical treatment of tumors are found in the Edwin Smith Papyrus from the Egyptian Middle Kingdom (approximately 1600 B.C.), the modern era of elective surgery for visceral tumors began in frontier America in 1809.[1,2] Ephraim MacDowell removed a 22-pound ovarian tumor from a patient, Mrs. Jane Todd Crawford, who survived for 30 years after the operation. This procedure, the first of 13 ovarian resections performed by MacDowell, was the first elective abdominal operation and provided a great stimulus to the development of elective surgery.

However, the treatment of most tumors depended on two subsequent developments in surgery. The first of these was the introduction of general anesthesia by two dentists, Dr. William Morton and Dr. Crawford Long. The first major operation using general ether anesthesia was an excision of the submaxillary gland and part of the tongue, performed by Dr. John Collins Warren on October 16, 1846, at the Massachusetts General Hospital. The second major development stimulating the widespread application of surgery resulted from the introduction of the principles of antisepsis by Joseph Lister in 1867. Based on the concepts of Pasteur, Lister introduced carbolic acid in 1867 and described the principles of antisepsis in an article in *The Lancet* in that same year.

These developments freed surgery from both pain and sepsis and greatly increased its use for the treatment of tumors. In the decade before the introduction of ether, only 385 operations were performed at the Massachusetts General Hospital. By the last decade of the 19th century, more than 20,000 operations per year were performed at that same hospital.[3]

Table 14-1 lists some selected milestones in the history of surgical oncology. Although this does not include all of the important developments, it does provide the tempo of the application of surgery to cancer treatment.[4] Major figures in the evolution of surgical oncology included Albert Theodore Billroth who, in addition to developing meticulous surgical techniques, performed the first gastrectomy, laryngectomy,

TABLE 14-1. Selected Historical Milestones in Surgical Oncology

Year	Surgeon	Event
1809	Ephraim McDowell	Elective abdominal surgery (excised ovarian tumor)
1846	John Collins Warren	Use of ether anesthesia (excised submaxillary gland)
1867	Joseph Lister	Introduction of antisepsis
1860–1890	Albert Theodore Billroth	First gastrectomy, laryngectomy, and esophagectomy
1878	Richard von Volkmann	Excision of cancerous rectum
1880s	Theodore Kocher	Development of thyroid surgery
1890	William Stewart Halsted	Radical mastectomy
1896	G. T. Beatson	Oophorectomy for breast cancer
1904	Hugh H. Young	Radical prostatectomy
1906	Ernest Wertheim	Radical hysterectomy
1908	W. Ernest Miles	Abdomenoperineal resection for rectal cancer
1912	E. Martin	Cordotomy for the treatment of pain
1910–1930	Harvey Cushing	Development of surgery for brain tumors
1913	Franz Torek	Successful resection of cancer of the thoracic esophagus
1927	G. Divis	Successful resection of pulmonary metastases
1933	Evarts Graham	Pneumonectomy
1935	A. O. Whipple	Pancreaticoduodenectomy
1945	Charles B. Huggins	Adrenalectomy for prostate cancer

and esophagectomy. In the 1890s, William Stewart Halsted elucidated the principles of en bloc resections for cancer, as exemplified by his development of the radical mastectomy. Examples of radical resections for cancers of individual organs include the radical prostatectomy by Hugh Young in 1904, the radical hysterectomy by Ernest Wertheim in 1906, the abdominoperineal resection for cancer of the rectum by W. Ernest Miles in 1908, and the first successful pneumonectomy performed for cancer by Evarts Graham in 1933. Modern technical innovations continue to extend the surgeon's capabilities. Recent examples include the development of microsurgical techniques that enable the performance of free grafts for reconstruction, automatic stapling devices, sophisticated endoscopic equipment that allows for a wide variety of "incisionless" surgery, and major improvements in postoperative management and critical care of patients that have extended the safety of major surgical therapy.

Many critics who feel that the application of surgery has reached a plateau beyond which it will not progress should remember the words of a famous British surgeon, Sir John Erichsen, who in his introductory address to the medical institutions at University College, said,

> . . . there must be a final limit to the development of manipulative surgery, the knife cannot always have fresh fields for conquest and although methods of practice may be modified and varied and even improved to some extent, it must be within a certain limit. That this limit has nearly, if not quite, been reached will appear evident if we reflect on the great achievements of modern operative surgery. Very little remains for the boldest to devise or the most dextrous to perform.

These comments, published in *The Lancet* in 1873, preceded the majority of important developments in modern surgical oncology.

THE OPERATION

ANESTHESIA

Modern anesthetic techniques have greatly increased the safety of major oncologic surgery. Both regional and general anesthesia play important roles in a wide variety of diagnostic techniques and local therapeutic maneuvers, as well as in major surgery, and these should be understood by all oncologists.

Anesthetic techniques may be divided into regional and general anesthesia. Regional anesthesia involves a reversible blockade of pain perception by the application of local anesthetic drugs. These agents generally work by preventing the activation of pain receptors or by blocking nerve conduction. A variety of agents commonly used for regional anesthesia are shown in Table 14-2.[5] Topical anesthesia refers to the application of local anesthetics to the skin or mucous membranes. Good surface anesthesia of the conjunctiva and cornea, the oropharynx and nasopharynx, esophagus, larynx, trachea, urethra, and anus can result from the application of these agents.

Local anesthesia involves injecting anesthetic agents directly into the operative field. Field block refers to injection of local anesthetic by circumscribing the operative field with a continuous wall of anesthetic agent. Lidocaine (Xylocaine) in concentrations from 0.5% to 1% is the most common anesthetic agent used for this purpose. Peripheral nerve block results from the deposition of a local anesthetic surrounding major nerve trunks. It can provide local anesthesia to entire anatomic areas.

Major surgical procedures in the lower portion of the body can be performed using either epidural or spinal anesthesia. Epidural anesthesia results from the deposition of a local anesthetic agent into the extradural space within the vertebral canal. Catheters can be left in place in the epidural

TABLE 14-2. Regional Anesthetic Agents

Technique	*Local Anesthetic*	*Concentration Range (%)*	*Duration of Action*	*Maximal Safe Dose (mg)*
Topical anesthesia (mucous membranes)	Lidocaine	2–4	15 min	100
	Cocaine	4–10	30 min	100–200
	Tetracaine	1–2	45 min	40
	Benzocaine	2–10	several hours	
Local infiltration	Procaine	0.5	¼–½ h	1000
	Lidocaine	0.5–1	½–1 h	500
	Mepivacaine	0.5–1	½–1 h	500
	Tetracaine	0.025–0.1	2–3 h	75
Major nerve block	Lidocaine	1–2	1–2 h	500
	Mepivacaine	1–2	1–2 h	500
	Tetracaine	0.1–0.25	2–3 h	75

Adapted from Brunner EA, Eckenhoff JE: Anesthesia. In Sabiston DC Jr (ed): Textbook of Surgery. Philadelphia, WB Saunders, 1977.

space, allowing the intermittent injection of local anesthetics for prolonged operations. The major advantage of epidural over spinal anesthesia is that it does not involve puncturing the dura, and thus the injection of foreign substances directly into the cerebrospinal fluid is avoided.

Spinal anesthesia involves the direct injection of a local anesthetic into the cerebrospinal fluid. Puncture of the dural sac generally is performed between the L2 and L4 vertebrae. Spinal anesthesia provides excellent anesthesia for intra-abdominal operations, operations on the pelvis, or procedures involving the lower extremities. Because the patient is awake during spinal anesthesia and is breathing spontaneously, it often has been thought that spinal anesthesia is "safer" than general anesthesia. There is, however, no difference in the incidence of intraoperative hypotension with spinal anesthesia compared with general anesthesia, and thus there is no clear benefit in using spinal anesthesia for patients with ischemic heart disease.[6] Because patients are awake during spinal anesthesia and can become agitated during the surgical procedure, spinal anesthesia actually can cause more myocardial stress than general anesthesia. The health status of patients with preoperative evidence of congestive heart failure is more likely to be worsened by general anesthesia than by spinal anesthesia. In one series, heart failure developed de novo in 4% of adults over the age of 40 years who were undergoing major surgery, and worsened in 22% of patients who had a history of heart failure.[6] Spinal anesthesia was not associated with any new or worsened heart failure. Because of local irritating effects of general anesthesia on the lung, it has been suggested that spinal anesthesia may be safer for patients with severe pulmonary disease.

General anesthesia refers to the reversible state of loss of consciousness produced by a variety of chemical agents that act directly on the brain. Most major oncologic procedures are performed under general anesthesia, which can be induced using either intravenous or inhalational agents. The advantages of intravenous anesthesia are the extremely rapid onset of unconsciousness and improved patient comfort and acceptance. Ultrashort-acting barbiturates, such as sodium thiopental, or tranquilizers, such as the benzodiazepines or droperidol, are the most frequently used intravenous agents for general anesthesia or for sedation during regional anesthesia.

A variety of inhalational anesthetic agents are in clinical use. The most popular is nitrous oxide, usually in combination with narcotics and muscle relaxants. This technique provides a safe form of general anesthesia with the use of nonexplosive agents. Two other agents in widespread use are the fluorinated hydrocarbons, halothane (Fluothane) and enflurane (Ethrane). Although they are used frequently, the fluorinated hydrocarbons have a variety of side-effects. Halothane depresses myocardial function, reduces cardiac output, causes significant vasodilation, and sensitizes the myocardium to both endogenous and administered catecholamines, which can lead to life-threatening cardiac arrhythmias. In rare instances, halothane can cause severe hepatotoxicity, which begins 2 to 5 days after surgery. Enflurane also depresses myocardial function but does not appear to sensitize the myocardium to catecholamines and has not been associated with hepatic toxicity. The newest of the halogenated hydrocarbons is isoflurane, which was introduced in 1980. Isoflurane depresses the myocardium less than halothane or enflurane, but it has more potent vasodilatory properties.

Virtually all general anesthetics affect various biochemical mechanisms, including depression of bone marrow, alteration of the phagocytic activity of macrophages, and exhibition of various immunosuppressive properties. General anesthetic agents, such as cyclopropane and diethyl ether, are rarely used in current practice because of their explosive potential.

Intravenous neuromuscular blocking agents, called muscle relaxants, are commonly used during general anesthesia. These agents are either nondepolarizing (*e.g.*, curare), preventing access of acetylcholine to the receptor site of the myoneural junction, or depolarizing (*e.g.*, succinylcholine) acting in a manner similar to that of acetylcholine by depolarizing the motor end-plate. These agents induce profound muscle relaxation during surgical procedures but have the obvious disadvantage of inhibiting spontaneous respiration because of paralysis of respiratory muscles. Succinylcholine is short acting (3–5 minutes) with a rapid recovery phase. Curare-induced paralysis lasts for 30 to 40 minutes after usual clinical doses of 0.3 to 0.5 mg/kg. Pancuronium is a newer nondepolarizing agent that has fewer side-effects than curare but can induce tachycardia by means of sympathetic stimulation.

DETERMINATION OF OPERATIVE RISK

As with any treatment, the potential benefits of surgical intervention in cancer patients must be weighed against the risks of surgery. The incidence of operative mortality is of major importance in formulating therapeutic decisions and varies greatly in different patient situations (Table 14-3). The incidence of operative mortality is a complex function of the basic disease process that involves surgery, anesthetic technique, operative complications, and, most importantly, the general health status of the patient and his ability to withstand operative trauma.

In an attempt to classify the physical status of patients and their surgical risks, the American Society of Anesthesiologists has formulated a General Classification of Physical Status that appears to correlate well with operative mortality.[7] Patients are classified into five groups depending on their general health status.

Class 1. The patient has no organic, physiologic, biochemical, or psychiatric disturbance. The pathologic process for which the operation is to be performed is localized and does not entail a systemic disturbance. (Examples: a fit patient with a lipoma or an otherwise healthy woman with a fibroid uterus)

Class 2. Mild to moderate systemic disturbance caused by either the condition to be surgically treated or the pathophysiologic processes. The extremes of age are included here, either the neonate or the octogenarian, even though no discernible systemic disease is present. Extreme obesity and chronic bronchitis also are included in this category. (Examples: nonlimiting or only slightly limiting organic heart disease, mild diabetes, essential hypertension, or anemia)

Class 3. Severe systemic disturbance or disease from whatever cause, even though it may not be possible to define firmly the degree of disability. (Examples: severely limiting organic heart disease, severe diabetes with vascular complications, moderate to severe degrees of pulmonary insufficiency, angina pectoris, or healed myocardial infarction)

Class 4. Indicative of the patient with severe systemic disorders that already are life-threatening and not always correctable by an operation. (Examples: severely cachectic patients with metastatic cancer; patients with organic heart disease showing marked signs of cardiac insufficiency, persistent anginal syndrome, or active myocarditis; advanced degrees of pulmonary, hepatic, renal, or endocrine insufficiency; severe neutropenia or thrombocytopenia in cancer patients)

Class 5. The moribund patient who has little chance of survival but who submitted to operation in desperation. Most of these patients require an operation as a resuscitative measure with little, if any, anesthesia. (Examples: burst abdominal aneurysm with profound shock, major cerebral trauma with rapidly increasing intracranial pressure, massive pulmonary embolus)

Emergency Operation (E). Any patient in classes 1 through 5 who is operated on as an emergency is considered to be in poorer physical condition. The letter *E* is placed beside the numerical classification. (Examples: perforation of a viscus, major hemorrhage from a gastrointestinal mass, or hitherto uncomplicated hernia now incarcerated and associated with nausea and vomiting)

TABLE 14-3. Determinants of Operative Risk

General health status
Severity of underlying illness
Degree to which surgery disrupts normal physiologic functions
Technical complexity of the procedure (related to incidence of complications)
Type of anesthesia required
Experience of personnel

Operative mortality usually is defined as mortality that occurs within 30 days of a major operative procedure. In oncologic patients, the basic disease process will be a major determinant of operative mortality. Patients undergoing palliative surgery for widely metastatic disease have a high operative mortality even if the surgical procedure can alleviate the symptomatic problem. Examples of these situations include surgery for intestinal obstruction in patients with widespread ovarian cancer and surgery for gastric outlet obstruction in patients with cancer of the head of the pancreas. These simple palliative procedures are associated with mortality rates of 20% to 30% in most series because of the debilitated state of the patient and the rapid progression of the basic disease.

Mortality caused by anesthetic administration alone is directly related to the physical status of the patient. In a review of 32,223 operations, Dripps and co-workers determined the mortality thought to be related to anesthetic administration alone (Table 14-4).[8] It is extremely difficult to differentiate the mortality caused by anesthesia from that resulting from other contributors to operative mortality. However, this analysis indicates that operative mortality due to anesthesia in physical status class 1 patients is extremely low, less than 1 in every 16,000 operations. The anesthetic mortality increased with worsened physical status. Most cancer patients

TABLE 14-4. Anesthetic Mortality Related to Physical Status

Physical Status	*Number of Patients*	*Number of Deaths*	*Anesthetic Mortality (%)*
Class I	16,192	0	<.006
Class II	12,154	7	0.058
Class III	4,070	11	0.27
Class IV	720	17	2.4
Class V	87	4	4.6
Total	33,223	39	0.12

(Adapted from Dripps RD, Lamont A, Eckenhoff JE: The role of anesthesia in surgical mortality. JAMA 178:261, 1961)

undergoing elective cancer surgery fall somewhere between physical status 2 and 3. An anesthetic mortality rate of 0.1% to 0.2% is a realistic estimate for this group.

In an attempt to determine the operative mortality from anesthesia alone, similar estimates to that found by Dripps and co-workers have been obtained. For example, Moir found the fatality rate for women undergoing cesarean sections in Great Britain to be 1 in 1250 to 2000 deliveries.[9] The mortality thought to be caused by anesthesia alone was 1 patient in every 6000 to 7500 deliveries. A similar estimate was obtained by Collins and associates, who estimated that the mortality resulting from general anesthesia alone was approximately 1 in 3000 to 5000 in otherwise healthy patients.[10] Several health factors can increase the risks of the operative procedure. If the patient recently had a myocardial infarction, the risk of cardiac death associated with surgery increases significantly.[11] A recurrent myocardial infarction or cardiac death will occur in approximately 30% of patients who have surgery within 3 months after a myocardial infarction and in about 15% of patients who have surgery 3 to 6 months after an infarction. The risk of a recurrent infarction or cardiac death decreases to about 5% after 6 months and remains approximately constant regardless of how much longer the patient survives. Operative risks are similar following either subendocardial and transmural infarctions.

Patients with a preoperative history of pulmonary edema or with clinical evidence of congestive heart failure by preoperative physical examination and chest x-ray films have a markedly increased risk for developing perioperative pulmonary edema. In a study of patients over the age of 40 undergoing major surgery, 23% of patients with a history of pulmonary edema developed cardiogenic pulmonary edema in the postoperative period, compared with 2% of patients with no history of congestive heart failure.[6,11] Because of the complexities of evaluating the general health status of a patient, multivariate analyses have been performed to determine which factors independently predict the development of complications. An example of one such multivariate analysis is presented in Table 14-5.[11] In this series of 1001 patients over the age of 40 years who had major noncardiac surgical procedures performed, nine separate factors were used to group the patients into categories with substantially different risks of cardiac complications. Each factor listed in Table 14-5 was associated with a number of points, and the total number of points determined the risk class. For patients in class I (0–5 points), 0.7% of patients had cardiac complications from the surgical procedure, and 0.2% of patients died of cardiac causes. The risk of cardiac complications and death in class II patients (6–12 points) was 5% and 2%, respectively. In class III patients (13–25 points), the probability of nonfatal complications was 11%, but the risk of death remained at 2%. In class IV risk patients (26 or more points), 56% of patients died of cardiac causes, and an additional 22% had life-threatening, nonfatal complications.

The impact of general health status on operative mortality is seen when operative mortality as a function of age is analyzed. Palmberg and co-workers studied the postoperative mortality of 17,199 patients undergoing general surgical procedures.[12] The overall mortality rate of patients under 70 years old was 0.25%, compared with 9.2% for patients over 70 years of age. In these elderly patients, the operative mortality rate for emergency operations was 36.8%, compared with 7.8% for elective surgical procedures. The four leading causes of operative mortality that accounted for approximately 75% of all postoperative deaths in this age group were pulmonary embolism, pneumonia, cardiovascular collapse, and the primary illness itself.

Reports of most surgical series include an account of oper-

TABLE 14-5. Correlation Between Signs and Symptoms of Preoperative Heart Failure and Risk of Perioperative Pulmonary Edema After Major Surgery in Patients over Age 40

Signs and Symptoms	*Total Patients (no.)*	*Percentage Developing Cardiogenic Pulmonary Edema (%)*
No history of congestive heart failure	853	2*
History of left heart failure but not evident on preoperative examination or chest roentgenogram	87	6*
Left heart failure by preoperative physical examination or chest roentgenogram	66	16*
Preoperative NYHA functional class for congestive heart failure		
I	935	
II	15	7
III	34	6
IV	17	25†
History of pulmonary edema	22	23‡
S3 gallop	17	35‡
Jugular venous distention and signs of left heart failure	23	30‡

Goldman L: Cardiac risks and complications of noncardiac surgery. Ann Surg 198:780–791, 1983.

*$p < 0.01$ for all pairs.

†$p < 0.001$ for class IV versus all others.

‡$p < 0.01$ when comparing patients to those without these findings.

ative mortality and operative complications. These results, combined with a consideration of the general health status of the patient, allow a reasonable estimate of the operative mortality for any given surgical intervention in the treatment of cancer.

ROLES FOR SURGERY

PREVENTION OF CANCER

Because the surgeon is often the primary provider of medical care, he is responsible for educating patients about carcinogenic hazards and about direct surgical intervention for the prevention of cancer. All surgical oncologists should be aware of the high-risk situations that require surgery to prevent subsequent malignant disease.

A variety of underlying conditions or congenital or genetic traits are associated with an extremely high incidence of subsequent cancer. When these cancers are likely to occur in nonvital organs, it is necessary to remove the offending organ to prevent subsequent malignancy.[13] Examples of diseases associated with a high incidence of cancer that can be prevented by prophylactic surgery are presented in Table 14-6. An excellent example is presented by patients with the genetic trait for multiple polyposis of the colon. If colectomy is not performed in these patients, approximately half will develop colon cancer by the age of 40. By the age of 70, virtually all patients with multiple polyposis will develop colon cancer.[13] It is therefore advisable for all patients containing the mutant gene for multiple polyposis to undergo prophylactic colectomy before the age of 20 in order to prevent these cancers.

In this situation, as for many of the other familial conditions associated with a high incidence of cancer, the surgeon has a responsibility for alerting the family to the hereditary nature of the disorder and its possible occurrence in other family members. Another disease associated with a high incidence of cancer of the colon is ulcerative colitis. Approximately 40% of patients with total colonic involvement will ultimately die of colon cancer if they survive the ulcerative colitis.[14] Three percent of children with ulcerative colitis will develop cancer of the colon by the age of 10, and 20% will develop cancer during each ensuing decade.[15] Colectomy is indicated for patients with cancer of the colon if the chronicity of this disease is well established.

Other disorders that require early treatment in order to prevent subsequent cancers include cryptorchidism and multiple endocrine neoplasia. Cryptorchidism is associated with a high incidence of testicular cancer that probably can be prevented by early prophylactic surgery. Patients with multiple endocrine neoplasia (types II and III) should be screened for the presence of C-cell hyperplasia using pentagastrin-stimulation tests. If thyrocalcitonin levels are increased following this provocative test, thyroidectomy should be performed to prevent the subsequent clinical occurrence of medullary cancer of the thyroid gland.

A more complex example of the role of surgery in cancer prevention involves women at high risk for breast cancer. Because the risk of cancer in some women is substantially increased over the normal risk (but does not yet approach 100%), counseling is required. Women in this situation must carefully balance the benefits and risks of prophylactic mastectomy. A careful understanding of the factors involved in increased breast cancer incidence is essential for the surgical oncologist to provide sound advice in this area. Statistical techniques can provide approximations of the risk for patients depending on the frequency of disease in the family history, the age at the first pregnancy, and the presence of fibrocystic disease. For example, a woman with a family history of breast cancer in a sister or mother, who has fibrocystic disease, and either is nulliparous or had a first pregnancy at a late age has an approximately 18% probability of developing breast cancer over a 5-year period.[13] These estimates can be of value in advising women about prophylactic mastectomy.

DIAGNOSIS OF CANCER

The major role of surgery in the diagnosis of cancer lies in the acquisition of tissue for exact histologic diagnosis. The principles underlying the biopsy of malignant lesions vary depending on the natural history of the tumor under consideration. A variety of techniques exist for obtaining tissues suspected of malignancy, including aspiration biopsy, needle biopsy, incisional biopsy, and excisional biopsy.

Aspiration biopsy involves the aspiration of cells and tissue

TABLE 14-6. Surgery That Can Prevent Cancer

Underlying Condition	*Associated Cancer*	*Prophylactic Surgery*
Cryptorchidism	Testicular	Orchiopexy
Polyposis coli	Colon	Colectomy
Familial colon cancer	Colon	Colectomy
Ulcerative colitis	Colon	Colectomy
Multiple endocrine neoplasia, types II and III	Medullary cancer of the thyroid	Thyroidectomy
Familial breast cancer	Breast	Mastectomy
Familial ovarian cancer	Ovary	Oophorectomy

Adapted from Mulvihill JJ: Cancer control through genetics. In Arrighi FE, Rao PN. Stubblefield E (eds): Genes, Chromosomes, and Neoplasia. New York, Raven Press, 1980.

fragments through a needle that has been guided into the suspect tissue. Cytologic analysis of this material can provide a tentative diagnosis of the presence of malignant tissue. However, major surgical resections should not be undertaken solely on the basis of the evidence of aspiration biopsy. Even the most experienced cytologist can mistake inflammatory or benign reparative changes for malignant cells. This error is inherent in the uncertainties of individual cell analysis and, even in the best of hands, provides an error rate substantially higher than that of standard histologic diagnosis.

Needle biopsy refers to obtaining a core of tissue through a specially designed needle introduced into the suspect tissue. The core of tissue provided by needle biopsies is sufficient for the diagnosis of most, but not all, tumor types. Soft-tissue and bony sarcomas often present major difficulties in differentiating benign and reparative lesions from malignancies and often cannot be diagnosed accurately. If these latter lesions are considered in the diagnosis, attempts should be made to obtain larger amounts of tissue than are possible from a needle biopsy.

Incisional biopsy refers to removal of a small wedge of tissue from a larger tumor mass. Incisional biopsies often are necessary for diagnosing large masses that require major surgical procedures for even local excision. Incisional biopsies are the preferred method of diagnosing soft-tissue and bony sarcomas because of the magnitude of the surgical procedures necessary to extirpate these lesions definitively. The treatment of many visceral cancers cannot be undertaken without an incisional biopsy, but be aware of opening new tissue planes contaminated with tumor by performing excisional biopsies for large lesions. An inappropriately performed excisional biopsy can compromise subsequent surgical excision. When this is a possibility, incisional biopsies should be performed.

In excisional biopsy, an excision of the entire suspected tumor tissue with little or no margin of surrounding normal tissue is done. Excisional biopsies are the procedure of choice for most tumors if they can be performed without contaminating new tissue planes or further compromising the ultimate surgical procedure.

There is little evidence that differences exist between incisional and excisional biopsies with respect to tumor spread. Several studies comparing incisional and excisional biopsies of suspected melanoma lesions found no differences in ultimate outcome in these patients, but the surgeon should avoid cutting directly into suspected tumor if it is not necessary to do so.[16,17]

The following principles guide the performance of all surgical biopsies.

1. Needle tracts or scars should be placed carefully so that they can be conveniently removed as part of the subsequent definitive surgical procedure. Placement of biopsy incisions is extremely important, and misplacement often can compromise subsequent care. Incisions on the extremity generally should be placed longitudinally so as to make the removal of underlying tissue and subsequent closure easier.
2. Care should be taken not to contaminate new tissue planes during the biopsy. Large hematomas after biopsy can lead to tumor spread and must be scrupulously avoided by securing excellent hemostasis during the biopsy. For biopsies on extremities, the use of a tourniquet may help in controlling bleeding. Instruments used in a biopsy procedure are another potential source of contamination of new tissue planes. It is not uncommon to take biopsy samples from several suspected lesions at one time. Care should be taken not to use instruments that may have come in contact with tumor when obtaining tissue from a potentially uncontaminated area.
3. Choice of biopsy technique should be selected carefully in order to obtain an adequate tissue sample for the needs of the pathologist. For the diagnosis of selected tumors, electron microscopy, tissue culture, or other techniques may be necessary. Sufficient tissue must be obtained for these purposes if diagnostic difficulties are anticipated.
4. Handling of the biopsy tissue by the pathologist is also important. When the orientation of the biopsy specimen is important for subsequent treatment, the surgeon should mark distinctive areas of the tumor carefully in order to facilitate subsequent orientation of the specimen by the pathologist. Different fixatives are best for different types or sizes of tissue. If all biopsy specimens are immediately placed in formalin, the opportunity to perform valuable diagnostic tests may be lost. The handling of excised tissue is the surgeon's responsibility. Biopsy tissue obtained from breast cancer lesions, for example, should be saved for estrogen receptor studies and placed in cold storage until ready for processing.

Surgery also has a role in diagnosing pathologic states in cancer patients that do not directly involve the diagnosis of cancer. Cancer patients often are immunosuppressed by either their disease or their treatment and are subject to a variety of opportunistic infections not commonly seen in most general surgical patients. Open lung or liver biopsies are often important in diagnosing these lesions adequately and in planning suitable therapy.

Oncologists are becoming increasingly aware of the need for precise staging of patients when planning treatment. Lack of proper staging information can lead to poor treatment planning and compromise the ability to cure patients. Staging laparotomy can be important in determining the exact extent of spread of lymphomas. (This is considered in more detail in Chapter 50.)

In performing accurate surgical staging, the surgeon must be familiar with the natural history of the disease under consideration. The development of ovarian cancer treatment is an excellent example. The tendency of ovarian cancer to metastasize to the undersurface of the diaphragm is a good example of the need to biopsy an anatomic site that would not normally be biopsied by most surgeons. Extensive surgical staging may be required before undertaking other major surgical procedures with curative intent. For example, biopsy of the celiac and para-aortic lymph nodes in patients with cancer of the esophagus is often important so that unnecessary esophageal resections can be avoided.

Placement of radio-opaque clips during biopsy and staging

procedures is important in order to delineate areas of known tumor and as a guide to the subsequent delivery of radiation therapy to these areas.

TREATMENT OF CANCER

Surgery can be a simple, safe method to cure patients with solid tumors when the tumor is confined to the anatomic site of origin. Unfortunately, when patients with solid tumors present to the physician for the first time, approximately 70% already will have micrometastases beyond the primary site. The extension of the surgical resection to include areas of regional spread can cure some of these patients, although regional spread often is an indication of undetectable distant micrometastases.

The emergence of effective nonsurgical therapies has had profound impact on the treatment of cancer patients and on the role and responsibilities of the surgeon treating the cancer patient. John Hunter, a brilliant 18th century surgeon, characterized surgery as being "like an armed savage who attempts to get that by force which a civilized man would get by strategem."

Although surgery continues to be the most important aspect of the treatment of most patients presenting with solid tumors, modern clinical research in oncology has been devoted to applying other adjuvant "strategems" to improve the cure rates of those 70% who ultimately will fail surgical therapy alone.

The role of surgery in the treatment of cancer patients can be divided into six separate areas. In each area, interactions with other treatment modalities can be essential for a successful outcome.

1. Definitive surgical treatment for primary cancer, selection of appropriate local therapy, and integration of surgery with other adjuvant modalities
2. Surgery to reduce the bulk of residual disease (Examples: Burkitt's lymphoma, ovarian cancer)
3. Surgical resection of metastatic disease with curative intent (Examples: pulmonary metastases in sarcoma patients, hepatic metastases from colorectal cancer)
4. Surgery for the treatment of oncologic emergencies
5. Surgery for palliation
6. Surgery for reconstruction and rehabilitation

Surgery for Primary Cancer

There are three major challenges confronting the surgical oncologist in the definitive treatment of solid tumors:

1. Accurate identification of patients who can be cured by local treatment alone
2. Development and selection of local treatments that provide the best balance between local cure and the impact of treatment morbidity on the quality of life
3. Development and application of adjuvant treatments that can improve the control of both local and distant invasive and metastatic disease

The selection of the appropriate local therapy to be used in cancer treatment varies with the individual cancer type and the site of involvement. In many instances, definitive surgical therapy that encompasses a sufficient margin of normal tissue is sufficient local therapy. The treatment of many solid tumors falls into this category. Including the wide excision of primary melanomas in the skin that can be cured locally by surgery alone in approximately 90% of cases. The resection of colon cancers with a 5-cm margin from the tumor results in anastomotic recurrences in less than 5% of cases.

In other instances, surgery is used to obtain histologic confirmation of diagnosis, but primary local therapy is achieved through the use of a nonsurgical modality such as radiation therapy. Examples of this include the treatment of Ewing's sarcoma in long bones and the treatment of selected primary malignancies in the head and neck. In each instance, selection of the definitive local treatment involves careful consideration of the likelihood of cure balanced against the morbidity of the treatment modality.

The magnitude of surgical resection is modified in the treatment of many cancers by the use of adjuvant treatment modalities. Rationally integrating surgery with other treatments requires a careful consideration of all effective treatment options. The surgical oncologist must be thoroughly familiar with adjuncts and alternatives to surgical treatment. It is a knowledge of this rapidly changing field that separates the surgical oncologist from the general surgeon most distinctly.

In some instances, effective adjuvant modalities have led to a decrease in the magnitude of surgery. The evolution of childhood rhabdomyosarcoma treatment is a striking example of the successful integration of adjuvant therapies with surgery in the treatment of cancer (Table 14-7).[18,19]

Childhood rhabdomyosarcoma is the most common soft tissue sarcoma in infants and children. Before 1970, surgery alone was used almost exclusively, and 5-year survivals of from 10% to 20% were commonly reported. Local surgery alone failed in patients with rhabdomyosarcomas of the prostate and extremities because of both extensive invasion of surrounding tissues and the early development of metastatic disease. The failure of surgery alone to control local disease in patients with childhood rhabdomyosarcoma led to the introduction of adjuvant radiation therapy. This resulted in a marked improvement in local control rates that was further improved dramatically by the introduction of combination chemotherapy with vincristine, actinomycin D, and cyclophosphamide. Long-term cure rates are now in the range of 80%. Further consideration of this disease and of the impor-

TABLE 14-7. Treatment of Childhood Rhabdomyosarcoma

Treatment	*5-Year Survival (%)*
Surgery alone	10–20
Surgery + radiotherapy	40–50
Surgery + radiotherapy + chemotherapy	80–90

Adapted from Kilman JW, Clatworthy HW Jr, Newton WA, et al: Reasonable surgery for rhabdomyosarcoma: A study of 67 cases. Ann Surg 3:346, 1973; and from Heyn RM, Holland R, Newton WA, et al: The role of combined chemotherapy in the treatment of rhabdomyosarcoma in children. Cancer 34:2128–2142, 1974.

tance of adjuvant therapy in its treatment can be found in Chapter 47. Current investigations are exploring the use of preoperative radiation therapy to see if the magnitude of surgery can be reduced further or perhaps even eliminated by using radiation and chemotherapy as the primary treatment modalities, with surgery reserved for elimination of residual disease. This latter approach has been successful in treating Ewing's sarcoma and has largely replaced surgery as the primary therapy. Many other examples of the integration of surgery with other treatment modalities appear throughout this book.

Surgery for Residual Disease

The concept of cytoreductive surgery has received much attention in recent years.[20] In some instances, the extensive local spread of cancer precludes the removal of all gross disease by surgery. The surgical resection of bulk disease in the treatment of selected cancers may well lead to improvements in the ability to control residual gross disease that has not been resected. Studies will be discussed that suggest the merit of this approach in Chapters 48 and 33 (Burkitt's lymphoma and ovarian cancer, respectively).

Enthusiasm for cytoreductive surgery has led to the inappropriate use of surgery for reducing the bulk of tumor in some cases. Clearly, cytoreductive surgery will be of benefit only when other effective treatments are available to control the residual disease that is unresectable. Except in rare palliative settings, there is no role for cytoreductive surgery in patients in whom little other effective therapy currently exists.

Surgery for Metastatic Disease

The value of surgery in the cure of patients with metastatic disease tends to be overlooked. As a general principle, patients with a single site of metastatic disease that can be resected without major morbidity should undergo resection of that metastatic cancer. Many patients with few metastases to lung or liver or brain can be cured by surgical resection (see Chap. 62, sects. 1, 2, and 3). This approach is especially true for cancers that tend not to be highly responsive to systemic chemotherapy. The resection of pulmonary metastases in patients with soft tissue and bony sarcomas can cure up to 30% of patients. As effective systemic therapy is developed for the treatment of these diseases, cure rates may increase. Studies have shown that similar cure rates occur in patients with adenocarcinomas when resected metastatic disease to the lung is the sole clinical site of metastases. Small numbers of pulmonary metastases often are the only clinically apparent metastatic disease in patients with sarcomas. However, this is rare in the natural history of most adenocarcinomas. If solitary metastases to the lung do occur in patients with carcinoma of the colon or other adenocarcinomas, then surgical resection is indicated.

Similarly, there is increasing enthusiasm for the resection of hepatic metastases, especially from colorectal cancer, in patients in whom the liver is the only site of known metastatic disease. In patients with solitary hepatic metastases from colorectal cancer, resection can lead to long-term cure in approximately 25% of patients. This far exceeds the cure rates of any other available treatment.

The resection for cure of solitary brain metastases should also be considered when the brain is the only site of known metastatic disease. The exact location and functional sequelae of resection should be considered when making this treatment decision.

SURGERY FOR ONCOLOGIC EMERGENCIES

As in the treatment of all patients, emergencies arise for oncologic patients that require surgical intervention. These generally involve the treatment of exsanguinating hemorrhage, perforation, drainage of abscesses, or impending destruction of vital organs. Each category of surgical emergency is unique and requires an individual approach. These are considered in detail in Chapter 58, section 4.

The oncologic patient often is neutropenic, thrombocytopenic, and has a high risk of hemorrhage or sepsis. Perforations of an abdominal viscus can result from direct tumor invasion or from tumor lysis resulting from effective systemic treatments. Perforation of the gastrointestinal tract following effective treatment for lymphoma involving the intestine is not uncommon. The ability to identify patients at high risk for perforation may lead to the use of surgery to prevent this problem. Surgery to decompress cancer invading the CNS represents another surgical emergency that can lead to preservation of function.

Surgery for Palliation

Surgical resection often is required for the relief of pain or functional abnormalities. The appropriate use of surgery in these settings can improve the quality of life for cancer patients. Palliative surgery may include the relief of mechanical problems such as intestinal obstruction or the removal of masses that are causing severe pain or disfigurement.

Surgery for Reconstruction and Rehabilitation

Surgical techniques are being refined that aid in the reconstruction and rehabilitation of cancer patients following definitive therapy. The ability to reconstruct anatomic defects can substantially improve both function and cosmetic appearance. The development of free flaps using microvascular anastomotic techniques is having a profound impact on the ability to bring fresh tissue to resected or heavily irradiated areas. Loss of function (especially of extremities) often can be rehabilitated by surgical approaches. This includes lysis of contractures or muscle transposition to restore muscular function that has been damaged by prior surgery or radiation therapy.

THE SURGICAL ONCOLOGIST

Several factors have led to a recent increase in the development of surgical oncology and to the organization of separate sections of surgical oncology in large hospitals and departments of surgery within universities. This enthusiasm derives from the recognition that modern oncologic management requires levels of expertise in cancer surgery, chemotherapy, and radiation therapy that are not common to most general surgeons, as well as a desire to use effectively the resources being committed to cancer care and research by hospitals, private foundations, and the federal government. A sense of urgency has existed because some surgical leaders believe that the surgeon is experiencing a declining intellectual role in modern cancer treatment and research and that steps must be taken to reassert the surgeon's role in modern oncology.

Many surgeons, however, have resisted the development of surgical oncology as a specialty area because of the fear of fragmenting the field of general surgery. A survey of 124 university surgery departments in the United States between January and July, 1985, revealed that 38% had formal divisions of surgical oncology compared with divisions of medical oncology present in 95%, radiation oncology in 94%, pediatric oncology in 76%, and gynecologic oncology in 79% of university medical institutions.[21] Of the 47 divisions of surgical oncology that did exist, only 13 (28%) had formal clinical training programs in surgical oncology.[21] This lack of emphasis on surgical oncology at universities may be a factor in the decreasing success of surgeons in obtaining grant support from the National Cancer Institute. For the six years from 1980 through 1985, an analysis of 6407 applications submitted from clinical departments of medical schools for peer-reviewed grants revealed that 44% were submitted from departments of medicine and only 16% from departments of surgery.[22] Thirty-four percent of applications submitted from departments of medicine were awarded, compared with 25% from departments of surgery.[22]

The development of surgical oncology as a specialty area of surgery depends on a clear delineation of its role. There are six major areas in which the modern surgical oncologist can play a valuable role in the care of cancer patients at major treatment centers:[23]

1. Organize surgical oncology teaching programs for staff, residents, and students
2. Provide expert consultation for unusual or difficult oncologic patient problems
3. Provide unique surgical expertise in surgical cases unfamiliar to general surgeons (*e.g.*, major soft tissue resections, exenterations, head and neck resections, isolation-perfusions)
4. Organize clinical research protocols for surgical oncology patients
5. Coordinate surgical oncology efforts with medical and radiation oncologists
6. Conduct experimental research programs in oncology where possible

The rapid development of new information in surgery, chemotherapy, and medical oncology, in addition to newer disciplines of immunotherapy, hyperthermia, and phototherapy, requires the continuing education of all surgical staff. Surgical oncologists maintain close contact with all of these areas and should be responsible for teaching programs for general surgical staff, residents, and students in these different areas.

Because of the unique training and exposure to oncologic problems, the surgical oncologist has expertise in dealing with unusual or difficult oncologic patient problems, and thus can provide expert consultation in these areas. The surgical oncologist is trained to perform many types of surgical procedures not commonly performed by most general surgeons. Although most surgeons are able to perform many of the standard cancer resections, some operations are not performed frequently by general surgeons and can be performed better by a specialist in surgical oncology.

In most hospital settings, a variety of general surgeons operate on cancer patients. It is often essential, however, that patients receiving care for a variety of cancers enter clinical protocols that will help answer important questions related to the treatment of that cancer. The surgical oncologist can help organize clinical research protocols for surgical oncology patients treated by all surgeons at that institution. A large surgical group should have a surgical specialist capable of coordinating efforts with medical and radiation oncologists. Successful coordination with these nonsurgical specialists requires expertise in medical oncology and radiation therapy that is not common among most general surgeons.

The surgical oncologist can also be involved in administering and defining the need for a variety of adjuvant treatments. Adjuvant chemotherapy commonly is administered by surgeons when the chemotherapy regimens use well-known single or combination agents. The future development of immunotherapies and other new adjuvant treatments can be logically administered by the surgical oncologist to his patient following recovery from the surgical procedure.

Finally, the surgical oncologist, when the situation allows, is in a position to perform experimental research in oncology that can lead to the introduction of new diagnostic and treatment regimens in clinical care. Laboratory research programs that contribute to basic knowledge of cancer biology also provide an important source of stimulation to residents and students.

The emergence of a subspecialty of surgical oncology within general surgery requires that special attention be given to the training of surgeons interested in pursuing this area of clinical care. Although it is generally agreed that all surgical oncologists should be well-trained general surgeons, attempts have been made to define additional areas of expertise that must be studied. In 1978, a group of surgical oncologists met under the sponsorship of the Society of Surgical Oncology and the Division of Cancer Research, Resources, and Centers of the National Cancer Institute to develop guidelines for the training of surgical oncologists.

The guidelines adopted by this meeting included a variety of suggestions for such training.[24,25]

1. Two-year training program on a surgical oncology service after completion of eligibility for general surgical certification by the American Board of Surgery or other surgical specialty board
2. Training at an institution whose cancer program is approved by the Commission on Cancer of the Ameri-

can College of Surgeons and whose clinical resources provide a sufficient variety and volume of clinical material to assure exposure to a broad variety of clinical cancer problems
3. Training at a center with sufficient basic science resources to provide education in these areas, with exposure to both basic and clinical research
4. Training at an institution that will provide adequate operative experience, including standard curative and palliative procedures, with broad exposure to surgical procedures unique to the oncologic patient
5. A full-time assignment during the training period to both radiation oncology and chemotherapy services to allow the trainee to gain confidence and knowledge in these nonsurgical disciplines

These training recommendations are designed to provide general surgeons with the expertise in oncology and nonsurgical disciplines necessary to bring the best aspects of all disciplines of modern oncology to the care of the cancer patient.

REFERENCES

1. Brested JH: The Edwin Smith Surgical Papyrus. Chicago, University of Chicago Press, 1930
2. Thorwald J: Science and the Secrets of Early Medicine. New York, Harcourt, Brace, and World, 1962
3. Wangensteen OH: Has medical history importance for surgeons? Surg Gynecol Obstet 140:434, 1975
4. Hill GJ: Historic milestones in cancer surgery. Semin Oncol 6:409–427, 1979
5. Brunner EA, Eckenhoff JE: Anesthesia. In Sabiston DC Jr (ed): Textbook of Surgery. Philadelphia, WB Saunders, 1977
6. Goldman L, Caldera DL, Nussbaum SR, et al. Multifactorial index of cardiac risk in noncardiac surgical procedures. N Engl J Med 297:845–850, 1977
7. Dripps RD, Eckenhoff JE, Vandam LD: Introduction to Anesthesia. Philadelphia, WB Saunders, 1977
8. Dripps RD, Lamont A, Eckenhoff JE: The role of anesthesia in surgical mortality. JAMA 178:261, 1961
9. Moir DD: Maternal mortality and anesthaesia. Br J Anaesth 52:1–3, 1980
10. Collins VJ: Principles of Anesthesiology. Philadelphia. Lea & Febiger, 1976
11. Goldman L: Cardiac risks and complications of noncardiac surgery. Ann Surg 198:780–791, 1983
12. Palmberg S, Hirsjarvi E: Mortality in geriatric surgery. Gerontology 25:103–112, 1979
13. Mulvihill JJ: Cancer control through genetics. In Arrighi FE, Rao PN, Stubblefield E (eds): Genes, Chromosomes, and Neoplasia. New York, Raven Press, 1980
14. MacDougall IPM: The cancer risk in ulcerative colitis. Lancet 2:655, 1964
15. Devroede GJ, Taylor WF, Sauer WG: Cancer risk and life expectancy of children with ulcerative colitis. N Engl J Med 285:17, 1971
16. Epstein E, Bragg K, Linden GJ: Biopsy and prognosis of malignant melanoma. JAMA 208:1369, 1969
17. Knutson CO, Hori JM, Spratt JS Jr: Melanoma. Curr Probl Surg, Dec 1971
18. Kilman JW, Clatworthy HW Jr, Newton WA, et al: Reasonable surgery for rhabdomyosarcoma: A study of 67 cases. Ann Surg 3:346, 1973
19. Heyn RM, Holland R, Newton WA, et al: The role of combined chemotherapy in the treatment of rhabdomyosarcoma in children. Cancer 34:2128–2142, 1974
20. Silberman AW: Surgical debulking of tumors. Surg Gynecol Obstet 155:577–585, 1982
21. Lawrence W Jr, Wilson RE, Shingleton WW, et al: Surgical oncology in university departments of surgery in the United States. Arch Surg 121:1088–1093, 1986
22. Avis FP, Ellenberg S, Friedman MA: Surgical oncology research—a disappointing status report. Ann Surg 207:262–266, 1988
23. Rosenberg SA: The organization of surgical oncology in university departments of surgery. Surgery 95:632–634, 1984
24. Leffall LD Jr: Presidential address. Surgical oncology—expectations for the future. Cancer 42:2925–2928, 1980
25. Schweitzer RJ, Edwards MH, Lawrence W et al: Training guidelines for surgical oncology. Cancer 48:2336–2340, 1981

SAMUEL HELLMAN

CHAPTER 15 *Principles of Radiation Therapy*

To understand the practice of radiation therapy, one must seek its roots in principles derived from three separate areas. The first is practical radiation physics. This must be understood much as the surgeon understands the use of the equipment available in the operating room and as the internist understands the pharmacologic basis of therapeutics. The basic concepts of physics necessary to consider radiation therapy in the disease-related chapters are introduced in this chapter.

The second important discipline to be understood is cell, tissue, and tumor biology. This chapter describes the fundamental principles of radiation biology and cell kinetics; cell kinetics in relation to both chemotherapy and radiation therapy is discussed in Chapter 1. These two discussions provide the rudiments of cell biology necessary to understand the uses of radiation.

Finally, a large clinical experience in radiation use has resulted in certain principles of treatment. These are discussed separately and related to the physical and biologic concepts that may underlie their success.

PHYSICAL CONSIDERATIONS

Only the most important concepts of the physics of ionizing radiation can be discussed in this chapter. If more detailed information is needed, a standard textbook of radiation physics is a more appropriate source of information.[1]

Ionizing radiation is energy that, during absorption, causes the ejection of an orbital electron. A large amount of energy is associated with ionization. Ionizing radiation can be electromagnetic or particulate, and electromagnetic radiation can be considered both as a wave and as a packet of energy (a photon). It is the particulate nature of electromagnetic radiation that explains much of its biologic activity. The packet of energy is large enough to cause ionizations, and these are distributed unevenly through tissue. Examples of particulate radiation are the subatomic particles: electrons, protons, alpha particles, neutrons, negative pimesons, and atomic nuclei. All of these have been experimentally considered or are being used in radiation therapy.

ELECTROMAGNETIC RADIATION

Electromagnetic radiation consists of roentgen and gamma radiation. They differ only in the way in which they are produced: gamma rays are produced intranuclearly, and roentgen rays are produced extranuclearly. In practice, this means that gamma rays used in radiation therapy are produced by the decay of radioactive isotopes and that almost all of the roentgen rays used in radiation therapy are made by electrical machines. Exceptions are roentgen rays produced by orbital electron rearrangements, as in the decay of ^{125}I, which is a radioactive isotope but produces photons by extranuclear processes. Iodine-125 also emits a small number of gamma rays from the nucleus.

The intensity of electromagnetic radiation dissipates as the inverse square of the distance from the source. Thus, the dose of radiation 2 cm from a point source is 25% of the dose at 1 cm.

The relative prevalence of the three dominant absorption mechanisms of electromagnetic radiation depends on the energy of the radiation. The first is photoelectric absorption, which predominates at lower energies. In this circumstance, the photon interaction results in the ejection of a tightly bound orbital electron. The vacancy left in the atomic shell is then filled by another electron falling from an outer shell of the same atom or from outside the atom. All or most of the photon energy of the transition is lost in this process. Photoelectric absorption varies with the cube of the atomic number (Z^3). This has significant practical implications because it explains why materials with high atomic numbers, such as lead, are such effective shielding materials. It also means that bones will absorb significantly more radiation than soft tissues at lower photon energies, the basis for conventional diagnostic radiology.

The second type of radiation absorption is the Compton type. In this process, the photon interaction is with a distant orbital electron that has a very low binding energy. In this absorptive process, the photon does not give up all its energy to a single electron; an appreciable portion reappears as a secondary photon, which is created in the interaction. In contrast to the photoelectric effect, the probability of Compton absorption does not depend much on atomic number, but rather on electron density. This explains why films made at supervoltage energy to not show much difference between bone and soft tissue, but air cavities are clearly distinguished.

The third type of absorption is the pair production process. This type of absorption requires an incident photon energy greater than 1.02 MeV. In this process, positive and negative electrons are produced at the same time.

The fundamental quantity necessary to describe the interaction of radiation with matter is the amount of energy absorbed per unit mass. This quantity is called *absorbed dose*, and the *rad* was the most commonly used unit. In current nomenclature, absorbed dose is measured in joules per kilogram. Another name for 1 joule/kg is the Gray (1 Gray = 100 rad). This is now the recommended unit. The roentgen (R) is a unit of roentgen rays or gamma rays based on the ability of radiation to ionize air. At the energies used in radiation therapy, 1 R of roentgen rays or gamma rays results in a dose of somewhat less than 1 rad (0.01 Gy) in soft tissue.

The different ranges of electromagnetic radiations used in clinical practice are *superficial radiation* or roentgen rays from approximately 10 to 125 KeV; *orthovoltage* radiation or electromagnetic radiation between 125 and 400 KeV; and *supervoltage* or megavoltage radiation for energies above 400 KeV. There are important differences between these classes. As energy increases, the penetration of the roentgen rays increases, as shown in Figure 15-1, and at supervoltage energies, absorption in bone is not higher than that in surrounding soft tissues, as is the case with lower energies. This is because at supervoltage energies, Compton absorption predominates. Compared with orthovoltage, supervoltage radiation is "skin sparing," meaning that the maximum dose is not reached in the skin, but instead occurs below the surface. The electrons created in the interaction travel some distance and do not attain full intensity until they reach some depth, resulting in a reduced dose to the skin. With orthovoltage radiation, the skin frequently is the dose-limiting normal tissue.

RADIATION TECHNIQUES

Two general types of radiation techniques are used clinically —*brachytherapy* and *teletherapy*. In brachytherapy, the radiation device is placed either within or close to the target volume. Examples of this are interstitial and intracavitary radiation used in the treatment of many gynecologic and oral tumors. Teletherapy uses a device quite removed from the patient, as is the case in most orthovoltage or supervoltage machines.

Because the radiation source is close to or within the target volume with brachytherapy, the dose is determined largely by inverse-square considerations. This means that the geometry of the implant is very important. Spatial arrangements have been determined for different types of applications based on the particular anatomic considerations of the tumor and important normal tissues. An example of isotope distribution around an intracavitary application for carcinoma of the cervix is shown in Figure 15-2. The dose decreases rapidly as the distance from the applicator increases. This emphasizes the importance of proper placement. The applica-

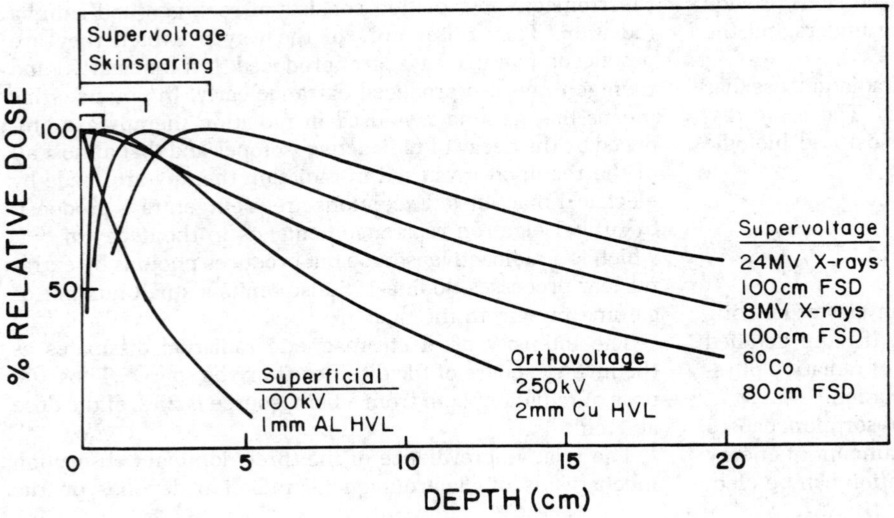

FIG. 15-1. Relative dose at different depths for various types of ionizing radiation.

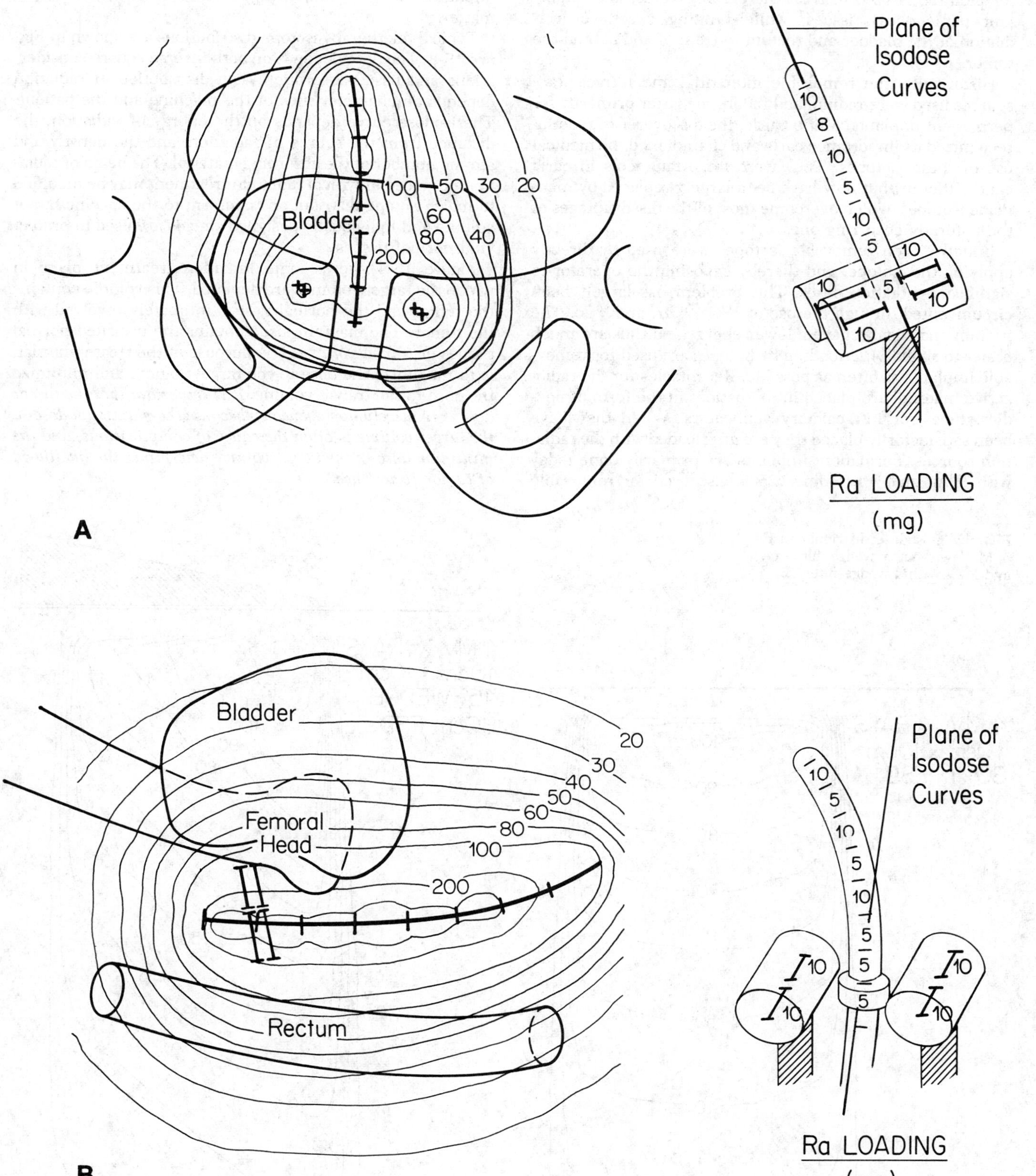

FIG. 15-2. **A**. AP view of isodose distribution around an intrauterine radium applicator. **B**. Lateral view.

tor pictured is used to treat the cervix, uterus, and important paracervical tissues, while limiting excessive irradiation of the bladder and rectum in front of and behind the tumor.

Historically, the removable interstitial and intracavitary sources used were radium and radon, the latter primarily for permanent implants. Marie Curie, the discoverer of radium, recognized its importance early and championed the medical use of these isotopes. They were important tools in early cancer therapy but now have been largely replaced by man-made isotopes, which overcome most of the disadvantages of the naturally occurring ones.

Initially, even removable isotopes were used by directly applying the isotope, and thereby exposing the operator to significant radiation doses. This problem has largely been circumvented through the use of ^{137}Cs, ^{192}Ir, and ^{60}Co. The iridium and cesium have a lower energy and thus are much easier to shield. *Afterloading* techniques are used for removable implants as often as possible. Receptacles for the radioactive material are placed in the patient in the form of needles, tubes, or intracavitary applicators. When they have been satisfactorily placed they are afterloaded with the radiation sources. Permanent implants are primarily done today with ^{198}Au and ^{125}I. Iodine-125 is also used for removable implants. Its very low energy makes shielding a simple matter.

Typical teletherapy isotope distributions are shown in Figure 15-3. The dose depends on both inverse-square considerations and tissue absorption. The distribution of radiation depends on characteristics of the machine and the patient. The isodose curve depends on the energy of radiation, the distance from the source of radiation, and the density and atomic number of the absorbing material. The beam of radiation produced in typical radiation treatment may be modified to make isotope distributions conform to the specific target volume and individually designed shields are used to protect vital normal tissues.

Figure 15-4 shows some radiation treatment plans in which the target volumes are depicted. This volume contains the tumor and the normal tissues intimately involved with the tumor. The diagram also contains the transited normal tissues or *transit volume*. The purpose of the treatment plan is to maximize the dose to the target volume and minimize the dose to the transit volume. *It is important that the tumor dose is relatively homogeneous, because the maximum dose in the target volume is often the cause of complications, and the minimum dose in the target volume determines the likelihood of tumor recurrence.*

FIG. 15-3. Isodose distributions for 4 MeV without a wedge filter (**A**) and MeV with a wedge filter (**B**).

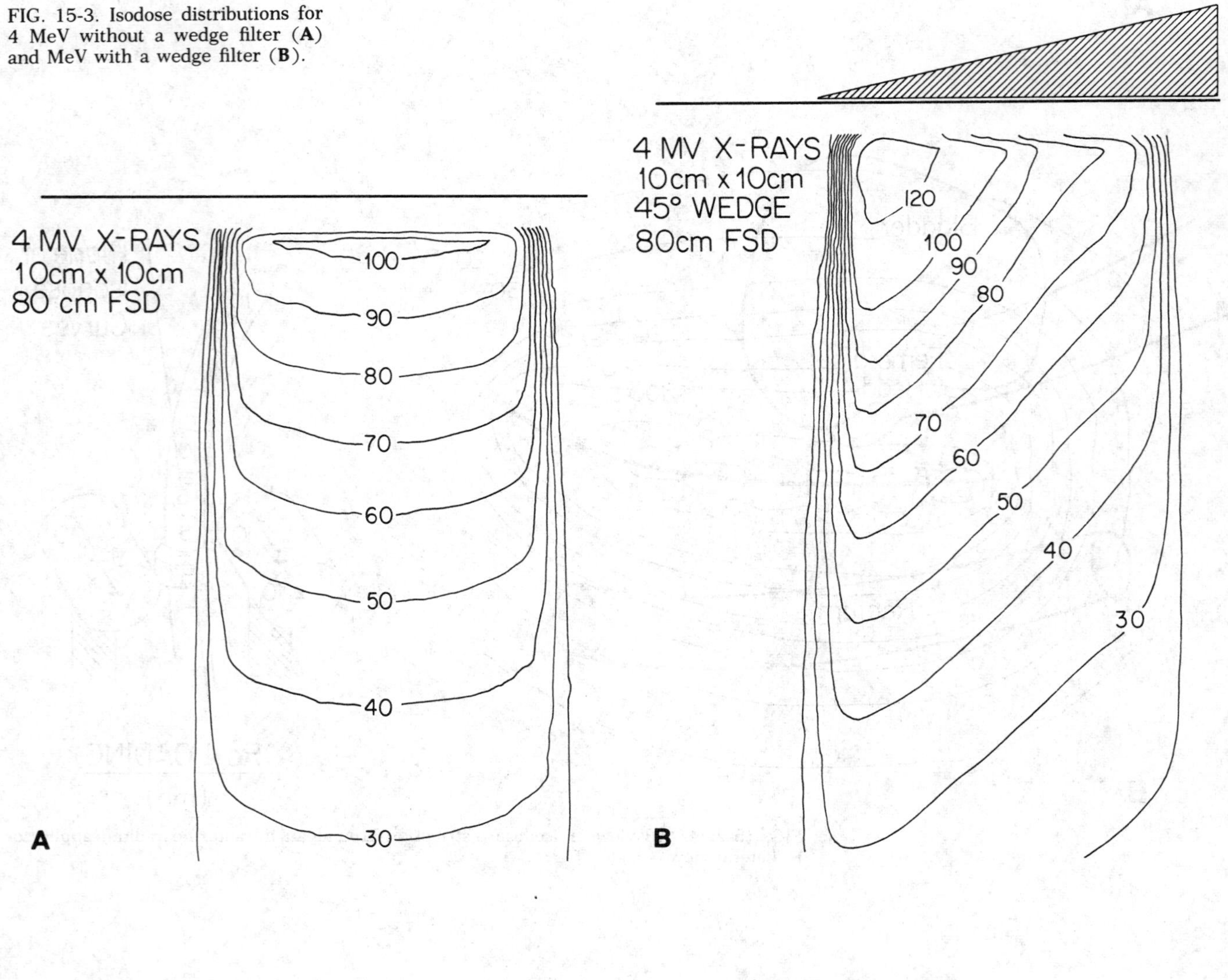

Beam-Modifying Devices

In modern radiation therapy, teletherapy is given almost exclusively with supervoltage equipment. These radiations are produced by the decay of radioactive cobalt or with the production of roentgen rays in the range of 2 to 35 MeV (the most common are 4–8 MeV). Higher-energy photons and electrons can be made by various electrical machines, of which the most common are linear accelerators.

Regardless of the radiation source, the beam must be modified for clinical use. With electrical machines, the beam tends to have a much greater intensity in the center than on the sides. Modification to give a uniform dose of radiation across the beam is done with a *flattening filter* (unnecessary in cobalt units). For the beam to be limited to the designated size, collimators are placed in the head of the machine. These usually are made of materials that have a high Z value and can be varied to conform to the exact rectangular beam dimensions desired.

It is sometimes desirable for the beam to be more intense on one side than the other. This is especially important when fields at angles to each other are to be used. To modify the beam in this fashion, wedge filters are used (Fig. 15-3B). These are literally wedge-shaped pieces of metal that absorb the beam differentially, depending on the thickness that produces the desired angled isodose curves. Depending on the anatomic volume being treated, it is often desirable to outline the beam differently from that which can be constructed by rectangular collimators. In these circumstances, certain areas within the beam should be shielded. To do this, individually fashioned blocks are made to conform to the individual distributions desired for each patient and each beam. They are made of material with a high Z, such as lead or the commercial product Libowitz metal, composed of bismuth, lead, tin, and cadmium.

The primary radiation beam is rectangular. This rectangle may be varied for individual patients, using the secondary collimators in the head of the machine. These can then be further modified by individually constructed blocks made to the contour of the normal tissue, an example of which is shown in Figure 15-5. The newest equipment has multileaf collimators, which permit the collimator to follow closely the desired portal contour, rather than being restricted to a rectangular shape.

RADIATION TREATMENT

Once the decision has been made to treat a patient with radiation, a number of pretreatment procedures must be performed. First, there must be accurate localization of the target volume and determination of the dose-limiting, transited normal tissues. This localization requires physical examination, radiography, ultrasonography, computed tomography (CT), and other diagnostic procedures. Before this, the clinician must understand the natural history of the disease and its patterns of spread. CT has greatly changed the process of tumor localization by allowing much greater accuracy in determining the location of normal tissues, as well as tumor.

Once localization has been completed, the treatment-planning process begins, in which alternative techniques of treatment are considered. The selection of the appropriate treatment plan is made by the clinician consulting with the radiologic physicist and dosimetrist. This team effort must consider the best beam distribution, homogeneity within the target volume, and appropriate minimizing of dose in the transit volume.

Once the appropriate treatment plan has been accepted, the technique is tested using a radiation simulator. This device mimics the treatment machine but produces superficial radiation that can be used for direct imaging with an image intensifier and for producing radiographs that delineate exactly the beam location. Treatment simulation often causes modifications to be made in the treatment plan, thus allowing further sparing of normal tissues. Examples of simulator films are shown in Figure 15-5. These must be compared with the check or portal films made with the supervoltage machine, which confirm the treatment plan (Fig. 15-5). Image quality is poor because they do not distinguish bone from soft tissue. This is because supervoltage radiation is absorbed primarily by the Compton process, which does not depend on Z. In contrast, the simulator films are made with radiations of 80 to 110 KeV, which are in the photoelectric range and therefore dependent on Z^3.

In order for the treatment to be applied as designed on the radiation simulator, proper immobilization and marking techniques must be used. These also ensure that daily treatments are given to the same volume. Markings on the patient's skin may be temporary or permanent. Usually temporary marks are used to supplement the permanent small dots or "tattoos," ensuring that the treatment will be given to the same volume each day. In addition, should the patient require further therapy at a later date, these markings will accurately indicate the location of previous treatment portals. Within the treatment room, light localizers describe the outline of the field, and small laser dots are used to check whether the patient is in the correct position. Immobilization of the patient usually is achieved by devices made of foam, plastic, plaster, and a variety of other materials that can be made to conform to each patient's anatomy. It is most important that the patient be put in a position that is comfortable and easily reproduced from day to day.

Electron Therapy

With the development of betatrons and high-energy accelerators, electron beam therapy has become available for teletherapy. Electrons differ greatly in their characteristic depth-dose distributions (Fig. 15-6). The maximum dose is reached followed by a very prompt fall. There is little skin sparing with electron beam therapy, but it is the most useful radiation in the treatment of superficial tumors because the deeper tissues will be spared by the prompt fall in the radiation dose. With higher electron energy, the penetration is greater and the fall in depth dose is not as steep.

A major problem with electrons is that absorption can be modified greatly by bone or air-containing tissues. Bone will cause the depth dose to be greatly reduced because it will absorb much more of the radiation; the contrary is true for air-containing spaces.

(Text continues on p. 254.)

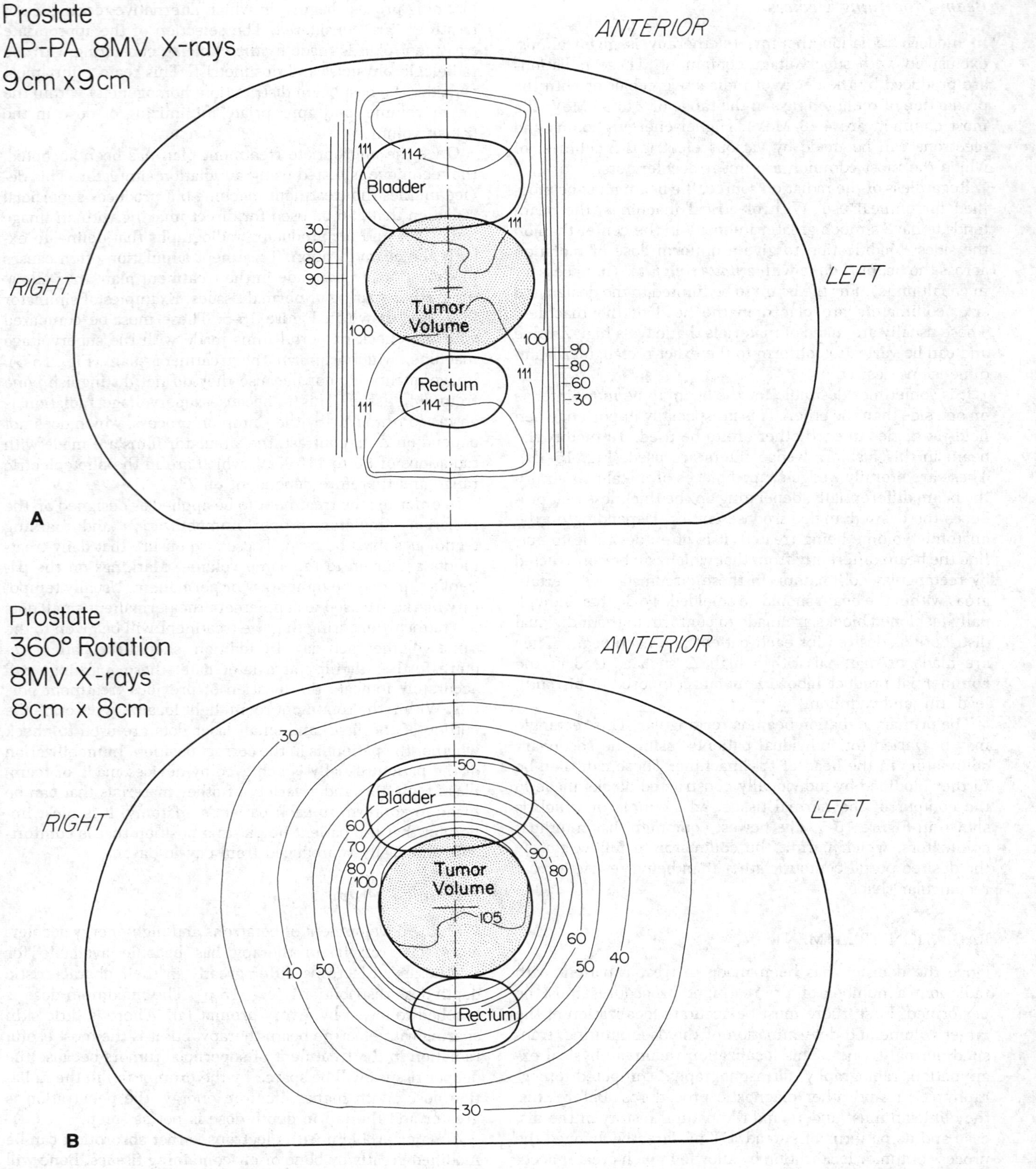

FIG. 15-4. Typical supervoltage treatment plans for opposing fields (**A**), rotation (**B**). C. Three field. D. Wedge rotation.

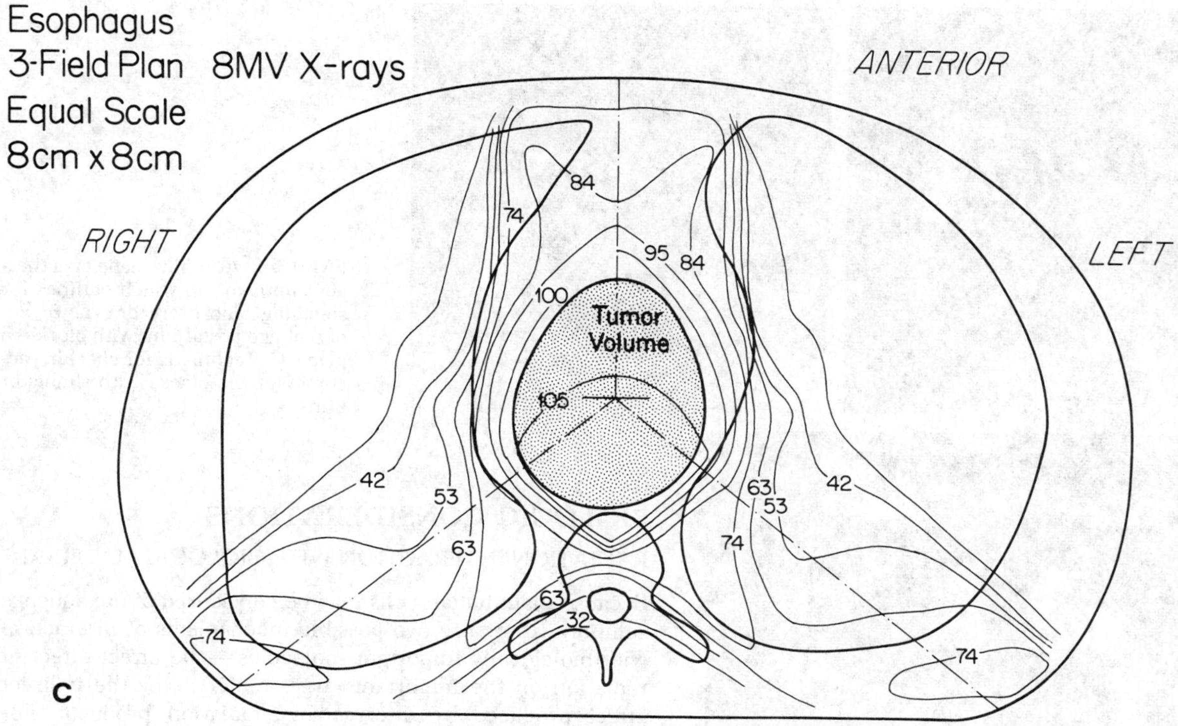

FIG. 15-4. (*continued*). Three field (*C*).

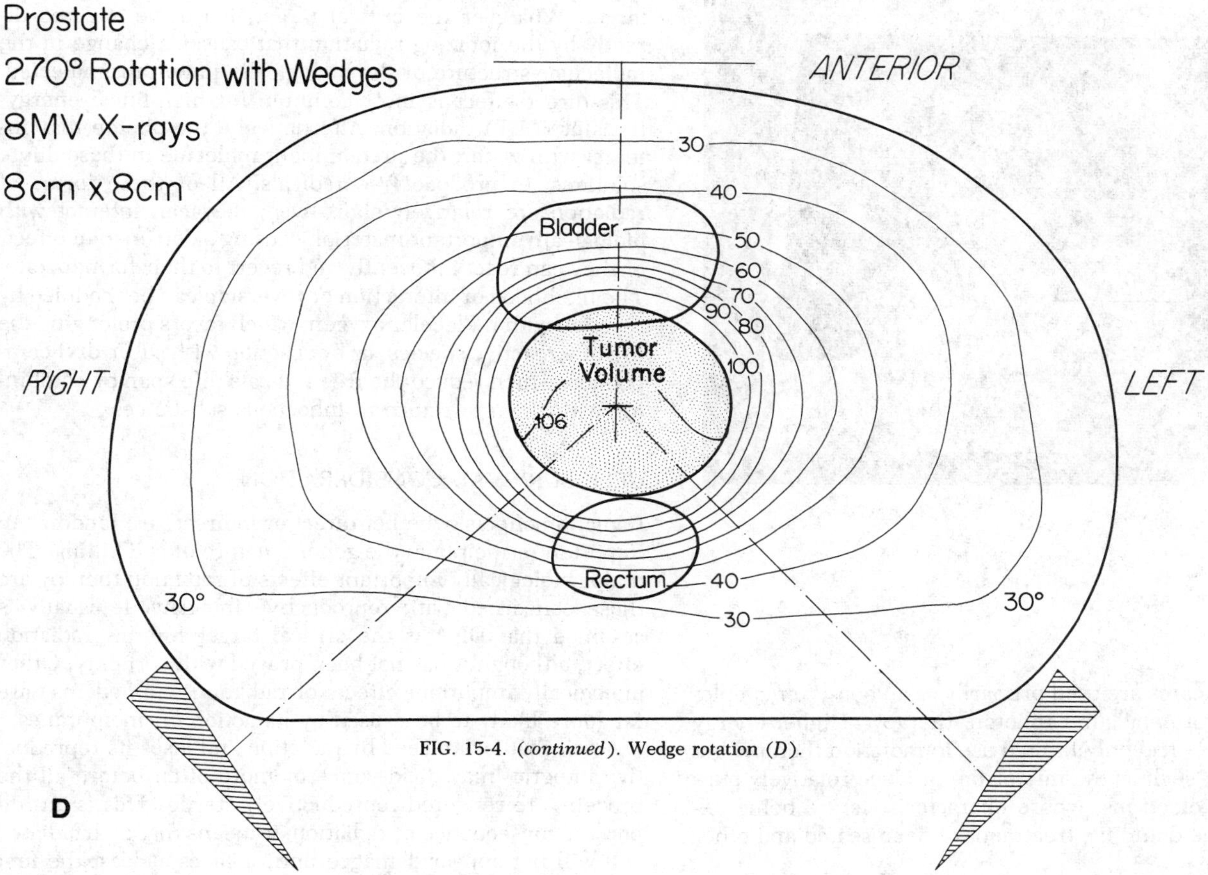

FIG. 15-4. (*continued*). Wedge rotation (*D*).

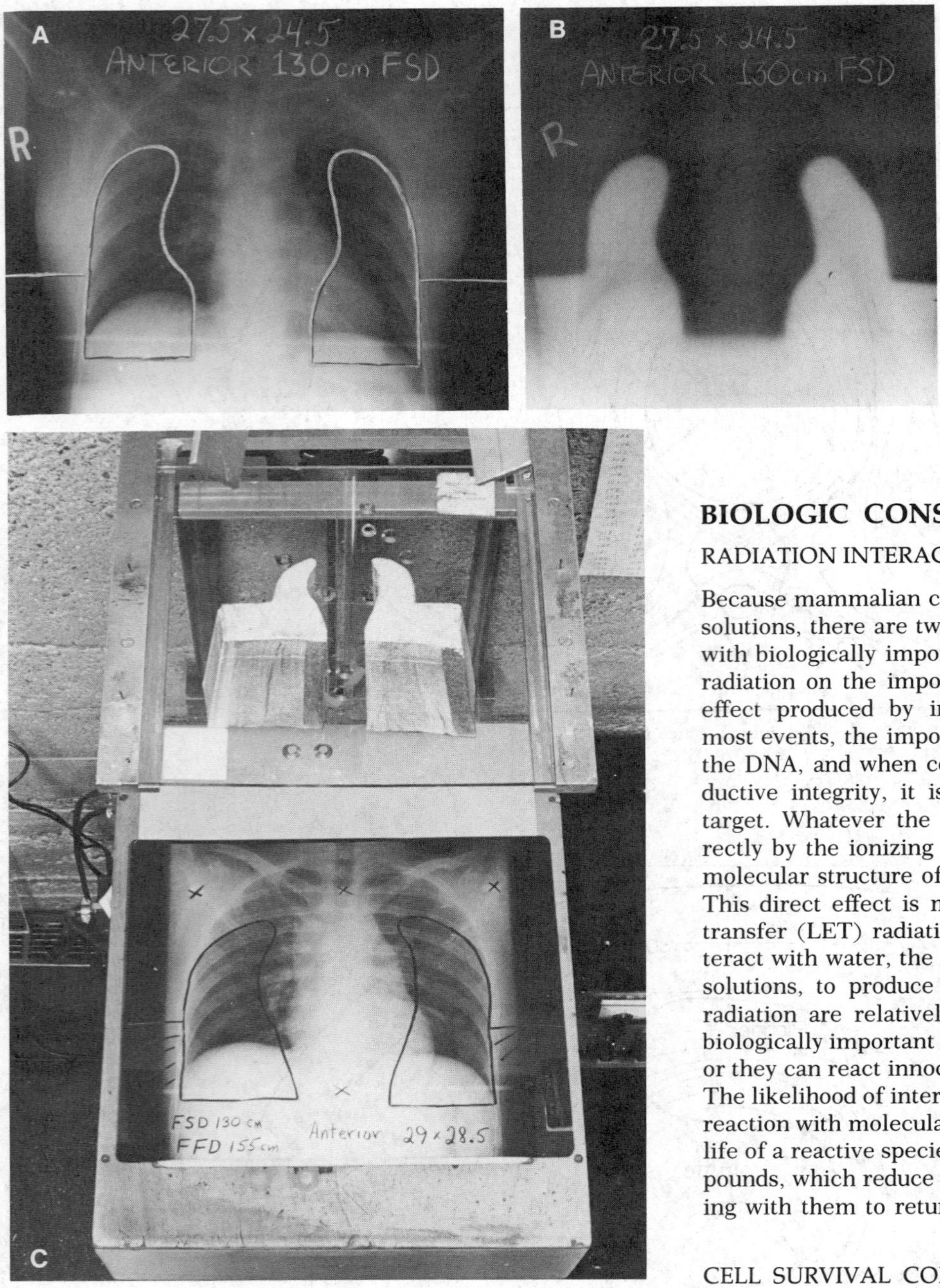

FIG. 15-5. **A**. A film made on a therapy simulator on which outlines for shielding blocks are drawn. **B**. Supervoltage portal film with blocks in place. **C**. Technique for checking accuracy of the blocks with simulator films.

Electron beams are used primarily as a "boost" or supplementary treatment after photon therapy. Higher-energy electrons have had only limited use in radiation therapy, but new devices, such as the microtron, produce relatively pure high-energy electrons, whose characteristics are being explored for the definitive treatment of deep-seated and other tumors.

BIOLOGIC CONSIDERATIONS

RADIATION INTERACTION WITH BIOLOGIC MATERIALS

Because mammalian cells may be considered dilute aqueous solutions, there are two possible mechanisms of interaction with biologically important molecules—the direct effect of radiation on the important target molecule or the indirect effect produced by intermediary radiation products. For most events, the important target molecule is thought to be the DNA, and when considering the maintenance of reproductive integrity, it is useful to assume that DNA is the target. Whatever the critical target, it can be affected directly by the ionizing radiation that causes a change in the molecular structure of the biologically important molecule. This direct effect is most common for high-linear-energy-transfer (LET) radiation. Alternatively, the photon may interact with water, the predominant molecule in these dilute solutions, to produce free radicals. All of these forms of radiation are relatively short-lived; they can interact with biologically important material, causing a detrimental effect, or they can react innocently and revert to their former state. The likelihood of interaction or reversion can be modified by reaction with molecular oxygen, which favors prolonging the life of a reactive species, or by reaction with sulfhydryl compounds, which reduce the free radicals' life span by combining with them to return to innocuous substances.

CELL SURVIVAL CONSIDERATIONS

Radiation effects, whether direct or indirect, are random, an important principle in the general nature of cell killing. The major biologically important effects of radiation therapy are those concerned with reproductive integrity. It usually is assumed that DNA is the critical target for this radiation effect, although it has not been proved with certainty. Other biologically important effects of radiation (*e.g.*, edema) are far more likely to be caused by its action on membranes.

A cell that is damaged by radiation and loses its reproductive integrity may divide once or more often before all the progeny are rendered reproductively sterile. This is an important consequence of radiation; it means that an irradiated cell will not appear damaged until it faces at least the first

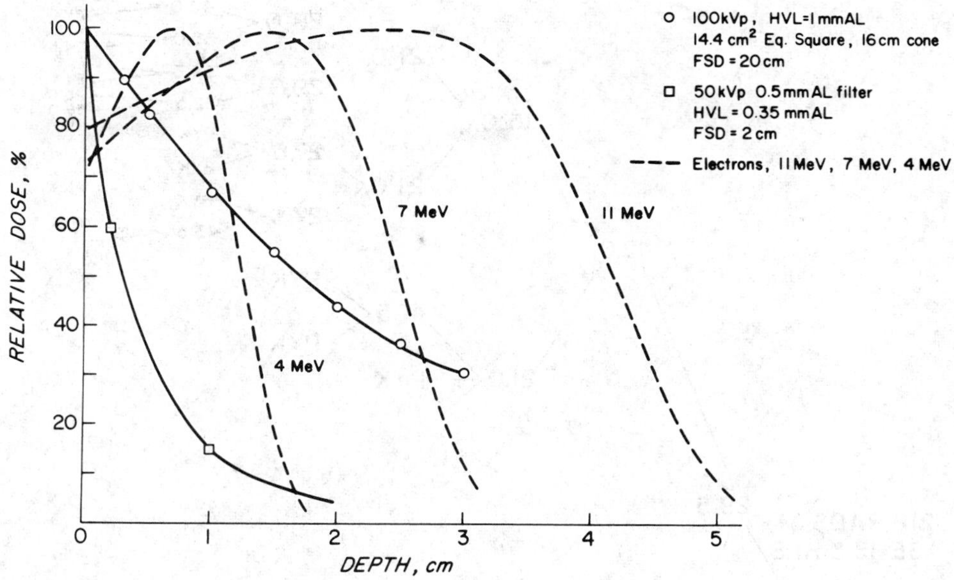

FIG. 15-6. Electron and superficial roentgen ray depth dose curves.

division. At the time of reproduction, there are a number of possible paths for this cell:

1. It may die while trying to divide.
2. It may produce unusual forms as a result of aberrant attempts at division.
3. It may stay as it is, unable to divide, but physiologically functional for a long period of time. Such functional but sterile cells will not appear different from fertile cells.
4. It may divide, giving rise to one or more generations of daughter cells before some or all of the progeny become sterile. Those colonies in which some reproductively viable progeny emerge may then regrow.
5. The cell may suffer no alterations in the divisional process or only minor ones.

Usually some delay in division is produced, even in cells that are not damaged lethally. An example of cellular pedigrees photographed in vitro is shown in Figure 15-7.[2]

Survival Curves

Survival curves plot the fraction of cells surviving radiation against the dose given. Survival is determined by the ability to form a macroscopic colony. The simplest relationship can be seen for bacteria in which survival is a constant exponential function of dose. The importance of this exponential relationship is that for a given dose increment, a constant proportion, rather than a constant number, of cells is killed. Because of the randomness of radiation damage, if there is on average one lethal lesion per cell, some cells will have one lesion, some more than one, and some less than one. Under such circumstances the proportion of cells that have less than one, that is, no lethal events, is e^{-1}, or a survival fraction of 0.37. The dose required to reduce the survival fraction to 37% on the exponential curve is known as the D_0. This term, therefore, is related to the slope of the exponential survival curve. Thus if a smaller dose is required to reduce the survival fraction to 37%, then the cells are more sensitive to radiation.

Survival curves of most mammalian cells differ from those of bacterial cells by having a "shoulder" in the low-dose region and the exponential relationship at higher doses. This shoulder indicates a reduced efficiency of cell killing. Such an idealized curve is shown in Figure 15-8 with the important shorthand terminology used to describe survival curves. The terminal exponential portion is described by the D_0, whereas the initial shoulder region can be described by the extrapolation number n or the D_q, the quasi-threshold dose. The former is the number on the ordinate found when the exponential portion is extrapolated to 0 dose, whereas D_q is the dose at which the straight portion of the survival curve extrapolated backward intersects the line where the survival fraction is unity. If any two of these are known, the third can be calculated. The survival curve is described as follows: $\log e^n = D_q/D_0$. This curve is best described by a linear quadratic model with the formula $S = e^{-(\alpha D + \beta D^2)}$.[3]

Survival curves have been determined for a variety of benign or neoplastic mammalian cells in culture. There are no general characteristics of tumor cells that make them different from normal cells in culture. The survival curves for various human tumors thought to be both sensitive and resistant to radiation were studied by Weichselbaum and coworkers, who failed to show any survival curve characteristics that allow these two to be separated.[4] Therefore, the differences in clinical response cannot be explained by simple acute differences in survival curves.

Normal tissues also have been studied using clonogenic survival as an endpoint, with survival curves determined analogously to those for cells in tissue culture. The simplest clonal system, as originally described by Till and McCulloch, is that used for murine bone marrow stem cells.[5] When bone marrow cells are injected into lethally irradiated recipient animals, colonies are formed in the animals' spleens. These

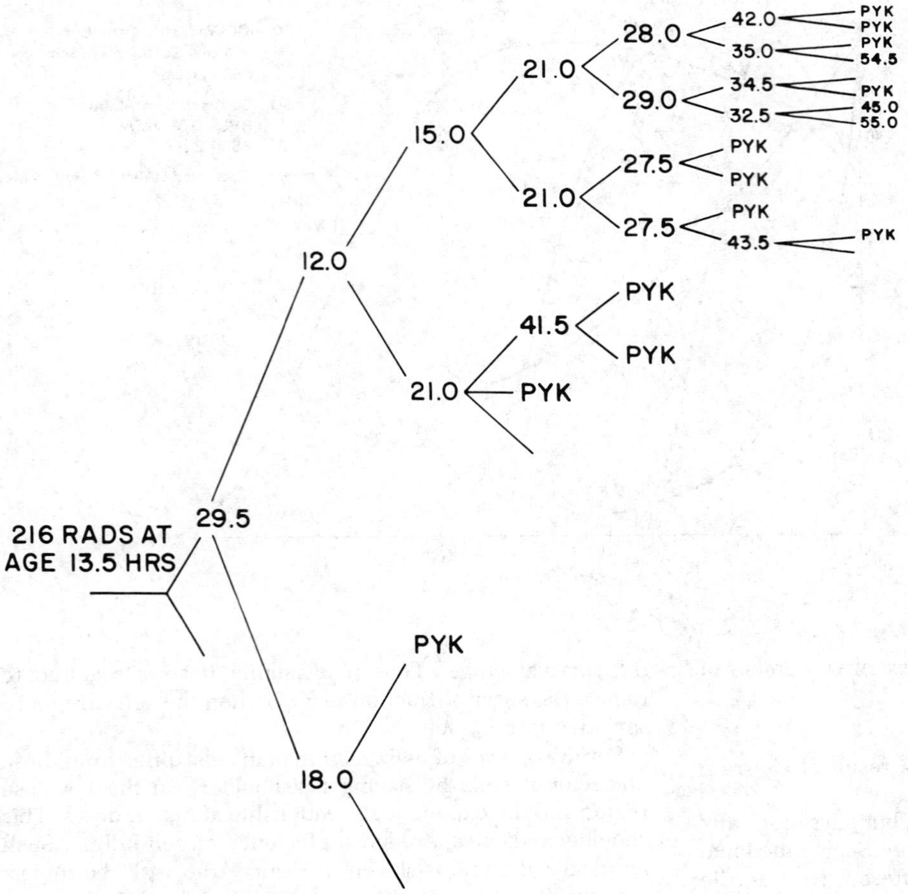

FIG. 15-7. Two cell pedigrees indicating cell cycle times and the outcome of cells irradiated in vitro. *PYK* = pyknosis. (Thompson LH, Suit HD: Proliferation kinetics of x-irradiated mouse L cells studied with time lapse photography: II. Int J Radiat Biol 15:347–362, 1969)

can be used to assess the reproductive integrity of the injected cells. The viability of the small intestinal clonogenic mucosal cells can be assessed by looking at sections of the small intestine at various times after irradiation and determining the appearance of colonies derived from cells surviving this radiation.[6] Using these and other techniques, the general properties of survival curves of both normal and tumor cells are shown in Table 15-1. There are no characteristic differences in survival curves between normal tissues and tumors. Tumors generally resemble their normal tissue of origin in this respect.

Repair of Radiation Damage

When cells are irradiated, lethal damage can occur, or the damage may be modified and not lead irrevocably to cell death. Such amelioration of radiation damage is called repair. Repair can be divided into potentially lethal damage repair and sublethal damage repair.

Potentially lethal damage, under certain circumstances, leads to cell death. However, if postirradiation conditions are modified to allow repair, cells that would have died can be salvaged. In general, postirradiation conditions that suppress cell division are the ones most favorable to repair of potentially lethal damage. The simplest example of this was shown first in bacteria for both ultraviolet and X-radiation.[7] A similar effect was seen in mammalian cells and persists into the first few postirradiation generations.[8–10] Potentially lethal damage repair may be most important in relating the cell culture studies of human tumors to their clinical response. Weichselbaum and co-workers have shown that osteogenic sarcoma, a tumor characteristically thought to be quite resistant to radiation, has a great capacity for potentially lethal damage repair compared with tumors that may be much more responsive to radiation.[11] After irradiation in the clinical circumstance, the tumor cell may not be faced with the necessity of rapid cell division, and it may have the opportunity for potentially lethal damage repair.

One explanation for the shoulder of the radiation survival curve is that the cell can repair some of the radiation damage, including a great proportion of the damage incurred with low doses of radiation. This is called *sublethal damage*. Elkind and colleagues have studied the shoulder and its return by using divided doses of radiation.[12] They have shown that if the dose of radiation is divided into two fractions and a few hours elapse between radiation doses, the shoulder will

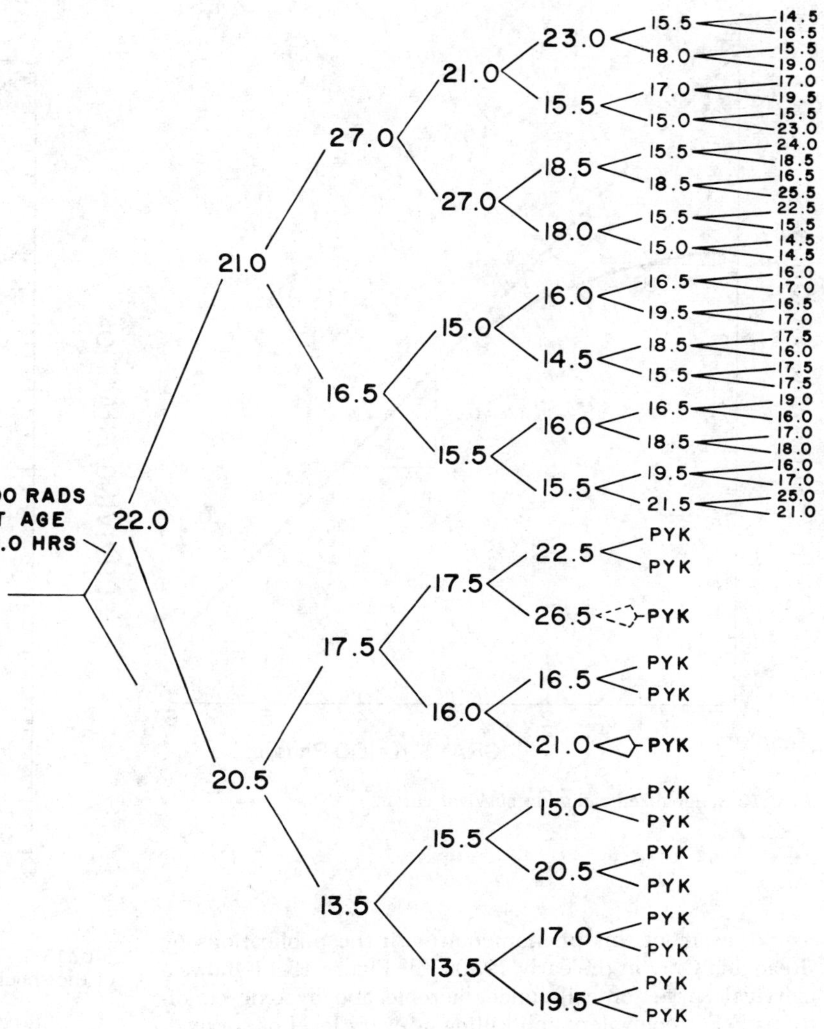

FIG. 15-7. (*continued*)

return. Therefore, two doses of radiation separated in time are less effective than the same total dose given as a single dose. The difference between a single dose and the divided dose that produce equivalent cell kills is the D_q if all the doses are sufficiently large to cause the loss in cell survival to extend to the exponential portion of the survival curve (Fig. 15-9).

The D_q is a measure of sublethal damage repair. Table 15-2 shows the D_q for bone marrow, skin, lung, and gastrointestinal mucosa. The contrast is striking. Bone marrow stem cells have a very small D_q, whereas the others have considerable sublethal damage repair capacity. This suggests that multiple small fractions of radiation can preserve these tissues, but not bone marrow. Radiation fractionation schemes must account for whether or not the fraction size is sufficient to be off the shoulder. If all of the variations are on the shoulder, there will be little difference in cell kill. With such small fractions, essentially all the damage that can be repaired is being repaired already, and fractionation becomes much less important. However, if the fractions are large enough to include a portion of the steeper part of the survival curve, then differences in fraction size are very important, because the proportion of shoulder-to-steep-exponential portion varies for different fraction sizes.

Varying the dose rate of radiation may be considered a form of radiation fractionation. When the dose rate is quite low, such as during interstitial or intracavitary irradiation, it can be considered as a large number of small doses on the shoulder of the survival curve.[12] Therefore, differences between the dose-limiting normal tissues and the tumor in their shoulder characteristics and differences in the break point between shoulder and steep exponential will have great clinical implications for such continuous radiation. An example of this for cells in culture is shown in Figure 15-10.

Importance of Oxygen

The most important modifier of the biologic effect of ionizing irradiation is molecular oxygen. This was noted in the 1920s, but it was not understood, nor was its importance realized, until Mottram and colleagues studied it systematically.[14-16] The general scientific community be-

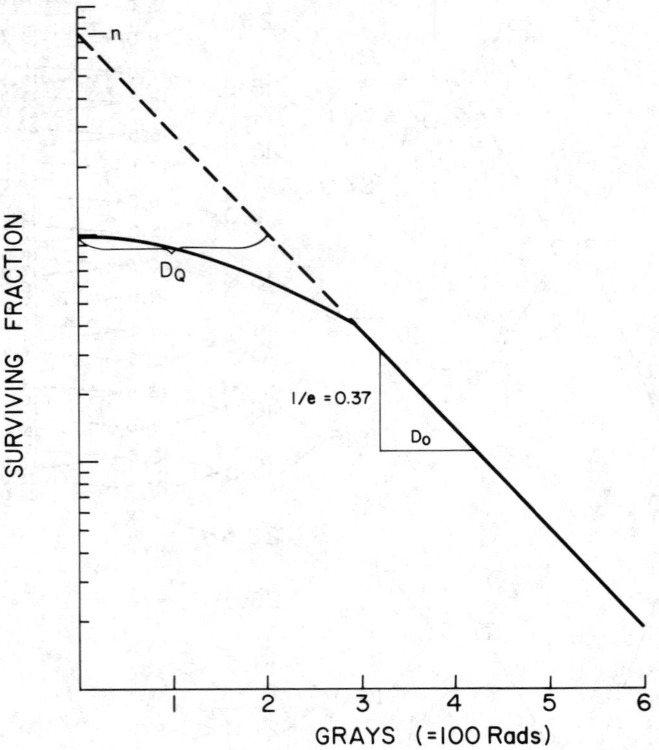

FIG. 15-8. Idealized radiation survival curve.

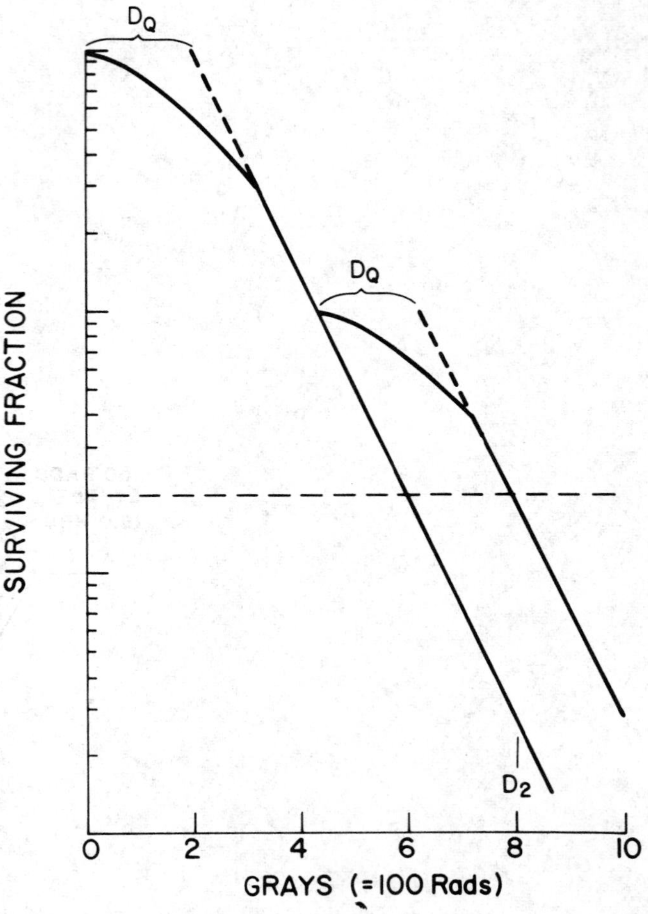

FIG. 15-9. Two dose radiation survival curves demonstrating return of the shoulder.

came aware of this phenomenon with the publications by Read and Gray in the early 1950s.[15,16] Figure 15-11 shows a survival curve for cells under aerobic and hypoxic conditions.[17] For equivalent cell killing at every level of survival, greater doses are required under hypoxic conditions compared with oxic conditions. There is some disagreement in the literature as to whether the dose ratio is the same throughout the survival curve. Most data suggest a smaller difference when low doses are used. A shorthand term, the oxygen enhancement ratio (OER), often is used. OER is the ratio of dose required for equivalent cell killing in the absence compared with the dose required in the presence of oxygen. This term has most relevance on the exponential

TABLE 15-2. D_q Determination for Some Normal Tissues

Normal Tissue	*D_q (Gy)**
Mouse skin	~4.00
Mouse intestine	3.50–4.00
Mouse lung	~3.75
Mouse bone marrow	0–0.60

*Average calculated from literature.

TABLE 15-1. Survival Curve Parameters for Some Mammalian Cells In Vivo or In Vitro

Cell Type	*How Determined*	*D_0 (Rad)*	*n*	*D_q (Rad)*
Hamster V-79 fibroblast	in vitro	~160	~7	250–300
Chang liver	in vitro	150	2	150
HeLa	in vitro	130	4	180
P 388 leukemia	in vivo	130	8.5	280
Mouse bone marrow	in vivo	90–100	1.5–2.0	~60
Mouse small intestine	in vivo	100	50	390
Mouse chondroblast	in vivo	160	9	350
Rat endothelium	in vivo	170	7	340

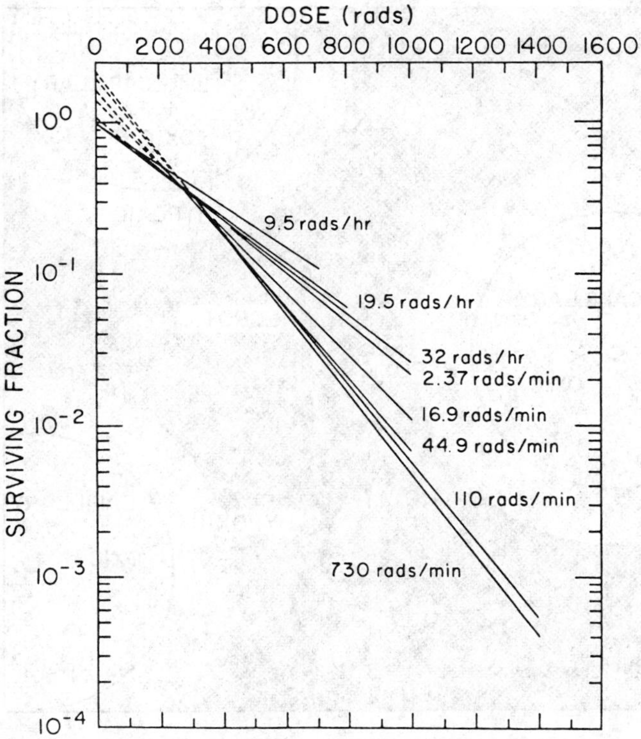

FIG. 15-10. In vitro survival curves for cells irradiated at different dose rates. (Hall EJ: Radiation dose-rate: A factor of importance in radiobiology and radiotherapy. Br J Radiol 45:81–97, 1972)

portion of the curve, because there appears to be a reduced shoulder on the survival curve of cells under hypoxic conditions.[17] As shown in Figure 15-12, tumor cells allowed to grow into physiologic hypoxia have reduced capacity to repair sublethal damage.

The OER range for different cells that have been studied varies from about 2.5 to 3.5. This means that for reduction to a given survival level, three times as much radiation is required under hypoxic conditions as under oxic conditions. Because the curves are exponential, the ratio of survival fractions may be much greater at a given dose and will increase with dose. For example, in Figure 15-11, at 1000 rad the ratio of survival is 30.

Study of the phenomenon reveals that oxygen must be present during irradiation. Figure 15-13 shows the relative radiosensitivity of cells as a function of the oxygen tension at the time of irradiation. A very low oxygen tension must be reached before there is a protective effect of hypoxia. The exact mechanism of the oxygen effect has not been determined definitively. It is believed that oxygen affects the initial chemical products of the interaction of radiation with biologic material. The important free radicals have short half-lives. A useful way to think about them is that they may either return to an innocuous state or remain highly reactive molecules. Oxygen appears to favor the latter, whereas the presence of high levels of sulfhydryl compounds favors the former.

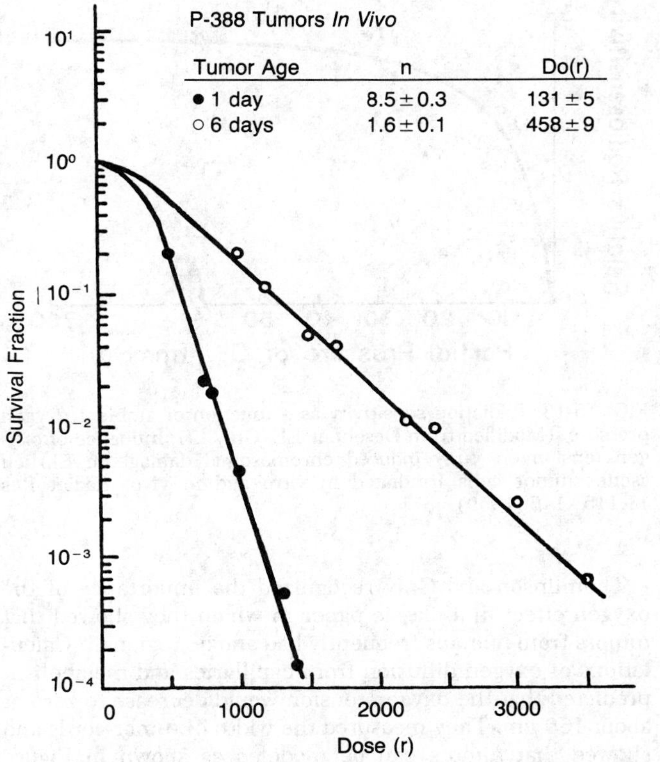

FIG. 15-11. In vivo survival curves for oxic and hypoxic tumor cells. (Belli JA, Dicus GJ, Bonte FJ: Radiation response of mammalian tumor cells: 1. Repair of sublethal damage in vivo. JNCI 38:673–682, 1967).

FIG. 15-12. In vivo curves comparing two dose survival to single dose survival for oxic and hypoxic tumor cells. (Belli JA, Dicus GJ, Bonte FJ: Radiation response of mammalian tumor cells: 1. Repair of sublethal damage in vivo. JNCI 38:673–682, 1967)

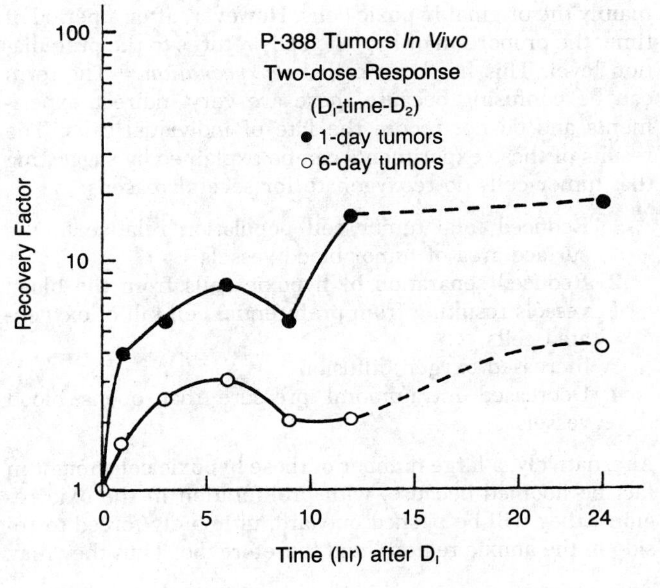

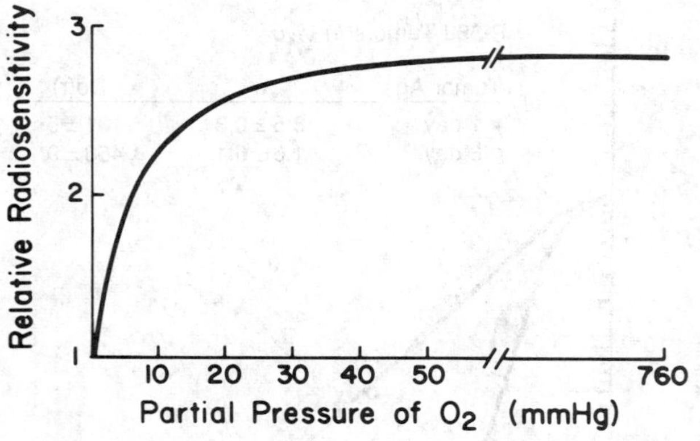

FIG. 15-13. Radiation sensitivity as a function of ambient oxygen pressure. (Modified from Deschner EE, Gray LH: Influence of oxygen tension on x-ray induced chromosomal damage in Ehrlich ascites tumor cells irradiated in vitro and in vivo. Radiat Res 11:115–146, 1959)

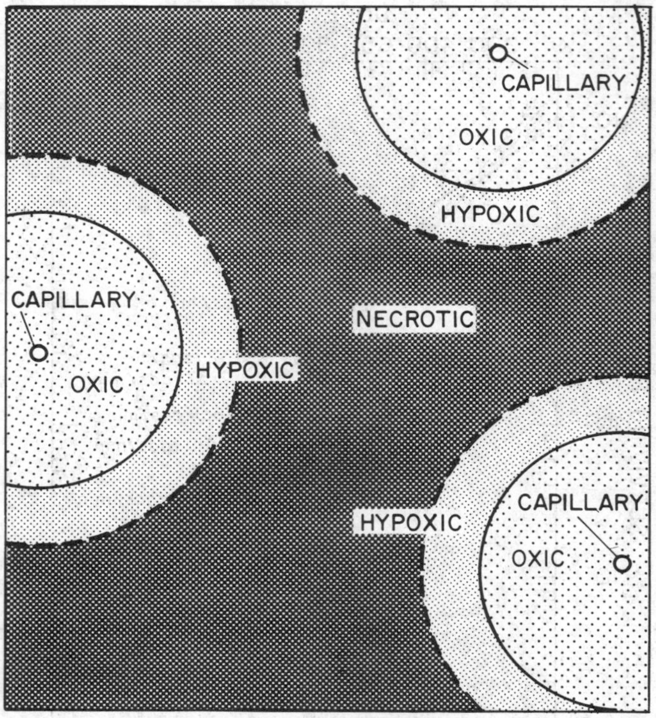

FIG. 15-14. Diagrammatic representation of a tumor.

Thomlinson and Gray recognized the importance of the oxygen effect in a classic paper in which they showed that tumors from humans frequently had anoxic regions.[19] Calculations of oxygen diffusion from capillaries and metabolism predicted that the oxygen tension would decrease to zero at about 150 μm. They measured the width of tumor cords and showed that tumors can be modeled as shown in Figure 15-14. Those cells within about 100 μm of the capillary are well oxygenated; those beyond 150 μm are anoxic and necrotic; and those between 100 and 150 μm are hypoxic at an oxygen tension that might protect cells from radiation. This model has had a profound influence on radiobiologic and radiotherapeutic thinking. If all tumors look this way and such hypoxic regions contain cells that ultimately could cause tumor regrowth, then no clinically apparent tumor would be cured by radiation therapy. Because this obviously is not the case, this paradox must be explained.

Laboratory experiments have indicated that immediately after a single dose of radiation, the surviving tumor cells are mainly the original hypoxic cells. However, after a period of time, the proportion of hypoxic cells returns to the preradiation level. This has been called *reoxygenation*.[20] The term can be confusing because these are very indirect experiments and do not record the fate of individual cells. The results of these experiments can be explained by suggesting that tumor cells do reoxygenate for several reasons:

1. Reduced total tumor cell population relative to the surface area of tumor blood vessels
2. Reduced separation of hypoxic cells from the blood vessels resulting from preferential cell kill of oxygenated cells
3. Increased oxygen diffusion
4. Decreased intratumoral pressure that opens blood vessels

Alternatively, a large number of these hypoxic cells might in fact be doomed because, with proliferation in the oxic regions, they will be pushed outward, ultimately forced to reside in the anoxic regions, and therefore die. Thus they may have only a limited clinical importance in determining tumor curability. It is likely that different mechanisms occur under different circumstances, both in the laboratory and in the clinic.

The obvious clinical importance of the oxygen effect has led to a number of clinical and laboratory experiments, including the use of high-pressure oxygen with radiation therapy to improve results. These studies have indicated that with a small number of radiation fractions, hyperbaric oxygen will increase curability. However, when normal fractionation schemes are used, hyperbaric oxygen often has failed to show an advantage. There are, however, some reports of tumors of the head, neck, and uterine cervix that indicate that hyperbaric oxygen with 10 fractions of radiation results in greater cure than does conventional daily fractionation.[21–23] Table 15-3 depicts the results with head and neck cancers. Despite these promising studies, the hyperbaric oxygen technique is cumbersome, difficult for the

TABLE 15-3. Results of a Randomized Prospective Trial of Hyperbaric Oxygen in the Radiation Treatment of Head and Neck Cancer

	Local Control	*Survival at 4 Years*
HP O_2	61%	56%
Conventional treatment	40%	27%

Henk JM, Kindler PB, Smith CW: Radiotherapy and head and neck cancer: Final report on the first clinical trial. Lancet 2:101–103, 1977.

patient, and prohibits the use of the careful beam definition and beam modification so important in radiation therapy. Thus, the technique has been abandoned in most radiotherapy centers.

A more attractive alternative has been the development of *hypoxic cell sensitizers*. In the 1960s, Adams and colleagues began searching for compounds that would mimic oxygen in its effect.[24,25] They sought agents that would be metabolized slowly and reach all portions of the tumor. This is an important distinction, because high-pressure oxygen increases diffusion only slightly, whereas slowly metabolized sensitizers can reach all areas of the tumor. Although newer methods were based on replacing molecular oxygen, there are other effects of the nitroimidazoles, the most well-studied class of these agents. They appear to be quite cytotoxic to hypoxic cells and may sensitize cells to chemotherapeutic agents.[26,27] How important these last two points are in their use remains to be seen. However, this general class of agents offers a whole new approach to the chemical treatment of tumors based on a known tumor-normal tissue difference (*i.e.*, the presence of hypoxic cells in tumors). These agents and agents designed to protect normal tissue are discussed specifically in Chapter 66, section 3.

A practical clinical concern is whether the presence of anemia affects tumor response to radiation. Historic review and a prospective study from the Princess Margaret Hospital (Table 15-4) appear to indicate that anemia results in an adverse effect on tumor curability by radiation, presumably because it increases the hypoxic component of tumor cells.[28]

A recent review of intercapillary distance and tissue oxygen tension correlates local recurrence with evidence of hypoxia using these parameters in studying carcinoma of the cervix.[29] These studies emphasize the promise of techniques that improve tissue oxygenation in the treatment of epithelial cancers. In vitro measurement of hypoxia using radioactively labelled hypoxic sensitizers may alter selection of appropriate tumors for such therapeutic manipulation.[30,31]

Variable Radiation Response During the Division Cycle

As described in Chapter 1, the cell cycle can be divided into four phases: G1, S, G2, and M. Terasima, Tolmach, and Sinclair studied relatively synchronized populations to determine whether there is a difference in response to radiation as a function of the cell's position in the division cycle.[32,33] They found that generally the mitotic phase (M) is most sensitive and G2 almost as sensitive. G1 is relatively sensitive in cells with a short G1. Cells gradually increase in resistance as they proceed through the late G1 and S phases, reaching a maximum of resistance in the late S phase. In cells with a long G1, there appears to be a peak of resistance early in G1. These findings in vitro seem to be true in vivo as well for both normal and tumor cells.[34,35]

The changes in radiation response are reflected in changes in the shoulder of the survival curve, as well as in the terminal slope. These differences can be quite large. The difference between the most resistant and the most sensitive can show slope ratios equal to that of the oxygen effect. The clinical consequence of a dose of 200 rad is shown in Table 15-5 for two different radiation fractionation schemes: one used in Hodgkin's disease (20 fractions) and one used in epithelial cancer (32 fractions).[36] Note how small differences in survival fractions following a single dose may change the final survival level achieved. All of these fractional survivals are within the range seen for cells in different parts of the cell cycle.

A second consequence of differential cell killing and the mitotic delay induced by radiation is a tendency to partially synchronize the cells. Thus the timing of the second dose of a fractionated scheme may be critical. However, this synchronization is short-lived because cells desynchronize rapidly and redistribute themselves according to the original cell age distribution. This phenomenon, which could pose a clinical problem or a clinical advantage, does not seem to be important unless there is incomplete redistribution between fractions.

CELL PROLIFERATION. During a course of fractionated radiation, the ultimate response of the tumor and normal tissue will depend on whether there has been cell proliferation between the fractions, thereby increasing the number of cells exposed to radiation. This may be caused by cell proliferation within the irradiated volume (*i.e.*, within the tumor or normal cell renewal tissue) or by cells that immigrate from unirradiated adjacent areas. The latter situation is seen in the skin, oral gastrointestinal mucosa, or from great distances, as found with bone marrow and lymph node repopulation. The balance between radiation-induced cell killing and repopulation is responsible for most of the clinical findings seen during fractionated radiotherapy treatment.

TABLE 15-4. Effect of Anemia on Pelvic Recurrence in Stage IIB–III Cervical Cancer

	Control		*Transfused*
Hemoglobin (g/dl)	<12	>12	>12
Pelvic recurrence	50% (10/20)	23% (11/48)	16% (11/67)

Bush RS, Jenkin RP, Allt WE et al: Definitive evidence for hypoxic cells influencing cure in cancer therapy. Br J Cancer 37:302–306, 1978.

TABLE 15-5. Calculated Cumulative Survival Fraction*

Survival Fraction	X^{32} X =	X^{20} X =
10^{-11}	0.45	0.28
10^{-10}	0.49	0.32
10^{-9}	0.52	0.35
10^{-8}	0.56	0.40
10^{-7}	0.60	0.45
10^{-6}	0.65	0.50
10^{-5}	0.70	0.56

Hellman S: Cell kinetics, models, and cancer treatment: Some principles for the radiation oncologist. Radiology 114:219–223, 1975.

*Calculated cumulative survival fraction for either 32 or 20 equal fractions when the fractional survival is varied.

In addition to spontaneous repopulation, there may be an induced cell proliferation or *recruitment* of cells.[37,38] Physiologically, many tissues of the body respond to trauma by being recruited into rapid proliferation (*e.g.*, following a wound in the skin, a break of the bone, or a partial hepatectomy). The reparative process requires proliferation of the undamaged cells. Similarly, when the oral mucosa is irradiated, there is strong evidence that the cell cycle time is decreased and that net cell proliferation increases. This also may occur in some tumors but appears to be of less magnitude than that in normal tissues.[39] Part of the differential effect of fractionated radiation may lie in differential recruitment of normal versus tumor cells.

Pharmacologic Modification of Radiation Effects

A number of pharmacologic agents can modify the basic parameters of radiation response. Figure 15-15 shows a radiation survival curve for cells that have semiconservatively incorporated the halogenated pyrimidine, BUDR, into their DNA. Under such circumstances, these cells are more sensitive to radiation, their survival curve having both the slope and the shoulder modified.[40] This occurs only when the halogenated pyrimidines BUDR or IUDR are incorporated into the DNA; their presence at the time of radiation is not sufficient (Fig. 15-15). Sublethal damage repair also is markedly inhibited under these circumstances. Clinical experiments using these agents are discussed in Chapter 66, section 3.

FIG. 15-15. Radiation survival curve for cells incorporating halogenated pyrimidines. (Szybalski W: X-ray sensitization by halopyrimidines. Cancer Chemother Rep 58:539–557, 1974)

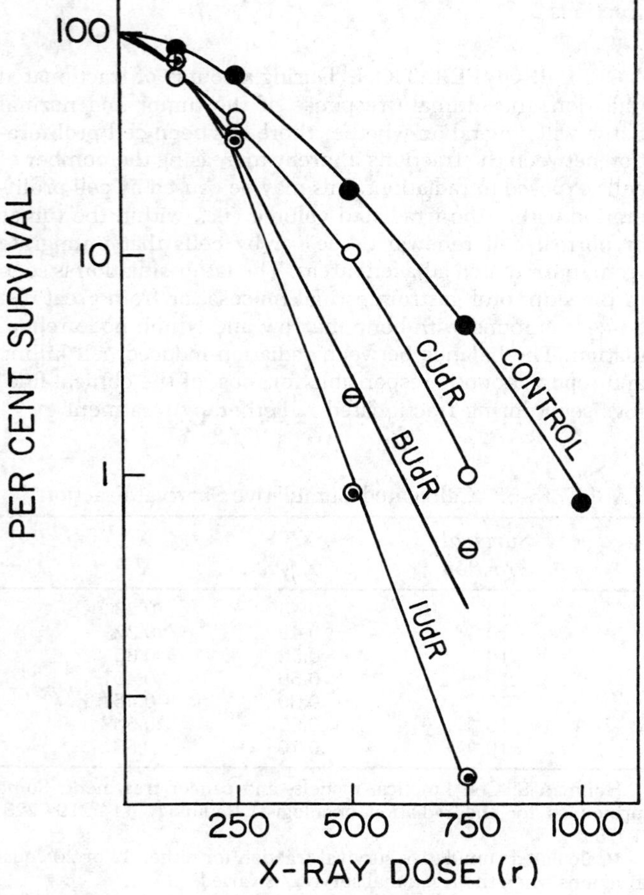

A second class of agents includes those that primarily affect the shoulder and only slightly affect the slope. The two most important agents here are actinomycin D and Adriamycin. Sublethal damage apparently is inhibited by actinomycin D but not by Adriamycin.[41–47] The mechanisms by which these drugs affect radiation response are complicated. From a clinical standpoint, however, there appears to be strong evidence that these drugs can and do modify radiation effects when given simultaneously. Further, when given after radiation therapy, they can "recall" the irradiated volumes by erythema on the skin or by producing pulmonary reactions.[42,45,48,49] It is not known whether this is due to interaction between the damage done by radiation and that by drug or whether it represents only additivity of the effects.

Chemicals may also interact with radiation by preferentially killing cells that are more resistant to radiation. For example, agents that preferentially destroy cells in the most resistant phase of the cell cycle (S), along with radiation, will increase the cell kill; an example of this is hydroxyurea.[50] Hypoxic sensitizers also kill hypoxic cells and therefore act similarly in destroying a population of cells that is resistant to radiation. Radioprotective agents such as sulfhydryl-containing compounds act in the reverse fashion and tend to make cells more resistant.[51]

Agents with dose-limiting normal tissue toxicities different from radiation may be used very effectively with radiation. This is one of the basic principles of multiple-drug chemotherapy—add agents with nonoverlapping toxicities. This also works well with radiation.

The combined effects of drugs and radiation, or of two drugs, can be divided into the following types:

1. Independent—the agents act independently, their mechanisms of action are independent, and their damage is independent.
2. Additivity—the agents act on the same loci, and therefore their sublethal damage and their lethal damage are additive. Because of additive sublethal damage, the lethality of the two together may be greater than the lethality of each alone added together.
3. Synergism—the two agents have a result that is more effective than pure additivity.
4. Antagonism—the cell killing is less than independent action.

The most important parameter for the clinician is the therapeutic index. The sigmoid curve of tumor cure and that of dose-limiting toxicity are portrayed in Figure 15-16. If both curves are moved but their relative place (one to the other) is not changed, then the proportion cured for a given level of toxicity is unchanged. Drug–roentgen-ray interac-

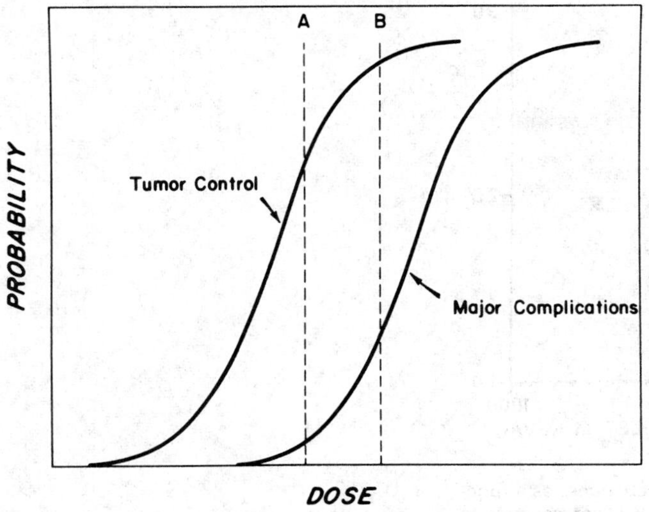

FIG. 15-16. Sigmoid curves of tumor control and complications. **A.** Dose for tumor control with minimum complications. **B.** Maximum tumor dose with significant complications.

tion is useful only when the curves are separated and not merely displaced.

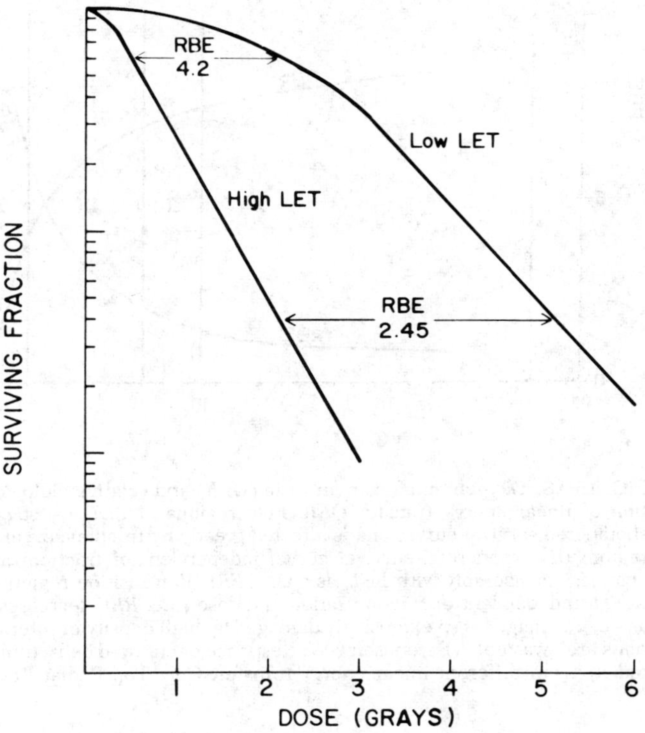

FIG. 15-17. Survival fractions for high and low *LET* radiations.

HIGH LINEAR ENERGY TRANSFER RADIATION

Most of the previous discussion has been concerned with sparsely ionizing radiation, such as that produced by photons or high-energy electrons. More densely ionizing radiation is produced by larger atomic particles. The biologic actions of these two types of radiation are quite different and relate to the density of ionization. LET is the rate of energy loss along the path of the particle (de/dl). High LET radiations are very densely ionizing, with de/dl being very high. In general, the density of ionization depends on Z^2/v^2, where Z equals the atomic number and v is the particle velocity. Photons and electrons are characterized by high energy and very low mass. Therefore, the density of ionization will be low until the secondary electrons come to rest at the very end of their path. Particulate radiation ionizes directly. Alpha particles and stripped nuclei have a high LET; neutrons have an intermediate LET due to recoil protons. The Z^2 is quite large for large particles, intermediate for protons, and low for photons.

RELATIVE BIOLOGIC EFFECTIVENESS

Relative biologic effectiveness (RBE) is a commonly used parameter in radiation biology. It is the dose ratio of different average LET beams required to produce the same biologic effect. This term generally is a descriptive one, but its numerical value is fraught with many difficulties because it varies with the biologic endpoint used. High LET radiation differs from low LET radiation in affecting both the shoulder and the slope of the radiation survival curves (Fig. 15-17). If the biologic endpoint of interest is one associated with a high survival fraction, then the RBE will be large because it considers shoulder differences as well as those of the terminal slope. However, if the biologic endpoint involves a very low survival fraction, the RBE will be less because it primarily considers slope differences. In general, RBE increases as the dose decreases. Not only is the shoulder reduced, but other measures of sublethal damage repair or potentially lethal damage repair are markedly reduced with high LET radiation.

A general explanation is that the ionization is so dense that when a cell is hit, the damage is so great that it cannot be repaired. It is also true that the oxygen effect decreases as the LET increases. With very high LET radiation, there is no oxygen effect. Figure 15-18 plots both RBE and OER as a function of LET.[52] With very high LET radiation, there is a fall in RBE because these very densely ionizing radiations deposit more than one lethal event per cell. Thus, some of the absorbed dose is redundant and becomes less efficient.

Although this obvious advantage in RBE and OER would suggest the possible therapeutic use of these radiations, a cautionary note should be made. Increasing RBE in itself does not afford a therapeutic advantage. It is the therapeutic gain factor that is important—the RBE of the tumor compared with the RBE of the normal tissue. This is quite complicated and greatly depends on the specific tumor and the dose-limiting normal tissue being considered.[53] These forms of radiation will be discussed further in Chapter 66, section 5.)

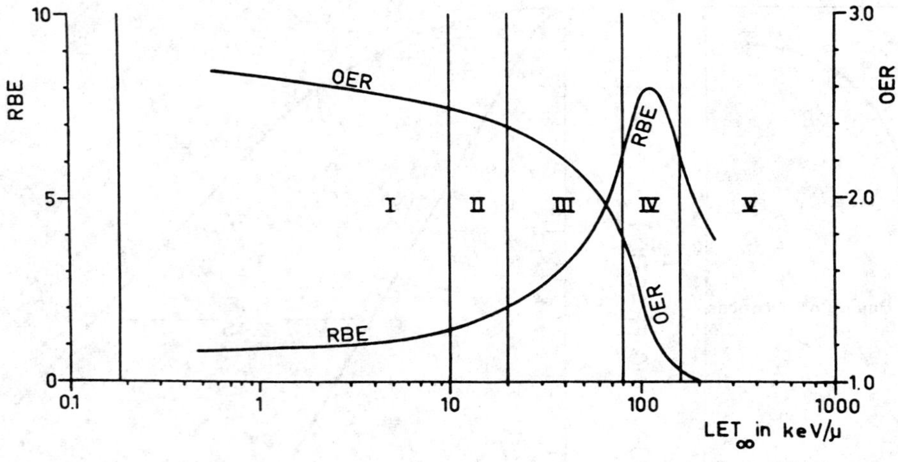

FIG. 15-18. Oxygen enhancement ratio *(OER)* and relative biologic effectiveness as a function of linear energy transfer *OER*. Five regions of *LET* are suggested: *I*, corresponds to shouldered survival curves and is affected greatly by fraction size and dose rate; *II*, transition region; *III*, exponential survival curve, independent of fractionization and dose rate. *RBE* changes considerably with *LET*, as does *OER*; *IV*, transition region; *V*, *LET* in excess of 160 *KeV/u* independent of fractionization and dose rate. *RBE* decreases as *LET* increases, since any cell damaged is so extensively damaged by high density of interactions that some interactions are "wasted." (Barendsen GW: Response of cultured cells, tumors and normal tissues to radiations of different linear energy transfer. Curr Top Radiat Res 4:293–356, 1968)

TUMOR RADIOBIOLOGY

Many experiments have been done using a variety of animal tumors. In general, these tumors are either spontaneous tumors occurring with reasonably high frequency in certain strains of mice (*e.g.*, mammary carcinoma in C3H mice) or tumors induced by carcinogens. Such primary tumors of animals are difficult to use experimentally because their production is time-consuming, and numbers of tumors of the same size and location are limited, restricting some experimental designs. A much more common technique is the use of transplanted tumors. These are tumors that may have occurred spontaneously or from the application of a carcinogen but have now been transplanted from animal to animal. They grow with predictable and known kinetics. Although this is a great advantage in experimental work, it does increase the likelihood that the application of the results may be somewhat limited. Because these tumors are selected for rapid growth and for the ability to transplant serially, they may not represent tumors that occur spontaneously in the host animal.

Tumors can be used in radiobiologic experiments and assayed in a number of ways. The simplest is to study the likelihood for cure. A researcher implants a tumor into animals, allows it to grow to palpable size, treats it with a specific regimen, and then determines how many tumors of this type in various host animals are cured. If the dose of radiation is plotted against the likelihood for cure, a sigmoid curve is generated, as seen in Figure 15.19.[54] There is insufficient cell kill to cause tumor cure at very low doses. However, as the dose is raised (to about one lethal event per cell, the statistics of random cell kill become important. Occasionally, tumors will have zero viable cells and are cured. The likelihood of cure rises rapidly with dose at this portion of the curve; it starts to plateau when the maximum effect of the particular technique is reached. The dose required to increase a 10% likelihood of tumor control to 90% is about three times the D_0 dose. This sigmoid relationship is very important, because it is true not only for tumors in experimental animals, but also for clinical situations.

FIG. 15-19. Sigmoid curve of tumor control.

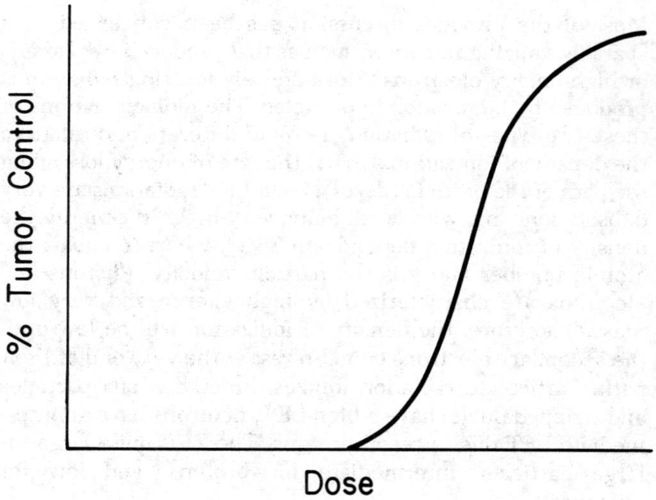

The shape and steepness of the sigmoid dose–response relationship for tumors can be affected by many factors. If the radiation survival curve is quite shallow for individual tumor cells (*i.e.*, the D_0 is large), then the dose–response curve will also be shallow. It will also be affected by host defense mechanisms. This curve is quite steep with nonimmunogenic tumors or when the immune response is abrogated, but it is significantly shallower in immunogenic tumors.[55] The shallowness means that there will be occasional cures at low doses and occasional failures at very high doses.

A similar sigmoid relationship is seen when plotting the likelihood for complications against tumor control. Figure 15-16 shows the two sigmoid curves, one for cure and one for complications. This is presented optimistically—the important complication curve is placed to the right of the tumor cure curve. The difference between these curves is a measure of therapeutic gain. Much of clinical medicine and research in cancer treatment is concerned with separating these curves.[53] Once the curves are separated, for a given level of complications, the likelihood of cure can be increased. Or, for a high likelihood of cure, the likelihood of complications can be decreased.

Another method of measuring tumors' response to treatment is to determine their growth delay following treatment. The longer the time for regrowth, the more effective was the treatment. If it is assumed that tumors grow and regrow with the same kinetics when they are at similar sizes, then the separation between the original curve and the regrowth curve is a direct measure of cell kill.[56] A direct measure of tumor cell kill is to remove the tumor after treatment, separate the cells, and score the surviving colony-forming cells, either in vivo or in vitro. Assay techniques include transplantation and measurement in recipient animals of death, tumor growth, or the number of colonies in the lung, liver, or brain. In vitro techniques require tumors to adapt to grow both in vivo and in vitro.

It is important to realize that tumors, like normal tissues, have certain physiologic characteristics. We associate some of these with the definition of malignancy: continued growth and extension into surrounding tissues and the ability to metastasize. In addition, growing tumors must induce a blood supply to meet their increasing metabolic needs. The production of these blood vessels appears to result from the release of a substance described by Folkman and colleagues as "tumor angiogenesis factor." This may have very important clinical implications. If tumors can be prevented from producing such substances, then they could not grow beyond a size supported by diffusion alone.[57–59] From the radiobiologic point of view it also means that when irradiating a tumor, both the radiobiology of the tumor and the vascular endothelial cells are important. Complete destruction of the tumor blood vessels' ability to proliferate will effectively limit tumor growth.

As tumors grow, they often exceed their blood supply and develop areas of necrosis and hypoxia (Fig. 15-14). The proportion of hypoxic cells in a tumor can be determined by studying the radiation survival curves. In Figure 15-20, curve A represents a well-oxygenated cell population, curve B describes hypoxic cells, and curve C represents a mixture of oxic and hypoxic cells (as in a tumor). Extrapolation of the curves to the ordinate gives the proportion of hypoxic cells within a tumor, first described by Powers and Tolmach.[60] In most experimental tumors studied, the percentage of hypoxic cells is 10% to 20%.

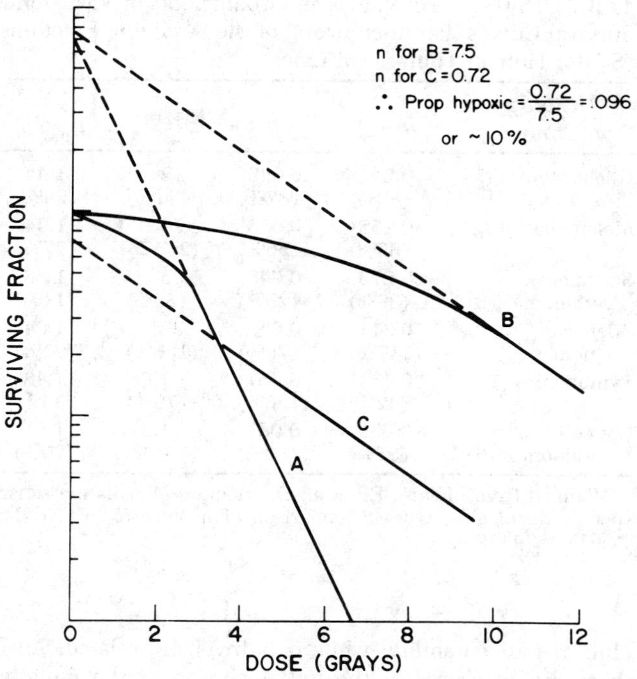

FIG. 15-20. Idealized survival curves for (**A**) oxic tumor cells; (**B**) hypoxic tumor cells; (**C**) a tumor containing both oxic and hypoxic tumor cells.

Calculation of the likelihood to cure tumors based on D_0, n, repopulation, repair, and hypoxia indicates that, because each fraction of radiation increases the proportion of hypoxic cells, the currently used treatment regimens should not be effective. Because radiotherapy cures a large number of tumors that have hypoxic components and show necrosis on pathologic examination, then this conclusion must be erroneous. After multiple fractions of radiation, a marked increase in the proportion of the more resistant hypoxic cells could be expected, but in fact, the proportion remained constant when observed 72 hours after the last of five radiation fractions. Kallman has called this *reoxygenation*.[20] Hypoxic cells may not be important in tumors that are cured but may be important in some tumors that are not cured. Clinical evidence that this is significant includes the benefits of correcting anemia, hyperbaric oxygen, and the hypoxic sensitizers. All appear to favorably influence tumor curability in certain clinical circumstances.

There has been a renaissance in trying to determine whether there are appropriate laboratory correlates for clinical radiation treatment.[61,62] Table 15-6 shows a number of important parameters found by in vitro survival determinations for six histologic groups of human tumor cells.[63] The first four parameters have been described earlier. S_2 and S_8 are the survival fractions found with 2 Gy and 8 Gy, respectively. $\overline{D}$ is the mean inactivation dose, a mathematically determined characteristic of the initial portion of the survival curve. It appears that S_2 and $\overline{D}$ correlate directly with

TABLE 15-6. Mean Values and Coefficients of Variation (in parentheses) of the Survival Curves' Parameters and of the Surviving Fractions at 2 Gy (S_2) and at 8 Gy (S_8) for Human Tumor Cell Lines

Histologic Groups	α	β	n	D_0 (Gy)	S_2 (%)	S_8 (%)	$\bar{D}$ (Gy)
Glioblastomas (5)	0.241 (86%)	0.029 (37%)	12 (71%)	1.44 (28%)	58 (34%)	4.98 (111%)	3.10 (38%)
Melanomas (19)	0.255 (69%)	0.053 (56%)	73 (265%)	1.04 (27%)	51 (28%)	1.11 (109%)	2.43 (25%)
Squamous cell carcinomas (6)	0.273 (39%)	0.045 (25%)	5 (38%)	1.28 (11%)	49 (18%)	0.88 (49%)	2.35 (25%)
Adenocarcinomas (6)	0.311 (117%)	0.055 (79%)	37 (166%)	1.04 (26%)	48 (37%)	0.39 (130%)	2.22 (28%)
Lymphomas (7)	0.451 (42%)	0.051 (126%)	1.8 (79%)	1.48 (34%)	34 (27%)	0.57 (121%)	1.77 (22%)
Oat cell carcinomas (6)	0.650 (37%)	0.081 (183%)	1.8 (104%)	1.51 (70%)	22 (42%)	0.14 (85%)	1.33 (21%)

Modified from Malaise EP et al: Distribution of radiation sensitivities for human tumor cells of specific histological types: Comparison of in vitro to in vivo data. Int J Radiat Oncol Biol Phys 12:617–624, 1986.

clinical radiocurability, while α is inversely related. All of these are measures of the initial portion of the radiation survival curve; S_2 is the most closely correlated with clinical practice, because doses between 1.5 and 2.5 Gy are used most often in patient care.

Because doses are repeated, small differences in S_2 can have very large consequences. Table 15-5 shows that, in a typical 32-fraction radiation treatment, the difference between survival fractions of 0.45 and 0.60 results in an ultimate survival fraction of 10^{-11} compared with 10^{-7}, respectively. Also, certain tumors that are known to be difficult to cure by radiation have been shown to have great capacity to repair radiation damage, as measured by allowing the cells time for repair before plating them for in vitro growth.[64] That these two simple laboratory determinations correlate with clinical results gives hope that in vitro techniques can be used to determine mechanisms of modifying clinical parameters. This does not mean that the other biologic parameters such as oxygenation, position in the cell cycle, and cell proliferation are not important; no doubt all add to the complexity of correlating the clinical response with in vitro determinations.

NORMAL TISSUE RADIATION BIOLOGY

To understand normal tissue radiation biology, an appreciation of the cell kinetics of cell renewal tissues is vital (see Chap. 1). The effects on organ function very much depend on the reproductive requirements of the irradiated cells. Tissues, (*e.g.*, muscle and neurologic tissue) whose functional activity does not require cell renewal are "resistant" to radiation. Both muscle and neurologic tissue also have important vasculoconnective tissue stroma that support them.[65] These stromal cells may be required to divide, and therefore determine the organ response to radiation. The radiation response of endothelial cells demonstrates a $D_q = 340$ rad, $n = 7$, and a $D_0 = 170$ rad, values similar to those of epithelial cells.[66]

Many tissues of the body require continued cellular proliferation for their function, and they promptly demonstrate the effects of radiation. These cell renewal tissues include the skin and its appendages, the gastrointestinal mucosa, bone marrow, reproductive tissues, and many exocrine glands. Clonogenic survival curves for bone marrow stem cells, gastrointestinal epithelial cells, and skin are all available. In slowly proliferating tissues (*e.g.*, lung), the effects of radiation are seen much later, but the effects depend on radiation damage to proliferating cells.

Tissues such as the liver and bone require little or no proliferation during the steady state, and normal function can be maintained despite large doses of radiation. However, both of these respond to injury with rapid cell renewal. If trauma (fracture or partial hepatectomy) occurs, then the cells die when they attempt repair. Irradiation of the liver has few consequences in moderate doses, but if this is followed by a partial hepatectomy, then hepatic failure can occur. This has been of clinical importance in the preoperative irradiation of right-sided Wilms' tumors attached to the liver, in which a significant amount of liver must be removed.[67] Under such circumstances it is far better to operate, allow the liver to regenerate, and then irradiate.

Patients who have received large amounts of radiation to the bone do perfectly well unless the bone is fractured. Such damaged bones will either fail to be reconstituted or will heal slowly, causing a significant deformity and disability to the patient. These examples are included to stress that it is not the different cells that have such great differences in radiation response, but rather that the proliferative requirements of different tissues largely determine the radiation effects. When the proliferative requirements are low, the organ will be considered relatively resistant to radiation. When the proliferative requirements are high, it will be considered very radiosensitive. There may be some common limitations on all systems based on the radiosensitivity of the vascular connective tissue and endothelial cells.[65] Stem cells of the cell renewal tissues may have a limited proliferative capacity, and stem cell exhaustion appears to be a cause of late organ failure following irradiation.[68]

Many other effects of radiation that do not depend on reproductive viability may have clear clinical relevance. For example, radiation is quite damaging to the cell membrane and changes membrane transport. Subsequent radiation-induced edema is seen with moderate doses of radiation. These nonreproductive effects of radiation are far less well understood but may be important in understanding the effects of radiation on nondividing tissue — most importantly, the central nervous system.

Large doses of whole-body irradiation have obvious clinical consequences, which generally are not relevant to conventional radiation therapy. However, because whole-body irradiation has been used in low doses in treating the lymphomas and in high doses in treating metastatic carcinoma, this will be discussed briefly.

Following large doses of radiation, the prodromal syndrome of nausea, vomiting, diarrhea, cramps, fatigue, sweating, fever, and headache occurs. Three distinct modes of death may occur. The first, with very high doses of radiation ($> 10,000$ rad), is seen within hours and appears to result from neurologic and cardiovascular damage. Because this occurs so quickly, it probably is not caused by failure of a proliferating cell system but rather by extranuclear events within these organs. At intermediate doses of radiation (500–1000 rad), death occurs within days. It is associated with extensive gastrointestinal mucosal damage, resulting in prolonged, severe, bloody diarrhea, dehydration, and secondary infection occurring as the gastrointestinal mucosa is denuded. At lower doses of radiation (around the LD_{50}), death is caused by hematopoietic failure. This has a latency period because the formed blood elements are nondividing and bone marrow failure does not occur until the progeny of the proliferating cells are required to maintain the patient. The lymphocyte level falls promptly as some of these cells die without dividing. The granulocyte level will fall on about day 5 or 6, and thrombocytopenia will occur later. Anemia does not occur as a direct result of a failure of red cell production because of the long life of the red cell, but it may be caused by hemorrhage.

Whole-body irradiation appears to have significant antitumor activity exceeding that seen when the same dose is given to the tumor alone.[69,70] Very low doses of whole-body radiation in humans (10–15 rad, two to three times per week for 6–10 fractions) may be effective treatment for lymphomas and may cause marked depression of the formed blood elements. The mechanism of action of this type of treatment is not understood. The effects on both tumor and normal tissue are greater than can be explained by the typical survival curve.

ADVERSE EFFECTS OF RADIATION

Some biologic considerations of localized radiation may decrease the likelihood for tumor control. First and most discussed is the effect of radiation on the *immune response*. High-dose, whole-body irradiation has a well-known and profound effect on the immune response. However, this generalized treatment rarely is used in clinical radiation therapy, except as preparation for bone marrow transplantation.

Shortly after the discovery of roentgen rays, whole-body irradiation before the administration of antigens was found to suppress the production of antibodies. After whole-body irradiation, there is a prompt fall in the lymphocyte count. The lymphocytes appear to have two types of radiation response: About 80% die a prompt, intermitotic death, but some lymphocytes survive the radiation. When assayed on the basis of reproductive capacity by either exposure to mitogens after irradiation or other functional endpoints, their radiation survival curves looked similar to that of hematopoietic cells with a D_0 of about 70 to 80 rad and an n of about 1.[71] Response depends on the classes of lymphocytes involved, the extent of cell proliferation required, cell traffic, and the balance between suppressor and helper systems. In general, the following conclusions concerning the effect of radiation on the immune response can be made:[71]

1. B lymphocytes are radiosensitive and undergo both interphase and mitotic death following irradiation.
2. All functional T-cell subpopulations have sensitive precursor cells. Suppressor T-cell precursors may undergo interphase death.
3. The homing potential of cells is affected by radiation.
4. Resting cells are more sensitive to interphase death than are the same cells when stimulated to divide before irradiation. (In the latter case they have an n and D_0 similar to those of hematopoietic stem cells.)
5. The effects of whole-body irradiation are qualitatively and quantitatively different from those caused by localized or regional irradiation.

Whole-body irradiation is more effective in preventing response to new antigens than in modifying response to a previously encountered antigen. Survival of second-set skin grafts are affected much less than are initial grafts. Localized radiation, as used in radiation therapy, affects the immune response by decreasing the number of circulating lymphocytes, presumably by irradiating and destroying them as they pass through the irradiated volume. The consequences of this irradiation appear to be small if the tumor has been in place for a significant time before the irradiation and if the irradiated volume is relatively small. If the animal is irradiated at the time the tumor is implanted, the immune response will be inhibited. However, this rarely is the clinical situation. There have been reports suggesting the deleterious effects of localized radiation on the immune response affecting survival in breast cancer, but this does not appear to be the case in either the original series studied or in subsequent studies.[72–74]

It is clear that localized radiation, despite producing a chronic lymphopenia of both T and B cells, does not affect the immune response to bacterial or viral agents because treated patients do not seem to be more susceptible. This is the case with the immune suppression produced by whole-body irradiation or systemic chemotherapy. Clearly, regional irradiation of the lymph nodes adjacent to tumors has been associated with increased curability in head and neck tumors in adults without adverse effects.[75]

There also may be adverse effects of radiation on the patient other than those on host-defense mechanisms. Radiation-induced *mutagenesis* is of concern for both germ line and somatic cells. If the gonads are irradiated, then there is an increased likelihood of mutation with increasing doses, without any evidence of a threshold dose or of an ameliorating effect of fractionation. At higher doses, however, there is significant cell killing, and the dose–response curve is no longer linear, presumably because the cells that mutated received sufficient radiation to become sterile. Abnormal live births are uncommon after gonadal irradiation because most radiation-induced mutations are recessive. Further, dominant mutations, when they occur, usually are lethal. There is some evidence in the mouse that the risk of mutation decreases with time after ovarian irradiation. Whether this is true in humans and the mechanism by which it occurs in animals are not known. It does not appear to be true for irradiation of the testes.

The mutagenic effects of radiation depend on the type of irradiation. The RBE for high LET radiation can be extremely high for mutations. It is very difficult to quantify the risk because experiments with mice indicate a large difference in the mutation rate for different loci, with as much as a 1000-fold variation in the mutation rate.[76] In general, the prudent figure used is that the mutation rate doubles with approximately every 50 rad.

Perhaps of even greater concern are somatic mutations, especially those that may lead to tumors. A great deal of evidence indicates that low doses of radiation increase the incidence of tumors after significant latent periods. This information comes largely from whole-body exposures to the atomic bomb and experience with patients irradiated for a variety of benign diseases.[77–79] In general, there appears to be a linear increase in tumor incidence with dose until high doses are reached, at which point the incidence reaches a plateau or even falls.[80–81] Presumably, this is true again because of cell killing. Figure 15-21 is an example of this biphasic dose–response curve. Such tumor induction is associated with a latent period of 3 to 5 years for leukemia but is much longer for solid tumors. There are different ages at which tumor induction is most likely. For example, the induction of breast cancer by radiation appears primarily with exposure in the first and second decades of life and decreases with radiation later in life.[82]

Except for irradiation of children, it is difficult to demonstrate a significantly increased incidence of tumors in patients receiving therapeutic radiation for malignant disease. This may be an example of the biphasic nature of the tumor induction curve. For example, long-term studies of patients with carcinoma of the cervix do not show increased incidence of pelvic cancer.[82,83] In contrast, when patients are irradiated to the same volume for benign diseases with much lower doses of radiation, an increased tumor incidence can be seen.[78] Thus there appears to be a difference between the tumorigenicity of radiation doses used for benign disease (200–1000 rad) and that seen when therapeutic doses of radiation are used.

Clearly radiation is a teratogen when a woman is exposed during the rapidly proliferating period of embryogenesis, between weeks 2 and 16.

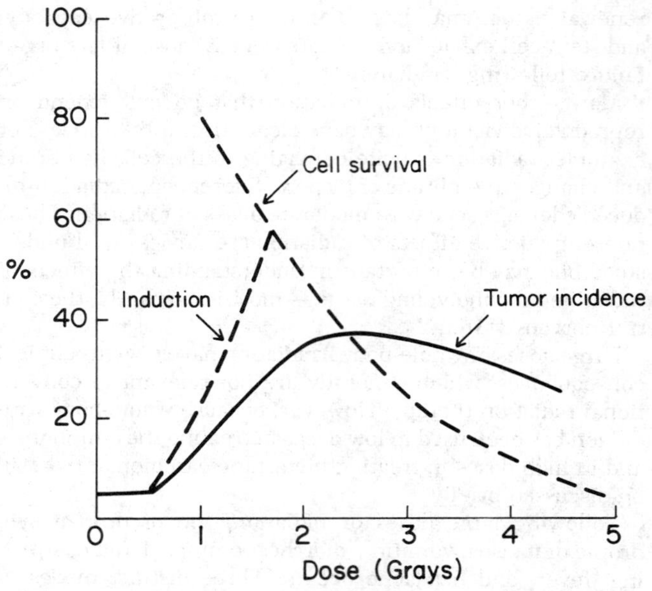

FIG. 15-21. Biphase curve of tumor incidence. (Redrawn from Gray LH: Radiation biology and cancer. In Cellular Radiation Biology, pp 7–25. M. D. Anderson Hospital and Tumor Institute 18th Symposium on Fundamental Cancer Research. Baltimore, Williams & Wilkins, 1965; and Upton AC, Randolph ML, Conklin JW: Late effects of fast neutrons and gamma rays in mice as influenced by the dose rate of irradiation: Induction of neoplasia. Radiat Res 41:467–491, 1970)

CLINICAL CONSIDERATIONS

It is often suggested that the goal of treatment is the greatest probability of uncomplicated cure. Although this is desirable, circumstances actually may dictate a different policy. Consider Figure 15-16, in which the curve for complications is to the right of the sigmoid curve for tumor control. The ideal dose would be that which gives as many cures as possible before the steep portion of the complication curve, as shown by line A. This, however, may not be the optimal dose. It depends very much on the consequences of both tumor failure and the nature of the complications. If tumor failure can be salvaged by subsequent surgery but complications are severe, long-lived, and difficult to manage, then line A is indeed the optimal line.[53] An example of this would be the treatment of T2 and T3 glottic cancer. On the other hand, if complications are either not severe or remediable, but cancer failure is fatal, then line B would be appropriate. This is the case in stage II and III carcinoma of the uterine cervix. Thus, there is no simple answer. Often the worst complication of treatment is tumor recurrence.

There are many clinical examples of sigmoid dose–response curves. An example for tumors of the head and neck is shown in Figure 15-22 and for Hodgkin's disease in Figure 15-23.[84,85] In Figure 15-22, the ordinate is arranged to convert a sigmoid curve to a straight line. These are simple because they do not consider time–dose relationships or tumor volume. An instructive clinical experience is described by Stewart and Jackson in which a consistent ~10% change in dose was used.[86] Figure 15-24 shows the results in

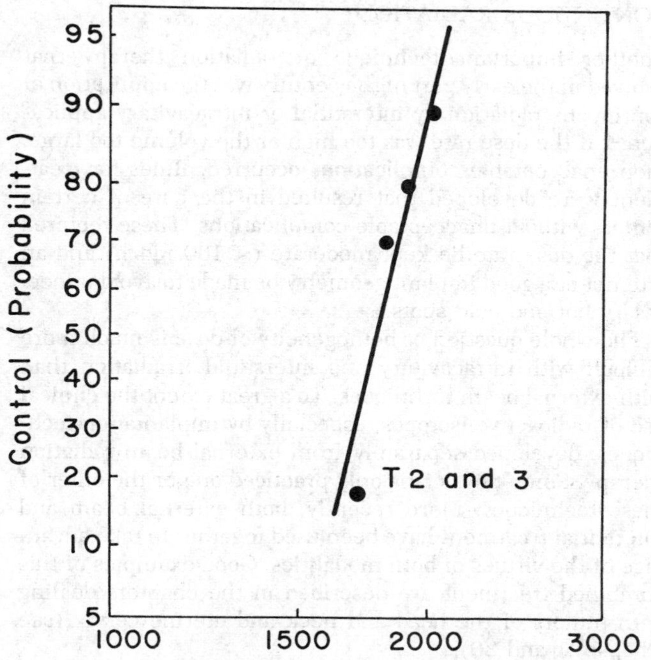

FIG. 15-22. Tumor control versus dose for supraglottic carcinoma. (Shukovsky LJ: Dose, time, volume relationships in squamous cell carcinoma of the supraglottic larynx. Am J Roentgenol Rad Ther Nucl Med 108:27–29, 1970)

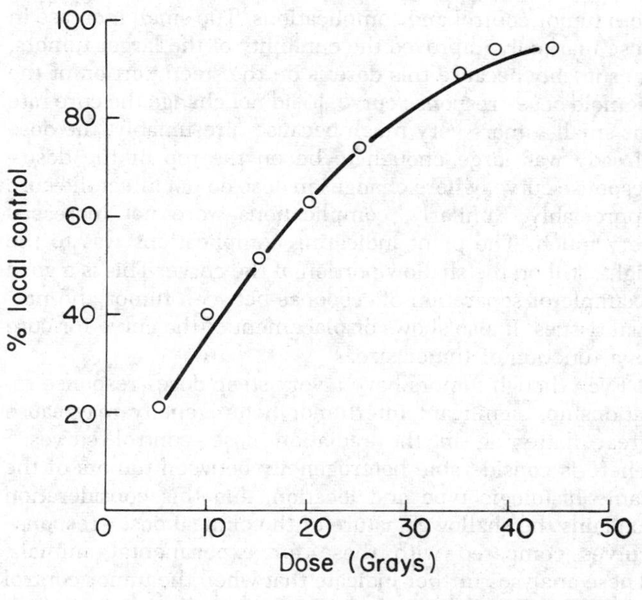

FIG. 15-23. Tumor control versus dose. (Kaplan HS: Evidence for a tumoricidal dose level in the radiotherapy of Hodgkin's disease. Cancer Res 26:1221–1224, 1966)

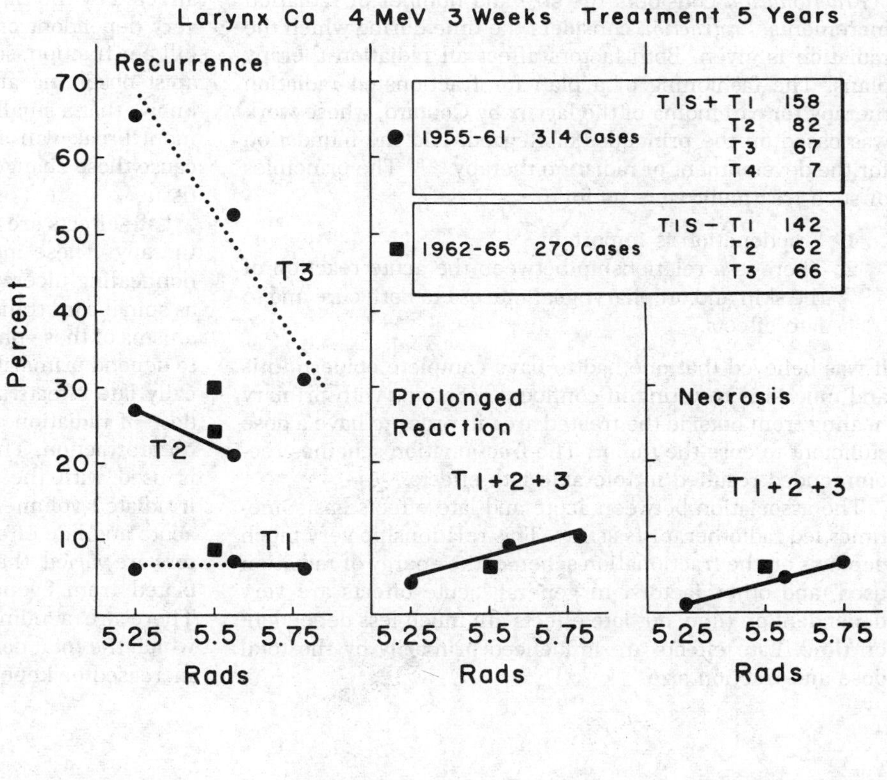

FIG. 15-24. Tumor control versus dose for cancer of the larynx. (Stewart JG, Jackson AW: The steepness of the dose response curve both for tumor and normal tissue injury. Laryngoscope 85:1107–1111, 1975)

both tumor control and complications. The small increase in dose markedly improved the curability of the larger tumors, presumably because this dose is on the steep portion of the sigmoid dose–response curve. It did not change the cure rate for small tumors very much because, presumably, the dose already was large enough to be on the top of the dose–response curve, where changes in dose do not affect the cure appreciably. Similarly, complications were not increased very much. The point indicating complications was to the right, still on the shallow portion of the curve. This is a good example of separation of response between tumor and normal tissues. It also shows displacement of the curve for cure as a function of tumor size.

Even though tumors have a very steep dose–response relationship, significant intertumor heterogeneity may cause great flattening in the radiation dose–control curves.[87] There is considerable heterogeneity between tumors of the same histologic type and location, and this consideration explains the shallower nature of the clinical dose–response curves compared with those for experimental animals. These analyses further indicate that when the tumor control probability is relatively low, the major reason is the high survival fraction associated with the initial fraction, that is, a high S_2. This emphasizes the importance of identifying prospectively tumors that have a high S_2.

FRACTIONATION

Early in this century, as the practice of radiation therapy evolved, the virtues of dividing the radiation into small fractions were noticed. The reasons given were often incorrect, but the clear observation was that fractionation of the dose allowed more effective tumor cure without excessive complications.

Fractionation considers the size and number of radiation increments. *Protraction* considers the time during which the radiation is given. Both factors affect all radiation therapy plans. The fashioning of a plan for fractionated radiation therapy for carcinoma of the larynx by Coutard, whose work was based on the principles of Regaud, laid the foundation for the development of radiation therapy.[88,89] The principles of such treatment were as follows:

1. Fractionation is important.
2. There is a relationship between the acute reaction of the skin and oropharyngeal mucosa to both cure and to late effects.

It was believed that one had to have complete epidermitis and mucositis resulting in confluent reactions with primary healing from outside the treated area in order to have a dose sufficient to cure the tumor. The fractionation schemes recommended resulted in tolerable late effects.

The association between acute and late effects has sometimes led radiotherapists astray. This relationship very much depends on the fractionation scheme, the energy of radiation used, and other factors. In general, acute effects are very dependent on time, but late effects are much less dependent on time. Late effects are influenced primarily by the total dose and fraction size.

CONTINUOUS RADIATION

Another important technique of radiation therapy that evolved in the early part of the century was the application of continuous radiation by interstitial or intracavitary application.[90] If the dose rate was too high or the volume too large, then unacceptable complications occurred. Rules for treatment were developed that resulted in the cure of certain tumors without unacceptable complications. These required that the dose rate be kept moderate (< 100 rad/h) and an attempt at a good implant geometry be made to avoid unnecessary hot and cold spots.

The whole question of homogeneity of dose is much more difficult with intracavitary and interstitial irradiation than with external beam techniques. To a great extent the clinical use of radioactive isotopes, especially by implantation techniques, developed separately from external beam radiation therapy. Some physicians only practiced one or the other of these techniques. More recently, both external beam and interstitial treatment have been used together to take advantage of the virtues of both modalities. Good examples of this combined treatment are described in the chapters dealing with tumors of the head and neck and uterine cervix (see Chaps. 21 and 36).

ACUTE AND LATE NORMAL TISSUE EFFECTS

Acute radiation effects occur largely in renewing tissues, such as skin, oropharyngeal mucosa, small intestine, rectum, bladder mucosa, and vaginal mucosa. These cell-renewing tissues are rapidly proliferating, and as they are confronted with fractionated radiation, the processes of repair, repopulation, and recruitment all obtain. Because the response of rapidly renewing tissues depends on the balance between cell birth and cell death, acute tissue reaction is crucially affected by the time allowed for repopulation, and therefore very dependent on protraction. It also depends on the cell kill per fraction, so fraction size is important. The radiotherapist observing an excessive reaction by the oral mucosa knows that a small decrease in fraction size or a small treatment break will allow rapid resolution of the problem because these changes will permit reconstitution of the normal tissue.

Late effects are really the dose-limiting factor in radiation therapy. These include necrosis, fibrosis, fistula formation, nonhealing ulceration, and damage to specific organs, such as spinal cord transection and blindness. Although the mechanisms of these phenomena are not clear, they do not appear to depend primarily on the rapid proliferation of cells. Clinically late effects appear to depend much more on the total dose of radiation and the size of the radiation fraction than on protraction. Thus, only if the same fractionation scheme is used with the same normal tissue endpoint, the same irradiated volume, and the same treatment technique, can acute and late effects be correlated. If any of these parameters are varied, the acute reactions to radiation may be dissociated from eventual late effects and will be misleading. There are a number of examples in radiation therapy in which the total dose was increased and the fraction size was increased or kept the same, but the time was protracted to minimize acute effects. Such techniques have resulted in unacceptable late complications.

Two hypotheses for late effects are worth discussion. One theory holds that all late effects result from damage to vasculoconnective stroma. Because this is common throughout the body, it would suggest a common mechanism for the late effects in any organ.[65] A variation on this hypothesis is that it is damage to the endothelial cells, ubiquitous throughout the body, that determines late effects.[66] An alternative hypothesis suggests that both the acute and the late effects of radiation and cytotoxic chemotherapy are caused by cell depletion of the targeted cell-renewal tissues. Acute effects depend on the balance between cell killing and compensatory replication of both the stem and proliferative cells. The development of late effects requires that stem cells have only a limited proliferative capacity.[91,92] Compensation for extensive or repeated cell killing may exhaust this capacity, resulting in eventual tissue failure.[64,93]

ALTERING THE THERAPEUTIC INDEX

Goodman and Gilman define the therapeutic index as the relationship between desired and undesired effects of therapy.[94] Clearly for the oncologist, separation of the sigmoid curve of complications from that of local control (Fig. 15-16) is the graphic representation of manipulation of the therapeutic index. Some techniques of time–dose relationships used by the radiotherapist to take advantage of this are fractionation, protraction, split-course technique, interstitial treatment, and manipulation of the target volume. Although fractionation has been discussed, the use of multiple small fractions two, three, or more times a day, *hyperfractionation*, is just beginning to be explored, with some good results.[95–97]

Another technique to reduce complications is the use of normal-sized fractions given more than once a day. This is referred to as multifraction, multiple daily fractions, or *accelerated fractionation*.[98] In the experiments that stimulated the recent interest, the investigators administered two daily fractions of radiation separated by 6 hours, and compared this to daily radiation given as a single fraction.[99] Six hours is believed to be long enough to allow complete sublethal damage repair but not long enough for significant proliferation. Because both methods are daily treatments, repair can be separated from repopulation and recruitment. The general results of the experiments were presented as the recovered radiation, the difference between the dose obtained when the radiation is given in two divided doses separated by 6 hours and that when it is given in one fraction. When the single fraction was 200 rad or less, there was little recovered dose. The recovered dose increased rapidly between 200 and 800 rad; then, with very large fractions, the recovered dose tended to level off. Thus, in clinical situations, when typical radiation doses of about 200 rad are divided into two smaller fractions, only a little more should be given because the recovered dose is small. This has been confirmed in a number of clinics.[100] The use of such hyperfractionation is being tried for several tumors; however, it is too soon to determine whether it will be useful.

When tumor cells are proliferating rapidly, accelerated fractionation makes sense. Waiting 24 hours between each fraction may allow significant proliferation. Perhaps the best example of the changing therapeutic index obtained with accelerated fractionation is the enhanced success in treating Burkitt's lymphoma.[101]

In general, most radiotherapists administer conventional radiation in fractions between 180 and 250 rad each day. This allows tumor control without excessive acute or late effects. The fraction size that is tolerated in terms of acute effects depends on the volume irradiated (the larger the volume, the smaller the fraction size), the amount and type of dose-limiting normal tissue, the age of the patient, and other clinical factors.

Small changes in fraction size will make a big difference in tolerance. Patients often are given small breaks during the treatment. These rest periods usually are caused by weekend interruptions of daily fractionation. This protraction of the treatment allows for repopulation and recruitment. The days of rest also allow amelioration of many acute effects, and they may allow time for tumor regression, resulting in reoxygenation.

An attempt to formalize and extend treatment breaks is the so-called *split course technique*.[102–104] Two to 3 weeks are allowed in the middle of treatment for recovery from the acute effects, as well as to permit tumor regression. When the dose of radiation is not increased, there is some evidence that this treatment (although clearly better tolerated) may be associated with less tumor control.[105] When the split course is administered with an increase in total dose, the results seem to be comparable to conventional fractionation but perhaps with greater late effects.

Interstitial irradiation is administered in radium needle implants, gold and radon seed implants, iridium wire implants, and a variety of other techniques for either permanently or temporarily placing radioactive material into tissues. It requires both biologic and physical considerations. Clearly there is great inhomogeneity in even the most geometrically perfect implant. There is large inhomogeneity of dose and a similar variation in dose rate; the dose rate of radiation is greater in areas of high dose. With temporary implants, the radiologist attempts to administer a calculated dose of between 30 and 100 rad per hour to the minimum tumor location. This is impossible with permanent implants because isotopes decrease their radiation intensity as they decay. The most commonly used isotopes have been radon and ^{198}Au. More recently, ^{125}I has been used and has created unusual new considerations. The half-life of ^{125}I is quite long (60 days), resulting in a significant amount of the dose being given so slowly that there may be significant cell division occurring in both the tumor and some normal cells. Therefore the important dose may not be the total dose, but rather the dose per cell cycle, which is different for each cell type and different as the isotope decays. Also, ^{125}I irradiates primarily by the emission of very low energy photons, some of which are absorbed by the seeds themselves, leading to even further inhomogeneity.[106]

When implants can be used alone or in combination with external irradiation, the results tend to be better in terms of the therapeutic index than with external beam techniques alone. The high local dose, continuous radiation, and even inhomogeneity allowing normal tissue regrowth all contribute to better cosmetic and functional results and cure of the tumor. Examples are breast cancer and tumors of the tongue and other head and neck sites.[107]

Tumor volume also is quite important in clinical radiotherapy. Although the gross tumor extent can be determined, most clinicians recognize that a characteristic of tumors is to extend far beyond those macroscopically identifiable borders. Determination of the target volume must include this consideration, but if a larger volume must be irradiated, then a smaller dose is tolerated. Conversely, if the volume of the tumor is larger, then a larger dose is required. This dilemma limited the success of early radiotherapy of certain tumors by reducing the target volume, resulting in recurrences at the treatment margins, or by causing significant complications in the treatment of large target volumes. Today, distinctions are made between gross tumor and the subclinical extensions into apparently normal tissues. Subclinical disease means small numbers of cells, perhaps favorable to irradiation (well-oxygenated), which can be controlled with modest doses of radiation (Table 15-7). The large number of cells present in the clinically evidenced tumor requires higher doses, as noted in the curves shown in Figures 15-22 and 15-23. This difference has led to the development of a variety of techniques for administering different doses to microscopic tumor extensions and to the gross tumor. These include shrinking field techniques, boost treatments, and certain strategies of combined surgery and radiotherapy to be described later in this chapter.

Shrinking field technique means giving the largest potential tumor bed a moderate dose of radiation, then reducing the target volume to the tumor and its immediate confines, raising the dose. This can be done by reducing the fields, by changing the treatment technique and target volume, or by using a treatment technique that gives both the desired moderate dose to the larger volume and a higher dose to the smaller volume. A modification of this is the *boost technique*, in which the maximum tolerated dose is given to a volume and then very localized radiation is used to raise the dose to the tumor bed. An implant or an electron boost can be used for this. A number of attempts have been made to consider fractionation, protraction, and even implantation used with external beam in some form of some mathematical formulae, all of which tend to simplify complex clinical circumstances and can be very misleading.

The normal tissues that limit the dose of radiation given may be so close to the tumor that any target volume that includes a tumor must include these normal tissues. Dose-limiting normal tissues are distinguished from these normal tissue transited by the radiation but not in the target volume, although both may contribute to the production of complications and thus be dose-limiting. Radiotherapy with detailed treatment planning, CT scanning, and a variety of techniques, the ultimate of which is computer-controlled radiation therapy, may reduce the dose to the transit volume, possibly changing the therapeutic index.[109] However, it is unlikely that there will be significant physical techniques for reducing the dose to normal tissues in the target volume. This can be done only by some biologic mechanism that distinguishes tumor from normal tissues.

TABLE 15-7. Control (%) of Subclinical Disease

Dose (Gy)	*Adenocarcinoma of the Breast*	*Carcinoma of Upper Aerodigestive Tract*
30–35	60–70%	60–70%
40	80–90%	>90%
50	>90%	>90%

Fletcher GH: Clinical dose–response curves of human malignant epithelial tumours. Br J Radiol 46:1–12, 1973.

RADIOSENSITIVITY

The term radiosensitivity is used in a number of different ways in the literature and can mean what we define as radiosensitivity, radioresponsiveness, or radiocurability. Each is a somewhat different concept. *Radiosensitivity* means the innate sensitivity of the cells to radiation. For cells that die a reproductive death, this is related to the slope of the survival curve or the D_0.

Radioresponsiveness means the clinical appearance of tumor regression promptly following moderate doses of radiation. This may be a function of the cell's radiosensitivity, but it also may be a function of the active cell kinetics of a tumor. Bergonie and Tribondeau first established an association between the rate of proliferation and the response of normal tissues, although they considered this to be radiosensitivity.[110] A similar relationship was presumed to apply to tumors. Because cells will not die until they face mitosis, some tumors that proliferate rapidly will regress rapidly, but they also may regrow rapidly. This is often confused with radiosensitivity. An excellent example of this is the adenoid-cystic tumor of the salivary gland or cylindroma. Such tumors are quite radioresponsive; however, they require very large doses to be cured.

Radiocurability means that the tumor–normal tissue relationships are such that curative doses of radiation can be applied regularly without excessive damage to normal tissues. Examples of such radiocurable tumors are carcinomas of the cervix, larynx, breast, and prostate, in addition to Hodgkin's disease and seminomas. Some of these are radioresponsive, some are radiosensitive, and some are neither.

RADIATION AND SURGERY

Radiation and surgery can be combined in many different ways. The general rationale for combining surgery and radiation is that the mechanism of failure for the two techniques is quite different. Radiation rarely fails at the periphery of tumors, where cells are small in number and well vascularized. When radiation fails, it usually does so in the center of the tumor where there are large volumes of tumor cells often under hypoxic conditions. Surgery, in contrast, is limited by the required preservation of vital normal tissues adjacent to the tumor. In resectable cancers the gross tumor can be removed, but it is these vital normal tissues that limit the anatomic extent of the dissection. When surgery fails under these circumstances, it is usually due to microscopic tumor cells left behind. It seems logical, therefore, to consider combining the two techniques.

Radiation can be given before or after surgery. Preoperative radiation has the advantages of sterilizing cells at the edges of the resection, sterilizing cells that perhaps would be dislodged and seeded at the time of surgery, and in the special circumstance of unresectable tumors, reducing the tumor volume sufficiently to allow resection. It is not clear how often this really results in a cure, because it may only change gross tumor to microscopic tumor and still result in tumor recurrence. It does seem to benefit selected cases of large unresectable cancers.[111]

There are disadvantages in the use of preoperative irradiation. The pathology reports are not evaluable because, if sufficient time is allowed between the radiation and the surgery, the destruction of tumor caused by preoperative radiation prevents ascertainment of the tumor's initial anatomic extent. In contrast, if the tumor is slow-growing or if the surgery is done shortly after the radiation, the consequences of the radiation will not be represented in the pathologic evaluation of the material because sufficient time was not allowed for tumor destruction and regression.

Another disadvantage is that the patient is irradiated before the careful staging available at surgical exploration, and thus some patients who would not benefit from preoperative radiation are given this treatment (*e.g.*, preoperative radiation to a colorectal carcinoma in a patient with occult liver metastases). Metastases may be found only at the time of surgery.

A disadvantage often mentioned is the delay before surgical resection. This may not be a disadvantage, because as long as the patient's tumor is being treated, the order of treatments should make no difference. The radiation dose usually is moderate (4000–5000 rad) and given in conventional 200-rad fractions 5 days a week or in smaller total doses given more quickly in larger fractions. If the total dose of radiation is kept small (≤ 2000 rad), then the delay between radiation and surgery is small. When the dose reaches approximately 4000 rad, it is valuable to delay the surgery (usually 4–6 weeks) to allow the tissues to recover from the radiation. If the total dose is greater than 5000 rad, then the surgery often will be more difficult. However, with moderate doses of radiation and some time allowed between radiation and surgery, the resection can proceed without difficulty.

The use of smaller doses of radiation over short periods of time, without surgical delay, has many advantages and is becoming the preferred technique. With this technique the pathology is less distorted, tumor reduction does not occur significantly, and the surgeon is not lulled into doing too small an operation. If the major value of the preoperative radiation is to prevent seeding, then large doses of radiation are not necessary. For example, preoperative use of intrauterine radium before surgical treatment of carcinoma of the endometrium is an effective way of preventing seeding. This can be done immediately before surgery.

Postoperative radiation has a number of advantages as well. The subgroup of patients who may be helped by radiation can be defined very accurately as a consequence of the surgical exploration and pathologic review. Unnecessary irradiation to patients who are not likely to benefit can be avoided, and the target volumes are tailored to meet what is found at surgery. Time can be allowed for wound healing so that the radiation will not interfere with this process. A disadvantage of such treatment is that it has no effect on seeding at the time of surgery. Surgery also may alter the physiology of the tumor left behind because of reduction of the vascular supply. Cells that were well-oxygenated may be rendered physiologically hypoxic and thus more resistant to radiation. Another disadvantage in the peritoneal cavity is that the surgery will cause loops of bowel to be fixed in specific positions and thus will increase the likelihood of small intestinal damage by radiation.

There is some uncertainty as to which technique is better for particular clinical circumstances. Both preoperative and postoperative radiation appear to be valuable and the choice of the method, the dose of radiation, and time between radiation and surgery should be considered in terms of the goals planned.

An additional technique for combining surgery with radiation is limited surgical removal of the gross tumor. Because the gross tumor limits the radiotherapeutic treatment, new interest has been raised in using surgery as the boost technique. Full courses of radiation combined with tumorectomy are given. This surgery can be done either before or after the irradiation. An example of this is the "lumpectomy" used in the treatment of breast masses before definitive radiation (see Chap. 38).[112,113] In the latter there appears to be evidence that the removal of gross tumor both displaces the sigmoid curve of cure to lower radiation doses and makes it change more steeply with dose (Fig. 15-25).

FIG. 15-25. Tumor control versus dose for breast cancer Stages II and III. (Hellman S: Improving the therapeutic index in breast cancer treatment. Cancer Res 40:4335–4342, 1980)

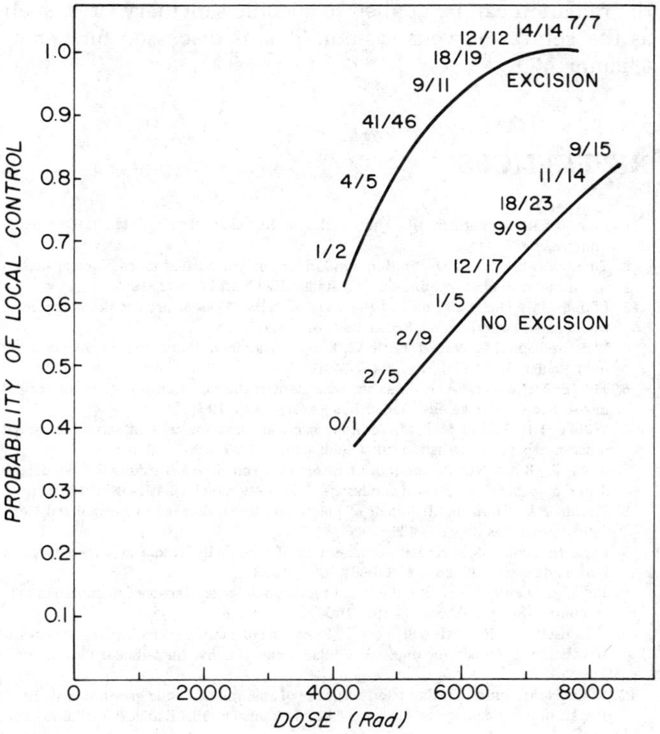

RADIATION AND CHEMOTHERAPY

The principles of combination radiation and chemotherapy were discussed earlier and emphasized that the purpose of such combined treatment is not to decrease the dose of radiation to gain the same effect, but rather to increase the therapeutic index. This may be achieved using a number of techniques that take advantage of the different mechanisms of action of systemic chemotherapy and regional irradiation. Chemotherapeutic agents that directly modify the radiation survival curve may be used. A good example of this is the use of actinomycin D in the treatment of childhood rhabdomyosarcoma or Wilms' tumor. A second way to increase the therapeutic index is to use drugs that specifically affect tumor response to radiation; the most exciting of these are the hypoxic sensitizers because they affect hypoxic cells that usually are restricted to tumors.

A third mechanism is the combination of drugs and roentgen rays with either independent action or additivity. This is just beginning to be explored but appears to be of value in increased local control achieved in head and neck cancer when chemotherapy is given before radiation.[114] Also, enhanced local control is obtained when radiotherapy is followed by or administered concomitantly with adjuvant chemotherapy in locally advanced breast cancer.[115]

Because the major advantage of chemotherapy is that it is distributed widely throughout the body, the combination of radiation and chemotherapy may improve the therapeutic index because, like the combination of surgery and irradiation, the target volumes are different. Adjuvant chemotherapy with radiation for breast cancer, or with surgery and radiation for colon cancer, may improve survival because the chemotherapy is effective against occult micrometastases outside the radiation field. Similarly, radiation may be of value in the treatment of leukemia by chemotherapy because the radiation can be applied to specific sanctuary sites, such as the central nervous system. This is discussed further in Chapter 47.

REFERENCES

1. Johns HE, Cunningham JR: The Physics of Radiology. Springfield, IL, Charles C Thomas, 1977
2. Thompson LH, Suit HD: Proliferation kinetics of x-irradiated mouse L cells studied with timelapse photography: II. Int J Radiat Biol 15:347–362, 1969
3. Elkind MM: The initial part of the survival curve: Does it predict the outcome of fractionated radiotherapy? Radiat Res (in press)
4. Weichselbaum RR, Nove J, Little JB: X-ray sensitivity of human tumor cells *in vitro*. Int J Radiat Oncol Biol Phys 6:437–440, 1980
5. Till JE, McCulloch EA: A direct measurement of the radiation sensitivity of normal mouse bone marrow cells. Radiat Res 14:213–222, 1961
6. Withers HR, Elkind MM: Microcolony survival assay for cells of mouse intestinal mucosa exposed to radiation. Int J Radiat Biol 17:261–267, 1970
7. Alper T, Gillies NE: Restoration of *Escherichia coli* Strain B irradiation: Its dependence on suboptimal growth conditions. J Gen Microbiol 18:461–472, 1958
8. Phillips RA, Tolmach LJ: Repair of potentially lethal damage in x-irradiated HeLa cells. Radiat Res 29:413–432, 1966
9. Little JB, Hahn GM, Frindel E et al: Repair of potentially lethal radiation damage *in vitro* and *in vivo*. Radiology 106:689–694, 1973
10. Belli JA, Shelton M: Potentially lethal radiation damage: Repair of mammalian cells in culture. Science 165:490–492, 1969
11. Weichselbaum R, Little JB, Nove J: Response of human osteosarcoma in vitro to irradiation: Evidence for unusual cellular repair activity. Int J Radiat Biol 31:295–299, 1977
12. Elkind MM, Sutton H: Radiation response of mammalian cells grown in culture: 1. Repair of x-ray damage in surviving Chinese hamster cells. Radiat Res 13:556–593, 1960
13. Hall EJ: Radiation dose-rate: A factor of importance in radiobiology and radiotherapy. Br J Radiol 45:81–97, 1972
14. Mottram JC: Factors of importance in radiosensitivity of tumors. Br J Radiol 9:606–614, 1936
15. Read J: The effect of ionizing radiation on the broad beam root: The dependence of the x-ray sensitivity on dissolved oxygen. Br J Radiol 25:89–99, 1952
16. Gray LH, Coger AD, Ebert M et al: The concentration of oxygen dissolved in tissues at the time of irradiation as a factor in radiotherapy. Br J Radiol 26:638–648, 1953
17. Belli JA, Dicus GJ, Bonte FJ: Radiation response of mammalian tumor cells: 1. Repair of sublethal damage *in vivo*. JNCI 38:673–682, 1967
18. Deschner EE, Gray LH: Influence of oxygen tension on x-ray induced chromosomal damage in Ehrlich ascites tumor cells irradiated *in vitro* and *in vivo*. Radiat Res 11:115–146, 1959
19. Thomlinson RH, Gray LH: The histological structure of some human lung cancers and possible implications for radiotherapy. Br J Cancer 9:539–549, 1955
20. Kallman RF: The phenomenon of reoxygenation and its implications for fractionated radiotherapy. Radiology 105:135–142, 1972
21. Henk JM, Kindler PB, Smith CW: Radiotherapy and head and neck cancer: Final report of the first clinical trial. Lancet 2:101–103, 1977
22. Henk JM, Smith CW: Radiotherapy and head and neck cancer: Interim report of second clinical trial. Lancet 2:104–105, 1977
23. Watson ER, Halman KE, Dische S et al: Hyperbaric oxygen and radiotherapy: A Medical Research Council trial in carcinoma of the cervix. Br J Radiol 51:879–887, 1978
24. Adams GE, Dewez DL: Hydrated electrons and radiobiological sensitization. Biochem Biophys Res Commun 12:473–477, 1963
25. Adams GE, Ahmed L, Fielden EM et al: The development of some nitromidazoles as hypoxic cell sensitizers. Cancer Clin Trials 3:37–42, 1980
26. Stratford LJ, Adams GE: Effect of hyperthermia on differential cytotoxicity of a hypoxic cell radiosensitizer RO-07-0582 on mammalian cells *in vitro*. Br J Cancer 35:307–313, 1977
27. Rose CM, Millar JL, Peacock JH et al: Differential enhancement of toxicity in tumors and normal tissues by misonidizole. Proceedings of the Key Biscayne Conference on Hypoxic Cell Sensitizers and Radioprotectors. New York, Masson, 1980
28. Bush RS, Jenkin RP, Allt WE et al: Definitive evidence for hypoxic cells influencing cure in cancer therapy. Br J Cancer 37:302–306, 1978
29. Kolstad P: Intercapillary distance, oxygen tension, and local recurrence in cervix cancer. Scan J Clin Lab Invest [Suppl] 106:145–157, 1968
30. Urtasun RC, Koch CJ, Franko AJ, et al: A novel technique for measuring human tissue pO_2 at the cellular level. Br J Cancer 54:453–457, 1986
31. Urtasun RC, Chapman JD, Raleigh JA et al: Binding of ^3H-misonidazole to solid human tumors as a measure of tumor hypoxia. Int J Rad Oncol Biol Phys 12:1263–1267, 1986
32. Terasima R, Tolmach LJ: X-ray sensitivity and DNA synthesis in synchronous populations of HeLa cells. Science 140:490–492, 1963
33. Sinclair WK, Morton RA: X-ray sensitivity during the cell generation cycle of cultured Chinese hamster cells. Radiat Res 29:450–474, 1966
34. Chaffey JT, Hellman S: Differing responses to radiation of murine bone marrow stem cells in relation to the cell cycle. Cancer Res 31:1613–1615, 1971
35. Madoc-Jones H, Mauro F: Age response to x-rays vinca alkaloids and hydroxyurea of murine lymphoma cells synchronized in vivo. JNCI 45:1131–1143, 1970
36. Hellman S: Cell kinetics, models, and cancer treatment: Some principles for the radiation oncologist. Radiology 114:219–223, 1975
37. Chaffey JT, Hellman S: Radiation fractionation as applied to murine colony-forming units in differing proliferative states. Radiology 93:1167–1172, 1969
38. Chaffey JT, Hellman S: Studies on dose fractionation as measured by endogenous spleen colonies in the mouse. Radiology 90:363–365, 1968
39. Hermens AF, Barendson GW: Changes in cell proliferation characteristics in a rat rhabdomyosarcoma before and after x-irradiation. Eur J Cancer Clin Oncol 5:173–189, 1969
40. Szybalski W: X-ray sensitization by halopyrimidines. Cancer Chemother Rep 58:539–557, 1974
41. Piro AJ, Taylor CC, Belli JA: Interaction between radiation and drug damage in mammalian cells: 1. Delayed expression of actinomycin D/x-ray effects in exponential and plateau phase cells. Radiat Res 63:346–362, 1975
42. D'Angio GJ, Farber S, Maddock CL: Potentiation of x-ray effects by actinomycin D. Radiology 73:175–177, 1959
43. Bases RE: Modification of the radiation response determined by single-cell techniques: Actinomycin D. Cancer Res 19:1223–1229, 1959
44. Elkind MM, Whitmore GF, Alescio T: Actinomycin D: Suppression of recovery in x-irradiated mammalian cells. Science 143:1454–1456, 1964
45. Pinkel D: Actinomycin D in childhood cancer: A preliminary report. Pediatrics 23:342–347, 1959
46. Hellman S, Hannon E: Effects of adriamycin on the radiation response of murine hematopoietic stem cells. Radiat Res 67:162–167, 1976
47. Belli JA, Piro AJ: The interaction between radiation and adriamycin damage in mammalian cells. Cancer Res 37:1624–1630, 1977
48. Cassady JR, Richter MP, Piro AJ et al: Radiation–adriamycin interactions: Preliminary clinical observations. Cancer 36:946–949, 1975
49. Donaldson SC, Glick JM, Wilbur JR: Adriamycin activating a recall phenomenon after radiation therapy. Ann Intern Med 81:407–408, 1974
50. Sinclair WK: Hydroxyurea: Effects on Chinese hamster cells grown in culture. Cancer Res 27:297–308, 1967

51. Yuhas JM, Yurconic M, Kligerman MM et al: Combined use of radioprotective and radiosensitizing drugs in experimental radiotherapy. Radiat Res 70:433–443, 1977
52. Barendsen GW: Response of cultured cells, tumours, and normal tissues to radiations of different linear energy transfer. Curr Top Radiat Res 4:293–356, 1968
53. Bloomer WD, Hellman S: Normal tissue responses to radiation therapy. N Engl J Med 293:80–83, 1975
54. Holthusen H: Erfahrungen über die Vertaglichkeitsgrenze fur Röntgenstrahler und deren Nutzanwendung zur Verhutung von Schaden. Strahlentherapie 57:254–269, 1936
55. Suit HD, Goitein M: Rationale for use of charged-particle and fast-neutron beams in radiation therapy. In Meyn RE, Withers HR (eds): Radiation Biology in Cancer Research. New York, Raven Press, 1980
56. Thomlinson RH: An experimental method for comparing treatments of intact tumors in animals and its application to the use of oxygen in radiotherapy. Br J Cancer 14:555–576, 1960
57. Folkman J, Tyler K: Tumor angiogenesis: Its possible role in metastasis and invasion. In Day B, Myers WP, Stans Garattini S et al (eds): Cancer Invasion and Metastasis: Mechanisms and Therapy, vol 5, pp 95–103. New York, Raven Press, 1977
58. Folkman J: Tumor angiogenesis: A possible control point in tumor growth. Ann Intern Med 82:96–100, 1975
59. Folkman J, Langer R, Linhardt RJ et al: Angiogenesis inhibition and tumor regression caused by heparin or a heparin fragment in the presence of cortisone. Science 221:719–725, 1983
60. Powers WE, Tolmach LV: A multicomponent x-ray survival curve for mouse lymphosarcoma cells irradiation *in vitro*. Nature 197:710–711, 1963
61. Fertil B, Malaise EP: Inherent cellular radiosensitivity as a basic concept for human tumor radiotherapy. Int J Radiat Oncol Biol Phys 7:621–629, 1981
62. Deacon J, Peckham MJ, Steel GG: The radioresponsiveness of human tumours and the initial slope of the cell survival curve. Radiother Oncol 2:317–323, 1984
63. Malaise EP, Fertil B, Chavaudra N et al: Distribution of radiation sensitivities for human tumor cells of specific histological types: Comparison of *in vitro* to *in vivo* data. Int J Radiat Oncol Biol Phys 12:617–624, 1986
64. Weichselbaum RR, Dahlberg W, Little JB: Inherently radioresistant cells exist in some human tumors. Proc Natl Acad Sci USA 82:4732–4735, 1985
65. Rubin P, Casarett GW: Clinical Radiation Pathology. Philadelphia, WB Saunders, 1968
66. Reinhold HS, Buisman GH: Radiosensitivity of capillary endothelium. Br J Radiol 46:54–57, 1973
67. Filler RM, Tefft M, Vawter GF et al: Hepatic lobectomy in childhood: Effects of x-ray and chemotherapy. J Pediatr Surg 4:31–41, 1969
68. Reincke U, Hannon EC, Rosenblatt M, Hellman S: Proliferative capacity of murine hematopoietic stem cells in vitro. Science 215:1619–1622, 1982
69. Medinger FG, Craver LF: Total-body irradiation. Am J Roentgenol Radium Ther Nucl Med 48:651–671, 1942
70. Hellman S, Chaffey JT, Rosenthal DS et al: Place of radiation therapy in the treatment of non-Hodgkin's lymphomas. Cancer 39:843–851, 1977
71. Anderson RE, Warner NL: Ionizing radiation and the immune response. Adv Immunol 24:215–335, 1976
72. Stjernsward J: Decreased survival related to irradiation postoperatively in early operable breast cancer. Lancet 2:1285–1286, 1974
73. Levitt SH, McHugh RB: Early breast cancer and postoperative irradiation. Lancet 2:1258–1259, 1975
74. Cancer Research Campaign (Kings/Cambridge) Trial for Early Breast Cancer. Lancet 2:55–60, 1980
75. Fletcher GH: Clinical dose–response curves of human malignant epithelial tumours. Br J Radiol 46:1–12, 1973
76. Kohn HI, Melvold RW: Divergent x-ray-induced mutation rates in the mouse for Hand "7 locus" groups of loci. Nature 259:209–210, 1976
77. Folley JH, Borges W, Yamawaki T: Incidence of leukemia in survivors of the atomic bomb in Hiroshima and Nagasaki, Japan. Am J Med 13:311–321, 1952
78. Smith PG, Doll R: Late effects of x-irradiation in patients healed for metropathia hemorrhagica. Br J Radiol 49:224–232, 1976
79. Court Brown WM, Doll R: Mortality from cancer and other causes after radiotherapy for ankylosing spondylitis. Br Med J 2:1327–1332, 1965
80. Gray LH: Radiation biology and cancer. In Cellular Radiation Biology, M.D. Anderson Hospital and Tumor Institute 18th Symposium on Fundamental Cancer Research, pp 7–25. Baltimore, Williams & Wilkins, 1965
81. Upton AC, Randolph ML, Conklin JW: Late effects of fast neutrons and gamma rays in mice as influenced by the dose rate of irradiation: Induction of neoplasia. Radiat Res 41:467–491, 1970
82. Boice JD, Hutchinson GB: Leukemia in women following radiotherapy for cervical cancer: Ten-year follow-up of an international study. JNCI 65:115–129, 1980
83. Zippen C, Bailar JC III, Kohn HI et al: Radiation therapy and cervical cancer: Late effects on life span and leukemia incidence. Cancer 28:937–942, 1971
84. Shukovsky LJ: Dose, time, volume relationships in squamous cell carcinoma of the supraglottic larynx. Am J Roentgenol Rad Ther Nucl Med 108:27–29, 1970
85. Kaplan HS: Evidence for a tumoricidal dose level in the radiotherapy of Hodgkin's disease. Cancer Res 26:1221–1224, 1966
86. Stewart JG, Jackson AW: The steepness of the dose–response curve both for tumor and normal tissue injury. Laryngoscope 85:1107–1111, 1975
87. Zagars GK, Schultheiss TE, Peters LJ: Inter-tumor heterogeneity and radiation dose-control curves. Radiother Oncol 8:353–362, 1987
88. Coutard H: Roentgen therapy of epitheliomas of the tonsillar region, hypopharynx, and larynx from 1920 to 1926. Am J Roentgenol 28:313–331, 1932
89. Regaud C, Ferroux R: Discordance des effets des rayons X, d'une part dans la peau, d'autre part dans le testicule par le fractionement de la dose: Diminution de l'efficacite dans le peau, maintien de l'efficacite dans le testicule. Compt Rend Soc Biol 97:431–434, 1927
90. Danlos H: Quelques considerations sur le traitement des dermatoses par le radium. J Physiotherapie (Paris) 3:98–106, 1905
91. Botnick L, Hannon EC, Hellman S: Multisystem stem cell failure after apparent recovery from alkylating agents. Cancer Res 38:1942–1947, 1978
92. Hellman S, Botnick LE: Stem cell depletion: An explanation of the late effects of cytotoxins. Int J Radiat Oncol Biol Phys 2:181–184, 1977
93. Harris JR, Recht A, Almaric R, et al: Time course and prognosis of local recurrence following primary radiation therapy for early breast cancer. J Clin Oncol 2:37–41, 1984
94. Goodman LS, Gilman A: The Pharmacological Basis of Therapeutics, p 21. London, Macmillan, 1970
95. Withers HR, Peters LJ, Thames HD et al: Hyperfractionation. Int J Radiat Oncol Biol Phys 8:1807–1809, 1982
96. Withers HR, Thames HA, Peters LJ: Dose fractionation and volume effects in normal tissues and tumors. Cancer Treat Symp 1:75–83, 1984
97. Shank B, Chu FCH, Dinsmore R et al: Hyperfractionated total body irradiation for bone marrow transplantation. Results in seventy leukemia patients with allogeneic transplants. Int J Radiat Oncol Biol Phys 9:1607–1611, 1983
98. Thames HD Jr, Peters LJ, Withers HR et al: Accelerated fractionation vs hyperfractionation: Rationales for several treatments per day. Int J Radiat Oncol Biol Phys 9:127–138, 1983
99. Dutreix J, Wambersie A, Bounik C: Cellular recovery in human skin reactions: Application to dose, fraction number, overall time relationship in radiotherapy. Eur J Cancer Clin Oncol 9:159–167, 1973
100. Marks RD, Witherspoon BJ, Davis LW et al: Hyperfractionation—where do we stand: A preliminary report. Int J Radiat Oncol Biol Phys 4(suppl):139–140, 1978
101. Norin T, Onyango J: Radiotherapy in Burkitt's lymphoma: Conventional or superfractionated regime—early results. Int J Radiat Oncol Biol Phys 2:399–406, 1977
102. Scanlon P: Split-dose radiotherapy: The original premise. Int J Radiat Oncol Biol Phys 6:527–528, 1980
103. Sambrook DK: Split-course radiation therapy in malignant tumors. Am J Roentgenol 91:37–45, 1964
104. Parsons JT, Thar TL, Bova FJ et al: An evaluation of split-course irradiation for pelvic malignancies. Int J Radiat Oncol Biol Phys 6:175–181, 1980
105. Parsons JT, Bova FJ, Million RR: A re-evaluation of the University of Florida split-course technique for squamous carcinoma of the head and neck. Int J Radiat Oncol Biol Phys 6:1645–1652, 1980
106. Ling CC, Anderson LL, Shipley WU: Dose inhomogeneity in interstitial implants using ^{125}I seeds. Int J Radiat Oncol Biol Phys 5:419–425, 1979
107. Pierquin B, Chassagne D, Baillet F et al: Clinical observations on the time factor in interstitial radiotherapy using iridium-192. Clin Radiol 24:506–509, 1973
108. Beadle GF, Silver B, Botnick L et al: Cosmetic results following primary radiation therapy for early breast cancer. Cancer 54:2911–2918, 1984
109. Levene MB, Kijewski PK, Chin LM et al: Computer controlled radiation therapy. Radiology 129:769–775, 1978
110. Bergonie J, Tribondeau L: Interpretation of some results of radiotherapy and an attempt at determining a logical technique of treatment. Radiat Res 11:587–588, 1959
111. Kligerman MM: Radiotherapy and rectal cancer. Cancer 39:896–900, 1977
112. Harris JR, Beadle GF, Hellman S: Clinical studies on the use of radiation therapy as primary treatment of early breast cancer. Cancer 53:705–711, 1984
113. Hellman S: Improving the therapeutic index in breast cancer treatment. Cancer Res 40:4335–4342, 1980
114. Ervin TJ, Weichselbaum RR, Fabian RL et al: Advanced squamous carcinoma of the head and neck: A preliminary report of neoadjuvant chemotherapy with cisplatin, bleomycin, and methotrexate. Arch Otolaryngol 110:241–245, 1984
115. Harris JR, Sawicka J, Gelman R et al: Management of locally advanced carcinoma of the breast. Int J Radiat Oncol Biol Phys 9:345–349, 1983

VINCENT T. DEVITA, JR.

CHAPTER 16 *Principles of Chemotherapy*

Benign tumors compress tissue in their immediate environment but rarely kill patients unless located in strategic sites, such as the brain. Malignant tumors consist of cells that possess the capability of invading their surrounding stroma, passing through basement membranes, and establishing a metastatic clone even before the primary tumor reaches a clinically detectable level. When localized malignancies are controlled by surgery or radiation therapy, the capacity to cure a patient is limited by the presence of viable micrometastases outside the treatment field, a fact not fully appreciated until the last two decades. The chemotherapy of cancer is thus the treatment of metastases.[1–4]

One of the most important advances in tumor biology in recent years has been the discovery that the metastatic process itself is, in effect, an aberration of normal embryogenesis, and that the steps of this process are under genetic control. This information opens up the possibility of controlling expansion of both the primary tumor and its metastases by interfering with the steps in the metastatic process at the molecular level. A detailed discussion of this subject can be found in Chapter 7.

Systemic treatment had its roots in the work of Paul Ehrlich, who coined the word *chemotherapy.* Ehrlich's use of rodent models of infectious diseases to develop antibiotics led George Clowes, at Roswell Park Memorial Institute in Buffalo, New York, to develop, in the early 1900s, inbred rodent lines that could carry transplanted tumors.[5] These models served as the testing ground for potential cancer chemotherapeutic agents and have only recently been effectively supplemented by human cells grown in culture. Alkylating agents, the first modern chemotherapeutic agents, were a product of the secret war gas program in both world wars. An explosion in Bari Harbor during World War II[6,7] and the exposure of seamen to mustard gas led to the observation that alkylating agents caused marrow and lymphoid hypoplasia and led to their use in humans with Hodgkin's disease and other lymphomas, first attempted at Yale–New Haven Medical Center in 1943. Because of the secret nature of the gas warfare program, this work was not published until 1946.[1,5] The demonstration of dramatic regressions of advanced cancers with chemicals caused much excitement and later much disappointment as the tumors invariably grew back. After Farber's observation on the effects of folic acid on leukemic cell growth in children with lymphoblastic leukemia, and the development of the antifols as cancer drugs, the chemotherapy of cancer began in earnest.

THE RESPONSE TO CHEMOTHERAPY IS AFFECTED BY THE BIOLOGY OF TUMOR GROWTH

In the early 1960s Skipper and his colleagues laid down the guiding principles of present-day chemotherapy, using the rodent leukemia L1210 as a model.[8–10] Applying these principles to the drug treatment of human cancers required an understanding of the differences between the growth characteristics of this rodent leukemia and of human cancers, and the differences in growth rates of normal target tissues in mice and man. For example, L1210 leukemia is a rapidly growing tumor with a high percentage of cells synthesizing DNA (the labeling index) as measured by the uptake of tritiated thymidine (see Chapter 1). Because it has a growth fraction of 100% (that is, all of its cells are actively progressing through the cell cycle), its life cycle is consistent and predictable.[11] On the other hand, the cell cycles of human tumors are heterogeneous and prolonged[12–15]; their growth fraction is small, and many cells contributing to measurable tumor masses are not clonogenic and cannot form metastases.[16–19]

The relationship between cell number and survival in L1210 leukemia is linear, as shown in Figure 16-1. The time to death of animals bearing L1210 leukemia is the interval required to achieve a population size of about one billion (10^9) cells. With a growth fraction of 100% and a doubling time of 12 hours, 10^9 cells will accumulate by 19 days after the injection of a single cell, by 10 days after the injection of 10^5 cells, and by 5 days after the administration of 10^8 cells. Skipper postulated that the increase in host life span after cytotoxic chemotherapy of L1210 leukemia was largely due to the cytocidal effect of treatment on the tumor cell population. In these early elegant mouse experiments he calculated the residual number of cells after treatment by extrapolating back from the duration of prolongation of life after a single treatment. An increase of 2 days in life would be equivalent to a 90% destruction of tumor cells (a 1-log kill), or a reduction in the cell number from 10^6 to 10^5. A 99.999% destruction of tumor cells, a figure that seems enormous to most clinicians, represents only a 5-log kill and will not cure animals unless the initial inoculum is small, perhaps 10^4 cells or less. If multiple treatments are given, the net tumor cell kill per treatment is the sum of the surviving cells plus the regrowth of the tumor cell population before the next treatment.

FIG. 16-1. Relationship between size of tumor cell inoculation and time to death of the host in L1210 leukemia in CDF_1 mice.

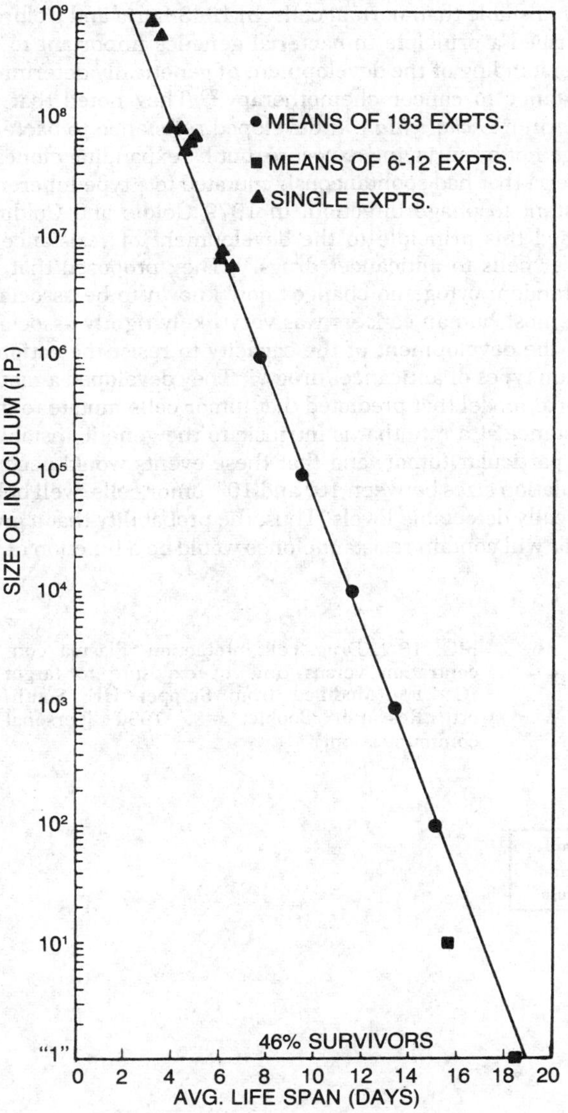

The killing effects of cancer drugs thus follow log kill kinetics, that is, if a particular dose of an individual drug kills 3 logs of cells and reduces tumor burden from 10^{10} to 10^7 cells, the same dose used at a tumor burden of 10^5 cells will reduce the tumor mass to 10^2. The cell kill is therefore proportional regardless of tumor burden. This model fits the response of L1210 murine leukemia to chemotherapy. When treatment failed in Skipper's experiments, it was because the initial tumor burden was too high to allow delivery of enough doses of chemotherapy to eradicate the last cell. The cardinal rule of chemotherapy, the invariable inverse relationship between cell number and curability, was established. Skipper went on to show that with an understanding of these basic facts, this rodent leukemia could be cured by specifically designed doses and schedules tied to tumor volume and growth characteristics.[8]

Although murine leukemias seemed to follow exponential kinetics, available data suggested that most human tumors did not appear to grow exponentially. For example, the concept of log kill would have predicted that some large tumors in the clinic should have been more sensitive to treatment than has been experienced. In vitro chemosensitivity studies have shown that the surviving fraction of tumor cells exposed to a particular dose of drug is frequently not constant regardless of the starting population size, as would be expected if the tumor grew exponentially. Larger starting populations have consistently showed a higher surviving fraction. Also, in several studies metastases have been documented to grow faster than primary tumors. In toto, the available data support a Gompertzian model of tumor growth and regression. The critical distinction between Gompertzian and exponential growth is that in Gompertzian kinetics, the growth fraction of the tumor is not constant but decreases exponentially with time (exponential growth is matched by exponential retardation of growth). The growth fraction peaks when the tumor is about 37% of its maximum size. As the tumor enlarges the growth fraction falls exponentially, the growth rate slows, and the tumor volume begins to plateau. In a Gompertzian model, when a patient with advanced cancer is treated the tumor mass is larger, its growth fraction is low, and the fraction of cells killed is therefore small. Gompertzian kinetics also make predictions about the behavior of small tumors, such as tumor burdens that might be present after primary surgical therapy. When the tumor is clinically undetectable, its growth fraction would be at its largest and the fractional cell kill from a "known to be effective" therapeutic dose of chemotherapy would be higher than at later times in the tumor course. Thus, experimental observations imply that there are kinetic reasons for failure of chemotherapy to cure large tumors. This information has been useful in the application of chemotherapy to patients with smaller tumor volume in the clinic since it should be possible to overcome cell kinetic reasons for chemotherapy failure.

BIOCHEMICAL RESISTANCE TO CHEMOTHERAPY IS THE MAJOR IMPEDIMENT TO SUCCESSFUL TREATMENT

Unlike most cellular drug targets, the cancer cell presents a variable and moving target to anticancer drugs. The interrelationship of pharmacokinetics and tumor and normal target cell kinetics is the fulcrum of clinical cancer chemotherapy. The therapeutic and toxic effects of chemotherapeutic agents are related to the time the active principle is exposed in an effective concentration to its target (Fig. 16-2). The same degree of cytotoxicity can be achieved, on different schedules, from the same concentration of drug multiplied by the time of exposure ($C \times T$). This relationship obtains across different species when the drugs are both metabolized and excreted in a similar fashion. This principle has made it possible to translate doses of drugs devised in animals to humans for early clinical testing[23,24] (see Early Clinical Trials of Antitumor Agents, below). A given $C \times T$ will generally be equally cytotoxic in populations of cells with equivalent growth characteristics and sensitivity to the agent(s) in question.

When the active principles of anticancer drugs reach their target, another obstacle to the capacity to kill the cancer cell appears: specific and permanent biochemical resistance to anticancer drugs. Resistance to drugs either occurs de novo in cancer cells or is concomitant to the process of replication.[21,24–32]

Many specific mechanisms of primary drug resistance have been revealed whereby cancer cells demonstrate the ability to circumvent a well-defined pathway of attack by a given cytotoxic agent. These mechanisms are summarized in Table 16-1 and discussed in detail in Chapter 18. Mechanisms of primary drug resistance include decreased uptake caused by changes in drug-specific transport mechanisms, decreased activation of prodrugs, alteration in the drug's target enzymes, alterations in cellular metabolism and repair mechanisms, and increased inactivation of drugs.[33] Gene amplification of an enzyme target has been documented to occur in a tumor as a result of exposure to the drug[34] with the attendant development of chromosomal homogeneous staining regions or double-minute chromosomes representing an increased copy number of the target gene.

A fundamental property of DNA is spontaneous mutation; there is also evidence that tumor cells may be more genetically unstable than normal cells. In 1943 Luria and Delbruck described a principle in bacterial genetics important to our understanding of the development of genetically determined resistance to cancer chemotherapy.[20] They noted that the bacterium *Escherichia coli* developed resistance to bacteriophage not by surviving exposure, but by expanding clones of bacteria that had spontaneously mutated to a type inherently resistant to phage infection. In 1979 Goldie and Coldman applied this principle to the development of resistance by cancer cells to anticancer drugs.[21] They proposed that the nonrandom cytogenic changes now known to be associated with most human cancers was very likely tightly associated with the development of the capacity to resist the action of certain types of anticancer drugs.[22] They developed a mathematical model that predicted that tumor cells mutate to drug resistance at a rate that is intrinsic to the genetic instability of a particular tumor, and that these events would occur at population sizes between 10^3 and 10^6 tumor cells, well below clinically detectable levels. Thus, the probability that a given tumor will contain resistant clones would be a function of the

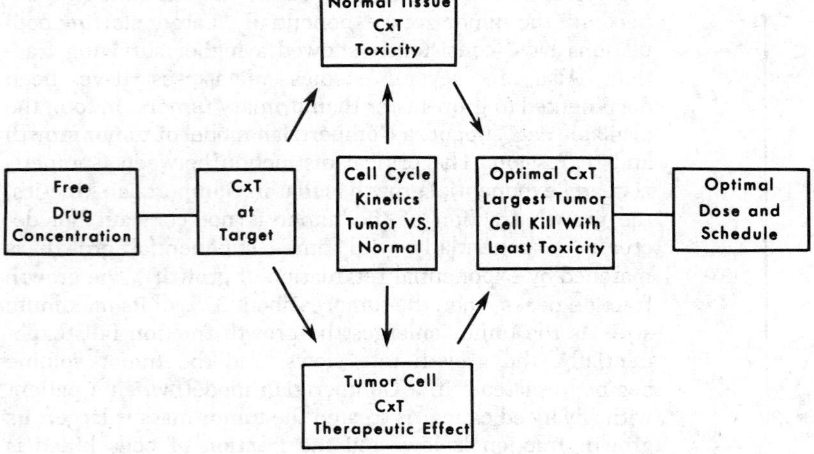

FIG. 16-2. Drug–cell interaction. Plasma concentration versus time of exposure to target ($C \times T$) (Modified from Skipper HE: Southern Research Booklet #9, 1980 [personal communication])

TABLE 16-1. Mechanisms of Drug Resistance

General Mechanism	*Drug*	*Result*
Multidrug resistance	Vinca alkaloids	
	Antitumor antibiotics	Drug actively pumped out
	Etoposide	
Transport defect	Methotrexate	
	Melphalan	Low carrier-mediated uptake
	Nitrogen mustard	
	Cytosine arabinoside	Low membrane binding
Poor activation	Cytosine arabinoside	Low deoxycytidine kinase
	5-Azacytidine	Low uridine-cytidine kinase
	5-Fluorouracil	Low uridine kinase, orotic acid PRT, uridine phosphorylase
	6-Thioguanine	Low hypoxanthine–guanine PRT
	6-Mercaptopurine	
	Methotrexate	Low polyglutamation
	Doxorubicin	Low P-450 enzymes
Drug inactivation	Cytosine arabinoside	High cytidine deaminase
	Alkylating agents	High glutathione
	6-Thioguanine	High alkaline phosphatase
	6-Mercaptopurine	
Improved DNA repair	Alkylating agents	
	Antitumor antibiotics	High efficiency repair of strand breaks, ligase
	Cisplatin	
Gene amplification	Methotrexate	Dihydrofolate reductase
	PALA	Aspartate transcarbamylase
	2-Deoxycoformycin	Adenosine deaminase
	5-Fluorouracil	? Thymidylate synthetase
Alternate pathways	Methotrexate	Increased thymidine salvage
	5-Fluorouracil	Increased thymidine kinase
Altered pools of competing substrate	Cytosine arabinoside	High CTP and dCTP
	5-Fluorouracil	
Target alterations	Vincristine	Tubulin
	Methotrexate	Dihydrofolate reductase
	5-Fluorouracil	Thymidylate synthetase
	Hydroxyurea	Ribonucleotide reductase
	Steroids	Receptor or receptor–DNA binding

PRT = phosphoribosyl transferase, PALP = *N*-phosphomacetyl-L-aspartic acid, CTP = cytidine triphosphate, dCTP = deoxycytidine triphosphate.

mutation rate and the size of the tumor. If the mutation rate is only around 10^{-6}, a tumor composed of 10^9 cells (a mass only 1 cm in size) would be virtually certain to have at least one drug-resistant clone. However, if the mutation rate is around 10^{-6}, the *absolute number* of resistant cells in a tumor composed of 10^9 cells would be relatively small. In the clinic, such tumors would appear to respond initially to treatment with a complete or partial remission, but then reappear as the resistance clone(s) expanded. Such a pattern is seen with the use of chemotherapy in many cancers in the clinic.

However, some tumors are not responsive to chemotherapeutic agents at all, even when diagnosed with minimal tumor volume, which suggests that they are either inherently resistant or are largely made up of clones that have mutated to resistance. There is a cell kinetic explanation for this phenomenon in some slowly growing visceral tumors. For example, as tumor masses grow, there is considerable cell loss from shedding of cells, say into the lumen of the bowel, or actual cell death, which can amount to 90% of the total tumor volume. In such a setting, a tumor 1 cm in size and consisting of 10^9 cells, while appearing to be an early tumor, might have gone through 1200 doublings to reach that size to compensate for cell loss, instead of the expected 32 doublings. Such a kinetic history together with the expected genetic instability could well be associated with a very high probability that the entire mass consists of resistant cell lines.

The Goldie–Coldman hypothesis presumed that resistance to drugs occurred in a single step. Another pattern of resistance has emerged. When malignant cell lines are made resistant to a single chemotherapeutic agent by stepwise incubation in increasing amounts of drug, some such lines are curiously found to be resistant to structurally unrelated cytotoxic compounds. This finding has been repeated for many different cell lines initially exposed to many different drugs. This phenomenon of broad resistance was termed *pleiotropic drug resistance,* or *multidrug resistance* (MDR).[35] Cell lines that display the MDR phenotype are generally resistant to natural product cytotoxic agents such as the anthracyclines, vinca alkaloids, epipodophyllotoxins, and actinomycin D.

Since all of these agents are believed to have different mechanisms of action, investigation of MDR has not focused on specific enzymes but rather on the cell's basic defense mechanism against toxic agents found naturally in the environment.

Multidrug resistance was shown to be associated with decreased intracellular drug accumulation and the presence of a 170,000-dalton plasma membrane–associated glycoprotein (P-glycoprotein) that was not detectable in parenteral drug-sensitive lines.[36,37] P-glycoprotein content was shown to directly correlate with both the degree of decrease in intracellular accumulation of the toxins and the degree of drug resistance exhibited by the cell.[38,39] These observations suggested that the P-glycoprotein conferred resistance by regulating transport of toxins in or out of the cell. Most cell lines with the MDR phenotype that have since been established show increased expression of the gene encoding P-glycoprotein, the *mdr* gene.[40–44] A great deal of evidence now suggests that the P-glycoprotein is, in fact, an energy-dependent drug efflux pump. The ability of the P-glycoprotein to bind natural product type drugs has also been demonstrated. It has been shown to bind photoaffinity analogs of vinblastine, a reaction that is competitively inhibited by unlabeled vinblastine as well as by anthracyclines.[45,46] Furthermore, several agents, including the calcium channel blocker verapamil, as well as quinidine and nifedipine, can also bind to the P-glycoprotein and can compete with the vinblastine analogs for binding with the P-glycoprotein.[47] Full-length cDNA sequences encoding the mouse[48] and human[49] P-glycoprotein gene have been isolated and their nucleotide sequences determined. The deduced amino acid sequence of this protein shows structural similarities to a well-characterized bacterial membrane transport protein, diagrammed in Figure 16-3.[48–50a] P-glycoprotein RNA expression has been found in high levels in normal adrenal and kidney tissue and in moderate levels in hepatic and colon tissue.[51] Since colon, kidney, and liver tissues are exposed to naturally occurring environmental toxins, the role of the P-glycoprotein in health may be one of protecting, by facilitating efflux of these toxins. There is evidence that the P-glycoprotein may be a member of a multigene family. At least two different classes of P-glycoprotein cDNAs have been identified in hamster,[52] mouse,[53] and human[54] cells.

In some cell lines the phenomenon of multidrug resistance is associated with more than the production and function of the P-glycoprotein alone. This was suggested by the fact that each MDR cell line displays a slightly different pattern of cross-resistance,[55,56] and the degree of resistance does not always directly correlate with the degree of intracellular accumulation of drugs.[57–59] In addition, despite the relative

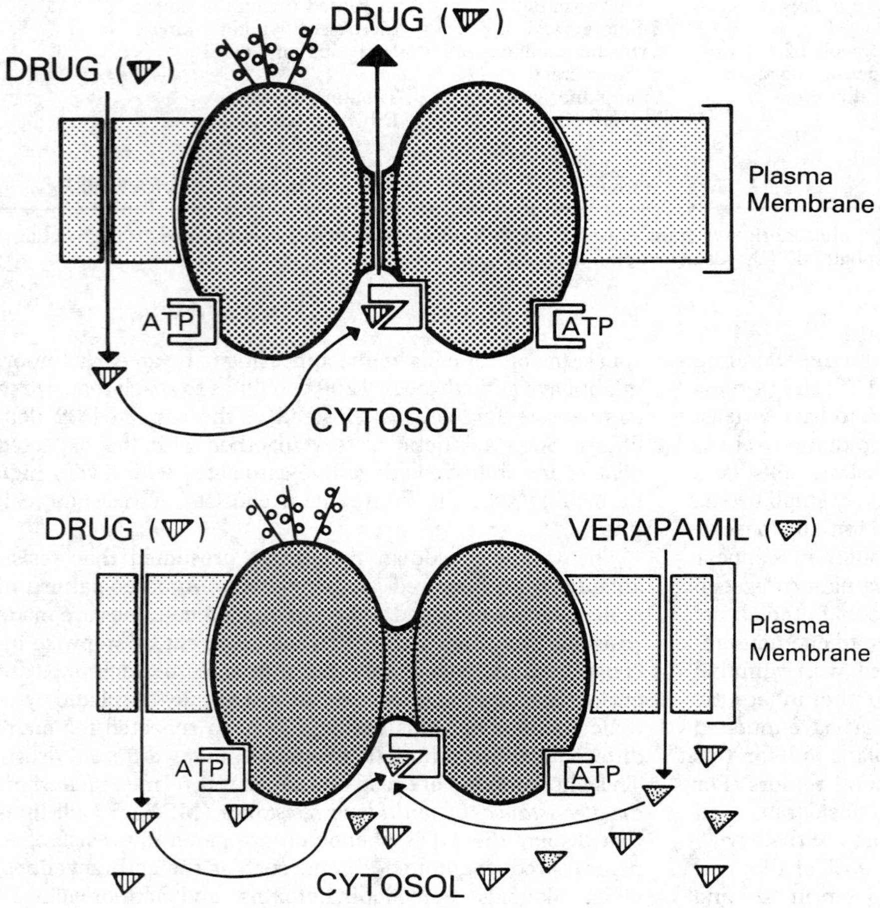

FIG. 16-3. Model of how P-glycoprotein might be involved in transporting cytotoxic drugs, such as vinblastine, out of cells (*top*) and how drugs such as verapamil that reverse multidrug resistance compete with vinblastine to block the pump (*bottom*). (Pastan IH, Gottesman MM: Molecular biology of multidrug resistance in human cells. In DeVita VT Jr, Hellman S, Rosenberg SA [eds]: Important Advances in Oncology 1988, p 9. Philadelphia, JB Lippincott, 1988)

ease with which the *mdr* gene expression is found in resistant cell lines, there have been relatively few reports relating P-glycoprotein expression in vivo to clinical drug resistance.

A model of chemical carcinogenesis proposed by Solt, Medline, and Farber[60] has helped shed some light on a second set of mechanisms associated with MDR. Chemical carcinogenesis is believed to be a two-step process consisting of an irreversible initiation event, followed by exposure to promoting agents. In the Farber model, laboratory rats are exposed to carcinogens and then subjected to partial hepatectomy, which, since it stimulates cell growth in the residual liver, serves as a promoting event. This procedure consistently results in liver nodules, some of which develop into frank hepatocellular carcinomas. The cells in these nodules are found to be more resistant to the toxic effects of the initiating carcinogens than normal hepatocytes,[61] and the hepatocytes in the hepatic nodules are resistant not only to the agent that precipitated their transformation but, like MDR cell lines associated with the P-glycoprotein, also to other structurally dissimilar cytotoxic chemicals.[62] In these nodules, while there is overexpression of the *mdr* gene, there is also decreased activity of several drug-activating microsomal cytochrome P-450 phase I enzymes, including aryl hydrocarbon hydroxylase, increased activities of several drug-conjugating enzymes, including the anionic isoenzyme of glutathione S-transferase, and increased activity of other enzymes involved in drug metabolism, including DT-diaphorase and glucuronyl transferase.[63,64] Each of these changes may play a role in providing the cell with the ability to withstand toxic agents. This complex set of changes, observed in two very different models of broad resistance to xenobiotics, indicates that cells have the capacity to call upon an adaptive, coordinated defense mechanism when assaulted by cytotoxins. Once this program is turned on by one agent, it appears to be effective against others. Such a system may protect normal cells against environmental assault, but in cancer patients it appears to protect neoplastic cells against chemotherapeutic agents, which are also derived from environmental sources.

A third type of MDR has recently been elucidated that is not associated with P-glycoprotein gene expression at all.[65,66] In some cells, drug influx and steady-state intracellular concentrations are no different than in the parenteral drug-sensitive cells; by contrast, cells with the classic MDR phenotype invariably show changes in drug transport. Although the precise defect in the resistant cells that do not show changes in transport is not yet known, there is strong evidence implicating altered topoisomerase activity.[67] Topoisomerases are enzymes necessary for DNA replication that catalyze changes in the secondary and tertiary structures of DNA. Topoisomerase II appears to be the enzyme that is the target of antineoplastic drugs that act as DNA-intercalating agents, such as etoposide and the anthracyclines. An etoposide-resistant Chinese hamster ovary cell line that was cross-resistant to the structurally dissimilar agent m-AMSA, mitoxantrone, and the anthracycline doxorubicin demonstrated altered topoisomerase II activity.[68] In addition, alteration of the topoisomerase I-like activity was found in Chinese hamster cells selected for resistance to elipticine and cross-resistance to m-AMSA and etoposide.[69] Topoisomerases, therefore, may represent the final common pathway of cytotoxicity of several different classes of antineoplastic agents. However, no studies have been able to show that altered topoisomerase activity plays a role in clinical drug resistance.

As a result of these data there is considerable excitement over the prospect of improving the effectiveness of chemotherapy by preventing the development of MDR or by interfering with the mechanism itself. Drugs that reverse MDR are being tested. The first such drug to reach clinical trial was verapamil, a drug that has reversed acquired drug resistance in a variety of in vitro systems. This calcium channel blocker enhances cytotoxicity by increasing intracellular accumulation of drugs, which suggests that it acts on P-glycoprotein or other transport proteins, as illustrated in Figure 16-3.[47,70] Unfortunately, the verapamil concentrations required to reverse resistance in vitro result in excessive clinical toxicity. Quinidine, a drug that also binds to P-glycoprotein, has also reached clinical trial as an inhibitor of drug resistance, but no definitive results are available. Monoclonal antibodies have also been developed against the P-glycoprotein. In addition to a role in targeting toxins to P-glycoprotein–containing tumor cells,[71] such antibodies should prove useful as a diagnostic tool to identify cells with the MDR phenotype in vivo, and to allow the selection of drugs for treatment that can circumvent the pump.

Buthioninesulphoxamine (BSO) is a synthetic amino acid that inhibits γ-glutamyl-cysteine synthetase, which in turn leads to marked reduction of intracellular concentrations of glutathione, the substrate for the glutathione-S transferase isozymes and glutathione peroxidase involved in some forms of MDR.[72] Several studies of different tumor cell lines have shown reversal of drug resistance after treatment with BSO, corresponding with decreases in intracellular glutathione concentration.[73–75] In vitro toxicity studies on mouse and human bone marrow cells indicate that normal cells may be less susceptible to the toxicity of chemotherapeutic agents than tumor cells when also exposed to BSO. Phase I clinical trials are in progress in which BSO is given with an antineoplastic agent in refractory cancer.

FOR DRUG-SENSITIVE CANCERS IN FAVORABLE KINETIC CIRCUMSTANCES, THE FACTOR LIMITING THE CAPACITY TO CURE IS PROPER DOSING: THE CONCEPT OF DOSE INTENSITY

The dose–response curve in biologic systems is usually sigmoidal in shape with a threshold, a lag phase, a linear phase, and a plateau phase. For both radiation therapy and chemotherapy it is the difference between the dose–response curves of normal and tumor tissue that must be exploited during treatment. In experimental models, the dose–response curve is usually steep in the linear phase. Almost without exception, reduction of doses in the linear phase of the dose–response curve results first in a loss of the capacity to cure the tumor before there is a diminution in the response rate. That is, complete remissions will continue to be observed in animals bearing palpable tumors, but the last few residual cells will not be ablated, and relapse becomes inevitable. There is an extremely important lesson in these animal data for clinicians who, in their daily practice, judge the adequacy of their therapy by measuring response rate of visible or palpable tumor masses. This point is illustrated in Table 16-2, which summarizes data from numerous experiments conducted by Skipper and his colleagues at the Southern Research Institute using the transplantable and palpable Ridgway osteosarcoma tumor model.[76,77] Reduction in the average dose intensity of the two-drug combination of L-phenylalanine mustard (L-PAM) and cyclophosphamide causes a marked decrease in the cure rate *before a significant reduction in the complete remission rate is noted.* On the average, a dose reduction of approximately 20% will lead to a loss in the cure rate in excess of 50%. The converse is also true. In high growth fraction tumors a twofold increase in dose often leads to a tenfold increase (1 log) in tumor cell kill. Although animal models are not the perfect analogue for human cancers, the invariable nature of these data indicate that the general principle is transferable to the clinic and is ignored at great peril. Because anticancer drugs are toxic, it is very appealing to reduce toxicity by diminishing the dose or increasing the intervals between cycles of treatment. This kind of ad hoc adjustment of dosing is probably the main reason for treatment failure in patients with *drug-sensitive human tumors* undergoing their first chemotherapy treatment. If so, the most toxic effect of treatment may be premature death from insufficient dosing.

It has been difficult to compare the impact of different dosing practices in treatment programs. Recently, Hyrniuk and his colleagues analyzed treatment outcome in a number of different tumors as a function of what they have termed dose intensity.[78-83] They defined dose intensity as the amount of drug delivered per unit time, expressed as $mg/m^2/wk$, regardless of the schedule or route of administration. Relative dose intensity (RDI) is the amount of drug delivered per unit time relative to an arbitrarily chosen standard single drug, or, for a combination regimen, the decimal fraction of the ratio of the test regimen to the standard regimen. To compare the dose intensity of combinations of drugs, the average dose intensity of the combination is calculated as the average amount of drugs delivered per unit time compared to an arbitrarily chosen standard. A sample calculation of the RDI for a commonly used regimen, the CMF combination (cyclophosphamide, methotrexate, 5-fluorouracil) for breast cancer is provided in Table 16-3.[78] To calculate average RDI for a regimen containing fewer drugs than the standard regimen, a dose intensity of zero is assigned to the missing drug(s), and the average RDI of the test regimen is divided by the total number of drugs in the standard.[79] The dose intensity of various programs is compared over whatever time frame the treatment programs are administered. Calculations can be made of intended dose intensity, the dose intensity as described in the treatment protocol, or actual or received dose intensity. Received dose intensity reflects the impact of dose reductions and necessary treatment delays imposed in actual practice because of toxicity and is thus the more important datum.

Since calculations are made on the basis of the amount of drugs given per week regardless of schedule, treatment delays are given equal weight to dose reductions. Calculations of the dose intensity, therefore, require the assumption that scheduling does not determine treatment outcome. While at first this appears to be heretical, close scrutiny of all available data in humans and rodents shows that scheduling influences outcome largely by affecting toxicity, in this way allowing greater doses to be administered over the same time frame. An example can be found in the use of methotrexate both in rodents and in humans. Daily administration of low doses of methotrexate is very toxic and severely limits the dose and duration of therapy with this drug. A twice-weekly schedule, which is much more effective in rodents and in humans, allows much greater doses to be delivered for longer durations, because this schedule is associated with less toxicity. The dose intensity of the twice-weekly schedule is therefore far greater than that of the daily oral schedule when calculated on a basis of $mg/m^2/wk$ of delivered drug. In practice, the impact of scheduling on the calculation of dose intensity can be neutralized by comparing programs in which drugs with toxicities affected by scheduling, such as the antimetabolites, are given in like schedules.

Calculation of an average RDI of a drug combination also assumes equivalency of the affects of all the drugs in the combination. The impact of any single drug, or combinations of two or three drugs in a multidrug combination, can, however, be assessed separately. This has been done by Hyrniuk to show the greater impact of cisplatin in a drug combination for ovarian cancer.[78,84] This kind of analysis can help iden-

TABLE 16-2. Ridgway Osteogenic Sarcoma: Response to Different Dose Intensity of Two-Drug Combination of Cyclophosphamide and L-PAM*

RDI				
CPA	*L-PAM*	*Average*	*% CR*	*% Cures*
0.38	0.82	0.60	100	60
0.75	0.18	0.47	100	44
0.25	0.55	0.44	100	10
0.50	0.12	0.31	10	0
0.17	0.36	0.27	0	0

RDI = relative dose intensity, CPA = cyclophosphamide, L-PAM=L-phenylalanine, CR = complete response. Tumors weighed 2 to 3 g.

* Modified from Skipper HE: Booklet No. 5, Southern Research Institute, 1986.

TABLE 16-3. Sample Calculations: Dose Intensity, Relative Dose Intensity, and Average Relative Dose Intensity*

	Dose Intensity	*Relative Dose Intensity*
Calculation of Dose Intensity		
Test Schedule		
Cyclophosphamide 80 mg/m²/day (continuously)	560 mg/m²/wk	
Calculation of Relative Dose Intensity		
Standard		
Cyclophosphamide 80 mg/m²/day (continuously)	560 mg/m²/wk	
Test Schedule		
Cyclophosphamide 100 mg/m²/day (days 1–14, q 28 days)	350 mg/m²/wk	350/560 = 0.62
Calculation of Average Relative Dose Intensity		
Standard†		
Cyclophosphamide 2 mg/kg/day	560 mg/m²/wk	
Methotrexate 0.7 mg/kg/wk	28 mg/m²/wk	
5-Fluorouracil 12 mg/kg/wk	480 mg/m²/wk	
Test Regimen		
Cyclophosphamide 100 mg/m²/day (days 1–14)	350 mg/m²/wk	350/560 = 0.62
Methotrexate 40 mg/m²/days 1, 8	20 mg/m²/wk	20/28 = 0.71
5-Fluorouracil 600 mg/m²/days 1, 8	300 mg/m²/wk	300/480 = 0.62
Repeat cycles every 28 days		*Average* 0.65

* Hryniuk WM: The importance of dose intensity in the outcome of chemotherapy. In DeVita VT, Hellman S, Rosenberg SA (eds): Important Advances in Oncology, pp 121–142. Philadelphia, JB Lippincott, 1988.

† Assume standard regimen to be CMF content of CMFVP regimen of Cooper and associates. To convert mg/kg to mg/m², multiply by 40.

tify the most effective drug in a combination, and it is important because such data can influence how doses and schedules are adjusted to avoid adjustments that radically alter the effectiveness of a program. Alterations in dose intensity of the most effective drug in a combination of drugs has greatest impact, as illustrated in Table 16-4, which displays the effects of the two-drug combination of L-PAM and the antimetabolite 6-mercaptopurine (6-MP) against the Ridgway osteogenic sarcoma model. In this case, L-PAM is the more effective drug. The relationship of average dose intensity of the two drugs to outcome is erratic, but the relationship of the dose intensity of L-PAM to outcome is linear, as in Table 16-2. Decreases in the dose intensity of L-PAM reduce the effect of the combination even when the dose of 6-MP is increased to compensate for these reductions. In fact, any decrease in the dose intensity of L-PAM below 55% of the

TABLE 16-4. Ridgway Osteogenic Sarcoma: Effect of Varying Dose Intensity of More Effective Drug, L-PAM*

Relative Dose Intensity				*Observed*	
L-PAM	*6-MP*	*Ratio (L-PAM/6-MP)*	*Average*	*% CR*	*% Cures*
0.82	0.49	1.7	0.66	100	60
0.73	1.3	0.56	1.0	90	50
0.55	1.0	0.55	0.78	90	20
0.55	0.33	1.7	0.44	80	20
0.36	0.67	0.54	0.52	56	0
0.36	0.21	1.7	0.29	30	0
0.27	1.5	0.18	0.89	70	0
0.24	0.44	0.57	0.35	0	0
0.24	0.15	1.6	0.20	0	0
0.18	1.0	0.18	0.59	0	0
0.12	0.67	0.18	0.50	0	0
0.08	0.44	0.18	0.26	0	0

L-PAM = L-phenylalanine mustard; 6-MP = 6-mercaptopurine. Tumors weighed 2 to 3 g. Varying the dose intensity of L-PAM has a greater impact on outcome than can be overcome by increasing the dose of 6-MP.

* Skipper HE: Booklet No. 4, Southern Research Institute, 1986.

optimal single dose schedule results in loss of the capacity of this combination to cure animals, regardless of the dose of 6-MP.

Two additional pieces of information could increase the precision and usefulness of these data: the total dose of each drug administered, and a cumulative dose plot of each drug on a week by week basis for each patient. Collection of such data is not part of routine practice, and these data are not generally available in the literature. It is the opinion of this author, however, that in order to assess the impact of dosing schedules in practice and in clinical trials, such data should be required before papers are accepted for publication. Practicing physicians would also find such data useful in assessing the benefits and limitations of the use of chemotherapy.

A clear-cut relationship between dose intensity and response rate has been demonstrated in advanced ovarian cancer, breast cancer, colon cancer, and in the lymphomas.[77,78,80,81] Hyrniuk is conducting a prospective trial in which the dose intensity of the combination of cyclophosphamide, doxorubicin, and fluorouracil (CAF) used in advanced breast cancer is increased to a point on the dose–response curve calculated to produce response rates superior to the published results with standard CAF.[78] In a preliminary analysis, the data fit on the plotted dose–response curve. This approach has practical implications.

Calculations of the impact of dose intensity on outcome are particularly important in estimating the value and exploring some of the pitfalls of adjuvant chemotherapy. A significant effect of dose intensity on relapse-free survival after the use of drugs or adjuvant therapy has been found for breast cancer (Fig. 16-4). The correlation between dose intensity and outcome is all the more significant since almost all the drugs in the programs shown are used at the low end of their dose–response curve. The invariable inverse relationship between cell number and curability and the steep dose–response curve for anticancer drugs clearly indicate that dose reductions in adjuvant drug treatment programs are likely to be associated with significantly less therapeutic effect. Dose reduction has, however, been the norm in the design of adjuvant trials. An example is given in Table 16-5 for the standard CMF regimen. The model for the regimen was published in 1974 by Canellos et al.[85] It produced an impressive complete remission rate, but its toxicity was considerable. As a result, when it was advanced for use in a cooperative group setting for advanced disease,[84] and later for adjuvant trials by the Milan group,[86] its doses were arbitrarily reduced without pretesting the impact of such reductions on outcome. In addition, further reduction was made, a priori, for patients over the age of 60 years. When the impact of these reductions is related to outcome, there is a strong suggestion of a negative impact. In Table 16-5 dose intensity is compared using the National Cancer Institute (NCI) CMF+P program as the reference standard. A zero is assigned to the value of prednisone in the calculations. In the cooperative group study,[84] the reduced program resulted in a substantial reduction of the complete remission rate; also, the results in women less than 60 years old were significantly better than in women more than 60 years old, which could be the result of the a priori dose reductions, although

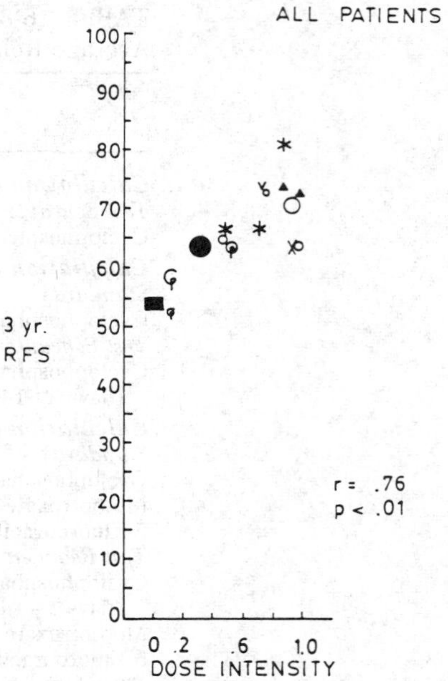

FIG. 16-4. Three-year relapse-free survival (*RFS*) versus average relative dose intensity for adjuvant chemotherapy trials containing all four prognostic subgroups (<50 years; 1–3 or >3 positive nodes; >50 years; 1–3 or >3 positive nodes). The size of the symbols is proportional to the number of cases at each dose intensity. ■, control; ▲, CMFVP; X, CMFP; ●, C_pF; . . . , trial with radiotherapy added; *, levels of CMF chemotherapy according to Bonadonna; [25]V, CMFV; ○, CMF; ⚲, C_pMF; ♀, phenylalanine mustard. (Hryniuk WM: The Importance of dose intensity in the outcome of chemotherapy. In DeVita VT Jr, Hellman S, Rosenberg SA [eds]: Important Advances in Oncology 1988, p 129. Philadelphia, JB Lippincott, 1988)

the dose effect cannot be completely separated from other variables.

In a later analysis of the effect of dose on the outcome in the Milan trial, Bonadonna et al divided the delivered doses of CMF into three levels and determined the impact of dosing at these levels on outcome.[87] The doses at these levels have been converted in Table 16-5 to their dose intensity relative to the NCI CMF+P regimen. In advanced cases, a substantial dose–response effect seems apparent. Since complete responses were not reported, the impact of dose reductions on the quality of response cannot be assessed. In the adjuvant situation, a dose–response effect was also noted. In premenopausal woman the differences in relapse-free survival at the high and low doses are statistically significant. The most important point, however, is that the average dose intensity of CMF as used in clinical trials and in the community is probably only a little more than half the dose intensity of the original program. These dose reductions exceed the levels that animal models predict would lead to a loss in the capacity to cure.

An example of the potential impact dose intensity can have on the design of clinical trials has been provided by Hyrniuk in Figure 16-5.[78] The dose intensity of 5-fluorouracil is plotted against response rate for advanced colorectal

TABLE 16-5. Ad Hoc Dose Modifications of the CMF Program Used for Breast Cancer: Impact of Dose Intensity on Outcome

A. Advanced Breast Cancer

*Study/Doses**	*Intended Dose Intensity*	*Actual Dose Intensity*	*Response Rate*	
			CR	*CR + PR*
CMF − P (NCI, 1974): 100/60/700	1	. . .	28	68
CMF − P (ECOG, 1976):				
Age < 60 yr: 100/40/600	0.84	. . .	15	53
Age < 60 yr: 100/30/400	0.69	. . .	<60 vs. > 60 yr: $p < 0.01$	
CMF − P (Milan, 1976)†				
Level I:	>0.71	0.74	. . .	67
Level II:	0.55−0.71	0.58	. . .	53
Level III:	<0.55	0.42	. . .	35

B. Adjuvant Therapy

*Study**	*Intended Dose Intensity*	*Actual Dose Intensity*	*Relapse-Free Survival*	
			Premenopausal	*Postmenopausal*
CMF − P (Milan, 1976)†				
Level I:	>0.71	0.74	79‡	75§
Level II:	0.55−0.71	0.58	56	56
Level III:	<0.55	0.42	46	49

Intended actual dose intensities are calculated using NCI's CMF − P, the program with the highest dose intensity, as the reference standard according to the method of Hryniuk.[78] ECOG = Eastern Cooperative Oncology Group.

* CMF+P = cyclophosphamide, methotrexate, 5-fluorouracil, +prednisone. Numbers refer to the doses of each drug respectively in mg/m² BSA.

† The Milan trial used the same dose modifications as ECOG, reducing the doses of CMF, a priori, for patients older than 60 years. When reporting results they divided doses into three levels and reported responses by dose level regardless of age. These doses have been recalculated to determine their dose intensity relative to the original NCI CMF+P program.

‡ Differences in RFS of Level I vs. II for premenopausal patients is significant at $p < 0.06$. Level I vs. Level III is significant at $p < 0.05$.

§ For postmenopausal patients, $p < 0.23$, Level I vs. II, $p < 0.17$, Level I vs. Level III.

cancer in panel *A*. Points indicated by the asterisks are from a single study in which response was reported for actual delivered doses at three different levels.[88] The steep nature of the dose–response curves should be noted. Panel *B* of Figure 16-5 plots the same three points from the single study, but adds the doses used in four published adjuvant studies.[88–93] The doses in all of these studies are well below the level that most investigators would consider the threshold for producing useful responses in advanced colorectal cancer.

The effect of dose intensity on the capacity to cure advanced Hodgkin's disease and diffuse large cell lymphomas is also striking and described in detail in Chapters 49 and 50.

Increasing the dose intensity can be a useful way to improve the effect of certain drugs or combinations of drugs, but it is not useful in all clinical circumstances. Large tumor burdens tend to shift the dose–response curve to the right. At the low end of the curability curve (*i.e.*, in the presence of the highest tumor burdens), increasing the dose intensity to unacceptable toxicity, therefore, may not produce more impressive treatment outcomes because the curve is flat. In addition, regimens that are already curing 100% of a subset of patients, such as the combination of platinum, vinblastine, and bleomycin in low-burden testicular cancer and MOPP in Stage IIIA Hodgkin's disease, cannot be expected to be improved upon by augmenting dose intensity. However, for most drugs and most tumors there appears to be a threshold dose that produces responses, and the remarkable success of high-dose chemotherapy programs with marrow support in refractory lymphomas, breast cancer, childhood sarcomas, and neuroblastomas suggests that maximizing dose intensity can improve the chances of cure.

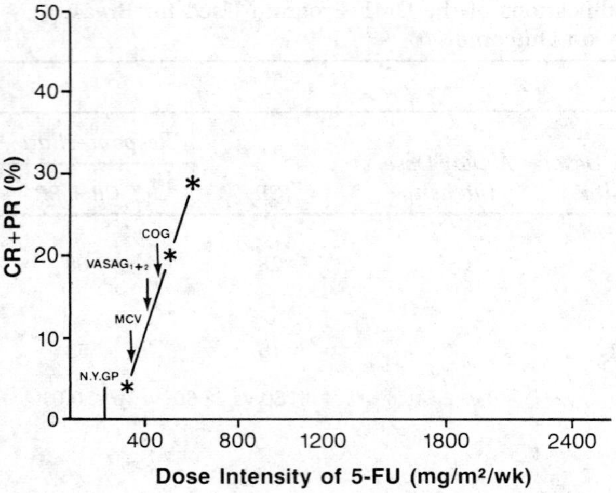

A

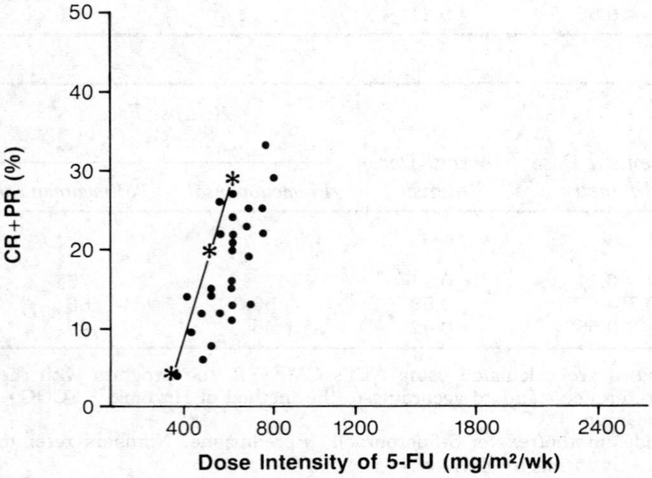

B

FIG. 16-5. **A.** Response rate at various intended dose intensity of 5-fluorouracil in advanced colorectal cancer. Each point represents results from one arm of a randomized trial. Asterisks indicate results of three doses from a single study, and solid circles indicate received dose intensity. **B.** Dose intensities of 5-fluorouracil used in four adjuvant studies of colorectal cancer superimposed on the dose response line for advanced disease shown in panel **A.** Asterisks represent received dose intensity from single study (see text). (Hryniuk WM: The importance of dose intensity in the outcome of chemotherapy. In DeVita VT Jr, Hellman S, Rosenberg SA [eds]: Important Advances in Oncology 1988, p 125. Philadelphia, JB Lippincott, 1988)

PRINCIPLES OF COMBINATION CHEMOTHERAPY

In the early days of chemotherapy, drug combinations were developed based on known biochemical actions of available anticancer drugs rather than on their clinical effectiveness. These programs were largely ineffective.[94–98] The era of effective combination chemotherapy began when an array of effective drugs became available for use in combination in the treatment of leukemias and lymphomas. Combination chemotherapy has now been extended to the treatment of most other malignancies as described throughout this text.

With the exception of choriocarcinoma and Burkitt's lymphoma, combination chemotherapy is required to cure all drug-sensitive human cancers. The relationship of tumor cell number to the likelihood of the presence of resistant cell lines provides a firm basis for the invariable inverse relationship between cell number and curability and is the most reasonable explanation for the effectiveness of combination chemotherapy. Omission of a drug from a combination may allow overgrowth by a cell line sensitive to that drug alone and resistant to other drugs in the combination. Also, arbitrarily reducing the dose of an effective drug to add other, less effective drugs may reduce the dose below the threshold of effectiveness and destroy the capacity of the combination to cure that particular cancer.

Combination chemotherapy, then, accomplishes three important things not possible with single agent treatment: (1) it provides maximal cell kill within the range of toxicity tolerated by the host for each drug; (2) it provides a broader range of coverage of resistant cell lines in a heterogeneous tumor population; and (3) it prevents or slows the development of new resistant lines.

Several principles have been useful in the selection of drugs in the most effective drug combinations and guide the development of new programs.

1. Only drugs known to be partially effective when used alone should be selected for use in combination. If available, drugs that produce some fraction of complete remission are preferred to those that produce only partial responses.
2. When several drugs of a class are available, a drug should be selected on the basis of toxicity that does not overlap with the toxicity of other drugs used in the combination. Although such selection leads to a wider range of side-effects and greater general discomfort to the patient, it minimizes the risk of a lethal effect caused by multiple insults to the same organ system by different drugs.
3. Drugs should be used in their optimal dose and schedule.
4. Drug combinations should be given at consistent intervals. The treatment-free interval between cycles should be the shortest possible time period necessary for recovery of the most sensitive normal target tissue, which is usually the bone marrow.

Bone marrow has a storage compartment that can supply mature cells to the peripheral blood for 8 to 10 days after the stem cell pool has been damaged by cytotoxic drugs. Thus, events measured in the peripheral blood are usually a week behind events occurring in the bone marrow. In previously untreated patients, leukopenia and thrombocytopenia are discernible on the ninth or tenth day after initial dosing. Nadir blood counts are noted between days 14 to 18, with recovery apparent by day 21 and usually complete by day 28. Prior treatment with drugs or x-irradiation may alter this sequence by depleting the stem cell pool, shortening the time to the appearance of leukopenia and thrombocytopenia, and prolonging the recovery time. Curiously, when the second half of a combination given in the clinic on a day 1, day 8 schedule is omitted, leukopenia and thrombocytopenia comparable to that seen with the full combination usually occur, suggesting that the second set of doses does not cause an equal increment in toxicity, possibly because the stem cell compartment has entered a quiescent state. This also suggests that in most cases, the day 8 doses can be given safely even if leukopenia and thrombocytopenia have already become evident. The cytotoxic effect of greatest importance in the clinic is the duration of the nadir level of white cells and platelets. The highest risk of infection or bleeding occurs with granulocyte counts of less than 500/ml^3 and platelet counts of less than 20,000/ml^3. If this nadir lasts only 4 to 7 days it is tolerated by most patients without supplemental support. Increasing doses of most anticancer drugs, within the range of the maximally tolerated dose, usually does not ablate the marrow or even prolong the time to recovery. Repeated dosing during the phase of early recovery of the marrow (days 16–21) may cause more severe toxicity in the second treatment cycle in patients whose marrow is not the source of, or involved with, tumor.

These kinds of data led to the familiar 2-week interval between cycles of the most effective drug combinations (new cycles begin on day 28 after the first dose) to accommodate the recovery time of human bone marrow. Although this treatment schedule is suitable for some tumors, the regrowth characteristics of others, such as diffuse histiocytic lymphoma, Burkitt's lymphoma, and leukemia, often permit the tumor mass to return to pretreatment levels in the interval required for bone marrow recovery, and other approaches to cycling drug combinations are being explored. One approach has been to use non-marrow-toxic chemotherapeutic agents, cycled with marrow-toxic agents, to permit the bone marrow to recover despite continuous treatment. This has been useful in patients with the rapidly growing diffuse large cell lymphomas. It is limited by the sensitivity of the tumor in question to the available non-marrow-toxic agents. The availability of colony-stimulating factors (CSF) as supportive tools (discussed in Chapter 59, Section 4) is altering the design of clinical trials as well. CSF have been coupled with cytotoxic combination chemotherapy, and in the first such report in which G-CSF were used with the combination of methotrexate, vinblastine, Adriamycin, and cisplatin (M-VAC) for treatment of advanced bladder cancer, the nadir leukopenia and thrombocytopenia have been ablated.[99]

The Goldie–Coldman hypothesis also has had a major impact on the design of clinical studies employing combination chemotherapy. Since it suggests that resistance is a problem even with small tumor burdens, it predicts a maximal chance of cure if all available effective drugs are given simultaneously. This approach has not been tested in the clinic because of the fear that the simultaneous use of more than five cytotoxic drugs at full doses would not be possible. Alternatives to using all available effective drugs simultaneously, such as using alternating cycles of equally effective, non-cross-resistant drug combinations, are being tested. Unfortunately, many studies reported to test the Goldie–Coldman hypothesis have been poorly designed. Usually inadequate testing has been done to determine whether the alternate combination is truly non-cross-resistant and equally effective as the primary treatment, which it must be to fulfill the hypothesis. A more recent approach is the use of half of the drugs of each effective combination on days 1 and 8, respectively (hybrid combinations). This approach is being tried in patients with Hodgkin's disease and diffuse large cell lymphomas. At this juncture, the use of alternating cycles of combination chemotherapy has not yet proved to be more effective than full doses of a single effective combination program.

In reality, no rigid schedule can accommodate all the variables assumed to be important for maximum effectiveness of combination chemotherapy and the requirements of the patients in the practice of medical oncology. Physicians often must adjust doses at intervals to administer drugs safely. The surety that the therapeutic effect of a drug or drug combination can be lost if the dose or schedule is drastically altered should temper these judgments. Reductions in dose rates also often result only in minimal decreases in toxicity. Both the physician and the patient must consider the risk of dying from cancer along with the transient benefits of reducing the side-effects of treatment. Adhering to the standard sliding scale for dose adjustments, usually published with most new treatments, is the most useful approach to follow. In addition to providing guidelines for dose reduction, these sliding scales provide consistency between patients and between studies by preserving both the intervals between cycles and the integrity of the drug combination. These points should be made clear to patients as part of the informed consent process if they are to share intelligently in decisions about dose modifications made by their physicians.[100]

USES OF CHEMOTHERAPY AS PART OF THE INITIAL TREATMENT OF CANCER

There are four ways chemotherapy is generally used[101]: (1) as induction treatment for advanced disease, (2) as an adjunct to the local methods of treatment, (3) as the primary treatment of patients who present with localized cancer, and (4) by direct installation into sanctuaries or by site-directed perfusion of specific regions of the body most affected by the cancer.

INDUCTION CHEMOTHERAPY. The term *induction chemotherapy* has been used to describe the drug therapy given as the primary treatment for patients who present with advanced cancer for which no alternative treatment exists.[102] Selection of treatment is based on the effectiveness of the cancer drugs in rodent models. Combinations of drugs are fashioned based on the effectiveness, level of cross-resistance, and limiting toxicity of the available drugs when used alone in similar patient populations. Patients who fail after one drug treatment and require further chemotherapy pose a particularly difficult treatment problem because of the volume of tumor, their poor general health, and drug resistance. Induction chemotherapy in these patients is referred to as *salvage treatment.*

ADJUVANT CHEMOTHERAPY. Adjuvant chemotherapy denotes the use of systemic treatment after the primary tumor has been removed by an alternative method. The selection of adjuvant treatment program is based on response rates in separate groups of patients with advanced cancers of the same histologic type; the selection of suitable population of patients for adjuvant treatment is based on their risk of recurrence after local treatment alone and on disease variables known to adversely influence prognosis.

PRIMARY CHEMOTHERAPY. Primary chemotherapy denotes the use of chemotherapy as initial treatment for patients who present with localized cancer for which there is an alternative but less than completely effective treatment. This has been described as *neoadjuvant chemotherapy,*[103] but the term *primary chemotherapy*[104] is more accurate. Since the likelihood of development of spontaneous resistant cell lines relates to tumor mass, earlier drug treatment in the form of primary chemotherapy may have the advantage of treatment in the presence of fewer drug-resistant lines, although this point is questionable because the time interval, in practice, between chemotherapy used as adjuvant treatment, after tumor has been removed, or as primary treatment at the time of diagnosis can sometimes be only a few weeks.[105] Primary chemotherapy does have the potential to downstage tumors by decreasing the size and extent of the presenting tumor mass. This can influence both the need for, and radical nature of, the subsequent alternative treatment by influencing operability and/or decreasing tumor hypoxia, and by increasing the effectiveness of a given dose of radiation therapy or decreasing the size of the radiation therapy field. The theoretical disadvantages of primary chemotherapy are that by leaving the primary tumor mass in place, even temporarily, the tumor volume faced by chemotherapy is actually larger than if surgery or radiation therapy were used first and chemotherapy were used as an adjunct. Also, the favorable influence of resection of the primary tumor on the kinetics of proliferation of the residual micrometastases may be lost.[106] In addition, the toxicity of chemotherapy may impair the effectiveness and increase the side-effects of subsequent alternative treatments, and may delay the use of an alternative treatment sufficiently to have an impact on the outcome. As in the case of adjuvant chemotherapy, patients who would otherwise be cured by local treatment alone are exposed to the acute and chronic side-effects of chemotherapy in combined modality programs.

CLINICAL END POINTS IN EVALUATING RESPONSE TO CHEMOTHERAPY

In induction chemotherapy for advanced cancer it is possible to determine the response to drugs on a case by case basis. The partial response rate, usually defined as the fraction of patients who demonstrate a 50% or greater reduction in measurable tumor mass, usually is not of much clinical value because such responses are usually short in duration, but it is useful in the testing of new drug programs to determine whether the particular experimental approach is worth pursuing further. The most important indicator of effectiveness of chemotherapy is the complete response rate. It is the prerequisite for cure. When new programs consistently produce more than an occasional complete remission, they have invariably later proved of practical value in medical practice. The qualitative and quantitative differences in the clinical value between a complete and partial response is such that complete responses should always be reported separately. The most important indicator of the quality of a complete remission is the relapse-free survival from the time all treatment is discontinued. This is the only clinical counterpart of the quantifiable cytoreductive effect of drugs in rodent systems. The current trend in many clinical protocols to use freedom from progression in complete and partial responders combined as an indicator of the practical potential of a new treatment obscures the value of a relapse-free survival of complete responders as the major determinant of the quality of remission. Other end points such as median response duration or median survival are of little practical value until treatment results have been refined to the point that the complete response rate is over 50%.

There was great excitement concomitant with the move to the use of chemotherapy as an adjunct to local treatments, or adjuvant chemotherapy. The promise was great because tumor volume is at a minimum when adjuvant therapy is initiated, and it was assumed that either a much higher cure rate could be achieved or treatment intensity could be reduced and side-effects thereby diminished. Failure to appreciate the circumstances surrounding the assessment of response to adjuvant chemotherapy is the source of some of the current disillusionment with the positive but less than dramatic results achieved with adjuvant chemotherapy of common tumors such as breast and colorectal cancer.[107,108] The major indicator of effectiveness, the complete remission rate, is lost in the adjuvant setting, since the primary tumor has already been removed. Treatment is selected for individual patients based on response rates in entirely different populations of patients with advanced disease with the same histologic type. While relapse-free survival remains the major end point, the micrometastases in treated patients could consist of tumor cells either sensitive or resistant to chemotherapy. The relapse-free survival in the adjuvant setting, therefore, measures the equivalent of the duration of remission of both complete and partial responders as well as the interval of regrowth in patients who would have been classified as nonresponders, and is similar to the use of freedom from progression in patients with advanced disease. Attempts to use in vitro assays of drug sensitivity from biopsy material of primary tumors (see below) to overcome the shortcomings of the absence of an indicator of individual response have not proved practical.

The unique feature of primary chemotherapy in patients with localized tumor is preservation of the presenting tumor mass as a biologic marker of responsiveness to anticancer drugs. Thus, as with induction chemotherapy, it is possible to determine, on a case by case basis, the potential effectiveness of a new treatment program. By definition, the presenting tumor mass is also the largest aggregate of tumor in the body and historically the oldest, and thus the aggregate mass of tumor cells most likely to contain one or more resistant cell lines.[105] It is also a mass with the least favorable cell kinetics. It is reasonable to assume, then, that whatever the effect of chemotherapy the physician sees on the primary tumor, a similar or greater effect is occurring fairly uniformly in micrometastatic deposits, unless a metastasizing cell line phenotypically is one that spontaneously develops drug resistance. Although there is no direct evidence for the latter occurrence, such an event would explain the clinical observation of control of the primary tumor with chemotherapy, with death resulting from uncontrolled metastases at a distant site. A poor response of the primary tumor to chemotherapy clearly indicates a group of patients for which alternative methods of treatment should be used and used quickly. Another feature of primary chemotherapy is the ability to delineate partial responders with varying degrees of prognosis, as determined by the state of the residual tumor mass after an initial good but partial response. Removal and histologic examination of residual masses allows determination of the viability of remaining tissue. Obviously, the response duration of these categories of responders must be determined separately.

The most important issue facing investigators of primary chemotherapy is whether or not an effective primary chemotherapy treatment, pursued flexibly and intensively to the point of the complete remission, plus two or more additional cycles of treatment, will define a significant fraction of patients whose disease is cured by chemotherapy, with or without the addition of alternative treatments. In carefully selected patients with some stages of the most common tumors for which there is less than satisfactory standard treatment, such studies are ethically and theoretically sound and are being pursued. Such an approach could result in shorter duration, less morbid, and more effective treatment programs. In some tumor types such as localized diffuse large cell lymphomas, limited-stage small cell cancers, some pediatric malignancies, and some subsets of head and neck cancers, primary chemotherapy has already become the standard of treatment.[101]

SPECIAL USES OF CHEMOTHERAPY

Special uses of chemotherapy include the installation of drugs into the spinal fluid, either directly through a lumbar puncture needle or into an implanted Ommaya reservoir, to treat meningeal leukemia and lymphoma; the installation of drugs into the pleural or pericardial space to control effusions; splenic infusion to control spleen size; hepatic artery infusion to treat hepatic metastases selectively; carotid artery infusion to treat head and neck cancers and brain tumors; and the intraperitoneal installation of drugs using dialysis techniques. These uses are discussed throughout this book in relation to specific cancers. In all cases the rationale for directed chemotherapy is based on achieving a greater $C \times T$ against the target tumor tissue, and the sparing of normal tissue. The place of intracerebrospinal fluid and intrapleural administration of drugs is already established. Hepatic infusion of chemotherapy has been simplified and improved by the development of technology for infusion of drugs sufficient to reevaluate these approaches (see Chap. 64). It is now possible to measure both the active principle of cancer drugs and their targets, within the biologic range, and drugs can be infused in timing with the body's circadian rhythm.

The intraperitoneal administration of drugs to treat ovarian cancer, a disease that kills almost exclusively by local effects in the abdomen, is now commonly used because it allows wide distribution of antitumor drugs in the smallest interstices of the abdominal cavity, and a greater $C \times T$ at the tumor is achieved (see Chaps. 34 and 64).[109–111] The concentration of drug available in the peritoneal cavity for some drugs with this "belly bath" technique far exceeds the plasma level achievable with systemic administration. The effects are particularly marked for drugs like 5-fluorouracil, which is metabolized in the liver as well as excreted by the kidney, and drugs like Adriamycin and cisplatin, which, because of their molecular size, diffuse more slowly across the peritoneal membrane.

Drugs can also be encompassed in lipid bilayer droplets called liposomes.[112–114] The surface characteristics of liposomes can be altered to direct their delivery to specific organ sites or into resistant cell lines. Labile liposomes that dissolve at temperatures of 41°C can deposit drugs selectively in preheated areas.[113] A drawback to liposomes, however, is their failure to leave the vascular system except in the sinusoids of the liver and the spleen, and thus far liposome encapsulation of drugs for targeted delivery has been of limited value.[114]

IN VITRO TESTS TO SELECT CHEMOTHERAPEUTIC AGENTS FOR INDIVIDUALIZED TREATMENT

Short-term assays are not useful for determining the primary treatment for patients for whom a known effective treatment exists. They are of minimal value for the remainder of newly diagnosed patients and for those with drug-sensitive tumors who fail the first trial of chemotherapy. They can be of use to avoid patient exposure to the toxicity of drugs that are unlikely to be effective, but in general, the tests are too cumbersome and expensive for routine practice. No convincing reports in the literature have indicated that short-term assays provide additional benefit over what the clinician can provide by using good judgment and a knowledge of the effectiveness of the limited number of available single agents.

In vitro assays can be divided into three types: (1) clonogenic assays, usually conducted in soft agar media, (2) short-term culture techniques performed in defined media, and (3) short-term biochemical assays, which include histologic, or radioautographic measurements on cells exposed to chemotherapy on a short-term basis.

CLONOGENIC ASSAYS. Clonogenic assays have the advantage that they measure the response of those cells that theoretically have the capacity to reproduce themselves and ultimately kill the host.[115,116] They suffer from the disadvantage that single-cell suspensions are required, with the resulting loss of normal cell–cell interactions. Plating efficiency is also low, and cells already committed to differentiate may also form colonies. In addition, cells in the G_0 growth phase, capable of reentering the growth cycle, are not assayed, and the limited range of clonogenic assays (1- to 2-log kill) is insufficiently sensitive to predict drug sensitivity.[115-118]

In numerous reports the value for true predictions of sensitivity of the clonogenic assay is consistently around 65%, and the figure for true prediction of resistance is consistently about 90%. Two thirds of tumors predicted to be sensitive ultimately respond to the drug selected, and 10% of those predicted to be resistant respond to drugs predicted to be ineffective. An interesting illustration of problems with the use of the clonogenic system has been provided by Twentyman,[119] using data of Von Hoff.[120,121] In Von Hoff's reports, of 8000 tumors cultured, only 2480 (31%) grew enough colonies for testing; therefore, no prediction was possible in 6320 patients whose samples were sent for testing. In only 198 (8%) of the patients whose tissues proved sufficient for testing was the prediction of sensitivity made; of these, 139 responded in vivo but 59 did not. Another 2280 tumors were predicted to be resistant, 228 of these incorrectly so. No survival benefit was found for patients whose tumor cells responded in short-term clonogenic assay over those whose cells did not respond. Therefore, for the vast majority of patients, the assay was of little use in selecting a usable treatment.

DYE EXCLUSION ASSAY. A simple dye exclusion assay has been used by Weisenthal and associates on cells in short-term culture. Cells are stained with the fast green dye and counterstained with hematoxylin–eosin.[122-125] The true response rate is equivalent to that of the clonogenic assay.[124] The major advantages of this assay are its short duration and the fact that relatively unskilled personnel can be trained to read the slides and evaluate the majority of specimens. In a prospective trial it has been used as the assay to determine the potential effectiveness of drugs for small cell lung cancer in permanently derived cell lines.[126] In the experimental arm of this study patients are treated with a predetermined program while cell lines are established, and switched at week 13 of treatment, if response has been less than complete, to three drugs selected on the basis of the dye exclusion assay. Preliminary results suggest some benefit in patients whose continued treatment was selected from results of this in vitro assay.

HUMAN–MURINE XENOGRAFTS. Human xenografts implanted under the renal capsule of athymic mice have been used by Bogden and co-workers as a rapid 6-day screening method.[127] A retrospective and prospective clinical trial has been performed with this assay in 837 patients who contributed 1,000 specimens; 858 (85%) of the specimens resulted in an evaluable assay.[128] The test predicted clinical response in 82% of tumors and clinical resistance in 94%, and thus was comparable to the clonogenic assay. The advantage of this assay is that it retains the spatial relationships of the tumor because cell–cell contact is maintained in the whole fragments that are implanted under the renal capsule. Multiple assays can also be done on tissue from the same patient in 6 days. While this test has a high assay evaluability rate, and allows testing of compounds requiring in vivo activation, it is expensive, particularly since a histologic end point is used, and the testing facility must maintain a very large mouse colony.

Recently, the human–murine xenograft assay was performed with surgical specimens from about 400 patients. In heavily treated patients with drug-resistant, far-advanced cancer, the test identified some active drugs yielding good responses.[129] However, use of surgical specimens for the xenograft assay depends critically on the selection of tumor for implantation and requires long experience.

MICROENCAPSULATION ASSAY. A microencapsulation technique has been recently described[115,130-132] in which human tumor cells encapsulated in 1-mm microcapsules with semipermeable membranes are injected intraperitoneally into nude mice.[130] Chemotherapeutic agents are administered intravenously, and the microcapsules are harvested to determine cell survivability in the treated animals compared to untreated controls. Several properties of the tumor microencapsulation assay make it attractive as a potential future test for drug selection. The antitumor activity of drugs can be tested against human tumor cells under conditions that provide for three-dimensional growth and an in vivo supply of nutrients; the sensitivity of tumor cells can be assessed following exposure to drugs in concentrations achievable in vivo; compounds requiring in vivo metabolic activation can be tested; the effect of each drug injection can be quickly evaluated; the inhibition of tumor cell proliferation versus the cytoreductive effects of drugs can be discriminated; the test is applicable to virtually all histologic types of tumor cells; and the assay is short term, simple, and relatively inexpensive. In the studies reported, the antitumor effects were consistent with the relative therapeutic efficacy or level of resistance to drugs detected by other in vitro and in vivo tests.

OTHER ASSAYS. Other tests have included use of monolayer cultures of cell maintained in short-term cultures in defined medium.[133-135] Further evaluation of newer assays will be required to determine if any of these tests can provide practical assistance to physicians in their choice of treatment, but the usefulness of all tests will likely remain limited as long as the pool of available drugs remains small.

CANCER DRUG DEVELOPMENT

The steps in the development of anticancer drugs are shown in Figure 16-6 and discussed below.

SCREENING

The most important step in the drug selection process is mass screening, the mechanism used to narrow the universe of chemicals potentially useful for the treatment of human cancers to a manageable number of high priority drugs for clinical testing.[136-139]

From its inception in 1955 until 1975, the mainstay of NCI's screening program was the murine L1210 leukemia.

ACQUISITION
↓
SCREENING
↓
PRODUCTION AND FORMULATION
↓
TOXICOLOGY
↓
PHASE I CLINICAL TRIALS
↓
PHASE II CLINICAL TRIALS
↓
PHASE III—IV CLINICAL TRIALS
↓
GENERAL MEDICAL PRACTICE

FIG. 16-6. Steps in cancer drug development.

Drugs found to be active against L1210 were evaluated in other rodent tumors for dose and schedule dependency, but entrance into the clinic was almost exclusively based on the antitumor effect in L1210. Many currently available anticancer drugs active against human leukemias and lymphomas were identified and developed as a result of this system. The input to this type of screening program reached its maximum of 40,000 compounds screened per year in 1975. In 1975 a major change was made in the NCI's screening program because of the availability of new rodent models. More rational selection of compounds was coupled with a panel of transplantable rodent tumor screens designed to match the histologic type of common visceral cancers. These rodent solid tumor screens were matched to human tumor cell lines of the same type grown in nude mice. This panel posed the question of the clinical specificity of the preclinical models. Because of the expense of high volume screening in such a panel, however, a prescreening system was necessary, and prescreening was performed in the rodent P388 mouse leukemia, a leukemia more sensitive to natural products than L1210. An agent shown to have activity against P388 leukemia was passed to the tumor panel where, if antitumor effect was noted, the agent was advanced to clinical trial. The prescreen had the effect of biasing selection of compounds toward those traditionally selected by rodent leukemias. The panel of tumors was changed periodically to pose additional questions to the screening process.[140] Later, human tumors grown in soft agar, and under the renal capsule, were also introduced into the screening program to further test the hypothesis that the use of human tissue in short-term assays could better select compounds more active in the clinic than could simpler rodent tumor models. Problems with the technical details of these in vitro systems led to their discontinuation.[140,143]

As it became possible to maintain human tumor cells in defined media, the screening program was again changed by developing disease-oriented panels of human tumor cell lines grown in defined media.[144,145] The initial selection of cell lines for this screening panel was based on several considerations, including (1) representatives of major histologic subtypes, (2) utilization of multiple cell lines for each tumor type, and (3) utilization of cell lines that retain appropriate features of the tumor of origin. The cell lines now in use include lung, ovarian, and renal cancer, malignant melanoma, brain tumors, and leukemia. Because of the interest in the phenomenon of multidrug resistance and the likelihood that it is one of the factors limiting the effectiveness of chemotherapy, the MCF-7 cell line, a human breast cancer line, and an MDR variant of MCF-7 selected for resistance to Adriamycin are included, along with a P388 murine leukemia and a comparable Adriamycin-induced MDR variant of P388. These cell lines provide the potential for identifying new agents with particular activity against MDR cell populations.

A key element in screening strategy is to maintain the capacity for high volume screening. The most promising assay available to do this is a colorimetric growth inhibition assay that is based on the metabolic reduction of the tetrazolium salt formazan inside viable cells. Under appropriate conditions, a linear relationship is obtained between viable cell number and formazan optical density, measured using a standard ELISA plate reader.[147] Automation of this assay has made it possible to maintain an adequate volume of in vitro screening (10,000 compounds per year) at less expense. Preliminary analysis of screening results indicate that individual cell lines show characteristic degrees of in vitro chemosensitivity to individual test compounds with known patterns of clinical activity. Ease of automation of the colorimetric assay and the stability of the cell lines have largely overcome the technical problems associated with clonogenic or subrenal capsular assays.[143,148] The central goal of the in vitro–based disease-oriented screening program is to identify new antitumor drug candidates that would not have been discovered by the previously available screening program. Clinical testing of these new leads, as with previous versions of preclinical screening, will ultimately be the only way to establish or disprove the validity of the new screen for identifying new drugs active against the common refractory human solid tumors.

In the early days of screening, acquisition of agents was purely random. Random acquisition of chemicals for screening was associated with two major problems: repetitious screening of compounds already tested, and screening of analogs of drugs already known to be active, rather than the identification of new structures. Modern molecular biologic techniques present an unusual opportunity to select materials, defined at the molecular level, that might prove useful in inhibition of vital cell functions. To take advantage of new technology and to reduce the randomness of screening, the NCI has established drug discovery groups, consortia of investigators in academia, government, and industry funded to deal with the development of potential new types of chemicals such as those that inhibit polyamine biosynthesis, oncogene products, the sense message of DNA (antisense message compounds), and inhibitors of topoisomerase II. Still, some collection of compounds on a random basis is required, and the NCI's chemical collection program for screening also emphasizes the collection of natural products from a wide variety of terrestrial and marine sources over collection of synthetic chemicals. This emphasis follows directly from the realization that many of the most useful agents in the therapy of human diseases of all kinds are natural products and that the microbial, plant, and marine worlds are a virtually inexhaustible source of biologically active novel compounds that provide important leads for subsequent structural modification. Also, with the introduction of high-speed computers capable of performing 100 million calculations per second and possessing sophisticated graphics capability, the possibility of designing compounds based on known characteristics of presumed targets has now become a realistic goal. These supercomputers can graphically illustrate the nature of chemicals capable of binding to specific receptors, and chemical synthesis can be simulated through computer programs developed to synthesize complex molecules based on known synthetic reactions. The future of the design of new anticancer drugs may lie in the capacity of these high-speed computers to offer compounds designed on a rational basis for later biologic testing.

Inherent in all screening systems is the tenet that biologic activity in some preclinical system must be demonstrated before human testing is performed. To date, no currently marketed, useful anticancer agent is devoid of such preclinical antitumor effect. Workers in cancer drug development often face advocates for various anticancer agents who, by reason of theory or personal interest, believe their material shows great promise as a human cancer treatment. Whether compounds selected for theoretical reasons, without demonstrated biologic activity in rodent systems, might be effective in human tumors has never been adequately tested. Without demonstrated activity in an in vitro system or in one of the many rodent systems available, the decision usually is not to initiate clinical testing of such materials. Given the need to use some selection criteria to narrow the choice of drugs for clinical trials, screening systems are likely to remain the mainstay for decision-making.

FORMULATION AND TOXICOLOGY TESTING

Formulation and production of anticancer drugs, required before anticancer drugs can proceed to toxicology studies and clinical trials, often present formidable obstacles for chemists. Anticancer agents with considerable activity in rodents have been discarded for lack of an adequate formulation for human use. This is particularly true of the more complicated products extracted from plants. Once these formulation problems have been solved, however, preclinical testing for toxicity is a requirement of development. Then, the Food and Drug Administration (FDA) will approve an investigational new drug application (INDA) that permits clinical testing.

Toxicology testing has evolved over the last decade from complicated testing in rodents, dogs, and monkeys to a less expensive and simpler system that relies on toxicity testing primarily in mice. Large amounts of data accumulated since the beginning of anticancer drug development have allowed comparisons to be made across species with respect to common toxicity of chemicals. These data have shown that there is no real safety advantage in using larger animal species instead of rodents. In the current system, implemented in 1980, the dose–response curve of a new drug is first developed in mice. The lethal dose (LD) in 10%, 50%, and 90% of animals is determined and the reproducible lethal dose in 10% of tested animals (LD_{10}) is used as the basis for establishing the initial dose in clinical trials. Usually, 10% of the LD_{10} dose in rodents is selected for the initial human dose; this dose is first tested for toxicity in dogs, prior to use in humans, to minimize the risks associated with administering an unknown compound to humans. Although correlation of toxic effects on rapidly dividing normal tissue among rodents, dogs, monkeys, and humans is good, correlation of other toxic effects is not as consistent.[149] Therefore routine pathologic examination of rodent tissue is not always performed prior to clinical testing.

TRANSLATION OF DOSES ACROSS SPECIES. All drugs should be given in reference to either body weight or surface area. The preferable reference point is body surface area, because better cross-species comparisons can be made and because doses calculated from body surface area allow doses to be determined for adults and children without further adjustment. The assumptions leading to the dose conversion factors have been described in detail by Freireich and coworkers[24] and are shown in Table 16-6, which is useful in converting doses in milligrams per kilogram to the comparable milligram per square meter dose. Table 16-7 shows the procedure for conversion of a milligram per kilogram dose in rodents, monkeys, or dogs to the equivalent dose in man.

TABLE 16-6. Representative Surface Area to Weight Ratios (km) of Various Species*

Species	*Body Weight (kg)*	*Surface Area*	*Surface Area to Weight Ratio (km)*
Mouse	0.02	0.0066	3.0
Rat	0.15	0.025	5.9
Monkey	3	0.24	12
Dog	8	0.40	20
Human			
Child	20	0.80	25
Adult	60	1.6	37

* To express a mg/kg dose in any given species as the equivalent mg/m^2 dose, multiply the dose by the appropriate *km*. In the adult human, for example, 100 mg/kg is equivalent to 100 mg/kg× 37 kg/m^2 = 3700 mg/m^2.

TABLE 16-7. Equivalent Surface Area Dosage Conversion Factors*

	Mouse, 20 g	*Rat, 150 g*	*Monkey, 3.0 kg*	*Dog, 8 kg*	*Man, 60 kg*
Mouse	1	½	¼	⅙	1/12
Rat	2	1	½	¼	1/7
Monkey	4	2	1	⅗	⅓
Dog	6	4	⁵⁄₃	1	½
Man	12	7	3	2	1

* This table gives approximate factors for converting doses expressed in terms of mg/kg from one species to an equivalent *surface area* dose expressed in the same terms mg/kg in the other species. For example, given a dose of 50 mg/kg in the mouse, what is the appropriate dose in man assuming equivalency on the basis of mg/m^2?

$$50 \text{ mg/kg} \times 1/12 = 4.1 \text{ mg/kg}$$

EARLY CLINICAL TRIALS OF ANTITUMOR AGENTS

Antitumor agents go through four phases of clinical testing before they are accepted for general medical practice, marketed, or discarded (Fig. 16-6).[137,150–153] The average time from discovery of an effective antitumor agent to marketing of that agent is quite long, in the range of 10 to 12 years. To facilitate access to drugs for desperately ill cancer patients before the drugs are marketed, anticancer drugs with known efficacy are made available to physicians by the NCI in the premarketing phase (Tables 16-8 and 16-9).

Table 16-10 details the phases of clinical testing and the main purpose of each step. Phase I trials are done on small groups of patients, usually no more than 15 to 30 per study. Although the main purpose of Phase I trials is to identify a maximally tolerated dose (MTD) in one of several schedules suggested by the preclinical data, patients are entered into Phase I trials with therapeutic intent. For most of the effective anticancer drugs, some therapeutic effect was often seen even in Phase I trials. Because a limited number of patients with a variety of diseases are treated in Phase I trials, and doses may be below the ultimate therapeutic range in a fraction of the patients, the absence of any positive effect in a Phase I trial is not sufficient reason to discontinue testing of a drug. The only reason not to proceed to a Phase II study is prohibitive toxicity in Phase I trials. Escalation of doses in Phase I trials is usually done by a modified Fibonacci system.[150] Doses are first doubled and then increased at decreasing increments of 66%, 50%, and 33% in succeeding groups of patients (usually three at a time) until limiting toxicity is noted. Recently, attempts have been made to rationalize and accelerate dose escalation by the systematic use of preclinical pharmacologic data.[154] This approach has relied on the assumption that the elimination rate of a drug determines its C × T, and further assumes that for agents showing no major differences in target cell sensitivity, schedule dependence, or toxicity between mouse and man, the C × T at the mouse LD_{10} and the human MTD should be similar. These assumptions lead naturally to a simple algorithm for escalating doses by targeting the human C × T in a Phase I trial to the mouse C × T at LD_{10}.[155] The steps are as follows: (1) determine the mouse LD_{10} (part of the routine preclinical toxicology testing discussed earlier), (2) determine the

TABLE 16-8. National Cancer Institute Classification of New Anticancer Drugs in Clinical Testing

Group A Drugs
This group includes drugs in Phase I clinical trials and Phase II clinical trials in specified tumors. Protocol acceptance and drug distribution are limited to clinical investigators.

Group B Drugs
This group includes drugs already tested in initial Phase II studies and of clinical interest. Protocol acceptance and drug distribution are extended more broadly to clinical cooperative groups, NCI contractors, and cancer centers.

*Group C Drugs**
Group C includes drugs that demonstrate efficacy within a tumor type in more than one study, that alter the pattern of care of the disease in question, and that are administered safely by properly trained physicians without requiring specialized supportive care facilities. This group includes the following:

1. Azacytidine (NSC 102816)—for refractory acute myelogenous leukemia
2. Ervinia asparaginase (NSC 106977)—for acute lymphatic leukemia in patients sensitive to *E. coli* L-asparaginase
3. Hexamethylmelamine (NSC 13875)—for ovarian carcinoma
4. Amsacrine (NSE 249992)—for refractory myelogenous leukemia

* Drugs in Group C are available for use by physicians for specific indications.

TABLE 16-9. Procedure for Obtaining Drugs in Group C of the National Cancer Institute New Anticancer Drug Classification

A physician must be registered with the NCI as an investigator having completed an FDA-Form 1573.
A written request for the drug, indicating the disease to be treated, must be submitted.
Use of the drugs shall be limited to indications outlined in the guidelines that will be provided to the physician.
All adverse reactions must be reported to the Investigational Drug Branch, DCT, NCI.
Office of the Chief, Investigational Drug Branch, CTEP*, DCT, National Cancer Institute, 7910 Woodmont Avenue, Landow Building, Room 4A22, Bethesda, MD 20892 (301-496-6138).

* CTEP = Cancer Therapy Evaluation Program.

TABLE 16-10. Stages in the Clinical Testing of New Anticancer Agents

Stage of Drug Testing	*Objectives*	*Patient Population Studied*
PHASE I	*Determine Tolerance*	
	Maximally tolerable dose (MTD)	Histologically confirmed advanced malignancy
	Limiting toxicity	No longer amenable to conventional therapy
	Reversibility of toxicity	
	Proper schedule	Physiologically well compensated
		A variety of tumor types per study permissible
	Pharmacology	
	Bioavailability	
	Plasma clearance	
	Biotransformation	
	Excretion	
	Therapeutic Effect	
	Secondary	
PHASE II	*Therapeutic Effect*	
	Determine effectiveness in a panel of human tumors	Histologically confirmed advanced malignancy
	Dose-response relationships	Measurable tumor masses
		No longer amenable to conventional therapy
		A variety of tumor types in groups of 15 to 30
		Physiologically well compensated
	Nontherapeutic Effects	
	Toxicity in relationship to therapeutic effect	
PHASE III	*Therapeutic Effectiveness*	
	Compare experimental therapy to existing standard therapy	Histologically confirmed malignancy Patient sample must be of adequate size and uniformity Usually previously untreated
	Nontherapeutic Effects	
	Are toxic effects tolerable in the context of observed therapeutic effect and in comparison to standard therapy?	Controls usually are selected randomly, but on occasion historical controls are used
PHASE IV	*Therapeutic Effectiveness*	
	Integration of drug therapy into primary treatment in combination with surgery or radiation therapy (*e.g.,* postoperative drug treatment in breast cancer)	Histologically confirmed malignancy Patient sample must be of adequate size and uniformity Controls usually randomized
	Compared to current standard program	
	Nontherapeutic Effects	
	Are toxic effects sufficiently minimal to risk giving drug to patients whose tumor will not necessarily recur?	
	Long-term toxic effects require monitoring (second tumors, sterility, marrow aplasia)	

mouse C × T at LD_{10}, (3) begin human testing at a safe starting dose (currently one-tenth of the mouse-equivalent LD_{10}), (4) determine the human C × T at the starting dose in Phase I, and (5) escalate doses in subsequent patients based on how close the C × T at the starting dose is to the target C × T. Preliminary studies have suggested that application of this procedure may save 20% to 50% of escalation steps for many agents. This approach is now being tested prospectively in NCI's Phase I testing program.

The definition of a dose as maximally tolerated depends on how much toxicity the patient and physician are willing and able to tolerate. It has been amply demonstrated that for several drugs such as cyclophosphamide, thiotepa, BCNU, and etoposide, the MTD as determined from toxic effects other than bone marrow suppression is 3 to 10 times higher than the conventional MTD determined by granulocytopenia. The fact that the response rates are commonly a function of dose gives strong impetus to further trials exploring the upper end of the dose curve. As a result, an alternative approach to Phase I testing is under consideration, that is, to redefine the MTD as the dose beyond which unacceptable non-marrow-related toxicity supervenes despite deployment of all modern aspects of care. At the moment it seems prudent to delay decisions on escalation of new agents past the conventionally determined MTD until more information about their clinical characteristics is at hand. This approach should be greatly facilitated by the availability of colony-stimulating factors if they succeed in eliminating bone marrow suppression as the rate-limiting step in early testing.

The purpose of Phase II studies is to develop estimates of the response rate of patients with specified tumor types to a particular drug. Phase II studies determine activity, rather than efficacy, and answer a biologic as well as a clinical question. However, since Phase II study results do determine whether a new treatment should be pursued further, the outcome of the Phase II trial is clearly a decisive point in a drug's development. Specifically, a Phase II testing program should be constructed so as to (1) minimize the chance of a false negative result, (2) maximize the chance of benefit to the individual study patient, and (3) minimize the number of patients treated with drugs that turn out to be inactive. During the 1970s the NCI created a clinical Phase II panel to match the preclinical screening panel in histologic types to create a sufficiently large data base to permit validation of the transplantable murine screen as predictive of clinical activity in corresponding tumor types. An analysis of these data is currently in progress but reveals little correlation between murine and clinical activity for corresponding histologies.

When a drug enters Phase II testing in individual diseases, it should be tested in the patient group that is most likely to show a favorable effect, provided it is ethically permissible to do so. Failure to do this increases the chance of missing potentially useful activity. Obviously, this criterion is best fulfilled by enrolling patients with advanced cancer but who have maximum performance status, minimal heterogeneity of metastatic sites, and a minimal amount of prior chemotherapy.[156] This means that for tumors sensitive to chemotherapy, patients who have failed no more than one prior regimen are ideal for study. For the less sensitive epithelial cancers in many cases previously untreated patients can be entered into Phase II studies. In view of the poor track record of the large majority of single agents in heavily pretreated patients with advanced disease, such a strategy seems sensible, since for patients with advanced drug-resistant cancer, the likelihood of toxicity is vastly greater than the likelihood of therapeutic benefit.

The number of patients accrued to Phase II trials should be appropriate for the scientific goals of the study. Under the best of circumstances, a drug that produces no antitumor effect in 14 patients with the same tumor type, particularly if the heterogeneity of the distribution of metastases is minimized, has a greater than 95% chance of being ineffective against that tumor and could reasonably be dropped from further studies against that specific cancer. One or two responses, however, increase the chance of efficacy sufficiently to dictate an expansion of the trial to 30 or more patients, in order not to miss a drug with a response rate in the 20% range. In general, partial response rates in excess of 20% place the agent in a category of potential clinical usefulness to be determined in further studies. Response rates in the range of 5% to 10% are consistent with observer variation in Phase II trials. Response rates below 20% can be meaningful, however, if the quality of the response is good. For example, a few complete remissions, even if the overall frequency of complete response is low, should lead to a decision to proceed with further testing in that disease since complete disappearance of disease, however infrequent, is an important sign of a potentially effective new treatment. Because multiple doses and schedules may be tested, a Phase II trial for each drug, schedule, and tumor type is required before a drug can be disqualified from further clinical use. Given all these confounding variables, a complete Phase II trial often requires 600 or more patients.

At the completion of a Phase II trial, a decision is made to proceed with or discard the agent. This decision is based on lack of efficacy or excessive or intolerable toxicity, given the observed therapeutic effect. Because it is not possible to test each new agent against every tumor type, the potential for discarding agents that might be useful in rare tumors is significant. The early testing results of cisplatin are particularly instructive. Cisplatin showed very little activity against the common tumors in its early testing, its use was associated with considerable toxicity, and it was almost discarded. Incidental testing in patients with testicular cancer, who were not generally part of major Phase II studies, revealed interesting activity, and cisplatin was very quickly advanced to inclusion with other drugs to treat testicular cancer with curative intent. As a result, very little data on its single agent activity was available to the FDA in its appraisal of the new drug application, and marketing was delayed. This drug has now proved to be not only the mainstay of curative treatment of advanced testicular cancer, but an important part of the therapy of bladder cancer, head and neck cancer, ovarian cancer, and other common tumors.

If a drug is found effective in Phase II trials, Phase III and IV testing establishes its place in the therapeutic armamentarium. These clinical trials usually require large numbers of

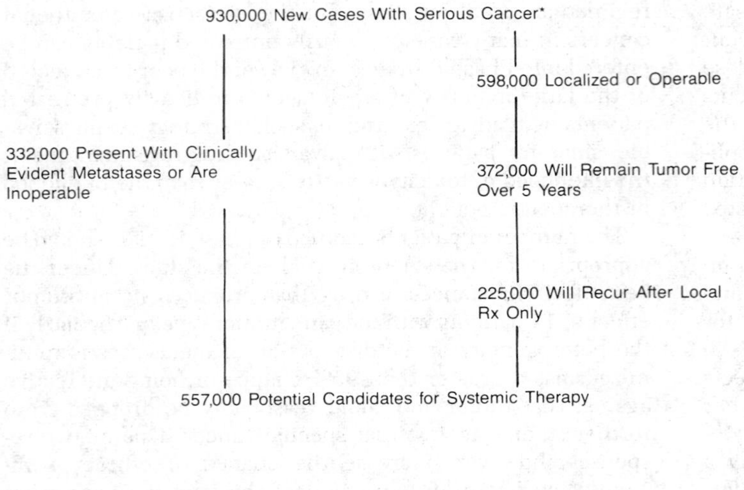

*Total is 1,531,000; 580,000 cases of skin and in situ cervix and breast cancer are excluded.

FIG. 16-7. Distribution of cancer patients according to presentation and type of treatment. (Derived from 1986 data from the NCI's Surveillance, Epidemiology and End Results [SEER] Program)

patients and are difficult to perform. The issue of randomized versus historical controls in Phase III and IV trials is an important one and is discussed in detail in Chapter 19.

THE IMPACT OF CANCER CHEMOTHERAPY

Figure 16-7, using 1986 data, shows an estimate of the distribution of localized and advanced cancers in the United States. The majority of newly diagnosed cancer patients in 1986 (598,000) presented with what appeared to be localized cancers. These patients are primarily managed by surgeons and radiation therapists, with or without the help of medical and pediatric oncologists, and the goal of treatment at this stage is cure. Those who present with either clinically evident metastases (320,000 in 1986) or with recurrences after local treatment for localized tumor (225,000) are usually seen by medical oncologists because the correct treatment is systemic therapy. Thus, the total number of patients per year who might receive systemic therapy (557,000, based on 1986 data) is sizable. In recent years some patients in the latter two groups have also become candidates for treatment with surgery for metastases with curative intent.[157]

Survival rates have improved as new treatments have been introduced into practice, and national mortality has declined. The relative survival rate has been used as an indicator of improvements in management and curability of cancer because it is a comparison of the survival of cancer patients 5 years after diagnosis with survival of an age- and sex-matched control population without cancer.[5] Relative survival rates are good predictors of ultimate outcome since 20-year figures are about 85% of 5-year figures, the decrease largely accounted for by late recurrences in patients with breast, renal, and prostate cancers. Early surgical techniques and crude kilovoltage radiation therapy equipment led to about a 25% 5-year survival rate by the 1930s; this rose to about 33% in the 1950s.[5] Almost all of the improvement was attributable to improvements in surgical techniques and supportive care. The introduction of cobalt radiation therapy units in 1953 and linear accelerators in 1957 gave radiation therapists the proper tools to compete with surgeons in treating some forms of localized cancers. The improvement in relative survival rates from about 33% in the 1950s to 37% by the mid-1960s can be largely attributed to widespread use of improved radiation therapy technology.

The impact of chemotherapy at a national level has appeared only recently. Chemotherapy was not introduced until the late 1950s and was not a consistent part of medical practice until the specialty of medical oncology was established in the early 1970s. By 1973 the U.S. 5-year relative survival rates had risen to 40%, and the most recent figures for the period ending in 1984 (Fig. 16-8) show a relative survival rate of 50% for the white population and 37% for blacks. This 30% improvement in survival rates in the past two decades can be attributed to further improvements in radiation therapy and to the rapid expansion of the use of

FIG. 16-8. Five-year relative survival rates for males and females, with all sites combined. (Data derived from the NCI's SEER Program)

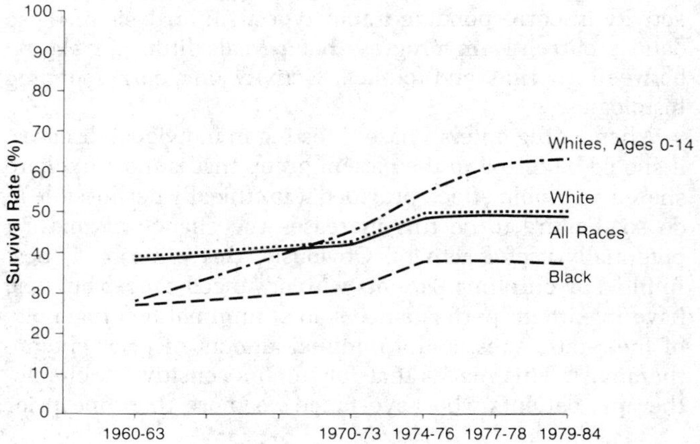

TABLE 16-11. Thirty-five-Year Trends in Cancer Mortality per 100,000 Persons, All Races, Both Sexes

	All Sites			All Sites Minus Lung		
Age	*1950*	*1984*	*% Change*	*1950*	*1984*	*% Change*
0–4	11.1	3.7	−66.7	11.0	3.7	−66.4
5–14	6.7	3.7	−44.8	6.6	3.6	−45.5
15–24	8.6	5.3	−38.4	8.4	5.2	−38.1
25–34	20.0	12.8	−36.0	19.1	12.2	−36.1
35–44	62.7	47.8	−23.8	57.6	39.9	−30.7
45–54	175.1	174.5	−0.3	152.2	121.8	−20.0
55–64	392.9	439.9	12.0	337.7	293.5	−13.1
65–74	692.5	835.9	20.7	623.2	582.6	−6.5
75–84	1,153.3	1,290.9	11.9	1,084.0	1,011.9	−6.7
85+	1,451.0	1,592.1	9.7	1,387.0	1,403.2	1.2
All Ages	157.7	170.7	8.2	144.7	125.1	−13.5

chemotherapy alone or added to surgery and radiation therapy.

A decrease in national mortality rates for cancer for which there is effective treatment also occurred steadily for the period 1950 to 1984 (Table 16-11). National mortality from cancer for patients below the age of 55 decreased most impressively owing to the development of successful treatment in younger patients with lymphomas, ovarian cancer, leukemias, and an array of childhood cancers. One point in Table 16-11 is worthy of emphasis. The impact of lung cancer, a disease that is not effectively treated but is almost totally preventable, is clearly demonstrated by the observation that a decrease in mortality from other cancers occurs up to age 85 when lung cancer mortality rates are examined separately.

Chemotherapy can cure some fraction of patients with advanced cancer of the types listed in Table 16-12. These cancers make up approximately 12% of human tumors. The impact in person-years of life saved is, however, disproportionately large because the younger average age at diagnosis results in a highly significant salvage of person-years of productive life. Other tumor types shown in Table 16-12 are treated for metastatic cancer with chemotherapy with substantial benefit, and in many cases, new treatments described elsewhere in this text offer the prospect of cure.

Systemic treatment bears a special burden of fear of toxicity in the minds of both doctors and patients, beyond that associated with surgery or radiation therapy, because its effects cannot be limited precisely to the region involved by tumor. Even though more sophisticated techniques of delivering systemic therapy to target organs have been developed, systemic toxicity is always a concomitant of systemic treatment. The same is true of biologicals. The promise of diminished side-effects with the use of biologic materials because they were natural products has not been fulfilled. A general principle is that all chemicals, natural or xenobiotic, when used in pharmacologic doses will produce significant side-effects. Patients cured of cancer by any modality generally find the toxicity associated with the treatment a justifiable expe-

TABLE 16-12. Tumors Responsive to Chemotherapy

Tumors Curable in Advanced Stages by Chemotherapy	
Choriocarcinoma	Wilms' tumor
Acute lymphocytic leukemia (in children and adults)	Burkitt's lymphoma
Hodgkin's disease	Embryonal rhabdomyosarcoma
Diffuse large cell lymphoma	Ewing's sarcoma
Lymphoblastic lymphoma (in children and adults)	Peripheral neuroepithelioma
Follicular mixed lymphoma	Neuroblastoma
Testicular cancer	Small cell cancer of the lung
Acute myelogenous leukemia	Ovarian cancer
Tumors Curable in the Adjuvant Setting by Chemotherapy	
Breast cancer	Soft tissue sarcoma
Osteogenic sarcoma	Colorectal cancer
Tumors Responsive in Advanced States But Not Yet Curable by Chemotherapy	
Bladder cancer	Head and neck cancer
Chronic myelogenous leukemia	Endometrial cancer
Chronic lymphocytic leukemia	Adrenocortical carcinoma
Hairy cell leukemia	Medulloblastoma
Multiple myeloma	Polycythemia rubra vera
Follicular small-cleaved cell lymphoma	Prostate cancer
Gastric carcinoma	Glioblastoma multiforme
Cervical carcinoma	Insulinoma
Soft tissue sarcoma	Breast cancer
	Carcinoid tumors
Tumors Poorly Responsive in Advanced Stages to Chemotherapy	
Osteogenic sarcoma	Colorectal cancer
Pancreatic cancer	Non-small cell lung cancer
Renal cancer	Melanoma
Thyroid cancer	Hepatocellular carcinoma
Carcinoma of the vulva or penis	

rience. For those with advanced unresponsive cancers, however, who have the burden of progressive tumor and impending death, the risks and side-effects of treatment should be carefully balanced against the potential benefits. Patients who are offered systemic therapy with a potential for cure should be treated aggressively; those for whom palliation is the only choice should not be overly burdened with very toxic treatments that may prolong life in an uncomfortable fashion. In practice this means that patients with metastatic cancer for whom there is no known effective systemic treatment are best advised to take part in one of the many clinical trials testing new treatments, or should be treated minimally to avoid undue side-effects.

To expand the benefits of chemotherapy, greater use of anticancer drugs before and after surgery and radiotherapy will be required, when tumor burden is at a minimum, kinetic features of cell growth are favorable, and drug resistance is less likely. Because patients sometimes feel themselves free of tumor after surgery, however, they may be less willing to accept the additional trauma of chemotherapy unless the benefits are carefully explained and accurately and honestly balanced against the chances of recurrence.

REFERENCES

1. DeVita VT: The evolution of therapeutic research in cancer. N Engl J Med 298:907–910, 1978
2. DeVita VT, Henney JE, Hubbard SM: Estimation of the numerical and economic impact of chemotherapy in the treatment of cancer. In Bruchenal JH, Oettgen HS (eds): Cancer Achievements, Challenges, and Prospects for the 1980s, pp 857–880. New York, Grune & Stratton, 1981
3. Steel GG: Cell loss from experimental tumors. Cell Tissue Kinet 1:193–207, 1968
4. Tannock IF: Biology of tumor growth. Hosp Pract, pp 81–93, 1983
5. Marshall EK Jr: Historical perspectives in chemotherapy. In Goldin A, Hawking IF (eds): Advances in Chemotherapy, vol 1, pp 1–8. New York, Academic Press, 1964
6. Hersh SM: Chemical and biological warfare: America's hidden arsenal. New York, Bobbs Merrill, 1968
7. Alexander SF: Final report of Bari mustard casualties. Allied Force Headquarters, Office of the Surgeon, APO 512, June 20, 1944
8. Skipper HE, Schabel FM Jr, Wilcox WS: Experimental evaluation of potential anticancer agents: XII. On the criteria and kinetics associated with "curability" of experimental leukemia. Cancer Chemother Rep 35:1–111, 1964
9. Skipper HE: Reasons for success and failure in treatment of murine leukemias with the drugs now employed in treating human leukemias. Cancer Chemotherapy, vol 1, pp 1–166. Ann Arbor, MI, University Microfilms International, 1978
10. Skipper HE, Schabel FM Jr, Mellet LB et al: Implications of biochemical, cytokinetic, pharmacologic, and toxicologic relationships in the design of optimal therapeutic schedules. Cancer Chemother Rep 54:431–450, 1950
11. Yankee RA, DeVita VT, Perry S: The cell cycle of leukemia L1210 cells in vivo. Cancer Res 27:2381–2385, 1968
12. Young RC, DeVita VT: Cell cycle characteristics of human solid tumors in vivo. Cell Tissue Kinet 3:285–295, 1970
13. Clarkson B, Ohkita T, Ota K et al: Studies of the cellular proliferation in human leukemia: I. Estimation of growth rates of leukemia and normal hematopoietic cells in two adults with acute leukemia given single injections of tritiated thymidine. J Clin Invest 46:506–529, 1967
14. Whang-Peng J, Perry S, Knutsen TA et al: Cell cycle characteristics, maturation and phagocytosis in vitro in blast cells from patients with chronic myelocytic leukemia. Blood 38:153–161, 1971
15. Tannock I: Cell kinetics and chemotherapy: A critical review. Cancer Treat Rep 62:1117–1133, 1978
16. Perry S, Moxley JH, Weiss GH et al: Studies of leukocyte function by liquid scintillation counting in normal individuals and in patients with chronic myelocytic leukemia. J Clin Invest 45:1388–1399, 1966
17. DeVita VT, Denham C, Perry S: Relationship of normal CDF_1 mouse leukocyte kinetics to growth characteristics of leukemia L1210. Cancer Res 29:1067–1071, 1969
18. Simpson-Herren L, Sanford AH, Holmquist JP: Cell population kinetics of transplanted Lewis lung carcinoma. Cell Tissue Kinet 7:349–361, 1974
19. Mendelsohn ML: The growth fraction: A new concept applied to tumors. Science 132:1496, 1960
20. Luria SE, Delbruck M: Mutations of bacteria from virus sensitivity to virus resistance. Genetics 28:491–511, 1943
21. Goldie JH, Coldman AJ: A mathematic model for relating the drug sensitivity of tumors to the spontaneous mutation rate. Cancer Treat Rep 63:1727–1733, 1979
22. Yunis J: The chromosomal basis of human neoplasia. Science 221(4607):227–236, 1983
23. Schabel FM Jr, Simpson-Herren L: Some variables in experimental tumor systems which complicate interpretation of data from in vivo kinetic and pharmacologic studies with anticancer drugs. Antibiot Chemother 23:113–127, 1978
24. Freireich EJ et al: Quantitative comparison of toxicity of anticancer agents in mouse, rat, dog, monkey and man. Cancer Chemother Rep 50:219–244, 1966
25. Brockman RW: Circumvention of resistance: Pharmacologic basis of cancer chemotherapy. In Proceedings of the 27th Annual Symposium on Fundamental Research, pp 691–711. Baltimore, Williams & Wilkins, 1975
26. DeVita VT Jr, Young RC, Canellos GP: Combination versus single agent chemotherapy: Review of the basis of selection of drug treatment of cancer. Cancer 35:98, 1975
27. Hutchinson DJ, Schmid FA: Cross-resistance and collateral sensitivity. In Mihich E (ed): Drug-Resistance and Selectivity: Biochemical and Cellular Basis, pp 73–126. New York, Academic Press, 1973
28. Brockman RW: Resistance to therapeutic agents. In Bruchenal JH, Oettgen HS (eds): Cancer Achievements, Challenges, and Prospects for the 1980s. New York, Grune & Stratton (in press)
29. Hutchinson DJ: Cross-resistance and collateral sensitivity studies in cancer chemotherapy. In Haddow A, Weinhouse S (eds): Advances in Cancer Research, vol 7, pp 235–350. New York, Academic Press, 1963
30. Klein M: A mechanism for the development of resistance to streptomycin and penicillin. J Bacteriol 53:463–467, 1947
31. Furth J, Kahn MC: The transmission of leukemia of mice with a single cell. Am J Cancer 31:276–282, 1937
32. Goldin A, Venditti JM, Humphries SR et al: Influences of the concentration of leukemic inoculum on the effectiveness of treatment. Science 123:840, 1956
33. Vickers PJ, Townsend AJ, Cowan KH: Mechanisms of resistance to antineoplastic drugs. CRC Crit Rev Dev Cancer Chemother (in press)
34. Ozols RJ, Cowan KH: New aspects of clinical drug resistance: The role of gene amplification and the reversal of drug refractory cancer. In DeVita VT Jr, Hellman S, Rosenberg SA (eds): Important Advances in Oncology 1986, pp 129–157. Philadelphia, JB Lippincott, 1986
35. Biedler JL, Riehm H: Cellular resistance to actinomycin D in Chinese hamster cells in vitro: Cross-resistance, radioautographic and cytogenic studies. Cancer Res 30:1174–1184, 1970
36. Juliano RL, Ling V: A surface glycoprotein modulating drug permeability in Chinese hamster ovary cell mutants. Biochem Biophys Acta 455:152–162, 1976
37. Bech-Hanson NT, Till JE, Ling V: Pleiotropic phenotype of colchicine-resistant CHO cells: Cross-resistance and collateral sensitivity. J Cell Physiol 88:23–32, 1976
38. Ling V, Thompson LH: Reduced permeability in CHO cells as a mechanism of resistance to colchicine. J Cell Physiol 83:103–116, 1973
39. Kartner N, Riordan JR, Ling V: Cell surface P-glycoprotein as associated with multidrug resistance in mammalian cell lines. Science 221:1285–1288, 1983
40. Fojo AT, Whang-Peng J, Gottesman MM et al: Amplification of DNA sequences in human multidrug resistant KB carcinoma cells. Proc Natl Acad Sci USA 82:7661–7665, 1985
41. Gros P, Croop J, Roninson I et al: Isolation and characterization of DNA sequences amplified in multidrug-resistant hamster cells. Proc Natl Acad Sci USA 83:337–341, 1986
42. Fairchild CR, Ivy SP, Kao-Shan CS et al: Isolation of amplified DNA sequences associated with pleiotropic drug resistance from human breast cancer cells. Cancer Res 47:5141–5148, 1987
43. Scotto KW, Biedler JL, Melera PW: Amplification and expression of genes associated with multidrug resistance in mammalian cells. Science 232:751–755, 1986
44. Roninson IB, Abelson HT, Housman DE et al: Amplification of specific DNA sequences correlates with multidrug resistance in Chinese hamster cells. Nature 309:2070–2076, 1984
45. Corwell MM, Safa AR, Felsted RL et al: Membrane vesicles from multidrug-resistant human cancer cells contain a specific 150 to 170-kDa protein detected by photoaffinity labelling. Proc Natl Acad Sci USA 83:3847–3850, 1986
46. Safa AR, Glover CI, Meyers CB et al: Vinblastine photoaffinity labeling of a high molecular weight surface membrane glycoprotein specific for multidrug-resistant cells. J Biol Chem 261:6137–6140, 1986
47. Cornwell MM, Pastan I, Gottesman MM: Certain calcium channel blockers bind specifically to multidrug-resistant human KB carcinoma membrane vesicles and inhibit drug binding to P-glycoprotein. J Biol Chem 262:2166–2170, 1987
48. Gros P, Croop J, Housman D: Mammalian multidrug-resistance gene: Complete cDNA sequence indicates strong homology to bacterial transport proteins. Cell 47:371–374, 1986
49. Chen C-J, Chin JE, Ueda K et al: Internal duplication and homology to bacterial transport proteins in the mdrl (P-glycoprotein) gene from multidrug-resistant human cells. Cell 47:381–389, 1986
50. Gerlach JH, Endicott JA, Juranka PF et al: Homology between P-glycoprotein and a bacterial haemolysin transport protein suggests a model for multidrug resistance. Nature 324:485–489, 1986

50a. Pasten IH, Gottesman MM: Molecular biology of multidrug resistance in human cells. In DeVita VT, Hellman S, Rosenberg SA (eds): Important Advances in Oncology 1988, pp 3–16. Philadelphia, JB Lippincott, 1988

51. Fojo AT, Ueda K, Slamon DJ et al: Expression of a multidrug-resistant gene in human tumors and tissues. Proc Natl Acad Sci USA 84:265–269, 1987
52. Endicott JA, Juranka PF, Sarangi F et al: Simultaneous expression of two P-glycoprotein genes in drug sensitive Chinese hamster ovary cells. Mol Cell Biol 7:4075–4081, 1987
53. Gros P, Ben Neriah Y, Croop JM et al: Isolation and expression of a complementary cDNA that confers multidrug resistance. Nature 323:728–731, 1986
54. Van Der Bliek AM, Baas F, Ten Houte de Lange T et al: The human mdr3 gene encodes a novel P-glycoprotein homologue and gives rise to alternatively spliced mRNAs in liver. EMBO J 6:3325–3331, 1987
55. Beck WT, Mueller TJ, Tanzer LR: Altered surface membrane glycoproteins in vinca alkaloid–resistant human leukemia lymphoblasts. Cancer Res 39:2070–2076, 1979
56. Riordan JR, Deuchars K, Kartner N et al: Amplification of P-glycoprotein genes in multidrug resistant mammalian cell lines. Nature 316:817–819, 1985
57. Louie KG, Hamilton TC, Winker MA et al: Adriamycin accumulation and metabolism in Adriamycin-sensitive and -resistant human ovarian cancer cell lines. Biochem Pharmacol 35:476–472, 1986
58. Chang BK, Gregory JA: Comparison of cellular pharmacology of doxorubicin in resistant and sensitive models of pancreatic cancer. Cancer Chemother Pharmacol 14:132–134, 1985
59. Seigfried JM, Tritton TR, Sartorelli AC: Comparison of anthracycline concentrations in S180 cell lines of varying sensitivity. Eur J Clin Oncol 19:1133–1141, 1983
60. Solt DB, Medline A, Farber E: Rapid emergence of carcinogen-induced hyperplastic lesions in a new model for the sequential analysis of liver carcinogenesis. Am J Pathol 88:595–618, 1977
61. Farber E, Parker S, Gruenstein M: The resistance of putative premalignant liver cell populations, hyperplastic nodules, to the acute cytotoxic effect of some hepatocarcinogens. Cancer Res 36:3879–3887, 1976
62. Fairchild CR, Ivy SP, Rushmore T et al: Carcinogen-induced mdr overexpression is associated with xenobiotic resistance in rat preneoplastic liver nodules and hepatocellular carcinomas. Proc Natl Acad Sci USA 84:7701–7705, 1987
63. Cowan KH, Batist G, Tulpule A et al: Similar biochemical changes associated with multidrug resistance in human breast cancer cells and carcinogen-induced resistance to xenobiotics in rats. Proc Natl Acad Sci USA 83:9328–9332, 1986
64. Moscow JA, Cowan KH: Multidrug resistance. JNCI 80:14–20, 1988
65. Marsh W, Center MS: Adriamycin resistance in HL60 cells and accompanying modifications of a membrane protein contained in drug-sensitive cells. Cancer Res 47:5080–5086, 1987
66. Danks MK, Yalowich JC, Bech WT: Atypical multiple drug resistance in a human leukemic cell line selected for resistance to teniposide (VM-26). Cancer Res 47:1297–1301, 1987
67. Ross WE, Sullivan DM, Chow KC: Altered function of DNA topoisomerases as a basis for antineoplastic drug action. In DeVita VT, Hellman S, Rosenberg S (eds): Import Advances in Oncology 1988, pp 65–81. Philadelphia, JB Lippincott, 1988
68. Glisson B, Gupta R, Hodges P et al: Cross resistance to intercalating agents in an epipodophyllotoxin-resistant Chinese hamster ovary cell line: Evidence for a common intracellular target. Cancer Res 46:1939–1942, 1986
69. Pommier Y, Kerrigan D, Schwartz RE et al: Altered DNA topoisomerase II activity in Chinese hamster cells resistant to topoisomerase II inhibitors. Cancer Res 46:3075–3081, 1986
70. Tsuruo T, Iida H, Tsukagoshi S et al: Increased accumulation of vincristine and Adriamycin in drug-resistant P388 tumor cells following incubation with calcium antagonists and calmodulin inhibitors. Cancer Res 42:4730–4733, 1982
71. Fitzgerald DJ, Willingham MC, Cardarelli CO et al: A monoclonal antibody-*Pseudomonas* toxin conjugate that specifically kills multidrug resistant cells. Proc Natl Acad Sci USA 84:4288–4292, 1987
72. Meister A: Selective modification of glutathione metabolism. Science 220:472–477, 1983
73. Kramer RA, Greene K, Ahmad S et al: Chemosensitization of L-phenylalanine mustards by the thiol-modulating agent buthionine sulfoximine. Cancer Res 47:1593–1597, 1987
74. Ozols RF, Louie KG, Plowman J et al: Enhanced melphalan toxicity in human ovarian cancer in vitro and in tumor-bearing nude mice by buthionine sulfoximine depletion of glutathione. Biochem Pharmacol 36:147–153, 1987
75. Russo A, Mitchell JB: Potentiation and protection of doxorubicin cytotoxicity by cellular glutathione modulation. Cancer Treat Rep 69:1293–1296, 1985
76. Skipper H: Data and Analyses Having To Do with the Influence of Dose Intensity and Duration of Treatment (Single Drugs and Combinations) on Lethal Toxicity and the Therapeutic Response of Experimental Neoplasms. Southern Research Institute, Booklets 13, 1986, and 2–13, 1987
77. DeVita VT, Hubbard SM, Longo DL: The chemotherapy of lymphomas: looking back, moving forward. The Richard and Hinda Rosenthal Foundation Award Lecture. Cancer Res 47:5810–5824, 1987
78. Hryniuk WM: The importance of dose intensity in the outcome of chemotherapy. In DeVita VT, Hellman S, Rosenberg SA (eds): Important Advances in Oncology 1988, pp 121–142. Philadelphia, JB Lippincott, 1988
79. Hryniuk W, Levine MN: Analysis of dose intensity for adjuvant chemotherapy trials in stage II breast cancer. J Clin Oncol 4:1162–1170, 1986
80. Hryniuk WM: Average relative dose intensity and the impact on design on clinical trials. Semin Oncol 14:65–74, 1987
81. Levin L, Hryniuk W: Dose intensity analysis of chemotherapy regimens in ovarian carcinoma. J Clin Oncol 5:756–767, 1987
82. Hryniuk W, Bush H: The importance of dose intensity in chemotherapy of metastatic breast cancer. J Clin Oncol 2:1281–1288, 1984
83. Hryniuk W: Editorial: Is more better? J Clin Oncol 4:621–622, 1986
84. Canellos GP, Pocock SJ, Taylor SG III et al: Combination chemotherapy for metastatic breast cancer: Prospective comparison of multiple drug therapy with L-phenylalanine mustard. Cancer 38:1882–1886, 1976
85. Canellos GP, DeVita VT, Gold GL et al: Cyclical combination chemotherapy for advanced breast cancer. Br Med J 1:218–220, 1974
86. Bonadonna G, Brusamalino MP, Valagussa R et al: Combination chemotherapy as an adjuvant treatment in operable breast cancer. N Engl J Med 298:405–410, 1976
87. Bonadonna G, Valagussa R: Dose response effect of adjuvant chemotherapy in breast cancer. N Engl J Med 304:10–15, 1981
88. Horton J, Olson KB, Sullivan J et al: 5-Fluorouracil in cancer: An improved regimen. Ann Intern Med 78:897–900, 1970
89. Grage TB, Moss SE: Adjuvant chemotherapy in cancer of the colon and rectum: Demonstration of effectiveness of prolonged 5-FU chemotherapy in a prospectively controlled randomized trial. Surg Clin North Am 61:1321–1329, 1981
90. Higgins GA, Dwight RW, Smith JV et al: Fluorouracil as an adjuvant to surgery in carcinoma of the colon. Arch Surg 102:339–343, 1971
91. Higgins GA Jr, Humphrey E, Juler GL et al: Adjuvant chemotherapy in the surgical treatment of large bowel cancer. Cancer 38:1461–1467, 1976
92. Lawrence W Jr, Terz JJ, Horsley JS et al: Chemotherapy as an adjuvant to surgery for colorectal cancer. Arch Surg 113:164–168, 1978
93. Grossi CE, Wolff WI, Nealon TF Jr et al: Intraluminal fluorouracil chemotherapy adjunct to surgical procedures for resectable carcinoma of the colon and rectum. Surg Gynecol Obstet 145:549–554, 1977
94. Nathanson L, Hall TC, Schilling AC et al: Concurrent combination chemotherapy of human solid tumors: Experience with three-drug regimen and review of the literature. Cancer Res 29:419–425, 1969
95. Potter VR: Sequential blocking of metabolic pathways in vivo. Proc Soc Exp Biol Med 76:41–46, 1951
96. Elion GB, Singer S, Hitchings GH: Antagonists of nucleic acid derivatives: VIII. Synergism in combinations of biochemically related antimetabolites. J Biol Chem 208:477–488, 1954
97. Sartorelli AC: Approaches to the combination chemotherapy of transplantable neoplasms. Prog Ext Tumor Res 6:228–288, 1965
98. DeVita VT, Schein PS: The use of drugs in combination for the treatment of cancer: Rationale and results. N Engl J Med 288:998–1006, 1973
99. Yagoda A: Use of M-VAC on colony stimulating factors. In DeVita VT, Hellman S, Rosenberg S (eds): Important Advances in Oncology 1988. Philadelphia, JB Lippincott, 1988
100. DeVita VT: Only if you believe in magic. In Jones SE, Salmon SE (eds): Adjuvant Therapy of Cancer IV, pp 3–16. Orlando, Fla, Grune & Stratton, 1984
101. DeVita VT: On the value of response criteria in therapeutic research. In: Proceedings of the 2nd International Congress on Neoadjuvant Chemotherapy. Bull Cancer Colloque INSERM (in press)
102. Holland JF: Induction chemotherapy: An old term for an old concept. In: Neoadjuvant Chemotherapy. Colloque INSERM 137:45–47, 1986
103. Frei A III, Clark JR, Miller D: The concept of neoadjuvant chemotherapy. In: Adjuvant Therapy of Cancer V, p 67. Orlando, Fla, Grune & Stratton, 1987
104. Muggia FM: Primary chemotherapy: Concepts and issues. In: Primary Chemotherapy in Cancer Medicine, pp 377–383. New York, Alan R Liss, 1985
105. Goldie JH: Scientific basis for adjuvant and primary (neoadjuvant) chemotherapy. Semin Oncol 14:1–7, 1987
106. Simpson-Herron L, Sanford AH, Holmquist JP: Effects of surgery on the cell kinetics of residual tumor. Cancer Treat Rep 60:1749–1760, 1976
107. DeVita VT: The relationship between tumor mass and resistance to treatment of cancer. Cancer 51:1209–1220, 1983
108. Skipper HE: Critical variables in the design of combination chemotherapy regimens to be used alone or in adjuvant setting. In: Neoadjuvant Chemotherapy. Colloque INSERM 137:11–12, 1986
109. Dedrick RL, Myers CE, Bungay PM et al: Pharmacokinetic rationale for peritoneal drug administration in treatment of ovarian cancer. Cancer Treat Rep 62:1–11, 1978
110. Jones RB, Myers CE, Guarino AM et al: High volume intraperitoneal chemotherapy ("belly bath") for ovarian cancer: Pharmacologic basis and early results. Cancer Chemother Pharmacol 1:161–166, 1978
111. Jones RB, Collins JM, Myers CE et al: High volume intraperitoneal chemotherapy with methotrexate in patients with cancer. Cancer Res (in press)
112. Papahadjopoulos D, Poste G, Vail WJ et al: Use of lipid vesicles as carriers to introduce actinomycin D into resistant tumor cells. Cancer Res 36:2988–3012, 1976
113. Weinstein JM, Magin RL, Cysyk RL et al: Treatment of solid L1210 murine tumors with local hyperthermia and temperature-sensitive liposomes containing methotrexate. Cancer Res 40:1388–1396, 1980
114. Weinstein JN: Liposomes as drug carriers in cancer therapy. Cancer Treat Rep 68:127–135, 1984
115. Weisenthal LM, Lippman ME: Clonogenic and non-clonogenic in vitro chemosensitivity assays. Cancer Treat Rep 69:615–632, 1985
116. Von Hoff DD, Weisenthal L: In vitro methods to predict patient response to chemotherapy. Adv Pharmacol Chemother 7:133–156, 1980
117. Von Hoff DD, Clark GM, Stogdill BJ et al: Prospective clinical trial of a human tumor cloning system. Cancer Res 43:1926–1931, 1983
118. Alberts DS, Leigh SA, Moon TE et al: Improved survival for relapsing ovarian cancer

patients using the human clonogenic assay to select chemotherapy, p 31. In: Proceedings of the 4th Conference on Human Tumor Cloning, 1984
119. Twentyman PR: Predictive chemosensitivity testing. J Cancer 51:295–299, 1985
120. Von Hoff DD: "Send this patient's tumor for culture and sensitivity." N Engl J Med 308:154, 1983
121. Von Hoff DD, Clark GM: Drug sensitivity of primary versus metastases. In: Salmon SE, Trent JN (eds): Human Tumor Cloning. Orlando, Fla, Grune & Stratton, 1984
122. Weisenthal LM, Marsden JA, Dill PL et al: A novel dye exclusion method for testing in vitro chemosensitivity of human tumors. Cancer Res 43:749–757, 1983
123. Weisenthal LM, Dill PL, Kurnick NB et al: Comparison of dye exclusion assays with a clonogenic assay in the determination of drug-induced cytotoxicity. Cancer Res 43:258–264, 1983
124. Weisenthal LM, Marsden JA, Macaluso CK et al: In vitro chemosensitivity assay based on the concept of total tumor cell kill. Recent Cancer Res (in press)
125. Bosanquet AG, Bird MC, Price WJP et al: An assessment of a short-term tumour chemosensitivity assay to chronic lymphocytic leukemia. Br J Cancer 74:781–789, 1983
126. Ihde D, Russell E, Oic HK et al: Prospective clinical trial of individualized chemotherapy based on in vitro drug sensitivity testing in extensive stage small cell lung cancer. In: Adjuvant Therapy of Cancer V, pp 201–207. Orlando, Fla, Grune & Stratton, 1987
127. Bodgen AE, Kelton DE, Cobb WR et al: A rapid screening method for testing chemotherapeutic agents against human tumor xenografts. In Houchens DP, Ovejera AA (eds): Proceedings of the Symposium on the Use of Athymic (Nude) Mice in Cancer Research, pp 231–250. New York, Gustav Fisher, 1978
128. Griffin TW, Bodgen AE, Reich SD et al: Initial clinical trials of the subrenal capsule assay as a predictor of tumor response to chemotherapy. Cancer 52:2185–2192, 1983
129. Pihl A: UICC study group on chemosensitivity testing of human tumors: Problems—applications—future prospects. Int J Cancer 37:1–5, 1986
130. Gorelik E, Ovejera A, Shoemaker R et al: Micro-encapsulated tumor assay: New short-term assay for in vivo evaluation of the effects of anticancer drugs on human tumor cell lines. Cancer Res 47:5739–5747, 1987
131. Schroy III PC, Cohen A, Winowar SJ et al: New chemotherapeutic drug sensitivity assay for colon carcinomas in monolayer culture. Cancer Res 48:3236–3244, 1988
132. Ajani JA, Baker FL, Spitzer G et al: Comparison between clinical response and in vitro drug sensitivity of primary human tumors in the adhesive tumor cell culture system. J Clin Oncol 5:1912–1921, 1987
133. Gazdar AF, Carney DN, Russel EK et al: Small cell carcinoma of the lung: Establishment of continuous, clonable cell lines having APUD properties. Cancer Res 40:3502–3507, 1980
134. Carney DN, Mitchell JB, Kinsella TJ: In vitro radiation and chemosensitivity of established cell lines of human small cell lung cancer and its large cell morphological variants. Cancer Res 43:2806–2811, 1983
135. Kornblith PL, Smith BH, Leonard LA: Response of cultured human brain tumors to nitrosourceas: Correlation with clinical data. Cancer 47:255–265, 1981
136. Goldin A, Schepartz SA, Venditti JM et al: Historical development and current strategy of the National Cancer Institute Drug Development Program. In DeVita VT, Busch H (eds): Methods of Cancer Research, vol XVI, Cancer Drug Development, Part A, pp 165–247. New York, Academic Press, 1979
137. DeVita VT, Oliverio VT, Muggia FM et al: The Drug Development Program and Clinical Trials Programs of the Division of Cancer Treatment, National Cancer Institute. Cancer Clin Trials 2:195–216, 1979
138. Zubrod CG, Schepartz S, Leiter J et al: The Chemotherapy Program of the National Cancer Institute: History, analysis, and plans. Cancer Chemother Rep 50:349–540, 1966
139. Hirschberg E: Patterns of response of animal tumors to anticancer agents. Cancer Res 23 (suppl 5, Part 2):521–980, 1963
140. Driscol JS: The preclinical new drug research program of the National Cancer Institute. Cancer Treat Rep 68:63–76, 1984
141. Shoemaker RH, Wolpert-DeFilippes MK, Venditti JM: Potentials and drawbacks of the human tumor stem cell assay. Behring Inst Mitt 74:262–272, 1984
142. Rockwell S: Effects of clumps and clusters on survival measurements with clonogenic assays. Cancer Res 45:1601–1607, 1985
143. Shoemaker RH, Wolpert-DeFilippes MK, Kern DH et al: Application of a human tumor colony-forming assay to new drug screening. Cancer Res 45:2145–2153, 1985
144. Boyd M, Shoemaker R, Alley M et al: New NCI disease-oriented drug screening program. In: Proceedings of the 5th NCI-EORTC Symposium on New Drugs in Cancer Therapy. Amsterdam, 1986
145. Boyd MR, Shoemaker RH, McLemore TL et al: New drug development. In Roth JA, Ruckdescel JC, Weisenburger THE (eds): Thoracic Oncology. Philadelphia, WB Saunders, 1987
146. Alley MC, Scudiero DA, Monks A et al: Feasibility of drug screening with panels of human tumor cell lines using a microculture tetrazolium assay. Cancer Res 48:589–601, 1988
147. Mosmann T: Rapid colorimetric assay for cellular growth and survival: Application to proliferation and cytotoxicity assays. J Immunol Methods 65:55–63, 1983
148. Shoemaker RH: New approaches to antitumor drug screening: The human tumor colony forming assay. Cancer Treat Rep 70:9–12, 1986
149. Rozencweig M, Von Hoff DD, Staquet MJ et al: Predictive value of animal toxicology with anticancer agents prior to early clinical trials (abstr). Clin Res 27(2):391A, 1979
150. Muggia FM, Rozencweig M, Chiuten DF et al: Phase II trials: Use of a clinical tumor panel and overview of current resources and studies. Cancer Treat Rep 64:1–9, 1980
151. Wooley PV, Schein PS: Clinical pharmacology and phase I trial design. In DeVita VT, Busch H (eds): Methods in Cancer Research. XVII. Cancer Drug Development, part B, pp 177–199, 1979
152. Muggia FM, McGuire WP, Rozencweig M: Rationale, design and methodology of phase II clinical trials. In DeVita VT, Busch H (eds): Methods in Cancer Research. XVII. Cancer Drug Development, part B, pp 199–215, 1979
153. Von Hoff DD, Rozencweig M, Soper WT et al: Commentary: Whatever happened to NSC---? An analysis of clinical results of discontinued anticancer agents. Cancer Treat Rep 61:759–768, 1977
154. Collins JM, Zaharko DS, Dedrick RL et al: Potential roles for preclinical pharmacology in phase I clinical trials. Cancer Treat Rep 70:73, 1986
155. Goldin A, Venditti JM: Progress report on the screening program at the Division of Cancer Treatment, National Cancer Institute. Cancer Treat Rev 7:167, 1980
156. Marsoni S, Hoth D, Simon R et al: Clinical drug development: An analysis of phase II trials, 1970–1985. Cancer Treat Rep 71:71, 1987
157. Rosenberg SA (ed): Surgical Treatment of Metastatic Cancer. Philadelphia, JB Lippincott, 1987

STEVEN A. ROSENBERG
DAN L. LONGO
MICHAEL T. LOTZE

CHAPTER 17 *Principles and Applications of Biologic Therapy*

"Biologic therapy" refers to cancer treatment that produces antitumor effects primarily through the action of natural host defense mechanisms or by the administration of natural mammalian substances. Biologic therapy has emerged in the last several years as an important fourth modality for the treatment of cancer. This growth has resulted from an increased understanding of the basic aspects of host defense mechanisms against cancer and the rapid development of biotechnologies that have made molecules, previously obtainable only in minute amounts, available in quantities large enough for use in manipulating in vivo biologic processes. Although this field is still in the infancy of its development, many examples now exist of the successful application of biologic therapy to the treatment of cancer in humans.

BASIC PRINCIPLES OF TUMOR IMMUNOLOGY

Most efforts to utilize biologic therapy for the treatment of cancer have involved attempts to stimulate immune defense mechanisms. The immune system evolved as a means to detect and eliminate substances that are recognized as "nonself" and thus eliminate foreign molecules or pathogens yet not react to host (self) tissues. Thus, many biologic immune therapies have involved attempts to cause the tumor to appear more "foreign" compared with normal tissues or to find means for magnifying relatively weak host immune reactions to growing tumors.

The immune system differs from most other organ systems because its cells are not in constant contact with each other. Rather, they circulate freely throughout the body both in and out of the circulatory and lymphatic systems. Immune reactivity involves the integrated action of a large number of different cell types, including lymphocytes, monocytes, macrophages, basophils, eosinophils, dendritic cells, endothelial cells, and many others throughout the body. Although separate functions have been assigned to these cell types, it is now clear that they interact in many ways and can regulate each others' activities.

Immune cells secrete two major classes of soluble protein. The first of these lymphocyte products to be recognized was the antibody. Antibodies are a group of proteins composed of one or several units, each of which is composed of two pairs of different polypeptide chains (heavy and light chains). Each unit possesses two recognition sites, which are capable of combining with the immunizing antigen. The unique bond between antigen and antibody is part of the basis for the exquisite specificity that is the hallmark of immunologic reactivity. The existence of circulating antibodies was first demonstrated in 1890, and until recently, scientific studies of antibodies monopolized the study of immune reactions.

Over the past two decades, it has become clear that selected subpopulations of lymphoid cells can secrete a second (nonantibody) class of protein molecules. These molecules are not biochemically similar to antibodies, are produced in tiny amounts, and are not normally detectable in the circulation. Collectively called cytokines, they represent a new class of hormones with actions on many different target cells both within and outside the immune system. Increasing knowledge of a wide variety of cytokines has dramatically altered our understanding of the functions of the immune system and has opened new possibilities for the immunotherapy of human cancer.

CELLS OF THE IMMUNE SYSTEM

The central cell in immune function is the lymphocyte. Lymphocytes constitute approximately 20% of blood leukocytes and fall into three major classes — B cells, T cells, and null cells — on the basis of ontogeny and function. Recently, however, analysis of cell-surface molecules, usually using monoclonal antibodies, has revealed substantial heterogeneity in human leukocytes and lymphocytes. In November 1982, the First International Workshop on Human Leukocyte Differentiation Antigens was held in Paris to attempt to codify the proliferating number of cell-surface determinants detected on leukocytes and the antibodies used to detect them. As a result of the testing of large numbers of antibodies on target cells of many different leukocyte types, cluster analysis permitted the definition of groups of antigens that are similar and those that are clearly different on each type of target cell. This workshop led to the definition of "clusters of differentiation" (CD), which are now used to define cell-surface components on leukocytes. A summary of selected CD classifications, the cells on which they are found, and the principal antibodies that are used to detect them is shown in Table 17-1.

In birds, B cells develop in a special organ called the bursa of Fabricius. There is no anatomical counterpart of this bursa in man; instead, it is thought that human B cells develop in the bone marrow and acquire surface immunoglobulin, which acts as their antigen receptor. B cells also develop receptors for lymphokines, which enable their regulation by T-cell products. B cells require both the presence of antigen and help from antigen-specific T cells to produce and secrete antibodies.

The term "T cells" was derived from the role of the thymus in the differentiation of these lymphocytes. Lymphoid cells produced in the bone marrow traffic to the thymus late in fetal life, differentiate there, and then seed secondary lymphoid tissues. In the thymus, T cells are thought to acquire antigen-specific receptors and to differentiate into the various T-cell subpopulations. Death of many lymphocytes occurs in the thymus during ontogeny, which is thought to be, in part, the mechanism for the loss of self-reactive clones. T cells are involved in cellular immune reactions and recognize antigen via receptor molecules quite distinct from the immunoglobulin found on B cells. The T-cell receptor is generated from the recombination of germ-line genes to produce a wide diversity of receptors that can bind antigen together with self-MHC (major histocompatibility complex) molecules. Thus the generation of diversity in T-cell receptors is similar to that of antibodies. The T-cell receptor for antigen is associated with a glycoprotein complex, T3, present on all mature human T cells. Whereas B cells can recognize antigen alone, T cells recognize antigen in association with MHC molecules.

Although T cells were initially subtyped by functions (helper, suppressor, cytotoxic), it has now been possible to identify two major T-cell subsets, each of which is restricted to recognizing one of the two major classes of major histocompatibility molecules. Class I molecules (serologically defined as HLA-A, B, or C) are involved with the presentation of processed antigen to T cells expressing the CD8 molecule. Similarly, Class II molecules (currently recognized as DP, DQ, and DR) present antigen to T cells expressing the CD4 molecule. Interestingly, this molecule is the cellular target for HIV, and the profound immunodepression observed in AIDS is probably related to the destruction of this T-cell subset. Both helper and cytotoxic functions can be ascribed to cells of each lineage, and other antigens have been useful to further delineate functional subsets within each of these T-cell populations.

Recently, a third population of lymphocytes, null cells, has been identified that express neither T nor B cell-surface markers. These cells appear to be a distinct lineage of lymphoid cells that bear some T-cell markers early in differentiation and later acquire markers also present on macrophages and neutrophils. Although the principal function of null cells is not known, recent studies have shown that natural killer (NK) cells and lymphokine-activated killer (LAK) cells are derived from this subpopulation. NK cells are cells that can lyse a select group of cultured cell lines without a known prior exposure to an immunizing stimulus. LAK cells are cells that develop the ability to kill fresh tumor cells following exposure of these lymphoid precursors to the lymphokine interleukin-2 (IL-2). Cells mediating antibody-dependent cellular cytotoxicity (see below) also are found in this null cell population.

Other important cells in the immune system are the reticuloendothelial cells, predominantly monocytes and macrophages. Monocytes are long-lived circulating cells that develop into tissue macrophages. Macrophages are highly phagocytic cells that possess a variety of physiologic protective functions. They are also capable of presenting antigen to lymphocytes and may play a role in carrying antigen from the periphery to other immune sites. A variety of other cell types derived from bone-marrow stem cells play a similar antigen-presenting role, including the Langerhans' cells of the skin, follicular dendritic cells in lymph nodes, B cells, and endothelial cells.

IMMUNE EFFECTOR MECHANISMS RESULTING IN CELL DESTRUCTION

A variety of immune effector mechanisms can cause destruction of vascularized tissue or of circulating tumor cells (Table 17-2).

Antibodies can mediate cell destruction either via the binding of complement or by action as an opsonin to facilitate

TABLE 17-1. Selected CD Classifications of Leukocytes

Cluster of Differentiation (CD)	*Antibodies Reactive with CD*	*Cellular Distribution of Determinant*
CD1	OKT6, T6, Leu 6	80% of thymocytes
CD2	LFA-2, OKT11, T11, Leu 5	95% of thymocytes, 100% of T cells, and a variable percentage of LGLs; E-rosette receptor
CD3	OKT3, T3, Leu 4	20–80% of thymocytes and 100% of T cells; associated with T-cell antigen receptor *(T1)*
CD4	OKT4, T4, Leu 3	80% of thymocytes and 65–70% of T cells ("helper/inducer" subset)
CD5	OKT1, T1, Leu 1	Thymocytes, most T cells, and some B cells
CD7	3A1, Leu 9	Thymocytes, 100% of T cells, and some LGLs
CD8	OKT8, T8, Leu 2	50–80% of thymocytes, 30–35% of T cells ("cytotoxic/suppressor"), and some LGLs (low density)
CD9	BA2	Monocytes, pre-B cells, and platelets
CD10	CALLA, J5, BA3	Some bone-marrow pre-B cells and >90% of common ALL
CD11a	LFA-1	T cells, B cells, LGLs, monocytes, and granulocytes
CD11b	CR3 (C3bi), OKM1, Mo1, Leu 15	CD8 T cells, LGLs, monocytes, and granulocytes
CD11c	Leu M5	100% of monocytes and granulocytes
CD14	Leu M3, Mo3	70–93% of monocytes
CD15	Leu M1, My 1	100% of monocytes and >95% of mature granulocytes
CD16	Leu 11a,b,c and Vep 13	LGLs (NK cells) and granulocytes; Fc IgG receptor
CD18	See CD11	T cells, B cells, LGLs, monocytes, and granulocytes
CD19	B4, Leu 12	100% of B cells
CD21	CR-2 (C3d), B2	Mature B cells; EBV receptor
CD22	Leu 14, to 15	B cells
CD25	IL-2R, Tac	T cells, B cells, and LGLs; 9.3-negative T cell appears to function as a suppressor cell
CDw29	4B4	Thymocytes, 40% of T cells (appears to identify helper/inducers); some B cells, LGLs, and monocytes
CD35	CR1 (C3b receptor)	B cells, some T cells, monocytes
CD38	OKT10, T10, Leu 17	LGLs, B cells, some T cells, monocytes, thymocytes, bone marrow cells, and activated T cells
CD45	Antileukocyte	>95% of lymphocytes; monocytes and granulocytes
CD45R	2H4, Leu 18	40% of T cells (appears to identify suppressor/inducers); some B cells, LGLs, monocytes, and granulocytes
Leu 8, TQ 1		7% of thymocytes, >50% of T cells (appears to identify suppressor/inducers), some B cells and monocytes
Transferrin receptor, OKT9		Activated T cells and B cells; found on 10% of thymocytes and monocytes
4F2		Activated T cells, B cells, and monocytes
HNK-1, Leu 7		Some T cells and 50% of LGLs
NKH-1, Leu 19		Small percentage of T cells (cytotoxic), most LGLs and monocytes
LFA 3		T cells (100% CTLs), B cells, LGLs, and monocytes
Class I MHC	HLA A,B,C	Thymocytes, T cells, B cells, LGLs, and monocytes
Class II MHC	HLA DP, DQ, DR (Leu 10, 12)	B cells, monocytes, and activated T cells
Surface Ig		B cells
PCA-1		Plasma cells (weakly positive on monocytes)

phagocytosis by macrophages or by other phagocytic cells bearing Fc receptors.

The direct interaction of an immune cell with a target cell can also result in lysis, and a variety of immune cytotoxic cells have been described. The best-characterized lytic immune cell is the cytotoxic T lymphocyte (CTL). These T cells can interact with specific cell-surface antigens via an interaction with the T-cell receptor and a Class I or II MHC molecule. This lysis appears to involve direct cell contact and can occur quickly, with the initial lytic events initiated within minutes of the adhesion of the target cell to the lymphocyte. Although binding of the CTL to the tumor target occurs via the T-cell receptor, other means for binding lytic cells to targets also can result in lysis. One such mechanism

TABLE 17-2. Immune Effector Mechanisms Resulting in Cell Destruction

Antibody-mediated lysis (plus complement or antibody as an opsonin for macrophages and other Fc-receptor-positive cells).
Direct cell-mediated lysis
Cytotoxic T lymphocytes (CTL)
Antibody-dependent cellular cytotoxicity (ADCC)
Lectin-dependent cellular cytotoxicity (LDCC)
Natural killer cells (NK)
Lymphokine-activated killer cells (LAK)
Macrophage lysis
Release of toxic mediators from lymphocytes and other immune cells

has been referred to as antibody-dependent cellular cytotoxicity (ADCC). In this lysis, antibody bound to immune cells serves as a cross-link to a cytolytic cell bearing an Fc receptor. The Fc receptor on the immune effector binds to the free Fc portion of the antibody on the target cell; following this cross-linkage, lysis of the target cell occurs. Similarly, the phenomenon of lectin-dependent cellular cytotoxicity (LDCC) involves the association of a lytic cell with a target using a lectin such as concanavalin A or phytohemagglutinin as the cross-linking agent.

Recently, much has been learned of NK cells. These lymphocytes can lyse selected cultured target cells in the absence of a previous sensitizing stimulus. The most common target for NK cells is the K562 leukemia cell line. NK cells have little, if any, ability to kill fresh tumor cells, and therefore their physiologic role as an antitumor effector mechanism is unclear.

LAK cells are lymphocytes that acquire the ability to lyse a broad array of fresh tumor targets following incubation in IL-2. The precursor of LAK cells is a null lymphocyte, and most mature LAK cells do not bear T- or B-cell markers. A subpopulation of LAK cells, however, has been shown to be CD3 positive, and both precursor and effector LAK cells appear to bear the Leu-19 cell-surface marker. LAK cells can lyse a broad array of malignant, but not normal, fresh target cells in 4-hour chromium-release assays. LAK cells also can lyse both normal and malignant cultured lines. Thus, LAK cells appear capable of lysing most cells that have their membranes perturbed by either malignant transformation, culture, or other activation processes.

Activated macrophages also can recognize and lyse tumor cells. Whereas most lymphocyte-mediated lysis can easily be detected in 4 hours, the measurement of significant macrophage-mediated lysis often requires 48 to 72 hours.

Many of the cytokines secreted by immune cells can mediate toxicity of tissue, either directly or via the recruitment of other inflammatory processes. For example, tumor necrosis factor (TNF) and lymphotoxin are two cytokines capable of direct destruction of tumor cells. Gamma-interferon has an antiproliferative effect against some tumor cells. In addition, a wide variety of chemotactic and vascular permeability factors that are involved in inflammatory responses also can indirectly mediate tumor destruction and may play a role in tumor immune phenomena.

CYTOKINES

Cytokines are soluble proteins produced by mononuclear cells of the immune system (usually lymphocytes or monocytes) that have regulatory actions on other cells of the immune system or target cells involved in immune reactions. Cytokines produced by lymphocytes are referred to as lymphokines and cytokines produced by monocytes are referred to as monokines. Cytokines are true hormones, acting on other cells at a distance from the secreting cells.

For the past 25 years, it has been realized the soluble substances produced by immune cells are involved in immune function and regulation. Until recently, these cytokines were identified by the function they exhibit in in vitro assays. Thus, lymphokines that inhibit the migration of macrophages were known as migration-inhibition factor (MIF), and other factors that activate macrophages were known as macrophage-activation factor (MAF). This identification of cytokines on the basis of function led to a confusing situation in which the same molecules were often described by various investigators using different assays for their detection.

Substantial recent progress in this field resulted from the use of molecular biologic techniques to clone the genes for these cytokines, express them in bacteria, and purify them to homogeneity so that large amounts of homogeneous cytokines were available for detailed study. A new nomenclature referring to cytokines as interleukins (meaning "between leukocytes") has been introduced that supplants the acronyms based on functional properties. A meeting of the Second International Lymphokine Workshop in Ermatingen, Switzerland, in 1979 reached a consensus that a variety of lymphokines that had been referred to as T-cell growth factor (TCGF), thymocyte-stimulating factor (TSF), thymocyte mitogenic factor (TMF), killer-cell helper factor (KHF) costimulator, and secondary cytotoxic T-cell-inducing factor were all the same molecule and should be referred to as IL-2. The term "interleukin-1" was adopted to refer to a monocyte product previously called lymphocyte-activating factor (LAF). Since that time, many cytokines have been described, and a list of some of these is presented in Table 17-3. This list is rapidly expanding as new hormones produced by cells of the immune system are described.

Cytokines are proteins or glycoproteins, mostly with molecular weights in the range of 15,000 to 40,000, and many are glycosylated, although it appears that the glycosylation is often not essential for function. In many cases, the cytokines described in both mouse and man are structurally related. For example, IL-1 alpha shows a 61% to 65% amino acid homology between human, rabbit, and mouse. Some lymphokines exhibit species specificity; for example, IL-1, IL-2, IL-5, and IL-6 derived from man are active on cells from both mouse and man, whereas IL-3, IL-4, and gamma-interferon derived from man are active only on human cells and not on mouse cells.

Each cytokine presumably reacts with receptors specific for that cytokine on the cell surface. Little is known about most cytokine receptors with the exception of the IL-2 receptor, which is present in low-, intermediate-, and high-affinity forms, depending on the specific aggregation of a 55- and a 75-kd polypeptide chain receptor.

TABLE 17-3. Cytokines: Sources and Physiological Effects

Cytokine	*Other Names*	*Sources*	*Effects*
IL-1	Endogenous pyrogen (EP) Lymphocyte-activating factor (LAF) Leukocyte endogenous mediator (LEM) Catabolin Mononuclear cell factor (MCF)	Monocyte and macrophage lines Dendritic cells Natural killer cells B-cell lines T-cell lines Endothelial cells Epithelial cells Fibroblasts Astrocytes Keratinocytes	Induces Lymphokine release from activated T cells and fibroblasts Growth of fibroblasts, synovial cells, endothelial cells Tissue catabolism Release of PGE_2, collagenase, acute-phase proteins Fever Chemotactic for neutrophils, macrophages, lymphocytes Increases NK cell activity Differentiation of activated B cells with B-cell differentiation factor Proliferation of activated B cells with B-cell growth factor
IL-2	T-cell growth factor (TCGF) T-cell maturation/stimulating factor (TMF/TSF) Killer helper factor (KHF) T-cell replacing factor (TRF)	Activated T cells	Induces Growth of activated T cells, thymocytes Lymphokine production by T cells Cytotoxic T lymphocyte activity Lymphokine-activated killer-cell activity Increases NK cell activity Monocyte cytotoxicity Proliferation of Tonsillar B cells with BCGF SAC-activated splenic, tonsillar, PBLB cells Chronic lymphocytic leukemic B cells Differentiation of Small and large tonsillar B cells
IL-3	Multiple colony-stimulating factor (multi-CSF) Most-cell growth factor (MCGF)	Lectin-stimulated peripheral blood lymphocytes (PBL) Activated T-cell clones Gibbon cell line MLA 144	Gibbon MLA 144 supports growth of erythroid and myeloid progenitor cells Stimulates growth of multipotential stem cells
IL-4	B-cell growth factor (BCGF) B-cell stimulatory factor (BSF1) B-cell stimulatory factor pl (BSFpl)	Activated T cells	Growth factor for T cells Proliferation of tonsillar and splenic activated B cells FceR and HLA DR on B-cell lines FceR on PBL and tonsillar B cells IgE secretion by PBLB cells Induces release of CD23 (FceR) from normal B cells
IL-5	Eosinophil differentiation factor (EDF) B-cell growth factor II (BCGF II) Killer helper factor (KHF)	T cells	Induces differentiation of eosinophils IgM secretion by SAC-stimulated PBL and splenic B cells IgA secretion by SAC-stimulated PBLB cells
IL-6	Hybridoma growth factor (HGF) Interferon B_2 B-cell stimulatory factor-2 (BSF-2) B-cell differentiation factor (BCDF)	Monocytes HTLV-transformed T-cell lines Fibroblasts Bladder carcinoma cells Osteosarcoma cells Cardiac myxoma cells Carcinoma cells	Induces Class I HLA expression on fibroblasts Production of acute-phase proteins by hepatocytes/hepatoma cells Growth of plasmacytomas and hybridoma Ig secretion by EBV-transformed B cells

(continued)

TABLE 17-3. Cytokines: Sources and Physiological Effects *(continued)*

Cytokine	*Other Names*	*Sources*	*Effects*
Tumor necrosis factor-alpha	TNF-alpha Cachectin	Macrophages T cells Thymocytes Endothelial cells	Cytotoxic or cytostatic for selected cell lines Induces Fever Cachexia Chemotaxis of neutrophils Endothelial cell procoagulant activity Endothelial-cell adhesion molecules Bone resorption In vivo injection can cause necrosis of selected subdermal mouse tumors
Tumor necrosis factor-beta	TNF-beta Lymphotoxin	T cells	Cytotoxic or cytostatic for selected cell lines Increases phagocytosis by neutrophils
Interferon-alpha	INF-alpha Type I interferon	Leukocytes Macrophages	Antiviral Antiproliferative Class I MHC expression Synergizes with other lymphokines
Interferon-beta	IFN-beta Type I interferon	Fibroblasts Epithelial cells	Antiviral Antiproliferative Class I MHC expression Synergizes with other lymphokines
Interferon-gamma	IFN-gamma Type II interferon Macrophage activating factor	T cells LGL	Antiviral Antiproliferative Increases HLA DR on endothelial cells, fibroblasts, myelomonocytic cells Antimicrobial and tumoricidal activity of monocytes/macrophages FcYR on myelomonocytic cells NK cell activity Proliferation of anti-Ig-stimulated tonsillar PBL, splenic B cells Proliferation and differentiation of SAC-activated PBL, splenic, lymph node B cells + IL-2 only

Adapted from O'Garra A: Immunology Today, February 1988.

Most research on cytokines has involved in vitro studies or studies in experimental animals. Many cytokines, such as alpha-, beta- and gamma-interferon, IL-2, tumor necrosis factor, and the colony-stimulating factors, have reached clinical application in patients with cancer. The clinical use of colony-stimulating factors will be presented in depth in Chapter 59, section 3. Clinical application of the interferons and of IL-2 is presented in this chapter in more detail.

TUMOR ANTIGENS

The central tenet of tumor immunology is that there are immunologically recognizable molecules at the tumor-cell surface that are qualitatively or quantitatively different from those on normal cells. Operationally, these immunologically detectable differences or "tumor antigens" are the reciprocal counterparts of what are thought to be highly specific immunologic reagents, namely immunoglobulins and specific cellular receptors found on T lymphocytes. The ability of the immune system to recognize an immense variety of novel antigens is determined by these unique molecules.

Since the successful demonstration of immunization to bacterial and mycobacterial antigens as protective measures against disease, many attempts have been made in both humans and murine tumor models to immunize the host with tumor. The most convincing evidence of tumor immunity is the ability to reject a subsequent tumor challenge. This has been demonstrated with a variety of animal tumors induced by viruses or chemical carcinogens. However, the ability to demonstrate tumor antigens convincingly in humans has been difficult.

The development of two new approaches has made it possible to demonstrate convincingly the differential expression of certain molecules on human tumor cells in concentrations greater than that found on normal cells. The first of these was the description of murine monoclonal antibodies in 1975 by Kohler and Milstein and, more recently, of similar human monoclonal antibodies that recognize tumor antigens (discussed later in this chapter). In addition, the demonstration that the lymphokine IL-2 could be used to expand polyclonal and monoclonal T-cell populations in the human allowed the production of cellular reagents with both specific and nonspecific antitumor reactivity.

The major antigenic class defined on human tumors using monoclonal antibodies are oncofetal antigens, products normally expressed early in embryonic development and subsequently expressed in normal cells only in small amounts or on the surface of dedifferentiated tumor cells. There are also murine monoclonal antibodies that recognize differentiation antigens unique for cells of an individual tissue. These have perhaps best been defined for B and T cells as well as other hematopoietic cell types and have been useful both in classifying normal differentiation stages and also in allocating cells to separate functional subgroups. A limited number of antibodies have also been developed that recognize tumor antigens unique to an individual tumor and absent from others of identical histology, best exemplified by anti-idiotypic antibodies reactive with B-cell lymphoma. Finally, histocompatibility antigens present on many somatic tissues and initially defined by the ability of inbred strains of animals to reject normal tissues such as skin and kidney allografts, play an important role in immune recognition and are especially important for cell-mediated recognition by T cells.

If one posits the presence of tumor antigens in humans, one must also explain the absence of an immunologic response in the individual tumor-bearing host. It is usually assumed that tumor antigens are "weak," especially when compared to histocompatibility or microbial antigens. The methods to increase the antigenicity of tumors include modification of the tumor-cell surface by chemicals and enzymes (such as neuraminidase treatment to strip sialic acid residues), use of "viral oncolysates," which take advantage of the immunogenicity of associated viral proteins, and more traditional immune adjuvants such as Freund's or attenuated or inactivated organisms such as bacillus Calmette-Guerin (BCG) or *Corynebacterium parvum*.[1] Although many clinical trials have been conducted with such active immunization, the actual identity of many of the constituents of the vaccines has not been well defined. Both serologic and cellular reactivity to tumor antigens have been reported with[2-4] or without[5-10] active immunization.

EVIDENCE FOR THE EXISTENCE OF A HOST RESPONSE TO TUMORS IN HUMANS

Probably the earliest evidence suggesting the existence of an immune response to tumors was the spontaneous regression occasionally observed in a variety of malignancies, most frequently in melanoma and renal cell carcinoma.[11,12] Spontaneous regressions occur in about 1% to 2% of patients with melanoma and renal cell carcinoma. In addition, it has been claimed that during periods of immune activation by an acute bacterial infection, tumor regressions occasionally occur.[13,14] Subsequently, the search for autologous serologic and cellular reactivity was carried out. Many of these studies were done at a time when immunologic techniques were less sophisticated and the ability to address questions of cross-reactivity was somewhat limited. Still, in many tumors, evidence of a host humoral response, especially to melanoma, neuroblastomas, and osteogenic sarcomas, was claimed.[5,7-10,15-17] Most of the antibodies demonstrated were of relatively low titer and, although sometimes capable of immune reactivity via ADCC or complement-mediated cytotoxicity, were of questionable significance. In large part, the search for autologous serologic reactivity has been supplanted by the development of murine monoclonal antibodies. Recent claims for the development of a host anti-idiotypic response to passively transferred murine monoclonal antitumor antibodies, which themselves evoke a host response to the original antigen, have renewed interest in this area.[18]

The earliest claims of specific cell-mediated immunity to human tumors were made in the early 1970s by the Hellstroms and their collaborators.[19-22] These studies, done before the recognition of natural effectors mediating natural and lymphokine-activated killing, were difficult for other investigators to repeat.[23] Subsequent studies reported by Vanky, Vose, Argov, and Klein[24-26] found that both specific proliferative and cytotoxic reactivity could be demonstrated against fresh tumors. These studies helped to demonstrate cell-mediated recognition of the antigens presumed to exist on tumors in their fresh (noncultured) state. Subsequent studies extended these observations,[27,28] demonstrated correlation of antitumor activity with survival,[29] and introduced the use of IL-2 to culture reactive T cells for long periods.[30,31] The use of autologous controls was suggested by the recognition that T cells capable of reacting with both autologous fibroblasts and lymphocytes could be demonstrated in normal patients as well as in those with cancer.[32-34] Autologous normal cells, such as those derived from normal lung, liver, colon, and bowel, proved capable of stimulating comparable responses in mixed lymphocyte–tumor interactions.[35] Subsequent studies focused on the more restricted antigens recognized by cloned T cells selected by limiting dilution culture.[36-50] In addition, these studies used autologous controls and could demonstrate restricted (and presumably specific) killing of tumor by some clones. The most convincing evidence of restricted recognition came with the use of cloned T cells that could recognize only autologous tumor cells and not autologous normal cells or allogeneic targets.

The possibility that active suppression of an immune response to tumor existed has also been explored using cellular reagents in the human.[51-54] Most recently, cultured T cells, derived directly from human tumors (both lines and clones) or tumor-infiltrating lymphocytes (TIL), have been obtained that have tumor specificity and are entering clinical trials.[55,56] Thus, the demonstration of unique tumor antigens using cellular reagents has progressed gradually (Table 17-4) over the last two decades with further understanding of the processes of natural killing, reactivity to autologous normal cells, and technical advances allowing the long-term culture and cloning of human lymphoid cells. Absolute proof of specific cellular recognition of tumor-cell antigens will require the biochemical isolation of such antigens and the successful adoptive transfer of cells that can mediate specific antitumor responses in humans. One of the apparent requirements for T-cell-mediated recognition of antigen is that

TABLE 17-4. Evidence for Autologous Cellular Reactivity to Human Tumor Antigens*

Year	*Tumor(s)*	*Source of Cells*	*Autologous Controls*	*Tumor Targets*	*Assay*	*Reference*	*Notes*
1968–73	Bladder, melanoma, neuroblastoma, colorectal	PBL	Fibroblasts, lymphocytes	C	Colony inhibition assays; MCA	15–22	Activity of "natural effectors" (NK, LAK) not recognized at time of these studies
1977	Lung, sarcoma, nasopharyngeal, renal, melanoma	TIL, LN, PBL	None	F	MLTI; MCA	26	Less activity in tumor than PBL and LN; less activity against allogeneic tumors
1981, 1982	Various	Cultured PBL from MLTI	PHA, IL-2 PBL blasts	F	MCA	24–25 30–31	Modest relative specificity by MCA and cold target studies for autologous tumor
1982	Lung, breast, melanoma	Cultured PBL from MLTI	None	F	MCA, MLTI	27–28	Cultured cells lysed autologous targets preferentially
1983	Sarcoma, lung	PBL	None	F	MCA, MLTI	29	Survival correlated with PBL antitumor reactivity; positive tests in 25%–70% of tumors
1984	Various	PBL	Liver, lung, colon, bladder	F	MLTI	35	19/37 (+) MLT1; in 14 with autologous controls, tumor stimulation was no better
1983	Melanoma	Cloned PBL	None	C	MCA	36	Relative specificity for autologous tumor
1984	B-cell lymphoma	Cloned PBL	None	F	MTLI	37	Relatively specific for B-cell lymphomas. Not restricted by MHC; antibodies to CD3, CD4 could not block
1984	Melanoma	Cloned PBL from MLTI	Fibroblasts, T-cell blasts	C	MCA	38	Cloned lines could kill allogeneic melanoma as well; not inhibited by antibody to Class I MHC
1984	Melanoma	Cultured PBL from MLTI	Fibroblasts, EBV-B cells	C	MCA	39,40	7/13 patients with autologous antimelanoma reactivity; activity lost with prolonged culture; some killing of autologous B-cell line
1985	Ovarian	Cloned cells from ascites	None	F	MCA	41	Relative specificity for autologous tumor with 5/6 clones
1985	Melanoma	Cloned PBL from MLTI	IL-2 PBL blasts	C	MCA	42–45	No clones absolutely restricted to autologous tumor; blocked by Class I MHC-directed antibodies; heterogeneity of lysis of cloned tumor cells
1986	Soft-tissue and osteogenic sarcomas	Cloned PBL from MLTI	PBL blasts, fibroblasts	F,C	MCA	46	Cloned lines could kill allogeneic sarcoma as well; one killed only if HLA-2 shared on target
1986	Melanoma	Cloned PBL from MLTI	EBV-B cells	C	MCA	47	Cold target inhibition studies suggest cross-reactivity with other cells
1986	Lung, breast, ovarian, renal	Cloned PBL from MLTI	None	F	MCA, MLTI	48,49	Restricted killing by some clones to autologous tumor; no restriction in MLTI

(continued)

TABLE 17-4. Evidence for Autologous Cellular Reactivity to Human Tumor Antigens* *(continued)*

Year	*Tumor(s)*	*Source of Cells*	*Autologous Controls*	*Tumor Targets*	*Assay*	*Reference*	*Notes*
1987	Melanoma	Cloned PBL from MLTI and after in vivo stimulation	EBV-B cells	C	MCA, cell growth	50	Restricted killing and cell growth by autologous tumor; definition of antigens by cloned reagents
1987	Melanoma	Cultured TIL	EBV-B cells PBL blasts, lung	F	MCA	55	Restricted killing in 3/6 patients with melanoma
1987	Melanoma	Cloned PBL from TIL	EBV-B cells, fibroblasts PBL	F	MCA, MLTI	56	Restricted killing of fresh autologous tumor by cloned TILs

*F, fresh; C, cultured; MCA, microcytotoxicity assay; PBL, peripheral blood lymphocytes; NK, natural killer; LAK, lymphokine activated killer; MTLI, mixed lymphocyte–tumor interaction; EBV-B, Epstein–Barr virus-transformed B cells; TIL, tumor-infiltrating lymphocytes; LN, lymph nodes; MHC, major histocompatibility complex; IL-2, interleukin-2.

it occur in the context of restriction elements encoded for within the MHC.[57] This presumably would restrict the use of immortalized cell lines to the individual from which they were derived or, at best, to a small number of others.

Less restricted and more broadly reactive cells that can mediate lysis of fresh tumor cells but not of normal cells have been defined over the last decade.[58] These cells, which are demonstrable following brief culture with IL-2, have been termed LAK cells and are non-MHC restricted in their cytotoxicity.[59] When adoptively transferred in murine tumor models in conjunction with IL-2, they have mediated the regression of a variety of different tumors.[60] Recently, clinical trials have similarly demonstrated an apparent role in the treatment of human tumors.[61,62] No unique tumor antigen or restricted killing has been noted. The tumor-related determinant that is recognized has not yet been defined, and it has been suggested that destruction of tumor cells follows the recognition of a defect in the expression of some otherwise universally expressed determinant. MHC Class I molecules have been suggested as a candidate.[63]

Finally, the suggestion that transferred immunocompetent allogeneic lymphoid cells might mediate direct antitumor effects (graft versus tumor) was initially tested in animal models. The earliest studies, performed in leukemia models in guinea pigs, demonstrated that allogeneic transfer significantly decreases the development of leukemia in these animals.[64] In addition, protection against subsequent leukemic challenge suggested some long-lived immunologic response. Subsequent studies revealed separable graft-versus-host disease and graft-versus-leukemia effects.[65-69] In addition, the ability to stimulate or produce such effects could be demonstrated with donors that were identical at MHC loci.[70] It was subsequently recognized that graft-versus-host disease also had an antileukemic effect in humans receiving allogeneic bone-marrow grafts.[71,72] Methods to decrease graft-versus-host disease in both animals and humans have been associated with increased relapse rates.[73-75] For example, in a recent prospective, randomized, double-blind trial in which monoclonal anti-T-cell antibody and complement depletion of T lymphocytes from donor bone marrow was carried out before treatment, only 3 episodes of acute graft-versus-host disease in 20 patients were demonstrated, whereas this reaction appeared in 13 of 20 untreated controls.[75] Marrow in five patients in the T-cell-depleted group failed to engraft, whereas all the control patients had successful transplants. Relapse of leukemia occurred in 7 of 20 in the T-cell-depletion group and in two controls. Although this is not definitive evidence that tumor-specific antigens are recognized, such transplants are currently being done in patients with advanced-stage solid tumors, and the demonstration of specific antitumor reactivity could be sought in that setting.

OTHER TUMOR-CELL PRODUCTS POTENTIALLY APPLICABLE TO IMMUNOLOGIC THERAPY

Histologic and serum markers have been sought for cancer diagnosis and therapy for many years (reviewed in reference 76). It is clear that many of the "tumor" markers such as carcinoembryonic antigen[77,78] (CEA) and alpha-fetoprotein[79] (AFP) initially demonstrated are not tumor specific, as they also are expressed on early embryonic or fetal cells. However, this does not preclude their use as either diagnostic markers or potential targets for immune recognition and destruction. In fact, it is likely that most available "tumor-specific" monoclonal antibodies detect antigens expressed at some point in normal human somatic development but reexpressed only on malignant tissue (see discussion below of monoclonal antibodies). In addition, certain blood group antigens have been found to be deleted on a growing tumor cell population and, conversely, that additional antigens, present on normal epithelial cells, are sometimes expressed. Many of these are likely neoantigens, expressed subsequent to the altered glycosylation of normal proteins on the cell membrane.[80,81]

A variety of tumor markers have been used in the serologic diagnosis of cancer, some of which are expressed at the cell surface and are potentially exploitable for therapy. This subject was extensively reviewed recently.[76] The list includes the classically described oncofetal antigens, CEA[82,83] and AFP,[84-86] and enzymes specific for individual tumors such as prostatic acid phosphatase[87] and lactic dehydrogenase,[88] proteins such as ferritin,[89] hormones such as calcitonin[90] and bombesin,[91] or more recently described oncofetal antigens identified by monoclonal antibody preparation techniques.[92-106] There also appears to be differential expression of more universal antigens such as histocompatibility antigens[107-111] on tumor cells, which may be critical to recognition by cellular reagents. Presumably, virtually every novel cell-surface determinant recognized by monoclonal antibodies could be investigated as a shed antigen useful in serodiagnosis. The most recent examples of this are shed IL-2 receptors, which are released after antigen stimulation.[112] Concentrations are elevated in individuals with T- and B-cell tumors[113] and cancer patients undergoing IL-2 therapy.[114]

Even an antigen that is not necessarily specific for tumor might be targeted with cellular or serologic reagents. Examples of this include antibodies to the IL-2 receptors or epidermal growth factor receptors, which have entered or are being developed for clinical trials.[115-120]

MONOCLONAL ANTIBODIES

Shortly after the demonstration that neutralizing substances exist in the serum that can bind to microbes, a similar notion developed that serologic reactivity to tumor cells might be demonstrated and that such sera might be useful in the treatment of cancer.[121] Although evidence steadily accumulated, both in murine tumor models and in humans, that serologically detectable differences between tumors and normal cells exist, there were multiple problems in exploiting these observations. Much of the difficulty arose because putative tumor antigens had in most cases not been characterized biochemically. For this reason, the generation of xenogeneic antiserum required the immunization of animals, such as goats or rabbits, with crude membrane digests or whole tumor cells. Most of the reactivity thus generated was against antigenic moieties present on normal human cells, and serologic evidence of specific antitumor reactivity required multiple absorptions against normal human tissues. Similarly, most of the reactivity found in humans to their own tumors was of low titer and difficult to characterize. Also, many xenogeneic sera varied from batch to batch and animal to animal, and this variability inherent in polyclonal antisera representing presumably hundreds, if not thousands, of different antibody molecules frustrated investigators for many years.

The development of techniques to produce monoclonal antibodies in 1975 by Kohler and Milstein[122] allowed the identification, selection, and production of antibodies to specific antigens in theoretically unlimited quantities. Although this monoclonal approach is new, considerable work has already been done in developing these reagents for both diagnostic and therapeutic applications.

Before considering in detail the clinical studies that have been performed, some analysis of the factors important to successful use of monoclonal antibodies will be reviewed.

MOLECULAR BIOLOGY, STRUCTURE, AND FUNCTION OF IMMUNOGLOBULINS

Immunoglobulins are the second most prevalent species in human serum after albumin. These glycoproteins are found in every mammal and in their monomeric form are com-

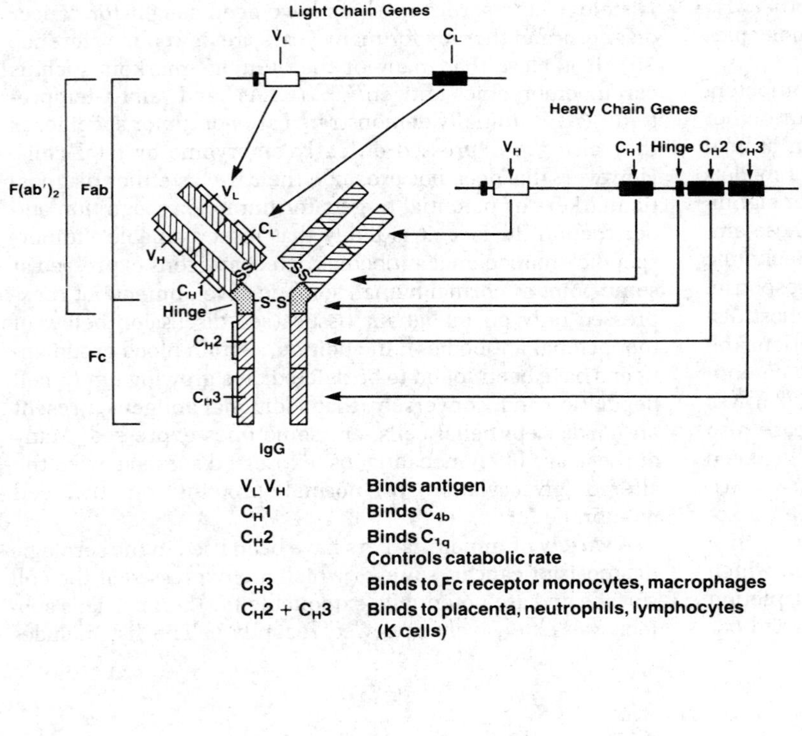

FIG. 17-1. Molecular biology, structure, and functional aspects of an immunoglobulin molecule. The genes for the human bearing chain are located on chromosome 14, the kappa light chain on 2, and the lambda light chain on 22. In mice they are located on chromosomes 12, 6, and 16, respectively. The k : λ ratio in humans is 70 : 30 and in mice 95 : 5. Each chain is encoded for by multiple introns with both variable (*V*) and constant (*C*) regions providing the antigen binding and functional domains of the antibody molecule, respectively. Multiple allelic copies of V and J segment genes within the variable region of the light chain and of V, D, and J segment genes of the heavy chain exist. Immunoglobulin diversity occurs by selection and "shuffling" of these genetic elements with varying recombinations, somatic mutations, and association of different heavy and light chains. The hinge region provides some molecular flexibility and serves as the site for disulfhydryl bonds between the heavy chains and with the light chain of IgG1. For the other IgG subclasses the light and heavy chains are joined at the intersection of the variable and constant portions. Enzymatic cleavage by papain will split the molecule into Fab and Fc portions, respectively. Pepsin splits just distal to the hinge heavy chain linkage and maintains a dimeric antigen binding structure [*F(ab')*$_2$]. The individual constant regions of the heavy chain as shown provide the functional characteristics of the molecule and may become "activated" following antigen binding. Antibody fragments have been used for radioimmunodiagnosis and have been coupled to toxins or radionuclides for therapy.

posed of two heavy and two light chains (Fig. 17-1). The molecular weight of these molecules ranges from 146,000 (IgG) to the 970,000 of the pentameric IgM. The mature molecule consists of globular domains that serve as antigen-binding sites as well as regions involved in antibody effector function.[123,124] The immense diversity within immunoglobulins is generated through variation in isotype (several different subclasses of light and heavy chains), allotype (variability normally encoded in the constant portion of the light or heavy chains), and idiotype (which accounts for most of the heterogeneity in this system). Idiotypic variation has recently been demonstrated to occur through a unique process of gene shuffling, recombination, and somatic mutation.

The predominant immunoglobulin molecule in the serum is IgG, which is represented by four subclasses with somewhat different functions (Table 17-5). Although the earliest molecule to be produced after immunization is usually pentameric IgM, this species cannot bind to effector cells. Consequently, most efforts have been devoted to selecting antibodies of the IgG isotype, and within this isotype, multiple subclasses and enzyme-derived fragments have been prepared from monoclonal sources. For example, the murine IgG3 subclass has been identified as a good mediator in human cells of ADCC, an important effector mechanism in antibody action. Similarly, IgG4 murine antibodies have been selected because of their lack of binding to Fc receptors, making them suitable for use as diagnostic reagents.

Each antibody molecule in its native state is composed of a number of homologous domains which are related to different functions. For example, the Cγ1 and Cγ2 regions bind C4b and C1q (see Fig. 17-1). Complement-mediated lysis of tumor cells is one of the mechanisms by which tumor-cell destruction by antibodies takes place. However, most of the currently available antitumor human monoclonal antibodies interact with human complement components poorly. The terminal domain Cγ3 is important in binding to cellular effectors, such as monocytes, macrophages, neutrophils, and lymphocytes. In addition to its ability to bind antigen, an antibody molecule (because it usually does not subserve an enzymatic function) can also readily dissociate from its target structure without altering it. The relative strength of the interaction between an antibody molecule and the site on a molecule that it recognizes (the epitope) is defined by a dissociation constant or K_d. The K_d of most monoclonal antibodies ranges from 10^{-6} to 10^{-10} M/L. The portions of a molecule that are recognized and bind to an antibody is in a large part determined by the molecular conformation, with regions deep within the three-dimensional structure being less accessible to antigen.[126,127] The ability to engineer an antibody-combining site, or Fab, using molecular biologic techniques to enhance its affinity or specificity[128] or to subserve enzymatic functions[129] is an interesting future direction in the development of antibodies as therapeutic and diagnostic reagents.

PREPARATION OF MONOCLONAL ANTIBODIES

Although others had demonstrated that somatic cells could be fused and that monoclonal antibodies could be produced from murine and human myelomas, it was not until the experiments of Kohler and Milstein[122,130,131] that antibodies of predetermined specificity were obtained. This finding revolutionized biology, and its general application to producing serologic reagents of high affinity, specificity, and reproducibility became widely apparent. It was widely applied to the development of antitumor monoclonal antibodies against melanoma,[132-135] colorectal carcinoma,[136-138] carcinoma of the lung,[139,140] and most other tumors.

The general strategy for the derivation of murine monoclonals[141] is demonstrated in Figure 17-2. In brief, a mouse is immunized with an appropriate antigen, usually whole tumor cells or cell-membrane digests. Reactive B cells are usually obtained from the immunized mouse's spleen or lymph nodes and immortalized by fusing with an enzyme-marked

TABLE 17-5. Human Antibody Subclasses Mediating Biologic Functions

Variable	IgG				IgA					
	IgG1	IgG2*	IgG3	IgG4	IgA1	IgA2	sIgA	IgM	IgD	IgE
Allotypes (number)		Gm(20)				Am(2)		Mm(2)		
Molecular weight (kD)	146	146	170	146	160	160	385	970	184	188
Sediment. constant	6.75	6.65	6.65	6.65	75	75	115	195	75	85
Mean serum level (mg/dl)	9	3	1	0.5	3.0	0.5	0.05	1.5	0.03	0.00005
Carbohydrate (%)	2–3	2–3	2–3	2–3	7–11	7–11	7–11	12	9–14	12
Total circulating pool (mg/kg body wt)		494.0			95.0			37.0	1.1	0.019
Half-life (days)		23.0			5.8			5.1	2.8	2.5
Rate of synthesis (mg/kg/day)		33.0			24.0			6.7	0.4	0.016
Placental transfer	+	+	+	+	+	+	–	–	–	–
Monocytes	+	–	+	–	–	–	–	–	–	–
Neutrophils	+	+	+	±	+	+	+	–	–	–
Lymphocytes (K, NK, LAK)	+	+	+	±	–	–	–	–	–	–
Platelets	+	+	+	+	–	–	–	–	–	–
Complement Fixation	++	+	+++	±†	+	+	–	+	+†	–

*Associated with immune response to carbohydrate antigens (in the mouse mediated by IgG3).
†Alternative pathway.
Modified from Roitt I, Brostoff J, Male D: Immunology. St Louis, CV Mosby, 1985, and Jeske DJ, Capra JD: Immunoglobulins: Structure and function. In Paul WE (ed): Fundamental Immunology, pp 131–165. New York, Raven Press, 1984.

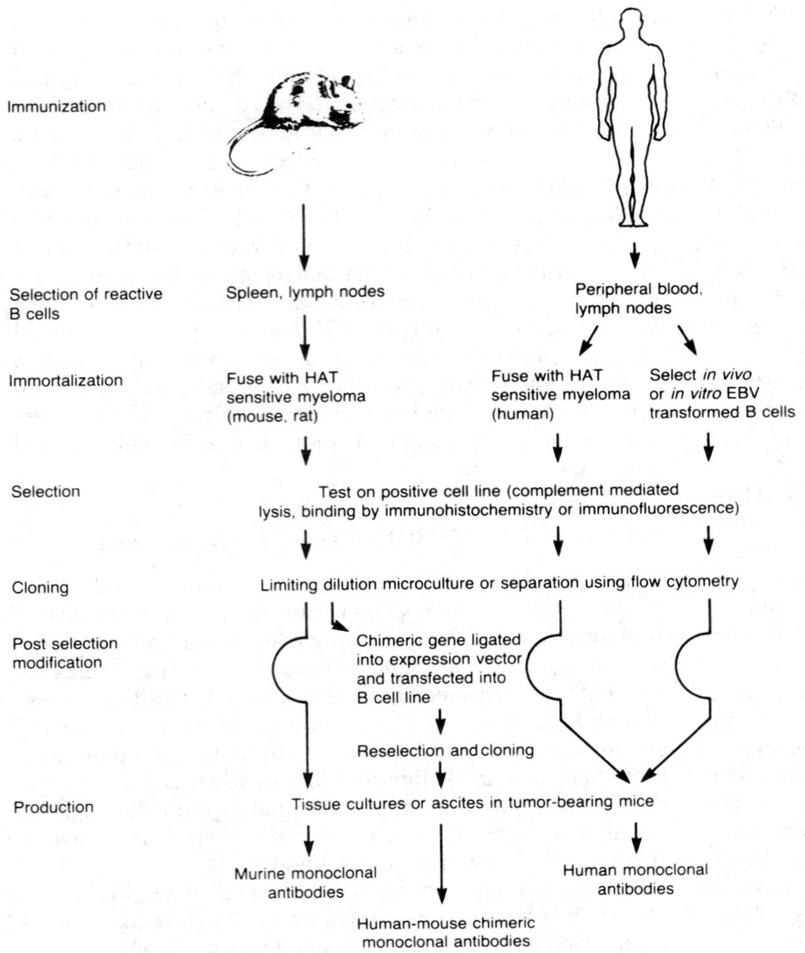

FIG. 17-2. Mechanism for preparing monoclonal antibodies. Shown are the usual procedures used to produce monoclonal antibodies from human or murine sources. Human mouse chimeric genes have been produced by ligation of the mouse variable region to a human constant region. They are produced in transfected B-cell lines using conventional molecular biologic techniques. The procurement of large quantities of antibody for clinical trials usually involves production and purification from ascites of hybridoma bearing mice or in tissue culture. The latter produces 10 to 100 μg/ml, whereas ascitic fluid yields as much as 1 to 25 mg/ml.

myeloma. These enzyme-marked cells lack enzymes critical for growth or detoxification of certain compounds. In the usual technique, these myeloma cells lack either thymidine kinase or hypoxanthine guanosine phosphoribosyl transferase (HGPRT). Thus, when the parent and fused cells are grown in hypoxanthine, aminopterine, and thymidine (HAT) medium, the principal synthetic pathway for ribonucleotides is blocked by the aminopterin, and the ability to incorporate these nucleotides is possessed only by hybrid cells, which contain normal levels of HGPRT from the normal B cells derived from the spleen or lymph node. Consequently, the nonfused myeloma cells die, and only the HAT-resistant (fusion) products survive. Individual small groups of cellular supernatant fluids are tested on a tumor cell line either for complement-mediated lysis or for binding (immunohistochemical or immunofluorescence). After identification of an appropriate antibody-secreting hybridoma, limiting-dilution microculture is carried out, and the cloned, immortalized B cell can then be placed either in tissue culture or into the peritoneal cavity of mice to produce large quantities of murine monoclonal antibodies. A similar procedure can be used, although much less successfully, to produce human monoclonal antibodies. Alternatively, Epstein–Barr virus can be used to transform B cells that are making appropriate antibody (see below). Most recently, chimeric genes and protein products have been produced using molecular biologic techniques[142] to ligate the genes for the variable portion of both the heavy and light chains to constant portions encoded by human genes. As noted below, such chimeric antibodies are entering clinical trials. The original technique of murine monoclonal antibody preparation, although relatively straightforward, has thus been extended to produce a variety of protein products, some of which differ substantially from the original antibody molecule.

IN VIVO MECHANISMS OF ANTIBODY ACTION

In vivo mechanisms of antibody-mediated tumor inhibition and destruction are listed in Table 17-6. The ability of antibodies to coat targets and, in association with other serum opsonins, to cause phagocytosis or lysis by leukocyte effectors in the human is mediated largely by the IgG1 and IgG3 subclasses.[123,124] The Fc portion of the antibody (Fc: crystallizable fragment) can bind to any one of three different FC receptors that have been defined both in mice and humans. The subset of lymphocytes that expresses Fc receptors with effector function includes large granular lymphocytes, which

TABLE 17-6. Possible in Vivo Mechanisms of Antibody-Mediated Tumor Inhibition and Destruction

Complement-mediated lysis after interaction with antigen
Antibody-dependent cellular cytotoxicity with lymphocytes (K cells), polymorphonuclear leukocytes or monocytes
Organization with normal serum constituents and elimination by reticuloendothelial cells
Radiotoxicity or chemotoxicity secondary to conjugated reagents
Block receptor for autocrine growth products or normal hormones, cytokines
Induction of host antitumor response subsequent to development of anti-idiotypic antibodies (appearing similar to original tumor antigen)

can manifest natural killing, lymphokine-activated killing, and ADCC. The Fc_gRIII Fc receptor, defined by the antibodies 3G8 and Leu 11 (CD16), is a receptor for polymeric IgG and is also present on polymorphonuclear leukocytes (PMNs) and differentiated monocytes.[143,144] This is the major Fc receptor on lymphoid cells. Monocytes express additional receptors known as Fc_gRI and Fc_gRII.[145] Fc_gRI, recognized by the murine monoclonal antibodies 32.2 and 62.2, identifies a receptor with high affinity for monomeric IgG1. This receptor and its mediation of ADCC are increased on monocytes by the lymphokine gamma-interferon, which also causes de novo expression of this molecule on PMNs. The Fc_gRII receptor identified by the antibody IV-3 appears to have relatively low affinity for monomeric antibody and appears to have as its principal role the clearing of heavily opsonized particles. The Fc_gRII has also been identified on human platelets.[146] The identity of Fc receptors on lymphocytes[147] and granulocytes[148] in the human and their susceptibility to modulation by cytokines has now been carefully defined and the genes encoding these molecules cloned in the mouse.[149,150] Other serum proteins, including activated complement components such as C5a and C-reactive protein,[151-155] also appear to have a role in Fc-receptor function and expression. It is presumed that the therapeutic role of native unaltered monoclonal antibodies involves ADCC or opsonization with removal by the reticuloendothelial system.

When various human and murine effector cells are tested for their ability to mediate killing of human tumors using monoclonal antibodies of different isotypes,[138] the cells that can mediate the greatest killing prove to be murine monocytes followed in turn by human lymphocytes and human monocytes. The murine antibody that can mediate the greatest lysis by these cells is IgG3, followed by IgG2a and IgG2b. Other antigens might elicit other isotypes effectively in a different hierarchy. Antibodies recognizing a colorectal antibody and the disialogangliosides GD2 and GD3 effectively target human killer cells.[135,156-158] Certain lymphokines can also activate these lymphoid killers, including alpha- and gamma-interferon and IL-2.[159-161]

ANTIBODY CONJUGATES

The earliest development of antibodies against murine and human tumors was done in the context of using these antibodies coupled to other, more toxic reagents to fashion a magic bullet that would seek out tumor cells and destroy them uniquely, leaving uninjured the cells to which they did not bind.[162] A large variety of cytotoxic agents have been described for possible conjugation to monoclonal antibodies (Table 17-7) (summarized in Ref. 163). These include different radioisotopes producing alpha and beta emissions.[164] The one used in most clinical trials currently is ^{131}I, employed therapeutically as a beta-particle emitter (Figure 17-4). The limitations of using antibody-coupled radioisotopes include irradiation of adjacent tissues, even in the absence of specific antibody binding.[165] In spite of the great specificity of available antibodies, the maximum tumor-to-normal tissue ratios, in terms of delivered dose, have been only about 10 to 20. One of the advantages, however, associated with the use of such radiolabeled antibodies is that they do not require internalization of the antibody complex as is necessary for toxins or coupled chemotherapeutic agents.

The selection of an individual radionuclide is dependent on a number of factors. Because antibodies require percolation through tissues, it has been estimated that 1 to 3 days will be required for adequate delivery of antibody to tumor sites. This is in large part based on preliminary radiolabeling studies (see below). For that reason, radionuclides with relatively short biologic half-lives—on the order of 24 hours to 5 to 7 days—have been recommended. The range of the toxic-

TABLE 17-7. Cytotoxic Agents for Conjugation to Monoclonal Antibodies

Beta-particle emitters
Iodine-131
Scandium-47
Palladium-109
Yttrium-90
Alpha-particle emitters
Bismuth-212
Astatine-211
Auger electron generators
Iodine-125
Bromine-77
Fissionable nuclides
Boron-10
Actinides
Protein toxins and cytotoxins
Ricin
Diphtheria
Purothionine
Pseudomonas exotoxin
Alpha amanitin
Chemotherapeutic drug
Vindesine
Methotrexate
Daunorubicin
Doxorubicin
Cytosine arabinoside
5-Fluorouridine
Biologic agents
Interleukin-2
Interferon
Cobra venom factor
Liposomes
Antibody to lymphocyte surface structures (antibody heteroconjugates)
Photosensitive agents (hematoporphyrin)

Adapted from Houghton AN, Scheinberg DA: Monoclonal antibodies: Potential applications to the treatment of cancer. Semin Oncol 13:165–179, 1986.

ity of the radionuclides is also important, and it is estimated that up to 0.5 mm will be required for sufficient radiation to penetrate all tumor cells.[166] Radionuclides producing high-energy gamma rays are thus excluded. For example, one of the major deficiencies of ^{131}I as a radiopharmaceutical, in spite of its sufficiently energetic beta ray, is the presence of significant high-energy gamma rays. In addition, iodine radionuclides frequently are stripped from the antibody molecules through a process of dehalogonization. Finally, the radionuclide must be available at reasonable cost and be accessible to clinical centers. Other recently evaluated radionuclides include boron-11(^{11}B)[162], useful as a neutron target[167], palladium-109 (^{109}Pd)[168], Yttrium-90, and Astatine-211.

An alternative to coupling an antibody to a radionuclide is to conjugate it to a chemical toxin, many of which are plant or bacterial products that are extremely toxic at doses of only a few molecules per cell. The antibody–toxin conjugate is presumably endocytosed after binding to the cell surface via coated pits and vesicles and thereafter causes toxicity. For example, the toxins derived from ricin,[118,169-171] diphtheria, and the pseudomonas endotoxin[172] all interrupt ribosomal processes with extremely high efficiency. One of the major problems associated with the use of bacterial or plant toxins is that they can themselves bind directly to the cell surface without antibody coupling. It has therefore been necessary to strip the toxin of this characteristic either by enzyme treatment or by removing a second, B, chain that binds to the cell surface. Most recently, the toxin molecule has been linked to the monoclonal antibody by direct ligation of the antibody gene to the toxin gene using molecular biologic techniques.[142] This same procedure can be used to link toxin molecules to ligands other than antibodies, including hormones and cytokines such as IL-2.[173] These antibody–toxin conjugates have proved active in vitro as toxic molecules and have entered clinical trials. In addition, allogeneic bone marrow has been cleared of T cells using anti-T-cell monoclonal antibody–ricin conjugates.[170] Similarly, other toxins have been developed, including chemotherapeutic agents bound directly to the antibody[174-176] or incorporated into liposomes containing staphylococcal protein A coupled to a chemotherapeutic agent.[177] Hematoporphyrin derivatives have also been coupled directly to antibodies without losing their ability to cause phototoxicity of the relevant target when exposed to light.[178]

Antibodies have been used to block the receptor for autocrine growth products or normal hormones or cytokines. For example, the IL-2 receptor is present on a variety of T-cell leukemias associated with infection by the human T-cell lymphotrophic virus (HTLV-I).[179-181] Antibodies to the IL-2 receptor coupled to diphtheria toxin have been used to treat patients with T-cell leukemia.[182-183] This anti-IL-2 receptor (anti-Tac) has also been coupled to alpha-emitters including ^{212}bismuth.[184] More recently, antibodies to the epidermal growth factor receptor[120,185,186] have been used in murine models to define human glioma xenografts and to modulate their growth as well as that of epidermal, colorectal, and cervical carcinoma-derived cell lines.[120] An immunotoxin prepared from the monoclonal antibody reactive with the human transferrin receptor coupled with the ricin A chain has shown tumoricidal activity in an intraperitoneal nude-mouse model.[187]

Finally, it is possible that murine monoclonals act by inducing a host response to the murine antibody or anti-idiotype, which itself bears resemblance to the original tumor antigen and elicits a host response.[188-191] Thus, an initial antibody (antibody-1) may elicit a second host antibody (antibody-2), which in turn elicits a third host antibody (antibody-3), forming a network of interacting antibodies. Antibody-3 and antibody-1 presumably both recognize the same tumor antigen. This network theory, originally proposed by Jerne,[192] has been clearly demonstrated in murine models and has been suggested to be related to the efficacy of murine monoclonal antibodies administered in clinical trials.[188] Administration of anti-idiotypic antibodies has been explored as a means to immunize humans against viruses[193] and to elicit an antitumor response.[194]

ANTIBODY HETEROCONJUGATES

An alternative approach to exploiting the ability of antibodies to target tumor cells is to couple them directly to other antibodies that bind an effector cell.[195] Antibodies directed to cell-surface determinants such as those that bind to T3, associated with the T-cell receptor for antigen or with antibodies to the Fc-gamma receptor, have been effective in vitro. These "heteroaggregates" or "heteroconjugates" will lyse targets such as tumor cells to which one limb of the conjugate is directed.[196-199] These cross-links have been used to lyse murine tumor targets and, more recently, human tumor targets with a demonstration that they can prevent tumor growth in an intraperitoneal nude-mouse model using both anti-T3 and anti-Fc receptor conjugates.[200,201] The utility of such unique heteroconjugates in the treatment of human tumors is now being evaluated. The major advantage of this approach is that it bypasses the requirement for cytolytic T cells or PMNs to interact directly with the tumor through a specific receptor. One of the limitations of such an approach is related to the generation of a host response to these artificial heteroconjugates. Chimeric antibodies could be produced using molecular biologic techniques to overcome this problem in part.

HUMAN ANTIBODIES

Because autologous reactivity in the sera of patients against their own tumor can be demonstrated, attempts have been made to derive human monoclonal antibodies from such individuals. An obvious approach would be to generate a monoclonal antibody from the fusion of human B-cells with a human or murine B-cell fusion partner, which would allow immortalization of this immunoglobulin producing cell. In practice, however, derivation of human monoclonals in this fashion has been extremely difficult.[202] An alternative approach has been to transform cells directly with Epstein–Barr virus to immortalize their secretion of antitumor antibodies. This can be done by transforming them in vitro or by selecting from in vivo sites cells that have already been transformed by endogenous Epstein–Barr virus.[203,204] Most of the antibodies that have been derived from patients with melanoma or colorectal carcinoma have been IgMs, which makes them less suitable for coupling to radionuclides or toxins. Trials have been initiated using these antibodies by injecting them directly into lesions or systemically.[205] Techniques have been developed to select such antigen-specific B-cells using cell-sorting techniques.[206]

An alternative approach to obtaining human antibody molecules with reactivity against human tumors has been to produce genetically engineered antibody molecules combining the variable-region genes for both the heavy and light chain from the mouse, which are in turn directly ligated to the genes encoding the Fc portion of the immunoglobulin molecule from the human[142] (Fig. 17-3). The ability to transfect immunoglobulin genes into lymphoid cells has been demonstrated with production of these unique molecules. Such recombinant monoclonal antibodies have been obtained against the common acute lymphocytic leukemia antigen[207] and three others with broad reactivity against adenocarcinomas 17-1A,[208] L6.[209] and B72.3[210]. These unique molecules can be engineered to be coupled at the genetic level directly to genes encoding other proteins such as toxins or metal-binding proteins. Whether these primary antibodies will be less antigenic is currently unclear, but preliminary human trials are encouraging; both a long half-life and decreased immunogenicity have been noted.

FIG. 17-3. Construction of a human–mouse chimeric immunoglobulin. Shown are the steps used to create chimeric L6, an antibody recognizing a variety of adenocarcinomas. The unshaded variable regions from the mouse heavy (V_H) and light chains (V_K) have been ligated to the appropriate constant portion of the human genes in separate plasmids prior to combinational ligation. Alternatively separate plasmids for each chain could be transfected into a B-cell line. Chimeric antibodies such as these have entered clinical trials. (Modified from reference 209)

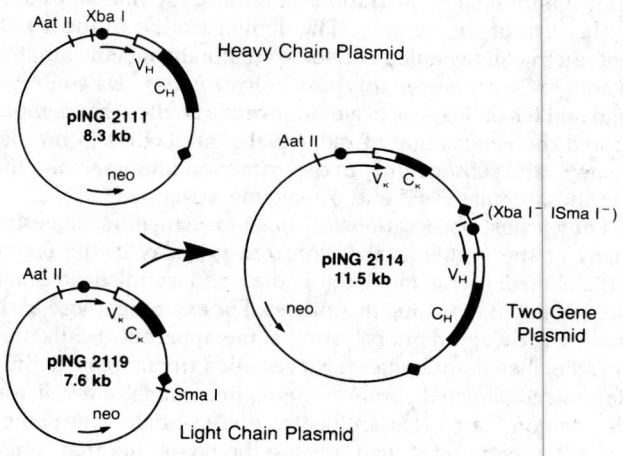

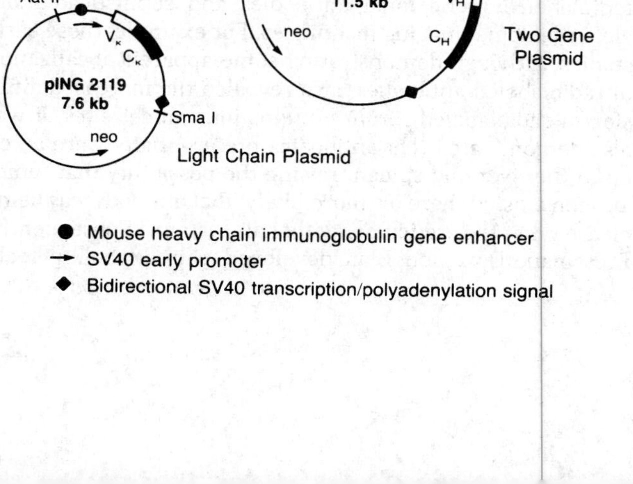

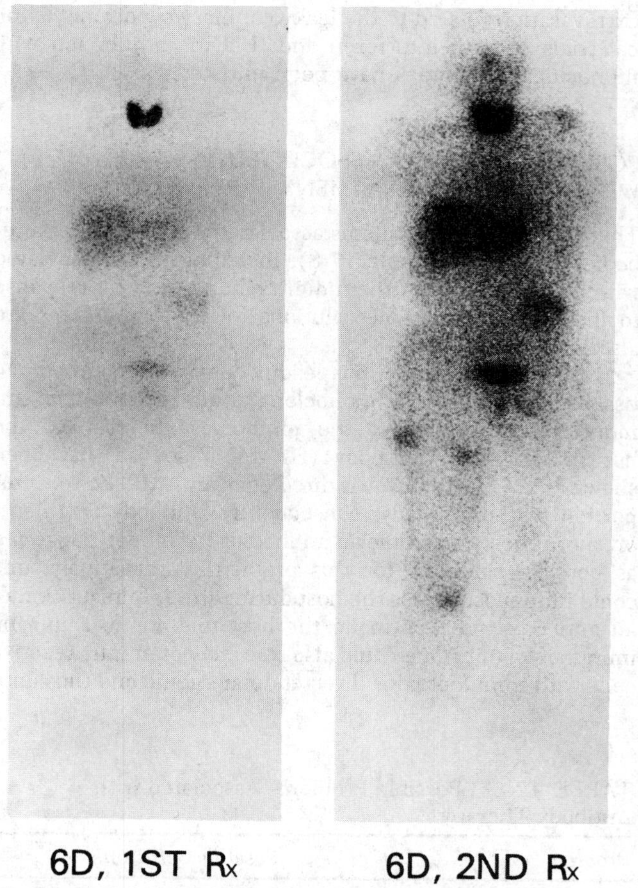

FIG. 17-4. Radioimaging and therapy with ^{131}I-coupled antimelanoma Fab. Treatment of a patient with 50 mg of antibody labeled with 6.4 mCi of ^{131}I is shown at the end of 6 days following the first and second treatments. Uptake by cutaneous deposits of tumor is apparent, with nonspecific uptake in thyroid, liver, and excretion of radiolabel into the urinary bladder.

ADMINISTRATION IN COMBINATION WITH RECOMBINANT HUMAN CYTOKINES

That cytokines such as interferon could modulate the lysis of tumor cells by immune effectors has been known for some time.[211] Interferon and, more recently, TNF have been demonstrated to markedly increase MHC Class I and Class II antigens and many tumor-associated antigens.[212,213] This ability to augment the expression of MHC antigens is thought to be important in enhancing the therapeutic potential of antibodies in murine models. Anti-idiotypic antibodies in conjunction with alpha-interferon in treatment of murine lymphomas and antibodies to adenocarcinomas in human colon tumor xenograft models have been administered with synergistic effects.[214,215] Recently, IL-2 has been demonstrated to synergize with antitumor antibodies in murine models of melanoma[216] and lymphoma.[217] Presumably, its function is to enhance MHC expression through the secondary elaboration of gamma-interferon, to activate cytolytic effectors with Fc receptors, and to increase the delivery of antibodies to tumor sites secondary to the increased protein extravasation related to the leaky capillary syndrome. Clinical trials of both interferon and IL-2 in conjunction with monoclonal antibodies have been initiated.

POSSIBLE PROBLEMS ASSOCIATED WITH ANTIBODY TREATMENT

There are multiple problems associated with the use of antibodies in therapy (Table 17-8), including those associated with characteristics of the tumor cell and the host response to the antibody. Possible solutions for these problems are also listed in Table 17-8.

Murine immunoglobulin is readily demonstrated in human tissues after infusion of monoclonal antibody,[218] and an immune response against the antibodies themselves, the human antimouse antibody (HAMA) response, has been shown.[219-221] Most HAMA is directed against the Fc receptor portion of the antibody; consequently, antibody fragments or, more recently, chimeric antibodies have been suggested as possible solutions for this problem. Alternatively, one could immunosuppress the host during the administration of an antibody and thus make the host tolerant to a murine immunoglobulin. One could also lyse any potentially reactive cells with immunotoxins directed to antigenic and thus anti-idiotypic determinants.[219] The ability to give different antibodies recognizing the same specificity but different idiotypes and potentially different isotypes has also been suggested. Preexisting human antimouse immunoglobulin reactivity has been demonstrated. It appears to be primarily of an IgM type and to be related to polyclonal rheumatoid factors that can be demonstrated in certain cancer patients, in patients with rheumatoid arthritis, and in some normal individuals.[222] Anti-idiotypes and anti-anti-idiotypes have been demonstrated against murine antibodies in mice as well as in humans.[189]

TABLE 17-8. Possible Problems Associated with Antibody Therapy

Problem	*Possible Solutions*
Antigenic modulation	Use multiple monoclonal antibodies recognizing same or different antigens; choose nonmodulating antigen
Release of free antigen	Plasmapheresis; varying schedule of monoclonal antibody treatments
Antimouse antibodies	Develop human chimeric antibodies, immunosuppressive drugs, plasmapheresis with immunospecific absorption, large dose of antibody to induce tolerance
Tumor heterogeneity	Treat with multiple antibodies that react with different antigens
Lack of in vivo cytotoxicity of antibody alone	Conjugate monoclonal antibody to drugs, toxins, or radionuclides
Neoplastic cells not accessible to blood supply	Conjugate monoclonal antibody to radionuclides that "emit" radiation beyond a single cell. Produce capillary "leak" with IL-2.
Bone-marrow toxicity from toxin-labeled antibody	Use in association with bone marrow transplantation
Lack of in vivo expression of antigen	Treat with cytokines that induce expression of tumor antigens (interferon, tumor necrosis factor)
Absence of effectors capable of mediating antibody-directed cytotoxicity	In vitro activation and transfer of effectors or direct in vivo activation (Il-2, GM-CSF)

Adapted from Foon KA, Morgan AC: Monoclonal antibody therappy of cancer: Animal models and human trials. In Roth JA (ed): Monoclonal Antibodies in Cancer. Mt Kisco, Futura Publishing, 1986.

Most, if not all, of the antitumor monoclonals recognize oncofetal antigens, that is, these antibodies recognize products that are normally expressed early in fetal life but which are not expressed, or are expressed only in small amounts, in adults. Consequently, they cannot be considered true tumor-specific transplantation antigens but rather are only preferentially expressed on neoplastic cells. The potential cross-reactivity of these monoclonal reagents is of some concern. For example, several groups of investigators have defined the expression of the melanoma-associated gangliosides (such as G_{D2} and G_{D3}) and have developed antibodies to them.[36-38] These antibodies have antitumor reactivity even though such antigens also can be demonstrated on certain normal cells, such as a subset of human T cells.[223] The administration of antibodies in both murine and human studies has also demonstrated novel findings that were not unexpected, including the ability to induce tolerance by monoclonal antibody therapy[224] and the induction of immunosuppression with immune complexes formed in antibody excess.[225]

IMAGING STUDIES WITH RADIOLABELED ANTIBODIES

EARLY STUDIES

The suggestion that therapy or localization of tumor might be carried out with radiolabeled antibodies was made shortly after the initial demonstrations of antibody to human tumors at the turn of the century. The demonstration in the 1930s that chemically coupled antibodies maintain specific binding to antigen[226] supported this possibility. In 1948, David Pressman and his colleagues began innovative studies that demonstrated the localization of radiolabeled antibodies in normal tissue[227] and subsequently in experimental tumors, including lymphosarcomas[228,229] and osteogenic sarcoma.[230]

The earliest observations of these investigators suggested many of the problems that confront us today in the use of radiolabeled monoclonal antibodies and sophisticated nuclear medicine imaging techniques. For example, these early studies, although demonstrating some apparent localization of radiolabeled antibodies, also revealed the increased diffusion of radiolabeled serum proteins into cancer sites. It was also demonstrated that antibodies preferentially were taken up in the liver and spleen, raising the possibility that tumor antigen existed there or, more likely, that antibody was being cleared by the reticuloendothelial system. Subsequently, Pressman, Day, and Blau developed paired-labeling tech-

(Text continues on page 320.)

TABLE 17-9. Diagnostic Studies with Radiolabeled Antibodies

Year	Institution (ref.)	Route of Injection*	Tumor	No. of Patients	Antigen/ Antibody/ Class	Isotope	Dose mCi	Dose mg	%ID/g	Identification of Lesions
Gliomas										
1965	Duke Univ.[232]	IA	Gliomas	8	Rabbit anti-autologous glioma	$^{131}I/^{125}I$	0.1–0.2	0.05	0.001–0.010	11/11 pts and 38/39 clinically positive sites
1968	Duke Univ.[233]	IA	Gliomas	2	Rabbit antimyelin	^{125}I	0.170	0.01	–	2/2 glioma pts confirmed higher localization in tumor
Adenocarcinoma										
1974	Tufts Univ.[237]	IV,IA	Colorectal	1	CEA/rabbit Ig	^{131}I	0.1–1.59	0.42–480	–	No imaging of lesion, transient drop in CEA with each of three injections
1975	Dalhousie Univ., Nova Scotia[235]	IV	Renal carcinoma	1	Autologous/goat	^{131}I	4.2	100	–	1/1 pt and 1/1 lesion; more in tumor, less in liver/spleen at 48 hours
			Melanoma	2	autologous/ rabbit goat Ig		1.95–3.48	100–120		0/2 pt; serum sickness in one patient
			Squamous cell cancer, lung		Autologous/goat		5.6	120		1/1 pt and 1/1 lesions
1978	Dalhousie[236]	IV	Renal carcinoma	6	Renal Ca/goat Ig	^{131}I	3.5–4.0	100	–	7/7 lesions observed
1978	Univ. Kentucky[238,240]	IV	Adeno-carcinoma	18	CEA/goat Ig	^{131}I	0.6–1.6	100–200	–	15/18 pts; 30/40 affinity-purified, hyper-immune goat antisera
1980	Univ. Kentucky[267,268]	IV	Hepatocellular, embryonalca, seminoma, ovarian, Endometrial, adenocar-cinoma of lung	16	AFP/goat Ig	^{131}I	1.0–2.5	0.13–0.35	–	12/12 pts with AFP-containing tumors; 16/38 lesions image enhancement factor 2.28; required subtraction to enhance differences
1980	Ludwig Inst., Geneva[239]	IV	Colorectal	27	CEA/goat Ig	^{131}I	1.0	0.5–1.0	–	11/27 pts; some given F(ab')2 fragments; 4 pts given ^{125}I-labeled goat immuno-globulin con-comitantly with ratios of 5–6 less than specific radiolabeled antibody
1981	Ludwig Inst.[241]	IV	Colorectal Pancreatic	28	CEA/VII 23/IgG1 and F(ab')2	^{131}I ^{125}I nonspecific	1.0	0.5–1.0	–	14/28 pts positive and six equivocal studies

(continued)

TABLE 17-9. Diagnostic Studies with Radiolabeled Antibodies *(continued)*

Year	Institution (ref.)	Route of Injection*	Tumor	No. of Patients	Antigen/ Antibody/ Class	Isotope	Dose mCi	Dose mg	%ID/g	Identification of Lesions
1982	Univ. Nottingham[242]	IV	Colorectal	11	791T/36/IgG2b	^{131}I	1.0	0.2	–	10/11 pts; image enhancement factor 4.4; after subtraction studies and before 1.2–2.0; resected specimens 1.1–5.8 tumor-to-nontumor
1982	Institut Gustave Roussy/ Ludwig Institute[243]	IV	Colorectal and medullary	17	CEA/III-23e, VII-37a/IgG1, IgG2	^{131}I	0.1–0.2 1.0–1.5	0.05–3.33 0.3	0.001–0.010 –	16/17 sites detected; used tomographic techniques to increase visibility of lesions
1983	Ludwig Inst., Cancer Research Centre Rene Gaudu-cheau[244]	IV	Colorectal and others	52 15	/17-1A/IgG2a F(ab′)2 and whole Ab	^{131}I	1.0–2.0	0.01–0.5	–	34/63 colorectal tumor sites imaged and 0/20 other tumors; 3.6–6.3-fold higher uptake in tumor compared with normal tissue; specific uptake limited to 2.1–5.1-fold increase
1984	Fox Chase Cancer Center[245]	IV	Colorectal and breast	9	/171A-F(ab′) 2/IgG2a	^{131}I	NS	NS	0.0047	7/8 pts; 22/32 lesions (69%) detected
1984	Fox Chase Cancer Center[246]	IV	Colorectal	1	/171A-F(ab′) 2/IgG2a	^{131}I	2.6	0.376	–	1/1 pts; lesion not detected abnormal by CT seen in a lymph node by radiolabeled study
1986	Hammersmith Hospital[247]	IV	GI, breast and ovarian	19	Human milk fat globule protein/ HMFG2/ IgG1 "proliferating cells"/AUA1/ IgG1 L-phenyl-alanine/ placental alkaline phosphatase H317/IgG1	^{131}I specific; ^{125}I nonspecific	0.05–.10	0.01–0.5	0.015	No imaging; maximal tumor:blood ratios 35.8:1 at 12 days 0.026% ID/g in normal lymph nodes
1986	City of Hope[248,249]	IV	Colorectal	45	CEA/T84.66/ NS	^{111}In	2.0	0.20	0.002–0.008	11/16 primary, 10/29 metastatic; increased uptake in liver with liver-to-tumor ratio of 5:6; normal lymph nodes had higher

(continued)

TABLE 17-9. Diagnostic Studies with Radiolabeled Antibodies *(continued)*

Year	*Institution (ref.)*	*Route of Injection**	*Tumor*	*No. of Patients*	*Antigen/ Antibody/ Class*	*Isotope*	*Dose mCi*	*Dose mg*	*%ID/g*	*Identification of Lesions*
										uptake (10.8 ± 2.2% ID/kg) than tumor-bearing lymph nodes (3.47 ± 0.54%)
1987	St. Bartholomew's Hospital London[250]	IP,IV	Ovarian	18	Human milk fat globule protein/ HMFG2/ IgG1	$^{123}I/^{125}I/^{131}I$	0.5–2	0.5	0.0001–0.0030	Not examined; 4–71-fold greater localization in ascites when given IP compared with IV
1987	NCI, NIH[251]	IV	Colorectal	27	TAG72/ B72.3/IgG1	^{131}I	0.8–10.0	0.16–20.0	NS	14/27 pts; 17/20 with "specific" uptake in tumor tissue (> × control) 70% of all lesions (99/142)
1987	NCI, NIH[252]	IV,IP	Colorectal	10	TAG72/ B72.3/IgG1	$^{131}I/^{125}I$	5–10	0.76–1.2	0.003–0.017	7/10 pts; peritoneal implants were targeted most efficiently by IP compared with IV injection
Lymphoma										
1986	NIH[253]	IV	Cutaneous T-cell lymphoma	11	CD5/T101/ IgG2a	^{111}In	3.8–5.1	1–50	0.01–0.03	11/11 pts and 38/39 clinically positive sites
Hepatoma										
1982–1986	Johns Hopkins[254,257]	IV	Hepatoma, cholangiocarcinoma	18	Ferritin/ polyclonal antisera	^{131}I	37–157	NS	NS	6/9 evaluable pts respond to this in combination with radiation and chemotherapy
Melanoma										
1983	Univ. Washington[258]	IV	Melanoma	6	p97/96.5; 8.2/IgG2a, IgG1	^{131}I, ^{125}I (nonspecific)	5	1–10	NS	6/6 specific uptake in 22/25 lesions ≥ 1.5 cm
1983	Univ. Washington[259,260]	IV	Melanoma	33	p97/96.5, 8.2/Fab IgG1, IgG2a	^{131}I, ^{125}I (nonspecific)	5	1–10	NS	20/22; specific uptake and clearance correlated with cancer fraction of p97 in tumor; treated 7 pts with high dose Fabs
1985	Univ. Calif., San Diego[261]	IV	Melanoma	21	p97/96.5/ IgG2a	^{111}In	5	1–20	NS	21/21; 56% of lesions ≥ 1.5 cm detected
1986	NCI, NIH[262]	IV, SubQ	Melanoma	59	p97/HMW/ 96.5, 48.7/IgG2a/ IgG1 9.2.27	^{131}I, ^{111}In	0.2–12	0.2–50	NS	2/8 pts injected subcutaneously had nodes imaged specifically; 22/38 pts injected systemically had lesions imaged

(continued)

TABLE 17-9. Diagnostic Studies with Radiolabeled Antibodies *(continued)*

Year	*Institution (ref.)*	*Route of Injection**	*Tumor*	*No. of Patients*	*Antigen/ Antibody/ Class*	*Isotope*	*Dose*		*%ID/g*	*Identification of Lesions*
							mCi	*mg*		
1986	Milan and others[263,264]	IV	Melanoma	254	HMW/225.285/ IgG2a, F(ab')2	^{99m}Tc; ^{111}In	10–30; 2–6	NS	NS	159/191 pts known to have melanoma; 250/412 lesions including 95 occult lesions; Tc had superior charac- teristics
1986	Univ. Calif., San Francisco[265]	SubQ	Melanoma	6	HMW/ XMMME-01/ IgG2a	^{111}In	1	1	NS	6/6 pts imaged whether in the tumor or not; 1/2 pts had proliferative uptake in tumor- bearing nodes
1987	Univ. Utah[266]	IV	Melanoma	12	HMW/ZME- a8/IgG2a	^{111}In	5	2.5–10	NS	9/12 pts and 26/33 lesions ≥ 1 cm
Choriocarcinoma										
1980	NCI, NIH; Univ. Kentucky[269]	IV	Choriocar- cinoma, embryonal	3	hCG/goat polyclonal	^{131}I	1.2–1.8	2–3 g/kg	NS	3/3 pts with (+) hCG
1984	Vancouver Gen. Hospital[270]	IV	Choriocar- cinoma, lung	14	hCG/NS/NS, $F(ab')_2$	^{99m}Tc	50	0.150	NS	12/14 pts and 15/28 lesions
Thyroid Carcinoma										
1983	Queen Elizabeth Hospital/ Birming- ham[271]	IV	Thyroid		Thyroglobulin/ sheep polyclonal IgG	^{131}I	0.5–1.0	0.100	NS	12/12 and 34/41 lesions; better than ^{131}I scans
Insulinoma										
1982	Queen Elizabeth Hosp[272]	IV	Insulinoma	3	Insulin, antitumor C peptide/NS	^{131}I	1.0	NS	NS	2/3 localized

*IV, intravenous; IP, intraperitoneal; IA, intra-arterial; Subq, subcutaneous; NS, not stated.

niques to demonstrate tumor-specific localization.[231] These investigators speculated that tumors pick up some of the injected antibodies nonspecifically. These studies were also the first to express results as a percentage of injected dose per gram of tissue, terminology that has been widely adopted to express the results in a variety of different trials.

The first reported clinical trials of radiolabeled antibodies were those of Eugene Day and colleagues from Duke University. They initially used xenogeneic antisera from rabbits immunized with a patient's glioma and subsequently absorbed against normal human tissues.[232] It is clear from these and subsequent studies that vascularity and blood flow are of major importance in the localization of antibody in the differential uptake in tumors.

Subsequent studies were performed using antibodies to myelin.[233] Many of the theoretical aspects for these studies were developed by Bales and Spar.[234] Similar studies were carried out using preparations against renal cell carcinoma at Dalhousie University, with successful imaging of this tumor with goat antibodies.[235,236] Subsequently, the demonstration that CEA is recognizable in the serum and on the tumor-cell surface of a large number of adenocarcinomas suggested that such broadly expressed antigens could be targeted. The first attempt at using radiolabeled CEA, involving a rabbit polyclonal immunoglobulin preparation,[237] was unsuccessful. However, using specialized subtraction techniques and a purified goat antiserum to CEA, tumor was clearly imaged, and these studies, performed by Goldenberg and associates at the University of Kentucky,[238] stimulated further development of murine monoclonal antibodies, as well as their use as radiolabeled reagents in cancer diagnosis. These and subsequent studies are summarized in Table 17-9. Much of the information derived from these studies has been helpful in the design of therapeutic protocols using these antibodies and in the evaluation of concepts with regard to better monoclonal antibody preparation.

RADIONUCLIDE SELECTION AND SPECIALIZED NUCLEAR MEDICINE TECHNIQUES

Radioimmunoscintigraphy, or the detection of lesions using antibodies coupled to radionuclides, has been studied for some time. Which radionuclide is selected is dependent on the ease of conjugation and availability to clinical centers. The vast preponderance of studies have used ^{131}I because it has a gamma ray (364 keV) that is readily detectable externally and because it is widely available. On the other hand the high-energy gamma ray that is produced requires specialized collimating devices, which necessarily decreases the sensitivity. In addition, the isotope releases beta particles, which provide additional, unwanted radiation dosing in the setting of radioimaging. For this reason, other radionuclides have been investigated. Iodine-123 has some favorable characteristics (159 keV gamma ray and no production of beta particles). It has a relatively short half-life, however, which has made it difficult to employ in imaging trials, and it is expensive to prepare. Most trials have demonstrated superior imaging 2 to 4 days after injection of the radiolabeled antibody, as clearance of blood pool radiolabel and of nonspecific uptake by nontumor tissues leaves residual radiolabeled antibody at presumably greatest concentrations only in the tumor at these times. Another isotope that has been used is ^{111}In, which has a low-energy gamma ray (173 and 240 keV), is readily detectable by external imaging, and has a short half-life (67 hours). In comparative studies, ^{111}In appears to be superior to ^{131}I but requires specialized chelating agents for its use. Technetium-99m (^{99m}Tc) has been employed only in limited studies because of the problems of coupling it to antibody.

The ability to detect radiolabeled antibodies has been significantly improved by the development of more sophisticated external imaging equipment.[273] Tomographic and computerized gamma detectors have been used to create superior images. Single-photon emission computed tomography (SPECT) has been reported to have greater sensitivity in the detection of lesions. In addition, the ability to subtract images obtained with nonspecific radionuclides, such as technetium, has allowed greater detection of some lesions. As a rule, the sensitivity of external imaging devices is still limited to 1.0 to 1.5 cm, which is well within the range of currently available CT scanning and magnetic resonance imaging techniques.

ROUTES OF ADMINISTRATION OF ANTIBODY

The earliest clinical studies of antibody delivery used intraarterial administration[232] and subsequently intravenous, intraperitoneal, and intralymphatic routes.[233] Murine and human models have enabled evaluation of therapies[275,276] and suggested the superiority of imaging of nodal metastatic disease after delivery into the lymphatics.[277,278] The high background uptake, probably related to reticuloendothelial-cell processing, even of Fab fragments, has been a significant limitation. In a recent study evaluating these techniques in 20 patients undergoing nodal dissection for melanoma, only two had specific uptake in nodes when radiolabeled antibody was delivered into the subcutaneous tissues.[262] More encouraging has been the delivery of antibodies directly into visceral spaces, such as the peritoneal cavity, which has provided some of the highest tumor-to-normal tissue ratios yet observed.[252,277] In most human studies, the tumor:nontumor ratios with intravenously administered antibodies have ranged from 1 to 10, with most studies reporting ratios between 1 and 4. Very high ratios (greater than 20) have been demonstrated with intraperitoneal administration in a number of studies. This is currently being exploited in the development of specific radiation therapy protocols using highly radiolabeled antibodies delivered directly into the peritoneal cavity.

Great enthusiasm has been generated for the use of radioimaging techniques, and steady improvements have been made in our ability to identify lesions. Most of the lesions that have been identified, however, are those readily apparent using conventional techniques. Improvements would be required to make radioimaging a generally clinically useful technique (which it currently is not). The development of more specific monoclonal antibodies, perhaps chimeric antibodies, used either alone or in combination with radioisotopes with more favorable imaging characteristics coupled with better external detection systems will be required to increase the utility of these techniques.

TREATMENT WITH MONOCLONAL ANTIBODIES

The central problems in using monoclonal antibodies in therapy have been to define the appropriate target structure that is represented uniquely or in a limited fashion on the malignant cells (and to a much lesser extent on normal cells) and to define the conditions under which such antibodies could be made to eradicate tumor.[279] Although some of the earliest imaging studies were conducted with antibodies to CEA, an oncofetal antigen, no major effort has yet been reported in which antibodies to this antigen are used in therapy. To date, most studies of antibody therapy have reported only minor responses and used relatively small amounts of antibody, whereas murine models suggest that gram quantities would be required. Thus, these studies represent very early efforts in the evolution of these treatments. Major efforts in the therapy of cancer with monoclonal antibodies are summarized in Table 17-10.

Some of the first efforts were devoted to producing tumor-specific antibodies unique to an individual's own tumor. This is best represented by B-cell lymphomas. The immunoglobulin molecule expressed on the cell surface of the lymphoma represents a unique target for antibody action with recognition of a specific idiotype. Several studies have been conducted with anti-idiotypic antibodies with up to gram quantities being used.[281-285] The first patient reported to have been given such therapy had a dramatic complete response and remained in complete remission many years later.[281] These innovative studies, begun at Stanford University by Levy, Miller, and colleagues, were continued in a second series of patients, in which only half demonstrated some evidence of an antitumor response.[282] It appears on subsequent analysis that those individuals who "escaped" this therapy did so by developing idiotype-negative tumor variants. Of those who responded partially, most demonstrated an endogenous host T-cell response within residual tumor.

Other studies in the hematologic malignancies used antibodies to differentiation antigens such as CD5 and CD10. Most of the patients obtained only transient reductions in circulating tumor cells. The treatment appeared to have somewhat greater efficacy in some of the cutaneous T-cell lymphomas.[291-295] The most extensively studied antibody to adenocarcinoma has been 17-1A.[292-295] Although minor and partial responses have been reported, long-term follow-up of these individuals has not yet appeared. Combinations of this antibody with autologous lymphocytes or "armed" cells, as well as with gamma-interferon, have also been given. A number of studies have been conducted at the National Institutes of Health (NIH) and the University of Washington using antibodies directed to a transferrin-like molecule, p97, present on 70% to 80% of melanomas and to a similarly prevalent high-molecular weight antigen.[258,259,262,305] These studies, employing relatively low doses of antibody, have not produced significant responses.

Certain gangliosides are expressed at much higher con-

TABLE 17-10. Therapeutic Studies Using Monoclonal Antibodies*

Year	*Institution (Ref.)*	*Tumor*	*No. of Patients*	*Antigen/ Antibody/ Class*	*Human Antimouse Antibody*	*Maximum Total Dose (mg)*	*Tumor Regression*
1980	Sidney Farber[280]	B lymphoma	1	AB89/IgG2a	NR	1580	0/1; brief decrease in circulatory cells
1982	Stanford[281]	B lymphoma	1	Anti-idiotype/ IgG2b	0/1	501	1/1; complete remission 60+ months
1984	Dana Farber[282]	B lymphoma	8	CD20/B1/ IgG2a	NR	50	6/8; bone marrow treated ex vivo with antibody
1985	Stanford[283]	B lymphoma	10	Anti-idiotype/ IgG1, IgG2a, IgG2b	5/10	3183	6/10; transient responses
1985	Netherlands Cancer Inst.[284]	B lymphoma	2	Anti-idiotype/ NS	0/2	5800	0/2; no significant response
1984	NCI, NIH[285]	B CLL	1	Anti-idiotype/ IgG2b, IgG1	NR	1500	0/1; transient reduction in circulating tumor cells
1982, 1984	Univ. California San Diego[286,287]	B CLL	4	CD5/T101/ IgG2a	0/4	200	0/4; transient drop in circulating tumor cells
1984	NCI, NIH[288]	B CLL	13	CD5/T101/ IgG2a	0/13	140	0/13; Transient decrease in circulating cells
1981	Dana Farber[289]	ALL	4	CD10/J5/ IgG2a	NR	170	0/4; Transient reduction in circulating cells
1981	Stanford[290]	ALL (T-cell)	1	CD5/L17/F12/ IgG2a	0/1	164	1/1; partial response
1983	Stanford[291]	ALL (T-cell)	8	CD5 & others, IgG2a, IgG1	NR	50	0/8; transient reduction in circulating tumor cells
1981, 1983	Stanford[292,293]	CTCL	6	CD5/L17F12/ IgG2a, IgG1	4/6	100	5/6; minor response
1984	Univ. California San Diego[287,294]	CTCL	4	CD5/T101/ IgG2a	2/4	200	4/12; minor response
1985	NCI, NIH[295]	CTCL	12	CD5/T101/ IgG2a	NR	100	4/4; minor response
1983	Dartmouth[296]	AML	3	Multiple/PMN6/ PMN29/PM8/ AML2-23/ IgG2b and IgM	1/1 tested	930	0/3; transient reduction in circulating tumor cells
1984	Hammersmith Hospital[297]	Squamous and adenocarcinoma	3	HMFG2/IgG1	NR	NR	3/3 (local only); direct injection of radiolabeled (^{131}I) antibody into pericardial, pleural, or peritoneal cavity
1984, 1985	Wistar Inst.[298,299]	Colon, gastrointestinal	40	17-1A/IgG2a	19/38	1000	5/40; minor responses only; some given with cells
1986	NCI, NIH[300]	Pancreas	25	17-1A/IgG2a	23/25	1200	0/25; some minor responses noted; also combined with cells in 15/25 patients

(continued)

TABLE 17-10. Therapeutic Studies Using Monoclonal Antibodies* *(continued)*

Year	*Institution (Ref.)*	*Tumor*	*No. of Patients*	*Antigen/ Antibody/ Class*	*Human Antimouse Antibody*	*Maximum Total Dose (mg)*	*Tumor Regression*
1986	Fox Chase[301]	Gastrointestinal	27	171A/IgG2a	8/11 (tested)	400	0/27; gamma-interferon pretreatment
1982	Univ. Calif., San Diego[302]	Melanoma	3	p97,p240/ IgG1, IgG2a	NR	50	0/3
1982	Fred Hutchinson Cancer Center, Veterans Admin.[303]	Melanoma	1	p97/IgG1, Fab	NR	1	0/1; labeled with ^{131}I
1984	NCI, NIH[304]	Melanoma	8	gp240/9.2.27/ IgG2a	3/8	250	0/8
1985	Fred Hutchinson Cancer Center[305]	Melanoma	5	p97, gp240/96.5, 48.7	4/5	424	0/5
1985	Mainz Universität[306]	Melanoma, apudoma	3	GD3/R24/ IgG3	NR	440	0/3; inflammatory cutaneous responses around lesions noted
1985	Memorial Sloan Kettering[307]	Melanoma	12	GD3/R24/ IgG3	12/12	400	5/12; both partial and mixed responses; inflam- matory responses noted
1987	Children's Hosp., San Francisco[308]	Melanoma	22	p220/XMMME-01/ IgG2a	22/22	300	5/22; ricin-coupled antibody; 1 complete response, 4 mixed responses; significant antibody response to ricin
1987	R.L. Ireland Cancer Center, Case Western Reserve Univ.[309]	Melanoma, neuroblastoma	17	GD2/3F8/ IgG3	17/17	100/m²	7/17 responses with 2 complete responses in patients with neuroblastoma and 2 partial responses in patients with melanoma
1987	Jefferson Univ., Philadelphia[310]	Multiple	20	CD8/Leu 2a/IgG1	20/20	100	0/20; aimed at decreasing "suppressor cells" in cancer patients

*ALL, acute lymphocytic leukemia; G1, gastrointestinal; B-CLL, B-cell chronic lymphocyte leukemia; CTCL, cutaneous T-cell lymphoma; NR, not reported; AML, acute myelogenous leukemia.

centrations on melanoma cells and tumors of neural crest origin. Antibodies to the gangliosides GD_2 and GD_3 have elicited both inflammatory responses within lesions[306,307] and objective antitumor responses at Memorial Sloan-Kettering[307] and, more recently, at Case Western Reserve.[309] Direct injection of a human antibody to GD_2 has been reported to cause regression of cutaneous metastases.[205] Limited responses to a ricin-conjugated antibody to a high-molecular-weight antigen have recently been reported also.[208]

Toxicity associated with the infusion of murine monoclonal antibodies has been tolerable. Fever, chills, pruritus, chest tightness, dyspnea, rash, arthralgia, myalgia, and hypotension have been noted in individual patients and may be related to the rate of infusion of the antibody. Anaphylactoid responses are distinctly unusual. Far more frequent is the subsequent development of a HAMA response, which is associated with more rapid clearance of the antibody and thus presumedly a lesser likelihood of response. Houghton and colleagues at Memorial Sloan-Kettering have administered an anti-GD_3 antibody after the development of significant HAMA and still observed significant antitumor responses.[307] Serum sickness is distinctly uncommon.

It is likely that the immediate future of monoclonal antibodies as cancer treatments will be determined by the success of trials employing large quantities of antitumor antibodies alone or in conjunction with other biologic response modifiers, such as interferon and IL-2. The use of antibodies conjugated to radionuclides or toxins and the further development of anti-idiotypic antibodies will be areas of great interest and clinical activity. Antibodies have also been used to clear bone marrow of malignant cells before reinfusion into the host[310] in transplantation studies. Ex vivo application of these antibodies is being pursued at a number of centers and is suggested by the ability to maximally clear tumor using high doses of chemotherapy in vivo and toxin or complement-mediated lysis of tumor present in the harvested marrow. In addition, the continuous development of novel chimeric antibodies for use either alone or in conjunction with toxins will likely be the major areas of interest over the next decade. The fact that objective antitumor responses have been observed suggests that these approaches will have greater applicability in the future.

IMMUNOTHERAPY

INTRODUCTION

Strategies for the immunotherapy of cancer can be divided into active and passive approaches (Table 17-11). "Active immunotherapy" refers to the immunization of the tumor-bearing host with materials designed to elicit an immune reaction capable of eliminating or retarding tumor growth. Active immunotherapy can be further subdivided into nonspecific or specific immunization. Most early attempts at the immunotherapy of cancer utilized nonspecific active approaches to immune stimulation with adjuvants such as BCG, *C. parvum*, levamisole, and a variety of other substances. Specific attempts at immunotherapy utilized immunization with tumor cells or tumor-cell extracts either alone or in vaccines, often in conjunction with immune stimulators such as BCG. These early approaches were almost uniformly unsuccessful in man and have largely been abandoned. More recently, the advent of recombinant cytokines has provided a more selective means for stimulating the immune system. Treatment with the interferons or with IL-2 is a form of nonspecific active immunotherapy, although the selective action of these purified lymphokines provides a greater ability to manipulate immune responses than was previously possible.

Many studies have demonstrated that the tumor-bearing host is immunosuppressed by growing tumor and thus attempts at active immunotherapy may have intrinsic disadvantages. More recent efforts have concentrated on passive approaches to immunotherapy, which involve the transfer to the tumor-bearing host of previously sensitized immunologic reagents such as cells or antibody that have the ability, either directly or indirectly, to mediate antitumor responses. The term "adoptive immunotherapy" is usually used to denote passive immunotherapy with cells (lymphocytes or macrophages). Recent efforts have been devoted to developing adoptive immunotherapies utilizing LAK cells, TIL, or other means for in vitro stimulation of cells with antitumor reactivity.

The development of techniques for generating monoclonal antibodies has greatly improved the ability to obtain preparations with specific reactivity to human tumor-associated antigens. Considerable effort is being devoted to the utilization of these antibodies either alone or conjugated with toxins or radiolabels for use in cancer treatment, as discussed earlier.

In addition to these active and passive approaches, the immune system can be used in a variety of indirect ways to mediate antitumor responses. Included in this category are approaches such as the removal of blocking factors from serum or the inhibition of essential tumor growth factors.

TABLE 17-11. Classification of Cancer Immunotherapies

Classification	*Examples*
Active immunotherapy	
Nonspecific	Immune adjuvants such as BCG, *C. parvum*, levamisole
	Interferon
	IL-2
Specific	Immunization with tumor-cell vaccines
Passive immunotherapy	
Antibodies	Monoclonal or polyclonal antibodies either alone or conjugated with toxins or radiolabels
Cells	LAK cells
	Tumor-infiltrating lymphocytes (TIL)
Indirect	Removal of blocking factors
	Inhibition of growth factors or angiogenic factors

ACTIVE NONSPECIFIC IMMUNOTHERAPY

Any agent that can alter host–tumor relationships in favor of the host can be considered a biologic response modifier. Most biologic response modifiers stimulate the immune system.[311] The earliest modifiers were discovered accidentally when clinicians noted rare cases of significant tumor regression after a patient with cancer survived a nearly fatal septic episode with a bacterial organism, or a systemic viral illness such as herpes zoster. Microorganisms are now known to elicit a wide range of host responses that activate neutrophils, macrophages, NK cells, T cells, and B cells and their products, many of which can mediate tumor-cell killing. Thus, initial attempts at boosting the immune system of cancer-bearing humans have used a variety of microorganisms or fractions of microbial products.

Table 17-12 gives a partial list of biologic response modifiers. The largest body of knowledge has been accumulated from the use of microorganisms and their products. Initial experimental use of such reagents in animal tumor models has demonstrated prolongation of survival under certain conditions: the tumor burden is low (immunotherapy given early or used as adjuvant with other cytoreductive treatment; never effective alone against large established tumors), the host is immunocompetent (young animals freshly inoculated with tumor), and the tumor is immunogenic. The immune stimulation appears to work best in the setting where the immunostimulant is in direct contact with the tumor.

There are two implications of these findings. First, the mechanism of tumor-cell killing appears to be an "innocent bystander" effect mediated by a vigorous local immune response; there is little evidence for effective boosting of systemic reactions. Second, it is difficult to relate the conditions for successful experimental immunotherapy in animals to any clinical circumstance in man. Local control of human cancer is rarely an important clinical problem with the judicious application of modern surgical and radiation therapy techniques. Rather, the principal problem in cancer patients is effective treatment of metastatic disease, a setting in which nonspecific active immunotherapies have been largely unsuccessful in animals and are unlikely to be successful in humans. In addition cancer-bearing patients often have demonstrable defects in their immune responses,[312] yet it appears that intact cell-mediated responses are critical to the therapeutic effect of many biologic response modifiers.[2]

TABLE 17-12. Biologic Response Modifiers

Microorganisms
Bacille Calmette-Guerin (BCG)
Corynebacterium parvum
Salmonella typhimurium
Mycobacterium tuberculosis
Viruses (vaccinia, Newcastle disease, influenza)
Brucella abortus
Bordetella pertussis
Listeria monocytogenes
OK-432 (Picibinil)
Mixed bacterial vaccines
Microbial components
Methanol-extractable residue of BCG (MER)
Nocardia rubra cell-wall skeleton
Glucan (from *Saccharomyces*)
Lentinan (from *Basidiomycetes*)
Krestin (from *Basidiomycetes*)
Other glucans
BCG cell walls
Endotoxin
Muramyl dipeptide
Trehalose dimycolate
Schizophillan
Staphylococcal protein A
Immunomodulators from miscellaneous sources
Levamisole
Cyclophosphamide
Polyribonucleotides
Doxorubicin
Alkyl lysophospholipids
Maleic anhydride divinyl ether (MVE-2)
Liposomes
Many natural products
Bestatin
Tuftsin
Flavone acetic acid
Cimetidine
Swainsonine
Prostaglandin inhibitors
Dinitrochlorobenzene (DNCB)
Physiologic mediators
Cytokines
Colony-stimulating factors
Neuropeptides
Antibodies (*e.g.*, anti-CD8)
Complement
LFA 1, LFA 3
Lymphokines (IL1-6, IFNs, NKCF, leukoregulin, etc.)
Endorphins
Thymic hormones
Perforins
Leukocyte dialysates

Finally, as discussed elsewhere in this chapter, spontaneous human tumors may not be very immunogenic. Thus, the application of this animal research to humans was unlikely to be useful, and this has certainly proved to be the case.

Since the 1960s, a large number of clinical studies have attempted to achieve systemic immune stimulation employing BCG or the methanol-extractable residue of BCG (MER); fewer studies have used *C. parvum* or levamisole.[313] Usually, immunotherapy was used in an adjuvant setting after conventional treatment with surgery, radiation, or combination chemotherapy had produced clinical complete remission. In general, initial trials suggested positive results and raised hopes for therapeutic benefit, but such studies often were not properly controlled, involved small numbers of patients, or both. When well-controlled prospective randomized trials were performed with adequate numbers of carefully staged patients, interim analyses of end-points such as disease-free survival at 1 or 2 years of follow-up often demonstrated a trend that favored the immunotherapy arm of the study in a magnitude that was not quite statistically significant. However, when the study matured with reasonable numbers of patients followed for reasonable periods of time, the disease-free or overall survival curves usually were not significantly different. Hersh recently analyzed the more than 175 studies of active nonspecific immunotherapy reported in the literature in the 2-year period 1982–1984.[314] Among 26 studies of BCG-MER administered intravenously or subcutaneously that were either randomized or were thought to have appropriately well-matched historical controls, only six studies (23%) had positive results. Another 150 studies reported results with other agents designed to boost host immunity, but only 60 of these were thought to be analyzable. Twenty-three of the studies (38%) demonstrated therapeutic effects from systemic active nonspecific immunotherapy.

The possible reasons for the failure of so many studies are numerous. Little effort has been devoted to finding a dose and schedule that optimizes in vivo immune responses. Thus, simple inadequate administration of an immunomodulating agent could explain some failures. However, some investigators have carefully documented that the agent, as delivered by them, is capable of boosting host immunity. For example, Hersh and associates demonstrated augmentation of NK activity, monocyte-mediated ADCC, in vitro lymphocyte proliferation, and delayed-type hypersensitivity responses after single or multiple doses of BCG-MER.[315] However, they observed no consistent effects on clinical end-points such as disease-free or overall survival rate. Therefore, it would appear that a significant limitation of systemic immunotherapy is that the available biologic response modifiers do not appear capable of including enough systemic immune augmentation to accomplish clinically significant tumor cytoreduction. This finding does not imply that immune-mediated tumor-cell destruction is not significant in magnitude. However, it must be kept in mind that, like the physiologic mechanisms regulating most organ systems, the immune system is subject to both positive and negative homeostatic influences. Immune stimulation without accompanying downregulation of the immune response would be dangerous, and in the healthy state never occurs. It is clear from the histopathology of the thyroid gland from a patient with Hashimoto's thyroiditis or the pannus of a patient with rheumatoid arthritis that the destructive power of the immune system is enormous. A key limitation to harnessing this power and using it against tumors is our extensive ignorance about the negative control points in an immune response. We intuitively know there are limits on in vivo lymphocyte proliferation and activation (how large was the largest lymph node you have ever seen?); however, the nature of those limits is unknown. We know that lymphocytes become desensitized to stimulation if called upon to act too frequently or if given too much antigen.[316,317] We know that some antigens and some tumors elicit suppression of immune responses.[318] When basic science provides us with an understanding of the physiologic controls of the immune response, we may be able to intervene to remove those controls temporarily so that the nonspecific immune stimulants can turn on the system and it is not turned off until the physician replaces the negative control elements after the therapeutic effect has been achieved. Of course, such a strategy is likely to create a problem similar to that faced in the use of other treatment modalities: how to protect the normal tissues and preserve an appropriate therapeutic index.

Unlike the disappointing results obtained with systemic immunotherapy, the local or regional use of nonspecific immunostimulants more commonly achieves local or regional antitumor responses.[319] The injection of cutaneous metastases of malignant melanoma has been the most common form of local immunotherapy. BCG, MER, and dinitrochlorobenzene (DNCB) have been the agents most commonly injected into tumor masses. The following conclusions can be drawn from the accumulated clinical experience. First, the induction of a local inflammatory – immune response can cause the regression of large tumor masses. Injected lesions regress in 70% to 90% of the cases, and the regressions appear to be clinically useful. Second, histologic study of regressing lesions supports the idea that the tumor is killed as an innocent bystander of a granulomatous inflammatory response. There is the suggestion that local immunity is common, since regrowth of completely regressing injected lesions is rare but recurrence at noninjected sites is common. Third, in about 5% to 15% of cases, noninjected distal cutaneous lesions or, more rarely, organ metastases were documented to regress; therefore, systemic immunity is elicited rarely.[320] However, systemic toxicity was seen and was sometimes fatal.[321] In one series, intralesional injection of BCG followed by surgical excision appeared to result in an unexpectedly large fraction of long-term disease-free survivors.[322] Whether this result was secondary to the elicitation of systemic immunity is unclear; however, it should be noted that successful nonspecific therapy in animal models has followed surgical resection of an injected lesion.[323]

Intralesional injection of primary lung tumors[324] and chest wall recurrences of breast cancer[325] have produced local antitumor responses, but none of the intralesional approaches to the treatment of any cancer has produced long-term disease-free survival of patients with metastatic disease. Intralesional therapy can be palliative in certain instances.

Perhaps the most impressive success of active nonspecific immunotherapy has been in the instillation of agents into tumor-bearing body cavities such as the pleura, the peritoneum, and the bladder. About 75% to 85% of newly identified patients with bladder cancer have superficial tumors, and, even with complete resection, recurrence is common. At least two prospective randomized studies have documented that intravesical BCG results in apparently permanent complete responses in about 70% of patients, including those whose tumors have advanced during intravesical chemotherapy (usually with thiotepa).[326,327] BCG appears to be significantly better than thiotepa in patients with superficial bladder cancer and is viewed as the treatment of choice by many urologists, although the Food and Drug Administration has not yet approved it for routine use. BCG also has been instilled into the pleural cavity to control malignant effusions with some success, but superiority to other methods of effusion control has not been demonstrated. Intrapleural BCG as a surgical adjuvant in the treatment of lung cancer has in some studies been superior to surgery alone;[328] however, the capacity of such therapy to prevent systemic recurrences is unclear. Because the major clinical problem in bladder cancer is local control, the data justify the use of intravesical BCG. Because the major problem in lung cancer is not local control, its role in this disease is less certain.

Corynebacterium parvum is another bacterium that has been used for regional immunotherapy. Unlike BCG, *C. parvum* appears to be able to induce antitumor effects in animals without T cells, a fact that suggests its effects may be more dependent on macrophage-mediated tumor killing. It has been installed into the pleural[329] and peritoneal[330] cavities for the control of malignant ascites and has been used in the treatment of ovarian cancer with some evidence of response.[331,332] Unfortunately, the inflammatory response in the peritoneal cavity can lead to serious medical complications from adhesions compressing the bowel and vasculature. Therefore, the use of *C. parvum* is restricted to palliation of symptoms in these settings.

Another strategy in active nonspecific immunotherapy has been the paring down of bacteria to the smallest subunit capable of eliciting a potent immune response. Trehalose dimycolate (also known as cord factor) is a disaccharide esterified to two long-chain fatty acids that has potent adjuvant effects. However, the smallest structure that retains immune stimulatory capacity is N-acetylmuramyl-L-alanine-D-isoglutamine, also known as muramyl dipeptide. These compounds are undergoing preclinical studies,[333] and a study of muramyl tripeptide enclosed in liposomes is being conducted in man; however, there are not obvious reasons for them to be superior to the organisms from which they were derived in obtaining systemic immune stimulation.

ACTIVE SPECIFIC IMMUNOTHERAPY

The word "immune" is derived from the Greek root meaning memory, the critical attribute of the immune system shared only with the central nervous system. Perhaps the ideal approach to immunologic cancer treatment would be to resect the primary tumor and immunize the patient against his own tumor so that any recurrence in any site at any time thereafter would be remembered, recognized, and rejected. The concept of memory is critical, for it implies the development of *antigen-specific* recognition by cells of the immune system: by B cells that will make tumor-specific antibodies, and by T cells that will make tumor-specific cell-mediated responses. Cells with NK, K, and LAK activity and neutrophils and macrophages can kill tumor cells but have no memory and no antigen-specific tumor recognition capacity.

This principle of vaccination or immunization has ample precedent in infectious diseases and has been pursued for many years in connection with cancer. However, there are several problems that have prohibited a simple direct approach to active specific immunotherapy. First, tumor-associated or tumor-specific antigens are very difficult to demonstrate in man: most of the putative tumor-associated antigens are also expressed to some degree on some normal tissue(s). Second, there is substantial heterogeneity in tumor cells, and there is some evidence that metastatic cells differ antigenically from primary tumors. Thus, the development of immunity to some component of the primary tumor may not be protective against the metastatic deposits. Third, some tumors have managed to escape immune detection by the ingenious mechanism of decreasing or eliminating their expression of MHC antigens, structures that are required for antigen-specific recognition by cytotoxic T lymphocytes. This change renders T cells blind to the tumor. Furthermore, tumors express certain soluble factors that may interfere with or suppress the action of immune cells. Finally, the positive animal models that have been developed have rarely been suitably analyzed to discern what aspect of immunity is critical to the therapeutic effect. Is it critical that the vaccine induce measurable levels of antibody? If so, what antibody class is most important? Does one need to demonstrate delayed-type hypersensitivity to the tumor or its antigens? Are MHC-restricted cytotoxic T cells involved in the effect? What role, if any, is played by antigen-specific helper–inducer-phenotype T cells? What are the critical technical features of vaccine preparation that are associated with the optimal clinical effects?

A variety of strategies have been taken to vaccine development; however, all have employed one or more sources of antigen and an adjuvant of some sort. The antigen source is usually either cells or cell extracts. When cells are used, they may be varied in several ways: autologous or allogeneic tumor cells, living or inactivated by radiation, freeze–thaw alteration, heat alteration, or drug inactivation (*e.g.*, mitomycin C), and often immunogenicity is enhanced in vitro by a process called xenogenation. Xenogenation involves altering the expression of membrane proteins through the use of viruses (xenogenation),[334,335] physical treatment of the cells with, for example, ultraviolet (UV) light or heat (physical xenogenation),[336] or chemical treatment of the cells with enzymes, mutagens, and cancer chemotherapeutic agents (chemical xenogenation).[337] Influenza, Newcastle disease, and vaccinia viruses have all been employed in human clinical trials of tumor vaccines, but study design has not permitted straightforward interpretation of results. Physically altered cells have been examined recently by Edelson and his colleagues.[338] After administering psoralen to 37 patients with cutaneous T-cell lymphoma refractory to local treatments, the investigators leukopheresed the patients and treated the cells with UV light ex vivo before returning the cells to the patients. The psoralen was designed to sensitize any circulating tumor cells to the effects of the UV light. Twenty-seven of these patients with refractory disease experienced clinically significant tumor regressions with this treatment, presumably related to the induction of an antitumor immune response by the UV-damaged infused tumor cells. Chemical xenogenation has been employed in a study in which patients undergoing curative resection of colon cancer were given allogeneic tumor cells treated with neuraminidase before being used as a vaccine.[339] It was said that the vaccinated patients with Dukes' Stage C colon cancer had a significantly increased probability of survival, but the nature of the immunity induced was not studied. It would be presumed that the immune effector mechanism in this instance, if any, is tumor-specific antibody, because MHC-restricted T-cell responses probably would not be elicited by an allogeneic tumor-cell vaccine. Morton and his colleagues used an allogeneic melanoma cell vaccine plus BCG in a prospective randomized study of patients with Stage II melanoma. Although there were no significant differences in the 5-year survival rates of vaccinated and nonvaccinated patients, among the 37% of vaccinated patients who made IgM antibodies reactive with membrane antigens of cultured melanoma cells there was a highly significant prolongation of survival.[340] Thus, patients who responded to the vaccine appeared to benefit, but most patients made no specific response (although most were alloimmunized to the vaccine's MHC antigens).

Chemical xenogenation appears to have potential clinical applications. The drugs employed to show this effect in animal models are the agents clinicians use to treat patients with cancer. Could our treatments be inducing xenogenation in vivo? It is of interest that at least one membrane change that has been thought to occur in vivo in response to treatment is the expression of the p170 glycoprotein associated with the phenotype of multidrug resistance.[341] Many structurally distinct drugs with different mechanisms of action can elicit this response from tumor cells, which appears to be a stereotyped reaction to xenobiotic toxins. Interestingly, cells induced to express p170 in vitro by drug exposure appear to be more immunogenic. Paired cell lines in which one expresses p170 and the other does not often differ in their capacity to induce tumors in nude mice: the one expressing p170 loses tumorigenicity (because of increased immunogenicity?). Such findings lead to the intriguing notion that cells expressing the multidrug-resistant phenotype may be more susceptible to immune attack. Experiments to test this notion are under way.

Extracts of tumor cells and purified components of tumor-cell membranes given together with immune adjuvants have been explored for their capacity to protect patients from tumor relapse. A series of trials by Hollinshead and her colleagues appear to show consistent therapeutic benefit for patients with Stage I squamous cell carcinoma given a vaccine consisting of membrane proteins from a few primary lung cancer specimens plus Freund's complete adjuvant:[342] The 5-year survival rate for patients receiving the vaccine was 69% compared with 49% for control patients. Vaccinated patients often developed skin-test reactivity to the immunizing proteins. However, there is some variability in the data analysis of a control group that receive Freund's adjuvant alone; sometimes, such patients are considered to have been vaccinated when they undergo repeated skin tests. Furthermore, some surgical series report a 5-year survival rate of 58% in Stage I squamous cell carcinoma of the lung, a result that may not be significantly different from the 69% achieved by vaccinated patients. Thus, it is not clear that patients have benefited specifically from the vaccine.

The most impressive clinical trial to date of active specific immunotherapy was performed by Hoover and Hanna and their colleagues. In this study, patients with Dukes' Stage B2 and C colon cancer were randomized to receive no postoperative treatment or immunization with 10^7 irradiated autologous tumor cells at weekly intervals for 3 weeks with 10^7 BCG organisms given with the first two injections.[3,343,344] The vaccinated group has significantly fewer recurrences and significantly fewer deaths than the control group. About two-thirds of the vaccinated patients made impressive delayed-type hypersensitivity responses upon skin testing with their own tumor. Some patients also made antibody responses, but most of these were the IgM isotype. It is not clear what immune mechanism is responsible for the observed improvement in clinical outcome, but a larger prospective study is under way that will address some of the questions about mechanism. This highly encouraging result obviously hinges on having a primary tumor that can be dispersed to provide adequate numbers of viable tumor cells for the vaccine. If the larger study can shed light on the critical component of the immune response associated with the therapeutic effect, one could imagine further boosting or prolonging cell-mediated mechanisms perhaps by adding IL-2 to the vaccination schedule or by augmenting antibody responses with concomitant administration of some other lymphokines, perhaps IL-4 or IL-6.

There is a suggestion that specific immunity can be obtained in the course of treatment. For example, in the study by Morton and associates of BCG as a nonspecific immunostimulant injected directly into metastatic melanoma lesions, the regression of distant noninjected skin nodules implies that the BCG primed the host immune system to tumor-associated antigens that were recognized at a distance by the cells.[2] Furthermore, it has been proposed that electrosurgery[345] or cryosurgery[346] of primary tumors results in some fraction of patients developing antibodies to the tumor.

Finally, some experimental data have suggested that signals that are normally activation signals for T cells (*e.g.*, antigen, anti-CD3, anti-CD2) can be associated with T-cell tumor regression and the simultaneous development of tumor immunity.[347] The mechanism of this antigen-specific effect is under investigation.

INTERFERONS

BIOLOGIC EFFECTS OF INTERFERONS

Interferon was discovered in 1957 as an activity made in response to viral infection that appeared to protect cells from such infection.[348] In the 30 years since that discovery, much has been learned about the interferon system, and today interferon has been found useful against a number of infectious and immune disorders and is the treatment of choice for at least one malignant disease.[349] There are three types of interferon: alpha, beta, and gamma. Alpha- and beta-interferons are stable to exposure to pH 2 and are sometimes referred to together as type I interferons. Gamma-interferon is labile at pH 2 and is sometimes called type II interferon. There is at least one form of alpha-interferon that is acid-labile, but it has been detected only in the setting of disease (*e.g.*, lupus erythematosus, AIDS).[350] Alpha- and beta-interferons appear to be able to be made by virtually all cells; gamma-interferon is made only by T lymphocytes and large granular lymphocytes. To date, there have been 15 genes identified that encode for alpha-interferon species, two genes for beta-interferon (although beta-2 interferon appears to be identical to a B-cell differentiation factor), and one gene for gamma-interferon.[351] The human alpha-interferon genes and the beta-1-interferon gene are free of introns, and it appears that their synthesis is induced by release of the genes from repression.[352] A large number of stimuli can induce interferon synthesis, including viruses, double-stranded RNA, synthetic polyribonucleotides (*e.g.*, poly ICLC, poly AU, ampligen), pyran copolymers (*e.g.*, maleic vinyl ether or MVE-2), low-molecular-weight amines, fluorenones (*e.g.*, tilorone), antibiotics (*e.g.*, kanamycin), microorganisms (bacteria [*C. parvum*, mycoplasma, mycobacteria], rickettsiae, fungi, protozoa), microbial components (endotoxin, OK432), drugs (pyrimidinones, flavone acetic acid), and, most recently, certain growth factors and cytokines (*e.g.*, platelet-derived growth factor, TNF, GM-CSF, M-CSF). The best-studied interferon inducer is poly ICLC, a hydrophilic complex formed between poly-1-lysine, carboxymethylcellulose, and the polyribonucleotide composed of inosinic and cytidylic acids. Poly ICLC appears to interact with a cellular gene (a trans-acting factor whose absence from certain cell types limits the inducibility of the interferon gene[353] to release repressors from the control sites of interferon gene transcription. In addition, poly ICLC can stabilize interferon mRNA;[354] thus, inducers act at both the transcriptional and post-transcriptional level.

In contrast to alpha- and beta-interferon genes, the single gamma-interferon gene has four exons and three introns. The mRNA appears to contain an AU-rich region in the 3′ untranslated portion of the message, a feature common to lymphokine genes that enhances mRNA stability. The precise mechanisms involved in the tissue-specific expression of gamma-interferon are not yet clear. Recently, some tissues and cells (*e.g.*, placenta) have been found to produce interferons constitutively.[355] The role of such interferons is unknown.

Interferons mediate a wide range of biologic responses: antiviral effects, antiproliferative effects, cytotoxic effects, immunomodulation, gene activation, and differentiation. The individual alpha-interferons differ in their capacity to mediate the various effects and are expressed to different degrees in distinct cell types.[356-358] All the diverse effects of interferons appear to be mediated through distinct receptors: alpha- and beta-interferons can compete with one another for binding to one type of receptor; gamma-interferon has a distinct receptor.[359] The interferon effects on target cells require internalization of the interferon–receptor complex.[360] Interferon appears to enhance the transcription of a large number of genes, at least a few of whose products are responsible for mediating some of the effects attributed to interferon action. Interferon-inducible genes include those encoding for enzymes (*e.g.*, 2′,5′ oligoadenylate synthetases, RNase L, indoleamine 2,3-dioxygenase, dsRNA-activated initiation factor 2 [eIF2] kinase), proteins with known functions (*e.g.*, Class I and Class II MHC antigens, beta-2 microglobulin, Fc receptors, metallothionein IIA, Mx protein), and a number of proteins whose functions are not yet known. The genes induced by interferons are located all over the genome, but several of them share homologous sequences that may be the target of interferon regulation.[361] The types of interferon vary in their induction of different gene products; for example, the Mx protein is induced only by alpha- or beta-interferon, not by gamma-interferon, and Class II MHC antigens and Fc receptors are more effectively induced by gamma-interferon than by alpha- or beta-interferon.

The mechanisms of some of the effects of interferon have been established. For example, the Mx protein, a 75 kD-protein located in the nucleus of alpha- or beta-interferon-treated cells, is sufficient to mediate resistance to influenza virus and acts by blocking transcription of the viral genome.[362] Furthermore, the gamma-interferon-induced enzyme, indoleamine 2,3-dioxygenase, is responsible for the interferon-related killing of *Toxoplasma gondii* because it breaks down the tryptophan of the host cell, upon which this parasite is exquisitely dependent.[363] The precise mechanisms involved in the effects of interferons on cell proliferation and differentiation are not known, but interferons have been demonstrated to affect the expression of a number of proto-oncogenes including *myc*, *ras*, *mos*, and *abl* and growth factor receptors,[364] and certain data suggest that the level of 2′,5′ oligoadenylate synthetase induced by interferon may be inversely related to cell proliferation. For example, levels of the enzyme decrease when liver cells start to regenerate after partial hepatectomy and increase when regeneration is complete.[365] All stages of the cell cycle are lengthened by interferons, but cells in G_0 are the most sensitive to the antiproliferative effects. Thus interferon effects are greater on resting than on dividing cells.

The immunomodulatory effects of the interferons are numerous and affect every cell type involved in host defense including NK cells, T cells, B cells, macrophages, PMNs, and other effector cells derived from the bone marrow. In general, the dominant effect of interferons on the immune system depends on the assay, the timing of interferon administration, the length of exposure, and the type and dose of interferon used. Cell-mediated responses are more affected than are the antibody responses. Even some interferon effects on the tumor cell enhance its susceptibility to cell-mediated lysis; for example, the induction of Class I and II MHC antigens and other cell-surface proteins facilitates the recognition of the tumor by T cells and may also enhance the number of monoclonal antibody molecules that might recognize the tumor. Interferon activates NK cells and can increase NK cell migration into tissues. Interferon can enhance ADCC, mediated by killer (K) cells, that mediate by monocytes by augmenting lytic activity and numbers of Fc receptors expressed on the cell surface, and that mediated by PMNs.

There is a burgeoning literature on the interaction of interferons with other biologic agents. For example, the effects of gamma-interferon on PMN-mediated ADCC is increased when used together with GM-CSF,[366] and the antitumor effects of TNF factor are enhanced when it is used in combination with gamma-interferon.[367] There are no doubt many more salutary interactions among the lymphokines, and it is hoped that some of them will be useful in the treatment of cancer.

Gamma-interferon is much more potent in its effects on the immune system than alpha- or beta-interferon, and most of the changes follow a bell-shaped dose–response curve. This is in contrast to the antiproliferative effects of the interferons, which are directly related to the dose used. Thus, the clinical use of interferons in cancer therapy is complicated. If the primary goal of interferon treatment is to affect tumor proliferation directly, the interferon should be used at the maximal tolerated dose, analogous to any antitumor agent. On the other hand, if the goal of treatment is a maximal boost of an immune response to the tumor, lower doses may be necessary because the optimal immunomodulatory dose can be substantially below the maximum tolerated dose in man.[368]

The mechanisms by which tumors may be affected by the interferons go beyond direct antiproliferative effects on the tumor cells and the manifold effects on the immune system. Interferons also can inhibit tumor angiogenesis.[369] A significant problem with the clinical application of interferons to cancer treatment is that we do not know which of the many effects are the most important for obtaining tumor responses. Because some of the effects occur at disparate doses and most of the effects are not easily assessed or monitored in vivo in man, many of the clinical trials that have been performed over the last 6 years, since an interferon gene was cloned, have been empiric. Despite these difficulties, substantial progress has been made.

CLINICAL APPLICATION OF INTERFERONS

It follows from the above discussion that there are substantial difficulties associated with attempting to use interferons and other biologic response modifiers in humans. The multitude of effects of such agents and the inadequate information about what effects are critical to obtaining in vivo antitumor responses interfere with the development of an optimal dose schedule. Such lack of information minimally interferes with the clinical application of cancer chemotherapeutic agents because the sequence of clinical testing of these drugs is based on the assumption that the agents are poisons with some therapeutic index and that more is better. Thus, clinical trials with drugs seek to establish the therapeutic index by determining the maximum tolerated dose (Phase I), determining the antitumor activity of the maximum tolerated dose in a variety of malignancies (Phase II), and integrating the drug into combinations of drugs and comparing these combinations with standard therapies (Phase III). For biologicals, however, animal models and some human studies[368,370] have suggested that there may be an extraordinarily wide disparity between the maximum tolerated dose and the optimal antitumor dose. Because some of the interferon's effects are direct antiproliferative actions on the tumor, it is conceivable that more is better. However, other interferon effects are immunomodulatory, and when these effects are more important the optimal antitumor does may be closer to the optimal immunomodulatory dose.

Unfortunately, the clinical development of the interferons has proceeded according to the precedent established for cancer chemotherapeutic agents, and at this writing an optimal immunomodulatory dose for alpha- and beta-interferon has not been established. The impact of gamma-interferon on the immune system is greater than that of alpha- and beta-interferon, and an optimal immunomodulatory dose of gamma-interferon has recently been established.[368] Clinical trials of gamma-interferon administered at its optimal immunomodulatory dose are just beginning.

Another factor complicating the use of interferons and other biologic agents, particularly cytokines, is that the physiological role of these agents cannot be easily duplicated by systemic administration in pharmacologic doses. Most of these agents are physiologically elicited in tissues, and they are meant to act locally or over short distances and in concert with a number of other molecules produced by other cells of the immune system. Separating a lymphokine from other mediators, removing it from its physiological compartment, and using it systemically may make it much less effective or even useless. Furthermore, in the process of altering host immunity systemically with these agents, it is possible that the intricate mechanisms that maintain self-tolerance may be altered or broken and deleterious autoimmune phenomena induced. Fortunately, to date, such problems have been rare in the treatment of cancer patients with interferons.

Despite these caveats and concerns, interferons (particularly the alpha species) have been found to be active in patients bearing a variety of tumor types. Table 17-13 lists the tumor types in which alpha-interferons have been most active, the overall response rates, and the doses at which those responses have occurred. The most common solid tumors—lung, colorectal, and breast cancers—have not been highly responsive to alpha-interferon used as a single agent; however, such tumors are refractory to most single-agent treatments. Interferon has been most active in certain hematopoietic tumors. The antitumor activity of interferon in patients with solid tumors is usually obtained with treatment near the maximum tolerated dose. Treatment experience with beta- and gamma-interferon is considerably smaller. As might be expected by the fact that alpha- and beta-interferons share a receptor, it does not appear that they have a different spectrum of single-agent activity. Gamma-interferon is also still under investigation in Phase II studies; however, it seems to differ from the alpha and beta species in that patients with hairy cell leukemia respond poorly to gamma-interferon. However, gamma-interferon appears to have some activity in chronic lymphocytic leukemia, a disease in which alpha- and beta-interferons are inactive.

Because in vitro studies suggest that the antiproliferative effects of interferon are related to the duration of exposure, pharmacokinetics in humans may be an important determinant of response. Interferons are filtered through the glomeruli, but more than 90% of the filtered molecules are reabsorbed and catabolized in the renal tubules.[371] Intravenous infusions result in clearance with a half-life of about 4 to 8 hours, whereas after intramuscular or subcutaneous injection, peak serum levels occur at about 6 to 8 hours with complete clearance by 16 to 24 hours.[372] Thus, longer exposure follows subcutaneous or intramuscular injection, and most responses have been obtained in patients so treated.

The most dramatic clinical antitumor effects from interferon have been seen in patients with hairy cell leukemia, an uncommon tumor of mature B cells characterized by pancytopenia secondary to marrow fibrosis, splenomegaly, and fatigue and associated with serious or fatal infectious and bleeding complications. Before the advent of interferon therapy, the treatment of hairy cell leukemia had been splenectomy, to which 65% to 75% of patients responded. However, for the patients who did not respond and for the one-third to one-half of responding patients whose disease worsened within the first 5 years after splenectomy, there was no effective treatment. Doses of alpha-interferon as low as 3 million units per day have been associated with some evidence of benefit in as much as 95% of patients[370,373] Complete remissions are rare, but 75% or more of patients have partial responses, and it appears that even the patients with apparently stable disease experience a survival advantage, with a dramatic reduction in the incidence of opportunistic infections. There are no differences in the response rates of patients with and without prior splenectomy. Expression of interferon receptors on hairy cells is heterogeneous and does not appear to correlate with responsiveness.[374] The median time to response is 4 to 6 months. Initially, the peripheral blood hairy-cell count falls, and there is often a slight decrease in erythrocyte, platelet, and granulocyte counts before these three cell types begin to increase. Generally, granulocyte counts improve before platelet and erythrocyte counts (within 2 months versus 2–3 months, and 3–6 months, respectively). Monocytopenia is the last peripheral blood abnormality to be corrected. Marrow fibrosis may be slow to clear, and even the patients with the most impressive

TABLE 17-13. Response Rates and Durations of Tumors Responsive to Alpha-Interferon

Tumor	*Dose (mU) and Schedule*	*Response Rate (%)*	*Response Duration (mo)*
Hairy cell leukemia	3/day or three times weekly	75–90	3–24+
Chronic myelogenous leukemia	5/day	45–85*	6–15+
Cutaneous T-cell lymphoma	$50/m^2$/day × 5 q 3 weeks	45	3–36+
Low-grade lymphocytic lymphoma	$50/M^2$ three times weekly	37–40	4–36+
Ovarian cancer	50 IP q week × 3	45	12–30+
Kaposi's sarcoma	$20/M^2$/day	28	4–31+
Glioma	$3–54/M^2$/day	22–35	1–9+
Multiple myeloma	$12/M^2$/day	17	3–26+
Melanoma	$12/M^2$ three times weekly	11–17	1–36+
Renal cell carcinoma	$20/M^2$/day	13–15	1–12+

*The 85% response rate includes peripheral blood responses.

clinical responses usually have residual marrow disease detectable morphologically or monoclonal cells detectable by flow cytometry (the tumor cells are the only marrow cells positive for both Leu M5 and Leu 14) or Southern analysis revealing clonal immunoglobulin-gene rearrangements. The concentration of soluble IL-2 receptor in the serum is a reliable noninvasive measure of tumor burden.[375] Responses to alpha-interferon are not sustained for long periods after interferon is stopped; therefore, most patients remain on maintenance doses of interferon (2–3 million units three times a week) essentially indefinitely.

Recently, a study of hairy cell leukemia patients receiving chronic treatment with interferon-alpha 2a (Roferon; Hoffman–LaRoche) revealed that 31 of 51 (59%) developed antibodies to the interferon. In half the patients, the antibodies neutralized the in vitro antiviral effects of alpha-2a-interferon.[376] However, the neutralizing antibodies were specific for the alpha-1-interferon and did not neutralize a mixed preparation of alpha-interferons (Cantell preparation). In this study, nine patients developed clinical resistance to interferon, and all of these patients had antibody to interferon ($p2 < 0.0001$). Whether such patients would respond to higher doses or a different preparation of interferon is under investigation. At the moment, the treatment of choice for interferon-resistant hairy cell leukemia is 2-deoxycoformycin, an adenosine deaminase inhibitor effective in 80% to 90% of patients[377] including those resistant to interferon.[377] Unfortunately, 2-deoxycoformycin is associated with significant depression of CD4+ T cells, similar to the defect in AIDS patients, and some opportunistic infections have been seen in hairy cell leukemia patients receiving the drug.[379] Studies are under way to evaluate the roles of splenectomy, interferon, and 2-deoxycoformycin in the management of hairy cell leukemia.

Remarkably high response rates to low doses of alpha-interferon are also seen in patients with chronic myelogenous leukemia. With the use of 5 million units a day, 75% of patients appear to clear the malignant cells from the peripheral blood, and around 5% have a cytogenetically complete remission in the marrow, a finding extremely rare with any known treatment including aggressive chemotherapy and radiation with bone marrow transplantation.[380] It has not yet been determined whether these responses in patients in the chronic phase of disease will result in either a longer disease-free survival or a longer chronic phase with a survival advantage; however, the remarkable effect of interferon on the expression of the translocated *abl* oncogene is extremely encouraging. Nevertheless, a number of conventional cytotoxic agents can induce transient tumor responses in the chronic phase of the disease; therefore, a cautious interpretation is in order until a survival advantage has been shown for interferon-treated patients.

Another experimental use for interferon in chronic myelogenous leukemia is in conjunction with the chemotherapeutic agent busulfan. This drug usually produces a decrease in the leukemic blood counts, but discontinuation of the drug is usually followed by a slow return of the leukemic cells. A second course of busulfan can result in a second response of similar magnitude, but the interval until the peripheral leukemic cells return to pretreatment levels is shorter and will continue to shorten with each subsequent cycle of busulfan treatment. It is thought that the busulfan increases the tumor growth fraction and causes a recruitment of tumor stem cells into cell cycle. Because interferons decrease the self-renewing capacity of myeloma and acute myeloid leukemia cells, the administration of interferon after busulfan cycles might prolong the busulfan-induced remissions. Preliminary results suggest that interferon is indeed capable of prolonging the effects of busulfan.[381] Further studies are needed to evaluate the role of interferon with and without other treatment modalities in patients with chronic myelogenous leukemia.

Clinically meaningful response rates to alpha-interferon used near the maximum tolerated doses have been obtained in patients with low-grade lymphoma, cutaneous T-cell lymphoma, AIDS-associated Kaposi's sarcoma, melanoma, myeloma, renal cell carcinoma, ovarian cancer, and glioma.[349] By and large, the responses are partial and continue only as long as interferon is administered. However, the fact that any activity has been identified is encouraging. Interferon may be useful in the local setting; for example, in the treatment of bladder cancer or intraepithelial cervical neoplasia. It is still under evaluation in patients with Hodgkin's disease and nasopharyngeal carcinoma, two malignancies with hinted viral contributions to pathogenesis. Interferon is useful in the management of patients with carcinoid tumors and certain secreting malignant endocrine pancreas tumors through its capacity to reduce the secretion of mediators from the tumor, although tumor shrinkage is rare.[382,383]

Efforts to improve response rates to interferon by antagonizing its toxic effects with indomethacin have failed,[384] but it appears that the response rates of renal cell carcinoma to interferon may be significantly augmented by aspirin.[384a] A variety of attempts at integrating interferon into chemotherapy, radiation therapy, and biologic therapy programs have begun,[385] but these are largely empiric combinations with Phase I end-points that have not yet produced dramatic antitumor results. There are myriad ways interferon could be used together with other modalities, and, based on exciting in vitro and in vivo animal model synergy, it seems probable that therapeutic advances will follow.

A major limitation to progress is the lack of methods for measuring the important biologic effects. To date, responses in human tumors have not correlated well with the expression of interferon receptors on the tumor, the induction of NK activity in the peripheral blood, the induction of 2′,5′ oligoadenylate synthetase levels in peripheral blood cells, or any other interferon-related biologic effect. A second significant limitation to progress is the toxicity associated with the use of interferon therapy. Dose-limiting toxicity is usually manifest as fatigue, weakness, anorexia, weight loss, lethargy, and disordered mentation, all symptoms that are difficult to quantitate. Nearly all patients experience flu-like illness, myalgias, fever, and chills, but tachyphylaxis of these symptoms prevents them from becoming dose limiting. Fatigue, inability to concentrate, and depression usually worsen with continued treatment. Table 17-14 lists the toxicities associated with interferon treatment at the maximum tolerated doses.[386] There is anecdotal evidence that administration of interferon at night results in less toxicity,[387] and there are suggestions that biologic response modifiers and other

TABLE 17-14. Toxicities Associated with Alpha-Interferon Treatment

Symptoms	*Laboratory Abnormalities*
Frequent	
Fever/chills	
Myalgias	
Fatigue/weakness	
Anorexia/weight loss	
Lethargy/lack of concentration	
Neutropenia	
Mild thrombocytopenia	
Elevated transaminases	
Proteinuria	
Less Frequent	
Gastrointestinal	
Nausea/vomiting	
Altered taste	
Diarrhea	
Cardiovascular	
Hypotension	
Hypertension	
Atrial and ventricular arrhythmias	
Myocardial infarction	
Neurologic	
Headaches	
Mood alterations (depression)	
Dizziness/lightheadedness	
Peripheral neuropathy	
EEG abnormalities (including seizures rarely)	
Mucocutaneous	
Inflammation at injection site	
Urticaria	
Stomatitis	
Reactivation of Herpes simplex	
Exacerbation of psoriasis	
Radiation recall	
Mild alopecia	
Increased eyelash growth	
Hematologic	
Normocytic normochromic anemia	
Coagulation abnormalities	
Renal/Metabolic	
Hypercalcemia	
Hypocalcemia	
Hyperkalemia	
Hypertriglyceridemia	
Nephrotic syndrome	
Elevated urea nitrogen	
Hepatic	
Elevated alkaline phosphatase	
Elevated lactic dehydrogenase	

chemotherapeutic agents may have enhanced therapeutic ratios and greater biologic effects if delivered in a fashion that accounts for normal biologic rhythms.[388] Such ideas are only beginning to be carefully studied.

INTERFERON INDUCERS

As noted above, a large number of compounds have been shown to be interferon inducers. The polyribonucleotides, especially poly ICLC, have been the most extensively evaluated in man.[389] The initial clinical trials in the 1970s determined a maximum tolerated dose; however, there was little evidence that interferon was induced. However, it is now clear that lower doses of poly ICLC may be more effective at inducing interferon, as well as other biologic mediators, that interferon-inducible proteins may be detected in the serum even when interferon is not measurable, and that patient-related variables such as age and tumor burden may affect responses. Thus, it is not clear that there is enough information available to evaluate poly ICLC fully as a therapeutic agent. Enthusiasm for taking a closer look at interferon inducers comes from a prospective randomized trial of patients with breast cancer who received either placebo or six weekly intravenous injections of 30 mg of polyadenylic–polyuridylic acid (poly AU) after definitive local therapy.[390] In patients with tumorous axillary lymph nodes, only 19% of controls were alive at 7 years compared with 60% of those receiving poly AU. Such results are similar to those obtained with adjuvant chemotherapy in node-positive breast cancer and suggest that further study is warranted.

Recently, it has been shown that flavone-8-acetic acid, a new agent from the drug development program of the National Cancer Institute, has potent interferon-inducing properties in both animals[391] and humans.[392] In vivo synergy of the drug with IL-2 has been demonstrated in animals,[391] and a clinical trial in humans is under way.

INTERLEUKIN-2 AND ADOPTIVE IMMUNOTHERAPY

BIOLOGIC ASPECTS OF IL-2

Interleukin-2, a lymphokine produced by activated T cells, has a wide variety of actions and plays a central role in immune regulation (reviewed in reference 393). The interaction of antigen in conjunction with IL-1 stimulates T cells to release IL-2, which is the second signal in lymphocyte mitogenesis. The primary action of IL-2 is its ability to stimulate the growth of activated T cells that bear IL-2 receptors,[394] although IL-2 has a variety of other actions on T cells (see Table 17-3),[395-397] B cells,[398,399] macrophages,[400,401] epidermal Langerhans' cells,[402] and oligodendroglial cells.[403] Human IL-2 was first isolated from supernatant fluids of cultured mitogen- or alloantigen-activated T cells.[394] The leukemic cell line Jurkat[404] was found to produce high concentrations of human IL-2,[405] and using this cell line, the gene coding for human IL-2 was isolated and expressed in *E. coli*.[406-408]

Human cells contain a single copy of the IL-2 gene, which consists of four exons and three introns on chromosome 4. The cDNA consists of a single open reading frame coding for 153 amino acids. The first 20 N-terminal amino acids are hydrophobic and are cleaved to give the mature protein, which consists of 133 amino acids and a predicted molecular weight of 15,420. The residue at position 3 of the mature molecule is O-glycosylated, and size and charge heterogeneity are attributable to this post-translational modification. The IL-2 molecule contains a single disulfide bond between residues 58 and 105 that appears to be essential for the full activity of the molecule. One form of IL-2 in clinical use contains a site-specific mutation with a serine-for-cysteine substitution that allows the production of a stable molecule containing the full biologic activity of native IL-2.[407,408]

IL-2 interacts with cells by binding to specific receptors on the cell surface (reviewed in references 117 and 393). High-affinity receptors with a K_d of 10^{-11} M are the principal ones that mediate the physiologic response of T cells to IL-2 and comprise about 10% of the IL-2 receptors. A second group of receptors bind IL-2 with low affinity (K_d 10^{-8} M). It now appears that a 55-kD protein recognized by the anti-Tac monoclonal antibody mediates low-affinity IL-2 binding. A 75-kD IL-2 receptor protein of intermediate affinity has also been identified,[409] and it appears that high-affinity receptors involve the interaction of IL-2 with a combination of the 55-kD and the 75-kD IL-2 receptor molecules.

Many of the actions of IL-2 suggested that this molecule might be of value in cancer therapy.[410] IL-2 causes lymphoid proliferation and, in some cases, reverses immune deficiency both in vitro and in vivo. For example, in vivo administration of IL-2 restores depressed allogeneic responses in cyclophosphamide-treated mice,[411] restores allograft responses in T-depleted rodents,[412] and can restore the cytotoxic response of lymphoid cells from patients with AIDS to cultured NK-sensitive tumor cells.[413] IL-2 also causes proliferation of endogenous and adoptive transferred lymphoid cells in vivo.[414,415]

Lymphoid cells incubated with IL-2 develop a capacity to lyse fresh tumor cells.[59,416-420] This generation of LAK cells occurs both in vitro and in vivo and has served as the basis for the development of adoptive immunotherapies for the treatment of cancer in humans (see section on adoptive immunotherapy below). Moreover, the direct administration of IL-2 to tumor-bearing animals mediates the regression of established hepatic, pulmonary, and subdermal metastases in a variety of murine tumor models.[421-425] Table 17-15 presents some of the characteristics of the effects of IL-2 in these animal studies.

Other actions of IL-2 that suggest an ability to alter tumor growth include its augmentation of the therapeutic effect of the adoptive transfer of lymphoid cells[415,426-430] and its effects on the emigration of lymphoid cells from the peripheral blood.[431] Finally, the administration of IL-2 causes the in vivo release of other lymphokines and hormones that themselves can mediate physiologic effects, often in concert with IL-2.[432]

CLINICAL APPLICATIONS OF IL-2 IN CANCER PATIENTS

The variety of physiologic effects of IL-2 noted above led to explorations of its use for mediating the immunotherapy of advanced cancers in humans. Initial clinical studies used IL-2 derived from the high-producer Jurkat cell line, although only small quantities of purified IL-2 could be obtained. Expression of the gene for IL-2 in *E. coli* has led to the availability of virtually unlimited amounts of recombinant IL-2, and most clinical trials have used this material.

TABLE 17-15. Immunotherapy of Murine Tumors with IL-2 Alone

Liver and lung micrometastases (3-day) from a variety of immunogenic and nonimmunogenic sarcomas, melanomas, and adenocarcinomas can be inhibited by IL-2 administration.
Lung macrometastases (10-day) from two immunogenic sarcomas, but not from two nonimmunogenic sarcomas, can be inhibited by IL-2 administration.
A direct relation exists between the dose of IL-2 and the therapeutic effect.
High-dose IL-2 administration leads to in vivo lymphoid proliferation in visceral organs, and these cells have LAK activity in vitro.
The immunotherapeutic effect of IL-2 on 3-day micrometastases is mediated by asialo-GM1-positive LAK cells. In immunogenic tumors, Lyt 2-positive cells also participate.
The immunotherapeutic effect of IL-2 on 10-day macrometastases is mediated by Lyt 2-positive cells.
Immunosuppression with radiation or cyclophosphamide can inhibit IL-2 activity against 3-day metastases but can enhance the effects of IL-2 on 10-day macrometastases.
The sensitivity of macrometastases to therapy with IL-2 appears to be directly related to the expression of MHC antigens (Class I) on the tumor.
The administration of IL-2 can enhance the therapeutic effect of concomitantly administered LAK cells, TIL, and specifically sensitized T lymphocytes.

A variety of schedules of IL-2 administration have been explored in humans.[61,62,432-437] Most studies have used the bolus administration of IL-2 at doses between 10,000 and 100,000 U/kg intravenously every 8 hours. IL-2 can also be administered by continuous infusion at doses from 1,000,000 to 7,000,000 U/m^2/per day. After the administration of IL-2, a lymphopenia occurs, but the lymphocytes rebound substantially after IL-2 administration is discontinued. If small amounts of IL-2 are administered for more than a week, lymphocytosis may occur as well. There is depletion of LAK precursor cells from the circulation within minutes after IL-2 administration.[431,432] Increases in serum levels of gamma-interferon and other hormones are also seen. After intravenous bolus administration, recombinant IL-2 is cleared from the circulation with an alpha distribution phase of 6.9 minutes and a second beta clearance phase of approximately 70 minutes.[432]

In the treatment of patients with advanced cancer, IL-2 has been used either alone or in conjunction with the adoptive transfer of LAK cells. Clinical results using IL-2 and the toxic side effects of this material will be considered in the next section on adoptive immunotherapy.

ADOPTIVE IMMUNOTHERAPY

Adoptive immunotherapy—the transfer to the tumor-bearing host of cells with antitumor activity—has substantial therapeutic attractiveness as an approach to treating human cancer.[421,438,439] Early cell-transfer experiments in animals demonstrated that the cellular arm of the immune response is crucial in mediating the rejection of allogeneic grafts and syngeneic tumor. In most experimental systems, the transfer of immune cells, but not of antibody directed against cellular antigens, produces immunity to tissue transplants.

The major obstacle to the development of successful adoptive immunotherapies for the treatment of cancer in humans has been the inability to develop immune cells with specific reactivity for human tumors that could be obtained in large enough numbers for transfer to tumor-bearing patients. However, several new approaches have been developed for generating human cells with reactivity to tumor, and the initial clinical experience with the adoptive transfer of these cells has been encouraging.[61,62,421]

Lymphokine-Activated Killer Cells

Beginning in 1980, Rosenberg and colleagues described a technique for generating lymphoid cells from both mice and humans that were capable of lysing fresh tumor but not normal cells.[416-421] The incubation of resting murine splenocytes or human peripheral-blood lymphocytes with the lymphokine IL-2 for 3 to 4 days results in the generation of cells that can lyse fresh tumor but not fresh normal cells. These killer cells have been referred to as lymphokine activated killer (LAK) cells. LAK cells differ from NK cells in their ability to kill fresh human tumor preparations.

The characteristics of LAK cells have been extensively studied.[416-421,440-441] These cells represent a lytic population quite distinct from NK cells or cytolytic T lymphocytes, and their phenotypic surface markers are characteristic of non-MHC-restricted killer cells. LAK cells can be either CD3 positive or negative, are nonadherent and E-rosette negative, and bear NK-like markers such as CD11 and NKH-1 (Leu 19). IL-2 is the sole signal required for the generation of LAK cells, as demonstrated by experiments using purified homogeneous recombinant IL-2.[407] The nature of the determinants recognized on fresh tumor targets by LAK cells is not known, although the determinants appear to be broadly expressed, not only on fresh and cultured tumor cells, but also on cultured normal cells as well. Fresh normal cells, with the possible exception of monocytes, do not appear to bear cell-surface determinants recognized by LAK cells.

Following the description of the LAK cell phenomenon, a variety of studies were undertaken in rodent models to evaluate the use of LAK cells in the adoptive immunotherapy of established tumors. These studies demonstrated that the adoptive transfer of LAK cells in conjunction with IL-2 can mediate the regression of established pulmonary, hepatic, and subdermal metastases from a variety of animal tumor models.[60,423,425,442-445] IL-2 appeared to stimulate the in vivo expansion of LAK cells with maintenance of cellular function.[414,415] A summary of the results of studies in animal models is shown in Table 17-16. In these systems, significant antitumor effects are seen with the administration of IL-2 alone that generally are improved by the adoptive transfer of LAK cells.

Based on these animal models, clinical trials using IL-2 and LAK cells plus IL-2 for the treatment of advanced cancer in humans were developed. A chronology of the development of these studies by Rosenberg and colleagues is shown in

TABLE 17-16. Immunotherapy of Murine Tumors with LAK Cells Plus IL-2

Liver and lung micrometastases (3-day) from a variety of immunogenic and nonimmunogenic sarcomas, melanomas, and adenocarcinomas can be inhibited by treatment with LAK cells plus IL-2.
A direct relation exists between therapeutic effect and the dose of IL-2 and the number of LAK cells.
The precursor of the LAK cell effective in vivo is Thy 1^{-}Ig^{-}Ia^{-} asialo-GM1.
Three-day incubation of splenocytes appears optimal for the generation of LAK cells effective in vivo.
Immunotherapy of micrometastases with LAK cells and IL-2 is effective in hosts suppressed by total-body irradiation or treatment with cyclophosphamide. Therapy is also effective in "B" mice (thymectomized, lethally irradiated, reconstituted with T-cell-depleted bone marrow).
Immunotherapy of micrometastases with allogeneic LAK cells plus IL-2 is effective.
LAK cells effective in immunotherapy can be generated from the splenocytes of tumor-bearing mice.
Metastases that persist after in vivo therapy with LAK cells plus IL-2 are sensitive to LAK cell lysis both in vitro and in subsequent in vivo experiments. We have been unable to generate LAK-resistant tumor cells.
Administration of IL-2 leads to in vivo proliferation of transferred LAK cells.
Diffuse intraperitoneal carcinomatosis can be treated successfully with intraperitoneal LAK cells plus IL-2.
LAK cells can mediate antibody-dependent cellular cytotoxicity, and administration of IL-2 alone or LAK cells plus IL-2 can enhance the in vivo therapeutic efficiency of monoclonal antibodies with antitumor reactivity.

Table 17-17. Early studies of the use of activated killer cells began with the use of phytohemagglutinin-activated killer (PAK) cells because sufficient amounts of IL-2 were not available to generate LAK cells.[446,447] Similarly, clinical trials of IL-2 alone began with the use of natural Jurkat-derived IL-2.[448] When recombinant IL-2 became available, studies with LAK cells alone or with recombinant IL-2 alone were attempted.[432,447] No antitumor responses were seen in any of these early studies using activated killer cells alone. After these Phase I studies, a combination of LAK cells and recombinant IL-2 was administered to patients with advanced cancer, and regression of tumor was seen in some patients.[61,62]

An outline of the protocol using IL-2 plus LAK cells is shown in Figure 17-5. Patients receiving IL-2 alone received it on a schedule similar to this but without the administration of LAK cells. In the Surgery Branch, National Cancer Institute, 177 patients were treated with IL-2 in conjunction with LAK cells, and 119 patients received IL-2 alone. The results of immunotherapy in these 296 patients are shown in Table 17-18. Most experience with this treatment approach has been obtained in patients with renal cell cancer and melanoma. In these diseases, approximately 10% of patients will obtain a complete regression of metastatic cancer, and about 20% will have objective partial regressions. About 15% of patients with metastatic colorectal cancer will experience an objective regression of tumor. There has been little experience with other tumor types.

Regression of metastatic cancer has been seen at a variety of sites, including lung, liver, bone, skin, subcutaneous tis-

TABLE 17-17. Chronology of Clinical Trials of IL-2 and LAK Cells

Year	Clinical Study	No. of Patients	Findings
1980	Adoptive transfer of long-term-cultured peripheral blood lymphocytes[58]	3	Small numbers (up to 5×10^8) of long-term-cultured PBL can be infused safely
1981	Adoptive transfer of phytohemagglutinin-activated killer (PAK) cells[446]	10	Large numbers (up to 1.7×10^{11}) of activated killer cells, obtained from up to 15 successive leukophoreses, can be infused safely
1982	Adoptive transfer of PAK cells plus cyclophosphamide[447]	6	Activated killer cells can be infused safely in conjunction with high-dose cyclophosphamide (50 mg/kg)
1983	Adoptive transfer of PAK cells plus activated macrophages[447]	5	Activated killer cells plus activated macrophages can be infused safely
1983	Administration of natural (Jurkat-derived) IL-2[448]	16	Natural (Jurkat-derived) IL-2 can be infused safely at doses up to 2 mg
1984	Adoptive transfer of LAK cells[447]	6	LAK cells (activated with recombinant IL-2) can be infused safely
1984	Administration of recombinant IL-2[432]	23	Recombinant IL-2 (from *E. coli*) can be administered safely, though significant toxicity is seen at high doses
1985	Administration of LAK cells plus recombinant IL-2[61]	25	Regression of metastatic cancer of a variety of types in some patients
1986	Administration of high-dose bolus IL-2 alone[433]	10	Regression of metastatic cancer in 3 patients with melanoma
1987	Administration of IL-2 alone or with LAK cells[62]	157	Complete and partial regression of cancer of several histologic types
1988	Administration of IL-2 alone or with LAK cells*	296	Complete and partial regression of cancer of several histologic types

*Unpublished data.

sue, and circulating tumor cells. When tumor regression is seen at one site, it tends to occur at all sites; mixed responses are unusual. The duration of responses of these patients is shown in Table 17-19. Of 18 patients who achieved complete regression, 10 have remained in complete remission for as long as 42 months follow-up. Examples of patient responses are shown in Figures 17-6 through 17-9. Because these trials began in November 1984, follow-up is short, and the ability of these approaches to cure patients with metastatic cancer has not yet been established.

Because meaningful clinical responses have been seen in patients given high-dose IL-2 and in patients receiving LAK cells and IL-2, Rosenberg and colleagues have conducted a prospective randomized trial in patients with advanced cancer comparing high-dose IL-2 alone and in conjunction with LAK cells. Early results from this trial reveal that both treatments can produce partial and complete responses, although the incidence of complete responses is higher when LAK cells are administered concomitantly with IL-2.

(text continues on page 338)

TABLE 17-18. Results of Immunotherapy in Patients with Advanced Cancer (accrued by 5/1/88)

Diagnosis	LAK/IL-2			IL-2		
	Total Evaluable*	No. of CR†	No. of PR	Total Evaluable‡	No. CR	No. PR
Renal	72	8	17	52	4	7
Melanoma	48	4	6	37	0	9
Colorectal	30	1	4	12	0	0
Non-Hodgkin's lymphoma	5	1	2	6	0	0
Sarcoma	6	0	0	1	0	0
Lung adenocarcinoma	5	0	0	1	0	0
Breast	1	0	0	2	0	0
Brain	1	0	0	2	0	0
Esophageal	1	0	0	0	0	0
Hodgkin's lymphoma	1	0	0	0	0	0
Ovarian	1	0	0	1	0	0
Testicular	1	0	0	0	0	0
Hepatoma	0	0	0	1	0	0
Gastrinoma	1	0	0	0	0	0
Thyroid	1	0	0	0	0	0
Unknown primary	1	0	0	0	0	0
Total	175	14	29	115	4	16

*Two treated patients not included; one (melanoma) died of complications of therapy, and one (breast) was lost to follow-up.
†CR = complete response; PR = partial response.
‡Four treated patients (renal) not included; died of therapy.

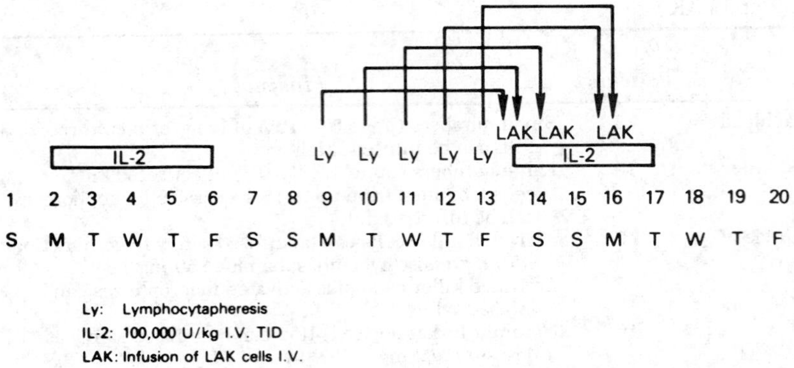

FIG. 17-5. Clinical protocol for the immunotherapy of human cancer with LAK cells plus recombinant IL-2. IL-2 is administered for 4 to 5 days, resulting in a marked lymphocytosis that increases the yield of lymphocytes obtained from daily lymphocytophereses. Lymphocytes are put into culture to produce LAK cells, and these are then reinfused into patients along with the simultaneous administration of IL-2.

TABLE 17-19. Duration of Response (months) to Immunotherapy

	LAK/IL-2		*IL-2*	
Diagnosis	*CR*	*PR*	*CR*	*PR*
Renal	20+,17+,15,13+,13, 11,9,6	26+,17+,13, 11,10+, 10+,10,9,7,7,6,6, 6,6,3,1,1	24+,18+,17+,15+	17+,17+,15+,11+,11, 9+,5+
Melanoma	42+,22+,13,8+	20+,6,5+,3,2,2	–	31+,15,10,8,7+,7,5, 3,2
Non-Hodgkin's lymphoma	10	21+,18+	–	–
Colorectal	21	7+,6,6,2	–	–

Note: 10 of 18 patients achieving CR remain in CR at 11 to 42 months.

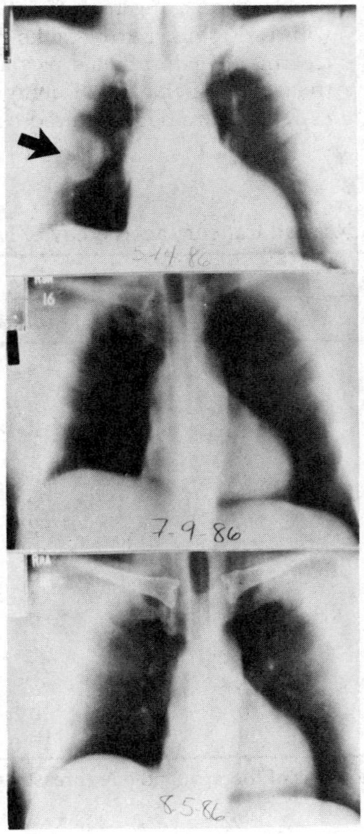

FIG. 17-6. Complete regression of pulmonary metastasis in a patient with renal cell cancer treated with high dose IL-2 alone. **Upper Panel**. Pretreatment. **Middle and Lower Panels**. Post-treatment.

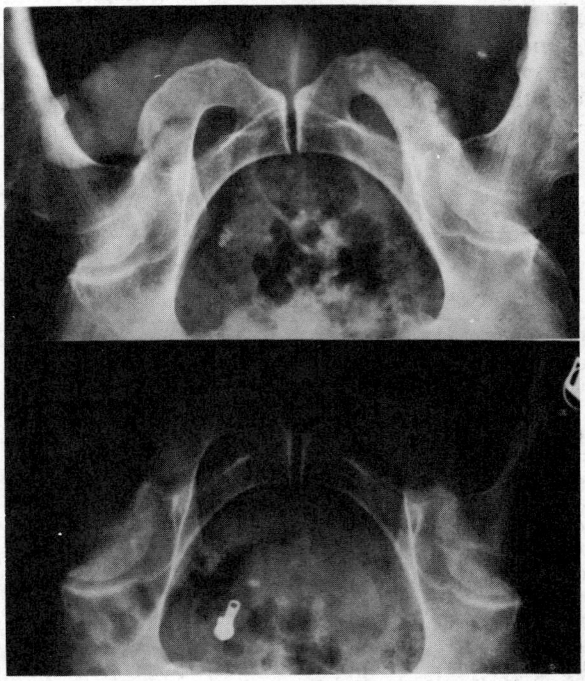

FIG. 17-7. Complete regression of a bony metastasis of the pubic ramus in a patient with renal cell cancer treated with LAK cells and IL-2. **Upper Panel**. Pretreatment. **Lower Panel**. Post-treatment. This patient also underwent complete regression of multiple pulmonary metastases.

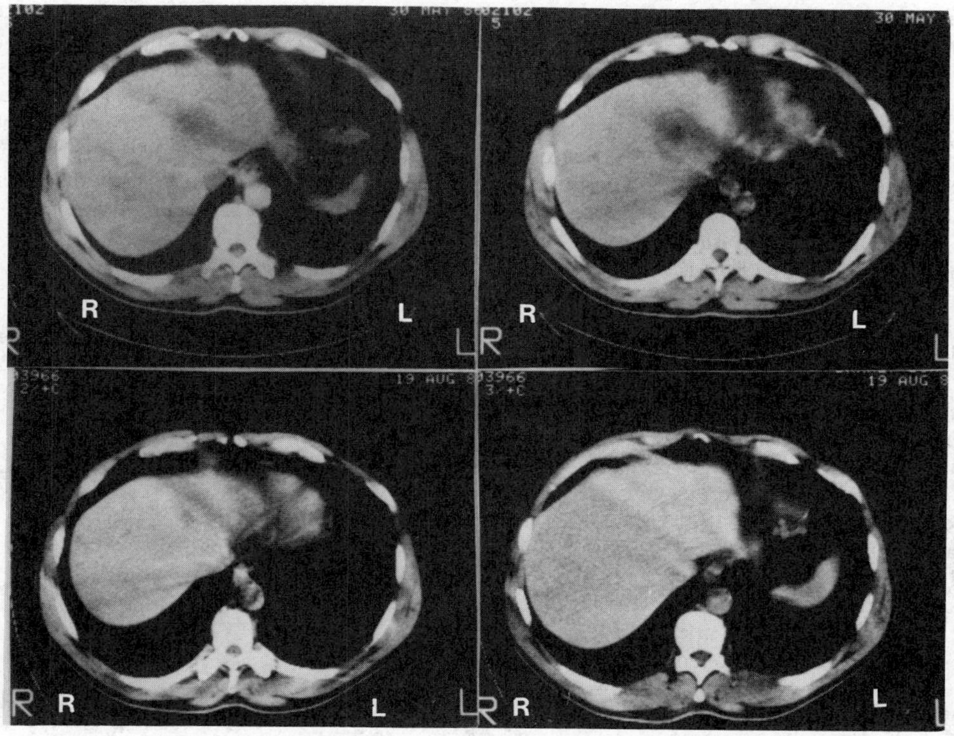

FIG. 17-8. Regression of a liver metastasis in a patient with melanoma treated with high dose IL-2. **Upper Panels**. Pretreatment. **Lower Panels**. Post-treatment.

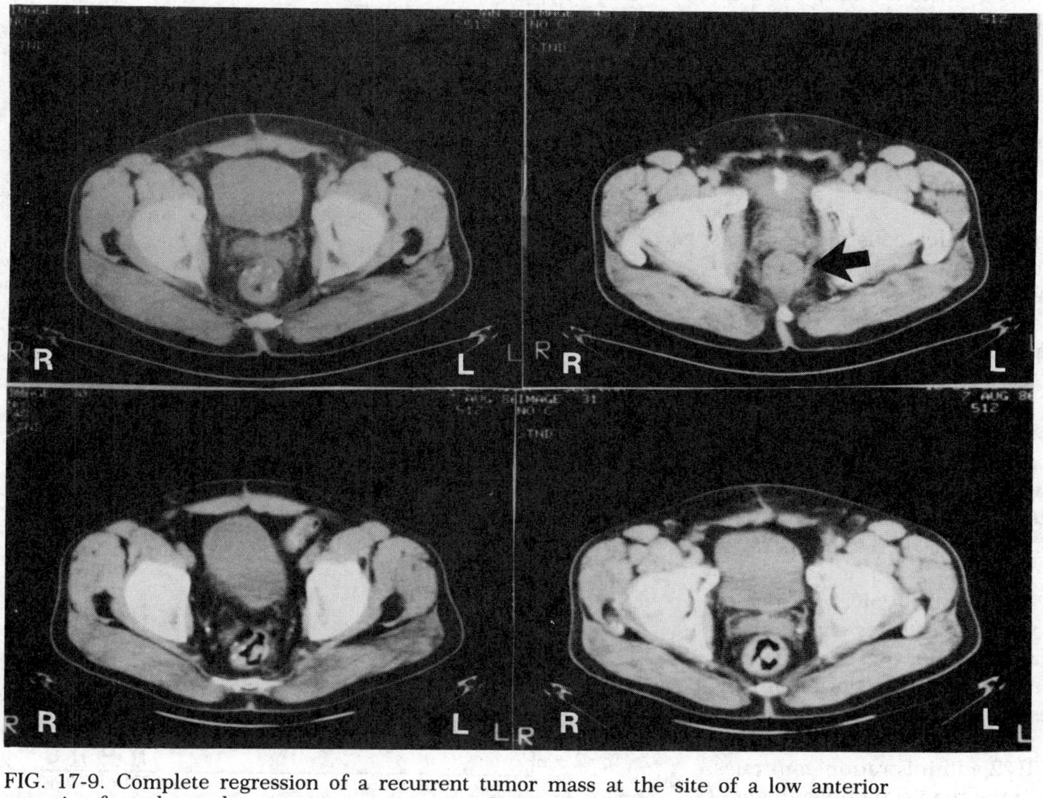

FIG. 17-9. Complete regression of a recurrent tumor mass at the site of a low anterior resection for colorectal cancer in a patient treated with LAK cells and IL-2. **Upper Panels**. Pretreatment. Arrow points to the mass at the site of the anastomosis. **Lower Panels**. Post-treatment. This patient also underwent complete regression of lung and liver metastases.

Other investigators have confirmed both the clinical responses and the toxicities of this treatment regimen. West and co-workers utilized continuous infusion of IL-2 in conjunction with LAK cells and reported 13 partial responses in 40 evaluable patients with advanced cancer.[435] These workers reported that the toxicity resulting from the continuous intravenous infusion of IL-2 was less than that seen with bolus administration, although it is likely that the decreased toxicity was at least in part due to the administration of less IL-2. Using IL-2 bolus administration along with LAK cells, Dutcher and associates saw six partial responses in 32 patients with advanced melanoma, including response of tumor in liver, spleen, kidney, and lymph nodes and of subcutaneous lesions.[449] Similarly, Fisher and colleagues reported five responses in 34 patients with metastatic renal cell cancer.[450] Steiss and co-workers have utilized LAK cells plus IL-2 intraperitoneally to cause partial regression of cancer in patients with intraperitoneal, ovarian, and colorectal cancer.[451] Using a modified procedure for producing LAK cells, Paciucci and co-workers also reported partial responses in patients with advanced cancer.[452]

A variety of questions remain concerning the use of IL-2 and LAK cells in cancer therapy. The dose–response and schedule-dependent characteristics of IL-2 have not been established. Are higher response rates obtained with higher doses? What is the optimal administration schedule of IL-2 and cells? A need exists to test this immunotherapy approach in patients with a variety of cancers at different sites. Are brain metastases affected? A need exists for simpler means of raising more potent cells for use in adoptive immunotherapy. Studies of the pathophysiology of IL-2 toxicities and means for decreasing these toxicities are needed.

Toxicity of Treatment

The adoptive transfer of activated killer cells alone causes little toxicity,[446,447] but the administration of high-dose recombinant IL-2 can be associated with substantial dose-limiting toxic side-effects in a variety of organ systems.[61,62] Many of the side-effects of IL-2 are probably attributable to lymphoid infiltrates in vital organs; to a vascular permeability leak induced by IL-2 that leads to fluid retention and interstitial edema which can compromise organ function,[453] and to the ability of IL-2 to lead to the secretion of other lymphokines such as gamma-interferon, which have a range of physiologic effects and toxicities of their own.[432] The side-effects of IL-2 appear to be completely reversible when administration ceases.

A summary of the clinical course of a typical patient receiving IL-2 and LAK cells, which illustrates many of the physiologic side-effects encountered in these patients, is shown in Figure 17-10.[454] Soon after administration of IL-2, a drop in systemic vascular resistance is seen associated with tachycardia, decreased mean arterial blood pressure, and an increase in cardiac index. As IL-2 administration continues, weight gain occurs secondary to the requisite replacement of fluid lost from the intravascular space by the capillary leak. Urine output drops and serum creatinine rises, probably from prerenal azotemia.[455,456] Vasopressors are often used early in treatment in an attempt to limit the need for fluid replacement, as exogenous fluid contributes to the interstitial edema, which can lead to respiratory compromise and a decrease in arterial oxygenization. Weight gain, renal dysfunction, and hepatic dysfunction can occur. These toxicities and others seen in 296 patients treated by Rosenberg and associates are summarized in Table 17-20.[61,62,454-458] The treatment-related mortality rate in these 296 patients given high-dose IL-2 either alone or with LAK cells was 2%.

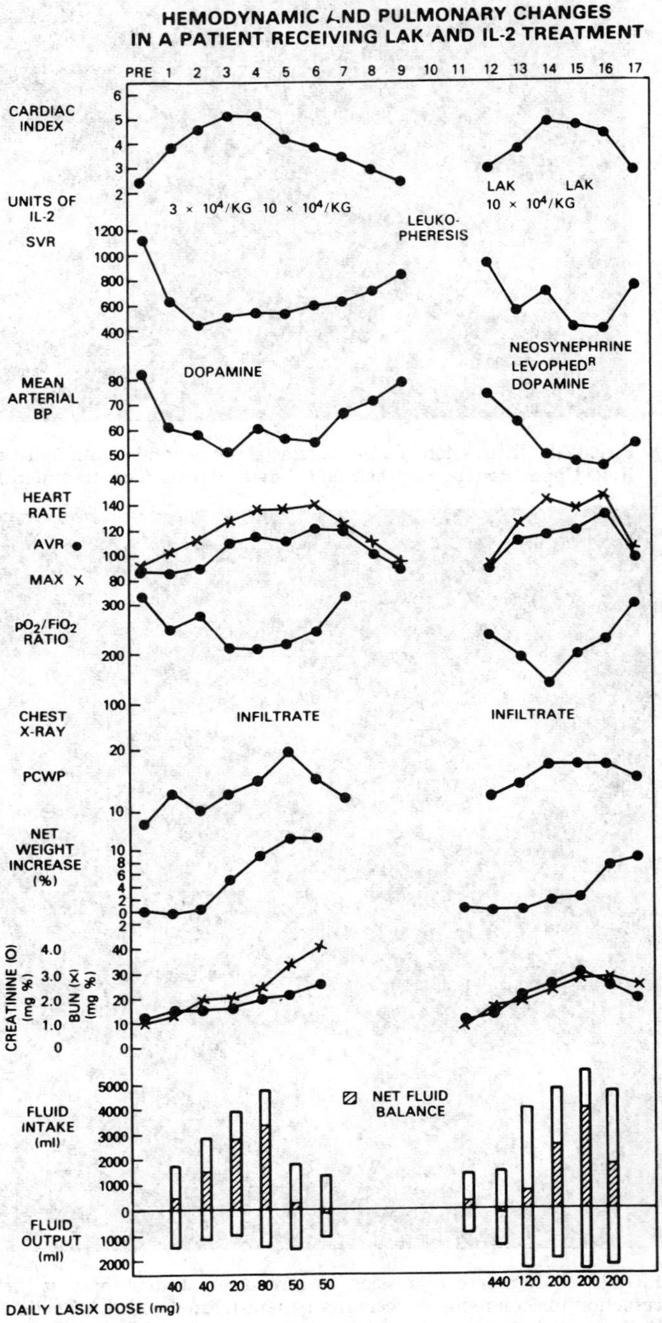

FIG. 17-10. Sequential clinical measurements in a patient receiving treatment with LAK cells and IL-2.

Tumor-Infiltrating Lymphocytes

Considerable efforts are under way to find cells with potent antitumor reactivity for use in adoptive immunotherapy. Rosenberg and colleagues recently described a subpopulation of lymphocytes termed TIL that appear to have far greater efficacy than LAK cells in the treatment of experimental tumors.[429,430] TIL are lymphocytes that infiltrate growing tumors and can be isolated by growing single-cell suspensions from the tumor in IL-2. In experimental animal models, these TIL can be 50 to 100 times as potent as LAK cells in mediating the regression of micrometastases.[429]

TIL have now been isolated from virtually all human tumors.[459-464] The human TIL are T cells and can exhibit specific MHC-restricted lysis of tumor. From approximately half of patients with malignant melanoma, TIL with specific reactivity for the tumor from which they were derived can be obtained. An example of the lytic specificity of TIL is shown in Figure 17-11.[459] Such specificity provides the best available evidence that at least some patients manifest immune reactions to their growing cancers. Clinical trials with TIL are being pursued in the treatment of advanced cancer in humans. Rosenberg and co-workers reported objective remissions in 11 of 20 patients with metastatic melanoma treated with TIL.[465]

TABLE 17-20. Number of Courses in Which Various Toxicities of Treatment with LAK/IL-2 (N = 271) or IL-2 (N = 179) Alone Were Seen

	LAK/IL-2 (177 Pts)	*IL-2 (119 Pts)*	*Total*
Chills	160	59	219
Pruritis	74	44	118
Necrosis	0	3	3
Anaphylaxis	0	0	0
Mucositis (requiring liquid diet)	9	4	13
Alimentation not possible	1	1	2
Nausea and vomiting	208	128	336
Diarrhea	197	118	315
Hyperbilirubinemia (maximum mg/dl)			
2.1–6.0	148	89	237
6.1–10.0	51	41	92
≥10.0	32	21	53
Hepatitis A (due to LAK infusion)	5	—	5
Oliguria			
<80 m/8 hours	85	58	143
<240 m/24 hours	11	18	29
Weight gain (% body weight)			
0.0–5.0	85	79	164
5.1–10.0	118	59	177
10.1–15.0	50	32	82
15.1–20.0	14	7	21
20.1+	4	2	6
Elevated creatinine (maximum mg/dl)			
2.1–6.0	188	117	305
6.1–10.0	29	16	45
≥10.0	2	5	7
Hematuria (gross)	2	0	2
Edema (symptomatic nerve or vessel compression)	6	4	10
Tissue ischemia	1	0	1
Respiratory distress			
Not intubated	24	15	39
Intubated	12	14	26
Bronchospasm	4	1	5
Pleural effusion requiring thoracentesis	8	4	12
Somnolence	41	26	65
Coma	8	8	16
Disorientation	76	50	126
Hypotension requiring pressors	196	102	298
Angina	6	4	10
Myocardial infarction	1	4	5
Arrhythmias	29	13	42
Anemia requiring transfusion (No. of units)			
1–5	137	61	198
6–10	49	22	71
11–15	15	4	19
≥16	10	1	11
Thrombocytopenia (minimum per mm³)			
≤20,000	50	24	74
21,000–60,000	110	65	175
61,000–100,000	65	37	102
Central-line sepsis	32	12	44
Death	2	4	6

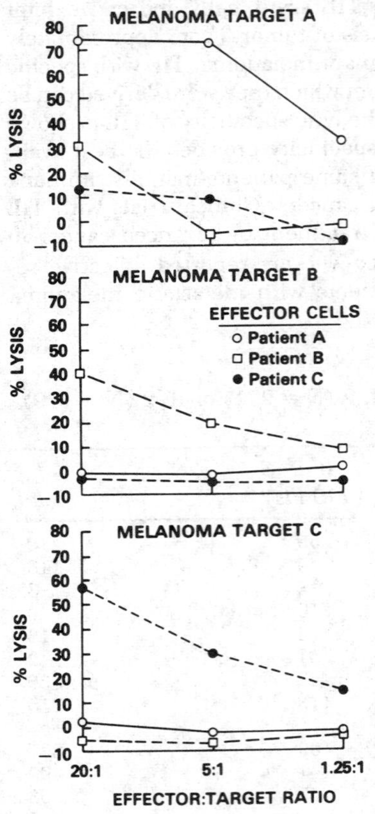

FIG. 17-11. Lytic specificity of TILs from three patients with melanoma tested simultaneously against fresh melanoma cells. Note that TILs exhibit strong preferential lysis for the target from which they were derived (reference 459).

REFERENCES

1. Morton DL: Active immunotherapy against cancer: Present status. Semin Oncol 180–185, 1986
2. Morton DL, Eilber FR, Malmgren RA et al: Immunological factors which influence response to immunotherapy in malignant melanoma. Surgery 68:158–164, 1970
3. Hoover HC Jr, Surdyke MG, Dangel RB et al: Delayed cutaneous hypersensitivity to autologous tumor cells in colorectal cancer patients immunized with an autologous tumor cell: Bacillus Calmette-Guerin vaccine. Cancer Res 44:1671–1676, 1984
4. Morton DL: Active immunotherapy against cancer: Present status. Sem Oncol 13:180–185, 1986
5. Hellstrom I, Hellstrom KE, Warner GA: Increase of lymphocyte-mediated tumor-cell destruction by certain patient sera. Int J Cancer 12:348–353, 1973
6. Roth JA, Holmes EC, Reisfeld RA et al: Isolation of a soluble tumor-associated antigen from human melanoma. Cancer 37:104–110, 1976
7. Ferrone S, Pellegrino MA: Cytotoxic antibodies to cultured melanoma cells in the sera of melanoma patients. J Natl Cancer Inst 58:1201–1204, 1977
8. Brown JM, Thorpe WP, Rosenberg SA: A sensitive assay for the detection of cytotoxic antibodies to mammalian cell surface antigens. J Immunol Meth 30:23–35, 1979
9. Ueda R, Shiku H, Pfreundschuh M et al: Cell surface antigens of human renal cancer defined by autologous typing. J Exp Med 150:564–579, 1979
10. Curry RA, Quaranta V, Pellegrino MA et al: Serologically detectable human melanona-associated antigens are not genetically linked to HLA-A and B antigens. J Immunol 122:2630–2632, 1979
11. Everson TC, Cole WH: Spontaneous Regression of Cancer. Philadelphia, WB Saunders, 1966
12. Montie JE, Stewart BH, Straffon RA et al: The role of adjunctive nephrectomy in patients with metastatic renal cell carcinoma. J Urol 117:272–275, 1977
13. Coley WB: The treatment of malignant tumors by repeated inoculations of erysipelas: With a report of ten original cases. Am J Med Sci 105:487–511, 1893
14. Gressler I: A. Chekhov and Coley's toxins (letter). N Engl J Med 317:457, 1987
15. Hellstrom I, Hellstrom KE, Pierce GE et al: Demonstration of cell-bound and humoral immunity against neuroblastoma cells. Proc Natl Acad Sci USA 60:1231–1238, 1968
16. Hellstrom I, Hellstrom KE, Pierce GE et al: Cellular and humoral immunity to different types of human neoplasms. Nature 220:1352–1354, 1968
17. Hellstrom I, Hellstrom KE: *In vitro* demonstration of cell-bound immunity against autologous MCA and plastic disc-induced mouse tumors. Science 156:981–983, 1967
18. Houghton AN, Scheinberg DA: Monoclonal Antibodies: Potential applications to the treatment of cancer. Sem Oncol 13:165–179, 1986
19. Hellstrom I, Hellstrom KE, Bill AH et al: Studies on cellular immunity to human neuroblastoma cells. Int J Cancer 6:172–188, 1970
20. Hellstrom I, Hellstrom KE, Sjogren HO et al: Demonstration of cell-mediated immunity to human neoplasma of various histological types. Int J Cancer 7:1–16, 1971
21. Hellstrom I, Hellstrom KE, Shepard TH: Cell-mediated immunity against antigens common to human colonic carcinomas and fetal gut epithelium. Int J Cancer 6:346–351, 1970
22. Hellstrom I, Hellstrom KE: Some recent studies on cellular immunity to human melanomas. Fed Proc 32:156–159, 1973
23. Hellstrom I, Hellstrom KE: Cell-mediated reactivity to human tumor-type associated antigens: Does it exist? J Biol Response Mod 2:310–320, 1983
24. Vanky F, Argov S, Klein E: Tumor biopsy cells participate in systems in which cytotoxicity of lymphocytes is generated: Autologous and allogeneic studies. Int J Cancer 28:273–280, 1981
25. Vanky F, Klein E: Human T-cell cultures with selective autotumor reactivity. Cancer Immunol Immunother 14:73–77, 1982
26. Vose BM, Vanky F, Klein E: Human tumour–lymphocyte interaction in vitro V: Comparison of the reactivity of tumour-infiltrating, blood and lymphnode lymphocytes with autologous tumour cells. Int J Cancer 20:895–902, 1977
27. Voss BM, Bonnard GD: Human tumour antigens defined by cytotoxicity and proliferative responses of cultured lymphoid cells. Nature 296:359–361, 1982
28. Vose BM, Bonnard GD: Specific cytotoxicity against autologous tumour and proliferative responses of human lymphocytes grown in interleukin-2. Int J Cancer 29:33–39, 1982
29. Vanky F, Willems J, Kreicbergs A et al: Correlation between lymphocyte-mediated auto-tumor reactivities and clinical course. Cancer Immunol Immunother 16:11–16, 1983
30. Vanky F, Gorsky T, Gorsky Y et al: Lysis of tumor biopsy cells by autologous T lymphocytes activated in mixed cultures and propagated with T cell growth factor. J Exp Med 155:83–95, 1982
31. Vanky F, Klein E: Human T-cell cultures with selective autotumor reactivity. Cancer Immunol Immunother 14:73–77, 1982
32. Parkman R, Rosen FS: Identification of a subpopulation of lymphocytes in human peripheral blood cytotoxic to autologous fibroblasts. J Exp Med 144:1520–1530, 1976
33. Tomonari K: Cytotoxic T cells generated in the autologous mixed lymphocyte reaction I: Primary autologous mixed lymphocyte reaction. J Immunol 124:1111–1121, 1980
34. Uchida A, Micksche M: Autologous mixed lymphocyte reaction in the peripheral blood and pleural effusions of cancer patient. J Clin Invest 70:98–104, 1982
35. Grimm EA, Voss BM, Chu EW et al: The human mixed lymphocyte–tumor cell interaction test: I: Positive autologous lymphocyte proliferative responses can be stimulated by tumor cells as well as by cells from normal tissues. Cancer Immunol Immunother 17:83–89, 1983
36. Mukherji B, Guha A, Loomis R et al: Cell-mediated amplification and down regulation of cytotoxic immune response against autologous human cancer. J Immunol 138:1987–1991, 1987
37. Yssel H, Spits H, de Vries JE: A cloned human T cell line cytotoxic for autologous and allogeneic B lymphoma cells. J Exp Med 160:239–254, 1984
38. de Vries JE, Spits H: Cloned human cytotoxic T lymphocyte (CTL) lines reactive with autologous melanoma cells I: In vitro generation, isolation and analysis to phenotype and specificity. J Immunol 132:510–519, 1984
39. Knuth A, Danowski B, Oettgen HF et al: T-cell-mediated cytotoxicity against autologous malignant melanoma: Analysis with interleukin-2 dependent T-cell cultures. Proc Natl Acad Sci USA 81:3511–3515, 1984
40. Knuth A, Dippold W, Meyer zum Bueschenfelde K-H: Target level blocking of T-cell cytotoxicity for human malignant melanoma by monoclonal antibodies. Cell Immunol 83:398–403, 1984
41. Ferrini S, Biassoni R, Moretta A et al: Clonal analysis of T lymphocytes isolated from ovarian carcinoma ascitic fluid: Phenotypic and functional characterization of T-cell clones capable of lysing autologous carcinoma cells. Int J Cancer 36:337–343, 1985
42. Anichini A, Fossati G, Parmiani G: Clonal analysis of cytotoxic T-lymphocyte response to autologous human metastatic melanoma. Int J Cancer 35:683–389, 1985
43. Anichini A, Mortarini R, Fossati G et al: Phenotypic profile of clones from early cultures of human metastatic melanomas and its modulation by recombinant interferon-gamma. Int J Cancer 38:505–511, 1986
44. Anichini A, Fossati G, Parmiani G: Heterogeneity of clones from a human metastatic melanoma detected by autologous cytotoxic T lymphocyte clones. J Exp Med 163:215–220, 1986
45. Fossati G, Anichini A, Parmiani G: Melanoma cell lysis by human CTL clones: Differential involvement of T3, T8, and HLA antigens. Int J Cancer 39:689–694, 1987
46. Slovin SF, Lackman RD, Ferrone S et al: Cellular immune response to human sarcomas: Cytotoxic T cell clones reactive with autologous sarcomas. J Immunol 137:3042–3048, 1986
47. Hersey P, MacDonald M, Schibeci S et al: Clonal analysis of cytotoxic T lymphocytes (CTL) against autologous melanoma. Cancer Immunol Immunother 22:15–23, 1986

48. Roberts TE, Shipton U, Moore M: Proliferative and cytotoxic responses of human peripheral blood lymphocytes to autologous malignant effusions: An analysis at the clonal level. Cancer Immunol Immunother 22:107–113, 1986
49. Roberts TE, Shipton U, Moore M: Role of MHC Class-I antigens and the CD3 complex in the lysis of autologous human tumours by T-cell clones. Int J Cancer 39:436–441, 1987
50. Herin M, Lemoine C, Vessiere F et al: Production of stable cytolytic T-cell clones directed against autologous human melanoma. Int J Cancer 39:390–396, 1987
51. Mukherji B, Guha A, Loomis R et al: Cell-mediated amplification and down regulation of cytotoxic immune response against autologous human cancer. J Immunol 138:1987–1991, 1987
52. Mukherji B, Nashed AL, Guha A et al: Regulation of cellular immune response against autologous human melanoma: II. Mechanism of induction and specificity of suppression. J Immunol 138:1893–1898, 1986
53. Hoon DSB, Bowker RJ, Cochran AJ: Suppressor cell activity in melanoma-draining lymph nodes. Cancer Res 47:1529–1533, 1987
54. Berd D, Mastrangelo MJ: Depletion of suppressor–cytotoxic T-lymphocytes by administration of a murine monoclonal antibody. Cancer Res 47:2727–2732, 1987
55. Muul LM, Spiess PJ, Director EP et al: Identification of specific cytolytic immune responses against autologous tumor in humans bearing malignant melanoma. J Immunol 138:989–995, 1987
56. Tomita S, Lotze MT, Rosenberg SA: Clonal analysis of tumor infiltrating lymphocytes (TIL) against human malignant melanoma. Fed Proc 46:1195, 1987
57. Pellegrino MA, Ferrone S, Reisfeld RA et al: Expression of histocompatibility (HLA) antigens on tumor cells and normal cells from patients with melanoma. Cancer 40:36–41, 1977
58. Lotze MT, Line BR, Mathisen DJ et al: The *in vivo* distribution of autologous human and murine lymphoid cells grown in T cell growth factor (TCGF): Implications for the adoptive immunotherapy of tumors. J Immunol 125:1487–1493, 1980
59. Grimm EA, Mazumder A, Zhang HZ et al: Lymphokine-activated killer cell phenomenon: Lysis of natural killer-resistant fresh solid tumor cells by interleukin-2-activated autologous human peripheral blood lymphocytes. J Exp Med 155:1823–1841, 1982
60. Mule JJ, Shu S, Schwarz SL et al: Adoptive immunotherapy of established pulmonary metastases with LAK cells and recombinant interleukin-2. Science 225:1487–1489, 1984
61. Rosenberg SA, Lotze MT, Muul LM et al: Observations on the systemic administration of autologous lymphokine-activated killer cells and recombinant interleukin-2 to patients with metastatic cancer. N Engl J Med 313:1485–1492, 1985
62. Rosenberg SA, Lotze MT, Muul LM et al: A progress report on the treatment of 157 patients with advanced cancer using lymphokine-activated killer cells and interleukin-2 or high-dose interleukin-2 alone. N Engl J Med 316:889–897, 1987
63. Wiebke EA, Custer MC, Rosenberg SA, Lotze MT: Cytokines alter target cell susceptibility to lysis I: Evaluation of non-MHC restricted effectors reveals differential effects on natural and lymphokine-activated killing (submitted)
64. Katz DH, Ellman L, Paul WE et al: Resistance of guinea pigs to leukemia following transfer of immunocompetent allogeneic lymphoid cells. Cancer Res 32:133–140, 1972
65. Borton MM, Rimm AA, Saltzstein EC et al: Graft versus leukemia III: Apparent independent antihost and antileukemic activity of transplanted immunocompetent cells. Transplantation 16:182–187, 1973
66. Chester SJ, Esparza AR, Flinton LJ et al: Further development of a successful protocol of graft versus leukemia without fetal graft-versus-host disease in AKR mice. Cancer Res 37:3494–3496, 1977
67. Putman DL, Kind PD, Goldin A et al: Adoptive immunochemotherapy of a transplantable AKR leukemia (K36). Int J Cancer 21:230–233, 1978
68. Bortin MM, Truitt RL, Rimm AA et al: Graft-versus-leukaemia reactivity induced by alloimmunisation without augmentation of graft-versus-host reactivity. Nature 281:490–491, 1979
69. Bortin MM, Truit RL, Shih C-Y et al: Alloimmunization for induction of graft-versus-leukemia reactivity in H-2 compatible donors: Critical role for incompatibility of donor and alloimmunizing strains at non-H-2 loci. Transplant Proc 15:2114–2117, 1983
70. Meredith RF, Okunewick JP: Possibility of graft-vs-leukemia determinants independent of the major histocompatibility complex in allogeneic marrow transplantation. Transplantation 35:378–385, 1983
71. Weiden PL, Flournoy N, Thomas ED, et al: Antileukemic effect of graft-versus-host disease in human recipients of allogeneic-marrow grafts. N Engl J Med 300:1068–1073, 1979
72. Weiden PL, Sullivan KM, Flournoy N et al: Antileukemic effect of chronic graft-versus-host disease. N Engl J Med 304:1529–1532, 1981
73. Denham S, Attridge S, Barfoot RK et al: Effect of cyclosporin A on the anti-leukaemia action associated with graft-versus-host disease. Br J Cancer 47:791–795, 1983
74. Gratama JW, Jansen J, Lipovich RA et al: Treatment of acute graft-versus-host disease with monoclonal antibody OKT3. Transplantation 38:469–473, 1984
75. Mitsuyasu RT, Champlin RE, Gale RP et al: Treatment of donor bone marrow with monoclonal anti-T-cell antibody and complement for the prevention of graft-versus-host disease. Ann Intern Med 105:20–26, 1986
76. Bates SE, Longo DL: Use of serum tumor markers in cancer diagnosis and management. Semin Oncol 14:102–138, 1987
77. Gold P, Freedman SO: Demonstration of tumor specific antigens in human colonic carcinomata by immunologic tolerance and absorption techniques. J Exp Med 121:439–462, 1965
78. Gold P, Freedman SO: Specific carcinoembryonic antigens of the human digestive system. J Exp Med 122:467–481, 1965
79. Braunstein GD, McIntire KR, Waldmann TA: Discordance of human chorionic gonadotropin and alpha-fetoprotein in testicular teratocarcinomas. Cancer 31:1065–1068, 1973
80. Springer GF, Desai P, Murthy M et al: Precursors of the blood group NM antigens as human carcinoma associated antigens. Transfusion 19:233–249, 1979
81. Coon JS, Weinstein RS: Blood group antigens in tumor cell membranes. Biomembranes 11:173–205, 1983
82. Wanebo HJ, Rao B, Pinsky CM et al: Preoperative carcinoembryonic antigen level as a prognostic indicator in colorectal cancer. N Engl J Med 299:448–451, 1978
83. Sugarbaker PH, Zamcheck N, Moore FD: Assessment of serial carcinoembryonic antigen (CEA) assays in postoperative detection of recurrent colorectal cancer. Cancer 38:2310–2315, 1976
84. Waldmann TA, McIntire KR: The use of radioimmunoassay for alpha-fetoprotein in the diagnosis of malignancy. Cancer 34:1510–1515, 1974
85. Heyward WL, Lanier AP, McMahon BJ et al: Early detection of primary hepatocellular carcinoma: Screening for primary hepatocellular carcinoma among persons infected with hepatitis B virus. JAMA 254:3052–3054, 1985
86. Catalona WJ: Tumor markers in testicular cancer. Urol Clin North Am 6:613–628, 1979
87. Gutman AB, Gutman EB: An "acid" phosphatase occurring in the serum of patients with metastasizing carcinoma of the prostate gland. J Clin Invest 17:473–478, 1938
88. Zondag HA, Klein F: Clinical applications of lactate dehydrogenase isozymes: Alterations in malignancy. Ann NY Acad Sci 151:578–586, 1968
89. Jones PAW, Miller FM, Worwood M et al: Ferritinaemia in leukemia and Hodgkin's disease. Br J Cancer 27:212–217, 1973
90. Melvin KEW, Miller HH, Tashjian AH: Early diagnosis of medullary carcinoma of the thyroid gland by means of calcitonin assay. N Engl J Med 285:1115–1120, 1971
91. Said JW, Vimadalal S, Nash G et al: Immunoreactive neuron-specific enolase, bombesin, and chromogranin as markers for neuroendocrine lung tumors. Hum Pathol 16:236–240, 1985
92. Haagensen DE Jr, Kister SF, Panic J et al: Comparative evaluation of carcinoembryonic antigen and gross cystic disease fluid protein as plasma markers for human breast carcinoma. Cancer 42:1646–1652, 1978
93. Foon KA, Schroff RW, Gale RP: Surface markers on leukemia and lymphoma cells: Recent advances. Blood 60:1–19, 1982
94. Koprowski H, Steplewski Z, Mitchell et al: Colorectal carcinoma antigens detected by hybridoma antibodies. Somat Cell Genet 5:957–972, 1979
95. Magnani JL, Steplewski Z, Koprowski H et al: Identification of the gastrointestinal and pancreatic cancer-associated antigen detected by monoclonal antibody 19-9 in the sera of patients as a mucin. Cancer Res 43:5489–5492, 1983
96. Del Villano BC, Brennan S, Brock P et al: Radioimmunometric assay for a monoclonal antibody-defined tumor marker, CA 19-9. Clin Chem 29:549–552, 1983
97. Bast RC Jr, Klug TL, St John E et al: A radioimmunoassay using a monoclonal antibody to monitor the course of epithelial ovarian cancer. N Engl J Med 309:883–887, 1983
98. Greaves MF, Hariri G, Newman RA et al: Selective expression of the common acute lymphoblastic leukemia (gp100) antigen on immature lymphoid cells and their malignant counterparts. Blood 61:628–639, 1983
99. Benson MD, Lurain JR, Newton M: Ovarian tumor antigens. J Reprod Med 28:17–23, 1983
100. Ashall F, Bramwell ME, Harris HJ: A new marker for human cancer cells 1: The Ca antigen and the Ca1 antibody. Lancet 2:1–6, 1982
101. McGee JO'D, Woods JC, Ashall F et al: A new marker for human cancer cells 2: Immunohistochemical detection of the Ca antigen in human tissues with the Ca1 antibody. Lancet 2:7–10, 1982
102. Dippold WG, Lloyd KO, Li LTC et al: Cell surface antigens of human malignant melanoma: Definition of six antigenic systems with mouse monoclonal antibodies. Proc Natl Acad Sci USA 77:6114, 1980
103. Gelder FB, Reese CJ, Moossa AR et al: Purification, partial characterization, and clinical evaluation of pancreatic oncofetal antigen. Cancer Res 38:313–324, 1978
104. Sorenson GD, Bloom SR, Ghatel MA et al: Bombesin production by human small cell carcinoma of the lung. Regul Pept 4:59–66, 1982
105. Staab HJ, Brummendorf T, Hornung A et al: The clinical validity of circulating tumor-associated antigens CEA and CA 19-9 in primary diagnosis and follow-up of patients with gastrointestinal malignancies. Klin Wochenschr 63:106–115, 1985
106. Gupta MK, Arciaga R, Bocci, L: Measurement of a monoclonal-antibody-defined antigen (CA 19-9) in the sera of patients with malignant and nonmalignant diseases. Cancer 56:277–283, 1985
107. Allen CA, Hogg N: Association of colorectal tumor epithelium expressing HLA-D/DR with CD8-positive T-cells and mononuclear phagocytes. Cancer Res 47:2919–2923, 1987
108. van den Ingh HF, Ruiter DJ, Griffioen G et al: HLA antigens in clorectal tumours—Low expression of HLA Class I antigens in mucinous colorectal carcinomas. Br J Cancer 55:125–130, 1987
109. Yamashita K, Nakamura T, Shimizu T et al: Expression of HLA Class I and Class II antigens in human choriocarcinoma cell lines. Int J Gynaecol Obstet 24:301–307, 1986
110. Pesando JM, Graf L: Differential expression of HLA-DR, -DQ, and -DP antigens on malignant B cells. J Immunol 136:4311–4318, 1986
111. Drewinko B, Lichtiger B: Full expression of blood group-related, transplantation-re-

lated, and carcinoembryonic antigens in human colorectal cancer cells with different degrees of phenotypic differentiation. Cancer Res 45:1560–1564, 1985

112. Wagner DK, York-Jolley J, Malek TR et al: Antigen-specific murine T cell clones produce soluble interleukin-2 receptor on stimulation with specific antigens. J Immunol 137:592–596, 1986

113. Medina-Ibarrondo C, Lahuerta-Palacios JJ, Lahuerta-Palacios M: Soluble interleukin-2 receptors in B-cell leukemia and the acquired immunodeficiency syndrome. Ann Intern Med 106:774, 1987

114. Lotze MT, Custer MC, Sharrow SO et al: *In vivo* administration of purified human interleukin-2 to patients with cancer: Development of interleukin-2 receptor positive cells and circulation soluble interleukin-2 receptors following interleukin-2 administration. Cancer Res 47:2188–2195, 1987

115. Soulillou JP, LeMauff B, Olive D et al: Prevention of rejection of kidney transplants by monoclonal antibody directed against interleukin-2. Lancet 1339–1343, 1987

116. Waldmann TA: The interleukin-2 receptor on malignant cells: A target for diagnosis and therapy. Cell Immunol 99:53–60, 1986

117. Waldmann TA: The structure, function, and expression of interleukin-2 receptors on normal and malignant lymphocytes. Science 232:727–732, 1986

118. Kronke M, Depper JM, Leonard WJ et al.: Adult T cell leukemia: A potential target for ricin A chain immunotoxins. Blood 65:1416–1421, 1985

119. Takahashi H, Herlyn D, Atkinson B et al: Radioimmunodetection of human glioma xenografts by monoclonal antibody to epidermal growth factor receptor. Cancer Res 47:3847–3850, 1987

120. Rodeck U, Herlyn M, Herlyn D et al: Tumor growth modulation by a monoclonal antibody to the epidermal growth factor receptor: Immunologically mediated and effector cell-independent effects. Cancer Res 47:3692–3696, 1987

121. Ranz E: Über Komplimentablenkung durch Serum und Organe. Wien Klin Wochenschr 19:1552–1555, 1906

122. Kohler G, Milstein C: Continuous cultures of fused cells secreting antibodies of predefined specificity. Nature 256:495–497, 1975

123. Jeske DJ, Capra JD: Immunoglobulins: Structure and function. In Paul WE (ed): Fundamental Immunology, pp 131–165. New York, Raven Press, 1984

124. Roitt I, Brostoff J, Male D: Antibody structure and function. In Roitt I, Brostoff J, Male D (eds): pp 5.1–5.8 Immunology, St Louis, CV Mosby, 1986.

125. Berzofsky JA, Berkower IJ: Antigen–antibody interaction. In Paul WE (ed): Fundamental Immunology, pp 595–644. New York, Raven Press, 1984

126. Geysen HM, Tainer JA, Rodda SJ et al: Chemistry of antibody binding to a protein. Science 235:1184–1190, 1987

127. Getzoff ED, Geysen HM, Rodda SJ et al: Mechanisms of antibody binding to a protein. Science 235:1191–1196, 1987

128. Roberts S. Cheetham JC, Reese AR: Generation of an antibody with enhanced affinity and specificity for its antigen by protein engineering. Nature 328:731–734, 1987

129. Massey RJ: Catalytic antibodies catching on. Nature 328:457–458, 1987

130. Kohler G, Howe SC, Milstein C: Fusion between immunoglobulin secreting and non-secreting myeloma cells lines. Eur J Immunol 6:292–298, 1976

131. Kohler G, Howe SC, Milstein C: Derivation of specific antibody producing tissue culture and tumor lines by cell fusion. Eur J Immunol 6:611–617, 1976

132. Brown JP, Woodbury RG, Hart CE et al: Quantitative analysis of melanoma-associated antigen p97 in normal and neoplastic tissues. Proc Natl Acad Sci USA 78:539–543, 1981

133. Morgan AC, Galloway DR, Reisfeld RA: Production and characterization of monoclonal antibody to a melanoma specific glycoprotein. Hybridoma 1:17–36, 1981

134. Hellstrom I, Garrigues HJ, Cabasco L et al: Studies of a high molecular weight human melanoma-associated antigen. J Immunol 130:1467–1472, 1983

135. Hellstrom I, Brankovan V, Hellstrom KE: Strong antitumor activities of IgG3 antibodies to a human melanoma-associated ganglioside. Proc Natl Acad Sci USA 82:1499–1502, 1985

136. Johnson VG, Schlom J, Paterson AJ et al: Analysis of a human tumor-associated glycoprotein (TAG-72) identified by monoclonal antibody B72.3. Cancer Res 46:850–857, 1986

137. Muraro R, Wunderlich D, Thor A et al: Definition by monoclonal antibodies of a repertoire of epitopes on carcinoembryonic antigen differentially expressed in human colon carcinoma versus normal adult tissues. Cancer Res 45:5769–5780, 1985

138. Herlyn D, Herlyn M, Steplewski Z et al: Monoclonal anti-human tumor antibodies of six isotypes in cytotoxic reactions with human and murine effector cells. Cell Immunol 92:105–114, 1985

139. Fargion S, Carney D, Mulshine J et al: Heterogeneity of cell surface antigen expression of human small cell lung cancer detected by monoclonal antibodies. Cancer Res 46:2633–2638, 1986

140. Hellstrom I, Horn D, Linsley P et al: Monoclonal mouse antibodies raised against human lung carcinoma. Cancer Res 46:3917–3923, 1986

141. Kearney JF: Hybridomas and monoclonal antibodies. In Paul WE (ed): Fundamental Immunology, pp 751–766. New York, Raven Press, 1984

142. Morrison SL: Transfectomas provide novel chimeric antibodies. Science 229:1202–1207, 1985

143. Graziano RF, Fanger MW: FcgRI and FcgRII on monocytes and granulocytes are cytoxic trigger molecules for tumor cells. J Immunol 139:3536–3541, 1987

144. Shen L, Guyre PM, Fanger MW: Polymorphonuclear leukocyte function triggered through the high affinity Fc receptor for monomeric IgG. J Immunol 139:534–538, 1987

145. Looney RJ, Abraham GN, Anderson CL: Human monocytes and U937 cells bear two distinct Fc receptors for IgG. J Immunol 136:1641–1647, 1986

146. Rosenfeld SI, Looney RJ, Leddy JP et al: Human platelet Fc receptor for immunoglobulin G: Identification as a 40,000-molecular-weight membrane protein shared by monocytes. J Clin Invest 76:2317–2322, 1985

147. Titus JA, Sharrow SO, Segal DM: Analysis of Fc (IgG) receptors on human peripheral blood leukocytes by dual fluorescence flow microfluorometry II: Quantitation of receptors on cells that express the OKM1, OKT3, OKT4, and OKT8 antigens. J Immunol 130:1152–1158, 1983

148. Perussia B, Kobayashi M, Rossi ME et al: Immune interferon enhances functional properties of human granulocytes: Role of Fc receptors and effect of lymphotoxin, tumor necrosis factor and granulocyte–macrophage colony stimulating factor. J Immunol 138:765–774, 1987

149. Ravetch JV, Luster AD, Weinshank R et al: Structure heterogeneity and functional domains of murine immunoglobulin G Fc receptors. Science 234:718–725, 1986

150. Lewis VA, Koch T, Plutner H et al: A complementary DNA clone for a macrophage–lymphocyte Fc receptor. Nature 324:372–375, 1986

151. Deodhar SD, James K, Chiang T et al: Inhibition of lung metastases in mice bearing a malignant fibrosarcoma by treatment with liposomes containing human C-reactive protein. Cancer Res 42:5084–5088, 1982

152. Muller H, Fehr J: Binding of C-reactive protein to human polymorphonuclear leukocytes: Evidence for association of binding sites with Fc receptors. J Immunol 136:2202–2207, 1986

153. Yancey KB, Hammer CH, Harvath L et al: Studies of human C5a as a mediator of inflammation in normal human skin. J Clin Invest 75:486–495, 1985

154. Yancey KB, O'Shea J, Chused T et al: Human C5a modulates monocytes Fc and C3 receptor expression. J Immunol 135:465–470, 1985

155. Huey R, Hugli TE: Characterization of a C5a receptor on human polymorphonuclear leukocytes (PMN). J Immunol 135:2063–2068, 1985

156. Mujoo K, Cheresh DA, Yang HM et al: Disialoganglioside G_{D2} on human neuroblastoma cells: Target antigen for monoclonal antibody-mediated cytolysis and suppression of tumor growth. Cancer Res 47:1098–1104, 1987

157. Hersey P, MacDonald M, Burns C et al: Enhancement of cytotoxic and proliferative responses of lymphocytes from melanoma patients by incubation with monoclonal antibodies against ganglioside GD_3. Cancer Immunol Immunother 24:144–150, 1987

158. Thurin J, Thurin M, Kimoto Y et al: Monoclonal antibody-defined correlations in melanoma between levels of GD_2 and GD_3 antigens and antibody-mediated cytotoxicity. Cancer Res 47:1229–1233, 1987

159. Shiloni E, Eisenthal A, Sachs D et al: Antibody-dependent cellular cytotoxicity mediated by murine lymphocytes activated in recombinant interleukin-2. J Immunol 138:1992–1998, 1987

160. Anasetti C, Martin PJ, Morishita Y et al: Human large granular lymphocytes express high affinity receptors for murine monoclonal antibodies of the IgG3 subclass. J Immunol 138:2979–2981, 1987

161. Ortaldo JR, Woodhouse C, Morgan AC et al: Analysis of effector cells in human antibody-dependent cellular cytotoxicity with murine monoclonal antibodies. J Immunol 138:3556–3572, 1987

162. Ghose T, Tai J, Aquino J et al: Tumor localization of ^{131}I-labeled antibodies by radionuclide imaging. Radiology 116:445–448, 1976

163. Houghton AN, Scheinberg DA: Monoclonal antibodies: Potential applications to the treatment of cancer. Semin Oncol 13:165–179, 1986

164. Carrasquillo JA: Radioimmunoscintigraphy with polyclonal or monoclonal antibodies. In Zalutsky M (ed): Antibodies in Radiodiagnosis and Therapy. Boca Raton, FL, CRC Press, 1989

165. Bradwell AR, Fairweather DS, Dykes PW et al: Limiting factors in the localization of tumors with radiolabelled antibodies. Immunol Today 6:163-170, 1985

166. Jungerman JA, Yo K-HP, Zanelli CI: Radiation absorbed dose estimates at the cellular level for some electron-emitting radionuclides for radioimmunotherapy. Int J Appl Radiat Isot 35:883–888, 1984

167. Barth RF, Alan F, Soloway AH et al: Boronated monoclonal antibody 17-1A for potential neutron capture therapy of colorectal cancer. Hybridoma 5:S43–S50, 1986

168. Fawwaz RA, Wang ST, Srivastava SC et al: Potential of palladium-109-labeled antimelanoma monoclonal antibody for tumor therapy. J Nucl Med 25:796–799, 1984

169. Bumol TF, Wang QC, Reisfekd RA et al: Monoclonal antibody and an antibody–toxin conjugate to a cell surface proteoglycan of melanoma cells suppress in vivo tumor growth. Proc Natl Acad Sci USA 80:529–533, 1983

170. Leonard JE, Wang QC, Kaplan NO et al: Kinetics of protein synthesis inactivation in human T-lymphocytes by selective monoclonal antibody–ricin conjugates. Cancer Res 45:5263–5269, 1985

171. Kronke M, Depper JM, Leonard WJ et al: Adult T cell leukemia: A potential target for ricin A chain immunotoxins. Blood 65:1416–1421, 1985

172. Waldmann TA, Tsudo M: Interleukin-2 receptors: Biology and therapeutic potentials. Hosp Pract January 15, 1987, pp 77–94

173. Strom TB: The cellular and molecular basis of allograft rejection: What do we know? Transport Proc 20:143–146, 1988

174. Dillman RO, Shawler DL, Johnson DE et al: Preclinical trials with combinations and conjugats of T101 monoclonal antibody and doxorubicin. Cancer Res 46:4886–4891, 1986

175. Endo N, Kato Y, Takeda Y et al: *In vitro* cytotoxicity of a human serum albumin-mediated conjugate of methotrexate with anti-MM46 monoclonal antibody. Cancer Res 47:1076–1080, 1987
176. Tsukada Y, Ohkawa K, Hibi N: Therapeutic effect of treatment with polyclonal or monoclonal antibodies to alpha-fetoprotein that have been conjugated to duanomycin via a dextran bridge: Studies with an alpha-fetoprotein-producing rat hepatoma tumor model. Cancer Res 47:4293–4295, 1987
177. Matthay KK, Heath TD, Badger CC et al: Antibody-directed liposomes: Comparison of various ligands for association, endocytosis, and drug delivery. Cancer Res 46:4904–4910, 1986
178. Mew D, Lum V, Wat C-K et al: Ability of specific monoclonal antibodies and conventional antisera conjugated to hematoporphyrin to label and kill selected cell lines subsequent to light activation. Cancer Res 45:4380–4386, 1985
179. Waldmann TA: The structure, function, and expression of interleukin-2 receptors on normal and malignant lymphocytes. Science 232:727–732, 1986
180. Waldmann TA, Longo DL, Leonard WJ et al: Interleukin-2 receptor (Tac antigen) expression in HTLV-I-associated adult T-cell leukemia. Cancer Res 45:4559s–4562s, 1985
181. Greene WC, Leonard WJ, Depper JM et al: The human interleukin-2 receptor: Normal and abnormal expression in T cells and in leukemias induced by the human T-lymphotropic retroviruses. Ann Intern Med 105:560–572, 1986
182. Waldmann TA: Use of monoclonal antibody to the interleukin-2 receptor in therapy of patients with adult T-cell leukemia. In Singhal SK, Delovitch (eds): Mediators of Immune Regulation and Immunotherapy, New York, Elsevier Science, 1986
183. Waldmann TA: The interleukin-2 receptor on malignant cells: A target for diagnosis and therapy. Cell Immunol 99:53–60, 1986
184. Kozak RW, Atcher RW, Gansow OA et al: Bismuth-212-labeled anti-Tac monoclonal antibody: Alpha-particle-emitting radionuclides as modalities for radioimmunotherapy. Proc Natl Acad Sci USA 83:474–478, 1986
185. Takahashi H, Herlyn D, Atkinson B et al: Radioimmunodetection of human glioma xenografts by monoclonal antibody to epidermal growth factor receptor. Cancer Res 47:3847–3850, 1987
186. Masui H, Kawamofo T, Sato JD et al: Growth inhibition of human tumor cells in a thymic nude mouse by antiepidermal growth factor receptor monoclonal antibodies. Cancer Res 44: 1002–1007, 1984
187. Griffin TW, Richardson C, Houston LL et al: Antitumor activity of intraperitoneal immunotoxins in a nude mouse model of known malignant mesothelioma. Cancer Res 47:4266–4270, 1987
188. Koprowski H, Herlyn D, Lubeck M et al: Human anti-idiotypic antibodies in cancer patients: Is the modulation of the immune response beneficial for the patient? Proc Natl Acad Sci USA 81:216–219, 1984
189. Herlyn D, Ross AH, Koprowski H: Anti-idiotypic antibodies bear the internal image of a human tumor antigen. Science 232:100–102, 1986
190. DeShambo RM, Krolick KA: Selective in vitro inhibition of an antibody response to purified acetylcholine receptor by using anti-idiotypic antibodies coupled to the A chain of ricin. J Immunol 137:3135–3139, 1986
191. Kusama M, Kageshita T, Tsujisaki M et al: Syngeneic antiidiotypic antisera to murine antihuman high-molecular-weight melanoma-associated antigen monoclonal antibodies. Cancer Res 47:4312–4317, 1987
192. Jerne NK: Towards a network theory of the immune system. Ann Immunol [Paris] 125C:373–389, 1974
193. Burdette S, Schwartz RS: Current concepts: Immunology: Idiotypes and idiotypic networks. N Engl J Med 317:224, 1987
194. Mittelman A, Ferone S, Kageshita T et al: A Phase I clinical trial of murine anti-idiotypic monoclonal antibodies to anti human high molecular weight-melanoma associated antigen monoclonal antibodies in patients with malignant melanoma (abstract). Proc Am Assoc Cancer Res 28:390, 1987
195. Karpovsky B, Titus JA, Stephany DA et al: Production of target-specific effector cells using hetero-cross-linked aggregates containing anti-target cell and anti-Fc receptor antibodies. J Exp Med 160:1686–1701, 1984
196. Staerz UD, Kanagawa O, Bevan MJ: Hybrid antibodies can target sites for attack by T cells. Nature 314:628–631, 1985
197. Staerz UD, Bevan MJ: Use of anti-receptor antibodies to focus T-cell activity. Immunol Today 8:241–245, 1986
198. Perez P, Titus JA, Lotze MT et al: Specific lysis of human tumor cells by T cells coated with anti-T3 cross-linked to anti-tumor antibody. J Immunol 137:2069–2072, 1986
199. Lotze MT, Roberts K, Custer MC et al: Specific binding and lysis of human melanoma by IL-2-activated cells coated with anti-T3 or anti-Fc receptor cross-linked to antimelanoma antibody: A possible approach to the immunotherapy of human tumors. J Surg Res 42:580–589, 1987
200. Titus JA, Garrido MA, Hecht TT et al: Human T cells targeted with anti-T3 cross-linked to antitumor antibody prevent tumor growth in nude mice. J Immunol 138:4018–4022, 1987
201. Titus JA, Perez P, Kaubisch A et al: Human K/natural killer cells targeted with hetero-cross-linked antibodies specifically lyse tumor cells in vitro and prevent tumor growth *in vivo*. J Immunol 139:3153–3158, 1987
202. Yamaguchi H, Furukawa K, Fortunato SR et al: Cell-surface antigens of melanoma recognized by human monoclonal antibodies. Proc Natl Acad Sci USA 84:2416–2420, 1987
203. Watson DB, Burns GF, Mackay IR: *In vitro* growth of B lymphocytes infiltrating human melanoma tissue by transformation with EBV: Evidence for secretion of anti-melanoma antibodies by some transformed cells. J Immunol 130:2442–2447, 1983
204. Haspel MV, McCabe RP, Pomato N et al: Generation of tumor cell-reactive human monoclonal antibodies using peripheral blood lymphocytes from actively immunized colorectal carcinoma patients. Cancer Res 45:3951–3961, 1985
205. Irie RF, Morton DL: Regression of cutaneous metastatic melanoma by intralesional injection with human monoclonal antibody to ganglioside GD2. Proc Natl Acad Sci USA 83:8694–8698, 1986
206. Casali P, Inghirami I, Nakamura M et al: Human monoclonals from antigen-specific selection of B lymphocytes and transformation by EBV. Science 234:476–479, 1987
207. Nishimura Y, Yokoyama M, Araki K et al: Recombinant human–mouse chimeric monoclonal antibody specific for common acute lymphocytic leukemia antigen. Cancer Res 47:999–1005, 1987
208. Shaw DR, Khazaeli MB, Sun LK et al: Characterization of a mouse/human chimeric monoclonal antibody (17-1A) to a colon cancer tumor-associated antigen. J Immunol 138:4534–4538, 1987
209. Liu AY, Robinson RR, Hellstrom KE et al: Chimeric mouse–human IgG1 antibody that can mediate lysis of cancer cells. Proc Natl Acad Sci USA 84:3439–3443, 1987
210. Whittle N, Adair J, Lloyd C et al: Expression in COS cells of a mouse-human chimaeric B72.3 antibody. Protein Engineering 1:499–505, 1987
211. Ng AK, Imai K, Pellegrino A et al: Modulation of immune lysis of tumor cells by interferon. Biomembranes 11:313–339, 1983
212. Houghton AN, Thomson TM, Gross D et al: Surface antigens of melanoma and melanocytes: Specificity of induction of Ia antigens by human gamma-interferon. J Exp Med 160:255–269, 1984
213. Pfizenmaier K, Scheurich P, Schluter C et al: Tumor necrosis factor enhances HLA-A,B,C and HLA-DR gene expression in human tumor cells. J Immunol 138:975–980, 1987
214. Basham TY, Kaminski MS, Kitamura K et al: Synergistic antitumor effect of interferon and anti-idiotype monoclonal antibody in murine lymphoma. J Immunol 137:?3019–3024, 1986
215. Greiner JW, Guadagni F, Noguchi P et al: Recombinant interferon enhances monoclonal antibody-targeting of carcinoma lesions in vivo. Science 235:895–898, 1987
216. Eisenthal A, Lafreniere R, Lefor AT et al: Effect of anti-B16 melanoma monoclonal antibody on established murine B16 melanoma liver metastases. Cancer Res 47:2271–2776, 1987
217. Berinstein N, Levy R: Treatment of a murine B cell lymphoma with monoclonal antibodies and IL 2. J Immunol 139:971–976, 1987
218. Ernst CS, Sears HF, Herlyn M et al: Detection of murine immunoglobulin in human tissues following therapeutic infusion of monoclonal antibody. Hybridoma 5:S79–S85, 1986
219. Chatenoud L, Junker M, Villemain F et al: The human immune response to the OKT3 monoclonal antibody is oligodonal. Science 232:1406–1408, 1986
220. Reynolds JC, Carrasquillo JA, Keenan AM et al: Human antimurine antibodies following immunoscintigraphy or therapy with radiolabeled monoclonal antibodies. J Nucl Med 21:16, 1986
221. Courtenay–Luck NS, Epenetos AA, Moore R et al: Development of primary and secondary immune responses to mouse monoclonal antibodies used in the diagnosis and therapy of malignant neoplasms. Cancer Res 46:6489–6493, 1986
222. Courtenay–Luck NS, Epenetos AA, Winearls CG et al: Preexisting human anti-murine immunoglobulin reactivity due to polyclonal rheumatoid factors. Cancer Res 47:4520–4525, 1987
223. Welte K, Miller G, Chapman PB et al: Stimulation of T lymphocyte proliferation by monoclonal antibodies against GD3 ganglioside. J Immunol 139:1763–1771, 1987
224. Benjamin RJ, Waldmann H: Induction of tolerance by monoclonal antibody therapy. Nature 320:449–451, 1986
225. Caulfield MJ, Shaffer D: Immunoregulation by antigen/antibody complexes I: Specific immunosuppression induced in vivo with immune complexes formed in antibody excess. J Immunol 138:3680–3683, 1987
226. Marrack J: Nature of antibodies. Nature 133:292, 1934
227. Pressman D, Kerghley G: The zone of activity of antibodies as determined by the use of radioactive tracers: The zone of activity of nephritoxic anti-kidney serum. J Immunol 59:140–141, 1948
228. Korngold L, Pressman D: The localization of antilymphosarcoma antibodies in the Murphy lymphosarcoma of the rat. Cancer Res 14:96–99, 1954
229. Day ED: Myelin as a locus for radioantibody absorption *in vivo* in brain tumors. Cancer Res 28:1335–1343, 1968
230. Pressman D, Korngold DL: The *in vivo* localization of anti-Waagner-osteogenic sarcoma antibodies. Cancer 6:619–623, 1953
231. Pressman D, Day ED, Blau M: The use of paired labeling in the determination of tumor-localizing antibodies. Cancer Res 17:845–850, 1957
232. Day ED, Lassiter S, Woodhall B et al: The localization of radioantibodies in human brain tumors: I. Preliminary exploration. Cancer Res 25:773–778, 1965
233. Day ED, Plannisek J, Korngold L et al: Tumor localizing antibodies purified from antisera against Murphy rat lymphosarcoma. J Natl Cancer Inst 17:517–532, 1956
234. Bale WF, Spar IL: Studies directed toward the use of antibodies as carriers of radioactivity for therapy. Adv Biol Med Phys 5:285–356, 1957
235. Ghose T, Tai J, Aquino J et al: Tumor localization of ^{131}I-labeled antibodies by radionuclide imaging. Radiology 116:445–448, 1975
236. Belitsky P, Ghose T, Aquino J, Tai J et al: Radionuclide imaging of metastases from renal cell carcinoma by ^{131}I-labeled antitumor antibody. Radiology 126:515–517, 1978

237. Reif AE, Curtis LE, Duffield R et al: Trial of radiolabeled antibody localization in metastases of a patient with a tumor containing carcinoembryonic antigen (CEA). J Surg Oncol 6:133–150, 1974
238. Goldenberg DM, Kim EE, DeLand F et al: Clinical studies on the radioimmunodetection of tumors containing alpha-fetoprotein. Cancer 45:2500–2500, 1980
239. Mach J-P, Carrel S, Forni M et al: Tumor localization of radiolabeled antibodies against carcinoembryonic antigens in patients with carcinoma: A critical evaluation. N Engl J Med 303:5–10, 1980
240. Kim EE, DeLand FH, Casper S et al: Radioimmunodetection of colorectal cancer. Cancer 45:1243–1427, 1980
241. Mach J-P, Buchegger F, Forni M et al: Use of radiolabelled monoclonal anti-CEA antibodies for the detection of human carcinomas by external photoscanning and tomoscintigraphy. Immunol Today 2:239–249, 1981
242. Farrands PA, Pimm MV, Embleton MJ et al: Radioimmunodetection of human colorectal cancers by an anti-tumour monoclonal antibody. Lancet 397–400, 1982
243. Berche C, Mach J-P, Lumbruso J-D et al: Tomoscintigraphy for detecting gastrointestinal and medullary thyroid cancers: First clinical results using radiolabelled monoclonal antibodies against carcinoembryonic antigen. Br Med J 285:1447–1451, 1982
244. Mach J-P, Chatal J-F, Lumbroso J-D et al: Tumor localization in patients by radiolabeled monoclonal antibodies against colon carcinoma. Cancer Res 43:5593–5600, 1983
245. Moldofsky PJ, Powe J, Mulhern CB et al: Metastatic colon carcinoma detected with radiolabeled F9ab′) monoclonal antibody fragments. Radiology 149:549–555, 1983
246. Moldofsky PJ, Sears HF, Mulhern CB et al: Detection of metastatic tumor in normal-sized retroperitoneal lymph nodes by monoclonal-antibody imaging. N Engl J Med 311:106–107, 1984
247. Epenetos AA, Snook D, Durbin H et al: Limitations of radiolabeled monoclonal antibodies for localization of human neoplasms. Cancer Res 46:3183–3191, 1986
248. Beatty JD, Duda RB, Williams LE et al: Preoperative imaging of colorectal carcinoma with ^{111}In-labeled anticarcinoembryonic antigen monoclonal antibody. Cancer Res 46:6494–6502, 1986
249. Duda RB, Beatty JD, Sheibani K et al: Imaging of human colorectal adenocarcinoma with indium-labeled anticarcinoembryonic antigen monoclonal antibody. Arch Surg 121:131–1319, 1986
250. Ward BG, Mather SJ, Hawkins LR et al: Localization of radioiodine conjugated to the monoclonal antibody HMFG2 in human ovarian carcinoma: Assessment of intravenous and intraperitoneal routes of administration. Cancer Res 47:4719–4723, 1987
251. Colcher D, Esteban J, Carrasquillo JA et al: Quantitative analyses of selective radiolabeled monoclonal antibody localization in metastatic lesions of colorectal cancer patients. Cancer Res 47:1185–1189, 1987
252. Colcher D, Esteban J, Carrasquillo JA et al: Complementation of intracavitary and intravenous administration of a monoclonal antibody (B72.3) in patients with carcinoma. Cancer Res 47:4218–4224, 1987
253. Carrasquillo JA, Bunn PA, Keenan AM et al: Radioimmunodetection of cutaneous T-cell lymphoma with ^{111}In-labeled T101 monoclonal antibody. N Engl J Med 315:673–680, 1986
254. Ettinger DS, Order SE, Wharam MD et al: Phase I–II study of isotopic immunoglobulin therapy for primary liver cancer. Cancer Treat Rep 66:289–297, 1982
255. Leichner PK, Klein JL, Siegelman SS et al: Dosimetry of ^{131}I-labeled antiferritin in hepatoma: Specific activities in the tumor and liver. Cancer Treat Rep 67:647–658, 1983
256. Order SE, Stillwagon GB, Klein JL et al: Iodine 131 antiferritin, a new treatment modality in hepatoma: A Radiation Therapy Oncology Group study. J Clin Oncol 3:1573–1582, 1985
257. Order SE, Klein JL, Leichner PK: Hepatoma: Model for radiolabeled antibody in cancer treatment. NCI Mongr 3:37–41, 1987
258. Larson SM, Brown JP, Wright PW et al: Imaging of melanoma with ^{131}I-labeled monoclonal antibodies. J Nucl Med 24:123–129, 1983
259. Larson SM, Carrasquillo JA, Krohn KA et al: Localization of ^{131}I-labeled p97-specific Fab fragments in human melanoma as a basis for radiotherapy. J Clin Invest 72:2101–2114, 1983
260. Carrasquillo JA, Krohn KA, Beaumler P et al: Diagnosis of and therapy for solid tumors with radiolabeled antibodies and immune fragments. Cancer Treat Rep 68:317–328, 1984
261. Halpern SE, Sillman RO, Witztum KF et al: Radioimmunodetection of melanoma utilizing In-111 96.5 monoclonal antibody: A preliminary report. Radiology 155:493–499, 1985
262. Lotze MT, Carrasquillo JA, Weinstein JN et al: Monoclonal antibody imaging of human melanoma: Radioimmunodetection by subcutaneous or systemic injection. Ann Surg 204:223–235, 1986
263. Siccardi AG, Buraggi GL, Callegaro L et al: Multicenter study of immunoscintigraphy with radiolabeled monoclonal antibodies in patients with melanoma. Cancer Res 46:4817–4822, 1986
264. Buraggi GL, Callegaro L, Mariani G et al: Imaging with ^{131}I-labeled monoclonal antibodies to a high-molecular weight melanoma-associated antigen in patients with melanoma: Efficacy of whole immunoglobulin and its $F(ab')_2$ fragments. Cancer Res 45:3378–3387, 1985
265. Engelstad BL, Spitler LE, Del Rio MJ et al: Phase I immunolymphoscintigraphy with an In-111-labeled antimelanoma monoclonal antibody. Radiology 161:419–422, 1986
266. Taylor Jr A, Milton W, Eyre H et al: Radioimmunodetection of human melanoma with indium-111-labeled monoclonal antibodies. NCI Monogr 3:25–31, 1987
267. Goldenberg DM, DeLand F, Kim E et al: Use of radiolabeled antibodies to carcinoembryonic antigen for the detection and localization of diverse cancers by external photoscanning. N Engl J Med 25:1384–1388, 1978
268. Kim WW, DeLand FH, Nelson MO et al: Radioimmunodetection of cancer with radiolabeled antibodies to alpha-fetoprotein. Cancer Res 40:3008–3012, 1980
269. Goldenberg DM, Kim EE, DeLand FH et al: Radioimmunodetection of cancer using radioactive antibodies to human chorionic gonadotropin. Science 208:1284–1286, 1980
270. Monison RT, Lyster DM, Alcorn L et al: Radioimmunoimaging with ^{99m}Tc monoclonal antibodies: Clinical studies. Int J Nucl Med & Biol 11:184–188, 1984
271. Fairweather DS, Bradwell AR, Watson–James SF: Detection of thyroid tumors using radiolabeled anti-thyroglobulin. Clin Endocrinol 18:563–570, 1983
272. Fairweather DS, Bradwell AR, Dykes PW: Monoclonal antibodies for *in vivo* localisation. Lancet 2:660, 1982
273. Nimmon CC, Carroll MJ, Flatman W: Partial probability mapping of temporal change: Application to gamma quality control and immunoscintigraphy. Nucl Med Commun 5:231, 1984
274. Order SE, Bloomer WB, Jones AG et al: Radionuclide immunoglobulin lymphangiography: A case report. Cancer 35:1487–1492, 1975
275. Weinstein JN, Steller MA, Covell DG et al: Monoclonal antitumor antibodies in the lymphatics. Cancer Treat Rep 68:257–264, 1984
276. Eger RR, Covell DG, Carrasquillo JA et al: Kinetic model for the biodistribution of an ^{111}In-labeled monoclonal antibody in humans. Cancer Res 47:3328–3336, 1987
277. Parker RJ, Keenan AM, Dower SK et al: Targeting of murine radiolabeled monoclonal antibodies in the lymphatics. Cancer Res 47:2073–2076, 1987
278. Weinstein JN, Black CDV, Barbet J et al: Selected issues in the pharmacology of monoclonal antibodies. In Tomlinson E (ed): Site-Specific Drug Delivery. New York, John Wiley, 1986
279. Schlom J: Basic principles and applications of monoclonal antibodies in the management of carcinomas: The Richard and Hinda Rosenthal Foundation Award Lecture. Cancer Res 46:3225–3238, 1986
280. Nadler LM, Stashenko P, Hardy R et al: Serotherapy of a patient with a monoclonal antibody directed against a human lymphoma-associated antigen. Cancer Res 40:3147–3154, 1980
281. Miller RA, Maloney DG, Warnke R et al: Treatment of B-cell lymphoma with monoclonal anti-idiotype antibody. N Engl J Med 306:517–522, 1982
282. Miller RA, Oseroff AR, Stratte PT et al: Monoclonal antibody therapeutic trails in seven patients with T-cell lymphoma. Blood 62:988, 1983
283. Meeker TC, Lowder JN, Maloney DG et al: A clinical trial of anti-idiotype therapy for B cell malignancy. Blood 65:1349–1363, 1985
284. Rankin EM, Hekman A, Somers R et al: Treatment of two patients with B cell lymphoma with monoclonal anti-idiotypic antibodies. Blood 65:1373–1381, 1985
285. Giardina SL, Schroff RW, Kipps TJ et al: The generation of monoclonal anti-idiotype antibodies to human B cell-derived leukemias and lymphomas. J Immunol 135:653–658, 1985
286. Dillman RO, Shawler DL, Sobel RE et al: Murine monoclonal antibody therapy in two patients with chronic lymphocytic leukemia. Blood 59:1036–1045, 1982
287. Dillman RO, Shawler DL, Dillman JB et al: Therapy of chronic lymphocytic leukemia and cutaneous T-cell lymphoma with T101 monoclonal antibody. J Clin Oncol 2:881–891, 1984
288. Foon KA, Schroff RW, Bunn PA et al: Effects of monoclonal antibody therapy in patients with chronic lymphocytic leukemia. Blood 64:1085–1094, 1984
289. Ritz J, Pesando JM, Sallan SE et al: Serotherapy of acute lymphoblastic leukemia with monoclonal antibody. Blood 58:141–152, 1981
290. Miller RA, Maloney DG, McKillop J et al: *In vivo* effects of murine hybridoma monoclonal antibody in a patient with T-cell leukemia. Blood 58:78–86, 1981
291. Miller RA, Oseroff AS, Stratte PT et al: Monoclonal antibody therapeutic trials in seven patients with T-cell lymphoma. Blood 62:988–995, 1983
292. Miller RA, Levy R: Response of cutaneous T cell lymphoma to therapy of hybridoma monoclonal antibody. Lancet 2:225–230, 1981
293. Levy R, Miller RA: Tumor therapy with monoclonal antibodies. Fed Proc 42:2650–2656, 1983
294. Foon KA, Schroff RW, Bunn PA: Monoclonal antibody therapy for patients with leukemia and lymphoma. In Foon KA, Morgan AC (eds): Monoclonal Antibody Therapy of Human Cancer, pp 85–101. Boston, Martinus Nijhoff, 1985
295. Rosen ST, Zimmer AM, Goldman-Leikin R et al: Radioimmunodetection and radioimmunotherapy of cutaneous T cell lymphomas using ^{131}I-labeled monoclonal antibody: An Illinois Cancer Council study. J Clin Oncol 5:562–573, 1987
296. Ball ED, Bernier GM, Cornwell GG et al: Monoclonal antibodies to myeloid differentiation antigens: In vivo studies of three patients with acute myelogenous leukemia. Blood 62:1203–1210, 1983
297. Courtenay–Luck N, Epenetos AA: Antibody-guided irradiation of malignant lesions: Three cases illustrating a new method of treatment. Lancet 1:1441–1443, 1984
298. Sears HF, Atkinson B, Mattis J et al: The use of monoclonal antibody in Phase I clinical trial of human gastrointestinal tumors. Lancet 1:762–765, 1982
299. Sears HF, Herlyn D, Steplewski Z et al: Phase II clinical trial of a murine monoclonal antibody cytotoxic for gastrointestinal adenocarcinoma. Cancer Res 45:5910–5913, 1985
300. Sindelar WF, Maher MM, Herlyn D et al: Trial of therapy with monoclonal antibody

17-1A in pancreatic carcinoma: Preliminary results. Hybridoma 5:S125–S132, 1986

301. Weiner LM, Steplewski Z, Koprowski H et al: Biologic effects of gamma interferon pre-treatment followed by monoclonal antibody 17-1A administration in patients with gastrointestinal carcinoma. Hybridoma 5:S65–S77, 1986
302. Sobol RE, Dillman RO, Smith JD: Phase I evaluation of murine monoclonal anti-melanoma antibody in man: Preliminary observations. In Mitchell MS, Oettgen HF (eds): Hybridomas in Cancer Diagnosis and Treatment, pp 199–206, New York, Raven Press, 1982
303. Larson SM, Carrasquillo JA, Krohn KA: Radiotherapy with "anti-p97" iodinated monoclonal antibodies in melanoma. In Raynaud C (ed): Proceedings of the Third World Congress of Nuclear Medicine and Biology, pp 3666–3669. New York, Pergamon Press, 1982
304. Oldham RK, Foon KA, Morgan C et al: Monoclonal antibody therapy of malignant melanoma: In vivo localization in cutaneous metastasis after intravenous administration. J Clin Oncol 2:1235–1244, 1984
305. Goodman GE, Beaumier P, Hellstrom I et al: Pilot trial of murine monoclonal antibodies in patients with advanced melanoma. J Clin Oncol 3:340–352, 1985
306. Dippold WG, Knuth KRK, zum Buschenfelde K-HM: Inflammatory tumor response to monoclonal antibody infusion. Eur J Cancer Clin Oncol 21:907–912, 1985
307. Houghton AN, Mintzer DM, Corden-Cardo C et al: Mouse monoclonal antibody detecting GD3 ganglioside: A phase I trial in patients with malignant melanoma. Proc Natl Acad Sci USA 82:1242–1246, 1985
308. Spitler LE, Del Rio M, Khentigan A et al: Therapy of patients with malignant melanoma using a monoclonal antimelanoma antibody-ricin A chain immunotoxin. Cancer Res 47:1717–1723, 1987
309. Cheung N-KV, Lazarus H, Miraldi FD et al: Ganglioside G_{D2} specific monoclonal antibody 3F8. A Phase I study in patients with neuroblastoma and malignant melanoma. J Clin Oncol 5:1430–1440, 1987
310. Nadler L, Takvorian T, Botnick et al: Anti-B1 monoclonal antibody and complement treatment in autologous bone marrow transplantation for relapsed B cell non-Hodgkin's lymphoma. Lancet 2:427–433, 1984
311. Longo DL: Biological therapy of cancer. In Fortner JG, Rhoads JE (eds): Accomplishments in Cancer Research, p 233. Philadelphia, JB Lippincott, 1986
312. Karavodin LM, Golub SH: Immunocompetence in cancer patients. In Herberman RB (ed): Basic and Clinical Tumor Immunology, p 215. Boston, Martinus Nijhoff, 1983
313. Terry WD, Rosenberg SA (eds): Immunotherapy of Human Cancer. New York, Elsevier-North Holland, 1982
314. Hersh EM: Current status of active non-specific immunotherapy. In Reif AE, Mitchell MS (eds): Immunity to Cancer, p 443. Orlando, Academic Press, 1985
315. Hersh EM, Murphy SG, Quesada JR et al: Effect of immunotherapy with Corynebacterium parvum and methanol extraction residue of BCG administered intravenously on host defense function in cancer patients. JNCI 66:993, 1981
316. Ashwell JD, Fox BS, Schwartz RH: Functional analysis of the interaction of the antigen-specific T cell receptor with its ligands. J Immunol 136:757, 1986
317. Talmadge JE, Herberman RB, Chirigos MA et al: Hyporesponsiveness to augmentation of murine natural killer cell activity in different anatomical compartments by multiple injections of various immunomodulators including recombinant interferons and interleukin-2. J Immunol 135:2483, 1985
318. Rollinghoff M, Starzinski-Powitz A, Pfizenmaier K et al: Cyclophosphamide-sensitive T-lymphocytes suppress the in vitro generation of antigen-specific cytotoxic T lymphocytes. J Exp Med 145:455, 1977
319. Pinsky CM: Local administration of immunomodulators. Semin Oncol 13:141, 1986
320. Bast RC Jr, Zbar B, Borsos T et al: BCG and cancer. N Engl J Med 290:1413, 1974
321. McKhann CF, Hendrickson CG, Spitler LE et al: Immunotherapy of melanoma with BCG: Two fatalities following intralesional injection. Cancer 35:514, 1975
322. Rosenberg SA, Rapp H, Terry W et al: Intralesional BCG therapy of patients with primary stage I melanoma. In Terry WD, Rosenberg SA (eds): Immunotherapy of Human Cancer, p 239. New York, Excerpta Medica, 1982
323. Zbar B, Canti G, Ashley M et al: Eradication by immunization with mycobacterial vaccines and tumor cells of microscopic metastases remaining after surgery. Cancer Res 39:1597, 1979
324. Holmes EC, Ramming KP, Bein ME et al: Intralesional BCG immunotherapy of pulmonary tumors. J Thorac Cardiovasc Surg 77:362, 1979
325. Pardridge DH, Sparks FC, Goodnight JE Jr et al: Intratumor Bacillus Calmette-Guerin therapy for chest wall recurrence of carcinoma of the breast. Surg Gynecol Obstet 148:867, 1979
326. Schellhammer PF, Ladaga LE, Fillion MB: Bacillus Calmette-Guerin for superficial transitional cell carcinoma of the bladder. J Urol 135:261, 1986
327. Herr HW, Pinsky CM, Whitmore WF Jr et al: Long-term effect of intravesical Bacillus Calmette-Guerin on flat carcinoma in situ of the bladder. J Urol 135:265, 1986
328. McKneally MF, Maver C, Kausel HW: Regional immunotherapy of lung cancer with intrapleural BCG. Lancet 1:377, 1976
329. Miller JW, Hunter AM, Horne NW: Intrapleural immunotherapy with Corynebacterium parvum in recurrent malignant pleural effusions. Thorax 35:856, 1980
330. Webb HE, Oaten SE, Pike CP: Treatment of malignant ascitic and pleural effusions with Corynebacterium parvum. Br Med J 1:338, 1978
331. Mantovani A, Sessa C, Peri G et al: Intraperitoneal administration of Corynebacterium parvum in patients with ascitic ovarian tumors resistant to chemotherapy: effects on cytotoxicity of tumor associated macrophages and NK cells. Int J Cancer 27:437, 1981
332. Bast RC Jr, Berek JS, Obrist R et al: Intraperitoneal immunotherapy of human ovarian carcinoma with Corynebacterium parvum. Cancer Res 43:1385, 1983
333. Warren HS, Vogel FR, Chedid LA: Current status of immunological adjuvants. Annu Rev Immunol 4:369, 1986
334. Kobayashi H: Viral xenogenization of intact tumor cells. Adv Cancer Res 30:279, 1979
335. Schirrmacher V, Ahlert T, Heicappell R et al: Successful application of non-oncogenic viruses for antimetastatic cancer immunotherapy. Cancer Rev 5:19, 1986
336. Peppoloni S, Herberman RB, Gorelik E: Induction of highly immunogenic variants of Lewis lung carcinoma tumor by ultraviolet irradiation. Cancer Res 45:2560, 1986
337. Boon T: Antigenic tumor cell variants obtained with mutagens. Adv Cancer Res 39:121, 1983
338. Edelson R, Berger C, Gasparro F et al: Treatment of cutaneous T-cell lymphoma by extracorporeal photochemotherapy: Preliminary results. N Engl J Med 316:297, 1987
339. Wunderlich M, Schiessel R, Rainer H et al: Effect of adjuvant chemo- or immunotherapy on the prognosis of colorectal cancer operated for cure. Br J Surg 72:107, 1985
340. Jones PC, Sze LL, Liu PY et al: Prolonged survival for melanoma patients with elevated IgM antibody to oncofetal antigen. J Natl Cancer Inst 66:249, 1981
341. Bell DR, Gerlach JH, Kartner N et al: Detection of P-glycoprotein in ovarian cancer: A molecular marker associated with multidrug resistance. J Clin Oncol 3:331, 1985
342. Hollinshead A, Stewart THM, Takita H et al: Adjuvant specific active lung cancer immunotherapy trials: Tumor-associated antigens. Cancer 60:1249, 1987
343. Hoover HC Jr, Surdyke MG, Dangel RB et al: Prospectively randomized trial of adjuvant active specific immunotherapy for human colorectal cancer. Cancer 55:1236, 1985
344. Hanna MG, Brandhorst JS, Peter LC: Active specific immunotherapy of residual micrometastasis: An evaluation of sources, doses and ratios of BCG with tumor cells. Cancer Immunol Immunother 7:165–173, 1979
345. Straus AA, Appel M, Saphir J et al: Immunologic resistance to carcinomas produced by electrocoagulation. Surg Gynecol Obstet 121:989, 1965
346. Moore FT, Blackwood J, Sanzenbacker L et al: Hypotherapy for malignant tumors: Immunologic response. Arch Surg 96:527, 1968
347. Ashwell JD, Longo DL, Bridges SH: T-cell tumor elimination as a result of T-cell receptor-mediated activation. Science 237:61, 1987
348. Isaacs A, Lindenmann J: Virus interference. Proc Soc [Biol] 147:258, 1957
349. Clark JW, Longo DL: Interferons in cancer therapy. In DeVita VT Jr, Hellman S, Rosenberg SA (eds): Cancer: Principles and Practice of Oncology Updates, 2nd ed, p 1. Philadelphia, JB Lippincott, 1987
350. Preble OT, Black RJ, Friedman RM et al: Systemic lupus erythematosus: Presence in human serum of an unusual acid-labile leukocyte interferon. Science 216:429, 1982
351. Weissmann C, Weber H: The interferon genes. Prog Nucl Acid Res 33:251, 1986
352. Zinn K, Maniatis T: Detection of factors that interact with the human beta-interferon regulatory region in vivo by DNAase I footprinting. Cell 45:611, 1986
353. Enoch T, Zinn K, Maniatis T: Activation of the human beta-interferon gene requires an interferon-inducible factor. Mol Cell Biol 6:801, 1986
354. Nir U, Cohen B, Chen L et al: A human IFN-beta 1 gene deleted of promoter sequences upstream from the TATA box is controlled post-transcriptionally by dsRNA. Nucl Acid Res 12:6979, 1984
355. Duc-Goiran P, Robert-Galliot B, Lopez J et al: Unusual apparently constitutive interferons and antagonists in human placental blood. Proc Natl Acad Sci USA 82:5010, 1985
356. Week PK, Apperson S, May L et al: Comparison of the antiviral activities of various cloned human interferon-alpha subtypes in mammalian cell cultures. J Gen Virol 57:233, 1981
357. Ortaldo JR, Herberman RB, Harvey C et al: A species of human alpha-interferon that lacks the ability to boost human natural killer activity. Proc Natl Acad Sci USA 81:4926, 1984
358. Hiscott J, Cantell K, Weissmann C: Differential expression of human interferon genes. Nucl Acid Res 12:3727, 1984
359. Branca AA, Faltynek CR, D'Allesandro S et al: Interaction of interferon with cellular receptors. J Biol Chem 257:13291, 1982
360. Faltynek CR, Princler G, Ruscetti FR et al: Lectins modulate the internalization of recombinant interferon alpha and the induction of 2′5′-oligo(A) synthetase (submitted).
361. Friedman RL, Stark GR: Alpha-interferon-induced transcription of HLA and metallothionein genes containing homologous upstream sequences. Nature 314:637, 1985
362. Staeheli P, Maller O, Boll W et al: Mx protein: Constitutive expression in 3T3 cells transformed with cloned Mx cDNA confers selective resistance to influenza virus. Cell 44:147, 1986
363. Pfefferkorn ER: Interferon gamma blocks the growth of Toxoplasma gondii in human fibroblasts by inducing the host cells to degrade tryptophan. Proc Natl Acad Sci USA 81:908, 1984
364. Friedman RM, Merigan T, Sreevalsan T (ed): Interferons as Cell Growth Inhibitors and Antitumor Factors. UCLA Symposia on Molecular and Cellular Biology, New Series Volumn 50, New York, Alan R Liss, 1986
365. Smekens-Etienne M, Goldstein J, Ooms HA et al: Variation of (2′5′) oligo (adenylate) synthetase activity during rat liver regeneration. Eur J Biochem 130:209, 1983
366. Perussia B, Kobayashi M, Rossi ME et al: Immune interferon enhances functional properties of human granulocytes: Role of Fc receptors and effect of lymphotoxin,

tumor necrosis factor, and granulocyte–macrophage colony stimulating factor. J Immunol 138:765, 1987
367. Stone–Wolff DS, Yip YK, Kelker HC et al: Interrelationships of human interferon-gamma with lymphotoxin and monocyte cytotoxin. J Exp Med 159:828, 1984
368. Maluish AE, Urba WJ, Longo DL et al: The determination of an immunologically active dose of interferon gamma in patients with melanoma. J Clin Oncol 6:434, 1988
369. Sidky YA, Borden EC: Inhibition of angiogenesis by interferons: effects on tumor- and lymphocyte-induced vascular responses. Cancer Res 47:5155, 1987
370. Quesada JR, Hersh EM, Manning J et al: Treatment of hairy cell leukemia with recombinant alpha interferon. Blood 68:493, 1986
371. Bocci V, Pacini A, Muscetti OM et al: The kidney is the main site of interferon catabolism. J Interferon Res 2:309, 1982
372. Gutterman JU, Fine S, Quesada J et al: Recombinant leukocyte A interferon: Pharmacokinetics, single-dose tolerance, and biologic effects in cancer patients. Ann Intern Med 96:549, 1982
373. Golomb HW, Jacobs A, Fefer A et al: Alpha-2 interferon therapy of hairy cell leukemia: A multicenter study of 64 patients. J Clin Oncol 4:900, 1986
374. Faltynek CR, Princler GL, Rossio JL et al: Relationship of the clinical response and binding of recombinant interferon alpha in patients with lymphproliferative disease. Blood 67:1077, 1986
375. Steis RG, Marcon L, Urba WJ et al: Serum soluble IL2 receptor levels as a tumor marker in patients with hairy cell leukemia. Blood 71:1304, 1988
376. Steis RG, Smith JW, Urba WJ, et al: Resistance to recombinant interferon alpha 1 in hairy cell leukemia associated with neutralizing anti-interferon antibodies. N Engl J Med 318:1409, 1988
377. Spiers ASD, Moore D, Cassileth PA et al: Hairy cell leukemia: Complete remission with pentostatin (2′-deoxycoformycin). N Engl J Med 316:825, 1987
378. Foon KA, Nakano GM, Koller CA et al: Response to 2′-deoxycoformycin after failure to interferon alpha in nonsplenectomized patients with hairy cell leukemia. Blood 68:297, 1986
379. Urba WJ, Steis RG, Clark JW et al: Immune effects of treating hairy cell leukemia patients with deoxycoformycin (submitted)
380. Talpaz M, Kantarjian HM, McCredie K et al: Hematologic remission and cytogenetic improvement induced by recombinant human interferon alpha A in chronic myelogenous leukemia. N Engl J Med 314:1065, 1986
381. Bergsagel DE, Haas RH, Messner HA: Interferon alfa-2b in the treatment of chronic granulocytic leukemia. Semin Oncol 13:29, 1986
382. Oberg K, Funa K, Alm G et al: Effects of leukocyte interferon on clinical symptoms and hormone levels in patients with mid-gut carcinoid tumors and carcinoid syndrome. N Engl J Med 309:129, 1983
383. Anderson JV, Bloom SR: Treatment of malignant endocrine pancreatic tumors with human leukocyte interferon. Lancet 1:97, 1987
384. McKnight J, Clark J, Miller R et al: Randomized trial of recombinant interferon alpha with or without indomethacin in patients with metastatic malignant melanoma (abstr). Proc Am Soc Clin Oncol 6:250, 1987
384a. Creagan ET, Kovach JS, O'Connell MJ et al: Improved response of renal cell carcinoma to alpha interferon by the addition of aspirin. Cancer 61:1787, 1988
385. Borden EC, Hawkins MJ: Biologic response modifiers as adjuncts to other therapeutic modalities. Semin Oncol 13:144, 1986
386. Quesada JR, Talpaz M, Rios A et al: Clinical toxicity of interferons in cancer patients: A review. J Clin Oncol 4:234, 1986
387. Abrams PG, McClamrock E, Foon KA: Evening administration of alpha interferon. N Engl J Med 312:443, 1985
388. Hrushesky WJM: The rationale for non-zero-order drug delivery using automatic, computer-based drug delivery systems (chronotherapy). J Biol Response Mod (in press)
389. Herberman RB, Pinsky CM: Polyribonucleotides for cancer therapy: summary and recommendations for further research. J Biol Response Mod 4:680, 1985
390. Lacour J, Lacour F, Spira A et al: Adjuvant treatment with polyadenylic–polyuridylic acid in operable breast cancer: Updated results of a randomized trial. Br Med J 288:489, 1984
391. Wiltrout RH, Boyd MR, Back TT et al: Flavone-8-acetic acid augments systemic natural killer cell activity and synergizes with interleukin 2 for treatment of murine renal cancer. J Immunol 140:3261, 1988
392. Urba WJ, Longo DL, Lombardo F et al: Flavone acetic acid (NSC 347512) enhances natural killer activity in human peripheral blood. J Natl Cancer Inst 80:521, 1988
393. Smith KA: Interleukin-2: Inception, impact and implications. Science 240:1169–1175, 1988
394. Morgan DA, Ruscetti FW, Gallo RG: Selective *in vitro* growth of T lymphocytes from normal human bone marrow. Science 193:1007–1008, 1976
395. Stern JB, Smith KA: Interleukin-2 induction of T-cell G_1 progression and c-*myb* expression. Science 233:203–206, 1986
396. Kornfeld H, Berman JS, Beer DJ et al: Induction of human T lymphocyte motility by interleukin 2. J Immunol 134:3887–3890, 1985
397. Nedwin GE, Svederdky LP, Bringman TS et al: Effect of interleukin 2, interferon-x, and mitogens on the production of tumor necrosis factors x and x. J Immunol 135:2492–2497, 1985
398. Waldmann TA, Goldman CK, Robb RJ et al: Expression of interleukin-2 receptors on activated human B cells. J Exp Med 160:1450–1466, 1984
399. Jung LKL, Toshiro H, Fu SM: Detection and functional studies of p60–65 (Tac antigen) on activated human B cells. J Exp Med 160:1597–1602, 1984
400. Malkovsky M, Loveland B, North M et al: Recombinant interleukin-2 directly augments the cytotoxicity of human monocytes. Nature 325:262–264, 1987
401. Hancock WW, Muller WA, Cotran RS: Interleukin 2 receptors are expressed by alveolar macrophages during pulmonary sarcoidosis and are inducible by lymphokine treatment of normal human lung macrophages, blood monocytes, and monocyte cell lines. J Immunol 138:185–191, 1987
402. Steiner G, Tschachler E, Tani M et al: Interleukin 2 receptors on cultured murine epidermal Langerhans cells. J Immunol 137:155–159, 1986
403. Benveniste EN, Merrill JE: Stimulation of oligodendroglial proliferation and maturation by interleukin-2. Nature 321:610–613, 1986
404. Kaplan J, Tilton J, Peterson WD: Identification of T-cell lymphoma tumor antigens on human T-cell lines. Am J Hematol 1:219–226, 1976
405. Gillis S, Watson J: Biochemical and biological characterization of lymphocyte regulatory molecules: V. Identification of an interleukin-2 producing human leukemia T cell line. J Exp Med 152:1709–1715, 1980
406. Taniguchi T, Matsui H, Fujita T et al: Structure and expression of a cloned cDNA for human interleukin-2. Nature 302:305–307, 1983
407. Rosenberg SA, Grimm EA, McGrogan M et al: Biological activity of recombinant human interleukin-2 produced in *E. coli*. Science 223:1412–1415, 1984
408. Doyle MV, Lee MT, Fong S: Comparison of the biological activities of human recombinant interleukin-2_{125} native interleukin-2. J Biol Response Mod 4:96–109, 1985
409. Sharon M, Klausner RD, Cullen BR et al: Novel interleukin-2 receptor subunit detected by cross-linking under high affinity conditions. Science 234:859–863, 1987
410. Rosenberg SA, Lotze MT, Mule JJ: New approaches to the immunotherapy of cancer. Ann Intern Med 108:853–864, 1988
411. Merluzzi VJ, Walker MM, Fananes RB: Inhibition of cytotoxic T-cell clonal expansion by cyclophosphamide and the recovery of cytotoxic T-lymphocyte precursors by supernatants from mixed lymphocyte cultures. Cancer Res 41:850–853, 1981
412. Clason AE, Duarte AJS, Kupiec–Weglinski JW et al: Restoration of allograft responsiveness in B rats by interleukin-2 and/or adherent cells. J Immunol 129:252–259, 1982
413. Rook AH, Masur H, Lane HC et al: Interleukin-2 enhances the depressed natural killer and cytomegalovirus specific cytotoxic activities of lymphokines from patients with the acquired immune deficiency syndrome. J Clin Invest 72:398–407, 1983
414. Ettinghausen SE, Lipford EH III, Mule JJ et al: Systemic administration of recombinant interleukin-2 stimulates *in vivo* lymphoid cell proliferation in tissues. J Immunol 135:1488–1497, 1985
415. Ettinghausen SE, Lipford EH III, Mule JJ et al: Recombinant interleukin-2 stimulates *in vivo* proliferation of adoptively transferred lymphokine activated killer (LAK) cells. J Immunol 135:3623–3635, 1985
416. Yron I, Wood TA, Spiess P et al: *In vitro* growth of murine T cells V: The isolation and growth of lymphoid cells infiltrating syngeneic solid tumors. J Immunol 125:238–245, 1980
417. Lotze MT, Grimm E, Mazumder A et al: *In vitro* growth of cytotoxic human lymphocytes IV: Lysis of fresh and cultured autologous tumor by lymphocytes cultured in T cell growth factor (TCGF). Cancer Res 41:4420–4425, 1981
418. Grimm EA, Ramsey KM, Mazumder A et al: Lymphokine-activated killer cell phenomenon II: The precursor phenotype is serologically distinct from peripheral T lymphocytes, memory CTL, and NK cells. J Exp Med 157:884–897, 1983
419. Rosenstein M, Yron I, Kaufman Y, Rosenberg SA: Lymphokine activated killer cells: Lysis of fresh syngeneic NK-resistant murine tumor cells by lymphocytes cultured in interleukin-2. Cancer Res 44:1946–1953, 1984
420. Rayner AA, Grimm EA, Lotze MT et al: Lymphokine-activated killer (LAK) cell phenomenon: Analysis of factors relevant to the immunotherapy of human cancer. Cancer 55:1327–1333, 1985
421. Rosenberg SA: Adoptive immunotherapy of cancer using lymphokine activated killer cells and recombinant interleukin-2. In DeVita VT Jr, Hellman S, Rosenberg SA (eds): Important Advances in Oncology 1986, pp 55–91. Philadelphia, JB Lippincott, 1986
422. Rosenberg SA, Mule JJ, Speiss PJ et al: Regression of established pulmonary metastases and subcutaneous tumor mediated by the systemic administration of high dose recombinant IL-2. J Exp Med 161:1169–1188, 1985
423. Lafreniere R, Rosenberg SA: Successful immunotherapy of murine experimental hepatic metastases with lymphokine-activated killer cells and recombinant interleukin-2. Cancer Res 45:3735–3741, 1985
424. Mule JJ, Yang JC, Lafreniere R et al: Identification of cellular mechanisms operational *in vivo* during the regression of established pulmonary metastases by the systemic administration of high-dose recombinant interleukin-2. J Immunol 139:285–294, 1987
425. Papa MZ, Mule JJ, Rosenberg SA: The anti-tumor efficacy of lymphokine-activated killer cells and recombinant interleukin-2 *in vivo*: Successful immunotherapy of established pulmonary metastases from weakly and non-immunogenic murine tumors of three distinct histologic types. Cancer Res 46:4973–4978, 1986
426. Donohue JH, Rosenstein M, Chang AE et al: The systemic administration of purified interleukin-2 enhances the ability of sensitized murine lymphocyte lines to cure a disseminated syngeneic lymphoma. J Immunol 132:2123–2128, 1984
427. Shu S, Chou T, Rosenberg SA: *In vitro* sensitization and expansion with viable tumor cells and interleukin-2 in the generation of specific therapeutic effector cells. J Immunol 136:3891–3898, 1986

428. Shu S, Chou T, Rosenberg SA: Generation from tumor-bearing mice of lymphocytes with *in vivo* therapeutic efficacy. J Immunol 139:295–304, 1987
429. Rosenberg SA, Spiess P, Lafreniere R: A new approach to the adoptive immunotherapy of cancer with tumor-infiltrating lymphocytes. Science 223:1318–1321, 1986
430. Spiess PJ, Yang JC, Rosenberg SA: The in vivo anti-tumor activity of tumor infiltrating lymphocytes expanded in recombinant interleukin-2. J Natl Cancer Inst 79:1067–1075, 1987
431. Lotze MT, Custer MC, Rosenberg SA: Interleukin 2 (IL-2) administration to humans results in the rapid emigration of a specific lymphokine subset ($CD2^+$, 3^-, 11^+, 16^+) from the peripheral blood (submitted)
432. Lotze MT, Matory YL, Ettinghausen SE et al: *In vivo* administration of purified human interleukin-2 II: Half life, immunologic effects and expansion of peripheral lymphoid cells in vivo with recombinant IL-2. J Immunol 135:2865–2875, 1985
433. Lotze MT, Chang AE, Seipp CA et al: High-dose recombinant interleukin-2 in the treatment of patients with disseminated cancer: Responses, treatment-related morbidity and histologic findings. JAMA 256:3117–3124, 1986
434. Lotze MT, Custer MC, Rosenberg SA: Intraperitoneal administration of interleukin-2 in patients with cancer. Arch Surg 121:1373–1379, 1986
435. West WH, Tauer KW, Yannelli JR et al: Constant-infusion recombinant interleukin-2 in adoptive immunotherapy of advanced cancer. N Engl J Med 316:898–905, 1987
436. Hank JA, Kohler PC, Weil–Hillman G et al: *In vivo* induction of the lymphokine-activated killer phenomenon: Interleukin-2 dependent human non-major histocompatibility complex-restricted cytotoxicity generated *in vivo* during administration of human recombinant interleukin-2[1]. Cancer Res 48:1965–1971, 1988
437. Thompson JA, Lee DJ, Lindgren CG et al: Influence of dose and duration of infusion of interleukin-2 on toxicity and immunomodulation. J Clin Oncol 6:669–678, 1988
438. Rosenberg SA, Terry W: Passive immunotherapy of cancer in animals and man. Adv Cancer Res 25:323–388, 1977
439. Rosenberg SA: The adoptive immunotherapy of cancer: Accomplishments and prospects. Cancer Treat Rep 68:233–255, 1984
440. Roberts K, Lotze MT, Rosenberg SA: Separation and functional studies of the human lymphokine-activated killer cell. Cancer Res 47:4366–4371, 1987
441. Phillips LL: Dissection of the LAK phenomenon. J Exp Med 164:814–825, 1986
442. Lafreniere R, Rosenberg SA: Adoptive immunotherapy of murine hepatic metastases with lymphokine activated killer (LAK) cells and recombinant interleukin-2 (RIL-2) can mediate the regression of both immunogenic and non-immunogenic sarcomas and an adenocarcinoma. J Immunol 135:4273–4280, 1985
443. Mule JJ, Ettinghausen SE, Spiess PJ et al: The anti-tumor efficacy of lymphokine-activated killer cells and recombinant interleukin-2 in vivo: An analysis of survival benefit and mechanisms of tumor escape in mice undergoing immunotherapy. Cancer Res 46:676–683, 1986
444. Mule JJ, Yang J, Shu S et al: The anti-tumor efficacy of lymphokine-activated killer cells and recombinant interleukin-2 *in vivo*: Direct correlation between reduction of established metastases and cytolytic activity of lymphokine-activated killer cells. J Immunol 136:3899–3909, 1986
445. Shiloni E, Lafreniere R, Mule JJ et al: Effect of immunotherapy with allogeneic lymphokine-activated killer cells and recombinant interleukin-2 on established pulmonary and hepatic metastases in mice. Cancer Res 46:5633–5640, 1986
446. Mazumder A, Eberlein TJ, Grimm EA: Phase I study of the adoptive immunotherapy of human cancer with lectin-activated autologous mononuclear cells, Cancer 53:896–905, 1984
447. Rosenberg SA: Immunotherapy of cancer by the systemic administration of lymphoid cells plus interleukin-2. J Biol Response Mod 3:501–511, 1984
448. Lotze MT, Frana LW, Sharrow SO et al: *In vivo* administration of purified human interleukin-2 I: Half life and immunologic effects of the Jurkat cell line-derived IL-2. J Immunol 134:157–166, 1985
449. Dutcher JP, Creekmore S, Weiss GR et al: Phase II study of high dose interleukin-2 (JIL-2) and lymphokine activated killer (LAK) cells in patients (PTS) with melanoma (abstr). Proc Am Soc Clin Oncol 6:246, 1987
450. Fisher, RI, Coltman CA, Doroshow JH et al: Phase II clinical trial of interleukin II plus lymphokine activated killer cells (IL-2/LAK) in metastatic renal cancer (abstr). Proc Am Soc Clin Oncol 6:244, 1987
451. Steis R, Bookman M, Clark J et al: Intraperitoneal lymphokine activated killer (LAK) cell and interleukin-2 (IL-2) therapy for peritoneal carcinomatosis: Toxicity, efficacy, and laboratory results (abstr). Proc Am Soc Clin Oncol 6:250, 1987
452. Paciucci PA, Konefal R, Ryder J et al: Phase I–II study of adoptive immunotherapy with rIL-2 activated cells and escalating continuous infusion rIL-2 in patients with disseminated cancer (abstr). Proc Am Soc Clin Oncol 6:248, 1987
453. Rosenstein M, Ettinghausen SE, Rosenberg SA: Extravasation of intravascular fluid mediated by the systemic administration of recombinant interleukin-2. J Immunol 137:1735–1742, 1986
454. Lee RE, Lotze MT, Skibber JM et al: Cardiorespiratory effects of immunotherapy with interleukin-2. J Clin Oncol (in press)
455. Belldegrun A, Webb DE, Austin HA et al: Effects of interleukin-2 on renal function in patients receiving immunotherapy for advanced cancer. Ann Intern Med 106:817–822, 1987
456. Webb DE, Austin HA, Belldegrun A, Vaughan E, Linehan WM, Rosenberg SA: Metabolic and renal effects of interleukin-2 immunotherapy for metastatic cancer. Clin Nephrology 30:141–145, 1988
457. Ettinghausen SE, Moore JG, White DE et al: Hematologic effects of immunotherapy with lymphokine-activated killer cells and recombinant interleukin-2 in cancer patients. Blood 69:1654–1660, 1987
458. Denicoff KD, Rubinow DR, Papa MZ et al: The neuropsychiatric effects of interleukin-2/lymphokine activated killer cell treatment. Ann Intern Med 107:293–300, 1987
459. Muul LM, Spiess PJ, Director EP et al: Identification of specific cytolytic immune responses against autologous tumor in humans bearing malignant melanoma. J Immunol 138:989–995, 1987
460. Itoh K, Tilden AB, Balch CM: Interleukin-2 activation of cytotoxic T-lymphocytes infiltrating into human metastatic melanomas. Cancer Res 46:3011–3017, 1986
461. Topalian SL, Muul LM, Rosenberg SA: Growth and immunologic characteristics of lymphocytes infiltrating human tumor. Surg Forum 37:390–391, 1987
462. Kurnick JT, Kradin RL, Blumberg R et al: Functional characterization of T lymphocytes propagated from human lung carcinomas. Clin Immunol Immunopathol 38:367–380, 1986
463. Anderson TM, Ibayashi Y, Holmes EC et al: Enhancement of natural interleukin-2. Surg Forum 37:392–393, 1986
464. Belldegrun A, Muul LM, Rosenberg SA: Interleukin-2 expanded tumor-infiltrating lymphocytes in human renal cell cancer: Isolation, characterization and antitumor activity. Cancer Res 48:206–214, 1988
465. Rosenberg SA, Packard BS, Aebersold PM et al: Immunotherapy of patients with metastatic melanoma using tumor infiltrating lymphocytes and interleukin-2. Preliminary report. N Engl J Med 319:1676–1680, 1988

BRUCE A. CHABNER

CHARLES E. MYERS

CHAPTER 18 *Clinical Pharmacology of Cancer Chemotherapy*

The primary goal of clinical pharmacology is to develop a rational basis for the treatment of disease. Unfortunately, the required information often comes many years after the empirical discovery of active pharmacologic agents, and only then are important drug actions and interactions understood. In dealing with highly toxic agents that possess a narrow therapeutic index, such information is all the more important. The effective use of chemotherapeutic agents in oncology requires a higher level of pharmacologic understanding than in any other subspecialty of internal medicine.

The objective of this chapter is to provide the fundamental information on drug action, metabolism, disposition, and toxicity in humans that will allow optimal clinical use of anticancer drugs. This discussion assumes that the reader has a basic understanding of cell constituents, the general scheme of synthesis of DNA, RNA, and protein, and the fundamental principles of drug transport, metabolism, and excretion. The synthesis of DNA and its precursors is summarized in Figure 18-1. For a review of these latter topics, refer to primary texts in biochemistry and pharmacology.[1,2]

Safe drug use requires a few initial steps: (1) determination of safe dosage range; (2) choice of an appropriate route of administration; (3) awareness of the incidence and course of potentially life-threatening toxicity; (4) awareness of routes of drug elimination and adjustment of dose to accommodate organ dysfunction; and (5) knowledge of drug interactions as influenced by dose and schedule to maximize favorable interactions and minimize toxicity. Each of these points should be considered in developing a new protocol or in using an unfamiliar protocol for the first time. In addition, each new patient brings unique disease-related or preexisting problems to the therapeutic trial, requiring careful consideration of the choice of drugs and dosage. Every effort should be made to employ the best protocol in full doses, but the oncologist must always be aware of the unique challenges presented by each patient.

A few tables are provided to allow a rapid confirmation of the essential drug characteristics. Dose, toxicity, and pharmacokinetics of the most important agents are summarized in Table 18-1. Table 18-2 provides dose adjustment guidelines for agents affected by organ dysfunction. The indicated dose adjustments, particularly those for hepatic dysfunction, are only approximations, and doses should be calibrated against dose-limiting toxicity, such as myelosuppression. In Table 18-3, a summary of indications for drug-level monitoring of anticancer agents is given. The only routine indication for drug-level monitoring in clinical chemotherapy is for high-dose methotrexate regimens. The other uses indicated are associated with experimental protocols. Table 18-4 contains information on the new drugs that entered clinical trials from 1984 to 1987, under sponsorship of the National Cancer Institute. The reader is referred to Chapter 64 for a practical guide to the administration of chemotherapy and its complications.

Not all agents listed or discussed in this chapter are available commercially. However, a number of "group C" agents are available for specific diseases under protocols of the National Cancer Institute, and upon request for specific pa-

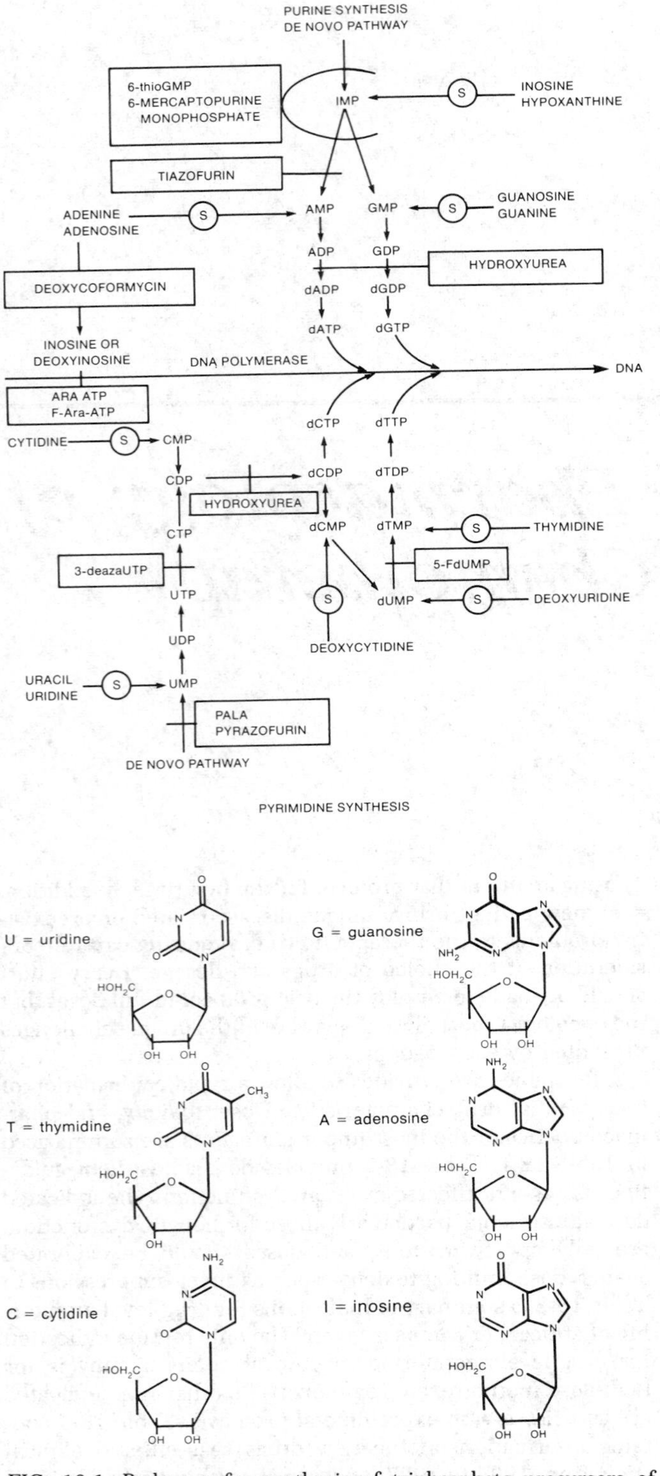

FIG. 18-1. Pathways for synthesis of triphosphate precursors of DNA and site of action of antimetabolites. Salvage pathways of nucleotide biosynthesis are indicated by –(S)→. Agents, or their metabolites, that inhibit specific synthetic reactions are enclosed in box: □. The inhibited pathway is indicated by ∔. d = deoxyribose; MP = monophosphate; DP = diphosphate; TP = triphosphate.

tients, they will be distributed to private physicians in the United States. Limited reporting of side-effects is required in conjunction with group C drug use (Table 18-5).

ANTIMETABOLITES

ANTIFOLATES

Antimetabolites are fraudulent agents that, by virtue of structural similarity with physiologic intermediates, are accepted as substrates for vital biochemical reactions and thus interfere with a required cell process. The first agent in the antifolate class of antimetabolites to find clinical application was aminopterin, a 4-NH_2 analogue of folic acid. Aminopterin has since been replaced in common use by the 4-NH_2,N^{10}-methyl analogue, amethopterin or methotrexate (Fig. 18-2). The latter, although a less-potent antifolate, has more predictable clinical toxicity and at least equal clinical activity.

In the past 20 years, new antifolate compounds such as the diaminopyrimidines and quinazolines have entered clinical trials. The most recent of these is trimetrexate, a more lipid-soluble quinazoline antifolate, which circumvents the requirement of folates and methotrexate for active transport into cells. Trimetrexate has potent antiparasitic activity and antineoplastic effects and is undergoing advanced trials in both clinical subspecialty areas.[3] Another folate of growing interest is 10-EDAM (10-ethyl-5-deaza-aminopterin), a potent inhibitor of dihydrofolate reductase, but with improved transport and polyglutamylation compared with methotrexate.[4] Trimetrexate and 10-EDAM have shown evidence of antitumor activity against carcinomas of the bowel and lung, respectively, in preliminary clinical trials.

Mechanism of Action

Methotrexate exerts its cytotoxic effects through inhibition of the enzyme dihydrofolate reductase (Fig. 18-3). This enzyme is responsible for maintaining the intracellular pool of folates in a reduced state as tetrahydrofolates, which function as carriers of one-carbon groups that are required for synthesis of the purine nucleotides and of thymidylate. In the thymidylate synthesis reaction (catalyzed by thymidylate synthase), N^{5-10} methylene tetrahydrofolate is relieved of its one-carbon methylene group and at the same time is oxidized to dihydrofolate, an inactive form of folic acid. Thus, in the presence of ongoing thymidylate synthesis, an intact dihydrofolate reductase pathway is needed to recycle oxidized folates to their active tetrahydrofolate form.

As a result of inhibition of reductase, methotrexate causes an accumulation of cellular folates in the inactive oxidized form, and a cessation first of thymidylate and then of purine nucleotide synthesis. Thymidylate synthesis inhibition appears to be more sensitive to methotrexate and occurs at free extracellular methotrexate concentrations of 1×10^{-8} M, whereas inhibition of purine synthesis takes place at somewhat higher free drug concentrations (above 1×10^{-7} M).

Cell killing proceeds somewhat more efficiently at higher drug levels, presumably because of the greater lethality of the antipurine effects.[5]

The precise mechanism by which methotrexate produces its toxicity is uncertain. Although inhibition of dihydrofolate reductase would be expected to lead to depletion of intracellular reduced folates, the depletion is only partial. For example, the key folate cofactor for purine biosynthesis, 10-formyl tetrahydrofolate, is present at 60% or more of its baseline concentration at a time when purine biosynthesis is totally inhibited.[6]

Exposure of cells to methotrexate generates a number of toxic metabolites (polyglutamate derivatives) of the parent compound. These compounds have an extended intracellular half-life and have potent, direct inhibitory effects on thymidylate synthase, as well as on the enzymes of de novo purine biosynthesis. In addition, dihydrofolate, which accumulates behind the blocked dihydrofolate reductase, directly inhibits the same distal metabolic sites.[7] Thus, the toxic effects of methotrexate are probably the result of both depletion of reduced folates and direct inhibition of other folate-dependent enzymes (Fig. 18-3).

The requirement for an excess of free (unbound) drug to produce inhibition of nucleotide biosynthesis is thought to result from the reversible nature of methotrexate binding to dihydrofolate reductase. Although methotrexate is bound very tightly in its complex with reductase, a measurable off-rate of inhibitor from enzyme is found in living cells. When there is an excess of dihydrofolate (FH_2), which builds up "behind" the inhibited reaction, an excess of free drug is required to compete for unoccupied binding sites. In addition, the inhibition of thymidylate synthase and inhibition of de novo purine biosynthesis require methotrexate polyglutamates in concentrations ($>10^{-8}$ M) sufficient to compete with intracellular folates.

The biochemical effects of methotrexate can be reversed by administering a reduced folate. The most commonly used rescue agent, leucovorin or DL-N^5-formyl-tetrahydrofolic acid, effectively prevents methotrexate toxicity to bone marrow and gastrointestinal epithelium if it is administered in sufficient doses following 6-hour to 36-hour infusions of high doses of methotrexate. Longer exposures to methotrexate lead to clinically significant toxicity.

The dose of leucovorin required to reverse methotrexate toxicity depends on the antifolate concentration at the time of antidote administration. The reason for this competitive relationship is unclear, but it may relate to competition between reduced folates and FH_2 or methotrexate polyglutamates at thymidylate synthase, or to competition between FH_2 and methotrexate at dihydrofolate reductase.

Other rescue measures used clinically include administration of thymidine, which restores intracellular pools of thymidine triphosphate (TTP), and administration of carboxypeptidase G_1, an enzyme that hydrolyzes and inactivates methotrexate. These measures are not available for general use.

Methotrexate enters cells by a carrier-mediated, active transport mechanism shared by the physiologic, reduced folates, and it reaches equilibrium concentrations in most cells in less than 30 minutes.[8] The affinity constant of the transport system lies in the range of 1 to 10 μM for most mammalian cells. At higher drug concentrations, methotrexate enters cells by passive diffusion, an inefficient process compared with active transport. Methotrexate efflux is blocked by vincristine in concentrations above those found in clinical use.

Methotrexate undergoes transformation to polyglutamate forms by a process analogous to the polyglutamation of physiologic folates.[9] The methotrexate polyglutamates, consisting of the parent molecule plus one to four additional glutamates in γ-peptide linkage, are formed in tumor cells, bone marrow, and other normal tissues and, in a matter of hours, become the predominant form of drug found intracellularly. The polyglutamates bind to dihydrofolate reductase with the same affinity as the parent drug and inhibit enzymes (thymidylate synthase, GAR, and AICAR transformylase) not affected by the parent compound. After removal of free drug, the polyglutamates of 3 to 5 glutamyl chain length persist intracellularly for a longer period than does the parent compound. Thus, polyglutamate formation may be an important determinant of the duration and site of drug action in both normal and malignant cells.

The kinetic aspects of methotrexate cytotoxicity are important in clinical chemotherapy. For bone marrow granulocyte precursors and for experimental tumors, cell kill is proportional to the duration of exposure to methotrexate. Greater cell kill also is seen with increases in drug concentration above the threshold required for inhibition of DNA synthesis, but in this relationship cell kill is approximately correlated with the log of drug concentration. The dependence on duration of exposure can be explained best by the S-phase specificity of cell kill by antifolates; nonproliferating cells are extremely resistant to this class of compounds. In addition, polyglutamate formation is enhanced by long periods of incubation and may increase toxicity.

In experimental systems, resistance of tumor cells to antifolates results from several different biochemical mechanisms, including deletion of the reduced folate transport system, an increased concentration of dihydrofolate reductase, an altered reductase with decreased affinity for methotrexate, and decreased formation of polyglutamates.[10,11] The increase in enzyme concentration results from amplification of the gene coding for this enzyme. Resistant mutants can be selected by exposing cells to stepwise increases in drug concentrations in cell culture systems. The amplified genes may be present on bits of extrachromosomal material called double minutes or may exist within the chromosome as broad new bands of homogeneously staining genetic material on the long arm of chromosome 10.[12] Gene amplification associated with double-minute chromosomes is unstable and is lost gradually without the selective pressure of methotrexate, but integrated genetic material is heritable and becomes a stable characteristic of the resistant cell lines. Gene amplification has been identified as the cause of increased enzyme levels in resistant human tumor cells from patients treated with methotrexate.[13]

Other clinical studies have yielded examples of resistance

(*Text continues on page 354.*)

TABLE 18-1. Dose, Toxicity, and Pharmacokinetics of Major Antineoplastic Agents

Acute Toxicity					
Class	*Route**	*Dose (mg/m^2)*	*Injection Vehicle*	*Infusion Duration*	*Dose Frequency*
Plant Alkaloids					
Vincristine	IV	1.0	10 ml NS	1–5 min	qwk
Vinblastine	IV	6.0	10 ml NS	1–5 min	qwk
	IV	2.0	NS	24 h × 5 d	q3wk
Vindesine	IV	2.0	10 ml NS	1–5 min	qwk
VP-16	IV	86	20 ml NS/ml reconstituted drug	1–5 min	2 d qwk
	PO	200			2 d qwk
VM-26	IV	67	20 ml NS/ml reconstituted drug	1–5 min	qwk
Antibiotics					
Actinomycin D	IV	0.6	500 μg/ml SW	1–5 min	qd × 5
Doxorubicin	IV	75	5 mg/ml SW	1–5 min	q3wk
	IV	20	5 μg/ml SW	1–5 min	qwk
Daunorubicin	IV	30	1 mg/ml SW	1–5 min	3d, q3wk
Mithramycin	IV	1.75	500 μg/ml SW, then add to 100 ml D_5W	15–30 min	qod to toxicity
for high Ca^{++}	IV	0.75	500 μg/ml SW	1–5 min bolus	qd × 3–4 d
Mitomycin C	IV	2.0	500 μg/ml SW	1–5 min bolus	qd × 3, q3wk
Bleomycin	IV	10	5 U/ml NS	1-min test dose then IV bolus	qwk
	IM	10	15 U/ml NS		qwk
	SC	10	15 U/ml NS		qwk
Antimetabolites					
Methotrexate (high-dose)	IV	>500	100 ml D_5W or NS	10 min–1 h	q3wk
w/leucovorin	IV	15	In vehicle	Bolus	q6 h × 7 doses
Methotrexate	IV	25	10–25 ml D_5W or NS	Bolus	Twice weekly
	IM	25	2 ml NS		Twice weekly
	IT	12 (total dose)	10 ml Elliott's B	1–5 min	q4 d
5-Fluorouracil	IV	500	Any convenient volume NS	Bolus	qwk or qd × 5
	IV	800–1200	Any convenient volume NS	24 h × 5 d	q 3–4 wk
	IA	800–1200	Any convenient volume NS	24 h	qd × 14–21 d
5-Fluorouracil	IV	375	Any convenient volume NS	Bolus	qwk × 6
w/leucovorin	IV	500	200 ml D_5W	2–h infusion begin 1 h before 5-FU	qwk × 6
5-Fluorodeoxyuridine	IA	5–20	Any convenient volume NS	24 h	qd × 14–21 d
6-Mercaptopurine	PO	100			qd × 5
6-Thioguanine	IV	100	15 mg/ml NS	Bolus	qd × 5
Cytarabine (cytosine arabinoside)	IV	100	20 mg/ml NS	Bolus	q12 h × 5–10 d
	IV	2000–3000	50 mg/ml SW then dilute in 150 ml D_5W	1 h	q12 h × 6 d
5-Azacytidine	IV	200	Reconstitute vial in 20 ml SW, dilute in 150 ml D_5W	15–30 min	qd × 5
Hydroxyurea	IV	1000–1500	100 mg/ml SW	1–5 min	qd × 5
	PO	1000			qd
Deoxycoformycin	IV	4	Any volume NS	Bolus	qowk
Alkylating Agents					
Cyclophosphamide	IV	400	20 mg/ml SW	Bolus	qd × 5
	PO	100			qd × 14
Ifosfamide and	IV	1800–2400	Any volume D_5W or NS	24 h	qd × 5
Mesna	IV	1800–2400	With ifosfamide	24 h	qd × 5.5
Melphalan	PO	4			qd
	IV	8	Reconstituted vial dilute in 100–200 ml D_5W	30–45 min	qd × 5

Acute Toxicity					
Plasma WBC	*Platelet*	*Nausea/ Vomiting*	*Other Toxicity*	*Elimination†*	*Plasma Half-Life (h)**
Mild	Mild	Mild	Distal neuropathy, inappropriate ADH	M	2.6
Marked	Marked	Mild	Mucositis	M	3.1
Marked	Marked	Mild	Mucositis	M	3.1
Moderate	Mild	Mild	Neurotoxicity	M	1.6
Moderate	Mild	Mild	Distal neuropathy	M, R	6
Moderate	Mild	Moderate			
Moderate	Mild	Mild	Distal neuropathy	M, R	3
Marked	Marked	Moderate	Alopecia, Mucositis	M, R	?
Marked	Marked	Moderate	Alopecia, Cardiomyopathy	M	3/25
Moderate	Moderate	Moderate	Alopecia, less cardiomyopathy	M	3/25
Marked	Marked	Moderate	Alopecia, cardiomyopathy	M	3/?
Mild	Marked	Severe	Renal, hepatic, neurologic, fever, rash	M	?
Mild	Mild	Mild			
Marked	Marked	Moderate	Renal, pulmonary	M	?
Rare	Rare	Mild	Skin, pulmonary fibrosis, fever, allergic reactions	R	0.4/2
Mild	Mild	Moderate	Hepatic dysfunction, renal failure	R	2/8
				M	
Moderate-marked	Moderate-marked	Mild	Stomatitis	R	2/8
Moderate-marked	Moderate-marked	Mild	Stomatitis	R	2/8
Mild	Mild	None	Fever, motor dysfunction	R	12 (CSF)
Moderate-marked	Moderate-marked	Mild	Cerebellar, conjunctivitis	M	0.3
Mild	Mild	Moderate	Mucositis, diarrhea	M	0.3
Mild	Mild	Moderate	Catheter-related	M	0.3
Marked	Marked	Mild	Diarrhea	M	0.3
Mild	Mild	Moderate	Catheter-related	M	0.3
Moderate-marked	Moderate-marked	Mild	Cholestasis	M	0.3–0.6
Moderate-marked	Moderate-marked	Mild	Cholestasis	M	1.5
Marked	Marked	Moderate	Cholestasis, mucositis	M	0.15
Marked	Marked	Marked	Cholestasis, mucositis, sedation, cerebellar, conjunctivitis	M, R	
Marked	Marked	Severe	Neurotoxicity, mucositis	M	Rapid
Marked	Moderate	Moderate	None	R, M	1.7
Marked	Marked	Mild		R, M	1.7
Mild	Mild	Mild	None	R	1/10
Marked	Mild	Moderate }	Cystitis, water retention, alopecia	M	1–4
Moderate	Mild	Mild }			
Moderate	Moderate	Mild	Neurotoxicity, urothelial toxicity	M	5–6
None	None	None	None	M	?
Moderate	Moderate	Mild	Leukemia	M	2
Marked	Marked	Moderate			

*Slash indicates multiple half-lives.

(continued)

TABLE 18-1. Dose, Toxicity, and Pharmacokinetics of Major Antineoplastic Agents *(continued)*

Acute Toxicity					
Class	*Route**	*Dose (mg/m^2)*	*Injection Vehicle*	*Infusion Duration*	*Dose Frequency*
Busulfan	PO	2–6			qd
CCNU	PO	100–150			q6 wk
MeCCNU	PO	150–200			q6 wk
BCNU	IV	200–225	Reconstituted vial diluted to 100 mg/ml D_5W	30–45 min	q6 wk
Streptozotocin	IV	500	Reconstituted vial diluted to 100 mg/ml D_5W	10–15 min	qd × 5 q 3–4 wk
Chlorambucil	PO	1–3			qd
cis-diamminedi-chloroplatinum	IV	50–100	1000 ml/m²NS‡	6 h	q 3–4 2 wk
		20	150 ml NS	1 h	qd × 5
	IV	40	250 ml 3% saline	1 h	qd × 5
CBDCA (carboplatin)	IV	300	Any volume D_5W	Bolus	qd × 5
Aziridinylbenzoquinone (AZQ)	IV	18–20	150 ml NS	10–15 min	Days 1 and 8 of 28-d cycle
	IV	8	150 ml NS	10–15 min	qd × 5
Miscellaneous					
DTIC (Dacarbazine)	IV	200	10 mg/ml D_5W	10–15 min	qd × 5
mAMSA	IV	120	250 ml D_5W	2 h	qd × 5
Procarbazine	PO	100			qd × 10–14 d
Hexamethylmelamine	PO	150			qd × 14 d
Mitoxantrone	IV	14	10 ml NS	30 min	q3 wk

*IV = intravenous; PO = per os; SC = subcutaneous; IM = intramuscular; IT = intrathecal; IA = intra-arterial; NS = normal saline; D_5W = dextrose (5 g/dl) in water; and SW = sterile water.

†R = renal; M = metabolic; F = fecal.

‡See chapter for details.

related to decreased polyglutamate formation and decreased thymidylate synthase activity (with decreased need for recycling oxidized folates). Two clinical examples of transport deficiency have been reported.[14]

Clinical Pharmacology and Pharmacokinetics

Because of the common use of methotrexate in high-dose regimens and the well-understood relationship between extracellular drug concentration and inhibition of DNA synthesis, monitoring of methotrexate concentrations in plasma has become important for guiding drug dosage, detecting patients at high risk of toxicity, and allowing institution of rescue measures in high-risk situations. At least four methods are available for methotrexate assay, and all provide rapid and sensitive analysis.[15] These include an enzyme inhibition assay using dihydrofolate reductase (most cumbersome assay); a competitive protein-binding assay that uses reductase as the binding protein; a commercial radioimmunoassay that uses an antibody to the methotrexate-albumin conjugate; and an enzyme-linked immunoassay.[16] The competitive protein-binding assay is specific for ligands that bind tightly to the enzyme active site, whereas the immunoassays show degrees of cross-reactivity with a methotrexate metabolite, 2,4-diamino-N^{10} methylpteroic acid (DAMPA). This metabolite may produce spuriously high assay results. High-pressure liquid chromatographic (HPLC) assay systems can be used to produce clean separation of methotrexate from contaminants and metabolites, with quantitation of the various peaks by spectral or other assay methods, but HPLC is not practical for routine clinical monitoring. Methotrexate undergoes metabolic conversion to 7-OH methotrexate through the action of aldehyde oxidase. The product becomes the predominant compound in plasma within 6 hours, and 7-OH levels exceed the parent compound by tenfold or more at 12 hours.[17] The metabolite weakly inhibits dihydrofolate reductase, but its polyglutamates do inhibit thymidylate synthase and AICAR transformylase and compete for the folate transport mechanism.

Oral methotrexate is well absorbed in doses less than 25 mg/m^2, but bioavailability becomes erratic for larger doses. Except in maintenance regimens, the drug usually is administered intravenously. The plasma pharmacokinetics after intravenous administration vary from patient to patient, but over the clinical dose range of 25 to 1500 mg/m^2, the drug generally follows a three-phase disappearance pattern. A brief distributional phase is followed by a primary elimination half-life of 2 to 3 hours and a final phase of elimination with a half-life of 8 to 10 hours.

Drug excretion occurs primarily through renal elimination. Rapid rates of drug clearance have been correlated with

Acute Toxicity					
Plasma WBC	*Platelet*	*Nausea/ Vomiting*	*Other Toxicity*	*Elimination†*	*Plasma Half-Life (h)**
Marked	Marked	Mild	Pulmonary fibrosis	M	?
Marked	Marked	Moderate	Leukemia, pulmonary fibrosis, renal failure	M	?
Marked	Marked	Moderate	Leukemia, pulmonary fibrosis, renal failure	M	?
Marked	Marked	Marked	Leukemia, pulmonary fibrosis, renal failure	M	1.0
Mild	Mild	Moderate-marked	Renal failure, hyperglycemia, hepatic enzyme elevation	R	0.25
Moderate	Moderate	Mild	Leukemia	M	1.5
Moderate	Moderate	Severe	Renal failure, Mg** wasting, peripheral neuropathy	R, M	0.3
Mild	Mild	Moderate			
Moderate	Moderate	Marked	Neurotoxicity, ototoxicity	M	0.3
Marked	Marked	Mild		R	
Moderate	Moderate	Moderate	Cumulative myelosuppression	M	0.5
Moderate	Moderate	Moderate	Cumulative myelosuppression	M	0.5
Mild	Mild	Marked	Flulike syndrome	M	0.65
Moderate	Moderate	Mild	Cardiac arrhythmias	M	7
Moderate	Moderate	Mild	Sensitivity to amines	M	?
Mild	Mild	Moderate	Neurotoxicity	M	5
Moderate	Moderate	Mild	Cholestasis	M	0.25/37

*Slash indicates multiple half-lines.

a high risk of relapse in childhood acute lymphocytic leukemia. Methotrexate is filtered by the glomerulus, reabsorbed in the proximal tubule (a process blocked by probenecid), and secreted by the distal tubule. Its clearance equals or exceeds creatinine clearance but is not entirely predictable on the basis of clinical measures of renal function. In patients with compromised renal function or in those receiving potentially lethal doses (above 1000 mg/m²), plasma concentration should be monitored to avoid serious toxicity. In high-dose therapy, small test doses may be used to establish pharmacokinetic characteristics in an individual patient, allowing calculation of a safe dose.[19]

Methotrexate distributes slowly into third-space accumulations of fluid, such as ascites or pleural effusions, but also exists slowly from these spaces. The reentry of the drug into the systemic circulation from these spaces prolongs the terminal phase of plasma drug disappearance and causes unexpected toxicity. It is advisable to evacuate effusions or to monitor drug levels in patients with ascites or massive pleural effusions.

Methotrexate also enters the cerebrospinal fluid (CSF) slowly and produces concentrations that are (during continuous intravenous infusion) approximately 1/30 the concentration found simultaneously in plasma. Cytotoxic drug concentrations can be achieved in the spinal fluid by giving a high dose of methotrexate; peak levels approach 1×10^{-5} M in regimens that use 500 to 1500 mg/m². However, doses of 20 to 30 g/m² are required to achieve the peak concentrations and the concentration × time product resulting from direct installation of small doses of methotrexate into the intrathecal space, and efficacy of systemic high-dose regimens in preventing or treating meningeal leukemia or carcinomatosis is not confirmed.

The pharmacokinetics of trimetrexate are quite different from those of methotrexate. The drug undergoes demethylation and glucuronidation of the O-methoxy groups, with elimination of the glucuronide metabolites in the urine. The primary half-life of the parent compound in plasma is 11 hours.[3] High doses of trimetrexate can be effectively "rescued" with leucovorin, but such regimens have been used only for antiparasitic therapy.[3]

Dose Adjustment

Special emphasis must be given to the rationale, methods, and results of monitoring drug levels during therapy with high doses of methotrexate. These are summarized in Table 18-3. Methotrexate infusions for 6 to 36 hours, in total dosages of 1000 mg/m² or greater, can be given without toxic consequences if preceded by intensive hydration and urinary

TABLE 18-2. Drugs Requiring Dose Modification for Organ Dysfunction

Agent	*Organ Dysfunction*	*Suggested Dose Modification*
Methotrexate	Renal failure or ↓ creatinine clearance	In proportion to ↓ creatinine clearance (normal 60 ml/min/m²)
cis-Platinum (cisplatin)	Renal failure	In proportion to creatinine clearance
Cyclophosphamide	Renal failure (creatinine clearance below 25 ml/min)	50% decrease
Bleomycin	Renal failure (creatinine clearance below 25 ml/min)	50–75% decrease
Streptozotocin	Renal failure (creatinine clearance below 25 ml/min)	50–75% decrease
Carboplatin Hydroxyurea VP-16 Deoxycoformycin	Renal failure	In proportion to creatinine clearance
mAMSA Vincristine Vinblastine	Hepatic dysfunction	1. Only approximate guidelines can be offered and are probably inaccurate. See text. 2. For bilirubin of >1.5 mg/100 ml, reduce initial dose by 50%. 3. For bilirubin of >3.0 mg/100 ml, reduce initial dose by 75%.

alkalinization and if followed by a series of leucovorin doses. Because of the competitive relationship between leucovorin and methotrexate, the actual dose of leucovorin required to provide rescue depends on the plasma concentration of antifolate at the time of rescue. Doses of leucovorin in the range of 15 to 25 mg/m² usually provide plasma levels of 1×10^{-6} M and are adequate to prevent toxicity of similar concentrations of antifolate. However, in patients with altered renal function, either induced by methotrexate or antedating this treatment, methotrexate excretion is delayed, plasma concentrations are higher than anticipated, and conventional doses of leucovorin are inadequate for rescue. Nonsteroidal anti-inflammatory drugs also inhibit renal excretion and the plasma clearance of methotrexate, increasing the risk of inadequate rescue.[20]

Severe myelosuppression and mucositis in patients receiving high dosages of methotrexate have been correlated directly with delayed drug elimination and elevated drug levels in plasma.[21] This relationship has dictated critical guidelines for leucovorin administration based on drug-level monitoring

TABLE 18-3. Drug Monitoring in Cancer Therapy

Agent	*Assay**	*Uses*
Methotrexate	Competitive binding to enzyme or to antibody HPLC	1. Early detection of patients at high risk of toxicity in high-dose therapy. Drug level $>5 \times 10^{-7}$ M at 48 h alerts to need for increased and prolonged leucovorin. In toxic patients, tailor leucovorin dosage to plasma methotrexate level. 2. Aid in differential diagnosis of neurotoxicity. High drug level in cerebrospinal fluid favors drug reaction. 3. Predict drug clearance in patients with altered renal function. Allow choice of safe dose.
5-Fluorouracil	HPLC	Design intra-arterial and intraperitoneal chemotherapy regimens with acceptable systemic toxicity. Detect inappropriately elevated ($>10^{-5}$ M) venous blood levels.
6-Mercaptopurine Hexamethylmelamine L-Phenylalanine mustard	HPLC HPLC HPLC	Determine plasma levels after oral therapy to assure adequate bioavailability (experimental).

*See text for references to specific drug assays.

TABLE 18-4. Drugs in Phase I and II Trials, 1984–1987

Drug	*Mechanism of Action*	*Maximum-Tolerated Dose (mg/m²)*	*Toxicities*
Acodazole		1370, each 3 wk	Cardiac arrhythmias
Amonafide	DNA strand breaks	300, 5 d each 3 wk	Myelosuppression
Curacemide	DNA synthesis inhibition	650 CI, 5 d each 3 wk	Neurotoxicity
Didemnin B	DNA synthesis inhibition	3.5, weekly	Nausea, vomiting, hepatotoxicity
Echinomycin	DNA cross-linker	1.5, each 4 wk	Nausea, vomiting, myelosuppression
Flavone acetic acid	DNA binder	2,300 CI, 1 h weekly (×4)	
		10,000 CI, 3 h each 3 wk	Hypotension neurotoxicity
Menogaril	DNA binder, anthracycline	160, each 4 wk	Myelosuppression
Merbarone	DNA strand breaks	Uncertain	Uncertain
Taxol	Tubulin binder	250 CI, 24 h each 3 wk	Myelosuppression, anaphylaxis, peripheral neuropathy
Trimetrexate	Antifolate	8–12, 5 d each 3 wk	Myelosuppression
Hexamethylene bisacetamide	Differentiation	2400 CI, 5 d	Neurotoxicity
Pibenzimol	DNA binder	15 CI, 5 d each 3 wk	Hyperglycemia
Gallium nitrate	Not known	300, 7 d each 3 wk	
		300, 3 d each 2 wk	Renal, ototoxicity, anemia, neurotoxicity
Dihydro-5-azacytidine	Incorporated into RNA and DNA	2500, 5 d each 3 wk	Chest pain, nausea and vomiting

TABLE 18-5. Restricted Drugs

Drugs	*Indication*
*Group C Drugs**	
Azacytidine (5-aza)	Refractory acute leukemia single-agent treatment
Amsacrine (mAMSA)	Refractory acute leukemia single-agent treatment
Erwinia asparaginase	Patients allergic to *E. coli* asparaginase
Hexamethylmelamine	Refractory ovarian cancer single-agent treatment
Pentostatin (Deoxycoformycin)	Hairy cell leukemia
Modified Group C Drugs†	
Interleukin-2 (IL-2) with or without lymphokine-activated killer (LAK) cells	Metastatic or unresectable renal cell carcinoma
	Metastatic or unresectable melanoma

*Available as of 1988 to authorized physicians upon request to Investigational Drug Branch, Executive Plaza North, National Cancer Institute, Bethesda, Maryland 20892.

†Restricted for use in cancer centers.

at specific times following infusion and has allowed adjustment of leucovorin dosage to compensate for elevations of plasma methotrexate levels. For the commonly used Jaffe regimen (50–250 mg/kg methotrexate given over 6 hours, followed by eight doses of leucovorin, 15 mg/m² every 6 hours), a plasma methotrexate level above 9×10^{-7} M at 48 hours is associated with a high risk of severe myelosuppression (Table 18-6).[21] Increased leucovorin dosage (100 mg/m² for levels of 10^{-6} M, with proportional increases for higher antifolate concentrations) is effective in preventing myelosuppression.

Alternate high-dose regimens have been used. Infusions of equivalent doses of methotrexate (1.5–7.5 g/m²) over an infusion period of more than 6 hours produce lower plateau concentrations of drug in the range of 10 to 100 μM, but for longer periods. A typical 36-hour regimen used for preoperative chemotherapy of head and neck carcinoma is given in Table 18-6. In this regimen, extreme precautions were taken to assure the adequacy of hydration, urinary alkalinization, and leucovorin rescue in treating a high-risk patient population. A comparison of the pharmacokinetics of high-dose methotrexate given as a 6-hour infusion and 36-hour infusion is shown in Figure 18-4.

There are no known effective means for removing methotrexate from body fluids without normal renal function. Drug can be bound in the intestinal lumen by cholestyramine and removed from the enterohepatic circulation, but the efficacy of this method has not been established.[22] Hemodialysis produces clearance rates of only 35 to 40 ml/min. Circulating drug can be effectively hydrolyzed and inactivated by a bacterial enzyme, carboxypeptidase G_1, but this enzyme is not available for general clinical use.[23]

Only a small fraction of administered drug is metabolized to inactive products. However, two metabolites, DAMPA and 7-OH methotrexate, tend to accumulate in plasma at later

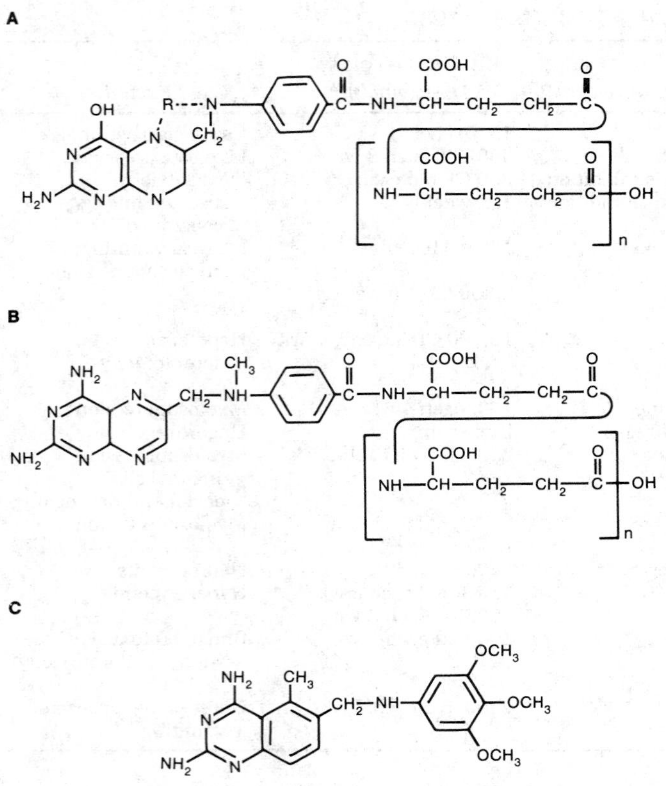

FIG. 18-2. Structure of folic acid (**A**), methotrexate (**B**), and trimetrexate (**C**). Note potential for addition of glutamyl groups to methotrexate and folic acid.

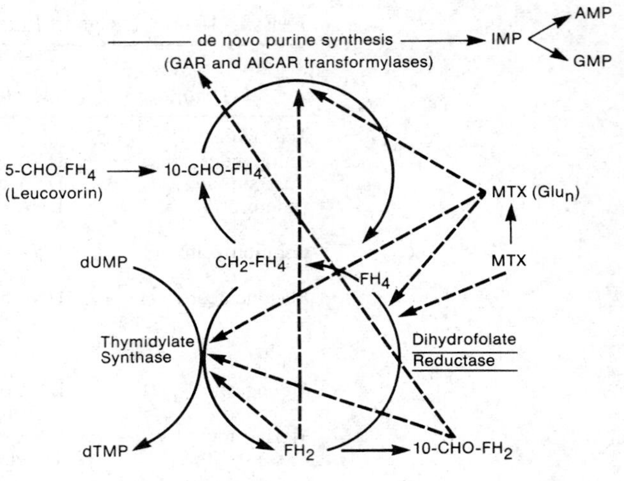

Compound	Inhibits
MTX	Dihydrofolate reductase
MTX (Glu$_n$)	Dihydrofolate reductase; Thymidylate synthase; AICAR transformylase
FH_2 (Glu$_n$)	Thymidylate synthase; AICAR transformylase
10-CHO-FH_2 (Glu$_n$)	Thymidylate synthase; GAR transformylase

FIG. 18-3. Sites of action of methotrexate (MTX), its polyglutamated metabolites [MTX(Glu$_n$)], and folate byproducts of the inhibition of dihydrofolate reductase, including dihydrofolate (FH_2) and 10-formyl-dihydrofolate (10-CHO-FH_2). Also shown are 5-10-methylene tetrahydrofolic acid (CH_2-FH_4), the folate cofactor required for thymidylate synthesis, and 10-formyl-tetrahydrofolate (10-CHO-FH_4), the required intermediate in the synthesis of purine precursors. (Other abbreviations as in Figure 18-1.)

times in patients receiving high doses of methotrexate. Neither has potent antifolate activity, but both are less soluble than is the parent compound and may contribute to the renal precipitation of methotrexate-derived material observed in high-dose therapy.

The pharmacokinetics of methotrexate in the CSF have an important bearing on both therapeutic and toxic effects. Drug injected in the lumbar intrathecal space is distributed poorly in the ventricular spinal fluid, a factor that may contribute to the high incidence of relapse of meningeal leukemia.[24] For patients with known meningeal leukemia, direct intraventricular injection through an indwelling reservoir is recommended. Peak drug concentrations of approximately 10^{-3} M are reached in the CSF by injection of 12-mg doses; the major half-life in patients without active meningeal disease is approximately 12 hours, but this may be prolonged considerably in patients without active leukemic meningitis. Delayed methotrexate elimination from the CSF is associated with methotrexate neurotoxicity.[25]

Toxicity

The toxicities observed in humans as a consequence of methotrexate therapy fall into two categories: those related to the action of the drug on rapidly proliferating tissues (bone marrow and intestinal and oral epithelium) and those manifested by nondividing tissues, which are less predictable in their incidence. Myelosuppression and mucositis reach

TABLE 18-6. High-Dose Methotrexate Therapy

1. *Prehydration*
   In 12 h before treatment establish diuresis with 1.5 liters/m² D_5W with 100 mEq HCO_3^- and 20 mEq KCl per liter. Test urine *p*H to assure neutrality (*p*H 7 or >) at time of drug infusion.
2. *Drug Infusion*
   a. Jaffe regimen: 50 to 250 mg/kg methotrexate (MTX) over 6-h infusion. Continue hydration (3 liters/m²) for 24 h. Begin leucovorin 2 h after end of drug infusion, 15 mg/m² 1 M q6h × 7 doses.
   b. Alternative: bolus administration of 50 mg/m² MTX intravenously followed by infusion of MTX over 36-h period at dose of 1.5 g/m². At 36 h, begin leucovorin infusion 200 mg/m² for 12 h. At 48 h, give leucovorin 25 mg/m² q6h × 6 doses 1 M.
3. *Monitor Points*
   For Jaffe regimen and for 36-h infusion, drug levels above 5×10^{-7} M at 48 h require additional leucovorin rescue.

Drug Level	*Dose Leucovorin*
5×10^{-7} M	15 mg/m² q6h × 8 doses
1×10^{-6} M	100 mg/m² q6h × 8 doses
2×10^{-6} M	200 mg/m² q6h × 8 doses

Drug levels should be repeated every 48 h and leucovorin dose adjusted until drug concentration is less than 5×10^{-8} M.

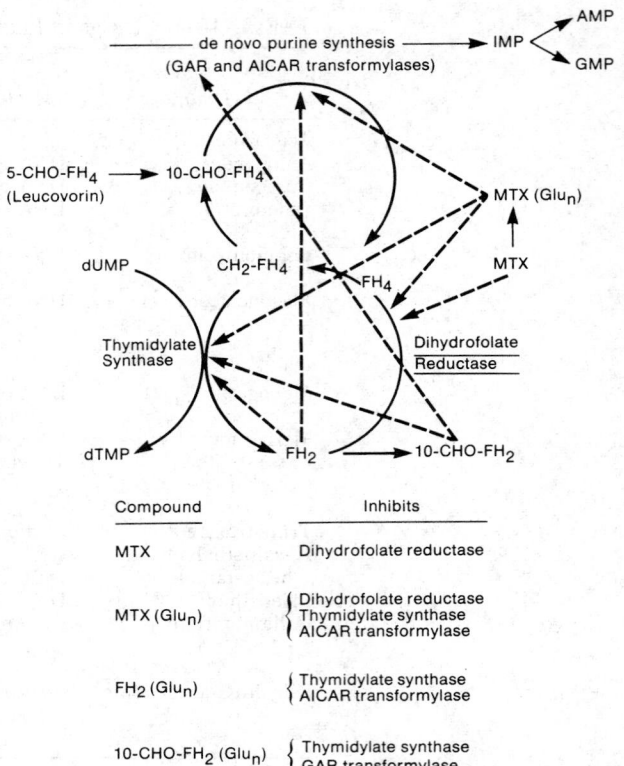

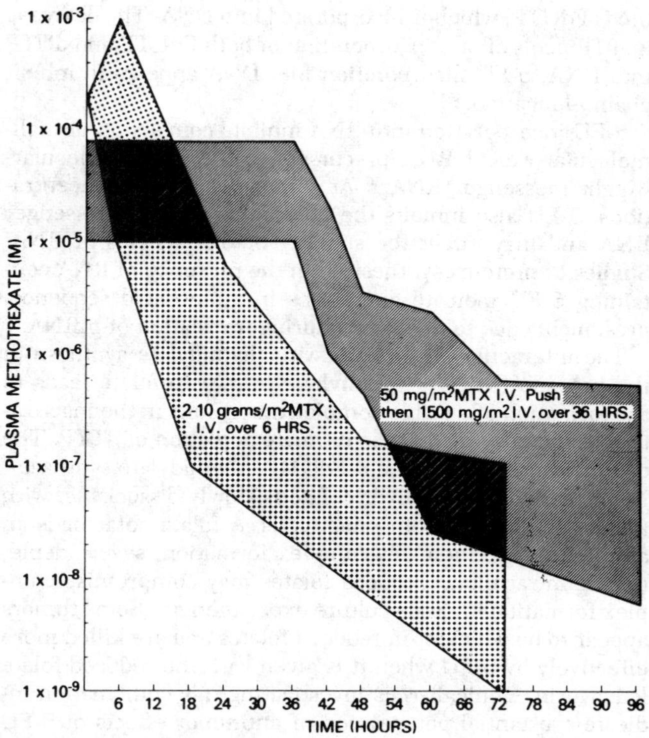

FIG. 18-4. Comparison of methotrexate pharmacokinetics in two high-dose regimens, the first a 6-hour infusion of 50 to 250 mg/kg, the second a bolus dose of 50 mg/m² followed by a 36-hour infusion of 1500 mg/m².

their maximum in 5 to 14 days after a bolus dose or short-term infusion, and recovery usually is rapid thereafter. More prolonged and severe toxicity has been observed in patients who receive high doses of methotrexate and seems to be related to the long exposure (>48 hours) of these sensitive tissues to the circulating drug. These toxicities can be prevented through administration of adequate doses of leucovorin or of thymidine, although the latter form of rescue is less reliable than is rescue with leucovorin.[26] It should be remembered that in patients with renal dysfunction, even small doses of methotrexate may cause serious or fatal myelosuppression.

Renal tubular injury is another serious toxic effect of methotrexate. Conventional doses of methotrexate rarely cause renal injury, but high-dose therapy without adequate hydration (3 liters/m² for 24 h) and urinary alkalinization (pH 7 or higher), is associated with at least a 10% incidence of acute renal injury, as indicated by a rise in BUN and serum creatinine and a decrease in urine volume. In most cases, renal toxicity is believed to be caused by renal precipitation of methotrexate or of methotrexate-derived material; however, other causes of renal damage are suggested by the finding that 30-fold lower doses of aminopterin, a more potent antifolate, cause similar deterioration in renal function.[27,28] These adverse renal effects can be prevented by vigorous pretreatment hydration, by urinary alkalinization, and by dose reduction in patients with underlying renal disease (see Tables 18-2 and 18-3).

Both acute and chronic hepatotoxicity are caused by methotrexate. Acute rises in hepatic enzyme levels often are observed during high-dose therapy, but the levels return to normal within 1 week. Hyperbilirubinemia is occasionally observed in high-dose treatment. Long-term administration of daily oral methotrexate, as used for treatment of psoriasis, is associated with hepatic fibrosis in up to 30% of these patients and with an infrequent occurrence of cirrhosis. The cause of hepatic lesions is unknown. A much lower rate of hepatic fibrosis is seen in patients with rheumatoid arthritis treated with methotrexate on weekly or intermittent schedules.[29] The results of animal experiments suggest impairment of choline synthesis and consequent inhibition of lipid mobilization, which is supported by the finding of fatty infiltration in biopsy material of patients who exhibit acute hepatotoxicity.[30]

Acute pneumonitis is observed occasionally in patients who receive methotrexate.[31] When biopsied, the lung often shows granuloma formation and eosinophilia, suggesting a hypersensitivity reaction. However, retreatment of such patients has not caused a recurrence of this syndrome.

Various manifestations of neurotoxicity are observed in almost 30% of patients receiving intrathecal methotrexate. Symptoms include motor dysfunction of the extremities, cranial nerve palsies, coma, or seizures. This syndrome is different from the acute arachnoiditis often seen during the 48 hours following drug injection. Neurotoxicity usually occurs after the third or fourth course of intrathecal therapy and is found most often in adult patients and in those who have active meningeal leukemia. Symptoms may be accompanied by an increase in spinal fluid pressure, an elevated protein concentration, and a reactive pleocytosis. When the syndrome is recognized, a change in therapy to cytarabine (cytosine arabinoside) or thiotepa is indicated. Continued treatment may be fatal. Chronic brain injury is believed to occur in the many children treated prophylactically with the standard combination of intrathecal methotrexate and cranial irradiation. In these children, computed tomography (CT) reveals intracerebral calcification, thinning of the cerebral cortex, and ventricular dilatation. High-dose systemic methotrexate appears to be an effective alternative to intrathecal methotrexate for prophylaxis of meningeal leukemia in average-risk patients.[32]

FLUOROPYRIMIDINES

Few of the active antitumor agents used clinically have resulted from rational design; rather, most are the product of serendipitous observations or screening. 5-Fluorouracil (5-FU), conceived and synthesized by Dr. Charles Heidelberger at the University of Wisconsin, represents a notable exception (Fig. 18-5).[33] Heidelberger observed that certain malignant cells used the base uracil more efficiently than did rat intestinal mucosa, and he designed a series of uracil analogues with fluorine substitutions at the 5 position. This substitution, after suitable intracellular transformation of the derivative, yields a nucleotide, 5-fluorodeoxyuridylate (5-FdUMP), which inhibits the thymidylate synthase reaction and DNA synthesis (Fig. 18-6).

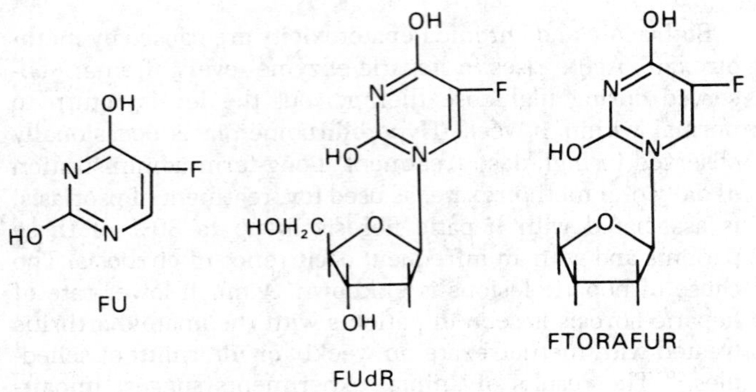

FIG. 18-5. Structures of clinically useful 5-fluoropyrimidines.

5-FU has antitumor activity against many types of solid tumors, including breast, colon, and ovarian carcinomas. In these tumors, the response rates vary from 10% to 40%, but complete remissions are unusual. The drug now is used frequently in combination therapy and has interesting biochemical interactions with methotrexate, physiologic nucleosides like thymidine, and leucovorin, all of which have become the subject of new clinical trials.

Mechanism of Action

5-FU has multiple biochemical actions that may be responsible for its cytotoxicity. It is converted by one of several possible pathways (Fig. 18-6) to the nucleotide fluorouridine monophosphate (FUMP); from this point, two "active" nucleotides may be formed: fluorouridine triphosphate (FUTP), which is incorporated into RNA and inhibits RNA processing and function, and 5-FdUMP, which binds tightly to thymidylate synthase and inhibits the eventual formation of deoxythymidine triphosphate (dTTP), one of the four necessary precursors of DNA. Although interest initially was focused on 5-FdUMP action, evidence from both in vitro and in vivo experiments suggests that the toxicity of 5-FU cannot be accounted for completely by thymidine, a direct precursor of dTMP. Also, manipulations that increase 5-FU incorporation into RNA increase cytotoxicity.[34] A third toxic metabolite is FdUTP, which is incorporated into DNA. The decrease in TTP pools allows incorporation of both FdUTP and dUTP into DNA. 5-FU incorporation into DNA appears to inhibit chain elongation.[35]

5-FU incorporation into RNA inhibits conversion of high-molecular-weight RNA precursors to the lower-molecular-weight messenger RNA.[36] At somewhat higher concentrations, 5-FU also inhibits the polyadenylation of messenger RNA and may affect the stability of this species of RNA. Studies of proteins synthesized in the presence of RNA containing 5-FU indicate alterations in amino acid sequence, presumably due to miscoding during translation of mRNA.[37]

The interaction of FdUMP with thymidylate synthase in the presence of N^{5-10} methylene tetrahydrofolate leads to the formation of a stable complex and results in the inactivation of the enzyme and the ultimate depletion of dTTP. The complex formed between 5-FdUMP–thymidylate synthase–N^{5-10} methylene tetrahydrofolate is slowly dissociable, with a half-life of 6 hours in intact cells. A folate cofactor is an absolute requirement for complex formation; severe depletion of intracellular reduced folates may compromise complex formation in tissue culture experiments.[38] Some tumors appear to be deficient in reduced folates and are killed more effectively by 5-FU when it is given with the reduced folate leucovorin. Clinical trials investigating this combination indicate substantial potentiation of antitumor effects of 5-FU by leucovorin, with some increased gastrointestinal toxicity.

Because the active forms of 5-FU are nucleotides, resistance to 5-FU can develop through deletion of one of the key enzymes required for its activation. In murine tumors, resistance has been associated with deletion of uridine kinase, uridine phosphorylase, or orotic acid phosphoribosyl transferase. In addition, an increase in thymidylate synthase has been seen in resistant cells and is related to amplification of the thymidylate synthase gene.[39]

Resistant mutants have been described that have increased cytidine triphosphate pools, with enhanced feedback inhibition of 5-FU conversion to its active nucleotide forms.[40] It is not known which of these mechanisms is responsible for resistance in humans. Inhibition of tumor thymidylate synthase, a function of the ratio of FdUMP to dUMP, predicted response to therapy in one study of colon cancer patients.[41] In a second clinical study, the drug-activating enzymes were

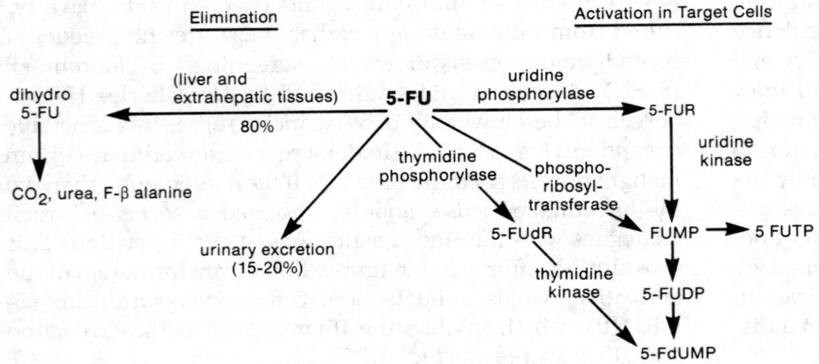

FIG. 18-6. Pathways of 5-fluorouracil elimination and activation.

uniformly high in malignant tissues and did not correlate with response; nor did thymidylate synthase activity, suggesting that fluoropyrimidine incorporation into DNA or RNA might be the important determinant.[42]

In an effort to enhance 5-FU activation and overcome resistance, various antitumor agents and nucleosides have been used in combination with the fluoropyrimidine. When given before 5-FU, methotrexate increases 5-FU nucleotide formation by increasing the intracellular content of phosphoribosylpyrophosphate (PRPP), a substrate required in the orotic acid phosphoribosyltransferase reaction.[43] A metabolite of allopurinol inhibits this enzyme, which appears to be the preferred pathway for 5-FU activation in normal tissues but not in all tumors, and thus improves the therapeutic index of 5-FU against some experimental tumors. However, the combination of 5-FU and allopurinol does not improve antitumor activity in humans.[44] Thymidine and other nucleosides enhance 5-FU incorporation into RNA by unknown mechanisms. In addition, thymidine and uridine delay 5-FU breakdown by the hepatic enzyme dihydrouracil dehydrogenase, and thus prolong 5-FU plasma half-life and increase its toxicity for both normal and malignant cells.[45] The combination of 5-FU and thymidine in humans has not improved clinical results.

Clinical Pharmacology and Pharmacokinetics

A variety of methods may be used to measure 5-FU levels in biologic specimens. The most rapid and sensitive of these methods are those using HPLC, either with anion exchange resins or with reverse-phase columns.[46] The sensitivity of this method, with appropriate sample cleanup, is less than 0.1 μM, or less than the threshold for bone marrow toxicity (probably 1 μM). The sensitivity of HPLC can be enhanced by derivatization of 5-FU with fluorescent conjugates.[47] Gas chromatographic–mass spectrophotometric methods, which are equally sensitive and specific, require derivatization and additional processing time.

An understanding of 5-FU pharmacokinetics is required in order to choose the proper route, schedule, and dose of administration. The alternative routes of administration (oral, intravenous, intraarterial, and intraperitoneal) have unique advantages and disadvantages that determine their usefulness in clinical chemotherapy. The clinical effectiveness and pattern of toxicity seen with each of these routes can be explained largely by pharmacokinetic considerations.

5-FU usually is administered intravenously (IV). Plasma levels vary considerably after oral administration, probably because of erratic absorption and variable first-pass metabolism in the transit from the intestinal tract through the portal system and liver to the systemic circulation.[48] After IV delivery, the drug penetrates well into the CSF and extracellular "third space" fluids, such as ascites or pleural fluid. Following conventional single doses of 10 to 15 mg/kg, peak plasma concentrations reach 0.1 mM to 1.0 mM, but rapid metabolic breakdown to dihydrofluorouracil in the liver and other tissues leads to an abrupt fall in plasma concentrations. The primary plasma half-life of about 10 minutes varies considerably from patient to patient, but its correlation with clinical tests of hepatic function is not clear. Within 6 hours of injection, plasma concentrations of 5-FU fall below 1 μM, the approximate threshold for exerting cytotoxic effects in tissue culture, thereafter they decline more slowly.

Because it is metabolized by the liver, 5-FU can be infused into the hepatic artery or portal vein for treatment of hepatic metastases, and only limited amounts of drug reach the systemic circulation. Preliminary data indicate that infusion of 30 mg/kg/day produces plasma levels of 0.13 to 0.35 μM, although these figures are likely to depend on catheter position and hepatic function.[49] At this infusion rate, more than 50% of the infused drug is cleared in its first pass through the liver.[50] This route is most useful in the treatment of isolated hepatic metastases.

5-FU also has been administered by peritoneal instillation for treatment of ovarian cancer.[51] This route takes advantage of the high intraperitoneal concentration of the drug (4mM), the slow absorption of the drug into the portal circulation, its rapid metabolism in the liver, and the minute amounts of drug that ultimately reach the systemic circulation. Minimal systemic toxicity occurs if drug concentrations are maintained at or below 4 mM in the peritoneal cavity, because a 100:1 to 1000:1 gradient in drug concentration is established between the peritoneal fluid and plasma. The therapeutic effects of this type of regimen have not been evaluated conclusively.

More than 80% of administered 5-FU (by IV or intraarterial route) is eliminated by metabolic conversion to dihydrofluorouracil; the remainder is excreted intact in the urine. The primary metabolite, dihydro-5-FU, is cleaved further to yield α-fluoro-β-ureidoproprionic acid, α-fluoro-β-alanine, and CO_2. The liver, kidney, and gastrointestinal mucosa are the primary sites of metabolism; it is not known whether neoplastic cells also degrade 5-FU. Doses do not have to be modified in the presence of hepatic dysfunction because metabolism occurs in extrahepatic tissues. Cimetidine, the H_2-histamine receptor antagonist, enhances the total drug exposure, as measured by the product of concentration $\times$ time, by inhibiting hepatic blood flow and hepatic drug metabolism.[52]

The active intracellular nucleotides 5-FdUMP and FUTP have prolonged half-lives intracellularly; their decay rates vary among tissues, and their persistence may be an important determinant of the duration and, ultimately, of the magnitude of drug effect.

Clinical Toxicity

The primary clinical toxicity of 5-FU results from its effects on rapidly dividing tissues, specifically intestinal and oral mucosa and bone marrow. After bolus IV administration, using either a 5-day course or single, weekly doses, suppression of the leukocyte and platelet counts occurs in 4 to 7 days, with full recovery within 2 weeks after the last dose. Stomatitis and diarrhea also are frequent side-effects, particularly in patients who receive a 5-day course of treatment. Repeated episodes of watery diarrhea (more than three movements per day) for several days should alert the oncologist to the danger of dehydration, sepsis, and death and should generate dose adjustments in subsequent courses of therapy.

An alternative regimen using continuous IV infusion of

5-FU at doses of 30 mg/kg/day for 5 days gives equivalent therapeutic results but a different pattern of toxicity. Myelosuppression usually is mild, and gastrointestinal symptoms such as stomatitis and diarrhea are the predominant toxicities. Continuous intrahepatic infusion of 5-FU also is a useful alternative to IV therapy in patients with liver metastases. In patients with colonic carcinoma with hepatic metastases, response rates of 50% or greater have been achieved with this mode of therapy. Because at least 50% of the drug is cleared in its first pass through the liver, systemic toxicity is mild, consisting primarily of mucositis and, less frequently, myelosuppression. The primary complications are related to catheter slippage into the gastroduodenal artery, with resultant necrosis of the intestinal epithelium, hemorrhage, or perforation. The physician must be alert to sudden onset of epigastric pain or ileus in the patient as early signs of catheter displacement into a feeding artery of the stomach or small bowel. Thrombosis of the extremity vessel used for insertion of the cannula can be anticipated if the catheter is inserted into a brachial artery. Hepatic portal perfusion is a less favorable form of local therapy because most large hepatic metastases derive their blood supply from the arterial circulation; it may be useful in the adjuvant setting.

Less common adverse effects caused by 5-FU include acute neurologic symptoms (somnolence, ataxia, and upper motor neuron signs) seen primarily in patients receiving intracarotid infusions; this syndrome is thought to be caused by a neurotoxic metabolite, 5-fluorocitrate. A syndrome of chest pain, serum enzyme elevations consistent with myocardial necrosis, and electrocardiographic findings consistent with myocardial ischemia has been described in patients undergoing 5-FU infusion. The reason for these episodes is unclear.

5-FU causes acute and chronic conjunctivitis that may lead to tear-duct stenosis and ectropion. The acute inflammatory response is reversible when the drug is discontinued, but surgical correction of tear-duct stenosis may be required.

Other Fluoropyrimidines

Two other fluoropyrimidines (Fig. 18-5), 5-fluoro-2-deoxyuridine (FUdR) and ftorafur (1-2-tetrahydrofuranyl)-5-fluorouracil, have undergone extensive clinical trials but have not replaced 5-FU in general clinical use. FUdR is converted to 5-FdUMP by a nucleoside kinase and functions primarily as an inhibitor of thymidylate synthase, with lesser effects than 5-FU on RNA. The deoxyribose group is removed readily by the ubiquitous enzyme thymidine phosphorylase, and the resulting 5-FU undergoes metabolic degradation as outlined previously. More than 90% of FUdR is removed in its first pass through the liver.[50] Its pattern of toxicity and the advantages of its use in hepatic perfusion closely parallel the characteristics of 5-FU (Table 18-1).

Ftorafur acts as a depot form of 5-FU and produces little myelosuppression. However, significant diarrhea, nausea, vomiting, and neurotoxicity in the form of altered mental status and ataxia are the usual dose-limiting complaints.[53] It is administered IV in doses of 1.5 g/m^2/day for 5 days and is absorbed well orally. The parent compound, ftorafur, has a prolonged plasma half-life of 6 to 16 hours and is eliminated by conversion to hydroxylated metabolites. The circulating concentrations of 5-FU produced are low (less than 0.1 mg/ml), suggesting that conversion to 5-FU may occur predominantly in tumor cells and the liver and that the circulating level of 5-FU may not adequately reflect the extent of this conversion.[54] Another analogue, 5′ deoxy-5-fluorouridine, functions as a prodrug, which is cleaved to yield 5-FU in tumor cells by action of the enzyme pyrimidine nucleoside phosphorylase.[55] It has no obvious advantage over 5-FU in clinical practice.

CYTOSINE ARABINOSIDE (CYTARABINE)

Cytosine arabinoside (ara-C) is one of several arabinose nucleosides first isolated from the sponge, *Cryptothethya crypta*, differing from its physiologic counterpart deoxycytidine by the presence of an OH group in the β-configuration at the 2′ position (Fig. 18-7). Since this initial discovery, many arabinose nucleosides have been synthesized or isolated from bacterial broths, and a few have been tested as antitumor agents. The most prominent of these are the purine analogues ara-adenine and fludarabine. However, neither of these compounds has as potent clinical activity against human acute myeloblastic leukemia as does ara-C. As a single agent, ara-C induces remission in 50% of patients with acute myeloblastic leukemia (AML) and is the standard agent in combination with anthracyclines for treatment of this disease. It has activity against other human tumors, including the blastic crisis of chronic granulocytic leukemia (CGL), acute lymphoblastic leukemia (ALL), and non-Hodgkin's lymphoma, but its selective activity against rapidly growing tumors and its pharmacokinetic features have

FIG. 18-7. Structure of physiologic cytidine nucleosides and related antimetabolites.

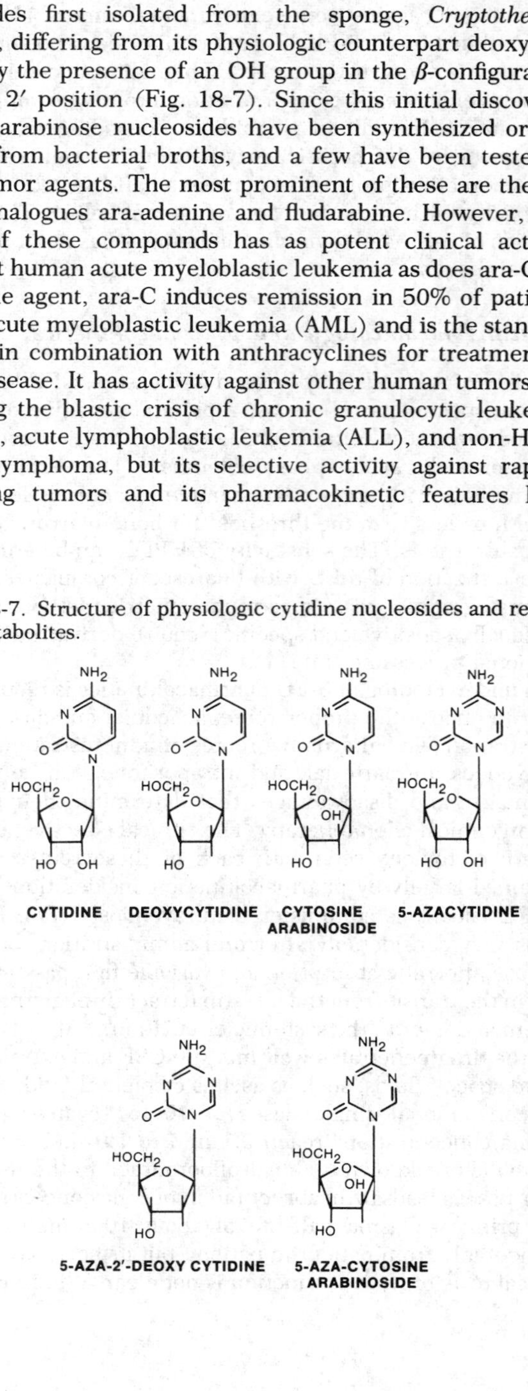

rendered this agent less useful in treating most solid malignancies.

Structure and Mechanism of Action

Because of the absence of a 2′-OH group in the α position, ara-C is recognized enzymatically as an analogue of 2′-deoxycytidine and is metabolized by salvage pathway enzymes to its active form, ara-CTP (Fig. 18-8). This nucleotide acts as an inhibitor of DNA polymerase in competition with deoxycytidine triphosphate (dCTP) and has a K_1 of approximately 0.1 μM.[56] Repair of ultraviolet light damage to DNA is inhibited by ara-C—presumably through polymerase inhibition—but not repair of radiation-induced damage.[57] A more important action of ara-C appears to be its incorporation into DNA, leading to a marked slowing of the elongating chain of DNA and a defect in ligation of fragments of newly synthesized DNA.[58] There also is evidence indicating that cells exposed to ara-C during the S, or DNA synthetic, phase of the cell cycle can reinitiate DNA synthesis when ara-CTP levels fall below inhibitory levels, resulting in an abnormal duplication of early portions of the DNA strand.[59]

Ara-C penetrates cells by a carrier-mediated process that allows the rapid achievement of steady-state intracellular drug concentrations.[60] Entry is an important determinant of ara-C sensitivity of human leukemic cells; for example, there is a strong correlation between the number of transport sites and the formation of the ultimate toxic metabolite ara-CTP.[61] At high drug concentrations (> 100 μM), ara-C enters cells by passive diffusion, a less efficient mechanism.

Intracellular metabolism of ara-C by three sequential phosphorylation reactions, mediated by deoxycytidine kinase, deoxycytidine monophosphate (dCMP) kinase, and nucleoside diphosphate kinase, leads to formation of ara-cytidine triphosphate (CTP). Two inactivating enzymes, cytidine deaminase and dCMP deaminase, also may act on ara-C or ara-CMP, respectively.[62] These deaminating enzymes are found in high concentrations relative to the activating enzymes and are thought to limit drug action (see Fig. 18-8).

FIG. 18-8. Metabolism of cytosine arabinoside by tumor cells. The names of important enzymes are in italics. The conversion of ara-UMP to a triphosphate has not been demonstrated in mammalian cells. d = deoxyribose; MP = monophosphate; DP = diphosphate; TP = triphosphate; NDP = nucleoside diphosphate. See legend to Figure 18-1 for other abbreviations.

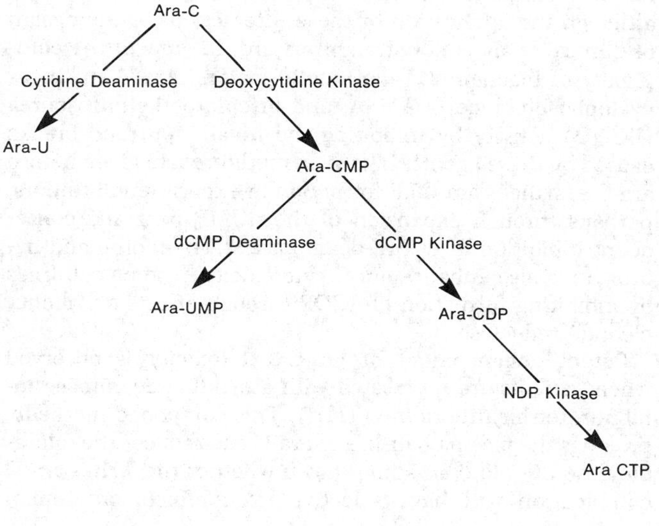

The biochemical changes responsible for resistance to ara-C have not been clearly defined in humans. Deletion of deoxycytidine kinase often is observed in resistant murine leukemia cells and has been implicated by at least one study in AML.[63] A second mechanism of resistance, documented only in preclinical studies, is an increased intracellular pool of dCTP (the nucleotide that competes with ara-CTP). Increased activity of cytidine deaminase has been correlated with resistance in a single study in AML but has not been confirmed subsequently.[64] In separate work, transport capacity of acute nonlymphocytic leukemia cells correlated with achievement of complete remission.[61] All of these changes ultimately decrease ara-CTP concentration. It is possible to predict clinical response to ara-C by a test incubation of leukemic cells with the drug *in vitro*; the ability of cells to retain ara-CTP after exposure to ara-C can be used to predict the duration of a subsequent remission.[65] These studies require the separation and quantitation of ara-C nucleotides by HPLC and are not adapted easily to routine clinical use.

As an inhibitor of DNA synthesis, ara-C kills cells selectively during the S phase of the cell cycle, although exposure of cells during other phases may lead to chromatid deletions and to a failure to repair strand breaks induced by other agents. The cytotoxicity of ara-C is not only cell-cycle specific, but also depends on the rate of DNA synthesis. Cytotoxic effects are greatest if cells are exposed to ara-C during periods of rapid DNA synthesis, for example, during the recovery phase after treatment with an initial dose of ara-C or another S-phase-specific drug. Thus the timing of the second dose of ara-C may have a critical impact on the therapeutic outcome. Karp and coworkers have demonstrated a marked increase in DNA synthetic rate in residual leukemic cells one week after an initial dose of ara-C and have advocated the use of sequential ara-C doses spaced 1 week apart to take advantage of this change.[66]

In addition to its cytotoxic effects, which are exerted at low concentrations (10 nM maintained continuously in culture will kill 50% of human marrow myeloid progenitors), ara-C is capable of inducing terminal differentiation of leukemic cells. Differentiation is associated in some instances with decreased oncogene (c-*myc*) expression.[67] Low-dose ara-C regimens induce remission both in leukemic patients and in patients with preleukemic states, and in both instances it has been possible in some cases to demonstrate persistence of chromosomal markers of the leukemic cell line in the mature cells, suggesting differentiation as a mechanism.[68] However, fewer than 20% of preleukemic patients achieve remission, and the dosage of ara-C used (20 mg/m²/day) achieves cytotoxic concentrations in plasma, leading to severe myelosuppression.

Clinical Pharmacology and Pharmacokinetics

The measurement of ara-C in biologic fluids presents significant problems. Because it is structurally similar to the physiologic nucleosides (deoxycytidine, cytidine), it is difficult to separate ara-C from these endogenous compounds. Further, ara-C is subject to deamination by cytidine deaminase, an enzyme found in plasma and in granulocytes; thus a deaminase inhibitor, such as tetrahydrouridine, must be included in samples at the time of their collection. Various chemical and microbiologic assays for ara-C have been developed and applied to clinical pharmacokinetic studies. The best of these uses HPLC with a cation-exchange column and cleanly separates ara-C from its primary metabolite ara-U.[69] The sensitivity of this method approaches 0.1 μM in plasma. An easier, more rapid method is the radioimmunoassay based on a sheep antibody to an ara-C conjugate with albumin.[70] This assay, which is more sensitive than HPLC, is highly specific for ara-C (and its nucleotides, which are not found in plasma), takes less than 3 hours to complete, and is applicable to routine pharmacokinetic monitoring and other clinical uses.

Because of the presence of cytidine deaminase in gastrointestinal epithelium and first-pass elimination in the liver, the drug is not given orally. When administered by IV infusion, it distributes rapidly into total-body water; concentrations in the CSF reach 50% of simultaneous plasma levels after 2 hours of continuous IV administration. Peak plasma concentrations reach 1×10^{-5} M after a 100-mg dose and thereafter fall with a primary half-life of 7 to 20 minutes.[71] A second half-life of 0.5 to 2.6 hours has been detected by more sensitive assay procedures but is probably of little clinical significance at standard doses. More than 70% of the clinical dose is excreted in the urine, primarily in the form of the inactive metabolite ara-U. Within minutes of injection, ara-U becomes the predominant form of the drug found in plasma; its formation takes place in the liver, plasma, peripheral granulocytes, and other sites. High-dose ara-C regimens (2–3 g/m^2 twice daily for 6 days) produce proportionately higher peak plasma concentrations, and ara-C disappears from plasma with a terminal half-life of 6 hours. In high-dose regimens, cerebrospinal fluid concentrations of drug reach a peak of 8 μM and decline with a half-life of 2 hours.[72]

Constant IV infusion of 5 to 10 mg/hour ara-C yields an average plasma concentration of about 3×10^{-7} M; a loading dose of three times the hourly infusion rate should be given before infusion to allow rapid achievement of the steady-state level.

The increases in plasma ara-C are proportional for infusion rates up to 2 g/m^2/d, or about 150 mg/hour, but at higher rates of infusion, the deamination capacity is saturated and ara-C levels rise sharply.[73] A maximum-tolerated infusion rate of 2 g/m^2/d for 3 days has been recommended and yields steady-state levels of 5 μM.

Schedules of Administration

Because of the rapid inactivation of ara-C by cytidine deaminase and its phase-dependent killing, the drug usually is administered as a continuous infusion or in bolus doses of 100 mg every 8 to 12 hours for 5 to 10 days. Single bolus doses of 4 g/m^2 produce minimal toxicity because of rapid drug inactivation, whereas the continuous infusion of 2 g/m^2/d over a 72-hour period produces severe myelosuppression.

The primary toxic side-effects of ara-C are myelosuppression and gastrointestinal epithelial injury. With the conventional dosage of 200 mg/m^2/day for 5 to 7 days, leukopenia and thrombocytopenia reach their maximum in 7 to 14 days. The duration of myelosuppression depends on the dose of ara-C, rate of achievement of remission, the nature of concomitant therapy, and prior treatment experience.

Gastrointestinal toxicity is prominent in patients receiving ara-C. The most frequent complaints include nausea, vomiting, and diarrhea: a spectrum of pathologic changes is observed in the intestinal mucosa, ranging from superficial ulceration to intramural hematoma formation and perforation. Patients receiving ara-C often develop elevated levels of serum enzymes consistent with mild hepatocellular damage, but hepatotoxicity necessitates discontinuation of treatment in fewer than 25% of patients.

High-dose ara-C regimens, using 2 to 3 g/m^2 given as a 2-hour infusion twice daily for 6 days, have been used to treat patients with refractory forms of acute leukemia. Toxicity in the form of myelosuppression, ataxia, and confusion is tolerable in most patients.

In addition to conventional administration by IV injection or infusion, ara-C may be given by subcutaneous (SC) injection or infusion on an outpatient basis, and total drug exposure (concentration $\times$ time) is twofold greater than is achieved by the same doses given by the IV bolus route.[74]

Ara-C also may be administered intrathecally for treatment of meningeal leukemia or carcinomatosis. Because deamination is minimal in the CSF, doses of 50 mg/m^2 yield peak levels of 1 mM, which decline slowly with a half-life of approximately 2 hours. Cytotoxic concentrations of greater than 0.1 μM are maintained for 24 hours. Ara-C often is used intrathecally as a substitute for methotrexate in patients experiencing antifolate neurotoxicity; however, ara-C also may cause neurotoxic side-effects, including seizures and alteration in mental status.[75]

Drug Interactions

Ara-C has shown synergistic interaction with many other antitumor agents, including alkylating agents, thiopurines, uridine analogues, and antifolates. Each of these interactions has been explained on a biochemical or cellular kinetic basis, although the application of these interactions to the design of clinical trials is not straightforward, in view of the complexity of biochemical and kinetic factors. Ara-C enhances cyclophosphamide, mAMSA, and bischloroethylnitrosourea (BCNU) activity by inhibiting the repair of strand breaks caused by these agents. Likewise, methotrexate given before ara-C enhances ara-CTP formation in experimental tumors, perhaps through expansion of the dUMP pool and consequent inhibition of dCMP deaminase.[76] Thymidine and hydroxyurea also enhance ara-C cytotoxicity in some cell lines by inhibiting formation of dCDP through effects on ribonucleotide reductase.[77]

Potent enhancement of ara-C cytotoxicity is observed when patients are pretreated with a cytidine deaminase inhibitor, tetrahydrouridine (THU). This compound markedly prolongs the plasma half-life of ara-C and reduces the tolerable dose 30-fold.[78] It is not known whether the THU–ara-C combination will have selective toxic effects on human tumor cells, but on the basis of experimental work, this combination would be expected to have synergistic activity only against cells with high deaminase levels, as are found in a fraction of patients with AML.

Other Cytidine Analogues

Because of the rapid metabolism of ara-C, attempts have been made to develop alternate therapies that would resist deamination. Ara-C enclosed in lipid vesicles, or liposomes, has increased potency, probably because of the prolonged half-life of the vesicles in plasma, but this increased potency has not been translated into improved therapeutic efficacy, compared with optimal use of free ara-C.[79] Various conjugates of ara-C, including N^4-acyl analogues, ara-C or ara-CMP esters, and the anhydro compound, cyclocytidine, have shown subject to deamination, but they do not have a superior therapeutic index. Most of these derivatives owe their activity to ara-CTP, and thus have the same mechanism of action as ara-C.

Other nucleosides with distinctly different mechanisms of cytidine antagonism have been developed, and two—5 azacytidine (5-azaC) and 3-deazauridine—have received clinical trial (Fig. 18-7). 5-AzaC has significant activity in the treatment of leukemia. As with ara-C, it is subject to deamination in plasma, in the liver, and in tumor cells, but its activation proceeds by a separate pathway. It is phosphorylated by uridine-cytidine kinase and then follows the same pathways as ara-CMP to reach its active form, 5-azaCTP. The latter is a substrate for RNA polymerase, and when it is incorporated into RNA, it causes defective protein synthesis and polyribosomal degradation.[80] 5-AzaC also is incorporated into DNA and inhibits methylation of DNA; the latter action may explain its ability to induce differentiation of both normal and malignant cells. It has been used clinically to induce fetal hemoglobin synthesis in patients with beta-thalassemia.[81] Resistance to 5-azaC in murine leukemic cells develops through deletion of uridine-cytidine kinase.

The 5-azaC ring system is unstable in solution; this instability may contribute to its lethal effects after incorporation into RNA. The rapid decomposition of 5-azaC in alkaline or neutral solution necessitates either fresh mixing before administration or formulation at a slightly acid *p*H in Ringer's lactate (*p*H 6.2), in which it has a half-life of 65 hours at 25°C.

5-AzaC is removed rapidly from the plasma, through both metabolic clearance and chemical decomposition. Less than 2% of an administered dose remains in plasma as the parent compound 30 minutes after administration. The compound is a substrate for cytidine deaminase, but the product, 5-azauridine, is chemically unstable and has not been identified in the urine or plasma of humans.

The primary adverse reactions to 5-azaC are myelosuppression and severe and prolonged nausea and vomiting. The latter symptoms are ameliorated if the drug is administered by prolonged or continuous infusion, which does not change its therapeutic efficacy or myelosuppressive effects. Patients sometimes develop abnormal liver function, myalgias, transient temperature elevation, or rash following 5-azaC therapy.

Other uridine and cytidine analogues have shown antitumor activity. 3-Deaza-uridine, an inhibitor of CTP synthesis, enhances the cytotoxicity of ara-C by diminishing intracellular dCTP. However, clinical trials of this compound as a single agent or in combination with ara-C indicated little antileukemic activity. Two new analogues, 5-azadeoxycytidine and 5-azacytosine arabinoside, are undergoing initial clinical evaluation (Fig. 18-7). The former is incorporated into DNA and, like 5-azacytidine, inhibits DNA methylation. 5-Azacytosine arabinoside acts as a potent inhibitor of DNA synthesis and has a broader spectrum of activity against experimental solid tumors than does either ara-C or 5-azacytidine.

PURINE ANALOGUES

The development of purine analogues for treatment of cancer has been one of the most fruitful endeavors in rational antitumor drug synthesis. Not only have effective antileukemic agents such as 6-mercaptopurine (6-MP) and 6-thioguanine (6-TG) resulted from these efforts, but potent immunosuppressive agents such as azathioprine, the xanthine oxidase inhibitor allopurinol, and the antiviral compounds ara-adenine and acyclovir have proved to be important in nononcologic fields.[82] A new area of great potential has been opened by the discovery of adenosine deaminase inhibitors such as deoxycoformycin, which have selective action against T-lymphocytes and promise to be useful in the treatment of hairy cell leukemia and other lymphoid tumors. This chapter deals with established and potentially important new antipurine agents in cancer chemotherapy.

Structure and Mechanism of Action of 6-Thiopurines

6-MP and 6-TG are used commonly in treating childhood ALL and AML, respectively, but do not have appreciable activity against human solid malignancies. Because of the similarities in their mechanisms of action, pharmacokinetic properties, and patterns of clinical toxicity, these two agents are considered jointly.

The 6-thiopurine analogues have the single substitution of a thiol group in place of the 6-hydroxyl group found in guanine or in the basic purine nucleus (Fig. 18-9). Both 6-MP and 6-TG are inactive compounds in their native state and require activation to the nucleotide level by the enzyme hypoxanthine-guanine phosphoribosyl transferase (HGPRT'ase).

FIG. 18-9. Purine analogues and their physiologic counterparts, hypoxanthine and guanine.

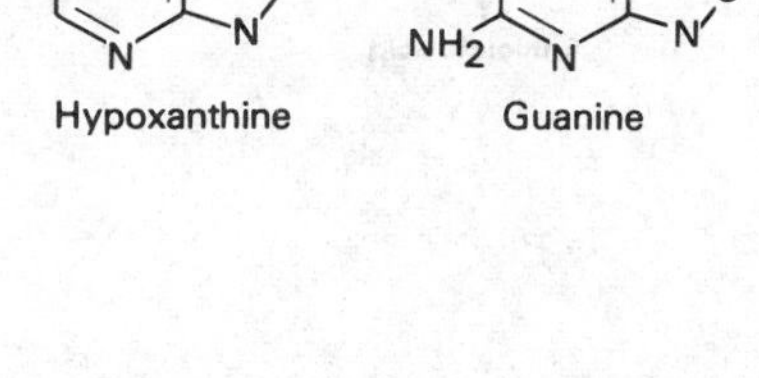

As monophosphate nucleotides, these analogues inhibit *de novo* purine biosynthesis at its first step (phosphoribosylpyrophosphate amidotransferase) and also block the conversion of inosinic acid to adenylic acid or to guanylic acid. The triphosphate nucleotides of 6-TG and 6-MP are incorporated into DNA and produce toxicity that is manifested in a delayed manner after drug exposure.[83] 6-TG incorporation into DNA leads to strand breaks, the frequency of which correlates with cytotoxicity.[84] Incorporation of the nucleophilic 6-TG base also renders DNA more susceptible to alkylation.[85]

Biochemical resistance to these agents has been ascribed to the absence of the activating enzyme (HGPRT'ase) in experimental tumors, but in human leukemic cells, resistance also is associated with increased concentrations of a degrading enzyme, a membrane-bound alkaline phosphatase, and the conjugating enzyme 6-thiopurine methyltransferase.[86,87]

The purine analogues readily penetrate cells. Their intracellular metabolism proceeds in several phases (Fig. 18-10).[88] Substantial quantities are converted to the inactive products 6-thiouric acid and 6-methylmercaptopurine; in the activation pathway, the thiopurines are converted to monophosphate nucleotides, which inhibit de novo purine synthesis, and to the triphosphate nucleotides, which are incorporated into DNA. It is believed that the initial inhibition of purine synthesis allows a buildup of PRPP pools and thus increases conversion of 6-MP and 6-TG to nucleotides. Inhibitors of de novo purine biosynthesis, such as methotrexate, are synergistic with 6-thiopurines because the block in purine synthesis leads to an expansion of the PRPP pool required for thiopurine activation. 6-MP-resistant cells, which lack HGPRT'ase, depend completely on the de novo pathway for purines and are thus highly sensitive to methotrexate.

Clinical Pharmacology and Pharmacokinetics

Although initial information on 6-MP pharmacokinetics came from the use of radiolabeled drug, this approach is impractical for routine monitoring or for repetitive studies in a single patient. Improved analytic techniques using HPLC have been described. The most sensitive of these new methods used derivatization of the thiopurines to phenyl mercury derivatives or oxidation to sulfonates with alkaline permanganate, followed by column separation and fluorometric detection.[89,90] The level of sensitivity of these procedures is approximately 0.1 μM in plasma.

When taken orally, both 6-MP and 6-TG are absorbed erratically; less than 50% of a dose reaches the systemic circulation, but this varies considerably among patients.[91] Both feeding and the antibiotic cotrimoxazole decrease 6-MP absorption.[92,93] The influence of erratic bioavailability on clinical response has not been determined.

The plasma half-lives are approximately 80 to 90 minutes for 6-TG and 20 to 45 minutes for 6-MP. The major determinants of drug elimination are metabolic alteration by several pathways (Fig. 18-10). 6-MP is oxidized to 6-thiouric acid by xanthine oxidase, a reaction sequence inhibited by allopurinol. In the presence of allopurinol, 6-thioxanthine, an intermediate oxidation product, becomes the predominant elimination product of 6-MP.

There is clinical evidence of increased 6-MP toxicity in patients receiving oral 6-MP concomitant with allopurinol but not in those treated with IV 6-MP. A dose reduction of 75% is recommended for patients receiving oral 6-MP and allopurinol. 6-MP also undergoes S-methylation to yield 6-methylmercaptopurine, which on phosphorylation becomes an active antipurine. However, the 6-methylmercaptopurine nucleotides are less cytotoxic than 6-MP nucleotides, and the activity of the methylation enzyme, which is quite variable among patients, has been correlated inversely with 6-MP nucleotide content of erythrocytes.[87] It has been suggested that 6-MP dosage be judged by toxicity (myelosuppression) rather than depend on a fixed dosage.

The catabolism of 6-TG is somewhat different than that of 6-MP. Methylation of the sulfur substituent plays a major role, leading ultimately to oxidation and elimination of the sulfur molecule. 6-TG also is converted to 6-thioxanthine in a reaction catalyzed by the enzyme guanase. This intermediate is oxidized further to 6-thiouric acid by xanthine oxidase, but because the substrate for this reaction, 6-thioxanthine, is inactive, no reduction in 6-TG dosage is required for patients who are also receiving allopurinol.

Dose, Schedule, and Toxicity

6-MP, given orally, and 6-TG, given IV, are well tolerated in doses of approximately 100 mg/m². These doses usually are given for at least 5 days in leukemic induction therapy or, in the case of 6-MP, for longer courses at slightly reduced doses for maintenance of remission. A 6-MP dosage reduction of 75% is indicated for patients also receiving allopurinol. Extremely high doses of 6-MP have been used (up to 1000 mg/m²/day for 5 days by IV infusion) without effectively increasing antitumor activity.[94]

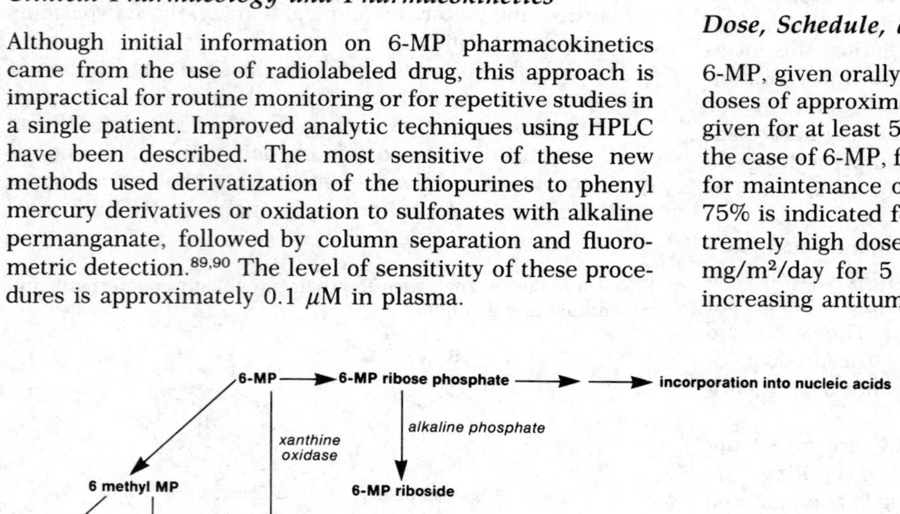

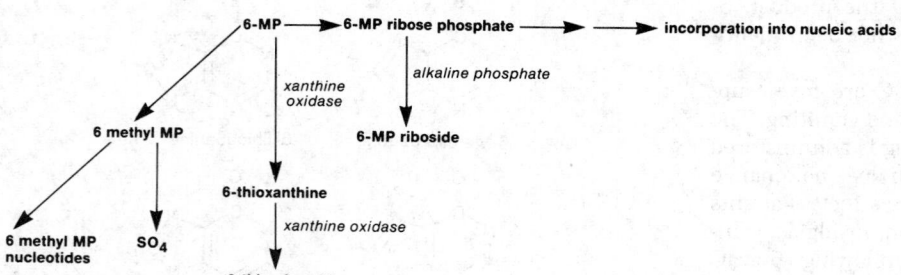

FIG. 18-10. Pathways for activation and degradation of 6-mercaptopurine (6-MP).

Because both 6-MP and 6-TG produce cytotoxicity by virtue of their incorporation into DNA, it follows that their primary toxicity would be exerted against the rapidly dividing precursor cells of the bone marrow and intestinal epithelium. After single doses, myelosuppression is maximal within 7 days of drug administration; the time to recovery is dose-dependent but usually is complete 14 days after the last dose. Reversible hepatotoxicity occasionally is observed after treatment with either thiopurine or, more frequently, after 6-MP. Serum alkaline phosphatase, direct bilirubin, and transaminase levels are elevated during this acute toxicity in a pattern consistent with cholestatic jaundice. Mucositis, esophagitis, and gastrointestinal complaints usually are mild and not a significant hindrance to antipurine therapy.

The 6-thiopurines and the related compound azathioprine, which releases 6-MP through hepatic metabolism following oral administration, are potent suppressors of cell-mediated immunity and are used to suppress rejection of transplanted organs or to treat autoimmune diseases such as Crohn's disease, ulcerative colitis, or rheumatoid arthritis.[95] Therapeutic immunosuppression will occur at doses of 100 mg/day (1.5 mg/kg), which cause only a small decrease in the leukocyte count. Long-term immunosuppressive therapy with azathioprine increases the risk of squamous carcinomas of the skin, histiocytic lymphoma, and Kaposi's sarcoma; these complications have not been reported after chronic 6-MP therapy. Other complications of chronic 6-thiopurine treatment include predispositions to bacterial and parasitic infections.

FIG. 18-11. Adenosine antimetabolites (ara-A and 2-fluoro-ara-AMP) and inhibitors of adenosine deaminase [2′-deoxycoformycin (2′-DCF) and EHNA].

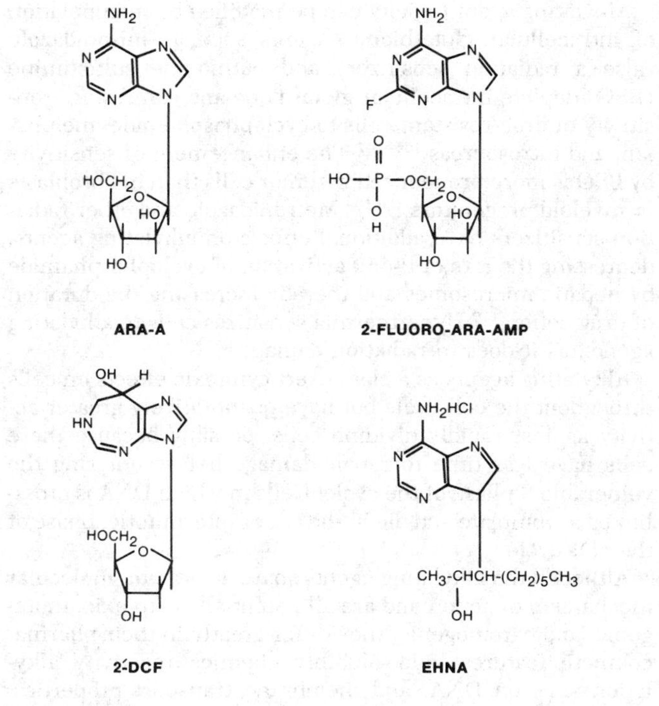

ADENOSINE ANALOGUES

In addition to the 6-thiopurines which act as guanine analogues, a number of analogues of adenosine have been synthesized or isolated from fermentation broths. The most prominent among these is 9-β-D-arabinofuranosyladenine (ara-A), which, as a triphosphate, inhibits DNA polymerase (Fig. 18-11). This compound has antiviral activity against DNA viruses, particularly those of the herpes group.[96] Although ara-A has shown potent antitumor activity in animal tumors, its clinical usefulness has been hindered by its limited aqueous solubility and its rapid deamination by adenosine deaminase. Its 2-fluoro monophosphate analogue (2-fluoro-AMP) is not susceptible to deamination and is highly toxic to both normal and malignant lymphoid and myeloid cells.[97] Its clinical utility is compromised by severe, late-onset neurotoxicity, including seizures, dementia, coma, and blindness.[98] It is highly active against chronic lymphocytic leukemia.

Inborn deficiency of adenosine deaminase is highly toxic for T-lymphocytes, an observation that has prompted interest in inhibitors of this enzyme for treatment of human T-cell tumors (Fig. 18-11). Two potent inhibitors of adenosine deaminase, 2′-deoxycoformycin and erythro-9-(2-hydroxy-3-nanyl)adenine(EHNA), enhance antitumor potency of ara-A and other adenosine analogues, such as tubercidin, xylosyl adenine, and 3′-deoxyadenosine.[99] The increase in intracellular ara-ATP produced by deoxycoformycin is greatest in tumor cells that contain adenosine deaminase; the decrease is smaller in bone marrow or gastrointestinal epithelium. Deoxycoformycin is highly toxic when given in daily schedules or weekly doses exceeding 10 mg/m^2 per week; azotemia, confusion, hepatic enzyme elevation, and nausea and vomiting are frequent side-effects. At lower doses (4 mg/m^2 biweekly), the incidence of side effects is low, but activity against hairy cell leukemia is preserved. Between 30% and 50% of a dose is excreted unchanged in the urine. In patients with normal renal function, sequential plasma half-lives are 1 and 10 hours.[100]

ALKYLATING AGENTS

Two primary classes of cytotoxic compounds have proven useful in the treatment of cancer: those that interfere with the synthesis of DNA precursors and those that chemically interact with DNA itself. Most prominent among the latter compounds are drugs known as alkylating agents because of their ability to form covalent bonds with nucleic acid. It is not fully understood how the alkyl groups that become attached to DNA in this reaction interfere with the integrity or function of DNA, but the alkylation process is known to have significant cytotoxic, mutagenic, and carcinogenic effects.

The biochemical process of alkylation is shown in Figure 18-12. Most alkylating agents form positively charged carbonium ions in aqueous solution. In the cases of the chloroethyl alkylating groups, a preliminary cyclization to form an unstable imonium ion takes place, with spontaneous opening of the three-member ring to yield the alkylating intermediate $R-CH_2-CH_2^+$. This charged group then attacks nucleo-

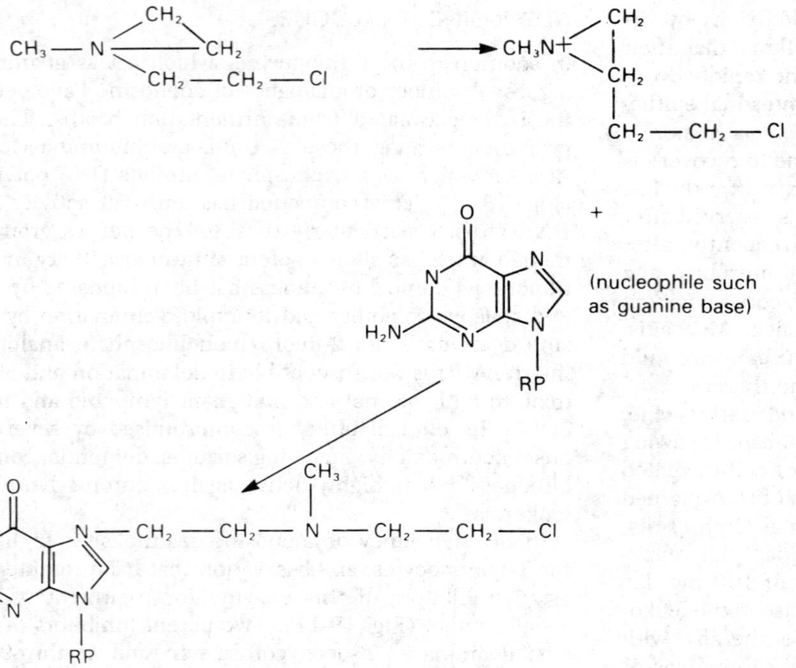

FIG. 18-12. Spontaneous activation of nitrogen mustard to an imonium ion that forms a covalent bond with nucleophilic sites such as the N-7 position of guanine. The remaining free chloroethyl arm of nitrogen mustard can repeat the same sequence of reactions to form DNA cross-links.

philic (electron-rich) sites on nucleic acids, proteins, and small molecules, such as sulfhydryls (glutathione) and amino acids. It seems likely that the primary cytotoxic and mutagenic effects of alkylating agents are caused by their interactions with DNA.[101] The favored sites of DNA attack are the N^7 position of guanine, which accounts for about 90% of alkylated sites; the 1 position of guanine; the 1, 3, and 7 positions of adenine; and the N^3 position of cytosine. It is not clear which of these sites of attack is the most important in producing the pharmacologic action of this class of compounds; alkylation of the N^7 position of guanine has less of an effect on misreading the DNA template than does alteration of the N^3 position of cytidine or the O^6 position of guanine, both of which interfere with accurate base pairing.

The consequences of base alkylation include not only misreading of the DNA code but also cross-linking of DNA and single-strand and double-strand breaks. Additional effects include inhibition of DNA, RNA, and protein synthesis in rapidly dividing tissues. Single-strand breakage occurs primarily as a consequence of the enzymatic processes of repair; the alkylated base is excised by endonuclease enzymes that specifically open the DNA strand at sites of base alkylation. The resulting gap can be repaired by a ligase enzyme if such an enzyme is present in the affected cell. Both alkylation and repair occur preferentially at sites of active DNA transcription.

Cross-linkage of DNA occurs when so-called bifunctional alkylating agents are used. For example, the prototype drug nitrogen mustard possesses two chloroethyl groups, each of which can form a carbonium ion. The establishment of cross-strand covalent binding correlates closely with the lethality of alkylating agents and nitrosourea derivatives.[102]

Repair of alkylated DNA depends on enzymes with highly specific action; for example, the guanine-O-alkyl transferase that repairs alkylation by nitrosoureas does not remove the alkyl groups fixed to DNA by other agents or platinum-DNA adducts. The intracellular action of alkylating agents may be aborted by their conjugation to glutathione or to thiol-containing proteins such as glutathione transferases (nitrosoureas) or metallothionine (cisplatin). Increased glutathione appears to be a general mechanism of alkylating agent resistance, but mechanisms specific for each agent have also been identified.[103,104]

Alkylating agent toxicity can be modified by manipulation of intracellular glutathione. Agents such as misonidazole (also a radiation sensitizer) and buthionine sulfoximine (BSO) deplete intracellular glutathione and can restore sensitivity of drug-resistant cells to cyclophosphamide, melphalan, and nitrosoureas.[105-107] The enhancement of sensitivity by BSO is more pronounced in tumor cells than in fibroblasts or myeloid progenitors.[108,109] Metronidazole and other radiation sensitizers have additional effects on alkylating agents, depressing the rate of P-450 activation of cyclophosphamide by hepatic microsomes and thereby increasing the duration of drug action.[110] Hyperthermia sensitizes cells to alkylating agents, as it does to radiation damage.

Alkylating agents as a class exert cytotoxic effects on cells throughout the cell cycle but have quantitatively greater activity against rapidly dividing cells, possibly because these cells have less time to repair damage before entering the vulnerable S phase of the cycle. Cells in which DNA is cross-linked accumulate and die in the G_2, or intermitotic, phase of the cell cycle.

Although the alkylating agents share a common molecular mechanism of action and are all potentially cytotoxic, mutagenic, and carcinogenic, they differ greatly in their pharmacokinetic features, lipid solubility, chemical reactivity, alkylation sites on DNA, and membrane transport properties, and thus do not uniformly share cross-resistance in experimental or clinical chemotherapy.[111] Thus the nitrosoureas and cyclophosphamide are not cross-resistant clinically in the treatment of lymphomas. Therefore, a consideration of the pharmacology of individual agents is necessary to understand their unique properties and optimal clinical use. The structures of commonly used alkylating agents are shown in Figure 18-13.

NITROGEN MUSTARD

Nitrogen mustard, or mechlorethamine, was the first alkylating agent to receive clinical trial and was found to produce responses in patients with lymphomas. This agent is highly reactive in aqueous solution and must be administered by IV injection. It also is effective as a topical solution for treatment of mycosis fungoides but produces hypersensitivity to its chloroethyl side-chain when used in this way. Nitrogen mustard penetrates cells through an active transport mechanism shared with the physiologic amine choline.[112] Resistance to the agent is poorly understood; it is believed to result from enhanced ability to repair DNA alkylation, but other mechanisms, such as defective transport or increased inactivation of the carbonium ion by enzymatic conjugation with intracellular sulfhydryl groups, may play a role.[113]

The primary clinical toxicities of nitrogen mustard are shown in Table 18-1 and consist of myelosuppression, nausea, and vomiting. Minor cholinergic side-effects are present at high doses and include lacrimation, diarrhea, and diaphoresis. Because of the high chemical reactivity of this compound, it is a potent vesicant and causes severe local tissue injury when infiltrated into the skin. Thus it is useful for ablating the pleural space in patients with chronic pleural effusion caused by malignant disease. Nitrogen mustard has been replaced to a great extent in clinical use by more stable agents, as described below.

CYCLOPHOSPHAMIDE

In an attempt to improve the selectivity of alkylating agents, cyclophosphamide was designed based on the fact that tumor cells possess a high concentration of enzyme activity that can cleave the P–N bond and liberate the potent phosphoramide mustard. In fact, activation of the drug is a multistep process. The first metabolite, hydroxycyclophosphamide, is produced by hepatic microsomal metabolism (Fig. 18-14).[114] 4-OH cyclophosphamide reenters plasma and is transported to peripheral target tissues, where it crosses the cell membrane and undergoes sequential conversion to aldophosphamide and its ultimate active principles, phosphoramide mustard and acrolein. Aldophosphamide is also subject to inactivation by aldehyde dehydrogenase, an enzyme elevated in some resistant tumor cells.[115] Although phosphoramide mustard is believed to be the primary active product, acrolein is a highly reactive compound capable of depleting gluta-

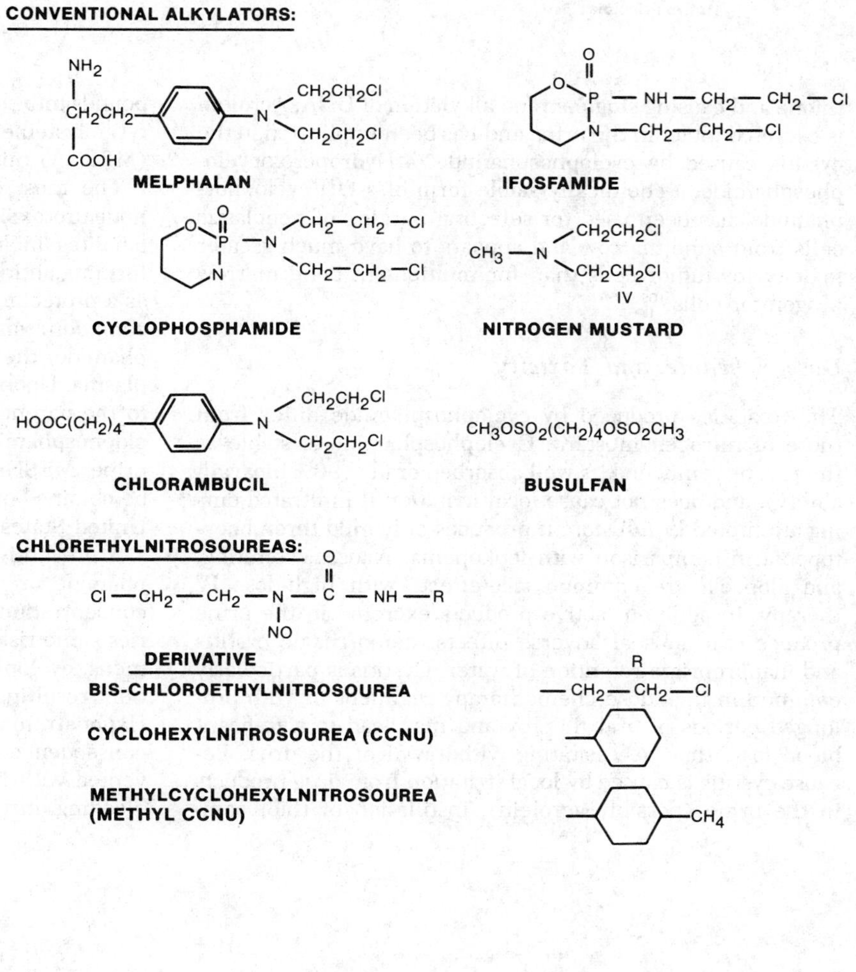

FIG. 18-13. Structures of commonly used alkylating agents and chloroethylnitrosoureas.

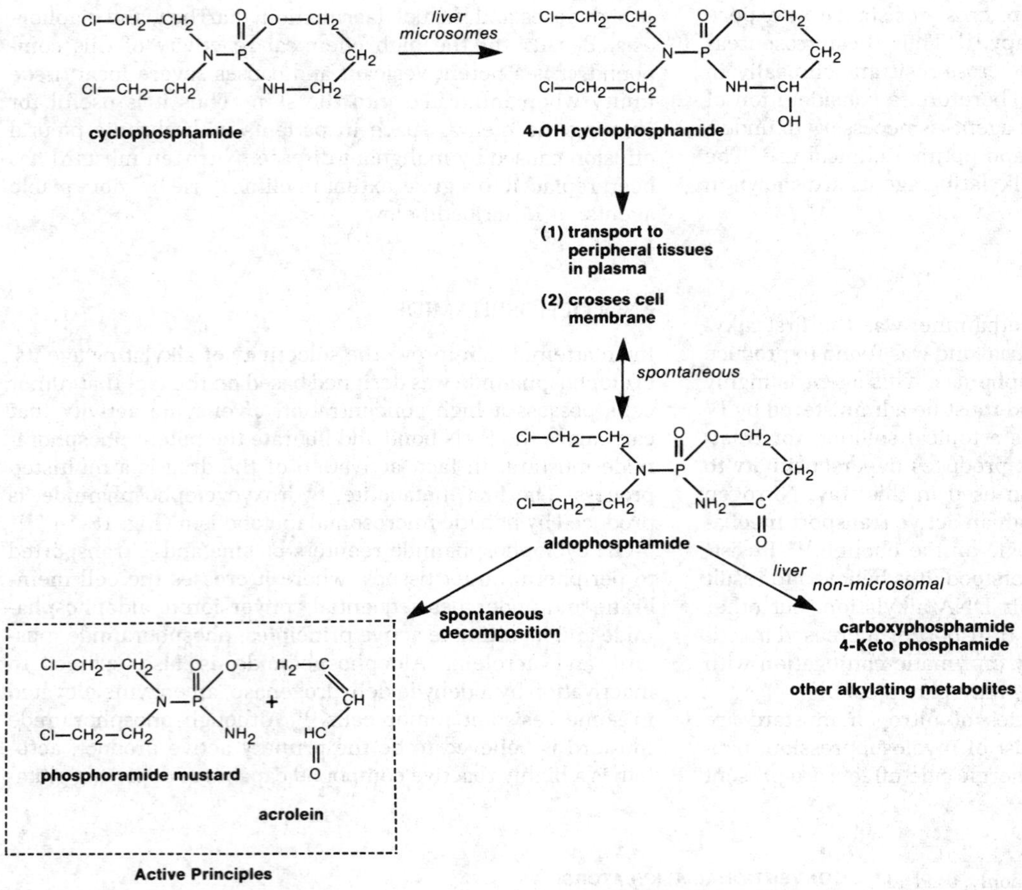

FIG. 18-14. Metabolism of cyclophosphamide by hepatic mixed-function oxidase, and transformation into active intermediates.

thione and causing single-strand alkylation of DNA. Acrolein is excreted intact in the urine and has been implicated in the cystitis caused by cyclophosphamide. 4-Hydroperoxicyclophosphamide, a chemically stable form of 4-OH cyclophosphamide, has been used for selecting purging of neoplastic cells from bone marrow and appears to have much greater toxicity for tumor cells than for multipotent bone marrow progenitor cells.[109]

Dose, Schedule, and Toxicity

The toxicities produced by cyclophosphamide differ from those of nitrogen mustard. Cyclophosphamide is stable as the parent compound, is well absorbed orally (90% bioavailability), and does not cause local irritation if infiltrated during attempted IV infusion. It produces only mild thrombocytopenia in comparison with leukopenia. Nausea, vomiting, and alopecia are common side-effects with high-dose IV therapy. In addition, active products excreted in the urine produce two unusual adverse effects: hemorrhagic cystitis and inappropriate retention of water. Cystitis is particularly common in high-dose chemotherapy regimens or with prolonged periods of oral therapy and may lead to significant blood loss, thus necessitating withdrawal of the drug. Because cystitis is caused by local irritation from drug products in the urine (possibly acrolein), instillation of thiol compounds into the bladder or systemic administration of N-acetyl cysteine or sodium-2-mercapto-ethane sulfonate (MESNA) mitigates this toxicity.[116]

The most effective agent for preventing cyclophosphamide urotoxicity is MESNA, which inactivates alkylating metabolites, including acrolein and phosphoramide mustard, by forming an inert thioether. MESNA is particularly attractive as a protectant because it dimerizes in serum to an inactive compound and thus does not inactivate hydroxycyclophosphamide, the essential metabolite of cyclophosphamide, in plasma. Upon excretion into the urine, the dimer hydrolyzes to the parent, mercaptan, which effectively neutralizes cyclophosphamide and ifosfamide alkylating species in the urine. MESNA is available commercially in Europe, but can be obtained only under individual patient exemptions in the United States.

A preventive maneuver for patients receiving cyclophosphamide or ifosfamide is to reduce alkylating metabolite concentration by diuresis.[117] Hydration of such patients carries some risk, however, because in high-dose infusion regimens, cyclophosphamide causes inappropriate water retention resulting from direct effects on the renal tubule. Hyponatremia, seizures, and death have been reported as a consequence of water retention. This toxicity can be prevented with furosemide.[118] In cases of severe or prolonged bleeding, installation of a dilute alum solution (1%) directly into the bladder may be required to stop the hemorrhage; the extreme measure of cystectomy may also be necessary if other measures fail. Chronic bladder inflammation due to cyclophosphamide may ultimately lead to malignant transitional cell tumors of the urothelium.[119]

Other toxicities include potent suppression of both humoral and cell-mediated immunity, although in low doses, cyclophosphamide is preferentially toxic to suppressor cells and thereby enhances cell-mediated immunity.[120] In low-dose schedules, it also enhances natural killer cell activity and macrophage activation and is synergistic with lymphokine-activated killer cells (LAK cells). These effects are highly dependent on dose and schedule of administration.[121]

Cyclophosphamide is carcinogenic in animals and leukemogenic in humans. It causes sterility that is potentially reversible in males and possibly reversible in females, and on rare occasions, it causes interstitial pulmonary fibrosis.[122] Renal and bladder tumors have been reported in patients receiving long-term therapy for both malignant and nonmalignant diseases. Acute myocardial necrosis also has been observed in patients receiving extremely large doses (> 100 mg/kg) of cyclophosphamide before bone marrow transplantation; most instances of cardiac toxicity occur at total doses of greater than 1.55 g/m^2. Other predisposing factors are age greater than 50 years and prior anthracycline therapy.[123]

Pharmacokinetics

The pharmacokinetics of cyclophosphamide and its metabolites have been studied to a limited extent; because the active metabolites are generated intracellularly from 4-hydroxycyclophosphamide, it is difficult to relate these studies to clinical toxicity. Cyclophosphamide and its 4-OH metabolite can be assayed in plasma by gas chromatography with nitrogen-phosphorous detection.[124] The half-life of the parent compound is 5.3 hours in adults, with somewhat more rapid clearance in children. The half-life for 4-OH cyclophosphamide is 1.5 to 6.0 hours and is primarily a function of its rate of formation in liver.[125] Of possible relevance to the selective action of cyclophosphamide is the longer half-life for repair of phosphoramide mustard adducts to DNA (8.5 hours) compared with 1.6 hours for nitrogen mustard adducts.[126] In patients with renal or hepatic failure, the serum half-life of cyclophosphamide is prolonged and correlates with increased myelosuppression.[127]

IFOSFAMIDE

Ifosfamide, a drug closely related to cyclophosphamide by virtue of its oxazaphosphorine ring structure, differs in its pattern of toxicity, causing less myelosuppression but dose-limiting cystitis. Like cyclophosphamide, it is activated by hepatic P-450 mixed-function oxidase, and alkylating metabolites are excreted in the urine. MESNA effectively prevents cystitis, even in patients with a history of cyclophosphamide-related or ifosfamide-related cystitis.[128] Other significant toxicities include cerebellar dysfunction, seizures, and altered mental status in as many as 30% of patients treated with high doses of ifosfamide (1.6 g/m^2/d for 5 days, or >5 g/day as a single dose). The risk of neurotoxicity appears related to hepatic dysfunction.[129] High levels of a potentially neurotoxic metabolite, chloroacetaldehyde, have been detected in patients by gas chromatography.[130]

The drug is well-absorbed orally (100% bioavailability) and has a plasma half-life of 5 to 6 hours after either oral or intravenous administration.[131] It is usually administered as a continuous 5-day infusion in doses up to 2400 mg/m^2/day, with equivalent mg doses of MESNA, or in doses up to 3 g/m^2 daily for two doses every 14 to 28 days, with 600 mg/m^2 MESNA every 4 hours for 48 hours. Patients should be hydrated, with a urine specific gravity below 1.010 before drug administration.

MELPHALAN

Melphalan, a phenylalanine derivative, was conceived as a compound that would localize preferentially in tumors, such as melanin-producing malignancies, that actively use phenylalanine or tyrosine. The resulting compound has a broad spectrum of antitumor activity similar to that of cyclophosphamide (lymphomas, breast and ovarian cancers, multiple myeloma) but has the added advantage of not causing hemorrhagic cystitis.

Melphalan enters cells by active transport, using a high-affinity carrier—the "L" amino acid transport system, which also transports the amino acids leucine and glutamine. In some tumor cells, a second transport system (which also carries alanine, cysteine, and serine) promotes melphalan uptake but is less effective than the L system at high drug concentrations.[132] High concentrations of leucine and glutamine can reduce melphalan toxicity in both bone marrow colony-forming units in vitro and in tumor cells.[133] Thus, amino acid concentration in plasma or ascitic fluid may influence the uptake and cytotoxicity of melphalan. The antiestrogen tamoxifen inhibits melphalan uptake by breast cancer cells.[134]

The drug shows variable bioavailability when given orally, and thus doses must be adjusted by this route according to bone marrow tolerance.[135] Food slows its absorption. After oral administration, between 20% and 50% of the oral drug is excreted in the stool. After IV administration, the parent compound disappears from plasma with a half-life of approximately 1 to 2 hours, a rate consistent with the rate of hydrolysis of the chloride groups in plasma, with little influence of dose. Monohydroxy and dihydroxy metabolites, as well as alkylated proteins, are found in plasma soon after IV drug administration. About 15% of the drug is excreted intact in the urine.[136] The drug should be used cautiously in patients with severe renal failure, and doses should be reduced initially in patients with greater than 50% reduction in creatinine clearance.

Because the parent compound does not irritate peritoneal surfaces and does not require hepatic activation, melphalan has been employed for treatment of intraperitoneal malignancy by direct intraperitoneal installation.[137] A 100:1 gradient in drug concentration between peritoneal fluid and plasma is achieved by this route, with little systemic toxicity. This schedule produces antitumor responses, but its ultimate usefulness in ovarian cancer and other intraperitoneal tumors has not been established.

Melphalan causes equal suppression of granulocyte and platelet production. These effects are reversed in 10 to 14 days. Alopecia is also common during extended courses of treatment. Melphalan appears to be more carcinogenic than cyclophosphamide. An analysis of acute leukemia in women with ovarian cancer revealed a 93-fold increase in incidence compared with the general, age-matched population and a twofold to threefold increase compared with patients treated with cyclophosphamide.[138]

CHLORAMBUCIL

Chlorambucil, a close structural congener of melphalan, has similar stability in aqueous solution because of the electron-withdrawing properties of its unsaturated ring. Chlorambucil is given orally and is a convenient alkylating agent for treatment of malignancies such as chronic lymphocytic leukemia (CLL), nodular lymphomas, or multiple myeloma, which require long-term management. It has predictable myelosuppressive effects on both granulocytes and platelets but few other side-effects. Like other alkylating agents, chlorambucil has been implicated in late occurrences of AML and in pulmonary fibrosis.[139,140] Its pharmacokinetics are poorly understood, but the drug appears to be eliminated by metabolic transformation.

BUSULFAN

Busulfan consists of two labile methane-sulfonate groups attached at opposite ends of a four-carbon alkyl chain (Fig. 18-13). This compound is stable enough to allow oral administration but rapidly forms carbonium ions after systemic absorption through release of the methane-sulfonate group, leading to alkylation of DNA.[141] Although the potential for interstrand cross-linkage exists in the bifunctional structure of busulfan, such cross-linkage has not been demonstrated.

This agent is used primarily in schedules of daily oral administration for the treatment of chronic granulocytic leukemia, where its strongly myelosuppressive action provides smooth, long-term regulation of the leukocyte count. However, myelosuppression produced by busulfan is not quickly reversible; bone marrow "burn out" may last indefinitely if excessive doses are used, and close monitoring of blood counts is essential. The relationship between drug concentration in plasma and myelotoxicity is not known.

In addition to myelosuppression, busulfan causes two unusual side-effects: diffuse pulmonary fibrosis and an Addisonian-like state characterized by cutaneous hyperpigmentation and weakness, but without abnormalities of adrenal function.

NITROSOUREA

The chloroethylnitrosoureas are highly lipid-soluble and chemically reactive compounds that are clinically active against the lymphomas, malignant melanomas, brain neoplasms, and gastrointestinal carcinomas. Many derivatives that incorporate this basic structure but differ in their lipid solubility, side-group substitution, and aqueous stability have been synthesized in an effort to improve their therapeutic index.[142] Chlorozotocin, streptozotocin, and other glycosylated nitrosoureas (Fig. 18-13) have less bone marrow toxicity but have unproven clinical usefulness.

Chemical decomposition of these agents in aqueous solution (Fig. 18-15) yields two reactive intermediates, a chloroethyldiazohydroxide (II) and an isocyanate group (III). The former decomposes further to yield a reactive chloroethyl carbonium ion (IV) that forms a single-strand adduct with DNA and then, through a dehalogenation step, forms a second reactive site and cross-links DNA. Thus, cross-links are produced by both the monofunctional and bifunctional nitrosoureas.[143]

In distinction to the classic alkylating agents, decomposition of nitrosoureas also yields isocyanates (III) that react with amine groups in a carbamoylation reaction. The isocyanates are believed to deplete glutathione, inhibit DNA repair, and alter maturation of RNA. However, although carbamoylation may contribute to the overall effects of the nitrosoureas, compounds such as chlorozotocin that lack significant carbamoylating activity still preserve antitumor activity. Thus alkylation seems to be a more important feature of nitrosourea action.[144,145]

The nitrosoureas have many of the same features as classical alkylating agents. Their activity is enhanced by nitroimidazoles, hyperthermia, and glutathione depletion. They do not, in many experimental systems, share cross-resistance

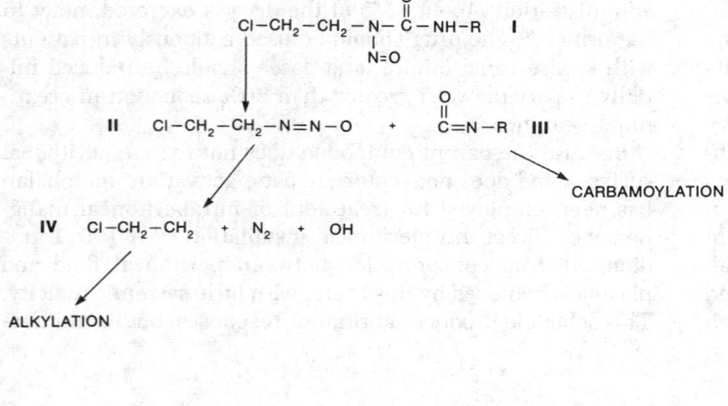

FIG. 18-15. Decomposition of chloroethylnitrosoureas to form chloroethyl carbonium ion and a carbamoylating isocyanate group.

with the classical alkylators. Nitrosourea resistance has been ascribed to increased levels of glutathione-S-transferase and to a specific repair enzyme, guanine-O^6-methyl transferase (found in 80% of tumor cells).

As a result of the extreme clinical reactivity of these compounds in aqueous solution, they disappear rapidly from the blood after absorption or IV infusion. BCNU has a half-life of 22 minutes, while the orally administered CCNU is not detectable as parent drug in plasma.[146] The cyclohexylnitrosoureas undergo ring hydroxylation by hepatic microsomes, resulting in decreased carbamoylating potential but increased alkylating activity.[147] The high lipid solubility of the nitrosoureas may account for their excellent activity against experimental and clinical intracranial tumors; the chloroethyl portion of CCNU crosses readily into the CNS, reaching concentrations that are 30% of those of combined parent and metabolites in plasma.

The toxicities of the clinically useful nitrosoureas are listed in Table 18-1. The most notable and consistent toxicity is delayed myelosuppression, which reaches a nadir 4 to 6 weeks after treatment and prevents the repetition of cyclic therapy at intervals shorter than 6 to 8 weeks. Severe and protracted leukopenia and thrombocytopenia may occur in patients receiving conventional doses of BCNU, CCNU, or methyl-CCNU, particularly in those who have received extensive prior chemotherapy. Prolonged use of these drugs leads to cumulative bone marrow toxicity and, in some patients, to an aplastic bone marrow. AML has been reported following methyl-CCNU treatment.[148]

Prolonged courses of treatment with BCNU and with methyl-CCNU have been associated with pulmonary fibrosis. The total dose of BCNU was 1000 mg/m^2 or greater in all cases reported and was 2733 mg/m^2 for the one reported case of pulmonary fibrosis induced by methyl-CCNU.[149] Chronic renal failure has been reported in children receiving methyl-CCNU for the treatment of brain tumor.[150] Azotemia or elevated serum creatinine levels developed after treatment was stopped in five of six patients who received more than 1500 mg/m^2 methyl-CCNU, and a decrease in kidney size was observed in all six patients. Total doses greater than 1200 mg/m^2 of either BCNU or methyl-CCNU are associated with an increased risk of renal failure.

CISPLATIN

Cis (II) platinum diamminedichloride (cis-DDP) is the only heavy metal compound used as a cancer chemotherapeutic agent and has a spectrum of unique biologic effects. The biologic activity of platinum coordinate compounds was first recognized in 1965.[151,152] Cis-DDP subsequently entered clinical trials in 1971 and since then has become established as a highly effective drug for treating testicular tumors, ovarian carcinoma, bladder carcinoma, and head and neck cancer.

The antitumor activity of cis-DDP is best understood in terms of its chemical properties in aqueous solution (Fig. 18-16). The tetravalent heavy metal platinum (Pt) binds two potential leaving groups, its chloride ions; in transposition to the chlorides are bound two NH groups in a firm linkage. Only the cis-dichloro structure is an active antitumor agent; the trans-DDP isomer lacks cytotoxic activity, possibly because of its inability to form stable intrastrand DNA cross-links.[153] Both chloride ions undergo a slow displacement by water, a process that may be accelerated in an environment of low chloride concentration (e.g., inside the cell or in urine), generating a positively charged, aquated complex. This activated complex then can interact with a nucleophilic site on DNA, RNA, or protein to form bifunctional covalent links analogous to alkylating reactions. Favored sites of attack are the N^7 position of guanine and the N^3 position of cytosine.[154] A variety of bifunctional and monofunctional covalent bonds are possible, including intrastrand cross-links, interstrand links, and DNA–protein complexes.[155] The formation of intrastrand cross-links, a type of bond not formed by *trans*-DDP, may be an important feature of cis-DDP action, particularly those links that form between the N^7, N^1, or O^6 of one guanine base and the N^3 of a neighboring cytosine.

The consequences of cis-DDP attack on DNA include changes in DNA conformation and inhibition of DNA synthesis.[156] The formation of cross-links is a slow process that continues for hours after drug exposure and is opposed by enzymatic repair processes that excise and rebuild damaged segments of DNA and ultimately determine cytotoxicity.[157,158] DNA cross-links also may be prevented by preincubating the drug with thiourea, which combines readily with the aquated platinum binding sites.[159] Thiourea also can reverse interstrand cross-links in isolated DNA, but the concentrations of thiol required for this reversal cannot be achieved within intact cells.

Other thiols, including sodium thiosulfate, which decreases cis-DDP systemic toxicity, and diethyl dithiocarbamate, which specifically prevents cis-DDP renal toxicity, are potentially of clinical value, particularly in conjunction with

FIG. 18-16. Cis-diamminedichloroplatinum: generation of a reactive complex in aqueous solution.

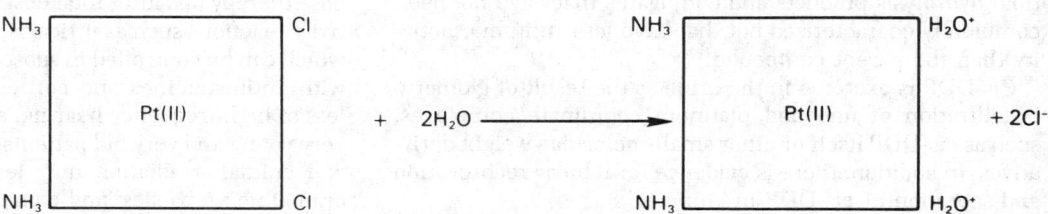

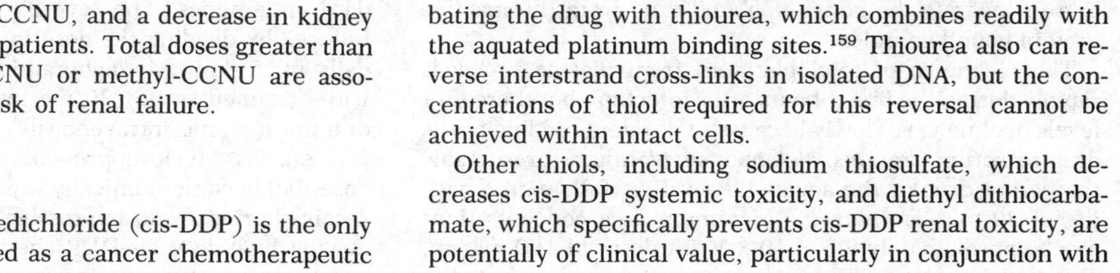

intraperitoneal cis-DDP, or during high-dose cis-DDP therapy.[160] The radioprotector WR2721 also ameliorates platinum toxicity by conjugation with the reactive aquated drug; this combination is undergoing clinical evaluation.[161]

The cell-cycle dependence of cis-DDP is poorly understood. It appears that some cells are most sensitive to cis-DDP when exposed during the G_1 (intermitotic) phase of the cycle, possibly because of the delay in cross-link formation, which would then be maximal during the following S phase.[162] A delay in transit through S phase and the succeeding cell cycle is induced by drug treatment.

Little is known about the mechanisms of resistance to cis-DDP. Resistance to cis-DDP in some experimental studies has been linked to elevated levels of intracellular glutathione or the thiol-rich protein metallothionine.[163] It is likely that the ability to prevent (through sulfhydryl reaction) or repair DNA cross-links plays an important role in determining sensitivity to this drug.[158] Platinum compounds do not share cross-resistance with nitrosoureas or classic alkylating agents in most experimental systems. Although specific processes that repair DNA-platinum adducts have not been identified, it has been possible to quantitate adduct formation with extreme sensitivity and to correlate the level of adducts in peripheral blood leukocytes with the dose of cis-DDP and response to treatment in patients with ovarian cancer.[164] These findings imply that pharmacogenetic or metabolic characteristics common to tumor and peripheral tissues determine response to cis-DDP.

Clinical Pharmacology

Cis-platinum is measured readily in biologic fluids by flameless atomic absorption spectroscopy, a technique that has high sensitivity (about 0.3 μg/ml) and specificity but is not routinely available in pharmacology laboratories.[165] HPLC allows separation and quantitation of the parent drug and its hydrolysis products.[166] Because of the high rate of covalent binding to protein, plasma samples must undergo ultrafiltration to separate the active unbound drug from the inactive protein-bound complex.

The clearance of total platinum from plasma proceeds rapidly during the first 2 hours after injection, but thereafter levels decline very slowly because of covalent binding of the drug to serum proteins.[167] Unbound platinum, presumably the parent drug or the aquated derivative, falls with a half-life of 30 to 40 minutes.[168] Maximum drug concentrations reach approximately 2.5×10^{-5} M for doses of 100 mg/m^2. Twenty percent to 75% of administered drug is excreted in the urine in the 24 hours after administration, the remainder representing drug bound to tissues or plasma protein.[169] Cis-DDP penetrates poorly into the central nervous system.[170] Even after simple incubation in plasma, the drug forms multiple hydrolysis products and conjugates that have not been completely characterized but that have less antitumor activity than the parent compound.[171]

Cis-DDP is excreted in the urine as the result of glomerular filtration of unbound platinum coordinate complexes, such as cis-DDP itself or other small-molecular-weight derivatives. In addition, there is evidence for tubular reabsorption and secretion of cis-DDP in animals.[172]

Dose, Schedule, and Toxicity

The mode of clinical administration of cis-DDP is determined largely by its primary toxicities. Because of its nephrotoxic potential, cis-DDP usually is administered after a 4-hour to 6-hour period of hydration with 1 liter of fluid and 25 to 50 g of mannitol.[173] Mannitol or furosemide diuresis does not alter the pharmacokinetics of cis-DDP. The total dose administered in most regimens usually is between 40 and 120 mg/m^2 per cycle of therapy but depends on the frequency of cycles and individual patient tolerance. A common schedule is 20 mg/m^2/day for 5 days, a regimen that causes little nephrotoxicity and tolerable nausea.

Renal toxicity of high-dose cis-DDP may be prevented by saline diuresis. The regimen consists of 250 ml normal saline/hour for 12 hours before cis-DDP, continuing for 12 hours after cis-DDP. Furosemide is given with each dose of drug. cis-DDP is administered in 250 ml of 3% hypertonic saline. This regimen allows a dosage as high as 40 mg/m^2/day for 5 days with no significant decrease in creatinine clearance.[174]

Without hydration, the incidence of nephrotoxicity reaches 30% in patients treated with 50 to 75 mg/m^2 per course.[175] Although both the proximal and distal tubules are pathologically affected in animals, in humans the primary finding is coagulative necrosis of the distal tubular epithelium and collecting ducts.[176] A reduction in renal blood flow and glomerular filtration rate occurs within hours of cis-DDP administration, as does a series of changes in tubular function, including magnesium and potassium wasting and the excretion of various high-molecular-weight proteins.[177,178] Asymptomatic hypomagnesemia is a common finding in patients treated with cis-DDP, but magnesium loss may lead to symptomatic tetany. With adequate hydration, repeated cycles of treatment can be tolerated by most patients without clinical impairment of renal function.

Nausea and vomiting are frequent and persistent in patients taking cis-DDP and are relieved only partially by standard antiemetics. The severity of these symptoms can be reduced by dividing the dose into smaller doses given once daily for 5 days. Metoclopramide (3 mg/kg intravenously) with dexamethasone (20 mg intravenously) and diphenhydramine (50 mg intravenously) ameliorate but do not prevent emesis. Myelosuppression is moderate at usual clinical doses but becomes clinically significant in patients who have received prior myelosuppressive treatment or in patients receiving high-dose cis-DDP chemotherapy. Both leukopenia and thrombocytopenia occur; significant anemia, occasionally caused by hemolysis, may develop after extended periods of treatment.

Other toxicities include a distal sensory neuropathy that develops after prolonged treatment, particularly after high-dose therapy and after total doses of 300 mg/m^2, hypersensitivity reactions such as urticaria, wheezing, and hypotension, which can be controlled in subsequent doses by pretreatment with antihistamines and corticosteroids; and a progressive loss of high-frequency hearing, an effect found most often in very young and very old patients.[179,180] Concomitant cis-DDP and cranial irradiation may lead to enhanced ototoxicity, cranial nerve palsies, and coma in pediatric patients.[181] cis-

DDP is mutagenic to mammalian cells and is carcinogenic in animals.

cis-DDP has been administered by intraperitoneal instillation in patients with intraperitoneal malignancy; 200 mg/m^2 cis-DDP is diluted in 2 liters of dialysate and instilled in the peritoneal cavity. Residual peritoneal fluid is withdrawn after 4 hours. Systemic toxicity can be prevented by simultaneous administration of sodium thiosulfate (7.5 gm/m^2 by bolus followed by 2.13 gm/m^2 over 12 hours). The half-life of intraperitoneal cis-DDP is approximately 1 hour, and most drug is inactivated before it reaches the systemic circulation. Thus, high local concentrations of cis-DDP (approaching 1 mM) can be achieved in the peritoneal cavity with minimal systemic toxicity. A 20 : 1 gradient in free cis-DDP concentration is established between the peritoneal fluid and plasma. Although responses have been observed in patients with ovarian cancer refractory to systemic cis-DDP, the value of this therapy remains uncertain.[182]

Other experimental approaches to the prevention of cis-DDP toxicity have been considered, including the development of new analogues. Two analogues, CHIP (cis-dichlorotranshydroxy-bis-isopropylamine platinum IV) and CBDCA (carboplatin), produced myelosuppression but little renal toxicity or ototoxicity in initial trials. CBDCA has the most promising antitumor activity (ovarian cancer, testicular cancer, and head and neck cancer). It is less reactive in solution than cis-DDP and is limited by thrombocytopenia and leukopenia, with minimal or no toxicity to the kidneys, hearing, and peripheral nerves. CBDCA is eliminated by renal excretion; dose adjustment should be based on creatinine clearance.[183]

ANTITUMOR ANTIBIOTICS

BLEOMYCIN

One of the most unusual structures that has antitumor activity is bleomycin, a mixture of small-molecular-weight (1500 daltons) peptides isolated from the fungus *Streptomyces verticullus*. Bleomycin is one of a family of antibiotic peptides that possess both antitumor and antimicrobial activity. The bleomycin mixture contains mostly the A_2 peptide, the unique pharmacologic properties of which have been characterized extensively.

The structure of the A_2 compound consists of a DNA-binding fragment and an iron-binding portion located at the opposite end of the molecule. The primary action of bleomycin is to produce single-strand and double-strand breaks in DNA.[184] The sequence of events leading to DNA breakage begins with the binding to DNA, preferentially to G-T or G-C sequences. Ferrous ion (Fe^{2+}), which is bound intimately to the imidazole, pyrimidine, and other nitrogen-containing groups of bleomycin, undergoes spontaneous or enzymatic oxidation to the Fe^{3+} state. The electron that is liberated in this reaction is accepted by oxygen and forms active oxygen intermediates, such as the superoxide or hydroxyl radicals. These radicals, in turn, attack the 4′-H of deoxyribose, leading to cleavage of the sugar and release of its attached base, usually thymine, cytosine, or their propenal adducts.[185] The action of bleomycin is specific for DNA and is not exerted against RNA.

There appears to be some cytokinetic specificity to bleomycin cell kill.[186] Cells in synchronized culture systems are most susceptible during the premitotic or G_2 phase, or in the mitotic phase of the cell cycle. However, cells exposed during G_1; also are killed, and it is not known whether rapid cell division predisposes to cytotoxicity. The possibility of increasing cell kill by exposing cells during the G_2 phase has prompted trials of bleomycin administration by continuous infusion.

The DNA lesions produced by bleomycin are visible as chromosomal breaks and deletions. It seems likely that repair processes play an important role in determining the lethality of these lesions because repair of potentially lethal damage occurs in cultured cells exposed to this agent.[187] There is indirect evidence that the same processes required to repair ionizing radiation damage also are used in bleomycin repair. The repair process is inhibited by calmodulin antagonists such as trifluoperazine.[188] Glutathione enhances bleomycin cytotoxicity, as does misonidazole.[189] Enhancement by glutathione likely relates to the need to recycle the Fe^{3+} ion to its active Fe^{2+} state with each oxidation–reduction cycle.

Little is known about the determinants of bleomycin resistance in tumor cells. A bleomycin-inactivating enzyme has been detected in both normal and malignant cells and is particularly prominent in the liver.[190] The enzyme is found in low concentrations in lung and skin; its concentration in lung varies from one species to another and appears to determine the susceptibility to pulmonary injury.[191] Increased degradative activity has been found in resistant experimental tumors.[192]

Clinical Pharmacology and Pharmacokinetics

The most sensitive and reliable technique for assay of bleomycin is radioimmunoassay; ^{125}I or ^{57}Co-bleomycin is used in this assay.[193]

Bleomycin is administered by parenteral injection, either subcutaneously (SC), intramuscularly (IM), or IV. There are no obvious differences in clinical response rates associated with the different routes, although continuous IV infusion has been used widely in the curative treatment of testicular cancer (see Chap. 35). Bleomycin has a two-phased plasma disappearance curve with half-lives of 24 minutes and 2 to 4 hours. Peak plasma concentrations reach 1 to 10 mU/ml after IV bolus doses of 15 U/m^2. The postinfusion half-life is approximately 3 hours, a value similar to the β-half-life following bolus administration. Most bleomycin is excreted unchanged in the urine in patients with normal renal function.[194]

Bleomycin pharmacokinetics are altered markedly in patients with abnormal renal function. A half-life of 21 hours has been observed in a patient with a creatinine clearance of 11 ml/min. It thus would be wise to decrease the dosage of bleomycin by 50% to 75% in patients with severely compromised renal function, who are at high risk for pulmonary toxicity, probably because of altered drug-excretion rates.

In addition to conventional routes of administration, bleomycin may be injected into the pleural or peritoneal space to control malignant effusions.[195] Intracavitary doses of 60 mg/m^2 provide high-effusion concentrations of up to 50 mU/ml, or approximately tenfold higher levels than in plasma. About 50% of an intracavitary dose enters the systemic circulation; the remaining fraction either is metabolized in the pleural or peritoneal cavity or is eliminated in its first pass through the portal circulation.

Clinical Toxicity

In contrast to most antitumor agents, bleomycin has little myelosuppressive toxicity. Only at high doses (> 25 mg/m^2) or in patients with severely compromised bone marrow is a decrease in white blood cell count or platelet count observed. The primary toxicity of bleomycin is subacute or chronic pneumonitis that progresses to interstitial fibrosis.

The first signs are cough, dyspnea, and fever. The carbon monoxide diffusion capacity of the lung is decreased progressively with increased total doses of the drug, particularly above 250 mg, and the incidence of clinically significant pulmonary toxicity reaches 10% at total doses of 450 mg or greater.[196] Carbon monoxide diffusion capacity does not appear to be a reliable predictor of impending pulmonary toxicity in asymptomatic patients, most of whom will experience a steady, dose-related decrease of 10% to 15% in this sign over the course of treatment.[197] Toxicity is most frequent in older patients (over 70 years of age), in those with underlying lung disease such as emphysema, and in those previously treated with pulmonary or mediastinal irradiation. Although there appears to be a close relationship between total dose and risk of toxicity, well-documented cases have been observed at total doses below 100 mg.

There are anecdotal cases to suggest that pulmonary fibrosis can be prevented with corticosteroid.

The clinical symptoms and x-ray findings of bleomycin-induced pulmonary toxicity are not distinguished easily from other syndromes commonly found in cancer patients, including progressive metastatic tumor (especially lymphangitic tumor), infectious processes such as *Pneumocystis carinii* or cytomegalovirus, and radiation injury. Radiologic abnormalities, including linear and nodular densities, which may become confluent, are detectable by CT scanning in approximately 40% of asymptomatic patients receiving bleomycin, even though routine chest films are usually negative.[198] Symptomatic patients usually show bibasilar pulmonary infiltrates on chest x-ray film, although symptoms may precede the appearance of obvious radiologic findings. Gallium scans may detect drug-induced effects before routine chest x-ray films. Open lung biopsy often is required, and it reveals an acute inflammatory infiltrate, interstitial and intra-alveolar edema, pulmonary hyaline membrane formation, and intra-alveolar and interstitial fibrosis. In addition, squamous metaplasia of the alveolar lining cells often is found. Radiologic evidence of pulmonary toxicity and abnormalities in carbon monoxide diffusion resolve in most asymptomatic patients after therapy is discontinued. Resolution of abnormalities is often incomplete in symptomatic patients.

Bleomycin frequently produces an unusual cutaneous adverse reaction. Almost 50% of patients develop erythema, induration, thickening, and eventual peeling of the skin on the fingers, palms, and extremity joints. In addition, most patients develop hyperpigmentation of skin creases and a general darkening of the skin. Some patients also may develop Raynaud's phenomenon during bleomycin therapy.

Less frequent side-effects include acute hypertension, primarily in patients receiving doses greater than 25 mg/day, and hyperbilirubinemia. Fever often is observed in the first 48 hours after drug administration, and occasional hypersensitivity reactions, with urticaria and bronchospasm, have been observed. These reactions usually do not necessitate withdrawal of the drug, but pretreatment with antihistamines and corticosteroids is recommended for patients who have a history of allergic reactions to bleomycin.

In addition to its conventional systemic use, bleomycin has been administered by intraarterial infusion and by direct instillation into the urinary bladder.[199,200] The latter route causes a predictable and, at times, severe cystitis. Neither of these routes has proved to be beneficial in the treatment of cancer.

ANTHRACYCLINES

The first anthracyclines in clinical use, daunomycin and doxorubicin, are antibiotics produced from the *Streptomyces* species. These antibodies are, in fact, part of a large group of highly colored bacterial products known as the rhodomycins. There are exhaustive reviews of the structure and properties of the rhodomycins.[201,202] In general, these compounds, like daunomycin and doxorubicin, have a planar anthraquinone nucleus attached to an amino sugar (Fig. 18-17). Within this group, or closely related to it, are compounds that have a wide range of biologic activity, which include antibacterial and antitumor agents.

As antitumor agents, anthracyclines are matched only by alkylating agents in terms of their clinical usefulness. Daunorubicin is one of the most effective agents in the treatment of acute lymphocytic and myelocytic leukemia. Doxorubicin, on the other hand, is used to treat solid tumors, such as carcinomas of the breast, lung, thyroid, and ovary, and soft tissue sarcomas. As a result of this clinical activity, more

FIG. 18-17. Structure of anthracyclines.

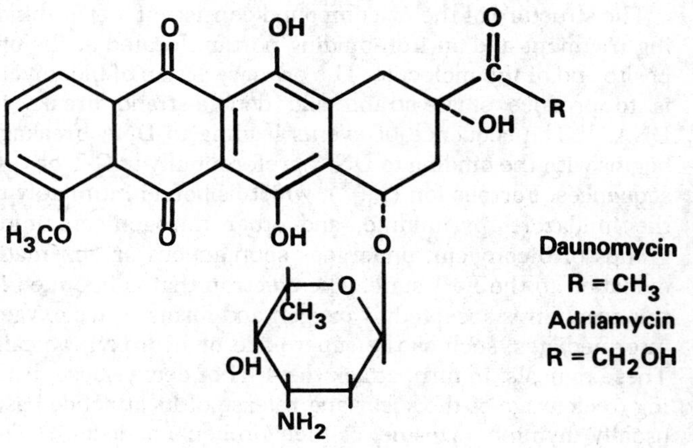

than 500 analogues have been synthesized or isolated from *Streptomyces*. It is likely these will provide the clinician with a number of new anthracyclines with different therapeutic spectra or altered toxicity. For this reason, we shall place some emphasis in this section on pertinent structure–activity relationships.

Mechanism of Action

There is no single, clearly defined mechanism of action for the anthraquinones. Anthraquinones, of which the anthracyclines are a subset, exhibit a wide range of biologic, biochemical, and chemical properties.[203] They are known to chelate divalent cations, especially calcium, and as a result can alter bone metabolism and dissolve kidney stones. Other anthraquinones have laxative effects. Because of the quinone-hydroquinone functionalities characteristic of the anthraquinones, these compounds can participate in oxidation–reduction reactions. Because of the size and planar nature of the anthraquinones, many agents in this group intercalate between strands of the DNA double helix.

Doxorubicin and daunorubicin are known to intercalate DNA, chelate transition metal ions, such as iron or copper, and engage in oxidation–reduction reactions.[204,205] In addition, these agents react directly with cell membranes at low concentrations, with resultant alterations in membrane function.[206,207]

Of these actions, we know most about the interaction with DNA. Both doxorubicin and daunorubicin act as intercalators with the planar anthracycline ring structure that lies perpendicular to the long axis of the DNA double helix. The B and C rings appear to be buried within the helix, with the A and D rings projecting out on either side. The amino sugar appears to add stability to the binding through its interaction with the sugar-phosphate backbone of DNA. DNA intercalation has been shown to block DNA replication and RNA and protein synthesis. However, the drug concentrations required to do so are far greater than those that are clinically relevant. It is now clear that these effects have nothing to do with the clinical utility of these drugs as anticancer agents. DNA intercalation does appear to trigger DNA cleavage by topoisomerase-II, an enzyme critical in the maintenance of DNA tertiary structure.[208] There is now strong circumstantial evidence that supports this topoisomerase-II-mediated antitumor effect in murine cell lines such as L1210.[209] This effect can be demonstrated within a clinically useful drug concentration range.[210]

Another school of thought advocates that the antitumor effect is due to the formation of drug free radicals.[211,212] A wide range of NADPH-dependent reductases, such as cytochrome P-450 reductase, xanthine oxidase, and cytochrome B_5 reductase, are able to reduce doxorubicin and daunomycin to semiquinone free radicals that, in turn, can react with molecular oxygen to yield superoxide, hydrogen peroxide, and the hydroxyl radical.[213] Several workers have shown that this process is the mechanism by which doxorubicin kills human breast cancer cells in vitro. Superoxide dismutase and catalase both protect the MCF-7 human breast cancer cell line at doxorubicin concentrations as low as 10 nM.[211,212]

Doxorubicin may kill tumor cells by either mechanism, depending upon the biochemistry of the tumor being treated. For example, the finding of free-radical formation in breast cancer cells may be conditioned by the high levels of microsomal enzyme activity in that tissue.[212] There are other factors as well. Drug free-radical formation is NADPH-dependent. NADPH is predominantly the product of the pentose phosphate shunt and is also used for such key biochemical processes as fatty acid synthesis. Perhaps because it must produce milk fat, breast tissue is second only to the adrenal gland in the activity of its pentose shunt. This elevated pentose shunt activity is also found in breast cancer cell lines and guarantees adequate NADPH for doxorubicin free-radical formation.[214]

One of the most unusual aspects of the anthracyclines is the ability of these agents to cause cardiomyopathy. Most of the existing evidence supports free-radical formation as the basis for this toxicity. Other hypotheses have been put forward over the years, but none has survived experimental scrutiny for very long. It is now clear that heart tissue is able to activate doxorubicin to a free radical at multiple sites, including the cytosol, mitochondria, and sarcoplasmic reticulum.[215] In addition, cardiac tissue has very low levels of catalase, a key enzyme in the detoxification of hydrogen peroxide.[216] In addition, doxorubicin destroys glutathione peroxidase activity, a second major mechanism of peroxide removal. Thus, doxorubicin stimulates oxygen-radical formation in the heart muscle while simultaneously abrogating the major mechanism by which the heart defends itself against oxygen radicals.

The major criticism of the free-radical hypothesis was that free-radical scavengers, such as tocopherol and N-acetylcysteine, have not been successful in preventing the cardiac toxicity in man. However, at the time these studies were run, the unique involvement of iron in doxorubicin biochemistry was not appreciated.[217] We now know that in most experimental systems involving cells or subcellular organelles, iron must be present for doxorubicin free-radical formation to result in significant damage. Doxorubicin is a remarkably active iron chelator, with measured binding affinities of 10^{28} to 10^{33}. The resulting iron–doxorubicin complex is very reactive in catalyzing a variety of free-radical reactions, such as the conversion of hydrogen peroxide to hydroxyl radical. Neither tocopherol nor thiols such as N-acetylcysteine are very effective in blocking this chemistry.

The logical conclusion of all of this work on doxorubicin chemistry is that the most critical step in the reactions leading up to free-radical-induced cardiac injury is the reaction between doxorubicin, iron, and peroxide. Thus, it is no surprise that the first clinically successful cardioprotective agent is an effective iron chelator, ICRF-187.[218]

This EDTA derivative was originally synthesized as an anticancer agent (Fig. 18-18). The initial phase I clinical trial showed that this drug was a remarkably effective iron chelator, causing a greater than tenfold increase in urinary iron clearance.[219] Preclinical studies had documented that this agent also prevented doxorubicin cardiac toxicity in a wide range of animal species.[220] More recently a randomized clinical trial has demonstrated that ICRF-187 is able to dramatically lessen the cardiac toxicity of doxorubicin in man

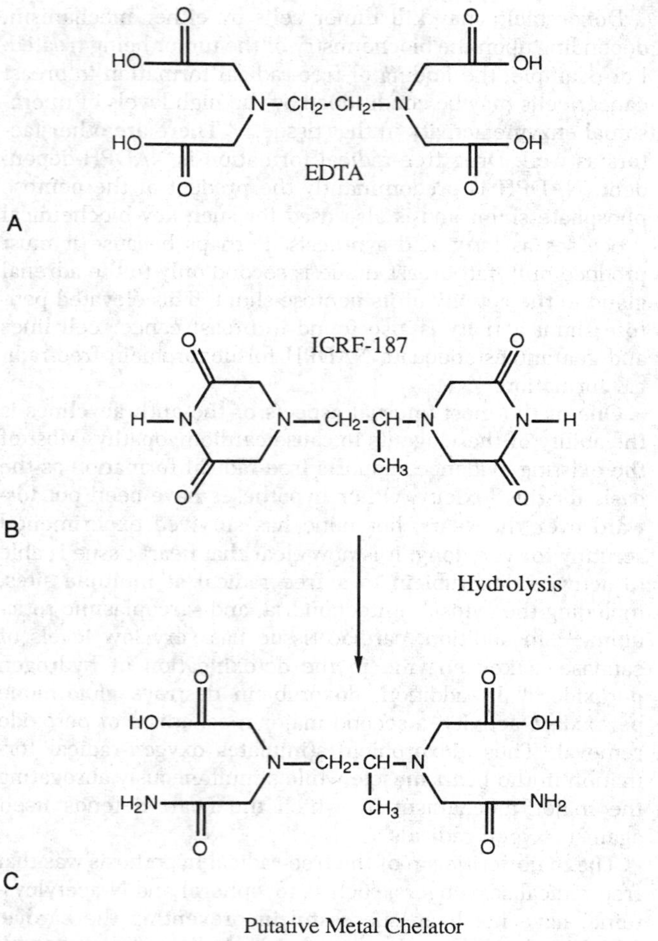

FIG. 18-18. **A.** A strongly charged anion at physiologic pH. Enters cells poorly. **B.** Nonpolar and should enter cells well, but a weak chelator. **C.** A better metal chelator, but will be highly charged like EDTA.

without seriously compromising antitumor activity.[218] While this study obviously needs confirmation, the result is entirely consistent with the biochemistry and preclinical toxicology of the drug.

Clinical Pharmacology and Pharmacokinetics

The clinical pharmacology of the anthracyclines is in its infancy. Only within the past few years has adequate assay methodology become available. For many years, thin-layer chromatography was the method used to separate the parent drug from its metabolites. It now is known that many anthracyclines (*i.e.*, doxorubicin) are unstable on thin-layer chromatographic plates and that significant artifacts resulted from this process. Currently, the only valid assay methodology is with HPLC, which allows rapid resolution of doxorubicin and its metabolites.[221,222]

The major metabolites of daunorubicin and doxorubicin are doxorubicinol and daunorubicinol, the products of reduction by means of aldo-keto reductase. These compounds exhibit antitumor activity, although not as much as the parent drug. The parent drug and these metabolites also predominate in bile and urine. The deoxyalglycones, other metabolites of interest, are one of the by-products of semiquinone radical formation and thus are markers for this process in vivo. Other minor metabolites have been described, the importance of which is not known at present.[223] Although the pharmacokinetics of doxorubicin are undoubtedly complex, its disappearance curves can be fit to a three-compartment model with half-lives of 11 minutes, 3 hours, and 25 to 28 hours.[224] Clearance of doxorubicinol and daunorubicinol does not always parallel that of the parent drug.

The effects of renal and hepatic failure on doxorubicin and daunomycin clearance are important to the clinician because this information may provide a basis for rational modification of drug dosage in cases of malfunction of these organs. Renal clearance of anthracyclines is minor in magnitude, and there is no need to modify drug dosages because of renal failure. Both doxorubicin and daunorubicin are metabolized significantly in the liver. As a result, drug doses often are modified because of abnormal liver function, especially elevated bilirubin. Precise guidelines based on sound pharmacokinetic information, however, are completely lacking, and this subject warrants careful study. Nevertheless, existing information on the pharmacology of doxorubicin suggest that mild-to-moderate liver function abnormalities do not alter the pharmacokinetics of the drug. Furthermore, administration of full doses of doxorubicin in the face of abnormal liver function has not been associated with increased drug toxicity.[225] Because the liver is the major site of doxorubicin clearance, these observations are somewhat surprising. It may be that the prolonged terminal phase of doxorubicin clearance (half-life of 730 hours) is a function of the rate at which the drug dissociates from DNA, rather than a function of liver metabolism.

Toxicity

Both doxorubicin and daunorubicin cause bone marrow suppression and mucositis, which are dose-limiting. Alopecia is a nearly universal adverse effect that, although not life-threatening, often causes significant patient distress. Extravasation of these agents leads to severe local reaction. Erythema and pain usually develop within 24 hours and can progress over weeks, resulting in deep ulceration that can reach tendon and bone. These lesions heal very slowly and are difficult to skin graft. Multiple local measures used to manage this complication include ice packs and local injections of steroids, bicarbonate, or saline solution. Clearly, the best approach is to take all possible precautions to avoid extravasation.

Perhaps the most perplexing reaction these agents cause is cardiac toxicity. Clinically, two aspects are involved. First is an acute syndrome that can be seen for hours to days after a dose of doxorubicin or daunorubicin; it is unrelated to cumulative dose and can manifest as either disturbances in conduction and rhythm or pump failure. Electrocardiographic (ECG) studies have revealed supraventricular arrhythmias, heart block, and ventricular tachycardia. In addition, ECG-gated pool scans have shown major drops in ejection fraction that reach a nadir within 24 to 48 hours after drug administration. In certain patients, this can cause congestive heart failure. Some of these patients develop pericardial effusions, and this whole complex has been called the myocarditis–pericarditis syndrome. It can be severe enough to cause the sudden demise of the patient.

The other aspect of this toxicity is a cumulative, dose-dependent cardiomyopathy that can lead to congestive heart failure in 1% to 10% of the patients who receive a total dose of 550 mg/m^2 of doxorubicin. The pathologic features of this lesion are unique and can be quantitated readily by endocardial biopsy. This technique is valuable both in diagnosing the cause of congestive heart failure in patients who may have received doxorubicin and in detecting subclinical cardiac damage, which contraindicates further doxorubicin treatment. ECG-gated pool scan measurement of ejection fraction has proved valuable in detecting heart damage. It may be more practical than endocardial biopsy for widespread clinical use.

The mechanism of this cardiac toxicity was discussed in part earlier. It is important to note that three independent investigations suggest that this toxicity may not be related to the antitumor activity of these agents. First, antidotal agents such as ICRF-187 have lessened cardiac toxicity without affecting tumor response in animals. Second, new anthracyclines have been developed that, in animals, possess significantly less cardiac toxicity while preserving antitumor activity.[226,227] Third, alterations in drug schedule affect cardiac toxicity without changing antitumor efficacy.

Importance of Dose and Scheduling

The traditional method of administering doxorubicin was as a bolus at a dosage of 45 to 75 mg/m^2 every 3 to 4 weeks. It is with this dosage that the risk of cardiac toxicity as a function of total dose was developed. It is now clear that this method of drug administration is not optimal. Repeated small doses (every week) or prolonged infusions (>96 hours) are associated with a much lower risk of cardiac toxicity, without significantly compromising antitumor activity. On these schedules, gastrointestinal toxicity does, however, become a more significant problem.[228] Also, little has been done to work out how prolonged infusions of doxorubicin might be integrated into combination chemotherapy programs.

Analogues

While enormous effort has been expended on anthracycline analogue development, very few agents that have seen clinical trial offer any advantage over daunomycin or doxorubicin (Fig. 18-19). Epirubicin (4′-epidoxorubicin) has been claimed to be less cardiotoxic for equivalent therapeutic doses.[229] However, the advantage is not quantitatively impressive and may merely reflect differences in potency.

Idarubicin (4-demethyoxydaunomycin) has considerable activity in acute leukemia and may find limited use in that disease.[229] In addition, this drug also shows impressive activity in non-Hodgkin's lymphoma, with response rates of 55%, with a median duration of 6 months.[229] This drug has also

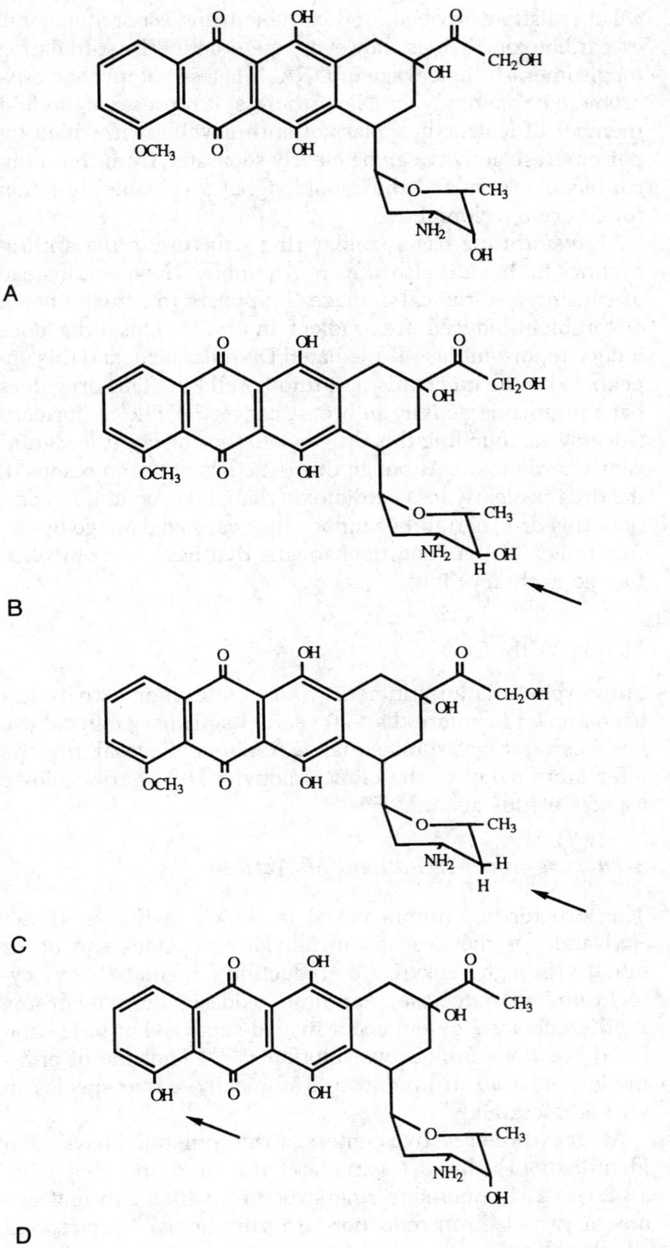

FIG. 18-19. **A.** Doxorubicin. **B.** Epirubicin. **C.** Esorubicin. **D.** Idarubicin.

exhibited very little cardiac toxicity in animal models and in clinical trials.

Esorubicin (4′-deoxydoxorubicin) has shown activity in melanoma, renal cancer and colon cancer. In colon cancer, one complete response and three partial responses occurred in 30 patients.[229] This relatively negative outcome to analogue development may reflect a genuine narrow range of opportunity in this drug class. However, it must be pointed out that several very interesting analogues have never been subjected to clinical trial.

5-Iminodaunomycin is quite inactive in all of the free-radical chemistry described for doxorubicin and is not mutagenic or cardiotoxic.[230] It is, however, quite active in stimulating topoisomerase-II cleavage of DNA. It is less potent than doxorubicin or daunomycin. Nevertheless, it represents the first member of a structural class of anthracyclines in which topoisomerase activity can be clearly separated from free-radical biochemistry and thus could signal a valuable direction for future development.

Mitoxanthrone has a similar ring structure to the anthracyclines in that it is also a hydroxyquinone. However, instead of causing free-radical damage, it appears to actually block doxorubicin-induced free-radical injury.[231] This drug does induce topoisomerase-II-mediated DNA damage, and this appears to be the mechanism of tumor cell kill. This drug does have promising activity in breast cancer.[232] The major controversy surrounding this drug is whether or not it is significantly cardiotoxic. Although this issue has not been resolved, the drug is clearly less cardiotoxic than doxorubicin. In addition, this drug certainly cannot cause cardiac damage by the free-radical-dependent mechanisms that have been invoked for the anthracyclines.

MITOMYCIN C

Mitomycin C is an antibiotic whose antitumor activity has been known for more than 20 years. Its primary clinical use has been for gastrointestinal carcinoma. Several reviews offer more detail of the clinical activity and pharmacologic aspects of this agent.[233,234]

Structure and Mechanism of Action

The structure of mitomycin C is shown in Figure 18-20. Activation of the drug to an alkylating species can occur either through enzymatic reduction, mediated by cytochrome C reductase, xanthine oxidase, or cytochrome P-450 reductase, or can occur in acid-catalyzed or base-catalyzed reactions in aqueous solution.[235,236] The role of enzymatic reduction in producing a clinically active species in vivo is uncertain.[237]

At least three reactive centers of the compound have been identified: (1) the C-1 carbon of the mitosane ring (Fig. 18-20); (2) the quinone ring structure, which can undergo one or two electron reduction to form reactive species; and (3) the urethane group, which can open to form an alkylating site. Once activated, mitomycin C alkylates and cross-links DNA at the N^6 atom of adenine and the O^6 and N^2 atoms of guanine of DNA.[238] Cross-links result in inhibition of DNA synthesis and cell death. Mitomycin C also induces lipid peroxidation through the intermediate of oxygen radicals.[239]

Although some investigators have found evidence for preferential "bioreductive" activation in hypoxic tumor cells, which have high intracellular NADPH concentrations, a comprehensive examination of human cell lines under hypoxic and euoxic conditions has not substantiated this preferential activity under hypoxic conditions.[240] Resistance to mitomycin C is poorly characterized. In some, but not all, cell lines that demonstrate broad-base multidrug resistance against natural-product drugs, mitomycin C resistance is associated with amplification of the P-170 glycoprotein.[241]

Clinical Pharmacology

After bolus IV administration of 22.5 to 45 mg/m^2, plasma levels peak at an average of 0.4 μg/ml. The drug appears to have a volume of distribution that approaches that of total-body water.

Metabolic activation by reduction appears to occur in all tissues. It does not, therefore, explain the selectivity of this agent for tumor tissue. As a result of this ubiquitous metabolism, clearance of the drug is rapid. As with the anthracyclines, renal clearance is minor, and the role of the liver is defined so poorly that no guidelines can be given for dose modification in the presence of liver or renal disease. The drug may be measured in biological fluids by HPLC. The primary half-life is 54 minutes.[242] The plasma disappearance rate is uniform over the dose range of 15 to 60 mg/m^2.[243] The drug may be used for treatment of carcinoma in situ of the bladder by direct intravesicular installation; after 2 hours, 50% is recoverable in the bladder fluid, but none is measurable in plasma.[244]

Toxicity

The major dose-limiting toxicity of mitomycin C is myelosuppression. This myelosuppression is delayed and cumulative in a fashion similar to that of the nitrosoureas. After a single bolus dose, leukocyte and platelet counts usually reach a nadir between weeks 4 and 6. Typically, by the third course of treatment, doses have to be modified, usually to 50% or less of the initial dose.

Mitomycin C has been implicated as the cause of renal failure, often associated with microangiopathic hemolytic anemia in a syndrome called the hemolytic-uremic syndrome (HUS). Both hemolysis and renal failure appear to be precipitated by renal endothelial injury by the drug, as demonstrated by isolated renal perfusion experiments.[245] Mitomycin-C-induced renal failure is rarely reversible; corticosteroids, plasmapheresis to remove circulating immune complexes, or aspirin are ineffective in patients with HUS. The incidence of renal failure increases strikingly with the total dose of drug administered, being less than 2% at 50 mg/m^2 and rising to 28% at 70 mg/m^2 or higher.[246] The syndrome is exacerbated by blood transfusion, which may precipitate pulmonary edema. Hypertension and neurologic abnormalities frequently supervene in patients with HUS.[247]

Less commonly, this drug has been associated with interstitial pneumonitis and cardiomyopathy. The pneumonitis is uncommon, not dose-related, and exhibits pathologic characteristics similar to those of busulfan lung.[248] The incidence of pneumonitis is higher in patients receiving both mitomycin C and a vinca alkaloid.[249] Pneumonitis is enhanced by raised oxygen tension and appears to be mediated by lipid peroxidation resulting from the generation of reactive oxygen species.[250] It may progress to extensive pulmonary fibrosis. The cardiomyopathy has been reported in patients receiving doxorubicin and mitomycin C in combination and manifests itself as accelerated appearance of cardiac toxicity at doses of doxorubicin that, by themselves, are not associated with significant damage. This phenomenon is not surprising because both doxorubicin and mitomycin C can be activated to radicals by reduction, and in the former case,

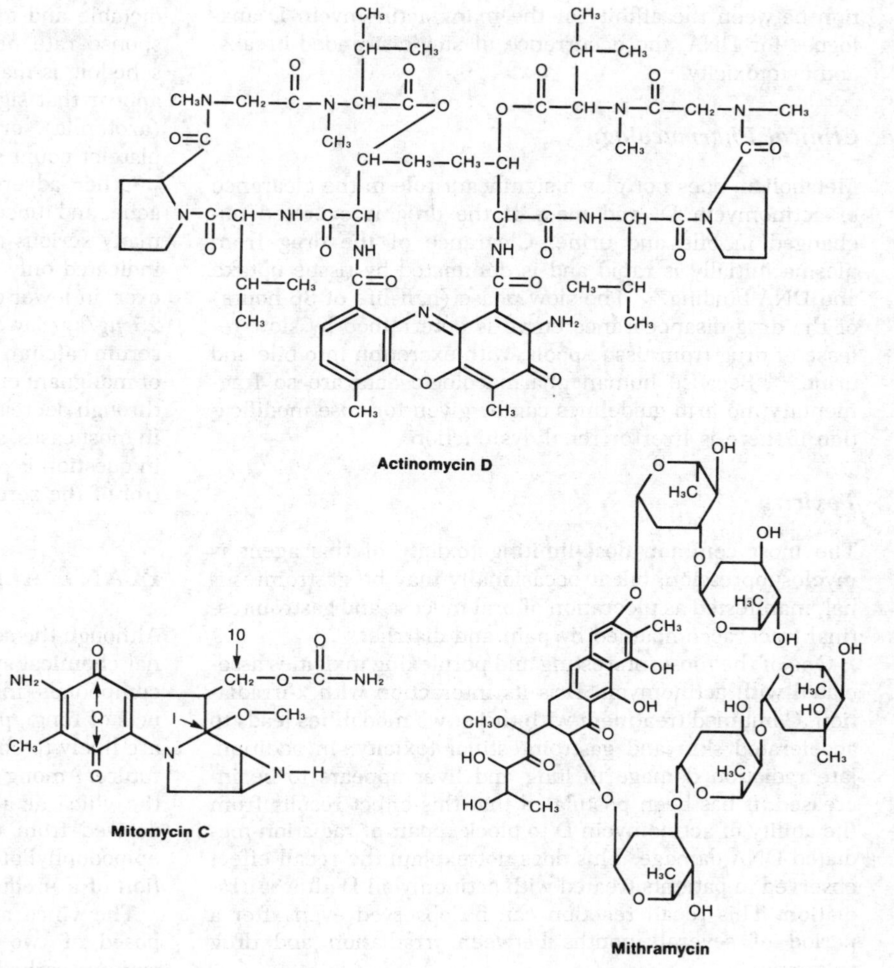

FIG. 18-20. Antitumor antibiotics. Potential sites of activation of mitomycin C are indicated by arrows and include the carbon linked to a labile methoxy group (1), the C-10 carbon (10), and the quinone ring system (Q).

this radical production has been proposed to be the cause of the cardiac toxicity.[251] Extreme caution should be exercised in preparing for the intravenous infusion of mitomycin C, because extravasation leads to local tissue injury and ulceration.

ACTINOMYCIN D

Actinomycin D is a member of a large class of similar drugs that were first isolated from *Streptomyces* species.[252] It is the only member of the class to achieve significant clinical use. Actinomycin D is effective in the treatment of Wilms' tumor, Ewing's sarcoma, embryonal rhabdomyosarcoma, and gestational choriocarcinoma.[253] Responses also are seen in testicular cancer, Kaposi's sarcoma, and lymphoma.

Structure and Mechanism of Action

Actinomycin D has an interesting structure. It is composed of a phenoxazone ring chromophore that gives a red color to the drug. Two identical cyclic polypeptides are bound to the chromophore (Fig. 18-20). This antibiotic binds to DNA by intercalation, with the phenoxazone ring inserted perpendicularly to the long axis of the DNA double helix and the polypeptide chains extending along the minor groove. This intercalation depends on a specific interaction between the polypeptide chains and deoxyguanosine and blocks the ability of DNA to act as a template for both RNA and DNA synthesis. At low drug concentrations, inhibition of RNA synthesis predominates, whereas at higher concentrations both RNA and DNA syntheses are affected.[254,255]

In addition to these effects, actinomycin D causes single-stranded DNA breaks in a manner similar to that of doxorubicin.[256] As with doxorubicin, there are several possible explanations for this observation. Actinomycin D can be reduced by means of cytochrome P-450 reductase to a radical intermediate; this has been postulated as the cause of the single-strand breakage. Another hypothesis is that intercalation causes sufficient strain on the three-dimensional topography of the double helix to trigger enzymatic nicking and strand breakage by topoisomerase-II. However, the role of single-strand breaks is unclear because there is no correlation between the affinity of the many actinomycin D analogues for DNA, the occurrence of single-stranded breaks, and cytotoxicity.

Clinical Pharmacology

Metabolism does not play a significant role in the clearance of actinomycin D, and most of the drug is excreted unchanged in bile and urine. Clearance of the drug from plasma initially is rapid and is dominated by tissue uptake and DNA binding.[257] The slow phase (half-life of 36 hours) of the drug disappearance curve is determined by slow release of drug from tissue pools, with excretion into bile and urine.[258] Because human pharmacologic data are so fragmentary, no firm guidelines can be given for dose modification if there is liver or renal dysfunction.

Toxicity

The most common dose-limiting toxicity of this agent is myelosuppression, but it occasionally may be gastrointestinal, manifested as ulceration of oral mucosa and gastrointestinal tract, accompanied by pain and diarrhea.

One of the most interesting and perplexing toxicities associated with actinomycin D is its interaction with x-irradiation. Combined treatment with these two modalities leads to accelerated skin and gastrointestinal toxicity. In addition, late radiation damage to lung and liver appears to be increased. It has been postulated that this effect results from the ability of actinomycin D to block repair of radiation-mediated DNA damage. This does not explain the recall effect observed in patients treated with actinomycin D after x-irradiation. This recall reaction can be observed even after a period of several months between irradiation and drug treatment.

MITHRAMYCIN

Mithramycin, an antibiotic isolated from *Streptomyces plicatus*, not only has antitumor activity against testicular carcinoma, but also has a specific hypocalcemic effect that is valuable in the treatment of malignant hypercalcemia.[259]

Mithramycin is an inhibitor of DNA-directed RNA synthesis. It is administered IV. Little is known about its pharmacokinetics and disposition in humans. There are no suitable assays for this drug at present. It is known to produce differentiation of human myeloid leukemia cells in culture and to produce remissions in the blastic phase of chronic myelogenous leukemia in man, possibly through differentiation.[260] This agent has a number of unusual side-effects in addition to its antitumor activity. It causes acute nausea and vomiting and occasionally diarrhea and stomatitis. More important, a hemorrhagic diathesis often is seen with daily treatment and is manifested as a fall in platelet count, a lengthening of the prothrombin time, and a depression of clotting factors II, V, VII, and X. Deaths resulting from uncontrolled gastrointestinal hemorrhage have been reported with this schedule of administration. Mithramycin also has serious renal and hepatic toxicities, the mechanisms of which are unclear. An alternate-day regimen of 50 μg/kg/day appears to cause predictable and tolerable toxicity and is associated with a response rate of nearly 50% in testicular carcinoma. This schedule is maintained on an alternate-day basis until signs appear that signal hepatic (LDH > 2000 U/100 ml), renal (azotemia), or clotting (prothrombin time > 15 seconds, platelet count < 100,000 cells/mm³) dysfunction.

Other adverse reactions include fever, myalgias, headache, and, uncommonly, vascular thrombosis. Because of its many serious toxic side-effects, mithramycin at present is indicated only for treatment of testicular neoplasms. However, in lower doses and for brief courses of treatment (15–25 μg/kg/day for 3 days), mithramycin effectively lowers serum calcium concentration in patients with hypercalcemia of malignant or nonmalignant origin. Its effects are mediated through decreased bone resorption and last for 7 to 21 days. In most cases, specific therapy directed against the neoplasm in question is required to produce permanent, effective control of the serum calcium level.

PLANT ALKALOIDS

Although the search for new anticancer drugs through rational chemical synthesis of antimetabolites has yielded useful compounds, many more antitumor agents are natural products of fungi, plants, and marine animals, and these sources are likely to be the primary resources for compounds of the future. Among plant products, the most important have been the vinca alkaloids, vincristine and vinblastine, which are derived from the ornamental shrub *Vinca rosea*, and the epipodophyllotoxins, VM-26 and VP-16, derived by modification of a product of the mandrake plant.

The vinca alkaloids are closely related structures composed of two complex multiringed systems linked by a carbon–carbon bridge. A single modification on the catharanthine ring, as shown in Figure 18-21, is the only difference in structure between the two, but the two compounds are significantly different in their spectrum of clinical action and toxicity. A third analogue, vindesine (deacetylvin-

FIG. 18-21. Structure of vinblastine and vincristine.

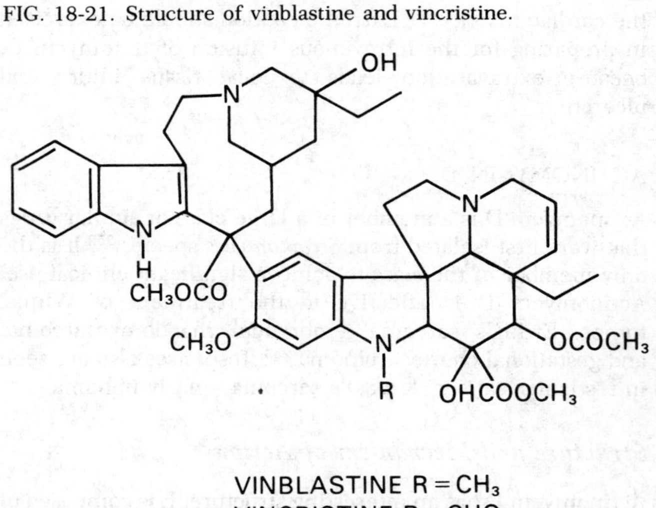

VINBLASTINE R = CH_3
VINCRISTINE R = CHO

blastine), which is also a metabolic product of vinblastine in humans, has activity against lung cancer and hematologic malignancies, but its future clinical development is uncertain.[261]

The vinca alkaloids possess cytotoxic activity by virtue of their binding to tubulin. The latter is a dimeric protein found in the soluble fraction of the cytoplasm of all cells; it exists in equilibrium with a polymerized form, the microtubular apparatus, which forms the spindle along which chromosomes migrate during mitosis. In addition, microtubules play a vital role in maintaining cell structure, providing a conduit for cellular secretions and for neurotransmitter transit along axons. Through their high-affinity binding to tubulin, the vinca alkaloids inhibit the assembly of microtubules and lead to the dissolution of the mitotic spindle.[262] A separate site for binding on tubulin is shared by two other spindle poisons, colchicine and podophyllotoxin.[263] A new spindle poison, taxol (Table 18-4), acts by promoting the assembly of microtubules.[264]

The primary action of the vinca alkaloids is an arrest of cells in the metaphase of mitosis. However, cells in vitro appear to be most sensitive to the cytotoxic effects of these compounds when exposed to drug during the late S phase of the cell cycle.[265] The vinca alkaloids bind strongly to tubulin in their parent form, but evidence is growing that these compounds may undergo oxidative metabolism to potentially reactive intermediates.[266] Ceruloplasmin, a protein found in high concentration in plasma of patients with Hodgkin's disease, can effect this transformation.

The mechanism by which the vinca alkaloids permeate cells is uncertain. There is evidence that they cross the cell membrane by a saturable process.[267] However, these experiments were conducted at drug levels well above those achieved clinically, or those required to kill cells in culture (1×10^{-8} M).[268] Resistance to the vinca alkaloids may result from mutations in tubulin, which leads to decreased drug binding, and from decreased ability of cells to accumulate drug. These latter cells have increased capacity to efflux drug and concomitantly are resistant to taxol, anthracyclines, actinomycin D, and other natural products.[269] This type of pleiotropic drug resistance may be accompanied by amplification of a specific membrane glycoprotein, called the P-170 protein.[270] This protein, an ATP-requiring transport molecule, can be competitively inhibited by calcium channel-blocking drugs, which reverse resistance in culture and animals.[271] There appears to be some specificity in the molecular form of P-170 induced by each vinca alkaloid, in that cells selected for resistance to vincristine, in early passages in culture, may not share complete cross-resistance to vinblastine or taxol.[272] This observation, perhaps explained by the structural heterogeneity of P-170, has its parallel in the lack of cross-resistance of vinca alkaloids in some patients with lymphoma.[273]

CLINICAL PHARMACOLOGY

The development of a comprehensive understanding of the pharmacokinetics of vinca alkaloids has been hindered by the lack of sufficiently sensitive and specific methods for drug assay. Most information has been obtained using radiolabeled drug, supplemented with chromatographic separation of the parent drug from metabolites.[274] Radioimmunoassays for vincristine and vinblastine have been described, although their specificity for parent compound versus metabolites is not known.[275] A highly sensitive immunosorbent assay that can detect as little as 5 pg of vincristine has been developed and may permit more detailed pharmacokinetic studies.[276]

The primary pharmacokinetic characteristics of vincristine and vinblastine are similar and include peak plasma concentrations of approximately 0.4 μM, followed by a multiphasic plasma disappearance with half-lives of 164 minutes for vincristine, and 190 minutes for vinblastine.[274,275,277] A terminal velban half-life of 20 hours has been observed using the radioimmunoassay. Little vincristine permeates into the CSF.[278] A minimal amount of either drug is excreted in the urine. Almost 70% of a vincristine dose is excreted in the feces, primarily as metabolites resulting from hepatic metabolism and biliary excretion.[279,280] The fecal excretion of vinblastine is only 10%, as measured by radioimmunoassay, although drug metabolites may not be measured by this technique.[281]

Vinblastine may also be administered by continuous infusion, in which the cytotoxicity of the spindle poisons is greater for cells in the S phase of the cell cycle and the rapid efflux from tumor cells is faster than with vincristine.[282] Continuous infusion of 2 mg/m^2/d for 5 days, a commonly used regimen, produces vinblastine plasma concentrations of 2 ng/ml or about 2 nM, a concentration well within the cytotoxic range for this agent.[283] Serum levels above 1 nM are maintained for 4 days by doses of vinblastine of 6 mg/m^2 at 0 and 48 hours.

Vincristine and vinblastine are usually administered by IV bolus in doses of 1 to 1.4 mg/m^2 and 0.1 mg/kg, respectively. Vincristine doses may be repeated at weekly or longer intervals. A progressive and disabling neurotoxicity may occur with vincristine therapy, particularly in older patients, in patients with neuromuscular disorders such as Charcot-Marie-Tooth disease or polio, and in patients receiving weekly treatment.[284,285] The first signs of neuropathy are a decrease in deep tendon reflexes and paresthesias of the fingers and lower extremities. More advanced neurotoxicity may lead to cranial nerve and laryngeal nerve palsy and profound weakness of the dorsiflexors of the foot and extensors of the wrist. At higher doses of vincristine (above a 3-mg total dose), constipation, obstipation, and paralytic ileus may occur because of autonomic neuropathy. Alterations in mental status rarely accompany signs and symptoms of peripheral neuropathy; rarely, seizures may occur.[286] Direct intrathecal injection of vincristine is absolutely contraindicated, and if it occurs by accident, it leads to coma, seizures, and death. There is no effective antidote for vincristine neurotoxicity.[287] Although the motor and sensory changes and reflex changes may improve when vincristine is withdrawn, deficits may be permanent.

Vincristine causes little myelosuppression. As the result of inhibition of mitosis, megakaryocytes undergo endoreduplication, and, at low doses of vincristine, the platelet count actually may rise during treatment. In contrast, the primary toxicity of vinblastine is found in the bone marrow. Leukopenia usually is dose-limiting. Mucositis is another frequent side-effect, and neurotoxicity rarely is observed at conventional doses. Vindesine causes both myelosuppression and mild, but consistent, neurotoxicity similar to that caused by vincristine.[261,288]

In addition to the more common adverse effects, vincristine stimulates the release of antidiuretic hormone and, in rare instances, may lead to symptomatic dilutional hyponatremia.[289] This syndrome is self-limited and, if recognized early, can be treated with simple fluid restriction. Vigorous hydration should be used cautiously in patients receiving high doses of vincristine (> 2-mg total dose).

Although specific pharmacokinetic information is not available as the basis for dose modification in patients with hepatic dysfunction, it is advisable to reduce the dose of either vincristine or vinblastine in these patients. A reduction of 50% is recommended in patients with bilirubin above 3 mg/100 ml. No modification is recommended for patients with impaired renal function. Extravasation of the vinca alkaloids leads to local tissue ulceration and necrosis, a process that can be ameliorated by warming the affected area of drug infiltration.[290] Surgical debridement of affected tissue may be required.

The only well-documented drug interaction of importance is the inhibition of the efflux of methotrexate by the vinca alkaloids. However, this effect requires relatively high concentrations of the vinca alkaloids ($\geq 0.1\ \mu M$), and the combination of methotrexate following vincristine has not been shown to improve treatment results in experiments with murine leukemia.[291]

THE EPIPODOPHYLLOTOXINS

Podophyllotoxin, an extract of the mandrake plant, has been used as a folk remedy for treatment of poisoning, parasites, and warts. Like vincristine and vinblastine, it binds to tubulin and inhibits microtubular assembly, but it failed initial clinical trials because of prohibitive toxicity. However, two glycosidic derivatives, VP-16 and VM-26, have been synthesized and have important clinical activity in the treatment of lymphomas, small-cell carcinoma of the lung, leukemia, and testicular cancer. These derivatives differ only in a single substitution (Fig. 18-22) and have basic similarities in their pharmacodynamics, toxicity, and spectrum of clinical action.[292]

The mechanism of action of these synthetic derivatives is incompletely understood. They have no discernible effect on microtubular assembly and arrest cells in G_2 rather than in mitosis.[293] A more important effect is the production of single-strand and double-strand breaks in DNA.[294] Strand breakage correlates closely with cytotoxicity and may be due to the formation of free-radical derivatives of the parent compound by one-electron oxidation catalyzed by intracellular peroxidases.[295] Unlike the anthracyclines and actinomycins, the epipodophyllotoxins do not intercalate between the DNA strands, but they do form a stable terniary complex with DNA and topoisomerase-II. The enzyme then attaches covalently to DNA, forming single-strand, protein-associated breaks. It is not known which of these mechanisms is most crucial to the cytotoxic action. As with many other agents

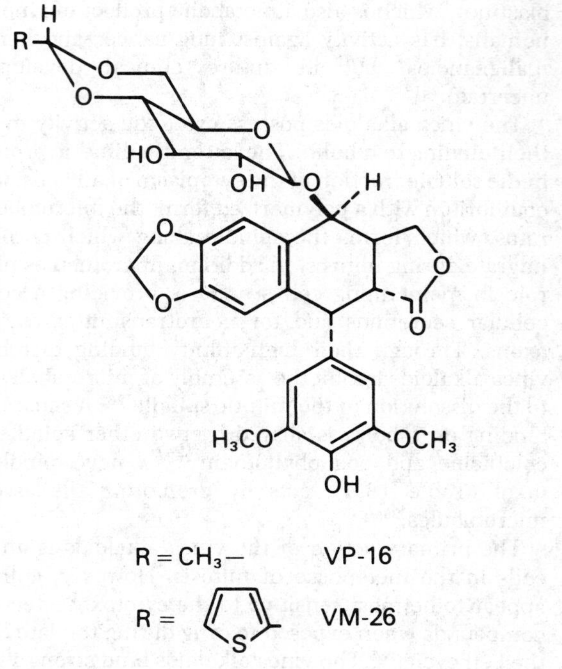

FIG. 18-22. Structure of VP-16 and VM-26.

that cause DNA strand breaks, sensitivity to VP-16 is augmented in experimental systems by inhibition of polyamine biosynthesis, by drugs that inhibit DNA repair or synthesis, or by inborn defects in DNA repair, such as in patients with ataxia-telangiectasia.[296]

In experimental studies, resistance to VP-16 and VM-26 develops through amplification of the multidrug resistance exit pump (the P-170 glycoprotein) and through alterations in formation or repair of strand breaks.[297] The epipodophyllotoxins likely undergo significant intracellular metabolism and detoxification, although these processes are poorly understood.

The primary features of epipodophyllotoxin disposition in humans are given in Table 18-7.[298] VP-16 is administered either in the form of capsules or a drinking ampule or by IV infusion, whereas VM-26 is given only IV. VP-16 has a more rapid renal clearance, shorter terminal half-life, and undergoes less metabolism than does VM-26. Both drugs penetrate poorly into the CSF despite their high lipid solubility. The primary route of elimination for VM-26 is metabolic, although the products have not been identified; at least 30% of VP-16 is excreted unchanged. Doses of VP-16 should be modified in proportion to changes in creatinine clearance. Doses of both drugs should not be reduced for patients with hepatic dysfunction.[299,300]

TABLE 18-7. Pharmacokinetics of VP-16 and VM-26

Characteristics	*VM-26*	*VP-16*
Plasma half-life	3.85 h	6 h
Urinary excretion (% dose)	45	45
% excreted as metabolite	79	33

VP-16 has been used in a variety of schedules and administered by both oral and IV routes. At least a twofold increase in dose is required if the drug is given orally in order to compensate for decreased bioavailability. Bioavailability by the oral route varies from 30% to 100% but averages 50% for the drinking ampules.[301] Maximum tolerated IV doses are 45 mg/m^2/day for 7 days, 86 mg/m^2/day for twice-weekly doses, and 290 mg/m^2 once weekly. VM-26 usually is given in weekly doses of 67 mg/m^2.

In standard doses, the dose-limiting toxicity for both drugs is leukopenia. Thrombocytopenia occurs in fewer than 25% of patients. Mild gastrointestinal complaints such as nausea and vomiting are reported by fewer than 20% of patients receiving IV VP-16 or VM-26, but increase to a 55% incidence in those receiving oral VP-16. A mild peripheral neuropathy, usually paresthesias or tenden reflex depression, is observed in fewer than half the patients receiving these drugs but may be severe in patients previously treated with vincristine. High-dose VP-16 (2400 mg/m^2 over 3 days) has been administered with autologous bone marrow reinfusion 64 hours after the end of chemotherapy infusion and produces severe mucositis and leukopenia.[302]

HEXAMETHYLMELAMINE AND PENTAMETHYLMELAMINE

Hexamethylmelamine (HMM) and pentamethylmelamine (PMM) belong to a unique class of antitumor agents that have uncertain mechanisms of action but significant antineoplastic activity against ovarian cancer, breast cancer, the lymphomas, and small cell carcinoma of the lung. Despite partial elucidation of the complex metabolism of HMM, the active intermediate has not been identified, and the drug has no clear relationship with conventional classes of chemotherapeutic agents. Its relatively mild myelosuppressive effects make this agent a good candidate for combination therapy.

HMM consists of a symmetric, 6-member triazene ring, with three attached dimethylamine groups (Fig. 18-23). PMM, a more water-soluble analogue, has one less methyl side-group. These methyl substitutions are removed readily by microsomal metabolism to yield various possible methylmelamine derivatives, and corresponding quantities of formaldehyde, a weakly cytotoxic compound.[303,304] None of the melamine metabolites is cytotoxic in vitro in the absence of microsomes. HMM and several of its demethyl metabolites can be converted by enzymatic hydroxylation to methylol ($R—CH_2OH$) analogues, which are cytotoxic in vitro.

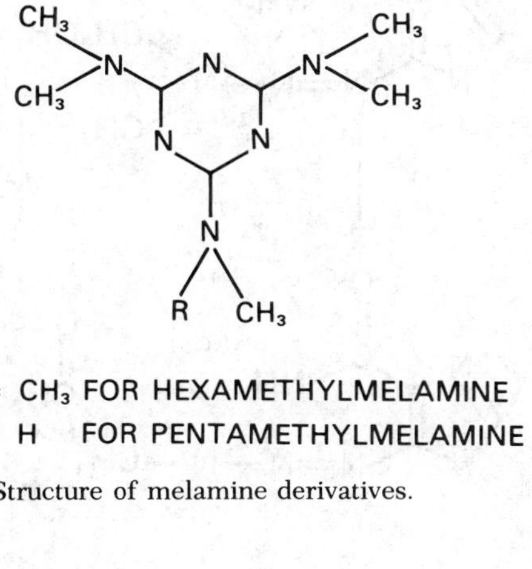

FIG. 18-23. Structure of melamine derivatives.

Experimental studies with HMM labeled in either the triazene ring or in the methyl groups have demonstrated covalent binding of both types of labeled compound to acid-insoluble material in both tumor cells and normal tissues, indicating possible alkylating action.[305] However, HMM is not consistently cross-resistant with classic alkylating agents in rodent tumors or in human cancer.

As in rodents, both HMM and PMM undergo extensive and rapid N-demethylation in humans. The S-triazene ring is excreted intact, whereas the methyl groups appear as respiratory CO_2, undergo metabolic reuse by the intermediate formaldehyde, or remain attached to the ring system of partially demethylating metabolites.

Following concentration steps, PMM and HMM are best measured by gas chromatography with a nitrogen detector or by gas chromatography–mass spectrometry.[306,307] Both of these methods can detect concentrations as little as 0.1 μM of either compound in plasma.

Because of its limited aqueous solubility, HMM can be given only by the oral route. Usual doses of 4 to 12 mg/kg/day are given for courses of 14 to 21 days. The bioavailability of HMM by this route is highly variable, yielding peak blood levels of 0.2 to 0.8 mg/ml.[308] This variability results from either variable absorption or variable first-pass metabolism in the liver. The parent compound has a half-life of 4.7 to 10.2 hours in plasma. PMM, given IV, has half-lives of 27 and 133 minutes, and therefore is eliminated somewhat faster than HMM.

Both HMM and PMM produce nausea and vomiting as their dose-limiting toxicity. These symptoms, produced by bolus administration of PMM, are particularly severe and have led to the use of more protracted infusion of PMM, which causes less emesis. Oral administration of HMM leads to a gradual increase in these symptoms over a period of days, limiting therapy to 2 to 3 weeks. Higher daily doses of HMM (above 12 mg/kg/day) are tolerated for shorter periods. No standard schedule of PMM dosage has been established in preliminary clinical trials, although single doses of 1500 mg/m^2 repeated every week produce dose-limiting gastrointestinal symptoms in most patients.

Both PMM and HMM also produce neurotoxic symptoms. HMM treatment may lead to mood alterations, hallucinations, and peripheral neuropathy; these effects appear gradually during a protracted course of treatment and disappear when the drug is withdrawn. PMM has caused convulsive death in preclinical trials and acute coma after rapid IV injection in humans.

DACARBAZINE

Dacarbazine (DTIC) 5-(3,3-dimethyl-1-triazeno)-imidazole-4-carboxamide is the product of a fortuitous misadventure in drug design. This compound resulted from efforts to synthesize analogues of 5-amino-imidazole-4-carboxamide, an intermediate in purine biosynthesis. DTIC actually functions as an alkylating agent. It is active against a broad spectrum of murine solid and ascitic tumors, but its clinical effectiveness is limited to Hodgkin's disease, malignant melanoma, and soft tissue sarcomas.

The probable pathway of metabolic activation of this agent is shown in Figure 18-24 and consists of hepatic microsomal-mediated demethylation, followed by spontaneous rearrangement of the product, which leads to elimination of a methyl diazonium cation ($^{+1}N = NCH_3$). This cation further yields an active methyl cation (CH_3^{1+}) and N_2. Methylation of nucleic acids has been observed in both experimental systems and in urinary excretion products in humans, but the active species of drug and the route of its generation are still not known.[309] In addition to the alkylating activity generated as described above, the metabolite methyltriazinoimidazole carboxamide (MTIC) inhibits purine nucleoside incorporation into DNA.[310]

In addition to its microsomal metabolism, DTIC undergoes spontaneous decomposition when exposed to light, yielding diazoimidazole carboxamide and azahypoxanthine, an active antimetabolite in its own right. This light-activation pathway may account of the antitumor effects of DTIC in vitro in the absence of microsomes, but there is little evidence to support any relevance of this reaction sequence to in vivo toxicity.

The effects of DTIC on cell cycle progression and its cycle specificity are uncertain. It appears to kill cells in all phases of the cell cycle and shows little schedule dependency in experimental studies.

Triazine compounds, in addition to cytotoxicity, induce differentiation of malignant cells at sublethal concentrations.[311]

The parent compound disappears from plasma, with a terminal half-life of 41 minutes. Up to 50% of the parent compound is excreted unchanged in the urine.[312]

Preliminary information indicates that the drug is absorbed adquately when given orally, but a similar dose given IV yields fivefold higher peak blood levels. Its disappearance half-life from plasma is about 3 hours. An ultimate metabolite, aminoimidazolecarboxamide, has been detected in humans.[312]

A variety of schedules of administration are used in humans. Intravenous doses vary from 150 to 300 mg/m²/day for 5 to 10 days, depending on treatment history, concurrent therapy, and patient tolerance. The drug also has been given by intraarterial infusion, but this route lacks rationale because of the likely requirement for hepatic microsomal activation.

The most significant side-effects are nausea and vomiting, which are most severe during the first few days of treatment and which may be lessened by reducing the initial dose and gradually increasing the dose during the course of treatment. Moderate myelosuppression may occur during the second or third week following treatment but usually is not dose-limiting. Other toxicities include a flu-like syndrome and possible enhancement of doxorubicin cardiac toxicity.[313] Fulminant hepatic venoocclusive disease, associated with fever, eosinophilia, and acute hepatic necrosis, has been reported in patients receiving DTIC as adjuvant therapy for malignant melanoma, and it may cause death.[314]

PROCARBAZINE

Procarbazine N-isopropyl-α-(2-methylhydrazino)-*p*-toluamide hydrochloride was discovered during a search for new monoamine oxidase inhibitors; it also was found to have antitumor activity and has since become an important agent in the treatment of Hodgkin's disease, brain tumors, and lung cancer.

The mechanism of action and metabolism of procarbazine are not understood completely; it is likely, however, that the drug requires microsomal metabolite activation and that the end-product is an alkylating agent, probably a methyldiazonium ion.[315–317]

FIG. 18-24. Metabolic activation of dacarbazine (DTIC). The initial step is enzymatically mediated, but the mechanism of subsequent reactions has not been clarified.

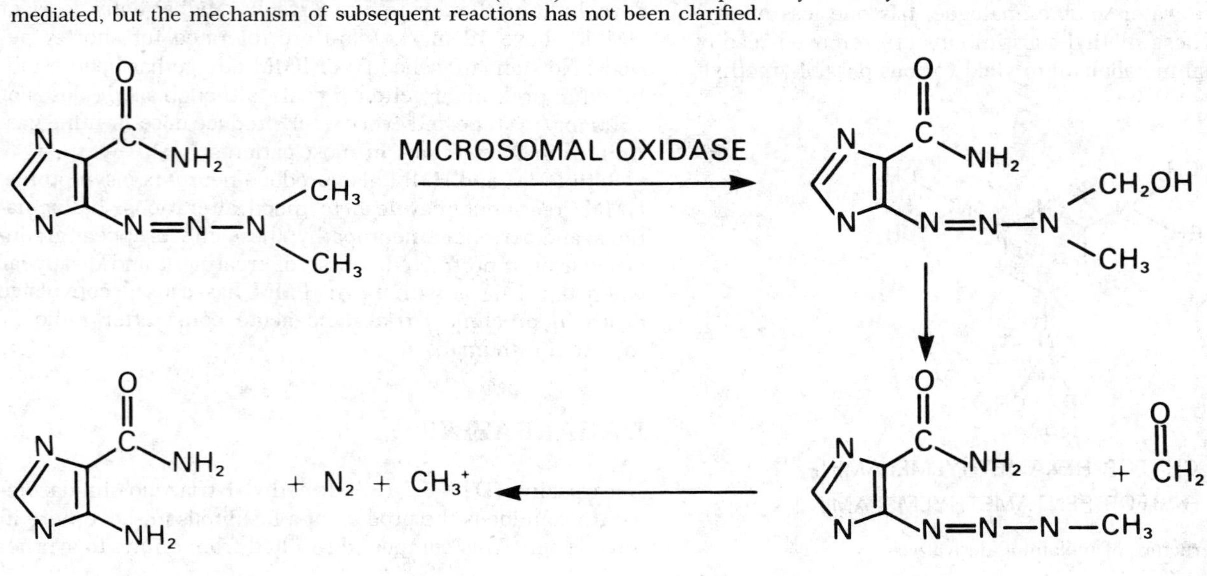

There is no reliable information on the mechanisms of cellular resistance to procarbazine.

The pharmacokinetics of procarbazine in humans have not been characterized completely. The parent drug disappears rapidly from plasma with a half-life of 7 minutes following IV administration. The primary excretion product is N-isopropylterephthalamic acid. Procarbazine-derived radioactivity in the CSF reaches equilibrium with plasma within 15 minutes after injection; the highly lipophilic azoxy metabolites also have been found in rat brains 10 to 30 minutes after IV administration.

The antitumor activity and the rate of microsomal metabolism of procarbazine are increased in rodents by pretreatment with phenobarbital, a microsomal enzyme inducer.[318] However, procarbazine itself inhibits microsomal biotransformation of pentobarbital and aminopyrene, indicating that it may have important interactions with antitumor drugs that undergo microsomal metabolism in humans, such as DTIC and cyclophosphamide.

Procarbazine usually is administered orally in daily doses of 100 mg/m^2 for 10 to 14 days. When given orally, procarbazine causes moderate nausea and a decrease in appetite, mild-to-moderate leukopenia and thrombocytopenia, and, less frequently, neurotoxicity, which is manifested by paresthesias of the extremities, drowsiness, or depression. These changes in mental status may be related to its inhibition of monoamine oxidase. Patients receiving procarbazine should be warned to avoid foods that contain significant quantities of tyramine, such as wine, bananas, yogurt, and ripe cheese, because these may provoke a hypertensive crisis. Other monoamine oxidase inhibitors such as tricyclic antidepressants and sympathomimetic drugs should not be used concomitantly with procarbazine. Potent hypnotics also should not be used, because procarbazine causes mild hypnotic effects and is known to depress the microsomal inactivation of other agents.

The neurotoxicity of procarbazine is the most prominent and disabling side-effect when the drug is given IV.[319] Total doses of 2 g/m^2 by this route produce confusion or coma in patients but little myelosuppression. Clinical benefit is uncertain.

Procarbazine has a disulfiram (Antabuse)-like action that may lead to sweating, flushing, and headache after ingestion of alcohol by patients receiving procarbazine. Hypersensitivity reactions also have been observed and frequently include a maculopapular rash and pulmonary infiltrates. In our experience, the development of a rash is not cause for withdrawal of procarbazine. The rash usually abates with concurrent use of corticosteroids, and continued treatment with procarbazine plus corticosteroids does not lead to progressive cutaneous reaction or anaphylaxis.

Procarbazine is a potent immunosuppressant in rodents; it prolongs the survival of the first or second set skin grafts across major histocompatibility barriers.[320] It has been used as an immunosuppressant in patients with lupus erythematosus and for suppression of graft-versus-host disease in bone marrow transplantation. Procarbazine also is a highly teratogenic and carcinogenic agent in rodents.[321] When exposed to the drug in utero, fetal rats acquire a variety of skeletal and nervous system abnormalities. The compound is highly mutagenic in the Ames' assay and produces both adenocarcinomas and AML in rodents and monkeys. An increased incidence of both solid tumors and acute leukemias has been observed in patients receiving MOPP combination chemotherapy with irradiation for Hodgkin's disease (see Chap. 49), and it is believed that procarbazine is the responsible carcinogen. Thus its use in treating nonneoplastic diseases should be considered carefully because of these late toxicities. It also is highly toxic to the reproductive organs, producing azospermia and anovulation.

mAMSA

Amsacrine (mAMSA), a 9-anilino derivative of the DNA binding dye acridine, was synthesized by Bruce Cain and colleagues in New Zealand in 1974 and was found to have potent clinical activity against human acute nonlymphocytic leukemia.[322,323] It is particularly valuable because of its synergy with ara-C, its activity in anthracycline-resistant patients, and its lower incidence of cardiotoxicity than anthracyclines.[324]

MECHANISM OF ACTION

Like other acridine dyes, mAMSA intercalates between strands of DNA and produces single-stranded and double-stranded breaks in DNA. Its cytotoxicity correlates closely with the formation of these breaks.[325] The DNA-cleaving enzyme topoisomerase-II has been implicated in the action of the drug, in that the enzyme forms a tight complex with mAMSA and DNA. Although the normal action of topoisomerase-II is to break and reseal DNA at points of torsion, in the presence of mAMSA, resealing of breaks does not take place and the protein remains bound to the free 5′ ends of the broken DNA strand.[326–328] Another hypothesis has been proposed by Crooke and colleagues, who offer evidence that mAMSA in the presence of Cu(II) undergoes oxidation, leading to the formation of oxygen radicals and DNA strand breaks.[329] Evidence from the examination of a number of mAMSA-resistant cell lines supports the role of topoisomerase-II because the enzyme extracted from resistant cells cannot mediate strand breakage in the presence of mAMSA.[330,331]

mAMSA-induced strand breakage and cytotoxicity are greatest during the S phase of the cell cycle, when topoisomerase levels within the cell increase to a maximum.[332] Slowly dividing cells, such as fibroblasts or cells at confluence, are less sensitive to the drug. Resistance to mAMSA has been completely characterized but appears related to altered topoisomerase-II, which no longer cleaves DNA in the presence of mAMSA. Other agents, such as VP-16 and various anthracycline derivatives, that also cleave DNA through activation of topoisomerase-II share cross-resistance with mAMSA in some mAMSA-resistant cell lines.[333–335] There is little evidence to indicate that mAMSA is affected by multidrug resistance related to P-170 amplification, although verapamil, a calcium channel blocker that reverses multidrug resistance, does enhance sensitivity to mAMSA in some cell lines.[336]

CLINICAL PHARMACOLOGY AND PHARMACOKINETICS

mAMSA is administered IV in doses of 100 to 150 mg/m² per day for 5 days. It is concentrated in the liver, where it undergoes conjugation to glutathione and excretion in bile.[337] Its primary plasma half-life is 7.4 hours, but it is prolonged to 17 hours in patients with hepatic dysfunction, leading to recommendation of a 40% dose reduction in patients with serum bilirubin greater than 2 mg/100 ml. Less than 20% of drug is excreted unchanged in urine, and the need to reduce the dose in patients with renal failure is uncertain.[338]

Within liver cells and other tissues, including tumor cells, the parent drug undergoes microsomal metabolism to an oxidized derivative (mAQDI) that may undergo hydrolysis to form mAQI (Fig. 18-25) or may be conjugated to glutathione in a detoxification reaction.[339] Both mAQDI and mAQI are considerably more cytotoxic than the parent compound. Interestingly, the oxidation of mAMSA to mAQDI can also occur in the presence of Cu(II) and may be the mechanism underlying strand breakage mediated by the Cu(II)–mAMSA combination.[329]

mAMSA is highly protein-bound in human plasma, with less than 5% of the drug in its free state in the therapeutic range of 1 to 100 μM.[340] Its ability to penetrate the blood–brain barrier is likely limited by this high degree of protein binding.

The primary toxicity caused by mAMSA is pancytopenia, which reverses within two weeks of drug administration. It also causes acute and chronic cardiac toxicity.[341] The acute effects on the heart are a prolongation in the Q-T interval, atrial and ventricular arrhythmias, and, rarely, acute heart failure, all of which may occur within the first hour after drug administration. Although anecdotal cases suggest that prior anthracycline therapy may predispose to mAMSA-induced cardiac toxicity, the incidence of cardiac events appears to be approximately 1% in both previously treated and previously untreated patients. Toxicity may occur with the first dose of mAMSA, and in most affected patients there is no prior history of cardiac disease. Because of the frequent occurrence of Q-T prolongation with mAMSA therapy, investigators have warned that caution be exercised in treating hypokalemic patients.

In preparing an IV injection of mAMSA, the drug should be diluted in dextrose and water, rather than saline, because free chloride ions lead to mAMSA precipitation.[342]

L-ASPARAGINASE

The growth of malignant and normal cells depends on the availability of specific nutrients used in the synthesis of proteins, nucleic acids, and lipids. Some of these nutrients can

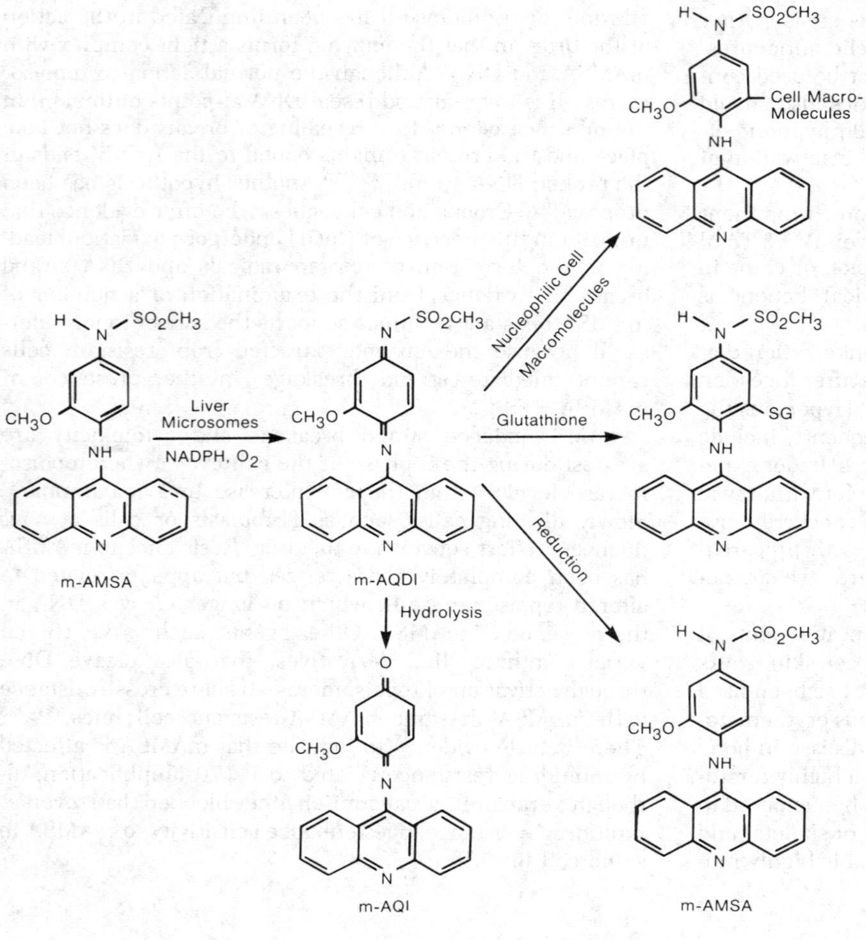

FIG. 18-25. Pathways of microsomal activation of mAMSA to a reactive, alkylating intermediate (mAQDI). mAQDI is inactivated by spontaneous hydrolysis, conjugation with glutathione, or reduction back to the parent compound.

be synthesized within the cell, but others are needed from external sources, such as another organ (liver) or from food sources (essential amino acids). Nutritional therapy of cancer has been directed toward identifying the differences between the host and malignant cells that might be exploited in treatment; these attempts, for the most part, have been unsuccessful because of difficulties in producing a deficiency state by dietary means and a lack of clear differences between the rapidly proliferating host cells and the tumor. The only exception has been the use of L-asparaginase in the treatment of childhood acute leukemia.

L-asparagine is a nonessential amino acid that is synthesized by transamination of L-aspartic acid (Fig. 18-26). The amine group in this reaction is donated by glutamine, and the reaction is catalyzed by the enzyme L-asparagine synthase. This enzyme is constitutive in many tissues, thus accounting for the lack of toxicity of asparagine depletion, but is present in low concentrations in certain human malignancies, particularly lymphocytes. In tumor cells lacking L-asparagine synthase, the amino acid can be obtained only from the circulating pool of amino acids.

In 1953, Kidd observed that the serum of guinea pigs had antileukemic effects when administered to mice.[343] Ten years later, Broome and co-workers demonstrated that the responsible factor copurified with the enzyme L-asparaginase.[344] Subsequently, highly purified preparations of enzyme from *E. coli* and *Erwinia* species have shown significant activity against childhood ALL and have become standard components of induction and maintenance regimens in this disease. Their antitumor effects result from the rapid and complete depletion of circulating pools of L-asparagine, whereas resistance to this treatment is caused by an increase in L-asparagine synthase activity in tumor cells. This increase occurs either by a process of mutation or by enzyme induction in response to the fall in intracellular asparagine levels.

Purified L-asparaginase enzyme has a molecular weight of 133,000 daltons and is composed of four subunits that each have one active catalytic site.[345] Enzyme from different bacterial strains have slight differences in specific activity, isoelectric point, and substrate specificity and affinity. Of greater clinical importance, enzymes prepared from *Erwinia* do not cross-react immunologically with *E. coli* preparations, and therefore may be used in patients who are hypersensitive to the *E. coli* L-asparaginase.[346] The clinical preparations have an affinity constant for L-asparagine of approximately 1×10^{-5} M, a figure tenfold higher than the minimum L-asparagine concentration at which the growth of sensitive tumors is retarded in vitro.[347] Thus a considerable excess of enzyme is required to degrade L-asparagine to sufficiently low concentrations.

FIG. 18-26. Pathways for synthesis of L-asparagine intracellularly and effect of L-asparaginase on circulating L-asparagine.

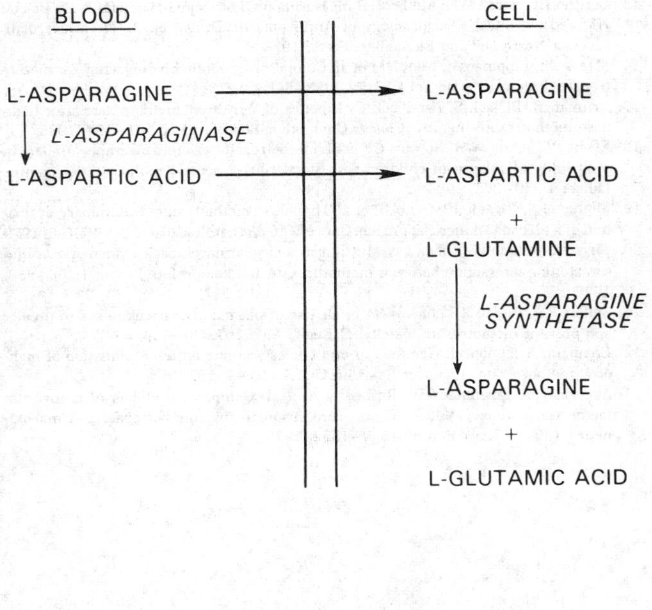

The cytotoxicity of L-asparaginase results from inhibition of protein synthesis and correlates with effects of the enzyme on the incorporation of an amino acid such as ^{3}H-valine into protein. Inhibition of nucleic acid synthesis also is observed in sensitive cells but is believed to be secondary to the block in protein synthesis. As might be expected, resistant cells have high endogenous activity of asparagine synthase.

Most bacterial L-asparaginase preparations contain low, but significant, L-glutaminase activity (<5% of the L-asparaginase activity). The enzymes from mammalian sources and from certain bacterial sources (*Vibrio succinogenes*) lack L-glutaminase activity but have lesser affinity for L-asparagine.[348] Evidence suggests that the immunosuppressive properties of *E. coli* L-asparaginase may be caused by L-glutamine depletion and that cerebral dysfunction observed in patients may be the result of degradation of L-glutamine.[349]

In an effort to circumvent hypersensitivity reactions, bacterial L-asparaginase has been extensively modified by conjugation to dextran or polyethylene glycol; the PEG-modified enzyme has a much prolonged plasma half-life and, based on preliminary clinical results, is active against disease and well-tolerated by patients hypersensitive to unmodified enzyme.[350]

CLINICAL PHARMACOLOGY

L-asparaginase levels are measured easily in biologic fluids by assays that detect ammonia release or by a coupled enzymic assay.[351,352] The drug is given IV or IM; the latter route produces peak drug levels that are 50% lower than the former, but may produce fewer hypersensitivity reactions. The usual doses are 6000 IU/m^2 every other day for 3 to 4 weeks, or daily doses of 1000 to 20,000 IU/m^2 for 10 to 20 days. Widely spaced schedules of administration are used infrequently because of the increased risk of anaphylaxis.[353] Blood concentrations of L-asparagine fall below 1 μM within minutes of enzyme injection and cannot be measured for 7 to 10 days after completion of therapy.[354]

The concentration of L-asparaginase in plasma is proportional to the dose for doses up to 200,000 IU/m^2 and falls with a primary half-life of 14 to 22 hours. L-asparaginase is detectable in blood for 1 to 3 weeks after these doses. (The preparation of L-asparaginase manufactured by Merck & Co. has a somewhat longer half-life than does the preparation made by Bayer.) In patients who are hypersensitive to the enzyme, plasma clearance is accelerated greatly and enzyme activity may be undetectable in plasma as soon as 4 hours after administration.[355] The enzyme distributes primarily within the intravascular space. However, the concentration of asparagine in CSF falls rapidly, and an antileukemic effect is exerted here despite the poor penetration of enzyme into the CSF. The drug can be given directly into the CSF but exits rapidly from this site, and there appears to be no clear therapeutic advantage for this route.

TOXICITY

The primary toxicities of L-asparaginase fall into two main groups: those related to immunologic sensitization to the foreign protein and those resulting from decreased protein synthesis. Positive skin tests to L-asparaginase rarely are observed before drug administration, but anaphylaxis may occur with the initial dose of drug. More commonly, hypersensitivity phenomena, such as urticaria, laryngeal edema, bronchospasm, hypotension, and abdominal pain, occur after multiple courses of the enzyme. Passive hemagglutinating antibodies are observed in patients who subsequently develop anaphylaxis, and complement-fixing antibodies are found in serum after an anaphylactic episode.[355] The reason for the relatively low incidence of hypersensitivity reactions (< 30%) in patients receiving L-asparaginase may be related to the immunosuppressive properties of the drug itself or to the concomitant administration of other immunosuppressive agents. Patients hypersensitive to the *E. coli* enzyme can usually tolerate the *Erwinia* preparation, although about 20% ultimately become sensitive to the second enzyme.[356]

Other adverse effects are related to the inhibition of protein synthesis, the most important being the inhibition of synthesis of clotting factors. Either thrombosis or hemorrhage may result from L-asparaginase therapy, probably resulting from the depletion of vitamin-K-dependent factors, including protein C and its cofactor protein S, which inhibit clotting; antithrombin III, also an inhibitor of clotting; and factors II, VII, IX and X, which are essential for coagulation. Decreases in protein C occur within the first few days of treatment and have been implicated in early thrombotic events.[357,358] Other effects include hypoalbuminemia; decreased serum insulin with hyperglycemia; decreased serum lipoproteins; decreased thyroxin-binding globulin; and in 25% of the patients, cerebral dysfunction with confusion, stupor, or coma.[354] The latter syndrome resembles ammonia toxicity and in some patients correlates with marked elevations in serum ammonia.[359] Alternative explanations include low concentrations of either L-asparagine or L-glutamine in the brain.[354]

Other toxicities are not as easily explained by the mode of action of the drug; the most important of these is acute hyperamylasemia, which occurs in fewer than 15% of patients, but which may progress to severe hemorrhagic pancreatitis. L-asparaginase frequently causes abnormal liver function test findings, including increased serum bilirubin, SGOT, and alkaline phosphatase. Histologic examination reveals fatty metamorphosis.

Approximately two thirds of patients receiving L-asparaginase experience nausea, vomiting, and chills as an immediate reaction, but these side-effects can be mitigated by antiemetics, antihistamines, or, in extreme cases, corticosteroids.

L-asparaginase has no known effects on gastrointestinal mucosa or bone marrow and thus is a favorable agent for combination chemotherapy. The only well-established drug interaction is its ability to terminate methotrexate action, because it inhibits protein synthesis and thus blocks cells in G_1.[360] Polyglutamylation of methotrexate is inhibited by L-asparaginase pretreatment.[361] When the enzyme is given after methotrexate administration, the action of the antifolate is abbreviated. Large doses of the antifolate are well-tolerated if followed by L-asparaginase rescue.

REFERENCES

1. Chabner BA (ed): Pharmacologic principles of cancer treatment. Philadelphia, WB Saunders, 1982
2. Pratt WB, Ruddon RW: The anticancer drugs. New York, Oxford Press, 1979
3. Allegra CJ, Chabner BA, Tuazon CU et al: Trimetrexate, a novel and effective agent for the treatment of *Pneumocystis carinii* pneumonia in patients with acquired immunodeficiency syndrome. N Engl J Med 79:478–782, 1987
4. Sirotnak FM, DeGraw JI, Schmid FA et al: New folate analogs of the 10-deaza-aminopterin series. Further evidence for markedly increased antitumor efficacy compared to methotrexate in ascites and solid murine tumor models. Cancer Chemother Pharmacol 12:2630, 1984
5. Zaharko DS, Fung W-P, Yang F-H: Relative biochemical aspect of low and high doses of methotrexate in mice. Cancer Res 37:1602–1607, 1977
6. Allegra CJ, Fine RL, Drake JC et al: The effect of methotrexate on intracellular folate pools in human MCF-7 breast cancer cells: evidence for direct inhibition of purine synthesis. J Biol Chem 261:6478–6485, 1986
7. Allegra CJ, Hoang K, Yeh GC et al: Evidence for direct inhibition of de novo purine synthesis in human MCF-7 breast cells as a principal mode of metabolic inhibition by methotrexate. J Biol Chem 262:13520–13526, 1987
8. Kane MA, Portillo RM, Elwood PC et al: The influence of extracellular folate concentration on methotrexate uptake by human KB cells. Partial characterization of a membrane-associated methotrexate-binding protein. J Biol Chem 261:44–49, 1986
9. Schilsky RL, Bailey BD, Chabner BA: Methotrexate polyglutamate synthesis by cultured human breast cancer cells. Proc Natl Acad Sci USA 77:2919–2922, 1980
10. Dedhar S, Hartley D, Goldie JH: Increased dihydrofolate reductase activity in methotrexate-resistant human promyelocyte-leukaemia (HL-60) cells. Biochem J 225:609–617, 1985
11. Curt GA, Jolivet J, Carney DN et al: Determinants of the sensitivity of human small-cell lung cancer cell lines to methotrexate. J Clin Invest 76:1323–1329, 1985
12. Meltzer PS, Cheng YC, Trent JM: Analysis of dihydrofolate reductase gene amplification in a methotrexate-resistant human tumor cell line. Cancer Genet Cytogenet 17:289–300, 1985
13. Curt GA, Carney DN, Cowan KH et al: Unstable methotrexate resistance in human small-cell carcinoma associated with double-minute chromosomes. N Engl J Med 308:199–202, 1983
14. Rodenhuis S, McGuire JJ, Narayanan R et al: Development of an assay system for the detection and classification of methotrexate resistance in fresh human leukemic cells. Cancer Res 46:6513–6519, 1986
15. Bertino JR, Isacoff WH: Methods of measuring methotrexate in body fluids. In Pinedo HM (ed): Clinical Pharmacology of Antineoplastic Drugs, pp 3–11. Amsterdam, Elsevier-North Holland Biomedical Press, 1978
16. Myers CE, Lippman M, Eliot HM et al: Competitive protein binding assay for methotrexate. Proc Natl Acad Sci USA 72:3683–3686, 1975
17. Erttman R, Bielack S, Landbeck G: Kinetics of 7-hydroxy-methotrexate after high-dose methotrexate therapy. Cancer Chemother Pharmacol 15:101–104, 1985
18. Evans WE, Crom WR, Stewart CF et al: Methotrexate systemic clearance influences probability of relapse in children with standard-risk acute lymphocytic leukaemia. Lancet 1:359–362, 1984
19. Monjanel S, Rigault JP, Cano JP et al: High-dose methotrexate: Preliminary evaluation of a pharmacokinetic approach. Cancer Chemother Pharmacol 3:189–196, 1979
20. Thyss A, Milano G, Kubar J et al: Clinical and pharmacokinetic evidence of a life-threatening interaction between methothrexate and ketoprofen. Lancet 1:256–258, 1986
21. Stoller RG, Hande KR, Jacobs SA et al: Use of plasma pharmacokinetics to predict and prevent methotrexate toxicity. N Engl J Med 297:630–634, 1977
22. Erttmann R, Landbeck G: Effect of oral cholestyramine on the elimination of high-dose methotrexate. J Cancer Res Clin Oncol 110:48–50, 1985
23. Abelson HT, Ensminger W, Rosowsky A et al: Competitive effects of citrovorum factor and carboxypeptidase G_1 on cerebrospinal fluid methotrexate pharmacokinetics. Cancer Treat Rep 62:1549–1552, 1978

24. Shapiro WR, Young DG, Mehta BM: Methotrexate distribution in cerebrospinal fluid after intravenous, verticular, and lumbar injection. N Engl J Med 293:161–166, 1975
25. Bleyer WA: The clinical pharmacology of methotrexate. Cancer 41:36–51, 1978
26. Tattersall MHN, Brown B, Frei E III: The reversal of methotrexate toxicity by thymidine with maintenance of antitumor effects. Nature 253:198–200, 1975
27. Jacobs SA, Stoller RG, Chabner BA et al: 7-Hydroxymethotrexate as a urinary metabolite in human subjects and Rhesus monkeys receiving high-dose methotrexate. J Clin Invest 57:534–538, 1976
28. Glode LM, Pitman SW, Ensminger WD et al: A phase I study of high-dose aminopterin with leucovorin rescue in patients with advanced metastatic tumor. Cancer Res 39:3707–3714, 1979
29. Wilke WS, Mackenzie AH: Methotrexate therapy in rheumatoid arthritis: Current status. Drugs 32:103–113, 1986
30. Dahl MGC, Gregory MM, Scheuer PJ: Liver damage due to methotrexate in patients with psoriasis. Br Med J 1:625–630, 1971
31. Sostman HD, Matthay RA, Putman C et al: Methotrexate-induced pneumonitis. Medicine 55:371–388, 1976
32. Brouwers P, Moss H, Reaman G et al: Central nervous system preventive therapy with systemic high-dose methotrexate versus cranial radiation and intrathecal methotrexate: Longitudinal comparison of effects of treatment on intellectual function of children with acute lymphoblastic leukemia. Proc Am Soc Clin Oncol 6:158, 1987
33. Heidelberger C, Chandhari NK, Dannenberg P et al: Fluorinated pyrimidines: A new class of tumor inhibitory compounds. Nature 179:663–666, 1957
34. Mandel HG: Incorporation of 5-fluorouracil into RNA and its molecular consequences. Prog Mol Subcell Biol 1:82–135, 1969
35. Schuetz JD, Collins JM, Wallace HJ et al: Alteration of the secondary structure of newly synthesized DNA from murine bone marrow cells by 5-fluorouracil. Cancer Res 46:119–123, 1986
36. Kanamaru R, Kakuta H, Sato T et al: The inhibitory effects of 5-fluorouracil on the metabolism of peribosomal and ribosomal RNA in L1210 cells in vitro. Cancer Chemother Pharmacol 17:43–46, 1986
37. Dolnick BJ, Pink JJ: Effects of 5-fluorouracil on dihydrofolate reductase and dihydrofolate reductase mRNA from methotrexate-resistant KB cells. J Biol Chem 260:3006–3014, 1985
38. Evans RM, Laskin JD, Hakala MT: Effect of excess folates and deoxyinosine on the activity and site of action of 5-fluorouracil. Cancer Res 41:3288, 1981
39. Jenh CH, Geyer PK, Baskin F et al: Thymidylate synthase gene amplification in fluorodeoxyuridine-resistant mouse cell lines. Mol Pharmacol 28:80–85, 1985
40. Kaufman ER: Resistance to 5-fluorouracil associated with increased cytidine triphosphate levels in V79 Chinese hamster cells. Cancer Res 44:3371–3376, 1984
41. Spears CP, Gustavsson BG, Mitchell MS et al: Thymidylate synthase inhibition in malignant tumors and normal liver of patients given intravenous 5-fluorouracil. Cancer Res 44:4144–4150, 1984
42. Finan PJ, Koklitis PA, Chisholm EM et al: Comparative levels of tissue enzymes concerned in the early metabolism of 5-fluorouracil in normal and malignant colorectal tissue. Br J Cancer 50:711–716, 1984
43. Cadman EC, Heimer R, Davis L: Enhanced 5-fluorouracil nucleotide formation following methotrexate: Biochemical explanation for drug synergism. Science 205:1135–1137, 1979
44. Schwartz PM, Handschumacher RE: Selective antagonism of 5-fluorouracil cytotoxicity by 4-hydroxypyrazolopyrimidine (Allopurinol) in vitro. Cancer Res 39:3095–3101, 1979
45. Vogel SJ, Presant CA, Ratkin GA et al: Phase I study of thymidine plus 5-fluorouracil infusions in advanced colorectal carcinoma. Cancer Treat Rep 63:1–5, 1979
46. Peters GJ, Kraal I, Laurensse E et al: Separation of 5-fluorouracil and uracil by ion pair reversed-phase high-performance liquid chromatography on a column with porous polymeric packing. J Chromatogr 307:464–468, 1984
47. Iwamoto M, Yoshida S, Hirosi S: Fluorescence determination of 5-fluorouracil and 1-(tetrahydro-7-furanyl-5-fluorouracil) in blood serum by high-pressure liquid chromatography. J Chromatogr 310:151–157, 1984
48. Christophidis N, Vajda FJE, Lucas I et al: Fluorouracil therapy in patients with carcinoma of the large bowel: A pharmacokinetic comparison of various rates and routes of administration. Clin Pharmacokinet 3:330–336, 1978
49. Jones RB, Buckpitt AR, Londer H et al: Potential clinical application of a new method for quantitation of plasma levels of 5-fluorouracil and 5-fluorodeoxyuridine. Bull Cancer (Paris) 66:75–78, 1979
50. Ensminger WD, Rosowsky A, Raso V: A clinical pharmacological evaluation of hepatic arterial infusion of 5-fluoro 2′-deoxyuridine and 5-fluorouracil. Cancer Res 38:3784–3792, 1978
51. Speyer JL, Collins JM, Dedrick RL et al: Phase I and pharmacologic studies of intraperitoneal 5-fluorouracil. Cancer Res 40:567–572, 1980
52. Dow RT, Fritz WL: 5-Fluorouracil. In Dow RT, Fritz WL (eds): Cancer Chemotherapy Handbook, pp 435–454. New York, Elsevier-North Holland, 1980
53. Valdivieso M, Bodey GP, Gottlieb JA et al: Clinical evaluation of ftorafur (pyrimidine-deoxyyribose N,-2′-furanidyl-5-fluorouracil). Cancer Res 36:1821–1824, 1976
54. Au JL, Wu AT, Friedman MA et al: Pharmacokinetics and metabolism of ftorafur in man. Cancer Treat Rep 63:343–350
55. Armstrong RD, Diasio RB: Metabolism and biological activity of 5′-deoxy-5-fluorouridine, a novel fluoropyrimidine. Cancer Res 40:3333–3338, 1980
56. Cohen SS: The lethality of ara nucleotides. Med Biol 54:299–326, 1976
57. Fram RJ, Kufe DW: Effect of 1-β-D-arabinofuranosyl cytosine and hydroxyurea on the repair of x-ray-induced DNA single-strand breaks in human leukemic blasts. Biochem Pharmacol 34:2557–2560, 1985
58. Fridland A: Inhibition of DNA chain initiation by 1-β-D-arabinofuranosylcytosine (ara-C) in human lymphoblasts. J Supramol Struct 771:331, 1978
59. Woodcock DM, Fox RM, Cooper IA: Evidence for a new mechanism of cytotoxity of 1-β-D-arabinofuranosyl cytosine. Cancer Res 39:1418–1424, 1979
60. Wiley JS, Jones SP, Sawyer WH et al: Cytosine arabinoside influx and nucleoside transport sites in acute leukemia. J Clin Invest 69:479, 1982
61. Wiley JS, Taupin J, Jamieson GP et al: Cytosine arabinoside transport and metabolism in acute leukemias and T-cell lymphoblastic lymphoma. J Clin Invest 75:632–642, 1985
62. Chabner BA, Hande KR, Drake JC: Ara-C metabolism: Implications for drug resistance and drug interactions. Bull Cancer 66:89–92, 1979
63. Tattersall MNH, Ganeshagura K, Hoffbrand AV: Mechanisms of resistance of human acute leukaemia cells to cytosine arabinoside. Br J Haematol 27:39–46, 1974
64. Steuart CD, Burke PJ: Cytidine deaminase and the development of resistance to arabinosyl cytosine. Nature 233:109–110, 1971
65. Preisler HD, Rustum Y, Priore RL: Relationship between leukemic cell retention of cytosine arabinoside triphosphate and the duration of remission in patients with acute nonlymphocytic leukemia. Eur J Cancer Clin Oncol 21:23–30, 1985
66. Karp JE, Donehower RC, Dole GB et al: Direct relationship of marrow cell growth and 1-β-D-arabinofuranosylcytosine metabolism. Cancer Res 44:5046–5050, 1984
67. Mitchell T, Sariban E, Kufe D: Effects of 1-β-D-arabinofuranosylcytosine on protooncogene expression in human U-937 cells. Mol Pharmacol 30:398–402, 1986
68. Tilly H, Bastard C, Bizet M et al: Low-dose cytarabine persistance of a clonal abnormality during complete remission of acute nonlymphocytic leukemia (letter). N Engl J Med 314:246–247, 1986
69. Zimm S, Collins JM, Miser J et al: Cytosine arabinoside cerebrospinal fluid kinetics. Clin Pharmacol Ther 35:826–830, 1984
70. Shimada N, Ueda T, Yokoshima T et al: A sensitive and specific radioimmunoassay for 1-β-D-arabinofuranosylcytosine. Cancer Lett 24:173–178, 1984
71. Ho DHW, Frei E III: Clinical pharmacology of 1-β-D-arabinofuranosylcytosine. Clin Pharmacol Ther 12:944–954, 1971
72. Early AP, Preisler HD, Slocum H et al: A pilot study of high-dose 1-beta-D-arabinofuranosylcytosine for acute leukemia and refractory lymphoma: Clinical response and pharmacology. Cancer Res 42:1587, 1982
73. Donehower RC, Karp JE, Burke PJ: Pharmacology and toxicity of high-dose cytarabine by 72-hour continuous infusion. Cancer Treat Rep 70:1059–1065, 1986
74. Moloney WC, Rosenthal DS: Treatment of early acute nonlymphocytic leukemia with low-dose cytosine arabinoside. Haematol Blood Transfus 26:59–62, 1981
75. Aden OB, Goldie W, Wood T et al: Seizures following intrathecal cytosine arabinoside in young children with acute lymphoblastic leukemia. Cancer 42:53–58, 1978
76. Cadman E, Eiferman F: Mechanism of synergistic cell killing when methotrexate precedes cytosine arabinoside. Study of L1210 and human leukemic cell. J Clin Invest 64:788–797, 1979
77. Harris AW, Reynolds EC, Finch LR: Effect of thymidine on the sensitivity of cultured mouse tumor cells to 1-β-D-arabinofuranosylcytosine. Cancer Res 39:538–541, 1979
78. Kreis W, Wokcock TM, Gordon CS et al: Tetrahydrouridine physiologic disposition and effect upon deamination of cytosine arabinoside in man. Cancer Treat Rep 61:1347–1353, 1977
79. Rustum YM, Dave C, Mayhew E et al: Role of liposome type and route of administration in the antitumor activity of liposome-entrapped 1-β-D-arabinofuranosylcytosine against mouse L1210 leukemia. Cancer Res 39:1390–1395, 1979
80. Lu LJW, Randerath K: Effects of 5-azacytidine on transfer RNA methyltransferases. Cancer Res 39:940–948, 1979
81. Ley TJ, DeSimone J, Anagnon NP et al: 5-Azacytidine selectively increases gamma-globin synthesis in a patient with beta-thalassemia. N Engl J Med 307:1469, 1982
82. Elion GB: Biochemistry and pharmacology of purine analogs. Fed Proc 26:898–904, 1967
83. Tidd DM, Paterson ARP: Distinction between inhibition of purine nucleotide synthesis and the delayed cytotoxic reaction of 6-mercaptopurine. Cancer Res 34:733–737, 1974
84. Christie NT, Drake S, Meyn RE et al: 6-Thioguanine-induced DNA damage as a determinant of cytotoxicity in cultured Chinese hamster ovary cells. Cancer Res 44:3665–3672, 1984
85. Bodell WJ, Morgan WF, Rasmussen J et al: Potentiation of 1,3-bis(2-chloroethyl)-1-nitrosourea (BCNU)-induced cytotoxicity in 9L cells by pretreatment with 6-thioguanine. Biochem Pharmacol 34:515–520, 1985
86. Lee MH, Huang Y-M, Sartorelli AC: Alkaline phosphatase activities of 6-thiopurine-sensitive and -resistant sublines of sarcoma 180. Cancer Res 38:2413–2418, 1978
87. Lennard L, Lillyman JS: Are children with lymphoblastic leukemia given enough 6-mercaptopurine? Lancet 2:785–787, 1987
88. Breter HJ, Zahn RK: Quantitation of intracellular metabolites of [^{35}]-6-mercaptopurine in L5178Y cells grown in time-course incubates. Cancer Res 39:3744–3748, 1979
89. Ding TL, Benet LZ: Determination of 6-mercaptopurine and azathioprine in plasma by high-performance liquid chromatography. J Chromatogr 163:281–288, 1979
90. Tidd DM, Dedhar S: Specific and sensitive combined high performance liquid chromatographic-flow fluorometric assay for intracellular-6-thioguanine metabolites of 6-mercaptopurine and 6-thioguanine. J Chromatogr 145:237–246, 1978
91. Zimm S, Collins JM, Riccardi R et al: Variable bioavailability of oral 6-mercaptopur-

ine: Is maintenance chemotherapy in acute lymphoblastic leukemia being optimally delivered. N Engl J Med 308:1005–1009, 1983
92. Burton NK, Barnett MJ, Aherne GW et al: The effect of food on the oral administration of 6-mercaptopurine. Cnacer Chemother Pharmacol 18:90–91, 1986
93. Burton NK, Aherne GW: The effect of cotrimoxazole on the absorption of orally administered 6-mercaptopurine in the rat. Cancer Chemother Pharmacol 16:81–84, 1986
94. Esterhay RJ, Aisner J, Levi JA et al: High-dose 6-mercaptopurine in advanced refractory cancer. Cancer Treat Rep 62:1229–1231, 1978
95. Present DH, Korelitz BI, Wisch N et al: Treatment of Crohn's disease with 6-mercaptopurine. N Engl J Med 302:981–986, 1980
96. Pavan-Langston D, Buchanan RA, Alford CA Jr (eds): Adenine arabinoside: An antiviral agent. New York, Raven Press, 1979
97. Brockman RW, Schabel FM, Montgomery JH: Biologic activity of 9-β-arabinofuranosyl-2-fluoro adenine, a metabolically stable analog of 9-β-D-arabinofuranosyladenine. Biochem Pharmacol 26:2193–2196, 1977
98. Weiss GR, Arteaga CL, Brown TD et al: New anticancer agents. In Pinedo HM, Chabner BA, Longo DL (eds): Cancer chemotherapy, annual 9, pp 93–120. Amsterdam, Elsevier, 1987
99. Plunkett W, Alexander L, Chubb S et al: Biochemical basis of the increased activity of 9-beta-D-arabinofuranosyladenine in the presence of inhibitors of adenosine deaminase. Cancer Res 39:3655–3660, 1979
100. Smyth JF, Paine RM, Jackman AL et al: The clinical pharmacology of the adenosine deaminase inhibitor 2′-deoxycoformycin. Cancer Chemother Pharmacol 5:93–101, 1980
101. Ludlum DB: Alkylating agents and the nitrosoureas. In Becker FF (ed): Cancer: A comprehensive treatise, Vol 5, pp 285–307. New York, Plenum Press, 1977
102. Kohn KW: Interstrand cross-linking of DNA by 1,3-bis(chlorethyl)-1-nitrosourea and other 1-(2-haloethyl)-1-nitroureas. Cancer Res 37:1450–1454, 1977
103. Wang AL, Tew KD: Increased glutathione-S-transferase activity in a cell line with acquired resistance to nitrogen mustards. Cancer Treat Rep 69:677–682, 1985
104. Tobey RA, Tesmer JG: Differential response of cultured human normal and tumor cells to trace-element-induced resistance to the alkylating agent melphalan. Cancer Res 45:2567–2571, 1985
105. Crook TR, Souhami RL, Whyman GD et al: Glutathione depletion as a determinant of sensitivity of human leukemia cells to cyclophosphamide. Cancer Res 46:5035–5038, 1986
106. Somfai-Relle S, Suzukake K, Vistica BP et al: Reduction in cellular glutathione by butathionine sulfoximine and sensitization of murine tumor cells resistant to L-phenylalanine mustard. Biochem Pharmacol 33:485–489, 1984
107. Mulcahy RT, Dembs NL, Ublacker GA: Enhancement of nitrosourea cytotoxicity by misonidazole in vitro: Correlation with carbamoylating potential. Br J Cancer 49:307–313, 1984
108. Henner WD, Peters WP, Eder JP et al: Pharmacokinetics and immediate effects of high-dose carmustine in man. Cancer Treat Rep 70:877–880, 1986
109. DeJong JP, Nikkels PGJ, Brockbank KGM et al: Comparative in vitro effects of cyclophosphamide derivatives on murine bone marrow-derived stromal and hemopoietic progenitor cell classes. Cancer Res 45:4001–4005, 1985
110. Lee FYF, Workman P: Interaction of nitroimidazole sensitizers with drug metabolizing enzymes—spectral and kinetic studies. Int J Radiat Oncol Biol Phys 13:1383–1387, 1986
111. Bergsagel DE: Treatment of plasma cell myeloma with cytotoxic agents. Arch Intern Med 135:172–176, 1975
112. Lyons RM, Goldenberg GJ: Active transport of nitrogen mustard and choline by normal and leukemic human lymphoid cells. Cancer Res 32:1679–1685, 1972
113. Lawley PD, Brookes P: Molecular mechanisms of the cytotoxic action of difunctional alkylating agents and of resistance to this action. Nature 206:480–483, 1965
114. Colvin M: A review of the pharmacology and clinical use of cyclophosphamide. In Pinedo HM (ed): Clinical pharmacology of antineoplastic drugs. pp 245–261. Amsterdam. Elsevier-North Holland, 1978
115. Hilton J: Role of aldehyde dehydrogenase in cyclophosphamide-resistant L1210 leukemia. Cancer Res 44:5156–5160, 1984
116. Brock N, Pohl J, Stekar J: Detoxification of urotoxic oxazaphosphorines by sulfhydryl compounds. J Cancer Res Clin Oncol 100:311, 1981
117. Cox PJ: Cyclophosphamide cystitis. Identification of acrolein as the causative agent. Biochem Pharmacol 28:2045–2049, 1979
118. Green TP, Mirken BL: Prevention of cyclophosphamide-induced antidiuresis by furosemide infusion. Clin Pharmacol Ther 29:634, 1981
119. Manohoran A: Carcinoma of the urinary bladder in patients receiving cyclophosphamide. Aust NZ J Med 14:507–512, 1984
120. Connors TA: Alkylating drugs, nitrosourea and dialkyl triazenes. In Pinedo HM (ed): Cancer chemotherapy, pp 25–55. Amsterdam, Elsevier-North Holland, 1979
121. Hengst JCD, Kempf RA: Immunomodulation by cyclophosphamide. Clin Immunol Allergy 4:199–216, 1984
122. Alvarado CS, Boat TF, Newman AJ: Late onset pulmonary fibrosis and chest deformity in two children treated with cyclophosphamide. J Pediatr 92:443–446, 1978
123. Steinherz LJ, Steinherz PG: Cyclophosphamide cardiotoxicity. Cancer Bull 37:231–234, 1985
124. El-Yazigi A, Martin CR: Improved analysis of cyclophosphamide by capillary gas chromatography with thermionic (nitrogen-phosphorus)-specific detection and silica sample purification. J Chromatogr Biomed Appl 374:177–182, 1986
125. Sladek NE, Powers JF, Grage GM: Half-life of oxazaphosphorines in biological fluids. Drug Metab Dispos 12:553–559, 1984
126. Kallama S, Hemminki K: Stabilities of 7-alkylguanosines and 7-deoxyguanosines formed by phosphoramide mustard and nitrogen mustard. Chem Biol Interact 57:85–96, 1986
127. Juma FD: Effect of liver failure on the pharmacokinetics of cyclophosphamide. Eur J Clin Pharmacol 26:591–593, 1984
128. Andriole GL, Sandlund JT, Miser JS et al: The efficacy of MESNA (2-mercaptoethane sodium sulfonate) as a uroprotectant in patients with hemorrhagic cystitis receiving further oxazaphosphorine chemotherapy. J Clin Oncol 5:799–803, 1987
129. Meanwell CA, Blade AE, Kelly KA et al: Prediction of ifosfamide/MESNA-associated encephalopathy. Eur J Clin Oncol 22:815–819, 1986
130. Goren MP, Wright KR, Pratt CB et al: Dechloroethylation of ifosfamide and neurotoxicity. Lancet 2:1219–1220, 1986
131. Carny T, Margison JM, Thatcher N et al: Bioavailability of ifosfamide in patients with bronchial carcinoma. Cancer Chemother Pharmacol 18:261–264, 1986
132. Vistica DT, Toal JN, Rabinovitz M: Amino-acid-conferred protection against melphalan. Biochem Pharmacol 27:2865–2870, 1978
133. Vistica DT, Toal JN, Rabinovitz M: Amino-acid-conferred protection against melphalan: Interference with leucine protection of melphalan cytotoxicity by the basic amino acids in cultured murine L1210 leukemic cells. Mol Pharmacol 14:1136–1142, 1978
134. Goldenberg GJ, Froese EK: Antagonism of the cytocidal activity and uptake of melphalan by tamoxifen in human breast cancer cells in vitro. Biochem Pharmacol 34:763–770, 1985
135. Tattersall MN, Jarman M, Newlands ES et al: Pharmacokinetics of melphalan following oral or intravenous administration in patients with malignant disease. Eur J Cancer 14:507–514, 1978
136. Alberts DS, Chang SY, Chen HSG et al: Kinetics of intravenous melphalan. Clin Pharmacol Ther 26:73–80, 1979
137. Howell SB, Pfeifle CE, Olshen RA: Intraperitoneal chemotherapy with melphalan. Ann Intern Med 101:14–20, 1984
138. Green MH, Harris EL, Gershenson DM et al: Melphalan may be a more potent leukemogen than cyclophosphamide. Ann Intern Med 105:360–367, 1986
139. Fiere D, Felman P, Vivian H et al: Acute myeloid leukemia following the administration of chlorambucil. Two cases. Nouv Presse Med 7:756, 1978
140. Cole SR, Myers TJ, Klatsky AU: Pulmonary disease with chlorambucil therapy. Cancer 41:455–459, 1978
141. Nedkarni MV, Trams EG, Smith PK: Preliminary studies on the distribution and fate of TEM, TEPA, and myleran in the human. Cancer Res 19:713–718, 1959
142. Heal JM, Franza BR, Schein PS: Pharmacology of nitrosourea antitumor agents. In Pinedo HM (ed): Clinical pharmacology of antineoplastic drugs, pp 263–275. Amsterdam, Elsevier-North Holland, 1978
143. Ewig RAG, Kohn KW: DNA damage and repair in mouse leukemia L1210 cells treated with nitrogen mustard, 1,3-bis(2-chloroethyl)-1-nitrosourea, and other nitrosoureas. Cancer 37:2114–2122, 1977
144. Kann HE Jr: Comparison of biochemical and biological effects of four nitrosoureas with differing carbamoylating activities. Cancer Res 38:2363–2366, 1978
145. Tew KD, Sudhakar S, Schein PS, Smulson ME: Binding of chlorozotocin and 1-(2-chlorethyl)-3-cyclohexyl-1-nitrosourea to chromatin and nucleosomal fractions of HeLa cells. Cancer Res 38:3371–3378, 1978
146. Lee FYF, Workman P, Roberts JT et al: Clinical pharmacokinetics or oral CCNU (Lomustine). Cancer Chemother Pharmacol 14:125–128, 1985
147. Reed DJ, May HE: Cytochrome P-450 interactions with the 2-chloroethylnitrosoureas and procarbazine. Biochimie 60:989–995, 1978
148. Greene MH, Boile JD, Strike TA: Carmustine as a cause of acute nonlymphocytic leukemia. N Engl J Med 313:579, 1985
149. Hundley R, Lukens JN: Nitrosourea-associated pulmonary fibrosis. Cancer Treat Rep 63:2128–2130, 1979
150. Harmon WE, Cohen HJ, Schneeberger EE et al: Chronic renal failure in children treated with methyl CCNU. N Engl J 300:1200–1203, 1979
151. Rosenberg B, Van Camp L, Krigas T: Inhibition of cell division in *Escherichia coli* by electrolysis products from a platinum electrode. Nature 205:698–699, 1965
152. Rosenberg B, Van Camp L, Trosko JE et al: Platinum compounds: A new class of potent antitumor agents. Nature 222:385–386, 1969
153. Filipski J, Kohn KW, Bonner WM: The nature of inactivating lesions produced by platinum(II) complexes in phase DNA. Chem Biol Interact 32:321–330, 1980
154. Scovell WM, O'Connor T: Interaction of aquated *cis*-[$(NH_3)_2$PtII] with nuclei acid constituents: 1. Ribonucleosides. J Am Chem Soc 99:120–126, 1977
155. Zwelling LA, Kohn KW: Mechanism of action of *cis*-dichlorodiammineplatinum(II). Cancer Treat Rep 63:1439–1444, 1979
156. Cohen GL, Bauer WR, Barton JK, Lippard SJ: Binding of *cis*- and *trans*-dichlorodiammineplatinum(II) to DNA: Evidence for unwinding and shortening of the double helix. Science 203:1014–1016, 1979
157. Roberts JJ, Thomson AJ: The mechanism of action of antitumor platinum compounds. Prog Nucleic Acid Res Mol Biol 22:71–133, 1979
158. Meyn RE, Jenkins SF, Thompson LH: Defective removal of DNA cross-links in a repair-deficient mutant of chinese hamster cells. Cancer Res 42:3106, 1982
159. Burchenal JH, Kalaher K, Dew K et al: Studies of cross-resistance, synergistic combination and blocking activity of platinum derivatives. Biochimie 60:961–965, 1978
160. Borch RF, Katz JC, Lieder, PH et al: Effect of diethyldithiocarbamate rescue on tumor

response to cis-platinum in a rat model. Proc Natl Acad Sci USA 77:5441–5444, 1980
161. Glover D, Glick JH, Weiler C et al: Phase I trials of WR-2721 and cis-platinum. Int J Radiat Oncol Biol Phys 10:1781–1784, 1984
162. Fraval HNA, Roberts JJ: G_1 phase Chinese hamster V79-379A cells are inherently more sensitive to platinum bound to their DNA than mid S phase or asynchronously treated cells. Biochem Pharmacol 28:1575–1580, 1979
163. Endressen L, Schjerven L, Rugstad HE: Tumours from a cell strain with a high content of metallothionein show enhanced resistance against *cis*-dichlorodiammineplatinum. Acta Pharmacol Toxicol 55:183–187, 1984
164. Reed E, Yuspa SH, Zwelling LA et al: Quantitation of cis-diamminedichloroplatinum(II) (cisplatin)-DNA-intrastrand adducts in testicular and ovarian cancer patients receiving cisplatin chemotherapy. J Clin Invest 77:545–550, 1986
165. LeRoy AF, Wehling ML, Sponseller HL et al: Analysis of platinum in biological materials by flameless atomic absorption spectrophotometry. Biochem Med 18:184–191, 1977
166. Marsh KC, Sternson LA, Repta AJ: Post-column reaction detector for platinum(II) antineoplastic agents. Anal Chem 56:491–497, 1984
167. Litterst CL, LeRoy AF, Guarino AM: The disposition and distribution of platinum following parenteral administration to animals of *cis*-dichlorodiammineplatinum(II). Cancer Treat Rep 63:1485–1492, 1979
168. Vermorken JB, Van der Vijgh WJF, Klein I et al: Pharmacokinetics of free and total platinum species after short-term infusion of cisplatin. Cancer Treat Rep 68:505–513, 1984
169. Patton TF, Himmelstein KJ, Belt R et al: Plasma levels and urinary excretion of filterable platinum species following bolus injection and i.v. infusion of *cis*-dichlorodiammineplatinum(II) in man. Cancer Treat Rep 63:1359–1361, 1979
170. Gormley P, Poplack D, Pizzo P: The cerebrospinal fluid pharmacokinetics of *cis*-diamminedichloroplatinum(II) and several platinum analogues. Proc Am Assoc Cancer Res 20:279, 1979
171. Daley-Yates PT, McBrien DCH: Cisplatin metabolites in plasma, a study of their pharmacokinetics and importance in the nephrotoxic and antitumour activity of cisplatin. Biochem Pharmacol 33:3063–3070, 1984
172. Jacobs C, Kalman SM, Tretton M et al: Renal handling of *cis*-diamminedichloroplatinum(II). Cancer Treat Rep 64(12):1223–1226, 1980
173. Chary KK, Higby DJ, Henderson ES et al: Phase I study of high-dose *cis*-dichlorodiammineplatinum(II) with forced diversis. Cancer Treat Rep 61:367–370, 1977
174. Ozols RF, Corden BF, Jacob J et al: High-dose cisplatin in hypertonic saline. Ann Intern Med 100:19–24, 1984
175. Madias NE, Harrington JT: PLatinum nephrotoxicity. Am J Med 65:307–314, 1978
176. Gonzalez-Vitale JC, Hayes DM, Cvitkovic E et al: The renal pathology in clinical trials of *cis*-platinum (II) diamminedichloride. Cancer 39:1362–1371, 1977
177. Schilsky RL, Anderson T: Hypomagnesemia and renal magnesium wasting in patients receiving *cis*-platin. Ann Intern Med 90:929–931, 1979
178. Jones B, Mladek J, Bhalla R et al: Enzymuria and beta$_2$ microglobulinuria as a sensitive index of *cis*-platinum nephrotoxicity. Proc Am Soc Clin Oncol 20:336,1979
179. Roelofs RI, Hrushersky W, Rogin J et al: Peripheral sensory neuropathy and cisplatin chemotherapy. Neurology 34:934–938, 1984
180. Wiesenfeld M, Reinders E, Corder M et al: Successful retreatment with *cis*-DDP after apparent allergic reactions. Cancer Treat Rep 63:219–221, 1979
181. Granowetter L, Rosenstock JG, Packer RJ: Enhanced cis-platinum neurotoxicity in pediatric patients with brain tumors. J Neurooncol 1:293–297, 1983
182. Howell SB, Pfeifle CL, Wang WE et al: Intraperitoneal cisplatin with systemic thiosulfate protection. Ann Intern Med 97:845–851, 1982
183. Egorin MJ, Van Echo DA, Tipping SJ et al: Pharmacokinetics and dosage reduction of cis-diammine(1,1-cyclobutanedicarboxylato) platinum in patients with impaired renal function. Cancer Res 44:5432–5438, 1984
184. Takeshita M, Grollman AP, Ohtsubo E et al: Interaction of bleomycin with DNA. Proc Natl Acad Sci USA 75:5983–5987, 1978
185. Wu JC, Stubbe J, Kozarich JW: Mechanism of bleomycin: evidence for 4′-ketone formation in poly(dA-dU) associated exclusively with free base release. Biochemistry 24:7569–7573, 1985
186. Barranco SC, Humphrey RM: The effects of bleomycin on survival and cell progression in Chinese hamster cells *in vitro*. Cancer Res 31:1218–1223, 1971
187. Barranco SC, Novak JK, Humphrey RM: Studies on recovery from chemically induced damage in mammalian cells. Cancer Res 35:1194–1204, 1975
188. Chafouleas JG, Bolton WE, Means AR: Potentiation of bleomycin lethality by anticalmodulin drugs: a role for calmodulin in DNA repair. Science 224:1346–1348, 1984
189. Russo A, Mitchell JB, McPherson S et al: Alteration of bleomycin cytotoxicity by glutathione depletion or elevation. Int J Radiat Oncol Biol Phys 10:1675–1678, 1984
190. Umezawa H, Hori S, Sawa T, et al: A bleomycin-inactivating enzyme in mouse liver. J Antibiot 27:419–424, 1974
191. Sehti SM, Lazo JS: Separation of the protective enzyme bleomycin hydrolase from rabbit pulmonary aminopeptidases. Biochemistry 26:432–437, 1987
192. Akiyama S, Kuwano M: Isolation and preliminary characterization of bleomycin-resistant mutants from Chinese hamster ovary cells. J Cell Physiol 107:147, 1981
193. Broughton A, Strong JE: Radioimmunoassay of bleomycin. Cancer Res 36:1418–1421, 1976
194. Alberts DS, Chen HSG, Liu R et al: Bleomycin pharmacokinetics in man: I. Intravenous administration. Cancer Chemother Pharmacol 1:177–181, 1978
195. Alberts DS, Chen HSG, Mayersohn M et al: Bleomycin pharmacokinetics in man: II. Intracavitary administration. Cancer Chemother Pharmacol 2:127–132, 1979
196. Blum RH, Carter SK, Agre K: A clinical review of bleomycin—a new antineoplastic agent. Cancer 31:903–914, 1973
197. Bell MR, Meredith DJ, Gill PG: Role of carbon monoxide diffusing capacity in the early detection of major bleomycin-induced pulmonary toxicity. Auts NZ J Med 15:235–240, 1985
198. Bellamy EA, Husband JE, Blaquiere RM et al: Bleomycin-related lung damage: CT evidence. Radiology 156:155–158, 1985
199. Morrow CP, DiSaia PJ, Mangan CF et al: Continuous pelvic arterial infusion with bleomycin for squamous carcinoma of the cervix recurrent after irradiation therapy. Cancer Treat Rep 61:1403–1405, 1977
200. Bracken RB, Johnson DE, Rodriquez L, Samuels ML, Ayala A: Treatment of multiple superficial tumors of bladder with intravesical bleomycin. Urology 9:161–163, 1977
201. Thompson RH: Naturally Occurring Quinones, pp 536–575. London, Academic Press, 1971
202. DiMarco A, Galtani M, Orezzi PO: Daunomycin, a new antibiotic of the rhodomycin group. Nature 201:706–707, 1964
203. Friedmann CA: Structure–activity relationships of anthraquinones in some pathological conditions. Pharmacology 20:113–122, 1980
204. Handa K, Sato S: Generation of free radicals of quinone group containing anticancer chemicals in NADPH-microsome system as evidenced by initiation of sulfite oxidation. Gann 66:43–47, 1975
205. Pigram WJ, Fuller W, Amilton LDH: Stereochemistry of intercalation: Interaction of daunomycin with DNA. Nature 235:17–19, 1972
206. Murphree SA, Cunningham LS, Hwang KM et al: Effects of adriamycin on surface properties of sarcoma 180 ascites cells. Biochem Pharmacol 25:1227–1231, 1976
207. Mikkelsen RB, Lin PS, Wallach DF: Interaction of adriamycin with human red blood cells: A biochemical and morphologic study. J Mol Med 2:33–40, 1977
208. Liu LF, Rowe TC, Yang L et al: Cleavage of DNA by mammalian DNA topoisomerase-II. J Biol Chem 258:15365–15370, 1983
209. Tewey KM, Chen GL, Nelson EM et al: Intercalative antitumor drugs interfere with the breakage-reunion reaction of mammalian DNA topoisomerase II. J Biol Chem 259:9182–9187, 1984
210. Potmesil M, Kirshenbaum S, Isreal M et al: Relationship of adriamycin concentrations to the DNA lesions induced in hypoxic and euoxic L1210 cells. Cancer Res 43:3528–3532, 1983
211. Doroshow JH: Prevention of doxorubicin-induced killing of MCF-7 human breast tumor cancer cells by oxygen radical scavengers and iron chelating agents. Biochem Biophys Res Commun 135:330–337, 1986
212. Sinha BK, Katki AG, Batist G et al: Differential formation of hydroxyl radicals by adriamycin in sensitive and resistant MCF-7 human breast cells: implication for the mechanism of action. Biochemistry 26:3776–3781, 1987
213. Myers CE, Gianni L, Zweier J et al: The role of iron in adriamycin biochemistry. Fed Proc 45:2792–2797, 1986
214. Yeh GC, Occhipinit SJ, Cowan KH et al: Adriamycin resistance in human tumor cells associated with marked alterations in the regulation of the hexose monophosphate shunt and its response to oxidant stress. Cancer Res 47:5994–5999, 1987
215. Doroshow JH: Role of reactive oxygen production in doxorubicin cardiac toxicity. In Hacker MP, Lazo JS, Tritton TR (eds): Organ directed toxicities of anticancer drugs, pp 31–40. The Hague, Martinus Nijhoff, 1988
216. Doroshow JH, Locker GY, Myers CE: The enzymatic defenses of the mouse heart against reactive oxygen metabolites. J Clin Invest 65:128–135, 1980
217. Myers CE: Role of iron in anthracycline action. In Hacker MP, Lazo JS, Tritton TR (eds): Organ directed toxicities of anticancer drugs, pp 17–30. The Hague, Martinus Nijhoff, 1988
218. Speyer JL, Green MD, Ward C et al: A trial of ICRF-1878 to selectively protect against chronic adriamycin cardiac toxicity: rationale and preliminary result of a clinical trial. In Hacker MP, Lazo JS, Tritton TR (eds): Organ directed toxicities of anticancer drugs, pp 64–76. The Hague, Martinus Nijhoff, 1988
219. Von Hoff DD, Howser D, Lewis BJ et al: Phase I trial of ICRF-187. Cancer Treat Rep 65:249–252, 1981
220. Ferrans VJ, Herman EH, Hamlin RL: Pretreatment with ICRF-187 protects against the chronic cardiac toxicity produced by very large cumulative doses of doxorubicin in beagle dogs. In Hacker MP, Lazo JS, Tritton TR (eds): Organ directed toxicities of anticancer drugs, pp 56–63. The Hague, Martinus Nijhoff, 1988
221. Israel M, Pegg WJ, Wilkinson PM et al: Liquid chromatographic analysis of adriamycin and metabolites in biological fluids. J Liquid Chromatogr 1:795–809, 1978
222. Eksborg S: Reversed-phase liquid chromatography of adriamycin and daunorubicin and their hydroxyl metabolites, adriamycinol, and daunorubicinol. J Chromatogr 149:225–232, 1978
223. Takanashi S, Bachur NR: Adriamycin metabolism in man: Evidence from urinary metabolites. Drug Metab Disp 4:79–87, 1976
224. Benjamin RS: Pharmacokinetics of adriamycin in patients with sarcomas: Cancer Chemother Rep 58:271–273, 1974
225. Sulkes A, Collins JM: Reappraisal of some dosage adjustment guidelines. Cancer Treat Rep 71:229–233, 1987
226. Dantchev D, Slioussantchouk V, Paintrand M et al: Electron microscopic studies of the heart and light microscopic studies of golden hamsters with adriamycin, doxorubicin, AD 32, and aclacinomycin. Cancer Treat Rep 63:875–888, 1979
227. Tong GL, Wu HY, Smith TH et al: Adriamycin analogues: 3. Synthesis of N-alkylated

anthracyclines with enhanced efficacy and reduced cardiotoxicity. J Med Chem 22:912–918, 1979
228. Benjamin RS, Chawla SP, Ewer MS et al: Adriamycin cardiac toxicity—an assessment of approaches to cardiac monitoring and cardioprotection. In Hacker MP, Lazo JS, Tritton TR (eds): Organ directed toxicities of anticancer drugs, pp 41–55. The Hague, Martinus Nijhoff, 1988
229. Myers CE: Anthracyclines. In Pinedo HM, Longo DL, Chabner BA (eds): Cancer chemotherapy and biological response modifiers, annual 9, pp 36–49. Amsterdam, Elsevier, 1987
230. Myers CE, Muindi JR, Zweier J et al: 5-Iminodaunomycin: An anthracycline with unique properties. J Biol Chem 262:11571–11577, 1987
231. Sinha BK, Motten AD, Hanck K: The electrochemical reduction of 1,4-bis-(2-hydroxyethyl)-amino-(ethylamino)-anthracenedione and daunomycin: Biochemical significance of superoxide formation. Chem Biol Inter 43:371–377, 1983
232. Shenkenberg TD, Von Hoff DD et al: Mitoxantrone: A new anticancer drug with significant clinical activity. Ann Intern Med 105:67–70, 1986
233. Crooke ST, Bradner WT: Mitomycin C: A review. Cancer Treat Rev 3:121–139, 1976
234. Reich SD: Clinical pharmacology of mitomycin C. *In* Carter SK, Crooke ST (eds): Mitomycin C: Current status and new developments, p 243. New York, Academic Press, 1979
235. Keyes SR, Fracasso PM, Heimbrook DC et al: Role of NADPH: cytochrome C reductase and DT-diaphorase in the biotransformation of mitomycin C. Cancer Res 44:5638–5643, 1984
236. Iyengar BS, Remers WA: A comparison of mechanism proposed for the conversion of mitomycins into mitosenes. J Med Chem 28:963–967, 1985
237. den Hartigh J, Verweij J, Pinedo HM: Mitomycin C. In Pinedo HM, Chabner BA (eds): Cancer chemotherapy, annual 7, pp 83–90. Amsterdam, Elsevier, 1985
238. Dorr RT, Bowdan GT, Alberts DS et al: Interactions of mitomycin C with mammalian DNA detected by alkaline elution. Cancer Res 45:3510–3516, 1985
239. Nakano H, Siugoka K, Nakano M et al: Importance of Fe^{2+}-ADP and the relative unimportance of OH in the mechanism of mitomycin C-induced lipid peroxidation. Biochim Biophys Acta 796:285–293, 1984
240. Ludwig CU, Peng YM, Beaudry JN et al: Cytotoxicity of mitomycin C on clonogenic human carcinoma cells is not enhanced by hypoxia. Cancer Chemother Pharmacol 12:146–150, 1984
241. Tsuruo T, Iida-Saito H, Kawabata H et al: Characteristics of resistance to adriamycin in human myelogenous leukemia K562 resistant to adriamycin and in isolated clones. Jpn J Cancer Res 77:682–692, 1986
242. den Hartigh J, McVie JG, Van Oort WJ et al: Pharmacokinetics of mitomycin C in humans. Cancer Res 43:5017–5021, 1983
243. Schilcher RB, Young JD, Ratanatharathorn V et al: Clinical pharmacokinetics of high-dose mitomycin C. Cancer Chemother Pharmacol 13:186–190, 1984
244. Hopkins SC, Robert GB, Matheny R et al: The stability and antitumor activity of recycled (intravesical) mitomycin C. Cancer 53:2063–2068, 1984
245. Cattell V: Mitomycin-induced hemolytic uremic kidney. An experimental model in the rat. Am J Pathol 121:88–95, 1985
246. Valavaara R, Nordman E: Renal complications of mitomycin C therapy with special reference to the total dose. Cancer 55:47–50, 1985
247. Cantrell JE, Phillips TM, Schein PS: Carcinoma-associated hemolytic uremic syndrome: a complication of mitomycin C chemotherapy. J Clin Oncol 3:723–734, 1985
248. Oswoll ES, Kiessling PJ, Patterson JR: Interstitial pneumonia from mitomycin. Ann Intern Med 89:352–355, 1978
249. Kuedke D, McLaughlin TT, Daughaday C et al: Mitomycin C and vindesine associated pulmonary toxicity with variable clinical expression. Cancer 55:542–547, 1985
250. Trush MA, Mimnaugh EG, Ginsburg E et al: Studies on the in vitro interaction of mitomycin C, nitrofuantoin and paraquat with pulmonary microsomes. Stimulation of reactive oxygen-dependent lipid peroxidation. Biochem Pharmacol 31:805, 1982
251. Bachur NR, Gordon SL, Gee RV: A general mechanism for microsomal activation of quinone anticancer agents to free radicals. Cancer Res 38:1745–1750, 1978
252. Selman Waksman Conference on actinomycins: Their potential for cancer chemotherapy. Cancer Chemother Rep 58:1–123, 1974
253. Frei E: The clinical use of actinomycin. Cancer Chemother Rep 58:49–54, 1974
254. Sobell HM, Jain SC, Sakere TD et al: Stereochemistry of actinomycin-DNA binding. Nature (New Biol) 231:200–205, 1971
255. Reich E, Franklin RM, Shatkin AJ et al: Action of actinomycin D on animal cells and viruses. Proc Natl Acad Sci USA 48:1238–1245, 1962
256. Ross WE, Glaubiger DL, Kohn KW: Quantitative and qualitative aspects of intercalator-induced DNA damage. Biochim Biophys Acta 562:41–50, 1979
257. Galbraith WM, Mellett LB: Tissue disposition of ^3H-actinomycin D in rat, monkey and dog. Cancer Chemother Rep 59:1061–1069, 1975
258. Tattersall NHM, Sodergren JE, Segupta SK et al: Pharmacokinetics of actinomycin D in patients with malignant melanoma. Clin Pharmacol Ther 17:701–708, 1975
259. Kennedy BJ: Mithramycin therapy in testicular cancer. J Urol 107:429–433, 1972
260. Koller C, Miller DM: Preliminary observations on the therapy of the myeloid blast phase of chronic granulocytic leukemia with plicamycin and hydroxyurea. N Engl J Med 315:1433–1437, 1986
261. Mathe G, Misset JL, de Vassal F et al: Phase II clinical trial with vindesine for remission induction in acute leukemia, blastic crisis of chronic myeloid leukemia, lymphosarcoma, and Hodgkin's disease: Absence of cross-resistance with vincristine. Cancer Treat Rep 62:805–809, 1978
262. Owellen RJ, Hartke CA, Dickerson RM et al: Inhibition of tubulin-microtubule polymerization by drugs of the vinca alkaloid class. Cancer Res. 36:1499–1502, 1976
263. Lapinjoki SP, Verajankowa HM, Huhtikangas AE et al: An enzyme-linked immunosorbent assay for the antineoplastic agent vincristine. J Immunoassay 7:113, 1986
264. Horwitz SB, Lothstein L, Manfredi JJ et al: Taxol: mechanisms of action and resistance. Ann NY Acad Sci 466:733–744, 1986
265. Madoc-Jones H, Mauro F: Interphase action of vinblastine and vincristine: Differences in their lethal action through the mitotic cycle of cultured mammalian cells. J Cell Physiol 72:185–196, 1968
266. Rosazza JPN, Duffel MW: Metabolic transformation of alkaloids. Alkaloids 27:323–405, 1986
267. Bleyer WA, Frisby SA, Oliverio VT: Uptake and binding of vincristine by murine leukemia cells. Biochem Pharmacol 24:633–639, 1975
268. Jackson DV, Bender RA: Cytotoxic thresholds of vincristine in L1210 murine leukemia and a human lymphoblastic cell line *in vitro*. Cancer Res 39:4346–4349, 1979
269. Dan K: Development of resistance to daunomycin (NSC 83151) in Ehrlich ascites tumor. Cancer Chemother Rep 55:133–141, 1971
270. Kartner N, Shales M, Riordan JR et al: Daunorubicin-resistant Chinese hamster ovary cells expressing multidrug resistance and a cell-surface P-glycoprotein. Cancer Res 43:4413–4419, 1983
271. Tsuruo T: Reversal of acquired resistance to vinca alkaloids and anthracycline antibiotics. Cancer Treat Rep 67:889–893, 1983
272. Conter V, Beck WT: Acquisition of multiple drug resistance by CCRF-CEM cells selected for different degrees of resistance to vincristine. Cancer Treat Rep 68:831–836, 1984
273. Greenberger LM, Williams SS, Horwitz SB: Biosynthesis of heterogeneous forms of multidrug resistance—associated glycoproteins. J Biol Chem, in press
274. Bender RA, Castle MC, Margileth DA et al: The pharmacokinetics of ^3H-vincristine in man. Clin Pharmacol Ther 22:430–438, 1977
275. Owellen RJ, Root MA, Hains FO: Pharmacokinetics of vindesine and vincristine in humans. Cancer Res 37:2603–2607, 1977
276. Lapinjoki SP, Verajankorva HM, Huhtikangas AE et al: An enzyme-linked immunosorbent assay for the antineoplastic agent vincristine. J Immunoassay 7:113–128, 1986
277. Sethi VS, Kimball JC: Pharmacokinetics and vincristine sulfate in children. Cancer Chemother Pharmacol 6:111, 1981
278. Jackson DV, Sethi VS, Spurr CL et al: Pharmacokinetics of vincristine in the cerebrospinal fluid of humans. Cancer Res 41:1466, 1981
279. Castle MC, Margileth DA, Oliverio VT: Distribution and excretion of ^3H-vincristine in the rat and the dog. Cancer Res 36:3684–3689, 1976
280. Jackson DV, Castle MC, Bender RA: Biliary excretion of vincristine. Clin Pharmacol Ther 24:101–107, 1978
281. Owellen RJ, Hartke CA, Hains FO: Pharmacokinetics and metabolism of vinblastine in humans. Cancer Res 37:2567–2602, 1977
282. Ferguson PJ, Phillips JR, Selner M et al: Differential activity of vincristine and vinblastine against cultured cells. Cancer Res 44:3307–3312, 1984
283. Zeffren J, Yagoda A, Kelsen D et al: Phase I-II trial of a 5-day continuous infusion of vinblastine sulfate. Anticancer Res 4:411–413, 1984
284. Griffiths JD, Stark RJ, Ding JC et al: Vincristine neurotoxicity in Charcot-Marie-Tooth syndrome. Med J Aust 143:305–306, 1985
285. Miller BR: Neurotoxicity and vincristine. J Am Med Assoc 253:2045, 1985
286. Weiss HD, Walker MD, Wiernik PH: Neurotoxicity of commonly used antineoplastic agents. N Engl J Med 291:127–133, 1974
287. Williams ME, Walker AN, Bracikowski JP et al: Ascending myeloencephalopathy due to intrathecal vincristine sulfate. A fatal chemotherapeutic error. Cancer 51:2041–2047, 1983
288. Dyke RW, Nelson RL: Phase I anticancer agents. Vindesine (desacetyl vinblastine amide sulfate). Cancer Treat Rep 4:135–142, 1977
289. Robertson GL, Bhoopalam N, Zelkowitz LJ: Vincristine neurotoxicity and abnormal secretion of antidiuretic hormone. Arch Intern Med 132:717–720, 1973
290. Dorr RT, Alberts DS: Vinca alkaloid skin toxicity: antidote and drug disposition studies in the mouse. JNCI 74:113–120, 1985
291. Bender RA, Nichols AP, Norton L et al: Lack of therapeutic synergism of vincristine and methotrexate in L1210 murine leukemia *in vivo*. Cancer Treat Rep 62:997–1003, 1978
292. Radice PA, Bunn PA, Ihde DC: Therapeutic trials with VP-16-213 and VM-26: Active single agents in small cell lung cancer, non-Hodgkin's lymphoma, and other malignancies. Cancer Treat Rep 63:1231–1239, 1979
293. Drewinko B, Barlogie B: Survival and cycle-progression delay of human lymphoma cells *in vitro* exposed to VP-16-213. Cancer Treat Rep 60:1295–1306, 1976
294. Wozniak AJ, Ross WE: DNA damage as a basis for 4′-demethylepipodophyl-lotoxin-9-(4,6-0-ethylidene-beta-D-glucopyranoside (etoposide) cytoxicity. Cancer Res 43:120, 1983
295. Haim N, Roman J, Nemec J et al: Peroxidative free radical formation and o-demethylation of etoposide (VP-16) and teniposide (VM-26). Biochem Biophys Res Commun 135:215–220, 1986
296. Dorr RT, Liddil JD, Gerner EW: Modulation of etoposide cytotoxicity and DNA strand scission in L1210 and 8226 cells by polyamines. Cancer Res 46:3891–3895, 1986
297. Pommier Y, Schwartz RE, Zwelling LA et al: Reduced formation of protein-associated DNA strand breaks in Chinese hamster cells resistant to topoisomerase II inhibitors. Cancer Res 46:611–616, 1986
298. Allen LM, Creaven PJ: Comparison of the human pharmacokinetics of VM-26 and VP-16, two antineoplastic epipodophylotoxin glucopyranoside derivatives. Eur J Cancer 11:697–707, 1975

299. Cunningham D, McTaggart L, Soukop M et al: Etoposide: a pharmacokinetic profile including an assessment of bioavailability. Med Oncol Tumor Pharmacother 3:95–100, 1986
300. Arbuck SG, Douglass HO, Crom WR et al: Etoposide pharmacokinetics in patients with normal and abnormal organ function. J Clin Oncol 4:1690–1695, 1986
301. D'Incalci M, Farina P, Sessa C et al: Pharmacokinetics of VP16-123 given by different administration methods. Cancer Chemother Pharmacol 7:141, 1982
302. Littlewood TJ, Spragg BP, Bentley DP: When is autologous bone marrow transplantation safe after high-dose treatment with etoposide? Clin Lab Haematol 7:213–218, 1985
303. Worzalla JF, Kaima BD, Johnson BM et al: N-demethylation of the antineoplastic agent hexamethylmelamine by rats and man. Cancer Res 33:2810–2815, 1972
304. Lake LM, Grunden EE, Johnson BM: Toxicity and antitumor activity of hexamethylmelamine and its N-demethylated metabolites in mice with transplantable tumors. Cancer Res 35:2858–2863, 1975
305. Rutty CJ, Connors TA, Nguyen-Hoang-Nam et al: *In vivo* studies with hexamethylmelamine. Eur J Cancer 14:713–720, 1978
306. Ames MM, Powis G: Determination of pentamethylmelamine and hexamethylmelamine in plasma and urine by nitrogen-phosphorous gas–liquid chromatography. J. Chromatogr 174:245–249, 1979
307. Dutcher JS, Jones RB, Boyd MR: A sensitive and specific assay for pentamethylmelamine in plasma: Applicability to clinical studies. Cancer Treat Rep 64:99–104, 1980
308. D'Incalci M, Bolis G, Mangioni C et al: Variable oral absorption of hexamethylmelamine in man. Cancer Treat Rep 62:2117–2119, 1978
309. Montgomery JA: Experimental studies at Southern Research Institute with DTIC (NSC-45388). Cancer Treat Rep 60:125–134, 1976
310. Hayward IP, Parson PG: Epigenetic effects of the methylating agent 5-(3-methyl-1-triazeno) imidazole-4-carboxamide in human melanoma cells. Austr J Exp Biol Med Sci 62:597–606, 1984
311. Tisdale MJ: Induction of haemoglobin synthesis in the human leukaemia cell line K562 by monomethyltriazenes and imidazotetrazinones. Biochem Pharmacol 34:2077–2082, 1985
312. Breithaupt H, Dammann A, Aigner K: Pharmacokinetics of decarbazine and its metabolite 5-aminoimidazole-4-carboxamide following different dose schedules. Cancer Chemother Pharmacol 9:103, 1982
313. Smith PJ, Ekert H, Waters KD et al: High incidence of cardiomyopathy in children treated with adriamycin and DTIC in combination chemotherapy. Cancer Treat Rep 61:1736–1738, 1977
314. Feaux de Lacroix W, Runne U, Hauk H et al: Acute liver dystrophy with thrombosis of hepatic veins: a fatal complication of dacarbazine treatment. Cancer Treat Rep 67:779–784, 1983
315. Weinkam RJ, Shiba DA: Metabolic activation of procarbazine. Life Sci 22:937–945, 1978
316. Kreis W, Yen Y: An antineoplastic ^{14}C-labeled methyl hydrazine derivative in P815 mouse leukemia. A metabolic study. Experentia 21:284–285, 1965
317. Dost F, Reed D: Methane formation *in vivo* from N-isopropyl-alpha-(2-methylhydrazino)-*p*-toulamide hydrochloride, a tumor-inhibiting methyl hydrazine derivative. Biochem Pharmacol 16:1741–1746, 1967
318. Shiba DA, Weinkam RJ: Metabolic activation of procarbazine: Activity of the intermediates and the effects of pretreatment. Proc Am Assoc Cancer Res 20:139, 1979
319. Chabner BA, Sponzo R, Hubbard S et al: High-dose intermittent intravenous infusion of procarbazine. Cancer Chemother Rep 57:361–363, 1973
320. Liske R: A comparative study of the activity of cyclophosphamide and procarbazine on the antibody production in mice. Clin Exp Immunol 15:271–280, 1973
321. Lee IP, Dixon RL: Mutagenicity, carcinogenicity, and teratogenicity of procarbazine. Mutat Res 55:1–14, 1978
322. Cozzarelli NR: DNA topoisomerases. Cell 22:327–328, 1980
323. McCredie KB: Amsacrine: A new drug for hematological malignancies. Eur J Cancer 21:1–3, 1985
324. Minford J, Kerrigan D, Nichols M et al: Enhancement of the DNA breakage and cytotoxic effects of intercalating agents by treatment with sublethal doses of 1-β-D-arabinofuranosylcytosine or hydroxyurea in L1210 cells. Cancer Res 44:5583–5593, 1984
325. Pommier Y, Zwelling LA, Kao-Shan CS et al: Correlations between intercalator-induced DNA strand breaks and sister chromatid exchanges, mutations, and cytotoxicity in Chinese hamster cells. Cancer Res 45:3143–3149, 1985
326. Rowe TC, Chen GL, Hsiang YH et al: DNA damage by antitumor acridines mediated by mammalian DNA topoisomerase-II. Cancer Res 46:2021–2026, 1986
327. Pommier Y, Minford JK, Schwartz RE et al: Effects of the DNA intercalators 4'-(9-acridinylamino)methanesulfon-*m*-anisidide and 2-methyl-9-hydroxyellipticinium on topoisomerase-II-mediated DNA strand cleavage and strand passage. Biochemistry 24:6410–6416, 1985
328. Zwelling LA, Silberman L, Estey E: Intercalator-induced, topoisomerase-II-mediated DNA cleavage and its modification by antineoplastic antimetabolites. Int J Radiat Oncol Biol Phys 12:1041–1047, 1986
329. Wong A, Huang CH, Crooke ST: Mechanism of deoxyribonucleic acid breakage induced by 4'-(9-acridinylamino)methanesulfon-*m*-anisidide and copper: role for cuprous ion and oxygen free radicals. Biochemistry 23:2946–2952, 1984
330. Pommier Y, Kerrigan D, Schwartz RE et al: Altered DNA topoisomerase-II activity in Chinese hamster cells resistant to topoisomerase-II inhibitors. Cancer Res 46:3075–3081, 1986
331. Bakic M, Beran M, Anderson BS et al: The production of topoisomerase II-mediated DNA cleavage in human leukemia cells predicts their susceptibility to 4'-(9-acridinylamino)methanesulfon-*m*-anisidide (m-AMSA). Biochem Biophys Res Commun 134:638–645, 1986
332. Markovits J, Pommier Y, Kerrigan D et al: Topoisomerase-II-mediated DNA breaks and cytotoxicity in relation to cell proliferation and the cell cycle in NIH 3T3 fibroblasts and L1210 leukemia cells. Cancer Res 47:2050–2055, 1987
333. Pommier Y, Schwartz RE, Zwelling LA et al: Reduced formation of protein-associated DNA strand breaks in Chinese hamster cells resistant to topoisomerase-II inhibitors. Cancer Res 46:611–616, 1986
334. Estey EH, Silberman L, Beran M et al: The interaction between nuclear topoisomerase-II activity from human leukemia cells, exogenous DNA, and 4'-(9-acridinylamino)methanesulfon-*m*-anisidide (m-AMSA) or 4'-(4,6-0-ethylidene-β-D-glucopyranoside) (VP-16) indicates the sensitivity of the cells to the drug. Biochem Biophys Res Commun 144:787–783, 1987
335. Glisson B, Gupta R, Smallwood-Kentro S et al: Characterization of acquired epipodophyllotoxin resistance in a Chinese hamster ovary cell line: loss of drug-stimulated DNA cleavage activity. Cancer Res 46:1934–1938, 1986
336. Darkin S, Ralph RK: Potentiation of 4'-(9-acridinylamino)methanesulphon-*m*-anisidine) action by verapamil. Cancer Lett 30:25–33, 1986
337. Shoemaker DD, Cysyk RL, Padmanabhan S et al: Identification of the principal biliary metabolite of m-AMSA in rats. Drug Metab Dispos 10:35–39, 1982
338. Hall SW, Friedman J, Legha SS et al: Human pharmacokinetics of a new acridine derivative, 4'-(9-acridinylamino)methanesulfon-m-anisidide (NSC 249992). Cancer Res 43:3422–3426, 1983
339. Shoemaker DD, Cysyk RL, Gormley PE et al: Metabolism of 4'-(9-acridinylamino) methanesulfon-*m*-anisidide by rat liver microsomes. Cancer Res 44:1939–1945, 1984
340. Paxton JW, Jurlina JL, Foote SE: The binding of amsacrine to human plasma proteins. J Pharm Pharmacol 38:432–438, 1986
341. Weiss RB, Grillo-Lopez AJ, Marsoni S et al: Amsacrine-associated cardiotoxicity: an analysis of 82 cases. J Clin Oncol 4:918–928, 1986
342. Engelking C, Sullivan P, Agoliati G et al: Amsacrine administration: a precautionary note (letter). Cancer Chemother Pharmacol 13:150, 1984
343. Kidd JG: Regression of transplanted lymphomas induced in vivo by means of normal guinea pig serum. I. Course of transplanted cancers of various kinds in mice and rats given guinea pig serum, horse serum, or rabbit serum. J Exp Med 98:565–582, 1953
344. Broome JD: Evidence that the L-asparaginase of guinea pig serum is responsible for its antilymphoma effects. I. Properties of the L-asparaginase of guinea pig serum in relation to those of the antilymphoma substance. J Exp Med 118:99–120, 1963
345. Jackson RC, Handschumacher RE: *Escherichia coli* L-asparaginase. Catalytic activity and subunit nature. Biochemistry 9:3585–3590, 1970
346. Ohnama T, Holland JF, Meyer P: *Erwinia carotovora* asparaginase in patients with prior anaphylaxis to asparaginase from *E. coli*. Cancer 30:376–381, 1972
347. Haley EE, Fischer GA, Welch AD: The requirement for L-asparagine of mouse leukemia cells L5178Y in culture. Cancer Res 21:532–536, 1961
348. Distasio JA, Neederman RA, Kafkewitz D et al: Purification and characterization of L-asparaginase with antilymphoma activity from *Vibrio succinogenes*. J Biol Chem 251:6929–6933, 1976
349. Haw T, Ohnuma T: L-asparaginase: *In vitro* inhibition of blastogenesis by enzyme from *Erwinia carotovora*. Nature 239:50–51, 1972
350. Yoshimoto T, Nishimura H, Saito Y et al: Characterization of polyethylene-glycol-modified L-asparaginase from *Escherichia coli* and its application to therapy of leukemia. Jpn J Cancer Res 77:1264–1270, 1986
351. Meister A, Levintow L, Greenfield RE et al: Hydrolysis and transfer reactions catalyzed by amidase preparations. J Biol Chem 215:441–460, 1955
352. Cooney DA, Capizzi RI, Handschumacher RE: Evaluation of L-asparagine metabolism in animals and man. Cancer Res 30:929–935, 1970
353. Nesbitt M, Chard R, Evans A et al: Intermittent L-asparaginase therapy for acute childhood leukemia. Proc 10th Int Cancer Cong, p 447, 1970
354. Ohnuma T, Holland JF, Sinks LF: Biochemical and pharmacological studies with L-asparaginase in man. Cancer Res 30:2297–2305, 1970
355. Peterson RC, Handschumacher RF, Mitchell MS: Immunological responses to L-asparaginase. J Clin Invest 50:1080–1090, 1971
356. Clavell LA, Gelber RD, Cohen HJ et al: Four-agent induction and intensive asparaginase therapy for treatment of childhood acute lymphoblastic leukemia. N Engl J Med 315:657–663, 1986
357. Homans AC, Rybak ME, Baglini RL et al: Effect of L-asparaginase administration on coagulation and platelet function in children with leukemia. J Clin Oncol 5:811–817, 1987
358. Bezeaud A, Drouet L, Leverger G et al: Effect of L-asparaginase therapy for acute lymphoblastic leukemia on plasma vitamin-K-dependent coagulation factors and inhibitors. J Pediatr 108:698–701, 1986
359. Leonard JV, Kay JDS: Acute encephalopathy and hyperammonaemia complicating treatment of acute lymphoblastic leukaemia with asparaginase. Lancet 1:162–163, 1986
360. Capizzi R: Improvement in the therapeutic index of L-asparaginase by methotrexate. Cancer Chemother Reps 6 (Pt 3):37–41, 1975
361. Jolivet J, Cole DE, Holcenberg JS et al: Prevention of methotrexate cytotoxicity by asparaginase inhibition of methotrexate polyglutamate formation. Cancer Res 45:217–220, 1985

RICHARD M. SIMON

CHAPTER 19 *Design and Conduct of Clinical Trials*

The purpose of this chapter is to highlight principles for the design and conduct of valuable therapeutic clinical trials in oncology. Many such studies are one of the following types.

1. *Phase I studies*. Determine the relationship between toxicity and dose-schedule of treatment
2. *Phase II studies*. Identify tumor types for which the treatment appears promising
3. *Phase III studies*
   a. Determine the effects of a treatment relative to the natural history of the disease
   b. Determine whether a new treatment is more effective than a standard therapy
   c. Determine whether a new treatment is as effective as a standard therapy but is associated with less morbidity

These classes of studies include evaluation of surgical procedures, radiotherapeutic treatments, chemotherapeutic drugs, immunostimulants, biologic response modifiers, antibiotics, antiemetics, and pain control agents. Each of the objectives stated above is meaningful, however, only within the context of a clearly defined patient population.

The experimental approach plays an important role in clinical oncology today. By the experimental approach, I refer to roughly two components: first, clinical results, rather than deductive reasoning, are required for the evaluation of a treatment[1]; and second, the experimental approach requires that preplanned therapeutic interventions be administered to specified types of patients under conditions that are controlled to enable well-defined medical questions to be answered directly. Comparing the survival rates of breast cancer patients treated with mastectomy to those of patients receiving mastectomy plus postoperative radiotherapy based on regional tumor registry data is an example of a nonexperimental survey. In such surveys, the investigator is a passive observer and abstracts records that he hopes will provide information about the phenomena he wishes to study. Treatment assignments, diagnostic tests, and follow-up procedures are determined by the patients and physicians independently of the investigator. The statistical associations resulting from such studies are in themselves a weak basis for causal inferences about the relationship between treatment administered and results observed. Treatments usually are selected based on subjective assessment of prognosis for the patient, capabilities of the physician, and variable diagnostic evaluations. It is generally impossible to identify and eliminate all the biases inherent in survey data.

Surveys are sometimes called "observational studies," although this is inaccurate because all knowledge is based on observations. Surveys generally are the only feasible mechanisms for epidemiologic assessment of disease etiology, and when performed by highly trained and critical investigators can contribute greatly to public welfare.[2,3] Acute observations in poorly structured therapeutic settings can also lead to immensely valuable ideas to be pursued and tested in the laboratory and planned clinical trials. Surveys are, however, sometimes proposed as an easy alternative to planned clinical trials for the evaluation of treatments.[4,5] For this purpose, the survey is distinctly inferior with regard to inherent reliability of conclusions concerning therapeutic effects. MacMahon and Pugh[3] point out that

> Only a minority of statistical associations are causal. . . . Once a statistical association has been demonstrated, how can it be determined whether or not it is causal. . . . The most satisfactory procedure is direct experiment. . . . The evaluation of the causal nature of a relationship, in the absence of direct experiment, is neither easy nor objective. . . . The field of cancer therapy is replete with examples of new modalities that were taken up with enthusiasm and proved worthless only after they had resulted in many years of futile cost and suffering.

The difficult problems in analysis of survey data are discussed elsewhere.[6–8] Improvements in computer technology have increased the ease of conducting medical surveys but have not had a major role in solving the basic weaknesses of this approach.

This chapter addresses principles for the design and conduct of therapeutic clinical trials in oncology. Such studies can be direct and easily interpretable mechanisms for answering important medical questions. To achieve this objective, however, certain principles must be followed in planning the study. The following sections address certain key aspects of this planning process.

The first result of the planning process is a written protocol. Typical subject headings for the protocol are shown in Table 19-1. This document should be self-contained, consistent, and carefully prepared. It should define uniform treatment and evaluation policies for a well-defined set of patients and should not leave important decisions to the discretion of the physician or the study chairperson. The protocol should clearly define the questions to be answered by the study and should directly justify that the number of patients and nature of controls are adequate to answer these questions definitively. It is very easy to embark on a futile or trivial study and to write the protocol merely as a guideline for clinical management supplemented by lofty objectives of no scientific meaning. Rushing the protocol development process and not being sufficiently critical of what is written or omitted contributes to this tendency. From the presentation of scientific background through the definition of data forms, the protocol should show clear, precise, and practical thinking.

TABLE 19-1. Subject Headings for a Protocol

1. Introduction and scientific background
2. Objectives
3. Selection of patients
4. Design of study (including schematic diagram)
5. Treatment programs
6. Procedures in event of toxicity
7. Required clinical and laboratory data
8. Criteria for evaluating the effect of treatment
9. Statistical considerations
10. Informed consent
11. Data forms
12. References
13. Study chairperson, collaborating participants, addresses, and telephone numbers

STUDY OBJECTIVES

It is important to describe the study objectives specifically in the protocol. This helps orient the protocol to represent a clearly thought-out research plan rather than merely a guide for clinical management. Clearly stated objectives are necessary to ensure that size of the study, nature of controls, and plans for patient management are adequate and unbiased with regard to the questions posed.

Many studies in the social sciences are fishing expeditions that include numerous batteries of tests and result in exhaustive analyses. Such unstructured investigations are likely to result in some erroneous conclusions owing to the multiplicity of the questions addressed.[9] Therapeutic studies in oncology generally have a more specific natural focus. Nevertheless, it is useful to describe the objectives in terms of specific questions to be answered by the study. Some protocols state that the objective is to "improve treatment" and some list numerous objectives that are not feasible within the size of study planned or for which there are inadequate controls. These characteristics often are an indication that insufficient critical thinking has been done in the planning stage to permit clear interpretation of the results that will be obtained.

The realities of numbers of patients required dictate that most studies should be restricted to one major question. It is best when either positive or negative results are informative for patient management and for developing better treatments. Two examples of such studies are comparison of mastectomy to tumor resection for patients with stage I breast cancer and comparison of high-dose versus conventional-dose therapy with an effective drug. Many current studies provide no leads to build on when the results are negative.

Many current studies also fail to address the most important medical questions. The most important studies are often the most difficult to initiate. They may involve withholding a treatment established by tradition, potential transfer of patient management responsibility across specialties, standardization of procedures among individuals who believe their way is best, and sharing recognition with a large group of collaborators.

PATIENT ELIGIBILITY

Phase I studies generally are conducted with previously treated patients. However, the organ systems that are the expected targets of toxicity should be competent in patients selected for the study. Otherwise, the relationships between dose-schedule and toxicity found in the study will not be relevant to the treatment of less debilitated patients.

Whereas phase I studies need not be performed separately by histologic tumor type, this is not the case for phase II studies. In phase II studies the biologic response of major interest is that of the tumor itself. Because cytosensitivities vary among histologic types, it is important to study enough patients so that evaluation of tumor response can be made separately by type.

Some kinds of advanced cancer have no known therapy that prolongs survival (*e.g.*, melanoma, esophageal, pancreatic). For such sites, phase II studies should consist of nonpreviously treated patients. The chance of tumor response generally decreases with prior treatment. Consequently, the inclusion of previously treated patients in phase II studies of diseases in which treatment does not prolong survival constitutes a decrease in the potential sensitivity of the study and a reduction in the likelihood of patient benefit.[9a]

For phase III studies, determination of eligibility criteria involves a trade-off between broad applicability of conclusions and addressing the study to those patients most likely to benefit from the new treatment. In a study with broad eligibility requirements, a conclusion of no difference between the treatments may result from a positive effect in one subset being cancelled by a negative effect in another or a positive effect in one subset being hidden in the overall comparison by the variability introduced by including patients less likely to benefit. For most studies, the basic analysis should include all patients; thus broad eligibility requirements may entail a loss of sensitivity.

Some statisticians advise that the eligibility criteria be very broad because subset analyses can always be performed later.[10,11] This approach has certain risks, however: misleading conclusions may result from multiple subset analyses, and one must be careful to plan the study so that adequate numbers of patients within each major subset are available for separate analysis.

Studies with relatively narrow eligibility criteria may not yield results that are generalizable to patients of the types excluded. Such studies have been criticized for this.[11a] But if the narrow eligibility criteria provide improved homogeneity of prognosis, then such studies can yield more clearcut answers to therapeutic questions with reasonable numbers of patients of a well-defined type.

In general, clearcut evidence of benefit for a well-defined class of patients is likely to be more valuable than a finding of no effect for a mixed population. Although often it is not obvious which patients are most likely to benefit, some studies of intensive treatment include debilitated patients for whom reduced doses are planned from the outset. Generally, their inclusion is detrimental to the study and not beneficial to the patient. The added numbers they represent are more than compensated for by the increase in variability of response and uncertainty of to whom the conclusions apply. Sir Bradford Hill made this point in discussing a clinical trial of streptomycin for respiratory tuberculosis:[12]

> . . . for it was realized that no two patients have an identical form of the disease and it was desired to eliminate as many of the obvious variations as possible. This planning . . . is a fundamental feature of the successful trial. To start out upon a trial with all and sundry included, and with the hope that the results can be sorted out statistically in the end is to court disaster.

ENDPOINT

The term *endpoint* refers to the criterion by which patient benefit is measured. A meaningful and reliable endpoint is essential for a worthwhile study. In some of the social sciences, lack of an adequate endpoint is a major impediment to progress. For clinical oncology this generally is not a severe problem. Nevertheless, explicit definition of the endpoint(s) is important for determining the size and duration of the trial and for ensuring that the proper measurements are taken and that follow-up evaluations are performed without bias.

The major endpoints of evaluating the effectiveness of a treatment should be measures of patient welfare. Duration of survival and quality of life are two such endpoints. Quality of life is used infrequently because sufficiently simple and reproducible measures of important aspects of quality of life have not been developed. The development of such measures that can be used broadly by clinicians in the conduct of therapeutic evaluations is an important area that warrants research.

Survival generally is the most meaningful measure of benefit for phase III studies. For a variety of reasons, it generally is not the endpoint upon which sample sizes are planned or ultimate therapeutic recommendations are made. The endpoints commonly used instead of or in addition to survival are degree of tumor shrinkage and duration for which the tumor is below the level of clinical detection. These are basically subjective measures. Whether a patient has a partial response depends on who is doing the measuring and what the response criteria are.[13–16]

The more closely one looks, the fewer complete remissions are obtained and the more rapidly recurrent disease is detected. Consequently, it is important that follow-up procedures be standardized in the protocol to ensure that the study is not jeopardized by biased evaluation of response. Lack of standardization of response assessment is a major cause of confusion in communication of results.

It cannot be assumed that response rates, duration of response, or disease-free intervals are proper endpoints for drawing conclusions about therapeutic efficacy because they are not direct measures of patient welfare. There are obvious examples in which survival extensions and cure rates have followed major improvements in complete response rates and complete response durations. The situation is more mixed, however, with regard to partial responses.

A treatment that causes partial responses is not necessarily beneficial to the patient. Even if one demonstrates that partial responders live longer than nonresponders, one cannot conclude that the treatment is beneficial.[17–19] Comparisons of survivals between responders and nonresponders are biased in two ways. First, responders by definition have lived long enough to achieve that status. Second, responders may have more favorable prognostic factors that would result in their living longer than nonresponders even in the absence of any treatment. Finally, one cannot assume that the difference in survival does not result from the treatment's shortening survival for the nonresponders. To demonstrate that treatment extends survival, the comparison of survival between responders and nonresponders is not relevant. One must demonstrate that the treated group as a whole lives longer than an appropriate control group of similar prognosis.

For some kinds of cancer, partial responses are of substantial duration, are clearly associated with improved palliation, and have been demonstrated to represent the effect of treatment on prolonging life by comparison to an appropriate untreated or single agent control group. For other kinds of cancer, however, partial responses are of minimal duration and have not been demonstrated to represent a beneficial therapeutic effect for the patient. Increases in partial response rates without corresponding improvements in survival or palliation for the treated group should not be viewed as therapeutic improvements. However, partial responses are useful indicators of biologic activity for phase II studies, even in diseases where direct patient benefit cannot be demonstrated.

TREATMENT ALLOCATION

PHASE I STUDIES

The simplest phase I studies involve estimation of the relationship between dose and toxicity for a single schedule and mode of administration. Such studies usually are performed by starting with a low dose not expected to produce serious toxicity in any patients and increasing the dose for subsequent patients according to a series of preplanned steps. Several patients are treated at each dosage level, often three patients per step when no toxicity is encountered and six patients per step thereafter.[20,21] The initial dose selection generally is based on animal toxicity data. A starting dose of one tenth the LD_{10} expressed as milligrams per square meter of body surface area in the mouse usually is used.[21a-25]

Dose escalation for subsequent patients occurs only after sufficient time has passed to observe acute toxic effects for patients treated at lower doses. Insufficient attention has been given to quantitative methods of determining dose steps. One commonly used is based on a modified Fibonacci series.[26,27] The second step is twice the starting dose, the third step is 67% greater than the second, the fourth step is 50% greater than the third, the fifth step is 40% greater than the fourth, and each subsequent step is 33% greater than that preceding it. In some cases this procedure may result in an insufficiently rapid escalation,[28] and other methods of dose escalation have been proposed.[29,30]

Escalating doses for subsequent courses in the same patient generally is not carried out except at low doses because it may mask the presence of cumulative toxicity. An escalated second dose for a patient may be toxic because it is a higher dose or because it is a second dose. Many phase I studies that escalate doses within patients are not analyzed in a way that distinguishes patients from courses of therapy.

Some phase I studies evaluate several schedules or modes of administration. If study of the second schedule is begun after evaluation of the first has been completed or is well under way, the accumulated information can be used to establish a starting dose. Otherwise, it may be useful to allocate the schedules randomly to newly eligible patients. This is not crucial but serves to eliminate bias in selecting patients for one schedule or other based upon their condition. Such randomization is not for the purpose of directly comparing the schedules but to better ensure that the maximum tolerable dose determined for one schedule is not misleadingly high or low because of patient selection.

For any phase I study, and particularly for studies of combinations, criteria for dose reductions should be specified clearly in the protocol and monitored closely. Active monitoring of results by the study chairperson is essential for a safe trial.

PHASE II STUDIES

The results of phase II studies can be misleading in two ways.[9a,31] First, little antitumor effect may be seen, but the patients may be so debilitated or extensively pretreated that the results do not reflect true potential usefulness of the agent; and second, because of patient selection or inadequately rigorous response criteria, more favorable results are obtained than will be substantiated by further trials. Both types of results are undesirable.

To deal with these potential problems, it has been suggested that phase II studies involve a randomization between the experimental agent and a treatment known to have antitumor value.[11,32-34] The purpose of randomization would not be for determining which treatment was better, but for having a baseline response rate of similar patients treated with a known therapy. The known therapy would not be a "standard therapy" in the sense of being the treatment of choice. Peto[11] has suggested that two thirds of the patients should be randomized to the new treatment. For phase II studies of previously treated patients, it often is not possible to identify an active control treatment. When it is possible, this design can deal effectively with the false-positivity problem. Adequate standardization of response criteria usually would be just as effective, however. The randomized design appears to have less value for dealing with the false-negativity problem. The control therapy generally will have a low response rate for such patients, and it will not serve as a sensitive control. A better safeguard against false-negative results is to use nonpreviously treated patients in phase II studies when it is ethically possible.

For cooperative groups with sufficient patients to conduct simultaneously several phase II studies in a disease, randomization among the new agents is desirable.[31] There is no question that patient selection can influence results.[35] Such selection can lead to bias in the ranking of new agents. Differences among institutions in evaluation of response can make the problem even more severe. The conduct of one master phase II study with randomized treatment assignment helps alleviate these problems.

Phase II trials may be designed with cross-over to a specified treatment (either another experimental agent or an established drug) when the patient fails the initial therapy. This aspect of the design usually supplies little information because so few patients make it through the secondary treatment, because there are so few responses, and because the condition of the patient has changed.

PHASE III STUDIES

Controls

The interpretation of most phase III studies involves some type of comparison of results. In some cases the basis of comparison will be the natural history of the disease, and in others it will be another treatment. We shall use the term "control" to represent the basis against which a treatment is to be evaluated. Rarely, if ever, do we just want to know whether a treatment is better or worse than the control. We want to estimate the degree of difference. All measurement ultimately is comparative, however, and the categorization of a treatment as "good" or "bad" involves an implicit comparison to the natural history of the disease.

To determine whether a new treatment cures any patients with a disease that is uniformly and rapidly fatal, history is a satisfactory control. In this situation the patient population is completely homogeneous with regard to cure in the absence of the new therapy. If 20% of patients are cured by conventional therapy and we can identify them by patient and tumor characteristics measured at diagnosis, we can restrict a study to the remaining 80% and have complete homogeneity. Once we leave the setting of complete homogeneity with regard to the chosen endpoint, the definition of an adequate nonrandomized control becomes problematical.

In many studies the controls are either numbers determined from publications or patients treated in nonexperimental settings in which the information is abstracted from tumor registries, data banks, or medical records. The meaningfulness of such controls is questionable. Often diagnostic and staging procedures, supportive care, secondary treatments, and methods of evaluation and follow-up are different for the controls and the current treatment group. There generally is differential bias in the selection of patients to be treated resulting from judgments by the physicians, self-selection by the patients, and differences in referral patterns. There may be bias in treatment ineligibility rates.[36] Current patients are sometimes excluded from analysis for not meeting eligibility criteria, not receiving "adequate" treatment, refusing treatment, or a major protocol violation. The controls, on the other hand, generally contain all the patients. There may be differences in the distribution of known and unknown prognostic factors between the controls and the current treatment group. Often there is inadequate information to determine whether such differences are present, and current known prognostic factors may not have been measured or recorded for the controls. It generally is difficult to tell whether the controls would have been eligible for the current study and in what way they represent a selection of all eligible patients.

In the best of circumstances historical controls will be patients treated within the previous few years at the same institution or institutions performing the new study. The controls would be treated on a protocol having exactly the same eligibility requirements, work-up, follow-up, and response evaluation procedures as the current study, referral patterns and accrual rates would be static, no patients in either group would be excluded from analysis because of ineligibility or nonevaluability, and an exhaustive demonstration of similarity in distribution of all suspected prognostic factors would be presented. These circumstances rarely are encountered in practice. Pocock[37] has reported 19 unselected instances under circumstances approaching these where a collaborative group carried one treatment over for two successive studies. Even here, for 4 of the 19 pairs of trials the differences in outcome were statistically significant at the $p < 0.02$ level.

Formation of the control group by random assignment of treatment as an integral part of the planned study can avoid most of the systematic biases mentioned above.[38-41] The random assignment should not be performed until the patient is found eligible, and then a truly random or nondecipherable mechanism should be used. Alternation, day of the week, or other predictable procedures are not adequate because they allow bias in the decision of whether to enter a patient into a study based on knowledge beforehand of what treatment the patient will receive. Randomization does not ensure that the study will include a representative sample of all patients with the disease, but it does help to ensure an unbiased evaluation of the relative merits of the two treatments for the types of patients entered.

Some of the advantages of randomization are subtle and not widely understood. For example, it is sometimes said that randomization is unnecessary because matched historical or concurrent controls can be selected. But one can match only with regard to known prognostic factors, and these generally explain only a minor portion of the heterogeneity in prognosis among patients.[42] Matching with regard to known factors gives no assurance that the distributions of unknown factors are similar between the treatment groups. It also is sometimes said that randomization is not effective in ensuring that the treatment groups are similar with regard to unknown prognostic factors unless the number of patients is large. This is true but reflects a misunderstanding of randomization. Randomization does not ensure that the groups are medically equivalent, but it distributes the unknown biasing factors according to a known random distribution so that their effects can be rigorously allowed for in significance tests and confidence intervals.[43] This is true regardless of the study size. A significance level represents the probability that differences in outcome are due to random fluctuations. Without randomized treatment allocation, a "statistically significant difference" may be due to a nonrandom difference in the distribution of unknown prognostic factors.

Randomization (or stratified randomization, to be discussed later) is inherently the method of treatment assignment that results in the most reliable basis for inference.[44,45] This is not to say that all randomized studies are good or that all nonrandomized studies are bad, but that, everything else being equal, randomization adds considerably to the ease of interpretability of the study since one need not worry about conscious or inadvertent systematic biases in patient selection or treatment assignment. Gehan and Freireich[46] and Pocock[47] have listed conditions under which nonrandomized studies can be considered reliable. The majority of nonrandomized studies do not meet these conditions. The oncology literature is filled with reports of nonrandomized studies in which scant attention is paid to comparability with regard to known prognostic factors. At this point the major advantages of randomization are not the subtle aspects mentioned but avoidance of the major biases of the majority of poorly done, nonrandomized studies. If nonrandomized studies were scrupulously conducted and critically reported under the conditions described above for consecutive trials, the subtle advantages that randomization will always have might be less decisive. Modern alternative approaches based on nonexperimental data bases and tumor registries[4] having concurrent nonrandomized controls are a poor alternative to either method.

Are randomized trials necessary for identifying major advances in treatment? No. There are many examples of therapeutic breakthroughs that were recognized without randomized trials. For the most part, however, these occurred in diseases where the prognosis was 100% predictable before the advent of the new therapy, and hence there was no possibility of bias with regard to patient selection. False innovations are much more numerous than real breakthroughs, however, and it is difficult to distinguish one from the other.[48] There certainly is a role for innovative nonrandomized studies in diseases with uniformly bleak prognoses.

Some physicians are uncomfortable with the notion of randomization, believing that they have an obligation to develop an opinion about the relative merits of alternative possible treatments and to recommend a therapy to their patients accordingly.[49] This position is understandable but must be tempered by the following considerations: different competent physicians often hold widely divergent opinions about the relative merits of alternative treatments for the same patient;[50] the little research done indicates that experienced, well-educated adults are likely to overrate the correctness of their opinions and hunches;[51] and the experimental treatment generally is neither much better nor much worse than the control, and we have little real basis for selecting between the treatments before the trial. As Gilbert, McPeek, and Mosteller point out,[51]

> Much of current popular discussion of the ethical issue takes the position that physicians should use their best judgment in prescribing for a patient. To what extent the physician is responsible for the quality of the judgment is not much discussed, except to say that he must keep abreast of the times. Some physicians will feel an obligation to find out that goes beyond the mere holding of an opinion. Such physicians will feel a responsibility to contribute to the research. In similar fashion, some current patients may feel a responsibility to contribute to the better care of future patients. The current model of the passive patient and the active outgoing physician is not the most effective one for a society that not only wants cures rather than sympathy, but insists on them—a society that has been willing to pay both in patient cooperation and material resources for the necessary research.

If randomization is used, it generally should take place as late as possible before effecting treatment of the patient.[10] For example, in evaluating a chemotherapeutic regimen as a postsurgical adjuvant treatment, randomization should take place after the surgery has been completed and the patient has recovered sufficiently to begin receiving chemotherapy. This approach serves to reduce bias in the surgery administered and possible bias in disqualifications of randomized patients owing to surgical findings, morbidity, or mortality.

Protocols for nonrandomized phase III studies should describe the control group to be used. The control group should consist of patients for whom individual records are available for detailed evaluation of comparability.

Stratified Randomization

When there are known major prognostic factors for patients in a randomized study, it often is advisable to stratify the randomization to assure equal distribution of these factors.[52] This usually is accomplished by preparing a separate randomization list (or set of cards in sealed envelopes) for each distinct subset of patients (stratum). Each list must be balanced so that after each block of four to ten patients within the stratum the treatment groups contain equal numbers of patients. Within the blocks, the sequence of treatment assignments is random. The stratification factors must, of course, be known for each patient at the time of randomization.

For example, as shown in Figure 19-1, in a comparison of treatments for testicular cancer the factors may be histology and stage. These two stratification factors determine six patient strata. For a comparison of two treatments, designated A and B, the sequence of treatment assignments for a stratum can be determined in the following manner. We shall assume that is has been decided that the sequence for each stratum will be balanced in blocks of six patients. One obtains a table of two-digit random numbers and starts reading the table down an arbitrarily selected column. Random numbers in the range 00 to 49 will indicate treatment A, and random numbers in the range 50 to 99 will indicate treatment B. If no more than 30 patients are anticipated in the stratum, the tentative treatment assignments are determined by the first 30 random numbers read. This determines a sequence of a total of 30 As and Bs. This list must be modified in the following way to ensure balance after each block of six patients in the stratum. If the random sequence is

ABAAAABBABABBBBAAAABBAABBAAABB

then it is modified to

ABAABB AABBAB ABBBAA BAAABB ABBAAB.

FIG. 19-1. Example of stratification for a randomized clinical trial.

Histology	*Stage* II	*Stage* III
Teratocarcinoma with or without seminoma		
Embryonal carcinoma with or without seminoma		
Either of above with elements of choriocarcinoma		

If three As occur in a block before three Bs, the remainder of the block is automatically filled in with Bs before the random sequence is continued. Similarly, if three Bs occur in a block before three As, the remainder of the block is automatically filled in with As. This procedure is performed separately for each stratum. The sequence of treatment assignments for each stratum is then transferred to a randomization list or to sealed and numbered randomization envelopes. The randomization sequences should be prepared by someone who will not be entering patients into the study. Generally, the blocksize should not be known to the participants, and they should not be permitted to examine the partially used randomization sequences. These procedures are easily generalized to more than two treatments or to block sizes other than six. For unstratified randomizations, the sequence of treatment assignments can be prepared in exactly the same way except that the block size is often larger.

The number of strata increases multiplicatively with the number of stratification factors because the patient subsets are defined by combinations of these factors. Although limited stratification often is desirable, overstratification is detrimental to the trial. If there is extensive stratification, numerous strata will contain very few patients. Consequently, balance with regard to the most important factor or factors may be seriously impaired by the inclusion of factors of secondary importance. Even the total numbers of patients assigned to each of the treatments may be very unequal. Extensive overstratification becomes equivalent to randomization with no stratification at all.[53]

It generally is best to limit stratification to those factors definitely known to have important independent effects on response. If two factors are closely correlated, one, at most, should be included in the stratification. Peto and others[10] believe that stratification is an unnecessary complication because adjustment for imbalances of known factors can be made in the analysis. For small studies, however, such adjustments should not be relied on. Stratification may obviate the chance of gross imbalances that cannot be adjusted for and ensures that the treatment comparisons are not totally dependent on statistical adjustment methods.[54,55] Simon[56] and Kalish and Begg[57] have reviewed the various stratification methods available. Kalish and Begg[57a] studied analytic aspects of adaptive stratification methods.

Cross-over Designs

Cross-over designs have been discussed in the context of phase II studies but also are used in other settings, such as the comparative evaluation of antiemetics and antipain treatments. For example, patients might be randomized to receive either an antiemetic during the first course of chemotherapy and a placebo during the second, or the alternate sequence. This design is motivated by the desire to increase the sensitivity of a study by using each patient as his own control, and thereby to reduce the number of patients required. The usefulness of this approach is limited because the condition of the patient changes with time and the effect of a treatment may be influenced by previous treatments or conditioned by previous responses.

Cross-over designs in which there are more than two treatment episodes per patient are almost always difficult or impossible to interpret clearly. Frequently such studies are analyzed and reported in a manner that fails to distinguish distinct patients from multiple treatment episodes of the same patient.

Useful methods for analyzing a two-period cross-over design are described by Hills and Armitage[58] and by Koch.[59] Use of the cross-over design is controversial and has been discouraged by the Biometric and Epidemiologic Advisory Committee of the Food and Drug Administration.[60] If the relative efficacy of the treatments in the second period differs from that in the first period or is conditioned by first period response, it is not possible to use each patient as his own control. To determine whether such an interaction exists requires as many patients as a non-cross-over design, and one should seriously weigh these considerations before adopting the cross-over design.[61,61a,62]

It is always best to administer a treatment in a clinical trial the way that it would be recommended for administration in general medical practice. The cross-over design is artificial in this regard. Less structured designs that repeatedly rerandomize the same patients are subject to this criticism and suffer from the introduction of additional correlations that generally are impossible to account for properly in the analysis.

Common Control Designs

In randomized multi-institution studies, it is sometimes difficult to obtain agreement among all participants concerning the treatments to be used. A compromise design sometimes suggested is to allow each institution to select between doing randomized study of treatments A and C or doing a randomized study of treatments B and C. These two studies are conducted simultaneously, but at different institutions. It usually is recognized that this design is inferior to a simple randomization among all treatments A, B, and C within each institution, but it is hoped that it is better than a totally nonrandomized design. Schoenfeld and Gelber[63] have shown that unless one can assume that there are no differences among institutions in response to treatment, this design is very inefficient. With three treatments (one being the common control), this design requires twice as many patients as a straightforward three-way randomized design. Makuch and Simon[64] have pointed out that similar results for the common control treatment between the sets of institutions selecting the two options do not ensure that the other two treatments can be validly compared. Systematic differences among the institutions may be manifested only in intensively treated patients. Consequently, the common control design is not a good alternative unless the experimental treatments are minor variants of each other. In general, it is best to standardize the treatments rigorously in order to eliminate extraneous causes of variability and bias.

Factorial Designs

In a 2×2 factorial design there are actually four treatments under study. The first factor represents two alternative treatment interventions, such as amputation or resection. The second factor represents two other alternative interventions superimposed on the first factor, such as adjuvant chemotherapy or no further treatment. Although there are actually four treatment groups (amputation alone, resection alone, amputation plus chemotherapy, resection plus chemotherapy), proponents of such designs[11,45,65] suggest that the effect of each treatment factor can be addressed using all of the patients and pooling with regard to the other factor (or with the influence of the other factor accounted for in the analysis, but not separate analysis for each level of the other factor). The validity of such an analysis depends on the following types of assumptions: if adjuvant chemotherapy is beneficial for amputees, it is also beneficial for resected patients, and the difference in efficacy of the two surgical procedures is either concurrently positive, negative, or zero, both for patients receiving adjuvant chemotherapy and for those not receiving further treatment. If these assumptions are not satisfied, the study must be analyzed by the simultaneous comparison of all four treatment groups. The risk in planning such a study is that the number of patients established will be sufficient only for pooled two-group comparisons, yet the data may suggest that such an analysis is not adequate. Also, the number of patients required to determine whether such an interaction is present is greater than the number required to perform two group comparisons. Thus the factorial design offers the possibility of answering two questions for the price of one, but there is a risk of difficulty in interpretation.[66]

Combining Randomized and Historical Controls

Randomized studies are sometimes conducted weighted 2:1 in favor of the new treatment with the intent of incorporating historical controls in the analysis if their outcomes are similar to those of the randomized controls.[10] This design rarely provides enough randomized controls for an adequate comparison with results for the historical control group.[67] Pocock[47] has investigated other methods of combining controls from two successive studies, but he assumes that the expected difference between outcomes from the control groups is zero. As discussed in the next section, a 2:1 randomization often is reasonable but not for the purpose of including historical controls.

SIZE AND DURATION OF THE STUDY

PHASE I AND PHASE II TRIALS

The size of phase I studies cannot be completely determined in advance. Guidelines that exist for planning the size of such studies have been presented in a previous section.

Simon[68] has recently reviewed the statistical designs that have been developed for phase II trials. With any of the proposed designs, the accrual plan and decision rules are applied seaparately to each subset of patients for whom inferences are to be made (*e.g.*, nonpreviously treated advanced colon cancer patients). The oldest approach is Gehan's two-stage design.[69] If the target activity level of interest is 20%, then 14 patients are accrued in the first stage. If no responses are obtained, the trial is terminated for such patients and the drug is considered inactive for that subset. The basis for this conclusion is that a drug with a 20% response rate probability has a 95% chance of causing at least 1 response in 14 patients. Thus if we reject the drug for this subset when no responses are seen in the first 14 patients, the rejection error is 5% for a true effectiveness of 20%. Table 19-2 shows the number of patients to be treated in the first stage as a function of the rejection error and true effectiveness proportion. If no responses are seen in the tabulated number of patients, the drug is rejected for this subset.

For a rejection error of 5% and a true activity level of 20%, if at least one response is obtained in the first 14 patients, a second stage of the trial is conducted to better estimate the response rate of the drug. The number of patients required for the second stage depends strongly on the precision desired for the estimated response rate. For a standard error of 10%, about 25 total patients are required (*e.g.*, 14 in the first stage, 11 in the second). For a standard error of 5%, the required total number of patients is generally in the range of 50 to 90. Gehan's design is often applied with 14 patients in the first stage and 25 total if any responses are obtained. A sample of 25 patients, however, generally provides a poor estimate of the true response probability, and a study of 35 to 40 patients is often preferable.

Gehan's plan frequently is misapplied by having too heterogeneous a set of patients in the first stage. If no responses are observed among 14 patients of diverse tumor types or previous treatment experiences, no conclusion can be reached for any single well-defined class of patients. One usually should strive for separate evaluation of results by whether or not the patient has previously received chemotherapy. If nonpreviously treated patients are to be included in order to minimize the number of patients exposed to an ineffective drug, it is advisable to delay entry of previously treated patients until the drug has demonstrated activity.

Gehan's plan also is frequently misapplied by failure to conduct the second stage for strata that exhibit at least one response in the first 14 patients. The second stage usually is essential because even a drug with a 5% response rate has a 51% chance of producing at least one response in 14 patients.

Simon[68] has developed an optimized modification of Gehan's design. It is a two-stage design with n_1 patients in the first stage and n patients total. If the observed response rate at the end of the first stage is $\leq r_1/n_1$, then the trial terminates and the drug is rejected as being of little interest. Otherwise, accrual continues to a total of n patients. At the

TABLE 19-2. Sample Size (n_1) Required for Preliminary Trial of a New Agent for Given Levels of Therapeutic Effectiveness and Rejection Error

Rejection	*Therapeutic Effectiveness (%)*									
Error (β)	5	10	15	20	25	30	35	40	45	50
5%	59	29	19	14	11	9	7	6	6	5
10%	45	22	15	11	9	7	6	5	4	4

end of the second stage, the drug is rejected if the observed response rate is ≤ r/n.

Table 19-3 shows some of these optimized designs. To select a design one must specify a target activity level p_1 of interest, and also a lower activity level p_0. The optimal designs in Table 19-3 provide probability ≥ 0.90 of rejecting drugs worse than p_0 and probability ≥ 0.90 of not-rejecting drugs better than p_1. Subject to these two constraints the optimal designs minimize the average sample size as functions of n_1,r_1,n,r.

The average sample size is calculated at the activity level p_0. Hence the optimal designs are optimized for screening out poor drugs. Table 19-3 shows for each design the decision criteria, the average sample size, and the probability of stopping after the first stage for a drug with activity level p_0.

Table 19-3 also shows the "minimax" design for each situation. The minimax design is that design with the smallest maximum sample size n that satisfies the two constraints described above. If there are several such designs, the one with the minimum average sample size (calculated at activity level p_0) is shown. Although minimax designs have somewhat larger average sample sizes than optimal designs, in some cases they are preferable because the small increase in average sample size is more than compensated for by a large reduction in maximum sample size.

PHASE III TRIALS

The protocol for a phase III study should specify the number of patients and duration of follow-up planned. These plans should be based on the specific study objectives and endpoints used. In many cases, the same protocol will include plans for treating very distinct subsets of patients (*e.g.*, stage I and stage II breast cancer patients). In such instances, plans should be made for accruing sufficient numbers of patients of each type for separate analyses because the relative merits of the treatments may vary substantially. Because of unforeseen complications or larger than expected treatment differences, patient accrual may have to be terminated prematurely. Nevertheless, target sample sizes are essential to ensure that the study is feasible and to know when to stop in the absence of premature termination. If too few patients are studied, the results may be ambiguous or erroneous, which commonly happens.[70–73] It is equally undesirable to have more patients studied than is necessary to reliably answer the questions posed by the study. The protocol should document that the target sample size can be accrued within a reasonable period of time (usually 3–4 years).

The usual statistical methods of sample size determination in comparative trials are oversimplified as rigid models of the complete analysis but are useful for planning purposes. These methods are based on the assumption that at the conclusion of the trial, a statistical significance test will be performed comparing the treatment groups with regard to the major endpoint(s). A statistical significance level of 0.05 resulting from a treatment comparison has the following meaning: if there is no true difference in treatment efficacy, the probability of obtaining a difference in outcomes as extreme as that observed in the data is 0.05. The significance level does not represent the probability that the null hypothesis is true, it represents a probability of an observed difference, assuming that the null hypothesis is true. Conventional statistical theory ascribes no probabilities to hypotheses, only to data.

With few patients in each of the treatment groups being compared, the difference in observed outcomes must be very extreme in order for the significance level to be as small as 0.05. As the sample size increases, smaller differences in response will be statistically significant at the 0.05 level. In comparing proportions, 10 of 10 compared to 7 of 10 (a difference of 30%) is not statistically significant at the 0.05 level, whereas 40 of 40 compared to 35 of 40 (a difference of 12%) is.

For comparing two proportions, the usual method of sample size determination is as follows. It is assumed that after n patients have been observed on treatment A and n patients have been observed on treatment B, a statistical significance test will be performed. One wishes to determine n to be just large enough so that if the true response rate for A is p_A% (*i.e.*, the response rate that would be observed in an infinite number of patients receiving A) and the true response rate for B is p_B%, 80% of the time the significance level will be no greater than 0.05. The 80% figure is called the power of the test.

If we think of a study resulting in a significance level of less than 0.05 for the major comparison as a positive study, the power represents the probability of getting a true positive result when the actual response rates are p_A and p_B. The power is a design parameter that usually is specified between 80% and 95%. Whereas performing a significance test does not require knowledge of the unknown p_A and p_B, these parameters are an integral part of determining n to achieve a

TABLE 19-3. Optimum and Minimax Two-Stage Phase II Designs

		Optimum Design				*Minimax Design*			
p_0	p_1	r_1/n_1*	r/n	PET†	ANP††	r_1/n_1	r/n	PET	ANP
0.05	0.25	0/9	2/24	0.63	14.55	0/13	2.20	0.51	16.41
0.05	0.20	0/12	3/37	0.54	23.50	0/18	3/32	0.40	26.44
0.10	0.25	2/21	7/50	0.65	31.20	2/27	6/40	0.48	33.70
0.20	0.40	3/17	10/37	0.55	26.0	3/19	10/36	0.46	28.26

*Reject drug if observed response rate is ≤ r_1/n_1 or ≤ r/n.
†Probability of early termination, after the first stage, when the true response probability is p_0.
††Average number of patients when the true response probability is p_0.

preplanned power. If treatment A is a standard treatment, p_A is estimated from past data. The absolute magnitude $|p_B - p_A|$ is viewed as a difference that we wish to have a power of 80% (say) for detecting.

For comparing two proportions, Tables 19-4 and 19-5 can be used to determine the number of patients to be assigned each of two treatments in order to achieve a specified power as a function of the true response rates. Table 19-4 is for obtaining one-sided significance levels less than 0.05, and Table 19-5 is for two-sided significance levels of less than 0.05. A two-sided significance level represents the probability by chance alone of obtaining a difference in either direction as large as the one actually observed. A one-sided significance level represents the probability by chance alone of obtaining a difference as large as and in the same direction as that actually observed. Controversy exists over the appropriateness of one-sided or two-sided significance levels. This will be discussed later in the chapter. A conservative approach is to use two-sided significance levels. Suppose that based on past data we estimate the response rate for treatment A to be 30% and that we wish to have 80% power for detecting a true response rate of treatment B of 55%. For a two-sided statistical significance test, we find from Table 19-5 that 68 patients for each of the two treatments are needed (136 patients total). If we wish power of 80% for detecting a true response rate of treatment B of 50%, 103 patients per treatment are needed. The required number of patients increases rapidly as size of the difference to be detected decreases. Almost all phase III studies should be large enough to detect reliably a difference of 20% to 25% in success rate. The "not significantly different" results of smaller comparative studies often are mistakenly interpreted as saying something about the treatments, whereas they may be just a consequence of the inadequate numbers of patients.[70–73]

Tables 19-4 and 19-5 were constructed according to the methods of Casagrande, Pike, and Smith,[74] and are considered more accurate than tables previously published based on other approximations.[75] When the smaller response rate is thought to exceed 50%, the tables given here should be used to compare failure rates (100% minus response rate).

When an unbalanced $K/1$ randomization is contemplated for comparing two treatments, the total sample size obtained from Tables 19-4 and 19-5 should be multiplied by $(K + 1)^2/4K$. For example, a 2:1 randomization requires 12.5% more total patients than an equally weighted design of the same power. Weightings more extreme than 2:1 are rarely desirable.

For comparative trials of proportions using historical controls, appropriate tables are given by Makuch and Simon,[76] and are reproduced here as Tables 19-6, 19-7, and 19-8. These tables are more bulky because the number of patients to be given the experimental treatment depends on the size of the historical control group. Tables 19-6, 19-7, 19-8 are for achieving 80% power with a one-sided significance level of 0.05. If our historical control group of 50 patients showed a response rate of 30% and we want 80% power for detecting a true response rate of 50% for the new treatment, Table

TABLE 19-4. Number of Patients in Each of Two Treatment Groups (One-Sided Test)

Smaller Success Rate	*Larger Minus Smaller Success Rate*									
	0.05	*0.10*	*0.15*	*0.20*	*0.25*	*0.30*	*0.35*	*0.40*	*0.45*	*0.50*
0.05	512*	172	94	62	45	35	28	23	19	16
	381†	129	72	48	35	27	22	18	15	13
0.10	786	236	121	76	54	40	31	25	21	17
	579	176	91	58	41	31	24	20	16	14
0.15	1026	292	144	88	60	44	34	27	22	18
	752	216	108	66	46	34	26	21	17	14
0.20	1231	339	163	98	66	48	36	29	23	19
	900	250	121	73	50	37	28	22	18	15
0.25	1402	377	178	105	70	50	38	29	23	19
	1024	278	132	79	53	38	29	23	18	15
0.30	1539	407	189	111	73	52	38	30	23	19
	1122	300	141	83	55	39	30	23	18	15
0.35	1642	429	197	114	74	52	38	29	23	18
	1196	315	146	85	56	40	30	23	18	14
0.40	1711	441	201	115	74	52	38	29	22	17
	1246	324	149	86	56	39	29	22	17	14
0.45	1745	446	201	114	73	50	36	27	21	16
	1271	327	149	85	55	38	28	21	16	13
0.50	1745	441	197	111	70	48	34	25	19	15
	1271	324	146	83	53	37	26	20	15	12

*Upper figure: Significance level 0.05, power 0.90.
†Lower figure: significance level 0.05, power 0.80.

TABLE 19-5. Number of Patients in Each of Two Treatment Groups (Two-Sided Test)

Smaller Success Rate	*Larger Minus Smaller Success Rate*									
	0.05	*0.10*	*0.15*	*0.20*	*0.25*	*0.30*	*0.35*	*0.40*	*0.45*	*0.50*
0.05	620*	206	113	74	54	42	33	27	23	19
	473†	159	88	58	43	33	27	22	18	16
0.10	956	285	146	92	64	48	38	30	25	21
	724	218	112	71	50	38	30	24	20	17
0.15	1250	354	174	106	73	53	41	33	26	22
	944	269	133	82	57	42	32	26	21	18
0.20	1502	411	197	118	79	57	44	34	27	22
	1132	313	151	91	62	45	34	27	22	18
0.25	1712	459	216	127	84	60	45	35	28	23
	1289	348	165	98	65	47	36	28	22	18
0.30	1880	495	230	134	88	62	46	36	28	22
	1414	375	175	103	68	48	36	28	22	18
0.35	2006	522	239	138	89	63	46	35	27	22
	1509	395	182	106	69	49	36	28	22	18
0.40	2090	537	244	139	89	62	45	34	26	21
	1571	407	186	107	69	48	36	27	21	17
0.45	2132	543	244	138	88	60	44	33	25	19
	1603	411	186	106	68	47	34	26	20	16
0.50	2132	537	239	134	84	57	41	30	23	17
	1603	407	182	103	65	45	32	24	18	14

*Upper figure: significance level 0.05, power 0.90.
†Lower figure: significance level 0.05, power 0.80.

19-6 indicates that 69 new patients should be treated with the new experimental therapy. If there were 100 appropriate historical controls, Table 19-7 indicates that 48 new patients should be treated with the experimental therapy. Tables 19-6, 19-7, and 19-8 assume that all new patients will be given the experimental therapy. Mixtures of historical and concurrent controls have not been studied in this way.

Tables for comparing proportions are useful when the endpoint can be dichotomized as success or failure. This can be done for response rate or complete response rate. The tables also can be used when survival or continuous disease-free survival is to be compared. In such cases, the table is used with regard to the proportion of patients who survive (or remain without evidence of disease) for some meaningful time period (*e.g.*, 5 years). The number of patients required must then be observed for this time period. The final analysis of such studies generally will consist of a comparison of the entire survival curves, rather than just the proportions surviving 5 years. It is not possible, however, to produce general tables of required number of patients for comparing survival curves because the results depend on the form of the survival distributions. For example, fewer patients are needed to detect a 50% increase in median survival when the variability in survival time among similarly treated patients is smaller than would be required to detect the same 50% increase if variability were large.

Rubinstein, Gail, and Santner[77] have developed useful methods for determining the required number of patients and duration of follow-up when the survival distributions have an exponential form. Exponential survival corresponds to a constant force of mortality, that is, a constant percentage of the remaining patients die each month. For exponential survivals, the number of deaths required to achieve a specified power depends only on the ratio of median survivals to be detected, not on the actual median values. In using the tables presented here to plan survival studies, it must be remembered that the tabulated entry represents the number of patients per group followed for the specified period of time. George[78] has reviewed methods of sample size planning for phase III studies.

The kinds of methods described are useful for ensuring that sufficient numbers of patients are treated so that an improvement in response is not erroneously missed owing to the random fluctuations of small numbers. For studies comparing a standard treatment to a more conservative or less invasive therapy, it is particularly important that the sample size be large because with few patients it is unlikely that the difference in outcomes will be statistically significant at a level as small as 0.05 even though the conservative treatment may be truly inferior. In the usual statistical formulation, the null hypothesis specifies that the two treatments are equivalent. Acceptance of the null hypothesis may result in erroneous adoption of a new, more conservative therapy. The burden of proof for studies of this type should be on showing that results are similar, not on demonstrating that they are dissimilar. Consequently, accepting the null hypothesis based on a significance test of low power is very inappropriate. Large numbers of patients are required to ensure that

TABLE 19-6. Number of Patients Needed in an Experimental Group for a Given Probability of Obtaining a Significant Result (One-Sided Test) with Significance Level $\alpha = 0.05$ and Power $(1-\beta) = 0.80$ When $n_c = 20, 30, 40$, and 50 Historical Controls Are Used for Comparison

Proportion of Success for Experimental Patients	*Proportion of Success for Historical Control Patients*							
	0.1	*0.2*	*0.3*	*0.4*	*0.5*	*0.6*	*0.7*	*0.8*
0.2	*†							
	*‡							
	>40,000§							
	944‖							
0.3	116	*						
	53	*						
	40	*						
	35	*						
0.4	22	385	*					
	17	98	*					
	15	67	*					
	14	55	*					
0.5	11	31	882	*				
	9	23	137	*				
	9	21	87	*				
	8	19	69	*				
0.6	7	13	37	913	*			
	6	12	27	147	*			
	6	11	24	92	*			
	6	10	22	74	*			
0.7	5	8	14	36	455	*		
	4	7	13	27	122	*		
	4	7	12	24	83	*		
	4	7	11	22	68	*		
0.8	4	5	8	14	30	179	*	
	3	5	8	12	24	83	*	
	3	5	7	12	22	63	*	
	3	5	7	11	20	55	*	
0.9	3	4	5	8	12	22	68	*
	3	4	5	7	11	19	47	>40,000
	3	4	5	7	10	17	40	745
	3	4	5	7	10	17	37	355

*No solution.
†Sample size for $n_c = 20$ historical controls.
‡Sample size for $n_c = 30$ historical controls.
§Sample size for $n_c = 40$ historical controls.
‖Sample size for $n_c = 50$ historical controls.

important differences can be ruled out in the analysis by calculating confidence intervals for the true difference in efficacy. The confidence interval provides a much clearer picture of what differences in efficacy are consistent with the data that does a significance test. Makuch and Simon[65] discuss this approach for planning the size and duration of studies evaluating a conservative therapy.

INTERIM ANALYSES OF PHASE III TRIALS

The methods described above for determining the required number of patients assume that statistical analysis will be performed only at the conclusion of the trial. If statistical significance tests are performed repeatedly throughout the trial, the probability that the difference in outcomes will be statistically significant at the 0.05 level at some point is greater than 5% by chance alone.[79] This probability is called the type 1 error of the design. Fleming et al[80] have shown that the type 1 error can be as great as 26% or more if one performs a significance test every 3 months of a 3-year trial comparing two identical treatments. If the times of the analyses are determined by visual trends in the accumulating data, this error may be even greater. If we think of a study that reports a significance level of less than 0.05 for the major comparison as a positive study, the type 1 error represents the probability of getting a false-positive result.

Interim analyses can be misleading because they may be dominated by differences in treatment efficacy for minor subsets of patients of poorer prognosis and by transient differences in the distribution of prognostic factors.[72] Interim analyses also may influence the types and numbers of patients subsequently entered and even cause undesirable changes in patient management and evaluation of response. For these reasons, it is common in fields other than oncology to review interim results only by a monitoring board rather

TABLE 19-7. Number of Patients Needed in an Experimental Group for a Given Probability of Obtaining a Significant Result (One-Sided Test) with Significance Level $\alpha = 0.05$ and Power $(1 - \beta) = 0.80$. When $n_c = 75, 100, 125$, and 150 Historical Controls Are Used for Comparison

Proportion of Success for Experimental Patients	*Proportion of Success for Historical Control Patients*							
	0.1	*0.2*	*0.3*	*0.4*	*0.5*	*0.6*	*0.7*	*0.8*
0.2	232*							
	156*							
	129‡							
	115§							
0.3	29	907						
	27	383						
	26	271						
	25	223						
0.4	13	44	3373					
	13	40	702					
	12	38	424					
	12	36	327					
0.5	8	18	54	8392				
	8	17	48	949				
	8	16	46	525				
	8	16	44	390				
0.6	5	10	20	58	6016			
	5	10	19	52	893			
	5	10	19	49	511			
	5	9	18	47	385			
0.7	4	7	11	21	55	1944		
	4	6	11	20	50	609		
	4	6	10	19	47	398		
	4	6	10	19	45	316		
0.8	3	5	7	11	19	46	596	
	3	5	7	11	18	42	331	
	3	5	7	10	18	40	253	
	3	5	7	10	18	39	217	
0.9	3	4	5	7	10	16	33	187
	3	4	5	7	10	15	31	146
	3	4	5	6	9	15	30	129
	3	4	5	6	9	15	30	119

*Sample size for $n_c = 75$ historical controls.
†Sample size for $n_c = 100$ historical controls.
‡Sample size for $n_c = 125$ historical controls.
§Sample size for $n_c = 150$ historical controls.

than by the participating physicians. Several cancer cooperative groups blind treatment identification on interim reports. More groups are adopting this or more restrictive policies in response to the potential damage resulting from overinterpretation of interim results. For these same reasons, it generally is inappropriate to present interim results at national meetings.[81]

A number of useful statistical designs have been developed for monitoring and interpreting interim results. Perhaps the simplest is that due to Haybittle[82] and Peto.[11] They suggest that interim differences be discounted unless the difference is statistically significant at the two-sided $p < 0.0025$ level or the one-sided 0.005 level. If the interim differences are not significant at this level, the trial continues until its originally intended size. The final analysis is performed without regard to the interim analyses and the type 1 error is affected little by the monitoring.

Pocock,[83] O'Brien and Fleming,[84] Fleming, Harrington, and Green,[85] and others have developed group-sequential methods for assessing whether one treatment is superior to another based on a prespecified number of interim analyses. The critical p value for determining whether an interim difference should be judged statistically significant depends on the number of analyses that will be performed during the study. For a five-stage trial, four interim analyses and one final analysis, the critical p values are shown in Table 19-9. These designs are further discussed by Geller.[86]

The group-sequential methods are based on the assumption that interim-analyses are performed after equal amounts of information are accumulated during the trial. When survival or disease-free survival is the endpoint, this means that there are equal numbers of "failures" between interim analyses. Simulations by DeMets and Gail[87] have indicated that the boundaries are also valid if the log-rank significance test is used and interim analyses are performed at equal intervals of time.

Extreme treatment differences at an interim analysis are unusual in cancer clinical trials. It is more common to find that interim results do not support the hypothesis that the experimental treatment is substantially better than the con-

TABLE 19-8. Number of Patients Needed in an Experimental Group for a Given Probability of Obtaining a Significant Result (One-Sided Test) with Significance Level $\mu = 0.05$ and Power $(1 - \beta = 0.80$, When $n_c = 200$, 250, 300, and 500 Historical Controls Are Used for Comparison

Proportion of Success for Experimental Patients	*Proportion of Success for Historical Control Patients*							
	0.1	*0.2*	*0.3*	*0.4*	*0.5*	*0.6*	*0.7*	*0.8*
0.2	101*							
	94†							
	90‡							
	82§							
0.3	24	181						
	24	162						
	23	151						
	23	133						
0.4	12	35	250					
	12	34	217					
	12	33	199					
	12	32	170					
0.5	7	16	42	289				
	7	16	41	248				
	7	16	40	226				
	7	15	38	190				
0.6	5	9	18	44	288			
	5	9	18	43	248			
	5	9	18	42	226			
	5	9	17	41	191			
0.7	4	6	10	19	43	248		
	4	6	10	18	42	218		
	4	6	10	18	41	201		
	4	6	10	18	40	174		
0.8	3	5	7	10	17	38	182	
	3	5	7	10	17	37	166	
	3	5	7	10	17	36	156	
	3	5	7	10	17	35	139	
0.9	3	4	5	6	9	15	29	108
	3	3	5	6	9	15	28	102
	3	3	5	6	9	15	28	99
	3	3	5	6	9	14	28	92

*Sample size for $n_c = 200$ historical controls.
†Sample size for $n_c = 250$ historical controls.
†Sample size for $n_c = 300$ historical controls.
§Sample size for $n_c = 350$ historical controls.

TABLE 19-9. Some Sequences of Nominal Significance Levels for Two-Sided Five-Stage Group Sequential Trials Maintaining an Overall Significance Level of 0.05

Pocock[7]	*Peto et al.*[8] *and Haybittle*[9]	*O'Brien nd Fleming*[10]	*Fleming et al.*[11]
0.016	0.001	0.00001	0.0051
0.016	0.001	0.0013	0.0061
0.016	0.001	0.008	0.0073
0.016	0.001	0.023	0.0089
0.016	0.049	0.041	0.0402

trol. The method of stochastic curtailment[88] was developed for evaluating such a circumstance. At any interim analysis one calculates the probability of rejecting the null hypothesis at the end of the trial. This probability is calculated conditional on the data already obtained and on the assumption that the alternative hypothesis of superiority of the experimental treatment, used in designing the trial, is true. If this "conditional power" is less than about 0.20, then the trial may be terminated without rejecting the null hypothesis of treatment equivalence. Stochastic curtailment can also be used as a basis for early rejection of the null hypothesis of equivalence if the probability of rejecting the null hypothesis at the end, conditional on the current data and calculated under the null hypothesis, exceeds 0.80. With stochastic curtailment, interim analyses need not be equally spaced and the number of interim analyses need not be specified in advance; in fact, monitoring may be continuous. Stochastic curtailment is also useful for indicating when the actual failure rate in the control group is so much less than the planned failure rate that the clinical trial is no longer feasible.

DeMets and Ware,[88a] Ellenberg and Eisenberger,[88b] and Thall, Simon and Ellenberg[88c] have also developed designs for early termination of the clinical trial if results are not promising for the experimental treatment. Jennison and

Turnbull[88d] have presented methods for calculating confidence intervals for treatment differences at interim analyses. Such confidence intervals can be very informative.

The sequential designs that have been developed are useful tools for the difficult decisions sometimes presented by interim monitoring. Important clinical trials can be easily ruined by poorly based decisions to terminate early. Such errors are sometimes due to inadequate recognition of the variability of sequentially accumulating data and sometimes due to incomplete or poor quality data. Resulting publications foist unreliable conclusions on the medical community. As discussed above, the protocol should generally specify the target number of patients to be accrued, the duration of follow-up, and an interim monitoring plan that is soundly based statistically. It is usually inappropriate to present interim results at professional meetings or to publish results before accrual is complete and sufficient patient follow-up has occurred to ensure stability of conclusions.

EPIDEMIOLOGY OF CLINICAL TRIALS

Staquet and associates[89] and Zelen[90] have claimed that many of the positive results reported from small trials can be expected to be false-positives. Of the many small trials performed, at least 5% will by chance alone yield differences significant at the 0.05 level when there is no true difference in treatment efficacy. Journal publication policies are biased toward accepting positive results. These individuals believe that there are few true treatment differences of sufficient magnitude to be detected in small clinical trials. Hence they claim that the literature of positive results from small trials is dominated by false-positive claims. For example, Peto states,[11]

> My interpretation is that, having done what resections we can, almost all past claims or hopes of great therapeutic improvements have been mistaken, and so, despite appearances, almost all current therapeutic suggestions will likewise eventually be found to yield either small or no benefits. . . . Because the need is to distinguish between small benefits and no benefits, historically controlled comparisons will not suffice, nor will small randomized trials suffice. . . .

The elimination of moderate sized innovative clinical trials conducted by one or a few cooperating major research centers would eliminate much of the possibility of real breakthrough as well as the false-positive claims.[91] Such studies generally need substantiation, however, on a larger scale.[92] There are so few effective therapies that failure to examine promising intensive treatments may be more troublesome than false-positives. Staquet and associates[89] and Zelen,[90] however, are correct in pointing out that the proportion of false-positive claims in the literature is probably much greater than 5%. For many studies it is clear at the outset that a large number of patients are necessary. Single institutions with inadequate accrual do a disservice by initiating such trials, for misleading results are likely.

DATA MANAGEMENT

Data management is a very important part of the conduct of a clinical trial, particularly for multi-institution studies. Obtaining reliable data requires the same planning and professional expertise as do the other aspects of the study. Some general guidelines for data management follow, although these are not applicable to all situations.

1. Data forms should be as simple and unambiguous as possible.
2. Relatively extensive initial information about patients should be collected, but follow-up information to the major endpoints and acute complications should be limited severely.
3. Details of treatment administration should be reviewed continuously so that errors and misinterpretations can be corrected for future patients quickly.
4. Forms should be filled out only by fully qualified persons. Uniformity of subjective evaluations should be ensured.
5. Epidemiologic, psychosocial, and optional laboratory data should not be included for addressing peripherally related questions. These should be viewed as independent studies to be reviewed critically and requiring additional resource allocation.
6. Whenever possible, an existing computerized data management system should be used rather than hiring programmers to start from scratch.
7. Data management should be treated seriously and problems quickly resolved.

Generally, physicians are tempted to design more elaborate data collection than is really useful. This results in unnecessary complexity in the conduct of the study, increased effort on the part of all involved in data collection, and reduced reliability of the most important data elements. For multi-institution studies, data management can be very complex, expensive, and time consuming. The development of good forms and procedures should occupy a prominent role in the planning process. If it is not treated with due respect by the trial organizers or supported adequately, the consequences are severe. Wright and Haybittle[93] have described specific considerations for the design of data forms.

ETHICS

INFORMED CONSENT

The basic principle of a clinical trial is to give patients the best known treatment in a preplanned manner that allows reliable conclusions to be drawn that can benefit future patients. Medical experiments have been performed by the Nazis and others that were clearly not in the interest of the human subjects. The United States and some other countries have adopted regulations for the protection of human subjects in research.[94] One of the regulations of the U.S. Department of Health and Human Services is that the investigator obtain informed consent of the patient or the patient's legally authorized representative. The three major elements of informed consent are information, comprehension, and voluntariness. The regulation specifies that the consent must be sought under conditions that provide the patient opportunity to consider whether or not to participate and that minimize the possibility of coercion. The information must be in language understandable to the patient. Informed consent must be documented by use of a form signed by the patient. The basic required elements of informed consent are as follows.

1. A statement that the study involves research, an explanation of the purposes and procedures of the research, and identification of experimental procedures to be used
2. A description of reasonably foreseeable risks to the patient
3. A description of any benefits to the patient or others that may result from the research
4. A disclosure of appropriate alternative procedures or treatments
5. A statement concerning confidentiality of records and the possibility that the Food and Drug Administration may inspect the records
6. An explanation of whether compensation or treatment is available if injury occurs
7. An explanation of whom to contact concerning further information on the research or patients' rights and whom to contact in the event of a research-related injury
8. A statement that participation is voluntary and that refusal will involve no loss of benefits to which the patient is otherwise entitled

Informed consent is required today in the United States for clinical trials. Some physicians believe that the process may be detrimental to the mental health of patients who do not want to know all of the potential, although perhaps unlikely, complications of therapy. For randomized studies, informed consent should be sought before the randomization is performed. Consequently, the patient must agree to accept any of the treatments being compared. This makes clear to the patient that the physician does not reliably know which treatment is best. This may be embarrassing to the physician and unsettling to the patient. However, for best reliability of conclusions drawn from a randomized study, the randomization should occur after the patient agrees to receive any of the treatments; otherwise the informed consent process may serve, consciously or unconsciously, to select patients for one treatment or another based on their prognosis. For example, some patients with relatively poor prognosis may refuse to participate in a surgical adjuvant study unless they know beforehand that they will be in the chemotherapy group.

It has been pointed out by many people that informed consent is not really informed because most patients have neither the educational background nor the psychologic composure to be truly informed. Research is being conducted on ways of more effectively informing patients. Some individuals, however, believe that the process of informed consent is "a legalistic trick to devolve what should properly be the doctor's responsibility onto the patient."[11] It is likely that most abuses of good medical treatments today occur outside clinical trials.

PRERANDOMIZATION

Zelen[95] proposed a design in which patients are randomized after being found eligible for the protocol but before consent to participate is sought. With one version of his proposal, consent is sought only for patients randomized to an experimental therapy. This version was controversial with regard to ethical considerations. The other version of Zelen's proposal involves seeking consent for both randomized groups of patients. Since the treatment assignment is known and can be presented at the time consent is sought, it was thought that physicians would approach more patients for participation in the trial and patients would be more likely to participate. To avoid the possibility of bias in analysis of results, patients must be compared "as randomized" rather than "as treated," that is, a patient randomized to treatment A who refuses and received treatment B must be considered in the A group for analysis. Otherwise, the treatment comparison can be biased by a possible relationship between prognosis, treatment, and refusal rate. Since the analysis must be performed "as randomized," refusals dilute the differences in outcome that can be observed. To counteract this effect, the number of patients must be increased compared to a conventional trial in which most refusals occur before randomization and thus can be excluded from analysis. The relationship between refusal rate and increased sample size required for a prerandomization design is dramatic and is shown in Table 19-10. For a 15% refusal rate, the number of patients required is double that of a conventional randomized trial. Even though the informed consent process may be more comfortable for the physician and patient, it seems infrequent that prerandomization would result in a doubling of accrual.

Two other concerns have been expressed about preran-

TABLE 19-10. Sample Size Inflation Factor According to Overall Refusal Rate[96]

Refusal Rate	*Inflation Factor*
0.02	1.09
0.05	1.23
0.10	1.56
0.15	2.04
0.20	2.78
0.25	4.00
0.30	6.25
0.35	11.11
0.40	25
0.45	100
0.50	*

*If half the patients on each arm refuse and receive the other treatment, determination of differences in treatment effect is impossible regardless of the sample size.

domization.[96] First is the ethical issue of whether patients are really fully informed about possible alternative treatments when randomization has already occurred. The second issue is that there will be demand to analyze results both "as randomized" and "as treated." The results may differ, ruining credibility of the trial.

Prerandomization is attractive to many physicians, although there is a lack of awareness of the above-mentioned problems. The limited experience to date with this design has given mixed results. Refusal rates have ranged from 10% to 30%. Accrual generally has increased but not always by an amount sufficient to compensate for the inefficiency of the design. Prerandomization has been abandoned in one large multicenter trial. The prerandomization design needs to be evaluated more carefully before it can be considered as an acceptable alternative.[96]

ACCUMULATING INFORMATION

Many have struggled with the following question: Although it may be ethical to initiate a randomized clinical trial, does not the accumulation of interim results favoring one treatment make it unethical for a physician to continue entering patients? If the rate of patient entry is rapid compared to the time required to observe the major endpoints (*e.g.*, survival or duration of remission), this problem does not arise. A strong impetus for the development of sequential analysis methods has been to enable a reliable conclusion to be reached as early as possible for trials with slower accrual. Statistical methods of sequential analysis are not in themselves, however, substitutes for the human monitoring of interim results. Chalmers and others[81,97] have suggested that the decision of when a trial should stop should be in the hands of a small monitoring committee that contains individuals who are not themselves entering patients into the study. The physicians entering patients would not see interim results, and hence, in a multi-institution study, their opinions about the relative value of the treatments essentially would remain unchanged. Although the concept of ethical behavior inherent in this plan seems controversial, it is likely that the patients in general would benefit. Clinical trials would not be terminated prematurely or accrual reduced when results remain questionable, causing ambiguity to persist or new trials of the same treatments to be required. This approach is used widely in fields other than oncology.

The focus on ethical problems of accumulating information in randomized clinical trials derives to some extent from an oversimplified view of such studies. Most major trials are complex, requiring long-term follow-up for evaluation of survival and complications and warranting subset analyses to determine which treatment is best for which patients. It is often difficult to evaluate the treatments thoroughly after adequate follow-up and to interpret the results in the context of other studies. This type of reliable evaluation usually is impossible during accrual with limited follow-up on limited numbers of patients. In addition, few randomized studies result in treatments that differ so greatly in efficacy and with such slow accrual as to require early termination.

ANALYSIS

In this section we shall address several general aspects of analysis that are important for interpreting your own results and those of others.

SIGNIFICANCE LEVELS AND HYPOTHESIS TESTS

Medical decision-making is complicated, and clinicians frequently misinterpret statistical significance tests in search of clear-cut answers from ambiguous data. A statistical significance test for comparing outcomes of two treatment groups is performed in the following way. We define a test statistic, for example, difference in response rates, and then calculate the probability of getting a difference as large as that actually obtained if the treatments are actually of equal efficacy and differences occur merely by chance. That probability is called the *significance level*. If we calculate the probability of getting a difference in either direction as large in absolute value as the one we actually obtained, the significance level is called *two-sided*. If the probability is calculated only for differences in the same direction as that actually obtained, the significance level is called *one-sided*. Generally the two-sided significance level is twice the one-sided level.

After significance tests had been used for many years, Neyman and Pearson[98] formalized a mathematical theory of "hypothesis testing." In this theory, before conducting the study you rigidly specify a null statistical hypothesis, an alternative statistical hypothesis, and a decision rule for accepting one hypothesis and rejecting the other, based on the data obtained. The fraction of the time that the null hypothesis will be rejected in hypothetical repetitions of the experiment when it is in fact true is called the *type I error*. Similarly, the *type 2 error* is the fraction of the time that the alternative hypothesis would be rejected when it is true. The study involves collecting the data, applying the decision rule, and announcing whether you accept or reject the null hypothesis. This theory had great appeal to mathematical statisticians because its tight structure opened fields of statistical research devoted to finding decision rules having minimum type 2 errors for a given type 1 error and specified probability distribution.

This hypothesis testing framework has dominated introductory statistical courses, in large part because academic statisticians liked its mathematical niceties. The theory also appealed to clinicians because it simplified complex medical decision-making by providing yes or no answers: either the difference is "statistically significant" or it is not, period. With this theory the value of 0.05 for type 1 error has become very special. The distinction between one-sided and two-sided decision rules becomes crucial because a one-sided $p = 0.05$ is simply "nonsignificant" if a type 1 error of 0.05 based on a two-sided decision rule is prespecified (the two-sided $p = 0.10$). Within this theory the interpretation of results critically depends on what was written in the experimental plan, because the specific statistical hypotheses, type 1 and 2 errors, monitoring plan, and decision rules must be prespecified. Consideration of hypotheses suggested by the data is strictly forbidden in this framework.

It is ironic that so many physicians accept the theory of hypothesis testing as the ultimate model of a scientific study, whereas it has been questioned by so many prominent statisticians as a basis for inference in research.[81,88,98–104] Sir Ronald Fisher, a pioneer of modern statistics, dismissed this approach as being applicable only to routine assembly line testing:[99]

> Neyman, thinking that he was correcting and improving my own early work on tests of significance, as a means to the "improvement of natural knowledge," in fact reinterpreted them . . . as an acceptance procedure. . . . I am casting no contempt on acceptance procedures . . . but the logical differences between such an operation and the work of scientific discovery . . . seem to me so wide that the analogy between them is not helpful, and the identification of the two sorts of operations is decidedly misleading. . . . The conclusions drawn by a scientific worker from a test of significance are provisional and involve an intelligent attempt to understand the experimental situation. . . . We have the duty of formulating, of summarising, and of communicating our conclusions, in intelligible form, in recognition of the right of other free minds to utilize them in making their own decisions.

Other prominent statisticians have expressed similar views. Anscombe says of this approach,[101]

> The concept of error probabilities of the first and second kinds . . . has no direct relevance to experimentation. The formation of opinions, decisions concerning further experimentation and other required actions, are not dictated in a simple prearranged way by the formal analysis of the experiment, but call for judgment and imagination. . . . Sequential rules are simultaneously two things, stopping rules and decision rules. . . . When the experiment has been completed, the number of observations taken is an unalterable fact. The verdict, on the other hand, is no better than an opinion of the experimenter, and if anyone considers it to be a mistaken opinion he can form a different opinion of his own. . . . The primary aim of the statistical analysis of the experiment should be to present as clearly and accurately as possible the evidence concerning relative effectiveness. . . .

Cox and Hinkley comment,[102]

> An approach to the analysis of data that confines us to questions and a model laid down in advance would be seriously inhibiting. . . . The relation of the decision problem with significance testing is no more than a crude resemblance.

Greenhouse and colleagues comment,[103]

> . . . the classical precepts of the specifications of the two possible types of error and their relationship to the determination of sample size should serve as a guide . . . in the planning stage of the study. . . . But, it should not bind the investigator or the statistician in the analysis of the data. . . .

It is not the intention here to imply that one should adopt an "anything goes" attitude in the analysis of data. But the hypothesis testing framework is not entirely satisfactory and should not be viewed as a rigid prescription for good science. Significance levels play a prominent role in the reporting of clinical trial results, but they often cannot be interpreted as type 1 errors. Determination of type 1 error is virtually impossible unless a rigid decision rule is used for monitoring interim results. Significance levels can serve as useful aids to interpretation of results, but quibbling about whether a one-sided $p = 0.04$ is significant makes little sense. Significance levels are influenced by sample sizes, and failure to reject the null hypothesis does not mean that the outcomes are not different. In almost all cases, confidence intervals are more informative than significance levels. There is no simple index of truth for interpreting results. Many physicians attempt to use the notion of statistical significance in this way, but the attempt has an unsound basis. Thorough presentation, skeptical evaluation, and cautious interpretation of results are always required.

EXCLUSIONS

Excluding patients from analysis because of treatment deviations, early death, or patient withdrawal for other reasons may seriously bias the results.[10,11] Often, excluded patients have poorer outcomes than those not excluded. One can rationalize that patients not receiving treatment as specified in the protocol did worse because of that fact, but this is just a rationalization, which may be erroneous. The poor prognosis of these patients may have led directly or indirectly to their exclusion. There may be more potential exclusions in one treatment group, or the reasons for potential exclusion may differ among treatments. Excluding patients (or "analyzing them separately," which is equivalent to excluding them) for reasons other than that they did not satisfy the eligibility criteria of the study is a major problem in interpreting many studies. If the conclusions of a study depend on exclusions, then these conclusions are suspect. Eligibility criteria for both patients and collaborators should be established in such a way that there will be few protocol deviations. Generally the treatment plan should be viewed as a policy to be evaluated. This policy cannot be applied completely to all patients, but all patients should generally be evaluable in phase III studies.

PROGNOSTIC FACTORS AND MULTIPLE ANALYSES

The results of a clinical trial are often multifaceted and require analysis with regard to several endpoints. If major prognostic factors are known beforehand, it will frequently be desirable to incorporate these factors into the analysis either to correct for imbalances or to improve the precision of the estimates of treatment differences. Ignoring major prognostic factors in the analysis unnecessarily increases background patient variability and obscures comparisons between the treatments.[105,106] The identification and careful utilization of major prognostic factors can increase the sensitivity of clinical trials considerably. For some major patient or tumor characteristics, it may be desirable to evaluate the treatments separately by the determined subsets.

Multiple analyses can be carried too far, however, and can result in erroneous conclusions caused by ransacking the data. The subsets and adjusting variables preferably should represent characteristics known to be of major prognostic importance before the analysis is begun. They should represent characteristics measurable at the time of patient entry to the protocol and the major subset hypotheses, few in number, should be specified in the protocol. Statistical methodology for performing subset analyses has been described by Simon[106,107] and by Gail and Simon.[108] Generally, it is not valid to subset or to adjust the analysis by characteristics measured after the start of treatment (*e.g.*, treatment compliance, dose delivered or toxicity). Analyses not restricted to the widely recognized endpoints and the few major subset hypotheses specified at the outset should be interpreted generally as hypothesis generation to be tested in a subsequent study.

As mentioned previously, it often is important to perform interim monitoring of results, even though interim results may be misleading and affect the subsequent conduct of the study adversely. In reporting the results of a study, it is desirable to specify whether, when, and on what basis interim analyses were performed, to describe the nature of the interim analyses, and to specify how it was decided to terminate the trial. To some statisticians and clinicians, interpretation of results will be independent of these factors and based solely on the data, which should be summarized clearly and thoroughly. Some readers, however, may wish to revise their assessment of the results based on such information, and adequate information should be presented to permit them to do this. For either type of reader, your conclusions and significance levels are no substitute for extensive data presentations and descriptions of the conduct of the trial.

ESTIMATION OF SURVIVAL FUNCTIONS

Representation of the distribution of survivals for a group of patients is a commonly encountered problem. The problem of representing the distribution of remission duration or time until disease progression is mathematically identical, although we will refer to survivals here. The usual elementary methods of plotting histograms or calculating means and medians generally are not applicable because some patients will not have died at the time of analysis. Thus the data contain censored observations in the sense that survivals are known only to be at least as great as the observed values for the living patients.

The most satisfactory way of representing such data is to estimate the survival function $S(t)$. This function represents the probability of surviving more than t time units. Time t is measured from diagnosis, start of treatment, or some other meaningful time-point. For randomized studies, it is best to measure time from the date of randomization. There are basically two satisfactory methods for estimating $S(t)$. The first is the life table or actuarial method. It frequently is attributed to Berkson and Gage[109] or Cutler and Ederer[110] and is appropriate when the number of patients is large. The other method is the product limit method of Kaplan and Meier.[111] This method is appropriate for any number of patients, but it involves more effort than the life table method when the number of patients is large.

The first step in the application of either method is the calculation of survival time for all patients. Survival is the duration from the chosen baseline (*e.g.*, date of randomization) until either death or date last known to be alive for patients who are not known to have died. To use the life table method, one determines intervals for the grouping of survival times. The life table, shown in Table 19-11, is then filled out. This sample life table is prepared with yearly intervals in the first column. The number of patients alive at the beginning of the interval is entered in column 2. The number who died in the interval is entered in the fourth column. Patients dying exactly at a time that represents a boundary between two intervals (*e.g.*, 365 days) are considered to have died in the preceding interval (*e.g.*, 0–1 year). The third column contains the number of patients who either are lost to follow-up during the interval or are alive with maximum follow-up duration included in the interval. This last set of patients are referred to as "withdrawn alive" in the conventional life table terminology. The life table method assumes that patients lost to follow-up or withdrawn alive during the interval are at risk of death for half of the

TABLE 19-11. Life Table Method for Estimating a Survival Distribution

(1) Years After Randomization $x - 1$ to x	*(2) Number Alive at Beginning of Interval* 1_x	*(3) Number Lost to Follow-up or Withdrawn Alive During Interval* w_x	*(4) Number Died During Interval* d_x	*(5) Effective Number Exposed to Risk of Dying During Interval (Col 2 − ½ Col 3)* 1_x	*(6) Proportion Dying (Col 4/Col 5)* q_x	*(7) Proportion Surviving (1 − Col 6)* p_x	*(8) Cumulative Proportion Surviving from Randomization Through End of Interval* $(p_2 \times p_2 \times \ldots \times p_x)$ S_x
0–1	252	38	94	233	0.40	0.60	0.60
1–2	120	34	10	103	0.10	0.90	0.54
2–3	76	30	4	61	0.07	0.93	0.50
3–4	42	18	4	33	0.12	0.88	0.44
4–5	20	12	0	14	0.00	1.00	0.44
5–6	8	8	0	4	0.00	1.00	0.44

interval. Hence column 5, the number alive at the start of the interval minus half the number lost or withdrawn during the interval, represents an approximate number of patients at risk of death during the interval. Column 6 gives the ratio of the number dying in the interval to the number at risk, which is an estimate of the probability of dying during the interval for patients who are alive at the start of the interval. Column 7 gives the estimated probability of surviving the interval for patients alive at the start of the interval. Column 8 should be studied carefully because it provides the life table estimate of the survival distribution and indicates the logic behind the method. The probability of surviving more than 3 years after randomization, for example, equals the entry in the third row of column 8 (0.50). The logic is as follows. In order to survive 3 full years, you must survive through the first year, and given that you have survived the first year you must survive the second year, and given that you have survived second year you must survive the third year. Consequently, the probability of surviving for at least 3 years is estimated by the product $p_1 \times p_2 \times p_3$ of factors in column 7. By using this product, the life table method takes maximal advantage of the mortality experience of patients with limited follow-up. The entry S_x in column 8, row x, represents the life table estimate of the probability of surviving more than x years from randomization. Computational shortcuts to observe are that for column 8, S_x equals p_x times S_{x-1}, and for column 2, $l_{x+1} = l_x - w_x - d_x$.

The product limit method of Kaplan and Meier is similar in concept to the life table method. With the Kaplan-Meier approach, however, the intervals are defined by the actual survival times of patients who have died. Suppose, for example, that the survivals are 3, 3, 3+, 5, 6, 8+, 8+, 10, 10, and 12+ months, where a plus follows survivals for patients still alive. Then the intervals are 0 to 3, 3 to 5, 5 to 6, and 6 to 10 months, as shown in Table 19-12. With the Kaplan-Meier method, deaths occur only at the end of intervals. The entry l'_x in column 5 equals $l_x - w_x$ rather than $l_x - ½\,w_x$ for the life table method. This is because deaths occur only at the ends of intervals here, and the number of patients at risk of death just before the interval end is $l_x - w_x$. In the entry w_x in column 3 for the Kaplan-Meier method, patients who are lost to follow-up or withdrawn alive at the end of an interval are considered not lost or withdrawn until the following interval. These differences between the Kaplan-Meier and life table methods render the former more appropriate for studies with smaller numbers of patients.

Once the values S_x have been calculated for the Kaplan-Meier method, they may be graphed with time on the horizontal axis. The graph is a step function that starts at time zero and ordinate 1.0. It drops to value S_x at time x, where x is the time at the right end of an interval. The survival curve corresponding to Table 19-11 is shown in Figure 19-2. The tic marks are placed on the curve at 3, 8, and 12 months to represent the follow-up times of living patients. The step function is extended horizontally out to 12 months to represent follow-up of the last patient. The estimator S_x is approximately normally distributed in large samples. If m patients remain alive at time x, the standard error of S_x can be conservatively estimated as

$$S_x\sqrt{(1 - S_x)/m}.$$[10]

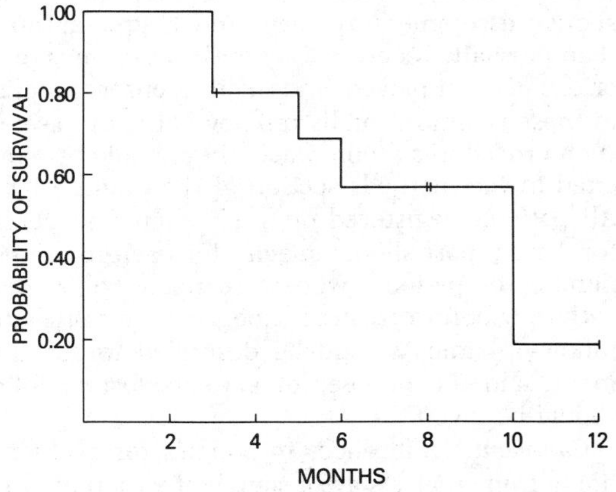

FIG. 19-2. Example of estimated survival distribution.

TABLE 19-12. Kaplan-Meier Method for Estimating a Survival Distribution

(1) Months After Randomization	(2) Number Alive at Beginning of Interval l_x	(3) Number Lost to Follow-up or Withdrawn Alive During Interval w_x	(4) Number Died During Interval d_x	(5) Effective Number at Risk of Dying Just Before End of Interval (Col 2 − Col 3) l_x	(6) Proportion Dying (Col 4/Col 5) q_x	(7) Proportion Surviving (1 − Col 6) p_x	(8) Cumulative Proportion Surviving from Randomization Through End of Interval $(P_1 \times p_2 \times \ldots \times p_x)$ S_x
0–3	10	0	2	10	0.2	0.8	0.8
3–5	8	1	1	7	0.14	0.86	0.68
5–6	6	0	1	6	0.17	0.83	0.57
6–10	5	2	2	3	0.67	0.33	0.19

REPORTING RESULTS OF CLINICAL TRIALS

Effective reporting of results is an integral part of good research. Unfortunately numerous surveys have indicated that the quality of reporting of clinical trial results is poor. Simon and Wittes[112] developed a set of methodologic guidelines for reports of clinical trials and these guidelines have been adopted by major cancer journals worldwide. The nine guidelines are listed below with brief comments.

1. Authors should discuss briefly the quality control methods used to ensure that the data are complete and accurate. A reliable procedure should be cited for ensuring that all patients entered on study are actually reported upon. If so such procedures are in place, their absence should be noted. Any procedures employed to ensure that assessment of major endpoints is reliable (*e.g.*, second-party review of responses) should be mentioned or their absence noted.

   Comment: The intent here is that a report make clear the extent to which the major data of the study rest on a firm and verifiable foundation. To ensure that all patients entered on a study are in fact included in the final report, there should be a formal registration mechanism for study entry. Quality control of response assessment requires much greater attention than it usually receives. Currently, numerous response criteria are employed, and the interobserver reliability of these is almost totally unknown. In any case, where such procedures are in place, they should be explicitly cited in the methods section of the manuscript.
2. All patients registered on study should be accounted for. The report should specify for each treatment the number of patients who were not eligible, died, or withdrew before treatment began. The distribution of follow-up times should be described for each treatment, and the number of patients lost to follow-up should be given.

   Comment: Differences in policies for excluding patients from analysis are a source of variation in results among similar studies. Regardless of how response rates are calculated, all patients must be accounted for. This will permit the reader to recalculate rates as he or she wishes.
3. The study should not have an inevaluability rate for major endpoints of greater than 15%. Not more than 15% of eligible patients should be lost to follow-up or considered inevaluable for response due to early death, protocol violation, missing information, or other reasons.

   Comment: The 15% figure is obviously somewhat arbitrary, but inevaluability rates of ≥20% usually reflect inappropriate patient selection. For phase III studies, disqualifications are a source of potential bias; when the disqualification rate approaches the magnitude of the difference in outcomes being tested, the results are not sufficiently reliable.
4. In randomized studies, the report should include a comparison of survival and other major endpoints for all eligible patients as randomized, that is, with no exclusions other than those not meeting eligibility criteria.

   Comment: Comparisons of outcomes in randomized studies that exclude eligible randomized patients are subject to potential bias. Patients who refuse further treatment, for example, may be prognostically favorable or unfavorable. This has been clearly demonstrated for placebo patients in major cardiovascular trials. Consequently, the analysis of randomized trials should contain comparisons of all eligible randomized patients. The report may also contain other comparisons.
5. The sample size should be sufficient to either establish or conclusively rule out the existence of effects of clinically meaningful magnitude. For "negative" results in therapeutic comparisons, the adequacy of sample size should be demonstrated by either presenting confidence limits for true treatment differences or calculating statistical power for detecting differences.

   Comment: The point here is basic but frequently not recognized. Small studies that find no statistically significant differences between treatments are generally indeterminate, not negative. Unfortunately, such studies are usually erroneously interpreted as negative. The problem is that the statistical power of small studies (*i.e.*, the probability of obtaining a statistically significant difference if the two treatments are truly different) is low. Reporting confidence limits in addition to or instead of significance levels clarifies the distinction between indeterminate and negative results.[71] For example, suppose the response rate for treatment A is 10 of 20 (50%) and for treatment B is 8 of 20 (40%). This difference is not significant ($p = 0.75$). But approximate 95% confidence limits for the true differences in response rates are −20.7% to +40.7%. So the data are consistent with both a moderate difference favoring treatment B and a tremendous difference favoring treatment A. The trial is not negative but rather indeterminate; the p value is misleading, and the number of patients is inadequate.

   A sample size that is insufficient to answer the question originally posed by the trial is a serious problem. Oncologists and cancer patients are not well served by the publication of results that are inconclusive because of avoidable flaws in trial execution. The trial that does not accrue an adequate number of patients is a failed experiment; unless the reason for the poor accrual is itself illuminating, the field is no wiser after the trial than before.
6. Authors should state whether there was an initial target sample size and, if so, what it was. They should specify how frequently interim analyses were performed and how the decisions to stop accrual and report results were arrived at.

   Comment: This refers to the sequential analysis of data as they are accumulating. It is not appropriate to interpret significance levels and confidence intervals at face value if one repeatedly analyzes accumulating data. That is, stopping accrual and publishing results as soon as a p value falls below 0.05 is a procedure with a high probability of producing erroneous conclusions. Generally it is necessary to perform interim evaluation of results. But premature termination and reporting of the study should be based upon p values much smaller than 0.05 if unreliable results are to be avoided.

7. All claims of therapeutic efficacy should be based upon explicit comparisons with a specific control group, except in special circumstances where each patient is his own control. If nonrandomized controls are used, the characteristics of the patients should be presented in detail and compared to those of the experimental group. Potential sources of bias should be adequately discussed. Comparison of survival between responders and nonresponders does not establish efficacy and should not generally be included. Reports of phase II trials which draw conclusions about antitumor activity but not therapeutic efficacy generally do not require a control group.

   Comment: Controls are generally not required for single agent phase II trials because no claims of therapeutic efficacy are (or should be) made. Such trials attempt to evaluate only antitumor activity. Phase III trials, however, require controls. Nonrandomized studies should be performed as well as possible using explicit controls for which comparability can be thoroughly evaluated on a patient-by-patient basis. Comparison of survival between responders and nonresponders is not a valid way of establishing therapeutic efficacy.[113,114] This comparison can be biased in several ways. First, patients who die quickly are by definition nonresponders. Hence, there is a time bias. Second, responders may have more favorable prognoses regardless of treatment. They may have less disease, less prior treatment, and better performance status. They may also be more favorable with regard to unknown prognostic factors. To evaluate the impact of a treatment on survival or disease-free survival, outcomes for all of the treated patients should be compared to those for an appropriate control group.

8. The patients studied should be adequately described. Applicability of conclusions to other patients should be carefully dealt with. Claims of subset-specific treatment differences must be carefully documented statistically as more than the random results of multiple-subset analyses.

   Comment: Care should be employed in extrapolating results to the general population of patients. Only a small fraction of patients enter clinical trials, and they are not a random sample. Proper statistical methodology is necessary to distinguish true subset-specific treatment differences from the random results of multiple-subset analyses. It is not generally recognized that, by chance alone, there is a 40% probability of finding at least one statistically significant false-positive treatment difference in the evaluation of ten disjoint subsets.

9. The methods of statistical analysis should be described in detail sufficient that a knowledgeable reader could reproduce the analysis if the data were available.

META-ANALYSIS

A meta-analysis is a quantitative summary of research in a particular area. It is distinguished from the traditional literature review by its emphasis on quantifying results of individual studies and on combining results across studies. Meta-analysis arose in the social sciences. It has become extremely popular in psychology and education, but the value of the approach remains controversial.[115] A major point of concern is the tendency to combine dissimilar studies and to overemphasize average results. For example, Eysenck[116] objected to the inclusion of all studies on a given topic, regardless of quality: "(Smith and Glass) advocate and practice the abandonment of critical judgments of any kind. A mass of reports—good, bad, and indifferent—are fed into the computer . . . If their abandonment of scholarship were to be taken seriously, a daunting but improbable likelihood, it would mark the beginning of a passage into the dark age of scientific psychology."

Research reviews in medical therapeutics are often limited by unavailability of actual study data to compare, reanalyze, and perhaps combine. Within the past few years a new type of review method has appeared in the medical literature.[117] Key components of this method are to include only randomized clinical trials, include all relevant randomized trials that have been initiated anywhere in the world whether completed, published or not, exclude no randomized patients from analysis, and assess therapeutic effectiveness based upon the average results pooled across trials.

With this approach, attention is restricted to randomized trials because potential bias from nonrandomized comparisons may swamp out small to moderate therapeutic effects. Including all relevant randomized trials that have been initiated anywhere in the world represents an attempt to avoid publication bias and ensures that all relevant evidence is available. Publication bias results from the tendency of journals to accept positive rather than negative studies. Avoiding exclusion of any randomized patient for reasons such as protocol compliance is also to avoid bias because patients excluded from one treatment may be prognostically different than those excluded from another. Assessing therapeutic effectiveness based upon average pooled results is an attempt to make recommendations based on the totality of evidence rather than upon extreme but irreproducible isolated reports. In calculating average results, a measure of difference in outcome between treatments is calculated separately for each study. A weighted average of these study-specific differences is then computed.

A major issue of concern is the reasonableness of the calculation of average effect. When the studies being pooled are similar with regard to the therapy delivered, patient population, and data quality, then averaging of results makes sense. In this situation pooling could be quite valuable for detecting moderate treatment effects and may be essential for examining patient subsets. Often, however, the studies will not be very similar. The studies will differ with regard to the therapeutic interventions compared. In general, even if two studies plan to employ the same interventions, the doses actually delivered may differ grossly. Such differences may be accentuated by including all worldwide studies. Studies may also differ with regard to the kinds of patients included and these differences can influence results. For example, old patients may tolerate intensive chemotherapy less well and have higher rates of death from other causes. Studies may also differ greatly with regard to degree of protocol compliance, adequacy of follow-up and reliability of data.

When the studies differ substantially, one must recognize that the average results may not be representative of the components making up the average. For example, substantial effectiveness of one treatment or one class of patients may be masked by pooling with ineffective treatments or unresponsive types of patients. Peto[118] has argued that although the degree of effectiveness may vary, unanticipated reversals of outcome differences ("qualitative interactions") are unlikely. That is, if one subset of patients benefits from the experimental treatment, then the other subsets may benefit more or less but will not be harmed by the treatment. When dealing with toxic or expensive treatments, however, differences of degree, even without reversals, severely limit the extent to which the results are useful for patient care purposes.

Unfortunately, the database available in an overview will often be insufficient to answer the question of whether different classes of treatments have different levels of effects relative to a control or whether effects differ substantially among subsets of patients. This should not necessarily be viewed as a license to pool results across classes of treatments or patients on grounds of practicality. Although the average result can be of interest in itself, the overview should identify where the data are inadequate as a basis for reaching strong conclusions. For example, in evaluating adjuvant chemotherapy for primary breast cancer, it would seem important to treat intensive CMF (cyclophosphamide, methotrexate, and 5-fluorouracil) combinations separately. If results are inconclusive because of lack of data or substantial interstudy variability, then that should be a primary conclusion.

In reporting a meta-analysis it is important to display the results of individual trials in a manner that permits assessment of whether they are consistent with one another or whether there are outliers that dominate the averages. Although formal interaction tests may not be sufficiently powerful to test homogeneity of results, graphic display is very important. The apparent outliers provide leads to follow-up and may be much more important than the averages in some cases. The overview should attempt to understand major interstudy differences in results, not just average the outcomes. This process requires substantial knowledge of the disease and therapeutic modalities involved.

The overview method described can be very useful in certain circumstances. It may permit one to have sufficiently large samples from randomized trials to identify small to moderate treatment effects and to examine relative treatment efficacy for subsets of patients. Some investigators dismiss this approach as important only for identifying trivial differences. But a 10% difference in long-term survival rate for breast cancer is clinically important yet requires larger sample sizes than are common for even multi-institution phase III clinical trials. For diseases such as primary breast cancer where there are several subsets that warrant separate analysis, the sample size problem is even more severe. Meta-analysis is not a substitute for properly designed and sized clinical trials, but when several very similar major trials have been performed, evaluating and perhaps combining their results in a uniform manner can be quite useful. Some investigators also dismiss pooling results as trivial because even miniscule differences are statistically significant if the sample sizes are large enough. This is a valid criticism of statistical significance testing and emphasizes the importance of focusing attention on the size of the treatment differences found.[71]

Meta-analysis can be a useful tool when several very similar trials have been conducted and methodologic aspects of meta-analysis in medicine have been recently discussed in depth.[117] Often, however, the studies themselves will differ grossly. In such circumstances the average effect only provides an indication of whether or not there is a benefit or detriment of a class of treatments. The ability to answer questions about what treatments are actually effective, how effective they are, and what subsets of patients benefit depends on the existence of well-designed and well-conducted major clinical trials.

REFERENCES

1. Bull JP: The historical development of clinical therapeutic trials. J Chronic Dis 10:218–248, 1959
2. Doll R, Hill AE: A study of the aetiology of carcinoma of the lung. Br Med J 2:1271–1286, 1952
3. MacMahon B, Pugh TF: Epidemiology: Principles and Methods. Boston, Little, Brown & Co, 1970
4. Starmer CF, Rosati RA, McNeer JF: Data bank use in the management of chronic disease. Comput Biomed Res 7:111–116, 1974
5. McShane DJ, Porta J, Fries JF: Comparison of therapy in severe systemic lupus erythematosus employing stratification techniques. J Rheumatol 5:51–58, 1978
6. Cochran WG: The planning of observational studies of human populations. JR Stat Soc A 128:234–250, 1965
7. Byar DP: Why data bases should not replace randomized clinical trials. Biometrics 36:337–342, 1980
8. Dambrosia JM, Ellenberg JH: Statistical considerations for a medical data base. Biometrics 36:323–332, 1980
9. Tukey JW: Some thoughts on clinical trials, especially problems of multiplicity. Science 198:679–684, 1977

9a. Wittes RE, Marsoni S, Simon R, et al: The phase-II trial. Cancer Treat Rep 69:1235–1239, 1985

10. Peto R, Pike MC, Armitage P, et al: Design and analysis of randomized clinical trials requiring prolonged observation of each patient. 1. Introduction and design. Br J Cancer 34:585–612, 1976; 2. Analysis and examples. Br J Cancer 35:1–39, 1977
11. Peto R: Clinical trial methodology. Biomedicine 28:24–36, 1978

11a. Begg CA, Engstrom PF: Eligibility and extrapolation in cancer clinical trials. J Clin Oncol 5:962–968, 1987

12. Hill AB: The clinical trial. Br Med Bull 7:278–282, 1951
13. Schneiderman M: Non-objective art and objective evaluation in cancer chemotherapy. In Brodsky I, Kahn SB, Moyer JH (eds): Cancer Chemotherapy, pp 67–76. New York, Grune & Stratton, 1969
14. Schneiderman MA: The clinical excursion into 5-fluorouracil. Cancer Chemother Rep 16:107–118, 1962
15. Moertel CG, Hanley JA: The effect of measuring error on the results of therapeutic trials in advanced cancer. Cancer 38:388–394, 1976
16. Gurland J, Johnson RO: How reliable are tumor measurements? JAMA 29:973–978, 1965
17. Weiss GB, Bunce H, Hokanson JA: Comparing survival of responders and non-responders after treatment. A potential source of confusion in interpreting cancer clinical trials. Controlled Clin Trials 4:43–52, 1983
18. Anderson JR, Cain KC, Gelber RD: Analysis of survival by tumor response. J Clin Oncol 1:710–719, 1983
19. Simon R, Makuch RW: A non-parametric graphical representation of the relationship between survival and the occurrence of an event: Application to responder versus non-responder bias. Stat Med 3:1–9, 1984

20. Carter SK, Selawry O, Slavik M: Phase I clinical trials. In Saunders JP, Carter SK (eds): Methods of Development of New Anticancer Drugs, pp 75–80. Natl Cancer Inst Monogr 45, Bethesda, US Dept HEW, 1977
21. Woolley PV, Schein PS: Clinical pharmacology and phase I trial design. In DeVita VT Jr, Busch H (eds): Methods in Cancer Research, vol XVII, Cancer Drug Development Part B, pp 177–198. New York, Academic Press, 1979
21a. Freireich EJ, Gehan EA, Rall DP, et al: Quantitative comparison of toxicity of anticancer agents in mouse, rat, hamster, dog, monkey, and man. Cancer Chemother Rep 50:219–244, 1966
22. Shein PS, David RD, Carter S, et al: The evaluation of anticancer drugs in dogs and monkeys for the prediction of qualitative toxicities in man. Clin Pharmacol Ther 11:3–40, 1970
23. Homan ER: Quantitative relationships between toxic doses of antitumor chemotherapeutic agents in animals and man. Cancer Chemother Rep 3:13–19, 1972
24. Shein PS: The prediction of clinical toxicities of anticancer drugs. In The Pharmacologic Basis of Cancer Chemotherapy, pp 383–399. Baltimore, Williams & Wilkins, 1975
25. Guarino AM: Pharmacologic and toxicologic studies of anticancer drugs: of sharks, mice, and men (and dogs and monkeys). In DeVita VT Jr, Busch H (eds): Methods in Cancer Research, vol XVII. Cancer Drug Development Part B, pp 91–174. New York, Academic Press, 1979
26. Schneiderman MA: Mouse to man: Statistical problems in bringing a drug to clinical trial. In Proc Fifth Berkeley Symp Math Statis Prob, Univ of California 4:855–866, 1967
27. Hansen H, Selawry OS, Muggia FM et al: Clinical studies with 1-(2-chloroethyl)-3-cyclohexyl-1-nitrosourea (NSC 79037) Cancer Res 31:223–227, 1971
28. Goldsmith MA, Slavik M, Carter SK: Quantitative prediction of drug toxicity in humans from toxicity in small and large animals. Cancer Res 35:1354–1364, 1975
29. Storer BE: Design and analysis of phase I clinical trials: Preliminary studies using a markov chain representation and monte carlo simulations. Wisconsin Clinical Cancer Center Biostatistics Technical Report # 36, 1986
30. Gottlieb JA: Phase I and II clinical trials: A critical reappraisal. In The Pharmacological Basis of Cancer Chemotherapy, pp 485–498. Baltimore, Williams & Wilkins, 1974
31. Simon R, Wittes RE, Ellenberg SS: Randomized phase II clinical trials. Cancer Treat Rep 69:1375–1381, 1985
32. Herson J, Carter SK: Calibrated phase II clinical trials in oncology. Stat Med 5:441–447, 1986
33. Chalmers TC: Randomization of the first patient. Med Clin North Am 59:1035–1038, 1975
34. Lee YJ, Wesley RA: Statistical considerations to phase II trials in cancer: Interpretation, analysis and design. Semin Oncol 8:403–416, 1981
35. Moertel CG, Schutt AJ, Hahan RG, et al: Effects of patient selection on results of phase II chemotherapy trials in gastrointestinal cancer. Cancer Chemother Rep 59:257, 1974
36. Zelen M: Statistical options in clinical trials. Semin Oncol 4:441–446, 1977
37. Pocock SJ: Randomized clinical trials (letter). Br Med J 1:1161, 1977
38. Lasagna L: The controlled clinical trial: Theory and practice. J Chronic Dis 1:353–367, 1955
39. Ingelfinger FJ: The randomized clinical trial. N Engl J Med 287:100–101, 1972
40. Chalmers TC, Block JB, Lee S: Controlled studies in clinical cancer research. N Engl J Med 287:75–78, 1972
41. Schneiderman MA: Looking backward: Is it worth the crick in the neck? Or: Pitfalls in using retrospective data. Am J Roentgen Rad Ther Nucl Med 96:230–235, 1966
42. Simon R: The importance of prognostic factors in cancer clinical trials. Cancer Treat Rep 68:185–192, 1984
43. Wendel HA: Randomization in clinical trials. Science 199:368, 1979
44. Byar DP, Simon RM, Friedewald WT, et al: Randomized clinical trials: perspectives on some recent ideas. N Engl J Med 295:74–80, 1976
45. Pocock SJ: Allocation of patients to treatment in clinical trials. Biometrics 35:183–197, 1979
46. Gehan EA, Freireich EJ: Non-randomized controls in cancer clinical trials. N Engl J Med 290:198–203, 1974
47. Pocock SJ: The combination of randomized and historical controls in clinical trials. J Chronic Dis 29:175–188, 1976
48. Silverman WA: The lesson of retrolental fibroplasia. Sci Am 236(6):100–107, 1977
49. Hellman S: Editorial: Randomized clinical trials and the doctor-patient relationship. Cancer Clin Trials 2:189–193, 1979
50. Shapiro AR: The evaluation of clinical predictions. N Engl J Med 296:1509–1514, 1977
51. Gilbert JP, McPeek B, Mosteller F: Statistics and ethics in surgery and anesthesia. Science 198:684–689, 1977
52. Zelen M: Aspects of the planning and analysis of clinical trials in cancer. In Srivastava JN (ed): A Survey of Statistical Design and Linear Models, pp 629–645. New York, North-Holland, 1975
53. Pocock SJ, Simon R: Sequential treatment assignment with balancing for prognostic factors in the controlled clinical trial. Biometrics 31:103–115, 1975
54. Brown BW Jr: Statistical controversies in the design of clinical trials. Controlled Clin Trials 1:13–27, 1980
55. Simon R: Heterogeneity and standardization in clinical trials. In Tagnon HJ, Staquet MJ (eds): Controversies in Cancer. Design of Trials and Treatment, pp 37–49. New York. Masson Publishing, 1978
56. Simon R: Restricted randomization designs in clinical trials. Biometrics 35:503–512, 1979
57. Kalish LA, Begg CB: Treatment allocation methods in clinical trials: A review. Stat Med 4:129–144, 1985
57a. Kalish LA, Begg CB: The impact of treatment allocation procedures on nominal significance levels and bias. Controlled Clin Trials 8:121–135, 1987
58. Hills M, Armitage P: The two period cross-over clinical trial. Br J Clin Pharmacol 8:7–20, 1979
59. Koch GG: The use of non-parametric methods in the statistical analysis of the two-period change-over design. Biometrics 28:577–584, 1972
60. Brown BW Jr: The crossover experiment for clinical trials. Biometrics 36:69–79, 1980
61. Willan AR, Pater JL: Carryover and the two-period crossover clinical trial. Biometrics 42:593–599, 1986
61a. Olver IN, Simon RM, Aisner J: Antiemetic studies: A methodological discussion. Cancer Treat Rep 70:555–564, 1986
62. Koch GG, Gitomer SL, Skalland L, et al: Some nonparametric and categorical data analyses for a change-over design study and discussion of apparent carry-over effects. Stat Med 2:397–412, 1983
63. Schoenfeld DA, Gelber RD: Designing and analyzing clinical trials which allow institutions to randomize patients to a subset of the treatments under study. Biometrics 35:825–830, 1979
64. Makuch RW, Simon R: A note on the design of multi-institution three-treatment studies. Cancer Clin Trials 1:301-303, 1978
65. Byar DP, Piantadosi S: Factorial designs for randomized clinical trials. Cancer Treat Rep 69:1055–1064, 1985
66. Simon R: A critical assessment of approaches to improving the efficiency of cancer clinical trials. In Baum M, Kay R, Scheurlen H (eds): Recent Results in Cancer Research, vol III. Heidelberg, Springer Verlag, 1988
67. Makuch R, Simon R: Sample size requirements for evaluating a conservative therapy. Cancer Treat Rep 62:1037–1040, 1978
68. Simon R: How large should a phase II trial of a new drug be? Cancer Treat Rep 71:1079–1085, 1987
69. Gehan EA: The determination of the number of patients required in a preliminary and follow-up trial of a new chemotherapeutic agent. J Chronic Dis 13:346–353, 1961
70. Simon R: The size of phase III cancer clinical trials. Cancer Treat Rep 69:1087–1092, 1985
71. Simon R: Confidence intervals for reporting results of clinical trials. Ann Intern Med 105:429–435, 1986
72. Pocock SJ: Size of cancer clinical trials and stopping rules. Br J Cancer 38:757–766, 1978
73. Freiman JA, Chalmers TC, Smith H Jr, et al: The importance of beta, the type II error and sample size in the design and interpretation of the randomized control trial: Survey of 71 "negative" trials. N Engl J Med 299:690–694, 1978
74. Casagrande JT, Pike MC, Smith PG: An improved formula for calculating sample sizes for comparing two binomial distributions. Biometrics 34:483–486, 1978
75. Gehan EA, Schneiderman MD: Experimental design of clinical trials. In Holland JF, Frei E (eds): Cancer Medicine. Philadelphia, Lea & Febiger, 1973
76. Makuch RW, Simon R: Sample size considerations for nonrandomized comparative studies. J Chronic Dis 33:171–175, 1980
77. Rubinstein LV, Gail MH, Santner TJ: Planning the duration of a comparative clinical trial with loss to follow-up and a period of continued observation. J Chronic Dis 34:469–479, 1981
78. George SL: The required size and length of a phase III clinical trial. In Buvse ME, Staquet MJ, Sylvester RJ (eds): Cancer Clinical Trial: Design, Practice and Analysis. New York, Oxford University Press, 1983
79. McPherson K: Statistics: The problem of examining accumulating data more than once. N Engl J Med 290:501–502, 1974
80. Fleming TR, Green SJ, Harrington DP: Considerations of monitoring and evaluating treatment effects in clinical trials. Controlled Clin Trials 5:55–66, 1984
81. Green SJ, Fleming TR, O'Fallon JR: Policies for study monitoring and interim reporting of results. J Clin Oncol 5:1477–1484, 1987
82. Haybittle JL: Repeated assessment of results in clinical trials of cancer treatment. J Radiol 44:793–797, 1971
83. Pocock SJ: Interim analyses for randomized clinical trials: The group sequential approach. Biometrics 38:153–162, 1982
84. O'Brien PC, Fleming TR: A multiple testing procedure for clinical trials. Biometrics 35:549–556, 1979
85. Fleming TR, Harrington DP, O'Brien PC: Designs for group sequential tests. Controlled Clin Trials 5:348–361, 1984
86. Geller N: Planned interim analysis and its role in cancer clinical trials. J Clin Oncol 5:1485–1490, 1987
87. DeMets DL, Gail MH: Use of logrank tests and group sequential methods at fixed calendar times. Biometrics 41:1039–1044, 1985
88. Lan KKG, Simon R, Halperin M: Stochastically curtailed tests in long-term clinical trials. Commun Stat Sequent Anal 1:207–219, 1982
88a. DeMets DL, Ware JH: Group sequential methods in clinical trials with a one-sided hypothesis. Biometrics 67:651–660, 1980
88b. Ellenberg SS, Eisenberger MA: An efficient design for phase III studies of combination chemotherapies. Cancer Treat Rep 10:1147–1152, 1985

88c. Thall PF, Simon R, Ellenberg SS: Optimal two-stage designs for clinical trials with binary response. Stat Med (in press)

88d. Jennison C, Turnbull BW: Repeated confidence intervals for group sequential clinical trials. Controlled Clin Trials 5:33–45, 1984

89. Staquet MJ, Rozencweig M, Von Hoff DD, et al: The delta and epsilon errors in the assessment of cancer clinical trials. Cancer Treat Rep 63:1917–1921, 1979

90. Zelen M: Strategy and alternate randomized designs in cancer clinical trials. Cancer Treat Rep 66:1095–1100, 1982

91. Williams CJ, Whitehouse JMA: Cancer trials. Lancet 2:909, 1979

92. Simon R: Randomized clinical trials and research strategy. Cancer Treat Rep 66:1083–1087, 1982

93. Wright P, Haybittle J: Design of forms for clinical trials. Br Med J 2:529–530, 590–592, 650–651, 1979

94. Fed Register, vol 46, no 17, 8951, January 27, 1981

95. Zelen M: A new design for randomized clinical trials. N Engl J Med 300:1242–1245, 1979

96. Ellenberg SS: Randomization designs in comparative clinical trials. N Engl J Med 310:1404, 1984

97. Chalmers TC, Block JB, Lee S: Controlled studies in clinical cancer research. N Engl J Med 287:75–78, 1972

98. Neyman J, Pearson ES: On the use and interpretation of certain test criteria. Biometrika 20A:175–240, 263–294, 1928

99. Fisher RA: Statistical methods and scientific induction. J R Stat Soc B 17:69–78, 1955

100. Cox DR: Some problems connected with statistical inference. Ann Math Stat 29:357–372, 1958

101. Anscombe F: Sequential medical trials. J Am Stat Assoc 58:365–382, 1963

102. Cox DR, Hinkley DV: Theoretical Statistics. New York. Halsted Press, 1974

103. Cutler SJ, Greenhouse SW, Cornfield J, et al: The role of hypothesis testing in clinical trials. J Chronic Dis 19:857–882, 1966

104. Zelen M: Importance of prognostic factors in planning therapeutic trials. In Staquet MJ (ed): Cancer Therapy: Prognostic Factors and Criteria of Response. New York, Raven Press, 1975

105. Simon R: Importance of prognostic factors in cancer clinical trials. Cancer Treat Rep 68:185–192, 1984

106. Simon R: Patient subsets and variation in therapeutic efficacy. Br J Clin Pharmacol 14:473–482, 1982

107. Simon R: Statistical tools for subset analysis in clinical trials. In Baum M, Kay R, Scheurlen H (eds): Recent Results in Cancer Research, vol III. Heidelberg, Springer-Verlag, 1988

108. Gail M, Simon R: Testing for qualitative interactions between treatment effects and patient subsets. Biometrics 41:361–372, 1985

109. Berkson J, Gage RP: Calculations of survival rates for cancer. Proc Mayo Clin 25:270–286, 1950

110. Cutler SJ, Ederer F: Maximum utilization of the life table method in analyzing survival. J Chronic Dis 8:699–712, 1958

111. Kaplan EL, Meier P: Nonparametric estimation from incomplete observations. J Am Stat Assoc 53:457–481, 1958

112. Simon R, Wittes RE: Methodologic guidelines for reports of clinical trials. Cancer Treat Rep 69:1–3, 1985

113. Anderson JR, Cain KC, Gelber RD: Analysis of survival by tumor response. J Clin Oncol 1:710–719, 1983

114. Simon R, Makuch RW: A nonparametric graphical representation of the relationship between survival and the occurrence of an event. Stat Med 3:35–44, 1984

115. Slavin R: Meta-analysis in education: How has it been used? Educ Res 6–15, 1984

116. Eysenck HJ: An exercise in mega-silliness. Am J Psychol 33:517, 1978

117. Yusuf S, Simon R, Ellenberg S: Proceedings of the workshop on methodologic issues in overviews of randomized clinical trials. Stat Med 6:217–409, 1987

118. Peto R: Statistical aspects of cancer trials. In Halnan KE (ed): Treatment of Cancer, pp 867–871. London, Chapman and Hall, 1982

PART 2 *Practice of Oncology*

CHAPTER 20 *Specialized Techniques of Cancer Management*

PAUL H. SUGARBAKER
JACK A. ROTH

SECTION 1

Endoscopy

Endoscopy is one of the few medical technological advances that has resulted in a simultaneous decrease in patient morbidity and mortality as well as in cost. These advances have been made possible by the delivery of high-intensity cold light and high-resolution images through fiberoptic light bundles. Direct visual inspection of many internal organs and structures is now possible, permitting tissue histologic diagnosis, assessment of operability, and endoscopic surgery without requiring major exploratory procedures. Photography, biopsy, and excision of many pathologic processes are now possible. In this section we shall explore the indications and results, techniques and complications of diagnostic procedures often useful to oncologists. Throughout the discussion we shall emphasize proper techniques, for only with meticulous attention to technical detail can these diagnostic procedures be used repeatedly without appreciable morbidity or mortality. Endoscopic techniques for treatment are discussed in other chapters.

PERITONEOSCOPY (CELIOSCOPY, LAPAROSCOPY)

INDICATIONS AND RESULTS

DETECTION OF PERITONEAL TUMOR IMPLANTS IN PATIENTS WITH ADVANCED CANCER. Peritoneoscopy frequently provides information traditionally obtained only by exploratory laparotomy. It enables the physician to assess operability without making an abdominal incision; consequently, many patients can be spared exploratory surgery. Peritoneal and pelvic tumor implants can be visualized and biopsied to determine the stage of intra-abdominal malignant neoplasms.[1] Suitable candidates include patients with advanced primary gastric and pancreatic cancers, and those with advanced endometrial or rectal cancer. Patients with primary colonic or ovarian cancer do not require preoperative peritoneoscopy, since colonic cancer (and occasionally gastric cancer) requires resection for accurate staging of the disease and to prevent intestinal obstruction and bleeding. Abdominal computed tomography (CT) is notoriously inaccurate in the assessment of low-volume cancer on peritoneal surfaces.[2]

DETECTION OF LIVER METASTASES. Few items of clinical information change patient management more than the presence or absence of hepatic metastases. Several tests can be used to detect hepatic disease; however, all the noninvasive techniques can provide clues only to the presence or absence of hepatitic metastases. Only histologic examination of liver biopsy specimens provides reliable proof of hepatic metastases. Blind percutaneous liver biopsy sometimes can provide this information, but biopsies taken under peritoneoscopic control detect hepatic neoplastic disease nearly twice as frequently.[3-6] In a majority of patients, CT- or ultrasound (US)-guided biopsy is less invasive than biopsy performed under peritoneoscopic control.

STAGING AND FOLLOW-UP OF OVARIAN CANCER. Ozols and co-workers[7] recently reviewed their experience with 159 peritoneoscopic examinations in the management of 99 patients with ovarian cancer. In these patients, all of whom had undergone prior abdominal surgical procedures, peritoneoscopy was reported to be safe and feasible. It could not be technically performed in only 6% of patients. Peritoneoscopy disclosed sites of cancer spread undetected by conventional radiologic and nuclear medicine studies in 64% of examinations and provided the only evidence of followable disease in 38% of patients. Twenty-one percent of patients referred with Stage I or II disease were upstaged to Stage III on the basis of diaphragmatic disease detected at peritoneoscopy. In 66 restaging examinations, residual intra-abdominal disease was found in 33 patients (50%), and peritoneoscopic findings were the only evidence of disease in 24 patients (36%). Twenty-two patients with negative restaging peritoneoscopy went on to exploratory laparotomy; in 12 (55%), residual ovarian cancer was found. Ozols and coworkers urge that a negative peritoneoscopy be followed by a laparotomy before a patient with ovarian cancer can be considered disease free. However, most patients in whom recurrent or persistent intra-abdominal disease was present were spared an exploratory laparotomy by peritoneoscopy.

TECHNIQUES

Examinations are done in the operating room and usually under general anesthesia. In women with an intact uterus and cervix, the legs should be in stirrups, with the buttocks 5 cm off the end of the table. A Cohen-Eder cannula is placed in the uterus and secured with a tenaculum to allow elevation of the uterus out of the pelvis.

A 2- to 3-cm incision is made through the skin only at the lower edge of the umbilicus; the subcutaneous tissue is spread with a large hemostat until the fascia is seen clearly. If a patient has had a midline abdominal incision with possible diffuse fibrous adhesions, the puncture site is made just lateral to the rectus muscle, or the peritoneum is exposed surgically and a Verres needle is introduced under direct vision. After the peritoneum has been punctured, 2 liters of nitrous oxide are introduced into the abdominal cavity under manometric control. Uncontrolled insufflation of gas by syringe or hand pump should not be performed because it exposes patients to a needless risk of air embolism.

The trocar in the sleeve is introduced at an angle of 45° to the abdominal wall. It is passed through the abdominal incision and toward the pouch of Douglas. During penetration, the anterior abdominal wall is stabilized by grasping a fold of skin midway between the umbilicus and the os pubis and pulling upward. As the trocar is removed from its sleeve, a rush of air from the abdominal cavity is noted. The operating peritoneoscope is advanced through the sleeve; and a second puncture can now be made in other parts of the abdomen under direct vision.

When the peritoneal cavity is entered, it is visualized by a standard routine, starting at the pelvis and proceeding clockwise around the abdominal cavity. A percutaneous needle biopsy of most intra-abdominal organs can be performed under direct vision. Biopsy of less stationary lesions or organs is performed with forceps introduced through the peritoneoscope. Irrigation and aspiration for recovery of cytologic specimens frequently is indicated.

We have found it useful to tilt the table to examine different abdominal quadrants; the reverse Trendelenburg position is used to look into the upper part of the abdomen and the Trendelenburg position to look into the pelvis. The spleen is seen only with the patient in a sharp reverse Trendelenburg position and with the right side down. In women, the entire pelvis is visualized if the uterus is moved inward and upward. Rotation and elevation of the uterus with the tenaculum placed to the opposite side of the abdomen improves visualization of a fallopian tube. All gas should be evacuated from the abdomen at the end of the procedure. The skin incision is closed with absorbable subcuticular sutures.[1,6]

COMPLICATIONS

In the study by Ozols and associates,[7] severe complications included bleeding, wound infection, hypotension, and pneumothorax. These complications occurred in only 3% of examinations. Bleeding was most frequently from a biopsy site. If bleeding occurs after a needle biopsy of the liver, there may be hemorrhage into the free peritoneal cavity or into the bile (hemobilia). This blood loss can sometimes be controlled by hepatic angiography and clot embolization. Bleeding from other more accessible biopsy sites usually is controlled easily by electrocoagulation through the peritoneoscope. Bleeding from the anterior abdominal wall as a result of the trocar puncture can be controlled without surgery. A large Foley catheter is inserted into the abdominal cavity through the bleeding puncture wound, the Foley balloon is inflated, and traction is exerted until bleeding stops.

Introduction of the trocar into the abdominal cavity rarely causes bowel perforation. A more common cause of perforation is full-thickness heat necrosis occurring inadvertently during biopsy using electrocautery. Perforations almost always involve small bowel. These are difficult to detect because free air is introduced into the peritoneal cavity by peritoneoscopy, and the onset of symptoms may be delayed. Surgical repair of a perforation immediately after diagnosis is indicated.

The fear of bowel perforation when the trocar is inserted through the abdominal wall has kept peritoneoscopy from being used more widely. Unless the procedure is performed by highly experienced personnel, patients who have had prior abdominal surgery usually do not undergo peritoneoscopy.

COLONOSCOPY

INDICATIONS AND RESULTS

COLONOSCOPIC POLYPECTOMY. Colonoscopy has had its greatest impact in reducing the morbidity, mortality, and cost of medical care by allowing colonic polypectomy without laparotomy.[8,9] All but the largest and most sessile benign lesions can be removed in toto.

DIFFERENTIAL DIAGNOSIS OF DIVERTICULITIS AND CANCER. Not infrequently, diverticulitis and colon cancer produce similar clinical and radiologic findings. Colonoscopy has been found useful in making this differential diagnosis.[10–13] Cancer can be ruled out if the colonoscope can be passed through the entire segment of colon in question and no neoplasm is seen. A diagnosis of cancer is made if biopsy or cytologic brushing reveals malignancy.[11]

DETECTION OF DYSPLASIA IN PATIENTS WITH ULCERATIVE COLITIS. In ulcerative colitis, in situ carcinoma (dysplasia) is thought to precede the development of colon cancer. Several authors have suggested that sampling the colonic mucosa in multiple areas at frequent intervals may enable the clinician to predict when a colitic colon is undergoing malignant degeneration. Prophylactic colectomy may no longer be necessary, since selection of patients for surgery may be based on histopathologic study of biopsy specimens obtained at colonoscopy.[14,15] However, the problems with sampling error in this approach to the long-term management of ulcerative colitis have not yet been determined. Studies to assess the number of cancers that progress to invasive malignancy despite colonoscopic follow-up must be performed. The colitic colon often contains many abnormalities, and proper histopathologic sampling of all lesions may be impossible. In some instances, total colectomy is advisable on clinical grounds even though biopsies may not show dysplasia.

EVALUATION OF SUTURE LINES. Following resection and anastomosis for colon cancer, tumor cells may implant on the suture line and result in recurrent disease (see Chap. 29, section on Natural History of Colon Cancer). These mucosal recurrences are difficult to diagnose by barium enema and often are too far from the anus to visualize by sigmoidoscopy. Colonoscopy and suture line biopsy may lead to a diagnosis of local recurrence and result in a curative repeat resection.

CLARIFICATION OF CONFUSING FINDINGS SEEN ON BARIUM ENEMA. The ileocecal valve and midsigmoid areas often are not defined clearly even with the most meticulous radiologic techniques. Colonoscopy often may complement barium enema, especially if the radiologic findings are confusing.[16–19] Barium enema examination is the indicated procedure after a careful history, physical examination, rectal examination, and stool test for occult blood. The endoscopist should not undertake colonoscopy before a barium enema examination is performed, for several reasons: (1) Colonoscopy with biopsy delays barium enema examination by at least 10 days to allow healing of the mucosal and submucosal damage produced by biopsy. This prevents submucosal dissection of barium or perforation at the time of barium enema. (2) The barium enema examination reveals whether diverticuli are present. If they are, special precautions must be taken so that the colonoscope is not moved into a diverticulum and then through the colon wall, causing perforation. (3) The barium enema examination, by identifying pathology, gives the endoscopist a definite area within the colon to reach and then to inspect and photograph. A narrowed or obstructing lesion presents a serious risk for perforation if not recognized before examination. Sometimes a segment of colon that appears questionable on the barium enema examination may look entirely normal on colonoscopy. Success rates in reaching lesions known to exist are much better than success rates in reaching undefined lesions. (4) A barium enema examination defines the anatomy of the colon so that the endoscopist knows the length and configuration of the bowel. (5) Patients whose barium enema examination suggests inflammatory bowel disease should have multiple biopsies performed.

IDENTIFICATION OF A LESION IN PATIENTS WITH OCCULT RECTAL BLEEDING. Colonoscopy may show a lesion in about 50% of patients with occult blood in the stool and a negative sigmoidoscopy and single contrast barium enema examination.[20]

SURVEILLANCE OF PREMALIGNANT CONDITIONS OF THE LARGE BOWEL IN HIGH-RISK GROUPS AND IN THE NORMAL POPULATION. Shinya[21] has followed patients with serial colonoscopic examinations after resection of a large bowel malignancy or snare polypectomy of an adenomatous polyp or polypoid cancer. These patients have been kept polyp free by subsequent endoscopic follow-up, and second primary large bowel cancers have virtually been eliminated. Apparently the polyp-cancer transition has been eliminated, and therefore invasive malignancy has been prevented. The same type of large bowel cancer surveillance may be applicable in the general population.[22] If individuals are kept polyp free by endoscopy, colorectal cancer can be prevented. The development of self-advancing endoscopy instruments that would allow visualization of the entire large bowel needs to be pursued vigorously.

TECHNIQUES

Advancement of the Colonoscope Tip

The most difficult aspect of colonoscopy is the most fundamental maneuver—advancement of the colonoscope tip up into the colon. Experience indicates that a definite sequence of maneuvers repeated in every patient allows most rapid advancement.[23] A barium enema image is displayed and is used as a road map.

Localization of the Colonoscope Tip

The tip of the colonoscope can be located with fluoroscopy. However, colonoscopy without fluoroscopy is more versatile because examinations can then be performed in the operating room, at the patient's bedside, or in the physician's office, replacing the use of the rigid sigmoidoscope. Guidance for locating the tip of the colonoscope is available from the light transmitted through the abdominal wall, the internal appearance of the colon, and certain gross anatomical landmarks.

EXTERNAL LOCALIZATION BY MEANS OF TRANSMITTED LIGHT. As the colonoscope is passed from the anus to the ileocecal valve, the transilluminated intracolonic light on the abdominal wall can be located at key check points in a darkened room in most patients. The patient initially is positioned in the right lateral decubitus position. As the colonoscope is passed up into the midportion of the sigmoid colon, transmitted light first appears in the left lower quadrant; then the light disappears as the junction of the sigmoid and descending colon is transversed. As the tip of the colonoscope moves up the descending colon, transmitted light appears in the left flank at the level of the splenic flexture. At this point the patient is turned onto his back. Light travels across the abdomen at the level of the umbilicus during navigation of the transverse colon and then disappears behind the liver to reappear at McBurney's point when the cecum is entered.

LOCALIZATION USING INTERNAL APPEARANCE OF COLON. Often the internal appearance of the colon is sufficient to allow the tip of the colonoscope to be located, but overinsufflation of air may distort characteristic anatomical features. The rectum is a smooth-walled cavity partially divided by transverse rectal folds, the valves of Houston. The inferior fold lies left and posterior in the patient; the middle fold lies right and anterior; the superior fold lies left and posterior. The sigmoid colon is characterized by low-profile, irregular mucosal folds, tubular lumen, and, if the colonoscopic examination is prolonged, forceful peristaltic waves. Acute angulations from pelvic adhesions or from overdistention with air may occur upon insertion, for the mesentery allows great mobility of the sigmoid colon within the abdominal cavity. The transverse colon is characterized by a triangular lumen with prominent, repetitive, draperylike mucosal folds, the interhaustral septa. Deep pockets, the haustra, separate triangular interhaustral septa at regular intervals. In the ascending colon and cecum, the lumen is capacious and circular in outline; the folds between irregular haustra are widely separated and deep. Small mucosal lesions may be especially difficult to locate. The appendicular orifice may be patulous, a mere dimple if the lumen of the appendix is scarred shut, or a shallow diverticulum if an appendectomy has been done. When viewed from the ascending colon, the ileocecal valve appears merely as a mound of mucosa projecting from an interhaustral fold. Often it is recognized by a fleck of ileal contents within it. In the terminal ileum the delicate mucosa is arranged in closely spaced folds around the oval lumen. Peristalsis is continuous and makes further advancement of the colonoscope difficult.

LOCALIZATION USING GROSS ANATOMICAL LANDMARKS. A major landmark may be the obstruction to easy advancement encountered at the junction of the sigmoid and descending colons, which may be navigated using the alpha maneuver. At the splenic flexure, respiratory excursions are seen. Beneath the left hemidiaphragm, motion imparted by cardiac contractions is first noted. A darkened indentation caused by the spleen frequently is seen at the splenic flexure, and a similar darkened area is produced by the liver at the hepatic flexure. Both cardiac and respiratory movements disappear as the instrument enters the hepatic flexure. The cecum usually is close enough to the anterior abdominal wall that the application of local pressure at McBurney's point can be seen from within this part of the colon.

Once navigation from anus to cecum is complete, the colonoscope is slowly withdrawn to visualize, biopsy, or remove diseased areas. Usually, locating the lesion seen on barium enema is not difficult. However, certain portions of the colon just beyond acute angulations should be considered blind spots and require special effort to visualize (junction of sigmoid and descending colon, splenic flexure, hepatic flexure).

Biopsy is seldom difficult, although problems in passing the biopsy forceps through the biopsy channel do occur unless this channel is kept well cleaned and lubricated. If difficulty arises during a procedure, 10 to 20 ml of mineral oil injected down the biopsy channel will facilitate passing the biopsy forceps.

TECHNIQUE OF COLONOSCOPIC POLYPECTOMY. Few recent technical advances have had a more favorable impact on the standard of medical practice than colonoscopic polypectomy. Wolff and Shinya developed and popularized the technique in the United States. The technique is basically simple.[24,25] A wire loop is passed over the head of a polyp and secured loosely around the stalk. The loop is pulled into its catheter as electrocautery is applied. However, no two polyps are the same, and multiple technical details must be practiced to keep complications to a minimum (Fig. 20-1). For some very small lesions, excision should not be attempted, since hot biopsy can be used to sample and destroy the lesion simultaneously.[26]

COMPLICATIONS. Complications resulting from diagnostic colonoscopy have been few (0.3%) and usually occur in patients with underlying colorectal pathology that weakens the colon wall.[27] Diverticular disease causes problems because increased intracolonic air pressure can result in a "blowout." In addition, the orifice of a large diverticulum can be mistaken for the colon lumen and the colonoscope passed into the free peritoneal cavity. These problems are magnified greatly in patients with diverticular disease who are taking corticosteroids. Active ulcerative colitis results in a weak colon wall, making examination and biopsy more hazardous. Active granulomatous colitis usually does not weaken the bowel wall, but patients experience severe pain if traction is placed on the involved segment of bowel. A narrowed segment of bowel caused by adenocarcinoma may be extremely friable, and minimal pressure from the colonoscope tip may result in free perforation.

The management of colonoscopic complications rarely requires laparotomy. Bleeding occurs at the time of polypectomy in about 2% of patients; it usually can be controlled with the hot-biopsy forceps. Not infrequently, bleeding may

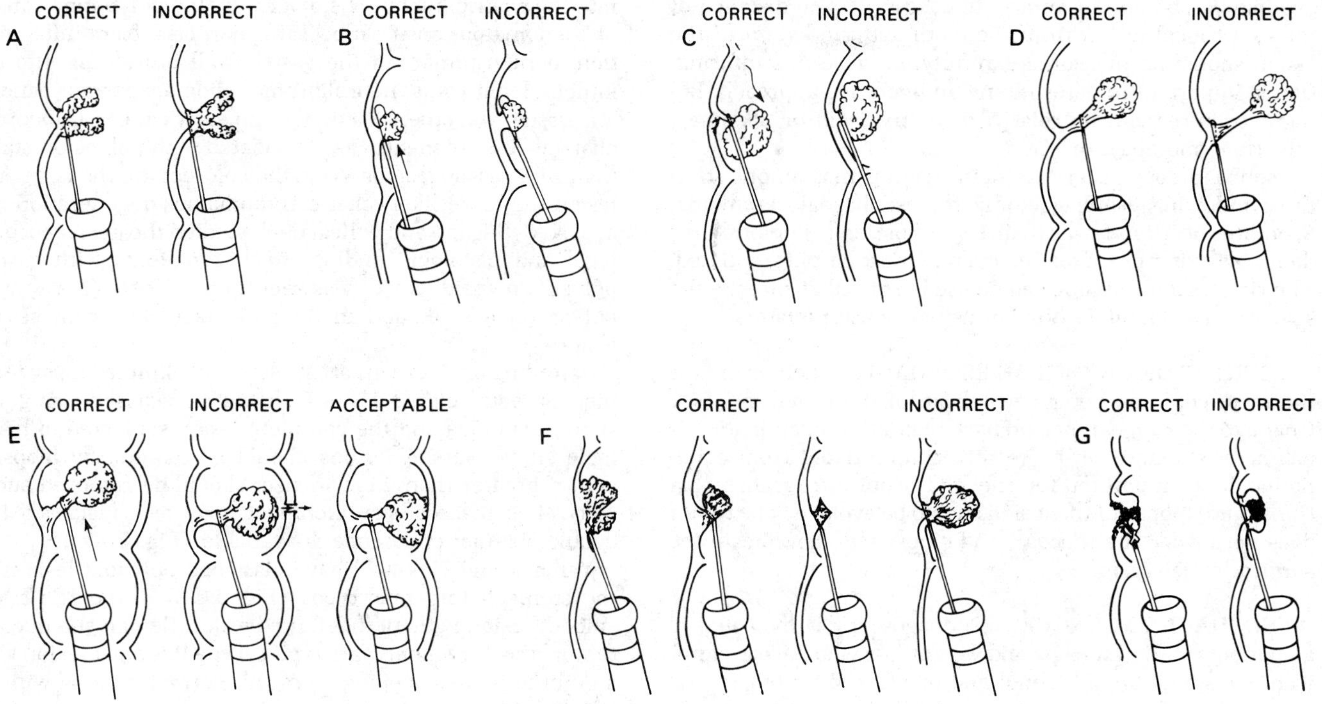

FIG. 20-1. Techniques of colonoscopic polypectomy. **A**. Sessile multilobed polyps. Sessile multilobed polyps should be excised piecemeal. En bloc excision may include bowel wall in the specimen, especially if the polyp occurs on an interhaustral fold. **B**. Excision of small polyps. In excising small sessile or small pedunculated polyps, the catheter should be advanced to the base of the polyp before beginning to even up on the snare wires. If this is not done, the polyp will slip out of the snare as the wires are manipulated to secure the polyp (Shinya maneuver). **C**. Minimally pedunculated polyps. Many polyps that do not appear pedunculated grossly will, on microscopic examination, be shown to be completely excised. Small sessile polyps can be lifted gently away from the colon wall by tenting up the mucosa. **D**. Polyps with long stalks. Excision of polyps with long stalks at their base incurs unnecessary risk of full thickness heat necrosis of the colon wall. Division of the stalk at its midpoint should always be attempted. **E**. Minimizing sparking. Sparking to the bowel wall has caused perforation and should be avoided. The profile of a polyp may be lowered by pushing out on the tightened snare, or sparking may be avoided if a large portion of the opposite colon wall is in contact with the polyp head. **F**. Piecemeal excision of sessile polyps. Sessile polyps, if they are to be removed by colonoscopic polypectomy, should be excised piecemeal. Snare excision of a large tissue mass allows the colon wall to be included in the specimen. If the snare wire is tightened slowly while (not before) electrocautery is applied, hemostasis will be better and the colon wall less likely to be puckered into the resected specimen. **G**. Carcinoma in sessile polyps. Because of distortion and retraction of tissue surrounding invasive cancer, perforation or bleeding has occurred frequently with excision of carcinomatous polyps. A suspicious sessile lesion should be biopsied before excision is attempted.

start 3 to 5 days after polypectomy. Early or late after polypectomy, persistent bleeding usually is controlled by blood replacement and peripheral venous vasopressin infusion, if necessary. If this is unsuccessful, arteriography should be used to identify the bleeding point, and Gelfoam sponge or blood clot should be used to occlude the bleeding vessel.

Perforations occur in about 1% of polypectomies. This is a more serious problem and requires good surgical judgment to prevent a life-endangering situation. Perforations through a segment of diseased bowel or those caused by the colonoscope's being pushed through the colon wall are unlikely to close spontaneously. The danger of bacterial contamination of the peritoneal cavity by bowel flora is great, and laparotomy to close the leak is indicated. If the patient has suspected carcinoma, biopsy confirmation on an emergency basis should be obtained and definitive surgery undertaken. If a small perforation has occurred through a segment of healthy colon, expectant management is indicated. This can be recommended only if the bowel preparation at the time of endoscopy was excellent.

ESOPHAGOSCOPY

INDICATIONS AND RESULTS

ESOPHAGEAL STRICTURES. Differentiation of esophageal strictures as benign or malignant by biopsy and brush cytology is possible in almost all cases.[28,29] The distance of the esophageal lesion from the teeth and the extent of the lesion should be measured carefully, because this information is important in determining an operative approach. Benign strictures can be related to reflux (acid or alkaline), infection (monilia), or scar.

Esophagoscopy also is useful in treating anastomotic strictures following esophagectomy for esophageal carcinoma. Strictures occur in fewer than 10% of patients, but strictures due to scarring or tumor recurrence must be differentiated. The rigid esophagoscope can be used to visualize directly the stricture and facilitate dilation using Jackson dilators.

BENIGN TUMOR OF THE ESOPHAGUS. Leiomyoma is the most common benign neoplasm of the esophagus (see Chap. 24). Its appearance on barium swallow examination is characteristic and can be readily differentiated from carcinoma. It is important for the endoscopist to realize that transmural biopsy of the lesion should be avoided. The tumor does not invade the mucosa, and biopsy will complicate the surgical enucleation.

ESOPHAGEAL CANCER. Esophagoscopy is indicated in all patients with dysphagia and weight loss who have a significant consumption of alcohol and tobacco. With biopsy and cytology added to visual inspection, the accuracy of diagnosis approaches 100%.

Endoscopic ultrasonography is being investigated as a tool for determining the stage and resectability of esophageal carcinoma. In one series, local resectability was correctly demonstrated in five of six patients because a clearly demarcated intramural mass without deep infiltration into surrounding tissues could be identified. Palliative resection was accurately predicted in 11 of 13 patients because abnormal distant lymph nodes were detected with a clearly demarcated tumor mass. However, some difficulty was encountered in distinguishing reactive inflammatory lymph nodes from those infiltrated with tumor.[30]

UPPER GASTROINTESTINAL ENDOSCOPY

Upper gastrointestinal (UGI) endoscopy is a clinical skill shared by the surgeon and gastroenterologist. However, the nature of the disease process usually indicates who should manage a particular patient. The gastroenterologist is asked to consult on those patients whose problems require medical management. On the other hand, cancer patients who are likely to need surgical intervention in the near future usually are directed to the surgeon.

UGI endoscopy is of great use in a preoperative setting. Visualization and biopsy of pathologic lesions allow the surgeon to define better the type and extent of the operation to be performed. Preoperative endoscopy leads to more accurate histopathologic diagnosis and allows the pathophysiology of the lesion to be defined better.

INDICATIONS AND RESULTS

GASTRIC POLYP. A gastric polyp is a local proliferation of abnormal gastric mucosa producing a lesion that protrudes into the gastric lumen. Histologically, the polyp may consist of adenomatous tissue, mucosal hyperplasia from inflammation, benign tumors of the gastric wall protruding into the lumen (leiomyoma, neurofibroma, lipoma, aberrant pancreatic tissue, and others), a cyst, or an early cancer. Cancerous changes less frequently are associated with polyps on stalks than with sessile lesions. As in the colorectum, the larger the lesion the more likely that carcinomatous degeneration has occurred. Sugano and colleagues[31] studied the gross morphologic and histologic findings in 154 patients with gastric polyps. Polypoid cancer was seen in 5 patients (3.2%) with polyps on a stalk and in 39 patients (36%) with sessile lesions.

Sampling error is a great problem with simple biopsy technique. Pedunculated lesions should be excised using the snare technique and the complete lesion subjected to histologic study. Sessile lesions should be generously biopsied and, if greater than 2 cm in size, should be removed surgically. The macrobiopsy technique may be considered if a double-channel endoscope is available (Fig. 20-2).[32]

Yamada and Hukuto[33] have classified polypoid lesions of the stomach into four types (Fig. 20-3). Type I is a flat smooth lesion without a definite border. Benign submucosal tumors most frequently are type I. Type II is a flat lesion with a definite border, sloping from the normal mucosa without indentation. This is the type of lesion frequently seen with early gastric cancer. Type III is a protruding lesion with a definitive indentation at the mucosal margin but not containing a definitive stalk. A Borrmann type II polypoid cancer would have this appearance (see Gastric Cancer, below). A type IV polypoid lesion is a pedunculated polyp with a definitive stalk. This endoscopic classification of gastric polypoid lesions is important because there is a definite relationship between the type of protrusion and the histologic finding.

GASTRIC ULCER. Gastric ulcers usually can be visualized radiologically. Their appearance suggests a benign lesion if mucosal folds radiate into a flat punched-out ulcer. In a malignant ulcer the mucosal folds terminate before they reach a shaggy ulcer bed with raised edges. Other features that tend to differentiate benign and malignant gastric ulcers both radiologically and endoscopically are listed in Table 20-1. However, whether the gross appearance of the ulcer is

FIG. 20-2. Macrobiopsy of gastric mucosa. (Martin TR, Onstad GR, Silvis SE et al: Lift and cut biopsy technique for submucosal sampling. Gastrointest Endosc 23:29–30, 1976)

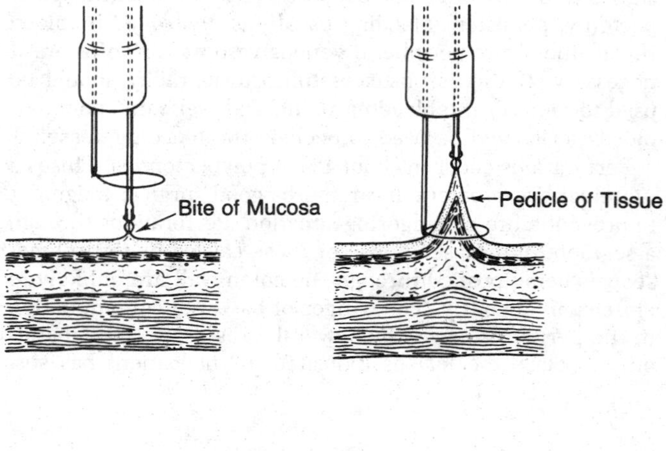

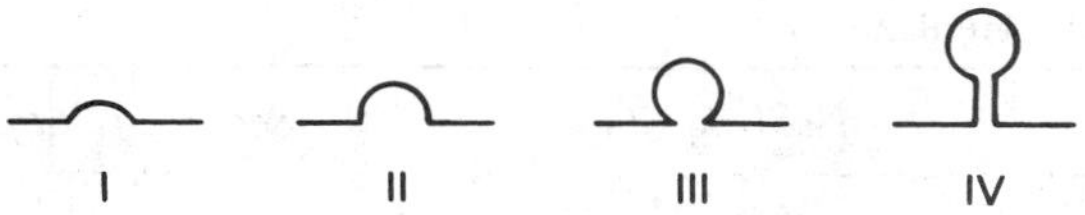

FIG. 20-3. Classification of polypoid lesions of the stomach. Type I lesions are flat; type II appear raised from the surrounding mucosa; type III lesions represent sessile polyps; and type IV lesions are stalked polyps. (Yamada T, Hukuto MI: Gastric polyp. Gastrointest Endosc 7:448–454, 1965)

benign or malignant, multiple biopsies from each quadrant of the ulcer must be secured,[34,35] and specimens from the depths of the ulcer crater may sometimes be helpful. Cytologic brushings from the ulcer and cytology specimens obtained with a water pick are sometimes necessary to confirm the diagnosis of suspected malignancy.[36] Radiologically benign-appearing ulcers can harbor malignancy.[37–40] If the gross appearance of the tumor, the biopsy specimens, and the histologic preparations suggest a benign process, a second endoscopic study 3 to 4 weeks after a medical regimen for ulcer disease should be performed. If, at the second endoscopy, malignancy is not suggested, cancer is highly unlikely; the accuracy of diagnosis approaches 100% when this management plan is followed.[37–39]

A benign gastric ulcer may be seen at different stages of the healing process. Realizing that benign ulcer disease is a dynamic process with expanding or healing lesions may make interpretation of endoscopic findings much clearer.[41] Table 20-2 shows the changes in the endoscopic picture of an ulcer as described by Tsuneoka and colleagues.[41] The irregular appearance of the healing ulcer may cause it to be confused with a malignant process.

GASTRIC CANCER. Gastric cancer has been classified endoscopically according to two different systems that reflect the degree of disease progression at the time of gastroscopy. The macroscopic classification of early gastric carcinoma (mucosal and submucosal malignancy) was agreed on at a meeting of the Japan Gastrointestinal Endoscopy Society in 1962.[42] Early gastric cancer was divided into three main groups and three subgroups on the basis of the macroscopic appearances at endoscopy and in gastrectomy specimens. Figure 20-4 shows these types. The classification system may become complex when a lesion has features of more than one endoscopic type. Some combinations of types are more common than a single type, and all possible combinations of the five types have been described. The dominant macroscopic feature is placed first; therefore, early gastric cancer can be described as type I plus IIc or type IIc plus III. Combinations of more than two types are not seen often.

The rationale for endoscopic classification of gastric cancer is obvious. Unless one has a high index of suspicion and watches carefully for these subtle lesions, they will be missed. An endoscopically trained eye is needed to detect early gastric cancer. However, the 5-year survival rate after surgical treatment of early gastric carcinoma is about 95%.[43,44] In cases of intramucosal carcinoma, lymph node involvement is exceptionally rare but can occur. In advanced gastric cancer, the frequency of lymph node involvement is 60% to 70%.

In the United States and Europe, gastric cancer rarely is seen endoscopically in its earliest stages. Unfortunately, the Japanese classification of malignancy limited to the gastric mucosa is seldom needed. The endoscopic findings in advanced gastric cancer are described by the Borrmann classification.[45] Type I is a polypoid carcinoma characterized by a localized protuberance of varying size. It is similar in appearance to Yamada's type III polypoid lesion of the stomach (see Fig. 20-3). Type II consists of a noninfiltrating malignant-appearing ulcer. The ulcer's edges are raised and nodular but limited sharply by surrounding mucosa. Type III gastric cancer is an infiltrative carcinomatous ulcer in which the tumor is grossly invading into the surrounding stomach wall. The edge of the ulcer crater is not maintained but is broken down at one or more sites. In type IV cancer, the stomach wall is grossly infiltrated by cancer and becomes rigid. The mucosa may have healed over the cancer in some cases so that deep biopsy may be necessary to make a diagnosis.

The Borrmann classification of gastric cancer endoscopically describes two aspects of this disease: First, the extent of local spread, as suggested by the tumor's endoscopic appearance, indicates that the tumor has been diagnosed early or late in its natural history; second, the biologic nature of the tumor may be reflected in its tendency to grow intraluminally as a polypoid mass or to invade through the gastric wall

TABLE 20-1. Endoscopic and Radiologic Features Useful for Distinguishing Benign from Malignant Gastric Ulcers

Endoscopic Finding	*Benign Ulcer*	*Malignant Ulcer*
Ulcer crater	Punched out	Irregular
Base of ulcer crater	Clear	Shaggy
Mucosal folds around ulcer	To edge of crater	Interrupted short of crater
Mucosal surface around ulcer	Smooth and edematous	Heaped up; crater within a mass
Gastric wall surrounding crater	Pliable with peristalsis	Rigid without peristalsis
Depth of crater	Deep, may hold fluid	Shallow with rolled edges
Associated duodenal ulcer or inflammation	Common	Almost never
Evidence of healing with medical management	Rapid healing	Healing slow
Peristalsis in ulcer area	Present	Absent
Size	No indication	No indication
Location	No indication	Greater curvature

TABLE 20-2. Changes in Endoscopic Picture of a Gastric Ulcer with Healing*

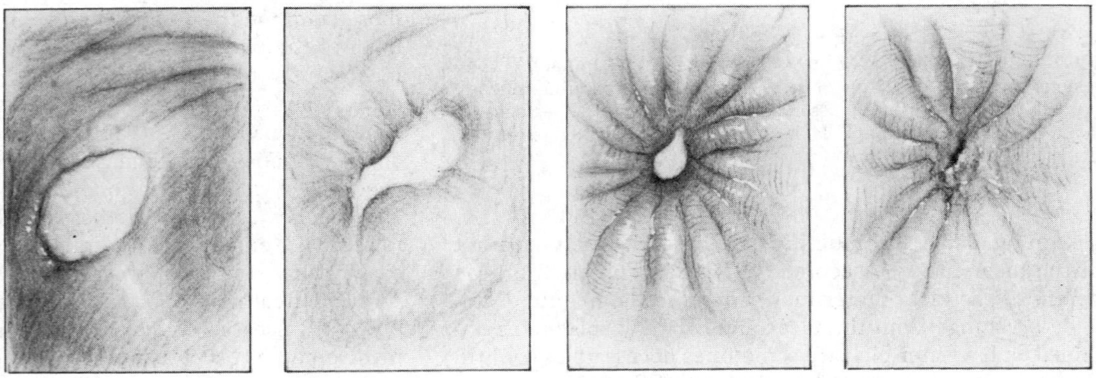

	Acute Active Stage	*Regressive Stage*	*Healing Stage*	*Scarring Stage*
Shape	*Round or Oval*	*Round or Oval*	*Round, Irregular Linear, or Dumbbell-Shaped*	*Point, Linear, or Irregular*
Edema	++	+	−	−
Diffuse erythema	+	−	−	−
Red halo	−	+	++	+++
Overriding of coating	+(−)	+	−	−
Ulcer bottom	Thick white coating, occasionally mingled with brown or black tint	White or yellow coating	Thin gray or yellowish white coating	No coating
Convergence of folds	−	+	++	+++

* Modified from Tsuneoka K, Tadayoski T, Sotaro F: Fiberoscopy of Gastric Diseases, p 139. Tokyo, Igaku-Shoin, 1973.

as a high-grade malignancy. These correlations of gross pathology and prognosis were noted by Borrmann in 1926 and still have meaning for the UGI endoscopist today.

A not uncommon problem in differential diagnosis occurs in patients seen to have remarkably thickened gastric mucosal folds by UGI radiologic examination. These patients may have hypertrophic gastritis, Menetrier's disease, gastric lymphoma, or superficial spreading carcinoma of the stomach. As shown in Figure 20-2, endoscopy with macrobiology is the procedure of choice to differentiate these entities.

SURVEILLANCE OF PREMALIGNANT CONDITIONS OF THE UPPER GASTROINTESTINAL TRACT

During the last two decades there has been a growing awareness that cancer of the esophagus and stomach may arise in association with several underlying diseases. Definitive guidelines for the use of endoscopy in the long-term management of these diseases cannot be formulated precisely. However, some recommendations can be made that are likely to benefit the patient and yet not lead to untoward medical costs.

ACHALASIA. In patients with achalasia, esophageal cancer is seen in 2% to 8% of the patients with untreated disease. These cancers occur only after many years of symptomatic disease.[46–51] With effective balloon dilation or myotomy, the cancer risk seems to fall to that of the general population. However, in patients who remain symptomatic for many years or in patients treated late in the course of their disease, an increased risk of malignancy may remain for years. A yearly UGI endoscopy is recommended to follow the course of the disease and to rule out the development of esophageal cancer.

BARRETT'S ESOPHAGUS. With Barrett's esophagus there is a columnar epithelial lining of the lower esophagus. Retrospective studies suggest that the incidence of developing adenocarcinoma may be as high as 10%.[52,53] The cancer may be microinvasive and multifocal in character.[54,55] Although long-term benefits of endoscopic surveillance have not been determined, at least an annual endoscopic examination with biopsies and brushings for cytology in the columnar portion of the esophagus is recommended.

ADENOMATOUS POLYPS. Adenomatous polyps of the stomach have a well-defined risk for malignancy. As lesions become increasingly sessile and of increasing size, the risk of cancer increases.[56–60] Gastric polyps should be excised endoscopically if possible. Polyps smaller than 2 cm in size may be followed with repeated biopsy. Even if all polyps can be removed, the gastric lining has demonstrated a malignant potential, and endoscopic follow-up is indicated on a yearly basis.

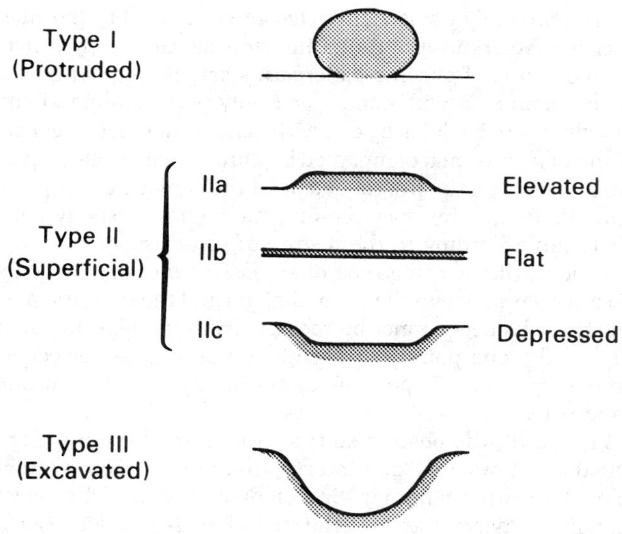

FIG. 20-4. Macroscopic classification of early (mucosal and submucosal) gastric carcinoma.

Type I—the protruded type. The tumor projects clearly into the lumen and includes all polypoid, nodular, and villous tumors. Perhaps the best nomenclature for the English literature would be protuberant or polypoid, rather than protruded.

Type II—the superficial type. This is further subdivided into three subgroups.

Type II(a)—elevated above surrounding mucosa. In carefully prepared gastrectomy specimens, this is seen as a flat, plaque-like lesion, well circumscribed, and raised up above surrounding mucosa only by a few millimeters.

Type II(b)—flat. No abnormality is visible macroscopically, although some color change may be visible endoscopically and in very carefully prepared gastrectomy specimens.

Type II(c)—depressed. The surface is slightly depressed below adjacent mucosa for not more than the thickness of the submucosa. Surface erosion may be apparent from a thin covering of exudate.

Type III—the excavated type. This essentially is ulceration of variable depth into the gastric wall. It rarely is seen in pure form and almost always is combined with any of the other types. (Modified from Morson BC, Dawson IMP: Gastrointestinal Pathology. Oxford, Blackwell Scientific Publications, 1979)

PERNICIOUS ANEMIA. Pernicious anemia and the associated atrophic gastritis were previously thought to be a precursor of gastric malignancy. One recent population study suggests that the incidence of gastric cancer in patients with pernicious anemia is only slightly increased over that of the general population and does not justify the cost of periodic surveillance.[61]

SURGICAL FOLLOW-UP AFTER GASTRIC SURGERY. UGI endoscopy is useful for follow-up after surgery for benign gastric or duodenal ulcer disease. The incidence of gastric cancer in patients who have undergone gastric resection for peptic ulcer may range from 2% to 9%.[62–64] A recent large population base study suggested that the risk of gastric cancer in patients previously operated on for benign disease is no greater than the risk of developing a spontaneous gastric cancer in the same population.[65,66] However, patients with any symptoms deserve annual examination with UGI endoscopy.

After excision of a gastric cancer, frequent repeat endoscopy is indicated. Gastric cancer often may first recur at a previous suture line. Anastomoses traditionally are difficult to evaluate radiologically because postoperative changes distort the normal anatomy. The size and shape of an anastomotic channel, marginal ulceration, and inflammatory changes can be evaluated best with endoscopy. One must be cautioned that endoscopy can detect the presence of recurrent cancer intrinsic to the gut wall, but recurrent disease extrinsic to the intestinal lumen is difficult or impossible to evaluate. Radiologic examination is more accurate than endoscopic examination in assessing progressive recurrent extrinsic disease of a hollow viscus.

UPPER GASTROINTESTINAL BLEEDING. A role for emergency UGI endoscopy in patients with UGI bleeding has not been firmly established as yet. A published summary statement from a National Institutes of Health consensus conference suggested that endoscopy was an excellent tool for the differential diagnosis of UGI bleeding.[67] However, the lack of demonstrated effect on overall morbidity and mortality suggested that the diagnostic information gleaned from emergency UGI endoscopy did not significantly affect the overall prognosis.

ENDOSCOPY IN PATIENTS WITH PANCREATIC CANCER

THE JAUNDICED PATIENT. Obstructive jaundice is likely to be caused by biliary tract stones, pancreatic cancer, or pancreatitis. Percutaneous transhepatic cholangiography with the Chiba needle usually is the simplest procedure that results in a diagnosis in most patients.[68,69] Interventional radiology has the additional advantage of providing temporary preoperative decompression of the obstructed biliary tree by means of percutaneous intubation of the biliary ducts. However, endoscopic retrograde cholangiopancreatography (ERCP) is an additional diagnostic tool in patients in whom the diagnosis cannot be determined from the percutaneous cholangiogram. Duodenoscopy is performed simultaneously with ERCP; this is critical for duodenal cancer and tumors of the ampulla of Vater. Pancreatography and retrograde cholangiography can be performed simultaneously with ERCP and may help greatly in defining the existing pathology accurately.[70,71]

Ogoshi[72] maintains that endoscopic retrograde pancreatography renders a diagnosis of pancreatic cancer in most cases. About 80% of the patients in his experience had pancreatic cancer of ductal orgin that caused some kind of ductal abnormality. Patients with acinar cell carcinoma, which constituted the remaining 20% of cases, had ductal abnormalities less frequently; nevertheless, pancreatography suggested a malignancy in most patients. However, one must always remember that some findings on the pancreatogram strongly suggestive of chronic pancreatitis can be caused by pancreatic cancer.

Changes in the pancreatic duct are extremely varied but can be categorized into three major types (Fig. 20-5). Type I represents a stenotic lesion of the pancreatic duct. In the area of stenosis, the main pancreatic duct is thin and has a beaded border. Branch ducts around the stenotic area disap-

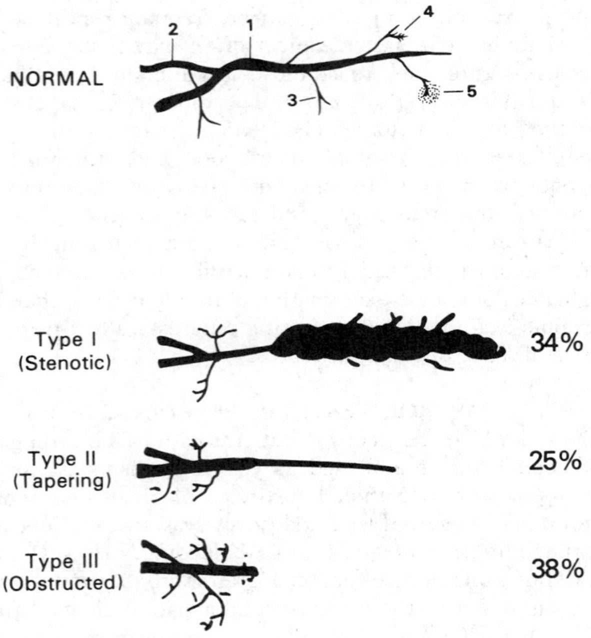

FIG. 20-5. Normal and abnormal appearing pancreatic duct radiographs with cancer of the pancreas. The normal pancreatic duct runs a smooth, tapering, slightly wavering course from the ampulla of Vater to the tail of the pancreas (*1*). The accessory pancreatic duct divides from the main duct in the head of the pancreas and runs superior to the main pancreatic duct, ending at the accessory papilla (*2*). Branch ducts (*3*) and fine ducts (*4*) arise from accessory ducts in an angular fashion. The smallest ducts are called fine pancreatic ducts (*5*). Pancreatic duct cancer gives four types of pancreatographic findings: type I (stenotic), type II (tapering) and type III (obstructed) include most patterns; type IV or unclassified type of pancreatic duct radiograph represents only 3% of the total. (Modified from Kizu M: Normal endoscopic cholangiopancreatogram. In Takemoto T, Casugai T: Endoscopic Retrograde Cholangiopancreatography. Tokyo, Igaku-Shion, 1979; also modified from Ogoshi K: Diseases of the pancreas and biliary system. In Takemoto T, Casugai T: Endoscopic Retrograde Cholangiopancreatography. Tokyo, Igaku-Shion, 1979)

pear completely or partially. Ogoshi suggests that the most decisive factors in differentiating stenosis caused by cancer from stenosis of chronic pancreatitis are the regular border of the main duct with cancer and only partial filling of surrounding branch ducts by dye with cancer. In cases of cancer of the pancreas unaccompanied by chronic pancreatitis, pancreatic ducts on the proximal side of the stenotic area appear normal. Peripheral ducts behind the stenosis usually show dilatation according to the degree of stenosis.

Type II, the tapering type of stenosis, generally has a distinct border between the normal gland and the tapering part, and branch ducts cannot be recognized in the tapering area. This is the one point that permits differentiation of cancer producing this type of abnormality from chronic pancreatitis.

In type III, the obstructed type, the normal main pancreatic duct shows a sudden interruption at one point, with an irregular sawtooth border. Branch ducts may be fully visualized in the normal area of the main pancreatic duct, but in the obstructed area irregularity in arrangement or interruption usually is observed. In cases of chronic pancreatitis accompanied by a high degree of fibrosis or when a pancreatic calculus exists in the main pancreatic duct, obstruction of the main pancreatic duct in the same manner may be recognized. Differential diagnosis may be obtained by observation of the obstructed main duct and surrounding branch ducts.

Ogoshi[72] reports nearly equal frequency of the three main types of pancreatic duct changes with pancreatic cancer. As shown in Table 20-3, he has summarized the differences that can be used to distinguish pancreatic cancer from chronic pancreatitis. Ogoshi emphasizes that if clear pancreatograms are obtained, differential diagnosis usually is not difficult. However, to obtain such clear radiologic findings in all patients requires extreme skill. He suggests that chronic pancreatitis may overlap with cancer of the pancreas in about 10% of patients, so that in some patients a clear differentiation is impossible. A major problem is that pancreatitis may result in cyst formation. The pancreatic cyst or pseudo-

TABLE 20-3. Differential Diagnosis of Carcinoma of the Pancreas and Chronic Pancreatitis from Endoscopic Retrograde Pancreatography*

Condition of Main Pancreatic Duct	*Carcinoma*	*Pancreatitis*
Strictured	Localized stricture with irregular mucosal pattern within strictural segment	Elongated stricture lined by smooth mucosa
	Irregular pattern of branch ducts	Branch ducts absent
Dilated	Dilatation diffuse and limited to the distal pancreas, main duct distensible	Multiple chain-of-lakes dilation
Tapered	Irregular and rigid tapered segment, irregular pattern to branch ducts	Not seen
Obstructed	Irregular branch ducts in proximal pancreas	Absence of branch ducts

* Modified from Ogoshi K: Diseases of the pancreas and the biliary system. In Takemoto T, Kasugai T (eds): Endoscopic Retrograde Cholangiopancreatography. Tokyo, Igaku-Shoin, 1979.

cyst may cause a mass effect that clearly resembles a cancerous lesion. Conversely, pancreatic cancer may undergo necrosis so that the demonstration of a cyst in or around the pancreas by ERCP does not necessarily rule out the presence of a pancreatic cancer.

Yasuda and colleagues have reported on their experience with endoscopic ultrasonography in the diagnosis of pancreas cancer.[73] They found that small tumors within the pancreas are readily detected with endoscopic ultrasonography. This examination may be superior to conventional radiologic techniques such as CT, ERCP, and extracorporeal ultrasonography. Finally, they suggested that endoscopic ultrasound may help in determining which tumors are operable. The possibility that endoscopes may be used not only to examine the bowel wall, but also, with the aid of ultrasound, to see through it is of great interest.

ENDOSCOPICALLY OBTAINED PANCREATIC DUCT CYTOLOGY AND TUMOR ANTIGENS. In the patient whose radiographs are nondiagnostic, pancreatic duct carcinoembryonic antigen (CEA), pancreatic duct pancreatic oncofetal antigen (OFA), and pancreatic duct cytology may be helpful in differentiating pancreatitis from pancreatic cancer. Estimates of cytology positivity range from 10% to 60%.[72,74,75] More efforts to determine the usefulness of pancreatic duct cytology need to be undertaken.

TECHNIQUES

Rigid esophagoscopy is accomplished most easily under general anesthesia. A small endotracheal tube is used for general anesthesia so that the lumen of the pharynx is not compromised. The eyes must be covered and the upper teeth protected with a moist gauze pad. The scope is held in the right hand and guided by the thumb and index finger of the left hand. Under direct vision, the scope is inserted into the posterior pharynx with the bevel up. The tip is guided into the pharynx where the opening of the esophagus (cricopharyngeal sphincter) is visible. The endoscope is advanced slowly under direct vision down the esophagus. Usually some resistance is met at the seventh cervical vertebra, an area in which perforation commonly occurs. The rigid esophagoscope is useful to visualize and biopsy middle and upper third esophageal tumors. Flexible UGI endoscopy allows better visualization of lower third esophageal tumors and the cardioesophageal junction as well as visualization of the stomach.

Flexible UGI endoscopy is the least technically demanding of the endoscopy procedures discussed thus far. An exception to this is ERCP, which demands meticulous endoscopic technique. For routine UGI endoscopy, the sedated patient is given an anesthetic to the posterior pharynx while seated. Then, with the patient in the right lateral decubitus position, the endoscope tip is passed on the forefinger into the pharynx. Before insertion of the endoscope, the patient is given a generous intravenous dose of meperidine and diazepam. Alternatively, the endoscopist may pass the instrument through the mouth guard and over the tongue to the back of the mouth. Then, with blind tip manipulation, the tip is deflected so that it curls over the back of the tongue and into the midpharynx. While the operator applies slight forward pressure, the patient is asked to swallow to relax the cricopharyngeal sphincter, which lies 15 cm to 18 cm from the teeth. The endoscope passes easily down the esophagus. If the endoscope tip just below the cardioesophageal sphincter is flexed 45° to the patient's left, the greater curvature comes into view. Rotation of the endoscope clockwise scans the anterior surface of the stomach; rotation counterclockwise scans the posterior surface of the stomach. If the endoscope tip is repositioned just below the cardioesophageal sphincter and extended 45° to the patient's right, the lesser curvature is visualized. The cardioesophageal sphincter is visualized from above and then from below by retroflexing the endoscope. The lesser curvature is followed to the antrum and then through the pylorus into the duodenum. Persistent advancement will move the tip to the ligament of Treitz and even beyond.

The techniques involved in UGI endoscopy and colonoscopy are very different. The esophagus, stomach, and duodenum are structures whose positions within the abdominal cavity are fixed; therefore, as the hollow viscus is inflated with air, the endoscope is moved readily ahead under direct vision. This is not so with the colon. The sigmoid, transverse colon, and often ascending colon are free to move nearly anywhere within the abdominal cavity. Therefore, maneuvers to reduce bowel loops by accumulating collapsed colon on the endoscope are required.

COMPLICATIONS

The first rule for esophagoscopy and UGI endoscopy is "Don't push." The incidence of esophageal perforation is reported to be 0.074% with the rigid esophagoscope and 0.093% with the fiberoptic esophagoscope.[76] Treatment should be instituted as soon as the perforation is recognized. If the perforation occurs through a pathologic lesion, surgery must be performed immediately and the lesion resected. If a perforation occurs through normal esophagus, more conservative treatment should be considered. Perforation usually is evidenced by a spiking fever, substernal or upper abdominal pain, subcutaneous emphysema in the neck, and pneumothorax.

A water-soluble contrast esophagogram is indicated but may not demonstrate extravasation. Treatment depends on location of the perforation, time of recognition, status of the esophagus, condition of the patient, and severity of sepsis.[77] Cervical perforations can be managed by no oral feeding, antibiotics, and observation.[78] If an abscess forms, it is easily drained. If a thoracic esophageal perforation is recognized during the first 24 hours and there is evidence of sepsis, closure with adequate chest tube drainage should be attempted. Small perforations or perforations that drain well into the esophagus without sepsis may be managed with pharyngeal suction, antibiotics, and total parenteral alimentation. Perforation proximal to or through an obstructing tumor requires resection of the tumor and perforated segment of esophagus. If recognized very early when inflammation is minimal, a primary gastroesophageal anastomosis may be attempted. Late recognition of perforation in patients with infection requires exclusion of the esophagus by oversewing the esophagogastric junction, creating a diverting cervical esophagostomy and a gastrostomy.[79]

If a perforation occurs through normal stomach or through a benign duodenal ulcer, nasogastric suctioning, intravenous antibiotics, and careful observation usually are enough. However, perforation through a gastric cancer requires immediate surgical intervention. If this occurs, tumor cells are likely to be disseminated throughout the peritoneal cavity, and healing across the perforated malignancy is unlikely to occur.

BRONCHOSCOPY

INDICATIONS AND RESULTS

Bronchoscopy is one of the most useful modalities in the diagnosis and staging of thoracic neoplasms. Bronchoscopy may be indicated for the diagnosis and staging of pulmonary, esophageal, and mediastinal lesions. It is indicated in determining the extent of surgical resection necessary for pulmonary and esophageal tumors. When lung cancer patients have centrally located thoracic masses, bronchoscopy must be performed to assess involvement of mainstem and lobar bronchi. Invasion of tumor into the mainstem bronchi or carina will necessitate pneumonectomy or tracheal reconstruction following resection. Patients with more peripheral lesions generally do not require bronchoscopy before exploration unless there is some indication that the lesions may be multifocal and involve the opposite lung.

Bronchoscopy also may be useful in the localization of hemoptysis that occurs in patients with pulmonary neoplasms, and in the evaluation of diffuse interstitial infiltrates, which are frequently seen in cancer patients undergoing aggressive chemotherapy.

FLEXIBLE VERSUS RIGID BRONCHOSCOPES. Both the flexible and rigid instruments have features that may make one or the other particularly suitable for certain problems (Table 20-4). Thus any physician dealing with thoracic neoplasms must have a working knowledge of both instruments. Different caliber rigid bronchoscopes are available with side arms for ventilation. The Storz model has a fiberoptic optical magnification system and angled lenses that allow direct viewing of all lobar bronchi. Flexible bronchoscopes are available with differing external diameters (3.6–6.5 mm) and interchannel widths (0.8–2.6 mm). The larger flexible bronchoscope requires a minimum of 8 mm of endotracheal tube for convenient passage, whereas the smaller scopes may be passed through small-diameter endotracheal tubes and are useful for pediatric patients and endoscopy through double-lumen endotracheal tubes. The flexible bronchoscope can be used comfortably under local anesthesia and allows direct visualization and biopsy of lesions in subsegmental locations. Peripheral lesions can be biopsied effectively by using either the rigid scope with flexible biopsy forceps and fluoroscopic control or the flexible bronchoscope. The visualization of primary, secondary, and even tertiary bronchi with the fiberoptic instrument is shown in Figure 20-6.

The rigid bronchoscope, especially with the fiberoptic system, provides excellent magnification and clarity. It allows one to obtain larger biopsy specimens than can be obtained through even the largest flexible bronchoscope. In addition, it is considerably more effective in suctioning thick secretions and blood. Finally, use of the rigid instruments allows the operator to judge fixation of the carina, an important prognostic sign indicating advanced unresectable tumor.

BRONCHOSCOPY VERSUS OTHER TECHNIQUES IN THE DIAGNOSIS OF PARENCHYMAL LESIONS. In comparison with other diagnostic techniques, bronchoscopic biopsy will make the diagnosis of malignancy in a lower percentage of cases but with more accurate histologic diagnosis. Payne and co-workers[80] noted that a diagnosis of malignancy was made in 88% of specimens obtained by percutaneous lung biopsy, but the accuracy of the histologic diagnosis was only 48%. Malignant tissue was obtained in 69% of cases with bronchial biopsy, with the correct histologic type predicted in 80% of cases. In the diagnosis of diffuse interstitial pulmonary infiltrates, transbronchial biopsy can be accurate in a high percentage of cases but generally is less accurate than open lung biopsy. Feldman and co-workers[81] achieved 84% accuracy in the diagnosis of

TABLE 20-4. Comparison of Rigid and Flexible Fiberoptic Bronchoscopy Technique

	Rigid Bronchoscopy	*Flexible Fiberoptic Bronchoscopy*
Biopsy	Generous specimen	Minute specimen
Visualization of bronchi	Excellent	Excellent
Visualization of segmental bronchi	With angled lenses only	Excellent
Biopsy of peripheral lesions	No	Yes
Anesthesia required	General	Local
Performed through orotracheal tube	No	Yes
Suctioning secretions	Excellent	Good
Complications	Perforation and bleeding reported	Very unusual
Durability of instrument	Durable	Delicate
Training to perform examination	Extensive	Minimal

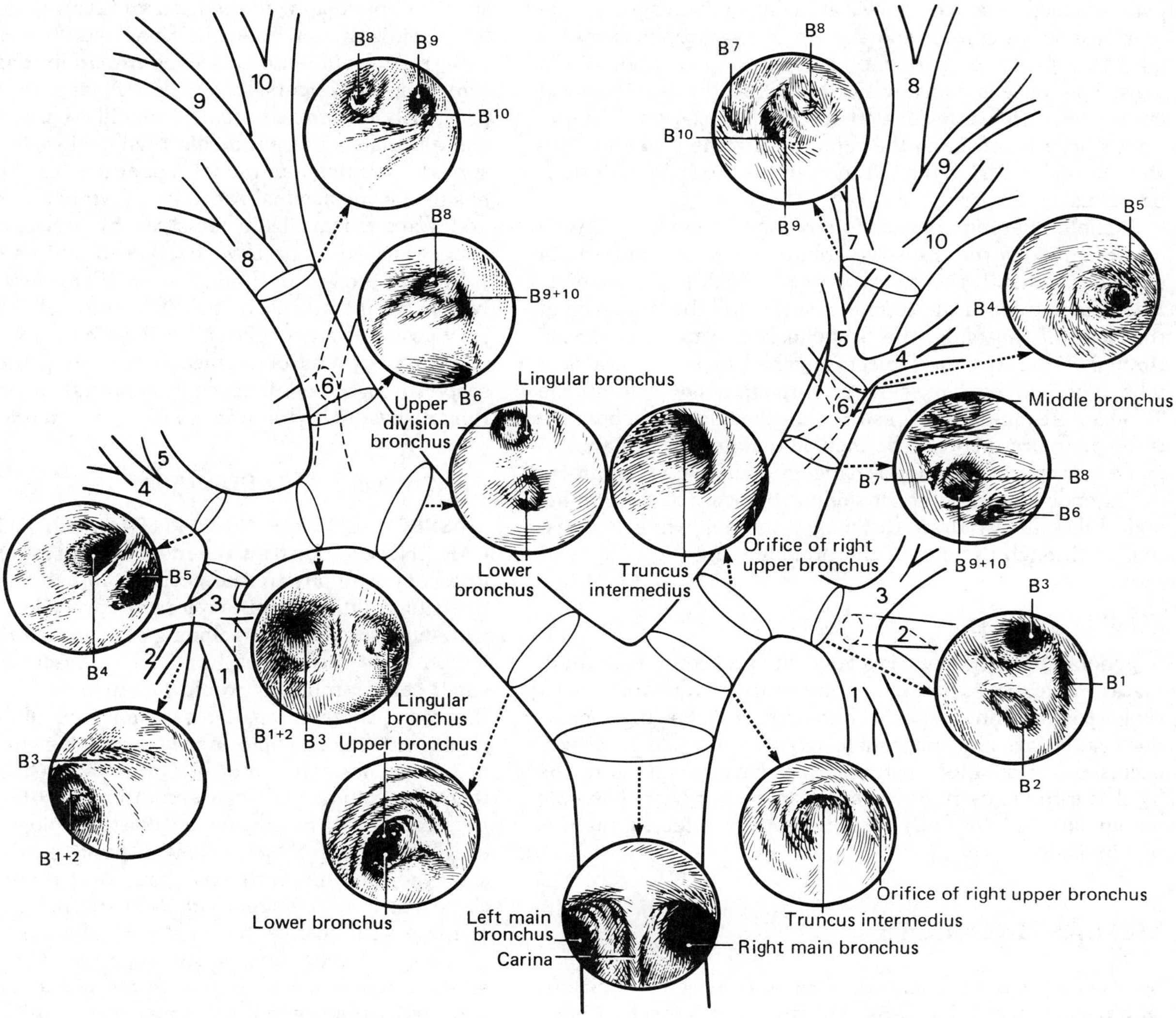

FIG. 20-6. Anatomy of the bronchial tree as seen through the flexible bronchoscope. The diagram shows the tracheobronchial tree; the insets reproduce the bronchoscopic picture obtained at important positions. Checkpoints include the carina and right and left main-stem orifices; major bifurcations on the right into upper, middle, and lower lobes; and major bifurcations on the left into the upper, lingula, and lower lobes. A standard nomenclature for designating tertiary bronchi within lung segments is indicated. Because of variations in the segmental anatomy, endoscopists have found that this simplified nomenclature expedites a thorough description of the endoscopic findings. The letters correspond to the following anatomic segments: Right upper lobe — B^1 apical, B^2 posterior, B^3 anterior; right middle lobe — B^4 lateral, B^5 medial; right lower lobe — B^6 superior segment, B^7 medial basal, B^8 anterior basal, B^9 lateral basal, B^{10} posterior basal; left upper lobe — B^{1+2} apical posterior, B^3 anterior; lingula — B^4 superior, B^5 inferior; left lower lobe — B^6 superior, B^8 anterior basal, B^9 lateral basal, B^{10} posterior basal. (Modified from Ikeda S: Atlas of Flexible Bronchofiberoscopy, p 63. Tokyo, Igaku-Shion, 1974)

diffuse pulmonary infiltrates by transbronchial biopsy compared to only a 43% diagnostic yield in localized infiltrates. In a prospective study, Burt and co-workers[82] compared aspiration needle biopsy, cutting needle biopsy, transbronchial biopsy, and open lung biopsy. They found open lung biopsy to be the most accurate technique, although in two patients a diagnosis was obtained by transbronchial biopsy that could not be obtained by open lung biopsy.

TECHNIQUES

Rigid bronchoscopy can be performed under local anesthesia, but generally the patient is more comfortable and the examination is facilitated when general anesthesia is used. The patient is placed in the supine position with the head extended. The bronchoscope is supported by the examiner's index finger and thumb. A moist gauze is placed over the patient's teeth to avoid undue trauma to teeth and gums. The epiglottis is visualized, and the tip of the bronchoscope is used to lift up the epiglottis, bringing the vocal cords into view. The scope is then advanced carefully through the vocal cords. The carina is evaluated to note its fixation. The patient's head is moved to the right to examine the left mainstem bronchus and to the left to examine the right mainstem bronchus.

Flexible fiberoptic bronchoscopy may be performed with equal facility by the transnasal route under local anesthesia or under general anesthesia through an orotracheal tube. With the patient in the supine position and the physician at the head of the table, the bronchoscope can be advanced through the end of a T-piece attached to the orotracheal tube. The patient is oxygenated through a side arm off the T-piece. Advantages of using the flexible bronchoscope through an orotracheal tube include maintenance of an adequate airway, ability to interchange bronchoscopes, ability to do extended procedures, including biopsy and suctioning, and ability to withdraw the biopsy forceps while it is extended through the end of the bronchoscope.

COMPLICATIONS

In general, bronchoscopy is a very safe procedure with minimal complications. Potential complications may include laryngospasm, bronchospasm, hemorrhage following biopsy, pneumothorax, and inadequate oxygenation due to airway occlusion. In addition, patients may have reactions to the local anesthetic used. Fever may occur after bronchoscopic manipulations, especially when necrotic or infected tumor is manipulated.

MEDIASTINOSCOPY

Mediastinoscopy as practiced today was devised by Carlens, with results reported in 1959. The midline approach through a small, low cervical incision made biopsy of lymph nodes on both sides of the superior mediastinum possible. Through this technique, visualization and biopsy of nearly all paratracheal and hilar lymph nodes in the middle and lower portions of the superior mediastinum were possible. However, Pearson[83] has pointed out that the surgeon is anatomically limited in sampling anterior mediastinal, subaortic, and subcarinal nodes posterior to the trachea. The subcarinal nodes anterior to the tracheal bifurcation are important nodes for visualization and sampling at the lowermost extent of the endoscopic dissection.

Two important anatomical features of the lymphatic drainage of the lung should be noted. First, lymphatic crossover from a lung on one side of the mediastinum to lymph nodes on the opposite side is not unusual. Goldberg and co-workers[84] reported that 28 of 46 patients (60%) with positive mediastinal nodes from lung carcinoma in the right upper lobe had bilateral spread of disease within the mediastinum. One patient (3%) had only contralateral spread. Similarly, 5 of 20 patients (25%) with positive mediastinal nodes from left upper lobe cancer had bilateral mediastinal nodal spread, and 6 (30%) had only contralateral spread. Bilateral spread in patients with mediastinal involvement from lower lobe lesions was 37% on the right and 25% on the left.

Borrie[85] documented a second important anatomical fact. Cancer in the upper lobe of the left lung, in addition to its previously recognized tracheobronchial lymphatic drainage, has alternate anterior mediastinal pathways of lymphatic spread. Carcinoma of the left upper lobe can spread directly to anterior mediastinal pathways of lymphatic spread. These nodes are not available for study by cervical mediastinoscopy. However, as shown by Bowen and colleagues[86] and Jolly and Anderson,[87] anterior mediastinoscopy revealed lymphatic metastasis in nearly a third of patients having previously negative cervical mediastinoscopy. Anterior mediastinoscopy was performed by inserting the mediastinoscope through the left second intercostal space so that anterior mediastinal lymph nodes could be evaluated.

INDICATIONS AND RESULTS

ASSESSMENT OF MEDIASTINAL SPREAD OF LUNG CARCINOMA. Perhaps the most widespread use of mediastinoscopy is to obviate thoracotomy in patients who are unlikely to profit from this exploratory procedure. For patients with lung carcinoma, the finding of contralateral mediastinal lymph node metastases, tracheal or vascular invasion, or small cell morphology would preclude resection. However, the role of surgery in patients with non-small-cell lung carcinoma with microscopic involvement of mediastinal lymph nodes remains controversial. The study of Gibbons[88] showed that thoracotomy and an attempt to resect tumors curatively in patients with a positive mediastinal biopsy is rarely, if ever, possible. In 28 patients with positive mediastinal biopsies, thoracotomy with resection was attempted; none of these 28 survived longer than 2½ years, and, at 1 year, only 3 of those with positive biopsies were alive.

In general, most studies have reported 10% to 30% 5-year survival figures for patients with resectable lung carcinoma and mediastinal lymph node metastases. Squamous lesions have a better prognosis than other non-small-cell histologic types, but extrapulmonary extension or subcarinal node involvement is a poor prognostic feature. Kirsh and co-workers[89] reported a 34.4% 5-year survival for patients with squamous cell carcinoma and mediastinal lymph node metastases. Martini and co-workers[90] observed a 29% actuarial 5-year survival for patients with non-small-cell lung carcinoma. Thus the presence of mediastinal lymph node metastases alone should not exclude patients from surgery if their disease is otherwise resectable. Mediastinoscopy is therefore useful primarily to determine unresectability in patients with lung carcinoma.

Some authors have presented data to suggest that not all lung cancer patients need mediastinoscopy before thoracotomy; size, location (peripheral versus central), and cell type of the primary tumor influence the incidence of positive mediastinal nodes. Hutchinson and Mills[91] found a high incidence of mediastinal metastases associated with central tumors (63%—100%) of all cell types and with peripheral lesions (63%) of undifferentiated cell types. However, only 8.6% of peripheral carcinomas of adenosquamous or squamous type with a radiographically normal mediastinum were found to have mediastinal metastases. Baker and co-workers[92] found only 3 of 40 patients with T1 lesions (3 cm in size or smaller) to have mediastinal node metastases detected by mediastinoscopy. All 3 patients had large cell undifferentiated tumors. Therefore, in patients with small, peripherally located tumors of well-differentiated histology and a normal mediastinum by radiologic examination, mediastinoscopy need not precede thoracotomy. In this group of patients, the slight risk of mediastinoscopy can be avoided.

The use of CT scans of the chest may eliminate routine mediastinoscopy in patients with lung cancer. The absence of abnormally enlarged mediastinal lymph nodes on CT correlates well with the absence of lymph node metastases and with resectability. However, enlarged lymph nodes detected on CT do not necessarily indicate metastases. Nodal enlargement may be due to inflammatory changes caused by a coexisting infectious process in the lung. Thus, if the presence of nodal metastases would influence the operative decision, histologic confirmation by mediastinoscopy or some other technique is indicated.[93]

DIAGNOSIS OF MEDIASTINAL HODGKIN'S DISEASE. Vaeth and colleagues[94] reviewed a group of patients with Hodgkin's disease limited to the mediastinum at the time of initial presentation. From their experience, they suggested that if bone marrow biopsy was negative, a tissue diagnosis was best established by mediastinoscopy rather than thoracotomy. An attempt to resect mediastinal Hodgkin's disease is not indicated. However, Redding and co-workers[95] found that the routine use of mediastinoscopy as a staging procedure in all patients with Hodgkin's disease was not indicated.

TECHNIQUES

The patient is placed on his back with the neck hyperextended by a cushion beneath the scapulae (Fig. 20-7). Under general anesthesia, a 4-cm incision is made in the suprasternal notch about 2 cm above the manubrium. The strap muscles are separated in the midline so that the loose areolar tissue anterior to the trachea can be dissected bluntly and bloodlessly using the index finger. The exploring finger

FIG. 20-7. Technique of mediastinoscopy. **A**. Make a 3- to 4-cm incision just above the manubrium. **B**. Use the finger to dissect bluntly the loose fibrofatty tissue in front of the trachea down to the level of the pulmonary artery. **C**. Introduce the endoscope and take biopsies of suspicious tissues. Needle aspiration of structures before biopsy will help to reduce hemorrhagic complications. (Modified from Kerschner PA: Transcervical approach to the superior mediastinum. Hosp Pract, June 1970)

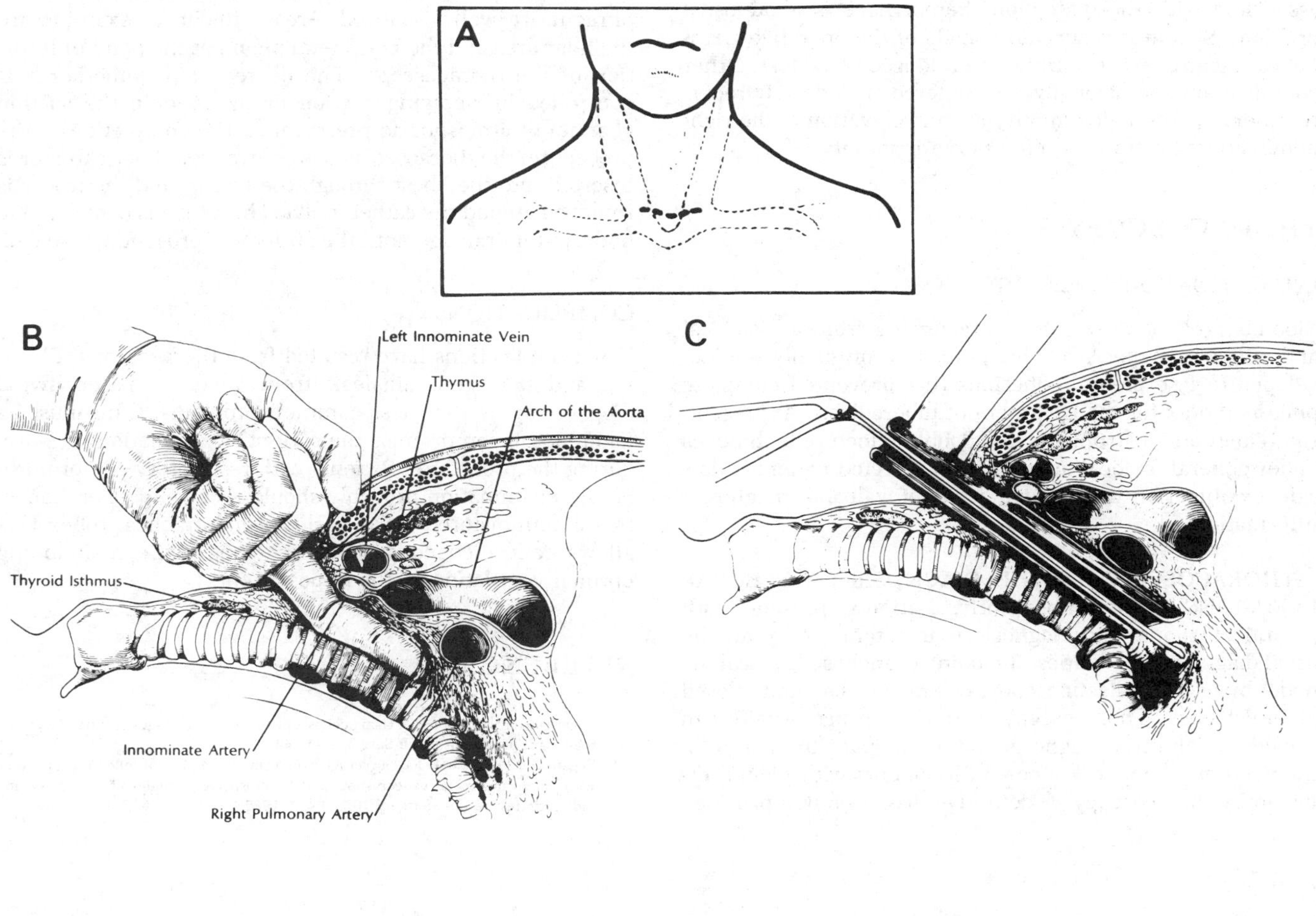

moves along the anterior surface of the trachea beneath the innominate vein, innominate artery, and aortic arch to the level of the tracheal bifurcation. During this dissection, the surgeon should note the position of nodes that feel pathologic for possible later biopsy.[96]

After a tunnel has been prepared, the mediastinoscope is introduced and advanced, with the anterior tracheal wall kept in view. Further dissection is accomplished through the endoscope using a blunt suction apparatus and gauze pledgets. In a complete exploration, which may not be necessary in every patient, both main bronchi, the azygos vein, paratracheal and parabronchial lymph nodes, the right pulmonary artery, the undersurface of the aortic arch, and the left recurrent nerve are visualized.

Biopsy sampling or removal of suspicious lymph nodes is performed; needle aspiration of sutures to be removed may prevent subsequent hemorrhage as a result of damage to vascular channels. Metal clips are useful for hemostasis and to mark biopsy sites. Preparation for emergency thoracotomy should always be made before mediastinoscopy is begun, so that complications may be dealt with quickly.

COMPLICATIONS

Foster and colleagues[97] reviewed 14 mediastinoscopy series published between 1968 and 1970; 3 (0.08%) deaths and 60 (1.6%) complications among 3742 examinations were reported. Postoperative respiratory insufficiency in 2 patients and cardiac arrest in 1 accounted for the 3 deaths. Despite the large number of major vascular structures immediately associated with the dissection, hemorrhage is an unusual problem. Should it occur, tamponade of the operative channel with gauze seems to prevent prolonged blood loss. Other complications occasionally encountered include left recurrent nerve paresis, pneumothorax, and elevation of the right hemidiaphragm from phrenic nerve irritation.[98,99]

THORACOSCOPY

INDICATIONS AND RESULTS

Bloomberg[100] has reviewed thoracoscopy from a historical and clinical perspective. This procedure originally was developed to lyse pleural adhesions that prevented complete pneumothorax for the treatment of tuberculosis. At present, rigid fiberoptic instruments and double-puncture techniques under general or local anesthesia in selected patients allow safe examination and a high yield of valuable diagnostic information.

THORACOSCOPY IN THE DIAGNOSIS OF PLEURAL EFFUSIONS. Not infrequently, patients present with pleural effusions, and diagnosis is unobtainable by all the usual diagnostic modalities, including bronchoscopy, scalene node biopsy, mediastinoscopy, thoracentesis, and closed pleural biopsy. Thoracoscopy in these settings usually can provide a definitive diagnosis and often spare the patient a thoracotomy. Pepper[101] studied 39 patients with pleural effusion by thoracoscopy. A definitive diagnosis was provided in 31 patients by thoracic endoscopy, and in 22 of these the cause of the pleural effusion was malignancy. Lewis and co-workers[102] reported similarly good results in this group of patients.

PREOPERATIVE SCREENING OF PATIENTS WITH BRONCHIAL CARCINOMA. LeRoux[103] found that 7% of patients with bronchial carcinoma had pleural fluid. Because pulmonary resection is always likely to fail in the presence of pleural metastases, LeRoux recommended preoperative thoracoscopy for patients with pleural fluid. In 82 of 139 patients, pleural metastases were found and a needless thoracotomy was averted.

TECHNIQUES

Oldenburg and Newhouse[104] described the preferred method for performing thoracoscopy. The procedure is performed under local anesthesia in the operating room with adequate premedication. Patients are placed in the lateral decubitus position, the skin is prepared, local anesthesia is administered, and a 1.5-cm incision is made in the midaxillary line of the sixth to eighth intercostal space. The pleural space is entered bluntly, and, after an adequate cavity is ensured, the trocar and sleeve are inserted. A rigid 11-cm-diameter thoracoscope (Stortz) is used for visualization; biopsy, cytologic brushing, and photography of all pleural and some parenchymal lesions are possible. Except where adhesions interfere, the parietal pleura, visceral pleura, mediastinum, and diaphragm are well visualized. Areas difficult to examine are the hilar area and the peripheral pleura at the point of insertion of the thoracoscope. The degree of pneumothorax is controlled by applying suction or by opening the suction channel to atmospheric pressure. At the completion of the procedure, the thoracoscope is removed, a rubber catheter is inserted into the chest through the trocar, and the trocar is removed around the catheter. The chest tube is connected to underwater drainage until the air leak, if present, has sealed.

COMPLICATIONS

Few complications have resulted from thoracoscopy. Bleeding and persistent air leak from generous parenchymal biopsy may be the most common problems. Care must be taken not to compromise the patient's oxygenation seriously during the procedure. Patients with respiratory compromise before examination probably should receive a general anesthetic administered via a Carlen's endotracheal tube. This allows controlled collapse of one lung while maintaining optimal ventilation of the opposite one.

REFERENCES

1. Sugarbaker PH, Wilson RE: Using celioscopy to determine stages of intra-abdominal malignant neoplasms. Arch Surg 111:41–44, 1976
2. Sugarbaker PH, Gianola FJ, Duryer AJ et al: A simplified plan for follow up of patients with colon and rectal cancer supported by prospective studies of laboratory and radiologic test results. Surgery 102:79–83, 1982

3. Jori GP, Peshle C: Combined peritoneoscopy and liver biopsy in the diagnosis of hepatic neoplasm. Gastroenterology 63:1016–1019, 1972
4. Czaja AJ, Steinberg AS, Saldana M et al: Peritoneoscopy: Its value in the diagnosis of liver disease. Gastrointest Endosc 20:23–25, 1973
5. McCallum RW, Berci G: Laparoscopy in hepatic disease. Gastrointest Endosc 23:20–24, 1976
6. Sugarbaker PH: Double peritoneoscopy. Surg Gynecol Obstet 152:655–657, 1981
7. Ozols RF, Fisher RI, Anderson T et al: Peritoneoscopy in the management of ovarian cancer. Am J Obstet Gynecol 140:611–619, 1981
8. Goldhaber Z, Bloom BS, Sugarbaker PH et al: Effects of the fiberoptic laparoscope and colonoscope on morbidity and cost. Ann Surg 179:160–162, 1974
9. Knutson CO, Schrock LG, Polk HC: Polypoid lesions of the proximal colon: Comparison of experiences with removal at laparotomy and by colonoscopy. Ann Surg 179:567–662, 1974
10. Dean ACB, Newell JP: Colonoscopy in the differential diagnosis of carcinoma from diverticulitis of the sigmoid colon. Br J Surg 60:633–635, 1973
11. Sugarbaker PH, Vineyard GC, Lewicki AM et al: Colonoscopy in the management of diseases of the colon and rectum. Surg Gynecol Obstet 139:341–349, 1974
12. Glerum J, Agenant D, Tytgat GN: Value of colonoscopy in the detection of sigmoid malignancy in patients with diverticular disease. Endoscopy 9:228–230, 1977
13. Warwick RRG, Sumerling MD, Gilmour HM et al: Colonoscopy and double contrast barium enema examination in chronic ulcerative colitis. AJR 117:292–296, 1973
14. Dobbins WO, Stock M, Ginsberg AL: Early detection and prevention of carcinoma of the colon in patients with ulcerative colitis. Cancer 40:2542–2548, 1977
15. Riddel RH: Dysplasia in inflammatory bowel disease. Clin Gastroenterol 9:439–458, 1980
16. Wolff WI, Shinya H, Geffen A et al: Comparison of colonoscopy and barium enema in five hundred patients with colorectal disease. Am J Surg 129:181–186, 1975
17. Leinicke JL, Dodds WJ, Hogan WJ et al: A comparison of colonoscopy and roentgenography for detecting polypoid lesions of the colon. Gastrointest Radiol 2:125–128, 1977
18. Amberg JR, Berk RN, Burhenne J et al: Colonic polyp detection: Role of roentgenography and colonoscopy. Radiology 125:255–257, 1977
19. Thoeni RF, Menuck L: Comparison of barium enema and colonoscopy in the detection of small colonic polyps. Radiology 124:631–635, 1977
20. Teague RH, Salmon PR, Read AE: Fiberoptic examination of the colon: A review of 255 cases. Gut 14:139–142, 1973
21. Shinya H: Colonoscopy: Diagnosis and Treatment of Colonic Diseases, pp 163–164. New York, Igaku-Shoin, 1982
22. Gilbertsen VA, Nelms JM: The prevention of invasive cancer of the rectum. Cancer 41:1137–1139, 1978
23. Sugarbaker PH, Vineyard GC, Peterson LM: Anatomic localization and step by step advancement of the fiberoptic colonoscope. Surg Gynecol Obstet 143:457–462, 1976
24. Shinya H, Wolff WI: Colonoscopic polypectomy: Technique and safety. Hosp Pract 10:71–78, 1975
25. Sugarbaker PH, Vineyard GC: Snare polypectomy with the fiberoptic colonoscope. Surg Gynecol Obstet 138:581–583, 1974
26. Williams CB: Diathermy-biopsy—A technique for the endoscopic management of small polyps. Endoscopy 5:215–218, 1973
27. Shamir M, Schuman BM: Complications of fiberoptic endoscopy. Gastrointest Endosc 26:86–91, 1980
28. Kobayashi S, Yoshii Y, Kasugai T: Selective use of brushing cytology in gastrointestinal strictures. Gastrointest Endosc 2:76–77, 1972
29. Winawer S, Posner G, Belladonna J et al: Application of panendoscopic directed brush cytology to the diagnosis of esophageal cancer. Gastrointest Endosc 21:188, 1974
30. Totio TL, Den Hartog Jager CA, Tytgat GNJ: The role of endoscopic ultrasonography in assessing local resectability of oesophagogastric malignancies. Scand J Gastroenterol 21 (suppl 22):78–86, 1900
31. Sugano H, Nakamura K, Takagi K: Pathomorphogical study of polyp, polypogenic cancer and polypoid cancer. Stomach Intest 3:729, 1968
32. Martin TR, Onstad GR, Silvis SE et al: Lift and cut biopsy technique for submucosal sampling. Gastrointest Endosc 23:29–30, 1976
33. Yamada T, Hukuto MI: Gastric polyp. Gastrointest Endosc 7:448–454, 1965
34. Dekker W, Tytgat G: Diagnostic accuracy of fiberendoscopy in the detection of upper intestinal malignancy. Gastroenterology 73:710, 1977
35. Littman A (ed): The VA cooperative study on gastric ulcer. Gastroenterology 61(Part II):567, 1971
36. Kasugai T, Kobayashi S: Evaluation of biopsy and cytology in the diagnosis of gastric cancer. Am J Gastroenterol 62:199, 1974
37. Montgomery R, Richardson B: Gastric ulcer and cancer. Q J Med 44:591, 1975
38. Kukrai JC: Gastric ulcer: An appraisal. Surgery 63:1024, 1968
39. Gear M, Truelove S, Williams G et al: Gastric cancer simulating benign gastric ulcer. Br J Surg 56:739, 1969
40. Myren J, Dybdahl J, Serck-Hanssen A et al: Gastroscopy with directed biopsy and routine x-ray in the diagnosis of malignancies of the stomach. Scand J Gastroenterol 10:193, 1975
41. Tsuneoka K, Tadayoshi T, Sotaro F: Fiberoscopy of Gastric Diseases. Tokyo, Igaku-Shoin, 1973
42. Murakami T: Pathomorphological diagnosis: Definition and gross classification of early gastric cancer. In Murakami T (ed): Early Gastric Cancer, Gann Monograph on Cancer Research II, pp 53–55. Tokyo, University of Tokyo Press, 1971
43. Comfort M, Priestly J, Dockerty M et al: The small benign and malignant gastric lesion. Surg Gynecol Obstet 105:435, 1957
44. Hayashida T, Kidokoro T: End results of early gastric cancer collected from 22 institutions. Stomach Intest 4:1077, 1969
45. Borrmann R: Geschwulste des Magens und Duodenums. Handbuch d. spez. pathol. Anatomie U Histologie 4:812, 1926
46. Just-Viera JO, Haight C: Achalasia and carcinoma of the esophagus. Surg Gynecol Obstet 128:1081–1095, 1969
47. Seliger G, Lee T, Schwartz S. Carcinoma of the proximal esophagus: A complication of longstanding achalasia. Am J Gastroenterol 57:20–25, 1972
48. Pierce WS, MacVaugh III H, Johnson J: Carcinoma of the esophagus arising in patients with achalasia of the cardia. J Thorac Cardiovasc Surg 59:355–359, 1970
49. Hankins JR, McLaughlin JS: The association of carcinoma of the esophagus with achalasia. J Thorac Cardiovasc Surg 69:355–360, 1975
50. Carter R, Brewer III LA: Achalasia and esophageal carcinoma. Am J Surg 130:114–120, 1975
51. Wychulis AR, Woolam GL, Anderson HA et al: Achalasia and carcinoma of the esophagus. JAMA 215:1638–1641, 1971
52. Naef A, Savary M, Ozzello P: Columnar-lined lower esophagus: An acquired lesion with malignant predisposition. J Thorac Cardiovasc Surg 70:826–835, 1975
53. Berenson MM, Riddell RH, Skinner DB et al: Malignant transformation of esophageal columnar epithelium. Cancer 41:554–561, 1978
54. McDonald GB, Brand DL, Thorning DR: Multiple adenomatous neoplasms arising in columnar-lined (Barrett's) esophagus. Gastroenterology 72:1317–1321, 1977
55. Sjogren RW Jr, Johnson LF: Barrett's esophagus: A review. Am J Med 74:313–321, 1983
57. Tomasulo J: Gastric polyps: Histologic types and their relation to gastric carcinoma. Cancer 27:1346–1355, 1971
58. Hay LJ: Surgical management of gastric polyps and adenomas. Surgery 39:114–119, 1956
59. Huppler EG, Priestley JT, Morlock CG et al: Diagnosis and results of treatment in gastric polyps. Surg Gynecol Obstet 110:309–313, 1960
60. Marshak RH, Feldman F: Gastric polyps. Am J Dig Dis 10:909–935, 1965
61. Elsborg L, Mosbech J: Pernicious anemia as a risk factor in gastric cancer. Acta Med Scand 206:315–318, 1979
62. Helsingen N, Hillestad L: Cancer development in the gastric stump after partial gastrectomy for ulcer. Am Surg 143:173–179, 1956
63. Stalsberg H, Taksdal S: Stomach cancer following gastric surgery for benign condition. Lancet 2:1175–1177, 1971
64. Domellof L, Janunger KG: The risk of gastric carcinoma after partial gastrectomy. Am J Surg 134:581–584, 1977
65. Schafer LW, Larson DE, Melton LF III et al: The risk of gastric carcinoma following surgical treatment for benign ulcer disease: A population-based study in Olmsted County, Minnesota. N Engl J Med 309:1210–1213, 1983
66. Ross AHM, Smith MA, Anderson JR et al: Late mortality after surgery for peptic ulcer. N Engl J Med 307:519–522, 1982
67. National Institutes of Health Consensus Development Conference Summary: Endoscopy in upper GI bleeding, Vol 3, No 5, 1980
68. Ferrucci JT, Wittenberg J, Sarns RA et al: Fine needle transhepatic cholangiography: A new approach to obstructive jaundice. AJR 127:403–407, 1976
69. Elias E, Hamlyn AN, Jain S et al: A randomized trial of percutaneous transhepatic cholangiography with the Chiba needle versus endoscopic retrograde cholangiography for bile duct visualization in jaundice. Gastroenterology 71:439–443, 1976
70. Kasugai T, Kuno N, Kobayashi S et al: Endoscopic pancreatocholangiography: I. The normal endoscopic pancreatocholangiogram. Gastroenterology 63:217–226, 1972
71. Kasugai T, Kuno N, Kizu M et al: Endoscopic pancreatocholangiography: II. The pathological endoscopic pancreatocholangiogram. Gastroenterology 63:227–234, 1972
72. Ogoshi K: Diseases of the pancreas and the biliary system. In Takemoto T, Kasugai T (eds): Endoscopic Retrograde Cholangiopancreatography. Tokyo, Igaku-Shoin, 1979
73. Yasuda K, Mukai H, Fujimoto S et al: The diagnosis of pancreatic cancer by endoscopic ultrasonography. Gastrointest Endosc 34:1–8, 1988
74. Mackie CR, Cooper MJ, Lewis MH et al: Non-operative differentiation between pancreatic cancer and chronic pancreatitis. Ann Surg 189:480–487, 1979
75. Cotton PB, Williams CB: Practical Gastrointestinal Endoscopy. Oxford, Blackwell, 1980
76. Katz D: Morbidity and mortality in standard and flexible gastrointestinal endoscopy. Gastrointest Endosc 15:134–138, 1969
77. Michel L, Grillo HC, Malt RA: Esophageal perforation. Ann Thorac Surg 33:203–210, 1982
78. Triggiani E, Belsey R: Oesophageal trauma: Incidence, diagnosis and management. Thorax 32:241–249, 1977
79. Mayer JE Jr, Murray CA, Varco RL: The treatment of esophageal perforation with delayed recognition and continuing sepsis. Ann Thorac Surg 23:568–573, 1977
80. Payne CR, Stovin PGI, Baker V et al: Diagnostic accuracy in primary bronchial carcinoma. Thorax 34:294–299, 1979
81. Feldman NT, Pennington JE, Ehrie MG: Transbronchial lung biopsy in the compromised host. JAMA 238:1377–1379, 1977
82. Burt ME, Flye MW, Webber BL et al: Prospective evaluation of aspiration needle, cutting needle, transbronchial and open lung biopsy in patients with pulmonary infiltrates. Ann Thorac Surg 32:146–153, 1981

83. Pearson FG: An evaluation of mediastinoscopy in the management of presumably operable bronchial carcinoma. J Thorac Cardiovasc Surg 55:617–625, 1968
84. Goldberg EM, Shapiro CM, Glicksman AS: Mediastinoscopy for assessing mediastinal spread in clinical staging of lung carcinoma. Semin Oncol 1:205–215, 1974
85. Borrie J: Lung Cancer Surgery and Survival. New York, Appleton-Century-Crofts, 1965
86. Bowen TE, Zajtchuk R, Green DC et al: Value of anterior mediastinotomy in bronchogenic carcinoma of the left upper lobe. J Thorac Cardiovasc Surg 79:269–271, 1980
87. Jolly PC, Li W, Anderson RP: Anterior and cervical mediastinoscopy for determining operability and predicting resectability in lung cancer. J Thorac Cardiovasc Surg 79:366–371, 1980
88. Gibbons JRP: The value of mediastinoscopy in assessing operability in carcinoma of the lung. Br J Dis Chest 66:162–166, 1972
89. Kirsh MM, Rotman H, Argenta L et al: Carcinoma of the lung: Results of treatment over ten years. Ann Thorac Surg 21:371–377, 1976
90. Martini N, Flehinger BJ, Zaman MB et al: Results of resection in non-oat cell carcinoma of the lung with mediastinal lymph node metastases. Ann Surg 198:386–397, 1983
91. Hutchinson CM, Mills NL: The selection of patients with bronchogenic carcinoma for mediastinoscopy. J Thorac Cardiovasc Surg 71:768–773, 1976
92. Baker RR, Lillemoe KD, Tockman MS: The indications for transcervical mediastinoscopy in patients with small peripheral bronchial carcinoma. Surg Gynecol Obstet 148:860–862, 1979
93. Daily BDT Jr, Failing LJ, Pugatch RD et al: Computed tomography an effective technique for mediastinal staging and lung cancer. J Thorac Cardiovasc Surg 88:486–494, 1900
94. Vaeth JM, Moskowitz SA, Green JP: Mediastinal Hodgkin's disease. AJR 126:123–126, 1976
95. Redding ME, Anagnostopoulos CE, Ultmann JE: The possible value of mediastinoscopy in staging Hodgkin's disease. Cancer Res 31:1741–1745, 1971
96. Kirschner PA: Transcervical approach to the superior mediastinum. Hosp Pract, June 1970
97. Foster ED, Munro DD, Dobell ARC: Mediastinoscopy. A review of anatomical relationships and complications. Ann Thorac Surg 13:273–286, 1972
98. Bacsa S, Czaro Z, Vezendi S: The complications of mediastinoscopy. Panminerva Med 74:402–406, 1974
99. Kliems G, Savic B: Complications of mediastinoscopy. Endoscopy 1:9–12, 1979
100. Bloomberg AE: Thoracoscopy in perspective. Surg Gynecol Obstet 147:433–443, 1978
101. Pepper JR: Thoracoscopy in the diagnosis of pleural effusions and tumors. Br J Dis Chest 72:74–75, 1978
102. Lewis RJ, Kunderman PJ, Sisler GE et al: Direct diagnostic thoracoscopy. Ann Thorac Surg 21:536–539, 1976
103. LeRoux BT: Bronchial Carcinoma, p 127. Edinburgh, E & S Livingston, 1968
104. Oldenburg FA, Newhouse MT: Thoracoscopy: A safe, accurate diagnostic procedure using the rigid thoracoscope and local anesthesia. Chest 75:45–50, 1979

DAVID G. BRAGG
H. RIC HARNSBERGER
WILLIAM M. THOMPSON

SECTION 2

Radiologic Techniques in Cancer

Tumor imaging in its entirety is too broad to cover in the few pages that follow. We have chosen to focus on the controversial anatomical sites, cancers that commonly occur in these sites, and the selection of an appropriate imaging modality for evaluating such cancers. For a more complete discussion of the many challenges and applications for tumor imaging procedures, the reader is referred to the textbook *Oncologic Imaging,* edited by Bragg, Rubin, and Youker.[1]

Tumor imaging has become more complex and controversial as the number of available technologies has increased. In most body sites, imaging is used primarily to detect, stage, and follow the cancer rather than as a screening method. Notable exceptions are certain radiologic screening programs for breast and gastrointestinal tract cancers. One should critically analyze reports concerning the accuracy of imaging procedures in any given tumor site, paying particular attention to the type of equipment used, the date of the report, and the unique challenges posed by each body site. The rapid evolution of imaging technologies has made obsolete many of the earlier reports on the accuracy of various modalities for staging neoplasms, particularly with regard to neoplasms of the central nervous system, chest, and abdomen. The complex changes in magnetic resonance (MR) imaging equipment have further confounded a thoughtful analysis of this technology. The recently completed consensus conference on MR imaging established the dominance of this imaging technique in the central nervous system and reported preliminary advantages in musculoskeletal tumor staging. To date, MR imaging has not been shown to have a clear advantage over computed tomography (CT) in most other thoracoabdominal sites. MR imaging and CT appear to be nearly equivalent in the detection of most brain tumors; however, because of the absence of bone artifacts, MR imaging is the preferred modality for detecting lesions near the skull vertex, posterior fossa, skull base, and orbit.[2]

DAVID G. BRAGG

Thorax

Current controversies in imaging of thoracic cancer largely focus on the relative accuracy and efficacy of CT versus MR imaging and the appropriate use of these modalities for staging neoplasms and guiding biopsy procedures. This discussion briefly considers the application of these modalities and the use of biopsy procedures in tumors of the chest wall, pleura, lung, and heart.

CHEST WALL

The imaging approach to the individual with a chest wall neoplasm is summarized in Table 20-5. This simplified algorithm does not attempt to consider the variety of different tumor cell types or tumorlike abnormalities that may affect the thoracic cage. The initial step in imaging the chest wall should always be plain radiography, with films showing rib detail. This examination will allow the clinician to determine whether the lesion is destructive or is one of the multitude of traumatic and acquired benign lesions that can mimic tumors. If, based on the plain films, tumor continues to be a diagnostic possibility, a radionuclide bone scan should be the next step to determine whether the lesion is monostotic or polyostotic. If the neoplasm is localized to a single rib or a group of contiguous ribs, consideration of a primary tumor should be paramount. The decision to proceed with CT or

TABLE 20-5. Algorithm of Imaging Approach to Patient with Chest Wall Neoplasm

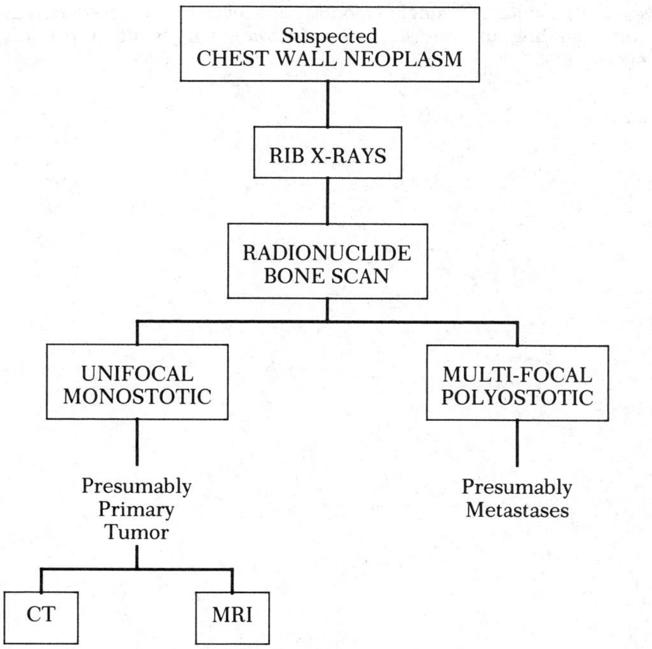

MR imaging to analyze and stage the tumor may be a local option, contingent on the availability of the technology. MR imaging better defines the muscle compartments and provides the surgeon with the information necessary to plan the appropriate surgical procedure and to determine the resectability of the lesion. In addition, T2-weighted MR images are more useful than CT in determining the presence of chest wall invasion with peripheral primary lung cancers.[3,4]

In general, plain radiographs seldom show an associated soft tissue mass with metastatic rib lesions. When a presumed, surrounding soft tissue mass is seen in association with a destructive rib lesion, consideration should be given to multiple myeloma and non-Hodgkin's lymphoma. If MR imaging, CT, or ultrasound is used to further characterize the metastatic rib lesions, a much higher percentage of associated soft tissue masses will be found with metastatic rib lesions, a feature not generally visible on plain radiographs.

MR imaging with both T1- and T2-weighted images is the recommended procedure for staging a variety of primary chest wall neoplasms prior to definitive treatment. Limited post-treatment MR imaging can be used to monitor tumor response to radiation therapy and chemotherapy (Fig. 20-8).

PLEURA

A suspected mesothelioma is often better evaluated by imaging than by microscopic review of the excised tissue. In diffuse malignant mesothelioma the affected pleura exhibits a lobular pleural thickening that often extends into the interlobar fissures, reducing the volume of the hemithorax. The tumor subsequently encases the involved hemithorax, progressively reducing lung volume, yet rarely breaks through the pleura to invade contiguous ribs. Radiographic findings of associated asbestosis are usually lacking. Often, a limited tissue biopsy sample may make a specific pathologic diagnosis very difficult and differentiation from a metastatic adenocarcinoma impossible. Radiographic signs favoring metastatic adenocarcinoma over mesothelioma include bilateral disease, hilar or mediastinal lymphadenopathy, and nodular pulmonary parenchymal disease.[5] Either MR imaging or CT will demonstrate the extent of the mesothelioma before and after treatment. Both of these techniques afford the opportunity to access contiguous invasion, particularly of the mediastinum, pericardium, and diaphragm.[6-8]

Metastatic involvement of the pleural compartment almost invariably manifests as pleural effusion on routine chest radiographs. Rarely are the tumor deposits of sufficient size to be imaged directly by any modality. Neoplasms responsible for secondary pleural involvement represent one of two general categories: either direct extension from primary lung tumors, or metastatic involvement, usually from a primary in the breast or subdiaphragmatic sites. Individuals with ascitic fluid accumulations not infrequently have pleural effusions, due to the communications through the diaphragm with the peritoneum. Pleural effusions in patients with lymphoproliferative disorders are usually secondary manifestations of disease in the mediastinum or lung parenchyma.

LUNG

The three national lung cancer screening trial programs in the United States that used serial chest radiography and sputum cytology to evaluate heavy smokers found an insufficient survival benefit with these procedures to lead to their recommended use in a routine screening protocol. These studies also demonstrated the difficulty in recognizing the low-contrast object represented by a primary lung cancer on a routine chest radiograph. Nearly 90% of the peripheral lung cancers and 75% of the more central lesions could be seen in retrospect on earlier 4-month screening radiographs in one of the trials.[8-11]

It is thought that the majority of primary lung cancers arise distal to a segmental bronchus and undergo approximately 30 doublings before reaching a size of 1.0 cm, the accepted threshold for detection on plain radiographs. Squamous cell carcinomas invariably occur as central lesions and have a tendency to excavate and generally metastasize later than other non-oat cell lung cancers. In contrast, small cell carcinomas have spread outside the thorax in 70% to 90% of patients at the time of diagnosis. These small cell carcinomas often resemble squamous cell cancers on chest radiographs, as both arise as central lesions. Adenocarcinoma, a more frequent peripheral primary lung cancer, tends to metastasize early and has an apparent predilection to spread to the central nervous system and adrenal glands. Large cell carcinomas resemble adenocarcinomas in terms of their peripheral presentation and metastatic characteristics.[12,13] An appreciation of these more common presenting characteris-

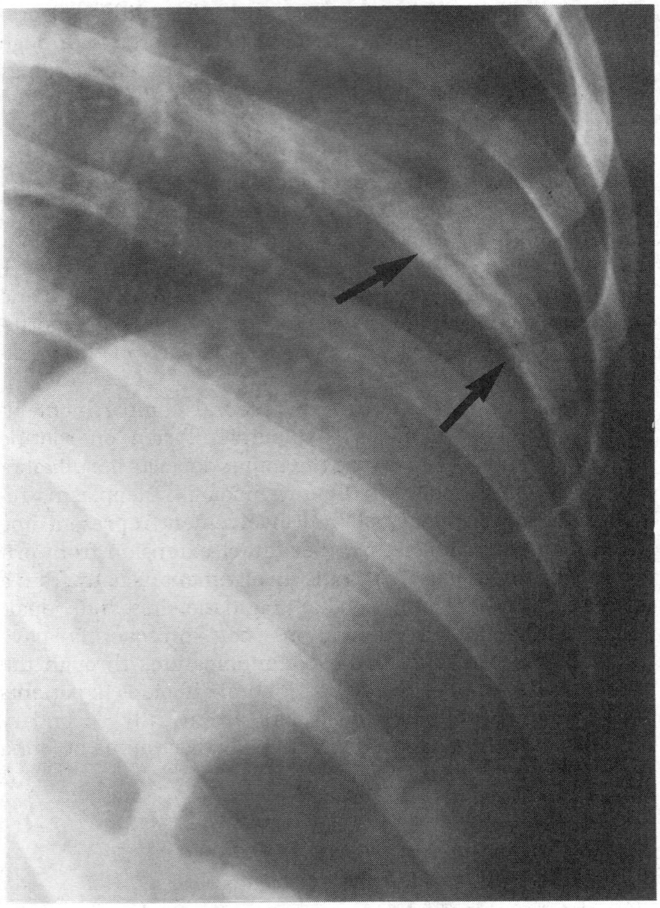

A

FIG. 20-8. An 18-year-old girl had complained of left chest pain for several months but denied a history of trauma. The rib detail films (**A**) show the destructive permeative process (*black arrows*) typical of the changes of an aggressive neoplasm. The radionuclide bone scan (**B**) identifies a single (monostotic) focus of increased activity corresponding to the rib lesion (*arrow*), suggesting a primary neoplasm.

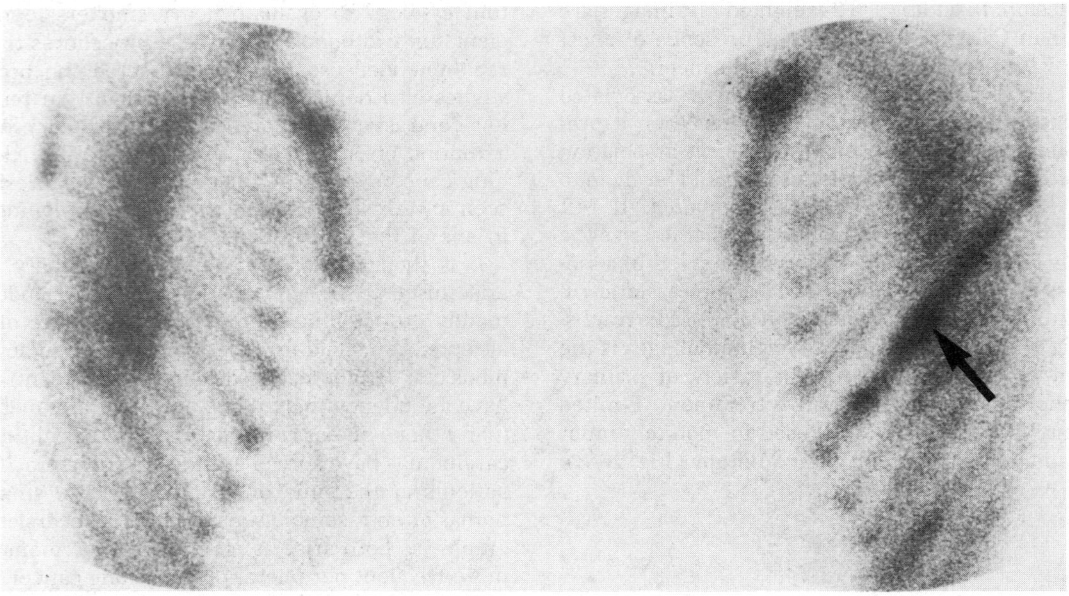

B

(*continued*)

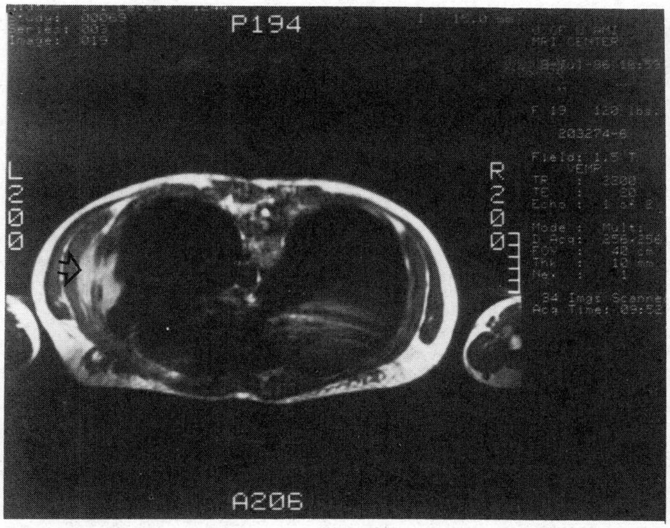

C

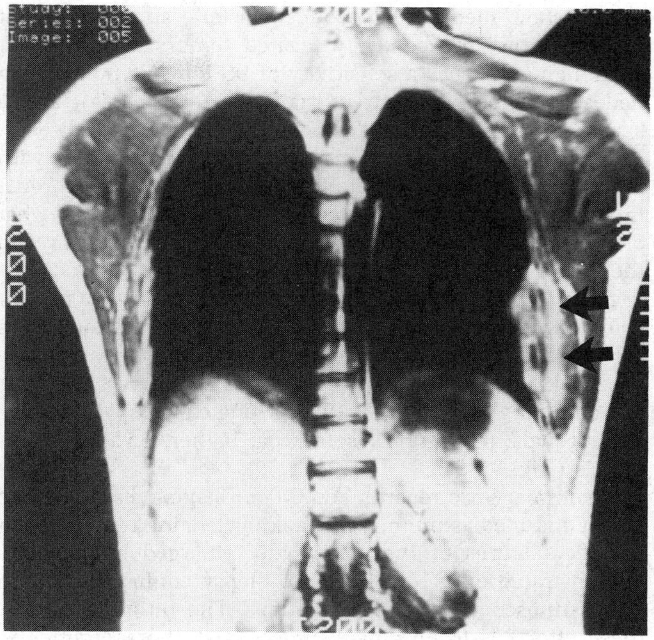

D

(*FIG. 20-8 continued*)
The axial (**C**) and coronal (**D**) MRI scans, T-1 weighted, demonstrate the higher signal, white tumor (*arrows*) displacing but not invading contiguous chest wall musculature. The neoplasm was excised and found to be a high-grade non-Hodgkin's lymphoma.

tics of the primary lung cancers can help the clinician understand both imaging features and radiologic staging protocols.

A CT evaluation of the solitary pulmonary nodule was suggested by Siegelman et al in 1980 as a means of discriminating benign from malignant pulmonary masses. Lesions with high CT numbers in excess of 164 Hounsfield units were presumed to contain calcium and therefore to be benign.[14] Other investigators had difficulty confirming these findings, leading to a multi-institutional trial program in which several different CT scanners and a standardization phantom were used. As a result of these trials it was found that an absolute CT number could not be used as a threshold to separate benign from malignant lesions; however, the characteristics of the tumor margin and its size have helped to unify the recommendations for the potential application of CT in evaluating the solitary pulmonary nodule.[15] In our opinion, the use of CT in this setting will be limited, as it requires an expensive phantom, various imaging procedures, and education of surgeons not familiar with this technique.

The selection of an appropriate imaging procedure to evaluate and further characterize a thoracic neoplasm must be tailored to the anatomical compartment, the presumed or known histology of the neoplasm, and the anticipated treatment. Chest wall invasion cannot be accurately assessed with either CT or MR imaging unless there is frank bone invasion. The mere contact and effacement of fat planes is insufficient evidence from which to infer chest wall invasion. In comparisons of film tomography, CT, and MR imaging in the evaluation of nodular pulmonary lesions, CT was the most sensitive and accurate; however, it suffers from a lack of specificity. The size threshold for recognition on plain films of the solitary pulmonary nodule representing a primary lung cancer is generally thought to be between 5 and 10 mm.[16] Film tomography is no longer used to screen for lung nodules. Data reported in earlier studies, in which less sophisticated CT instrumentation was used than is currently employed, showed that 35% more pulmonary nodules were detected with CT than with film tomography in a group of 91 patients. CT is considerably more accurate than either plain radiography or film tomography in demonstrating the actual size of pulmonary nodules.[17]

The major controversy in the application of imaging techniques to lung cancer relates to staging. A recent article reported a survey of thoracic surgeons in North America and their opinion regarding the role of CT in the preoperative assessment of the patient with lung cancer. Some 85% of the 329 respondents used CT selectively for the patient with an abnormal hilum or mediastinum on routine chest radiographs, whereas only 10% requested CT in the presence of a "normal" hilum and mediastinum on plain chest radiographs.[18]

Because approximately 50% of patients with lung cancer can be expected to have metastatic nodal involvement at the time of initial presentation, the goal of imaging should be to identify those patients with an abnormal mediastinum who should be further evaluated with mediastinoscopy or mediastinotomy with biopsy prior to thoracotomy. Plain chest radiographs show mediastinal nodal metastatic sites only about half the time; the centrally located tumors are the most challenging. CT has a sensitivity of 95% for demonstrating nodes in excess of 1 cm in diameter (short axis), and a specificity of 65% for nodes containing metastatic disease. The sensitivity and specificity obviously are different with increasing lymph node size. No significant advantage for MR imaging over CT has been shown, other than a somewhat clearer separation of lymph nodes and vascular structures in the hilum with MR imaging.[19,20]

The CT protocol for imaging the mediastinum in a patient prior to initial treatment entails contrast agent infusion, with a bolus injection if sections through the hilum are to be obtained. The examination should also encompass the liver and adrenal glands. Nearly 12% of lung cancers will involve the adrenals; the figure is somewhat higher for adenocarcinomas (Fig. 20-9).

In summary, we recommend CT for staging disease in the hilum and mediastinum, while acknowledging that the nonspecific features of the abnormally enlarged lymph node demonstrated on CT will require biopsy confirmation with mediastinoscopy or mediastinotomy. The ultimate goal of these efforts is to eliminate unnecessary thoracotomies in patients with unresectable disease. MR imaging affords no advantage over CT in the evaluation of the hilum or mediastinum but does appear superior in the assessment of the chest wall and lung apex. Gallium radionuclide scanning, film tomography, and fluoroscopy no longer have a meaningful role in the workup of the patient with primary lung cancer.

The percutaneous biopsy of parenchymal, hilar, or mediastinal abnormalities is a safe and reliable technique for the diagnosis of pulmonary, pleural, or chest wall mass lesions. The technique is firmly based on the experience of both radiologists and pathologists, with accuracies in excess of 95% reported. The incidence of complications is related to patient factors (*e.g.*, his or her ability to cooperate), the location of the lesion (a higher incidence of pneumothorax occurs with apical lesions), and the number of times the needle punctures the pleural surface. In an effort to minimize the latter complication, a "coaxial technique" has been suggested, in which a thin (no. 22 or 23) needle is inserted and a larger 19-gauge needle is passed over the thinner needle. Subsequent biopsies are performed through the larger needle to avoid multiple pleural punctures.[21]

Fluoroscopic guidance is usually all that is required to perform the percutaneous biopsy. Lesions more difficult to biopsy, such as indistinct or central lesions, may require CT guidance, even though complications have been reported to be higher when CT is used, probably due to the longer procedure time and patient characteristics. A postprocedure pneumothorax is usually evident within 4 hours; the vast majority are visible immediately after the biopsy. This complication is reported following approximately 20% of lung biopsies. Local hemorrhage is the only other important complication. Only approximately 10% of these pneumothorax complications require treatment, which often entails the placement of a small, 9-F chest tube attached to a Heimlich valve.[22]

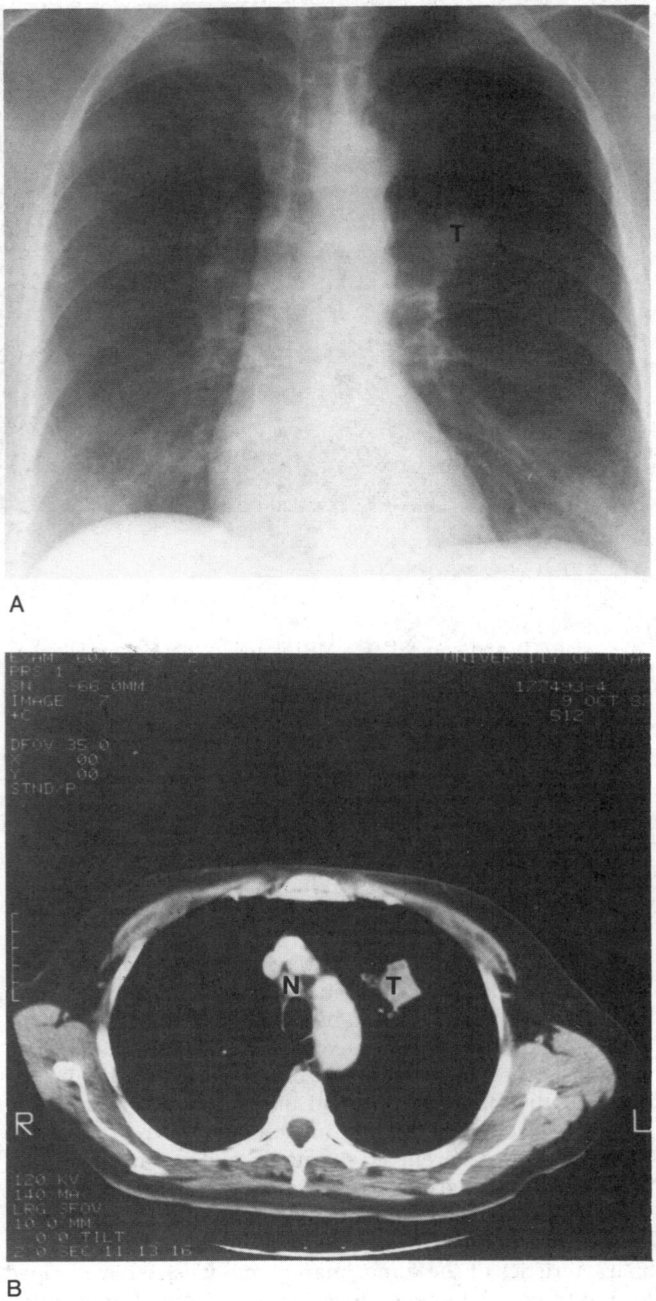

FIG. 20-9. A mass lesion was discovered on a routine chest radiograph (**A**) of a 63-year-old female smoker, which was found to be an adenocarcinoma by lung biopsy (labeled T). A staging CT scan (**B**) shows the T-1 tumor (*T*) and pretracheal nodes (*N*), indicating a stage N-2 lung cancer.

HEART

A discussion of the uncommon primary intracardiac tumors is beyond the scope of this chapter. The extension of contiguous mediastinal or lung parenchymal tumors to the heart can now be elegantly imaged with cardiac and respiratory gated MR imaging. The extent of the tumor to or through the pericardium and into the chambers of the heart can be quite accurately assessed with MR imaging. Tumors with a propensity to extend through the great vessels to the heart, such as renal cell cancers, can also be noninvasively imaged with MR imaging techniques, particularly those with reconstruction algorithms that create a positive image of flowing blood (Fig. 20-10). The MR imaging characteristics of a variety of intracardiac masses have recently been reported, illustrating this potential for cardiac imaging.[23] MR images in coronal projections are useful to the radiation oncologist in treatment planning. Some centers have reported predictable changes on T2-weighted images of mediastinal neoplasms, especially lymphomas, after treatment. A controlled imaging

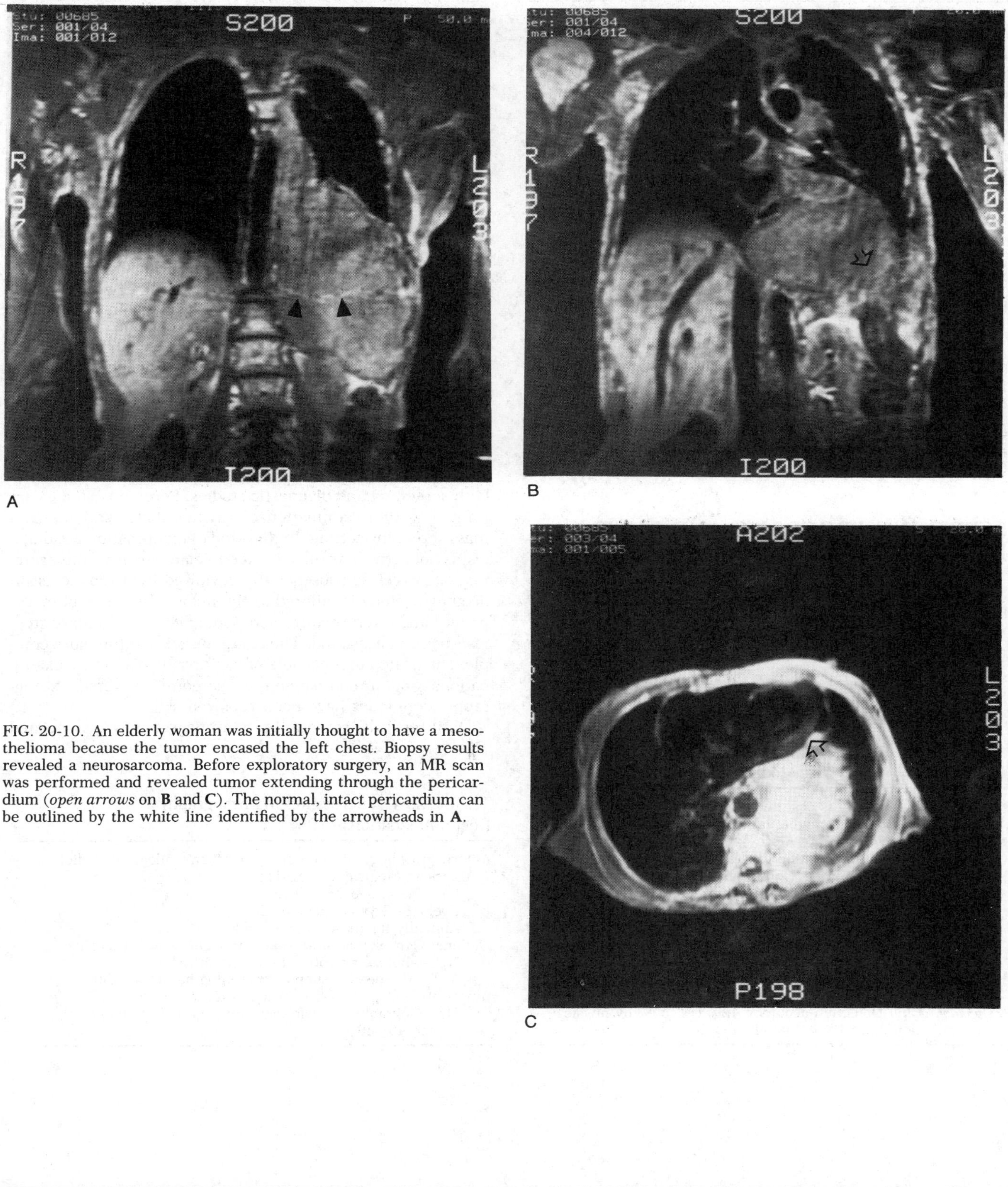

FIG. 20-10. An elderly woman was initially thought to have a mesothelioma because the tumor encased the left chest. Biopsy results revealed a neurosarcoma. Before exploratory surgery, an MR scan was performed and revealed tumor extending through the pericardium (*open arrows* on **B** and **C**). The normal, intact pericardium can be outlined by the white line identified by the arrowheads in **A**.

study of a large number of tumors will be required to confirm these observations, as we have not found these changes to be reliable indicators of disease regression.

DAVID G. BRAGG

Breast

Initial reports on roentgenography of the breast appeared more than 50 years ago, but it was not until the 1960s that dedicated mammographic systems became available and the concept of screening mammography came of age.[24] These initial mammographic studies were flawed by an unacceptably high radiation exposure dose, long exposure times, and less than optimal image quality. Soon after the introduction of dedicated mammographic units in the mid-1960s, alternative imaging techniques were suggested, the first of which was thermography. These alternative screening techniques are summarized in Table 20-6. Xeromammography was introduced in 1972 as a technique to improve breast imaging by providing edge enhancement to structures of differing radiographic contrast density and calcifications.[25]

In the United States, virtually all breast imaging entails either screen-film mammography or xeroradiography. There is no significant difference in the diagnostic yield of these two techniques.[26] Other screening techniques have not proved suitable for stand-alone screening and have a limited role as ancillary diagnostic procedures in certain clinical circumstances.

SCREENING PROGRAMS AND THEIR JUSTIFICATION

The initial study documenting the role of mammography in breast cancer detection was the Health Insurance Plan of New York City (HIP), completed in the 1960s. Long-term follow-up of patients enrolled in these controlled trials has shown a significant reduction in breast cancer mortality that is limited to patients over age 50.[27] Similar results were reported from a controlled, randomized trial in Sweden, with survival advantage also limited to individuals over age 50. The Swedish study used a longer interval of nearly 3 years between screening examinations. The investigators also employed a single oblique mammogram, an imaging strategy that has since been shown to be cost-ineffective and has been discontinued in the United States. The Swedish investigators reported a 31% reduction in breast cancer mortality and a 25% reduction in the incidence of Stage II or more advanced cancers.[28] The Breast Cancer Detection Demonstration Projects (BCDDP) validated the effectiveness of mass mammographic screening through multiple separate screening centers in an uncontrolled trial. Reports from the BCDDP demonstrated the ability of modern mammography to detect early breast cancer before it becomes palpable. In this study, nearly 42% of the proven cancers were seen only with mammography.[29]

The results of these and other mammographic screening programs support a role for screening mammography in the patient over age 50 and suggest the application of this technique as an effective means to detect preclinical breast cancer in the patient under age 50. These data form the basis for the recommendations of the American Cancer Society and American College of Radiology, summarized in Table 20-7.

TECHNICAL ASPECTS, RADIATION DOSES, AND LOCALIZATION PROCEDURES

Dedicated mammography installations using screen-film or xerographic techniques are divided into those facilities dedicated to screening examinations and those which perform both screening and diagnostic studies. Screening studies are limited to the examination of asymptomatic patients in a mass screening setting. In this kind of examination a radiologist is not actively involved; a technician performs the examination, which is subsequently reviewed by a radiologist. A diagnostic study is tailored to the needs of the symptomatic patient and often requires additional views or ancillary studies, such as ultrasound. The characteristics of the more complex, dedicated unit capable of performing diagnostic examinations and a comparison of screen-film versus xerography techniques have been reported.[30,31]

Until recently, screen-film mammography was associated

TABLE 20-6. Screening Modalities

- *Screen-film* (1960): Less cost and lower radiation dose (0.1 rad to midbreast); less technical latitude; misses chest wall
- *Xeromammography* (1972): More expensive, higher radiation dose (0.8 rad to midbreast); greater technical latitude; images chest wall; new toner-developer will decrease dose
- *Digital Mammography:* Early results not encouraging
- *Ultrasound:* Small-part—only for symptomatic patient with dense breast and palpable mass; resolution poor for lesions <1 cm; dedicated—poor with fatty breasts; not adequate for screening
- *Diaphanography* (cancer absorbs more near infrared radiation than benign): Poor for deep lesions
- *Thermography:* Detection accuracy 42% (vs. 57% by physical examination and 91% by mammography)

TABLE 20-7. Screening Mammography Recommendations (1987)

American College of Surgeons, American College of Radiology, American Medical Association:
- Baseline at age 35–40 yr
- Every 1–2 yr at ages 40–50
- Annually for those over age 50

National Cancer Institute, American College of Physicians:
- NCI—before age 50 *only* if at high risk
- ACP—no data to support screening before age 50

American College of Obstetrics and Gynecology:
- Mammography "considered" for high-risk patients aged 40–49 yr

with a considerably lower radiation exposure than xeromammography for a two-view examination. The average midbreast glandular dose should be less than 0.1 rad with screen-film studies and five to eight times that amount for xeromammography. More recent developments in the xerography technique are claimed to improve image resolution at a reduced radiation dose.

Dedicated ultrasound units have not proved effective as they are incapable of resolving lesions less than 1 cm in diameter and seldom image clinically occult masses. Ultrasound waves do not adequately penetrate fatty breast tissue, making the technique more effective in imaging the dense, nonfatty breast of the premenopausal woman. Small-part ultrasound examination is occasionally useful in characterizing the palpable mass lesion in the symptomatic young patient with dense breasts. Breast transillumination (diaphanography) is based on the principle that cancers absorb more near infrared radiation than benign lesions. This technique is still experimental and has not been shown to be effective as a stand-alone screening technique. It is also not sensitive for the deeper lesions in the breast.

Digital mammography, the registration of mammographic images with a digital rather than an analog technique, shows promise, but at present only prototype systems are available. Digital recording affords the viewer unlimited flexibility in the contrast–recording mode.

Magnetic resonance imaging vividly displays some of the unique characteristics of certain breast neoplasms. Earlier, CT was shown to have a potential ability to discriminate benign and malignant breast cancers. At present MR imaging is of a research rather than practical interest in the imaging, detection, and characterization of breast cancer. The logistics, cost, and patient numbers make the widespread application of MR imaging or CT to breast diagnosis impractical.

Mammographic signs of cancer are based on the detection of an ill-defined mass, microcalcifications, or one or more indirect signs (Table 20-8). Clusters of microcalcifications less than 0.5 mm in size are visible radiologically in nearly 50% of all breast cancers. "Clustering" refers to a number of these microcalcifications, which should be more than five per square centimeter to qualify as "suspicious." The greater the number of calcifications and the more diverse their form, the more likely they are to be associated with a cancer. The linear or branching forms are the most suspicious; however, there is an overlap in the appearance of benign and malignant microcalcifications, and biopsy is often needed to distinguish them. These calcifications are presumed to develop within necrotic materials found in the obstructed lumen of ducts in the vicinity of the cancer.[32–34]

The most important of the indirect signs of cancer is asymmetry of the two breasts, with a nonspecific increase in breast tissue density on the abnormal side. Although this sign is nonspecific, it should stimulate additional scrutiny of that involved breast. Architectural distortion is a nonspecific finding in which the normal breast tissue components are distorted or drawn together, in contrast to the usual radial pattern of normal breast tissue oriented toward the nipple. A developing density refers to an area of increased breast tissue density not present in an earlier examination. The breasts should become progressively more atrophic with time, particularly in the postmenopausal patient. The most nonspecific of the indirect signs is a single dilated duct or large vessel, both usually nonspecific and not clinically relevant. A recent review of the mammographic characteristics of 512 consecutive occult mammographic abnormalities showed that the positive predictive value of an ill-defined or stellate mass was 0.75, and that for strongly suspicious microcalcifications, described above, 0.56. An ill-defined mass with poorly defined but not stellate margins had a positive predictive value for cancer of 0.35. None of the other findings had a sufficiently large positive predictive value to warrant a recommendation for biopsy.[35]

TABLE 20-8. Mammographic Signs of Cancer

Direct	
Microcalcifications	
Mass	
Indirect	
Architectural distortion	
Developing density	
Asymmetry	
Large duct or vessel	
% Primary Abnormality	
~40%	
~40%	
~20%	

LOCALIZATION AND BIOPSY TECHNIQUES

Because nearly 50% of breast cancers will be visible mammographically but not palpable clinically, localization techniques are necessary to identify these abnormalities before biopsy. Many techniques have been proposed; the ideal one remains elusive. Most techniques use a wire placed through a needle, with the coordinates previously established by mammography. Either a visible dye or a hooked wire is introduced through the localizing needle and its placement is confirmed with 90° verification mammograms. The surgeon then excises the lesion that has been localized. If microcalcifications were present, specimen radiographs should be obtained to verify that the abnormality has been excised, and follow-up mammograms should be obtained 4 to 6 months after the procedure (Fig. 20-11).[36]

Localization under radiographic control should enable the radiologist to place the needle–wire system within less than 1 cm from the mammographic abnormality. Newer stereoscopic and computer-aided localization techniques should allow aspiration biopsy and cytologic analysis of mammographic abnormalities in the near future. This should decrease the cost and morbidity associated with breast biopsy procedures.

Galactography is occasionally useful in the patient with persistent nipple discharge, following initial cytologic evalu-

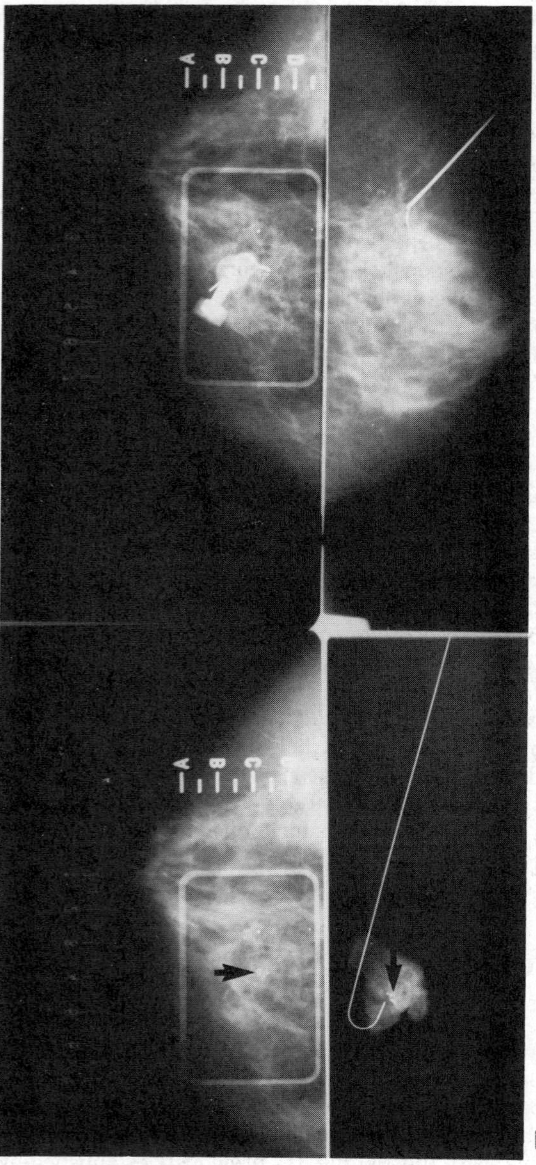

FIG. 20-11. Mammographic localization—homer technique. **A.** The rectangular square is centered on a small cluster of white microcalcifications (*arrow*) which can be localized with the letter and numerical coordinates. A needle with a curved wire is then inserted into the microcalcifications and verification films are obtained (**B** and **C**), showing the curved wire to be surrounding the microcalcifications. **D.** The specimen radiograph with the wire in place identifies that the clustered microcalcifications (*arrow*) indeed have been removed. Verification postbiopsy mammograms should be obtained within 4 to 6 months after the biopsy procedure.

ation of the expressed discharge. Contrast material can be locally instilled and radiographs obtained to analyze the ducts responsible for the discharge, and to help characterize the major duct abnormality. Occasionally, the offending duct can be adequately localized with this technique for surgical biopsy.[37]

H. RIC HARNSBERGER

Head, Neck, and Spine

CENTRAL NERVOUS SYSTEM NEOPLASMS: BRAIN

For most of the last decade, CT has functioned as the principal imaging modality for the detection and follow-up of neoplasms of the central nervous system (CNS).[38–43] Although CT represents a vast improvement over previously available techniques for imaging the CNS, it has multiple blind spots in the search for CNS cancers.[44] In areas of high bone content such as the posterior fossa and the supratentorial brain adjacent to the calvaria, streak artifacts often distort the image and may conceal small neoplasms. Additionally, smaller CNS tumors that lack either significant blood–brain barrier disruption or mass effect often are not visible on CT (Fig. 20-12). Today, MR imaging has emerged as the radiologic method of choice for investigating CNS tumors. MR imaging has inherently greater sensitivity for brain pathology than CT, and it displays the brain in regions adjacent to areas of high bone content with relatively few artifacts.[45–48] This section considers first the advantages of MR imaging over CT for lesions of the head, neck, and spine, and then the profound impact of MR imaging on the diagnosis, treatment, and follow-up of lesions in these areas. The details of MR imaging are beyond the scope of this chapter but are well delineated elsewhere.[49–53] In brief, MR imaging is based on the principle that static tissue protons subjected to an intense external magnetic field will emit a characteristic relaxation signal when perturbed by a specific radiofrequency pulse. This characteristic signal can be spatially localized into an image with the aid of computers. The image may be obtained in the sagittal, coronal, or axial plane. No signal will be detected from moving protons (blood), allowing images to be obtained with clear identification of blood vessels without the use of intravascular contrast medium.[50] Bone generates a weak signal without artifact because of its low proton content; for this reason MR images are superior to CT scans in imaging the skull base, posterior fossa, and cerebellopontine angle.

When MR imaging is compared with CT, several advantages of the former become apparent. The most important advantage of MR imaging is its ability to demonstrate abnormal water content in brain tissue caused by tumor or inflammation, before a blood–brain barrier leak or mass effect is produced. As a result, MR imaging is more sensitive to smaller CNS tumors than CT. MR imaging can display tumors in the range of 3 to 5 mm; these tumors are not visible on CT (see Fig. 20-12). Other advantages of MRI include the use of magnetic fields and radiowaves, rather than x-rays, to produce images; the ability to generate multiplaner (axial, sagittal, and coronal) images without patient repositioning; and no need for intravenous or intrathecal contrast agents in routine screening examinations. Since bone is "proton poor," the bone artifacts ordinarily seen on CT scans are not present on MR images. These qualities of

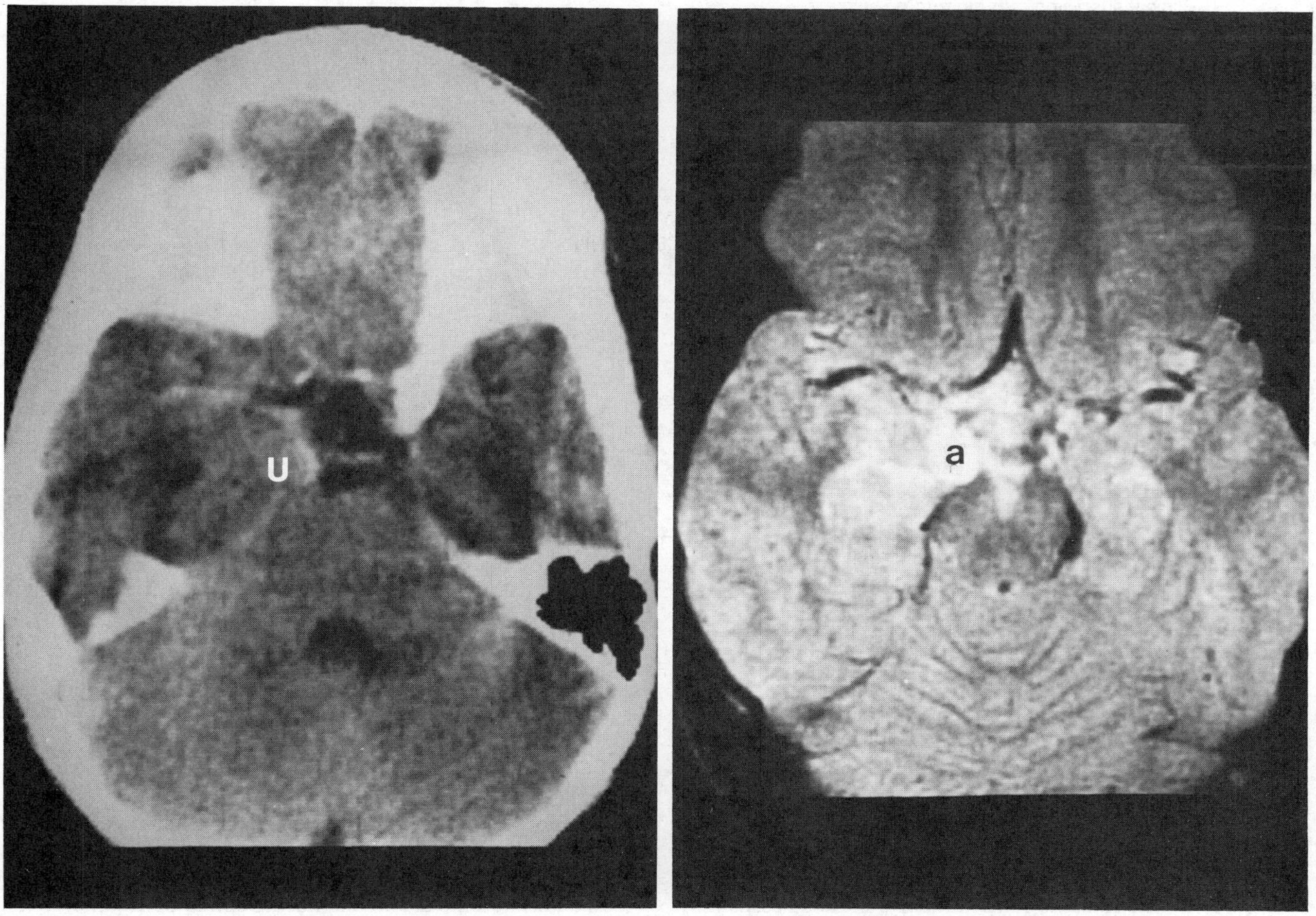

A B

FIG. 20-12. Comparative CT and MR brain images in a patient with a temporal lobe astrocytoma. **A**. Enhanced, axial CT scan through the suprasellar cistern shows an enlarged uncus (*U*) with no evidence for contrast enhancement (blood-brain barrier leak). **B**. T-2 weighted axial MR image through the same level is streak-artifact free and graphically delineates the temporal lobe astrocytoma (*a*).

MR imaging make it a highly sensitive radiologic tool that detects smaller CNS tumors than CT, without subjecting the patient to radiation, iodinated contrast agents, or uncomfortable body positions.

MR imaging has emerged as the examination of choice in the search for CNS mass lesions. Figure 20-13 shows a decision tree for use in imaging patients thought to have brain tumors; the decision tree acknowledges the principal role of this modality in the diagnostic and follow-up phases of brain tumor evaluation.

Because MR imaging can now demonstrate subcentimeter brain lesions that are possibly cancerous but may instead result from demyelination, stroke, or infection, the need for a safe tissue biopsy technique has dramatically increased. Stereotaxic biopsy guided by CT, therefore, has become an important diagnostic and therapeutic technique (Fig. 20-14A).[54-56] The stereotaxic placement of the biopsy needle has become an extremely accurate technique. Successful biopsies of 5-mm lesions are now routine. Although CT guidance is presently required for stereotaxic biopsy, nonferromagnetic, stereotaxic frames that use MR imaging guidance are being developed (Fig. 20-14B).

MR imaging has also had a major impact on the approach to the treatment of CNS neoplasia with radiation therapy. The superior spatial and contrast resolution and multiplaner capability of MR imaging permit more precise planning of radiation therapy ports than was previously possible with CT. The graphic delineation of tumor margins in sagittal and coronal views allows the information obtained with MR imaging to be translated with high precision onto external beam radiation therapy simulation films. Both the stereotaxic technology and the precise anatomical information available from multiplaner images have greatly improved radiation therapy implant techniques as well.[57]

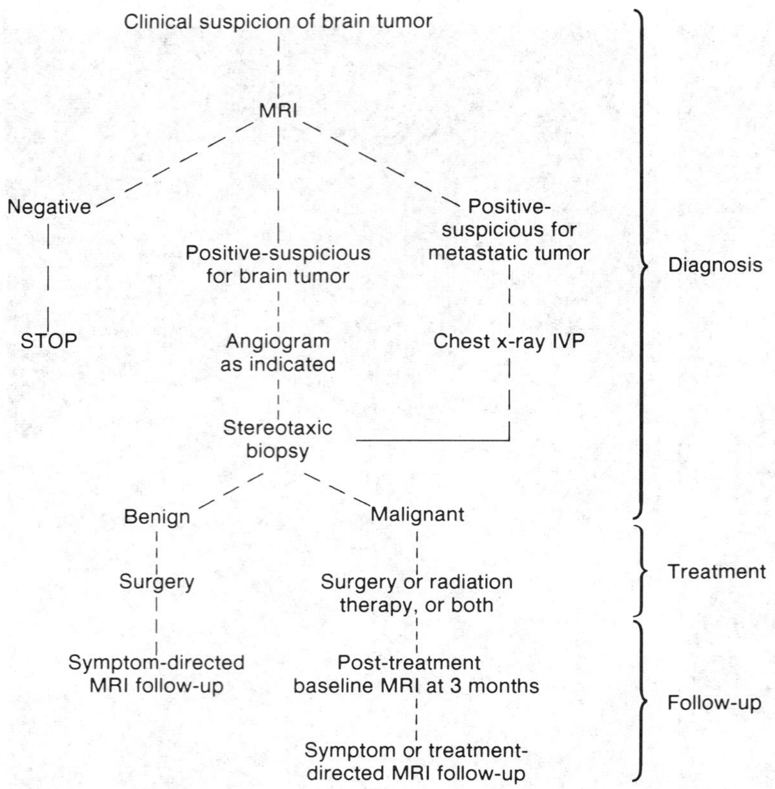

FIG. 20-13. Imaging decision algorithm for patients suspected of having a brain tumor. MRI, magnetic resonance imaging; IVP, intravenous pyelogram.

There are at least three drawbacks to the use of MR imaging for diagnosing CNS tumors. The first drawback becomes evident when the tumor-associated edema is extensive. Planning surgical margins and radiation ports in these cases may be difficult because of poor tumor-nidus definition. Intravenous administration of the paramagnetic contrast agent gadolinium-DTPA, which will be available in the near future, will solve the problem of tumor-nidus identification.[58–60] A second disadvantage is the inability of MR imaging to depict smaller deposits of calcification within the tumor. This shortcoming has proved to be more theoretical than real and has not caused particular problems in clinical practice. A third disadvantage, and one shared by both MR imaging and CT, is that neither modality easily differentiates radiation necrosis from recurrent tumor. Radiation necrosis of the CNS may occur from 1 month to 16 years after treatment, with the peak period of occurrence falling 1 to 3 years after radiation treatment.[61,62] At times, only biopsy can distinguish recurrent CNS tumor from radiation necrosis.

CENTRAL NERVOUS SYSTEM NEOPLASMS: SPINAL CORD

A second anatomical region of the CNS where MR imaging has replaced CT as the preferred method for evaluating suspected tumor is the spinal cord.[63,64] Patients presenting with myelopathy thought to be related to spinal cord neoplasia should now be initially evaluated with MR imaging (Fig. 20-15). This modality directly images the spinal cord, allowing tumors to be detected before an associated mass effect develops. A suggested decision tree for imaging patients with possible spinal cord cancer is given in Figure 20-16.

In addition to its use in diagnosing spinal cord tumors, MR imaging can, at times, distinguish tumor from secondary syringomyelia; this information can be used to plan the surgical margins and radiation therapy ports for each spinal cord tumor. MR imaging also demonstrates the level and extent of encroachment of metastatic epidural tumor on the spinal cord without the need for extensive patient repositioning or intrathecal contrast agent injection.[65] However, drop metastases (tumor deposits within the subarachnoid space of the spine that have spread from more central CNS tumors, such as medulloblastoma and pineal cancers), although occasionally identifiable with MR imaging, usually must still be evaluated with traditional CT/myelographic techniques because of their small size.

EXTRACRANIAL HEAD AND NECK CANCERS

The following discussion considers the issues surrounding the use of CT or MR imaging in the staging of head and neck neoplasms. Additional details on this subject, subdivided by major anatomical areas in the upper aerodigestive tract and neck, can be found in a text by Mancuso and Hanafee.[66]

The introduction of CT vastly expanded the role of radiology in the management of head and neck neoplasms. The radiologist's knowledge of the intricate CT anatomy of

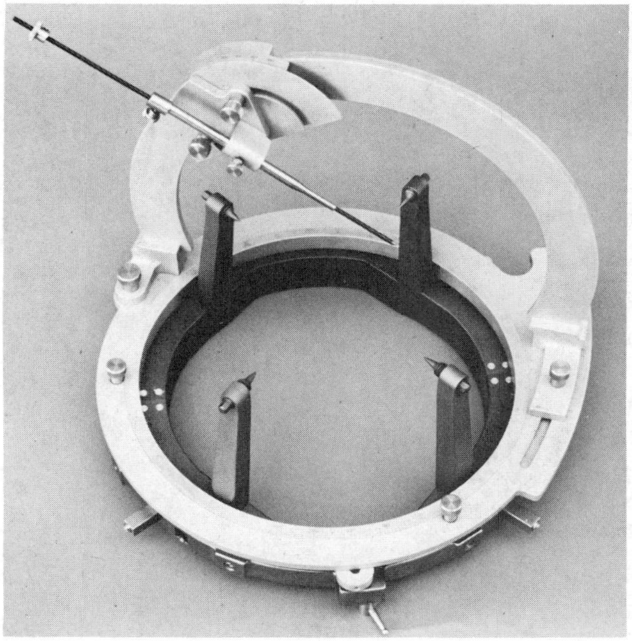

A

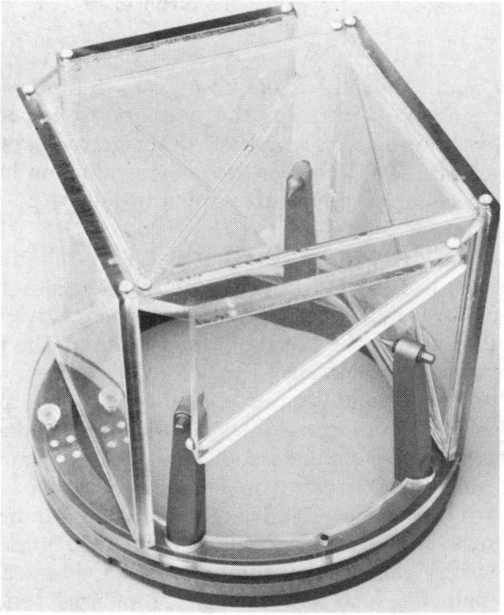

B

FIG. 20-14. Stereotaxic localization frames. **A**. Brown-Roberts-Wells frame, when placed on the patient's head, allows CT coordinates to be defined for placement of a percutaneous biopsy needle or localization of a brain lesion for treatment by interstitial techniques. **B**. Nonferromagnetic MR-compatible frame accomplishes the same goals for lesions identified by magnetic resonance imaging.

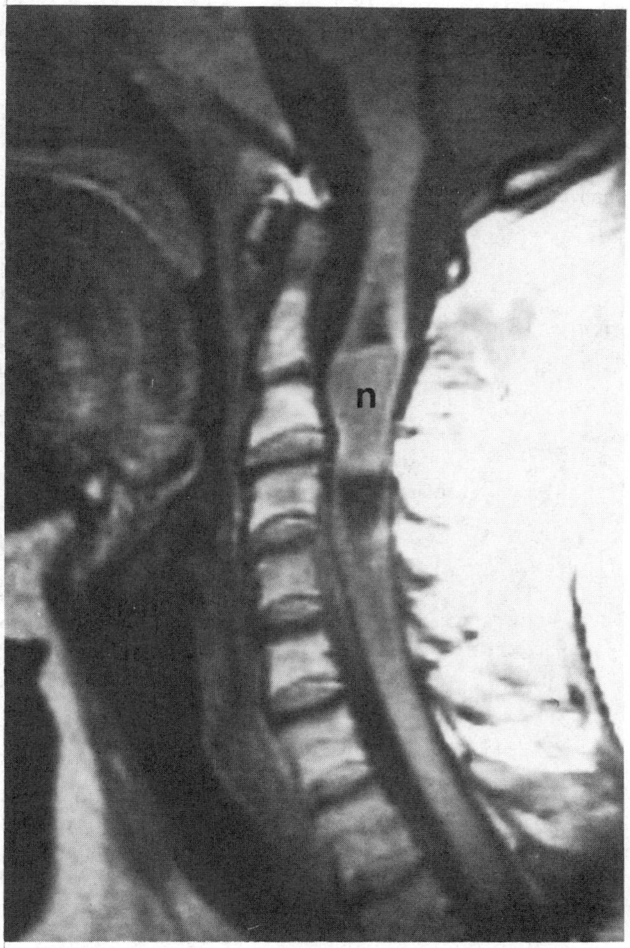

FIG. 20-15. Cervical cord astrocytoma. Sagittal MR image of the spinal cord diagnoses the intramedullary neoplasm (*n*).

the head and neck, coupled with his or her understanding of the routes of tumor spread by primary site location, allows tumor stage and extent to be determined accurately. As a result, the endoscopic demonstration of the mucosal extent of primary squamous carcinoma can be combined with CT mapping of the deep tissue and regional nodal involvement for a more specific pretreatment assessment of tumor stage.

As in the brain, MR imaging holds great promise for staging tumors of the upper aerodigestive tract and neck.[67-69] Clinical experience with MR imaging of the neck is limited, but the benefits of examining this area without the use of iodinated contrast agent or ionizing radiation are obvious. The routine use of direct sagittal and coronal imaging in tumors with known extensive craniocaudal spread patterns (nasopharynx and tongue base) will allow more complete pretreatment assessment of tumor extent. Early indications suggest that MR imaging will be more sensitive to cartilaginous invasion than will CT, which should prove extremely useful in staging laryngeal carcinoma.[68,70,71] Because of the potential of MR imaging to demonstrate tumor deposits in normal-sized lymph nodes, the detection of malignant lymph nodes may improve, especially with the use of Gd-DTPA. Soft tissue interfaces also are identified better on MR imaging, allowing the primary tumor mass to be differentiated from adjacent nodal involvement.[72]

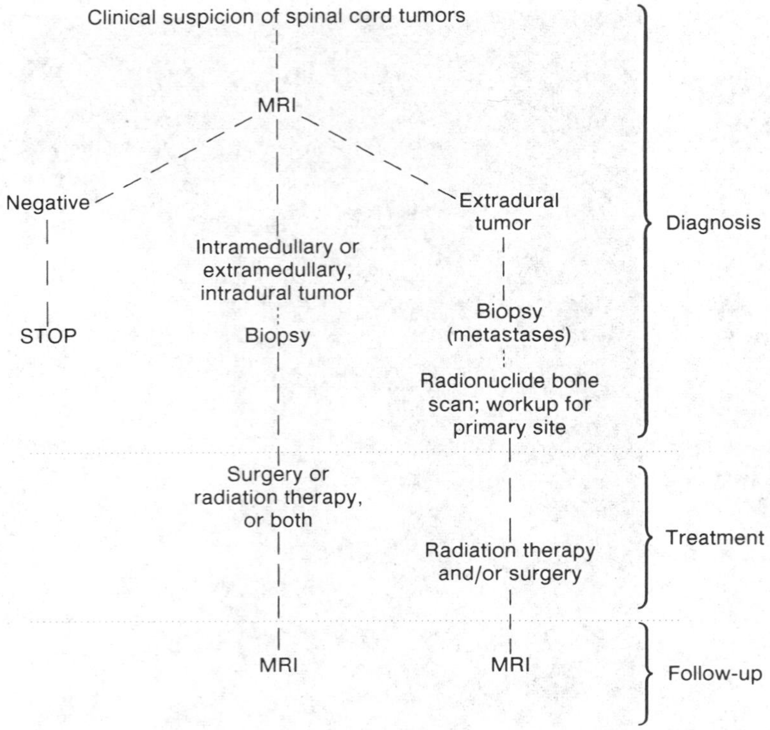

FIG. 20-16. Imaging decision algorithm for patients suspected of having a spinal cord cancer.

The principal disadvantage of MR imaging in the evaluation of head and neck cancer arises from the longer acquisition times necessary. Patients with head and neck squamous cell carcinoma often have obstructive pulmonary disease and an associated exaggerated respiratory motion that degrades MR images. The swallowing motion induced by bulky tumor may also degrade the MR image. Nevertheless, both CT and MR imaging can be effectively applied to this clinical problem.

Although the American Joint Committee's *TNM Staging Manual* currently recommends the use of CT in head and neck cancer only as an adjunctive procedure, extensive clinicopathologic correlation has shown CT to be a powerful imaging modality in evaluating head and neck neoplasms.[70,71,73] CT or MR imaging should be used as the oncologic imaging procedure of choice for the staging and follow-up of nearly all head and neck cancers. The primary role for CT or MR imaging is in staging the primary tumor site and in demonstrating regional nodal disease (Figs. 20-17 and 20-18). CT may also be occasionally helpful when an occult primary tumor of the head and neck is suspected.[74]

GENERAL NECK CT TECHNIQUE. Each CT examination is tailored to the area of the known primary tumor and regional lymphatics. Intravenous contrast agent is administered through a 19-gauge needle in the antecubital fossa vein with an initial 50-ml bolus of 60% meglumine iothalamate, followed by rapid drip infusion of 300 ml of 30% meglumine iothalamate. This rapid drip technique is mandatory for two reasons: (1) it allows neck vessels to be distinguished from lymph nodes (which do not enhance); and (2) extranodal disease and primary tumor extent are delineated best with contrast agent enhancement. Contiguous 5-mm-thick sections are obtained through the primary tumor site and throughout the regional lymphatic drainage routes. General guidelines on the CT format for nodal evaluation based on initial clinical impressions are shown in Figure 20-19.

STAGING THE PRIMARY TUMOR WITH CT. The overall purpose of using CT to stage the primary site of upper aerodigestive tract tumors is to obtain an objective impression of the actual extent of the primary lesion. The primary tumor extent classification (T) used by the American Joint Committee on Cancer is based entirely on size and anatomical extent of the tumor mass. This initial clinical–diagnostic stage is estimated from endoscopic and physical examination results; subsequent treatment decisions are based on this subjective impression. CT gives the clinician a more objective picture of the primary tumor's actual anatomical extent.[70,71,73,75,76] Submucosal tumor and tumor in areas difficult to palpate, such as the high oropharynx and nasopharynx, often will have more extensive deep tissue components on CT examination than are clinically apparent.[77,78] CT findings have been shown to alter treatment planning in up to 35% of patients as a result of changes in primary tumor extent (T) and nodal involvement (N) (Fig. 20-20).[79]

STAGING NECK NODES WITH CT. The reported frequency of cervical nodal metastases from squamous cell carcinoma in the head and neck has a wide variation that relates to the rich system of venous channels and lymphatics at the site of the primary tumor. The detection of cervical nodal metastases, either by clinical examination or with CT, will affect the mode of treatment and the general prognosis.[80]

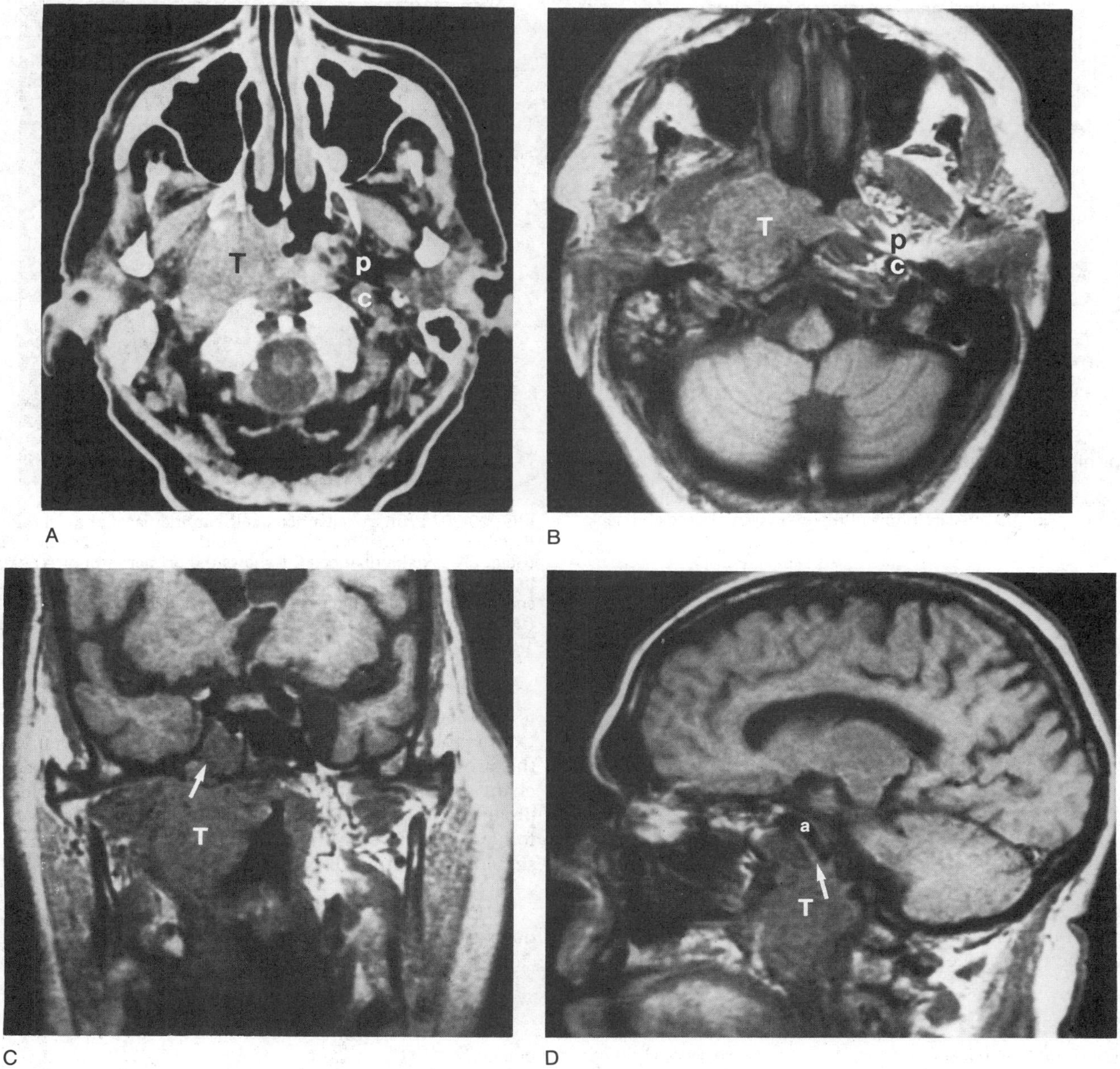

FIG. 20-17. CT and MR staging of nasopharyngeal carcinoma. **A**. Axial, enhanced CT through the nasopharynx shows the tumor (T) invading the parapharyngeal (*p*) and carotid (*c*) spaces. **B**. T-1 weighted axial MR image contains the same information. **C**. Direct sagittal and coronal (**D**) T-1 MR images display the exact craniocaudad extent of the tumor (T). In the sagittal image (**C**), perivascular spread (*arrow*) into the skull base along the internal carotid artery (*a*) is seen. On the coronal image (**D**), the tumor is seen invading (*arrow*) the sphenoid sinus (s).

The overall 5-year survival rate for patients with malignant cervical adenopathy at tumor diagnosis is less than 30%, regardless of primary tumor location.[81] The American Joint Committee's nodal staging criteria are based on the subjective evaluation, by neck palpation, as to the side, size, and extent of nodal disease in the neck. CT can give objectivity to the staging of cervical metastasis if strict criteria are applied.[73] Lymph nodes in the deep cervical chain larger than 1.5 cm, especially those with central necrosis (see Fig. 20-20), should be considered malignant. Extranodal disease is diagnosed when soft tissue planes around the abnormal lymph node are obscured.

The use of CT for tumor staging is limited by its lack of tissue specificity and reliance on size criteria to diagnose malignant adenopathy. Reactive hyperplasia has been shown to enlarge cervical lymph nodes, but generally the nodes will

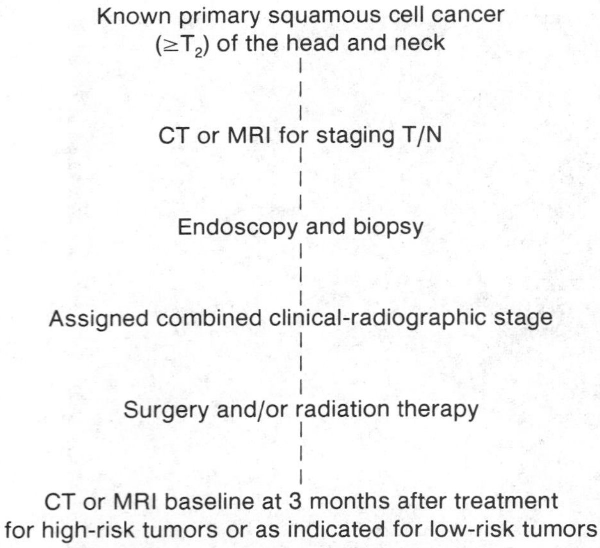

FIG. 20-18. Imaging decision algorithm for patients with known primary squamous cell carcinoma of the extracranial head and neck. T/N, tumor/nodal stage.

remain less than 1.5 cm in size.[72] Fine-needle aspiration biopsy in select cases can minimize false-positive results. Small tumor deposits in normal-sized lymph nodes will be missed on both clinical examination and CT.

RECURRENT TUMOR EVALUATION. CT can be a vital tool for evaluating tumor recurrence in the upper aerodigestive tract and neck.[78-82] Because of alterations in the normal deep tissue planes resulting from surgical or radiation therapy, such recurrences often are difficult to evaluate clinically. Subtle symptoms signaling recurrence often remain undiagnosed for months after their onset. In about 25% of cases of suspected tumor recurrence, CT will be the only means of diagnosis (Fig. 20–21). In one third of patients in whom the recurrence is clinically apparent, CT will show it

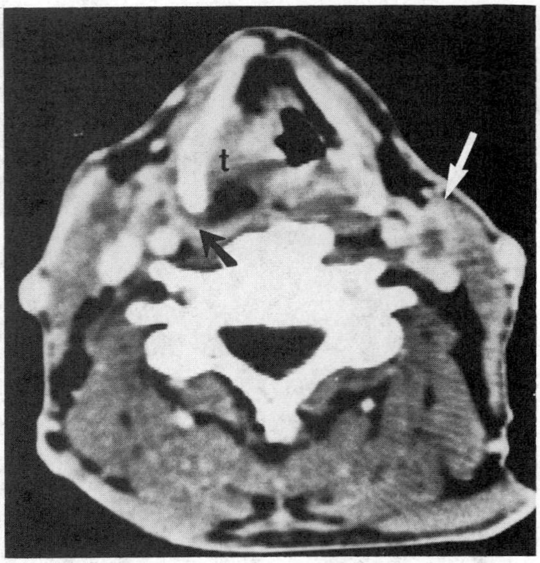

FIG. 20-20. Primary squamous cell carcinoma of the supraglottis. By clinical examination, this supraglottic tumor was labelled T2NO (Stage II). Axial, enhanced CT shows the primary tumor (*t*) extending into the soft tissues of the neck (*dark arrow*) and an 8 mm contralateral nodal metastasis in the middle, deep cervical chain (*white arrow*). CT upgraded this tumor from T2NO (Stage II) to T4N3C (Stage IV).

to be more extensive than was appreciated from physical examination alone.[78] The information available from CT on the presence and extent of recurrent tumor may lead to a change in the radiation therapy ports and the surgical approach.[78] As CT is applied more widely in post-treatment follow-up, delays in the diagnosis of tumor recurrences should be minimized.

THE UNKNOWN PRIMARY TUMOR. CT primarily functions as a staging tool in the workup of head and neck cancers. CT also plays a role in evaluating a small but trou-

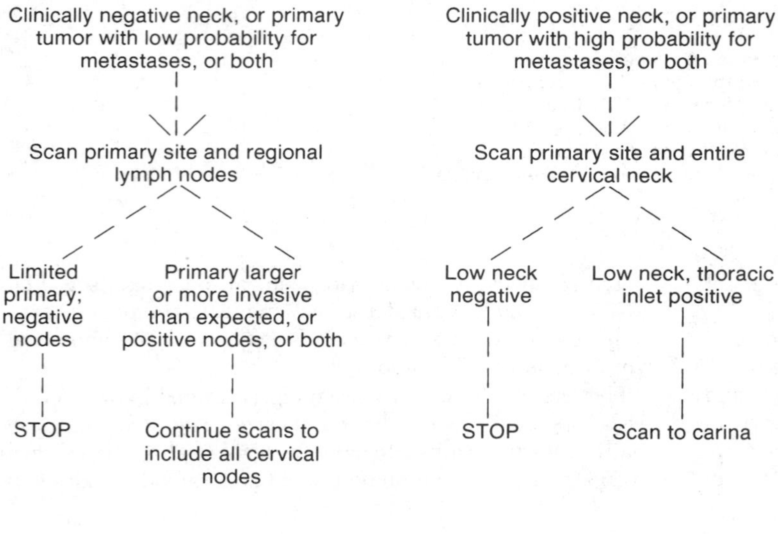

FIG. 20-19. CT protocol for studying neck adenopathy in patients with known primary squamous cell carcinoma of the head and neck. (Modified from Mancuso AA: Cervical lymph node metastases. In Bragg DG, Rubin P, Youker JE [eds]: Oncologic Imaging. Elmsford, New York, Pergamon Press, 1985)

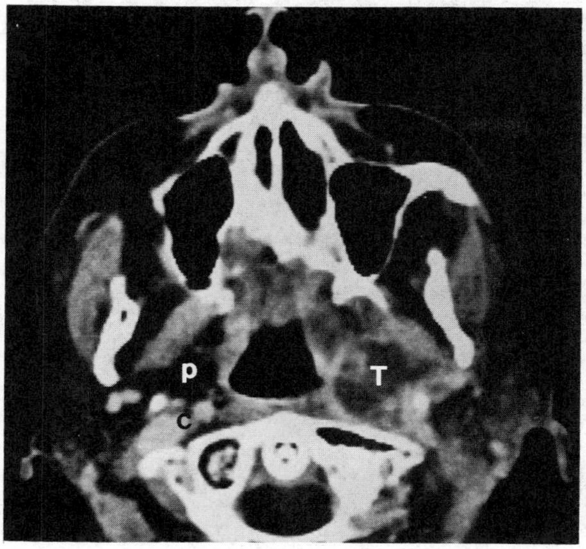

FIG. 20-21. Recurrent squamous cell carcinoma. Eighteen months after radiotherapy for Stage II (T2) carcinoma of the oropharyngeal tonsil, this patient presented with left ptosis and vocal cord paralysis. No mucosal tumor was seen on physical examination. Axial CT through the superior alveolar ridge demonstrates a deeply invasive recurrent tumor (*T*) that involves these parapharyngeal (*p*) and carotid (*c*) spaces on the left.

blesome group of patients in whom malignant adenopathy is present but the primary tumor is clinically occult. When fine-needle aspiration biopsy reveals a neck mass to be a metastatic squamous cell carcinoma in lymphatic tissue, and no primary source is found on endoscopy, the nodal disease may have originated outside the head and neck region or from an occult primary within the head and neck region.[73,81,84] In the case of an occult head and neck primary tumor, there are three possible explanations for the tumor's apparent absence: the primary tumor site may be very small; the tumor may have regressed after metastasizing to cervical lymph nodes; or the tumor is primarily submucosal in location.[77] In the last case, CT of the upper aerodigestive tract may identify the primary site when endoscopy is negative.[74] Careful attention to the nasopharynx, base of tongue, and piriform sinus is required because these are the areas in which occult carcinoma is commonly found.[83,84] CT is used in this setting to identify the primary tumor (when possible), to locate suspicious areas for deep tissue biopsy at the time of endoscopy, and to help stage the neck for additional nodal disease, extranodal tumor spread, and fixation to critical neck structures, such as the carotid artery. If no primary tumor is found to explain the patient's cervical disease, follow-up CT in 3 to 6 months to reevaluate the upper aerodigestive tract for occult submucosal malignancy is recommended.[74]

WILLIAM M. THOMPSON

Gastrointestinal and Genitourinary Systems

The newer imaging modalities of ultrasound (US), CT, and MR imaging provide exquisite multiplanar anatomical detail of the gastrointestinal (GI) and genitourinary systems. Based on this detail, specific information about tumor location, size, and extent can be obtained before surgery. This information, coupled with percutaneous biopsy results, provides meaningful staging data not previously available except through surgical and pathologic evaluation.[85,86]

Although not enough experience has accrued to define the advantages and disadvantages of the new imaging modalities in relation to the traditional radiologic techniques, or for that matter in relation to each other, some conclusions can be drawn from current data. Only the more recent and more consequential developments are discussed.

GASTROINTESTINAL TRACT CANCER

Although the cross-sectional imaging modalities play a relatively minor role in the detection of GI cancers, they have a major role in the preoperative staging and follow-up of certain tumors.[87–91] Unfortunately, these new imaging modalities cannot be used to stage GI tumors with the standard tumor-node—metastasis (TNM) system because they are limited in their ability to demonstrate the depth of bowel wall penetration, the T component of the TNM system; accurate demonstration of metastases in lymph nodes, the N criterion, is also beyond their capability.[88,89] Local invasion and distant metastases, especially to the liver, can be demonstrated accurately.

CT has been shown to be accurate in staging squamous cell carcinoma of the esophagus.[87,88,90] Although the barium swallow examination is more precise than CT for determining tumor length, local invasion (Fig. 20-22A) and distant metastases in the liver and subdiaphragmatic lymph nodes can be accurately detected with CT. One group reported poor results using CT for staging,[92] but there were some differences in their study compared with other reports.[87,88,90] CT has been shown to be helpful in evaluating patients who have had an esophagogastrectomy for esophageal cancer.[93]

Although the initial reports were favorable,[87,94] more recent studies[89,95] have shown that CT cannot be reliably used to stage gastric carcinoma (Fig. 20-22B) or colorectal adenocarcinoma (Fig. 20-22C)[89,96,97]; nor does CT accurately demonstrate the exact depth of bowel wall penetration or the presence of metastases in normal-sized lymph nodes, two major criteria in the TNM and Duke's staging systems. Many patients with gastric and colorectal adenocarcinoma have metastases in normal-sized (<1 cm) lymph nodes.[88,89,96,97] Thus, most recent reports do not recommend CT for routine preoperative staging in patients with adenocarcinoma of the stomach, colon, or rectum.[96,97] When indicated, CT can be used to accurately evaluate the liver and can demonstrate the

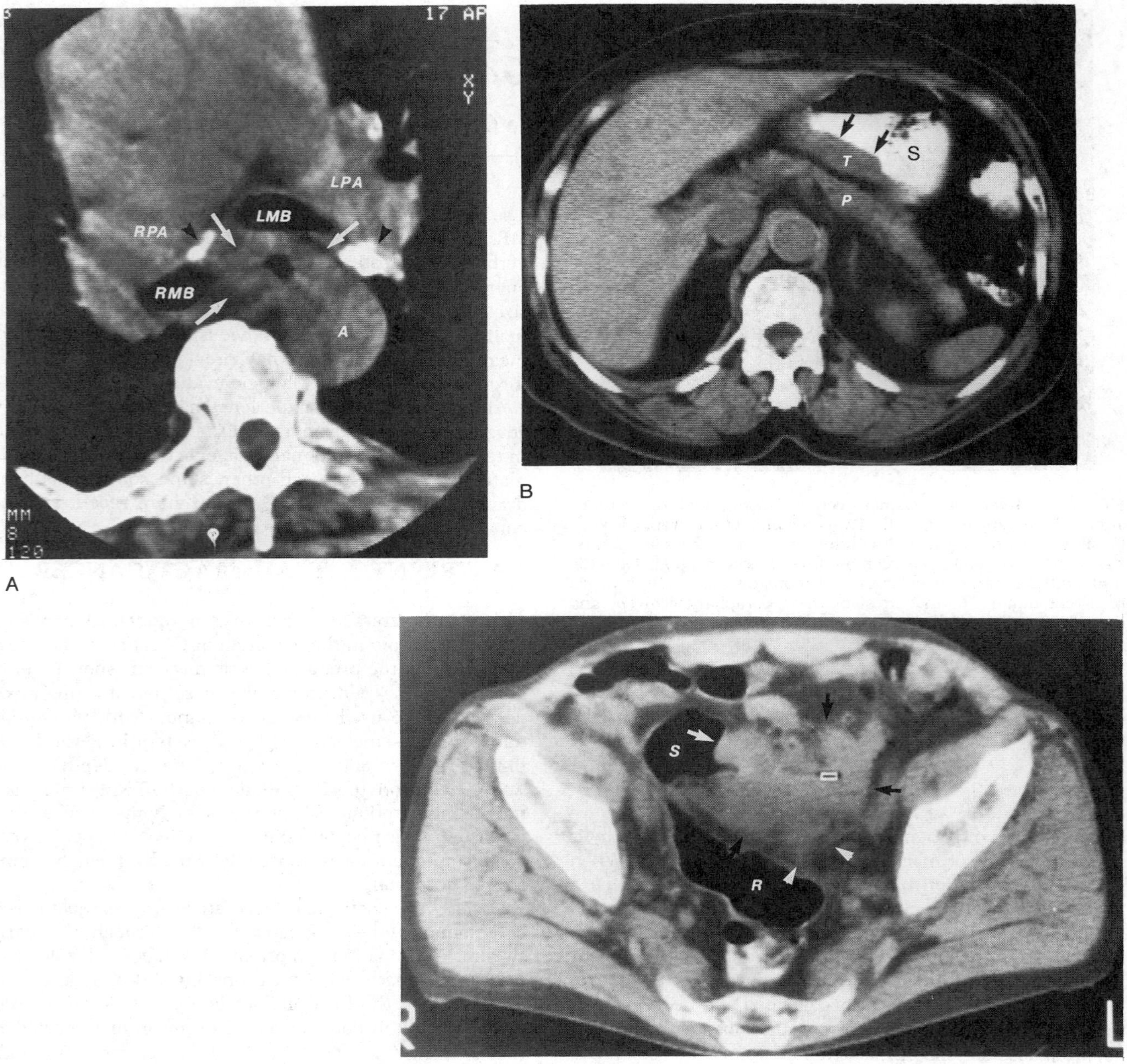

A

B

C

FIG. 20-22. CT imaging gastrointestinal malignancies. **A**. Esophageal carcinoma. CT section through level of carcinoma demonstrating a squamous cell carcinoma (*arrows*) locally invading the left main-stem bronchus (*LMB*) and aorta (*A*). Right main-stem bronchus (*RMB*), right pulmonary artery (*RPA*) and left pulmonary artery (*LPA*). Note calcification in mediastinal lymph nodes (*arrowheads*). **B**. Gastric carcinoma. CT through distal stomach (*S*) showing moderate thickening of posterior gastric wall (*arrows*) because of adenocarcinoma. The fat plane between the tumor (*T*) and the pancreas (*P*) is preserved. At operation the tumor did not extend into the pancreas; however, there were lymph nodes containing metastases in the surgical specimen which were not identified by CT. **C**. Sigmoid carcinoma. Dukes C—CT through level of midpelvis showing air in the rectum (*R*) and sigmoid (*S*). A large adenocarcinoma in the sigmoid (*arrows*) was partially obstructing the bowel lumen (cursor box). The tumor had extended through the bowel wall, which is suggested by the increased density in the pericolic fat (*arrowheads*). A number of lymph nodes in the resected specimen contained metastatic tumor. These were not identified by CT.

(continued)

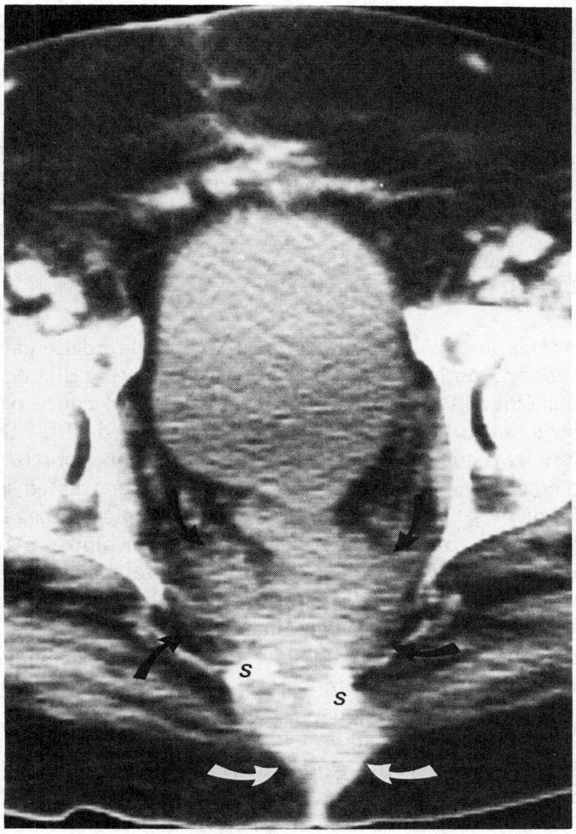

D

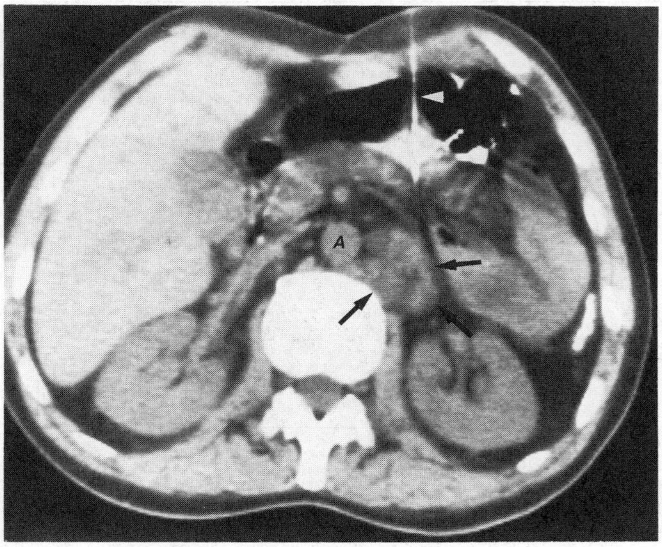

E

FIG. 20-22. *continued*
D. Recurrent rectal carcinoma. CT through pelvis in a 50-year-old man who had a rectal carcinoma resected 2 years earlier. A large soft tissue mass (*arrows*) is demonstrated in the presacral space and is extending from the bladder through the sacrum (*S*) to the subcutaneous tissues dorsal to the sacrum. The sacrum is being destroyed by the recurrent tumor. **E**. Recurrent rectosigmoid carcinoma in paraaortic lymph nodes. CT through level of kidneys during a percutaneous needle biopsy (needle, *arrowhead*) of enlarged lymph nodes (*arrows*) in the left paraaortic region. Cytologic evaluation confirmed metastatic adenocarcinoma. The patient's primary tumor had been resected 2 years earlier. A, aorta.

amount of extracolonic involvement in large tumors and those that have perforated.

CT has been shown to be effective in monitoring patients who have undergone surgical resection of rectosigmoid carcinoma.[89,96,97] Both postoperative changes and recurrent tumor (Fig. 20-22D) can be detected. In some cases, a percutaneous needle biopsy is required to distinguish between the two.[96-] However, if a baseline scan is obtained 3 to 4 months after surgery and the patient is rescanned periodically, postoperative changes can usually be distinguished from recurrent tumor. Since the majority of local rectosigmoid recurrences occur within 2 years of the primary resection, most authors recommend obtaining a postoperative baseline CT scan and then performing CT at 6-month intervals for at least 2 years. After 2 years, annual follow-up CT is adequate. All suspect lesions should be biopsied percutaneously.[85,86,96–98] Metastatic lymph nodes can be biopsied to confirm recurrence (Fig. 20-22E).

The few studies reported to date suggest that MR imaging is not likely to overcome the limitations of CT in evaluating patients with GI carcinoma.[92,99] One preliminary report has suggested that MR imaging may be able to distinguish postoperative fibrosis from recurrent tumor after resection of rectosigmoidal carcinoma.[100] However, no large series has been reported.

Figure 20-23 shows an imaging scheme for the workup of patients with known or suspected GI cancer. This scheme applies primarily to patients with squamous cell carcinoma of the esophagus, and adenocarcinoma of the stomach, small bowel, colon, and rectum. MR imaging is not included because of the current lack of data.

HEPATIC MALIGNANCIES — PRIMARY AND METASTATIC

Several imaging modalities are available to evaluate the liver. CT has been shown to be more sensitive and specific than the radionuclide liver–spleen scan or US for demonstrating both primary and metastatic lesions, especially if CT is coupled with a percutaneous fine-needle aspiration biopsy.[85,86,101,102] The radionuclide liver–spleen scan is still used by some as a screening study because of its lower cost and greater availability. However, it has low spatial resolution, is unable to detect lesions less than 2 cm in diameter, and rarely provides any etiologic information about the space-occupying lesion in the liver. Thus, both the false-negative and the false-positive rates for radionuclide scintigraphy are higher than for US or CT.

US has been shown to be less accurate than CT for detect-

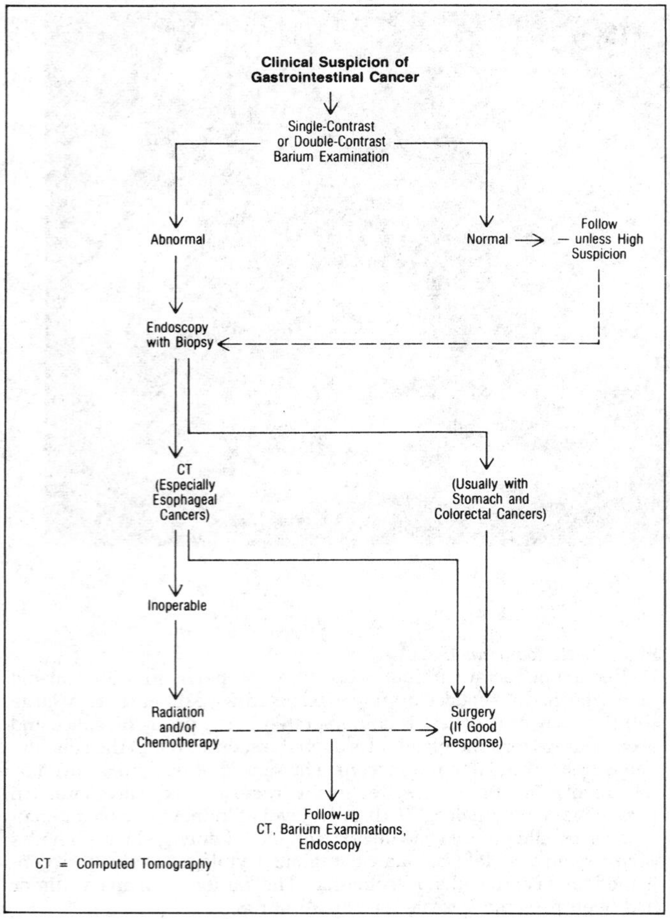

FIG. 20-23. Imaging decision tree for patients with suspected gastrointestinal cancer: Squamous cell carcinoma of the esophagus and adenocarcinoma of the stomach, small bowel, colon, and rectum. Most patients with stomach and colorectal tumors require surgery, so routine preoperative staging with CT is not recommended. CT may help define the extent of small bowel tumors prior to surgery. CT is best for follow-up of GI tumors. (Thompson WM: Imaging strategies for tumors of the gastrointestinal system. CA 37:165–186, 1987)

ing hepatic tumors.[101] Nevertheless, some investigators do advocate the use of US for detecting hepatic masses because of its lower cost and greater availability compared with CT. Also, tumors can be percutaneously biopsied under US guidance. Recently, investigators have used US in the operating room during hepatic resections and have found it is particularly useful for detecting hepatic tumors less than 3 cm in size. Operative US has been found to demonstrate more tumors than preoperative US, CT, or angiography.[103] This technique will be used with increasing frequency, especially in patients undergoing partial hepatectomy for metastatic disease.

Although CT has been the preferred technique for evaluating the liver for the past 6 to 8 years, MR imaging may demonstrate hepatic lesions not shown by even the most advanced CT scanning techniques.[104,105] Some tumors are more easily demonstrated by MR imaging than by CT (Fig. 20-24). MR imaging performed using specific tissue variables and higher resolution may lead to specific diagnoses and thus may replace CT as the reference standard for detecting and evaluating focal hepatic lesions. Whether percutaneous biopsy of hepatic tumors can be easily performed under MR imaging guidance is unknown at this time. An imaging scheme for hepatic tumors is shown in Figure 20-25. MR imaging is not included due to lack of experience with this modality.

PANCREATIC CANCER

For jaundiced patients thought to have a pancreatic cancer, US is frequently the best modality for detecting dilated bile ducts (Fig. 20-26).[106–108] If the location and cause of the obstruction cannot be adequately demonstrated with US, CT is usually recommended. If the cause and level of obstruction can be determined with CT, the patient can be treated surgically or by percutaneous drainage; endoscopic drainage can also be performed. A fine-needle aspiration biopsy may be needed to confirm the diagnosis. If the level or cause of the obstruction cannot be determined with US or CT, then endoscopic retrograde cholangiopancreatography (ERCP) or percutaneous transhepatic cholangiography (PTC) should be performed to clearly demonstrate the site of obstruction.

The new percutaneous radiologic techniques have had their greatest impact in cases of obstructive jaundice due to malignancy, especially pancreatic carcinoma. Not only can the radiologist confirm the level of obstruction with US and CT[106–108] and establish the diagnosis with a fine-needle aspiration biopsy,[85,86] he or she can now treat the malignant obstruction with percutaneous transhepatic biliary drainage.[109–112] This technique has been used most commonly to decompress the biliary system and allow the serum bilirubin level to decline before operative intervention. Chemotherapeutic agents and local radiation therapy can also be administered through the catheter. In some patients with advanced disease or who refuse an operation, the bile ducts can be permanently drained by converting the external percutaneous transhepatic biliary drainage system to an internal drainage system. Ring and Kerlan have used an endoprosthesis in some patients and have found that the larger endoprosthetic devices remain patent for at least 6 months, thereby functioning beyond the survival of most patients with pancreatic cancer.[111] There is a higher complication rate associated with the endoprosthesis than with the external catheter, and some authors have abandoned its use.[112] Others continue to use an endoprosthesis but take the high complication rate into consideration when deciding what type of drainage should be performed.[111,113]

MR imaging is not included in the imaging scheme in Figure 20-25 because to date it has not been shown to be more accurate than CT.[114]

GENITOURINARY TRACT CANCERS

RENAL CARCINOMA

Despite the greater accuracy of CT, excretory urography, which is more available, costs less, and has an acceptable accuracy, continues to be considered the best imaging mo-

FIG. 20-24. **A**. Contrast-enhanced CT scan through liver in a 30-year-old man with a hepatoma involving left lobe of liver. Note calcification in center of lesion *(arrowhead)*, subtle fullness of left lobe of liver *(arrows)*, and extension of tumor to local nodes *(curved arrows)*. S, stomach containing contrast; SP, spleen; K, left kidney; A, aorta. **B**. MR image of same patient at similar location in liver. This T_1-weighted (TR 2000 MSEC TE 160 MSEC) image shows the hepatoma involving the left lobe of liver. Note fullness of left lobe *(arrows)*, tumor extension *(curved arrows)*, and no evidence of the calcification (a limitation of MRI). PV, portal veins; IVC, inferior vena cava; A, aorta; S, stomach; SP, spleen. **C**. The tumor *(arrows)* is shown much better on the T_2-weighted (TR 2000 TE 20) image, because it has a stronger signal than the remainder of the liver. (Thompson WM: Imaging strategies for tumors of the gastrointestinal system. 37:165–186, 1987)

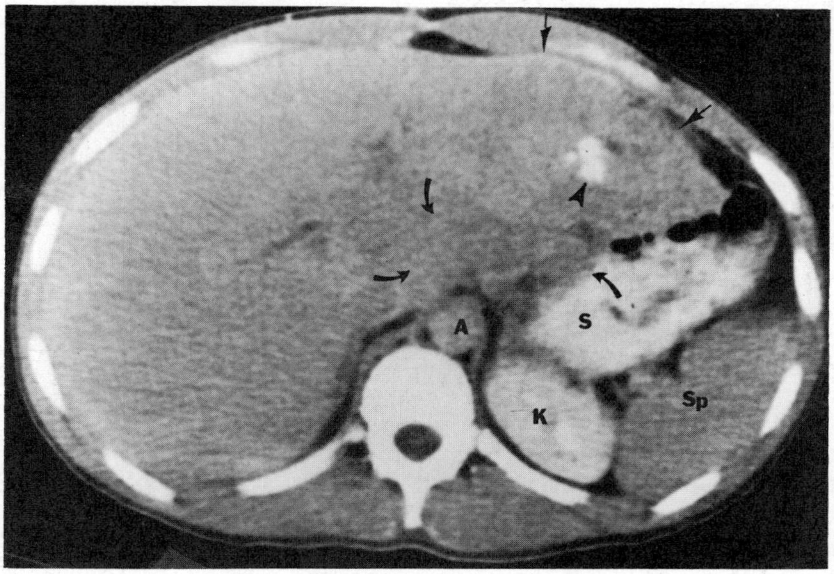

A

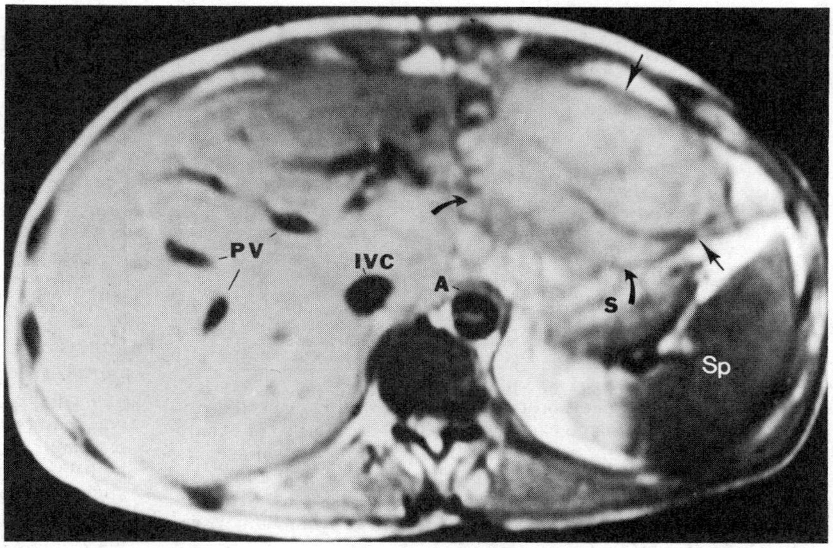

B

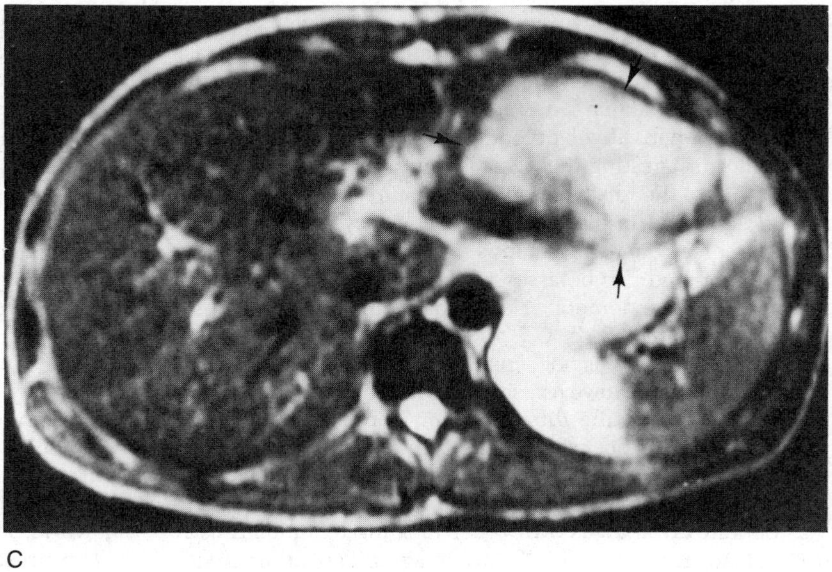

C

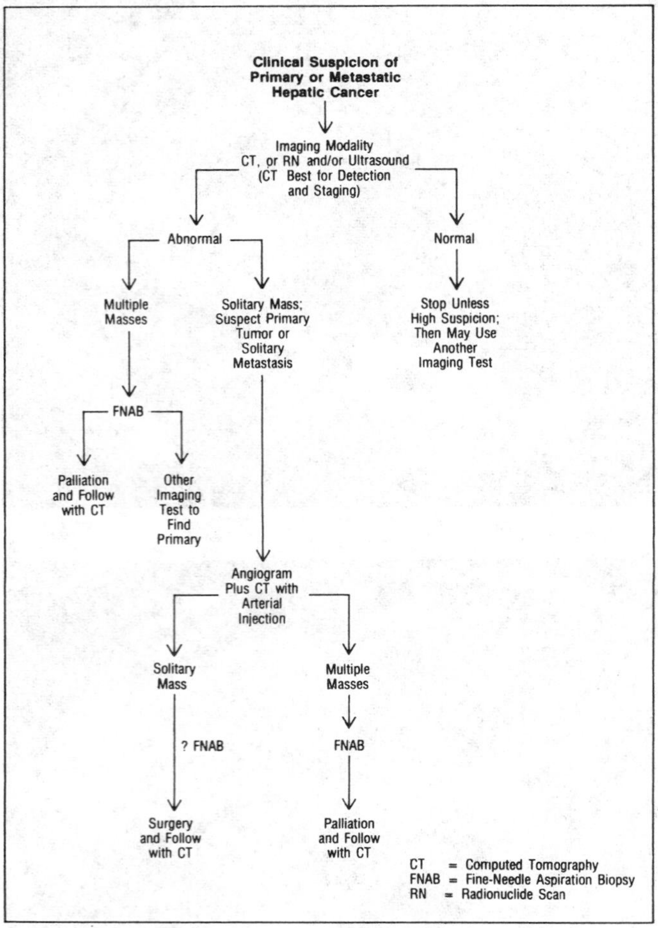

FIG. 20-25. Imaging decision tree for patients with suspected primary or metastatic hepatic cancer. CT is the best method of examination for detection, but cost and limited availability in some cases will dictate use of radionuclide scan or ultrasound, or both. Fine-needle aspiration biopsy is helpful in confirming metastases. (Thompson WM: Imaging strategies for tumors of the gastrointestinal system. CA 37:165–186, 1987)

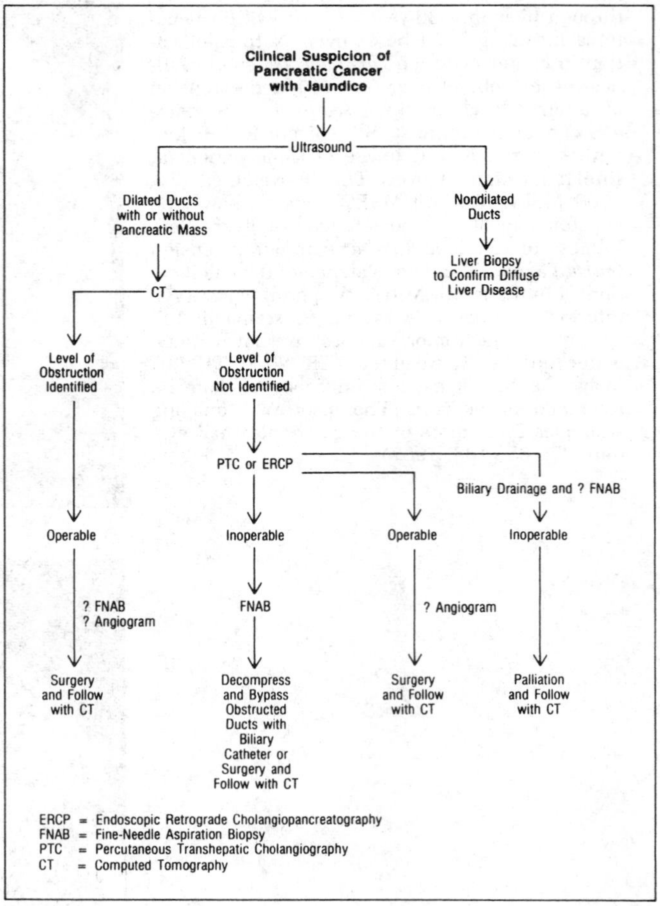

FIG. 20-26. Imaging decision tree for jaundiced patients suspected of having pancreatic cancer. If CT confirms obstructive jaundice and shows the level of obstruction and pancreatic head mass, many patients can go to surgery from CT. Some surgeons may request both fine needle aspiration biopsy to confirm the diagnosis and an angiogram to define the peripancreatic blood vessels. Follow-up of pancreatic tumors is best performed by CT. (Thompson WM: Imaging strategies for tumors of the gastrointestinal system. CA 37:165–186, 1987)

dality for screening patients suspected of having a renal carcinoma.[115] Once a solid renal mass is identified, contrast agent–enhanced CT is of major value in confirming the solid nature of the mass, in staging, in detecting contralateral kidney or venous involvement, and in detecting fat within the tumor, suggesting that it is benign.[115,116] CT is useful in determining the distribution of calcium within a lesion, which is helpful in distinguishing benign cysts from malignant tumors. Venous invasion is of particular importance to the surgeon and can be assessed during CT with bolus contrast agent enhancement. If the renal veins cannot be completely evaluated with CT, US or angiography may be necessary.[115–117] CT is not sensitive in the evaluation of perinephric invasion. However, since most patients undergo radical nephrectomy, the differentiation between Stage I and Stage II tumors is not critical. The overall accuracy of CT for staging renal carcinoma is 90%.[118]

Although much more experience is needed, MR imaging has definite advantages over other imaging techniques used to evaluate renal tumors.[119] MR imaging can differentiate solid masses from benign cystic lesions and can demonstrate major blood vessels and vascular invasion without administration of contrast medium (Fig. 20-27). Limited availability, high cost, long imaging times, inability to demonstrate calcium, and motion artifacts are current disadvantages of MR imaging in the evaluation of renal carcinoma.

Since a number of modalities can identify a solid mass in the kidney, no specific imaging scheme has been developed.[115] Some patients may go directly to surgery after excretory urography. Currently, CT provides the best overall staging information.[118]

PROSTATIC CARCINOMA

The digital rectal examination of the prostate has been the reference standard for the evaluation of prostatic carcinoma with respect to detection, tumor size, prognosis, and response to therapy.[120] However, this examination has been shown to be relatively inaccurate.[121]

The prostate has a central zone and a peripheral zone;

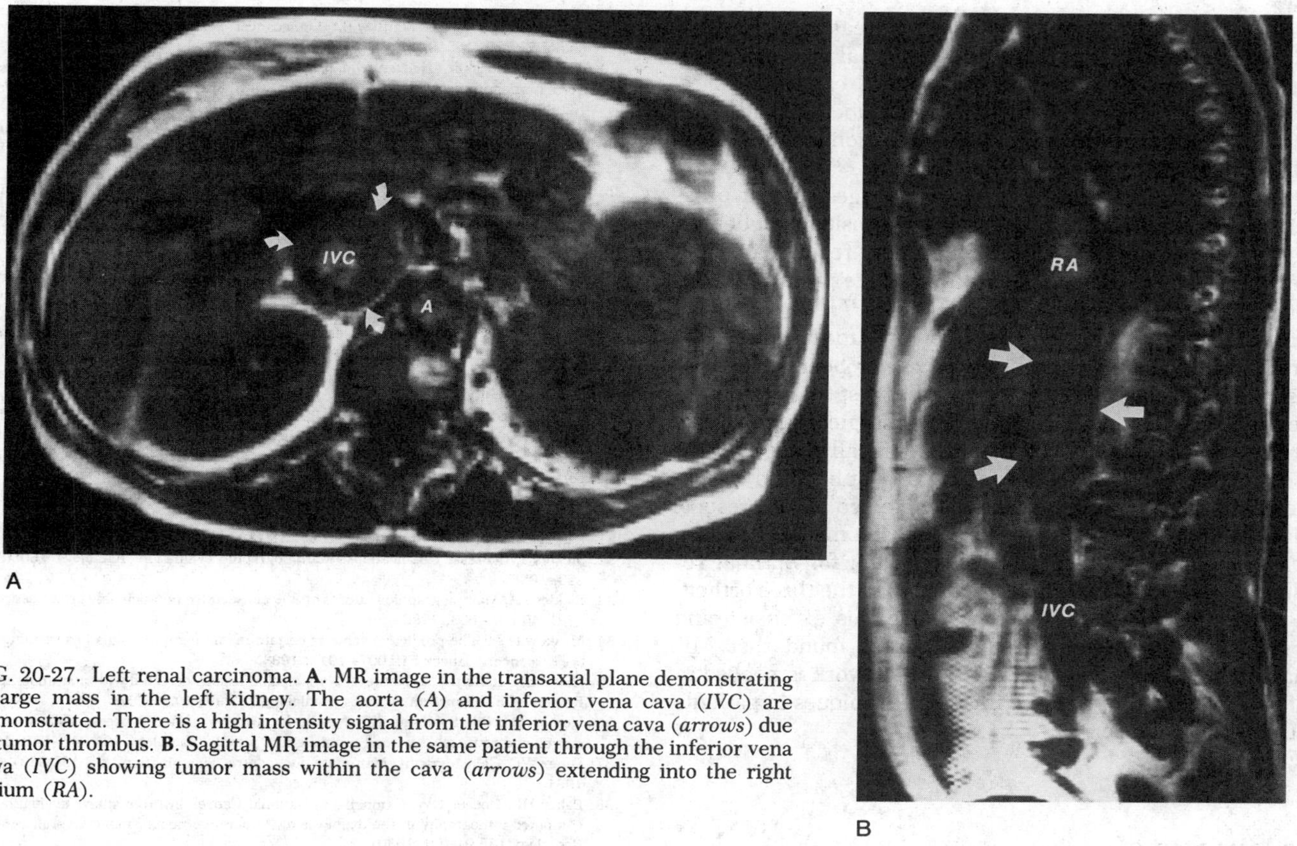

FIG. 20-27. Left renal carcinoma. **A**. MR image in the transaxial plane demonstrating a large mass in the left kidney. The aorta (*A*) and inferior vena cava (*IVC*) are demonstrated. There is a high intensity signal from the inferior vena cava (*arrows*) due to tumor thrombus. **B**. Sagittal MR image in the same patient through the inferior vena cava (*IVC*) showing tumor mass within the cava (*arrows*) extending into the right atrium (*RA*).

tumors commonly originate in the latter, within a few millimeters of the prostate capsule, and spread by infiltrating adjacent tissue just beneath the capsule and by extending toward the central gland. A variety of imaging techniques have been used to detect and stage prostatic carcinoma.

Transrectal US has recently been developed for evaluating the prostate and has proved more sensitive than digital examination for detecting abnormalities.[122-124] Certain sonographic features suggest benign disease, including areas of increased echogenicity that lie entirely within the prostate.[122] Areas of decreased echogenicity purely within the peripheral zone are highly suggestive of cancer (Fig. 20-28).[122-124] There is some overlap, and most investigators believe that all suspect lesions should be biopsied.[123] Rifkin et al, in the largest series reported to date, found no specific US characteristics that differentiated between many cases of benign prostatic disease and malignancy. Transrectal US may help determine which areas should be biopsied.[123] Also,

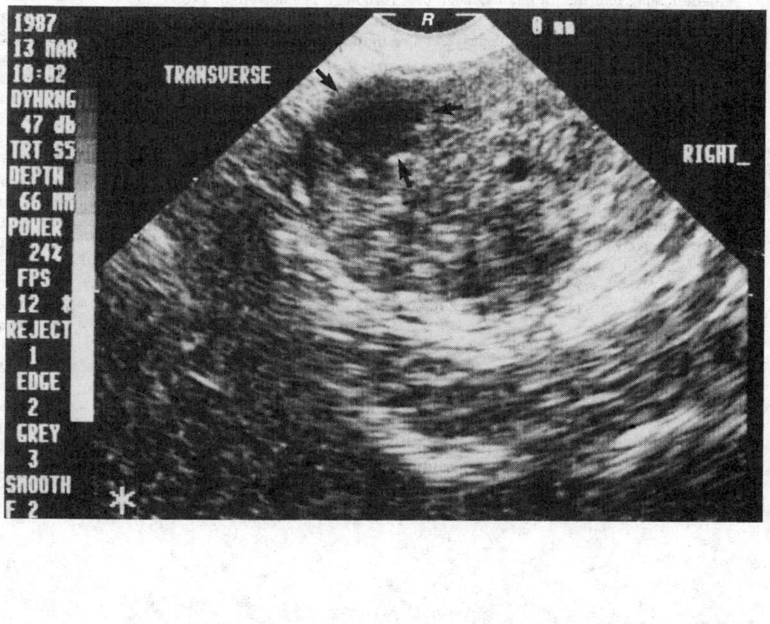

FIG. 20-28. Prostatic cancer: transrectal ultrasound. Transrectal ultrasound through level of prostate, a hypoechoic area is demonstrated in the peripheral zone to the right of midline (*arrows*), rectal lumen (*R*). Ultrasound guided needle biopsy of the lesion was positive for adenocarcinoma.

transrectal US can accurately delineate areas that are difficult to palpate, or sonographically abnormal areas that are not palpable. At this time, transrectal US cannot be used alone as a screening technique. In conjunction with US-guided biopsy, however, it allows the detection of many clinically nonpalpable, subtle prostatic cancers.[123]

Initial experience with MR imaging suggested that prostatic carcinoma had a different signal intensity than benign prostatic hypertrophy[125,126]; however, more recent data have shown that MR imaging cannot differentiate prostatic carcinoma from benign prostatic hypertrophy.[127,128]

Both CT and MR imaging have been used to stage prostatic carcinoma. The results with CT have not been favorable. Based on their experience, Platt et al suggest that CT not be used to influence decisions concerning surgical versus nonsurgical treatment in patients with clinically staged local disease. CT has been useful for staging only when unsuspected metastatic nodal disease was detected.[129] At present, MR imaging is the most accurate diagnostic modality for the local staging of carcinoma of the prostate; for optimal results, multiple sequences and at least two of the three orthogonal imaging planes are needed. Using this extensive and time-consuming technique, Hricak et al found that MR imaging had an 83% accuracy.[130] Further work is needed to define the exact role of these imaging techniques in patients with prostatic cancer.

REFERENCES

1. Bragg DG, Rubin P, Youker J (eds): *Oncologic Imaging.* Elmsford, NY, Pergamon Press, 1985
2. Marx JL: Imaging technique passes muster. *Science* 238:888–889, 1987
3. Haggar AM, Pearlberg JL, Froelich JW et al: Chest-wall invasion by carcinoma of the lung: Detection by MR imaging. AJR 148:1075–1078, 1987
4. Wetzel LH, Levine E, Murphey MD: A comparison of MR imaging and CT in the evaluation of musculoskeletal masses. RadioGraphics 7:851–874, 1987
5. Adams V, Krishnan KU, Muhm JR et al: Diffuse malignant mesothelioma of pleura: Diagnosis and survival in 92 cases. Cancer 58:1540–1551, 1986
6. Mirvis S, Dutcher JP, Haney PJ et al: CT of malignant pleural mesothelioma. AJR 140:665–670, 1983
7. Dedrick CG, McCloud TC, Shepard JO et al: Computed tomography of localized pleural mesothelioma. AJR 144:275–280, 1985
8. Muhm JR, Miller WE, Fontana RS et al: Lung cancer detected during a screening program using four-month chest radiographs. Radiology 148:609–615, 1983
9. Frost JK, Ball WC, Levin ML et al: Early lung cancer detection: Results of the initial (prevalence) radiologic and cytologic screening in the Johns Hopkins study. Am Rev Respir Dis 130:549–554, 1984
10. Flehinger BJ, Melamed MR, Zaman MB et al: Early lung cancer detection: Results of the initial (prevalence) radiologic and cytologic screening in the Memorial Sloan-Kettering study. Am Rev Respir Dis 130:555–560, 1984
11. Fontana RS, Sanderson DR, Taylor WF et al: Early lung cancer detection: Results of the initial (prevalence) radiologic and cytologic screening in the Mayo Clinic study. Am Rev Respir Dis 130:561–565, 1984
12. Filderman AE, Shaw C, Matthay RA: Lung cancer: Part I. Etiology, pathology, natural history, manifestations and diagnostic techniques. Invest Radiol 21:80–90, 1986
13. Armstrong JD, Bragg DG: Thoracic neoplasms: Imaging requirements for diagnostic and staging. In Bragg DG, Rubin P, Youker J (eds): Oncologic Imaging, chap 10. Elmsford, NY, Pergamon Press, 1985
14. Siegelman SS, Zerhouni EA, Leo FP et al: CT of the solitary pulmonary nodule. AJR 135:1–13, 1980
15. Heitzman ER: The Lung: Radiologic–Pathologic Correlations. St Louis, CV Mosby, 1984
16. Muhm JR, Brown LR, Crowe JK et al: Comparison of whole lung tomography and computed tomography for detecting pulmonary nodules. AJR 131:981–984, 1978
17. Zerhouni EA, Stitik FP, Seigelman SS et al: CT of the pulmonary nodule: Cooperative study. Radiology 160:319–327, 1986
18. Epstein DM, Stephenson LW, Gefter WB et al: Value of CT in the preoperative assessment of lung cancer: A survey of thoracic surgeons. Radiology 161:423–427, 1986
19. Filderman AE, Shaw C, Matthay RA: Lung cancer: Part II. staging and therapy. Invest Radiol 21:173–185, 1986
20. Poon PY, Bronskill MJ, Henkelman RM et al: Mediastinal lymph node metastases from bronchogenic carcinoma: Detection with MR imaging and CT. Radiology 162:651–656, 1987
21. vanSonnenberg E, Lin AS, Deutsch AL et al: Percutaneous biopsy of difficult mediastinal, hilar and pulmonary lesions by computed tomographic guidance and a modified coaxial technique. Radiology 148:300–302, 1983
22. Perlmutt LM, Braun SD, Newman GE: Transthoracic needle aspiration: Use of a small chest tube to treat pneumothorax. AJR 148:849–851, 1987
23. Winkler M, Higgins CB: Suspected intracardiac masses: Evaluation with MR imaging. Radiology 165:117–122, 1987
24. Egan RL: Experience with mammography in a tumor institution: Evaluation of 1,000 studies. Radiology 75:894–900, 1960
25. Wolfe JN: Xerography of the breast. Radiology 91:231–240, 1968
26. Pagani JJ, Bassett LW, Gold RH et al: Efficacy of combined film-screen/xeromammography: Preliminary report. AJR 135:144–146, 1980
27. Shapiro S, Venet W, Strax P et al: Ten to fourteen year effect of screening on breast cancer mortality. JNCI 69:349–355, 1982
28. Tabar L, Gad A, Holmberg LH et al: Reduction in mortality from breast cancer after mass screening with mammography. Lancet 1:829–832, 1985
29. Baker LH: Breast Cancer Detection Demonstration Project: Five-year summary report. CA 32:196–225, 1982
30. Gold RH, Bassett LW, Kimme-Smith C: Breast imaging: State-of-the-art. Invest Radiol 21:298–304, 1986
31. Paulus D: Imaging in breast cancer. CA 37:133–150, 1987
32. Sickles EA: Breast calcifications: Mammographic evaluation. Radiology 160:289–293, 1986
33. Sickles EA: Mammographic features of 300 consecutive non-palpable breast cancers. AJR 146:661–663, 1986
34. Moskowitz M: The predictive value of certain mammographic signs in screening for breast cancer. Cancer 51:1007–1011, 1983
35. Ciatto S, Cataliotti L, Distante V: Nonpalpable lesions detected with mammography: Review of 512 consecutive cases. Radiology 165:99–102, 1987
36. Homer MJ, Pile-Spellman ER: Needle localization of occult breast lesions with a curved-end retractable wire: Technique and pitfalls. Radiology 161:547–548, 1986
37. Diner WC: Galactography: Mammary duct contrast examination. AJR 137:853–856, 1981
38. Baker HL, Houser OW, Cambell JK: National Cancer Institute study: Evaluation of computed tomography in the diagnosis of intracranial neoplasms. I. Overall results. Radiology 136:91–96, 1980
39. Bismar J, Stromblad LG, Stanford LG: Impact of CT in the neurosurgical management of intracranial tumors. Neuroradiology 16:506–509, 1978
40. Davis DO: CT in the diagnosis of supratentorial tumors. Semin Roentgenol 12:97–108, 1977
41. Enzmann DR, Norman D, Levin V et al: Computed tomography in the follow-up of medulloblastomas and ependymomas. Radiology 128:57–63, 1978
42. Marks JE, Gado M: Serial computed tomography of primary brain tumors following surgery, irradiation, and chemotherapy. Radiology 125:119–125, 1977
43. Norman D, Enzmann DR, Levin VA et al: Computed tomography in the evaluation of malignant glioma before and after therapy. Radiology 121:85–88, 1976
44. Anderson R: Brain and spinal cord neoplasms. In Bragg DG, Rubin P (eds): Oncologic Imaging. New York, John Wiley & Sons, 1984
45. Weinstein MA, Modic MT, Pavlicek W et al: Nuclear magnetic resonance for the examination of brain tumors. Semin Roentgenol 19:139–147, 1984
46. Brant-Zawadzki M, Norman D, Newton TH et al: Magnetic resonance of the brain: The optimal screening technique. Radiology 152:71–77, 1984
47. Brant-Zawadzki M, Badami JP, Mills CM et al: Primary intracranial tumor imaging: A comparison of magnetic resonance and CT. Radiology 150:435–440, 1984
48. Zimmerman RA: Magnetic resonance of cerebral neoplasms. Magnetic Resonance Annual, New York, 1985
49. Partain CL, James AE, Rollo FD et al: Nuclear Magnetic Resonance (NMR) Imaging. Philadelphia, WB Saunders, 1983
50. Mills CM et al: Nuclear magnetic resonance: Principles of blood flow imaging. AJNR 4:1161–1166, 1983
51. Brant-Zawadski M: Magnetic resonance imaging principles: The bare necessities. In Brant-Zawadski M, Norman D (eds): Magnetic Resonance Imaging of the Central Nervous System, pp 1–12. New York, Raven, 1987
52. Bradley W, Newton T, Crooks LE: Physical properties of NMR. In Newton TH, Potts DG (eds): Modern Neuroradiology, Vol 2, Advanced Imaging Techniques, pp 15–61. San Francisco, Clavadel Press, 1983
53. Young IR, Burl M, Clarke G et al: Magnetic resonance properties of hydrogen: Imaging the posterior fossa. AJR 137:895–901, 1981
54. Brown RA, Roberts TS, Osborn AG: Simplified CT guided stereotactic biopsy. AJNR 2:181–184, 1981
55. Kelly PJ, Alker GJ: A method for sterotactic laser microsurgery in treatment of deep-seated CNS neoplasms. Appl Neurophysiol 43:210–215, 1980
56. Sheldon CA, McCann G, Jacques S et al: Development of a computerized microstereotaxic method for localization and removal of minute CNS lesions under direct 3-D vision. J Neurosurg 52:21–27, 1900
57. Sapozink MO, Moeller JH, McDonald DN et al: Improved precision of interstitial brain tumor irradiation using the BRW CT stereotactic guidance system (unpublished)

58. Graif M, Bydder GM, Steiner RE et al: Contrast-enhanced MR imaging of malignant brain tumors. AJNR 6:855–862, 1985
59. Carr DH, Brown J, Bydder GM et al: Gadolinium-DTPA as a contrast agent in MRI: Initial clinical experience in 70 patients. AJR 143:215–224, 1984
60. Claussen C, Laniado M, Schorner W et al: Gadolinium-DTPA in MR imaging of glioblastomas and intracranial metastases. AJNR 6:699–674, 1985
61. Kingsley DP, Kendall BE: CT of the adverse effects of therapeutic radiation of the central nervous system. AJNR 2:453–460, 1981
62. Kramer S, Lee KF: Complications of radiation therapy: The central nervous system. Semin Roentgenol 9:75–83, 1974
63. DiChiro G, Doppman JL, Swyer AJ et al: Tumors and arteriovenous malformations on the spinal cord: Assessment using MR. Radiology 156:689–697, 1985
64. Norman D: The spine. In Brant-Zawadski M, Norman D (eds): Magnetic Resonance Imaging of the Central Nervous System, pp 289–328. New York, Raven, 1987
65. Smoker WRK, Godersky C, Knutson RK et al: The role of MRI in the evaluation of metastatic spinal disease. AJNR 8:901–908, 1987
66. Mancuso AA, Hanafee WN: Computed Tomography of the Head and Neck. Baltimore, Williams & Wilkins, 1982
67. Dillon WP, Mills CM, Kjos B et al: Magnetic resonance imaging of the nasopharynx. Radiology 152:731–738, 1984
68. Lufkin RB, Hanafee WN, Wortham D et al: Larynx and hypopharynx: MR imaging with surface coils. Radiology 158:747–754, 1986
69. Lufkin RB, Larssan SG, Hanafee WN: NMR anatomy of larynx and tongue base. Radiology 148:173–175, 1983
70. Archer CR, Yeager VL: Computed tomography of laryngeal cancer with histopathological correlation. Laryngoscope 92(20):1173–1180, 1982
71. Mafee MF, Schild JA, Valvassori GE et al: Computed tomography of the larynx: Correlation with anatomic and pathologic studies in cases of laryngeal carcinoma. Radiology 147:128, 1983
72. Mancuso AA: Cervical lymph node metastases. In Bragg DG, Rubin P, Youker J (eds): Oncologic Imaging. Elmsford, NY, Pergamon Press, 1985
73. Mancuso AA, Harnsberger HRN et al: Computed tomography of cervical and retropharyngeal lymph nodes: Normal anatomy, variants of normal, and applications in staging head and neck cancer. Parts I and II. Radiology 148:709–714, 1983
74. Muraki AS, Mancuso AA, Harnsberger HR: Metastatic cervical adenopathy from tumors of unknown origin: The role of computed tomography. Radiology 152:749–753, 1984
75. Silver JA, Mawad ME, Hilal SK et al: Computed tomography of the nasopharynx and related spaces: Part II. Pathology. Radiology 147:733–738, 1983
76. Muraki AS, Mancuso AA, Harnsberger HR et al: The upper aerodigestive tract and neck: CT evaluation of recurrent tumors. Radiology 149:725–731, 1983
77. Mancuso AA, Hanafee WN: Elusive head and neck tumors beneath intact mucosa. Laryngoscope 93:133–139, 1983
78. Harnsberger JR, Mancuso AA, Muraki AS et al: The upper aerodigestive tract and neck: CT evaluation of recurrent tumors. Radiology 149:503–509, 1983
79. Gatenby RA, Mulhern CB, Strawitz J et al: Comparison of clinical and CT staging of head and neck tumors. AJNR 6:399–401, 1985
80. Rouvier H: Anatomy of the Human Lymphatic System. Ann Arbor, Edwards Brothers, 1938
81. Blady JV: The present status of treatment of cervical metastases from carcinoma arising in the head and neck region. Am J Surg 111:56, 1971
82. Som PM, Shugar JM, Biller HF: The early detection of antral malignancy in the postmaxillectomy patient. Radiology 143:509–512, 1982
83. Leipsiz B, Winter ML, Hokanson JA: Cervical nodal metastases of unknown origin. Laryngoscope 91:593–598, 1981
84. Templer J, Perry MC, Davis SE: Metastatic cervical adenocarcinoma from unknown primary tumor. Arch Otolaryngol 107:45–47, 1981
85. Ferrucci JT, Wittenburg J, Mueller PR et al: Diagnosis of abdominal malignancy by radiologic fine-needle aspiration biopsy. AJR 134:323–330, 1980
86. Bernadino ME: Percutaneous biopsy. AJR 142:41–45, 1984
87. Moss AA: Computed tomography in the staging of gastrointestinal carcinoma. Radiol Clin North Am 20:761–780, 1982
88. Halvorsen RA Jr, Thompson WM: CT for staging gastrointestinal malignancies: Part I. Esophagus and stomach. Invest Radiol 22:2–16, 1987
89. Thompson WM, Halvorsen RA Jr: CT for staging gastrointestinal malignancies: Part II. Small bowel and colon. Invest Radiol 22:96–105, 1987
90. Thompson WM: Imaging strategies for tumors of the gastrointestinal system. CA 37:165–185, 1987
91. Thompson WM: Esophageal cancer. Int J Radiat Oncol Biol Phys 9:1533–1565, 1983
92. Quint LE, Glazer GM, Orringer MB: Esophageal imaging by MR and CT: Study of normal anatomy and neoplasms. Radiology 156:727–731, 1985
93. Heiken JP, Balfe DM, Roper CL: CT evaluation after esophagogastrectomy. AJR 143:555–560, 1984
94. Moss AA, Schnyder P, Marks WM et al: Gastric adenocarcinoma: A comparison of the accuracy and economics of staging by computed tomography and surgery. Gastroenterology 80:45–50, 1981
95. Sussman SK, Halvorsen RA, Illescas FF et al: Gastric adenocarcinoma: CT vs surgical staging. Radiology 167:335–340, 1988
96. Freeny PC, Marks WM, Ryan JA et al: Colorectal carcinoma evaluation with CT: Preoperative staging and detection of postoperative recurrence. Radiology 158:347–353, 1986
97. Thompson WM, Halvorsen RA, Foster WL Jr et al: Preoperative and postoperative CT staging of rectosigmoid carcinoma. AJR 146:703–710, 1986
98. Butch RJ, Wittenberg J, Muller PR et al: Presacral masses after abdominoperineal resection for colorectal carcinoma: The need for needle biopsy. AJR 144:309–312, 1985
99. Butch RJ, Stark DP, Wittenberg J et al: Staging rectal cancer by MR and CT. AJR 146:1155–1160, 1986
100. Gomberg JS, Friedman AC, Radecki PD et al: MRI differentiation of recurrent colorectal carcinoma from postoperative fibrosis. Gastrointest Radiol 11:361–363, 1986
101. Zeman RK, Paushter DM, Schiebler ML et al: Hepatic imaging: Current status. Radiol Clin North Am 23:473–487, 1985
102. LaBerge JM, Laing FC, Federle MP et al: Hepatocellular carcinoma: Assessment of resectability by computed tomography and ultrasound. Radiology 152:485–490, 1984
103. Castaing D, Emond J, Kunstlinger F et al: Utility of operative ultrasound in the surgical management of liver tumors. Ann Surg 204:600–605, 1986
104. Moss AA, Goldberg HI, Stark DB et al: Hepatic tumors: Magnetic resonance and CT appearance. Radiology 150:141–147, 1984
105. Stark DD, Wittenberg J, Butch RJ et al: Hepatic metastases: Randomized, controlled comparison of detection with MR imaging and CT. Radiology 165:399–406, 1987
106. Freeny PC, Lawson TL: Adenocarcinoma of the pancreas, In Freeney PC, Lawson TL (eds): Radiology of the Pancreas, pp 397–496. New York, Springer-Verlag, 1982
107. Clark LR, Jaffe MH, Choyke PL et al: Pancreatic imaging. Radiol Clin North Am 23:489–501, 1985
108. Ferrucci JT Jr, Adson MA, Mueller PR et al: Advances in the radiology of jaundice: A symposium and review. AJR 141:1–20, 1983
109. Gobien RP, Stanley JH, Soucek CK et al: Routine preoperative biliary drainage: Effect on management of obstructive jaundice. Radiology 152:353–356, 1984
110. Bonnel D, Ferrucci JT Jr, Muller PR et al: Surgical and radiological decompression in malignant biliary obstruction: A retrospective study using multivariate risk factor analysis. Radiology 152:347–351, 1984
111. Ring EJ, Kerlan RK: Interventional biliary radiology. AJR 142:31–34, 1984
112. Mendez G Jr, Russell E, Le Page JR et al: Abandonment of endoprosthetic drainage technique in malignant biliary obstruction. AJR 143:617–622, 1984
113. Mueller PR, Ferrucci JT Jr, Teplick SK et al: Biliary stent endoprosthesis: Analysis of complications in 113 patients. Radiology 156:637–639, 1985
114. Tashdakoff D, Hricak H, Thoeni R et al: MR imaging in the diagnosis of pancreatic disease. AJR 148:703–709, 1987
115. Davidson AJ, Hartman DS: Imaging strategies for tumor of the kidney, adrenal gland, and retroperitoneum. CA 37:151–164, 1987
116. Cronan JJ, Zeman RK, Rosenfield AT: Comparison of computed tomography, ultrasound and angiography in staging renal cell carcinoma. J Urol 127:712–714, 1982
117. Schwerk WB, Schwerk WN, Rodeck G: Venous renal tumor extension: A prospective US evaluation. Radiology 156:491–495, 1985
118. Johnson CD, Dunnick NR, Cohan RH et al: Renal adenocarcinoma: CT staging of 100 tumors. AJR 148:59–63, 1987
119. Karstaedt N, McCullough DL, Wolfman NT et al: Magnetic resonance imaging of the renal mass. J Urol 136:566–570, 1986
120. Stamey TA: Cancer of the prostate: Analysis of some important contributions and dilemmas. Monogr Urol 4:68–92, 1983
121. Siegelman SS, McNeal JE, Freiha FS et al: Rectal examination in volume determination of carcinoma of the prostate: Clinical and anatomic correlations. J Urol 136:1228–1230, 1986
122. Lee F, Gray JM, McLeary RD et al: Prostatic evaluation by transrectal sonography: Criteria for diagnosis of early carcinoma. Radiology 158:91–95, 1986
123. Rifkin MD, Friedland GW, Shortliffe L: Prostatic evaluation by transrectal endosonography: Detection of carcinoma. Radiology 158:85–90, 1986
124. Lee F, Littrup PJ, McLeary RD et al: Needle aspiration and core biopsy of prostatic cancer: Comparative evaluation with biplanar transrectal US guidance. Radiology 163:515–520, 1987
125. Steyn JH, Smith FW: Nuclear magnetic resonance imaging of the prostate. Br J Urol 54:726–728, 1982
126. Hricak H, Williams RD, Spring DB et al: Anatomy and pathology of the male pelvis by magnetic resonance imaging. AJR 141:1101–1110, 1983
127. Poon PY, McCallum RW, Henkelman MM et al: Magnetic resonance imaging of the prostate. Radiology 154:143–149, 1985
128. Ling D, Lee JKT, Heiken JP et al: Prostatic carcinoma and benign prostatic hyperplasia: Inability of MR imaging to distinguish between the two diseases. Radiology 158:103–107, 1986
129. Platt JF, Bree RL, Schwab RE: The accuracy of CT in the staging of carcinoma of the prostate. AJR 149:315–318, 1987
130. Hricak H, Dooms GC, Jeffrey RB et al: Prostatic carcinoma: Staging by clinical assessment, CT, and MR imaging. Radiology 162:331–336, 1987

DONALD L. MILLER
RICHARD CHANG
JOHN L. DOPPMAN

SECTION 3

Interventional Radiology in Oncology

Interventional radiology may be loosely defined as comprising those procedures in which radiologic guidance is used to direct needles or catheters for the invasive diagnosis or treatment of various disorders. In large measure, interventional radiologic procedures represent an alternative to surgery for either diagnosis or treatment. Whereas the surgeon uses direct vision as a guide, the radiologist relies on indirect vision through the use of a variety of imaging methods.

Interventional radiology is a very young field that essentially began in the 1960s.[1] The term itself was first used by Margolis in 1967.[2] Developments in this area have depended on technological innovations, such as Seldinger's development of a practical method of percutaneous vascular catheterization[3] and Grüntzig and Hopff's development of the balloon dilation catheter,[4] but even more so on the imagination of radiologists such as Dotter, who first conceived of transluminal angioplasty,[5] and Baum and others, who developed catheter techniques for localizing and managing gastrointestinal bleeding.[6]

The techniques of the interventional radiologist can be divided into five categories: diagnostic procedures, performed to obtain material for histologic, cytologic, or other laboratory analysis, and four broad categories of therapeutic intervention (as suggested by White[1]): drainage procedures (biliary, urinary, and abscesses), vascular and nonvascular balloon dilatation, chemotherapy administration, and embolotherapy. All the various paraphernalia and procedures used in modern interventional radiology can be considered as adaptations or applications of these basic concepts.

With regard to the application of interventional radiology to oncology, a simpler classification is more appropriate and will be used in this chapter. Oncologic interventional radiology may be divided into procedures used for cancer diagnosis, procedures used for cancer therapy, and procedures used as adjuncts in the management of cancer patients. This classification excludes several types of procedures, such as stone extraction and transluminal angioplasty, that have no direct application in oncologic practice. This chapter is not intended as a guide to the full extent of interventional radiology, but is narrowly focused on oncologic interventions.

CANCER DIAGNOSIS—PERCUTANEOUS BIOPSY

Percutaneous needle biopsy has become a technique of major importance in the diagnosis and staging of cancer.[7,8] Increased utilization of this technique is a consequence of the availability of safer needles, newer imaging techniques, and advances in cytology.[9]

Technique

Radiologically guided percutaneous needle biopsy is usually performed with thin ("skinny") needles of 20 to 23 gauge, which are designed to yield aspirates of cells for cytologic examination. Some of these needles are also designed to yield small cores of tissue.[10-13] Regardless of which of these needles is used, the technique is usually referred to as fine-needle aspiration biopsy (FNAB).[8,14,15] Larger needles can be used to obtain larger cores of tissue and are most commonly used in the evaluation of bone tumors, hepatic lesions, and lymphomas.[9] In these areas, the larger needles produce more tissue, yield higher accuracy rates, and do not appear to have a higher complication rate.[9,12,16-21] The choice of needle type and size depends on the size, type, and location of the lesion and the preferences of the radiologist and cytopathologist.[22] Pathologists with less experience in cytology may require larger tissue samples for confident diagnosis.

The role of the pathologist is critical, since skill and experience in cytology is the most important factor in reaching an accurate diagnosis. Pathologists vary in their preference for different methods of tissue sampling, tissue fixation, and sample handling.[8,9,23,24] It is wise to follow the pathologist's preferences in this regard. Often it is possible to arrange for the cytologist to be present during the biopsy, and this is extremely helpful: The cytologist can prepare the specimens on the spot and can provide the radiologist with virtually instant information as to their adequacy.[9,25] Although the immediate cytologic assessment of biopsy specimens does not seem to increase accuracy rates or decrease complication rates,[26] it does provide benefits for patient care. This is principally because preliminary results are rapidly available and the selection of further diagnostic tests may be made immediately.

A variety of imaging techniques can be used for needle guidance during biopsy. Fluoroscopy is useful for lesions that are visible on plain films, such as pulmonary nodules, some bone lesions, and lymph nodes opacified by lymphangiography. Ultrasound (US) and computed tomography (CT) have extended our ability to visualize lesions in the mediastinum, abdomen, pelvis, and head and neck and are commonly used to guide biopsies of these areas (Fig. 20-29).[14,15,27,28] It was initially thought that magnetic resonance (MR) imaging would be much less useful to guide percutaneous biopsy, and that nonferrous needles would be required to avoid the creation of the severe artifact commonly seen with ferromagnetic materials and to prevent needle motion due to magnetic field effects. However, Mueller et al have shown that biopsy needles fabricated from a specific stainless steel (SS 316) do not produce artifacts on MR imaging–guided percutaneous biopsies and do not move in a magnetic field. They have performed liver biopsies in humans with these needles.[29] Virtually any imaging technique that provides three-dimensional localization of a lesion can be used to guide a biopsy needle, but the choice of modality is based on lesion size, position, and visibility; equipment availability; and the skills and preference of the individual radiologist. The radiologist who performs the biopsy must be the final arbiter in the choice of imaging modality.

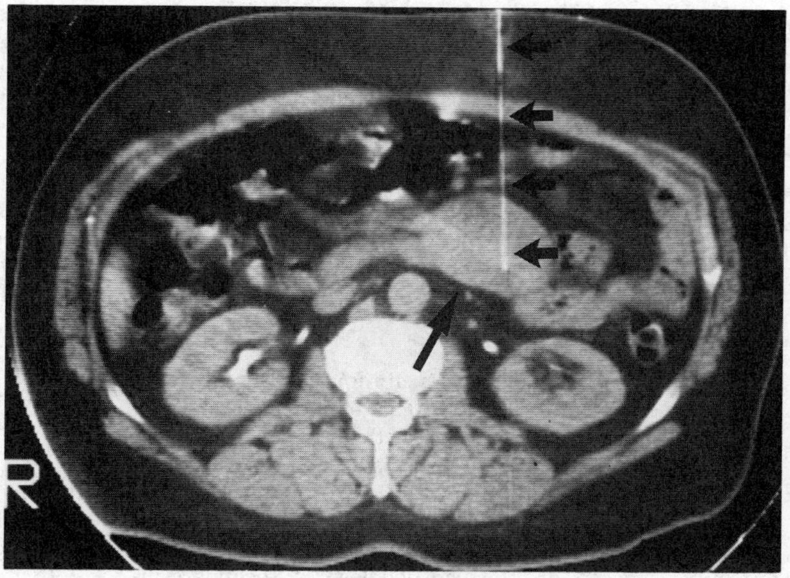

FIG. 20-29. CT-guided biopsy of an abdominal mass. The needle is visible as a thin white line (*short black arrows*) that terminates in the mass (*long black arrow*). Note that the needle passes through gas-containing bowel. With thin needles, this is quite safe. The patient had no complications from the biopsy.

Clinical Advantages

Much of the appeal of percutaneous biopsy is based on the use of this technique as a substitute for surgical biopsy, with an attendant decrease in patient morbidity and decrease in costs.[8,30] In a review of 82 percutaneous biopsies performed in patients with gynecologic malignancies and extrapelvic lesions, biopsy proved highly cost-effective and permitted surgery to be avoided in a number of patients.[31] In 72 patients undergoing percutaneous biopsy of thoracic lesions, biopsy reduced the need for the diagnostic thoracotomy, shortened the time from admission to diagnosis, reduced the total number of thoracotomies, shortened the length of hospital stay, and resulted in a significantly reduced average and total hospitalization charge.[32] In a series of 422 patients with 400 proven pulmonary lesions, Westcott found that percutaneous biopsy established the diagnosis in 191 patients and made mediastinoscopy and/or thoracotomy unnecessary.[33] In 53 patients with a clinical diagnosis of carcinoma of the pancreas, 30 laparotomies were avoided in 37 patients with positive biopsies.[34]

Most biopsies in adults can be performed as outpatient procedures and require only local anesthesia to the skin. Percutaneous biopsy procedures are also appropriate for pediatric patients. Although some form of sedation or regional anesthesia may be necessary, general anesthesia is usually not required in children.[35] In one series of 69 percutaneous diagnostic procedures in children aged 2 days to 17 years, general anesthesia was never necessary.[25] In another series of 14 pediatric patients, general anesthesia was necessary for percutaneous biopsy in three patients.[36]

Accuracy

The accuracy of percutaneous biopsy depends on the radiologist's skill in directing the needle, the size of the specimen, and the cytopathologist's skill in interpreting the specimen. Large masses should be biopsied near their periphery to avoid possible areas of necrosis. Accuracy varies according to the specific biopsy site, as different organs present different problems in terms of access and interpretation. A single needle pass into a malignant lesion will yield a specimen containing malignant cells approximately 75% of the time.[37] Additional needle passes will increase the sensitivity, but more than four passes are rarely necessary.

In general, a negative biopsy report does not necessarily mean that malignancy has been excluded; the wrong site may have been sampled, or the sample may be inadequate. Only positive biopsies should influence therapeutic decisions.

The sensitivity of percutaneous biopsy for the detection of malignancy in lung nodules is as high as 95% to 97%, with accuracies of 96% to 98% reported.[33,38,39] Biopsy of the hila and mediastinum is equally sensitive.[40]

In the abdomen, FNAB of the liver has an accuracy of 84% to 99%.[11,16,23,28] There is some evidence that use of larger needles (14 or 18 gauge) increases sensitivity and accuracy.[12,16,17] Pancreatic biopsy is somewhat less useful, with a sensitivity ranging from 77% to 86% and an accuracy of 80% to 89%.[11,28,34,41] It may be more appropriate to biopsy associated liver metastases or abdominal masses in patients with pancreatic lesions than to biopsy the pancreas directly.[9] Adrenal biopsy is safe in the absence of pheochromocytoma. An adrenal mass in a patient with a malignancy should be biopsied to exclude the presence of a nonfunctioning adenoma, or "incidentaloma." These are seen as serendipitous findings on approximately 1% of abdominal CT scans.[42,43] Adrenal FNAB is successful in 83% to 93% of enlarged glands.[44,45]

The diagnostic accuracy of retroperitoneal and pelvic lymph node biopsy varies from 65% to 90%.[9] Accuracy is higher in patients with nodal metastases from carcinoma than in patients with lymphoma, because the diagnosis of lymphoma requires a much larger tissue sample for accurate evaluation of cell patterns. It was initially thought that biopsy of pelvic nodes that appeared normal on lymphangiography might aid in the staging of prostatic carcinoma, but this appears not to be the case.[46,47]

Percutaneous bone biopsy has an overall accuracy of about 79% in the diagnosis of primary bone tumors and 95% in the diagnosis of osseous metastases.[18,21] Large needles are usually required for the diagnosis of primary bone tumors and for biopsy of blastic lesions.[9] The blood from a bone biopsy specimen should also be sent for cytologic analysis, especially in patients with osseous metastases.[48]

Complications

Fine-needle aspiration biopsy is a remarkably safe technique. The complications of FNAB are summarized in Table 20-9. The risk of hemorrhage is less than 1% and the risk of death is less than 0.01%.[8,49] Deaths have been reported from hemorrhagic pancreatitis following FNAB of the pancreas, and from asphyxiation due to hemoptysis after lung biopsy. Even hepatic hemangiomas can be biopsied with relative impunity using 20- or 22-gauge needles.[50,51] Secondary infection is rare.[52] Despite the theoretical risk of seeding tumor cells along the needle tract, reports of needle tract tumor implants are very uncommon,[53–55] and animal studies have shown the phenomenon to be highly unlikely.[56,57] Further, survival rates for patients with breast, lung, and kidney cancers diagnosed by FNAB have been shown to be similar to those of patients with these cancers diagnosed by open surgical biopsy.[8]

The most common complication of FNAB is pneumothorax, associated with biopsy of lesions in the lung and mediastinum. Pneumothorax occurs in 20% to 41% of these patients, with chest tube drainage required in 5% to 13% of patients undergoing biopsy.[38,40,58–60] The use of a blood patch does not reduce this frequency.[61] In one series of 673 transthoracic needle biopsies, 98% of all pneumothoraces were detected on chest radiographs obtained 1 hour after biopsy, and all pneumothoraces were apparent on chest radiographs obtained 4 hours after biopsy. All pneumothoraces requiring treatment were evident within 1 hour of biopsy, and 88% of these were evident immediately after biopsy.[59] With 4 hours of observation following biopsy, the procedure can be safely performed on an outpatient basis.[58,59] Many pneumothoraces can also be managed on an outpatient basis, with a small, 9-F chest tube placed percutaneously by the radiologist.[58,60,62]

Although biopsy of most adrenal masses is no more dangerous than biopsies of other parts of the body,[44,45,63] inadvertent FNAB of pheochromocytomas is potentially lethal. Several cases of severe hypertension, hypotension, and massive hemorrhage have been reported.[64,65] Since pheochromocytoma is not always clinically evident, caution is in order when adrenal biopsy is performed. Preliminary evidence suggests that MR imaging can distinguish pheochromocytomas from other adrenal masses such as metastases and cortical adenomas.[66]

TABLE 20-9. Complications of Fine Needle Aspiration Biopsy (FNAB)

Complication (Refs.)	*Frequency*
Death* [8,49]	<0.01%
Hemorrhage[49]	<1%
Infection[52]	Rare
Tumor seeding[53–57]	Rare
Pneumothorax (biopsy of lung and mediastinum)[38,40,58–60]	20%–41%
Pneumothorax requiring treatment (biopsy of lung and mediastinum)[38,40,58–60]	5%–13%

* Markedly increased risk with fine-needle aspiration biopsy of pheochromocytoma.[64,65]

CANCER TREATMENT

The application of intravascular catheter techniques to the therapy of tumors can be divided into two major modalities, regional chemotherapy delivered through selectively positioned catheters, and infarction of tumor by embolization. Both modalities have benefited from the development of highly selective catheter techniques and suitable embolizing agents. The most recent development is chemoembolization, a combination of both methodologies in which the blood supply to the tumor is occluded with a mixture of embolic material and a chemotherapeutic agent, thereby providing both an ischemic and a chemotherapeutic component to the therapy.

INTRA-ARTERIAL CHEMOTHERAPY

Selective intra-arterial infusion of chemotherapeutic agents is based on the principle that tumor response increases with drug exposure. The narrow therapeutic index of many anticancer drugs limits the systemic dose of chemotherapeutic agent and provides a rationale for selective intra-arterial chemotherapy.[67–69] Infusion of chemotherapeutic agents directly into the arterial supply of a neoplasm can produce higher drug concentrations in the tumor-bearing region without corresponding increases in systemic concentration. The most common target has been metastatic disease in the liver,[70–73] but primary bone sarcomas,[74] pelvic tumors,[75–77] and head and neck tumors[78,79] have all been treated in this way.

Broad experience, meticulous technique, and persistent efforts are required of the angiographer to complete many of these treatment courses. Prior to treatment of hepatic tumors, angiographic occlusion of accessory hepatic arteries or the gastroduodenal artery may be required (Fig. 20-30).[80–83] Occlusion of the hepatic artery frequently complicates prolonged or repeated infusions, and collateral vessels may have to be used for later cycles.[84] Narrowing of the extrahepatic and intrahepatic biliary ducts due to cholangitis induced by the chemotherapeutic agent occurs with distressing frequency.[85–89] In the brain, severe unilateral retinal toxicity complicates internal carotid artery infusions proximal to the ophthalmic artery, and specialized catheters have been designed to permit perfusion distal to the carotid siphon.[90–91]

Because infusion rates for chemotherapeutic agents are

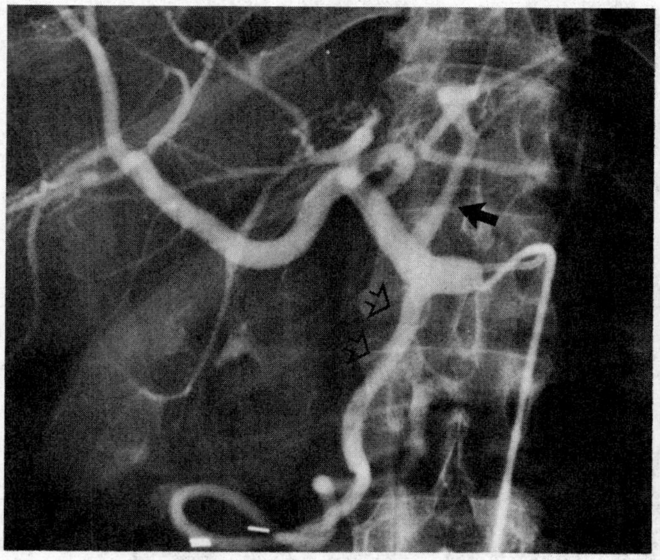

A

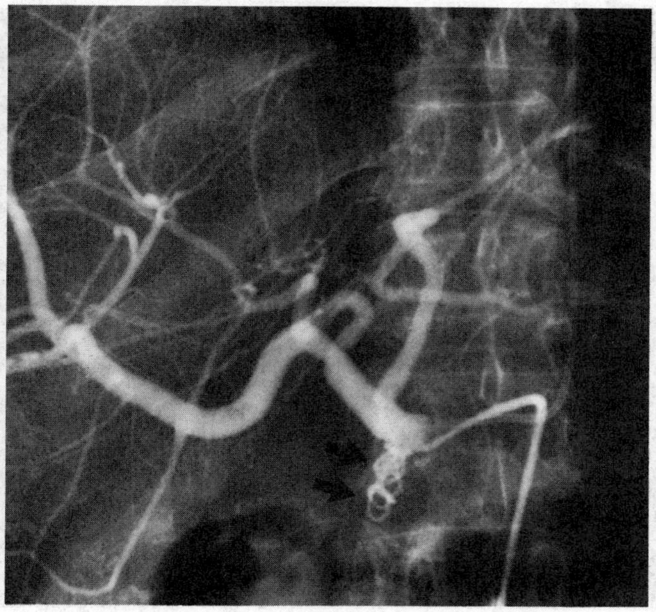

B

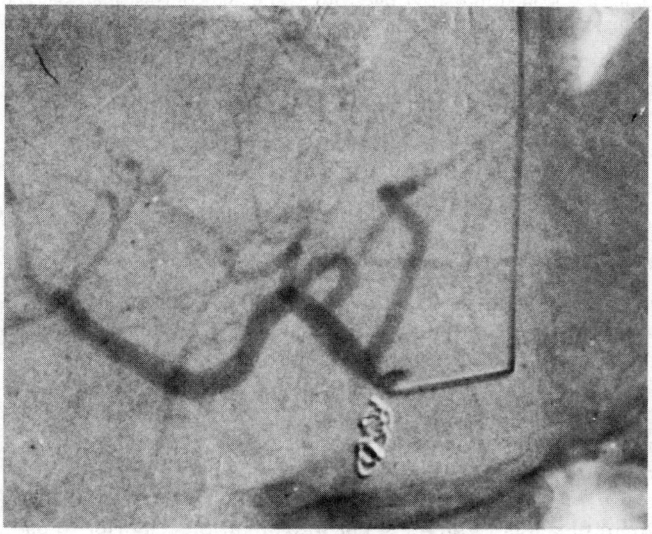

C

FIG. 20-30. Hepatic artery infusion chemotherapy may require the use of interventional radiologic techniques. **A**. A preinfusion, common hepatic artery angiogram reveals that the gastroduodenal artery (*open arrows*) arises nearly opposite the left hepatic artery (*solid arrow*). The origin of the gastroduodenal artery must be blocked or drug will enter its vascular territory and cause gastric, duodenal, and pancreatic toxicity. **B**. The gastroduodenal artery has been occluded at its origin with Gianturco-Wallace-Anderson coils (*arrows*) delivered through the angiographic catheter. Retrograde filling of the gastroduodenal artery from the superior mesenteric artery via the pancreatic arcades will maintain blood supply to the duodenum and pancreas. **C**. Contrast material administered through the infusion catheter fills the right and left hepatic arteries but not the gastroduodenal artery. The effect is equivalent to surgical ligation of the gastroduodenal artery.

invariably very slow, uniform perfusion may not occur, due to the tendency for streaming when slow infusions are performed into a rapidly moving bloodstream.[92,93] Techniques for determining perfusion patterns have been developed, and various pumps have been devised in an attempt to improve the uniformity of distribution of the chemotherapeutic agent.[94–96]

EMBOLIZATION

General Principles

Transcatheter embolization seeks to induce necrosis of tumor by obstructing its arterial supply. This usually entails deliberate sacrifice of the organ of origin, as in embolization of hypernephromas. In the liver, with its dual blood supply, tumor can be embolized via the hepatic artery while the normal hepatic parenchyma is sustained by portal venous inflow.

Embolizing agents can be categorized on the basis of the duration of vascular occlusion (temporary versus long-acting) and site of occlusion (peripheral versus proximal). Temporary agents, such as absorbable gelatin sponge (Gelfoam dental packs) (Fig. 20-31), microfibrillar collagen hemostat (Avitene), and autologous clot, are resorbed over a period of days to weeks. Permanent agents, such as polyvinyl alcohol foam (Ivalon) and Gianturco-Wallace-Anderson coils

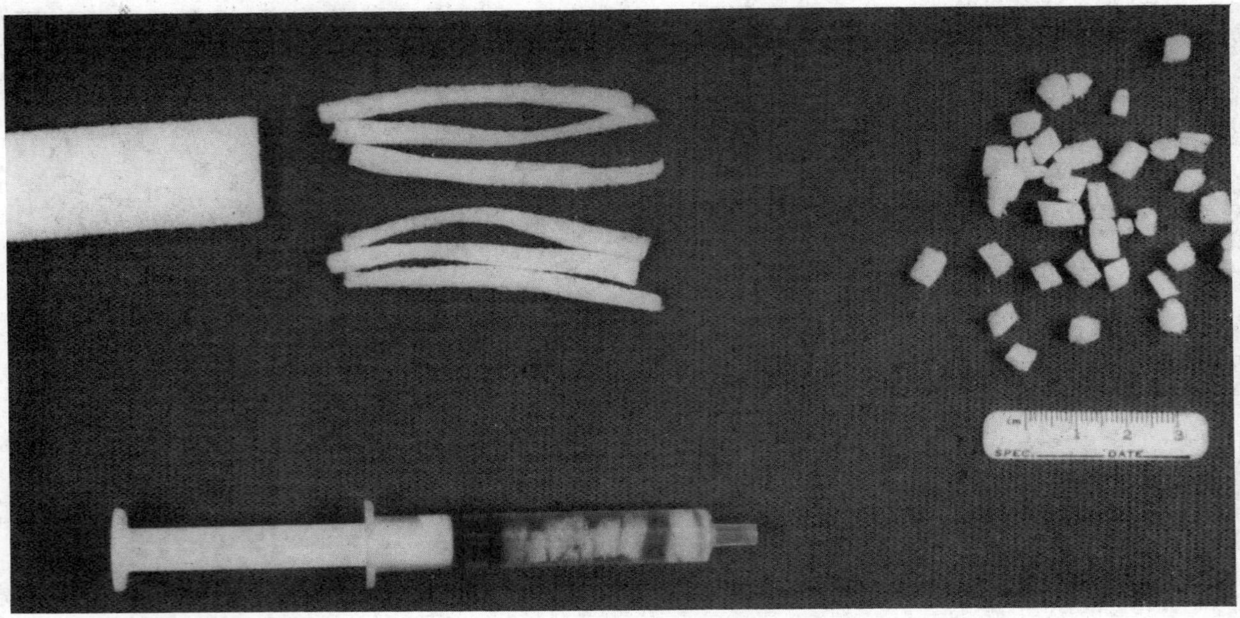

FIG. 20-31. Gelfoam is cut into segments and cubes for arterial embolization. Five to ten cubes are loaded into a syringe with saline and contrast material and injected into the artery for peripheral embolization. They are guided by blood flow in the vessel (flow-guided embolization). (Reprinted from Wallace S, Charnsangavej C, Carrasco CH: Transcatheter management of the cancer patient. In DeVita VT Jr, Hellman S, Rosenberg SA [eds]: Cancer: Principles and Practice of Oncology, 2nd ed, p 2305. Philadelphia, JB Lippincott, 1985)

(Fig. 20-32) are not metabolized, although the embolic effects may not be permanent in all cases.[97]

Even more important than the choice between temporary and permanent agents is the choice between peripheral and proximal occluding agents. Alcohol (dehydrated alcohol injection, USP), which acts as far peripherally as the capillary level, and absorbable gelatin powder (Gelfoam sterile powder), which lodges in arterioles, both cause vascular occlusion at a level distal to any possible collateral anastomoses, and cause necrosis of the embolized territory. Gelfoam pledgets (which are cut into small pieces prior to use, and fragment further as they pass through the angiographic catheter) and Ivalon both cause occlusion proximal to the most distal level of vascular anastomoses. They produce a peripheral embolic effect without infarction. At the most proximal level, coils occlude vessels 2 to 8 mm in diameter. In action and effect they are identical to surgical ligation.

Temporary agents are rarely used as the sole agent for tumor embolization. Also, proximal occlusion of major feeding arteries is generally ineffective in tumor embolization because of the rapidity with which collateral channels develop. Peripheral embolizing agents occlude the arterial bed of a tumor and delay the development of collateral flow. Most angiographers seek to achieve peripheral occlusion of the vascular bed of the tumor with a permanent agent and, if indicated, follow with proximal large-vessel occlusion in an effort to prolong the efficacy of the peripheral occlusion.

Applications

In many respects, tumors of the liver are ideal targets for embolic therapy. The liver has a dual blood supply from the hepatic artery (30%) and the portal vein (70%). Since primary and secondary hepatic neoplasms receive their blood supply exclusively from the hepatic artery with minimal peripheral contributions from the portal vein[98] and since the liver can survive on its portal venous inflow alone, the hepatic artery can be embolized with a great margin of safety. Carrasco et al have listed relative contraindications to hepatic artery embolization.[99] However, the major contraindication is the presence of main portal vein occlusion due to tumor or thrombus.[100] When first- or second-order branches of the portal vein are occluded, hepatic artery embolization increases the risk of segmental hepatic infarction, but there is less risk of hepatic failure. Recently, Nakao et al have sought to produce complete tumor ischemia by deliberately embolizing both the segmental hepatic arterial and portal venous branches leading to a tumor, deliberately infarcting the hepatic segment in an attempt to achieve more complete tumor necrosis.[101]

Embolization of hypernephromas is performed preoperatively to facilitate surgical resection and decrease intraoperative blood loss. It may also be used to control massive hematuria or to reduce the bulk of inoperable tumors, thereby controlling pain. No convincing evidence exists that emboli-

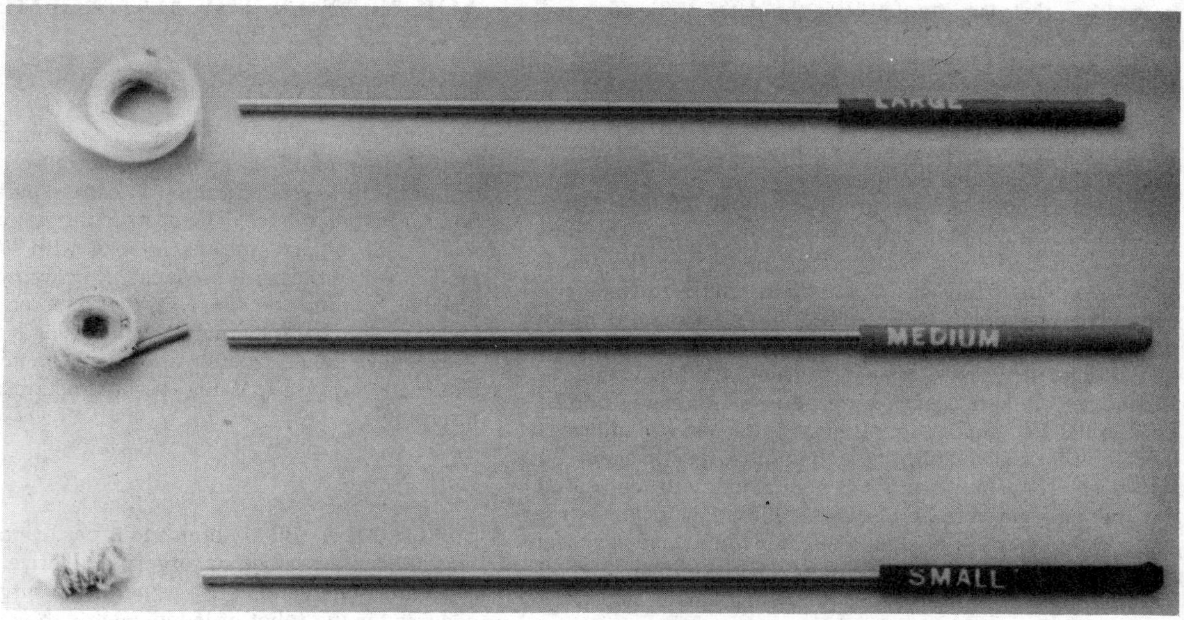

FIG. 20-32. Stainless steel coils are housed inside metal cartridges. When pushed out of the cartridge with a guidewire, the coil resumes a helical configuration. Strands of synthetic fiber are attached to the coil and help promote thrombus formation. The common sizes of coils are 3 mm, 5 mm, and 8 mm. (Reprinted from Wallace S, Charnsangavej C, Carrasco CH: Transcatheter management of the cancer patient. In DeVita VT Jr, Hellman S, Rosenberg SA [eds]: Cancer: Principles and Practice of Oncology, 2nd ed, p 2306. Philadelphia, JB Lippincott, 1985)

zation of renal tumor stimulates an immune response.[102] Infarction with absolute alcohol has replaced particulate embolization in many institutions.[103,104] Reflux of ethanol into the adrenal artery or the aorta may lead to complications.[105,106] Infusion through an occluding balloon catheter in the renal artery is essential.

Control of pain from bony metastases may be achieved with some success with selective embolization.[107,108] Transcatheter embolization has also been recommended to control massive hematuria from radiation cystitis,[109] to reduce vascularity of metastatic renal carcinoma in bone before stabilization operations,[108] and to treat bony tumors of the spine and pelvis, particularly unresectable giant cell tumors or aneurysmal bone cysts.[110]

Complications

All embolization procedures involve the risk of inadvertently embolizing nontargeted, often critical, organs. Cutaneous and mucosal injury during embolization of external carotid or internal iliac arteries has occurred, as has nerve damage, particularly when peripheral occluders such as cyanoacrylate or neurotoxic agents such as alcohol are used. The use of intra-arterial digital subtraction arteriography to monitor the embolic process has reduced the incidence of renal failure associated with excessive doses of contrast agent.

In addition to complications of the embolization procedure itself, about 50% of patients will experience a postembolization syndrome consisting of pain, fever, and sometimes nausea and vomiting.[110a] Narcotics will control the pain, and the syndrome is self-limited (24–48 hours). Delayed complications such as abscess formation in the infarcted tumor or organ are surprisingly rare but usually require percutaneous or surgical drainage. Gas within the infarcted tumor or organ, usually demonstrated by CT, occurs routinely either due to tumor necrosis or to air introduced at the time of embolization. In the absence of clinical signs of sepsis, the demonstration of gas is not indicative of infection and antibiotic therapy is not required.[111,112]

CHEMOEMBOLIZATION

Chemoembolization combines the benefits of intra-arterial high-dose chemotherapy with obstruction of the tumor vascular bed.[113] The goal is both to prolong exposure time of the tumor to the chemotherapeutic agent and to add an ischemic component to enhance tumor necrosis.[114] The Japanese have refined this technique and directed it principally at hepatomas, first by incorporating chemotherapeutic agents into ethylcellulose microcapsules[113] and most recently by taking advantage of the prolonged sequestration of intra-arterially injected iodized oil within both primary and secondary hepatic tumors. The iodinated ethyl ester of poppyseed oil (Lipiodol, Ethiodol) is sequestered in both primary and secondary hepatic tumors when injected selectively into the hepatic artery.[115,116] This technique was originally developed to increase the visibility and thus the detectability of small hepatomas and metastases on CT. The mechanism of prolonged retention of these iodized oils within tumors has not been fully explained. Miller et al have demonstrated that in hepatic tumor models in rabbits, iodized oil accumulates within both the tumor vasculature and the abnormal hepatic sinusoids surrounding the tumor.[117]

Regardless of mechanism, the contact time between tumor and chemotherapeutic agent can be increased by combining cytotoxic drugs with iodized oil.[118,119] Takayasu et al[120] mixed Lipiodol with doxorubicin, and Konno et al[121] combined Lipiodol with SMANCS (co-poly[styrene-maleic acid] conjugated neocarzinostatin). In Takayasu's series of 99 patients, the results suggest that iodized oil by itself is an ineffective embolizing agent despite its prolonged persistence in hepatocellular carcinomas.[120] Efficacy was improved by combining iodized oil with a chemotherapeutic agent, but the most promising results were obtained with iodized oil, doxorubicin, and peripheral embolization. Particularly striking was the necrosis of small daughter tumor nodules, seen only when doxorubicin was combined with Gelfoam embolization. Although this therapy is promising, not all hepatocellular carcinomas retain iodized oil.

There is still little experience with chemoembolization in the therapy of liver metastases, although preliminary reports indicate that metastases do retain iodized oil in some instances.[115] If vascularity determines efficacy, as suggested with hepatocellular carcinomas, metastases may prove less susceptible to this interesting new modality.

DIRECT TUMOR ABLATION BY PERCUTANEOUS TECHNIQUES

Several groups[122,122a] have investigated direct intratumoral injections of alcohol. Burgener and Steinmetz injected absolute alcohol percutaneously into adenocarcinomas implanted in the hind leg of rabbits.[123] Local coagulation necrosis was produced with minimal side-effects. Sheu et al treated six patients with hepatocellular carcinomas by direct percutaneous alcohol injection.[124] Serum α-fetoprotein levels decreased in all patients in whom the initial levels were elevated, and returned to normal in two. CT demonstrated necrosis of the tumor, and in five patients follow-up biopsy showed no evidence of viable cancer cells. The role of direct intratumoral injection of alcohol or other cytotoxic agents has not been established. Particularly for avascular tumors that respond poorly to embolization and chemoembolization, such a technique may have application.

Phototherapy of tumors sensitized by the preliminary administration of a photosensitizer (hematoporphyrin derivative—H_pD) is an evolving intervention. Intravesical[125] and transbronchial[126] applications of this technique have been described. Gattenby et al treated a variety of presacral and cervical malignant masses by direct injection of a hematoporphyrin sensitizer (H_pD) followed by laser therapy through a clear plastic sheath percutaneously inserted directly into the tumor under CT control.[127] Reduction of tumor mass was observed.

ADJUNCTS IN THE MANAGEMENT OF CANCER PATIENTS

BILIARY INTERVENTIONS

While interventional radiology has a prominent role in the management of biliary stones and strictures, the major indication for biliary intervention in cancer patients is obstruction of the biliary tree. The obstructing lesion may be proximal in the biliary tree, as is seen with Klatskin tumors, metastases to the porta hepatis, and carcinoma of the gallbladder, or it may be distal, as in carcinoma of the pancreas and carcinoma of the ampulla. The intent is always the same —to relieve the obstruction and divert the flow of bile, either externally or, by bypassing the obstruction with a catheter, internally.

Indications

PALLIATION. Biliary drainage is performed either for palliation or as a prelude to surgery. Palliative biliary drainage procedures are as effective as palliative surgical bypass procedures for the relief of jaundice, and the choice of therapy (surgery versus interventional drainage) does not appear to affect survival. In two large retrospective studies[128,129] and one prospective study[130] there was no difference in mortality at 30 days or in median survival.

Biliary drainage performed as a palliative procedure should be reserved for patients with symptoms related to jaundice (pruritus, anorexia, nausea) and for patients with biliary sepsis, in whom it is a relatively low-risk procedure and potentially lifesaving.[131,132] The procedure is associated with discomfort, and an external catheter, if one is left in place, is a visible reminder to the patient of the underlying malignancy. Some patients find an external catheter psychologically unbearable. For the patient with minimal symptoms due to biliary obstruction, it is wise to remember the maxim that is difficult to make an asymptomatic patient feel better.

PREOPERATIVE DRAINAGE. Guidelines for the use of biliary drainage as a prelude to surgical bypass, rather than as the sole palliative procedure, are much less clear. Two retrospective studies[133,134] report a reduction in surgical mortality and morbidity when preoperative biliary drainage is used, while two prospective studies[132,135] conclude that the addition of preoperative biliary drainage has no effect on mortality and morbidity but does increase hospital costs. In an animal study, external biliary drainage had no effect on mortality in jaundiced rats, but internal drainage did reduce mortality significantly.[136] Another study suggests that preoperative biliary drainage is warranted when the obstructing lesion is located distally in the biliary tree and is inadvisable when the obstructing lesion is proximal.[137] There is no consensus on the appropriateness of preoperative biliary drainage,[138,139] and little guidance can be offered, save to abide by local surgical philosophy. Unfortunately, we are not yet in a position to define subsets of patients who will benefit from preoperative biliary drainage and those who will not.

CHOICE OF TECHNIQUE. The various methods of nonoperative therapy of the biliary tree were extensively discussed in a 1987 review by McLean and Burke.[140] Access to the biliary tree may be obtained percutaneously, with percutaneous transhepatic biliary drainage (PTBD), or endoscopically, with endoscopic retrograde biliary drainage (ERBD). The choice of endoscopic versus percutaneous approach to the biliary tree is affected by several factors, not the least of which is the skill and experience of the local radiologist and endoscopist. ERBD requires specialized equipment and is not universally available. In patients with unfavorable anatomy due to previous gastric or duodenal surgery, the endoscopist may be unable to pass the endoscope to the level of the papilla of Vater. Very distal common bile duct obstruction may sometimes prevent cannulation of the biliary tree, and firm proximal lesions in the common hepatic duct may not permit passage of an endoprosthesis.[141] Overall, in experienced hands, ERBD is successful in approximately 90% of patients.[140–142]

PTBD has an initial success rate close to 100%, and the anatomical problems that make ERBD difficult or impossible in some patients are not a factor with PTBD.[128,142] However, ERBD is associated with fewer bleeding complications than PTBD and better patient acceptance.[142] Ascites, coagulopathies, and intrahepatic metastases are relative contraindications to PTBD but not to ERBD.

A final consideration is the use of an endoprosthesis (an entirely internal biliary stent) versus a catheter which extends outside the patient. Endoprostheses can be placed via both PTBD and ERBD, and occasionally both techniques are used simultaneously.[143] Catheters, which can be used for both internal and external drainage, must be placed percutaneously. Endoprostheses have the major advantage of providing relief of obstruction without a protruding external catheter, which may be uncomfortable and psychologically unsettling.[144] However, since access to the biliary tree is lost when the endoprosthesis is placed, ERBD or PTBD must be repeated to remove and replace the endoprosthesis when it becomes occluded.[145,146] Catheters can be irrigated daily to maintain patency, and changing them is a relatively simple matter since access to the biliary tree is available.

An additional factor is that endoprostheses placed endoscopically are usually smaller than those placed by PTBD.[138] While even 6-F catheters permit adequate bile flow in vitro, clinical observation has demonstrated that 10- to 12-F catheters are necessary for adequate drainage in some patients.[147] Endoprostheses of this size often cannot be placed endoscopically, but require a percutaneous approach.[138]

In general, patients with malignant disease and a life expectancy of less than 4 months may be best served by placement of an endoprosthesis with ERBD, if possible.[138,141,144,148] A randomized prospective trial of endoprosthesis placement via ERBD versus PTBD in 75 patients with malignant obstructive jaundice demonstrated a statistically significant higher success rate for relief of jaundice and a significantly lower 30-day mortality for ERBD.[149] In other patients, the choice between endoprosthesis and catheter drainage depends mostly on the individual patient's preference and the technical feasibility and availability of ERBD.

Technique

Before any type of biliary drainage is considered, the diagnosis of biliary obstruction must be made. In patients with an elevated total bilirubin level (>5 mg/dl), dilation of the intrahepatic biliary tree is usually obvious on US. Nonetheless, both obstruction without dilation and dilation without obstruction are well-recognized though uncommon phenomena.[150,151] CT, radionuclide hepatobiliary scintigraphy, and endoscopic retrograde cholangiopancreatography (ERCP) are useful in patients with equivocal US findings.[139,152] Percutaneous transhepatic cholangiography (PTC) with a fine needle is both safe and diagnostic[153] but is more invasive than the other diagnostic studies. When PTC is performed on an obstructed biliary system, an immediate drainage procedure should be considered to prevent leakage of bile along the needle track and into the peritoneum, which may otherwise occur and may cause bile peritonitis.[140]

The first step in biliary drainage is cholangiography, to opacify the biliary tree. Biliary anatomy and the number, location, and appearance of all obstructing lesions must be defined. Cholangiography may be done via either PTC or ERCP, depending on whether drainage is to be performed percutaneously or endoscopically.

For PTBD, a guide wire is then advanced into the biliary tree, and a drainage catheter is placed either proximal to or past the obstruction. If the catheter has not been placed through the obstruction, bile must be drained externally into a collecting bag (external drainage). If the obstruction has been negotiated, bile can pass through proximal sideholes in the catheter and exit distal to the obstruction, reestablishing a physiologically normal bile pathway and draining internally into the duodenum (internal drainage) (Fig. 20-33). If extensive manipulation is required to negotiate the obstruction or if the patient is septic, external drainage is instituted initially, followed 1 to 3 days later by negotiation of the obstruction. The delay permits the ducts to return to normal caliber and allows inflammation in the area of the obstruction to subside.[140] Subsequently, an entirely internal endoprosthesis may be placed across the obstruction, if desired.[148]

With ERBD, the entire procedure is performed endoscopically. Temporary external drainage can be instituted with a nasobiliary catheter, or an endoprosthesis can be placed at the initial sitting. ERBD often requires endoscopic sphincterotomy or papillotomy to ease catheter or endoprosthesis insertion into the common bile duct, but this is not invariably necessary.[140,141,146]

Regardless of the method used to enter the biliary tree, bile samples are obtained for culture and cytology. In the setting of biliary obstruction, Suzuki et al demonstrated infected bile in 89% of patients with fever and 39% of afebrile patients.[154] *Escherichia coli* and *Klebsiella* were the most frequent aerobic species. Anaerobes were much less frequent. In another study, Muro et al obtained 10-ml samples of bile during the course of PTBD.[155] Bile cytology was positive in 34% of 100 patients with malignant obstruction of the biliary tree. If desired, brush, screw, and core biopsies of the obstructing lesion can also be obtained via the biliary tree.[156]

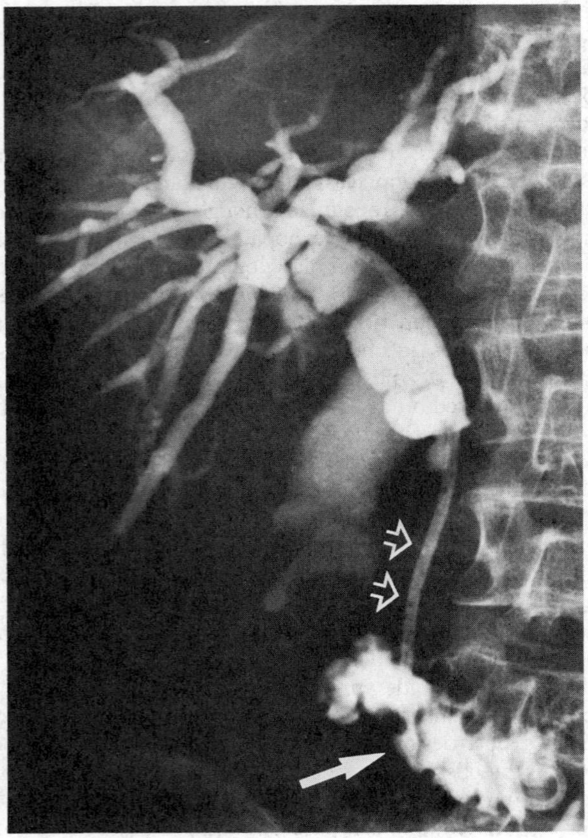

FIG. 20-33. Internal drainage with a percutaneously placed transhepatic biliary drainage catheter. The catheter traverses the area of obstruction in the common bile duct (*open arrows*) and terminates in the duodenum (*long arrow*). Bile enters the catheter through sideholes proximal to the obstruction and exits through sideholes in the duodenum.

Efficacy

Biliary drainage procedures (both PTBD and ERBD) are unquestionably effective for the relief of obstruction and cholestasis. In one series, the mean serum bilirubin level decreased from 15.7 mg/dl before drainage to 4.9 mg/dl 10 days after drainage.[148] In another study, the decrease in bilirubin showed a negative exponential correlation with the duration of drainage.[128] In a third study, the rate of decrease in bilirubin ranged from 0.23 to 4.9 mg/dl/day (mean, 1.4 mg/dl/day) and had no relation to the initial bilirubin value.[157] In patients with proximal obstruction of the biliary tree at or above the level of the bifurcation of the common hepatic duct, relief of jaundice will still occur even if only a portion of the biliary tree is drained. However, cholangitis may develop in the undrained segment, and placement of a second catheter may be required.

Complications

PTBD and ERBD are associated with different types of complications that occur with different frequencies.[142] PTBD results in death in 2% to 9% of patients.[128,158–160] Major complications, including septic shock, pleural effusions, bile peritonitis, hepatic abscess and major hemorrhage, occur in an additional 5% to 17%.[128,158,160] Cholangitis is the most common complication, occurring acutely in approximately 20% of patients. (In debilitated cancer patients, cholangitis may occur, either early or late, in up to 47% of those undergoing PTBD.[159]) Overall, between 20% and 69% of patients will eventually experience some kind of complication.[128,158,159,161] Tumor spread as a result of PTBD has been reported.[161,162]

In contrast, ERBD is considerably safer. Mortality is 4% or less. Major acute complications are seen in 3% to 10% of patients. The overall complication rate is 10% to 18%, and bleeding complications are far less likely with ERBD than with PTBD.[141,142,146] ERBD is safer because it is not necessary to transgress the liver capsule or push catheters through the hepatic parenchyma. The primary risk is that associated with endoscopic sphincterotomy, which has a mortality of 1% to 2% and a major complication rate of 7%.[140]

Intervention in the Gallbladder

In some critically ill, high-risk patients, standard surgical therapy for cholecystitis, gallbladder abscess, and malignant obstruction of the gallbladder may carry high morbidity and mortality.[163] These patients are candidates for percutaneous cholecystostomy. The gallbladder can be punctured percutaneously with a fine needle, and bile obtained for culture.[164] The gallbladder may be opacified with contrast material to diagnose obstruction, and drainage can be instituted for empyema, acute calculous or acalculous cholecystitis, or common bile duct obstruction (Fig. 20-34).[164,165] The procedure may be guided by US or CT. If a portable real-time US unit is used, the entire intervention can be performed as a bedside procedure. The complication rate is low, with no major complications in one series of 17 high-risk patients.[163] Serious vagal reactions have been reported in some patients, especially those with acutely inflamed gallbladders.[164] Although this procedure does not provide access to the entire biliary tree, it is a useful and minimally invasive adjunct in critically ill patients with gallbladder disease.

URINARY TRACT INTERVENTIONS

Since the first report of percutaneous nephrostomy (PCN) in 1955,[166] the number of conditions treated in this fashion has greatly expanded as a result of the development of interventional radiology and endourology.[167–169] Nonetheless, the primary indication for PCN in the oncology patient continues to be urinary diversion, and it has largely replaced operative nephrostomy tube placement for this purpose.

Guidance for PCN can be provided by fluoroscopy, US, CT, or a combination of these methods.[167] Generally, the skin entry site is along the posterior axillary line, below the 12th rib, and the needle is directed toward the posterolateral cortex of the kidney. More cephalad entry sites risk pneumothorax and injury to the spleen or liver. Adjustments in technique are required for splenomegaly, scoliosis, and anomalous rotations and positions of the kidney.

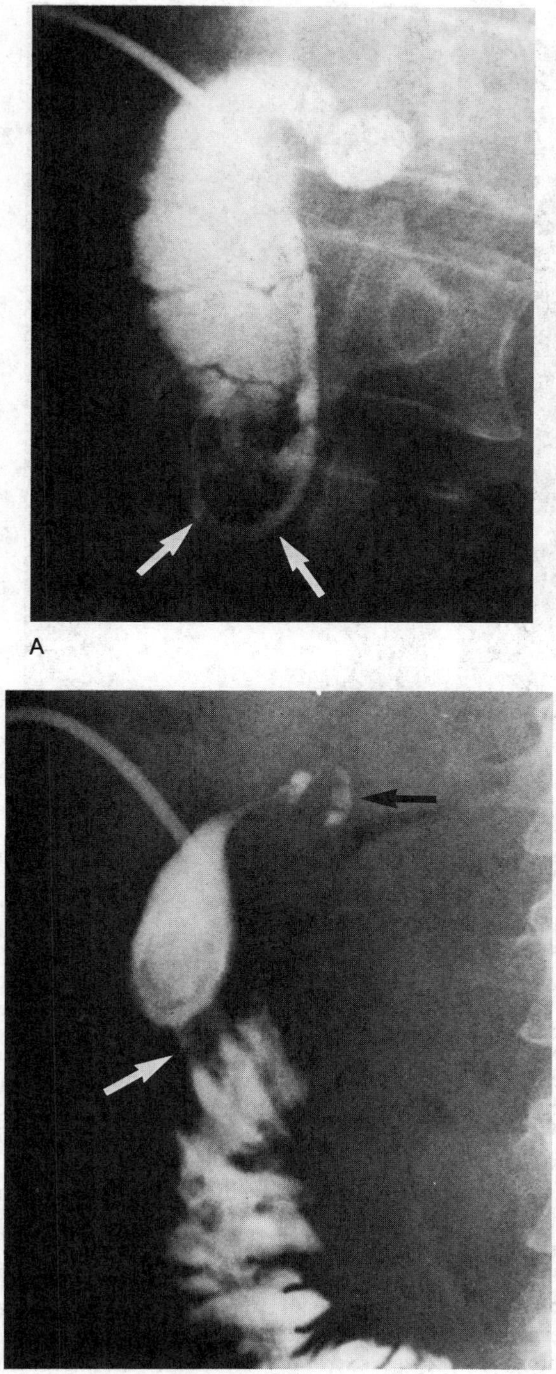

A

B

FIG. 20-34. Percutaneous cholecystostomy for empyema of the gallbladder. Obstruction of the common bile duct was also present because of a malignant islet cell tumor. **A**. Percutaneous cholecystostomy was performed with ultrasound and fluoroscopic guidance. The catheter tip (*arrows*) is seen in the fundus of the partially opacified gallbladder. **B**. The patient subsequently underwent surgical cholecystoenterostomy as a permanent bypass procedure. The cholecystostomy catheter was left in place in the immediate postoperative period. A contrast study demonstrates the anastomosis (*white arrow*) and reflux of contrast material into the cystic duct (*black arrow*).

Types of Urologic Prostheses

There are three basic types of prostheses for urinary drainage: nephrostomy catheters, internal stents, and external stent catheters. Nephrostomy catheters are short catheters placed in the renal pelvis or upper collecting system to divert urine externally. They do not stent the ureter and cannot be used for internal drainage. They are the simplest devices to place and to change.

Double-J or double-pigtail stents have largely replaced other designs for entirely internal ureteral stents.[170,171] Both the end in the renal pelvis and the end in the bladder have a J or pigtail shape to reduce mucosal irritation and prevent migration (Fig. 20-35). These catheters can be placed using either an antegrade (percutaneous) approach or a retrograde (cystoscopic) approach.[172,173]

The third general type of urologic prosthesis is the ureteral stent with external drainage or access port (nephroureterostomy).[170] In some ways this is the most versatile of the urologic prostheses. The external port may be used for external drainage or can be capped off for internal drainage, and it provides easy accessibility when the catheter needs to be changed.

Each type of urologic prosthesis has advantages and disadvantages. Simple nephrostomy diversion uses a urine collection appliance that requires daily maintenance and is unsuitable for patients who are poorly motivated or who have altered mental status. Some patients find it socially unacceptable. Internal stents obviate many of these inconveniences, but cystoscopy is required for removal or replacement of the stent. Because there is no outward indicator of stent function, stent failure can be insidious and permanent renal damage may occur before it is recognized (see Fig. 20-35). In contrast, nephrostomy tube failure is readily identified by decreased urine volume, leakage around the catheter, fever, or flank pain that leads the patient to seek prompt attention. All urologic prostheses should be changed prophylactically on a regular basis.[171,174,175]

Complications

The mortality associated with PCN is less than 0.2%, and significant complications occur at the rate of only 4% to 5%.[167,176] By contrast, mortality for surgical urinary diversion in the oncology patient is about 3% to 8%, and the complication rate is 25% to 45%.[177,178]

Serious complications associated with PCN are primarily related to septicemia and hemorrhage. Septicemia, including septic shock, occurs in 1% to 2% of patients, most often those with preexisting infection.[179] Minor bleeding is common but clears within a few days. Clinically significant hemorrhage occurs at a rate of 1% to 2%.[167,180] Bleeding may be into the collecting system, the renal parenchyma and subcapsular tissue, or the perinephric space and retroperitoneum.[181,182] Hemorrhage may be delayed rather than immediate, since the nephrostomy tube may initially tamponade the injured vessel.[183]

Permanent injury to the kidney from PCN is rare. In a study of 36 patients 3 years or more after PCN, only one patient had a focal cortical scar that appeared to be related to

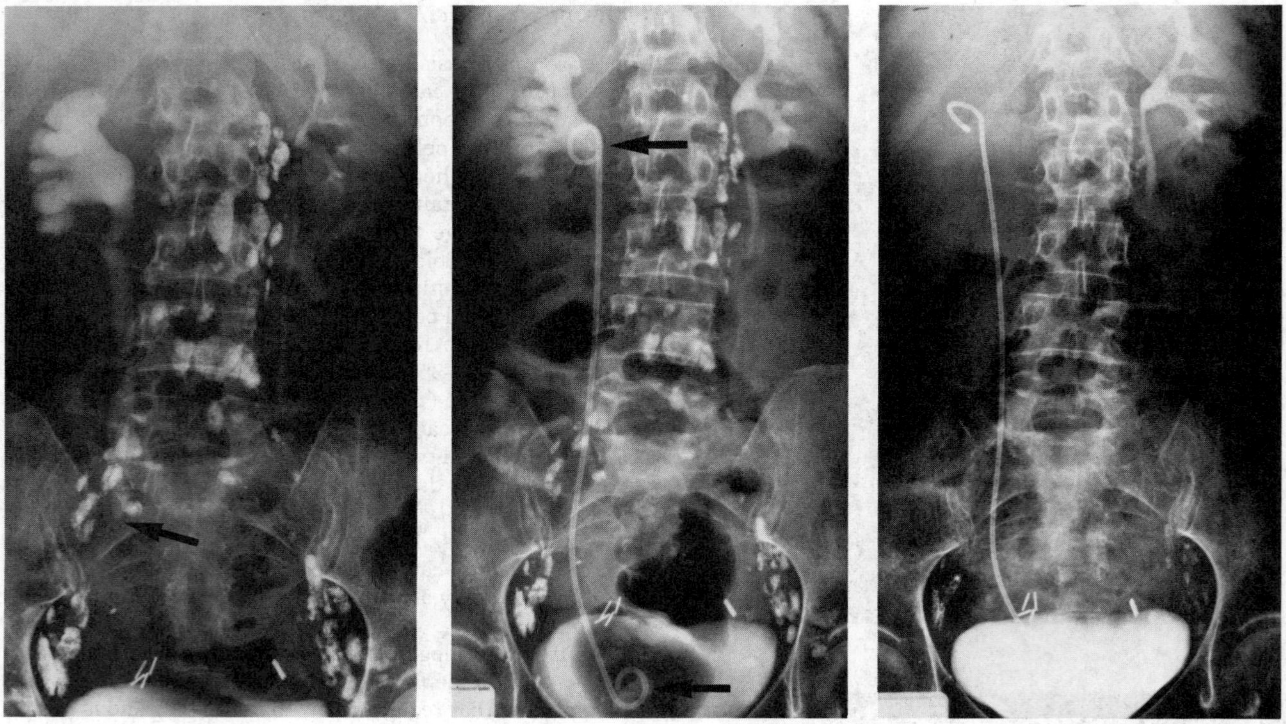

FIG. 20-35. Complete obstruction of the right ureter in a woman with ovarian carcinoma. **A**. The initial intravenous urogram demonstrates hydronephrosis of the right kidney and complete obstruction of the right ureter (*arrow*). **B**. The patient refused any drainage device that was not completely internal. A double pigtail internal ureteral stent was placed percutaneously. One pigtail is in the renal pelvis and the other in the bladder (arrows). **C**. The patient returned for a routine follow-up intravenous urogram 2 months later. She was asymptomatic, but the urogram revealed complete obstruction of the right kidney. The internal stent was removed cystoscopically and a new one placed. The lumen of the original stent was completely blocked by encrustations.

PCN.[184] (For additional information, see Chapter 58, section 5).

OTHER INTERVENTIONS

PERCUTANEOUS PLACEMENT OF INFERIOR VENA CAVA FILTERS. Cancer is a frequent underlying cause of pulmonary embolic disease and a common indication for placement of inferior vena cava (IVC) filters.[185,186] A number of filters have been developed.[187-191] Of these, only two —the Mobin-Uddin filter and the Greenfield filter (Fig. 20-36)—have been in general clinical use. Both can be inserted percutaneously.[192-194] The Mobin-Uddin filter had a high rate of IVC occlusion,[195] and is no longer available.[191]

The Greenfield filter can be inserted surgically or percutaneously through either the femoral vein or the jugular vein, using a carrier system (see Fig. 20-36). Percutaneous insertion avoids the necessity of venotomy and a large surgical incision. The entire procedure can be performed in the radiology department, and much of the discomfort and expense of surgery is avoided. Although metastatic cancer may be a relative contraindication to surgical placement of an IVC filter,[185] the use of the percutaneous technique eliminates much of this objection since an experienced angiographer can insert a Greenfield filter percutaneously in 10 to 20 minutes with little discomfort to the patient.[193]

In two small series, no complications were observed after percutaneous filter placement.[192,196] In other larger series, the incidence of femoral vein thrombosis after percutaneous filter placement via the femoral route was 2% to 10%.[197-199] In one series of 17 patients, 41% had venographic evidence of femoral vein thrombosis, but only 12% had significant symptoms.[200] Lower extremity swelling, when present, is usually transient.

PERCUTANEOUS ENTEROSTOMY. Percutaneous gastrostomy is a valuable adjunct in patients who require enteral alimentation. It is also occasionally useful for chronic gastrointestinal decompression.[201,202] Percutaneous gastrostomy may be performed by a radiologist, using a trocar or the Seldinger technique,[203-207] or by a surgeon or gastroenterologist using an endoscope.[201,208,209] In either case, local anesthesia is all that is usually required. Fixation and adherence of the stomach to the anterior abdominal wall usually occurs

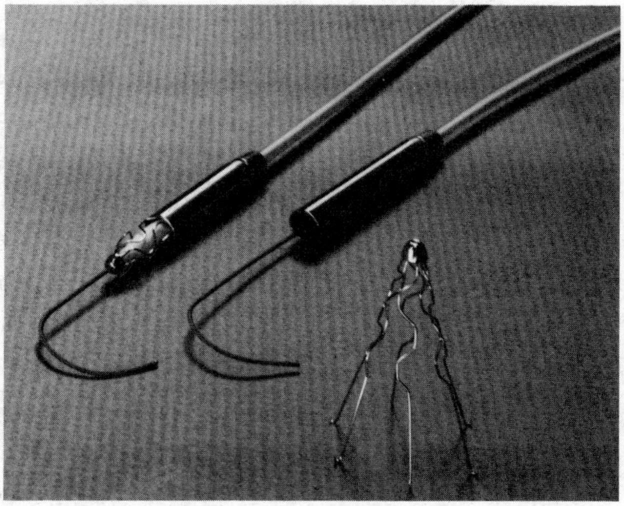

FIG. 20-36. The Greenfield filter (*foreground*) is a conical device designed to be inserted using a special carrier. Different carriers are available for insertion through the femoral vein (*left*) or the jugular vein (*center*). (Courtesy of Medi-tech, Inc., Watertown, MA)

within days.[205,208] In two series totaling 637 endoscopic percutaneous gastrostomies there was a 0.3% to 1.0% mortality and a 3% to 6% rate of major complications.[208,209] There were no major complications in one series of 32 patients who underwent radiologic percutaneous gastrostomy, two major complications in another series of 40 patients, and two major complications in a third series of 72 radiologic procedures.[204,206,207] The endoscopic technique cannot be used in patients with esophageal obstruction, and previous gastric surgery (*e.g.*, Billroth II procedure) may make either approach difficult or impossible.

Percutaneous radiologic techniques can also be used for enterostomy elsewhere in the gastrointestinal tract. There are reports of percutaneous cecostomy for drug instillation and for therapy of Ogilvie's syndrome (adynamic ileus of the colon).[210,211] Leakage of fecal material into the peritoneal cavity does not appear to be a problem. This technique has also been used for nonsurgical relief of a closed-loop small bowel obstruction.[212] As of 1988, these procedures must still be considered experimental.

MISCELLANEOUS PROCEDURES. The patient with cancer often has other medical problems as well, and radiologic interventions of many types may occasionally be useful. New forms of radiologic intervention and new methods for better accomplishing existing interventions are being developed on an almost daily basis. Abscess drainage, management of gastrointestinal bleeding, transluminal angioplasty, intra-arterial and intravenous thrombolysis, treatment of biliary and urinary stones and strictures, and removal of intravascular foreign bodies may all be accomplished by a well-trained radiologist. Radiologic intervention has had and will continue to have a major impact on the practice of oncology.

REFERENCES

1. White RI Jr: Interventional radiology: Reflections and expectations. The 1985 Eugene P. Pendergrass New Horizons Lecture. Radiology 162:593–600, 1987
2. Margolis AR: Interventional diagnostic radiology: A new subspecialty. AJR 99:761–762, 1967
3. Doby T: A tribute to Sven-Ivar Seldinger. AJR 142:1–3, 1984
4. Grüntzig A, Hopff H: Perkutane Rekanalization chronischer Arteriellar verschlüsse mit einem neuen Dilationskatheter: Modification der Dotter-technik. Dtsch Med Wochenschr 99:2502–2505, 1974
5. Dotter CT, Judkins MP: Transluminal treatment of arteriosclerotic obstruction: Description of a new technique and a preliminary report of its application. Circulation 30:654–670, 1964
6. Baum S, Nusbaum, M, Blakemore W: Demonstration of intraabdominal bleeding by selective arteriography. JAMA 191:389–390, 1965
7. Husband JE, Golding SJ: The role of computed-tomography guided needle biopsy in an oncology service. Clin Radiol 34:255–260, 1983
8. Bottles K, Miller TR, Cohen MB et al: Fine needle aspiration biopsy: Has its time come? Am J Med 81:525–531, 1986
9. Bernardino ME: Percutaneous biopsy. AJR 142:41–45, 1984
10. Lieberman RP, Hafez GR, Crummy AB: Histology from aspiration biopsy: Turner needle experience. AJR 138:561–564, 1982
11. Wittenberg J, Mueller PR, Ferrucci JT Jr et al: Percutaneous core biopsy of abdominal tumors using 22 gauge needles: Further observations. AJR 139:75–80, 1982
12. Haaga JR, LiPuma JP, Bryan PJ et al: Clinical comparison of small- and large-caliber cutting needles for biopsy. Radiology 146:665–667, 1983
13. Weisbrod GL, Herman SJ, Tao L-C: Preliminary experience with a dual cutting edge needle in thoracic percutaneous fine-needle aspiration biopsy. Radiology 163:75–78, 1987
14. Grant EG, Richardson JD, Smirniotopoulous JG et al: fine-needle biopsy directed by real-time sonography: Technique and accuracy. AJR 141:29–32, 1983
15. Harter LP, Moss AA, Goldberg HI et al: CT-guided fine-needle aspirations for diagnosis of benign and maligant disease. AJR 140:363–367, 1983
16. Pagani JJ: Biopsy of focal hepatic lesions: Comparison of 18 and 22 gauge needles. Radiology 147:673–675, 1983
17. Martino CR, Haaga JR, Bryan PJ et al: CT-guided liver biopsies: Eight years' experience. Work in progress. Radiology 152:755–757, 1984
18. Ayala AG, Zornosa J: Primary bone tumors: Percutaneous needle biopsy. Radiologic-pathologic study of 222 biopsies. Radiology 149:675–679, 1983
19. Pais MJ, Lightfoote JB, Burnett K et al: Trephine bone biopsy system: A refined needle for radiologists. Radiology 153:253–254, 1984
20. Larédo J-D, Bard M: Thoracic spine: Percutaneous trephine biopsy. Radiology 160:485–489, 1986
21. Mink J: Percutaneous bone biopsy in the patient with known or suspected osseous metastases. Radiology 161:191–194, 1986
22. Hall-Craggs MA, Lees WR: Fine needle biopsy: Cytology, histology, or both? Gut 28:233–236, 1987
23. Kasugai H, Yamamoto R, Tatsuta M et al: Value of heparinized fine-needle aspiration biopsy in liver malignancy. AJR 144:243–244, 1985
24. Zajdela A, Zillhardt P, Voillemot N: Cytological diagnosis by fine needle sampling without aspiration. Cancer 59:1201–1205, 1987
25. vanSonnenberg E, Wittich GR, Edwards DK et al: Percutaneous diagnostic and interventional radiologic procedures in children: Experience in 100 patients. Radiology 162:601–605, 1987
26. Miller DA, Carrasco CH, Katz RL et al: Fine needle aspiration biopsy: The role of immediate cytologic assessment. AJR 147:155–158, 1986
27. Axel L: Simple method for performing oblique CT-guided needle biopsies. AJR 143:341–342, 1984
28. Sundaram M, Wolverson MK, Heiberg E et al: Utility of CT-guided abdominal aspiration procedures. AJR 139:1111–1115, 1982
29. Mueller PR, Stark DD, Simeone JF et al: MR-guided aspiration biopsy: Needle design and clinical trials. Radiology 161:605–609, 1986
30. Bret PM, Fond A, Casola G et al: Abdominal lesions: A prospective study of clinical efficacy of percutaneous fine-needle biopsy. Radiology 159:345–346, 1986
31. Fortier KF, Clarke-Pearson DL, Creasman WT et al: Fine-needle aspiration in gynecology: Evaluation of extrapelvic lesions in patients with gynecologic malignancy. Obstet Gynecol 65:67–73, 1985
32. Gobien RP, Bouchard EA, Gobien BS et al: Thin-needle aspiration biopsy of thoracic lesions: Impact on hospital charges and patterns of patient care. Radiology 148:65–67, 1983
33. Westcott JL: Direct percutaneous needle aspiration of localized pulmonary lesions: Results in 422 patients. Radiology 137:31–35, 1980
34. Mitty HA, Efremidis SC, Yeh H-C: Impact of fine-needle biopsy on management of patients with carcinoma of the pancreas. AJR 137:1119–1121, 1981
35. Diament MJ, Boechat MI, Kangarloo H: Interventional radiology in infants and children: Clinical and technical aspects. Radiology 154:359–361, 1985
36. Towbin RB, Strife JL: Percutaneous aspiration, drainage and biopsies in children. Radiology 157:81–85, 1985
37. Ferrucci JT Jr, Wittenberg J, Mueller PR et al: Diagnosis of abdominal malignancy by radiologic fine-needle aspiration biopsy. AJR 134:323–330, 1980
38. Khouri NF, Stitik FP, Erozan YS et al: Transthoracic needle aspiration biopsy of benign and malignant lung lesions. AJR 144:281–288, 1985

39. Stanley JH, Fish GD, Andriole JG et al: Lung lesions: Cytologic diagnosis by fine-needle biopsy. Radiology 162:389–391, 1987
40. Westcott JL: Percutaneous needle aspiration of hilar and mediastinal masses. Radiology 151:301–304, 1981
41. Hall-Craggs MA, Lees WR: Fine-needle aspiration biopsy: Pancreatic and biliary tumors. AJR 147:399–403, 1986
42. Mitnick JS, Bosniak MA, Megibow AJ et al: Nonfunctioning adrenal adenomas discovered incidentally on computed tomography. Radiology 148:495–499, 1983
43. Belldegrun A, Hussain S, Seltzer SE et al: Incidentally discovered mass of the adrenal gland. Surg Gynecol Obstet 163:203–208, 1986
44. Heaston DK, Handel DB, Ashton PR et al: Narrow gauge needle aspiration of solid adrenal masses. AJR 138:1143–1148, 1982
45. Bernardino ME, Walther MM, Philips VM et al: CT-guided adrenal biopsy: Accuracy, safety, and indications. AJR 144:67–69, 1985
46. Kidd R, Crane RD, Dail DH: Lymphangiography and fine-needle aspiration biopsy: Ineffective for staging early prostate cancer. AJR 141:1007–1012, 1984
47. Kidd R, Correa R Jr: Fine needle aspiration biopsy of lymphangiographically normal lymph nodes: A negative view. AJR 141:1005–1006, 1984
48. Hewes RC, Vigorita VJ, Freiberger RH: Percutaneous bone biopsy: The importance of aspirated osseous blood. Radiology 148:69–72, 1983
49. Rose JS: Invasive Radiology: Risks and Patient Care, p 122. Chicago, Year Book Medical Publishers, 1983
50. Solbiati L, Livraghi T, De Pra L et al: Fine-needle biopsy of hepatic hemangioma with sonographic guidance. AJR 144:471–474, 1985
51. Cronan JJ, Esparza AR, Dorfman GS et al: Cavernous hemangioma of the liver: Role of percutaneous biopsy. Radiology 166:135–138, 1988
52. Martin CR, Haaga JR, Bryan PJ: Secondary infection of an endometrioma following fine-needle aspiration. Radiology 151:53–54, 1984
53. Ferrucci JT Jr, Wittenberg J, Margolies MN et al: Malignant seeding of the tract after thin needle aspiration biopsy. Radiology 130:345–346, 1979
54. Smith FP, MacDonald JS, Schein S et al: Cutaneous seeding of pancreatic cancer by skinny needle aspiration biopsy. Arch Intern Med 140:855, 1980
55. Sinner WN, Zajicek J: Implantation metastasis after percutaneous transthoracic needle aspiration biopsy. Acta Radiol [Diagn] 17:473–480, 1976
56. Eriksson O, Hagmar B, Ryo W: Effects of fine-needle aspiration and other biopsy procedures on tumor dissemination in mice. Cancer 54:73–78, 1984
57. Mühlberger G, Gottschalk A, Gericke D: Needle biopsy and metastasis: Investigations in rats. Radiologe 23:185–188, 1983
58. Stevens GM, Jackman RJ: Outpatient needle biopsy of the lung: Its safety and utility. Radiology 151:301–304, 1984
59. Perlmutt LM, Braun SD, Newman GE et al: Timing of chest film follow-up after transthoracic needle aspiration. AJR 146:1049–1050, 1986
60. Perlmutt LM, Braun SD, Newman GE et al: Transthoracic needle aspiration: Use of a small chest tube to treat pneumothorax. AJR 148:849–851, 1987
61. Bourgouin PM, Shepard J-AO, McCloud TC et al: Transthoracic needle aspiration biopsy: Evaluation of the blood patch technique. Radiology 166:93–95, 1988
62. Casola G, vanSonnenberg E, Keightley A et al: Pneumothorax: Radiologic treatment with small catheters. Radiology 166:89–91, 1988
63. Pagani JJ: Normal adrenal glands in small cell lung carcinoma: CT-guided biopsy. AJR 140:949–951, 1983
64. McCorkell SJ, Niles NL: Fine-needle aspiration of catecholamine-producing adrenal masses: A possibly fatal mistake. AJR 145:113–114, 1985
65. Casola G, Nicolet V, vanSonnenberg E et al: Unsuspected pheochromocytoma: Risk of blood-pressure alterations during percutaneous adrenal biopsy. Radiology 159:733–735, 1986
66. Reining JW, Doppman JL, Dwyer AJ et al: MRI of indeterminate adrenal masses. AJR 147:493–496, 1986
67. Eckman WW, Patlak CS, Fenstermacher JD: Critical evaluation of principles governing the advantages of intra-arterial infusion. J Pharmacokinet Biopharm 102:221–229, 1974
68. Chen HG, Gross JK: Intra-arterial infusion of anticancer drugs: Theoretical aspects of drug delivery and review of response. Cancer Treat Rep 64:31–40, 1980
69. Dedrick RI, Oldfield EH, Collins JM: Arterial drug infusions with extracorporeal removal: I. Theoretical basis with particular reference to brain. Cancer Treat Rep 68:373–380, 1984
70. Sullivan RD, Norcross JW, Watkins E Jr: Chemotherapy of metastatic liver cancer by prolonged hepatic artery infusion. N Engl J Med 270:321, 1964
71. Patt YZ, Chuang VP, Wallace S et al: The palliative role of hepatic artery infusion and arterial occlusion in colorectal carcinoma metastatic to the liver. Lancet 1:349–351, 1981
72. Patt YZ, Peters RE, Chuang VP et al: Effective retreatment of patients with colorectal cancer and liver metastases. Am J Med 75:237–240, 1983
73. Patt YZ, Chuang VP, Wallace S: Hepatic arterial chemotherapy and occlusion for palliation of primary hepatocellular and unknown primary neoplasm in the liver. Cancer 51:1359–1363, 1983
74. Benjamin RS, Murray JA, Wallace S et al: Intra-arterial preoperative chemotherapy for osteosarcoma: A judicious approach to limb salvage. Cancer Bull 36:32–36, 1984
75. Wallace S, Chuang VP, Samuels ML et al: Transcatheter intra-arterial infusion of chemotherapy in advanced bladder cancer. Cancer 49:640–645, 1982
76. Logothetis CJ, Samuels ML, Wallace S et al: Management of pelvic complication of malignant urothelial tumors with combined intra-arterial and IV chemotherapy. Cancer Treat Rep 66:1501–1507, 1982
77. Scarabelli C, Tumolo S, De Paoli A et al: Intermittent pelvic arterial infusion with peptichemo, doxorubicin and cisplatin for locally advanced and recurrent carcinoma of the uterine cervix. Cancer 60:25–30, 1987
78. Molinori R: Present role of intra-arterial regional chemotherapy in head and neck cancer. Drugs Exp Clin Res 7:491–504, 1983
79. Lee YY, Wallace S, Dimery I et al: Intra-arterial chemotherapy of head and neck tumors. AJNR 7:343, 1986
80. Kuribayashi S, Phillips DA, Harrington DP et al: Therapeutic embolization of the gastroduodenal artery in hepatic artery infusion chemotherapy. AJR 137:1169, 1981
81. Granmayeh M, Wallace S, Schwarten D: Catheter occlusion of the gastroduodenal artery. Radiology 131:59–64, 1979
82. Michels NA: Blood Supply and Anatomy of the Upper Abdominal Organs, p 581. Philadelphia, JB Lippincott, 1955
83. Chuang VP, Wallace S: Hepatic arterial redistribution for intra-arterial infusion for hepatic neoplasms. Radiology 135:295–299, 1981
84. Charnsangavej C, Chuang VP, Wallace S et al: Angiographic classification of hepatic arterial collaterals. Radiology 144:485, 1982
85. Makuuchi M, Sukigara M, Mori T et al: Bile duct necrosis: Complication of transcatheter hepatic arterial embolization. Radiology 156:331–334, 1985
86. Botet JF, Watson RC, Kemeny N et al: Cholangitis complicating intra-arterial chemotherapy in liver metastases. Radiology 156:335–337, 1985
87. Pien EH, Zeman RK, Benjamin SB et al: Iatrogenic sclerosing cholangitis following hepatic arterial chemotherapy infusion. Radiology 156:329–330, 1985
88. Shea WJ, Demas BE, Goldberg HI et al: Sclerosing cholangitis associated with hepatic arterial FUDR chemotherapy: Radiographic/histiologic correlation. AJR 146:717, 1986
89. Anderson SD, Holley HC, Berland LL et al: Causes of jaundice during hepatic artery infusion chemotherapy. Radiology 161:439, 1986
90. Chrousos G, Oldfield EH, Doppman JL et al: Prevention of ocular toxicity by carmustine (BCNU) with supraophthalmic intracarotid infusion. Ophthalmology 93:1471–1475, 1986
91. Doppman JL, Dedrick RL, Shook DR et al: Glioblastoma catheter techniques for isolated chemotherapy perfusion. Radiology 159:477–483, 1986
92. Blacklock JB, Wright DC, Dedrick R et al: Drug streaming during intra-arterial chemotherapy. J Neurosurg 64:284–291, 1986
93. Lutz RJ, Dedrick RL, Boretos JW et al: Mixing studies during intracarotid artery infusions in an in vitro model. J Neurosurg 64:277–283, 1986
94. Bledin AG, Kim EE, Haynie TP: Technetium Tc 99m macroaggregated albumin angiography and perfusion: Intra-arterial chemotherapy for neoplasms. JAMA 250:941–943, 1983
95. Wright KC, Wallace S, Kim EE et al: Pulsed arterial infusions: Chemotherapeutic considerations. Cancer 57:1952–1956, 1986
96. Shook DR, Beaudet LM, Doppman JL: Uniformity of intracarotid distribution with diastole-phased pulsed infusions. J Neurosurg 67:721–725, 1987
97. Miller DL: Failure of Ivalon to provide permanent hepatic arterial occlusion. Cardiovasc Intervent Radiol 10:111–113, 1987
98. Lin G, Hagerstrand I, Lunderquist A: Portal blood supply of liver metastasis. AJR 143:53, 1984
99. Carrasco CH, Charnsangavej C, Ajani J et al: The carcinoid syndrome: Palliation by hepatic artery embolization. AJR 147:149–154, 1986
100. Yamada R, Sato M, Kawabata M et al: Hepatic artery embolization in 120 patients with unresectable hepatoma. Radiology 148:397–401, 1983
101. Nakao N, Miura K, Takahashi H et al: Hepatocellular carcinoma: combined hepatic arterial and portal venous embolization. Radiology 161:303, 1986
102. Wallace S, Charnsangavej C, Carrasco CH: Transcatheter management of the cancer patient. In DeVita VT, Hellman S, Rosenberg SA (eds): Cancer: Principles and Practice of Oncology, 2nd ed, pp 2304–2320. Philadelphia, JB Lippincott, 1986
103. Ekelund L, Ek A, Forsberg L et al: Occlusion of renal arterial tumor supply with absolute ethanol: Experience with 20 cases. Radiology 155:275, 1985
104. Klinberg I, Hunter P, Hawkins IF et al: Preoperative angioinfarction of localized renal cell carcinoma using absolute ethanol. Radiology 156:271, 1985
105. Fink IJ, Girton M, Doppman JL: Absolute ethanol injection of the adrenal artery: Hypertensive reaction. Radiology 154:357–358, 1985
106. Cox GC, Lee KR, Price HI et al: Colonic infarction following ethanol embolization of renal cell carcinoma. Radiology 145:343, 1982
107. Chuang VP, Wallace S, Swanson D et al: Arterial occlusion in the management of pain from metastatic renal carcinoma. Radiology 133:611–614, 1979
108. Bowers TA, Murray JA, Charnsangavej C et al: Bone metastasis from renal carcinoma. J Bone Joint Surg [AM] 64:749–754, 1982
109. Kobayashi I, Kusano S, Matsubayashi T et al: Selective embolization of the vesical artery in the management of massive bladder hemorrhage. Radiology 136:345–348, 1980
110. Wallace S, Granmayeh M, de Santos LA et al: Arterial occlusion of pelvic bone tumors. Cancer 43:322–328, 1979
110a. Hemingway AP, Allison DJ: Complications of embolization: Analysis of 410 procedures. Radiology 166:669–672, 1988
111. Carroll BA, Walter JF: Gas in embolized tumors: An alternate hypothesis for its origin. Radiology 147:441–444, 1983
112. Rankin RN: Gas formation after renal tumor embolization without abscess: A benign occurrence. Radiology 130:317–320, 1979
113. Kato L, Nemoto R, Mori H et al: Arterial embolization with microencapsulated anticancer drug. JAMA 245:1123–1127, 1981

114. Kerr DJ: Microparticulate drug delivery systems as an adjunct to cancer treatment. Cancer Drug Deliv 4:55–61, 1987
115. Nakakuma K, Tashiro S, Hiraoka T et al: Hepatocellular carcinoma and metastatic cancer detected by iodized oil. Radiology 154:15–17, 1985
116. Yumoto Y, Jino K, Tokuyama K et al: Hepatocellular carcinoma detected by iodized oil. Radiology 154:19–24, 1985
117. Miller DL, O'Leary TJ, Girton M: Distribution of iodized oil within the liver after hepatic arterial injection. Radiology 162:849–852, 1987
118. Ohnishi K, Tsuchiya S, Nakayama T et al: Arterial chemoembolization of hepatocellular carcinoma with mitomycin-C microcapsules. Radiology 152:51–55, 1984
119. Ohishi H, Uchida H, Yoshimura H et al: Hepatocellular carcinoma detected by iodized oil: Use of anti-cancer agents. Radiology 154:25–29, 1985
120. Takayasu K, Shima Y, Muramatsu Y et al: Hepatocellular carcinoma: Treatment with intra-arterial iodized oil with and without chemotherapeutic agents. Radiology 162:345–351, 1987
121. Konno T, Maeda H, Iwai K et al: Effect of arterial administration of high molecular-weight anticancer agent SMANCS with lipid lymphangiographic agent on hepatoma. Eur J Cancer Clin Oncol 19:1053–1065, 1983
122. Livraghi T, Festi D, Monti F et al: US-guided percutaneous alcohol injection of small hepatic and abdominal tumors. Radiology 161:309, 1986
122a. Shiina S, Yasuda H, Muto H et al: Percutaneous ethanol injection in the treatment of liver neoplasms. AJR 149:949–952, 1987
123. Burgener FA, Steinmetz SD: Treatment of experimental adenocarcinomas by percutaneous tumor injection of absolute alcohol. Invest Radiol 22:472–478, 1987
124. Sheu J-C, Huang GT, Chen DS et al. Small hepatocellular carcinoma: Intratumoral ethanol treatment using new needles and guidance system. Radiology 160:43–48, 1987
125. Misaki T, Hizazumi H, Miayoski N: Photoradiation therapy of bladder tumors. In Doiron DR, Gomer CJ (eds): Porphyrin Localization and Treatment of Tumors, pp 795–804. New York, Alan R Liss, 1987
126. Hayata Y, Kato H, Konaka C et al: Hematoporphyrin derivative in laser photoradiation and treatment of lung cancer. Chest 81:269–277, 1982
127. Gattenby RA, Hartz WH, Engstrom PF et al: CT-guided laser therapy in resistant tumors: Phase I clinical trials. Radiology 163:172–175, 1987
128. Passariello R, Pavone P, Rossi P et al: Percutaneous biliary drainage in neoplastic jaundice: Statistical data from a computerized multicenter investigation. Acta Radiol [Diagn] 26:681–688, 1985
129. Bonnel D, Ferrucci JT Jr, Mueller PR et al: Surgical and radiological decompression in malignant biliary obstruction: A retrospective study using multivariate risk factor analysis. Radiology 152:347–351, 1984
130. Bornman PC, Harries-Jones EP, Tobias R et al: Prospective controlled trial of transhepatic biliary endoprosthesis versus bypass surgery for incurable carcinoma of the head of the pancreas. Lancet 1:69–71, 1986
131. Pessa ME, Hawkins IF, Vogel SB: The treatment of acute cholangitis: Percutaneous transhepatic biliary drainage before definitive therapy. Ann Surg 205:389–392, 1987
132. Thomas JH, Connor CS, Pierce GE et al: Effect of biliary decompression on morbidity and mortality of pancreaticoduodenectomy. Am J Surg 148:727–731, 1984
133. Gobien RP, Stanley JH, Soucek CD et al: Routine preoperative biliary drainage: Effect on management of obstructive jaundice. Radiology 152:353–356, 1984
134. Gundry SR, Strodel WE, Knol JA et al: Efficacy of preoperative biliary tract decompression in patients with obstructive jaundice. Arch Surg 119:703–708, 1984
135. Pitt HA, Gomes AS, Lots JF et al: Does preoperative percutaneous biliary drainage reduce operative risk or increase hospital cost? Ann Surg 201:545–553, 1985
136. Gouma DJ, Coelho JCU, Schlegal JF et al: The effect of preoperative internal and external biliary drainage on mortality of jaundiced rats. Arch Surg 122:731–734, 1987
137. Lygidakis NJ, Brummelkamp WH, Huibregtse K et al: Different response to preliminary biliary drainage in proximal versus distal malignant biliary obstruction. Surg Gynecol Obstet 164:159–162, 1987
138. McLean GK, Jordan HA: Percutaneous transhepatic biliary drainage: Comments and recommendations. Semin Intervent Radiol 2:69–73, 1985
139. Lokich JJ, Kane RA, Harrison DA et al: Biliary tract obstruction secondary to cancer: Management guidelines and selected literature review. J Clin Oncol 5:969–981, 1987
140. McLean GK, Burke DR: Nonoperative therapy of biliary obstruction. In DeVita VT Jr, Hellman S, Rosenberg SA (eds): Important Advances in Oncology 1987, pp 279–292. Philadelphia, JB Lippincott, 1987
141. Marks WM, Freeny PC, Ball TJ et al: Endoscopic retrograde biliary drainage. Radiology 152:357–360, 1984
142. Stanley J, Gobien RP, Cunningham J et al: Biliary decompression: An institutional comparison of percutaneous and endoscopic methods. Radiology 158:195–197, 1986
143. Tsang T-K, Crampton AR, Bernstein JR et al: Percutaneous-endoscopic bilary stent placement: A preliminary report. Ann Intern Med 106:389–392, 1987
144. Dick R, Platts A, Gilford J et al: The Carey–Coons percutaneous biliary endoprosthesis: A three-centre experience in 87 patients. Clin Radiol 38:175–178, 1987
145. Adam A: Use of the modified Cope introduction set for transhepatic removal of obstructed Carey-Coons biliary endoprosthesis. Clin Radiol 38:171–174, 1987
146. Walta DC, Fausel CS, Brant B: Endoscopic biliary stents and obstructive jaundice. Am J Surg 153:444–447, 1987
147. Kerlan RK Jr, Stimac G, Pogany AC et al: Bile flow through drainage catheters: An in vitro study. AJR 143:1085–1087, 1984
148. Lammer J, Neumayer K: Biliary drainage endoprostheses: Experience with 201 placements. Radiology 159:625–629, 1986
149. Speer AG, Cotton PB, Russel RCG et al: Randomised trial of endoscopic versus percutaneous stent insertion in malignant obstructive jaundice. Lancet 2:57–62, 1987
150. Ferrucci JT Jr, Adson MA, Mueller PR et al: Advances in the radiology of jaundice: A symposium and review. AJR 141:1–20, 1983
151. Beinart C, Efremidis S, Cohen B et al: Obstruction without dilatation: Importance in evaluating jaundice. JAMA 245:353–356, 1981
152. Zeman RK, Lee C, Jaffe MH et al: Hepatobiliary scintigraphy and sonography in early biliary obstruction. Radiology 153:793–798, 1984
153. Pereiras R Jr, Chiprut RO, Greenwald RA et al: Percutaneous transhepatic cholangiography with the "skinny" needle: A rapid, simple and accurate method in the diagnosis of cholestasis. Ann Intern Med 86:562–568, 1977
154. Suzuki Y, Kobayashi A, Ohto M et al: Bacteriological study of transhepatically aspirated bile: Relation to cholangiographic findings in 295 patients. Dig Dis Sci 29:109–115, 1984
155. Muro A, Mueller PR, Ferrucci JT Jr et al: Bile cytology: A routine addition to percutaneous biliary drainage. Radiology 149:846–847, 1983
156. Portner WJ, Koolpe HA: New devices for biliary drainage and biopsy. AJR 138:1191–1195, 1982
157. Clark RA, Mitchell SE, Colley DP et al: Percutaneous catheter biliary decompression. AJR 137:503–509, 1981
158. Yee ACN, Ho C-S: Complications of percutaneous biliary drainage: Benign vs malignant diseases. AJR 148:1207–1209, 1987
159. Carrasco CH, Zornoza J, Becthel WJ: Malignant biliary obstruction: Complications of percutaneous biliary drainage. Radiology 152:343–346, 1984
160. Joseph PK, Bizer LS, Sprayregen SS et al: Percutaneous transhepatic biliary drainage: Results and complications in 81 patients. JAMA 255:2763–2767, 1986
161. Cutherell L, Wanebo HJ, Tegtmeyer CJ: Catheter tract seeding after percutaneous biliary drainage for pancreatic cancer. Cancer 57:2057–2060, 1986
162. Anschuetz SL, Vogelzang RL: Malignant pleural effusion: A complication of transhepatic biliary drainage. AJR 146:1165–1166, 1986
163. Klimberg S, Hawkins I, Vogel SB: Percutaneous cholecystostomy for acute cholecystitis in high-risk patients. Am J Surg 153:125–129, 1987
164. vanSonnenberg E, Wittich GR, Casola G et al: Diagnostic and therapeutic percutaneous gallbladder procedures. Radiology 160:23–26, 1986
165. Teplick SK, Haskin PH, Sammon JK et al: Common bile duct obstruction: Assessment by transcholecystic cholangiography. Radiology 161:135–138, 1986
166. Goodwin WE, Casey WC, Woolf W: Percutaneous trocar (needle) nephrostomy in hydronephrosis. JAMA 157:891–894, 1955
167. Reznek RH, Talner LB: Percutaneous Nephrostomy. Radiol Clin North Am 22:393–406, 1984
168. Coleman CC, Kimura Y, Lange PH et al: Percutaneous nephrostomy: Indications, contraindications, preparation, and complications. Semin Intervent Radiol 1:38–41, 1984
169. Lee WJ, Smith AD, Cubelli V et al: Percutaneous nephrolithotomy: Analysis of 500 consecutive cases. Urol Radiol 8:61–66, 1986
170. Brazzini A, Castaneda-Zuniga WR, Coleman CC et al: Urostent designs. Semin Intervent Radiol 4:26–35, 1987
171. Finney RP: Double-J and diversion stents. Urol Clin North Am 9:89–94, 1982
172. Mazer MJ, LeVeen RF, Call JB: Permanent percutaneous antegrade ureteral stent placement without transurethral assistance. Urology 14:413–419, 1979
173. Rozenblit G, Tarasov E, Srur MF et al: Druy ureteral stent set: Clinical experience in 25 patients. Radiology 160:737–740, 1986
174. Mardis HK: Evaluation of polymeric materials for endourologic devices: Emerging importance of hydrogels. Semin Intervent Radiol 4:36–45, 1987
175. LeRoy AJ, Williams HJ Jr, Segura JW et al: Indwelling ureteral stents: Percutaneous management of complications. Radiology 158:219–222, 1986
176. Stables DP, Ginsberg NJ, Johnson ML: Percutaneous nephrostomy: A series and review of the literature. AJR 130:75–82, 1978
177. Holden S, McPhee M, Grabstald H: The rationale of urinary diversion in cancer patients. J Urol 121:19–21, 1979
178. Sharer W, Grayhack JT, Graham J: Palliative urinary diversion for malignant ureteral obstruction. J Urol 120:162–164, 1978
179. Barbaric ZL: Percutaneous nephrostomy for urinary tract obstruction. AJR 143:803–809, 1984
180. Cope C, Zeit RM: Pseudoaneurysms after nephrostomy. AJR 139:255–261, 1982
181. Cronan JJ, Dorfman GS, Amis ES et al: Retroperitoneal hemorrhage after percutaneous nephrostomy. AJR 144:801–803, 1985
182. Harris RD, Walther PC: Renal arterial injury associated with percutaneous nephrostomy. Urology 23:215–217, 1984
183. Gavant ML, Gold RE, Church JC: Delayed Rupture of renal pseudoaneurysm: Complication of percutaneous nephrostomy. AJR 138:948–949, 1982
184. Hruby W, Marberger M: Late sequelae of percutaneous nephrostomy. Work in progress. Radiology 152:383–385, 1984
185. Walsh DB, Downing S, Nauta R et al: Metastatic cancer: A relative contraindication to vena cava filter placement. Cancer 59:161–163, 1987
186. Maxwell RJ, Greenfield LJ: Effect of pulmonary embolism on survival of patients with Greenfield vena caval filters. Surgery 101:389–394, 1987

187. Günther RW, Schild H, Fries A et al: Vena caval filter to prevent pulmonary embolism: Experimental study. Work in progress. Radiology 156:315–320, 1985
188. Darcy MD, Cardella JF, Hunter DW et al: Experience with the Amplatz Retrievable vena caval filter. Work in progress. Radiology 161:611–614, 1986
189. Günther RW, Schild H, Hollman JP et al: First clinical results with a new caval filter. Cardiovasc intervent Radiol 10:104–108, 1987
190. Burke PE, Michna BA, Harvey CF et al: Experimental comparison of percutaneous vena caval devices: Titanium Greenfield filter versus bird's nest filter. J Vasc Surg 6:66–70, 1987
191. Katsamouris AA, Waltman AC, Delichatsios MA et al: Inferior vena cava filters: In vitro comparison of clot trapping and flow dynamics. Radiology 166:361–366, 1988
192. Denny DF, Cronan JJ, Dorfman GS et al: Percutaneous Kimray-Greenfield filter placement by femoral vein puncture. AJR 145:827–829, 1985
193. Tadavarthy SM, Castaneda-Zuniga W, Salomonowitz E et al: Kimray-Greenfield vena cava filter: Percutaneous introduction. Radiology 151:525–526, 1984
194. Knight L, Rizk G, Amplatz K: Percutaneous introduction of inferior vena cava filter: Human experience. Radiology 111:61–63, 1974
195. Cimochowski GE, Evans RH, Zarins CK et al: Greenfield filter versus Mobin-Uddin umbrella. J Thorac Cardiovasc Surg 79:358–365, 1980
196. Zeit RM: Greenfield filter placement via the femoral vein: Improved technique with extra-long sheath and purse-string suture. Radiology 163:575–576, 1987
197. Pais SO, Mirvis SE, De Orchis DF: Percutaneous insertion of the Kimray-Greenfield filter: Technical considerations and problems. Radiology 165:377–381, 1987
198. Rose BS, Simon DC, Hess ML et al: Percutaneous transfemoral placement of the Kimray-Greenfield vena cava filter. Radiology 165:373–376, 1987
199. Denny DF Jr, Dorfman GS, Cronan JJ et al: Greenfield filter: Percutaneous placement in 50 patients. AJR 50:427–429, 1988
200. Kantor A, Glanz S, Gordon DH et al: Percutaneous insertion of the Kimray-Greenfield filter: Incidence of femoral vein thrombosis. AJR 149:1065–1066, 1987
201. Stellato TA, Gauderer MWL: Percutaneous endoscopic gastrostomy for gastrointestinal decompression. Ann Surg 205:119–122, 1987
202. Picus D, Marx MV, Weyman PJ: Chronic intestinal obstruction: Value of percutaneous gastrostomy tube placement. AJR 150:295–297, 1988
203. Wills JS, Oglesby JT: Percutaneous gastrostomy: Further experience. Radiology 154:71–74, 1985
204. Ho C, Gray RR, Goldfinger M et al: Percutaneous gastrostomy for enteral feeding. Radiology 156:349–351, 1985
205. vanSonnenberg E, Wittich GR, Brown LK et al: Percutaneous gastrostomy and gastroenterostomy: 1. Techniques derived from laboratory evaluation. AJR 146:577–580, 1986
206. vanSonnenberg E, Wittich GR, Cabrera OA et al: Percutaneous gastrostomy and gastroenterostomy: 2. Clinical experience. AJR 146:581–586, 1986
207. Gray RR, St Louis EL, Grosman H: Percutaneous gastrostomy and gastro-jejunostomy. Br J Radiol 60:1067–1070, 1987
208. Ponsky JL, Gauderer MWL, Stellato TA et al: Percutaneous approaches to enteral alimentation. Am J Surg 149:102–105, 1985
209. Larson DE, Burton DD, Schroeder KW et al: Percutaneous endoscopic gastrostomy: Indications, success, complications, and mortality in 314 consecutive patients. Gastroenterology 93:48–52, 1987
210. Casola G, Withers C, vanSonnenberg E et al: Percutaneous cecostomy for decompression of the massively distended cecum. Radiology 158:793–794, 1986
211. Haaga JR, Bick RJ, Zollinger RM Jr: CT-guided percutaneous catheter cecostomy. Gastrointest Radiol 12:166–168, 1987
212. Bezreh JS: Percutaneous catheter drainage of closed-loop small-bowel obstruction. AJR 141:797–798, 1983

SECTION 4 ANTHONY B. MILLER

Cancer Screening

Of the approaches to cancer control that can reduce mortality from cancer—prevention, treatment, and screening—screening holds perhaps the greatest promise for a rapid major impact, but for a number of practical and organizational difficulties its potential may not be achieved. Further, there are several scientific reasons why the early detection of cancer does not automatically guarantee reduced cancer mortality.[1] This chapter first reviews the scientific basis for screening and then considers the evidence on screening for a number of major cancer sites.

GENERAL PRINCIPLES OF SCREENING

There are both benefits and disadvantages to screening for cancer.[2] The benefits include an improved prognosis for some patients whose disease is detected by screening, but not for all. Those who benefit are primarily those who in the absence of screening would have died. This is the major benefit sought in screening programs. A second benefit of screening, related to early detection, is that less radical treatment may be needed to cure some cases of disease. This is a potentially important benefit of screening for breast cancer, for example. A third benefit is reassurance for those with negative test results. Indeed, many people participate in screening programs for just this reassurance. A fourth benefit is resource savings, in particular a lower treatment cost if less radical treatment can be instituted, and lower costs for treating patients who otherwise would have died, as these costs for cancer can often be substantial.

The list of disadvantages is somewhat longer. The first is a longer period of morbidity, due to the lead time from screening, for patients whose prognosis is unaltered. A second disadvantage, potentially critical in the case of breast cancer screening, is overtreatment of borderline abnormalities. Many abnormalities brought to light by screening programs might never have been recognized without screening. A third disadvantage is false reassurance for those with false-negative test results. In such cases, the development of symptoms after a false-negative screening test may be ignored, leading to postponement of the diagnosis and consequently a poorer prognosis. A fourth disadvantage is unnecessary morbidity for those with false-positive test results. False-positive results may precipitate a cascade of complex investigations and varying diagnoses, a critical factor influencing the cost-effectiveness of screening for certain cancers, such as colorectal cancer.[3] A fifth disadvantage is the potential hazards of a screening test, a particular concern in mammography,[4] although for several screening tests the concern may be more theoretical than real. Finally, there are resource costs, particularly those resulting from the overtreatment of borderline abnormalities and the investigation and diagnosis of persons with false-positive screening tests.

Because of the potential disadvantages of screening programs, it is appropriate to insist on definitive evaluation of the effectiveness of screening. A number of approaches can be used for evaluating screening programs. These include geographical comparisons, time trends in defined populations, studies in which such trends are correlated with intensity of screening, and quasi-experimental comparisons of trends in different areas based on identification of individuals, but all of these are inferior to the randomized controlled trial.[2] A new approach to which much thought is being devoted is the use of case–control studies to evaluate screening programs.[2,5] Case–control studies should be designed to resemble as far as possible the controlled clinical trial. Thus, cases should be deaths from cancer, or advanced disease as a surrogate for death, and controls should be drawn at random from the same population as the cases and should include living persons (who may or may not have disease, depending on the population sampled) and those without advanced disease.[1]

The preferred evaluation approach, the randomized controlled trial, avoids the biases that are inherent in the assessment of screening if less perfect measures are used. These four screening biases are lead time, or the time by which diagnosis is advanced through screening; length bias, or the tendency of the screening process to detect cases of disease with a more prolonged natural history and thus a better prognosis than normal; selection bias, reflecting the dependence of screening programs on volunteer populations, who inevitably have a different incidence of disease than the general population; and overdiagnosis bias, or the tendency for screening to bring to light and label as disease lesions that might never have been diagnosed in the lifetime of the screenee.[1] These biases must be borne in mind in deciding the end points for evaluation of screening programs. If the screening test used is of any validity, counts of cases, the disease stage distribution of cases, and case fatality (survival) assessments are all influenced by these biases and inevitably result in better indices than for cases detected in the usual fashion in the absence of screening. Disease incidence is appropriate as an end point only if a precursor is removed as a result of using the screening test, as is the case for cancer of the cervix. Mortality is the only absolute measure, although in some circumstances the absolute number of cases of advanced disease could be substituted for deaths.[1]

Once screening programs are in place, continued evaluation is required. Screening programs may fail for many reasons, none of which may necessarily represent an inherent fault in the approach. Such reasons include failure to reach the population at risk, lack of sensitivity of the screening test, too infrequent rescreening to detect rapidly growing disease, and inadequate treatment of the abnormalities detected on screening.[6] Thus, for many cervical cancer screening programs, one should now be concerned with operational issues that could explain relative failure, rather than with the efficacy of the approach itself.

SCREENING FOR CERVICAL CANCER

Several years ago we established a strong correlation between the intensity of screening in Canada and a reduction in mortality from uterine cancer in the 1960s.[7] The correlation was strongest at the census district or county level and persisted when various census-derived socioeconomic status variables were incorporated in a multivariate analysis. This evidence was reviewed by the first Canadian Task Force on the evaluation of screening programs, which concluded that screening for cervical cancer had significantly contributed to the reduced mortality from the disease in Canada.[8] Since then, although mortality has continued to decline in Canada, the correlation has largely disappeared: in practice, screening has not had the anticipated effect of eliminating mortality from the disease, and the areas of country that were less intensely screened in the mid-1960s have largely caught up in terms of screening intensity.[9] There is still some evidence, however, that screening is making an important contribution to the control of cervical disease in Canada.[10] In the meantime, important evidence on the effect of screening on the incidence of and mortality from cervical cancer has come from the Nordic countries.[11] The organized screening programs developed in Iceland and Finland resulted in a fairly rapid and important reduction in incidence; the less organized programs in Sweden and in Denmark have made a delayed but similarly important contribution. Norway, however, which used to have an incidence similar to that of all the other Nordic countries (with the exception of high-incidence Denmark), failed to introduce an organized program, and there was no reduction in incidence.

In Canada, we have noted a reduction in incidence in nearly all age groups until recently, when the incidence appears to have risen in the younger age groups.[12] This change, which reflects differences in expression of risk factors in younger birth cohorts, was regarded with some concern by the second Canadian Task Force on the evaluation of screening programs[12] and resulted in recommendations that more attention should be paid to screening younger women and ensuring that individuals at risk for the disease were brought into screening programs. The second Canadian Task Force's approach to the evaluation of periodicity of rescreening depended rather heavily on mathematical models,[13] as did the American Cancer Society in recommending rescreening at 3-year intervals,[14] based on the model of Eddy.[15] The Canadian Task Force[12] recommended that registers be established to ensure the following: (1) that appropriate follow-up systems were in place so that women with normal test results would be recalled at regular intervals for repeat testing, (2) that action was taken following discovery of an abnormality, and (3) that long-term follow-up was provided for patients treated for an abnormality. In 1982 they reinforced their previous recommendation for centralized registries throughout the country.[8]

This belief in the organization of screening programs to ensure that those at risk enter into the program and that all at risk are rescreened at an appropriate interval was echoed in the deliberations of an International Union Against Cancer (UICC) workshop.[16] This group had available the results of a study coordinated by the International Agency for Research on Cancer (IARC) which documented from a number of screening programs the degree of protection conferred by a negative screening test. Protection was maximal in the first 3 years after a negative test and persisted to some degree for at least 5 years. On the basis of this analysis, it was possible to compute the expected degree of benefit from different intensities of rescreening (Table 20-10). It seems clear that annual schedules are wasteful of resources and that almost as much benefit can be obtained from tests conducted at 3-year intervals, beginning at about age 25 and continuing through age 60.

The UICC group assessed the state of the art of screening for cervical cancer and concluded that the effectiveness of screening programs was established but that within each country a consensual policy was required to ensure that the target population was identified, that individual women were identifiable, that measures were available to guarantee high coverage, that there were adequate field facilities for carry-

TABLE 20-10. Effect of Different Screening Policies for Cervical Cancer, Starting at Age 20

Screening Schedule	*Cumulative Rate per 100,000 Women Aged 20–64*	*% Reduction in Cancer Rate*	*Number of Tests*
1. No screening	1575		
2. Screening every 5 yr, ages 20–64	257.6	83.6	9
2a. Screening every 5 yr, ages 25–64	286.7	81.8	8
2b. Screening every 5 yr, ages 35–64	478.8	69.6	6
2c. Screening every year, ages 20–34, then every 5 yr, ages 35–64	232.3	85.5	21
2d. Screening at age 25, 26, 30, then every 5 yr	274.5	82.6	9
3. Screening every 3 yr, ages 20–64	137.8	91.2	15
3a. Screening every 3 yr, ages 26–64	161.0	89.8	13
3b. Screening every 3 yr, ages 35–64	352.8	77.6	10
3c. Screening every year, ages 20–34, then every 3 yr, ages 35–64	131.2	91.7	25
3d. Screening at age 25, 26, 29 then every 3 yr	156.6	90.1	14
4. Screening every year, ages 20–64	105.0	93.3	35

ing out cervical cytology examinations, that organized quality control programs were available in the laboratories, and that there were adequate facilities for diagnosis and treatment, with carefully designed referral systems and with an overall program for evaluation and monitoring trends in the population.[16]

Research is still needed on appropriate strategies for screening in developing countries, and on whether or not the natural history in high-incidence areas such as South America and Asia reflects current knowledge of the natural history of the disease from studies in technically advanced countries. Continued research on etiology is desirable to identify markers of high risk, while the long-term effects of therapy for precancerous lesions, especially the use of colposcopically assisted procedures, should be further assessed.

The UICC group recommended that policies be developed for each population, though noting that variation in the rate of progression and in the risk of preinvasive lesions does not currently appear to warrant differences in screening policies.[16] They noted that it appeared cost-effective to start screening at age 25, to rescreen at intervals of 3 years, and to stop after age 60, and that screening only high-risk groups does not seem to have general applicability.

Many of these recommendations were echoed by an expert group convened by the World Health Organization (WHO),[18] though their recommendations were tailored to the lesser resources available in most developing countries. Even a single smear applied to a substantial proportion of the population at an appropriate age (35–40 years) could achieve an important benefit.

Some of the concerns expressed by the Canadian Task Force regarding the changes in disease incidence in younger women[12] were also expressed by many physicians and professional groups in the United States. The working guidelines issued by the National Cancer Institute (NCI) for physicians state that "all women who are, or have been sexually active, or have reached 18 years, [should] have an annual Pap test and pelvic examination. After a women has had three or more consecutive satisfactory normal annual examinations, the Pap test may be performed less frequently at the discretion of her physician." [19] This issue has been addressed by other countries also. European countries, including the United Kingdom,[20] continue to recommend, largely on the grounds of cost-effectiveness, that screening should be offered not more frequently than every 3 years.

The other difference between many recommendations is the age at which women should enter screening programs. This recommendation varies from the age at which a female becomes sexually active, in the Canadian[12] and NCI[19] guidelines, to not before the age of 25, in the UICC guidelines.[16] The recommendation by the Canadian Task Forces that screening should start at age 18 for sexually active girls was based on the premise that those with detectable precancerous lesions and who are less than 25 years old may form an ultra-high-risk group. Thus, if the opportunity presents itself (by their attendance for oral contraceptives or for antenatal or postnatal care) to include them in screening programs, they can be placed on special surveillance if lesions have already developed. However, for countries that have the mechanisms to identify all women potentially at risk from the age of 25, offering screening before that age would not be cost-effective.[16] Clearly more research is needed into the natural history of the disease in younger high-risk birth cohorts; some of this research is ongoing in Canada.

SCREENING FOR BREAST CANCER

United States

Much is known about screening for breast cancer, largely because this is the only entity for which a controlled clinical trial has been completed, that of the Health Insurance Plan of Greater New York (HIP). Other clinical trials are in progress. Although the final report from the HIP study has yet to appear, it is clear that the mortality reduction noted initially at 5 years[21] and confirmed through 14 years[22] for the combination of mammography and physical examination persisted throughout 18 years of follow-up.[23]

The long-term follow-up in the HIP study has emphasized some aspects of breast cancer detection programs that were beginning to be appreciated 4 years earlier.[22] The early lack of a demonstrable effect of screening in women under the age of 50[21] was later replaced by an almost equivalent degree of benefit to that for women aged 50 years or older (Table 20-11). The benefit for those aged 45 to 49 years first became apparent after 5 years of follow-up, and that for women aged 40 to 44 years became apparent after 8 years of follow-up. The early benefit (noted after 3 years) for those aged 50 to 59 years maximized at 5 years and later decreased somewhat. None of the benefits for individual age groups are statistically significant of themselves, but from the results now available it seems likely that screening benefits all ages, with a longer delay in benefit for younger women—perhaps because of a different natural history of breast cancer in premenopausal and postmenopausal women.

The other aspect of the study that deserves emphasis is the question as to which of the two screening modalities used annually for 4 years contributed to the mortality reduction. Again, the design of the HIP study does not allow resolution of this issue, but a clue is derived from the case detection rates (Table 20-12), which emphasize the contributions of both modalities, especially physical examination in younger women.

The HIP study was followed in the United States by the Breast Cancer Detection Demonstration Projects (BCDDP). These projects used mammography, thermography, and physical examination of the breasts in 280,000 women aged 35 years or older, but there was no control group, so the effectiveness of the screening program could not be established.[24] Further, thermography proved to be of low sensitivity and specificity. Mammography, however, seemed to be of higher sensitivity than physical examination in the BCDDP than in the HIP study, especially in women aged 40 to 49 years.[25]

Recently, survival data have become available on the cancers diagnosed in the BCDDP.[26] These are of considerable interest, as they show almost equivalent survival whether or not the breast cancers were diagnosed by screening, irrespective of age. The data have been interpreted as confirming the benefit of screening in women aged 40 to 49 years, but clearly they do not, as the effects of screening biases related to survival cannot be corrected. However, they do raise the possibility that in self-selected women who attend screening programs, the benefit may not be as great as has been assumed.

The controversy that surrounded the BCDDP[27] resulted in a lack of interest in further large-scale research to evaluate the effects of screening for breast cancer in the United States. The focus therefore shifted to Europe and Canada, where major projects were initiated in the 1970s and 1980s.

The European Studies

Three programs, two in the Netherlands[28,29] and one in Florence,[30] have been assessed by the case–control approach. All three show important reductions in deaths from breast cancer in women over the age of 50, two as a result of programs using mammography alone (in Nijmegen and Florence) and one using the combination of mammography plus physical examination (in Utrecht). The results of the Nijmegen study indicate no benefit so far for women less than 50 years old. There was a nonsignificant reduction in mortality in women less than 50 in the Florence study, possibly reflecting a longer follow-up time.

In the large Swedish WE randomized trial, the initial results again showed no benefit for women aged 40 to 49 years but an important benefit for women more than 50 years old.[31] In this trial, single-oblique-view mammography was used.

In all these studies, the lack of benefit from screening in women less than 50 years old may be explained by the same factors that led to the delayed appearance of benefit in the

TABLE 20-11. Percentage Reduction in Deaths from Breast Cancer in the HIP Study

Age at Entry (yr)	% Reduction in Breast Cancer Deaths* At 5 Years	At 18 Years	Year Reduction Began
40–44	(18)	36	9
45–49	(0)	16	6
50–54	65	22	3
55–59	(30)	24	3
60–64	(50)	17	3

* Parentheses indicate observations based on 20 or fewer breast cancer deaths in study and control groups combined.

TABLE 20-12. Breast Cancer Cases Histologically Confirmed in HIP Study, by Screening Modality

			% Detected by:	
Age at Entry (yr)	*Total No.*	*No. Detected by Mammography Alone*	*Clinical Alone*	*Mammography and Clinical*
40–49	40	25	58	18
50–59	67	39	40	21
60–64	25	32	36	32
All ages	132	33	45	22

HIP study. If so, these studies may all be on the verge of showing mortality reduction in the under 50 age group, although there could be other explanations for a lack of effect in younger women. One possible explanation could be a relative lack of sensitivity of the screen. All of the studies have incorporated mammography, but so far no reported study on European women less than 50 years old has used physical examination. In Utrecht the study was originally planned with objectives other than demonstrating benefit,[32] and therefore women less than 50 years old were not screened initially, as it was expected that little benefit would accrue to them. The absence of physical examination in the European studies could have contributed to a lower sensitivity of the screening program. That the screening was less sensitive in women aged 40 to 49 years than in women over the age of 50 has in fact been demonstrated for the Swedish WE trial,[33] and by a different analysis for the Nijmegen study.[34]

A second possible explanation is that the periodicity of rescreening was too low in women aged 40 to 49 years. There was no difference in the periodicity of rescreening by age in the Nijmegen and Florence studies, but in the Swedish study the younger women were screened every 21 months, compared to every 33 months and then every 24 months in the older cohorts. An attempt to assess the sojourn time of preclinical lesions in the Swedish study (*i.e.*, the total time that a lesion is potentially detectable before clinical presentation) has suggested that this period is not much less in younger women than in older women.[33] Thus, too infrequent a repeat screen in younger women may not be the reason for a lack of demonstrable effect in them.

Ongoing Studies

Three important studies in progress should provide further guidance on screening for breast cancer. The first is the United Kingdom study incorporating women aged 45 to 64; biennial mammography and annual physical examination are used in two centers and breast self-examination (BSE) alone in two more, with four control districts.[35] In one of the mammography screening centers there is randomization by family practices. Time will tell whether this study is sufficiently powerful to provide much additional evidence on the benefits to be expected from this screening approach. For example, it is not clear whether we can expect any elucidation of the age issue, as women aged 40 to 44 were not enrolled in the study. Nor is it clear whether the study will be sufficiently powerful to provide any information on the effectiveness of BSE. Mortality results should be available in 1989–1990.

The National Breast Screening Study in Canada was designed specifically to provide additional information on the benefit of the combination of annual mammography, physical examination, and regular BSE in women aged 40 to 49 years, and the incremental effect of mammography over and above physical examination and BSE in women aged 50 to 59 years.[36] This study should have the power to answer both objectives. So far the women enrolled have had the expected numbers of breast cancers but a much lower mortality from breast cancer than expected. Some of the reduced mortality might reflect a benefit of physical examination in women aged 50 to 59 years and the single physical examination with the teaching of BSE in women aged 40 to 49 years. If the trend continues, follow-up will have to be extended for at least an additional 3 years before mortality results can be reported.

The third ongoing study of critical importance to those countries that have tended to rely on BSE is a randomized trial being conducted in factories in Moscow and polyclinics in Leningrad, evaluating team teaching of BSE in Moscow and individual instruction in Leningrad.[37] This trial will eventually include more than 200,000 women, but results will probably not be available for 8 to 10 years. A geographically controlled comparison of BSE is underway in East Germany, and there are plans to attempt to evaluate the BSE program introduced by Dr. Gastrin in Finland, the "Mama" program, about 14 years ago.[38] Some evidence on effectiveness of BSE could, therefore, become available within the next few years.

The UICC project on screening evaluation concluded that in countries where breast cancer is common and where the necessary resources are available, screening with mammography alone or mammography plus physical examination is applicable as public health policy.[39] However, the greatest initial benefit will be obtained by concentrating screening on women aged 50 to 69 years. The ambiguity of the modality to be used is obvious in this recommendation. Although most people tend to concentrate on mammography, we and others maintain that the benefit of physical examination, either with mammography or in partial substitution for mammography, could be considerable. The experience in Canada, in contradistinction to that of the United Kingdom,[40] is that a policy based on physical examination could be less expensive rather than more (Table 20-13). Whether or not this is

TABLE 20-13. Preliminary Data on Cost-Effectiveness of Mammography Compared to Physical Examination in Detecting Invasive Cancers (NBSS Study), According to Size of Tumor.*

	Women Aged 40–49		*Women Aged 50–59*	
Size of Tumor	*Mammography*	*Physical Examination*	*Mammography*	*Physical Examination*
All sizes	$18,340	$ 8,290	$ 8,890	$ 5,950
>1 cm	23,390	9,620	11,850	7,380
>2 cm	43,220	19,620	23,130	13,960

* Based on cost per examination of $12 for physical examination and $30 for mammography in Canadian dollars.

confirmed by a full cost-benefit analysis is likely to be resolved by the Canadian trial within the next few years.

POLICIES FOR BREAST CANCER SCREENING

The American Cancer Society[14,41] and the American College of Radiology[42] have both recommended that mammography and physical examination be offered to all women over the age of 40, with a baseline mammogram obtained at ages 35 to 40. The rationale for the baseline mammogram has not been established. Mammography is recommended every 1 or 2 years for women aged 40 to 49 years, and annually for those over age 50. The same periodicity is recommended in the NCI working guidelines.[19] The European studies, however, suggest that these frequencies be reversed.[39] Other countries have recommended policies based on mammography only—such as mammography every 3 years for women more than 50 years old in the United Kingdom.[43] All recognize the need for adequate training and attention to the technical aspects of mammography.[44] This has been confirmed by the experience in the National Breast Screening Study in Canada. Care must be taken in many aspects of technique, including type of machine, appropriate focal spot film distance, processing, positioning of the patient, and adequate compression of the breast.[45] Mammography quality and dosimetry should be monitored on a regular basis. The dosage required for mammography has fallen substantially from the 8-rad surface dose used in the HIP study, to 3 to 1 rad used in the BCDDP, to 0.6 to 0.2 rad used in the National Breast Screening Study with screen-film technology. The low dose achievable in screen-film mammography, better film quality, and the opportunity for batch processing of films make screen-film mammography preferable to xerography for screening. However, these are not the only aspects that must be taken into account when the use of mammography as a screening tool is contemplated. Many lesions can be identified on breast cancer screening, including cysts, mammary dysplasia, benign atypical hyperplasias, borderline abnormalities, in situ cancers with or without microinvasion, and small invasive cancers.[45] For those not palpable, both benign and malignant, considerable care is required for localization, diagnosis, and management. This usually requires specimen radiography and particularly the availability of skilled radiologists, surgeons, and pathologists. For a national program, special training would be required.[44] These requirements should not be taken lightly. In each Canadian city in which the National Breast Screening Study has been introduced, considerable care has been taken with these aspects of breast screening. The medical profession must be assured it is appropriate to biopsy impalpable abnormalities, and family physicians must be encouraged to refer patients to institutions where the necessary skills are available. Even so, in the National Breast Screening Study currently about one in six biopsies conducted for impalpable abnormalities visible on mammography result in a diagnosis of in situ or invasive cancer. Yet, although mammography is clearly more sensitive than physical examination, the lesions found on mammography alone that potentially have a good prognosis may never surface clinically, whereas the lesions found on physical examination alone tend to be small and infiltrating cancers, possibly with one or two micrometastases, and of a type which, if detected early, might result in better prognosis. Hence, it may be inappropriate to base breast screening policies entirely on considerations of mammography.

BSE as an alternative approach to breast screening may have wider applicability than mammography and physical examination.[46] This conclusion of a WHO-supported meeting reinforces the need for better teaching and more careful evaluation of the effectiveness of BSE. Experience in the National Breast Screening Study shows how women's skills in BSE can be improved by annual reinforcement.[47]

Because only BSE can contribute to the early detection of the interval cancers that occur in all screening programs, BSE reinforcement should be combined with physical examination, whether given by a physician or, as in the Canadian study, by a nurse.

SCREENING FOR COLORECTAL CANCER

Colorectal cancer is an importance cause of morbidity and mortality in both sexes, and its natural history may make it amenable to control by screening.[48] There are two screening tests available, sigmoidoscopy and tests for occult blood in the feces. The American Cancer Society recommends that screening with both should start at age 50, at which time tests for occult blood should be performed annually and sigmoidoscopy every 5 years.[14] The NCI working guidelines call for annual tests for occult blood and sigmoidoscopy every 3 to 5 years from the age of 50.[19]

Unfortunately, the patients at risk are relatively old. Both patients and physicians dislike sigmoidoscopy, and there may have to be major public and professional educational programs to persuade individuals to accept even flexible sigmoidoscopy. However, the scientific basis for recommendations is slight. Gilbertsen et al[49,50] performed annual proctosigmoidoscopy on 21,150 men and women. Of 27 carcinomas found on initial examination, 25 were followed at least 5 years, with a 5-year survival rate of 64%. Though better than usual, this survival rate would be expected from screening biases. Of 13 patients in whom carcinomas were subsequently found, 11 have survived 5 years. Thus, there are 11 known deaths from colorectal cancer over a 5-year period in this population. Although it is difficult to derive an expected survival figure, as the age and sex distribution of the participants is not known, the figure may not be very low: all persons with preexisting colorectal cancers were ineligible for the screen, and it is known that most of the deaths from cancer in any one year occur in people diagnosed in previous years. Once the selective nature of the population screened is considered, it becomes apparent that the survival results may simply reflect a common selection bias in screening.[51]

In the randomized trial reported by Dales et al,[52] digital rectal examination and sigmoidoscopy were included as part of a multiphasic screen provided annually in the study group; the control group was offered "usual care." In an 11-year follow-up period there were 5 deaths from colorectal cancer in the study group and 18 in the control group ($p < 0.05$). However, this study had multiple end points, and thus a p-value of 0.05 cannot be given the usual weight. Further, only 6 cases (out of 20) in the study group were diagnosed after sigmoidoscopy.

The sensitivity of the tests for occult blood in the stool is relatively low, not only for potential precursors of cancer such as adenomatous polyps but also for relatively early, less advanced cancers.[3] The specificity of the tests currently available is also low, increasing costs in terms of the diagnosis and treatment of benign abnormalities and also the potential risk of applying screening tests.

Thus, to date no reduction in the mortality from colorectal cancer has been demonstrated with screening, even though two controlled trials have been in progress for many years in the United States.[53,54] Additional trials have been initiated in the United Kingdom, Denmark, and Sweden.[3] The UICC project on the evaluation of screening[3] concluded that there is as yet no firm evidence that screening for colorectal cancer can result in reduced mortality, and therefore that screening for colorectal cancer or its precursors cannot be recommended as public health policy. This conclusion was largely endorsed by a committee on screening charged to develop the NCI's year 2,000 goals.[55]

SCREENING FOR OTHER CANCERS

The UICC project has evaluated screening programs for cancer in several other sites.[2,3,16] A number of problems have been identified, and no program is currently recommended as public health policy.

LUNG CANCER. Several early studies suggested that screening for lung cancer by means of 6-month chest radiographs with or without sputum cytology did not improve the prognosis of lung cancer in the populations studied.[2] In the 1970s, three randomized trials of lung cancer screening were initiated in the United States, and it now seems clear that although chest radiographs and sputum cytology are capable of detecting cases in high-risk males, sputum cytology at 4-month intervals adds a small proportion of cases to those discovered on annual chest radiographs and does not demonstrably reduce mortality. Further, chest radiographs at 4-month intervals confer no mortality advantage over routine care that includes annual chest radiographs. The UICC group[2] recommended assessing the value of the annual chest radiograph and suggested that case–control studies may have promise in this regard. One such study has since been performed in the German Democratic Republic, evaluating the role of mass miniature radiographs obtained at 2-year intervals, and found no evidence that such radiologic screening reduced the mortality from lung cancer.[56] This may not satisfy those who advocate full-size chest radiographs for screening. However, it seems unlikely that the annual chest radiograph is beneficial when the 4-month chest radiograph conferred no mortality advantage over routine care that included chest radiographs obtained only when symptoms became apparent.

BLADDER CANCER. Urinary cytology is clearly capable of detecting urinary bladder cancers in persons in high-risk occupations, as well as those living in areas where urinary schistosomiasis is endemic. Improved survival of patients with screening-detected bladder cancer has been demonstrated, but it is not known if a reduction in mortality will follow. Screening-detected cases in areas where urinary schistosomiasis is endemic are at an earlier stage and require less extensive therapy than those diagnosed by routine measures. However, if bladder cancer screening is to play a role in cancer control, further research is needed. Critically, the role of urinary cytology in reducing mortality from bladder cancer in high-risk occupational groups and in areas of endemic urinary schistosomiasis must be evaluated. An important prerequisite to such evaluation is to undertake treatment trials of early lesions found by screening.[57]

ORAL CANCER. Visual examination is capable of identifying presymptomatic oral cancers. Exfoliative cytology is less sensitive than visual examination.[2] Neither test has yet been shown to reduce mortality from oral cancer. Thus, research on oral cancer screening programs is clearly needed. In technically advanced countries it will be difficult to evaluate the place of routine dental examinations, as these tend to be restricted to those at low risk, high-risk individuals often avoiding dental care. Evaluation of mortality reduction following screening is needed in areas of high incidence; the role of screening in the primary prevention of oral cancer in persons with oral epithelial dysplasia might be evaluated concurrently. The NCI working guidelines for oral cavity cancer recommend that "oral examination including palpation of the tongue, floor of the mouth, salivary glands and lymph nodes of the neck be performed as part of the periodic health examination," and that "special attention should be given those at high risk due to tobacco and alcoholism."[19]

OVARIAN CANCER. Ovarian cancer is common in Western countries and has a relatively high mortality, often exceeding that for cervical cancer. Several screening tests are under development.[16]

ENDOMETRIAL CANCER. For endometrial cancer, although the disease is relatively common in Western countries, the person-years saved by screening may be limited because it is largely a disease of elderly women. Available screening tests are based on endometrial samples subjected to cytologic analysis. These are not simple tests, requiring considerable care in their application.[16] If endometrial cancer screening is to play a role in cancer control, much further research into its effectiveness is required.

STOMACH CANCER. Considerable mass radiologic screening for stomach cancer has been undertaken in Japan, but its contribution to reduced mortality is unclear. Although Hirayama has demonstrated a correlation between the rate of mass screening for stomach cancer at different ages and the percentage change in death rates from stomach cancer since 1960, he concluded that much of the reduction in mortality has been due to changes in diet rather than to mass screening.[58]

One case–control study performed in Japan provided suggestive evidence that screening reduces mortality from stomach cancer.[59] The UICC group concluded that screening in Japan had contributed to the reduced mortality from stomach cancer, but that its contribution was small in relation to the concomitantly diminishing incidence.[3]

LIVER CANCER. Screening by means of serum α-fetoprotein levels is being evaluated in some parts of China where the risk of liver cancer is very high.[3] There is some evidence that small liver cancers can be successfully treated. However, pending further research, screening for liver cancer cannot be recommended as public health policy.[3]

ESOPHAGUS. A similar conclusion was reached by the UICC group for esophageal cancer screening.[3] Although a possible screening test is available that involves cytologic examination of cells obtained by esophageal intubation and withdrawal, with a scrape obtained with the aid of a balloon, there are difficulties associated with the cytologic diagnosis of esophageal dysplasia (a possible precancerous lesion); another concern is the availability of suitable treatment for any abnormalities found. Research into chemoprevention might provide a solution to the latter problem.

OTHER CANCERS. Screening might be attempted for skin, prostate, and pancreatic cancer, which may potentially benefit from advances in monoclonal antibody technology. The NCI working guidelines recommend that "annual digital rectal examination of the prostate be performed on all males over 40 years of age."[19] Some have advocated screening for melanoma, particularly to search for dysplastic nevi[60]; so far this approach has not been definitively evaluated. However, the NCI working guidelines state that "all individuals should be encouraged to examine their skin thoroughly on a regular basis. That primary care physicians be encouraged to examine the skin as part of the periodic health examination. That further public and professional education be promoted on the early detection of skin cancers and in particular malignant melanoma."[19]

FUTURE PERSPECTIVES

There are many obstacles to a major contribution of screening to cancer control. For some sites, lung cancer being a particular example, the natural history of the disease may make it unamenable to screening. For other sites the potential for screening has so far been poorly evaluated; in this regard it should be noted that case finding is not equivalent to mortality reduction. Poor organization of screening programs has probably prevented the full utilization of cervical cancer screening, yet even for this cancer, the potential for reduction in mortality by screening may be less than assumed.[10] Many screening tests are costly; this seems to be a barrier to accepting mammographic screening in the United States.[61] For other screening programs, persons at risk may be less willing to participate than those not at risk; cervical cancer screening is one example. The cost of and morbidity from treatment consequent on false-positive tests may continue to plague screening for colorectal cancer until new tests are available. Overtreatment in the case of true-positive results may be a psychological barrier to screening for breast cancer, but with increasing support for less radical surgery,[62] mastectomy seems inappropriate unless it is absolutely necessary.

Table 20-14 lists the speculative potential for reduction in mortality from cancer following screening by the year 2000; the figures are mine.[63] Some may find a 60% speculative reduction in mortality from cervical cancer too pessimistic, but this figure is probably realistic, in light of the current epidemiologic situation. Even a 25% reduction in mortality from breast cancer could be overly optimistic, however, un-

TABLE 20-14. Speculative Potential for Reduction in Mortality from Cancer with Screening by Year 2000

Cancer Site	*% Reduction in Mortality*
Cervix	60
Breast	25
Lung	0
Colon/rectum	20
Bladder	5
Oral	5
Stomach (Japan)	30
Ovary	(10)
Endometrium	0
Other	(5)

less acceptance of screening by women and their physicians improves. For the remaining cancers on the list, the figures are less precisely derived. The NCI has estimated that screening might contribute 11% to 15% to the reduction in cancer mortality by the year 2000, part of the 50% overall reduction in cancer mortality by this time.[55] These figures assume acceptance of breast and cervical cancer screening by a large part of the population.

Screening can be an expensive use of health care resources. There are many barriers to its use, not the least of which is that its mere introduction does not solve the problem. Maintaining some level of effectiveness requires continued application of the screening program. For this reason, screening seems a less optimal approach to cancer control than primary prevention. Nevertheless, primary prevention may require many decades to achieve its full potential, except possibly for cancer of the colon and rectum, and under these circumstances screening appears to offer a fairly rapid return. Wherever it is shown to be effective, it should be included as part of the armamentarium for cancer control.

REFERENCES

1. Miller AB: General principles of evaluation of screening. In Miller AB (ed): Screening for Cancer, pp 3–24. Orlando, Fla, Academic Press, 1985
2. Prorok PC, Chamberlain J, Day NE et al: UICC workshop on the evaluation of screening programmes for cancer. Int J Cancer 34:1–4, 1984
3. Chamberlain J, Day NE, Hakama M et al: UICC workshop of the project on evaluation of screening programmes for gastrointestinal cancer. Int J Cancer 37:329–334, 1986
4. Miller AB: Screening cancer of the breast. In Miller AB (ed): Screening for Cancer, pp 325–345. Orlando, Fla, Academic Press, 1985
5. Morrison AS: Screening in Chronic Disease. Monographs in Epidemiology and Biostatistics, Vol 7. New York, Oxford University Press, 1985
6. Chamberlain J: Reasons that some screening programmes fail to control cervical cancer. In Hakama M, Miller AB, Day NE (eds): Screening for Cancer of the Uterine Cervix. IARC Sc Publ 76:161–168, 1986
7. Miller AB, Lindsay J, Hill GB: Mortality from cancer of the uterus in Canada and its relationship to screening for cancer of the cervix. Int J Cancer 17:602–612, 1976
8. Task Force: Cervical cancer screening programs: The Walton Report. Can Med Assoc J 114:1003–1033, 1976
9. Miller AB, Visentin T, Howe GR: The effect of hysterectomies and screening on mortality from cancer of the uterus in Canada. Int J Cancer 27:651–657, 1981
10. Miller AB: Evaluation of the impact of screening for cancer of the cervix. In Hakama M, Miller AB, Day NE (eds): Screening for Cancer of the Uterine Cervix. IARC Sci Publ 76:149–160, 1986
11. Hakama M: Trends in the incidence of cervical cancer in the Nordic countries. In Magnus K (ed): Trends in Cancer Incidence: Causes and Practical Implications, pp 279–292. New York, Hemisphere, 1982
12. Task Force: Cervical cancer screening programs: Summary of the 1982 Canadian Task Force Report. Can Med Assoc J 127:581–589, 1982
13. Yu SJ, Miller AB, Sherman GJ: Optimising the age, number of tests and test-interval for cervical screening in Canada. J Epidemial Community Health 36:1–10, 1982
14. American Cancer Society: Guidelines for the cancer-related check-up: Recommendations and rationale. CA 30:193–240, 1980
15. Eddy D: Screening for Cancer: Theory, Analysis, and Design. Englewood Cliffs, NJ, Prentice-Hall, 1980
16. Hakama M, Chamberlain J, Day NE et al: UICC workshop on the evaluation of screening programmes for gynecological cancer. Br J Cancer 52:669–673, 1985
17. IARC Working Group on Cervical Cancer Screening: Summary Chapter. In Hakama M, Miller AB, Day NE (eds): Screening for Cancer of the Uterine Cervix. IARC Sci Publ 76:133–142, 1986
18. Control of cancer of the cervix uteri. Bull WHO 64:607–618, 1986
19. National Cancer Institute, Early Detection Branch: Working guidelines for early cancer detection: Rationale and supporting evidence to decrease mortality. Bethesda, Md, National Cancer Institute, Division of Cancer Prevention and Control, 1987
20. Draper GJ: Screening for cervical cancer: Revised policy. The recommendations of the DHSS committee on gynecological cytology. Br J Family Planning 8:95–100, 1982
21. Shapiro S, Strax P, Venet L: Periodic breast cancer screening in reducing mortality from breast cancer. JAMA 215:1777–1785, 1971
22. Shapiro S, Venet W, Strax P et al: Ten to fourteen year effect of screening on breast cancer mortality. JNCI 69:349–355, 1982
23. Shapiro S, Venet W, Strax P et al: Current results of the breast cancer screening randomized trial: The Health Insurance Plan (HIP) of greater New York study. In Day NE, Miller AB (eds): Screening for Breast Cancer, pp 3–15. Toronto, Hans Huber, 1988
24. Beahrs OH, Shapiro S, Smart C et al: Report of the Working Group to Review the National Cancer Institute-American Cancer Society Breast Cancer Demonstration Projects. JNCI 62:640–709, 1979
25. Baker LH: Breast Cancer Detection Demonstration Project: Five year summary report. CA 32:194–225, 1982
26. Seidman H, Gelb SK, Silverberg E et al: Servival experience in the Breast Cancer Detection Demonstration Project. CA 37:258–290, 1987
27. Thier SO: Breast cancer screening: A view from outside the controversy. N Engl J Med 297:1063–1065, 1977
28. Collette HJA, Day NE, Rombach JJ et al: Evaluation of screening for breast cancer in a non-randomized study (the Dom project) by means of a case–control study. Lancet 1:1224–1226, 1984
29. Verbeek ALM, Hendriks JHCL, Holland R et al: Mammographic screening and breast cancer mortality: Age-specific effects in Nijmegen project, 1975-82. Lancet 1:865–886, 1985
30. Palli D, Del Turco MR, Buiatti E et al: A case–control study of the efficacy of a non-randomized breast cancer screening program in Florence (Italy). Int J Cancer 38:501–504, 1986
31. Tabar L, Fagerberg CJG, Gad A et al: Reduction in mortality from breast cancer after mass screening with mammography. Lancet 1:829–832, 1985
32. de Waard F, Collette HJA, Rombach JJ et al: The DOM project for the early detection of breast cancer, Utrecht, the Netherlands. J Chronic Dis 37:1–44, 1984
33. Day NE, Walter SD, Tabar L et al: The sensitivity and lead time of breast cancer screening: A comparison of the results of different studies. In Day NE, Miller AB (eds): Screening for Breast Cancer, pp 105–109. Toronto, Hans Huber, 1988
34. Verbeek ALM, Straatman H, Hendricks JHCL: Sensitivity of mammography in Nijmegen women under age 50. In Day NE, Miller AB (eds): Screening for Breast Cancer, pp 29–32. Toronto, Hans Huber, 1988
35. U.K. Trial of Early Detection of Breast Cancer Group: Trial of early detection of breast cancer: Description of method. Br J Cancer 44:618–627, 1981
36. Miller AB, Howe GR, Wall C: The national study of breast cancer screening. Clin Invest Med 4:227–258, 1981
37. World Health Organization: The USSR/WHO study: Protocol of the study of the role of breast self-examination in reduction of mortality from breast cancer (in preparation)
38. Gastrin G: Breast Cancer Control. Stockholm, Almqvist & Wiksell, 1981
39. Day NE, Baines CJ, Chamberlain J et al: UICC project on screening for cancer: Report on the workshop on screening for breast cancer. Int J Cancer 38:303–308, 1986
40. Chamberlain J, Clifford RE, Nathan BE et al: Error-rates in screening for breast cancer by clinical examination and mammography. Clin Oncol 5:135–146, 1979
41. American Cancer Society: Mammography guidelines 1983: Background statement and update of cancer related check-up guidelines for breast cancer detection in asymptomatic women age 40–49. CA 33:255, 1983
42. American College of Radiology: New ACR guidelines on mammography. ACR Bull 38:6–7, 1982
43. Working Group: Breast cancer screening: Report to the Health Ministers of England, Wales, Scotland and Northern Ireland. London, Her Majesty's Stationery Office, 1987
44. Miller AB, Tsechovski M: Imaging technologies in breast cancer control: Summary of a World Health Organization meeting. AJR 148:1093–1094, 1987
45. Miller AB, Bulbrook RD: Screening, detection and diagnosis of breast cancer. Lancet 1:1109–1111, 1982
46. Miller AB, Chamberlain J, Tsechkovski M: Self-examination in the early detection of breast cancer: A review of the evidence, with recommendations for further research. J Chronic Dis 38:527–540, 1985
47. Baines CJ, Wall C, Risch HA et al: Changes in breast self-examination behaviour in a cohort of 8214 women in the Canadian National Breast Screening Study. Cancer 57:1209–1216, 1986
48. Winawer SJ, Fath RB, Schottfeld D et al: Screening for colorectal cancer. In Miller AB (ed): Screening for Cancer, pp 347–366. Orlando, Fla, Academic Press, 1985
49. Gibertsen VA: Proctosigmoidoscopy and polypectomy in reducing the incidence of rectal cancer. Cancer 34:936–939, 1974
50. Gilbertsen VA, Nelms JM: The prevention of invasive cancer of the rectum. Cancer 41:1137–1139, 1978
51. Miller AB: Review of sigmoidoscopic screening for colorectal cancer. In Chamberlain J, Miller AB (eds): Screening for Gastro-intestinal Cancer, pp 3–7. Toronto, Hans Huber, 1988
52. Dales LG, Friedman GD, Collen VIF: Evaluating periodic multiphasic health checkups: A controlled trial. J Chronic Dis 32:385–404, 1979
53. Gilbertsen V, McHugh RB, Schuman LM et al: The colon cancer control study: An interim report. In Winawer SJ, Schottenfeld D, Sherlock P (eds): Colorectal Cancer: Prevention, Epidemiology and Screening, pp 261–266. New York, Raven, 1980
54. Winawer SJ, Andrews M, Flehinger B et al: Progress report on controlled trial of fecal occult blood testing for the detection of colorectal neoplasia. Cancer 43:2959–2964, 1980

55. National Cancer Institute, Division of Cancer Prevention and Control: Cancer Control Objectives for the Nation 1985–2000. NCI Monogr 2, 1986
56. Ebeling K, Nischan P: Screening for lung cancer: results from a case–control study. Int J Cancer 40:141–144, 1987
57. Cartwright RA: Screening for bladder cancer with particular reference to individual groups. In Prorok PC, Miller AB (eds): Screening for Cancer: 1. General Principles on Evaluation of Screening for Cancer and Screening for Lung, Bladder and Oral Cancer, pp 144–160. Geneva, International Union Against Cancer, 1984
58. Hirayama T: Screening for gastric cancer. In Miller AB (ed): Screening for Cancer, pp 367–376. Orlando, Fla, Academic Press, 1985
59. Oshima A, Hirata N, Ubukata T et al: Evaluation of a mass screening program for stomach cancer with a case–control study design. Int J Cancer 38:829–833, 1986
60. National Institutes of Health: Consensus Conference: Precursors to malignant melanoma. JAMA 251:1864–1866, 1984
61. American Cancer Society: Survey of physicians' attitudes and practices in early cancer detection. CA 35:197–213, 1985
62. Fisher B, Bauer M, Margolese R et al: Five-year results of a randomized clinical trial comparing total mastectomy and segmental mastectomy with or without radiation in the treatment of breast cancer. N Engl J Med 312:665–673, 1985
63. Miller AB: Screening for cancer: Issues and future directions. J Chronic Dis 39:1067–1077, 1986

RODNEY R. MILLION
NICHOLAS J. CASSISI
JOHN R. CLARK

CHAPTER 21 *Cancer of the Head and Neck*

EPIDEMIOLOGY OF HEAD AND NECK CANCER

The estimated number of new head and neck cancer cases (excluding skin cancer) in the United States for 1987 is 41,900; this represents 4.3% of the total new cancer cases.[1] The male-to-female ratio is approximately 4:1. The usual time of diagnosis is past the age of 40, except for salivary gland and nasopharyngeal tumors, which may occur in younger age groups. There has been no major change in the incidence of head and neck cancer over the past three decades in either the male or female population, which is somewhat surprising since a common etiologic factor (cigarette smoking) has resulted in a large increase in lung cancer. Cigarette smokers have an increased risk for multiple head and neck primary cancers as well as for lung cancer. Alcohol has also been implicated as a causative factor for certain head and neck cancers, and the effects of alcohol and tobacco seem to be additive. The smoking of marijuana has been reported to be a cause of head and neck cancer; it occurs in a younger age group.[2] We have observed several cases in marijuana users who were in their late 20s or early 30s at the time of diagnosis. Patients with pharyngeal cancer have an increased risk for developing esophageal cancer, and patients with major salivary gland tumors may have an increased risk for breast cancer.

ANATOMY

The regional anatomy is described separately under specific sites.

LYMPHATIC SYSTEM

There are no capillary lymphatics in the epithelium. Tumor must penetrate the lamina propria before lymphatic invasion can occur. One can predict the richness of the capillary network in any given head and neck site by the relative incidence of lymph node metastases at presentation. The nasopharynx and pyriform sinus have the most profuse networks of capillary lymphatics. The paranasal sinuses, middle ear, and vocal cords have few or no capillary lymphatics, based on their low rate of lymph node metastases when tumor is confined to these sites. Muscle and fat contain few capillary lymphatics. Bone and cartilage are thought to have a few capillary lymphatics in the periosteum or perichondrium. There are no capillary lymphatics in the eye, and few in the orbit. The arrangement of the important lymph nodes in the head and neck is shown in Fig. 21-1.[3]

PATHOLOGY

The vast majority of head and neck malignant neoplasms arise from the surface epithelium and are therefore squamous cell carcinoma or one of its many variants, including lymphoepithelioma, spindle cell carcinoma, verrucous carcinoma, and undifferentiated carcinoma. Lymphomas and a wide variety of other malignant and benign neoplasms make up the remaining cases (discussed under the appropriate section or chapter).

Lymphoepithelioma is a carcinoma with a lymphoid stroma. The lymphoid stroma may or may not be present in regional lymph node or distant metastases. Lymphoepithe-

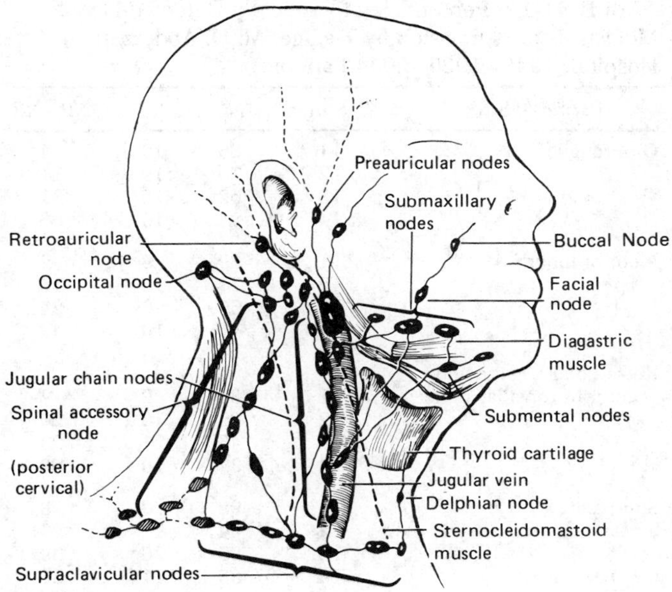

FIG. 21-1. The cervical lymphatics. (Redrawn from Rouvière H: Anatomy of the Human Lymphatic System, p 27. Ann Arbor, Edwards Brothers, 1938)

lioma occurs at anatomical sites with lymphoid aggregates in the submucosa, namely, the nasopharynx, tonsil, and base of tongue; it may also occur in the major salivary glands. This carcinoma has a higher rate of cure by radiation therapy than does squamous cell carcinoma.

In the spindle cell variant, found in 2% to 5% of malignant specimens taken from the upper aerodigestive tract, there is a component of spindle cells that resemble sarcoma intermixed with squamous cell carcinoma. This picture is variously described in the literature as pleomorphic carcinoma, sarcomatoid squamous cell carcinoma, squamous cell carcinoma with spindle cell variant, pseudosarcoma, and spindle cell squamous cell carcinoma, among others. For the most part, these lesions cannot be distinguished grossly from the usual squamous cell carcinoma. In some, the spindle cell component is relatively minor; in others, it dominates the picture and the squamous cell component is difficult to find. The sarcomatoid component may have features that are consistent with malignant fibrous histiocytoma. The lymph node metastases may show only the spindle cell component, only the carcinomatous element, or a mixture of both. This pattern may be seen anywhere that squamous cell carcinoma is found in the head and neck area.

Leventon and Evans reported 20 cases of spindle cell carcinoma.[4] All of the patients with superficially invasive tumors were cured, whereas only 1 of the 10 patients with deep invasion was cured. The tumors responded both to surgery and to radiation therapy, with six of the survivors being treated by operation, three by irradiation only, and two by combined treatment. Six of the tumors were said to have occurred in previously irradiated areas, and five of these patients eventually died. There are no data to compare the effectiveness of surgery and radiation therapy. It is our policy to consider the spindle cell variant as a high-grade carcinoma, but otherwise to disregard the spindle cell element in treatment decisions.

Verrucous carcinoma is a "grade one-half" squamous cell carcinoma found most often in the oral cavity, particularly on the gingiva and buccal mucosa. It usually has an indolent growth pattern and often is associated with the chronic use of snuff or chewing tobacco. Verrucous tumors resemble a wart: white or pink, exophytic, with distinct margins and multiple filiform processes that produce a roughened, cobblestone surface. The lesion may be soft or firm to palpation depending on the degree of keratinization and associated inflammation. The patient with verrucous carcinoma very often has multiple biopsies of an obvious lesion, but the pathologist returns a diagnosis of hyperkeratosis or pseudoepitheliomatous hyperplasia. Eventually one may recommend cancer therapy based only on the appearance of the lesion and observation of its continued growth. If the pathologist can readily make a diagnosis of invasive carcinoma from histologic examination, the diagnosis of verrucous carcinoma is suspect. De novo verrucous carcinomas rarely develop lymph node metastases.

Small cell carcinoma occurs rarely throughout the head and neck region and is managed by radiation therapy and chemotherapy.

Lymphoma occurring in the upper aerodigestive tract almost always shows a diffuse non-Hodgkin's histologic pattern; nodular non-Hodgkin's lymphoma and Hodgkin's disease rarely involve the mucosal sites. Undifferentiated lymphomas and undifferentiated carcinoma may appear similar under the microscope. If lymphoma is suspected, fresh tissue should be given to the pathologist immediately for preparation for cell membrane studies. Lymphoma cells are quite susceptible to crush artifact, and the specimen should be obtained by sharp dissection rather than with punch biopsy forceps.

NATURAL HISTORY OF SQUAMOUS CELL CARCINOMA

PATTERNS OF SPREAD

Primary Lesion

Epidermoid carcinomas usually begin as surface lesions, but occasionally arise from ducts of minor salivary glands and therefore originate below the surface of the visible mucosa; this latter phenomenon is more likely to occur in the floor of the mouth, base of the tongue, and nasopharynx. The very early surface lesions may show only erythema and a slightly elevated, slightly roughened mucosa. These are the so-called red lesions and always deserve consideration for biopsy.

Spread is dictated by local anatomy, and each anatomical site has its own peculiar spread patterns. Muscle invasion is a common feature, and tumor may spread along muscle or fascial planes for a surprising distance from the palpable or visible lesion. Tumor may attach to periosteum or perichondrium quite early, but actual bone or cartilage invasion is usually a late event.

Bone and cartilage generally act as a barrier to spread, and these structures generally are spared until the neoplasm has explored easier avenues of growth. Tumor that encounters cartilage or bone in its path usually will be diverted and spread along a path of less resistance. Slow-growing neoplasms of the gingiva may produce a smooth pressure defect or saucerization of the underlying bone without actual bone invasion.

Entrance of tumor into the parapharyngeal space allows superior or inferior spread from the base of the skull to the root of the neck.

Spread inside the lumen of the sublingual, submandibular, and parotid gland ducts is not a prevalent pattern. The nasolacrimal duct, however, frequently is invaded in ethmoid sinus and nasal carcinoma.

Perineural spread is an important pathway for tumor spread; no site or histology is immune to this growth pattern. Squamous cell carcinoma and its variants and minor salivary gland tumors, especially adenoid cystic carcinoma, may show this pattern. The presence of perineural invasion predicts a poorer rate of local control when managed by surgery[5]; there are no specific data for success when the management is by radiation therapy. Local recurrence increases the likelihood of perineural involvement, and tumors may track along a nerve to the base of the skull and the central nervous system (CNS). Peripheral perineural spread, that is, growth away from the CNS, is also observed. Patients with perineural invasion often develop neurologic symptoms. Some nerve palsies are probably secondary to compression or entrapment rather than actual nerve invasion.

The risk of perineural spread is related to the anatomic site and diameter of the lesion.[6]

Vascular space invasion is associated with an increased risk for regional and distant metastases.

Lymphatic Spread

The risk of lymph node metastasis may be predicted by the differentiation of the tumor (the more poorly differentiated, the greater the risk), by the size of the primary lesion, by the presence of vascular space invasion, and by the availability of capillary lymphatics. Recurrent lesions likewise have an increased risk.

There is no exclusion of a particular histology from lymphatic spread; mere access to the capillary lymphatics determines the opportunity. In other words, minor salivary gland tumors and sarcomas assume a risk of lymphatic metastasis commensurate with the particular mucosal site.

A patient may present with squamous cell carcinoma in a cervical lymph node, and despite an extensive work-up, the site of origin may remain undetermined. If only the neck is treated, a primary lesion may appear at a later date, but some may never show a primary site.

The risk of subclinical disease in the patient with a clinically negative neck may be obtained either by studying the incidence of positive nodes found in elective neck dissection specimens or by counting the number of necks that become positive when the neck is not treated. The relative incidence of clinically positive lymph nodes on admission by anatomical site and T stage is given in Table 21-1.[7]

Well-lateralized lesions spread to ipsilateral neck lymph nodes. Lesions on or near the midline and lateralized tongue and nasopharyngeal lesions may spread to both sides but tend to spread to the side occupied by the bulk of the lesion. Patients with clinically positive lymph nodes in the ipsilateral neck are at risk for contralateral disease, especially if the nodes are large or multiple. Obstruction of the lymphatic pathways by surgery or radiation therapy will also shunt the lymphatic flow to the opposite neck. This shunting is mainly through anastomotic channels that cross through the submental space.[8]

TABLE 21-1. Percentage of Clinically Detected Nodal Metastasis on Admission by T stage: M. D. Anderson Hospital, 1948–1965 (2044 Patients)

Primary Site	*T Stage*	*N0*	*N1*	*N2–N3*
Oral tongue	T1	86	10	4
	T2	70	19	11
	T3	52	16	31
	T4	24	10	66
Floor of mouth	T1	89	9	2
	T2	71	18	10
	T3	56	20	24
	T4	46	10	43
Retromolar trigone and anterior tonsillar pillar	T1	88	2	9
	T2	62	18	20
	T3	46	21	33
	T4	32	18	50
Soft palate	T1	92	0	8
	T2	64	12	24
	T3	35	26	39
	T4	33	11	56
Tonsillar fosa	T1	30	41	30
	T2	32	14	54
	T3	30	18	52
	T4	10	13	76
Base of tongue	T1	30	15	55
	T2	29	14	56
	T3	26	23	52
	T4	16	8	76
Oropharyngeal walls	T1	75	0	25
	T2	70	10	20
	T3	33	22	44
	T4	24	24	52
Supraglottic larynx	T1	61	10	29
	T2	58	16	26
	T3	36	25	40
	T4	41	18	41
Hypopharynx	T1	37	21	42
	T2	30	20	49
	T3	21	26	54
	T4	26	15	58
Nasopharynx	T1	8	11	82
	T2	16	12	72
	T3	12	9	80
	T4	17	6	78

Modified from Lindberg R: Distribution of cervical lymph node metastases from squamous cell carcinoma of the upper respiratory and digestive tracts. Cancer 29:1446–1449, 1972.

When contralateral metastases occur from well-lateralized lesions, the subdigastric node is the most commonly involved but may be bypassed, with the midjugular or low jugular next affected. When lymph node metastases appear at an unusual site, a careful search must be made for a second primary.

Although there is usually an orderly progression of lymph node involvement, there are examples of skips and random involvement. Rarely one will see retrograde lymph node metastases in the ipsilateral axilla associated with involvement of the lower neck nodes.

Distant Spread

Stage for stage, the risk of distant metastases is the same for patients treated by radiation therapy alone and those treated by surgery alone. The risk of distant metastasis is more related to neck stage than primary stage. The risk is less than 10% for N0–N1 and rises to approximately 30% for N2 and N3.[9,10] Vascular space invasion is associated with an increased risk of distant metastasis. Lung is the most common site, accounting for 52% of the first recognized sites. Mediastinal metastases are uncommon, occurring in only 3%. Almost one half of the metastases are recognized by 9 months, 80% by 2 years, and 90% by 3 years. The risk of distant metastasis doubled in patients developing a recurrence above the clavicles: 16.7% for those having a recurrence, even if salvaged, and 7.9% for those never developing a recurrence.[11]

STAGING

The staging for the primary lesions (T) is given in the appropriate section. The AJCC (1983) neck staging (N) is common to all head and neck sites except the major salivary glands.[12]

- NX Minimum requirements to assess the regional nodes cannot be met
- N0 No clinically positive node
- N1 Single clinically positive homolateral node 3 cm or less in diameter
- N2a Single clinically positive homolateral node more than 3 cm but not more than 6 cm in diameter or multiple clinically positive homolateral nodes, none more than 6 cm in diameter
- N2a Single clinically positive homolateral node more than 3 cm but not more than 6 cm in diameter
- N2b Multiple clinically positive homolateral nodes, none more than 6 cm in diameter
- N3 Massive homolateral node(s), bilateral nodes, or contralateral node(s)
- N3a Clinically positive homolateral node(s), one more than 6 cm in diameter
- N3b Bilateral clinically positive nodes (each side of the neck should be staged separately; *e.g.*, N3b: right, N2a; left, N1)
- N3c Contralateral clinically positive node(s) only

The format for combining T and N stages into a total stage is shown in Figure 21-2.[13] Distant metastasis automatically places the patient into Stage IV. Stage IV represents a wide spectrum of disease. A patient may have a T1, T2, or T3 lesion with treatable N2 or N3A neck disease (Stage IVA) and represent a reasonable candidate for curative therapy, whereas another may have either a far-advanced primary (T4) or far-advanced neck disease (N3B), or both (Stage IVB). The 5-year disease-free survival rate is about twice as high for some sites for Stage IVA as for Stage IVB when radiation therapy is the initial treatment for the primary tumor.[13] A comparison of the results for Stages IVA and IVB when the initial treatment of the primary site is surgical has not been reported.

PRINCIPLES OF TREATMENT

GENERAL PRINCIPLES FOR SELECTION OF TREATMENT

Surgery and radiation therapy are the only curative treatments for carcinoma arising in the head and neck. Chemo-

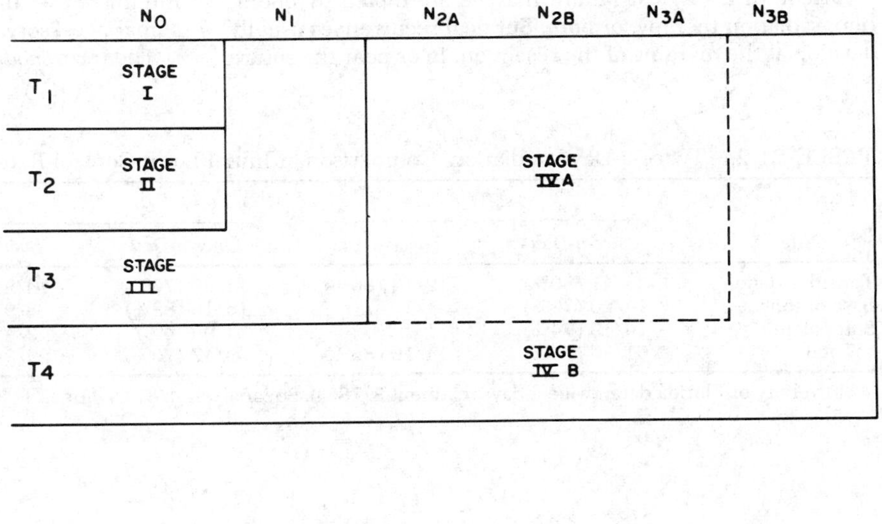

FIG. 21-2. American Joint Committee on Cancer stage grouping, as modified by Mendenhall et al.[12] (Mendenhall WM, Parsons JT, Million RR, et al: A favorable subset of AJCC stage IV squamous cell carcinoma of the head and neck. Int J Radiat Oncol Biol Phys 10:1841–1843, 1984)

therapy must be considered investigational at present; used alone, it is not curative, and its role as an adjunct to surgery, radiation therapy, or both is in a state of flux.

The advantages of an operation compared with radiation therapy, assuming similar cure rates, may include the following:

1. A limited amount of tissue is exposed to treatment.
2. Treatment time is shorter.
3. The risk of immediate and late radiation sequelae is avoided.
4. Irradiation is reserved for a subsequent head and neck primary tumor, which may not be as suitable for an operation.
5. Pathologic examination of tissues permits identification of patients with more extensive disease than originally determined, in whom immediate postoperative irradiation can be added.

The advantages of irradiation may include the following:

1. The threat of the major operation is avoided. An operative mortality of only 1% to 2% may seem high to the patient compared with no immediate threat from radiation therapy.
2. No tissues are removed. Resection of even a relatively small lesion may produce a functional or cosmetic defect. This risk must be weighed against the risk of a radiation necrosis.
3. Elective irradiation of the lymph nodes can be included with little added morbidity, whereas the surgeon either must adopt a "watch and wait" attitude or must proceed with elective neck dissection. This is important for lesions with a high rate of spread to the lymph nodes, especially where there is a high opportunity for bilateral spread (*i.e.*, floor of mouth, base of tongue, soft palate, hypopharynx, and some larynx lesions).
4. The surgical salvage of irradiation failure is more likely than the salvage of a surgical failure. When a primary lesion recurs after irradiation, the recurrence is almost always in the center of the original lesion; marginal failures are uncommon. A rescue operation would be similar in scope had the patient been managed initially by operation, albeit with a greater risk for a serious complication.

Rescue of a surgical failure may be attempted by operation, radiation therapy, or both. Surgical recurrences usually develop at the margins of the resection, in or near the suture line. It is difficult to distinguish the normal surgical scarring from recurrent disease, and diagnosis of recurrence is often delayed. Tumor response to radiation therapy under these circumstances is poor. Small mucosal recurrences and some neck recurrences, however, may be salvaged by an operation, radiation therapy, or both.

MANAGEMENT

PRIMARY SITE

The management of the primary site will be considered separately for each anatomical site. Since radiation therapy has the advantage of preserving anatomical integrity, the local control rates for radiation therapy must be known in order to select either curative radiation therapy with surgery reserved for local failure or initial surgical resection. The initial local control rates with once-a-day treatment and twice-a-day treatment for T2-T4 carcinomas of the oropharynx, larynx, and hypopharynx are compared in Tables 21-2 and 21-3. Patients treated with the twice-a-day scheme have received 120 cGy at each session with a 4-hour gap between treatments.[14] The total dose currently varies between 7440 cGy and 8100 cGy for oropharynx lesions and is limited to 7440 cGy to 7680 cGy when the larynx is in the reduced volume. Local control rates are at least as good or up to 10% to 15% improved with the twice-a-day treatment. Regional control rates are improved and complications fewer.

THE NECK

Management of the neck is closely tied to management of the primary site, but certain general principles may be outlined. Death due only to failure to control neck disease, with the primary tumor controlled, should be an uncommon event if surgery and radiation therapy are used to their maximum advantage.

In a standard *radical neck dissection*, the superficial and deep cervical fascia with its enclosed lymph nodes is removed in continuity with the sternocleidomastoid muscle, the omohyoid muscle, the internal and external jugular veins, the spinal accessory nerve, and the submandibular gland. The incisions used by the surgeon will be governed largely by the primary lesion. Proper physical therapy may minimize the functional changes associated with loss of the spinal accessory nerve and sternocleidomastoid muscle.

The term *modified neck dissection* refers to any neck node

TABLE 21-2. Twice-a-Day Irradiation: Comparison of Initial Local Control Rates for Oropharynx

	T2		*T3*		*T4*	
Site	*Once-a-Day*	*Twice-a-Day*	*Once-a-Day*	*Twice-a-Day*	*Once-a-Day*	*Twice-a-Day*
Tonsillar region	33/41 (80%)	12/14 (86%)	14/20 (70%)	14/21 (67%)	4/11 (36%)	4/9 (44%)
Base of tongue	14/20 (70%)	1/1	15/18 (83%)	8/9 (89%)	2/12 (17%)	3/6 (50%)
Soft palate	14/19 (74%)	1/1	4/9 (44%)	2/4	n.d.	n.d.
Total	61/80 (76%)	14/16 (88%)	33/47 (70%)	24/34 (71%)	6/23 (26%)	7/15 (47%)

University of Florida data; twice-a-day treatment 3/78–4/85; analysis 4/87 by James T. Parsons, M.D. n.d., no data.

TABLE 21-3. Twice-a Day Irradiation: Comparison of Initial Local Control Rates for Larynx/Hypopharynx

	T2		*T3*		*T4*	
Site	*Once-a-Day*	*Twice-a-Day*	*Once-a-Day*	*Twice-a-Day*	*Once-a-Day*	*Twice-a-Day*
Supraglottic larynx	18/23 (78%)	9/11 (82%)	3/5 (60%)	12/17 (71%)	1/7	0/1
True vocal cord	n.d.	n.d.	7/13 (54%)	10/14 (71%)	n.d.	1/5
Pyriform sinus	12/16	3/3	1/3	1/2	0/2	0/1
Pharyngeal wall	8/17	4/4	8/21 (38%)	5/7 (71%)	1/8	1/2
Total	38/56 (68%)	16/18 (89%)	19/42 (45%)	28/40 (70%)	2/17 (12%)	2/9 (22%)

University of Florida data; twice-a-day treatment 3/78–4/85; analysis 4/87 by James T. Parsons, M.D. n.d., no data.

resection that is less than the radical neck dissection. A modified neck dissection is tailored to remove those groups of lymph nodes at highest risk for metastatic disease while also attempting to reduce the sequelae by selectively preserving certain muscles, nerves, and vessels. A modified neck dissection sparing normal tissues (*e.g.*, the functional neck dissection) is usually recommended for the clinically negative neck, for selected clinically positive necks (mobile, 1–3 cm lymph nodes), and for removing residual disease after radiation therapy when there has been excellent regression of N2 or N3 disease.

Complications after radical neck dissection include hematoma, seroma, lymphedema, wound infections and dehiscence, damage to the 7th, 10th, and 12th cranial nerves, carotid exposure, and carotid rupture. The last-mentioned can be minimized by covering the carotid artery with a dermal graft at the time of surgery.

CLINICALLY NEGATIVE NECK. The risk for subclinical disease for any particular patient may be estimated based on the primary site, the T stage or size of the primary lesion, the differentiation of the neoplasm, and the presence of lymphatic invasion. The incidence of subclinical disease in the regional lymphatics when the neck is clinically negative is presented in Table 21-4.[15] The use of contrast-enhanced CT will improve the diagnostic ability and decrease the chance of underestimating disease in the neck in 5% to 10% of patients.[45] Both irradiation and neck dissection are approximately 90% efficient in eradicating subclinical disease in the neck lymph nodes. A policy of "wait and see" may be adopted for the clinically negative neck to avoid unnecessary treatment, and the neck may then be managed by surgery, radiation therapy, or both only if cervical metastases develop. Even though the salvage neck treatment may be regionally successful, these patients are at an increased risk to develop distant metastasis and therefore have a poorer prognosis compared with patients who have immediate control of neck disease from the beginning. The salvage rate for patients developing clinically positive lymph nodes with the primary lesion controlled is only 60% in the University of Florida experience.[46]

When a neck node does appear, the diagnosis often may be delayed so that the morbidity of the salvage procedure is considerably greater than one would experience with elective treatment.

The physician and patient must adhere to a schedule of very close observation and examination if they choose the policy of observation.

Elective neck treatment has the added advantage of giving complete treatment at the initial point of management and

TABLE 21-4. Incidence of Lymph Node Metastasis by Site of Primary in Head and Neck Squamous Cell Carcinoma

Site	*Percentage N+ at Presentation (Reference)*	*Percentage N0 Clinically, N+ Pathologically (Reference)*	*Percentage N0− > N+ with No Neck Treatment (Reference)*
Floor of mouth	30–59 (16–18)	40–50 (19, 20)	20–35 (21–23)
Gingiva	18–52 (16, 24–26)	19 (24)	17 (21, 24)
Hard palate	13–24 (26–28)		22 (21)
Buccal mucosa	9–31 (16, 18)		16 (21)
Oral tongue	34–65 (16–18, 29)	25–54 (20, 25, 30–32)	38–52 (23, 29, 31, 33)
Nasopharynx	86–90 (9, 10, 34)		19*–50 (35, 36)
Anterior tonsillar pillar/ retromolar trigone	39–56 (37–39)		10–15 (40)
Soft palate/uvula	37–56 (37–39)		16–25 (39)
Tonsillar fossa	58–76 (9, 10, 17, 34, 38)		22† (41)
Base of tongue	50–83 (34, 38, 40, 42)	22 (42)	
Pharyngeal walls	50–71 (34, 38, 40, 42)	66 (42)	
Supraglottic larynx	31–54 (17, 40)	16–26 (42, 43)	33 (43, 44)
Hypopharynx	52–72 (9, 40, 42)	38 (42)	

Mendenhall WM, Million RR, Cassisi NJ: Elective neck irradiation in squamous cell carcinoma of the head and neck. Head Neck Surg 3:15–20, 1980.

*T1N0 patients only.

†Patients received preoperative irradiation.

simplifying the follow-up neck examinations because of its high success rate. The relative effectiveness of irradiation and surgery in the management of the N0 neck is shown in Tables 21-5, 21-6, and 21-7.[15,48] Partial neck treatment is inefficient for primary lesions of the oropharynx, supraglottic larynx, or hypopharynx (Tables 21-6 and 21-7), and treatment of the entire neck is advised for sites with a high rate of subclinical disease.

When the primary tumor is to be treated surgically, it is our recommendation to add elective neck treatment when the risk of regional lymph node metastasis is 10% to 15% or greater. In some cases elective neck treatment is added when the risk is less; it is relatively easy to add elective neck treatment with either radiation therapy or surgery because of the type of operation or irradiation being delivered to the primary site. If the primary lesion is to be treated with external beam irradiation, then elective neck irradiation adds no cost and, if properly done, little additional morbidity.

When the primary lesion is to be treated surgically, the surgeon has the responsibility to manage the neck unless postoperative irradiation is definitely planned. Most surgeons do not use radical neck dissection for the clinically negative neck so that there are fewer cosmetic or functional problems. Modified neck dissections have as good a rate of disease control as does the radical neck dissection if patients who are found to have multiple positive nodes or disease extending through the capsule are then referred for postoperative irradiation.[49]

Radiation therapy occasionally fails to eradicate subclinical disease. Most of the failures are due to geographic misses with nodes appearing near the edge or just outside the edge of the treatment field. Other causes of failure are low dose, selection of the wrong beam energy (which results in low dose), and failure to detect a clinically positive node.

Elective neck surgery occasionally fails because of a failure to remove all the lymph nodes at risk or because of extranodal extension.

CLINICALLY POSITIVE NECK LYMPH NODES. The rate of neck failure by N stage and therapeutic category reported from M. D. Anderson Hospital is shown in Tables 21-6 and 21-7.[48] The irradiation preceded the operation if the primary site was to be treated by radiation therapy or if the node was fixed. The operation preceded the irradiation if the primary site was to be treated surgically.

TABLE 21-5. Efficacy of Elective Neck Irradiation (ENI) with Primary Tumor Controlled—125 Patients

Primary Stage	*No. of Patients with Neck Controlled/ No. of Patients with Primary Controlled* — *No ENI*	*Partial ENI*	*Whole ENI*
T1	11/12	17/18	9/10
T2	6/8	17/17	22/22
T3	0/1	10/10	18/18
T4	1/1	5/5	3/3
Total	18/22 (82%)*	49/50 (98%)*	52/53 (98%)*

*Significance level = 0.01, using exact test procedures.[47]
Mendenhall WM, Million RR, Cassisi NJ: Elective neck irradiation in squamous cell carcinoma of the head and neck. Head Neck Surg 3:15–20, 1980.

Radical neck dissection is sufficient treatment for the ipsilateral neck for patients with N1 or N2A disease. Radiation therapy is added for N2B and N3 stages, for control of contralateral subclinical disease (Table 21-7), for invasion through the capsule of the node, and for the finding of multiple positive nodes in the specimen.

When the primary lesion is to be managed by irradiation, then radiation therapy alone is sufficient for patients with N1 (1–3 cm) disease. Neck dissection may be added in selected cases in which the 3 cm node is fixed or fails to regress completely. Radiation therapy is followed by a neck dissection for most N2A and nearly all N3A disease. The decision to add radical neck dissection for N2B and N3B disease is individualized, based on the diameter of the largest node or the multiplicity of palpable nodes. Large, fixed nodes require 6000 cGy to 8000 cGy before neck dissection; some of the specimens will show "no viable tumor," and a substantial number of patients will have the disease controlled in the neck. There will be less fibrosis in the neck by 5 years after treatment when large node masses are managed by radiation therapy followed by neck dissection compared with irradiation alone.

The neck disease control rate in patients managed between 1978 and 1984 with 120 cGy twice daily to doses of 7440 cGy to 8000 cGy to the primary lesion is shown in Table 21-8. At least a part of the upper neck received the same doses. When the primary lesion was controlled by radiation therapy, the rate of control of neck disease was very

TABLE 21-6. Failure of Initial Neck Treatment (596 Patients with Carcinoma of the Tonsillar Fossa, Base of Tongue, Supraglottic Larynx, or Hypopharynx, M. D. Anderson Hospital, 1948–1967)

	Stage							
	N0							
Treatment	*No Treatment*	*Partial*	*Complete*	*N1*	*N2A*	*N2B*	*N3A*	*N3B*
Radiation		15%	2%	15%	27%	27%	38%	34%
Surgery	55% (16/29)	35%	7%	11%	8%	23%	42%	41%
Combined		1/5	0/6	0	0	0	23%	25%

Adapted from Barkley HT Jr, Fletcher GH, Jesse RH et al: Management of cervical lymph node metastases in squamous cell carcinoma of the tonsillar fossa, base of tongue, supraglottic larynx, and hypopharynx. Am J Surg 124:462–467, 1972.

TABLE 21-7. Cervical Metastasis Appearing in the Contralateral Neck (596 Patients with Carcinoma of the Tonsillar Fossa, Base of Tongue, Supraglottic Larynx, or Hypopharynx, M. D. Anderson Hospital, 1948–1967)

Treatment	*N0*	*N1*	*N2A*	*N2B*	*N3A*
Radiation	2/50	1/52	2/22	2/27	0/21
Surgery	7/28	8/47	3/13	13/30	4/12
Combined	0/6	0/21	0/17	3/28	0/13

Barkley HT Jr, Fletcher GH, Jesse RH et al: Management of cervical lymph node metastases in squamous cell carcinoma of the tonsillar fossa, base of tongue, supraglottic larynx, and hypopharynx. Am J Surg 124:462–467, 1972.

high. There were only four neck failures in 30 patients selected for planned neck dissection; the patients selected for neck dissection were usually those with fixed masses, large masses, or a poor response to radiation therapy. These results have been updated to 1985. Forty-one ipsilateral and 4 bilateral planned neck dissections after twice-a-day therapy have been evaluated for complications. There have been no carotid ruptures and no operative deaths. There were 8 wound complications in 41 unilateral neck dissections and 1 minor wound complication in 4 bilateral neck dissections (JT Parsons, unpublished data, 1986). The average time to discharge was 6 days for non-Veterans Administration patients and 14 days for Veterans Administration patients.

Biopsy of a neck mass for diagnosis by excisional or incisional biopsy has been condemned by many. McGuirt and McCabe[50] compared results with and without open biopsy and concluded that the risks of neck failure, distant metastases, and complications of subsequent neck surgery were all increased. Their patients were managed by operation following open neck biopsy.

Parsons and co-workers[51] studied the results of therapy following incisional or excisional biopsy of a lymph node before treatment. In 25 patients with no gross residual disease after excisional biopsy (NX), the referring surgeons' and pathologists' reports showed that a single, clinically positive lymph node had been totally excised. These patients received irradiation to the primary site and neck. No other clinically positive lymph nodes were found upon referral, and no neck dissections were performed for this group of patients. The rate of control of neck disease was 96%, the absolute 5-year disease-free survival rate was 79%, and the 5-year determinate survival rate was 88%. These results are good, considering that all patients had Stage III or IV disease.

Fifty-five patients had gross residual neck disease after biopsy.[51] In some patients, only an incisional biopsy of a very large mass had been performed; in others, only one of several lymph nodes had been removed. The absolute 5-year disease-free survival rate in this group of patients was 31%, the 5-year determinate survival rate was 38%, and the overall rate of control of neck disease was 64%. All except three had Stage IV disease. The more consistent addition of a neck dissection in recent years had resulted in improved rates of neck disease control and survival in this latter group.

After open biopsy of the neck, it is recommended that radiation therapy be the initial treatment. If the primary tumor is to be managed by radiation therapy, no further neck treatment is needed if the neck node has been removed. If there is residual gross tumor in the neck after open biopsy, a planned neck dissection should be added. If the primary tumor is to be managed by operation, it is recommended that preoperative radiation therapy be used, followed by removal of the primary lesion plus an appropriate neck dissection.

Once the normal lymphatic pathways have been surgically interrupted by the open biopsy procedure, shunting of lymph to the contralateral side of the neck may occur, placing it at risk for lymph node spread when the opposite neck would not normally be at risk.[8,52]

CHEMOTHERAPY

The role of chemotherapy in the management of patients with squamous cell carcinoma of the head and neck has not

TABLE 21-8. Control of Disease in the Neck with Twice-a-Day Fractionation When the Primary Lesion Is Controlled (No. of Heminecks Controlled/No. Treated)

Hemineck Stage	*Radiation Therapy Alone*	*Radiation Therapy plus Neck Dissection*	*Total*
NX	1/1	n.d.	1/1
N0	82/84	n.d.	82/84
N1	21/22	6/7	27/29
N2A	1/1	4/5	5/6
N2B	9/12	11/12	20/24
N3A	0/2*	5/6	5/8
Total		26/30 (87%)	140/152 (92%)

University of Florida data; patients treated 3/78 – 4/84; analysis 4/86 by James T. Parsons, M.D.
n.d., no data.
*Lung metastases; neck dissections cancelled.

been adequately defined and remains an area of active investigation. For patients with metastatic or recurrent disease following maximal surgery and radiotherapy, chemotherapy can induce significant tumor regression in 20% to 50% of patients and provide palliation for the patient with symptomatic or life-threatening disease. For patients with potentially curable advanced local–regional disease (M0), the use of chemotherapy as induction, adjuvant, or synchronous treatment with surgery or radiotherapy remains an investigative approach.

Single-Agent Chemotherapy for Advanced Disease

Numerous individual drugs have demonstrable activity against squamous cell carcinoma of the head and neck (Table 21-9). These drugs belong to several major classes of antineoplastic compounds, including bifunctional alkylating agents, antimetabolites, antitumor antibiotics, plant alkaloids, and heavy metal coordination complexes. The response rates recorded in Table 21-9 must be interpreted with caution, as they are derived from pooled data from a large number of individual trials using different criteria for patient entry, variable drug doses and schedules, and often discrepant criteria for response.

Methotrexate was one of the earliest and most thoroughly evaluated single agents in the treatment of squamous cell cancers of the head and neck. By virtue of its documented activity, acceptable toxicity, convenience of administration, and low cost, it remains the standard of therapy for patients with recurrent or metastatic disease. Methotrexate has been given in a wide variety of doses and schedules (Table 21-10). Weekly or twice-weekly conventional dose administration may be more effective than loading doses once every 3 to 4 weeks or daily administration of small doses. Moderate to high doses of methotrexate with leucovorin can be safely administered to patients with head and neck cancer and may limit the myelosuppression, alopecia, nephrotoxicity, and mucositis associated with lower doses of methotrexate without leucovorin. However, the use of moderate to high doses of methotrexate with leucovorin rescue adds cost, inconvenience, and risk of toxicity in noncompliant patients with no apparent increase in antitumor activity, duration of response, or overall survival.[57,59,61,64,65] For palliation of patients with advanced, incurable disease and acceptable renal function, it is appropriate to begin oral or intravenous methotrexate with weekly doses of 40 to 50 mg/m² or biweekly doses of 15 to 20 mg/m² and escalate the dose in weekly increments until either mild toxicity or therapeutic response is achieved. Moderate-dose methotrexate with leucovorin may be appropriate for the patient with treatment-limiting mucositis or myelosuppression on low-dose methotrexate or as a nonmyelosuppressive addition to combination chemotherapy.

Bleomycin is another single agent with activity against squamous cell carcinomas. Response rates from trials in the United States, however, have been consistently lower than those from the initial Japanese studies.[66–72] Experimental data in animals[99,100] support the clinical impression[101–103] that bleomycin's clinical activity and therapeutic index are greater when given by continuous infusion than when administered by intermittent bolus. Despite the potential of skin and mucosal toxicity and severe interstitial pulmonary disease, bleomycin has been employed in many regimens of

TABLE 21-9. Single-Agent Activity in Patients with Recurrent or Metastatic Head and Neck Cancer

Drug	*No. of Patients*	*Response Rate (%)**
Methotrexate[53–65] (doses <200 mg/m²)	447	36
Bleomycin[66–72]	386	26
Cisplatin[73–78]	194	32
5-Fluorouracil[79–87]	115	27
Cyclophosphamide[88]	77	36
Doxorubicin[89–90]	88	13
New or Inadequately Studied Agents		
Hydroxyurea[91]	22	23
Carboplatin[92–95]	115	26
Iproplatin[95]	34	12
Mitozantrone[96–98]	113	4

*Includes subjective, <50%, or unquantified responses.

TABLE 21-10. Methotrexate Given Parenterally in Doses Less Than 200 mg/m² for Head and Neck Cancer

Investigator	*Schedule**	*No. of Patients*	*Percentage of Patients with >50% Tumor Regression*
Papac et al.[53]	0.8 mg/kg every 4 days IV	15	53
Lane et al.[54]	25 to 50 mg every 4 to 7 days	27	52
Leone et al.[55]	60 mg/m² weekly IV or 40 mg/m² biweekly IV	35	57
DePalo et al.[56]	40 or 60 mg/m² weekly IV	23	35
Levitt et al.[57]	80 mg/m² for 30 h every 2 wk with escalation to toxicity	16	44
DeConti and Schoenfeld[59]	40 mg/m² weekly IV	81	26
Kirkwood et al.[60]	40 to 200 mg/m² IV on days 1, 4 weekly; leucovorin on days 2, 5	19	63
Woods et al.[61]	50 mg/m² bolus; leucovorin 15 mg PO every 6 h × 12 doses	23	26
Hong et al.[62]	40 to 60 mg/m² IV weekly	17	23
Grose et al.[63]	15 mg/m² IM on days 1 through 3 every 3 wk	44	18
Vogler et al.[64]	60 mg/m² IV weekly	61	35
Total		361	35

*PO, by mouth.

combination chemotherapy for head and neck cancer because of its lack of significant myelosuppression.

The experience with cisplatin suggests that this agent has antitumor activity that is comparable to methotrexate.[73–78] Two relatively small randomized studies comparing cisplatin to methotrexate have shown similar response rates; however, cisplatin produced more nephrotoxicity and emesis, whereas methotrexate resulted in more mucositis and myelosuppression.[62,63] Cisplatin has also been compared to "symptomatic care," infusion bleomycin, or a combination of cisplatin and bleomycin in a randomized trial of patients with recurrent or metastatic disease.[104] In this study, patients treated with cisplatin had significantly prolonged survival in comparison to the control group. In addition, the combination of cisplatin and bleomycin was no more effective than cisplatin alone, and bleomycin offered no benefit over symptomatic care.

Two cisplatin analogues, iproplatin and carboplatin, have recently been evaluated in Phase I and II trials and offer the potential for decreased renal and gastrointestinal toxicity and the advantage of outpatient administration. Both drugs can be administered without prior hydration or mannitol diuresis. Preliminary studies of iproplatin and carboplatin have demonstrated significant antitumor activity with myelosuppression as the principal side-effect. In a single study of 34 patients, a 12% response rate to iproplatin was recorded,[95] and in three studies with 115 total patients, a response rate of 26% to carboplatin was noted.[92–95]

Cyclophosphamide and 5-fluorouracil have also demonstrated substantial antitumor activity as single agents in patients with metastatic or recurrent head and neck cancer. Of particular interest is a recent report of four partial responses in seven such patients treated with infusion 5-fluorouracil.[105]

Numerous other drugs have been evaluated in patients with recurrent or metastatic head and neck cancer. Unfortunately, an encouraging preliminary study of mitoguazone[106] has not been reproduced.[107–109] In addition, clinically significant activity has not been demonstrated in recent studies of mitozantrone,[96–98] m-AMSA,[110–111] dibromodulcitol,[96,112,113] VP-16,[114–116] vindesine,[117–119] and triazinate.[120]

Biologic response modifiers, especially interferon, have also been used in the treatment of patients with advanced head and neck cancer.[121–123] Mendenica and Slack,[122] using human leukocyte interferon, reported 3 complete and 4 partial responses in 12 patients with refractory head and neck cancer. In this study, the duration of response was approximately 10 months. Connors and co-workers[123] similarly evaluated human leukocyte interferon in 12 patients with advanced nasopharyngeal carcinoma and noted measurable responses in 4 patients and stabilization of disease in 3 additional patients.

Combination Chemotherapy for Advanced Disease

Over the past 10 to 15 years, numerous Phase II trials have evaluated combinations of active single agents in patients with advanced head and neck cancer. The majority of published regimens of combination chemotherapy for head and neck cancer have been two- or three-drug schedules of cisplatin, bleomycin, methotrexate, or vincristine. Recent combinations include cisplatin and 5-fluorouracil and sequential methotrexate and 5-fluorouracil. Cisplatin with infusion 5-fluorouracil has been shown to be more effective than cisplatin with bolus 5-fluorouracil.[124] While several studies of patients with recurrent or metastatic disease have suggested modest increases in the rates of complete or total response to combination chemotherapy (Table 21-11), the toxicity of some combinations is formidable, with no obvious therapeutic gain over single-agent cisplatin or methotrexate.

The clinical significance of such Phase II studies is limited by the absence of a control group and the possibility of selection bias. Given the impact of various prognostic factors in treatment outcome, a definitive analysis of combination chemotherapy requires a prospective, randomized study.

To date, six randomized trials have been published that directly compare combination to single-agent chemotherapy in the treatment of patients with metastatic or recurrent squamous cell carcinoma of the head and neck (Table 21-12). As noted, five of the six studies compared combination chemotherapy to single-agent methotrexate. Although combination chemotherapy was associated with a higher total response rate in five of six studies, a statistically significant difference was apparent in only two. More importantly, the use of combination chemotherapy was not associated with an improved duration of response or median survival in any of the six trials.

GENERAL PRINCIPLES OF COMBINING MODALITIES

Surgery Plus Radiation Therapy

Either preoperative or postoperative radiation therapy may be used; there are advocates of each. Analysis of available data suggests that there is no difference in local-regional control or survival rates comparing the two sequences.

Combined modality therapy should be avoided for lesions with a high cure rate (70% or greater) by either surgery or radiation therapy alone. The increased morbidity from combined treatment does not increase the control rate significantly, and many patients with local or regional failure can be salvaged by secondary procedures.

The advantages of postoperative compared with preoperative radiation therapy include less operative morbidity, more meaningful margin checks at the time of the operation, a knowledge of tumor spread for radiation treatment planning, safe use of a higher radiation dose, and no chance that the patient will refuse surgery.

The disadvantages of postoperative radiation therapy include the larger treatment volume necessary to cover surgical dissections and scars, a delay in the start of radiation therapy with possible growth of tumor (especially contralateral neck nodes), and the higher dose required to accomplish the same rate of local-regional control.

PREOPERATIVE RADIATION THERAPY. Preoperative radiation therapy is recommended for the following situations:

1. A trial of radiation therapy (5000 cGy) is given to judge the response of the primary lesion. The patient

TABLE 21-11. Recent Drug Combinations

Investigator	Dosage and Schedule*	No. of Patients†	Response Rate (%) Total	Response Rate (%) Complete	Duration of Response (mo)
Kish et al.[125]	Cisplatin 100 mg/m² on day 1 5-FU 1000 mg/m²/d on days 1 through 4	30 (5)	70	27	11.3 (if CR) 6.5. (if PR)
Merlano et al.[126]	Cisplatin 20 mg/m²/d on days 1 through 5 5-FU 200 mg/m²/d on days 1 through 5	30 (29)	53	13	6.5 (survival)
Bitran et al.[127]	Doxorubicin 40 mg/m² Cyclophosphamide 750 mg/m²	26 (26)	46	0	6.5
Scherlacher et al.[128]	Methotrexate 250 mg/m² at hour 0 5-FU 600 mg/m² at hour 1	28 (17)	39	18	6.5
Pitman et al.[129]	Methotrexate 250 mg/m² at hour 0 5-FU 600 mg/m² at hour 1	23 (5)	65	13	3.6
Lester et al.[130]	Cisplatin 50 mg/m² on day 1 Bleomycin 7 mg/m² on days 1, 8, 15 Methotrexate 120 mg/m² at hour 0 on days 8, 15, 22 followed by leucovorin 5-FU 600 mg/m² at hour 1 on days 8, 15, 22	74(19)	52	18	16 (survival CR) 9 (survival PR)
Vogl et al.[131]	Cisplatin 50 mg/m² on day 4 Bleomycin 10 mg/d on days 1, 8, 15 Methotrexate 40 mg/m² at hour 0 on days 1, 15 5-FU 600 mg/m² at hour 1 on days 1, 15	46 (NA)	50	4	3.5
Cognetti et al.[132]	Bleomycin 10 mg/wk Vincristine 2 mg/wk Methotrexate 40 mg/m²/d on days 1, 15 Cisplatin 50 mg/m² on day 4	43 (19)	74	21	6

*5-FU, 5-fluorouracil.
†Number of patients with prior chemotherapy in parentheses; NA, not available.

is reevaluated with the surgeon, and a decision is made to continue for cure by radiation therapy or to stop the irradiation and proceed in 4 to 6 weeks to an operation. This philosophy is selected for moderately advanced lesions that have a reasonable chance of responding favorably to radiation therapy, thereby avoiding a major ablative procedure. The pyriform sinus and larynx are common primary sites for use of this strategy.

2. Solitary neck nodes that are fixed or on the borderline of resectability are a reason to give radiation therapy before surgery. The preoperative dose to the primary lesion is 5000 cGy, but treatment of the major neck mass is continued to a dose of 6000 cGy to 8000 cGy through a reduced tangential portal. Most large nodes will become resectable, and in approximately 50% of the specimens no tumor is seen. A fibrous capsule forms around the neck mass that facilitates dissection from the neurovascular bundles.
3. If the reconstruction and rehabilitation will delay the start of postoperative radiation therapy by more than 6

TABLE 21-12. Chemotherapy for Metastatic or Recurrent Squamous Cell Carcinoma of the Head and Neck—Randomized Trials

Investigator	Drugs Used	No. of Patients	Total Response (%)	Median Survival (mo)
DeConti and Schoenfeld[59]	Methotrexate	81	26	5.0
	Methotrexate/leucovorin	80	24	4.4
	Methotrexate/leucovorin, cyclophosphamide, cytosine arabinoside	76	18	3.2
Kaplan et al.[133]	Methotrexate	61	26*	5.0
	Cisplatin, bleomycin, methotrexate	61	46*	5.5
Jacobs et al.[134]	Cisplatin	41	18	6.2
	Cisplatin, methotrexate	39	33	6.9
Drelichman et al.[135]	Methotrexate	20	33	5.5
	Cisplatin, vincristine, bleomycin	20	41	3.5
Vogl et al.[136]	Methotrexate	83	35†	5.6
	Cisplatin, bleomycin, methotrexate	80	48†	5.6
Williams et al.[137]	Methotrexate	98	16	7.3
	Cisplatin, vinblastine, bleomycin	92	24	6.8

*$p = 0.04$.
†$p = 0.07$.

to 12 weeks, then consideration should be given to preoperative radiation therapy.

4. If an operative procedure is planned that includes use of the gastric pull-up for pharyngeal or esophageal reconstruction, preoperative irradiation is preferred because the tolerance limit of the stomach is thought to be 4000 cGy.
5. If a neck mass has been excisionally or incisionally biopsied and the primary lesion is to be resected, preoperative radiation therapy is advised.[50,51]

The dose for preoperative radiation therapy is usually 5000 cGy in 5 to 6 weeks. Short treatment schemes using a few large fractions followed immediately by surgery have shown little or no advantage over surgery alone.[138–141] Moderate-dose schemes, 3000 cGy to 4000 cGy, have not resulted in any great increase in control rates. A dose of 5000 cGy will control a large percentage of subclinical disease in lymph nodes and also reduce the recurrence rates for the primary site. A few venturesome groups have tried higher doses (6000 cGy), but the morbidity may exceed the gain. A reduced volume encompassing a large node may receive a high dose.

POSTOPERATIVE RADIATION THERAPY. Postoperative radiation therapy is considered when the risk of recurrence above the clavicles exceeds 20%. The operative procedure should be one-stage and of such magnitude that irradiation is started no later than 6 to 12 weeks after surgery. The operation should be undertaken only if it is believed to be highly likely that all gross disease will be removed and margins will be negative. It is fashionable to talk about "debulking" operations prior to radiation therapy. This term has no precise meaning and should be avoided because it may imply partial removal of gross disease ("cut-through"), a maneuver that probably reduces the chance of control by radiation therapy rather than enhancing it.

The radiation therapist is frequently called upon to make a decision regarding further treatment based on the pathologist's report following a cancer operation. Positive margins or close margins are an indication for radiation therapy. Looser and co-workers[142] compared the clinical significance of negative and positive margins for 1775 previously untreated squamous cell carcinomas of the head and neck (excluding glottic and skin). Only 3.5% were scored as positive margins. The incidence of recurrence at the primary site was 31.7% for patients with negative margins and 71% for those with positive margins. There was no difference whether the positive margin was due to carcinoma in situ, invasive tumor, or close margin (within 5 mm). Other indications for postoperative irradiation may be cartilage or bone invasion, perineural spread, and high-grade histology.

The findings in the neck dissection frequently are the indication for postoperative radiation therapy. Multiple positive nodes, invasion through the capsule, and high-grade histology predict a high risk of recurrence in both the dissected and the contralateral neck.

Amdur and co-workers[143] analyzed the results of radical surgery and postoperative radiation therapy in 161 patients with advanced, previously untreated squamous cell carcinoma of the oral cavity, oropharynx, hypopharynx, or larynx. Ninety-six percent had Stage III or IV cancer, and none had evidence of gross disease at the start of irradiation. The majority of recurrences above the clavicles occurred in the primary field (84%) as opposed to the posterior neck area (8%) or low neck (8%). Five factors were found to be significantly important for predicting disease control above the clavicles: treatment course (continuous course, 77%, versus split course, 33%; $p < 0.001$), surgical margin (invasive cancer at the margin, 50%, versus margin free of invasive cancer, 81%; $p = 0.01$), primary site (oral cavity, 64%, versus other sites, 83%; $p = 0.029$), multiple positive nodes in the surgical specimen (presence being worse than absence of this finding), and number of indications for irradiation (1–3 indications, 85%, versus ≥4 indications, 61%; $p = 0.06$).[144,145] The rate of disease control above the clavicles did not correlate well with AJCC pathologic stage. The interval between surgery and the start of radiation therapy up to 3 months also was not prognostically important.

At 5 years the actuarial survival rate was 33% for the entire group; for patients with invasive cancer at the margin, the survival rate was approximately half that of those whose margins were free of invasive cancer (17% versus 37%). Three factors were found to significantly influence survival rates: course of irradiation (continuous better than split), nodal status (negative better than positive), and extension of the primary tumor into the soft tissues of the neck (absence better than presence of this finding). Overall, 7% of patients experienced a severe complication of combined therapy, including pharyngeal stricture, stomal stenosis, bone or soft tissue necrosis, laryngeal edema, infection, and fistula.

Contrary to an earlier report,[146] there was no obvious dose response (excluding split course) when patients with similar risk factors were compared (Table 21-13). We continue to recommend 6000 cGy in 6 weeks to 6500 cGy in 7 weeks for patients with negative margins and fewer than three indications for radiation therapy. For patients with close (<5 mm) or positive margins we recommend 7000 cGy in 7 to 7.5 weeks or 7440 cGy at 120 cGy twice a day. Oral cavity lesions have a higher failure rate in our experience and may receive the higher doses even with negative margins.

Chemotherapy Plus Local–Regional Treatment

INDUCTION CHEMOTHERAPY. Contrary to the experience with combination chemotherapy for patients with recurrent or metastatic disease, combination chemotherapy may hold special promise for the patients with previously untreated squamous cell carcinoma of the head and neck. Recent studies evaluating combination chemotherapy in this setting have reported significant tumor regression in 70% to 90% of patients, with complete clinical disappearance of tumor in 20% to 50%.[147–172]

Given the apparent sensitivity of previously untreated squamous cell carcinoma of the head and neck to chemotherapy, numerous pilot studies and a few controlled trials have used induction chemotherapy, either single agent or combination, before surgery or radiation therapy with the intent that such treatment will promote tumor regression of primary and nodal disease and enhance local–regional con-

TABLE 21-13. Squamous Cell Carcinoma of the Head and Neck Treated with Postoperative Radiation Therapy: Control Above the Clavicles by Surgical Margin and Tumor Dose (Continuous-Course Versus Split-Course Irradiation)

	Split Course (19 Patients)	*Continuous Course (108 Patients)*	*p Value*[144,145]
Surgical margin			
Invasive cancer	1/4	8/16 (50%)	0.375
CIS or close (≤5 mm)	1/4	19/22 (86%)	0.028
Negative	5/11 (45%)	56/70 (80%)	0.023
Tumor dose (cGy)			
<5000	1/2	0/2	
5000–5900	2/9	17/18 (94%)	<0.001
6000–6500	2/5	48/61 (79%)	0.087
6600–7200	2/3	18/27 (67%)	
All eligible patients	7/19 (37%)	83/108 (77%)	<0.001

Amdur RJ, Parsons JT, Mendenhall WM, et al: Postoperative irradiation for squamous cell carcinoma of the head and neck: An analysis of treatment results and complications. Presented at the 29th Annual Meeting of the American Society for Therapeutic Radiology and Oncology, Boston, 1987

Number controlled/number eligible for analysis of control above the clavicles. CIS, carcinoma in situ.

trol of tumor with subsequent surgery or irradiation; reduce the tumor bulk of initially unresectable lesions and allow eventual surgical resection; identify a patient population for whom, after significant tumor regression by chemotherapy, extensive and radical surgical procedures could be deferred or revised in favor of more conservative procedures; identify a patient population with tumors that responded to induction chemotherapy who may benefit from additional adjuvant chemotherapy following surgery or irradiation; and provide the earliest possible treatment for small foci of subclinical disease (micrometastases), which may be present in 30% to 50% of patients with advanced head and neck cancer.

The experience with induction chemotherapy for patients with squamous cell carcinoma of the head and neck began in the early 1960s when several trials evaluated sequential single-agent chemotherapy and radiation therapy. The earliest trials were uncontrolled and used methotrexate in a variety of doses and schedules before local treatment.[173–176] To date, four randomized trials of single-agent induction chemotherapy have been published, and none has shown that such an approach improves disease-free or overall survival rates.[177–180]

Since the late 1970s, numerous trials of induction chemotherapy for patients with previously untreated, advanced disease have been performed (Table 21-14). Findings from the uncontrolled experience can be summarized:

1. Induction combination chemotherapy causes significant tumor regression in 70% to 90% of patients and complete clinical regression of tumor in 20% to 50% prior to local–regional treatment.[147–156]
2. Tumor regression continues and response rates increase through at least three cycles of induction treatment.[154,157]
3. A complete response to induction chemotherapy is associated with optimal local–regional control of tumor and survival rates.[149,154,155,158,159]
4. Following a complete clinical response to induction chemotherapy, a complete pathologic regression of tumor has been documented in 30% to 70% of patients undergoing subsequent biopsies of the primary site or definitive surgical resection[153,155,159–161]
5. Single-modality radiation therapy or surgery may be sufficient to achieve adequate local–regional control of tumor in selected patients with a complete response to induction chemotherapy.[150,155]
6. An initially unresectable lesion may become resectable after a response to chemotherapy; however, whether such a resection enhances local–regional control rates beyond those achieved with chemotherapy and radiotherapy alone remains uncertain.[149,162]
7. Initial tumor extent as defined by overall stage, T stage, N stage, or resectability predicts for response to chemotherapy and survival.[154,156,159,162,163]
8. The histologic subtype of squamous cell carcinoma of the head and neck does not predict for response to induction chemotherapy or survival when all patients are considered[158,164,165]; however, when only patients achieving a complete response are analyzed, those with poorly differentiated tumors are at greater risk for relapse.[165]
9. The toxicity of local treatment is not significantly increased by initial chemotherapy.[149,150,160,166]
10. Survival rates after induction chemotherapy are improved compared with historical controls treated with conventional surgery or irradiation alone.[149,150,156]
11. The optimal regimen of induction chemotherapy has not been defined, and when the extent of disease and duration of treatment are controlled, the activity of present cisplatin-containing combination chemotherapy regimens may be comparable.[157]

While the results from uncontrolled studies are encouraging and strongly suggest a role for chemotherapy in the treatment of patients with advanced, previously untreated head and neck cancer, the true value of chemotherapy can

TABLE 21-14. Induction Combination Chemotherapy for Advanced Squamous Cell Carcinoma of the Head and Neck—Uncontrolled Trials

Institution	No. of Patients	Regimen	Response (%) Complete (CR)	Response (%) Partial (PR)	Findings
Boston Veterans Administration[149]	41 (unresectable)	Cisplatin, bleomycin	17	53	Increased survival in CR group; increased resectability without apparent survival advantage if resected; increased disease-free survival compared with institutional controls
Buffalo Veterans Administration[150]	47 (resectable)	Cisplatin, vincristine, bleomycin	22	66	Postoperative radiotherapy deferred in 39 of 43 patients; increased disease-free survival compared with historical controls
Wayne State[153]	61	Cisplatin, 5-fluorouracil	54	39	Increased survival in CR group; pathologic CR in 9 of 13 resected specimens from CR group
Stanford[155]	30 (resectabe)	Cisplatin, 5-fluorouracil	43	40	Increased survival in the CR group; adequate local control with radiotherapy alone in 10 patients with pathologic CR
Dana-Farber[156]	114	Cisplatin, bleomycin, methotrexate, leucovorin	26	52	Increased survival in CR group; increased disease-free survival compared with historical controls; positive randomized study of adjuvant chemotherapy

only be determined by prospective, randomized, controlled trials. To date, the results of five such trials of induction combination chemotherapy have been published. While none has reported an improved survival rate with induction chemotherapy (Table 21-15), critical analysis indicates that these studies cannot be considered definitive.

Stell and co-workers[167] and the Head and Neck Contracts Program[172] utilized only one cycle of induction chemotherapy and recorded complete response rates of only 3% and 5%, respectively. Holoye and co-workers[169] administered either one or two cycles of an induction regimen that did not contain cisplatin, failed to note the percentage of patients receiving only one course of treatment, and reported a complete response rate of only 10%. Haas and co-workers[170] used up to three cycles of cisplatin with infusion 5-fluorouracil, but reported a complete response rate of only 17%. This low rate of complete response is in sharp contrast to the complete response rate of 54% achieved with an identical induction regimen in an uncontrolled trial at another institution. Martin and co-workers[171] also recorded an unexpectedly low complete response rate of 7% with a four-drug cisplatin-based regimen. Schuller and co-workers[168] evaluated a 9-week, three-course regimen of induction combination chemotherapy in 73 patients with advanced disease. In

TABLE 21-15. Induction Combination Chemotherapy for Advanced Squamous Cell Carcinoma of the Head and Neck—Controlled Trials

Author	No. of Patients	Regimen	Response (%) Complete (CR)	Response (%) Partial (PR)	Findings
Stell et al.[167]	86	Vincristine, bleomycin, methotrexate, 5-fluorouracil, hydrocortisone			No survival advantage with induction chemotherapy
Schuller et al.[168]	146 (resectable)	Cisplatin, vincristine, methotrexate, bleomycin	20	45	Same
Holoye et al.[169]	83 (resectable)	Bleomycin, cyclophosphamide, methotrexate, 5-fluorouracil	5	64	Same
Haas et al.[170]	50 (resectable)	Cisplatin, 5-fluorouracil	17	70	Same
Martin et al.[171]	60	Bleomycin, methotrexate, 5-fluorouracil, cisplatin	7	57	Same
NCI Head and Neck Contracts Program[172]	462 (resectable)	Cisplatin, bleomycin	3	34	Same

their trial, total and complete response rates of 65% and 20% were achieved, but an improved survival rate was not associated with chemotherapy. This study may have been compromised by the use of less than maximal doses of cisplatin in the induction regimen and the administration of only 5000 cGy of postoperative radiation therapy.

In addition to problems with experimental design, limited follow-up evaluation, and inadequate patient accrual, the inability to document an improved survival rate with induction chemotherapy may relate to attenuations of local–regional treatment delivered to patients receiving chemotherapy. In general, the randomized trials of induction chemotherapy have not reported whether surgery or irradiation was limited in selected patients who had a response to induction chemotherapy. Such reductions were present in the study by Stell and co-workers[167] and may have compromised the survival rate in patients treated with induction chemotherapy.

ADJUVANT CHEMOTHERAPY. Adjuvant chemotherapy after local-regional treatment has been used in relatively few studies of patients with advanced head and neck cancer. The objective of these trials has been to treat subclinical persistent disease after surgery or irradiation and decrease the risk of relapse. Huang and co-workers[181] administered a combination of bleomycin, methotrexate, and CCNU to 31 patients (8 with Stage III, 12 with Stage IV, and 12 with recurrent local–regional disease) after surgery or radiation therapy. With a minimum follow-up of 14 months, only 5 (16%) of 31 patients developed recurrent disease, and none of these 5 patients relapsed prior to 18 months. These survival data were thought to be superior to those of a nonrandomized control group of patients who did not receive adjuvant chemotherapy. In the latter group of 24 patients, 16 patients (67%) relapsed, with most recurrences developing within the first 18 months after treatment.

Johnson and co-workers[182] similarly evaluated a combination of weekly sequential methotrexate and 5-fluorouracil after surgery and irradiation in 50 patients who had histologic evidence of extracapsular spread in cervical lymph nodes at the time of surgical resection. Their regimen of adjuvant chemotherapy was remarkably well tolerated, and the estimated 2-year disease-free survival of 66% was superior to that of a retrospective control group of patients treated with surgery and irradiation alone.

The most remarkable experience with adjuvant chemotherapy was reported by Bitter,[183] who compared postoperative combination chemotherapy to postoperative radiation therapy in a small randomized trial of 33 patients with resectable oral cavity lesions. In this study, significantly improved disease-free and overall survival rates were associated with postoperative chemotherapy.

INDUCTION PLUS ADJUVANT CHEMOTHERAPY. Induction and adjuvant chemotherapy have been administered together in several multidisciplinary studies. Three studies of induction chemotherapy have specifically addressed the use of additional adjuvant treatment by randomized comparison with a control group that received only induction chemotherapy and local–regional treatment. Neither Tejada and Chandler[184] nor the Head and Neck Contracts Program[172] reported a survival benefit with adjuvant chemotherapy. However, both of these trials reported significant toxicity with adjuvant chemotherapy, which led to periodic interruptions of treatment and poor drug compliance.

Contrasting results have recently been reported by Ervin and co-workers.[156] In a study of 114 patients with advanced disease, 89 patients (78%) responded to induction chemotherapy, and after local–regional treatment, 46 of these patients entered a randomized trial of additional adjuvant cisplatin, bleomycin, and methotrexate. Those patients receiving both induction and adjuvant chemotherapy had an improved disease-free survival rate in comparison with those receiving only induction chemotherapy and local-regional treatment. The apparent success of this trial may have been related to the specific dose-attenuated regimen of adjuvant chemotherapy used, to the acceptable performance status of patients consenting to the randomized trial, or to the fact that patient eligibility was restricted to those who responded to initial chemotherapy.

SYNCHRONOUS CHEMOTHERAPY AND RADIATION THERAPY. The simultaneous administration of chemotherapy and radiation therapy may offer distinct therapeutic advantages over the administration of either modality alone. Potentiation of the cytotoxic effects of radiation by chemotherapy, that is, 5-fluorouracil, cisplatin, bleomycin, and mitomycin-C, has been well documented in preclinical studies. Direct extrapolation of these results to the clinic is impossible, however, given the potential for synergistic enhancement of normal tissue injury by simultaneous chemotherapy and radiation therapy.

Numerous studies of radiation therapy and various single agents have been performed with mixed results. Enhanced mucositis with combined treatment has been a common finding, and many studies have found it necessary to reduce the dose of chemotherapy administered or the use of split-course fractionation schedules of radiation therapy. The majority of randomized trials noting improved local–regional control of disease with synchronous treatment have used bleomycin,[185–188] bolus 5-fluorouracil,[189–190] or mitomycin-C.[191] Randomized trials reporting no advantage with synchronous therapy have frequently employed hydroxyurea[192,193] or methotrexate[178,194–196] with radiation therapy. Several uncontrolled trials of synchronous cisplatin and radiation therapy have been performed and a randomized study has recently been completed by the Radiation Therapy Oncology Group in patients with unresectable advanced head and neck cancer.[197–200]

Synchronous combination chemotherapy and radiation therapy has also been evaluated in patients with advanced head and neck cancer. After a favorable preliminary experience with simultaneous radiation therapy and infusion 5-fluorouracil,[201] the addition of cisplatin[202,203] or mitomycin-C[204] was evaluated. The latter studies utilized split-course fractionation of radiation therapy with chemotherapy, and all reported high initial response rates. Taylor and co-workers[203,205] have reported 34 patients treated "curatively" (5 Stage III, 24 Stage IV, 6 recurrent) with a biweekly regimen of synchronous cisplatin, infusion 5-fluorouracil, and radiation therapy. Initial disease control was achieved in all patients. With a median follow-up of 36 months (range, 24–58 months), four patients have developed recurrent tumor within the field of irradiation and seven additional patients have recurrence at distant sites. Recurrences developed only in those patients with T4 or N3 disease. In addition to the low rate of recurrence, the pattern of recurrence appears affected by this approach. Local–regional failure developed in only 12% of patients and composed only 36% of failures.

REGIONAL CHEMOTHERAPY. Most studies of intra-arterial chemotherapy prior to or with irradiation or surgery may have yielded some short-term control of disease, but randomized trials have not demonstrated a significant increase in long-term survival.[88,196,206,207] Present efforts are directed toward defining the activity of intra-arterial cisplatin and combinations of intra-arterial and systemic therapy against advanced head and neck cancers, as well as toward developing intra-arterial chemoembolization as a therapeutic modality. Further advances await clarification of the pharmacologic advantage of intra-arterial therapy and ultimately the comparison of intra-arterial and systemic chemotherapy by controlled trial.

ORAL CAVITY

The oral cavity consists of the lip, floor of mouth, oral tongue (the anterior two thirds of the tongue), buccal mucosa, upper and lower gingiva, hard palate, and retromolar trigone. Squamous cell carcinomas of the oral cavity mostly occur after the age of 45 and are associated with the use of tobacco and alcohol.

The AJCC staging system for all primary tumors of the oral cavity is as follows:[12]

TX	Minimum requirements to assess the primary tumor cannot be met
T0	No evidence of primary tumor
Tis	Carcinoma in situ
T1	Greatest diameter of primary tumor 2 cm or less
T2	Greatest diameter of primary tumor more than 2 cm but not more than 4 cm
T3	Greatest diameter of primary tumor more than 4 cm
T4	Massive tumor more than 4 cm in diameter with deep invasion to involve antrum, pterygoid muscles, base of tongue, or skin of neck

LIP

The ratio between men and women with cancer of the lip is approximately 15:1.[208] Persons with light-colored skin or with prolonged exposure to sunlight are most prone to develop lip carcinoma; tobacco has not been definitely implicated as a causative agent.

Anatomy

The lips are composed of the orbicular muscle with skin on the external surface and mucous membrane on the internal surface. The transition from skin to mucous membrane of the oral cavity is the lip vermilion, where the muscle is covered by a very thin layer of squamous epithelium that allows the underlying vasculature to show, giving the lips their reddish color. The blood supply is by way of the labial artery, a branch of the facial artery. The motor nerves are branches of the seventh cranial nerve. The sensory nerve to the upper lip is the infraorbital branch of the maxillary nerve, and the lower lip is supplied by the mental nerve.

Pathology

The most common neoplasms are squamous cell carcinomas. Basal cell carcinomas start on the skin of the lip and may secondarily invade the vermilion. Benign lesions such as hemangiomas, fibromas, and cysts may involve the lips. Keratoacanthoma occurs on the skin of the lips and may be mistaken grossly and histologically for squamous cell carcinoma.

Leukoplakia and carcinoma in situ are common problems on the lower lip and may precede the appearance of carcinoma by many years. Primary lesions arising from the moist mucosa of the lip are considered under the section on the buccal mucosa.

Patterns of Spread

Squamous cell carcinoma starts on the vermilion of the lip and invades adjacent skin and the orbicular muscle. Advanced lesions invade the adjacent commissures of the lip, the buccal mucosa, the skin and wet mucosa of the lip, the adjacent mandible, and eventually the mental nerve. Perineural invasion occurred in 2% of the cases reported by Byers and co-workers[209] and was related to recurrent lesions, large tumor size, mandibular invasion, and poorly differentiated histology. Lymphatic spread is to the submental and submandibular lymph nodes and then to the jugular chain. The risk for lymph node metastases is approximately 5% on admission. Bilateral involvement may occur.[210] The risk of lymphatic involvement is increased by high-grade histology, large lesions, spread to involve the wet mucosa of the lip and buccal mucosa, and especially for patients with recurrent disease.

Clinical Picture

The vermilion is the most common site of origin. Squamous cell carcinoma of the red lip may present as an enlarging, discrete lesion that is not tender until it ulcerates and becomes infected. There will be occasional minor bleeding. These lesions are diagnosed easily by their appearance. However, some lesions develop very slowly on a background of leukoplakia and present as superficially ulcerated lesions with little or no bulk and a history of repeated episodes of scab formation without complete healing. These lesions are not so easy to diagnose clinically, and only biopsy provides the answer. An obvious carcinoma is often accompanied by leukoplakia or carcinoma in situ of the remaining lower lip.

Erythema of the adjacent skin suggests dermal lymphatic invasion. Palpation of the lip will reveal the extent of induration. Anesthesia or paresthesias of the skin of the lip indicate nerve invasion.

Methods of Diagnosis and Staging

The diagnosis is readily established by biopsy, or if the lesion is not discrete, a lip shave may be done. Mandible films are requested when bone or mental nerve involvement is suspected.

The AJCC staging for oral cavity cancer includes only those lesions arising from the vermilion.

Treatment

SELECTION OF TREATMENT MODALITY. Early lesions may be cured equally well with surgery or radiation. The length of the relaxed lower lip is approximately 5 cm but tends to be shorter in edentulous patients. Surgical excision is preferred for the majority of lower lip lesions up to 2.0 cm in diameter that do not involve the commissure; the treatment is simple and the cosmetic result quite satisfactory. Removal of more of the lip with simple closure usually results in a poor cosmetic and functional result and therefore requires reconstructive procedures. Irradiation is often preferred for lesions involving the commissure, for lesions over 2.0 cm in length, and for high-grade carcinomas. Upper lip carcinomas may require complex reconstruction and radiation therapy may be preferred. Advanced lesions with bone, nerve, or node involvement frequently require a combined approach. Surgery is preferred for the younger patient who will have years of climatic exposure and for previously irradiated persons.

The regional lymphatics are not treated electively for early cases. Advanced lesions, high-grade lesions, and especially recurrent lesions should be considered for either elective neck irradiation or elective neck dissection, depending on the treatment selected for the primary lesion. Clinically positive nodes are managed according to policies outlined in "Principles of Treatment."

SURGICAL TREATMENT. Surgical treatment for early lesions (0.5–1.5 cm) involves a W or V excision (see Fig. 21-3). V excisions may be used for very small lesions but do not give as good a margin for the larger tumors. Larger lesions (>1.5 cm) may be closed with an Abbe flap from the upper lip to reconstruct the lower lip defect. If the vermilion is diffusely involved with little or no involvement of the muscle, then a vermilionectomy (lip shave) may be done and the mucosa from the oral cavity advanced to cover the defect. Excision of a carcinoma may be combined with vermilionectomy. If the commissure must be sacrificed, it must be reconstructed to prevent microstomia and to allow the patient to continue to wear dentures.

IRRADIATION TECHNIQUE. Lip cancer may be successfully treated by external beam, interstitial implants, or a combination of both.

Interstitial implants may be accomplished with removable sources such as radium or cesium needles or ^{192}Ir.

External beam techniques use orthovoltage or electrons with lead shields behind the lip to limit exit irradiation. The dose schemes are similar to those used for skin cancer.[174] Fractionation schemes of 4 to 6 weeks are preferred over the shorter regimens for the larger lesions to decrease the normal-tissue effects.

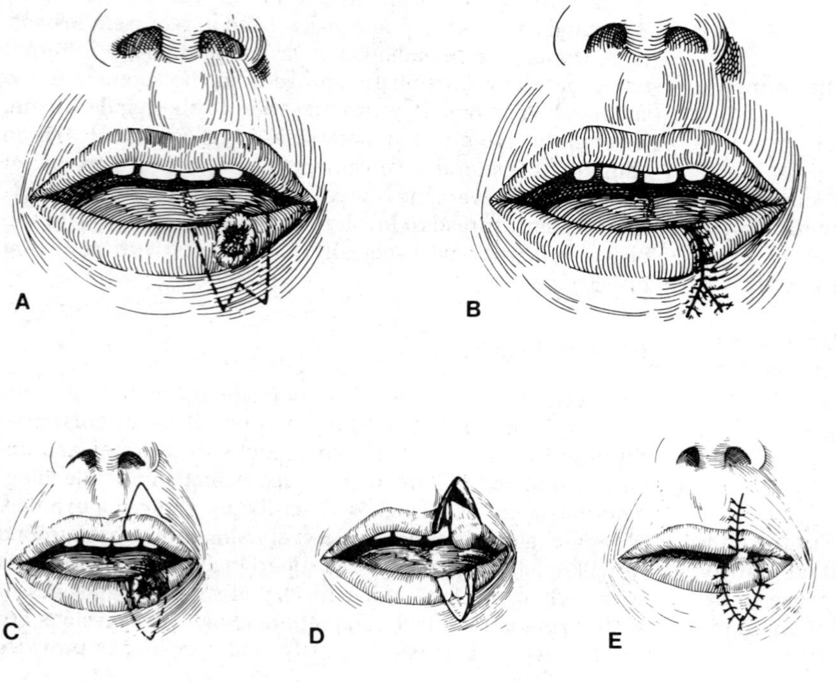

FIG. 21-3. Small lip lesions that do not involve the oral commissure can be removed using a "W" excision (**A**) and can be closed primarily (**B**). Larger lesions of the lip may be removed in a "V" fashion (**C**), and the defect can be closed using an Abbe flap from the upper lip (**D, E**). A second procedure to release the flap also can be performed 2 weeks later.

Results of Treatment

MacKay and Sellers[210] reviewed 2854 patients with all stages of lip cancer, of whom 92% were managed initially by radiation therapy. The primary lesion was controlled by the initial treatment in 84% of cases, and an additional 8% were saved by later treatment for an overall local control rate of 92%. Fifty-eight percent of those who presented with clinically involved nodes had control of disease, but only 35% had control of disease when neck nodes appeared later. The determinate 5-year survival rate was 89%; the absolute 5-year survival rate was 65%. Death resulting from intercurrent disease occurred in 17% of patients.

The M.D. Anderson Hospital local control rates for 444 previously untreated patients are shown in Table 21-16.[212] The 3-year and 5-year determinate survival rate was 94%.

Fitzpatrick[208] reviewed the Princess Margaret Hospital results for 361 lip carcinomas seen between 1971 and 1976. Surgery alone (85 patients) controlled 89%, surgery with postoperative radiation therapy (70 patients) controlled 93%, and radiation therapy alone (206 patients) controlled 94%. Regional node metastasis occurred in only 7%. Only 3% of the entire group died of lip cancer. Radiation necrosis of soft tissues requiring surgical intervention occurred in 3%. There were no cases of osteoradionecrosis.

Heller and Shah[213] reported the Memorial Sloan-Kettering Cancer Center results for 171 squamous cell carcinomas treated initially by surgery between 1955 and 1969. The sites of initial recurrence and 5-year determinate survival rates by stage are given in Table 21-17.

Hendricks and co-workers[214] reviewed the Mayo Clinic surgical results for 613 patients seen between 1950 and 1969. The lip recurrence rate was 5% for lesions less than 1 cm, 4% for lesions 1 cm to 3 cm, and 17% for lesions greater than 3 cm.

Mohs[215] reported the results for microscopically controlled surgical treatment for squamous cell carcinomas of the lower lip. Between 1936 and 1976, 1448 patients with squamous cell carcinoma were managed by microscopically controlled surgery. Eighty-three percent had cancers less than 3 cm in diameter, and they had a 5-year cure rate of 96.6%. For patients with cancers that measured 2 cm or greater, the cure rate dropped to 60% for 192 patients. For patients with Grade I or II carcinoma, the 5-year cure rate was 96%, as contrasted with 67% for 81 patients with Grade III or IV carcinoma.

Complications of Treatment

Microstomia and drooling secondary to oral incompetence may occur when a large flap reconstruction is necessary. If the oral opening is too small, the patient may not be able to insert a denture. Speech is not often affected.

There will be some atrophy of the irradiated tissues; this progresses with time. Continued exposure to the elements may result in a soft-tissue necrosis; this problem is reduced by schemes that prolong the treatment. The irradiated lip must be carefully protected from sun exposure by use of hats and UV protectants. Fishermen may wear a surgical face mask while on the water, because the various UV protectants are insufficient.

FLOOR OF THE MOUTH

Anatomy

The floor of mouth is a U-shaped area bounded by the lower gum and the oral tongue; it terminates posteriorly at the insertion of the anterior tonsillar pillar into the tongue. The paired sublingual glands lie immediately below the mucous membrane; they are separated by the paired genioglossus and geniohyoid muscles. Bony protuberances, the genial tubercles, occur at the point of insertion of these two muscle groups at the symphysis. The genial tubercles may be prominent and extend a centimeter or so from the inner rim of the mandible and would interfere with the placement of interstitial sources. The mylohyoid muscle arises from the mylohyoid ridge of the mandible and is the muscular floor for the oral cavity. The mylohyoid muscle ends posteriorly at about the level of the third molars. The normal submandibular gland is about the size of a walnut. Most of the gland rests on the external surface of the mylohyoid muscle in the niche between the mandible and the insertion of the mylohyoid. A tongue-like process wraps around the posterior border of the

TABLE 21-16. Cancer of the Lip in Previously Untreated Patients (M. D. Anderson Hospital)

Size of Lesion	*Treatment**	*No. of Patients*	*No. with Local Recurrence*	*No. Salvaged*
0–1 cm	RT	30	0	
	S	239	6	6
1–2 cm	RT	36	2	1
	S	116	3	1
>2 cm	RT	7	0	
	S	7	3	0
Massive	RT	1	0	
	S	8	1	0

MacComb WS, Fletcher GH, Healey JE Jr: Intra-oral cavity. In MacComb WS, Fletcher GH (ed): Cancer of the Head and Neck, pp 89–151. Baltimore, Williams & Wilkins, 1967.

*RT, radiotherapy; S, surgery.

TABLE 21-17. Squamous Cell Carcinoma of the Lip: Sites of Initial Recurrence and 5-Year Determinate Survival (171 Patients Treated at Memorial Sloan-Kettering Cancer Center, 1955–1969)

	Clinical Stage			
Result	*I*	*II*	*III*	*IV*
Site of recurrence				
No recurrence	106	24	13	3
Lip	10	1	3	0
Ipsilateral neck	4	1	0	0
Contralateral neck	0	1	1	1
Distant metastasis	0	1	0	0
5-year determinate survival	94%	83%	93%	50%

Modified from Heller KS, Shah JP: Carcinoma of the lip. Am J Surg 138:600–607, 1979.

mylohyoid muscle and extends forward on the internal surface of the mylohyoid. This process is absent in 10% to 20% of cases. The submandibular duct (Wharton's duct) is about 5 cm long. It courses between the sublingual gland and the genioglossus muscle and exits in the anterior floor of mouth near the midline. The relationships of the lingual nerve, hypoglossal nerve, and submandibular duct are shown in Figure 21-4.

Pathology

Most neoplasms are squamous cell carcinoma, usually of moderate grade. Adenoid cystic and mucoepidermoid carcinomas account for about 5% of malignant tumors in this area.

Patterns of Spread

PRIMARY. Approximately 90% of neoplasms originate within 2 cm of the anterior midline floor of the mouth, penetrating quite early beneath the mucosa into the sublingual gland and eventually into the midline genioglossus and geniohyoid muscles. The mylohyoid muscle acts as an effective barrier until the lesion becomes very advanced. Extension toward the gingiva and periosteum of the mandible occurs early and frequently. Even small lesions become attached to the periosteum. The periosteum is an effective barrier to mandibular invasion; when tumor reaches the periosteum, the tumor usually spreads along the periosteum rather than through it. Mandible invasion is usually a late manifestation. Tumor sometimes will grow over the alveolar ridge before grossly invading bone. The skin of the lower lip may be involved in advanced cases. Posterior extension occurs into the muscles of the root of the tongue; this pattern of extension is usually associated with ulceration of the floor of the mouth and undersurface of the tongue.

One or both submandibular ducts frequently are obstructed by tumor or after biopsy. An enlarged duct may be palpated through the floor of mouth, and it may be difficult to distinguish between tumor extension and low-grade infection in an obstructed duct. Tumor rarely grows inside the duct but may grow along the path of the duct. The submandibular gland frequently will enlarge and become firm and occasionally painful when the duct is obstructed. It is difficult to distinguish between tumor directly invading the gland and chronic infection related to obstruction.

Tumors arising in the lateral floor of the mouth are less common but have the same general spread patterns. Extensive lesions may escape the oral cavity by following the anatomic plane of the mylohyoid muscle to its posterior extremity, emerging in the submandibular space of the neck.

LYMPHATIC. Approximately 30% of patients will have clinically positive nodes on admission; 4% will have bilateral nodes. The reported incidence of conversion from N0 to N+ with no neck treatment varies from 20% to 35%.[21–23] For T1 or superficial T2 lesions, the risk for occult metastasis is probably 10% to 15% (see Table 21-4).[15]

The first nodes involved are the submandibular and the subdigastric nodes (Fig. 21-5). The midline submental nodes

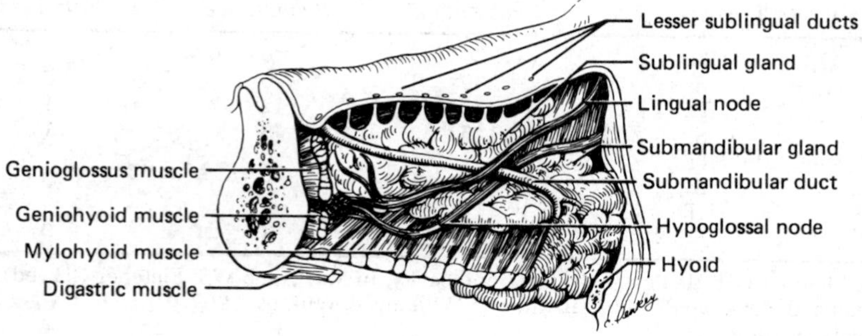

FIG. 21-4. Anatomic relationships of the floor of the oral cavity.

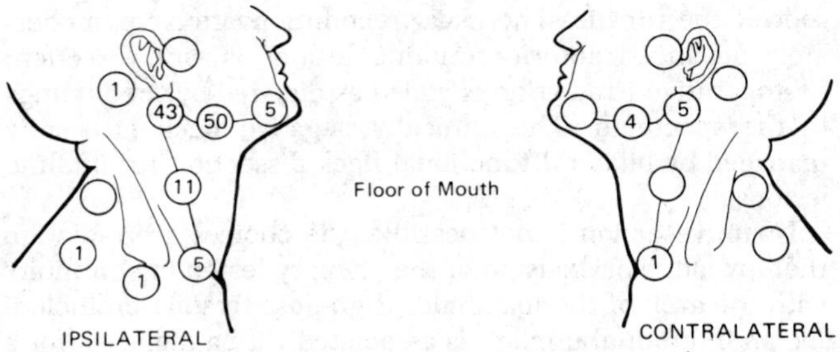

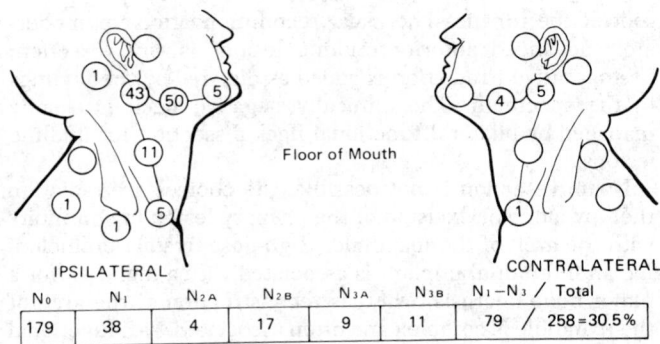

N_0	N_1	N_{2A}	N_{2B}	N_{3A}	N_{3B}	N_1–N_3 / Total
179	38	4	17	9	11	79 / 258 = 30.5%

FIG. 21-5. Floor of mouth cancer: nodal distribution on admission, M.D. Anderson Hospital, 1948–1965. (Lindberg RD: Distribution of cervical lymph node metastases from squamous cell carcinoma of the upper respiratory and digestive tracts. Cancer 29:1446–1450, 1972)

are bypassed; Lindberg[7] reported 2% clinically positive submental nodes in 258 cases. Because most lesions either approach or cross the midline, the risk for bilateral spread is fairly high. Fletcher[44] reported that 47% of patients (9 of 19) with ipsilateral positive necks (N1 or N2) developed contralateral neck disease if no elective neck treatment was given. This rate was reduced to 10% (3 of 28) after 3000 cGy to 4000 cGy to the upper neck.

Clinical Picture

The earliest carcinomas are asymptomatic, red, slightly elevated mucosal lesions with ill-defined borders. A background of leukoplakia may be present. White lesions (leukoplakic) are less likely to be malignant, but 10% eventually become cancer. These lesions are usually diagnosed by the dentist or physician on routine oral examination.

As the carcinoma progresses, the tumor is first noticed when the patient feels a lump in the floor of mouth with the tip of his tongue. There is mild soreness when eating or drinking that is usually thought by the patient (and sometimes the physician) to be due to a canker or denture sore. Dentures may not fit properly. Advanced lesions produce pain, bleeding, foul breath, loose teeth, change in speech owing to fixation of the root of the tongue, and a submandibular mass that is often painful.

On physical examination, the earliest lesions appear as a red area, slightly elevated, with ill-defined borders and very little induration. As the lesion enlarges, the edges of the tumor become distinct, elevated, and "rolled," with a central ulceration and induration. Some lesions start with a background of leukoplakia. If the leukoplakia is extensive, it is difficult to know where or when to biopsy.

Bimanual palpation will determine the extent of the induration and the degree of fixation to the periosteum. Large lesions bulge into the submental space and rarely grow through the mylohyoid muscle into the soft tissues of the neck and even the skin. Gross invasion of the mandible may be detected, especially when the anterior teeth have been removed; tumor may be seen growing through the mandible to involve the gingivolabial sulcus and lip.

The submandibular duct and gland are evaluated by bimanual palpation.

Methods of Diagnosis and Staging

The occlusal view (dental film) of the arch or ramus of the mandible is the best technique for determining early invasion. A Panorex examination of the entire mandible is not useful for determining early bone invasion but may be obtained to evaluate the teeth and to determine the extent of invasion if extensive bony destruction is obviously present. The Panorex also assists the surgeon in evaluating whether enough mandible exists in edentulous patients for a rim resection.

Submandibular gland sialograms are not useful in determining the presence or absence of cancer in the gland. A bone scan will be positive when tumor is attached to the periosteum but is not an accurate method to detect early bone invasion. CT with bone windows is the preferred method for determining bone invasion and extent of local spread in advanced lesions.

Small (5 mm) discrete lesions may be excised. Larger lesions have an incisional or punch forceps biopsy.

Treatment

SELECTION OF TREATMENT MODALITY. *Leukoplakia.* Patches of thin leukoplakia usually are observed. Biopsy is done if the area becomes symptomatic or if the appearance changes and malignancy is suspected. Localized areas of leukoplakia may be excised, but many patients have extensive or scattered areas of leukoplakia that preclude complete excision. Cryotherapy or the laser may be tried in these cases. Radiation therapy is not recommended for treatment of leukoplakia; however, when leukoplakia is inadvertently irradiated along with an adjacent carcinoma, the leukoplakia may disappear. In most cases it will reappear at a later time.

Early Lesions. Operation or radiation therapy is equally effective treatment for T1 or T2 lesions; therefore, treatment decisions are based on rather subtle differences in the expected functional result and on the management of the neck. The status of the teeth and mandible and the age of the patient also enter into the decision.

A few patients are seen after excisional biopsy of a tiny lesion, and the only finding is a surgical scar with varying degrees of induration or nodularity under the scar (TX). The margins are stated to be free, close, or positive. If the excisional biopsy is judged inadequate, these patients are usually treated with an interstitial implant or intraoral cone, because the surgeon has difficulty knowing where to start and stop the reexcision. The use of margin checks is essentially useless under these conditions because there are very few tumor cells present and the pathologist is in effect looking for a needle in a haystack. Additionally, a few tumor cells may be spread at some distance from the excision site by way of the hematoma. The radiation therapist can be generous with the treatment volume and cover potential spread without functional loss. The neck is usually observed. A review of six patients treated in this manner at M.D. Anderson Hospital revealed a 100% local control rate; similar patients treated at the University of Florida had a 100% local control rate.[216] None of the patients developed neck nodes. If the margins of the excisional biopsy are free and there is little or no induration or nodularity, 5500 cGy is delivered. If the margins are positive or if there is slight induration or nodularity, the dose is raised to 6500 cGy. In cases in which gross cut-through is suspected, one may wish to use external beam to a dose of 5000 cGy to include the regional nodes prior to the interstitial implant. A high index of suspicion is important in these cases to avoid undertreatment.

Small lesions (<1 cm) may be excised transorally if there is a margin between the lesion and the gingiva. If the submandibular duct is surgically obstructed, then the submandibular gland also must be removed. A common presentation is an anterior midline lesion, 2 cm to 3 cm in diameter, which abuts the gingiva, with a clinically negative neck; there is a risk for subclinical disease in one or both sides of the neck in 10% to 30% of cases. Most of these lesions are managed by wide local excision with rim resection of the mandible. Either the neck is observed or bilateral elective functional neck dissections are done. If it is necessary to remove one or both salivary ducts, then the submandibular glands are removed or the ducts reimplanted. If the submandibular glands are to be removed, a modified neck dissection is done at the same time. Although radiation therapy produces similar cure rates, there is a lifelong risk of bone and soft tissue necrosis. The ideal candidate for radiation therapy is an edentulous patient in whom the lesion does not approximate the mandible. These patients receive about one third of their dose by an intraoral cone so that the mandible is spared high doses. The primary site and the neck (and thus the mandible) receive 4500 cGy from external beam, which electively treats the lymph nodes. Well-lateralized floor of mouth lesions usually are treated by an operation with an in-continuity ipsilateral neck dissection. These lesions usually abut the mandible and require either a rim resection or a partial mandibulectomy. If the gingiva is uninvolved, radiation therapy is an alternative.

Moderately Advanced Lesions. These lesions usually involve the periosteum and gingiva and frequently involve the root of the tongue. The usual recommendation for moderately advanced anterior midline lesions is rim resection; postoperative irradiation is added as dictated by the findings in the specimen. The clinically negative neck is usually managed by bilateral functional neck dissection for midline lesions.

If rim resection is not possible, the choices are radiation therapy alone or excision of the primary lesion in continuity with the arch of the mandible. High-dose irradiation including an interstitial implant is associated with a high risk for a major bone necrosis, whereas reconstruction of the arch of the mandible is complex and often associated with functional and cosmetic deficits. The local control rate and complications for T2–T3 lesions that extended to the periosteum and gingiva, managed by external beam irradiation plus interstitial implant, are shown in Table 21-18.

Advanced Lesions. Massive lesions are usually associated with bone invasion and extension into the root of the tongue and have a small chance of cure with combined surgery and radiation therapy. The entire arch of the mandible must usually be removed. Only palliation can be offered in some cases.

SURGICAL TREATMENT. *Wide Local Excision.* Small lesions (5 mm or less in size) may be excised transorally with a 1-cm margin with primary closure or a skin graft. If the duct is involved, the submandibular gland and duct are removed in continuity.

Rim Resection. Rim (coronal) resection of the mandible in continuity with excision of the primary lesion preserves the arch and usually gives an adequate surgical margin; the procedure may be combined with postoperative radiation therapy (Figs. 21-6 and 21-7). Invasion of the periosteum is often an indication for this procedure. Patients who have been edentulous for a long time may have a thin, atrophic mandible and are not suitable for rim resection because the mandible is likely to fracture. Rim resection is not recommended for treatment of radiation failures because of the risk of bone necrosis and pathologic fracture. If rim resection is attempted for radiation failure, hyperbaric oxygen should be added before and after the operation.

Mandibulectomy ("Jaw-Neck"). Lateral floor of mouth: a

TABLE 21-18. Floor of Mouth Cancer: Local Control (Radiation Therapy Alone) Related to Gingival Extension (Stage T2–3)

Extent of Disease	*Local Control*	*Surgical Salvage*	*Ultimate Local Control*	*Complications Requiring Surgery*
Minimal gingiva/periosteal extension	4/8	3/4	7/8	1
Tethered to gingiva/periosteum	4/6	1/2	5/6	0
Fixed to gingiva	6/11	1/2	7/11	4
Total			19/25 (76%)	

University of Florida data: 10/64–12/77; analysis 12/79 by W. M. Mendenhall, M.D.

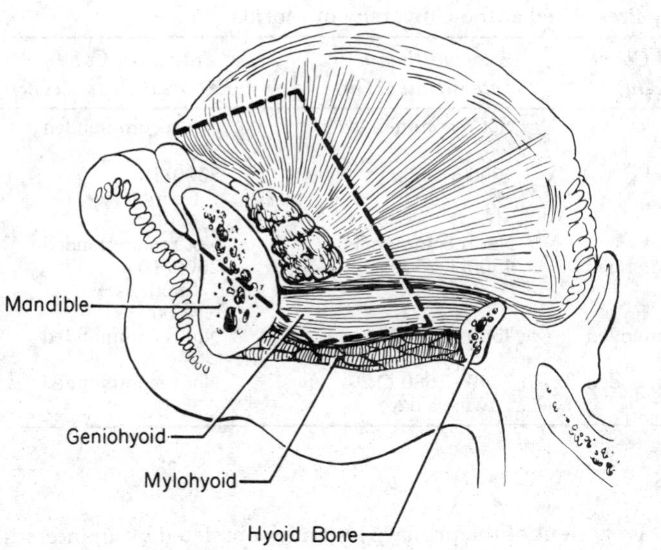

FIG. 21-6. Borders of rim resection for early carcinoma of the floor of the mouth.

radical neck dissection is performed and the specimen remains attached to the mandible. Partial mandibulectomy with resection of the floor of the mouth is done through a lip-splitting incision or by using a visor flap. A cheek flap is elevated to the level of the mandibular condyle to provide exposure. The mandible is separated at the mental foramen anteriorly and the neck of the condyle posteriorly. The primary lesion and neck specimen are then removed in continuity. Primary closure is usually feasible, unless a sizable portion of the oral tongue must be removed, in which case a myocutaneous flap is necessary to repair the defect.

The cosmetic and functional result is acceptable to patients, and very few request mandibular reconstruction. The mandible shifts to the opposite side, and if the patient has teeth, chewing may be impaired but can be corrected with a glide plane. Edentulous patients cannot wear a lower denture.

FIG. 21-7. Schematic for rim resection of the arch of the mandible. **Left**. Anterior view. **Right**. Lateral view.

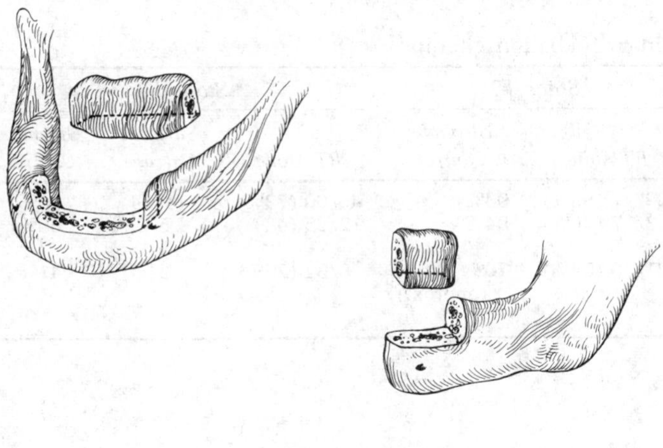

Anterior floor of mouth: a full-thickness resection of the anterior mandible (arch) is required. This operation results in major cosmetic and functional loss and is usually reserved for advanced lesions with bone invasion or for irradiation failures. New techniques for reconstruction include the use of a trapezius myocutaneous flap with a portion of the scapular spine to bridge the bony gap, or the use of a free flap such as the radial forearm flap or the iliac crest flap. The technique currently used at the University of Florida to reconstruct the mandible employs a spacer (such as a cobalt-chromium alloy [Vitallium] tray) for 3 to 6 months. The tray is removed, freeze-dried bone is shaped to fit the defect, and the graft is then packed with bone chips harvested from the iliac crest.

IRRADIATION TECHNIQUE. The current treatment guidelines at the University of Florida are shown in Table 21-19. Prominent geniohyoid tubercles and tori and undesirable teeth should be removed if present prior to radiation therapy. A minimum of 3 weeks for healing is needed before starting treatment.

External Beam Irradiation. External beam portals for anterior floor of mouth carcinoma are opposed lateral portals. The entire width of the mandibular arch is included in the portal. The superior border is shaped to spare part of the parotid and minor salivary glands. The submandibular and subdigastric nodes are included to the level of the thyroid notch if the neck is clinically negative; the lower neck may be electively irradiated on an individual basis. If the neck is clinically positive, the portals are enlarged to include all of the upper neck nodes, and an en face lower neck field is added.

Interstitial Irradiation. The availability of interstitial therapy (or intraoral cone therapy) is essential if maximum local control rates are to be obtained. External beam alone gives inferior local control results even for T1N0 lesions (Table 21-20).[217–219]

Implantation of small lesions confined to the floor of the mouth with minimal extension to the mucosa of the tongue or minimal extension to the gingiva or periosteum can be accomplished with either radium or cesium needles or iridium in the form of ribbons or "hairpins."

A preloaded, custom-designed implant device for radium needles has been in use at the University of Florida since 1976.[220] It holds the radium needles in a fixed position and is used only for T1 or T2 lesions. The arrangement of the needles for early lesions is usually a modified, curved, teardrop-shaped, two-plane implant with a single needle crossing the top of the implant. The arrangement of the needles for an early T2 lesion is shown in Figure 21-8; the needles are shown on a roentgenogram in Figure 21-9.

Implants for late T2 and T3 lesions are usually modified volume or multiplane arrangements. Needles or wires are usually inserted through the tongue.

Intraoral Cone Irradiation. Intraoral cone therapy is preferable to interstitial irradiation since there is little or no irradiation of the mandible. An intraoral cone can be used for

TABLE 21-19. Floor of Mouth Cancer: Dose Scheme Currently Prescribed at the University of Florida

	Interstitial Only (cGy)	*Intraoral Cone Only (cGy)*	*External Beam + Interstitial (cGy)*	*Intraoral Cone + External Beam (cGy)*
TX—No visible or palpable tumor	5500	5000/4 weeks	Not recommended	Not recommended
TX—Palpable induration or positive margins	6500	5500/4 weeks	4500 + 2500	2500/10 fractions + 4500
Early, superficial	6000–6500	5500/4 weeks	Not recommended	Not recommended
Early, 1–3 cm, induration	Not recommended	Not recommended	4500 + 2500	2500/10 fractions + 4500
Moderately advanced (3–5 cm, induration)	Not recommended	Not recommended	4500 + 3000	Not recommended
Advanced	Not recommended	Not recommended	7440–7680 (120 twice a day)	Not recommended

well-circumscribed anterior superficial lesions; this technique is easiest to perform in the edentulous patient. Minimal extension to the gingiva can sometimes be encompassed with the cone as well as early extension to the undersurface of tongue. The orthovoltage cones in use at the University of Florida are 2 cm to 6 cm in diameter; they are poured from lead and can be trimmed individually to adapt the cone to the anatomy. Electron beam cones can be fabricated individually as described by Tapley.[221] Intraoral cone therapy requires daily positioning by the physician.

Intraoral cone therapy may be used for the entire treatment or as a reduced field treatment in which 2500 cGy is given in conjunction with external beam portals (see Table 21-19). It is preferable to complete the intraoral cone therapy prior to starting the external beam, because the mouth becomes sore and the lesion disappears.

Management of the Neck When the Primary Tumor is Treated by Irradiation Alone. N0: Small superficial lesions are treated by interstitial or intraoral cone irradiation alone; the neck is not treated unless the histology is poorly differentiated. Patients with lesions that are more deeply invasive and have palpable induration received radiation therapy to the primary site and the upper neck lymph nodes on both sides, 4500 cGy to 5000 cGy, to include the submandibular and subdigastric nodes to the level of the thyroid notch. Treatment of the primary lesion is completed by an interstitial implant or intraoral cone therapy. The lower neck is electively treated through an anteroposterior portal when the risk for occult disease is judged to be significant.

N+: Guidelines for management of the patient with clinically positive neck nodes is outlined in "Principles of Treatment."

COMBINED TREATMENT POLICIES. The results of combined surgery and irradiation may be better than those for single-modality therapy in the large, infiltrative, ulcerative lesions. If rim resection is possible, postoperative irradiation is preferred, since the risk of bone complications and fistulae is higher with preoperative irradiation. Preoperative irradiation may be used if the patient has a large fixed node. The dose for postoperative radiation therapy is 6000 cGy in 6 weeks to 6500 cGy in 7 weeks. If the tongue margins were close or positive, the dose should be 7000 cGy in 7 to 7.5 weeks or 7440 cGy, 120 cGy twice a day, in 6.5 weeks, using reducing fields when possible.

MANAGEMENT OF RECURRENCE. Radiation failures are treated by an operation. The salvage rate is good for patients with early lesions and moderately good for the more advanced lesions (see Tables 21-18 and 21-20). Rim resection may be tried for selected radiation therapy failures, but

TABLE 21-20. Floor of Mouth Cancer: Local Control with Primary Radiation Therapy

		Stage T1		*Stage T2*		*Stage T3*		
Institution	*RT Technique**	*RT Alone*	*Ultimate Control*	*RT Alone*	*Ultimate Control*	*RT Alone*	*Surgical Salvage*	*Ultimate Control*
M. D. Anderson[217]	Mixed†	48/49 (98%)	100%	68/77 (88%)	93%	46/60 (73%)	11/14	95%
University of Florida[218]	Mixed	14/16 (88%)	88%	13/17 (76%)	94%	12/25 (48%)	5/9	68%
University of California (San Francisco)[219]	External beam	29/38 (76%)	90% (approx.)	21/39 (54%)	70% (approx.)	8/32 (25%)	3	41%

*RT, radiation therapy.
†Mixed, external beam irradiation and interstitial implant.

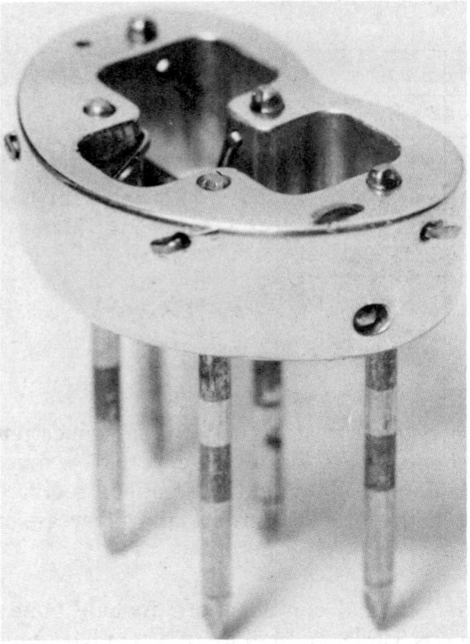

FIG. 21-8. Custom-made implant device for stage T1-T2 carcinoma of the floor of mouth. (Marcus RB Jr, Million RR, Mitchell TP: A preloaded, custom-designed implantation device for stage T1-T2 carcinoma of the floor of mouth. Int J Radiat Oncol Biol Phys 6:111–113, 1980)

the risk of a bone necrosis is significant; hyperbaric oxygen before and after the operation may reduce the risk of necrosis.

Surgical failures may be treated by a repeat operation, radiation therapy, or both on an individual basis. Radiation therapy alone is not likely to succeed.

Results of Treatment

Survival rates at 2 and 5 years for patients initially treated with radiation are shown in Table 21-21.[218] The local control rates for patients with stage III–IV disease treated by combined surgery and radiation therapy are shown in Table 21-22.[218,219,222]

Guillamondegui and Jesse[223] reported 20 patients treated by rim resection. All patients had invasion of the periosteum and 7 had early bone invasion on examination of the specimen. With 1-year follow-up, there was only one local recurrence. Four patients, however, developed recurrence in the neck, and for this reason the authors recommended postoperative radiation therapy.

Atkins and Cassisi[224] reviewed the University of Florida experience for rim resection in 20 patients with squamous cell carcinoma of the floor of the mouth (Table 21-23). Postoperative radiation therapy was added in 3 patients, and preoperative radiation therapy was used in one. Two of the patients had evidence of bone invasion on examination of the specimen, and treatment failed locally in both despite postoperative irradiation. Four rim resections were attempted in patients who had a recurrence after radiation therapy; the disease was controlled in 3 of 4 patients, but all developed a bone complication and loss of mandibular continuity. The local control and salvage rates were nearly identical to those shown in Table 21-12 for irradiation.

Wang and co-workers[225] reported the results for 33 patients with T1–T2 lesions treated by intraoral cone, sometimes combined with external beam radiation therapy. The local control rate was 94% and the 2-year disease-free survival rate was 97%. Soft-tissue ulceration occurred in 23% and osteoradionecrosis occurred in two patients.

FOLLOW-UP POLICY. Patients are seen at 4 to 6 week intervals for the first 2 years. There are two major difficul-

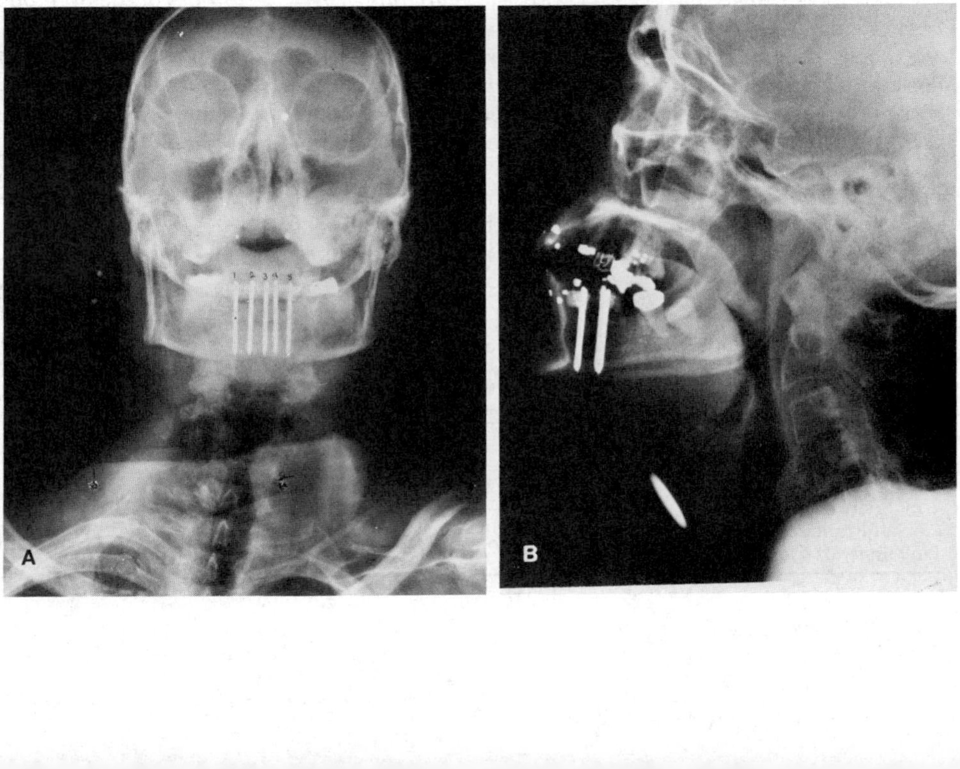

FIG. 21-9. Roentgenograms of an implant in place in the floor of the mouth. (**A**) AP view. (**B**) Lateral view. (Marcus RB Jr, Million RR, Mitchell TP: A preloaded, custom-designed implantation device for Stage T1-T2 carcinoma of the floor of mouth. Int J Radiat Oncol Biol Phys 6:111–113, 1980)

TABLE 21-21. Floor of Mouth Carcinoma: Survival for Patients Treated Initially by Irradiation ± Radical Neck Dissection with Surgery for Salvage

	Absolute Survival		*Determinate Survival**	
Stage	*2 Years*	*5 Years*	*2 Years*	*5 Years*
I	14/17 (82%)	6/8	14/14 (100%)	6/6
II	11/14 (79%)	4/7	11/13 (85%)	4/4
III	20/28 (71%)	11/27 (41%)	20/24 (83%)	11/19 (58%)
IV	4/14 (29%)	0/7	4/11 (36%)	0/6
Total	49/73 (67%)	21/49 (43%)	49/62 (79%)	21/35 (60%)

University of Florida data.[218] Patients treated 10/64–12/77; analysis 12/79 by W. M. Mendenhall, M.D.

*Excludes patients dead of intercurrent disease.

ties in follow-up after irradiation: soft tissue ulcers and enlarged submandibular glands. An ulcer in the floor of the mouth within 2 years of treatment can be either recurrence or necrosis. If the lesion appears to be soft-tissue necrosis, a trial of conservative therapy and observation at close intervals is adequate. The soft-tissue necroses are notoriously slow to heal. Failure to stabilize or show some indication of healing is an indication for biopsy. A negative biopsy does not rule out recurrence, and if the lesion remains suspicious, repeat deep biopsies are in order.

An enlarged submandibular gland(s) may be a sequel to obstruction of the submandibular duct. The gland may be enlarged on initial examination, or it may enlarge during or after treatment. It is difficult to distinguish between an enlarged submandibular gland and tumor in a lymph node. CT scan with contrast and needle biopsy are useful, but only removal will clarify the situation in most instances.

Follow-up of surgical cases may be difficult if skin grafts or flaps have been used because of the associated induration and thickness of the flaps. If the submandibular ducts have been reimplanted, stenosis may occur with subsequent enlargement of the submandibular glands. This enlargement must be distinguished from cancer metastatic to the neck.

COMPLICATIONS OF TREATMENT. *Radiation Therapy.* A small soft-tissue necrosis may develop in the floor of the mouth, usually in the site of the original lesion where the dose is highest. These ulcers are moderately painful and respond to local anesthetic, antibiotics, and tincture of time.

If the ulceration develops on the adjacent gingiva, then the underlying mandible is exposed. These areas are mildly painful. They are managed by discontinuing dentures, local anesthetic, antibiotics, and smoothing of the bone by filing if needed. These small bone exposures do not often progress to full-blown osteonecrosis. They either sequestrate a small piece of bone or are simply re-covered by mucous membrane. Healing is slow, and the patient requires constant reassurance that the discomfort and ulcer are not due to cancer.

TABLE 21-22. Floor of Mouth Cancer, Stage III–IV: Local Control with Primary Combined Treatment (Surgery + Radiation Therapy)

Institution	*Local Control*	*Ultimate Control*
University of Louisville[222]	13/15	13/15 (87%)
University of California (San Francisco)[219]	9/10	9/10 (90%)
University of Florida[218]	5/11	5/11 (46%)

Surgical. Surgical complications include bone exposure, orocutaneous fistula, and failure of osteomyocutaneous flaps. Salvage procedures after radiation therapy are associated with an increased risk of complications.

ORAL TONGUE

Anatomy

The circumvallate papillae locate the division between oral tongue and base of tongue. The papillae foliatae may be recognized as 2 mm to 4 mm, slightly elevated, irregular areas on the dorsum at the junction with the anterior tonsillar pillar.

The arterial supply is mainly by way of paired lingual arteries that are branches of the external carotid. One lingual artery may be sacrificed without danger of necrosis, but sacrifice of both lingual arteries results in an increased risk for loss of the oral tongue and almost certain loss of the base of tongue.

The sensory pathway is by way of the lingual nerve to the gasserian ganglion.

Pathology

More than 95% of oral tongue lesions are squamous cell carcinomas. Coexisting leukoplakia is common. Verrucous carcinoma and minor salivary gland tumors are quite uncommon. Granular cell myoblastoma is a benign tumor of uncertain origin that commonly occurs on the dorsum of the tongue and may be confused histologically with carcinoma because of the associated pseudoepitheliomatous hyperplasia. Granular cell myoblastoma does not respond to radiation therapy.

Patterns of Spread

PRIMARY. Nearly all oral tongue squamous cell carcinomas occur on the lateral and undersurfaces of the tongue.

TABLE 21-23. Carcinoma of the Floor of the Mouth: Results of Treatment by Rim Resection in 20 Patients*

Stage	*No of Patients*	*Local Recurrence*	*No. Salvaged/ No. Attempted*	*Ultimate Control*
T2	11	3	1/2	9/11 (81%)
T3	8	4	2/2	6/8 (75%)
T4	1	1	0/0	0/1 (0%)

Million RR, Cassisi NJ: Oral cavity. In Million RR, Cassisi NJ [eds]: Management of Head and Neck Cancer: A Multidisciplinary Approach, p 264. Philadelphhia, JB Lippincott, 1984.

*University of Florida data. Patients treated 6/73–6/81, analysis 3/83 by J. S. Atkins, Jr, M.D., and N. J. Cassisi, D.D.S., M.D.

A few lesions appear on the dorsum. Most of the carcinomas occur on the middle and posterior thirds of the oral tongue. Oral tongue carcinomas tend to remain in the tongue until large unless they originate near the junction with the floor of the mouth. Perineural invasion and vascular space invasion occur.

Anterior third (tip) lesions usually are diagnosed early. Advanced lesions invade the floor of the mouth and root of the tongue, producing ulceration and fixation.

Middle third lesions invade the musculature of the tongue and later invade the lateral floor of the mouth.

Posterior third lesions grow into the musculature of the tongue, the floor of the mouth, anterior tonsillar pillar, base of the tongue, and glossotonsillar sulcus. Posterior third lesions behave more like base of tongue cancer with a higher incidence of lymph node metastasis compared to the anterior two thirds of the oral tongue.

LYMPHATICS. The first-echelon nodes are the subdigastric and submandibular nodes (Fig. 21-10).[7] The submental and spinal accessory lymph nodes are seldom involved. Rouviere[3] describes lymphatic trunks that bypass the subdigastric and submandibular nodes and terminate in the midjugular lymph nodes. One seldom sees this pattern clinically. The lymphatic vessels of the tongue anastomose freely, allowing contralateral lymph flow. Thirty-five percent of patients with oral tongue cancer have clinically positive nodes on admission; 5% are bilateral. The incidence of occult disease is approximately 30% (see Table 21-4).[15] The incidence of positive nodes increases with T stage (see Table 21-1).[7]

Patients with N1 or N2 ipsilateral nodes have a 27% risk of developing node metastasis in the opposite neck.

Clinical Picture

Mild irritation of the tongue is the most frequent complaint. The patient frequently thinks he has bitten his tongue. The pain may occur only during eating or drinking. As ulceration develops, the pain becomes progressively worse and is referred to the external ear canal. Extensive infiltration of the muscles of the tongue affects speech and deglutition. Patients with advanced lesions have a foul mouth odor.

The extent of disease is determined by visual examination and palpation. The tongue protrudes incompletely and toward the side of the lesion as fixation develops. Posterior oral tongue lesions may grow inferiorly, behind the mylohyoid, and present as a mass in the neck at the angle of the mandible; the mass may be confused with an enlarged lymph

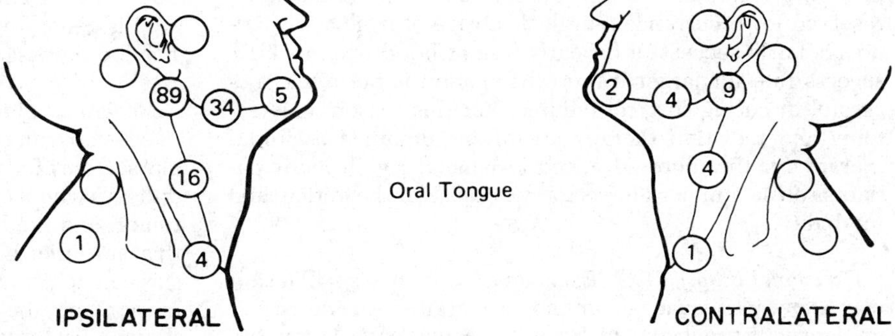

N_0	N_1	N_{2A}	N_{2B}	N_{3A}	N_{3B}	$N_1 - N_3$ / Total
197	40	9	32	8	16	105 / 302 = 35 %

FIG. 21-10. Nodal distribution at admission, M.D. Anderson Hospital, 1948–1965. (Lindberg RD: Distribution of cervical lymph node metastases from squamous cell carcinoma of the upper respiratory and digestive tracts. Cancer 29:1446–1450, 1972)

node. Invasion of the hypoglossal nerve is rare and may cause atrophy. Posterolateral lesions may be difficult to evaluate because of pain; examination with the patient under anesthesia may be required.

Methods of Diagnosis and Staging

The differential diagnosis includes granular cell myoblastomas, which are usually slow-growing, nontender masses, 0.5 cm to 2.0 cm in size. The lesions are well circumscribed, firm, and slightly raised; they may be multiple. Malignant behavior is either nonexistent or rare, and wide local excision is the treatment of choice. Pyogenic granulomas mimic small exophytic carcinomas. Tuberculous ulcer and syphilitic chancre are rare considerations.

CT scan with contrast is useful to determine the extent of disease in the more advanced lesions and will help define mandible invasion when tumor abuts the jaw; the neck lymph nodes and submandibular gland can also be evaluated when indicated.

A Panorex film may be useful to evaluate dentition and the extent of tumor invasion and to determine if the mandible is large enough for rim resection in edentulous patients. Occlusal dental films are helpful for early bone invasion and dental evaluation. Bone scans are often falsely positive and are not recommended.[226]

Biopsy is by punch forceps or incisional biopsy. Small lesions are excised and margins checked.

Treatment

SELECTION OF TREATMENT MODALITY. Both glossectomy and irradiation are curative for oral tongue cancer, and reported cure rates are similar for similar stages. For this reason, selection of treatment is individualized. The management of the neck may dictate the management of the primary lesion. The disadvantages of surgery include removal of part of the tongue and the decision on whether or not to do a neck dissection for the N0 neck. The disadvantage of radiation therapy is the risk of radiation necrosis. For irradiation to produce satisfactory control rates, the use of interstitial or intraoral cone therapy is essential. When hemiglossectomy is predicted to produce some degree of speech impediment and difficulty in swallowing, irradiation may be selected as the initial treatment, with glossectomy reserved for recurrence. Surgical salvage of irradiation failures is fairly successful for early lesions but drops to a 50% success rate for larger lesions. Irradiation is not often successful in curing surgical failures. For this reason, glossectomy and radiation therapy are often combined as initial therapy for the more advanced lesions, although many patients refuse a major glossectomy because of the anticipated morbidity.

Excisional Biopsy (TX). Excisional biopsy of a small lesion may show inadequate or unknown margins. An interstitial implant will produce a high rate of control and is favored over reexcision.[216]

Early Lesions (T1 or T2). Operation and irradiation produce similar local control rates, and treatment decisions are based on anticipated functional loss, management of the neck, and patient preference. A limited glossectomy with primary closure may be done transorally in an outpatient setting and is usually the preferred therapy. Postoperative radiation therapy would only be added for positive margins or perineural invasion.

Glossectomy is the treatment of choice for small, well circumscribed, well to moderately differentiated lesions that can be excised transorally, small lesions on the tip of the tongue, and the rare lesion on the dorsum of the tongue. Irradiation may be selected for larger T1 and the T2 lesions in order to preserve speech and swallowing for poorly differentiated carcinomas, and for lesions that have a high risk for bilateral lymph node metastases.

Moderately Advanced Lesions (T2 or T3). Lesions that have a large surface involvement but minimal infiltration are favorable lesions and are managed with radiation therapy alone. Those lesions that are deeply infiltrative will have a higher control rate with combined surgery and radiation therapy, but the patient must be willing to accept glossectomy, possibly mandibulectomy, and flap reconstruction. Postoperative radiation therapy should be considered when the initial margins are microscopically positive even though the margins are ultimately negative.[227] Radical radiation therapy with surgery reserved for salvage is a reasonable alternative.

Advanced Lesions (T4). Combined treatment with surgery and radiation therapy will cure a very few patients, especially those with minimal neck disease. We have never cured a true T4 oral tongue cancer with radiation therapy alone. Operation usually implies total glossectomy, mandibulectomy, neck node dissection on one or both sides, laryngectomy, and postoperative radiation therapy. The chances of cure are slim to none, and the treatment produces major morbidity at enormous cost. Most patients in this category will receive palliative therapy.

SURGICAL TREATMENT. *Early Lesions.* Examples of two lesions and the amount of tongue to be removed are shown in Figure 21-11. Speech impediment and difficulty swallowing would be unlikely in these cases. Glossectomy offers the advantage of a short treatment time. Primary closure is generally done, although with large resections a flap may be necessary.

Moderately Advanced Lesions (T2 or T3). Deeply infiltrative lesions not suitable for irradiation alone are managed by glossectomy followed by postoperative radiation therapy. It is difficult when cutting the tongue to judge projections of tumor, and the likelihood of cutting across tumor is greater than for other head and neck sites. It is an advantage to the surgeon to be able to feel the tumor mass so that a wide margin may be gained, which is not as easy if radiation therapy has preceded the glossectomy. Frozen section control is an essential part of the procedure. Positive margins are an indication for excision of additional tissue. Scholl and co-workers[227] reported that no tumor will be found in 73% of

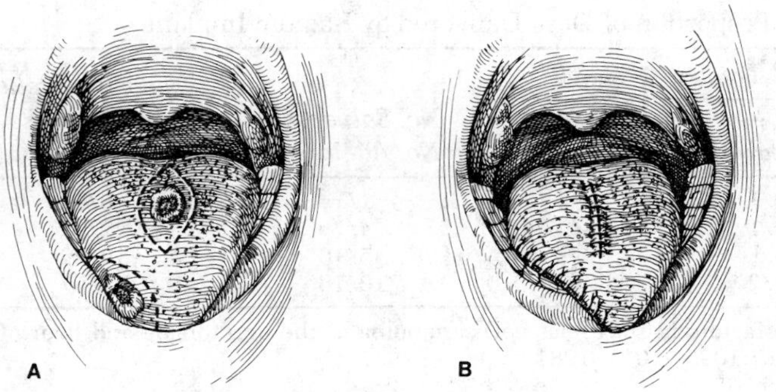

FIG. 21-11. Small lesions on the anterior free margin of the tongue or in the midline of the tongue can be excised (**A**) and the defect closed primarily (**B**).

cases when the reexcision specimen is examined. Finally, if a mandibulotomy or mandibulectomy is done after preoperative radiation therapy, the likelihood of exposed bone, nonunion, and radionecrosis is increased.

Advanced Lesions (T4). Advanced lesions would require a total glossectomy and usually a laryngectomy combined with postoperative radiation therapy. The procedure would only be offered to patients in good general condition and with minimal neck disease.

IRRADIATION TECHNIQUE. The dose schemes currently prescribed at the University of Florida are given in Table 21-24.

The ability to control the primary lesion is enhanced by giving all or part of the treatment by interstitial radiation therapy or by intraoral cone.[29,217,218,228,229] The time factor is thought to be critical for oral tongue cancer, and the external beam portion of the treatment is shortened to 3000 cGy in 2 weeks in order to increase the proportion of the therapy given by either interstitial or intraoral cone therapy. The interstitial therapy may be given before or after the external beam treatment, but the intraoral cone therapy should be done prior to the external beam treatment. The major advantage of intraoral cone therapy is to avoid irradiation of the adjacent mandible and to avoid the trauma of the implant. The disadvantage of intraoral cone therapy is the technical difficulty in avoiding a geographic miss due to tongue mobility. The local control rate by T stage and the rate of salvage by operation at the University of Florida are shown in Table 21-25.[218] Treatment of the neck is an integral part of the treatment plan. The authors favor elective neck irradiation for nearly all lesions.

COMBINED TREATMENT POLICIES. When glossectomy is selected for the treatment, postoperative irradiation is considered for positive or close margins, poorly differentiated lesions, vascular space invasion, perineural invasion, and recurrent lesions. If the initial margins (either mucosal or muscular) are positive on frozen section and then become negative on reexcision, radiation therapy is advised.[227] If the indication for postoperative radiation therapy is on account of neck node metastases, the area of primary resection should be included in the fields of irradiation.

Interstitial implants are not used in postoperative radiation therapy because recurrences may appear at any point along the surgical dissection. If the margins in the tongue are positive, the chances of local control are poor; high doses should be tried. Preoperative radiation therapy is advised only when fixed nodes are present.

MANAGEMENT OF RECURRENCE. Most recurrences appear in the first 2 years. Local recurrence after radiation therapy or surgery is heralded by ulceration, pain, or increased induration. A trial of antibiotics such as tetracycline will often reduce the pain of either radiation necrosis or recurrent tumor. Recurrences have a slightly elevated or rolled border, whereas necroses do not. The induration associated with necrosis is usually less than with recurrence. Biopsy should be done as soon as ulceration appears, if the ulcer is within the original tumor site. Ulcers that appear on adjacent normal tissues (*e.g.*, the gingiva) are due to radiation effect and not cancer. Outpatient biopsies with a local anesthetic may miss the tumor. If suspicion remains high for local recurrence after a negative biopsy, generous biopsies with the patient under a general anesthetic are required, and even this maneuver occasionally will miss persistent tumor.

Radiation failure is managed by glossectomy. Surgical failure occasionally is salvaged by radiation therapy or an operation, if the recurrence is limited to the mucosa. Recurrence in soft tissues of the neck is rarely eradicated by any procedure.

Nodes appearing in a previously untreated neck are managed by neck dissection with or without postoperative radiation therapy.

TABLE 21-24. Irradiation Policies for Oral Tongue Cancer at the University of Florida

	Interstitial Alone (cGy)	*External Beam + Interstitial (cGy)*
TX—No visible or palpable tumor	6000	Not recommended
TX—Palpable induration or nodularity	7000	Not recommended
TX—Tumor at margins; gross residual	7500	5000 + 3000
Early—<1 cm	6500	Not recommended
Early—1–3 cm	Not recommended	3000/2 weeks + 3500
Moderately advanced—3–5 cm	Not recommended	3000/2 weeks + 4000
Advanced	Not recommended	5000 ± 3500
Postoperative radiation therapy, negative margins	Not recommended	6000 to 6500/6 to 7 weeks
Preoperative radiation therapy, fixed nodes	Not recommended	5000/6 weeks

TABLE 21-25. Oral Tongue Carcinoma: Local Control Versus Proportion of Dose Delivered by Radium Implant

	No. of Patients with Local Control/No. Treated					
Stage	Radium or Radium + <3000 cGy	Radium + ≥3000 cGy	External Beam	RT Alone (Total)	No. Salvaged/ No. Attempted	No. Ultimately Controlled/No. Treated
T1	5/5	2/2	0/1	7/8	1/1	8/8
T2	10/11*	7/15*	1/1	18/27	4/7	22/27
T3	0/2	7/20	n.d.	7/22	5/10	12/22
Total	15/18	16/37	1/2	32/57	10/18	42/57

Mendenhall WM, VanCise WS, Bova FJ, et al: Analysis of time-dose factors in squamous cell carcinoma of the oral tongue and floor of mouth treated with radiation therapy alone. Int J Radiat Oncol Biol Phys 7:1005–1011, 1981.

*Significance: $p = 0.02$, Fisher's exact test.[145]

RESULTS OF TREATMENT. The ultimate control rate above the clavicles (*i.e.*, local plus regional) for a series of 117 patients is shown in Table 21-26. The 2-year survival rate is presented in Table 21-27. Approximately 20% will die of intercurrent disease; 10% will die of distant metastases.

COMPLICATIONS OF TREATMENT. *Surgical.* Orocutaneous fistula, flap necrosis, and dysphagia are the three most common complications of surgery of the tongue. Damage to the lingual nerve or the hypoglossal nerve during the course of surgery, although rare, increases the difficulty that the patient may have in swallowing and in speaking.

Fistula and flap necrosis must be handled judiciously because the danger of carotid artery hemorrhage increases with either of these complications.

Enunciation difficulties occur whenever the tongue is bound down by scarring. The incidence of complications increases for surgical salvage attempts after radiation failure, and multiple procedures may be necessary to obtain satisfactory healing.

Radiation Therapy. Many patients will complain of a sensitive tongue for many months after completion of treatment, even when the mucosa is well healed. The effect disappears with time.

Taste will reappear from 1 week to several months after treatment. Taste may return to normal, but more frequently it is "not quite as keen" as before. The dryness of the mouth may contribute to the poorer sense of taste.

Return of saliva is variable, depending on the treatment volume and the dose to the salivary glands. Patients treated with interstitial therapy alone eventually will have nearly normal saliva. Patients treated with 4500 cGy external beam therapy plus interstitial therapy will eventually have 25% to 50% return of saliva if one parotid receives 3000 cGy or less.

Soft-Tissue Necrosis. A minor soft-tissue necrosis is fairly common. Once recurrence has been ruled out, considerable patience is required for healing. The patient associates pain with recurrence of the cancer, because the original lesion frequently caused a similar pain. He needs to be reassured constantly that the ulcer will heal slowly and that there is no evidence of recurrence. Patients who develop a necrosis rarely get a recurrence, so in a sense, there is some good news associated with the pain.

There is no good, simple treatment for soft-tissue necrosis. The treatment plan is mainly to rule out recurrent cancer, provide local anesthesia, and reduce local infection. The patient is placed on a biweekly or monthly examination schedule. Broad-spectrum antibiotics (*e.g.*, tetracycline, 1 g/day), local anesthetic to be applied with a cotton-tipped applicator, and analgesics as needed are prescribed. Chewable aspirin (*e.g.*, Aspergum) will give good analgesia if the patient can chew gum. Frequently, pain will be reduced dramatically in 1 to 3 days after starting antibiotics, but sometimes the response is nil. Lidocaine (Xylocaine viscous) can be applied to the ulcer with a cotton swab for local analgesia. The authors have had little success with alcohol nerve blocks. Hyperbaric oxygen treatment may be tried in difficult cases. The authors have tried local fulguration with silver nitrate to attempt pain relief but with little success; they also have a variable experience with cryotherapy. When all else fails, however, and necrosis is persistent and pain uncontrollable, the necrosis must be resected.

TABLE 21-26. Oral Tongue Carcinoma: Ultimate Control Above the Clavicles by Treatment Technique (117 Patients)

AJCC Stage	Surgery with RT Salvage	RT ± RND with Surgical Salvage*	Postoperative RT	Preoperative RT
I	6/7 (86%)	11/14 (79%)		
II	4/4 (100%)	19/26 (73%)		
III	3/3 (100%)	13/27 (48%)	1/4	1/2
IVA		8/17 (47%)	2/2	0/2
IVB		3/7 (43%)	1/1	0/1

University of Florida data. Patients treated 10/64–3/83; analysis 3/85 by Tim R. Williams, M.D. (2-year minimum follow-up).

*RT, radiation therapy; RND, radical neck dissection.

TABLE 21-27. Oral Tongue Carcinoma: Two-Year Survival Rates by Treatment Technique

AJCC Stage	*Surgery with RT Salvage*		*RT ± RND with Surgical Salvage**		*Postoperative RT*		*Preoperative RT*	
	Abs.	*Det.*	*Abs.*	*Det.*	*Abs.*	*Det.*	*Abs.*	*Det.*
I	56%	71%	72%	93%				
II	67%	80%	70%	78%	0/1	0/1		
III	100%	100%	68%	70%	20%	20%	50%	50%
IVA			55%	65%	100%	100%	50%	50%
IVB			27%	43%	100%	100%	0/1	0/1

University of Florida data. Patients treated 10/64–3/83; analysis 3/85 by Tim R. Williams, M.D. (2-year minimum follow-up).
*RT, radiation therapy; RND, radical neck dissection; Abs., absolute survival; Det., determinate survival.

The key word for management of radiation necroses is patience.

Radiation-Induced Bone Disease. The endentulous person is less likely to develop serious radiation-induced disease of the mandible than is a person with teeth. There are several ways in which the mandible may be affected.

The most frequent problem involving the mandible is termed bone exposure. The gingiva disappears, exposing the underlying bone, with the exposed area or areas usually varying from 2 mm to 2 cm in diameter. If the exposed area is small, the patient is often unaware of the problem. There may be modest discomfort. The bone appears intact. Biopsy is not needed unless there was tumor at that location on the gingiva prior to treatment. If the patient has dentures, they should be discontinued, or in certain cases altered by the dentist to relieve the denture over the exposed bone. If sharp bony edges appear, they are filed to a smooth contour and the bone edge lowered to speed healing. The bone exposure may become more or less stationary at this point. Healing may require months or even years. Healing occurs when the gingiva regrows over the exposed area; a small, superficial piece of bone may sequestrate first, and then the gingiva regrows to cover the exposed area. Again, patience is the major requirement.

In some instances the bone exposure may progress so that a large area of bone is exposed. Pain is usually intermittent, mild to moderate, and occasionally severe. Antibiotics will usually reduce pain when it does occur. Local care is similar to that used for early bone exposures. It is amazing that rampant osteomyelitis rarely develops in the exposed, relatively avascular bone.

In some cases, the bone becomes frankly necrotic with intermittent sequestration. Hyperbaric oxygen treatment has been used with some success. It is a matter of individualization when surgical intervention should be instituted. Conservative measures should be given a fair trial, but if pain becomes a problem an operative procedure must be considered. The dead bone is removed and replaced with tissue such as myocutaneous flap, carrying its own blood supply.

BUCCAL MUCOSA

Epidemiology

Squamous cell carcinoma is relatively uncommon in the United States. In southern India it is common and is related to chewing a combination of tobacco mixed with betel leaves, areca nut, and shell lime.[230]

Anatomy

The buccal mucosa is the mucous membrane covering the inner surface of the cheeks and lips, ending above and below with a transition to the gingiva. It ends posteriorly at the retromolar trigone. The parotid duct opens into the buccal mucosa opposite the second upper molar. The blood supply is a branch of the facial artery. The long buccal nerve, a branch of the mandibular nerve (V), is sensory to the buccal mucosa and the skin of the check that covers the buccinator muscle.

Pathology

Most malignant tumors are low-grade squamous cell carcinoma, frequently appearing on a background of leukoplakia. Verrucous carcinoma occurs and may be particularly difficult to diagnose histologically because of associated inflammatory changes. Minor salivary gland tumors and malignant melanoma occur rarely.

Patterns of Spread

Almost all of the squamous cell carcinomas originate on the mucosa lining the cheeks; primary lesions seldom originate from the wet mucosa of the lips. Early lesions are usually discrete, elevated tumors, often exophytic. As they enlarge, they penetrate the underlying muscles and eventually penetrate to the skin. Peripheral growth occurs into the gingivobuccal gutters and eventually onto the gingiva and underlying bone.

The lymphatic spread is first to the submandibular and subdigastric nodes. The incidence of positive nodes on admission is 9% to 31%, and the risk of occult disease is 16% (see Tables 21-1 and 21-4).[7,15]

Clinical Picture

Early, asymptomatic lesions may be discovered by the dentist or physician. A background of leukoplakia is common and sometimes quite extensive. Small lesions produce the sensation of a lump that is felt with the tongue. Pain is minimal even when the lesion becomes large, unless there is posterior extension to involve the lingual and dental nerves. Pain may be referred to the ear. Obstruction of Stensen's duct will produce parotid enlargement. Extension posteriorly, behind the pterygomandibular raphe or into the buccinator and masseter muscles, eventually will cause trismus. Intermittent bleeding occurs when the lesion is irritated by chewing or is ulcerated by growing against the teeth.

Methods of Diagnosis and Staging

The differential diagnosis includes lues and tuberculosis, both of which are quite uncommon. If the first biopsy report is chronic inflammation or pseudoepitheliomatous hyperplasia and there is an obvious neoplasm present, repeat biopsy is in order. Sometimes multiple repeat biopsies are required to establish the diagnosis and the physician must be persistent.

CT or MRI is used to evaluate the larger lesions.

Treatment

SELECTION OF TREATMENT MODALITY. Small lesions (≤1 cm) may simply be excised with primary closure; small lesions that involve the anterior commissure are best treated by radiation therapy. Lesions 2 cm to 3 cm in size usually are treated by radiation therapy. These lesions can be excised and grafted, but the graft tends to shrink and become irregular and firm; this makes detection of recurrence difficult, and the cheek feels tight and uncomfortable to the patient. Larger lesions are treated by either radical surgical excision, radiation therapy, or a combination of both on an individualized basis. Preference is given to radiation therapy when the tumor invades near the commissure. Preference is given to an operation when there is invasion of the mandible or maxilla.

Surgical Treatment. Lesions that invade the mandible or maxilla require that an appropriate amount of bone be resected along with the soft tissues. Repair may require a maxillary prosthesis. Full-thickness removal of the cheek is repaired by a myocutaneous flap.

Irradiation Technique. Buccal mucosa lesions are suited for treatment with electrons, intraoral cone, and interstitial techniques to spare the contralateral normal tissues. When tumors extend into one of the gingivobuccal gutters or onto bone, treatment must be entirely by external beam. A lead block placed in the mouth will help decrease transit irradiation.

RESULTS OF TREATMENT. MacComb and co-workers[212] reported the results for 115 patients treated between 1947 and 1962. Irradiation was the initial treatment in 69 patients, surgery was used in 44 patients, and combined therapy was used in 2 patients. The local recurrence rate was 10% for Stage I, 12% for Stages II and III, and 38% for Stage IV. The 3-year absolute survival rate was 49% and the 5-year absolute survival rate was 48%. The determinate 3-year and 5-year survival rates were 71% and 70%, respectively. The same authors reported a 35% cure rate for 40 patients referred after failure of initial treatment given elsewhere.

Ash[21] reported 35% absolute 5-year survival for 374 patients with carcinoma of the buccal mucosa for all stages. The primary lesion was controlled initially in 53% of patients with early lesions and in 25% with advanced lesions; salvage raised the ultimate control rates to 69% and 34%. The initial treatment to the primary lesion was radiation therapy in 97% of the patients.

Bloom and Spiro[231] reported the surgical results for 90 patients with buccal mucosal cancer. They reported a 43% local recurrence rate, 37% neck failures, and 22% incidence of distant metastases. The overall failure rate was 42%. The 5-year survival rate by stage was Stage I, 77%; Stage II, 65%; Stage III, 27%; and Stage IV, 18%. The rate of complications was 24%.

Nair and co-workers[230] reported the radiation therapy results for 234 cases of buccal mucosa cancer treated in southern India by radical radiation therapy during a single year, 1982. Treatment was either small-volume external beam (33 patients), single-plane radium implant (45 patients), or single lateral field (106 patients). The disease-free survival rate at 3 years by stage was Stage I, 85%; Stage II, 63%; Stage III, 41%; and Stage IV, 15%. Thirty-two patients had verrucous carcinoma; the 3-year disease-free survival rate was 47%, similar to that for other grades of squamous cell carcinoma.

COMPLICATIONS OF TREATMENT. The buccal mucosa is quite tolerant of high-dose radiation therapy, and complications are uncommon. Bone exposure may appear on the mandible or maxilla. Trismus may develop if the muscles of mastication receive high doses.

Surgical injury of Stensen's duct may cause obstruction and parotitis. The parotid gland will eventually atrophy. Injury to branches of the seventh nerve may occur. Split-thickness skin grafts may shrink and produce partial trismus. Resection of the lip commissure may produce oral incompetence with drooling.

GINGIVA AND HARD PALATE (INCLUDING RETROMOLAR TRIGONE)

Carcinomas arising from the upper and lower gingiva have a similar clinical picture and require a similar approach to diagnosis. Primary squamous cell carcinoma of the hard palate is uncommon, the majority of hard palate neoplasms being minor salivary gland tumors. Some authors include the retromolar trigone with the anterior tonsillar pillar, but in their natural history and management, these lesions are more similar to lesions of the lower gingiva.

Anatomy

The lower gingiva includes the mucosa covering the mandible from the gingivobuccal gutter to the origin of the mobile mucosa on the floor of the mouth. Behind the third molar is a small triangular surface called the retromolar trigone; it is continuous above with the maxillary tuberosity.

Beneath the mucosa of the retromolar trigone is the tendinous pterygomandibular raphe, which is attached to the pterygoid hamulus and the posterior mylohyoid ridge of the mandible and serves as the insertion of the buccinator, orbicular oris, and superior pharyngeal constrictor muscles. Just behind the pterygomandibular raphe and between the medial pterygoid muscle and the ascending ramus is the pterygomandibular space, which contains the lingual and dental nerves. The pterygomandibular space is related posteriorly to the deep lobe of the parotid and the contents of the parapharyngeal space.

There are no minor salivary glands in the attached mucous membrane over the alveolar ridges.

Pathology

Most neoplasms of the lower gum and retromolar trigone are squamous cell carcinoma; squamous cell carcinoma is relatively uncommon on the upper gum and hard palate, where minor salivary gland tumors, usually adenoid cystic carcinoma, are more frequent. Verrucous lesions occur, usually on the lower gingiva. Melanoma is reported. Metastatic lesions to the underlying bone may be confused with primary mucosal tumors.

Epidermoid carcinoma may arise within the body of the mandible or maxilla (intra-alveolar epidermoid carcinoma) either from odontogenic epithelium or from epithelium trapped during embryonic development. It is more frequent in the mandible than the maxilla, and is most common in the molar regions. It must be distinguished from metastatic squamous cell carcinoma and ameloblastoma.

Ameloblastoma is a rare tumor with an incidence of about 1% of all tumors of the maxilla and mandible. Most patients are in the age range of 20 to 50 years. Some 80% of cases of ameloblastoma occur in the mandible with the molar–ramus region most commonly involved. No appreciable differences are found by sex or race.[232] Histologically, the ameloblastoma is an epithelial tumor histologically similar to basal cell carcinoma.[233] The lesion may appear histologically benign, but should be considered a low-grade malignancy.[234] Ameloblastoma may arise in the gingiva without bone involvement.

Patterns of Spread

LOWER GUM. Squamous cell carcinoma invades the periosteum and the adjacent buccal mucosa and floor of the mouth. Slow-growing, low-grade lesions tend to produce atrophy of adjacent bone and produce a smooth, saucerized defect before invading the mandible. Moderate-grade to high-grade lesions invade the bone directly or through recently opened dental sockets and produce a lytic defect.

Lymphatic spread is to the submandibular and subdigastric nodes. Eighteen percent to 52% have clinically positive nodes on admission; occult disease occurs in 17% to 19% (see Tables 21-1 and 21-4).[7,15]

Ameloblastoma is a rather indolent tumor that usually arises in bone, expands, and destroys the bone, slowly extending to adjacent areas by contiguous growth. Regional and even distant metastasis may occur in a few cases, but even when present is compatible with a long natural course. Metastatic disease usually is reported in the lungs, but bone and liver metastases have been reported.[235]

UPPER GUM AND HARD PALATE. Most squamous cell carcinomas originate on the gingiva and spread secondarily to the hard palate, soft palate, buccal mucosa, and underlying bone; the maxillary antrum is invaded quite late unless there are recent extractions that provide an open pathway. Primary carcinoma of the maxillary antrum must be excluded because it frequently presents in the upper gum and hard palate. The risk for positive lymph nodes is 13% to 24% on admission, and the incidence of occult disease is 22% (see Tables 21-1 and 21-4 and "Minor Salivary Gland Tumors").

RETROMOLAR TRIGONE. The retromolar trigone is a small area, and spread to adjacent buccal mucosa, anterior tonsillar pillar, and maxilla occurs early. Posterior spread occurs early into the pterygomandibular space and the medial pterygoid muscle. Posterolateral spread occurs into the buccinator muscle and fat pad.

The submandibular and subdigastric lymph nodes are the first to be involved.

The incidence of clinically positive nodes on presentation is about 30% and the risk for occult disease is about 15% to 25%.[236]

Clinical Picture

The patient with squamous cell carcinoma may present first to the dentist with ill fitting dentures, dental pain, loose teeth, or a sore that will not heal. A history of inappropriate dental extractions or root canal therapy is common. Intermittent bleeding and mild pain occur when the lesion is traumatized. Invasion into the mandible may involve the inferior dental nerve and produce paresthesias or anesthesia of the lower lip. A background of leukoplakia is frequently present.

Retromolar trigone lesions may have pain referred to the external auditory canal and preauricular area. Invasion of the pterygoid muscle produces trismus, usually accompanied by severe pain.

Intra-alveolar epidermoid carcinoma presents with a submucosal mass and dental symptoms. Roentgenograms show a lytic lesion in the mandible.

Ameloblastoma is a slow-growing neoplasm with few symptoms in the early stages. Patients may notice a gradually increasing facial deformity or loosening of teeth in the area of tumor.[237] An intraoral submucosal mass may be present initially. Ulceration occurs as the mass increases in size. On roentgenograms, a radiolucent area is seen with some of the following features: expansion of the overlying cortical plate, a scalloped margin, a multilocular appearance, or resorption of the roots of adjacent teeth.[238]

Minor salivary gland tumors start as a submucosal mass, enlarge slowly, and may present with a central ulceration (see "Minor Salivary Gland Tumors").

Methods of Diagnosis and Staging

The differential diagnosis includes dental disease and underlying bony cysts or tumors, including metastatic tumors.

Dental roentgenograms should be used where fine detail is needed to look for early mandible invasion. It may be difficult to exclude early bone invasion when recent extractions have been done. A CT scan is useful to detect bone invasion, to show posterior extension of retromolar trigone lesions, and to outline the soft-tissue extent of upper gum and hard palate lesions.

The AJCC staging system for oral cavity lesions is difficult to apply to gum lesions. In fact, the presence of mandible invasion is not even included as a staging factor. Evidence of lytic bone invasion should qualify for T4. Because even small lesions (less than 2 cm) may invade bone, there will be a wide prognostic range for T4 tumors. Swearingen and co-workers[239] reported a 56% incidence of mandible involvement for gum lesions and 10% for retromolar trigone lesions.

Treatment

SELECTION OF TREATMENT MODALITY. *Lower Gum.* The majority of lesions are managed by operation. Early lesions may be resected intraorally, removing only soft tissue or a margin of bone (*i.e.,* rim resection) and closing primarily or with a split-thickness skin graft. When bone invasion is present, removal of a segment of mandible is required; a neck dissection is usually included with mandibulectomy since the neck is entered in any event. Irradiation may be used for small lesions or those with only a pressure defect in the bone with good curative results, but the functional results are generally better after operation. Postoperative irradiation may be advised for close or positive margins, nerve involvement, large extensive lesions with bone invasion, recurrent lesions, and multiple node involvement or extracapsular extension.

Ameloblastoma. The initial treatment of ameloblastoma is an operation, but local recurrence is a problem. Sehdev and co-workers[235] reported that curettage was followed by local recurrence in 90% of mandibular and in all maxillary ameloblastomas. Subsequent resection controlled 80% of the mandibular but only 40% of the maxillary tumors. The initial use of segmental mandibular resection controlled 78% (18 of 23) with subsequent resection controlling those that recurred. The use of partial maxillectomy as the first treatment controlled 100% (7 of 7) of maxillary ameloblastomas as opposed to only 40% when partial maxillectomy was performed for recurrence. Hemimandibulectomy controlled 100% of curettage failures in one series.[240]

The lesions respond quite readily to irradiation. However, because radiation therapy has generally been applied to patients only after multiple operative failures and in cases of advanced disease, the curative ability is not clear.

Retromolar Trigone. Small retromolar trigone lesions may appear innocuous and easily cured, but often are more extensive than they seem. For early, well-localized lesions without detectable bone invasion, a rim or marginal resection of mandible may be done to preserve continuity of the mandible. If rim resection is not feasible, consider initial treatment with radiation therapy, reserving partial mandibulectomy for radiation therapy failure. Radiation therapy is recommended for lesions involving a rather large surface area, such as lesions with superficial extension to the anterior tonsillar pillar, soft palate, and buccal mucosa.[224] Evidence of bone invasion is an indication for partial mandibulectomy. Preference is given to surgical treatment unless the cosmetic and functional result would be unacceptable to the patient, in which case operation is reserved for radiation therapy failure. Moderately advanced lesions usually are managed by resection followed by postoperative radiation therapy.

Upper Gum and Hard Palate. Surgical resection is the usual treatment for most lesions of the upper gum. Postoperative radiation therapy is added as needed. However, if the lesion is superficial and extensively involves the hard palate or involves a significant portion of the soft palate, then radiation should be the initial therapy. If the lesion is small and discrete and there is no bone involvement, the resection includes the periosteum or occasionally some underlying bone. Bone invasion requires a partial maxillectomy. The defect usually is repaired with a prosthesis.

SURGICAL TREATMENT. *Rim Resection (Coronal).* See the section on surgical treatment of floor of mouth lesions.

Segmental Mandibulectomy. For small lesions with minimal bone invasion, a short section of mandible is removed in continuity with the tumor (*e.g.,* removal of the mandible from the angle to the mental foramen).

Partial Mandibulectomy. The mandible and tumor usually are resected from the mental foramen to the coronoid process, usually leaving the head of the condyle. The remaining mandible is stabilized by a cobalt-chromium alloy (Vitallium) mesh spacer if there are teeth; if there are no teeth, no spacer is used. In certain cases, the mandible may be reconstructed at a later date, but few patients actually request the procedure.

Hemimandibulectomy. Extensive lesions may require removal of the mandible from symphysis to condyle on one side. Massive anterior lesions require removal of the mandible from angle to angle. This produces a major cosmetic and functional loss and is reconstructed with flaps and metal trays. A composite osteomyocutaneous flap is also available for reconstruction.

IRRADIATION TECHNIQUE. Small lesions of the lower gum and retromolar trigone may be treated by intraoral cone for all or part of their therapy. Well lateralized lesions of the retromolar trigone and posterior gum may be treated by either an ipsilateral mixed beam or angled wedge portal technique with a lead intraoral stent. Anterior gum lesions are treated by parallel opposed portals.

The usual indication for irradiation of hard palate lesions is a carcinoma that involves nearly the entire hard palate and upper gums with little or no bone invasion. These lesions may be treated by external beam, but an intraoral surface brachytherapy applicator is preferred.

The dose for retromolar trigone lesions is usually 6000 cGy in 6 weeks to 6500 cGy in 7 weeks for T1, 6500 cGy to 7000 cGy for T2, and 7500 cGy in 7.5 weeks for T3. The dose for gum lesions is similar.

TABLE 21-28. Carcinoma of the Lower Gum: Local Control (26 Patients)*

Stage	Initial Treatment by Radiation Therapy: Initial Control (No. Controlled/ No. Treated)	Initial Treatment by Radiation Therapy: Surgical Salvage (No. Salvaged/ No. Attempted)	Initial Treatment by Surgery (No. Controlled/ No. Treated)	Initial Treatment by Surgery Plus Radiation Therapy (No. Controlled/ No. Treated)
T1	1/1		2/2	0
T2	1/5	0/2	3/5†	0
T3	0		0	0
T4	1/2	0/1	3/4†	4/7†

Million RR, Cassisi NJ: Oral cavity. In Million RR, Cassisi NJ (eds): Management of Head and Neck Cancer: A Multidisciplinary Approach, p 295. Philadelphia, JB Lippincott, 1984).

*University of Florida data. Patients treated 10/64–12/80; analysis 4/83 by G. R. Ayers, M.D.

†Salvage not attempted in any failures.

MANAGEMENT OF RECURRENCE. Radiation therapy failures are managed by operation. Surgical failures may be managed by surgery, radiation therapy, or a combination of both (see Tables 21-28, 21-29, and 21-30).[224] Salvage procedures frequently are not attempted, however, because of the advanced nature of the recurrence.

Results of Treatment

Byers and co-workers[241] reported the results for 61 patients with squamous cell carcinoma of the lower gum managed between 1970 and 1975 at the M. D. Anderson Hospital. Fifty-seven patients were treated by surgical resection and radiation therapy was added in six. The disease was controlled above the clavicles in 96%. There was one operative mortality. The incidence of neck disease was 29%, and the neck disease was controlled in all but two patients. At 2 years, the absolute survival rate was 67% and the determinate rate was 90%.

Byers and co-workers[236] reported the M. D. Anderson Hospital results for 110 previously untreated patients with squamous cell carcinoma of the retromolar trigone treated between 1965 and 1977, with a minimum 5-year follow-up. Surgery was often selected for patients with leukoplakia, poor teeth, mandible invasion, large neck nodes, or trismus. Radiation therapy was selected for poorly differentiated tumors, for lesions that were mainly exophytic, involved the faucial arch or soft palate, or had ill defined borders, and for poor surgical risk cases. Local control rates by treatment modality are shown in Table 21-31. In spite of the high local and regional control rates, the absolute 5-year survival rate was only 26% due to a high incidence of death due to intercurrent disease, including a 33% risk for second cancers.

Shibuya and co-workers[242] reported the results for 38 cases of carcinoma of the hard palate and 82 cases of carcinoma of the upper gum treated between 1953 and 1982 in Japan. Sixty-six patients were managed initially by radiation therapy alone to the primary lesion, and 54 patients were managed by radiation therapy and surgery. The 5-year actuarial survival rate by stage was Stage I, 56%; Stage II, 41%; Stage III, 32%; and Stage IV, 12%. There was no difference in survival when comparing hard palate versus upper gum, squamous cell carcinoma versus minor salivary gland tumors, or radiation therapy alone versus radiation therapy plus surgery as initial therapy. The overall risk for metastatic lymph nodes was 47% for hard palate and 49% for the upper gum. Thirty patients recorded as having "slight bone invasion" and no metastases had a 5-year survival rate of 75% when treated by radiation therapy. Major bone involvement was an indication for partial maxillectomy.

TABLE 21-29. Carcinoma of the Retromolar Trigone: Local Control (42 Patients)

Stage	Initial Treatment by Radiation Therapy: Initial Control (No. Controlled/ No. Treated)	Initial Treatment by Radiation Therapy: Surgical Salvage (No. Salvaged/ No. Attempted)	Initial Treatment by Surgery: Initial Control (No. Controlled/ No. Treated)	Initial Treatment by Surgery: Radiation Therapy or Surgical Salvage (No. Salvaged/ No. Attempted)	Initial Treatment by Surgery Plus Radiation Therapy
T1	4/4		1/2	1/1*	0
T2	2/8	0/3	2/2		3/4
T3	2/2		3/4	0/0	2/3†
T4	0/4	0/1	2/3	0/1	3/6†

Million RR, Cassisi NJ: Oral cavity. In Million RR, Cassisi NJ (eds): Management of Head and Neck Cancer: A Multidisciplinary Approach, p 295. Philadelphia, JB Lippincott, 1984.

University of Florida data. Patients treated 10/64–12/80; analysis 4/83 by G. R. Ayers, M.D.

*Follow-up 10 months after salvage by radiation therapy.

†Salvage not attempted in any failures.

TABLE 21-30. Carcinoma of the Upper Gum: Local Control (Nine Patients)

	Initial Treatment by Radiation Therapy			
Stage	*Initial Control (No. Controlled/ No. Treated)*	*Surgical Salvage (No. Salvaged/ No. Attempted)*	*Initial Treatment by Surgery (No. Controlled/No. Treated)*	*Initial Treatment by Surgery Plus Radiation Therapy (No. Controlled/No. Treated)*
T1	0		0	1/1
T2	0/2	1/1	0	0
T3	0		0	0
T4	0/1	0	3/5*	0

Million RR, Cassisi NJ: Oral cavity. In Million RR, Cassisi NJ (eds): Management of Head and Neck Cancer: A Multidisciplinary Approach, p 296. Philadelphia, JB Lippincott, 1984.
University of Florida data. Patients treated 10/64–12/80; analysis 4/83 by G. R. Ayers, M.D.
*Salvage not attempted in any failures.

The analysis of local control for lower gum, retromolar trigone, and upper gum lesions is shown in Tables 21-28, 21-29, and 21-30.[224] The high rate of local failure for retromolar trigone carcinoma treated with radiation therapy alone (except for T1 lesions) is not explained by low dose or marginal failure. The absolute survival rate for 42 patients was 56% at 2 years and 34% at 5 years.

Fayos[243] reported that local control by radiation therapy alone for lesions with early bone invasion was approximately 50% and for extensive invasion about 25% (Fayos JV: Personal communication, 1973).

Cady and Catlin[24] reported an absolute 5-year survival rate of 43% for patients with lower gum lesions and 40% for upper gum lesions treated by surgery.

Complications of Treatment

Surgical complications include orocutaneous fistula, bone exposure with sequestration, extrusion of a metal tray, and loss of graft or flap. Following hemimandibulectomy, the edentulous patient usually cannot wear dentures and the patient with teeth cannot chew because of shifting of the remaining mandible.

The complications of radiation therapy include soft tissue necrosis with bone exposure and subsequent osteoradionecrosis. The risk is greatest for patients with advanced lesions of the lower gum and retromolar trigone. Byers and coworkers[236] reported that 14% of patients treated by radiation therapy for retromolar trigone lesions required a partial mandibulectomy for mandible necrosis. The risk was greatest for patients having preirradiation extraction for poor dentition or impacted molars.

TABLE 21-31. Retromolar Trigone Carcinoma: Local Control by Treatment Modality for 110 Patients Treated 1965–1977 (No. Controlled/No. Treated)

Stage	*Surgery*	*Radiation Therapy*	*Surgery + Radiation Therapy*	*Total*
T1	5/5	5/6	2/2	12/13
T2	20/22	26/31	4/4	50/57
T3	10/10	6/7	2/3	18/20
T4	6/9	5/6	4/5	15/20

Data from Byers et al.[236]

OROPHARYNX

The oropharynx includes four areas: the base of the tongue, the tonsillar region (tonsillar fossa and tonsillar pillars), the soft palate, and that portion of the pharyngeal wall between the pharyngoepiglottic fold and the nasopharynx. The pharyngeal walls will be considered in the section on the hypopharynx.

ANATOMY

The base of the tongue is bounded anteriorly by the circumvallate papillae, laterally by the glossotonsillar sulci, and posteriorly by the epiglottis. The vallecula is a short, smooth strip of mucosa that is the transition from the base of the tongue to the epiglottis; it is considered part of the base of the tongue. The surface of the base of the tongue appears irregular and bumpy due to scattered submucosal lymphoid follicles; the mucous membrane itself is smooth.

The musculature of the base of the tongue is continuous with that of the oral tongue. A midsagittal section through the oropharynx showing important relationships with neighboring sites is presented in Figure 21-12. A cross-section through the oropharynx (Fig. 21-13) shows relationships to the lateral pharyngeal space.

The tonsillar area is a triangular region bounded anteriorly by the anterior tonsillar pillar (palatoglossal muscle), posteriorly by the posterior tonsillar pillar (palatopharyngeal muscle), and inferiorly by the glossotonsillar sulcus and pharyngoepiglottic fold. The palatine tonsil lies within the triangle. The tonsillar region is bounded laterally by the pharyngeal constrictor muscle and its fascia, the mandible, and the lateral pharyngeal space.

The tonsillar area is separated from the base of the tongue by the glossotonsillar sulcus. The sulcus extends from the

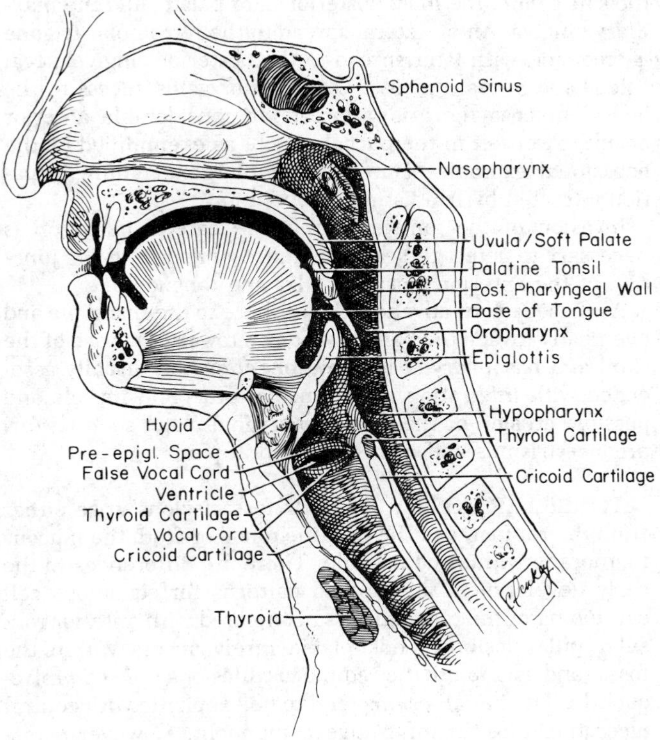

FIG. 21-12. Sagittal section of the upper aerodigestive tract. (Redrawn from Sabotta drawings in Clemente CD: Anatomy: A Regional Atlas of the Human Body. Philadelphia, Lea & Febiger, 1975. Copyright 1975, Urban & Schwarzenburg, Munich, Berliin, Vienna)

anterior tonsillar pillar to the pharyngoepiglottic fold. Beneath the mucous membrane of the sulcus are the styloglossal muscle and the stylohyoid ligament.

The soft palate is a thin, mobile muscle complex that separates the nasopharynx from the oral cavity and oropharynx. The epithelium of the oral side of the soft palate is squamous and the epithelium of the nasopharyngeal surface is respiratory. The soft palate is continuous laterally with the tonsillar pillars.

PATHOLOGY

Squamous cell carcinoma or one of its variants accounts for 95% of malignant lesions. Lymphoepitheliomas occur in the tonsil and base of tongue. Verrucous carcinomas occur rarely. Malignant lymphomas account for approximately 5% of tonsillar and 1% to 2% of base-of-tongue malignancies. Minor salivary gland malignancies, plasmacytomas, and other rare tumors make up the remainder of the malignancies.

PATTERNS OF SPREAD

Base of the Tongue

PRIMARY. Squamous cell carcinoma of the base of the tongue tends to early, silent, deep infiltration. The tumor tends to remain in the tongue unless it begins at the very peripheral margin. Vallecular lesions spread along the mucosa to the lingual surface of the epiglottis, laterally along the pharyngoepiglottic fold, and then to the lateral pharyngeal wall and anterior wall of the pyriform sinus. Vallecular lesions frequently penetrate through the thin mucous membrane of the vallecula; tumor spread is contained for a while by the hyoepiglottic ligament, but this thin, often incomplete structure eventually is breached and cancer enters the preepiglottic space.

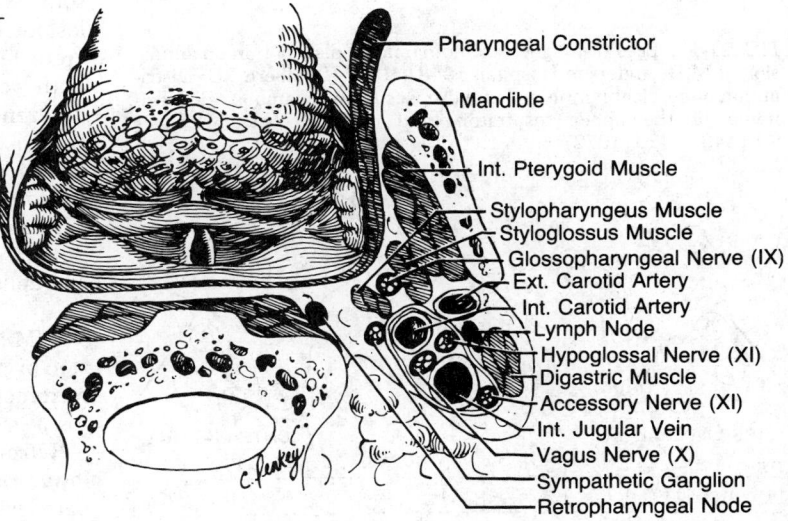

Lesions that begin on the lateral base of the tongue may invade the glossotonsillar sulcus. Deep penetration in the glossotonsillar sulcus allows tumor to escape into the neck, because there is no effective muscular barrier at this point. The mylohyoid muscle is an effective barrier for oral tongue lesions, but the mylohyoid terminates near the angle of the mandible. The primary tumor mass may be palpable below

FIG. 21-13. Section at the level of the midoropharynx, depicting relationships in the parapharyngeal area.

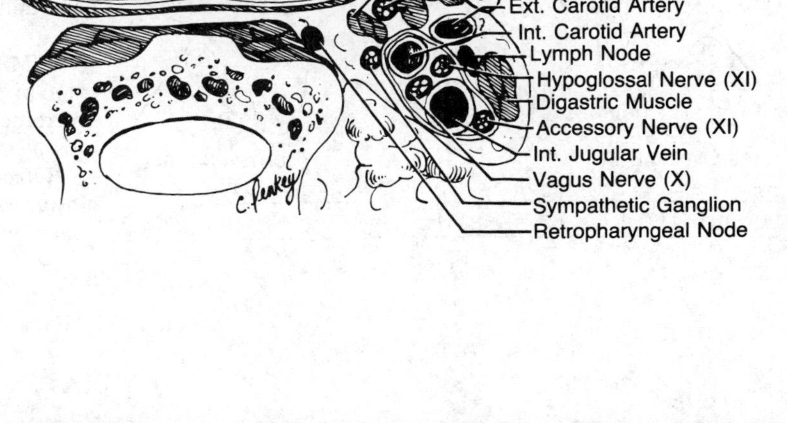

the angle of the mandible and be confused with an involved lymph node.

Advanced lesions tend to spread toward the larynx, oral tongue, and parapharyngeal space. There is a tendency to underestimate the extent of disease.

LYMPHATIC. The first-echelon nodes are the subdigastric; the path of spread is then along the jugular chain to the midjugular and lower jugular nodes. The submandibular nodes may become involved if tumor extends anteriorly into the oral tongue or if massive upper neck disease is present. The posterior cervical nodes are involved often enough to be included in treatment plans.

Approximately 75% of patients with base-of-tongue cancer will have clinically positive neck nodes on admission; 30% will have bilateral nodes (Fig. 21-14).[7] The incidence of occult disease in clinically negative necks is reported at 22% in one series, but this figure is undoubtedly low, considering the selection of these patients for operation and the use of preoperative irradiation.[42] The risk for occult disease is probably 40% to 50%.

Tonsillar Area

The tonsillar area includes the anterior and posterior tonsillar pillars and the tonsillar fossa. Some authors group retromolar trigone lesions with those of the anterior tonsillar pillar. However, the retromolar trigone lesions more appropriately are considered as oral cavity lesions and grouped with the gingival (gum) lesions.

ANTERIOR TONSILLAR PILLAR. Almost all malignant tumors arising on the anterior tonsillar pillar are squamous cell carcinomas. The lesions tend to be early when diagnosed and have relatively little bulk or infiltration and therefore a good prognosis. Asymptomatic lesions are common and may be red lesions, white lesions, or a mixture of both. Their borders are usually indistinct. As the lesions progress they may develop a central ulcer with a rolled margin and infiltrate the palatoglossus. Superior medial spread occurs onto the soft palate, the most posterior hard palate, and the maxillary gingiva. Anterolateral spread to the retromolar trigone is frequent, with later spread to the posterior gingivobuccal sulcus and buccal mucosa. Once tumor gains access to the buccal mucosa there is a threat for considerable anterior occult extension in the buccal pouch, as exemplified by the occasional example of an anterior marginal failure in patients treated by irradiation or operation.

Invasion of the tongue is frequent; careful palpation is necessary to detect the early submucosal nodule at the junction of the anterior tonsillar pillar and tongue.

As these lesions advance, they adhere to the mandible and eventually invade the bone. Extension toward the base of the skull and nasopharynx is a late phenomenon, usually associated with infiltration of the medial pterygoid muscle and possible erosion of the medial pterygoid plate; such lesions produce trismus and marked temporal pain.

FIG. 21-14. Base-of-tongue carcinoma: nodal distribution on admission at M.D. Anderson Hospital, 1948–1965. (Lindberg RD: Distribution of cervical lymph node metastases from squamous cell carcinoma of the upper respiratory and digestive tracts. Cancer 29:1446–1450, 1972)

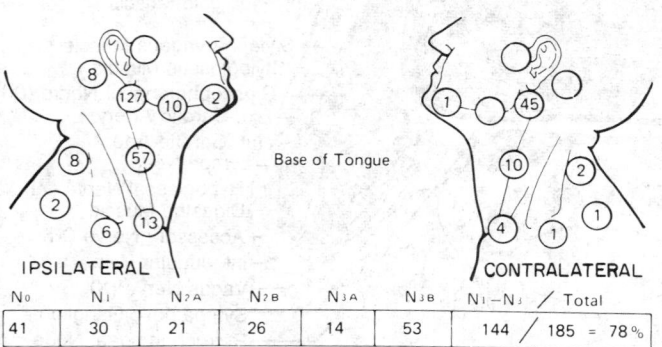

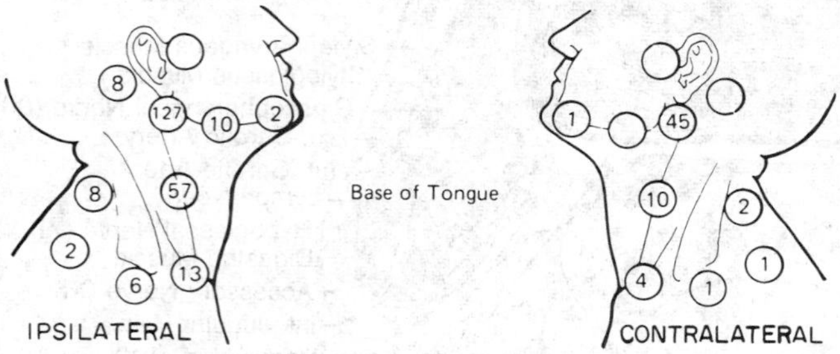

N_0	N_1	N_{2A}	N_{2B}	N_{3A}	N_{3B}	N_1–N_3 / Total
41	30	21	26	14	53	144 / 185 = 78%

TONSILLAR FOSSA. Tonsillar fossa lesions arise either from the remnants of the palatine tonsil or from the mucous membrane within the triangle. There are differences in the early development and spread patterns for squamous cell carcinoma of the tonsillar fossa compared with anterior tonsillar pillar lesions. Leukoplakia rarely occurs within the fossa, and asymptomatic red mucosal lesions are seen infrequently. The initial lesions tend to be exophytic with central ulceration plus an infiltrative component. However, some lesions develop submucosally and present with neck nodes and no obvious tonsillar lesion. Extension to the posterior tonsillar pillar and the oropharyngeal wall occurs early. Invasion into the glossotonsillar sulcus and base of the tongue occurs in approximately 25% of cases. As the lesions advance, they penetrate to the parapharyngeal space and gain access to the base of the skull superiorly. Cranial nerve involvement is uncommon, however. Advanced lesions invade the mandible, nasopharynx, and base of the tongue and may extend below the pharyngoepiglottic fold into the pyriform sinus.

POSTERIOR TONSILLAR PILLAR. Early lesions arising from the posterior tonsillar pillar are uncommon and for some unknown reason have an evil reputation. The only two lesions the authors have seen were 1.0 cm to 1.5 cm, discrete lesions with a raised border and central ulceration. Both were cured by radiation therapy. There are two major differences in their potential spread patterns. They may spread inferiorly along the palatopharyngeal muscle to its insertions into the middle pharyngeal constrictor, the pharyngoepiglottic fold, and the posterior border of the thyroid cartilage. Also, the lymphatic trunks of the posterior tonsillar pillar are theoretically more likely to spread to the junctional (parapharyngeal) and spinal accessory lymph nodes.

LYMPHATIC. The distribution and N staging on admission prior to treatment for previously untreated patients with retromolar trigone/anterior tonsillar pillar and tonsillar fossa squamous cell carcinomas are shown in Figure 21-15.[7]

Retromolar trigone/anterior tonsillar pillar lesions have a lower risk of clinically positive lymph nodes (45%) compared with the tonsillar fossa (76%). The distribution for the

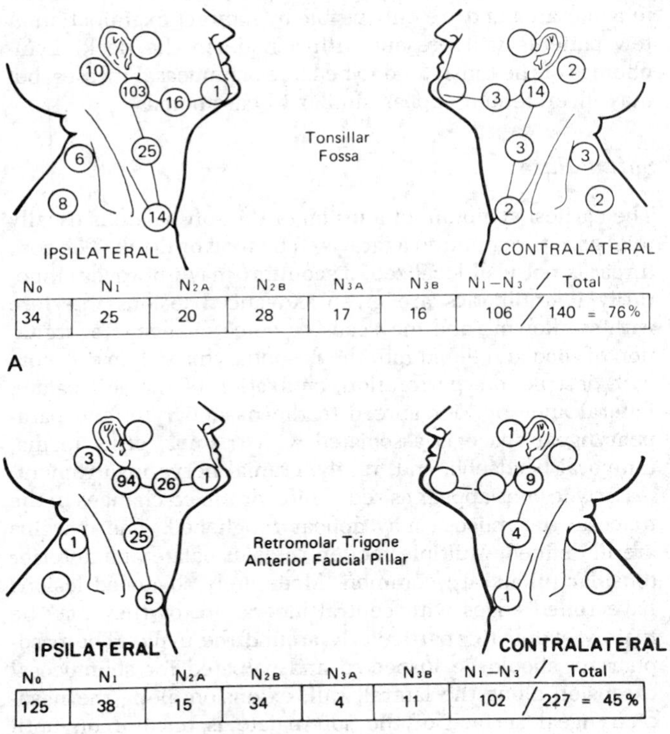

A

N_0	N_1	N_{2A}	N_{2B}	N_{3A}	N_{3B}	N_1–N_3 / Total
34	25	20	28	17	16	106 / 140 = 76%

B

N_0	N_1	N_{2A}	N_{2B}	N_{3A}	N_{3B}	N_1–N_3 / Total
125	38	15	34	4	11	102 / 227 = 45%

FIG. 21-15. Nodal distribution on admission at M.D. Anderson Hospital, 1948–1965. **A.** Carcinoma of the retromolar trigone and anterior tonsillar pillar. **B.** Carcinoma of the tonsillar pillar. (Lindberg RD: Distribution of cervical lymph node metastases from squamous cell carcinoma of the upper respiratory and digestive tracts. Cancer 29:1446–1450, 1972)

retromolar trigone/anterior tonsillar pillar on the ipsilateral side is to the jugular and submandibular lymph nodes with a very low risk for junctional and spinal accessory lymph nodes. Contralateral spread is uncommon (5%) and is confined to the jugular chain. The risk of occult disease in the clinically negative neck (N0) is 10% to 15%.[40] The incidence of positive nodes increases with T stage.

Tonsillar fossa lesions have a high risk of clinically positive lymph nodes (76%) on admission. The lymph node distribution for tonsillar fossa lesions on the ipsilateral side includes the jugular, junctional, spinal accessory, and the more posterior submandibular lymph nodes. Contralateral spread occurs in only 11% of patients and is mainly to the jugular chain lymph nodes, but there is some risk for spinal accessory and submandibular involvement. The risk of contralateral spread is related to invasion of the tongue, spread near or across the midline of the soft palate, and large lymph nodes in the ipsilateral neck that produce lymphatic obstruction; when these features are present, treatment of the opposite neck must be considered. The incidence of occult disease after preoperative irradiation is 22%[41]; the actual risk is probably closer to 50% to 60%.

There is no information about lymphatic spread for posterior tonsillar pillar lesions.

Soft Palate

PRIMARY. Nearly all soft palate squamous cell carcinomas occur on the oral side of the palate. The nasopharyngeal side seems nearly immune to tumor production. Even large tumors of the nasopharynx avoid secondary invasion of the soft palate.

The earliest tumors are red lesions with ill-defined borders. White lesions are common on the soft palate and may be leukoplakia, carcinoma in situ, or early invasive carcinoma. Multiple sites of involvement with normal-appearing intervening mucosa are a common finding, dramatically demonstrated during the first week of radiation therapy when a tumoritis "lights up" the tumor sites, some of which are unsuspected.

The majority of soft palate carcinomas are diagnosed while still confined to the soft palate and adjacent pillars. Spread from the soft palate occurs first to the tonsillar pillars and hard palate. Lateral spread eventually may penetrate the superior constrictor muscle with subsequent invasion of the medial pterygoid muscle and base of skull, and rarely compression or invasion of cranial nerves in the parapharyngeal space. Involvement of the lateral wall(s) of the nasopharynx is common in advanced lesions. Perforation of the palate may occur in advanced cases.

LYMPHATIC. The spread pattern is first to the subdigastric node and then along the jugular chain. The submandibular, submental, and spinal accessory nodes are less commonly involved.

Approximately 56% of patients will have clinically positive nodes on admission; 16% will have bilateral nodes (Figure 21-16).[7] The incidence of occult disease is not well-established because the first-echelon nodes are usually irradiated in all but the earliest lesions. Lindberg and co-workers[39] noted an approximately 20% incidence of occult disease following either no or partial neck irradiation with the primary lesion controlled. The incidence of clinically positive nodes increases with T stage (Table 21-1).

FIG. 21-16. Soft palate carcinoma: nodal distribution on admission at M.D. Anderson Hospital, 1948–1965. (Lindberg RD: Distribution of cervical lymph node metastases from squamous cell carcinoma of the upper respiratory and digestive tracts. Cancer 29:1446–1450, 1972)

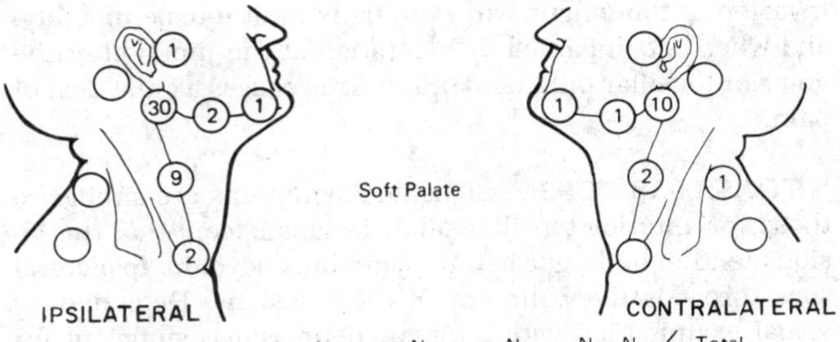

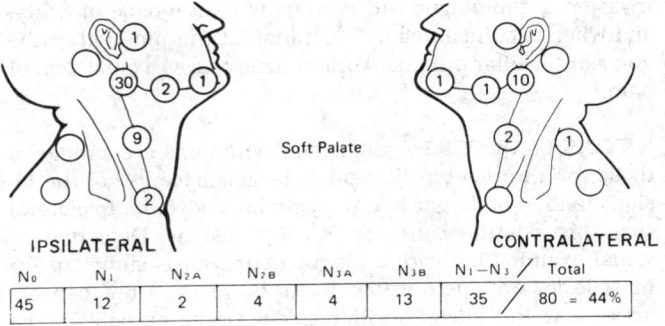

N_0	N_1	N_{2A}	N_{2B}	N_{3A}	N_{3B}	N_1–N_3 / Total
45	12	2	4	4	13	35 / 80 = 44%

CLINICAL PICTURE

Base of the Tongue

Asymptomatic lesions are rarely diagnosed because the base of tongue is visualized only by indirect mirror examination.

Often, the earliest symptom is a mild sore throat. The patient may sense a lump in the back of the tongue and actually feel it by digital palpation; the patient is not amused by the physician who cannot see the lesion with a tongue depressor and fails to palpate the base of tongue. Because many of the early lesions are relatively silent, a subdigastric neck mass, often quite large, is often the first sign. The patient may insist that a 5 cm or larger neck mass "came about overnight." In a sense, the patient is correct. Small clinically positive lymph nodes, 1 cm to 4 cm in diameter, are almost always asymptomatic. Sudden enlargement occurs because of necrosis or internal bleeding with rapid increase in size and mild tenderness. Difficulty swallowing, a nasal voice quality, and deep-seated ear pain occur as the lesion enlarges. Far-advanced lesions fix the tongue. Deep ulceration and necrosis result in foul breath.

Indirect mirror examination, digital palpation, and a high level of suspicion are the ingredients for diagnosis of early lesions of the base of tongue. Because early lesions are often submucosal and relatively soft and the base of tongue is irregular, diagnosis is often a challenge. The rigid fiberoptic telescope will allow examination in some patients not easily examined by indirect mirror examination, and the flexible fiberoptic laryngoscope allows outpatient examination by way of the nose. A small lesion originating in the glossotonsillar sulcus area may ulcerate and produce symptoms quite early; it may be overlooked unless the area is critically examined.

Lymphomas are usually large, mostly submucosal masses, and the diagnosis can be suspected by their appearance. Minor salivary gland tumors are also usually submucosal, but more discrete and firm than lymphomas.

Tonsillar Area

ANTERIOR TONSILLAR PILLAR. Asymptomatic lesions may be found on routine examination by both dentists and physicians. Early symptoms include sore throat, usually aggravated by food or drink. Pain is referred to the ear as soon as ulceration takes place. If the lesion involves the hard palate or posterior upper gum, dentures may fit improperly or cause irritation. Advanced lesions invade the pterygoid or buccinator muscle and produce trismus and temporal pain. Invasion of the tongue will eventually limit tongue mobility, and when accompanied by ulceration at the junction of the anterior tonsillar pillar and oral tongue causes a great deal of pain.

TONSILLAR FOSSA. Signs and symptoms are similar to those for anterior tonsillar pillar lesions except that the lesions tend to be larger before symptoms develop. Ipsilateral sore throat is the hallmark of these lesions. Detection by visual examination with a tongue depressor is sufficient for most lesions of the tonsillar fossa; however, a few cancers arise near the glossotonsillar sulcus or lower pole of the tonsillar area and are only visible by indirect examination. A few patients will present with a node in the neck. Lymphomas of the tonsil tend to be large submucosal masses, but may ulcerate and appear similar to carcinomas.

Soft Palate

The earliest symptom of a lesion of the soft palate is usually mild sore throat, often aggravated by food or drink. The sore throat is not well localized; discomfort may improve temporarily if antibiotics are given. Advanced lesions interfere with swallowing and may cause a voice change. Regurgitation of food and liquid into the nasopharynx and nose occurs with destruction, perforation, or fixation of the soft palate. Lateral and superior spread to the nasopharynx and parapharyngeal space is associated with trismus, otitis media, temporal headache, and, rarely, cranial nerve involvement.

Early lesions appear as red, white, or mixed changes in the mucosa; the mucosa may appear roughened. The margins are ill-defined. Multiple foci on the soft palate and anterior tonsillar pillars are common. Moderately advanced lesions have rolled edges with central ulceration, or they may be mainly exophytic, particularly around the uvula. The nasopharynx should be inspected and palpated for submucosal extension along the lateral wall; extension along the nasopharyngeal surface of the soft palate is uncommon until quite late. Extension to the posterior nasal cavity is seen only in advanced lesions that erode the posterior hard palate.

Carcinoma of the soft palate is associated with an exceptionally high rate of second head and neck primary carcinomas.

METHODS OF DIAGNOSIS AND STAGING

Most lesions of the oropharynx can be biopsied by incisional or punch forceps biopsy under local anesthesia in the outpatient clinic. Base of tongue lesions may require general anesthesia. Frozen section control is helpful in base of tongue lesions since it is sometimes difficult to obtain representative tissue. Fresh tissue is sent to the pathologist if lymphoma is suspected.

Early lesions are staged by physical examination; direct laryngoscopy under general anesthesia may be required for base of tongue or vallecula lesions. CT scan is obtained in the more advanced lesions and used to determine the extent of lymphatic spread.

The AJCC staging system is used:[12]

- Tis Carcinoma in situ
- T1 Tumor 2 cm or less in greatest diameter
- T2 Tumor more than 2 cm, but not more than 4 cm in greatest diameter
- T3 Tumor more than 4 cm in greatest diameter
- T4 Massive tumor more than 4 cm in diameter with invasion of bone, soft tissues of neck, or root (deep musculature) of tongue

T1 and T2 are simply measurements of size and are easy to apply. There is a tendency to overestimate the size of lesions in the oropharynx; insertion of a measuring device will help to judge the maximum diameter. The difference between T3 and T4 is not so easily determined. Bone involvement is uncommon but must be seen on roentgenograms to qualify. Invasion of soft tissues of the neck requires some judgment. Tumors of the tonsillar area or base of the tongue that penetrate the glossotonsillar sulcus frequently can be palpated as a deep mass just under the angle of the jaw and qualify as T4 if the mass is larger than 4 cm in diameter. Invasion of the root or deep musculature of the tongue is easy to diagnose if the tongue is partially fixed. If a base-of-tongue cancer can be palpated easily through the floor of mouth or in the submentum, then invasion of deep muscle has probably occurred. Lesions that produce trismus or cranial nerve palsy or grossly invade the nasopharynx usually are classified as T4.

TREATMENT: BASE OF THE TONGUE

Selection of Treatment Modality

Operation and irradiation produce similar cure rates for early (T1) base-of-tongue lesions, but because excision of the base of tongue generally causes greater disability and because of the high risk for bilateral lymphatic involvement, radiation therapy is the treatment of choice for the majority of lesions, with operation reserved for salvage of radiation therapy failures and to help control the neck disease. The local–regional control and survival rates are better for radiation therapy for T2–T4 lesions. Radiation therapy automatically encompasses the neck nodes on both sides of the neck. Extended supraglottic laryngectomy may be used for limited vallecular lesions and lateralized base-of-tongue lesions, but there are definite anatomical criteria that must be satisfied, and this selection limits its usefulness. The following conditions must be met: no gross involvement of the pharyngo-epiglottic fold, preservation of one lingual artery, resection of less than 80% of the base of the tongue, pulmonary function suitable for supraglottic laryngectomy, and medical condition suitable for a major operation. At least an ipsilateral neck dissection is indicated, but with the high risk of bilateral neck disease even in the N0 patient, this represents incomplete treatment. Postoperative irradiation may have to be administered in any event for close margins or for fear of neck failure. Therefore, radiation therapy is usually the treatment of choice for the primary lesion, with neck dissection added as needed (see "Principles of Treatment").

Surgical Treatment

The surgical approach for neoplasms of the base of the tongue is either by splitting the lip, mandible, and tongue in the midline to reach the base of the tongue, or by dividing the horizontal mandible and swinging it outward to expose the tongue base. Suprahyoid, transhyoid, and infrahyoid approaches also can be used to resect small lesions at the base of the tongue. After the tumor has been removed, the mandible is wired together. Only one lingual artery may be sacrificed. A neck dissection is done in continuity with excision of the base-of-tongue lesion. Removal of a large base-of-tongue tumor requires simultaneous removal of part or all of the larynx.

Irradiation Technique

Irradiation of base-of-tongue cancer is accomplished by parallel opposed external beam portals that also encompass the regional nodes on both sides. Interstitial implants may be used for part of the treatment if the lesion is small, discrete, and located in the anterolateral base of the tongue. Implants of posterior lesions are technically difficult; these implants are usually accomplished with a flexible source (*e.g.*, ^{192}Ir ribbons), which allows through-and-through implantation from the base of the tongue to the skin. There is no proven advantage in local control for interstitial boosts as opposed to external beam treatment alone. (For oral tongue cancer, there is no doubt that interstitial treatment significantly improves local control compared with external beam therapy alone.) Base-of-tongue lesions have a good local control rate with external beam therapy alone. The base of the tongue has a good vascular supply and tolerates high doses of radiation without soft-tissue necrosis.

A boost of 1000 cGy to 1500 cGy may be delivered to the base of the tongue by way of the submental route without traversing the mandible. The submental boost may be given with high-energy electrons or a photon beam that is angled superiorly to avoid the previously irradiated spinal cord. The submental boost has proven successful, partly because of the high dose achieved and the relatively small volume irradiated. It is selected for those base-of-tongue lesions that are central and posterior. Large lesions that extend into the oral tongue near the junction with the anterior tonsillar pillar area are not suited for submental boost because the distance from the skin to the tongue surface is several centimeters and the portal is inefficient; an interstitial boost or reduced lateral portals are considered in these cases.

One of the common errors in planning external beam portals is failure to recognize anterior growth of neoplasm as measured by palpation through the lateral floor of the mouth.

The inferior border of the lateral portals is usually the thyroid notch unless tumor has extended into the upper pyriform sinus, lateral pharyngeal wall, or pre-epiglottic space.

The skin and subcutaneous fat in the submental area should be shielded, if possible, because high-dose radiation therapy to this area produces considerable fibrosis. Shielding this area may not be possible if the patient is thin or if tumor is bulging into the mylohyoid muscle.[244]

Management of the lymphatics is critical. One of the major advantages of radiation therapy is the ease of irradiating all the nodes at risk. Even small, well-lateralized base-of-tongue lesions will spread to the opposite neck, and both sides are always treated.

The primary portals include the upper jugular, posterior submandibular, and posterior upper cervical node(s) when the neck is clinically negative. The superior border is approximately 2 cm above the tip of the mastoid even with clinically negative nodes to ensure coverage of the nodes near the base of the skull.

The lower neck nodes on both sides are always treated. If the upper neck is clinically negative, the lower neck portals are carefully tailored to exclude as much normal tissue as possible; the midjugular nodes are the major risk area in this situation. If the upper neck is clinically positive, the lower neck portals become more generous.

The dose for T1 lesions is usually 6000 to 6600 cGy in 6 to 6.5 weeks. Since 1978, T2–T4 lesions have been treated with 120 cGy twice daily with 4 hours between fractions to a total dose of 7440 cGy to 7920 cGy.[245]

Combined Treatment Policies

Combined treatment is seldom selected because an operation for moderately advanced lesions usually implies major functional loss, and few patients are willing to accept the morbidity and possible immediate mortality. The most common indication for offering glossectomy and laryngectomy is a lesion that simply fails to respond to irradiation after 5000 cGy. However, if the patient is offered and accepts a glossectomy-laryngectomy, the authors prefer an operation followed by postoperative radiation therapy.

Management of Recurrence

Radiation failures are treated surgically, but salvage is infrequent except for T1 lesions. Fletcher[246] reported surgical salvage of radiation failure in 2 of 9 patients with T1 disease, 1 of 13 with T3 disease, and 2 of 15 with T4 disease.

Surgical failures are rarely salvaged by either an operation or radiation therapy, except for the early lesion with a discrete local recurrence in the base of tongue.

Recurrence of a small, discrete primary tumor may be managed by a wide local excision. The remaining recurrences require either a jaw-tongue-neck resection or glossectomy-laryngectomy.

RESULTS OF TREATMENT: BASE OF THE TONGUE

Surgical Results

Whicker and co-workers[247] of the Mayo Clinic reported 102 patients selected for curative attempts by operation; 23 received preoperative or postoperative radiation therapy. Eleven were irradiation failures. Some 23% required partial or total laryngectomy; 56% had positive nodes in the specimen. The operative mortality was 4%, with a 27% local recurrence rate and 10% neck failure rate. The 5-year survival rate was 37%.

The Memorial Sloan-Kettering Cancer Center[248] reported the results for 160 squamous cell carcinomas of the base of tongue treated between 1969 and 1978. Radiation therapy alone was used in 33% of cases; radiation therapy was given as an adjunct in 60 patients, but the dose was greater than 5000 cGy in only 14 cases. The 5-year determinate survival for Stages I and II was 33% and for Stages III and IV was 6%.

Irradiation Results

The initial local control rates are shown in Table 21-32 for patients treated for cure with continuous-course external beam irradiation.[245] The actuarial survival curves by stage are shown in Figure 21-17 for a group of 114 patients treated between 1964 and 1981. These survival curves include 24 patients managed by the split-course scheme and 24 patients who had an interstitial boost, two treatment schemes that had much poorer results.

TABLE 21-32. Base of Tongue Carcinoma: Initial Local Control by Radiation Therapy (Continuous Course)

	*One Fraction/Day**	*Two Fractions/Day†*
T1	2/3	1/1
T2	12/14 (86%)	1/1
T3	12/13 (92%)	8/9
T4	3/12 (25%)	3/6

* Modified from Gardner et al.[245] Excludes split course and radium boost cases.

† Unpublished University of Florida data. Patients treated 3/78–4/85; analysis 4/87 by J. T. Parsons, M.D.

FOLLOW-UP POLICY: BASE OF THE TONGUE

Surgical or radiation therapy, or both, will occasionally salvage the failure of an early lesion. Radiation failures may present as an ulcer and must be distinguished from radiation necrosis. Most radiation ulcers will appear in the vallecula or glossotonsillar sulcus, not on the base of tongue proper. Biopsies usually must be done with the patient under general anesthetic to obtain adequate tissue and control of bleeding.

COMPLICATIONS OF TREATMENT: BASE OF THE TONGUE

Surgical Complications

The complications of surgery include an operative mortality of about 5%; fistula, mandibular necrosis, dysphagia, hoarseness, trismus, and carotid rupture are nonfatal complications. Pneumonia is frequent due to aspiration when the glottis is preserved.

FIG. 21-17. Base-of-tongue carcinoma: survival by AJCC stage (actuarial method[249]). University of Florida data; patients treated 10/64 to 9/81. (Analysis 9/83 by K. E. Gardner, M.D.)

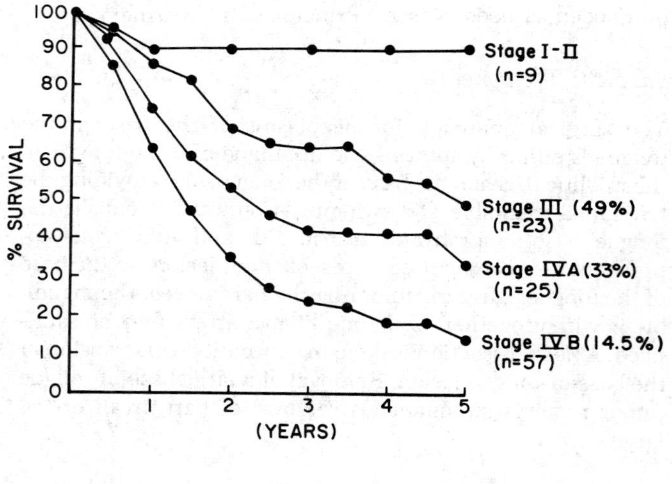

Complications of Irradiation

Bone exposure and osteoradionecrosis are uncommon. Soft-tissue necrosis of mild to moderate degree occurs in approximately 10% and bone exposure of mild to moderate degree occurs in 5% of patients treated solely by external beam irradiation.[245] Severe necroses requiring an operation or hospitalization have not been observed at the University of Florida. The rate of complications has been even less since 1978 with the twice-daily fractionation schedule. Treatment of necrosis requires patience and reassurance to the patient, who assumes the pain is due to cancer. Antibiotics often will reduce pain. The patient will lose weight because of dysphagia and will require nutritional support. Many necroses persist several months. Serious hemorrhage is uncommon.

Hypoglossal nerve palsy occurred in two patients and is reported in other series. It usually is associated with an ulcer in the posterior glossotonsillar sulcus. Unilateral hypoglossal nerve palsy does not produce serious morbidity because the opposite side compensates very nicely.

An occasional patient cured of advanced base-of-tongue cancer by radiation therapy may have difficulty swallowing solid foods. The action of the base of the tongue is to force the bolus of food into the hypopharynx, and loss of full motion impedes swallowing. This is probably a result of some fibrosis of the base of the tongue compounded by a dry mouth. The addition of a radical neck dissection to radiation therapy increases the risk of this problem. Aspiration is unusual, however, even if the tip of the epiglottis has been amputated by tumor.

Complications of Combined Treatment

Preoperative irradiation will increase the risk of fistula, delayed healing, and carotid exposure. Postoperative irradiation increases the amount of fibrosis in the neck. Radiation necrosis of the soft tissues or bone is uncommon. The added effect of xerostomia further worsens the swallowing defect produced by glossectomy.

TREATMENT: TONSILLAR AREA

Selection of Treatment Modality

EARLY (T1 OR T2). Early lesions are generally treated by irradiation with a high rate of success and relatively low morbidity. A small lesion may be cured by wide local excision or tonsillectomy. A surgical attack for larger lesions usually implies removal of the mandible, the tonsillar area including both pillars, a part of the soft palate, and a part of the tongue; additionally, an ipsilateral neck dissection is performed even with a clinically negative neck. The functional loss from this operation is not justified in view of the high success rate with irradiation, which leaves the patient intact; even a dry mouth may be avoided when well-lateralized lesions are treated by techniques that allow at least partial salivary recovery. An operation often will salvage the few radiation treatment failures. The local control, surgical salvage, and ultimate control rates by T stage for tonsillar area lesions treated by continuous-course radiation therapy are shown in Table 21-33. The local control rate is better for T1–T2 tonsillar fossa lesions than for anterior tonsillar pillar lesions.[250–252]

MODERATELY ADVANCED (LATE T2 OR T3). There are advocates of combining surgery and radiation therapy as the initial therapy and advocates of radical radiation therapy with or without neck dissection, with surgery reserved for radiation therapy failure.[250,251,253–257] The local failure rate with radiation therapy is approximately 20% for T2 lesions and 30% for T3 lesions when adequate doses are prescribed; therefore, radiation therapy has been the choice for initial therapy at the University of Florida. Preoperative irradiation followed by an operation has shown better results in some nonrandomized series and no difference in other series compared to radiation therapy with surgical salvage.[258–260] Surgical salvage works better for anterior tonsillar pillar failures than for those of the tonsillar fossa.

ADVANCED (T4). If the lesion is assigned to stage T4 only because of mandible invasion, then combined therapy

TABLE 21-33. Squamous Cell Carcinoma of the Tonsillar Region: Local Control with Radiation Therapy as a Function of Tonsillar Region Site* (No. Controlled/No. Treated)

T Stage	*Excluded*†	*Tonsillar Fossa*	*Tonsillar Pillars*		*Overall Control with Irradiation*	*No. Salvaged/ No. Attempted*	*Ultimate Control*
			Anterior	*Posterior*			
T1	4	4/4	5/7	1/1	10/12 (83%)	2/2	12/12
T2	9	17/18 (94%)	18/26 (69%)	1/2‡	36/46 (78%)	5/7	41/46 (89%)
T3	8	23/31 (74%)	5/8		28/39 (72%)	0/3	28/39 (72%)
T4	5	3/12 (25%)	2/4		5/16 (31%)	0/1	5/16 (31%)

Mendenhall WM, Parsons JT, Cassisi NJ, et al: Squamous cell carcinoma of the tonsillar area treated with radical irradiation. Radiother Oncol 10:23–30, 1987.

*A total of 136 patients treated 10/64–8/83 with continuous course, once-a-day or twice-a-day fractionation.

†A total of 110 patients eligible for local control analysis with 113 evaluable primary lesions; 26 patients excluded from local control analysis because they died in less than 2 years of intercurrent disease with primary lesion controlled.

‡Failure at 4700 cGy.

should be considered. Mandible invasion usually is associated with extensions that contraindicate surgical removal, however.

Radical irradiation using a hyperfractionation technique will control about 30% of T4 lesions. Combined treatment may be recommended in selected cases.

Surgical Treatment

Surgical treatment for very early cancers of the tonsillar pillars consists of a wide local excision, including tonsillectomy, through a transoral approach. Larger lesions may require removal of the adjacent mandible as well as a portion of the tongue and soft palate. Depending on the size of the defect, a tongue, deltopectoral, or myocutaneous flap may be required to close the defect. Flaps are usually necessary for extensive lesions or after radiation therapy failure. Deglutition is not generally a problem, but some patients remain on liquid diets. Chewing is difficult since a portion of the mandible has been removed and the patient will be unable to wear dentures. Speech may be impaired if a significant portion of the tongue or palate has been removed. A prosthesis may be needed for the palatal defect.

Irradiation Technique

The basic portal arrangement depends to a large degree on the extent of the local lesion and presence or absence of positive lymph nodes. The risk for contralateral lymph node metastases is very small unless there is tongue invasion, invasion of the soft palate within 1 cm to 2 cm of the midline, or clinically positive nodes in the ipsilateral neck. If these risk features are absent, a technique with both photon and electron beams is used to reduce the dose to the contralateral mucosa and salivary glands, if the medial extent of the primary lesion is no more than 4.5 cm from the ipsilateral skin surface. The major advantage of this technique is not a greater cure rate but a lower incidence of xerostomia secondary to partial preservation of minor and major salivary gland function on the contralateral side. An intraoral lead block also may be added, which further protects the minor salivary glands and a portion of the parotid. Because the tonsillar area lesions lie behind the mandible, an extra 1.0 cm to 1.5 cm is added to the depth-dose calculations for the electron portion of the treatment.[244,261]

Lesions with a medial extent greater than 4.5 cm or clinically positive neck nodes are at risk for bilateral neck disease and are treated with parallel opposed photon portals, usually weighted 2:1 or 3:2 to the involved side; if there are positive contralateral nodes or extension across the midline, the portals usually are equally weighted. Small, discrete lesions of the anterior tonsillar pillar may have part of the treatment by intraoral cone.

The dose prescribed for tonsillar area lesions is critical if a high rate of control is to be achieved. An interstitial boost frequently is added to the tongue extension when present; if there is also suspicion of residual tumor in the tonsillar area, the tonsil is implanted at the same time (tongue/pterygoid implant). The local control and complication rates are increased by the implant (Table 21-34).[250]

The dose for tonsillar fossa lesions is 6000 cGy in 6 weeks for T1 lesions, 7440 cGy to 7680 cGy (120 cGy twice a day) with or without an interstitial boost for T2–T3 lesions, and 7920 cGy (120 cGy twice a day) with or without an interstitial boost for T4 lesions. The dose for anterior tonsillar pillar lesions is higher: T1 lesions, 6500 cGy to 7000 cGy with or without an interstitial boost; T2–T3 lesions, 7440 cGy to 7680 cGy (120 cGy twice a day) with or without an interstitial boost; T4 lesions, 7920 cGy to 8160 cGy (120 cGy twice a day) with or without an interstitial boost. Intraoral cone may be substituted for part of the external beam or implant dose for discrete lesions of the anterior tonsillar pillar.

Combined Treatment Policies

Preoperative radiation therapy has been favored by many centers, but surgery followed by radiation therapy is a satisfactory option for those favoring combined therapy.

Management of Recurrence

An operation will salvage a good proportion of T1 or T2 radiation therapy failures, but only an occasional advanced lesion is salvaged (see Table 21-33).

RESULTS OF TREATMENT: TONSILLAR AREA

The results and the complications for 136 patients treated by continuous-course radiation therapy (with planned neck dissection in 32) at the University of Florida are shown in

TABLE 21-34. Carcinoma of the Tonsillar Region: Soft Tissue and/or Bone Complications by Severity (No. Complications/No. Treated)*

	Mild (1+)		*Moderate (2+)*		*Severe (3+)*	
T Stage	*E*	*E + R*	*E*	*E + R*	*E*	*E + R*
T1	3/15 (20%)		0/15		0/15	
T2	10/41 (24%)	4/12 (33%)	2/41 (5%)	0/12	0/41	0/12
T3	4/23 (17%)	10/24 (42%)	1/23 (4%)	2/24 (8%)	4/23 (17%)	0/24
T4	2/14 (14%)	2/7	0/14	1/7	0/14	1/7

Mendenhall WM, Parsons JT, Cassisi NJ, et al: Squamous cell carcinoma of the tonsillar area treated with radical irradiation. Radiother Oncol 10:23–30, 1987.
*A total of 136 patients.
E, external beam alone; E + R, external beam plus radium needle implant.

TABLE 21-35. Carcinoma of the Tonsillar Region: Control of Neck Disease as a Function of Treatment* (No. Heminecks Controlled/No. Treated)

Hemineck Stage	*Radiation Therapy Alone*	*Ratiation Therapy + Neck Dissection*	*Overall Control with Initial Treatment*	*No. Salvaged/ No. Attempted*	*Overall Ultimate Control*
N0†	33/34	0/0	33/34	0/1	33/34
N1	18/18	4/4	22/22		22/22
N2A	1/2	3/4	4/6	0/1	4/6
N2B	9/12	12/12	21/24	1/2	22/24
N3A	0/1	2/3	2/4		2/4

Modified from Mendenhall WM, Parsons JT, Cassisi NJ, et al: Squamous cell carcinoma of the tonsillar area treated with radical irradiation. Radiother Oncol 10:23–30, 1987.

* Primary site continuously disease-free; 43 patients with 56 evaluable heminecks.

† For N0 patients, figures represent the number of patients with neck disease controlled/number of patients treated.

Tables 21-33 through 21-36. The local control rate for T3 lesions was 76% when an interstitial boost was added compared with 56% without the boost.[250] The local control rate for patients treated since 1978 with twice-a-day treatment are given in Table 21-2.

The poorer local control for T1–T2 anterior tonsillar pillar lesions is difficult to explain. An interstitial implant is currently being used as part of the treatment to try to reduce the overall time and increase the local control rates.[262]

Fourteen patients were selected for combined treatment. Eight were treated with preoperative radiation therapy; only one had no evidence of disease over 2 years after treatment. Six were treated by resection and postoperative radiation therapy, and four had no evidence of disease for greater than 2 years.

Dasmahapatra and co-workers[253] compared the results for combined surgery and radiation therapy versus radiation therapy alone for patients with cancer of the tonsil treated between 1962 and 1982. For Stage III, the 5-year survival rate with radiation therapy plus surgery was 31% versus 11% for radiation therapy alone, and for Stage IV, the results for radiation therapy plus surgery were 15% at 5 years compared with 0 for radiation therapy alone.

Shrewsbury[254] compared radiation therapy alone to combined radiation therapy and surgery. The 2-year survival rate for radiation therapy alone by T stage was T1, 78%; T2, 50%; T3, 15%; and T4, 0. The results for combined treatment were T1, 100%; T2, 82%; T3, 76%; and T4, 33%.

Perez and co-workers[257] compared the results of radiation therapy alone, preoperative irradiation, and surgery alone for 144 patients with carcinoma of the tonsil. They concluded that combined surgery and radiation treatment produced the same rates of local and regional control and 3- and 5-year survival as radiation therapy alone, and that radiation therapy was the best initial treatment, with surgery reserved for salvage of radiation failures.

TABLE 21-36. Carcinoma of the Tonsillar Region: Five-Year Survival by Modified AJCC Stage (No. Alive/No. Treated)*

	5-Year Survival	
Modified AJCC Stage	*Absolute*	*Determinate*
I	3/9	3/3
II	13/22 (59%)	13/14 (93%)
III	14/22 (64%)	14/17 (82%)
IVA	6/17 (35%)	6/14 (43%)
IVB	4/24 (17%)	4/19 (21%)

Mendenhall WM, Parsons JT, Cassisi NJ, et al: Squamous cell carcinoma of the tonsillar area treated with radical irradiation. Radiother Oncol 10:23–30, 1987.

*Ninety-four patients eligible for 5-year survival analysis.

COMPLICATIONS OF TREATMENT: TONSILLAR AREA

Radiation Therapy

The rate of bone or soft tissue necrosis following radiation therapy is shown in Table 21-34.[250] The risk for a severe complication requiring surgical intervention was 3%. Improved management of the teeth and use of twice-daily fractionation have reduced the incidence of serious complications. Other complications included laryngeal edema (1), hypoglossal nerve palsy (3), and trismus (2). The complication rate for 83 patients with oropharyngeal tumors (tonsil, base of tongue, soft palate) managed by twice-a-day therapy, of which 28 with tonsil lesions had an interstitial boost after external beam doses of 7440 cGy to 8160 cGy, is shown in Table 21-37.

Surgery

Complications of operation include oropharyngeal dysfunction (limited or no ability to swallow, and drooling), fistula, failure of flaps, complications of neck dissection, and aspiration occasionally leading to laryngectomy.

TREATMENT: SOFT PALATE

Selection of Treatment Modality

Recommendations for management of soft palate cancer must consider the primary lesion and both sides of the neck. Very small (2–5 mm), well-defined lesions may be excised and the neck observed, but the multifocal nature of soft palate lesions predicts marginal recurrence after limited treatment unless patients are very carefully selected. Tiny lesions confined to the uvula may be treated by surgical excision with little morbidity. Irradiation is the modality most often selected for early and advanced soft palate carci-

TABLE 21-37. Oropharynx Cancer: Complications According to Dose for 83 Patients Treated with Twice-a-Day Fractionation

		Complications		
Dose (cGy)	*No. of Patients*	*Mild*	*Moderate*	*Severe*
≤7440	17	1	0	0
7680	20	3	1	0
7920	11	2	0	2*
8160	7	0	1	0
7440–8160 + 1000–1500 Ra	28	4	1	1*

University of Florida data. Patients treated 3/78–4/85; analysis 4/87 by J. T. Parsons, M.D.
*Severe complications: permanent gastrostomy tube, 1 (7920 cGy); bone necrosis, 2 (7920 cGy; 7800 + 1000 cGy implant).

nomas; neck dissection is added as needed. The initial success rate with irradiation for early lesions is high, leaving the patient functionally intact without the need for a prosthesis or elaborate reconstruction. The local control rate for T3 and T4 lesions treated by radiation therapy is about 50% to 60%, and combined treatment may be considered, but the extent of the surgical resection required usually precludes that option. Elective irradiation of both sides of the neck is included for stage N0, and neck dissection is added in selected patients with clinically positive neck nodes. Fletcher[263] reported a very high rate of success for patients treated by radiation therapy alone.

Surgical Treatment

Small, discrete lesions can be managed by transoral excision and repaired by a pharyngeal flap to prevent any velopharyngeal incompetence. Tonsillectomy may also be necessary in order to obtain an adequate margin. If full-thickness resection is required, however, then a prosthesis generally is required to restore velopharyngeal competence. Operations for salvage after failure of radiation therapy should generally include full-thickness removal of the soft palate.

Irradiation Technique

The basic irradiation technique for early and advanced lesions involves parallel opposed external beam portals that include the primary lesion and the first relay of upper neck nodes on both sides, because even very tiny lesions are at some risk for occult lymph node disease. If the primary lesion is discrete, a portion of the treatment may be given by way of intraoral cone or an interstitial implant. If intraoral cone therapy is to be used, it should be given prior to external beam when the lesion is clearly visible and the mouth is not yet sore from the radiation reaction. Intraoral cone therapy requires meticulous care to avoid geographic miss.

A single-plane implant (*e.g.*, iridium hairpins) is an effective reduced-field technique. The implant is usually done after external beam therapy.[264]

The external beam technique usually is equally weighted, parallel opposed portals. The minimum treatment volume for early lesions includes the entire soft palate and the adjacent tonsillar areas. If the neck is clinically negative, high-energy photons (17–22 MV) will produce an ideal isodose distribution, allowing a tumor dose at the soft palate of 7000 cGy while maintaining the lymph node dose at 5000 cGy. If the lymph nodes are clinically positive, then cobalt-60 or a 4 MV to 6 MV photon beam is preferred on the involved side(s).

Combined Treatment Policies

Combined therapy is seldom planned because of the success rate with radiation therapy and the morbidity associated with resection of the soft palate.

Management of Recurrence

Soft tissue necrosis is uncommon after radiation therapy; thus a persistent ulcer is the hallmark of recurrent disease following irradiation. Recurrence following irradiation is treated by surgical removal when feasible, and a few patients are salvaged.

RESULTS OF TREATMENT: SOFT PALATE

Surgical Results

Ratzer and co-workers[265] reported the Memorial Sloan-Kettering results for 299 patients with squamous cell carcinoma of the soft palate; 112 were treated by surgery, 139 by radiation therapy, and 22 by combined treatment. The 5-year absolute survival rate was 21% and the determinate survival rate was 30%. The determinate survival rate for the group treated by surgery alone was 38%. The main cause of failure was recurrence at the primary site.

Irradiation Results

Weller and co-workers[266] reported a local failure rate of 50% in 30 patients with soft palate lesions. Only 5 of the patients had T1 lesions.

Seydel and Scholl[267] reviewed the results of 41 patients with previously untreated soft palate malignancies, including 4 nonsquamous carcinomas. Thirty-one patients were treated with doses between 6000 cGy and 7000 cGy, and 10 (32%) developed local recurrence.

The local control rate and the 2- and 5-year determinate survival rates for 55 patients treated with radiation therapy at the University of Florida are given in Tables 21-38 and 21-39.[268]

TABLE 21-38. Soft Palate Carcinoma: Control of Disease at the Primary Site with Continuous-Course Irradiation — 55 Patients* (No. Controlled/No. Treated)

T Stage	*Excluded†*	*Initial Control*	*No. Salvaged/ No. Attempted*	*Ultimate Control*
T1	2	8/8		8/8
T2	7	14/19 (74%)	2/5	16/19 (84%)
T3	3	5/11 (45%)	0/2	5/11 (45%)
T4	1	1/4		1/4

Amdur RJ, Mendenhall WM, Parsons JT, et al: Carcinoma of the soft palate treated with irradiation: Analysis of results and complications. Radiother Oncol 9:185–194, 1987.

*Once-a-day or twice-a-day fractionation. Includes two patients who received most or all of their treatment with an interstitial implant.

†Excludes patients who died of other causes <2 years after treatment with no recurrence at primary site.

TABLE 21-39. Soft Palate Carcinoma: Determinate Survival Rates with Continuous-Course Irradiation

Modified AJCC Stage	*2-Year Survival*	*5-Year Survival*
I	7/8	5/6
II	13/13	7/9
III	10/12	3/8
IVA	1/2	0/2
IVB	4/10	2/8

Modified from Amdur RJ, Mendenhall WM, Parsons JT, et al: Carcinoma of the soft palate treated with irradiation: Analysis of results and complications. Radiother Oncol 9:185–194, 1987.

Lindberg and Fletcher[269] reported a high rate of control for soft palate lesions (T1, 100%; T2, 88%; T3, 77%; T4, 83%). A few failures were salvaged by operation. A compilation of nine treatment series for squamous cell carcinoma of the soft palate is given in Table 21-40.[268]

COMPLICATIONS OF TREATMENT: SOFT PALATE

Surgical Complications

Nasal speech and regurgitation of food into the nasopharynx are sequelae of full-thickness resection of the soft palate. A prosthesis is only partially successful in correcting the functional defect when the defect is large. Oropharyngeal dysfunction may occur.

Complications of Irradiation

Complications of irradiation are few. Soft-tissue necrosis of the soft palate is uncommon; an ulcer must be considered to be a possible recurrence. The soft palate may become retracted following successful treatment of advanced lesions; this may result in regurgitation into the nasopharynx and slight alteration in speech. Small perforations may persist after successful treatment at sites where tumor has grown through the soft palate. Bone necrosis requiring surgical management occurred in 1 of 55 patients treated at the University of Florida.[268]

LARYNX

Cancer of the larynx represents about 2% of the total cancer risk. The estimated number of new cases in 1987 in the United States was 12,100 — 9800 in men and 2300 in women, with an estimated 3800 deaths because of laryngeal cancer.

A study of trends in cancer incidence in the United States from 1935 to 1970 showed that cancer of the larynx increased by 33% in white men but was 3.5 times increased in nonwhite men. The incidence in women showed only a very minimal increase in spite of the fact that lung cancer in women quadrupled in the same period.

Cancer of the larynx seems to be related primarily to cigarette smoking. The risk of tobacco-related cancers of the upper alimentary and respiratory tract declines among ex-smokers after 5 years and is said to approach the risk of nonsmokers after 10 years of abstention.[273]

A 12-year American Cancer Society study showed that low-tar and low-nicotine cigarettes (<15 mg of tar and <1 mg of nicotine) resulted in slightly lower death rates from lung cancer, but whether they affect the risk of laryngeal cancer is unknown.

The importance of alcohol in the etiology of laryngeal cancer remains unclear, but it is probably less important than in the other head and neck sites, for which alcohol can be shown to be synergistic to tobacco.[274]

The geographic distribution for laryngeal cancer in the United States shows excess occurrence in the northeast, particularly in northern New Jersey, New York City, and along the Hudson River. The rates are also higher along the southeastern Atlantic Coast and the Gulf Coast, a distribution that closely resembles the high-risk areas for lung cancer.[275]

ANATOMY

The larynx is composed of several cartilages connected by ligaments and muscles, divided anatomically into the supraglottic, glottic, and subglottic regions. The supraglottic larynx consists of the epiglottis, the false vocal cords, the ventricles, the aryepiglottic folds, and the arytenoids; the arytenoids are cartilages that articulate on the cricoid (Fig. 21-18). The glottis includes the true vocal cords and the

TABLE 21-40. Literature Review for Squamous Cell Carcinoma of the Soft Palate

Series	No. of Patients (Follow-up)	Primary Treatment	Staging System	Ultimate Control of Disease at Primary Site*	5-Year Determinate Survival†
Amdur et al.,[268] University of Florida, 1986	55 (≥2 yr)	RT alone	AJCC	T1, 100%; T2, 84%; T3, 45%; T4, 1/4	I, 83%: II, 78%; III, 38%; IV, 20%
Chung and Constable,[270] University of Virginia, 1979	63 (≥2 yr)	Individualized; RT alone in 51%	AJCC	T1, 100%; T2, 83%; T3, 52%; T4, 2/5	T1–T2, 70%; T3–T4, 25%
Lindberg and Fletcher,[269] M. D. Anderson Hospital, 1978	NS (≥2 yr)	Individualized; RT alone in 70%	AJCC	T1, 100%; T2, 100%; T3, 82%; T4, 83%	NS
Garrett and Beale,[271] Princess Margaret Hospital, 1984	70 (≥2 yr)	RT alone	UICC	T1, 90%; T2, 95%; T3, 56%	T1, 65%; T2, 84%; T3, 28%
Seydel and Scholl,[267] Fox Chase Center, Philadelphia; 1974	41 (NS)	Individualized; RT alone in 73%	AJCC	T1, 83%; T2, 87%; T3, 46%; T4, no data‡	Overall 54%
Eneroth et al.,[28] Karolinska Institute, 1972	112§ (≥5 yr)	Individualized	NS	Overall 86%	Overall 37%
Weller et al.,[266] Stanford, 1976	30 (≥2 yr)	RT alone	UICC	Overall 50%	Overall 38%**
Fee et al.,[272] Stanford and UC(SF), 1979	106 (NS)	Individualized; RT alone in 75%	AJCC	NS	I, 75%; II, 29%; III, 30%; IV, 18%
Ratzer et al.,[265] Memorial Sloan-Kettering, 1970	299†† (≥5 yr)	Individualized; RT alone in 39%	NS	NS	Overall 30%‡‡

Amdur RJ, Mendenhall WM, Parsons JT, et al: Carcinoma of the soft palate treated with irradiation: Analysis of results and complications. Radiother Oncol 9:185–194, 1987.

NS, Not specified; AJCC, American Joint Committee on Cancer; UICC, International Union Against Cancer.

*Includes the results of salvage therapy.

†Excludes deaths from intercurrent disease.

‡Control with initial treatment, not ultimate results. Two additional patients were successfully salvaged with surgery.

§Includes lesions of hard palate as well as soft palate.

**Absolute, not determinate, survival figure.

††Eighteen percent of patients had recurrent lesions following prior treatment at another institution.

‡‡Disease-free survival figure.

anterior commissure. The subglottic area is located below the vocal cords and ends at the upper margin of the first tracheal ring. The transition from the vocal cord to subglottis is ill-defined, but is considered clinically to begin 5 mm below the free margin of the vocal cord. The subglottic larynx is therefore about 2 cm in length.

The preepiglottic space is an important anatomic region because of frequent direct extension to this area.

Anatomically, the preepiglottic space is bounded by the epiglottis posteriorly, the hyoepiglottic ligament and vallecula superiorly, and the thyroid cartilage and thyrohyoid membrane anteriorly and laterally. It can be seen as a low-density area on a CT scan.

The supraglottic structures have a moderately rich capillary lymphatic plexus. The lymphatic trunks pass through the preepiglottic space and the thyrohyoid membrane to the subdigastric nodes. A few trunks drain directly to the middle or lower jugular chain.

There are essentially no capillary lymphatics of the true vocal cords; as a result, lymphatic spread from glottic cancer rarely occurs unless tumor extends to supraglottic or subglottic areas.

The subglottic area has relatively few capillary lymphatics. The lymphatic trunks pass through the thyrocricoid membrane to the pretracheal (Delphian) node(s) in the region of the thyroid isthmus, or the trunks may carry the tumor to the lower jugular nodes. The pretracheal nodes are midline in position and even when clinically positive are small (1–5 mm to rarely >1–2 cm). The subglottic area also drains posteriorly through the cricotracheal membrane with some trunks going to the paratracheal nodes while others pass to the inferior jugular chain.

PATHOLOGY

The laryngeal surfaces of the epiglottis and vocal cords are lined with stratified squamous epithelium and the remainder of the larynx is lined with pseudostratified ciliated columnar epithelium. Nearly all malignant tumors of the larynx arise from the surface epithelium and therefore are squamous cell carcinoma or one of its variants.

Minor salivary gland tumors arise from the mucous glands, but are rare; even more rare is the appearance of a soft-tissue sarcoma, malignant lymphoma, small cell carcinoma, or

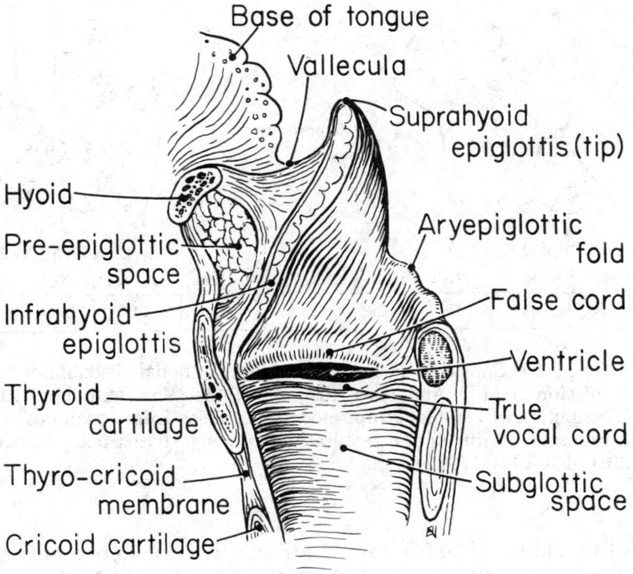

FIG. 21-18. Diagrammatic sagittal section of the larynx. (Million RR, Cassisi NJ: The management of local and regional laryngeal cancer. In Carter SK, Glatstein E, Livingston RB: Principles of Cancer Treatment. New York, McGraw-Hill, 1981)

plasmacytoma. Benign hemangiomas, chondromas, and osteochondromas are reported, but their malignant counterparts are rare.[276]

Carcinoma in situ is common on the vocal cords. Distinction between dysplasia, carcinoma in situ, squamous cell carcinoma with microinvasion, and true invasive carcinoma is a problem frequently confronting the pathologist and the physician. In patients with minimal lesions, the cord is biopsied by stripping the mucosa; the specimen tends to curl or fold, creating difficulty in orientation of the basement membrane. However, the precise distinction among carcinoma in situ, microinvasion, and invasive carcinoma is a bit academic. The authors recommend treatment, usually irradiation, in most patients. The local recurrence rate after irradiation for carcinoma in situ or microinvasive or invasive carcinoma is, surprisingly, about the same within the T1 category; the recurrences are almost always invasive carcinoma.

Most of the vocal cord carcinomas are either well-differentiated or moderately well-differentiated. In a few cases there is an apparent carcinoma and sarcoma occurring together, but most of these are, in reality, a carcinoma with a spindle cell stroma. The term pseudosarcoma is applied to a rare laryngeal lesion, usually polypoid or pedunculated with a stringlike umbilical cord. It has a favorable prognosis.

Verrucous carcinoma occurs on the vocal cords in about 1% to 2% of patients with carcinoma. The histologic diagnosis is difficult and must correlate with the gross appearance of the lesion.

Supraglottic carcinomas are less differentiated than those of the vocal cord; verrucous lesions are rare. Carcinoma in situ is rarely diagnosed as a distinct entity in the supraglottic larynx, although a zone of carcinoma in situ is seen at the margin between invasive tumor and normal mucosa. Small cell or oat cell carcinomas are reported to occur in the supraglottic larynx and have an aggressive behavior similar to that of oat cell carcinomas of the lungs.

PATTERNS OF SPREAD

Supraglottic Larynx

The majority of lesions are epiglottic in origin. It is difficult to assign a site of origin for advanced lesions.

SUPRAHYOID EPIGLOTTIS. Lesions of the suprahyoid epiglottis may grow like a mushroom, producing a huge exophytic mass with little tendency to destruction of cartilage or spread to adjacent structures. Others may infiltrate the tip and produce destruction of cartilage and eventual amputation of the tip. The latter lesions tend to invade the vallecula and preepiglottic space, the lateral pharyngeal walls, and the remainder of the supraglottic larynx.

INFRAHYOID EPIGLOTTIS. Lesions of the infrahyoid epiglottis tend to produce irregular outgrowths of tumor nodules with simultaneous invasion through the porous epiglottic cartilage into the preepiglottic space. These lesions grow circumferentially to involve the false cords, aryepiglottic folds, and eventually, the medial wall of the pyriform sinus and the pharyngoepiglottic fold. Invasion of the anterior commissure and cords is usually a late phenomenon, and subglottic extension occurs only in advanced lesions. Infrahyoid epiglottic lesions that extend onto or below the vocal cords are at a high risk for cartilage invasion, even if the cords are mobile.[277] Tumor may burrow through the epiglottic cartilage and preepiglottic fat space and present in the vallecula and base of tongue without involving the suprahyoid epiglottis. This anterior and superior extension is difficult to appreciate clinically; CT scan is of assistance in outlining this spread pattern.

FALSE CORD. Early false cord carcinomas usually have the appearance of a submucosal mass and are difficult to delineate accurately by indirect examination. Direct laryngoscopy and CT scan are important for staging. They extend toward the thyroid cartilage and medial wall of the pyriform sinus quite early. Extension to the infrahyoid epiglottis is common. Initial invasion of the vocal cord may occur submucosally and may be difficult to detect at this stage. Gross invasion of the vocal cord is usually associated with thyroid cartilage invasion. Subglottic extension is uncommon until the lesion is advanced.

ARYEPIGLOTTIC FOLD AND ARYTENOID. Early lesions are usually exophytic growths. It is often difficult to decide whether they start on the medial wall of the pyriform sinus or the aryepiglottic fold. As the lesions advance, they extend to adjacent sites and eventually cause fixation of the larynx. Fixation is often secondary to involvement of the cricoarytenoid muscle and joint. It is often impossible to distinguish the cause of fixation at the time therapeutic decisions are made; CT scan may suggest the cause of fixation.

Advanced lesions invade the base of the tongue, pharyngeal wall, and postcricoid pharynx.

Vocal Cord

The majority of lesions begin on the free margin and upper surface of the vocal cord and are easily visible. When diagnosed, about two thirds are confined to one cord. The anterior portion of the cord is the most common site, and extension to the anterior commissure is frequent. Anterior commissure involvement is said to occur when no tumor-free cord can be seen anteriorly; when the lesion crosses to the opposite cord, anterior commissure invasion is certain. Small lesions isolated to the anterior commissure account for only 1% to 2% of all cases.

As vocal cord lesions enlarge, they extend to the ventricle, false cord, vocal process of the arytenoid, and subglottic region. Infiltrative lesions invade the vocal ligament and thyroarytenoid muscles, eventually reaching the thyroid cartilage. As cancers reach the cartilage, they tend at first to grow up or down along the paraglottic fat space rather than attacking the cartilage. The conus elasticus acts initially as a barrier to subglottic penetration. Advanced glottic lesions eventually penetrate through the thyroid cartilage or thyrocricoid membrane to enter the neck and often invade the thyroid gland.

A fixed cord with less than 1 cm of subglottic extension and no false cord involvement does not predict invasion of the thyroid cartilage; if the false cord is also involved, cartilage invasion is likely.[278]

Subglottic Larynx

The epithelium changes from squamous to respiratory about 5 mm below the free margin of the cord, and this is considered the beginning of subglottic area; the inferior border corresponds to the inferior border of the cricoid cartilage.

Subglottic cancers are uncommon. It is difficult to define whether a tumor started on the undersurface of the vocal cord or in the true subglottic larynx with extension to the cord. These lesions involve the cricoid cartilage quite early, because there is no intervening muscle layer. Involvement of the undersurface of the vocal cord is usually present, and fixation of a cord is the rule.

Lymphatic Spread

SUPRAGLOTTIC. The incidence of clinically positive nodes is 55% at the time of diagnosis; 16% are bilateral (Fig. 21-19).[7] Elective neck dissection will show pathologically positive nodes in 16% to 26% of cases; observation of the neck will be followed by the appearance of positive nodes in 33% of cases (see Table 21-4). Extralaryngeal spread to the pyriform sinus and vallecula or base of tongue increases the risk of node metastases. Delphian node involvement is rare and associated with extension to the anterior commissure or subglottic area.

GLOTTIC. The incidence of clinically positive nodes at diagnosis approaches zero for lesions confined to the cords

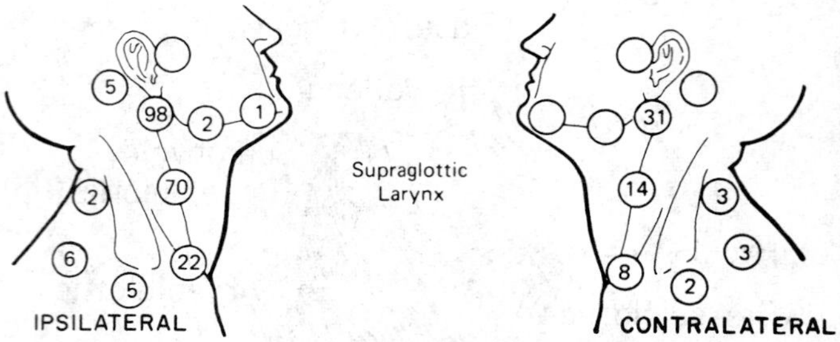

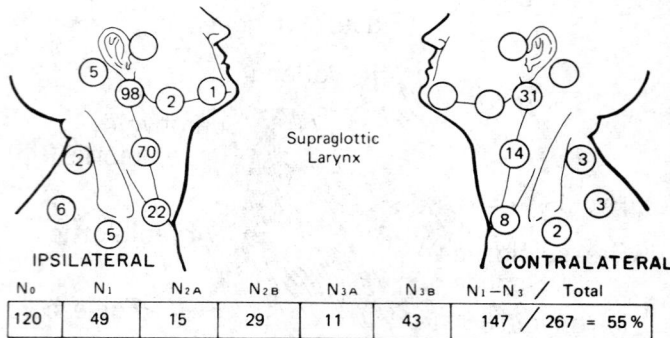

N_0	N_1	N_{2A}	N_{2B}	N_{3A}	N_{3B}	$N_1 - N_3$ / Total
120	49	15	29	11	43	147 / 267 = 55%

FIG. 21-19. Supraglottic larynx carcinoma: nodal distribution on admission at M.D. Anderson Hospital, 1948–1965. (Lindberg RD: Distribution of cervical lymph node metastases from squamous cell carcinoma of the upper respiratory and digestive tracts. Cancer 29:1446–1450, 1972)

(T1) and is 2% to 5% for T2 lesions. The incidence of neck metastases increases to 20% to 30% for T3 and T4 lesions. Supraglottic spread is associated with metastasis to the jugulodigastric nodes. Anterior commissure and anterior subglottic invasion is associated with midjugular, lower jugular, and midline pretracheal (Delphian) node involvement. Delphian node involvement is associated with spread to the lower neck nodes on both sides and a high rate of neck failure when treated by surgery alone.[279]

SUBGLOTTIC. Lederman[280] reported a 10% incidence of clinically positive lymph nodes on admission. Spread is primarily to the Delphian nodes and the lower jugular chain.

CLINICAL PICTURE

Presenting Symptoms

VOCAL CORDS. Carcinoma arising on the true vocal cords produces hoarseness at a very early stage. Pain or sore throat is a symptom of advanced lesions. Dysphagia and airway obstruction producing respiratory distress are features of advanced lesions and are rarely seen even with bulky early-stage lesions.

SUPRAGLOTTIC LARYNX. Hoarseness is not a prominent symptom for cancer of the supraglottic larynx until the lesion becomes quite extensive. Changes in voice quality are often subtle and described as having a "hot potato" quality, the voice quality associated with unexpectedly swallowing a bite of very hot food. Pain on swallowing, usually mild, is the most frequent initial symptom. The pain is often described as a mild, persistent irritation or sore throat, and often the patient can point to the area with one finger. Mild difficulty in swallowing is frequent; some patients report a sensation of a lump in the throat. Cancer of the epiglottis may be quite large before symptoms are produced. Pain is referred to the ear by way of the vagus nerve and auricular nerve of Arnold. A mass in the neck may be the first sign of a supraglottic cancer. Late symptoms include weight loss, foul breath, dysphagia, and aspiration.

Physical Examination

In addition to the simple, inexpensive laryngeal mirror, there are rigid and flexible fiberoptic illuminated endoscopes that are now used routinely as a complement to the laryngeal mirror examination. The Hopkins rod with a right-angle lens gives excellent visualization of the infrahyoid epiglottis and anterior commissure, areas that may be difficult, if not impossible, to visualize with the laryngeal mirror. The mirror gives a larger image of the larynx and hypolarynx than that obtained by direct laryngoscopy or by fiberoptic endoscopes. The flexible fiberoptic laryngoscope is inserted through the nose and is useful in the more difficult cases. Sedation with diazepam (Valium) intramuscularly usually will allow outpatient examination of the patient with the most active gag reflex.

A horseshoe-shaped epiglottis may prohibit adequate laryngeal examination for even the most skilled examiner. The tip of the epiglottis may be amputated with a biopsy forceps to facilitate indirect examination of the larynx. Loss of the tip of the epiglottis does not result in functional problems.

Determination of the mobility of the larynx frequently requires multiple examinations because the subtle distinctions between mobile, partially fixed, and fixed cords are often difficult and in fact seem to change from examination to examination. A cord that appeared mobile to the surgeon prior to direct laryngoscopy may show sluggish motion or even fixation after biopsy.

Invasion of the preepiglottic space occurs more frequently than one can diagnose clinically. Early invasion of the preepiglottic space is impossible to diagnose clinically. Ulceration of the infrahyoid epiglottis or fullness of the vallecula is an indirect sign of preepiglottic space invasion. Palpation of diffuse, firm fullness above the thyroid notch with widening of the space between the hyoid and thyroid cartilages signifies invasion of the preepiglottic space. Lateral soft-tissue roentgenograms of the neck may show the presence of irregular air cavities inferior to the vallecula in patients with lesions of the suprahyoid epiglottis that invade into the preepiglottic space by way of the vallecula. CT scan is excellent to show involvement of the prepiglottic space; the hyoepiglottic ligament often causes a shadow, which must not be confused with tumor.[281]

Postcricoid extension may be suspected when the laryngeal "crackle" or "click" disappears on physical examination. The diagnosis is confirmed by direct laryngoscopy and CT scan.

Early invasion of the thyroid cartilage is another difficult clinical diagnosis. Localized pain or tenderness to palpation over one ala of the thyroid cartilage is suggestive. Advanced tumors may actually penetrate through the thyroid ala and be felt as a small bulge on the thyroid ala. Cartilage invasion may be diagnosed by roentgenographic examination, but the cartilage must be calcified to show destructive changes.[282] CT scan of the larynx is of help in detecting catilage invasion, but irregular calcification of the cartilage, coupled with volume-averaging of the CT slice, creates technical problems in interpretation of early cartilage invasion.[281] MRI examination of the larynx has not been helpful as of 1987 due to motion artifact associated with long scanning times (Mancuso AA: Personal communication, 1987).

METHOD OF DIAGNOSIS AND STAGING

The differential diagnosis of laryngeal lesions includes papillomas, polyps, vocal nodules, fibromas, and granulomas. Papillomas can involve the epiglottis or false or true cords and can extend subglottically. They generally occur in children and young adults, possibly persisting into adulthood. Vocal polyps and nodules occur at the junction of the middle and anterior one third of the true vocal cords. There is usually a history of voice abuse followed by hoarseness.

Granulomas of the larynx usually occur as a result of intubation and are located on the posterior one third of the vocal cords, near the posterior commissure. Endoscopic removal is the definitive treatment.

Tuberculosis of the larynx, although rare, still occurs. Generally, the lesion is destructive in nature and occurs at the posterior commissure of the glottis, but the epiglottis and false cords may be involved. The appearance mimics cancer; pulmonary tuberculosis is usually present.

Direct laryngoscopy for biopsy with frozen section is usually performed with the patient under a general anesthetic. A generous biopsy, taken from the bulk of the lesion, will help the pathologist to make the diagnosis. For staging purposes, biopsies should be obtained from suspicious areas as well as areas grossly involved.

Staging

The AJCC staging system for laryngeal primary cancer is as follows:[12]

Supraglottis

- Tis Carcinoma in situ
- T1 Tumor confined to region of origin with normal mobility
- T2 Tumor involving adjacent supraglottic site(s) or glottis without fixation
- T3 Tumor limited to the larynx with fixation or extension to involve postcricoid area, medial wall of pyriform sinus, or preepiglottic space
- T4 Massive tumor extending beyond the larynx to involve oropharynx, soft tissues of neck, or destruction of thyroid cartilage

Glottis

- Tis Carcinoma in situ
- T1 Tumor confined to vocal cord(s) with normal mobility (includes involvement of anterior or posterior commissures)
- T2 Supraglottic or subglottic extension of tumor with normal or impaired cord mobility, or both
- T3 Tumor confined to the larynx with cord fixation
- T4 Massive tumor with thyroid cartilage destruction or extension beyond the confines of the larynx, or both

Subglottis

Tis Carcinoma in situ
T1 Tumor confined to the subglottic region
T2 Tumor extension to vocal cords with normal or impaired cord mobility
T3 Tumor confined to larynx with cord fixation
T4 Massive tumor with cartilage destruction or extension beyond the confines of the larynx, or both

Staging Procedures

Staging procedures for laryngeal cancer include the following:

Indirect laryngoscopy (with photography)
CT scan with contrast prior to biopsy
Direct laryngoscopy with multiple biopsies
Chest roentgenogram

Direct laryngoscopy with multiple biopsies is required to assess extent of tumor and confirm the diagnosis. The ventricles, subglottic area, apex of the pyriform sinus, and postcricoid area must be examined carefully, because these areas are not consistently seen by any other method.

Indirect laryngoscopy actually gives a better panorama and allows better evaluation of function than can be obtained at direct laryngoscopy.

CT scans have replaced conventional tomography and contrast laryngography. CT scan is not useful for early vocal cord lesions.

CT scan may show invasion of the thyroid and cricoid cartilage, cricoarytenoid joint, or preepiglottic fat space, and soft-tissue extension into the neck. CT scan is especially useful for examination of the subglottic space.[45,281,283]

TREATMENT

Vocal Cord Carcinoma

SELECTION OF TREATMENT MODALITY. The goal is cure with the best functional results and the least risk of a serious complication. External beam irradiation and operation are the only curative modalities available.

Dysplasia, Hyperkeratosis, Leukoplakia. Complete stripping of the mucosa of the cord is often curative for lesions classified as leukoplakia, hyperkeratosis, or dysplasia. Careful observation is essential since regrowth often occurs. While repeated stripping may seem a satisfactory plan of management, the cords may become thickened and the voice harsh, and it becomes increasingly difficult to tell whether invasive tumor is present. Irradiation may be recommended when there are repeated recurrences at short intervals.[284]

Carcinoma in situ. Lesions diagnosed as carcinoma in situ may sometimes be controlled by stripping the cord. However, it is difficult to exclude the possibility of microinvasion in these specimens. Recurrence is frequent, and the cord may become thickened and the voice hoarse with repeated stripping.

We recommend irradiation for carcinoma in situ in patients with multiple recurrences that appear in rapid succession.

Many of the patients treated in the past as carcinoma in situ have had obvious residual gross lesions that probably contained invasive carcinoma. We have sometimes proceeded with radiation therapy rather than put the patient through a repeat biopsy.

Early Vocal Cord Lesions (T1, T2). In most centers, irradiation is the initial treatment prescribed for early lesions, with operation reserved for salvage of irradiation failures. While cordectomy or hemilaryngectomy will produce comparable cure rates for selected T1 or T2 vocal cord lesions, irradiation is generally the preferred initial therapy. The major advantages of irradiation compared to cordectomy or hemilaryngectomy are that a major operation is avoided and the voice quality is likely to be better. The voice after hemilaryngectomy remains hoarse; most physicians tell the patient that his voice will be as hoarse as it is now or even worse. After successful irradiation, the voice is usually better than before therapy, but occasional cases are seen in which there is no improvement or, uncommonly, a worsening of voice quality. Hemilaryngectomy may be used as a salvage operation in suitable cases after irradiation failure. Even if the patient has a local recurrence after a salvage hemilaryngectomy, there is a third chance with total laryngectomy, which may still be successful. Hemilaryngectomy is also used in patients who have had prior head and neck irradiation and for the patient who cannot afford 6 weeks away from home or job for the irradiation series.[285]

Although there have been reports that anterior commissure involvement predicts for radiation therapy failure or necrosis, we find no evidence in our data to support this finding.[286]

Currently, there is an increasing use of the carbon dioxide laser in removing benign lesions and very early carcinomas involving the true vocal cords. Although this is being tried in some centers, the experience has not been great enough at this point to determine the long-term results, and the experience of the laserist is most important. If laser is used, it should be used as a cutting instrument rather than to vaporize the tumor. Using this technique, small midcord lesions might be treated with the laser, but the voice would not be as good as expected after radiation therapy.

Verrucous lesions have the reputation of being unresponsive to irradiation and in some instances of losing their verrucous nature to convert into invasive, often anaplastic, metastasizing lesions after unsuccessful irradiation. The authors, however, have observed typical verrucous lesions that have disappeared with radiation therapy and not recurred. Burns and co-workers[287] have also made this observation. The authors favor hemilaryngectomy for early verrucous carcinoma of the glottis, but do not hesitate to use radiation therapy if the alternative is total laryngectomy.

Advanced Vocal Cord Lesions (T3, T4). The mainstay of treatment in most centers is total laryngectomy with or without postoperative irradiation. In some centers, radiation therapy is the initial modality for T3 lesions, with surgery reserved for the failures. The most frequent sites of local failure after total laryngectomy are around the tracheal stoma, in the base of the tongue, and in the neck nodes. If the neck is clinically negative prior to operation and if postoperative irradiation is planned, no neck dissection is done and irradiation is used to treat both sides of the neck. If nodes are clinically positive, a radical neck dissection is done with total laryngectomy. Postoperative irradiation may be used to control subclinical disease in the opposite neck as well as to help prevent recurrence in the dissected neck.

Fixed cord lesions (T3) treated by irradiation fall into two groups. One group consists of patients with fixed, bulky, bilateral, advanced lesions who either refuse laryngectomy or are medically inoperable. Irradiation of these lesions is seldom successful; about 10% to 20% are cured. The second group includes patients with a fixed cord but minimal total tumor bulk. They usually have subglottic extension and minor supraglottic extension confined to one side of the larynx; the airway is adequate and the larynx relatively easy to visualize. An attempt at irradiation in this group is worthwhile. The patient must be willing to return for follow-up every month for the first 2 years and understand that total laryngectomy may be recommended purely on clinical grounds without biopsy-proven recurrence. The reported local control rate for fixed cord lesions (T3N0) varies from 30% to 70%.[14,288,289]

The major difficulty in the use of irradiation for advanced lesions is in distinguishing between radiation edema and local recurrence during follow-up examinations. Progressive edema, increased hoarseness, pain, and immobility of a formerly mobile cord are all signs of recurrence. If the edema is stable or limited to the arytenoids, the patient may be watched, especially if there is no pain. The detection of recurrence is difficult because the surface epithelium may be intact, with tumor growing submucosally. Deep biopsies are necessary, but may aggravate the radiation damage if no tumor is found. The patient must be apprised that total laryngectomy may be recommended if suspicion of recurrence is very high, even without proof of recurrence.

SURGICAL TREATMENT. Stripping of the cord implies transoral removal of the mucosa of the edge of the cord. The operating microscope assists the surgeon in total stripping of the mucosa.

Cordectomy is an excision of the vocal cord. Its use usually is confined to small lesions of the middle one third of the cord. Cordectomy is generally reserved for the uncommon situation in which there is a postirradiation recurrence limited to the middle one third of the cord with normal mobility. Following cordectomy a pseudocord is formed, and the patient has a useful, if somewhat harsh, voice. A portion of the adjacent thyroid cartilage may be removed with the cord.

Hemilaryngectomy is a partial, "vertical" laryngectomy that allows removal of limited cord lesions with voice preservation. There are definite restrictions with this operation. One entire cord plus 5 mm of the opposite cord is the maximum cordal involvement suitable for the operation in men; generally the operation is reserved for lesions involving one cord. Partial fixation of one cord is not a contraindication to hemilaryngectomy, but only a few surgeons have attempted hemilaryngectomy for fixed cord lesions. The maximum subglottic extension allowable is 9 mm to 10 mm anteriorly and 5 mm posteriorly, because the cricoid cartilage must be preserved. Extension to the epiglottis, false cord, or interarytenoid area is a contraindication to hemilaryngectomy. One arytenoid may be sacrificed, but the vocal cord must be fixed in the midline or postoperative aspiration is a possibility, and therefore the patient must have a satisfactory pulmonary status.

The last surgical alternative is total laryngectomy with or without radical neck dissection. Total laryngectomy is used as a salvage procedure for radiation failure in the early lesions that are not suited for conservative operations. It is the operation of choice for advanced lesions. The entire larynx is removed, the pharynx is reconstituted, and a permanent tracheostomy is required.

Artificial speech is created by a number of techniques. Electronic devices may be used immediately after the operation. Esophageal speech is accomplished by belching swallowed air that is used to produce phonation. Only 10% of patients develop satisfactory esophageal speech.

There have been numerous attempts to recreate the larynx after total laryngectomy, with very few producing predictable results. There have been attempts to surgically create a fistula between the trachea and esophagus to shunt air to the pharynx. The problem has been one of aspiration in a large number of cases. Recently, prosthetic devices (*e.g.*, the Singer-Blom valve) have been developed for insertion into a tracheoesophageal fistula; the prosthesis allows the patient to speak without the problem of aspiration.[290–293] This simple innovation has made the impact of total laryngectomy less devastating. Most patients can learn to speak with this technique since it does not require the training and motivation needed for esophageal speech.[294]

IRRADIATION TECHNIQUE. Irradiation for early vocal cord cancer is delivered by small portals covering only the primary lesion. The incidence of lymph node involvement is so small (0–1%) that elective irradiation of nodes usually is recommended only for T3 or T4 lesions or for T2 lesions with poorly differentiated histology.[289] Radiation portals for T1 lesions usually extend from the thyroid notch superiorly to the inferior border of the cricoid; the posterior border depends on posterior extension of the tumor. The field size ranges from 4 × 4 cm to 5 × 5 cm. Portals larger than this increase the risk of edema without increasing the cure rate. Because the portals are small and the skin of the neck is mobile, it is the authors' practice to have the physician check the portal on the treatment table each day by palpation of the anatomic landmarks. The portals for T2 lesions are slightly larger, depending on the anatomical extent of the lesion. The dose scheme used at the University of Florida for T1 and T2 lesions is shown in Table 21-41.

Treatment plans for T3 and T4 lesions include the primary lesion and the subdigastric, midjugular, low jugular, and Delphian lymph nodes. The initial treatment with once-a-day fractionation is delivered at 200 cGy/day to a total of 4600 cGy. The portal then is reduced to include only the primary lesion, and the dose per fraction is increased to 225 cGy; the final tumor dose is 6600 cGy to 7000 cGy. The low

TABLE 21-41. Vocal Cord Cancer: Radiation Treatment Plan at the University of Florida (September 1980)

Stage	*Description*	*External-Beam Irradiation (cGy Tumor Dose)*
T1	Early, no visible tumor	5625/25 fractions/5 weeks
T1	Moderate size	6300/28 fractions/5.5 weeks
T2	Early, normal motion	6300/28 fractions/5.5 weeks
T2	Moderate size, reduced motion	6525/29 fractions/6 weeks
T3–T4	Fixed cord	See text

neck is treated through a separate anterior portal.[289] Since 1978, T3 or T4 lesions (and since 1986, T2 lesions) have been managed with 120 cGy twice a day, to a total tumor dose of 7440 cGy to 7680 cGy.[14]

MANAGEMENT OF RECURRENCE. Most recurrences appear within 24 months, but late recurrences may appear after 5 years.[295] Additionally, these patients are prone to develop second primaries in the head and neck area, and 5% to 10% develop lung cancer; for this reason the authors recommend a chest roentgenogram every 6 months.

With careful follow-up, recurrence often is detected before the patient notices return of hoarseness. Edema of the larynx, particularly the false cords and arytenoids, suggests recurrence. Fixation of the cord usually implies local recurrence; the authors have observed two patients who developed a fixed cord with an otherwise normal-appearing larynx and have not shown evidence of recurrence. A paralyzed left vocal cord should also suggest the possibility of lung cancer.

Irradiation failures (T1–T2) are almost always salvaged by cordectomy, hemilaryngectomy, or total laryngectomy. The salvage rate for T3 lesions recurring after radiation therapy is approximately 60%.

Salvage by radiation therapy for recurrences or new tumors that appear after hemilaryngectomy is about 50%. Lee and co-workers[296] reported 7 successes in 12 patients; one lesion subsequently was controlled by total laryngectomy. Isolated recurrences at the trachael stoma may be managed by radiation therapy or surgery. Balm and co-workers[297] reported the results for radiation therapy in conjunction with simultaneous chemotherapy (vincristine, bleomycin, and methotrexate) for 8 patients treated between 1978 and 1985. Three patients had been disease-free for 7, 3, and 2.5 years and 2 patients for less than 1 year after treatment. Only 1 patient developed recurrent disease at the stoma.

A multi-institutional surgical experience in the management of stomal recurrence for the years 1970–1985 was reported by Gluckman and co-workers.[298] Forty-one came to operation. The 2-year determinate survival was 24%. Patients with localized recurrences had a 45% 5-year survival rate.

Supraglottic Larynx Carcinoma

SELECTION OF TREATMENT MODALITY. For purposes of treatment planning, patients may be considered to be in either an early or favorable group suitable for radiation therapy or supraglottic laryngectomy, or a late or unfavorable group managed either by total laryngectomy (with or without radiation therapy) or by radiation therapy with laryngectomy reserved for recurrence at the primary site.

The division of lesions into early and late is arbitrary. T1 and T2 lesions are nearly always early or favorable cases, but T2 lesions, and occasionally T1 lesions, can be quite extensive and still not produce fixation yet not be technically or medically suitable for voice-sparing surgery. Lesions can be staged T3 without fixation and with minimal extension to the postcricoid area, medial wall of the pyriform sinus, preepiglottic space, or base of tongue, and be very suitable for radiation therapy with surgical salvage or extended supraglottic laryngectomy. Fixation and cartilage invasion do not preclude attempted cure with radiation therapy.

EARLY SUPRAGLOTTIC LESIONS. Treatment of the primary lesion is either by external beam irradiation or supraglottic laryngectomy. Total laryngectomy would rarely be indicated as the initial treatment for this group of patients and is reserved for those in whom the initial treatment fails.

Irradiation and supraglottic laryngectomy are both highly successful modes of therapy for the early lesions, and for this reason it is seldom necessary to combine radiation therapy and surgery for initial management of the primary lesions; however, combined treatment may be indicated to control the neck disease. Approximately 50% of patients having a supraglottic laryngectomy at the University of Florida have received postoperative radiation therapy.

The following paragraphs outline our guidelines for selection of either supraglottic laryngectomy or radiation therapy. The patient and family are often instrumental in making the decision, and should be apprised of the alternative modes of therapy.

Approximately one half of the patients seen in our clinic whose lesions are anatomically suitable for treatment by a supraglottic laryngectomy are not suitable for medical reasons (*e.g.*, inadequate pulmonary status or other major medical problems) and are managed by radiation therapy. When the patient is both technically and medically suitable for supraglottic laryngectomy, the patient is apprised of the alternative and makes the decision. The decision process is best described as whimsical most of the time.

The only absolute contraindication to radiation therapy is prior radiation therapy to the laryngeal area. Analysis of local disease control by anatomical subsite within the supraglottic larynx shows no obvious differences in local control by radiation therapy when comparing similar stages (Table 21-42).[301] Similarly, analysis of local control by anatomical subsite shows no obvious difference in local control by supraglottic laryngectomy when comparing similar stages. Transglottic lesions are not suitable for conventional supraglottic laryngectomy, but they may be managed by radiation therapy. Invasion of the preepiglottic space is not a contraindication to supraglottic laryngectomy or radiation therapy.

Lesions that are mainly exophytic are usually suitable for radiation therapy. Extensive submucosal disease predicts a less favorable result; these patients often have partial airway obstruction prior to treatment. Unilateral vocal cord fixation due to invasion of the cricoarytenoid joint is not a contraindication to radiation therapy, but fixation due to extension to the vocal cord or subglottic area predicts a poor result with radiation therapy. Women tend to have a better cure rate than men, and the indications for radiation therapy can be extended.

The status of the neck often determines the selection of treatment for the primary lesion. Patients with clinically negative neck nodes and a high risk for occult bilateral neck disease may be treated by radiation therapy because of the ease of bilateral elective neck irradiation (*e.g.*, poorly differentiated carcinoma of the suprahyoid epiglottis with midline base of tongue extension). Alternatively, supraglottic laryngectomy and bilateral conservative neck dissections may be done.

When a patient presents with an early-stage primary lesion but advanced neck disease (N2B or N3), combined treatment is frequently necessary to produce a high rate of control of the neck disease. In these cases, the primary lesion is preferably treated for cure by irradiation, with neck dissection(s) added to the involved side(s) of the neck. If such a patient is managed with supraglottic laryngectomy followed by a neck dissection and postoperative radiation therapy, the functional result is expected to be poorer, as it is impossible to irradiate both sides of the neck and not irradiate the primary site. This means that the primary site, which was adequately treated by supraglottic laryngectomy, is unnecessarily irradiated, and the resulting edema may produce an unsatisfactory functional result.

If the patient has early, resectable neck disease (N1 or N2A) and surgery is elected for the primary site, postoperative irradiation is only added because of unexpected findings (*e.g.*, positive margin, multiple positive nodes, or extracapsular spread). We prefer to avoid routine high-dose preoperative or postoperative irradiation in conjunction with a supraglottic laryngectomy because the lymphedema of the remaining larynx may be considerable, although it will partially or completely subside with time.

LATE SUPRAGLOTTIC LESIONS (LATE T3, T4). Selected T3 and T4 lesions of the upper supraglottic larynx that are mainly exophytic can be treated by irradiation, since the control rate is fairly high. Borderline lesions are given a trial of irradiation to 4500 cGy to 5000 cGy and if response is good, irradiation is continued for cure. If response is unsatisfactory, irradiation is stopped and total laryngectomy is done 4 to 6 weeks later. There is no proof that one may select patients by this therapeutic trial, but many of the T3 and T4 successes were culled out in this fashion.

Lesions unsuitable for irradiation are managed by total laryngectomy. If the neck disease is resectable, then operation is the initial treatment, and postoperative irradiation is added if needed. If the neck disease is unresectable or borderline, preoperative irradiation is used.

Surgical Treatment

SUPRAGLOTTIC LARYNGECTOMY. Supraglottic laryngectomy is a voice-sparing operation that can be tailored to the individual supraglottic lesion. Because the patient has an increased tendency to aspirate, it is essential that adequate pulmonary reserves be present, as determined by blood gases, pulmonary function tests, chest roentgenogram, and a work test (walking the patient up two flights of stairs to determine tolerance to pulmonary stress). The voice quality is generally good following supraglottic laryngectomy. All patients have some difficulty swallowing in the immediate postoperative period, but almost all learn to swallow in a short time; motivation is the key factor in learning to swallow.

Supraglottic laryngectomy can be used successfully for lesions involving the epiglottis, a single arytenoid, the aryepiglottic fold, and false vocal cords. Extension of the tumor

TABLE 21-42. Supraglottic Larynx Carcinoma: Comparison of Control of Primary Lesion by Irradiation by Subsites in Two Series

	T1		*T2*		*T3*		*T4*	
	*MDAH**	*UF†*	*MDAH*	*UF*	*MDAH*	*UF*	*MDAH*	*UF*
Suprahyoid epiglottis	3/4	4/4	7/7	6/8	13/15	3/3	3/5	2/8
Infrahyoid epiglottis	5/5	2/2	11/12	8/11	3/4	2/3	1/1	0/2
Aryepiglottic folds	5/5	1/1	6/7	2/2	3/4	4/6	3/6	0/1
False cords	2/2	3/4	8/10	4/5		0/2	1/1	
Arytenoids	2/2	1/1	1/1					

Million RR, Cassisi NJ, Parsons JT, et al: Radiation therapy in the management of carcinoma of the larynx. In Fried MP: The Larynx. Boston, Little, Brown (in press)

*MDAH: University of Texas M. D. Anderson Hospital and Tumor Institute (1964–1972); data from Fletcher and Goepfert.[299]

†UF: University of Florida (1964–1981); data from Mendenhall et al.[300]

to the true vocal cords, anterior commissure, or both arytenoids, fixation, or cartilage invasion excludes supraglottic laryngectomy. The extended supraglottic laryngectomy may be used to include the base of the tongue to the level of the circumvallate papillae as long as one lingual artery is preserved. A neck dissection on one or both sides may be added as part of the supraglottic laryngectomy; about 35% of patients will have histologically positive nodes even when the neck is negative to clinical appraisal. Postoperative irradiation is added only as needed, based on the surgical and pathologic findings. The incision is usually a modified Schobinger, a half-H, or a hockey stick incision. If the likelihood of a total laryngectomy is high, than an apron flap is used. The neck dissection is completed and left attached to the thyrohyoid membrane. The perichondrium of the larynx is then elevated in continuity with the strap muscles. This is very important because it will be used to close the surgical defect. Saw cuts are made through the thyroid cartilage and the hyoid bone so that the preepiglottic space is included in the specimen. The pharynx is entered above the hyoid through the vallecula. The specimen is removed, leaving only the arytenoids and true vocal cords. If one arytenoid has to be sacrificed, the cord must be fixed in the midline to prevent aspiration. The defect is closed by suturing the previously saved perichondrium and muscle into the base of the tongue. After the tracheostomy is removed, usually within seven days, the patient is retrained in the act of swallowing. The patient is then discharged when he can swallow 2000 cc or more without significant coughing.

TOTAL LARYNGECTOMY. The entire larynx and preepiglottic space are resected en bloc and a permanent tracheostomy is fashioned. A portion of the thyroid gland usually is included with the specimen. The pharynx is sutured to the base of tongue.

Irradiation Technique

The primary lesion and both sides of the neck are included with opposed lateral portals. The dose for T1 lesions is 6000 cGy in 6 weeks to 6500 cGy in 7 weeks. The dose for T2–T3 lesions is 6500 cGy to 7000 cGy in 6.5 to 7 weeks (1 fraction per day). Since 1978 the T2–T3 lesions have been managed with 120 cGy twice a day to a total dose of 7460 cGy to 7680 cGy. The lower neck nodes are irradiated through a separate anterior portal. An anterior "boost" portal may be used for the last 1000 cGy for suprahyoid epiglottic lesions that invade the vallecula (see the section on the base of the tongue). It is important to spare a small strip of anterior midline skin, which helps to reduce the degree of lymphedema.[283,300]

Patients develop a sore throat, loss of taste, and moderate dryness during irradiation. Edema of the arytenoids may occur and produce the sensation of a lump in the throat. Tracheostomy is seldom necessary before the start of therapy, even for bulky lesions.

Edema of the larynx may persist for several months to a year. Radical neck dissection increases the degree of lymphedema on the side of the operation. The lymphedema of the larynx and submental space resolves together. Patients who continue to smoke and drink heighten the side-effects of dryness, dysphagia, and hoarseness.

Combined Treatment Policies

Either surgery or irradiation alone is preferred for the early primary lesions.

If total laryngectomy is required and the lesion is resectable, postoperative irradiation is preferred, since there is no evidence that preoperative irradiation produces any better local–regional control or survival rates. Radiation therapy is added for close or positive margins, invasion of soft tissues of the neck, cartilage invasion, and N2 or N3 neck disease. The high-risk areas are usually the base of the tongue and neck. The stomal area is at risk only when subglottic extension is present or there is tumor in the low neck lymph nodes. Complications related to postoperative irradiation are relatively uncommon in this group.

Irradiation is used prior to total laryngectomy for patients with technically unresectable neck nodes, as a trial of radiation therapy prior to deciding on radiation therapy alone or total laryngectomy, or when scheduling problems require a long delay to operation.

A number of patients either refuse laryngectomy or are medically unsuitable for the operation; hence, irradiation is the treatment by default. However, a few of these patients can be cured, and one should not take a hopeless attitude.[295]

MANAGEMENT OF RECURRENCE. Failures after supraglottic laryngectomy or irradiation frequently can be salvaged by further treatment; recognition of recurrence should be pursued vigorously. Salvage of recurrences that develop after total laryngectomy and preoperative or postoperative irradiation is quite uncommon.

Subglottic Larynx Carcinoma

Early lesions are treated with radiation therapy, and advanced lesions are usually managed by total laryngectomy and postoperative radiation therapy.

RESULTS OF TREATMENT

Vocal Cord Cancer

SURGICAL RESULTS. Ogura and co-workers[302] reported a 3-year determinate survival without disease of 86% for patients treated by hemilaryngectomy. The local-regional recurrence rate was 6%. The 3-year determinate survival rate without disease for patients treated by total laryngectomy with or without radical neck dissection was 70%. The local–regional recurrence rate was 22%.

RADIATION THERAPY RESULTS. The results of irradiation for 304 patients with T1 and T2 squamous cell carcinoma of the vocal cord treated by irradiation are presented in Table 21-43. The results are grouped by the operation that would have been required as determined by the anatomical extent of disease. Voice preservation for the same group is shown in Table 21-44.[286]

TABLE 21-43. Carcinoma of the Glottic Larynx: Local Control — 304 Patients (No. Controlled/No. Treated)

*T Stage**	*Subgroup*	*Size*	*Excluded†*	*Local Control*	*No. Salvaged/No. Attempted*		*Ultimate Local Control*
					Hemilaryngectomy	*Total Laryngectomy*	
T1a	C	<5 mm	1	12/12 (100%)			12/12 (100%)
		5–15 mm	6	73/78 (94%)	3/4	0/1	76/78 (97%)
		>15 mm	2	45/50 (90%)		4/5	49/50 (98%)
T1b	HL	All	0	14/15 (93%)		0/1	14/15 (93%)
	TL	All	2	15/16 (94%)	0/1		15/16 (94%)
T2a	HL	All	5	23/27 (85%)		4/4	27/27 (100%)
	TL	All	2	27/38 (71%)	2/3	7/8	36/38 (95%)
T2b	HL	All	3	13/18 (72%)	1/2	2/3	16/18 (89%)
	TL	All	2	18/25 (72%)		4/6	22/25 (88%)

Mendenhall WM, Parsons JT, Stringer SP, et al: T1–T2 vocal cord carcinoma: A basis for comparing the results of irradiation and surgery. Head Neck Surg 10:373–377, 1988.

C, suitable for cordectomy; HL, suitable for hemilaryngectomy; TL, suitable for total laryngectomy.

*T1 lesions were subdivided as T1a, involvement of one true vocal cord with or without involvement of the anterior commissure; T1b, involvement of both true vocal cords. T2 lesions were subdivided according to mobility of the vocal cord(s): T2a, normal mobility; T2b, reduced mobility.

†Excludes 23 patients who died of intercurrent disease <2 years after treatment with vocal cord cancer controlled.

TABLE 21-44. Glottic Larynx Carcinoma: Voice Preservation in 304 Patients Treated with Radiation Therapy (No. Patients with Voice Preservation/No. Treated)

T Stage	*Subgroup*	*Size*	*Proportion with Voice Preservation*
T1a	C	<5 mm	13/13
		5–15 mm	83/86 (97%)
		>15 mm	47/52 (90%)
T1b	HL	All	14/15 (93%)
	TL	All	17/18 (94%)
T2a	HL	All	28/32 (88%)
	TL	All	31/40 (78%)
T2b	HL	All	17/21 (81%)
	TL	All	20/27 (74%)

Mendenhall WM, Parsons JT, Stringer SP, et al: T1–T2 vocal cord carcinoma: A basis for comparing results of irradiation and surgery. Head Neck Surg 10:373–377, 1988.

C, suitable for cordectomy; HL, suitable for hemilaryngectomy; TL, suitable for total laryngectomy.

A few local failures continue to appear after 5 years of follow-up. Some of these late failures occur on the opposite cord and undoubtedly represent new cancers. The same pattern of late recurrence is also seen after hemilaryngectomy.

The reported results for T3 carcinoma of the vocal cord according to treatment modality are shown in Table 21-45. Irradiation was generally selected for fixed lesions with involvement of one vocal cord and with an adequate airway. The current local control rate for T3 lesions managed with 120 cGy twice a day is 70% (10 of 14).[289]

Treatment results for T3 glottic carcinomas for seven series are shown in Table 21-46 and the results for T4 lesions in Table 21-47.

Supraglottic Larynx Cancer

A comparison of irradiation and surgical results for 195 patients managed at the University of Florida over a period of 20 years (1964 to 1984) is presented in Tables 21-48 through 21-54.[315] Selection of therapy was individualized. Supraglottic laryngectomy became a surgical option in 1975. The local control rate for radiation therapy alone, with the use of twice-daily fractionation (since 1978), is 82% for T2 and 71% for T3 lesions.

The absolute survival rates obtained with surgery alone or with combined operation and radiation therapy for stage IV disease are shown in Table 21-55.[299]

COMPLICATIONS OF TREATMENT

Surgical

Repeated stripping of the cord may result in a thickened cord and hoarse voice. Neel and co-workers[316] reported a 26% incidence of nonfatal complications for cordectomy. Imme-

TABLE 21-45. Vocal Cord Carcinoma, Stage T3: Results of Treatment

	No. of Patients	*Initial Local Control (%)*	*Ultimate Local Control (%)*	*Control Above the Clavicles (%)*	*5-Year Survival (%)*	
					Absolute	*Determinate*
Irradiation + surgical salvage	22	61	83	79	53	67
Surgery ± irradiation*	46	84	89	87	50	68

Data from Mendenhall et al.[289]

*Preoperative, 7 patients; postoperative, 14 patients.

TABLE 21-46. T3 Glottic Cancer: Results of Treatment with Irradiation Alone

Reference	*No. of Patients*	*Percentage of All Glottic Cancers Irradiated*	*Minimum Follow-up (yr)*	*Local Control (%)*		*5-Year Survival (%)*	
				Initial	*Ultimate**	*Actuarial*	*Determinate*
Harwood et al.,[288] Toronto, 1980	112	12†	3	51	77	55	74‡
Wang,[303] Mass. General, 1974	56	10	3	52	73		
Mills,[304] University of Cape Town, 1979	18	18	2	44	78	67§	
Fletcher et al.,[305] MDAH, 1969	17	4	2	76			
Stewart et al.,[306] Manchester, 1975	67	23	10	57	69		57
Mendenhall et al.,[289] University of Florida, 1984	22	8**	2	61††	83††	53‡‡	67

Mendenhall WM, Million RR, Sharkey DE, et al: Stage T3 squamous cell carcinoma of the glottic larynx treated with surgery and/or radiation therapy. Int J Radiat Oncol Biol Phys 10:357–363, 1984.

*After surgical salvage of irradiation failures.

†Percentage of glottic cancers treated from 1/65 through 12/74.[307,308]

‡Five-year actuarial determinate survival.

§Crude disease-free survival.

**Percentage of glottic cancers, stage T1–T3, treated from 10/64 through 10/77.[309]

††Excludes 4 patients who were not evaluable for control at the primary site.[289]

††Absolute survival.

diate postoperative complications included atelectasis and pneumonia, severe subcutaneous emphysema in the neck, bleeding from the tracheotomy site or larynx, wound complications, and airway obstruction requiring tracheotomy. Late complications included removal of granulation tissue by direct laryngoscopy to exclude recurrence, extrusion of cartilage, laryngeal stenosis, and obstructing laryngeal web.

The postoperative complications of hemilaryngectomy include aspiration, chondritis, wound slough, inadequate glottic closure, and anterior commissure webs.

The postoperative complications of total laryngectomy may include operative death, hemorrhage, fistula, chondritis, wound slough, carotid rupture, dysphagia, and pharyngeal/esophageal stenosis.

The complication rate following supraglottic laryngectomy is about 10%, including fistula formation, aspiration, chondritis, dysphagia, dyspnea, and carotid rupture.

Radiation Therapy

After irradiation, the quality and volume of the voice tend to diminish at the end of the day. Many patients report changes in voice with changes in weather, upper respiratory infections, and the like. Edema of the larynx is the most common sequela following irradiation for glottic or supraglottic lesions. The rate of clearance of the edema is related to dose of radiation, volume of tissue irradiated, addition of a neck dissection, continued use of alcohol and tobacco, and the size and extent of the original lesion. Edema is accentuated by a radical neck dissection; it may require 6 months to as long as 2 years for the lymphedema to disappear. Steroids (*e.g.*, Decadron) have been used to reduce edema secondary to radiation effect after recurrence has been ruled out by biopsy. If ulceration and pain occur, antibiotics are used.

Soft-tissue necrosis leading to chondritis occurs in about

TABLE 21-47. T4 Glottic Cancer: Results of Treatment

Author	*Stage*	*No. of Patients*	*Method of Treatment*	*Results (NED)*
Jesse[310]	T4 N0–N+	48	Laryngectomy	54% at 4 years
Ogura et al.[302]	T4 N0	11	Laryngectomy	45% at 3 years
Skolnick et al.[311]	T4 N0	7	Laryngectomy	30% at 5 years
Vermund[312]	T4 N0	31	Laryngectomy	35% at 5 years
Stewart and Jackson[313]	T4 N0	13	Irradiation with surgery for salvage	38% at 5 years
Harwood et al.[314]	T4 N0	56	Irradiation with surgery for salvage	49% at 5 years*

Modified from Harwood AR, Beale FA, Cummings BJ, et al: T4N0M0 glottic cancer: An analysis of dose-time volume factors. Int J Radiat Oncol Biol Phys 7:1507–1512, 1981.

NED, no evidence of disease.

*Actuarial survival, uncorrected for deaths due to intercurrent disease.

TABLE 21-48. Supraglottic Larynx Carcinoma: Local Control Following Initial Treatment as a Function of T Stage — 152 Patients (No. Controlled/No. Treated)

T Stage	*Irradiation Alone*	*Surgery ± Adjuvant Irradiation*	*Significance Levels*[144,145]
T1	12/13 (92%)	9/9	0.591
T2	29/36 (81%)	20/25 (80%)	0.603
T3	12/20 (60%)	17/18 (94%)	0.015
T4	4/13 (31%)	15/18 (83%)	0.005

Weems DH, Mendenhall WM, Parsons JT, et al: Squamous cell carcinoma of the supraglottic larynx treated with surgery and/or radiation therapy. Int J Radiat Oncol Biol Phys 13:1483–1487, 1987.

1% of patients. Soft-tissue and cartilage necroses mimic recurrence with hoarseness, pain, and edema; a laryngectomy may be recommended in desperation for fear of recurrent cancer, even though biopsies show only necrosis.

Mendenhall and co-workers[317] recorded a serious complication rate of 0.54% in 184 T1 lesions and 3.36% in 119 T2 lesions (Table 21-56). Complications were related to use of a single portal, T stage, and high total dose.

Combined Treatment

Most surgeons agree that preoperative irradiation is generally associated with an increased risk of an operative complication and slightly prolonged hospitalization. The increased risk is not prohibitive by any means, but if the same goal can be accomplished by postoperative irradiation, the overall complication rates are reduced. The major late effects of combined treatment are an increased fibrosis of soft tissues, stomal stenosis, and pharyngeal stricture.

HYPOPHARYNX: PHARYNGEAL WALLS, PYRIFORM SINUS, AND POSTCRICOID PHARYNX

Both the oropharyngeal and hypopharyngeal walls will be considered together because there is no distinct difference in the presentation, treatment, or prognosis. The great majority of hypopharyngeal lesions originate in the pyriform sinus. Postcricoid carcinomas fortunately are quite uncommon in the United States.

ANATOMY

The epithelium of the pharyngeal mucous membrane is squamous. It is continuous with the mucous membrane of the nasopharynx; there is no visible point or line of transition. The dividing point between the nasopharynx and posterior pharyngeal wall is actually Passavant's ridge, a muscular ring that contracts to close the nasopharynx during swallowing. The posterior and lateral walls are surrounded by the thin constrictor muscles. Between the constrictor muscle and the prevertebral fascia that covers the longitudinal spine muscles (longus colli and longus capitis) is a thin layer of loose areolar tissue, the retropharyngeal space. The entire thickness of the posterior pharyngeal wall from the mucous membrane to the anterior vertebral body is no more than 1 cm in the midline. Lateral to the pharyngeal wall are the vessels, nerves, and muscles of the parapharyngeal space (see Fig. 21-13). The constrictor muscles are relatively thin, especially the superior constrictor, and do not present much of an obstacle to tumor penetration. There is a variable weak spot in the lateral pharyngeal wall just below the hyoid where the middle and the inferior constrictor muscles fail to overlap. The lateral wall in this area is composed of the thin thyrohyoid membrane, which is penetrated by the vessels, nerves, and lymphatics of the laryngopharynx.

The pharyngeal walls are continuous with the cervical esophagus below. The hypopharyngeal walls are visible by indirect mirror examination; the transition to cervical esophagus is below the arytenoids (C4) and invisible to mirror examination. The transition zone, 3 cm to 4 cm in length, is referred to as the postcricoid pharynx and will be dealt with

TABLE 21-49. Supraglottic Larynx Carcinoma: Ultimate Local Control After Salvage Therapy - 152 Patients (No. Controlled/No. Treated)

T Stage	*Irradiation Alone*	*Surgery ± Adjuvant Irradiation*	*Significance Levels*[144,145]
T1	13/13 (100%)	9/9	1.00
T2	32/36 (89%)	21/25 (84%)	0.426
T3	15/20 (75%)	18/18 (100%)	0.031
T4	7/13 (54%)	15/18 (83%)	0.084

Weems DH, Mendenhall WM, Parsons JT, et al: Squamous cell carcinoma of the supraglottic larynx treated with surgery and/or radiation therapy. Int J Radiat Oncol Biol Phys 13:1483–1487, 1987.

TABLE 21-50. Supraglottic Larynx Carcinoma: Ultimate Local Control with Voice Preservation—195 Patients (No. Controlled with Voice Preservation/No. Treated)

T Stage	*Irradiation Alone*	*Surgery ± Adjuvant Irradiation*	*Significance Levels*[144,145]
T1	15/16 (94%)	8/9	0.600
T2	38/45 (84%)*	12/31 (39%)	<0.001
T3	17/25 (68%)	6/26 (23%)	0.002
T4	14/21 (67%)	3/23 (13%)	<0.001

Weems DH, Mendenhall WM, Parsons JT, et al: Squamous cell carcinoma of the supraglottic larynx treated with surgery and/or radiation therapy. Int J Radiat Oncol Biol Phys 13:1483–1487, 1987.

*One patient had two T2 primary lesions and was thus counted twice.

separately, since tumors of this area present a special clinical picture.

The lateral pharyngeal wall is a rather narrow, ill-defined strip of mucosa. It lies behind the posterior tonsillar pillar in the oropharynx, is partially interrupted by the pharyngoepiglottic fold, and then continues into the hypopharynx, where it becomes the lateral wall of the pyriform sinus. The lateral pharyngeal wall has a maximum width of no more than 2 cm. The posterior cornu of the hyoid bone occasionally will protrude into the lateral pharyngeal wall on one or both sides, producing a submucosal bulge.

The posterior pharyngeal wall is about 4 cm to 5 cm wide and about 6 cm to 7 cm in height. Submucosal bulges, caused by osteophytes on the anterior lips of the cervical vertebrae, may be mistaken for submucosal tumor.

The pyriform sinus is created by the intrusion of the larynx into the anterior aspect of the pharynx, which creates pharyngeal grooves lateral to the larynx. The superior margin of the pyriform sinus is the pharyngoepiglottic fold and the free margin of the aryepiglottic fold. The superolateral margin of the pyriform sinus is considered to be an oblique line along the lateral pharyngeal wall just opposite the aryepiglottic fold. The pyriform sinus is therefore made up of three walls: the anterior, lateral, and medial (there is no posterior wall). The pyriform sinus tapers inferiorly to the apex and usually terminates at the level of the cricoid cartilage. The superior limit of the pyriform sinus is opposite the hyoid. The thyrohyoid membrane is lateral to the upper portion of the pyriform sinus (membranous pyriform sinus), and the thyroid cartilage, cricothyroid membrane, and cricoid cartilage are lateral to the lower portion (cartilaginous pyriform sinus). The internal branch of the superior laryngeal nerve, a branch of the vagus, lies under the mucous membrane on the anterolateral wall of the pyriform sinus. The auricular branch is sensory to the skin of the back of the pinna and the posterior wall of the external auditory canal.

The postcricoid pharynx is funnel-shaped, to direct food into the gullet. There is no discrete superior margin, but it may be considered to begin just below the arytenoids. The anterior wall lies behind the cricoid cartilage and is the posterior wall of the lower larynx; this wall is often called the "party wall." The posterior wall is merely a continuation of the hypopharyngeal walls. The recurrent laryngeal nerve lies between the lateral wall and the deep surface of the thyroid gland.

PATHOLOGY

More than 95% of malignant tumors are squamous cell carcinoma or one of its variants. Carcinoma in situ is commonly seen in surgical specimens at the edge of neoplasms of the pharyngeal wall, and multifocal skip areas of carcinoma in situ may make it difficult to obtain clear margins if excision is done. Minor salivary gland tumors are rare.

TABLE 21-51. Supraglottic Larynx Carcinoma: Control Above the Clavicles Following Initial Treatment—156 Patients (No. Controlled/No. Treated)

Modified AJCC Stage	*Irradiation Alone*	*Surgery ± Adjuvant Irradiation*	*Significance Levels*[144,145]
I	9/10	9/9	0.526
II	13/17 (76%)	13/15 (87%)	0.392
III	11/18 (61%)	9/10	0.116
IVA	7/10	5/11 (45%)	0.245
IVB	10/28 (36%)	20/28 (71%)	0.008

Weems DH, Mendenhall WM, Parsons JT, et al: Squamous cell carcinoma of the supraglottic larynx treated with surgery and/or radiation therapy. Int J Radiat Oncol Biol Phys 13:1483–1487, 1987.

TABLE 21-52. Supraglottic Larynx Carcinoma: Ultimate Control Above the Clavicles — 156 Patients (No. Controlled/No. Treated)

Modified AJCC Stage	*Irradiation Alone*	*Surgery ± Adjuvant Irradiation*	*Significance Levels*[144,145]
I	10/10	9/9	1.00
II	16/17 (94%)	14/15 (93%)	0.726
III	15/18 (83%)	10/10	0.249
IVA	8/10	6/11 (55%)	0.221
IVB	14/28 (50%)	23/28 (82%)	0.012

Weems DH, Mendenhall WM, Parsons JT, et al: Squamous cell carcinoma of the supraglottic larynx treated with surgery and/or radiation therapy. Int J Radiat Oncol Biol Phys 13:1483–1487, 1987.

PATTERNS OF SPREAD

Posterior Pharyngeal Wall

Carcinomas of the posterior pharyngeal wall have a strong tendency to remain on the posterior wall, grow up or down the wall, and infiltrate posteriorly; they seldom spread circumferentially to the lateral walls, even when quite advanced. Early lesions are red lesions, sometimes with white areas sprinkled over the involved area. As the lesion progresses, the tumor bulges into the pharyngeal cavity and a ragged, midline, linear ulceration appears. The posterior tonsillar pillars may become involved, and tumor may spread up the pillars, eventually reaching the palate. Advanced lesions tend to terminate inferiorly at the level of the arytenoids without growing into the postcricoid region. Superiorly they may extend into the nasopharynx. Direct invasion of the cervical vertebrae or base of skull is uncommon.

Lateral Pharyngeal Wall

Early tumors may be well-defined exophytic lesions. As they advance, they have a tendency to lateral penetration through the constrictor muscle, thus entering the lateral pharyngeal space or the soft tissue of the neck. A mass may become palpable in the neck just below the hyoid and be confused with a lymph node.

The muscles of the pharynx originate from the base of skull, eustachian tube, styloid process, pterygomandibular raphe, and hyoid bone; tumor may spread along muscle and fascial planes to all muscular points of origin.[318] Tumor also follows a course along cranial nerves IX and X and the sympathetic chain. The thyroid gland is adjacent to the lower walls and often is invaded. Tumor secondarily invades the pharyngoepiglottic fold, the vallecula, and the anterior and lateral walls of the pyriform sinus.

Pyriform Sinus

Early lesions usually appear as nodular mucosal irregularities. Medial wall lesions may grow superficially along the aryepiglottic fold and arytenoids, or invade directly into the false cord and aryepiglottic fold. Medial wall lesions also extend posteriorly to the postcricoid region. Extensive submucosal spread is a characteristic feature. There is frequently an area of central ulceration for lesions larger than 1 cm to 2 cm.

Large bulky exophytic lesions may arise on the upper medial wall and appear similar to primary lesions of the aryepiglottic fold. The vocal cord becomes fixed because of infiltration of the intrinsic muscles of the larynx, the cricoarytenoid joint or muscle, or less commonly, the recurrent laryngeal nerve. These lesions grow posteriorly to involve the postcricoid pharynx and cricoid cartilage and may extend to the opposite pyriform sinus. Spread into the cervical esophagus is a late event.

Lesions arising on the lateral wall tend toward early inva-

TABLE 21-53. Supraglottic Larynx Carcinoma: Incidence of Severe Complications — 195 Patients

Initial Treatment	*No. Patients with Severe Complications/ No. Initially Treated*	*No. Patients with Severe Complications/No. Attempted Salvage Procedures*
Irradiation alone	5/106 (5%)	2/20 (10%)
Surgery alone	6/26 (23%)	1/4
Preoperative irradiation + surgery	6/28 (21%)	0/1
Surgery + postoperative irradiation	6/35 (17%)	1/4

Weems DH, Mendenhall WM, Parsons JT, et al: Squamous cell carcinoma of the supraglottic larynx treated with surgery and/or radiation therapy. Int J Radiat Oncol Biol Phys 13:1483–1487, 1987

TABLE 21-54. Supraglottic Larynx Carcinoma: Determinate 5-Year Survival—105 Patients (No. Alive/No. Treated)

Modified AJCC Stage	*Irradiation Alone*	*Surgery ± Adjuvant Irradiation*	*Significance Levels*[144,145]
I	6/6	8/8	1.00
II	7/7	8/9	0.562
III	3/6	8/8	0.055
IVA	4/7	3/7	0.500
IVB	5/26 (19%)	11/21 (52%)	0.019

Weems DH, Mendenhall WM, Parsons JT, et al: Squamous cell carcinoma of the supraglottic larynx treated with surgery and/or radiation therapy. Int J. Radiat Oncol Biol Phys 13:1483–1487, 1987.

TABLE 21-55. Squamous Cell Carcinoma of the Supraglottic Larynx: Absolute Survival Rates* in Patients with Stage IV† Disease

Absolute Survival	*Surgery Only‡*	*Surgery and Radiation Therapy*
2 years	39.1% (34/87)§	68.5% (37/54)§
5 years	24.4% (19/78)**	42.1% (16/38)**

Fletcher GH, Goepfert H: Larynx and pyriform sinus. In Fletcher GH: Textbook of Radiotherapy, 3rd ed, pp 330–363. Philadelphia, Lea & Febiger, 1980.

M. D. Anderson Hospital data; patients treated 1954–1972.

*Living, free of cancer.

†Stage IV: T4 N0–N1, T1–T4 N2–N3.

‡All patients had a total laryngectomy.

§$p < 0.005$.

**$p < 0.08$.

sion of the posterior thyroid cartilage and the posterior superior cricoid cartilage. The ipsilateral superior lobe of the thyroid gland may be invaded after tumor penetrates the cartilage, but thyroid invasion can occur in cases with no cartilage invasion when tumor penetrates behind the thyroid cartilage or through the cricothyroid membrane. Kirchner[319] reported that thyroid cartilage invasion was associated with involvement of the apex of the pyriform sinus, and the extent of invasion could not be predicted on the extent of visible disease.

Lesions of the lateral walls tend to spread submucosally to the posterior pharyngeal wall. It is often difficult to estimate the extent of posterior pharyngeal wall or postcricoid invasion except at direct laryngoscopy, since these areas are often impossible to visualize indirectly. Even with direct endoscopy, invasion may be underestimated.

Advanced lesions of the pyriform sinus invade all three walls, fix the larynx, involve the ipsilateral posterior pharyngeal wall, invade the thyroid cartilage and thyroid gland, and often escape into the soft tissues of the neck. The preepiglottic space often is involved. Perineural invasion of the recurrent laryngeal nerve may be seen in whole organ sections.

Postcricoid Pharynx

Early lesions of the postcricoid area are rarely diagnosed. Lesions arising from the posterior wall tend to remain on the posterior wall. Lesions arising from the anterior wall tend to invade the posterior cricoarytenoid muscle and the cricoid and arytenoid cartilages. Advanced tumors eventually encircle the lumen. Because the apex of the pyriform sinus terminates in the postcricoid area, some lesions secondarily invade the apex of the pyriform sinus very early.

Lymphatics

PHARYNGEAL WALLS. The lymphatics of the pharyngeal walls terminate primarily in the jugular chain with a secondary avenue by way of the spinal accessory chain. The jugulodigastric node is the most commonly involved node.

TABLE 21-56. T1–T2 Glottic Larynx Carcinoma: Incidence of Serious Complications by Radiation Dose—303 Patients* (No. Complications/No. Patients Treated)

Total Dose (cGy)	*T1 Dose/Fraction*		*T2 Dose/Fraction*		*Total Dose/Fraction*	
	225–255 cGy†	*<185–245 cGy*	*225–245 cGy†*	*<175–224 cGy*	*225–255 cGy*	*175–224 cGy*
>7000				0/3		0/3
6700–7000		0/2	2/7 (29%)	0/12	2/7 (29%)	0/14
6000–6600	0/86	1/58 (1.7%)	1/61 (1.6%)	1/34 (2.9%)	1/147 (0.7%)	2/92 (2.2%)
5400–5700	0/36	0/2		0/2	0/36	0/4

Mendenhall WM, Parsons JT, Million RR, et al: T1–T2 squamous cell carcinoma of the glottic larynx treated with radiation therapy: Relationship of dose-fractionation factors to local control and complications. Int J Radiat Oncol Biol Phys (in press).

*Patients treated with once-a-day fractionation.

†Only one patient was treated at >235 cGy/fraction.

Lindberg[7] reported 59% clinically positive nodes on admission; 17% were bilateral (Fig. 21-20). Wang[320] reported 55% positive nodes for lesions of the posterior pharyngeal wall, of which 10% were bilateral. At the University of Florida, the incidence of clinically positive nodes for posterior pharyngeal wall lesions was 65%.

Retropharyngeal lymph node involvement occurs and is diagnosed by CT or MRI scan.

PYRIFORM SINUS. The capillary lymphatics of the pyriform sinus are profuse. The distribution of lymph node metastases is mainly to the jugular chain with a relatively small proportion to the spinal accessory chain. The subdigastric node is the most commonly involved, but midjugular involvement occurs without subdigastric node involvement.

On admission, 75% of patients have clinically positive nodes and at least 10% have bilateral nodes (see Fig. 21-20). There is no difference in the risk of lymph node metastases by T stage (see Table 21-1). Ogura and co-workers[42] reported a 62% incidence of subclinical disease; some of the patients had 1500 cGy to 3000 cGy of preoperative irradiation. Biller and co-workers[321] reported a 9% incidence of delayed-appearing contralateral nodes after an ipsilateral pathologically positive neck dissection. The risk for late-appearing contralateral lymph nodes was independent of whether the positive ipsilateral lymph nodes were palpable.

FIG. 21-20. Nodal distribution on admission at M.D. Anderson Hospital, 1948–1965. **A.** Oropharyngeal walls. **B.** Hypopharynx. (Lindberg RD: Distribution of cervical lymph node metastases from squamous cell carcinoma of the upper respiratory and digestive tracts. Cancer 29:1446–1450, 1972)

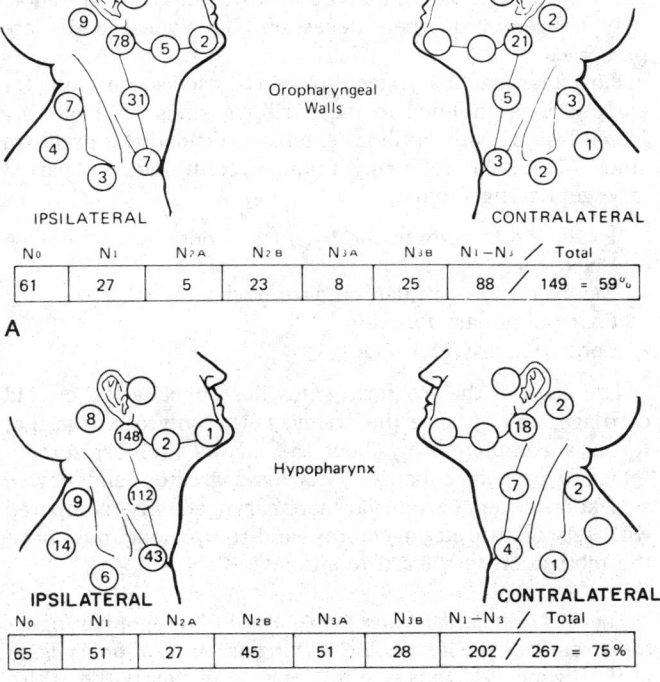

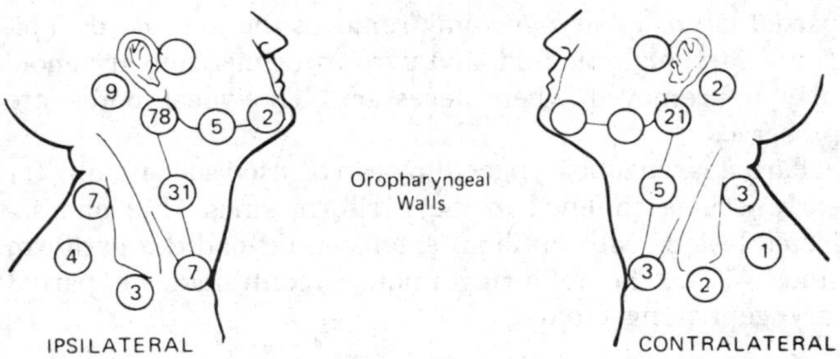

N_0	N_1	N_{2A}	N_{2B}	N_{3A}	N_{3B}	N_1-N_3 / Total
61	27	5	23	8	25	88 / 149 = 59%

A

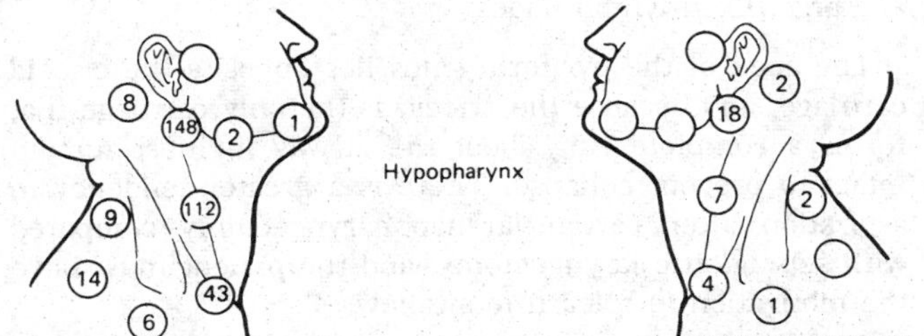

N_0	N_1	N_{2A}	N_{2B}	N_{3A}	N_{3B}	N_1-N_3 / Total
65	51	27	45	51	28	202 / 267 = 75%

B

Retropharyngeal lymph node involvement occurs and is diagnosed by CT or MRI scan.

CLINICAL PICTURE

Tumors that are lateralized to the lateral pharyngeal wall or pyriform sinus produce a unilateral sore throat, a symptom rather specific for cancer since infectious sore throat is bilateral. The patient with cancer can point to the painful site with one finger, whereas the patient with inflammatory sore throat cannot. Dysphagia, sensation of foreign body, ear pain, blood-streaked saliva, and voice change occur later. A neck mass may be the presenting complaint.

Lesions of the posterior pharyngeal wall are often overlooked even by competent physicians because of failure to examine the posterior pharyngeal wall routinely during indirect laryngoscopy.

Small lesions of the pyriform sinus are easily missed unless very careful examinations are done. Many of these patients have active gag reflexes, and complete topical anesthesia is required, coupled with patience on the part of the examiner.

Lesions of the apex of the pyriform sinus or postcricoid area produce indirect findings that are clues to tumor not visible by indirect laryngoscopy. Pooling of secretions in the pyriform sinus and arytenoid area indicates obstruction of the upper gullet. Edema of the arytenoids and inability to see into the apex of the pyriform sinus are clues to postcricoid or low-lying pyriform sinus tumors. Invasion of the palatopharyngeal muscle at its insertion into the inferior constrictor can cause shortening of the muscle and asymmetry of the posterior tonsillar pillars. As the postcricoid tumor enlarges it pushes the larynx anteriorly. This produces a full, expanded neck appearance. The thyroid click or crackle is produced by the superior thyroid cornu hitting against the spine while rocking the thyroid cartilage back and forth; this is lost when the larynx and thyroid cartilage protrude anteriorly.

METHODS OF DIAGNOSIS AND STAGING

Lesions of the oropharyngeal wall can sometimes be biopsied in the outpatient clinic with topical anesthetic. Hypopharyngeal lesions usually require general anesthetic and biopsy under direct visualization.

Direct laryngoscopy and esophagoscopy are needed to map the extent of low pharyngeal wall, pyriform sinus, and postcricoid lesions.

CT scans are useful in demonstrating invasion of the preepiglottic space, invasion of the thyroid and cricoid cartilages, invasion of the soft tissues of the neck, and the extent of lymph node metastases. CT scan should be done prior to biopsy.

Staging

The AJCC staging for the hypopharynx is satisfactory for the pyriform sinus, but unsatisfactory for the pharyngeal wall.[12]

TX Minimum requirements to assess the primary tumor cannot be met

T0	No evidence of primary tumor
Tis	Carcinoma in situ
T1	Tumor confined to one site
T2	Extension of tumor to adjacent region or site without fixation of hemilarynx
T3	Extension of tumor to adjacent region or site with fixation of hemilarynx
T4	Massive tumor invading bone or soft tissues of neck

If there is definite decrease in mobility, the lesion should be assigned to the T3 stage.

Lesions of the posterior pharyngeal wall tend to stay on the posterior pharyngeal wall rather than invade the larynx or lateral walls; therefore, fixation does not enter into staging. Posterior pharyngeal wall lesions would be staged more appropriately by tumor diameter.

TREATMENT

Selection of Treatment Modality

POSTERIOR PHARYNGEAL WALL. Most lesions on the posterior pharyngeal wall are treated by radiation therapy, although the results are far from outstanding. Attempts have been made to combine surgery and radiation therapy for selected, moderately advanced lesions, with limited success.

All aspects considered, high-dose radiotherapy will produce cure rates similar to those produced by either surgery alone or combined surgery plus radiation therapy, and with lesser morbidity. A few selected patients who fail to respond to radiation therapy or whose lesions recur after irradiation will be salvaged by pharyngectomy.

LATERAL PHARYNGEAL WALL. There is very little local control information specifically related to the lateral walls. Small lesions (1–2 cm) are usually exophytic and are usually managed by irradiation. Larger lesions tend to be deeply infiltrative, and the control rate by irradiation, surgery, or both is only modest at best. An operation for a large lesion usually implies a laryngectomy in combination with pharyngectomy.

PYRIFORM SINUS. The pyriform sinus is the most common primary site in the hypopharynx. Lesions confined to the pyriform sinus with normal mobility (T1) are locally controlled in 85% to 90% of cases by irradiation or partial laryngopharyngectomy.[322] Irradiation is the preferred choice of the authors because it leaves the patient with nearly normal swallowing and speech while permitting wider coverage of the regional lymphatics. Irradiation is more generally applicable, whereas there are certain anatomical and medical restraints on use of partial laryngopharyngectomy.

Lesions that extend outside the pyriform sinus with normal or reduced mobility (T2–T3) represent the group of cases in which treatment selection is more complex. The local control rate with radiation therapy for selected cases is approximately 60%; some of the failures will be rescued by operation, although the operative mortality and morbidity are considerable after high-dose irradiation.

Invasion of the pyriform sinus apex is a contraindication to partial laryngopharyngectomy, but these same patients do poorly with radiation therapy also; these patients usually are selected for total laryngopharyngectomy plus postoperative radiation therapy, but they may be treated for cure with radiation therapy if apex involvement is minimal. Fixation is a relative indication for total laryngopharyngectomy and postoperative radiation therapy. If the lesion is mainly exophytic and in the upper pyriform sinus, a trial of radiation therapy is offered as an alternative to total laryngopharyngectomy. If the disease disappears at 4500 cGy to 5000 cGy and mobility is returning, radical irradiation is a reasonable choice, with total laryngopharyngectomy reserved for failure. A select group of early T2 lesions with minimal extension beyond the pyriform sinus and a normal apex are also suitable for partial laryngopharyngectomy. However, these are the very patients that do well with radiation therapy only.

The more advanced, infiltrative lesions are best treated with total laryngopharyngectomy, radical neck dissection, and postoperative radiation therapy. Those patients presenting with an extensive primary lesion and extensive neck metastases (and usually accompanied by major medical problems) are frequently offered palliative therapy.

Surgical Treatment

POSTERIOR PHARYNGEAL WALL. If the lesion is high on the posterior wall, then a transoral approach can be used; however, for lower lesions the midline mandibulolabial glossotomy approach may be used. Alternatives are the transhyoid approach or a lateral pharyngotomy approach. The lesion is removed down to the prevertebral fascia, and no skin graft is placed.

PYRIFORM SINUS. *Partial laryngopharyngectomy.* A partial laryngopharyngectomy removes the false cords, epiglottis, aryepiglottic fold, and pyriform sinus; one arytenoid may be removed when necessary. The vocal cords are preserved.

Partial laryngopharyngectomy can be used successfully for early lesions confined to the pyriform sinus (T1) and selected lesions with minimal extension beyond the pyriform sinus (T2). The following findings contraindicate partial laryngopharyngectomy:

- Extension to apex of the pyriform sinus
- Fixed cord
- Extension to contralateral arytenoid
- Poor pulmonary function
- Large, fixed lymph nodes

The apex of the pyriform sinus lies opposite the cricoid cartilage, and because the cricoid is the only cartilage that forms a complete ring about the airway, it must remain intact to prevent collapse. There is a greater tendency to aspiration after partial laryngopharyngectomy compared with supraglottic laryngectomy, and the patient must have the motivation to relearn to swallow.

Total Laryngopharyngectomy. Total laryngopharyngectomy removes the larynx and varying amounts of pharyngeal wall. Advanced lesions require excision of nearly the entire circumference. The pharynx is reestablished by primary closure after a partial pharyngectomy, but a flap is required after total pharyngectomy. Because almost all these patients received postoperative radiation therapy, the operation should be planned for one-stage reconstruction in order to start radiation therapy within 6 weeks. A planned controlled fistula speeds the healing process and largely eliminates the occurrence of an uncontrolled fistula, which delays healing and the start of radiation therapy. If a myocutaneous flap is used, a controlled fistula is unnecessary.

POSTCRICOID PHARYNX. Postcricoid carcinoma generally requires a total laryngopharyngectomy with immediate reconstruction, generally using a pectoralis major myocutaneous flap. Before undergoing the surgery, however, the patient must undergo direct laryngoscopy and esophagoscopy to determine the extent of the lesion. If the lesion extends into the cervical esophagus, then reconstruction becomes more difficult and often stomach will be used for reconstruction. If irradiation is to be used in conjunction with gastric pull-up, preoperative radiation therapy is preferred.

Irradiation Technique

In selected cases, patients expected to have a poor nutritional status will have placement of a gastrostomy tube prior to irradiation.

POSTERIOR PHARYNGEAL WALL. The irradiation technique for lesions of the posterior pharyngeal wall is opposed lateral fields to include the primary lesion and the regional nodes. Because these lesions tend to have "skip" areas, the entire posterior pharyngeal wall is included initially. If the lesion extends near the arytenoids, the postcricoid pharynx, pyriform sinus, and upper cervical esophagus are included. The retropharyngeal nodes will be included within these fields. The spinal accessory nodes are included even if the neck nodes are negative.

The critical portion of the treatment occurs when the field is reduced at 4500 cGy to 5000 cGy to avoid the spinal cord. The posterior border of the portal is placed just anterior to the spinal cord (*i.e.*, posterior edge of the bodies of the cervical vertebrae).[323] Daily imaging films and precision setups are required.

The dose for T1 lesions (0–2 cm) is 6000 cGy in 6 weeks. The dose for T2–T4 lesions is 7440 cGy to 7680 cGy with 120 cGy twice a day.

PYRIFORM SINUS. Parallel opposed lateral portals are used to encompass the primary lesion and regional nodes on both sides. The superior border is placed 2 cm above the tip of the mastoid to cover the most superior jugular chain and the retropharyngeal lymph nodes. The posterior border encompasses the spinal accessory nodes. Clinically positive nodes behind the plane of the spinal cord require the addition of a neck dissection or electron boosts. The anterior border usually is placed about 1 cm behind the anterior skin edge. When the anterior border is shielded, the radiotherapist checks the setup daily because the margin for error is rather slim. However, protection of this narrow anterior segment reduces irradiation of the anterior arch of the thyroid and cricoid cartilages, anterior commissure of the glottis, and anterior midline skin. The inferior border is 2 cm below the inferior border of the cricoid. The inferior recess or apex of the pyriform sinus varies, but generally terminates at the upper to middle cricoid. The remaining lower neck lymph nodes are treated through an en face portal.

Dosimetry is individualized, using wedges, compensators, and unequal loadings as needed. The doses are the same as for the posterior pharyngeal wall.

Combined Treatment Policies

POSTERIOR PHARYNGEAL WALL. Operation usually should precede radiation therapy when a combination is selected, unless a gastric pull-up is planned. There is a high incidence of operative mortality and complications with a preoperative dose of 2500 cGy to 3000 cGy.[324] When postoperative irradiation is used, a dose of 6000 cGy to 6500 cGy is used with negative margins.

PYRIFORM SINUS. Following total laryngopharyngectomy with or without radical neck dissection, radiation therapy is recommended if there are close or positive margins, multiple or large positive nodes, extension of nodal disease through the capsule, or cartilage invasion. In short, almost all patients receive postoperative radiation therapy. There is an increased risk of pharyngeal stenosis, especially if the pharyngeal closure is tight.

Irradiation is given before total laryngopharyngectomy in those T2 or T3 patients for whom a trial of radiation therapy is planned; the patients are reevaluated at 4500 cGy with the surgeon. Irradiation is also used prior to operation for patients with a large fixed node to reduce the size of the mass and to help obtain surgical margins. The preoperative dose to the node may be 6000 cGy to 7500 cGy, although the dose to the primary will be only 4000 cGy to 5000 cGy.

Management of Recurrence

POSTERIOR PHARYNGEAL WALL. Recurrence after radiation therapy may be limited to the posterior pharyngeal wall and suitable for surgical excision, with occasional salvage. There is frequently a persistent ulcer at the completion of radiation therapy for the more advanced lesions. If the ulcer does not heal in short order, it should be considered evidence of persistent disease. Surgical excision is limited posteriorly by the prevertebral fascia. Meoz-Mendez and co-workers[325] report 11 irradiation failures salvaged by an operation out of a total of 68 local failures. Irradiation salvage of a surgical failure would be unusual.

PYRIFORM SINUS. The hallmark of local recurrence after radical irradiation is persistent major edema with inability to visualize the pyriform sinus, pain on swallowing, and fixation of laryngeal structures. Direct laryngoscopy is required, but biopsy may be negative and misleading. Eventually a decision may be made to recommend total laryngopharyngectomy for salvage without a positive biopsy.

Recurrence after total laryngopharyngectomy is usually in

the soft tissues of the neck, the untreated opposite neck, the base of the tongue, or the stoma.

Surgical failures after partial laryngopharyngectomy for early lesions may be salvaged by total laryngopharyngectomy. Surgical failures after total laryngopharyngectomy are rarely salvaged.

Radiation failure occasionally may be salvaged by total laryngopharyngectomy with or without radical neck dissection. The risk of an operative mortality or major morbidity is high.

TABLE 21-57. Pharyngeal Wall Carcinoma: Local Control with Radiation Therapy—External Beam, Continuous Course (No. Controlled/No. Treated)

Stage	*Once-a-Day Treatment*	*Twice-a-Day Treatment*
T1 (0–2 cm)	2/3	1/1
T2 (>2–4 cm)	7/12	4/4
T3 (>4–6 cm)	8/19	4/6
T4 (>6 cm)	1/6	1/2

Data from Mendenhall et al.[323]

RESULTS OF TREATMENT

Pharyngeal Wall

The treatment policy at the University of Florida primarily has been radical irradiation with neck dissection added as necessary. The local control rates for once-daily versus twice-daily irradiation (external beam treatment only) are given in Table 21-57. The improvement in local control and survival rates with the twice-a-day regimen has been impressive to date.[323]

Wang[320] reported a 25% 3-year survival without recurrence for 36 patients with carcinoma of the posterior pharyngeal wall treated by radiation therapy alone; the 3-year survival rate was 47% for patients with clinically negative nodes. Sixteen of 24 patients (66%) with T1 or T2 lesions had their disease controlled by radiation therapy, as did 3 of 13 patients with T3 lesions.

Meoz-Mendez and co-workers[325] reported the results of radiation therapy alone for 164 patients with lesions arising from the pharyngeal walls. The rates of local control by T stage and salvage of radiation therapy failures are shown in Table 21-58. The cause of death was local failure in 38%, neck recurrence in 6%, distant metastases in 10%, and second primary cancer in 16%.

Marks and co-workers[324] compared low-dose preoperative radiation therapy (2500-3000 cGy) followed by operation to radiation therapy alone (Table 21-59). The local control was slightly better for the combined group, but the 3-year actuarial survival rate was 17%, and the 3-year absolute survival rate was 14%. An operative mortality of 14% and a high risk of major surgical complications offset any gain in local control. M. D. Anderson Hospital reported a group of 25 patients (5 Stage T2, 10 Stage T3–T4) treated by combined surgery and radiation therapy.[325] Nineteen patients received postoperative radiation therapy, 7 had positive margins, and 3 had close margins. Fifteen patients were dead at 5 years: 6 died of local recurrence or neck recurrence, 5 of distant metastasis, 1 of intercurrent disease, and 3 of uncertain causes. The 5-year absolute survival was 4 of 19 (21%).

Pyriform Sinus

The results of treatment for 80 patients with carcinoma of the pyriform sinus treated at Washington University, St. Louis, by preoperative radiation therapy followed by partial laryngopharyngectomy are given in Table 21-60.[326] Seventy patients had the equivalent of AJCC T1 lesions (disease limited to the pyriform sinus) and 10 patients had disease ex-

TABLE 21-59. Local Control in Carcinoma of the Posterior Pharyngeal Wall (Washington University, St. Louis)

Treatment	*Local Control* T1	T2	T3	T4
Surgery (31 patients)*	6/8	7/12	4/12	0/1
Radiation therapy alone	1/1	3/6	0/5	1/1

Adapted from Marks JE, Freeman RB, Lee F, et al: Pharyngeal wall cancer: An analysis of treatment results complications and patterns of failure. Int J Radiat Oncol Biol Phys 4:587–593, 1978.

*Twenty-nine patients had preoperative radiation therapy; 2 patients had postoperative radiation therapy.

TABLE 21-58. Squamous Cell Carcinoma of the Pharyngeal Walls: Local Control (164 Patients: M. D. Anderson Hospital, 1954–1974)

Stage	*Local Control with RT* Alone (No. controlled/ No. treated)*	*Surgical Salvage (No. salvaged)*	*Ultimate Local Control (No. controlled/ No. treated)*
T1 (0–2 cm)	10/11 (91%)	1	11/11 (100%)
T2 (2–4 cm)	33/45 (73%)	2	35/45 (78%)
T3 (>4 cm)	38/62 (61%)	6	44/62 (71%)
T4 (massive)	15/46 (37%)	2	17/46 (41%)

Adapted from Meoz-Mendez RT, Fletcher GH, Guillamondegui OM, et al: Analysis of the results of irradiation in the treatment of squamous cell carcinomas of the pharyngeal walls. Int J Radiat Oncol Biol Phys 4:579–585, 1978.

*RT, radiation therapy.

TABLE 21-60. Carcinoma of the Pyriform Sinus: Results of Treatment by Low-Dose Radiation Therapy plus Partial Laryngopharyngectomy (PLP) or Low-Dose Radiation Therapy plus Total Laryngectomy and Partial Pharyngectomy (TLP) (Washington University, St. Louis, 1964–1974)

Result	*PLP (80 Patients)**	*TLP (57 Patients)†*
Local recurrence ± neck recurrence	14%‡	14%
Neck recurrence ± distant metastases (primary controlled)	9%	23%
Distant metastases alone	11%	21%
5-year actuarial survival (no evidence of disease)	40%	22%

Data from Marks et al.[326]
*T1, 70 patients; T2–T4, 10 patients (AJC staging).
†T1, 35 patients; T2–T4, 22 patients (AJC staging).
‡Four patients salvaged.

tending beyond the pyriform sinus. None had invasion of the apex of the pyriform sinus, as determined before surgery. The cause of death was cancer in 26%, complications of treatment in 14%, and intercurrent disease in 20%. The 2-year absolute survival rate was 45 of 80 (56%) and the 5-year absolute survival was 25 of 66 (38%) (Marks JE: Personal communication, 1979).

Table 21-60 also shows the results of treatment for 57 patients from the same institution who were treated by preoperative radiation therapy followed by total laryngectomy and partial pharyngectomy.[326] Thirty-five patients had lesions confined to the pyriform sinus (AJCC T1) and the remainder had extension beyond the pyriform sinus (AJCC T2–T4). The cause of death was cancer in 56%, complications of treatment in 11%, and intercurrent disease in 18%.

The results of radiation therapy for carcinoma of the pyriform sinus with neck dissection added in selected cases are shown in Tables 21-61 through 21-64.[327] Most patients with T1 and T2 lesions were selected for radiation therapy; T3 lesions were irradiated if they were exophytic and in the upper pyriform sinus or because the patient refused operation. All T4 lesions were irradiated by default. Patients with stage IVA represent a relatively favorable group with early primary lesions and N2 or N3 neck disease; the neck disease is usually managed by adding a neck dissection after radiation therapy.

El-Badawi and co-workers[328] compared results for 203 patients treated by surgery alone, and 125 patients treated by surgery (total laryngopharyngectomy) followed by 6000 cGy of postoperative irradiation or preceded by 4500 cGy to 5000 cGy of preoperative irradiation. The stages of the three groups were comparable. There was a minimum follow-up of 4 years. The patients treated with combined therapy showed approximately a 15% improvement in survival at 5 years (Table 21-65).

The ultimate control rate above the clavicles for 65 patients treated by total laryngopharyngectomy and 2 patients

TABLE 21-62. Pyriform Sinus Carcinoma: Initial Control of the Clinically Positive Hemineck with Radiation Therapy ± Neck Dissection (No. Controlled/No. Treated)*

Stage	*Irradiation Alone*	*Irradiation and Neck Dissection*
N1	6/6	1/1
N2A	1/2	3/3
N2B	3/3	5/6
N3A	0/2	1/2

Mendenhall WM, Parsons JT, Cassisi NJ, et al: Squamous cell carcinoma of the pyriform sinus treated with radical radiation therapy. Radiother Oncol 9:201–208, 1987.
*Twenty-three patients, continuously disease-free at the primary site, with 25 evaluable clinically positive heminecks. None of the neck failures were controlled by subsequent treatment.

TABLE 21-61. Pyriform Sinus Carcinoma: Local Control with Continuous-Course Radiation Therapy ± Neck Dissection (No. Controlled/No. Treated)

Stage	*Excluded**	*Once-a-Day Fractionation*	*Twice-a-Day Fractionation†*	*Total Local Control with Radical Radiation Therapy*	*No. Salvaged/ No. Attempts*	*Ultimate Control*
T1	2	8/9		8/9	0/0	8/9
T2	10	12/16	3/4	15/20	3/4	18/20
T3	2	1/3	1/2	2/5	1/2	3/5
T4	2	0/2	0/1	0/3	0/1	0/3

Mendenhall WM, Parsons JT, Cassisi NJ, et al: Squamous cell carcinoma of the pyriform sinus treated with radical radiation therapy. Radiother Oncol 9:201–208, 1987.
*Patients were excluded from the local control analysis if they died within 2 years of treatment of other causes with the primary site continuously disease-free.
†University of Florida data. Patients treated 3/78–4/85; analysis 4/87 by J. T. Parsons, M.D.

TABLE 21-63. Pyriform Sinus Carcinoma: Control Above the Clavicles (No. Controlled/No. Treated)

Modified AJCC Stage	*Excluded**	*Control with Initial Treatment*	*No. Salvaged/ No. Attempts*	*Ultimate Control*
I	0	1/1	0/0	1/1
II	1	5/6	1/1	6/6
III	3	5/10	1/2	6/10
IVA	6	12/16†	1/2	13/16‡
IVB	2	1/9†	0/2	1/9‡

Mendenhall WM, Parsons JT, Cassisi NJ, et al: Squamous cell carcinoma of the pyriform sinus treated with radical radiation therapy. Radiother Oncol 9:201–208, 1987.

*Patients excluded from analysis of control above the clavicles if they died within 2 years after treatment of other causes, continuously free of disease above the clavicles.

†12/16 versus 1/9, $p = 0.003$.[145]

‡13/16 versus 1/9, $p = 0.001$.[145]

TABLE 21-64. Pyriform Sinus Carcinoma: Five-Year Survival (No. Alive/No. Treated)

Modified AJCC Stage	*5-Year Survival*	
	Absolute	*Determinate*
I	1/1	1/1
II	3/5	3/3
III	5/13	5/8
IVA	7/17*	7/12†
IVB	2/10*	2/8†

Mendenhall WM, Parsons JT, Cassisi NJ, et al: Squamous cell carcinoma of the pyriform sinus treated with radical radiation therapy. Radiother Oncol 9:201–208, 1987.

*7/17 versus 2/10, $p = 0.187$.[145]

†7/12 versus 2/8, $p = 0.132$.[145]

treated by partial laryngopharyngectomy at the University of Florida is presented in Table 21-66.[329] The patients with more advanced lesions in Stages T2 and T3 were selected for an operation. Preoperative or postoperative radiation therapy was added in 54 of the patients. The ultimate control rate above the clavicles for T3 lesions treated by operation was 21 of 36 (58%) and for T4 lesions was 3 of 7. The survival figures are presented in Table 21-67.[329]

TABLE 21-66. Pyriform Sinus Carcinoma: Ultimate Control Above the Clavicles (Including Salvage) for 67 Patients* Treated by Surgery ± Radiation Therapy (No. Controlled/No. Treated)

Stage	*Preoperative Radiation Therapy*	*Postoperative Radiation Therapy*	*Surgery Alone*
T1	0/1		
T2	1/1	1/1	2/3
T3	8/15	10/15	3/6
T4	1/5	2/2	0/0

Million RR, Cassisi NJ: Hypopharynx: Pharyngeal walls, pyriform sinus, and postcricoid pharynx. In Million RR, Cassisi NJ (eds): Management of Head and Neck Cancer: A Multidisciplinary Approach, pp 373–391. Philadelphia, JB Lippincott, 1984.

University of Florida data. Patients treated 10/64–12/80 (2-year to unlimited follow-up); analysis 2/83 by J. W. Devine, M.D.

*Excludes 16 patients who died of intercurrent disease less than 2 years after treatment with no recurrence above the clavicles.

COMPLICATIONS OF TREATMENT

Posterior Pharyngeal Wall

SURGICAL COMPLICATIONS. Marks and co-workers[324] reported a 14% operative mortality plus major complications

TABLE 21-65. Carcinoma of the Pyriform Sinus: Results of Treatment

Treatment Modality	*No. of Patients*	*Failure Above Clavicles (%)*	*2-Year NED (%)*	*Cause of Death (>2 Year)*
Surgery	203	39*	40†	DM—8 ID—23
Surgery and postoperative irradiation	125	11*	50†	N—1 DM—6 ID—7
Preoperative irradiation and surgery	17	29	47	DM—2 ID—2

Adapted from El-Badawi SA, Goepfert H, Fletcher GH, et al: Squamous cell carcinoma of the pyriform sinus. Laryngoscope 92:357–364, 1982.

M. D. Anderson Hospital data. Patients treated 1949–1976; analysis 1/81.

NED, no evidence of pyriform sinus cancer; DM, distant metastasis; ID, intercurrent disease; N, neck nodes.

*$p = <0.001$.

†$p = 0.04$.

TABLE 21-67. Pyriform Sinus Carcinoma: Survival Free of Disease in 67 Patients Treated by Surgery ± Radiation Therapy

Modified AJCC Stage	*Absolute Survival*		*Determinate Survival*	
	2 Years	*5 Years*	*2 Years*	*5 Years*
I,II	0/2	0/2	0/2	0/2
III	9/14 (64%)	2/9	9/12 (75%)	2/7
IVA	2/4	2/4	2/4	2/4
IVB	18/47 (38%)	7/41 (17%)	18/42 (43%)	7/35 (20%)
Total	29/67 (43%)	11/56 (20%)	29/60 (48%)	11/48 (23%)

Million RR, Cassisi NJ: Hypopharynx: Pharyngeal walls, pyriform sinus, and postcricoid pharynx. In Million RR, Cassisi NJ (eds): Management of Head and Neck Cancer: A Multidisciplinary Approach, pp 373–391. Philadelphia, JB Lippincott, 1984.

University of Florida data. Patients treated 10/64–12/80 (to 12/77 for 5-year figures); analysis 2/83 by J. W. Devine, M.D.

including pharyngocutaneous fistula (31%) and carotid rupture (14%) for patients treated with preoperative radiation therapy, 2500 cGy to 3000 cGy.

RADIATION THERAPY COMPLICATIONS. Meoz-Mendez and co-workers[325] analyzed the complications for 164 patients with carcinoma of the pharyngeal wall treated by radiation therapy alone. There was a 5% incidence of fatal complications. In 7 patients the fatality was secondary to carotid rupture, associated with attempts at surgical salvage. Only 2 patients developed severe laryngeal edema. Radiation myelitis was documented in 2 patients. The overall incidence of radiation therapy–related complications was 12%; the complication rate increased with rising T stage.

Mendenhall and co-workers[323] reported that 8 of 75 patients developed severe complications secondary to radiation therapy. The incidence of severe complications by stage is as follows: Stage I, 0 of 2; Stage II, 1 of 16; Stage III, 2 of 22; Stage IVA, 2 of 14; Stage IVB, 3 of 20. Four patients developed inability to swallow requiring a permanent gastrostomy tube. One patient developed severe laryngeal edema that required a permanent tracheostomy. One patient developed a unilateral vocal cord palsy, Horner's syndrome, brachial plexopathy, and a stricture requiring a permanent gastrostomy; although recurrent disease was initially suspected, she survived for 5 years after treatment without evidence of recurrent cancer before dying of intercurrent disease. Finally, two patients developed severe soft-tissue necrosis of the posterior pharyngeal wall, which was fatal in one case.

Pyriform Sinus

SURGICAL COMPLICATIONS. The complications of partial laryngopharyngectomy include a 12% operative mortality, fistula, aspiration, and dysphagia.[326]

The complications of total laryngopharyngectomy include a treatment-related mortality of 11%, fistula, and pharyngeal stenosis.[326]

The complication rate is increased by the addition of radiation therapy.

RADIATION THERAPY COMPLICATIONS. The major radiation therapy complication is laryngeal necrosis. Laryngeal edema occurs temporarily in most cases and is increased by radical neck dissection.

COMPLICATIONS OF SALVAGE TREATMENT. Attempted surgical salvage of radiation therapy failures has a significant operative morbidity and mortality even in the best of hands, but a few cures are produced.

NASOPHARYNX

Malignant tumors of the nasopharynx are uncommon in the United States. The Chinese have a high frequency; American-born second-generation Chinese maintain the risk of nasopharynx cancer. It is undecided whether the risk is reduced by moving away from China. Nasopharynx cancer has also been shown to have an association with elevated titers of Epstein-Barr virus; this finding is independent of geography.[35]

There is a 3:1 ratio of predominance in men. The age distribution for carcinoma is much younger than for other head and neck sites; about 20% of patients are younger than 30 years of age.

ANATOMY

The nasopharynx is roughly cuboidal in shape. It is in direct continuity with the nasal cavity, inferiorly with the oropharynx, and laterally with the middle ears by way of the eustachian tubes.

The mucosa of the roof and posterior wall is often irregular because of the pharyngeal bursa, pharyngeal tonsil (adenoids), and pharyngeal hypophysis. The mucosa tends to become smooth with age, but many folds may remain in the later years of life, adding to the examiner's confusion as to whether tumor is present. Adenoids may persist well past puberty and may even be present in elderly people. Following successful irradiation, these irregularities are usually replaced by a smooth, atrophic appearance.

The lateral walls include the eustachian openings with the fossa of Rosenmuller (pharyngeal recess) located behind the torus tubarius. The superolateral muscular wall of the nasopharynx is incomplete and provides a meager barrier to tumor spread. Once tumor has penetrated the lateral wall, it enters the lateral pharyngeal space and its contents. The floor of the nasopharynx is incomplete and consists of the upper surface of the soft palate, which is rarely the origin of nasopharyngeal tumors and is invaded infrequently even with the extensive local disease.

Lymphatics

There is an extensive submucosal lymphatic capillary plexus, attested to by the high incidence of neck metastases. Tumor cells spread along three different lymph node pathways: the jugular chain, the spinal accessory chain, and the retropharyngeal pathway.

The lateral retropharyngeal nodes lie in the retropharyngeal space and medial to the carotid artery. Directly behind the nodes are the lateral masses of C1 and C2. Marked nodal enlargement, such as that which occurs in lymphoma, may distort the posterior tonsillar pillar, shifting it medially and anteriorly. Otherwise, diagnosis depends on contrast-enhanced CT or MRI. The involved lymph nodes may have the characteristic CT appearance of metastatic carcinoma: rim enhancement and central necrosis.

Inconstant lymphatic vessels are described as draining directly to the midjugular nodes and to the spinal accessory nodes.[3]

PATHOLOGY

Most histologic varieties of malignant tumor have been reported to arise from the nasopharynx and its immediate supporting structures. Carcinomas compose about 85% and lymphomas about 10% of the malignant lesions. Lymphoepithelioma and transitional cell carcinoma are considered variants within the epithelial group; the incidence of lymphoepithelioma varies from about 30% to 50% in various series. A miscellaneous group of malignant tumors includes melanoma, plasmacytoma, juvenile angiofibroma, carcinosarcoma, sarcomas, nonchromaffin paragangliomas, and unclassified tumors. Minor salivary gland tumors are nearly always adenocarcinomas.

PATTERNS OF SPREAD

Primary

The recognized spread to contiguous structures in 99 patients with epithelial lesions on admission prior to treatment is shown in Table 21-68.[330]

Inferior extension along the lateral pharyngeal walls and tonsillar pillars is recognized in almost one third of patients. Extension into the posterior nasal cavity is frequent but usually limited to <1 cm. Thorough shrinking of the nasal mucosa and examination with a small-diameter fiberoptic nasoscope is the best clinical method for detecting nasal extension. CT scan and MRI are best to determine soft-tissue extension into the nasal cavity, but inflammatory exudates or coagulated blood may give a false impression.

Invasion of the posterior ethmoids, the maxillary antrum, and the orbit occurs fairly often and is important to recognize because it dictates a modification of treatment techniques.

TABLE 21-68. Malignant Tumors of the Nasopharynx—Incidence of Spread to Contiguous Structures on Admission (M. D. Anderson Hospital, August 1948–December 1960)

*Site of Spread**	*No. of Cases*
Oropharyngeal wall	29
Base of skull (sphenoid sinus—11)	25
Tonsillar bed	15
Cranial nerves	12
Pterygoid fossa	9
Nasal cavity	5
Maxillary antrum	4
Orbit	3
Soft palate	3
Hard palate	2
Ethmoids	2
Hypopharynx	1

Fletcher GH, Million RR: Malignant tumors of the nasopharynx. AJR 93:44–55, 1965. © 1965, American Roentgen Ray Society.
*In several patients, more than one structure was involved.

Invasion into or through the base of the skull is recognized roentgenographically or clinically in at least 25% of patients before treatment.[330,331] Early, unrecognized invasion presumably occurs in a far greater number of patients, because the base of the skull, brain, and cranial nerves are frequently the site of local recurrence. The sphenoid sinus frequently is invaded. Tumor may erode through the foramen ovale, the foramen lacerum, and the foramen spinosum. Tumor eventually reaches the cavernous sinus area and has access to cranial nerves II to VI.

The lateral muscular wall of the nasopharynx is incomplete superiorly. This defect, termed the sinus of Morgagni, is traversed by the cartilaginous portion of the eustachian tube and the levator palatine muscle, providing an avenue of egress for cancer of the nasopharynx to the lateral pharyngeal space and base of skull.

Lymphatics

There is an 80% to 90% incidence of metastatic neck node disease on presentation; approximately 50% of patients have bilateral lymph node metastases (Figure 21-21).

Low-grade squamous carcinomas produce fewer metastases (73%) than high-grade carcinomas (92%). There is a curious inverse relationship of neck node metastases relative to T stage (see Table 21-1).

Metastases to submental and occipital nodes may appear when there is blockage of the common lymphatic pathways either by massive neck disease or by an untimely neck dissection.

CLINICAL PICTURE

The most common presenting complaint is a painless upper neck mass or masses, which may be quite large when first discovered. The neck mass may enlarge rapidly owing to necrosis or hemorrhage. A rare patient will report exquisite

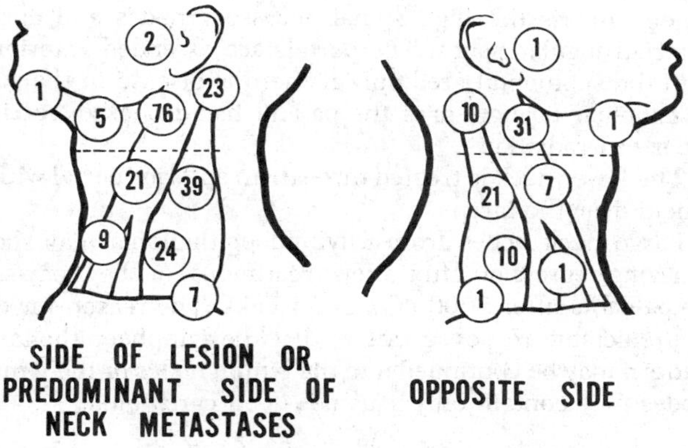

FIG. 21-21. Distribution of metastases to lymph node areas in epithelial tumors of the nasopharynx. The circled numbers indicate the number of times the particular lymph node is involved. Note the high incidence of involvement of the lymph nodes of the spinal accessory chain. Total cases = 99. No lymph nodes were involved in 10 patients (10%); lymph nodes were involved in 89 patients (89%). There was unilateral involvement in 38 patients (39%) and bilateral involvement in 51 patients (51%). (Fletcher GH, Million RR: Malignant tumors of the nasopharynx. Am J Roentgenol Radium Ther Nucl Med 93:44–55, 1965. Copyright © 1965, American Roentgen Ray Society)

tenderness of the nodes and will be unable to tolerate palpation of the masses.

Nasal obstruction, epistaxis, and otitis media are caused by local tumor effect.

Sore throat occurs in about 15% of patients and is related to spread into the oropharyngeal wall. Facial pain may be referred from any of the three divisions of the trigeminal nerve, usually the mandibular division. Occipital or temporal headache frequently is seen. Pain in the scalp over the left mastoid area is related to involvement of a high jugular lymph node that has become fixed to the skull and spine.

Pain in lifting the head and extending the neck is related to posterior infiltration of the prevertebral muscles. Proptosis occurs with posterior orbital invasion and usually displaces the eyeball straight forward. Trismus is related to the invasion of the pterygoid region.

Neurologic symptoms and signs occur in about 25% of patients. Involvement of cranial nerves II to VI indicates intracranial extension into the cavernous sinus and pituitary region. Cranial nerves IX to XII and the sympathetic chain are involved in the lateral pharyngeal space.

Examination of the nasopharynx will show a lesion on the lateral wall or roof; the nasopharyngeal surface of the soft palate is almost never the site of origin and not often invaded secondarily, even by advanced lesions. In early lesions, the findings may be quite subtle—only slight fullness in the fossa of Rosenmuller or a small submucosal bulge in the roof. Lymphomas tend to remain submucosal until quite large.

Nasoscopy may show tumor growing into the posterior and superior nasal cavity.

Tumor may be seen infiltrating submucosally along the posterior tonsillar pillars but infrequently grows very far down the posterior pharyngeal wall. The posterior tonsillar pillars may bulge into the oropharynx if an enlarged node develops in the lateral pharyngeal space.

The cranial nerves should be carefully evaluated; cranial nerve VI is the one most commonly involved. The eyes should be measured for proptosis. Ear examination may show findings of otitis media or, rarely, gross tumor.

METHODS OF DIAGNOSIS AND STAGING

Adults with large, easily visible masses may have a biopsy performed in the outpatient clinic while under local anesthetic. A straight biopsy forceps is placed through the nose and the procedure visualized indirectly from the nasopharynx, or a curved biopsy forceps may be inserted behind the retracted soft palate. Biopsy of a small lesion or random biopsies for suspected lesions require general anesthetic. The palate is retracted with a Yonkers speculum, providing direct visualization of the nasopharynx. Because some of these lesions tend to grow submucosally, random biopsies must be deep to detect an invisible lesion. A mucosal sample is taken and then the biopsy forceps is placed back into the biopsy site and a deeper sample is obtained. If a juvenile angiofibroma is suspected, the work-up should include contrast-enhanced CT.

All patients have a contrast-enhanced CT scan, MRI, or both. MRI has the advantage of obtaining images in sagittal and coronal planes. Involved retropharyngeal lymph nodes can be diagnosed by CT and MRI and are commonly diagnosed.

Staging

The AJCC staging system for nasopharyngeal primary tumors is as follows:[12]

Tis	Carcinoma in situ
T1	Tumor confined to one site of nasopharynx or no tumor visible (positive biopsy only)
T2	Tumor involving two sites (both posterosuperior and lateral walls)
T3	Extension of tumor into nasal cavity or oropharynx
T4	Tumor invasion of skull, cranial nerve involvement, or both

TREATMENT

Selection of Treatment Modality

The treatment of almost all malignancies of the nasopharynx is by radiation therapy since surgical resection is usually not feasible. Neck dissection is used less often in the management of neck disease in nasopharyngeal cancer because of the relatively high success rate with radiation therapy alone, particularly for lymphoepithelioma. Neck dissection should be added for large masses, persistence, or recurrence after irradiation. A small adenocarcinoma or sarcoma may be excised. Juvenile angiofibromas are preferably excised because of the young age of the patient, although the tumors are quite successfully cured by radiation therapy when surgical excision is impossible or dangerous.

Irradiation Technique

The anatomic planning is the same for squamous cell carcinoma, transitional cell carcinoma, and lymphoepithelioma. There is no place for small-volume irradiation even for an early epithelial tumor of the nasopharynx. If after complete clinical and roentgenographic workup the tumor is thought to be limited to the nasopharynx (T1–T2) or to have minimal soft-tissue extension (early T3), the following areas are included in the treatment volume:

1. Nasopharynx proper
2. Posterior 2 cm of the nasal cavity
3. Posterior ethmoid sinuses
4. Entire sphenoid sinus and basioccipital bone
5. Cavernous sinus
6. Base of skull (7–8 cm width encompassing the foramen ovale, carotid canal, and foramen spinosum laterally)
7. Pterygoid fossae
8. Posterior one third of maxillary sinus
9. Oropharyngeal wall to the level of the midtonsillar fossa
10. Retropharyngeal nodes
11. Neck nodes on both sides

Extension to the base of skull or involvement of cranial nerves II to VI requires that the superior border be raised to include all of the pituitary, the base of the brain in the suprasellar area, the adjacent middle cranial fossa, and the posterior portion of the anterior cranial fossa. Patients with anterior invasion into the orbit, ethmoids, or maxillary sinus require an individualized plan to produce a satisfactory volume distribution. The dose specified for the primary lesion is outlined in Table 21-69.[332] Patients are currently managed by irradiation with 120 cGy twice a day, but there are no reportable results to date.[14]

NECK NODES. A comprehensive en bloc plan must be developed to irradiate the neck to the level of the clavicles for both the epithelial lesions and the lymphomas. Even patients with no palpable disease in the neck have full neck irradiation.[9]

The retropharyngeal nodes are included in the treatment of the local lesion. The upper neck nodes are included in the primary fields to the level of the thyroid notch. In the case of no palpable nodes, the posterior margin is placed about 1 to 2 cm behind the posterior border of the sternocleidomastoid to encompass the high spinal accessory nodes and upper internal jugular nodes. The portals are extended anteriorly into the submental area only if there is disease in the submandibular triangle or if the patient had a neck dissection prior to irradiation.

The lower neck is treated through an anterior portal with a shield over the larynx.

Large neck nodes from a lymphoepithelioma may show amazing regression after a few treatments, or they may still be palpable after 5000 cGy in 5 weeks. The reason for the unpredictable response rate is that the lymphoepithelioma pattern may be continued into the lymph nodes or the lymph nodes may contain only squamous cell carcinoma.

ACUTE SEQUELAE. The large volume of mucosa irradiated produces unpleasant side-effects during treatment. Sore throat begins at the end of the second week of therapy and persists for 3 to 4 weeks after the completion of treatment. Dryness is always present and may be quite severe. Loss of taste and appetite is often quite profound, but both return 1 to 6 months after completion of treatment.

The auditory tube is in the high-dose area, and obstruction may occur with secondary otitis media and hearing loss. This condition can be corrected by polyethylene tubes inserted through the eardrums to drain the middle ears. The obstruction often improves or clears completely following mucosal healing of the nasopharynx. Politzerization of the eustachian tubes may reopen the canal.

Although mild nausea may occur, severe nausea and vomiting are uncommon. The overall effect of the treatment is quite wearing on the patient, and a period of several months may be required for successfully irradiated patients to regain a sense of well-being.

Management of Recurrence

The majority of recurrent squamous cell carcinomas are diagnosed within 2 years, but lymphoepithelioma may reappear many years after initial therapy. Recurrence in the base of skull or middle cranial fossa may be difficult to diagnose even with CT scan or MRI. Headache and cranial nerve palsies usually indicate recurrence.

Retreatment for recurrence may be rewarding, particularly in the lymphoepitheliomas. Patients have been kept free of local disease for varying lengths of time by irradiation to a limited portal with a high-energy beam or with brachy-

TABLE 21-69. Guide to Dosage for Primary Nasopharynx Tumors*

	Squamous Cell Carcinoma (cGy)	*Lymphoepithelioma* (cGy)	*Lymphocytic Lymphoma*† (cGy)	*Histiocytic Lymphoma*† (cGy)
T1, T2, early T3	6500	6000	3000	5000
Late T3, T4	7000	6500	3500	6000

Fletcher GH, Million RR: Nasopharynx. In Fletcher GH (ed): Textbook of Radiotherapy, 3rd ed, pp 364–383. Philadelphia, Lea & Febiger, 1980.

*850–900 cGy/week.

†See lymphoma chapter for additional information.

TABLE 21-70. Nasopharynx Cancer: Results of Radiation Therapy

Institution (Dates of Treatment)	*No. of Patients*	*5-Year Survival*	*Percentage of T4 Lesions*	*Percentage of Lymphoepithelioma*
M. D. Anderson Hospital[333] (1954–1977)	251	52% (actuarial)	30	45
University of Florida* (1964–1984)	69	53% (actuarial)	48	29
Stanford[334] (1956–1973)	74	59% (absolute)	11	36
University of California[36] (1940–1968)	146	37% (absolute)		25

*Analysis 1/87 by A. E. Spangler, M.D.

therapy sources inserted into the nasopharynx by mold technique.

RESULTS OF TREATMENT

The 5-year survival rate has improved considerably over the past 30 years. Survival rates of 10% to 30% were reported before the use of supervoltage techniques. Reports from the supervoltage era give encouraging 5-year survival rates in excess of 50% (Table 21-70).[36,333,334] The gains have not come from earlier diagnosis but from better staging of the primary lesion with tomography or CT scan, use of a larger treatment volume, higher doses, and comprehensive irradiation of the neck.

The actuarial local control curves for 69 patients treated at the University of Florida with a follow-up of 2 to 20 years are displayed in Figure 21-22. Eighty-eight percent of patients were Stage IV. The local control rate was better for lymphoepithelioma compared with similar-stage squamous cell carcinomas; the difference was especially noted for T4 lesions. The disease-free survival rate at 5 and 10 years was similar for lymphoepithelioma and squamous cell carcinoma when comparing similar stages (Figure 21-23). Distant metastasis was most closely related to neck stage and occurred in 18% of N0-N3A patients and 32% of N3B patients. The higher rate of local–regional control for lymphoepithelioma was offset by a higher rate of distant metastasis.

FIG. 21-22. Nasopharynx cancer: local control by stage and histology (actuarial method[249]). Lym, lymphoepithelioma; SCCa, squamous cell carcinoma. University of Florida data; patients treated 9/64 to 12/84. (Analysis 1/87 by A.E. Spangler, M.D.)

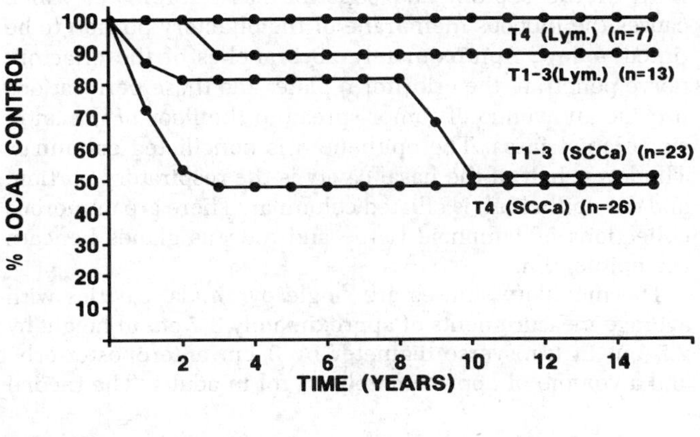

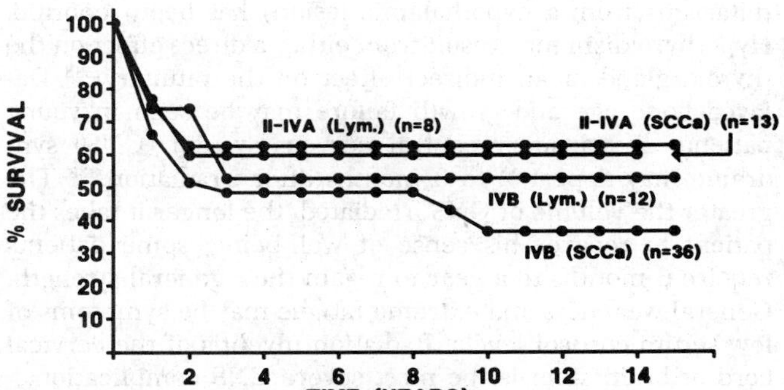

FIG. 21-23. Nasopharynx cancer: disease-free survival by AJCC stage and histology (actuarial method[249]). Lym, lymphoepithelioma; SCCa, squamous cell carcinoma. University of Florida data; patients treated 9/64 to 12/84. (Analysis 1/87 by A.E. Spangler, M.D.)

Operative results for juvenile angiofibroma have improved in recent years with the use of arteriography and CT to localize the tumor extent and preoperative arterial occlusion to reduce intraoperative blood loss. Biller and co-workers[335] reported a 93% cure rate with modern techniques.

Briant and co-workers[336] reported the results for irradiation of 45 patients with juvenile angiofibroma treated at the Princess Margaret Hospital. The disease was eventually controlled in all cases. Some 80% of the lesions were controlled by the initial treatment of 3000 cGy to 3500 cGy. Seven patients had their tumors controlled with a second course of radiation therapy and three by operation. No radiation-induced neoplasms have been observed with a follow-up of 2 to 20 years.[337]

FOLLOW-UP POLICY

Follow-up includes careful observation and laboratory testing for possible endocrine hypofunction of the thyroid and pituitary.

Dental care must be closely monitored because of the severe xerostomia.

The neck should be carefully observed because a patient with isolated neck recurrence may be salvaged by neck dissection. Documentation of local recurrence is important, but salvage is rarely possible if high-dose, large-volume treatment has been given initially. Localized recurrence of a lymphoepithelioma may be re-treated, especially if the initial doses were low.

COMPLICATIONS OF TREATMENT

The unavoidable irradiation of part of the brain including the hypothalamus, frontal and temporal lobes, and pituitary to doses between 6000 cGy and 7500 cGy has only rarely been associated with brain necrosis. Primary or secondary hypopituitarism (from a hypothalamic lesion) has been reported. Hypothyroidism may result from either a direct effect on the thyroid gland or an indirect effect on the pituitary.[338] Delayed bone age and growth failure may be seen in young patients. A transitory central nervous system (CNS) syndrome may appear 2 to 3 months after irradiation.[339] The greater the volume of CNS irradiated, the longer it takes the patient to recover his sense of well-being; some patients require 6 months to a year to regain their general strength. General weakness and extreme fatigue may be symptoms of low serum cortisol levels. Radiation myelitis of the cervical cord or brain stem is the most severe CNS complication.

Trismus occurs to varying degrees because of fibrosis and contracture of the pterygoid muscles rather than temporomandibular joint fibrosis. (This complication is more likely in those treated with two opposing portals for the entire course.)

Palsy of cranial nerves IX to XII may occur several years after treatment. This is a problem related to nerve entrapment in the lateral pharyngeal space.

Eye complications (*e.g.,* retrobulbar optic neuritis) may develop owing to irradiation of the optic nerve.

Irradiation of the posterior eyeball to high doses may produce a radiation retinopathy with decreased vision or even total loss of one eye.

NASAL VESTIBULE, NASAL CAVITY, AND PARANASAL SINUSES

Tumors of the nasal vestibule, the anterior entrance to the nasal cavity, are considered separately from nasal cavity tumors because they are essentially skin cancers and have a different natural history.

Primary tumors arising from the nasal cavity and paranasal sinuses are considered together because the lesions are frequently advanced when first seen and it is not always possible to determine the site of origin with certainty. Primary lesions of the lower half of the maxillary sinuses and Stage I lesions of the nasal cavity can be identified as such.

Cancer of the nasal cavity or paranasal sinuses is a relatively rare problem with a yearly risk factor estimated at approximately 1 case for every 100,000 people. These cancers occur more often in men (2:1) and usually appear after the age of 40 except for tumors of minor salivary gland origin or esthesioneuroblastomas, which may even appear before the age of 20.

Nasal cavity and ethmoid sinus adenocarcinomas have been linked to occupations associated with wood dust: the furniture industry, sawmill work, and carpentry. Other occupations with dust-filled work environments such as bootmaking and shoemaking, baking, and the flour milling industry also have been implicated as a cause of adenocarcinomas.[340–343]

Thorotrast, containing the radioactive metal thorium, is a known etiologic agent in maxillary sinus carcinomas. Thorotrast was used in past years as a contrast medium for roentgenographic study of the maxillary sinuses. The Thorotrast was retained in the sinus and was responsible for tumor induction.

Primary carcinomas of the sphenoid sinuses are said to be rare. They mimic nasopharyngeal carcinoma and most often are diagnosed after they penetrate the nasopharynx, at which time they are thought to be advanced nasopharyngeal cancer.

Frontal sinus neoplasms are rare.

ANATOMY

The nasal vestibule is the entrance to the nasal cavity. It is lined by skin in which there are numerous hair follicles and sebaceous glands. The vestibule is a three-sided, pear-shaped cavity about 1.5 cm in diameter that ends posteriorly at the limen nasi. The anterolateral wall is formed by the alar cartilages. The medial wall is the mobile columella, formed by the medial wing of the alar cartilage and the anterior portion of the cartilaginous septum. The floor is the superior surface of the hard palate (maxilla).

The nasal cavity begins at the limen nasi and ends at the posterior nares, where it communicates directly with the nasopharynx. Each lateral wall is composed of thin bony folds that project into the nasal cavity. These are the inferior, medial, and superior nasal turbinates. The nasolacrimal duct enters the nasal cavity beneath the inferior turbinate. The frontal sinus and ethmoid bullae connect to the nasal cavity with openings that lie under the middle turbinate. The sphenoid sinus communicates with the nasal cavity by an opening on the anterior wall of the sphenoid sinus. The olfactory nerves enter the nasal cavity through the cribriform plate and distribute nerve fibers over the upper one third of the septum and superior nasal turbinate, which causes the mucous membrane of the olfactory portion to be tinted yellow. Approximately 20 branches of the olfactory nerve penetrate the cribriform plate, and these perforations provide an avenue of tumor spread to the floor of the anterior cranial fossa. The epithelium is nonciliated columnar. The lower half of the nasal cavity is the respiratory portion, and the epithelium is ciliated columnar. There are numerous collections of lymphoid tissue and mucous glands beneath the epithelium.

The maxillary sinuses are single pyramidal cavities with average measurements of approximately 3.7 cm in height by 2.5 cm in transverse diameter by 3 cm anteroposteriorly, and a volume of approximately 15 ml in adults. The medial wall is the lateral wall of the nasal cavity and has one or two openings that communicate with the middle meatus under the medial turbinate. The inferior wall or floor is the hard palate. The roots of the teeth may penetrate into the cavity. The posterolateral wall is in relation to the zygomatic process and the pterygomaxillary space. The superior wall or roof separates the orbit from the sinus. All walls may be invaded and destroyed by cancer. The medial wall is breached easily by tumor because it is thin, with one or two large natural perforations, and the inferolateral wall may be traversed easily when the roots of the teeth provide partial bone disruption.

The frontal sinuses are two irregular, asymmetrical air cavities separated by a thin bony septum. They connect to the middle meatus of the nasal cavity by the frontonasal duct. Frontal sinus cells may extend far laterally in the orbital process of the frontal bone. They are separated from the anterior ethmoid cells by thin bony walls. The posterior wall separating the frontal sinus from the anterior cranial fossa is quite thick in most patients.

The ethmoid sinuses consist of a number of air cells lying between the medial walls of the orbits and the lateral wall of the nasal cavity. The lateral wall is the lamina papyracea, a very thin, porous bone easily penetrated by tumor. Medially, the ethmoid air cells bulge into the lateral wall of the nasal cavity and form the superior and medial turbinates. The ethmoid cells communicate with the nasal cavity in the middle meatus. These bony walls are thin and easily traversed by tumor. The ethmoid air cells extend quite far anteriorly, and for this reason ethmoid lesions may present as a subcutaneous mass at the inner canthus. The anterior cells actually are covered laterally by the lacrimal bone. The ethmoid bone is porous and presents little resistance to tumor spread. The right and left ethmoid cells are separated anatomically by the midline perpendicular plate of the ethmoid. There is no anatomic barrier between the anterior, middle, and posterior ethmoids.

The sphenoid sinus is a midline structure in the body of the sphenoid bone. The pituitary lies above, the cavernous sinuses laterally, the nasal cavity and ethmoid sinuses in front, and the nasopharynx beneath. The clivus and brain stem lie posteriorly. The pneumatization varies widely and can extend into all portions of the sphenoid bone. The right and left sinuses are partially separated by a septum, but are considered as one in treatment planning as the septum is said to be incomplete and easily penetrated. The sphenoid sinus connects anteriorly with the nasal cavity in the sphenoethmoidal recess.

Lymphatics

NASAL VESTIBULE. The lymphatic trunks run to the submaxillary nodes. There is a small risk for involvement of an intercalated facial node just behind the commissure of the lip along the course of a lymphatic vessel. In addition, preauricular nodes occasionally are involved, especially when tumor invades the lip or skin of the ala nasi.

NASAL CAVITY AND PARANASAL SINUSES. The lymphatics of the nasal cavity are separated into the olfactory group and the respiratory group. According to Rouviere,[3] they do not communicate with each other. There is a connection between the lymphatic network of the olfactory region and the subarachnoid spaces, which allows some absorption of cerebrospinal fluid (CSF) into the lymphatic system.

The lymphatics of the olfactory region of the nasal cavity run posteriorly to terminate in lymph nodes alongside the jugular vein at the base of the skull in the lateral pharyngeal space. The lymphatics of the respiratory nasal cavity also run posteriorly to terminate a bit lower, either in the lateral retropharyngeal node or the subdigastric node. The capillary lymphatic plexus of the nasal mucosa must not be very profuse, judged by the relatively small incidence of metastatic nodes even with advanced disease.

The mucosa of the paranasal sinuses has no capillary lymphatics or a very sparse number of capillary lymphatics. Metastases from carcinoma of the paranasal sinuses are uncommon, even though lesions frequently are quite advanced. It is literally unheard-of for a paranasal sinus tumor to present with cervical lymphadenopathy and an asymptomatic primary lesion confined to a sinus. Metastases probably only occur once tumor has extended beyond the paranasal sinuses to areas containing a supply of capillary lymphatics (*e.g.*, nasopharynx, buccal mucosa, nasal cavity, and skin).

PATHOLOGY

Benign Tumors

Many so-called benign tumors destroy bone and soft tissues and, if uncorrected, cause death. The management of some of these problems is not unlike cancer treatment.

Inflammatory polyps, giant cell reparative granulomas, benign mixed tumors of minor salivary gland origin, benign odontogenic tumors, and necrotizing sialometaplasia are some of the benign lesions appearing in this area.[344]

Malignant Tumors

NASAL VESTIBULE. Almost all malignant tumors arising in the nasal vestibule are squamous cell carcinoma; basal cell carcinoma and adnexal carcinomas are also reported.

NASAL CAVITY AND PARANASAL SINUSES. Squamous cell carcinoma or one of its variants is the most common neoplasm. Minor salivary gland tumors account for about 10% to 15% of neoplasms in this region. Malignant melanoma accounts for less than 1% of all neoplasms of the nasal cavity and paranasal sinuses. Malignant lymphoma, usually histiocytic, occurs in about 5% of cases. It is frequently a locally destructive lesion because it arises more often in bone than in soft tissue.

Esthesioneuroblastoma or olfactory neuroblastoma is a malignant neurogenic tumor that originates from the olfactory mucosa and has a histologic picture resembling adrenal neuroblastoma or retinoblastoma. The normal olfactory epithelium covers the undersurface of the cribriform plate, the upper surface of the middle turbinate, and the superior nasal septum.[276] Histologically, esthesioneuroblastoma may be confused with undifferentiated carcinoma or undifferentiated lymphoma. It occurs at all ages, with cases commonly seen in the second and third decades. A 3-year-old boy with an advanced lesion has been reported; the authors have treated a 12-year-old boy.[345]

A wide range of soft tissue and bone sarcomas is reported for the nasal cavity and paranasal sinus region, including chondrosarcoma, osteosarcoma, Ewing's sarcoma, and most of the soft-tissue sarcomas.

Inverting papilloma of the nasal cavity is a confusing condition often called benign, but for practical reasons it is best classified under malignant because it may have a rather aggressive clinical picture that requires cancer-type management and may be associated with a carcinoma. It is better approached as a "grade ½" neoplasm than as a benign polyp; it may be lethal if uncontrolled. The histologic picture is that of a papilloma that is growing into the stroma rather than growing outward. The histologic appearance does not predict the clinical course. The lesion occurs predominantly in men 40 to 70 years of age. Squamous cell or transitional cell carcinoma is reported in association with inverting papilloma in 5% to 15% of cases and may represent conversion of the papilloma to a more malignant tumor.[346]

Midline lethal granuloma is a rather mysterious, progressively destructive condition that involves the nose, paranasal sinuses, and hard palate, and produces secondary erosion of contiguous structures. Unchecked, the disease is fatal, usually after an extended illness. Death results from extension to the CNS, hemorrhage, sepsis, or inanition. Etiology is debatable. Midline lethal granuloma can be distinguished from Wegener's granulomatosis, which also produces inflammatory and destructive changes in the paranasal sinuses and nasal cavity. Wegener's granulomatosis also involves lung and kidney with a necrotizing vasculitis. Kassel and co-workers[347] subdivide midline lethal granuloma into three different histologic entities: midline malignant reticulosis, malignant lymphoma (usually histocytic lymphoma), and Wegener's granulomatosis.

PATTERNS OF SPREAD

Nasal Vestibule

PRIMARY. Lesions of the nasal vestibule invade the alar and septal cartilages and may extend to the skin surface of the nose. The upper lip is frequently invaded. Posterior growth into the nasal cavity is frequent. Early lesions originating on the columella and anterior septum are often superficial lesions that ulcerate and produce a crust or scab and often present with perforation of the membranous and cartilaginous septum.

LYMPHATIC. Lymph node spread is usually to a solitary ipsilateral submaxillary node, but may be unilateral. The facial, preauricular, and submental nodes are at small risk. Goepfert and co-workers[348] report only 1 of 26 patients with clinically positive lymph nodes on admission, but 7 patients later developed positive lymph nodes with 4 patients eventually showing bilateral disease. Mendenhall and co-workers[349] reported 2 patients with biopsy-proven lymph nodes out of 22 cases. Another two subsequently developed lymph node metastases. The neck disease was controlled in all 4 cases.

Nasal Cavity and Paranasal Sinuses

NASAL CAVITY. The routes of spread are essentially the same for various histologies, with the exception of esthesioneuroblastoma and minor salivary gland tumors. The latter have a greater propensity for perineural spread, although squamous carcinoma and esthesioneuroblastoma also may follow nerve pathways.

Lesions arising in the olfactory region invade the ethmoids and the orbit, spread through the sievelike cribriform plate to the anterior cranial fossa, and spread between bone and dura. Eventually they penetrate dura and invade the frontal lobes. These lesions also tend to destroy the septum and may invade through nasal bone to the skin. Lesions arising on the lateral wall of the respiratory portion of the nasal cavity invade the medial wall of the maxillary sinus, the ethmoids, and the orbit.

Esthesioneuroblastomas may show submucosal spread and may grow along olfactory nerves and penetrate through an intact dura to the frontal lobe.[350]

The nasopharynx and sphenoid sinus are secondarily invaded in advanced lesions. Tumor may follow the numerous nasal nerves posteriorly and then superiorly toward the sphenopalatine ganglion near the base of the skull or along the maxillary branch of the trigeminal nerve.

MAXILLARY SINUS. All walls of the sinus may be penetrated by tumor. The pattern of spread and bone destruction is largely dependent on site of origin within the sinus. Lesions arising in the anterolateral infrastructure tend to invade through the lateral inferior wall or grow through dental sockets. Cancer presents in the oral cavity when tumor erodes through the maxillary gingiva or into the gingival-buccal sulcus. When tumor erupts through into the oral cavity, the tumor is at first submucosal, causing elevation of the mucosa, loosening of the teeth, or improper seating of a denture. Ulceration follows, with the development of an oral-antral fistula.

Lesions arising on the medial infrastructure readily extend through the thin, porous medial wall into the nasal cavity.

Posterior infrastructure lesions erode through the posterolateral wall and into the infratemporal fossa. The extension is best seen on CT or MRI scan. Recognition of this route of spread is important because tumor escaping posteriorly has immediate access to the base of the skull and may defeat an operative attempt. Extension of lesions to the orbit occurs either directly through the roof of the maxillary sinus, by a circuitous route through the ethmoids and lamina papyracea, or by way of the infratemporal fossa and then through the infraorbital fissure.

Tumors arising in the upper half (suprastructure) of the antrum have two general patterns of development. One group develops laterally, invades the malar bone, and produces a mass just below the lateral floor of the orbit. The soft-tissue mass may become quite large and eventually ulcerate through to the skin, producing an antrocutaneous fistula. The orbit is invaded laterally and displaces the eye inward and upward. The temporal fossa is often involved, as is the zygomatic bone in very advanced lesions.

The suprastructural cancers that develop medially invade the nasal cavity, ethmoid and frontal sinuses, lacrimal apparatus, and medial inferior orbit. It is often impossible to determine whether the origin is maxillary antrum, nasal cavity, or ethmoid.

ETHMOID SINUSES. Lesions of the ethmoid sinuses have many options for local spread because of their location and thin, porous bony walls, none of which offers particular resistance to tumor penetration. The lamina papyracea is the lateral wall for the middle and posterior ethmoid air cells. Invasion through the lamina papyracea into the medial orbit is common. The anterior ethmoid cells are covered laterally by the small, thin lacrimal bone and the frontal process of the maxilla. Thus, the ethmoid air cells extend anteriorly within a centimeter of the inner canthus.[351]

The medial surfaces of the ethmoid labyrinth are the middle and superior nasal conchae, which are formed by thin, convoluted bone; spread into the nasal cavity is common. The more advanced lesions invade the maxillary antrum, nasopharynx, sphenoid sinus, and anterior cranial fossa.

SPHENOID SINUS. There is little information regarding spread patterns for tumors arising in the sphenoid sinus. It is probable that some of the advanced nasopharyngeal lesions are, in reality, primary sphenoid sinus lesions. The fact that a disproportionate number of advanced nasopharynx lesions have no neck metastases is suggestive of their origin in the sphenoid sinus, a site with sparse, if any, capillary lymphatics.

The sphenoid sinus is in close relationship with the cranial nerves in the cavernous sinus: III, IV, and VI, and the ophthalmic and maxillary branches of the trigeminal nerve (Fig. 21-24). Cranial nerve palsies and headache are frequently the first clinical evidence of a sphenoid sinus tumor. Diagnosis is usually made, however, when tumor eventually breaks through into the nasopharynx or nasal cavity where it can be seen and biopsied.

FIG. 21-24. Coronal section of the cavernous sinus.

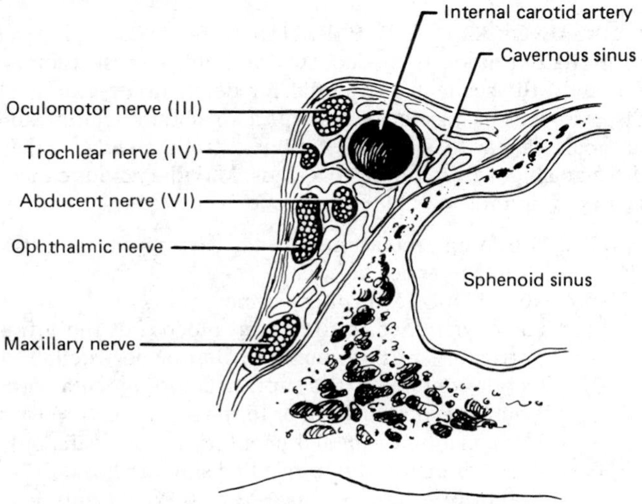

INVERTING PAPILLOMA. A report of 223 cases of inverting papilloma showed that the lateral nasal wall was the most commonly involved site (68%), with ethmoid and maxillary sinus involvement also common (57%), as was involvement of the septum (28%). However, ethmoid and maxillary sinus involvement without tumor of the lateral nasal wall occurred in only 4%. Intracranial extension was usually associated with a carcinoma. Tumor occurred bilaterally when there was spread through the nasal septum; multicentric sites of origin were reported.[352] There are two reports in the literature of cervical metastases from benign-appearing inverted papilloma; the metastases had the microscopic appearance of inverting papilloma.[353,354]

LYMPHATIC. The incidence of lymphatic metastases on admission is 10% to 15% for nasal cavity and ethmoid sinus tumors and probably even lower for antral and sphenoid tumors. The risk of lymphatic metastases is related to extension of tumor outside the sinus to areas with capillary lymphatics. Maxillary sinus tumors that invade the oral cavity and involve the buccal mucosa, maxillary gingiva, or hard palate may spread to the submandibular and jugulodigastric nodes. Lesions that invade the nasal cavity or naropharynx spread posteriorly to the parapharyngeal nodes and then to the jugulodigastric area. Esthesioneuroblastoma, minor salivary gland tumors, melanoma, and sarcomas have an unknown rate of lymph node metastasis.

CLINICAL PICTURE

Nasal Vestibule

These lesions present with symptoms of a slow-growing mass in the entrance to the nose with attendant crusting, scabbing, and occasional minor bleeding. Pain, if it occurs, is usually modest, even with destruction of cartilage or involvement of the lip. Secondary infection may occur, in which case the nose is painful on manipulation. Septal perforation may occur.

Nasal Cavity and Paranasal Sinuses

NASAL CAVITY. The earliest symptoms of nasal cavity neoplasm are a low-grade chronic infection with discharge, obstruction, and minor, intermittent bleeding. The symptoms mimic those associated with nasal polyps; because many of the patients with nasal neoplasms have a previous history of nasal operations for polyps, cancer is often missed in an early stage. The patient often complains of "sinus trouble" and intermittent anterior headache. Subsequent symptoms depend on pattern of growth. Lesions arising in the olfactory region may cause unilateral or bilateral nasal expansion of the bridge of the nose, and a submucosal mass may appear near the inner canthus and eventually ulcerate. Obstruction of the nasolacrimal system may be a presenting complaint, with the patient treated by incision and drainage for a dacryocystitis. Extension through the cribriform plate or onto the ethmoid sinuses is accompanied by frontal headache. Aberration of smell is rare.

Invasion of the medial orbit produces proptosis and diplopia; a mass may be palpated in the orbit. Indirect examination of the nasopharynx may show early submucosal invasion through the posterior nares.

MAXILLARY SINUS. These cancers develop silently when they are confined to the sinus and produce symptoms on extension through the walls. If the tumor invades toward the oral cavity, the presenting symptoms relate to pain associated with the upper teeth; there may be loosening and eventually loss of teeth. The dentist is often the first one consulted, and the patient may have dental extraction without pain relief. Tumor may penetrate into the gingivobuccal sulcus or upper gum and eventually progress to an oral-antral fistula. If the patient wears upper dentures, the first symptom will be an ill-fitting denture. Palpation and observation of the face may show a mass. Early invasion of the floor of the orbit may be detected by feeling both orbits simultaneously with the tips of the index fingers inserted between the bony rim and eyeball. Posterior invasion of the orbit will produce proptosis, diplopia, and edema of the conjunctiva. Invasion of the inferior orbital nerve or its branches in the floor of the orbit may cause paresthesias or anesthesia of the skin of the lower eyelid, side of the nose, and anterior premaxillary skin. Nasal obstruction and bleeding are common complaints, along with "sinus pain" or "fullness" over the involved antrum. Trismus and headache are associated with invasion posteriorly into the pterygopalatine fossa, pterygoid muscles, infratemporal fossa, and base of the skull.

Cancers developing in the medial suprastructure of the antrum present with nasal symptoms of discharge or bleeding, mild infraorbital pain, infected lacrimal sac, and displacement of the eye upward and laterally with proptosis, diplopia, and conjunctival edema.

Cancer developing in the lateral suprastructure produces a mass below the lateral canthus with associated pain. The eye may be deviated medially and upward when orbital invasion occurs. There is edema of the conjunctiva, narrowing of the palpebral opening, diplopia, and proptosis. Tumor may extend to the temporal fossa, producing a diffuse fullness.

ETHMOID SINUSES. Mild to moderate sinus ache or pain referred to the frontal-nasal area is an early symptom. A painless mass may present near the inner canthus; the mass may become infected and be interpreted as a boil or dacryocystitis, at which time an inappropriate incision and drainage procedure is done. Diplopia develops with invasion of the medial orbit. Proptosis is often present, and a mass may be felt by digital palpation of the orbit. Nasal discharge, epistaxis, and obstruction are frequent presenting complaints. Paresthesias may occur over the distribution of sensory nerves.

Physical examination includes anterior and posterior rhinoscopy after thorough shrinking of the nasal mucosa. A fiberoptic nasoscope is a great aid in visualizing the posterior and superior nasal cavity and the nasopharynx. Early invasion of the nasal cavity may produce only submucosal bulging into the superior or medial meatus, which is easily confused with allergic rhinitis, polyps, or inflammatory changes. Pus may be seen coming from beneath the superior, middle, or inferior turbinate.

Eye examination includes palpation of the orbit for masses. Palpation should be carried out simultaneously in both orbits because the changes in the involved orbit are frequently subtle. Extraocular movements are examined and proptosis is measured.

Invasion into the nasopharynx is usually submucosal and appears on the roof and lateral wall. Advanced lesions may obstruct the eustachian canal.

METHODS OF DIAGNOSIS AND STAGING

Biopsy Technique

Tumor in the nasal cavity is biopsied with punch forceps. Biopsy of tumor in the maxillary antrum is usually approached through a Caldwell-Luc procedure, which is an incision through the gingivobuccal sulcus opposite the premolars. The approach allows adequate visualization of the entire antrum.

Biopsy of ethmoid tumors is usually taken from the extension to the nasal cavity or inner canthus area. Tumor confined to the ethmoids may be found unexpectedly at the time of a lateral rhinotomy planned for diagnosis or treatment of benign disease.

An undiagnosed orbital mass occasionally may be the site of biopsy because of incomplete examination of other areas. Sphenoid sinus tumors are biopsied by way of the transnasal route for the rare localized disease, but biopsy is usually made of an extension to the nasopharynx or nasal cavity. Frontal sinus tumors are approached by supraorbital incision and osteotomy.

Staging

NASAL VESTIBULE. The staging used for skin cancer is appropriate for this area. CT and MRI scans are useful for advanced or recurrent lesions.

NASAL CAVITY AND PARANASAL SINUSES. Physical examination alone is inadequate for staging these tumors. CT and MRI scans are essential for determining extent of disease. MRI is particularly helpful to obtain sagittal and coronal planes, to eliminate artifacts from metals, and to distinguish pus from tumor in a sinus. Maxillary sinus cancer is staged as follows:[12]

- TX Minimum requirements to assess the primary tumor cannot be met
- T0 No evidence of primary tumor
- T1 Tumor confined to the antral mucosa of the infrastructure with no bone erosion or destruction
- T2 Tumor confined to the suprastructure mucosa without bone destruction, or to the infrastructure with destruction of medial or inferior bony walls only
- T3 More extensive tumor invading skin of cheek, orbit, anterior ethmoid sinuses, or pterygoid muscle

T4 Massive tumor with invasion of cribriform plate, posterior ethmoids, sphenoid, nasopharynx, pterygoid plates, or base of skull

There is no AJCC staging system for nasal cavity or ethmoid, sphenoid, or frontal sinus cancer. The following system, based on prognostic factors that seemed to correlate best with response to treatment, was adopted at the University of Florida:

I Limited to site of origin
II Extension to adjacent sites (*e.g.*, orbit, nasopharynx, paranasal sinuses, skin, pterygomaxillary fossa)
III Base of skull or pterygoid plate destruction, or intracranial extension, or both

TREATMENT

Nasal Vestibule

SELECTION OF TREATMENT MODALITY. Both surgical resection and radiation therapy produce a high degree of success in experienced hands.[348,355,356] Radiation therapy is usually the preferred treatment because of the deformity produced by excision. Excision is preferred for very small lesions, the removal of which will not produce cosmetic deformity or require reconstruction; few lesions fit this description. Radiation therapy is selected for the remainder, with surgery reserved for radiation failure. Radiation therapy has been successful in salvaging surgical failures, but the nasal deformity has already been produced and the value of irradiation lost.

SURGICAL TREATMENT. Excision of lesions in the nasal vestibule usually involves removal of cartilage as well as skin. Depending on the site of the lesion, either the columella, the septum, or the alar cartilages will have to be removed, with a resulting cosmetic deformity that is difficult to reconstruct. If the alar cartilage has been sacrificed, either a composite graft consisting of skin and cartilage from the ear or a nasolabial flap can be used to repair the defect. If the entire external nose is resected, a prosthesis is used.

IRRADIATION TECHNIQUE. External beam, interstitial, or a combination of both may be used.

There are two basic external beam treatment plans: opposed lateral portals and single anterior portal. When the tumor volume can be encompassed by lateral portals, there is an advantage in avoiding unnecessary exit irradiation to the nasal cavity, nasopharynx, and CNS. This technique confines irradiation to the anterior nasal area, but has the disadvantage of full skin reaction because a wax bolus nose block is necessary to ensure homogeneous irradiation. The portals may be angled posteriorly to ensure sufficient posterior coverage; wedges are added to compensate for the angle. Fractionation schemes are those used for orthovoltage because the bolus produces skin reactions comparable to orthovoltage therapy.

The anterior portal technique uses a single anterior portal with a combination of photons and electrons. A wax bolus is used to ensure a homogeneous dose. The advantages of this technique are that the portal may be shaped, it is easier to shield the eyes, and the skin of the tip of the nose and sometimes the bridge of the nose need not be covered by the wax and therefore some of the skin receives a lesser dose of radiation.[349,356]

Interstitial implants of the nasal vestibule and nasal cavity are highly individualized. The basic implant is usually composed of two, three, or four planes of sources inserted through the skin surface of the external nose. The basic arrangement to cover the entire nasal vestibule and upper lip is shown in Figure 21-25. The dose has varied, depending on the size of the lesion.[349,356]

Nasal Cavity

SELECTION OF TREATMENT MODALITY. The histology, extent, and location of the malignant tumor in the nasal cavity are all considered when treatment decisions are made.

Inverting papilloma is treated initially by surgical excision. The local recurrence rate is fairly high, and subsequent excisions may be required. When the lesion begins to act aggressively with rapid recurrences and invasion of the sinuses, orbit, and anterior cranial fossa, it should be considered a low-grade cancer and treated appropriately by more radical removal. Irradiation is recommended for lesions that are surgically unresectable, for patients with multiple recur-

FIG. 21-25. Diagram of interstitial implant for carcinoma of the nasal vestibule.

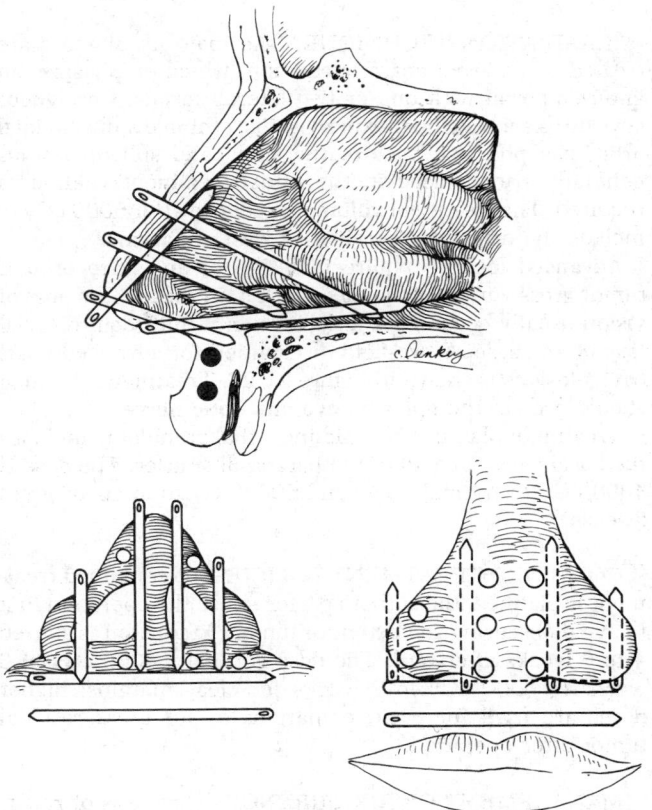

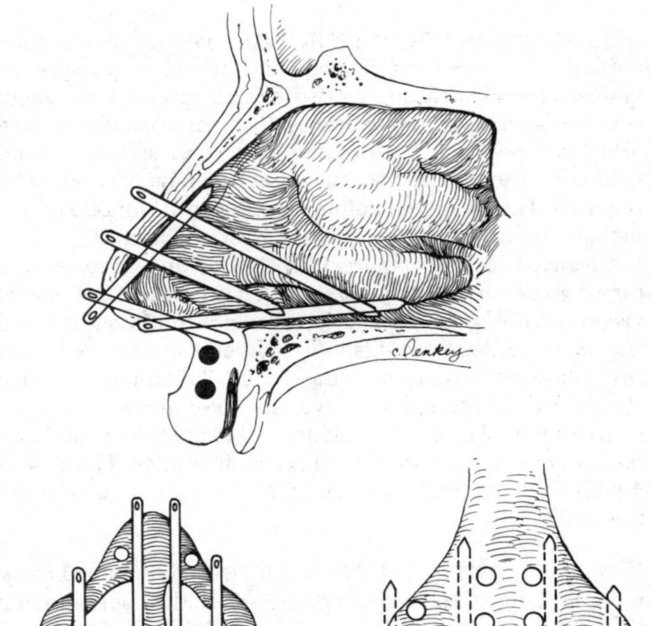

rences, and for those in which carcinoma is found in the specimen.[346,352]

Squamous cell carcinoma and adenocarcinoma of the nasal cavity can be treated with surgery, irradiation, or both. Most analyses of nasal cavity carcinomas are included with paranasal sinus cancer series. Because standardized staging is not applied, it is difficult to compare the results of various therapies. Regional and distant metastases are relatively uncommon, and therefore, local control is tantamount to cure.

Either surgery or radiation therapy is used for discrete early lesions. Operative management may be indicated for early lesions, in which good surgical margins can be expected without cosmetic or functional loss. Excision is also the treatment of choice for melanomas and sarcomas. Radiation therapy is used for the majority of nasal cavity carcinomas because of the difficulty in obtaining en bloc removal of the more advanced lesions and reasonably good results with irradiation. Combined therapy may be recommended in selected cases.

Midline lethal granuloma is treated by radiation therapy to the nasal cavity and all of the paranasal sinuses.

SURGICAL TREATMENT. Lateral rhinotomy provides the best access for resection of lesions of the nasal cavity. Generally reconstruction is not necessary unless the entire cartilaginous septum has been removed, in which case there will be a saddle deformity of the nose. The lateral wall of the nose may be removed by this approach for resection of inverting papilloma and other localized neoplasms. More advanced lesions require removal of involved sinuses and orbit. A craniofacial procedure may be required.

IRRADIATION TECHNIQUE. The majority of cases are treated by external beam irradiation, which emphasizes an anterior portal with one or two lateral portals. Contiguous structures such as the maxillary sinus, ethmoid sinus, medial orbit, nasopharynx, base of the skull, and sphenoid sinus generally are included in the initial treatment volume as required. The treatment volume is reduced after 5000 cGy to include the original gross disease with a margin.

Advanced lesions require inclusion of an entire orbit if tumor grossly invades the medial orbit; in these cases, loss of vision usually occurs, but an operation would require visual loss in any case. A two-field distribution for advanced nasal cavity lesions is shown in Figure 21-26. Treatment planning should protect the opposite eye and optic nerve.

Treatment planning for midline lethal granuloma includes the nasal cavity and all of the paranasal sinuses. The dose is 4000 cGy to normal areas and 5000 cGy to areas of gross disease.

COMBINED TREATMENT POLICIES. If combined treatment is planned, the authors prefer to use the operation first to avoid obscuring the extent of tumor. Irradiation is started 4 to 6 weeks afterward. The dose is usually 6000 cGy in 6 weeks to 6500 cGy in 7 weeks for clear margins; higher doses are used for positive margins or for gross residual tumor after operation.

MANAGEMENT OF RECURRENCE. Diagnosis of recurrent lesions is important because salvage may be possible.

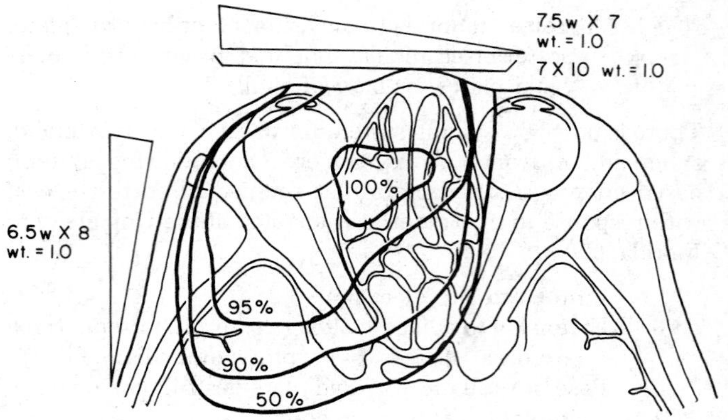

FIG. 21-26. Isodose distribution for carcinoma of the nasal cavity or ethmoid sinus with invasion of the orbit.

Once the patient has had an operation or irradiation, it is difficult to determine the extent of recurrent disease because of changes from the previous therapy. The most common situation for salvage is a radiation or surgical failure that can be treated successfully by a craniofacial resection. Tumor extension to the sphenopalatine fossa with definite destruction of a pterygoid plate is a relative contraindication to a craniofacial procedure. Cranial nerve involvement, invasion posteriorly near the optic chiasm, and sphenoid sinus or cavernous sinus invasion are absolute contraindications to resection. MRI can distinguish between exudate and gross tumor in a sinus, but surgical exploration may be necessary to exclude microscopic extension to the sinuses. The anterior wall of the sphenoid sinus may be removed, but the sinus itself cannot be resected.[357] Postoperative irradiation should be considered whether or not margins are positive. About 25% of patients may be saved by this approach.

Maxillary Sinus

SELECTION OF TREATMENT MODALITY. Surgical resection gives the best results. Early infrastructural lesions may be excised and cured by surgery alone, but for most other cases, irradiation is given postoperatively even if margins are negative. Extension of cancer to the base of the skull, nasopharynx, or sphenoid sinus contraindicates surgical excision. The pterygoid process below the foramen rotundum may be removed along with the attached pterygoid muscles, but destruction of the sphenoid bone above this point is a contraindication to operation. Operations to resect portions of the base of the skull are described for special clinical situations.

SURGICAL TREATMENT. Surgery for carcinoma of the maxillary sinus depends on which walls are involved. If the floor of the orbit is free of disease, then the eye and the orbital rim may be left undisturbed. If, however, there is involvement through the floor of the orbit, then a maxillectomy and orbital exenteration must be performed. If the posterior wall or the pterygoid plates are involved, they too must be included in the resection. A split-thickness skin graft is used to line the cavity, and a dental prosthesis then is used to fill the resulting deformity in the palate. The prosthesis is constructed prior to surgery so that it can be placed at the time of operation and act as a stent. The permanent prosthesis is constructed about 6 months after the operation.

IRRADIATION TECHNIQUE. Irradiation treatment planning includes the entire maxilla, the adjacent nasal cavity, ethmoid sinus, nasopharynx, and pterygopalatine fossa. All or part of the orbit is included in patients with extension into or near the orbital fossa; failure to include the orbital contents is one of the most common causes of failure. The prescribed dose is 6500 cGy to 7000 cGy for irradiation alone. The dose for preoperative irradiation varies from 5000 cGy to 6000 cGy, and the dose for postoperative irradiation varies from 6000 cGy to 7000 cGy. If radiation therapy alone is planned, localized drainage procedures can be done before, during, or after radiation therapy, as dictated by clinical necessity.

COMBINED TREATMENT POLICIES. Except for the early infrastructural lesion, surgical resection is usually followed by external beam radiation therapy.

Ethmoid Sinus

SELECTION OF TREATMENT MODALITY. Ethmoid sinus lesions are usually extensive when first diagnosed. Radiation therapy alone produces better results than surgery alone and is the preferred single treatment.[358] If resection is feasible with acceptable functional and cosmetic results, then the operation is carried out, followed by postoperative radiation therapy even if the margins are clear.

SURGICAL TREATMENT. Localized lesions require resection of the ethmoids and the ipsilateral maxilla and orbit. Extensive lesions are removed by a craniofacial procedure.

IRRADIATION TECHNIQUE. Radiation treatment is entirely by external beam, emphasizing treatment through an anterior field combined with one or two lateral fields. This field arrangement, weighted 2:1 or 3:1 in favor of the anterior field, provides adequate treatment of the tumor volume while avoiding excessive irradiation of the contralateral eye and optic nerve. Wedges are added to achieve a satisfactory dose distribution. Electrons should not be used for the anterior portal.

MANAGEMENT OF RECURRENCE. Recurrent disease is heralded by recurrent pain and cranial nerve palsies. Exploration of the sinuses is necessary for diagnosis.

Localized recurrence after surgery only may be managed by radiation therapy alone or craniofacial resection and postoperative radiation therapy. Radiation therapy failures may be suitable for maxillectomy or craniofacial resection.

Sphenoid Sinus

The treatment is with radiation therapy, and the technique is similar to that for advanced carcinoma of the nasopharynx.

RESULTS OF TREATMENT

Nasal Vestibule

Goepfert and co-workers[348] reviewed the M. D. Anderson Hospital experience of 26 patients with squamous cell carcinoma of the nasal vestibule. The absolute 5-year survival was 78%. Ten patients were treated initially by surgery; one developed a local recurrence and was salvaged by radiation therapy. Sixteen patients were treated by radiation therapy; three developed local recurrence, and two were salvaged by an operation.

Mendenhall and co-workers[349] reviewed 22 patients treated by irradiation at the University of Florida for squamous cell carcinoma of the nasal vestibule; 7 had recurrent disease after one to four previous surgical excisions, and 15 had had no prior treatment. Eleven patients had obvious cartilage invasion, two had bone destruction, and three had massive infiltration of the soft tissues of the face (Table 21-71). Two patients had biopsy-proven lymph node metastases on admission, and both were cured by radiation therapy. Two patients subsequently developed a single submandibular node that was controlled by radical neck dissection; they were alive at 9 and 16 years postsurgery. Radiation therapy complications were minor. There was no example of persistent chondritis or soft-tissue necrosis. The 5-year actuarial determinate survival rate was 95%, and the 10-year and 15-year rate was 82%.

Nasal Cavity and Ethmoid Sinus

INVERTING PAPILLOMA. Weissler and co-workers[352] reported 233 cases of inverting papilloma seen over a 35-year period. One hundred thirty-four patients had at least 1 year of follow-up. The risk of recurrence was 71% in patients who had an intranasal procedure. The recurrence rate was 56% for those having a Caldwell-Luc approach. Patients having a lateral rhinotomy had the smallest incidence of recurrence (29%). Reports from more modern series show an even lower incidence of recurrence when a lateral rhinotomy approach was used.[359]

TABLE 21-71. Nasal Vestibule Carcinoma: Local Control by Radiation Therapy

	No. Controlled/No. Treated	
T Stage	*De novo*	*Recurrent*
Tx	1/1	
T1	4/4	2/2
T2	1/1	1/1
T3	1/1	1/1*
T4	6/8*†	2/3†
Total	13/15	6/7

Mendenhall NP, Parsons JT, Cassisi NJ, et al: Carcinoma of the nasal vestibule treated with radiation therapy. Laryngoscope 97:626–632, 1987.

University of Florida data. Patients treated 1964 to 1984; minimum 2-year follow-up.

*Two patients had biopsy-proven lymph node metastases on admission.

†None of the 3 failures was salvaged.

Weissler and co-workers[352] also reported 6 patients who received radiation therapy for benign inverting papilloma and 9 for inverting papilloma associated with malignant disease. Twelve of the 15 patients had a complete response to radiation therapy and were free of disease for long periods of follow-up.

Mendenhall and co-workers[346] also reported success with radiation therapy. Their series has been recently updated (Mendenhall WM: Personal communication, 1987), and there are a total of seven patients who received radiation therapy for inverting papilloma. All but one were treated for recurrent disease after one or more operations, and two had foci of carcinoma. Six of the 7 patients remained free of disease at 3, 5, 7, 7, 9, and 14 years. One patient died of persistent disease 17 months after radiation therapy. In one patient treated with preoperative radiation therapy followed by surgery, there was no tumor in the specimen. Two of the patients had surgery followed by immediate irradiation for residual disease and 4 patients were treated with radiation therapy alone.

CARCINOMA. Frazell and Lewis[360] reported a 56% 5-year cure rate for 68 nasal cavity neoplasms treated surgically. The 5-year cure rate by radiation therapy was 18% for 28 patients treated. The selection and stage of patients for each modality were not analyzed. Frazell and Lewis[360] reported that 40% of patients (4 of 10) with ethmoid sinus carcinoma treated by radiation therapy were cured at 5 years, but only 4 of 21 patients treated by an operation were cured. They concluded, however, that the operation was the treatment of choice.

Cheesman and co-workers[361] selected craniofacial resection for 54 patients with a variety of malignant tumors of the nasal cavity and paranasal sinuses; the majority were recurrent after surgery, radiation therapy, or chemotherapy. The operative mortality was 5%. Seven of 25 patients were free of disease with a minimum of 3 years of follow-up.

Bosch and co-workers[362] reported their experience with 40 cases of cancer of the nasal cavity. Eighty-five percent were treated by radiation therapy. The 5-year survival rate was 56% for the entire group and 50% for those treated by radiation therapy alone.

Boone and co-workers[363] reported the M. D. Anderson Hospital experience for 28 patients with nasal cavity carcinoma. The 5-year absolute cure rate was 64%; the local recurrence rate was 21%.

Parsons and co-workers[364] reviewed the results for 48 patients with malignant tumors of the nasal cavity, ethmoid sinus, and sphenoid sinus treated from October 1964 through December 1983 by radiation therapy. Forty-two patients were treated by radiation therapy only and 7 by combined surgery and radiation therapy. Of the 42 patients treated by radical courses of irradiation, 37 had de novo lesions and 5 had postsurgical recurrences. Twenty-one percent presented with clinical evidence of advanced orbital invasion, and 12 others had only radiographic evidence of orbital extension. The actuarial local control results at 5, 10, and 15 years by histology are shown in Table 21-72 and the local control rates[249] by stage are shown in Figure 21-27. Although adenoid cystic carcinomas were initially responsive, late-onset recurrence was the rule. The overall 10-year actuarial local control rate for 42 patients with histologies other than adenoid cystic carcinoma was 52% for all stages combined. Eight patients had evidence of intracranial extension prior to irradiation, and in three the disease remains locally controlled at 3.5, 4, and 9 years following treatment of adenocarcinoma (1 patient) or esthesioneuroblastoma (2 patients). Forty-four patients presented with a clinically neg-

FIG. 21-27. Carcinoma of the nasal cavity and paranasal sinuses: actuarial[249] local control according to tumor stage for all histologies combined. Failures after 5 years are due to minor salivary gland tumors. (Parsons JT, Mendenhall WM, Mancuso AA, et al: Malignant tumors of the nasal cavity and ethmoid and sphenoid sinuses. Int J Radiat Oncol Biol Phys Int J Radiat Oncol Biol Phys 14:11–22, 1988)

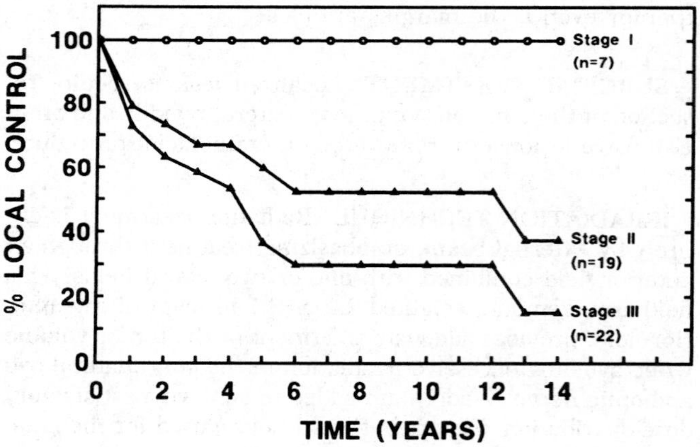

TABLE 21-72. Actuarial Local Control After Radiation Therapy in Nasal Cavity and Ethmoid/Sphenoid Sinus Cancer (All Stages; 2-Year Minimum Follow-up)

Type of Tumor	*No. of Patients*	*Actuarial Local Control (%)*		
		5 Years	*10 Years*	*15 Years*
Squamous cell carcinoma	21	45	45	45
Esthesioneuroblastoma	8	43	43	
Minor salivary gland tumors (excluding adenoid cystic)	8	75	75	45
Adenoid cystic	6	65	30	18
Miscellaneous (melanoma, sarcoma)	5	60	60	60

Data from Parsons et al.[364]

ative neck. Elective neck irradiation was given to 22 patients who were thought to be at risk for occult disease in the neck, and none developed recurrence in the neck. Of 22 patients who did not receive elective neck irradiation, 2 developed lymph node metastases in the absence of primary failure, and both were successfully salvaged with a radical neck dissection. Of 4 patients who presented with clinically positive lymph nodes, no neck failures occurred following high-dose radiotherapy alone. Four patients died of distant metastases alone with apparent disease control above the clavicles. Actuarial survival rates for the entire group at 5, 10, 15, and 20 years were 52%, 30%, 22%, and 22%. The 10-year continuously disease-free survival rate for Stage I was 86%, for Stage II, 42%, and for Stage III, 22%. The single failure among the Stage I patients was a submandibular lymph node metastasis at 10 months that was successfully salvaged by radical neck dissection, resulting in 100% survival for Stage I patients. Surgical salvage of local failure was successful in two of eight attempts.

ESTHESIONEUROBLASTOMA. Elkon and co-workers[365] reviewed the world literature on esthesioneuroblastoma and compiled the results of 78 cases (Table 21-73). They concluded that either radiation therapy or surgery was sufficient treatment for early-stage disease, but that combined treatment might be advantageous for late-stage presentations. The 5-year absolute survival rate was 75% for Stage A, 60% for Stage B, and 41% for Stage C.

The Mayo Clinic reviewed 21 cases of esthesioneuroblastoma seen between 1960 and 1980. The 5-year survival rate was 58% with only 4 of 19 patients being continuously free of disease for 7 to 16 years after initial surgery. Local recurrence occurred in 57%. Extension to the brain was noted in 10 patients, 3 at the time of diagnosis and 7 after the initial treatment. The overall rate of cervical metastases was 48%.[350]

Shah and Feghali[366] analyzed the Memorial Sloan-Kettering Cancer Center results for 31 patients seen between 1949 and 1975; there was a 5-year minimum follow-up. The 5-year survival rate was 52% with only 2 patients continuously free of disease. The 5-year survival rates by stage were Stage A, 5 of 6; Stage B, 2 of 6; and Stage C, 9 of 19. Fourteen were successfully salvaged to date after local or regional recurrence. Late recurrence after 5 years was seen.

Fauci and co-workers[367] reported the results of ten patients with midline lethal granuloma treated by high-dose irradiation. Long-term remissions occurred in seven patients. Four patients developed malignancies at other sites.

Maxillary Sinus

Jesse[368] reviewed 87 patients with squamous cell carcinoma of the maxillary antrum. The 3-year survival rate was about 30% for all cases, including 15 treated for palliation only and 9 that were too advanced for any treatment. Sixty-three were treated for cure with a 3-year survival rate of 44%. Three-year survival after surgery alone for selected lesions was 9 of 20 patients. Patients selected for combined treatment had either preoperative or postoperative irradiation; the results were similar for both techniques. The local recurrence rate with combined treatment was 38%. Patients with infrastructural lesions and superolateral lesions had a 3-year survival rate of 13 of 19 (68%), whereas those with superomedial or superoposterior lesions had a survival rate of only 29%.

Bataini and Ennuyer[369] reported Curie Foundation results for 31 patients with carcinoma of the maxillary antrum treated by supervoltage radiation therapy between 1959 and 1965. Only three patients had limited primary disease; 30% had clinically positive lymph nodes. The 3- and 5-year survival rates were 39% and 32%, respectively.

COMPLICATIONS OF TREATMENT

Surgery

Complications of maxillectomy include failure of the split-thickness skin graft to heal, trismus, cerebrospinal fluid leak, and hemorrhage.

Complications of ethmoid sinus surgery include hemorrhage, meningitis, CSF leak, cellulitis and pansinusitis, brain abscess, and stroke. Complications of the craniofacial procedure are reported by Ketcham and co-workers.[357] About one third of the patients had a life-threatening complication requiring intensive care and prolonged hospitalization. Opera-

TABLE 21-73. Esthesioneuroblastoma: Results of Treatment to Primary Tumor by Modality and Stage for 78 Patients with Follow-up of 6 Months to 32 Years (No. Controlled/No. Treated)

	Stage A—Confined to Nasal Cavity		*Stage B—Confined to Nasal Cavity and Paranasal Sinuses*		*Stage C—Beyond Nasal Cavity and Paranasal Sinuses*	
Modality	*Initial Treatment*	*For Recurrent Disease at Primary Site*	*Initial Treatment*	*For Recurrent Disease at Primary Site*	*Initial Treatment*	*For Recurrent Disease at Primary Site*
Radiation therapy alone	3/5	5/5	6/7	3/4	1/5	1/1
Surgery alone	5/9	2/2	3/6		1/1	0/0
Radiation therapy and surgery	9/10	0/0	15/20	0/1	7/15	0/0
Ultimate local control	24/24 (100%)		27/33 (82%)		10/21 (48%)	

Modified from Elkon D, Hightower SI, Lim ML, et al: Esthesioneuroblastoma. Cancer 44:1087–1094, 1979.

tive mortality was 4%. Complications included meningitis, subdural abscess, CSF leak, diplopia, and hemorrhage. Most of these patients had recurrent or far-advanced disease prior to surgery.

Radiation Therapy

Eye complications are the most frequent and bothersome of the complications of radiation therapy.[370,371] When only a portion of the ipsilateral eyeball is irradiated (medial one third), it is possible to preserve vision in the majority of patients. When there is gross disease in the orbit, however, the entire eyeball is irradiated to a high dose with almost certain loss of vision; however, these same patients would require orbital exenteration if treated by surgery. The actuarial probability of unilateral blindness at 10 years was 65% for 48 patients treated by radiation therapy for carcinomas of the nasal cavity or ethmoid or sphenoid sinus, and the probability of bilateral blindness was about 18% at 10 years.[364] The risk for bilateral blindness can be greatly reduced by use of CT and MRI scans for improved treatment planning and through knowledge of the tolerance of the optic nerve.[371]

A few patients will develop a transitory CNS syndrome that includes vertigo, headaches, decreased cerebration, and lethargy. This syndrome usually appears 2 to 3 months after completion of treatment, but has been seen as late as 12 to 15 months after completion of radiation therapy. The early-appearing CNS syndromes usually last 1 to 2 months, but the late-appearing syndromes last 6 to 12 months before slowly resolving.

Aseptic meningitis, chronic sinusitis, or serous otitis media can occur. High-dose irradiation of the nasal cavity can cause narrowing and synechiae of the nasal cavity. Douching with salt water and daily self-dilations with petrolatum-coated cotton swabs will reduce the problem.

Septal perforations occur when tumor has destroyed part of the septum. These do not usually require treatment and may heal spontaneously.

Destruction of the nasal bone and septum by tumor may result in cosmetic deformity. Two patients had successful reconstructive rhinoplasties after 7000 cGy.

Maxillary necrosis may develop if dental extraction is undertaken, but this can usually be successfully managed because the blood supply is much better than in the mandible.

CHEMODECTOMAS (GLOMUS BODY TUMORS)

Chemodectomas are a fascinating but uncommon group of neoplasms that may originate anywhere glomus bodies are found. The lesions are uncommon before the age of 20, there is a female predominance in some series, and the lesions may occur in multiple sites in about 10% to 20% of cases, especially in families with a history of this tumor. Carotid body tumors are associated with conditions producing chronic hypoxia, such as high altitude habitation, and chronic hypoxemia (as occurs in cyanotic heart disease).

ANATOMY

The normal glomus bodies in the head and neck vary from 0.1 mm to 0.5 mm in diameter. An autopsy study showed a correlation between carotid body size and increased right ventricular weight secondary to emphysema.[372] Because of their small size, the total distribution of glomus bodies in the head and neck remains speculative. Tumors arising in glomus bodies (*i.e.*, chemodectomas or nonchromaffin paragangliomas) arise most often from the carotid and temporal bone glomus bodies, with rare reports of tumors arising in the orbit, nasopharynx, larynx, nasal cavity, paranasal sinuses, tongue, and jaw.

The glomus bodies arising in relation to the temporal bone require special mention in regard to their distribution, because the site of origin of the tumor explains the different clinical pictures. Guild[373] reported an average of 2.82 glomera per temporal bone with a range of 0 to 12. The temporal bone glomus bodies are not found consistently in any location, but vary from person to person. At least one half of the glomus bodies are found in the general region of the jugular fossa and are located in the adventitia of the superior bulb of the internal jugular vein. The remainder are distributed along the course of the nerve of Jacobson (a branch of cranial nerve IX) and the nerve of Arnold (a branch of cranial nerve X). Approximately 20% of all temporal bone glomus bodies lie in the tympanic canaliculus and approximately 10% in relation to the cochlear promontory. A few glomus bodies are located in the descending part of the facial canal.

The carotid bodies are located in relation to the bifurcation of the common carotid. Orbit bodies are in relation to the ciliary nerve, and vagal bodies are adjacent to the ganglion nodosum of the vagus nerve.

PATHOLOGY

Chemodectomas are histologically benign tumors that resemble the parent tissue and consist of nests of epithelioid cells within stroma-containing, thin-walled blood vessels and nonmyelinated nerve fibers. The tumor mass is well circumscribed, but a true capsule is not seen. Dense fibrous bands occur in some tumors and account for the firmness of some masses. The histologic appearance varies, depending upon the relative amounts of epithelioid and vascular tissue present. The criterion of malignancy is based on the clinical progress of the disease rather than the histologic picture. Chemodectomas without cellular atypia may metastasize to regional nodes or to distant organ sites.

PATTERNS OF SPREAD

These lesions usually grow slowly; it is usual to have a history of symptoms for a few years and occasionally for 20 years or longer.

Carotid Body Tumors

Carotid body tumors are usually located at the bifurcation of the common carotid and, as they expand, tend to displace and encircle the internal and external carotid vessels. The tumor begins in the adventitia of the artery and initially derives its blood supply from the vaso vasorum. An accessory blood supply may come from branches of the vertebral artery and the ascending cervical artery.[374] The tumor is usually closely adherent to the wall of the carotid adjacent to the vascular pedicle, and there may be thinning of the arterial wall owing to pressure by the mass. Large masses extend toward the cervical spine, base of the skull, angle of the mandible, and the lateral pharyngeal space and its contents.

Temporal Bone Tumors

Glomus tympanicum lesions tend to be small when diagnosed because they produce symptoms quite early in their course. Tumor may involve the ossicles, tympanic membrane, mastoid, external auditory canal, semicircular canal, and the facial, Jacobson's, and Arnold's nerves.

Glomus jugulare tumors invade the base of skull, petrous apex, jugular vein, middle ear, and middle and posterior cranial fossae. Cranial nerves V to XII may be involved.

Lymphatic

Lymphatic metastases occur in about 5% of carotid body tumors but are very rare for temporal bone tumors. An upper neck mass may be an inferior extension of a jugular fossa or vagal tumor rather than a lymph node metastasis.

Distant Metastases

Distant metastases have been rarely reported for temporal bone tumors; carotid body tumors have a low risk for distant metastases, probably in the range of 5% or less.

CLINICAL PICTURE

Symptoms may be present from a few months to many years before diagnosis; the average is 3 to 4 years. Tumors are reported in children.

Carotid Body Tumors

The most common presenting symptom is an asymptomatic, slow-growing mass in the upper neck near the bifurcation of the carotid. Large masses may encroach on the parapharyngeal space and produce dysphagia, pain, and cranial nerve palsies. A carotid sinus syndrome may occur because of the pressure of the mass.

On examination, the mass usually lies deep to the sternocleidomastoid muscle and is tethered to surrounding structures. Fixation occurs only in large tumors that extend to the spine and base of skull. A submucosal bulge may be seen in the tonsillar area. A bruit may be heard. Steady compression of the mass may reduce its size, which recovers when the pressure is released.

Temporal Bone Tumors

Because glomus bodies are distributed throughout the temporal bone, the initial symptoms and signs depend on the site of origin.

Tumor arising in or near the middle ear presents with an insidious conductive hearing loss, pulsatile tinnitus, vertigo, and headache.

Patients with lesions developing in or around the jugular fossa develop headache, often pulsatile in nature, referred to the orbit or temple. Cranial nerves V to XII and the sympathetic nerves become affected.

Lesions developing in the facial canal present with facial nerve symptoms. Otorrhea and hemorrhage may occur when tumor breaks through into the external auditory canal.

A characteristic blue-red mass may be seen bulging the tympanic membrane or actually occupying the external auditory canal. A mass may be seen or felt in the upper neck between the mandible and mastoid and, at times, may be quite large.

Paralysis of cranial nerves V to XII and sympathetic nerves may occur.

METHODS OF DIAGNOSIS

Carotid Body Tumors

The differential diagnosis includes enlarged lymph nodes, aneurysm of the carotid artery, branchial cleft cyst, benign tumors (*e.g.*, lipoma), and direct extension of a lateral pharyngeal wall or pyriform sinus cancer into the soft tissues of the neck.

Carotid angiography and CT scan with contrast provide the preoperative diagnosis. Biopsy usually produces serious hemorrhage and is not recommended.

Temporal Bone Tumors

The differential diagnosis includes the presentation of an internal carotid artery in the middle ear either as an aberrant vessel or as an aneurysm, and these patients also present with hearing loss, pulsatile tinnitus, and a pulsatile mass behind the eardrum. Needless to say, biopsy may have a disastrous result.[375]

A high jugular bulb may present as a vascular mass in the middle ear and mimic a glomus tumor.[376]

Other diagnoses to be considered include the following:

- Polyp of ear canal
- Malignant tumor of the nasopharynx with extension to the temporal bone
- Acoustic neuroma
- Carcinoma of the middle ear
- Metastatic carcinoma (especially breast cancer)
- Cholesteatoma
- Histiocytosis
- Chronic serous otitis and mastoiditis

The diagnosis of glomus tumor is established by CT and MRI with contrast enhancement. Biopsy may be associated with serious or even fatal hemorrhage and is not essential if the diagnosis is characteristic by CT and MRI scans. If an operation is planned for a localized lesion of the tympanic cavity, then excision of the lesion is the biopsy.

Staging

There is no accepted staging scheme for chemodectomas. Patients are considered to have an early lesion when there is little or no bone destruction and to have an advanced lesion when there is extensive bone destruction or cranial nerve deficits. Tumors recurring after prior treatment usually are advanced because of the delay in diagnosis.

A 24-hour urine sample may be examined for vanillylmandelic acid (VMA) and metanephrines if hypertension is present, and for 5-hydroxyindoleacetic acid (5-HIAA) if a carcinoid picture is present.

TREATMENT

Selection of Treatment Modality

Although chemodectomas have a low potential for metastatic spread and a slow growth pattern, they can cause major disability and eventually death if unchecked. It may be appropriate to recommend no active treatment in selected cases, but the great majority should be treated.

TEMPORAL BONE TUMORS. Surgical excision is satisfactory for small lesions that can be removed without risk of operative death or damage to normal structures.

Early lesions of the tympanic cavity are managed successfully by excision without loss of hearing or vestibular function. The remainder of the lesions are managed best by irradiation, with a very high success rate and minimal morbidity with modern-day techniques. Partial removal of the tumor prior to irradiation does not improve the results but only increases the overall morbidity and puts the patient at risk for a fatal complication.

There remains a great deal of confusion regarding radiation treatment of chemodectomas.

A recent review by Kim and co-workers[377] of more than 200 patients showed that the recurrence rate after adequate radiation therapy for temporal bone chemodectomas was 2% with doses of 4000 cGy or greater. In some cases, examination of the temporal bone after radiation therapy has shown either no definable tumor or few microscopic residuals. However, in the majority of patients the tumor regresses but stable remnants may be seen for years. Success in these patients is equated with the lack of tumor regrowth and permanent improvement in signs and symptoms. It seems poor judgment to risk any operative resection that carries an operative mortality or morbidity when irradiation has been so successful.

CAROTID BODY TUMORS. Small lesions (1–5 cm) may be successfully removed with little risk to the patient. However, if ligation or replacement of the carotid vessels is anticipated or if a large lesion is fixed or unresectable because of size, radiation therapy is the preferred initial treatment. These lesions are identical histologically to temporal bone chemodectomas, and the response to radiation is similar. It is preferable to use radiation therapy rather than risk the possibility of a stroke or other operative calamity. A radiation dose of 4000 cGy to 4500 cGy does not exclude the possibility of surgical excision.

Surgical Treatment

TEMPORAL BONE TUMORS. Small glomus tympanicum lesions are approached through the eardrum or mastoid area and are removed. Hearing loss may occur from the operation, but if there is conductive hearing loss from the tumor, it may be correctable.

For the glomus jugulare tumors, surgery is reserved for radiation failure, in which case a radical mastoidectomy or a subtotal temporal bone resection would be required. Some surgeons advocate a base-of-skull approach.[378]

CAROTID BODY TUMORS. When an adequate work-up indicates that the most likely diagnosis is a carotid body tumor, hypertension, if present, should be treated. A standard neck incision is made in a skin crease at the level of the carotid bulb, and the carotid sheath and its contents are identified. The tumor mass is usually lying at the crotch of the internal and external carotid arteries, often displacing these vessels. Marked drops in blood pressure and bradycardia can be avoided by injecting the bulb area with lidocaine (Xylocaine). Troublesome bleeding may be avoided by using the bipolar electrode before excising the mass. The mass is then removed, preserving the carotid arteries.

Irradiation Technique

The current treatment plan is 4500 cGy in 5 weeks, 180 cGy/fraction, to the tumor volume. The dose is well below the tolerance of all normal tissues included, even if the brain stem and cord must be included for a large lesion.

Tumor-related symptoms may begin to improve during the first week of treatment, and the tumor mass, if visible, may show a decrease in size during the course of therapy; complete regression would be the exception.

Acute sequelae of treatment should be almost nil at 180 cGy/fraction. The patient will have temporary hair loss in the entrance and exit areas beginning about the third week. Mild nausea may occur.

Late sequelae are few. The hair should regrow over a period of 2 to 4 months but may show a slightly different texture or color. The patient may develop an otitis media, especially if the middle ear is involved with tumor.

Management of Recurrence

The diagnosis of recurrence often is delayed because of the inaccessibility to examination. Therefore, baseline CT or MRI scans should be obtained for reference.

Recurrence after irradiation is so uncommon that the diagnosis must be made only after complete reevaluation and evidence or progression of symptoms or an enlarging mass seen on CT or MRI. Pulsatile tinnitus may persist after irradiation because of incomplete regression of the vascular component of the tumor.[379,380]

Documented recurrence after operation usually is treated by irradiation; the complication rate in this group is higher than for those treated initially by irradiation. Recurrence after irradiation should be treated by operation if feasible; if operation is not possible, reirradiation may be considered. Although there are no reports of reirradiation for this tumor, there is experience with reirradiation of nasopharynx and brain tumors. The potential for a complication would be significant, but, in the face of advancing neoplasm, the risk probably would be acceptable.

RESULTS OF TREATMENT

Temporal Bone Tumors

The local control rates for five irradiation series of temporal bone chemodectomas in which adequate doses were prescribed and the treatment volumes adequate are listed in Table 21-74.[381-385] No patients had documented evidence of disease progression in 71 patients treated. In the University of Florida series, 9 patients have remained free of recurrence for ≥10 years and 5 patients for ≥15 years. Fifty-seven cranial nerve deficits were diagnosed before radiation therapy. Of these, 5 resolved completely, 14 partially improved, 36 were unchanged, and 2 deteriorated. The local control rates for operation for five series are listed in Table 21-75.[386-390]

Carotid Body Tumors

The local recurrence rates after complete excision are low, 0 to 10%.[391-396]

Mendenhall and co-workers[397] surveyed the radiation therapy results for carotid body and ganglion nodosum chemodectomas (Table 21-76). Two carotid body tumors treated at the University of Florida showed complete tumor regression, and the others stabilized with no progression. Five patients treated for de novo lesions remain free of regrowth at 1.5, 1.5, 3.5, 4, and 6 years (Mendenhall WM: Personal communication, 1987).

FOLLOW-UP POLICY

It is not unusual to have a persistent blue-red mass behind the eardrum after irradiation, even though the patient is clinically improved and there is no evidence of progression.

TABLE 21-75. Local Control of Chemodectomas with Surgery

Author	*Year*	*No. of Patients*	*No. with Recurrence*
Newman et al.[386]	1973	14	11
Grubb and Lampe[387]	1965	9	5
Hatfield et al.[388]	1972	16	8
Rosenwasser[389]	1967	8	3
Spector et al.[390]	1975	11 (GT)*	1
		45 (GJ)†	10

Adapted from Tidwell TJ, Montague ED: Chemodectomas involving the temporal bone. Radiology 116:147–149, 1975.
*GT, glomus tympanicum.
†GJ, glomus jugulare.

About 5% to 10% of patients will develop a second chemodectoma (often in the head and neck area), either a carotid body tumor or a contralateral temporal bone tumor. Baseline CT and MRI scans are recommended and are usually obtained about 6 months after therapy.

COMPLICATIONS OF TREATMENT

Surgery

Fatalities have been reported from biopsy and resection. The major risks during operation are hemorrhage and injury to cranial nerves. Other complications include hemiparesis, spinal fluid leak, and hearing loss.[376]

Irradiation

There have been isolated reports of brain necrosis; these cases were associated with high doses, high daily fractions, or repeat courses of irradiation. This complication should not occur at a dose of 4500 cGy or less given at 180 cGy a day, 5 days a week. Other complications include cholesteatoma and sequestrum of the mastoid and otitis media. Detectable damage to the hearing mechanism and vestibular apparatus does not occur at 4000 cGy to 4500 cGy to the normal temporal bone. Cranial nerves may regain complete or partial function, especially if the deficit is of recent onset. Cranial nerve palsy due to irradiation should not occur at 4500 cGy. The complication rate is greater when operation and irradiation are combined.

TABLE 21-74. Local Control of Temporal Bone Chemodectomas with Irradiation

Institution	*Tumor Dose (cGy)*	*Local Control**	*Follow-up (yr)*
M. D. Anderson Hospital[381]	4250–5000	17/17	4–18
University of Florida[382]	3750–5640	19/19	2–18
Baylor Medical Center[383]	4000–5000	9/9	1–7
Geisinger Medical Center[384]	4000–5000	11/11	1–12
Princess Margaret Hospital[385]	3500	20/20	2–20

*Local control: regression and absence of disease progression.

TABLE 21-76. Local Control of Carotid Body or Glomus Vagale Chemodectomas with Irradiation

Series	No. of Patients	No. of Lesions	Dose (cGy)	Results
Mitchell and Clyne[398]	6	6	3750–5500	5/6 controlled* at 1.5–8 years
Lybeert et al.[399]	9	11	4000–6000†	9/9 controlled at 1.5–18 years
Krupski et al.[400]	1	1	Not stated	Controlled at 8 years
Wilson[401]	1	1	Not stated	Controlled at 10 years
Endicott and Maniglia[402]	1	1	4500	Controlled at 1 year
Mendenhall et al.[397]	4	6	4000–4800	4/4 controlled at 2–4.5 years

Mendenhall WM, Million RR, Parsons JT, et al: Chemodectoma of the carotid body and ganglion nodosum treated with radiation therapy. Int J Radiat Oncol Biol Phys 12:2175–2178, 1986.

*Controlled = regression or stabilization of local disease; no evidence of lymph node or distant metastasis.

†200 cGy per fraction.

MAJOR SALIVARY GLANDS

Tumors of the major salivary glands account for 3% to 4% of all head and neck neoplasms. The average age of patients with malignant neoplasms is approximately 55 years; for benign tumors, about 40 years. Approximately one fourth of parotid tumors and one half of submandibular tumors are malignant.

ANATOMY

The parotid gland is a relatively simple structure with rather complex anatomic relationships. It is indented and formed by the muscles, bones, vessels, and nerves that come in contact with the gland. The major bulk of the parotid gland is superficial, extending superiorly to the zygomatic arch and anterior aspect of the external auditory canal. The anterior border is variable, but does not continue beyond the opening of the parotid duct into the oral cavity opposite the second molar. Inferiorly, the gland fills the gap between the mastoid and the angle of the mandible. The gland lies in front of and below the external auditory canal. A deep lobe extends into the parapharyngeal area, where it is in relationship to the lateral process of C1, the styloid process, and the contents of the parapharyngeal space.

The parotid gland is encompassed by fascia that is sufficient to contain most parotid infections in addition to benign and low-grade malignant tumors. However, the fascia between the parotid gland and the conchal and tragal cartilages is quite thin; this is a weak spot that tumor quickly traverses. The fascia separating the deep lobe from the parapharyngeal space (stylomandibular fascial membrane) may be sufficiently thin to allow tumor or infection easy access to the parapharyngeal space and pharynx.

The sensory nerve supply to the parotid area and part of the pinna is by way of the greater auricular nerve (C2–3). This nerve is severed in removal of the parotid gland with permanent loss of sensation. The facial nerve penetrates the parotid gland almost immediately upon leaving the stylomastoid canal. The seventh nerve forms an extensive anastomotic network within the gland and gives off branches to the muscles of expression.

The parotid gland is richly supplied from several arteries that freely anastomose and create arteriovenous bleeding during parotidectomy. The external carotid, internal maxillary, and superficial temporal arteries and the posterior facial vein lie deep to the seventh nerve; if these vessels require attention during an operation, the seventh nerve may be damaged.

The superficial preauricular nodes, usually one or two in number, lie outside the fascia of the parotid gland and immediately in front of the tragus. These nodes are important because they drain the skin of the anterior ear, temple, and upper face, including the eye and nose. They are involved most frequently by metastatic skin cancer and lymphoma, but not usually from parotid neoplasms. The preauricular nodes then empty into the superficial cervical nodes along the external jugular vein, or they may communicate with the jugular chain of nodes.

There are two groups of nodes within the fascia of the parotid gland. Within the substance of the parotid gland are numerous lymph follicles and four to ten small lymph nodes scattered along the posterior facial and external jugular veins. Thus, they may lie deep to the seventh nerve. Outside the gland but within the fascia are one or two nodes that lie in front of the tragus and one or two nodes that lie between the inferior aspect of the tail of the parotid and the anterior border of the sternocleidomastoid muscle. These are referred to as the subparotid nodes. When enlarged, the subparotid nodes are difficult to distinguish from a mass in the tail of the parotid gland.

PATHOLOGY

There is a large variety of benign and malignant neoplasms that occur in the major salivary glands. It is not at all unusual to have the diagnosis changed from that given at frozen section; the patient must be made aware of this risk.

Benign Tumors

BENIGN MIXED TUMORS. These slow-growing neoplasms are surrounded by an imperfect pseudocapsule that is traversed by fingers of tumor. Enucleation or removal of a narrow cuff of normal tissue usually results in recurrence. The histologic distinction between benign and malignant mixed tumor is often difficult. The age of appearance begins in the early 20s with a mean age of 40.

PAPILLARY CYSTADENOMA LYMPHOMATOSUM. This benign tumor, also called Warthin's tumor, probably arises from lymphoid elements. It is encased by a thin but complete capsule. It occurs predominantly in older men. It is bilateral in approximately 10% of cases and may be multiple on one or both sides.

BENIGN LYMPHOEPITHELIAL LESIONS. Benign lymphoepithelial lesions (Godwin's tumor) account for about 5% of benign lesions. The tumor may be bilateral and is more common in women. Excision may be followed by recurrence.

ONCOCYTOMA. Oncocytoma is a benign, slow-growing tumor found mostly in the older age group. The encapsulated tumor has a dark appearance similar to melanoma.

BASAL CELL ADENOMA. The basal cell adenoma is an uncommon benign lesion, usually appearing in older people. It is histologically and clinically benign and is cured by simple excision. Basal cell adenoma must be distinguished from basal cell carcinoma of the skin metastatic to parotid lymph nodes.

Malignant Tumors

LOW-GRADE MALIGNANCY. *Acinic Cell Tumor.* Acinic cell tumors typically are slow-growing, low-grade neoplasms that appear in all age groups and are most common in women. They will recur after inadequate removal, sometimes as long as 25 to 30 years after initial treatment. Metastases occur in a small percentage of cases but cannot be predicted by the histologic picture.

Mucoepidermoid Carcinoma, Low Grade. Most mucoepidermoid carcinomas are low-grade lesions readily cured by adequate excision. They may appear in any age group. They grow slowly; there is little or no capsule. They are usually well-circumscribed, but they may widely infiltrate the normal gland or become fixed to skin. The mucin produced by the neoplasm may incite inflammatory changes about the edge of the mass.

HIGH-GRADE MALIGNANCY. *Mucoepidermoid Carcinoma, High Grade.* A few of the mucoepidermoid carcinomas behave in a very aggressive fashion, widely infiltrating the salivary gland and producing lymph node and distant metastases. They may be difficult to distinguish from high-grade epidermoid carcinoma.

Adenocarcinoma; Poorly Differentiated Carcinoma; Anaplastic Carcinoma; Squamous Cell Carcinoma. These histologies tend to appear late in life and have an aggressive behavior. True squamous cell carcinoma arising from the salivary gland occurs rarely. Almost all of the so-called squamous cell carcinomas of the parotid are actually metastatic from skin cancer, especially from the temple area.[403,404]

Malignant Mixed Tumor. A small percentage of benign mixed tumors may develop into frank malignancy.

Adenoid Cystic Carcinoma. This neoplasm is uncommon in the major salivary glands. It varies in growth rate from slow to fast. Metastases to regional lymph nodes and distant sites occur; perineural involvement is characteristic; and recurrences may appear many years after initial treatment.

Lymphoepithelioma (Malignant Lymphoepithelial Lesion, "Eskimoma"). Lymphoepithelioma occurs rarely in the parotid and submandibular gland. Povah and co-workers[405] reported 17 cases from Winnipeg. Fifteen of the patients were Eskimo and 2 were white, with an age range of 17 to 65 years. The histologic picture was that of lymphoepithelioma with varying degrees of nonmalignant lymphoid stroma.

PATTERNS OF SPREAD

Benign Mixed Tumors

Benign mixed tumors of the parotid gland grow by expansion and local infiltration. Most tumors begin in the superficial lobe. Because of their slow growth they rarely cause seventh nerve palsy, although the nerve may be severely stretched by large masses. When incompletely excised, multiple tumor nodules develop within the tumor bed. Skin invasion may occur in recurrent lesions; bone invasion does not occur, but a mass may cause pressure defects of adjacent bone.

Malignant Tumors

The malignant neoplasms infiltrate the parotid gland, invade the seventh nerve and the auriculotemporal nerve, and spread along nerve sheaths. Tumor may invade the adjacent skin, muscles, and bone, depending on the site of origin. Deep lobe lesions invade the parapharyngeal space, infratemporal fossa, and base of skull, and compromise additional cranial nerves.

Malignant tumors of the submandibular gland invade the gland, fix the tumor to the adjacent mandible, and invade the mylohyoid muscle and eventually the tongue, hypoglossal nerve, and oral cavity or oropharynx. Skin invasion occurs in advanced cases.

Sublingual gland neoplasms usually present as a submucosal mass in the floor of the mouth. The advanced lesions show an ulcerated mass in the floor of the mouth with extension to the tongue, mandible, and submental soft tissues.

Lymphatic Spread

Lymph node metastases may occur from all of the malignant neoplasms. Approximately 20% to 25% of patients with malignant tumors will have clinically positive or occult metastases in lymph nodes at the time of diagnosis. Low-grade mucoepidermoid carcinoma and acinic cell adenocarcinoma have a low rate of lymph node metastasis. There is little difference in the rate of lymph node metastasis among the various high-grade lesions. The risk for lymph node metastasis increases with recurrent disease and increased size of the primary lesion.

CLINICAL PICTURE

Parotid Gland

The great majority of patients with either benign or malignant parotid tumors present with a mass that is easily seen and felt. Mild, intermittent pain is associated with a few of the masses, but does not distinguish between benign and malignant. Facial nerve palsy is an infrequent presenting complaint and indicates malignancy, since untreated benign tumors do not cause seventh nerve palsy. Tumors of the deep lobe may produce dysphagia.

The mobility of the mass depends on its size and location. Fixation or reduced mobility may occur in both benign and malignant neoplasms and does not distinguish the two. Tumors presenting in the deep lobe may cause bulging of the palate and tonsillar area.

Advanced malignant lesions may affect cranial nerve VII, and, more rarely, cranial nerves IX to XII and the sympathetic chain if the parapharyngeal space is invaded. The mandibular branch of cranial nerve V may be involved when tumor tracks along the auriculotemporal nerve to the base of the skull; pain is an associated finding.

Submandibular Gland

Both benign and malignant neoplasms present as a mass usually associated with mild pain. Nerve palsy is rarely seen with submandibular gland cases. These lesions may infiltrate the skin in advanced lesions. The tumor mass usually is partially fixed to the mandible unless quite small. Loss of mobility occurs with both benign and malignant lesions.

Sublingual Gland

Sublingual gland lesions are clinically similar to squamous cell carcinomas of the floor of the mouth. They produce a mass, submucosal at first, that may be felt by the tongue; they may displace dentures, and there is mild discomfort, if any, in the early stages.

METHODS OF DIAGNOSIS AND STAGING

Parotid Gland

DIFFERENTIAL DIAGNOSIS. It is often easy to distinguish non-neoplastic from neoplastic conditions by history, physical examination, and simple diagnostic tests. The distinction between benign and malignant neoplasms is more difficult unless there is obvious nerve palsy, pain, or metastatic cervical lymph nodes.

Gallia and Johnson[406] reviewed 140 patients who eventually underwent parotidectomy for diagnoses. Only 11% had malignant masses; the remainder had benign neoplasms (62%) or non-neoplastic conditions (27%).

Conditions that may be confused with a parotid tumor include the following:

- Metastatic cancer, lymphoma, or leukemia involving parotid area lymph nodes
- Fatty replacement, tail of parotid
- Chronic parotitis
- Boeck's sarcoid
- Stone in duct
- Cysts (branchial cleft, dermoid)
- Hypertrophy associated with diabetes
- Hypertrophy of masseter muscle, unilateral or bilateral
- Neoplasms of the mandible
- Prominent transverse process of C1 (atlas)
- Penetrating foreign bodies
- Hemangioma/lymphangioma
- Lipoma

RADIOLOGIC EXAMINATION. Radiologic examination of the parotid has progressed to the point that it is an essential tool in the differential diagnosis of parotid conditions and for determining disease extent in neoplastic conditions. MRI is comparable to CT with contrast for examination of the parotid gland; CT with sialography is no longer used. Sialography is reserved for nonacute inflammatory disease. Although one could argue that it is not necessary to perform a CT scan or MRI on every parotid mass (especially discrete, mobile, asymptomatic, slow-growing, superficial masses), observation of numerous diagnostic and surgical errors leads us to advise CT scan with contrast or MRI on a routine basis prior to biopsy or other operative procedures. CT scan and MRI will distinguish between intrinsic and extrinsic parotid masses and show the relationship of the mass to the facial nerve.[45] The characteristics of the mass as seen on CT or MRI scans will often predict for a malignant as opposed to a benign tumor. CT and MRI scans will assist the surgeon with the probable diagnosis, the proper approach to the facial nerve, the probable necessity to remove part or all of the nerve, the degree of invasion of the deep lobe, and the extension outside the parotid to the parapharyngeal space and base of skull. CT and MRI scans prior to surgery also greatly assist in radiation therapy treatment planning if radiation is used in a postoperative setting.

Submandibular Gland

DIFFERENTIAL DIAGNOSIS. The differential diagnosis of a submandibular mass centers around inflammatory disease, squamous cell carcinoma metastatic to a lymph node, and a primary neoplasm of the submandibular gland.

Episodic pain and mass are the hallmark of inflammatory disease, but approximately one third of inflammatory lesions will be asymptomatic.[407]

Obstructive sialadenitis is a common cause of submandibular gland enlargement. It is caused by stricture of the duct or stone in the duct. There is pain and swelling associated with eating that recedes after several hours. There may be erythema over the mass. A stone may be palpated in the duct, and occasionally pus can be stripped from the submandibular duct. A sialogram will show the site of the obstruction. Sialolithiasis may be found, however, in the presence of submandibular carcinoma.

A solitary squamous cell carcinoma metastatic to a submandibular lymph node in the absence of an obvious oral cavity primary lesion is uncommon. A primary submandibular neoplasm, benign or malignant, is a relatively rare event, but failure to recognize the possibility may result in an inappropriate and sometimes disastrous initial step in management.

Gallia and Johnson[406] reviewed 110 submandibular lesions in patients who underwent biopsy. Ninety-three (85%) were non-neoplastic, usually inflamed glands, and 9 (8%) were benign tumors. Eight patients (7%) had malignant lesions, of which 3 were lymphoma, 3 were metastatic carcinoma, and 2 were primary submandibular gland carcinoma.

RADIOLOGIC EXAMINATION. Radiologic examination plays an important part in the differential diagnosis of submandibular space masses of uncertain etiology. CT with contrast is usually the initial imaging procedure, although MRI may be used in selected circumstances. Plain films may reveal an opaque stone, or sialogram may show a nonopaque stone or other benign pathology. In masses that may be either a primary submandibular tumor or possibly a submandibular lymph node metastasis, CT scan with contrast will distinguish intrinsic versus extrinsic mass (*e.g.*, metastatic lymph node) and extent of disease spread to adjacent tissues when neoplasm is present. The diagnosis of malignant neoplasm may be strongly suggested in certain situations.

Biopsy Technique

PAROTID GLAND. The biopsy and the definitive surgical treatment are often the same for parotid masses. Lesions lying in the superficial lobe are biopsied best by performing a superficial parotidectomy. Lesions involving both the superficial and deep lobe or just the deep lobe are "biopsied" by total parotidectomy. This approach avoids contamination of the tumor bed. Incisional or excisional biopsy (*e.g.*, lumpectomy) increases the risk of tumor recurrence and facial nerve damage and increases the definitive surgical procedure by necessitating wide removal of the biopsy site.

There are several advocates of fine-needle aspiration for diagnosis; it is essential that the pathologist be familiar with this method. Fine-needle biopsies, even when correct, do not alter treatment decisions. There is a significant error rate in frozen section diagnoses, so that surgical decisions often rely heavily on clinical and radiographic findings for planning surgical resections. Needle biopsy can be used in the inoperable or recurrent lesion when radiation therapy is planned as the initial treatment.

SUBMANDIBULAR GLAND. Needle biopsy is helpful when positive for tumor, but may delay diagnosis when falsely negative. When needle biopsy is negative, but history, physical examination, and radiographic studies suggest neoplasm, and a careful search of the head and neck area fails to reveal a primary mucosal lesion, the submandibular triangle is dissected as the biopsy procedure. Incisional or excisional biopsy increases the risk of tumor recurrence, even when followed by appropriate treatment, and increases the surgical morbidity by requiring excision of the biopsy site.

Staging

The AJCC staging for salivary gland tumors is as follows:[12]

Primary tumor

- TX Minimum requirements to assess the primary tumor cannot be met
- T0 No evidence of primary tumor
- T1 Tumor 2.0 cm or less in greatest diameter without significant local extension*
- T2 Tumor more than 2.0 cm but not more than 4.0 cm in greatest diameter without significant local extension*
- T3 Tumor more than 4.0 cm but not more than 6.0 cm in greatest diameter without significant local extension*
- T4a Tumor over 6.0 cm in greatest diameter without significant local extension*
- T4b Tumor of any size with significant local extension*

Nodal involvement

- NX Minimum requirements to assess the regional nodes cannot be met
- N0 No evidence of regional lymph node involvement
- N1 Evidence of regional lymph node involvement

TREATMENT

Selection of Treatment Modality

PAROTID GLAND. The initial management of resectable superficial lobe parotid masses is exploration and en bloc superficial lobectomy for diagnosis and treatment. The tumor usually can be dissected free of the facial nerve. If the tumor involves the deep portion of the gland, the nerve is gently retracted and the deep portion excised (*i.e.*, total parotidectomy). If the tumor grossly involves the facial nerve, one or more branches may have to be sacrificed (*i.e.*, radical parotidectomy). Skin, bone, and muscle may also be resected as needed.

Low-grade malignant neoplasms are usually managed by operation only. Radiation therapy is given postoperatively for nearly all high-grade lesions. Radiation therapy is advised for low-grade malignant lesions that are recurrent and those with positive margins or narrow margins on the facial nerve. Tumor spill at the time of operation is a controversial indication for postoperative irradiation.[408] Postoperative radiation therapy is advised for selected benign mixed tumors when there is residual disease after operation, and for nearly all patients operated on for recurrent disease. Inoperable tumors are treated by radiation therapy with occasional success reported.

Chemotherapy has been reserved for patients with incurable disease or planned clinical trials.

SUBMANDIBULAR GLAND. Submandibular triangle dissection is used to make the diagnosis of lesions in this loca-

*Significant local extension is defined as evidence of tumor involvement of skin, soft tissues, bone, or the lingual or facial nerves.

tion. If frozen section diagnosis shows a malignant lesion and there is no involvement of nerves, mandible, or soft tissues, the operation is concluded, and postoperative irradiation is given to the submandibular bed and ipsilateral neck. If there is perineural invasion, bone invasion, a clinically positive node, or extension to contiguous soft tissues, then the resection is enlarged to encompass the necessary areas. This may include the mandible, mylohyoid muscle, digastric muscle, adjacent floor of the mouth or tongue, and involved nerves. Postoperative radiation therapy is added in nearly all cases.

Surgical Treatment

SUPERFICIAL PAROTIDECTOMY. The parotid gland is a unilobular gland but is artificially divided into superficial and deep portions by the seventh nerve. A superficial mass in the parotid gland is best approached by a superficial parotidectomy and frozen section diagnosis because this affords the best method of diagnosis and often is the definitive treatment. The facial nerve is not sacrificed unless it is grossly involved with disease.

The incision is made in the preauricular crease and then curves under the earlobe posteriorly and then into the neck. The facial nerve must be identified in all superficial and total parotidectomies. Once this is accomplished, the dissection is carried out between the mass and the facial nerve. A margin of at least 1 cm around the mass is necessary if a benign tumor is suspected, and a larger margin if the mass is malignant. The adequacy of treatment is determined by frozen sections.

TOTAL PAROTIDECTOMY. Total parotidectomy is recommended for tumors in the deep lobe of the parotid gland or for tumors that arise in the superficial lobe and extend into the deep lobe. A superficial parotidectomy generally is performed; then the nerve is dissected free from the underlying deep lobe and the deep lobe and tumor are removed. Occasionally, the mandible must be divided to gain access to the retromandibular portion of the deep lobe of the parotid gland. A partial mandibulectomy is required when the mandible is invaded by tumor. When pain is present, the auriculotemporal nerve should be explored to the base of the skull.

The paraparotid nodes are removed with the primary lesion. If the nodes are positive, a radical neck dissection is added. Radical neck dissection is always included for clinically positive nodes. Elective neck dissection is not done for low-grade lesions.

A radical parotidectomy implies removal of the entire parotid, the facial nerve, and other involved tissues such as skin, bone, or muscle. If a branch of the facial nerve or the entire nerve must be sacrificed, an immediate autologous nerve graft may be done. Postoperative radiation therapy is delayed for 6 weeks, and the chance of successful function is reported to be good.[409]

Radiation Therapy

Radiation therapy plays its major role as an adjunct to surgery and is usually given postoperatively, although preoperative treatment is advised in special situations. Postoperative irradiation is indicated for nearly all high-grade lesions, for low-grade neoplasms with close or positive margins, for tumors of the deep lobe, for perineural invasion, for recurrent tumors, and for multiple regional node metastases. According to Spiro and co-workers,[408] tumor spill at the time of operation may not be a single prognostic factor for recurrence.

The minimum treatment volume for parotid lesions includes the parotid bed and upper neck nodes. Perineural involvement indicates enlargement of the portals to cover the nerve pathways. The entire ipsilateral neck is included for high-grade lesions or for clinically positive nodes in the neck dissection specimen. The tumor dose to the primary area is 6000 cGy to 6500 cGy over 6 to 7 weeks if there is no gross residual disease. Higher doses including interstitial implants are used for gross disease. There are no good data to show a difference in dose required for the various histologies.[410,411]

Submandibular space external beam portals are tailored to the extent of disease found in the surgical dissection. The entire ipsilateral neck is included. The postoperative dose is 6500 cGy to 7000 cGy because the rate of recurrence even with combined treatment is substantial.

RESULTS OF TREATMENT

Parotid Gland

BENIGN MIXED TUMORS. Enucleation or excision with a narrow rim of normal tissue will result eventually in a local recurrence rate of approximately 20% after 10 to 15 years of follow-up.

Rafla[412] reported only a 2.7% recurrence rate when enucleation or excision was followed by postoperative radiation therapy. Superficial parotidectomy (or excision for selected small lesions) will result in a recurrence rate of approximately 5%. Spiro[413] reported a 7% recurrence rate, with a minimum of 10 years of follow-up, for 1342 benign parotid tumors treated by surgery.

The surgical success rate for recurrent lesions depends on the number of previous operations and the size and extent of recurrence. It may be necessary to sacrifice one or several branches of the seventh nerve and to repair the defect with a nerve graft. Postoperative irradiation of 6000 cGy to 6500 cGy is added in selected cases in which there are close margins or residual disease, or in cases in which a subsequent recurrence would be almost impossible to manage surgically or would result in loss of the facial nerve.

Death because of benign mixed tumor should be a rare event.

MALIGNANT TUMORS. Treatment results for parotid tumors have been analyzed by grade or histology, but results have not often been available by stage. The surgical results for low-grade malignant lesions are quite good, and radiation therapy is not often required. The local recurrence rate for operation alone is approximately 50% to 60% for high-grade tumors.[408,414]

McNaney and co-workers[415] reported the M. D. Anderson Hospital experience for 77 patients with malignant parotid tumors who received postoperative radiation therapy. Parotidectomy was performed for a de novo tumor in 70% and for a recurrent tumor in 30%. Patients with a history of more than two surgical procedures for parotid tumor were excluded. There was a minimum follow-up of 3 years; follow-up was greater than 5 years in 81% and greater than 10 years in 27% of the patients. The sites of local–regional failures according to the estimated extent of residual disease after parotidectomy are shown in Table 21-77. The overall incidence of local failure was 8%, and the incidence of neck failure alone was 5%. There were no failures after 4 years of observation. There were no local or regional failures in the 14 patients with low-grade lesions; the local failure rate for high-grade tumors was 10%. Analysis of local recurrence according to the extent of facial nerve sacrifice showed one local failure in 35 cases in which the nerve was preserved, one local failure in 21 cases after partial facial nerve resection, and three local failures in 21 cases after total resection of the nerve. Distant metastasis developed in 23%.

The 5-year absolute survival rate by histology for patients treated with surgery and postoperative radiation therapy added on a selective basis at M. D. Anderson Hospital is shown in Table 21-78.[411]

Theriault and Fitzpatrick[416] reviewed 271 patients with parotid cancer seen at the Princess Margaret Hospital between 1958 and 1980. The minimum follow-up was 5 years and the median follow-up was 10 years. Thirty-five patients had only radiation therapy, 67 had only surgery, and 169 had surgery plus postoperative radiation therapy, 4500 cGy to 5500 cGy in 20 fractions. Relapse-free survival and cause-specific survival (determinate survival) rates are compared to treatment modality in Table 21-79. Local–regional control at 10 years was obtained in 12% by radiation therapy, 22% by surgery, and 71% by surgery plus radiation therapy. Significant prognostic factors for survival were tumor stage, regional metastases, age (young better than old), histology, and facial nerve involvement.

Chemotherapy Results

The development of effective chemotherapy for patients with salivary gland carcinomas has been limited by the heterogeneity of this disease, the relative efficacy of surgery and radiotherapy, and the paucity of patients with recurrent or metastatic disease. Significant tumor regression has been reported with single-agent chlorambucil,[417] hydroxyurea,[418] hexamethylmelamine,[419] daunorubicin,[419] 5-fluorouracil,[420,421] doxorubicin,[419,422] and cisplatin.[423,424] The last three drugs appear to be the most active single agents, with partial response rates of 30% to 70% in patients with advanced local–regional or metastatic disease. Responses to single agents, however, are rarely complete or durable.

The experience with combination chemotherapy in this disease is similarly limited. Multiagent chemotherapy has included the aforementioned cytotoxic agents, as well as mitomycin-C, cyclophosphamide, methotrexate, bleomycin, and vincristine.[425–433] Regimens containing doxorubicin have been evaluated in numerous small series. A combination of cyclophosphamide and doxorubicin led to 5 partial but no complete responses in 13 patients with recurrent or metastatic salivary gland tumors.[427] Cisplatin, doxorubicin, and 5-fluorouracil resulted in 2 complete and 4 partial responses in 17 patients with advanced disease.[428] The combination of cyclophosphamide, doxorubicin, and cisplatin (CAP) is the most extensively studied regimen.[430–433] Dreyfuss and co-workers[433] recently summarized the published experience with CAP and noted 10 (28%) complete and 13 (36%) additional partial responses (median duration of response, 5–11 months) to chemotherapy in 36 patients with advanced disease.

The apparent activity of combinations containing cisplatin or doxorubicin in patients with recurrent or metastatic disease suggests a role for chemotherapy as induction or adjuvant treatment in patients with potentially curable lesions

TABLE 21-78. Parotid Cancer: Absolute 5-Year Survival (120 Patients)*

Histology	*No. of Patients*	*5-Year Survival (%)*
Acinic cell	12	92
Mucoepidermoid (low grade)	28	76
Adenocarcinoma	12	66
Malignant mixed	27	50
Adenoid cystic	10	50
Squamous cell	6	50
Mucoepidermoid (high grade)	13	46
Undifferentiated	12	33

Guillamondegui OM, Byers RM, Luna MA, et al: Aggressive surgery in treatment for parotid cancer. The role of adjunctive postoperative radiotherapy. AJR 123:49–54, 1975 © 1975, American Roentgen Ray Society.

*M. D. Anderson Hospital, 1944–1965.

TABLE 21-77. Postoperative Radiation Therapy in Malignant Tumors of the Parotid Gland: Local–Regional Failures by Extent of Residual Disease

		Site of Failure		
Residual Disease	*No. of Patients*	*Primary Site*	*Neck*	*Primary Site and Neck*
Gross (any grade)	14	1	1	0
Microscopic (any grade)	26	2	1	0
High grade (good margin)	16	1	2	0
Unknown grade (good margin)	17	1	0	1
Low grade (questionable margin)	4	0	0	0
Total	77	5	4	1

Adapted from McNaney D, McNeese MD, Guillamondegui OM, et al: Postoperative irradiation in malignant epithelial tumors of the parotid. Int J Radiat Oncol Biol Phys 9:1289–1295, 1983.

TABLE 21-79. Parotid Carcinoma: Survival in 269 Patients Treated at Princess Margaret Hospital, 1958–1980 (5-Year Minimum Follow-up)

	Relapse-Free		*Cause-Specific (Determinate)*	
	5-Year	*10-Year*	*5-Year*	*10-Year*
Surgery plus radiation therapy	69%	63%	78%	72%
Surgery	30%	23%	63%	48%
Radiation therapy	9%	9%	23%	18%

Data from Theriault and Fitzpatrick.[416]

that are at high risk for relapse (*e.g.*, tumors with high-grade histology or base of skull extension). To date, the use of combination chemotherapy in this setting has been anecdotal [427,429,432,433] and its true value awaits definition by multi-institutional cooperative trials.

Submandibular Gland

Byers and co-workers[434] reported the results of treatment for 22 malignant tumors of the submandibular gland with no prior therapy. Treatment was resection followed selectively by postoperative irradiation. The local control rate was 64% and the survival rate was 50%.

Spiro[413] reported the results of surgery for 129 malignant submandibular gland carcinomas seen between 1939 and 1973. All patients had a minimum of 10 years of follow-up. Adenoid cystic carcinoma occurred in 35%, mucoepidermoid carcinoma in 29%, and malignant mixed tumor in 19%. Cervical lymph nodes were malignant in 28%. The local–regional control rate was 40% and the determinate cure rate was 31% at 5 years and 22% at 10 years.

Benign tumors of the submandibular gland were resected in 106 patients; only 2 developed a local recurrence.[413]

COMPLICATIONS OF TREATMENT

Surgery

Temporary facial nerve palsy may occur due to manipulation of the nerve during operation, and function will gradually return over a few months' time. Persistent weakness of the lower lip may occur, even though the remainder of the nerve recovers. Tarsorrhaphy may be required to protect the eye until function returns. Spontaneous return of facial movement has been reported to occur after surgical division of the seventh nerve. Facial nerve palsy may be repaired by a nerve graft. If grafting is not possible, a nerve crossover technique may be used that connects the ipsilateral hypoglossal nerve to branches of the seventh nerve.

Gustatory sweating (Frey's syndrome) occurs in about 10% of patients after parotidectomy. This problem rarely requires treatment.

Persistent salivary fistula is a rare complication.

Radiation Therapy

Xerostomia is avoided by techniques that spare the contralateral salivary tissues.

There may be trismus due to fibrosis of the masseter and pterygoid muscles and the temporomandibular joint. It should be possible to exclude the temporomandibular joint from high doses in most situations.

Otitis media may occur if the ear is irradiated. Localized hair loss may occur with some techniques. Osteoradionecrosis may occur with high doses.

MINOR SALIVARY GLANDS

Tumors of minor salivary gland origin are uncommon, accounting for about 2% to 3% of all malignant neoplasms of the upper aerodigestive tract. They may appear at any age, but are uncommon before age 20 and rare under age 10. There is no known causative agent except for the adenocarcinomas of the nose. They tend to occur most often in the hard palate, nasal cavity, and paranasal sinuses, areas infrequently involved by squamous cell carcinomas. Thus, the site of origin is related more to the population density of the minor salivary glands in a particular tissue than to an environmental factor.

ANATOMY

Minor salivary glands are ubiquitous in the mucosa of the upper aerodigestive tract with the exception of the gingivae and the anterior portion of the hard palate, which are free of minor salivary glands. They are distributed on the undersurface of the anterior and lateral oral tongue and the base of the tongue. Aberrant salivary tissue sometimes is seen in lymph nodes, in the body of the mandible just behind the third molar teeth, in the vestigial remnant of the nasopalatine canal in the anterior maxilla, the middle ear, lower neck, sternoclavicular joint, thyroglossal duct, and other sites.

PATHOLOGY

Approximately one half of minor salivary gland tumors are malignant. The histologic varieties of malignant tumors include adenoid cystic carcinoma, mucoepidermoid carcinoma, adenocarcinoma, malignant mixed, acinic cell, and oncocytic carcinomas. About two thirds are adenoid cystic. The mucoepidermoid carcinoma and adenocarcinomas arise predominantly in the oral cavity.[435]

The benign tumors are benign mixed (pleomorphic adenoma) in the great majority of cases, with a few cases of intraductal papillomas, papillary cystadenomas, basal cell adenomas, and benign oncocytomas.[436]

PATTERNS OF SPREAD

Tongue lesions usually originate from the base of the tongue. There are no minor salivary glands in the anterior one half of the hard palate, so tumors arise on the posterolateral hard palate and all of the soft palate. The site of origin for floor-of-mouth salivary gland tumors is moot — either the sublingual gland or a minor salivary gland. The nasopharynx is an uncommon site of origin.

These tumors grow by local infiltration with eventual invasion of muscle, bone, and cartilage. Perineural spread is a common feature, particularly for adenoid cystic carcinoma. Tumor may track both centrally and peripherally along nerves, but the central spread is the more common event because most lesions arise near the terminations of the nerves. Extension along nerves eventually may traverse the base of skull and surface intracranially, although this spread pattern may not become manifest for several years after the original treatment. Tumor growth along a nerve may be characterized by skipped areas, so that a normal nerve segment is no assurance of free margins. Adenoid cystic carcinoma may grow along the Haversian systems of bone without showing bone destruction.[437]

The risk of positive lymph nodes is related to the site of origin and the histology. Lymph node metastases are most likely from sites with a dense capillary lymphatic network, similar to the pattern for squamous carcinoma. Adenoid cystic carcinoma, low-grade mucoepidermoid carcinoma, and acinic cell carcinoma are at low risk to spread to lymph nodes; about 20% of adenoid cystic carcinomas spread to lymph nodes, but this low incidence is related partly to their frequent site of origin in the hard palate and paranasal sinuses, areas that infrequently produce lymph node metastases. The high-grade tumors (high-grade mucoepidermoid carcinoma, adenocarcinoma, and malignant mixed tumor) have a 30% incidence of lymph node involvement on admission, and eventually 51% showed lymph node metastases. Schell and co-workers[435] reported a 17% incidence of positive nodes on admission for all histologies and grades and subsequent appearance in 11%. Most were staged N1 or N2A and were usually associated with lesions of the tongue or floor of mouth. At least 25% of patients will develop distant metastasis, usually to the lung.

CLINICAL PICTURE

The clinical picture obviously depends on the site of origin. The signs and symptoms differ somewhat from those of squamous cell carcinoma arising in the same area. Many of the lesions are indolent, and the history may go back many months or even years; about 25% will give a history of a mass being present over 10 years. Because the lesions develop under the epithelium, the initial lesion is a submucosal mass that is often painless until ulceration develops. Perineural involvement is expressed as pain or paresthesias. Otherwise, the clinical picture resembles that for squamous cell carcinomas for a given size and site. Lymph node metastases occur at predictable sites. The clinically positive nodes are usually small and mobile, but neck dissection on such a patient may show numerous small, clinically undetectable positive nodes.

METHODS OF DIAGNOSIS AND STAGING

The differential diagnosis includes lesions that produce an enlarging submucosal mass, such as an abscess, a stone in a duct, a cyst of soft tissue or bone, sarcoma, or lymphoma.

Because of the infrequency of these lesions, faulty histologic interpretation is not unusual and often leads to inappropriate therapy.

The same staging systems applied to squamous cell carcinomas may be used, although very few reported series bother to correlate size and extent of tumor with results by various treatment modalities. CT scan and MRI are useful for staging and treatment selection.

TREATMENT

Selection of Treatment Modality

Surgery and radiation therapy are the only curative therapies available. Because radiation therapy has often been used as a last-ditch effort for high-grade, advanced lesions after multiple surgical procedures, it is hardly surprising that results in some reports have been poor. Those series using radiation therapy alone for early lesions or as an immediate postoperative adjunct to surgical removal have had a favorable experience. After all, the histologies of the minor salivary gland tumors are the same as those of parotid tumors, and it is generally accepted that routine postoperative irradiation will decrease the local recurrence rate in high-grade parotid lesions and that irradiation alone will even control a few locally recurrent or inoperable tumors.[410] Similar responses have been observed for mucoepidermoid carcinoma and adenocarcinoma. The complete response rate of malignant minor salivary gland tumors to irradiation is similar to that of squamous cell carcinomas of the same size and same anatomic site, and the doses used are similar.

Benign mixed tumors are managed by operation; postoperative irradiation sometimes is advised in cases in which margins are close or positive. Inoperable lesions are treated with high-dose radiation therapy, and long-term control has been reported.

The low-grade lesions (low-grade mucoepidermoid carcinoma and acinic cell carcinoma) are treated initially by an operation when feasible, but irradiation is sometimes used as the primary treatment for inaccessible lesions or where the functional loss would be considerable. Postoperative irradiation is added for close margins or for those lesions that have recurred more than once. If the patient presents after excisional biopsy of a small lesion, irradiation is an alternative to reexcision, particularly if the procedure would produce significant cosmetic or functional loss.

The treatment of high-grade lesions varies immensely, depending on the site of origin, stage of disease, and willingness of the patient to accept a major cosmetic or functional change subsequent to an operation. Because the philosophy at the University of Florida is to accept radiation therapy as a curative therapy, the authors essentially approach most lesions as they would a squamous cell carcinoma of similar stage and similar anatomic site.

When combined treatment is indicated, the operation should precede radiation therapy to facilitate healing and to gain knowledge of tumor extent for radiation treatment planning.

Chemotherapy

Because of the rarity of these neoplasms, information about chemotherapy is almost entirely anecdotal. Some evidence of antitumor effects has been seen with 5-fluorouracil, hydroxyurea, methotrexate, cisplatin, and bleomycin, but the magnitudes of responses are often difficult to evaluate in the context of broad phase II studies or retrospective review of medical records.[417,419,422,438] Using a combination of methyl-CCNU, doxorubicin, and vincristine, Hayes and coworkers[439] have seen significant responses in adenoid cystic carcinoma.

Surgical Treatment

Benign tumors are removed by wide local excision that includes a cuff of normal tissue. Local excision or enucleation is insufficient treatment due to the high recurrence rate associated with limited procedures.

Small low-grade lesions with a long history of slow growth may be treated with a wide local excision including a shell of normal tissue. Large low-grade lesions and high-grade lesions require a more radical resection. When perineural invasion is present, it is not possible, of course, to remove all the nerves potentially involved, but the nerves that are involved should be sacrificed wherever it is reasonable to do so. As an alternative, postoperative irradiation may be used to cover the perineural routes of spread. Because unsuccessfully treated patients often live many years before they eventually die of the disease, careful planning must go into reconstruction and rehabilitation.

Irradiation Technique

The irradiation techniques are similar to those for squamous cell carcinomas of the same anatomic site and similar tumor size, with the exception that nerve pathways must be covered for adenoid cystic carcinomas. Subclinical perineural spread for adenoid cystic carcinomas must be considered to be present even though not seen on the biopsy or surgical sections. Recurrences frequently are manifested in and about the base of the skull at the termination of the cranial nerves.

A dose of 7000 cGy over 7 to 7.5 weeks to the area of gross disease is recommended for early lesions by radiation therapy alone. A dose of 6500 cGy is advised in the postoperative situation.[440] Low doses are inadequate.[440,441]

The regression rate of adenoid cystic carcinoma during treatment is similar to that of squamous cell carcinoma. Successfully treated adenocarcinomas or low-grade mucoepidermoid carcinomas may require several weeks or months to disappear after completion of treatment. The regional lymphatics are irradiated electively, depending on the site of origin and grade of the lesion. The response of benign mixed tumors is predictably slow and usually incomplete.

RESULTS OF TREATMENT

Spiro and co-workers[442] reported the Memorial Sloan–Kettering results for 434 malignant minor salivary gland tumors, of which 90% were treated surgically. The determinate 5-, 10-, and 15-year cure rates were 44%, 32%, and 21%; 51% died of the original cancer. Patients with adenoid cystic carcinoma had the poorest prognosis, with about 20% surviving without recurrence. Those with adenocarcinoma had an intermediate outlook, about 35% surviving without recurrence, and mucoepidermoid carcinomas had the best control rate with about 70% long-term cures. Local control rates differed considerably by site (Table 21-80), but this difference is partly explained by the higher incidence of advanced adenoid cystic carcinoma in the sinuses. Local control was also better for small lesions and those without bone or lymph node involvement. Previous treatment had little effect on cure rate.

Bardwil and co-workers[443] reported a similar series from M. D. Anderson Hospital with shorter follow-up (3–20 years) in which surgery was the sole treatment in 88% of cases (see Table 21-81). Local control was reported to be

TABLE 21-80. Results of Surgical Treatment of Minor Salivary Gland Tumors (267 Patients)*

Site	*No. of Patients*	*Local Control*
Oral cavity/oropharynx	198	68%
Sinus/nasal/nasopharynx	58	28%
Larynx	11	55%

Data from Spiro et al.[416]

*Memorial Hospital, 1939–1963. 60%—no prior treatment; 14%—clinically positive nodes on admission; 90%—treated surgically; 5 yr follow-up.

TABLE 21-81. Results of Treatment of Malignant Minor Salivary Gland Tumors (M. D. Anderson Hospital)

	No. of Patients	*No Prior Treatment*	*Follow-Up*	*Local Control*	*Distant Metastases*	*DOD or LWD**	*Methods of Treatment†*	
1945–1962 Bardwil et al.[443]	87	56%	3–20 years	75%	30%	47%	S	71
							S + RT	10
							RT	6
1970–1978 Schell et al.[435]	118	42%	2–10 years	79%‡	25%	36%	S	11
							S + RT	69
							RT	38

*DOD or LWD, dead of disease or living with disease.
†S, surgery; RT, radiation therapy.
‡Eleven patients salvaged by repeat operations for ultimate control rate of 88%.

TABLE 21-82. Malignant Minor Salivary Gland Tumors: Primary Recurrence Related to Treatment Modality (No. of Patients with Recurrence After Initial Treatment at M. D. Anderson Hospital/Total Patients Treated)

Histology	*Surgery Only*	*Surgery + Radiation Therapy*	*Radiation Therapy Only*	*Total*
High grade				
Adenoid cystic	3/4	9/40	0/23	12/67
Mucoepidermoid	0/1	0/6	4/7	4/14
Adenocarcinoma	3/4	3/14	1/4	7/22
Malignant mixed	0/0	0/1	0/0	0/1
Low grade				
Mucoepidermoid	1/2	0/7	1/4	2/13
Acinic cell	0/0	0/1	0/0	0/1
Total	7/11*	12/69†	6/38	25/118

Schell S, Barkley HT Jr, Chiminazzo H Jr: Treatment of malignant minor salivary gland tumors. Unpublished data, 1980.
*Five patients salvaged by repeated surgical resection(s).
†Six patients salvaged by surgery.

75%, but 47% died of their original cancer, a percentage similar to that in the Memorial Sloan–Kettering series.

Schell and co-workers[435] reported a group of 118 malignant salivary gland tumors of which only 10% were treated by operation alone, 58% by surgery plus radiation therapy, and 32% by radiation therapy alone (see Table 21-81). The group treated by radiation therapy alone included 15 early and 23 advanced lesions; follow-up was 2 to 10 years. The initial local control rate for the entire group was 79%; 11 patients were saved by subsequent operation for an ultimate control rate of 88%.

The risk of local recurrence by treatment category and histology is shown in Table 21-82.[432] The low incidence of recurrence with radiation therapy alone for adenoid cystic carcinoma indicates that this histology responds quite consistently to radiation. Surgery plus radiation therapy seems to provide better initial control than surgery alone for high-grade lesions.

Ellis and co-workers[440] compared the University of Florida results of radiation therapy alone versus combined surgery and radiation therapy for 52 patients with malignant minor salivary gland tumors with a follow-up of 2 to 20 years; 80% had a minimum follow-up of 5 years. Control at the primary site is shown in Table 21-83. Although permanent local control was never achieved in 7 patients with advanced adenoid cystic carcinoma treated with radiation therapy, the average time to local recurrence was 5 years and 7 months; in 2 patients the recurrence appeared at 9 and 13 years.

Benign mixed tumors of minor salivary gland origin have a good prognosis. Enucleation, however, is followed by recurrence, and a cuff of normal tissue is required. Spiro[413] reported on 81 benign tumors. Sixty occurred on the palate and 13 on the lip or cheek. With a minimum follow-up of 10 years, the local recurrence rate was 6%.

Bardwill and co-workers[443] reported 13 patients with benign mixed tumors, all of whom were cured, 12 by operation and 1 by radiation therapy alone.

Rafla-Demetrious[444] reported the Royal Marsden experience of 44 cases of benign mixed tumor (see Table 21-84). Eleven patients were treated by radiation therapy alone, and none of the tumors regrew, although not all had complete regression. Several photographs demonstrate the response to radiation therapy. Local recurrence of benign mixed tumor may appear after many, many years, and an occasional patient may eventually die of uncontrolled disease.

TABLE 21-83. Malignant Minor Salivary Gland Tumors: Initial Local Control at the Primary Site by Histology and Stage and Actuarial Survival Rates at 5 and 10 Years

	*Early Stage**		*Advanced Stage†*		*Actuarial Survival*	
Histology	*RT Alone*	*RT + Surgery*	*RT Alone*	*RT + Surgery*	*5 Years*	*10 Years*
Adenoid cystic	3/4‡	6/7	0/7§	3/5	63%	43%
Adenocarcinoma		3/3	1/4	3/4	43%	43%
Mucoepidermoid	2/2		1/1	3/3	72%	72%
Malignant mixed	1/1	1/1	0/1	1/1	100%	

Ellis ER, Million RR, Mendenhall WM, et al. The use of radiation therapy in the management of minor salivary gland tumors. Int J Radiat Oncol Biol Phys 15:613–617, 1988.
Follow-up, 2 to 23 years.
*Excludes 1 patient dead of intercurrent disease <2 years after treatment.
†Excludes 7 patients dead of intercurrent disease <2 years after treatment.
‡Ultimate control rate was 4 of 4 after surgical salvage.
§Average time to recurrence was 5 years 7 months.

TABLE 21-84. Incidence of Recurrence of Pleomorphic Adenoma of Minor Salivary Glands in the Royal Marsden Series Distributed According to the Method of Treatment

Method of Treatment	*No. of Patients*	*No. with Recurrence*	*Length of Follow-up*
Radiation alone	11	0	5 for 5+ years
Preoperative radiation and surgery	14	2	9 for 5+ years
Surgery and postoperative radiation	18	0	14 for 5+ years 9 for 10+ years
Surgery alone	1	0	5 years
Total	44	2	29 for 5+ years

Rafla-Demetrious SF: Mucous and Salivary Gland Tumours, p 118. Springfield, IL, Charles C Thomas, 1970.

REFERENCES

1. Silverberg E, Lubera J: Cancer statistics, 1987. CA 37:2–19, 1987
2. Donald PJ: Marijuana smoking—Possible cause of head and neck carcinoma in young patients. Otolaryngol Head Neck Surg 94:517—521, 1986
3. Rouviere H: Anatomy of the Human Lymphatic System, pp 1–70 (Tobias MJ trans). Ann Arbor, MI, Edwards Brothers, 1938
4. Leventon GS, Evans HL: Sarcomatoid squamous cell carcinoma of the mucous membranes of the head and neck: A clinicopathologic study of 20 cases. Cancer 48:994–1003, 1981
5. O'Brien CJ, Lahr CJ, Soong S-J, et al: Surgical treatment of early-stage carcinoma of the oral tongue: Would adjuvant treatment be beneficial? Head Neck Surg 8:401–408, 1986
6. Carter RL, Foster CS, Dinsdale EA. et al: Perineural spread by squamous carcinomas of the head and neck: A morphological study using antiaxonal and antimyelin monoclonal antibodies. J Clin Pathol 36:269–275, 1983
7. Lindberg RD: Distribution of cervical lymph node metastases from squamous cell carcinoma of the upper respiratory and digestive tracts. Cancer 29:1446–1449, 1972
8. Fisch U: Lymphography of the Cervical Lymphatic System. Philadelphia, WB Saunders, 1968
9. Berger DS, Fletcher GH, Lindberg RD, et al: Elective irradiation of the neck lymphatics for squamous cell carcinomas of the nasopharynx and oropharynx. Am J Roentgenol Radium Ther Nucl Med 111:66–72, 1971
10. Lindberg RD, Jesse RH: Treatment of cervical lymph node metastases from primary lesions of the oropharynx, supraglottic larynx, and hypopharynx. Am J Roentgenol Radium Ther Nucl Med 102:132–137, 1968
11. Merino OR, Lindberg RD, Fletcher GH: An analysis of distant metastases from squamous cell carcinoma of the upper respiratory and digestive tracts. Cancer 40:145–151, 1977
12. American Joint Committee on Cancer: Manual for Staging of Cancer, 2nd ed, pp 25–54. Philadelphia, JB Lippincott, 1983
13. Mendenhall WM, Parsons JT, Million RR: A favorable subset of AJCC stage IV squamous cell carcinoma of the head and neck. Int J Radiat Oncol Biol Phys 10:1841–1843, 1984
14. Parsons JT, Million RR, Cassisi NJ, et al: Hyperfractionation for head and neck cancer. Int J Radiat Oncol Biol Phys 14:649–658, 1988
15. Mendenhall WM, Million RR, Cassisi NJ: Elective neck irradiation in squamous cell carcinoma of the head and neck. Head Neck Surg 3:15–20, 1980
16. Fletcher GH, MacComb WS, Braun EJ: Analysis of sites and causes of treatment failures in squamous cell carcinomas of the oral cavity. Am J Roentgenol Radium Ther Nucl Med 83:405–411, 1960
17. Goffinet DR, Gilbert EH, Weller SA et al: Irradiation of clinically uninvolved cervical lymph nodes. Can J Otolaryngol 4:927–933, 1975
18. Jesse RH, Barkley HT, Lindberg RD et al: Cancer of the oral cavity: Is elective neck dissection beneficial? Am J Surg 120:505–508, 1970
19. Hardingham M, Dalley VM, Shaw HJ: Cancer of the floor of the mouth: Clinical features and results of treatment. Clin Oncol 3:227–246, 1977
20. Southwick HW, Slaughter DP, Trevino ET: Elective neck dissection for intraoral cancer. Arch Surg 80:905–909, 1960
21. Ash CL: Oral cancer: A twenty-five year study. Am J Roentgenol Radium Ther Nucl Med 87:417–430, 1962
22. Campos JL, Lampe I, Fayos JV: Radiotherapy of carcinoma of the floor of the mouth. Radiology 99:677–682, 1971
23. Million RR: Elective neck irradiation for TXN0 squamous carcinoma of the oral tongue and floor of mouth. Cancer 34:149–155, 1974
24. Cady B, Catlin D: Epidermoid carcinoma of the gum: A 20-year survey. Cancer 23:551–569, 1969
25. Del Regato JA, Spjut HJ: Ackerman and del Regato's Cancer: Diagnosis, Treatment, and Prognosis, 5th ed, pp 264, 281, 341, 342, 345. St Louis, CV Mosby, 1977
26. Martin CL, Craffey EJ: Cancer of the gums. Am J Roentgenol Radium Ther Nucl Med 67:420–427, 1952
27. Chung CK, Rahman SM, Lim ML et al: Squamous cell carcinoma of the hard palate. Int J Radiat Oncol Biol Phys 5:191–196, 1979
28. Eneroth CM, Hjertman L, Moberger G: Squamous cell carcinomas of the palate. Acta Otolaryngol (Stockholm) 73:418–427, 1972
29. Horiuchi J, Adachi T: Some considerations on radiation therapy of tongue cancer. Cancer 28:335–339, 1971
30. Beahrs OH, Devine KD, Henson SW Jr: Treatment of carcinoma of the tongue: End-results in one hundred sixty-eight cases. Arch Surg 79:399–403, 1959
31. Frazell EL, Lucas JC Jr: Cancer of the tongue: Report of the management of 1554 patients. Cancer 15:1085–1099, 1962
32. Kremen AJ: Results of surgical treatment of cancer of the tongue. Surgery 39:49–53, 1956
33. Spiro RH, Strong EW: Discontinuous partial glossectomy and radical neck dissection in selected patients with epidermoid carcinoma of the mobile tongue. Am J Surg 126:544–546, 1973
34. Million RR, Fletcher GH, Jesse RH Jr: Evaluation of elective irradiation of the neck for squamous cell carcinoma of the nasopharynx, tonsillar fossa, and base of tongue. Radiology 80:973–988, 1963
35. Ho JHC: An epidemiologic and clinical study of nasopharyngeal carcinoma. Int J Radiat Oncol Biol Phys 4:183–198, 1978
36. Moench HC, Phillips TL: Carcinoma of the nasopharynx: Review of 146 patients with emphasis on radiation dose and time factors. Am J Surg 124:515–518, 1972
37. Barker JL, Fletcher GH: Time, dose, and tumor volume relationships in megavoltage irradiation of squamous cell carcinomas of the retromolar trigone and anterior tonsillar pillar. Int J Radiat Oncol Biol Phys 2:407–414, 1977
38. Jesse RH, Fletcher GH: Metastases in cervical lymph nodes from oropharyngeal carcinoma: Treatment and results. Am J Roentgenol Radium Ther Nucl Med 90:990–996, 1963
39. Lindberg RD, Barkley HT Jr, Jesse RH et al: Evolution of the clinically negative neck in patients with squamous cell carcinoma of the faucial arch. Am J Roentgenol Radium Ther Nucl Med 111:60–65, 1971
40. Southwick HW: Elective neck dissection for intraoral cancer. JAMA 217:454–455, 1971
41. Rolander TL, Everts EC, Shumrick DA: Carcinoma of the tonsil: A planned combined therapy approach. Laryngoscope 81:1199–1207, 1971
42. Ogura JH, Biller HF, Wette R: Elective neck dissection for pharyngeal and laryngeal cancers: An evaluation. Ann Otol Rhinol Laryngol 80:646–651, 1971
43. Putney FJ: Elective versus delayed neck dissection in cancer of the larynx. Surg Gynecol Obstet 112:736–742, 1961
44. Fletcher GH: Elective irradiation of subclinical disease in cancers of the head and neck. Cancer 29:1450–1454, 1972
45. Mancuso AA, Hanafee WN: Computed Tomography and Magnetic Resonance Imaging of the Head and Neck, 2nd ed, pp 16, 139–151, 184. Baltimore, Williams & Wilkins, 1985
46. Mendenhall WM, Million RR: Elective neck irradiation for squamous cell carcinoma of the head and neck: Analysis of time-dose factors and causes of failure. Int J Radiat Oncol Biol Phys 12:741–746, 1986
47. Agresti A, Wackerly D: Some exact conditional tests of independence for T×C cross-classification tables. Psychometrika 42:111–125, 1977
48. Barkley HT Jr, Fletcher GH, Jesse RH et al: Management of cervical lymph node metastases in squamous cell carcinoma of the tonsillar fossa, base of tongue, supraglottic larynx, and hypopharynx. Am J Surg 124:462–467, 1972
49. Byers, RM: Modified neck dissection: A study of 967 cases from 1970 to 1980. Am J Surg 150:414–421, 1985
50. McGuirt WF, McCabe BF: Significance of node biopsy before definitive treatment of cervical metastatic carcinoma. Laryngoscope 88:594–597, 1978
51. Parsons JT, Million RR, Cassisi NJ: The influence of excisional or incisional biopsy of metastatic neck nodes on the management of head and neck cancer. Int J Radiat Oncol Biol Phys 11:1447–1454, 1985
52. Million RR, Cassisi NJ: General principles for treatment of cancers in the head and neck: Selection of treatment for the primary site and for the neck. In Million RR,

Cassisi NJ (eds): Management of Head and Neck Cancer: A Multidisciplinary Approach, pp 43–62. Philadelphia, JB Lippincott, 1984

53. Papac R, Lefkowitz E, Bertino JR: Methotrexate (NSC-740) in squamous cell carcinoma of the head and neck. II. Intermittent intravenous therapy. Cancer Chemother Rep 51:69–72, 1967
54. Lane M, Moore JE, Levin H, et al: Methotrexate therapy for squamous cell carcinoma of the head and neck: Intermittent intravenous dose program. JAMA 204:561–564, 1968
55. Leone LA, Albala MM, Rege VB: Treatment of carcinoma of the head and neck with intravenous methotrexate. Cancer 21:828–837, 1968
56. DePalo GM, DeLena M, Molinari R, et al: Sperimentazione clinica con alte dosi intermittendi di methotrexate nel carcinoma oro-faringeo in fase avanzata. [Clinical evaluation of high weekly intravenous dose of methotrexate in advanced oropharyngeal carcinoma.] Tumori 56:259–268, 1970
57. Levitt M, Mosher MB, DeConti RC, et al: Improved therapeutic index of methotrexate with "leucovorin rescue." Cancer Res 33:1729–1734, 1973
58. Tejada F, Murphy E, Zubrod CG: Proceedings of the International Head and Neck Oncology Conference. Abstract 2.14. National Cancer Institute, 1980
59. DeConti RC, Schoenfeld D: A randomized prospective comparison of intermittent methotrexate, methotrexate with leucovorin, and a methotrexate combination in head and neck cancer. Cancer 48:1061–1072, 1981
60. Kirkwood JM, Canellos GP, Ervin TJ, et al: Increased therapeutic index using moderate dose methotrexate and leucovorin twice weekly vs. weekly high dose methotrexate-leucovorin in patients with advanced squamous cell carcinoma of the head and neck: A safe new effective regimen. Cancer 47:2414–2421, 1981
61. Woods RL, Fox RM, Tattersall MHN: Methotrexate treatment of squamous-cell head and neck cancers: Dose-response evaluation. Br Med J [Clin Res] 282:600–602, 1981
62. Hong WK, Schaefer S, Issell B, et al: A prospective randomized trial of methotrexate versus cisplatin in the treatment of recurrent squamous cell carcinomas of the head and neck (Abstract C-787). Proc Am Soc Clin Oncol 1:202, 1982
63. Grose WE, Lehane DE, Dixon DO, et al: Comparison of methotrexate and cisplatin for patients with advanced squamous cell carcinoma of the head and neck region: A Southwest Oncology Group study. Cancer Treat Rep 69:577–581, 1985
64. Vogler WR, Jacobs J, Moffitt S, et al: Methotrexate therapy with or without citrovorum factor in carcinoma of the head and neck, breast, and colon. Cancer Clin Trials 2:227–236, 1979
65. Taylor SG, McGuire WP, Hauck WW, et al: A randomized comparison of high-dose infusion methotrexate versus standard-dose weekly therapy in head and neck squamous cancer. J Clin Oncol 2:1006–1011, 1984
66. Bonadonna G, Tancini G, Bajetta E: Controlled studies with bleomycin in solid tumors and lymphomas. Prog Biochem Pharmacol 11:172–184, 1976
67. Halnan KE, Bleehen NM, Brewin TB, et al: Early clinical experience with bleomycin in the United Kingdom in series of 105 patients. Br Med J [Clin Res] 4:635–638, 1972
68. Haas CD, Coltman CA, Gottlieb JA, et al: Phase II evaluation of bleomycin: A Southwest Oncology Group Study. Cancer 38:8–12, 1976
69. Yagoda A, Mukherji B, Young C, et al: Bleomycin, an antitumor antibiotic: Clinical experience in 274 patients. Ann Intern Med 77:861–870, 1972
70. Durkin WJ, Pugh RP, Jacobs E, et al: Bleomycin (NSC-125066) therapy of responsive solid tumors. Oncology 33:260–264, 1976
71. EORTC Clinical Screening Co-operative Group: Study of the clinical efficiency of bleomycin in human cancer. Br Med J [Clin Res] 2:643–645, 1970
72. Wasserman TH, Comis RL, Goldsmith M, et al: Tabular analysis of the clinical chemotherapy of solid tumors. Cancer Chemother Rep 6:399–419, 1975
73. Wittes RE, Cvitkovic E, Shah J, et al: Cis-dichlorodiammineplatinum (II) in the treatment of epidermoid carcinoma of the head and neck. Cancer Treat Rep 61:359–366, 1977
74. Jacobs C, Bertino JR, Goffinet DR, et al: 24-hour infusion of cis-platinum in head and neck cancers. Cancer 42:2135–2140, 1978
75. Panettiere FJ, Lehane D, Fletcher WS, et al: Cis-platinum therapy of previously treated head and neck cancer: The Southwest Oncology Group's two-dose-per-month outpatient regimen. Med Pediatr Oncol 8:221–225, 1980
76. Creagan ET, O'Fallon JR, Woods JE, et al: Cis-diamminedichloroplatinum (II) administered by 24-hour infusion in the treatment of patients with advanced upper aerodigestive cancer. Cancer 51:2020–2023, 1983
77. Sako K, Razack MS, Kalnins I: Chemotherapy for advanced and recurrent squamous cell carcinoma of the head and neck with high and low dose cis-diamminedichloroplatinum. Am J Surg 136:529–533, 1978
78. Randolph VL, Wittes RE: Weekly administration of cis-diamminedichloroplatinum (II) without hydration or osmotic diuresis. Eur J Cancer Clin Oncol 14:753–756, 1978
79. Gold GL, Hall TC, Shnider BI, et al: A clinical study of 5-fluorouracil. Cancer Res 19:935–939, 1959
80. Olson KB, Greene JR: Evaluation of 5-fluorouracil in treatment of cancer. JNCI 25:133–140, 1960
81. Weiss AJ, Jackson LG, Carabasi R: An evaluation of 5-fluorouracil in malignant disease. Ann Intern Med 55:731–741, 1961
82. Staley CJ, Kerth JD, Cortes N, et al: Treatment of advanced cancer with 5-fluorouracil. Surg Gynecol Obstet 112:185–190, 1961
83. Ansfield FJ, Schroeder JM, Curreri AR: Five years clinical experience with 5-fluorouracil. JAMA 181:295–299, 1962
84. White JE, Ricketts WN, Strudwick WJ: A clinical study of 5-fluorouracil in a variety of far advanced human malignancies. J Natl Med Assoc 54:315–317, 1962
85. Moore GE, Bross IDJ, Ausman R, et al: Effects of 5-fluorouracil (NSC 19893) in 389 patients with cancer: Eastern Clinical Drug Evaluation Program. Cancer Chemother Rep 52:641–653, 1968
86. Young CW, Ellison RR, Sullivan RD, et al: The clinical evaluation of 5-fluorouracil and 5-fluoro-2′-deoxyuridine in solid tumors in adults: A progress report. Cancer Chemother Rep 6:17–20, 1960
87. Jacobs EM, Luce JK, Wood DA: Treatment of cancer with weekly intravenous 5-fluorouracil. Cancer 22:1233–1238, 1968
88. Carter SK: The chemotherapy of head and neck cancer. Semin Oncol 4:413–424, 1977
89. Krakoff IH: Adriamycin (NSC-123127) studies in adult patients. Cancer Chemother Rep 6:253–257, 1975
90. Blum RH: An overview of studies with Adriamycin (NSC-123127) in the United States. Cancer Chemother Rep 6:247–251, 1975
91. Lee G, Pitman SW, Bertino JR: Weekly hydroxyurea in squamous head and neck cancer (abstract C-572). Proc Am Soc Clin Oncol 4:147, 1985
92. Hornedo-Muguiro J, So M, Spaulding MB, et al: Phase II trial of carboplatin (CBDCA) in aerodigestive malignancies (abstract C-350). Proc Am Soc Clin Oncol 4:136, 1985
93. Basauri L, Pousa AL, Alba E, et al: Carboplatin, an active drug in advanced head and neck cancer. Cancer Treat Rep 70:1173–1176, 1986
94. Eisenberger M, Hornedo J, Silva H, et al: Carboplatin (NSC-241-240): An active platinum analog for the treatment of squamous-cell carcinoma of the head and neck. J Clin Oncol 4:1506–1509, 1986
95. Al-Sarraf M, Metch B, Kish J, et al: Platinum analogs in recurrent and advanced head and neck cancer: A Southwest Oncology Group and Wayne State University Study. Cancer Treat Rep 71:723–726, 1987
96. Vogl SE, Ryan L, Wernz J, et al: Ineffective agents in the chemotherapy (CT) of head and neck cancer (HNCA): Mitoxantrone (DHAD), dibromodulcitol (DBD) and vinblastine (VLB): The Eastern Cooperative Oncology Group (ECOG) experience (abstract 679). Proc Am Assoc Cancer Res 26:171, 1985
97. Williams SD, Birch R, Velez-Garcia E, et al: Phase II study of mitoxantrone in advanced squamous cell carcinoma of the head and neck. A Southeastern Cancer Study Group trial. Invest New Drugs 3:311–313, 1985
98. DeJager R, Cappelaere P, Armand JP, et al: An EORTC phase II study of mitoxantrone in solid tumors and lymphomas. Eur J Cancer Clin Oncol 20:1369–1375, 1984
99. Sikic BT, Collins JM, Mimnaugh EG, et al: Improved therapeutic index of bleomycin when administered by continuous infusion in mice. Cancer Treat Rep 62:2011–2017, 1978
100. Peng Y-M, Alberts DS, Chen H-SG, et al: Antitumour activity and plasma kinetics of bleomycin by continuous and intermittent administration. Br J Cancer 41:644–647, 1980
101. Samuels ML, Johnson DE, Holoye PY: Continuous intravenous bleomycin (NSC-125066) therapy and vinblastine (NSC-49842) in stage III testicular neoplasia. Cancer Chemother Rep 59:563–570, 1975
102. Baker LH, Opipari MI, Wilson H, et al: Mitomycin C, vincristine and bleomycin therapy for advanced cervical cancer. Obstet Gynecol 52:146–150, 1978
103. Carlson RW, Sikic BI: Continuous infusion or bolus injection in cancer chemotherapy. Ann Intern Med 99:823–833, 1983
104. Morton RP, Rugman F, Dorman EB, et al: Cisplatinum and bleomycin for advanced or recurrent squamous cell carcinoma of the head and neck: A randomized factorial phase III controlled trial. Cancer Chemother Pharmacol 15:283–289, 1985
105. Tapazoglou E, Kish J, Ensley J, et al: The activity of a single-agent 5-fluorouracil infusion in advanced and recurrent head and neck cancer. Cancer 57:1105–1109, 1986
106. Perry DJ, Crain SM, Weltz MD, et al: Phase II trial of mitoguazone in patients with advanced squamous cell carcinoma of the head and neck. Cancer Treat Rep 67:91–92, 1983
107. Thongprasert S, Bosl GJ, Geller NL, et al: Phase II trials of mitoguazone in patients with advanced head and neck. Cancer Treat Rep 68:1301–1302, 1984
108. Luedke D, Maddox W, Birch R, et al: Phase II trial of methyl glyoxal bis (guanylhydrazone) (MGBG) in advanced head and neck squamous cell carcinoma (abstract C-506). Proc Am Soc Clin Oncol 4:130, 1985
109. Coninx P, Nasca S, Jezekova D, et al: Essai phase II de mitoguazone chez des patients porteurs de tumeurs cervico-faciales etendues en recidive [Phase II trial of mitoguazone in patients with recurrent head and neck cancer.] Bull Cancer (Paris) 72:153–154, 1985
110. Ratanatharathorn V, Drelichman A, Sexon-Porte M, et al: Phase II evaluation of 4′-(9-acridinylamino)-methanesulfon-m-anisidine (AMSA) in patients with advanced head and neck cancers. Am J Clin Oncol (CCT) 5:29–32, 1982
111. Forastiere AA, Young CW, Wittes RE: A phase II trial of m-AMSA in head and neck cancer. Cancer Chemother Pharmacol 6:145–146, 1981
112. Andrews NC, Weiss AJ, Ansfield FJ, et al: Phase I study of dibromodulcitol (NSC-104800). Cancer Chemother Rep 55:61–65, 1971
113. Andrews NC, Weiss AJ, Wilson W, et al: Phase II study dibromodulcitol. Cancer Chemother Rep 58:653–660, 1974
114. Nissen NI, Pajak TF, Leone LA, et al: Clinical trial of VP 16-213 (NSC 141540) IV twice weekly in advanced neoplastic disease. A study by the Cancer and Leukemia Group B. Cancer 45:232–235, 1980
115. Grunberg SM, Felman IE, Gala KV, et al: Phase II study of etoposide (VP-16) in the treatment of advanced head and neck cancer. Am J Clin Oncol (CCT) 8:393–395, 1985
116. Crivellari D, Veronesi A, Magri MD, et al: Phase II trial of oral VP 16-213 (etoposide) in patients with advanced head and neck cancer. Tumori 71:499–500, 1985

117. Cheng E, Young CW, Wittes RE: Phase II trial of vindesine in advanced head and neck cancer. Cancer Treat Rep 64:1141–1142, 1980
118. Kaplan BH, Vogl SE, Cinberg J, et al: Phase II trial of vindesine in squamous cancer of the head and neck (abstract C-775). Proc Am Soc Clin Oncol 1:199, 1982
119. Sledge GW, Clark GM, Griffin C, et al: Phase II trial of vindesine in patients with squamous cell cancer of the head and neck. Am J Clin Oncol (CCT) 7:209–211, 1984
120. Krasnow S, Eisenberger M, Green M, et al: Phase I–II study of triazinate (TCT) for advanced head and neck cancer (HNC) (abstract 682). Proc Am Assoc Cancer Res 26:172, 1985
121. Ikic D, Padovan I, Brodarec I, et al: Application of human leucocyte interferon in patients with tumours of the head and neck. Lancet 1:1025–1027, 1981
122. Medenica RN, Slack N: Clinical results of leukocytes interferon-induced tumor regression in resistant human metastatic cancer resistent to chemotherapy and/or radiotherapy-pulse therapy schedule. Cancer Drug Deliv 2:53–76, 1985
123. Connors JM, Andiman WA, Howarth CB, et al: Treatment of nasopharyngeal carcinoma with human leukocyte interferon. J Clin Oncol 3:813–817, 1985
124. Kish JA, Ensley JF, Jacobs J, et al: A randomized trial of cisplatin (CACP) + 5-fluorouracil (5-FU) infusion and CACP + 5-FU bolus for recurrent and advanced squamous cell carcinoma of the head and neck. Cancer 56:2740–2744, 1985
125. Kish JA, Weaver A, Jacobs J, et al: Cisplatin and 5-fluorouracil infusion in patients with recurrent and disseminated epidermoid cancer of the head and neck. Cancer 53:1819–1824, 1984
126. Merlano M, Tatarek R, Grimaldi A, et al: Phase I–II trial with cisplatin and 5-FU in recurrent head and neck cancer: An effective outpatient schedule. Cancer Treat Rep 69:961–964, 1985
127. Bitran JD, Goldman M: A phase II trial of cyclophosphamide and Adriamycin in refractory squamous cell carcinoma of the head and neck: An effective salvage regimen. Am J Clin Oncol (CCT) 8:61–64, 1985
128. Scherlacher A, Jaske R, Lehnert M: Therapie rezidivierender Plattenepithelkarzinome (rPECHN) im HNO-Bereich mit einem sequentiellen Methotrexat-(MTX)/5-Fluorouracil (5-FU)-Protokoll. Laryngol Rhinol Otol (Stuttg) 64:58–61, 1985
129. Pitman SW, Kowal CD, Bertino JR: Methotrexate and 5-fluorouracil in sequence in squamous head and neck cancer. Semin Oncol 10 (suppl 2):15–19, 1983
130. Lester EP, Johnson CM, Lester AK, et al: Head and neck advanced squamous carcinoma: Treatment with cis-platinum, bleomycin, and sequential methotrexate/5-fluorouracil (abstract C-707). Proc Am Soc Clin Oncol 3:182, 1984
131. Vogl SE, Komisar A, Kaplan BH, et al: Sequential methotrexate and 5-fluorouracil with bleomycin and cisplatin in the chemotherapy of advanced squamous cancer of the head and neck. Cancer 57:706–710, 1986
132. Cognetti F, Pinnaro P, Carlini P, et al: CABO treatment (cisplatin, methotrexate, bleomycin, vincristine) in advanced or recurrent squamous cell carcinoma of the head and neck. J Exp Clin Cancer Res 3:411–417, 1984
133. Kaplan BH, Schoenfeld D, Vogl SE: Treatment of recurrent (REC) or metastatic (MET) squamous cancer of the head and neck (SCH&N) with methotrexate (M), M plus *Corynebacterium parvum* (CP) or M plus bleomycin (B) plus diamminedichloroplatinum (D): A prospective randomized trial of the Eastern Cooperative Oncology Group (abstract C-780). Proc Am Assoc Cancer Res 22:532, 1981
134. Jacobs C, Meyers F, Hendrickson C, et al: A randomized phase III study of cisplatin with or without methotrexate for recurrent squamous cell carcinoma of the head and neck. A Northern California Oncology Group study. Cancer 52:1563–1569, 1983
135. Drelichman A, Cummings G, Al-Sarraf M: A randomized trial of the combination of cis-platinum, oncovin, and bleomycin (COB) versus methotrexate in patients with advanced squamous cell carcinoma of the head and neck. Cancer 52:399–403, 1983
136. Vogl SE, Schoenfeld DA, Kaplan BH, et al: A randomized prospective comparison of methotrexate with a combination of methotrexate, bleomycin, and cisplatin in head and neck cancer. Cancer 56:432–442, 1985
137. Williams SD, Velez-Garcia E, Essessee I, et al: Chemotherapy for head and neck cancer: Comparison of cisplatin + vinblastine + bleomycin versus methotrexate. Cancer 57:18–23, 1986
138. Ketcham AS, Hoye RC, Chretien PB, et al: Irradiation twenty-four hours preoperatively. Am J Surg 118:691–697, 1969
139. Lawrence WL, Terz JJ, Rogers C, et al: Preoperative irradiation for head and neck cancer: A prospective study. Cancer 33:318–323, 1974
140. Strong EW: Preoperative radiation and radical neck dissection. Surg Clin North Am 49:271–276, 1969
141. Fletcher GH: Basic principles of the combination of irradiation and surgery. Int J Radiat Oncol Biol Phys 5:2091–2096, 1979
142. Looser KG, Shah JP, Strong EW: The significance of "positive" margins in surgically resected epidermoid carcinomas. Head Neck Surg 1:107–111, 1978
143. Amdur RJ, Parsons JT, Mendenhall WM, et al: Postoperative irradiation for squamous cell carcinoma of the head and neck: An analysis of treatment results and complications. Int J Radiat Oncol Biol Phys (in press)
144. Colton T: Statistics in Medicine, pp 163–167. Boston, Little, Brown, 1974
145. Mendenhall W, Ott L, Larson RF: Statistics: A Tool for the Social Sciences. North Scituate, MA, Duxbury Press, 1974
146. Marcus RB Jr, Million RR, Cassisi NJ: Postoperative irradiation for squamous cell carcinomas of the head and neck: Analysis of time-dose factors related to control above the clavicles. Int J Radiat Oncol Biol Phys 5:1943–1949, 1979
147. Peppard SB, Al-Sarraf M, Powers WE, et al: Combination of cis-platinum, oncovin and bleomycin (COB) prior to surgery and/or radiotherapy in advanced untreated epidermoid cancer of the head and neck. Laryngoscope 90:1273–1280, 1980
148. Elias EG, Chretien PB, Monnard E, et al: Chemotherapy prior to local therapy in advanced squamous cell carcinoma of the head and neck: Preliminary assessment of an intensive drug regimen. Cancer 43:1025–1031, 1979
149. Pennacchio JL, Hong WK, Shapshay S, et al: Combination of cis-platinum and bleomycin prior to surgery and/or radiotherapy compared with radiotherapy alone for the treatment for advanced squamous cell carcinoma of the head and neck. Cancer 50:2795–2801, 1982
150. Spaulding MN, Kahn A, DeLos Santos R, et al: Adjuvant chemotherapy in head and neck cancer: An update. Am J Surg 144:432–436, 1982
151. Randolph VL, Vallejo A, Spiro RH, et al: Combination therapy of advanced head and neck cancer: Induction of remission with diamminedichloroplatinum (II), bleomycin and radiation therapy. Cancer 41:460–467, 1978
152. Brown AW Jr, Blom J, Butler WM, et al: Combination chemotherapy with vinblastine, bleomycin, and cis-diamminedichloroplatinum (II) in squamous cell carcinoma of the head and neck. Cancer 45:2830–2835, 1980
153. Weaver A, Flemming S, Kish J, et al: Cis-platinum and 5-fluorouracil as induction therapy for advanced head and neck cancer. Am J Surg 144:445–448, 1982
154. Rooney M, Kish J, Jacobs J, et al: Improved complete response rate and survival in advanced head and neck cancer after three-course induction therapy with 120-hour 5-FU infusion and cisplatin. Cancer 55:1123–1128, 1985
155. Jacobs C, Goffinet DR, Goffinet L, et al: Chemotherapy as a substitute for surgery in the treatment of advanced resectable head and neck cancer: A report from the Northern California Oncology Group. Cancer 60:1178–1183, 1987
156. Ervin TJ, Clark JR, Weichselbaum RR, et al: An analysis of induction and adjuvant chemotherapy in the multidisciplinary treatment of squamous-cell carcinoma of the head and neck. J Clin Oncol 5:10–20, 1987
157. Clark J, Fallon B, Norris C, et al: A randomized trial of two induction regimens for advanced squamous cell carcinoma of the head and neck (SCCHN): Preliminary results (abstract 515). Proc Am Soc Clin Oncol 5:132, 1986
158. Weichselbaum RR, Clark JR, Miller D, et al: Combined modality treatment of head and neck cancer with cisplatin, bleomycin, methotrexate-leucovorin chemotherapy. Cancer 55:2149–2155, 1985
159. Kies MS, Gordon LI, Hauck WW, et al: Analysis of complete responders after initial treatment with chemotherapy in head and neck cancer. Otolaryngol Head Neck Surg 93:199–205, 1985
160. Norris CM Jr, Clark JR, Frei E III, et al: Pathology of surgery after induction chemotherapy: An analysis of resectability and locoregional control. Laryngoscope 96:292–302, 1986
161. Al-Kourainy K, Kish J, Ensley J, et al: Achievement of superior survival for histologically negative versus histologically positive clinically complete responders to cisplatin combination in patients with locally advanced head and neck cancer. Cancer 59:233–238, 1987
162. Clark J, Fallon B, Weichselbaum R, et al: The influence of resectability on response to induction chemotherapy and survival in advanced squamous cell carcinoma of the head and neck (SCCHN) (abstract C-542). Proc Am Soc Clin Oncol 4:139, 1985
163. Jacobs C, Wolf GT, Makuch RW, et al: Adjuvant chemotherapy for head and neck squamous carcinomas (abstract C-708). Proc Am Soc Clin Oncol 3:182, 1984
164. Fallon B, Clark J, Weichselbaum R, et al: Locoregional control in advanced squamous cell carcinoma of the head and neck after induction chemotherapy (abstract C-541). Proc Am Soc Clin Oncol 4:139, 1985
165. Ensley J, Crissman J, Kish J, et al: The impact of conventional morphologic analysis on response rates and survival in patients with advanced head and neck cancers treated initially with cisplatin-containing combination chemotherapy. Cancer 57:711–717, 1986
166. Posner MR, Weichselbaum RR, Fitzgerald TJ, et al: Treatment complications after sequential combination chemotherapy and radiotherapy with or without surgery in previously untreated squamous cell carcinoma of the head and neck. Int J Radiat Oncol Biol Phys 11:1887–1893, 1985
167. Stell PM, Dalby JE, Strickland P, et al: Sequential chemotherapy and radiotherapy in advanced head and neck cancer. Clin Radiol 34:463–467, 1983
168. Schuller DE, Wilson H, Hodgson S, et al: Preoperative reductive chemotherapy for stage III or IV operative epidermoid carcinoma of the oral cavity, oropharynx, or larynx, phase III: A Southwest Oncology Group study (abstract 185). Presented at the International Conference on Head and Neck Cancer, Baltimore, 1984
169. Holoye PY, Grossman TW, Toohill RJ, et al: Randomized study of adjuvant chemotherapy for head and neck cancer. Otolaryngol Head and Neck Surg 93:712–717, 1985
170. Haas C, Anderson T, Byhardt R, et al: Randomized neo-adjuvant study of 5-fluorouracil (FU) and cis-platinum (DDP) for patients (PTS) with advanced resectable head and neck squamous carcinoma (ARHNSC) (abstract 735). Proc Am Assoc Cancer Res 27:185, 1986
171. Martin M, Mazeron JJ, Glaubiger D, et al: Neo-adjuvant polychemotherapy of head and neck cancer: Preliminary results of a randomized study (abstract 551). Proc Am Soc Clin Oncol 5:141, 1986
172. Adjuvant chemotherapy for advanced head and neck squamous carcinoma: Final report of the Head and Neck Contracts Program. Cancer 60:301–311, 1987
173. Condit PT, Ridings GR, Coin JW, et al: Methotrexate and radiation in the treatment of patients with cancer. Cancer Res 24:1524–1533, 1964
174. Friedman M, DeNarvaes FN, Daly JF: Treatment of squamous cell carcinoma of the head and neck with combined methotrexate and irradiation. Cancer 26:711–721, 1970
175. Tarpley JL, Chretien PB, Alexander JC, et al: High dose methotrexate as a preoperative adjuvant in the treatment of epidermoid carcinoma of the head and neck: A feasibility study and clinical trial. Am J Surg 130:481–486, 1975

176. Ervin TJ, Kirkwood J, Weichselbaum RR, et al: Improved survival for patients with advanced carcinoma of the head and neck treated with methotrexate-leucovorin prior to definitive radiotherapy or surgery. Laryngoscope 91:1181–1190, 1981
177. von Essen CF, Joseph LBM, Simon GT, et al: Sequential chemotherapy and radiation therapy of buccal mucosa carcinoma in South India: Methods and preliminary results. Am J Roentgenol Radium Ther Nucl Med 102:530–540, 1968
178. Knowlton AH, Percarpio B, Bobrow S, et al: Methotrexate and radiation therapy in the treatment of advanced head and neck tumors. Radiology 116:709–712, 1975
179. Fazekas JT, Sommer C, Kramer S: Adjuvant intravenous methotrexate or definitive radiotherapy alone for advanced squamous cancers of the oral cavity, oropharynx, supraglottic larynx or hypopharynx: Concluding report of an RTOG randomized trial on 638 patients. Int J Radiat Oncol Biol Phys 6:533–541, 1980
180. Taylor SG, Applebaum E, Showel JL, et al: A randomized trial of adjuvant chemotherapy in head and neck cancer. J Clin Oncol 3:672–679, 1985
181. Huang AT, Cole TB, Fishburn R, et al: Adjuvant chemotherapy after surgery and radiation for stage III and IV head and neck cancer. Ann Surg 200:195–199, 1984
182. Johnson JT, Myers EN, Schramm VL, et al: Adjuvant chemotherapy for high-risk squamous-cell carcinoma of the head and neck. J Clin Oncol 5:456–458, 1987
183. Bitter K: Postoperative chemotherapy versus postoperative cobalt 60 radiation in patients with advanced oral carcinoma: Report on a randomized study (abst). Head Neck Surg 3:264, 1981
184. Tejada F, Chandler JR: Combined therapy for stage III and IV head and neck cancer (H&N) (abstract C-774). Proc Am Soc Clin Oncol 1:199, 1982
185. Shanta V, Krishramurthi S: The combined therapy of oral cancer. GANN Monogr Cancer Res 19:159–170, 1976
186. Abe M, Shigematsu Y, Kimura S: Combined use of bleomycin with radiation in the treatment of cancer. Recent Results Cancer Res 63:169–178, 1978
187. Kapstad B, Bang G, Rennaes S, et al: Combined preoperative treatment with cobalt and bleomycin in patients with head and neck carcinoma: A controlled clinical study. Int J Radiat Oncol Biol Phys 4:85–89, 1978
188. Fu KK, Phillips TL, Silverberg IJ, et al: Combined radiotherapy and chemotherapy with bleomycin and methotrexate for advanced inoperable head and neck cancer: Update of a Northern California Oncology Group randomized trial. J Clin Oncol 5:1410–1418, 1987
189. Gollin FF, Ansfield FJ, Brandenburg JH, et al: Combined therapy in advanced head and neck cancer: A randomized study. Am J Roentgenol Radium Ther Nucl Med 114:83–88, 1972
190. Ansfield FJ, Ramirez G, Davis HL Jr, et al: Treatment of advanced cancer of the head and neck. Cancer 25:78–82, 1970
191. Papac RJ, Weissberg JB, Son YH, et al: Prospective randomized trial of radiation therapy (RT) ± mitomycin C (MC) in head and neck cancer (abstract 492). Proc Am Soc Clin Oncol 6:126, 1987
192. Stefani S, Eells RW, Abbate J: Hydroxyurea and radiotherapy in head and neck cancer: Results of a prospective controlled study in 126 patients. Radiology 101:391–396, 1971
193. Richards GJ, Chambers RG: Hydoxyurea: A radiosensitizer in the treatment of neoplasms of the head and neck. Am J Roentgenol Radium Ther Nucl Med 105:555–565, 1969
194. Kramer S: Methotrexate and radiation therapy in the treatment of advanced squamous cell carcinoma of the oral cavity, oropharynx, supraglottic larynx, and hypopharynx: Preliminary report of a controlled clinical trial of the Radiation Therapy Oncology Group. Can J Otolaryngol 4:213–218, 1975
195. Condit PT: Treatment of carcinoma with radiation therapy and methotrexate. Mo Med 65:832–835, 1968
196. Bagshaw MA, Doggett RLS: A clinical study of chemical radiosensitization. Front Radiat Ther Oncol 4:164–173, 1969
197. Haselow RE, Adams GS, Oken MM, et al: Simultaneous cis-platinum (DDP) and radiation therapy (RT) for locally advanced unresectable head and neck cancer (Abstract C-780). Proc Am Soc Clin Oncol 1:201, 1982
198. Leipzig B, Wetmore SJ, Klug D, et al: Cis-platinum sensitization to radiotherapy of squamous cell carcinoma in the head and neck. In Vidockler HR (ed): Proceedings of the International Conference on Head and Neck Cancer, p 42. Baltimore, Lancaster Press, 1984
199. Coughlin CT, Grace M, LeMarbre P, et al: Combined modality therapy for advanced head and neck cancer (abstract C-776). Proc Am Soc Clin Oncol 1:200, 1982
200. Al-Sarraf M, Pajak TF, Marcial VA, et al: Concurrent radiotherapy and chemotherapy with cisplatin in inoperable squamous cell carcinoma of the head and neck: An RTOG study. Cancer 59:259–265, 1987
201. Byfield JE, Sharp TR, Frankel SS, et al: Phase I and II trial of five-day infused 5-fluorouracil and radiation in advanced cancer of the head and neck. J Clin Oncol 2:406–413, 1984
202. Adelstein DJ, Sharan VM, Earle AS, et al: Combined modality therapy (CMT) with simultaneous 5-fluorouracil (5FU), cis-platinum (DDP) and radiation therapy (RT) in the treatment of squamous cell cancer of the head and neck (Abstract C-511). Proc Am Soc Clin Oncol 4:131, 1985
203. Taylor SG IV, Murthy AK, Showel JL, et al: Improved control in advanced head and neck cancer with simultaneous radiation and cisplatin/5-FU chemotherapy. Cancer Treat Rep 69:933–939, 1985
204. Kaplan MJ, Hahn SS, Johns ME, et al: Mitomycin and fluorouracil with concomitant radiotherapy in head and neck cancer. Arch Otolaryngol 111:220–222, 1985
205. Taylor SG IV: Integration of chemotherapy into the combined modality therapy of head and neck squamous cancer. Int J Radiat Oncol Biol Phys 13:779–783, 1987
206. Goldsmith MA, Carter SK: The integration of chemotherapy into a combined modality of approach to cancer therapy. V. Squamous cell cancer of the head and neck. Cancer Treat Rev 2:137–158, 1975
207. Arcangeli G, Nervi C, Righini R, et al: Combined radiation and drugs: The effect of intra-arterial chemotherapy followed by radiotherapy in head and neck cancer. Radiother Oncol 1:101–107, 1983
208. Fitzpatrick PJ: Cancer of the lip. J Otolaryngol 13:32–36, 1984
209. Byers RM, O'Brien J, Waxler J: The therapeutic and prognostic implications of nerve invasion in cancer of the lower lip. Int J Radiat Oncol Biol Phys 4:215–217, 1978
210. Mackay EN, Sellers AH: A statistical review of carcinoma of the lip. Can Med Assoc J 90:670–672, 1964
211. Million RR, Cassisi NJ: Carcinoma of the skin. In Million RR, Cassisi NJ (eds): Management of Head and Neck Cancer: A Multidisciplinary Approach, pp 475–511. Philadelphia, JB Lippincott, 1984
212. MacComb WS, Fletcher GH, Healey JE Jr: Intra-oral cavity. In MacComb WS, Fletcher GH (eds): Cancer of the Head and Neck, pp 89–151. Baltimore, Williams & Wilkins, 1967
213. Heller KS, Shah JP: Carcinoma of the lip. Am J Surg 138:600–603, 1979
214. Hendricks JL, Mendelson BC, Woods JE: Invasive carcinoma of the lower lip. Surg Clin North Am 57:837–844, 1977
215. Mohs FE, Snow SN: Microscopically controlled surgical treatment for squamous cell carcinoma of the lower lip. Surg Gynecol Obstet 160: 37–41, 1985
216. Ange DW, Lindberg RD, Guillamondegui OM: Management of squamous cell carcinoma of the oral tongue and floor of mouth after excisional biopsy. Radiology 116:143–146, 1974
217. Chu A, Fletcher GH: Incidence and causes of failures to control by irradiation the primary lesions in squamous cell carcinomas of the anterior two-thirds of the tongue and floor of mouth. Am J Roentgenol Radium Ther Nucl Med 117:501–508, 1973
218. Mendenhall WM, VanCise WS, Bova FJ, et al: Analysis of time-dose factors in squamous cell carcinoma of the oral tongue and floor of mouth treated with radiation therapy alone. Int J Radiat Oncol Biol Phys 7:1005–1011, 1981
219. Fu KK, Lichter A, Galante M: Carcinoma of the floor of mouth: An analysis of treatment results and the sites and causes of failures. Int J Radiat Oncol Biol Phys 1:829–837, 1976
220. Marcus RB Jr, Million RR, Mitchell TP: A preloaded, custom-designed implantation device for stage T1-T2 carcinoma of the floor of mouth. Int J Radiat Oncol Biol Phys 6:111–113, 1980
221. Tapley N: Clinical Applications of the Electron Beam, pp 125–129. New York, John Wiley & Sons, 1976
222. Flynn MB, Mullins FX, Moore C: Selection of treatment in squamous carcinoma of the floor of the mouth. Am J Surg 126:477–481, 1973
223. Guillamondegui OM, Jesse RH: Surgical treatment of advanced carcinoma of the floor of the mouth. Am J Roentgenol 126:1256–1259, 1976
224. Million RR, Cassisi NJ: Oral cavity. In Million RR, Cassisi NJ (eds): Management of Head and Neck Cancer: A Multidisciplinary Approach, pp 239–297. Philadelphia, JB Lippincott, 1984
225. Wang CC, Doppke KP, Biggs PJ: Intra-oral cone radiation therapy for selected carcinomas of the oral cavity. Int J Radiat Oncol Biol Phys 9:1185–1189, 1983
226. Leipzig, B.: Assessment of mandibular invasion by carcinoma. Cancer 56:1201–1205, 1985
227. Scholl P, Byers RM, Batsakis JG, et al: Microscopic cut-through of cancer in the surgical treatment of squamous carcinoma of the tongue: Prognostic and therapeutic implications. Am J Surg 152:354–360, 1986
228. Fu KK, Ray JW, Chan EK, et al: External and interstitial radiation therapy of carcinoma of the oral tongue: A review of 32 years experience. Am J Roentgenol 126:107–115, 1976
229. Lees AW: The treatment of carcinoma of the anterior two-thirds of the tongue by radiotherapy. Int J Radiat Oncol Biol Phys 1:849–858, 1976
230. Nair MK, Sankaranarayanan R, Padmanabhan TK: Evaluation of the role of radiotherapy in the management of carcinoma of the buccal mucosa. Cancer (in press)
231. Bloom NO, Spiro RH: Carcinoma of the cheek mucosa: A retrospective analysis. Am J Surg 140:556–559, 1980
232. Small IA, Waldron CA: Ameloblastomas of the jaws. Oral Surg Oral Med Oral Path 8:281–297, 1955
233. Sinclair NA: Cysts and ameloblastomas: A relationship. Aust Dent J 22:27–30, 1977
234. Pandya NJ, Stuteville OH: Treatment of ameloblastoma. Plast Reconstr Surg 50:242–248, 1972
235. Sehdev MK, Huvos AG, Strong EW, et al: Proceedings: Ameloblastoma of maxilla and mandible. Cancer 33:324–333, 1974
236. Byers RM, Anderson B, Schwarz EA, et al: Treatment of squamous carcinoma of the retromolar trigone. Am J Clin Oncol 7:647–652, 1984
237. Goldberg SJ, Friedman JM: Ameloblastoma: Review of the literature and report of case. J Am Dent Assoc 90:432–438, 1975
238. McIvor J: The radiological features of ameloblastoma. Clin Radiol 25:237–242, 1974
239. Swearingen AG, McGraw JP, Palumbo VD: Roentgenographic pathologic correlation of carcinoma of the gingiva involving the mandible. Am J Roentgenol Radium Ther Nucl Med 96:15–18, 1966
240. Rankow RM, Hickey MJ: Adamantinoma of the mandible: Analysis of surgical treatment. Surgery 36:713–719, 1954
241. Byers RM, Newman R, Russell N, et al: Results of treatment for squamous carcinoma of the lower gum. Cancer 47:2236–2238, 1981
242. Shibuya H, Horiuchi J-I, Suzuki S, et al: Oral carcinoma of the upper jaw: Results of radiation treatment. Acta Radiol Oncol 23:331–335, 1984

243. Fayos JV: Carcinoma of the mandible: Result of radiation therapy. Acta Radiol Ther Phys Biol 12:378–386, 1973
244. Million RR, Cassisi NJ: Oropharynx. In Million RR, Cassisi NJ (eds): Management of Head and Neck Cancer: A Multidisciplinary Approach, pp 299–314. Philadelphia, JB Lippincott, 1984
245. Gardner KE, Parsons JT, Mendenhall WM, et al: Time-dose relationships for local tumor control and complications following irradiation of squamous cell carcinoma of the base of tongue. Int J Radiat Oncol Biol Phys 13:507–510, 1987
246. Fletcher GH: Oral cavity and oropharynx. In Fletcher GH (ed): Textbook of Radiotherapy, 2nd ed, pp 212–254. Philadelphia, Lea & Febiger, 1973
247. Whicker JH, DeSanto LW, Devine KD: Surgical treatment of squamous cell carcinoma of the base of the tongue. Laryngoscope 82:1853–1860, 1972
248. Callery CD, Spiro RH, Strong EW: Changing trends in the management of squamous carcinoma of the tongue. Am J Surg 148:449–454, 1984
249. Cutler SJ, Ederer F: Maximum utilization of the life table method in analyzing survival. J Chron Dis 8:699–712, 1958
250. Mendenhall WM, Parsons JT, Cassisi NJ, et al: Squamous cell carcinoma of the tonsillar area treated with radical irradiation. Radiother Oncol 10:23–30, 1987
251. Mizono GS, Diaz RF, Fu KK, et al: Carcinoma of the tonsillar region. Laryngoscope 96:240–244, 1986
252. Gelinas M, Fletcher GH: Incidence and causes of local failure of irradiation in squamous cell carcinoma of the faucial arch, tonsillar fossa, and base of tongue. Radiology 108:383–387, 1973
253. Dasmahapatra KS, Mohit-Tabatabai MA, Rush BF, et al: Cancer of the tonsil: Improved survival with combination therapy. Cancer 57:451–455, 1986
254. Shrewsbury D, Adams GL, Duvall AJ, et al: Carcinoma of the tonsillar region: A comparison of radiation therapy with combined preoperative radiation and surgery. Otolaryngol Head Neck Surg 89:979–985, 1981
255. Remmler D, Medina JE, Byers RM, et al: Treatment of choice for squamous carcinoma of the tonsillar fossa. Head Neck Surg 7:206–211, 1985
256. Amornmarn R, Prempree T, Jaiwatana J, et al: Radiation management of carcinoma of the tonsillar region. Cancer 54:1293–1299, 1984
257. Perez CA, Purdy JA, Breaux SR, et al: Carcinoma of the tonsillar fossa: A nonrandomized comparison of preoperative radiation and surgery or irradiation alone: Long-term results. Cancer 50:2314–2322, 1982
258. Weichert KA, Aron BS, Maltz R, et al: Carcinoma of the tonsil: Treatment by a planned combination of radiation and surgery. Int J Radiat Oncol Biol Phys 1:505–508, 1976
259. Perez CA, Lee FA, Ackerman LV, et al: Non-randomized comparison of preoperative irradiation and surgery versus irradiation alone in the management of carcinoma of the tonsil. Am J Roentgenol 126:248–260, 1976
260. Strong MS, Vaughan CW, Kayne HL, et al: A randomized trial of preoperative radiotherapy in cancer of the oropharynx and hypopharynx. Am J Surg 136:494–500, 1978
261. Bova FJ: Treatment planning for irradiation of head and neck cancer. In Million RR, Cassisi NJ (eds): Management of Head and Neck Cancer: A Multidisciplinary Approach, pp 209–230. Philadelphia, JB Lippincott, 1984
262. Mazeron JJ, Marinello G, Leung S, et al: Interstitial radiation therapy for squamous cell carcinoma of the tonsillar region: The Creteil experience (1971–1981). Int J Radiat Oncol Biol Phys 12:895–900, 1986
263. Fletcher GH: The Third Annual Lectureship of the Juan A. del Regato Foundation: Squamous cell carcinomas of the oropharynx. Int J Radiat Oncol Biol Phys 5:2073–2090, 1979
264. Pierquin B, Chassagne DJ, Chahbazian CM, et al: Brachytherapy, pp 104–108. St. Louis, WH Green, 1978
265. Ratzer ER, Schweitzer RJ, Frazell EL: Epidermoid carcinoma of the palate. Am J Surg 119:294–297, 1970
266. Weller SA, Goffinet DR, Goode RL, et al: Carcinoma of the oropharynx: Results of megavoltage radiation therapy in 305 patients. Am J Roentgenol 126:236–247, 1976
267. Seydel HG, Scholl H: Carcinoma of the soft palate and uvula. Am J Roentgenol Radium Ther Nucl Med 120:603–607, 1974
268. Amdur RJ, Mendenhall WM, Parsons JT, et al: Carcinoma of the soft palate treated with irradiation: Analysis of results and complications. Radiother Oncol 9:185–194, 1987
269. Lindberg RD, Fletcher GH: The role of irradiation in the management of head and neck cancer: Analysis of results and causes of failure. Tumori 64:313–325, 1978
270. Chung CK, Constable WC: Squamous cell carcinoma of the soft palate and uvula. Int J Radiat Oncol Biol Phys 5:845–850, 1979
271. Garrett PG, Beale FA: Carcinoma of the oropharynx: Soft palate. J Otolaryngol 13:165–168, 1984
272. Fee WE, Schoeppel SL, Rubenstein R, et al: Squamous cell carcinoma of the soft palate. Arch Otolaryngol 105:710–720, 1979
273. Wynder EL: The epidemiology of cancer of the upper alimentary and upper respiratory tracts. Laryngoscope 88 (suppl 8):50–51, 1978
274. Vincent RG, Marchetta F: The relationship of the use of tobacco and alcohol to cancer of the oral cavity, pharynx or larynx. Am J Surg 105:501–505, 1963
275. Fraumeni JF Jr: Geographic distribution of head and neck cancers in the United States. Laryngoscope 88 (suppl 8):40–44, 1978
276. Batsakis JG: Tumors of the Head and Neck, 2nd ed, pp 219–220, 342. Baltimore, Williams & Wilkins, 1979
277. Pillsbury HRC, Kirchner JA: Clinical vs histopathologic staging in laryngeal cancer. Arch Otolaryngol 105:157–159, 1979
278. Kirchner JA: Staging as seen in serial sections. Laryngoscope 85:1816–1821, 1975
279. Olsen KD, DeSanto LW, Pearson BW: Positive Delphian lymph node: Clinical significance in laryngeal cancer. Laryngoscope 97:1033–1037, 1987
280. Lederman M: Place de la radiotherapie dans le traitment du cancer du larynx [The place of radiotherapy in the treatment of cancer of the larynx.] Ann Radiol 4: 433–454, 1961
281. Mancuso AA, Hanafee WN, Juillard GJF, et al: The role of computed tomography in the management of cancer of the larynx. Radiology 124:243–244, 1977
282. Fletcher GH, Jing B-S: The Head and Neck, p 168. Chicago, Year Book, 1968
283. Million RR, Cassisi NJ: Larynx. In Million RR, Cassisi NJ (eds): Management of Head and Neck Cancer: A Multidisciplinary Approach, pp 315–364. Philadelphia, JB Lippincott, 1984
284. Harwood AR: Cancer of the larynx: The Toronto experience. J Otolaryngol (suppl 11) 3–21, 1982
285. Biller HF, Barnhill FR Jr, Ogura JH, et al: Hemilaryngectomy following radiation failure for carcinoma of the vocal cords. Laryngoscope 80:249–253, 1970
286. Mendenhall WM, Parsons JT, Stringer SP, et al: TI–T2 vocal cord carcinoma: A basis for comparing the results of irradiation and surgery. Head Neck Surg 10:373–377, 1988
287. Burns HP, van Nostrand AWP, Bryce DP: Verrucous carcinoma of the larynx: Management by radiotherapy and surgery. Ann Otol Rhinol Laryngol 85:538–543, 1976
288. Harwood AR, Beale FA, Cummings BJ, et al: T3 glottic cancer: An analysis of dose time-volume factors. Int J Radiat Oncol Biol Phys 6:675–680, 1980
289. Mendenhall WM, Million RR, Sharkey DE, et al: Stage T3 squamous cell carcinoma of the glottic larynx treated with surgery and/or radiation therapy. Int J Radiat Oncol Biol Phys 10:357–363, 1984
290. Singer MI, Blom ED: An endoscopic technique for restoration of voice after laryngectomy. Ann Otol Rhinol Laryngol 89:529–533, 1980
291. Singer MI, Blom ED, Hamaker RC: Further experience with voice restoration after total laryngectomy. Ann Otol Rhinol Laryngol 90:498–502, 1981
292. Panje WR: Prosthetic vocal rehabilitation following laryngectomy: The voice button. Ann Otol Rhinol Laryngol 90:116–120, 1981
293. Panje WR, VanDemark D, McCabe BF: Voice button prosthesis rehabilitation of the laryngectomee: Additional nodes. Ann Otol Rhinol Laryngol 90:503–505, 1981
294. Merwin GE, Goldstein LP: Speech rehabilitation after total laryngectomy. In Million RR, Cassisi NJ (eds): Management of Head and Neck Cancer: A Multidisciplinary Approach, pp 365–372. Philadelphia, JB Lippincott, 1984
295. Fletcher GH, Lindberg RD, Hamberger A, et al: Reasons for irradiation failure in squamous cell carcinoma of the larynx. Laryngoscope 85:987–1003, 1975
296. Lee F, Perlmutter S, Ogura JH: Laryngeal radiation after hemilaryngectomy. Laryngoscope 90:1534–1539, 1980
297. Balm AJM, Snow GB, Karim ABMF, et al: Long-term results of concurrent polychemotherapy and radiotherapy in patients with stomal recurrence after total laryngectomy. Ann Otol Rhinol Laryngol 95:572–575, 1986
298. Gluckman JL, Hamaker RC, Schuller DE, et al: Surgical salvage for stomal recurrence: A multi-institutional experience. Laryngoscope 97:1025–1029, 1987
299. Fletcher GH, Goepfert H: Larynx and pyriform sinus. In Fletcher GH: Textbook of Radiotherapy, 3rd ed, pp 330–363. Philadelphia, Lea & Febiger, 1980
300. Mendenhall WM, Million RR, Cassisi NJ: Squamous cell carcinoma of the supraglottic larynx treated with radical irradiation: Analysis of treatment parameters and results. Int J Radiat Oncol Biol Phys 10:2223–2230, 1984
301. Million RR, Cassisi NJ, Parsons JT, et al: Radiation therapy in the management of carcinoma of the larynx. In Fried MP: The Larynx. Boston, Little, Brown (in press)
302. Ogura JH, Sessions DG, Spector GJ: Analysis of surgical therapy for epidermoid carcinoma of the laryngeal glottis. Laryngoscope 85:1522–1530, 1975
303. Wang CC: Treatment of glottic carcinoma by megavoltage radiation therapy and results. Am J Roentgenol Radium Ther Nucl Med 120:157–163, 1974
304. Mills EED: Early glottic carcinoma: Factors affecting radiation failure, results of treatment and sequelae. Int J Radiat Oncol Biol Phys 5:811–817, 1979
305. Fletcher GH, Lindberg RD, Jesse RH: Radiation therapy for cancer of the larynx and pyriform sinus. EENT Digest 31:58–67, 1969
306. Stewart JG, Brown JR, Palmer MK, et al: The management of glottic carcinoma by primary irradiation with surgery in reserve. Laryngoscope 85:1477–1484, 1975
307. Harwood AR, Hawkins NV, Beale FA, et al: Management of advanced glottic cancer: A 10-year review of the Toronto experience. Int J Radiat Oncol Biol Phys 5:899–904, 1979
308. Harwood AR, Hawkins NV, Rider WD, et al: Radiotherapy of early glottic cancer–I. Int J Radiat Oncol Biol Phys 5:473–476, 1979
309. Dickens WJ, Cassisi NJ, Million RR, et al: Treatment of early vocal cord carcinoma: A comparison of apples and apples. Laryngoscope 93:216–219, 1983
310. Jesse RH: The evaluation of treatment of patients with extensive squamous cancer of the vocal cords. Laryngoscope 85:1424–1429, 1975
311. Skolnik EM, Yee KF, Wheatley MA, et al: Carcinoma of the laryngeal glottis: Therapy and end results. Laryngoscope 85:1453–1466, 1975
312. Vermund H: Role of radiotherapy in cancer of the larynx as related to the TNM system of staging: A review. Cancer 25:485–504, 1970
313. Stewart JG, Jackson AW: The steepness of the dose response curve both for tumor cure and normal tissue injury. Laryngoscope 85:1107–1111, 1975
314. Harwood AR, Beale FA, Cummings BJ, et al: T4N0M0 glottic cancer: An analysis of dose-time volume factors. Int J Radiat Oncol Biol Phys 7:1507–1512, 1981
315. Weems DH, Mendenhall WM, Parsons JT, et al: Squamous cell carcinoma of the

supraglottic larynx treated with surgery and/or radiation therapy. Int J Radiat Oncol Biol Phys 13:1483–1487, 1987
316. Neel H III, Devine KD, Desanto LW: Laryngofissure and cordectomy for early cordal carcinoma: Outcome in 182 patients. Otolaryngol Head Neck Surg 88:79–84, 1980
317. Mendenhall WM, Parson JT, Million RR, et al: T1–T2 squamous cell carcinoma of the glottic larynx treated with radiation therapy: Relationship of dose-fractionation factors to local control and complications. Int J Radiat Oncol Biol Phys (in press)
318. Ballantyne AJ: Principles of surgical management of cancer of the pharyngeal walls. Cancer 20:663–667, 1965
319. Kirchner JA: Pyriform sinus cancer: A clinical and laboratory study. Ann Otol Rhinol Laryngol 84:793–803, 1975
320. Wang CC: Radiotherapeutic management of carcinoma of the posterior pharyngeal wall. Cancer 27:894–896, 1971
321. Biller HF, Davis WH, Ogura JH: Delayed contralateral cervical metastases with laryngeal and laryngopharyngeal cancers. Laryngoscope 81:1499–1502, 1971
322. Million RR, Cassisi NJ: Radical irradiation for carcinoma of the pyriform sinus. Laryngoscope 91:439–450, 1981
323. Mendenhall WM, Parsons JT, Mancuso AA, et al: Squamous cell carcinoma of the pharyngeal wall treated with irradiation. Radiother Oncol 11:205–212, 1988
324. Marks JE, Freeman RB, Lee F, et al: Pharyngeal wall cancer: An analysis of treatment results complications and patterns of failure. Int J Radiat Oncol Biol Phys 4:587–593, 1978
325. Meoz-Mendez RT, Fletcher GH, Guillamondegui OM, et al: Analysis of the results of irradiation in the treatment of squamous cell carcinomas of the pharyngeal walls. Int J Radiat Oncol Biol Phys 4:579–585, 1978
326. Marks JE, Kurnick B, Powers WE, et al: Carcinoma of the pyriform sinus: An analysis of treatment results and patterns of failure. Cancer 41:1008–1015, 1978
327. Mendenhall WM, Parsons JT, Cassisi NJ, et al: Squamous cell carcinoma of the pyriform sinus treated with radical radiation therapy. Radiother Oncol 9:201–208, 1987
328. El-Badawi SA, Goepfert H, Fletcher GH, et al: Squamous cell carcinoma of the pyriform sinus. Laryngoscope 92:357–364, 1982
329. Million RR, Cassisi NJ: Hypopharynx: Pharyngeal walls, pyriform sinus, and postcricoid pharynx. In Million RR, Cassisi NJ (eds): Management of Head and Neck Cancer: A Multidisciplinary Approach, pp 373–391. Philadelphia, JB Lippincott, 1984
330. Fletcher GH, Million RR: Malignant tumors of the nasopharynx. Am J Roentgenol Radium Ther Nucl Med 93:44–55, 1965
331. Chen KY, Fletcher GH: Malignant tumors of the nasopharynx. Radiology 99:165–171, 1971
332. Fletcher GH, Million RR: Nasopharynx. In Fletcher GH (ed): Textbook of Radiotherapy, 3rd ed, pp 364–383. Philadelphia, Lea & Febiger, 1980
333. Mesic JB, Fletcher GH, Goepfert H: Megavoltage irradiation of epithelial tumors of the nasopharynx. Int J Radiat Oncol Biol Phys 7:477–453, 1981
334. Hoppe RT, Goffinet DR, Bagshaw MA: Carcinoma of the nasopharynx: Eighteen years' experience with megavoltage radiation therapy. Cancer 37:2605–2612, 1976
335. Biller HF, Sessions DG, Ogura JH: Angiofibroma: A treatment approach. Laryngoscope 84:695–706, 1974
336. Briant TDR, Fitzpatrick PJ, Berman J: Nasopharynx angiofibroma: A twenty-year study. Laryngoscope 88:1247–1251, 1978
337. Million RR, Cassisi NJ: Juvenile angiofibroma. In Million RR, Cassisi NJ (eds): Management of Head and Neck Cancer: A Multidisciplinary Approach, pp 467–474. Philadelphia, JB Lippincott, 1984
338. Samaan NA, Bakdash MM, Caderao JB, et al: Hypopituitarism after external irradiation: Evidence for both hypothalamic and pituitary origin. Ann Intern Med 83:771–777, 1975
339. Boldrey E, Sheline G: Delayed transitory clinical manifestations after radiation treatment of intracranial tumors. Acta Radiol Ther 5:5–10, 1966
340. Acheson ED, Cowdell RH, Hadfield EH, et al: Nasal cancer in woodworkers in the furniture industry. Br Med J [Clin Res] 2:587–596, 1968
341. Acheson ED, Cowdell RH, Jolles B: Nasal cancer in the Northamptonshire boot and shoe industry. Br Med J [Clin Res]1:385–393, 1970
342. Acheson ED, Hadfield EH, Macbeth RG: Carcinoma of the nasal cavity and accessory sinuses in woodworkers. Lancet 1:311–312, 1967
343. Ironside P, Matthews J: Adenocarcinoma of the nose and paranasal sinuses in woodworkers in the state of Victoria, Australia. Cancer 36:1115–1121, 1975
344. Maisel RH, Johnston WH, Anderson HA, et al: Necrotizing sialometaplasia involving the nasal cavity. Laryngoscope 87:429–434, 1977
345. Kadish S, Goodman M, Wang CC: Olfactory neuroblastoma: A clinical analysis of 17 cases. Cancer 37:1571–1576, 1976
346. Mendenhall WM, Million RR Cassisi NJ, et al: Biologically aggressive papillomas of the nasal cavity: The role of radiation therapy. Laryngoscope 95:344–347, 1985
347. Kassel SH, Echevarria RA, Guzzo FP: Midline malignant reticulosis (so-called lethal midline granuloma). Cancer 23:920–935, 1969
348. Goepfert H, Guillamondegui OM, Jesse RH, et al: Squamous cell carcinoma of the nasal vestibule. Arch Otolaryngol 100:8–10, 1974
349. Mendenhall NP, Parsons JT, Cassisi NJ, et al: Carcinoma of the nasal vestibule treated with radiation therapy. Laryngoscope 97:626–632, 1987
350. Olsen KD, DeSanto LW: Olfactory neuroblastoma. Arch Otolaryngol 109:797–802, 1983
351. Million RR, Cassisi NJ, Hamlin DJ: Nasal vestibule, nasal cavity, and paranasal sinuses. In Million RR, Cassisi NJ (eds): Management of Head and Neck Cancer: A Multidisciplinary Approach, pp 407–444. Philadelphia, JB Lippincott, 1984
352. Weissler MC, Montgomery WW, Turner PA, et al: Inverted papilloma. Ann Otol Rhinol Laryngol 95:215–221, 1986
353. Schoub L, Timme AH, Uys CJ: A well-differentiated inverted papilloma of the nasal space associated with lymph node metastases. S Afr Med J 47:1663–1665, 1973
354. Fechner RE, Sessions RB: Inverted papilloma of the lacrimal sac, paranasal sinus, and cervical region. Cancer 40:2303–2308, 1977
355. Haynes WD, Tapley N: Radiation treatment of carcinoma of the nasal vestibule. Am J Roentgenol Ther Nucl Med 120:595–602, 1974
356. Mendenhall NP, Parsons JT, Cassisi NJ, et al: Carcinoma of the nasal vestibule. Int J Radiat Oncol Biol Phys 10:627–637, 1984
357. Ketcham AS, Chretien PB, VanBuren JM, et al: The ethmoid sinuses: A re-evaluation of surgical resection. Am J Surg 126:469–476, 1973
358. Ellingwood KE, Million RR: Cancer of the nasal cavity and ethmoid/sphenoid sinuses. Cancer 43:1517–1526, 1979
359. Myers EN, Schramm VL, Barnes EL: Management of inverted papilloma of the nose and paranasal sinuses. Laryngoscope 91:2071–2084, 1981
360. Frazell EL, Lewis JS: Cancer of the nasal cavity and accessory sinuses: A report of the management of 416 patients. Cancer 16:1293–1301, 1963
361. Cheesman AD, Lund VJ, Howard DJ: Craniofacial resection for tumors of the nasal cavity and paranasal sinuses. Head Neck Surg 8:429–435, 1986
362. Bosch A, Vallecillo L, Frias Z: Cancer of the nasal cavity. Cancer 37:1458–1463, 1976
363. Boone ML, Harle TS, Highott HW, et al: Malignant disease of the paranasal sinuses and nasal cavity: Importance of precise localization of extent of disease. Am J Roentgenol Radium Ther Nucl Med 102:627–637, 1968
364. Parsons JT, Mendenhall WM, Mancuso AA, et al: Malignant tumors of the nasal cavity and ethmoid and sphenoid sinuses. Int J Radiat Oncol Biol Phys 14:11–22, 1988
365. Elkon D, Hightower SI, Lim ML, et al: Esthesioneuroblastoma. Cancer 44:1087–1094, 1979
366. Shah JP, Feghali J: Esthesioneuroblastoma. Am J Surg 142:456–458, 1981
367. Fauci AS, Johnson RE, Wolff SM: Radiation therapy of midline granuloma. Ann Intern Med 84:140–147, 1976
368. Jesse RH: Preoperative versus postoperative radiation in the treatment of squamous cell carcinoma of the paranasal sinuses. Am J Surg 110:552–556, 1965
369. Bataini J-P, Ennuyer A: Advanced carcinoma of the maxillary antrum treated by cobalt teletherapy and electron beam irradiation. Br J Radiol 44:590–598, 1971
370. Shukovsky LJ, Fletcher GH: Retinal and optic nerve complications in a high dose irradiation technique of ethmoid sinus and nasal cavity. Radiology 104:629–634, 1972
371. Parsons JT, Fitzgerald CR, Hood CI, et al: The effects of irradiation on the eye and optic nerve. Int J Radiat Oncol Biol Phys 9:609–622, 1983
372. Edwards C, Heath D, Harris P: The carotid body in emphysema and left ventricular hypertrophy. J Pathol 104:1–13, 1971
373. Guild SR: The glomus jugulare, a nonchromaffin paraganglion, in man. Ann Otol Rhinol Laryngol 62:1045–1071, 1953
374. Ward PH, Jenkins HA, Hanafee WN: Diagnosis and treatment of carotid body tumors. Ann Otol Rhinol Laryngol 87:614–621, 1978
375. Lapayowker MS, Liebman EP, Ronis ML, et al: Presentation of the internal carotid artery as a tumor of the middle ear. Radiology 98:293–297, 1971
376. Glasscock ME III, Harris PF, Newsome G: Glomus tumors: Diagnosis and treatment. Laryngoscope 84:2006–2032, 1974
377. Kim J-A, Elkon D, Lim M-L, et al: Optimum dose of radiotherapy for chemodectomas of the middle ear. Int J Radiat Oncol Biol Phys 6:815–819, 1980
378. Mischke RE, Balkany TJ: Skull base approach to glomus jugulare. Laryngoscope 90:89–94, 1980
379. Maruyama Y, Gold LHA, Kieffer SA: Clinical and angiographic evaluation of radiotherapeutic response of glomus jugulare tumors. Radiology 101:397–399, 1971
380. Myers EN, Newman J, Kaseff L, et al: Glomus jugulare tumor: A radiographic-histologic correlation. Laryngoscope 81:1838–1851, 1971
381. Tidwell TJ, Montague ED: Chemodectomas involving the temporal bone. Radiology 116:147–149, 1975
382. Friedland JL, Mendenhall WM, Parsons JT, et al: Chemodectomas arising in temporal bone structures. Head Neck Surg (in press)
383. Hudgins PT: Radiotherapy for extensive glomus jugulare tumors. Radiology 103:427–429, 1972
384. Cole JM: Glomus jugulare tumor. Laryngoscope 87:1244–1258, 1977
385. Smith PE: Management of chemodectomas (glomus jugulare). Laryngoscope 80:207–216, 1970
386. Newman H, Rowe JF Jr, Phillips TL: Radiation therapy of the glomus jugulare tumor. Am J Roentgenol Radium Ther Nucl Med 118:663–669, 1973
387. Grubb WB Jr, Lampe I: The role of radiation therapy in the treatment of chemodectomas of the glomus jugulare. Laryngoscope 75:1861–1871, 1965
388. Hatfield PM, James AE, Schulz MD: Chemodectomas of the glomus jugulare. Cancer 30:1164–1168, 1972
389. Rosenwasser H: Current management: Glomus jugulare tumors. Ann Otol Rhinol Laryngol 76:603–610, 1967
390. Spector GH, Fierstein J, Ogura JH: A comparison of therapeutic modalities of glomus tumors in the temporal bone. Laryngoscope 86:690–696, 1976
391. Bergdahl L: Carotid body tumours: A report of twelve cases. Scand J Thorac Cardiovasc Surg 12:275–279, 1978

392. Chambers RG, Mahoney WD: Carotid body tumors. Am J Surg 116:554–558, 1968
393. Farr HW: Carotid body tumors: A thirty year experience at Memorial Hospital. Am J Surg 114:614–619, 1967
394. Morris GC, Balas PE, Cooley DA, et al: Surgical treatment of benign and malignant carotid body tumors: Clinical experience with sixteen tumors in twelve patients. Am Surg 29:429–437, 1963
395. Parry DM, Li FP, Strong LC, et al: Carotid body tumors in humans: Genetics and epidemiology. JNCI 68:573–578, 1982
396. Westbrook KC, Guillamondegui OM, Medellin H, et al: Chemodectomas of the neck: Selective management. Am J Surg 124:760–766, 1972
397. Mendenhall WM, Million RR, Parsons JT, et al: Chemodectoma of the carotid body and ganglion nodosum treated with radiation therapy. Int J Radiat Oncol Biol Phys 12:2175–2178, 1986
398. Mitchell DC, Clyne CAC: Chemodectomas of the neck: The response to radiotherapy. Br J Surg 72:903–905, 1985
399. Lybeert MLM, Van Andel JG, Eijkenboom WMH, et al: Radiotherapy of paragangliomas. Clin Otolaryngol 9:105–109, 1984
400. Krupski WC, Effeney DJ, Stoney RJ, et al: Carotid body tumours. Aust NZ J Surg 53:539–543, 1983
401. Wilson H: Carotid body tumors. Surgery 59:483–493, 1966
402. Endicott JN, Maniglia AJ: Glomus vagale. Laryngoscope 90:1604–1611, 1980
403. Cassisi NJ, Dickerson DR, Million RR: Squamous cell carcinoma of the skin metastatic to parotid nodes. Arch Otolaryngol 104:336–339, 1978
404. Mendenhall NP, Million RR, Cassisi NJ: Parotid area lymph node metastases from carcinoma of the skin. Int J Radiat Oncol Biol Phys 11:707–714, 1985
405. Povah WB, Beecroft W, Hodson I, et al: Malignant lympho-epithelial lesion: The Manitoba experience. J Otolaryngol 13:153–159, 1984
406. Gallia LJ, Johnson JT: Incidence of neoplastic versus inflammatory disease in major salivary gland masses diagnosed by surgery. Laryngoscope 91:512–516, 1981
407. Fee WE Jr, Goffinet DR, Calcaterra TC: Recurrent mixed tumors of the parotid gland: Results of surgical therapy. Laryngoscope 88:265–273, 1978
408. Spiro RH, Huvos AG, Strong EW: Cancer of the parotid gland: A clinicopathologic study of 288 primary cases. Am J Surg 130:452–459, 1975
409. Gullane PJ, Havas TJ: Facial nerve grafts: Effects of postoperative irradiation. J Otolaryngol 16:112–115, 1987
410. King JJ, Fletcher GH: Malignant tumors of the major salivary glands. Radiology 110:381–384, 1971
411. Guillamondegui OM, Byers RM, Luna MA, et al: Aggressive surgery in treatment for parotid cancer: The role of adjunctive postoperative radiotherapy. Am J Roentgenol Radium Ther Nucl Med 123:49–54, 1975
412. Rafla S: Submaxillary gland tumors. Cancer 26:821–826, 1970
413. Spiro RH: Salivary neoplasms: Overview of a 35-year experience with 2,807 patients. Head Neck Surg 8:177–184, 1986
414. Woods JE, Chong GC, Beahrs OH: Experience with 1360 primary parotid tumors. Am J Surg 130:460–462, 1975
415. McNaney D, McNeese MD, Guillamondegui OM, et al: Postoperative irradiation in malignant epithelial tumors of the parotid. Int J Radiat Oncol Biol Phys 9:1289–1295, 1983
416. Theriault C, Fitzpatrick PJ: Malignant parotid tumors: Prognostic factors and optimum treatment. Am J Clin Oncol 9:510–516, 1986
417. Moore GE, Bross IDJ, Ausman R, et al: Effects of chlorambucil (NSC-3088) in 374 patients with advanced cancer: Eastern Clinical Drug Evaluation Program. Cancer Chemother Rep 52:661–666, 1968
418. Richards GJ, Chambers RG: Hydroxyurea in the treatment of neoplasms of the head and neck: A resurvey. Am J Surg 126:513–518, 1973
419. Rentschler R, Burgess MA, Byers R: Chemotherapy of malignant major salivary gland neoplasms: A 25-year review of M. D. Anderson Hospital experience. Cancer 40:619–624, 1977
420. Johnson RO, Lange RD, Kisken WA, et al: Infusion of 5-fluorouracil in cylindroma treatment. Arch Otolaryngol 79:625–627, 1964
421. Tannock IF, Sutherland DJ: Chemotherapy for adenocystic carcinoma. Cancer 46:452–454, 1980
422. Vermeer RJ, Pinedo HM: Partial remission of advanced adenoid cystic carcinoma obtained with Adriamycin: A case report with a review of the literature. Cancer 43:1604–1606, 1979
423. Schramm VL Jr, Srodes C, Myers EN: Cisplatin therapy for adenoid cystic carcinoma. Arch Otolaryngol 107:739–741, 1981
424. Creagan ET, O'Fallon JR, Woods JE, et al: Cis-platinum (P) by 24-hour infusion in advanced upper aerodigestive cancer (ADC) (abstract C-785). Proc Am Soc Clin Oncol 22:533, 1981
425. Skibba JL, Hurley JD, Ravelo HV: Complete response of a metastatic adenoid cystic carcinoma of the parotid gland to chemotherapy. Cancer 47:2543–2548, 1981
426. Budd GT, Groppe CW: Adenoid cystic carcinoma of the salivary gland: Sustained complete response to chemotherapy. Cancer 51:589–590, 1983
427. Posner MR, Ervin TJ, Weichselbaum RR, et al: Chemotherapy of advanced salivary gland neoplasms. Cancer 50:2261–2264, 1982
428. Venook AP, Tseng A Jr, Meyers FJ, et al: Cisplatin, doxorubicin, and 5-fluorouracil chemotherapy for salivary gland malignancies: A pilot study of the Northern California Oncology Group. J Clin Oncol 5:951–955, 1987
429. Triozzi PL, Brantley A, Fisher S, et al: 5-fluorouracil, cyclophosphamide, and vincristine for adenoid cystic carcinoma of the head and neck. Cancer 59:887–890, 1987
430. Alberts DS, Manning MR, Coulthard SW, et al: Adriamycin cis-platinum cyclosphosphamide combination chemotherapy for advanced carcinoma of the parotid gland. Cancer 47:645–648, 1981
431. Creagan ET, Woods JE, Schutt AJ, et al: Cyclophosphamide, Adriamycin, and cis-diamminedichloroplatinum (II) in the treatment of advanced nonsquamous cell head and neck cancer. Cancer 52:2007–2010, 1983
432. Eisenberger MA: Supporting evidence for an active treatment program for advanced salivary gland carcinomas. Cancer Treat Rep 69:319–321, 1985
433. Dreyfuss AI, Clark JR, Fallon BG, et al: Cyclophosphamide, Adriamycin and cisplatin combination chemotherapy for advanced carcinomas of salivary gland origin. Cancer (in press)
434. Byers RM, Jesse RH, Guillamondegui OM, et al: Malignant tumors of the submaxillary gland. Am J Surg 126:458–463, 1973
435. Schell S, Barkley HT Jr, Chiminazzo H Jr: Treatment of malignant minor salivary gland tumors (in preparation)
436. Thawley SE, Ward SP, Ogura JH: Basal cell adenoma of the salivary glands. Laryngoscope 84:1756–1766, 1974
437. Ranger D, Thackray AC, Lucas RB: Mucous gland tumors. Br J Cancer 10:1–16, 1956
438. Wittes RE, Brescia F, Young CW, et al: Combination chemotherapy with cis-diamminedichloroplatinum (II) and bleomycin in tumors of the head and neck. Oncology 32:202–207, 1975
439. Hayes DM, Magill GB, Golbey RB, et al: Methyl CCNU, Adriamycin, and vincristine (MAV) chemotherapy of adenoid cystic carcinoma. Proc Soc Surg Oncol 35, 1976
440. Ellis ER, Million RR, Mendenhall WM, et al: The use of radiation therapy in the management of minor salivary gland tumors. Int J Radiat Oncol Biol Phys 15:613–617, 1988
441. Vikram B, Strong EW, Shah JP, et al: Radiation therapy in adenoid-cystic carcinoma. Int J Radiat Oncol Biol Phys 10:221–223, 1984
442. Spiro RH, Koss LG, Jagdu SI, et al: Tumors of minor salivary origin: A clinicopathologic study of 492 cases. Cancer 31:117–129, 1973
443. Bardwil JM, Reynolds CT, Ibanez ML, et al: Report of one hundred tumors of the minor salivary glands. Am J Surg 112:493–497, 1966
444. Rafla-Demetrious S: Mucous and Salivary Gland Tumours, p 118. Springfield, IL, Charles C Thomas, 1970

JOHN D. MINNA,
HARVEY PASS,
ELI GLATSTEIN,
and DANIEL C. IHDE

CHAPTER 22 *Cancer of the Lung*

INCIDENCE AND MORTALITY RATES

Lung cancer is a major cause of death in the United States and throughout the world in both developed and developing countries (Table 22-1; Fig. 22-1). It is the leading cause of cancer death in men 35 years old or older. It also is the second leading cause of cancer deaths in women 35 to 74 years old[1] and if present trends continue will become the leading cancer killer of American women during the 1980s. The majority of cases for both sexes are seen in the age range of 35 to 75 years, with a peak at age 55 to 65 years for each sex. At the time of diagnosis, the disease has spread to regional nodes or distant sites in 70% of patients (Table 22-2).[2] However, even in patients with supposedly localized disease, 5-year survival is the exception rather than the rule. Because of the low rate of cure, the mortality rates are nearly identical to the incidence. In general, women have a better 5-year survival rate than men for as yet unknown reasons.

It is estimated that at current incidence rates, there will be 590,000 new cases of lung cancer each year in the world, of which 80% to 90% are caused by tobacco.[3] Unfortunately, the incidence has, in general, been increasing, contributing significantly to total cancer death rates around the world. In the United States, the age-adjusted incidence in men has increased 225%, from 27 per 100,000 in the 1940s to 89 per 100,000 in 1982, an increase of almost 3% per year.[4] Fortunately, the rate of increase has declined in the United States, and there has actually been a decline in the incidence in white men since 1984,[5] a change that appears to be related to a decrease in cigarette smoking in more recent cohorts of men. However, the incidence in women rose 400%, from 7 to 35 per 100,000, between 1940 and 1984.[5] Of additional concern, a higher percentage than expected of women than men with lung cancer are clustered in the lower pack-year categories ($p < 0.0003$).[6] Thus, women are developing primary lung cancer at a younger age after smoking for fewer years than men.[6] Also, whereas the rate of beginning to smoke is decreasing in the United States as a whole, there is evidence that smoking onset may be increasing among certain minority groups and in adolescents.[7] This is particularly disturbing because the smoking-attributable years of potential life lost and the mortality rates in blacks are probably twice those among whites.[8]

PREDICTIONS OF FUTURE LUNG CANCER MORTALITY RATES

There have been dramatic decreases in smoking prevalence in the United States over the past 20 years, leading to the expectation of falling lung cancer rates. In fact, declines in age-specific rates of lung cancer for younger persons have been seen as a result of lower smoking prevalence among new cohorts and probably as a result of the lower tar content of cigarettes.[9] Nevertheless, age-adjusted rates of lung cancer mortality have continued to increase for men albeit with a flattening of the curve. However, the incidence and mortality rates for U.S. women continue to increase significantly. Overall, because of the changes in smoking prevalence, the lower tar content of cigarettes, and the increasing

TABLE 22-1. Lung Cancer: Magnitude of the Problem

	Men	Women
Estimated new cases (1988)	100,000	52,000
Estimated proportion of		
Total cancer incidence (1988)	20%	11%
Total cancer deaths (1988)	93,000 (35%)	46,000 (20%)
Deaths by age (1985)		
All	83,854	38,839
35–54	8,926	4,960
55–74	53,756	24,322
75+	20,996	9,279

Data from Silverberg E: Cancer statistics, 1988. CA 38:5–22, 1988.

popularity of low-tar cigarettes, future trends in lung cancer are hard to predict.[9] Brown and Kessler have prepared an age-period-cohort model based on lung cancer mortality data, prevention objectives for smoking behavior established by the National Cancer Institute (NCI), and current smoking consumption data, for projecting lung cancer deaths through the year 2025. If there are no changes in the number of individuals starting or continuing to smoke and no changes in the tar content of cigarettes, those authors project age-adjusted rates in men to be flat through the 1990s and then to decline. The rates for women will peak in 2010, because the age-specific peaks for women lag 5 years behind those for U.S. men. Achieving the reduced smoking objectives will have little impact by the year 2000 but could reduce the male rate by 33% and the female rate by 40% by the period 2023–2027. Brown and Kessler conclude that "recent trends in lung cancer are unlikely to be affected by changes in cigarette composition and consumption in the near term, but increasing the effectiveness of anti-smoking campaigns can have a considerable effect on lung cancer rates in the more distant future."[9]

ETIOLOGY OF LUNG CANCER

Despite application of all our best current diagnostic and treatment modalities, including surgery, radiotherapy, and chemotherapy, the overall cure rate for lung cancer is only about 10%. Thus, any gains made in prevention or new methods of treating this disease, even if they affect only a small percentage of the total cases, would have a large impact in terms of total lives saved. These preventative efforts have to take into account data on the known etiologic factors, including cigarette and other types of smoking, exposures to other carcinogens such as asbestos and radon progeny, and the preventive role of diet. In addition, new approaches to prevention, diagnosis, staging, and treatment ultimately will be based rationally on a firm understanding of the molecular and cellular biology of lung cancer.

PATIENTS WITH LUNG CANCER HAVE BEEN HEAVILY EXPOSED TO CARCINOGENS

It is widely recognized that cigarette smoking (delivering large doses of carcinogens) is causally related to the development of lung cancer. In addition, recent evidence suggests that other carcinogens exist in the workplace and the home, such as alpha-particle-emitting radon daughters, which can increase the risk of lung cancer several-fold and probably act synergistically with cigarette smoke. Thus, there is ample exposure in lung cancer patients to agents that can damage DNA, creating the genetic lesions discussed below. Lowering this exposure provides our first target in preventative efforts.

The identification and characterization of the genetic events caused by this carcinogenic exposure has progressed rapidly over the past decade because of several factors that should have application to many other human tumors as well. These developments include methods to culture lung

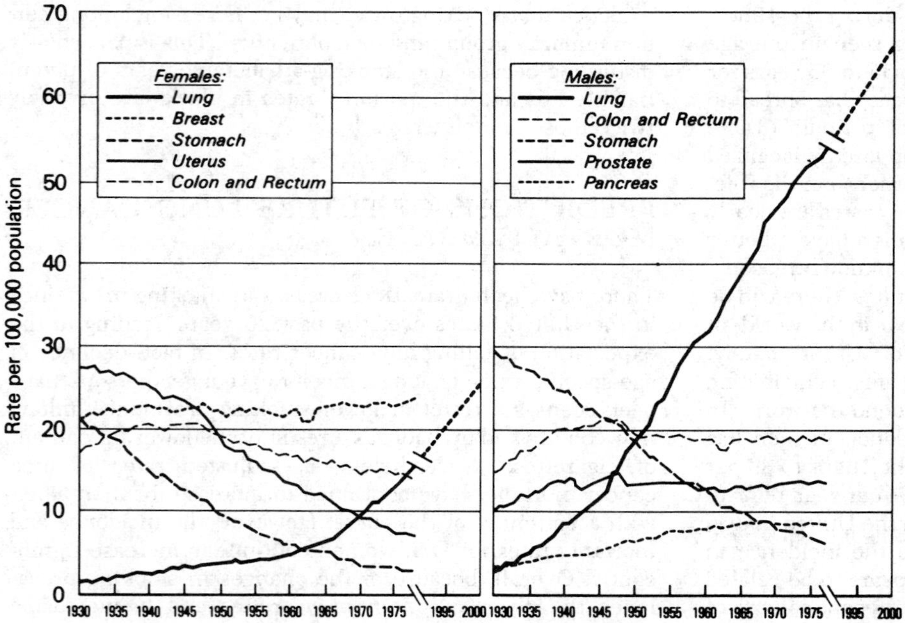

FIG. 22-1. Age-adjusted cancer death rates in the United States for lung cancer and other selected sites, with theoretical projections for lung cancer mortality in the year 2000. (Cancer Bull 32[3], 1980; CA 33[1], 1983. Sources of data cited are the U.S. National Center for Health Statistics and the U.S. Bureau of the Census)

TABLE 22-2. Extent of Disease at Time of Presentation and Overall 5-Year Survival Rate (%) for Lung Cancer

Stage of Disease (Cases Diagnosed 1970–1973)	%	5-Year Survival % (Cases Diagnosed 1965–1969) Male	Female
Local	17	28	51
Regional spread	22	10	15
Distant metastases	48	(<0.1)†	(<0.1)†
All stages*		8	13

Data from Cancer Patient Survival, Report No. 5, DHEW Publ. No. (NIH) 77-912, 1977.
* Not all patients classified according to stage.
† Not stated, but estimated from data on survival of all stages.

cancer cells in vitro, with the establishment of a large panel of lung cancer cell lines;[10–13] the field of cellular proto-oncogenes and chromosomal deletion analysis; and the identification of autocrine growth factors produced by tumor cells. The lung cancer cell lines have allowed the systematic characterization of cytogenetics, oncogenes, and growth factor production and responses, as well as development of in vitro drug and radiation sensitivity assays for lung cancer cells. As will become clear from the results of lung cancer prevention and treatment efforts, new strategies are urgently needed to approach this disease.

AUTOCRINE GROWTH FACTOR PRODUCTION, CHROMOSOMAL DELETIONS, AND ONCOGENE ACTIVATION IN THE PATHOGENESIS OF LUNG CANCER

Summary of a Current Working Model for the Pathogenesis of Lung Cancer

Evidence from several fronts suggest the following working model for the pathogenesis of lung cancer:[14,15]

1. Carcinogen exposure, probably enhanced by inheritance of a certain debrisoquine metabolic phenotype;
2. Production of gastrin-releasing peptide (GRP; mammalian bombesin) and other growth factors such as insulin-like (IGF) and transferrin-like (TGF) growth factors by neuroendocrine cells of the lung;
3. Autocrine growth stimulation of these neuroendocrine cells and thus increased growth factor production and probable paracrine growth stimulation of other bronchial epithelial cells, with resulting polyclonal proliferation;
4. Continued carcinogen exposure leading to the development of deletions and translocations in the replicating bronchial epithelial cells involving chromosome region 3p(14-23) to give clonal abnormalities exposing recessive oncogenes (which could have developed somatically or been inherited); as well as
5. Other genetic changes, including constitutive activation of *myc* family oncogenes and other nuclear-acting proto-oncogenes (such as *p53* and c-*jun*) potentially by alterations in oncogene transcription, resulting in locally invasive lesions;
6. Constitutive activation of the nuclear-acting proto-oncogenes, leading to increased transcription of a family of genes providing the malignant phenotype such as that for collagenase type IV by the c-*jun* (AP-1) transcription factor;
7. Addition of other genetic changes such as mutations of *ras* family, c-*raf-1*, and other oncogenes, some of which could involve growth factor or growth factor receptor genes, such as that for the epidermal growth factor receptor (EGFr); other chromosomal deletions (such as of the *rb* gene on chromosome 13 and other genes on chromosomes 10, 11, and 17); and further deregulation of *myc* family members by amplification and gene rearrangements to give progressive and metastatic lesions.

Thus, lung cancer cells produce factors capable of promoting their own growth early in pathogenesis, allowing accumulation of a series of genetic lesions involving both the dominant, classic cellular proto-oncogenes[16] and the newly described recessive (chromosomal deletion) or "tumor suppressor" genes,[17] which together account for the transformation to malignancy of lung cells.

Genetic Changes Underlie the Pathogenesis of Human Lung Cancer

Human lung cancer is not generally thought of as a genetic disease. However, a variety of recent experimental evidence (summarized below) leads inextricably to the conclusion that *lung cancer cells have accumulated a series of somatic genetic changes that activate the dominantly acting cellular proto-oncogenes* on the one hand, while another group of changes would seem to *inactivate a second class of genes* that appear to be recessive (deletion or tumor suppressor genes), both of which are likely to be necessary for the malignant transformation of lung cells. Experimental systems show that even the dominantly acting oncogenes required the cooperation of more than one oncogene to transform normal cells, (such as a combination of c-*myc* and a mutated *ras* gene,[18] and that cancer cells have used many different genetic motifs in activation or inactivation processes. Thus, we expect to find evidence of lesions in more than one of these genes and more than one type of lesion in any given gene in lung cancer cells.

Predisposition to Lung Cancer May Be Inherited

There is mounting circumstantial evidence that some of the genetic changes are inherited in a mendelian fashion.[19,20] Most notably, first-degree relatives of lung cancer probands have a strong (2.4-fold) excess risk for lung cancer[21] or other cancers, many of which are not smoking related.[22] This risk may be through inheritance of a predisposition to chronic obstructive pulmonary disease. In fact, there is a higher risk of lung cancer ($p = 0.024$) in persons with chronic obstructive pulmonary disease, of whom 8.8% develop lung cancer within 10 years.[23] Moreover, lung cancer risk in smokers is modified by characteristics of the smoker and the family history. For example, for smokers with lung cancer, there is a significantly increased frequency of a parent having had lung cancer (6.9%) ($p < 0.001$; odds ratio [OR] = 5.3; range 2.2–12.8), and there is a significantly increased lung cancer risk if there is a personal history of chronic bronchitis or emphysema (OR = 2.0; range 1.4–2.8).[24] The link to chronic obstructive pulmonary disease is strengthened by the finding that smokers with ventilatory obstruction are at greater risk for lung cancer than are smokers without obstruction.[25] Patients with systemic sclerosis carry a significantly increased relative risk (RR = 16.5) of lung cancer.[26] Finally, an abnormal c-*Ha-ras* allele distribution was found in non-small-cell lung cancer, suggesting a linkage of a chromosome 11p haplotype to this type of cancer.[27]

DEVELOPMENT OF A SECOND MALIGNANCY AFTER LUNG CANCER. In other inherited disorders, predispositions to multiple tumors are often seen. In lung cancer, it is difficult to sort out whether second cancers are related solely to carcinogen exposure from cigarette smoking or also to some inherited predisposition. Nevertheless, it is important to note that cured lung cancer patients have a very significant risk of a second malignancy such as another lung cancer[28-30] or an acute leukemia.[31-34] Conversely, patients cured of other malignancies outside the respiratory tree can have an increased risk of lung cancer.

Two very large series have looked at the risk of developing a second cancer. In 30,000 persons from Connecticut who had cancer at any site within the respiratory system diagnosed between 1935 and 1982, a 44% excess of all second cancers was seen following cancer of the lung.[35] These second cancers were in the respiratory tract, oral cavity, bladder, and kidney, all sites potentially associated with cigarette smoking. After 10 years of observation, the risk of a second cancer remained high, at 50% above expectation. In another study of 36,000 Danish persons with cancer of the respiratory system diagnosed between 1943 and 1980, there was a 10% increased risk of a second cancer. Elevated rates of second cancers were seen in the lung, buccal cavity, bladder, kidney; surprisingly, excess cancers in the breast and female genital organs, liver, and pancreas were also seen.[36] In both of these series, significant risks of lung cancers were noted after primary laryngeal cancers.

Acute nonlymphocytic leukemia was found in 2 of 377 patients with small cell lung cancer at 22 and 81 months after the start of therapy,[37] representing a highly significant ($p < 0.0001$) increased relative risk value (RR = 154; 95% confidence limit 38–293) for the development of leukemia. The Kaplan–Meier estimate of the cumulative probability of developing leukemia was $1.9 \pm 1.4\%$ 7 years after the start of treatment.

DEVELOPMENT OF LUNG CANCER AFTER CURE OF ANOTHER MALIGNANCY, PARTICULARLY LARYNGEAL CANCER. The association of lung cancer with upper aerodigestive cancers such as head and neck cancer is growing very strong, with the highest association being with laryngeal cancers. For example, 26% of 415 patients cured of laryngeal cancer developed lung cancer during the first 14 years of follow-up (RR = 6.73).[38] In another series of 748 laryngeal cancer patients, 9% had second primary lung cancers.[39] In one series of 1373 consecutive patients with head and neck or lung cancer, 2% had multiple primary cancers.[40] In another series of 1450 patients with upper airway cancers, 4% developed a lung cancer, nearly always after the head and neck cancer.[41] The mean interval between the diagnoses of the upper airway and the lung cancers was 6 years. In addition, the lung cancers can be of any histologic type (not only squamous cell cancer), and frequently, they occur in women. The post-thoracotomy management of patients who have had surgery or radiotherapy on their upper airways for head and neck cancer is challenging. If the lung and head and neck cancers occur synchronously, the lung cancer is usually dealt with first, as it appears to be the most life threatening.[41]

Evidence is beginning to accumulate of an increased risk (perhaps twofold to threefold) of lung cancer after treatment for non-Hodgkin's lymphoma or Hodgkin's disease.[42] Six patients among 288 with lymphoma developed lung cancer, suggesting that a lymphoma patient who is a smoker should be investigated thoroughly for lung carcinoma if there are signs or symptoms in the chest.

Correlation of Debrisoquine Metabolic Phenotype with Lung Cancer

There appears to be a strong association between the high metabolic phenotype for 4-debrisoquine hydroxylase and the development of lung cancer.[43] Extensive metabolizers of debrisoquine have a 10-fold increased risk of lung cancer, whereas the extensive metabolizers exposed to asbestos have a 22- to 30-fold increased relative risk, such that within the asbestos-exposed group, there is an approximately 10-fold increase in the risk for lung cancer among extensive metabolizers.[44] *These findings raise the question of whether some people are predisposed to get lung cancer, either by genes that determine how they handle carcinogens or by recessive genes that can also lead to the genesis of other tumors.* Identification of such genes would not only aid in targeting preventive effects for lung cancer but might also provide clues to the genetics of cancer as a whole.

Autocrine Growth Factor Production by Lung Cancer Cells Provides a Mechanism for Accumulation of Genetic Lesions

Lung cancer cells both produce and exhibit a mitogenic response to a variety of growth factors, so that these factors fit the definition of autocrine growth factors.[45,46] In fact, lung cancer cells can grow in medium supplemented with only a few or no added growth factors.[47,49] Other autocrine peptides produced by lung cancer cells include GRP and those with TGF- and IGF-1-like activities.[50–53] In some cases, lung cancer cells express multiple growth factors.[54]

The best-characterized autocrine growth factor in lung cancer is GRP, which is produced by small cell lung cancer[55–58] and acts through high-affinity receptors[59] to stimulate calcium mobilization[60] and phosphatidylinositol turnover, as well as constitutive activation of a protein-tyrosine kinase that phosphorylates a 115 kD protein associated with the GRP–receptor complex[61] and thereby functions as an autocrine growth factor for small cell lung cancer.[62] GRP is produced by the human fetal lung[63] and has known mitogenic effects in vitro and in vivo[64,65] as well as a multiplicity of other effects including induction of anorexia and the release of many other hormones.[66] Thus, it is likely that GRP is an important regulatory peptide for normal lung growth and development and that it may account for some of the paraneoplastic syndromes (see Chap. 55) associated with lung cancer. The complexity of the GRP system is underscored by the production of three mRNA forms from the pre-proGRP gene through alternative mRNA processing[67,68] to give a series of proteins, including three different GRP-gene-associated peptides, which are expressed in small cell lung cancer and human fetal lung.[69] These GRP-gene-associated peptides are further modified by post-translational processing into multiple other peptides,[70] all of which could have biologic activity. In addition to stimulating the growth of small cell lung cancer,[71,72] GRP can stimulate the growth of normal bronchial epithelial cells,[73] implying a role as a paracrine growth factor. Of great interest in this regard is the production of high levels of bombesin-like immunoreactivity detectable in the bronchial lavage fluid of smokers.[74] This observation, if substantiated, would place these growth factor-mediated events very early in the pathogenesis of lung cancer and provide a mechanism for promotion of the genetic lesions caused by carcinogens by allowing the accumulation of multiple lesions in individual cells through cell replication. One could also envision pulmonary neuroendocrine cells undergoing "autocrine" growth and thus expanding the number of cells producing such growth factors without themselves ultimately transforming but rather stimulating other bronchial epithelial cell populations to expand.

Future lines of investigation include testing for such growth factors in the pulmonary tree of smokers and clinical trials seeking to inhibit these growth factors. Antibodies and peptide antagonists against the biologically active portion of GRP inhibit the growth of small cell lung cancer in human tumor xenografts grown in nude mice, as well as in tissue culture.[62,75,76]

Evidence for Genetic Damage (Chromosomal and DNA Deletions) Involving the Recessive or Tumor Suppressor Genes

A variety of cytogenetic studies have indicated many chromosomal changes in lung cancer such as numerical and structural aberrations including deletions and translocations.[77–84] In addition, restriction fragment-length polymorphism (RFLP) technology has shown that many of these cytogenetic changes are associated with true loss of DNA from the tumor cell. The most prominent of these losses is deletion of material from chromosome region 3p(14–23), which shortest-region-of-overlap analysis would place at 3p21.[85–88] These changes in 3p21 are found in all types of lung cancer, suggesting they are either a common requirement for the development of lung cancer or an early step in the pathogenesis. Similar deletions have been seen in sporadic renal carcinomas,[89] and there are family pedigrees where the development of renal carcinoma segregates with cytogenetic abnormalities of chromosome region 3p.[90,91] It is of great interest that this region is a fragile site in the human genome, and increased fragility is seen in the normal cells of cigarette smokers.[92] More recently, DNA loss from other chromosomes has been identified, including chromosomes 13, 17, and 11.[93,94] Of great interest, in the case of chromosome 13, the DNA loss has been localized to the *rb* locus,[95] such that the large majority of small cell lung cancers have absent or dramatically reduced expression of the *rb* gene product.[96] *All of these changes raise the possibility of recessive mutations on the remaining chromosomal material being uncovered by the deletion.* Supportive evidence for this hypothesis comes from the lack of expression of aminoacylase (a gene assigned to chromosome region 3p21) in some small cell lung cancers.[97] These findings also raise the possibility of correcting the defect by introducing into the lung cancer cell a normal copy of the gene. That this may indeed be possible is suggested by the results of somatic cell hybrid experiments that show suppression of malignancy when a malignant non-small cell lung cancer line is fused to a nonmalignant mouse cell.[98] Candidate genes that reside on chromosome region 3p include a thyroid hormone receptor *ErbA* β[99] and retinoic acid-receptor-like genes, *Hap-1*.[100] Thus, one possibility is that the genes that are inactivated code for hormone receptor functions that transmit signals for differentiation.

Evidence for Genetic Damage of Dominant Genes: Oncogene Activation

Oncogenes of several families suffer changes in lung cancer cells (Table 22-3). These changes include point mutations in members of the *ras* family[101–108] and changes that predispose to the constitutive and often high-level expression of cellular proto-oncogenes that act in the nucleus, including c-*myc*, N-*myc*, L-*myc*, c-*myb*, and *p53*.[109–115] The changes in *myc* family member expression have been associated with gene amplification, gene rearrangement, and loss of intragenic pausing or the "attenuator" function.[116] Experimental studies show that transfecting a mutated *ras* gene into small cell lung cancer changes its phenotype to one suggesting a non-small cell lung cancer.[117] In addition, constitutive expression of c-*raf-1* has been found in all types of lung cancer.[118] This is particularly intriguing because c-*raf-1* is assigned to chromosome region 3p25, an area frequently involved in the terminal deletions of chromosome 3 in lung cancer.

The clinical relevance of the c-*myc* gene has been the first to be explored in any detail. Small cell lung cancer cell lines

TABLE 22-3. Chromosome Regions or Proto-Oncogenes Found to Have Genetic Alterations and/or Alterations of Expression in Human Lung Cancer

Chromosome regions frequently deleted in human lung cancer (putative recessive or tumor-suppressor genes)
3p(14–23)
11p
13q14 (*rb* locus)
17p
Cellular Proto-oncogenes activated in some lung cancers (dominantly acting genes)
c-*myc*
N-*myc*
L-*myc*
c-*myb*
p53
c-*jun*
H-*ras*
K-*ras-2*
N-*ras*
c-*raf-1*
c-*fms*

with high-level expression of the c-*myc* gene exhibit faster growth and higher cloning efficiency in vitro[119] and a change in the morphology to that characteristic of the large-cell "variants,"[120] and mark a poor prognosis in extensive-stage patients.[121] In addition, if a c-*myc* gene is transfected into a classic small cell lung cancer line initially not expressing the gene, the transfected cells take on the growth and morphologic characteristics of the c-*myc*-amplified small cell lung cancer lines,[122] demonstrating a direct relation between the expression of a particular oncogene and the cellular phenotype.

The L-*myc* gene was discovered in a small cell lung cancer, where it can be amplified and overexpressed. However, it is of particular interest because it can be expressed in both small cell and non-small cell lung cancer[123]; because it has a restricted pattern of expression during development (especially brain, kidney, and lung)[124]; and because it is associated with GRP-related signal transduction events. In addition, the L-*myc* gene undergoes a complex series of alternative mRNA processing and polyadenylation site selection to generate four different mRNAs,[125] which in turn generate a series of L-*myc* protein products.[126] These products transform primary rat embryo cells when cotransfected with a mutated *ras* gene. However, it is of great interest that they do this with 1% to 10% the efficiency of c-*myc*,[127] suggesting the need for other genetic lesions such as deletions or other oncogene activation or a more restricted cell type for action. Recently, certain L-*myc* haplotypes have been implicated in the metastatic behavior of lung cancer of several histologic types.[128]

Recently, another nuclear oncogene product, c-*jun*, has been found to be expressed at high levels in small cell and non-small cell lung cancer and normal lung.[129] This is of interest because c-*jun* lies in the same chromosomal region as L-*myc* (1p31–32),[130] and the c-*jun* product appears to be a proto-oncogene equivalent of the transcription factor AP-1 and thus intimately involved with regulation of transcription and mediation of tumor promotor effects such as those engendered by phorbol esters.[131] Thus, a scenario is established in normal lung and lung cancer cells where a transcription factor is activated, mimicking chronic stimulation by tumor promoters.

Because of the activation of dominant cellular proto-oncogenes, including those whose products act in the nucleus, as well as GTP-binding oncogene products, and phosphokinases, and because of the presence of the recessive tumor suppressor genes, it appears inescapable that new prevention and treatment strategies for lung cancer must ultimately be directed against the development of deregulated expression or functional outcome of these genes.

SMOKING AND LUNG CANCER

Cigarette smoking is the predominant cause of lung cancer in the United States and around the world (Tables 22-4 and 22-5). International data demonstrate that lung cancer death rates parallel cigarette smoking prevalence rates in both men and women.[132] Moreover, in all studies, there has been a clear dose–response relation between the amount of smoking and the development of lung cancer.[138] In addition, there is a significantly increased risk of lung cancer for pipe and cigar smokers whether or not they also smoke cigarettes (Table 22-4). Thus, effective control of lung cancer and other smoking-associated diseases can only be achieved by reducing smoking prevalence in the developed countries and stopping the increase in smoking in developing countries.[132] Lung cancer in underdeveloped countries is becoming a problem of large economic and political importance, and an epidemic of lung cancer is likely within a decade because of the rapidly increasing cigarette consumption in many of these countries.[138] This is true for blacks in South Africa[139] and Asians in Singapore[140] (67 to 73 cases per 100,000 persons). In China and India, 25% to 33% of all males are addicted to tobacco smoking by the time they are 18 to 20 years old.[138]

The latest in a long series of reports by the U.S. Surgeon General deals directly with cigarette smoking as a drug ad-

TABLE 22-4. Relationship of Smoking to the Development of Lung Cancer*

Cigarette smoking[132–136]
Lung cancer death rates parallel cigarette smoking prevalence[132]
Risk increases with each cigarette smoked per day[133]
Relative risk declines exponentially with duration of smoking cessation
Risk declines 5 years after cessation of smoking
Risk increased for all types of lung cancer,
Small cell lung cancer (RR = 17.5)
Adenocarcinoma (RR = 6.7)
Males OR = 4.49
Females OR = 3.95
Estimates of risk for other types of smoking[134,137]
Exclusive cigarette smoking: RR = 13.3
Exclusive cigar smoking: RR = 5.6
Exclusive pipe smoking: RR = 1.6
Mixed cigar and cigarette smoking: RR = 8.5
Mixed pipe and cigarette smoking: RR = 8.0
Dose–response relation for cigarette and pipe smoking

*RR = relative risk estimates; OR = odds ratio.

TABLE 22-5. Total Mortality, Weighted Smoking-Attributable Fractions, and Smoking-Attributable Mortality from Lung Cancer in the United States (1984)

	Males	*Females*	*Total*
Smoking-attributable fractions	0.80	0.75	
Smoking-attributable mortality	65,659	27,170	92,829
Total deaths	82,459	36,227	118,686
Involuntary smoking mortality estimate			3825

Data from Oncol Times December 1, 1987, p 8; Centers for Disease Control: Cigarette smoking in the United States, 1986. MMWR 36:581–585, 1987; National Academy of Sciences: Environmental tobacco smoke: Measuring exposures and assessing health effects (Appendix D). Washington, DC, National Academy Press, 1986.

diction.[141] The principal conclusions of this extensive data summary and analysis are:

1. Cigarettes and other forms of tobacco are addicting.
2. Nicotine is the drug in tobacco that causes addiction.
3. The pharmacologic and behavioral processes that determine tobacco addiction are similar to those that determine addiction to drugs such as heroin and cocaine.

This direct confrontation of the addictive properties of nicotine may provide the best method for dealing with the smoking problem.

It is estimated that 54,000,000 Americans smoke cigarettes, including 36% of the total work force or 37,000,000 workers (Table 22-6).[142] Because there appear to be multiple interactions between smoking and workplace carcinogens in the development of lung cancer, as well as effects of smoking on chronic obstructive pulmonary disease and heart disease that influence workplace performance, smoking creates a vast health and financial problem for the U.S. workplace.[143] Thus, there is a confluence of medical, epidemiologic, and economic reasons for focusing antismoking efforts on the workplace. Smoking control strategies include prevention of starting to smoke, efforts to get people to stop smoking, regulatory and legislative measures, and modifications in tobacco product composition. It is not clear how best to achieve a reduction in smoking, and thus the U.S. NCI has initiated intervention research programs to identify and assess the most promising strategies to reduce smoking prevalence in the general public and in high-risk populations (heavy smokers, blacks, Hispanics, women, youth, and smokeless tobacco users).[132]

Although modern cigarettes are usually low in tar and thus presumably in many toxic products and nicotine, epidemiology results have not shown much reduction in the mortality rate that can be attributed to lowering of tar.[143] Public health campaigns have sometimes appeared successful in getting the tobacco industry to reduce tar, but they have also been used by that industry to downplay the dangers of smoking.[143] The delivery of high levels of tar by the smoking products sold in the Third World is another area of serious concern.[143]

Early detection of lung cancer appears not to have a significant impact given current screening methods, as a large number of early detection studies have failed to show a significant impact on lung cancer mortality rates. In fact, analysis of the large population of cigarette smokers periodically screened by the Memorial Sloan-Kettering Cancer Center

TABLE 22-6. Smoking in the Workplace (United States)*

Group	*Estimated Prevalence (%)*	*Number of Persons Smoking*
White males	37	19,864,000
White females	33	13,478,000
Black males	42	2,180,000
Black females	34	1,750,000
Overall	35.6	37,258,000

	Percentage of the Group Smoking the Indicated No. of Cigarettes per Day		
Cigarettes per Day	≤15	15–24	≥24
White males	20	44	36
White females	31	48	22
Black males	49	39	12
Black females	61	34	5

	Smoking Prevalence (%) by Occupational Class and Sex	
	Blue Collar	*White Collar*
Male	47	33
Female	38	32

Data from LaRosa JH, Haines CM: A Guide to Heart and Lung Health at the Workplace. NIH Publication No. 86-2210, Washington, DC, September 1986.
*Estimated 104,658,000 employed persons in 1985.

(MSKCC) in New York has found, surprisingly, that the mean duration of the early stage of lung cancer is at least 4 years, the detectability less than 0.2, and the curability less than 0.5.[144] Thus, annual radiographic screening between the ages of 45 and 80 might decrease mortality rates from adenocarcinoma of the lung by less than 20%.[144] In contrast, there is significant evidence of a reduced risk of lung cancer beginning 5 years after cessation of smoking.[134]

PASSIVE SMOKING AND INCREASED RISK OF LUNG CANCER

Passive exposure to cigarette smoke and the development of lung cancer is an important issue with many social and political implications. The majority of lung cancers in nonsmoking women are probably related to environmental (passive) tobacco smoke, although passive exposures in utero and very early in life need to be considered.[145] The physicochemical nature of passive smoke (the smoke inhaled by nonsmokers) differs significantly from the mainstream smoke inhaled by the active smoker.[145]

Currently, the best means of assessing exposure to passive smoking is the urinary cotinine level.[145] A summary of 13 studies (10 case-controlled and 3 prospective) showed a highly significant (35% to 53%) increase in the risk of lung cancer among nonsmokers living with smokers compared with nonsmokers living with nonsmokers (RR = 1.35; 95% confidence interval 1.19–1.54, which rose after adjustment to an RR = 1.53, or a 53% increase).[146] Other individual studies confirm this. For example, wives of men who smoke have a twofold to threefold increased risk of lung cancer.[147,148] Also, there is a dose–response relation between the amount of smoking by the spouse and the risk of the nonsmoking spouse getting lung cancer that is significant for squamous cell and small cell lung cancer although not for other histologic types.[148,149] Thus, about one-third of lung cancer in nonsmokers who live with smokers and about 25% of lung cancer in nonsmokers in general comes from passive exposure to cigarette smoke.[146] However, one must beware of bias in passive smoking studies, because there is a strong tendency for smokers to marry smokers and for such "nonsmokers" to give false reports about their own smoking habits (2.5% to 10%).[150]

OTHER ETIOLOGIC AGENTS

Exposure to Asbestos

Mineral fibers, particularly asbestos, represent the greatest cause after cigarette smoking of respiratory cancer attributable to air pollutants.[151] The increased risk in asbestos workers account for about 8 excess cancers per 1000 exposed workers (RR = 1.4–1.7),[152] and for British asbestos workers followed over a long period of time, the relative risk was 1.4 to 2.6.[153] Past asbestos exposure accounts for 2000 mesothelioma deaths per year and 4000 to 6000 lung cancer deaths per year in the United States.[154] However, it is estimated that removal of asbestos from occupational exposure would reduce lung cancers by 23%.[155] All these studies show a strong dose–response effect with asbestos exposure.[156] Of great importance, the combination of occupational asbestos exposure and smoking further increases lung cancer risk; this association is strongest with small cell lung cancer and weakest with adenocarcinoma.[157,158] All common commercial types of asbestos (crocidolite, amosite, and chrysotile) can cause lung cancer of all histologic types. Most commonly, exposures occur in the workplace (*e.g.*, insulation, cement, shipyard workers). However, nonoccupational exposures are likely to be associated with malignant disease similar to that obtained through occupational exposure.[154]

Exposure to Radon Progeny

URANIUM MINING.[159,160]. All underground mining studies show an increased risk of lung cancer with radon (Rn) daughter exposure, and all cell types of lung cancer are increased with Rn exposure. Cumulative exposure to Rn and its alpha-emitting daughters is given by the "working level month" (WLM), which for historical reasons is defined as exposure to approximately 100 pCi of radon per liter of air in 170 hours. Occupational exposure to 4 WLM is estimated to increase lung cancer risk by 60% for the general population of people between 20 and 40 years of age.[161] Smokers are at 10-fold higher risk than nonsmokers of developing lung cancer after this occupational exposure.[160,161] The occupational standard for Rn exposure has been 4 WLM per year, whereas 2 WLM per year had been suggested as a threshold for remedial action in homes. Epidemiologic studies show that miners with cumulative Rn daughter exposures of even 100 WLM have an excess lung cancer mortality, with 3% to 8% of miners followed developing lung cancer attributable to Rn daughters.

A clear dose–response effect (RR increase of 3.3% per WLM) is seen for the development of lung cancer in uranium miners,[162] with an overall increase in relative risk of 2.3 per 100 WLM.[163] The National Institute for Occupational Safety and Health (NIOSH) has developed quantitative risk estimates of lung cancer after exposure to Rn daughters in the follow-up of the U.S. cohort of uranium miners.[164] These figures predict excess relative risks between 0.9 and 1.4 per 100 WLM in the lower cumulative exposure range. Of interest, low exposure rates appear more harmful per unit of cumulative exposure than higher rates. Relative risk increased with age at initial exposure, and the relative risk of lung cancer fell dramatically in the years following cessation of exposure.[164]

^{222}RN GAS PROGENY OUTSIDE THE WORKPLACE.[161,164,166]. Many of the general population also may be unknowingly exposed to Rn daughters. In fact, Rn exposure is the most serious cause of human irradiation, and excessive exposures may be readily avoidable. Human exposure to terrestrial gamma rays, cosmic rays, and natural radionuclides in diet is detectable but not highly variable,[166] with a basic background dose of about 1 mSv.[160] In contrast, indoor Rn levels have tremendous variability. In temperate latitudes, the average concentration is about 15 Bq m^{-3} of air, which is the equilibrium equivalent concentration of ^{222}Rn (conversion coefficient 10 Bq m^{-3} = 1 mSv per year).[166] This value can range from as little as one-tenth to 1000-fold higher in otherwise ordinary houses. Thus, annual doses range from 1 mSv or less through an average of 1.5 mSv to 1000 mSv or more.[166]

To relate general population exposure to miners' exposure, the potential risk of lung cancer appears to be between 1 and 2 per 10,000 persons per WLM, which yields a significant number of lung cancers, as some 220 million persons in the United States are exposed on average to 10 to 20 WLM in a life-time.[160] It is estimated that 10 ± 5% of the lung cancer rate in the general public is attributable to Rn daughters at an exposure rate of 10 to 20 Bq/m^{-3},[167] whereas 25% of lung cancers in nonsmokers and 5% of those in smokers are attributable to exposure to Rn daughters in the home.[168] Some homes have very high levels of Rn. In U.S. homes, the mean level is 1.5 pCi per liter (55 Bq/m^{-3}), but, 1% to 3% of homes exceed 8 pCi per liter. As 1.5 pCi per liter contributes about a 0.3% increased life-time risk of lung cancer, in the million homes with the highest concentrations, where annual exposures approximate or exceed those received by underground uranium miners, long-term occupants suffer an added life-time risk of at least 2%, reaching extraordinary values at the highest concentrations observed.[169]

Steady-state outdoor Rn concentration averages 200 pCi m^{-3}, whereas indoor levels are four times this.[160] The primary source of Rn in homes is the underlying soil, and levels in the homes depend on multiple variables such as reduced ventilation for energy conservation. Thus, high indoor levels are caused by the forced flow of Rn-laden soil gas into buildings.[166] Radon gas itself delivers only a very small dose of irradiation. However, the four immediate daughters of ^{222}Rn are radioactive isotopes of solid elements with short half-lives, two of which transform by emitting alpha particles.[166] The daughters create a radioactive aerosol with small particles in room air, which, inhaled, causes some daughters to be deposited and retained in the respiratory tract, where alpha particles irradiate bronchial epithelial cells, with the most significant result being lung cancer.[166] In addition, there is evidence for radioactive polonium in cigarettes.[170]

The International Commission on Radiological Protection (ICRP) has set the average life-time exposure at equilibrium equivalent concentrations of 15 Bq m^{-3} (to give a relative lifetime risk of lung cancer of 0.1%); the upper acceptable boundary at 100 Bq m^{-3} (to give a relative life-time risk of 0.5%); and the level at which action needs to be taken at 200 Bq m^{-3} (which would give a relative life-time risk of 1%). This action level was chosen because it would be expected to double the life-time risk of lung cancer.[166] This has been studied in Sweden, where women had increased relative risks (RR = 2.2; p = 0.01) for lung cancer associated with living in dwellings close to the ground in areas with an increased risk of Rn emanation. Actual measurements indicated increased Rn daughter concentrations in ground-level dwellings with Rn risk areas where patients had lived, suggesting that this exposure was of etiologic importance.[171]

Other Workplace Carcinogens

In assessing the risk of workplace carcinogens, it is important to estimate and exclude the role that smoking alone would play. However, these carcinogens could interact with smoking to increase lung cancer risk.[172] In the United States, blue collar workers have a higher smoking prevalence than white collar workers (see Table 22-6).[133] The occupations with the highest smoking rates include, for men, painters, construction and maintenance, truck drivers, carpenters, auto mechanics, and guards and watchmen, all of which have a 50% or higher smoking prevalence. For women, waitresses, cashiers, assemblers, nurses' aides, orderlies, machine operatives, practical nurses, packers, and wrappers all have a smoking prevalence exceeding 40%.[133] Thus, when both a high smoking prevalence and a workplace carcinogen exist, the potential for an occupation-associated lung cancer is probably greatly enhanced. In addition to asbestos and radioactive exposure, a variety of other carcinogens and occupations have been identified by epidemiologic studies in the workplace after subtracting the effect of smoking (Table 22-7). These include especially arsenic, cadmium, chromium, and certain chemicals such as chloromethyl ether.

That prevention could play a beneficial role is indicated by the finding of no increased risk of lung cancer in a group of

TABLE 22-7. Chemicals, Metals, Airborne Contaminants, and Occupations Contributing to Lung Cancer Risk[154,175,176]

Chemicals
Chloromethyl ether (chemical workers)[177]
Obs/Exp = 2.70; $p < 0.01$; a clear dose–response effect is seen with risk increased more than 10 fold with highest doses; latent period is 10–19 years
Cadmium (nickel–cadmium battery plant)[175,178]
EPA estimates risk from cadmium at 1.8×10^{-3} cases/μg/m^3, which results in more than 100,000 excess lung cancers (life-time)
Arsenic[175,178,180]
EPA estimates risk of 4.3 cases/1000 μg/m^3 to give more than 100,000 lung cancers (life-time). Smelter workers exposed to arsenic have lung cancer risk increased 2–9 times. Artesian well water high in arsenic gives 3-fold increased risk of lung cancer and shows dose–response relation (OR = 3.39)
Chromate[181]
Hexavalent chromium (masons)[182,183]
Formaldehyde[184]
Terpenes (wood industry[185]
Occupations[186,187]
Shipyard workers, truck drivers, plumbers (probably related to asbestos)[188]
Rubber curing and other rubber workers[189,190]
SMR = 133
Pottery workers[191]
talc exposure: 3.64 increased risk
Printers (typographers and lithographers in Sweden)[192]
Female cosmetologists[193]
Leather industry[194]
RR = 2.6; range 1.2–6.0
Building laborers[186]
RR = 1.7; range 1.0–2.9
Construction workers[186]
RR = 1.8; range 1.0–3.0
Bakers and pastry cooks[186,195]
RR = 3.6 range 1.3–10.4
Cooks
RR = 2.5, range 1.2–5.1
Truck drivers
Diesel exhaust (possible effect)[196]

iron-ore (hematite) miners where the lack of significant Rn exposure was demonstrated and there was strict smoking prohibition underground, an aggressive silicosis control program, and the absence of underground diesel fuel.[173] In contrast, nowhere has the combined effect of smoking and occupational carcinogen exposure been more dramatic than in the tin miners in the Yunnan province of south central China, who have had the highest lung cancer mortality rate in men in all of China.[174] These miners are exposed to extraordinarily high levels of Rn such that miners with 20 to 30 years of underground service before 1949 would have had 1600 to 2400 WLM of exposure. In addition, most of the miners have smoked, and arsenic trioxide is a by product of the smelting process and contaminates the local food and water supplies. The majority of the cancers have been squamous cell carcinomas, with the remainder mostly small cell carcinoma. The lung cancer incidence in this group of miners is 1% per year and among retired miners 2% to 3% per year.[174] This is some 10-fold greater then the SEER rate for U.S. men age 60 to 64, which is 0.3% per year.

PROTECTIVE EFFECTS OF DIET

Beta-carotene and other constitutents of green and yellow vegetables have strong potential as protective agents (Table 22-8).[197] Selenium also deserves attention as a potential chemopreventive nutrient, however, there are fewer data. Vitamin A intake is inversely associated with lung cancer risk, and this relation is strongest among cigarette smokers.[198] Analyses of index of carotenoids and of individual food items suggest that plant sources of vitamin A may play a more important role in producing the effect than do animal sources.[198] These findings have prompted chemoprevention trials with retinoids in persons at high risk.[199]

TABLE 22-8. Dietary Elements that Epidemiologic Evidence Suggests Decrease the Risk of Lung Cancer

Beta-carotene
Serum beta-carotene level inversely related to risk of squamous-cell lung cancer (relative odds 4.30; 95% confidence interval 1.38–13.41)[200]
Intake of dark green and, particularly, dark yellow-orange vegetables (RR = 1.7–2.2 for low intake after adjustment for smoking risk; beneficial effect only noted in current smokers, RR = 1.3 for low intake after adjustment for smoking)[201]
Current smokers who did not consume carrots showed a threefold risk of lung cancer compared with those who ate them more than once a week (OR = 2.9; $p < 0.01$); risk was independent of histologic type[202]
Vitamin A
Intake of vitamin A from fruits and vegetables (carotene) strongly associated with reduced cancer risk, more for males (RR = 1.8) than for females[203]
Decreased dietary vitamin A intake has increased risk of lung cancer (RR = 1.8)[204]
Vitamin A-deficient diet increases lung tumorigenesis in rats[205]
Selenium[192]
Vitamin E
Persons with low serum level had 2.5 times the lung cancer risk[200]

ANATOMICAL CONSIDERATIONS

Because the lungs are paired organs with a large reserve capacity, one lung may be sacrificed with little resultant disability in an otherwise-healthy person. The right lung is composed of three lobes—the upper, middle, and lower—and provides approximately 55% of the ventilatory capacity. The left lung consists of only two lobes—the upper and lower—with the lingular portion of the upper lobe corresponding to the middle lobe on the right. The lobes are separated by fissures that can be identified on roentgenograms, particularly the lateral views. On the right side, usually two fissures are present: the oblique or major fissure that separates the lower lobe from the upper and middle lobes and the horizontal or minor fissure that separates the upper and middle lobes. On the left side, the single fissure separates the upper and lower lobes, running obliquely from the level of the third rib posteriorly and forward, ending in the region of the sixth or seventh costochondral junction.

The bronchopulmonary segment is the basic anatomic unit (Figure 22-2 and Table 22-9). Although the anatomical relations of the pulmonary hilar structures, as well as the arrangement of the bronchopulmonary segments, are relatively constant, variations may be encountered frequently. Therefore, the thoracic surgeon must be alert for these anomalies.

The main structures of the primary pulmonary hilus are the main bronchus, the pulmonary artery, and the superior and inferior pulmonary veins (Fig. 22-2). The relations of these structures differ considerably on the two sides. On the left side, the pulmonary artery curves around the upper lobe bronchus, whereas on the right side, it remains anterior and below the upper lobe bronchus. The segmental arteries follow the segmental bronchi; the veins occupy an intersegmental position, converging to form segmental veins that empty into the superior and inferior pulmonary veins. On the right side, the middle lobe vein empties into the superior pulmonary vein. Variations are common; in order of frequency, they occur in the veins, arteries, and bronchi. The pulmonary arterial tree is a low-pressure system compared with the peripheral arteries, and these vessels are relatively thin-walled and fragile.

The regional lymph nodes and currently used lymph node map are discussed in the section on surgical staging of the mediastinum.

PATHOLOGY OF LUNG CANCER

HISTOLOGIC TYPES

The four major cell types of lung cancer are squamous cell (or epidermoid) carcinoma, small cell (also called oat cell) carcinoma, adenocarcinoma, and large cell (also called large cell anaplastic) carcinoma. However, for the many associated types of pleuropulmonary malignancies, the histologic classification of lung cancer recommended by the World Health Organization (WHO) in 1977 should be used as the current definitive classification (Table 22-10).[206] Carcinomas arising from the bronchial or bronchioloalveolar sur-

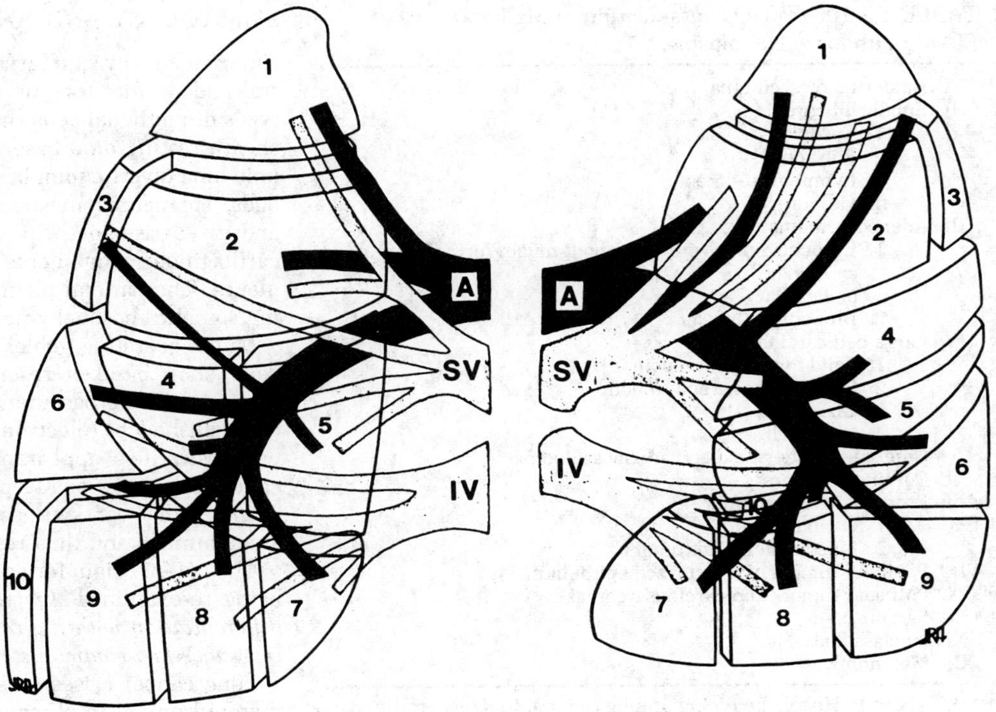

FIG. 22-2. Schematic diagram of segmental and vascular anatomy of the lung. The anatomical distribution of the bronchopulmonary segments is numbered according to the Boyden scheme (see text and Table 22-9 for description of bronchopulmonary segments). *A* = pulmonary artery; *SV* = superior pulmonary veins; *IV* = inferior pulmonary veins. (Redrawn from Sweet RH: Surgical anatomy of the thorax. In Thoracic Surgery. Philadelphia, WB Saunders, 1950)

face epithelium and from the bronchial mucous glands make up 90% to 95% of lung cancers.[207] Approximately 2% to 4% of these tumors will be a combination of squamous and glandular elements and are called adenosquamous cell carcinoma.

These various cell types have different natural histories and responses to therapy. Therefore, correct histologic identification of the cell type is a cornerstone of treatment planning. This is best accomplished by obtaining adequate amounts of tumor material for both histologic and cytologic evaluation. If discrepancies occur in these studies, it is important to have the material reviewed by a pathologist experienced in the histologic typing of lung cancer.

INCIDENCE OF TYPES

Estimates of the incidence of the four major cell types depend on the source of the pathologic materials reviewed (*e.g.*, biopsy, cytology, surgical resection, or autopsy) (Table 22-11). There appears to have been a shift in incidence of the histologic types over the past 20 years, with a fall in the fraction of cases of epidermoid cancer and a rise in the

TABLE 22-9. Bronchopulmonary Segments

Right Lung		*Left Lung*	
		Upper Lobe	
Jackson–Huber	Boyden	Jackson–Huber	Boyden
Apical	1	Apical–posterior	1–3
Anterior	2	Anterior	2
Posterior	3		
		Superior lingular	4
		Inferior lingular	5
		Middle Lobe	
Lateral	4	Medial	5
		Lower Lobe	
Superior	6	Superior	6
Medial basal	7	Anteriomedial	7–8
Anterior basal	8	Lateral basal	9
Lateral basal	9	Posterior basal	10
Posterior basal	10		

Jackson CL, Huber JF: Correlated applied anatomy of bronchial tree and lungs with system nomenclature. Dis Chest 9:319–326, 1943; Boyden EA: Segmental Anatomy of the Lungs. New York, McGraw-Hill, 1955.

TABLE 22-10. WHO Classification of Malignant Pleuropulmonary Neoplasms

I. Epidermoid carcinoma
II. Small cell carcinoma
    1. Fusiform
    2. Polygonal
    3. Lymphocyte-like
    4. Others
III. Adenocarcinoma
    1. Bronchogenic (with or without mucin formation)
        a. Acinar
        b. Papillary
    2. Bronchioloalveolar
IV. Large cell carcinoma
    1. Solid tumor with mucin
    2. Solid tumor without mucin
    3. Giant cell
    4. Clear cell
V. Combined epidermoid and adenocarcinomas
VI. Carcinoid tumors
VII. Bronchial gland tumors
    1. Cylindromas
    2. Mucoepidermoid tumors
VIII. Papillary tumors of the surface epithelium
IX. "Mixed" tumors and carcinosarcomas
X. Sarcomas
XI. Unclassified
XII. Melanoma

Kreyberg L: Histologic typing of lung tumors. In Kreyberg L (ed): International Histologic Classification of Tumors, No. 1, pp 19–26. Geneva, World Health Organization, 1967; Sobin LH: The World Health Organization's histological classification of lung tumors: A comparison of the first and second editions. Cancer Detect Prev 5:391–406; Yesner R, Gerstl B, Auerbach O: Application of the World Health Organization classification of lung carcinoma to biopsy material. Ann Thorac Surg 1:33–49, 1965; Matthews MJ: Morphologic classification of bronchogenic carcinoma. Cancer Chemother Rep 3:229–302, 1973.

percentage of adenocarcinomas.[208,209] This change is partly a result of the rise in the incidence of lung cancer in women, who have more adenocarcinomas than epidermoid cancers. However, an increase in adenocarcinomas also has been seen in men.

EMBRYOLOGY AND ANATOMY OF PATHOGENESIS

Embryologically, the laryngotracheobronchial tree is a ventral endodermal foregut derivative lined with five or more types of epithelial cells that form a pseudostratified mucosal sheath resting on a basement membrane.[210] As the embryonic lung diverticulum branches to form bronchopulmonary buds, splanchnic mesenchyme surrounds these structures and gives rise to the fibroelastic, vascular muscular, and cartilaginous components of the lung and forms the visceral pleura. The parietal pleura is derived from the corresponding somatic mesenchyme.

Mucus-secreting goblet cells, ciliated cells, brush border cells, short basal or reserve cells, and granular basal cells that rest on the basement membrane, all of which can be distinguished by electron microscopy, give the mucosa a pseudostratified appearance. The granular basal cells are called Kulchitsky or K-type cells. They have neurosecretory granules that can synthesize polypeptide hormones or biogenic amines and thus resemble small cell carcinomas.[211]

The cell of origin for each type of lung cancer is currently being re-examined. *In fact, the finding of several types of differentiation within a tumor or even within a given tumor cell suggests a common stem cell for all types of lung cancer.*

Lung cancer arises most often in segmental and subsegmental bronchi in response to repeated injury and chronic inflammation.[208] At segmental bronchial bifurcations, the epithelium is particularly susceptible to injury, and carcinogens may be deposited in these areas.[212] The carcinogens implicated in this process include the constituents of tobacco smoke, radioisotopes, asbestos, polycyclic hydrocarbons, haloethers, nickel, chromium, inorganic arsenic, iron ore, printing inks, and possibly other occupational and atmospheric pollutants discussed earlier.[213] Initially, basal cells respond to injury by proliferating to generate mucin-secreting goblet cells. When there is added injury, the columnar cells are replaced by orderly metaplastic stratified squamous epithelium. Finally, the epithelium becomes disorganized, and nuclear atypia and mitoses are seen in the basal half of the mucosa, findings that are called atypical metaplasia or

TABLE 22-11. Incidence of Major Histologic Types of Lung Cancer

Histologic Type	*Biopsy Cytology** *(n = 4107)*	*Surgical Specimens†* *(n = 1,206)*	*Autopsy‡* *(n = 1080)*	*Mayo Clinic§* *(n = 2926)*	*Johns Hopkins‖* *(n = 435)*
			% of cases		
Epidermoid carcinoma	45	64	33	34	39
Adenocarcinoma	22	16	25	26	19
Large cell carcinoma	11	9	16	16	20
Small cell carcinoma	19	19	25	22	19
Other (*e.g.*, bronchioloalveolar or mixed)	3	2	1	2	2

*Yesner R et al, Ann Thorac Surg 1:33–49, 1965; Matthews MJ, Gordon PR. In Straus MJ (ed): Lung Cancer Clinical Diagnosis and Treatment. New York: Grune & Stratton, 1977; Mountain CF et al, Am J Roentgenol Rad Ther Nucl Med 120:130–138, 1974; Feinstein AR et al, Chest 66:225–229, 1974.

†Matthews MJ, Gordon PR, In Straus MJ (ed): Lung Cancer Clinical Diagnosis and Treatment. New York: Grune & Stratton, 1977; Hinson KFW, Miller AB, Tall R, Cancer 35:399–405, 1975.

‡Matthews MJ, Gordon PR, In Straus MJ (ed): Lung Cancer Clinical Diagnosis and Treatment. New York: Grune & Stratton, 1977; Auerbach O, Garfinkel L, Parks UR, Chest 67:382–387, 1975.

§Rosenow EC III, Carr DT, CA 29:233–246, 1979.

‖Katlic M, Carter D, Prog Cancer Res Ther 11:143–150, 1979.

dysplasia. When this process occurs throughout the full thickness of the mucosa, a diagnosis of carcinoma *in situ* (intraepithelial carcinoma) is made. Finally, the basement membrane is violated by the neoplastic cells, and frank infiltration of neoplastic cells into the underlying stroma follows.[214-216] This process may take 10 to 20 years and represents the first phase of the natural history of lung cancer. The site of origin of a small cell cancer usually is difficult to identify. These tumors infiltrate the submucosa, while squamous metaplasia or dysplasia is seen in the overlying bronchial mucosa. In many cases, it also is difficult to distinguish whether adenocarcinomas or large cell carcinomas come from bronchial surface epithelium or the underlying mucous glands.

Marked atypia of cells in sputum cytology specimens has been felt to be highly suggestive of later appearances of lung cancer. However, this idea has recently been called into question.[217] Sixteen cases of marked atypia were found in 292 male smoking uranium miners. Four of these men had cells highly suspicious for malignancy, and three of these went on to develop lung cancer. However, the remaining 13 cases all reverted to mild atypia or normal cytologies with follow-up over an average period of 54 months. *These studies suggest that marked atypia will not by itself be useful as a marker in chemoprevention studies or early detection trials.* However, histologic evidence suggests that bronchial epidermoid metaplasia can regress with smoking cessation and retinoid treatment.[218] Forty heavy cigarette smokers had multiple fiberoptic bronchoscopy-directed biospies and were scored for a metaplasia index. They were then treated with a retinoid derivative orally (etretinate 25 mg/day) for 6 months and rebiopsied. Four of the patients stopped smoking, and they had complete regression of their metaplasia, whereas the remaining patients had significant reduction in the metaplasia despite their continuing to smoke.

Epidermoid and small cell carcinomas are usually central in location, whereas *adenocarcinomas and large cell tumors are often peripheral* and associated with pulmonary conditions that cause lung destruction, fibrosis, reconstruction of the airways into nonfunctional spaces, and hyperplasia of pneumocytes. Chronic interstitial lung diseases (*i.e.*, scleroderma, rheumatoid disease, sarcoidosis, interstitial pneumonitis, pulmonary scars and fibrosis from pulmonary infarcts, tuberculosis, chronic abscesses, and other necrotizing pulmonary diseases) have been noted as predisposing factors.[219-223] With progressive pulmonary fibrosis, avascularity, local tissue anoxia, and proliferation of the bronchioloalveolar epithelium are stimulated, resulting in adenomatous foci that frequently become metaplastic and mucus producing.[208] Exogenous agents involved in these processes include asbestos, cadmium, beryllium, gases, mineral oils, viruses, mycobacteria, and pneumoconiotic dusts.[213]

EPIDERMOID CARCINOMA

Epidermoid tumors grow centrally toward the main-stem bronchus and locally invade underlying bronchial cartilage, adjoining lung parenchyma, and lymph nodes. The bronchial mucosa usually shows squamous metaplasia, dysplasia, or frank intraepithelial neoplasia, processes that provide evidence for the primary nature of the tumor in the lung.[208]

ADENOCARCINOMA

Most adenocarcinomas are located peripherally, unrelated to bronchi except by contiguous growth or lymph node metastases. The tumors provoke a desmoplastic response, present as firm, localized, subpleural masses, and tend to invade the overlying pleura. Tumors arising from the bronchial epithelium present as thick, firm, gray–white pipestemmed structures with narrowed lumina. It may be difficult to distinguish the tumors in the lung from cancer of the pancreas, kidney, breast, or colon that metastasize to bronchi.[208] Adenocarcinomas arising from bronchia mucous glands form lobules of neoplastic glands that may produce mucin or exhibit a cribriform pattern.

BRONCHIOLOALVEOLAR CARCINOMA

Bronchioloalveolar carcinoma presents either as single nodules or in a multinodular pattern. The latter presentation has suggested that there are multiple primaries.[224,225] Papillary configurations may be seen in adenocarcinomas arising from bronchial surface epithelium and in tumors associated with scars, as well as in the classic bronchioloalveolar carcinoma. Psammoma bodies are noted in 5% to 15% of papillary tumors. Bronchioloalveolar cancer in the lung may be indistinguishable histologically from metastases to the lung from other adenocarcinomas, such as those of the kidney, ovary, thyroid, uterus, or colon, although ultrastructural studies suggest that the cell of origin is the bronchiolar lining cell, with subcellular features of the Clara and ciliated epithelial cells.[226] Some of these tumors have osmiophilic lamellar bodies and demonstrate surfactant production, relating them to the type II pneumocyte. The tumor is similar to the viral-induced pulmonary carcinoma of sheep.[227] Mice, horses, and guinea pigs have similar diseases as well.

Bronchioloalveolar carcinoma usually is reported to be associated with prior lung disease leading to fibrosis, including repeated pneumonias, idiopathic pulmonary fibrosis, granulomata, inflammation, asbestosis, fibrosing alveolitis, scleroderma, and Hodgkin's disease.[219,228,229] However, in some isolated reports, no antecedent lung damage has been found. The cancer also is found in families with other tumors and has been seen in identical twins.[230,231] Bronchioloalveolar carcinoma is not correlated with smoking.[232] Because of its association with fibrosing lung disease, any new roentgenographic mass or persistent infiltrate in such patients should be suspected of being bronchioloalveolar carcinoma.[233]

LARGE CELL CARCINOMA

Large cell carcinomas present as large peripheral subpleural lesions with necrotic or cavitary surfaces. These tumors usually are unrelated to bronchi except by contiguous growth, and they have a tendency to invade pulmonary parenchyma and the overlying pleura. In small foci, recognizable attempts at differentiation, usually glandular, may be identified, but the predominant anaplastic nature of the tumor is overwhelming. Microscopically, these tumors are a composite of all the anaplastic features of poorly differentiated squamous carcinomas and adenocarcinomas. A subtype of large cell carcinoma, giant cell carcinoma, is composed of bizarre cells with giant nuclei and very large quantities of cytoplasm that often show phagocytic activity or contain mucin vacuoles. Approximately 30% of lung cancers have areas of clear cell changes, whereas more than two-thirds of large cell carcinomas may show these changes, and almost one-third of adenocarcinomas and epidermoid carcinomas also will show these features.[234] The clear cells stain strongly for glycogen but weakly for mucin. However, it is rare to find a tumor composed solely of clear cells. The prognosis of tumors containing large areas of clear cells is no different from that of the other common lung cancer histologic types; the importance of recognizing the clear cell type of primary lung cancer is to differentiate it from metastatic renal carcinoma.

SMALL CELL CARCINOMA

Small cell carcinomas appear as submucosal infiltrates in the early phase of the disease. The mucosa may be normal or slightly lifted by a plaque that obliterates normal bronchial markings. In advanced stages, bronchial lumina may be obstructed by extrinsic compression or endobronchial tumor.[235] Silver stains are focally positive in approximately half the cases, and neurosecretory granules are usually found on electron micrographic studies.[208] However, electron microscopic findings, including absence of neurosecretory granules, do not predict responses to therapy so long as the light microscopic criteria for the diagnosis of small cell lung cancer are fulfilled.[236]

The 1981 WHO classification divides small cell lung cancer into three subtypes, including the oat cell or lymphocytelike, the intermediate, and the combined (oat cell combined with squamous or adenocarcinoma).[237] The classic oat cell type is characterized by small round or oval cells with darkly staining nuclei, indistinct or absent nucleoli, and scanty cytoplasm. The intermediate type is comprised of larger cells with a lower nuclear : cytoplasmic ratio and polygonal or fusiform nuclei. All subtypes of small cell carcinoma consist of cells that are at least two to three times the size of a mature lymphocyte and exhibit the characteristic features of "salt and pepper" distribution of chromatin, nuclear molding, areas of cellular necrosis, and deposition of DNA-derived material on elastic fibrils.[208] Numerous atypical mitoses may be identified. Mixtures of lymphocyte-like and intermediate subtypes of small cell cancer frequently are seen in a single tumor. The histologic distinction between small cell and non-small cell cancers is of great clinical importance. The intermediate subtype of small cell cancer may sometimes be confused with poorly differentiated epidermoid carcinoma, large cell cancer, or poorly differentiated adenocarcinoma, particularly in metastatic sites. Also, some tumors form distinct tubules as well as rosettes and can be confused with adenocarcinomas. In some small cell tumors, prominent clusters of anaplastic large cells may be seen; in others, nests of squamous cells may be found.

Despite their submucosal location, small cell carcinomas often have malignant cells exfoliated into sputa and cytologic washings, and bronchoscopy yields malignant cells in more than 90% of patients with clinically apparent disease.[235] With well-preserved material, cytologic diagnosis appears as accurate as tissue diagnosis.[238] Other features of clinicopathologic interest in small cell cancer include the presence of marked osteoblastic activity in a minority of patients with bony metastases, with new bone formation similar to that in prostate and breast cancer metastases; pancreatic involvement from peripancreatic nodal disease associated focal acute pancreatitis and possibly severe fat necrosis; and a significant number of metastases to endocrine organs (*i.e.*, thyroid in 8%, pituitary in 15%, testes in 7%, and parathyroid in 1%).[208,213,235–242]

CLINICOPATHOLOGIC CORRELATION WITH HISTOLOGIC TYPE

Differences in long-term survival rates according to the histologic type of lung cancer have been analyzed in a large number of patients (Table 22-12). In most instances, these patients have been treated with local modalities (*i.e.*, surgery and radiotherapy). The figures for small cell lung cancer have changed with the advent of intensive combination chemotherapy. At present, patients with epidermoid cancers have the best survival, followed by those with adenocarcinomas and large cell carcinomas. Until recently, it was rare for a patient with small cell carcinoma to survive for 5 years.

Epidermoid cancer is more common in males; adenocarcinoma is more common in females. An equal sex distribution exists for the other cell types. On the whole, females have a better survival rate than do males, independent of the stage of cancer.[243] Epidermoid and small cell cancers have a much higher incidence in smokers than nonsmokers, whereas adenocarcinoma is the predominant type in nonsmokers (Table 22-13). This may be accounted for in part by the inclusion of adenocarcinomas from an "unknown primary" with metastases to the lung in the nonsmoker group. *In any event, in women with a lung adenocarcinoma, it is important to rule out a primary breast or gynecologic tumor that would need different therapy than a primary lung cancer.*

The location of the primary tumor will determine the presenting signs and symptoms and dictate the methods for

TABLE 22-12. Overall 5-Year Survival (%) for Major Histologic Types of Lung Cancer

Histologic Type	*All Cases (n = 2155)*	*Resected (n = 835)*	*Per cent Resectable*
Epidermoid carcinoma	25	37	60
Adenocarcinoma	12	27	38*
Large cell carcinoma	13	27	38*
Small cell carcinoma	1	0	11

Matthews MJ, Gordon PR: Morphology of pulmonary and pleural malignancies. In Straus MJ (ed): Lung Cancer: Clinical Diagnosis and Treatment. New York: Grune & Stratton, 1977; Mountain CF, Carr DT, Martini N et al: Staging of lung cancer 1979. American Joint Committee for Cancer Staging and End Results Reporting, Task Force on Lung Cancer, Chicago, 1980.

*Combined in AJC report.

TABLE 22-13. Incidence According to Sex and Smoking Status of Major Histologic Types of Lung Cancer at the Mayo Clinic

Histologic Type	*Male* (*n* = 2411)	*Female* (*n* = 515)	*Smokers* (*n* = 2708)	*Never Smoked* (*n* = 218)
		% of cases		
Epidermoid carcinoma	37	18	36	9
Adenocarcinoma	22	44	23	64
Large cell carcinoma	17	12	16	14
Small cell carcinoma	22	20	23	3
Bronchioloalveolar	2	6	2	9

Rosenow EC III, Carr DT: Bronchogenic carcinoma. CA 29:233–246, 1979.

obtaining a histologic diagnosis (Table 22-14). Proximal tumors usually have histologic material obtained by bronchoscopy or sputum cytology, whereas distal lesions usually are detected on screening chest films and thus are diagnosed by transbronchial or percutaneous needle biospy or at the time of resection.

In surgically resected specimens, small cell cancer involves the lymph nodes in most cases, whereas the nonsmall cell cancers have lymph node involvement in approximately 40% of cases (see Table 22-14). Epidermoid carcinomas (28%) and large cell carcinomas (22%) cavitate more frequently than do adenocarcinomas (12%) or small cell carcinomas (8%).[244] In contrast, adenocarcinomas and large cell carcinomas show visceral pleural invasion more often than do other types of surgically resected tumors because of their peripheral location.

Approximately 20% to 30% of lung cancers studied histologically are associated with scars from other lung injury (called "pulmonary scar carcinoma").[245] The majority of these (58%–88%) are adenocarcinomas or bronchioloalveolar cancers and occur in peripheral locations. Chest roentgenographs often (50% of cases) are negative, and bronchoscopy and sputum cytology are ineffective as initial diagnostic tools. These patients frequently present with nonpulmonary symptoms of metastatic disease, and the chest lesion is clinically undetectable. However, when the primary is resectable, their survival rate is similar to that of other patients of similar postsurgical stage.[246]

The clinicopathologic correlation of therapeutic importance for bronchioloalveolar carcinoma relates to the number of nodules (solitary or multicentric) and the degree of differentiation.[247] Lymph node metastases occur in only 23% of patients with solitary nodules but in more than 77% of patients with multicentric lesions. A majority (84%) of patients with solitary nodules have well-differentiated tumors. In contrast, only 45% of multicentric tumors are as well differentiated. Some 80% of poorly differentiated tumors have lymph node metastases at presentation, whereas only 20% to 30% of the more highly differentiated tumors show this spread.

ACCURACY OF HISTOLOGIC DIAGNOSIS

The first principle of treatment is a correct histologic diagnosis. The quality and quantity of the samples are important for such diagnosis. Common problems for the clinical pathologist are crush artifact, poor fixation, overstaining, or inadequate amounts of materials. Crushing artifact in a needle aspiration must not be mistaken for small cell carcinoma, as sometimes occurs. A diagnosis of malignancy may be based on a cytologic sample, and differentiated malignancies and small cell carcinomas may be diagnosed as readily and as accurately in cytologic specimens as in small biopsies.[248,249] However, a histologic (tissue block) diagnosis is strongly preferred.

A significant problem in the use of histologic criteria when

TABLE 22-14. Anatomical Location of Primary Tumors in Relation to Histologic Type of Lung Cancer and Frequency of Early Regional Spread

Histologic Type	*Proximal Location*		*Resected Surgical Specimen* — *Lymph Node Involvement*		*Resected Surgical Specimen* — *Visceral Pleural Involvement*	
	n	*%*	*n*	*%*	*n*	*%*
Epidermoid carcinoma	275	81	158	42	109	33
Adenocarcinoma	140	29	109	41	59	59
Large cell carcinoma	113	49	65	42	27	52
Small cell carcinoma	96	83	29	72	13	15
Overall	641	63	631	48	211	41

Vincent RG, Pickren JW, Lane WW et al: The changing histopathology of lung cancer: A review of 1682 cases. Cancer 39:1647–1655, 1977; Rilke F, Carbone A, Clemente C et al: Surgical pathology of resectable lung cancer. Prog Cancer Res Ther 11:129–142, 1979.

determining prognosis and types of treatment is the degree of interobserver and intraobserver variability in reading the same specimens. In addition, there is heterogeneity within the tumor itself in both the primary and metastatic sites.[238,244,250,251] Tumors often show features of several histologic subtypes, suggesting a morphologic continuum. This is a particular problem with small cell carcinoma.[252,253] Some series have reported imperfect correlations between cytologic and subsequent histologic diagnosis of the cell type, and misleading results may be obtained from biopsy of cavitary lesions and necrotic tumors.[254] The distinction between small cell carcinoma and the non-small cell types is consistent in 90% of cases when adequate material is reviewed by well-trained observers experienced in lung cancer pathology.[244] The assignment of tumors to each of the major types of non-small cell cancer is less consistent (approximately 70%). Attempts to subdivide the four major types currently are subject to an even larger degree of interobserver variation.[255,256] This problem is particularly marked in the diagnosis of specimens of small cell carcinoma mixed with other major histologic types, especially large cell carcinoma. It may be necessary to obtain the opinion of several pathologists unless biochemical or immunologic markers of small cell cancer can be assessed. If several pathologists agree that a definite small cell component exists, the patient probably should be considered to have small cell carcinoma. *At present, we believe that the only treatment-related decisions that should be based on histologic type are the distinction between small cell cancer and the other, non-small cell, types and possibly identification of well-differentiated epidermoid lesions, which often appear amenable to aggressive local therapy.*

Epidermoid and adenocarcinoma have been subdivided in the WHO classification into groups that exhibit different degrees of histologic differentiation. Squamous tumors present with about equal frequency as well-, moderately, or poorly differentiated lesions, whereas adenocarcinomas present more frequently as poorly differentiated lesions.[244] At present, there appears to be a 5-year survival advantage for well- and moderately differentiated epidermoid carcinomas (20%–39%) compared with poorly differentiated lesions. There is no difference between well- and moderately differentiated (23%) and poorly differentiated (26%) adenocarcinomas.[256,257]

In studies of small cell carcinoma subtyping, large numbers of patients were evaluated extensively before therapy, then treated with intensive combination chemotherapy or with chemotherapy and radiotherapy. With one exception, no difference was seen between subtypes with respect to stage of disease, sites of metastases, response to therapy or number of complete responses, response duration, or survival.[252,253,258] When histologic subtypes in the primary biopsy specimen were compared with the subtype of other pathologic specimens from the same patient, concordance was present in only 71%, whereas two or three histologic subtypes were present in the remaining 29%.[259] The clinical implications of the combined subtype are unknown. At present, there appears to be no reason to base decisions on the presence of histologic subtypes of small cell carcinoma, with one exception: the mixed small cell–large cell carcinoma variant that occurs in approximately 6% to 14% of small cell lung cancer cases.[260,261] This type has a lower overall response to combination chemotherapy, a lower complete response rate, and a shorter median survival than small cell carcinoma without large cell components. The oat cell and intermediate subtypes have similar clinical features and prognosis, and because the oat cell subtype (which is never observed in vitro) may be an artifact of tissue fixation, a new subclassification of small cell carcinoma that combines these two subtypes as "classic small cell carcinoma" is in preparation. Cell biology and autopsy studies indicate that a transition can occur between small cell carcinoma and large cell carcinoma accompanied by a loss of expression of differentiated functions by the cells.[262–264] The cells with small cell carcinoma histology express the amine precursor uptake and decarboxylation (APUD) properties of high levels of DOPA decarboxylase (L-aromatic amino decarboxylase), formaldehyde-induced fluorescence after exposure to 5-hydroxytryptophane, and neurosecretory granules, whereas the large cell variants do not.[264] Recent molecular biology studies have shown that many of the large cell variants of small cell carcinoma (SCLC-*V* cells) have amplification of the c-*myc* oncogene and express large amounts of c-*myc* messenger RNA. Thus one mechanism of producing these histologic and biochemical variants with a poor prognosis may be oncogene amplification. Autopsy studies at Johns Hopkins and the NCI conducted on 131 patients after intensive chemotherapy or chemoradiotherapy for small cell carcinoma showed that 27% of the tumors also had a large cell, giant cell, squamous cell, tubular, or carcinoid component; 4% were pure squamous cell carcinoma without small cell elements; 3% were pure large cell tumors; and 1% were pure adenocarcinoma.[262,263,265] Thus, in a very large percentage of cases, other histologic types of lung cancer are found at autopsy. At the Finsen Institute (Copenhagen), the 13% of small cell carcinoma patients with non-small cell components at autopsy had shorter survival than patients with pure small cell lung cancer on postmortem microscopic examination.[266] The presence of the different histologic types of lung cancer could reflect the presence of separate primary tumors or the presence of a common stem cell that can differentiate along several pathways. These possibilities will have to be resolved by cell biology, cloning, and chromosome studies.

NEWER METHODS OF PATHOLOGIC DIAGNOSIS

New findings in cellular biology should eventually allow pathologists to distinguish small cell from non-small cell lung cancer, as well as subtype lung cancers by tests other than light microscopy. It has been demonstrated clearly that small cell tumors express the peptide hormone GRP, L-DOPA decarboxylase, neuron-specific enolase, and the BB isozyme of creatine kinase, as well as dense core granules by electron microscopy, whereas non-small cell tumors much less frequently express these markers. A list of these and other distinctions is provided in the section on the cellular biology of lung cancer. As biochemical and immunologic reagents become generally available, and as these markers are studied in prospective clinical trials, their utility in diagnosis and patient management can be assessed and documented.

New approaches for the identification of malignant cells

include isolation of antibodies reactive with lung cancer but not with normal respiratory epithelium or with products produced by lung cancer cells. Antisera against lung cancer antigens that react with antigens of apparent endodermal and neural crest derivation have been described.[267] Recently, monoclonal antibodies with specificity for lung cancer cells have been prepared.[268–270] Another approach involves identifying cells with increased DNA content, a condition frequently seen in malignant cells. There appears to be a progressive increase in the amount of DNA per cell in squamous metaplastic cells or in neoplastic cells exhibiting progressive amounts of atypia.[271] Combining DNA staining with new cell-sorting instruments will allow the screening of large numbers of cells by flow cytometry in individual sputum samples. Using flow cytometry, 83% of small cell and 85% of non-small cell patients' tumor specimens from metastatic sites were aneuploid.[272] A recent study utilizing flow cytometry of paraffin-embedded pathologic sections from 100 surgically treated patients with non-small cell lung cancer indicates that patients whose tumors had aneuploid DNA content had shorter survival.[273]

NATURAL HISTORY OF LUNG CANCER

Understanding the natural history of lung cancer is important for prevention, early detection, rationally planned initial curative or palliative therapy, anticipation of possible complications, and the institution of therapy at the time of relapse. The natural history of lung cancer begins with the exposure of a susceptible host to carcinogens, eventually leading to the cytologic changes of cellular atypia identifiable in cells exfoliated into the sputum. These changes progress to carcinoma *in situ*, then to frank invasion. Accurate definition of these early events is important to plan preventive therapy in future trials and for instituting surgery, radiotherapy, or chemotherapy in the patient with clinically occult disease. Information on early history will be provided from the mass screening program data described later in this chapter.

SIGNS AND SYMPTOMS OF LUNG CANCER

With the onset of local tumor growth and invasion, lung cancer can give rise to signs and symptoms as well as to chest radiograph or sputum cytology abnormalities (Table 22-15).[274] Findings may be the result of local tumor growth, invasion of adjacent structures, regional growth (from metastasis to peribronchial, hilar, mediastinal, and supraclavicular nodes) by way of lymphatic spread, growth in distant sites after hematogenous dissemination, or a remote effect of the tumor (paraneoplastic syndromes).

Unfortunately, by the time a sign, symptom, or visible nodule appears, dissemination to regional or distant lymph nodes or distant extranodal sites usually has occurred. This can be seen at autopsy when the patients die of other causes after a supposedly curative resection for lung cancer (Table 22-16). Patients with all histologic types of lung cancer sometimes had microscopic residual disease; these sites were frequently outside the areas where postoperative chest radiotherapy would have been directed. Small cell carcinoma in particular has a high frequency of extrathoracic metas-

TABLE 22-15. Common Signs and Symptoms of Lung Cancer

Symptoms secondary to central or endobronchial growth of the primary tumor
- Cough
- Hemoptysis
- Wheeze and stridor
- Dyspnea from obstruction
- Pneumonitis from obstruction (fever, productive cough)

Symptoms secondary to peripheral growth of the primary tumor
- Pain from pleural or chest wall involvement
- Cough
- Dyspnea on a restrictive basis
- Lung abscess syndrome from tumor cavitation

Symptoms related to regional spread of the tumor in the thorax by contiguity or by metastasis to regional lymph nodes
- Tracheal obstruction
- Esophageal compression with dysphagia
- Recurrent laryngeal nerve paralysis with hoarseness
- Phrenic nerve paralysis with hemidiaphragm elevation and dyspnea
- Sympathetic nerve paralysis with Horner's syndrome
- Eighth cervical and first thoracic nerves with ulnar pain and Pancoast's syndrome
- Superior vena cava syndrome from vascular obstruction
- Pericardial and cardiac extension with resultant tamponade, arrhythmia, or cardiac failure
- Lymphatic obstruction with pleural effusion
- Lymphangitic spread through lungs with hypoxemia and dyspnea

Cohen MH: Signs and symptoms of bronchogenic carcinoma. In Straus MJ (ed): Lung Cancer: Clinical Diagnosis and Treatment, pp 85–94. New York, Grune & Stratton, 1977.

TABLE 22-16. Incidence at Autopsy of Persistent Tumor After "Curative" Surgical Therapy for Lung Cancer in Patients Dying of Other Causes Within 30 Days Postoperatively

		Percentage with Persistent Tumor		
Cell Type	*No. of Patients*	*Total*	*Local Disease Only*	*Distant Metastases*
Epidermoid carcinoma	131	34	17	17
Adenocarcinoma	30	43	3	40
Large cell carcinoma	22	14	0	14
Small cell carcinoma	19	69	6	63

Matthews MJ, Kanhouwa S, Pickner J et al: Frequency of residual and metastatic tumors in patients undergoing curative surgical resection of lung cancer. Cancer Chemother Rep 3:63–67, 1973.

tases, followed by adenocarcinoma and then the other non-small-cell types. Often, these metastases were intra-abdominal.[275] Other data demonstrating the early metastatic behavior of lung cancer have been generated from analysis of surgical specimens. In non-small cell carcinoma, the approximate frequency of lymph node involvement in such specimens is 40%; invasion of veins occurs in 19%, invasion of arteries in 18%, and invasion of the visceral pleura in 44% (see Table 22-14).[244]

Excluding cases found by mass screening programs, most patients present with symptomatic disease. In 678 Yale-New Haven Hospital and Yale Veterans Administration patients, Feinstein found that 6% were asymptomatic, 27% had symptoms related to the primary tumor, 32% had symptoms of metastatic disease, and 34% had systemic symptoms that suggested tumor, such as anorexia, weight loss, and fatigue.[276] There was a significant difference in 5-year survival rate, with 18% of the asymptomatic, 12% of the primary symptomatic, 6% of the systemic symptomatic, and none of the patients with metastatic symptoms surviving 5 years.[276] Patients with a long history of symptoms related to their primary tumor had a better 5-year survival rate (16%) than those with a short duration of symptoms (9%), suggesting that some tumors may have an inherently more indolent course; this, in turn, may be related to their rate of growth. Of great interest was the correlation of symptomatic stage with anatomic stage. Here, there was an effect of symptoms independent of anatomic stage. *Thus, the accurate determination of signs and symptoms can be of prognostic value, and these features should be correlated with clinical and surgical pathologic evidence of disease when planning treatment and determining prognosis for individual patients.*

The frequency of the various presenting signs and symptoms will vary, depending on whether the series represents all patients presenting with lung cancer or the subpopulations selected for more limited disease, advanced disease, or from mass screening series. Recently, a large series of patients undergoing radical radiotherapy for cure contained a high incidence of asymptomatic patients with disease discovered on routine chest films and a lower percentage of patients with symptoms of regional spread or systemic symptoms compared with the Yale study (Table 22-17).[277]

Signs, symptoms, and radiographic findings in the chest are related to the central or peripheral location of the primary tumor, in addition to whether regional spread has occurred, both of which are related to the histologic type (Table 22-18, Fig. 22-3).[278] In general, epidermoid cancers have a central location, with atelectasis, pneumonitis (from bronchial obstruction), hilar adenopathy, and a tendency to cavitate; adenocarcinomas have a defined nodule in a periph-

TABLE 22-17. Manner of Presentation of Lung Cancer in 170 Patients Referred for Treatment with Radical Radiotherapy

Symptoms or Finding	*Percentage of Patients*
Routine chest radiograph (asymptomatic)	16
Primary tumor (total)	81
Hemoptysis	30
Cough	25
Dyspnea	11
Pneumonitis	8
Pain	6
Wheeze	2
Regional spread (total)	2
Dysphagia	1
Hoarseness	0.5
Systemic symptoms	
Weight loss	0.5

Coy P, Kennelly GM: The role of curative radiotherapy in the treatment of lung cancer. Cancer 45:698–702, 1980.

TABLE 22-18. Presenting Chest Roentgenologic Findings in Lung Cancer by T, N, and M Factor

Roentgen Finding	*Percentage with Finding*			
	Epidermoid Carcinoma	*Small Cell Carcinoma*	*Adenocarcinoma*	*Large Cell Carcinoma*
	(*n* = 338–585)	(*n* = 114–252)	(*n* = 135–301)	(*n* = 97)
Tumor (T) factor				
Nodule <4 cm	14	21	46	18
Nodule >4 cm	18	8	26	41
Peripheral location	29	26	65	61
Central location	64	74	5	42
Atelectasis	23	31	2	14
Pneumonitis	13	21	14	24
Cavitation	5	0	3	4
Pleural or chest wall	3	5	14	2
Lymph node (N) factor				
Hilar adenopathy	38	61	19 (40)*	32
Mediastinal adenopathy	5	14	9 (27)	10

Cohen MH: Signs and symptoms of bronchogenic carcinoma. In Straus MJ (ed): Lung Cancer: Clinical Diagnosis and Treatment, pp 85–94. New York, Grune & Stratton, 1977; Byrd RB, Carr DT, Miller WE et al: Radiographic abnormalities in carcinoma of the lung as related to histologic cell type. Thorax 24:573–575, 1969; Green N, Kurohara SS, George FW III et al: The biologic behavior of lung cancer according to histologic type. Radiol Clin Biol 41:160–170, 1972.

*Newer evidence suggests a large proportion of adenocarcinomas (numbers in parentheses) can present with hilar or mediastinal masses from involved lymph nodes on plain radiographs. (Woodring JH, Stelling CB, AJR 140:657–664, 1983.)

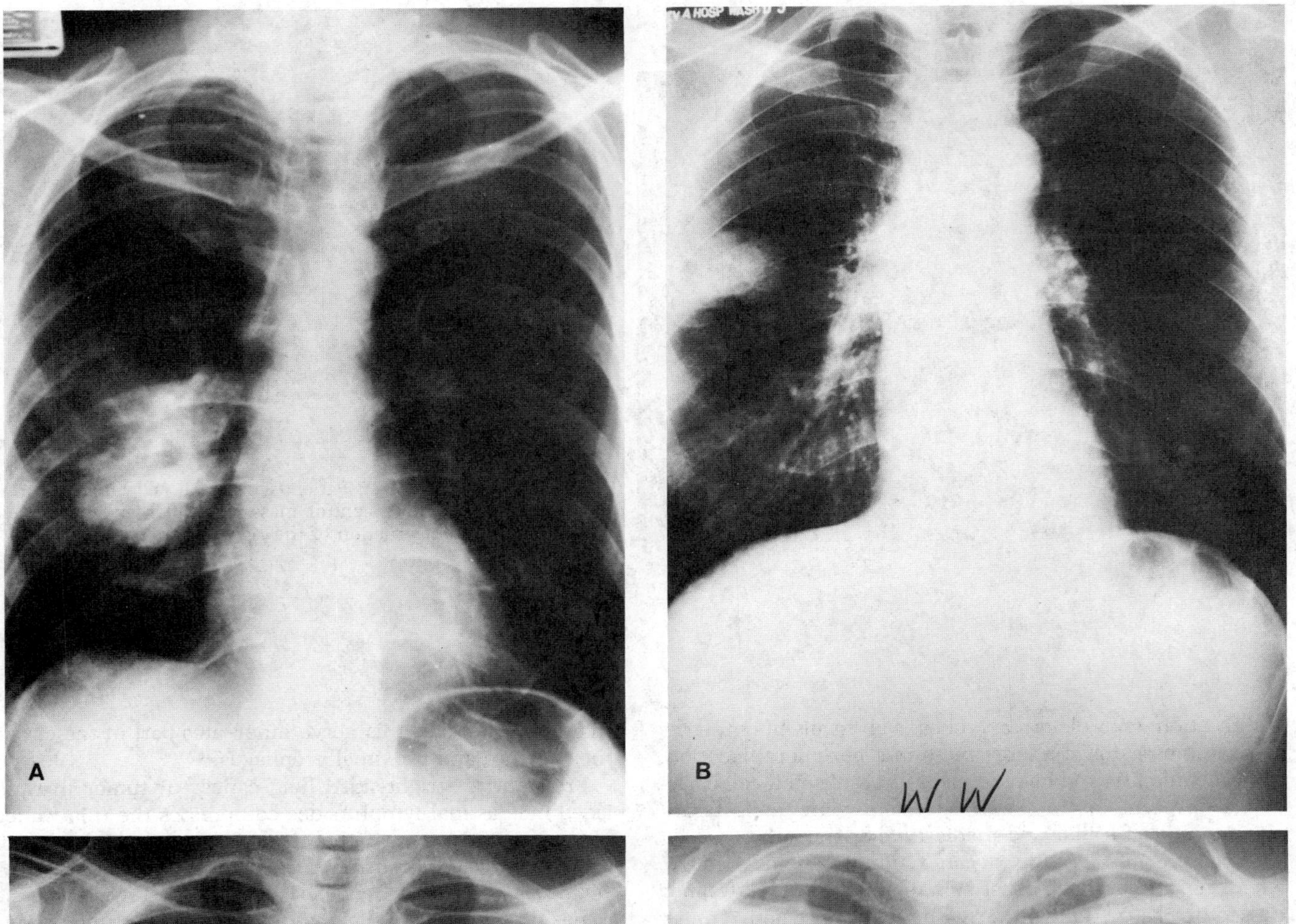

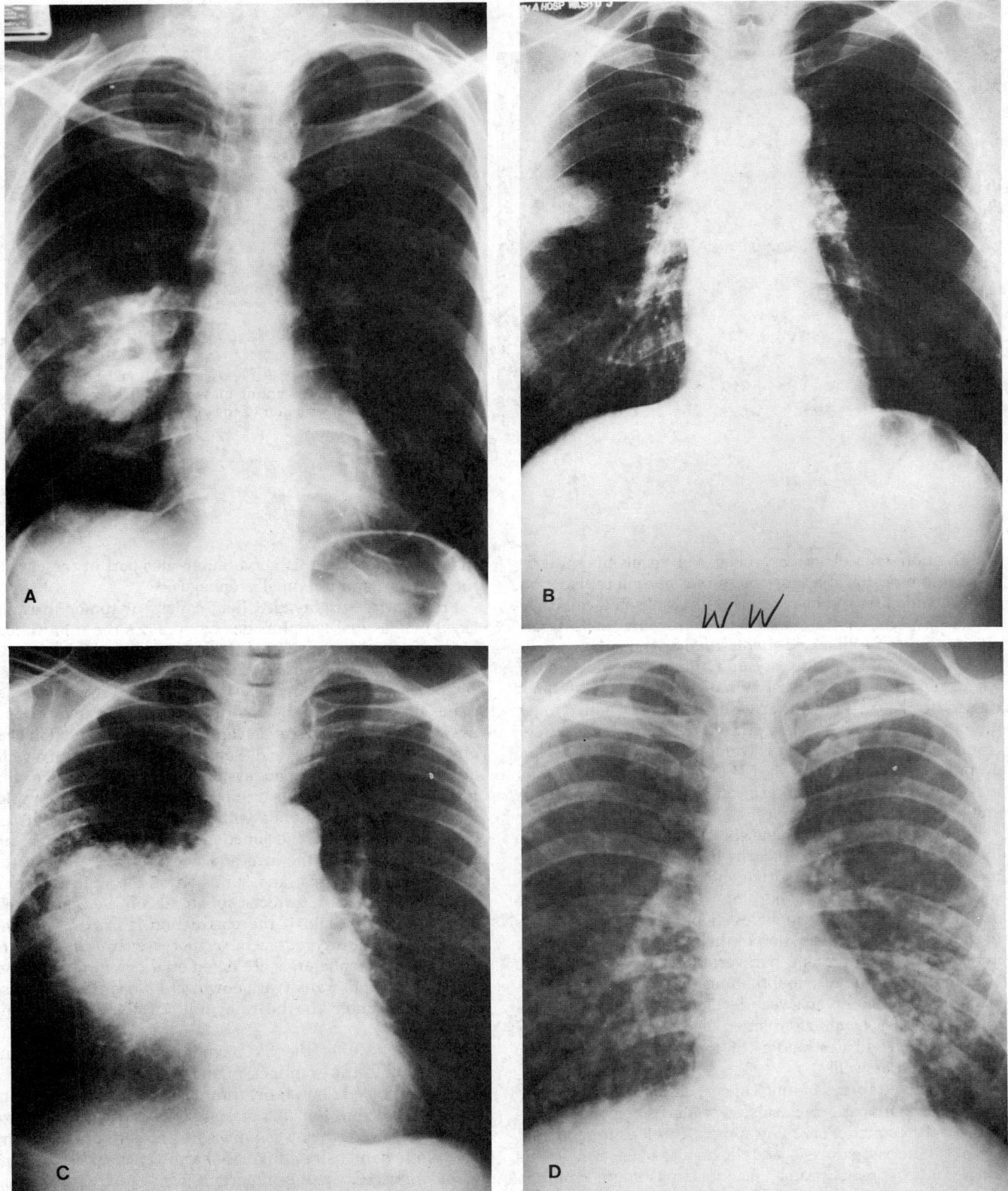

FIG. 22-3. Chest radiographs of patients with different histologic types of lung cancer. **A**. Patient with epidermoid lung cancer in which the tumor mass is centrally located, with beginning pneumonitis from bronchial obstruction, slight volume loss, and central cavitation. **B**. Patient with adenocarcinoma of the lung. The tumor denotes a peripherally located nodule with early pleural thickening suggesting involvement. **C**. Patient with large cell lung cancer containing a large mass with some peripheral pneumonitis. **D**. Patient with bronchioloalveolar carcinoma with multiple bilateral pulmonary nodules present for more than a year. (*Fig. 22-3 continues on p. 610*)

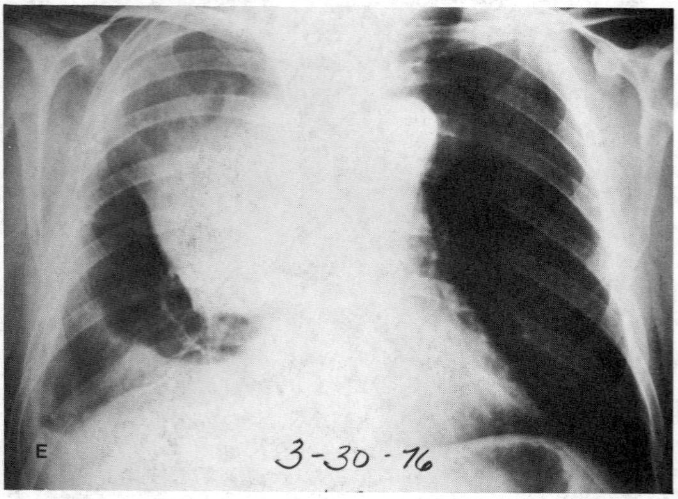

FIG. 22-3. *(continued)* **E** Patient with small cell lung cancer involving a large, bulky central mass with hilar and mediastinal adenopathy and obstruction of the right upper lobe.

eral location, with pleural and chest wall involvement; large cell carcinomas have a large mass in a peripheral location, with pneumonitis and hilar adenopathy; and small cell carcinomas present as a central lesion with atelectasis–pneumonitis and hilar and mediastinal adenopathy.

Symptoms of centrally located tumors include cough, wheezing, stridor, deep chest pain, hemoptysis, and dyspnea caused by obstruction with or without postobstructive pneumonitis. Peripheral lesions present with pain and cough from pleural or chest wall involvement, pleural effusion, and dyspnea on a restrictive basis.[274] Occasionally, large tumor masses, usually of epidermoid or large cell histology, cavitate and present as lung abscesses.

When a tumor (usually epidermoid carcinoma) presents in the apex of the lung and grows by local extension to involve the eighth cervical and first thoracic nerves, the Pancoast or superior sulcus tumor syndrome results.[278–281] The syndrome characteristically includes shoulder pain that radiates in the ulnar nerve distribution of the arm. With sympathetic nerve involvement from paravertebral tumor extension, Horner's syndrome of enophthalmus, ptosis, miosis, and ipsilateral loss of ability to sweat develops. With early involvement, mydriasis (pupillary dilation on the affected side) may result. Radiologic destruction of the first and second rib often is seen as well.

Intrathoracic spread of lung cancer, either by direct extension or by lymphatic metastases, produces regional symptoms in the thorax. Nerve entrapment can lead to recurrent laryngeal nerve paralysis and hoarseness. Because of its longer intrathoracic course, hoarseness is more common from involvement of the left than the right recurrent laryngeal nerve. Involvement of the phrenic nerve can lead to paralysis and elevation of the hemidiaphragm with resulting dyspnea. Compression of the esophagus by the tumor can lead to dysphagia. Also, with recurrent laryngeal nerve paralysis, dysphagia for both solids and liquids (and aspiration) may result because this nerve innervates part of the circoid musculature and proximal esophagus.[282]

Frequently, a right-sided lung cancer or tumor in right-sided mediastinal lymph nodes compresses the thin-walled, low-pressure system of the superior vena cava; hence, an obstructive vascular syndrome, *superior vena cava (SVC) syndrome* results.[274,283,284] The type of SVC syndrome depends on the level of the obstruction and the rapidity of its development. In epidermoid carcinoma, the obstruction usually develops gradually, and the patient presents with a well-developed collateral venous system visible on physical examination. With small cell carcinoma, the onset is more rapid, and frequently, collaterals will not have developed. If the obstruction is above the junction of the SVC and azygous veins, distention of the arm and neck veins; edema of the face, neck, and arms; and suffusion of the mucous membranes, with dilated, tortuous collaterals on the upper chest and back, will result. If the obstruction is proximal to the entrance of the azygous vein, a more severe clinical syndrome results: collaterals are noted on the anterior and posterior abdominal walls (with downward blood flow) because blood must enter the heart by way of the inferior vena cava.[284]

The diagnosis of the SVC syndrome usually is obvious from the physical examination and a review of chest films. Because of blood flow stasis, thrombosis occurs as a secondary phenomenon. For this reason, angiographic studies are not useful; although one can measure pressure in an arm and leg vein to demonstrate increased arm venous pressure, this is seldom necessary. It is important to be aware of the association of SVC syndrome with spinal cord compression from tumor extension and possibly vascular congestion.[285] A careful neurologic examination and review of roentgenographic films for bony abnormalities in this area are helpful because myelographic studies can be extremely difficult in these patients. Another association is that of SVC syndrome with tumor extension into the pericardium with resultant tamponade. It probably is useful to perform an echocardiogram in all patients with SVC obstruction as well as in those suspected of having pericardial tamponade. The treatment of SVC obstruction is discussed in Chapter 56, section 1.

Cardiac metastases occur in 15% to 35% of lung cancer patients.[286] Tumor extension into the pericardium and heart can result in pericardial tamponade, arrhythmias, and congestive heart failure. The exact frequency of these symptoms is unknown, largely because cardiac metastases only recently have been sought antemortem. One retrospective review showed that only 4% of patients who were proved pathologically to have cardiac metastases had both absence of clinical signs or symptoms related to the heart and a normal electrocardiogram.[287] Thus, the development of cardiac signs or symptoms in lung cancer patients should prompt consideration of heart involvement by tumor in the differential diagnosis. At autopsy, the pericardium is involved more frequently (88% of heart metastases) than the myocardium (45% of metastases, often by extension) for all cell types.[287] (Diagnosis and management of pericardial tamponade are discussed in Chapter 58). The development of arrhythmias, enlarging cardiac silhouette, increasing venous pressure, or congestive failure all can precede tamponade. The diagnosis is confirmed readily by echocardiography. The absence of the classic signs of tamponade (paradoxical pulse, grossly elevated venous pressure, distant heart sounds, friction rub, Kussmaul's sign, or low voltage on the electrocardiogram) should not stop the physician from obtaining an echocardiogram if there is any clinical reason to suspect cardiac involvement by tumor. The treatment and definitive diagnosis usually are accomplished together in the cardiac catheterization laboratory with pericardiocentesis and decompression followed by cytologic analysis of the pericardial fluid.

Bronchioloalveolar carcinoma can present on chest films as a solitary nodule, multiple nodules, persistent infiltrate, lobar consolidation, or a cavitary lesion.[233] Approximately 60% of cases present as solitary nodules and the remainder as multicentric disease.[225,227,232] However, what appears radiographically to be a single nodule is multifocal disease in 30% of cases. On chest films, 50% of these cancers have a "rabbit ear" or "tail" sign, with one or more fibrotic strands extending from the edge of a nodule toward the pleural surface.[288]

Patients with a persistent, unresolving, soft, fluffy infiltrate on chest films present a diagnostic problem as to whether this is inflammatory or neoplastic disease. Because the fluffy infiltrate represents alveolar involvement, an air bronchogram is seen on the film, and there is no airway obstruction or atelectasis.[233] True cavitation is rare, and what appears as cavities usually is alveolar spaces not involved by tumor.[233] Whereas a true solitary nodule is surgically curable, diffuse multinodular lesions represent an advanced stage of the disease, with survival being less than 1 to 2 years.[224,247]

Although bronchioloalveolar carcinomas can create signs and symptoms similar to those of other types of lung cancer (particularly adenocarcinoma), some findings particularly suggest this cell type. Oxygen transfer across capillary membranes may be impaired by the tumor cells growing along alveolar surfaces; hence, respiratory insufficiency with dyspnea and hypoxemia induces electrolyte disturbances and hypovolemia and predisposes to pneumonia.[233,286] In contrast to adenocarcinoma, pleura and chest wall invasion usually are not seen.[233]

EXTRATHORACIC METASTATIC DISEASE

Autopsy studies have found lung cancer metastases in nearly every organ system (Table 22-19). Again, there are differences in the frequency of metastases to different sites for each of the histologic types. At autopsy, extrathoracic metastases are epidermoid in 25% to 54%, adenocarcinoma in 50% to 82%, large cell carcinoma in 48% to 86%, and small cell carcinoma in 74% to 96%.[208,289] Common clinical problems related to distant metastatic disease are neurologic deficits, bone pain and pathologic fractures, and liver dysfunction and pain. Lymph node metastases usually occur in the supraclavicular region, but occasionally axillary and groin node lesions can be painful and break down and ulcerate if not treated. Except for the relatively small group of patients cured by primary treatment, lung cancer patients often will need therapy to palliate metastatic disease.

PARANEOPLASTIC SYNDROMES

The diagnosis, management, and pathophysiology of paraneoplastic syndromes are discussed in detail in Chapter 55. However, they frequently are encountered in the clinical management of lung cancer patients[290–295] and thus warrant comment here.

Table 22-20 lists the types and approximate frequencies of paraneoplastic syndromes.[296–300] In some cases, the syndrome is associated with a particular histologic type of lung cancer. Reversal of the clinical syndromes associated with successful treatment of the tumor in many cases provides documentation that the tumor caused the syndrome. The peptide hormones produced by lung cancer are the best understood mechanism underlying paraneoplastic syndromes, with classic examples being hyponatremia caused by production of arginine vasopressin and Cushing's syndrome secondary to excessive ACTH, both of which are associated with small cell lung cancer. Hypercalcemia related to the production of parathormone is associated with epidermoid carcinoma. However, some hormones such as GRP, documented in experimental animals to have many effects, as yet do not have a clinically associated syndrome.

Recently, the development of immune responses (best documented by detecting antibodies) in patients with lung cancer against normal tissue antigens that are also present on tumor cells have been described.[301] These include the Lambert–Eaton myasthenic syndrome, retinal blindness, and sensory neuronopathy. In the case of the Lambert–Eaton myasthenic syndrome (LEMS), this appears to be related to an antibody that blocks calcium-dependent voltage channels.[302]

The paraneoplastic syndromes sometimes are the first indication of a tumor's presence. In addition, many of the paraneoplastic syndromes can mimic metastatic disease and,

TABLE 22-19. Metastatic Patterns Found at Autopsy in Patients with Lung Cancer

Site of Metastasis	Percentage of Patients with Metastasis			
	Epidermoid Carcinoma	*Adenocarcinoma*	*Large Cell Carcinoma*	*Small Cell Carcinoma*
Number of patients studied	126	110	80	102
Hilar, mediastinal lymph nodes	77	80	84	96
Pleura	34	60	67	34
Chest wall	20	20	20	13
Diaphragm	9	11	15	14
Alternate lung	21	60	34	34
Cardiovascular system (total)	21	26	33	21
Pericardium	20	25	25	18
Myocardium	8	11	20	14
Limited to thorax	46	18	14	4
Liver	25	41	48	74
Adrenals	23	50	59	55
Bone	20	36	30	37
Kidney	21	23	28	22
CNS	18	37	25	29
Meninges	0	10	9	3
Dura	0	5	9	1
GI tract	12	5	20	14
Esophagus	13	8	3	14
Pancreas	4	12	22	41
Thyroid	4	2	6	18
Spleen	3	6	13	10
Parathyroid	1	0	0	1
Pituitary	1.6	4.5	3	15
Abdominal lymph nodes	10	24	30	52
Testes	0	0	0	7
Skin	0	0	6	0

Matthews MJ: Problems in morphology and behavior of bronchopulmonary malignant disease. In Israel L. Chahanian P (eds): Lung Cancer: Natural History, Prognosis, and Therapy, pp 23–62. New York, Academic Press, 1976.

unless detected, can lead to inappropriate palliative rather than curative treatment. For example, arterial emboli from *marantic endocarditis* can simulate brain metastases, as can cerebellar or cortical degeneration. *Hypertrophic pulmonary osteoarthropathy* with periostitis, in addition to clubbing, can cause pain, tenderness, and swelling over the affected bones and a positive bone scan, appearing as bone metastases. One of the most distressing syndromes is *weight loss and anorexia*, occurring in nearly one-third of patients and for which no mechanism currently is known. When noncachectic patients with non-small cell lung cancer are studied metabolically, they exhibit increases in protein turnover, glucose production, and muscle catabolism.[303] In addition, severe hypovitaminosis C, with values below the threshold for clinical scurvy, has been found in lung cancer patients.[304] Recent studies have shown that lung cancer patients with mild anemia have lower erythropoietin levels than control patients, supporting the concept of the lack of an appropriate erythropoietin response to anemia in these patients.[305]

OTHER MEDICAL PROBLEMS IN LUNG CANCER PATIENTS

Patients with lung cancer often have other medical problems, most commonly chronic obstructive pulmonary disease related to smoking, chronic bronchitis and emphysema, and cardiac problems related to coronary artery disease and pulmonary disease. In addition, it is not uncommon to see lung cancer patients in whom the disease is associated with ethanol abuse and related liver damage. All of these and the other medical problems commonly seen in the peak age range of lung cancer (55–65 years) have to be considered when planning and executing treatment. Often, the treatment (surgery, radiotherapy, or chemotherapy) can exacerbate these other medical problems. In addition, although lung cancer can metastasize and cause symptoms in many sites, new symptoms often are related to these nonmalignant medical problems. The challenge to the physician caring for such patients is to sort out these etiologies and institute the proper treatment.

As discussed earlier, multiple cancers frequently are seen in lung cancer patients, complicating treatment planning.[306,307] These cancers can be either synchronous or metachronous with the lung cancer. Common sites of secondary primary tumors include the lung, head and neck, esophagus, bladder, and pancreas (see earlier section for discussion).[306] These secondary neoplasms may have etiologies in common with lung cancer, such as smoking and possibly ethanol abuse.[308] *Because the development of a new primary cancer in a patient previously treated for lung cancer may simulate metastatic disease, it usually is important to document* (i.e., *biopsy*) *such a lesion, particularly if the patient could otherwise be cured of the first lung cancer.*

Conversely, a solitary lung shadow may appear either at the same time as or before or after a primary extrathoracic cancer. It should not be assumed automatically that this ab-

TABLE 22-20. Paraneoplastic Syndromes in Lung Cancer and the Histologic Type Predominantly Associated with the Syndrome*

- Systemic symptoms
  - Anorexia–cachexia (31%)
  - Fever (21%)
  - Suppressed immunity
- Endocrine (12%)
  - Ectopic parathyroid hormone: hypercalcemia (epidermoid)
  - Inappropriate secretion of antidiuretic hormone: hyponatremia (small cell)
  - Ectopic secretion of ACTH: Cushing's syndrome (small cell)
- Skeletal
  - Clubbing (29%)
  - Hypertrophic pulmonary osteoarthropathy: periostitis (1–10%) (adenocarcinoma)
- Neurologic–Myopathic (1%)
  - Myasthenic syndrome: Eaton–Lambert syndrome (small cell)
  - Peripheral neuropathy
  - Subacute cerebellar degeneration
  - Cortical degeneration
  - Polymyositis
  - Retinal blindness
- Coagulation–Thrombotic (1–4%)
  - Migratory thrombophlebitis, Trousseau's syndrome: venous thrombosis
  - Nonbacterial thrombotic (marantic) endocarditis: arterial emboli
  - Disseminated intravascular coagulation: hemorrhage
- Cutaneous (1%)
  - Dermatomyositis
  - Acanthosis nigricans
- Hematologic (8%)
  - Anemia
  - Granulocytosis
  - Leukoerythroblastosis
- Renal (<1%)
  - Nephrotic syndrome
  - Glomerulonephritis

* See Chapter 55 for a detailed discussion.

Odell WD, Wolfsen AR: Humoral syndromes associated with cancer. Ann Rev Med 29:379–406, 1978; Ayvazian LF: Extrapulmonary manifestations of tumors of the lung. Postgrad Med 63:93–99, 1978; Rassam JW, Anderson G: Incidence of paramalignant disorders in bronchogenic carcinoma. Thorax 30:86–90, 1975; Byrd RB, Divertie MB, Spittell JA: Bronchogenic carcinoma and thromboembolic disease JAMA 202:1019–1022, 1967; Greenfield GB, Schorsch HA, Shkolnik A: The various roentgen appearance of pulmonary hypertrophic osteoarthropathy. Am J Roentgenol Rad Ther Nucl Med 101:927–931, 1976; Croft PB, Wilkinson M: Carcinomatous neuromyopathy: its incidence in patients with carcinoma of the lung and breast. Lancet 1:184–188, 1965; Tyler HR: Paraneoplastic syndromes of nerve, muscle and neuromuscular junction. Ann NY Acad Sci 230:348–357, 1974; Heber D, Chlebowski RT, Ishibashi DE, Herrold JN, Block JB: Abnormalities in glucose and protein metabolism in noncachectic lung cancer patients. Cancer Res 42:4815–4819, 1982.

normality resulted from a metastasis from the extrathoracic cancer, because it frequently is a primary lung cancer. Because lung cancer has a worse prognosis than most other primary tumors, it is wise to approach a single pulmonary nodule (particularly in patients over 35 years of age who smoke) as though it were a primary lung cancer. Cahan, at the MSKCC, has studied this problem extensively and collected a large series of patients with multiple primaries, one of which was lung[309] (Table 22-21). Because of these data, the authors recommend vigorous evaluation for surgical resection of the lung nodule in patients with a single pulmonary nodule in addition to an extrathoracic primary neoplasm. This will establish a firm histologic diagnosis, potentially curing the patients of either the lung cancer or the other neoplasm. For example, after surgical treatment of patients with colon cancer and a single pulmonary nodule, the total 5-year survival rate free of cancer of either type was 22%; the total fraction of patients alive or dead with no evidence of cancer was 31%. Of interest was the fact that all of the primary group who survived later had a third primary tumor.[309]

SCREENING STUDIES FOR THE EARLY DIAGNOSIS OF LUNG CANCER

Although the overall incidence and mortality rates of lung cancer have been rising in parallel, the percentage of localized disease and overall resectability has remained approximately 20% over the past 30 years.[310] Local curative modalities (surgery and radiotherapy) have maintained an overall 5-year survival rate of 8% to 10% during the same period.[311] Staging studies have suggested that in the earlier stage of disease, more patients are likely to be cured of lung cancer, which has led to the hope that screening studies to detect early lung cancer will lead to earlier treatment and increased rates of cure. However, the actual survival benefits must be proved in prospective, controlled clinical trials.[311]

The highest incidence of lung cancer is seen in men over 40 years of age who have smoked 40 or more cigarettes a day for a long period.[308] Several mass roentgenographic screenings of such patients have been done at 4- to 6-month intervals. Early studies suggest that patients discovered by such screening have a 5-year survival rate of 15% to 18%, whereas control unscreened persons developing lung cancer have a 5-year survival rate of less than 10%.[312,313] The Philadelphia Pulmonary Neoplasm Research Project found lung cancer in 1.5% of the high-risk group they screened.[314] However, only 37% of the 94 lung cancers discovered were resectable; the 5-year survival rate for this group was 18% (7% for the entire group of cancers). Chest films and sputum cytology studies complement one another in early lung cancer diagnosis, detecting central tumors while cytologies and radiographs pick up peripheral lesions.[315] Following this lead, Johns Hopkins, the Mayo Foundation, MSKCC, and the University of Cincinnati have undertaken prospective randomized trials using chest films and sputum cytologies when screening men over 45 years of age who smoke one pack or more of cigarettes per day but who initially do not have signs or symptoms of lung cancer.[311,316,317]

The three radomized controlled trials conducted by Johns Hopkins Medical Institutions, the MSKCC, and the Mayo Clinic and sponsored by the NCI involving 31,360 men 45 years or older who smoked at least one pack of cigarettes daily and who were screened for early lung cancer have all shown that intensive screening with sputum cytology and chest films detects early lung cancer. However, this intense screening did not alter the mortality rate from lung cancer compared with standard recommendations for annual testing

TABLE 22-21. Probable Nature of a Solitary Lung Shadow with Known Cancer Elsewhere, MSKCC 1933–1972

Site of Other Primary Cancer	*No. of Cases*	*Ratio of New Lung Primary: Solitary Metastasis*
Head and neck (excluding skin)	168	15.8
Trachea and lung (all types)	51	11.8
Prostate	26	All new lung primaries
Urinary bladder	22	6.3
Stomach	7	All new lung primary
Breast	63	1.7
Colorectal	52	1.4
Kidney	20	1.2
Testicle	18	0.5
Bone sarcoma	23	0.13
Melanoma	36	0.24
Soft tissue sarcoma	37	0.06

Cahan WG: Multiple primary cancers of the lung, esophagus, and other sites. Cancer 40:1954–1960, 1977.

in such patients.[318,319] The Mayo Foundation first screened asymptomatic persons with chest films and sputum cytologies to detect prevalence cases (*i.e.*, cancer already present). They then randomized patients to an intensively screened group (chest film and sputum cytology every 4 months) and "unscreened" persons—those who were advised only to have a yearly chest film and sputum test.[311] The MSKCC group initially screened 10,400 men for signs and symptoms of lung cancer and then randomized patients to annual chest films with sputum cytologies every 4 months or to annual radiographs alone.[316] At the start of the study, the Mayo group found a prevalence of 8.4:1000 persons; MSKCC found a rate of 4 to 7:1000. At the Mayo Foundation, 62% of the prevalence cases were detected by radiographs, 18% by cytology, and 20% by both. For all prevalence cases, the overall curative resection rate was 57%, and the 5-year survival rate was 40%.[311] At MSKCC in the group screened by radiographs and cytology tests, 60% of the cancers were detected by radiographs, 33% by cytology tests, and 7% by both. The overall curative resection rate was 69%; survival data were not presented.[316]

After the prevalence cases were removed, the Mayo group screening studies identified lung cancer in 1.6% of the persons followed.[311] In the intensively screened group, 72% had lesions detected radiographically, 20% had cytologic detection, and 6% had tumors detected by both procedures (Table 22-22). In the screened group, fewer patients had symptoms at the time of detection than in the control group, and the frequencies of lung cancer cell types were similar in the two groups. More people in the screened group had resectable

TABLE 22-22. Early Results of the Mayo Foundation Randomized Controlled Trial to Detect Early Lung Cancer*

	Prevalence Cases (n = 87)	*Incidence Cases (n = 9223)*	
		Screened (n = 87)	*Control (n = 57)*
Cell type (%)			
Epidermoid	47	32	32
Adenocarcinoma	25	21	23
Large cell carcinoma	16	20	12
Small cell carcinoma	11	28	33
Symptoms at detection	?None	11	67
Resectability (%)	57	62	28
AJC postsurgical stage			
Occult	10	Not stated	Not stated
I	39	53	21
II	6	Not stated	Not stated
III	45	37	68
Probability of 5-year survival (rate/1000 persons/year)	40	45	19
Incidences of new cases	Not applicable	4.7	3.0
Deaths from lung cancer		1.8	2.1

Fontana RS: Early diagnosis of lung cancer. Am Rev Respir Dis 116:399–402, 1977; Sanderson D, Fontana R: Results of the Mayo lung project: An interim report. Recent Results Cancer Res 82:179–186, 1982.

*11,001 patients initially screened.

lesions, more had postsurgical Stage I cancer (American Joint Committee system; see below), and there was a greater actuarial 5-year survival rate. Sputum cytology has the added benefit of detecting upper airway (head and neck) cancers. In fact, by early 1978, in the screened group, 18 persons had had an upper airway cancer detected. Of these lesions, 44% were first detected by cytology.[320] Thus, screening a high-risk population with chest films and sputum cytology detects lung cancer at an earlier, more resectable stage than is found in prevalence or control cases. All of the patients detected in these screening studies who were postsurgical Stage I had the excellent 5-year survival expected for Stage I patients (80% plus). However, between 45% and 60% were postsurgical Stage II or III with corresponding inferior survival (5-year rate less than 15%), indicating that even this intensive screening failed to detect lung cancer before it had become incurable by surgery. In addition, all three centers concluded that mortality rates from lung cancer were not significantly different in the screened group than in the control group. Thus, there is no current justification for large-scale application of these screening methods, even in high-risk populations.[321] In considering the individual patient at risk, one approach may be to perform the screening follow-up in heavy smokers who have quit smoking.

BIOCHEMICAL MARKERS FOR EARLY DETECTION

At present, no biochemical markers should be used routinely to screen for lung cancer. However, some plasma or serum markers, such as polypeptide hormones (*e.g.*, ACTH, calcitonin) may be useful clinically. Of 74 patients with lung cancer, 72% had increased ACTH immunoreactivity.[322] In contrast, none of 24 patients with benign chest film abnormalities and 20% of patients with chronic obstructive pulmonary disease (COPD) had elevated levels; 10% of patients with granulomatous lung disease had elevated ACTH levels during an acute exacerbation of their disease, which returned to normal with recovery. Twenty-five percent of COPD patients with elevated ACTH levels and only 2% with normal ACTH levels developed lung cancer within 2 years.[322] Concentrations of the amino terminus of human pro-opiomelanocortin (pro-ACTH) were found to be elevated in 60% of patients with cancer. This immunoassay is simple and does not require plasma extraction before the assay, as does the assay for ACTH.[322]

Recently, a large number of serum markers were studied by radioimmunoassay in patients with localized lung cancer and compared with values from normal controls and patients with benign lung disease.[324] These substances included ferritin, lipid-bound sialic acid, total sialic acid, beta-2-microglobulin, lipotropin, alpha and beta subunits of human chorionic gonadotropin (hCG), calcitonin, parathyroid hormone, and carcinoembryonic antigen (CEA). A series of statistical methods were used to see which could distinguish lung cancer from control patients. Unfortunately, to achieve 95% specificity, the sensitivity rate was less than 40%.[324] It appears that markers with much greater tumor specificity are needed. CEA is not a sensitive indicator in the screening for lung cancer because 60% of 130 patients who had surgical resection of histologically proved lung cancer had normal levels (*i.e.*, values less than 2.5 ng/ml).[325] However, it may have prognostic value, as a CEA level greater than 15 ng/ml indicated a reduced possibility of a successful resection. In addition, patients who in follow-up appeared to be cured by surgery had significantly fewer elevated CEA measurements postoperatively than did patients who relapsed. Thus, a rising or persistently elevated CEA concentration appears to be a good indicator of relapse or a second primary tumor.[325] An elevated CEA level (720 ng/ml) also appears to be an excellent marker for monitoring the response to chemotherapy and tumor progression for all types of lung cancer.[326]

OCCULT (STAGE 0) LUNG CANCER

Sputum cytology screening has identified patients with cancer who have normal chest radiographs (discussed later as tumor stage Tx). In order for treatment involving surgery or radiotherapy to be instituted, the lesion or lesions must be located. Conversely, lesions detected by chest radiographs are localized, but appropriate treatment requires a histologic diagnosis. Although chemotherapy is the primary treatment for small cell lung cancer, there are as yet no data suggesting that such systematic therapy is appropriate for persons who have only malignant sputum cytology suggestive of small cell cancer but no radiographic or bronchoscopic evidence of the primary tumor and no metastatic lesions visible.

The groups at Johns Hopkins, the Mayo Foundation, and MSKCC have investigated patients with positive sputum cytologies and normal chest radiographs in order to locate their tumors (Table 22-23).[327–329] The method has been pioneered by Marsh at Johns Hopkins.[328,329] Smoking is discontinued before the procedure. In addition, bronchitis is treated, because inflammatory cells can interfere with cytologic interpretation. The patient first has a complete examination of the upper aerodigestive tract, particularly the nasopharynx, the base of the tongue, larynx, and hypopharynx, to detect an asymptomatic tumor by indirect and direct nasopharyngoscopy and laryngoscopy. A detailed fiberoptic bronchoscopic examination lasting up to 2 hours is then performed under general anesthesia with extensive examination of the bronchial tree out to the fifth-generation of bronchi. Suspicious areas, bronchial bifurcations (spurs), and prospective surgical margins are biopsied, and a series of differential brushings is collected. These biopsies are predictive that surgical margins will be clear or involved with in situ cancer.[327]

Additional endobronchial tumor markers are needed for the 10% of tumors that cannot be located bronchoscopically in order to assist in the initial localization and to detect multicentric lesions in patients with a lesion found by radiograph or bronchoscopy. The Johns Hopkins group has used tantalum powder bronchography, an experimental procedure.[327] Tantalum is instilled with a controlled catheter, bronchography is performed followed by a cine examination, and films are taken at 24 and 48 hours to detect delayed clearance of the tantalum. The tantalum bronchogram local-

TABLE 22-23. Findings and Management of Patients with Positive Sputum Cytology and Radiographically Occult Lung Cancer: Follow-up of ≥3 Years from Johns Hopkins and the Mayo Foundation

Number of patients	62
Age range	30–79 years (all men)
Upper aerodigestive cancer causing positive cytology	11%
In remaining 55 patients	
Fiberoptic bronchoscopic (FOB) localized the lesion	89% (49/55)
Squamous cancer found	98%
FOB gross lesion	48%
Carcinoma *in situ* found	43% (JH data only)
Multicentric *in situ* lesions or multiple tumors found	22% (6/27 patients with data)
Of those lesions localized	
Overall patients who had surgery	78% (38/49)
Tumor resected	98%
AJC Stage I	85%
AJC Stage III	15%
Lymph nodes positive	5%
Pneumonectomy required	24% (9/38)
Radiation therapy required instead of surgery for technical or medical reasons	11% (Mayo data only)
No treatment given for medical or technical reasons	13% (Mayo data only)

Baker RR, Ball WC Jr, Carter D et al: Identification and treatment of clinically occult cancer of the lung. Prog Cancer Res Ther 11:243–249, 1979; Sanderson DR, Fontana RS, Woolner LB et al: Bronchoscopic localization of radiographically occult lung cancer. Chest 65:608–612, 1974; Fontana RS: The needle in the haystack editorial. Mayo Clin Proc 53:616–617, 1978; Sanderson DR, Fontana RS: Early lung cancer detection and localization. Ann Otol Rhinol Laryngol 84:583–589, 1975.

ized lesions in more than 90% of cases and thus can direct the fiberoptic bronchoscopic examination.

The Mayo group has pioneered the use of a derivative of hematoporphyrin (an experimental procedure) that involves a photodynamically active dye that concentrates in cancer cells. It then exhibits a salmon-red fluorescence on excitation by ultraviolet (UV) light that is detected photoelectrically with a system that generates an audiosignal for the fiberoptic bronchoscopist.[330,331] Early results show the concentration of dye in areas where no mucosal abnormalities are seen through the fiberoptic bronchoscope, yet, biopsy reveals carcinoma in situ.[332] This method could greatly simplify bronchoscopic location of tumor in patients with occult cancer.

MANAGEMENT AND TREATMENT DECISIONS

Once the radiologically occult lung cancer has been located, treatment decisions can be made. These are complicated because of the multicentric nature of the lesions, the tendency for multiple primary lung cancers to develop, and reports of following patients with in situ lesions for several years without the appearance of invasive cancer.[327–330,333,334] Pathologically, the Johns Hopkins group found in situ carcinomas in only 43% of resected specimens but noted extensive glandular involvement in these cases.[325]

The Johns Hopkins and Mayo experiences in managing patients with radiographically occult lung cancer are similar (see Table 22-23).[327,328,330,333] Of the 55 patients in the combined group, nearly all had squamous carcinoma; 11% of the lesions could not be located. A large fraction had carcinoma in situ (including carcinoma in situ at the bronchial margins) or multicentric tumors, and new lung primaries already have started to appear in follow-up of resected cases.

Recently, the Mayo group has updated its 10-year experience with occult lung cancer.[335] The cancer eventually was located in all 54 patients studied, but this required three or more bronchoscopies in more than 90% of the patients over intervals of 1 year. Pulmonary resection was performed in all patients, and all tumors were squamous cell. Postsurgical pathologic staging revealed carcinoma in situ in 35% of the cases, Stage I lesions in 56%, Stage II lesions in 7%, and Stage III M0 in 2%. The overall 5-year survival rate was 90%. However, 22% of the patients subsequently developed an additional lung cancer (usually squamous cancer), half of which were again occult. Thus close surveillance is indicated.[336]

Current recommendations are for the most conservative surgical resection permitted to remove the cancer and to conserve lung parenchyma, even if the bronchial margins are positive for carcinoma in situ.[325,328,332,333] Because of the multicentric nature of so many of these tumors, there is a need for a local ablative procedure to deal with the multiple foci. Fontana estimates the projected 5-year survival rate of these patients with occult cancers detected by sputum cytology to be approximately 60% or greater, although follow-up is still short.

ESTABLISHING A TISSUE DIAGNOSIS OF LUNG CANCER

Once the signs and symptoms of lung cancer have developed or an abnormality has been detected on chest film or sputum cytology in a screening study, it is necessary to establish a histologic diagnosis of malignancy, determine the cell type, and stage the disease in order to select appropriate treatment. The procedures used depend on the individual clinical situation. In some cases (*i.e.*, patient with a solitary, asymptomatic pulmonary nodule), the tissue diagnosis will be made at the time of definitive surgical resection, whereas in others, it will be made at the time of bronchial biopsy or biopsy of a metastatic focus. In all cases, it is mandatory that a histologic diagnosis be made and the lung cancer cell type established.

A reasonable approach in the patient suspected of having lung cancer is first to review the patient's history and physical examination, looking specifically for signs or symptoms to direct a search for a tissue diagnosis. This involves careful examination of supraclavicular lymph node areas for palpable masses, the skin for subcutaneous nodules, and the chest for signs and symptoms of endobronchial tumor. If an obvious tumor-bearing lymph node or skin nodule is found, it should be biopsied. If a pleural effusion is present, it should be sampled and cytologic tests performed on a cytocentrifuge-prepared specimen. Also, needle biopsy of the pleura in patients with an effusion is a simple method to obtain a diagnosis and has a moderate positive yield. If the liver is grossly enlarged or if it has nodular lesions on physical examination or radionuclide scan, a biopsy may be done. In unexplained anemia, a bone-marrow biopsy may be performed. Occasionally, lytic or blastic bone lesions on radiograph or localized bone scan abnormalities in sites accessible to needle biopsy by an orthopedic surgeon may be investigated when no other tumor tissue is available. If there are no obvious distant lesions, it is best to proceed to a flexible fiberoptic bronchoscopic study, examining washings, brushing, and biopsies of suspicious lesions.

BRONCHOSCOPIC TECHNIQUES

Flexible Fiberoptic Bronchoscopy

Flexible fiberoptic bronchoscopy has largely replaced rigid bronchoscopy for the evaluation of patients with tracheobronchial disorders.[337–341] A greater area of the tracheobronchial tree can be examined with the fiberoptic instrument, and in several series, 13% to 39% of lesions not seen with the rigid instrument were seen with the fiberoptic one.[342] The efficacy of bronchoscopy in establishing a diagnosis of lung cancer will be influenced by the nature of the cancer itself as well as by the combination of techniques (forceps biopsy, bronchial brushing, washings) used to establish the diagnosis. The false-positive rate of bronchoscopic diagnostic biopsies is very low (0.8%), and most such errors are associated with squamous metaplasia in inflammatory lesions.[338] When a tumor is visible endoscopically, an accurate histologic diagnosis can be made in 71% to 94% of the cases.[338,343] When bronchial brushing and washings are added to forceps biopsy, the diagnostic yield of a centrally located tumor is increased to 94% and that of a peripheral tumor to 86%.[344] For peripheral lesions that cannot be biopsied with forceps, washings and brushing each have a diagnostic rate of about 55%, whereas the yield for central lesions from brushing and washing is close to 75%.[345] The estimated probability of obtaining cancer from an endobronchial lesion after one biopsy is 0.89, that after 2 biopsies 0.99, and that after three close to 0.999.[346]

When the lesion is visible endobronchially, forceps biopsy is usually performed. There may be a role, however, for needle biopsy of endobronchial lesions suspected to be excessively vascular or necrotic.[347–349] Submucosal lesions are difficult to biopsy with forceps, and bronchoscopic needle aspiration will increase the diagnostic yield over forceps biopsy alone.[350] By combining forceps with needle aspiration, the submucosal lesion can be diagnosed in 87% of the cases, and when washings and brushings are added, the yield is increased to 97%.[351]

For peripheral lesions not visible endoscopically, the yield of diagnosis for washings, brushings, and biopsy individually are 51%, 52%, and 61%.[352] Transbronchial biopsy and brush combined will have an average yield of 60%.[353–357] The yield of peripheral lesions will vary with the size of the lesion, with the lowest yields seen in tumors less than 2 cm (28%).[340] Bronchiographic mapping has been used with some success to increase the yield of diagnosis with these small lesions.[358]

Peripheral lesions not visible endoscopically merit fluoroscopically guided biopsies, either transbronchial or percutaneous. Brush biopsy under fluoroscopic guidance will produce a diagnosis in 63% to 90% of the cases.[340,344,359] The use of fluoroscopy itself will more than double the diagnostic yield. Transbronchial forceps biopsy of a peripheral lesion under fluoroscopy will be successful in 70% to 75% of the cases,[342,360] although four to six biopsies are necessary to prevent sampling error.[346,355] Recently, transbronchial needle aspiration has been shown to increase the yield of bronchoscopy in the diagnosis of peripheral carcinomas.[361,362] For lesions less than 2 cm, 33% positive biopsies will occur, whereas in lesions greater than 2 cm, the yield increases to 80%.[350] When passage of forceps for transbronchial biopsy is impossible because of extrinsic compression, needle aspiration has been associated with a positive diagnosis in 80% of the cases.[361]

Complications of fiberoptic bronchoscopy and related diagnostic procedures (including pneumothorax, bronchospasm, and hemoptysis) are minimal, with a mortality rate of less than 0.05% and morbidity of less than 0.15%.[363–365] Use of transbronchial biopsy increases the morbidity and mortality rates, with the most common cause of death being cardiac related. Modern-day use of fluoroscopy has decreased the rate of significant pneumothorax to less than 2%. Whereas correction of coagulation disorders prior to bronchoscopy will decrease the chance of bleeding, patients with moderate to severe coagulation disorders are not candidates for endoscopic biopsy. The use of oximetry and supplemental oxygen during the examination has decreased the incidence of hypoxemia and arrhythmia. Washings with large volumes should be avoided, as they have been associated with transient (<24 h) hypoxemia.[366]

Aspiration Biopsy of Mediastinal Lymph Nodes

The use of transcarinal needle biopsy for the evaluation of mediastinal adenopathy has been pioneered by Wang and associates[367] and by Shure.[350] Both flexible plastic and rigid steel needles that can be guided through the biopsy port of the flexible bronchoscope are available. Three aspiration sites are routinely sampled in the carina: anterior, mid portion, and posterior. Peritracheal aspirations are more difficult because of the tracheal rings.[368] In patients with suspicious adenopathy as defined by chest roentgenography or computed tomography (CT), a sensitivity of 50% and a specificity above 90% have been reported.[368] To avoid false-positive biopsies, the mediastinum should be aspirated before examination of the bronchi to prevent contamination of the specimen by bronchial secretions. The highest yield of positive transcarinal biopsies occurs in patients with visible endobronchial tumors or an abnormal-appearing carina, and approximately 15% of patients with lung cancer undergoing routine transcarinal biopsy will have positive aspirates.[369] The complication rate is low (0.3%); the complication is usually pneumomediastinum or pneumothorax.

TRANSTHORACIC PERCUTANEOUS FINE-NEEDLE ASPIRATION BIOPSY (PFNAB)

The ability to locate parenchymal and mediastinal lesions precisely by biplane fluoroscopy or CT has increased the ability to sample abnormalities by percutaneous insertion of a fine-bore needle. The use of PFNAB has been reported to reduce the need for diagnostic and all thoracotomy and to shorten the time from admission to diagnosis as well as the length of hospital stay.[370] Proper use involves coordination of the efforts of the radiologist, pathologist, and primary physician.

A 22-gauge Chiba needle attached to a stopcock and 20-ml syringe is inserted percutaneously into the lung or mediastinal mass with the patient adequately sedated and anesthetized.[371] Most biopsies can be performed with fluoroscopic guidance; CT-guided aspirations are performed in patients having prior unsuccessful fluoroscopic biopsies, for lesions not visible on fluoroscopy, to avoid puncturing necrotic areas of large lesions, or to define the safest route of biopsy in patients with severe pulmonary disease, especially when doing mediastinal biopsies.[371] The PFNAB can also be guided by real-time sonography, especially when lesions are located near the mediastinal, diaphragmatic, or apical lung surfaces. Smears are made for immediate fixation in 95% ethanol and stained by the Papanicolaou method. The remainder of the aspirate is suspended in medium for processing by membrane filters, direct smears, cytocentrifugation, and cell blocks. After rapid Pap staining with a 4% aqueous solution of toluidine blue and examination by the ctyopathologist, the radiologist can be notified immediately regarding the diagnostic suitability of the aspirate; if necessary, aspiration can be repeated.

Contraindications to the procedure include unconscious or uncooperative patients, hemorrhagic diathesis, severe respiratory distress, or high fever and uncontrollable cough. Patients with severe emphysema have a higher complication rate. Serious complications include pneumothorax (20%), but only 4% of all patients having PFNAB will require chest tube drainage.[371] Transient hemoptysis (2%–4%) and, rarely, air embolism can occur.[371] Implantation of tumor cells along the needle track has been reported in only two cases,[372,373] and seeding of tumor cells into the blood is similarly rare. Local bleeding around the lesion is seen by chest films in 4% to 11% of patients and usually requires only observation.

Sinner reported on 5300 transthoracic needle biopsies in 2726 patients and Sagel and coworkers reported on 1211 patients.[374,375] Final diagnosis was established in 91% of these patients, with 46% to 71% having cytologic evidence of malignancy (approximately 85% of which were primary lung cancers).[375,376] The false-positive rate was 2.4% and the false-negative rate 23%. One aspiration provided malignant cells in 87% of the patients subsequently proved to have malignant disease; this rose to 96% after two procedures.[375] In a recent series of 1518 PFNAB of the lung from Duke Medical Center, 653 specimens were interpreted as showing a primary malignant neoplasm.[377] Tumor types diagnosed by this method included squamous cell carcinoma in 37.7%, large cell carcinoma 30%, adenocarcinoma 13.2%, small cell carcinoma 11.6%, and adenosquamous carcinoma in 3.5%. No opinion regarding the classification of the malignancy could be reached in 3.8%. Of these 653 patients, 122 had confirmation of the diagnosis by open thoracotomy or biopsy within a week. Nineteen percent of the tissue specimens revealed a cancer that was not detected by PFNAB, and the false-positive rate was 1%. In a similar series of 132 patients whose needle aspiration showed no cancer, 29% ultimately were found to have malignancy.[378]

Agreement between the confirmed histologic diagnosis and the PFNAB diagnosis differs among cell types: squamous cell carcinoma 72%, adenocarcinoma 95%, large cell carcinoma 28%, and small cell carcinoma 98%.[377] In scanty specimens, crushing artifact may sometimes be misread as small cell carcinoma. The low concurrence rate with large cell carcinoma probably reflects the failure of the PFNAB specimen to permit correct recognition of adenomatous differentiation. However, PFNAB, is able to diagnose small cell cancers with high accuracy and should not falsely predict the presence of a carcinoid, atypical carcinoid, or lymphoma. The aspirate is able to confirm the diagnosis of maligancy in 45% of the patients whose preaspirate sputum or bronchoscopic material was suspicious or positive for malignancy, confirming that the diagnostic yield of routine sputa and bronchoscopic evaluations are higher than that of PFNAB, and in most cases the former should be used before resorting to PFNAB.

Although PFNAB is widely used, it does not provide a histologic diagnosis, and it is frequently falsely negative. Thus, the indications need to be carefully defined:

1. Pulmonary masses in the patient unsuitable for curative thoracotomy who needs a definitive tissue diagnosis. These cases would include patients with compromised pulmonary function or a medical contraindication to thoracotomy and those who refuse thoracotomy.
2. Identification of the patient with small cell lung cancer.[276] Although fiberoptic bronchoscopy provides cytologic or biopsy material for definitive diagnosis in a high percentage of proven cases of small cell lung

cancer,[337] recent adjuvant chemotherapy results after resection of small cell carcinoma pulmonary nodules are good enough (discussed later in this chapter) to recommend resection of a single peripheral nodule without mediastinal adenopathy, even if small cell lung cancer is proved.

3. Localized or worsening pneumonic infiltrate in an immunocompromised patient despite standard antibiotic therapy when an etiologic agent is not known.
4. A patient with a history of another malignancy, to allow the differentiation between a new primary, a metastatic lesion, or an inflammatory process.
5. During a thoracotomy, if excisional biopsy is judged to be hazardous or unlikely to yield a definite diagnosis.
6. Other masses identified on chest films or CT scan such as mediastinal masses that need to be evaluated histologically to develop a therapeutic plan.

CORE BIOPSY

Fine-needle or core biopsy with a 20-gauge needle can also be used for the sampling of anterior and central mediastinal lesions, including those in the paratracheal area, to evaluate suspicious lymphadenopathy. The sensitivity of this method in detecting metastatic carcinoma is 71%, and the technique is very accurate (90%) in the diagnosis of small cell carcinoma metastatic to the mediastinal nodes.[371] The subcarinal area, however, remains difficult to biopsy, and this almost always requires CT guidance.

STAGING OF LUNG CANCER

Efficient and appropriate staging can proceed once a tissue diagnosis of lung cancer is obtained. The purpose of staging is to aid in the selection of treatment, estimate the probability of cure and survival, facilitate accurate communication about a patient's status, and compare results from different clinical treatment series. Staging becomes more important with the development of multimodality treatment regimens and in evaluation of experimental clinical trials. For non-small cell lung cancer, only surgery or radiotherapy as single modalities offer the opportunity for long-term survival and cure for a significant number of patients, and selection of patients for a curative attempt by either of these modalities is determined by the anatomic stage of the disease and the technical and physiologic considerations concerning the patient's ability to tolerate the treatment and still be functional. Although there are biological differences between epidermoid carcinoma, adenocarcinoma, and large cell carcinoma, these differences at present probably should not be used in ruling out curative local therapy. However, there are great biologic differences between these non-small cell cancers and small cell carcinoma of the lung. Although anatomic considerations also are important in small cell cancer patients, the total tumor bulk and physiologic ability of the patient to tolerate chemotherapy with or without radiotherapy appear to be more important.

ANATOMICAL STAGING

The two major systems used for the staging of lung cancer have been those proposed by the American Joint Committee on Cancer (AJCC) and the Union Internationale contre Cancer (UICC), both of which use a TNM-based system as originally proposed by Denoix.[379] The TNM system is based on the primary tumor size and extent (*T factor*), regional lymph node involvement (*N factor*), and the presence or absence of distant metastases (*M factor*). Such TNM-based systems can incorporate different types of evidence available for classifying the extent of disease at different sites and at different times in the course of disease and patient evaluation. These types of evidence include (1) *clinical diagnostic staging* (all pretreatment information including that from endoscopy, mediastinoscopy, or other biopsies); (2) *surgical evaluative staging* (findings at exploratory thoracotomy), (3) *postsurgical pathologic staging* (surgical pathology report), (4) *retreatment staging* (staging at relapse), and, finally, (5) *autopsy staging.* Of greatest importance to the patients is the clinical diagnostic staging, which is used to select the mode of primary treatment, and the post-therapy staging, as an early indicator of potential success of therapy and the need for additional treatment.

The AJC system, developed in 1979,[380] was based on the analysis of 2155 cases of lung cancer in the United States and was in use until 1987. Currently, there are discrepancies between the AJC and UICC systems that need reconciliation, including:

1. Patients with N1 positivity (tumor in the peribronchial or the ipsilateral hilar lymph nodes or both including direct extension) and having T1 tumors (less than 3 cm in diameter) were classified as having Stage I disease according to the AJC criteria. This view was challenged by the Japanese Cancer Committee, which noted that the outcome for T1N1 patients was significantly worse than that of T1N0 patients and more closely resembled that of Stage II patients.
2. Subgroups of patients with N2 (mediastinal lymph node positivity) seemed to have different survival patterns.
3. Patients with T3 lesions needed to be reclassified to define those patients who could have complete resection. These patients included those with peripheral tumors invading the chest wall, tumor with direct extension to the mediastinum or pericardium, superior sulcus tumors in patients without a true Pancoast syndrome, and tumor involving the proximal main bronchus and carina that are amenable to sleeve resection.
4. Patients with N3 disease (contralateral and supraclavicular or scalene lymph nodes) needed reclassification with regard to potential radiotherapeutic curability. Nodal positivity at these sites indicated a subset of Stage III disease not amenable to surgical resection. However, tumor involvement of these nodes had been considered "regional disease" by the radiotherapists, and such nodal groups were routinely included in a "curative" radiation field.
5. The need to establish a role in the staging system for cytology-negative pleural effusions.

A new International Staging System (ISS) based on the records of 3753 patients from the M.D. Anderson Hospital and those treated under the auspices of the Lung Cancer Study Group (LCSG) was proposed in 1986[381] (Table 22-24). The ISS classification has been adopted by the LCSG and will, it is hoped, help in the prospective study of survival patterns after treatment with newer multimodality therapies. This system combines the UICC and AJC staging systems into one system consistent with international objectives, and we also recommend its use.

TABLE 22-24. TNM Definitions

	Primary Tumor (T)
TX	Tumor proved by the presence of malignant cells in bronchopulmonary secretions but not visible roentgenographically or bronchoscopically, or any tumor that cannot be assessed as in a retreatment staging
T0	No evidence of primary tumor
TIS	Carcinoma in situ.
T1	A tumor that is 3.0 cm or less in greatest dimension, surrounded by lung or visceral pleura and without evidence of invasion proximal to a lobar bronchus at bronchoscopy*
T2	A tumor more than 3.0 cm in greatest dimension, or a tumor of any size that either invades the visceral pleura or has associated atelectasis or obstructive pneumonitis extending to the hilar region. At bronchoscopy, the proximal extent of demonstrable tumor must be within a lobar bronchus or at least 2.0 cm distal to the carina. Any associated atelectasis or obstructive pneumonitis must involve less than an entire lung
T3	A tumor of any size with direct extension into the chest wall (including superior sulcus tumors), diaphragm, or the mediastinal pleura or pericardium without involving the heart, great vessels, trachea, esophagus, or vertebral body, or a tumor in the main bronchus within 2 cm of the carina without involving the carina
T4	A tumor of any size with invasion of the mediastinum or involving the heart, great vessels, trachea, esophagus, vertebral body, or carina or the presence of malignant pleural effusion.†
	Nodal Involvement (N)
N0	No demonstrable metastasis to regional lymph nodes
N1	Metastasis to lymph nodes in the peribronchial or the ipsilateral hilar region, or both, including direct extension
N2	Metastasis to ipsilateral mediastinal lymph nodes and subcarinal lymph nodes
N3	Metastasis to contralateral mediastinal lymph nodes, contralateral hilar lymph nodes, ipsilateral or contralateral scalene or supraclavicular lymph nodes
	Distant Metastasis (M)
M0	No (known) distant metastasis
M1	Distant metastasis present—specify sites(s)

Mountain CF: A new international staging system for lung cancer. Chest 89:225s–233s, 1986.

*The uncommon superficial tumor of any size with its invasive component limited to the bronchial wall that may extend proximal to the main bronchus is classified as T1.

†Most pleural effusions associated with lung cancer are secondary to tumor. There are, however, some patients in whom cytopathologic examination of pleural fluid on more than one specimen is negative for tumor and fluid is nonbloody and is not an exudate. In such cases, where these elements and clinical judgment dictate that the effusion is not related to the tumor, the patients should be staged T1, T2, or T3, excluding effusion as a staging element.

NEW TNM DEFINITIONS OF THE 1986 INTERNATIONAL STAGING SYSTEM

T: Primary Tumor

Four specific categories of primary tumors have been classified. The T1 tumor is a parenchymal nodule without invasion of the visceral pleural or proximal to a lobar bronchus. The T2 classification remains the same with the exception that it is now independent of the presence or absence of a pleural effusion. The T3 category is now reserved for operable resectable lesions, in which the areas of invasion to contiguous structures could be encompassed by either standard or tracheobronchial sleeve resection. The T4 category includes a superior sulcus lesion with vertebral body invasion (possibly resectable), lesions that are unresectable secondary to invasion of nonsacrificeable mediastinal contents, and tumors accompanied by a malignant pleural effusion.

N: Regional Lymph Nodes

The N1 category is unchanged from the previous classification. To identify objectively patients with limited mediastinal nodal involvement who could undergo resection, the N2 category has been restricted to ipsilateral mediastinal or subcarinal node involvement. Regional nodal spread outside the confines of the ipsilateral hemithorax (contralateral mediastinal or any supraclavicular scalene or node) is now classified as N3 and is by this definition unresectable.

M: Distant Metastases

Extrathoracic metastases exclusive of cervical regional nodal positivity has been classified as M1.

Stage Grouping

The changes in stage grouping include the reclassification of T1N1 disease as Stage II (Table 22-25) (Fig. 22-4). Stage III disease has been subdivided into Stage IIIa (T3N0N1, or any N2) and Stage IIIb (any N3 or any T4). Thus, Stage IIIa defines subsets of patients who may have a surgical option on

TABLE 22-25. Stage Grouping of the New International Staging System

Occult carcinoma	TX	N0	M0
Stage 0	TIS	Carcinoma in situ	
Stage I	T1	N0	M0
	T2	N0	M0
Stage II	T1	N1	M0
	T2	N1	M0
Stage IIIa	T3	N0	M0
	T3	N1	M0
	T1–3	N2	M0
Stage IIIb	Any T	N3	M0
	T4	Any N	M0
Stage IV	Any T	Any N	M1

Mountin CF: A new international staging system for lung cancer. Chest 89:225s–233s, 1986.

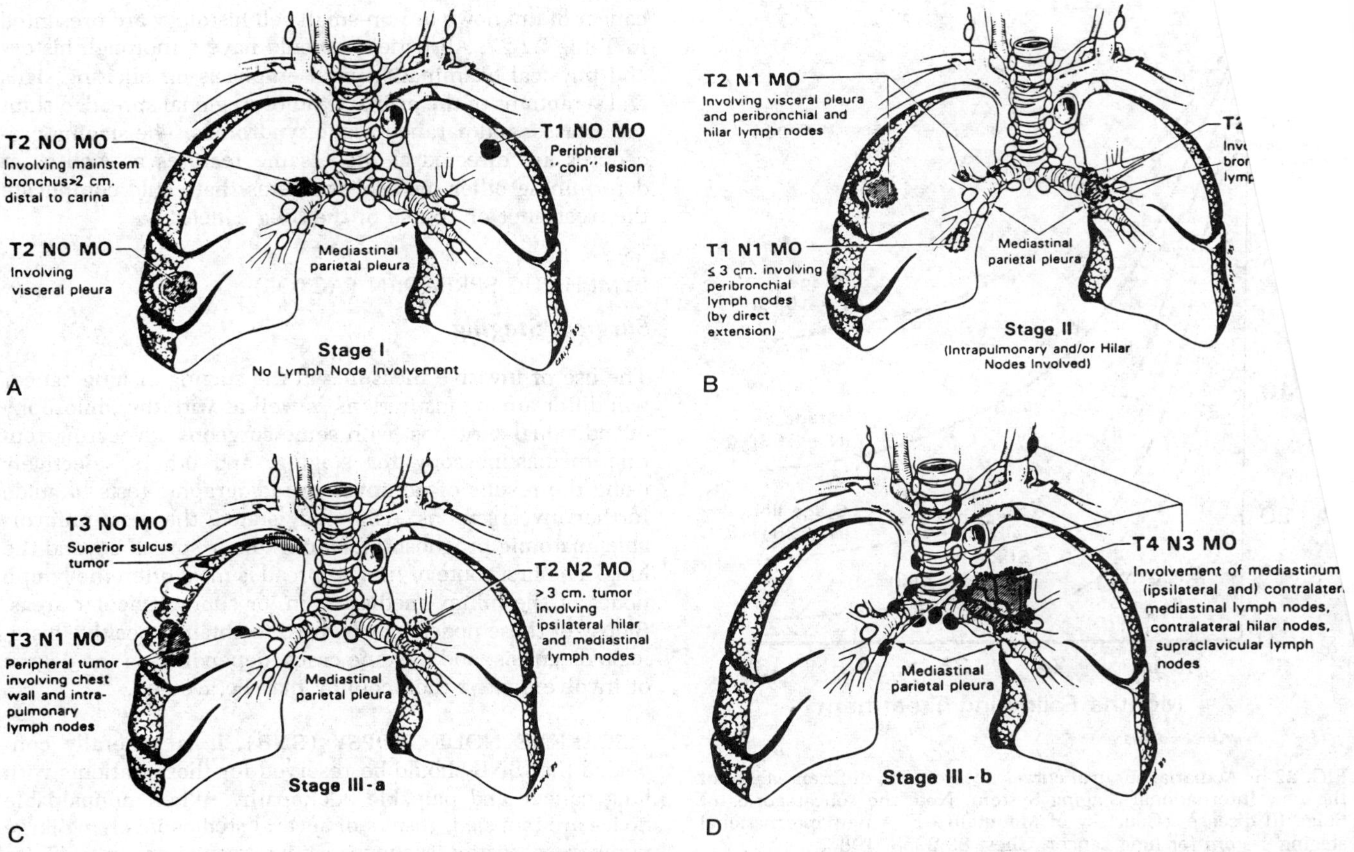

FIG. 22-4. New International Staging System (ISS): **A.** categories of Stage I disease; **B.** categories of Stage II disease; **C.** categories of Stage IIIa disease; **D.** categories of Stage IIIb disease. (Courtesy of Mountain CF: A new international staging system for lung cancer. Chest 89:225S, 1986)

presentation despite mediastinal disease or who may represent the upper limits of resectability for whom preoperative therapy may be indicated. At this time, Stage IIIb patients are considered to have nonresectable disease. The results according to the new staging system demonstrate the significant survival differences in the different stages (Fig. 22-5).

INFLUENCE OF HISTOLOGY AND LYMPHATIC AND BLOOD VESSEL INVASION

For patients with non-small cell cancers who have sufficiently limited disease permitting surgical resection, the overwhelming prognostic factor is whether the cancer has remained localized to the lung or has spread by local extension or metastases to the regional lymph nodes as determined by the postsurgical pathologic review. Histologic subtype has not in the past been of prognostic significance. Recently, however, in a prospective series of 282 patients with non-small cell cancer who were able to undergo a "curative resection," significant differences in survival were noted between those with epidermoid or adenocarcinoma histologies and those with large cell histologies.[382] The absence of lymph node involvement was associated with significantly longer survival, whereas the presence of peribronchial or mediastinal nodal involvement reduced median survival. Parenchymal lymphatic vessel invasion by itself without lymph node metastases indicated a poor prognosis, whereas blood vessel invasion identified by routine histologic examination did not provide any additional predictive information. When analyzed prospectively, in only patients with T3 lesions had inferior survival after resection when considered independent of lymph node involvement. In patients having a curative resection and in whom microscopic examination revealed no invasion of lymph nodes, lymphatic vessels, or blood vessels, the 3-year survival rate was 61%; with lymphatic vessel invasion and no nodal metastases, 42%; with lymph node invasion alone, 35%; and with both, 34%.

OVERALL APPROACH TO STAGING

By initial clinical diagnostic stage and postsurgical anatomic stage, the chances of a patient being cured by resection can be determined and compared with operative mortality rates and postoperative functional status. However, in practice, most clinicians want to know whether the chance of cure is within the general range of the operative mortality rate. Similar questions should be posed in discussions advocating curative radiotherapy or chemoradiotherapy for small cell lung cancer. The goal, thus, should be to identify that group of patients with non-small cell cancer who most surgeons,

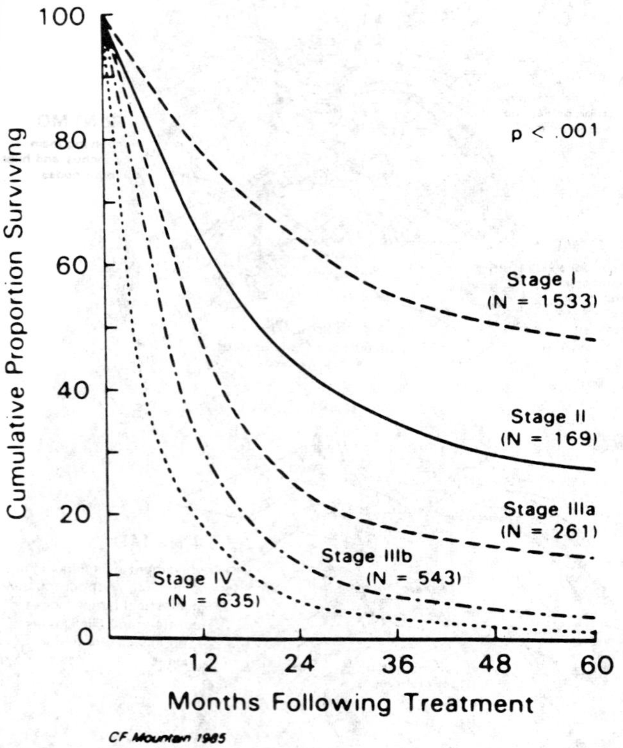

FIG. 22-5. Actuarial survival curves according to different stages of the new International Staging System. Note the subcategories of Stage III disease. (Courtesy of Mountain CF: A new international staging system for lung cancer. Chest 89:225S, 1986)

radiotherapists, and oncologists believe are essentially not curable by surgery or radiotherapy alone and that group with small cell carcinoma who are unlikely to gain long-term survival from intensive chemotherapy. When these patients are identified, the therapeutic approach should be directed at palliation. Because of the greater than 50% long-term survival prospects in patients with Stage I non-small cell cancer, trials of adjuvant therapy must enroll large numbers to detect significant differences. However, the 70% to 90% failure rate for patients with Stage II and Stage III disease means that newer approaches can be tested in fewer patients if cure is the end-point measured.

The first goal of staging is to obtain tumor tissue to confirm the diagnosis of cancer and determine the histologic type, particularly distinguishing non-small cell from small cell cancer. The next goal is to determine if the lesion is surgically resectable or can be encompassed within a tolerable radiotherapy port designed for cure. Obviously, the discovery of extrathoracic metastatic disease removes the curative potential of these local modalities. However, there are features generally agreed to be contraindications to attempts to cure lung cancer with surgery or radiotherapy alone (Table 22-26). Finally, assessment is made of the patients' physiologic status and ability to tolerate the treatment. A sensible plan is to proceed from simple and noninvasive procedures to more complex ones in as economic a fashion as possible.

Pretreatment staging procedures for patients with lung cancer of unknown or non-small cell histology are presented in Table 22-27. All patients should have a thorough history and physical examination with emphasis on eliciting signs and symptoms of the primary tumor, regional spread, distant metastases, and paraneoplastic syndromes. The staging procedures are directed at these same features as well as at determining other medical problems that could complicate the treatment or course of the lung cancer.

LYMPHATIC SPREAD (N FACTOR)

Surgical Staging

The use of invasive measures in the staging of lung cancer will differ among institutions as well as with the philosophy of individual surgeons, with some surgeons advocating routine mediastinoscopy for staging, and others selectively using the results of noninvasive radiographic tests to guide further investigations. As already stated, the most unfavorable anatomic prognostic factor is tumor spread beyond the lung. The first route of tumor spread is most often the lymph nodes of the hilum, mediastinum, or supraclavicular areas. Biopsy of these nodes may be used to obtain a positive histologic diagnosis, and in some cases, depending on the degree of involvement, a thoracotomy may be avoided.

SCALENE NODE BIOPSY (SNB). It is generally concluded that SNB should be reserved for those patients with lung cancer and palpable adenopathy. When nonpalpable nodes are biopsied, results of several studies involving large numbers of patients show positive results in only 4% to 10%.[383,384] Scalene node biopsy is performed under local anesthesia with a 3-cm incision over the lateral edge of the sternocleidomastoid muscle. The fat pad overlying the anterior scalene muscle is located and nodes sampled from this area. A 2% rate of complications is usually reported, including infection, pneumothorax, phrenic nerve injury, recurrent laryngeal nerve damage, and thoracic duct injury.

TABLE 22-26. Anatomical–Biologic Aspects of Tumor Involvement That Are Major Contraindications to Curative Attempts by Surgery or Radiotherapy Alone with Standard Methods

Extrathoracic distant metastases
Superior vena cava syndrome
Vocal cord paralysis
Malignant pleural effusion
Cardiac tamponade with pericardial involvement
Tumor within 2 cm of the carina*
Metastasis to the contralateral lung
Bilateral endobronchial tumor*
Metastasis to the supraclavicular lymph nodes
Lymph node metastasis in the contralateral mediastinum*
Involvement of mainstem pulmonary artery
Histologic diagnosis of small cell carcinoma†

*Depending on tumor location and physiologic factors, such tumors may be encompassed in a tolerable radiotherapy port and treated for cure.

†When an asymptomatic pulmonary nodule is resected and found to be small cell carcinoma, adjuvant chemotherapy is recommended.

TABLE 22-27. Pretreatment Staging Procedures for Lung Cancer Patients

All Patients

Complete history, physical examination, and evaluation of all medical problems, including determination of performance status and weight loss
Ear, nose, and throat examinations
Chest posterior-anterior and lateral roentgenograms
Complete blood count with platelet determination
Routine blood chemistries, including electrolytes, blood glucose, calcium, phosphorus, and renal and liver function tests
Electrocardiogram (ECG)
Pulmonary function studies and arterial blood-gas measurements if any signs or symptoms of minimal respiratory insufficiency are present
Skin tests for tuberculosis
CT or radionuclide scans of brain, liver, or bone if any of the above studies suggest presence of tumor in these organs; radiographs of any bony lesions suspicious by scan or symptom
Barium swallow radiographic examination if esophageal symptoms are present, followed by esophagoscopy if abnormalities are found
Biopsy of any accessible lesions suspicious for cancer if a histologic diagnosis is not yet made or if treatment or staging decisions would be based on whether or not the lesion contained cancer
Routine medical evaluation of any abnormalities detected in the first part of the screen not related to cancer

Patients Presenting with a Solitary Pulmonary Nodule

All of the above plus

Fiberoptic bronchoscopy with washings, brushings, and biopsy of suspicious areas
Pulmonary function tests, arterial blood-gas measurements
Coagulation tests
Transthoracic fine-needle aspiration biopsy or transbronchial forceps biopsy of peripheral lesions if material from routine fiberoptic bronchoscopy gives negative results and the patient is poor surgical candidate

Patients with a Mass Lesion in the Chest and No Obvious Contraindication to a Curative Local Approach (Surgery or Radiotherapy)

All of the above plus

CT or radionuclide scans of brain, liver, and bone if signs, symptoms, or laboratory abnormalities are detected in these systems
CT scans of areas where regular radionuclide scans are nondiagnostic
Mediastinoscopy or lateral mediastinotomy in individual patients (see text for discussion)

Patients with Disease Confined to the Chest but Not Resectable (Candidate for Curative Radiotherapy)

All of the above except mediastinoscopy plus

Transthoracic fine-needle aspiration biopsy or transbronchial forceps biopsy of peripheral lesion if material from routine fiberoptic bronchoscopy gives negative results

*Patients with Disease Not Curable by Either Surgery or Radiotherapy, Alone or Together**

All under first entry plus

Biopsy of accessible lesions suspicious for tumor to obtain histologic diagnosis or if therapy would be altered by findings of tumor
Fiberoptic bronchoscopy if indicated by hemoptysis, obstruction, pneumonitis, or no histologic diagnosis of cancer
Tap and cytologic examination of pleural effusion
Transthoracic fine-needle aspiration biopsy or transbronchial forceps biopsy of peripheral lesions if material from routine fiberoptic bronchoscopy gives negative results and no other material exists for a histologic diagnosis

* Extrathoracic metastatic disease or malignant pleural effusion.

MEDIASTINOSCOPY. Maasen and Greschuchner in 1975 reviewed the results of 1487 mediastinoscopies performed on patients with suspected or proved carcinoma of the lung and found that 36% of the nodes contained metastatic tumor, with central tumors having a higher rate of positivity than peripheral tumors (42% and 30%, respectively).[385] The pattern of mediastinal spread of tumor is not uniformly predictable, however, and thus one must sample the various nodal groups at the time of surgery.

Two recent series are representative of the results of mediastinoscopy in large numbers of patients at institutions where mediastinoscopic evaluation of lung cancer patients prior to surgery is routine.[386,387] Of 2259 mediastinoscopies, 624 (28%) found tumor in lymph nodes. With regard to primary cell type, 22% of the patients with squamous cell carcinomas had positive nodes, whereas 30% of those with large cell and adenocarcinomas had positive lymph node. Of 1510 patients who had negative mediastinoscopic findings, only 151 (10%) were found to have nodal tumor at thoracotomy. In fact, 88% of the patients with negative mediastinoscopic results were able to undergo "curative" resection. Complication rates of mediastinoscopy were lower than in earlier reports (hemorrhage 0.13%, pneumothorax 0.6%, recurrent nerve injury 0.3%, and tracheobronchial injury 0.09%). Both series also analyzed results of the subgroup of patients with metastatic cancer confined to ipsilateral nodes and discovered only by microscopic examination ("intranodal" disease). Only 98 (15%) of the 635 patients with nodal positivity qualified for this subanalysis, of which 81 (83%) had resectable disease with an estimated 5-year survival rate of 18%.

TECHNIQUE OF CERVICAL MEDIASTINOSCOPY. Cervical mediastinoscopy is usually performed under general anesthesia. After making a 2- to 4-cm incision in the suprasternal notch, dissection is continued in the pretracheal plane until the area of the carina is reached (Fig. 22-6). The mediastinoscope is then inserted and the lymph nodes sam-

FIG. 22-6. Transverse view of structures encountered during mediastinoscopy. Note the limited visualization of the left owing to the presence of the aortic arch.

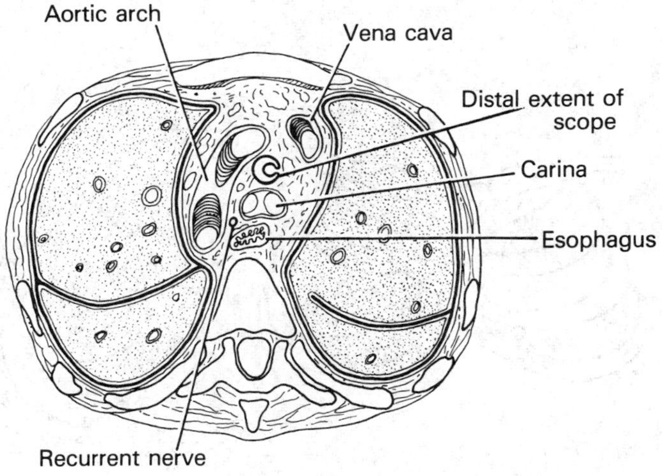

pled after aspiration to distinguish vascular from lymphatic structures.

The complication rate of standard mediastinoscopy is low, with a morbidity rate of 1.6% and a mortality rate of 0.08%.[388] The principal avoidable complication is hemorrhage from inadvertent biopsy of the right pulmonary artery, azygous vein, or aorta, all of which necessitate emergency thoracotomy. Other complications include vocal cord paralysis, esophageal perforation, mediastinitis, bradycardia, tumor seeding, myocardial infarction, stroke, and air embolism. Although SVC obstruction is a relative contraindication to mediastinoscopy, the procedure can be performed in such circumstances without death if there is a pressing clinical need to make a tissue diagnosis. The safety of repeat mediastinoscopy has also been detailed in two series of patients.[389-391]

ANTERIOR PARASTERNAL MEDIASTINOTOMY (CHAMBERLAIN PROCEDURE). Parasternal mediastinotomy is often performed instead of cervical mediastinoscopy when evaluating the left side of the mediastinum, because the subaortic and anterior hilar nodes cannot be evaluated by the suprasternal approach. However, anterior mediastinotomy also can be performed on the right. Other nodal groups inaccessible by cervical mediastinoscopy include those of the anterior mediastinum, subaortic area, and posterior subcarinal region.

A 6-cm incision is made over the second or third intercostal cartilages in a vertical fashion; alternatively, a horizontal incision in the interspace can be performed, obviating cartilage removal. Posterior dissection is carried past the internal mammary vessels, and the pleura can either be retracted or entered directly (Fig. 22-7). The mediastinum in the area of the aorticopulmonary window is thus accessible for biopsy of anterior and left-sided lesions, evaluation of extension of tumor, and biopsy of the aorticopulmonary nodes. Hiloscopy, as described in 1979 by Paris, adds direct mediastinoscopic evaluation of the hilum.[392] Greater access for evaluation of aortic or diaphramatic invasion, pleural metastases, and direct biopsy of the hilar, subaortic, or periaortic nodes is afforded by this technique. The procedure can be performed under the same anesthesia with standard mediastinoscopy. Mediastinotomy, with or without hiloscopy, is associated with low morbidity and mortality rates.[393]

Roentgenographic Evaluation of the Mediastinum

COMPUTED TOMOGRAPHY. Since the late 1970s, there has been enthusiasm for the use of CT scanning in the preoperative staging of lung cancer patients, particularly to interpret the mediastinal shadows seen on chest roentgenography with regard to nodal positivity. The original hope for the CT scan was that it would be able to predict noninvasively which patients had obvious mediastinal invasion or nodal involvement, rendering operative or other invasive staging unnecessary if its specificity and sensitivity was consistently high. In addition, the cross-sectional imaging, free from overlying shadows, made the mediastinal soft-tissue structures recognizable in their full transverse extent (Fig. 22-8). With the use of intravenous contrast medium, accurate differentiation between malignant deposits, fatty tissue, and vascular structures theoretically could be achieved. Various anatomic structures, specifically bronchial anatomy and lymph nodes, would be mapped, not only for staging purposes, but also to aid the surgeon in subsequent dissection.

In actual practice, there has been a learning process of the limitations of CT in the staging of the mediastinum. Misinterpretations can occur secondary to excessive slice intervals, poor contrast enhancement of vascular structures, and misreading.[394] Direct extension of tumor into the mediastinum is often convincingly demonstrated by CT, yet pitfalls exist, as simple abutment of tumor against mediastinal structures cannot be scored as invasion with great confidence. Circumferential narrowing of bronchovascular structures associated with a mass or the interdigitating of tumor mass with mediastinal fat is confidently recognized as tumor invasion, however.

When trying to evaluate nodal pathology by CT scans, one must measure the relative sizes of the nodes in order to classify them as abnormal. Mediastinal nodes greater than 1.5 cm in diameter in patients with bronchogenic carcinoma will harbor tumor in 94% to 97% of the cases, whereas lymph nodes ranging from 1 to 1.5 cm in diameter are involved with tumor in 50% of the cases and those less than

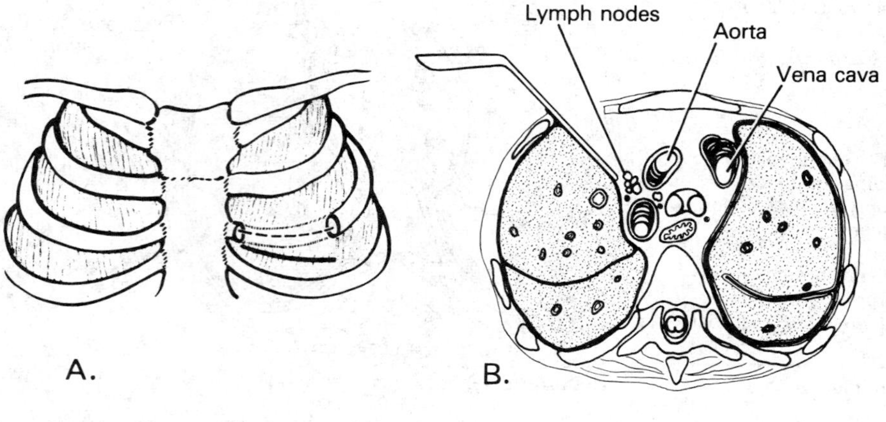

FIG. 22-7. Parasternal mediastinotomy (Chamberlain procedure). **A**. Transverse incision in second and third intercostal space. A vertical incision can also be used. **B**. Depiction of transverse anatomy encountered for access to anterior mediastinal nodes on the left (see text for description).

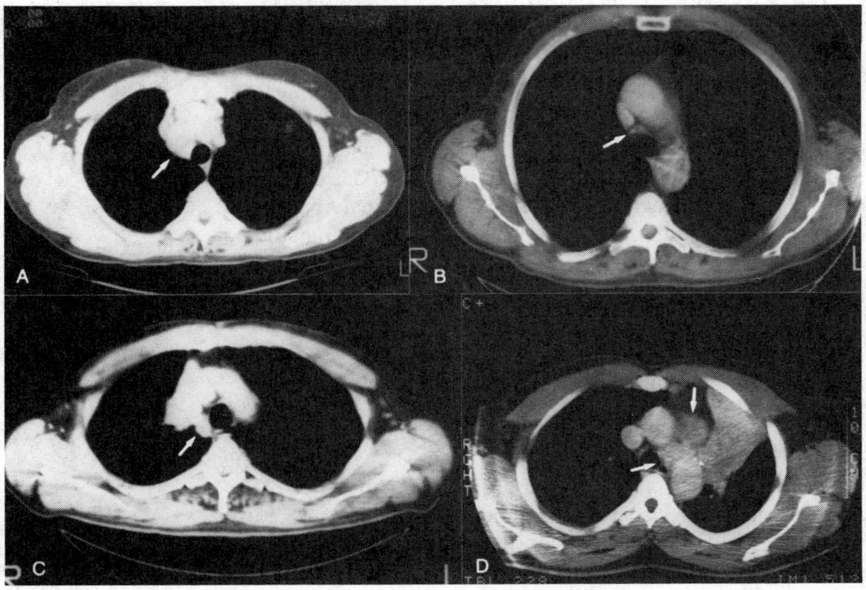

FIG. 22-8. Nodal basins in lung cancer (*arrows*) as visualized on computed tomography. **A**. High bulky tracheal nodes. **B**. Subtle 1.5-cm anterior tracheal node behind the vena cava. **C**. Posterior paratracheal node. **D**. Left-sided anterior mediastinal nodes and aorticopulmonary nodes with left upper lobe atelectasis.

1 cm are usually uninvolved.[395-397] Genereux and Howie found that 99% of normal nodes imaged by CT were less than 16 mm in diameter and 90% of the nodes in the precarinal and subcarinal area were in the 6- to 10-mm range.[398] Normal nodal size is influenced by location, with the largest nodes in the paratracheal regions and smaller nodes in the subcarinal and paraesophageal areas.[398] Nonpathologic lymph nodes in the region of the azygous vein commonly measure up to 1 cm.[397,399] Moreover, the size of the node will depend on the axis through which the node is imaged. Also, reactive nodes secondary to chronic infection accompanying atelectasis are larger than the upper limits of normal.

Usefulness of CT Scans in the Staging of Lung Cancer: Results of Various Series. There have been many conflicting reports regarding the efficacy of CT scans for preoperative staging of bronchogenic carcinoma. Table 22-28 summarizes the results in 1758 patients reported since 1978 correlating CT scan interpretation with histologic confirmation of nodal involvement. Nodes less than 1 cm in diameter have a low probability for tumor involvement, nodes 1 to 1.5 cm have an intermediate probability of tumor involvement, and those greater than 1.5 cm have a high probability of tumor involvement. Overall, those studies that use 1 cm as the upper limit of normal size have high sensitivity but low specificity, whereas the sensitivity is low and specificity high when nodes up to 2 cm are considered normal. The greatest accuracy with the highest specificity was seen with a cut-off size of 1.5 cm, with the positive predictive index, or chance of a CT-called positive being correct, and the negative predictive index reaching 82% and 92%, respectively (Table 22-29).

TABLE 22-28. Accuracy of CT Scans in Staging Lung Cancer 1978–1987[396,400-423]

Number of patients	1758
Overall sensitivity	73%
Overall specificity	80%
Accuracy	77%
Positive predictive index	72%
Negative predictive index	83%

Implications of CT for Selective Surgical Mediastinal Staging. The present CT studies indicate that patients with intermediate- or high-probability nodal sizes should have operative staging of the mediastinum by transcarinal needle biopsy, mediastinoscopy, or mediastinotomy. In patients with peripheral lesions and a normal-appearing mediastinum on chest roentgenography and CT, the possibility of

TABLE 22-29. Accuracy of CT Scans: Influence of Node Size*

				Prediction Index (%)	
Size (cm)	*Sensitivity (%)*	*Specificity (%)*	*Accuracy (%)*	*Positive*	*Negative*
<1	94	70	80	70	94
1.0	78	78	78	67	87
1.5	71	93	85	82	92
2.0	41	95	77	81	76

*Data derived from studies listed in Table 22-28 in which node size was specified.

performing a "curative" resection approaches 100%, obviating invasive preresection mediastinal staging. When an abnormal hilum or mediastinum is seen on routine chest radiography, CT can be used to identify patients with abnormally large nodes for selective mediastinal staging prior to resection, with 80% demonstrating nodal metastases histologically. Patients with obvious bulky bilateral nodal disease in the presence of a documented endobronchial lesion probably can proceed to radiotherapy without further staging studies.

Other Roentgenographic Techniques

^{67}GALLIUM SCANNING. Gallium-67 accumulates nonspecifically in lung lesions ranging from neoplasm to inflammation, and the detection of metastases in the hilum and mediastinum with gallium scanning has been investigated extensively with variable results.[424,425] Because of gallium's lack of sensitivity, as well as the greater availability of CT and the decreased cost effectiveness of gallium compared with other techniques, the enthusiasm for using gallium scanning to direct the management of patients with lung carcinoma has subsided. This view is reinforced by the lack of agreement regarding the implications that gallium scanning results have for mediastinoscopy among enthusiasts for the technique.

MAGNETIC RESONANCE IMAGING (MRI). A number of reports have compared MRI with CT (Fig. 22-9) in the staging of lung cancer, and the consensus is that MRI scans have been disappointing. Glazer and associates, comparing CT and MRI for the imaging of the hilum in 35 patients, found that MRI could not distinguish between benign and malignant enlarged nodes.[426] Webb and Levitt and their associates, in similar series of 33 and 37 patients, respectively, could distinguish lymph nodes from surrounding mediastinal tissues, but the imaging sequences could not distinguish lymph nodes that were involved by tumor from those that were uninvolved.[427,428] Similar information regarding the presence and size of lymph nodes was seen with CT or MRI. MRI was superior to CT, however, in distinguishing hilar structures, and in these series, collapsed peripheral lung gave a different image than the offending tumor. Webb and coworkers thought that MRI was qualitatively superior to CT in demonstrating mediastinal invasion. In a prospective study of 34 patients from MSKCC, equal sensitivity (61% and 65%) was seen in the imaging of lymph node metastases by CT and MRI, with equally low specificity (42%).[429] Neither method could distinguish contact from invasion by tumor. Poon and coworkers, in a series of 48 patients, confirmed that MRI was not superior to CT for lymph node staging.[430]

In summary, it is generally thought that further developments to improve tissue characterization will be necessary before MRI can supplant the CT scan in the mediastinal evaluation of bronchogenic carcinoma.

PULMONARY ANGIOGRAPHY. Pulmonary angiography may be able to assess pulmonary artery, pericardial, and arterial involvement in some patients.[431] However, a significant portion of patients with abnormal angiograms have re-

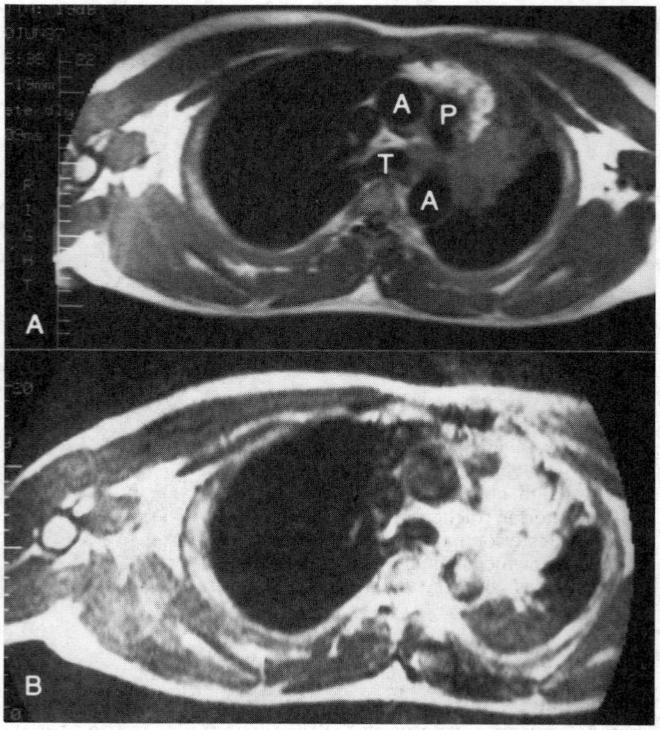

FIG. 22-9. Magnetic resonance image of patient whose CT scan is shown in Figure 22-8D. Image **A** is to be contrasted with Image **B**, which is an inversion recovery sequence that highlights the extent of tumor and the lymph nodes involved (shown in white). A = aorta; P = pulmonary artery; T = trachea.

sectable tumors, and thus an angiogram must always be used in conjunction with mediastinoscopy and CT scanning to make preoperative decisions regarding resectability.

Other Indirect Tests of Mediastinal and Hilar Nodal Involvement

The findings on mediastinal tomograms, esophagrams, azygograms, and perfusion lung scans correlate poorly with mediastinoscopy results, with false-positive and false-negative rates of 30% to 50%.[432–435] B-mode gray-scale sonography is useful in determining whether a large area of radiographic opacification is caused by fluid, tumor, or intrinsic pulmonary disease such as obstruction or consolidation.[436]

Monoclonal Antibody Imaging

Clinical studies of radiolabeled monoclonal antibodies recognizing specific determinants on cancer cells are just beginning in lung cancer (Figs. 22-10 and 22-11). So far, there have been relatively few antibodies shown to localize in lung tumors. Polyclonal anti-CEA antibodies[437] have been studied with mixed successes, as have polyclonal antibodies raised against alpha-fetoprotein.[438] Perkins and coworkers, using antibody 791T/36 labeled with ^{131}I reported imaging of three of eight primary lung tumors after blood pool subtraction and higher success rates (69%) when the antibody was linked

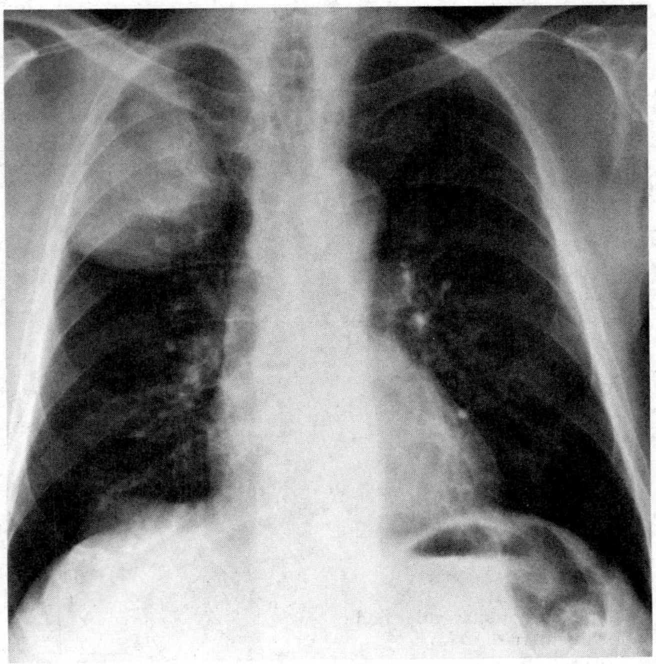

FIG. 22-10. Chest radiograph of a patient with a large right upper lobe mass invading the chest wall. This patient would require chest wall resection and en bloc lobectomy.

with indium-111.[439] Chan and associates, using radiolabeled antibodies directed against a c-*myc* oncogene product, had tumor localization in 12 of 14 patients with lung cancer, but success was dependent on the size of the tumor.[440]

FIG. 22-11. Monoclonal antibody scan performed on patient whose x-ray film is shown in Figure 22-10. Triangular arrows depict posterior and anterior views of the chest wall mass. Some cardiac blood pool is visualized, as is the thyroid.

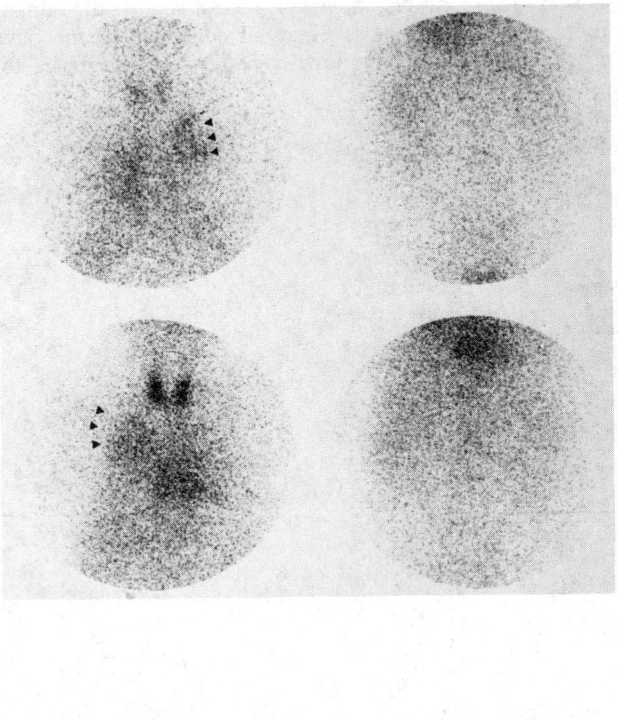

STAGING PROCEDURES FOR DISTANT METASTASES (M FACTOR)

The best screen for extrathoracic spread is a careful history and physical examination along with laboratory data including serum calcium, bilirubin, transaminases, lactate dehydrogenase (LDH), and alkaline phosphatase determination. The liver, bones, central nervous system, adrenal glands, and lymph nodes frequently harbor metastatic disease, yet the routine use of bone, brain, liver, and spleen scans is controversial.[441-447] Positive bone scans or liver scans may in fact represent areas of old inflammation or fracture and thus delay treatment unnecessarily. Moreover, in the absence of symptoms and signs, these tests will be positive in only 5% to 10% of patients. Thus, current recommendations by the authors are to perform brain, liver, and bone scans or skeletal surveys only if there is other clinical evidence that suggests the possibility of metastases. Biopsy of the bone marrow and liver in patients with non-small cell carcinomas and no other clinical evidence of metastases is positive in 10% to 15% or less of cases.[448-450] Therefore, we do not recommend routine biopsy of these sites unless some other clinical evidence suggests the possibility of metastases.

Whereas staging CT scans are vital in the conduct of clinical trials investigating new therapies, their cost effectiveness is low in the management of asymptomatic patients. Nevertheless, it would appear prudent to use head and upper-abdominal CT scans in all candidates for a curative approach with surgery or radiotherapy, as the finding of definitive evidence of brain or abdominal metastases would clearly alter the primary treatment plan. In a recent series of 63 patients screened with EEG, neurologic examination, and brain CT who were asymptomatic from a neurologic standpoint, five had silent brain metastases.[451] More routine use of upper-abdominal CT scanning at the time of chest CT has been advocated to evaluate the liver and adrenal glands. For example, 5 of 38 patients were found to have occult adrenal metastases in a recent series.[452]

PHYSIOLOGIC STAGING OF THE PATIENT

Assessment of the patient's physiologic and performance status is critical in order to determine his or her ability to tolerate thoracotomy and pulmonary resection, aggressive radiotherapy, or intensive chemotherapy. Patients with lung cancer often have cardiopulmonary problems related to chronic pulmonary disease or their age, and many studies have been performed to assess patients' ability to tolerate general anesthesia and pulmonary surgery, including whether pneumonectomy or lobectomy can be undertaken. The essence of preoperative physiologic evaluation is to determine which patients can undergo surgery with a reasonable operative mortality rate and still be functional. It is not always possible to predict whether a lobectomy or a pneumonectomy will be required until the time of surgery; thus, preoperative estimation of tolerance should always consider the possibility of pneumonectomy.

PERFORMANCE STATUS, AGE, AND SEX

Performance status (PS) is an important prognostic factor. Patients who are fully ambulatory and either asymptomatic (PS 0) or symptomatic (PS 1) tolerate surgery or aggressive chemoradiotherapy better than do those who are not fully ambulatory but are out of bed more than 50% of the time (PS 2). These patients, in turn, do better than those who are ambulatory less than 50% of the time (PS 3) and those who are bedridden (PS 4). When other medical problems are identified and corrected (including nutritional deficits, anemia, electrolyte disorders, dehydration, and infection), the performance status may improve and thus also improve prognosis and operability.[453–456]

The combination of a serious reduction in the patient's pulmonary reserve and significant cardiovascular, hepatic, or renal disease or poor performance status is a contraindication to resectional pulmonary surgery.[453,454] Stanley analyzed 77 prognostic factors in more than 5000 patients with lung cancer entered in Veterans Administration Lung Group (VALG) protocols between 1968 and 1978.[456] The most important prognostic factors, in order of importance, were initial performance status, extent of disease, weight loss greater than 10 pounds in the previous 6 months, and the presence of any systemic symptoms (Tables 22-30 and 22-31). In a similar study performed by Finkelstein and associates, looking at those pretreatment predictors of survival in 893 patients on Eastern Cooperative Oncology Group (ECOG) protocols, initial performance status, the absence of metastatic disease, female sex, and absence of weight loss in the previous 6 months all correlated with survival greater than 1 year.[457] The contributions of other factors such as tumor size and histologic type were minor after correction for the major prognostic features, particularly performance status. Interestingly, age does not seem to have a prognostic impact.[456,458] Although the operative mortality rate in general is greater for older patients, the rate in selected patients over 70 years old is no greater than the expected mortality rate for younger patients.[459] Thus, it is important to assess the patient's physiologic rather than chronologic age when making decisions about patients who are on the borderline of operability.

TABLE 22-31. Influence of Various Pretreatment Variables on the Survival of Patients with Inoperable Lung Cancer*

Variable	*Median Survival (wk)*	*% of Patients with Variable*
Stage of disease†		
Limited	28	21
Extensive	13	79
Weight loss (lb)		
Less than 10	22	52
More than 10	11	48
Presence of systemic symptoms		
No	28	49
Yes	15	51
Reduced appetite		
No	27	53
Yes	15	47
Initial lymphocyte count/ml		
>2000	16	42
<1000	8	19
Any metastatic disease symptoms		
No	22	64
Yes	15	36
Scalene or supraclavicular node involvement		
No	22	83
Yes	14	17

*Stanley KE: Prognostic factors for survival in patients with inoperable lung cancer. JNCI 65:25–32, 1980.

†Limited-stage disease is defined by VA Lung Group as disease confined to one hemithorax with or without scalene or supraclavicular node involvement; extensive-stage disease in all disease beyond one hemithorax and ipsilateral supraclavicular nodes.

In the United States, female patients with lung cancer tend to have better survival rates than do males. This difference is not explained by age, resectability, operative mortality rate, histopathology, location of the tumor, or differences in tumor stage.[460–462] The difference is particularly marked in female patients with localized disease who undergo surgical resection (Table 22-32). However, recent reports of younger women with bad-prognosis Stage III adenocarcinoma have appeared.[463] Also, for unknown reasons, the prognosis for

TABLE 22-30. Influence of Pretreatment Performance Status On Survival of 5022 Men with Inoperable Lung Cancer*

Performance Status Scale				
ECOG (Zubrod)†	*Karnofsky*	*Definitions*	*Median Survival (wk)*	*% of Patients In Group*
0	100	Asymptomatic	34	2
1	80–90	Symptomatic, fully ambulatory	24–27	32
2	60–70	Symptomatic, in bed <50% of day	14–21	40
3	40–50	Symptomatic, in bed >50% of day but not bedridden	7–9	22
4	20–30	Bedridden	3–5	5

*Stanley KE: Prognostic factors for survival in patients with inoperable lung cancer. JNCI 65:25–32, 1980.

†Eastern Cooperative Oncology Group (ECOG) or Zubrod performance status score.

TABLE 22-32. Comparison of Survival Rates of Men and Women with Lung Cancer*

Stage of Disease	*Time Period*	*5-Year Survival (%)* Male	Female
NCI SEER Program†			
All	1965–1969	8	13
Localized		28	51
Regional spread		10	15
Localized disease, postsurgical resection‡	1949–1962	29	49
	1950–1959	35	68

*The number of patients in each group is more than 1000.

†Silverberg E: Cancer statistics, 1984. CA 34:7–23, 1984; Cancer Patient Survival, Report No. 5, DHEW Publ. No. (NIH) 77-992, 1977.

‡Watson WLL, Schottenfeld D: Survival in cancer of the bronchus and lung 1949–1962: Comparison of men and women patients. Dis Chest 53:65–72, 1968; Ederer F, Mersheimer WL: Sex differences in the survival of lung cancer patients. Cancer 15:425–432, 1962; Connelly RR, Cutler SJ, Baylis P: End results in cancer of the lung: Comparison of male and female patients. JNCI 36:277–287, 1966.

women is worse than that for men in Wales and England and possibly in France even after surgical resection of localized disease.[464]

The observation that blood transfusion may deleteriously affect the survival of patients undergoing resection for colon cancer, breast cancer, and sarcoma has led to similar investigations in good-risk patients undergoing lung cancer resection. Perioperative blood transfusion was found to be a significant prognostic factor adversely affecting disease-free survival, with the prognosis being worse with intraoperative transfusion than postoperative transfusion.[465] The survival effected was long term and related to cancer recurrence, as patients receiving transfusions had a 62% disease-free rate at 5 years, whereas the other patients' rate was 76%. These findings were confirmed in a retrospective review by Hyman and associates,[466] and further cooperative studies are being analyzed to verify the deleterious survival impact of perioperative transfusion.

CARDIAC STATUS

The signs or symptoms of a myocardial infarction in the past 6 months in the patient with lung cancer should be sought and serial ECGs reviewed. An infarct in this period would be a contraindication to surgery and a documented infarct within the past 3 months an absolute contraindication to thoracic surgery. More than 20% of such patients will die of a complication related to reinfarction alone.[467] About 10% to 15% of all patients evaluated for lung cancer surgery will have ECG abnormalities, and all cardiac arrhythmias should be identified and, if possible, corrected. Serum potassium deficits and calcium excess should be identified and corrected as well, because these can potentiate digitalis toxicity and anesthetic hazard.[455,468] Uncontrolled major arrhythmias, such as multifocal premature ventricular contractions, carry a high risk and usually will contraindicate surgery. Bundle branch block is not a contraindication to surgery. However, in estimating risk, a right bundle-branch block or a left anterior fascicular block carries less risk than does a left posterior fascicular block, whereas combination and bifascicular blocks put the patient at greatest risk.[453] If the patient has a history of angina, cardiology evaluation should be obtained and noninvasive tests of myocardial function such as echocardiography performed. If the angina is progressive and not under treatment, evaluation with radionuclide multigated acquisition (MUGA) scans at rest and exercise may define high-risk groups (*i.e.*, triple coronary vessel disease and left main artery occlusive disease). Positive exercise multigated acquisition (MUGA) scans should be followed by coronary angiography, and if significant coronary occlusion is found, appropriate medical treatment with calcium-channel blockers or beta blockers (if underlying pulmonary disease permits) should be begun. For patients with significant coronary artery stenosis deemed better served by bypass grafting, this should be performed prior to or concomitantly with pulmonary resection. A series of 43 patients undergoing concomitant pulmonary cardiac operations requiring heart-lung bypass has been reported from the Mayo Clinic, of whom 10 had bronchogenic carcinoma.[469] Wedge resection, lobectomy, or pneumonectomy could be performed safely, and the resection was performed before commencing bypass or after the heparin was reversed with protamine to avoid hemorrhage, the cause for the two operative deaths (4.6%). Despite the technical ability to perform the operation via sternotomy, the ability to sample lymph node basins is compromised by this incision.

PULMONARY FUNCTION STATUS

Lung cancer surgery strenuously tests the patients' pulmonary reserve. Thus, patients must have pulmonary function testing to evaluate respiratory reserve before surgery. In lung cancer patients, in addition to chronic lung disease and cigarette abuse, the size of the primary tumor, its proximity to the hilum, and involvement of the ipsilateral hilar lymph nodes determine the extent of functional impairment. Thoracotomy is followed by postoperative chest pain with reduction in the depth of inspiration and inhibition of cough. Postoperative pain and the use of narcotics and other analgesics result in alveolar collapse, possibly leading to pneumonitis and respiratory failure. Postoperative respiratory complications are increased secondary to hypercarbia and ventilatory insufficiency if the patient's postoperative FEV_1 is less than 0.8 liters. Thus, preoperative attempts to improve pulmonary function should be aggressive and include cessation of smoking, bronchodilators, antibiotics in patients with bronchitis, inhalation of humidified air, segmental postural drainage, and chest physiotherapy. Preoperatively, if the FEV_1 is greater than 50% of the FVC and greater than 2.1 liters, the maximum voluntary ventilation is greater than 50% of predicted values, and the ratio of residual volume to total lung capacity is less than 50%, the patient is a reasonable candidate for surgery. If the FEV_1 is 2.5 liters or more, the patient can tolerate pneumonectomy; if the FEV_1 is less than 1 liter, the patient usually cannot tolerate any loss of functional lung tissue. However, if the FEV_1 falls between 1.1 and 2.4 liters of flow, the risk of any resection and the maximum tolerable resection are judgmental and require further study.[453,470–472]

The patient's postoperative pulmonary functional status will depend on the extent of resection and the functional contribution of the resected segments. A number of studies have indicated the ability of quantitative radionuclide ventilation scans to predict lung function following resection in patients with impaired pulmonary function and help plan the extent of resection in lung cancer patients.[473] Scintigraphic ventilation—perfusion studies may also provide serial data regarding radiation-induced changes to guide high-dose radiotherapy. Split function studies are carried out by summing the activity of each lung in the anterior and posterior view, and the postoperative function is predicted by multiplying the preoperative value by the ratio of the counts in the remaining lung to the total lung acitivity. Pneumonectomy is functionally tolerable if the percentage of ventilation to the nontumor-bearing lung when multiplied by the FEV_1 equals 1 liter or more of flow. If the volume of the normal lung exceeds its ventilation by more than 5%, there is a greater chance of postpneumonectomy ventilatory failure.[474] An estimated postoperative FEV_1 of less than 33% of the predicted value, when accompanied by evidence of severe generalized airway obstruction and abnormal V/Q distribution within the nontumor-bearing lung, indicates a high surgical risk.[474,475] The quantitative techniques are limited by the difficulty in predicting segmental or lobar contributions. Krypton scintigraphy and aerosol inhalation studies may provide better quantification of both regional ventilation and lobar ventilation–perfusion ratios.[476]

Preoperative blood gas analysis should also be performed for moderate to high-risk patients, with abnormalities ($PaCO_2$ exceeding 45 Torr or PaO_2 below 55 Torr) indicating a high risk of postoperative pulmonary insufficiency.[453] Abnormalities of CO_2 are more significant than abnormalities of PO_2 because the former can result only from alveolar hypoventilation, whereas the latter may result from an admixture of venous and arterial blood in the tumor area.[472] However, many patients who appear to be marginal surgical risks readily tolerate even extended resection if the burden of the ventilation defect is in the tumor-bearing area. If significant shunting occurs on the affected side, pulmonary function and arterial blood gases may improve after resection. Although hypoperfusion on the V/Q scan is not a sign of inoperability, a preoperative finding of less than 33% perfusion to the tumor-bearing lung suggests a pneumonectomy will be required for surgical cure.[477,478]

The measurement of preoperative pulmonary artery pressure as an indication of the development of postoperative pulmonary hypertension is rarely performed now, but criteria of mean pulmonary arterial pressure of 30 mm Hg or greater after unilateral occlusion, CO_2 greater than 45 mm Hg, and predicted postpneumonectomy FEV_1 above 0.8 liter still define patients who would not be able to tolerate pneumonectomy.

INFLUENCE OF OTHER FACTORS ON SURVIVAL

Lung Cancer in the Elderly

Lung cancer incidence increases with age in the United States, and analysis of nearly 23,000 cases from the Centralized Cancer Patient Data System showed that the percentage of patients with local-stage disease increases with age and that this is independent of sex, race, and histologic subtype.[479] At age 54 or younger, 15% present with local-stage disease, whereas the figure is 19% for those 55 to 64 years, 22% for those 65 to 74 years, and 25% for those 75 or older.[479] In addition, analysis of 6332 patients who underwent surgical staging showed a greater likelihood of local-stage disease with increasing age.[479]

Although elderly patients (over 70 years of age) with lung cancer do have other medical problems, they do not differ with respect to many presurgical variables such as smoking history, arterial blood gas values, degree of airflow obstruction, or cell type.[480] Although operative mortality rate in the elderly is greater (9% versus 4% in one series), there are no statistically significant differences in postoperative complication rates, length of postoperative hospital stay, or actuarial survival rates. Thus, elderly patients with reasonable cardiopulmonary function should not be denied potentially curative pulmonary resection simply because of concern about possible age-related complications.[480]

Effects of Socioeconomic Status on Lung Cancer Treatment

The role of socioeconomic factors in determining lung cancer treatment is not well defined. Studies conducted on patients treated between 1955 and 1964 found no significant difference between Veterans Administration status, whites, blacks, indigent versus nonindigent, income status, or private versus nonprivate patient status in the percentage of patients with localized disease or in survival.[481] Thus, the biology of the disease appeared to be more important than differences in natural history, detection, or treatment imposed by race or socioeconomic status. Recently, however, these observations have been challenged. Greenberg and associates studied 1403 cases of non-small cell cancer diagnosed between 1973 and 1976 in the regional tumor registries of New Hampshire and Vermont.[482] They found that the probability that patients would undergo potentially curative surgery was enhanced if they were younger, married, had private medical insurance, lived more than 39 km from a specialized center, had localized disease, or had a better functional status. Among the 1137 patients who did not undergo surgery, some form of cancer therapy (such as radiation or chemotherapy) was more frequently offered to patients who were younger, had private medical insurance, had a better functional status, or had no evidence of distant metastatic disease. Significantly, the probability of 3-year survival (about 11% in the 1403 patients) was unrelated to marital status, type of health insurance, or distance from a cancer treatment center. Those authors interpret their data as suggesting that physicians treat married patients and those with adequate medical insurance more aggressively, although these factors could also indicate these patients' better knowledge of the medical care system.[483]

TABLE 22-33. Frequency of TNM Findings at Diagnosis in the AJC Group of 368 Small Cell Lung Cancer Patients

	% of Patients
Asymptomatic at diagnosis	6
Tumor location	
Hilar	68
Peripheral	12
Apical	2
Mainstem bronchus	17
Tumor size	
<3 cm	20
>3 cm	80
Atelectasis/pneumonitis	
None	35
Segmental	43
Lobar	18
Entire lung	4
Pleural effusion	15
Clinical evidence of	
Mediastinal invasion	30
Metastases outside hemithorax of origin and mediastinum (M1)	48
Scalene or supraclavicular node involvement	30
Regional lymph node involvement clinically by radiography	
N0	27
N1 (hilar)	26
N2 (mediastinal)	47

Mountain CF: Clinical biology of small cell carcinoma: Relationship to surgical therapy. Semin Oncol 5:272–279, 1978.

STAGING AND PROGNOSTIC FACTORS IN PATIENTS WITH SMALL CELL LUNG CANCER

In patients who have histologic or cytologic evidence of small cell lung cancer, a different staging system and approach to staging are used because the primary treatment modality will be chemotherapy with or without radiotherapy, and no patients will receive solely locoregional therapy. In the uncommon case of a resected pulmonary nodule that proves to be small cell carcinoma, appropriate staging procedures should be employed postoperatively.

Mountain, in a review of 268 small cell lung cancer patients for the AJC staging system, found no difference in survival rate for small cell lung cancer for more than 40 characteristics, including sex; age; peripheral, central, or apical tumor location; radiographic appearance; size of the lesion (including tumors less than 3 cm in diameter); presence, absence, or degree of atelectasis; pneumonitis; pleural effusion; mediastinal invasion; regional lymph node involvement; or presence or absence of distant metastases (Table 22-33). There was no significant difference in 41 patients according to postsurgical Group (I, II, or III) in survival; none were cured.[484] Because the TNM factors did not appear to be prognostic for survival in small cell cancer patients treated predominantly with surgery or radiotherapy, the AJC initially recommended applying their system to small cell cancer only for purposes of later reference. With the recent recognition that a few small cell lung tumors can be extirpated surgically, detailed TNM staging has proved useful in identifying candidates for an operative approach and in estimating the prognosis in this infrequent clinical setting.[485] However, for the great majority of patients not undergoing thoracotomy for resection, nearly all investigators studying the treatment of small cell lung cancer have adopted the simple two-stage system of the VALG.[484]

In this two-stage system, limited disease is defined as that confined to one hemithorax and to the regional lymph nodes (including mediastinal and contralateral hilar and, usually, ipsilateral supraclavicular), whereas extensive disease is defined as that beyond this area, including distant lymph nodes, brain, liver, bone, bone marrow, and intra-abdominal and soft-tissue metastases. The definition of stage relates to whether the known tumor can be encompassed within a tolerable radiation port. Thus, ipsilateral pleural effusion, recurrent laryngeal nerve involvement, and SVC obstruction can still be considered limited-stage disease. However, pericardial effusion and bilateral pulmonary parenchymal involvement are scored as extensive-stage disease. Ipsilateral pleural effusion and various degrees of supraclavicular node involvement have been considered consistent with either limited or extensive disease by different authors. Among patients with otherwise limited tumors, neither of these factors appears to influence survival.[486,487]

PROGNOSTIC FACTORS

Limited-stage patients have both higher response rates and longer survival than do extensive-stage patients given identical or similar therapy.[487,488] In trials of combination chemotherapy with or without radiotherapy, patients classified as limited stage had a 86% total objective tumor regression rate, a 60% rate of complete clinical regression of tumor (complete response), and a median survival of 51 weeks. In contrast, patients scored as extensive stage had a 77% total response rate, a 25% complete response rate, and a median survival of 33 weeks.[488] Occasionally, similar response rates have been observed for both stages, with stage predicting only survival differences.[489,490] The durability of partial responses is only modestly affected by stage. However, complete response duration and long-term survival is markedly superior in limited-stage disease.[482,491,492]

Initial performance status strongly influences survival both in untreated patients and in patients receiving combination chemotherapy with or without radiotherapy.[486,493–496] Although more favorable performance status is found more frequently in limited-stage patients, within either stage, performance status is the most important variable.[486,487,491] Also, in extensive-stage patients, a strong correlation exists between worsening performance status and the number of sites of metastatic disease, suggesting that the prognostic effect of performance status may in some part be accounted for by its association with overall tumor burden.[486]

Stage of disease and performance status are the principal prognostic factors in previously untreated small cell lung cancer. In addition to stage (limited versus extensive), other tumor-related factors influence survival. For example, considerable variation in prognosis exists within extensive disease according to the distribution of tumor involvement. In an early review of 106 patients entered on NCI trials, extensive-disease patients with only a single site of metastases (outside areas of involvement included with limited stage) had survival rates that were not statistically distinguishable from those of patients with limited disease.[486] However, metastatic involvement of the liver, the central nervous system (CNS), or three or more extrathoracic organ systems presaged an especially unfavorable outcome. A more recent study of more than 800 patients from the Finsen Institute revealed that bone marrow, brain, and liver metastases, as well as the number of organ systems involved with metastatic cancer, significantly influenced prognosis in univariate analyses. In multivariate analysis, however, after stage of disease and probable "surrogate markers" of tumor burden such as performance status, plasma hemoglobin, and serum LDH were considered, specific sites of metastatic involvement no longer contributed significantly to prognosis.[497] When only 18-month disease-free survival rather than overall survival was the end-point, only stage of disease, and not performance status, hemoglobin, LDH, or specific sites of tumor, significantly influenced outcome.[498] The relatively favorable prognosis of one category of limited-disease patients, those whose tumor has been completely resected prior to initiation of chemotherapy or chemoradiotherapy, should be emphasized.[499–501] Whether this is attributable solely to the tumor resection or to the lesser tumor burden in patients whose cancers can be resected completely is not fully resolved.

In addition to performance status, other host-related factors, some of which correlate with performance status and others of which do not, affect prognosis. In some studies, weight loss is an unfavorable prognostic factor independent of stage and performance status for both untreated patients[493] and those given chemotherapy,[502] particularly for more ambulatory cases with a smaller tumor burden. Impaired immune status, as assessed by delayed hypersensitivity skin testing, also correlates with shorter survival, especially in patients with an otherwise favorable prognosis.[503] Sex and age were formerly thought to have little influence on prognosis,[486,504] but more recent studies of larger numbers of patients suggest that women[505] and younger patients[506] have better outcomes when receiving chemotherapy. A single study suggests that small cell lung cancer patients who discontinue cigarette smoking, particularly those who quit more than a year prior to diagnosis, have a better outcome that is independent of other prognostic factors.[507] Therefore, all such patients should be encouraged to stop smoking.

Finally, as in all other cancers, patients with small cell lung cancer who suffer tumor progression during or after administration of chemotherapy have an extremely poor prognosis, with a median survival of only 8 weeks in one large cooperative group study.[508]

Virtually all of the information on prognostic factors in small cell lung cancer has been derived from patients entered in prospective clinical trials. Although there is no reason to believe that such factors do not predict prognosis in the majority of patients who do not participate in these studies, survival differences might exist between patients who are and are not entered in clinical trials. In a recent study of 215 consecutive cases of small cell carcinoma, for various reasons, only 20% of patients were placed on available chemotherapy protocols.[509] Survival in extensive-stage patients placed on study was superior to that in patients who were managed "off protocol." In limited-stage patients, however, no survival differences were noted. These results are consistent with conventional wisdom that patients with poor performance status or those with severe non-neoplastic illnesses are less often entered in clinical trials. Because most limited-stage patients have their disease diagnosed while they are still in relatively good medical condition, however, their survival is much less affected by whether they are judged suitable for protocol entry.

CLINICAL PRESENTATION

Signs and symptoms of small cell lung cancer depend on the size and location of the primary tumor and the presence or absence of regional or distant metastases. With the exception of certain paraneoplastic syndromes, which are relatively uncommon, most clinical signs are no more specific for small cell carcinoma than for other types of lung cancer.[510] Because the primary tumor most often arises centrally, patients typically present with cough, dyspnea, wheezing, hemoptysis, chest pain, or postobstructive pneumonitis. The usual submucosal location of small cell carcinoma accounts for the relatively lower frequency of hemoptysis compared with squamous cell cancer.[511] Tumor extension to the mediastinum occurs almost invariably, accounting for the frequent occurrence of regional metastatic symptoms such as SVC syndrome, hoarseness from recurrent laryngeal nerve paralysis, and dysphagia. Almost 10% of patients will have SVC syndrome at diagnosis, and judicious invasive diagnostic procedures can usually be performed safely. Survival is similar to that in patients of the same stage without the syndrome.[512]

Patients may or may not be symptomatic from small cell carcinoma metastases. Radiographically detectable central nervous system (CNS) metastases are symptomatic in more than 90% of cases. Although bone metastases may be painful, they are not in most patients, and pathologic fractures are rare. Liver metastases cause (usually mild) dysfunction detectable by laboratory tests in 50% to 60% of cases with liver involvement, but liver function is impaired seriously in only a few of these cases. Usually, the liver involvement causes problems by its mass and overall contribution to tumor bulk and decreased performance status. In occasional patients, jaundice is secondary to extrahepatic biliary obstruction from pancreatic or nodal metastases rather than to tumor replacement of the liver; the prognosis is not so dire in the former group as in the latter.[513] Anemia, leukopenia, or thrombocytopenia related to bone marrow involvement is uncommon, and hemoglobin and white cell levels are not indicative of marrow involvement.[234,504] During intensive induction chemotherapy, patients with positive bone marrows have more severe infections and require more red blood cell transfusions than do patients without tumor in the marrow. However, leukopenia, thrombocytopenia, and the need for platelet transfusions during induction therapy do not appear to correlate with marrow involvement.[504]

Elevated plasma concentrations of immunologically detected polypeptide hormones are much more frequent in small cell lung cancer than are symptoms from the corresponding paraneoplastic syndromes.[514–516] The syndrome of inappropriate secretion of antidiuretic hormone (SIADH), ectopic Cushing's syndrome, and the Eaton–Lambert or myasthenia-like syndrome are relatively specifically associated with small cell carcinoma. The frequency of SIADH at presentation differs according to definition of the syndrome but in one recent large series was 11%. Only 27% of patients fulfilling the diagnostic criteria for SIADH, however, were symptomatic from hyponatremia. The presence of SIADH was not correlated with stage of disease, tumor involvement of specific metastatic sites, or prognosis.[517]

STAGING PROCEDURES

Staging procedures are of value in selecting individual patients who can benefit from therapy that is efficacious only in certain stages, most commonly patients who can be managed suitably with locoregional treatment alone; in assigning prognosis; and in identifying areas of tumor involvement that can be monitored to determine response. In groups of patients, the staging process documents patterns of failure with a given form of treatment, thus suggesting new therapeutic strategies and, through the use of staging systems derived from these procedures, permits uniform and more easily interpreted reporting of results of clinical trials. Because of overt or covert distant metastases at the time of diagnosis, all patients with small cell lung cancer will receive chemotherapy, and staging procedures do not identify patients who can be given solely locoregional treatment. However, the staging process does divide patients into limited- and extensive-stage disease, which is of clear prognostic significance, and in most cases will lead to the administration of chest radiation in addition to chemotherapy in the former group. In addition, documenting initially involved sites of tumor aids in the later evaluation of response to therapy and diagnosis of eventual tumor progression. Except for the CNS, initial local or metastatic tumor deposits are the areas in which relapse develops in most cases.

The extent of the initial staging evaluation depends on clinical circumstances. Our recommendations are given in Table 22-34. When distant metastases are obvious or treatment will not be affected by stage, simple screening tests followed by only those studies that have an increased likelihood of being positive[518,519] are performed outside a clinical trial setting. In a prospective clinical trial or when stage-specific therapy is to be administered, additional studies are appropriate. If the purpose of the staging is to exclude patients with extensive disease from receiving chest irradiation, then no further procedures need be done after an unequivocal site of distant metastases is documented. Because of the frequent involvement of mediastinal lymph nodes in small cell lung cancer and the poor prognosis of node-positive patients who undergo surgical resection,[485] additional staging tests to evaluate the mediastinum are recommended in patients with known small cell lung cancer in whom surgical removal of the primary tumor is being considered.

The timing of restaging to assess response and the tests that should be performed depend on the cost and availability of specific procedures and the philosophy of the treating physician. Clearly, tumor sites that were initially involved should be reevaluated.

Finally, it should be recognized that any set of staging recommendations is somewhat arbitrary and that individualization of the process in different clinical circumstances is often appropriate. The initial therapy (combination chemotherapy with or without radiotherapy) is, in many respects, as demanding as thoracotomy and pulmonary resection. Thus, physiologic as well as anatomic staging is required. The intensity of the initial therapy and the combined use of chemotherapy and aggressive radiotherapy produced treatment-associated mortality rates of 5% or more in many recent series. The most important risk factor for treatment-related death appears to be the initial performance status. Although there are few data from recent trials, it would appear prudent to submit to extremely aggressive induction therapy only those patients who are ambulatory more than 50% of the time and who have adequate cardiopulmonary, renal, and hepatic function.

The primary tumor and regional nodal spread are evaluated by chest posteroanterior and lateral roentgenograms. In addition, fiberoptic bronchoscopy with bronchial washings and biopsy is essential to document the extent of disease and may be used to determine the degree of tumor response during follow-up. Before treatment, fiberoptic bronchoscopy will reveal evidence of cancer in more than 90% of patients, including approximately 8% to 10% in whom the tumor is not evaluable on chest films.[235] In follow-up, patients with evidence of tumor by bronchoscopy after initial therapy have a much higher relapse rate in the chest within a 6-month period than do patients with normal bronchoscopy findings at this time.[235,520]

Computed tomographic scans of the thorax provide more precise definition of parenchymal, mediastinal, and pleural disease.[521] They are probably most useful in the design of radiotherapy portals and in assessing persistence or early relapse of chest tumor. In our experience, all patients with intrathoracic tumor resolution by chest roentgenography and persistent endobronchial disease on bronchoscopy are identified as not being in complete remission by chest CT scans; additional patients in only partial remission are also detected.

The common sites of extrathoracic metastatic disease detected during pretreatment staging are bone in 38%, liver in

TABLE 22-34. Staging Procedures for Small Cell Lung Cancer

Minimum Survey (Screening Tests)

Complete history and physical examination

Chest roentgenography (with CT to assist in portal design if other than palliative chest irradiation is to be given)

Liver function tests and physical examination of liver (with radionuclide or CT liver scan if results abnormal)

Bone pain/alkaline phosphatase (with radionuclide bone scan if results abnormal)

Neurologic history and examination (with CT scan of brain if results abnormal)

Platelet count or leukoerythroblastic peripheral blood smear (with bone marrow aspiration/biopsy if results abnormal; also recommended if no other unequivocal distant metastatic disease has been documented or if all initial sites of involvement are to be reassessed to determine response)

*Procedures for Patients in Clinical Trials or Receiving Stage-Dependent Therapy**

Complete history and physical examination

Chest roentgenography plus CT scan of chest to assist in portal design if chest irradiation (other than palliative) is to be employed; plus fiberoptic bronchoscopy if no evaluable tumor on chest film)

Liver function tests/radionuclide or CT liver scan

Liver biopsy (peritoneoscopy or ultrasound guided) if either liver function tests or scan abnormal and best information concerning liver status is required to select therapy

Radionuclide bone scan

CT scan of brain in presence or absence of neurologic abnormalities if brain irradiation is to be given to asymptomatic patients

Bone marrow aspiration/biopsy (bilaterally if best information concerning marrow status is required)

Procedures Prior to Attempted Surgical Resection if Patient Is Known to Have Small Cell Cancer

All staging procedures listed for patients in clinical trials

Fiberoptic bronchoscopy

Evaluation of mediastinum

    CT scan of chest

    Mediastinoscopy†

Modified from Ihde DC: Staging evaluation and prognostic factors in small cell lung cancer. In Aisner J (ed): Lung Cancer, pp 241–268. New York, Churchill Livingstone, 1985.

* Evaluation can be stopped after documentation of extensive disease if staging is being used only to identify candidates for stage-specific therapy.

† Unless thought unnecessary by operating surgeon.

22% to 28%, bone marrow in 17% to 23%, and the CNS in 8% to 14% (Table 22-35).[486,505] Radionuclide bone scans are more sensitive than skeletal roentgenograms in identifying osseous metastases; the latter should be employed principally to confirm or exclude potential metastatic sites detected on bone scan.[504,522] The greater the number of bone scan abnormalities, the more likely it is that sites of extraosseous metastatic disease will be found. Improvement or worsening on follow-up scans correlates with the extraosseous tumor response 70% of the time.[522] As in other cancers, however, the principal difficulty with bone scans in small cell lung cancer is false-positive examinations secondary to benign bone and joint disease. Therefore, bone scans should not serve as the sole basis for making therapeutic decisions but rather should alert the clinician to the need for further evaluation. After treatment, osteoblastic changes sometimes can be seen on bone radiographs, probably representing regeneration of bone, not new metastases.[504] Thus, unless some other evidence of tumor progression exists, such changes alone should not be an indication for changing therapy. Bone marrow involvement is found with marrow aspiration and biopsy; often, the two procedures are complementary, and thus aspiration may be positive when the biopsy is not, and vice versa.[504] An additional 10% of patients (30% of all with positive marrows) will be found to have marrow involvement if bilateral biopsies are done.[504]

Fewer than 5% of patients will have bone marrow involvement as the sole site of extensive-stage disease.[523] A positive marrow examination does, however, yield pathologic proof that extensive disease is present, providing assurance of extrathoracic metastases that cannot be obtained with equivocal imaging studies. The results of bone scans and marrow examinations are significantly correlated, but they are complementary as each can be positive when the other is unrevealing.[522,524] Interestingly, in patients receiving chemotherapy, the requirement for transfusion of blood products or drug dosage reductions does not predict that bone marrow metastases will be found at autopsy.[525]

Although liver function tests are abnormal in 93% of patients whose livers are histologically positive for tumor, they also are abnormal in 41% of patients with histologically negative livers.[504] Both false-positive and false-negative liver radionuclide scans are seen in small cell cancer. If patients have a filling defect on liver scan and abnormal liver function tests, histologic proof of liver involvement can be obtained in almost 90% of cases, whereas patients in whom both scan and function tests are negative will have positive liver biopsies less than 10% of the time. If either the scan or

TABLE 22-35. Results of Pretreatment Staging Procedures in Small Cell Lung Cancer*

	% of Patients with Finding
Final stage†	
Limited stage	31
Extensive stage	69
Chest staging	
Chest film mass‡	90
Fiberoptic bronchoscopy‡	
Visual endobronchial tumor	83
Washings/biopsy pathologically positive	87
Pleural effusion†	9
Ipsilateral supraclavicular node†	6
Contralateral lung†	7
Bilateral endobronchial tumor†	5
Bone (bone scan)†	38
Liver (histologically proven by biopsy)†§	22–28
Bone marrow*‖#**	17–23
Central nervous system†‡‡#	8–14
Brain	10
Spinal	5
Leptomeningeal	2
Retroperitoneal metastases (CT scan)§§	16
Soft tissue biopsy proven†	24

*Each category consists of between 100 and 600 patients.
†Ihde DC, Makuch RW, Carney DN et al, Am Rev Respir Dis 123:500–507, 1981.
‡Ihde DC, Cohen MH, Bernath AM et al, Chest 74:531–536, 1978.
§Dombernowsky P, Hirsch F, Hansen HH et al, Cancer 41:2008–2012, 1978.
‖Ihde DC, Simms EG, Matthews MJ et al, Blood 53:667–686, 1979.
#Hirsch FR, Hansen HH, Hainau B, Acta Pathol Microbiol Scand 87:59–62, 1979.
**Hirsch F, Hansen HH, Dombernowsky P et al, Cancer 39:2463–2567, 1977.
††Hansen HH, Dombernowsky P, Hirsch FR, Semin Oncol 5:280–287, 1978.
‡‡Bunn PA Jr, Nugenet JL, Matthews MJ, Semin Oncol 5:314–322, 1978.
§§Dunnick NR, Ihde DC, Johnston-Early A, AJR 133:1085–1088, 1979.

the function tests, but not both, is abnormal, the probability of liver involvement at biopsy is approximately 20%.[526] If it is deemed essential to prove or disprove liver involvement pathologically, the best method of detecting metastases is with multiple biopsies at peritoneoscopy.[504,526,527] Recent data suggest that ultrasound-guided fine-needle aspiration of the liver is approximately as sensitive as peritoneoscopy in yielding pathologic confirmation of liver involvement.[528] Contraindications to obtaining liver biopsy confirmation are bleeding disorders, a patient unable to cooperate, massive pleural effusion, or respiratory decompensation so that the procedure cannot be tolerated.

Metastases to the CNS are extremely common clinical problems, occurring in approximately 30% of patients at diagnosis or during the subsequent course of the disease.[529] CT scans of the brain are superior to radionuclide scans in documenting brain metastases in patients with neurologic symptoms or signs, but both tests are abnormal in the great majority of cases. As screening examinations in asymptomatic patients, the yield of both is low, in the range of 5% to 10% for CT scan and less than 5% for radionuclide scan.[518,530,531] However, the CT scan is clearly the examination of choice, with greater sensitivity and positive predictive accuracy.[532] Many clinicians advocate screening CT scans at diagnosis of small cell lung cancer in asymptomatic patients, because brain irradiation would be administered if the test were positive. In one series, however, there was no evidence that detection of brain metastases in asymptomatic patients is associated with survival rates superior to those in patients whose metastases are diagnosed because of neurologic symptoms or signs.[532] Patients with brain metastases as the only site of extensive-stage disease have a median survival not markedly different from that of patients with limited disease, although long-term survival is rare and relapse in the brain after irradiation is frequent.[530,532] At present, in asymptomatic patients with a negative, careful neurologic examination, a clear-cut indication for a head CT scan would be just before administration of prophylactic cranial irradiation. If asymptomatic lesions were discovered, a higher dose of radiotherapy would be delivered.[533,534]

Metastases to the CNS can be intracranial, spinal epidural with spinal cord compression, or leptomeningeal with carcinomatous meningitis.[533–535] Screening asymptomatic patients with cerebrospinal fluid (CSF) cytologies is unrewarding.[535,536] However, it is important to know that once one site of CNS metastatic disease is discovered, the probability of finding disease at other CNS sites is increased greatly. Clinically apparent multiple sites are present in 20% of patients with CNS metastases and are discovered in 73% of such patients at autopsy.[534] Patients suspected of having spinal cord compression should undergo a myelogram promptly. Likewise, patients with signs and symptoms of leptomeningeal involvement should have CSF cytologies performed. Brain imaging studies should also be performed in both situations. Back pain and abnormal spine findings on bone scan or radiographs or minimal neurologic abnormalities suggesting an epidural lesion in the presence of an intracranial metastasis or carcinomatous leptomeningitis should be an indication for a myelogram. Back pain and bone destruction on radiographs are found in most patients whose cord compression is present at diagnosis of small cell lung cancer but less often in patients whose epidural lesion is documented during the subsequent course of disease.[537] Occasional patients with symptoms of spinal cord dysfunction, often manifested as Brown-Sequard syndrome, will prove to have intramedullary rather than epidural tumor.[538]

Because of the high frequency of intra-abdominal metastases found at autopsy in the adrenals, pancreas, kidneys, and lymph nodes, pretreatment staging of these areas would be useful (see Table 22-19).[208] Abdominal CT scanning may be useful for such staging, but its general use in screening currently is not recommended, although CT scans are frequently used instead of radionuclide scans to image the liver. Upper abdominal CT scans performed prospectively reveal metastases in 36% of patients.[539] The most common site is the liver, whereas retroperitoneal metastases are found in 16%. The CT scan has a sensitivity of approximately 88% and a specificity of 94% as judged by biopsy results.[539] Although abdominal CT scans in small cell cancer can demonstrate metastatic dissemination that cannot be evaluated by other means, they provide relatively little therapeutically relevant information beyond that obtained with standard staging procedures,[536,540,541] because most positive studies occur in patients already known to have more extensive tumor dissemination.[536,540] However, in individual patients, CT scans may be excellent indicators of disease extent and response. When 24 patients with normal adrenal glands by CT scan underwent percutaneous thin-needle biopsy, 17% of the 29 glands sampled adequately contained metastases.[542] Thus, metastatic spread had occurred even to CT-negative organs.

POTENTIAL NEW METHODS FOR STAGING AND FOLLOW-UP OF LUNG CANCER PATIENTS

Although imaging studies provide excellent staging and follow-up data, they obviously are expensive and time consuming. Tumor markers that could be followed by blood tests would be highly desirable. Unfortunately, no such tests are as yet available. Potential candidates include neuron-specific enolase (NSE), creatine kinase BB (CK-BB), and chromogranin A (CGA, the matrix protein of neurosecretory granules) in small cell lung cancer and CEA for all types of lung cancer. Small cell lung cancer produces high levels of NSE, CK-BB, and CGA intracellularly, and with tumor cell breakdown, these products are released into the serum where they can be measured by radioimmunoassay.[543–547] Compared with normal adult controls, serum NSE was raised by more than 12 ng/ml in 69% of 94 newly diagnosed cases of small cell lung cancer. This included 39% of limited-stage and 87% of extensive-stage disease, and extensive-stage patients had higher NSE levels (59 ng/ml) than did limited-stage patients (13 ng/ml). Serial measurements in 23 patients receiving combination chemotherapy showed an excellent correlation between serum NSE and clinical response.[542,545,546] Thus, elevated serum NSE levels are associated with tumor cell bulk (and poor prognosis) and mirror tumor response in small cell lung cancer. A small number of reports indicate that the same observations hold for CK-BB and CGA.[544,545] There has been no demonstration, however, that utilization of any of these markers, including CEA (see below), can substitute for more conventional staging procedures or lead to improved therapeutic results.

CEA also is correlated with disease extent and clinical course. In small cell lung cancer, elevated levels (greater than 2.5 ng/ml) occurred in 88% of extensive-stage and 45% of limited-stage cases, whereas all patients with CEA levels exceeding 50 ng/ml had liver involvement.[548] CEA values provide prognostic information that is independent of stage and performance status,[549] and changes over time correlate with response to chemotherapy and relapse.[548,550] In addition, there is a strong correlation between positive staining of the tumor for CEA and plasma CEA elevation.[551] Thus, in the individual patient, an immunohistochemical stain can indicate whether CEA will be a followable marker.

TREATMENT OF LUNG CANCER BY SURGERY OR RADIOTHERAPY WITH CURATIVE INTENT

SURGICAL TREATMENT

Historical

The first successful total pneumonectomy for bronchogenic carcinoma was performed by Graham and Singer in 1933.[552] Up to that time, there were six cases in the literature in which a patient had survived the removal of a carcinoma for 1 year or more.[553] Rienhoff and colleagues described an individual ligation technique for pneumonectomy with improved management of the bronchial stump,[554] paving the way for the modern practice of individual venous, arterial, and bronchial ligation.

Overview

INFLUENCE OF RANDOMIZED TRIALS. Surgical resection currently offers the best hope of cure in non-small cell lung cancer (Tables 22-36 and 22-37). However, the disappointing results of surgical therapy alone in all stages have led to the investigation of multimodal therapies with the hope of improving survival. With historical study designs, it is not possible to establish unequivocally the extent of comparability between the cases investigated and the control groups. The advantage of prospective randomized trials in the investigation of treatment efficacy thus cannot be overemphasized, even in trials that answer only surgically related questions. Moreover, survival of patients participating in prospective randomized trials significantly exceeds that of nonparticipants,[555] and this survival advantage is not explained by differences in pretreatment disease status or factors of known prognostic significance to the extent to which such data are available. In other words, participation in controlled trials of cancer therapy seems to ensure an inherent advantage, regardless of whether trial patients received experimental therapy or standard therapy. Whatever the reason for this benefit, it should provide a strong impetus for patients to enter such trials.

The NCI LCSG was established in 1977 to carry out prospective randomized trials of adjuvant therapy in resectable lung cancer. The multicenter approach has assured that accrual of patients would not be a limiting factor in the performance of these trials. This group has been at the forefront, not only in the design of such protocols, but also in establishing the modern-day statistics on mortality and survival rates of resectional therapy for lung cancer. The LCSG has investigated the differences in the extent of resection with regard to survival and evaluated the extent and location of nodal positivity in relation to survival and treatment options, as well as serving as a source for pathologic evaluation of resected material. Because of the uniformly high quality of data representing nine institutions, we emphasize the current results of the LCSG over those from many other studies reported previously.

TECHNICAL CONSIDERATIONS. The selection of the appropriate surgical procedure in resectable cases is deter-

TABLE 22-36. Survival After Surgical Resection of Lung Cancer

	5- and 10-Year Survival (%)				
*Histologic Type**	*5-Year*	*Range*	*n*	*10-Year*	*n*
Epidermoid carcinoma	33	26–43	1643	17	1115
Adenocarcinoma	26	20–34	535	16	352
Large cell carcinoma	28	6–36	278	8	278
Bronchioloalveolar	51	48–61	76	24	76
Small cell carcinoma	1	0–20	125	<0.5	125
Total	30	26–36	2790	15	1946

Mountain CF: Assessment of the role of surgery for control of lung cancer. Ann Thorac Surg 24:365–373, 1977; Paulson DL, Reisch JS: Long-term survival after resection for bronchogenic carcinoma. Ann Surg 184:324–332, 1976; Wilkins WE Jr, Scannell JG, Crauer JG: Four decades of experience with resection for bronchogenic carcinoma at the Massachusetts General Hospital. J Thorac Cardiovasc Surg 76:364–368, 1978; Ashor GL, Kem WH, Meyer BW et al: Long term survival in bronchogenic carcinoma. J Thorac Cardiovasc Surg 70:581–589, 1975; Kirsch MM, Rotman H, Argenta L et al: Carcinoma of the lung: results of treatment over ten years. Ann Thorac Surg 21:371–377, 1976.

* Miscellaneous histologic types (*e.g.*, adenosquamous) had a 10-year survival rate of 14% for 87 patients.

mined by the size of the tumor, its anatomic extent, and the physiologic status of the patient. The actual extent of resection remains a matter of surgical judgment and experience based on the findings at exploration. The surgeon is guided by the principle of performing the procedure that will ensure removal of all known disease with maximum conservation of pulmonary tissue. Two decades ago, it was widely held that pneumonectomy with hilar node dissection should always be performed regardless of the size of the primary lesion. Now, lobectomy is considered the operation of choice by most surgeons when the lesion is confined to one lobe and no nodal positivity is suspected. In a large series of patients followed by the Veterans Administration Surgical Oncology Group, long-term survival was essentially the same after lobectomy as pneumonectomy.[556] The use of segmental resections or large wedge resections combined with lymph node sampling instead of lobectomy (even in patients with good pulmonary function) is now under investigation and will be discussed later in the chapter.

In all cases, the decision to resect for cure is based on the expectation that no gross residual disease would remain at the conclusion of the procedure. Thus, there is general agreement that candidates for curative surgical resection are those with Stage I and Stage II disease. Lobectomy is indicated for lesions totally confined within a lobe so as to permit 1 cm of more of normal lobar bronchus proximally. In addition, there should be no gross lymph node involvement central to the origin of the lobar bronchus. Careful attention is paid to en bloc dissection of the regional lymph nodes with frozen sections reviewed intraoperatively to ensure an adequate resection. It is with the Stage III lesions that controversy has always existed because of the finding of intraoperative mediastinal nodal positivity, which carries an unfavorable prognosis. The considerations for surgical resection in these situations revolve around the surgeon's findings at operation, including the extent and location of nodal positivity; the intactness of nodal capsules; the involvement of contiguous, sacrificeable structures; and the functional outcome predicted for the patient after an extended resection. These factors are discussed individually in a separate section of this chapter.

OTHER TECHNICAL CONSIDERATIONS. Anesthetic considerations for pulmonary resection involve the use of the safest inhalational and narcotic agents, proper airway control, and appropriate cardiovascular and respiratory

TABLE 22-37. Five-Year Survival (Cumulative %) After Surgical Resection of Lung Cancer by Postsurgical Stage (Old AJC System)*

Histology	*Stage I*	*Stage II*	*Stage III (M0)*	*Stage III-N2*
Epidermoid	54	35	19	13
	(231)†	(61)	(236)	(62)
Adenocarcinoma and large cell	51	18	10	2‡
	(99)	(42)	(165)	(45)
Small cell (41)	0	0	0	0

Carr DT, Mountain CF: The staging of lung cancer. Semin Oncol 1:229–234, 1974; Carr DT: Is staging of cancer of value? Cancer 51(12 Suppl):2503–2505, 1983.

* Figures in parentheses are numbers of patients.

†The fraction of these patients receiving postoperative radiotherapy is not reported.

‡The large cell cancer group had only a few patients but had an 11% 5-year survival rate.

monitoring. Patients with significant cardiac history or disease documented in the preoperative work-up benefit from on-line continuous arterial blood pressure monitoring as well as selective use of central venous catheterization. Highest-risk patients should have intraoperative Swan-Ganz catheterization, which can be used to optimize preload, afterload, and cardiac output to prevent an undue increase in myocardial oxygen consumption or fluid overload. For operations expected to be longer than 3 to 4 hours, urinary bladder catheterization is advised.

The routine use of disposable double-lumen endotracheal tubes and continuous digital oximetry have greatly facilitated inspection of the operative field for nodal mapping, defining fissures for transection, and permitting lung-sparing options, specifically sleeve lobectomies. Proper positioning of the tube prior to the start of the operation (to avoid upper lobe collapse by improper placement) can be achieved with the use of pediatric fiberoptic intubation bronchoscopes. On-line oximetry and measurement of end tidal P_{CO_2} will ensure that adequate oxygen tensions are being recorded without the need for multiple blood-gas measurements. The use of high-frequency ventilation, permitting reduced lung movements and lower airway pressures, is being evaluated at present and has been associated with improved oxygenation, increased hemodynamic stability, and better surgical access during major airway reconstruction.[557]

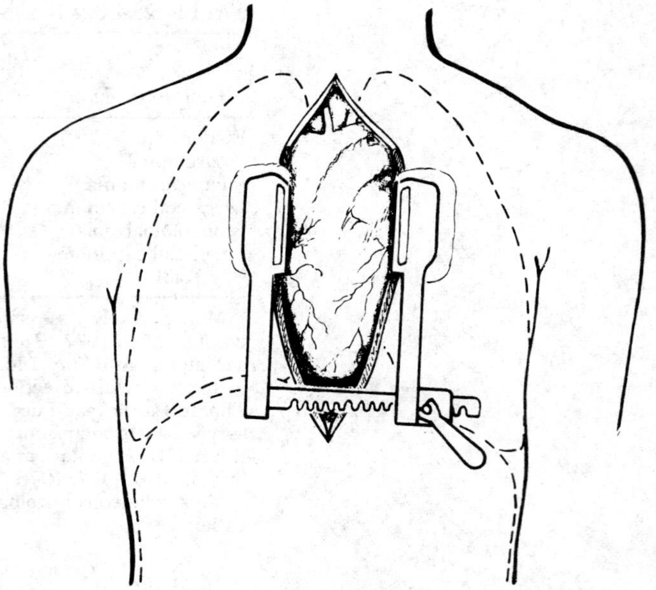

FIG. 22-12. Median sternotomy incision for pulmonary resection, allowing bilateral palpation of the lungs. However, left lower lobe resections are more difficult.

CHOICE OF INCISION. Pulmonary resection can be performed via a number of incisions: posterolateral, anterolateral, prone, or sternal splitting (Fig. 22-12). The most frequently used incision is the posterolateral thoracotomy beginning just below the nipple, curving posteriorly below the tip of the scapula, and extending cephalad to the vertebral column. The latissimus dorsi and serratus anterior muscles are divided and the chest entered usually via the resected fifth rib or through the fifth interspace (Fig. 22-13). This incision gives good visibility of both the bronchus and the blood vessels and improves management with the double-lumen tube by preventing spillage of secretions and blood into the opposite lung, collapsing the lung and expediting the manipulation and resection. However, it is a painful incision postoperatively. The anterolateral incision is less painful but does not provide the access needed for more difficult larger resections (Fig. 22-13). The prone incision, although providing ideal ventilation and drainage, has largely been abandoned because of the difficulty of performing cardiac resuscitation if necessary, inexperience of the anesthesiologists with it, and the resurgence of double-lumen technology. The median sternotomy has been championed by a number of surgeons as the incision of choice, citing decreased postoperative pain, quicker discharge from the hospital, and possible extension of pulmonary resection to patients with reduced pulmonary function who may not tolerate lateral thoracotomy.[558] However, experience with this technique is required to obtain maximum mediastinal

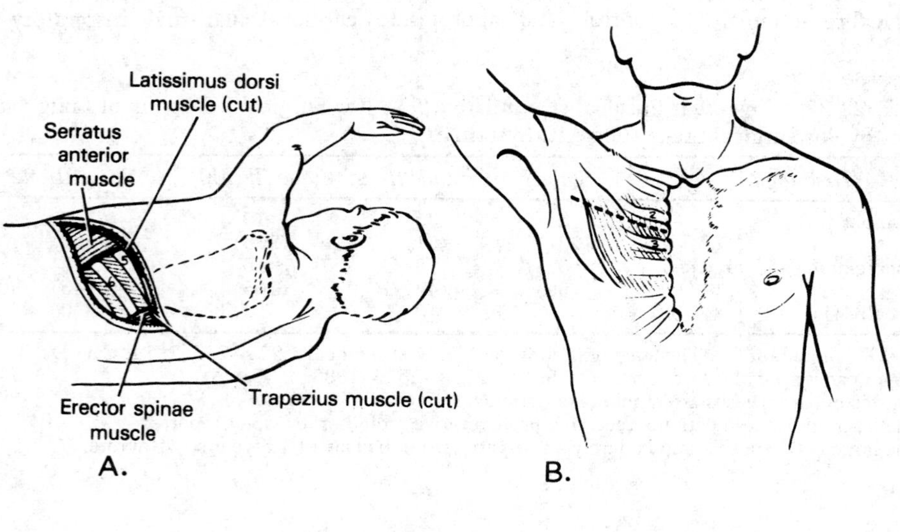

FIG. 22-13. **A.** Posterolateral thoracotomy incision for pulmonary resection. **B.** Anterior thoracotomy incision used for pulmonary resection.

exposure, and left lower-lobe resection may be difficult in obese individuals. Moreover, the median sternotomy incision cannot be used for resection of superior sulcus tumors or of posterior chest wall extensions. Finally, nodal sampling is compromised, especially access to the posterior subcarinal nodes.

DISSECTION, LIGATION, AND DIVISION OF PULMONARY VESSELS. Once the chest has been opened, the tumor and nodal basins must be assessed for resectability. Examination of the tumor will give an idea regarding the need for lobectomy, pneumonectomy, or sleeve resection. Palpation of the lesion should be performed, noting the position of the tumor with regard to the interlobar fissures and its proximity to the bronchovascular structures. Preoperative bronchoscopy will give the surgeon an idea of the proximal extent of the tumor with regard to its nearness to the carina. Intraoperative palpation and direct examination will reveal discrepancies from the preoperative findings if the tumor is densely adherent to the side wall of the main bronchus at a level higher than suspected from the preoperative bronchoscopy. The surgeon must then decide whether this T_3 lesion will require tracheal sleeve resection to remove it in its entirety (if a sleeve option is available) or if pneumonectomy at the level of the carina will suffice. The character and location of the nodal basins must be carefully investigated. Hilar nodes can be examined rapidly by sweeping back the pleura medially; subaortic and anterior mediastinal areas are palpated on the left, whereas paratracheal and azygous nodes are examined on the right.

Contiguous involvement of the pericardium, chest wall, or, rarely, the diaphragm must be assessed with regard to the ability to remove areas of invasion en bloc. When the hilum is difficult to evaluate, the pericardium can be opened for rapid examination of the pulmonary veins as well as the main pulmonary artery. This maneuver is critical when there is initial indecision regarding pulmonary artery involvement with tumor, because dissection without proximal control could lead to uncontrollable hemorrhage.

Once it is determined that the tumor is resectable, resection is accomplished in the most conservative manner that allows total tumor extirpation. The use of the stapling device has revolutionized pulmonary resection in all phases of the operation. Fissure division can be accomplished with the GIA stapling self-dividing device. The use of vascular staples can accomplish secure closure of the main pulmonary artery without suture reinforcement as well as division of the pulmonary veins; arterial division, however, is usually accomplished with the stapling device more easily in pneumonectomies than in lobectomies, necessitating double-ligation techniques for lobar arterial division with nonabsorbable suture ligature. Bronchial closure with the 4.8-mm stapler has been associated with a significantly lower incidence of bronchopleural fistula, yet the basic principle of maintaining a short bronchial stump without devascularization by nodal dissection must be upheld. Most surgeons prefer reinforcing the bronchial stump closure with a flap of mediastinal pleura, pericardium, or intercostal muscle pedicle flap, especially after right-sided pneumonectomy.

Careful intraoperative lymph node dissection and mapping must be performed in any resection for lung cancer and necessitates sampling of (at least) the paratracheal, subcarinal, hilar, and bronchopulmonary nodes. These nodes should be reported using the nomenclature for classification of pulmonary and mediastinal lymph nodes developed by the AJC.[380] Once the resection is completed, including lymph node dissection and sampling, the bronchus should be inspected and tested for air leak by sequentially subjecting it to airway pressures up to 40 cm H_2O. Any air leak should be repaired or the area reinforced.

Intraoperative measures aimed to decrease postoperative pain include intercostal blocks, yet these will last only 6 to 12 hours and will not block visceral pain or pain referred to the shoulder from the diaphragm. Placement of intercostal catheters for drug administration after surgery along four or five interspaces has had favorable results with regard to analgesia and improved pulmonary mechanics.[559] Other analgesic techniques include epidural local anesthetics, cryosurgery of intercostal nerves, or use of transcutaneous electrical nerve stimulation.[560]

The closure of the chest after pneumonectomy is performed without chest drainage; however, the mediastinum and intrathoracic pressures must be balanced by removing just enough air from the chest to establish a negative intrapleural pressure. After lobar or wedge resection, two intrapleural catheters are placed, one anteriorly for drainage of air and the other anteriorly for drainage of fluid. These are connected to closed underwater seal drainage and removed when they are no longer functional or when drainage of pleural fluid is less than 200 ml per 24 hours in the absence of a bronchopleural fistula.

Modern-day Mortality Rates After Pulmonary Resection

The majority of reports on 30-day operative mortality rate for the resection of lung cancer have been based on surgical series over the past 10 to 25 years, reporting rates of 2.1% to 12.4%.[561–566] With improvement in preoperative evaluation as outlined above, along with improvement in anesthetic techniques, the mortality rate for resectional surgery has decreased. Two recent reports, one from the LCSG and the other from a large university experience, have verified the lower death rates.[567,568] Between 1979 and 1981, 2200 resections for lung cancer were performed (1508 lobectomies, 569 pneumonectomies, and 143 lesser procedures) by the LCSG with mortality rates of 2.9%, 6.2%, and 1.4%, respectively. Three strata of risk according to the age of the patients were identified: patients under the age of 60 have a minimal risk (1.3%), those between 60 and 69 have a moderate risk (4.1%), and those 70 or older have a significant risk (7.1%), although in 85 patients over 70 years of age, the operative mortality rate was 5.9%. The most common causes of death following pulmonary resection were postoperative pneumonia and respiratory failure, bronchopleural fistula and empyema, myocardial infarction, and pulmonary embolus. In the university series covering the years 1972 to 1984, 19 of 476 patients (4.0%) died within the 30-day postoperative period. Risk factors included age greater than 60 years (7.4% versus 2.4%), extent of resection with pneumonectomy having an 11.7% mortality rate, and cardiac status as indicated by the presence of premature ventricular contractions. The causes of death were similar to those reported by the LCSG. Because of the greater number of pneumonectomies in the LCSG group, their lower mortality rate is probably more representative of modern-day standards. The causes of death during the immediate postoperative period include pulmonary thromboembolism (20%), myocardial infarction (24%), pneumonia and empyema (18%), bleeding (11%), and respiratory insufficiency (20%).

Specific Surgical Situations and Results

THE SOLITARY PULMONARY NODULE. Any patient in the lung cancer age group, particularly one who is a smoker, with an indeterminant nodular lung lesion, however small, on chest roentgenography that is undiagnosed by other methods should undergo thoracotomy. The Veterans Administration and Armed Services Hospitals (VA-ASH) conducted a combined study of asymptomatic solitary pulmonary nodules less than 6 cm in diameter;[569] considering all ages, 35% of the nodules were proved to be malignant, and 86% of these were primary bronchogenic carcinomas. In patients over 50 years of age, 56% of the nodules were malignant.

This same principle holds true in patients with suspected but unconfirmed pulmonary malignancies appearing different from a nodule. In a series of 303 patients over a 10-year period who did not have a diagnosis prior to thoracotomy but were suspected to have lung carcinoma, 102 had lobectomy, of whom 69% were found to have carcinoma.[570] However, a significant number of patients who appear preoperatively to have only a lung cancer nodule actually have disseminated disease, and the 5-year survival rate in patients with primary cancer in the VA-ASH study was only 38%.

OCCULT LUNG CANCER. "Occult" lung cancer describes the situation where sputum cytology examination is either diagnostic or highly suggestive of cancer but chest roentgenography and ear, nose, and throat examination reveal no lesion, and the patient has no history of aerodigestive cancer. The problem is to localize the lesion for definitive treatment. This is done by repeat bronchoscopic and ear, nose, and throat examinations and, often, selective bronchial washings.

The largest series of patients with roentgenographically occult lung cancer is an outgrowth of the Mayo Lung Project.[571] Fifty-four patients were found to have abnormal findings on sputum cytology, and all tumors were located by bronchoscopy requiring a mean of 1.5 examinations either by direct vision or by selective washings. All patients had complete resection. Nine (17%) were found to have N1 disease, and the overall 5-year survival rate was 74%. The continued follow-up of these patients is as important as the initial localization. In fact, a second cancer developed in 12 patients (22%), of which 11 were second primary lung cancers. Because of the possibility of second lesions, resection of the smallest amount of pulmonary tissue compatible with tumor extirpation should be considered. Interestingly, all of the patients in whom the lung cancer was not visible endoscopically had no evidence of extrabronchial invasion or metastatic involvement of lymph nodes. This subset of patients may be candidates for photodynamic therapy, and, in fact, long term survival has been reported in this situation. Patients in whom the cancer is seen, however, will have a 23% chance of metastatic involvement of regional lymph nodes and should be treated by conventional surgical resection.

T1-2N0M0 AND T1N1M0 DISEASE. To discuss current results of resection, the T1-2N0M0 and T1N1M0 categories should be considered separately, where formerly they were lumped together as Stage I disease. The LCSG has been able to analyze the prognostic factors in 392 patients with resected non-small cell cancer, and comment on freedom from recurrent lung cancer as well as the long-term survival. Patients with T1N0 squamous cell carcinoma had an 89% 3-year survival rate, whereas those with nonsquamous cell disease (adenocarcinoma and large cell carcinoma) in the same stage has a 79% 3-year survival rate.[572] This compares favorably with the 90% 3-year survival rate for 128 T1N0M0 patients from MSKCC.[573] For larger T2 lesions, survival was poorer. From the LCSG series, 73% of T2N0 patients with squamous histology were alive at 3 years compared with 65% of those with non-squamous histology. In the MSKCC series, a similar decrease in survival with T2 lesions (80%) compared with T1N0 lesions was noted. When death rates were compared in patients with N1 disease in the LCSG series, patients with non-squamous T1N1 disease had a significantly poorer 3-year survival rates than those with squamous histologies (55% versus 88%), and the presence of N1 disease seemed to have a greater impact on survival than the size of the primary lesion. A recent prospective analysis of 199 early-stage (T1-2 N0-1) patients also confirms the importance of N1 disease on survival, with no significant difference (72% versus 62%) in 2-year survival rates for T1N0 and T2N0 patients; patients with N1 disease had a 34% 2-year survival rate.[574]

CANCER RECURRENCE AFTER CURATIVE RESECTION. The presence of N1 disease also correlated with a higher risk of recurrence in the LCSG report, as did the presence of visceral pleural invasion.[572] Iascone and associates report that 64% of patients with resected N0 disease will be free of recurrence, compared with 19% of patients with resected N1 disease, at 5 years.[575] This has also been seen in a series from the Mayo Clinic, where the 5-year rates of freedom from recurrence after resection of T1N0, T2N0, and T1N1 disease were 70%, 58%, and 32%, respectively.[576] The overall rate of recurrence of cancer was 8.6% per year of observation and ranged from 15% the first year to 2.3% in the seventh or greater postoperative year. Fifty-six percent of the recurrences were distant metastases, and 26% of the cancers detected represented new primary lung cancers. A similar rate of 32% development of second primary cancers after resection of Stage I disease has been reported from MSKCC.[573] The management of second primary lung cancers should be resection, if possible, and will be discussed in a later section.

Overall Conclusions: Stage I Disease

The following conclusions can be arrived at concerning Stage I disease:

1. Stage I disease (T1-2N0M0) determined by postoperative pathologic staging is associated with 80% to 90% long-term survival rates following surgical resection.
2. Patients with Stage I disease are at great (20% to 30%) risk for the development of second primary lung cancers and need close surveillance.
3. The shift of the T1-2N1M0 category from Stage I to Stage II appears justified because of the poorer survival and increased recurrence rates in this group.

Results of Surgical Resection with Higher-Stage Disease: T3 Lesions and Mediastinal Nodal Positivity (N2 Disease)

The results of surgical resection in patients with Stage III lung cancer are disappointing, and many oncologists and thoracic surgeons feel that patients with such disease, as demonstrated by preoperative studies, are not candidates for surgical resection. In a noninvestigational situation, these patients are referred for radiotherapy or chemotherapy. There are reports in the literature of subsets of Stage III patients who may be curable, but, there is no consensus in the surgical community about how to identify this subset. The following sections represent an attempt by the authors to do this.

T3 DISEASE. The heterogeneous nature of T3 lesions, ranging from contiguous invasion of resectable mediastinal structures to proximity to the carina, makes it difficult for large series of such patients to be identified and analyzed independent of lymph node involvement. Mountain reported a series of 69 patients with either T3N0 or N1 disease who were felt to have had complete resection as defined by the encompassing of all gross disease, negative margins, freedom from tumor of the most distal node, and intact nodal capsules.[577] Although adjuvant chemotherapy was used in certain patients and could have played a role in survival, the 43% 5-year survival rate for squamous cell carcinomas and 23% rate for adenocarcinomas were excellent. Patients with tumor within 2 cm of the carina were treated by tracheobronchial resection and reconstruction, and those with chest wall involvement had en bloc chest wall resection with the tumor. The survival of 25 patients with chest wall resection was 35% at 5 years in this series. Although the majority of recurrences in these patients were distant, the T3 lesion also had a high rate of local recurrence, even without N2 involvement.

TRACHEAL SLEEVE PNEUMONECTOMY. In-continuity tracheal resection for large T3 lesions involving the trachea (tracheal sleeve pneumonectomy) has recently been popularized by various groups. DesLauriers and coworkers have published a large series involving tracheal sleeve pneumonectomies for patients with right and left upper-lobe tumors extending to the lower lateral tracheal wall[578] and thus unresectable by standard definition. Patients with mediastinal nodal positivity were not operated on. Five-year survival rates of 15% to 23% have been reported.[579] These operations were accomplished with jet ventilation via selective bronchial catheter placement. A high operative mortality rate (27%) was seen in these patients but was comparable to that in a similar series of patients with sleeve resection reported by Jensik and associates.[580] The most common cause of death was contralateral lung infection with respiratory failure, and long-term survivors usually had squamous cell tumors.

INTRATHORACIC ORGAN AND CHEST WALL INVOLVEMENT. Recent reports from the Mayo Clinic and MSKCC of the surgical and survival implications of invasion of intrathoracic structures by lung cancer emphasize the efficacy of extended resection and indicate that overall survival is influenced by nodal status, completeness of the resection, and, possibly, the age of the patient.[581–583] The importance of complete resection is stressed. In the absence of lymph node metastases, the depth of chest wall invasion does not significantly affect survival provided a complete resection is performed with negative microscopic margins. The 5-year actuarial survival rate was 54%: 56% in those patients without lymph node metastases and 21% in those with nodal metastases. The Mayo series also noted an improved survival rate for patients younger than 60 years of age. Operative mortality was tolerable at 4% to 12%.

The use of extrapleural versus full-thickness chest wall resection is controversial; however, with the low mortality rate of chest wall removal, as well as better methods of chest wall reconstruction either with muscle or with Marlex or Goretex sheets, the Mayo group urges chest wall resection and in fact found a survival advantage of full-thickness versus extrapleural resection. Despite higher morbidity (25%) than in standard resections, the Mayo group also feels that if complete resection can be performed, extended resection can be applied to other intrathoracic structures including the pericardium, phrenic or vagus nerve, left atrium, superior vena cava, and diaphragm. The role of the adjuvant therapy after chest wall resection is unanswered but is the subject of a LCSG randomized protocol.

MEDIASTINAL NODAL POSITIVITY (N2 DISEASE). The adverse prognostic implications of mediastinal nodal positivity in patients with lung cancer is pronounced, with only 25% of patients with N2 disease who undergo a "curative resection" alive at 5 years (Table 22-38). Resection strategies in this situation differ among surgeons, and several ways have been used to classify N2 disease morphologically, microscopically, and anatomically. It is only recently, with the use of mediastinoscopy for evaluation of disease, that the impact of the timing of the discovery of N2 positivity (*i.e.*, preresection versus at the time of thoracotomy) has become important. A detailed discussion of these subsets of N2 disease is presented in light of the ISS system of lung cancer, which would identify patients with ipsilateral mediastinal node and subcarinal node involvement as N2, placing them in Stage III, a category with a greater likelihood

TABLE 22-38. Five-Year Survival Rate (%) of Lung Cancer Patients with Resected N2 Disease

Year	*Histology*	*No. of Patients*	*5-Year Survival*
1972[584]	Squamous	110	37
	Adenocarcinoma	76	20
1977[585]		56	28.5
1978[586]	Squamous	110	29.5
	Adenocarcinoma	95	16.7
1982[587]		141	24
1983[588]	Squamous	46	26
	Adenocarcinoma	94	34
	Large cell	11	10
1983[589]		181	
	Squamous		24.2
	Adenocarcinoma		14.3
1984[577]	Squamous	36	39
	Adenocarcinoma	51	14
1985[590]	Squamous	43	48
	Adenocarcinoma	51	14
1987[574]		370	25
Overall totals		1741	
All histologies			26
Squamous			33
Nonsquamous			21

of 5-year survival compared with other sites of mediastinal node involvement.[381]

Influence of Primary Neoplasm Histology. In most reports of large series of patients who have had resection in the face of mediastinal node positivity, the importance of the primary tumor's histology has been emphasized, with patients with squamous cancer having better survival rates than those with adenocarcinoma or large cell carcinoma[574,577] (Table 22-38). It is probably reasonable to say that the prognosis after resection of large cell carcinoma in patients with N2 disease is worse than that of epidermoid or adenocarcinoma, whereas squamous histology may be more favorable than adenocarcinoma after resection of mediastinal nodes.

Primary Tumor Status. The size of the primary tumor as well as its location or invasion of contiguous structures seems to influence the long-term survival of patients who have undergone resection with N2 mediastinal nodes. Patients with T1N2 lesions have a greater survival rate than those with T2 or T3N2 disease.[586,591-593] In the study by Martini's group, survival was related to the size of the tumor as assessed after resection:[588] a better survival rate was noted in patients with small tumors (T1; 41% 5-year survival) than in those with large tumors (T2; 32% survival) or with extension outside the lung (T3; 29% survival), yet tumor size did not correlate with the number of levels of nodal involvement or with the location of the involved nodes. Naruke and coworkers likewise found significant decreases in survival as T stage increased with N2 positivity: 27.3% 5-year survival in T1, 18% in T2, and 0 in T4.[586,589]

Location or Level of the N2 Nodes. Naruke and coworkers were among the first to perform extensive lymph node mapping, such that levels of nodal involvement as well as the number of levels involved could be reported consistently.[586] This mapping is now a crucial element for all resections, regardless of the stage of the disease resected. It becomes even more crucial when different institutions belong to a cooperative group such as the LCSG and must standardize the reporting of nodal positivity, levels of nodes involved, and whether multiple levels are involved in any prognostic implications are to be investigated (Fig. 22-14).

Naruke's group found significantly decreased 5-year survival rates in patients who had positive subcarinal nodes compared with those with negative subcarinal nodes (9.1% versus 29%). Those authors found no significant difference in prognosis between patients with and without metastases to the superior mediastinal lymph nodes, tracheobronchial lymph nodes, or subaortic and para-aortic lymph nodes. This poor prognosis of subcarinal lymph node metastases probably stems from the high percentage of contralateral mediastinal node metastases.[586] Pearson and associates noted no

FIG. 22-14. Lymph node map showing mediastinal (N2) and hilar lobar nodes (N1) (see text for details).

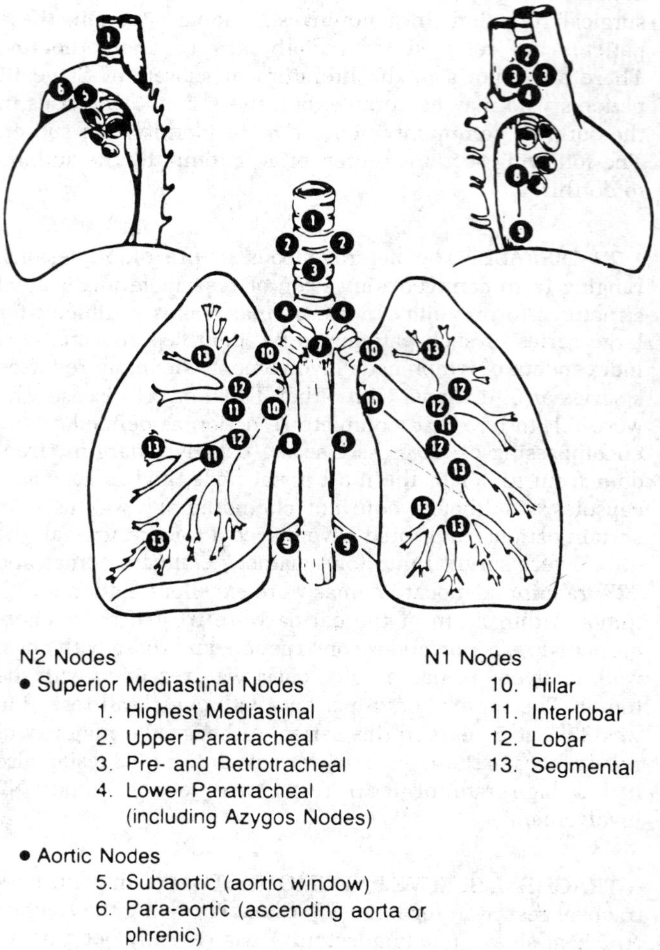

N2 Nodes
- Superior Mediastinal Nodes
  1. Highest Mediastinal
  2. Upper Paratracheal
  3. Pre- and Retrotracheal
  4. Lower Paratracheal (including Azygos Nodes)
- Aortic Nodes
  5. Subaortic (aortic window)
  6. Para-aortic (ascending aorta or phrenic)
- Inferior Mediastinal Nodes
  7. Subcarinal
  8. Paraesophageal (below carina)
  9. Pulmonary Ligament

N1 Nodes
10. Hilar
11. Interlobar
12. Lobar
13. Segmental

5-year survivors among patients with metastases to the highest paratracheal level.[587–590] Martini and coworkers found that 5-year survival was significantly poorer in patients with subcarinal node positivity compared with those with tumor in other lymph node stations (18% versus 34%, respectively).[588] Contrary to Pearson's findings, patients with involved nodes in the upper paratracheal region had no significant difference in survival from those without upper node positivity (25% versus 30%). The extent of lymph node involvement affected survival, with those patients with involvement at only one level doing better at 3 years than those with more than one positive level. At 5 years, however, the survival advantage of single-level positivity was less pronounced. A recent report from the Toronto group emphasizes the ability to obtain long-term survival in patients with isolated subaortic lymph node positivity (28%), with an even greater survival rate at 5 years if the resection is complete (42%).[594] The report excluded patients with tumor in other nodal sites.

Contralateral nodal positivity at this time is really the only agreed upon objective finding that would contraindicate exploration for resection. Some surgeons, on the basis of the above findings, believe that the presence of any positive mediastinal node, even ipsilateral, is a contraindication to resection, whereas others feel that in the presence of "favorable histology" (squamous) and easily resectable cancer confined to ipsilateral nodes, a resection should be performed. Other groups feel that independent of the level of nodal positivity, N2 positivity detected prior to thoracotomy mandates preoperative adjuvant treatment with resection if the patient has an objective response. This approach, in the authors' opinion, remains investigational.

Intranodal Versus Perinodal Disease. An important prognostic factor that is insufficiently emphasized in the analysis of mediastinal nodal positivity is the implication of microscopic disease confined to the lymph node without breaching of the capsule (intranodal) disease versus that in which tumor cells have escaped from the confines of the lymph node (perinodal or internodal disease). Perinodal involvement can be evident at the time of mediastinoscopy or at thoracotomy and can be subtle or associated with masses of contiguous lymph node groups with fixation and invasion of mediastinal structures. A series of studies show a significant survival advantage for patients with intranodal rather than perinodal mediastinal lymph node involvement.[591,595,596] The relative weight of intracapsular as opposed to extracapsular disease, however, has not been submitted to the necessary multivariate analysis to see if it functions as an independent predictor of survival distinguishable from the level of lymph node involvement, histology of the tumor, or completeness of resection.

Prognostic Implications of Mediastinal Lymph Node Involvement Found at Mediastinoscopy or at Thoracotomy

In patients with suspicious mediastinal lesions on chest roentgenography or CT scan who are otherwise good candidates for thoracotomy with possible resection, the use of mediastinoscopy is gaining popularity. In 1982, Pearson and associates reported a series of 141 mediastinal node-positive patients, all of whom had preoperative mediastinoscopy.[587] Of those, 79 patients were found to have tumorous nodes by mediastinoscopy. In all patients, the mediastinoscopic findings were correlated with thoracotomy findings. In the mediastinoscopy-negative group, 40% were able to undergo operation with curative intent. In contrast, only 15% of the positive-mediastinoscopy group were able to have curative resection. A significant difference in long-term survival was also seen between the two groups, with the 5-year survival rate being 9% for all cases of mediastinoscopy-positive patients and 24% for the patients with positive nodes found at surgery. In total, over 17 years, Pearson's group found that the group of mediastinal lymph node-positive patients able to undergo a complete resection represented only 4% of all patients. Thus, preoperative mediastinoscopy is extremely useful in identifying both those patients able to undergo a potentially curable resection and those likely to be cured by such a procedure.

Intraoperative Decision-making with Regard to Resecting Positive Mediastinal Nodes and Overall Conclusions

If the primary lesion can be extirpated by appropriate resection without impairing postoperative respiratory reserve or performed without undue mortality and morbidity, then the decision becomes limited by the extent of nodal involvement. A conservative approach would be to perform radical lymphadenectomy along with the pulmonary resection if the nodal disease is intranodal, regardless of the number of lymph node levels involved. In contrast, extranodal bulky disease, which might upgrade the necessary resection to a pneumonectomy without assuring curative intent, is associated with higher mortality and complication rates and offers no survival advantage. The real challenge, however, is in the prediction of those patients who will not benefit from thoracotomy prior to having to make these difficult intraoperative decisions. The authors believe that only by performing mediastinoscopy in all patients with the slightest suspicion of preoperative mediastinal abnormalities will such a uniform database be compiled. Once patients are found to have N2 disease on mediastinoscopy, they probably are best served by radiotherapy or enrollment in prospective trials studying multimodality therapy, such as neoadjuvant programs performed in a prospective randomized fashion.

Special Surgical Situations

PARENCHYMA-SPARING PROCEDURES. There has been increasing interest in lung-sparing resections, especially in older patients with compromised pulmonary function, patients with synchronous or second primary lung cancers, and patients whose primary tumors could be removed by a more limited procedure. There are two schools of thought with regard to elective resections in good-risk patients. First, some surgeons believe that the anatomic boundaries of lobectomy are arbitrary and that the patient should have the least amount of parenchyma removed. In their opinion, the removal of excess lung tissue will not affect long-term survival. The other school points to the increase in the local recurrence rate in patients with lesser resections, as well as the reported increase in operative morbidity from segmental resection. Iascone and associates, reviewing a series of patients with N0 and N1 disease who had been treated by lobectomy or pneumonectomy, reported local recurrence rates of 26% and 18%, respectively, arguing for even more aggressive resection in early-stage disease.[575]

The chief proponent of conservative resection is Jensik, who has reported a series of 467 segmental-type resections over a 26-year period, 274 in Stage I or II disease, 123 in Stage III cancer, and 70 in patients with a previous pulmonary resection.[597] Cumulative survival rates for the early-stage patients were 55% at 5 years, 27% at 10 years, and 21% at 15 years, which compare favorably with the results of standard resection. In the patients reoperated on, survival at 5 and 10 years after the second thoracotomy was 33% and 20%, respectively. Various segments were resected, the most frequent of which were the superior segments of the lower lobes, the anterior segment of the right upper lobe, and the superior division of the left upper lobe. The most common complication was persistent air leak (8%), some of which necessitated completion lobectomy, management of empyema, or changing of the chest tubes. The perioperative mortality rate was 1% for patients with Stage I or II disease, 4% for those with Stage III disease, and 6% for those with previous resection. Local recurrence was seen in 12%.

In another series of 197 patients with Stage I disease treated over a 17-year period, 100 received lobectomy, whereas 97 received wedge resection with lymph node sampling because of inferior preoperative pulmonary function.[598] Perioperative mortality (3% versus 2.1%) and morbidity were comparable in the two groups, and differences in 2-year (72% versus 74%) and 6-year survival (69% versus 75%) rates were not statistically significant. Unfortunately, recurrence patterns were not analyzed in detail in this study.

However, McCormack and Martini in a series of 61 patients undergoing segmentectomy or wedge resection for T1N0 or T2N0 lesions, reported a recurrence within the same lobe in 19% of the patients.[599] The perioperative mortality rate was acceptable (3.7%); the 5-year survival rate was lower than in the other series (50%). Their results with the use of lobectomy for Stage I disease (not performed as a prospective, randomized comparison with the wedge/segmentectomy group) were significantly better, with a 5-year survival rate of 72% and no local recurrences except for three patients developing regional lymph node metastases. Of this group of 135 patients who had lobectomies, 15 (11%) developed a second primary lung cancer, which is very close to the figure reported by Jensik. Currently, the LCSG is conducting a prospective randomized comparison of conservative resection and standard lobectomy or pneumonectomy in Stage I disease. Until the results of this trial are completed, either approach appears warranted.

SYNCHRONOUS LUNG CANCERS. If a preoperative evaluation indicates no evidence of an extrapulmonary source of malignancy or of extrapulmonary metastases, the appearance of two lesions strongly suggests synchronous lung cancers, the incidence of which is reported to be 1% to 7%.[600] If the CT evaluation reveals negative mediastinal nodes, evaluation for an extrathoracic primary lesion is indicated, including intravenous urography and a gastrointestinal series. Suspicious CT nodes must be confirmed by mediastinoscopy. If the mediastinal nodes are positive for tumor, the survival rate of the patients is so poor as not to warrant resection. In patients with two lesions on the same side (often located in separate lobes), pneumonectomy is the operation of choice. If pulmonary functions are limiting, lobectomy and wedge resection can be performed. In patients with lesions in both lungs, median sternotomy or staged thoracotomies can be performed. Segmental resection beginning with the most advanced lesion is done; preservation of lung tissue without compromise of the cancer resection is critical, but mediastinal or nodal dissection must be performed. Median survival for patients with resected synchronous Stage I cancers is 25 to 27 months and 11 months for those with Stage II or III cancers.

SECOND AND THIRD PRIMARY LUNG CANCERS. A 10% incidence of second bronchogenic lung cancers has been reported by the Mayo Clinic, which agrees with the reports of Jensik and Martini (see previous section).[597,599] Mathisen and colleagues defined the criteria for a second lung cancer as one of a histologic cell type different from the previous primary, a long interval between resections (metachronous tumors), location of the new lesion in the contralateral lung or a different ipsilateral lobe, or the presence of synchronous bilateral tumor.[601] Over a 23-year period, 90 patients met these criteria in those authors' series, of which 10 were synchronous lung cancers.

The majority of patients with second primary lung cancers will be asymptomatic, and the lesion will be discovered at the time of follow-up for their first cancer. The mean interval between the first and second cancers is 46 months, and the secondary or tertiary lesions can be handled with equal frequency by segmentectomy, lobectomy, sleeve lobectomy, pneumonectomy, or completion pneumonectomy. Survival was the worst in patients with synchronous cancers, whereas the 5- and 10-year survival rates for patients with metachronous tumor are 33% and 20%. Patients whose disease-free interval between separate tumors is greater than 3 years have significantly longer survival than those with shorter intervals. According to the Mathisen's group, the ability to salvage these patients over the long run is related to an initial conservative resection.

SLEEVE LOBECTOMY. The concept of segmental bronchial resection encompassing the involved main bronchial or tracheal segment in continuity with the involved lobe followed by reanastomosis of the bronchus in order to preserve pulmonary tissue is not new. The operation was popularized by Price Thomas,[602] Paulson and Shaw,[603] and Johnston and Jones[604] in the 1950s. The use of the operation in lung cancer resection is based on the anatomic principle that there is lymphatic drainage of the upper lobe to the ipsilateral hilar and low paratracheal areas, and the majority of resections performed involve tumors at the orifice of the right upper lobe. Weisel and coworkers reported 5- and 8-

year survival rates of 43% and 30% in patients with Stage I disease subjected to sleeve resection, with 31% (5-year) and 15% (8-year) survival in Stage II disease.[605] A review by Lowe and colleagues found an overall 5-year survival rate of 33% and a 10-year rate of 21%.[606]

The operation may be considered as an alternative to pneumonectomy if the tumor is centrally located and small and if it is anatomically possible to perform anastomosis with curative intent. Sleeve lobectomy also can serve as a limited resection in a patient with compromised pulmonary function. The procedure has been described with concomitant sleeve or patching of the ipsilateral pulmonary artery, and the presence of positive interlobar nodes is no longer considered a contraindication to its performance.[607] The operative mortality rate ranges from 0 to 7% in modern series,[608] chiefly from hemorrhage and bronchial anastomotic dehiscence. The latter complication can usually be prevented by wrapping the anastomosis with a pleural flap, but the chief factor is a meticulously performed air-tight anastomosis (Fig. 22-15). Postoperative atelectasis requires the liberal use of bronchoscopy to remove secretions, and bronchoscopy should be performed intraoperatively to assure removal of blood from the lung. The advent of double-lumen catheter anesthesia with reliably placed disposable tubes has also increased the use of sleeve lobectomy. Finally, late bronchial anastomotic stricture can usually be prevented with the use of absorbable suture material.

Local recurrence rates remain a problem with sleeve lobectomy, ranging from 7% to 16% in the literature.[605,608,609] This problem is usually related to nodal disease; a high anastomotic recurrence rate should be avoided by the compulsive use of frozen-section evaluation of the bronchial margins to assure completeness of resection (Fig. 22-15).

Complications of Pulmonary Resection

The primary complications of pulmonary resection have already been mentioned in previous sections. *Hemorrhage* is rare but can be from any site in the operative field, including the bronchovascular structures or the incision. Hemorrhage in excess of 100 ml per hour for 4 hours should alert the surgeon to check the patient's coagulation functions; if these are normal, mechanical bleeding necessitating reoperation is suggested. Patency of the pleural tubes must be maintained to prevent intrathoracic clot formation, which, if not drained, increases the chance of empyema or late fibrothorax with lung entrapment.

Pulmonary insufficiency is usually seen in patients with marginal pulmonary function and poor performance status prior to the operation. Positive-pressure ventilation with appropriate diuresis as well as optimizing cardiac output with guidance from a Swan-Ganz catheter is essential to reverse the insufficiency. These patients will also require nutritional support via enteral or intravenous alimentation while receiving respiratory support to try to prevent further muscle catabolism and inability to generate sufficient respiratory mechanics for ventilation. When secretions become a limiting factor and prevent safe extubation, the use of tracheostomy should be considered early in the patient's postoperative course. Vigorous clearing of airway secretions must be performed and cultures taken in order to guide antibiotic management of pneumonitis.

Management of *cardiac arrhythmia* will require treatment of pulmonary resection-induced atrial and ventricular tachyarrhythmias, management of hypokalemia, and digitalization. Patients with a cardiac disease history should have optimization of systemic blood pressure and volume management to prevent undue increases in myocardial oxygen requirements. This may necessitate the use of preload-reducing agents such as nitroglycerin or afterload reduction with nitroprusside.

A postoperative chest roentgenogram is examined to document complete expansion of the residual or contralateral lung, especially after pneumonectomy, to rule out *contralateral pneumothorax* or *inadequate expansion* secondary to the use of double-lumen catheter anesthesia. *Persistent air leakage* after pulmonary resection, either by lobectomy or segmentectomy, will usually respond to tube drainage with underwater seal suction. Expansion of the residual lung with adhesion formation will usually obliterate these peripheral bronchopleural fistulae.

Empyema after lobar resection can be treated with tube

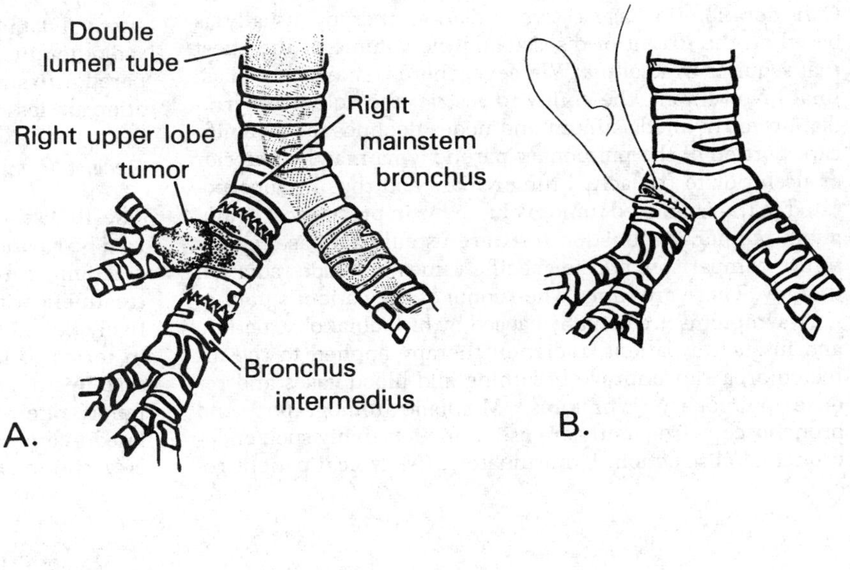

FIG. 22-15. Sleeve lobectomy, right upper lobe. **A.** Double-lumen anesthesia is used and the incision made in the right main-stem bronchus and the bronchus intermedius. **B.** The bronchus intermedius is anastomosed to the right main-stem bronchus after ensuring negative margins by frozen section analysis for tumor during surgery.

drainage and antibiotics. However, empyema after pneumonectomy, with or without associated bronchopleural fistula, remains the most morbid complication in these patients. Early empyema without associated bronchopleural fistula has been treated successfully with early catheter irrigation of the postpneumonectomy space either with iodine-containing solutions alone or with systemic antibiotics, but success with this technique is the exception rather than the rule. Most postpneumonectomy empyemas must be treated with early tube drainage to evacuate the space, with subsequent rib resection and conversion to open thoracostomy with irrigation of the cavity with bacteriostatic solutions when the mediastinum has stabilized. Closure of the thoracostomy at a later time, when the bacterial colony count is minimal, and institution of triple-antibiotic solution (Clagett's procedure) will succeed approximately 50% of the time. If empyema recurs, space obliteration with either muscle transposition or thoracoplasty will be necessary.

Empyema may signal the presence of a post*pneumonectomy bronchopleural fistula* and indeed contribute to its development in the early postoperative period. However, the cardinal sign of postpneumonectomy bronchopleural fistula is change in the air–fluid level by chest radiography with increasing amounts of air on the resected side. The acute development of a postpneumonectomy fistula will cause uncontrollable coughing secondary to the flooding of the opposite lung with the contents of the pneumonectomy space. Immediate placement of a chest tube to drain the pneumonectomy space must be performed, and usually the patient also requires tracheal intubation with isolation of the contralateral lung. Early postpneumonectomy fistulas are amenable to repair with a variety of muscle flaps, including those of intercostal muscle, serratus anterior, latissimus dorsi, or pectoralis. These muscle flaps have also made a tremendous impact in the closure of chronic or late-developing fistulae and at the same time can add bulk to the pneumonectomy space to obliterate it further.

RADIOTHERAPEUTIC TREATMENT

Determination of the Ability to Undergo Radical Radiation Therapy for a Cure

Consideration for aggressive radiation therapy usually is based on the extent of disease and the volume of the chest that requires irradiation. Whenever there is massive mediastinal involvement, the ability to restrict the volume of irradiation to the mediastinum and nodes declines, as a significant portion of the pulmonary parenchyma may lie anterior or posterior to the actual tumor mass and thus be incorporated in the irradiated tumor volume. As in presurgical evaluation, pulmonary function tests are useful as a baseline for future comparison, but no specific values preclude radiation therapy. There are times when some of the patient's pulmonary symptoms are actually caused by bronchial obstruction, and in such a patient, radiation therapy applied to the affected area can improve breathing and blood gases and reduce pulmonary symptoms. Midplane tomography and bronchoscopy frequently are useful in identifying such endobronchial obstruction. Unfortunately, the typical patient referred for radiation therapy has extensive disease that requires more than attention to relief of bronchial obstruction. The role of radiotherapy in the treatment of lung cancer has been summarized in several recent reviews.[610–612]

Radiotherapy Administered with Curative Intent

For patients who have non-small cell lung cancer that, after extensive evaluation, appears to be in Stage I or II, surgery is unequivocally the treatment of choice if the patient's underlying pulmonary status and other medical considerations suggest that he or she can tolerate a radical surgical procedure. Unfortunately, Stage I or Stage II disease is seen in only a minority of patients with carcinoma of the lung. In addition, many patients who appear clinically to have Stage I or II disease turn out at surgery to have microscopic involvement of lymph nodes in the mediastinum. Radiation therapy is considered an alternative to surgery for patients who either decline thoracotomy with its attendant risks or those whose underlying pulmonary and other medical problems make surgery excessively risky.[613] There are only limited data on primary radiotherapy in lieu of surgery for resectable disease in operable patients. The reported series from England, in which relatively low (4000–5000-rad) doses were used, suggest that modern high-dose radiotherapy is probably a reasonable approach for patients who decline surgery. Hilton and Smart reported more than 20% of patients surviving more than 5 years after radical radiotherapy for otherwise operable lung cancer.[614,615]

The vast majority of patients with lung cancer of the non-small cell varieties present with Stage III disease that is unresectable. Although it can be debated whether chest radiotherapy should be given to such patients,[615] we believe that in selected patients, it is beneficial in terms of local control (achieved in greater than 60% of patients) and possibility of cure.[616] Stage III patients who have clinically evident mediastinal adenopathy can be considered for curative radiotherapy, with or without surgery, although the long-term survival figures remain poor. Patients with distant metastases or positive supraclavicular nodes generally are not considered for curative radiation treatment. The median survival for patients with unresectable disease undergoing primary radiotherapy is less than 1 year; however, the 5-year survival data show about 6% of patients alive and well with radiotherapy alone (Table 22-39). This should not be compared with surgical results because patients selected for radiation are less favorable cases than those selected for surgery.

Recent Results of Curative Radiotherapy

The Radiation Therapy Oncology Group (RTOG) randomized 551 patients with unresectable or inoperable non-small cell lung cancer to different types of potentially curative treatment with radiation therapy.[617] These studies quantitatively define the limits for state of the art radiation therapy in terms of local tumor control and the need for effective systemic treatment for distant metastases. The intrathoracic failure rate within the irradiated volume varied in a dose-related manner: 48% for 4000 cGy continuous, 38% for 5000 cGy continuous (or 4000 cGy split course), and 27% for

TABLE 22-39. Five-Year Survival Data Following "Curative" Radiotherapy for Patients with Inoperable or Unresectable Lung Cancer

Series	*No. of Patients*	*5-Year Survival (%)*
Stanford*	284	6
Columbia†	253	5
Hammersmith‡	513	6
Pennsylvania§	171	6
Finland‖	158	6
Massachusetts General Hospital#	108	7

*Caldwell WL, Bagshaw MA: Cancer 22:999–1004, 1968.

†Guttman RJ: Am J Roentgenol Rad Ther Nucl Med 93:99–103, 1965; Guttman RJ: Carcinoma of the bronchus. In Deeley TJ (ed): Modern Radiotherapy, p 193. New York, Appleton-Century-Crofts, 1971.

‡Deeley TJ, Singh SP: Thorax 22:562–566, 1967.

§Katz HR, Alberts RW: Am J Clin Oncol 6:445–457, 1983.

‖Holsti LR, Mattson K: Int J Rad Oncol Biol Phys 6:977–981, 1980.

#Choi NCH, Doucette JA: Cancer 48:101–109, 1981.

6000 cGy continuous. The failure rate in the nonirradiated lung was 25% to 30% irrespective of the radiation dose. Seventy-five to eighty percent of all the patients developed distant metastases. Brain metastases ultimately occurred in 16% of those with squamous cell carcinomas and 30% of those with adenocarcinoma or large cell carcinoma.

It would clearly be an advantage if chest radiotherapy could be administered more conveniently. Thus, it is of interest that the University of Maryland found no differences in the preliminary analysis of a randomized trial in 100 patients comparing once-a-week radiotherapy (500-rad fractions given to a total dose of 6000 rad) with a 6000-rad total dose administered via 200-rad fractions given conventionally 5 days a week.[618]

When modern results of chest radiotherapy given with or without chemotherapy are compared for elderly (over 70 years) or younger patients, no significant differences are seen,[619] suggesting that older patients should be individually evaluated and, if they have a good performance status, be treated according to physiologic rather than chronologic age.

When curative treatment is planned with radiation, the intention is to take the known tumor volume to midplane doses of 5500 to 6000 rad. If the tumor is relatively small or the location favorable, one may consider boosting a small volume to an even higher dose. The principal concern is the amount of lung parenchyma that will be included within the treatment area. Organs that limit the amount of irradiation that can be applied to the thorax include the lung parenchyma, spinal cord, and heart. The esophagus, although frequently symptomatic from acute desquamation during the course of treatment, usually is not considered a dose-limiting organ in terms of long-term complications. For patients who have no significant degree of COPD, treatment plans may consist of opposing anterior and posterior fields, usually with a 2-cm margin around the entire tumor mass, for approximately 3000 rad before switching to a second treatment plan, which usually consists of an anterior field in conjunction with a posteriorly obliqued field to keep the spinal cord dose well within tolerance limits. In most cases, the entire upper mediastinum is included, whereas the inferior margin typically extends about 6 to 7 cm below the carina in the treatment position. Such treatment plans, which ideally require isocentric planning, have helped to improve dosimetry in these patients (Fig. 22-16). When such tools are available to assist in treatment planning, it is essential not only that the plan be documented at the tumor level, but also that a second treatment plan be obtained at the level of the thoracic inlet, where the chest is comparatively narrow compared with the lower level of the tumor itself. This discrepancy in

FIG. 22-16. **A**. Anterior port used in the treatment. **B**. Response to treatment after 5500 rad. Considerable tumor shrinkage has been achieved with good palliative results in terms of symptoms.

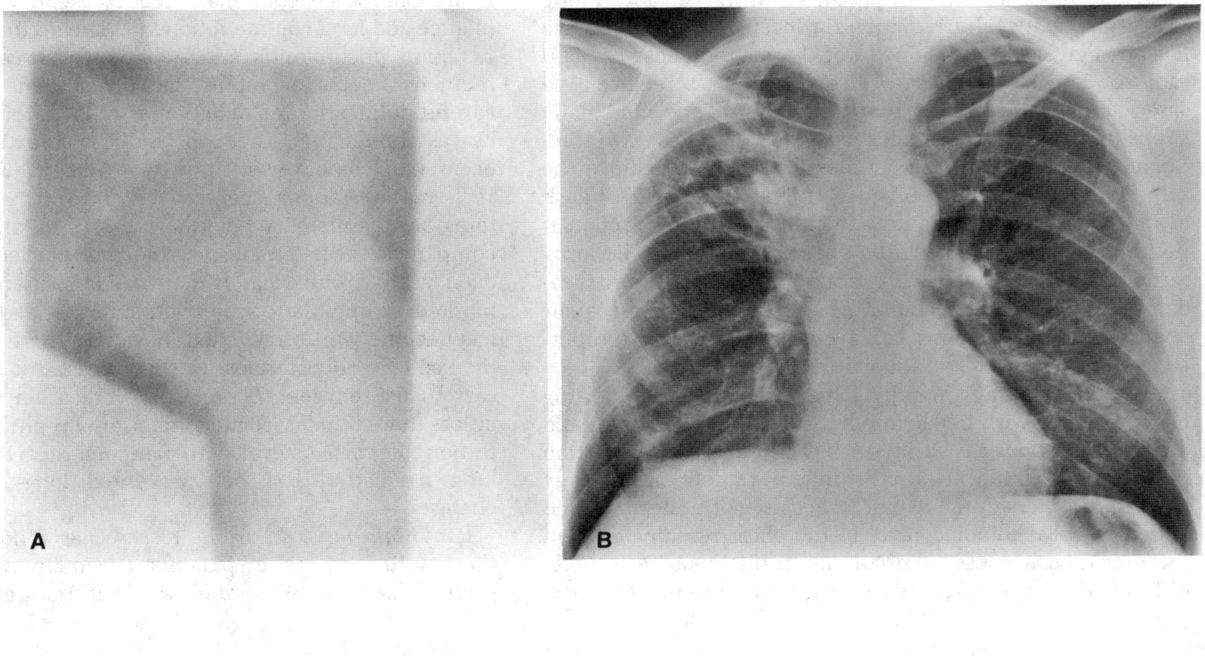

anterior–posterior chest thickness means that the spinal cord dose at the upper level of the treatment volume may be higher than the actual dose being delivered at the tumor level because there is less tissue at the upper level to attenuate the radiation. Knowledge of the exact dose being applied at the upper portion of the chest to the spinal cord will allow appropriate decisions to be made to minimize the dose to the upper thoracic spinal cord. Such consideration and meticulous execution of the dosimetric treatment plan should eliminate any concern about radiation myelitis.

For the patient who has a significant degree of restrictive pulmonary disease, the treatment plan usually is confined to opposing anterior–posterior fields with a spinal cord block inserted posteriorly somewhere between the 3000- and 4000-rad tumor dose to keep the total cord dose below 4500 rad. Such a treatment plan is considered a major compromise from optimal tumor treatment because the block may reduce the tumor dose as well. If possible, it is preferable to reduce the tumor volume at the time of shifting to the obliqued field, but this cannot always be done. Supraclavicular nodes usually are not included within the treatment volume in such patients, in contrast to the more typical patient with unresectable disease, in whom an anterior neck field ordinarily is used to treat the supraclavicular nodes routinely, regardless of their clinical status.

Time, Dose, and Fractionation

With time, dose, and fractionation schemes, the question of split-course treatment versus continuous therapy has been raised. No significant superiority in survival has been achieved by split-course treatment compared with continuous fractionation.[620,621] The case for split-course treatment (approximately 2500 to 3000 rad over 2 weeks followed by 2 to 3 weeks off treatment before a final 2500 to 3000 rad is delivered over 2 to 3 weeks) is predicated on better tolerance, simplicity for integration into combined-modality approaches, and an opportunity to reevaluate patients before their second half of treatment for any new manifestations of metastatic disease.[622–624] In patients with far-advanced lung cancer, once-a-week irradiation for locally advanced disease has been given (500 rad once weekly to a total dose of 6000 rad; 2050 ret) with success. If a tumor mass receives the same number of rad over a longer time with the same daily exposure, biologic differences exist between those two fractionation schemes. In the simplest concept, to achieve the same effect from split-course treatment, a higher total dose of radiation would be required to offset the tumor repopulation that may occur during the time of treatment. The long-term success achieved with radiation therapy alone (predominantly in unresectable Stage III disease or poor operative risks) remains relatively poor with either split-course treatment or continuous fractionation.

The poor survival generally achieved in patients with lung cancer treated with irradiation may have led to unwarranted conclusions about the utility of local control with radiation therapy. In addition, it often is difficult to define accurately the pretreatment tumor volume because of atelectasis and collapse. Local tumor control in the chest remains difficult to determine because of problems in distinguishing subtle differences between radiation changes and tumor on chest films. Inasmuch as metastatic disease has dominated the clinical course of these patients, it has been thought that local recurrence is not a significant problem.[624] This remains to be seen because local recurrence can be slow to manifest itself and certainly would predispose to further metastatic disease.[625]

Clinical Care of Patients During Radiotherapy

Most patients will tolerate daily doses of 200 to 300 rad midplane without significant problems during treatment. Approximately 3 weeks after their treatment has started, dysphagia caused by acute desquamation of the esophageal mucosa appears. This usually will persist (and can be severe in some patients, necessitating an unplanned break) for approximately 2 to 3 weeks after radiation therapy has been completed. Bronchial secretions will be altered by radiation therapy, becoming noticeably more tenacious. A nonproductive cough is common during and after radiation therapy; it may be present for the rest of the patient's life. Frank radiation pneumonitis does not occur during treatment; it is more likely to be seen in the first 1 to 3 months after completion of radiation therapy. Care should be taken to evaluate patients thoroughly before treatment to be sure that incipient obstructive pneumonia is not present. Such a problem may require antibiotics and can delay treatment until it clears, particularly if intensive chemotherapy is planned as part of the treatment.

Long-term Follow-up and Complications

Problems with *radiation pneumonitis* will depend on the dose and volume of lung incorporated within the radiation field.[624] *Pulmonary fibrosis* may take months to years to develop; it can be disabling or even fatal. However, such lethal complications are uncommon. The pathophysiology appears to represent both vascular and parenchymal cell injury. The diffusion capacity is reduced markedly, and interstitial fibrosis of pulmonary septa occurs. Whenever pulmonary fibrosis occurs, marked decrease in pulmonary compliance and lung volume follows.[626] The optimal approach to radiation pneumonitis and pulmonary fibrosis is to avoid them by means of sophisticated treatment planning and careful delineation of radiation portals. Often, patients will be asymptomatic although radiographic manifestations occur that coincide with the treatment volume. Typically, such manifestations decrease or disappear without symptoms or treatment. When shortness of breath or fever accompanies these radiologic changes, corticosteroids have been used; approximately half of the patients will report marked symptomatic improvement.[627] If radiation fibrosis has become well established, however, there is no value in the use of corticosteroids. In severe cases, it may be necessary to use oxygen. There is no indication for antibiotics unless there is an associated infection. Prophylactic administration of corticosteroids to patients receiving large-field lung irradiation has not prevented long-term radiation changes.

Radiation-induced cardiac disease has followed radiation therapy in lung cancer patients. It remains relatively rare, probably because of the short survival times of patients who have this disease. Again, elimination of most of the cardiac silhouette from the high-dose radiation volume avoids this problem for most patients. If the cancer is located close to the heart, this problem may be seen and can be difficult to distinguish from recurrent tumor. Paradoxical pulse may be present if pericardial constriction is present. Echocardiography, cardiac catheterization, and pericardiocentesis may be necessary for diagnostic and therapeutic purposes. Pericardial fluid must be evaluated cytologically to rule out a malignant effusion.

Acute radiation esophagitis usually occurs during treatment but proves self-limited once the mucosa has repopulated. During the acute esophagitis, viscous lidocaine often is helpful. Long-term esophageal problems are relatively rare, although stenosis has been reported occasionally, usually when relatively large (250- to 300-rad) daily fractions have been used. For most patients with this uncommon problem, simple esophageal dilatation will be adequate.

Spinal cord injury should be avoided by careful treatment planning. As noted above, careful delineation of dose distribution within the patient, not only at the level of the tumor but also in the upper thorax, should allow the therapist to avoid this problem. When the patient receives radiation to a posterior oblique field, care must be taken to ensure that the spinal cord is not included within the portal; if the location of the tumor makes the angle of the obliquity such that the spinal cord is included at the upper portion of the portal, an additional block must be inserted to reduce the exposure of the spinal cord.

INTEGRATION OF SURGERY, RADIOTHERAPY, AND CHEMOTHERAPY IN THE PRIMARY TREATMENT OF NON-SMALL CELL LUNG CANCER WITH CURATIVE INTENT

Non-small cell lung cancer accounts for 75% of all lung cancer, and roughly 30% of these patients present with extrathoracic metastatic disease, 30% present with clinical AJC Stage I and II disease and are treated with surgery or radiotherapy as described above, and 40% present clinically or at surgery with N2 (mediastinal) involvement. This group (about 41,000 patients in the United States) represents a significant therapeutic challenge, and many physicians have tried various combinations of surgery and radiotherapy, surgery and chemotherapy, or, recently, all three modalities. Combined-modality treatment appears appropriate for at least some of these patients.

Analysis of the failure patterns of current surgical and radiation treatment of lung cancer has been undertaken.[611,628–630] The results for surgical therapy have been summarized earlier (see Table 22-16).[629] For radiation therapy, 57% of epidermoid cancer patients will have their first failure in the chest area and 44% will have local failure only, whereas 33% will fail distantly and 20% will have distant failure only. For adenocarcinoma and large cell carcinoma, 25% will fail locally (19% local only), and 56% will fail in distant sites (40% distant sites only).[630] These results emphasize the importance of both local control and effective therapy for systemic metastases that are present early in the course of the disease. A significant therapeutic gain in either area would have an immediate impact on the disease.

ADJUVANT THERAPY: PREOPERATIVE, POSTOPERATIVE, AND INTRAOPERATIVE RADIATION THERAPY

Preoperative Radiation Therapy

The use of preoperative radiation therapy in the hope of modifying the survival results in early or locally advanced lung cancer began in the 1950s and has been reviewed by Faber.[631] Bromley and Szur, in a series of 66 patients, found that 47% could be sterilized of tumor, and a minority of patients who were thought to be inoperable could indeed have their disease resected after preoperative radiation therapy.[632] However, a high mortality rate (15%) and excessive rate of empyema and fistula were noted. Bloedorn and associates, in 1960, described similar results in 37 patients, with 46% sterilization of tumor using doses up to 6000 rad.[633] Nevertheless, a prohibitive mortality rate of 22% was noted, with a 5-year survival rate of 20%. Most of the studies that followed were nonrandomized and retrospective and differed in the radiation treatment plans used (Table 22-40). Some of these nonrandomized trials have suggested benefit, whereas others have not.

Randomized trials comparing surgery alone with preoperative radiation therapy followed by surgery have shown no benefit of preoperative radiotherapy (Table 22-40).[640,641] The VA cooperative study, supervised by Shields, randomized more than 300 patients who were all thought to have resectable disease to surgery alone or preoperative irradiation with 4000 to 5000 rad.[640] There was a predominance of squamous cell carcinoma, and most of the patients received pneumonectomy. The 4-year survival rate of the control group was 21% whereas that of the preoperative radiotherapy group was only 13%. Postoperative complications, including bronchopleural fistula, were more frequent in the radiation therapy group. In a 17-hospital collaborative study sponsored by the NCI in 1975 randomizing in excess of 550 patients, similar survival rates were noted for controls (14%) and irradiated patients (16%) at 5 years.[641] Similar smaller studies by Eichorn[642] and Tildon[643] and their coworkers revealed no survival advantage of preoperative radiation therapy in patients with resectable disease, and a randomized trial by Kazem and associates,[644] which revealed a modest survival advantage at 10 years using short-course radiotherapy (2000 rad in 1 week followed by immediate surgical resection) has never been corroborated.

At present, therefore, no study has established a survival benefit with the use of preoperative radiation therapy in patients with operable lung cancer. However, although its value is unconfirmed by prospective randomized studies, preoperative radiation therapy is routinely used in the management of superior sulcus tumors.

Diagnosis and Management of Carcinomas in the Superior Pulmonary Sulcus

Carcinomas in the superior pulmonary sulcus produce a characteristic clinical pattern known as Pancoast's syndrome.[279,281,645,646] The tumor occurs in the sulcus or groove made by the subclavian artery in the cupola of the pleura and apices of the upper lobes of the lungs. It produces pain in the

TABLE 22-40. Preoperative Radiation Therapy in Non-Small Cell Lung Cancer

Histology	*Pretherapy Resectability*	*Radiation Dose (Gy)*	*No. of Patients*	*Survival Advantage*	*Reference*
Nonrandomized Studies					
Mixed	78 yes +173 no	20–45	254	Yes: 45% vs 35% at 5 years	634
Mixed	36 yes +14 no	30–36	50	None apparent	635
Mixed	All no	30	107	None apparent	636
Mixed	54 yes +34 no	30–45	94	Yes: 47% vs 34% at 5 years	637
Mixed	Marginally yes	30	53	18% 5-year for all; 27% if resectable	638
Mixed	41/45 + mediastinoscopy (+20 postoperative)	35	48	18% at 5 years	639
Randomized Studies					
Mixed	Yes	40–50	166 treated; 165 controls	None: 13% vs 21% at 4 years	640
Mixed	Yes	40	290 treated; 278 controls	None: 14% vs 16% at 5 years	641
Mixed	Yes	55	99 treated; 97 controls	None: 28% vs 35% at 5 years	642
Mixed	Yes	45	21 treated; 16 controls	None: 6/21 vs 7/16 alive	643
Squamous	Yes	20	28	None: 58% vs 43% at 5 years	644

distribution of the eighth cervical and first and second thoracic nerve distribution and Horner's syndrome. A shadow is seen on chest films at the extreme apex of the lung; in 40% of patients, it appears only as an apical cap or thickening.[281] The pain is steady, severe, and unrelenting. At first, it is localized in the shoulder and vertebral border of the scapula and later extends down the ulnar distribution of the arm to the elbow (T1 distribution) and finally to the ulnar surface of the forearm and fourth and fifth fingers of the hand (C8 dermatome).[281] The first or second ribs or vertebrae and the related intercostal nerves also may be involved, increasing the pain and, in some cases, leading to spinal cord compression. With involvement of the sympathetic chain and stellate ganglion by direct extension, Horner's syndrome and anhidrosis develop on the same side of the face and arm. However, rib destruction and Horner's syndrome do not have to be present to diagnose a superior sulcus tumor.

Paulson has pioneered an aggressive approach to these patients that includes preoperative irradiation followed by extended resection.[281,646] (A review of results in the management of superior sulcus tumors from the various series is seen in Table 22-41). This approach was prompted by the observation that these tumors usually grow slowly and metastasize late. Patients should have the usual staging procedures done for any potentially resectable lung cancer lesion. However, there should be special emphasis on radionuclide bone scans, bone and cervical spine roentgenograms, and a CT scan of the area to determine tumor extent, as well as neurologic examination with electromyography. Mediastinoscopy usually is recommended because of the poor survival of patients with superior sulcus tumors even after radical procedures when these nodes are involved. However, scalene node biopsy is done only when palpable nodes are present or when the patient is of borderline operability.[281,647]

TABLE 22-41. Results of Preoperative Radiation and Resection for Pancoast Tumors

Series	*No. of Patients*	*Survival at 5 Years (%)*
Paulson[646]	78	35
Miller et al.[647]	25	40
Wright et al.[648]	21	27
Attar et al.[649]	19	23 (3 years)
Stanford et al.[650]	16	50
Shahian et al.[651]	18	56

In contrast to other situations, a histologic diagnosis often is not made before radiation and surgery because of the inaccessibility of the lesions, even to needle biopsy, and a desire not to violate tissue planes.[281,646] If the precise definition of a tumor mass in the extreme apex of the chest with pain down the ulnar distribution of the arm in T1 and C8 distribution is followed strictly, the diagnostic accuracy for cancer is better than 90%.[281,646] With inoperable or doubtful cases, open biopsy of the cupola of the pleura may be made through a supraclavicular scalenotomy incision if needed for histologic proof.[281]

Preoperative irradiation to a dose of 3000 rad in ten treatments over 12 days is given to the apex of the lung, upper ribs, upper mediastinum, ipsilateral hilum, and lower cervical spine.[646,647] This allows resection 3 to 6 weeks later. Standard higher doses have not been used routinely preoperatively because of the risk of increased radiotherapeutic and operative morbidity.[281] If surgery is not to be performed because of spread or underlying pulmonary risks, the dose to the spinal cord must be carefully limited. In these patients, shrinking-field techniques are used to achieve tumor doses of approximately 6000 rad. Pancoast tumors usually can be treated to high dose precisely because they are peripherally located, away from the midline. In fact, results with high-dose irradiation alone appear similar to those of combined-modality effort in selected patients without rib erosion.[652,653]

An extended en bloc resection of the chest wall often is carried out after radiotherapy and usually involves an extended radical lobectomy or segmental resection. The posterior portions of the first three ribs, portions of the upper thoracic vertebrae (including the transverse processes), the intercostal nerves, the lower trunk of the brachial plexus, the stellate ganglion, and a portion of the dorsal sympathetic chain are resected along with the involved lung.[281] Long-term complications include permanent ulnar nerve neurologic defects and Horner's syndrome, which do not appear to bother patients.[281] Immediate complications are respiratory in nature and include instability of the chest wall. They necessitate endotracheal tube ventilatory support for the first 3 postoperative days, bronchoscopy for removal of secretions in the immediate postoperative period, and Velpeau dressing to stabilize the chest wall.[646] There is debate about the number of patients who achieve pain relief, but at least two-thirds (and probably most long-term survivors) appear to do so.

Contraindications to resection generally include extensive invasion of the brachial plexus, subclavian artery, vertebral bodies, esophagus, or mediastinum and distant metastases.[646,647] Recent reports document successful arterial reconstruction when subclavian vessel resection was necessary.[648] Patients with hilar, mediastinal, or scalene node involvement have such a poor prognosis following the procedure that metastases in these sites also should be considered contraindications.[646,647] Only 50% of superior sulcus tumors are epidermoid; 30% are large cell or giant cell, and 15% are adenocarcinomas[649,650] Although the fraction of 3-year survivors was 42% for the epidermoid cancers and 21% for the large cell and adenocarcinomas, histology alone should not be used to determine resectability.[281] The use of postoperative radiation therapy for these tumors is controversial if complete resection can be accomplished.[651]

Innovative Radiotherapy Techniques

BRACHYTHERAPY. Brachytherapy or interstitial implantation has been championed by the MSKCC group and involves the placement of encapsulated radioactive sources within or close to the tumor or tumor residual at the time of surgical resection.[654–659] The MSKCC indications for brachytherapy include patients with limited pulmonary reserve, patients with hilar tumors adherent to the major vessels or extending to mediastinal structures where resection with negative margins is impossible, or patients with all gross primary or nodal tumor resected but where the margins of resection are involved. Iridium-192, ^{198}Au, or ^{125}I have been used. In theory, interstitial implantation allows delivery of a higher, more-uniform dose of radiation to the tumor, with less normal-tissue exposure than with external-beam therapy. The radioactive implants can be placed by the thoracic surgeon or afterloaded in intrathoracic catheters placed by the surgeon.[657] The disadvantages of such a technique include the necessity to keep the patient in specialized areas for radiation precautions and obligatory use of thoracotomy in a patient with potentially unresectable disease.

More than 1000 patients have been accumulated in the MSKCC experience since 1941. In 470 patients with non-small cell cancer treated by brachytherapy and thoracotomy, local control was obtained in 78% of those with Stage I or II disease, 71% with Stage III and negative nodes, and 63% of patients with involved lymph nodes.[657] However, the 5-year survival rate showed no improvement over that with other forms of therapy, with Stage I and II patients having a 33% 5-year survival rate and Stage III patients a 7% rate.

More recently, MSKCC has combined surgery with intraoperative brachytherapy and postoperative external-beam radiation in patients with residual gross disease or close resection margins.[660] A low complication rate, 7%, was observed. Despite good local control (53% for patients with positive margins and 89% for patients made free of disease), the actuarial 5-year survival rate was no different from that with other forms of treatment, and systemic disease accounted for cancer deaths. The absence of randomized comparisons of this therapy with surgery alone or external-beam radiation therapy alone, as well as the lack of survival improvement, currently relegates this unique methodology to an undefined role in the adjunctive management of locally advanced lung cancer. Moreover, it is unclear whether this technique can be applied outside a major cancer center, thus limiting its routine use.

Interstitial therapy has also been performed via bronchoscopic techniques for patients with malignant airway obstruction or hemorrhage or in patients with recurrent local disease such as stump recurrence.[661,662] The flexible or rigid bronchoscope can be used to deliver radon, ^{125}I or ^{198}Au. A dose of 3000 rad is delivered locally; however, problems include catheter dislodgment, airway obstruction, and hemoptysis. Currently, endobronchial brachytherapy has largely been replaced by the use of lasers.

INTRAOPERATIVE RADIATION THERAPY. Intraoperative radiation therapy delivered as a single large dose while the patient's chest is open has been described as a potentially useful adjunct to operation, external-beam irradiation postoperatively, or both in the treatment of locally advanced tumors.[663–668] Its utility in the treatment of lung cancer must be questioned, as severe toxicities have been noted at 2500 rad.[669] Only through further carefully designed clinical trials using lower doses will intraoperative radiotherapy ever be shown to have an appropriate risk : benefit ratio.

Postoperative Radiotherapy for Non-Small Cell Lung Cancer

RETROSPECTIVE TRIALS. The rationale for using postoperative radiation is to prevent locoregional relapse and hence increase the chance for cure and long-term survival. Unfortunately, there is scant scientific support for improved cure rate or survival despite the continued widespread use of this approach (Table 22-42). The use of postoperative radiation therapy in patients subjected to either curative or incomplete resection had been studied only in a retrospective fashion until the 1980s. Two widely quoted studies, by Green et

TABLE 22-42. Effect of Postoperative Radiation Therapy on Survival in Non-Small Cell Lung Cancer

Randomized Trials	*Control Arm*	*Radiotherapy Arm*
Van Houtte et al. 1980*		
"Completely resected" N2-negative, all histologies		
Number of patients	92	83
Radiation dose	–	60 Gy
5-year survival rate (%)	43	24
Lung Cancer Study Group 1978–1985†		
Stage II and III "completely resected" epidermoid carcinoma (20% N2+)		
Number of patients	108 (120)	102 (110)
Radiation dose	–	50 Gy
5-year survival rate (%)	38	38
Nonrandomized Trials	*Surgery Alone*	*Surgery + Radiation*
Green et al. 1954–1966‡		
Epidermoid and Adenocarcinoma		
Number of patients	38	52
Radiation dose	–	50–60 Gy
5-year survival rate (%)		
Epidermoid	6	21
Adenocarcinoma	14	50
Kirsh et al. 1959–1969§		
Epidermoid and Adenocarcinoma		
Number of patients	20	66
Radiation dose	–	Not specified
5-year survival rate (%)		
Epidermoid	0	34
Adenocarcinoma	0	12
Choi et al. 1971–1977‖		
Epidermoid and Adenocarcinoma		
Number of patients	50	86
Radiation dose	–	40–60 Gy
5-year survival rate (%)		
Epidermoid	33	33
Adenocarcinoma	8	43

*Van Houtte PV, Roemans P, Smets P et al: Postoperative radiation therapy in lung cancer: A controlled trial after resection of curative design. Int J Radiat Oncol Biol Phys 6:983, 1980.

†The Lung Cancer Study Group: Effects of postoperative mediastinal radiation on completely resected Stage II and Stage III epidermoid cancer of the lung. N Engl J Med 315:1377–1381, 1986.

‡Green N, Kurohara SS, George FW III, Crews QE Jr: Postresection irradiation for primary lung cancer. Radiology 116:405–407, 1975.

§Kirsh MM, Rotman H, Argenta L, et al. Carcinoma of the lung: Results of treatment over ten years. Ann Thorac Surg 21:371–377, 1976.

‖Choi NCH, Grillo HC, Gardiello M, Scannell JG, Wilkins EW Jr: Basis for new strategies in postoperative radiotherapy of bronchogenic carcinoma. Int J Radiat Oncol Biol Phys 6:31–35, 1980.

al[670] (52 patients with non-small cell cancer treated with surgery and postoperative irradiation for hilar and mediastinal nodes) conducted between 1954 and 1966 and Kirsh and associates[671] (66 patients treated with surgery and postoperative irradiation for the mediastinal nodes) conducted between 1959 and 1969, showed 5-year survival rates of 24% to 34% (depending on histology) compared with 0 to 22% with surgery alone (retrospective controls). In contrast, Choi and coworkers,[672] in a study of 86 patients, found 5-year survival rates of 33% to 43% compared with 8% (adenocarcinoma) to 33% (epidermoid carcinoma) historical controls with surgery alone. Thus, Green and Kirsh and their associates found an advantage for postoperative irradiation in both epidermoid carcinoma and adenocarcinoma, whereas Choi et al. found potential benefit only for adenocarcinoma. Both Cox,[673] a radiation oncologist, and Holmes,[674] a thoracic surgeon and chairman of the LCSG, have summarized the retrospective trials and their inconclusive results.

PROSPECTIVE RANDOMIZED TRIALS. Two randomized trials specifically examining the role of postoperative radiation therapy in resected non-small cell lung cancer have been reported, and both revealed no survival advantage of such adjuvant therapy. Van Houtte and associates randomized 175 patients with completely resected N2-negative disease to postoperative radiation therapy (6000 rad; 83 patients) or to no postoperative radiotherapy (92 patients).[669] The 5-year survival rate was actually lower in the postoperative radiation therapy group (24% versus 43%), although the difference was not statistically significant. Moreover, the radiation therapy group suffered more complications, including lung fibrosis, radiation pneumonitis, esophageal rupture, and constrictive pericarditis. Patients with squamous cell, large cell, and adenocarcinomas did equally poorly. Despite a small decrease in the local relapse rate in the radiation therapy group, this did not affect survival, with most patients dying from metastatic disease.

The LCSG[675] randomized 230 patients with "completely resected" Stage II (T2N1) and III (T3 tumor or any N2 disease) epidermoid lung cancer to receive postoperative adjuvant radiotherapy or no adjuvant treatment. Their patients were carefully staged intraoperatively, and the randomized groups were equally balanced as to prognostic factors. The mean follow-up time was 3.5 years. However, a relatively small fraction of patients had mediastinal node involvement, and this is the group traditionally receiving postoperative irradiation. Their 5-year survival rate was 38%, which was as good as any previously reported and may be related to the strict eligibility requirements and improved preoperative and intraoperative operative staging techniques in this study. The toxic effects of radiation included esophagitis (24%), other gastrointestinal symptoms (20%), dermatologic problems (11%), and neurologic problems (10%); interestingly, pulmonary toxicity was not significantly more common than in the control group (16% versus 9%). Their abstract summarizes the results of this important trial and their conclusions:

> There was no evidence that radiotherapy improved survival, and although recurrence rates appeared to be somewhat reduced among patients assigned to radiotherapy, these decreases were not statistically significant. However, radiotherapy did produce a striking and significant reduction in recurrences to the ipsilateral lung and mediastinum. Moreover, overall recurrence rates were reduced by radiotherapy in patients with N2 disease ($p < 0.05$), although even this subgroup had no evidence of improved survival. We conclude that radiotherapy can reduce local recurrences after resection of epidermoid carcinoma of the lung, but that it does not increase survival rates.

We concur with this analysis and believe that there is no mandated role for postoperative radiation therapy in carefully staged patients who have undergone potentially curative resection for lung cancer, as the reduction in the local recurrence rate does not translate into a survival advantage. However, insufficient patients with mediastinal node involvement (N2)—the group deriving the most benefit in retrospective studies—have been evaluated prospectively to exclude a small survival benefit in this category. No prospective trials to date have examined the efficacy of postoperative radiation therapy in higher-stage resected adenocarcinoma or large cell carcinoma.

POSTOPERATIVE ADJUVANT CHEMOTHERAPY

Studies of Historical Interest

Over the past 20 years, there have been a number of studies, a few of which were randomized, investigating the use of postoperative adjuvant chemotherapy in non-small cell lung cancer. Two large cooperative groups, one composed of VA hospitals and the second of university hospitals, began prospective randomized trials in which nitrogen mustard was administered at the end of the operation and in the immediate postoperative period.[676,677] There were no demonstrable survival benefits. A second trial, performed by the VA group, used chemotherapy administered during and immediately after the operation as well as a second course 5 weeks into the postoperative period. Again, there was no survival benefit compared with controls. A third trial compared postoperative cyclophosphamide with cyclophosphamide and methotrexate, both versus surgery alone.[678] Chemotherapy was given at 5-week intervals for 18 months. Survival was identical in all three arms. A fourth trial compared CCNU and hydroxyurea postoperatively with surgery alone. There was no demonstrable benefit from drug therapy.[679]

During this period, a number of reports from the United States from nonrandomized or partially randomized trials suggested improved survival with adjuvant chemotherapy.[680–682] However, all of the trials reporting beneficial survival figures were uncontrolled and involved small numbers or biased selection of patients. There also were a number of trials reported from outside the United States during this period, all indicating no benefit from adjuvant chemotherapy.[683–685] Some of these reports have been widely cited. Brunner et al.[686] administered cyclophosphamide for a 2-year period following surgical resection, and after a 9-year follow-up, the authors found that the rate of recurrence and death from lung cancer was significantly higher in the group receiving long-term chemotherapy. This finding raised the possibility that cyclophosphamide, a drug with strong immunosuppressive effects, impairs unspecified defense mechanisms against tumor cells. The British Medical Research Council conducted a large randomized trial of busulphan versus cyclophosphamide versus placebo and found no significant difference in survival at 5 years; however, the survival rates of 28%, 27%, and 34%, respectively, suggested a possible slight detriment to the chemotherapy-treated groups.[687] A cooperative group effort studied adjuvant CCNU therapy in postsurgical Stage I and II patients with non-small cell cancers.[688] More pronounced, even life-threatening, complications were found in the CCNU-treated arm, and if anything, the cancer relapse rate was higher, if not significantly so, with the chemotherapy.

Recent Adjuvant Chemotherapy Trials

Only with the recent discovery of drug combinations (many of which contain cisplatin) with better tumor response rates in patients with metastatic non-small cell lung cancer could the question of postoperative adjuvant chemotherapy be reinvestigated. The first evidence of the importance of cisplatin to drug combinations came from Eagan and coworkers, with the report of a 38% response rate with CAP chemotherapy (cyclophosphamide, Adriamycin [doxorubicin], and cisplatin).[689] Combination chemotherapy with cisplatin-containing regimens has produced initial response rates between 28% and 56%,[690–693] whereas in ECOG trials with larger groups of patients, such regimens have produced response rates of 23% to 31%, with the greatest 1-year survival rate (25%) seen with cisplatin and etoposide.[694]

The LCSG recently reported the results of a prospective randomized trial comparing surgery and immunotherapy with surgery and postoperative adjuvant chemotherapy in resected Stage II and Stage III non-small cell cancer.[695] Eligible patients had to undergo a complete resection of tumor with staging on the basis of lymph node mapping. Resection of subcarinal, paratracheal, hilar, and bronchopulmonary lymph nodes was required in all cases. The postoperative chemotherapy was CAP, whereas the control arm received BCG and levamisole immunotherapy. One hundred forty-one patients were randomized, of which 130 were eligible; of these 130, 23 did not receive the assigned treatment. There were no differences in the rates of postoperative complications. The usual side effects—gastrointestinal or hematologic toxicities—were noted with the CAP chemotherapy. Analysis of the data revealed a significantly lower recurrence and death rate in the chemotherapy group. With a mean time since randomization of 4 years and a mean observation period of 1.7 years among the 130 eligible patients, disease-free survival was longer, and deaths from cancer were significantly fewer, in the group receiving chemotherapy, and there was no evidence of a deleterious effect of the immunotherapy. Whether this early survival advantage will persist for 5 years or longer is unknown at this time and should be reported in the near future by the group. Although it appears unlikely that immunotherapy would have a deleterious effect, it would have been more conclusive to have a group treated by surgery alone.

The LCSG study is the first prospective randomized modern trial to show a survival advantage for adjuvant chemotherapy in non-small cell cancer. More trials with newer agents must be performed and carefully scrutinized to confirm the LCSG result before widespread application of such postoperative adjuvant chemotherapy becomes routine. At the present time, therefore, the addition of adjuvant chemotherapy after surgical resection should be considered investigational.

COMBINED-MODALITY TREATMENT WITH RADIATION AND CHEMOTHERAPY IN NON-SMALL CELL CARCINOMA OF THE LUNG WITH CURATIVE INTENT

Early Trials of Chemotherapy Added to Radiation

The addition of chemotherapy to high-dose radiation therapy given with curative intent could, in theory, kill tumor cells outside the treatment field and also act as a radiation sensitizer within the field. Cyclophosphamide, 5-fluorouracil (5-FU), nitrogen mustard, and vinblastine, when used as single drugs along with radiotherapy, have not improved survival over that obtained using radiotherapy alone.[696–704] In some cases, there actually appears to be a decrease in survival associated with radiochemotherapy. There have been several reports of nonrandomized trials that added combination chemotherapy to high-dose radiation with claims of improved median or long-term survival compared with historical controls treated with radiotherapy alone, with response rates in the 30% to 40% range.[705–711] Cox[712] and Cullen[713] and their coworkers, in two uncontrolled series, investigated the efficacy of cisplatin plus etoposide and radiation therapy in patients with limited-stage inoperable squamous cell carcinoma. The objective tumor response rates were 20% and 32%, yet the 1-year survival rates (47% and 40%, respectively) were not significantly different from historical controls given radiation therapy alone. Thus, patients given new drug combinations must be compared in a randomized fashion with a group of patients receiving the best current definitive radiation therapy with curative intent.

Recent Controlled Trials of Combined-Modality Therapy

Two recent controlled studies have evaluated the concomitant administration of cisplatin-containing chemotherapy regimens and high-dose radiotherapy (Table 22-43). Some

TABLE 22-43. Randomized Studies of Combined-Modality Therapy for Non-Small Cell Lung Cancer*

Series	*Patients (No. Evaluable)*	*Thoracic Irradiation Dose (Gy)*	*Chemotherapy*†	*Response Rate (%)*	*Median Survival (mo)*	*Statistical Analysis*
Radiotherapy With or Without Chemotherapy						
Wils et al.‡	14	60	None	50	5	
	19	60	P + A + VP-16	81	11	Significant
Van Houtte et al.§	32	50	None	55	12	
	27	45	P + VP-16 + VDS	20	9	Not significant
Incomplete Resection + Radiation With or Without Chemotherapy						
LCSG‖	164	40	none		12.7	Significant
		40	C + A + P		20	

*Adapted from Klastersky J: Therapy with cisplatin and etoposide for non-small cell lung cancer. Semin Oncol 13:104–111, 1986.

†C = cyclophosphamide, P = cisplatin, A = doxorubicin, VP-16 = etoposide, VDS = vindesine.

‡Wils JA, Utama I, Naus A, et al: Phase II randomized trial of radiotherapy alone vs the sequential use of chemotherapy and radiotherapy in Stage III non small cell lung cancer: Phase II trial of chemotherapy alone in Stage IV non small cell lung cancer. Eur J Cancer Clin Oncol 20:911–918, 1984.

§Van Houtte P, Klastersky J, Nguyen H et al: Comparative randomized study of chest radiotherapy preceded or not by chemotherapy with cisplatin, etoposide and vindesine for the treatment of non small cell lung cancer (NSCLC) (abstract). Proc Am Assoc Cancer Res 25:795, 1984.

‖Lad T, Rubinstein L, Sadeghi A: The benefit of adjuvant treatment for resected locally advanced non-small-cell lung cancer. J Clin Oncol 6:9–17, 1988.

of the studies showed modest improvement in survival in the patients receiving the combined-modality therapy.[714,715] Thus in the absence of significant numbers of controlled trials, and the lack of large increases in survival, *there remains no convincing evidence that chemotherapy added to appropriately delivered high-dose radiation therapy reproducibly and significantly increases the median survival or the fraction of long-term disease-free survivors.*

COMBINED-MODALITY TREATMENT WITH SURGERY, RADIATION, AND CHEMOTHERAPY OF NON-SMALL CELL LUNG CANCER

The use of both radiation therapy and chemotherapy after either "curative" or marginal resection of higher-stage non-small cell lung cancer has not been vigorously pursued in either controlled or uncontrolled studies. The rationale for such an approach posits radiation sterilization of residual microscopic disease after resection to prevent local recurrence with systemic adjuvant chemotherapy in the hope of preventing distant relapse. A nonrandomized retrospective study was performed by Newman and associates[716] over a 7-year period in which patients having resection of Stage II disease received either no adjuvant therapy, postoperative radiation therapy alone, or postoperative radiation therapy and CAMP (cyclophosphamide, doxorubicin, methotrexate, procarbazine). This study involved small numbers of patients in each subgroup, yet there was a significant survival advantage for those patients treated with postoperative multimodality therapy compared with those treated with surgery alone or surgery with postoperative radiotherapy alone: median survival 72^+ months with combined-modality therapy, 12 months with surgery alone, and 37^+ months with postoperative radiotherapy. Of note, there was a high rate of CNS relapse. In contrast, the LCSG,[717] in a prospective randomized trial, investigated postoperative chemoradiation therapy in 164 patients with non-small cell carcinoma who were able to have only incomplete resection of tumor. After resection, patients were randomized to receive either radiation therapy or 4000 rad of radiation plus CAP chemotherapy. Both recurrence and death rates were lower in the combined-modality arm. However, this difference was apparent only in the first year after randomization. Thus, longer follow-up is needed to see if the plateau values between the two arms are significantly different. From the paucity of data, *there seems to be no role at this time for routine chemoradiation therapy after resection of non-small cell cancer*, but future prospective randomized trials with more active agents are warranted in an investigational setting.

NEOADJUVANT (PREOPERATIVE) CHEMOTHERAPY OF NON-SMALL CELL LUNG CANCER

There is renewed interest in preoperative chemotherapy because of the more favorable tumor response rates (exceeding 50%) with the new drug combinations when given preoperatively to patients with disease confined to the ipsilateral hemithorax with lymph node positivity compared with the more typical 25% response rate seen in patients with extrathoracic disease (Table 22-44).[718] Thus, a major thrust of many investigative protocols at present in locally advanced disease involves the use of preoperative (also called neoadjuvant) chemotherapy with or without radiation therapy followed by attempted surgical resection (Table 22-45). The potential advantages of neoadjuvant therapy include increasing the incidence of complete resections by sterilizing local micrometastases, minimizing hematogenous or local seeding of cancer caused by surgical manipulation, and conservation

TABLE 22-44. Response to Combination Chemotherapy in Non-Small Cell Lung Cancer Related to Stage of Disease*

	Objective Tumor Response Rate (%)	
Chemotherapy Regimen	*Limited to the Chest*	*Metastatic*
Mitomycin-C + vinblastine + cisplatin	53	28
Cyclophosphamide + doxorubicin + cisplatin	47	23
Etoposide + cisplatin	56	27

*Adapted from Bonomi P: Brief overview of combination chemotherapy in non-small cell lung cancer. Semin Oncol 13:89–94, 1986.

TABLE 22-45. Use of Preoperative (Neoadjuvant) Chemotherapy and Radiotherapy in Non-Small Cell Lung Cancer

Year	*Histology/Stage*	*No. of Patients*	*Chemotherapy**	*No. with Pretherapy Resectability*	*No. of Responses (%)*	*No. (%) with Posttherapy Resectability*	*Survival Rate or Advantage*
1987[719]	Mixed/IIIA	41	Mito-C, VDS, P	0	30 (73)	21 (51)	>3.5 year median
1987[720]	Mixed/III	64	P, 5-FU, XRT	0	36 (56)	39 (60)	30% 2 years
1986[721]	Mixed/IIIB	20	V, P, VP16	7	14 (70)	7 (35)	34% 1 year
1984[722]	Squamous/I,II,III	32	P, Bleo, Mito-C	0	24 (75)	29 (91)	58% 1 year
1982[723]	Squamous/III	9	P, Mito-C	0	5 (56)	5 (56)	None
1982[724]	Squamous/I,II,III	16	P, Bleo	3	12 (75)	3 (19)	None
1982[725]	Mixed/III	12	C, A, P, XRT	0	6 (50)	11 (92)	None
1980[726]	Mixed/III	207	P	0	86 (43)	38 (18)	Yes
1979[727]	Squamous/III	27	Bronchial art Mito-C	0	18 (67)	15 (56)	None
1971[728]	Mixed/I,II,III	31	Bronchial art Mito-C	17	13 (42)	17 (55)	Yes

P = cisplatin; Mito-C = mitomycin C; Bleo = bleomycin; C = cyclophosphamide; VDS = vindesine; VP16 = etoposide; 5-FU = 5-fluorouracil; A = doxorubicin; XRT = radiation therapy; Bronchial art = bronchial artery infusion.

of normal lung by permitting less extensive resections. The potential hazards of neoadjuvant therapy include an increase in surgical morbidity or mortality related to the chemotherapy and loss of the surgical option if the tumor progresses during the chemotherapy. The patients for whom this approach seems particularly suited are those defined by the new staging system as having Stage IIIa disease.

The concept of neoadjuvant therapy is not new, with the earliest studies performed in mixed non-small cell histologies of various stages where mitomycin C was infused into the bronchial artery. Several recent studies have documented very high tumor response rates for neoadjuvant therapy and the conversion of unresectable tumors to resectable ones (Table 22-45). The impressive results of Martini and associates[719] have been confirmed in a series of 24 patients by R. Ginsberg (personal communication). In addition, recent reports of four ongoing studies of patients with unresectable Stage III non-small cell cancer who were treated with preoperative chemotherapy and in some cases radiotherapy showed 40 of 74 (54%) able to undergo a resection following the neoadjuvant therapy.[729–732]

NEOADJUVANT CHEMOTHERAPY REGIMENS AND TOXICITY

Three regimens appear to have the most activity in neoadjuvant studies: cisplatin plus etoposide, cisplatin plus 5-FU, and mitomycin C plus vinblastine (or vindesine) plus cisplatin (MVP). The cisplatin–etoposide combination has proved as good as any other regimen and was associated with a 30% overall response rate and the longest survival in metastatic disease in ECOG studies (Table 22-46).[694] However, toxicity in the ECOG studies included 3% deaths in 124 patients treated, with the most significant toxicities being hematologic and gastrointestinal. In fact, chemotherapy in the Martini study was associated with a 5% mortality rate, and the necessity for high-dose platinum required hospitalization.[719] Likewise, the study by Taylor and associates showed an 8% myocardial infarction rate and a 5% mortality rate attributable to the chemotherapy.[720] In investigating various adjuvant programs, it thus will be important to evaluate the ease of delivery, patient compliance, and toxicity in addition to survival and recurrence data. In this regard, the cisplatin plus etoposide combination can be administered in an outpatient setting, and in studies by Klastersky and associates,[733] there was no difference in the response rates between high- and low-dose cisplatin when combined with etoposide (Table 18-46).

Investigation of the role of neoadjuvant therapy in non-small cell lung cancer should be encouraged. However, such trials must be carefully designed with regard to the patient populations studied. The best population for such therapy would be those patients with locally advanced Stage IIIa disease. It is crucial that nodal disease be verified histologically in such patients prior to randomization to eliminate population heterogeneity caused by assumed nodal positivity based on CT scans alone. A neoadjuvant prospective randomized evaluation is in progress at the U.S. NCI comparing preoperative and postoperative cisplatin and etoposide chemotherapy and surgical resection with surgery and postoperative radiotherapy alone in Stage IIIa disease. Only after the completion of such trials can recommendations be made as to the standard use of neoadjuvant therapy for the management of locally advanced lung cancer.

PROPHYLACTIC CRANIAL IRRADIATION IN NON-SMALL CELL LUNG CANCER

The role of prophylactic cranial irradiation (PCI) in non-small cell cancer has not been defined. The frequency of brain metastases is less in this group than in those with small cell carcinoma of the lung both initially and during follow-up. However, patients with Stage III M0 adenocarcinoma of the lung receiving combined-modality therapy have been reported to have a very high rate (38%) of CNS metastases as the first site of relapse.[709] In N1 patients having an apparent complete surgical resection of non-small cell cancer, the brain was the most frequent site of recurrence (39%).[745] Likewise, in patients having a curative surgical resection for N2 disease, the brain was the most common site of distant metastases (19%).[746] In patients with Stage III M0 disease treated with curative radiation,[611,747] a large fraction relapsed with brain metastases, approaching 40% to 50% probability in patients living 3 years or more. In all of these studies, adenocarcinoma and large cell carcinoma spread to the brain more frequently than did epidermoid carcinoma (see also Table 22-19).

All of these studies suggest the possible utility of PCI to treat patients with non-small cell lung cancer (especially adenocarcinoma) potentially cured by surgery or radiotherapy.[611,747] The VALG conducted a prospectively randomized trial of PCI in all types of lung cancer and found a significant reduction in the frequency of clinically detectable brain metastases in those with non-small cell cancer (13% in the unirradiated and 6% in the irradiated group overall, and 29%

TABLE 22-46. Overview of Clinical Trials of Cisplatin plus Etoposide for Metastatic Non-Small Cell Lung Cancer*

Cisplatin Dose (mg/m²)	*Etoposide Dose (mg/m²)*	*No. of Studies*	*No. of Patients*	*Response Rate (%)*	
				Partial	*Complete*
60	100 or 120 × 3	4	273	27	1.8
80–90	50 × 4, 80 × 3, 100 × 3, 120 × 3	4	158	30	2.5
100	75 × 5, 80 × 3, 100 × 3, 120 × 3	5	158	35	2.5
120	120 × 3	1	93	29	NR†

*Adapted from Klastersky J: Therapy with cisplatin and etoposide for non-small cell lung cancer. Semin Oncol 13:104, 1986. Primary references are 734–744.

†NR = not reported.

versus 0 for adenocarcinoma).[748] Although there was no survival benefit of the PCI for these groups as a whole, patients exhibiting brain metastases had significantly shorter survival than those who did not. In a retrospective analysis of adenocarcinoma of the lung after potentially curative treatment, 5% of patients receiving PCI developed brain metastases compared with 24% of patients not receiving PCI.[749] Because of this information, many radiation oncology departments are starting to use PCI in potentially cured adenocarcinoma, particularly in patients with nodal involvement. Although this therapy must undergo further investigation, we believe it is reasonable to treat patients with adenocarcinoma or large cell carcinoma who are potentially cured but with high risk of relapse (N1, N2, and Stage III M0) with PCI. However, the long-term side-effects of PCI in adults with lung cancer, such as in those with small cell lung cancer, are only now being reported, and patients must be informed that there are potential long-term complications from PCI.[750,751]

LUNG CANCER IN YOUNG PERSONS

Lung cancer in patients under 40 years of age is uncommon and in children is rare.[753,754] The cancers in young adults occur in heavy smokers, and there is a higher frequency in female children. Adenocarcinomas and small cell cancers are much more common than epidermoid cancers. Survival after surgical resection is similar to that of adults; however, a more aggressive surgical resection and combined-modality therapy approach often is used.[752] In patients with unresectable disease, survival is short (6 months or less), and the disease is said to be more virulent than in older patients.[752]

APPROACH TO PATIENTS WITH DISSEMINATED NON-SMALL CELL LUNG CANCER

ALTERNATIVES

Patients with histologically documented, unresectable or inoperable non-small cell lung cancer should be evaluated first for radiotherapy. If it is believed the disease is sufficiently limited that it can be encompassed within a tolerable radiotherapy port and thus treated "for cure," or if there are pressing symptomatic needs for palliation such as, complete bronchial obstruction, hemoptysis, or upper airway or SVC obstruction, the initial treatment should be radiotherapy (with or without chemotherapy or surgery, if part of an experimental protocol). If a patient has more disseminated disease and there is no pressing need for radiotherapy, the approach can involve supportive therapy alone if the patient is reliable for follow-up or consideration of the use of chemotherapy.[493,754]

USE OF RADIOTHERAPY IN PALLIATION

Patients who have AJC Stage III cancer clearly have a poor prognosis, yet there is a small salvage rate with surgery or radiotherapy in those whose disease has not spread beyond the mediastinal nodes. In contrast, the question of whether the primary disease should be irradiated for palliation often arises in asymptomatic patients with poor prognostic features.[755,756] However, the argument is not so much to avoid treatment as to defer it to a time at which the patient becomes symptomatic. The case for palliative treatment of the asymptomatic patient is to prevent serious symptoms from occurring within the thorax. The case for delaying treatment really rests on the reliability of the patient.

The need for palliative chest radiotherapy was studied by following 134 inoperable patients not suitable for curative radiotherapy.[757] Immediate chest radiotherapy was believed to be necessary in 64% of the patients because of significant intrathoracic symptoms. The remaining patients were followed regularly without initial radiotherapy, and 54% of these (30% of the initial group) required radiotherapy within a median of 10 months because of progressive and significant symptoms of intrathoracic disease. Thus, more than 90% of the patients eventually needed to be irradiated.

If the patient can be followed closely, then deferring treatment until symptoms appear may very well be appropriate. However, patients with lung cancer often are followed infrequently, and these patients may present after a long interval with extreme symptoms (*e.g.*, SVC obstruction, obstructive pneumonia, or lobar collapse), all of which represent potentially life-threatening problems to the patient who has COPD in addition to lung cancer. In addition, when obstructive pneumonia complicates the patient's disease, the treatment often must be started with larger radiotherapy fields than would have been used at presentation or under emergency conditions, and sometimes must be delayed until sepsis can be controlled. The authors stress that if a decision is made not to irradiate asymptomatic tumors, *careful follow-up is required to avoid having a patient develop a highly symptomatic total bronchial obstruction that is difficult to relieve.*

When a patient relapses in the chest after primary surgical therapy, there may well be an indication for radiation therapy to the primary lesion. If prior radiation has not been used and the recurrence appears to be within the mediastinum, a course of low-dose palliative radiation (3000 rad in 2 weeks or slightly higher) often is given to the mediastinum to prevent progressive disease from obstructing the SVC or airway or from predisposing to pneumonia or sepsis. If the patient has a local relapse after surgery, careful restaging reveals no distant metastases, and the patient is in good shape physiologically, a course of high-dose radiotherapy can be attempted. However, no data from controlled trials demonstrate benefit in these cases. Retreatment with irradiation after prior palliative radiation also may be considered, depending on the previous volume and dose, the time course of symptoms after the first course, the progression of disease at other sites, and alternative treatment plans. The decision should be made by the radiotherapist in conjunction with other physicians taking care of the patient.

COMMON PROBLEMS IN THE MANAGEMENT OF LUNG CANCER

The general principles of diagnosis and management of metastatic disease, oncologic emergencies, and paraneoplastic syndromes (all common problems in lung cancer patients) are discussed in Chapters 55, 58, and 62. Other approaches to the primary therapy of small-cell lung cancer are discussed later. However, when lung cancer of any cell type presents as a localized problem that manifests symptoms, radiation therapy is frequently used (Table 22-47). A problem such as *SVC obstruction* usually can be relieved with a course of 3000 to 4000 rad over a 2- to 4-week period, with most patients achieving a response.[283,284,758,759] Recently, patients with SVC syndrome responded to radiotherapy in 50% to 70% of cases.[760] About 13% of patients will show a recurrence of the syndrome, and about 17% of those with non-small cell cancer and 24% of those with small cell lung cancer will survive for 1 year after such treatment. *Cardiac tamponade* also can be alleviated in many patients with pericardiocentesis and radiation therapy to the entire cardiac silhouette.[761] Such treatment usually is fractionated more slowly than standard treatment because of the possibility of later cardiac toxicity, interactions with chemotherapeutic agents, and the typically large volume of lung that has to be incorporated into the treatment volume behind the enlarged heart silhouette. Malignant pleural effusion usually does not respond well to radiation because the dose to the entire pleura is limited to about 2000 rad in order to spare the adjacent lung tissue. *Hemoptysis* as a symptom of tumor usually is relieved with radiation therapy.

Atelectasis from tumor obstruction is a common problem that is often difficult to relieve, responding in less than 25% of cases. However, recent data indicate that more than 60% of patients with non-small cell lung cancer presenting with atelectasis can have this problem relieved by appropriate radiotherapy.[762] When an entire lobe or lung has been collapsed by *bronchial obstruction*, radiation therapy frequently is used but with only modest success. In general, a lobe or lung has the greatest probability of being re-expanded if it has been collapsed only a short time (hours to few days); the longer the tissue has been collapsed, the less likely it is that radiation will be able to induce re-expansion.

TABLE 22-47. Local Symptomatic Relief Achieved by Radiation Therapy in Patients with Bronchogenic Carcinoma (All Cell Types)

Symptom	*Relief of Symptom (%)*
Hemopytsis*†	84
Cough*	60
Dyspnea*†	60
Atelectasis†‡	23
Superior vena caval obstruction†§‖	70–86
Vocal cord paralysis*	6
Pain*†	66
Brain metastasis#	70–90

**Philips TL, Miller RJ, Am Rev Respir Dis 117:405–410, 1978.
†Slawson RG, Scott RM, Radiology 132:175–176, 1979.
‡Majid OA, Lee S, Khushalani S, Seydel HG, Int J Radiat Oncol Biol Phys 12:231–232, 1986.
§Line D, Deeley TJ: Palliative therapy. In Deeley TJ (ed): Carcinoma of the Bronchus: Modern Radiotherapy, pp 298–306. New York, Appleton-Century-Crofts, 1972.
‖Armstrong BA, Perez CA, Simpson JR, Hederman MA, Int J Radiat Oncol Biol Phys 13:531–539, 1987.
#Perez CA, Presant CA, Van Ambury AL, Semin Oncol 5: 123–134, 1978.

Symptomatic *brain metastases* and *bone metastases* usually respond to palliative doses of radiation therapy (approximately 3000 rad in 2 weeks). Occasionally, such lesions will clear completely with treatment, but usually, careful evaluation of the site will show persistent neoplasm that is asymptomatic. If such a metastasis is the only site of distant spread, physicians occasionally decide to treat the metastasis and the primary with curative doses, hoping that the known sites of involvement can be controlled and that no other involvement exists.

MANAGEMENT OF BRAIN METASTASES IN NON-SMALL CELL LUNG CANCER

The median survival time of patients with brain metastasis is 3 to 4 months.[759] In addition to radiotherapy, dexamethasone is given. Seventy percent or more of patients have some relief of their symptoms; convulsions and headache usually are more thoroughly relieved than is motor loss or impaired mentation.[763] Patients whose CNS metastases respond to radiotherapy live twice as long as do those whose tumors do not respond.

Occasionally, patients are seen with a lung cancer and a solitary cerebral metastasis, which can present after or concurrent with the lung cancer.[764–766] When single brain metastases are found in patients with non-small cell carcinoma, surgical resection followed by radiotherapy may be undertaken when neurologically feasible. After careful staging to exclude other metastatic disease, if the brain lesion is a solitary peripheral (*i.e.*, neurosurgically accessible) lesion, these patients can be approached with surgical resection and then brain radiotherapy along with appropriate therapy of the primary lung cancer. Some 13% of these patients live for more than 1 year.[761] The MSKCC has compared the course of 43 such patients with an isolated brain metastasis treated with neurosurgical resection and radiotherapy with that of 43 patients treated with radiotherapy alone and found superior survival, lower recurrence rates, and fewer neurologically related deaths in the patients treated with surgical resection.[767]

SPINAL CORD COMPRESSION

Spinal cord compression should be suspected in patients complaining of back pain with or without lower-extremity weakness. In general, patients with spinal cord compression represent an emergency in which the best neurologic results are achieved by early diagnosis and treatment. Radiation usually will be the treatment of choice unless symptoms are rapidly progressive. Paralysis of the lower legs, with or without a radicular component of pain and with or without bowel or bladder dysfunction, makes the diagnosis obvious. When a spinal cord compression syndrome is suspected, a myelogram is essential to delineate the extent of the problem. Palliative irradiation usually is successful at alleviating the symptoms unless significant neurologic compromise has already occurred. Because lung cancer is the most common neoplastic cause of spinal cord compression, a low threshold for the diagnosis is the most important variable in achieving a good functional result.[768–770] The more extensive the neurologic deficit at the time of diagnosis, the more difficult it is to restore neurologic normality with radiation therapy.

Spinal cord compression can occur from extension into the spinal canal either from a vertebral metastasis or from a paravertebral mass invading through an intervertebral foramen. Because the compression may be occurring anywhere along the circumference of the spinal cord, decompressive laminectomy usually is reserved for patients whose symptoms are progressing so rapidly that there does not appear to be time for a response to irradiation; for those with recurrent cord compression in whom further irradiation cannot be delivered safely; and for those in whom a tissue diagnosis is not at hand. The more extensive the compression, the more difficult it is to return to normal neurologic function. Moreover, the more extensive the laminectomy, the greater is the instability of the spine that results. Because removal of the lamina only exposes the posterior aspect of the spinal cord, postoperative irradiation still is indicated in these patients because metastatic disease is rarely confined to the posterior aspect of the cord. With or without surgery, doses of 3000 to 4000 rad over 2 to 4 weeks are necessary for palliation, often starting with 300- to 400-rad fractions. Concomitantly, dexamethasone, 25 to 100 mg per day divided into four doses, is given initially and tapered rapidly to the lowest dosage that relieves the symptoms.[770] Again, the more extensive the neurologic deficit before treatment, the less recovery can be expected.

If the patient has had previous radiation therapy to the mediastinum and supraclavicular fossa, it can be difficult to distinguish between a brachial plexus syndrome caused by tumor and one caused by radiation injury. Typically, pain is more likely to be manifestation of tumor than of a radiation injury.[771] The presence of a supraclavicular mass is certainly suggestive of tumor. On the other hand, if the patient had radiation more than 6 months before the development of the brachial plexus syndrome, does not manifest pain, and has induration throughout the supraclavicular fossa without a discrete mass, then the chance of radiation injury is high. Correlation with careful dosimetric reconstruction is necessary, and a clinical diagnosis will often have to be made. When doubt exists and the patient is otherwise in good shape, surgical biopsy of the area may be necessary to plan treatment properly.

SELECTION OF PATIENTS FOR CHEMOTHERAPY OF METASTATIC NON-SMALL CELL LUNG CANCER

Everyone who has treated patients with small cell lung cancer using combination chemotherapy can readily appreciate both the prompt objective shrinkage of tumor and the relief of symptoms associated with the chemotherapy, which, in most cases, far outweigh any chemotherapy toxicity. In addition, many trials have demonstrated the survival benefit of such treatment and the cure of some of these patients (see later section). Such obvious clinical benefit is simply not seen with chemotherapy in the large majority of patients with non-small cell cancers.[772,773] Because of the strong correlation of tumor response with other significant prognostic factors such as performance status and bulk of disease (that is, the "best risk" patients have the best chance of responding to chemotherapy), there have been very few studies demonstrating a survival benefit from chemotherapy for metastatic non-small cell cancer. The median survival times for all patients treated are 5 to 6 months. Nevertheless, in nearly all studies, patients who show objective responses to chemotherapy have had significantly longer survival than those who do not respond.[772,774,775] Simply put, although response to chemotherapy is a significant prognostic factor in non-small cell cancer, *we do not know if this survival advantage is related to the chemotherapy or to some biologic feature of the disease that would permit increased survival independent of any treatment.* For this reason, it is generally accepted that *there is no "standard" regimen or chemotherapy treatment plan for non-small cell lung cancer.*[776–778]

RESPONSE TO SINGLE-AGENT CHEMOTHERAPY IN NON-SMALL CELL LUNG CANCER

No single-agent chemotherapy has significantly increased overall survival. The objective tumor responses that occur are usually brief, lasting 2 to 4 months, and complete responses are rare. Response rates are almost uniformly higher in patients who have not received prior chemotherapy of any type. Using relatively strict criteria for objective tumor response, Kris, Joss, and Bakowski and their colleagues have reviewed a large number of Phase II single-agent trials (Table 22-48).[776–778] More than 50 drugs were tested, but only six had significant antitumor activity in more than 15% of patients: *cisplatin, ifosfamide, mitomycin C, vindesine, vinblastine,* and *etoposide*. These agents were significantly different from the inactive drugs. For example, in 31% of the trials, no tumor responses of any kind were seen to the inactive drugs. Overall, the three reviews were in general agreement, although Kris et al[776] believed that etoposide was not as active as the other most active drugs. The response rates for these drugs were not related to tumor histology (squamous cell, adenocarcinoma, and large cell carcinoma). However, patients with prior chemotherapy had a lower response rate than did previously untreated patients.

Thus, only a few drugs have significant antitumor effects as single agents in non-small cell lung cancer. One of these drugs, ifosfamide, has been used more widely in European trials than in the United States. One of its serious side effects, urotoxicity, can be lowered by concomitant administration of the drug 2-mercaptoethane sulfonic acid (mesna) at 20% of the ifosfamide dose.[779] In addition to its activity as a single agent, ifosfamide is effective in combination with either etoposide or cisplatin. However, it is not yet clear to the authors whether it is superior to cyclophosphamide.

NEW DRUGS WITH POTENTIAL ACTIVITY AGAINST NON-SMALL CELL LUNG CANCER

The ECOG studied 676 patients in randomized trials comparing various combination chemotherapy regimens involving the platinum analogue *CBDCA* as a single agent.[780] The survival benefits and lesser toxicity of CBDCA led the ECOG to recommend further studies of this agent. A new antifolate, *10-EDAM* (10-ethyl-10-deaza-aminopterin), was found in

TABLE 22-48. Response Rates of Single-Agent Chemotherapy for Non-Small Cell Lung Cancer*

Drug	*No. of Patients*	*Response Rate (%)*†
Most active agents		
Cisplatin	305	16 (15, 20)
Ifosphamide	130	27 (25, 26)
Mitomycin-C	88	17 (17, 20)
Vinblastine	22	27
Vindesine	370	16 (19, 17)
Etoposide‡ (VP-16-213)		18
Agents with less activity		
Cyclophosphamide	405	12
Lomustine (CCNU)	216	10
Doxorubicin	296	12
5-FU	26	8
Methotrexate	105	11

*Data from Kris M, Cohen E, Gralla R: An analysis of 134 Phase II trials in non-small cell lung cancer (NSCLC). Proc. IV World Conference on Lung Cancer Cancer, Toronto 1985. Other agents reviewed with less than 15% response rates included the following commonly available drugs: cyclophosphamide, 5-FU, 6-mercaptopurine, methotrexate, PALA,BCNU, methyl-CCNU, CCNU, vincristine, teniposide, etoposide, L-asparaginase, dacarbazine, hexamethylmelamine, doxorubicin, and bleomycin as well as a series of other agents for a total of 51 drugs in 4340 patients. Note that these authors did not find etoposide to have activity equivalent to that of the other five agents.

†Response rates in parentheses correspond to the values obtained in the literature reviews by Joss RA, Cavalli F, Goldhirsch A et al: New agents in non-small cell lung cancer. Cancer Treat Rev 11:205–237, 1984; and Bakowski MT, Creech JC: Chemotherapy of non-small cell lung cancer: a reappraisal and look to the future. Cancer Treat Rev 10:159–172, 1983.

‡Etoposide (VP-16) data from Bakowski MT, Creech JC: Chemotherapy of non-small cell lung cancer: a reappraisal and look to the future. Cancer Treat Rev 10:159–172, 1983.

preclinical studies to have more selective entry into tumor cells and greater conversion to polyglutamate forms within tumor cells than its sister compound methotrexate.[781] A 33% tumor response rate was seen in 18 previously untreated patients by the MSKCC group, and stomatitis, rather than myelosuppression, was the limiting toxicity. Similarly, a nonclassical antifolate, *trimetrexate*, was found to have antitumor activity in 55 previously untreated patients.[782]

RESPONSES TO COMBINATION CHEMOTHERAPY IN NON-SMALL CELL LUNG CANCER

Over the past 15 years, several thousand patients with metastatic non-small cell cancer have been entered onto clinical studies testing various chemotherapy combinations (summarized in Tables 22-49 through 22-52) (for recent reviews, see Mulshine and Ruckdeschel[772] and Gralla[774]). Whereas tumor response rates of 50% to 70% are seen in the "neoadjuvant," preoperative setting (representing results in fully ambulatory patients with disease limited to the chest), the rates in patients with extrathoracic metastatic disease are significantly less: 20% to 40% objective response rates, with less than a 5% complete tumor remission rate.[772,774] Most studies have not found a difference in the response rates of the different histologic types of tumor, although occasional trials suggest such differences.[783]

TABLE 22-50. Pooled Results of Combination Chemotherapy with Cisplatin-Containing Regimens for Non-Small Cell Lung Cancer*

Combination†	*No. of Patients (No. of Trials)*	*Significant Response Rate (%)*
C + A + P	432 (5)	29
VDS + P	426 (9)	35
VP16 + P	384 (5)	29
VP16 + P (120 mg/m²) vs. P (60 mg/m²)	241 (1)‡	29 25
Mito-C + (VBL or VDS) + P	362 (7)	49
Total	1845 (27 trials)	

*Data from Gralla RJ: Issues and agents in the chemotherapy of non-small-cell lung cancer. Mediguide Oncol 5:1–5, 1985 covering randomized and nonrandomized trials.

†C = cyclophosphamide, A = doxorubicin, P = cisplatin, VDS = vindesine, VP16 = etoposide, Mito-C = mitomycin C, VBL = vinblastine.

‡Data on randomized high- vs. standard-dose cisplatin from Klastersky J, Sculier JP, Ravez P et al: A randomized study comparing a high and a standard dose of cisplatin in combination with etoposide in the treatment of advanced non-small-cell lung carcinoma. J Clin Oncol 4:1780–1786, 1986.

TABLE 22-49. Results of Combination Chemotherapy for Metastatic Non-Small Cell Lung Cancer*

Series	*Chemotherapy*†	*Objective Tumor Response Rate (%)*
Bitran et al.[784]	C + doxorubicin + MTX + procarbazine (CAMP)	48
Chahinian et al.[785]	MTX + doxorubicin + C + CCNU (MACC)	46
Vogl et al.[786]	MTX + doxorubicin + C + CCNU (MACC)	12
Eagan et al.[787]	C + doxorubicin + P (CAP)	39
Gralla et al.[788]	Vindesine + P (VP)	43
Longeval & Klastersky[789]	Etoposide + P (EP)	28
Mason & Catalono[790]	Mitomycin C + vinblastine + P (MVP)	53

*Adapted from Bonomi P: Brief overview of combination chemotherapy in non-small cell lung cancer. Semin Oncol 13:89, 1986.

†C = cyclophosphamide; MTX = methotrexate; CCNU = lomustine; P = cisplatin.

TABLE 22-51. Results of Combination Chemotherapy for Metastatic Non-Small Cell Lung Cancer in Eastern Cooperative Oncology Group Trials*

Trial and Regimen†	*No. of Patients*	*Response Rate (%)*	*Median Survival (wk)*
EST 2575 Generation III‡			
HEX + A + MTX vs.	77	13	22
C + A + MTX + PCZ	77	22	20
EST 2575 Generation IV§			
C + A + VP16 vs.	100	14	18
Mito-C + VBL	100	13	18
EST 2575 Generation V¶			
A + 5FU + P vs.	109	17	22
C + A + P vs.	107	23	24
C + Bleo + P vs.	112	20	22
Mito-C + VBL + P	104	26	24
*EST 1581***			
C + A + MTX + PCZ	15	17	24
vs. Mito-C + VBL + P vs.	121	31	22
VDS + P vs.	126	26	26
VP16 + P	124	23	26
Total	1272		

*Patients were stratified by histology (squamous, adenocarcinoma, large cell), performance status, and in some cases prior weight loss and randomly assigned to the different regimens. Exclusions included: small cell carcinoma histology, ECOG performance status of 3 or 4 (nonambulatory), prior radiotherapy to areas of evaluable disease, prior chemotherapy, inadequate laboratory values for renal, liver, and bone marrow function, brain metastases, and symptomatic cardiovascular disease.

†HEX = hexamethylmelamine; A = doxorubicin; MTX = methotrexate; C = Cyclophosphamide; PCZ = procarbazine; VP16 etoposide; Mito-C = mitomycin C; 5-FU = 5-fluorouracil; P = cisplatin; Bleo = bleomycin; VDS = vindesine.

‡Ruckdeschel JC, Mehta CR, Salazar OM, Creech RH, Sponzo RW: Chemotherapy for metastatic non-small cell bronchogenic carcinoma: EST-2575, generation III, HAM vs. CAMP. Cancer Treat Rep 65:959–963, 1981.

§Ruckdeschel JC, Day R, Weissman CH et al: Chemotherapy for metastatic non-small cell bronchogenic carcinoma: EST-2575, generation IV, cyclophosphamide, doxorubicin, and etoposide vs. mitomycin–vinblastine. Cancer Treat Rep 68:1325–1329, 1984.

¶Ruckdeschel JC, Finkelstein DM, Mason BA, Creech RH: Chemotherapy for metastatic non-small cell bronchogenic carcinoma: EST-2575, generation V: A randomized comparison of four cisplatin-containing regimens. J Clin Oncol 3:72–79, 1985.

**Ruckdeschel JC, Finkelstein DM, Ettinger DS et al: A randomized trial of the four most active regimens for metastatic non-small cell lung cancer. J Clin Oncol 4:14–22, 1986.

TABLE 22-52. Analysis of Long-Term Survivors in ECOG Combination Chemotherapy Trials for Metastatic Non-Small Cell Lung Cancer*

Total number of patients treated	893
Per cent surviving >1 year (N = 168)	19
Per cent surviving >2 years (N = 36)	4
Per cent suffering lethal complications	2
Overall major tumor response rate (per cent)	22
Overall complete tumor response rate (per cent)	2
Characteristics of patients surviving >1 year	
Major tumor response rate (per cent)	44
Complete tumor response rate (per cent)	8

*Finkelstein DM, Ettinger DS, Ruckdeschel JC: Long-term survivors in metastatic non-small cell lung cancer: An Eastern Cooperative Oncology Group study. J Clin Oncol 4:702–709, 1986.

RANDOMIZED TRIALS OF SINGLE-AGENT VERSUS COMBINATION CHEMOTHERAPY FOR METASTATIC NON-SMALL CELL LUNG CANCER

There have been several recent randomized trials that begin to provide information on the issue of the benefit or lack thereof from combination chemotherapy in non-small cell lung cancer. Overall, it appears that these trials demonstrate clinical benefit for combination chemotherapy. One type of trial randomized patients to single-agent chemotherapy versus a cisplatin combination. Elliot et al.[791] randomized 105 patients with metastatic cancer to treatment with vindesine alone or the combination of vindesine and cisplatin. More than 60% of patients in both treatment arms had tumor limited to the chest and thus had very favorable disease. The major tumor response rate to vindesine was 7%, with a 4-month median survival, whereas that to the combination was 33%, with an 11-month median survival, both highly significant differences. The Umbrian Lung Cancer Group trial also suggested benefits for combination chemotherapy.[792] It randomized 116 patients to cisplatin alone (4% response rate, 12% 1-year survival), cisplatin plus etoposide (38% response rate, 36% 1-year survival), or cisplatin plus etoposide plus mitomycin C (33% response rate, 24% 1-year survival).[792] The FONICAP trial in Italy randomized 124 patients to etoposide alone or etoposide plus cisplatin,[793] while the Southeastern Cooperative Group (SEG) randomized 453 patients to vindesine alone or vindesine plus mitomycin or vindesine plus cisplatin.[794] In the latter two trials, the combination chemotherapy resulted in a higher major tumor response rate, but no survival advantage despite increased toxicity. Indiana University randomized 124 patients with unresectable disease to therapy with vindesine alone (V; 14% response rate, 17 weeks' median survival), vindesine plus cisplatin (VP; 27% response rate, 26 weeks' median survival), or the two drugs plus mitomycin C (MVP; 20% response rate, 17 weeks' median survival).[795] There was no significant difference in overall survival, duration of remission, or survival of responders with the combination chemotherapy regimens compared with those receiving single-agent chemotherapy.

RANDOMIZED TRIALS OF COMBINATION CHEMOTHERAPY VERSUS SUPPORTIVE CARE FOR METASTATIC NON-SMALL CELL LUNG CANCER

Three studies have randomized patients with metastatic disease to treatment with combination chemotherapy and supportive care or supportive care alone, and thus compared survival and quality of life benefits from chemotherapy with those of supportive care alone.[796–798] The National Cancer Institute of Canada randomized 136 eligible patients to "best supportive care" or chemotherapy with vindesine and cisplatin (VP) (25% tumor responses) or CAP (16% tumor responses).[797] Although toxicity on the chemotherapy arms was significant, the median survival of the supportive-care group was 17 weeks, whereas it was 23 weeks for CAP and 31 weeks for VP, the latter being a significant improvement. The UCLA Solid Tumor Study Group randomized 63 patients with metastatic cancer to receive either supportive care, including palliative radiation, psychosocial support, analgesics, and nutritional support alone, or the same supportive care plus chemotherapy with VP.[798] Between 70% and 80% of the patients consented to the trial. The median survival time with supportive care only was 14 weeks compared with 20 weeks for chemotherapy plus supportive care (not significantly different). Differences in quality of life could not be determined because of difficulty in administering the test questionnaire to this population.

OUTPATIENT REGIMENS FOR CISPLATIN-COMBINATION CHEMOTHERAPY

Several chemotherapy regimens used to treat non-small cell lung cancer are described in Table 22-53. Hospitalization for chemotherapy obviously impacts on patients' lives, and it is desirable to keep this to a minimum when there are no curative or dramatic survival gains in sight. Whereas initial cisplatin-based combinations required hospitalization and intensive hydration, recently, programs of cisplatin and oral etoposide have been given safely in the outpatient setting with little toxicity and reasonable response rates.[801] Similarly, the Northern California Oncology Group divided the cisplatin dose between days 1 and 8 instead of administering the drug in the usual 5-day schedule.[802] Although the degree of nephrotoxicity was similar using this approach, the incidence and severity of myelosuppression and peripheral neuropathy were markedly reduced, while a high tumor response rate (47%) was maintained. The Institut Jules Bordet randomized 241 patients with advanced non-small cell lung cancer to chemotherapy with high-dose (120 mg/m^2 on day 1) or standard-dose (60 mg/m^2 on day 1) cisplatin therapy, both schedules given in combination with etoposide (120 mg/m^2 on days 3, 5, and 7). There was no significant response difference (25% versus 29%) or difference in overall survival or survival of responders between the two regimens.[803] As expected, toxicity (predominantly myelosupression), was significantly worse in the high-dose cisplatin arm. These results suggest using "standard-dose" cisplatin regimens.

PROGNOSTIC FEATURES IN THE SELECTION OF PATIENTS FOR CHEMOTHERAPY OF METASTATIC NON-SMALL CELL LUNG CANCER, PARTICULARLY THOSE PREDICTING LONG-TERM SURVIVAL

In many studies, the principal factors predicting a response to chemotherapy and survival in metastatic non-small cell cancer are performance status, disease extent, site of metastases, sex (females do better than males), and age.[772,776] In contrast, the histologic subtype appears to play little role. Quite often, medical oncologists give combination chemotherapy to patients with the hope of producing a dramatic response leading to significant prolongation of life (*e.g.* for a period of 1 to 2 years). Two large series, one from the ECOG[776] and the other from the MSKCC,[804] provide information on this question.

Eastern Cooperative Oncology Group Studies

The ECOG treated 893 good-performance-status patients using several combination chemotherapy regimens (listed in Table 22-51 and references 691 and 805) and obtained an overall median survival of 23 to 24 weeks, with no significant differences in survival among the seven different chemotherapy regimens. Nineteen percent of the patients survived for more than 1 year, and 4% survived for more than 2 years. The ECOG analyzed their multiple studies to identify characteristics associated with survival of 1 year or more (Table 22-52), finding that pretreatment characteristics most predictive of survival for more than 1 year were initial asymptomatic performance status (PS = 0); no bone, liver, or subcutaneous metastases; female sex; a histology other than large cell carcinoma; a prior weight loss of less than 5%; and no symptoms of shoulder or arm pain.[694] The 1-year survivors had a higher tumor response rate and complete regression rate than the population as a whole. Sixty-two percent of the complete responders and 34% of the partial responders, but only 14% of the nonresponders, lived for more than 1 year. The etoposide plus cisplatin combination had the highest proportion of 1-year survivors (25%), compared with 18% for the other regimens, whereas the mitomycin C plus vinblastine plus cisplatin combination had significantly fewer 1-year survivors (12%) than any of the other regimens despite having the highest tumor response rate (Table 22-51). The ECOG hypothesized that this was attributable to increased toxicity caused by long-term use of mitomycin.

Of interest, the ECOG found that those patients whose tumor took a long time to respond to chemotherapy maintained the response the longest. Thus, patients whose tumors took more than 90 days to exhibit the best response to ther-

TABLE 22-53. Sample Drug Regimens Used in the Treatment of Non-Small Cell Lung Cancer

CAP*

Cyclophosphamide	400 mg/m² IV
Doxorubicin	40 mg/m² IV
Cisplatin	40 mg/m² IV

All given day 1 and repeated every 4 weeks.

1. Patients must have normal cardiac and renal status (creatinine <1.5 mg/dl).
2. Doses are given by rapid IV, infusion with 1 liter of 5% glucose in half-normal saline over 1 to 2 hours; no special diuresis program is routinely used.
3. Doses are modified to obtain WBC nadirs of 1500–2500/μl or platelet nadirs of 75,000–100,000/μl measured at day 14. Before each subsequent treatment, WBC should be >4,000/μl and platelets >100,000/μl.
4. Stop cisplatin permanently if creatinine rises above 2.0 mg/dl or hearing loss develops.
5. Stop doxorubicin at a maximum cumulative dose of 450 mg/m² or if signs of congestive heart failure or arrythmias develop.

VP-16 + Cisplatin†

VP-16	120 mg/m² IV days 1, 3, 5. Repeat combination every 3 weeks.
Cisplatin	60 mg/ms², IV day 1

1. Patients must have normal renal function.
2. All patients will have nausea, vomiting, and alopecia.
3. Appropriate dose modifications are made for hematologic and renal toxicity. Omit cisplatin if creatinine is 2 mg/dl or higher until creatinine returns to less than 1.5 mg/dl.
4. Patients also should be monitored for hearing loss.
5. Hydration for cisplatin includes furosemide, 20 mg IV, given at the start of 2-hour infusion of 2 liters of 5% glucose in half-normal saline with 10 mEq of KCl/liter. Thirty minutes into infusion, 12.5 g of mannitol is given IV. If diuresis ensues, cisplatin is administered as an IV bolus. If no diuresis by 30 minutes, additional furosemide should be given.‡

Vinblastine + Cisplatin§

Vinblastine	6 mg/m² IV
Cisplatin	120 mg/m² IV or 60 mg/m² IV

1. Follow comments for VP-16 and cisplatin above.
2. In a comparison of cisplatin + vinblastine versus cisplatin + vindesine (3 mg/m²) there was no difference in response rates (41% versus 33%), median response durations (5.6 versus 8.6 months), or median survival times of responding patients (16.2 versus 18.4 months). However, more patients receiving vinblastine + cisplatin had WBC counts below 2100/μl whereas the vindesine-treated patients had more neurotoxicity.
3. Whether 120 mg/m² is better than 60 mg/m² for the cisplatin dose is not yet known. A randomized comparison in 85 patients between the same dose of another vinca alkaloid, vindesine, and either high-dose (120 mg/m²) or low-dose (60 mg/m²) cisplatin showed the same overall response rate of 43%, but the high-dose cisplatin regimen was superior to the low-dose regimen in median duration of response and in median survival for responding patients.[799] Patients receiving the high dose usually are hospitalized for hydration (150 ml/hour of 5% glucose normal saline with 20 mEq of KC1/liter) for 12 hours before therapy. Immediately before treatment, mannitol 12.5 g is given as a rapid IV infusion. The volume of fluid ordinarily requires either a large-bore Angiocath or a central venous line. Just before cisplatin is administered, 20 mg of furosemide is given IV. The high-dose cisplatin is mixed in 250 ml of 3% saline and infused over 30 min.[800] If patients cannot tolerate this fluid load for the full period of hydration despite appropriate medical management (diuretics), the hydration regimen can be altered to 5% glucose in half-normal saline at 150 ml/hour with KCl supplementation.

*Data from Eagan RT, Ingle JN, Frytak S et al: Platinum based polychemotherapy versus dianhydrogalacticol in advanced non-small cell lung cancer. Cancer Treat Rep 61:1339–1345, 1977; Ruckdeschel JC, Finkelstein DM, Mason BA, Creech RH: Chemotherapy for metastatic non-small cell bronchogeneic carcinoma: EST-2575, generation V: A randomized comparison of four cisplatin-containing regimens. J Clin Oncol 3:72–79, 1985

†Data from Klatersky J, Longeval E, Nicaise C, Weerts D: Etoposide and cisplatinum in non-small-cell bronchogenic carcinoma. Cancer Treat Rev 9(Suppl A):133–138, 1982; Longeval E, Klastersky J: Combination chemotherapy with cisplatin and etoposide in bronchogenic squamous cell carcinoma and adenocarcinoma: A study by the EORTC Lung Cancer Working Party (Belgium). Cancer 50:2751–2756, 1982; Goldhirsch A, Joss R, Cavalli F, Brunner KW: Etoposide as single agent and in combination chemotherapy of bronchogenic carcinoma. Cancer Treat Rev 9(Suppl A):85–90, 1982; Ruckdeschel JC, Finkelstein DM, Ettinger DS, et al: A randomized trial of the four most active regimens for metastatic non-small cell lung cancer J Clin Oncol 4:14–22, 1986.

‡Vogl SE, Zaravinos T, Kaplan BH et al: Safe and effective two hour outpatient regimen of hydration and diuresis for the administration of cis diaminedichloroplatinum(II). Eur J Cancer 17:345–350, 1981.

§Kris GM, Gralla RJ, Kalman LA et al: Randomized trial comparing vindesine plus cisplatin with vinblastine plus cisplatin in patients with non-small cell lung cancer, with an analysis of methods of response assessment. Cancer Treat Rep 69:387–395, 1985.

apy were more likely to be long-term survivors than were those whose tumors responded more quickly (less than 30 days). This result suggested a biologic difference between rapidly and slowly responding tumors.[694] Not surprisingly, long-term survivors were more likely to maintain or improve their performance status and serum albumin concentration during the first 3 months following therapy than patients living less than 1 year. However, the ECOG also noted that the 1-year survivors experienced more intense hematologic and gastrointestinal (vomiting) toxicity that was probably related to the longer duration of chemotherapy.[694]

Memorial Sloan-Kettering Cancer Center Study

The 554 patients with unresectable non-small cell cancer treated by the MSKCC group received cisplatin plus a vinca alkaloid (vindesine or vinblastine) with or without mitomycin C; 9.6% achieved a complete remission.[809] These patients, in general, had excellent pretreatment performance status and no weight loss, and 40% were women. A complete remission was achieved in 5.8% with chemotherapy alone, whereas another 3.8% where able to obtain a complete remission with surgical resection after a significant tumor response to chemotherapy. All of the patients improved or maintained their performance status while in a complete remission and lived a median of 28 to 36 months, compared with a median survival of 11 months for the overall series. In another multivariate analysis of 378 of these patients, the

Memorial group found that a good initial performance status (Karnofsky 80–100) was significantly related to achieving a significant tumor response to chemotherapy and increased survival, whereas bone metastases, elevated serum LDH, and male sex were associated with poorer response rate and shorter remission duration and survival, as was the presence of two or more extrathoracic metastatic organ sites.[775]

TOXICITIES IN THE TREATMENT OF NON-SMALL CELL LUNG CANCER WITH CHEMOTHERAPY

Most of the combination-chemotherapy trials in non-small cell lung cancer have produced significant treatment-related toxicities including death.[773] For example, of 65 consecutive patients treated with intensive induction chemotherapy by a major cancer center skilled in supportive care, more than half experienced an infectious episode, and 5% suffered drug-related infectious death.[806]

In addition, poor performance status patients were at significantly higher risk of developing an infectious complication.[806] Similarly, in trials reporting excellent objective response rates and increased survival for responders compared with nonresponders, significant chemotherapy toxicity was noted in more than half the patients, and both performance status and body weight dropped significantly during chemotherapy among all patients.[807]

Combination chemotherapy regimens that include repeated (more than three cycles) administration of mitomycin C, often with a vinca alkaloid, have been associated with pulmonary toxicity manifested by the clinical triad of progressive dyspnea, rales, and pulmonary infiltrates and associated with hypoxemia and profound reduction in diffusion capacity.[808] Transbronchial biopsy reveals characteristic but nonspecific changes. Treatment involves high-dose glucocorticoids, which have to be tapered gradually, and immediate discontinuation of mitomycin C when pulmonary toxicity is suspected. Most patients respond promptly to this therapy.

PERCEPTION OF RISK: BENEFIT RATIO FOR CHEMOTHERAPY IN THE MANAGEMENT OF NON-SMALL CELL LUNG CANCER

Such results cause many experienced physicians to feel that the deterioration in patients' well-being from chemotherapy offsets any potential survival advantage.[807] A dramatic testament to this clinical experience was provided in a study questionnaire administered to 118 Canadian physicians who treat lung cancer.[809,810] Whereas opinion was divided as to the role of immediate radiotherapy in operable cancer and the role of postoperative radiotherapy after incomplete resection, there was little debate as to the role of chemotherapy. Only 3% would want for themselves adjuvant chemotherapy after surgery for early disease, only 9% would want chemotherapy for advanced disease confined to the chest, and only 15% would want chemotherapy for symptomatic metastatic disease. Thus, experts in the field would not prescribe for themselves treatment currently given in many clinical trials for non-small cell lung cancer.

EXPERIMENTAL TREATMENT APPROACHES TO NON-SMALL CELL LUNG CANCER

Role of Combined-Modality Radiotherapy and Chemotherapy for Advanced Non-Small Cell Lung Cancer

Three trials indicate that combined-modality (chemoradiotherapy), now experimental, may hold some promise. Two hundred sixty-eight patients with localized unresectable epidermoid lung cancer were treated with cisplatin plus bleomycin and either mitomycin, vindesine, or etoposide followed by radiation therapy. There was a 62% objective tumor response rate.[811] The median survival for the group was 9 months. However, there was a 35% 1-year and a 13% 2-year survival rate. Sixty-four patients with Stage III locally unresectable cancer were given cisplatin plus 5-FU chemotherapy with simultaneous radiation therapy (40 Gy) followed by attempted surgical resection. Sixty-one percent underwent the resection, and 14% of the original group were found to have no tumor in the surgical specimens.[812] However, when 81 patients with inoperable cancer were randomized to receive split-dose irradiation alone or with cisplatin-based combination chemotherapy, the survival and quality of life measures were not different in the groups.[813]

New Types of Treatment

Chemoprevention trials using vitamin A (retinol palmitate), retinoids with or without beta-carotene, or N-acetylcysteine are being designed,[814,815] and thus it is of interest that clinically evident lung cancer has shown responses to these agents. A Phase II trial of *13-cis-retinoic acid* (100 mg/m^2 per day) in advanced non-small cell lung cancer produced one significant response among 23 evaluable patients that lasted 5 months,[816] whereas another trial showed one response in 10 patients and minor responses in two others.[817]

The RTOG randomized 117 patients to treatment with radiotherapy alone or with the hypoxic cell sensitizer *misonidazole*.[818] They found misonidazole did not enhance the effect of radiotherapy on either local tumor control or overall survival in patients with advanced lung cancer. In contrast, the Northern California Oncology Group, in a randomized trial of 100 patients, found that misonidazole did function as a chemosensitizer for the drug L-phenylalanine mustard in non-small cell lung cancer.[819]

Hydrazine sulfate, which is thought to improve the abnormal metabolism and reverse weight loss in patients with advanced cancer, was associated with significantly longer survival then was a placebo in a randomized trial of 65 patients with metastatic lung cancer receiving combination chemotherapy.[820] In a prospective double-blind trial, 12 malnourished lung cancer patients were randomized to receive placebo or hydrazine sulfate (60 mg three times daily). Fasting lysine flux was studied before and after treatment and revealed a significant improvement after 30 days of hydrazine sulfate administration.[821] In contrast, 102 patients with metastatic non-small cell cancer randomized to receive either ad lib diets or specific nutritional intervention during a 12-week period while receiving combination chemotherapy (vindesine and cisplatin) showed no difference in response rates, median time to progression, or overall duration of survival.[822]

Mopidamol (*RA-233*) is a derivative of dipyridamole (a phosphodiesterase inhibitor) that inhibits the progression of malignancy in experimental animal models. A Veterans Administration Cooperative Group randomized a large number of patients with small cell and non-small cell lung cancer to chemotherapy alone or chemotherapy with RA-233.[823] No significant difference in survival was found for small cell carcinoma patients (limited or extensive stage) or patients with disseminated non-small cell cancer. However, in the 71 patients with non-small cell disease limited to one hemithorax, the patients randomized to RA-233 and chemotherapy (with cyclophosphamide, doxorubicin, and methotrexate) had significantly longer survival than patients treated with chemotherapy and a RA-233 placebo (46 versus 29 weeks). This important trial needs to be confirmed with larger numbers of patients. However, it may be that RA-233 inhibits the breakdown of cyclic AMP and thus promotes the transduction of growth-inhibitory signals in tumor, possibly through effects on the function of the *ras* proto-oncogene.[824]

Immunotherapy

RANDOMIZED CLINICAL TRIALS. There is a large literature on impaired immune function in lung cancer patients, and this has stimulated many clinical trials of immunotherapy. Several randomized studies have evaluated immunotherapy, usually as an adjuvant to surgery, and over the past 10 years, there have been flurries of excitement about the benefits of such adjuvant immunotherapy. However, recent large-scale randomized trials suggest there is no standard role for such therapy at present. The Ludwig Lung Cancer Study Group prospectively randomized 303 patients with resected Stage I and II non-small cell cancer to receive intrapleural *Corynebacterium parvum* (*C. parvum*) and then subsequent intravenous *C. parvum* or a placebo.[825] They found no significant difference between the treatments with respect to disease-free interval or survival. In another trial, the Ludwig group prospectively randomized 441 patients with resected Stage I and II non-small cell cancer to adjuvant treatment with either intrapleural BCG (Tice strain) between postoperative days 6 and 12 or placebo.[826] There was no significant difference between the groups with respect to survival, but there was a high rate of pleural empyema in the BCG-treated group and a significant decrease in the disease-free interval for the patients who had undergone a pneumonectomy. In the Netherlands, the administration of intrapleural BCG actually appeared to enhance tumor growth.[827] Another study found significant survival advantages for patients with resected disease treated with the streptococcal preparation OK-432 and chemotherapy compared with those given chemotherapy alone.[828] However, until these observations are substantiated, these approaches should not be applied outside clinical trials.

RECENT FINDINGS OF IMMUNOLOGIC IMPORTANCE IN LUNG CANCER PATIENTS. The subpopulation of lymphocytes designated natural killer (NK) cells are capable of killing a variety of tumor cell targets. Despite high blood levels of NK cell activity, the NK activity of lymphocytes is significantly lower in lung specimens of patients undergoing a curative resection for lung cancer than in lymphocytes from normal lung specimens obtained from cadavers undergoing medicolegal autopsy.[829] This change appears to result from the release of inhibitors by pulmonary macrophages in lung cancer patients. Interleukin-2 (IL-2)-derived T lymphocytes were grown from explants of tumor tissues and given to lung cancer patients, where they were associated with tumor reduction in five of seven patients and an increase in delayed cutaneous hypersensitivity in three of these patients.[830] Intrapleural instillations of recombinant IL-2 in 11 patients with malignant pleural effusions resulted in clearing of the effusions and cancer cells in the effusions in nine patients, with side effects being fever, eosinophilia, and a transient increase in the effusion.[841]

NEW APPROACHES TO PALLIATIVE THERAPY

Neodynium: YAG Laser and Photodynamic (Hematoporphyrin) Therapy for Bronchial Obstruction

Management of intrabronchial lesions recurrent after surgery and radiotherapy, as well as of such lesions in patients with comprised pulmonary function, and treatment decisions about radiographically occult cancers are challenging. Two new forms of treatment offer promise in these arenas. *Neodynium: YAG (yttrium–aluminum–garnet) laser therapy* has been used increasingly in treating recurrent endotracheal and endobronchial lesions in lung cancer, usually in patients relapsing after several other therapies including surgery and radiotherapy.[832,833] Treatment can often be administered via a flexible fiberoptic bronchoscope, and usually, this is done under general anesthesia. Palliative improvement is seen in 80% to 90% of cases, and many patients have been treated. Serious complications include massive hemorrhage (usually related to high power settings), intrabronchial explosions, and damage to normal tissues.

After administration of *hematoporphyrin*, which may localize in tumors and which sensitizes tissues to light, *bronchoscopic phototherapy* has been administered to intrabronchial lesions.[834] Small, radiographically occult carcinomas treated this way will often regress completely for long periods of follow-up, whereas larger lesions will often show at least a partial response.

Malignant Pleural Effusions

The development of malignant pleural effusion in patients with lung cancer is an ominous sign. These effusions are usually recurrent and can be highly symptomatic, leading to shortness of breath and pain. The key to their management in lung cancer is prompt and complete chest tube drainage of all but the smallest effusions after appropriate physical examination and diagnostic tests to exclude congestive heart failure and infection. Although a variety of other treatments such as intrapleural instillation of tetracycline or chemotherapy, play a role, they are secondary to appropriate chest tube drainage.

Pain Control

Fortunately, severe, unrelenting pain is not a frequent problem in lung cancer compared with such problems as bronchial obstruction or brain metastases. Management of cancer-related pain is discussed in detail in Chapter 59, section 4. In a series of 221 lung cancer patients with intractable pain, the three chief causes were skeletal metastatic disease (34%), Pancoast's tumor (31%), and chest wall disease (21%), together accounting for 78% of the cancer-related pain problems.[835] The median interval between cancer diagnosis and the onset of pain was only 1 month, and the median survival after the onset of the pain was 10 months. A variety of treatment modalities have been employed, including local radiation, percutaneous cordotomy, regional deafferentation, and pharmacotherapy.

THERAPY OF SMALL CELL CARCINOMA OF THE LUNG

Small cell lung cancer differs from the other cell types in its more aggressive clinical course in the absence of treatment and in its superior responsiveness to chemotherapy and thoracic irradiation. Median survival of patients with surgically unresectable disease randomized to supportive care alone in a trial conducted during the 1960s was only 12 weeks for patients with limited-stage and 5 weeks for those with extensive-stage disease.[493] The disease's natural history is characterized by relentless progression and the early development of distant metastatic deposits. When compared with other types of lung cancer with a similar extent of tumor dissemination, a shorter duration of symptoms prior to diagnosis and reduced survival once a diagnosis is established are evident.[493,836] In a study of 19 patients subjected to potentially curative surgical resection and dying within 30 days of operation of noncancer-related causes, 70% had distant metastases at postmortem examination.[837] More than 70% of patients have mediastinal lymph node involvement at diagnosis, which in itself precludes surgical resection.[838,839] Approximately two-thirds of patients will have evidence of metastases beyond the hemithorax of origin.[839] At autopsy of patients managed without surgical extirpation of the primary tumor, only 4% will not demonstrate tumor dissemination beyond the thorax.[840]

These findings of frequent tumor spread to regional lymph nodes and distant extrathoracic sites by the time of initial clinical presentation indicate that small cell carcinoma is a systemic disease process very early after inception in almost all patients. Therefore, it is not surprising that reliance on solely locoregional forms of treatment fails in the vast majority of patients. In a British study performed in the 1960s, patients who were considered candidates for surgical resection by the standards of the time were randomized to thoracotomy with the intent of tumor removal or to definitive irradiation to the primary tumor and regional lymphatics.[841] Although radiotherapy proved superior to attempted surgical removal in terms of survival (Table 22-54), fewer than 4% of these apparently operable patients were alive 5 years after randomization. Today, these patients (if they had been appropriately staged) would represent a very favorable subset of limited-stage disease. Shortly thereafter, a review of the outcome of a large number of American small cell lung cancer patients who were thought to be operable revealed absolutely no differences in survival whether or not a thoracotomy was performed.[842] These data led to the abandonment of surgical therapy by many thoracic surgeons in patients with an established diagnosis of small cell carcinoma until the present decade.

In 1969, an important randomized trial by the Veterans Administration LCSG documented that three courses of cyclophosphamide more than doubled the median survival compared with supportive care alone in extensive-stage small cell lung cancer.[843] This finding sharply contrasted with the results of similar studies of single-agent chemotherapy in other cell types of lung cancer and led to the rapid investigation of the role of chemotherapy in patients with small cell carcinoma. Randomized studies (which employed what would today be considered suboptimal chemotherapy) in most instances demonstrated that adjuvant chemotherapy after surgical resection prolonged survival compared with no further treatment. Because of the small numbers of patients enrolled in most of these trials, this result becomes more obvious when the data are pooled (Table 22-55). Similarly, in most randomized clinical trials, the addition of chemotherapy to chest irradiation in patients with limited-stage small cell lung cancer yielded improved median or longer-term survival compared with a policy of irradiation as the sole initial treatment followed by chemotherapy at the time of tumor progression (Table 22-56). Once again, the chemo-

TABLE 22-54. Survival in Patients with Operable Small Lung Cancer Randomized to Surgery or Radiotherapy

Group	No. of Patients	Mean Survival (mo)	Survival Rate (%)		
			1-Year	2-Year	5-Year
Surgery	71	6.5	21	4	1†
Radiotherapy	73	10*	22	10	4

*Significant survival difference ($p = 0.04$) in favor of radiotherapy.
†One patient unable to receive surgery; given irradiation.
Modified from Fox W, Scadding JG: Medical Research Council comparative trial of surgery and radiotherapy for primary treatment of small-celled or oat-celled carcinoma of bronchus. Lancet 2:63–65, 1973.

TABLE 22-55. Pooled Results from Randomized Surgical Adjuvant Studies in Small Cell Lung Cancer

Adjuvant Therapy	*No. of Patients*	*2-Year Survivors (%)*
Chemotherapy	92	26
Placebo	61	8

Higgins GA, Shields TW: Experience of the Veterans Administration Surgical Adjuvant Group. Prog Cancer Res Ther 11:433–442, 1979; Shields TW, Humphrey EW, Eastridge CE et al: Adjuvant cancer chemotherapy after resection of carcinoma of the lung. Cancer 5:2057–2062, 1977; Wingfield HV: Combined surgery and chemotherapy for carcinoma of the bronchus. Lancet 1:470–471, 1970; Karrer K, Pridun N, Denck H: Chemotherapy as an adjuvant to surgery in lung cancer. Cancer Chemotherapy Pharmacol 1:145–159, 1978.

therapy used in these early trials, either as single agents or in combinations, was not optimal by current standards. Nevertheless, these early trials of chemotherapy as an adjuvant to locoregional treatments and multiple other studies employing chemotherapy as the sole form of therapy quickly established that small cell carcinoma was by far the most drug-responsive type of lung cancer.

The strategies of chemotherapy administration in small cell lung cancer are similar to the optimal methods of drug treatment in several adult cancers that can sometimes be cured with chemotherapy alone. For example, in small cell carcinoma, testicular carcinoma, Hodgkin's disease, and diffuse aggressive lymphomas, although numerous single agents induce objective responses, combination chemotherapy produces superior survival compared with single-agent treatment; responses to chemotherapy occur relatively quickly; increasing drug doses (up to a point) improves survival rates; and maintenance chemotherapy for responding patients is of little or no value. Over the past two decades, therapeutic research in small cell lung cancer has been built on the assumptions that this is fundamentally a systemic disorder that is usually responsive to chemotherapeutic agents and that combination chemotherapy is therefore the mainstay of treatment. Several detailed reviews summarizing the therapy of this neoplasm and critically evaluating which approaches yield optimal results have been published in the 1980s.[836,844–849]

PRETREATMENT EVALUATION

Several issues must be considered before therapy of the patient with small cell lung cancer is initiated: the pathologic diagnosis must be confirmed, the extent of tumor dissemination determined, and the ability of the patient to tolerate therapy assessed. Because the distinction of small cell carcinoma from other cell types of lung cancer has significant therapeutic implications, an experienced lung cancer pathologist should review the biopsy specimen. Although the oat cell subtype of small cell carcinoma is usually readily recognized, the intermediate subtype may be mistaken for non-small cell lung cancer by the less-experienced pathologist. Difficulties in diagnosis are most likely when the specimen is of poor quality, especially, in our experience, when the only material available for review is a fine-needle aspirate.

Staging procedures have already been discussed in detail. In brief, the purpose of staging is to assign prognosis, to identify tumor lesions that can be monitored to assess the

TABLE 22-56. Selected Randomized Trials of Radiotherapy Alone Versus Chemotherapy plus Radiation Therapy in Limited-Stage Disease*

Series	*2 Year Radiotherapy Dose (cGy)*	*Chemotherapy*†	*No. of Patients*	*Survival Median (mo)*	*Survival 1 Year (%)*	*Survival 2 Year (%)*
Seydel et al.	4500	None	110	10	NR	2
		C + CCNU	107	11‡	NR	8
MRC	3000	None	121	6	18	NR
		C + MTX + CCNU	115	10§	34	NR
Bergsagel	4000–5000	None	14	5	NR	NR
		C	27	10‖	NR	NR
Petrovich	5000–6000	None	33	5	28	12
		CCNU + HU	35	9§	28	5
Perez	4500	None	23	11	36	15
		C + A + DTIC	24	8‡	38	22

* Modified from Bunn PA, Ihde DC: Small cell bronchogenic carcinoma: A review of therapeutic results. In Livingston RB (ed): Lung Cancer 1, pp 169–208. Amsterdam, Martinus Nijhoff, 1981. Data from Seydel HG, Creech R, Pagano M et al: Small-cell carcinoma: Combined modality treatment of regional small cell undifferentiated carcinoma of the lung. Int J Radiat Oncol 9:1135–1141, 1983; Medical Research Council Lung Cancer Working Party et al: Radiotherapy alone or with chemotherapy in the treatment of small-cell carcinoma of the lung: The results at 36 months. Br J Cancer 44:611–617, 1981; Bergsagel D, Jenkin R, Pringle J et al: Lung cancer: Clinical trial of radiotherapy alone vs radiotherapy plus cyclophosphamide. Cancer 30:621–627, 1972; Petrovich Z, Ohanian M, Cox JD: Clinical research on the treatment of locally advanced lung cancer. Cancer 42:1129–1134, 1978; Perez CA, Krauss S, Bartolucci A et al: Thoracic and elective brain irradiation with concomitant or delayed multiagent chemotherapy in the treatment of localized small cell carcinoma of the lung. Cancer 47:2407–2413, 1981

†Abbreviations: NR = not reported, C = cyclophosphamide, CCNU = lomustine, MTX = methotrexate, HU = hydroxyurea, A = doxorubicin, DTIC = dacarbazine.

‡Survival differences between groups not statistically significant.

§Significantly improved survival with chemotherapy.

‖Survival differences not analyzed.

response to therapy, and to determine if treatment in addition to combination chemotherapy is required or desirable. In a clinical investigative setting, additional staging may be mandated. Patients with extensive-stage disease clearly have a worse prognosis, and those with limited-stage tumors or brain metastases will most often receive chest or brain irradiation, respectively. Ambulatory or performance status is not only an important prognostic factor, but bedridden patients and those with other serious illnesses tolerate intensive therapy poorly with increased morbidity and mortality rates. Pulmonary compromise secondary to cigarette abuse, which is often present, may limit the volume of lung that can be irradiated safely or render an otherwise-indicated surgical procedure inadvisable.

SINGLE-AGENT CHEMOTHERAPY

During the 1970s, seven chemotherapeutic agents that produced response rates of at least 30% when given to 30 or more patients with small cell lung cancer were identified (Table 22-57). Only two additional drugs fulfilling these criteria, carboplatin and teniposide, have been discovered since. Complete response rates to single-agent therapy are less than 5%, and the impact on survival is modest.[850,851] Furthermore, only vincristine and hexamethylmelamine among active drugs do not have myelosuppression as their dose-limiting toxicity, making it difficult to construct combination drug programs in which the full single-agent dose of each compound is employed. Cyclophosphamide, doxorubicin, vincristine, etoposide (VP-16), and cisplatin are probably the most commonly utilized agents. Vincristine is usually administered every 3 weeks because of neurotoxicity, although the best evidence for its single-agent activity was obtained with a weekly schedule.[852] In a randomized study comparing three schedules of etoposide as sole therapy, schedules with three or five doses per week produced higher response rates than a weekly schedule.[853] This drug is therefore most commonly administered several times per week, although when given with other active agents in combination regimens, a single dose every 3 weeks may be as effective.[854]

Highly active drugs in patients with no prior chemotherapy may exhibit only marginal activity in patients with relapsed small cell lung cancer. For example, etoposide has a response rate of more than 40% in previously untreated patients,[851] but when given to 116 patients relapsing after modern combination chemotherapy, it produced only a 9% response rate.[855] A similar situation is observed with the etoposide analogue teniposide (VM-26), which has a 90% response rate in untreated, and a 15% response rate in previously treated, patients.[856] In one of the few randomized studies designed to evaluate a dose–response relation for a single agent in small cell lung cancer,[857] too few responses to allow analysis were seen with etoposide at any of three dose levels up to 900 mg/m² in 77 previously treated patients.

Only five new drugs have been demonstrated to possess clear activity in Phase II trials in small cell lung cancer during the 1980s, and all of them are analogues of drugs already known to be useful. However, it is quite possible that some active drugs were among the 23 agents deemed inactive during the same era in studies that were conducted principally in previously treated patients. For example, whereas the single-agent response rate to cisplatin is only 15%,[858] placing it in the list of "less active" drugs in Table 22-57, it has been evaluated as a single drug almost exclusively in previously treated patients. Thus, it probably has significantly more activity, comparable to that of its analogue, CBDCA (carboplatin), which produced 60% response rate in 30 previously untreated patients.[859] These considerations have led to the suggestion that Phase II trials should be performed in previously untreated patients with a poor prognosis, that is, patients with extensive disease. If the disease fails to respond after a short time, a standard combination-chemotherapy regimen could be administered. Such a strategy is certainly acceptable when the Phase II agent is active, as already demonstrated with some drugs.[856,859] However, further experience is needed before this approach is generally adopted, as two recent Phase II studies in untreated extensive-stage patients, including one study utilizing a doxorubicin analogue, yielded shorter than anticipated survival.[860–862] Better drugs for the treatment of small cell lung cancer are clearly needed, and new agents, preferably those with novel mechanisms of action, will certainly continue to be tested in the setting of refractory disease. Any treatment that is useful in previously treated cases will immediately be evaluated in untreated patients.

TABLE 22-57. Chemotherapeutic Agents with Documented Activity Against Small Cell Lung Cancer

Group 1 (Confirmed response rate of >30% in at least 30 patients)
Cyclophosphamide
Mechlorethamine (nitrogen mustard)
Doxorubicin (Adriamycin®)
Methotrexate
Hexamethylmelamine†
Etoposide (VP-16-213)
Vincristine
Carboplatin (CBDCA)†
Teniposide (VM-26)†
Group 2 (Lesser or less well confirmed activity)
Cisplatin*
Ifosfamide†
Lomustine (CCNU)
Carmustine (BCNU)
Semustine (methyl-CCNU)†
Procarbazine
Vindesine†
Nimustine (ACNU, nitrosourea)†

*Adequate single-agent data only in previously treated patients.
†Not commercially available in the United States.

COMBINATION CHEMOTHERAPY

Treatment programs including aggressive combination chemotherapy regimens yield the best response rates (Fig. 22-17) and the highest percentage of long-term survivors.[836,847] In limited disease, optimal current regimens should produce 85% to 95% overall response rates, 50% to 60% complete response rates, median survival times of 12 to 16 months, and 2-year disease-free survival rates of 15% to 20%. Corresponding results in patients with extensive disease are overall response rates of 75% to 85%, complete

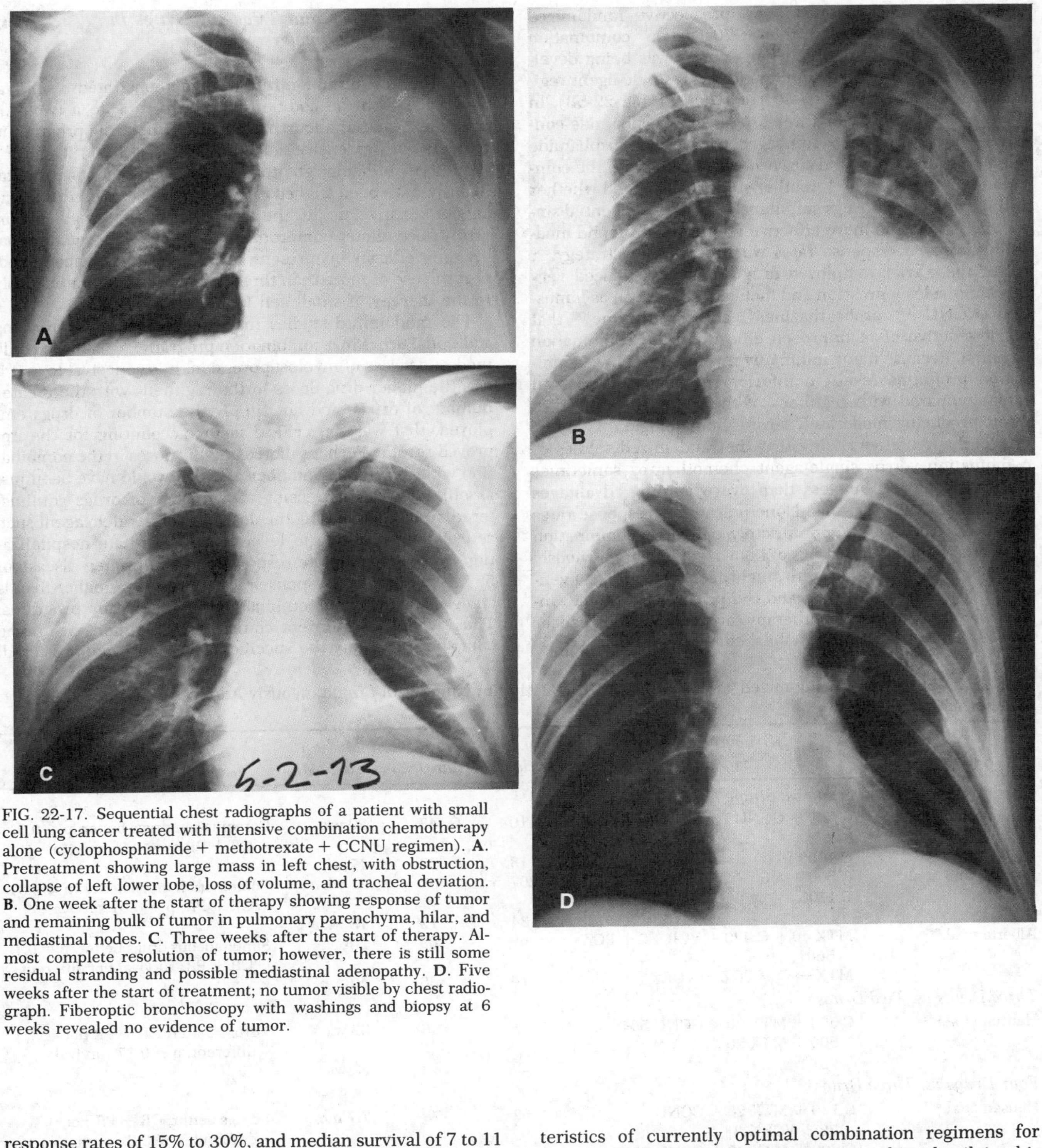

FIG. 22-17. Sequential chest radiographs of a patient with small cell lung cancer treated with intensive combination chemotherapy alone (cyclophosphamide + methotrexate + CCNU regimen). **A**. Pretreatment showing large mass in left chest, with obstruction, collapse of left lower lobe, loss of volume, and tracheal deviation. **B**. One week after the start of therapy showing response of tumor and remaining bulk of tumor in pulmonary parenchyma, hilar, and mediastinal nodes. **C**. Three weeks after the start of therapy. Almost complete resolution of tumor; however, there is still some residual stranding and possible mediastinal adenopathy. **D**. Five weeks after the start of treatment; no tumor visible by chest radiograph. Fiberoptic bronchoscopy with washings and biopsy at 6 weeks revealed no evidence of tumor.

response rates of 15% to 30%, and median survival of 7 to 11 months. Two-year disease-free survival in extensive disease is rare.

Although these therapeutic outcomes obviously leave substantial room for improvement, they do represent a four- to five-fold increase in median survival compared with that of untreated patients and have been made possible only by the effective combination chemotherapy programs. The characteristics of currently optimal combination regimens for small cell lung cancer will be discussed in detail in this section.

Superiority to Single Agents

Although, as just discussed, response rates routinely seen with current combination chemotherapy appear greatly superior to the rates observed with single agents in previously untreated patients,[863] only a few prospective randomized trials, conducted during the 1970s when combination chemotherapy for small cell lung cancer was being developed, directly compared combination with single-agent regimens in the absence of chest irradiation (Table 22-58). In two trials where two- or three-drug cyclophosphamide-containing programs were compared with cyclophosphamide alone, response rates and survival were better with the combination regimens.[490,864] Another study investigated whether administering four drugs simultaneously or as sequential single agents was the more effective approach and found modestly improved response rates with the former strategy.[865] All of these trials employed drug doses that induced very modest myelosuppression and included drugs such as lomustine (CCNU),[864] probcarbazine,[865] and dacarbazine[490] that are less active or of unproven efficacy in the combination regimen. Because many minimally myelosuppressive combination programs result in inferior response and survival rates compared with regimens of the same drugs given in doses producing moderately severe hematologic toxicity,[866] it is perhaps not surprising that the randomized studies of combination versus single-agent chemotherapy sometimes demonstrated real but less than overwhelming advantages for combination programs. Nonetheless, the response rates attained with current appropriately delivered combination programs utilizing only drugs of known activity are obviously superior to the early data with single agents given in conventional doses (Table 22-59), and the principle of the advantage of combination chemotherapy for small cell lung cancer can be considered firmly established.[847]

Optimal Number and Types of Drugs in Combination Regimens

Two prospective randomized trials demonstrated a survival advantage with the addition of a third drug to a two-drug program[867] and of a fourth agent to a three-drug program in patients with extensive stage disease (see Table 22-58).[253] Regimens utilizing greater numbers of agents simultaneously have been studied infrequently. Because most active agents are myelotoxic, the use of too many drugs concurrently necessitates compromises in dosage that would probably limit efficacy. At present, there is little evidence to support the use of more than three or four drugs simultaneously in the therapy of small cell lung cancer.[850]

The randomized studies that support the value of using additional drugs in a combination program[253,867] showed only modest degrees of myelosuppression. It is conceivable that it was the higher drug doses in the regimens with the greater number of drugs, and not simply the number of drugs employed, that was the critical factor accounting for the improved results. Perhaps increasing the doses in the combination with the smaller number of drugs would have been just as efficacious as increasing the number of drugs administered. In fact, escalating the dose of even a single agent such as cyclophosphamide to levels that necessitate hospitalization can yield complete response rates in limited disease of 55%,[868] a complete response rate as high as or higher than is achieved with many combination-chemotherapy programs. Thus, whenever different combination regimens are being compared, not only the specific agents being administered,

TABLE 22-58. Early Randomized Trials Evaluating the Optimum Number of Simultaneously Administered Chemotherapeutic Agents

Reference	*Drug and Dose (mg/m²)**	*No. of Patients*	*CR + PR Rate (%)*	*Median Survival*	*Comments*
Combination Chemotherapy vs. Single Agents					
Edmonson et al.[864]	C 700 + CCNU 70	110	43	20 wk	Combination drugs better, $p < 0.01$ CR + PR, $p = 0.07$ survival
	C 1000	118	22	17 wk	
Lowenbraun et al.[490]	C 500 + A 50 + DTIC 250	207	57	31 wk	Combination drugs better, $p < 0.01$ CR + PR, $p = 0.01$ survival
	C 1100	34	12	18 wk	
Alberto et al.[865]	MTX 40 + C 420 + VCR 1.2 + PCZ 560†	59	65	NR	Simultaneous drugs better, $p = 0.1$ CR + PR; survival not different
	MTX → C → PCZ → VCR‡	14	36	NR	
Three Drugs vs. Two Drugs					
Hansen et al.[253]	C 500 + MTX 20 + CCNU 50§	33	56	33 wk	3 drugs better, CR + PR not different, $p = 0.17$ survival
	C 500 + MTX 20	29	38	23 wk	
Four Drugs vs. Three Drugs					
Hansen et al.[867]	C 700 + MTX 20 + CCNU 70 + VCR 1.3‖	52	78	7.7 mo	4 drugs better, CR + PR not different, $p < 0.01$ survival
	C 700 + MTX 20 + CCNU 70	53	75	6.0 mo	

Modified from Ihde DC, Bunn PA: Chemotherapy of small cell bronchogenic carcinoma. In Williams CJ, Whitehouse JMA (eds): Recent Advances in Clinical Oncology, pp 305–323. Edinburgh, Churchill Livingstone, 1982.
*CR = complete response, PR = partial response, VCR = vincristine, PCZ = procarbazine; other drugs as in Table 22-56.
†Weekly doses given for 8 weeks.
‡Sequential single agents each given for 2 weeks.
§C every 3 weeks, MTX twice weekly, CCNU every 6 weeks.
‖C and CCNU every 4 weeks, MTX × 2 in week 3, VCR weekly first cycle.

TABLE 22-59. Summary of Objective Tumor Responses to Single-Agent or Combination Chemotherapy in Previously Untreated Patients with Small Cell Lung Cancer (No Radiation Therapy)

		Response (%)	
Drug Treatment	*No. of Patients*	*All Objective*†	Complete
Single agent‡	753	15–20	2.5
Combination	1236	70	31

*Adapted from Bunn PA Jr, Ihde DC: Small cell bronchogenic carcinoma: A review of therapeutic results. In Livingston RB (ed): Lung Cancer: Advances in Research and Treatment, pp 169–208. The Hague, Martinus Nijhoff, 1981.

†Objective tumor responses include partial and complete responses. Complete response rate data available for only 572 patients.

‡Includes only data for cyclophosphamide, nitrogen mustard, doxorubicin, methotrexate, etoposide, hexamethylmelamine, and vincristine.

but also the dose intensity with which they are delivered, must be considered. For example, a randomized study that found significantly improved response rates and survival in extensive-stage patients treated with cyclophosphamide, etoposide, and vincristine compared with those in patients receiving cyclophosphamide and vincristine more convincingly demonstrated the contribution of etoposide to the three-drug program, because the cyclophosphamide dose was doubled in the two-drug combination so that the myelosuppression associated with each regimen was similar.[869]

Although many combination-chemotherapy regimens for small cell lung cancer appear to possess similar efficacy, the CAV program (representative doses: cyclophosphamide 1000 mg/m^2, doxorubicin 45 mg/m^2, vincristine 2 mg) has been one of the most commonly used during the 1980s and reproducibly yields the current optimal response rates, median survival, and long-term survival outlined previously in both limited- and extensive-stage disease. It may reasonably be considered a "standard" regimen against which newer approaches can be compared. Etoposide is probably the most actively studied newer agent in recent years, and many randomized trials have attempted to determine whether adding etoposide to or substituting it for one of the components of CAV is of value.

Two studies compared CAV plus etoposide (CAVE) with CAV alone and found significantly greater response rates with CAVE. However, survival was not significantly improved in either study when results were adjusted for differences in pretreatment prognostic factors.[870,871] In an equitoxic comparison of standard-dose CAVE versus higher-dose CAV, there were no differences in response rates or survival.[872] Two other randomized trials addressed the utility of substituting etoposide for one of the drugs in CAV. Median survival in extensive-stage patients was prolonged by only 2 months when etoposide was substituted for either doxorubicin[869] (CEV versus CAV) or vincristine[873] (CAE versus CAV), although myelosuppression, and thus perhaps drug dose intensity, was greater with CAE in the latter trial. In neither study did the etoposide-containing program prove superior in limited-stage patients. In a large randomized study of 269 extensive-stage patients, etoposide was substituted for methotrexate at two different times in a 4-week cycle, four-drug regimen consisting of cyclophosphamide, methotrexate, CCNU, and vincristine.[874] Significantly improved survival was seen when etoposide was given early but not when it was given later in each cycle of chemotherapy. Increased myelosuppression, possibly correlating with increased antitumor effects, was observed with early etoposide. On balance, these studies adding etoposide to or substituting it in a standard combination program cannot be regarded as providing unequivocal evidence that etoposide-containing programs are superior to programs not containing this drug, although etoposide is clearly among the most active agents against small cell lung cancer.

The combination of etoposide and cisplatin exhibits therapeutic synergy in murine leukemia,[875] produces some long-term survivors in refractory testicular cancer,[876] and has recently been evaluated in many types of cancer. In previously treated small cell lung cancer, this two-drug program produced objective response rates of 50% or more in some recent studies,[877,878] which contrasts strikingly with the usual response rate of less than 10% for many other salvage regimens evaluated in the present decade. These encouraging results suggested the use of this combination as first-line therapy, either followed by other drugs[879,880] or as sole chemotherapeutic treatment.[881] The therapeutic results appear as good as or better than those with the standard CAV regimen in both limited and extensive disease, although results directly comparing CAV with etoposide–cisplatin are not yet available. In addition, etoposide–cisplatin is associated with less hematologic toxicity than most other active regimens,[882] suggesting an improved therapeutic index. One trial randomizing limited-stage patients to receive or not receive two cycles of etoposide–cisplatin after six cycles of CAV with or without chest irradiation demonstrated a 30-week improvement in median survival.[883] These data imply that etoposide–cisplatin may be able to eradicate tumor cells resistant to CAV.

Substitution of carboplatin for cisplatin in the etoposide–cisplatin program has yielded an active combination with reduced gastrointestinal toxicity.[884] In previously untreated patients, survival with etoposide–cisplatin was superior to that with etoposide–ifosfamide in a German study,[885] further supporting the value of the etoposide–cisplatin regimen.

Final definition of the role of this promising two-drug combination in the initial therapy of small cell lung cancer must await the results of ongoing clinical trials. Doses and schedules of some active combination regimens currently popular in the treatment of small cell carcinoma are provided in Table 22-60.

Intensity of Initial Chemotherapy

Most current chemotherapeutic programs for small cell lung cancer, with the possible exception of etoposide–cisplatin, are designed to produce moderately severe myelosuppression with leukopenia of 1000 to 2000 cells/μl in the majority of patients. Such regimens do not necessitate hospitalization but do mandate careful monitoring to avoid or ameliorate infectious or bleeding complications. One approach to the problem of drug resistance in this tumor has been to administer more intensive chemotherapeutic regimens, because the tenets of the dose–response relation in chemotherapy of cancer, both in animals and in humans, suggest that the dose rate may be critical to tumor cell kill, particularly in more responsive neoplasms.[886] Although increases in drug doses and frequency of administration might increase the response rate and duration, this approach is limited by toxicity to normal host tissues.

Several randomized (Table 22-61) and nonrandomized trials have studied the concept of dose–response relation in small cell lung cancer. The first randomized trial addressing this question administered two-fold higher doses of the CMC (cyclophosphamide–methotrexate–CCNU) regimen only for the initial 6-week induction period and demonstrated significantly improved response rates and survival with higher drug doses.[866] A much larger randomized trial of the CMC regimen studied the effects of a higher dose only of the cyclophosphamide component during the first 6 weeks and found modest but significant increases in response rate and survival, particularly in patients with limited-stage disease.[887] Nonrandomized trial results also suggest that extremely high doses of cyclophosphamide (4.8–8.0 g/m^2) as a single agent produce a substantially higher than anticipated fraction of complete responses in both limited[868] and extensive[888] disease.

Increasing the doses of other standard chemotherapy programs or drugs in an outpatient setting has yet to improve results. In two randomized studies of the CAV regimen, the doses of cyclophosphamide were increased 20% to 56% and those of doxorubicin 18% to 75% during the first 9 to 12 weeks of chemotherapy.[889,890] Although the complete response rate was modestly improved in one trial,[889] there was no effect on response duration or survival with higher doses of CAV in either study. Preliminary results of a smaller trial involving administration of 67% higher doses of etoposide and cisplatin for the first 6 weeks of therapy suggest no benefit for the high-dose program.[882] There appears to be no benefit of high-dose methotrexate with leucovorin rescue compared with standard-dose methotrexate when added to the CAV regimen.[891] It is conceivable that CMC is less effective than other regimens such as CAV or etoposide–cisplatin and that higher, more toxic doses of CMC are needed to produce the same therapeutic results that other programs

TABLE 22-60. Effective Commonly Used Combination Chemotherapy Programs for Small Cell Lung Cancer*

CAV		
Cyclophosphamide	1000	mg/m^2 IV day 1
Doxorubicin (Adriamycin®)	45	mg/m^2 IV day 1
Vincristine	2	mg IV day 1
Repeat cycle every 3 weeks		
CAVP16		
Cyclophosphamide	1000	mg/m^2 IV day 1
Doxorubicin	45	mg/m^2 IV day 1
Etoposide (VP-16)	50	mg/m^2 IV days 1–5
Repeat cycle every 3 weeks		
CAVVP-16		
Cyclophosphamide	1000	mg/m^2 IV day 1
Doxorubicin	50	mg/m^2 IV day 1
Vincristine	1.5	mg/m^2 IV day 1
Etoposide (VP-16)	60	mg/m^2 IV days 1–5
Repeat cycle every 3 weeks		
VP16-P		
Etoposide	100	mg/m^2 IV days 1–3
Cisplatin	25	mg/m^2 IV days 1–3
Repeat cycle every 3 weeks		
CMCcV		
Cyclophosphamide	700	mg/m^2 IV day 1
Methotrexate	20	mg/m^2 PO days 18, 21
Lomustine (CCNU)	70	mg/m^2 PO day 1
Vincristine	1.3	mg/m^2 IV days 1, 8, 15, 22 first cycle and then day 1.
Repeat cycle every 4 weeks		
CAV/VP-16P		
Cycle of CAV as above alternating every 3 weeks with cycle of VP-16P as above		

* Modified from Ihde DC: Chemotherapy in lung cancer. In Brain MC, Carbone PP (eds): Current Therapy in Hematology–Oncology 3, pp 213–217. Toronto, BC Decker, 1988.

TABLE 22-61. Completed Randomized Studies of Intensity of Initial Combination Chemotherapy in Small Cell Lung Cancer

Series	*Drug and Dose (mg/m²)*	*No. of Patients*	*CR + PR Rate (%)*	*Median Survival (mo)*	*Comments*
Cohen et al.[866]	C 1000 + MTX 15 + CCNU 100*	23	96	10.5	High doses better: $p < 0.05$ CR + PR, $p < 0.05$ survival
	C 500 + MTX 10 + CCNU 50	9	45	5.0	
Mehta et al.[887]	C 1500 + MTX 15 + CCNU*	175†	64	10.25	High dose better: $p = 0.04$ CR + PR, $p = 0.04$ survival
	700 + MTX 15 + CCNU 70	174	54	9	
O'Donnell[888a]	C 2000 + VCR total 2 + MeCCNU 100‡	14	73 (57 CR)	9	High dose better: $p < 0.05$ CR; CR + PR and survival not different
	C 750 + VCR total 2 + MeCCNU 75	14	43 (21 CR)	10.75	
Johnson et al.[889]	C 1200 + A 70 + VCR 1‡	101	63 (22 CR)	7	High dose better: $p = 0.04$ CR; CR + PR and survival not different
	C 1000 + A 40 + VCR 1	146	53 (12 CR)	8	
Figueredo et al.[890]	C 1560 + A 59 + VCR 0.9§	52	71 (21 CR LD, 8 ED‖)	14	No differences in CR, response duration, or survival
	C 990 + A 50 + VCR 1.0	51	61 (22 CR LD, 8 ED)	12	

*High-dose regimen for first 6 weeks.
†Approximate number.
‡High-dose regimen for first 9 weeks.
§Doses are actual doses given, not intended doses; high dose regimen for first 12 weeks.
‖LD = limited disease, ED = extensive disease.

achieve with less toxic doses. This could explain why improved antitumor effects can be demonstrated with dose escalation of one or more components of CMC.

Multiple nonrandomized trials involving even higher doses of cyclophosphamide, doxorubicin, etoposide, or cisplatin that necessitate hospitalization of most or all patients and are occasionally given with autologous bone-marrow transplant have been initiated in the hope of obtaining markedly increased tumor-cell kill, most often in patients with extensive-stage disease. Several earlier studies attempted to give higher individual doses or more frequent doses of cyclophosphamide, doxorubicin, and etoposide,[892-894] whereas more recent trials with similar philosophic intent utilized alternating drug combinations or regimens including high doses of etoposide and cisplatin.[895,896] Although high complete response rates sometimes have been observed, response duration and survival time appear similar to those attained with many standard, less intensive programs. Very high doses of initial chemotherapy with available agents have thus far produced substantially increased toxicity with only minimal additional therapeutic benefit. At present, such approaches are appropriate only in the setting of a clinical trial.

Late Intensification

Because most patients with small cell lung cancer ultimately relapse, several groups have proposed treating the smaller tumor burden in maximally responding patients with an intensive approach rather than awaiting overt tumor progression. This strategy would administer intensive treatment only to responders, those most likely to derive benefit; allow treatment to a reduced tumor bulk, which probably would be less resistant to treatment than at time of relapse; and apply intensive therapy only to patients in the best possible medical condition. Nine trials treating at least five patients each with such "late intensification" have been completed.[897-905] Most included patients with extensive-stage disease and did not restrict entry to patients in complete remission after standard therapy. The proportion of patients beginning standard therapy who received the late intensification ranged from only 18% to 38%. The late intensification programs were diverse and included both single-agent and combination chemotherapy with local field or total body irradiation in some cases. Autologous bone-marrow infusions were given to some or all patients, although this was probably unnecessary in many patients except for those receiving total body irradiation.

Treatment-associated death rates ranged from 15% to 30% in four of the nine trials. Although some patients not having a complete response to standard therapy achieved a complete response with the late intensification, these new complete responses were nearly always brief. The fraction of disease-free survivors among patients receiving late intensification has been small, and most such patients were in complete remission prior to the late intensive therapy. There has been no obvious improvement in the outcome of all patients beginning standard chemotherapy with the intent of administering late intensification compared with patients given standard therapy without late intensification.[900,906] The one randomized trial of late intensification found improved response duration but not survival in patients receiving it, but the 2-year survival rate for all patients beginning standard therapy was 7%, similar to that in many studies of conventional treatment.[899]

Late intensive therapies remain a suitable subject of clinical investigation, particularly in limited-stage patients who attain a complete response to standard therapy. However, because markedly superior results cannot be expected with this approach using currently available drugs, randomized trials will probably be required to demonstrate efficacy.

Cyclic Alternating Combination Chemotherapy

As might be predicted from its relatively rapid growth rate, responses to chemotherapy in small cell lung cancer occur quickly. Symptomatic improvement is usual with the first cycle of treatment, and it is uncommon for tumor masses to demonstrate further regression after 12 or sometimes even 6 weeks.[836,850,879] Thus, introduction of a new noncross-resistant drug program prior to tumor progression is conceptually attractive. Goldie and Coldman have provided a detailed mathematical model of the spontaneous origin of drug-resistant clones in malignant tumors at a mutation rate proportional to the number of actively dividing tumor cells.[907] This model predicts that as many active agents as possible should be given at full doses as quickly as possible to maximize the chance of eradication of the entire tumor cell population. Because myelosuppressive toxicity does not allow all possible drugs to be given simultaneously, another suitable strategy is to alternate the administration of two combination regimens that are equally effective and noncross-resistant.[908] This strategy has become common in the treatment of small cell lung cancer.

Although this point has not been rigorously demonstrated, many chemotherapy programs in small cell carcinoma appear to have approximately equal efficacy. If noncross-resistance is defined such that a second drug combination produces a substantial fraction of complete remissions when administered after tumor progression on a first drug combination, most, if not all, chemotherapy programs in small cell lung cancer are *not* noncross-resistant. Thus, it should not be surprising that there has not been a substantial survival benefit from alternation of two different combination regimes in small cell lung cancer, although new complete responses sometimes occur with initiation of the second combination and the duration of initial remission has been prolonged by this strategy in some randomized trials.[909–912] Occasional randomized studies have shown improved survival with alternating combinations, but the magnitude of the benefit has been extremely modest, requiring randomization of more than 500 patients to be detectable[913] or utilizing combinations that probably had unequal efficacy.[914]

Etoposide–cisplatin has recently been shown to be an active salvage regimen in patients failing CAV treatment and appears at least as efficacious as CAV when used as first-line therapy. Thus, it may be less cross-resistant with CAV than any combination studied to date. Although its complete response rate in CAV failures is still less than 10%,[877,878] several randomized trials alternating CAV and etoposide–cisplatin were recently initiated. A study of 289 patients with extensive-stage disease found an increased response rate, response duration, and survival time with an alternating CAV–etoposide/cisplatin program compared with CAV alone,[915] although the improvement in median survival was only 6 weeks. It is not clear whether the superiority of the cyclic alternating treatment was attributable to the alternating strategy or to the fact that etoposide–cisplatin is superior to CAV. This question should be resolved by ongoing clinical trials. Nonetheless, alternation of CAV and etoposide–cisplatin is an effective treatment program that produced excellent long-term survival results in a study began in 1979.[916]

At present, cyclic alternating administration of two active combination chemotherapy regimens is an acceptable but not mandatory treatment strategy in small cell lung cancer. At a minimum, this approach may reduce the toxicities of chemotherapy that are dependent on the total cumulative dose of a single drug, such as the cardiac toxicity of doxorubicin and the neurotoxicity of cisplatin and vincristine.

Duration of Chemotherapy Administration

Based on treatment strategies for acute lymphoblastic leukemia, chemotherapy in responding small cell lung cancer patients was often continued for up to 2 years in the 1970s. However, several early studies of CAV with chest irradiation for patients with limited-stage disease produced similar survival outcomes despite variations in the planned duration of chemotherapy from 3 or 4 to 24 months (Table 22-62). This suggests that a disproportionate fraction of the antitumor effects of chemotherapy occurs in the early cycles, consistent with the results of some randomized studies comparing

TABLE 22-62. Early Studies of Combined-Modality Therapy in (CAV + Chest RT) in Limited-Stage Disease with Various Durations of Maintenance Chemotherapy

Series	*Duration of Therapy (mo)**	*No. of Patients*	*CR Rate (%)*	*Median Survival (mo)*	*2-Year Disease-free Survival Rate (%)*
Johnson et al.†	3–4	36	75	18.5	28
Greco et al.‡	14	32	91	16	25
Einhorn et al.§	24	19	89	17	26

Modified from Ihde DC, Bunn PA: Chemotherapy of small cell bronchogenic carcinoma. In Williams CJ, Whitehouse JMA (eds): Recent Advances in Clinical Oncology, pp 305–323. Edinburgh, Churchill Livingstone, 1982.

* Total duration of chemotherapy planned in responding patients.

†Johnson RE, Brerton HD, Kent C, Ann Thorac Surg 25:509–515, 1978.

‡Greco FA, Richardson RL, Snell JD et al, Am J Med 66:625–630, 1979.

§Einhorn LH, Bond WH, Hornback N et al, Semin Oncol 5:309–313, 1978.

higher and lower doses of the same drugs (see Table 22-61) in which higher doses given for only the first 6 or 9 weeks produce superior response rates or survival. If most or all tumor regression is indeed accomplished within the first few cycles of therapy, continuation of chemotherapy (or "maintenance") would obviously be of minimal benefit.

Recently, treatment programs based on CAV and chest irradiation intended to last for 61 and 18 weeks had almost identical outcomes in consecutive large patient groups with respect to response rates and median and 2-year survival.[917] Many chemotherapy programs employed during the 1980s are intended to be discontinued after 4 to 6 months in responding patients, with therapeutic results that are similar to previously utilized 12- and 24-month regimens.

Few randomized trials have addressed the optimal duration of chemotherapy in small cell lung cancer. The results of almost all of them suggest that, as in most other cancers that are potentially curable with chemotherapy, there is very little role for maintenance therapy. A study of ten cycles of CAV following four cycles of etoposide–cisplatin with chest irradiation versus no further therapy showed no survival advantage for continued chemotherapy,[880] nor did another trial, in which complete responders with extensive disease who received maintenance chemotherapy had survival equivalent to that of patients in whom chemotherapy was discontinued.[913] A study that found superior median survival in extensive-stage patients with a complete or good partial response who continued to receive CAV compared to patients not given maintenance treatment also showed precisely the opposite result in limited-stage patients.[918] A preliminary report of a large European trial demonstrated a longer time to tumor progression in patients receiving twelve rather than five cycles of chemotherapy, but survival was modestly improved only in patients with extensive disease or a partial remission, the groups deriving the least benefit from therapy.[919] Administering chemotherapy for only 4 to 6 months in responding patients is recommended, as this approach produces at least similar survival, minimizes the toxicities of chemotherapy, and may be associated with a higher frequency of palliative responses to salvage chemotherapy programs (see below).

Toxicities

The principal acute toxicities produced by all combination chemotherapy programs utilized in small cell lung cancer are those related to myelosuppression, specifically neutropenia-associated fever and infection and, to a much lesser extent, thrombocytopenic bleeding. Patients with poor performance status or extensive-stage disease are at greater risk. Nausea, vomiting, and alopecia are also seen with many drugs. Toxicities peculiar to specific agents, such as cardiomyopathy with doxorubicin, neurotoxicity with vincristine and cisplatin, and hemorrhagic cystitis with cyclophosphamide, can also be observed.

With most currently employed standard chemotherapy programs, the duration of neutropenia is relatively short. Febrile episodes are reported in about 30% of patients, documented infections in about 5%, and infectious deaths in 2%.[920] Even much more intensive chemotherapy programs can be delivered in a hospital setting with a low frequency of treatment-related deaths provided there is strict adherence to meticulous supportive care.[921] In some randomized studies, the administration of prophylactic antibiotics such as trimethoprim–sulfamethoxazole significantly reduced the incidence of infection and time spent on antibiotics,[922] but this is not standard practice. Herpes zoster[923,924] and perirectal abscesses[925] occasionally develop during chemotherapy.

When chemotherapy is combined with chest irradiation, especially when the two modalities are given concurrently, the rate of infectious complications is increased because of the significantly greater myelosuppression.[920,926] The addition of chest radiotherapy to chemotherapy significantly reduces the frequency of circulating granulocyte–monocyte precursor colony-forming units in the peripheral blood,[927] and even the small radiation portals utilized for brain metastases can increase the degree of myelosuppression from concurrent chemotherapy.[928]

Acute myeloblastic leukemia has been reported in 17 long-term survivors who received chemotherapy for small cell lung cancer. The actuarial risk at 2 to 3 years is 2% to 4% in two large series,[929,930] and chromosomal deletions similar to those seen in treatment-associated leukemia after chemotherapy of Hodgkin's disease have been reported.[930,931] The majority of affected patients had received protracted chemotherapy including procarbazine or a nitrosourea or both; the current shorter durations of treatment and lesser utilization of nitrosoureas and procarbazine may reduce the frequency of this uncommon complication. Although several drugs administered to small cell carcinoma patients, including methotrexate, cyclophosphamide, and nitrosoureas, are associated with pulmonary toxicity, this problem occurs infrequently in patients not receiving chest irradiation. Serial pulmonary function studies in patients with tumor regression during chemotherapy alone generally show improvement.[932,933] Although acute tumor lysis syndrome, with hyperkalemia, hyperphosphatemia, and hypocalcemia, has been reported with initiation of chemotherapy in a single patient,[934] routine administration of allopurinol and frequent monitoring of serum electrolytes is not necessary.

Overall treatment-associated death rates of 0 to 4% in limited-stage and 2% to 8% in extensive-stage small cell lung cancer patients can be anticipated with standard chemotherapy regimens given with or without chest irradiation. This potential for major morbidity and occasional death emphasizes that chemotherapy for this neoplasm should be administered only by physicians experienced in avoiding and managing drug-related toxicities. However, the survival benefits of modern therapy greatly exceed the decrements in lifespan produced by its side effects.

COMBINED-MODALITY THERAPY

Chest Irradiation in Limited-Stage Small Cell Lung Cancer

The systemic nature of small cell lung cancer even when it appears localized after careful staging precludes sole reliance on a locoregional form of therapy. Most patients with limited-stage disease given chest irradiation alone rapidly die of distant metastases, emphasizing the need for primary systemic treatment. After combination chemotherapy began to be employed in the management of small cell carcinoma in the 1970s, the high response rates and improved survival led to speculation that chest radiotherapy added toxicities while contributing little or no therapeutic advantage in chemotherapy-treated patients. However, this neoplasm is the most responsive of all cell types of lung cancer to thoracic radiotherapy, with tumor regression in excess of 50% occurring in 90% of patients,[935] which is particularly important in that the primary tumor complex is a site of progression in as many as 80% of relapsing limited-stage patients treated with chemotherapy alone.[845,910] Thus, the premise that chest irradiation in conjunction with chemotherapy may improve therapeutic results, particularly in patients with limited disease, appears logical.

Retrospective review of numerous nonrandomized trials employing chemotherapy with or without chest irradiation for limited-stage disease suggested the following conclusions.[850,936] First, a lower rate of chest relapse is seen with combined-modality therapy, although the frequency of relapse still approaches 33%. Second, hematologic, pulmonary, and esophageal complications are increased with the employment of both modalities. Third, whereas the median survival time appears similar, the 2-year disease-free survival rate was superior for combined-modality therapy compared with that achieved with chemotherapy alone. Retrospective data, however, suffer from a number of deficiencies. Because chemotherapy alone is less toxic than combined-modality treatment, there may have been a consistent bias against giving combined modality therapy to poor-risk patients. If administration of radiotherapy is delayed until chemotherapy is completed, patients with the worst prognosis who suffer early failure are automatically excluded from combined-modality series. Analysis of local relapse rates can also be misleading, since only an isolated chest recurrence in a completely responding patient might be expected to compromise survival, and definitions of local relapse are far from uniform. Variations in dose and schedule of irradiation and specific chemotherapy programs employed further complicate comparison of chest relapse rates in different series. Less effective chemotherapy combined with effective irradiation will reduce the frequency of first failures in the chest (because distant metastases will be more prone to develop), whereas more effective chemotherapy combined with less efficacious irradiation will yield the opposite result. All these factors make it extremely difficult to determine the value of the addition of chest irradiation to combination chemotherapy from retrospective data.

In the past 5 years, this uncertainty has been clarified by the completion of several prospective randomized trials. Seven mature trials in which at least 80 patients with limited disease were randomized to receive chemotherapy alone or the same chemotherapy with chest irradiation are summarized in Table 22-63. The temporal relations between chemotherapy and irradiation have been far from uniform in these studies. In Table 22-63, "concurrent therapy" means combined-modality therapy in which chemotherapy and radiotherapy are given simultaneously. In "alternating therapy," radiotherapy is administered on days of the chemotherapy cycle in which no drugs are given, without any delay in the subsequent chemotherapy cycle. "Sequential therapy" is defined as administration of chemotherapy and radiotherapy separately in time, with delay in chemotherapy doses for delivery of irradiation or with one modality begun only after completion of the other. The trials also differed in the chemotherapy regimen employed, the time at which chest radiotherapy was begun, the dose and schedule of irradiation, whether it was given to all patients randomized to receive it or only to responders (or only complete responders) to chemotherapy, and whether PCI was administered.

Four of the seven studies reported significantly improved overall survival rates with combined-modality treatment; two employed concurrent radiotherapy,[926,937] one alternating radiotherapy,[938] and one sequential irradiation during a chemotherapy hiatus.[855] The magnitude of the survival benefit was relatively modest, ranging from 1 to 4 months' improvement in median survival and increases in 2-year survival from 7% to 17%. The two studies with the longest follow-up demonstrate much less advantage beyond 3 to 5 years for patients given radiotherapy,[926,935] at least partially because of intercurrent deaths and second lung cancers in the combined-modality arms. Of the three studies not demonstrating improved survival with added chest irradiation, two[939,940] employed sequential radiotherapy and one[941] a concurrent regimen in which only a single drug was given simultaneously with irradiation. The negative sequential trial conducted exclusively in patients in complete remission from chemotherapy[940] was initiated because of earlier data from uncontrolled trials suggesting marked improvement in disease-free survival when irradiation was given to complete responders at the completion of drug administration.[942] Combined-modality treatment also increased the complete response rate in three of the four trials for which this information was available and significantly reduced chest recurrence rates in five of seven trials.

Whether variables in delivery of the thoracic irradiation component of combined-modality therapy influence its antitumor efficacy is by no means resolved. Concurrent and alternating combined-modality programs that do not incorporate planned delays in chemotherapy for radiotherapy administration appear to possess superior antitumor efficacy. Among the randomized trials in Table 22-63, three of four concurrent or alternating programs yielded improved survival, whereas only one of the three sequential programs did so. The only positive sequential trial was able to demonstrate survival benefit only with multivariate statistical techniques.[943] This apparent superiority of concurrent or alternating programs is consistent with the known dominance of distant metastases as the principal determinant of survival in most patients and suggests that these methods should be employed in standard treatment. However, no randomized comparisons of concurrent or alternating versus sequential strategies have been reported.

The dose of thoracic irradiation needed to control locoregional small cell carcinoma was initially thought to be reduced when chemotherapy was also given.[944] As improved drug treatment allowed longer control of distant metastases, however, a high frequency of local failures with lower-dose schedules such as 3000 cGy (rad) in 2 weeks became appar-

TABLE 22-63. Randomized Prospective Trials of Combined-Modality Therapy Versus Chemotherapy Alone in Limited-Stage Small Cell Lung Cancer

Reference	Drugs*	Chest Radiotherapy	No. of Patients	Median Survival (mo)		Survival Differences	2-Year Disease-free or Overall Survival (actual or projected) (%)	
				CT	CMT		CT	CMT
Bunn et al.[926]	CML/VAP	40Gy/15Fx/wk 1/CONC/Cont	96	11.6	15.0	$p = 0.035$	12 6	28 (OS) 23 (DFS)
Perry et al.[937]	CAEV	I:50Gy/25Fx/wk 1/CONC/Cont II:50Gy/25Fx/wk 10/CONC/Cont	399	13.6	I: 13.1 II: 14.6	$p = 0.009$	8	I: 15 (DFS) II: 25
Perez et al.[938]	CAV	40Gy/14Fx/wk 5,8,11/ALT/Split	291	11.2	14.0	$p = 0.030$	19	28 (OS)
Fox[855,943]	CAV	40Gy/20Fx/wk10/SEQ/Cont	84	12.7	16.5	$p = 0.003$†	2	15 (DFS)
Østerlind et al.[941]	CMVL	40Gy/10Fx/wk 6,10/CONC/Split	125	11.5	10.5	$p = 0.240$	8	5 (DFS)
Souhami et al.[939]	AV/CM	40Gy/20Fx/wk 13/SEQ/Cont	130	R: 12.0 NR: 7.0	13.0 8.5	$p > 0.05$ $p > 0.05$	12 12	14 (OS) 4
Kies et al.[940]	VMEAC	48Gy/22Fx/wk 13,17/SEQ/Split/CR only	93	16.0‡	16.0‡	$p = 0.860$	25‡	35‡ (OS)

Modified from Seifter EJ, Ihde EJ, Ihde DC: Therapy of small cell lung cancer: A perspective on two decades of clinical research. Semin Oncol (in press).

*C = cyclophosphamide, M = methotrexate, L = lomustine, V = vincristine, A = doxorubicin, P = procarbazine, E = etoposide, P = cisplatin, CT = chemotherapy alone, CMT = combined-modality therapy, R = responders, NR = nonresponders, CR = complete responders, CONC = concurrent with chemotherapy, SEQ = sequential administration of two modalities with delay of chemotherapy to administer radiotherapy, ALT = alternating chemotherapy and radiotherapy without delay of chemotherapy, Cont = continuous radiotherapy five fractions per week, Split = split-course radiotherapy, Fx = fractions, wk = week(s), OS = overall survival, DFS = disease-free survival

†Influence of radiotherapy in a multivariate regression analysis.[943]

‡Survival values for complete responders only.

ent.[945] Most authorities now agree on the need for higher doses, in the range of 4500 to 5000 cGy or more with conventional fractionation, for optimal local control. Furthermore, simply because a radiotherapy program reduces local recurrences does not mean it is optimal. Even more effective irradiation might be able to eradicate chest tumor completely in additional patients with intrathoracic neoplasm as their only remaining cancer; this might be evident only if survival is the end-point analyzed. One randomized study by Cancer and Leukemia Group B[937] has evaluated whether radiation should be administered concurrently with the initiation of chemotherapy or given only after three cycles of drugs have been delivered (see Table 22-63). Delaying radiotherapy gave the best results in terms of response, disease-free survival, and overall survival, although these differences were of borderline significance. The delayed radiotherapy was associated with less hematologic toxicity and a greater percentage of projected chemotherapy doses actually administered, perhaps accounting for its greater effectiveness.

The optimal method for combining chemotherapy and chest radiotherapy in limited-stage small cell lung cancer has by no means been settled. Minimizing the toxicities of the approach without compromising therapeutic efficacy is one pertinent objective. Chest irradiation has added to toxicity in most studies. In addition to increased hematologic toxicities, particularly with concurrent regimens, pulmonary and esophageal complications of treatment are clearly increased with combined modality therapy. In the U.S. NCI trial[926,933] 26% of combined-modality recipients suffered severe pulmonary toxicity necessitating hospitalization a median of 2 months after the beginning of treatment, compared with 4% of patients given chemotherapy alone, and five combined-modality patients in complete remission died of this complication. In completely responding patients, pulmonary function tests improved in those given chemotherapy alone but not in combined-modality cases.[933] The Finsen Institute, which also employed concurrent chemotherapy and irradiation, reported a 7% death rate from pulmonary and pericardial complications in complete responders.[941] More than 70% of patients receiving 8.0 g/m² of cyclophosphamide followed by chest irradiation suffered symptomatic radiation pneumonitis.[946] This frequency of pulmonary complications in patients given combined-modality treatment is clearly higher than is seen, not only in patients given solely chemotherapy, but also in patients receiving chest irradiation alone. However, not all concurrent combined modality programs have noted excessive pulmonary toxicity,[934] suggesting that the specific drugs combined with irradiation may be important in this regard. Several trials report high rates of esophagitis (with occasional strictures) and weight loss in patients given combined-modality therapy.[926,934,941] Excess deaths from second malignancies, most often non-small cell lung cancer, have been noted in the combined-modality arm of two randomized trials,[926,941] possibly related to increased time at risk or to the treatment itself.

Although they have been utilized less often, alternating regimens with interdigitating chemotherapy and irradiation appear to have reduced pulmonary toxicity while maintaining a therapeutic advantage from radiotherapy.[938,947] Studies of radiation toxicity in animals suggest that concurrent chemotherapy programs might be expected to be more toxic than alternating or sequential designs, and available clinical data are consistent with this hypothesis, particularly with regard to pulmonary injury. Delivering chest irradiation in multiple daily fractions is another approach, which on experimental grounds might be expected to ameliorate pulmonary toxicity, and preliminary results from one pilot study are promising, with excellent survival rates and minimal pneumonitis.[948]

On balance, some programs incorporating chest irradiation in addition to chemotherapy in limited-stage small cell lung cancer improve survival, particularly when radiotherapy is given in a concurrent or alternating fashion. Combined-modality therapy is a technically complex undertaking requiring close coordination between medical and radiation oncologists. Custom-shaped radiation portals and shrinking field techniques (requiring repeated simulation) as the tumor regresses to attempt to preserve the maximum possible functional pulmonary tissue are recommended. Because not all combined-modality programs increase survival whereas essentially all increase toxicity, chest irradiation need not be considered mandatory in all patients, especially those with impaired pulmonary function or poor performance status. Investigational studies that do not include chest irradiation remain appropriate. Survival gains from greater antitumor efficacy of combined-modality programs are partially compromised by the toxicities of treatment, which can perhaps be modified, and by the tendency of cigarette abusers to develop second smoking-related cancers, which probably cannot. If the results of chemotherapy improve so that more patients have eradication of systemic but not of local tumor, chest radiotherapy could affect survival in larger numbers of cases. At present, however, most patients who are irradiated still die of their small cell carcinoma, and distant metastases remain the predominant cause of failure. Thus, improvements in systemic treatment currently have a much greater potential for producing survival gains in small cell lung cancer than does increased efficacy of locoregional therapy.

Chest Irradiation in Extensive-Stage Small Cell Lung Cancer

In retrospective reviews of the literature, the addition of chest irradiation to chemotherapy for extensive-stage small cell lung cancer reduced the frequency of progressive disease in the thorax but did not alter the overall response rates, median survival, or 2-year disease-free survival rate.[850,936] Because extensive-disease patients have complete response rates of only 15% to 30% with standard chemotherapy regimens and frequently relapse in distant sites, it is logical that a localized form of treatment would have little survival impact. Successive large studies by the Southwest Oncology Group confirm that although thoracic radiotherapy can substantially reduce the frequency of initial relapses at the primary tumor site, there is not apparent effect on survival.[949]

Three clinical trials have randomized patients with extensive disease to chemotherapy alone or chemotherapy with irradiation to the chest tumor and to some or all sites of overt distant metastases. In these studies as well, there were no worthwhile response or survival advantages with the addition of radiotherapy.[945,950,951] At present, other than as part of a clinical trial, there is no role for chest irradiation in extensive-stage small cell lung cancer except for symptomatic palliation.

Wide-Field Radiation Therapy

A number of pilot studies have examined the role of hemibody irradiation and total body irradiation in this radioresponsive malignancy. Hemibody irradiation is an active agent in small cell lung cancer, as it can induce some complete responses in patients in only partial response after combination chemotherapy.[952] The initial treatment is usually given to the upper hemibody, where the bulk of the tumor burden is located; in some studies, treatment of the lower hemibody is administered after hematologic recovery from the upper hemibody dose. In an early study employing what would today be considered suboptimal chemotherapy, patients who had received initial chest irradiation were randomized to receive chemotherapy or sequential upper and lower hemibody radiotherapy. Survival in limited-stage patients was similar, but in extensive disease, the addition of chemotherapy yielded superior results. As an adjunct to combination chemotherapy in both limited- and extensive disease, hemibody irradiation produced substantial toxicity in several pilot studies without obvious benefit in tumor response or survival.[952–955] There is no evidence that low doses of total body irradiation are of benefit as an adjuvant to chest irradiation or chemotherapy in limited- or extensive-stage patients.[952,956,957] In a large randomized trial in patients with limited disease given chemotherapy and chest irradiation,[958] additional radiotherapy to potential upper-abdominal sites of relapse produced no improvement in response duration or survival. Currently, wide field irradiation does not have a proven role in the management of small cell lung cancer.

Prophylactic Cranial Irradiation

Brain metastases are detected in approximately 10% of small cell lung cancer patients at the time of presentation and are subsequently diagnosed during life in another 20% to 25%, with an increasing likelihood of development with lengthening survival.[535,959] In the absence of therapy to the CNS, actuarial analysis reveals a probability of brain metastases of 50% to 80% in 2-year survivors.[535,960] At postmortem examination, such metastases are found in as many as 65% of cases.[961] Because these metastases are sometimes the sole site of clinical relapse from complete remission and are frequently disabling, PCI has been used for the past 10 to 15 years in an effort to curtail their development.

A review of 702 patients entered into seven prospective randomized trials assessed the benefit of PCI given at or within a few months of diagnosis to patients initially free of CNS involvement (Table 22-64). When the results of all these trials are considered together, doses of PCI ranging from 2000 to 4000 cGy reduced the frequency of clinically detected brain metastases from 20% to 6%.[967] In five of the seven trials, this reduced risk of intracranial tumor spread was statistically significant. However, no significant impact of PCI on survival could be appreciated. Retrospective analyses suggested that virtually all benefit in preventing intracranial metastases with PCI was confined to patients with a complete response to systemic therapy.[968,969] In actuarial analyses, partial responders or nonresponders had equivalent likelihoods of recurrence in the brain whether or not PCI was administered.[968] This is not surprising, as residual systemic cancer could readily metastasize to the CNS after completion of PCI.

It is also reasonable to predict that only complete responders could derive any survival benefit from PCI, because in patients without complete response, systemic tumor will likely be the predominant factor influencing survival. However, in both randomized and nonrandomized studies that addressed this question, there is no evidence that PCI influences survival in completely responding patients.[970,971] Thus, some investigators have proposed dispensing with PCI in favor of therapeutic brain irradiation when clinically indicated.[972] This policy assumes that cranial irradiation can effectively control symptoms from overt brain metastases for the duration of the patient's life in most instances. Because the duration of survival is short in most patients who develop brain metastases during therapy, this assumption is not unreasonable. However, other physicians[959,973] have questioned the durability of palliation following therapeutic brain radiotherapy (see below).

Even if survival were not improved, there would be no reason other than patient inconvenience and expense not to offer PCI to completely responding patients if it were free of toxicity. However, with the advent of greater numbers of long-term survivors with small cell lung cancer, it has become evident that some patients have neurologic and intellectual impairment and abnormalities on CT scan of the brain that are potentially related to PCI.[974–977] In one study, both CT scan and clinical CNS abnormalities were significantly more frequent in patients who had received PCI or therapeutic brain irradiation than in those who had not.[975] These findings are especially disturbing because complete responders—those most likely to benefit from PCI—also live longer and are at greater risk for complications. Many deficits on neuropsychologic testing are unsuspected on casual examination, but a few patients have obvious serious impairments. Neurologic abnormalities were most prominent in one series in patients who were given PCI concurrently with high-dose chemotherapy or in large radiation fractions of 400 cGy.[974] Certainly these abnormalities may not be attributable solely to PCI; chemotherapy, possible paraneoplastic syndromes, and the effects of chronic cigarette abuse are but some of the factors that might be contributory. In fact, administration of methotrexate and procarbazine was specifically associated with their occurrence in one study.[975]

Present opinion on whether PCI should be utilized in small cell carcinoma is widely divergent, and no consensus is possible. Current clinical trials randomizing completely responding patients to receive or not receive PCI should provide more conclusive documentation of toxicities and potential survival benefits. Until the results of such trials are available, we recommend the employment of PCI with the following guidelines: (1) only complete responders should be treated; (2) radiotherapy fractions of 200 to 300 cGy should be given over 2 to 3 weeks to a total dose of 2400 to 3000 cGy; and (3) PCI should not be administered on days when chemotherapy is given, and the interval between drug and radiation treatments should be as long as feasible. For patients with less than a complete response, cranial irradiation should be withheld until objective evidence of intracranial relapse supervenes.

TABLE 22-64. Randomized Trials of Prophylactic Cranial Irradiation

Series	No. of Patients	PCI Dose (cGy)	PCI Initiation	% of Patients with Brain Relapse: PCI	No PCI	p Value
Jackson et al.[962]	29	3000	Day 1	0	27	<0.05
Maurer et al.[487]	163	3000	Wks 8–12	4	18	<0.01
Hirsch et al.[963]	111	4000	Week 12	9	13	NS
Beiler et al.[964]	54	2400	Week 3	0	16	<0.05
Cox et al.[965]	45	2000	Day 1	17	24	NS
Seydel et al.[966]	271	3000	Day 1	5	21	<0.005
Aisner et al.[911]	29*	3000	AtCR	0	36	<0.02
Total	702			6	20	

Modified from Bleehan NM, Bunn PA, Cox JD et al: Role of radiation therapy in small cell anaplastic carcinoma of the lung. Cancer Treat Rep 67:11–19, 1983.

*Only those with complete response (CR) randomized.

Therapeutic Brain Irradiation

Brain metastases are a significant source of morbidity in patients with small cell lung cancer.[533] Furthermore, patients with brain metastases are at increased risk for spread to other areas of the CNS, especially for epidural and meningeal metastases.[534] Because the prognoses of patients with brain metastases differ widely, the therapeutic philosophy with which these metastases are approached is dependent on the clinical setting. In general, patients whose lesions are diagnosed at the time of presentation of small cell carcinoma have a relatively better prognosis,[978] with little difference in median survival in some series between patients with limited disease and those with brain metastases as the sole site of extensive disease at diagnosis.[532,979] Median survival is only 3 months, however, when metastases develop during treatment.[958,978] Not surprisingly, the prognosis is better if brain metastases are the only evidence of disease outside the thorax.[978] Two series report that neurologic symptoms at the time brain metastases are discovered have no impact on survival,[959,978] probably because many patients have successful short-term palliation and widespread systemic disease is present in most patients.

Radiotherapy is the treatment of choice for brain metastases in small cell lung cancer. Many radiation oncologists administer steroids (often dexamethasone 4 mg four times daily) with irradiation, especially if neurologic symptoms are present. After completion of irradiation, steroids are tapered to the lowest level that suppresses neurologic symptoms and often can be discontinued. Doses of cranial irradiation differ widely and are usually affected by performance status, life expectancy, extent of tumor dissemination, and the likelihood of meaningful response of systemic tumor. A common palliative dose schedule is 3000 cGy in 10 fractions over 2 weeks. Higher doses are often administered in appropriate clinical settings and are associated with better results, although patient selection factors probably explain much of this association.

Immediate response to brain irradiation is usually reported in terms of relief of neurologic symptoms, and the rate ranges from 60% to 85%.[958,972,978] In one series in which responses were confirmed by brain CT scans, complete and partial response rates were 32% and 31%, respectively.[978] Response duration can be disappointing, however. Brain metastases were said to be symptomatic or to be a continuing cause of death after irradiation in 45% and 54% of patients in two studies.[959,973] In another report,[978] 24 of 37 responding patients had clinical evidence of progressive intracranial tumor prior to death. The actuarial median response duration was 10 months in complete and 5 months in partial responders, with patients who died without evidence of intracranial tumor progression being censored at the time of death. The actuarial likelihood of remaining in response at 12 months for all responding patients was approximately 20%.

Despite these inadequacies in long-term control of brain metastases by irradiation, it remains true that small cell carcinoma is a widely disseminated disease in most patients afflicted with this problem, and that treatment of brain metastases will have little influence on survival in most patients. Therefore, short-term symptomatic control is an appropriate goal in most cases. It is patients with prospects for longer survival in whom the durability of therapeutic effects is relevant. These cases include those who are found to have brain metastases as the only site of disseminated disease at diagnosis and those whose complete response to systemic therapy is terminated solely by brain metastases. Although there is no conclusive evidence of better efficacy, more aggressive radiation dose schedules, such as 4000 to 5000 cGy in 4 to 5 weeks, are recommended in this setting.

Treatment of Spinal Cord and Leptomeningeal Metastases

Patients with small cell lung cancer can experience cancer dissemination throughout the neuraxis, including the spinal cord and leptomeninges.[534] At the time of diagnosis, approximately 2% will have spinal metastases and fewer than 0.5% will have meningeal tumor,[534,537,980] but a clinical diagnosis of spinal or meningeal cancer can be made at some time in the patient's course in an estimated 5% and 2.5% of cases, respectively.[529,534,537,980] As with brain metastases, the actuarial likelihood of developing spinal or meningeal tumor increases with lengthening survival but appears to plateau after approximately 3 years.[534,968,980]

The diagnostic evaluation and management of patients with spinal cord compression are outlined in detail in Chapter 58. In brief, early diagnosis is the key to successful therapy, as patients who are paraplegic by the time the diagnosis is established can only infrequently be restored to an ambulatory status with any form of treatment.[533] This is especially critical in small cell carcinoma, because a relatively high proportion of patients with spinal cord metastases present at initial diagnosis with a life expectancy of at least several months when chemotherapy is given.[534,537] Preservation of ambulation for this length of time is of obvious importance. Because of the increased risk of leptomeningeal carcinomatosis in patients with epidural or intramedullary small cell cancer of the spinal cord, cerebrospinal fluid obtained at myelography should always be submitted for cytologic analysis.

Median survival after the clinical diagnosis of carcinomatous leptomeningitis is less than 2 months. Eighty-six percent of patients have already been treated with chemotherapy and have either progressive or persistent systemic cancer at the time of diagnosis, so treatment has little influence on survival except in the minority of cases with meningeal involvement at initial diagnosis or as the sole site of relapse from complete remission.[981] Intrathecal methotrexate, often accompanied by irradiation to symptomatic areas of the neuraxis, is the most commonly utilized therapy. Patients treated with this combined approach are reported to clear their cerebrospinal fluid of malignant cells approximately 50% of the time but less often have complete resolution of neurologic symptoms and signs.[533,980] However, it is likely that only better-prognosis patients without rapidly advancing systemic tumor undergo this therapy. In the occasional patient with a life expectancy of 3 months or longer, we recommend placement of an Ommaya reservoir for intrathecal chemotherapy and monitoring of cerebrospinal fluid status. Because of the rarity of carcinomatous meningitis as the sole site of initial failure in completely responding patients, prophylactic therapy of the entire meningeal space is not indicated.

SURGICAL RESECTION

More than one-third of the rare patients who present with a solitary pulmonary nodule that upon surgical resection is diagnosed as small cell lung cancer will survive for 5 years or longer.[981] However, the inexorable development of distant metastases in most patients receiving surgical therapy alone, and the similar outcome of patients with apparently operable disease who did and did not undergo surgical resection in the early 1970s,[484] led many thoracic surgeons to forego any attempts at thoracotomy in patients with a confirmed pathologic diagnosis.

Several factors have recently caused this policy to be reappraised. First, patients undergoing resection of the primary tumor have relatively good survival. In 132 patients of the Veterans Administration Surgical Oncology Group surviving 30 days after complete resection, the actuarial 5-year survival rate was 23%; in patients with pathologically confirmed Stage I disease, constituting almost half the group, it was 41%.[982] Although adjuvant chemotherapy, usually with a single agent, was given to approximately half the patients, it had no effect on survival. Thus, these 5-year survival rates may legitimately be attributed to surgical therapy alone. A population-based study confirms the superior outcome of small cell cancer patients receiving initial surgical resection, often without subsequent adjunctive therapy.[983] Second, operative removal of the primary tumor favorably affects local tumor control. Relapse in the primary tumor site still occurs in completely responding limited-stage patients given chemotherapy, either alone or with chest irradiation,[936] whereas after surgical extirpation of the primary tumor, local relapse is infrequent.[984–986] Finally, excellent survival rates are observed in patients with thoroughly staged limited-stage tumor who have undergone surgical resection prior to the administration of chemotherapy (Table 22-65).[984,987,988] With various follow-up times, 42% of retrospectively identified patients who received postoperative combination chemotherapy with standard regimens (with or without chest irradiation) were alive and disease-free, including a small number of pathologically staged Stage I and II patients with an estimated 5-year survival rate of 80%.[989] Interestingly, patients who undergo an incomplete resection have a prognosis similar to that of operable cases who did not receive surgery.[988]

Current practice considers surgery as an adjunct to primary treatment with chemotherapy with or without thoracic radiotherapy. Resection of the primary tumor could be performed either before the initiation of chemotherapy or after response to treatment has been achieved. Fewer than 10% of patients with limited-stage small cell carcinoma have received combination chemotherapy after the primary tumor has been surgically removed.[984,987,988] Little data exist on how often surgical resection at the time of diagnosis is possible. Prospective studies of the feasibility of initial thoracotomy by their nature cannot include cases without a preoperative diagnosis who are discovered only at thoracotomy to have resectable small cell lung cancer. A large retrospective analysis of 435 limited-stage patients by Østerlind and associates[988] indicated that as many as 35% might have been considered operable. Of 96 operable patients actually subjected to thoracotomy, only 38% could have their tumors resected completely. This yields an estimated resectability rate of 13% (35% × 38%) in limited disease.

TABLE 22-65. Disease-Free Survival in Patients Undergoing Surgical Resection for Small Cell Lung Cancer in Conjunction with Chemotherapy or Chemoradiotherapy

Series	*No. Surgically Resected*	*No. Alive and Disease-free (%)*	*Comment*
Surgery Before Chemotherapy			
Friess et al.[987]	15	4 (27)	Retrospective, minimum 4-year follow-up
Shepherd et al.[984]	34	19 (56)	Retrospective, 1-year follow-up; includes 7 patients with chemotherapy before surgery
Meyer[989]	10	8 (80)	Retrospective, 2.5-year follow-up; Stages I and II patients
Østerlind et al.[988]	36	9 (25)	Retrospective, 3.5-year follow-up
Total	95	40 (42)	
Chemotherapy Before Surgery			
Prager et al.[985]	8	4 (50)	Prospective, 1-year follow-up
Johnson et al.[986]	24	4 (17)	Prospective, 1-year follow-up; no resection if biopsy negative
Baker et al.[992]	20	12 (60)	Prospective,† 10-month follow-up
Valdivieso[h]	13	6 (46)	Prospective, short follow-up
Williams et al.*	21	7 (33)	Prospective, 10-month follow-up
Total	86	33 (38)	

Table modified from Williams CJ, McMillan I, Lea R, et al: Surgery after initial chemotherapy for localized small cell carcinoma of the lung. J Clin Oncol 5:1579–1588, 1987.
*Prospectively identified patients from unknown population base.
†Valdivieso M, McMurtrey MJ, Farha P et al, Proc Am Soc Clin Oncol 3:220, 1984.

One important point concerning initial surgical resection of small cell carcinoma remains unresolved: is the superior outcome of limited-stage patients who undergo complete resection prior to initiation of chemotherapy attributable to the resection itself or to an inherently better prognosis for patients with a tumor burden small enough to permit resection? Retrospective data suggest much of the better prognosis of patients who are operated on is attributable to the latter factor. In Toronto, patients with "very limited" disease, defined as no evidence of mediastinal lymph node involvement on chest radiography or at mediastinoscopy, had a median and 5-year actuarial survival rate after chemoradiotherapy alone similar to that of surgically treated patients who then received chemoradiotherapy.[990] Danish patients with operable but nonresected limited-stage tumor had 18-, 30-, and 42-month survival rates of 17%, 13%, and 6%, respectively, compared with survival rates at identical time points of 22%, 18%, and 13% in patients receiving thoracotomy with the intent of complete resection. Although survival is better in operable patients subjected to thoracotomy, this degree of improvement cannot be regarded as conclusive from a retrospective study.[988]

In our opinion, resection of small cell lung cancer, if appropriate according to standard surgical criteria, should be performed in patients in whom the diagnosis is established only at thoracotomy. In patients with a known diagnosis preoperatively, a thoracotomy with intended complete tumor resection if possible is appropriate but not mandatory if complete staging, including evaluation of the mediastinum, reveals clinical Stage I or Stage II tumor. After resection, six cycles of adjuvant chemotherapy with a standard combination regimen should be administered, with or without chest irradiation.

Surgical resection in limited small cell carcinoma might be more effective if performed after initial chemotherapy rather than at diagnosis for several reasons. First, immediate chemotherapy would be given to attempt to eradicate occult distant metastatic disease. Only patients responding to chemotherapy—those most likely to benefit—would undergo thoracotomy. Second, comprehensive initial preoperative staging procedures could be avoided, because chemotherapy would be the first form of treatment. Finally, after response to chemotherapy, a larger fraction of patients might be surgical candidates.

Stringent criteria for operability after chemotherapy have allowed only 18% to 20%[985,986] to 37%[991] of limited-stage patients beginning induction chemotherapy to undergo eventual tumor resection in prospective trials, although this is still a potentially higher fraction than at the time of diagnosis. Among the factors preventing thoracotomy are poor response to chemotherapy, poor pulmonary function or other medical problems, presentation with SVC syndrome, and patient refusal.[991] No excessive operative morbidity or mortality compared with performing thoracotomy prior to chemotherapy is evident from most published series. Local recurrences are probably reduced in these patients.[986] No cancer is present in resected specimens in 5% to 20% of cases,[991,992] and not surprisingly, this patient subset enjoys a better prognosis. However, patients who have a negative biopsy of the primary tumor site and then do not have resection have a high frequency of local recurrence within a median of 5 months.[986] From 0 to 20% of resected or biopsied tumors after chemotherapy have contained non-small cell lung cancer or mixed small cell–non-small cell elements.[986,987,991–993] This frequency compares with an incidence of 25% of non-small cell components on biopsy of relapsing tumor following chemotherapy in one small series[994] and an incidence of 13% to 30% at autopsy.[266,995] Whether these pathologic findings are attributable to selection of non-small cell elements present in the original tumor, histologic changes induced by chemotherapy, the presence of a second lung cancer, or an incorrect initial diagnosis is not resolved. In any event, it is conceivable that surgery represents optimal treatment for residual non-small cell disease.

Data from the literature, summarized in Table 22-65, indicate that patients whose tumor can be surgically resected after response to modern combination chemotherapy have a better survival rate than all limited-stage patients beginning chemotherapy. In predominantly prospective series with various lengths of follow-up, the disease-free survival rate of patients whose disease was resected is 38%. Patient selection factors cloud interpretation of these results, however, and in the largest series,[991] survival of 38 patients beginning chemotherapy with the intent of performing later tumor resection if possible was no different from the survival of all 59 limited-stage cases seen during the interval of the study. The presence of lymph node involvement at prechemotherapy mediastinoscopy appears to be an especially poor prognostic factor.[996] This pretreatment staging procedure has not been performed in most series; hence, the definition of subsets of patients who may benefit from postchemotherapy surgery is not possible. In the absence of a clear-cut survival advantage for the policy of planned thoracotomy when possible after chemotherapy response, we do not recommend this approach outside the setting of a clinical trial. A current large LCSG trial of chemotherapy followed by surgery with postoperative radiotherapy versus chemotherapy followed by chest irradiation should help to resolve these issues.

TREATMENT OF RELAPSING OR PROGRESSIVE TUMOR

Although response rates to chemotherapy at diagnosis are high in small cell lung cancer, most patients eventually suffer tumor recurrence. The results of salvage therapy for disease relapsing or progressing after initial chemotherapy are poor, with infrequent objective responses and a median survival of 2 to 3 months.[836] Long-term disease-free survival after relapse is virtually nonexistent. Etoposide–cisplatin is currently the most commonly utilized salvage regimen in patients who have not received either of these agents previously. Although several studies have reported objective response rates of 50% or more with this treatment after failure of CAV chemotherapy,[877,878] complete responses are uncommon, and the impact on survival is uncertain. It is possible that the recent practice of administering initial chemotherapy for only 4 to 6 months has allowed the activity of etoposide–cisplatin in the relapse setting to be documented, because patients receiving this program in two studies that reported high response rates had not received any chemotherapy for a median of 3 to 5 months before relapse.[877,878] In contrast, another trial of etoposide–cisplatin in patients who had received six previous drugs with a median time off chemotherapy of only 3 weeks reported a 12% response rate.[997]

Although the usual practice in small cell carcinoma patients with relapsing disease is to administer agents to which the patient's tumor has not been previously exposed, it is important to recognize that patients who relapse after a long response, especially a complete response, demonstrate better response to salvage regimens, including those that consist of the same agents used for initial therapy,[998] than do patients with only a short remission. Similar results are noted in the therapy of relapsing multiple myeloma and Hodgkin's disease.

Radiotherapy is often the most useful palliative agent in patients with progressive symptomatic small cell carcinoma. The objective response rates of 60% or more to chest irradiation[999] are consistently higher than can be obtained with chemotherapeutic agents in this setting. Thoracic radiotherapy should be strongly considered in patients with pulmonary symptoms or in those who relapse solely in the chest. In a small pilot study in highly selected patients with relapse confined to the thorax after administration of chemotherapy alone, twice-daily chest irradiation followed by a new chemotherapy regimen was associated with a 67% complete response rate and a median survival of 6 months.[1000] Radiotherapy is the treatment of choice for SVC syndrome recurrent after chemotherapy, painful bone metastases, spinal cord compression, and brain metastases in patients without previous cranial irradiation and often provides short-term symptomatic relief. Unfortunately, patients with brain metastases following PCI or therapeutic cranial irradiation have an extremely poor prognosis and only occasionally derive palliative benefit.[978]

Relapsed patients frequently undergo testing with investigational chemotherapeutic agents in Phase I or Phase II trials. The difficulties in identifying new active drugs in this setting, in which most patients have poor prognostic factors such as impaired performance status and bulky advanced tumor, have already been discussed. New approaches to the development of useful salvage therapy for small cell carcinoma are sorely needed.

IMMUNOTHERAPY AND OTHER FORMS OF TREATMENT

Chemotherapy, radiotherapy, and, in selected cases, surgical resection are effective forms of therapy for small cell lung cancer. Other treatment modalities have been investigated but are not yet established. In early studies, lung cancer patients sometimes demonstrated both in vitro and in vivo evidence of immunosuppression, as manifested by depressed lymphocyte response to mitogens, low lymphocyte counts, and defective immunologic response to DNCB.[1001,1002] Impaired response to cutaneous delayed hypersensitivity testing has been associated with a poorer survival in small cell carcinoma.[503] These and other considerations led to a series of trials of immunotherapy as an adjunct to standard treatment modalities, beginning in the 1970s.

Nonspecific immunostimulation with both BCG vaccine and the methanol-extractable residue (MER) of BCG has been evaluated in several prospective randomized studies. In two large Southwest Oncology Group studies,[1003,1004] response rate, response duration, and overall survival were no different in patients given chemotherapy and chest irradiation who were randomized to receive or not receive BCG. There was a suggestion that long-term survival was improved with BCG in limited-stage, but impaired with BCG in extensive-stage, disease. At least three randomized trials demonstrated no benefit of the addition of MER-BCG to various standard treatments.[1005–1007]

Sixty-seven patients with small cell lung cancer were randomized to receive or not to receive calf thymosin fraction V (a modulator of T-cell function capable of correcting some immunologic defects in inherited T-lymphocyte disorders). Doses of 60 mg/m², 20 mg/m², or no thymosin were administered twice weekly during the first 6 weeks of chemotherapy with or without chest irradiation.[1008] Although no differences in complete response rates were noted, patients given thymosin 60 mg/m² had significantly improved survival, even after adjusting for other prognostic factors. However, a recent larger study conducted in 91 patients randomly assigned to thymosin 60 mg/m² twice weekly for 16 weeks or no thymosin during initial combined modality treatment could not confirm these findings.[1009] There was no evidence of effects on response rate, response duration, overall survival, long-term survival, or various serially studied immunologic parameters in the two patient groups. Interferon-alpha has not produced any objective responses in small Phase II trials.[858] In summary, there is no convincing evidence of therapeutic efficacy of any of the various forms of immunotherapy employed in any of these studies.

The nutritional status of small cell carcinoma patients is sometimes abnormal. Prior to treatment, patients can have preferential fat oxidation, ketogenesis, and changes in serum amino acid concentrations.[1010] Weight loss is also a negative prognostic factor in untreated patients.[502] Randomized trials have shown that some of these changes can be reversed with total parenteral nutrition during chemotherapy, but the weight gained with this maneuver is mostly fat or fluid and is not associated with improved total body nitrogen retention.[1011] No improvements in response rate or survival with total parenteral nutrition were noted in a randomized study of 119 patients.[1012]

Another adjunctive therapy evaluated because of antimetastatic effects in some animal tumor systems is systemic anticoagulation. A small randomized trial[1013] studied the effect of the addition of warfarin to combination chemotherapy and radiation and found improved time to tumor progression and survival. Results of larger studies designed to confirm or refute this observation are not yet mature.

SMALL CELL CARCINOMA ARISING IN EXTRAPULMONARY SITES

Four to five percent of small cell carcinoma patients present with no obvious pulmonary or mediastinal lesion on chest radiography and CT scan of the thorax and on bronchoscopy or sputum cytology.[1014,1015] These cases fall into two groups —those with an obvious primary extrapulmonary tumor arising in sites such as the larynx, esophagus, or uterine cervix, and a smaller fraction with lymph node or disseminated metastases without a detectable primary tumor in the lung or elsewhere.[1014-1016] These neoplasms resemble small cell lung cancer morphologically, usually contain neurosecretory granules on electron microscopy, and are occasionally associated with the same endocrine paraneoplastic syndromes (ectopic Cushing's syndrome, inappropriate antidiuretic hormone secretion) as pulmonary small cell lung cancer. Although there is some heterogeneity among different primary sites, their clinical behavior is also aggressive, with a median survival time of less than a year and a tendency for development of nodal and disseminated metastatic disease.[1014,1016] These unusual cancers are grouped collectively on morphologic grounds, but they probably represent several different neoplasms with variable biology, as suggested by the deletion of the short arm of chromosome 3 on karyotypic or genetic analysis of tumor cell lines (a finding present in more than 90% of pulmonary small cell carcinomas) in only a minority of extrapulmonary small cell lesions.[1017]

The most common sites of origin of extrapulmonary small cell carcinoma recorded in the literature are the uterine cervix (although many reports do not distinguish between neuroendocrine and squamous variants), esophagus, larynx and pharynx, colon and rectum, prostate, and paranasal sinuses.[1016] Merkel cell carcinoma of the skin, although not strictly a small cell carcinoma, is difficult to distinguish from small cell cancer morphologically, contains neurosecretory granules, and exhibits more aggressive clinical behavior than other skin carcinomas.[1018] Among all carcinomas arising in various organs where extrapulmonary small cell carcinoma has been observed, the frequency of small cell carcinoma is approximately 3.5% in the minor salivary glands, 1% in the pancreas, 0.9% in the esophagus, 0.3% in the larynx and pharynx, 0.2% in the colon and rectum, and extremely variable (from 0.2%–14%) in the uterine cervix, probably because of differing diagnostic criteria with inconsistent inclusion of the squamous cell variant.[1016]

Because of their low incidence and origin in diverse anatomic sites, uniform recommendations for therapy of these cancers cannot be made. In patients with a documented primary site and regional lymph node metastases, the prognosis is clearly worse.[1014] Partial and occasional complete responses to chemotherapy regimens utilized in small cell lung cancer are reported, although experience is insufficient to estimate response rates reliably.[1014-1016,1018] Patients with tumors arising in the esophagus, larynx and pharynx, and prostate have short median survival, and systemic chemotherapy as an adjunct to locoregional treatment should be considered. Although there is no clear documentation of survival benefit, complete responses to chemotherapy alone lasting as long as 12 months have been anecdotally reported in a few cases of esophageal tumors.[1014,1016] Because of the high frequency of nodal metastases, radiation therapy is recommended for tumors of the uterine cervix. There are few data on effects of chemotherapy in proved neuroendocrine small cell cervical carcinoma, but adjuvant chemotherapy in localized disease is sometimes suggested.[1016] Small cell carcinomas of the paranasal sinuses and minor salivary glands and colorectal tumors without nodal metastases have relatively good prognoses with locoregional therapy, and chemotherapy has not been utilized.[1016] In Merkel cell tumors originating in the skin of the head and neck, elective and therapeutic node dissections have been recommended; response to chemotherapy has been reported in a few cases of metastatic disease.[1018] In patients who present with distant metastatic and perhaps with regionally recurrent extrapulmonary small cell carcinoma, with or without a known primary tumor site, combination chemotherapy utilized for small cell lung cancer should be administered.

SUMMARY OF THE PRINCIPLES OF PRIMARY THERAPY OF SMALL CELL LUNG CANCER

The principles of initial treatment of the patient with small cell lung cancer and our recommendations for their implementation are outlined in Table 22-66. As in any malignant neoplasm, a correct pathologic diagnosis is imperative before therapy is initiated. Review of diagnostic material by an experienced pathologist is always appropriate, but especially so when the sole material available is from a fine-needle aspirate. The number of pretreatment staging procedures needed to determine the extent of tumor dissemination is dependent on the clinical situation, but sufficient procedures to identify tumor lesions to permit response assessment and to separate limited- from extensive-stage disease if therapy is to be affected by stage are required. Determination of the patient's ability to tolerate aggressive chemotherapy or combined-modality treatment is obviously important to avoid excessive morbidity and death in minimally ambulatory and other patients who derive little benefit from more toxic therapy. In patients believed to have Stage I or II tumor after thorough work-up that includes pathologic evaluation of the mediastinum, thoracotomy with attempted surgical resection may be considered. Moderately intensive combination chemotherapy (cyclophosphamide 750–1000 mg/m^2) with a published regimen of two to four drugs that is documented to produce at least 10% to 15% 2-year survival rates in limited-stage disease should be employed. This mandates the

TABLE 22-66. Principles of Initial Therapy for Small Cell Lung Cancer

Correct histologic diagnosis on adequate pathologic material
Appropriate initial staging to determine extent of tumor dissemination
Assessment of physiologic status and ability to tolerate therapy
Consideration of surgical resection in fully staged Stages I and II patients
Moderately intensive (cyclophosphamide doses 750–1000 mg/m^2) combination chemotherapy with a published regimen of proved efficacy consisting of two to four drugs
Capacity to provide good supportive care
Incorporation of chest irradiation into management of limited-stage disease
Restaging to assess response
Discontinuation of chemotherapy in responding patients after 4 to 6 months
Use of cyclic alternating combination chemotherapy appropriate but of unproved survival benefit
Consideration of prophylactic cranial irradiation in complete responders

capacity to provide supportive care of myelosuppressive complications, particularly infection and bleeding.

In limited-stage patients, concurrent or alternating combined-modality programs of chemotherapy and chest irradiation, preferably a program shown to increase survival in a prospective randomized trial, are recommended. Reevaluation of sites of initial disease to assess response should be performed after 12 to 18 weeks or possibly sooner. We believe that chemotherapy should be discontinued in responding patients after 18 to 24 weeks. Known effective cyclic alternating combination-chemotherapy regimens are certainly appropriate treatment and may well increase initial response duration, but their impact on survival is not clarified. Risk:benefit considerations for prophylactic cranial irradiation are far from defined. If PCI is to be administered, we recommend that it be given to complete responders shortly after documentation of response status, with avoidance of high doses per fraction of irradiation and of concurrent chemotherapy and cranial irradiation.

There is no question that current optimal treatments for small cell lung cancer have had a significant impact on survival (Table 22-67). Major gains in median survival occurred with the introduction of chemotherapy into the management of this disease, and this statistic has been improved fourfold to fivefold in both limited- and extensive-stage disease in comparison with results in patients receiving only supportive care. Furthermore, a fraction of patients with limited, and rare patients with extensive, disease attain 2- to 3-year disease-free survival and potential cure of their original neoplasm (see below). Nonetheless, it is also true that minimal improvement in therapeutic outcome has been documented since the early 1980s despite many modifications, combinations, and permutations of available agents and modalities, and approximately 95% of patients with small cell lung cancer will ultimately die of their affliction. Significant advances in understanding of the biology of this cancer have been forthcoming, however, at the same time that the pace of clinical advances has slowed. These advances may lead to novel and more effective approaches to the prevention, diagnosis, and therapy of small cell lung cancer.

LONG-TERM SURVIVAL AND CURE

Given the intensity and complexity of the staging and therapy of small cell lung cancer, it is reasonable to ask if any patients can be cured by applying the principles outlined in the preceding section. In the original publication describing the TNM staging system for lung cancer by the AJC,[1020] the outcome of small cell lung cancer patients treated during the 1960s at American university medical centers, some of which were centers devoted exclusively to the treatment of cancer patients, was reported. The 5-year survival rate in 368 patients was less than 1%. This figure amply documents the almost completely ineffective management of this neoplasm prior to the introduction of systemic chemotherapy.

In 1984, a compilation of nine reports covering 1343 small cell lung cancer patients treated with combination chemotherapy with or without chest irradiation revealed that 90 patients (7%) were alive and disease-free 2 years or more from the start of therapy.[836] These 2-year disease-free survivors represented 13% of patients presenting with limited, but only 2% of patients with extensive, stage disease. More than 80% of the 2-year survivors had received chest irradiation as part of their treatment, and almost all of the few extensive-stage patients had metatases confined to a single organ system. However, this duration of follow-up is not adequate to assess long-term survival, because relapses can still occur beyond this point.[836]

Sufficient time has now elapsed since the widespread utilization of chemotherapy for small cell lung cancer to permit assessment of survival at 5 years and beyond (Table 22-68). Overall calculations reveal that 72 patients (4%) of 2006 cases beginning what would today be regarded as standard treatment were alive 5 years later. One report excluded pa-

TABLE 22-67. Impact of Treatment on Survival in Small Cell Lung Cancer According to Extent of Disease

	Median Survival (mo)		*2–3 Year Survival (%)*	
Therapy	*LD**	*ED*	*LD*	*ED*
Supportive care	3	1.5	–	–
Surgery	5–6†	–	4–5†	–
	11‡	–	30–35‡	–
Thoracic radiotherapy	10†	–	10†	–
	3–9	–	2–7	–
Single-agent chemotherapy	6	4	–	–
Combination chemotherapy	10–14	7–11	5–15	1–3
Combination chemotherapy with chest irradiation	12–16	7–11	10–25	1–2

Modified from Morstyn G, Ihde DC, Lichter AS et al: Small cell lung cancer 1973–1983: Early progress and recent obstacles. Int J Radiat Oncol Biol Phys 10:515–539, 1984.
*LD = limited disease, ED = extensive disease.
†Operable patients in prechemotherapy era.
‡Selected, carefully evaluated, pathologically staged patients.

TABLE 22-68. Studies Reporting Small Cell Lung Cancer Patients Living 5 Years or Longer*

Series	*Stage*	*5-Year Survivors (%) (no./total)*	*% of Survivors at 5 Years (both stages)*
Smith et al.‡	Limited	417(24)	12
	Extensive	1/25 (4)	
Livingston et al.§	Limited	11/103 (11)	5
	Extensive	6/270 (2)	
Vogelsang et al.‖	Limited	5/94 (5)	2
	Extensive	0/131	
Johnson et al.#	Limited	17/103 (17)	8
	Extensive	4/149 (3)	
Jacobs et al.†**	Limited	2/102 (2)	1
	Extensive	0/138	
Østerlind et al.††	Limited	19/443 (4)	3
	Extensive	3/431 (1)	
Total	Limited	58/862 (7)	
	Extensive	14/1144 (1)	
Overall Total		72/2006 (4)	

*Modified from Seifter EJ, Ihde DC: Therapy of small cell lung cancer: A perspective on two decades of clinical research. Semin Oncol 15:278–299, 1988.

†Excluding patients with Stage I or II carcinomas.

‡Smith IE, Sappino P, Bondy P, Gilby ED: Long-term survival five years or more after combination chemotherapy and radiotherapy for small cell lung carcinoma. Eur J Cancer Clin Oncol 17:1249–1255, 1981.

§Livingston RB, Stephens RL, Bonnet JD et al: Long-term survival and toxicity in small cell lung cancer. Am J Med 77:415–417, 1984.

‖Vogelsang GB, Abeloff MD, Ettinger DS et al: Long-term survivors of small cell carcinoma of the lung. Am J Med 79:49–56, 1985.

#Johnson BE, Ihde DC, Bunn PA et al: Patients with small cell lung cancer treated with combination chemotherapy with or without irradiation: Data on potential cures, chronic toxicities, and late relapses after five- to eleven-year follow-up. Ann Intern Med 103:430–438, 1985.

**Jacobs RH, Greenberg A, Bitran JD et al: A ten-year experience with combined modality therapy for Stage III small cell lung carcinoma. Cancer 58:2177–2184, 1986.

††Østerlind K, Hansen HH, Hansen M et al: Long-term disease-free survival in small cell carcinoma of the lung: A study of clinical determinants. J Clin Oncol 4:1307–1313, 1986; Østerlind K, Hansen HH, Hansen M et al: Mortality and morbidity in long-term surviving patients treated with chemotherapy with or without irradiation for small cell lung cancer. J Clin Oncol 4:1044–1052, 1986.

tients with Stage I and II cancer, a prognostically more favorable group.[1020] The actual 5-year survival for limited-stage patients is 7%, and for extensive stage, it is 1%. These publications confirm that relapses of small cell lung cancer continue to occur between 2 and 5 years. However, approximately two-thirds of patients who are disease-free after 2 years will not relapse,[929,1021] and the likelihood of relapse is 26% and 14%, respectively, in patients who are disease free 30 months and 3 years from the beginning of treatment.[1021] Although a rare relapse can occur after 5 years, in small cell carcinoma, as in other types of lung cancer, 5 years of follow-up appears to be an appropriate time after which the curative potential of a therapy can be estimated.

Given a 5-year survival rate in limited disease of 7% when current treatment principles are applied, there is little question that modern therapy has had a quantitatively greater impact on median survival than on long-term survival. It is of some interest, therefore, to review older data on the long-term survival effects of surgical resection and chest irradiation when given to selected patient groups. In the large series of Shields and associates,[981] actuarial 5-year survival rate of completely surgically resected, pathologically staged patients who received either no or ineffective postoperative chemotherapy was 23%. In the majority with pathologically proved Stage I or II disease, an extremely uncommon presentation among all limited-stage small cell lung cancer, the estimated 5-year survival rate was 29%. In a small recent series of pathologically proved Stage I and II patients given postoperative combination chemotherapy, the 5-year survival rate was 80%.[485] In the 1960s, a Veterans Administration Lung Group study reported only 7% 1-year survival in limited-stage patients randomized to chest irradiation alone.[1022] In the 1960s British study of limited-stage patients who were thought to be operable,[841] 4% randomized to thoracic radiotherapy lived 5 years.

Few trials thereafter involved irradiation as the sole treatment for small cell lung cancer, and long-term survival with chest irradiation in the era of chemotherapy and of improving radiotherapy techniques can be assessed only in studies of patients who received radiotherapy alone, with chemotherapy often being administered when progressive disease developed. In this setting, reported survival rates for patients given radiotherapy as the sole initial treatment include 2% at 2 years,[1023] 7% at 30 months,[1024] 4% at 3 years,[1025] and 3% at

5 years.[1026] Given expected additional relapses up to the 5-year point and the heterogeneity in patient selection factors, the long-term survival results with a policy of chest irradiation alone for those with limited-stage disease at diagnosis must be considered inferior to those with initial chemotherapy or combined-modality therapy. There is no justification for the former policy, even when only potential cure rates are considered and overall survival disregarded.

Even though the original small cell lung cancer can be eradicated in a small fraction of patients, the risk of death from other causes in long-term survivors is far higher than in the age-matched population. Development of second malignancies, most notably non-small cell lung cancer and other smoking-related tumors, represents a significant threat to these patients.[929,1021] In the U.S. NCI series,[1027] non-small cell lung cancers appeared in most instances to be second primary cancers by virtue of their occurrence in pulmonary sites not involved with the initial small cell neoplasm. After 3 years of disease-free survival, subsequent pulmonary cancers were more likely to be of non-small cell than of small cell histology. In long-term survivors who present with a pulmonary mass, confirmation of the pathologic diagnosis is required, because an occasional patient will have a resectable non-small cell tumor. The risk of development of non-small cell lung cancer beyond 2 years from the diagnosis of small cell carcinoma was 4.4% per person–year, approximately 10 times higher than the rate found in screening studies in smoking men over the age of 45.[1027] As already discussed, long-term survivors of small cell lung cancer have a small but definite risk of treatment-associated acute myeloblastic leukemia and myelodysplastic syndromes.[930]

Chronic pulmonary, esophageal, and neurologic complications of treatment can also be present in long-term survivors of small cell lung cancer, as already mentioned. Between 50% and 70% of these patients, however, are able to resume a life-style similar to that which they led prior to the diagnosis of cancer.[929,1021] Although the increased risks of second malignancies and late toxicities can be devastating in individual patients, they clearly do not outweigh the benefits of prolonged survival for most patients and the small but real possibility of cure available with current therapeutic approaches. Nonetheless, it remains sobering that the vast majority of small cell lung cancer patients die of their disease despite the significant advances these approaches represent.

RESULTS OF RECENT STUDIES ON THE BIOLOGY OF LUNG CANCER

IN VITRO CHEMOTHERAPY AND RADIATION SENSITIVITY TESTING

With the advent of new tissue culture techniques and experience, and the identification of growth factor requirements, the past decade has seen rapid advances in the ability to grow lung cancer cells in vitro.[10–12,1028–1031] These cultures have opened up the possibility of drug[1032–1037] and radiation sensitivity testing, as well as testing of biologic response modifiers[1038,1039] and of differentiation-inducing agents[1040,1041] and antigrowth factors to identify new potentially beneficial treatments. It is possible that these tests could be used to select therapy for individual patients. The cell lines also provide material for biochemical analysis of the basis of drug resistance.[1042,1043] In fact, studies with methotrexate and doxorubicin in vitro have shown how complex and multifactorial drug resistance is in lung cancer cells. In the case of doxorubicin resistance, decreased intracellular drug levels, increased DNA repair, and altered drug–topoisomerase interaction were all noted.[1044]

Radiation sensitivity testing has revealed that lung cancer lines differ greatly in their sensitivity, with small cell tumor lines exhibiting greater sensitivity than non-small cell lines or the large cell variants of small cell lung cancer.[1045–1047] However, some of the small cell lines are more resistant, whereas some of the non-small cell lines are dramatically more sensitive. It will be important to know if these radiation response patterns for the individual tumors in vitro are the same as those the tumors exhibited in the patient. The results for the tumor cell lines showing small or no shoulders (low extrapolation numbers; $\tilde{n}$) on their radiation survival curves suggest the use of hyperfraction in treating patients.

Several assays, including tumor cloning, radiometric, and dye exclusion, have been used, and in other tumors, there is a good correlation between a tumor's response in vitro and that in vivo.[1048–1050] One hundred sixty-eight fresh lung cancer specimens were tested in the human tumor clonogenic assay, and 73% grew adequately for chemosensitivity testing. Most of the tumors were resistant to drugs, but the in vitro sensitivity varied markedly between specimens.[1051] The small cell lung cancer specimens were more sensitive than the non-small cell lung cancers, and the untreated patients' tumors were more sensitive than those whose tumors had relapsed during chemotherapy. In addition, primary and metastatic specimens from the same patient gave similar profiles. Recently, a tetrazolium dye-based semiautomated colorimetric assay (MTT assay)[1051] has been developed and applied to lung cancer cells for chemosensitivity and radiation sensitivity testing.[1053,1054] This assay appears to have several advantages over the clonogenic assays and allows the rapid and large-scale testing of large numbers of tumor cell lines against many different drugs, drug combinations, or combined-modality therapy. The assay has been applied to test the chemosensitivity to doxorubicin, melphalan [representing an alkylating drug], vincristine, vinblastine, VP-16, cisplatin, and BCNU [representing the nitrosoureas] of 30 lung cancer cell lines of all histologic types. These included untreated small cell lung cancers as well as those relapsing on chemotherapy and non-small cell lung cancer lines. The tumor lines derived from untreated small cell lung cancer patients were the most chemosensitive, whereas non-small cell and relapsed small cell tumors were significantly more resistant.[1055]

BIOLOGIC CHARACTERIZATION OF LUNG CANCER CELL TYPES AND STEM CELL OF ORIGIN

The development of human lung cancer cell lines has greatly facilitated the study of the cellular biology of lung cancer. Advances have been made in establishing markers that distinguish small cell from non-small cell lung cancer and,

TABLE 22-69. Comparison of the Biologic Properties of Lung Cancer Types[10-12,1030]

Property	*Small Cell*[1056]	*Small Cell Variant*	*Non-Small Cell*[1057]
L-DOPA decarboxylase activity	High	Absent/low	Absent
Dense core granules	Present	Absent/rare	Absent
Formaldehyde-induced fluoroescence	Present	Absent	Absent
Neuron-specific enolase	Present	Present	Absent
Creatine kinase-BB isozyme	High	High	Low/absent
Gastrin-releasing peptide	Present	Absent/low	Absent
Other peptide hormones	Present	Seldom	Seldom
HLA, B_2-microglobulin[1058,1059]	Absent-low	Absent/low	Present
Neurofilaments[1060,1061]	Present	Present	Absent
Intermediate filament pattern[1062]	"SCLC"	"Variant"	"NSCLC"
Leu-7, HNK-1 antigen[1063,1064]	Present	Present	Absent
Cell-surface protein phenotype[1065]	"SCLC"	"SCLC"	"NSCLC"
Macrophage–myeloid cell antigens[1066]	Present	?	?
Monoclonal antibody (MoAb) reactivity[1067]	"SCLC"		"NSCLC"
MoAb reactivity, epithelial antigens[1068]	Present?	Present	
Opioid peptides and receptors[1069]	Present	?	?
EGF receptors[1070,1071]	Low or absent?	Present	
Levels of high-energy phosphates[1072]	Diphosphodiesterphosphocreatine	Absent	
Glycolipid antigen expression[1073]	Unique	Unique	Unique

more recently, a non-small cell category with neuroendocrine features (Table 22-69). Although these studies have established markers that characterize these major types, nearly all investigators have found considerable heterogeneity in the expression of the markers within a tumor type and, in several cases, overlap of markers between the major divisions (such as some small cell lung cancers' expression of non-small cell lung cancer features, and vice versa). *This overlap suggests that there is a common stem cell for all types of lung cancer or that multiple programs of differentiation can be expressed in lung cancer cells.* Recently, Ruff and Pert proposed that the presence of macrophage and hematopoietic cell-surface markers indicates "that SCLC tumors are hemopoietic cells that arise from macrophages or their precursors . . . ."[1074] Although the expression of these cell-surface markers and their potential role in the pathogenesis of lung cancer has been noted by several investigators the extrapolation of lineage relation does not necessarily follow.

REFERENCES

1. Silverberg E: Cancer statistics, 1988. CA—A Cancer Journal for Clinicians 38:5–22, 1988
2. U.S. Department of Health, Education and Welfare: Cancer Patient Survival, Report Number 5. DHEW No. (NIH) 77-992. Washington, DC, 1977
3. Stanley KE: Lung cancer and tobacco: A global problem. Cancer Detect Prevent 9:83–89, 1986
4. Devesa SS, Silverman DT, Young JL Jr et al: Cancer incidence and mortality trends among whites in the United States, 1947–84. JNCI 79:701–770, 1987
5. Horm JWW, Kessler LG: Falling rates of lung cancer in men in the United States. Lancet 1:425–426, 1986
6. McDuffie HH, Klaassen DJ, Dosman JA: Female–male differences in patients with primary lung cancer. Cancer 59:1825–1830, 1987
7. Anonymous: Report calculates years lost, deaths attributable to smoking. Oncol Times, December 1, 1987, p 8 and Predictors of smoking examined among ethnic adolescent groups, p 10
8. Centers for Disease Control: Cigarette smoking among blacks and other minority populations. MMWR 36:404–407, 1987 and Cigarette smoking in the United States, 1986, pp. 581–585
9. Brown CC, Kessler LG: Projections of lung cancer mortality in the United States: 1985–2025. JNCI 80:43–51, 1988
10. Gazdar AF, Carney DN, Russell EK et al: Establishment of continuous clonable cultures of small-cell carcinoma of the lung which have amine precursor uptake and decarboxylation cell properties. Cancer Res 40:3502–3507, 1980
11. Carney DN, Gazdar AF, Bepler G et al: Establishment and identification of small cell lung cancer cell lines having classic and variant features. Cancer Res 45:2913–2923, 1985
12. Brower M, Carney DN, Oie HK, Gazdar AF, Minna JD: Growth of cell lines and clinical specimens of human non-small cell lung cancer in a serum-free defined medium. Cancer Res 46:798–806, 1986
13. Gazdar AF, Oie HK: Cell culture methods for human lung cancer. Cancer Genet Cytogenet 19:5–10, 1986
14. Minna JD, Battey JF, Brooks BJ et al: Molecular genetic analysis reveals chromosome deletion, gene amplification, and autocrine growth factor production in the pathogenesis of human lung cancer. Cold Spring Harbor Symp Quant Biol 51:843–853, 1986
15. Minna J, Battey J, Birrer M et al: Genetic changes involved in the pathogenesis of human lung cancer including oncogene activation, chromosomal deletions, and autocrine growth factor production. In Accomp Cancer Res—1987. General Motors Cancer Res Found. Fortner JG, Rhoads JE (Eds). Philadelphia: JB Lippincott Co, 155–182, 1988
16. Bishop JM: The molecular genetics of cancer. Science 235:305–311, 1987
17. Klein G: The approaching era of tumor suppressor genes. Science 238:1539–1545, 1987
18. Land H, Parada LF, Weinberg RA: Tumorigenic conversion of primary embryo fibroblasts requires at least two cooperating oncogenes. Nature 304:596–602, 1983
19. Kokuhata GK, Lilienfeld AM: Familial aggregation of lung cancer among hospital patients. Public Health Rep 78:277–283, 1963
20. Tokuhata GK, Lilienfeld AM: Familial aggregation of lung cancer in humans. J Natl Cancer Inst 30:289–312, 1963
21. Ooi WL, Elston RC, Chen VW, Bailey–Wilson JE, Rothschild H: Increased familial risk for lung cancer. JNCI 76:217–222, 1986
22. Lynch HT, Kimberling WJ, Markvicka SE et al: Genetics and smoking-associated cancers: A study of 485 families. Cancer 57:1640–1646, 1986
23. Skillrud DM, Offord KP, Miller RD: Higher risk of lung cancer in chronic obstructive pulmonary disease: A prospective, matched, controlled study. Ann Intern Med 105:503–507, 1986
24. Samet JM, Humble CG, Pathak DR: Personal and family history of respiratory disease and lung cancer risk. Am Rev Respir Dis 134:466–470, 1986
25. Tockman MS, Anthonisen NR, Wright EC, Donithan MG: Airways obstruction and the risk for lung cancer. Ann Intern Med 106:512–518, 1987
26. Peters–Golden M, Wise RA, Hochberg M, Stevens MB, Wigley FM: Incidence of lung cancer in systemic sclerosis. J Rheumatol 12:1136–1139, 1985
27. Heighway J, Thatcher N, Cerny T, Hasleton PS: Genetic predisposition to human lung cancer. Br J Cancer 53:453–457, 1986
28. Rohwedder JJ, Weatherbee L: Multiple primary bronchogenic carcinoma with a review of the literature. Am Rev Respir Dis 109:435–445, 1974
29. Martini N, Melamed MR: Multiple primary lung cancers. J Thorac Cardiovasc Surg 70:606–612, 1975
30. Johnson BE, Ihde DC, Matthews MJ et al: Non-small cell lung cancer: A major cause of late mortality in small cell lung cancer patients. Am J Med 80:1103–1110, 1986
31. Bradley EC, Schechter GP, Matthews MJ et al: Erythroleukemia and other hematologic complications of intensive therapy in long-term survivors of small cell lung cancer. Cancer 49:221–223, 1982
32. Markman M, Pavy MD, Abeloff MD: Acute leukemia following intensive therapy for small-cell carcinoma of the lung. Cancer 50:672–675, 1982

33. Whang-Peng J, Young RC, Lee EC, Longo DL, Schecter GP, DeVita VT Jr: Cytogenetic studies in patients with secondary leukemia/dysmyelopoietic syndrome after different treatment modalities. Blood 71:403–414, 1988
34. Dang SP, Liberman BA, Shepherd FA, Messner H et al: Therapy-related leukemia and myelodysplasia in small-cell lung cancer: Report of a case and results of morphologic, cytogenetic, and bone marrow culture studies in long-term survivors. Arch Intern Med 146:1689–1694, 1986
35. Boice JD Jr, Fraumeni JF Jr: Second cancer following cancer of the respiratory system in Connecticut, 1935–1982. Natl Cancer Inst Monogr 68:83–98, 1985
36. Olsen JH: Second cancer following cancer of the respiratory system in Denmark, 1943–1980. Natl Cancer Inst Monogr 68:309–324, 1985
37. Johnson DH, Porter LL, List AF, Hande KR, Hainsworth JD, Greco FA: Acute nonlymphocytic leukemia after treatment of small cell lung cancer. Am J Med 81:962–968, 1986
38. Christensen PH, Joergensen K, Munk J, Østerlind A: Hyperfrequency of pulmonary cancer in a population of 415 patients treated for laryngeal cancer. Laryngoscope 97:612–614, 1987
39. de Vries N, Snow GB: Multiple primary tumors in laryngeal cancer. J Laryngol Otol 100:915–918, 1986
40. Lyons MF, Redmon JD, Covelli H: Multiple primary neoplasia of the head and neck and lung: The changing histopathology. Cancer 57:2193–2197, 1986
41. Yellin A, Hill LR, Benfield JR: Bronchogenic carcinoma associated with upper aerodigestive cancers. J Thorac Cardiovasc Surg 91:674–683, 1986
42. Abernathy D, Beltran G, Stuckey W: Lung cancer following treatment for lymphoma. Am J Med 81:215–218, 1986
43. Ayesh R, Idle JR, Ritchie JC, Crothers MJ, Hetzel MR: Metabolic oxidation phenotypes as marker for susceptibility to lung cancer. Nature 312:169–170, 1984
44. Caporaso N, Hayes R, Dosemeci M, Hoover R, Idle J, Ayesh R: Debrisoquine metabolic phenotype (MP), asbestos exposure, and lung cancer (abstract). Proc Am Soc Clin Oncol 6:229, 1987
45. Minna JD, Cuttitta F, Battey JF et al: Gastrin-releasing peptide and other autocrine growth factors in lung cancer: Pathogenetic and treatment implications. In: DeVita VT Jr, Hellman S, Rosenberg SA (eds): Important Advances in Oncology 1988, pp 55–64. Philadelphia, JB Lippincott, 1988
46. Minna JD, Carney DN, Oie H, Bunn PA Jr, Gazdar AF: Growth of human small-cell lung cancer in defined medium. Cold Spring Harbor Conf Cell Prolif 9:627–639, 1982
47. Simms E, Gazdar AF, Abrams P. Minna JD: Growth of human small cell (oat cell) carcinoma of the lung in serum-free growth factor-supplemented medium. Cancer Res 40:4356–4363, 1980
48. Carney DN, Bunn PA, Gazdar AF, Pagan JF, Minna JD: Selective growth in serum-free hormone-supplemented medium of tumor cells obtained by biopsy from patients with small cell carcinoma of the lung. Proc Natl Acad Sci USA 78:3185–3189, 1981
49. Cuttitta F, Levitt M, Park J-G et al: Growth of human cancer cell lines in unsupplemented basal media as a means of identifying autocrine growth factors (abstract). Proc Am Assoc Cancer Res 28:27, 1987
50. Sherwin SA, Minna JD, Gazdar AF, Todaro GJ: Expression of epidermal and nerve growth factor receptors and soft agar growth factor production by lung cancer cells. Cancer Res 41:3538–3542, 1981
51. Nakanishi Y, Mulshine J, Kasprzyk PG et al: Small cell lung cancer cells autostimulate their growth via an insulin-like growth factor-1 activity: Evaluation of four cell lines. J Clin Invest 82:354–359, 1988
52. Natale RB, Cuttitta F, Nakanishi Y, Minna J, Gazdar A, Mulshine J: IGF-1 can stimulate proliferation of non-small cell lung cancer cell lines in vitro (abstract). Proc Am Soc Clin Oncol 7:197, 1988
53. Mucaulay V, Teale JD, Everard M, Joshi GP, Smith IE, Millar JL: Somatomedin-C (SM-C)/insulin-like growth factor 1 is a mitogen for human small cell lung cancer (abstract). Proc Am Assoc Cancer Res 28:54, 1987
54. Betsholtz C, Bergh J, Bywater M et al: Expression of multiple growth factors in a human lung cancer cell line. Int J Cancer 39:502–507, 1987
55. Moody TW, Pert CB, Gazdar AF, Carney DN, Minna JD: High levels of intracellular bombesin characterize human small cell lung carcinoma. Science 214:1246–1248, 1981
56. Wood SM, Wood JR, Ghatei MA, Lee YC, O'Shaughnessy D, Bloom SR: Bombesin, somatostatin and neurotensin-like immunoreactivity in bronchial carcinoma. J Clin Endocrinol Metab 53:1310–1312, 1981
57. Erisman MD, Linnoila RI, Hernandez O, DiAugstine RP, Lazarus LH: Human small-cell carcinoma of the lung contains bombesin. Proc Natl Acad Sci USA 79:2379–2383, 1982
58. Sorenson GD, Bloom SR, Ghatei MA, DelPrete SA, Cate CC, Pettengill OS: Bombesin production by human small cell carcinoma of the lung. Regul Pept 4:59–66, 1982
59. Moody TW, Carney DN, Cuttitta F, Quattrocchi K, Minna JD: High affinity receptors for bombesin/GRP-like peptides on human small cell lung cancer. Life Sci 37:105–113, 1985
60. Heikkila R, Trepel JB, Cuttitta F, Neckers LM, Sausville EA: Bombesin-related peptides induce calcium mobilization in a subset of human small cell lung cancer cell lines. J Biol Chem 262:16456–16460, 1987
61. Gaudino G, Cirillo D, Naldini L, Rossino P, Comoglio PM: Activation of the protein-tyrosine kinase associated with the bombesin receptor complex in small cell carcinomas. Proc Natl Acad Sci USA 85:2166–2170, 1988
62. Cuttitta F, Carney DN, Mulshine J, Moody TW, Fedorko J, Fischler A, Minna JD: Bombesin-like peptides can function as autocrine growth factors in human small-cell lung cancer. Nature 316:823–826, 1985
63. Wharton J, Polak JM, Bloom SR et al: Bombesin-like immunoreactivity in the lung. Nature 273:769–770, 1978
64. Rozengurt E, Sinnett–Smith J: Bombesin stimulation of DNA synthesis and cell division in cultures of Swiss 3T3 cells. Proc Natl Acad Sci USA 80:2936–2940, 1983
65. Lehy T, Accary JP, Labeille D, Dubrasquet M: Chronic administration of bombesin stimulates antral gastrin cell proliferation in the rat. Gastroenterology 84:914–919, 1983
66. Lezoche E, Basso N, Speranza V: Action of bombesin in man. In Bloom SR, Polak JM (eds): Gut Hormones, pp 419–424. London, Churchill Livingstone, 1981
67. Spindel ER, Chin WW, Price J, Rees LH, Besser GM, Habener JF: Cloning and characterization of cDNAs encoding human gastrin-releasing peptide. Proc Natl Acad Sci USA 81:5699–5703, 1984
68. Sausville EA, Lebacq–Verheyden A-M, Spindel ER, Cuttitta F, Gazdar AF, Battey JF: Expression of the gastrin-releasing peptide gene in human small cell lung cancer: Evidence for alternative processing resulting in three distinct mRNAs. J Biol Chem 261:2451–2456, 1986
69. Cuttitta F, Fedorko J, Gu J, Lebacq–Verheyden A-M, Linnoila RI, Battey J: Gastrin-releasing peptide gene associated peptide (GGAP) expressed in normal human fetal lung and small cell lung cancer. J Clin Endocrinol Metab 67:576–583, 1988
70. Lebacq–Verheyden AM, Kasprzyk P, Raum MG, Van Wyke, Coelingh K, LeBacq JA, Battey JF: Complex proteolytic processing of baculovirus expressed and of endogenous human gastrin-releasing peptide precursor. Mol Cell Biol 8:3129–3135, 1988
71. Carney DN, Cuttitta F, Moody TW, Minna JD: Selective stimulation of small cell lung cancer clonal growth by bombesin and gastrin-releasing peptide. Cancer Res 47:821–825, 1987
72. Weber S, Zuckerman JE, Bostwick DG, Bensch KG, Sikic BI, Raffin TA: Gastrin releasing hormone is a selective mitogen for small cell lung carcinoma in vitro. J Clin Invest 75:306–309, 1985
73. Willey JC, Lechner JR, Harris CC: Bombesin and the C-terminal tetradecapeptide of gastrin-releasing peptide are growth factors for normal human bronchial epithelial cells. Exp Cell Res 153:245–248, 1984
74. Aguayo SM, Kane M, Schwarz MI et al: Bombesin-like immunoreactivity in bronchoalveolar lavage from smokers and interstitial lung disease (abstract). Clin Res 35:530A, 1987
75. Sienhart D, Grauer L, Miller Y, Kane M, Bunn PA: A monoclonal antibody, BBC353, binds gastrin releasing peptide and inhibits growth of small cell lung cancer in vitro and in vivo (abstract). Clin Res 35:523A, 1987
76. Woll PJ, Rozengurt E: [D-Arg^{1},D-Phe^{5},D-Trp^{7,9},Leu^{11}] substance P, a potent bombesin antagonist in murine Swiss 3T3 cells, inhibits the growth of human small cell lung cancer cells *in vitro*. Proc Natl Acad Sci USA 85:1859–1863, 1988
77. Whang-Peng J, Kao-Shan CS, Lee EC et al: A specific chromosome defect associated with human small-cell lung cancer: Deletion 3p(14-23). Science 215:181–182, 1982
78. Whang-Peng J, Punn PA, Kao-Shan CS et al: A non-random chromosomal abnormality, del 3p(14-23), in human small cell lung cancer. Cancer Genet Cytogenet 6:119–134, 1982
79. Zech L, Bergh J, Nilsson K: Karyotypic characterization of established cell lines and short-term cultures of human lung cancers. Cytogenet Cell Genet 15:335–347, 1985
80. Yunis JJ: The chromosomal basis of human neoplasia. Science 221:227–236, 1983
81. Falor WH, Ward–Skinner R, Wegryn S: A 3p deletion in small cell lung carcinoma. Cancer Genet Cytogenet 16:175–177, 1985
82. de Leij L, Postmus PE, Buys CHCM, et al: Characterization of three new variant type cell lines derived from small cell carcinoma of the lung. Cancer Res 45:6024–6033, 1985
83. Graziano SL, Cowan BY, Carney DN et al: Small cell lung cancer cell line derived from a primary tumor with a characteristic deletion of 3p. Cancer Res 47:2148–2155, 1987
84. Morstyn G, Brown J, Novak U, Gardner J, Bishop J, Garson M: Heterogeneous cytogenetic abnormalities in small cell lung cancer cell lines. Cancer Res 47:3322–3327, 1987
85. Naylor SL, Johnson BE, Minna JD, Sakaguchi AY: Loss of heterozygosity of chromosome 3p markers in small-cell lung cancer. Nature 329:451–454, 1987
86. Brauch H, Johnson B, Hovis J et al: Molecular analysis of the short arm of chromosome 3 in small-cell and non-small-cell carcinoma of the lung. N Engl J Med 317:1109–1113, 1987
87. Kik K, Osinga J, Carritt B et al: Deletion of a DNA sequence at the chromosomal region 3p21 in all major types of lung cancer. Nature 330:578–581, 1987
88. Johnson BE, Sakuguchi AY, Gazdar AF et al: Restriction fragment length polymorphism studies show consistent loss of chromosome 3p alleles in small cell lung cancer patients' tumors. J Clin Invest 82:502–507, 1988
89. Zbar B, Brauch H, Talmadge C, Linehan M: Loss of alleles of loci on the short arm of chromosome 3 in renal cell carcinoma. Nature 327:721–724, 1987
90. Pathak S, Strong LC, Ferrell RE, Trindale A: Familial renal cell carcinoma with a 3;11 chromosome translocation limited to tumor cells. Science 217:939–941, 1982
91. Cohen AJ, Li FP, Berg S et al: Hereditary renal-cell carcinoma associated with a chromosomal translocation. N Engl J Med 301:592–595, 1979
92. Kao-Shan C-S, Fine RL, Whang-Peng J, Lee EC, Chabner BA: Increased fragile sites

and sister chromatid exchanges in bone marrow and peripheral blood of young cigarette smokers. Cancer Res 47:6278–6282, 1987
93. Yokota AJ, Wad M, Shimosato Y, Terada M, Sugimura T: Loss of heterozygosity on chromosomes 3, 13, and 17 in small cell carcinoma and on chromosome 3 in adenocarcinoma of the lung. Proc Natl Acad Sci USA 84:9252–9256, 1987
94. Shiraishi M, Morinaga S, Noguchi M, Shimosato Y, Sekiya T: Loss of genes on the short arm of chromosome 11 in human lung carcinomas. Jpn J Cancer Res 78:11302–11308, 1987
95. Friend SH, Bernards R, Rogelj S et al: A human DNA segment with properties of the gene that predisposes to retinoblastoma and osteosarcoma. Nature 323:643–650, 1986
96. Harbour JW, Lai S-L, Whang-Peng J, Gazdar AF, Minna JD, Kaye FJ: Abnormalities in structure and expression of the human retinoblastoma gene in small cell lung cancer. Science 241:353–357, 1988
97. Miller YE, Sullivan N, Kao B, Gazdar AF: Reduced or absent aminoacylase-1 activity in small cell lung cancer: Evidence for inactivation of genes encoded by chromosome 3p (abstract). Clin Res 34:568A, 1986
98. Carney DN, Edgell CJ, Gazdar AF, Minna JD: Suppression of malignancy in human lung cancer (A549/8) × mouse fibroblast (3T3-4E) somatic cell hybrids. JNCI 62:411–415, 1979
99. Weinberger C, Thompson CC, Ong ES, Lebo R, Gruol DJ, Evans RM: The c-*erb*-A gene encodes a thyroid hormone receptor. Nature 324:641–646, 1986
100. de The H, Marchio A, Tiollais P, Dejean A: A novel steroid thyroid hormone receptor-related gene inappropriately expressed in human hepatocellular carcinoma. Nature 330:667–670, 1987
101. Yuasa Y, Srivastava SK, Dunn CY, Rhim JS, Reddy EP, Aaronson SA: Acquisition of transforming properties by alternative point mutations within c-*bas/has* human proto-oncogenes. Nature 303:775–779, 1983
102. Capon DJ, Seeburg PH, McGrath JP et al: Activation of Ki-*ras* 2 gene in human colon and lung carcinomas by two different point mutations. Nature 304:507–513, 1983
103. Shimizu K, Birnbaum D, Ruley MA et al: Structure of the Ki-*ras* gene of the lung carcinoma cell line Calu-1. Nature 304:497–500, 1983
104. Santos E, Martin-Zanca D, Reddy EP, Pierotti MA, Della Porta G, Barbacid M: Malignant activation of a K-*ras* oncogene in lung carcinoma but not in normal tissue of the same patient. Science 223:661–664, 1984
105. Slamon DJ, deKernion JB, Verma IM, Cline MJ: Expression of cellular oncogenes in human malignancies. Science 224:256, 1984
106. Winter E, Yamamoto F, Almoguera C, Perucho M: A method to detect and characterize point mutations in transcribed genes: Amplification and overexpression of the mutant c-Ki-*ras* allele in human tumor cells. Proc Natl Acad Sci USA 82:7575–7579, 1985
107. Kurzrock R, Gallick GE, Gutterman JU: Differential expression of p21 *ras* gene products among histological subtypes of fresh primary human lung tumors. Cancer Res 46:1530–1534, 1986
108. Rodenhuis S, van de Wetering ML, Mooi WJ, Evers SG, van Zandwijk N, Bos JL: Mutational activation of the K-*ras* oncogene: A possible pathogenetic factor in adenocarcinoma of the lung. N Engl J Med 317:929–935, 1987
109. Little DC, Nau MM, Carney DN, Gazdar AF, Minna JD: Amplification and expression of the c-*myc* oncogene in human lung cancer cell lines. Nature 306:194–196, 1983
110. Griffin CA, Baylin SB: Expression of the c-*myb* oncogene in human small cell lung carcinoma. Cancer Res 45:272–275, 1985
111. Nau MM, Brooks JB, Carney DN et al: Human small-cell lung cancers show amplification and expression of the N-*myc* gene. Proc Natl Acad Sci USA 83:1092–1096, 1986
112. Nau MM, Brooks BJ, Battey J et al: L-*myc*: A new *myc*-related gene amplified and expressed in human small cell lung cancer. Nature 318:69–73, 1985
113. Brooks BJ, Battey J, Nau MM, Gazdar AF, Minna JD: Amplification and expression of the *myc* gene in small-cell lung cancer. Adv Viral Oncol 7:155–172, 1987
114. Kiefer PE, Bepler G, Kubassch M, Havemann K: Amplification and expression of proto-oncogenes in human small cell lung cancer cell lines. Cancer Res 47:6236–6242, 1987
115. Gu J, Linnoila RI, Seibel NC, Gazdor AF, Minna JD, Brooks BJ, Hollis GF, Kirsch IR: A study of myc-related gene expression in small cell lung cancer by in situ hybridization. Am J Path 132:13–17, 1988
116. Krystal G, Birrer M, Way J, Nau M, Sausville E, Thompson C, Minna J, Battey J: Multiple mechanisms for transcriptional regulation of the myc gene family in small-cell lung cancer. Mol Cell Biol 8:3373–3381, 1988
117. Mabry M, Nakagawak T, Gesell M, Nelkin BD, Eggleston JC, Ihle JN, Baylin SB: Introduction of Harvey murine sarcoma virus (Ha-MSV) into human small cell lung cancer (SCLC) is associated with phenotypic changes (abstract). Proc Am Assoc Cancer Res 28:39, 1987
118. Rapp UR, Huleihel M, Pawson T et al: Role of rat oncogenes in lung carcinogenesis. Lung Cancer (in press)
119. Gazdar AF, Carney DN, Nau MM, Minna JD: Characterization of variant subclasses of cell lines derived from small cell lung cancer having distinctive biochemical, morphological, and growth properties. Cancer Res 45:2924–2930, 1985
120. Radice PA, Matthews MJ, Ihde DC et al: The clinical behavior of "mixed" small cell/large cell bronchogenic carcinoma compared to "pure" small cell subtypes. Cancer 50:2894–2902, 1982
121. Johnson BE, Ihde DC, Makuch RW et al: *Myc* family oncogene amplification in tumor cell lines established from small cell lung cancer patients and its relationship to clinical status and course. J Clin Invest 79:1629–1634, 1987
122. Johnson BE, Battey J, Linnoila I et al: Changes in the phenotype of human small cell lung cancer cell lines following transfection and expression of the c-*myc* proto-oncogene. J Clin Invest 78:525–532, 1986
123. Vinocour M, Levitt M, Sausville EA, Nau MM, Seifter E, Minna JD: Expression of *myc* family members and p53 in human lung cancer cell lines. (in preparation)
124. Zummerman KA, Yancoupoulos GD, Collum RG et al: Differential expression of *myc* family genes during murine development. Nature 319:780–783, 1986
125. Kaye F, Battey J, Nau M et al: Structure and expression of the human L-*myc* gene reveal a complex pattern of alternative mRNA processing. Mol Cell Biol 8:186–195, 1988
126. De Greve J, Battey J, Fedorko J et al: The human L-*myc* gene encodes nuclear phosphoproteins from alternatively processed mRNAs. (submitted)
127. Birrer MJ, Segal S, De Greve JS, Kaye F, Sausville EA, Minna JD: L-*myc* cooperates with *ras* to transform primary rat embryo fibroblasts. Mol Cell Biol 8:2668–2673, 1988
128. Kawashima K, Shikama H, Imoto K et al: Close correlation between restriction fragment length polymorphism of the L-*myc* gene and metastasis of human lung cancer to the lymph nodes and other organs. Proc Natl Acad Sci USA 85:2353–2356, 1988
129. Schütte J, Nau M, Birrer M, Thomas F, Gazdar A, Minna J: Constitutive expression of multiple mRNA forms of the c-*jun* oncogene in human lung cancer cell lines (abstract). Proc Am Assoc Cancer Res 29:455, 1988
130. Haluska FG, Huebner K, Isobe M, Nishimura T, Croce CM, Vogt PK: Localization of the human *JUN* protooncogene to chromosome region 1p31-32. Proc Natl Acad Sci USA 85:2215–2218, 1988
131. Bohmann D, Bos TJ, Admon A, Nishimura T, Vogt PK, Tjian R: Human proto-oncogene c-*jun* encodes a DNA binding protein with structural and functional properties of transcription factor AP-1. Science 238:1386–1392, 1987
132. Cullen JW, McKenna JW, Massey MM: International control of smoking and the US experience. Chest 89(Suppl 4):2206S–2218S, 1986
133. National Academy of Sciences: Environmental Tobacco Smoke: Measuring Exposures and Assessing Health Effects, Appendix D. Washington, DC, National Academy Press, 1986
134. Damber LA, Larsson LG: Smoking and lung cancer with special regard to type of smoking and type of cancer: A case-control study in north Sweden. Br J Cancer 53:673–681, 1986
135. Vena JE, Byers TE, Cookfair D, Swanson M: Occupation and lung cancer risk: An analysis by histologic subtype. Cancer 56:9110–9117, 1985
136. Brownson RC, Reif JS, Keefe TJ, Ferguson SW, Pritzl JA: Risk factors for adenocarcinoma of the lung. Am J Epidemiol 125:25–34, 1987
137. Benhamou S, Benhamou E, Flamant R: Lung cancer risk associated with cigar and pipe smoking. Int J Cancer 37:825–829, 1986
138. Stanley KE: Lung cancer and tobacco: A global problem. Cancer Detect Prevent 9:83–89, 1986
139. McGlashan ND, Harington JS: Lung cancer 1978–1981 in the black peoples of South Africa. Br J Cancer 52:339–346, 1985
140. Lee HP: The epidemiology of lung cancer in Singapore. Ann Acad Med Singapore 14:485–490, 1985.
141. U.S. Department of Health and Human Services: The Health Consequences of Smoking: Nicotine Addiction: A Report of the Surgeon General. Washington, DC, DHHS Office on Smoking and Health, Publication No. (CDC) 88-8406, 1988
142. LaRosa JH, Haines CM: A Guide to Heart and Lung Health at the Workplace. Washington, DC, U.S. National Institutes of Health, Publication No. 86-2210, September 1986
143. Gray N: Low-tar cigarettes: Bane or benefit? Cancer Detect Prevent 10:187–192, 1987
144. Flehinger BJ, Kimmel M: The natural history of lung cancer in a periodically screened population. Biometrics 43:127–144, 1987
145. Kuller LH, Garfinkel L, Correa P et al: Contribution of passive smoking to respiratory cancer. Environ Health Perspect 70:57–69, 1986
146. Wald NJ, Nanchahal K, Thompson SG, Cuckle HS: Does breathing other people's tobacco smoke cause lung cancer? Br Med J 293:1217–1222, 1986
147. Garfinkel L, Auerbach O, Joubert L: Involuntary smoking and lung cancer: A case-control study. JNCI 75:4463–4469, 1985
148. Pershagen G, Hrubec Z, Svensson C: Passive smoking and lung cancer in Swedish women. Am J Epidemiol 125:17–24, 1987
149. Dalager NA, Pickle LW, Mason TJ et al: The relation of passive smoking to lung cancer. Cancer Res 46:4808–4811, 1986
150. Lee PN: Lung cancer and passive smoking: Association or an artefact due to misclassification of smoking habits? Toxicol Lett 35:157–162, 1987
151. Hughes JM, Weill H: Asbestos exposure: Quantitative assessment of risk. Am Rev Respir Dis 133:5–13, 1986
152. Kolonel LN, Yoshizawa CN, Hirohata T, Myers BC: Cancer occurrence in shipyard workers exposed to asbestos in Hawaii. Cancer Res 45:3924–3928, 1985
153. Hodgson JT, Jones RD: Mortality of asbestos workers in England and Wales 1971–1981. Br J Ind Med 43:1158–1164, 1986
154. Omenn GS, Merchant J, Boatman E et al: Contribution of environmental fibers to respiratory cancer. Environ Health Perspect 70:51–56, 1986
155. Kjuus H, Langard S, Skjaerven R: A case-referent study of lung cancer, occupational

exposure and smoking III: Etiologic fraction of occupational exposures. Scand J Work Environ Health 12:210–215, 1986
156. Seidman H, Selikoff IJ, Gelb SK: Mortality experience of amosite asbestos factory workers: Dose–response relationships 5–40 years after onset of short-term work exposure. Am J Ind Med 10:479–514, 1986
157. Kjuus H, Skjaerven R, Langard S, Lien JT, Aamodt T: A case-referent study of lung cancer, occupational exposures and smoking II: Role of asbestos exposure. Scand J Work Environ Health 12:203–209, 1986
158. Kjuus H, Skjaerven R, Langard S, Lien JT, Aamodt T: A case-referent study of lung cancer, occupational exposures and smoking I: Comparison of title-based and exposure-based occupational information. Scand J Work Environ Health 12:193–202, 1986
159. Saccomanno G, Yale C, Dixon W, Auerbach O, Huth GC: An epidemiological analysis of the relationship between exposure to Rn progeny, smoking and bronchogenic carcinoma in the U-mining population of the Colorado plateau—1960–1980. Heath Phys 50:605–618, 1986
160. Harley N, Samet JM, Cross FT, Hess T, Muller J, Thomas D: Contribution of radon and radon daughters to respiratory cancer. Environ Health Perspect 70:17–21, 1986
161. National Research Council: Health Risks of Radon and Other Internally Deposited Alpha-Emitters. Washington, DC, National Academy Press, 1988
162. Howe GR, Nair RC, Newcombe HB, Miller AB, Abbatt JD: Lung cancer mortality (1950–1980) in relation to radon daughter exposure in a cohort of workers at the Eldorado Beaverlodge uranium mine. JNCI 77:3357–3362, 1986
163. Thomas DC, McNeill KG, Gougherty C: Estimates of lifetime lung cancer risks resulting from Rn progeny exposure. Health Phys 49:825–846, 1985
164. Hornung RW, Meinhardt TJ: Quantitative risk assessment of lung cancer in U.S. uranium mines. Health Phys 52:417–430, 1987
165. Ginevan ME, Mills WA: Assessing the risks of Rn exposure. The influence of cigarette smoking. Health Phys 51:163–174, 1986
166. O'Riordan M: Natural radiation: How to live with radon. Nature 331:302, 1988
167. Jacobi W, Paaretzke HG: Risk assessment for indoor exposure to radon daughters. Sci Total Environ 45:551–562, 1985
168. Radford EP: Potential health effects of indoor radon exposure. Environ Health Perspect 62:281–287, 1985
169. Nero AV, Schwehr MB, Nazaaroff WW, Revzan KL: Distribution of airborne radon-22 concentrations in U.S. homes. Science 234:992–997, 1986
170. Marmorstein J: Lung cancer: Is the increasing incidence due to radioactive polonium in cigarettes? South Med J 79:145–150, 1986
171. Svensson C, Eklund G, Pershagen G: Indoor exposure to radon from the ground and bronchial cancer in women. Int Arch Occup Environ Health 59:123–131, 1987
172. Steenland K, Thun M: Interaction between tobacco smoking and occupational exposures in the causation of lung cancer. J Occup Med 28:110–118, 1986
173. Lawler AB, Mandel JS, Schuman LM, Lubin JH: A retrospective cohort mortality study of iron ore (hematite) miners in Minnesota. J Occup Med 27:507–517, 1985
174. Schatzkin A: Lung cancer in Yunnan mines. Cancer Prevention Studies Branch, Division of Cancer Control and Prevention, National Cancer Institute. Personal communication, 1988
175. Peters JM, Thomas D, Falk H, Oberdorster G, Smith TJ: Contribution of metals to respiratory cancer. Environ Health Perspect 70:71–83, 1986
176. Speizer FE: Overview of the risk of respiratory cancer from airborne contaminants. Environ Health Perspect 70:9–15, 1986
177. Maher KV, DeFonso LR: Respiratory cancer among chloromethyl ether workers. JNCI 78:839–843, 1987
178. Elinder CG, Kjellstrom T, Hogstedt C, Andersson K, Spang G: Cancer mortality in cadmium workers. Br J Ind Med 42:651–655, 1985
179. Lee–Feldstein A: Cumulative exposure to arsenic and its relationship to respiratory cancer among copper smelter employees. J Occup Med 28:296–302, 1986
180. Chen CJ, Chuang YCC, You SL, Lin TM, Wu HY: A retrospective study on malignant neoplasms of bladder, lung and liver in Blackfoot disease endemic area in Taiwan. Br J Cancer 53:399–405, 1986
181. Nishiyama H, Yano H, Nishiwaki Y et al: Lung cancer in chromate workers: Analysis of 11 cases. Jpn J Clin Oncol 15:489–497, 1985
182. Braver ER, Infante P, Chu K: An analysis of lung cancer risk from exposure to hexavalent chromium. Teratogen Carcinogen Mutagen 5:365–378, 1985
183. Rafnsson V, Johannesdottir SG: Mortality among masons in Iceland. Br J Ind Med 43:522–525, 1986
184. Nelson N, Levine RJ, Albert RE et al: Contribution of formaldehyde to respiratory cancer. Environ Health Perspect 70:23–35, 1986
185. Kauppinen TP, Partanen TJ, Nurminen MM et al: Respiratory cancers and chemical exposures in the wood industry: A nested case-control study. Br J Ind Med 43:84–90, 1986
186. Coggon D, Pannett B, Osmond C, Acheson ED: A survey of cancer and occupation in young and middle aged men I: Cancers of the respiratory tract. Br J Ind Med 43:332–338, 1986
187. Kvale G, Bjelke E, Heuch I: Occupational exposure and lung cancer risk. Int J Cancer 37:185–193, 1986
188. Blair A, Walrath J, Rogot E: Mortality patterns among U.S. veterans by occupation I: Cancer. JNCI 75:11039–11047, 1985
189. Deizell E, Monson RR: Mortality among rubber workers IX: Curing workers. Am J Ind Med 8:537–544, 1985
190. Sorahan T, Parkes HG, Veys CA, Waterhouse JA: Cancer mortality in the British rubber industry: 1946–1980. Br J Ind Med 43:363–373, 1986
191. Thomas TL, Stewart PA: Mortality from lung cancer and respiratory disease among pottery workers exposed to silica and talc. Am J Epidemiol 125:35–43, 1987
192. Malker HS, Gemmne G: A register-epidemiology study on cancer among Swedish printing industry workers. Arch Environ Health 42:73–82, 1987
193. Osorio AM, Bernstein K, Garabrant DH, Peters JM: Investigation of lung cancer among female cosmetologists. J Occup Med 28:291–295, 1986
195. Tuchsen F, Nordholm L: Respiratory cancer in Danish bakers: A 10 year cohort study. Br J Ind Med 43:516–521, 1986
196. Steenland K: Lung cancer and diesel exhaust: A review. Am J Ind Med 10:177–189, 1986
197. Colditz GA, Stampfer MJ, Willet WC: Diet and lung cancer: A review of the epidemiologic evidence in humans. Arch Intern Med 147:157–160, 1987
198. Bond GG, Thompson FE, Cook RR: Dietary vitamin A and lung cancer: Results of a case-control study among chemical workers. Nutr Cancer 9:109–121, 1987
199. Prentice RL, Omenn GS, Goodman GE et al: Rationale and design of cancer chemoprevention studies in Seattle. Natl Cancer Inst Monogr 69:249–258, 1985
200. Menkes MS, Comstock GW, Vuilleumier JP, Helsing KJ, Rider AA, Brookmeyer R: Serum beta-carotene, vitamins A and E, selenium and the risk of lung cancer. N Engl J Med 315:1250–1254, 1986
201. Ziegler RG, Mason TJ, Stemhagen A et al: Carotenoid intake, vegetables, and the risk of lung cancer among white men in New Jersey. Am J Epidemiol 123:1080–1093, 1986
202. Pisani P, Berrino F, Macaluso M, Pastorino U, Crosignani P, Baldasseroni A: Carrots, green vegetables and lung cancer: A case-controlled study. Int J Epidemiol 15:463–468, 1986
203. Byers TE, Graham S, Haugher BP, Marshall JR, Swanson MK: Diet and lung cancer risk: Findings from the western New York diet study. Am J Epidemiol 125:351–363, 1987
204. Kolonel LN, Hinds MW, Nomura AM, Hankin JH, Lee J: Relationship of dietary vitamin A and ascorbic acid intake to the risk for cancers of the lung, bladder, and prostate in Hawaii. Natl Cancer Inst Monogr 69:137–142, 1985
205. Dogra SC, Khanduja KL, Gupta MP: The effect of vitamin A deficiency on the initiation and postinitiation phases of benzo(a)pyrene-induced lung tumourigenesis in rats. Br J Cancer 52:931–935, 1985
206. Kreyberg L: Histologic typing of lung tumors. In Kreyberg L (ed): International Histologic Classification of Tumors, No. 1, pp 19–26. Geneva, World Health Organization, 1967
207. Yesner R, Gerstl B, Auerbach O: Application of the World Health Organization classification of lung carcinoma to biopsy material. Ann Thorac Surg 1:33–49, 1965
208. Matthews MJ, Gordon PR: Morphology of pulmonary and pleural malignancies. In Strauss MJ (ed): Lung Cancer: Clinical Diagnosis and Treatment. New York, Grune & Stratton, 1977
209. Vincent RG, Pickren JW, Lane WW et al: The changing histopathology of lung cancer: A review of 1682 cases. Cancer 39:1647–1655, 1977
210. Soroken SP: The respiratory system. In Greep RO, Weiss L (eds): Histology, 3rd Ed, pp 675–712. New York, McGraw-Hill, 1973
211. Tischler AS: Small cell carcinoma of the lung: Cellular origin and relationship to other neoplasms. Semin Oncol 5:244–252, 1978
212. Macholda F: Bronchogenic carcinoma: Study of growth and evolutionary dynamics of bronchogenic carcinoma: Its significance for early diagnosis. Acta Univ Carol 41(Suppl):39–62, 1970
213. Fraumeni JF Jr: Respiratory carcinogenesis: An epidemiologic appraisal. J Natl Cancer Inst 55:1039–1046, 1975
214. Auerbach O, Gere JB, Pawlowski JM: Carcinoma in situ and early invasive cancer occurring in the tracheobronchial tree in cases of bronchial carcinoma. J Thorac Surg 34:298–307, 1957
215. Valaitis JN, McGrew EA, Chomet B: Bronchogenic carcinoma in situ in asymptomatic high risk population of smokers. J Thorac Cardiovasc Surg 57:325–332, 1969
216. Auerbach O, Stout AP, Hammond EG et al: Changes in bronchial epithelium in relation to cigarette smoking and in relation to lung cancer. N Engl J Med 265:253–269, 1961
217. Band PR, Feldstein M, Saccomanno G: Reversibility of bronchial marked atypia: Implication for chemoprevention. Cancer Detect Prevent 9:157–160, 1986
218. Misset JL, Mathe G, Santelli G et al: Regression of bronchial metaplasia in heavy smokers with etretinate treatment. Cancer Detect Prevent 9:167–170, 1986
219. Meyer EC, Liebow AA: Relationship of interstitial pneumonia honeycombing and atypical epithelial proliferation to cancer of the lung. Cancer 18:322–350, 1965
220. Batsakis JG, Johnson HA: Generalized scleroderma involving lungs and liver with pulmonary adenocarcinoma. Arch Pathol 69:633–638, 1960
221. Moolten SE: Scar cancer of lung complicating rheumatoid lung disease. Mt Sinai J Med 40:736–743, 1973
222. Brincker H, Wilbek E: The incidence of malignant tumours in patients with respiratory sarcoidosis. Br J Cancer 29:247–251, 1974
223. Carroll R: The influence of lung scars on primary lung cancer. J Bacteriol 83:293–297, 1962
224. Liebow AA: Bronchiolar–alveolar carcinoma. Adv Intern Med 10:329–358, 1960
225. Hewlett TH, Gomez AC, Aronstam EM et al: Bronchiolar carcinoma of the lung: Review of 39 patients. J Thorac Cardiovasc Surg 48:614–624, 1964
226. Greenberg SD, Smith MN, Spjut HG: Bronchiolo–alveolar carcinoma: Cell or origin. Am J Clin Pathol 63:153–167, 1975

227. DeMartini JC, Rosadio RH, Sharp JM, Russell HI, Lairmore MD: Experimental coinduction of Type D retroviral-associated pulmonary carcinoma and lentivirus-associated lymphoid interstitial pneumonia in lambs. J Natl Cancer Inst 79:167–177, 1987
228. Beaver DL, Shapiro JL: A consideration of chronic pulmonary parenchymal inflammation and alveolar cell carcinoma with regard to a possible etiology relationship. Am J Med 21:879–887, 1956
229. Lutwyche VU: Another presentation of fibrosing alveolitis and alveolar cell carcinoma. Chest 70:292–293, 1976
230. Mulvihill JJ: Host factors in human lung tumors: An example of oncology. J Natl Cancer Inst 57:3–7, 1976
231. Joishy SK, Cooper RA, Rowley PT: Alveolar cell carcinoma in twins: Similarity in time of onset, histochemistry, and site of metastasis. Ann Intern Med 87:447–450, 1977
232. Watson WL, Farpour A: Terminal bronchiolar or "alveolar cell" cancer of the lung: Two hundred sixty-five cases. Cancer 19:776–780, 1966
233. Donaldson JC, Kaminsky DB, Elliott RC: Bronchiolar carcinoma: Report of 11 cases and review of the literature. Cancer 41:250–258, 1978
234. Katzenstein AA, Briolequ PG, Askin FG: The histologic spectrum and significance of clear-cell change in lung carcinoma. Cancer 45:943–947, 1980
235. Ihde DC, Cohen MH, Bernath AM et al: Serial fiberoptic bronchoscopy during chemotherapy of small cell carcinoma of the lung. Chest 74:531–536, 1978
236. Copple B, Wright SE, Moatamed E: Electron microscopy in small cell lung carcinoma: Clinical correlation. J Clin Oncol 2:910–916, 1984
237. World Health Organization: The World Health Organization histological typing of lung tumors. Am J Clin Pathol 77:123–136, 1982
238. Yesner R, Gerstl B, Auerbach O: Application of the World Health Organization classification of lung carcinoma to biopsy material. Ann Thorac Surg 1:33–49, 1985
239. Jett JR, Cortese DA, Fontana RS: Lung cancer: Current concepts and prospects. CA—A Cancer Journal for Clinicians 33:74–86, 1983
240. Saccomanno G, Archer VE, Auerbach O et al: Histologic types of lung cancer among uranium miners. Cancer 27:515–523, 1971
241. Gazdar AF, Carney DN, Guccion JE et al: Small cell carcinoma of the lung: Cellular origin and relationship to other tumors. In Greco FA, Oldham RK, Bunn PA (eds): Small Cell Lung Cancer. New York, Grune & Stratton, 1981
242. Ihde DC, Simms EG, Matthews MJ et al: Bone marrow metastases in small cell carcinoma of the lung: Frequency, description, and influence on chemotherapy toxicity and prognosis. Blood 53:667–686, 1979
243. Harley HRS: Cancer of the lung in women. Thorax 31:354–364, 1976
244. Rilke F, Carbone A, Clemente C et al: Surgical pathology of resectable lung cancer. Prog Cancer Res Ther 11:129–142, 1979
245. Bakris GL, Mulopulos GP, Korchik R, Ezdinli EZ, Ro J, Yoon BH: Pulmonary scar carcinoma: A clinicopathologic analysis. Cancer 52:493–497, 1983
246. Ochs RH, Katz AS, Edmunds LH, Miller CL, Epstein DM: Prognosis of pulmonary scar carcinoma. J Thorac Cardiovasc Surg 84:359–366, 1982
247. Tao LC, Delarue NC, Sanders D et al: Bronchiolo-alveolar carcinoma. Cancer 42:2759–2767, 1978
248. Kanhouwa SB, Matthews MJ: Reliability of cytologic typing of lung cancer. Acta Cytol 20:229–232, 1976
249. Cagneten CB, Geller CE, Saenz MDC: Diagnosis of bronchogenic carcinoma through the cytologic examination of sputum, with special reference to tumor typing. Acta Cytol 20:530–536, 1976
250. Hinson KFW, Miller AB, Tall R: An assessment of the World Health Organization classification of histologic typing of lung tumors applied to biopsy and resected material. Cancer 35:399–405, 1975
251. Feinstein AR, Gelfman NA, Yesner R: Observer variability in the histopathologic diagnosis of lung cancer. Am Rev Respir Dis 101:671–684, 1970
252. Burdon JGW, Sinclair RA, Henderson MM: Small cell carcinoma of the lung: Prognosis in relation to histologic subtype. Chest 76:302–304, 1979
253. Hansen HH, Dombernowsky P, Hansen M et al: Chemotherapy of advanced small cell anaplastic carcinoma. Ann Intern Med 89:177–181, 1978
254. Flower CD, Verney GI: Percutaneous needle biopsy of thoracic lesions: An evaluation of 300 biopsies. Clin Radiol 30:215–218, 1979
255. Hirsch FR, Matthews MJ, Yesner R: Histopathologic classification of small cell carcinoma of the lung: Comments based on an interobserver examination. Cancer 50:1360–1366, 1982
256. Yesner R: Observer variability and reliability in lung cancer diagnosis. Cancer Chemother Rep 4:55–57, 1973
257. Katlic M, Carter D: Prognostic implications of histology: Size and location of primary tumors. Prog Cancer Res Ther 11:143–150, 1979
258. Matthews MJ, Gazdar AF: Pathology of small cell carcinoma of the lung and its subtypes: A clinico-pathologic correlation. In Livingston RB (ed): Lung Cancer I, pp. 283–306. The Hague, Martinus Nijhoff, 1981
259. Carney DN, Matthews M, Ihde DC et al: Influence of histologic subtype of small cell carcinoma of the lung on clinical presentation, response to therapy and survival. JNCI 65:1225–1230, 1980
260. Hirsch FR, Østerlind K, Hansen HH: The prognostic significance of histopathologic subtyping of small cell carcinoma of the lung according to the classification of the World Health Organization: A study of 375 consecutive patients. Cancer 52:2144–2150, 1983
261. Radice RA, Matthews MJ, Idhe DC et al: The clinical behavior of "mixed" small cell/large cell bronchogenic carcinoma compared to "pure" small cell subtypes. Cancer 50:2894–2902, 1982
262. Matthews MJ: Effects of therapy on the morphology and behavior of small cell carcinoma of the lung—A clinicopathologic study. Prog Cancer Res Ther 11:155–165, 1979
263. Abeloff MD, Eggleston JC, Mendelsohn G et al: Changes in morphologic and biochemical characteristics of small cell carcinoma of the lung: A clinicopathologic study. Am J Med 66:757–764, 1979
264. Gazdar A, Carney D, Baylin S et al: Small cell carcinoma of the lung: Altered morphological, biologic and biochemical characteristics in long term cultures and heterotransplanted tumors (abstract). Proc Am Assoc Cancer Res Am Soc Clin Oncol 21:51, 1980
265. Little DC, Nau MM, Carney DM, Gazdar AF, Minna JD: Amplification and expression of the c-*myc* oncogene in human lung cancer cell lines. Nature 306:194–196, 1983
266. Sehested M, Hirsch FR, Østerlind K et al: Morphologic variations of small cell lung cancer: A histopathologic study of pretreatment and posttreatment specimens in 104 patients. Cancer 57:804–807, 1986
267. Bell CE, Seetharam S: Expression of endodermally derived and neural crest derived differentiation antigens by human lung and colon tumors. Cancer 44:13–18, 1979
268. Cuttitta F, Rosen S, Gazdar A et al: Monoclonal antibodies which demonstrate specificity for several types of human lung cancer. Proc Natl Acad Sci USA 78:4591–4595, 1981
269. Minna JD, Cuttitta F, Rosen S et al: Methods for production of monoclonal antibodies with specificity for human lung cancer cells. In Vitro 17:1068–1070, 1981
270. Mulshine JL, Cuttitta F, Bibro M et al: Monoclonal antibodies that distinguish non-small cell from small cell lung cancer. J Immunol 131:497–502, 1983
271. Nasiell MG, Kato H, Auer G et al: Cytomorphological grading and Feulgen DNA-analysis of metaplastic and neoplastic bronchial cells. Cancer 41:1511–1521, 1978
272. Bunn PA, Carney DN, Gazdar AF et al: Diagnostic and biologic implications of flow cytometric DNA content analysis in lung cancer. Cancer Res 43:5026–5032, 1983
273. Zimmerman PV, Bint MH, Hawson GAT et al: Ploidy as a prognostic determinant in surgically treated lung cancer. Lancet 2:530–533, 1987
274. Cohen MH: Signs and symptoms of bronchogenic carcinoma. In Straus MJ (ed): Lung Cancer: Clinical Diagnosis and Treatment, pp 85–94. New York, Grune & Stratton, 1977
275. Matthews MJ, Kanhouwa S, Pickner J et al: Frequency of residual and metastatic tumors in patients undergoing curative surgical resection of lung cancer. Cancer Chemother Rep 3:63–67, 1973
276. Carbone PP, Frost JK, Feinstein AR et al: Lung cancer: Perspectives and prospects. Ann Intern Med 73:1003–1024, 1970
277. Coy P, Kennelly GM: The role of curative radiotherapy in the treatment of lung cancer. Cancer 45:698–702, 1980
278. Paulson DL: Superior sulcus tumors: Results of combined therapy. NY State J Med 71:2050–2052, 1971
279. Pancoast HK: Superior pulmonary sulcus tumor: Tumor characterized by pain, Horner's syndrome, destruction of bone and atrophy of hand muscles. JAMA 99:1391–1396, 1932
280. Doehner GA, Marcus SS, Wolff WI: Pancoast's tumor: Five-year survival after combined radiotherapy and surgery. NY State J Med 67:2378–2380, 1967
281. Paulson DL: Carcinomas of the superior pulmonary sulcus. J Thorac Cardiovasc Surg 70:1095–1104, 1975
282. Henderson RD, Boszko A, Van Nostrand AWP: Pharyngoesophageal dysphagia and recurrent laryngeal nerve palsy. J Thorac Cardiovasc Surg 68:507–512, 1974
283. Salsali M, Cliffton EE: Superior vena cava obstruction with lung cancer. Ann Thorac Surg 6:437–442, 1968
284. Lokich JJ, Goodman R: Superior vena cava syndrome: Clinical management. JAMA 231:58–61, 1975
285. Rubin P, Hicks GL: Biassociation of superior vena cava obstruction and spinal cord compression. NY State J Med 73:2176–2182, 1973
286. Homma H, Kira S, Takahasi Y et al: A case of alveolar cell carcinoma accompanied by fluid and electrolyte depletion through production of voluminous amounts of lung liquid. Am Rev Respir Dis 111:857–862, 1875
287. Strauss BL, Matthews MJ, Cohen MH et al: Cardiac metastases in lung cancer. Chest 71:607–610, 1977
288. Rigler LG: Bronchiolo-alveolar carcinoma of lung with report on new roentgenologic sign. Int Congr Radio 1965
289. Matthews MJ: Problems in morphology and behavior of bronchopulmonary malignant disease. In Israel L, Chahanian P (eds): Lung Cancer: Natural History, Prognosis, and Therapy, pp 23–62. New York, Academic Press, 1976
290. Odell WD, Wolfsen AR: Humoral syndromes associated with cancer. Annu Rev Med 29:379–406, 1978
291. Blackman MR, Rosen SW, Weintraub BD: Ectopic hormones. Adv Intern Med x:85–113, 1978
292. Ayvazian LF: Extrapulmonary manifestations of tumors in the lung. Postgrad Med 63:93–99, 1978
293. Rassam JW, Anderson G: Incidence of paramalignant disorders in bronchogenic carcinoma. Thorax 30:86–90, 1975
294. Goldstraw P, Walbaum PR: Hypertrophic pulmonary osteoarthropathy and its occurrence with pulmonary metastases from renal carcinoma. Thorax 31:205–211, 1976
295. Green N, Kurohara SS, George FW III et al: The biologic behavior of lung cancer according to histologic type. Radiol Clin Biol 41:160–170, 1972
296. Byrd RB, Divertie MB, Spittell JA: Bronchogenic carcinoma and thromboembolic disease. JAMA 202:1019–1022, 1967
297. Sack GH, Levin J, Bell WR: Trousseau's syndrome and other manifestations of

chronic disseminated coagulopathy in patients with neoplasms. Medicine 56:1–37, 1977
298. Greenfield GB, Schorsch HA, Shkolnik A: The various roentgen appearance of pulmonary hypertrophic osteoarthropathy. Am J Roentgenol Rad Ther Nucl Med 101:927–931, 1976
299. Croft RB, Wilkinson M: Carcinomatous neuromyopathy: Its incidence in patients with carcinoma of the lung and breast. Lancet 1:184–188, 1965
300. Tyler HR: Paraneoplastic syndromes of nerve, muscle and neuromuscular junction. Ann NY Acad Sci 230:348–357, 1974
301. Anderson NE, Cunningham JM, Posner JB: Autoimmune pathogenesis of paraneoplastic neurologic syndromes. Crit Rev Clin Neurol 3:245–299, 1987
302. Kim YI, Neher I: IgG from patients with Lambert Eaton syndrome blocks calcium-dependent voltage channels. Science 239:405–408, 1988
303. Heber D, Chlebowski RT, Ishibashi DE, Herrold JN, Block JB: Abnormalities in glucose and protein metabolism in noncachetic lung cancer patients. Cancer Res 42:4815–4819, 1982
304. Anthony HM, Schorah CJ: Severe hypovitaminosis C in lung-cancer patients: The utilization of vitamin C in surgical repair and lymphocyte-related host resistance. Br J Cancer 46:354–367, 1982
305. Cox R, Musial T, Gyde OH: Reduced erythropoietin levels as a cause of anaemia in patients with lung cancer. Eur J Cancer Clin Oncol 22:511–514, 1986
306. Berg JW, Schottenfield D: Multiple primary cancers at Memorial Hospital 1949–1962. Cancer 40:1954–1960, 1977
307. Cahan WG: Multiple primary cancers of the lung, esophagus, and other sites. Cancer 40:1954–1960, 1977
308. Wynder EL, Muskinski MJ, Spivak JC: Tobacco and alcohol consumption in relation to the development of multiple primary cancers. Cancer 40:1872–1878, 1977
309. Cahan WG, Castro EB, Hajdu SI: The significance of solitary lung shadow in patients with colon carcinoma. Cancer 33:414–426, 1974
310. Enstrom JE, Austin DF: Interpreting cancer survival rates. Science 195:847–851, 1977
311. Fontana RS: Early diagnosis of lung cancer. Am Rev Respir Dis 116:399–402, 1977
312. Nash FA, Morgan JM, Tomkin JG: South London Lung Cancer Study. Br Med J 2:715–721, 1968
313. Brett GZ: Earlier diagnosis and survival in lung cancer. Br Med J 4:260–262, 1969
314. Weiss W, Boucot KE, Cooper DA: The Philadelphia Pulmonary Neoplasm Research Project: Survival factors in bronchogenic carcinoma. JAMA 216:2119–2123, 1973
315. Gryzbowski S, Coy P: Early diagnosis of carcinoma of lung: Simultaneous screening with chest x-ray and sputum cytology. Cancer 25:113–120, 1970
316. Melamed M, Flehinger B, Miller D et al: Preliminary report of the Lung Cancer Detection Program in New York. Cancer 39:369–382, 1977
317. Levin ML, Tockman MS, Frost JK, Ball WC: Lung cancer mortality in males screened by chest x-ray and cytologic sputum examination: A preliminary report. Recent Results Cancer Res 82:138–146, 1982
318. Fontana RS, Sanderson DR, Woolner LB, Taylor WF, Miller WE, Muhm JR: Lung cancer screening: The Mayo program. J Occup Med 28:746–750, 1986
319. Fontana RS: Screening for lung cancer: Recent experience in the United States. Cancer Treat Res 28:91–111, 1986
320. Neel HB III, Woolner LB, Sanderson DR: Sputum cytologic diagnosis of upper respiratory tract cancer. Ann Otol Rhinol Laryngol 87:468–473, 1978
321. Anonymous: Lung cancer mortality appears unaffected by roentgenographic and sputum screening in asymptomatic persons: Report from the NIH. JAMA 241:1582, 1979
322. Wolfsen AR, Odell WD: proACTH: Use for early detection of lung cancer. Am J Med 66:765–772, 1979
323. Chan JS, Seidah NG, Chretien M: Human NH_2 terminal of pro-opiomelanocortin as a potential marker for pulmonary carcinoma. Cancer Res 43:3066–3069, 1983
324. Gail MH, Muenz L, McIntire KR et al: Multiple markers for lung cancer diagnosis: Validation of models for localized lung cancer. JNCI 80:97–101, 1988
325. Vincent RG, Chu TM, Lane WW et al: Carcinoembryonic antigen as a monitor of successful surgical resection in 130 patients with carcinoma of the lung. Prog Cancer Res Ther 11:191–198, 1979
326. Mountain CF: Surgery of lung cancer including adjunctive therapy. In Hansen HH, Rorth M (eds): Lung Cancer 1980, pp 71–92. Amsterdam, Excerpta Medica, 1980
327. Baker RR, Ball WC Jr, Carter D et al: Identification and treatment of clinically occult cancer of the lung. Prog Cancer Res Ther 11:243–249, 1979
328. Sanderson DR, Fontana RS, Woolner LB et al: Bronchoscopic localization of radiographically occult lung cancer. Chest 65:608–612, 1974
329. Martini N, Beattie EJ, Cliffton EE et al: Radiologically occult lung cancer: Report of 26 cases. Surg Clin North Am 54:811–823, 1974
330. Fontana RS: The needle in the haystack (editorial). Mayo Clin Proc 53:616–617, 1978
331. Kinsey JH, Cortese DA, Sanderson DR: Detection of hematoporphyrin fluorescence during fiberoptic bronchoscopy to localize early bronchogenic carcinoma. Mayo Clin Proc 53:594–600, 1978
332. Cortese DA, Kinsey JH, Woolner LB, Sanderson DR, Fontana RS: Hematoporphyrin derivative in the detection and localization of radiographically occult lung cancer. Am Rev Respir Dis 126:1087–1088, 1982
333. Bell JW: Positive sputum cytology and negative chest roentgenogram: A surgeon's dilemma. Ann Thorac Surg 9:149–157, 1970
334. Sanderson DR, Fontana RS: Early lung cancer detection and localization. Ann Otol Rhinol Laryngol 84:583–589, 1975
335. Cortese DA, Pairolero PC, Bergstrahl EJ et al: Roentgenographically occult lung cancer: A ten-year experience. J Thorac Cardiovasc Surg 86:373–380, 1983
336. Ikeda S, Yanai T, Ishikawa S: Flexible bronchofiberscope. Keio J Med 17:1–18, 1968
337. Ihde DC, Cohen MH, Bernath AM et al: Serial fiberoptic bronchoscopy during chemotherapy of small cell carcinoma of the lung. Chest 74:531–536, 1978
338. Kvale PA, Bode FR, Kini S: Diagnostic accuracy in lung cancer: Comparison of techniques used in association with flexible fiberoptic bronchoscopy. Chest 69:752–757, 1976
339. Saltzstein SL, Harrell JH II, Cameron T: Brushings, washings or biopsy? Obtaining maximum value from flexible fiberoptic bronchoscopy in the diagnosis of cancer. Chest 71:630–632, 1977
340. Radke JR, Conway WA, Eyler WR et al: Diagnostic accuracy in peripheral lung lesions: Factors predicting success with flexible fiberoptic bronchoscopy. Chest 76:176–179, 1979
341. Mohsenifar Z, Chopra SK, Simmons DH: Diagnostic value of fiberoptic bronchoscopy in lung cancer presenting as mediastinal mass(es). Cancer 44:1894–1896, 1979
342. Khan MA, Whitcomb ME, Snider GL: Flexible fiberoptic bronchoscopy. Am J Med 61:151–155, 1976
343. Martini N, McCormack PM: Assessment of endoscopically visible carcinomas. Chest 73:718–720, 1978
344. Richardson RH, Zavala DC, Jukerjee PK et al: The use of fiberoptic bronchoscopy and brush biopsy in the diagnosis of suspected pulmonary malignancy. Am Rev Respir Dis 109:63–66, 1974
345. Zavala DC: Diagnostic fiberoptic bronchoscopy: Techniques and results of biopsy in 600 patients. Chest 68:12–19, 1975
346. Shure D, Astarita RW: Bronchogenic carcinoma presenting as an endobronchial mass: Optimum number of biopsy specimens for diagnosis. Chest 83:865–867, 1983
347. Givens CD Jr, Marini JJ: Transbronchial needle aspiration of a bronchial carcinoid tumor. Chest 88:152–153, 1985
348. Lundgren R, Bergman F, Angstrom T: Comparison of transbronchial fine needle aspiration biopsy, aspiration of bronchial secretion, bronchial washing, brush biopsy and forceps biopsy in the diagnosis of lung cancer. Eur J Respir Dis 64:378–385, 1983
349. Buirski G, Calverley PMA, Douglas NJ et al: Bronchial needle aspiration in the diagnosis of bronchial carcinoma. Thorax 36:508–511, 1981
350. Shure D: Fiberoptic bronchoscopy: Diagnostic applications. Clin Chest Med 8:1–13, 1987
351. Dhillon DP, Haslam PL, Townsend PJ et al: Bronchoalveolar lavage in patients with interstitial lung diseases: Side effects and factors affecting fluid recovery. Eur J Respir Dis 68:342–350, 1986
352. Lam WK, So SY, Hsu C et al: Fiberoptic bronchoscopy in the diagnosis of bronchial cancer: Comparison of washings, brushings and biopsies in central and peripheral tumours. Clin Oncol 9:35–42, 1983
353. Hanson RR, Zavala DC, Rhodes ML et al: Am Rev Respir Dis 114:67–72, 1976
354. Fletcher EC, Levin DC: Flexible fiberoptic bronchoscopy and fluoroscopically guided transbronchial biopsy in the management of solitary pulmonary nodules. West J Med 138:364–370, 1983
355. Popovich J Jr, Kvale PA, Eichenhorn MS et al: Diagnostic accuracy of multiple biopsies from flexible fiberoptic bronchoscopy: A comparison of central versus peripheral carcinoma. Am Rev Respir Dis 125:521–523, 1982
356. Teirstein AS, Chuang MT, Choy AR et al: Flexible bronchoscopy in nonvisualized carcinoma of the lung. Ann Otol 87:318–321, 1978
357. Zavala DC, Richardson RH, Mukerjee PK et al: Use of the bronchofiberscope for bronchial brush biopsy: Diagnostic results and comparisons with other brushing techniques. Chest 63:889–892, 1973
358. Ono R, Loke J, Ikeda S: Bronchofiberscopy with curette biopsy and bronchography in the evaluation of peripheral lung lesions. Chest 79:162–166, 1981
359. Solomon DA, Sollida NH, Gracey DR: Cytology in fiberoptic bronchoscopy: Comparison of bronchial brushings, washings and postbronchoscopy sputum. Chest 65:616–619, 1974
360. Ellis JH: Transbronchial lung biopsy via the fiberoptic bronchoscope: Experience with 107 consecutive cases and comparison with bronchial brushings. Chest 68:524–532, 1975
361. Shure D, Fedullo PF: Transbronchial needle aspiration of peripheral masses. Am Rev Respir Dis 128:1090–1092, 1983
362. Wang KP, Haponik EF, Britt EJ et al: Transbronchial needle aspiration of peripheral pulmonary nodules. Chest 86:819–823, 1984
363. Credle WF, Smiddy JF, Elliott RC: Complications of fiberoptic bronchoscopy. Am Rev Respir Dis 109:67–72, 1974
364. Simpson FG, Arnold AG, Purvis A et al: Postal survey of bronchoscopic practice by physicians in the United Kingdom. Thorax 41:311–317, 1986
365. Suratt PM, Smiddy JF, Gruber B: Deaths and complications associated with fiberoptic bronchoscopy. Chest 69:747–751, 1976
366. Burns DM, Shure D, Francoz R et al: The physiologic consequences of saline lobar lavage in healthy human adults. Am Rev Respir Dis 127:696–701, 1983
367. Wang KP, Haponik EF, Gupta PK et al: Flexible transbronchial needle aspiration: Technical considerations. Ann Otol Rhinol Laryngol 93:233–236, 1984
368. Schenk DA, Bower JH, Bryan CL et al: Transbronchial needle aspiration staging of bronchogenic carcinoma. Am Rev Respir Dis 134:146–148, 1986

369. Shure D, Fedullo PF: The rule of transcranial needle aspiration in the staging of bronchogenic carcinoma. Chest 86:693–696, 1984
370. Gobien RP, Bouchard EA, Gobien BS et al: Thin needle aspiration biopsy of thoracic lesions: Impact on hospital charges and patterns of patients care. Radiology 148:65–67, 1983
371. Weisbrod GL: Percutaneous fine needle aspiratory biopsy of the mediastinum. Clin Chest Med 8:27–41, 1987
372. Ferrucci JT, Wittenberg J, Margolies MN et al: Malignant seeding of the tract after thin needle aspiration biopsy. Radiology 130:345–346, 1979
373. Sinner WN, Zajicek J: Implantation metastases after percutaneous transthoracic needle aspiration biopsy. Acta Radiol [Diagn] 17:473–475, 1976
374. Sinner WN: Pulmonary neoplasms diagnosed with transthoracic needle biopsy. Cancer 43:1533–1540, 1979
375. Sagel SS, Ferguson TB, Forrest JV et al: Percutaneous transthoracic aspiration needle biopsy. Ann Thorac Surg 26:399–405, 1978
376. Sinner WN, Sandstedt B: Small cell carcinoma of the lung: Cytological, roentgenologic, and clinical findings in a consecutive series diagnosed by fine needle aspiration biopsy. Radiology 121:269–274, 1976
377. Johnston WW: Cytologic diagnosis of lung cancer: Principles and problems. Pathol Res Pract 181:1–35, 1986
378. Calhoun P, Feldman PS, Armstrong P et al: The clinical outcome of needle aspirations of the lung when cancer is not diagnosed. Ann Thorac Surg 41:592–596, 1986
379. Denoix PF: Enquete permanente dans les centres anticancereaux. Bull Inst Nat Hyg 1:70–80, 1946
380. Task Force on Lung Cancer: Staging of lung cancer 1979. In American Joint Committee for Cancer Staging and End Results Reporting: Manual for Staging of Cancer. Chicago, American Joint Committee, 1979
381. Mountain CF: A new international staging system for lung cancer. Chest 89:225S–232S, 1986
382. Kayser K, Bulzebruck H, Probst G et al: Retrospective and prospective tumor staging evaluating prognostic factors in operated bronchus carcinoma patients. Cancer 59:355–361, 1987
383. Yee J, Llewellyn GA, Williams PA, May IA, Dugan DJ: Scalene lymph node dissection: A study of 354 consecutive dissections. Am J Surg 118:596–601, 1969
384. Schatzlein MH, McAuliffe SE, Orriner MB, Kirsh MM: Scalene node biopsy in pulmonary carcinoma: When it is indicated? Ann Thorac Surg 31:322–324, 1981
385. Maasen W, Greschuchner D: Die endoskopische und bioptische Untersuchung des Mediastinums. Atem U Lungenkrankheit 3:161–169, 1975
386. Luke WP, Pearson FG, Todd TR et al: Prospective evaluation of mediastinoscopy for assessment of carcinoma of the lung. J Thorac Cardiovasc Surg 91:53–56, 1986
387. Coughlen M, Deslauriers J, Beaulieu M et al: Role of mediastinoscopy in pretreatment staging of patients with primary lung cancer. Ann Thorac Surg 40:556–560, 1985
388. Jepsen O: Mediastinoscopy. Copenhagen, Munksgaard, 1966
389. Lewis RJ, Siskler GE, Mackenzie JW: Mediastinoscopy in advanced superior vena caval obstruction. Ann Thorac Surg 32:458–462, 1981
390. Lewis RJ, Sisler GE, Mackenzie JW: Repeat mediastinoscopy. Ann Thorac Surg 37:147–149, 1984
391. Palva T, Palva A, Karja J: Re mediastinoscopy. Arch Otolaryngol 101:748–750, 1975
392. Paris F, Padilla J, Tarazona V et al: Results of surgical therapy for lung carcinoma. Cancer Clin Trials 2:71–76, 1979
393. Swain J: Surgical techniques in the diagnosis of pulmonary disease. Clin Chest Med 8:43–51, 1987
394. Martini N, Heelan R, Westcott J et al: Comparative merits of conventional, computed tomographic, and magnetic resonance imaging in assessing mediastinal involvement in surgically confirmed lung carcinoma. J Thorac Cardiovasc Surg 90:639–648, 1985
395. Nagaishi C: Functional Anatomy and Histology of the Lung, American Edition, p 102. Baltimore, University Park Press, 1972
396. Rea HH, Shevland JE, House AJ: Accuracy of computed tomographic scanning in assessment of the mediastinum in bronchial carcinoma. J Thorac Cardiovasc Surg 81:825–829, 1981
397. Hutchinson CM, Mills NL: The selection of patients with bronchogenic carcinoma for mediastinoscopy. J Thorac Cardiovasc Surg 71:768–773, 1976
398. Genereux GP, Howie JL: Normal mediastinal lymph node size and number: CT and anatomic study. AJR 142:1095–1100, 1984
399. James EC, Ellwood RA: Mediastinoscopy and mediastinal roentgenology. Ann Thorac Surg 18:531–538, 1974
400. Shevland JE, Chiu LC, Schapiro RL et al: The role of conventional tomography and computed tomography in assessing the resectability of primary lung cancer: A preliminary study. CT 2:1–19, 1978
401. Crowe JK, Brown LR, Muhm JR; Computed tomography of the mediastinum. Radiology 128:75–87, 1978
402. Underwood GH Jr, Hooper RG, Azelbaum SP, Goodwin DW: Computed tomographic scanning of the thorax in the staging of bronchogenic carcinoma. N Engl J Med 300:777–778, 1979
403. Mintzer RA, Malave SR, Neiman HL, Michaelis LL, Vanecko RM, Sanders JH: Computed vs. conventional tomography in evaluation of primary and secondary pulmonary neoplasms. Radiology 132:653–659, 1979
404. Ekholm S, Albrechtsson U, Kugelberg J, Tylen U: Computed tomography in preoperative staging of bronchogenic carcinoma. J Comput Assist Tomogr 4:763–765, 1980
405. Hirleman MT, Yiu-Chiu VS, Chiu LC, Shapiro RL: The resectability of primary lung carcinoma: A diagnostic staging review. CT 4:146–150, 1980
406. Richardson JV, Zenk BA, Rossi NP: Preoperative non invasive mediastinal staging in bronchogenic carcinoma. Surgery 88:382–385, 1980
407. Faling LJ, Pugatch RD, Jung Legg Y et al: Computed tomographic scanning of the mediastinum in the staging of bronchogenic carcinoma. Am Rev Respir Dis 124:690–695, 1981
408. Moak GD, Cockerill EM, Farber MO, Yaw PB, Manfredi F: Computed tomography vs standard radiology in the evaluation of mediastinal adenopathy. Chest 82:69–75, 1982
409. Osborne DR, Korobkin M, Ravin CE et al: Comparison of plain radiography, conventional tomography and computed tomography in detecting intrathoracic lymph node metastases from lung carcinoma. Radiology 142:157–161, 1982
410. Lewis JW, Madrazo BL, Gross St C et al: The value of radiographic and computed tomography in the staging of lung carcinoma. Ann Thorac Surg 34:553–558, 1982
411. Modini C, Passariello R, Jascone C et al: TNM staging in lung cancer: Role of computed tomography. J Thorac Cardiovasc Surg 84:569–574, 1982
412. Baron RL, Levitt RG, Sagel SS, White MJ, Roper CL, Marberger JP: Computed tomography in the preoperative evaluation of bronchogenic carcinoma. Radiology 145:727–732, 1982
413. Goldstraw P, Kurzer M, Edwards D: Preoperative staging of lung cancer: Accuracy of computed tomography versus mediastinoscopy. Thorax 38:10–15, 1983
414. Khan A, Khan FA, Garvey J et al: Oblique hilar tomography and mediastinoscopy. Chest 86:424–429, 1984
415. Richey HM, Matthews JI, Helsel RA, Cable H: Thoracic CT scanning in the staging of bronchogenic carcinoma. Chest 85:218–221, 1984
416. Frederick H, Bernardino ME, Baron M et al: Accuracy of chest computerized tomography in detecting hilar and mediastinal involvement by squamous cell carcinoma of the lung. Cancer 54:2390–2395, 1984
417. Daly DBT, Faling LJ, Pugatch RD et al: Computed tomography: An effective technique for mediastinal staging in lung cancer. J Thorac Cardiovasc Surg 88:486–494, 1984
418. Imhof E, Perruchoud AP, Tan KG et al: Mediastinal staging of bronchial carcinoma: Can computed tomography replace mediastinoscopy? Respiration 48:257–260, 1985
419. McKenna RJ, Libshitz HI, Mountain CE et al: Roentgenographic evaluation of mediastinal nodes for preoperative assessment in lung cancer. Chest 88:206–210, 1985
420. Graves WG, Martinez MJ, Carter PL et al: The value of computed tomography in staging bronchogenic carcinoma: A changing role for mediastinoscopy. Ann Thorac Surg 40:57–59, 1985
421. Doyle PT, Weir J, Robertson EM et al: Role of computed tomography in assessing "operability" of bronchial carcinoma. Br Med J 292:231–233, 1986
422. Ferguson MK, MacMahon H, Little AG et al: Regional accuracy of computed tomography of the mediastinum in staging of lung cancer. J Thorac Cardiovasc Surg 91:498–504, 1986
423. Matthews JI, Richey HM, Helsel RA et al: Thoracic computed tomography in the preoperative evaluation of primary bronchogenic carcinoma. Arch Intern Med 147:449–453, 1987
424. Santiago S, Houston D, Ezer J et al: Gallium scanning and tomography in the preoperative evaluation of lung cancer. Cancer 58:341–343, 1986
425. DeMeester TR, Golomb HM, Kirchner P et al: The role of gallium 67 scanning in the clinical staging and preoperative evaluation of patients with carcinoma of the lung. Ann Thorac Surg 28:451–464, 1979
426. Glazer GM, Gross BH, Aisen AM et al: Imaging of the pulmonary hilum: A prospective comparative study in patients with lung cancer. AJR 145:245–248, 1985
427. Webb WR, Jensen BG, Svelluto R et al: Bronchogenic carcinoma: Staging with MR compared with staging with CT and surgery. Radiology 156:117–124, 1985
428. Levitt RG, Glazer HS, Roper CL et al: Magnetic resonance imaging of mediastinal and hilar metastases: Comparison with CT. AJR 145:9–14, 1985
429. Martini N, Heelan R, Westcott J et al: Comparative merits of conventional computed tomographic and magnetic resonance imaging in assessing mediastinal involvement in surgically confirmed lung carcinoma. J Thorac Cardiovasc Surg 90:639–648, 1985
430. Poon PY, Bunnill MJ, Henkelman RM et al: Mediastinal lymph node metastases from bronchogenic carcinoma: Detection with MR imaging and CT. Radiology 162:651–656, 1987
431. Delarue NC, Sanders DE, Silverberg SA: Complementary role of pulmonary angiography and mediastinoscopy in individualizing treatment for patients with lung cancer. Cancer 26:1370–1378, 1970
432. Fishman NH, Bronstein MJ: Is mediastinoscopy necessary in the evaluation of lung cancer? Ann Thorac Surg 20:578–585, 1975
433. Benfield JE, Bonney H, Crummy AB et al: Azygograms and pulmonary arteriograms in bronchogenic carcinoma. Arch Surg 99:406–409, 1969
434. McLeod RA, Brown LR, Miller WE et al: Evaluation of the pulmonary hila by tomography. Radiol Clin North Am 14:51–83, 1976
435. Macumber HH, Calvin JW: Perfusion lung scan patterns in 100 patients with bronchogenic carcinoma. J Thorac Cardiovasc Surg 72:299–302, 1976
436. Cunningham JJ: Gray scale echocardiography of the lung and pleural space: Current applications of oncologic interest. Cancer 41:1329–1339, 1978

437. Biersach HJ, Bokisch A, Oehr P et al: Clinical results of immunoscintigraphy in a variety of malignant tumors with special reference to immunohistochemistry. Nuklearmedizin 25:167–171, 1986
438. Goldenberg DM, Kim EE, Deland F et al: Clinical studies on the radioimmunodetection of tumors containing alpha-fetoprotein. Cancer 48:2500–2502, 1980
439. Perkins AC, Perom MV, Morgan DAL et al: I^{131} and In^{111}-labeled monoclonal antibody imaged primary lung carcinoma. Nucl Med Commun 7:729–739, 1986
440. Chan SYT, Evan GI, Ritson A et al: Localisation of lung cancer by a radiolabelled monoclonal antibody against the c-myc oncogene product. Br J Cancer 54:761–769, 1986
441. Hansen HH, Muggia FM: Staging of inoperable patients with bronchogenic carcinoma with special reference to bone marrow examination and peritoneoscopy. Cancer 30:1395–1401, 1972
442. Muggia FM, Chervu LR: Lung cancer: Diagnosis in metastatic sites. Semin Oncol 1:217–228, 1974
443. O'Mara RE: Skeletal scanning in neoplastic disease. Cancer 37:480–486, 1976
444. Hansen HH, Muggia FM, Selawry OS: Bone marrow examination in 100 consecutive patients with bronchogenic carcinoma. Lancet 2:443–445, 1971
445. Newman SJ, Hansen HH: Frequency, diagnosis and treatment of brain metastases in 247 consecutive patients with bronchogenic carcinoma. Cancer 33:492–496, 1974
446. Ransdell JW, Peters RM, Taylor AT et al: Multiorgan scans for staging lung cancer: Correlation with clinical evaluation. J Thorac Cardiovasc Surg 73:653–659, 1977
447. Turner P, Haggith JW: Preoperative radionuclide scanning in bronchogenic carcinoma. Br J Dis Chest 75:291–294, 1981
448. Bell JW: Abdominal exploration in one-hundred lung carcinoma suspects prior to thoracotomy. Ann Surg 167:199–203, 1969
449. Yashar J: Transdiaphragmatic exploration of the upper abdomen during surgery for bronchogenic carcinoma. J Thorac Cardiovasc Surg 52:599–603, 1966
450. Hansen HH, Muggia FM: Staging of inoperable patients with bronchogenic carcinoma with special references to bone marrow examination and peritoneoscopy. Cancer 30:1395–1401, 1972
451. Mintz BJ, Tuhrim S, Alexander S: Intracranial metastases in the initial staging of bronchogenic carcinoma. Chest 86:850–853, 1984
452. Chapman GS, Kumar D, Redmond J et al: Upper abdominal computerized tomography scanning in staging non-small cell lung cancer. Cancer 54:1541–1543, 1984
453. Mountain CF: Biologic, physiologic, and technical determinants in surgical therapy for lung cancer. In Straus MJ (ed): Lung Cancer: Clinical Diagnosis and Treatment, pp 185–198. New York, Grune & Stratton, 1977
454. Mountain CF: Assessment of the role of surgery for control of lung cancer. Ann Thorac Surg 24:365–373, 1977
455. Tarhan S, Moffitt EA: Principles of thoracic anesthesia. Surg Clin North Am 53:813–826, 1973
456. Stanley KE: Prognostic factors for survival in patients with inoperable lung cancer. JNCI 65:25–32, 1980
457. Finkelstein DM, Ettinger DS, Ruckdeschel JC: Long term survivors in metastatic non small cell lung cancer: An Eastern Cooperative Oncology Group study. J Clin Oncol 4:702–709, 1986
458. Lee JY, Marks JE, Simpson JR: Age as a criterion for eligibility in a lung cancer trial. Am J Clin Oncol 5:449–452, 1982
459. Golebiowski A: Pulmonary resection in patients over 70 years of age. J Thorac Cardiovasc Surg 61:265–270, 1971
460. Watson WL, Schottenfeld D: Survival in cancer of the bronchus and lung 1949–1962: Comparison of men and women patients. Dis Chest 53:65–72, 1968
461. Ederer F, Mersheimer WL: Sex differences in the survival of lung cancer patients. Cancer 15:425–432, 1962
462. Connelly RR, Cutler SJ, Baylis P: End results in cancer of the lung: Comparison of male and female patients. JNCI 36:277–287, 1966
463. Kirsh MM, Tashian J, Sloan H: Carcinoma of the lung in women. Ann Thorac Surg 34:34–39, 1982
464. Harley HRS: Cancer of the lung in women. Thorax 31:254–264, 1976
465. Tartler PI, Burrirus L, Kirschner P: Perioperative blood transfusion adversely affects prognosis after resection of Stage I (subset N0) non oat cell lung cancer. J Thorac Cardiovasc Surg 88:659–662, 1984
466. Hyman NH, Fostes RS, DeMeules JE et al: Blood transfusions and survival after lung cancer resection. Am J Surg 149:502–507, 1985
467. Tarhan S, Moffitt EA, Taylor WF: Myocardial infarction after general anesthesia. JAMA 220:1451–1454, 1972
468. Robbins HM, Morrison DA, Sweet ME et al: Biopsy of the main carina: Staging lung cancer with the fiberoptic bronchoscope. Chest 75:484–486, 1979
469. Piehler JM, Trastek FV, Pairolero PL et al: Concomitant cardiac and pulmonary operations. J Thorac Cardiovasc Surg 90:662–667, 1985
470. Parker FB Jr: Surgery in chronic lung disease. Surg Clin North Am 54:1193–1202, 1974
471. Olsen GN, Block AJ, Swenson EW et al: Pulmonary function evaluation of the lung resection candidate: A prospective study. Am Rev Respir Dis 111:379–387, 1975
472. Legge JS, Palmer KN: Effect of lung resection for bronchial carcinoma on pulmonary function in patients with and without chronic obstructive bronchitis. Thorax 30:563–565, 1975
473. Alderson PO: Scintigraphic evaluation of patients with lung carcinoma. Chest 89:2455–2485, 1986
474. Block AJ, Olsen GN: Preoperative pulmonary function testing. JAMA 235:257–258, 1976
475. Ali MK, Mountain CF, Ewer MS et al: Predicting loss of pulmonary function after pulmonary resection for bronchogenic carcinoma. Chest 77:337–342, 1980
476. Ciofetta G, Silverman M, Hughes JMB: Quantitative approach to the study of regional lung function in children using krypton 81m. Br J Radiol 53:950–959, 1980
477. Ali ML, Ewer MS, Atallah MR et al: Regional and overall pulmonary function changes in lung cancer. J Thorac Cardiovasc Surg 86:1–8, 1983
478. Bria WF, Kanarek DJ, Kazemi H: Prediction of postoperative pulmonary function following thoracic operations. J Thorac Cardiovasc Surg 86:186–192, 1983
479. O'Rourke MA, Feussner JR, Feigl P, Laszlo J: Age trends of lung cancer stage at diagnosis: Implications for lung cancer screening in the elderly. JAMA 258:921–926, 1987
480. Sherman S, Guidot CE: The feasibility of thoracotomy for lung cancer in the elderly. JAMA 258:927–930, 1987
481. Page WF, Kuntz AJ: Racial and socioeconomic factors in cancer survival: A comparison of Veterans Administration results with selected studies. Cancer 45:1029–1040, 1980
482. Greenberg ER, Chute CG, Stukel T et al: Social and economic factors in the choice of lung cancer treatment: A population-based study in two rural states. N Engl J Med 318:612–617, 1988
483. Mayer RJ, Patterson WB: How is cancer treatment chosen? N Engl J Med 318:636–638, 1988
484. Mountain CF: Clinical biology of small cell carcinoma: Relationship to surgical therapy. Semi Oncol 5:272–279, 1978
485. Meyer JA: Effect of histologically verified TNM stage on disease control in treated small cell carcinoma of the lung. Cancer 55:1747–1752, 1985
486. Ihde DC, Makuch RW, Carney DN et al: Prognostic implication of sites of metastases in patients with small cell carcinoma of the lung given intensive combination chemotherapy. Am Rev Respir Dis 123:500–507, 1981
487. Maurer LH, Tulloh M, Weiss RB et al: A randomized combined modality trial in small cell carcinoma of the lung: Comparison of combination chemotherapy–radiation therapy versus cyclophosphamide–radiation therapy: Effects of maintenance chemotherapy and prophylactic whole brain irradiation. Cancer 45:30–39, 1980
488. Bunn PA Jr, Cohen MH, Ihde DC et al: Advances in small cell bronchogenic carcinoma. Cancer Treat Rep 61:333–342, 1977
489. Israel L, Depierre A, Choffel C et al: Immunochemotherapy in 34 cases of oat cell carcinoma of the lung with 19 complete remissions. Cancer Treat Rep 61:343–347, 1977
490. Lowenbraun S, Bartolucci A, Smalley RV et al: The superiority of combination chemotherapy over single agent chemotherapy in small cell lung carcinoma. Cancer 44:406–413, 1979
491. Livingston BR, Moore TN, Heilbrun L et al: Small cell carcinoma of the lung: Combined chemotherapy and radiation. Ann Intern Med 88:194–199, 1978
492. Østerlind K, Hansen HH, Dombernowsky P et al: Determinants of complete remission induction and maintenance in chemotherapy with or without irradiation of small cell lung cancer. Cancer Res 47:2733–2736, 1987
493. Zelen M: Keynote address on biostatistics and data retrieval. Cancer Chemother Rep 4:31–42, 1973
494. Einhorn LH, Bond WH, Hornback N et al: Long-term results in combined modality treatment of small cell carcinoma of the lung. Semin Oncol 5:309–313, 1978
495. Eagan RT, Carr DT, Lee RE et al: Phase II studies of polychemotherapy regimens in small cell lung cancer. Cancer Treat Rep 61:93–96, 1977
496. Cohen MH, Ihde C, Bunn PA et al: Cyclic alternating combination chemotherapy of small cell bronchogenic carcinoma. Cancer Treat Rep 63:163–170, 1979
497. Østerlind K, Andersen PK: Prognostic factors in small cell lung cancer: Multivariate model based on 778 patients treated with chemotherapy with or without irradiation. Cancer Res 46:4189–4194, 1986
498. Østerlind K, Hansen HH, Hansen M et al: Long-term disease-free survival in small cell carcinoma of the lung: A study of clinical determinants. J Clin Oncol 4:1307–1313, 1986
499. Østerlind K, Hansen M, Hansen HH et al: Treatment policy of surgery in small cell carcinoma of the lung: Retrospective analysis of a series of 874 consecutive patients. Thorax 40:272–277, 1985
500. Shepherd FA, Ginsburg RJ, Feld R et al: Reduction in local recurrence and improved survival in surgically treated patients with small cell lung cancer. J Thorac Cardiovasc Surg 86:498–506, 1983
501. Friess GG, McCracken JD, Troxell ML et al: Effect of initial resection of small cell carcinoma of the lung: A review of Southwest Oncology Group Study 7628. J Clin Oncol 3:964–968, 1985
502. DeWys WD, Begg C, Lavin PT et al: Prognostic effect of weight loss prior to chemotherapy in cancer patients. Am J Med 69:491–497, 1980
503. Johnston–Early A, Cohen MH, Fossieck BE et al: Delayed hypersensitivity skin testing as a prognostic indicator in patients with small cell lung cancer. Cancer 52:1395–1400, 1983
504. Hansen HH, Dombernowsky P, Hirsch FR: Staging procedures and prognostic features in small cell anaplastic bronchogenic carcinoma. Semin Oncol 5:280–287, 1978
505. Dearing MP, Steinberg SM, Phelps R et al: Women small cell lung cancer patients live longer than men (abstract). Proc Am Soc Clin Oncol 7:199, 1988
506. Poplin E, Thompson B, Whitacre M et al: Small cell carcinoma of the lung: Influ-

ence of age on treatment outcome. Cancer Treat Rep 71:291–296, 1987
507. Johnston–Early A, Cohen MH, Minna JD et al: Smoking abstinence and small cell lung cancer survival: An association. JAMA 244:2175–2179, 1980
508. Livingston RB, Trauth CJ, Greenstreet RL: Small cell carcinoma: Clinical manifestations and behavior with treatment. In Greco FA, Oldham RK, Bunn PA (eds): Small Cell Lung Cancer, pp 285–300. Orlando, Grune & Stratton, 1981
509. Quoix E, Finkelstein H, Wolkove N et al: Treatment of small cell lung cancer on protocol: Potential bias of results. J Clin Oncol 4:1314–1320, 1986
510. Seifter EJ, Ihde DC: Small cell lung cancer: A distant clinicopathologic entity. In Bitran JD, Golumb HM, Little AG, Weichselbaum RR (eds): Lung Cancer: A Comprehensive Treatise, pp 257–279. Chicago, Grune & Stratton, 1988
511. Cohen MH, Matthews MJ: Small cell bronchogenic carcinoma: A distinct clinicopathologic entity. Semin Oncol 5:234–241, 1978
512. Sculier JP, Evans WK, Feld R et al: Superior vena cava syndrome in small cell lung cancer. Cancer 57:847–851, 1986
513. Johnson DH, Hainsworth JD, Greco FA: Extrahepatic biliary obstruction caused by small cell lung cancer. Ann Intern Med 102:487–490, 1985
514. Gropp C, Havemann K, Scheuer A: Ectopic hormones in lung cancer patients at diagnosis and during therapy. Cancer 46:347–354, 1980
515. Hansen M, Hammer M, Hummer L: Diagnostic and therapeutic implications of ectopic hormone production in small cell carcinoma of the lung. Thorax 35:101–106, 1980
516. Hansen M, Hansen HH, Hirsch FR et al: Hormonal polypeptides and amine metabolites in small cell carcinoma of the lung, with special reference to stage and subtypes. Cancer 45:1432–1437, 1980
517. List AF, Hainsworth JD, Davis BW et al: The syndrome of inappropriate secretion of anti-diuretic hormone in small cell lung cancer. J Clin Oncol 4:1191–1198, 1986
518. Wittes RE, Yeh SDJ: Indications for liver and brain scans: Screening tests for patients with oat cell carcinoma of the lung. JAMA 238:506–507, 1977
519. Ihde DC: Staging evaluation and prognostic factors in small cell lung cancer. In Aisner J (ed): Lung Cancer, pp 241–268. New York, Churchill Livingstone, 1985
520. Nakhosteen JA, Niederle N: Small cell lung cancer: Serial bronchofiberscopy and photographic documentation—the bridge sign. Chest 83:12–16, 1983
521. Harper PG, Houang M, Spiro SG, Geddes D, Hodson M, Souhami RL: Computerized axial tomography in the pretreatment assessment of small-cell carcinoma of the bronchus. Cancer 47:1775–1780, 1981
522. Levenson RM, Sauerbrunn BJL, Ihde DC, Bunn PA Jr, Cohen MH, Minna JD: Small cell lung cancer: Radionuclide bone scans for assessment of tumor extent and response. AJR 137:31–35, 1981
523. Campling B, Quirt I, DeBoer G et al: Is bone marrow examination in small cell lung cancer really necessary? Ann Intern Med 105:508–512, 1986
524. Levitan N, Byrne RE, Bromer RH et al: The value of bone scan and bone marrow biopsy in staging small cell lung cancer. Cancer 56:652–654, 1985
525. Kristjansen PEG, Østerlind K, Hansen M: Detection of bone marrow relapse in patients with small cell carcinoma of the lung. Cancer 58:2538–2541, 1986
526. Mulshine JL, Makuch RW, Johnston–Early A et al: Diagnosis and significance of liver metastases in small cell carcinoma of the lung. J Clin Oncol 2:733–741, 1984
527. Dombernowsky P, Hirsch F, Hansen HH et al: Peritoneoscopy in the staging of 190 patients with small-cell anaplastic carcinoma of the lung with special reference to subtyping. Cancer 41:2008–2012, 1978
528. Hansen SW, Jensen F, Pedersen NT et al: Detection of liver metastases in small cell lung cancer: A comparison of peritoneoscopy with liver biopsy and ultrasonography with fine-needle aspiration. J Clin Oncol 5:255–259, 1987
529. Sculier JP, Feld R, Evans WK et al: Neurologic disorders in patients with small cell lung cancer. Cancer 60:2275–2283, 1987
530. Crane JM, Nelson MJ, Ihde DC et al: A comparison of computed tomography and radionuclide scanning for detection of brain metastases in small cell lung cancer. J Clin Oncol 2:1017–1024, 1984
531. Johnson DH, Windham WW, Allen JH, Greco FA: Limited value of CT brain scans in the staging of small cell cancer. AJR 140:37–40, 1983
532. Giannone L, Johnson DH, Hande KR et al: Favorable prognosis of brain metastases in small cell lung cancer. Ann Intern Med 106:386–389, 1987
533. Bunn PA Jr, Nugent JL, Matthews MJ: Central nervous system metastases in small cell bronchogenic carcinoma. Semin Oncol 5:314–322, 1978
534. Nugent JL, Bunn PA Jr, Matthews MJ et al: CNS metastases in small cell bronchogenic carcinoma: Increasing frequency and changing pattern with lengthening survival. Cancer 44:1885–1893, 1979
535. Rosen ST, Aisner J, Makuch RW et al: Carcinomatous leptomeningitis in small cell lung cancer: A clinicopathologic review of the National Cancer Institute experience. Medicine 61:45–53, 1982
536. Ihde DC, Dunnick NR, Johnston–Early A, Bunn PA, Cohen MH, Minna JD: Abdominal computed tomography in small cell lung cancer: Assessment of extent of disease and response to therapy. Cancer 49:1485–1490, 1982
537. Pedersen AG, Bach F, Melgaard B: Frequency, diagnosis, and prognosis of spinal cord compression in small cell bronchogenic carcinoma: A review of 817 consecutive patients. Cancer 55:1818–1822, 1985
538. Murphy KC, Feld R, Evans WK et al: Intramedullary spinal cord metastases from small cell carcinoma of the lung. J Clin Oncol 1:99–106, 1983
539. Dunnick NR, Ihde DC, Johnston–Early A: Abdominal CT in the evaluation of small cell carcinoma of the lung. AJR 133:1085–1088, 1979
540. Poon PY, Feld R, Evans WK, Ege C, Yeoh JL, McLoughlin ML: Computed tomography of the brain, liver, and upper abdomen in the staging of small cell carcinoma of the lung. J Comput Assist Tomogr 6:963–965, 1982
541. Lewis E, Bernardino ME, Valdivieso M, Farha P, Barnes PA, Thomas JL: Computed tomography and routine chest radiography in oat cell carcinoma of the lung. J Comput Assist Tomogr 6:739–745, 1982
542. Pagani JJ: Normal adrenal glands in small cell lung carcinoma: CT-guided biopsy. AJR 140:949–951, 1983
543. Carney DN, Ihde DC, Cohen MH et al: Serum neuron-specific enolase: A marker for disease extent and response to therapy of small-cell lung cancer. Lancet x:583–585, 1982
544. Carney DN, Zweig MH, Ihde DC et al: Elevated serum creatine kinase-BB levels in patients with small cell lung cancer. Cancer Res 44:5399–5403, 1984
545. Sobol RE, O'Connor DT, Addison J et al: Elevated serum chromogranin A concentrations in small cell lung carcinoma. Ann Intern Med 105:698–700, 1986
546. Johnson DH, Marangos PJ, Forbes JT et al: Potential utility of serum neuron-specific enolase in small cell carcinoma of the lung. Cancer Res 44:5409–5414, 1984
547. Ariyoshi Y, Kato K, Ishiguro Y, Ota K, Sato T, Suchi T: Evaluation of serum neuron-specific enolase as a tumor marker for carcinoma of the lung. Gann 74:219–225, 1983
548. Goslin RH, Skarin AT, Zamcheck N: Carcinoembryonic antigen: A useful monitor of therapy of small cell lung cancer. JAMA 246:2173–2176, 1981
549. Sculier JP, Feld R, Evans WK et al: Carcinoembryonic antigen: A useful prognostic marker in small cell lung cancer. J Clin Oncol 3:1349–1354, 1985
550. Woo KB, Waalkes P, Abeloff MD, Ettinger DS, McNutt KL, Gehrke CW: Multiple biologic markers in the monitoring of treatment for patients with small cell carcinoma of the lung: The use of serial levels of plasma CEA and serum carbohydrates. Cancer 48:1633–1642, 1981
551. Goslin RH, O'Brien MJ, Skarin AT, Zamcheck N: Immunocytochemical staining for CEA in small cell carcinoma of the lung predicts clinical usefulness of the plasma assay. Cancer 52:301–306, 1983
552. Graham EA, Singer JJ: Successful removal of an entire lung for carcinoma of the bronchus. JAMA 101:1371–1374, 1933
553. Carlson HA, Ballon HC: The operability of carcinoma of the lung. J Thorac Surg 2:323–340, 1933
554. Reinhoff WE Jr, Gannon J Jr, Sherman I: Closure of the bronchus following pneumonectomy. Ann Surg 116:481–531, 1942
555. Davis S, Wright PW, Schulman SF et al: Participants in prospective randomized trials for resected non small cell lung cancer have improved survival compared with nonparticipants in such trials. Cancer 56:1710–1718, 1985
556. Shields T, Higgins GA: Minimal pulmonary resection in the treatment of carcinomas of the lung. Arch Surg 108:420–422, 1974
557. Hildebrand PJ, Prakash D, Cosgrove J et al: High frequency ventilation: A method for thoracic surgery. Anaesthesia 39:1091–1095, 1984
558. Urschel HC, Razzuk MA: Median sternotomy as a standard approach for pulmonary resection. Ann Thorac Surg 41:130–134, 1986
559. Olivet RT, Nauss LA, Payne WS: A technique for continuous intercostal nerve block analgesia following thoracotomy. J Thorac Cardiovasc Surg 80:308–311, 1980
560. Danielson DR, Nauss LA: Post thoractomy analgesia. In Grillo HC, Eschapasse H (eds): International Trends in General Thoracic Surgery, Vol 2, pp 189–197. Philadelphia, WB Saunders, 1987
561. Vincent RG, Takita H, Lane WW et al: Surgical therapy of lung cancer. J Thorac Cardiovasc Surg 71:581–591, 1976
562. Fryjordet A, Klevmark B: Lung cancer. Scand J Thorac Cardiovasc Surg 5:92–102, 1971
563. Kirsh MM, Rotman H, Argenta L et al: Carcinoma of the lung: Results of treatment over 10 years. Ann Thorac Surg 21:371–377, 1976
564. Weiss W: Operative mortality and 5 year survival rates in men with bronchogenic carcinoma. Chest 66:483, 1974
565. Naruke T, Suemasu K, Ishikawa S: Lymph node mapping and curability at various levels of metastases in resected lung cancer. J Thorac Cardiovasc Surg 76:832–834, 1978
566. Nagasaki F, Flehinger BJ, Martini N: Complications of surgery in the treatment of carcinoma of the lung. Chest 82:25–29, 1982
567. Ginsberg RJ, Hill LD, Eagan RT et al: Modern thirty day operative mortality for surgical resection in lung cancer. J Thorac Cardiovasc Surg 86:654–658, 1983
568. Kohman LJ, Meyer JA, Ikins PM et al: Random versus predictable risks of mortality after thoracotomy for lung cancer. J Thorac Cardiovasc Surg 91:551–554, 1986
569. Steele JD: The solitary pulmonary nodule. J Thorac Cardiovasc Surg 46:21–39, 1963
570. Keagy BA, Starek PJ, Manay GF et al: Major pulmonary resection for suspected but unconfirmed malignancy. Ann Thorac Surg 38:314–316, 1984
571. Cortese DA, Pairolero PC, Bergstrahl EJ et al: Roentgenographically occult lung cancer. J Thorac Cardiovasc Surg 86:373–380, 1983
572. Gail MH, Eagan RT, Feld R et al: Prognostic factors in patients with resected Stage I non small cell lung cancer. Cancer 54:1802–1813, 1984
573. Martini N, Flehinger BJ, Nagasaki F et al: Prognostic significance of N1 disease in carcinoma of the lung. J Thorac Cardiovasc Surg 86:646–653, 1983
574. Kayser K, Bulzebruch H, Probst G et al: Retrospective and prospective tumor staging evaluating prognostic factors in operated bronchus carcinoma patients. Cancer 59:355–361, 1987
575. Iascone C, DeMeester TR, Albertucci M et al: Local recurrence of resectable non oat cell carcinoma of the lung. Cancer 57:471–476, 1986
576. Pariolero PC, Williams DE, Berstrahl EJ et al: Postsurgical Stage I bronchogenic carcinoma: Marked implications of recurrent disease. Ann Thorac Surg 38:331–338, 1984

577. Mountain CF: The biological operability of Stage II non small cell lung cancer. Ann Thorac Surg 40:60–64, 1985
578. DesLauriers J, Beaulieu M, Benuzera A et al: Sleeve pneumonectomy for bronchogenic carcinoma. Ann Thorac Surg 28:465–474, 1978
579. DesLauriers J: Discussion of survival in patients undergoing tracheal sleeve pneumonectomy for bronchogenic carcinoma. J Thorac Cardiovasc Surg 84:489–496, 1982
580. Jensik RJ, Faber LP, Kittle CF et al: Survival in patients undergoing tracheal sleeve pneumonectomy for bronchogenic carcinoma. J Thorac Cardiovasc Surg 84:489–496, 1982
581. Trastek FF, Pairolero PC, Piehler JM et al: En bloc (non chest wall) resection for bronchogenic carcinoma with parietal fixation. J Thorac Cardiovasc Surg 87:352–358, 1984
582. Piehler JM, Pairolero PC, Weiland LH et al: Bronchogenic carcinoma with chest wall invasion: Factors affecting survival following en bloc resection. Ann Thorac Surg 34:684–691, 1982
583. McCaughan BC, Martini N, Bains MS et al: Chest wall invasion in carcinoma of the lung. J Thorac Cardiovasc Surg 89:836–841, 1985
584. Kirsh MM, Prior M, Gago O et al: The effect of histological cell type on the prognosis of patients with bronchogenic carcinoma. Ann Thorac Surg 13:303–310, 1972
585. Abbey Smith R: The importance of mediastinal lymph node invasion by pulmonary carcinoma in selection of patients for resection. Ann Thorac Surg 25:5–11, 1978
586. Naruke T, Suemasu K, Ishikawa S: Lymph node mapping and curability of various levels of metastases in resected lung cancer. J Thorac Cardiovasc Surg 76:832–839, 1978
587. Pearson FG, Delarue NC, Ilves R et al: Significance of positive superior mediastinal nodes identified at mediastinoscopy in patients with resectable cancer of the lung. J Thorac Cardiovasc Surg 83:1–11, 1982
588. Martini N, Flehinger BJ, Zaman MB et al: Results of resection in non oat cell carcinoma of the lung with mediastinal lymph node metastases. Ann Surg 198:386–397, 1983
589. Naruke T: Staging of N2 disease. Chest 89:338S–339S, 1986
590. Pearson FG: Radical surgery for N2 disease. Chest 89:339S–340S, 1986
591. Bergh NP, Larsson S: The significance of various types of mediastinal lymph node metastases in lung cancer. In Jepsen O, Sorenson HR (eds): Mediastinoscopy: Proceedings of an International Symposium. Odense, Odense University Press, 1971
592. Martini N, Flehinger BJ, Zaman MB et al: Prospective study of 445 lung carcinomas with mediastinal lymph node metastases. J Thorac Cardiovasc Surg 80:390–399, 1980
593. Watanabe Y, Iwa T, Kobayashi H et al: Results of surgical treatment for lung cancer with N2 disease. Presented at the Third World Conference on Lung Cancer, Tokyo, Japan, 1982
594. Patterson GA, Pizza D, Pearson FG et al: Significance of metastatic disease in subaortic lymph nodes. Ann Thorac Surg 43:155–159, 1987
595. Bergh NP, Schersten I: Bronchogenic carcinoma: A follow up study of a surgically treated series with special references to prognostic significance of lymph node metastases. Acta Chir Scand (Suppl) 347:1–42, 1965
596. Larsson S: Pretreatment classification and staging of bronchogenic carcinoma. Scand J Thorac Cardiovasc Surg 7:1–130, 1973
597. Jensik RJ: The extent of resections for localized lung cancer: Segmental resection. In Kulle CF (ed): Current Controversies in Thoracic Surgery, pp 175–182. Philadelphia, WB Saunders, 1986
598. Errett LF, Wilson J, Chiu RC et al: Wedge resection as an alternative procedure for peripheral bronchogenic carcinoma in poor risk patients. J Thorac Cardiovasc Surg 90:656–661, 1985
599. McCormack PM, Martini N: Primary lung cancer: Results with conservative resection in treatment. NY State J Med 80:612–616, 1980
600. Ferguson MK, DeMeester TR, DesLauriers J et al: Diagnosis and management of synchronous lung cancers. J Thorac Cardiovasc Surg 90:378–385, 1985
601. Mathiesen DJ, Jensik RJ, Faber LP et al: Survival following resection for second and third primary lung cancers. J Thorac Cardiovasc Surg 88:502–510, 1984
602. Price Thomas C: Conservative resections of the bronchial tree. J Roy Coll Surg Edinburgh 1:169–171, 1956
603. Paulson DL, Shaw RR: Bronchial anastomosis and bronchoplastic procedures with interest of preservation of lung tissue. J Thorac Surg 29:238–259, 1955
604. Johnston JB, Jones PH: The treatment of bronchial carcinoma by lobectomy and sleeve resection of the main bronchus. Thorax 14:48–54, 1959
605. Weisel RD, Cooper JD, Dalarue NC et al: Sleeve lobectomy for carcinoma of the lung. J Thorac Cardiovasc Surg 78:839–849, 1979
606. Lowe JE, Bridgeman AH, Sabiston DC Jr et al: The role of bronchoplastic procedures in the surgical management of benign and malignant pulmonary lesions. J Thorac Cardiovasc Surg 83:227–234, 1982
607. Vogt Moykopf I, Toomes H, Heinrich ST: Sleeve resection of the bronchus and pulmonary artery for pulmonary lesions. Thorac Cardiovasc Surgeon 31:193–198, 1983
608. Eschapasse H, Gaillard J, Dahan M: Sleeve lobectomy for carcinoma of the lung. Chest 89:335S–336S, 1986
609. Bennett WF, Smith RA: A twenty year analysis of the results of sleeve resection for primary bronchogenic carcinoma. J Thorac Cardiovasc Surg 76:840–845, 1978
610. Kjaer M: Radiotherapy of squamous, adeno- and large cell carcinoma of the lung. Cancer Treat Rev 9:1–20, 1982
611. Cox JD, Byhardt RW, Komaki R: The role of radiotherapy in squamous, large cell, and adenocarcinoma of the lung. Semin Oncol 10:81–94, 1983
612. Choi NC: Curative radiation therapy of unresectable non-small-cell carcinoma of the lung: Indications, techniques, results, and Role of postoperative radiation therapy in lung cancer with either metastases to regional lymph nodes (N1 or unforeseen N2) or direct invasion beyond visceral pleura (T3). In Grillo H, Choi NC (eds): Thoracic Oncology, 163–199. New York, Raven Press, 1983
613. McNeil BJ, Weichselbaum RR, Parker SG: The fallacy of the five year survival in lung cancer. N Engl J Med 299:1397–1400, 1978
614. Hilton G: Present position relating to cancer of the lung: Results with radiotherapy alone. Thorax 15:17–18, 1960
615. Smart J: Can cancer of the lung be cured by radiation alone? JAMA 195:1034–1035, 1966
616. Cox JD, Komaki R, Byhardt RW: Is immediate chest radiotherapy obligatory for any or all patients with limited-stage non-small cell carcinoma of the lung? Yes. Cancer Treat Rep 67:327–331, 1983
617. Perez CA, Pajak TF, Rubin P et al: Long-term observations of the patterns of failure in patients with unresectable non-oat cell carcinoma of the lung treated with definitive radiotherapy: Report by the Radiation Therapy Oncology Group. Cancer 59:1874–1881, 1987
618. Salazar OM, Slawson RG, Poussin–Rosillo H, Amin PP, Sewchard W, Strohl RA: A prospective randomized trial comparing once-a-week vs daily radiation therapy for locally advanced, non-metastatic, lung cancer: A preliminary report. Int J Radiat Oncol Biol Phys 12:779–787, 1986
619. Kusumoto S, Koga K, Tsukino H, Nagamachi S, Nishikawa K, Watanabe K: Comparison of survival of patients with lung cancer between elderly (greater than or equal to 70) and younger age groups. Jpn J Clin Oncol 16:319–323, 1986
620. Katz HR, Alberts RW: A comparison of high-dose continuous and split-course irradiation in non-oat-cell carcinoma of the lung. Am J Clin Oncol 6:445–457, 1983
621. Holsti LR, Mattson K: A randomized study of split-course radiotherapy of lung cancer: Long term results. Int J Radiat Oncol Biol Phys 6:977–981, 1980
622. Caldwell WL, Bagshaw MA: Indications for and results of irradiation of carcinoma of the lung. Cancer 22:999–1004, 1968
623. Abramson N, Cavanaugh PJ: Short course radiation therapy in carcinoma of the lung: A second look. Radiology 108:685–687, 1973
624. Salazar OM, Rubin P, Brown JC et al: The assessment of tumor response to irradiation of the lung cancer. Int J Radiat Oncol Biol Phys 1:1107–1118, 1976
625. Eisert DR, Cox JD, Komaki R: Irradiation for bronchial carcinoma: Reasons for failure: Analysis of local control as a function of dose, time, and fractionation. Cancer 37:2665–2670, 1976
626. Salazar OM, Houtte V, Rubin P: Once-a-week irradiation for locally advanced lung cancer. Int J Radiat Oncol Biol Phys 9:923–930, 1983
627. Moss WT, Haddy FFJ, Sweany SK: Some factors altering the severity of acute radiation pneumonitis: Variation with cortisone, heparin, and antibiotics. Radiology 75:50–54, 1960
628. Stanley K, Cox JD, Petrovich Z et al: Patterns of failure in patients with inoperable carcinoma of the lung. Cancer 47:2725–2729, 1981
629. Shields TW: Treatment failures after surgical resection of thoracic tumors. Cancer Treat Symp 2:69–76, 1983
630. Alsner J. Forastiere A, Aroney R: Patterns of recurrence for cancer of the lung and esophagus. Cancer Treat Symp 2:87–105, 1983
631. Faber LP: Role of radiation and/or chemotherapy combined with surgery in advanced lung cancer. Presented at the 20th Postgraduate Program, Society of Thoracic Surgeons, 1986
632. Bromley LL, Szur L: Combined radiotherapy and resection of carcinoma of the bronchus: Experiences with 66 patients. Lancet 2:937–941, 1955
633. Bloedorn FG, Cowley RA, Cuccia CA et al: Combined therapy: Irradiation and surgery in the treatment of bronchogenic carcinoma. Am J Roentgenol Rad Ther Nucl Med 85:175–181, 1961
634. Perelman MI, Grigr'eva SP, Ivanov AN: [Surgical treatment of lung cancer after preoperative beta irradiation.] (Russ) Vopr Onkol 28:48–52, 1982
635. Klimenko AA, Kharchenko VP, Karibov I et al: [Fractionated operative irradiation in the combination therapy of lung cancer.] (Russ) Med Radiol (Mosk) 27:36–39, 1982
636. Paulson DL: Extended resection of bronchogenic carcinoma in the superior pulmonary sulcus. Surg Rounds 3:10–21, 1980
637. Grigr'eva SP, Ots ON: [Combined treatment of peripheral lung carcinoma.] (Russ) Vestn Rentgenol Radiol 4:80–85, 1980
638. Sherman DM, Neptune W, Weichselbaum RR et al: An aggressive approach to marginally resectable lung cancer. Cancer 41:2040–2045, 1978
639. Kirschner PA: Lung cancer: Preoperative radiation therapy and surgery. NY State J Med 81:339–342, 1981
640. Shields TW: Preoperative radiation therapy in the treatment of bronchial carcinoma. Cancer 30:1388–1393, 1972
641. Collaborative Study: Preoperative irradiation of cancer of the lung: Final report of a therapeutic trial. Cancer 36:914–925, 1975
642. Eichorn AJ, Eule H, Lessel A et al: Results of a controlled clinical trial for evaluation of intensive preoperative irradiation therapy for lung cancer. Arch Geschwulstforsch 45:376–380, 1975
643. Tildon TT, Hughes RK: Complications from preoperative irradiation therapy for lung cancer. Ann Thorac Surg 3:307–326, 1967
644. Kazen I, Jongerius CM, Lacquet LK et al: Evaluation of short course preoperative radiation in the treatment of resectable bronchus carcinoma: Long term analysis of a randomized pilot study. J Radiat Oncol Biol Phys 10:981–985, 1984
645. Paulson DL, Shaw RR, Kee JL et al: Combined preoperative irradiation and resec-

tion for bronchogenic carcinoma. J Thorac Cardiovasc Surg 44:281–294, 1962
646. Paulson DL: Carcinoma in the superior pulmonary sulcus. Ann Thorac Surg 28:3–4, 1979
647. Miller JI, Mansour KA, Hatcher CR: Carcinoma of the superior pulmonary sulcus. Ann Thorac Surg 28:44–47, 1979
648. Wright CD, Moneure AC, Shepherd JO et al: Superior sulcus lung tumors. J Thorac Cardiovasc Surg 94:69–74, 1987
649. Attar S, Miller JE, Satterfield J et al: Pancoast's tumor: Irradiation or surgery? Ann Thorac Surg 28:578–586, 1979
650. Stanford W, Barner RP, Tucker AR: Influence of staging in superior sulcus (Pancoast) tumors of the lung. Ann Thorac Surg 29:406–409, 1980
651. Shahian DM, Neptune WB, Ellis, FH: Pancoast tumors: Improved survival with pre and postoperative radiotherapy. Ann Thorac Surg 43:32–38, 1987
652. Komaki R, Roh J, Cox JD et al: Superior sulcus tumors: Results of irradiation in 36 patients. Cancer 48:1563–1568, 1981
653. Van Houtte P, MacLennon I, Poulter C, Rubin P: External radiation in the management of superior sulcus tumor. Cancer 54:223–227, 1984
654. Hilaris BS, Martini N, Batata M et al: Interstitial irradiation for unresectable carcinoma of the lung. Ann Thorac Surg 20:491–500, 1975
655. Martini N, Hilaris BS, Beattie EJ Jr: Interstitial vs. external irradiation combined with pulmonary resection in lung cancer. Cancer 26:638–641, 1970
656. Hilaris BS, Martini N: Interstitial brachytherapy in cancer of the lung: A 20 year experience. Int J Radiat Oncol Biol Phys 5:1951–1956, 1979
657. Hilaris BS, Nori D, Beattie EJ Jr, Martini N: Value of perioperative brachytherapy in the management of non oat cell carcinoma of the lung. Int J Radiat Oncol Biol Phys 9:1161–1166, 1983
658. Hilaris BS, Luomanen RK, Mahan DG, Henschke UK: Interstitial irradiation of apical lung cancer. Radiology 99:655–660, 1971
659. Hilaris BS, Martini N: Multimodality therapy of superior sulcus tumors. In Bonica JJ et al (eds): The Management of Lung Cancer, pp 113–122. New York, Raven Press, 1982
660. Hilaris BS, Gomez J, Dattatreyudu N et al: Combined surgery, intraoperative brachytherapy, and postoperative external radiation in Stage III non-small cell cancer. Cancer 55:1226–1231, 1985
661. Hilaris BS, Martini N, Luomanen RK: Endobronchial interstitial implantation. Clin Bull 9:17–20, 1979
662. Law MR, Henk JM, Goldstraw P et al: Bronchoscopic implantation of radioactive gold grains into endobronchial carcinomas. Br J Dis Chest 79:147–151, 1985
663. Tepper J, Sindelar W: Summary of the Workshop on Intraoperative Radiation Therapy. Cancer Treat Rep 65:911–930, 1981
664. Abe M, Yabumoto E, Takahashi M et al: Intraoperative radiotherapy of gastric cancer. Cancer 34:2034–2045, 1974
665. Wood WC, Shipley WU, Gunderson LL et al: Intraoperative irradiation for unresectable pancreatic carcinoma. Cancer 49:1271–1276, 1982
666. Cohen AM, Gunderson LL, Wood WC: Intraoperative electron beam radiation therapy boost in the treatment of recurrent rectal carcinoma. Dis Colon Rectum 23:453–458, 1980
667. Sindelar WF, Kinsella TJ, Tepper J et al: Experimental and clinical studies with intraoperative radiotherapy. Surg Gynecol Obstet 156:25–36, 1983
668. Pass HI, Sindelar WF, Kinsella T et al: Delivery of intraoperative radiation therapy after pneumonectomy: Experimental observations and early clinical results. Ann Thorac Surg 44:14–20, 1987
669. Van Houtte PV, Roemans P, Smets P et al: Postoperative radiation therapy in lung cancer: A controlled trial after resection of curative design. Int J Radiat Oncol Biol Phys 6:983–986, 1980
670. Green N, Kurohara SS, George FW III, Crews QE Jr: Postresection irradiation for primary lung cancer. Radiology 116:405–407, 1975
671. Kirsh MM, Rotman H, Argenta L et al: Carcinoma of the lung: Results of treatment over ten years. Ann Thorac Surg 21:371–377, 1976
672. Choi NCH, Grillo HC, Gardiello M, Scannell JG, Wilkins EW Jr: Basis for new strategies in postoperative radiotherapy of bronchogenic carcinoma. Int J Radiat Oncol Biol Phys 6:31–35, 1980
673. Cox JD: Non small cell lung cancer: Role of radiation therapy. Chest 89:284S–288S, 1986
674. Holmes EC: Surgical adjuvant therapy of non-small-cell lung cancer. Chest 89:295(s)–298(s), 1986
675. Lung Cancer Study Group: Effects of postoperative mediastinal radiation on completely resected Stage II and Stage III epidermoid cancer of the lung. N Engl J Med 315:1377–1381, 1986
676. Slack HH: Bronchogenic carcinoma: Nitrogen mustard as a surgical adjuvant and factors influencing survival: University Surgical Adjuvant Lung Cancer Project. Cancer 25:987–1002, 1970
677. Higgins GA, Humphrey EW, Hughes RA et al: Cytoxan as an adjuvant to surgery for lung cancer. Surg Oncol 1:211–228, 1969
678. Higgins GA, Shields TW: Experience of the Veterans Administration Surgical Adjuvant Group. Prog Cancer Res Ther 11:433–442, 1979
679. Shields TW, Higgins GW Jr, Humphrey EW, Matthews MJ, Keehn RJ: Prolonged intermittent adjuvant chemotherapy with CCNU and hydroxyurea after resection of carcinoma of the lung. Cancer 51:1713–1721, 1982
680. Pirogov AI, Trakhtenberg AK: Results and prospects of combined surgery and antitumor chemotherapy for lung cancer. Cancer Treat Rep 60:1489–1491, 1976
681. Wingfield HV: Combined surgery and chemotherapy for carcinoma of the bronchus. Lancet 1:470–471, 1970
682. Katsuki H, Shimada K, Koyama A et al: Long term intermittent adjuvant chemotherapy for primary, resected lung cancer. J Thorac Cardiovasc Surg 70:590–599, 1975
683. Crosbie WA, Kamdar HH, Belcher JR: A controlled trial of vinblastine sulphate in the treatment of cancer of the lung. Br J Dis Chest 60:28–35, 1986
684. Dolton EG: Combined surgery and chemotherapy for carcinoma of the bronchus. Lancet 1:40–41, 1970
685. Buyze EAC, Nelemans FA: A study of postoperative cytostatic medication in patients with operable carcinoma of the lung. Arzneimittelforschung 23:860–862, 1973
686. Brunner KW, Marthaler T, Muller W: Adjuvant chemotherapy with cyclophosphamide (NSC 26271) for radically resected bronchogenic carcinoma: 9 year follow up. Prog Cancer Res Ther 11:411–420, 1979
687. Stott H, Stephens WF, Roy DC: Five year follow up of cytotoxic chemotherapy as an adjuvant to surgery in carcinoma of the bronchus. Br J Cancer 34:167–173, 1976
688. Mountain CF, Vincent RG, Sealy R et al: A clinical trial of CCNU as surgical adjuvant treatment for patients with surgical Stage I and Stage II non small cell lung cancer: Preliminary findings. Prog Cancer Res Ther 11:421–431, 1979
689. Eagan RT, Ingle JN, Frytak S et al: Platinum based poly chemotherapy versus dianhydrogalactitol in advanced non-small cell lung cancer. Cancer Treat Rep 61:1339–1345, 1977
690. Ruckdeschel JC, Finkelstein DM, Ettinger DS: Chemotherapy of metastatic non small cell lung cancer (NSCLC): The Eastern Cooperative Group experience. Proc Fourth World Conference on Lung Cancer, p 39, 1985
691. Ruckdeschel JC, Finkelstein DM, Mason BA, Creech RH: Chemotherapy for metastatic non small cell bronchogenic carcinoma: EST 2575, generation V: A randomized comparison of four cisplatin-containing regimens. J Clin Oncol 3:72–79, 1985
692. Fram R, Skarin A, Balikian J et al: Combination chemotherapy followed by radiation therapy in patients with regional Stage III unresectable non small cell lung cancer. Cancer Treat Rep 69:587–590, 1985
693. Wagner H, Ruckdeschel J, Bonomi P et al: Treatment of locally advanced non small cell lung cancer (NSCLC) with mitomycin C, vinblastine, and cisplatin (MVP) followed by radiation therapy: An ECOG pilot study (abstract). Proc Am Soc Clin Oncol 4:183, 1985
694. Finkelstein DM, Ettinger DS, Ruckdeschel JC: Long term survivors in metastatic non small cell lung cancer: An Eastern Cooperative Group study. J Clin Oncol 4:702–709, 1986
695. Holmes EC, Gail M, Lung Cancer Study Group: Surgical adjuvant therapy for Stage II and Stage III adenocarcinoma and large-cell undifferentiated carcinoma. J Clin Oncol 4:710–715, 1986
696. Brouet D: Results of a trial using radiotherapy and chemotherapy in bronchial cancer. Eur J Cancer 4:437–445, 1968
697. Host H: Cyclophosphamide (NSC 26271) as an adjuvant to radiotherapy in the treatment of unresectable bronchogenic carcinoma. Cancer Chemother Rep 4:161–164, 1973
698. Kaung DT, Wolf J, Hyde L et al: Preliminary report on the treatment of nonresectable cancer of the lung. Cancer Chemother Rep 58:359–364, 1974
699. Holsti LR: Alternative approaches to radiotherapy alone and radiotherapy as part of a combined therapeutic approach for lung cancer. Cancer Chemother Rep 4:165–169, 1973
700. Hall TC, Dederick MM, Chalmers TC et al: A clinical pharmacologic study of chemotherapy and X-ray therapy in lung cancer. Am J Med 43:186–193, 1967
701. Benninghoff DL, Alexander LL: Treatment of lung carcinoma: Radiation versus radiation combined with 5-fluorouracil. NY State J Med 68(Pt 1):532–534, 1967
702. Krant MJ, Chalmers TC, Dederick MM et al: Comparative trial of chemotherapy and radiotherapy in patients with nonresectable cancer of the lung. Am J Med 35:363–373, 1963
703. Durrant KR, Ellis F, Black JM et al: Comparison of treatment policies in inoperable bronchial carcinoma. Lancet 1:715–719, 1971
704. Coy P: A randomized study of irradiation and vinblastine in lung cancer. Cancer 26:803–809, 1970
705. Hansen HH, Muggia FM, Andres R et al: Intensive combined chemotherapy and radiotherapy in patients with non-resectable bronchogenic carcinoma. Cancer 30:315–324, 1972
706. Samuels ML, Barkley HT Jr, Holoye PY et al: Combination chemotherapy with bleomycin (NSC 125066), vincristine (NSC 67574), and methotrexate (NSC 740), plus split course radiotherapy in the treatment of non oat cell bronchogenic carcinoma. Cancer Chemother Rep 59:377–383, 1975
707. Bitran JD, Desser RK, DeMeester T et al: Combined modality therapy for Stage III M0 non oat cell bronchogenic carcinoma. Cancer Treat Rep 62:327–332, 1978
708. Schultz HP, Overgaard M, Sell A: X ray therapy and combination chemotherapy in non small cell carcinoma of the lung: A pilot study. Abstracts Second World Conf Lung Cancer, Copenhagen, p 137. Amsterdam, Excerpta Medica, 1980
709. Bitran J, Golomb H, DeMeester T et al: Combined modality therapy for Stage II M0 non small cell bronchogenic carcinoma (abstract). Proc Am Assoc Cancer Res Am Soc Clin Oncol 21:446, 1980
710. Weshler Z, Sulkes A, Fuks Z et al: Combined modality treatment with radiation and chemotherapy in locally advanced bronchogenic carcinoma. Abstracts Second World Conf Lung Cancer, Copenhagen. Amsterdam, Excerpta Medica, 1980
711. Wils JA: Sequential combination chemotherapy and radiotherapy in metastatic non small cell cancer. Abstracts Second World Conf Lung Cancer, Copenhagen. Amsterdam, Excerpta Medica, 1980
712. Cox JD, Samson MK, Herskovic AM et al: Cisplatin and etoposide before definitive radiation therapy for inoperable carcinoma of the lung: A Phase II study of the RTOG. Cancer Treat Rep 70:1219–1220, 1986

713. Cullen MH, Latief TN, Spooner D et al: Cisplatin, etoposide, and radiotherapy in regional inoperable squamous cell carcinoma of the bronchus. Semin Oncol 12:14–16, 1985
714. Van Houtte P, Klastersky J, Nguyen H et al: Comparative randomized study of chest radiotherapy preceded or not by chemotherapy with cisplatin, etoposide and vindesine for the treatment of non small cell lung cancer (NSCLC) (abstract). Proc Am Assoc Cancer Res 25:795, 1984
715. Wils JA, Utama I, Naus A et al: Phase II randomized trial of radiotherapy alone vs the sequential use of chemotherapy and radiotherapy in Stage III non small cell lung cancer: Phase II trial of chemotherapy alone in Stage IV non small cell lung cancer. Eur J Cancer Clin Oncol 20:911–914, 1984
716. Newman SB, DeMeester TR, Golomb HM et al: The treatment of modified Stage II (T1N1M0, T2N1M0) non small cell bronchogenic carcinoma. J Thorac Cardiovasc Surg 86:180–185, 1983
717. Lung Cancer Study Group, Lad T, Rubinstein L, Sadeghi A: The benefit of adjuvant treatment for resected locally advanced non-small-cell lung cancer. J Clin Oncol 6:9–17, 1988
718. Bonomi P: Brief overview of combination chemotherapy in non small cell lung cancer. Semin Oncol 13:89–90, 1986
719. Martini N, Kris MG, Gralla RJ et al: The effects of preoperative chemotherapy on the resectability of non small cell lung carcinoma with mediastinal lymph node metastases (N2M0)(abstract). Proc Soc Thorac Surg 23:28, 1987
720. Taylor SG, Trybula M, Bonomi PD et al: Simultaneous cisplatin, fluorouracil infusion and radiation followed by surgical resection in regionally localized Stage III, non-small cell lung carcinoma. Ann Thorac Surg 43:87–91, 1987
721. Bitran JD, Golomb HM, Hoffman PC et al: Protochemotherapy in non small cell lung carcinoma. Cancer 57:44–53, 1986
722. Raul Y, Hui N, Claver J et al: Surgery and chemotherapy: A new method of treatment for squamous cell bronchial carcinoma. J Thorac Cardiovasc Surg 88:754–757, 1984
723. Fuller BL, Bonomi P, Reddy SG et al: Cisplatin and mitomycin C preceding local therapy in squamous cell bronchogenic carcinoma (abstract). Proc Am Soc Clin Oncol 1C:560, 1982
724. Israel L, Aquillera J, Breau JL: Potency of continuous infusion over 5 or 6 days of cis platinum and bleomycin on squamous cell carcinoma of the lung. Exerpta Medica Int Congr Ser 558:323, 1982
725. Skarin A, Veeder M, Malcolm A: Chemotherapy (CAP) prior to radiotherapy and surgery in marginally resectable non small cell lung cancer (NSCLC)(abstract). Proc Am Soc Clin Oncol 1C:544, 1982
726. Takita H, Edgerton F, Conway D et al: Reductive surgery of inoperable lung carcinoma (abstract). Proc Am Assoc Cancer Res 21:459, 1980
727. Hellekant C: Bronchial arteriography and intraarterial chemotherapy in bronchogenic carcinoma. Radiologe 19:521–524, 1979
728. Neyazaki T, Suzuki C: Bronchial artery infusion therapy for lung cancer in man. Panminerva Med 13:305–310, 1971
729. Strauss G, Sherman D, Schwartz J et al: Combined modality therapy for regionally advanced Stage III non small cell carcinoma of the lung (NSCLC) employing neoadjuvant chemotherapy (CT), radiotherapy (RT) and surgery (S) (abstract). Proc Fifth Int Conf Adjuvant Ther Cancer, March 1987, p 81
730. Sridhar SK, Thurer RJ, Raskin N, Beattie EJ: Multimodality treatment of non small cell lung cancer: Response to cisplatin, etoposide and 5 FU chemotherapy, surgery and radiation therapy (abstract). Proc Fifth Int Conf Adjuvant Ther Cancer, March 1987, p 81
731. Gralla RJ, Kris MG, Burke MT, Martini N: Adjuvant chemotherapy in non small cell cancer (abstract). Fifth Int Conf Adjuvant Ther Cancer, March 1987, p 36
732. Spain R, Jost J, Kircher T: Neoadjuvant mitomycin (M), cisplatin (P), and vinblastine (V) infusion (MPV) for Stage III limited, initially unresectable non small cell lung cancer (NSCLC): An analysis at 37+ month median follow up (abstract). Proc Fifth Int Conf Adjuvant Ther Cancer, March 1987, p 38
733. Klasterksy J, Sculier JP, Ravez P et al: A randomized study comparing a high and a standard dose of cisplatin in combination with etoposide in the treatment of advanced non-small cell lung carcinoma. J Clin Oncol 4:1780–1786, 1986
734. Klastersky J: Therapy with cisplatin and etoposide for non-small cell lung cancer. Semin Oncol 13:104–114, 1986
735. Dhingra HM, Valdivieso M, Booser DJ et al: Chemotherapy for advanced adenocarcinoma and squamous cell carcinoma of the lung with etoposide and cisplatin. Cancer Treat Rep 68:671–673, 1984
736. Goldhirsch A, Joss RA, Cavalli F et al: Cis-chlorodiaminepaltinum(II) and VP16 213 combination chemotherapy for non small cell lung cancer. Med Pediatr Oncol 9:205–208, 1981
737. Joss RA, Alberto P, Olbrecht JP et al: Combination chemotherapy for non small cell lung cancer with doxorubicin and mitomycin or cisplatin and etoposide. Cancer Treat Rep 68:1079–1084, 1984
738. Giaccone G, Musella R, Bertetto O et al: DDP VP16 combination chemotherapy in unresectable non small cell lung cancer (abstract). Proc Thirteenth Int Congr Chemother, Vienna, 1983
739. Scagliotti G, Lodico D, Gozzelino F: Clinical trial with high dose cisplatin and VP 16 213 in advanced non small cell lung cancer: Results after two years (abstract). Proc Thirteenth Int Congr Chemother, Vienna, 1983
740. Veronesi A, Zagonel V, Sanatarossa M et al: Cisplatinum and etoposide combination chemotherapy of advanced non oat cell bronchogenic carcinoma. Cancer Chemother Pharmacol 11:35–37, 1983
741. Rinaldi M, Venturo J, Tonachella R et al: Chemotherapy with DDP and VP16 213 in non small cell lung cancer: Results and toxicity (abstract). Proc Thirteenth Int Congr Chemother, Vienna, 1983
742. Mitrou PS, Graubner M, Berdel WE et al: Cisplatinum (DDP) and VP16 213 (etoposide) combination chemotherapy for advanced non small cell lung cancer: A Phase II clinical trial. Eur J Clin Oncol 20:347–351, 1984
743. Holsti LR, Mattson K, Grohn P et al: Cis platinum plus vindesine versus VP16 in combination with radiotherapy in the treatment of non small cell carcinoma of the lung (abstract). Proc World Conf Lung Cancer, Tokyo, 1982
744. Paccagnella A, Fiorentino MV, Brandes A et al: Cis platin (DDP) plus vindesine (VDS) versus DDP plus VP16 213 (VP) versus doxorubicin (DXR) plus Cytoxan (CTX): A randomized study in advanced non small cell carcinoma of the lung (NSCLC)(abstract). Proc Thirteenth Int Congr Chemother, Vienna, 1983
745. Martini N, Flehinger BJ, Nagasaki F, Hart B: Prognostic significance of N1 disease in carcinoma of the lung. J Thorac Cardiovasc Surg 86:646–653, 1983
746. Shields TW, Higgins GA Jr, Matthews MJ, Kühn RJ: Surgical resection in the management of small cell carcinoma of the lung. J Thorac Cardiovasc Surg 84:481–488, 1982
747. Komaki R, Cox JD, Stark R: Frequency of brain metastases in adenocarcinoma and large cell carcinoma of the lung: Correlation with survival. Int J Radiat Oncol Biol Phys 9:1467–1470, 1983
748. Cox JD, Stanley K, Petrovich Z et al: Cranial irradiation in cancer of the lung of all cell types. JAMA 245:469–472, 1981
749. Jacobs RH, Awan A, Bitran JD et al: Prophylactic cranial irradiation in adenocarcinoma of the lung: A possible role. Cancer 59:2016–2019, 1987
750. Johnson BE, Ihde DC, Lichter AS et al: Five to 10 year follow-up of small cell lung cancer (SCLC) patients disease free at 30 months: Chronic toxicities and late relapses (abstract). Proc Am Soc Clin Oncol 3:218, 1984
751. Looper JD, Einhorn LH, Garcia SA, Hornbach NB, Vincent B, Williams SD: Severe neurologic problems following successful therapy for small cell lung cancer (abstract). Proc Am Soc Clin Oncol 2:231, 1984
752. DeCaro L, Benfield JR: Lung cancer in young persons. J Thorac Cardiovasc Surg 83:372–376, 1982
753. Hartman GE, Shochart SJ: Primary pulmonary neoplasms of childhood: A review. Ann Thorac Surg 36:108–119, 1983
754. Hyde L, Wolf J, McCracken S et al: Natural course of inoperable lung cancer. Chest 64:309–312, 1973
755. Brashea RE: Should asymptomatic patients with inoperable bronchogenic carcinoma receive immediate radiotherapy? Am Rev Respir Dis 117:411–414, 1978
756. Phillips TL, Miller RJ: Should asymptomatic patients with inoperable bronchogenic carcinoma receive immediate radiotherapy? Yes. Am Rev Respir Dis 117:405–410, 1978
757. Carroll M, Morgan SA, Yarnold JR, Hill JM, Wright NM: Prospective evaluation of a watch policy in patients with inoperable non-small cell lung cancer. Eur J Cancer Clin Oncol 22:1353–1356, 1986
758. Slawson RG, Scott RM: Radiation therapy in bronchogenic carcinoma. Radiology 132:175–176, 1979
759. Perez CA, Presant CA, Van Ambury AL: Management of superior vena cava syndrome. Semin Oncol 5:123–134, 1978
760. Armstrong BA, Perez CA, Simpson JR, Hederman MA: Role of irradiation in the malignancy of superior vena cava syndrome. Int J Radiat Oncol Biol Phys 13:531–539, 1987
761. Katz RJ, Simms EB, DiBianco R et al: Pericardial tamponade in lung cancer: Diagnosis, management and response to treatment. (unpublished)
762. Majid OA, Lee S, Khushalani S, Seydel HG: The response of atelectasis from lung cancer to radiation therapy. Int J Radiat Oncol Biol Phys 12:231–232, 1986
763. Borgelt B, Gelber R, Kramer S et al: The palliation of brain metastases: Final results of the first two studies by the Radiation Therapy Oncology Group. Int J Radiat Oncol Biol Phys 6:1–9, 1980
764. Deviri E, Schachner A, Halevy A, Shalit M, Levy MJ: Carcinoma of lung with a solitary cerebral metastasis: Surgical management and review of the literature. Cancer 52:1507–1509, 1983
765. Sundaresan N, Galicich JH, Beattie EJ Jr: Surgical treatment of brain metastases from lung cancer. J Neurosurg 58:666–671, 1983
766. Hendrickson FR, Lee MS, Larson M, Gelber RD: The influence of surgery and radiation therapy on patients with brain metastases. Int J Radiat Oncol Biol Phys 9:623–627, 1983
767. Patchell RA, Cirrincione C, Thaler HT, Galicich JH, Kim JH, Posner JB: Single brain metastases: Surgery plus radiation or radiation alone. Neurology 36:447–453, 1986
768. Bruckman JE, Bloomer WD: Management of spinal cord compression. Semin Oncol 5:135–140, 1978
769. Raichle ME, Posner JB: The treatment of extradural spinal cord compression. Neurology 20:391–396, 1970
770. Gilbert RW, Kim JH, Posner JB: Epidural spinal cord compression from metastatic tumor: Diagnosis and treatment. Ann Neurol 3:40–51, 1978
771. Thomas JE, Colby MY Jr: Radiation-induced or metastatic brachial plexopathy? A diagnostic dilemma. JAMA 222:1392–1395, 1972
772. Mulshine J, Ruckdeschel JC: The role of chemotherapy in the management of disseminated non-small cell lung cancer. Roth JA, Ruckdeschel JC, Weisenburger TH (eds): Thoracic Oncology, 220–228. Philadelphia: WB Saunders, 1989
773. Hansen HH: Advanced non-small-cell lung cancer: To treat or not to treat? J Clin Oncol 5:1711–1712, 1987
774. Gralla RJ: Issues and agents in the chemotherapy of non-small-cell lung cancer.

Mediguide Oncol 5:1–5, 1985
775. O'Connell JP, Kris MG, Gralla RJ et al: Frequency and prognostic importance of pretreatment clinical characteristics in patients with advanced non-small-cell lung cancer treated with combination chemotherapy. J Clin Oncol 4:1604–1614, 1986
776. Kris M, Cohen E, Gralla R: An analysis of 134 Phase II trials in non-small cell lung cancer (NSCLC)(abstract). Proc Fourth World Conf Lung Cancer, Toronto, 1985
777. Joss RA, Cavalli F, Goldhirsch A et al: New agents in non-small cell lung cancer. Cancer Treat Rev 11:205–237, 1984
778. Babowski MT, Creech JC: Chemotherapy of non-small cell lung cancer: A reappraisal and look at the future. Cancer Treat Rev 10:159–172, 1983
779. Sakurai M, Saijo N, Shinkai T et al: The protective effect of 2-mercapto-ethane sulfonate (mesna) on hemorrhagic cystitis induced by high-dose ifosfamide treatment tested by a randomized crossover trial. Jpn J Clin Oncol 16:153–156, 1986
780. Bonomi P, Mehta C, Ruckdeschel J, Blum R, Mason B, Greene M: Phase II–III trial of mitomycin–vinblastine–cisplatin (MVP): vinblastine–cisplatin (VP); MVP alternating with cyclophosphamide–Adriamycin–methotrexate–procarbazine (MVP/CAMP); CBDCA followed by MVP; and CHIP followed by MVP in patients with metastatic non-small cell lung cancer (NSCLC): An ECOG study (abstract). Proc Am Soc Clin Oncol 6:A699, 1987
781. Shum KY, Kris MG, Gralla RJ et al: 10-ethyl-10 deaza-aminopterin (10-EDAM) in patients with non-small cell lung cancer (NSCLC): Trial of an active new agent (abstract). Proc Am Soc Clin Oncol 6:A698, 1987
782. Maroun J, Wiernik P, DeConti R et al: Phase 2 efficacy of trimetrexate (CI-898; TMTX) in patients (pts) with non-small cell lung cancer (NSCLC) (abstract). Proc Am Soc Clin Oncol 6:A669, 1987
783. Egan RT, Frytak S, Creagan ET, Richardson RL, Coles DT, Jett JR: Differing response rates and survival between squamous and non-squamous non-small cell lung cancer: Comparison of CAP versus MAP. Am J Clin Oncol 9:249–254, 1986
784. Bitran JD, Desser RK, DeMeester TR et al: Cyclophosphamide, Adriamycin, methotrexate, and procarbazine (CAMP): Effective four drug combination chemotherapy for metastatic non oat cell bronchogenic carcinoma. Cancer Treat Rep 60:1225–1230, 1976
785. Chahinian AP, Arnold DJ, Cohen JM et al: Chemotherapy for bronchogenic carcinoma: Methotrexate, doxorubicin, cyclophosphamide, and lomustine. JAMA 237:2392–2396, 1977
786. Vogl SE, Hemta CR, Cohen MH: MACC chemotherapy for adenocarcinoma and epidermoid carcinoma of the lung. Cancer 44:864–868, 1979
787. Eagan RT, Ingle JN, Frytak S et al: Platinum based poly chemotherapy versus dianhydrogalactictol in advanced non-small cell lung cancer. Cancer Treat Rep 61:1339–1345, 1977
788. Gralla RJ, Casper ES, Kelson DP et al: Cisplatin and vindesine combination chemotherapy for advanced carcinoma of the lung: A randomized trial investigating two dosage schedules. Ann Intern Med 95:414–420, 1981
789. Longeval E, Klastersky J: Combination chemotherapy with cisplatin and etoposide in bronchogenic squamous cell carcinoma and adenocarcinoma: A study for the EORTC Lung Cancer Working Party (Belgium). Cancer 50:2751–2756, 1982
790. Mason BA, Catalano RB: Mitomycin, vinblastine, and cisplatin combination chemotherapy in non small cell lung cancer (abstract). Proc Am Soc Clin Oncol 21:477, 1980
791. Elliot JA, Ahmedozcie S, Hole D et al: Vindesine and cisplatin combination chemotherapy compared with vindesine as a single agent in the management of non-small cell lung cancer: A randomized study. Eur J Cancer Clin Oncol 20:1025–1032, 1984
792. Crino L, Tonato M, Darwish S et al: A randomized trial of three cisplatin (CDDP)-containing chemotherapy regimens in advanced non-small cell lung cancer (NSCLC): A study of the Umbrian Lung Cancer Group (abstract). Proc Am Soc Clin Oncol 6:A716, 1987
793. Rosso R, Salvati F, Ardizzoni A et al: Etoposide (E) vs E plus cisplatin (P) in the treatment of advanced non small cell lung cancer (NSCLC): A FONICAP randomized trial (abstract). Proc Am Soc Clin Oncol 6:A732, 1987
794. Luedke DW, Sarma PR, Greco FA, Birch R, Prestridge K: Preliminary report of a randomized trial of vindesin (V) as V with mitomycin (M) or with cisplatin (C) in non-small cell lung cancer (NSCLC)(abstract). Proc Am Soc Clin Oncol 6:A670, 1987
795. Einhorn LH, Loehrer PJ, Williams SD et al: Random prospective study of vindesine versus vindesine plus high-dose cisplatin versus vindesine plus cisplatin plus mitomycin C in advanced non-small-cell lung cancer. J Clin Oncol 4:1037–1043, 1986
796. Woods RL, Levi JA, Page J et al: Non small cell cancer: A randomized comparison of chemotherapy with no chemotherapy (abstract). Proc Am Soc Clin Oncol 4:177, 1985
797. Rapp E, Pater J, Willan A et al: A comparison of best supportive care to two regimens of combination chemotherapy in the management of advanced non-small cell lung cancer (NSCLC): A report of a Canadian multicentre trial (abstract). Proc Am Soc Clin Oncol 6:168, 1987
798. Ganz PA, Giflin RA, Haskell CM et al: Supportive care (SC) vs supportive care plus chemotherapy (SCC) in advanced metastatic lung cancer: Response, survival, and quality of life (abstract). Proc Am Soc Clin Oncol 6:171, 1987
799. Gralla RJ, Casper ES, Kelsen DP et al: Cisplatin and vindesine combination chemotherapy for advanced carcinoma of the lung: A randomized trial investigating two dosage schedules. Ann Intern Med 95:414–420, 1981
800. Mitrou PS, Fischer M, Weissenfels I et al: Treatment of inoperable non-small-cell bronchogenic carcinoma with etoposide and cis-platinum. Cancer Treat Rep 9(Suppl A):139–142, 1982
801. Focan C, Le Hung S, Frere MH, Schallier D: Ambulatory combination chemotherapy with oral etoposide and cisplatin for advanced non small cell lung carcinoma patients: A Phase II study. Anticancer Res 6:977–981, 1986
802. Gandara DR, DeGregorio MW, Wold H et al: High-dose cisplatin in hypertonic saline: Reduced toxicity of a modified dose schedule and correlation with plasma pharmacokinetics: A Northern California Oncology Group pilot study in non-small-cell lung cancer. J Clin Oncol 4:1787–1793, 1986
803. Klastersky J, Sculier JP, Ravez P et al: A randomized study comparing a high and a standard dose of cisplatin in combination with etoposide in the treatment of advanced non-small-cell lung carcinoma. J Clin Oncol 4:1780–1786, 1986
804. Stampleman LV, Kris MG, Gralla RJ et al: Complete response (CR) in Stage III and IV non-small cell lung cancer (NSCLC) with chemotherapy (chemo) or chemotherapy plus surgery: An analysis of treatment in 554 patients (abstract). Proc Am Soc Clin Oncol 6:A696, 1987
805. Ruckdeschel JC, Finkelstein DM, Ettinger DS et al: A randomized trial of the four most active regimens for metastatic non-small cell lung cancer. J Clin Oncol 4:14–22, 1986
806. Fuks JZ, Patel H, Hornedo J, Van Echo DA, Moody M, Aisner J: Infections in patients with non-small-cell lung cancer treated with intensive induction chemotherapy. Med Pediatr Oncol 14:255–261, 1986
807. Bakker W, van Oosterom AT, Aaronson NK et al: Vindesine, cisplatin, and bleomycin combination chemotherapy in non-small cell lung cancer: Survival and quality of life. Eur J Cancer Clin Oncol 22:963–970, 1986
808. Chang AY, Kuebler JP, Pandya KJ et al: Pulmonary toxicity induced by mitomycin C is highly responsive to glucocorticoids. Cancer 57:2285–2290, 1986
809. Mackillop WJ, Ward GK, O'Sullivan B: The use of expert surrogates to evaluate clinical trials in non-small cell lung cancer. Br J Cancer 54:661–667, 1986
810. Mackillop WJ, O'Sullivan B, Ward GK: Non-small cell lung cancer: How oncologists want to be treated. Int J Radiat Oncol Biol Phys 13:929–934, 1987
811. Breau JL, Morere JF, Israel L: Response rates and survival for 268 unresectable epidermoid lung carcinoma patients treated with a cisplatin bleomycin based chemotherapy (abstract). Proc Am Soc Clin Oncol 6:A703, 1987
812. Taylor SG, Trybula M, Bonomi PD et al: Simultaneous cisplatin fluorouracil infusion and radiation followed by surgical resection in regionally localized Stage III non-small cell lung cancer. Ann Thorac Surg 43:87–91, 1987
813. Minet P, Bartsch P, Chevalier P et al: Quality of life of inoperable non-small cell lung carcinoma: A randomized Phase II clinical study comparing radiotherapy alone and combined radiochemotherapy. Radiother Oncol 8:217–230, 1987
814. Omenn GS, Goodman G, Rosenstock L et al: Cancer chemoprevention with vitamin A and beta-carotene in populations at high risk for lung cancer. In Nygaard OF, Simic M, Cerutti P (eds): Anticarcinogenesis and Radiation Protection. New York, Plenum Publishing, 1988
815. Pastorino U, deVries N, van Zandwijk N (coordinators): EUROSCAN (EORTC 24871, EORTC 08871) study on screening and chemoprevention with vitamin A and or N-acetylcysteine. EORTC Data Center, 125 Boulevard de Waterloo, 1000 Brussels, Belgium. Published October 1987
816. Grunberg SM, Itri L: Treatment of advanced non-small cell lung cancer with 13-cis-retinoic acid (abstract). Proc Fifth Int Conf Adjuvant Ther Cancer, March 1987, p 79
817. Uphouse W, Oishi N, Bernenberg J et al: Treatment of advanced non-small cell lung cancer with 13-cis retinoic acid (abstract). Proc Am Soc Clin Oncol 6:A712, 1987
818. Simpson JR, Bauer M, Wasserman TH et al: Large fraction irradiation with or without misonidazole in advanced non-oat cell carcinoma of the lung: A Phase II randomized trial of the RTOG (Radiation Therapy Oncology Group). Int J Radiat Oncol Biol Phys 13:861–867, 1987
819. Carlson RW, Coleman CN, Kohler M, Gribble MJ, Halsey J: A randomized Phase II study of L-PAM versus L-PAM + the chemosensitizer misonidazole (MISO) for non-small cell lung cancer (NSCLC): A Northern California Oncology Group study (abstract). Proc Am Soc Clin Oncol 6:A106, 1987
820. Chlebowski RT, Bulcavage L, Grosvenor M et al: Influence of hydrazine sulfate on survival in non-small cell lung cancer: A randomized, placebo-controlled trial (abstract). Proc Am Soc Clin Oncol 6:688, 1987
821. Tayek JA, Heber D, Chlebowski RT: Effect of hydrazine sulphate on whole-body protein breakdown measured by ^{14}C-lysine metabolism in lung cancer patients. Lancet 2:241–244, 1987
822. Evans WK, Nixon DW, Daly JM et al: A randomized study of oral nutritional support versus ad lib nutritional intake during chemotherapy for advanced colorectal and non-small-cell lung cancer. J Clin Oncol 5:113–124, 1987
823. Zacharski LR, Moritz TE, Baczek LA et al: Effect of RA-233 (Mopidamol) on survival in carcinoma of the lung and colon: Final report of Veterans Administration Cooperative Study No. 188. JNCI 80:90–96, 1988
824. Livingston RB: Mopidamol in non-small cell lung cancer: Antioncogene or accident? JNCI 80:77–78, 1988
825. Ludwig Lung Cancer Study Group: Intrapleural and intravenous Corynebacterium parvum in patients with resected Stage I and II non-small cell carcinoma of the lung. Cancer Immunol Immunother 23:1–4, 1986
826. Ludwig Lung Cancer Study Group: Immunostimulation with intrapleural BCG as adjuvant therapy in resected non-small cell lung cancer. Cancer 58:2411–2416, 1986
827. Bakker W, Nijhuis–Heddes JM, van der Velde EA: Post-operative intrapleural BCG in lung cancer: A 5-year follow-up report. Cancer Immunol Immunother 22:155–159, 1986
828. Watanabe Y, Iwa T: Clinical value of immunotherapy with the streptococcal prepara-

tion of OK-432 in non-small cell lung cancer. J Biol Response Modif 6:169–180, 1987

829. Weissler JC, Nicod LP, Toews GB: Pulmonary natural killer cell activity is reduced in patients with bronchogenic carcinoma. Am Rev Respir Dis 135:1353–1357, 1987
830. Kradin RL, Boyle LA, Preffer FI et al: Tumor-derived interleukin-2-dependent lymphocytes in adoptive immunotherapy of lung cancer. Cancer Immunol Immunother 24:76–85, 1987
831. Yasumoto K, Mivazaki K, Nagashima A et al: Induction of lymphokine-activated killer cells by intrapleural instillations of recombinant interleukin-2 in patients with malignant pleurisy due to lung cancer. Cancer Res 47:2184–2187, 1987
832. Gelb AF, Epstein JD: Neodymium-yttrium–aluminum–garnet laser in lung cancer. Ann Thorac Surg 43:164–167, 1987
833. Brutinel WM, Cortese DA, McDougall JC, Gillio RG, Bergstrahl EJ: A two-year experience with the neodymium–YAG laser in endobronchial obstruction. Chest 8:159–165, 1987
834. Edell ES, Cortese DA: Bronchoscopic phototherapy with hematoporphyrin derivative for treatment of localized bronchogenic carcinoma: A 5-year experience. Mayo Clin Proc 62:8–14, 1987
835. Watson PN, Evans RJ: Intractable pain with lung cancer. Pain 29:163–173, 1987
836. Morstyn G, Ihde DC, Lichter AS et al: Small cell lung cancer 1973–1983: Early prognosis and recent obstacles. Int J Radiat Oncol Biol Phys 10:515–539, 1984
837. Matthews MJ, Kanhouwa S, Pickner J et al: Frequency of residual and metastatic tumors in patients undergoing curative surgical resection of lung cancer. Cancer Chemother Rep 3:63–67, 1973
838. Hansen HH, Dombernowsky P, Hirsch FR: Staging procedures and prognostic features in small cell anaplastic bronchogenic carcinoma. Semin Oncol 5:280–287, 1978
839. Østerlind K, Ihde DC, Ettinger DS et al: Staging and prognostic factors in small cell carcinoma of the lung. Cancer Treat Rep 67:3–9, 1983
840. Matthews MJ: Problems in morphology and behavior of bronchopulmonary malignant diseases. In Israel L, Chahinian AP (eds): Lung Cancer: Natural History, Prognosis, and Therapy, pp 23–62. New York, Academic Press, 1976
841. Fox W, Scadding JG: Medical Research Council comparative trial of surgery and radiotherapy for primary treatment of small-celled or oat-celled carcinoma of bronchus: Ten-year follow-up. Lancet 2:63–65, 1973
842. Mountain CF: Clinical biology of small cell carcinoma: Relationship to surgical therapy. Semin Oncol 5:272–279, 1978
843. Green RA, Humphrey E, Close H et al: Alkylating agents in bronchogenic carcinoma. Am J Med 46:516–525, 1969
844. Greco FA, Einhorn LH: Small cell lung cancer. Semin Oncol 5:233–235, 1978
845. Johnson DH, Greco FA: Small cell carcinoma of the lung. CRC Crit Rev Oncol/Hematol 4:303–336, 1986
846. Seifter EJ, Ihde DC: Therapy of small cell lung cancer: A perspective on two decades of clinical research. Semin Oncol 15:278–299, 1988
847. Aisner J, Alberto P, Bitran J et al: Role of chemotherapy in small cell lung cancer: A consensus report of the International Association for the Study of Lung Cancer workshop. Cancer Treat Rep 67:37–43, 1983
848. Livingston RB: Small cell carcinoma of the lung. Blood 56:575–584, 1980
849. Comis RL: Small cell carcinoma of the lung. Cancer Treat Rev 9:237–258, 1982
850. Bunn PA Jr, Ihde DC: Small cell bronchogenic carcinoma: A review of therapeutic results. Cancer Treat Res 1:169–208, 1981
851. Ihde DC, Bunn PA Jr: Chemotherapy of small cell bronchogenic carcinoma. In Whitehouse JMA, Williams CJ (eds): Recent Advances in Clinical Oncology, vol 1, pp 305–323. Edinburgh, Churchill Livingstone 1982
852. Dombernowsky P, Hansen HH, Sorenson PG et al: Vincristine in the treatment of small cell anaplastic carcinoma of the lung. Cancer Treat Rep 60:239–242, 1976
852. Cavalli F, Sonntag R, Jungl F et al: VP-16-213 monotherapy for remission induction of small cell lung cancer: A randomized trial using three dosage schedules. Cancer Treat Rep 62:473–475, 1978
854. Mead GM, Thompson J, Sweetenham JW et al: Extensive stage small cell carcinoma of the bronchus: A randomized study of etoposide given orally by one-day or five-day schedule together with intravenous Adriamycin and cyclophosphamide. Cancer Chemother Pharmacol 19:172–174, 1987
855. Issell BF, Einhorn LH, Comis RL et al: Multicenter Phase II trial of etoposide in previously treated small cell carcinoma of the lung. Cancer Treat Rep 69:127–128, 1985
856. Bork E, Hansen M, Dombernowsky P et al: Teniposide (VM-26), an overlooked highly active agent in small cell lung cancer: Results of a Phase II trial in untreated patients. J Clin Oncol 4:524–527, 1986
857. Wolff SN, Birch R, Sarma P et al: Randomized dose–response evaluation of etoposide in small cell carcinoma of the lung. Cancer Treat Rep 70:583–587, 1986
858. Joss RA, Cavalli F, Goldhirsch A et al: New drugs in small cell lung cancer. Cancer Treat Rev 13:157–176, 1986
859. Smith IE, Harland SJ, Robinson BA et al: Carboplatin: A very active new cisplatin analog in the treatment of small cell lung cancer. Cancer Treat Rep 69:43–46, 1985
860. Aisner J: Identification of new drugs in small cell lung cancer: Phase II agents first? Cancer Treat Rep 71:1131–1133, 1987
861. Cullen M, Smith SR, Benfield GFA et al: Testing new drugs in untreated small cell lung cancer may prejudice the results of standard treatment: A Phase II study of oral idarubicin in extensive disease. Cancer Treat Rep 71:1227–1230, 1087
862. Malik STA, Rayner H, Fletcher J et al: Phase II trial of mitoxantrone as first-line chemotherapy for extensive small cell lung cancer. Cancer Treat Rep 71:1291–1292, 1987
863. Broder LE, Cohen MH, Selawry OS: Treatment of bronchogenic carcinoma II: Small cell cancer. Cancer Treat Rev 4:219–260, 1977
864. Edmonson JH, Lagako SW, Selawry OS et al: Cyclophosphamide and CCNU in the treatment of inoperable small cell carcinoma and adenocarcinoma of the lung. Cancer Treat Rep 60:925–932, 1976
865. Alberto P, Brunner KW, Martz G et al: Treatment of bronchogenic carcinoma with simultaneous or sequential combination chemotherapy, including methotrexate, cyclophosphamide, procarbazine, and vincristine. Cancer 38:2208–2216, 1976
866. Cohen MH, Creaven PJ, Fossieck BE et al: Intensive chemotherapy of small cell bronchogenic carcinoma. Cancer Treat Rep 61:349–354, 1977
867. Hansen HH, Selawry OS, Simon R et al: Combination chemotherapy of advanced lung cancer: A randomized trial. Cancer 38:2201–2207, 1976
868. Souhami RL, Finn G, Gregory WM et al: High-dose cyclophosphamide in small cell carcinoma of the lung. J Clin Oncol 3:958–963, 1985
869. Comis RL, Lawson R, Maroun J et al: Cytoxan, etoposide, vincristine versus Cytoxan, Adriamycin, vincristine versus Cytoxan, vincristine in the treatment of small cell lung cancer (abstract). Proc Am Soc Clin Oncol 6:168, 1987
870. Jackson DV, Case DL: Small cell lung cancer: A ten-year perspective. Semin Oncol 13(Suppl 3):63–74, 1986
871. Messieh AA, Schweitzer JM, Lipton A et al: Addition of etoposide to cyclophosphamide, doxorubicin, and vincristine for remission induction and survival in patients with small cell lung cancer. Cancer Treat Rep 71:61–66, 1987
872. Lowenbraun S, Birch R, Buchanan R et al: Combination chemotherapy in small cell lung cancer: A randomized study of two intensive regimens. Cancer 54:2344–2350, 1984
873. Einhorn L, Greco F, Wampler G et al: Cytoxan, Adriamycin, etoposide versus Cytoxan, Adriamycin, vincristine in the treatment of small cell lung cancer (abstract). Proc Am Soc Clin Oncol 6:168, 1987
874. Hirsch FR, Hansen HH, Hansen M et al: The superiority of combination chemotherapy including etoposide based on in vivo cell cycle analysis in the treatment of extensive small cell lung cancer: A randomized trial of 288 consecutive patients. J Clin Oncol 5:585–591, 1987
875. Schabel FM, Trader MW, Laster WK et al: Cisdichlorodiamineplatinum(II): Combination chemotherapy and cross-resistance studies with tumors of mice. Cancer Treat Rep 63:1459–1473, 1979
876. Hainsworth JD, Williams SD, Einhorn LH et al: Successful treatment of resistant germinal neoplasms with VP-16 and cisplatin. J Clin Oncol 3:666–671, 1985
877. Evans WK, Osoba D, Feld R et al: Etoposide (VP-16) and cisplatin: An effective treatment for relapse of small cell lung cancer. J Clin Oncol 3:65–71, 1985
878. Porter LL, Johnson DH, Hainsworth JD et al: Cisplatin and etoposide combination chemotherapy for refractory small cell carcinoma of the lung. Cancer Treat Rep 69:479–481, 1985
879. Sierocki JS, Hilaris BS, Hopfan S et al: cis-Dichlorodiamineplatinum(II) and VP-16-213: An active induction regimen for small cell carcinoma of the lung. Cancer Treat Rep 63:1593–1597, 1979
880. Woods RL, Levi JL: Chemotherapy for small cell lung cancer: A randomized study of maintenance chemotherapy with cyclophosphamide, Adriamycin, and vincristine after remission induction with cis-platinum, VP-16-213 and radiotherapy (abstract). Proc Am Soc Clin Oncol 3:214, 1984
881. Evans WK, Shepherd FA, Feld R et al: VP-16 and cisplatin as first-line therapy for small cell lung cancer. J Clin Oncol 3:1471–1477, 1985
882. Ihde DC, Johnson BE, Mulshine JL et al: Randomized trial of high dose versus standard dose etoposide and cisplatin in extensive stage small cell lung cancer (abstract). Proc Am Soc Clin Oncol 6:181, 1987
883. Einhorn LH, Crawford J, Birch R et al: Cisplatin plus etoposide consolidation following cyclophosphamide, doxorubicin, and vincristine in limited small cell lung cancer. J Clin Oncol 6:451–456, 1988
884. Bishop JF, Raghavan D, Stuart–Harris R et al: Carboplatin (CBDCA, JM-8) and VP-16-213 in previously untreated patients with small cell lung cancer. J Clin Oncol 5:1574–1578, 1987
885. Wolf M, Havemann K, Holle R et al: Cisplatin/etoposide versus isosfamide/etoposide combination chemotherapy in small cell lung cancer: A multicenter German randomized trial. J Clin Oncol 5:1880–1889, 1987
886. Frei E, Canellos GP: Dose: A critical factor in cancer chemotherapy. Am J Med 69:585–591, 1980
887. Mehta C, Vogl SE: High-dose cyclophosphamide in the induction chemotherapy of small cell lung cancer: Minor improvements in rate of remission and survival (abstract). Proc Am Assoc Cancer Res 23:155, 1982
888. Ettinger DS, Karp JE, Abeloff MD et al: Intermittent high-dose cyclophosphamide chemotherapy for small cell carcinoma of the lung. Cancer Treat Rep 62:413–422, 1978
888a. O'Donnell MR, Ruckdeschel JC, Baxter D et al: Intensive induction chemotherapy for small cell anaplastic carcinoma of the lung. Cancer Treat Rep 69:571–575, 1985
889. Johnson DH, Einhorn LH, Birch R et al: A randomized comparison of high-dose versus conventional-dose cyclophosphamide, doxorubicin, and vincristine for extensive stage small cell lung cancer. J Clin Oncol 5:1731–1738, 1987
890. Figueredo AT, Hryniuk WM, Straufmanis I et al: Co-trimoxazole prophylaxis during high-dose chemotherapy of small cell lung cancer. J Clin Oncol 3:54–64, 1985
891. Hande KR, Oldham RK, Fer MF, Richardson RL, Greco FA: Randomized study of high-dose low-dose methotrexate in the treatment of extensive small cell lung cancer. Am J Med 73:413–418, 1982
892. Abeloff MD, Ettinger DS, Order SE et al: Intensive induction chemotherapy with 54

patients with small cell carcinoma of the lung. Cancer Treat Rep 65:639–646, 1981
892a. Valdivieso M, Cabanillas F, Keating M et al: Effects of intensive induction chemotherapy for extensive disease small cell bronchogenic carcinoma in protected environment-prophylactic antibiotic units. Am J Med 76:405–412, 1984
893. Brower M, Ihde DC, Johnston–Early A et al: Treatment of extensive stage small cell bronchogenic carcinoma: Effects of variation in intensity of induction chemotherapy. Am J Med 75:993–998, 1983 and Valdivieso M, Cabanillas F, Keating M et al: Effects of intensive induction chemotherapy for extensive disease small cell bronchogenic carcinoma in protected environment–prophylactic antibiotic units. Am J Med 76:405–412, 1984
894. Farha P, Spitzer G, Valdivieso M et al: High-dose chemotherapy and autologous bone marrow transplantation for the treatment of small cell lung carcinoma. Cancer 52:1351–1355, 1983
895. Johnson DH, DeLeo MJ, Hande KR et al: High-dose induction chemotherapy with cyclophosphamide, etoposide, and cisplatin for extensive stage small cell lung cancer. J Clin Oncol 5:703–709, 1987
896. Markman M, Abeloff MD, Berkman AW et al: Intensive alternating chemotherapy regimen in small cell carcinoma of the lung. Cancer Treat Rep 69:161–166, 1985
897. Klastersky J, Nicaise C, Longeval E et al: Cisplatin, Adriamycin, and etoposide (CAV) for remission induction of small-cell bronchogenic carcinoma: Evaluation of efficacy and toxicity and pilot study of a "late intensification" with autologous bone-marrow rescue. Cancer 50:652–658, 1982
898. Stewart P, Buckner CD, Thomas ED et al: Intensive chemoradiotherapy with autologous bone marrow transplantation for small cell carcinoma of the lung. Cancer Treat Rep 67:1055–1059, 1983
899. Humblet Y, Symann M, Bosly A et al: Late intensification chemotherapy with autologous bone marrow transplantation in selected small cell carcinoma of the lung: A randomized study. J Clin Oncol 5:1864–1873, 1987
900. Ihde DC, Deisseroth AB, Lichter AS et al: Late intensive combined modality therapy followed by autologous bone marrow infusion in extensive stage small cell lung cancer. J Clin Oncol 4:1443–1454, 1986
901. Smith IE, Evans BD, Harland SJ et al: High-dose cyclophosphamide with autologous bone marrow rescue after conventional chemotherapy in the treatment of small cell lung carcinoma. Cancer Chemother Pharmacol 14:120–124, 1985
902. Spitzer G, Farha P, Valdivieso M et al: High-dose intensification therapy with autologous bone marrow support for limited small cell bronchogenic carcinoma. J Clin Oncol 4:4–13, 1986
903. Sculier JP, Klastersky J, Strychkmans P et al: Late intensification in small cell lung cancer: A Phase I study of high doses of cyclophosphamide and etoposide with autologous bone marrow transplantation. J Clin Oncol 3:184–191, 1985
904. Cunningham D, Banham SW, Hutcheon AH et al: High-dose cyclophosphamide and VP-16 as late dosage intensification therapy for small cell carcinoma of the lung. Cancer Chemother Pharmacol 15:303–306, 1985
905. Cornbleet M, Gregor A, Allan S et al: High-dose melphalan as consolidation therapy for good prognosis patients with small cell carcinoma of bronchus (abstract). Proc Am Soc Clin Oncol 3:210, 1984
906. Harper PG, Souhami RL: Intensive chemotherapy with autologous bone marrow transplantation in small cell carcinoma of the lung. Recent Results Cancer Res 97:146–156, 1985
907. Goldie JH, Coldman AJ: A mathematical model for relating drug sensitivity of tumors to their spontaneous mutation rate. Cancer Treat Rep 63:1727–1733, 1979
908. Goldie JH, Coldman AJ: Genetic origins of drug resistance in neoplasms. Cancer Res 44:3743–3653, 1984
909. Østerlind K, Sorenson H, Hansen HH et al: Continuous versus alternating combination chemotherapy for advanced small cell carcinoma of the lung. Cancer Res 43:6085–6089, 1983
910. Cohen MH, Ihde DC, Bunn PA et al: Cyclic alternating combination chemotherapy of small cell bronchogenic carcinoma. Cancer Treat Rep 63:163–170, 1979
911. Aisner J, Whitacre W, Van Echo DA, Wiernik PH: Combination chemotherapy for small cell carcinoma of the lung: Continuous versus alternating non-cross-resistant combinations. Cancer Treat Rep 66:221–230, 1982
912. Elliott JA, Østerlind K, Hansen HH: Cyclic alternating "non-cross resistant" chemotherapy in the management of small cell anaplastic carcinoma of the lung. Cancer Treat Rev 11:103–113, 1984
913. Ettinger DS, Mehta CR, Abeloff MD et al: Maintenance chemotherapy versus no maintenance chemotherapy in complete responders following induction chemotherapy in extensive disease small cell lung cancer (abstract). Proc Am Soc Clin Oncol 6:175, 1987
914. Daniels JR, Chak LY, Sikic BL et al: Chemotherapy of small cell carcinoma of the lung: A randomized comparison of alternating and sequential combination chemotherapy programs. J Clin Oncol 2:1192–1199, 1984
915. Evans WK, Feld R, Murray N et al: Superiority of alternating non-cross resistant chemotherapy in extensive small cell lung cancer. Ann Intern Med 107:451–458, 1987
916. Natale RB, Shank B, Hilaris BS et al: Combination cyclophosphamide, Adriamycin, and vincristine rapidly alternating with combination cisplatin and VP-16 in treatment of small cell lung cancer. Am J Med 79:303–308, 1985
917. Feld R, Evans WK, DeBoer G et al: Combined modality induction therapy without maintenance chemotherapy for small cell carcinoma of the lung. J Clin Oncol 2:294–304, 1984
918. Cullen M, Morgan D, Gregory W et al: Maintenance chemotherapy for anaplastic small cell carcinoma of the bronchus: A randomized controlled trial. Cancer Chemother Pharmacol 17:157–160, 1986
919. McVie JG, Dalesio O, Kirkpatrick A et al: Induction versus induction plus maintenance therapy in small cell lung cancer (abstract). Proc Am Soc Clin Oncol 5:188, 1986
920. Abeloff MD, Klastersky J, Drings PD et al: Complications of treatment of small cell carcinoma of the lung. Cancer Treat Rep 67:21–26, 1983
921. Markman M, Abeloff MD: Management of hematologic and infectious complications of intensive induction therapy for small cell carcinoma of the lung. Am J Med 74:741–746, 1983
922. De Jongh CA, Wade JC, Finley RS et al: Trimethoprim/sulfamethoxazole versus placebo: A double-blind comparison of infection prophylaxis in patients with small cell carcinoma of the lung. J Clin Oncol 1:302–307, 1983
923. Huberman M, Fossieck BE, Bunn PA Jr, Cohen MH, Ihde DC, Minna JD: Herpes zoster and small cell bronchogenic carcinoma. Am J Med 68:214–218, 1980
924. Feld R, Evans WK, DeBoer G: Herpes zoster in patients with carcinoma of the lung. Am J Med 73:795–801, 1982
925. Earle MF, Fossieck BE, Cohen MH, Ihde DC, Bunn PA Jr, Minna JD: Perirectal infections in patients with small cell lung cancer. JAMA 246:2464–2466, 1981
926. Bunn PA, Lichter AS, Makuch RW et al: Chemotherapy alone or chemotherapy with chest radiation therapy in limited stage small cell lung cancer: A prospective randomized trial. Ann Intern Med 106:655–662, 1987
927. Abrams RA, Lichter AS, Bromer RH et al: The hematopoietic toxicity of regional radiation therapy: Correlations for combined modality therapy with systemic chemotherapy. Cancer 55:1429–1435, 1985
928. Lee JS, Umsawasdi T, Dhingra HM et al: Effects of brain irradiation and chemotherapy on myelosuppression in small cell lung cancer. J Clin Oncol 4:1615–1619, 1986
929. Johnson BE, Ihde DC, Bunn PA et al: Patients with small cell lung cancer treated with combination chemotherapy with or without irradiation: Data on potential cures, chronic toxicities, and late relapses after five- to eleven-year follow-up. Ann Intern Med 103:430–438, 1985
930. Johnson DH, Porter LL, List AF et al: Acute nonlymphocytic leukemia after treatment of small cell lung cancer. Am J Med 81:962–968, 1986
931. Bradley EC, Schechter GP, Matthews MJ et al: Erythroleukemia and other hematologic complications of intensive therapy in long-term survivors of small cell lung cancer. Cancer 49:221–223, 1982
932. Sorensen PG, Østerlind K, Groth S et al: Effects of intensive chemotherapy on respiratory function in patients with small cell carcinoma of the lung. Eur J Cancer Clin Oncol 19:901–906, 1983
933. Brooks BJ, Seifter EJ, Walsh TE et al: Pulmonary toxicity with combined modality therapy for limited stage small cell lung cancer. J Clin Oncol 4:200–209, 1986
934. Vogelzang NJ, Nelimark RA, Nath KA: Tumor lysis syndrome after induction chemotherapy of small cell bronchogenic carcinoma. JAMA 249:513–514, 1983
935. Salazar OM, Rubin P, Brown JC et al: Predictors of radiation response in lung cancer: A clinico-pathobiologic analysis. Cancer 37:2636–2650, 1976
936. Lichter AS, Bunn PA, Ihde DC et al: The role of radiation therapy in the treatment of small cell lung cancer. Cancer 55:2163–2175, 1985
937. Perry MC, Eaton WL, Propert KJ et al: Chemotherapy with or without radiation therapy in limited small cell carcinoma of the lung. N Engl J Med 316:912–918, 1987
938. Perez CA, Einhorn L, Oldham RK et al: Randomized trial of radiotherapy to the thorax in limited small cell carcinoma of the lung treated with multiagent chemotherapy and elective brain irradiation: A preliminary report. J Clin Oncol 2:1200–1208, 1984
939. Souhami RL, Geddes DM, Spiro SG et al: Radiotherapy in small cell cancer of the lung treated with combination chemotherapy: A controlled trial. Br Med J 288:1643–1646, 1984
940. Kies MS, Mira JG, Livingston RB et al: Multimodal therapy for limited small cell lung cancer: A randomized study of induction combination chemotherapy with or without thoracic irradiation in complete responders, and with wide field versus reduced volume radiation in partial responders. J Clin Oncol 5:592–600, 1987
941. Østerlind K, Hansen HH, Hansen HS et al: Chemotherapy versus chemotherapy plus irradiation in limited small cell lung cancer: Results of a controlled trial with five years of follow-up. Br J Cancer 54:7–17, 1986
942. Cox JD, Holoye PY, Libnoch JA: The role of consolidation irradiation in combined modality therapy of small cell carcinoma of the lung. Int J Radiat Oncol Biol Phys 8:1271–1276, 1982
943. Smyth J, Hansen HH: Current status of research into small cell carcinoma of the lung: Summary of the Second Workshop of the International Association for the Study of Lung Cancer (IASLC). Eur J Cancer Clin Oncol 21:1295–1298, 1985
944. Cox JD, Byhardt R, Komaki R et al: Interaction of thoracic irradiation and chemotherapy on local control and survival in small cell carcinoma of the lung. Cancer Treat Rep 63:1251–1255, 1979
945. Williams C, Alexander M, Glatstein EJ et al: The role of radiation therapy in combination with chemotherapy in extensive oat cell cancer of the lung: A randomized study. Cancer Treat Rep 61:142–143, 1977
946. Trask CWL, Joannides T, Harper PG et al: Radiation-induced lung fibrosis after treatment of small cell carcinoma of the lung with very high dose cyclophosphamide. Cancer 55:57–60, 1985
947. Arriagada R, LeChevelier T, Baldeyrou P et al: Alternating radiotherapy and chemo-

therapy schedules in small cell lung cancer, limited disease. Int J Radiat Oncol Biol Phys 11:1461–1467, 1985
948. Turrisi AT, Glover DJ, Mason B et al: Concurrent twice-daily multifield radiotherapy and platinum–etoposide chemotherapy for limited small cell lung cancer: Update 1987 (abstract). Proc Am Soc Clin Oncol 6:172, 1987
949. Livingston RB, Mira JG, Chen TT et al: Combined modality treatment of extensive small cell lung cancer. J Clin Oncol 2:585–590, 1984
950. Wilson HE, Stanley K, Vincent RG et al: Comparison of chemotherapy alone versus chemotherapy and radiation therapy of extensive small cell carcinoma of the lung. J Surg Oncol 23:181–184, 1983
951. Livingston RB, Schulman S, Mira JG et al: Combined alkylators and multiple-site irradiation for extensive small cell lung cancer. Cancer Treat Rep 70:1395–1401, 1986
952. Urtasun RC, Belch A, Bodnar D et al: Radiation as a non-cross resistant systemic agent: Experience with hemibody and total body irradiation in patients with small cell lung cancer. Cancer Treat Symp 2:41–47, 1985
953. Mason BA, Richter MP, Catalano RB, Creech RB: Upper hemibody and local chest irradiation as consolidation following response to high-dose induction chemotherapy for small cell bronchogenic carcinoma: A pilot study. Cancer Treat Rep 66:1609–1612, 1982
954. Powell BL, Jackson DV, Scarantino CW et al: Sequential hemibody irradiation integrated into a chemotherapy–local radiotherapy program for limited disease in small cell lung cancer. Int J Radiat Oncol Biol Phys 12:1951–1956, 1986
955. Salazar OM, Creech RH, Rubin P et al: Half-body and local chest irradiation as consolidation following response to standard induction chemotherapy for disseminated small cell lung cancer. Int J Radiat Oncol Biol Phys 6:1093–1102, 1980
956. Dillman RO, Seagren SL, Taetle R: Failure of low-dose, total-body irradiation to augment combination chemotherapy in extensive-stage small cell carcinoma of the lung. J Clin Oncol 1:242–250, 1983
957. Byhardt RW, Cox JD, Wilson JF et al: Total body irradiation vs. chemotherapy as a systemic adjuvant for small cell carcinoma of the lung. Int J Radiat Oncol Biol Phys 5:2043–2048, 1979
958. Hansen HH, Dombernowsky P, Hirsch FR et al: Prophylactic irradiation in bronchogenic small cell anaplastic carcinoma: A comparative trial of localized versus extensive radiotherapy including prophylactic brain irradiation in patients receiving combination chemotherapy. Cancer 46:279–284, 1980
959. Cox JD, Komaki R, Byhardt RW et al: Results of whole-brain irradiation for metastases from small cell carcinoma of the lung. Cancer Treat Rep 64:957–961, 1980
960. Komaki R, Cox JD, Whitson W: Risk of brain metastases from small cell carcinoma of the lung related to length of survival and prophylactic irradiation. Cancer Treat Rep 65:811–814, 1981
961. Hirsch FR, Paulson OB, Hansen HH, Vraa-Henssen J: Intracranial metastases in small cell carcinoma of the lung: Correlation of clinical and autopsy findings. Cancer 50:2433–2437, 1982
962. Jackson DV, Richards F, Cooper MR et al: Prophylactic cranial irradiation in small cell carcinoma of the lung: A randomized study. JAMA 237:2730–2733, 1977
963. Hirsch FR, Hansen HH, Paulson OB et al: Development of brain metastases in small cell anaplastic carcinoma of the lung. In Kay J, Whitehouse J (eds): CNS Complications of Malignant Disease, pp 175–184. London, Macmillan Press, 1979
964. Beiler DD, Kane RC, Bernath AM et al: Low dose elective brain irradiation in small cell carcinoma of the lung. Int J Radiat Oncol Biol Phys 5:944–945, 1979
965. Cox JD, Petrovich Z, Paig C et al: Prophylactic cranial irradiation in patients with inoperable carcinoma of the lung. Cancer 42:1135–1140, 1978
966. Seydel HG, Creech R, Pagano M et al: Small cell carcinoma: Combined modality treatment of regional small cell undifferentiated carcinoma of the lung. Int J Radiat Oncol Biol Phys 9:1135–1141, 1983
967. Bleehen NM, Bunn PA, Cox JD et al: Role of radiation therapy in small cell anaplastic carcinoma of the lung. Cancer Treat Rep 67:11–19, 1983
968. Rosen ST, Makuch RW, Lichter AS et al: Role of prophylactic cranial irradiation in prevention of central nervous system metastases in small cell lung cancer: Potential benefit restricted to patients with complete response. Am J Med 74:615–624, 1983
969. Aroney RS, Aisner J, Wesley MN et al: Value of prophylactic cranial irradiation given at complete remission in small cell lung carcinoma. Cancer Treat Rep 67:675–682, 1983
970. Sargent EN, Turner AF, Gordonson J et al: Percutaneous pulmonary needle biopsy: Report of 350 patients. Am J Roentgenol Rad Ther Nucl Med 122:758–768, 1974
971. Seydel HG, Creech R, Pagano M et al: Prophylactic versus no brain irradiation in regional small cell lung carcinoma. Am J Clin Oncol (CCT) 8:218–223, 1985
972. Baglan JR, Marks JE: Comparison of symptomatic and prophylactic irradiation of brain metastases from oat cell carcinoma of the lung. Cancer 47:41–45, 1981
973. Lucas CF, Robinson B, Hoskin PJ et al: Morbidity of cranial relapse in small cell lung cancer and the impact of radiation therapy. Cancer Treat Rep 70:565–570, 1986
974. Johnson BE, Becker B, Goff WB et al: Neurologic, neuropsychologic, and computed cranial tomography scan abnormalities in 2- to 10-year survivors of small cell lung cancer. J Clin Oncol 3:1659–1667, 1985
975. Lee JS, Umsawasdi T, Lee YY et al: Neurotoxicity in long-term survivors of small cell lung cancer. Int J Radiat Oncol Biol Phys 12:313–321, 1986
976. Livingston RB, Stephens RL, Bonnet JD et al: Long-term survival and toxicity in small cell lung cancer. Am J Med 77:415–417, 1984
977. Licciardello JTW, Cersosimo RJ, Karp DD et al: Disturbing central nervous system complications following combination chemotherapy and prophylactic whole-brain irradiation in patients with small cell lung cancer. Cancer Treat Rep 69:1429–1430, 1985
978. Carmichael J, Crane JM, Bunn PA et al: Results of therapeutic cranial irradiation in small cell lung cancer. Int J Radiat Oncol Biol Phys 14:455–459, 1988
979. Van Hazel G, Scott M, Eagan RT: The effect of CNS metastases on the survival of patients with small cell cancer of the lung. Cancer 51:933–937, 1983
979a. Rosen ST, Aisner J, Makuch RW et al: Carcinomatous leptomeningitis in small cell lung cancer: A clinicopathologic review of the National Cancer Institute experience. Medicine 61:45–53, 1982
980. Van Hazel G, Scott M, Eagan RT: The effect of CNS metastases on the survival of patients with small cell cancer of the lung. Cancer 51:933–937, 1983
981. Higgins GA, Shields TW, Keehn RJ: the solitary pulmonary nodule: Ten-year follow-up of Veterans Administration–Armed Forces Cooperative Study. Arch Surg 110:570–575, 1975
982. Shields TW, Higgins GA, Matthews MJ et al: Surgical resection in the management of small cell carcinoma of the lung. J Thorac Cardiovasc Surg 84:481–488, 1982
983. Davis S, Wright PW, Schulman SF et al: Long-term survival in small cell carcinoma of the lung: A population experience. J Clin Oncol 3:80–91, 1985
984. Shepherd FA, Ginsburg RJ, Feld R et al: Reduction in local recurrence and improved survival in surgically treated patients with small cell lung cancer. J Thorac Cardiovasc Surg 86:498–506, 1983
985. Prager RL, Foster JM, Hainsworth JD et al: The feasibility of adjuvant surgery in limited stage small cell carcinoma: A prospective evaluation. Ann Thorac Surg 38:622–626, 1984
986. Johnson DH, Einhorn LH, Mandelbaum I et al: Postchemotherapy resection of residual tumor in limited stage small cell lung cancer. Chest 92:241–246, 1987
987. Friess GG, McCracken JD, Troxell ML et al: Effect of initial resection of small cell carcinoma of the lung: A review of Southwest Oncology Group Study 7628. J Clin Oncol 3:964–968, 1985
988. Østerlind K, Hansen M, Hansen HH et al: Influence of surgical resection prior to chemotherapy on the long-term results in small cell lung cancer: A study of 150 operable patients. Eur J Cancer Clin Oncol 22:589–593, 1986
989. Meyer JA: Effect of histologically verified TNM stage on disease control in treated small cell carcinoma of the lung. Cancer 55:1747–1752, 1985
990. Shepherd FA, Ginsberg R, Evans WK et al: "Very limited" small cell lung cancer: Results of non-surgical treatment (abstract). Proc Am Soc Clin Oncol 3:223, 1984
991. Williams CJ, McMillan I, Lea R et al: Surgery after initial chemotherapy for localized small cell carcinoma of the lung. J Clin Oncol 5:1579–1588, 1987
992. Baker RR, Ettinger DS, Ruckdeschel JD et al: The role of surgery in the management of selected patients with small cell carcinoma of the lung. J Clin Oncol 5:697–702, 1987
993. Valdivieso M, McMurtrey MJ, Farha P et al: Prospective evaluation of adjuvant surgical resection in small cell lung cancer. (abstract). Proc Am Soc Clin Oncol 3:220, 1984
994. Abeloff MD, Eggleston JC, Mendelsohn G et al: Changes in morphologic and biochemical characteristics of small cell carcinoma of the lung: A clinico-pathologic study. Am J Med 66:757–764, 1977
995. Matthews MJ: Effects of therapy on the morphology and behavior of small cell carcinoma of the lung: A clinicopathologic study. In Muggia F, Rozencweig M (eds): Lung Cancer: Progress in Therapeutic Research, pp 155–165. New York, Raven Press, 1979
996. Meyer JA, Gullo JJ, Ikins PM et al: Adverse prognostic effect of N2 disease in treated small cell carcinoma of the lung. J Thorac Cardiovasc Surg 88:495–501, 1984
997. Batist G, Carney DN, Cowan KH et al: Etoposide (VP-16) and cisplatin in previously treated small cell lung cancer: Clinical trial and in vitro correlates. J Clin Oncol 4:982–986, 1986
998. Batist G, Ihde DC, Zabell A et al: Small-cell carcinoma of lung: Reinduction therapy after late relapse. Ann Intern Med 98:472–474, 1983
999. Ochs JJ, Tester WJ, Cohen MH, Lichter AS, Ihde DC: "Salvage" radiation therapy for intrathoracic small cell carcinoma of the lung progressing on combination chemotherapy. Cancer Treat Rep 67:1123–1126, 1983
1000. Choi NC, Propert K, Carey R et al: Accelerated radiotherapy followed by chemotherapy for locally recurrent small cell carcinoma of the lung. Int J Radiat Oncol Biol Phys 13:263–266, 1987
1001. Holmes EC: Immunology and lung cancer. Ann Thorac Surg 21:250–258, 1976 and Chest 71:643–644, 1977
1002. Price-Evans DA: Immunology of bronchial carcinoma. Thorax 31:493–506, 1978
1003. McCracken JD, Chen T, White J et al: Combination chemotherapy, radiotherapy, and BCG immunotherapy in limited small cell carcinoma of the lung. Cancer 49:2252–2258, 1982
1004. McCracken JD, Heilbrun L, White J et al: Combination chemotherapy, radiotherapy, and BCG immunotherapy in extensive (metastatic) small cell carcinoma of the lung. Cancer 46:2335–2340, 1980
1005. Jackson DV, Paschal BR, Ferree C et al: Combination chemotherapy–radiotherapy with and without the methanol-extraction residue of Bacillus Calmette-Guerin (MER) in small cell carcinoma of the lung: A prospective randomized trial of the Piedmont Oncology Association. Cancer 50:48–52, 1982
1006. Maurer LH, Pajak T, Eaton W et al: Combined modality therapy with radiotherapy, chemotherapy, and immunotherapy in limited small cell carcinoma of the lung. J Clin Oncol 3:969–976, 1985
1007. Aisner J, Wiernik PH: Chemotherapy versus chemoimmunotherapy for small cell undifferentiated carcinoma of the lung. Cancer 46:2543–2549, 1980

1008. Cohen MH, Chretien PB, Ihde DC et al: Thymosin fraction V and intensive combination chemotherapy: Prolonging the survival of patients with small cell lung cancer. JAMA 241:1813–1815, 1979, and Cohen MH, Chretien PB, Early AJ et al: Thymosin fraction V prolongs survival of intensively treated small cell lung cancer patients. In Terry W, Windhorst D (eds): Immunotherapy of Cancer: Present Status of Trials in Man, Second International Conference. New York, Raven Press, 1980
1009. Scher HJ, Shank B, Chapman R et al: Randomized trial of combined modality therapy with and without thymosin fraction V in the treatment of small cell lung cancer. Cancer Res 48:1663–1670, 1988
1010. Evans WK, Russell DM, Shepherd FA et al: Changes in substrate–hormone profiles and amino acid metabolism in small cell lung cancer (abstract). Proc Am Assoc Cancer Res 24:651, 1983
1011. Shike M, Russell DM, Detsky As et al: Changes in body composition in patients with small cell lung cancer: The effect of total parenteral nutrition as an adjunct to chemotherapy. Ann Intern Med 101:303–309, 1984
1012. Clamon GH, Feld R, Evans WK et al: Effect of adjuvant central IV hyperalimentation on the survival and response to treatment of patients with small cell lung cancer: A randomized trial. Cancer Treat Rep 69:167–177, 1985
1013. Zacharski LR, Henderson WG, Rickles FR et al: Effect of warfarin on survival in small cell carcinoma of the lung: Veterans Administration Study No. 75. JAMA 245:831–834, 1981
1014. Levenson RM, Ihde DC, Matthews MJ et al: Small cell carcinoma arising in extrapulmonary sites: Response to chemotherapy. JNCI 67:607–612, 1981
1015. Fer MF, Levenson RM, Cohen MH et al: Extrapulmonary small cell carcinoma. In Greco FA, Oldham RK, Bunn PA (eds): Small Cell Lung Cancer, pp 301–325. New York, Grune & Stratton, 1981
1016. Remick SC, Hafez GR, Carbone PP: Extrapulmonary small cell carcinoma: A review of the literature with emphasis on therapy and outcome. Medicine 66:457–471, 1987
1017. Johnson BE, Naylor SL, Zbar B et al: Restriction fragment length polymorphism studies show loss of chromosome 3 alleles in small cell lung cancer but not in extrapulmonary small cell cancer (abstract). Proc Am Soc Clin Oncol 7:199, 1988
1018. Goepfert H, Remmler D, Silva E et al: Merkel cell carcinoma (endocrine carcinoma of the skin) of the head and neck. Arch Otolaryngol 110:707–712, 1984
1019. Mountain CF, Carr DT, Anderson WA: A system for the clinical staging of lung cancer. Am J Roentgenol Rad Ther Nucl Med 120:130–138, 1974
1020. Jacobs RH, Greenberg A, Bitran JD et al: A ten-year experience with combined modality therapy for Stage III small cell lung carcinoma. Cancer 58:2177–2184, 1986
1021. Østerlind K, Hansen HH, Hansen M et al: Mortality and morbidity in long-term surviving patients treated with chemotherapy with or without irradiation for small cell lung cancer. J Clin Oncol 4:1044–1052, 1986
1022. Roswit B, Patno ME, Rapp R et al: The survival of patients with inoperable lung cancer: A large-scale randomized study of radiation therapy versus placebo. Radiology 80:688–697, 1968
1023. Seydel HG, Creech R, Pagano M et al: Small cell carcinoma: Combined modality treatment of regional and small cell undifferentiated carcinoma of the lung. Int J Radiat Oncol Biol Phys 9:1135–1141, 1983
1024. Petrovich Z, Ohanian M, Cox JD: Clinical research on the treatment of locally advanced lung cancer. Cancer 42:1129–1134, 1978
1025. Carr DT, Childs DS Jr, Lee RE: Radiotherapy plus 5-FU compared to radiotherapy alone for inoperable and unresectable bronchogenic carcinoma. Cancer 29:375–380, 1972
1026. Choi CH, Carey RW: Small cell anaplastic carcinoma of the lung: Reappraisal of current management. Cancer 37:2651–2657, 1976
1027. Johnson BE, Ihde DC, Matthews MJ et al: Non-small cell lung cancer: Major cause of late mortality in patients with small cell lung cancer. Am J Med 80:1103–1110, 1986
1028. Baillie–Johnson H, Twentyman PR, Fox NE et al: Establishment and characterisation of cell lines from patients with lung cancer (predominantly small cell carcinoma). Cancer 52:495–504, 1985
1029. Klein JC, Zurcher C, Van Bekkum DW: Differential behavior of human bronchial carcinoma cells in culture. Cancer Res 47:3251–3258, 1987
1030. Bepler G, Jaques G, Neumann K, Aumuller G, Gropp C, Havemann K: Establishment, growth properties, and morphological characteristics of permanent human small cell lung cancer cell lines. J Cancer Res Clin Oncol 113:31–40, 1987
1031. Ruckdeschel JC, Oie HK, Gazdar AF: In vitro characterization of non-small cell lung cancer. Cancer Treat Res 28:49–59, 1986
1032. Kaiser LR, Kern DH, Campbell M, Mann PD, Holmes EC: In vitro assessment of antineoplastic therapy: New indication for thoracotomy? J Thorac Cardiovasc Surg 82:538–541, 1981
1033. Shorthouse AJ, Jones JM, Steel GG, Peckham MJ: Experimental combination and single-agent chemotherapy in human lung-tumor xenografts. Br J Cancer 46:35–44, 1982
1034. Ruckdeschel JC, Carney DN, Oie HK, Russell EK, Gazdar AF: In vitro chemosensitivity of human lung cancer cell lines. Cancer Treat Rep 71:697–704, 1987
1035. Douple EB, Cate CC, Curphey TJ et al: Evaluation of drug efficacy in vitro using human small cell carcinoma of the lung spheroids. Cancer 56:1918–1925, 1985
1036. Roed H, Vindelov LL, Spang–Thomsen M, Engelholm SA: Limitations and potentials of in vitro sensitivity testing of human small cell carcinoma of the lung. Cancer Treat Res 28:77–89, 1986
1037. Casero RA Jr, Go B, Theiss HW et al: Cytotoxic response of the relatively difluoromethylornithine-resistant human lung tumor cell line (NCI-H157 to the polyamine analogue N1,N8-bis(ethylo)spermidine. Cancer Res 47:3964–3967, 1987
1038. Munker M, Munker R, Sazton RE, Koeffler HP: Effect of recombinant monokines, lymphokines, and other agents on clonal proliferation of human lung cancer cell lines. Cancer Res 47:4081–4085, 1987
1039. Bepler G, Carney DN, Nau MM, Gazdar AF, Minna JD: Additive and differential biological activity of alpha-interferon A, difluoromethylornithine, and their combinations on established human lung cancer cell lines. Cancer Res 46:3413–3419, 1986
1040. Teraskai T, Shimosato Y, Nakajima T et al: Reversible squamous cell characteristics induced by vitamin A deficiency in a small cell lung cancer cell line. Cancer Res 47:3533–3537, 1987
1041. Doyle A, Giangiulio D, Hussain A, Park H, Borges M: Retinoic acid changes variant small cell lung cancer (SCLC) to a classic morphology (abstract). Proc Am Soc Clin Oncol 6:A57, 1987
1042. Curt GA, Jolivet J, Carney DN et al: Determinants of the sensitivity of human small-cell lung cancer cell lines to methotrexate. J Clin Invest 76:1323–1329, 1985
1043. Twentyman RP, Fox NE, Wright KA, Bleehen NM: Derivation and preliminary characterisation of Adriamycin resistant lines of human lung cancer cells. Br J Cancer 53:529–537, 1986
1044. Zijlstra JG, de Vries EG, Mulder NH: Multifactorial drug resistance in an Adriamycin-resistant human small cell lung carcinoma cell line. Cancer Res 47:1780–1784, 1987
1045. Carney DN, Mitchell JB, Kinsella TJ: In vitro radiation and chemotherapy sensitivity of established cell lines of human small cell lung cancer and its large cell morphological variants. Cancer Res 43:2806–2811, 1983
1046. Fox NE, Twentyman PR: A comparison of clonogenic and radionuclide uptake assays for determining the radiation response of human small-cell lung cancer xenografts and cell lines. Br J Radiol 60:381–388, 1987
1047. Duchesne GM, Peakcock JH, Steel GG: The acute in vitro and in vivo radiosensitivity of human lung tumour lines. Radiother Oncol 7:353–361, 1986
1048. Von Hoff DD, Casper H, Bradley E et al: Association between human tumor colony-forming assay results and response of an individual patient's tumor to chemotherapy. Am J Med 70:1027, 1981
1049. Von Hoff DD, Forseth B, Warfel LE: Use of a radiometric system to screen for antineoplastic agents: Correlation with a human tumor cloning system. Cancer Res 45:4032, 1985
1050. Weisenthal LM, Morsden JA, Dill PL, Macaluso CK: A novel dye exclusion method for testing in vitro chemosensitivity of human tumors. Cancer Res 43:749, 1983
1051. Kanzawa F, Matsushima Y, Ishihara J et al: In vitro chemosensitivity patterns of carcinoma of the lung in human tumor clongenic assay. J Pharmacobiodyn 9:715–721, 1986
1052. Cole SPC: Rapid chemosensitivity testing of human lung tumour cells using the MTT assay. Cancer Chemother Pharmacol 17:259, 1986
1053. Carmichael J, DeGraff WG, Gazdar AF, Minna JD, Mitchell JB: Evaluation of a tetrazolium-based semiautomated colorimetric assay: Assessment of chemosensitivity testing. Cancer Res 47:936–942, 1987
1054. Carmichael J, DeGraff WG, Gazdar AF, Minna JD, Mitchell JB: Evaluation of a tetrazolium-based semiautomated colorimetric assay: Assessment of radiosensitivity. Cancer Res 47:943–946, 1987
1055. Carmichael J, Mitchell JB, DeGraff WG et al: Chemosensitivity testing of human lung cancer cell lines using the MTT assay. Br J Cancer (in press)
1056. Carney DN: Recent advances in the biology of small cell lung cancer. Chest 89 Suppl:253S–257S, 1986
1057. Gazdar AF: Advances in the biology of non-small cell lung cancer. Chest 89 Suppl:277S–283S, 1986
1058. Funa K, Gazdar AF, Minna JD, Linnoila RI: Paucity of beta 2-microglobulin expression on small cell lung cancer, bronchial carcinoids and certain other neuroendocrine tumors. Lab Invest 55:186–193, 1986
1059. Doyle A, Martin J, Gazdar A et al: Markedly decreased or absent expression of class I histocompatibility antigens in human small cell lung cancer. J Exp Med 161:1135–1151, 1985
1060. Bernal SD, Baylin SB, Shaper JH et al: Cytoskeleton-associated proteins of human lung cancer cells. Cancer Res 43:1798–1808, 1983
1061. Lehto VP, Stenman S, Miettinen M et al: Expression of a neural type of intermediate filament as a distinguishing feature between oat cell carcinoma and other lung cancers. Am J Pathol 110:113–118, 1983
1062. Broers JL, Carney DN, Klein RM et al: Intermediate filament proteins in classic and variant types of small cell lung carcinoma cell lines: a biochemical and immunochemical analysis using a panel of monoclonal and polyclonal antibodies. J Cell Sci 83:37–60, 1986
1063. Bunn Pa, Linnoila I, Minna JD et al: Small cell lung cancer, endocrine cells of the fetal bronchus, and other neuroendocrine cells express the Leu-7 antigenic determinant present on natural killer cells. Blood 65:764–768, 1985
1064. Cole SP, Mirski S, McGarry RC et al: Differential expression of the Leu-7 antigen on human lung tumor cells. Cancer Res 45:4285–4290, 1985
1065. Baylin SB, Gazdar AF, Minna JD, Shaper JH: A unique cell surface protein phenotype distinguishes human small cell from non-small cell lung cancer. Proc Natl Acad Sci USA 79:4650–4654, 1982
1066. Ball ED, Sorenson GD, Pettengill OS: Expression of myeloid and major histocompatibility antigens on small cell carcinoma of the lung cell lines analyzed by cytofluorography: modulation by gamma-interferon. Cancer Res 46:2335–2339, 1986

1067. Hellstrom I, Horn D, Linsley P et al: Monoclonal mouse antibodies raised against human lung carcinoma. Cancer Res 46:3917–3923, 1986

1068. Moss F, Bobrow LG, Sheppard MN et al: Expression of epithelial and neural antigens in small cell and non small cell lung carcinoma. J Pathol 149:103–111, 1986

1069. Roth KA, Barchas JD: Small cell carcinoma cell lines contain opioid peptides and receptors. Cancer 57:769–773, 1986

1070. Cerny T, Barnes DM, Hasleton P et al: Expression of epidermal growth factor receptor (EGF-R) in human lung tumours. Br J Cancer 54:265–269, 1986

1071. Sakiyama S, Nakamura Y, Yasuda S: Expression of epidermal growth factor receptor gene in cultured human lung cancer cells. Jpn J Cancer Res 77:965–969, 1986

1072. Knop RH, Carney DN, Chen CW et al: Levels of high energy phosphates in human lung cancer cell lines by 31^P nuclear magnetic resonance spectroscopy. Cancer Res 47:3357–3359, 1987

1073. Spitalnik SL, Spitalnik PF, Dubois C et al: Glycolipid antigen expression in human lung cancer. Cancer Res 46:4751–4755, 1986

1074. Ruff MR, Farrar WL, Pert CB: Interferon gamma and granulocyte–macrophage colony-stimulating factor inhibit growth and induce antigens characteristic of myeloid differentiation in small-cell lung cancer cell lines. Proc Natl Acad Sci USA 83:6613–6617, 1986

J. C. ROSENBERG

CHAPTER 23 *Neoplasms of the Mediastinum*

Mediastinal masses are asymptomatic in a little less than half the patients who are discovered to have them (Fig. 23-1).[1] Asymptomatic masses are usually detected when a chest roentgenogram is obtained for a reason unrelated to the mediastinal tumor. One can expect asymptomatic patients to harbor a benign lesion, because 90% of the lesions occurring in asymptomatic patients are benign.[1–3] The most common symptoms produced by mediastinal masses are listed in Table 23-1.

Some patients with benign tumors of the mediastinum are at risk of disability or death if the lesion's size or position interferes with cardiopulmonary function. Because of this hazard and the high incidence of malignant tumors in the mediastinum, a mass in this location cannot be "passively observed or treated by radiation without benefit of a specific diagnosis," as was occasionally the practice in the past.[4] The lesion must be diagnosed with precision and treated appropriately.

ANATOMICAL CONSIDERATIONS

The boundaries of the mediastinum are the diaphragm inferiorly, the parietal pleura laterally, the sternum anteriorly, the vertebral column and adjacent ribs posteriorly, and the thoracic outlet superiorly. The thoracic outlet is the area encompassed by the superior extent of the thoracic cage, that is, the level of the first thoracic vertebra and the first ribs.

Because of the constancy with which anatomical structures are located within specific areas of the mediastinum and the predilection of different lesions to occur within certain mediastinal areas, it is clinically relevant to divide the mediastinum into compartments. The superior mediastinum is the area between the thoracic outlet and a line drawn from the sternal angle of Louis (the junction of the manubrium and body of the sternum) to the fourth intervertebral disc. Since the mediastinum is trapezoidal in shape, the superior mediastinum is narrowed by the approximation of its lateral boundaries and cannot easily be subdivided further. However, the remainder of the mediastinum can be subdivided into anterior, middle, and posterior divisions.

The anterior mediastinum extends from the sternum to the pericardium and great vessels. The posterior mediastinum is bounded by the posterior rib cage and spinal column and extends anteriorly for a variable distance. Some authors define the anterior extent of the posterior mediastinum as the pericardium (Fig. 23-2C). Others set it at a line drawn along the anterior borders of the bodies of the vertebrae (Figs. 23-2A and 23-2B). In the latter case, the posterior mediastinum would consist of the costovertebral (or paravertebral) areas.

The middle mediastinum includes the section between the anterior and posterior compartments. It is also referred to as the hilar or visceral area since it contains the heart and great vessels.

Burkell and colleagues have suggested a different map of the mediastinum.[5] They speak of only three areas, the

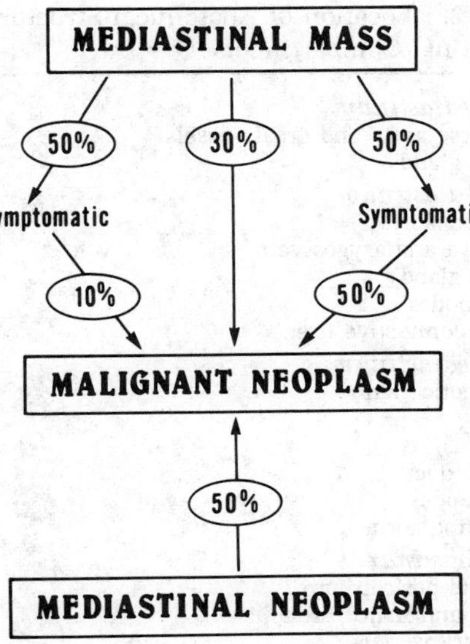

FIG. 23-1. Symptomatic mediastinal masses are often malignant neoplasms. Half of all new growths of the mediastinum are malignant.

anterosuperior, posterior, and the middle mediastinal divisions. They consider it impractical to designate the superior mediastinum as a distinct division of the mediastinum because many lesions that are found in the superior mediastinum are also found in the anterior mediastinum. Furthermore, superior mediastinal masses tend to extend down into the chest and also occupy the anterior mediastinum. Many posterior mediastinal lesions extend upwards, also occupying the superior mediastinum. Thus there is merit to their suggestion that the anterior and superior mediastinal compartments be combined into one division. Another way of looking at the mediastinum divided into three compartments is illustrated in Figure 23-2D.

TABLE 23-1. Mediastinal Masses: Signs and Symptoms

Nonspecific
- Chest discomfort — fullness, tightness, pain
- Anorexia
- Weight loss
- Malaise

Secondary to Compression or Displacement of Adjacent Mediastinal Structures
- Tracheo-bronchial compression — cough, wheezing, stridor, dyspnea, recurrent respiratory infections
- Esophageal compression — dysphagia
- Superior vena cava syndrome
- Horner's syndrome
- Vocal cord paralysis — dysphonia
- Pulmonic stenosis — murmurs
- Cardiac tamponade or arrhythmias

Secondary to Endocrine Function
- Cushing's disease
- Gynecomastia
- Hypertension
- Hypoglycemia

Systemic Syndromes
- Thymoma*
  - Myasthenia gravis
  - Red cell aplasia
  - Hypogammaglobulinemia
  - Autoimmune diseases
- Carcinoid of thymus
  - Multiple endocrine abnormalities (type I)
  - Cushing's syndrome
- Neurofibroma
  - Osteoarthritis
- Lymphoma
  - Alcohol-induced pain
  - Fever
- Teratoma
  - Hypoglycemia — insulin-producing tumor

* See Table 23-4 for a complete list of systemic syndromes associated with thymomas.

FIG. 23-2. Various recommendations for dividing the mediastinum into compartments.

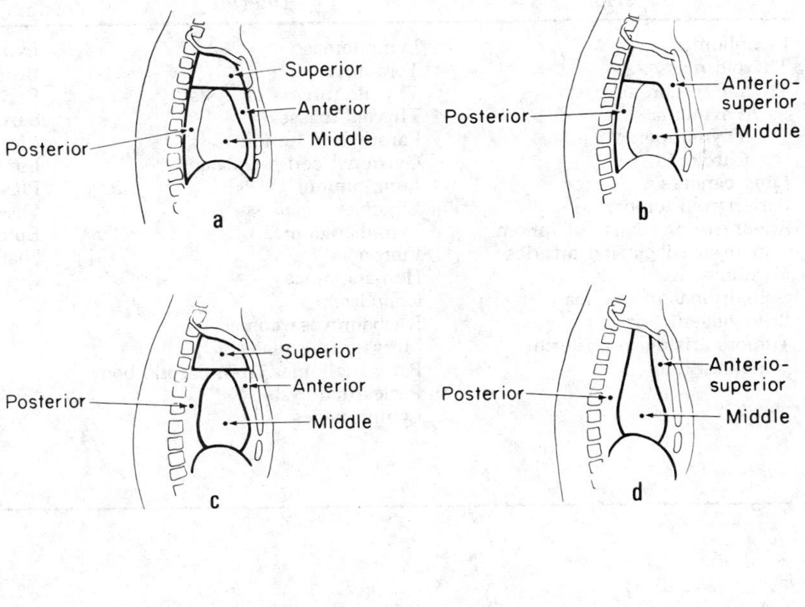

The anatomical structures normally found in the mediastinal compartments are listed in Table 23-2. Many of the lesions outlined in Table 23-3 can be derived from the list in Table 23-2. In addition to lesions arising from structures normally found in the mediastinum, abnormalities in the mediastinum may arise from adjacent anatomical areas, such as the abdomen, neck, lungs, and chest wall.

TABLE 23-2. Location of Anatomical Structures Within the Mediastinal Compartments

Superior Mediastinum
Transverse aorta and great vessels
Thymus gland
Anterior Mediastinum
Ascending aorta
Vena cava and azygos vein
Thymus gland
Lymph nodes
Fat and connective tissue
Posterior Mediastinum
Sympathetic chain
Vagus
Esophagus
Thoracic duct
Lymph nodes
Descending aorta
Middle Mediastinum
Heart and pericardium
Trachea and major bronchi
Pulmonary vessels
Lymph nodes
Fat and connective tissue

FREQUENCY OF MEDIASTINAL MASSES

Although lesions occur predominantly in one or another of the anatomic divisions of the mediastinum, there is an overlap in their distribution (Table 23-3). The most constant relationships are the thyroid masses, teratomas, and thymomas, which are located anteriorly and superiorly 90% of the time. Eighty percent of neurogenic tumors are located in the posterior mediastinum, and 50% of mediastinal lymphomas occur in the middle mediastinum.[6]

Mediastinal tumors and cysts in the adult are distributed throughout the mediastinal compartments in the following manner: 55% are in the anterior-superior compartment, 20% in the middle mediastinum, and 25% in the posterior mediastinum.[7] Some lesions cannot be localized because of their large size or indistinct margins. In children, the posterior mediastinum will contain 63% of the lesions; 26% occur in the anterior mediastinum, and 11% occur in the middle compartment.[8]

Tables 23-3 and 23-4 are fairly comprehensive lists of the lesions encountered in the mediastinum. Table 23-3 includes lesions arising outside the mediastinum that are located so close to it that they often extend into the mediastinum and may present as a primary mediastinal mass. In addition, physicians must be alert to the odd lesions that inevitably occur, such as an osteophyte of the spine protruding into the posterior mediastinum. Some spurious mediastinal masses that are on the surface of the patient appear on x-ray film to lie within the mediastinum. A considerable number of "mediastinal masses" will eventually not be found within the mediastinum or will be lesions that secondarily involve the mediastinum, such as lung cancers.

Because primary tumors of the mediastinum are infrequent and not readily classified in a tabulation of malignancies, the best approximation of their incidence is to determine how often a major referral center with an interest in mediastinal masses encounters these lesions. Approximately 1 in every 3400 admissions to Duke University Medical Center was found to have a primary mediastinal tumor or cyst.[1] At the University of Wisconsin, 7 to 10 patients with different kinds of mediastinal lesions were seen each year.[5]

TABLE 23-3. Mediastinal Masses and Their Distribution

Superior	*Anterior*	*Middle*	*Posterior*
Lymphomas	Lymphomas	Lymphomas	Neurogenic tumors
Thyroid masses	Teratomas	Bronchogenic cysts	Lymphomas
Thymic tumors or cysts	Thymic tumors or cysts	Pericardial cysts	Bronchogenic cysts
Thymoma	Thyroid masses	Sarcoidosis	Enteric cysts
Thymolipoma	Parathyroid tumors	Lipomas	Xanthogranulomas
Carcinoid	Germinal cell neoplasms	Lung cancers	Esophageal masses and diverticula
Lung cancers	Lung tumors	Plasma cell myeloma	Lung cancers
Parathyroid tumors	Lipomas	Vascular tumors	Thyroid masses
Aneurysm or ectasia of innominate or subclavian arteries	Lymphangiomas	Epicardial fat pads	Hiatal hernias
Myxomas	Fibromas	Hiatal hernias	Paravertebral abscesses
Cylindromas of trachea	Hemangiomas		Fibrosarcomas
Bronchogenic cysts	Chondromas		Meningoceles
Tumors arising in posterior mediastinum	Rhabdomyosarcomas		Myxomas
	Morgagni hernias		Chondromas
	Paragangliomas from carotid body		Pheochromocytomas
	Pericardial cysts		Aneurysms of descending aorta
	Lymph nodes		Enlargement of azygous and hemiazygous veins
			Thoracic duct cysts
			Tumors of spinal column

TABLE 23-4. Classification of Mediastinal Tumors

Neurogenic	*Mesenchymal Tumors*
Arising from peripheral nerves	Fibroma and fibrosarcoma
Neurofibroma	Lipoma and liposarcoma
Neurilemomma (Schwannoma)	Myxoma
Neurosarcoma	Mesothelioma
Arising from sympathetic ganglia	Leiomyoma and leiomyosarcoma
Ganglioneuroma	Rhabdomyosarcoma
Ganglioneuroblastoma	Xanthogranuloma
Neuroblastoma	Mesenchymoma
Arising from paraganglionic tissue	Hemangioma
Pheochromocytoma	Hemangioendothelioma
Chemodectoma (paraganglioma)	Hemangiopericytoma
Thymic	Lymphangioma
Thymoma	Lymphangiomyoma
Caarcinoid	Lymphangiopericytoma
Thymolipoma	*Endocrine Tumors*
Lymphoma	Thyroid
Hodgkin's disease	Parathyroid
Histiocytic lymphoma	*Cysts*
Undifferentiated	Pericardial
Germ Cell Tumors	Bronchogenic
Seminoma	Enteric
Nonseminomatous tumors	Thymic
Pure embryonal cell	Thoracic duct
Mixed embryonal cell	Meningoceles
with seminomatous elements	*Hernias*
with trophoblastic elements	Hiatal
with teratoid elements	Morgagni
with entodermal sinus elements	*Lymphadenopathy*
(yolk sac tumors)	Inflammatory
Teratoma, benign	Granulomatous
Aneurysms	Sarcoid

Overall, the rate of malignancy of mediastinal masses is estimated at about 40%.[7] The relative incidence of tumors and cysts in a large combined group of patients is shown in Table 23-5.

In the Mayo Clinic series (1064 patients from 1929 to 1968), the incidence of malignant tumors in children was approximately the same as that encountered in adults (25%).[9] Most of the cancers in children were of neurogenic, teratomatous, or vascular origin. The types of benign lesions found in children also differed from those seen in adults. Neurogenic and teratomatous tumors and enterogenous cysts made up approximately 78% of the mediastinal masses seen in the pediatric age group. Vascular tumors and cystic hygromas occurred more frequently in infants and children than in adults. Only 1 of the 206 patients with thymoma in the Mayo Clinic series was younger than 20 years of age.[9] Pericardial cysts and intrathoracic goiters were also rare in children.

The data presented in Table 23-5 differ significantly from those presented in earlier publications on this subject. In a series of 2251 mediastinal tumors collected from the literature from 1946 to 1971, neurogenic tumors were most frequently found (38%), followed by thymoma and thymic cysts (13.5%). Currently, the incidences of both are about 20%. This change is thought to be the result of the recent, more assiduous search for thymomas in patients with myasthenia gravis and autoimmune disorders.[1,7] Another factor that may distort these statistics is the criteria used for including lymphomas in tabulations of mediastinal tumors. Lymphomas presenting as a mediastinal mass should be included, but not all lymphomas with mediastinal involvement qualify as primary mediastinal neoplasms. Primary mediastinal lymphomas do have some unique characteristics, but they are not sufficiently unique to merit separate consideration in this chapter.[10]

TABLE 23-5. Relative Frequency (%) of Primary Mediastinal Tumors and Cysts

Tumor or Cyst	*Adults* ($n = 1950$)	*Children* ($n = 437$)
Neurogenic tumors	21	40
Thymomas	19	0
Lymphomas	13	18
Germ cell neoplasms	11	11
Mesenchymal tumors	7	9
Endocrine tumors (thyroid, parathyroid, and carcinoid)	6	0
Primary carcinomas	3	4
Cysts (pericardial, bronchogenic, enteric, and others)	20	18

Silverman NA, Sabiston NC Jr: Mediastinal masses. Surg Clin North Am 60:757, 1980.

A recent review of the frequency of primary anterior mediastinal tumors in a combined series of 702 adults and 179 children resulted in the data shown in Table 23-6.

TABLE 23-6. Relative Frequency (%) of Primary Anterior Mediastinal Tumors

Tumors	Adults (n=702)	Children (n=179)
Thymic lesions (cysts, hyperplasia, and thymoma)	47	17
Germ cell neoplasms	15	24
Lymphomas	23	45
Endocrine tumors (thyroid and parathyroid)	16	0
Mesenchymal tumors	0	15

Mullen B, Richardson JD: Primary anterior mediastinal tumors in children and adults. Ann Thorac Surg 42:338, 1986.

Only 5 cases of thymoma in children are included in this study.[11]

DIAGNOSIS

IMAGING TECHNICS

Roentgenographic examinations constitute the most important diagnostic studies that can be performed to define the location and extent of a mediastinal mass. Chest roentgenograms in posteroanterior and lateral projections can identify most lesions and localize the bulk of the mass to one of the mediastinal compartments (Fig. 23-3). The shape, size, and density of the mass as it is seen on the chest roentgenogram do not differentiate whether it is benign or malignant. Most malignant primary lesions are located in the anterosuperior compartment of the mediastinum. The value of comparing current films with previously obtained chest roentgenograms cannot be overemphasized, because growth rates can be estimated and indistinct lesions more clearly defined.

Small lesions located in front of or behind the heart may be missed on a routine roentgenographic examination of the chest, especially in those patients with a large amount of fat. Suspected mediastinal masses or those that are ill-defined can be best delineated and localized by computed tomography (CT). Before the introduction of this valuable diagnostic tool in 1975, a long list of procedures were recommended in the diagnostic evaluation of mediastinal masses, such as penetrated views in various projections and coned views looking for bony projections and erosions of the spine, tomograms in various projections, barium contrast studies of the esophagus (still valuable in detecting a hiatal hernia presenting as a mediastinal mass), fluoroscopy, aortograms (Fig. 23-4 and 23-5), pulmonary arteriograms, venograms, azygograms, selective thymic venography, angiocardiography, pneumomediastinography, myelography (for posterior mediastinal masses accompanied by neurologic abnormalities), ultrasonography, echocardiography, and nuclide imaging procedures, such as thyroid, bone, and gallium scans.[12,13] The information obtained by performing these procedures can usually be derived from CT of the mediastinum.[7,14-18]

CT of the mediastinum offers two great advantages over conventional radiographic procedures. First is the ability to examine the mediastinum's cross-sectional anatomy. CT is better than lateral or oblique views for visualizing the mediastinum. Some mediastinal tumors may blend in with adjacent mediastinal structures in chest roentgenograms. CT can more precisely identify the margins between the tumor and adjacent anatomic structures, and anatomy heretofore not visible by noninvasive technics can be examined by the clinician (Fig. 23-6).

Widening of the mediastinum because of physiologic fat deposition or by dilation or ectasia of the great vessels can be readily detected by CT. Cystic areas and areas of calcification in the mediastinum can be precisely identified. The extent of involvement by a tumor or structures within the mediastinum can also be assessed by CT.

Magnetic resonance imaging (MRI), unlike CT, can define vascular structures without the use of contrast material. Several publications have appeared comparing CT with MRI without clearly defining the role of each.[19,20] MRI can define

FIG. 23-3. Posteroanterior (**A**), lateral (**B**), and oblique (**C**) view of an anterior mediastinal mass that was found to be an encapsulated thymoma on exploration of the mediastinum (see Fig. 23-6).

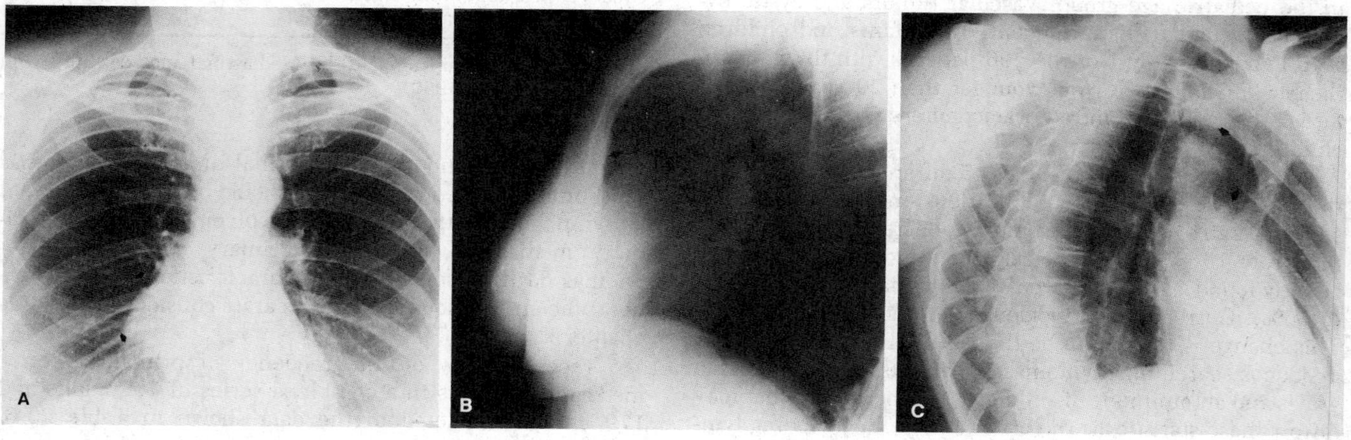

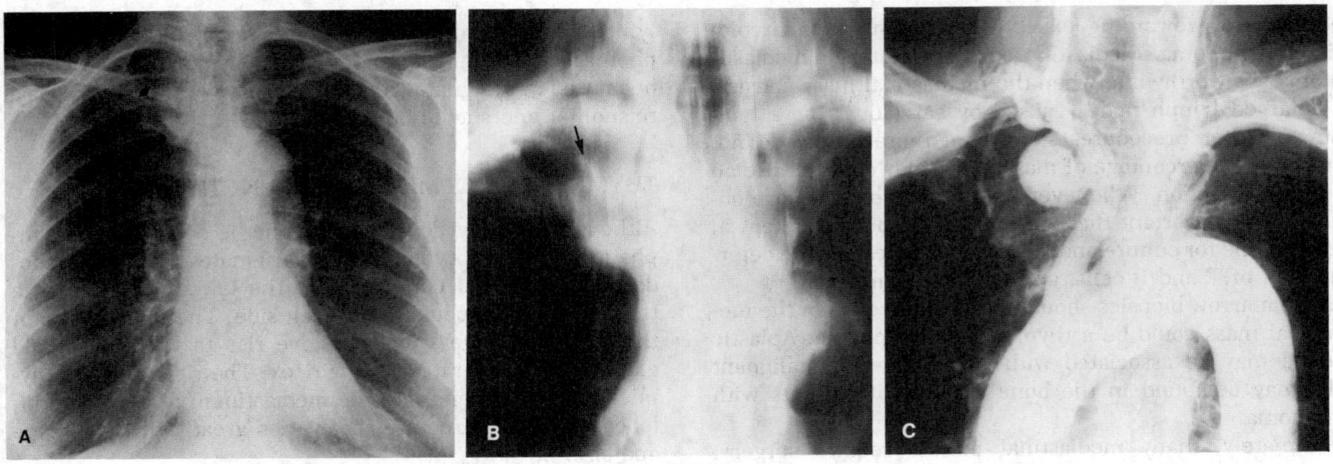

FIG. 23-4. Anterosuperior mediastinal mass seen on a plain film of the chest (**A**) and by tomography (**B**)was revealed to be a saccular aneurysm of the innominate artery when an arteriogram was obtained (**C**).

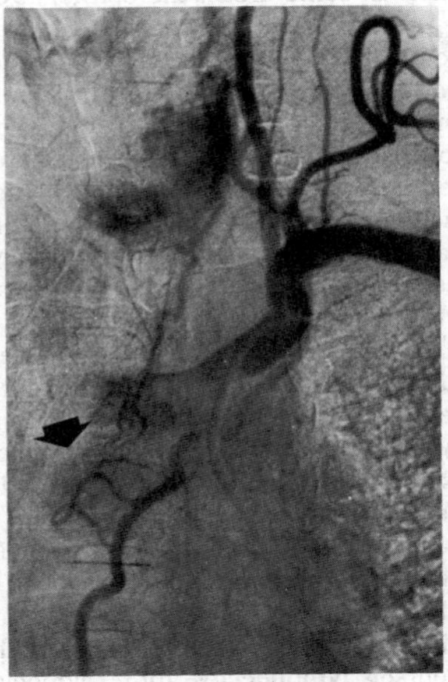

FIG. 23-5. Anteriograms delineate a parathyroid adenoma located within the thymus gland.

the mediastinal anatomy very well but has the disadvantage of requiring long scanning times, great expense, and limited availability.

If a thyroid scan is to be carried out to delineate a mass in the anterosuperior mediastinum, ^{131}I must be used rather than technetium pertechnetate, which will not identify mediastinal masses because of the high background of this nuclide in the vascular structures of the chest.[21] Iodine-131 will localize in the thyroid in most patients with mediastinal thyroid tissue. As many as 10% of mediastinal masses may be goiter, with as many as 25% in the posterior mediastinum.

ENDOSCOPY

Bronchoscopy and esophagoscopy should be performed whenever the radiographic abnormality could in any way be caused by a lung or esophageal tumor. The frequency of lung cancer requires that it be considered in patients with a smoking history who are 40 years of age or older.

BIOPSY PROCEDURES

If cervical or supraclavicular nodes are palpable, they should be biopsied. Scalene node biopsy in the absence of palpable

FIG. 23-6. Computed tomography of the patient with the thymoma depicted in Figure 23-3. The thymoma (*T*) is located immediately anterior to the base of the heart (*H*).

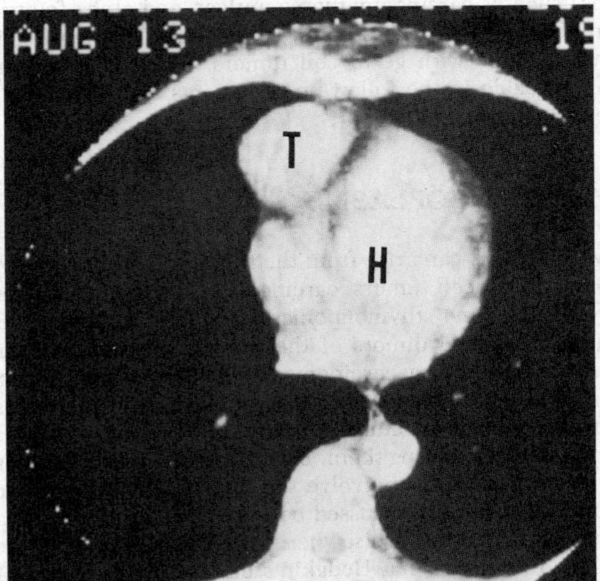

nodes is rarely rewarding, except when one suspects sarcoidosis or lymphoma. Mediastinoscopy and anterior mediastinotomy are worthwhile when the mediastinal mass consists of enlarged lymph nodes caused by sarcoidosis or a lymphoma. Other procedures short of a thoracotomy do not detect a high percentage of masses and may compromise an adequate resection. Whenever lymph node biopsies are obtained, it is important that portions of the node are kept in sterile saline for culture and sensitivity studies, for the determination of T and B cells, and for direct imprints.

Bone marrow biopsies should be considered when the mediastinal mass could be a thymoma or lymphoma. Aplastic anemia may be associated with thymoma, and malignant cells may be found in the bone marrow of patients with lymphoma.

Ultimately, many mediastinal masses require surgery. Thoracotomy will be required, using a median sternotomy or posterolateral incision. However, even under these circumstances, biopsy of a mass that cannot be completely removed occasionally leaves the pathologist confused if light microscopy alone is relied upon. Electron microscopy should be used in these instances.

If the patient with a mediastinal mass cannot tolerate a thoracotomy because of cardiopulmonary insufficiency, one of the limited biopsy procedures, an aspiration, or a needle biopsy of the mass may be attempted.[22] However, before this is done, be sure the structure being biopsied is not of vascular origin by using one or more of the imaging procedures.

HORMONAL ASSAYS AND TUMOR MARKERS

Hormonal assays and the determination of tumor markers may be of value in selected instances. Pheochromocytomas and some neurogenic tumors will be accompanied by elevated urinary catecholamine, homovanillic acid, or vanillyl mandelic acid levels. Germ cell tumors, teratomas, and some carcinomas will also elaborate glycoproteins (oncofetal antigens) such as carcinoembryonic antigen and alpha-fetoprotein. Chorionic gonadotrophin levels may be elevated in some patients with germ cell tumors. These markers are most valuable in the follow-up of patients and occasionally useful for diagnosis.

THYMIC NEOPLASMS

Several lesions can arise from the thymus: lymphomas, thymomas, germ cell tumors, carcinoids of the thymus, thymic carcinomas, and thymolipomas. Thymomas, germ cell tumors, carcinoid tumors of the thymus, mediastinal lymphomas, and primary carcinomas of the thymus may be confused with each other because of similarities in their gross and microscopic structure. Electron microscopy is of great value in differentiating them. Both Hodgkin's and non-Hodgkin's lymphomas may involve the thymus, but thymic lymphomas will not be discussed because they act the same as lymphomas that occur elsewhere (see Chap. 50). However, it should be noted that Hodgkin's disease of the thymus is almost always of the nodular sclerosis type and the most common non-Hodgkin's lymphomas of the thymus are the lymphoblastic lymphomas and the large-cell diffuse lymphomas. The term, "granulomatous thymoma," which has been used to designate Hodgkin's disease of the thymus, is a misnomer and should be discarded.[23]

THYMIC DEVELOPMENT AND FUNCTION

Although the fully developed thymus is considered a lymphatic organ, embryologically it originates from the endoderm as epithelial outgrowths of the lower portion of the third pharyngeal pouches on each side. The upper parts of the third pharyngeal pouches give rise to the parathyroid glands, which migrate into the neck. The right and left thymic anlagen descend into the mediastinum to become a bilobed glandular structure that varies greatly in both shape and size.[24-26]

The cords of epithelial cells that initially make up the thymus grow out into the surrounding mesenchyma. These cords subsequently constitute the medullary areas of the lobules of the thymus.[27] The epithelial cells in the cords eventually spread out to form a reticulum but never lose contact with each other. In some areas, the epithelial cells pile up and undergo keratinization and degeneration, forming distinctive structures known as Hassall's corpuscles. These structures are found in the medulla of the lobules.

As the epithelial cords proliferate and send out side branches into the mesenchyma, lymphocytes appear within the spaces between the epithelial cells of the cortex of the lobules. These lymphocytes are derived from hematopoietic stem cells that arise in the bone marrow and migrate to the thymus. The stem cells are concentrated in the periphery of the cortex of the thymic lobules. They give rise to the smaller lymphocytes, which are located in the deeper cortex of the lobule and fill the spaces between the epithelial cells. Medullary areas of the lobules in the mature thymus contain few lymphocytes and are largely epithelial in character. Germinal centers and lymphoid follicles are normally not found in the thymus.[26]

The process of lymphoblastic differentiation into mature thymocytes requires a humoral factor produced by the epithelial cells of the thymus. One preparation of this hormone (thymosine) is a polypeptide that can support the development of precursor lymphocytes into thymocytes.[28] This preparation and others, such as the thymic humoral factor of Trainin, are common to all mammals studied thus far.[29]

The differentiation of human lymphoblasts into thymocytes by the thymus takes place in fetal and early postnatal life. The thymocytes in the deeper cortex of the thymic lobules enter the circulation and populate all of the lymphatic tissue as thymus-derived lymphocytes (T lymphocytes). They have characteristic surface markers and specialized immunological functions, but are morphologically similar to the other major class of lymphocytes, the bone-marrow-derived lymphocytes (B lymphocytes).

Congenital absence of the thymus (DiGeorge syndrome) or its removal early in life results in a deficiency of cellular immune function. Thymectomy in the adult will also result in a decrease in immunological competence. However, because the half-life of thymus-derived lymphocytes in man is several years, the decrease in immunologic function due to the loss of T lymphocytes is gradual and less evident than when the thymus is removed at birth or shortly thereafter.

Although the mature thymus glands of individuals vary greatly with respect to size and shape, there is a relatively predictable pattern with respect to their size and the age of the patients. The thymus gland reaches a maximum size of 30 to 40 g in the adolescent, but its greatest size relative to the rest of the body is attained at about 4 years of age.[26] Following puberty, the thymus gradually involutes and the lymphoid component disappears. The parenchyma is largely replaced by fat. Hassell's corpuscles remain to identify the gland. The thymus never completely disappears.

A study of the morphology of the adult thymus by Bell and colleagues quantitated the variation in the dimensions and configuration of the thymus (Fig. 23-7).[24] The gland is generally situated beneath the upper part of the sternum. Its lower tip may end at any point between the first intercostal space and the costal cartilage of the seventh rib. In two thirds of the cases studied by Bell and colleagues, the caudal extremity of the thymus was between the third and fourth ribs. The thoracic portion of the thymus is usually thickest where it rests on pericardium. The cervical extent of the thymus is usually the least distinct of the gland's margins. The upper end of the thymus blends imperceptibly into the cervical fat and may extend up to the level of the sixth cervical vertebra.

THYMOMA

It is the epithelium of the thymus gland derived from the third pharyngeal pouches that may undergo neoplastic change to create a thymoma. Lymphocytic elements may be present and even dominate the histologic appearance of a thymoma. Nevertheless, a neoplasm of the thymus is not considered to be a thymoma unless the epithelial component is the neoplastic element. The immunologic characteristics of the lymphocytic component of thymomas are similar to the phenotype of immature lymphocytes (thymocytes) found in the normal thymus, thus supporting the contention that thymomas are strictly tumors of thymic epithelium.[30]

FIG. 23-7. The caudal tip of thymus gland was found between the third and fourth ribs in 66% of the 125 cadavers studied by Bell and colleagues.[24] Almost all of the glands terminated at some point above the xyphoid.

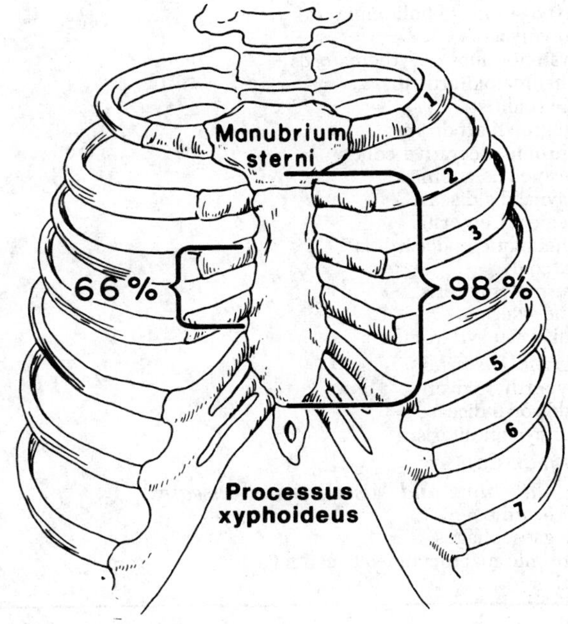

Pathology

Thymomas have fibrous septae on cut section. Cystic areas are seen in 40% to 60% of specimens.[26] Several classifications of thymomas have been devised, based on the histopathology of these tumors. Rosai and Levine have reviewed this aspect of thymomas completely in their monograph.[26] The simplest classification designates three types, based on the predominant cell type comprising the tumor: lymphocytic, epithelial, and mixed (lymphoepithelial). A cell type is considered predominant by Bergh and colleagues if more than 80% of the tumor is made up of that cell.[31] By their standards, 23% of 43 thymomas studied were lymphocytic; 35% were lymphoepithelial; and 42% were epithelial.

The pathologists at the Mayo Clinic reviewed 197 thymomas and classified them into four types: lymphocytic (35% of tumors), epithelial (18%), mixed (25%), and spindle cell (22%).[9] Spindle cell thymomas are considered variants of epithelial thymomas.

Another variant of the epithelial thymoma is the pseudorosette type characterized by a predominant pattern of pseudorosette formation by the neoplastic epithelial cells.

The Mayo Clinic group found that patients with thymomas of mixed or predominantly epithelial cell types had lower survival rates than patients with spindle cell or predominantly lymphocytic cell types.[9] At the University of Michigan, epithelial thymomas also tended to be more extensive and pursue a more aggressive course.[32]

Most researchers do not find a correlation between the histopathology of a specific thymoma and its invasive potential.[26] Nor is there a correlation between the histopathology of a thymoma and the coexistence of associated systemic syndromes.[26] The malignancy of a thymoma is determined by its invasive characteristics rather than the microscopic appearance of the tumor. The number of mitotic figures seen is low in all thymomas, regardless of the invasiveness of the tumor.[26,31-37]

In general, thymomas are slow-growing tumors. Some have stayed the same size for as long as 15 years.[26] This has led to the designation of some thymomas as benign and others as malignant. A "benign" thymoma has been defined as a tumor that is well-encapsulated and does not invade adjacent mediastinal structures. Fifty percent to 65% of the thymomas fit this definition (Fig. 23-8). However, the distinction between a benign and a malignant thymoma is artificial and should be replaced by the designation encapsulated and invasive.[1] All thymomas are potentially invasive, and therefore they should all be considered malignant.

The surgeon is usually in the best position to determine whether a thymoma has infiltrated the surrounding tissue. Frozen-section analyses of dense fibrous attachments between the thymoma and surrounding tissue may be neces-

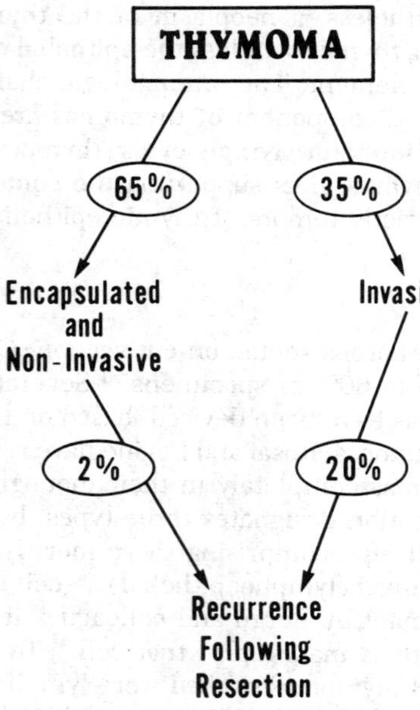

FIG. 23-8. Although figures vary from series to series, generally about two thirds of thymomas are "benign." The recurrence rate after removal of these tumors is low, in contrast to the higher recurrence rate after resection of invasive thymomas.

sary to be sure that the tumor is truly confined by its capsule. The capsule should be carefully examined for any discontinuity, which may represent an area of local invasion. The most common form of metastatic involvement is the occurrence of pleural or pericardial implants. They are thought to result from the shedding of tumor cells from the primary thymoma.

Staging of thymomas is based on the extent of invasiveness. The following staging system has been suggested by Bergh and colleagues:[31]

Stage I: Intact capsule or growth within the capsule
Stage II: Pericapsular growth into the mediastinal fat tissue
Stage III: Invasive growth into the surrounding organs, intrathoracic metastases or both

In the series from the University of Goteborg in Sweden, 40% of patients were stage I, 19% were stage II, and 41% were stage III. Thymomas over 500 g were all stage III tumors. Pleural metastases occurred in half of the patients with stage III thymomas. A more comprehensive staging system has been proposed, which subdivides the three stages based on additional pathologic findings at the time of surgery.[38] The drawback to these more detailed staging systems is the small number of patients available for analysis if they are classified into more than three groups.

Metastases to regional nodes or distant organs is uncommon. Only 30 instances of blood-borne metastases to extrathoracic sites were reported before 1976.[1] More have been reported since then. The organs involved were the liver, bone, colon, kidney, brain, and spleen. Epithelial thymomas gave rise to these metastases more often than other tumors. Thymomas, although rare in children, appear to run a more malignant course in them than in adults.[39]

Clinical Findings

Fortuitous discovery of a thymoma when a chest roentgenogram is obtained for reasons unrelated to the tumor occurs in 30% to 40% of patients with this neoplasm. Patients are usually between 40 and 60 years of age. No more than 10% of thymomas are found in patients younger than 20 years of age.[36] There is very little difference in the frequency with which men and women are affected, although some series report a slightly increased incidence in women.

Vague, nonspecific symptoms may be present, such as cough, dyspnea, dysphagia, chest tightness, and chest pain. Chest pain may be a sign of an advanced malignant lesion. A superior vena cava syndrome may also result from an advanced lesion.

Thymoma-associated Systemic Syndromes

The systemic syndromes that may be associated with a thymoma are listed in Table 23-7, and the three most common will be discussed. The occurrence of these syndromes often leads to the discovery of a thymoma.

Because both the parathyroid and thymus glands are derived from the third pharyngeal pouches, the group at the Mayo Clinic thought it would be reasonable to compare the incidence of diseases associated with thymomas and parathyroid adenomas, the latter acting as a control to the former.[40] They reviewed 146 of their own patients with thymoma and

TABLE 23-7. Syndromes and Diseases Associated with Thymomas

Autoimmune or Immune Phenomena
Myasthenia gravis
Cytopenias
Hypogammaglobulinemia
Polymyositis
Systemic lupus erythematosus
Rheumatoid arthritis
Thyroiditis
Sjögren's syndrome
Chronic ulcerative colitis
Pernicious anemia
Raynaud's disease
Regional enteritis
Rheumatic endocarditis
Sarcoid
Dermatomyositis
Scleroderma
Takayasu syndrome
Endocrine Disorders
Hyperthyroidism
Addison's disease
Panhypopituitarism
Nonthymic Cancer
Severe Infections and Miscellaneous Diseases
Myocarditis
Megaesophagus
Chronic macrocutaneous candidiasis
Other

452 found in the literature with sufficient data to evaluate whether or not an associated disease occurred. The incidence of other diseases with thymomas was 71%, compared with a 12% incidence in 177 patients with parathyroid adenomas. The diseases associated with thymomas were classified into categories (Table 23-7).

In some patients more than one disease was associated with the thymoma, such as myasthenia gravis and thrombocytopenia. Almost 70% of the patients with thymoma and other diseases will have immunologic disorders. About 10% will have a malignancy and 5% will have an endocrine disorder. The remaining 15% will have a severe infection or another seemingly unrelated condition, such as megaesophagus. The most frequent association is between thymoma and myasthenia gravis. Some 40% to 50% of patients with syndromes associated with thymoma have myasthenia gravis. Some of the endocrine disorders, such as Cushing's syndrome, are concomitants of carcinoid tumor of the thymus, which may be mistakenly diagnosed as a thymoma.

MYASTHENIA GRAVIS. The pathophysiologic characteristic of myasthenia gravis is the rapid exhaustion of voluntary muscular contractions, with a slow return to a normal state. Repetitive stimulation of the motor nerve to a muscle in patients with myasthenia gravis results in a progressive decrement of muscle action potentials. Thus, the major symptoms of patients with this disease are weakness and fatigability. Another characteristic is that these symptoms are relieved by drugs that inhibit acetylcholinesterase, an enzyme located within the synaptic junction (the end plate) between the motor neuron and striated muscle. Because of these features of myasthenia gravis, the disease is considered an abnormality of neuromuscular transmission.[41]

It is widely accepted that myasthenia gravis is an autoimmune disease caused by antibodies directed against acetylcholine receptors in voluntary muscle. A myasthenic state can be produced in rabbits by immunizing them with a purified protein having the properties of acetylcholine receptors.[42] The effect of the immune response is to eliminate acetylcholine receptors and impair postsynaptic structure and functions. Patients with myasthenia gravis have 70% to 90% fewer acetylcholine receptors per neuromuscular junction than do normal people.[41] Because there is a decreased number of acetylcholine receptors present within the end plate of patients with myasthenia gravis, acetylcholine, which is responsible for neuromuscular transmission across the synaptic junction, is less effective in transmitting the signal from nerve to muscle.

An association between the thymus and myasthenia was first suspected when pathologic changes were found in the thymus gland of 75% to 85% of patients with this neuromuscular disease (Fig. 23-9). Germinal centers are not normally present in the thymus gland; yet 70% of patients with myasthenia gravis and thymic abnormalities demonstrate this form of "thymic lymphoid (follicular) hyperplasia."[43] It is characterized by germinal center proliferation in the medullary and cortical areas of the thymus, without necessarily increasing the gross appearance or weight of the thymus. Furthermore, 15% to 50% of patients with myasthenia will have gross or microscopic (occult) thymomas, depending upon the frequency with which patients with myasthenia gravis have thymectomy or have an autopsy to search for this lesion. Follicular hyperplasia of the nonneoplastic portions of the thymus may accompany a thymoma.

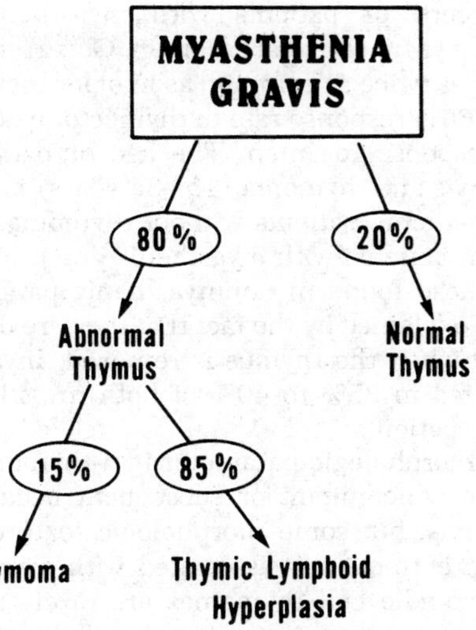

FIG. 23-9. Thymic abnormalities are frequent in patients with myasthenia. Both thymic lymphoid hyperplasia and thymoma may be present in the same patient.

Thymectomy in patients with myasthenia gravis can be effective in producing a complete remission of the disease in 20% to 36% of patients. An additional 57% to 86% will be improved (Fig. 23-10).[41] The presence of a thymoma in a patient with myasthenia carries a poorer prognosis than for myasthenia patients without thymomas. Improvement in muscle strength following thymectomy can be anticipated in only 25% of patients with myasthenia and a thymoma. A 40% to 60% response rate may result when myasthenic patients have a thymectomy and do not have a thymoma.

FIG. 23-10. Response to thymectomy varies depending on age and sex of the patient and whether a thymoma is present.

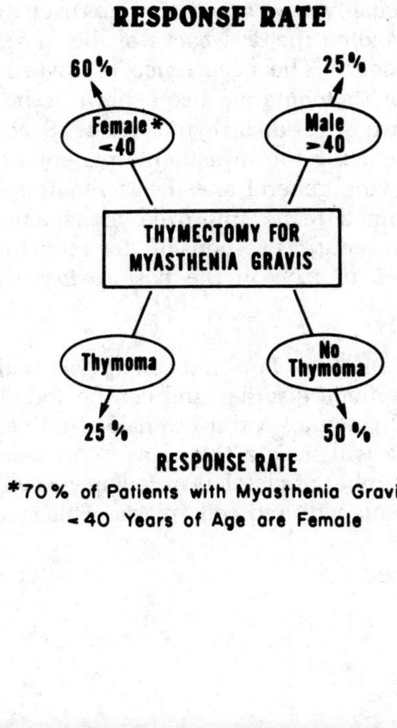

Seventy percent of patients with myasthenia gravis younger than 40 years of age are women. Occurrence of the disease in them is twice as common as in older men, and the women have a 60% response rate to thymectomy, compared with a 25% response for men. The age of patients with myasthenia gravis and thymoma (15–35 years) is generally older than myasthenic patients without thymoma.

Thymomas in patients with myasthenia gravis are usually smaller than those found in nonmyasthenic patients. This finding may be explained by the fact that they are discovered serendipitously when the thymus is removed. Invasive thymomas are found in 35% to 40% of both myasthenic and nonmyasthenic patients.

There is no morphologic parameter in a thymoma that is specific for the concomitant or subsequent occurrence of myasthenia gravis, but some morphologic features of thymomas are more frequently associated with myasthenia.[43] For example, spindle cell thymomas are rarely associated with myasthenia gravis. Another feature of thymomas and myasthenia gravis is the high frequency of lymphoid follicles with germinal centers in the thymic tissues surrounding the thymoma.[26]

The association of the thymus, thymomas, and myasthenia gravis remains an enigma despite all that has been learned in the past decade. There are data to suggest that myoid or muscle-like cells in the thymus and thymomas cross-react with antimuscle antibodies. These cells may be responsible for initiating the antibodies.[41] It has been suggested that a virally induced "thymitis" could trigger the process in which antigenic components within the thymus are recognized by the T lymphocytes and that these antigens cross-react with acetylcholine receptors.[41]

Myasthenic patients may show significant improvement after receiving immunosuppressive drugs, such as corticosteroids and azathioprine.[41,44] The salutory effect of thymectomy may also be explained by the immunosuppressive effect of extirpation of this gland.

Two important aspects of thymectomy for patients with thymomas and myasthenia gravis deserve mention. First, the entire thymus must be removed, along with the thymoma, and an aggressive surgical approach demands the wide resection of invaded structures if possible. Transcervical thymectomy may qualify as an acceptable approach to removing the thymus, avoiding the drawbacks of the more extensive thoracic approach.[45] The occurrence of myasthenia after thymectomy for thymoma has been shown to be related to recurrent disease of residual thymus tissue. Second, the intricacies of managing the myasthenic patient's respiratory problems following general anesthesia requires an experienced, well-trained team. Improved management of this phase of the procedure is responsible for reducing the mortality from 10% to 27% in the past to less than 6% at present.[41]

RED CELL APLASIA. Pure red cell aplasia is also considered an autoimmune disorder and can be found in 5% of patients with thymoma.[1] A third to half of all patients with red cell aplasia will have a thymoma.[46] An associated decrease in the number of platelets or leukocytes will be found in 30% of patients with red cell aplasia. This syndrome appears after the age of 40 in 96% of the patients who develop it. The diagnosis is based on examination of the bone marrow. Red cell precursors are absent, but platelet and leukocytic elements are normal. Thymectomy will result in a 25% to 30% remission of the disease.[46] The relationship between thymoma and red cell aplasia is not yet understood.

HYPOGAMMAGLOBULINEMIA. This abnormality is present in 5% to 10% of patients with thymoma.[40] Patients with hypogammaglobulinemia have a 10% incidence of thymoma. More than a third of those patients also have red cell hypoplasia. Combined humoral and cellular immunodeficiencies are present. Almost all patients are over the age of 40 years. Thymectomy has not proved beneficial in this condition.

Roentgenographic Features of Thymomas

Seventy-five percent of tumors are located in the anterior mediastinum and are the most frequent neoplasms found in this compartment (see Fig. 23-3). Approximately 15% occupy both the anterior and superior mediastinum, and 6% are primarily in the superior mediastinum. No more than 5% to 10% of thymomas occur in other locations, such as the neck and middle and posterior mediastinum. The lesion is characteristically located anterior to the junction of the great vessels, which may be displaced posteriorly by the tumor. Thymomas are round or oval, with smooth or lobulated margins. The mass may protrude to one or both sides of the mediastinum. Calcifications may be seen in as many as 20% of thymomas, either at the periphery of the tumor or throughout its substance.[26] Calcifications are best visualized by overpenetrated films, laminograms, or by CT (see Fig. 23-6).

CT allows precise definition of the extent of involvement and the nature of a tumor mass suspected of being a thymoma.[47] Among 19 patients with myasthenia gravis, CT was accurate in detecting 9 of the masses that were present but could not differentiate thymomas from nonthymomatous masses. Glands with thymic hyperplasia could not be differentiated from normal glands.[48] Cysts can be more easily differentiated from solid tumors by CT. By measuring the thickness of the thymic lobes, thymic hyperplasia and lymphoma can be diagnosed.[49] Pleural metastases are also more easily identified by CT than by conventional roentgenograms or laminograms of the chest.[47]

Treatment of Thymoma

SURGERY. The most effective therapy of a thymoma is its complete removal. When the thymoma is encapsulated and can be removed with the entire thymus, without disturbing the integrity of the capsule, virtually all patients will be cured of the tumor. As few as 2% will develop recurrences, which take the form of pleural, pericardial, or diaphragmatic implants or of a localized mediastinal tumor (Fig. 23-11).[37]

Poor prognostic determinants are invasiveness of the tumor and an associated syndrome such as myasthenia gravis.[34,50] Associated diseases are present in half of all patients who develop a recurrence following surgery. Fortu-

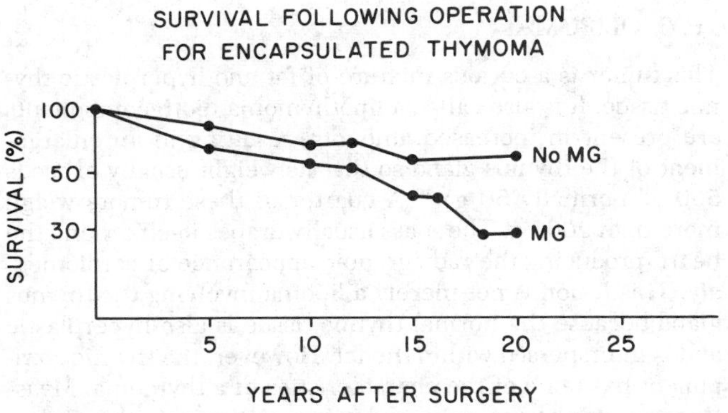

FIG. 23-11. Bernatz found that patients with thymoma and myasthenia gravis had a poorer prognosis than did those without myasthenia gravis (*MG*). (Bernatz PE, Khonsari S, Harrison EG et al: Thymomas: Factors influencing prognosis. Surg Clin North Am 53:885, 1973)

nately, 65% of thymomas are well-encapsulated and not associated with myasthenia gravis. As expected of patients with a neuromuscular disorder, survival following resection of encapsulated thymomas is also poor when myasthenia gravis is present (Fig. 23-11). However, recent experiences have shown that patients with thymoma and myasthenia gravis do as well as those without myasthenia.[51]

Because of the propensity of thymomas to recur or develop local metastases when the integrity of the capsule is violated, biopsy of these tumors should be avoided. The tumor should be removed intact whenever possible. Biopsy should be reserved for the patient who is unable to tolerate a resection. Needle aspiration is another option for such patients.[22]

Thymectomy and resection of a thymoma is best carried out using a midline sternal-splitting incision. A bilateral submammary incision transecting the sternum may provide a more cosmetic result. However, the exposure this incision provides is not optimal, and it may be more difficult to deal with any invasive lesions encountered. The poor exposure provided by a cervical incision renders this approach unsatisfactory, although it may be used for smaller lesions. Standard right or left thoracotomies have been performed if the tumor appears to be present largely on one side or the other.

Resection of encapsulated noninvasive thymomas presents few problems to the surgeon because they are easily removed.[34] Invasive tumors, on the other hand, can be difficult and challenging. An aggressive surgical approach should be adopted because these tumors are slow-growing and remain localized in the chest for long periods. In order to obtain sufficient exposure to resect all of the tumor, the median sternotomy may have to be combined with a thoracotomy. Pericardium, phrenic nerve, pleura, diaphragm, and lung can be resected if these structures are involved. Lobectomy and pneumonectomy may be required, depending upon the specific circumstances and extent of involvement. Resection of the innominate vein and portions or all of the superior vena cava has been performed when these vessels are invaded.[52] A patch graft of autogenous vein or prosthetic material or a vascular graft of Teflon or Dacron can be used to bridge the resulting venous defect, with expectation of a good functional result. When extensive involvement precludes complete resection, such as with invasion of the heart, great vessels, or trachea, as much tumor as can be safely resected should be removed to prevent cardiac tamponade or tracheal occlusion and asphyxiation. Resection should also be considered in the treatment of local recurrences and pleural and pericardial metastases.

RADIOTHERAPY. Thymomas are relatively radiosensitive. Radiation therapy constitutes excellent adjuvant therapy and is considered mandatory for all patients with invasive thymomas, whether or not a complete resection is performed.[53,54] The surgeon should therefore mark off the extent of the resected tumor and thymus with metallic radiopaque clips in order to facilitate treatment planning by the radiotherapist. Preoperative radiation therapy was used by several groups and was not helpful.[55] Investigative efforts are currently underway to determine if intraoperative radiation therapy may be of benefit.

There is some disagreement concerning the role of adjuvant radiotherapy for patients with encapsulated noninvasive thymomas. Because the recurrence rate is low (about 2%) and radiotherapy carries some morbidity, Rosai and Levine oppose the use of postoperative radiotherapy if these tumors are removed in toto.[26] At the other extreme is the view that no patient with thymoma can be considered to have been adequately treated unless he receives radiotherapy.[38] It is reasonable to adopt either course, depending upon the circumstances. If long-term follow-up is not possible or likely, and experienced radiotherapists are able to treat the area with minimal side effects, patients with noninvasive thymomas may be advised to undergo postoperative radiotherapy. On the other hand, easily followed patients with small, encapsulated tumors, which were removed with the entire thymus, can receive radiation if recurrences appear. Reresection should also be considered. In the absence of a prospective controlled randomized study, no definitive statement can be made concerning the role of adjuvant radiotherapy for Stage I thymomas.

Radiotherapy as adjuvant therapy, for the treatment of recurrences or to treat unresectable primary thymomas, usually consists of 3500 to 4500 rad given over 3 to 6 weeks. Dosages in excess of 4500 rad do not significantly increase response rates but do increase the risk of postirradiation complications if large fields are used. If the tumor is small, Penn and Hope-Stone recommend using two large anterior oblique wedge fields.[54] Field size in their experience was about 15 cm by 8 cm. More extensive lesions are treated with large parallel opposed fields, which can be supplemented with a wedge pair or an additional direct anterior field. Field sizes up to 20 cm by 15 cm are used. These techniques minimize exposure to the spinal cord.

In addition to irradiating the tumor, it is also often important to treat the entire thymus gland, which extends from the sixth cervical vertebra to the level of the fourth to seventh costal cartilage. Skeggs recommends a single anterior and two posterior oblique fields to provide satisfactory dose distribution.[56]

Marks and colleagues recommend a dose of 4000 rad to the tumor bed in 4 to 5 weeks if the invasive thymoma is completely removed. The last 1000 rad should be given with a pair of anterior oblique fields to reduce the total dose to the spinal cord. For unresectable or partially resectable disease, a dose of 4500 rad in 5 to 6 weeks is recommended. Shrinking fields should be used as the tumor responds. A split course of irradiation should be considered for large tumors in order to spare the spinal cord.[57] This approach has resulted in 100% local tumor control in 9 patients when used in conjunction with resection.

Pneumonitis is a frequent (40%) side effect of radiotherapy when large fields are used.[54] To minimize radiation damage to the lungs in patients with pleural implants, Ariaratnam and colleagues use a moving strip technique.[53] Mediastinitis, pericarditis, and myocarditis are additional infrequent complications of thymic radiation when unresectable or residual thymomas require large fields and high doses. However, if unresectable or residual tumor is carefully marked out at operation by the surgeon, it should be possible to treat a small tumor volume to a high dose without undue complications.

CHEMOTHERAPY. Corticosteroids have caused regression of some unresectable thymomas that do not respond to radiotherapy.[45] Chemotherapy for thymomas should be reserved for patients with advanced disease who respond neither to radiation nor steroids. Effective single drugs are cisplatin and doxorubicin.[58] Responses have also been reported with the use of alkylating agents.[45] Daugaard and colleagues reported complete responses, which lasted a median of 37 months, in four of nine patients treated with vincristine, cyclophosphamide, lomustine, and prednisone.[59] These are the best results in the largest series of patients treated with chemotherapy. The overall response rate was 56%. Partial remissions have been reported with combinations of cyclophosphamide, vincristine, prednisone, and procarbazine and with combinations of bleomycin, doxorubicin, cisplatin, and prednisone.[38,60,61]

RESULTS OF THERAPY. At the Mayo Clinic, the 10-year survival rate for noninvasive tumors was 65%, compared with 30% for invasive tumors.[50] The 5-year survival at the Memorial Hospital for encapsulated and invasive tumors was 83% and 54%, respectively.[36] Less than half of the patients with invasive thymomas who survived for 5 years were free of disease. Ten-year survival of patients with thymoma treated at the Massachusetts General Hospital are 57% overall; totally resected, 72%; encapsulated tumor without myasthenia gravis, 85%; and invasive tumor with myasthenia gravis, 8.7%. In France, patients with noninvasive thymomas had survival rates of 85% at 5 years and 80% at 10 years. Patients with invasive tumors had a survival rate of about 50% at 5 years and 35% at 10 years. In this series, associated autoimmune diseases had no influence on survival. All patients were treated with radiation postoperatively. Recurrences were found in 6% of patients with noninvasive tumors and in 36% of patients with invasive tumors. Slightly invasive, completely excised thymomas had the same rate of recurrence as largely invasive tumors in which only biopsy had been performed.[38]

THYMOLIPOMA

This tumor is a curious mixture of fat and hyperplastic thymic tissue. It is also called a lipothymoma. Both components are present in increased amounts, resulting in an enlargement of the thymus gland so that its weight usually exceeds 500 g (normally 50 g).[26] A quarter of these tumors weigh more than 2000 g. The mass usually drapes itself around the heart, producing the radiographic appearance of cardiomegaly. This lesion is not merely a lipoma involving the thymus gland because the normal thymic tissue is also hyperplastic and is interspersed within the fat. However, the thymic component has none of the characteristics of a thymoma. Myasthenia gravis has not occurred in association with this tumor. This is a rare, benign tumor that has never been reported to invade adjacent structures, to metastasize, or to recur following removal.

CARCINOID OF THE THYMUS

Until 1972, many carcinoid tumors of the thymus were not recognized as distinct lesions and were mistakenly labeled as variants of thymomas.[26,62–64] The fact that they have a similar morphology and similar biologic characteristics with respect to their malignant potential and that they respond to the same therapy probably accounts for the confusion between carcinoids and thymomas. However, significant morphological and biochemical differences exist between these two tumors, and they can be readily differentiated.

Thymic carcinoids develop from cells of neural crest origin, which differentiate into Kulchitsky cells. They can undergo malignant change to become carcinoid tumors. No more than 100 thymic carcinoids have been reported in the literature as of 1980.[64] Their gross appearance is similar to that of thymomas. The tumors may be encapsulated or invade adjacent structures. Invasiveness is seen in 50% of thymic carcinoids, compared with 35% of thymomas. Furthermore, thymomas rarely have extrathoracic metastases, but thymic carcinoids metastasize to bone, often forming blastic lesions, and other sites in up to 73% of patients with this tumor. Metastases may appear as long as 8 years after initial diagnosis.[64]

Fibrous compartmentalization and cystic changes seen in thymomas do not occur with thymic carcinoids. The two tumors may have similar appearances by light microscopy, but electron microscopy can accurately differentiate carcinoid tumors from thymomas. Carcinoids are characterized by numerous cytoplasmic neurosecretory granules, as are other foregut carcinoids. Thymomas will have desmosones, tonofilaments, and elongated cytoplasmic processes not seen in carcinoids. Carcinoids will also contain argyrophil cells that can be detected by appropriate staining techniques.

Thymic carcinoids have been classified among the "amine precursor uptake and decarboxylation" tumors (APUDomas), which are known to have the potential of elaborating peptides, amines, kinins, and prostaglandins. The only endocrine syndrome reported to be directly caused by thymic carcinoids is Cushing's syndrome. In these instances, the carcinoid produces elevated levels of ACTH. Patients with carcinoid syndrome caused by thymic carcinoids have not been reported, but other endocrine tumors have occurred with thymic carcinoids. Approximately one third to one half of thymic carcinoids have been associated with paraneoplastic syndromes. Although most of these have been Cushing's syndrome, patients with thymic carcinoids have been described with Type I multiple endocrine neoplasias (MEN I; Werner's syndrome; pituitary, parathyroid, and pancreatic islet cell tumors). In two thirds of these patients, the carcinoids have been malignant. Carcinoid tumors of the thymus have also been reported to coexist with medullary carcinomas of the thyroid (MEN II: Sipple's syndrome, medullary thyroid carcinoma, pheochromocytoma, and hyperparathyroidism). It has been postulated that the rare oat cell carcinomas of the thymus can arise from a carcinoid tumor of the thymus.[63,65]

Carcinoid tumors of the thymus are treated by wide excision of the thymus containing the tumor. The resection should include contiguous invaded structures that can be sacrificed or replaced. Postoperative radiation therapy has helped patients with persistent or recurrent tumor.

GERM CELL TUMORS

Much of the material covered in Chapter 35 on testicular tumors applies to this section as well since testicular and mediastinal germ cell tumors share many characteristics. All types of germinal tumors found in the testes have been reported in the mediastinum.[25] Approximately 10% of all mediastinal tumors are of germinal origin.

HISTOGENESIS

Extragonadal germ cell tumors are usually situated along the body midline in the cranium, the mediastinum, and the retroperitoneal and presacral areas. The histogenesis of these tumors is not clear. Those arising within the thymus presumably originate from germ cells that may have migrated into this gland during embryogenesis. Because the urogenital ridge extends from C6 to L4, its juxtaposition to the thymic anlage favors such a possibility. Alternatively, germ cell tumors may arise from a maldevelopment of a thymic anlage during embryogenesis or from potentially biphasic germ cells left within the thymus.

Germ cell tumors of the mediastinum are considered thymic neoplasms because they most likely arise within the gland. Many studies have demonstrated that they do not represent metastases from a primary gonadal site. Autopsies of patients with these tumors have enabled pathologists to examine multiple sections of the patient's gonads, and no evidence of testicular or ovarian involvement has been found in the vast majority of patients with mediastinal germ cell tumors.[26] Other autopsies of patients with germ cell tumors of the testes have shown that metastases solely to the anterior mediastinum do not occur.[66] If anterior mediastinal metastases are present from a testicular tumor, middle and posterior mediastinal nodes are also involved.[67]

INDICATIONS FOR TESTICULAR BIOPSY

Suggestions have been made to remove or biopsy the testes to exclude the possibility of an occult testicular primary tumor giving rise to mediastinal germ cell tumors. If the testes are abnormal on physical examination, these procedures are indicated. However, testes that appear normal on physical examination and on high-resolution ultrasonography need not be removed nor explored when a mediastinal germ cell tumor is present.[68] However, a testicular biopsy is indicated when lymphangiography or CT demonstrates involvement of pelvic or retroperitoneal lymph nodes or if an isolated retroperitoneal germ cell tumor is discovered.

CLASSIFICATIONS

Several classifications of germ cell tumors have been devised. Mediastinal germ cell tumors are often difficult to fit into any classification because they contain mixtures of various types. Rosai and Levine classify mediastinal germ cell tumors as germinomas (seminomas), adult teratomas, embryonal carcinomas, teratocarcinomas, choriocarcinomas, and yolk sac tumors (endodermal sinus tumors).[26] A simpler system of classification considers tumors as either pure seminomas or nonseminomatous carcinomas.[67] The latter may be pure embryonal carcinomas, pure teratocarcinomas, pure choriocarcinomas, pure entodermal sinus carcinomas, or mixtures of all these elements. Most often, the nonseminomatous tumors are of mixed composition, with or without seminomatous elements.

It is reasonable to classify mediastinal germ cell tumors into primary seminomas of the mediastinum and primary nonseminomatous germ cell tumors of the mediastinum. This division separates the tumors on the basis of their treatment and also by their prognosis. Seminomas have a better prognosis and are more responsive to therapy than the other pure and mixed malignant germ cell tumors of the mediastinum.

PRIMARY SEMINOMAS

Seminomas of the mediastinum make up half of all germ cell tumors of the mediastinum and occur in men 20 to 40 years of age. No more than 5% of these tumors occur in women.[69] They usually cause symptoms by impinging upon structures in the anterior mediastinum. Chest pain, cough, dyspnea, and superior vena caval obstruction are the most prominent symptoms. In a small percentage of patients, other germ cell elements are present in the malignancy in small amounts, resulting in elevated serum levels of alpha-fetoprotein or of the beta unit of human chorionic gonadotrophin (β-HCG). Radioimmunoassays may be required to detect these increases, because immunodiffusion techniques are not sufficiently sensitive. If the levels are very high, the pathologic diagnosis should be reevaluated and a diagnosis of a nonseminomatous tumor of the mixed type should be considered.

Most patients with mediastinal seminoma have extensive involvement of the great vessels when they are first seen. Only 20% of the tumors could be completely excised in the patients reported by the Memorial Hospital and the Mayo

Clinic.[67,70] The role of tumor reductive surgery (debulking) for mediastinal seminomas is questionable. If performed, it should be conservative and not add to the morbidity and mortality of the patient.

Because this tumor is extremely radiosensitive, local disease can usually be well-controlled. The excellent response of seminomas to radiation therapy is in marked contrast to the nonseminomatous germ cell tumors, which are relatively radioresistant. A recent review of the contribution of radiotherapy to the management of primary malignant mediastinal germ cell tumors revealed that the actuarial 5-year survival for seminomas was 100%, but it was only 8.8% for the remaining germ cell varieties.[71]

Megavoltage radiation therapy should be given to all patients. A shaped mediastinal field should be used with a midplane dose of up to 4500 rad over 5 to 6 weeks.[72] This dose is greater than that recommended for gonadal seminoma because it is the experience of some radiotherapists that lower doses may result in local recurrences.[72] A split course therapy with interruption after approximately 2000 to 3000 rad is a possible alternative. A more conservative dose of 3500 to 4000 rad is recommended by the Mayo Clinic group.[70]

It is important to emphasize that radiation therapy is the mainstay of curative therapy for primary mediastinal seminoma. Because the supraclavicular and infraclavicular low cervical lymph nodes can be easily included in the field of radiation, these areas should be treated as well. Prophylactic irradiation of the upper abdominal and para-aortic lymph nodes is recommended by some groups and not deemed necessary by others.

The combination of surgery and radiotherapy will result in a 58% to 82% 5-year survival rate.[72,73] Martini and colleagues reported that the local component of mediastinal seminomas could be controlled by resection and radiation in all patients with this tumor, regardless of the extent of mediastinal involvement.[67] Most patients in their series had disseminated disease, which caused their deaths. For this reason, they recommended early systemic chemotherapy even if there is no disease evident outside the mediastinum.

Metastases from the seminoma are commonly present. Involvement of bone, liver, spleen, tonsil, thyroid, skin, and the central nervous system has been reported. Factors that may predict the presence of distant metastases are age greater than 35 years, fever, superior vena caval obstruction, cervical and supraclavicular lymph node involvement, and hilar disease.[71]

A review of the management of primary mediastinal seminomas pointed out that combination chemotherapy with vinblastine, bleomycin, and cis-platinum (VBP) with or without doxorubicin can induce complete remissions (58%) and long-term disease-free survival.[73] Alkylating agents have also been recommended. A patient treated exclusively with chlorambucil and actinomycin D was free of disease 11 years after diagnosis. These observations and the results obtained in the treatment of testicular seminomas provide an encouraging outlook for patients with mediastinal seminoma.

NONSEMINOMATOUS PURE AND MIXED GERM CELL CARCINOMAS

Nonseminomatous tumors can be pure or mixed germ cell carcinomas. Mixed types contain seminomatous, embryonal, endodermal sinus, teratomatous, or trophoblastic elements. The latter subtype has the appearance and functional characteristics of a choriocarcinoma. Teratocarcinomas can be cystic or solid. All of these tumors occur most often in men. Of 20 patients with mixed germ-cell carcinomas of the mediastinum of various kinds treated at Memorial Sloan-Kettering Cancer Center from 1949 through 1971, 14 were men and 6 were women.[67] In many smaller series, all of the patients have been men. The majority of patients are between 15 and 35 years of age.

Pleuritic or substernal pain with dyspnea, cough, and hemoptysis are frequent presenting symptoms. Gynecomastia is present in 33% to 50% of men with choriocarcinoma. Patients with Kleinfelter's syndrome may be predisposed to the development of nonseminomatous extragonadal germ cell tumors and should be followed carefully.[74]

Elevated levels of β-HCG may be present in patients with choriocarcinoma and can be used to evaluate the efficacy of therapy and detect early recurrences and metastases. Elevated levels of β-HCG are present in 60% of patients with nonseminomatous germ cell tumors.[75] Serum levels of alpha-fetoprotein and carcinoembryonic antigen may also help in identifying some of these tumors preoperatively. If the tumors demonstrate a predominant pattern of endodermal sinus elements, serum alpha-fetoprotein levels are likely to be very high. Approximately 70% of patients with nonseminomatous germ cell tumors have elevated levels of alpha-fetoprotein.[75] These markers can also be used to follow the tumor's response to therapy and to detect recurrences.

Teratocarcinomas usually contain elements of embryonal cell carcinoma, but other malignant components, such as adenocarcinoma, squamous cell carcinoma, and sarcoma may be present.[76]

The mainstay of therapy for nonseminomatous germ cell tumors is intensive chemotherapy. VBP with or without doxorubicin resulted in complete remission in approximately 65% of patients with nonseminomatous germ cell tumors; choriocarcinomas showed the poorest response.[77] Patients with pure endodermal sinus tumors have poor prognoses also. The single most important prognostic indicator for mediastinal endodermal sinus tumors is whether they can be completely excised before or after chemotherapy.[78]

VBP is a toxic regimen, but attempts at lessening the drug dosages seem to reduce its efficacy.[79] A combination of vinblastine, actinomycin D, bleomycin, cis-platinum, and cyclophosphamide (VAB-3) has also been recommended.[80] There is some dissatisfaction with the results of these regimens, and several groups continue to search for better approaches to these tumors.[75,79,81] Some success has recently been achieved with VP-16, ifosfamide, and cisplatin as salvage therapy.[82] The benefit of radiation therapy for control of local and metastatic disease is questionable. Neither irradiation nor surgery can control the local disease for a significant length of time. Resection of the tumor after treatment with combination chemotherapy is recommended and may be beneficial.[75]

BENIGN (ADULT) TERATOMAS

Teratomas are neoplasms that originate in pluripotent cells, and are composed of a wide diversity of tissues foreign to the organ or anatomic site in which they arise. The tumors frequently occur in young adults, with equal incidence in both sexes. Approximately 20% of mediastinal teratomatous tumors are teratocarcinomas.[1] When they are malignant, they can contain any of the varieties of germ cell cancers. The subject of extragonadal teratomas has been comprehensively covered by Gonzalez-Crussi in the Armed Forces Institute of Pathology *Atlas of Tumor Pathology*, which contains a section on mediastinal teratomas.

In adults, the mediastinum is the second most frequent location of a teratoma, after the gonads. In children, the sacrococcygeal area is the most frequent site of teratomas, followed by the mediastinum. Teratomas are found almost exclusively in the anterosuperior mediastinum, at the junction of the heart and great vessels. Calcifications are present in 75% of the lesions. Occasionally, they occur in the pericardium or posterior mediastinum. The tumors contain representations of all three germ layers in a rather mature state. When the lesions are cystic and contain hair and teeth, they have been called dermoid cysts, but this is a misnomer because these tumors, like the ovarian dermoids, are not of ectodermal origin.

Most patients with teratomas are asymptomatic. Those with symptoms have them because of the size of the tumor and compression of adjacent structures. Tumors have reached 30 cm in diameter. Erosion into a bronchus is an uncommon complication, as is rupture into the pericardium. Insulin production by a teratoma may produce hypoglycemia.

Benign teratomas are easily excised after exposing them through a sternal-splitting or standard thoracotomy incision.

THYMIC CARCINOMA

The histogenesis of thymic carcinoma is indeterminate.[1] Wick and colleagues reviewed a large series of patients with this diagnosis and presented evidence suggesting that the tumors are more malignant variants of thymic epithelium, which differ from thymomas morphologically as well as biologically.[83] About half are highly undifferentiated. The others may have adenocarcinomatous, sarcomatous, or a squamous cell appearance. Some of the latter subtypes have the appearance of lymphoepitheliomas seen in the nasopharynx. This similarity in appearance has recently been shown to have a common cause—Epstein-Barr viral (EBV) penetration and replication in the epithelial elements of the thymus, which also occurs in the epithelial cells of the nasopharyngeal lymphoid tissue. A patient with a thymic carcinoma of the lymphoepithelioma type has recently been shown to have the serological profile of EBV, the presence of EBV-associated nuclear antigens in the carcinoma cells, and a high level of viral genomes of EBV detected in the DNA. All of this indicates that EBV is involved in the genesis of some thymic carcinomas and some undifferentiated nasopharyngeal carcinomas.[84]

Because these cancers are most common in the anterosuperior compartment, they probably arise from thymic epithelium or embryonic nests within the thymus. These tumors should not be classified with thymomas and, like the lymphomas of the thymus, should be considered a separate entity with a poorer prognosis than the true thymomas.[81] Rarely, an oat cell tumor may also arise from the thymus.[65]

NEUROGENIC TUMORS

Neurogenic tumors vie with thymomas as the most common primary neoplasm of the mediastinum in adults and are the most common neoplasms in children (Table 23-5).[1–6,9,85,86]

HISTOGENESIS

Neural crest tissue gives rise to the nerve cells and the supporting elements (Schwann cells) that surround them. The sheath cells undergo neoplastic transformation to become neurilemmomas or schwannomas. Neurofibromas arise from the Schwann cells also but contain neuronal elements.

In the transformation of neural crest cells into neurones (ganglion cells), there is a certain progression. Sympathogonia develop from the embryonic neural crest and can be identified as the cells of origin of the tumor called a sympathogonioma. Sympathogonia become neuroblasts, the cells of origin of neuroblastomas. The neuroblast can either develop into a sympathicoblast or a pheochromocyte. The latter gives rise to pheochromocytomas (chromaffin positive or chemodectomas) and paragangliomas (chromaffin negative). Sympathicoblasts give rise to ganglioneuroblastomas.

Mature ganglion cells are derived from sympathicoblasts and can give rise to ganglioneuromas. Both malignant neuroblastomas and ganglioneuroblastomas can revert to the benign, more differentiated ganglioneuroma in 25% of instances.

NEURILEMMOMAS AND NEUROFIBROMAS

Neurilemmomas (Schwannomas) and neurofibromas can arise from the intercostal nerves or the sympathetic ganglia in the posterior mediastinum. The vagus and phrenic nerves are very rarely the sites of this neoplasm. Neurilemmomas and neurofibromas make up at least 65% of all neurogenic tumors, and about 66% to 75% will be found in the upper half of the chest. These tumors will also be found on the right side 65% to 75% of the time.

Differentiation between neurilemmomas and neurofibromas by the pathologist may be difficult at times. In most series neurilemmomas predominate over neurofibromas and are thus considered the most frequently encountered neurogenic tumor.[87] Ganglioneuromas may also have a histopathologic picture similar to the nerve sheath tumors.

From 25% to 40% of patients with nerve sheath tumors will have multiple neurofibromatosis (von Recklinghausen's disease). However, if a patient with von Recklinghausen's disease presents with a posterior mediastinal mass, it will more often be a meningocele than a posterior mediastinal neurofibroma.

Neurofibrosarcomas and malignant neurilemmomas constitute 10% to 20% of the tumors and are more frequently seen in patients with von Recklinghausen's disease. Radiation therapy and chemotherapy for those lesions are outlined in Chapters 39 and 46. These neoplasms carry a poor prognosis. Recurrences may occur even when the lesion is originally thought to be benign. Because malignant degeneration and recurrence can take place, patients operated upon for neurogenic tumors should be followed closely for many years.[87]

TUMORS OF NERVE CELLS

Neuroblastomas and ganglioneuroblastomas are poorly differentiated malignant tumors found predominantly in children (see Chap. 46). If present in the posterior mediastinum, their treatment is the same as for those encountered elsewhere in the body. These tumors are often unresectable.

The benign ganglioneuroma is easily excised at the time of thoracotomy.

Intrathoracic pheochromocytomas do not differ from those arising in the abdomen. Chemodectomas (paragangliomas) of the thorax may be locally invasive, involving the aorta, aortic branches, and the pulmonary artery. The capacity to synthesize catecholamines is the distinguishing feature of pheochromocytomas, but it is not unique to these neurogenic tumors. Any of the cells derived from the neural crest can develop this ability.

It may be possible to use this property of neurogenic tumors in the follow-up of patients with these tumors. The urinary metabolites of the catecholamines, vanillyl mandelic acid and homovanillic acid, can be used as tumor markers. Metanephrine and normetanephrine, the metabolites of epinephrine and norepinephrine, can be similarly used.

INTRASPINOUS INVOLVEMENT

One unique aspect of neurogenic tumors of the posterior mediastinum is the possibility that they may extend through an intervertebral foramen to assume a dumbbell shape.[85] Among 706 patients with mediastinal neurogenic tumors seen at the Mayo Clinic, 10% presented in this manner. Sixty percent of patients with dumbbell-shaped neurogenic tumors had symptoms of spinal cord compression. Roentgenologic studies demonstrating erosion or vertebral pedicles or enlargement of the intervertebral foramina adjacent to a mediastinal mass suggest the possibility of a dumbbell tumor. A myelogram can establish whether there is an intraspinous component of the posterior mediastinal neurogenic tumor. If such is the case, a one-stage combined intrathoracic and intraspinal approach can completely excise the tumor. The spinal component should be dealt with first to minimize bleeding into the spinal canal. If this occurs, the patient can become paraplegic.[87] If a dumbbell-shaped tumor is inadvertently found during a thoracotomy, a two-stage procedure can be effective. Dumbbell tumors carry the same 10% to 20% malignancy rate that other neurogenic tumors of the posterior mediastinum do.

MESENCHYMAL TUMORS

Most of the connective tissue tumors found in the soft tissues and discussed in Chapter 40 can also be found in the mediastinum. They constitute 6% to 7% of mediastinal neoplasms, and about half are malignant.[1] Benign tumors are permanently eradicated by surgical excision. Malignant mesenchymal tumors should be treated, as other soft tissue sarcomas are, with combined resection, radiation, and chemotherapy.

Seventy-five percent of mediastinal lipomas are located anteriorly and may present the same roentgenographic appearance as a pericardial cyst in the right cardiophrenic angle. Large lipomas extend into adjacent mediastinal compartments in an unpredictable manner. Liposarcomas, on the other hand, tend to occur in the posterior compartment where they may be confused with neurogenic tumors and the rare xanthogranulomas. Lipomatous tumors can be easily recognized by CT.

Mediastinal lymphangiomas can be difficult tumors to completely excise because they grow in a budding fashion and become densely adherent to the great vessels and other mediastinal structures. They are most often found in the anterior mediastinum.

Mesotheliomas may also present as mediastinal masses arising from parietal or pericardium. When they are localized, resection is curative. Diffuse invasive lesions have a poorer prognosis. Histologic criteria cannot differentiate benign from malignant lesions.

OTHER MEDIASTINAL TUMORS

There are a wide variety of lesions in this category, all of which are infrequently encountered, except for cysts. Cysts can now be readily diagnosed by CT and ultrasonography. Cysts are of congenital origin, have no neoplastic elements, and are pertinent only in the context of their differential diagnosis from other tumors of the mediastinum. Substernal goiters presenting in the anterosuperior mediastinum, like mediastinal cysts, make up a relatively large number of mediastinal masses and are of interest in differential diagnosis. Like cysts, they are readily managed by excision in order to eliminate the danger of sudden, life-threatening compressive complications, which can occur in asymptomatic and symptomatic patients.[88]

Mediastinal hemangiomas are rare lesions, which have been reported in 103 patients.[89] They can be found in either the anterosuperior or posterior mediastinum. Radical resection of these tumors to achieve total excision is not recommended, but they can be removed without undue blood loss. Local recurrences are possible, but they cause few problems and have shown no evidence of malignant degeneration.[89]

Inflammatory pseudotumors of the mediastinum are another group of rare lesions. They are not neoplastic, consist of chronic inflammatory fibrous tissue, and have an obscure cause. They can appear in either of the two major mediastinal compartments, anterosuperior or posterior, and are similar to those described in the lung.[90]

REFERENCES

1. Silverman NA, Sabiston DC Jr: Mediastinal masses. Surg Clin North Am 60:757, 1980
2. Oldham HN Jr: Mediastinal tumors and cysts. Ann Thorac Surg 11:246, 1971
3. Hammon JW Jr, Sabiston DC Jr: The mediastinum. In Ellis HE, Goldsmith HS (eds): Thoracic Surgery. Hagerstown, MD, Harper & Row, 1979
4. Lyons HA, Calvy GL, Sammons BP: The diagnosis and classification of mediastinal masses: 1. A study of 782 cases. Ann Intern Med 51:897, 1959
5. Burkell CC, Cross JM, Kent HP et al: Mass lesions of the mediastinum. Curr Prob Surg (Chicago), 1969
6. Herlitzka AJ, Gale JW: Tumors and cysts of the mediastinum, Arch Surg 76:697, 1958
7. Davis RD Jr, Oldham HN Jr, Sabiston DC Jr: Primary cysts and neoplasms of the mediastinum: Recent changes in clinical presentation, methods of diagnosis, management and results. Ann Thorac Surg 44:229, 1987
8. Grosfeld JL, Weinberger M, Kilman JW et al: Primary mediastinal neoplasms in infants and children. Ann Thorac Surg 12:179, 1971
9. Wychulis AR, Payne WS, Clagett OT et al: Surgical treatment of mediastinal tumors. J Thorac Cardiovasc Surg 62:379, 1971
10. Lichtenstein AK, Levine A, Taylor CR et al: Primary mediastinal lymphomas in adults. Am J Med 68:509, 1980
11. Mullen B, Richardson JD: Primary anterior mediastinal tumors in children and adults. Ann Thorac Surg 42:338, 1986
12. Strother CM, Schett JS, Crummy AB et al: Clinical application of computerized fluoroscopy: the extracranial carotid arteries. Radiology 136:781, 1980
13. Sone S, Higashihara T, Morimoto S et al: Normal anatomy of thymus and anterior mediastinum by pneumomediastinography. Am J Roentgenol 134:81, 1980
14. Pugatch RD, Foling LJ: Computed tomography of the thorax: A status report. Chest 80:618, 1981
15. Livesay JJ, Mink JH, Fee HJ et al: The use of computed tomography to evaluate suspected mediastinal tumors. Ann Thorac Surg 27:305, 1979
16. Miller GA, Heaston DK, Moore AV et al: CT differentiation of thoracic aneurysm from pulmonary masses adjacent to the mediastinum. J Comput Assist Tomogr 8:437, 1984
17. McLoud TC, Wittenberg J, Ferrucci JT: Computed tomography of the thorax and standard radiographic evaluation of the chest: A comparative study. J Comput Assist Tomogr 3:170, 1979
18. Goldwin RL, Heitzman ER, Proto AV: Computed tomography of the mediastinum: Normal anatomy and indications for the use of CT. Radiology 124:235, 1977
19. Webb WR, Gamou G, Stark DD et al: Evaluation of magnetic resonance sequences in imaging mediastinal tumors. Am J Radiol 143:525, 1984
20. vonShulthess GK, McMurdo K, Tscholakoff D et al: Mediastinal masses: MR imaging. Radiology 158:289, 1986
21. Irwin RS, Braman SS, Arvanitidis AN et al: Thyroid scanning in preoperative diagnosis of mediastinal goiter. Ann Intern Med 89:73, 1978
22. van Sonnenberg E, Lin AS, Deutsch AL et al: Percutaneous biopsy of difficult mediastinal hilar and pulmonary lesions by computed tomographic guidance and a modified coaxial technique. Radiology 148:300, 1983
23. Keller AR, Castleman B: Hodgkin's disease of the thymus gland. Cancer 33:1615, 1974
24. Bell RH, Knapp BI, Anson BJ et al: Form, size, blood supply and relations of the adult thymus. Bull Northwest Univ Med Sch 28:156, 1954
25. Sloan HE Jr: The thymus in myasthenia gravis. Surgery 13:154, 1943
26. Rosai J, Levine GD: Tumors of the thymus. Atlas of Tumor Pathology, Second Series, Fascicle 13. Washington DC, Armed Forces Institute of Pathology, 1976
27. Ham AW, Cormack DH: Histology, 8th ed. Philadelphia, JB Lippincott, 1979
28. Schulof RS, Goldstein AL: Thymosin and the endocrine thymus. Adv Intern Med 22:121, 1977
29. Trainin N: Thymic hormones and the immune response. Physiol Rev 54:272, 1974
30. Lauriola L, Maggiano N, Marino M et al: Human thymoma: Immunologic characteristics of the lymphocyte component. Cancer 48:1992, 1981
31. Bergh NP, Gatzinsky P, Larsson S et al: Tumors of the thymus and thymic region: I. Clinicopathological studies of thymomas. Ann Thorac Surg 25:91, 1978
32. LeGolvan DP, Abell MR: Thymomas. Cancer 39:2142, 1977
33. Gray GF, Gutowski WT: Thymoma: A clinicopathologic study of 54 cases. Am J Surg Pathol 3:235, 1979
34. Gerein AN, Srivastava SP, Burgess J: Thymoma: A ten-year review. Am J Surg 136:49, 1978
35. Salyer WR, Eggleston JC: Thymoma: A clinical and pathological study of 65 cases. Cancer 37:229, 1976
36. Batata MA, Martini N, Huvos AG et al: Thymomas: Clinicopathologic features, therapy, and prognosis. Cancer 34:389, 1974
37. Fechner RE: Recurrence of noninvasive thymomas. Cancer 23:1423, 1969
38. Verley JM, Hollmann KH: Thymoma: A comparative study of clinical stages, histologic features, and survival in 200 cases. Cancer 55:1074, 1985
39. Welch KJ, Tapper D, Vawter GP: Surgical treatment of thymic cysts and neoplasms in children. J Pediatr Surg 14:691, 1979
40. Souadjian JV, Enriquez P, Silverstein MN et al: The spectrum of diseases associated with thymoma. Arch Intern Med 134:374, 1974
41. Drachman DB: Myasthenia gravis. N Engl J Med 298:136, 186, 1978
42. Lindstron J: Autoimmune response to acetylcholine receptors in myasthenia gravis and its animal model. Adv Immunol 27:1, 1979
43. Alpert LI, Papatestas A, Kark A et al: Histologic reappraisal of thymus in myasthenia gravis. Arch Pathol 91:55, 1971
44. Shellito J, Khandekar JD, McKeever WP et al: Invasive thymoma responsive to oral corticosteroids. Cancer Treat Rep 62:1397, 1978
45. Papatestas AE, Pozner J, Genkins G et al: Prognosis in occult thymomas in myasthenia gravis following transcervical thymectomy. Arch Surg 122:1352, 1987
46. Zeok JV, Todd EP, Dillon M et al: The role of thymectomy in red cell aplasia. Ann Thorac Surg 28:257, 1979
47. Zerhouni EA, Scott WW, Baker RR et al: Invasive thymomas: Diagnosis and evaluation by computed tomography. J Comput Assist Tomogr 6:92, 1982
49. Baron RL, Lee JKT, Sagel SS et al: Computed tomography of the abnormal thymus. Radiology 142:127, 1982
50. Bernatz PE, Khonsari S, Harrison EG et al: Thymoma: Factors influencing prognosis. Surg Clin North Am 53:885, 1973
51. Wilkins EW, Castleman B: Thymoma: A continuing survey at the Massachusetts General Hospital. Ann Thorac Surg 28:252, 1979
52. Tanabe T, Kubo Y, Hashimoto M et al: Patch angioplasty of the superior vena caval obstruction (case reports with long follow-up results). J Cardiovasc Surg 20:519, 1979
53. Ariaratnam LS, Kalnicki S, Mincer F et al: The management of malignant thymoma with radiation therapy. Int J Radiat Oncol Biol Phys 5:77, 1979
54. Penn CRH, Hope-Stone HF: The role of radiotherapy in the management of malignant thymoma. Br J Surg 59:533, 1972
55. Sellors TH, Thackray AC, Thompson AD: Tumors of the thymus. Thorax 22:193, 1967
56. Skeggs DBL: Complications associated with the radiotherapy of thymic tumors. Proc R Soc Med 66:155, 1973
57. Marks RD, Wallace KM, Petit HS: Radiation therapy control of 9 patients with malignant thymoma. Cancer 41:117, 1978
58. Boston B: Chemotherapy of invasive thymoma. Cancer 38:49, 1976
59. Daugaard G, Hansen HH, Rorth M: Combination chemotherapy for malignant thymoma. Ann Intern Med 99:189, 1983
60. Evans WK, Thompson DM, Simpson WJ et al: Combination chemotherapy in invasive thymoma: Role of COPP. Cancer 46:1523, 1980
61. Chahinian AP, Bhardroj S, Meyer RJ et al: Treatment of invasive or metastatic thymoma: Report of eleven cases. Cancer 47:1752, 1981
62. Levine GD, Rosai J: Thymic hyperplasia and neoplasia: A review of current concepts. Hum Pathol 9:495, 1978
63. Salyer WR, Salyer DC, Eggleston JC: Carcinoid tumors of the thymus. Cancer 37:958, 1976
64. Wick MR, Carney JA, Bernaty PE et al: Primary mediastinal carcinoid tumors. Am J Surg Pathol 6:195, 1982
65. Wick MR, Scheithauer BW: Oat cell carcinoma of the thymus. Cancer 49:1652, 1982
66. Luna MA, Valenzuela-Tamariz J: Germ-cell tumors of the mediastinum, postmortem findings. Am J Clin Pathol 65:450, 1976
67. Martini N, Golbey RB, Hajdu SJ et al: Primary mediastinal germ cell tumors. Cancer 33:763, 1974
68. Kirschling RJ, Krols LK, Charboneau JW et al: High-resolution ultrasonographic and pathologic abnormalities of germ cell tumors in patients with clinically normal testes. Mayo Clin Proc 58:648, 1983
69. Polansky SM, Barwick KW, Ravin CE: Primary mediastinal seminoma. Am J Roentgenol 132:17, 1979
70. Hurt RD, Bruckman JE, Farrow GM et al: Primary mediastinal seminoma. Cancer 49:1658, 1982
71. Kersh CR, Eisert DR, Constable WC et al: Primary malignant mediastinal germ-cell tumors and the contribution of radiotherapy: A southeastern multi-institutional study. Am J Clin Oncol 10:302, 1987
72. Bush SE, Martinez A, Bagshaw MA: Primary mediastinal seminoma. Cancer 48:1877, 1981
73. Clamon GH: Management of primary mediastinal seminoma. Chest 83:263, 1983
74. Nichols CR, Heerema NA, Palmer C et al: Klingfelter's syndrome associated with mediastinal germ-cell neoplasms. J Clin Oncol 5:1290, 1987
75. Economou JS, Trump PL, Holmes EC et al: Management of primary germ cell tumors of the mediastinum. J Thorac Cardiovasc Surg 83:643, 1982
76. Fox RM, Woods RL, Tattersall MH et al: Undifferentiated carcinoma in young men. The atypical teratoma syndrome. Lancet 1:1316, 1979
77. Hainsworth JD, Einhorn LH, Williams SD et al: Advanced extragonadal germ-cell tumors: Successful treatment with combination chemotherapy. Ann Intern Med 97:7, 1982
78. Truong LD, Harris L, Mattioli C et al: Endodermal sinus tumor of the mediastinum. A report of seven cases and review of the literature. Cancer 58:730, 1986
79. Feun LG, Samson MK, Stephens RL: Vinblastine, bleomycin, cis-diamminedichlorplatinum in disseminated extragonadal germ cell tumors: A Southwest Oncology Group study. Cancer 45:2543, 1980
80. Vugrin D, Martini N, Whitmore WF et al: VAB-3 combination chemotherapy in primary mediastinal germ cell tumors. Cancer Treat Rep 66:1405, 1982

81. Vogelzang HJ, Raghaven D, Anderson RW et al: Mediastinal nonseminomatous germ cell tumors: The role of combined modality therapy. Ann Thorac Surg 33:333, 1982
82. Loehrer PJ Sr, Einhorn LH, Williams SD: VP-16 plus ifosfamide plus cisplatin as salvage therapy in refractory germ cell cancer. J Clin Oncol 4:528, 1986
83. Wick MR, Weiland LH, Scheithauer BW et al: Primary thymic carcinomas. Am J Surg Pathol 6:613, 1982
84. Leyslraz S, Henle W, Chahinian AP et al: Association of Epstein-Barr virus with thymic carcinoma. N Engl J Med 312:1296, 1985
85. Akwari OE, Payne WS, Onofrio BM et al: Dumbbell neurogenic tumors of the mediastinum. Mayo Clin Proc 53:353, 1978
86. Gale AW, Jelihovsky T, Grant AF et al: Neurogenic tumors of the mediastinum. Ann Thorac Surg 17:434, 1974
87. Hajula A, Mattila S, Luosto R et al: Mediastinal neurogenic tumors. Early and late results of surgical treatment. Scand J Thorac Cardiovasc Surg 20:115, 1986
88. Katlic MR, Wang C, Grillo HC: Substernal goiter. Ann Thorac Surg 39:391, 1985
89. Cohen A, Sbaschnig RJ, Hochholzer L et al: Mediastinal hemangiomas. Ann Thorac Surg 43:656, 1987
90. Harpaz N, Gribety AR, Krellenstein DJ et al: Inflammatory pseudotumors of the thymus. Ann Thorac Surg 42:331, 1986

J. C. ROSENBERG
ALLEN S. LICHTER
LAWRENCE P. LEICHMAN

CHAPTER 24 *Cancer of the Esophagus*

Cancer of the esophagus was first recorded in China more than 2000 years ago when it was referred to as "Ye Ge," meaning dysphagia and belching.[1] Galen in the second century and Avenzoar (Ibn Zuhr), 1000 years later described the manifestations of what must have been a cancer of the esophagus. Avenzoar wrote about a condition "beginning with mild pain and difficulty in swallowing, and going on gradually to its complete prevention."[2] He treated these patients with silver sounds and nutritive enemas, palliative measures that were not improved upon for almost 750 years.

More aggressive attempts than those of Avenzoar at improving the outcome of a patient with malignant obstruction of the esophagus were undertaken in the middle of the 19th century. In 1849, Sédillot of Strasbourg performed the first gastrostomy for a patient suffering from severe dysphagia.[3] Unfortunately, the patient died less than 24 hours after the operation. At autopsy, an epithelial tumor of the esophagus was found. Bilroth, in 1871, wrote about resection of the esophagus for cancer after experimenting with animals, but it was Czerny, his co-worker in this project, who first attempted this surgery for a carcinoma of the cervical esophagus in 1877.[4]

The first successful resection of a thoracic esophageal malignancy was performed in 1913 in New York City by Franz Torek.[5] Like Czerny, he did not attempt to reconstruct the gastrointestinal tract but chose to allow the patient, a 67-year-old woman, to use an external rubber tube to connect a cervical esophagostomy to a gastrostomy tube while she ate. The patient survived for 13 years after this procedure. In 1920, Kirschner suggested that an esophagogastrostomy should be performed to reconstruct the esophagus after an esophagectomy.[6] It was not until 1932 that this was successfully carried out by Ohsawa in Japan.[7] Reconstruction was first performed in the United States by Adams and Phemister in 1938.[8]

Because of the high mortality following resection of the esophagus during the third and fourth decades of the 20th century, radiation therapy was often chosen as a means of controlling the growth and spread of these malignancies. Radiation therapy using radium bougies and external radiation for esophageal carcinoma was introduced in the 1920s. Radium bougies were applied intermittently with disappointing results.[9] Deep seated lesions such as carcinomas of the esophagus were poorly handled by external radiation (~250 KeV) using orthovoltage therapy. Skin reactions and damage to structures close to the esophagus were frequent. In 1945, Nielsen reported on the use of radiation as primary treatment for esophageal cancer and introduced the use of a rotating chair to limit the side-effects of the roentgen beam.[10]

The most recent innovation in the treatment of carcinoma of the esophagus has been the use of multimodality therapy, employing combinations of chemotherapy, radiotherapy, and surgery. Preliminary studies have suggested that this approach may enhance the outlook of patients with this disease.

BENIGN NEOPLASMS OF THE ESOPHAGUS

Non-neoplastic tumors of the esophagus that may present as neoplasms comprise small islands of gastric heterotopia, cysts of various types (inclusion cysts, retention cysts or duplication cysts), or granulomatous (fibrovascular) polyps.[11]

SQUAMOUS CELL PAPILLOMA

Benign neoplasms of epithelial origin are rare; the only type known is the squamous cell papilloma. Half the patients with squamous cell papillomas have multiple lesions, and most patients are asymptomatic. It is not known whether these lesions are precursors of squamous cell carcinoma. Occasionally, one may encounter difficulty in differentiating the squamous cell papilloma of the esophagus from a carcinoma or condylomata. Positive reactions to the human papillomavirus have been reported in these lesions. Treatment usually consists of endoscopic removal of the lesions.

BENIGN TUMORS OF MESODERMAL ORIGIN

The most common benign neoplasm of the esophagus is the leiomyoma, which accounts for 75% of all benign esophageal tumors.[12] The ratio of leiomyomas to leiomyosarcomas is 100:1. Leiomyomas are found in men two times more often than in women and are most often located in the lower third of the esophagus. Dysphagia is the most frequent presenting complaint, but half the patients with leiomyomas are asymptomatic. The treatment of choice is submucosal enucleation. Esophageal resection may be required for larger lesions. When resection is necessary, morbidity is increased; however, recurrences are rare.

Other benign nonepithelial neoplasms that occur in the esophagus are fibromyomas, lipomyomas, fibromas, lipomas, neurofibromas, giant cell tumors, osteochondromas, and granular cell myoblastomas.

SQUAMOUS CELL CARCINOMA OF THE ESOPHAGUS

PATHOLOGY

A list of malignant primary esophageal neoplasms based on the World Health Organization (WHO) classification is presented in Table 24-1.[11] More than 90% of malignant esophageal tumors are squamous cell carcinomas, arising from the squamous cell epithelium lining the lumen of the esophagus. The well-differentiated cancers have the characteristic features of keratin formation (epithelial pearls), intercellular bridges, and minimal pleomorphism. Poorly differentiated tumors do not contain keratin or demonstrate intercellular bridges, but they do have marked nuclear and cellular pleomorphism. The moderately differentiated tumors are intermediate between these two. The degree of differentiation has no prognostic value.

Spindle cell carcinoma, pseudosarcoma, carcinosarcoma, and verrucous carcinoma of the esophagus are pathologic variants of squamous cell carcinoma. They are discussed near the end of this chapter with other infrequent cancers of the esophagus.

TABLE 24-1. Malignant Esophageal Tumors

Epithelial Tumors
- Squamous cell carcinoma
  - Well differentiated
  - Moderately differentiated
  - Poorly differentiated
- Variants of squamous cell carcinoma
  - Spindle cell carcinoma
  - Pseudosarcoma and carcinosarcoma
  - Verrucous carcinoma
  - In situ carcinoma
- Adenocarcinoma
  - Adenoacanthoma
- Adenoid cystic carcinoma (cylindroma)
- Mucoepidermoid carcinoma
- Adenosquamous carcinoma
- Carcinoid
- Undifferentiated carcinoma
  - Oat cell carcinoma

Nonepithelial Tumors
- Leiomyosarcoma
- Malignant melanoma
- Rhabdomyosarcoma
- Myoblastoma
- Choriocarcinoma

EPIDEMIOLOGIC AND ETIOLOGIC CONSIDERATIONS

The age-adjusted incidence of cancer of the esophagus in the United States is low. In 1984, it was 3.5 per 100,000 for all races (5.6 per 100,000 men and 1.9 per 100,000 women).[13] The age-adjusted mortality rate in the United States in 1984 was 5.7 per 100,000 men and 1.5 per 100,000 women.[13] These data vary significantly according to race. A statistically significant ($p<0.05$) change of 0.6% has been observed in the average annual esophageal cancer mortality rate between 1975 and 1984. Esophageal cancer was responsible for approximately 8800 deaths in 1986, and during 1987, almost 9300 new cases were diagnosed. Cancer of the esophagus constitutes 1.5% of all cancers and 7% of all gastrointestinal carcinomas in the United States.[14]

The data from the United States are by no means representative of the incidence of this disease throughout the world or among different groups within a given country. Geographic variations in the incidence of squamous cell carcinoma of the esophagus are greater than for any other malignancy. Data obtained by WHO and published in 1977 show that mortality, standardized to the world population, was highest in China. Puerto Rico and Singapore were second and third (Fig. 24-1).[1]

There is also great variation in the geographic distribution of esophageal cancer in China. A 700-fold difference in mortality exists between the highest and lowest incidence areas. The highest rates in China were found in the north along the Taihang Mountain range. Honan Province is in this area. The age-adjusted mortality from esophageal cancer in Honan Province is 436 per 100,000 men and 22.5 per 100,000 women. In Yunan Province, on the southern border of China, the rates are 1.4 and 0.7 per 100,000, respectively. The Linxian county in Honan Province has the highest mortality rate from esophageal carcinoma (131.8 per

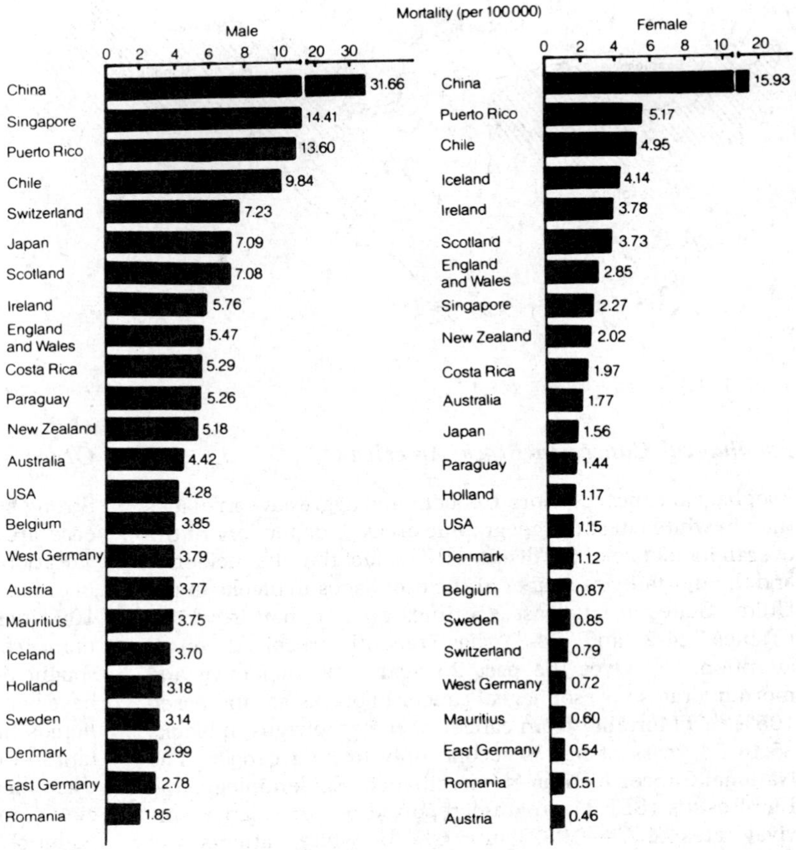

FIG. 24-1. Age-adjusted mortality for esophageal cancer as determined by the World Health Organization and published in 1977.[1]

100,000).[15] Chickens in Honan Province were also found to have esophageal cancer. When residents of Honan moved to the Hobei Province, both they and their chickens retained their high esophageal cancer rate. This observation led to the discovery of nitrosamines in food samples from areas of high incidence.[15] It is postulated that esophageal carcinoma is the end result of the combined effects of several etiologic factors.

Examples of variations in the geographic distribution of esophageal cancer can also be found in Africa, where the incidence has changed with time.[16] The incidence of esophageal cancer increased dramatically between 1940 and 1950 in the Transkei region of the Cape Province in South Africa. Before 1940, the disease was unknown, but the incidence is now 246 per 100,000 black men 35 to 64 years of age. In Nigeria (West Africa), the incidence is similar: 3 per 100,000.[17] The sex ratio (males : females) is also much higher among the black population of Cape Province than among the white people (9 : 1 for blacks and 4 : 1 for whites). Environmental factors seem to be responsible for these phenomena. Certain alcoholic drinks (kachosu, home-brewed from sugar and maize husks rather than the kafir beer made from sorghum), homegrown tobacco smoked in homemade pipes, and nutritional deficiencies may be responsible for the increased incidence. The etiologic relationships in the Transkei and in China are not clear.

Perhaps the area of the world with the highest incidence and most obscure etiologic relationships is in Iran and the Soviet Union around the Caspian Sea.[18] There is no significant alcohol or tobacco consumption among the Moslem population in this area. Dietary factors are most suspect. The Caspian littoral forms part of an "Asian esophageal cancer belt" which extends through northern China (Fig. 24-2). However, within this area there are striking variations in the frequency and sex incidence of esophageal carcinoma. The age-standardized incidence rates in Gorgan and Gonbad in the northeastern parts of the province of Mazandaran in Iran are approximately 108 per 100,000 men and 174 per 100,000 women.[18]

Cancer of the esophagus is common in France, Switzerland, Finland, Iceland, and Puerto Rico. The disease is less frequently seen in Norway, Britain, and Australia and among the white population of the United States. Alcohol consumption is thought to be a carcinogenic agent in the United States, Britain, France (Brittany), Sweden, and Japan. Tobacco consumption may be a factor in the United States, France, Britain, Sweden, India, and South Africa. Tobacco and excessive alcoholic intake are widely accepted as the major reason why squamous cell carcinoma of the esophagus is seen in many western countries. Each increases the risk of developing esophageal cancer, and, when combined, as is often the case, the risks are multiplied. The risk of developing esophageal cancer in smokers is increased ten-fold for beer drinkers and about 25-fold for whiskey drinkers compared with smoking matched nondrinkers.[19] Racial and genetic factors have been studied with inconclusive results.

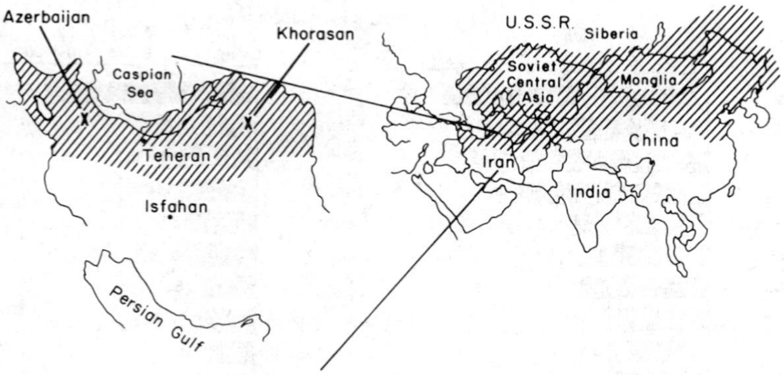

FIG. 24-2. An "esophageal cancer belt" extends across Asia from the southern shore of the Caspian Sea in Iran, through Soviet Central Asia and Mongolia, to Northern China. The incidence of cancer of the esophagus in the area around the Caspian Sea is higher than in any other area of the world. (Kmet J, Mahboudi E: Esophageal cancer in the Caspian littoral of Iran: Initial studies. Science 175:846, 1972)

Esophageal Cancer in Black Americans

Esophageal cancer is more frequent and aggressive in blacks than in whites in some geographic areas, independent of the overall incidence of the disease.[20] The fact that the incidence and the mortality of cancer of the esophagus in blacks in the United States are at least 3.5 times greater than in whites (Tables 24-2 and 24-3) has recently received much attention.[21–23] Over the past 25 years, the incidence and mortality rates for esophageal cancer in blacks has increased 105%.[20,23] Mortality from cancer of the esophagus in blacks 35 to 54 years of age is second only to lung cancer. The National Cancer Institute's Surveillance, Epidemiology, and End-Results (SEER) program reported 5-year relative survival rates (1974–1983) of 5.6% for white patients and 4.1% for black patients with esophageal cancer. The difference is statistically significant ($p<0.05$).[13]

It has been postulated that increased tobacco consumption among blacks or nutritional deficiencies may account for this increased risk. Alcohol potentiates the risk of developing esophageal cancer among smokers, and more black Americans smoke than white Americans (40% and 30%, respectively). More white Americans are former smokers than black Americans. However, nutritional surveys do not show that blacks are heavier drinkers than whites. The Health and Nutrition Survey carried out from 1971 to 1974, which included 20,749 persons, 20% of whom were black, showed that a smaller proportion of black men report heavy drinking than do white men of comparable age.[24]

In contrast to the higher incidence of squamous cell carcinoma of the esophagus in blacks than in whites is the higher incidence of adenocarcinomas of the esophagus in whites than in blacks. This relationship is discussed in the section on adenocarcinoma of the esophagus.

Other Risk Factors

Strong suspicions of nutritional factors involved in this disease are derived from the observation that there is a wide variation in the rates for men and women (from 5 : 1 to 1 : 1). Because the Plummer-Vinson syndrome is associated with a 10% incidence of esophageal or pharyngeal cancer and is more frequent in women, nutritional deficiencies have been sought as predisposing factors. No clear-cut relationships have been found. Heavy seasoning of foods and hot foods and liquids have been implicated, as have the use of betel nut, tannin-rich foods, contamination of food with silica particles, trace metal deficiencies and excesses, and vitamin deficiencies. Consideration has been given to poor oral hygiene, air pollution, radiation, exposure to asbestos, and previous gastric surgery as etiologic factors. These are speculations with little evidence to support them.

A recent review of dietary factors influencing esophageal cancer suggested that a high-risk diet depended on corn or wheat as staples, with marginal or deficient amounts of riboflavin, nicotinic acid, magnesium, and zinc.[25,26] Silica particles contaminating millet bran have also been implicated as an etiologic agent in areas with a high incidence of esophageal cancer.[27]

Predisposing Conditions

TYLOSIS. Attempts at correlating genetic factors with an increased incidence of esophageal cancer have failed to reveal a significant relationship, with the exception of patients with tylosis. In a classic article on this obscure condition, Howel-Evans described the occurrence of esophageal cancer in patients with this disease characterized by changes of the skin of the palms and soles (hyperkeratosis palmaris et plantaris) and papillomata of the esophagus. The syndrome is the

TABLE 24-2. Age-Adjusted Incidence of Cancer of the Esophagus, 1984*

	Race	*Male*	*Female*
Black	17.2	5.4	
White	4.6	1.5	

* 1986 Annual Cancer Statistics Review, incidence per 100,000; age-adjusted to the 1970 U.S. standard population.

TABLE 24-3. Age-Adjusted Mortality Rate for Cancer of the Esophagus, 1984*

	Race	*Male*	*Female*
Black	16.4	4.1	
White	4.7	1.3	

* 1986 Annual Cancer Statistics Review, incidence per 100,000; age-adjusted to the 1970 U.S. standard population.

result of an autosomal dominant gene. In some families, 95% of patients with tylosis will develop squamous cell carcinoma of the esophagus by the age of 65 years.[28]

ACHALASIA. Approximately 5% of patients with achalasia have developed squamous cell carcinomas of the esophagus. The cancers are located equally in the middle third and lower third of the esophagus.[29,30] Carcinomas occur after the achalasia has been present for 20 years or longer. In some instances, the cancer has been thought to be the cause of the achalasia.[31] Rarely, an adenocarcinoma may be found in the dilated esophagus.[32] Joske and Benedict suspected that the obstructive process somehow led to the squamous cell carcinoma, and literature continues to implicate retention esophagitis as a premalignant condition.[33,34] The esophagitis is thought to arise from stagnating retained food in the megaesophagus. The advent of fiberoptics for flexible endoscopy has promoted the use of esophagoscopy, which should generate increased reports of squamous cell cancer in patients with achalasia. The discovery of early lesions should improve survival rates.[35]

Treatment is the same as for any squamous cell carcinoma. Patients with this unusual association have as poor an outcome as do patients with esophageal cancer.[36]

ESOPHAGEAL DIVERTICULA. Isolated case reports constitute the basis of this uncommon association of conditions. As of 1976, 35 cases were collected from the literature. Two-thirds of the cancers occurred in pharyngoesophageal diverticula and the remainder at the epiphrenic level. Epithelial cysts of the esophagus do not develop cancers.[37] Of 1249 patients with a pharyngoesophageal diverticulum, 0.4% had an associated squamous cell carcinoma.[38] These cancers are treated as any other squamous cell carcinoma. In one series, diverticulectomy alone was curative in the absence of full-thickness penetration, nodal metastasis, or extension to the line of resection.[38]

LYE STRICTURE. Squamous cell carcinomas have occurred in esophageal strictures secondary to lye ingestion. The cancer occurs at the site of the stricture, which is frequently located at the level of the tracheal bifurcation.[39] The interval between the detection of the carcinoma and the ingestion of lye is between 30 and 45 years. The later in life that the lye is ingested, the shorter the interval before carcinoma develops.[40] The similarity of this lesion to squamous cell carcinomas occurring in chronic, draining sinus tracts and chronic skin ulcers suggests a common etiologic mechanism. These instances of carcinoma are less aggressive, have a slightly higher resectability rate, and may have a better prognosis than the usual forms of squamous cell carcinoma.

Resection of an extensively strictured esophagus not involved with cancer is a formidable procedure. Because the mortality may be higher than the risk of developing cancer in the esophagus, resection of the excluded esophagus is not advised, and a bypass procedure to relieve dysphagia may be the preferred procedure.

PLUMMER-VINSON (PATERSON-KELLY) SYNDROME. Sideropenic anemia, glossitis, and esophagitis are associated with a 10% incidence of pharyngeal or esophageal cancer, which is usually located in the upper esophagus. The syndrome and the cancers are more frequent in women than men. Nutritional deficiencies have been postulated as etiologic factors. The syndrome is seen less often now than when it was first described more than 65 years ago.[41] When strictures are present, dysplastic changes and in situ carcinoma can be found at the site of the narrowed esophagus.[42]

ANATOMIC CONSIDERATIONS OF CLINICAL SIGNIFICANCE

The esophagus begins at the level of C6, below the cricoid cartilage, where the cricopharyngeus muscle separates it from the pharynx. The length of the esophagus, from pharynx to stomach, is between 23 and 30 cm.

Endoscopists localize lesions in the esophagus by measuring the lesion's distance from the central incisor teeth. By this method of measurement, the esophagus begins 15 cm from the central incisors and terminates 38 to 45 cm distally, beneath the diaphragm. The thoracic inlet, the dividing line between the cervical and thoracic esophagus, is located 20 cm from the central incisors, at the level of T1 (Fig. 24-3).

The cervical esophagus is about 5 cm long. It extends down to the thoracic inlet, at the level of T1. The first 3 cm are located behind the larynx. This segment is the postcricoid portion of the cervical esophagus. Malignancies in this area present a special problem and are fully discussed in Chapter 21.

The thoracic esophagus begins at the thoracic inlet at the level of the clavicles and ends at T10. As the esophagus passes down the posterior mediastinum toward the left of the midline, it lies close behind the tracheal bifurcation and left main stem bronchus. This occurs at the level of T4 or T5, about 23 cm from the central incisors. The arch of the aorta passes in front of the left side of the esophagus at this level, producing a shallow depression that pulsates during endoscopy. These close anatomic relationships are demonstrated in Fig. 24-4. Because of the juxtaposition of these organs, malignant lesions can involve vital structures early in the

FIG. 24-3. Anatomic relationship and major subdivisions of the esophagus.

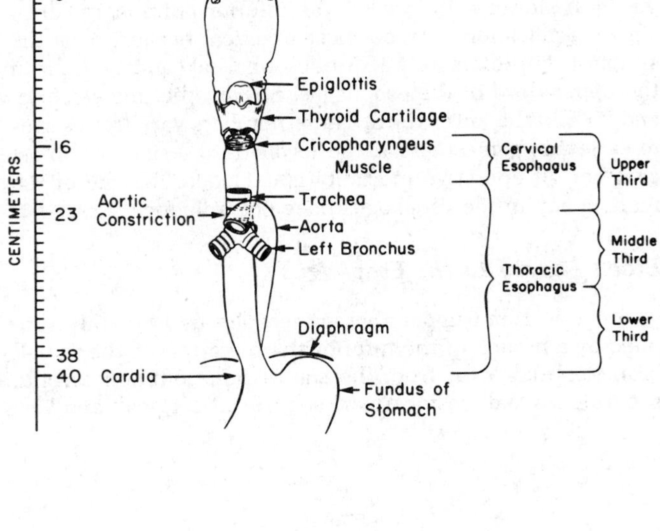

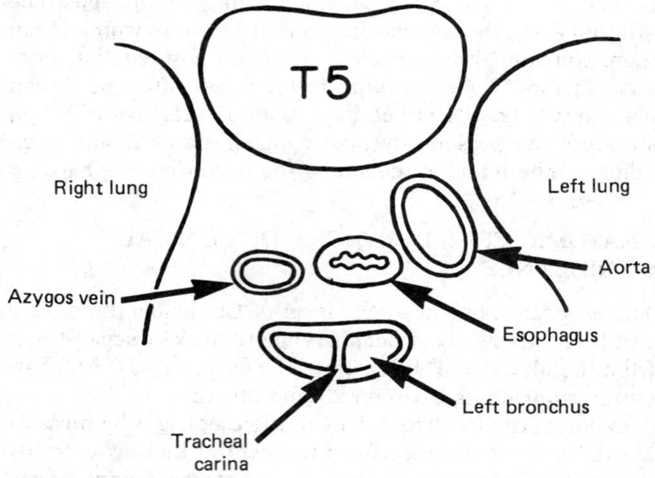

FIG. 24-4. Diagrammatic cross-sectional anatomy depicting the close relationship of the thoracic esophagus to the aorta, trachea, left mainstem bronchus, and azygos vein at the midthoracic (T4 and T5) level, 23 cm from the central incisors.

course of the disease. Tracheoesophageal fistulae are the most common problems encountered. These anatomic relationships contribute significantly to the higher operative mortality following resection of lesions at the midesophageal level.

The American Joint Committee for Cancer Staging and End-Results Reporting divides the esophagus into three principal regions: The cervical esophagus; the upper and midthoracic esophagus, extending from the thoracic inlet (18 cm from the upper incisor teeth) to a point 10 cm above the esophagogastric junction, usually located at T8 (31 cm from the upper incisor teeth); and the lower thoracic esophagus, which is the distal 10 cm of esophagus.[43] The Japanese Society for Esophageal Diseases has a similar system of dividing the esophagus into regions but further subdivides the upper and midthoracic esophagus and the lower esophagus each into two subdivisions.[44]

The esophagus can also be divided into thirds (Fig. 24-3). The cervical esophagus and upper thoracic esophagus are the upper third (above the aortic arch); the middle thoracic esophagus is the middle third (between the aortic arch and the inferior pulmonary vein); and the lower thoracic esophagus is the lower third (below the inferior pulmonary vein). This classification may be most practical because it is the simplest. Approximately 15% of esophageal cancers occur in the upper third of the esophagus, 50% in the middle third, and 35% in the lower third. These numbers vary from series to series. In some reports, the lower-third lesions are most common. If operative mortality is excluded, the site of the malignancy in the esophagus does not influence survival.[45]

Blood Supply to the Esophagus

The cervical and upper thoracic esophagus is mainly supplied by a branch of the inferior thyroid artery. Other small branches may arise from the subclavian, common carotid, superior thyroid, costocervical superficial cervical, and vertebral arteries. The bronchial arteries and occasionally direct branches from the aorta supply the midesophagus, which is the most vascularized portion of the esophagus. Below the bifurcation of the trachea, the esophagus is supplied by arteries arising from the aorta.[46] The veins emanating from the thoracic esophagus drain directly into the azygos and hemiazygos systems and the intercostal veins, which are also tributaries of the azygos system.

Lymphatic Drainage of the Esophagus

A closely knit plexus of small lymphatic vessels in the mucosa merge with a less-dense network located in the submucosa.[47,48] Both of these plexuses communicate with five widely spaced lymphatic channels in the muscular layers of the esophagus, which, in turn, communicate with a network of cooperative lymphatics that extend throughout the esophagus (Fig. 24-5). Thus, lymphatic fluid can follow any one of a great number of pathways before emerging from the esophagus to drain into a lymph node. Because of the longitudinal course of the lymphatics and the interconnections between the mucosal, submucosal, and muscular lymphatics draining the esophagus, the pattern of flow to lymph nodes is unpredictable. Flow may be in the direction of adjacent lymph nodes or through the aforementioned network to more distant nodes. The pattern of lymphatics favors the flow of lymph in the direction of the long axis of the esophagus rather than in a circumferential direction.

Afferent lymphatics leaving the esophagus to drain into a lymph node tend to follow the arteries, which, as a rule, course longitudinally rather than radially. The lymphatics

FIG. 24-5. Lymphatics extend throughout the esophagus, draining the esophageal wall and passing to collections of lymph nodes that extend from the neck to the abdomen. Lymph node chains, which also may receive lymphatics from the esophagus, that are not illustrated are the cervical and supraclavicular lymph nodes.

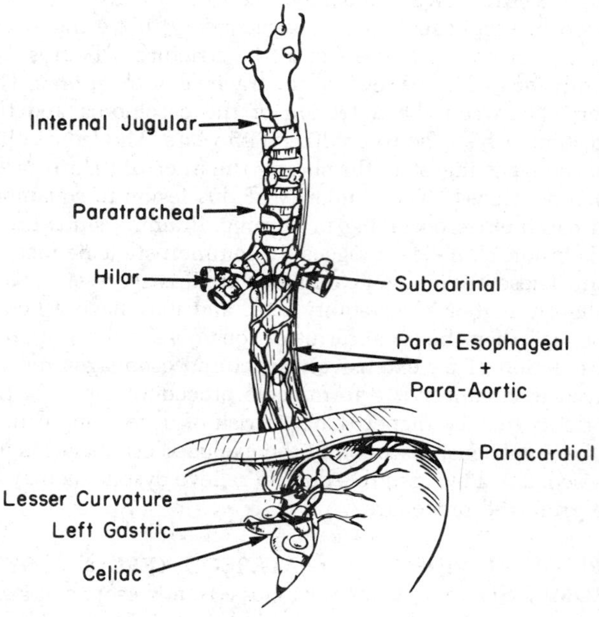

drain into the following lymph node chains: internal jugular, cervical, supraclavicular, paratracheal, hilar, subcarinal, paraesophageal, para-aortic, paracardial, lesser curvature, left gastric, and celiac (Fig. 24-5). Involvement of the paratracheal nodes on the right is more common than involvement of those on the left. The lowest right paratracheal lymph node is the azygos node. The posterior hilar lymph nodes are more frequently involved than the other hilar nodes. The paraesophageal and para-aortic group of lymph nodes are part of a chain of lymphatics extending from the inferior pulmonary vein to the diaphragm. Similarly, the celiac nodes are part of an extensive group of retroperitoneal lymph nodes.

Celiac node involvement occurs in 10% of the esophageal cancers located in the cervical and upper thoracic esophagus (up to the tracheal bifurcation). The middle third of the esophagus (up to the distal 10 cm of esophagus) may have celiac node involvement in 44% of patients.[49] The peculiar lymphatic drainage of the esophagus is responsible for the phenomenon of "skip areas" of involvement.[50] As much as 8 cm of normal esophagus may be interposed between the site of gross tumor and micrometastases within lymphatic vessels or the esophageal wall.

CLINICAL PRESENTATION

The patient with esophageal cancer will usually be a man between 55 and 65 years of age with a long-standing history of cigarette smoking and heavy alcohol intake. Dysphagia and weight loss are the initial symptoms of carcinoma of the esophagus in 90% of patients. Difficulty swallowing does not occur until the circumference of the esophagus is narrowed to a third or half of normal. Occasionally, the onset is sudden; most often symptoms have been present for 3 to 4 months. Pain on swallowing (odynophagia) is seen in about half the patients with cancer of the esophagus. When the pain radiates to the back, spinal column involvement should be suspected (Table 24-4). Regurgitation or vomiting and a discomfort in the throat, substernal area, or epigastrium may be additional symptoms. Aspiration pneumonia can be another presenting or concomitant feature of the disease. Advanced lesions may present with hematemesis, hemoptysis or melena, persistent cough caused by an esophagotracheobronchial fistula, dysphonia caused by involvement of the left recurrent laryngeal nerve with laryngeal paralysis, Horner's syndrome, or superior vena caval obstruction. Exsanguinating bleeding may occur if the cancer erodes into the aorta. Other ominous findings are pleural effusion, palpable cervical or supraclavicular lymph nodes, and hepatomegaly. Hematuria can occur with renal involvement. Pain is prominent if there are metastases to the bones.

TABLE 24-4. Signs and Symptoms Produced by Advanced Carcinoma of Esophagus

Pain radiating to the back on swallowing
Dysphonia (laryngeal paralysis)
Diaphragmatic paralysis (involvement of phrenic nerve)
Coughing when swallowing (tracheoesophageal fistula)
Superior vena cava syndrome
Palpable supraclavicular or cervical nodes
Malignant pleural effusion
Malignant ascites
Bone pain

Occasionally a paraneoplastic syndrome is produced by an esophageal tumor. The most common is hypercalcemia unrelated to bone involvement.[51] Gonadotropin-producing and ACTH-producing tumors have been described but are rare.[52]

The gross appearance of an advanced carcinoma of the esophagus is best depicted by an esophagram. There are few lesions that can simulate the appearance of an esophageal carcinoma. Most confusion arises with lesions at the distal end of the esophagus. Adenocarcinoma of the esophagus or stomach, benign tumors, other malignant tumors, peptic strictures, and achalasia may have an appearance similar to squamous cell carcinoma radiographically and esophagoscopically.

DIAGNOSIS

Obtaining tissue for histopathologic confirmation of the diagnosis may not be easy when visualizing an esophageal tumor through an esophagoscope. Often, the submucosal extension of the tumor will push normal mucosa in front of it, and the biopsy forceps will not bite deeply enough to reach the malignant tissue. Brushings of the tumor will be diagnostic 90% of the time, compared with only 70% of the biopsies.[53,54] When both techniques are used and multiple biopsies (up to 7) obtained, a diagnosis can most often be established.[55] Exfoliative cytology also has diagnostic value.[56]

The Linxian County Hospital in the Honan Province of China developed the technique of abrasive cytology, using a catheter with a balloon covered by a cotton net to scrape loose esophageal mucosal cells. Cytologic examination has been 90% accurate in patients with very early cancer of the esophagus.[15] Dowlatshaki developed a similar technique using a brush passed through a nasogastric tube.[56]

EVALUATING THE PATIENT WITH ESOPHAGEAL CARCINOMA

Noninvasive Studies

The history and physical examination can provide important clues to the local extent and metastatic involvement of a cancer of the esophagus. The findings produced by advanced esophageal cancers were described above and are listed in Table 24-4.

The length of involvement of the esophagus by cancer, as determined by the esophagram, does not correlate well with resectability, cure, or the extent of involvement as determined by direct measurement of surgical or autopsy specimens.[45] The high frequency of metastases to the lungs, liver, adrenals, kidney, and bones has been used to justify computed tomography (CT) scans of the chest and upper abdomen, bone scans, and skeletal surveys.

Small esophageal carcinomas (<3.5 cm long) are not easily identified as malignant lesions by esophagrams.[57] Diagnostic accuracy approaches only 60% under these circumstances. A thickened posterior strip or band (wider than 4.5 cm) can be identified on the lateral chest x-ray film of patients with carcinoma of the esophagus. The thickened area is caused by periesophageal lymphatic involvement and can be seen as early as 6 months before the development of symptoms.[15,58]

Endosonography, also referred to as endoscopic ultrasonography, is valuable in diagnosing early lesions and contributes to the preoperative staging of esophageal carcinomas. Cancers of the esophagus appear as a hypoechoic mass or a mass containing heterogeneous echo spots. The length of the esophagus involved by the cancer, the infiltration by the cancer into adjacent organs, and the lymph node involvement can also be assessed by this technique.[59,60]

The results of several studies involving CT in esophageal cancer have recently been reviewed.[61,62] Those using preoperative CT, followed by surgical confirmation of stage, have shown that CT is best at assessing local extension of disease and at delineating liver or adrenal metastases. It is less accurate in assessing the degree of periesophageal lymph node involvement. In three different studies, CT underestimated the length of the esophageal lesion by 1 to 6 cm.[62–64] The current recommendation for staging purposes is to obtain both a barium esophagram and a CT scan to assess tumor length; the longer of the two measurements can be used. In addition to staging the tumor, CT has also proved helpful in radiation therapy planning and may be useful in assessing tumor response to both radiation and chemotherapy.[65]

Nuclear magnetic resonance imaging is used for precisely determining the extent of involvement of esophageal cancer. Experience with it thus far indicates that it has many of the same drawbacks as CT.[66]

Invasive Studies

Endoscopy, using the flexible esophagoscope, is best for evaluating esophageal cancers. Because of the high frequency of other malignancies within the upper and lower respiratory passageways, a careful examination of the mouth, pharynx, larynx, and tracheobronchial tree must be performed. Another compelling reason for performing laryngoscopy and bronchoscopy is the frequency of extension of midesophageal lesions into the tracheobronchial tree. Special attention should be given to the posterior wall of the left main stem bronchus and trachea where the esophagus crosses these structures. Narrowing in this area or infiltration of tumor, as evidenced by edema, prominent longitudinal folds, and bleeding upon contact are ominous findings.

Mediastinoscopy is used only if the patient is inoperable and a tissue diagnosis is required. Laparoscopy is helpful in identifying patients with malignant ascites, liver metastases, and extensive involvement of the stomach. All enlarged cervical or supraclavicular lymph nodes should be biopsied.

Biopsy of the celiac and lesser curvature lymph nodes is of great significance in planning therapy and providing prognostic data. Therefore, biopsy of these lymph nodes during laparotomy should be part of every therapeutic plan. Celiac node involvement occurs in 10% of patients with upper esophageal malignancies. With lower esophageal cancers, the incidence increases at least fivefold.[49]

STAGING

Because the esophagus is not an accessible organ, its clinical evaluation leaves a great deal to be desired. The use of invasive techniques, including biopsy procedures, is more appropriate. However, these techniques should be carried out before radiotherapy or chemotherapy is used if they are to be reliable. Because many esophageal cancers are being treated with preoperative radiation or chemotherapy, postsurgical evaluation may not accurately define the stage of the diagnosed cancer. The TNM staging system for the cervical and thoracic esophagus is outlined in Table 24-5. Stage grouping is given in Table 24-6.[43,67]

NATURAL HISTORY AND PATTERNS OF SPREAD

Esophageal cancers are characterized by extensive local growth and lymph node involvement before becoming widely disseminated. Follow-up of early asymptomatic patients with in situ carcinoma has demonstrated that it takes 3 to 4 years before advanced cancer develops.[68] Other studies of early superficial squamous cell carcinomas have resulted in estimates of 5 months for the doubling time of the longitudinal growth of these malignancies.[69] The unique lymphatic drainage of the esophagus and the long interval during which the tumor is asymptomatic account for the extensive involvement of lymph nodes and structures adjacent to the esophagus at the time of diagnosis. The poor prognosis of these patients is influenced by the proximity of the aorta and trachea and by the absence of a serosal covering.

The length of esophagus involved by the neoplasm is di-

TABLE 24-5. TNM Staging for Esophageal Cancer

Primary Tumor (T)	
T0	No demonstrable tumor
TIS	Carcinoma in situ
T1	Tumor involves 5 cm or less of esophageal length with no obstruction nor complete circumferential involvement nor extraesophageal spread.
T2	Tumor involves more than 5 cm of esophagus and produces obstruction with circumferential involvement of the esophagus but no extraesophageal spread.
T3	Tumor with extension outside the esophagus involving mediastinal structures.
Regional Lymph Nodes (N)	
Cervical esophagus (cervical and supraclavicular lymph nodes)	
N0	No nodal involvement
N1	Unilateral involvement (moveable)
N2	Bilateral involvement (moveable)
N3	Fixed nodes
Thoracic esophagus (nodes in the thorax, not those of the cervical, supraclavicular or abdominal areas)	
N0	No nodal involvement
N1	Nodal involvement
Distant Metastases	
M0	No metastases
M1	Distant metastases. Cancer of thoracic esophagus with cervical, supraclavicular, or abdominal lymph node involvement is classified as M1.

TABLE 24-6. Stage Grouping for Esophageal Cancer

Stage I	
T1N0M0	Tumor that involves less than 5 cm of esophagus without obstruction and no circumferential, extraesophageal or nodal involvement and no metastases.
Stage II	
T1N1M0 T1N2M0 T2N0M0 T2N1M0 T2N2M0	Cervical esophagus: No extraesophageal involvement with moveable regional lymph nodes but no metastases or a tumor more than 5 cm in size without lymph node involvement.
T2N0M0	Thoracic esophagus: Any tumor that is greater than 5 cm in length or produces obstruction or involves the entire circumference of the esophagus without extraesophageal spread.
Stage III	
Any M1 Any T3	Any esophageal cancer with extraesophageal spread or distant metastases. Cervical esophagus: fixed nodes (Any N3) Thoracic esophagus: regional lymph node involvement (Any N1)

rectly correlated with the extent of involvement of adjacent structures and inversely related to curability. If the resected tumor (with no pretreatment) is 5 cm long or less, approximately 40% of the specimens demonstrate localized disease, 25% are locally advanced, and 35% have distant metastases or are unresectable. If the length exceeds 5 cm, as determined by pathologic examination, only 10% are localized, 15% are locally advanced, and 75% have distant metastases or exceed curative resection.[69–71]

Distant metastases do not usually dominate the initial clinical course of patients with esophageal cancer, but autopsies have shown that widespread distant metastases are almost always present at the time of death.[72,73] Esophageal carcinoma can spread to virtually any site, including lung, pleura, stomach, peritoneum, kidney, adrenal gland, brain, and bone; it is most likely present as subclinical metastatic tumor when the patient is first diagnosed.[74]

Autopsy studies have shown that disseminated tumor is frequently found in patients with disease that was thought to be limited to the local-regional area. In one review, 94% had residual cancer at postmortem.[75] Nine percent had local tumor only, and 85% had extensive disease, including residual local cancer. The most common sites of metastases were lymph nodes, lung, and liver, with the last two sites involved in approximately 50% of patients. Because the median survival of this group was only 4 months, the extensive disease found at autopsy cannot be ascribed to a prolonged interval between diagnosis and death. In a similar study of 113 autopsies, 73% had metastases.[76] In a third analysis, Bosch and his colleagues found that 32% had no residual local disease; however, more than half of these patients had died in the immediate postoperative period. Autopsies disclosed that 51% of their patients had nodal or visceral metastases.[77]

ASSOCIATED MALIGNANCIES AT OTHER SITES

Synchronous or metachronous malignant tumor of the aerodigestive tract occurs in 5% to 12% of patients with cancer of the esophagus.[78–81] The oral cavity, pharynx, larynx, and lung are the most frequent sites. About half can be found in the head and neck areas, on the floor of the mouth, the tongue, tonsil, and larynx. Oral and pharyngeal cancers are most often associated with cancer of the esophagus, and laryngeal cancers are most often associated with cancer of the lung. Direct laryngoscopy, bronchoscopy, and esophagoscopy carried out in patients with head and neck cancer show that 5.5% of patients have synchronous lung or esophageal cancer, or both. Most of these patients (75%) are symptomatic.

At the Memorial Sloan-Kettering Cancer Center, 25% of patients with two primary cancers of the oral cavity, pharynx, larynx, or esophagus had synchronous cancers.[79] In 68%, the cancers appeared within 2 years of each other. The 60 patients with the multiple primary tumors came from a pool of 7000 patients seen during the same period for one of these malignancies.

TREATMENT

Despite all that surgeons have accomplished in recent years and the advances that have been made in radiation therapy and chemotherapy, the outlook for patients with squamous cell cancer of the esophagus remains poor. From 1974 to 1983, the average 5-year survival rate was 5%.[13]

Lack of progress in curing esophageal cancer has reinforced pessimism when considering the treatment of this disease. Many oncologists emphasize palliation rather than cure. Palliation is important because patients suffer greatly with malignant esophageal obstruction and tracheoesophageal fistulae. However, palliation and cure can be integrated into a management plan that can accomplish both objectives and compromise neither. The philosophy of this approach was most succinctly stated by Burdette, who advocated a plan of management for carcinoma of the esophagus "in which palliative measures were a part of the sequence leading to cure rather than a separate route of management."[82]

It is futile to attempt to determine which therapeutic approach is most likely to result in either cure or palliation because there are very few randomized comparisons of therapeutic approaches. Comparisons of reports from single institutions and historical data are not valid. Survival rates from both surgical and radiotherapy series can be markedly altered by reducing the denominator from which the survival percentage is determined.[83a,b] Surgical cure rates can be determined from the total number of patients evaluated, the number operated on, the number operated for attempted cure, the number successfully resected, or the number successfully resected who survive the immediate postoperative period. Similarly, radiation series can report survival based on various patient populations. The lack of standardized reporting continues to thwart an accurate assessment of 5-year survival rates, which range from 1% to 20%. These factors frustrate interpreting any report on therapy for carcinoma of the esophagus.

Although the three major modalities of therapy are discussed separately, the most important approach is combined modality therapy. Local eradication of squamous cell tumors will not suffice to improve the long-term survival of patients.

Effective chemotherapy in combination with surgery or radiation, or both, is the most promising approach to the treatment of esophageal malignancies.

Surgical Therapy

It must first be established whether the patient can withstand a thoracotomy and laparotomy. Advanced age is itself not a contraindication to surgical therapy. Inadequate cardiopulmonary function is the most frequent reason for declining to operate. Impaired cardiac and respiratory reserves frequently result from prolonged alcohol abuse and cigarette smoking, which are characteristic of patients with squamous carcinoma of the esophagus in the western hemisphere.

Because of the frequency of alcohol abuse, liver function tests are an important part of the preoperative assessment. Portal hypertension may also be severe enough to contraindicate an operation for esophageal cancer.

PREOPERATIVE PREPARATIONS. Debilitation from nutritional deficits should be corrected before considering surgery or any other therapy. Patients have fewer postoperative complications if they receive at least 5 days of preoperative nutritional support.[84] Protein and electrolyte derangements require immediate attention. Skin testing to determine whether the patient is anergic may be worthwhile. However, intense nutritional therapy with restoration of positive nitrogen balance may not suffice to correct anergy, and the ultimate benefits of nutritional supplementation have been questioned.[85,86] There is clear indication that prognosis can be related to the degree of weight loss. Patients with less than 10% weight loss do better than those with greater than 10% weight loss, but there is no evidence that correction of the weight loss improves prognosis.[87]

If the alimentary tract cannot be used, intravenous hyperalimentation should be employed. Gastrostomy should be avoided because the stomach is often used to replace or bypass the esophagus, but a feeding jejunostomy is acceptable. An excellent controlled randomized study has shown that the beneficial effects of enteral nutritional support are the same as by the venous parenteral route.[88]

Pulmonary function can be improved by eliminating cigarette smoking and by instituting chest physiotherapy and respiratory therapy in the form of intermittent positive-pressure breathing, incentive spirometry, bronchodilators, and antibiotics. Eliminating aspiration of oral secretions by placing a nasogastric tube above the malignant obstruction and attaching it to suction may be necessary for complete esophageal obstruction. Digitalization may be required, along with diuretics, to correct congestive heart failure.

Because the microbial flora of the esophagus of patients with cancer consist of many aerobic and anaerobic organisms, prophylactic antibiotics are used.[89] A third-generation cephalosporin or a combination of an aminoglycoside with clindamycin should be suitable.

These measures, vigorously applied, and equally effective postoperative care allow at least 50% of patients with cancer of the esophagus to undergo resection for either palliation or cure.

OPERATIVE CONSIDERATIONS. Patients who are operable should undergo a laparotomy to determine the extent of lymph node involvement and local (extraesophageal) spread. This information is vital in planning therapy. The surgeon should try to remove as much tumor as possible, leaving radiotherapy and chemotherapy the task of eliminating tumor that defies surgical removal. Radiopaque clips should be placed around the site of the tumor. This optimistic approach depends on the isolated case reports or the experience of surgeons who have struggled with the problem of esophageal cancer for many years. Wangensteen reported an 11-year cure for a patient with a cancer of the esophagus who had involvement of a lymph node on the greater curvature of the stomach.[4] Recent results reported by Ong and colleagues indicate that 10-year survival is possible even when a bronchoesophageal fistula is present from a lobar bronchus to the esophagus. Ong's patient had an esophagectomy and lobectomy.[90]

Ong cautions that if the main bronchus, trachea, or aorta is infiltrated by the malignancy, resection of these involved adjacent structures carries a high mortality and should not be performed. Patching the trachea or bronchus with pericardium is rarely successful. Most often the repair breaks down or infection causes the patched pericardium to slough.

Lymph node involvement following esophagectomy results in half of the 5-year survival rate of patients with negative regional lymph nodes. Even with positive regional lymph nodes, 10% to 15% of patients who have survived esophagectomy can be cured. However, 5-year survival rates may not be a valid basis for deciding whether a patient with esophageal cancer has been cured. After 5 years, as many as 78% of survivors may die of recurrences.[91]

Another cogent argument for proceeding with an esophageal resection whenever operable criteria are met is that this operation constitutes excellent palliation. Operative mortality for esophageal resection varies from 5% to 30%.[90] More recent reports have indicated that an operative mortality of less than 5% can be attained.[91]

ESOPHAGECTOMY. Because of the unusual lymphatic drainage of the esophagus, malignant cells can be found as far as 8 cm from the site of gross tumor with intervening skip areas free of tumor.[50] Lymph node involvement can also occur some distance from the site of the primary. The anatomic bases for these phenomena deserve emphasis because they support the generally accepted principle that the only adequate resection for a carcinoma of the thoracic esophagus is its complete removal. Esophagectomy should include a generous margin of the lesser curvature of the stomach, including the adjacent lymph node areas, and extend up to the cervical esophagus or the uppermost portion of the thoracic esophagus. The preferred method of reestablishing gastrointestinal continuity in most of these patients is an esophagogastrostomy. The mobilized stomach is brought up to the cervical esophagus or pharynx through a retrosternal tunnel or through the posterior mediastinum in the bed of the excised esophagus.

Watson's papers in the mid-1950s adequately documented the "case against segmental resection for esophageal carcinoma" and emphasized these principles.[50] Scanlon reported

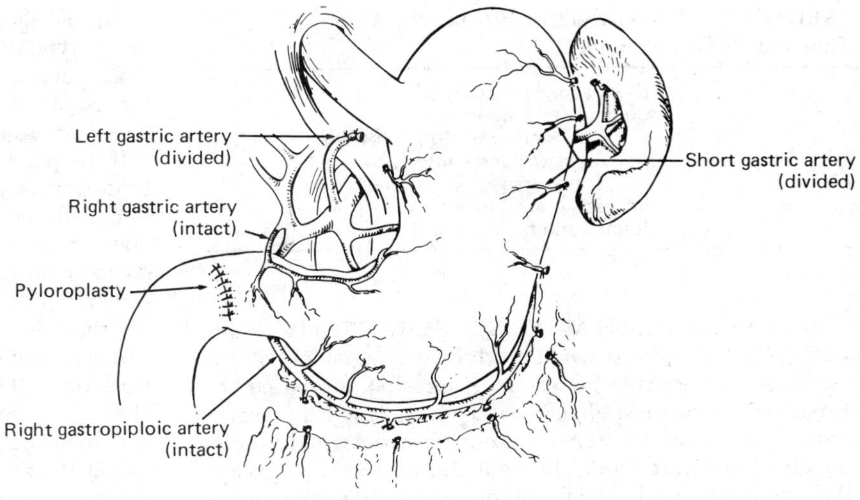

FIG. 24-6. Mobilization of the stomach for reconstruction of the esophagus involves division of the short gastric and left gastric arteries. The right gastric and gastroepiploic artery suffice to vascularize the stomach adequately. Since the vagus nerves are divided when the esophagus is resected, a pyloroplasty is required for adequate gastric drainage.

a 45% incidence of recurrence at the anastomotic site when a segmental resection of the esophagus was performed for carcinoma.[92] Wu and colleagues found cancerous tissue present at the margins in 14% of the resected specimens when they confined resection to 5 cm of esophagus above the cancer.[93] They advocate resection of the lower two-thirds of the esophagus for cancers of the lower third, and they perform an esophagogastrostomy in the chest above the level of the aortic arch. For midesophageal cancers, esophagogastrostomy is performed at the level of the dome of the pleural cavity. When the cancer extends above the level of the aortic arch, they perform an esophagogastrostomy in the neck. In one report, 43% of patients with cancer of the esophagus had cancer cells in the submucosa 5 cm above the tumor.[94] Thus, a resection that is less than a total thoracic esophagectomy will often be inadequate.

In addition to longitudinal resection of an esophageal cancer, a wide margin of surrounding normal tissues and as many as possible of the regional lymphatic channels, including the lymph nodes, should be removed. This is difficult in the upper thoracic esophagus because of the proximity of vital structures, including the aorta, the heart, the left main bronchus, and the inferior pulmonary veins. Skinner has advocated a radical en bloc resection of the esophagus, which was originally described by Logan.[95] This procedure aims to vacate the posterior mediastinum. It carried an 11% operative mortality and a complication rate of 52% in Skinner's hands. The difficulties encountered in performing an adequate resection of the upper esophagus provides a rationale for the use of radiotherapy or chemotherapy, or both, as adjuncts to local control of the tumor.

There are three approaches to esophageal resection: through a right thoracotomy, combined with a laparotomy; through a left thoracotomy, using a thoracoabdominal incision; and without thoracotomy, using separate abdominal and cervical incisions.

Esophagectomy through the right chest is the most widely accepted approach. During the same anesthetic, it is preceded by a laparotomy, during which the celiac and lesser curvature lymph nodes are biopsied and the stomach is mobilized if it is to be used to replace the esophagus (Fig. 24-6).[96,97]

The esophagus can also be removed by blunt dissection through abdominal (transhiatal) and cervical incisions, thus avoiding thoracotomy (Fig. 24-7). This operation was first described in England during the 1930s and was reintroduced by Kirk in 1974.[98] It has been used in the United States with acceptable results.[99–102] However, it does not allow for a wide resection of adjacent tissues and can be followed by disastrous complications.[103,104] It may be that esophagectomy without thoracotomy will suffice as a low-risk tumor reductive procedure, allowing radiotherapy and chemotherapy to eliminate the cancer that is left behind. It is most applicable for distal esophageal lesions and cervical esophageal lesions that can be mobilized adequately under direct vision.[105]

FIG. 24-7. The esophagus can be bluntly and blindly dissected free of surrounding structures through the esophageal hiatus and a cervical incision and thus removed.

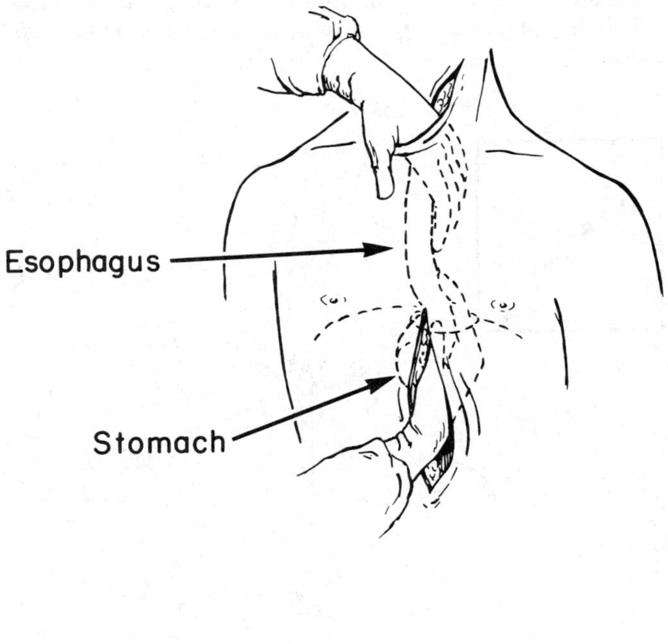

TABLE 24-7. Reconstructive Procedures After Thoracic Esophagectomy

Esophagogastrostomy
Colon interposition
Left (antiperistaltic)
Right (isoperistaltic)
Transverse
Reverse gastric tube
Jejunal interposition

RECONSTRUCTION AFTER ESOPHAGECTOMY. Table 24-7 lists the options available for reconstruction of the esophagus. Esophagogastrostomy, as first proposed by Kirschner, is the most effective and widely practiced form of reconstructive procedure.[6] The stomach is mobilized as demonstrated in Figure 24-6. The right chest is then opened and the tumor removed. A right anterolateral thoracotomy has been used by some surgeons rather than the right posterolateral thoracotomy demonstrated in the illustrations.[106] The stomach is then brought up through the hiatus and anastomosed to the proximal esophagus (Figs. 24-8 and 24-9). Alternatively, the stomach can be brought up to the neck through the esophageal hiatus, or behind the sternum, and anastomosed to the esophagus in the neck.[107]

Emphasis should be placed on the anastomosis between the esophagus and stomach because its disruption is a major cause of the morbidity and mortality following esophagogastrostomy. In addition to anastomotic disruption, strictures can occur at the anastomotic site and gastroesophageal regurgitation can cause discomfort and disability resulting from aspiration. Stapling devices can be used for this anastomosis with great success (Fig. 24-8).[108,109] An inkwell-type anastomosis or fundoplication is performed if possible, bringing the stomach around the esophagus, surrounding the anastomosis with the stomach. This reinforces the anastomosis and diminishes the possibility of gastroesophageal reflux (Fig. 24-9).[110] Gastroesophageal reflux can be controlled by avoiding recumbency and by eating small meals.[111] An innovative form of anastomosis developed by Shao and associates in China is the intraluminal esophagogastrostomy, which did not develop an anastomotic leak in more than 200 cases.[15]

The anastomosis should be free of tension. In order to assure this, the stomach should be tacked to the prevertebral fascia. Because a vagectomy is inevitable when removing the esophagus, delayed gastric emptying can occur postoperatively unless a pyloroplasty is performed (Fig. 24-10).[112]

If the patient has had a previous gastrectomy, an esophagogastrostomy cannot be performed following esophagectomy. In such instances, a colon interposition will be required to provide a conduit to the stomach (Fig. 24-11).[113,114] A preoperative barium enema is mandatory for a colon interposition. The left colon is best suited for this procedure, but the right or transverse colon can also be used. Two surgical teams should be used to limit operative time, with one team working in the abdomen while the other team works in the chest. Because this procedure requires three anastomoses and involves the colon, which has a less adequate blood supply than the stomach, the incidence of anastomotic leaks is higher than after esophagogastrostomy.

Two other options exist for reconstruction of gastrointestinal continuity after a subtotal esophagectomy. A gastric tube can be fashioned from the greater curvature of the stomach (Fig. 24-12) or a jejunal loop can be used to bridge the esophageal defect.[115,116] They have no advantages over esophagogastrostomy and carry a higher rate of complications.

Based on a review of several surgical series, the portion of 5-year survivors varies from 2% to 21%.[117] The average survival after the operation ranges from 7 to 28 months. Results are generally better for smaller and more distally located cancer.

The operative mortality with esophagogastrostomy ranges from 4% to 30%.[117] Extremes of operative mortality for all kinds of operations are 0.8% to 57%.[118] However, there appears to be a trend in recent years to lower operative mortality rates which should be less than 5%.[119] Cardiopulmonary complications and anastomotic leaks lead the list of causes of postoperative death.[120–123] Other complications are listed in Table 24-8.

Radiation Therapy

Radiotherapy is rarely associated with acute mortality and, when used by itself, frequently provides prompt relief of

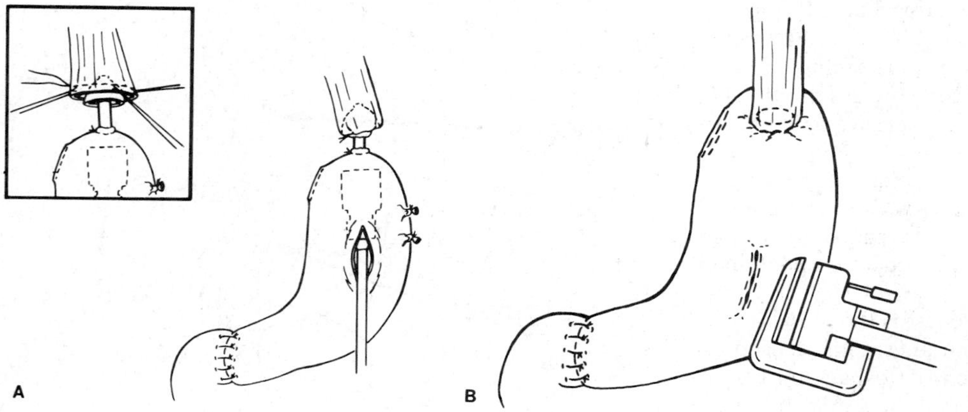

FIG. 24-8. **A**. Esophagogastrostomy is performed using an end-to-end anastomosis stapler. The stapler may also be inserted at the site of the pyloroplasty. The completed anastomosis is shown in **B**. (Steichen FM, Ravitch MM: Mechanical sutures in esophageal surgery. Ann Surg 191:373, 1980)

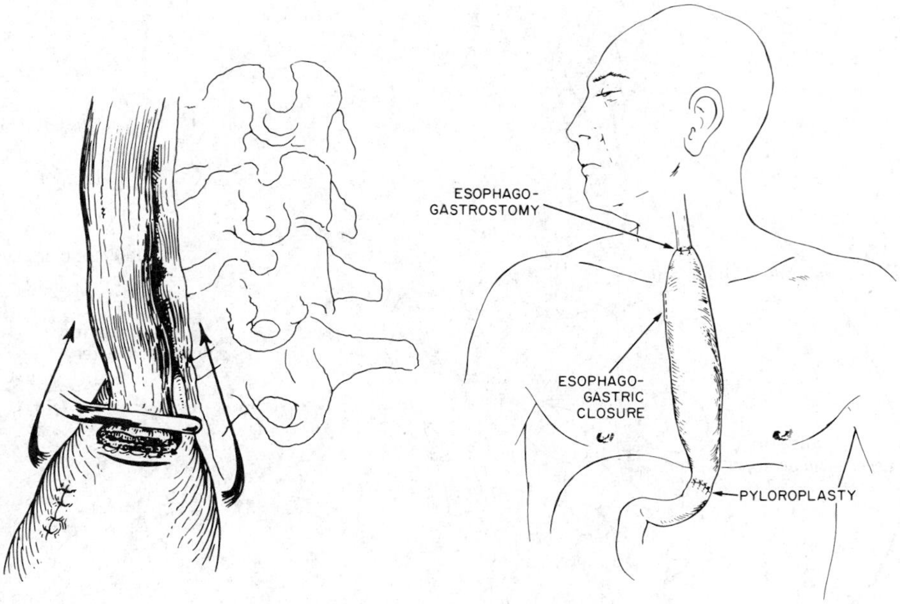

FIG. 24-9. A two-layered, end-to-side anastamosis is performed. After completion of the anastomosis, the stomach is wrapped around the esophagogastrostomy (*arrows*). **A**. The stomach also is sutured to the prevertebral fascia to prevent tension on the anastomosis. **B**. The finished operation.

FIG. 24-10. Barium contrast study following esophagogastrostomy.

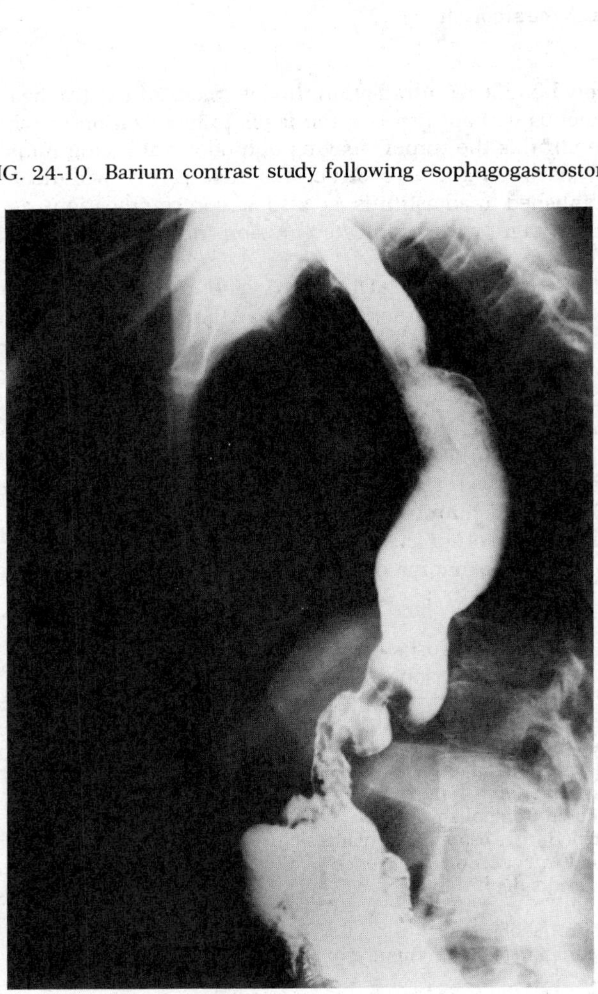

esophageal obstruction. However, definitive radiotherapy is a complex and demanding treatment, often requiring 6 to 8 weeks to complete. In a disease in which the median survival is measured in months, this is a substantial investment in time and resources for many of these patients. Furthermore, swallowing relief is only short-term in more than 50% of cases.

Radiotherapy alone is being used less frequently because newer techniques have been introduced that combine radiation with chemotherapy, with or without surgery. The radiotherapy is used to enhance local control and to control disease that may be difficult to resect, such as in mediastinal lymph nodes and periesophageal soft tissues.

PROGNOSTIC FACTORS AND PATIENT SELECTION. It is likely that radiotherapy alone will become confined to the elderly or infirm patient who is not a candidate for aggressive combined modality therapy, and radiation for palliation will be used in patients who present with metastatic disease. The optimal combined therapy for esophageal carcinoma has yet to be devised, but those in use are reviewed. Potential complications of surgery or chemotherapy still render many patients unsuitable for treatment with aggressive combined modality therapy, and radiotherapy alone will continue to play a role in the management of esophageal cancer.

A list of prognostic factors relevant to the radiotherapeutic treatment of esophageal cancer is presented in Table 24-9. In general, patients with small lesions (≤5 cm) are potentially curable with radiation, but those with lesions longer than 10 cm are rarely cured.[124] Although some institutions have not found tumor size to correlate with response, data from a large series of cases at The Princess Margaret Hospital indicate that response to radiation is 100% for lesions less than 5 cm, 66% for lesions 5 to 10 cm, and only 29% for tumors greater than 16 cm.[125,126] Circumferential lesions re-

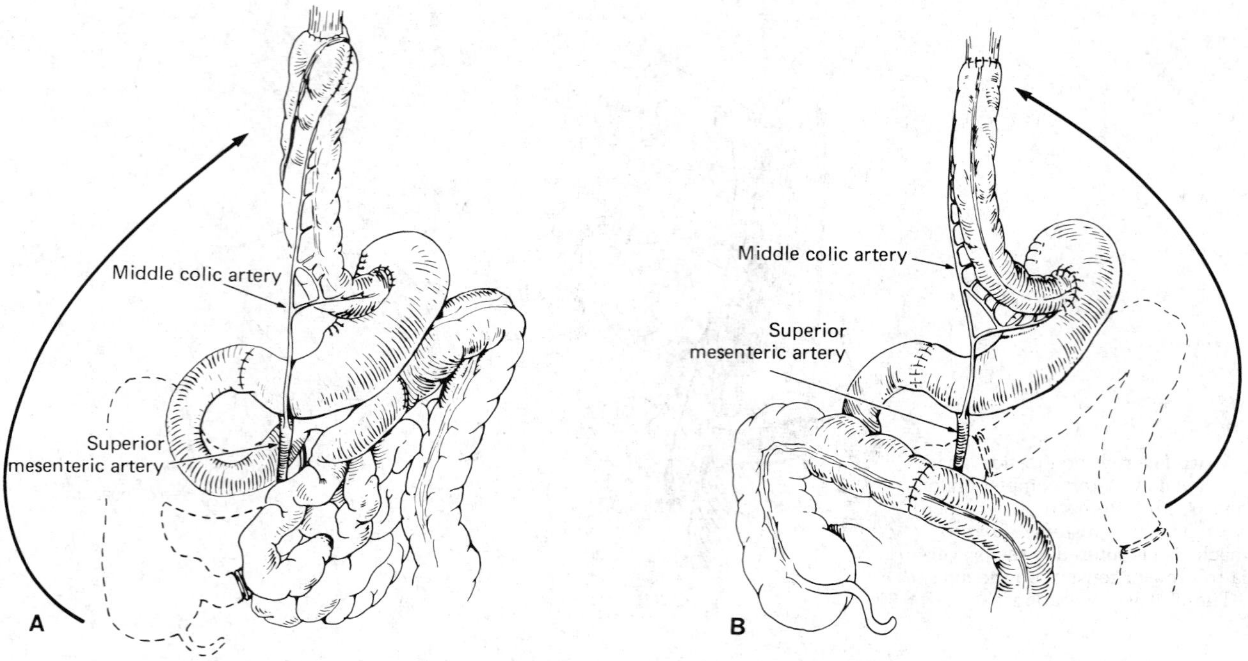

FIG. 24-11. Mobilization of the right colon to form an isoperistaltic conduit to the stomach (**A**) or the left colon to form an antiperistaltic esophageal substitute (**B**).

spond less well than do longitudinal tumors, probably a covariable with size.[127] Women respond better than men; exophytic lesions respond better than ulcerative ones; older patients respond more frequently than younger patients; and upper-third lesions respond somewhat better than lesions in other areas of the esophagus.[124–128]

Several factors are relative contraindications to radiotherapy. Patients with a communication from the esophagus into the tracheobronchial tree have extremely short survivals and rarely benefit from radiation. Involvement of the trachea or bronchus without fistula often leads to fistulization as radiation shrinks the tumor, leaving behind a frank communication between the two structures that rarely will heal.[124] Established mediastinitis is also a contraindication, as is hemorrhage, which indicates erosion into a major vessel.

TECHNIQUE OF RADIATION. The intent of curative radiotherapeutic treatment is to treat the primary tumor, its potential microscopic extension, and the appropriate regional nodes to a cancericidal dose while respecting the tolerance of adjacent normal tissue. The radiotherapist must arrange the treatment fields and the patient's treatment position so that the setup can be reproduced accurately each treatment day for 6 to 7 weeks. Reproducibility is greatly facilitated by immobilization on the treatment table by a body cast or other customized molded support system. Patients with carcinoma of the esophagus often will be treated

FIG. 24-12. A gastric tube constructed from the greater curvature of the stomach can be used to reconstruct or bypass the esophagus. The gastric tube depicted here is isoperistaltic with the blood supply coming from the right gastroepiploic artery. A reverse gastric tube can be fashioned with the blood supply based at the fundus. (Postlethwait RW: Technique for isoperistaltic gastric tube for esophageal bypass. Ann Surg 189:673, 1979)

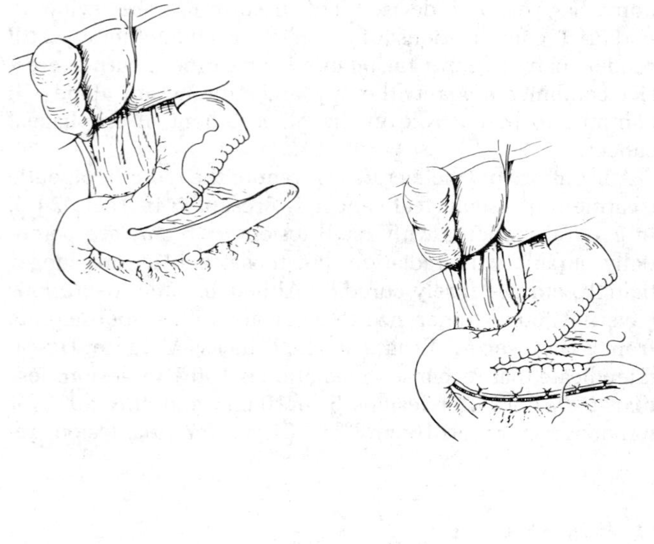

TABLE 24-8. Causes of Morbidity After Esophageal Resection

Anastomotic leak
Anastomotic stricture
Respiratory insufficiency
Congestive heart failure
Pulmonary embolism
Obstruction at esophageal hiatus
Wound infection or dehiscence
Ruptured spleen
Phlebitis
Subphrenic abscess
Torsion, gangrene or rupture of gastrointestinal replacement
Hemorrhage

TABLE 24-9. Prognostic Factors for Radiation Treatment of Esophageal Cancer

Better	*Worse*
Female	Male
<5 cm length	>10 cm length
Less than circumferential	Circumferential
Upper one-third	Lower one-third
Older age	Younger age
Exophytic	Ulcerative

in the prone position to maximize the separation between the esophagus and spinal cord.[129–131] Many elderly patients find they cannot hold this treatment position long enough to accomplish simulation and subsequent treatment. In that case, patients are treated in the supine position. Arms are raised overhead to allow for access into the CT scanner in the treatment position.

Normal structures must be taken into account during esophageal irradiation to minimize complications. In esophageal carcinoma, the major dose-limiting structure is the spinal cord, which lies close to the esophagus. The radiation tolerance of the spinal cord is usually regarded as 4500 cGy, less than the dose required to eradicate the tumor. Therefore, some of the radiation treatment must be administered through oblique fields that avoid the spinal cord. These oblique fields, coupled with anterior or posterior fields, make up the commonly used three-field or four-field esophageal treatment plan (Fig. 24-13).[132]

The radiation therapy field is designed to encompass the gross and microscopic extensions of tumor, as well as regional lymph nodes. The radiographic extent of the tumor is covered with a 5-cm to 6-cm margin in the cephalad-caudad direction. Although esophageal cancer can spread more than 6 cm from the primary site in approximately 15% of cases, such patients are rarely cured with radiation therapy alone.[133] There is little evidence that radiation response or cure is associated with field size.[126] Pearson achieved the best results ever reported using a relatively limited field size.[134] Even when a 5- to 6-cm margin is taken around the tumor, field sizes will be 15 cm or longer, which is substantial (Fig. 24-14).

For treatment with radiation therapy alone, the field width is usually 7 to 8 cm, enough to cover the esophagus and nearby structures such as periesophageal lymph nodes. CT scans can detect significant amounts of periesophageal soft tissue extension that are difficult, if not impossible, to recognize on plain x-ray films taken with barium contrast.[62–65] CT scans display the location, size, and density of pulmonary tissue, which allows treatment to be performed with a correction built in for the increased radiation transmission that occurs through low-density lung tissue.[135]

CT scans can be used as a basis for radiotherapy treatment planning. The scan can be brought up on the treatment planning screen (Fig. 24-15A) and beams superimposed on this image. Dose calculations can be made, and the region of the esophagus and periesophageal soft tissues can be seen as encompassed within the high-dose volume (Fig. 24-15B). Furthermore, CT scans can be reformatted in the sagittal

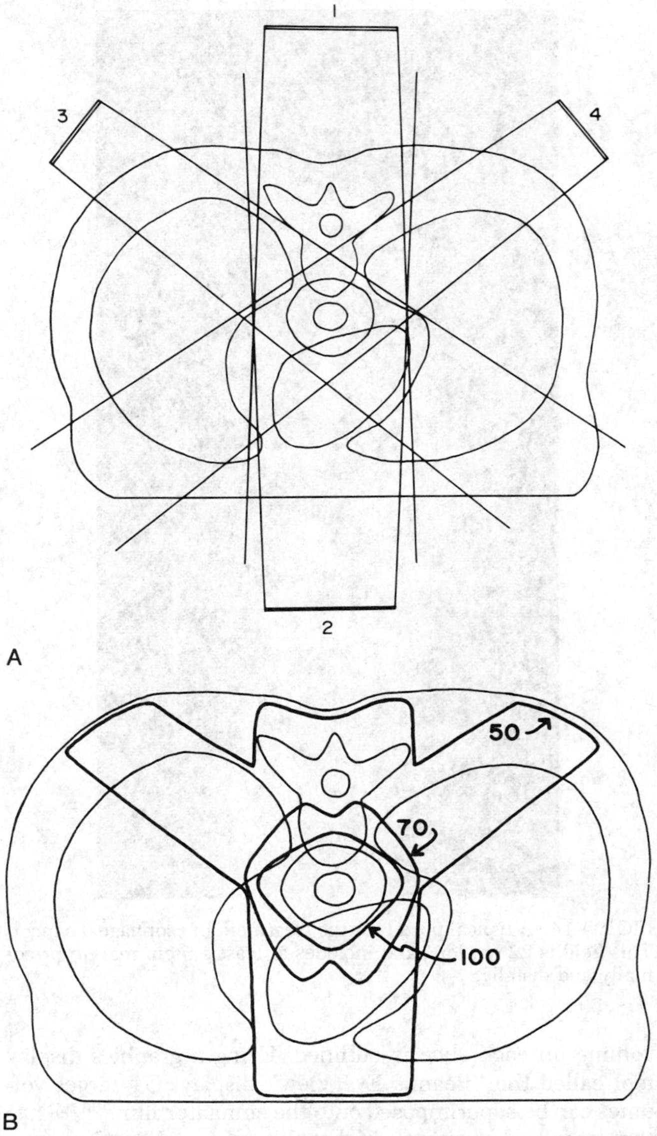

FIG. 24-13. **A**. The classic radiation field configuration for treatment of esophagus cancer. Two oblique fields are used matched to an anterior field, with or without a posterior field. This three- or four-field plan produces a high dose volume around the esophagus. The oblique fields spare the spinal cord so that dose to this structure can be kept below tolerance levels. **B**. Isodose curves for this treatment technique. The 100% volume encompasses the tumor while the spinal cord receives less than 70% of the dose.

plane. This allows a view of the region of the esophagus and the spinal cord throughout the treatment length. These displays are extremely valuable in planning treatment (Fig. 24-15C).

The CT scan can also verify the adequacy of the radiotherapy portals. First, the patient is simulated and films of each treatment port are taken using barium contrast (Fig. 24-14). The patient is then taken to the CT scanner, and CT slices throughout the esophageal tumor volume are obtained while the patient is positioned in a fashion to duplicate the treatment position. The CT scans are then viewed and the target

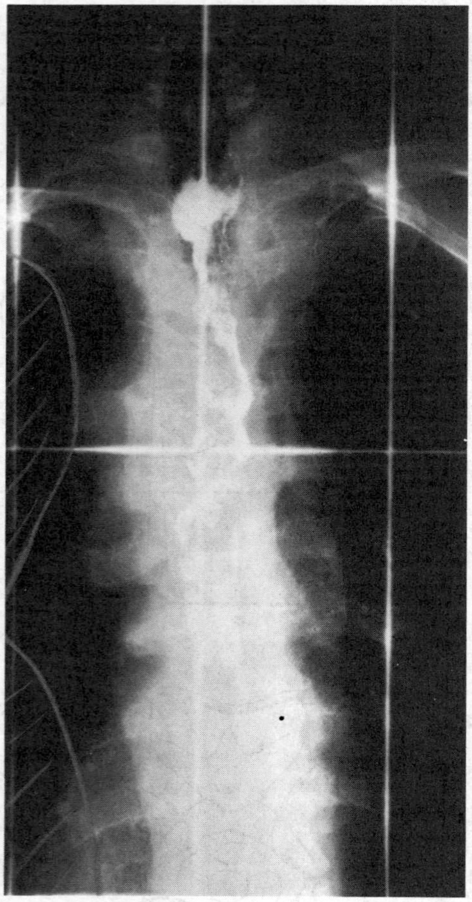

FIG. 24-14. A typical portal for the treatment of esophageal cancer. This field is 22 cm long and includes at least a 5 cm margin proximally and distally.

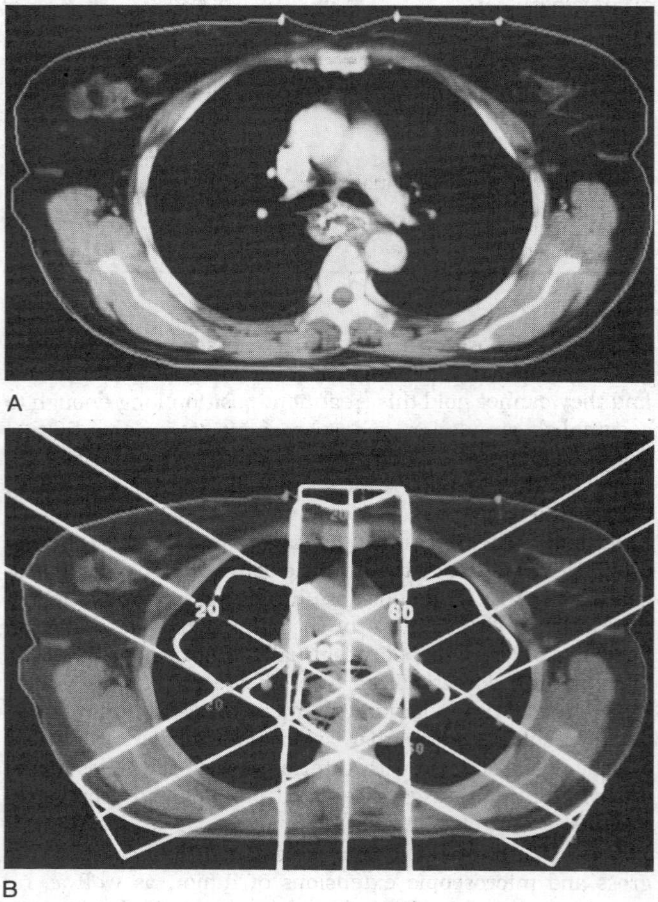

FIG. 24-15. **A.** CT scan of a patient with esophageal cancer. The patient is in the supine position on a flat couch that duplicates the treatment couch. The esophageal tumor with thickening of the esophageal wall can be clearly seen. **B.** Three-field plan (anterior and two posterior obliques) superimposed on the CT scan. The esophageal tumor is encompassed in the high dose zone, and the spinal cord is partially spared radiation with the oblique portals.

volume on each slice is outlined. Using a graphics display tool called the "Beam's Eye View" display, CT target volumes can be superimposed onto the simulator film.[136,137] It is then easy to determine whether the target volumes are adequately included in the radiation field and whether shielding blocks can be safely added to protect normal tissue (Fig. 24-16).[138]

The ability to see tumor and normal tissue anatomy on CT scans and the increasing use of combined modality therapy have refocused attention on regional lymph node treatment. Spread to regional nodes occurs in 40% to 70% of esophageal cancer patients, and sterilization of these areas is critical in the curative treatment of this disease. Many institutions now routinely include radiotherapy for supraclavicular nodes in their patients with upper esophageal lesions and for celiac nodes in their patients with middle and lower esophageal lesions.[138,140,141]

The dose of radiation varies from one institution to another and also depends on whether chemotherapy or surgery will be added to the treatment. Definitive doses of radiation range between 5000 cGy in 20 treatments over 4 weeks to 6600 cGy in 33 treatments over 7 weeks. In many instances, these doses are reduced when concurrent chemotherapy is administered. No dose regimen has proved superior to any other, but, as combined modality therapy becomes more effective and systemic micrometastases are controlled, local control in the esophagus itself will take on increasing importance. In general, higher doses of radiation lead to higher local control rates.[142]

CLINICAL COURSE AFTER IRRADIATION. The squamous epithelium of the esophagus has approximately the same radiosensitivity as that of the oral mucosa.[143] Deepithelialization leads to clinical symptoms of esophagitis that begin 1 to 2 weeks after the start of treatment and can be severe in some patients. Tumor response usually begins during the second or third week. Improvement in swallowing and relief of tumor pain can make the discomfort of esophagitis more tolerable. Measures that reduce the symptoms of esophagitis include systemic analgesics and viscous lidocaine. The possibility of monilial esophagitis should always be considered, and antimonilial agents can benefit some patients. The radiation tolerance of the esophagus is usually

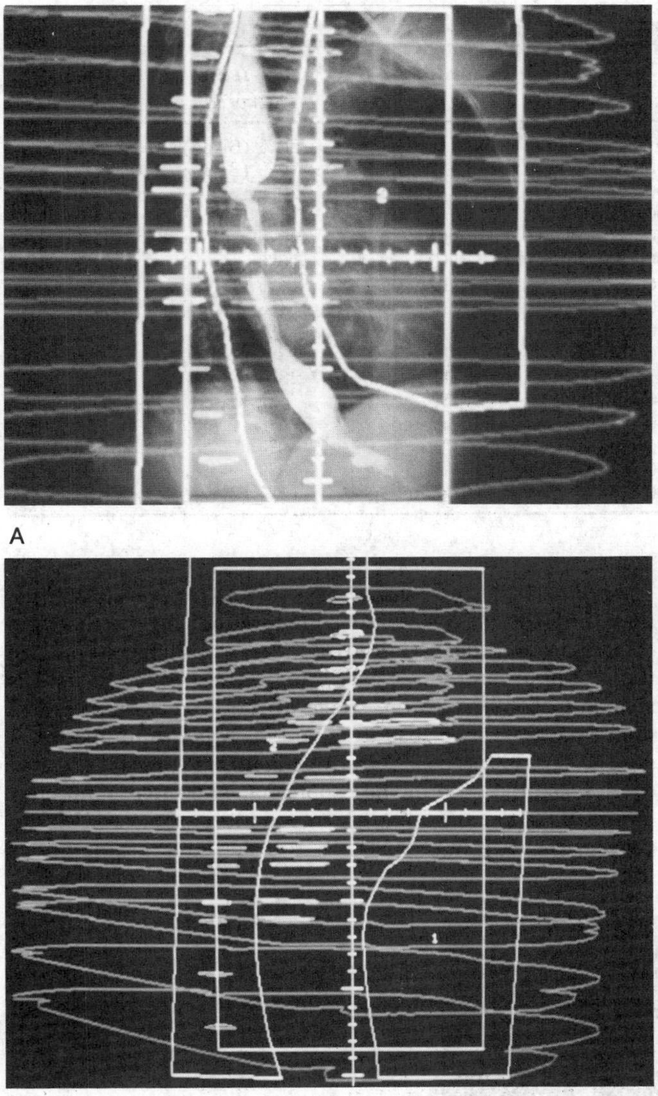

A

B

FIG. 24-16. **A**. Beam's eye view display for esophageal treatment. The CT target volumes and the spinal cord are superimposed on the simulator film with a barium esophagram. The shielding blocks treat the esophagus but can clearly be seen to encroach on the target volumes anteriorly. **B**. The blocks can be modified to better include the target volume. Here the spinal cord is protected by the posterior block, and the anterior block allows a generous margin around the target volume.

between 6000 and 6500 rad.[144] However, chemotherapeutic agents, especially doxorubicin, can dramatically increase the radiation sensitivity of the esophagus, and care must be exercised in the concurrent administration of drugs and radiation.[145]

RESULTS OF RADIATION THERAPY ALONE. Table 24-10 summarizes the result of radiation therapy alone and includes survival data for untreated patients. There is a suggestion that modern high-energy x-ray treatment produces an improvement compared with the natural history of the disease. Between 60% and 80% of irradiated patients will have their dysphagia partially or completely relieved by irradiation (Fig. 24-17). This response is often rapid and in many patients occurs during treatment. In about one-third of treated patients, this restoration of swallowing will persist for the duration of their illness. This correlates reasonably well with the 15% to 30% complete tumor regression seen when radiation is used preoperatively in the treatment of esophageal cancer (Table 24-11).

COMPLICATIONS OF RADIATION THERAPY. Death or serious long-term morbidity caused by esophageal irradiation is uncommon. Occasionally, patients have been reported with radiation pneumonitis, pericarditis, myocarditis, or spinal cord damage. The most frequent complications from esophageal irradiation are stricture, fistula, and hemorrhage. Many of these complications are related to regrowth of the cancer itself. Although more than 50% of irradiated patients will develop stricture, many of these are due to persistent cancer.[125,126,150] Fistulas and hemorrhage following irradiation occur in 10% to 20% of cases and usually result from resolution of cancer that has invaded the neighboring trachea, bronchus, or aorta.[150,155,156] However, not all complications are tumor related, and benign esophageal stricture from radiation or infectious complications have been reported.[125]

INTRACAVITARY RADIATION. The concept of implanting radioactive sources within or around a tumor has a long history. The first cancer to be treated in this fashion was probably carcinoma of the cervix in which the cervical canal was a natural holder for the radium tube. In the early 1900s, Exner recognized that the lumen of the esophagus represented a natural opening for the introduction of radioactive material into the center of an esophageal cancer.[158] Since that time, several intraluminal applicators have been tried. In 1969, Rider reported on a series of patients treated with external radiation followed by an insertion of an intraluminal radium bougie.[159] These early results were encouraging, with a 37% 3-year survival. Since that time, a number of reports have appeared concerning intraluminal radiation, the most recent of which used remote after-loading sources to eliminate exposure of hospital staff.[160–165] The esophageal lesion suitable for such therapy is relatively small because the esophagus must be able to accept intubation and the dose distribution is about 1 to 1.5 cm. For these reasons, intraluminal therapy is being used in many cases after external-beam treatment has shrunk the primary tumor. The intraluminal treatment is then used as a boost dose, much as a radioactive implant of seeds is used in the head and neck or breast. Early reports of intraluminal therapy for rapid palliation of obstruction are encouraging.[165]

CONFORMATIONAL THERAPY. When the esophagus and periesophageal tissues are irradiated, a substantial amount of normal tissue is also irradiated. To reduce the dose to normal tissues, many radiotherapy centers have tried rotational therapy in which the treatment volume describes a tight circle around the target, with a rapid falloff in dose reaching the adjacent normal structures. However, the

TABLE 24-10. Studies of Radiation Alone for Esophageal Cancer

Author	*Reference*	*Dates*	*Patients Treated**	*Dose (rad)*	*Median Survival (mo)*	*2-Year Survival*	*5-Year Survival*
Roberts	146		975	Untreated	Not stated	20% (6 mo)	6% (1 yr)
Applequist	147	1965–74	50	5100–6800	12	12% (3 yr)	4%
Beatty	126	1969–75	146	4000–6000	9	20%	6%
Cedarquist	91	1945–69	388	4500–7000	8	11%	4%
Elkon	148	1968–73	50	5000–7000	11	28%	2%
Hussey	124	1945–75	69	5500–6500	10	16%	10%
Jobsen	149	1978–81	38	5500–6500	12	14%	4%
Lewinsky	130	1966–71	85	5000–6000	8	11%	4%
Lowe	150	1958–69	244	Not stated	5	7%	1%
Newaisky	151	1956–74	444	5000–5500	12	18%	9%
Pearson	134	1949–69	388	5000	12	28%	20%
Schuchmann	152	1950–78	77	4500	10	Not stated	0%
Van Andle	153	1970–78	115	6000–6600	Not stated	4%	1%
Van Houtte	154	1962–72	81	6000–7500	8	9%	3%
Wara	155	1950–73	103	5000–6000	7	8%	1%
Wei-Bo Yin	156	1968–69	1212	6000–7000	Not stated	11% (3 yr)	7%

* With curative doses; some data extracted from survival curves.

esophagus is rather difficult to treat in this fashion because the tissue that needs treatment is of different widths in different areas of the esophagus and because the esophagus has a curved shape.

Conformational therapy is a way around this dilemma. In this technique, the conventional radiation collimator is replaced by a device made up of 20 or 30 separate pairs of leaves. These leaves can independently be adjusted to any width, allowing the tumor to be treated with a shaped field that conforms to the tumor configuration. As the machine rotates around the patient, the leaves continuously change their position so that at every angle the treatment field is shaped to conform to the shape of the target volume. This creates a very tight dose distribution, which minimizes the dose to normal tissues.[166] In this manner, it may be possible to increase the dose of the esophagus while maintaining or diminishing the dose to the surrounding tissues.[127,166] Because increasing dose is usually related to increasing tumor

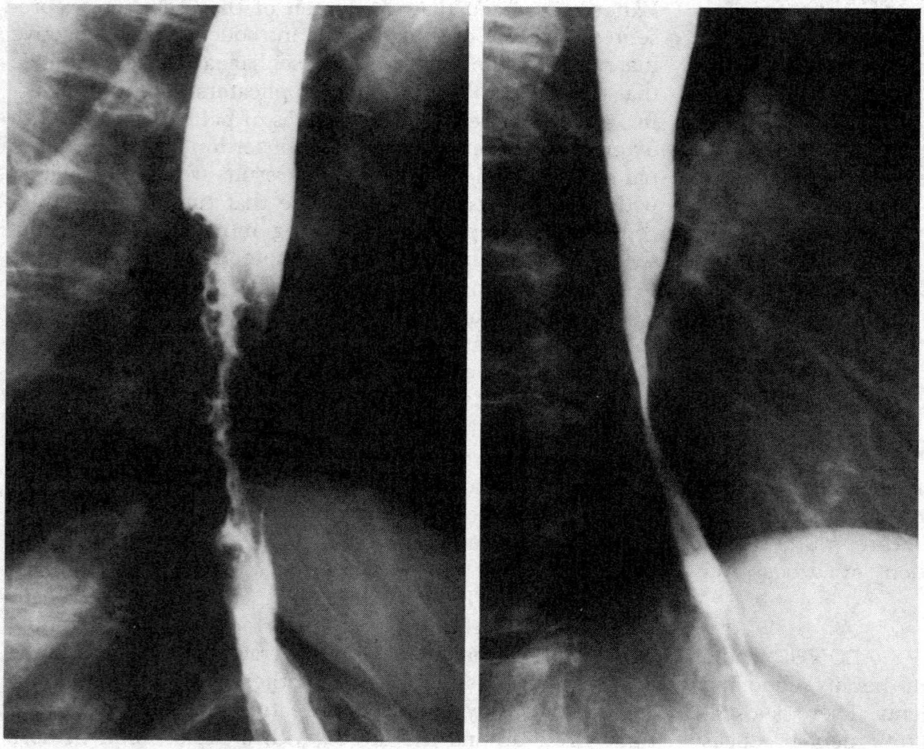

A B

FIG. 24-17. **A**. Midesophageal lesion before treatment. **B**. Post-treatment esophagram. Swallowing was restored, and the surgical specimen was negative on pathologic examination.

TABLE 24-11. Ability of Radiation to Sterilize Esophageal Cancer

Reference	*Dose (rad)*	*% Tumor-Free Specimen*
4000	21	213
5000	23	
4500	13	214
4000	30	127
3000	14	217

control, this therapy promises improved local control of esophageal cancer.

Chemotherapy

Autopsy studies of patients who died of locally controlled esophageal cancer indicate that treatment of the primary tumor and regional lymph nodes is insufficient.[72–77] The search for useful systemic therapies for squamous cell carcinoma of the esophagus has become an important goal because chemotherapy is no longer used solely as a treatment of last resort but has become a vital component of multimodality approaches.

Unfortunately, accurately assessing the effect of chemotherapy as part of initial treatment of esophageal lesions has posed special problems for clinical investigators. At best, measurement by CT of the chest, barium swallow, or endoscopy allows independent observers to declare a lesion improved. The classic partial response (50% reduction of the perpendicular diameters) as determined by barium swallow or endoscopy criteria is more likely to involve investigator bias than are measurements of pulmonary, soft tissue, and liver nodules. A clinically complete response demonstrated by x-ray film or endoscopy is far more elusive than a complete response confirmed by examination of the resected esophagus.[167,168] Despite their deficiencies, these diagnostic methods can determine partial responses with some reliability.

Data generated during the past decade have convincingly demonstrated that epidermoid tumors of the esophagus are relatively responsive to chemotherapy. Kelsen's review showed that nine adequately tested chemotherapeutic agents have modest but defined response rates for patients with measurable lesions.[169] Combinations of the active single agents have consistently yielded higher response rates than the single agents alone.[169]

Initial reports of clinical trials using single agents against epidermoid tumors of the esophagus concentrated on measurable lesions outside the esophagus itself. The modestly active agents, employed after esophagectomy or radiation therapy, produced responses lasting less than 3 months. Furthermore, palliation of symptoms was minimal. Occasionally, patients treated with chemotherapy who were not candidates for surgery or primary radiation experienced improvement of dysphagia, even if the distant measurable disease had not responded.[170,171]

It is no longer uncommon for investigators to report that chemotherapy given as first-line treatment before radiation or surgery improves dysphagia.[172,173] Subjective clinical improvement may or may not correlate with improvement in barium or endoscopy studies.[172,173] A complete response of the primary tumor to chemotherapy does not mean complete eradication of metastatic cancer of the esophagus.[174,175] Thus, current chemotherapy takes on some of the palliative properties of localized surgery and radiation.

SINGLE-AGENT CHEMOTHERAPY. Recent reviews outline the results of single-agent therapy for cancer of the esophagus, and Table 24-12 summarizes these data.[167,176,177] Most clinical trials of single agents enrolled patients whose disease was progressing after surgery or radiation. New Phase II chemotherapeutic agents are not commonly tested

TABLE 24-12. Standard Single Agents Against Squamous Cell Carcinoma of the Esophagus

*Drug**	*Dose*	*No. of Patients Treated*		*Response (%)*		*Dysphagia Relief*	*Reference*
		1st Line	*2nd Line*	*PR*	*CR*		
Bleo	15 mg/m² 1V, twice weekly	15	0	3	1 (27)	?	178
Bleo	20 mg/m², IV, every day to 280 mg	0	14	0	0	?	179
Bleo	0.25 mg/kg, IV, every day to toxicity	0	4	0	0		180
Bleo	15 mg/m², IV, twice weekly × 4	?	?	1	1 (20)	40%	181
DDP	90 mg/m², every 3 weeks	0	10	2	2 (40)	?	182
DDP	2 mg/kg, every 4 weeks	17	0	1	0 (6)	35%	183
DDP	50 mg/m², IV, days 1 and 8, every 3 weeks	0	35	6	3 (26)	?	184
DDP	50 mg/m², IV, every 3 weeks	15	9	6	0 (25)	?	185
5-FU	500 mg/m², IV, every day × 5	0	23	4	0 (17)	?	186
5-FU	300 mg/m², continuous infusion every 6 weeks	11	0	0	11 (82)	100%	187
MMC3	0.05 mg/kg, IV, every day × 10	0	7	1	0 (14)	?	188
MMC	20 mg/m², IV, every 4 weeks × 2, then every 6 weeks	11	13	10	0 (42)	?	185
Dox	40 mg/m², IV, for 2 days	15	0	4	1 (33)	?	189
Dox	60 mg/m², IV, every 3 weeks	0	16	0	0	?	186
MTX	40 mg/m², IV, weekly	0	26	3	0 (12)	?	186
MTX	200 mg/m², IV, every 10 days × 2	44	0	20	1 (48)	73%	173

* Bleo = bleomycin; DDP = cisplatin; 5-FU = 5-fluorouracil; MMC = mitomycin C; Dox = doxorubicin; MTX = methotrexate.

against squamous cell tumors of the esophagus because the tumor is less common and less easy to measure than the classic signal tumors. Nevertheless, modest responses to bleomycin, mitomycin C, doxorubicin, 5-fluorouracil, and cisplatin were considered in designing combinations of chemotherapeutic agents used in initial treatments with surgery or radiation, or both. Investigational drugs, such as vindesine or mitoguazone (MGBG), were found to have modest but reproducible activity against advanced disease treated with other therapies.[190,191] A different picture might have emerged if intact, untreated primary tumors were studied rather than advanced disseminated disease. Based on experience garnered from preoperative and preradiation chemotherapy regimens, single-agent therapy can produce responses in intact, untreated primary tumors in more than 50% of patients treated, and perhaps it is in this context that new and promising phase II agents should be tested.

COMBINATION CHEMOTHERAPY. Data reported for single-agent chemotherapy have been used to rationally combine agents. Table 24-13 is a partial listing of the combinations used to treat disseminated esophageal cancer. Most

TABLE 24-13. Combination Chemotherapy Trials for Disseminated Squamous Cell Carcinoma of the Esophagus

*Chemotherapy**	*No. of Patients*	*PR*	*CR*	*%*	*Median Survival†*	*Reference*
DDP + Bleo DDP = 3 mg/kg day 1 Bleo = 10 mg/m², IV, load day 3 10 mg/m², 24-h infusion days 3–6	18	2	1	17	4 mo	192
DDP + Bleo DDP = 20 mg/day × 8 Bleo = 10 mg, infusion each day × 8	17	1	3	24	?	193
DDP + Bleo + Vind DDP = 3 mg/kg, day 1 Bleo = 10 mg/m², IV, load day 3 10 mg/m², 24-h infusion days 3–6 Vind = 3 mg/m², IV, weekly	24	8	0	33	4 mo	194
DDP + Bleo + Vind DDP = 50 mg/m², day 1 Bleo = 15 mg/m² , day 1 Vind = 3 mg/m² weekly Recycle every 3 weeks	27	7	0	29	3.5 mo	195
DDP + Bleo + MTX DDP = 50 mg/m², day 3 Bleo = 10 mg/m², IM, weekly MTX = 40 mg/m², IV, days 1 and 15 Recycle every 3 weeks	31	7	1	26	5 mo	196
DDP + Bleo + MTX DDP = 50 mg/m², day 4 Bleo = 10 U, IM, weekly MTX = 40 mg/m², days 1 and 14 Recycle every 3 weeks	10	4	1	50	7.5 mo	197
DDP + Vind + MGBG DDP = 120 mg/m², day 1 Vind = 3 mg/m², weekly MGBG = 500 mg/m², days 1 and 14 Recycle every 29 days × 1	20	8	0	40	4.8 mo	198
DDP + Vind + MGBG DDP = 100 mg/m², day 2 Vind = 1.6 mg/m², IV, days 1,2,3,4 MGBG = 500 mg/m², IV, days 1 and 14 Recycle every 29 days	4	2	0	50	?	199
DDP + MGBG + MTX + Bleo DDP = 50 mg/m², day 4 MGBG = 500 mg/m², days 1 and 14 MTX = 40 mg/m², days 1 and 14 Bleo = 10 U, IM, days 1 and 14 Recycle every 21 days	8	4	1	63	?	200
DDP + 5-FU + Dox DDP = 75 mg/m², day 1 Dox = 30 mg/m², day 1 5-FU = 600 mg/m², days 1 and 8 Recycle every 29 days	21	2	5	33	?	201

* DDP = cisplatin; Bleo = bleomycin; Vind = vindesine; MTX = methotrexate; MGBG = mitoquazone; 5-FU = 5-fluorouracil; Dox = doxorubicin.
† Median survival from time on study.

of the relatively successful regimens outlined in Table 24-13 have been used as first-line treatment for esophageal tumors in combination with radiation or surgery; because combined chemotherapy is used as primary therapy, its effect on survival becomes more important than its effect on tumor response. The signal contributions of Kelsen and colleagues at the Memorial Sloan-Kettering Cancer Center deserve special notation: they carefully defined partial and complete clinical responses, separated clinical and pathologic responses, and always kept sight of the ultimate aim of improving overall survival. They investigated the use of cisplatin and bleomycin infusion, basing their study on the work of Wittes and colleagues, which indicated that this combination had substantial activity in head and neck cancers.[202] Sixty-one patients were treated, producing a 15% complete and partial response rate, with a median duration of response of 6 months in patients with metastatic disease.[203]

After their initial studies had indicated activity for both bleomycin and doxorubicin, Kolaric and co-workers combined the two agents.[189] Of 16 patients, 3 had partial responses. Although the response rate observed was lower than that seen with doxorubicin alone, the 95% confidence limits overlap.

Using a combination of cisplatin, methotrexate, MGBG, and bleomycin, which had shown activity in head and neck cancers, Vogel and colleagues treated ten patients, nine of whom had metastatic disease.[200] Five patients had complete or partial responses, with remissions lasting 3.5 to 7 months.

Because their patients had different mechanisms of action and toxicities and appeared to lack cross-resistance, Kelsen and colleagues studied the three-drug combination of cisplatin, vindesine, and bleomycin (DVB).[204] Sixty-eight patients were treated. The response rate of patients with metastatic disease was 33%, and the median response for patients with extensive disease receiving chemotherapy alone was 7 months. Although DVB was fairly well tolerated, myelosuppression was dose-limiting. The median leukocyte nadir was 1700 cells/mm^3. Other major toxicities were nephrotoxicity, nausea, vomiting, and a peripheral neuropathy.

Gisselbrecht and coworkers, treated 21 patients with advanced esophageal cancer, using a three-drug combination of 5-fluorouracil (5-FU), doxorubicin, and cisplatin.[201] Objective responses were seen in seven patients, including two complete remissions. The overall response rate was 33%. Cardiotoxicity was seen in one patient. Other toxicities included nausea, vomiting, myelosuppression, and occasional nephrotoxicity.

In the most recent studies, patients with poor Karnofsky performance status (*e.g.*, bedridden patients) have been excluded. Because responses are rare and toxicity is substantial in patients with severely impaired performance status, they should probably not receive aggressive therapy. For patients with a Karnofsky performance status of 50 or better, response rates between 15% and 80% have been reported, with response durations averaging 5 to 9 months. The complete response rate ranged from 0 to 20%. The lowest complete response rates were reported by investigators who restaged patients aggressively using endoscopy or surgery. Some patients have more durable remissions. However, for the smaller series, the 95% confidence limits are quite large.

Combined Modality Therapy

PREOPERATIVE RADIATION THERAPY. Several groups of radiation oncologists and surgeons have tested the hypothesis that for esophageal cancer treatment results improve by giving radiation therapy before resection (Table 24-14). The researchers hoped the two used together would cancel the disadvantages of each and reinforce their benefits. Radiation therapy carries a low mortality and morbidity and can, in higher doses, produce a marked regression in tumor bulk and sterilize microscopic disease in unresected areas (Table 24-11). It is possible to treat a wider area surrounding the esophageal cancer by radiation therapy than can be reasonably accomplished by surgery (Fig. 24-18). On the other hand, esophagectomy can treat a greater length of esophagus, contributing to local control of the tumor and providing a better chance of long-term palliation and possible cure. Reduction in tumor bulk from radiation can, in some cases, increase resectability rates and decrease operative mortality by making surgical procedures easier to perform. Preoperative radiation can prevent metastases and local recurrences that stem from clonogenic tumor cells being liberated by the surgical manipulations.

A variety of radiation dosages and schedules have been used (Table 24-14). In most studies, dosages of 3000 to 6000 cGy over 3 to 6 weeks have been employed. Surgery is undertaken 4 to 6 weeks after completion of the radiotherapy. Alternatively, some studies have used concentrated or large doses of radiation therapy consisting of 2000 to 3000 cGy over 7 to 10 days, with the operation taking place within a week. In most cases, difficulties encountered in operating in areas that received radiation did not increase morbidity and mortality. However, in some instances, the morbidity of preoperative radiation has been as high as either surgery or radiation therapy alone. Mortality rates have ranged from 4% to 33%.

Long-term survival from preoperative radiation correlates with the extent of tumor destruction seen in the operative specimen. For example, Morita found 44% 2-year and 28% 5-year survival rates when preoperative radiation showed extensive tumor destruction.[127] Survival rates were cut in half when this destructive effect was not seen histologically in the resected specimen. Sugimachi reports virtually identical findings.[217] However, Liu reported that long-term survival rates were unrelated to the degree of histologic destruction caused by preoperative radiation. In general, the disappearance of tumor is a significant goal in preoperative radiation, and most long-term survivors come from the groups whose tumor was nearly or completely eradicated by radiation. The fact that combined treatments of radiation plus chemotherapy increases this tumor-free rate is a possible explanation for the increased benefits of chemoradiation compared with radiation only before surgery.

The results of studies of preoperative radiation therapy must be interpreted with caution because many authors do not specify whether survival rates are based on the total number of patients examined, the total number of patients treated, the total number of patients taken to surgery, the total number of patients resected, or the total number of patients who survived the operation. If patients are omitted

TABLE 24-14. Studies of Preoperative Radiation Therapy for Esophageal Cancer

Author	*Reference*	*Dates*	*Proprative Dose (cGy)*	*No. Treated**	*No. Operated on*
Akakura	206	1963–68	5000–6000	117	117
Anderson	207	1977–81	3500	59	36
Doggett	208	1962–68	5000–6600	42	29
Gignoux	209	1976–81	3300	102	97
Groves	210	1964–71	2400	70	Not stated
Hussey	124	1944–75	3000–4000	56	41
Jobson	149	1978–81	4000	91	81
Huang	205	1977–82	4000	89	79
Kelsen	211	1965–76	2000–4500	76	66
Launois	212	1973–76	4000	67	62
Liu	213	1966–82	3000–7000	Not stated	74
Marks	214	1960–73	4500	332	137
Mortia	127	1971–80	3000–4000	130	Not stated
Nakayama	215	1959–79	2000–3000	Not stated	Not stated
Parker	216	1965–75	4500	75	75
Sugimachi	217	1972–83	2500–3000	Not stated	104
Van Andel	153	1970–77	4000	133	133

* Usually taken from larger series. Screening criteria often not specified.
† Distinction is often not made between curative and palliative resections.
‡ Many authors do not specify whether survival rates are calculated based on total number treated, number operated, or number surviving operation. Some data extracted from survival curves.

at each one of these branch points, thus reducing the denominator, long-term survival figures can be artificially inflated.

Two randomized studies involving preoperative radiation have been reported. Launois and colleagues studied 124 patients treated between 1973 and 1976.[212] In this trial, only middle-third or lower-third primary tumors were included. The two groups were similar in age, sex, tumor localization, and surgical approach. The resection rates for the two groups were similar, as was the operative mortality, which was substantial. Most disappointing were the median and long-term survival rates. When operative deaths were excluded from the analysis, the average survival was only 4.5 months for those receiving preoperative radiation and 8.2 months for those treated by surgery alone. There was no statistically significant difference for the two arms of the study or for the 5-year survival rates: 9.5% for combined treatment group and 11.5% for the patients treated by surgery alone. Although the preoperative radiation group had a higher operative mortality rate for patients with middle-third lesions, it was also not significant statistically.

A multi-institutional trial was performed by the European Organization for Research on Treatment of Cancer on 208 patients with resectable lesions.[209] The radiation regimen was 3300 cGy given in 10 fractions over 12 days. Resection was performed within 8 days. The control arm underwent surgery alone. The cure rate for resection alone was 57.5%. It was 49.5% in the group treated with preoperative radiation. There was no difference in resectability between the two treatment groups. The operative mortality was 24.7% for the group treated with preoperative radiation and 17.9% for the patients treated only with surgery. There was no difference in the 2-year survival or median survival for these groups.

Both studies used radiation doses that were relatively concentrated compared with the regimens used by others. In addition to the use of intense radiation, resection was undertaken 8 days after completion of radiation therapy, when the inflammatory response to therapy was still present and before maximal shrinkage of the tumor took place. Despite these criticisms, the standard preoperative approach to esophageal carcinoma now frequently involves both radiation therapy and chemotherapy.

POSTOPERATIVE RADIATION THERAPY. When an exploratory thoracotomy or laparotomy reveals an unresectable advanced carcinoma of the thoracic esophagus, postoperative radiation therapy is often used to control the cancer. Radiation therapy under these circumstances should be considered palliative therapy. An unresectable lesion is unlikely to be cured by radiation therapy, although the possibility always exists.

The rationale for radiation therapy following curative resections of esophageal cancers is that irradiation will eradicate residual macroscopic or microscopic disease, which

FIG. 24-18. Portions of esophagus and adjacent tissues best treated by radiation and resection. (Adapted from Pearson JG: The present status and future potential of radiotherapy in the management of esophageal cancer. Cancer 39:882, 1977)

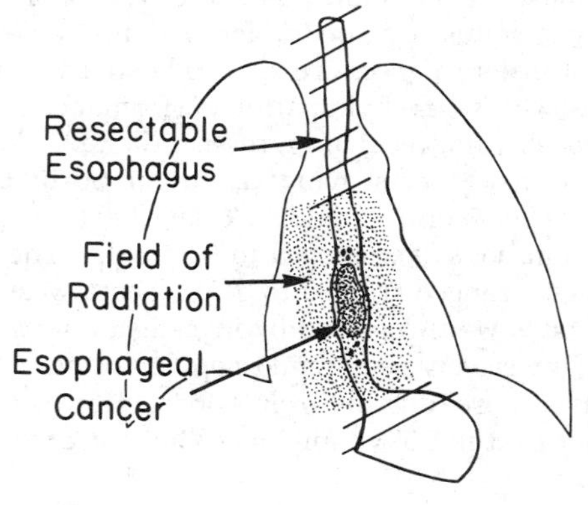

No. Resected	Operative Mortality (%)	Median Survival (mo)	2-Year Survival (%)*	5-Year Survival (%)*
96	21	11	32	25
19	6	7	19	Not stated
24	33	Not stated	12	5
75	25	Not stated	25	10
46	20	Not stated	11	Not stated
30	18	10	13	Not stated
69	20	18 (resected patients)	45	Not stated
79	4	Not stated	Not stated	Not stated
41	12	9	10	5
47	20	10	20	10
59	9	Not stated	70	60
101	18	25 (resected patients)	23	14
Not stated	Not stated		35	23
542	6	Not stated	Not stated	13
75	19	Not stated	15	10
104	6	Not stated	28	17
81	21	Not stated	Not stated	14

could be located within the unresected esophagus, at the margins of resection, or in regional lymphatics and lymph nodes that were not removed. Postoperative radiation may also be effective in controlling implantation or seeding of tumor cells, which may have occurred at the time of operation.

More effective radiation is possible postoperatively because the surgeon can demarcate the extent of the tumor with radiopaque clips at the time of operation, allowing the radiotherapist to direct the treatment accurately to the involved area. However, if the stomach or colon is brought up into the area formerly occupied by the esophagus, radiation therapy must be limited to 4500 to 5000 cGy to avoid radiation injury. Furthermore, the anatomy has been so distorted by these surgical procedures that it is difficult to delineate the volume that is at risk for tumor spread even with the aid of surgical clips and CT scans.

Of seven patients who underwent esophagectomy and postoperative radiation for the reasons enumerated above, Fraser and colleagues reported two 10-year survivors.[218] Both had cancer at the resected margins of the esophagus. Goodner reported 25 patients who had esophagectomy and esophagogastrostomy with postoperative irradiation.[219] Two patients survived for 5 years; the average survival was 9.9 months. At the Mayo Clinic, 14 patients with cancer of the upper thoracic esophagus were treated with postoperative radiation. Five of these patients were 3-year survivors.[220]

Hankins reported a doubling of median survival (7–13 months) for Stage III patients given postoperative irradiation.[221] Langer reported a 28% 2-year survival for nine patients treated with postoperative radiation.[222] Giuli and Gignoux found little effect if doses were less than 3000 cGy; at higher doses the rate of recurrence decreased.[223] In the only large-scale report concerning the use of irradiation after resection for cure, Stage I patients were excluded from this trial.[224] Treatment consisted of 6000 cGy to the mediastinum and neck. Patients with involved nodes at the time of surgery did not benefit, but patients with uninvolved nodes had an extraordinary survival rate (Table 24-15).

There is a paucity of data on the efficacy of postoperative radiation. The advantages of this approach over preoperative radiation are that an accurate anatomic staging of the disease is possible, surgery is not delayed, and it has no influence on operative mortality. On the other hand, esophageal reconstruction often requires lower doses of radiation. This combination of radiation and surgery is probably best used after low-dose preoperative radiation along with chemotherapy. Patients whose tumors are resectable but who have positive

TABLE 29-15. Survival After Postoperative Irradiation for Esophageal Carcinoma

Nodes	Mediastinal 1 Year	2 Years	5 Years
Negative (39)			
Radiation (20)	19/20 (95%)	17/18 (94.4%)	7/8 (87.5%)
No radiation (19)	10/19 (53%)	8/17 (47%)	3/11 (27%)
Positive (72)			
Radiation (32)	20/32 (63%)	11/30 (37%)	2/18 (11%)
No radiation (40)	21/40 (51%)	9/36 (24%)	4/22 (18%)
Overall Survival*			
Radiation		58%	35%
No radiation		30%	20%

* Not actuarial. Follow-up is 1 to 6 years.

or close tumor margins can have this area clipped and postoperative irradiation added through oblique portals.

PREOPERATIVE CHEMOTHERAPY. The rationale for using chemotherapy before and after surgery for squamous cell carcinoma of the esophagus has been described in the section on chemotherapy and is similar to that described for the use of preoperative radiation. Surgery following chemotherapy provides not only the potential of definitive treatment, but also an opportunity to assess pathologic responses to the chemotherapy program. Following resection of the esophageal cancer, chemotherapy can prevent recurrence and inhibit metastases.

Single-drug therapy with bleomycin, given daily or every other day to a total dose of 300 mg, followed by surgery resulted in a resectability rate of 47% and a 2-year survival of 21%.[225] Similar results were reported with this regimen from other centers in Japan.[226] Miller and colleagues used cisplatin as a single agent preoperatively and followed the resection with 4500 to 6000 cGy. More than half of these patients showed partial responses to cisplatin, but no patient had a complete response.[227]

Bleomycin was used as a continuous 3-day infusion after administration of cisplatin (Table 24-16).[192] Although approximately half the patients experienced subjective improvement in swallowing, only 14% were judged to have a partial response by barium swallow, and no patient had complete disappearance of all the cancer after esophagectomy. The median survival for those with local-regional cancer of the esophagus was 10 months.

After finding modest activity for the experimental vinca alkaloid, vindesine, Kelsen and his colleagues added it to bleomycin and cisplatin.[228] After the first 23 patients had been treated, two courses of chemotherapy were instituted before esophagectomy. Postoperative radiation was planned at 5000 cGy over 5 to 6 weeks for patients with T3 or N1 cancer found at operation. Nine percent of patients taken to resection were found to have no cancer in the resected esophagus. The median survival for the group was 16.2 months.

The report by Schlag and colleagues using the same regimen had similar results. Only one patient had a complete response. Fewer than half of the treated patients could be resected for cure.[229]

In the only prospectively randomized trial testing the efficacy of chemotherapy before surgery, 36 patients were randomly assigned to either immediate surgery or chemotherapy with cisplatin, vindesine, and bleomycin, using the dose and schedule recommended by Kelsen.[230] Although 8 (47%) of 17 patients treated before surgery responded to chemotherapy, no significant difference in resectability and survival was found between the two groups. Median survival was 9 months. When the eight patients responding to chemotherapy were compared with the cohort undergoing surgery without chemotherapy, a highly significant difference in median survival was detected.

After retesting an older drug, MGBG, with a new schedule, several investigators found modest activity against disseminated cancer of the esophagus.[231,232] Kelsen and colleagues hoped to be able to eliminate the bleomycin pulmonary toxicity by substituting MGBG.[198] The median duration of survival was greater than 2 years for all those having an operation after receiving MGBG, cisplatin, and vindesine.

After receiving preoperative vinblastine, cisplatin, and MGBG for 2 cycles scheduled 3 weeks apart, 9% of the patients treated had a pathologically confirmed complete response.[199] The median survival for the entire group of patients was 14 months.

Based on previous reports of the efficacy of 5-fluorouracil (5-FU) combined with cisplatin, Shields and colleagues used three courses of cisplatin and 5-FU before surgery for cancer of the esophagus.[233,234] Thirteen (76%) of 17 patients responded to the chemotherapy. No patient had a complete response. Postsurgical treatment consisted of three additional courses of chemotherapy. Those judged to have disease remaining after chemotherapy were offered radiation. Median survival reported for this group of patients is 17.3 months, with projected survival at 3 years of 36%.[234]

Carey and colleagues reported on 24 patients treated preoperatively with 5-FU and cisplatin.[235] Patients with tumor invading the mediastinum or with positive lymph nodes had postoperative radiation. Patients with complete clinical responses were offered four more courses of 5-FU and cisplatin. At the time of surgery 10 (43%) of 24 patients had no visible cancer; four patients who responded still had visible tumor. Only one patient was found pathologically to be free of cancer. Median survival for patients responding to the chemotherapy was projected at 20.4 months compared with 6.7 months for those patients who did not respond to the preoperative therapy.[234]

TABLE 24-16. Preoperative Chemotherapy

*Combination**	*Patients Operated on/ Patients on Study†*	*(%)*	*PR (%)*	*CR (%)‡*	*Median Survival§*	*Reference*
DDP-Bleo	34/43	(79)	6 (14)	0	10.0 mo	192
DDP-Bleo-Vind	34/44	(77)	28 (63)	1 (2)	16.2 mo	194
DDP-Vind-MGBG	14/19	(74)	8 (42)	1 (5)	8.5 mo	198
DDP-Vind-MGBG	11/11	(100)	6 (55)	1 (9)	14.0 mo	199
DDP-5-FU	6/17	(35)	13 (76)	0	17.6 mo	233
DDP-5-FU	22/24	(92)	14 (58)	1 (4)		234

* For doses, see references listed. DDP = cisplatin; Bleo = bleomycin; Vind = vindesine; MGBG = mitoguazone; 5-FU = 5-fluorouracil.
† Patients operated on; all patients treated on study.
‡ Pathologic CR.
§ Median survival from time on study.

These experiences clearly indicate that combination chemotherapy can affect primary tumors in the esophagus (Table 24-16). Whether survival is enhanced by using chemotherapy before surgery awaits a randomized, controlled trial or more striking data than are available.

PREOPERATIVE CHEMORADIATION THERAPY. The earliest experiences with preoperative chemoradiation therapy used single agents. Fujimaki treated 76 patients with radiation and bleomycin before surgery.[225] Their results, as other reports from Japan, were encouraging.[226,236] Thirty percent of the 27 patients at risk for 3 or more years were still alive at the time of the report. A multi-institutional randomized trial from the Scandinavian countries involved 63 patients treated with preoperative radiation and 70 patients treated with preoperative radiation plus bleomycin. No significant differences in median survival or 2-year survival rates were observed.[207] Other studies of bleomycin combined with radiation have not been impressive either.[237]

Werner reviewed the results of a combination of methotrexate, leucovorin, and radiation.[238] Thirty-one percent of the resected patients had no tumor in the resected specimen. Operative mortality was 14%. The average survival reported for patients undergoing surgery was 2 years and 2 months. In a much smaller series from India, the results were similar.[173]

Beginning in 1976, Franklin and colleagues at Wayne State University (WSU) treated epidermoid tumors of the esophagus by using 5-FU and mitomycin C with radiation.[239] Franklin's study contained 30 patients judged to have resectable esophageal cancer.[240] The 23 patients (77%) who subsequently underwent surgery had preoperative barium swallows interpreted as "improved." Six patients (26%) who underwent esophagectomy did not have tumor in the resected esophagus. Four (13%) of these patients survived 5 or more years after their treatment ended. The median survival for the entire group treated was 12 months. Seven patients (30%) died after the operation. One of the patients who died in the postoperative period had no cancer in the resected esophagus.

Parker and colleagues reported on 34 patients treated with either one or two cycles of preoperative 5-FU and mitomycin C plus external-beam radiation of 3000 cGy over 3 weeks.[241] Thirty-four patients were treated in 3 years; 21 (62%) underwent surgery. Eleven had no cancer in the resected esophagus. Although the median survival for the group was not given, Parker clearly documented the problem of distant recurrence for patients rendered free of localized cancer by the preoperative treatment.

The WSU group attempted to decrease protocol mortality by eliminating the potential pulmonary complications of mitomycin C and, in its place, using cisplatin. Cisplatin was chosen as an alternative to mitomycin C because it had caused complete remissions in phase II trials.[184] Furthermore, there was a developing literature on cisplatin's radiation sensitizing properties.[242,243] Cisplatin is not initially toxic to the bone marrow, a property that allowed it to be combined with other chemotherapeutic agents, radiation, or surgery.

Leichman and colleagues reported on 21 patients treated with cisplatin and 5-FU.[233] Radiation and surgery were planned as in the 5-FU–mitomycin trial. Follow-up treatment was included only if cancer remained in the esophagus. Fifteen patients had esophageal resections; 7 (33%) patients were free of all cancer in the esophagus, but 2 of these patients had tumor within the celiac lymph nodes. The median survival for the entire group was 18 months. The median survival for those who could undergo resection was 24 months. Five patients (23%) survived for more than 3 years; three of these patients had no cancer in the resected esophagus and two had microscopic tumor in the resected esophagus.

Although these investigators believed that the patients who survived 3 years or more were cured, Leichman has reported that all these patients have died of recurrent esophageal cancer 3.5 to 5.5 years after treatment was completed. All patients who survived 2 or more years from the completion of surgery had documented distant recurrence of their cancer.

Several researchers reported data on 33 patients treated preoperatively with cisplatin, 5-FU, and radiation.[244,245] They compared the neoadjuvant patients with recent historical controls treated by surgery alone. Each group found a 2-year survival of more than 50% for those treated with neoadjuvant chemotherapy and radiation. Campbell reported no 2-year survivors for surgery alone, but Austin reported that 18% of those receiving surgery were alive at 2 years.

The Southwest Oncology Group (SWOG) and the Radiation Therapy Oncology Group (RTOG) treated patients with the WSU protocol.[175] The group was able to evaluate 106 patients; of this group, 71 (67%) underwent surgery. Eighteen (17%) of the patients (25% of those who underwent resection) were found to have no cancer in the resected esophagus. Operative mortality was 11%. Median survival for all patients who completed the protocol was 14 months. The median survival for those 18 without cancer in the resected esophagus was 32 months. When all patients are considered, 28% had 2-year survivals and 16% had 3-year survivals. In analyzing patterns of failure for patients treated on the SWOG and RTOG trials, Leichman found that 68% of the patients had distant recurrences, 20 had local (within the radiation field) and distant recurrences, and 12% had local recurrences only.[168]

Popp and colleagues used a combination of preoperative 5-FU, cisplatin, and vincristine sulfate with radiation.[246] They had utilized 5-FU mitomycin, and 5-FU–cisplatin on previous series of patients. Because of the small numbers of patients in each group, all patients treated by multimodality therapy are presented as a unit. Twenty-one percent of their combined modality group survived at least 30 months from treatment, compared with 4.8% of their patients treated with surgery alone. There were no long-term survivors who did not achieve a complete remission from preoperative chemoradiation. Their overall impression of multimodality therapy was that it was an improvement over previously used therapy.

Wolfe and co-workers used 5-FU, etopside, and radiation preoperatively.[247] At least 40% of the patients with squamous cell cancer of the esophagus resected had no tumor in the specimen. The 2-year survival for 17 patients completing the full course of treatment was 30%.

TABLE 24-17. Preoperative Chemoradiation

*Drugs**	*Radiation Dose (cGy)‡*	*Total No. of Patients*	*Patients Operated on*	*CR*	*Median Survival*	*Reference*
5-FU-Mito C	3000	30	23 (77)	6 (20)	12 mo	218
5-FU-Mito C	3000	34	21 (62)	11 (32)		241
5-FU-DDP	3000	21	15 (71)	5 (24)	18 mo	232
5-FU-DDP or Mito C	3000	27	27 (100)	6 (24)		174
5-FU-DDP	3000	13	5 (38)	3 (23)		244
5-FU-DDP	3000	11	11 (100)	6 (55)	26 mo	245
5-FU-DDP	3000	106	71 (67)	18 (17)	14 mo	174
MTX with leucovorin	2000	58	58 (100)	18 (18)	26 mo	246

* 5-FU = 5-fluorouracil; Mito C = mitomycin C; DDP = cisplatin; MTX = methotrexate.
† Radiation given before surgery.

Clinical trials using chemotherapy and radiation before surgery for patients with untreated primary esophageal tumors can produce a partial response in at least half of the patients treated if the barium swallow and endoscopic improvement are used as indicators of response (Table 24-17). Fifteen percent to 30% of those treated will show a pathologically confirmed complete response upon review of the surgical specimen. Although it is true that radiation biologists have demonstrated that cisplatin and 5-FU enhance ionizing radiation, the degree of this sensitization has yet to be defined clinically.[52] Yet, Parker, Leichman, and Poplin have independently shown that distant recurrences are the rule, even for the patient with a pathologically proven complete response. No trial to date has shown a 5-year survival for even 20% of those treated. Moreover, toxicity and mortality from combining chemotherapy, radiation, and surgery have remained very troubling aspects of these trials.[249]

CHEMORADIATION THERAPY WITHOUT SURGERY. Surgery has been a very useful guidepost to instruct investigators as to the efficacy of chemotherapy alone or with radiation and may be indicated in clinical trials for this purpose. However, as a modality offering only local control for a disease that tends to disseminate early, surgery may be the modality most easily eliminated without sacrificing overall survival. Poplin's report on combined modality therapy found that the median survival for 113 patients entered on the SWOG trial was 12 months, and the median survival for the 71 patients undergoing surgery was only 2 months more.[175] Furthermore, because surgery and radiation therapy seem to have equal long-term results and their combination offers no apparent benefit, it seems worthwhile to attempt to treat esophageal cancer with chemoradiation without surgery to avoid the morbidity and mortality that occasionally follow esophagectomy.[85]

It must be stressed that in this discussion of therapy without surgery, we are referring to a combined modality approach that is designed as primary therapy for esophageal cancer. In the past, chemoradiation without surgery was considered only for patients who were unsuitable for operation because of advanced disease. The earlier literature reflects this latter approach and must be evaluated from this perspective.

As early as 1972, single-agent chemotherapy with irradiation was employed in a limited number of patients as primary treatment for esophageal carcinoma with encouraging results.[250] Kolaric evaluated the use of bleomycin, doxorubicin, and bleomycin–doxorubicin, in addition to radiation, in three sequential studies.[178,189,251] In each trial, a control group received chemotherapy alone. The number of patients in each arm was small (15–20 patients). In each study, the objective response rate to chemotherapy and radiation was superior to that seen with chemotherapy alone. Toxicity was, however, significant. The median duration of response for the radiation and chemotherapy group ranged from 5 to 9 months.

The results of a randomized trial involving bleomycin plus radiation or radiation alone were not encouraging.[252] Patients were given 5000 to 6000 cGy over 5 to 6 weeks; bleomycin was given at a dose of 15 units/day to a total dose of 210 mg. There was no improvement in swallowing function (objective regressions were not quantitated) or in survival for the bleomycin–radiation group compared with those receiving radiation alone.

A combination of methotrexate, bleomycin, 5-FU, and vincristine, followed by radiation, was used in a group of 26 patients.[253] After one to two cycles of chemotherapy, 55% had some degree of tumor shrinkage. After radiation, 66% had complete remissions; however, it was not clear how this evaluation was performed. There was one drug-related death. The median survival was 11 months.

Using cisplatin and bleomycin or cisplatin, vindesine, and bleomycin, Kelsen and co-workers treated 20 patients with local-regional tumor who either refused surgery or were poor surgical risks.[203,204] The response rates were similar to those seen in the larger group treated preoperatively (22% for cisplatin and bleomycin, 55% for cisplatin, vindesine, and bleomycin); radiation was well tolerated by most patients. Of the 20 patients, 5 were long-term survivors.

Abitbol and colleagues treated nine patients with radiation plus 5-FU, cisplatin, and methotrexate.[254] The median survival was 29 weeks.

Berenzweog and colleagues used a combination of cisplatin, methotrexate, bleomycin, and MGBG before radiation in 5 patients.[255] They were part of a larger group of 18 patients receiving this combination. The average survival of the whole group was 8 months.

The combination of vincristine, methotrexate, and cisplatin plus 5800 cGy did not appear to be an improvement over radiation alone. However, these studies were not carried out in a controlled fashion and can be compared only with historical controls.

Leichman and colleagues initiated a combined modality trial using criteria identical to those of the WSU studies in which surgery followed chemotherapy and radiation.[174] This group of patients received 5-FU, cisplatin, and radiation without intention to operate. Following the second course of 5-FU and cisplatin, mitomycin C and bleomycin were added. A second course of bleomycin was given 3 weeks after completion of the first cycle of mitomycin and bleomycin. Patients then received a follow-up radiation course of 2000 cGy over 2 weeks. Those with improvement in dysphagia were followed without further therapy.

The WSU group treated 20 patients on this protocol. The median lesion size was 7 cm; four patients were older than 80 years of age. Sixteen patients (80%) had an excellent clinical response as shown by subjective improvement in dysphagia and objective increase in body weight. Four patients who did not respond received esophagectomy without complication. The median survival for all patients treated had not been reached after 30 months. Pulmonary toxicity (presumably from bleomycin and radiation) necessitated steroids for 8 of the first 16 patients treated. The last 4 patients received cisplatin and 5-FU instead of bleomycin and radiation.

Lokich and co-workers reported the results of primary treatment of epidermoid tumors of the esophagus for 11 patients treated with 300 mg/m^2 of 5-FU continuously for 6 weeks.[187] All the patients treated reported symptomatic improvement. Nine (81.8%) of 11 had measurable improvement confirmed independently by barium swallow and endoscopy. These patients had further therapy with radiation and 5-FU. Two solid tumor trials have shown the superiority of this schedule for 5-FU compared with the bolus schedule.[256,257] Lokich's schedule may allow clinicians to take further advantage of Byfield's hypothesis that the best infusion schedule is the one that best potentiates the radiation sensitizing properties of 5-FU.[258] Lokich and colleagues have confirmed that low-dose continuous-infusion 5-FU without radiation is cytotoxic and can cause significant damage to the primary tumor without radiation.

Coia and colleagues treated 30 patients with squamous cell carcinoma of the esophagus with 5-FU, mitomycin C, and 6000 cGy of radiation over 6 to 7 weeks.[259] Some patients required breaks in their radiation therapy because of esophagitis, but no severe hematologic problems developed with this regimen. Complete responses based on clinical criteria were obtained in 84% of their patients. Two-year and 5-year actuarial survival rates were 47% and 32%, respectively.

Keane and colleagues from The Princess Margaret Hospital reported on 35 patients treated with 5-FU, mitomycin C, and radiation.[260] This group found significant improvement in both local disease-free survival and overall survival when compared with their own historical controls. The actuarial 2-year relapse-free rate was 47%, and the rate of local tumor control at 2 years was 54%, which was twice as long as their historical group.

John and co-workers treated 21 patients with inoperable cancer of the esophagus with infusion 5-FU, mitomycin C, and radiation followed by infusion 5-FU, cisplatin, and radiation.[261] Dysphagia was relieved within 7 to 14 days of starting therapy for 15 patients (71%), and the median survival for the entire group was 16 months. Six were alive 3 to 40 months after treatment.

Advani and colleagues, noting a paucity of data on the use of methotrexate in good-performance patients with squamous cell carcinoma of the esophagus, reported their experience with methotrexate as a single, first-line agent without leucovorin rescue.[173] Forty-eight percent of patients treated showed "good" responses by barium swallow criteria. When methotrexate was combined with cisplatin, response rates were increased to 76.2%. Twenty-nine of these 42 patients then received 6000 cGy of radiation. Twenty-three obtained further improvement in swallowing capability and esophagram changes. The median duration of response, however, was limited to 12 months, and a significant number of patients developed local-regional recurrences.

These reports indicate that little is lost in terms of survival if aggressive chemotherapy and radiation are used without surgical intervention in the primary treatment of epidermoid tumors of the esophagus. Nevertheless, the scientific rationale for combined radiation and chemotherapy needs refining. The definition of radiation sensitization should be clarified, because the chemotherapeutic agents once used as "sensitizers" for external-beam radiation possess cytotoxic properties against the primary tumor. Finally, a clearer understanding of why microscopic disseminated cancer is resistant to chemotherapy while gross esophageal mucosal tumors usually exhibit partial responses would be most helpful in designing regimens to overcome the differences in the sensitivities of the primary and metastatic cancers of the esophagus.

The past decade of clinical research in cancer of the esophagus has been the decade of emergence of chemotherapy as a primary modality in the therapeutic armamentarium. The clinical trials outlined have defined reproducible clinical and pathologic responses that radiation or surgery alone have not been able to produce in most series. The combined modality trials using chemotherapy with radiation or surgery, or both, have commonly reported median 2-year survivals between 25% and 30%, with median 3-year survivals between 12% and 25%. Unfortunately, there are only a few long-term survivors in each of these trials, and cure remains elusive.

Neither surgery alone nor radiation alone has been adequate. Nevertheless, it is incumbent on investigators to define a survival advantage for patients prospectively randomized to treatments of radiation with or without chemotherapy or surgery with or without chemotherapy. Without such proof, chemotherapy will join surgery and radiation as another toxic, inadequate therapy for primary cancer of the esophagus.

Treatment of Cervical Esophageal Carcinoma

Because of its intimate relationship to the larynx, cervical esophageal carcinomas present special kinds of problems. A recent review of 71 patients, seen from 1965 through 1980,

TABLE 24-18. Reconstructive Procedures After Cervical Esophagectomy

Pharyngogastrostomy
Reverse gastric tube
Skin tubes and skin grafts
Wookey procedure
Deltopectoral flap (Bakamjian)
Others
Intestinal grafts with vascular anastomoses
Jejunum
Sigmoid
Gastric antrum
Colonic interposition

revealed that extramural penetration was present in 77% of the patients. Tracheal invasion was found in 35% and vocal cord paralysis occurred in 24% of the patients.[262] These findings carry a poor prognosis. Resection of a carcinoma of the cervical esophagus usually requires removal of portions of the pharynx, the entire larynx, the thyroid, and the proximal esophagus.[263] If cervical lymph nodes are involved and the lesion is localized to that side, a unilateral radical neck dissection may be included. This is a formidable procedure; it leaves a large defect that is difficult to reconstruct and that is followed by a high mortality and morbidity.[221] Table 24-18 outlines the techniques that can be used to reestablish pharyngoesophageal continuity.

The operation of choice is currently a pharyngogastrostomy.[263,264] The stomach is brought up through the posterior mediastinum after it has been adequately mobilized. The entire thoracic esophagus is bluntly dissected free of the surrounding mediastinal structure and resected (Fig. 24-7). Alternatively, a gastric tube may be constructed from the greater curvature of the stomach to reestablish gastrointestinal continuity (Fig. 24-12). These extensive reconstructive procedures further compromise the patient who has already been stressed by the resection of the carcinoma. Harrison has reported a 12% operative mortality for pharyngolaryngoesophagectomy with gastric anastomosis.[263] A review of the mortality and morbidity of this operation was published by Ong, who first described this operation in 1958.[265]

The surgical treatment of cervical esophageal malignancies carry a significant morbidity, leave the patient with a great disability, and provide little hope for cure. Most recent reports cite a 20% 2-year survival rate. However, if an esophagogastrostomy is uncomplicated, significant palliation is achieved, and the patient may swallow food and saliva without difficulty.

Lesions in the cervical esophagus represent a particularly vexing problem for the radiation therapist also. Generally, these lesions are too low to allow good coverage with parallel, opposed lateral fields because irradiation would take place through the patient's shoulders. Conversely, they are often too high to allow treatment with posterior oblique fields. However, it is possible to use anterior oblique fields, often with wedges, to obtain satisfactory treatment. It must be stressed that the proximity of dose-limiting structures such as the spinal cord to the esophagus makes treatment of this disease technically challenging in all patients.

Like squamous cell carcinomas in the thoracic esophagus, multimodality therapy for these patients offers excellent palliation, and the potential for cure exists when chemoradiation therapy is employed. Because of the disfigurement and disability resulting from surgery, resection is best kept in reserve as a salvage procedure.

ADENOCARCINOMA OF THE ESOPHAGUS

The literature on adenocarcinoma of the esophagus is difficult to summarize because so many authors include gastric lesions that invade the esophagus. The rationale for doing so is that the prognosis and treatment are the same. This may be true for the advanced lesions, but, as diagnostic techniques such as esophagogastroscopy improve, early lesions of the esophagus are found and a distinction can be made between primary adenocarcinoma of the esophagus and those that involve it by direct extension from the stomach. Detection of the less-advanced lesion may be accompanied by a better understanding of the factors responsible for the emergence of these cancers and, hopefully, a better approach to their cure. Curative approaches also produce the best palliation.

Until recently, many authorities doubted the existence of primary adenocarcinoma of the esophagus because it was so rare.[266] The Mayo Clinic reported 19 patients with this diagnosis who constituted 3.3% of the 1312 patients with cancer of the esophagus or cardia seen from 1946 to 1963. Turnbull and co-workers found an incidence of 2.3% among the 1918 patients with esophageal cancer seen from 1926 to 1968 at the Memorial Hospital for Cancer in New York.[267] In a series of 163 patients with esophageal cancer seen between 1975 and 1982, 6.7% had a primary adenocarcinoma of the esophagus.[268] This figure is close to the one reported from Denmark, in which 6.9% of the esophageal carcinomas were found to be of the glandular type.[269]

HISTOGENESIS OF PRIMARY ADENOCARCINOMA

Three possible sources exist for the development of an adenocarcinoma of the esophagus: the superficial and deep glands of the esophagus, persistence of embryonic remnants of glandular epithelium in the esophagus, and metaplastic glandular epithelium.

The superficial and deep glands of the esophagus are mucus-secreting cells which are indistinguishable in appearance from the cardiac glands of the stomach. Secretions from the superficial glands located within the mucosa enter the lumen of the esophagus through ducts lined by a single layer of mucus cells. The terminal portion of the ducts from these glands is lined with squamous cells. The deep esophageal glands are thought to give rise to the mucoepidermoid carcinomas occasionally found in the esophagus.[270]

Congenital persistence of columnar lining the esophagus is possible because during early embryonic life the esophagus is a tube of stratified columnar cells that develops a lumen and then becomes lined with ciliated columnar cells. During the 14th week of embryonic life, squamous cells appear in the middle third of the esophagus. They spread craniad and caudad, gradually lining the entire lumen of the esophagus by the 7th month of gestation. If this process is arrested during fetal life, segments of the esophagus could remain lined with glandular epithelium rather than squamous epithelium. Another possible explanation for small patches of fundic gastric mucosa in the esophagus is that they represent heterotopic deposits of displaced embryonic tissue, as are occasionally seen in a Meckel diverticulum.[270]

A columnar-lined esophagus resulting from glandular mucosa replacing the squamous cell mucosa occurs in some patients with reflux esophagitis (Barrett's esophagus). Although currently accepted, this explanation was not appreciated when Barrett first drew attention to the columnar-lined lower esophagus in 1950. He originally attributed the phenomenon to a congenitally short esophagus. He discarded the possibility that the shortened esophagus was acquired as a result of "reflux esophagitis," a term he coined. By 1957, he changed his views on the subject and postulated that the lower esophagus lined by columnar epithelium was most probably "the result of a failure of the embryonic lining of the gullet to achieve normal maturity," meaning that it was of congenital origin.[271]

As early as 1953, Allison and Johnstone pointed out the relationship between a hiatal hernia, reflux esophagitis, and the columnar-lined esophagus, but they did not understand that the reflux esophagitis was responsible for the appearance of the columnar epithelium. Indeed, it was thought that the "gastric mucosa" in the esophagus contributed to the esophagitis. One of the seven patients reported by Allison and Johnstone had an adenocarcinoma in the glandular ("gastric") lining of the esophagus.[272]

Barrett's explanation of the presence of a columnar-lined lower esophagus held sway for the next 20 years, and a columnar-lined esophagus is still commonly known as a "Barrett's esophagus."

Allison accumulated extensive experience with peptic esophagitis, recognizing that there was incompetence of the esophagogastric sphincter mechanism resulting in reflux. However, he focused on the anatomical abnormality rather than on the physiologic one, and he concentrated on repairing the hiatal hernia. He did not recognize that this did not correct the reflux. By 1970, he still considered the columnar-lined esophagus to be a failure of complete development but did recognize that it was inclined to malignant degeneration.[273] Others began to suspect as early as 1960 that reflux esophagitis could be responsible for the presence of the columnar epithelium. Adler's outstanding studies published in 1963 gave great credibility to this explanation—one that was subsequently substantiated and is now widely held.[274,275] It was also at this time that Nissen described his operation, the fundoplication, which effectively prevented reflux esophagitis and has become the standard operation for this condition.[276]

ADENOCARCINOMA IN BARRETT'S ESOPHAGUS

Etiologic and Pathologic Considerations

Barrett's esophagus is emphasized because 59% to 86% of adenocarcinomas of the esophagus arise in a Barrett's esophagus. It is thus possible that common factors are involved in the causation of both lesions.[277] The constituents of the refluxed material that are responsible for the conversion of the squamous epithelium to columnar epithelium are not known. It is difficult to reproduce the lesion in experimental animals.[278] Because it has been observed in 9 of 17 patients who had total gastrectomy with esophagojejunostomy, the alkaline small bowel contents have been suspected in its pathogenesis.[279]

Several explanations exist for the replacement of the squamous cell lining by the glandular epithelium. Epithelial cells from the stomach may grow up into an esophagus denuded of its mucosa. Submucosal esophageal glands or the cardiac glands in the lamina propria may proliferate and cover the denuded luminal surface of the esophagus. The squamous cell epithelium may undergo metaplasia under the influence of the esophagitis, which is the generally accepted explanation. However, there is a possibility that the columnar-lined esophagus can be of congenital origin. Ransom and colleagues considered the extended form of Barrett's esophagus (extending to 30 cm or more from the incisors) to be of congenital origin and to have a greater predilection for malignant degeneration. This group made up half of the 34 patients whom they studied.[280]

The microscopic changes that characterize a Barrett's esophagus have been carefully studied by both light and electron microscopy and by immunohistochemical techniques.[281–283] The mucosa can assume one of three forms, and there is usually a mixture of them in any given patient. There is a predilection of the gastric type of epithelium to be located distally. This type of tissue resembles the mucosa seen in the fundus of the stomach and contains parietal and chief cells. It has an atrophic appearance, and the functional status of the acid and pepsinogen secreting cells is unclear. Located proximally in the columnar-lined esophagus is intestinal-type epithelium, with villae lined by columnar and goblet cells. The changes in this type of mucosa closely resemble the process of "intestinalization" that is seen in the stomach of patients with atrophic gastritis. Unlike normal intestinal absorptive cells, the columnar cells of this specialized epithelium contain glycoprotein secretory granules, usually lack brush borders, and do not absorb lipids. Paneth and neuroendocrine cells can also be found in this tissue. The third type of epithelial cells seen in a Barrett's esophagus is cardiac-type glands, which tend to be found between the gastric-type and the proximal intestinal-type cells.

Barrett's esophagus has been found in 8% to 20% of patients who undergo esophagoscopy for evaluation of esophagitis. The frequency rises to 44% if a stricture complicates the esophagitis.[275] The percentage of patients with Barrett's esophagus who subsequently develop adenocarcinoma ranges from 0 to 46.5%.[277] Very little is known about the factors responsible for the malignant degeneration of this tissue. However, the finding of a progression of changes from dysplasia to in situ neoplasia to invasive malignancy is consistent with a metaplasic process that accounts for the presence of the columnar epithelium in the esophagus. The component of the Barrett's mucosa most often associated with the malignancy is the intestinal-type tissue, which is characterized by large numbers of goblet cells. Detailed studies of the adenocarcinomas in Barrett's esophagus reveal many cell types, including keratin-producing cells.[44] These investigations support the theory that adenocarcinoma, like the Barrett's esophagus itself, is an example of multidirectional differentiation.

Other important features of the adenocarcinoma are multiple foci of malignancy. There could be genetic components to both the occurrence of Barrett's esophagus and the adenocarcinoma arising from it because these lesions are rarely seen in blacks, but squamous cell carcinoma is far more common in blacks than in whites.[268,275,277] Because cigarette smoking and alcohol ingestion are thought to be related to the cause of squamous cell carcinoma, investigators have looked for this relationship in patients with adenocarcinoma in a Barrett's esophagus. Some reports suggest such a relationship; others do not.[277]

Clinical Features

Patients with adenocarcinoma that developed in a Barrett's esophagus are usually white men in the fifth and sixth decades of life with histories of esophagitis, hiatal hernias, and strictures who often smoke and may have a heavy alcohol intake (see Fig. 24-19). The higher frequency of cancer of all cell types of the esophagus in men is well established. Skinner and colleagues found that the male–female ratio among patients with Barrett's esophagus was 2:1. When adenocarcinoma complicated the columnar-lined esophagus, the ratio increased to 9:1.[285] Patients with reflux esophagitis caused by scleroderma and those with reflux caused by cardiomyotomy for achalasia may also be at risk. Peptic ulcer disease and extraesophageal tumors are other conditions frequently associated with Barrett's esophagus.

FIG. 24-19. Esophagram showing a deep ulcer (*arrow*) and a stricture of the distal esophagus in a patient with a columnar-lined esophagus and in situ adenocarcinoma.

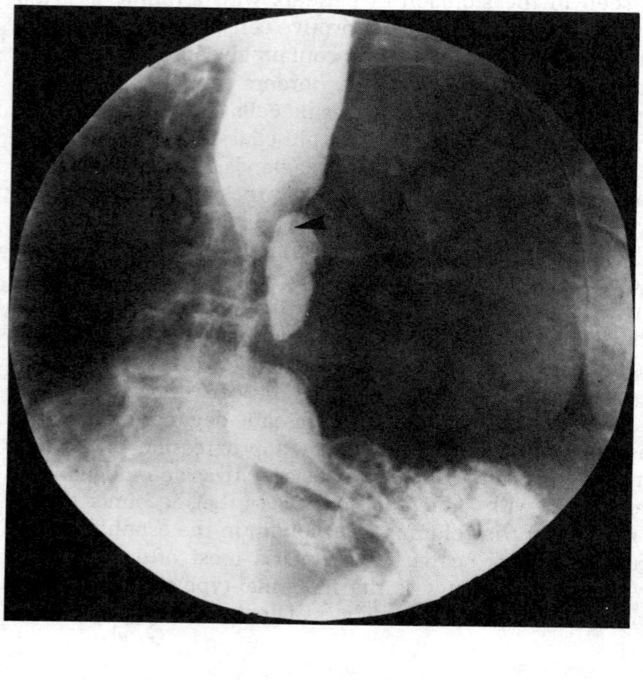

The absence of a history of Barrett's esophagus among patients found to have an adenocarcinoma in a columnar-lined esophagus is significant and underscores difficulty in recognizing the abnormally located epithelium in the esophagus. Its appearance on endoscopy is not strikingly different from that of squamous cell epithelium, and radiologic differentiation is unreliable. Pertechnetate scintigraphy has been recommended for the diagnosis of Barrett's esophagus, but this radionuclide will be concentrated by the columnar epithelium only if it is the gastric type.[286]

Barrett's mucosa may be granular with a salmon-pink color or have the velvety appearance of gastric mucosa. Biopsies must be taken to verify the diagnosis. Close surveillance of patients with reflux esophagitis and Barrett's esophagus may detect adenocarcinomas before they become extensive. Once adenocarcinomas cause symptoms, they are usually far advanced and have the same poor prognosis as squamous cell carcinomas.

Treatment

Patients with Barrett's esophagus who do not have dysplastic or neoplastic alterations in the columnar-lined esophagus may benefit from fundoplication, because some patients have experienced regression or stabilization of this process when the reflux of gastric contents was prevented.[285,287]

When patients show evidence of in situ or invasive malignancy in a Barrett's esophagus, esophagectomy followed by adjuvant chemotherapy of the type used for gastric adenocarcinoma is recommended.[277]

Dysplastic changes present within the Barrett's mucosa present a difficult therapeutic problem. It is difficult to recommend radical surgery under these circumstances, but evidence strongly indicates that dysplastic changes are the first stages of invasive carcinoma. This is especially true of "high-grade" dysplasia, which is considered a morphologic marker and precursor of adenocarcinoma.[275,288] Patients with this form of dysplasia are candidates for esophagectomy.[277,285]

The esophagectomy required is an extensive one, more extensive than can be performed using the Ivor Lewis approach. The columnar mucosa can extend quite high in the esophagus. By using an operation that places the esophagogastric or esophagocolic anastomosis in the neck, the sur-

TABLE 24-19. Staging of Adenocarcinoma Involving Barrett's Esophagus

Stage I
Carcinoma limited to the mucosa (including in situ carcinoma), not extending beyond the muscularis mucosa, with negative nodes
Stage II
Carcinoma limited to the esophageal wall but not extending to the adventitia, with negative nodes
Stage III
Any of the above with involved regional lymph nodes or full-thickness wall penetration of the tumor to the adventitia, without invasion of adjacent organs
Stage IV
Carcinoma invading adjacent organs or with distant metastases

geon can be more confident that all of the involved mucosa has been removed. A modification of the technique described by McKeown is recommended.[107]

The prognosis of patients with adenocarcinoma in a Barrett's esophagus depends on the pathologic stage of the tumor. The staging system proposed in Table 24-19 is similar to Duke's system of staging colon carcinoma and may more accurately predict the prognosis and progression than the TNM system. However, there have not been sufficient data available to prove this hypothesis.

PALLIATIVE THERAPY FOR CANCER OF THE ESOPHAGUS

RADIATION THERAPY

For patients not treated with a curative approach because of tumor extent, metastasis, or general medical condition, palliation of dysphagia and pain and the maintenance of a patent food passage are the goals of therapy. In some patients, this palliation is best achieved through surgery, but for many patients radiation continues to offer a reasonable expectation of symptom relief.[219] Dysphagia is relieved partially or completely in almost 80% of patients, resulting in stabilization or weight gain.[148,155,290] Simple anterior and posterior radiation fields can be used for the first 4000 cGy. If the patient is improving and tolerating treatment well, additional radiation may be administered through oblique or lateral fields that avoid the spinal cord. Fraction sizes are usually increased so that the overall time of treatment is kept to a minimum and the patient can spend the maximal time away from the hospital. Up to 5000 cGy have been delivered in 4 weeks of 250 cGy fractions.[126,134] In some cases, 400 cGy fractions have been used successfully.[291]

A significant percentage of patients whose symptoms are relieved by radiation will experience local tumor regrowth and a recurrence of their symptoms.[290] Pearson reported that 50% of irradiated patients will have a local recurrence, frequently within 6 months.[292] Beatty and colleagues studied 152 patients treated with "radical" radiation alone at The Princess Margaret Hospital.[126] Patients received at least 4000 cGy. Eighty-four percent of the patients had a shrinkage of their tumor. Only 28% (33% of responders) maintained their swallowing intact until death. Beatty also documented the high incidence of malignancy in esophageal strictures that were clinically judged to be benign. Of the 50 strictures that were diagnosed antemortem to be malignant, 24 were originally thought to be from "fibrosis," and 14 of these had an initial benign biopsy. Furthermore, autopsies on five patients who died with supposedly benign strictures revealed four who had tumor at the site of the stricture. These authors conclude that most benign strictures that do not resolve with dilation are related to persistent local tumor.

Wara and co-workers reported on a series of patients who received 5000 to 6000 cGy in 5.5 to 6.5 weeks.[155] The median survival was 7 months, whereas the median duration of palliation was only 3 months. Although 89% of patients had improvement in their dysphagia, most had recurrence of their symptoms.

TABLE 24-20. Palliative Procedures for Carcinoma of the Esophagus

Resect and reconstruct
Intrathoracic
Extrathoracic
Presternal
Retrosternal
Bypass
Intrathoracic
Extrathoracic
Presternal
Retrosternal
Colon
Stomach
Intraluminal intubation
Gastrostomy and cervical esophagogastrostomy with or without an external tube
Dilatation

These studies underscore the importance of proper identification of target volume and administration of an aggressive radiation dose even when palliation is the only goal. To deliver a low dose to an inadequate tumor volume may provide only temporary relief for a patient and may necessitate potentially hazardous surgery while the patient is in a reobstructed condition following radiation. In many respects, there is relatively little difference between the dose and field size that should be used for palliative or curative radiation. It may be worth taking an extra week or two to raise the radiation dose to a high level and taking an extra hour to plan the radiation with great care, even when the chances of cure are slim. Short-course, high-fraction radiotherapy should be reserved for patients whose life expectancy is extremely short because of metastatic disease or general physical condition.

SURGERY

The palliative operations available for patients with advanced carcinoma of the thoracic esophagus are outlined in Table 24-20 and have been reviewed by Orringer.[293]

A palliative esophagectomy should be performed only if the risk of morbidity and mortality are minimal and if at least a year of survival is reasonable. Patients who are not good candidates for palliative resection are those with the findings outlined in Table 24-21.

The rationale for esophageal resection to palliate esophageal cancer resides in the hope that the procedure can contribute to the patient's cure as well as palliation. If doubt

TABLE 24-21. Contraindications to Palliative Esophagectomy for Cancer of Thoracic Esophagus

Advanced inanition and debilitation
Inadequate cardiopulmonary function
Widespread (visceral) metastases
Malignant pleural effusion
Malignant ascites
Recurrent laryngeal, phrenic, or sympathetic nerve involvement
Superior vena cava obstruction
Tracheoesophageal fistula
Extension into the aortic wall or spinal column

exists about the removal of an esophageal lesion for cure, and the patient is judged to be a good surgical risk, the esophagus should be resected. The justification for this philosophy is twofold: occasionally, residual tumor may be successfully eliminated by radiotherapy and chemotherapy, and esophageal resection constitutes satisfactory palliative therapy. Payne said that "most efforts in the management of this condition [esophageal cancer] are palliative for most patients but not prejudicial to cure for the few.[294]

At the Mayo Clinic, more than 90% of patients undergoing resection had unobstructed swallowing throughout their subsequent survival.[294] Hankins and colleagues adapted a vigorous approach to palliation, a concept challenged by Orringer.[295,296]

The prognosis of patients with advanced esophageal cancer is so poor that the surgeon may question whether an undertaking of the magnitude of an esophageal resection is reasonable. When esophageal resection carries a prohibitive risk to the patient with concomitant cardiopulmonary disease or when resection cannot be performed because of technical reasons, a better palliative procedure is one that bypasses the malignant esophageal obstruction (Fig. 24-20).[297,298] Although this approach has had many advocates, more recent reports do not support bypass procedure as reasonable palliation because of the high mortality and morbidity that follow it, such as anastomotic leaks, mucocele formation, and infection in the excluded esophagus.[299–301] Orringer's patients with this operation had a postoperative mortality of 24%; 19% had anastomotic leaks, and 17% had disruptions of the divided distal thoracic esophagus, a condition that frequently leads to an intra-abdominal abscess.[299] Major postoperative complications occurred in 59% of his patients. The average survival time of those leaving the hospital was 5.9 months. Blunt transhiatal esophagectomy has become his palliative procedure of choice. Gastric bypass of the esophagus is reserved for the occasional patient with a tracheoesophageal fistula who is capable of withstanding this operation.

INTRALUMINAL INTUBATION

Intubation of the esophagus with a prosthetic tube has been used for many years to allow patients with malignant esophageal obstruction to swallow. This procedure is successful for 4 to 6 months in 40% to 85% of patients.[117,302]

Patients who are candidates for this procedure are those who have such advanced malignant obstruction of the esophagus that no other therapy is possible. These are patients who are very debilitated and who have tracheoesophageal fistulae or invasion of the trachea, bronchus, or aorta. Patients who have malignant strictures after a course of chemoradiation and are not candidates for operative palliation may also benefit from intraluminal esophageal tubes. Another category of patients who have received endoesophageal tubes are those whose obstructing cancers are treated with laser vaporization.[303]

Two types of tubes are used: pulsion or push-through tubes, which depend entirely on being pushed blindly

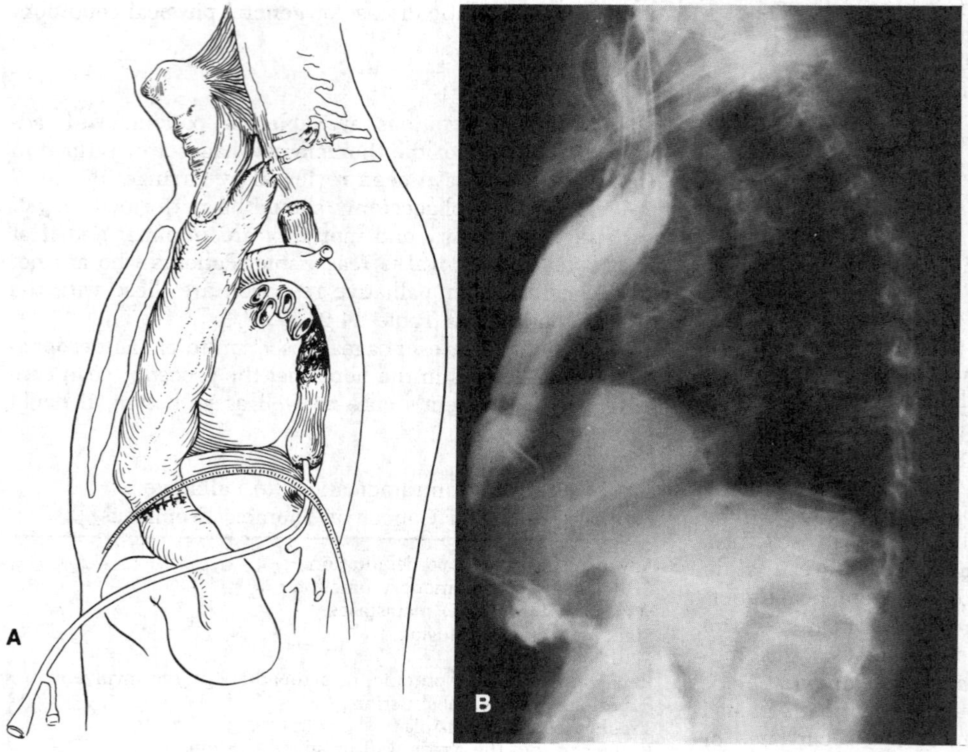

FIG. 24-20. **A.** The stomach is brought up behind the sternum and anastomosed to the esophagus. **B.** Radiographic appearance of a retrosternal gastric bypass.

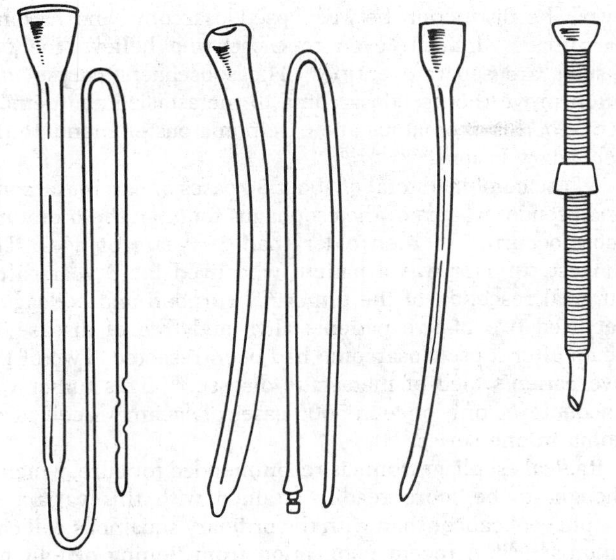

FIG. 24-21. Diagrammatic depiction of four commonly used intraluminal tubes.

through the area of obstruction, and traction tubes, which are pulled by a guide wire or string through the esophagus into the stomach. Pulsion tubes are usually limited to 10-cm segments and are best suited for middle-third and upper-third lesions. Traction tubes are best suited for middle-third or lower-third lesions. They are anchored to the stomach by a suture after being placed in proper position (Fig. 24-21). The use of introducers, such as the Nothingham introducer, and newer endoesophageal tubes, such as the Proctor-Livingston tube or Atkinson tube, has resulted in a preference for pulsion intubation over traction intubation and retrosternal gastric bypass for palliation of unresectable carcinoma of the esophagus.[304–306]

Endoesophageal tubes have several drawbacks as palliative procedures. A mortality of 10% to 40% accompanies placement of intraluminal tubes.[117,302] Perforation of the esophagus with mediastinitis may occur. Aspiration of gastric contents is frequent because the lower esophageal sphincter mechanism is blocked by the tube. Patients with this type of tube must be instructed to sleep with the head of the bed elevated. The tubes become dislodged and migrate in about 25% of patients; they also frequently become obstructed, and patients must be instructed to chew their food well or confine their diet to pureed foods.

Very often the malignant esophageal obstruction has to be dilated before an endoesophageal tube can pass through it.[307] Boyce has described his technique in detail.[308] The Eder-Peustow dilator is used for strictures that are very tight. When the lumen can take a 15-mm-dilator, Maloney bougies (tapered rubber tubes filled with mercury) are used. When a 15-mm dilator can be passed, the patient will no longer experience dysphagia. Dilatation with the mercury-filled bougies are continued daily or on alternate days for 1 week to 10 days, until the lumen of the esophagus will accept a 17-mm bougie. An endoesophageal tube can then be inserted and radiation given if indicated. Most patients (85%) can be maintained without a prosthesis by repeat dilatation. There was no increased incidence of perforation of the esophagus when radiation was combined with esophageal dilatation. During 5-years, 151 patients were treated by this technique with successful palliation in most of them.

Several precautions must be observed if dilatation of a malignant esophageal obstruction is to be used. The guide wire, as required with the Eder-Peustow dilator, should be passed under fluoroscopic control. Dilatation should not be carried out too rapidly. Physicians should never use more than three different-sized dilators during a single session. Patient discomfiture with this procedure is brief. Once the lumen is stretched to 17 mm, redilatation may be required no more than weekly or monthly. Intubation is necessary when dilatation cannot maintain a patent lumen for more than a day.

LASER THERAPY

Recently, endoscopic Nd:YAG and argon laser therapies have been used to reestablish esophageal continuity through malignant obstruction of the esophagus.[309–311] Fourteen patients were treated an average of five times to achieve luminal patency within a mean of 12 days.[309] Esophageal dilatation can be used after laser therapy. The mean survival was 14 weeks, but more than 75% of the patients could leave the hospital able to swallow. Nd:YAG laser equipment was used in this study, which employed an average of 4615 watt-seconds per treatment. Rather than using many treatments of lower energy to vaporize the tumor, some investigators advocate a single session of laser therapy to achieve luminal patency.[311] Complications of laser therapy are perforation of the esophagus, bleeding, and fistula formation. Occasionally, the lumen of the esophagus cannot be opened because of the distortion and twisting of the esophagus.

A tunable dye–argon laser system has been used in conjunction with the administration of sensitizing hematoporphyrin derivatives to destroy tumor tissue, using endoscopic techniques to deliver the light. This has been labeled photodynamic therapy and may be an additional modality of therapy available to patients with malignant obstruction of the esophagus.[310]

GASTROSTOMY AND CERVICAL ESOPHAGOSTOMY

The simplest palliative procedure is the creation of a gastrostomy to supply nutrition and a cervical esophagostomy to prevent aspiration of upper airway secretions or their passage into the tracheobronchial tree by a fistula to the esophagus. The cervical esophagostomy is of marginal benefit to the patient because there is a constant trickle of saliva through the esophagostomy that is difficult to collect. Personal hygiene and appearance are difficult to maintain. Eating or drinking is not possible with this form of palliation, unless a tube is fashioned to connect the cervical esophagostomy with the gastrostomy. Devices to accomplish this are not very effective.

OTHER CANCERS OF THE ESOPHAGUS

VARIANTS OF SQUAMOUS CELL CARCINOMAS OF THE ESOPHAGUS

Spindle Cell Carcinoma

This manifestation of squamous cell carcinoma is characterized histopathologically by spindle-shaped cells that resemble fibroblasts. It is a poorly differentiated squamous cell carcinoma that can be confused with a sarcoma. The spindle cells, however, have been studied by electron microscopy and have been shown to contain numerous tonofibrils and occasional well-developed desmosomes.[312] Desmosomes are characteristically found at the intercellular junction of epithelial cells. Tonofibrils radiate from them and contribute to the "stiffness" or cytoskeleton of this cell type. However, except for their large size and irregular shape, the spindle cells also resemble actively synthesizing fibroblasts and are closely associated with collagen fibrils. Battifora believes that the spindle cells originate from mesenchymal metaplasia of squamous cells and that collagen is produced by these metaplastic cells.[312] Similar tumors in the skin have shown a gradual transition of the spindle cells to typical squamous cells. This view has received support from others.[313]

Pseudosarcoma and Carcinosarcoma

Several observers argue that these two designations refer to the same lesion and should be referred to as polypoid carcinomas of the esophagus.[270,314,315] They both have the gross appearance of a polypoid lesion. Adenocarcinomas, inflammatory granulomas, smooth muscle tumors, and melanomas may also present as polypoid lesions.

In the case of pseudosarcomas or carcinosarcomas, the barium esophagram will usually reveal a large polypoid mass in the middle or lower third of the esophagus. The esophagus is usually distended at the site of the tumor, but the degree of esophageal obstruction is considerably less than one would expect from the size of the mass.

Histopathologically, they appear to be spindle cell carcinomas, which present a varying picture—from nests of squamous cells (which may or may not appear malignant) in a spindle cell stroma (referred to as pseudosarcoma) to an intimate mixture of carcinomatous- and sarcomatous-appearing cells growing together as a single tumor (carcinosarcoma). Although it is convincingly argued that these malignancies most likely arise from two different cell lines, carcinomatous and sarcomatous, that commingle, we regard them as highly undifferentiated squamous cell carcinomas of the spindle-cell type.[270]

Most carcinosarcomas do not invade very deeply into the underlying tissue. The carcinomatous elements are limited and may be found only at the base of the polypoid mass. Metastases from these tumors are usually sarcomatous in appearance.

According to authors who made a distinction between carcinosarcomas and pseudosarcomas, the latter differ from the former in that the seemingly sarcomatous tissue is considered nonmalignant because metastases do not occur. However, the distinction between pseudosarcoma and carcinosarcoma is difficult, even to those who believe the two lesions are separate entities. The subsequent course may often prove the pseudosarcoma to metastasize and demonstrate both sarcomatous and carcinomatous elements in the secondary lesions.[270,314,315]

Of the combined total of about 80 cases of carcinosarcoma and pseudosarcoma of the esophagus found in the literature, most occurred in men older than 50 years of ages. The longest survivor was a patient who lived for 6 years after surgical resection of the tumor.[270] Turnbull and colleagues reported two of five patients alive and free of disease 10 years after a pseudosarcoma had been resected. Two of the five patients died of metastatic disease.[267] This tumor was encountered only once in 5000 cases of squamous cell carcinoma in one series.[316]

Radical esophagectomy is recommended for cure, which is thought to be more readily attained with this variant of esophageal cancer than with the ordinary squamous cell carcinoma[317,318] A recent publication from Beijing of four patients with carcinosarcoma reported them all well 3 to 19 years after radical excision and esophagogastrostomy.[319]

Verrucous and Varicoid Carcinomas of the Esophagus

Verrucous and varicoid lesions are variants of fungating squamous cell carcinomas.[270,320] They may be confused with esophageal varices when an esophagram is obtained, which is their distinguishing feature. This lesion may also be confused with benign squamous cell papillomas of the esophagus.

ADENOID-CYSTIC CARCINOMA (CYLINDROMA)

Adenoid-optic carcinomas or cylindromas show histologic features that are identical with those found in the salivary glands, but they act more aggressively and have a poorer prognosis than do the relatively indolent salivary gland cylindromas.[270] Epstein and colleagues studied six cases of esophageal adenoid-cystic carcinomas and concluded that they were distinct morphologically and clinically from the adenoid-cystic carcinomas of salivary gland origin.[321] These tumors have the typical cystic or cribriform configuration of the tumor cells with some areas of solid or basaloid patterns. In the esophagus, the basaloid pattern predominates; the cells are more pleomorphic, and the overlying squamous mucosa contains focal areas of dysplasia and in situ carcinoma.

Based on a review of the 29 patients with this lesion who were reported in the literature before 1984, Epstein and colleagues found that 76% of the tumors occur in men during their sixth decade, in contrast to the salivary gland cylindromas, which predominate in women in the fourth and fifth decades of life.[321] The cancer's aggressive behavior is reflected in the 9-month median survival after diagnosis. It has been suggested that these lesions should be resected as is done for squamous cell carcinoma of the esophagus.[322] Recently, a combination of radiation therapy and cisplatin, cyclophosphamide, vincristine, and doxorubicin produced a complete response in a patient with metastases to the lung from an esophageal adenoid-cystic carcinoma. The 44 cases culled from the literature before 1986 confirmed the poor prognosis of these cancers, and further exploration of this combination chemotherapy has merit.[323]

MUCOEPIDERMOID CARCINOMA (ADENOCANTHOMA)

A mucoepidermoid carcinoma is an adenocarcinoma that contains squamous elements. The relative proportion of the two components varies both within and among these cancers. Ming suggests that when the tumor is a well-differentiated adenocarcinoma, some cells undergo squamous metaplasia and are surrounded by the unaffected glandular cells.[270] These lesions are typically referred to as adenocanthomas. They may arise from aberrant gastric epithelium; however, there are mucoepidermoid cancers of the esophagus that are thought to arise from the deep mucus glands of the esophagus. They are similar to those found in the salivary glands. In 1978, Woodard and colleagues collected only eight cases of this esophageal lesion, attesting to its rarity.[324]

Esophageal mucoepidermoid carcinomas are characterized by small groups of mucus cells scattered among large groups of squamous cells. These are very aggressive malignancies and are most often found at the lower end of the esophagus, although the tumor reported by Turnbull and co-workers was located in the upper thoracic esophagus.[267] Resection failed to cure this patient, and the poor prognosis was similar to that in patients with mucoepidermoid cancers arising from the bronchial glands.

CANCERS OF NEUROENDOCRINE ORIGIN

Primary Oat Cell Carcinoma

Various names are given to this cancer, which is similar in appearance and behavior to its counterpart in the lung. It is also referred to as a small cell carcinoma, a small cell undifferentiated carcinoma, or an apudoma (amine precursor uptake and decarboxylation tumor). A total of 88 cases of this lesion were recently collected from the literature.[325]

The tumors are thought to be of neuroectodermal origin because most investigators find them to be argyrophilic and on electron microscopy the cells contain neurosecretory granules.[326] Immunohistochemical studies have also revealed the presence of ACTH and calcitonin within some of the tumors that have been studied for their capacity to synthesize polypeptide hormones.[327] Evidence of Cushing's disease was not present in the patient found to have ACTH in the tumor. However, other patients have been reported with paraneoplastic syndromes, such as inappropriate antidiuretic hormone secretion and hypercalcemia.[328]

Because these tumors occasionally also have areas of squamous cell carcinoma within them, and even less often adenocarcinomatous elements, earlier authors had doubts about the origin of this malignancy. The accumulated evidence, however, leaves little doubt that it is of neuroectodermal origin.[329]

Like squamous cell carcinomas, most oat cell carcinomas are equally located in the middle and lower thirds of the esophagus. Men are more frequently affected than women (3:2) and the tumor is most common in the 50- to 70-year-old group.[325,328]

All of the patients with oat cell carcinoma of the esophagus have a very poor prognosis. All have died of disseminated disease. Overall survival is 4 to 5 months; the longest was 24 months.[325] Treatment has consisted of resection, radiation, and chemotherapy.[325,326,330] Combination chemotherapy used for patients with oat cell cancer of the lung has provided dramatic, albeit temporary, responses[330,331]

Carcinoid Tumors

Further evidence of the neuroendocrine basis of oat cell cancers is the rare carcinoid tumor, which is presumed to arise from the same cell type but which is a far less aggressive tumor. Resection of the esophagus is effective therapy.[332,333]

PRIMARY MALIGNANT MELANOMAS

Malignant melanomas are derived from neural crest tissue, as are apudomas and carcinoids. A review of the world literature revealed 110 patients with this infrequently encountered lesion of the esophagus.[334] The tumor is often polypoid and lymphatic and hematologic metastases are common, resulting in a 5-year survival rate of 4%. Resection is recommended and has resulted in a 10-year survival in one patient. Average survival, however, is only 13.4 months. Patients with secondary esophageal melanoma outnumber the patients with primary melanoma of the esophagus.

ESOPHAGEAL SARCOMAS

Leiomyosarcoma

This is the most common malignant nonepithelial tumor in the esophagus. Nonetheless, Choh and colleagues could find only 44 patients in the English literature with leiomyosarcoma of the esophagus.[335] Well-differentiated polypoid lesions respond best to surgical therapy. Radical excision may not be necessary in these extreme instances. Overall, the prognosis of patients with this rare cancer is poor, but resection has resulted in several 5-year survivors.

Rhabdomyosarcoma

These sarcomas, derived from striated muscle, are extremely rare. Resection can result in long-term survival.[336] Occasionally a granular cell myoblastoma may exhibit malignant characteristics.

CHORIOCARCINOMA

Three cases of choriocarcinoma of the esophagus were summarized in 1979.[337] The diagnosis was easily made by brush biopsy because the characteristic cytotrophoblastic and syncytotrophoblastic cells can be readily identified.

PRIMARY LYMPHOMA

Non-Hodgkin's and Hodgkin's lymphoma arising in the esophagus have been reported.[337-339] The radiographic appearance is characterized by a diffuse nodularity as a result of lymphomatous infiltration of the mucosa. This tumor is being seen increasingly in immunocompromised patients.[340]

METASTASES TO THE ESOPHAGUS

The esophagus is not a frequent site of metastatic disease. As indicated above, metastatic melanomas involve the esophagus more frequently than do primary melanomas. Lymphoma involving the esophagus as part of diffuse disseminated disease has also been reported. Direct extension from a tumor or its nodal involvement is responsible for 80% of the involvement of the esophagus by a malignancy arising in another organ.[341] Microscopic foci of tumor are seen at autopsy in 3% to 4% of patients dying of cancer and in 9% of women dying of breast cancer.[342,343] The relative frequency of involvement of the esophagus by metastatic breast cancer has resulted in recognition of the syndrome of postmastectomy dysphagia.[344,345] Fifty-eight cases of esophageal involvement in the course of breast cancer have been reported in the literature. Radiotherapy and chemotherapy may be beneficial in these instances.[345] Because the lesion often causes dysphagia by extrinsic compression, care must be taken during esophagoscopy that the esophagus is not perforated.[344] Biopsy by exploration of the neck or posterior mediastinum or by needle aspiration using CT can provide tissue for a definitive diagnosis. These lesions can mimic primary esophageal cancers. Other sites of cancer that have been reported to give rise to metastases to the esophagus are the kidneys, pancreas, cervix, and bladder.[343]

REFERENCES

1. Huang GJ, Wu YK: Carcinoma of the Esophagus and Gastric Cardia. New York, Springer-Verlag, 1984
2. Long ER: A History of Pathology. Baltimore, Williams & Wilkins, 1928
3. Wangensteen OH, Wangensteen SD: The Rise of Surgery: From Emperic Craft to Scientific Discipline. Minneapolis, University of Minnesota Press, 1978
4. Wangensteen OH: Cancer of the Esophagus and Stomach, 2nd ed. New York, American Cancer Society, 1956
5. Torek F: The first successful case of resection of the thoracic portion of the esophagus for carcinoma. Surg Gynecol Obstet 16:614, 1913
6. Kirschner H: Ein Neues Verfahren der Oesophagsplastik. Arch Klin Chir 114:606, 1920
7. Ohsawa T: The surgery of the esophagus. Arch Jpn Chir 10:605, 1933
8. Adams WE, Phemister DB: Carcinoma of the lower thoracic esophagus. Report of successful resection and esophagogastrostomy. J Thorac Surg 7:621, 1939
9. delRegato JA, Spjut HJ: Cancer: Diagnosis, Treatment and Prognosis, 5th ed. St. Louis, CV Mosby, 1977
10. Nielsen J: Clinical results with radiation therapy in cancer of the esophagus. Acta Radiol 26:361, 1945
11. Ota K, Shin LH: Histological typing of gastric and oesophageal tumors. Geneva, World Health Organization, 1977
12. Seremetic MG, Lyons WS, deGuzman VC et al: Leiomyomata of the esophagus: An Analysis of 838 cases. Cancer 38:2166, 1976
13. National Cancer Institutes: 1986 Annual Cancer Statistics Review. Division of Cancer Prevention and Control, NIH Publication No. 87-2889, Bethesda, MD, 1987
14. Cutler SJ, Devesa SS: Trends in cancer incidence and mortality in the USA. In Doll R, Vodopija I (eds): Host Environment Interactions in the Etiology of Cancer in Man. Lyon, France, World Health Organization International Agency for Research Cancer, 1973
15. Wu YK, Huang GJ, Shao LF et al: Progress in the study and surgical treatment of cancer of the esophagus in China, 1940–1980. J Thorac Cardiovasc Surg 84:325, 1982
16. Rose EF: A review of factors associated with cancer of the esophagus in Transkei. Prog Clin Biol Res 53:67–75, 1981
17. McGlashan ND: Oesophageal cancer and alcoholic spirits in central Africa. Gut 10:643, 1969
18. Kmet J, Mahboubi E: Esophageal cancer in the Caspian littoral of Iran: Initial studies. Science 175:846, 1972
19. Auerbach O, Stout AD, Hammond EC et al: Histologic changes in esophagus in relation to smoking habits. Arch Environ Health 11:4, 1965
20. Schoenberg BC, Bailar JC, Fraumeni JF: Certain mortality patterns of esophageal cancer in the United States, 1930–67. J Natl Cancer Inst 46:63, 1971
21. Potten LM, Morris LE, Blot WJ et al: Esophageal cancer among black men in Washington DC: I. Alcohol, tobacco and other risk factors. JNCI 67:777, 1981
22. Ziegler RG, Morris LE, Blot WJ et al: Esophageal cancer among black men in Washington DC: II. Role of nutrition. JNCI 67:1199, 1981
23. Rogers EL, Goldkind L, Goldkind SF: Increasing frequency of esophageal cancer among black male veterans. Cancer 49:610, 1982
24. Mettlin C: Nutritional habits of blacks and whites. Prev Med 9:601, 1980
25. vanRensburg SF: Epidemiologic and dietary evidence for a specific nutritional predisposition to esophageal cancer. JNCI 67:243, 1981
26. Munoz N, Crespi M, Grassi A et al: Precursor lesions of esophageal cancer in high-risk populations in Iran and China. Lancet 1:876, 1982
27. O'Neill C, Rani Q, Clarke G et al: Silica fragments from millet bran in mucosa surrounding oesophageal tumors in patients in northern China. Lancet 1:1202, 1982
28. Harper PS, Harper RMJ, Howel-Evans AW: Carcinoma of the oesophagus with tylosis. Q J Med 34:317, 1970
29. Lortat-Jacob JL, Richard CA, Fekete F et al: Cardiospasm and esophageal carcinoma: Report of 24 cases. Surgery 66:969, 1969
30. Just-Viera GO, Haight C: Achalasia and carcinoma of the esophagus. Surg Gynecol Obstet 128:1081, 1969
31. Rock LA, Latham PS, Hankins JR et al: Achalasia associated with squamous cell carcinoma of the esophagus: A case report. Am J Gastroenterol 80:526, 1985
32. Sigurgeirsson B, Johannson KB, Haroarson S et al: Acute thoracic inlet obstruction in achalasia with adenoid cystic and squamous cell carcinoma. Ann Thorac Surg 40:516, 1985
33. Joske RA, Benedict EB: The role of benign esophageal obstruction in the development of carcinoma of the esophagus. Gastroenterology 36:749, 1959
34. Hankins J Jr, McLaughlin JS: The association of carcinoma of the esophagus with achalasia. J Thorac Cardiovasc Surg 69:355, 1975
35. Lamb RK, Edwards CH, Pattison CW et al: Squamous carcinoma in situ of the esophagus in a patient with achalasia. Thorax 40:795, 1985
36. Wychulis AR, Woolam GL, Andersen HA et al: Achalasia and carcinoma of the esophagus. JAMA 215:1638, 1971
37. McGregor DH, Mills G, Boudet RA: Intramural squamous cell carcinoma of the esophagus. Cancer 37:1556, 1976
38. Huang B, Unni KK, Payne WS: Long-term survival following diverticulectomy for cancer in pharyngoesophageal (Zenker's) diverticulum. Ann Thorac Surg 38:207, 1984
39. Hopkins RA, Postlethwaite RW: Caustic burns and carcinoma of the esophagus. Ann Surg 194:146, 1981
40. Appelquist R, Salmo M: Lye corrosion carcinoma of the esophagus: A review of 63 cases. Cancer 45:2655, 1980
41. Ahlbom HE: Simple achlorhydric anaemia, Plummer-Vinson syndrome, and carcinoma of the mouth, pharynx and oesophagus in women: Observations at Radiumhemmet, Stockholm. Br Med J 2:331, 1936
42. Entwistle CC, Jacobs A: Histological findings in the Paterson-Kelly syndrome. J Clin Pathol 18:408, 1965
43. American Joint Committee for Cancer Staging and End-Results Reporting: Manual for Staging of Cancer. Chicago, American Joint Committee for Cancer Staging and End-Results Reporting, 1978
44. Japanese Society for Esophageal Diseases: Guidelines for the clinical and pathologic studies on carcinoma of the esophagus. Jpn J Surg 6:69, 1976
45. Younghusband JD, Aluwihare APR: Carcinoma of the oesophagus: Factors influencing survival. Br J Surg 57:442, 1970
46. Shapiro AL, Robillard GL: The esophageal arteries. Ann Surg 131:171, 1950
47. Haagenson CD, Feind CR, Herter FP et al: The Lymphatics in Cancer. Philadelphia, WB Saunders, 1972
48. Sarrazin R, Voilin C, Bade B et al: L'anatomie du drainage lymphatique de l'oesophage et so lymphologie sont encore mal connues. In Giuli R: Les Cancers de l'Oesophage en 1984: 135 Questions. Malonie SA, 1984
49. Guernsey JM, Knudsen DF: Abdominal exploration in the evaluation of patients with carcinoma of the thoracic esophagus. J Thorac Cardiovasc Surg 59:62, 1970
50. Watson WL, Goodner JT, Miller TP et al: Torek esophagectomy: The case against segmental resection for esophageal cancer. J Thorac Cardiovasc Surg 32:347, 1956
51. Stephens RL, Hansen HH, Muggia Fm: Hypercalcemia in epidermoid tumors of the head and neck and esophagus. Cancer 31:1487, 1973
52. Lohrenz FN, Custer GS: ACTH-producing metastases from carcinoma of the esophagus. Ann Intern Med 62:1017, 1965
53. Kobayashi S, Kasugai T: Brushing cytology for the diagnosis of gastric cancer involving the cardia of the lower esophagus. Acta Cytol 22:155, 1978
54. Winaiwer SJ, Sherlock P, Belladonna JA et al: Endoscopic brush cytology in esophageal cancer. JAMA 232:1358, 1975
55. Graham DY, Schwartz JT, Cain GD et al: Prospective evaluation of biopsy number in the diagnosis of esophageal and gastric carcinoma. Gastroenterology 81:228, 1982

56. Skinner DB, Dowlatshaki K, Delmeester TR: Potentially curable cancer of he esophagus. Cancer 50:2571, 1982
57. Moss AA, Koehler RE, Margulis AR: Initial accuracy of esophagograms in detection of small esophageal carcinoma. Am J Roentgenol 127:909, 1976
58. Putnam CE, Curtis AM, Westfried M et al: Thickening of the posterior tracheal strip: A sign of squamous cell carcinoma of the esophagus. Radiology 121:533, 1976
59. Murata Y, Muroi M, Yoshida M et al: Endoscopic ultrasonography in the diagnosis of esophageal carcinoma. Surg Endosc 1:11, 1986
60. Heyder N: Endoscopic ultrasonography of tumors of the esophagus and stomach. Surg Endosc 1:17, 1986
61. Halvorsen RA, Thompson W: Computed tomographic evaluation of esophageal carcinoma. Semin Oncol 11:1013, 1984
62. Moss AA, Schnyder P, Thoeni RF et al: Esophageal carcinoma: pre-therapy staging by computed tomography. AJR 136:1051, 1981
63. Lea JW, Prager RL, Bender H: The questionable role of computed tomography in preoperative staging of esophageal cancer. Ann Thorac Surg 38:479, 1984
64. Picus D, Balfe DM, Koehler R et al: Computed tomography in staging esophageal carcinoma. Radiology 146:433, 1983
65. Lichter AS, Fraass BA, van de Geijn J et al: An overview of clinical requirements and clinical utility of computed tomography based radiotherapy treatment planning. In Ling C, Rogers C, Morton R (eds): Computed Tomography in Radiation Therapy, p 1–22. New York, Raven Press, 1983
66. Quint LE, Glazer L, Orringer MB: Esophageal imaging by MR and CT: Study of normal anatomy and neoplasms. Radiology 156:727, 1985
67. Clinical staging system for carcinoma of the esophagus. CA 25:50, 1975
68. Guanrei Y, He H, Sunghong Q et al: Endoscopic diagnosis of 115 cases of early esophageal carcinoma. Endoscopy 14:157, 1982
69. Takagi I, Karasawa K: Growth of squamous cell esophageal carcinoma observed by serial esophagographies. J Surg Oncol 21:57, 1982
70. Merendino KA, Merk VJ: An analysis of 100 cases of squamous cell carcinoma: II. With special reference to its theoretical curability. Surg Gynec Obstet 94:110, 1952
71. Clayton ES: Carcinoma of the esophagus. Surg Gynecol Obstet 46:52, 1928
72. Mantravadi R, Lad T, Briele H et al: Carcinoma of the esophagus: Sites of failure. Int J Radiat Oncol Biol Phys 8:1897, 1982
73. Mandard AM, Chasle J, Marnay J et al: Autopsy findings in 111 cases of esophageal cancer. Cancer 48:329, 1981
74. Arbitol A, Straus M, Franklin G et al: Infusional chemotherapy and cyclic chemotherapy inoperable esophageal and gastric cardia carcinoma. Am J Clin Oncol 6:195, 1983
75. Anderson L, Lad T: Autopsy findings in squamous cell carcinoma of the esophagus. Cancer 50:1587, 1982
76. Attah E, Hadju S: Benign and malignant tumors of the esophagus at autopsy. J Thorac Cardiovasc Surg 55:396, 1980
77. Bosch A, Frias Z, Caldwell W et al: Autopsy findings in carcinoma of the esophagus. Acta Radiol Oncol 18:103, 1979
78. Cahan WG: Multiple primary cancers of the lung, esophagus and other sites. Cancer 40:1954, 1977
79. Goldstein HM, Zornoza J: Association of squamous cell carcinoma of the head and neck with cancer of the esophagus. Am J Roentgenol 131:791, 1978
80. Shibuya H, Tahogi M, Horiuchi J, et al: Carcinomas of the esophagus with synchronous or metachronous primary carcinoma in other organs. Acta Radiol Oncol 21:39, 1982
81. Shons AR, McQuarrie DG: Multiple primary epidermoid carcinomas of the upper aerodigestive tract. Arch Surg 120:1007, 1985
82. Burdette WJ: Palliative operation for carcinoma of cervical and thoracic esophagus. Ann Surg 173:714, 1971
83a. Earlam R, Cunha-Melo JR: Oesophageal squamous cell carcinoma: I. A critical review of surgery. Br J Surg 67:381, 1980
83b. Earlam R, Cunha-Melo JR: Oesophageal squamous cell carcinoma: II. A critical review of radiotherapy. Br J Surg 67:457, 1980
84. Daly JM, Massar E, Giacco G et al: Parenteral nutrition in esophageal cancer patients. Ann Surg 196:203, 1982
85. Haffejee AA, Angorn IB: Nutritional status and the nonspecific cellular and humoral immune response in esophageal carcinoma. Ann Surg 189:475, 1979
86. Brister SJ, Chin RCJ, Brown RA et al: Clinical impact of intravenous hyperalimentation on esophageal carcinoma: Is it worthwhile? Ann Thorac Surg 38:617, 1984
87. Pedersen H, Hansen HS, Cederquist C et al: The prognostic significance of weight loss and its integration in stagegrouping of oesophageal cancer. Acta Chir Scand 148:363, 1982
88. Burt ME, Gorschboth CM, Brennan MF: A controlled prospective randomized trial evaluating the metabolic effects of enteral and parenteral nutrition in the cancer patient. Cancer 49:1092, 1982
89. Finlay IG, Wright PA, Menzies T et al: Microbial flora in carcinoma of oesophagus. Thorax 37:181, 1982
90. Ong GB, Lam KH, Wong J et al: Factors influencing morbidity and mortality in esophageal carcinoma. J Thorac Cardiovasc Surg 76:745, 1978
91. Cedarquist C, Nielsen J, Berthelsen A et al: Cancer of the esophagus. II. Therapy and outcome. Acta Chir Scand 144:233, 1978
92. Scanlon EF, Morton DR, Walker JM et al: The case against segmental resection for esophageal carcinoma. Surg Gynecol Obstet 101:290, 1955
93. Wu Y, Chen P, Fang J et al: Surgical treatment of esophageal carcinoma. Am J Surg 139:805, 1980
94. Maillet P, Baulieux J, Boulez J et al: Carcinoma of the thoracic esophagus: Results of one-stage surgery (271 cases). Am J Surg 143:629, 1982
95. Skinner DB: En bloc resection for neoplasms of the esophagus and cardia. J Thorac Cardiovasc Surg 85:59, 1983
96. Lewis I: The surgical treatment of carcinoma of the esophagus. With special reference to a new operation for growths of the middle third. Br J Surg 34:18, 1946
97. Carey JS, Plested WG, Hughes RK: Esophagogastrectomy: Superiority of the combined abdominal-right thoracic approach (Lewis operation). Ann Thorac Surg 14:59, 1972
98. Kirk RM: Palliative resection of esophageal carcinoma without formal thoractomy. Br J Surg 61:689, 1974
99. Orringer MB, Sloan H: Esophagectomy without thoractomy. J Thorac Cardiovasc Surg 76:643, 1978
100. Szentpetery S, Wolfgang T, Lower R: Pull-through esophagectomy without thoractomy for esophageal carcinoma. Ann Thorac Surg 27:399, 1979
101. Stewart JR, Starr MG, Sharp KW, et al: Transhiatal (blunt) esophagectomy for malignant and benign esophageal disease: Clinical experience and technique. Ann Thorac Surg 40:343, 1985
102. Hankins JR, Miller JE, Attar S et al: Transhiatal esophagectomy for carcinoma of the esophagus: Experience with 26 patients. Ann Thorac Surg 44:123, 1987
103. Postlethwait RW: Esophagectomy without thoractomy. Ann Thorac Surg 27:395, 1979
104. Shakian DM, Neptune WB, Ellis FH et al: Transthoracic versus extrathoracic esophagectomy: Mortality, morbidity and long-term survival. Ann Thorac Surg 41:237, 1986
105. Steiger Z, Wilson RF: Comparison of the results of esophagectomy with and without a thoractomy. Surg Gynecol Obstet 153:653, 1981
106. Fisher RD, Brawley RK, Kieffer RF: Esophagectomy in the treatment of carcinoma of the distal two-thirds of the esophagus. Ann Thorac Surg 14:658, 1972
107. McKeown KC: Total three-stage oesophagectomy for cancer of the esophagus. Br J Surg 63:259, 1976
108. Steichen FM, Ravitch MM: Mechanical sutures in esophageal surgery. Ann Surg 191:373, 1980
109. Wong J: Stapled esophagogastric anastomosis in the apex of the right chest after subtotal esophagectomy for carcinoma. Surg Gynecol Obstet 164:569, 1987
110. Pearson FG, Henderson RD, Parrish RM: An operative technique for the control of reflux following esophagogastrostomy. J Thorac Cardiovasc Surg 58:668, 1969
111. Ward AS, Collis JL: Late results of oesophageal and oesophagogastric resection in the treatment of oesophageal cancer. Thorax 26:1, 1971
112. Cheung HC, Siu KF, Wong J: Is pyloroplasty necessary in esophageal replacement by stomach? A prospective, randomized controlled trial. Surgery 102:19, 1987
113. Wilkins EW, Burke JF: Colon esophageal bypass. Am J Surg 129:394, 1975
114. Postlethwait RW: Colonic interposition for esophageal substitution. Surg Gynecol Obstet 156:377, 1983
115. Postlethwait RW: Technique for isoperistaltic gastric tube for esophageal bypass. Ann Surg 189:673, 1979
116. Griffen WO, Daugherty ME, McGee EM et al: Unified approach to carcinoma of the esophagus. Am Surg 183:511, 1976
117. Cukingman RA, Carey JS: Carcinoma of the esophagus. Ann Thorac Surg 26:274, 1978
118. Mannell A: Carcinoma of the esophagus. Curr Probl Surg 19:554, 1982
119. Morstyn G, Thomas RJ, Mullerworth M et al: Improved survival in esophageal cancer in the period 1978 to 1983. J Clin Oncol 4:1062, 1986
120. Wilson SE, Stone R, Scully M et al: Modern management of anastomotic leak after esophagogastrectomy. Am J Surg 144:95, 1982
121. Isono K, Onoda S, Ishikawa T et al: Studies on the causes of deaths from esophageal carcinoma. Cancer 49:2173, 1982
122. Postlethwait RW: Complications and deaths after operation for esophageal carcinoma. J Thorac Cardiovasc Surg 85:827, 1983
123. Giuli R, Sancho-Garnier H: Diagnostic, therapeutic, and prognostic features of cancers of the esophagus: Results of the international prospective study conducted by the OESO group (790 patients). Surgery 99:614, 1986
124. Hussey DH, Barkley HT Jr, Bloedorn FG: Carcinoma of the esophagus. In Fletcher GH (ed): Textbook of Radiotherapy. pp 688–703. Philadelphia, Lea & Febiger, 1980
125. Levine MS, Langer J, Laufer I et al: Radiation therapy of esophageal carcinoma: Correlation of clinical and radiographic findings. Gastrointest Radiol 12:99, 1987
126. Beatty JD, DoBoer G, Rider WD: Carcinoma of the esophagus—pretreatment assessment, correlation of radiation treatment parameters with survival and identification and management of radiation treatment failure. Cancer 43:2254, 1979
127. Morita K, Takagi I, Watanabe M et al: Relationship between the radiologic features of esophageal cancer and the local control by radiation therapy. Cancer 55:2668, 1985
128. Hishikaw Y, Kamikonya N, Tanaka S et al: A multiple regression analysis for predicting local control of esophageal carcinoma treated by intracavitary irradiation. Radiat Med (Suppl 3)4:97, 1986
129. Smoron GL, O'Brien CA, Sullivan CA: Tumor localization and treatment technique for cancer of the esophagus. Radiology 111:735, 1974
130. Lewinsky BS, Annes GP, Mann SG et al: Carcinoma of the esophagus: An analysis of results and of treatment techniques. Radiol Clin North Am 44:192, 1975
131. Vijayakumar S, Muller-Runkel R: Irradiation of the thoracic esophagus: Prone versus supine treatment positions. Acta Radiol Oncol 25:187, 1986
132. Kagan AR, Wollin M, Rao AR et al: Treatment planning of esophagus, stomach, rectum and pancreas. Front Radiat Ther Oncol 21:236, 1987
133. Miller C: Carcinoma of the thoracic oesophagus and cardia. Br J Surg 49:507, 1962

134. Pearson JG: The present status and future potential of radiotherapy in the management of esophageal cancer. Cancer 39:882, 1977
135. McKenna WG, Yeakel K, Klink A et al: Is correction for lung density in radiotherapy treatment planning necessary? Int J Radiat Oncol Biol Phys 13:273, 1987
136. McShan DL, Fraass BA, Lichter AS: Treatment plan verification using portal images and beam's eye view treatment planning. Int J Radiat Biol Phys (in press)
137. Fraass BA, McShan DL, Weeks KJ: 3-D treatment planning: III. Complete beam's eye view planning capabilities. In Bruinvis IAD (ed): The Use of Computers in Radiation Therapy, pp 193–196. Amsterdam, Elsevier North-Holland, 1987
138. Bruso C, Perez-Tamayo C, McShan D et al: Results of beam's eye view treatment planning for esophageal carcinomas (abstr). Int J Radiat Oncol Biol Phys (Suppl 1) 13:195, 1987
139. Akiyama H, Tsurumaru M, Kawamara T et al: Principles of surgical treatment for carcinoma of the esophagus. Analysis of lymph node involvement. Ann Surg 194:438, 1981
140. Richmond J, Seydel HG, Bae Y et al: Comparison of three treatment strategies for esophageal cancer within a single institution. Int J Radiat Oncol Biol Phys 13:1617, 1987
141. Fisher SA, Brady LW: Carcinoma of the esophagus. In Perez CA, Brady LW (eds): Principles and Practice of Radiation Oncology, pp 700–722. Philadelphia, JB Lippincott, 1987
142. Fletcher DH: Clinical dose-response curves of human malignant epithelial tumors. Br J Radiol 46:1, 1973
143. Fajardo LF: Pathology of Radiation Injury, pp 50–53. New York, Masson, 1982
144. Seaman WB, Ackerman LV: The effect of radiation on the esophagus. Radiology 68:534, 1957
145. Phillips TL, Fu KK: Acute and late effects of multimodal therapy on normal tissues. Cancer 40:489, 1977
146. Roberts JG: Cancer of the oesophagus—How should tumor biology affect treatment? Br J Surg 78:791, 1980
147. Appelquist O, Silvo J, Rissanen P: The results of surgery and radiotherapy in the treatment of small carcinomas of the thoracic oesophagus. Ann Clin Res 11:184, 1979
148. Elkon D, Lee MS, Hendrickson FR: Carcinoma of the esophagus: Sites of recurrence and palliative benefits after definitive radiotherapy. Int J Radiat Oncol Biol Phys 4:615, 1978
149. Jobsen JJ, van Andel JG, Eijkenboom WMH et al: Carcinoma of the esophagus: Treatment results. Radiother Oncol 5:101, 1986
150. Lowe WC: Survival with carcinoma of the esophagus. Ann Intern Med 77:915, 1972
151. Newaishy GA, Read GA, Duncan W et al: Results of radical radiotherapy of squamous cell carcinoma of the esophagus. Clin Radiol 33:347, 1982
152. Schumann GF, Heydorn WH, Hall RV et al: Treatment of esophageal carcinoma. J Thorac Cardiovasc Surg 79:67, 1980
153. Van Andel JG, Dees J, Diskhuis CM et al: Carcinoma of the esophagus—results of treatment. Ann Surg 190:684, 1979
154. Van Houtte P: Radiotherapie du Cancer l'oesophage. Acta Gastroenterol Belg 40:121, 1977
155. Wara WM, Mauch PM, Thomas AN, Phillips TL: Palliation for carcinoma of the esophagus. Radiology 121:717, 1976
156. Yin W, Zhang LJ, Miao Y et al: The results of high-energy electron therapy in carcinoma of the oesophagus compared with telecobalt therapy. Clin Radiol 34:113, 1983
157. Robertson R, Coy P, Mokkhavesa S: The results of radical surgery compared with radical radiotherapy in the treatment of squamous carcinoma of the thoracic esophagus. J Thorac Cardiovasc Surg 53:430, 1967
158. Exner A: Veber die behandlung von oesophagus Karzinomen mit radiumstrahlen. Wien Klin Wochenschr 17:96, 1904
159. Rider W, Mendoza R: Some opinions on the treatment of cancer of the oesophagus. Am J Radiol 105:514, 1969
160. Moorthy CR, Nibhanupudy JR, Ashayeri E et al: Intraluminal radiation for esophageal cancer: A Howard University technique. J Natl Med Assoc 74:261, 1982
161. Bottrill DO, Plane JH, Newaishy GA: A proposed afterloading technique for irradiation of the esophagus. Br J Radiol 52:573, 1979
162. George FW: Radiation management in esophageal cancer. Am J Surg 139:795, 1980
163. Abe M, Kitagawa T: Treatment of esophageal cancer with high dose rate intracavitary irradiation. Tohoku J Exp Med 134:159, 1981
164. Hishikawa Y, Tanaka S, Miura T: Early esophageal carcinoma treated with intracavitary irradiation. Ther Radiol (Suppl 2)156:519, 1985
165. Rowland CG, Pagliero KM: Intracavitary irradiation in palliation of carcinoma of oesophagus and cardia. Lancet:981, 1985
166. Tate T, Brace JA, Morgan H, Skeggs DBL: Conformation therapy: A method of improving the tumour treatment volume ratio. Clin Radiol 37:267, 1986
167. Kelsen D, Bains M, Hilaris B et al: Combined-modality therapy of esophageal cancer. Semin Oncol 11:169, 1984
168. Leichman L, Steiger Z, Seydel HG et al: Combined preoperative chemotherapy and radiation therapy for cancer of the esophagus: The Wayne State University, Southwest Oncology Group and Radiation Therapy Oncology Group experience. Semin Oncol 11:178, 1984
169. Kelsen D: Chemotherapy of esophageal cancer. Semin Oncol 11:159, 1984
170. Folke S, Edsmyr F: Treatment of oesophagus carcinoma in Africa. Gann Monogr Cancer Res 19:187, 1976
171. Nabeya K: The use of bleomycin in the treatment of carcinoma of the esophagus. Gann Monogr Cancer Res 19:177, 1976
172. Resbeut M, Prise-Fleury E, Ben-Hassel M et al: Squamous cell carcinoma of the esophagus: Treatment by combined vincristine-methotrexate plus folinic acid rescue and cisplatin before radiotherapy. Cancer 56:1246, 1985
173. Advani SH, Saikia TK, Swaroop S: Anterior chemotherapy in esophageal cancer. Cancer 56:1502, 1985
174. Leichman L, Werskovic A, Leichman G et al: Non-operative therapy for squamous cell cancer of the esophagus. J Clin Oncol 5:365, 1987
175. Poplin E, Fleming T, Leichman L et al: Combined therapies for squamous cell cancer of the esophagus: A Southwest Oncology Group (SWOG 8037) Study. J Clin Oncol 5:633, 1987
176. Falkson G, Ckoetzer BJ, Terblanch AP: Oesophageal cancer—chemotherapy overview. S Afr Med J 71:21, 1987
177. Leichman L, Lokich JJ, Leichman CG: Esophageal and anal cancer. In Lokich JJ (ed): Cancer Chemotherapy by Infusion. Precept Press, 1987
178. Kolaric K, Moricic Z, Dujmovic I et al: Therapy of advanced esophageal cancer with bleomycin, irradiation and combination bleomycin and irradiation. Tumori 62:255, 1976
179. Ravry M, Moertel CG, Schutt AJ et al: Treatment of advanced squamous cell carcinoma of the gastrointestinal tract with bleomycin (NSC 125066). Cancer Chemother Rep 57:493, 1973
180. Yagoda A, Mukherji B, Young C et al: Bleomycin, an antitumor antibiotic: Clinical experience in 274 patients. Ann Intern Med 77:861, 1972
181. Bonnadonna G, de Lena M, Monfardini S et al: Clinical trial with bleomycin in lymphomas and solid tumors. Eur J Cancer Clin Oncol 8:205, 1972
182. Ravry M, Moore M: Phase II pilot study of cisplatinum (II) in advanced squamous cell esophageal cancer. Proc ASCO 21:353, 1980
183. Davis S, Shanmugathasa M, Kessler W: Cis-dichlorodiammine platinum (II) in the treatment of esophageal carcinoma. Cancer Treat Rep 64:709, 1980
184. Panettiere F, Leichman L, Tilchen E et al: Chemotherapy for advanced epidermoid carcinoma of the esophagus with single agent cisplatin: Final report on Southwest Oncology Group Study. Cancer Treat Rep 68:1023, 1984
185. Engstrom P, Lavin P, Lassen D: Phase II evaluation of mitomycin and cisplatin in advanced esophageal carcinoma. Cancer Treat Rep 67:713, 1983
186. Ezdinli E, Gelber R, Desai et al: Chemotherapy of advanced esophageal carcinoma: Eastern Cooperative Oncology Group experience. Cancer 46:2149, 1980
187. Lokich J, Shea M, Chaffey J: Sequential infusional 5-fluorouracil followed by concomitant radiation for tumors of the esophagus and the gastroesophageal junction. Cancer 60:275, 1987
188. Whitington R, Clos H: Clinical experience with mitomycin C. Cancer Chemother Rep 54:195, 1970
189. Kolaric K, Maricic Z, Roth A et al: Combination of bleomycin and adriamycin with and without radiation in the treatment of inoperable esophageal cancer. Cancer 45:2265, 1980
190. Bezwoda WR, Derman DP, Weaving A et al: Treatment of esophageal cancer with vindesine: An open trial. Cancer Treat Rep 68:783, 1984
191. Kelsen DR, Chapman R, Bains M: Phase II study of methyl-GAG in the present treatment of esophageal carcinoma. Cancer Treat Rep 66:1427, 1982
192. Coonley DJ, Bains M, Hilaris B et al: Cisplatin and bleomycin in the treatment of esophageal carcinoma: A final report. Cancer 54:2341, 1984
193. Bosset J, Hurteloup P, Bontemas P et al: A phase II trial of bleomycin and cisplatin in advanced oesophagus carcinoma (abstr). Proceedings of the 13th International Cancer Congress, 1982, p. 41.
194. Kelsen DP, Bains M, Hilaris B et al: Combination chemotherapy of esophageal carcinoma using cisplatin, vindesine and bleomycin. Cancer 49:1174, 1982
195. Dinwoodie WR, Bartolucci AA, Lyman GH et al: Phase II evaluation of cisplatin, bleomycin and vindesine in advanced squamous cell carcinoma of the esophagus: A Southeastern Study Group trial. Cancer Treat Rep 70:533, 1986
196. DeBasi P, Salvagno L, Endrizzi L et al: Cisplatin, bleomycin and methotrexate in the treatment of advanced oesophageal cancer. Eur J Cancer Clin Oncol 20:743, 1984
197. Vogl SE, Greenwald E, Kaplan BH: Effective chemotherapy for esophageal cancer with methotrexate, bleomycin, and cis-diamminedichloroplatinum II. Cancer 48:2555, 1981
198. Kelsen DP, Fein R, Coonley C et al: Cisplatin, vindesine and mitoguazone in the treatment of esophageal cancer. Cancer Treat Rep 70:255, 1986
199. Forastiere A, Gennis M, Orringer M et al: Cisplatin, vinblastine and mitoguazone chemotherapy for epidermoid and adenocarcinoma of the esophagus. J Clin Oncol 5:1143, 1987
200. Vogl SE, Camacho F, Berenzweig et al: Chemotherapy for esophageal cancer with mitoguazone, methotrexate, bleomycin and cisplatin. Cancer Treat Rep 69:21, 1985
201. Gisselbrecht C, Calvo F, Mignot L et al: Fluorouracil, adriamycin and cisplatin combination chemotherapy of advanced esophageal carcinoma. Cancer 52:974, 1983
202. Wittes R, Brescia F, Young CW: Combination chemotherapy with cis-diamminedichloroplatinum (II) and bleomycin in tumors of the head and neck. Oncology 32:202, 1975
203. Kelsen DP, Cvitkovic E, Bains M et al: Cis-diamminedichloroplatinum (II) and bleomycin in the treatment of esophageal carcinoma. Cancer Treat Rep 62:1041, 1978
204. Kelsen DP, Hilaris B, Coonley C et al: Cisplatin, vindesine and bleomycin combination chemotherapy of local-regional and advanced esophageal carcinoma. Am J Med 75:645, 1983
205. Huang GJ, Gu XZ, Wang LJ et al: Experience with combined preoperative irradiation and surgery for carcinoma of the esophagus. Gann Monogr Cancer Res 31:159, 1986
206. Akakura I, Nakamura Y, Kakegawa T et al: Surgery for carcinoma of the esophagus with preoperative irradiation. Chest 57:47, 1970

207. Andersen AP, Berdal P, Edsmyr F et al: Irradiation, chemotherapy and clinical study. Radiother Oncol 2:179, 1984
208. Doggett RLS, Guernsey JM, Bagshaw MA: Combined radiation and surgical treatment of carcinoma of the thoracic esophagus. Front Radiat Ther Oncol 5:147, 1970
209. Gignoux M, Roussel A, Paillot B et al: The value of preoperative radiotherapy in esophageal cancer: Results of a study of the EORTC. World J Surg 11:426, 1987
210. Groves LK, Rodriguez-Antunez A: Treatment of carcinoma of the esophagus and gastric cardia with concentrated preoperative irradiation followed by early operation. Ann Thorac Surg 15:333, 1973
211. Kelsen DP, Ahuja R, Hopfan S et al: Combined modality therapy of esophageal carcinoma. Cancer 48:31, 1981
212. Launois B, DeLaRue D, Campion JP et al: Preoperative radiotherapy for carcinoma of the esophagus. Surg Gynecol Obstet 153:690, 1981
213. Liu G, Huang Z, Rong T et al: Measures for improving therapeutic results of esophageal carcinoma in stage III: Preoperative radiotherapy. J Surg Oncol 32:248, 1986
214. Marks RD Jr, Scruggs HJ, Wallace KM: Preoperative radiation therapy for carcinoma of the esophagus. Cancer 38:84, 1976
215. Isono K, Onoda S, Ishikawa T et al: Studies on the causes of deaths from esophageal carcinoma. Cancer 49:2173, 1982
216. Parker EF, Gregorie HB, Prioleau WH Jr et al: Carcinoma of the esophagus—observations of 40 years. Ann Surg 195:618, 1982
217. Sugimachi K, Matsufuji H, Kai H et al: Preoperative irradiation for carcinoma of the esophagus. Surg Gynecol Obstet 162:174, 1986
218. Fraser RW, Wara WM, Thomas AN et al: Combined treatment methods for carcinoma of the esophagus. Radiology 128:461, 1978
219. Goodner JT: Surgical and radiation treatment of cancer of the thoracic esophagus. Am J Roentgenol Rad Ther Nucl Med 105:523, 1969
220. Gunnlaugsson GH, Wychulis AR, Roland et al: Analysis of the records of 1657 patients with carcinoma of the esophagus and cardia of the stomach. Surg Gynecol Obstet 130:997, 1970
221. Hankins JR, Cole FN, Ahar S et al: Carcinoma of the esophagus: Twelve years' experience with a philosophy for palliation. Ann Thorac Surg 33:464, 1982
222. Langer M, Choi NC, Orlow E et al: Radiation therapy alone or in combination with surgery in the treatment of carcinoma of the esophagus. Cancer 58:1208, 1986
223. Giuli R, Gignoux M: Treatment of carcinoma of the esophagus—retrospective study of 2400 patients. Ann Surg 192:44, 1980
224. Kasai M, Mori S, Watanabe T: Follow-up results after resection of thoracic esophageal carcinoma. World J Surg 2:543, 1980
225. Fujimaki M et al: Role of preoperative administration of bleomycin and radiation in the treatment of esophageal cancer. Jpn J Surg 5:48, 1975
226. Wada T, Matoumoto Y, Amano T: Chemotherapy of esophageal cancer with bleomycin. Prog Antimicrob Anticancer Chemother 2:696, 1970
227. Miller JJ, McIntyre B, Hatcher CR: Combined treatment approach in surgical management of carcinoma of the esophagus: A preliminary report. Ann Thorac Surg 40:289, 1985
228. Kelsen DP, Bains MS, Cvitkovic E et al: Vindesine in the treatment of esophageal carcinoma: A phase II study. Cancer Treat Rep 63:2019, 1979
229. Schlag P, Hermann R, Fritze D et al: Preoperative chemotherapy in localized cancer of the esophagus with cis-platinum, vindesine and bleomycin. Primary chemotherapy. In Cancer Medicine, pp 253–258. New York, Alan R Liss, 1985
230. Roth JA, Pass HI, Flanagan MM et al: Clinical trials with cisplatin, vindesine and bleomycin: Neoadjuvant chemotherapy for epidermoid carcinoma of the esophagus. In Levin B (ed): Gastrointestinal Cancer: Current Approaches to Diagnosis and Treatment. Austin, University of Texas Press, 1988
231. Falkson G: Methyl-GAG (NSC-32946) in the treatment of esophagus cancer. Cancer Chemother Rep 55:209, 1971
232. Kelsen DP, Yagoda A, Warrell R et al: Phase II trials of methyl-glyoxal bis [guanylhydrazone] (methyl-GAG). Am J Clin Oncol 5:221, 1982
233. Leichman L, Steiger Z, Seydel HG et al: Preoperative chemotherapy for patients with cancer of the esophagus: Potentially curative approach. J Clin Oncol 2:75, 1984
234. Shields TW, Rosen ST, Hellerstein SM et al: Multimodality approach to treatment of carcinoma of the esophagus. Arch Surg 119:558, 1984
235. Carey RW, Hilgenberg AD, Wilkens EW et al: Preoperative chemotherapy followed by surgery with possible postoperative radiotherapy in squamous cell carcinoma of the esophagus: Evaluation of the chemotherapy component. J Clin Oncol 4:697, 1986
236. Karasawa K, Okada Y, Akamire Y et al: The result of surgical treatment for esophageal cancer in combination with preoperative irradiation and bleomycin therapy (abstr). Nippon Gan Chiryo Gakkai Shi 12:209, 1975
237. Pedersen H, Hansen HS, Bertelsen S et al: Combined modality therapy for oesophageal squamous cell carcinoma. Acta Oncol 26:175, 1987
238. Werner ID: The multidisciplinary approach in the management of squamous carcinoma of the esophagus: The Groote Schmit Hospital experience. Front Gastrointest Res 5:130, 1979
239. Rosenberg JC, Franklin R, Steiger Z: Squamous cell carcinoma of the thoracic esophagus. Curr Probl Cancer 5:1–52, 1981
240. Franklin R, Steiger Z, Vaishanapayan G et al: Combined modality therapy for esophageal squamous cell carcinoma. Cancer 51:1062, 1983
241. Parker FP, Marks RD, Kratz JM et al: Chemoradiation therapy and resection for carcinoma of the esophagus: Short-term results. Ann Thorac Surg 40:121, 1985
242. Douple EB: Therapeutic potentiation in a mouse mammary tumor and an intracerebral rat brain tumor by combined treatment with cis-dichloroplatinum II and radiation. Hematol Oncol 7:585, 1977
243. Leipzig B, Wetmore SJ, Putzeys R et al: Cisplatin potentiation of radiotherapy. Arch Otolaryngol Head Neck Surg 11:114, 1985
244. Campbell WR, Taylor SA, Pierce GE et al: Therapeutic alternative in patients with esophageal cancer. Am J Surg 150:665, 1985
245. Austin JC, Postier RG, Elkins RC: Treatment of esophageal cancer: The continued need of surgical resection. Am J Surg 152:592, 1986
246. Popp MB, Hawley D, Reising J et al: Improved survival in squamous esophageal cancer. Arch Surg 121:1330, 1986
247. Wolfe WG, Burton GV, Seigler HF et al: Early results with combined modality therapy for carcinomas of the esophagus. Ann Surg 205:563, 1987
248. Vietti T, Eggerding F, Valeriote F: Combined effect of x-irradiation and 5-fluorouracil on survival of transplanted leukemic cells. J Natl Cancer Inst 47:865, 1971
249. Kelsen DP: Editorial: Multimodality therapy of esophageal carcinoma: Still an experimental approach. J Clin Oncol 5:530, 1987
250. Mathews CP: Results of combined chemo and radiotherapy in carcinoma oesophagus. Indian J Cancer 9:160, 1972
251. Kolaric K, Maricic Z, Roth A et al: Adriamycin alone and in combination with radiotherapy in the treatment of inoperable esophageal cancer. Tumori 63:485, 1977
252. Earle J, Gelbar R, Moertel C et al: A controlled evaluation of combined radiation and bleomycin therapy for squamous cell carcinoma of the esophagus. Int J Radiat Oncol Biol Phys 6:821, 1980
253. Marcial V, Velez-Garcia E, Clintron J et al: Radiotherapy preceded by multi-drug chemotherapy in carcinoma of the esophagus. Cancer Clin Trials 3:127, 1980
254. Abitbol A, Straus M, Franklin G et al: Infusional chemotherapy and cyclic radiation therapy in inoperable esophageal and gastric cardia carcinoma. Am J Clin Oncol 6:195, 1983
255. Berenzweig M, Vogl S, Camacho F et al: Esophageal squamous cancer chemotherapy with MGBG, methotrexate, bleomycin and dichlorodiammine platinum-MGBG-MBD. Pro Am Soc Clin Oncol 2:125, 1983
256. Seifert P, Baker LH, Reed ML et al: Comparison of continuously infused 5-fluorouracil with bolus injection in treatment of patients with colorectal adenocarcinoma. Cancer 36:123, 1975
257. Kish J, Ensley J, Weaver A et al: Superior response rates with 96-hour 5-fluorouracil infusional versus 5-FU bolus combined with cisplatinum (CACP) in a randomized trial for recurrent and advanced squamous head and neck cancer (HNC) (abstr). Proc Am Soc Clin Oncol 3:179, 1984
258. Byfield JE, Barone R, Mendelsohn J et al: Infusional 5-fluorouracil (5-Fu): Molecular and clinical scheduling implications. Proc Am Assoc Cancer Res 18:74, 1977
259. Coia LR, Engstrom PF, Paul A: Nonsurgical management of esophageal cancer. Report of a study of combined radiotherapy and chemotherapy. J Clin Oncol 5:1783, 1987
260. Kean TJ, Harwood AR, Tahany E et al: Radical radiation therapy with 5-fluorouracil infusion and mitomycin C for oesophageal squamous carcinoma. Radiother Oncol 4:205, 1985
261. John M, Flam M, Wittlinger P et al: Inoperable esophageal carcinoma: Results of aggressive synchronous radiotherapy and chemotherapy. Am J Clin Oncol 10:310, 1987
262. Collin CF, Spiro RH: Carcinoma of the cervical esophagus: Changing therapeutic trends. Am J Surg 148:460, 1984
263. Harrison DFN: Surgical repair in hypopharyngeal and cervical esophageal cancer: Analysis of 162 patients. Ann Otol Rhinol Laryngol 90:372, 1981
264. Ujiki GT, Pearl GJ, Poticha S et al: Mortality and morbidity of gastric pull-up for replacement of the pharyngoesophagus. Arch Surg 122:644, 1987
265. Lam KH, Wong J, Lim STK et al: Pharyngogastric anastomosis following pharyngolaryngoesophagectomy: Analysis of 157 cases. World J Surg 5:509, 1981
266. Raphael HA, Ellis HF, Dockerty MB: Primary adenocarcinoma of the esophagus: 18-year review and review of literature. Ann Surg 164:785, 1966
267. Turnbull AD, Rosen P, Goodner JT et al: Primary malignant tumors of the esophagus other than typical epidermoid carcinoma. Ann Thorac Surg 15:463, 1973
268. Steiger Z, Wilson RF, Leichman L et al: Primary adenocarcinoma of the esophagus. J Surg Oncol 36:68, 1987
269. Cedarquist C, Nielsen J, Berthelsen A et al: Adenocarcinoma of the esophagus. Acta Chir Scand 146:411, 1980
270. Ming SC: Tumors of the esophagus and stomach. In: Atlas of Tumor Pathology, 2nd series, fascile 7, Washington DC, Armed Forced Institute of Pathology
271. Barrett N: The lower esophagus lined by columnar epithelium. Surgery 41:881, 1957
272. Allison PR, Johnstone AS: The oesophagus lined with gastric mucous membrane. Thorax 8:87, 1953
273. Allison PR: Peptic oesophagitis and oesophageal stricture. Lancet 2:199, 1970
274. Adler RH: The lower esophagus lined by columnar epithelium: Its association with hiatal hernia, ulcer, stricture and tumor. J Thorac Cardiovasc Surg 45:13, 1963
275. Spechler SJ, Goyel RK: Barrett's esophagus. N Eng J Med 315:362, 1986
276. Nissen R: Eine einfache operation zur beinflussung der Refluxoesophagitis. Schweiz Med Wochenschr 86:590, 1956
277. Rosenberg JC, Budev H, Edwards RC et al: Analysis of adenocarcinoma in Barrett's esophagus utilizing a staging system. Cancer 55:1353, 1985
278. Bremner CG, Lynch VP, Ellis FH: Barrett's esophagus: Congenital of acquired? An experimental study of esophageal mucosal regeneration in the dog. Surgery 68:309, 1970
279. Hamilton SR, Yardley JG: Regeneration of cardiac type mucosa and acquisition of Barrett mucosa after esophagogastrostomy. Gastroenterology 72:669, 1977
280. Ranson JM, Patel GK, Clift SA et al: Extended and limited types of Barrett's esophagus in the adult. Ann Thorac Surg 33:19, 1982

281. Paull A, Trier JS, Dalton D et al: The histologic spectrum of Barrett's esophagus. N Engl J Med 295:576, 1976
282. Berenson MM, Herbst JJ, Freston JW: Enzyme and ultrastructural characteristics of esophageal columnar epithelium. Dig Dis Sci 19:895, 1974
283. Jass JR: Mucin histochemistry of the columnar epithelium of the oesophagus: A retrospective study. J Clin Pathol 34:866, 1981
284. Banner BF, Memoli VA, Warren WH et al: Carcinoma with multidirectional differentiation arising in Barrett's esophagus. Ultrastruct Pathol 4:205, 1983
285. Skinner DB, Walther BC, Riddell RH et al: Barrett's esophagus: Comparison of benign and malignant cases. Surgery 198:554, 1983
286. Mangla JC: Barrett's esophagus: An old entity rediscovered. J Clin Gastroenterol 3:347, 1981
287. Brand DL, Ylvisaker JT, Gelfand M et al: Regression of columnar esophageal (Barrett's) epithelium after anti-reflux surgery. N Engl J Med 302:844, 1980
288. Lee RG: Dysplasia in Barrett's esophagus: Clinicopathologic study of 6 patients. Am J Surg Pathol 9:845, 1985
289. Stoller JL, Brumwell ML: Palliation after operation and after radiotherapy for cancer of the esophagus. Can J Surg 27:491, 1984
290. Marcial VA, Tome JM, Ubinas J et al: The role of radiation therapy in esophageal cancer. Radiology 87:231, 1966
291. Schwade JG, Kinsella TJ, Kelly B et al: Clinical experience with intravenous misonidazole for carcinoma of the esophagus. Cancer Invest 2:91, 1984
292. Pearson JG: The value of radiotherapy in the management of esophageal cancer. Am J Roentgenol 105:500, 1969
293. Orringer MB: Palliative procedures for esophageal cancer. Surg Clin North Am 63:941, 1983
294. Payne WS: Palliation of esophageal carcinoma. Ann Thorac Surg 28:208, 1979
295. Hankins JR, Cole FN, Attar S et al: Carcinoma of the esophagus: Twelve years' experience with a philosophy for palliation. Ann Thorac Surg 33:464, 1982
296. Orringer MB: Esophageal carcinoma: What price palliation? Ann Thorac Surg 36:377, 1983
297. Orringer MB, Sloan H: Substernal gastric bypass of the excluded thoracic esophagus for palliation of esophageal carcinoma. J Thorac Cardiovasc Surg 70:836, 1975
298. Steiger Z, Nickel WD, Wilson RF et al: Improved surgical palliation of advanced carcinoma of the esophagus. Am J Surg 125:782, 1978
299. Orringer MB: Substernal gastric bypass of the excluded esophagus—Results of an ill-advised operation. Surgery 96:467, 1984
300. Olsen CO, Hopkins RA, Poltlethwait RW: Management of an infected mucocele occurring in a bypassed excluded esophageal segment. Ann Thorac Surg 40:73, 1985
301. Kamath MV, Ellison RG, Rubin JW et al: Esophageal mucocele: A complication of blind loop esophagus. Ann Thorac Surg 43:263, 1987
302. Angorn IB: Intubation in the treatment of carcinoma of the esophagus. World J Surg 5:535, 1981
303. Ghazi A, Nussbaum M: A new approach to the management of malignant esophageal obstruction and esophagorespiratory fistula. Ann Thorac Surg 41:531, 1986
304. Unruh HW, Pagliero KM: Pulsion intubation versus traction intubation for obstructing carcinoma of the esophagus. Ann Thorac Surg 40:337, 1985
305. Angorn IB, Haffegee AA: Pulsion intubation v. retrosternal gastric bypass for palliation of unresectable carcinoma of the upper thoracic oesophagus. Br J Surg 70:335, 1983
306. Rose JDR, Smith PM: Fibre endoscopic insertion of palliative oesophageal tubes with the Nottingham introducer. J R Soc Med 76:266, 1983
307. Celestin LR, Campbell WB: A new and safe system for oesophageal dilatation. Lancet 1:74, 1981
308. Boyce HW: Medical management of esophageal obstruction and esophageal-pulmonary fistula. Cancer 50:2597, 1982
309. Fleischer D, Kessler F, Hage O: Endoscopic Nd:YAG laser therapy for carcinoma of the esophagus: A new form of palliative treatment. Gastroenterology 85:600, 1983
310. McCaughan JS, Williams TE, Bethel BH: Palliation of esophageal malignancy with photodynamic therapy. Ann Thorac Surg 40:113, 1985
311. Pietrafitta JJ, Dwyer RM: Endoscopic laser therapy of malignant esophageal obstruction. Arch Surg 121:395, 1986
312. Battifora H: Spindle cell carcinoma: Ultrastructural evidence of squamous origin and collagen production by the tumor cells. Cancer 37:2275, 1976
313. Agha FP, Keren DF: Spindle-cell squamous carcinoma of the esophagus: A tumor with biphasic morphology. AJR 145:541, 1985
314. Osamura RY, Shinamura K, Hata J et al: Polypoid carcinoma of the esophagus: A unifying term for "carcinosarcoma" and pseudosarcoma. Am J Surg Pathol 2:201, 1978
315. Matsusaka T, Watanabe H, Enjoji: Pseudosarcoma and carcinosarcoma of the esophagus. Cancer 37:1546, 1976
316. Fennell WM, Perold JI: Pseudosarcoma of the esophagus: A case report. S Afr Med J 52:37, 1977
317. Postlethwait RW, Wechsler AS, Shelburne JD. Pseudosarcoma of the esophagus. Ann Thorac Surg 19:198, 1975
318. DeMeester TR, Skinner DB: Polypoid sarcomas of the esophagus: A rare but potentially curable neoplasm. Ann Thorac Surg 20:405, 1975
319. Xu LT, Sun CF, Wu LH et al: Clinical and pathological characteristics of carcinosarcoma of the esophagus: Report of 4 cases. Ann Thorac Surg 37:197, 1978
320. Yates CW, LeVine MA, Jensen KM: Varicoid carcinoma of the esophagus. Radiology 122:605, 1977
321. Epstein JI, Sears VL, Tucker RS et al: Carcinoma of the esophagus with adenoid cystic differentiation. Cancer 53:1131, 1984
322. Pourzand A, Freant L, Levin R et al: Primary adenoid cystic carcinoma of the esophagus: Report of a case and review of the literature. J Thorac Cardiovasc Surg 69:785, 1975
323. Petersson SR: Adenoid cystic carcinoma of the esophagus: Complete response to combination chemotherapy. Cancer 57:1464, 1986
324. Woodard BA, Shelburne JD, Vollmer RT et al: Mucoepidermoid carcinoma of the esophagus: A case report. Hum Pathol 9:352, 1978
325. Sabnathan S, Graham GP, Salama FD: Primary oat cell carcinoma of the esophagus. Thorax 41:318, 1986
326. Imai T, Sannoke Y, Okano H: Oat cell carcinoma (APUDOMA) of the esophagus: A case report. Cancer 41:358, 1978
327. Johnson FE, Clawson MC, Bashiti HM et al: Small cell undifferentiated carcinoma of the esophagus. Cancer 53:1746, 1984
328. Doherty MA, McIntyre M, Arnott SJ: Oat cell carcinoma of the esophagus: A report of six British patients with a review of the literature. Int J Radiat Oncol Biol Phys 10:147, 1984
329. Reyes CV, Chejfec G, Jao W et al: Neuroendocrine tumors of the esophagus. Ultrastruct Pathol 1:367, 1980
330. Kelsen DP, Weston E, Kurty R et al: Small cell carcinoma of the esophagus: Treatment by chemotherapy alone. Cancer 45:1558, 1980
331. Rosenthal SN, Lemkin JA. Multiple small cell carcinomas of the esophagus. Cancer 51:1944, 1983
332. Rankin R, Nirodi NS, Browne MK: Carcinoid tumor of the esophagus: Report of a case. Scott Med J 25:245, 1980
333. Siegel A, Swartz A: Malignant carcinoid of oesophagus. Histopathology 10:761, 1986
334. Chalkiadokis G, Wihlm JM, Morand G et al: Primary malignant melanoma of the esophagus. Ann Thorac Surg 39:472, 1985
335. Choh JH, Khazei AH, Ihm JH: Leiomyosarcoma of the esophagus: Report of a case and review of the literature. J Surg Oncol 32:223, 1986
336. Wobbes T, Rinsma SG, Holla AT et al: Rhabpdomyosarcoma of the esophagus. Arch Chir Neerl 27:69, 1975
337. Trillo AA, Accettulo LM, Yecter TL: Choriocarcinoma of the esophagus: Histologic and cytologic findings. A case report. Acta Cytol 23:69, 1979
338. Matsuura H, Saito R, Nakajing S et al: Non-Hodgkin's lymphoma of the esophagus. Am J Gastroenterol 80:941, 1985
339. Agha FP, Schnitzer B: Esophageal involvement in lymphoma. Am J Gastroenterol 80:412, 1985
340. Gedgaudos-McClees RK, Maglinte DD: Lymphomatous esophageal nodules: The difficulty in radiological differential diagnosis. Am J Gastroenterol 80:529, 1985
341. Agha FP: Secondary neoplasms of the esophagus. Gastrointest Radiol 12:187, 1987
342. Marshall ME: Gastrointestinal metastasis from carcinoma of the breast. J Ky Med Assoc 81:154, 1973
343. Anderson MF, Harrell GS: Secondary esophageal tumors. Am J Radiol 135:1243, 1980
344. Laforet EG, Kondi ES: Postmastectomy dysphagia. Am J Surg 121:368, 1971
345. Boccardo F, Merlano M, Canobbio L et al: Esophageal involvement in breast cancer: Report of six cases Tumori 68:149, 1982

JOHN S. MACDONALD
GLENN STEELE, JR.
LEONARD L. GUNDERSON

CHAPTER 25 *Cancer of the Stomach*

Cancer of the stomach is the eighth most common cause of cancer deaths in the United States. In 1986 25,000 new cases occurred, and 14,000 deaths resulted from stomach cancer. Although gastric cancer still remains a major health problem in the United States, the death rate from this disease in males has decreased from approximately 22.8:100,000 in 1950 to 9:100,000 in the 1980s. The corresponding changes in women are from 12.3 to 4.3:100,000. This represents a 59% and 65% decrease in age-adjusted mortality due to stomach cancer in men and women, respectively. This decline is steepest in older persons and in whites.[1,2] The decreasing mortality is a result of the decreasing incidence of stomach cancer. There has been no adequate explanation for the decreasing incidence of gastric adenocarcinoma in the United States.

This unexplained decrease in a highly lethal malignancy has intrigued and stimulated epidemiologists. The decline in gastric cancer in the United States is particularly striking when considered in the context of the very high incidence rates of the disease in such countries as Japan (78:10,000) and Chile (70:100,000).[3] In the United States the approximate incidence of gastric cancer is 10:100,000. The fact that populations emigrating from high- to low-incidence countries experience a significant decrease in the occurrence of the disease clearly suggests that the cause of this cancer must be related to the environment.[3] The first-generation immigrants have a higher risk of stomach cancer than do natives of the host country. This finding suggests an etiological factor that may persist in the migrant population for some time[4,5]—perhaps a learned dietary practice that disappears as migrant groups are assimilated into the host culture. A variety of environmental factors have been associated with a high incidence of gastric cancer, including consumption of smoked foods, salted foods, and foods contaminated with aflatoxin.[6]

In the United States and Western Europe, stomach cancer is twice as frequent in the lower as in the highest socioeconomic groups. Increased stomach cancer rates have been associated with a number of occupations, including coal mining, farming (in Japan), and nickel refining (in the Soviet Union). Rubber workers and workers who process timber also have been reported to have an increased risk of stomach cancer. Whether these occupations are truly associated with an increased risk for gastric cancer or merely reflect the socioeconomic characteristics of the employees is not clear.[7] Stomach cancer also is more common in asbestos workers, and it is likely that this increase is due to exposure to asbestos fibers.[8]

Familial occurrence of gastric cancer is rare, and associations between gastric cancer and blood group A and intestinal metaplasia are discussed in subsequent sections of this chapter.[9,10] There appears to be no increased risk of gastric cancer in persons using alcohol or tobacco.

PATHOLOGY

Of the malignant neoplasms of the stomach, 95% are adenocarcinomas, and generally when the term gastric cancer is used, it refers to adenocarcinoma of the stomach. Although adenoacanthoma, squamous cell carcinoma, and carcinoid tumors do occur in the stomach, they each represent less than 1% of gastric malignancies.[11] Leiomyosarcomas of the stomach may account for 1% to 3% of malignant gastric tumors.[12,13] The stomach is the most common site for lymphoma of the gastrointestinal (GI) tract.[6] With the relative decrease in incidence of carcinoma of the stomach, lymphomas represent a larger proportion of malignancies diagnosed.[14] Pathologists and clinicians must be alert to the possibility that a gastric neoplasm represents lymphoma rather than carcinoma.

In evaluating the pathology of gastric cancer, several factors have important clinical significance. The gross appearance, site, and degree of local invasion of the tumor all bear on prognosis, as does the histology of the cancer. The macroscopic appearance of gastric cancer has been described according to several schemes.[11,15] Fifty years ago, the German pathologist Borrmann developed a classification scheme that divided gastric cancer into five types, according to macroscopic appearance.[15] Type 1 represented polypoid or fungating cancers, type 2 encompassed ulcerating lesions surrounded by elevated borders, type 3 represented ulcerating lesions infiltrating the gastric wall, type 4 tumors were diffusely infiltrating carcinomas, and type 5 were unclassifiable cancers. In the United States, a less formalized descriptive classification of gastric cancers generally is used.[11] This scheme divides the gross pathologic features of stomach cancer into four categories. Most lesions are ulcerative. The lesions may have the appearance of a benign gastric ulcer, or they may exhibit the findings classically attributed to malignant gastric ulcers, including a diameter greater than 2 cm and heaped-up borders, making the ulcer appear raised above the level of the surrounding stomach. Approximately 10% of gastric cancers can be classified grossly as polypoid. These lesions may be large without showing evidence of significant invasion or metastases. This may result from the fact that, histologically, these tumors are well differentiated. In the European literature, such well-differentiated types of stomach cancers have been classified as being of the intestinal type and have a better prognosis than tumors with diffuse anaplastic histopathology.[16] The third type of gross appearance of gastric cancer is the scirrhous pattern. Approximately 10% of cancers fall into this category. Scirrhous tumors result in thickening and rigidity of the gastric wall owing to diffuse infiltration with anaplastic cancer cells. These malignant cells produce a marked fibrous reaction in the gastric wall, leading to a stiffened stomach, giving the appearance of linitis plastica. Scirrhous carcinoma is almost invariably fatal. In a series of 504 patients with resectable gastric cancer reported by the Veterans Administration Surgical Oncology Group, the 5-year survival rate after gastric resection for patients with scirrhous carcinoma was 2%.[17] The fourth type of gastric cancer, the superficial variety, is uncommon in the United States. This tumor, found in fewer than 5% of surgical specimens, is characterized by sheet-like collections of cancer cells replacing the normal mucosa.

Gastric cancer does not arise from all sites in the stomach with equal frequency.[11,18] Most tumors develop in the antrum, or lower third of the stomach. Cancers are generally less common in the body of the stomach and least common in the cardia. However, recent information in the United States[19,20] suggests a slight increase in the incidence of cardioesophageal junction carcinomas and a decrease in the incidence of more distal lesions. These proximal lesions may invade the distal esophagous. Gastric cancers are more common in the lesser curvature than in the greater curvature of the stomach. Berkson, in reviewing the site of origin in 587 cases of gastric cancer, noted that the tumors arose in the lesser curvature in 18% of cases but from the greater curvature in only 3% of cases.[21] Multicentric involvement of the stomach has also been reported in patients with stomach cancer. Moertel reported that 2.2% of 1835 patients with gastric cancer showed gross evidence of having more than one primary gastric tumor.[11] If the stomachs of patients with gastric cancer are carefully examined histologically for the presence of multicentric tumor, in as many as 22% tumors will be found arising from several sites.[22] This phenomenon is more common in patients with gastric cancer following pernicious anemia.

Adenocarcinoma occurring in the stomach may be classified according to degree of histologic differentiation. Although not an independent prognostic variable, differentiation is important because prognosis is worse in the poorly differentiated lesions.[23] If Broder's classification is used, which grades tumor cells from 1 (well differentiated) to 4 (anaplastic), patients with unresectable stomach cancer and well-differentiated lesions (Grades 1 and 2) have a median survival of 7 months. Patients with Grade 3 or 4 tumor histology have a median survival of only 4 months. It should be emphasized that histologic grade of the tumor and the gross pathology are not independent variables. For example, linitis plastica is never seen with well-differentiated tumors, occurring only with the more undifferentiated cancer. Conversely, polypoid tumors are very likely to have well-differentiated histology.

ANATOMICAL RELATIONSHIPS OF THE STOMACH

From the oncologist's point of view, the important features of the stomach relate to the other viscera with which it comes in contact, its vascular supply, its lymphatic supply, and which surgical procedures may be performed on the stomach without endangering patient survival (Fig. 25-1).

Since the stomach begins at the gastroesophageal junction and ends at the pylorus, direct spread to the esophagus or the duodenum or so-called skip submucosal metastases must be taken into account when determining appropriate visual as well as microscopic margins in planning resections of tumors at the proximal or distal ends of the stomach. In addition, the stomach is in contact with the diaphragm, the anterior abdominal wall, the liver, the transverse colon and mesocolon, the spleen, the left adrenal, the left kidney, the pancreas, the splenic flexure of the colon, the greater omentum, and various loops of small intestine.

The blood supply to the stomach is derived from the celiac axis. The major vessels involved are the left gastric artery, the right gastric artery, and the gastroduodenal artery (all branches of the hepatic artery), the right and left gastroepiploic vessels, and the short gastric or vasa brevia (branches of the splenic artery). Other arteries of concern in terms of dissemination of gastric carcinoma or in terms of operative procedures on the stomach include the splenic, the hepatic,

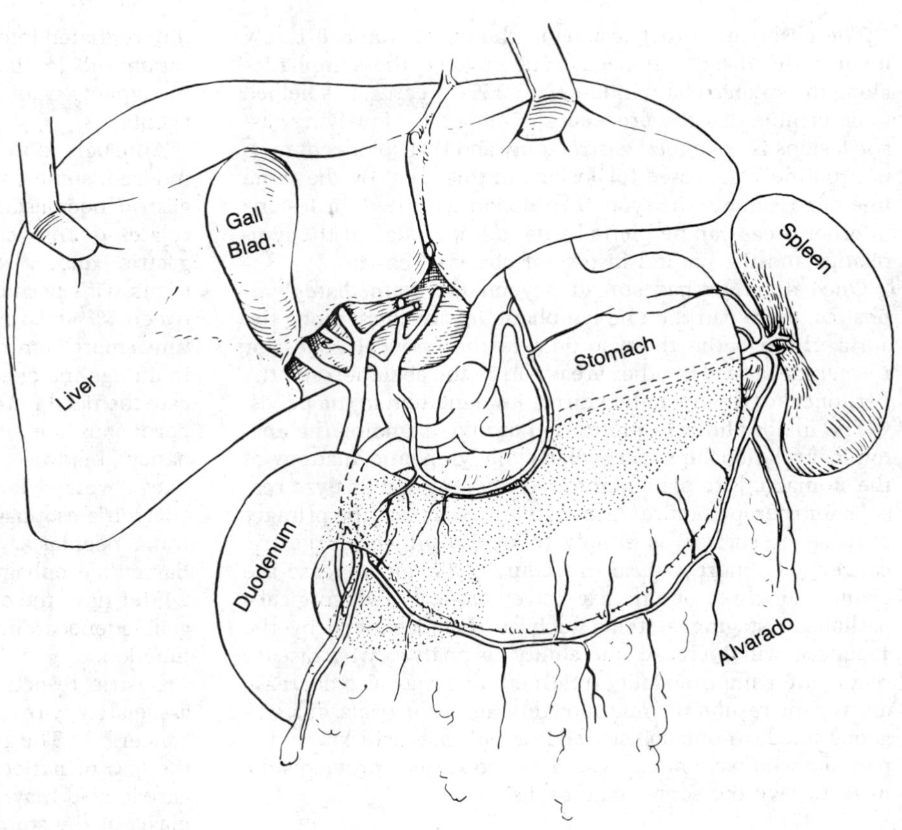

FIG. 25-1. Major anatomical relationships of the stomach, showing its blood supply, and the other organs most likely to be involved by primary malignant lesions in the stomach.

and the middle colic, any of which might be involved by an extensive tumor arising within the stomach or might be encountered during surgical procedures to remove these lesions.

In general, the venous drainage of the stomach parallels the arterial supply. The major additional vein is the coronary vein, which runs along the lesser curvature of the stomach and eventually drains into the portal vein.

The lymphatics of the stomach have been described in greater detail by Rouviere, and reference to his work is essential for anyone interested in the routes of potential spread of carcinoma of the stomach (Table 25-1).[18] Although there is a rich interconnecting lymphatic network within the stomach, the more important pathways with respect to gastric carcinoma are those that deal with the collecting trunk. Rouviere has divided these into three major systems: the region of the left gastric chain, the region of the splenic chain, and the region of the hepatic chain. The lymphatic pathways are complex and highly interconnected but, in general, follow the pathways of the major vascular supply to the stomach. It is clear from this that lymphatics can be involved along both the lesser and the greater curvatures of the stomach, extending to the hilum of the spleen on the left side and up the portal triad on the right side, across the surface of the pancreas, and down along the course of the duodenum inferiorly. The highly complex nature of the lymphatic pathways explains, to a certain extent, the problems with early and extensive spread of tumors from the stomach to other areas.

The gastric lymphatic pathways have been defined (see Table 25-1) to show that lesions in particular areas of the stomach generally follow a given direction, but this is not an invariable rule; if there is early blockage of the normal pathway, lymphatic drainage can then go in a different direction, thus causing even more extensive retrograde lymphatic blockage. The relatively rich lymphatic supply of the stomach makes accurate prediction of lymphatic spread of tumor more difficult, for example, than in colon or rectal cancer.

TABLE 25-1. Lymphatic Drainage of the Stomach

The lymphatic networks
The mucous network
The submucous network
The muscular network
The subserous or subperitoneal network
The collecting trunks
Left gastric chain
Left gastropancreatic fold
Lesser curvature nodes
Parietal group
Juxtacardiac nodes
Splenic chain
Suprapancreatic nodes
Infrapancreatic nodes
Afferent and efferent lymph vessels
The hepatic chain
Hepatic group
Right gastroepiploic and infrapyloric group
Right gastric group, suprapyloric nodes
Pancreaticoduodenal group
Afferent and efferent vessels

The observation that lesions in the distal stomach rarely involve the distal esophagus, and involve the lymphatics along the splenic chain in less than 25% of cases, has helped to determine that the procedure of choice for low-lying gastric lesions is not a total gastrectomy and that splenectomy is not routinely indicated for lesions in this area. By the same line of reasoning, the type of resection indicated for lesions in other areas can be plotted from a knowledge of the lymphatics and the natural history of observed cases.

Once a tumor has spread beyond the immediate lymphatics, there can then be lymphatic involvement along the aorta, through the thoracic duct to the cervical nodes, or retrograde spread to other areas within the abdomen and the peritoneal cavity, including direct implantation in the pelvis.

The major clinical ramification of understanding the anatomical relationships, particularly the lymphatic anatomy of the stomach, is to plan appropriate therapy and analyze reasons for therapy failure. Although it is clear that the primary purpose of surgery is simply to excise all visible gastric cancer (*i.e.*, more radical procedures will not increase the chance of cure), more extensive surgical and surgical–pathologic staging systems such as that described by the Japanese will increase our ability to analyze why disease recurs after multimodality treatment and may also decrease discrepant results of multimodality adjuvant trials, for surgeons, medical oncologists, and pathologists will know that patients who have been treated by the various protocols do, in fact, have the same stage of disease.

NATURAL HISTORY

PREMALIGNANT LESIONS

The premalignant histology of the normal stomach may have an important influence on the occurrence of gastric cancer. For example, intestinal metaplasia of the stomach is more frequent in countries where the incidence of stomach cancer is high.[24–26] This lesion is defined as a replacement of stomach epithelium by intestinal epithelium containing goblet and paneth cells. In Japan, where gastric cancer causes 40% of all deaths from malignancy, intestinal metaplasia is found in 80% of stomachs resected for gastric cancer.[26,27] The type of stomach cancer associated with intestinal metaplasia is well differentiated.[28,29] In cases in which metaplasia is not observed, the tumor is poorly differentiated and frequently has a scirrhous carcinoma pattern.[27] The scirrhous histologic pattern is more common in Western countries, where intestinal metaplasia is less frequent than in Japan.

Experimental evidence suggests that the metaplastic change in intestinal metaplasia is a carcinogen-induced precursor lesion of gastric cancer.[28–30] In studies done in rats, Japanese workers have shown that nitro-*N*-nitrosoguanidines, known gastric carcinogens, first induce gastric intestinal metaplasia, which is followed by gastric cancer. Tumors did not occur in rats that did not develop intestinal metaplasia after carcinogen exposure. The relationship between a well-defined premalignant pathologic finding (intestinal metaplasia) induced by a known carcinogen and predisposition of the stomach to a specific type of adenocarcinoma (well-differentiated intestinal type) clearly deserves further exploration and implies that intestinal metaplasia is capable of malignant transformation when exposed to promoting agents.

Although most gastric cancers appear to be carcinogen induced, some conditions predispose to the development of gastric neoplasia. The firmest, most convincing evidence relates to the association between pernicious anemia and gastric cancer.[11,31] The incidence of gastric cancer in patients with pernicious anemia has been reported to be between 5% and 10%, and gastric cancer is estimated to be 20 times more common in patients with pernicious anemia than in an age-matched control population.[32] These results indicate the need for careful monitoring of patients with chronic pernicious anemia for the development of gastric malignancy. Likewise, patients with chronic reflux esophagitis may develop glandular metaplasia of the distal esophagus (Barrett's esophagus), which may progress to dysplasia and frank neoplasia. Malignancies developing in patients with Barrett's esophagus are discussed in more detail in Chapter 24; for now, the clinician should be aware that these esophageal adenocarcinomas may involve the cardioesophageal junction.

Gastric resection for benign peptic ulcer disease is also associated with an increased risk of subsequent stomach cancer.[33,34] The reason for this association is not clear, but the loss of parietal cell mass and the resulting decrease in gastric acid may favor the development of intestinal metaplasia of the stomach,[33] which may be a premalignant precursor to stomach cancer. The typical lag time between gastric resection and the manifestations of carcinoma is 15 to 40 years.[32] Giarelli and associates,[34] in an autopsy study of 480 patients who had undergone gastric resection for benign conditions, found a 6.5% incidence of gastric stump carcinomas. The long-term risk of developing gastric cancer was 2.45 times increased in persons who had undergone gastric resection before age 45.

The relationship between gastric polyps and gastric ulcers and malignancy has been debated in the literature for many years.[35–37] In general, it is agreed that polyps are rarely precursor lesions to gastric cancer.[36,38] There are three histologic types of gastric polyps: hyperplastic adenomatous polyps, hamartomatous adenomatous polyps, and villous adenomas. The hyperplastic adenomatous polyps are the most common type and appear to have no malignant potential. Hamartomatous adenomatous polyps are composed of normal gastric mucosal cells and are identical to the lesions seen in the Peutz-Jeghers syndrome. These polyps are the rarest form of gastric polyps and do not become malignant. The lesion that does appear to have malignant potential is the villous adenoma.[36,39,40] These polyps are ten times less common than hyperplastic polyps but are clearly premalignant, since foci of carcinoma are found in approximately 40%.

The experience at the Aichi Cancer Center in Japan confirms the importance of polyp histologic type in relationship to malignant potential.[40] On histologic examination of 198 consecutive cases of gastric polyps, 87.8% were found to be hyperplastic, and only 2% were villous adenomas. In 10 of 198 cases in which cancers of the stomach were present, villous adenomatous pathology was found in 9, and hyperplastic polyps in only 1. Thus, 69% of the villous adenomas but only 0.6% of the hyperplastic polyps were associated with malignancy.

There is controversy between U.S. and Japanese investigators concerning the association between gastric ulcer and malignancy.[11,35–37] The U.S. data can be shown to support the hypothesis that gastric cancer may commonly ulcerate but benign gastric ulcers rarely, if ever, become cancers. In the United States, carcinoma has been found in only 3% of resected gastric ulcers.[41] Conversely, in Japan, the experience at the Yokohama Cancer Hospital initially suggested a very high correlation between chronic gastric ulcer and cancer.[42] In the 1950s, 70% of the early cancers resected consisted of a deep chronic ulcer surrounded by a narrow cancerous lesion, suggesting a preexisting chronic ulcer with malignancy developing at its border. Interestingly, this pathologic entity has been identified progressively less frequently in Japan coincident with the introduction of fiberoptic gastroscopy. In 1974, only 10% of gastric cancers were associated with chronic gastric ulcers, whereas 75% of resected tumors consisted of a primary malignant tumor with ulceration. This finding may be explained in part by the fact that the frequency of chronic gastric ulcer also decreased in Japan by 50% during the period 1958 to 1974.[42]

In general, it appears that now, even in Japan, the risk of gastric cancer occurring in conjunction with gastric ulcer disease is small. This is borne out by the experience of Larson and associates in the United States.[43] These workers followed the course of 664 patients with clinically benign gastric ulcers less than 4 cm in diameter. All patients were treated medically. Only 21% of the patients experienced healing, and 40% eventually required surgery for persistent symptoms or acute problems, such as hemorrhage. The overall incidence of gastric cancer in this group after 5 to 10 years of follow-up was small. Malignancy was demonstrated in 60 (9%) of 664 cases.

Fiberoptic endoscopy now permits safe and rapid inspection and biopsy of gastric ulcers to rule out malignancy. It would seem prudent to follow carefully patients with apparently benign gastric ulcers and to consider prompt surgical intervention if healing does not occur rapidly. The clinician should understand, however, that the likelihood of finding malignancy at surgery is small.

Several conditions once thought to be associated with gastric cancer now appear to have at best a tenuous relationship with that entity. For example, a number of epidemiologic studies seem to have suggested that gastric cancer is more common in persons with blood group A than in those with blood group O.[9,11] More than 55 studies from around the world have supported this finding. However, the risk ratio for gastric cancer in persons with blood group A compared to those with blood group O is only a modest 1.2. In addition, several large studies from the Scandinavian countries have found no correlation between gastric cancer and blood group A.

For many years, a relationship between atrophic gastritis and gastric cancer has been postulated.[11,36] Atrophic gastritis is very commonly associated with gastric malignancy, but it does not follow that atrophic gastritis is a precursor to gastric carcinoma. In the older age group in which gastric cancer occurs, approximately 80% to 95% of individuals have some degree of atrophic gastritis. Thus a large percentage of older patients without stomach cancer have atrophic gastritis, making untenable the hypothesis that atrophic gastritis is a definite precursor of gastric cancer. It is possible that atrophic gastritis is a condition that is permissive for the development of gastric cancer, just as removing parietal cell mass by gastrectomy for benign disease may increase the risk of subsequent gastric carcinoma.[33,34]

PATTERN OF SPREAD

The choice of treatment for any given lesion of the stomach presupposes knowledge of the natural history of the disease and the more common routes of spread.[44] The TNM staging system, which is gaining increasing acceptance, should be used as a baseline to allow appropriate comparisons to be made among series reported from different institutions or at different times. Determination of disease stage requires careful definition by the surgeon and pathologist of local and regional spread during surgical staging.

Complete surgical resection in which all resection margins are rendered free of microscopic disease is possible in only 30% of patients. The tumor stage as determined at surgery will depend on the surgeon's experience and knowledge, and the thoroughness of the surgical and pathologic staging criteria. Nevertheless, multiple studies have confirmed the Charity Hospital series in which only 11% of 423 patients operated on were found to have lesions grossly limited to the stomach.[45,46] In an additional 11%, the only evidence of disease beyond the stomach was clinically positive nodes. Contiguous extension was found in 27% and distant metastatic disease in 31%. Although clinical assessment suggested that only 11% of patients had lymphatic metastases, histologic studies demonstrated nodal involvement in 52% of cases. When the gross surgical or autopsy findings are compared with the final diagnoses based on histologic examination, it is apparent that the surgeon's and the pathologist's gross observations are inadequate. There is a need to stress increased detail in the surgical–pathologic correlation.

The routes of spread of gastric carcinoma are similar to those for other GI lesions.[44] They include (1) direct spread within the involved stomach and into the adjacent esophagus or pylorus, or both; (2) spread to adjacent viscera; (3) spread through lymphatic chains; (4) spillage of tumor cells either from the serosal surface of the stomach or from the lumen at the time of an operative procedure; and (5) blood-borne metastases (Table 25-2).

Studies by Arhelger et al[47] and Coller et al[48] have demonstrated that although the size and location of the primary tumor have some bearing on the frequency and location of lymphatic metastases, these factors are not significantly predictive.

The pattern of distant organ involvement was recorded in the Charity Hospital experience with 348 autopsy cases, and this experience[46] is tabulated along with the reports of Clarke and co-workers,[49] Warren,[50] and Warwick[51] in Table 25-3. In all these studies the liver was the most frequent site of metastasis, being involved almost twice as frequently as the peritoneum or omentum, which are the next two in

TABLE 25-2. Patterns of Spread of Gastric Cancer

- Direct extension
  - Lesser and greater omentum
  - Liver and diaphragm
  - Pancreas
  - Spleen
  - Biliary tract
  - Transverse colon
- Nodal metastases
  - Local
  - Distant
    - Virchow's node
    - Left axillary (Irish's) node
    - Umbilical node
- Vascular metastases
  - Liver
  - Pulmonary system
  - Bone
  - Brain
- Peritoneal metastases
  - Disseminated
  - Pelvic
    - Krukenburg tumor—ovary
    - Blumer's rectal shelf

sequence. The distant organs most commonly involved were the lungs, followed by the adrenals. Histologic involvement of the spleen was relatively uncommon, accounting for less than 10% of the entire series, in contrast to the received opinion that the spleen is involved in a large proportion of the patients with gastric carcinoma.[11] The infrequent involvement of the spleen indicates that routine splenectomy is not necessary and, for lesions originating in the distal stomach without gross involvement of either the spleen or the lymph nodes adjacent to it, that splenectomy is valuable only because it facilitates a more complete lymph node dissection.

PATTERNS OF FAILURE

Although disseminated disease can be found in 75% of patients at autopsy (see Table 25-3), the importance of locoregional failure should not be underestimated. The magnitude of the problem has been demonstrated in clinical,[52] autopsy,[53-55] and reoperation series.[56] McNeer and colleagues[53] have presented complete information on 92 patients autopsied after subtotal gastrectomies performed with curative intent. Some component of local failure was found in 74 (80%) patients, as follows: in 46 (50%), disease in the stomach wall or site or gastroenterostomy; in 14 (15%), tumor in the duodenum, in 5 cases associated with recurrence in the gastric remnant; and in 48 (52%), disease in the perigastric lymph nodes and stomach bed. Thomson and Robins[54] analyzed 28 cases with previous subtotal resection. In 5 (18%) cases disease recurred in the gastric stump alone, in 3 (11%) in the duodenal stump, in 13 (46%) in the gastric bed, and in 6 (21%) in the gastric bed and gastric stump. In a more recent autopsy analysis from the University of Washington, findings in 85 patients who died of gastric cancer were analyzed.[55] Of 16 who had undergone potentially curative resection, 15 (94%) had a locoregional component of failure. The liver was involved in 7 (44%), and peritoneal seeding was found in 8 (50%). Peritoneal seeding occurred in 7 of 10 patients with initial serosal involvement versus 1 of 6 with less extensive disease. Extra-abdominal spread occurred in 9 (69%) of 13 patients with primary lesions involving the gastroesophageal junction versus 35 (49%) of 72 patients with more distal lesions.

Gunderson and Sosin[56] approached the problem of defining sites of failure differently. These workers analyzed patterns of failure in a prospective study in which patients who had undergone gastric resection were subjected to periodic reoperation at the University of Minnesota. After the initial operative procedure, 109 patients underwent one or more reoperations. Since 2 had residual disease after the first procedure, 107 were evaluable for purposes of assessing sites of failure. All patients were treated by operation alone without preoperative or postoperative adjuvant therapy. The extent of the operative procedure was at the discretion of the surgeon, with a large group of patients undergoing a radical procedure, including splenectomy, omentectomy, and radical lymph node dissection in addition to some form of gastrectomy. Of the 107 evaluable patients, 86 (80%) had later evidence of cancer. Incidence and patterns of failure were analyzed in detail (Tables 25-4 and 25-5; Fig. 25-2). Distant

TABLE 25-3. Metastasis at Autopsy or Operation

Site	*Warwick*[51] (*n* = 176)	*DuPont et al*[46] (*n* = 348)	*Warren*[50] (*n* = 67)	*Clark et al*[49] (*n* = 250)
Liver	38	54	34	40
Peritoneum	20	24	28	17
Omentum	13	21		
Lungs	12	22	9	19
Mesentery	9			
Pleura	8		4	
Pancreas	7	29	10	
Adrenals	5	15	3	12
Intestine	4		6	
Genitourinary		3		8
Spleen	2	13	1	
Gallbladder/biliary tract	2	4	6	
Bone	6	1	6	9
Central nervous system	1	0.2		2
No metastasis	23	11	24	22

TABLE 25-4. Patterns of Failure in Reoperation Series After Curative Resection*

Pattern of Failure†	*Only Failure*‡			*Any Component*‡		
	No.	*%*	*(%)*	*No.*	*%*	*(%)*
LF-RF	24	29.3	(22.9)	72	87.8	(68.6)
+ Localized PS (20 patients)	44	53.7	(41.2)			
PS	3	3.7	(2.9)	44	53.7	(41.9)
Localized				20	24.4	(19)
Diffuse				24	29.3	(22.9)
DM	5	6.1	(4.8)	24	29.3	(22.9)

* Gunderson LL, Sosin H: Adenocarcinoma of the stomach—areas of failure in a reoperation series, second or symptomatic looks. Clinicopathologic correlation and implications for adjuvant therapy. Int J Radiat Oncol Biol Phys 8:1–11, 1982.

† Of the 107 evaluable patients, 86 had failure, which was totally documented in 82. LF-RF = locoregional failure, PS = peritoneal spread, DM = distant metastases.

‡ Open figures represent number and percentage of the failure group of 82 patients, and figures in parentheses represent percentage of the 107 patients with complete follow-up.

metastases alone were uncommon but occurred as some component of failure in 29% of the failure group. Nearly half of the peritoneal failures were localized. Of those that had a diffuse component, nearly all also had a fairly massive local recurrence. Locoregional failure occurred as the only failure in 29% of the failure group (53% if localized peritoneal seeding was included) and as any component of failure in 88%. Locoregional failure was primarily limited to lymph nodes and organs and structures of the gastric bed, with a smaller but significant number of failures in the anastomosis, gastric remnant, or duodenal stump. Very few failures occurred in the abdominal incision or stab wounds. Distant metastases were primarily to the liver.

In the reoperative series, the extent of the initial operative procedure had little if any effect on either the incidence or type of subsequent failure (Tables 25-6 and 25-7). Lymph node failures were found in a fairly high percentage of patients who supposedly had undergone radical lymph node dissections. Table 25-8 lists sites of failure according to histopathologic stage of the primary tumor. Patterns of failure by stage were analyzed in detail in a recent series of 130 patients who underwent resection performed with curative intent at the Massachusetts General Hospital.[57] Locoregional failure occurred as any component of failure in 49 patients (38%) and as the sole failure in 21 (16% of 130 at risk and 24% of 88 with any disease progression). The incidence of locoregional failure by stage was in excess of 35% for Stages B_2, B_3, C_2, and C_3 (see Table 25-8); the locations at highest risk for locoregional failure were the gastric bed (27 of 130 patients, 21%) and the anastomosis or stump (33 of 130 patients, 25%). Distant metastases occurred as any component of relapse in 52% (67 of 130 patients) and exceeded 50% for Stage B_2, B_3, C_2, and C_3 lesions. A majority of such failures were confined to the abdomen (61 of 67 patients, or 91%) with a liver component in 39 (30%) of 130 and peritoneal seeding in 30 (23%). A 20% or greater incidence of peritoneal seeding was found with only C_2 and C_3 lesions but if liver metastases were present, a 20% or greater incidence of peritoneal seeding was seen with all but Stage A lesions. The true incidences of gastric bed, nodal, and peritoneal failures may be higher, as this was not a reoperative or autopsy series (see comparative findings in Table 25-5).

All these data suggest that although systemic therapy is clearly important, the development of an effective therapy for regional disease as an adjuvant to surgery could potentially benefit at least 20% of patients.

CLINICAL PRESENTATION

Articles on cancer of the stomach stress the vague, nondiagnostic symptoms and the fact that patients are likely to be

TABLE 25-5. Patterns of Locoregional Failure in Clinical, Reoperative, and Autopsy Series

Site	*Incidence—Any Component*							
	MGH[57] *(clinical) (N = 130)**		*University of Minnesota*[56] *(reoperation) (N = 105)**		*McNeer et al*[53] *(autopsy) (N = 92)**		*Thomson and Robins*[54] *(autopsy) (N = 28)**	
	No.	*%*	*No.*	*%*	*No.*	*%*	*No.*	*%*
Gastric bed	27	(21)	58	(55)	48	(52)	19	(68)
Anastomosis or stumps	33	(25)	28	(27)	55	(60)	15	(54)
Abdominal or stab wounds	. . .	. . .	5	(5)	. . .	. . .	. . .	. . .
Lymph node(s)	11	(8)	45	(43)	48	(52)	. . .	. . .

*Number at risk.

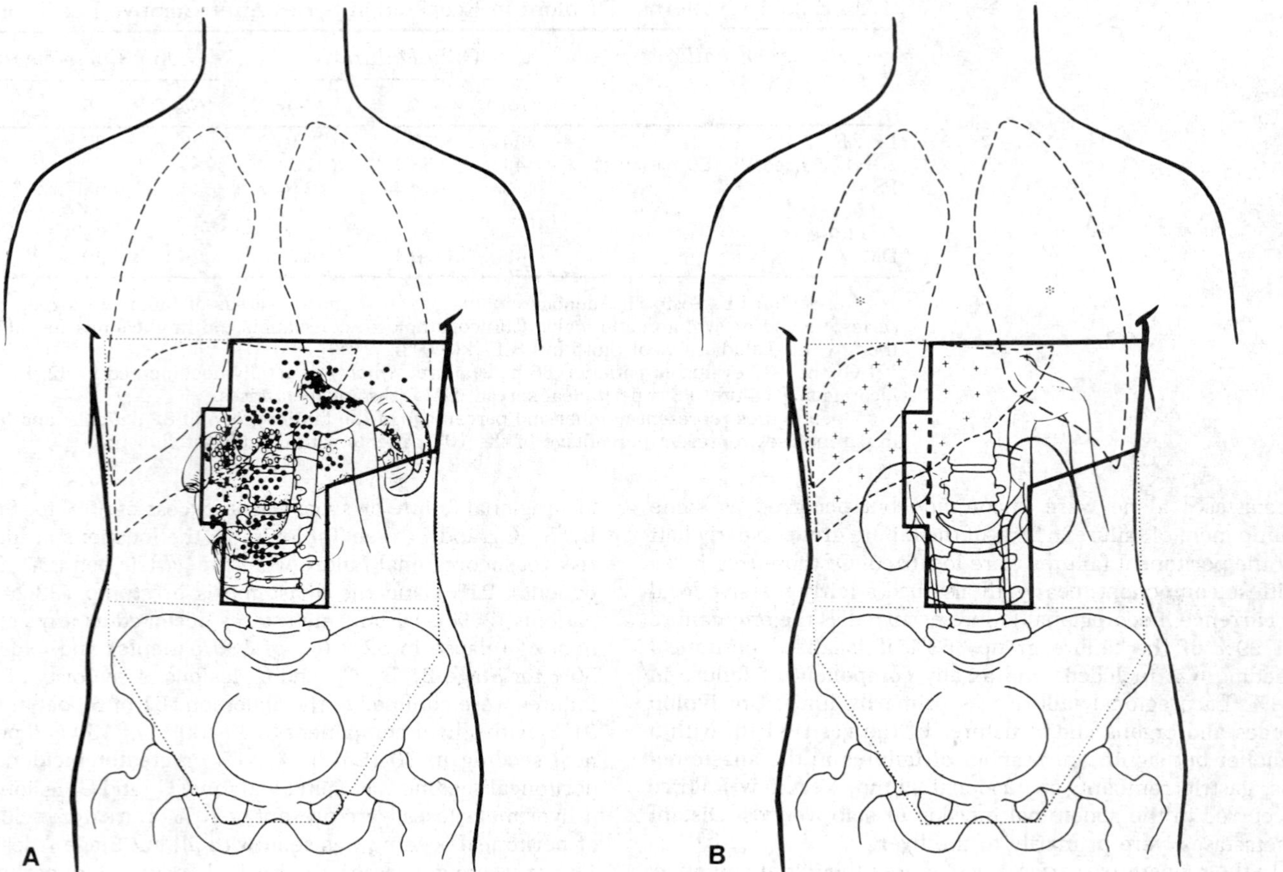

FIG. 25-2. Patterns of failure in the University of Minnesota reoperation series of 82 evaluable patients with evidence of gastric carcinoma after the initial operative procedure. Superimposed radiation portals: postsurgical gastric remnant, anastamoses, duodenal stump, gastric bed structures, and primary and secondary areas of lymph node drainage (*solid lines*), upper or total abdomen fields (*interrupted lines*), **A** • = local failures in surrounding organs or tissues; **B**, 0 = lymph node failures; * = lung metastasis; + = liver metastasis. Each marking indicates a single instance of such failure occurring alone or as any component except for lymph node failures where each major area of involvement is indicated.

unaware of their disease. Often patients present with a clinical picture that fails to trigger the proper diagnostic impressions in the physician's mind. Article after article stresses the "vague," "indefinite," "nonspecific" symptoms and then proceeds to list such things as epigastric uneasiness, mild anemia, fatigability, ulcer history, and weight loss. Clearly, none of these symptoms unequivocably indicates gastric cancer, and unless the clinician is alert to that possibility, the patient may be treated empirically for ulcer disease, not treated at all, or allowed to think there are no serious problems.[58-62]

Five different reviews covering the years 1950 to 1970 show essentially no change in the incidence of the key symptoms and show the vague, nonspecific nature of all of the findings in each individual study (Table 25-9).[49,58-61] The fact that the major presenting finding in some series could be a palpable mass in one third of the patients, ascites, or the less frequent findings of metastases to supraclavicular nodes or jaundice suggests that extensive disease can exist before the patient seeks medical help.

One study compared the incidence of the various symptoms in resectable versus nonresectable cases and found very little difference.[63] The same study evaluated extent of weight loss, duration of symptoms, and location of the tumor in the stomach in relation to symptoms. There were no differences in any of these parameters except for the relatively higher incidence of dysphagia and regurgitation with lesions located in the proximal stomach. Specific symptoms may indicate complicating factors in individual cases. For example, a patient with dysphagia may have a cardioesophageal junction lesion with partial obstruction from involvement of the distal esophagus. Patients with persistent nausea and vomiting, indicating bowel obstruction, may have several syndromes associated with gastric cancer.[11] An antral carcinoma may produce obstruction and gastric dilation. Gastric cancer occasionally invades the transverse mesocolon directly, result-

TABLE 25-6. Extent of Gastrectomy and Node Dissection Versus Patterns of Failure, Reoperation Series

		*Patterns of Failure**																	
		LF-RF						*PS*						*DM*					
		Alone			*Component*			*Alone*			*Component*			*Alone*			*Component*		
Operative† Procedure	*No. of Failure/ Total at Risk*	*No.*	*%*	*(%)*	*No.*	*%*	*(%)*	*No.*	*%*	*(%)*	*No.*	*%*	*(%)*	*No.*	*%*	*(%)*	*No.*	*%*	*(%)*
Subtotal gastrectomy	53/72	16	30	(22)	45	85	(63)	3	6	(4)	27	51	(38)	4	8	(6)	17	32	(24)
Method 1	25/36	9	36	(25)	23	92	(64)	1	4	(3)	12	48	(33)	0			7	28	(19)
Method 2	15/17	3	20	(18)	11	73	(65)	1	7	(6)	8	53	(47)	3	20	(18)	5	33	(29)
Method 3	13/19	4	31	(21)	11	85	(58)	1	8	(5)	7	54	(37)	1	8	(5)	5	39	(26)
Total gastrectomy	27/33	7	26	(21)	25	93	(76)	0			17	63	(52)	1	4	(3)	6	22	(18)
Method 1	0																		
Method 2	14/15	3	21	(20)	13	93	(87)	0			9	64	(60)	0			4	29	(27)
Method 3	13/18	4	31	(22)	12	92	(67)	0			8	62	(44)	1	8	(6)	2	15	(11)
Total	80/105	23	29	(22)	70	88	(67)	3	4	(3)	44	55	(42)	5	6	(5)	23	29	(22)

*Of the 86 patients with failure, 80 were evaluable by all parameters. Open figures represent number and percentage of the failure group, and figures in parentheses represent percentage of patients with complete follow-up. LF-RF, local-regional failure; PS, peritoneal spread; DM, distant metastases.

†Method 1 (pre-1950), subtotal or total gastrectomy, greater omentectomy, regional node dissection; method 2 (1950–1954), method 1 plus splenectomy, total omentectomy, additional node dissection regarding splenic suprapancreatic and central celiac axis; method 3 (1954 on), methods 1 and 2 plus extension of node dissection to porta hepatis and pancreaticoduodenal (intent: total lymph node dissection of all primary node areas).

ing in transverse colon obstruction. Patients who develop peritoneal dissemination with gastric cancer may have distal bowel obstruction. A Blumer's shelf resulting from metastatic gastric carcinoma can cause rectal obstruction.

By the time physical signs of gastric cancer are present, the disease is incurable. The commonly found physical findings with stomach cancer are direct manifestations of the pattern of spread of this disease, as outlined in Table 25-2. Gastric adenocarcinoma disseminates by both lymphatic and hematogenous routes. The earliest sites of lymphatic metastases are the regional nodes and clearly cannot be detected by physical examination. However, three sites of nodal metastases are detectable by examination. Careful evaluation of the supraclavicular fossae is necessary in cases of suspected gastric cancer. The finding of a firm left supraclavicular (Virchow's) node may allow a tissue diagnosis without abdominal exploration. Two less common sites of metastases are worth noting. Patients with systemic symptoms consistent with stomach cancer should undergo careful digital examination of the periumbilical area and left axilla. Gastric

TABLE 25-7. Extent of Gastrectomy and Node Dissection Versus Type of LF-RF, Reoperation Series

		*Any Component of LF-RF**											
		Gastric Bed			*Anastomosis or stumps*			*Abdomen or Stab Wound*			*Lymph Nodes*		
Operative† Procedure	*No. of Failure/ Total at Risk*	*No.*	*%*	*(%)*	*No.*	*%*	*(%)*	*No.*	*%*	*(%)*	*No.*	*%*	*(%)*
Subtotal gastrectomy	53/72	36	68	(50)	18	34	(25)	3	6	(4)	29	55	(40)
Method 1	25/36	18	72	(50)	13	52	(36)	0			11	44	(31)
Method 2	15/17	9	60	(53)	4	27	(24)	1	7	(6)	9	60	(53)
Method 3	13/19	9	69	(47)	1	8	(5)	2	15	(11)	9	69	(47)
Total gastrectomy	27/33	20	74	(61)	8	30	(24)	2	7	(6)	15	56	(45)
Method 1	0												
Method 2	14/15	10	71	(67)	5	36	(33)	1	7	(7)	11	79	(73)
Method 3	13/18	10	77	(56)	3	23	(17)	1	8	(6)	4	31	(22)
Total	80/105‡	56	70	(53)	26	33	(25)	5	6	(5)	44	55	(42)

*Open figures represent number and percent of the failure group, and numbers in parentheses represent percent of patients with complete follow-up. LF-RF, local-regional failure; PS, peritoneal spread; DM, distant metastases.

†For operative procedure, see Table 25-6.

‡An additional 6 patients had failure, but only 80 of 86 were evaluable for operative method and pattern of failure.

TABLE 25-8. Incidence and Patterns of Failure by Stage After Resection with Curative Intent, MGH Single Institution Study*

Stage†	*No. of Patients*	*Local Regional Failure*				*Distant Failure*					
		Only		*Total*		*Only*		*Total*		*Abdominal*‡	
		No.	*%*	*No.*	*%*	*No.*	*%*	*No.*	*%*	*No.*	*%*
A	4	0	(6)	0	(0)	0	(0)	0	(0)	0	(0)
B_1	16	1	(6)	3	(19)	3	(19)	5	(31)	5	(31)
B_2	12	1	(8)	6	(50)	1	(8)	6	(50)	6	(50)
B_3	5	0	(0)	2	(40)	1	(20)	3	(60)	3	(60)
C_1	17	2	(12)	4	(24)	3	(18)	5	(29)	4	(24)
C_2	44	10	(23)	16	(36)	18	(41)	24	(55)	21	(48)
C_3	32	7	(22)	18	(56)	13	(41)	24	(67)	22	(61)
Total	130	21	(16)	49	(38)	39	(40)	67	(52)	61	(47)

*Modified from Landry J, Tepper JE, Wood WL et al: Patterns of failure following curative resection of gastric carcinoma: ASTRO Proceedings 1986. Int J Radiat Oncol Biol Phys 12(1):119, 1986.
†Gunderson Sosin modification of Astler Coller system (see Ref. 56).
‡Abdominal = liver and peritoneal seeding.

cancer has been reported to metastasize to both these areas.[11] Nodular metastases to the umbilical area and left axillary lymph node metastases (Irish's node) should be searched for assiduously, since their presence allows a simple tissue diagnosis to be made in the patient with gastric cancer. Umbilical metastases may not be in lymph nodes but rather may represent peritoneal dissemination.

The most common site of hematogenous metastases in stomach cancer is the liver. Firm, smooth, or nodular hepatomegaly may be apparent on physical examination as an indication of hepatic metastases. Patients with locally extensive stomach cancer may have a palpable epigastric mass that may be mistaken for the left lobe of an enlarged liver, when it actually represents the gastric tumor itself.

Rarely does the patient with gastric carcinoma present with significant bleeding. Although minor blood loss that may be detected as occult blood in the stool is common in gastric cancer, massive upper GI bleeding is uncommon. In fact, the patient with a gastric mass and upper GI hemorrhage is more likely to have gastric leiomyosarcoma than adenocarcinoma of the stomach.[6,11] Hemorrhage in the absence of a gastric mass suggests benign gastric ulcer.

TABLE 25-9. Symptons of Gastric Carcinoma

Symptom	*La Due et al*[61] *(n = 1,121)*	*Adashek et al*[58] *(n = 501)*	*Goldsmith et al*[59] *(n = 270)*	*Clarke et al*[49] *(n = 250)*	*Kelsey*[60] *(n = 245)*
Weight loss	85	24	58	68	56
Pain	69	38	48	67	56
Vomiting	43	24	21	47	
Bowel symptoms	41		5		
Anorexia	30	4	21		
Dysphagia	20	13	17		9
Nausea	20		4	65	
Nausea and vomiting					38
Weakness	19	17			
Eructation	17				
Hematemesis	6	16	13	18	
Regurgitation	6				
Rapid satiation	5		2		
No symptoms	0.4			5	6

Syndromes of remote effects of carcinoma are rare with stomach cancer. This disease, however, does represent the most common visceral malignancy associated with acanthosis nigricans.[11] This syndrome is characterized by hypertrophic pigmented skin lesions, particularly noted in the axilla. Glucose intolerance also may be present. The syndrome of thrombotic nonbacterial endocarditis has been associated with gastric cancer but is not specific and may be seen in any patient with advanced wasting from malignant disease.

STAGING

As more sophisticated combined modality approaches have been used in the treatment of gastric cancer, staging has become more important. In the past, an informal staging scheme was used by physicians treating this disease. Thus, the surgeon at the time of operation determined the stage of the cancer, and this stage determined which treatment option might be useful. Therapy was dictated by stage: (1) completely resectable, (2) locally unresectable or only par-

TABLE 25-10. TNM Classification*

Primary Tumor (T)	
T_x	Minimum requirements to assess the primary tumor cannot be met.
T_0	No evidence of primary tumor.
T_{is}	Tumor limited to mucosa without penetration into the lamina propria.
T_1	Tumor limited to mucosa or mucosa and submucosa regardless of its extent (or location).
T_2	Tumor involves the mucosa and the submucosa (including the muscularis propria), and extends to or into the serosa but does not penetrate through the serosa.
T_3	Tumor penetrates through the serosa without invading contiguous structures.
T_{4a}	Tumor penetrates through the serosa and involves immediately adjacent tissues, such as lesser omentum, perigastric fat, regional ligaments, greater omentum, transverse colon, spleen, esophagus, or duodenum by way of intraluminal extension.
T_{4b}	Tumor penetrates through the serosa and involves the liver, diaphragm, pancreas, abdominal wall, adrenal glands, kidney, retroperitoneum, small intestine or esophagus, or duodenum by way of serosa.
Nodal Involvement (N)	
N_x	Minimum requirements to assess the regional nodes cannot be met.
N_0	No metastases to regional lymph nodes.
N_1	Involvement of perigastric lymph nodes within 3 cm of the primary tumor along the lesser or greater curvature.
N_2	Involvement of the regional lymph nodes more than 3 cm from the primary tumor, which are removed or removable at operation, including those located along the left gastric, splenic, celiac, and common hepatic arteries.
N_3	Involvement of other intra-abdominal lymph nodes, such as the para-aortic, hepatoduodenal, retropancreatic, and mesenteric nodes.
Distant Metastasis (M)	
M_x	Minimum requirements to assess the presence of distant metastasis cannot be met.
M_0	No (known) distant metastasis.
M_1	Distant metastasis present. Specify sites according to the following notations:
	Peritoneal PER
	Pulmonary PUL
	Osseous OSS
	Hepatic HEP
	Brain BRA
	Lymph nodes (above diaphragm or nonabdominal) LYM
	Bone marrow MAR
	Pleura PLE
	Skin SKI
	Eye EYE
	Other OTH
Stage Grouping	
Stage 0	T_{is}, N_0, M_0
Stage I	T_1, N_0, M_0
Stage II	T_2, T_3, N_0, M_0
Stage III	T_1–T_3, N_1, N_2, M_0
	T_{4a}, N_0–N_2; M_0
Stage IV	T_1–T_3, N_3, M_0
	T_{4b}, any N, M_0
	Any T, any N, M_1
Tumor Grade (G)	
G_1	Well differentiated
G_2	Moderately well differentiated
G_3–G_4	Poorly to very poorly differentiated.
Postgastrectomy Residual Tumor (R)	
R_0	No residual tumor
R_1	Microscopic residual tumor
R_2	Macroscopic residual tumor —Specify ________

Performance Status of Host (H)

	AJCC Performance	*ECOG Scale*	*Karnofsky Scale (%)*
H_0	Normal activity	0	90–100
H_1	Symptomatic but ambulatory, cares for self	1	70–80
H_2	Ambulatory more than 50% of time, occasionally needs assistance	2	50–60
H_3	Ambulatory 50% or less of time, nursing care needed	3	30–40
H_4	Bedridden, may need hospitalization	4	10–20

*Beahrs OH, Myers MH (eds): Manual for Staging of Cancer, p 67. Philadelphia, JB Lippincott, 1983.

tially resectable, indicating the use of radiation therapy, and (3) disseminated disease requiring chemotherapy.

More formal staging plans have been attempted during the last 50 years. In 1941, Coller and associates[48] reviewed 53 cases in detail in order to correlate lymphatic metastases and other features of primary lesions in the stomach. They divided the lymphatics into four zones, all four of which they recommended should be removed in all resectable cases. Their lymph node classification has served as the background for much that has been written about the staging of gastric cancer.

A suggestion for gross surgical classification of lesions of the stomach was advocated by Hoerr.[64,65] His original presentation and the subsequent reviews based on that classification have provided an additional means for studying the clinical significance of lesions in the stomach. This classification is based on the extent of invasion of the wall of the stomach and adjacent viscera, plus the extent of lymph node and distant involvement. Overall classification by this technique assists in determining whether a tumor is likely to be resectable and whether there is clear-cut evidence of distant spread. Another more recently proposed pathologic staging system is a modification of the Astler Coller system for stag-

TABLE 25-11. Five-Year Survival and Initial Stage of Gastric Cancer*

Extent of Disease	*5-Year Survival (%)*
Lymph nodes (−)	
Mucosa only	85
Mucosa and gastric wall	52
Through gastric wall	47
Lymph nodes (+)	
Extent of lymph node involvement	
Regional only	17
Other areas	5

*Data from Kennedy BJ: TNM classification for stomach cancer. Cancer 26:971, 1970.

ing colon cancer. This system, elaborated by Gunderson and Sosin,[56] gives the same type of information as the Hoerr[64,65] system and predicts failure rates after surgery.

The importance of the TNM classification (Table 25-10) has been established, and a review by Kennedy (Table 25-11) of 1241 patients demonstrated correlations between extent of disease (lymph node involvement, depth of penetration of the stomach by the lesion, presence of distant metastases) and survival.[66,67] More detailed clinicopathologic correlations have been provided by several large Japanese studies.[68,69] The system used by the Japanese as a basis for operative and adjuvant treatment staging should perhaps be considered for wider use in the United States in order to limit discrepancies in surgical staging. Such staging discrepancies may explain conflicting results in recently completed adjuvant multimodality treatment protocols.

Careful understanding of the patterns of dissemination as defined by staging systems may be helpful in dictating primary surgical therapy. Desmond[70] reviewed findings in 1363 cases and divided lymphatic drainage into seven different groups, with recommendations on appropriate surgical measures to be used for lesions involving any or all of these groups. The value of this approach will need to be confirmed in prospective studies. However, it should be emphasized that, although the simple staging of disease into "resectable," "locally advanced," and "disseminated" still has some descriptive value, use of a formalized staging plan such as the TNM system allows much more accurate comparison of different treatment results.

PROGNOSIS

The prognosis for patients with gastric cancer depends on the extent of the disease and on treatment. Extension of disease, whether local or regional, adversely affects survival. Until recently, only patients who had undergone complete excision of localized cancer had any potential for long-term survival. Lymph node involvement is an adverse prognostic factor. However, most important is the extent of nodal metastases. Minimal lymphatic involvement adjacent to the tumor has little if any adverse prognostic effect. Extensive and distant nodal metastases are very poor prognostic factors.

Experience with 1497 cases at a single hospital provides the background for a number of different evaluations of survival based on various forms of operative treatment.[45,46] The 5-year survival rate for all patients observed 5 years or more in this study was 7.45%. The best 5-year survival figure in the entire study — 30.3% — was in the relatively small group of 149 patients with localized disease. Dupont and associates[46] reviewed survival data in 18,767 gastric cancer patients from 11 series and found disappointing results. The 5-year survival rate varied from 4.7% to 16.9%, but only 4 of 11 series reported 5-year survival rates greater than 10%.

A detailed statistical study of 11,817 patients at the Mayo Clinic by ReMine and co-workers[71] demonstrated relationships among survival, size of lesion, age of patient at operation, operative mortality, year of operation, pathologic stage of the disease, and other features. An additional prognostic factor noted in recent trials is location of the tumor. The more proximal or gastroesophageal junction tumors are more ominous, stage for stage, than are body or distal gastric adenocarcinomas.[72] Since tumors with an intestinal (or glandular) histologic pattern are known to be less aggressive than those with a less differentiated structure, and since proximal gastric cancers may be more frequently composed of poorly differentiated tumor cells than the distal lesions,[73] it is difficult to distinguish the prognostic importance of site versus histologic variability. Prognosis is more clearly related to resectability. Recent data from the combined chemotherapy and radiation therapy regional treatment for locally advanced gastric carcinoma of the Gastrointestinal Tumor Study Group[74] implied that surgical resection of bulk disease may be the most important criterion for better patient survival with combined modality treatment. Approximately 25% of patients with known cancer who underwent resection for bulk disease were long-term survivors after continued radiation therapy and chemotherapy. Patients with unresected bulk disease had no survival benefit. Naturally, it is impossible to determine if the benefit in patients who had most of their tumor removed surgically was due simply to biologic selection or if the surgery itself improved the effectiveness of subsequent combined modality therapy. The keys to significant improvements in survival in the future will be more reliable diagnostic tests allowing the diagnosis to be established at a time when the disease is still confined to the stomach, and the application of aggressive combined modality therapy for earlier disease. The effects of the various forms of therapy on prognosis in gastric cancer will be dealt with in detail in other sections of this chapter. In addition, more recent survival data obtained from the various nontreatment control arms of completed and ongoing multi-institutional combined modality adjuvant trials will provide more updated survival figures on patients who are well staged.

DIAGNOSIS

A sequence of diagnostic procedures for gastric cancer is outlined in Table 25-12. In the past, the keystone of diagnosis of stomach cancer was the barium upper GI series.[11,75,76] Although most patients with gastric cancer present with relatively advanced disease, which should be detected by the conventional upper GI series, recently reported studies indicate this is not the case. Current information suggests that the barium upper GI series is now most useful as a tool to direct the endoscopist to the area of the

TABLE 25-12. Sequence of Diagnostic Procedures in Suspected Gastric Cancer

1. Physical examination
    - ? Lymph node metastasis → biopsy
    - ? Hepatomegaly → biopsy
    - ? Abdominal mass
2. Double contrast barium upper gastrointestinal series
3. Fiberoptic endoscopy with biopsy and cytology
4. Diagnostic/therapeutic laparotomy

stomach requiring careful examination and biopsy. A review of contemporary series that correlated roentgenographic findings with findings on endoscopic biopsy demonstrated that 9% to 40% of endoscopically positive lesions are not detected on previous barium studies.[76] These results suggest that, on the average, 10% of symptomatic carcinomas are missed in barium studies. An older study raised the question of faulty interpretation of abnormal findings on upper GI roentgenography.[75] This series reported data showing that 15% of malignant abnormalities may be misinterpreted as benign findings.

The diagnostic accuracy of barium roentgenography may be improved by the use of a double-contrast technique (Figs. 25-3 and 25-4).[76,77] This procedure makes use of high-density barium combined with an effervescent agent and glucagon administration to induce gastric atony. A double-contrast study allows careful evaluation of the proximal stomach, where malignant lesions are most likely to be missed by conventional barium studies. It should be emphasized that the vast majority of gastric ulcers should be examined endoscopically and biopsied. It is inappropriate to diagnose a gastric ulcer as benign solely on the basis of a barium study unless there is some compelling reason why upper GI endoscopy should not be performed.

With the advent of the flexible fiberoptic gastroscope, the preferred way to make a tissue diagnosis of gastric cancer has been by endoscopy to obtain material for either tissue biopsy or exfoliative cytology. Older studies reported wide variation in the success rate of endoscopic biopsy and cytology in gastric cancer.[11] In a review of several series, Bockus[78] reported positive cytologic findings in 37% to 97% of gastric cancer patients, with false-positive rates of 0.5% to 13%.[78] With improvement in both endoscopic technique and pathologic examination procedures, the success rate has improved. Winawer and colleagues[79,80] have pointed out several factors that bear on the likelihood of making a successful endoscopic tissue diagnosis. If the tumor mass is exophytic, endoscopy usually is successful in establishing a tissue diagnosis. In 24 (92%) of 26 such patients, Winawer et al obtained positive biopsy or cytologic brush pathology.[80] However, in 24 patients with infiltrative gastric cancer, the diagnosis was made in only 12 (50%). Other factors reducing the success of endoscopic biopsy are tumor diameter less than 3 cm, tumor location at the cardia or on the lesser curvature, and recurrent disease. In such unfavorable situations, lavage cytology may increase the accuracy of brush cytology or biopsy.[79] The use of endoscopic techniques in gastric cancer is described in greater detail in Chapter 20.

The recommended sequence for establishing a tissue diagnosis in the patient thought to have gastric cancer is the following: (1) careful physical examination for pathologic findings amenable to biopsy (nodal or liver involvement), (2) upper GI series with double contrast to establish the site of abnormality in the stomach, (3) endoscopy with biopsy and cytology, and (4) diagnostic/therapeutic laparotomy.

Other procedures that may be of ancillary use in cases of

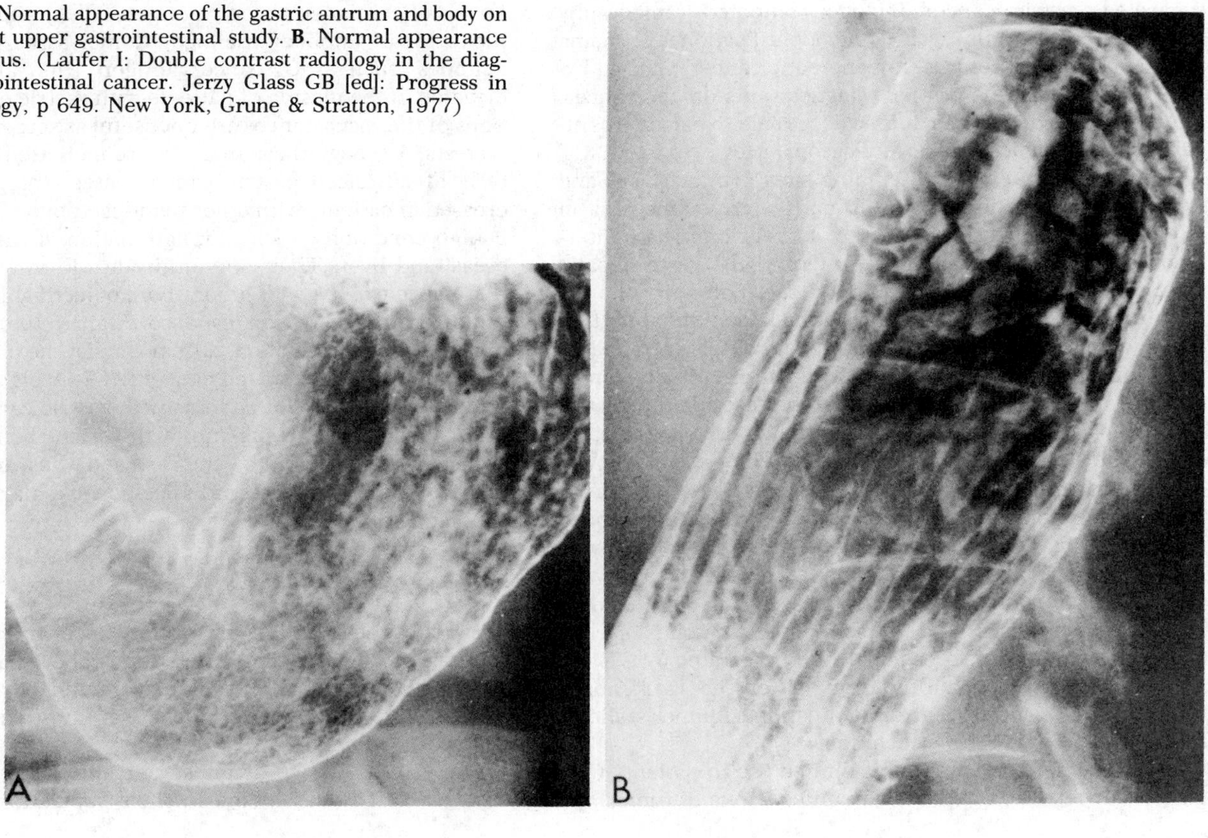

FIG. 25-3. **A**. Normal appearance of the gastric antrum and body on double-contrast upper gastrointestinal study. **B**. Normal appearance of gastric fundus. (Laufer I: Double contrast radiology in the diagnosis of gastrointestinal cancer. Jerzy Glass GB [ed]: Progress in Gastroenterology, p 649. New York, Grune & Stratton, 1977)

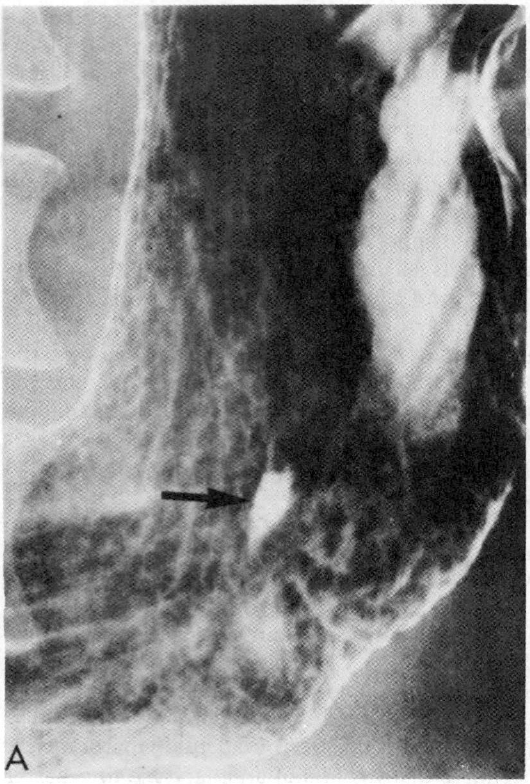

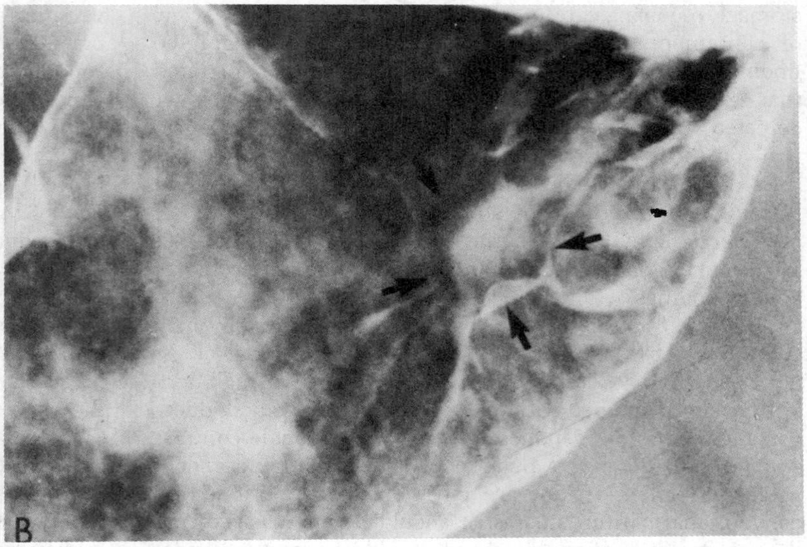

FIG. 25-4. **A**. Benign gastric ulcer on double-contrast UGI. The ulcer crater has smooth, sharply defined borders. **B**. Malignant gastric ulcer. Elevated irregular borders are present, and the ulcer crater is poorly circumscribed. (Laufer I: Double contrast radiology in the diagnosis of gastrointestinal cancer. In Jerzy Glass GB [ed]: Progress in Gastroenterology, p 652. New York, Grune & Stratton, 1977. By permission)

suspected gastric cancer include computed tomography (CT), ultrasonography (US), and identification of plasma tumor markers. In contrast to pancreatic cancer, CT and US are of little use in the primary diagnosis of stomach cancer, largely because the stomach is so accessible to barium roentgenographic studies and to endoscopy. However, both CT and US may be helpful in defining sites of metastases and extragastric extension.[81] This is particularly important in attempting to define surgical resectability. Complete obliteration of the lesser sac or involvement of the gastrohepatic tissues by direct extension of gastric carcinoma may be determined with CT or US. Tumors of the lesser curvature that encircle the left gastric and celiac vessels are also reasonably well defined by these techniques. This information is important for any surgeon attempting to circumscribe the gastric cancer, particularly in a patient known to have distant spread. For instance, in a patient with a biopsy-proven Virchow's node and CT evidence of extensive lesser sac tumor, palliative surgical attempts might not be appropriate prior to the use of chemotherapy or combined modality therapy to improve resectablity. The liver may also be evaluated with CT or US, along with radionuclide scanning, to elucidate suspected metastases. More disseminated peritoneal spread of gastric carcinoma is occasionally demonstrated by CT and US. Pelvic masses resulting from either the Krukenberg tumor or pelvic peritoneal dissemination (Blumer's shelf) may be detected by these techniques.

Plasma tumor markers are of limited use in patients with gastric cancer who have other manifestations of tumor.[82,83] Levels of carcinoembryonic antigen (CEA) and some newer monoclonal antibody–defined, tumor-associated antigen epitopes, such as GI cancer antigen 19-9, are frequently elevated in the plasma of patients with gastric cancer. Elevations of these substances are not useful as screening diagnostic tests. Although these markers are increased in more than 50% of advanced gastric cancer cases, they are also increased in patients with other manifestations of tumor and in benign conditions, such as inflammation of the bowel, pancreas, and liver. Their only utility lies in serial evaluations that may correlate with other, more objectifiable evidence of tumor growth or tumor response. Alpha-fetoprotein (AFP), another oncofetal protein, does not assist the clinician in the early diagnosis of stomach cancer. AFP levels are increased in only 15% to 20% of patients with gastric carcinoma; they are also increased in patients with various benign diseases, including cirrhosis and hepatitis, and thus are associated with both false-negative and false-positive diagnoses of gastric cancer.

SCREENING

Because of the extent of the gastric cancer problem in some countries other than the United States, there has been interest in developing techniques of screening to detect early lesions. Screening methods have been most extensively developed in Japan.

The Japanese have demonstrated the value of mass surveys for gastric carcinoma in their population. They have detected early cancers through mass upper GI surveys using sophisticated endoscopic and radiologic techniques.[84] These techniques undoubtedly are useful in a cancer-prone population such as exists in Japan.

The ultimate aim of screening programs is to decrease the mortality from gastric cancer. The Japanese have succeeded in this endeavor. Operative attempts are highly successful when gastric cancer is limited to the mucosa, but the incidence of such early lesions is less than 5% in most U.S. series. In Japan, the incidence of lesions initially confined to the mucosa or submucosa was only 3.8% in the years 1955 to 1956, but, because of screening procedures, this figure had increased to 34.5% by 1966, with a corresponding survival rate of 90.9%.[85]

TREATMENT

Gastric cancer treatment uses three therapeutic modalities: surgery, radiation therapy, and chemotherapy. The choice of an individual treatment and the appropriate combination of treatments depends on the stage of disease. Patients with localized gastric cancer are candidates for surgery with curative intent with or without adjunctive chemotherapy or irradiation. Patients with unresectable, partially resectable, or disseminated cancer require treatment designed around chemotherapy with or without irradiation or palliative surgery. The treatment section of this chapter examines the therapeutic options in the management of the patient with gastric cancer in relation to the stage of disease with which the patient presents.

SURGICAL MANAGEMENT OF LOCALIZED GASTRIC CANCER

The most favorable gastric cancer is a fully resectable tumor confined to the stomach. The major treatment modality in such cases is surgery.

Surgical procedures for gastric cancer should be based on anatomical considerations, knowledge of the natural history of the disease, and specific surgical goals—curative or palliative—in a particular case. Increased demands for more detailed surgical–pathologic correlation, particularly in the setting of adjuvant multimodality treatment protocols, will increase the need for appropriate staging as exemplified by the extensive surgical staging procedures of the Japanese protocols. Because the stomach is not vital to a normal life span, the surgical procedure can involve anything up to and including a total gastrectomy (Fig. 25-5). Resection also can entail removal of the omentum, removal of the spleen, removal of the distal portion of the esophagus, removal of the proximal portion of the duodenum, and even simultaneous removal of a portion of the transverse colon. Although such an extensive procedure is not recommended as a routine, experience has indicated that any or all of these structures can be removed without jeopardizing the patient's long-term survival. Lesser resections of the stomach are anatomically, surgically, and oncologically possible, and the extent of the resection can be determined partly by the extent of the lesion and partly by knowledge of its usual pathways of extension.

For most of the 20th century the preferred treatment for gastric carcinoma has been some form of radical subtotal gastrectomy (Fig. 25-6). There have been significant swings in opinion toward and away from total gastrectomy as the

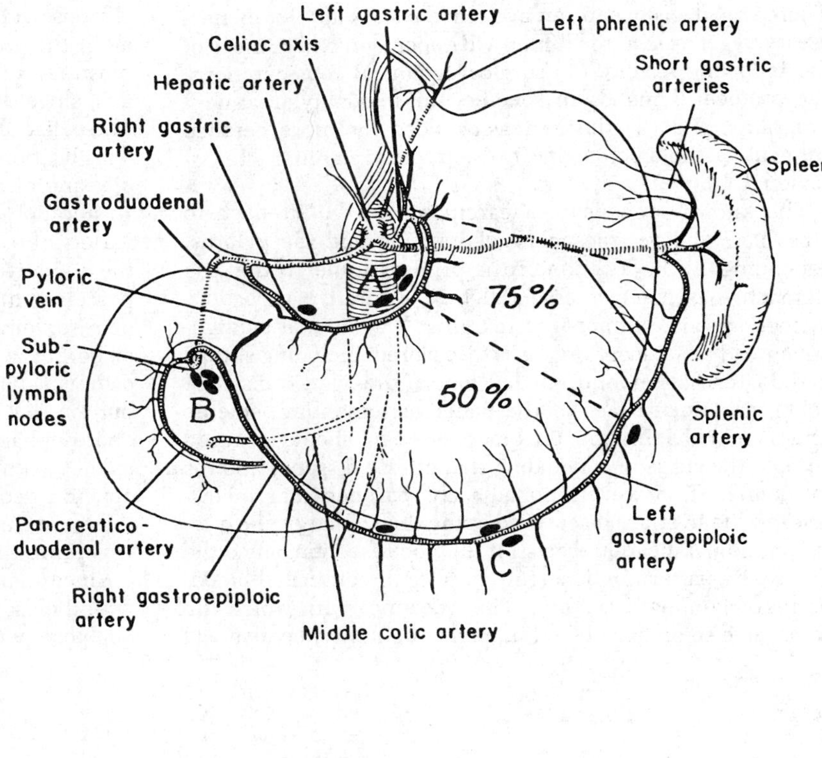

FIG. 25-5. Vascular supply and lymphatic drainage of the stomach in relation to the extent of gastrectomy commonly used in gastric cancer. Proximal resection margins for 50% and 75% subtotal gastrectomies are indicated. (Zollinger RM, Zollinger RM Jr: Atlas of Surgical Operations, 4th ed, plate XIX, no 1. New York, Macmillan, 1977. Copyright ©, 1975 by Macmillan Publishing Co., Inc.)

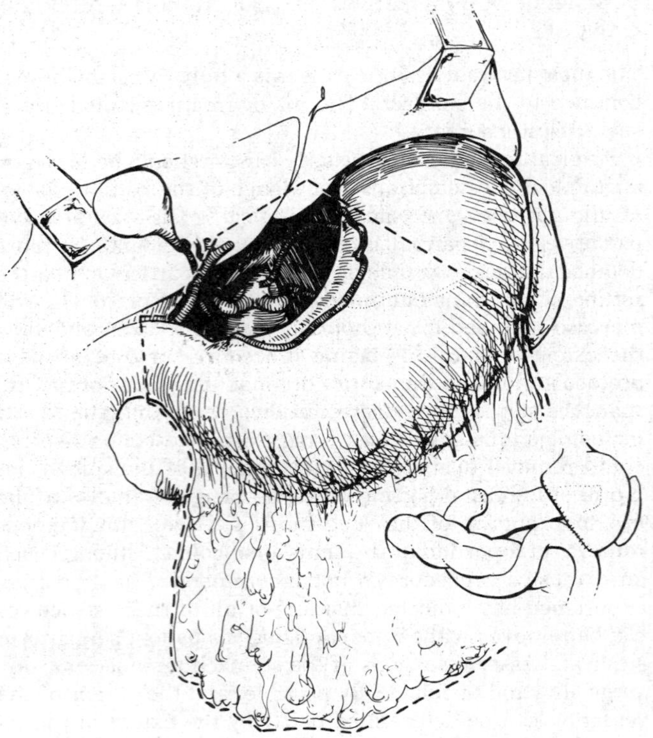

FIG. 25-6. Extent of resection margins of radical subtotal gastrectomy for distal gastric carcinoma. Inset shows appearance after anastomoses have been performed.

treatment of choice, and this has been coupled with various extensions of total gastrectomy that have been advocated from time to time.[86–92] At present, there is no evidence that surgery beyond that necessary to encompass all gross and microscopic disease will increase the chances of cure. Therefore, decisions to remove more than is absolutely necessary to get around the tumor will depend on one or more of the following factors: (1) surgical technical considerations, (2) protocol demands in specific multimodality treatment programs, and (3) the increasing need for more detailed surgical–pathologic staging to help analyze initial sites of regional failure.

The known propensity of carcinoma of the stomach to cross both the gastroesophagael junction and the pylorus, depending on the location of the primary tumor within the stomach, has made it essential that a curative procedure include adequate tumor-free margins. If additional contiguous spread to adjacent organs is discovered, including spread to the lateral segment of the left lobe of the liver, transverse colon, anterior surface of the pancreas, omentum, splenic hilum, and diaphragm, en bloc resection should proceed without the surgeon concluding that diffuse dissemination is inevitable. If, however, nonadjacent parenchymal metastases in the liver are discovered at the time of surgical exploration, no justification exists for en bloc resection, since the metastatic pattern undoubtedly implies disseminated bloodborne or lymphatic seeding. The frequency with which the transverse colon or its blood supply, or both, may be involved makes it mandatory that the colon be appropriately prepared before any elective procedure on a patient suspected of having carcinoma of the stomach.

Almost every retrospective study on the surgical treatment of patients with gastric carcinoma has found that the morbidity and mortality are higher than expected, which emphasizes the importance of careful preoperative evaluation and patient preparation. In addition to all the standard studies that one should do before any major abdominal procedure, certain other considerations are of major importance in the patient with gastric cancer. Appropriate studies, beyond history and physical examination, should be completed to determine if there is any evidence of distant metastases. Chest roentgenography and physical examination for hepatic and splenic enlargement should be followed by scans of the liver or spleen if there is any suggestion of involvement of these organs. Since anemia and weight loss are common accompaniments of gastric cancer, appropriate blood cell counts, serum protein studies, and evaluations of liver function should be completed. Replacement of blood volume, red cell mass, and protein stores should be accomplished insofar as possible. Depending on the patient's preoperative cancer-related cachexia, hyperalimentation may be considered as a part of the preoperative preparation. However, parenteral or enteral alimentation should be reserved only for the patient who will be undergoing an appropriate palliative or curative surgical attempt. Under no circumstances should nutritional support be considered if no appropriate palliative or curative therapy is contemplated.

The major procedures used for curative attempts in gastric cancer are total gastrectomy and some modification of a radical subtotal gastrectomy. A brief outline of the operative and postoperative problems associated with each of these procedures follows.

A total gastrectomy should entail removal of the entire stomach, as much of the adjacent duodenum or esophagus as is indicated by the location of the primary tumor and by obvious evidence of its spread into the organ in question, and all of the greater omentum. The spleen may be removed in most cases if the lesion is in the proximal half of the stomach, since this results in the most complete node dissection. The celiac axis should be dissected as completely as possible, with ligation of the major vessels at as high a level as possible, and dissection of the hepatic artery as far as possible. Restoration of GI continuity can be achieved by any one of a variety of techniques, depending on the patient's response to the operative procedure, the length of the operation, and the perceived importance of providing a substitute gastric pouch or reservoir at the time of the initial procedure. If it is decided not to make a pouch, an end-to-end esophagoduodenostomy can be fashioned in some cases, or, if this appears to put too much tension on the anastomosis, either an end-to-end esophagojejunostomy or an end-to-side esophagojejunostomy with or without a Roux-en-Y loop should be carried out. If a decision is made at the outset to fashion a pouch, there are a number of pouches which can be utilized, some of which are illustrated in Figure 25-7.

Since many of these procedures involve an anastomosis with the esophagus, a major problem is leak. Leak is a serious postoperative complication and can be avoided by pre-

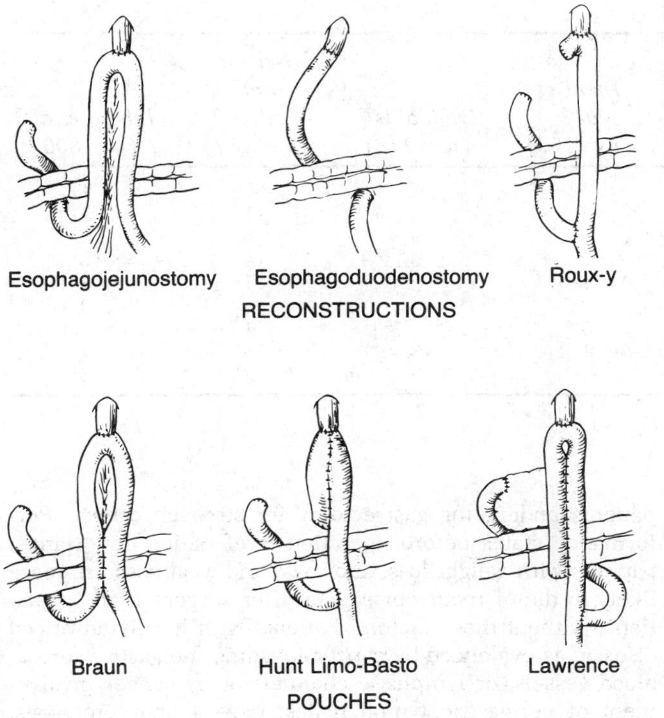

FIG. 25-7. Major variations in types of reconstructions possible after total gastrectomy. Examples of gastric reservoir pouches that can be used to increase the capacity of the substitute stomach after a total gastrectomy.

serving a rim of proximal stomach if the gross and microscopic examination of margins confirms that the tumor has been completely resected. Additional techniques for decreasing the probability of a leak have to do with good surgical technique, regardless of whether hand-sewn anastomoses or automatic stapling devices are used for reconstructing GI continuity. If a gastric cancer involves a sufficient portion of the stomach to require a total gastrectomy, that is the procedure of choice. It must be emphasized, however, that the extent of operation is determined by the surgical goal: resection of all of the tumor. Increasing the amount of stomach or adjacent tissue removed when excising a small tumor has not demonstrated superior curative potential compared to a resection that simply encompasses the tumor.[45] If frozen section examination of surgical margins has shown microscopic clearance but permanent histologic evaluation contradicts the earlier results, the surgeon should not reoperate to obtain microscopically clear disease. There is no evidence that such a reoperation will increase the curative potential in such a setting, and the morbidity and mortality of a second procedure will not be justified.

The preferred treatment for gastric carcinoma, particularly for a lesion located in the distal half of the stomach, is a subtotal resection of the stomach that adequately removes the tumor (see Fig. 25-6). This often includes removal of 80% to 85% of the stomach, the omentum, the first portion of the duodenum, and node-bearing tissue of the hepaticoduodenal pedicle, the gastrohepatic omentum, and the gastrocolic omentum. The spleen should be removed only if there is direct evidence of spread to the spleen or to the splenic nodes, or if the lesion is encroaching on the proximal half of the stomach. For cancers involving the proximal stomach or cardioesophageal junction, a variant of the radical subtotal gastrectomy, the proximal subtotal gastrectomy, should be performed.[6] This procedure may require an abdominal or thoracoabdominal surgical approach.

Many individual investigators have attempted to determine whether one or another type of surgical procedure gives the best curative result. Almost all of these experiences are retrospective or, at best, prospective nonrandomized studies. The evaluation of survival figures in such trials is biased, and conclusions concerning a best surgical approach will reflect mainly the contribution of biologic selection. Thus, such trials as reported from the Charity Hospital indicating that radical subtotal gastrectomy gives the best survival results (Fig. 25-8)[45] should be cautiously interpreted. No randomized trials have shown that one or another type of surgical resection will increase the cure rate as long as all the gastric cancer is removed. Design of surgery should be based on techniques that allow safe removal of all tumor, meet the specific demands of combined modality treatment or surgical staging protocols, palliate the patient's symptoms (bleeding, obstruction), and produce the least surgical mortality and morbidity (Table 25-13).[93–98]

Since there is often involvement of the transverse colon or its blood supply, and since this involvement does not contraindicate resection, adequate mechanical and antibiotic preparation of the large bowel should be performed preoperatively in every patient undergoing an elective procedure for removal of stomach cancer. Additional adjacent organs may be involved by contiguous extension of the tumor, not neces-

FIG. 25-8. Survival, computed by the life-table method, after various procedures for adenocarcinoma of the stomach. (Dupont JB, Cohn I: Gastric adenocarcinoma. Curr Probl Cancer 4:25, 1980)

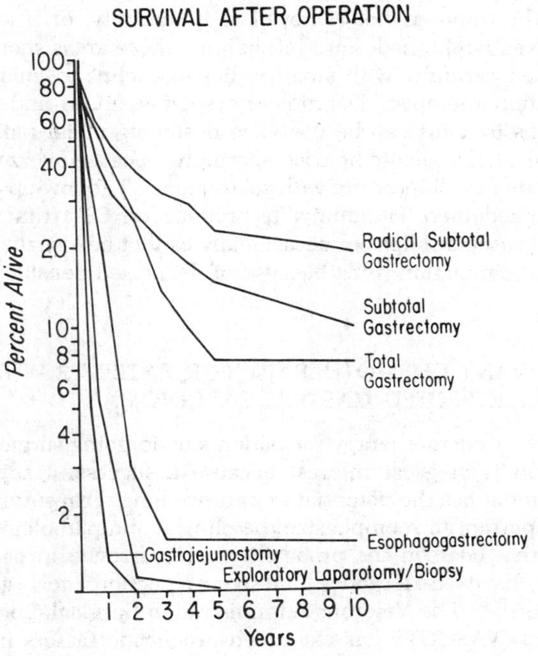

TABLE 25-13. Postoperative Complications

Complication	*CHNO** (*n* = 130)	*Adashek et al*[58] (*n* = 369)	*Ekbom and Gleysteen*[94] (*n* = 144)	*Diehl et al*[95] (*n* = 150)	*Lygidakis*[96] (*n* = 118)	*Nelson and Collier*[97] (*n* = 187)	*Inberg et al*[98] (*n* = 305)
	%	%	%	%	%	%	%
Pulmonary	55	11		3	3	11	9
Infectious	22		3	5	9	5	9
Anastomotic	21	9	18	3	8	14	12
Cardiac	10	6		1		1	3
Renal	8	1		0.5			0.3
Bleeding	5	4	4	0.5		1	0.3
Pulmonary embolus	4	1		1	3	3	4
Miscellaneous	5	1	6		3	2	3

* Charity Hospital of Louisiana at New Orleans.

sarily implying disseminated blood-borne or lymphatic metastases. En bloc resection of these structures should be part of the curative or palliative approach, and appropriate preoperative preparation, according to results of noninvasive staging procedures, should be individualized. Only in the case of complete obliteration of the lesser sac, as defined by CT or US, should the symptomatic gastric cancer be considered inoperable or unresectable prior to a laparotomy.

A specific point of surgical concern is the finding of disease in the lateral segment of the left lobe of the liver. If disease in this location is thought to represent contiguous extension, it is reasonable to remove the segment of the involved liver during the gastric resection. Attention must be paid to the aberrant arterial anatomy in a minority of patients whose left hepatic blood flow occurs from the left gastric artery. If this is not noted at the time of surgery, the lateral and medial segments of the left lobe may necrose, resulting in abscess formation, a long postoperative convalescence, and often multiple reoperations.

If the tumor is not removed in its entirety, or if known involved lymph nodes are left behind, these areas should be marked carefully with small radiopaque clips to guide the radiation therapist. Defining the splenic hilum and porta hepatis by clips can be useful in designing nodal radiation portals. Clips should be used sparingly, because overzealous placement will interfere with subsequent CT follow-up of the upper abdomen. Titanium clips produce less CT artifact than small vascular clips but occasionally cannot be visualized on lateral simulation films because of decreased density.

ADJUVANT CHEMOTHERAPY FOR PATIENTS WITH FULLY RESECTED GASTRIC CARCINOMA

Adjuvant chemotherapy for patients undergoing surgical resection is of great interest because a successful adjuvant treatment has the potential to improve long-term survival. It is important to reemphasize the clinical and pathologic factors that bear on the probability of recurrence in patients who have undergone curative resection for gastric cancer.[17,93] The Veterans Administration Surgical Oncology Group (VASOG)[93] has examined prognostic factors in 503 patients undergoing gastrectomy for stomach cancer. Performance status before operation is of major importance: patients with weight loss, anorexia, and weakness are more likely to die of recurrent cancer after surgery than are patients without these factors. Patients with locally advanced disease, as evidenced by cancer invading the gastric serosa, blood vessels, or lymphatic channels or by cancer involvement of perigastric lymph nodes, have a poor prognosis. Patients with extensive evidence of such local invasion have a less than 20% probability of being cured by gastric resection. A proximal location of the primary tumor in the stomach, necessitating a total gastrectomy, is an adverse prognostic factor. In the Veterans Administration studies,[93] only 15% of patients requiring proximal or total gastrectomies for resectable gastric cancer survived 5 years, as opposed to approximately 30% of those who had distal gastrectomies. The pathologic characteristics of the primary tumor are important in predicting survival. Only 2% of patients with linitis plastica survived 5 years after resection.

Most well-designed adjuvant chemotherapy studies that have been reported have failed to show significant benefit for treatment with chemotherapy. Table 25-14 describes a series of studies in which a large number of patients were evaluated.[72,99–104] In an adjuvant therapy study it is exceedingly important that a prospectively randomized design be used. Only in this way can one be assured of balancing prognostic factors between treatment and control groups. All of the studies detailed in Table 25-14 were prospectively randomized controlled trials of chemotherapy versus surgery alone. In the United States, VASOG was a pioneer in performing these studies. The data from this group have shown that single-agent chemotherapy with thiotepa or fluorodeoxyuridine (FUdR) fails to influence disease-free survival at 5 years after resection.[99,100] In the thiotepa study, treatment with chemotherapy appeared to influence survival adversely; however, the difference was not significant.[99]

Because of the high incidence of gastric cancer in Japan, there has been great interest in the surgical adjuvant therapy of the disease in that country. Table 25-14 describes a recent randomized controlled trial in which 223 patients were entered. Patients treated with adjuvant chemotherapy had a better disease-free survival rate than those treated with sur-

TABLE 25-14. Surgical Adjuvant Chemotherapy of Gastric Cancer

Group	*No. of Patients*	*Treatment*	*Randomized Untreated Controls*	*Survival Benefit for Treated Group*	*Reference*
VASOG	73	Thiotepa vs. control	Yes	No 5-Year Survival: *Treated* 25.5% *Control* 33.7%	99
	276	FudR vs. control	Yes	No 5-Year Survival: *Treated* 23.9% *Control* 21.3%	100
	134	5-FU + methyl-CCNU vs. control	Yes	No 4-Year Survival: *Treated* 37.8% *Control* 38.9%	101
GITSG	142	5-FU + methyl-CCNU vs. control	Yes	Survival (4-year median follow-up): *Treated* 59% *Control* 44% ($p < 0.03$)	72
ECOG	160	5-FU + methyl-CCNU vs. control	Yes	Survival (4-year median follow-up): *Treated* 44% *Control* 47% ($p = 0.68$)	102
SWOG	180	FAM vs. control	Yes	See text	103
MAOP	300	FAM vs. control	Yes	See text	
International gastric adjuvant study NCCTG	120	5-FU + doxorubicin vs. control	Yes	Survival (4-year median follow-up): *Treated* 52% *Control* 51% ($p = 0.49$)	103a
Cancer Institute of Toyko	73	Mitomycin C + Ara-C + 5-FU vs.	Yes	68% 5-yr survival	104
	76	Mitomycin-C + Ftorafur Ara-C vs.		63% 5-yr survival	
	74	Control		51% 5-yr survival	

VASOG = Veterans Administration Surgical Oncology Group; GITSG = Gastrointestinal Tumor Study Group; ECOG = Eastern Cooperative Oncology Group; SWOG = Southwest Oncology Group; HAOP = Mid-Atlantic Oncology Program; NCCTG = North Central Cancer Treatment Group. 5-FU = 5-fluorouracil; FudR = fluorodeoxyuridine.

gery alone. This result is at odds with results of other studies, and it is important to be aware that the biology of gastric cancer, the stage at diagnosis, and the natural history of this disease may differ between the United States and Japan. Thus, the benefits of Japanese treatment strategies must be confirmed in U.S. studies before treatments are adopted for noninvestigational use.

Both the Gastrointestinal Tumor Study Group (GITSG)[72] and the Eastern Cooperative Oncology Group (ECOG)[102] have reported adjuvant chemotherapy studies using 5-fluorouracil (5-FU) + methyl-CCNU. Both of these studies were prospectively controlled randomized clinical trials initiated in the mid-1970s when 5-FU + methyl-CCNU was thought to produce objective remission in approximately 40% of patients with advanced gastric cancer. The current analysis of these two studies reveals differing results. The GITSG program showed statistical benefit for treatment, the ECOG study did not. The VASOG also performed a Phase III study of 5-FU + methyl-CCNU as adjuvant therapy for gastric cancer and found no benefit with such treatment.[101] It is not clear why the GITSG trial demonstrated benefit and the ECOG and VASOG studies did not.

Table 25-14 also shows that two randomized comparisons of 5-FU, doxorubicin (Adriamycin), and mitomycin C (FAM), an active treatment in advanced gastric cancer, have been performed. The Middle Atlantic Oncology Group (MAOP) study has 300 patients enrolled and evaluable. The Southwest Oncology Group (SWOG) study has 180 patients enrolled. An interim report of the SWOG trial showed no significant differences in relapse rate and survival between patients receiving postoperative FAM and those receiving no additional therapy.[103] This study is ongoing and will require more time for data accrual. The value of adjuvant therapy for gastric cancer is unproved at present, and such treatment cannot be recommended as a routine in patients who have undergone surgical resection.

The adjuvant therapy studies that have been completed have demonstrated the need to have a surgery-only control group. It may be noted from the 5-FU + methyl-CCNU studies that the surgery-only groups have disease-free survival rates of 39% to 47%. If the 20% survivals of "historical controls" in these studies were compared with survival in the treatment arms, all three would be considered to demonstrate improved survival.

MEDICAL MANAGEMENT OF PATIENTS WITH GASTRIC RESECTION

Patients with stomach cancer have all had major disruptions of the GI tract. Patients who have undergone significant gastric resection may have special metabolic problems. The syndromes associated with gastric resection have been reviewed by Lawrence.[105] The most common complication of total gastric resection is the dumping syndrome. This symptom complex results from lack of antral function and includes epigastric fullness, hyperperistalsis, borborygmi, cramps, and occasionally nausea, vomiting, and diarrhea. Other subjective postprandial complaints include diaphoresis, tachycardia, weakness, and dizziness. The mechanisms of the dumping syndrome are due to major fluid shift out of the intravascular space and into the bowel after the sudden dumping of hypertonic foodstuffs into the small bowel in gastrectomized patients.

High-carbohydrate meals, which are most likely to be hyperosmolar, increase symptoms. Many of the symptoms of the dumping syndrome may be produced by the release of serotonin, and antiserotonin agents occasionally may ameliorate the syndrome. Symptomatic therapy for the patient with the dumping syndrome centers on decreasing the osmotic load presented to the small bowel. Small, frequent feedings of low-carbohydrate, high-protein meals usually will improve symptoms. A high fat content in the diet is useful because the high caloric value of fat makes it easier to provide the patient with adequate calories.

All patients who have undergone gastric resection eventually become deficient in vitamin B_{12}, since the stomach produces the intrinsic factor necessary for distal ileal absorption of this vitamin. Because of liver storage of vitamin B_{12}, megaloblastic anemia may not occur for up to 4 years after gastric resection. The administration of 100 μg of this vitamin every month will prevent deficiency.

Less commonly, patients who have undergone a gastrectomy may manifest malabsorption from the afferent or blind loop syndrome.[105] A blind loop of bowel is one that allows ingress of bowel contents but not adequate egress. Bacterial overgrowth may occur, with bacterial metabolism of bile acids resulting in malabsorption. Antibiotic therapy may be helpful in this situation.

All patients with gastric cancer who are undergoing active treatment by surgery, radiation therapy, or chemotherapy and who are manifesting significant malnutrition ($>10\%$ weight loss, albumin < 2.5 g/100 ml) should be considered for nutritional support. It makes no sense to support nutritionally a patient with advanced gastric cancer who has failed to respond to appropriate therapy. However, if poor nutritional status itself prevents the optimal application of a potentially useful treatment, nutritional support should be provided. Either parenteral or enteral hypernutrition may be used; both are described in Chapter 59, section 1.

TREATMENT OF LOCALLY UNRESECTABLE OR LOCALLY RECURRENT GASTRIC CANCER

Patients with stomach cancer frequently have advanced local tumors that are either unresectable or only partially resectable. Patients with completely resected gastric cancer may also have a tumor recur in the gastric bed and require management of locally advanced stomach carcinoma. The major issues facing clinicians dealing with locally advanced or recurrent gastric tumors are (1) what is the role of surgery in these patients, (2) how does one coordinate surgery with radiation therapy and cytotoxic chemotherapy in the management of these patients?

Because surgical resection is the curative treatment for gastric carcinoma, the disease should be considered operable and potentially resectable until proved otherwise. The patient whose stomach is involved with extensive local tumor on roentgenographic examination, one with evidence of widespread metastatic involvement, or one with ascites on the basis of peritoneal carcinomatosis should be considered to have an inoperable cancer. The presence of a Virchow's node or other evidence of lymphatic dissemination does not make the cancer inoperable, although it is likely to be incurable with present methods of therapy. The gastric lesion should not be considered unresectable until operation proves it so. As long as the stomach is mobile or the stomach and the organs to which it has become adherent can be removed without compromising the patient's survival, every attempt should be made to resect the primary lesion regardless of its size and the other organs involved. Leaving behind a mass lesion in the stomach is an open invitation to bleeding, perforation, or further obstruction and greatly diminishes the likelihood of success with adjuvant therapy.[106] Not only can removal of the primary tumor reduce the bulk and thereby improve the chances for chemotherapy, it also diminishes the likelihood of the other complications just named. Thus, whenever possible, a lesion in the stomach should be removed, even if this is done for purposes of palliation. Both the surgeon and the patient or the patient's family should be aware of the difference between an attempted curative procedure and a palliative one; nevertheless, a vigorous attempt at palliation is justified.

Many investigators have proved the inefficacy of various bypass procedures if the tumor cannot be removed. The surgeon should be wary of being pressured to "do something" surgically in patients with obstructing unresectable gastric cancer. A recent review of the Charity Hospital experience in New Orleans has concluded correctly that palliative bypass procedures do not increase survival and probably do not increase the quality of life.[45,46,66] The physiologic mechanism of inadequate relief of obstruction is not understood, but results are unsatisfactory regardless of the surgical techniques utilized to bypass unresectable gastric carcinomas.

Although as previously described, palliative gastrectomy is reasonable, a total gastrectomy should not be undertaken as a palliative procedure. The palliation achieved with a total gastrectomy is not good, and the mortality and morbidity of the procedure are too high to justify its use as a palliative procedure.

RADIATION THERAPY

Radiation therapy, usually in conjunction with chemotherapy, plays a major role in patients with locally advanced or recurrent stomach cancer. The effective use of radiation in patients with gastric cancer depends on defining in which clinical situation this modality will be most useful and on developing plans of treatment with tolerable morbidity. This section addresses considerations in planning and executing the radiotherapeutic management of gastric cancer, then reviews the results of existing studies.

The patterns of locoregional failures in the University of Minnesota reoperative group[56] were in a distribution suitable for inclusion within a shaped radiation portal (see Fig. 25-2), which should be modified according to the initial extent of the disease. In Figures 25-9 and 25-10, these portals are superimposed on the limiting organs of tolerance. With accurate field definition, aided by clip placement in the splenic hilum and porta hepatis, one half to two thirds of the left kidney could be spared in many patients, and inclusion of the porta hepatis and retroduodenal areas would include only a minor portion of the right kidney.

Dose-limiting organs and structures in the upper abdomen (stomach, small intestine, liver, kidneys, and spinal cord) are numerous. Because of the posterior extent of the gastric fundus, it is impractical to use lateral portals routinely for a portion of treatment, as is done with tumors of the head of

FIG. 25-9. Potential radiation portals are superimposed on organs and structures of tolerance (gastric remnant, duodenal stump, jejunum, liver, kidneys, spinal cord, and spinal and pelvic marrow).

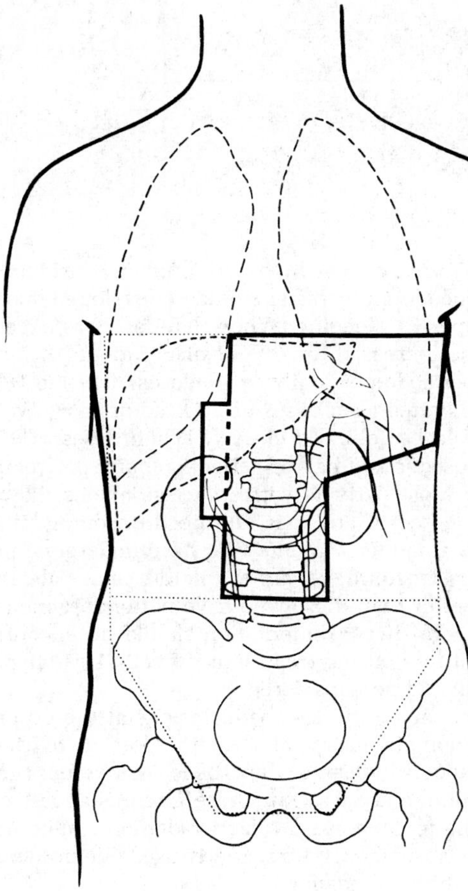

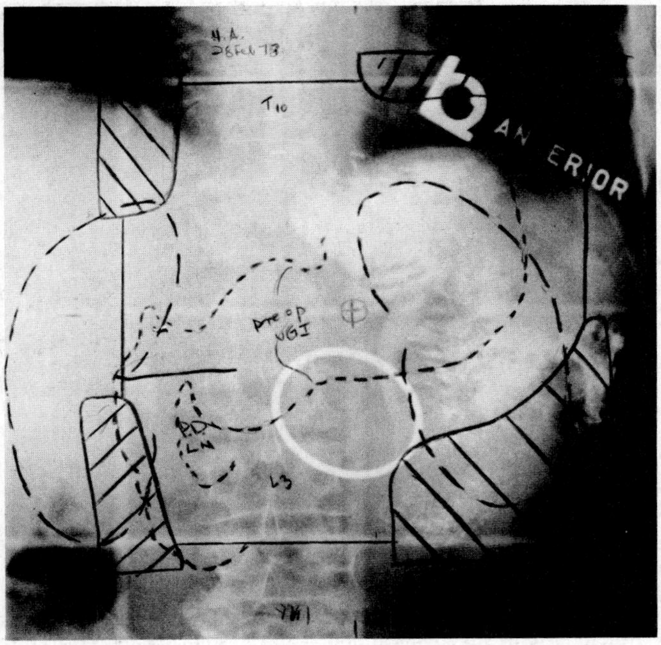

FIG. 21-10. Portals for radiation showing inclusion of the gastric bed plus 70% of the left kidney but excluding 75% or more of the right kidney.

the pancreas, in order to spare the spinal cord or kidney. Since parallel opposed portals are the most practical field arrangement for delivering most tumor and nodal radiation, one must limit either the volume of normal tissue included or the upper dose level. Multiple-field techniques should be considered when this would improve long-term normal tissue tolerance. (For example, with unresectable lesions at the level of the esophagogastric junction, if moderate lateral extension is noted on CT, lateral fields can be useful in decreasing the volume of heart within the radiation field.)

The exact tolerance of kidneys, when portions of both are included in the radiation field, is somewhat uncertain. When both kidneys are to be included in their entirety, Luxton and Kunkler[107] prefer to limit the dose to the upper third of each kidney to 1700 rad but believe their experience suggests that a dose of 2300 rad delivered over 5 weeks to the whole of both kidneys may be acceptable. When portions of both kidneys are to be included in the radiation field, the preference is to exclude two thirds to three fourths of one kidney.[108,109] For proximal gastric lesions, at least one half of the left kidney usually lies within the radiation portal (see Fig. 25-11), and the right kidney must be appropriately spared. For distal lesions with narrow or positive duodenal margins, a similar amount of right kidney often is included (Fig. 25-11), and then every effort must be made to spare enough left kidney. When this approach is followed, problems with radiation nephritis have not been encountered.[109,110] In a series reported from the Massachusetts General Hospital,[110] renal tolerance was evaluated in a group of 86 patients with upper abdominal malignancies who received irradiation with curative intent. At least 50% of the unilateral kidney received 300 rad or more, and all patients survived 1 year or

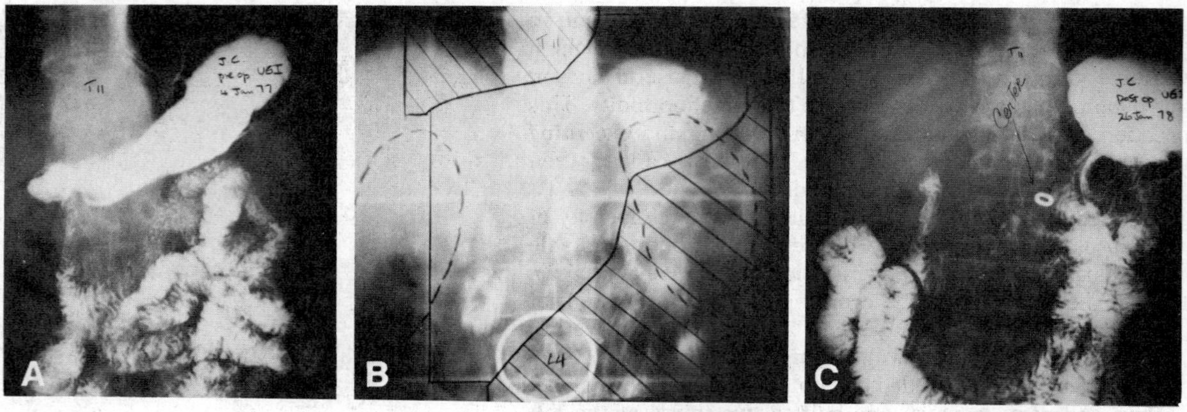

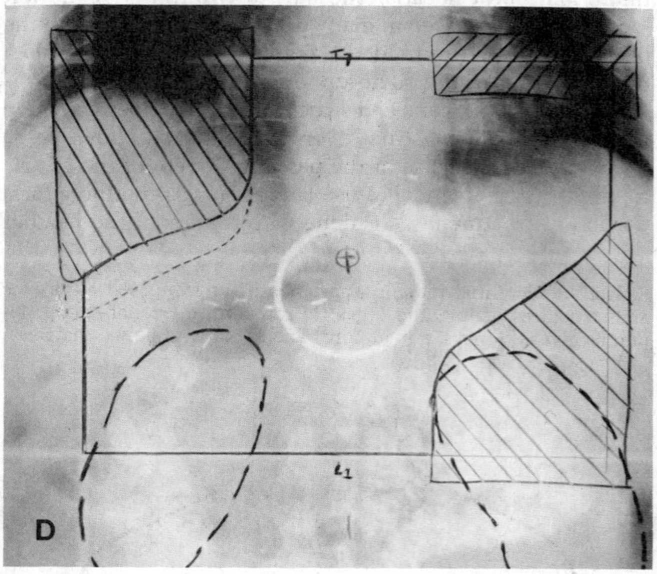

FIG. 25-11. Patient J.C. (**A–C**) had a subtotal gastrectomy with gastrojejunostomy for adenocarcinoma of the stomach and was referred to MGH for postoperative radiation. The initial intent was inclusion of the duodenal stump, a portion of the duodenal loop, the tumor bed and nodal areas, yet sparing 75 + % of the left kidney with blocks (*cross-hatched areas*). **A**. Position of the duodenum in the preoperative UGI. **B**, **C**. Good visualization of both the duodenal stump and gastric pouch in both the radiation planning film (**B**) and the postoperative diagnostic UGI (**C**).

Patient A.X. had an unresectable carcinoma of the stomach. (**D**) The lesion's extent was marked with clips at exploratory laparotomy. Since the radiation therapy portal included nearly 50% of the right kidney, cerrobend blocking was used to exclude the left kidney. Other blocks (*cross-hatched areas*) were used to exclude portions of liver and heart. Additional liver blocking was added after 3500 rad. (Parts **A–C** from Gunderson L: Part IX. In Alimentary Tract Radiology, p 606. St. Louis, C V Mosby, 1979)

longer. No patient developed acute or chronic renal failure. Of 73 patients who were normotensive before irradiation, 2 became hypertensive (easily controlled with medication in one; malignant hypertension required nephrectomy in the second).

The most commonly used dose schedules of 4000 to 5000 rad delivered over 4 to 5 weeks as continuous irradiation for various upper abdominal malignancies have been tolerated by the stomach and small intestine, with a complication rate ranging from 0 to 8.3% in recent series.[111,112] Roswit and co-workers[113] summarized the older Walter Reed Hospital testicular data, which showed a higher incidence of gastric and intestinal complications. This may have resulted from the following factors: lower voltage radiation (maximum 1 MeV), short fractionation schedules (4500 to 5400 rad delivered over 3 to 4 weeks), and treatment of one field per day. Duodenal and distal gastric tolerance were evaluated in a series of 36 patients treated with curative intent at Mayo Clinic with irradiation ± 5-FU for locally advanced biliary duct cancer.[114] Multiple-field techniques and 180-rad fraction size were used in most patients, and specialized irradiation supplements were used in 18 (transcatheter iridium in 10, IORT electrons in 8). Two (11%) of 19 patients who received 5500 rad or less by external beam ± iridium to a portion of duodenum or distal stomach developed duodenal ulcers or upper GI bleeding. When that dose was exceeded, the incidence increased to 33% (2 of 6 patients).

In the upper abdomen, daily single doses of 170 to 180 rad are better tolerated than doses of 200 rad or more. Weekly weights should be followed closely. When doses of 170 to 180 rad are used, about half of patients require pretreatment antiemetics. Most patients with intact stomachs, however, have some degree of anorexia and need encouragement to eat adequate amounts. Patients who have undergone partial or subtotal gastrectomies seem to tolerate upper abdominal irradiation better than those who have not undergone resection. Use of oral hyperalimentation should be encouraged, and if weight loss during treatment exceeds 10%, hyperalimentation should be considered.

With proximal gastric lesions or lesions at the esophagogastric junction, inclusion of a major portion of the left hemidiaphragm is indicated when the lesion extends through the entire alimentary wall. In these circumstances, cerrobend blocking to decrease cardiac irradiation can be important, since doxorubicin is a frequently used chemotherapeutic agent in this malignancy.

Method of Radiation

Differences of opinion may exist on the preferred way to combine surgery and irradiation for gastric carcinoma. Preoperative, intraoperative, and postoperative radiation therapy have been used to some degree in the past, mainly in Japan.[115-119] The main problem with using intraoperative radiation as the sole method of radiation, as is done in Japan, is that the pathologic extent of disease is not known and radiation portals cannot be individualized. A possible advantage is that dose-limiting tissues, such as the small intestine, colon, and liver, can be retracted outside the radiation field. Such retraction, however, might result in margin failures, since a significant number of locoregional failures in the Minnesota reoperative series involved those organs. A preferred method may be to combine external beam and intraoperative irradiation.

The direct controversy of preoperative versus postoperative radiation therapy versus a combination thereof is probably of greatest interest, since intraoperative irradiation is not feasible in most institutions. Theoretical considerations in this regard are discussed in Chapter 15. Since 30% to 50% of gastric lesions are technically unresectable, some preoperative irradiation to alter implantability or to shrink disease would be attractive. Because the routine diagnostic techniques often reveal only the "tip of the iceberg" regarding extent of disease, CT should be performed to define extragastric disease extent, and peritoneoscopy or minilaparotomy could be considered to rule out peritoneal seeding or minimal disease on the surface of the liver. If moderate-dose preoperative irradiation (4500–5000 rad) were used in an attempt to shrink disease to improve resectability, risks of anastomotic leaks probably would increase unless resections were wide and at least one of the limbs of the anastomosis was not irradiated.

With postoperative irradiation, field setup (portals) and dose could be individualized to some degree with potential portals according to extent of disease, as follows:

1. Negative lymph nodes, extension beyond mucosa but confined to gastric wall. Small field irradiation to the anastomotic area, including duodenal stump if it was a distal lesion. If only a small number of lymph nodes were sectioned, consider inclusion of primary lymph nodes.
2. Negative lymph nodes, extension beyond gastric wall. Moderate field radiation therapy to cover the stomach bed structures with or without nodal areas. Entire left hemidiaphragm should be considered for inclusion, especially in proximal lesions.
3. Positive lymph nodes, confined to gastric wall. Cover both the primary and secondary nodal drainage areas. Do not need to include the entire left hemidiaphragm, and therefore treat less lung and heart.
4. Positive lymph nodes, extension beyond gastric wall. Cover entire gastric bed plus primary and secondary lymph node drainage areas (major solid line field as shown in Figs. 25-2 and 25-9).

The nodal areas considered at risk for primary spread include the gastric and gastroepiploic nodes (usually resected), and the entire celiac axis, including porta hepatis, subpyloric, gastroduodenal, splenic suprapancreatic, and retropancreaticoduodenal nodes (paraesophageal nodes if the tumor is proximal). Secondary chains at risk include the superior mesenteric and para-aortic nodes.

The usual dose aim is 4500 to 5000 rad in 5 to 6 weeks delivered in 170 to 180 rad fractions to the initial field. A boost field can be safely carried to 5000 rad and occasionally is brought to 5500 rad for unresected or residual disease. Some European and Scandinavian centers use upper dose levels of 6000 rad in 6 to 9 weeks for unresected or residual disease, but these centers have provided only minimal information on long-term tolerance. Parallel opposed fields usually are necessary for the initial large field to the tumor or tumor bed and lymph node areas. Doses greater than 4500 to 5000 rad are discouraged with treatment energies of 4 MeV or less unless multiple-field techniques can be used for a portion of the treatment. If residual or unresected disease is marked with clips, that possibility exists. On rare occasions, the dose for residual disease in lymph nodes or tumor bed may be boosted to 6000 rad if clips are placed and an upper GI study is done to define the relationship of residual disease to the gastric pouch and small intestine.

Results

RADIATION WITH OR WITHOUT CHEMOTHERAPY. Radiation alone has been shown to have curative potential in a small percentage of patients with resected but residual[115] or with unresectable but localized disease.[119,120] Its greatest benefit has been when used in combination with chemotherapy, as noted for some time in studies from the Mayo Clinic[109,121] and a number of foreign centers.[116-120]

Adjuvant radiation alone or in combination with chemotherapy would be attractive for high-risk subgroups of patients with resected gastric carcinoma. Local failure after curative resection is common. Although some cures have been obtained with irradiation alone,[119,120] indicating that gastric cancer is radiosensitive, this is not a viable single-modality approach because the bulk of disease and the limited tolerance of the stomach and surrounding organs prevent a suitable therapeutic ratio between cure and complications. The preferred use of radiation as an aid to local regional control would be in combination with operative removal of all gross disease in the primary area and lymph nodes, with radiation usually in combination with chemotherapy being used to treat microscopic or subclinical residual disease.

RADIATION AND SURGERY. Available literature supports the concept that adenocarcinoma of the stomach is a radioresponsive lesion.[115-120] Wieland and Hymmen[120] used 6000 rad when feasible (150 to 200 rad daily) with 11% (9 of 82) 3-year and 7% (5 of 72) 5-year survivals. Takahashi[119] compared historical controls with patients with inoperable disease or patients who had undergone palliative procedures and received postoperative irradiation (no mention of chemotherapy). The average survival for the group treated by radiation therapy was longer by 9 to 10 months, with 74% survival (32 of 43 patients) at 1 year and 28% survival (12 of 43 patients) at 2.5 years. In a preoperative series, Hoshi[118] found histologic changes of tumor necrosis in 28% of patients with doses less than 2000 rad, in 74% with doses of 2000 rad, and in 88% with higher doses. Asakawa and associates[116,117] found a greater than 50% decrease in the size of tumor in 60% and total regression in 10% of 40 patients treated with radiation alone or in combination with chemotherapy prior to surgery.

CONVENTIONAL RADIATION AND CHEMOTHERAPY. Most reports on combined treatment deal with results in the patient with unresectable cancer and show suggestive improvement for irradiation plus 5-FU over that achieved with either irradiation alone or 5-FU alone.[121–123] In the Mayo Clinic series,[121] a randomized double-blind study of patients with unresectable disease, 5-FU was used during the first 3 days of radiation (3500–4000 rad at 900–1200 rad/week). For the combined therapy versus radiation therapy groups, mean survival was 12 versus 5.9 months, and 5-year survival rate was 12% (3 of 25 patients) versus 0% (0 of 23). Asakawa and co-workers[116,117] reported treatment results in 54 patients, of whom 42 received some 5-FU. At the 2-year interval, 3 of 33 patients treated without surgical resection and 4 of 8 treated with partial resection were alive (6000 rad over 6 to 9 weeks was the aim).

In a recent report of the randomized GITSG study (protocol 8274), including 90 patients with unresectable or residual disease,[74] the combination of radiation therapy plus 5-FU followed by maintenance 5-FU plus methyl-CCNU was statistically superior to 5-FU plus methyl-CCNU alone with regard to long-term survival, with a plateau of 20% reached after 3 years of follow-up ($p < 0.05$). The short-term advantage to 5-FU plus methyl-CCNU (median survival, 70 versus 36 weeks) was believed due to early tumor-related and toxicity deaths with the 5-FU–radiation therapy combination during the first 26 weeks of treatment. Irradiated patients received 5000 rad in 8 weeks in split-course fashion (2500 rad in 3 weeks, followed by 2 weeks' rest, followed by an additional 2500 rad in 3 weeks; 500 mg/m^2 of 5-FU was given on days 1, 2, and 3 of each radiation therapy sequence, followed by 5-FU plus methyl-CCNU maintenance chemotherapy). Patients with residual disease after resection had better long-term survival rates than those whose cancers were never resected.

In a series of 46 patients with localized gastric cancer treated with radiation alone (6 patients) or in combination with chemotherapy at the Massachusetts General Hospital,[109] toxicity-related deaths were not encountered. The numbers of patients by disease category were as follows: recurrent disease, 4; medically inoperable, 4; surgically unresectable, 9; resected but residual, 15; and resected but high risk for local recurrence, 14. Patients treated with radiation therapy plus chemotherapy followed two sequences: radiation therapy plus 3 days of 5-FU followed by maintenance 5-FU or combined drugs (26 patients); and single course of 5-FU plus *bis*-chloroethylnitrosourea (BCNU) or FAM, followed by radiation therapy and maintenance combination chemotherapy (14 patients). Radiation with 10 or 25 MeV photons was delivered to tightly contoured portals, sparing as much bone marrow and bowel as possible and delivering 4500 to 5200 rad in 25 to 29 fractions over 5 to 6 weeks. Only 4 patients (9%) had poor tolerance, and 2 of those completed radiation therapy. Hematologic parameters delayed the radiation therapy or chemotherapy course in 11 patients. The difference in treatment-related toxicity in the GITSG versus Massachusetts General Hospital series may in part be due to the use of tightly contoured portals in the latter series, an aspect of technique more difficult to coordinate in a multi-institution study.

Although patterns of failure and lack of positive chemotherapy trials help justify the incorporation of radiation therapy into future adjuvant trials, data from pilot trials are minimal. In the initial publication from the Massachusetts General Hospital,[109] 14 of the 46 patients had curative resection but were at high risk for locoregional failure and received postoperative irradiation + 5-FU. Local progression as any component of failure was subsequently documented in 2 (14%), and the 4-year actuarial survival rate was 46%. In a randomized trial from the Mayo Clinic,[124] 62 patients with involved nodes were randomized to no further treatment or postoperative irradiation (3750 rad over 4–5 weeks) plus 5-FU (15 mg/kg IV bolus on days 1–3). The 5-year survival rate in patients assigned to receive additional treatment was 23%, versus 4% in those treated by surgery alone ($p < 0.05$). However, 10 patients who refused additional treatment had a 5-year survival rate of 30%, compared to the 23% rate in patients given additional treatment. Local failure was documented as a component of initial progression in 39% of treated patients versus 55% of those treated with surgery alone. In view of the high rate of nonacceptance to assigned treatment, end results are difficult to interpret but suggest a decrease in local failure. It would be reasonable to evaluate further the combination of external radiation + 5-FU in subsequent randomized trials (alone or in combination with more aggressive chemotherapy).

RADIATION AND FAM. Combinations of FAM and radiation have been used in pilot studies for unresectable gastric or pancreatic cancer (MGH, Middle Atlantic Oncology Program [MAOP]), as well as in resected but high-risk (MGH) or resected but residual gastric cancer (MGH, SWOG). In the SWOG pilot study,[125] 12 patients were treated with concomitant FAM and radiation. The MGH trial used a sequential FAM plus irradiation plus FAM regimen (1 cycle of FAM, radiation therapy of 4500 to 5000 rad delivered over 5 to 5½ weeks in 180-rad fractions, FAM for 5 cycles).[109] Although some patients with pancreatic cancer have been treated at Massachusetts General Hospital, the major focus has been on gastric cancer, with 24 gastric patients having completed treatment as of a September 1985 report.[126] In a MAOP trial of 42 patients reported by Schein and colleagues[127] (gastric cancer, 21 patients; pancreatic cancer, 21 patients), FAM was used before and after a course of split-course radiation combined with 5-FU (4500 rad over 7 weeks: 2250 rad per sequence plus 5-FU, 350 mg/m^2, on days 1, 2, and 3 of each X-irradiation sequence). Both the MGH and MAOP trials used 1 cycle of FAM before radiation and 5 to 6 cycles afterward, with radiation instituted in week 7 in the MGH pilot and in week 10 in the MAOP pilot (5-FU was added to the X-irradiation course in the MAOP pilot but not at MGH). In the MGH and MAOP trials, GI tolerance was acceptable

TABLE 25-15. Component of Failure After Radiation and Chemotherapy*†

Treatment Group	*No. of Failures/ Total Group‡*	*Local*			*Liver*			*Peritoneal*			*Lung*		
		No.	*%*	*(%)*	*No.*	*%*	*(%)*	*No.*	*%*	*(%)*	*No.*	*%*	*(%)*
Curative	8/14	2	25	(14)	5	63	(36)	2	25	(14)	2	25	(14)
Residual microscopic	8/8	1	13	(13)	3	38	(38)	2	25	(25)	1	13	(13)
Gross	6/7	1	17	(14)	1	17	(14)	2	33	(29)	4	67	(58)
Unresectable	9/9	6	67	(67)	3	33	(33)	2	22	(22)	4	44	(44)

*Modified from Gunderson LL, Hoskins B, Cohen AM et al: Combined modality treatment of gastric cancer. Int J Radiat Oncol Biol Phys 9:965–975, 1983.

†Open figures represent number and percentage of failure group, and numbers in parentheses represent percentage of total evaluable patients.

‡An additional 8 patients were treated in this series (medically inoperable, 4; recurrent, 4), and 6 of the 16 local failures occurred in these 8 patients.

(mild to moderate nausea and vomiting), with myelosuppression representing the dose-limiting toxicity. In the larger MAOP trial, the median white blood cell nadir was $2.3 \times 10^3/mm^3$ (range, $0.2-6.6 \times 10^3/mm^3$) and the platelet nadir was 84 $10^3/mm^3$ (range, $20-288 \times 10^3/mm^3$). Median survival was 13+ months (range, 1+ to 15 months) for gastric patients in the MAOP trial and 19 months at MGH. In the MGH analysis, 2-year actuarial survival was 41%. While these trials indicate that such treatment combinations can be used with acceptable toxicity, randomized trials will be needed to determine whether the therapeutic effect of such combined treatment is better than that achieved with either irradiation plus 5-FU or multiple drug chemotherapy alone.

PATTERNS OF FAILURE. Sites of failure were analyzed in the group of 46 patients treated with combined radiation and chemotherapy for gastric cancer at MGH (Table 25-15). Disease progression was identified in 70 sites in 37 patients. Most sites were intra-abdominal (47 of 70 sites, or 67.2%; 32 of 46 patients, or 70%), with frequent liver metastases and peritoneal seeding (21 of 46 patients, or 46%, had either or both, 17 with a single component, 4 with both). A component of local or regional failure was noted in 16 patients (23% of sites and 35% of total patient group). Such failures were outside the irradiation field in 1 patient and possibly at the margin of the failed in 1 additional patient. Three failures were associated with peritoneal seeding. Pleural or pulmonary failure was noted in approximately 18% of sites or 28% of the total patient group.

In Table 25-15, the four major causes of failure are analyzed by treatment group. Although tissue confirmation of failure was available in 18 of the 37 patients, confirmation of failure sites by reoperation or autopsy was available in only 7. Interestingly, only 4 (14%) of 29 patients with curative resection or resection but residual disease had any evidence of failure within the radiation field, as opposed to 6 (66%) of 9 with unresectable disease. In 2 of the 4 patients in the former group, such failure probably was due to the use of a posterior cord block during irradiation, which was not used by the senior author of the MGH series and is thought not to be necessary at the dose levels in that series (4500 rad in 25 fractions to the large field, 5000 rad to the boost field). Of the 24 patients treated with FAM plus irradiation at MGH, 20 died with disease.[126] Local control was maintained in 16. Distant metastases were found in all 20 patients.

RADIATION (MULTIPLE DAILY FRACTIONS) PLUS CHEMOTHERAPY. In view of major local and systemic problems with gastric cancer identified in various series, a pilot study was instituted at the Mayo Clinic in an attempt to optimize the use of combination chemotherapy and irradiation.[128] The intent was to sequence combined drug regimens before and after radiation therapy and to use two fractions a day of irradiation with or without 5-FU. This was an attempt to shorten intervals from operative intervention to the institution of combined drug chemotherapy and between chemotherapy regimens, and to improve the radiation response of patients with poorly differentiated lesions (a majority of patients with gastric cancer) on the basis of less repopulation between radiation fractions. Such a schema contrasts markedly with the use of split-course irradiation regimens, which may be inappropriate with poorly differentiated lesions.

Eighteen patients with unresectable or residual regional gastric cancer without evident distant metastases were treated with an intensive combined modality regimen to determine patient tolerability (16 of 18 received irradiation and 12 had some maintenance chemotherapy).

1. Induction chemotherapy: 5-FU, 350 mg/m^2 IV on days 1 through 5, plus doxorubicin, 50 mg/m^2 IV on day 1.
2. Radiation therapy: beginning on day 21, 4500 rad given in two 165-rad fractions daily, plus 5-FU, 500 mg/m^2 IV on days 28 through 30.
3. Maintenance chemotherapy: beginning 4 weeks from the end of radiation therapy, 5-FU, 225 mg/m^2 IV on days 1 through 5 every 5 weeks; doxorubicin, 30 mg/m^2 IV on day 1 every 5 weeks; methyl-CCNU, 80 mg/m^2 PO on day 1 every 10 weeks.

Six of 7 patients treated with the combined regimen experienced prolonged anorexia and nausea during radiation therapy and for several weeks thereafter, requiring a delay in instituting maintenance chemotherapy in 5 of 6 patients.

Three of 6 patients also experienced leukopenia (white blood cell count ≤ 2500), one of whom was unable to receive maintenance chemotherapy because of prolonged leukopenia. Increasing the rest interval after induction chemotherapy by 1 week and decreasing the radiation dose per fraction to 150 rad did not reduce the severe nutritional effects in 2 of 3 patients thus treated. Nine additional patients have received either hyperfactionated radiation without 5-FU (6 patients) or single daily doses of radiation plus 5-FU (3 patients) with improved tolerance. At the last evaluation, disease in 11 patients had progressed (time to progression in weeks: median, 19; range, 4–49). All 13 patients evaluable for patterns of progression developed distant metastases. Only 2 of 11 who received radiation therapy also had initial local progression.

INTRAOPERATIVE RADIATION. Most information on the use of intraoperative radiation therapy (IORT) for the treatment of gastric cancer is based on data reported by Abe and Takahashi from Japan.[129] Abe has been treating gastric carcinoma with a relatively constant technique of IORT alone after gastrectomy (no external beam irradiation). A pentagonal treatment field, designed to cover the tumor bed and major nodal sites, receives 2800 to 4000 rad in a single fraction (measured at the 100% isodose line) with high-energy electrons.

Although formal randomization has not been performed, patients are selected for IORT on the basis of the day they are admitted to the hospital. In a prospective study, 110 patients were treated by surgery alone and 84 patients by surgery plus IORT.

Abe's results are shown in Table 25-16. Five-year survival is very similar in both treatment groups for Stage I disease, but there is a suggestion of a survival advantage for both Stage II (77.6% versus 54.5%) and Stage III (44.6% versus 36.8%) for the IORT group. The most impressive difference, however, is seen in patients with Stage IV disease who had direct local extension posteriorly or residual disease without distant metastases. In this subset, there were no survivors among 18 patients treated with operation alone, compared to a 19.5% 5-year survival rate among 27 patients treated with surgery plus IORT. This percentage is similar to the incidence of locoregional failure occurring as the only failure in the University of Minnesota reoperative series (29% of failure group, or 23% of total group at risk) and indicates that radiation therapy may add to survival in a subset of patients who are at high risk for local failure. There has been a small (less than 40 patients) randomized IORT study in resected gastric cancer performed at the National Cancer Institute. Neither disease-free nor overall survival was improved by IORT.

TABLE 25-16. Gastric Cancer—Surgery and IORT, Japan

	5-Year Survival			
	Surgery		*Surgery + IORT*	
	No.	*%*	*No.*	*%*
Stage I	43	93	20	88.1
Stage II	11	54.5	18	77.6
Stage III	38	36.8	19	44.6
Stage IV (no distant metastases)	18	0	27	19.5

Recommendations for Nonprotocol Radiation plus Chemotherapy

The major role of radiation therapy today in the treatment of gastric cancer is in the management of locally unresectable, partially resectable, or recurrent disease. The recommended nonprotocol therapy is the radiation plus 5-FU plus methyl-CCNU regimen previously outlined in this chapter, or continuous radiation plus 5-FU, possibly followed by FAM (4500–5000 rad in 180-rad fractions over 5–5½ weeks with a 500 mg/m² IV 5-FU push for 2 consecutive days in weeks 1 and/or 5, depending on blood cell counts and GI tolerance). With the 5-FU + methyl-CCNU program, the drugs are given in the following schedule: 5-FU, 325 mg/m² on days 1 through 5, 375 mg/m² on days 36 through 40; methyl-CCNU, 150 mg/m² on day 1. The schedule is repeated every 9 to 10 weeks, depending on tolerance, and is not initiated until radiation therapy has been completed and radiation-associated acute toxicities have cleared. Methyl-CCNU is currently not available for other than investigational use. Also, caution should be exercised in using methyl-CCNU in patients who may be long-term survivors. Boice and colleagues[130] have demonstrated that methyl-CCNU increases the incidence of acute leukemia (relative risk: 12.4) in patients with GI cancer who had received this drug as adjuvant therapy. It should be emphasized that there are no combined modality regimens that are dramatically successful, and there is continued need for active investigation in the use of combined radiation plus chemotherapy.

TREATMENT OF PATIENTS WITH DISSEMINATED CANCER

The major treatment modality currently available for metastatic gastric cancer is chemotherapy. The chemotherapy of advanced gastric cancer has aroused considerable interest[106,131–133] because several studies have documented response rates of 40% to 50% with combination chemotherapy. Whether currently available therapies result in improved survival for treated patients is not clear.

In evaluating the reported results of chemotherapy in advanced gastric cancer, several prognostic factors are important. Available data suggest that patients who have a good performance status, who are only minimally symptomatic, and who have evaluable disease confined to the abdomen are more likely to respond to chemotherapy than are patients with either widely disseminated metastatic disease or poor performance status.[106] Therefore, it becomes important in evaluating the results of chemotherapy studies that data on performance status and sites of metastatic disease be analyzed carefully. Clearly, any chemotherapy regimen used in totally asymptomatic patients with limited disease would appear to be more effective than a treatment program used in significantly symptomatic patients with widely disseminated cancer.

In evaluating the results of chemotherapy trials in gastric cancer, the following criteria for response are used. A complete response consists in the disappearance of all objective evidence of cancer. A partial response is defined as a greater than 50% decrease in the products of the two largest perpendicular diameters of clearly measurable metastatic lesions. An alternative, stricter interpretation of partial response requires a greater than 50% decrease in all metastatic lesions. A minimal response is defined as a less than 50% but greater than 25% decrease in measurable metastatic lesions. In general, lesion diameters may be measured physically or from radiographs. Radionuclide scans of the liver may be used if perfusion defects are clearly measurable and greater than 3 cm in diameter.[132] Similarly, large abnormalities on CT or US occasionally may serve as measurable disease. However, further clinical correlation with the changes in CT or US tumor images after chemotherapy is necessary. When response to chemotherapy is referred to in this chapter, only partial and complete responses are meant. Minimal responses will not be considered as objective disease regression.

Study design is another factor that must be evaluated carefully when assessing results of chemotherapy trials in patients with stomach cancer. Study design is particularly important when claims of improved survival with a particular regimen are made. The only proper way to demonstrate improved survival with a chemotherapy regimen is to evaluate that treatment program prospectively in a Phase III trial. In advanced gastric carcinoma, a disease in which complete remissions secondary to chemotherapy are exceedingly rare, it is difficult to sustain the claim that chemotherapy improves survival in partially responding patients. It may be entirely possible that response to a chemotherapy program does not result in prolongation of survival, but rather that the patients who will have the longest survival if untreated are the ones most likely to respond to chemotherapy. Thus response to chemotherapy may merely be another indication of good prognosis, as are other factors such as good performance status, relatively minimal disease, and well-differentiated histology.[106] With the above caveats firmly established, this section reviews the results of single-agent chemotherapy and combination chemotherapy of gastric cancer.

Single-Agent Chemotherapy

The use of systemic chemotherapy for disseminated gastric cancer has depended on documentation of antitumor activity of various single agents against this disease. Table 25-17 reviews objective response rates reported for single agents in patients with stomach cancer.[106,131,134–148] Many other agents have been reported anecdotally in the literature, but Table 25-17 reports studies in which 18 or more patients were evaluated.

The fluorinated pyrimidine 5-fluorouracil (5-FU), which has been tested in almost 400 patients, is the most completely evaluated single agent.[134] The dosage schedule most frequently used is the loading course method in which the drug is administered IV for 4 to 5 days, followed by half-doses every other day until toxicity is produced. Various maintenance schedules have been used; the most common are weekly IV doses or repeated loading courses at monthly intervals. The objective partial response rate with 5-FU is a disappointing 21%. Complete responses are exceedingly rare, and the median duration of 5-FU response can be expected to range from 3 months to 6 months.

The antibiotic mitomycin C, first developed in Japan, has been evaluated in gastric cancer. The original reports of Japanese clinical trials suggested an overall objective response rate of 35%.[134] The initial experience in the United States was considerably less impressive, however. Administration of mitomycin C on a daily schedule was found to produce significant delayed myelosuppression and a cumulative, persistent bone marrow injury.[149] In addition, inadvertent extravasation during IV administration resulted in a severe inflammatory reaction, with potential skin slough. Drug-related deaths occurred in 11% of the patients, and the objective response rate was only 18%. More recent experi-

TABLE 25-17. Single-Agent Chemotherapy in Advanced Gastric Cancer

Drug	*No. of Responses/ No. of Patients*	*% Response*	*Reference*
5-Fluorouracil	84/392	21	134
Mitomycin C	63/211	30	134
Adriamycin	17/68	25	135–137
Hydroxyurea	6/31	19	138
BCNU	6/33	18	131
Chlorambucil	3/18	17	139
Mechlorethane	3/23	13	140
Methyl-CCNU	3/37	8	106
Cisplatin	8/36	22	141,142
Triazinate	4/26	15	143
Methotrexate	3/28	11	143
Razoxane	0/19	0	143
4′-Epidoxorubicin	8/22	36	144
Carboplatin (CBDCA)	0/22	0	145
Bisantrene	1/26	4	146
m-AMSA	0/125	0	147
Ftorafur	5/19	27	148

TABLE 25-18. Combination Chemotherapy in Advanced Gastric Cancer

Drug Combination	*No. of Responses/ No. of Patients*	*% Responses*	*Median Duration of Survival (Months)*	*Reference*
Adriamycin + mitomycin C	13/46	29	3.5	151
5-FU + methyl-CCNU	12/30	40 (20% CR, 20% PR)	5.0	106
	6/44	14	3.0	151
	5/54	9	4.5	152
	6/29	21	4.5	153
	12/49	24	4.5	137
	1/18	6	5.5	154
Total	42/224	19		
5-FU+mitomycin C	6/43	14	6.0	152
	17/53	32	4.0	137
Total	23/96	24		
5-FU + Adriamycin	3/11	27	7.0	155
	1/19	5	6.0	156
Total	4/30	13		
5-FU + BCNU	14/34	41	7.7	131
	5/28	18	3.0	157
	2/18	11	4.0	158
Total	21/80	26		
Triazinate + mitomycin C	8/28	29	5.5	159
5-FU + high-dose folinic acid	13/27	48 (4% CR, 44% PR)	11 *	160
FAM	6/11	55	16.5*	161
(5-FU + Adriamycin + mitomycin C)	26/62	42	12.5*	132
	20/45	44	11.5*	163
	6/27	22	5.5	164
	28/81	35	17.0*	165
	7/33	21	5.5	166
	4/22	18	6.2	167
	25/83	30	5.8	168
	3/12	25	6.8	154
	3/18	17	6.2	156
	18/46	39	6.4	151
	5/13	38	7.2	155
Total	151/453	33		

(continued)

ence has shown an overall response rate for mitomycin C in gastric cancer of 15% to 30%.[134] There has been renewed interest in the use of this drug with the demonstration that single treatments of 10 mg/m^2 to 20 mg/m^2, at 6- to 8-week intervals, result in manageable hematologic toxicity while retaining therapeutic activity.[150]

The anthracycline antibiotic doxorubicin (Adriamycin) is a drug with a wide range of antitumor activity in human solid tumors that has recently been evaluated in gastric cancer. Early trials reported a response rate of 36% with doxorubicin.[135] More recently, the GITSG[138] and the ECOG have performed Phase II trials testing the efficacy of doxorubicin.[137] Both of these studies confirm the activity of this drug. Doxorubicin was administered at 60 mg/m^2 every 3 to 4 weeks, and objective responses were demonstrated in 4 of 17 cases (24%) and 8 of 37 cases (22%).[136,137] The median duration of response to doxorubicin was 4 months. These studies have demonstrated that doxorubicin is at least as active as the fluorinated pyrimidines and indicated a need to test this drug in combination chemotherapy regimens. Another anthracycline, 4′-epidoxorubicin,[144] which may cause fewer or less severe cardiac toxic effects than doxorubicin, has been evaluated in Phase II trials in stomach cancer. One small study reported 8 (36%) of 22 patients achieving a partial response.[144] This result will require confirmation.

The chloroethylnitrosoureas BCNU and methyl-CCNU represent another class of single agents evaluated in advanced gastric cancer patients.[106,131] BCNU produced objective partial remissions in 6 (18%) of 33 patients treated, with a 4-month duration of response. The methylated chloroethylnitrosourea, methyl-CCNU, also has been tested by ECOG and produced responses in 3 (8%) of 37 patients.[106] Median survival of patients receiving this drug was less than 15 weeks. Other single agents that have been reported to have minimal activity (<20%) in gastric cancer include hydroxyurea, carboplatin, bisantrene, and the alkylating agents mechlorethamine and chlorambucil (see Table 25-17).

Cisplatin[141,142] is reported to produce response in 22% of patients and its role in combination chemotherapy regimens will be discussed later in this chapter. Triazinate is of interest because it is a folate antagonist that has demonstrated modest activity (15% partial response) in heavily pretreated

TABLE 25-18. *(continued)*

Drug Combination	*No. of Responses/ No. of Patients*	*% Responses*	*Median Duration of Survival (Months)*	*Reference*
FAMtx (5-FU + Adriamycin + methotrexate)	22/62	35 (15% CR, 20% PR)	6.0	169
	59/100	59 (12% CR, 47% PR)	9.0	170
Total	81/162	50		
FAMe (5-FU + Adriamycin + methyl-CCNU)	7/15	47	6.0	136
	3/10	30	8.5	154
	4/16	25	7.1	156
	11/39	29	5.5	151
Total	25/80	31		
FAP (5-FU + Adriamycin + cisplatin)	10/35	29	5.5	171
	8/16	50	10.5	172
	13/26	50 (11% CR, 39% PR)	9.0	173
	5/16	31	13.0	174
Total	36/93	39		
5-FU + mitomycin C + cytosine arabinoside	3/18	17	3.2	136
5-FU + Adriamycin + BCNU	18/35	51	12 *	175
	4/17	24	5.5	157
	40/94	43	8.2	176
Total	62/146	42		
FAM + triazinate	4/22	18	NA	177
FAM + BCNU	9/41	22	6	178
FAM + methyl-CCNU	2/18	11	6.2	179
	12/31	39	7.1	180
Total	14/49	29		

CR = complete response, PR = partial response.
* Survival duration in responders only.

patients with gastric cancer (see Table 25-17).[143] The response rate may be significantly higher in previously untreated patients. Triazinate may be useful in investigational combination therapy programs because it has single-agent activity and also may synergize with fluorinated pyrimidines. Although some single agents do have activity in stomach cancer, it should be emphasized that all the single agents have the shared liability of low response rates and short duration of response (3–5 months); also, complete responses to single agents are very rare. Therefore, single-agent chemotherapy for gastric cancer is of minimal practical benefit to the patient. For this reason, the polychemotherapy of stomach cancer is being pursued with increasing intensity.

Combination Chemotherapy

There have been numerous attempts to develop effective combination chemotherapy regimens using both single-agents known to be active and agents that have not been evaluated for single-agent activity. Table 25-18 reviews the published results of 16 combination chemotherapeutic regimens tested in patients with gastric cancer.

Two of the most extensively evaluated regimens in the United States have used 5-FU in combination with either BCNU or methyl-BCNU.[106,131] In a study reported by Kovach et al,[131] the combination of 5-FU and BCNU was compared with each drug alone in a randomized Phase III trial. All drugs were given IV in the following doses: 5-FU alone, 13.5 mg/kg/day for 5 days; BCNU alone, 50 mg/m²/day for 5 days; 5-FU + BCNU, 10 mg/kg/day and 40 mg/m²/day, respectively, for 5 days. Objective responses to therapy were 29% for 5-FU alone, 17% for BCNU alone, and 41% for 5-FU + BCNU. Median survival for patients treated with the combination was 7 months and was not significantly different from that seen with the single agents alone. However, there was a significant improvement in survival at 18 months for the patients treated with 5-FU + BCNU. At that point, 25% of the group receiving combination chemotherapy were alive, compared to fewer than 10% of those receiving either single agent.

The ECOG conducted a controlled randomized trial in advanced gastric cancer comparing the combination of 5-FU + methyl-CCNU with methyl-CCNU used alone.[106] The dosages in the combination were as follows: 5-FU, 300 mg/m²/day IV for 5 days with methyl-CCNU, 175 mg/m² given orally on the first day; this regimen was repeated at 7-week intervals. The dosage of methyl-CCNU alone was 200 mg/m² given in a single oral dose and repeated at 7-week intervals. The combination produced a 40% response rate and definitely was superior to methyl-CCNU alone, which produced an 8% response ($p < 0.05$).[106] A significant survival benefit was reported for the patients treated with 5-FU + methyl-CCNU in this trial. The median survival of patients treated with the combination was 20 weeks, whereas patients treated with methyl-CCNU lived a median of 13 weeks. The differences in survival may reflect the inferior response rate produced by methyl-CCNU (8%). Also, this modest improvement in survival may be secondary to the relatively high order of complete response in the patients treated with 5-FU plus methyl-CCNU (see Table 25-18).

An ECOG study reported in 1979 also brings into question the high response rate originally reported for 5-FU + methyl-CCNU.[137] This study compared 5-FU + methyl-CCNU, 5-FU + mitomycin C, and doxorubicin used as a single agent. The 5-FU + methyl-CCNU was used in a dosage schedule identical to that which had earlier produced a 40% response.[106] That response rate was not confirmed in the more recent study. Twelve (24%) of 49 patients receiving 5-FU + methyl-CCNU responded in this study, compared to 17 (32%) of 53 responding to 5-FU + mitomycin C. The patients in all arms of this study were similar as to sites of disease, extent of disease, and performance status. The survival curves for all arms were identical, with a median survival of 17 weeks. Finally, an ECOG study published in 1984 showed only a 14% response rate in 44 patients with advanced gastric cancer treated with 5-FU + methyl-CCNU.[151] The median survival for patients in this study was only 8 months.

The regimen of 5-FU + doxorubicin + methyl-CCNU has been shown to be active in gastric cancer.[136,154] This treatment produced an average response of 31% (see Table 25-18) and is well tolerated. Levi and associates[175] reported a 52% response in 35 patients treated with 5-FU + doxorubicin + BCNU. Two other studies performed with this combination reported response rates of 24% and 43%.[157,176] The overall experience with 5-FU + Adriamycin + BCNU has yielded a response rate of 42% (62 of 146 patients). The combination of 5-FU + Adriamycin + cisplatin has been evaluated in advanced gastric cancer.[171–174] Two studies report response rates of 31%[174] and 29%[171]; two other studies report response rates of 50%. The clinical trial reported by Moertel et al[173] is of particular interest since 11% of patients had complete responses. This treatment program is currently undergoing confirmation in a Phase III trial.

Triazinate in combination chemotherapy may have a role in the treatment of patients with advanced stomach cancer. A recent Phase III trial performed by the GITSG[162] has shown that the combination of 5-FU + Adriamycin + triazinate (FAT) produces significantly prolonged median survival (29 weeks) when compared to that produced by FAM (24 weeks). The respective year survival rates are 28% for FAT and 15% for FAM.

The combination of 5-FU + doxorubicin (Adriamycin) + mitomycin C (FAM) has been tested in 520 patients in 12 separate clinical trials with a cumulative response rate of 33% (173 of 520 patients). A large Phase II evaluation of FAM in 62 patients[132] reported an overall response rate of 42%. There was significant response in patients with major metastatic liver disease and large abdominal masses. Response was correlated with palliation of symptoms, and responding patients had marked improvement in performance status. In this Phase II trial responding patients survived a median of 13 months, compared to 3 months for nonresponding patients; however, there were no complete responses. FAM was well tolerated, with the only significant toxic effect being moderate myelosuppression.

The activity of the FAM regimen has been confirmed in both Phase II and Phase III trials.[161,168] Bitran and coworkers[161] in a small study found that 6 (55%) of 11 patients responded to FAM. In an ECOG Phase III study published in 1984,[151] 18 (39%) of 46 patients treated with FAM responded. This result is consistent with the order of response seen with FAM in Phase II studies. In a Phase III trial, the SWOG compared two dose schedules of FAM. The drugs given in the simultaneous schedule developed at Georgetown[132] were superior to the same drugs given sequentially. With the simultaneous schedule, 8 (40%) of 20 patients responded. With the sequential schedule, the response rate was 11% (4 of 26 patients). Differences in survival between these two treatment regimens were not significant. Of interest, the substitution of the furanyl derivative of 5-FU, Ftorafur, which may have less myelosuppressive toxicity than the other fluorinated pyrimidines, decreased the activity of FAM. Woolley and associates[181] reported responses in 3 (20%) of 15 patients with advanced gastric cancer treated with the regimen. The toxicity seen with the Ftorafur-substituted FAM regimen was significant and qualitatively different, since the Ftorafur caused major transient cerebellar dysfunction.

The North Central Cancer Therapy Group (NCCTG)[155] has reported results of a Phase III trial comparing 5-FU, 5-FU + doxorubicin, and the FAM regimen. Patients with both gastric and pancreatic cancer were included in the study. In gastric cancer, median survivals were between 6 and 7 months for all regimens. However, in the small number of patients with measurable cancer, FAM produced a superior response rate. Five (38%) of 13 patients treated with FAM had objective tumor regression, whereas the response rates for 5-FU + doxorubicin and 5-FU alone were 27% and 18%, respectively. It is not surprising that median survival was not improved with any of these regimens because fewer than 50% of patients responded.

Although partial response will not improve median survival, this outcome does result in palliation of symptoms. Combination chemotherapy produces partial response more frequently than single-agent treatment. Although FAM produces a consistent, if modest, response rate with tolerable toxic effects, FAM is far from ideal therapy. The major problem with FAM is that this regimen only rarely produces complete responses. In an analysis of 302 patients treated with FAM, only 7 (2%) had complete regression of disease.[182] It is clear that without a high rate of complete remission, no chemotherapy program will produce prolonged survival in patients with any form of advanced cancer.

Presently there has been interest in chemotherapy regimens utilizing biochemical modulation of antimetabolites in the treatment of gastric cancer. Machover et al[160] used 5-FU + folinic acid to treat 27 patients with advanced gastric cancer. Reduced folates stabilize the fluorodioxyuridylate (Fdump) thymidylate synthetase enzyme complex and thereby increase the effective cytotoxicity of 5-FU. Thirteen (48%) of 27 patients responded to 5-FU + folinic acid. One patient evidenced complete response. The value of fluorinated pyrimidine plus folinic acid in gastric cancer therapy must be confirmed in subsequent clinical trials. Another biochemical modulation of potential interest in stomach cancer is the use of methotrexate-"directed" 5-FU. Table 25-18 reports two studies[169,170] in which methotrexate, 5-FU, and Adriamycin produced responses in 81 (50%) of 162 patients. This response rate is particularly impressive, since 27% of patients had complete responses. These protocols used high-dose methotrexate (1.5 g/m^2) with folinic acid rescue and were associated with considerable methotrexate-related toxicity, including treatment-related deaths. The results of these two European studies are of interest and will require confirmation.

The most important observation about the combination chemotherapy of advanced gastric cancer is the high order of activity evidenced by several regimens in this disease.[106,131,169,170,177] Response rates of 40% to 50% are distinctly uncommon in advanced GI adenocarcinomas, and the apparent responsiveness of gastric cancer has encouraged active investigation of polychemotherapy. In reviewing Table 25-18, however, it is apparent that not all studies with FAM, FAP, FAMe, or 5-FU + methyl-CCNU report response rates of 40% to 50%. Clinical oncologists must evaluate clinical trial design carefully for similarity of response criteria, prognostic factors, and other factors relating to patient selection to ensure that differences in response to the same regimens are not artifactual. It is hoped that confirmation of active combination chemotherapy regimens in advanced disease will translate into effective treatment for earlier stages of disease.

Recommendations

The first option in the treatment of any eligible patient with advanced gastric cancer should be entrance into a clinical trial. If this is not feasible, one could consider the use of a combination chemotherapy regimen such as FAM or FAP, because this approach may increase the probability of attaining partial remission and palliation of symptoms.

FUTURE CONSIDERATIONS

A major effort toward early diagnosis of gastric cancer is a necessity in countries with a high incidence of this disease. This chapter has described the success the Japanese have had with such an approach.[84] However, in the United States, where stomach cancer is not a major public health problem and, if anything, has been decreasing in incidence, massive screening programs for early diagnosis would hardly be cost-effective. Therefore, the future direction in gastric cancer management that the American clinician will deal with will concern attempts to improve therapy of this disease.

SURGERY

Complete surgical resection of the tumor remains the major curative therapy modality in patients with stomach cancer. There has also been interest in reoperation for attempted curative resection of recurrent disease in gastric cancer patients. The curative benefit of planned reoperations for gastric carcinoma was minimal in the University of Minnesota series—four conversions to disease-free status, but three operative deaths.[56] There is no justification for reoperation unless it has specific palliative intent. However, in future aggressive regional treatment protocols, reoperation may be indicated. At present, there is no indication that conventional treatment should include reoperation aimed at cure.

CHEMOTHERAPY PLUS RADIATION

In view of the patterns of treatment failure in gastric cancer, it appears that innovative combinations of chemotherapy plus radiation therapy versus polychemotherapy alone may be necessary to alter both short- and long-term survival in resectable as well as unresectable disease. Even after so-called curative resection, locoregional failure is a significant problem, as noted in both the University of Minnesota reoperative series[52] and autopsy series.[52,54] This knowledge must be tempered, however, by the fact that distant failures (distant metastases plus peritoneal spread occur more commonly than with colorectal cancer and the natural history is much shorter, perhaps because of the much higher incidence of poorly differentiated gastric lesions. Early tumor-related deaths in the GITSG study (protocol 8274) may be related to the fact that combined drug chemotherapy was not instituted until at least day 71 after onset of treatment, which may have been 4 to 6 weeks after operative resection or exploration (overall time after diagnosis, 13–17 weeks or more). If one saves the best chemotherapy for 3 to 4 months from the time of diagnosis in such a disease, the systemic component, if present, may then be beyond control.

In view of the major systemic failure problem with gastric cancers, there is a need to optimize the use of combination chemotherapy and irradiation. This may involve idealized sequencing of combined drug regimens before or concomitantly with irradiation in a manner that will result in acceptable toxicity, yet shorten intervals from operative intervention to the institution of combined drug chemotherapy, and the time between chemotherapy courses. The problem with systemic failures, however, was not alleviated in pilot programs at the MGH and the Mayo Clinic that used combined drug chemotherapy before and after either conventional radiation therapy (MGH: 5-FU + BCNU, or FAM) or radiation therapy given in two fractions per day (Mayo: FA + XRT + FAMe).

Since chemotherapy has not been shown to have definite

curative potential for advanced disease, the only patients with curable disease may be those without occult dissemination at initiation of treatment. Therefore, an alternate treatment approach is to provide the most effective locoregional treatment "up front" (x-irradiation, one or two daily fractions ± 5-FU, combined with resection whenever this can be accomplished before or after irradiation), followed by the most effective systemic treatment, such as FAM, FAP, or perhaps 5-FU + folinic acid if initial promising results are confirmed with this biochemical modulation. Other more recent approaches to chemotherapy with fluorinated pyrimidines may be useful in gastric cancer combined modality programs. Lokich et al[183] have demonstrated in a Phase III study in patients with advanced colon cancer that continuous IV infusion of 5-FU at 300 mg/m²/day is superior to bolus IV administration of the drug. The response rate in the infusion patients was 31%, versus 8% in patients treated with bolus 5-FU. Continuous low-dose infusion of 5-FU through a central catheter has minimal toxicity (mainly hand/foot syndrome) and is not associated with myelosuppression or GI toxicity. Such low-dose continuous fluorinated pyrimidine therapy may have a role in combination with radiation therapy in patients with stomach cancer.

Since liver metastases and peritoneal seeding are common both after resection and in patients with unresectable or residual disease treated with radiation therapy plus chemotherapy, such failures could possibly be prevented or delayed by extending external beam radiation portals to include the entire upper abdomen or total abdomen for a portion of treatment, or by treating the peritoneal surfaces with intraperitoneal radiocolloids or chemotherapy (of less potential value in lesions at or extending to the esophagogastric junction or beyond, since failures in the lung are also common). An external beam upper abdomen portal has an advantage over a total abdomen beam in that it would not significantly increase the amount of bone marrow included in the irradiation field, yet it potentially alters both liver failures (distant metastases) and upper abdomen peritoneal disease. In the Minnesota reoperative series,[52] peritoneal seeding was localized in 20 of 44 patients and, on the basis of serial reoperations in several other patients, was seen to progress from upper abdominal involvement to diffuse abdominal involvement. In a Japanese gastric cancer series by Nakajima and co-workers,[184] of 96 patients who had peritoneal seeding, 29 (30%) had implants only in the upper abdomen (above the transverse colon mesentery). In that series, the finding of positive peritoneal cytology was an independent negative prognostic factor with regard to survival, and peritoneal cytology might be used to make decisions on upper versus total abdomen prophylaxis. With either approach, the risks of radiation-induced hepatitis or nephritis may be increased, and tolerance problems should be worked out with residual or unresected disease before being considered in an adjuvant setting.

RADIATION TECHNIQUES AND DOSE MODIFIERS

The limited tolerance of the stomach and surrounding organs and tissues prevents a major increase in dose levels above 5000 to 5500 rad. With residual, unresectable, or recurrent disease, the most likely gains will come from combined radiation therapy and chemotherapy (chemotherapy plus radiation therapy plus chemotherapy), dose modifiers (sensitizers, protectors, hyperthermia), or, in selected cases, dose localization and increased doses with external beam or intraoperative irradiation.

For patients found to have locally unresectable cancers at initial exploration, it would be worthwhile to obtain a baseline CT study, deliver 4500 to 5000 rad, and restage the patient 3 to 4 weeks later. If the patient is without evidence of metastases and the lesion has shrunk or is stable on repeat CT, it would be justifiable to consider operative exploration and resection with an intraoperative or postoperative boost dose of irradiation. This sequence may in fact be preferable to the alternative of resecting lesions found to have disease adherence or fixation at the initial exploration, since this usually results in cutting through tumor and may produce an increased incidence of peritoneal or hematogenous failure.

The Japanese experience of achieving some long-term cures after partial resection with the addition of a single large dose of intraoperative radiation supports continued use of intraoperative irradiation alone or in combination with fractionated external beam irradiation or chemotherapy in Japan and other countries. In the latter circumstance, a dose of 1000 to 2000 rad could be delivered as a boost to the tumor bed and primary nodal areas after resection, or to areas of residual disease plus primary nodal sites after subtotal resection. Postoperative radiation therapy would then be used to deliver 4500 to 5000 rad to the areas at risk, based on both operative findings and pathologic reconstruction.

SUMMARY

Gastric malignancies present us with many challenges. Innovative combined modality approaches will be needed if survival is to be improved and toxic effects of treatment are to be acceptable. Careful and detailed intraoperative staging is imperative if seminal clinical trials are to be designed that will provide the information necessary for developing appropriate treatment strategies for this disease. Such strategies may include combinations of external beam and intraoperative irradiation plus resection for the local component, and systemic or intraperitoneal chemotherapy or wide-field irradiation, or a combination of these three, for therapy of intra-abdominal or systemic disease. The role of biological response modifiers (cytokines, adoptive immunotherapy, and differentiating agents) in gastric cancer needs to be defined. The possibilities for clinical research in stomach cancer therapy are manifold.

REFERENCES

1. Silverberg E, Lubera J: Cancer Statistics. CA 36:9–25, 1986
2. Devesa SS, Silverman DT: Cancer incidence and mortality trends in the United States 1935–1974. JNCI 60:545–561, 1978
3. Dunham LJ, Bailar JC III: World maps of cancer mortality rates and frequency ratios. JNCI 41:155–203, 1968
4. Staszewski J: Migrant studies in alimentary tract cancer. Recent Results Cancer Res 39:85–97, 1971

5. Haenszel W, Kurihara M, Segi M et al: Stomach cancer among Japanese in Hawaii. JNCI 49:969–988, 1972
6. Moertel CG: The stomach. In Holland JF, Frei E III (eds): Cancer Medicine, pp 1760–1774. Philadelphia, Lea & Febiger, 1982
7. Haas JF, Schottenfeld D: Epidemiology of gastric cancer. In Lipkin M, Good RA (eds): Gastrointestinal Tract Cancer. Sloan-Kettering Cancer Series. New York, Plenum Medical, 1978
8. Selikoff IJ: Cancer risk of asbestos exposure. In Hiatt HH, Watson JD, Winsten JA (eds): Origins of Human Cancer, Book C, pp 1765–1784. New York, Cold Spring Harbor Laboratory, 1977
9. Aird I, Benthall HH, Roberts JAF: A relationship between cancer of the stomach and the ABO blood groups. Br Med J 1:799–801, 1953
10. Imai T, Kubo T, Watanabe H: Chronic gastritis in Japanese with reference to high incidence of gastric carcinoma. JNCI 47:179–195, 1971
11. Moertel CG: The stomach. In Holland JH, Frei E III (eds): Cancer Medicine, pp 1527–1541. Philadelphia, Lea & Febiger, 1973
12. Pack GT: Unusual tumors of the stomach. Ann NY Acad Sci 114:985, 1964
13. Phillips JC, Linsay JW, Kendall JA: Gastric leiomyosarcoma: Roentgenologic and clinical findings. Am J Dig Dis 15:239, 1970
14. Macon WL: Gastric lymphoma vs adenocarcinoma. A diagnostic problem. Arch Surg 114:305–306, 1979
15. Piper SW (ed): Stomach Cancer, p 41. Geneva, UICC Technical Report Series, 1978
16. Morson BC: Carcinoma arising from areas of intestinal metaplasia in the gastric mucosa. Br J Cancer 9:377, 1955
17. Higgins GA, Serlin O, Amadeo JH et al: Gastric cancer factors in survival. Surg Gastrointest 10:393, 1976
18. Rouviere H: Anatomy of the Human Lymphatic System, pp 183–187. Ann Arbor, Edwards Bros, 1938
19. Cady B, Choed DS: Changing patterns of gastric cancer. In Nieburgs HE (ed.): Third International Symposium on Detection and Prevention of Cancer, pp 2041–2049. New York, Decker, 1980
20. O'Brien MJ, Bunakoff R, Robbins EA et al: Early gastric cancer: Clinicopathologic study. Am J Med 78:195–202, 1985
21. Berkson J: Statistical smmary. In ReMine JH, Priestley JT, Berkson J (eds): Cancer of the Stomach, p 207. Philadelphia, WB Saunders, 1964
22. Collins WT, Gall EA: Gastric carcinoma, multicentric lesion. Cancer 5:62, 1952
23. Moertel CG, Reitemeier RJ: Advanced Gastrointestinal Cancer: Clinical Management and Chemotherapy, pp 3–21. New York, Harper & Row, 1969
24. Correa P: IAP Maude Abbott Lecture. Geographic pathology of cancer in Colombia. Int Pathol 11:16, 1970.
25. Correa P, Cuello C, Duque E: Carcinoma and intestinal metaplasia of the stomach in Colombian migrants. J Natl Cancer Inst 44:297, 1970
26. Piper DW (ed): Stomach Cancer, p 16. Geneva, UICC Technical Report Series, 1978
27. Kawachi T, Sugimura T: Abnormal differentiation of stomach epithelium: Intestinalization as the possible beginning of neoplastic change. In Ebert J, Okada T (eds): Mechanisms of Cell Change. New York, John Wiley & Sons, 1979
28. Piper DW (ed): Stomach Cancer, p 27. Geneva, UICC Technical Report Series, 1978
29. Matsukura N, Kawachi T, Sasajima K et al: Induction of intestinal metaplasia in the stomach of rats by N-methyl-N′-nitro-N-nitrosoguanadine. J Natl Cancer Inst 61:141, 1978
30. Sasajima K, Kawachi T, Matsukura N et al: Intestinal metaplasia and adenocarcinoma induced in the stomach of rats by N-propyl-N′-nitro-N-nitrosoguanidine. J Cancer Res Clin Oncol 94:201, 1979
31. Hofman NR: The relationship between pernicious anemia and cancer of the stomach. Geriatrics 25:90, 1970
32. Hitchcock CR, Schneiner SL. Early diagnosis of gastric cancer. Surg Gynecol Obstet 113:655, 1961
33. Lygidakis NJ: Gastric stump cancer after surgery for gastroduodenal ulcer. Ann R Coll Surg Engl 63:203–205, 1981
34. Giarelli L, Melato M, Stauta G et al: Gastric resection a cause of high frequency of gastric carcinoma. Cancer 52:1113–1116, 1983
35. Kuru M: On cancers developed upon ulcerative lesions of the stomach: A study of the regeneration of the mucous membrane of the stomach with special reference to its malignant transformation. Gann 44:47, 1953
36. Ming SC: Histogenesis and premalignant lesions. JAMA 228:886, 1974
37. Oota K: On the nature of the ulcerative changes in early carcinoma of the stomach. Gann Monogr 3:141, 1968
38. Tomaslo J: Gastric polyps. Histologic types and their relationship to gastric carcinoma. Cancer 27:1346, 1971
39. Ming SC, Goldman H: Gastric polyps: A histogenetic classification and its relation to carcinoma. Cancer 18:721, 1965
40. Piper DW (ed): Stomach Cancer, p 30. Geneva, UICC Technical Report Series, 1978
41. Thunold S, Wetteland P: Ulcer-carcinoma of the stomach in a 10-year biopsy series. A follow-up study of 19 patients. Arch Pathol Microbiol Scand 56:155, 1962
42. Piper DW (ed): Stomach Cancer, p 31. Geneva, UICC Technical Report Series, 1978
43. Larson NE, Cain JC, Bartholomew LG: Prognosis of the medically treated small gastric ulcer; comparison of follow-up data in two series. N Engl J Med 164:119, 1961
44. Cohn I Jr: The meaning of lymph node metastases and their treatment: Cancer of the stomach, pancreas, and small bowel. In Weiss L, Gilbert HA, Ballon SG (eds): Lymphatic System Metastases, p 262. Boston, GK Hall, 1980
45. Dupont JB Jr, Cohn I Jr: Gastric adenocarcinoma. Curr Probl Cancer 4:25, 1980
46. Dupont JB Jr, Lee JR, Burton GR et al: Adenocarcinoma of the stomach: Review of 1497 cases. Cancer 41:941, 1978
47. Arhelger SW, Lober PH, Wangensteen OH: Dissection of the hepatic pedicle and retropancreaticoduodenal areas for cancer of the stomach. Surgery 38:675, 1955
48. Coller FA, Kay EB, McIntyre RS: Regional lymphatic metastases of carcinoma of the stomach. Arch Surg 43:748, 1941
49. Clarke JS, Cruze K, El Farra S et al: The natural history and results of surgical therapy for carcinoma of the stomach: An analysis of 250 cases. Am J Surg 102:143, 1961
50. Warren S: Studies on tumor metastasis: IV. Metastases of cancer of the stomach. N Engl J Med 209:825, 1933
51. Warwick M: Analysis of one hundred and seventy-six cases of carcinoma of the stomach submitted to autopsy. Ann Surg 88:216, 1928
52. Papachristou DN, Fortner JG: Local recurrence of gastric adenocarcinomas after gastrectomy. J Surg Oncol 18:47–53, 1981
53. McNeer G, Vandenberg H, Donn FY et al: A critical evaluation of subtotal gastrectomy for the cure of cancer of the stomach. Ann Surg 134:2, 1951
54. Thomson FB, Robins RE: Local recurrence following subtotal resection for gastric carcinoma. Surg Gynecol Obstet 95:351, 1952
55. Wisbeck WA, Becker EM, Russell AH: Adenocarcinoma of the stomach: Autopsy observations with therapeutic implications for the radiation oncologist. Radiother Oncol 7:13–18, 1986
56. Gunderson LL, Sosin H: Adenocarcinoma of the stomach—areas of failure in a reoperation series (second or symptomatic looks): Clinicopathologic correlation and implications for adjuvant therapy. Int J Radiat Oncol Biol Phys 8:1–11, 1982
57. Landry J, Tepper JE, Wood WL et al: Patterns of failure following curative resection of gastric carcinoma: ASTRO Proceedings 1986. Int J Radiat Oncol Biol Phys vol 12(1):119, 1986
58. Adashek K, Sanger J, Longmire WP Jr: Cancer of the stomach. Review of consecutive ten-year intervals. Ann Surg 189:6, 1979
59. Goldsmith HS, Ghosh BC: Carcinoma of the stomach. Am J Surg 120:317, 1970
60. Kelsey JR Jr: Cancer of the Stomach: A Clinical Guide for Diagnosis and Treatment. Springfield, Ill, Charles C Thomas, 1967
61. LaDue JS, Murison PJ, McNeer G et al: Symptomatology and diagnosis of gastric cancer. Arch Surg 60:305, 1950
62. Shahon DB, Hdorowitz S, Kelly WD: Cancer of the stomach: An analysis of 1,152 cases. Surgery 39:204, 1956
63. McNeer G, Pack GT: Malignant tumors of the stomach. In Pack GT, Ariel IM (eds): Treatment of Cancer and Allied Diseases, vol 5, pp 111–268. New York, Paul B Hoeber, 1962
64. Hoerr SO: Prognosis for carcinoma of the stomach. Surg Gynecol Obstet 137:205, 1973
65. Hoerr SO, Hodgman RW: Carcinoma of the stomach: An interpretive review. Am J Surg 107:620, 1964
66. Beahrs OH, Myers MH (eds): Manual for Staging of Cancer, p 67. Philadelphia, JB Lippincott, 1983
67. Kennedy BJ: TNM classification for stomach cancer. Cancer 26:971, 1970
68. Japanese Research Society for Gastric Cancer: The general rules for the gastric cancer study in surgery. Jpn J Surg 3:61, 1973
69. Okajima K: Surgical treatment of gastric cancer with special reference to lymph node removal. Acta Med Okayama 31:3269, 1977
70. Desmond AM: Radical surgery in treatment of carcinoma of the stomach. Proc R Soc Med 69:867, 1976
71. ReMine WH, Priestley JT, Berkson J: Cancer of the Stomach. Philadelphia, WB Saunders, 1964
72. Gastrointestinal Tumor Study Group: Controlled trial of adjuvant chemotherapy following curative resection for gastric cancer. Cancer 49:1116–1122, 1982
73. Antoniolli DA, Goldman H: Changes in the location and type of gastric adenocarcinoma. CA 50:775–781, 1982
74. Gastrointestinal Tumor Study Group: A comparison of combination chemotherapy and combined modality therapy for locally advanced gastric carcinoma. Cancer 49:1771–1777, 1982
75. Cooley RN: The diagnostic accuracy of upper gastrointestinal radiologic studies. Am J Med Sci 242:628, 1961
76. Laufer I: Double contrast radiology in the diagnosis of gastrointestinal cancer. In Glass J (ed): Progress in Gastroenterology, pp 643–669. New York, Grune & Stratton, 1977
77. Laufer I: A simple method for routine double contrast study of the upper gastrointestinal tract. Radiology 117:513, 1975
78. Bockus HL: Gastroenterology, 2nd ed, vol I, pp 743–801. Philadelphia, WB Saunders, 1963
79. Winawer SJ, Melamed M, Sherlock P: Potential of endoscopy, biopsy, and cytology in the diagnosis and management of patients with cancer. Clin Gastroenterol 5:575, 1976
80. Winawer SJ, Sherlock P, Hajdu SI: The role of upper gastrointestinal endoscopy in patients with cancer. Cancer 37:440, 1976
81. Wittenberg J: Computed tomography of the body. N Engl J Med 309:1224–1230, 1983
82. Nathanson L: Remote effects of cancer in the host. In Horton J, Hill L (eds): Clinical Oncology, pp 49–85. Philadelphia, WB Saunders, 1977

83. Schein PS: Tumor markers. In Beeson P, McDermott W, Wyngaarden J (eds): Textbook of Medicine, pp 1411–1413. Philadelphia, WB Saunders, 1979
84. Kaneko E, Nakamura T, Umeda N et al: Outcome of gastric carcinoma detected by gastric mass survey in Japan. Gut 18:6–26, 1977
85. Prolla JC, Kobayashi S, Kirsner JB: Gastric cancer: Some recent improvements in diagnosis based upon the Japanese experience. Arch Intern Med 124:238, 1969
86. Longmire WP Jr: Total gastrectomy for carcinoma of the stomach. Surg Gynecol Obstet 84:21, 1947
87. Miwa K: Advances in treatment of stomach carcinoma in Japan. In Hirayama T (ed): Epidemiology of Stomach Cancer: Key Questions and Answers, pp 105–110. Tokyo, WHO, 1977
88. Pack GT, McNeer G: Total gastrectomy for cancer. A collective review of the literature and an original report of twenty cases. Int Abstr Surg 77:265, 1943
89. Paulino F. Roselli A: Carcinoma of the stomach, with special reference to total gastrectomy. Curr Probl Surg, pp 1–72, Dec 1973
90. Ransom HK: Cancer of the stomach. Surg Gynecol Obstet 96:275, 1953
91. Rush BF Jr, Brown MW, Ravitch MM: Total gastrectomy: An evaluation of its use in the treatment of gastric cancer. Cancer 13:643, 1960
92. Lumpkin WM, Crow RL Jr, Hernandez CM et al: Carcinoma of the stomach: Review of 1,035 cases. Ann Surg 159:919, 1964
93. Serlin O, Keehn RJ, Higgins GA et al: Factors related to survival following resection for gastric carcinoma. Cancer 40:1318, 1977
94. Ekbom GA, Gleysteen JJ: Gastric malignancy: Resection for palliation. Surgery 88:476, 1980
95. Diehl JT, Hermann RE, Cooperman AM, Hoerr SO: Gastric carcinoma. A ten-year review. Ann Surg 198:9, 1983
96. Lygidakis NJ: Total gastrectomy for gastric carcinoma: A retrospective study of different procedures and assessment of a new technique of gastric reconstruction. Br J Surg 68:649, 1981
97. Nelson PG, Collier N: Carcinoma of the stomach: The need for a new approach. Aust NZJ Surg 52:358, 1982
98. Inberg MV, Heinonen R, Lauren P et al: Total and proximal gastrectomy in the treatment of gastric carcinoma: A series of 305 cases. World J Surg 5:249, 1981
99. Dixon WJ, Longmire WP, Holden WD: Use of triethylenethiophosphoramide as an adjuvant to the surgical treatment of gastric and colorectal carcinoma: Ten year follow-up. Ann Surg 173:16, 1971
100. Serlin O, Wolkoff JS, Amadeo JM et al: Use of 5-fluorodeoxyuridine (FudR) as an adjuvant to the surgical management of carcinoma of the stomach. Cancer 24:223, 1969
101. Higgins GA, Amadeo JH, Smith DE et al: Efficacy of prolonged intermittent therapy with combined 5-FU and methyl-CCNU following resection for gastric carcinoma. Cancer 52:1105, 1983
102. Engstrom P, Lavin P: Post-operative adjuvant therapy for gastric cancer patients. Proc Am Soc Clin Oncol 2:114, 1983
103. Galiano R, McCracken JD, Chen T: Adjuvant chemotherapy with 5-fluorouracil, adriamycin, and mitomycin (FAM) in gastric cancer. Proc Am Soc Clin Oncol 2:114, 1983
103a. Krook JE, O'Connell MJ, Wieand HS et al: Adjuvant therapy of gastric cancer with doxorubicin and 5-fluorouracil. Proc Am Soc Clin Oncol 7:93, 1988
104. Nakajima T, Takahashi T, Takagi K: Comparison of 5-FU with Ftorafur in adjuvant chemotherapies with combined inductive and maintenance therapies for gastric cancer. J Clin Oncol 2:1366–1371, 1984
105. Lawrence W: Nutritional consequences of surgical resection of gastrointestinal tract for cancer. Cancer Res 37:2379, 1977
106. Moertel CG, Mittelman JA, Bakermeier RF et al: Sequential and combination chemotherapy of advanced gastric cancer. Cancer 38:678, 1976
107. Luxton RW, Kunkler PB: Radiation nephritis. Acta Radiol 2:169, 1964
108. Goffinet DR, Glatstein E, Zuks Z, Kaplan HS: Abdominal irradiation in non-Hodgkin's lymphoma. Cancer 37:2797, 1976
109. Gunderson LL, Hoskins B, Cohen A et al: Combined modality treatment of gastric cancer. Proc ASTR Int J Radiol Oncol 5:118, 1979
110. Willett C, Tepper JE, Orlow EL et al: Renal complications secondary to treatment of upper abdominal malignancies. ASTRO Proceedings, 1985
111. Goldstein HM, Rogers LF, Fletcher GH, Dodd GD: Radiological manifestations of radiation-induced injury to the normal upper gastrointestinal tract. Radiology 117:135, 1975
112. Nordman E, Kauppinen C: The value of megavolt therapy in carcinoma of the stomach. Strahlentherapie 144:635, 1972
113. Roswit B, Malsky SJ, Reid CB: Radiation tolerance of the gastrointestinal tract. Radiat Ther Oncol 6:160–181, 1972
114. Buskirk SJ, Gunderson LL, Nagorney DM et al: Analysis of failure following curative radiation of extrahepatic bile duct cancers. Int J Radiat Oncol Biol Phys 12:120, 1986
115. Abe M, Yabumoto E, Takahashi M, Adachi H, Yoshi M, Mori K: Intra-operative radiotherapy of gastric cancer. Cancer 45:40, 1980
116. Asakawa H, Otawa K, Watarai J: High energy x-ray therapy for stomach carcinoma, second report: The evaluation of radiotherapy for the early and the inoperable stomach carcinoma. Nippon Acta Radiol 31:505, 1971 (English tables and extended summary)
117. Asakawa H, Takeda T: High energy x-ray therapy of gastric carcinoma. J Jpn Soc Cancer Ther 8:362, 1973
118. Hoshi H: Histologic study on the effect of preoperative irradiation on gastric cancer. Tohoku J Exp Med 96:293, 1968
119. Takahashi T: Studies on preoperative and postoperative telecolbalt therapy in gastric cancer. Nippon Acta Radiol 24:129, 1964 [English tables and abstract]
120. Wieland C, Hymmen U: Megavoltage therapy for malignant gastric tumors (abstr). Strahlentherapie 140:20, 1970
121. Childs DS, Moertel CG, Holbrook MA et al: Treatment of unresectable adenocarcinomas of the stomach with a combination of 5-fluorouracil and radiation. AJR 102:541, 1968
122. Falkson G, Falkson HC: Fluorouracil and radiotherapy in gastrointestinal cancer. Lancet 2:1252, 1969
123. Lagunova IG, Cybulskij BA, Kornev II et al: Ausseinander folgende Strahlentherapie mit einem 25-meV Betatron and Chemotherapie mit Fluoruracil zur Behandlung von Kranken mit fortgeschrittenem Krebs des oberen Magenabschnittes (abstr). Radiobiol Radiother (Berl) 13:307, 1978
124. Moertel CG, Childs DS, O'Fallon JR et al: Combined 5-fluorouracil and radiation therapy as a surgical adjuvant for poor prognosis gastric carcinoma. J Clin Oncol 2:1249, 1984
125. Haas L, Vaikevicius V, Bukowski R et al: Southwest Oncology Group (SWOG) pilot study of radiotherapy (R) + 5-fluorouracil (F) + adriamycin (A) + mitomycin C (M) in patients with minimal residual gastric cancer (abstr). Proc Am Soc Clin Oncol 21:342, 1980
126. Lingos T, Tepper JE, Gunderson LL et al: Adjuvant FAM–Rad–FAM after resection of high risk gastric carcinoma. Int J Radiat Oncol Biol Phys 11:110, 1985
127. Schein PS, Smith FP, Dritschillo A et al: Phase I-II trial of combined modality FAM plus split-course radiation (FAM-RT-FAM) for locally advanced gastric and pancreatic cancer: A Mid-Atlantic Oncology Program study. Abstr Am Soc Clin Oncol 1983:126, 1983
128. O'Connell MJ, Gunderson LL, Moertel CG et al: A pilot study to determine clinical tolerability of intensive combined modality therapy for locally unresectable gastric cancer. Int J Radiat Oncol Biol Phys 11:1827, 1985
129. Abe M, Takahashi M: Intraoperative radiotherapy: The Japanese experience. Int J Radiat Oncol Biol Phys 5:863–868, 1981
130. Boice JD, Greene MH, Killen JY et al: Leukemia and preleukemia after adjuvant treatment of gastrointestinal cancer with Semustine (methyl-CCNU). N Engl J Med 309:1079–1084, 1983
131. Kovach JS, Moertel CG, Schutt AJ: A controlled study of combined 1, 3-bis-2-chloroethyl-l-nitrosourea and 5-flurouracil therapy for advanced gastric and pancreatic cancer. Cancer 33:563, 1974
132. Macdonald JS, Schein PS, Woolley PV et al: 5-Fluorouracil, mitomycin-C, and adriamycin (FAM): A new combination chemotherapy program for advanced gastric carcinoma. Ann Intern Med 93:533, 1980
133. Schein PS, Smith FP, Woolley PV et al: Current management of advanced and locally unresectable gastric carcinoma. Cancer 50:2590–2596, 1982
134. Comis RL, Carter SK: Integration of chemotherapy into combined modality treatment of solid tumors: III. Gastric cancer. Cancer Treat Rev 1:221, 1974
135. Moertel CG: Chemotherapy of gastrointestinal cancer. Clin Gastroenterol 5:777, 1976
136. Gastrointestinal Tumor Study Group: Phase II–III chemotherapy studies in advanced gastric cancer. Cancer Treat Rep 63:1871, 1979
137. Moertel CG, Lavin PT: Phase II–III chemotherapy studies in advanced gastric cancer. Cancer Treat Rep 63:1863, 1979
138. Livingston RB, Carter SK: Single Agents in Cancer Chemotherapy. New York, IFI/Plenum, 1970
139. Moore G, Bross I, Ausman R et al: Effects of chlorambucil (NSC 3088) in 374 patients with advanced cancer. Cancer Chemother Rep 52:661, 1968
140. Hurley JD, Ellison EH, Carey LL: Treatment of advanced cancer of the gastrointestinal tract with antitumor agents. Gastroenterology 41:557, 1961
141. Lacave A, Izarzugaza I, Aparicio L et al: Phase II clinical trial of cisdichlorodiamminеplatinum in gastric cancer. Am J Clin Oncol 6:35–38, 1983
142. Beer M, Cocconi G, Ceci G et al: A phase II study of cisplatin in advanced gastric cancer. Eur J Cancer Clin Oncol 19:717–720, 1983
143. Bruckner HW, Lokich JJ, Stablein DM: Studies of Baker's antifol, methotrexate, and Razoxane in advanced gastric cancer: A gastrointestinal tumor study group report. Cancer Treat Rep 66:1713–1717, 1982
144. Cazap E, Bruno M, Levy D et al: Phase II trial of 4′-epi-doxorubicin (4′-epi-dx) in advanced gastric cancer. Proc Am Soc Clin Pathol 5:91, 1986
145. Kelsen D, Sternberg C, Einzig A et al: Phase II study of carboplatin (CBDCA) in advanced upper gastrointestinal tract malignancy. Proc Am Soc Clin Oncol 3:141, 1984
146. Panettiere F, Jones S, Oishi N et al: Bisantrene hydrochloride in gastric adenocarcinoma: A Southwest Oncology Group study. Med Pediatr Oncol 14:78–80, 1986
147. The Southeastern Cancer Study Group: m-AMSA treatment of advanced colorectal, pancreatic, and gastric carcinoma. Proc Am Soc Clin Oncol 22:454, 1981
148. Bjerkeset T, Fjosne H: Comparison of oral ftorafur and intravenous 5-fluorouracil in patients with advanced cancer of the stomach, colon or rectum. Oncology 43:212–215, 1986
149. Jones R: Mitomycin-C: A preliminary report of studies of human pharmacology and initial therapeutic trial. Cancer Chemother Rep 2:3, 1959
150. Baker IH, Caoili EM, Izbick VK: A comparative study of mitomycin-C and profiromycin. Proc Am Soc Clin Oncol 15:182, 1974

151. Douglass H, Lavin P, Goudsmit A et al: An Eastern Cooperative Oncology Group evaluation of combinations of methyl-CCNU, mitomycin-C, Adriamycin, and 5-fluorouracil in advanced measurable gastric cancer (Est 2277). J Clin Oncol 2:1372–1381, 1984
152. Buroker T, Kim P, Grappe C et al: 5-FU infusion with mitomycin-C versus 5-FU infusion with methyl-CCNU in the treatment of advanced upper gastrointestinal cancer. Cancer 44:1215–1221, 1979
153. The Southwest Oncology Group: Randomized prospective trial comparing 5-fluorouracil (NSC-19893) to 5-fluorouracil and methyl-CCNU (NSC-95441) in advanced gastrointestinal cancer. Cancer Treat Rep 60:733–737, 1976
154. The Gastrointestinal Tumor Study Group: A comparative clinical assessment of combination chemotherapy in the management of advanced gastric carcinoma. Cancer 49:1362–1366, 1982
155. Cullinan S, Moertel C, Fleming T et al: A comparison of three chemotherapeutic regimens in the treatment of advanced pancreatic and gastric carcinoma. JAMA 253:2061–2067, 1985
156. The Gastrointestinal Tumor Study Group: randomized study of combination chemotherapy in unresectable gastric cancer. Cancer 53:13–17, 1984
157. Jamieson G, Gill P: A prospective trial of 5-FU and BCNU in the treatment of advanced gastric cancer. Aust NZ J Surg 5:16–19, 1981
158. Schnitizler G, Queisser W, Heim M et al: Phase III study of 5-FU and carmustine versus 5-FU, carmustine and doxorubicin in advanced gastric cancer. Cancer Treat Rep 70:477–479, 1986
159. O'Connell M, Schutt A, Moertel C et al: Phase II clinical trial of triazinate in combination with mitomycin-C for patients with advanced gastric cancer. Proc Am Soc Clin Oncol 5:82, 1986
160. Machover D, Goldschmidt E, Chollet P et al: Treatment of advanced colorectal and gastric adenocarcinomas with 5-fluorouracil and high dose folinic acid. J Clin Oncol 4:685–696, 1986
161. Bitran JD, Desser RK, Kozloff MF et al: Treatment of metastatic pancreatic and gastric adenocarcinomas with 5-fluorouracil, Adriamycin, and mitomycin-C (FAM). Cancer Treat Rep 63:2049, 1979
162. Bruckner HW, Stablein DM (for the Gastrointestinal Tumor Study Group): A randomized study of 5-FU, methyl-CCNU, cis-platinum, or triazinate for treatment of advanced gastric cancer. Proc Am Soc Clin Oncol 5:90, 1986
163. Benetta G, Fraschini P, Labianca R et al: The value of FAM polychemotherapy in advanced gastric cancer. Proc Am Soc Clin Oncol 1:103, 1982
164. The Southwest Oncology Group: 5-Fluorouracil, Adriamycin, and mitomycin-C ± vincristine (FAM vs V-FAM) compared to chlorozotocin, mAMSA and dihydroxyanthracenedione with unimpressive differences. Proc Am Soc Clin Oncol 2:122, 1983
165. Cummingham D, Soukop M, McArdle C et al: Advanced gastric cancer: Experience in Scotland using 5-fluorouracil, Adriamycin, and mitomycin-C. Br J Surg 71:673–676, 1984
166. Haim N, Cohen Y, Honigman J et al: Treatment of advanced gastric carcinoma with 5-fluorouracil, Adriamycin, and mitomycin-C (FAM). Cancer Chemother Pharmacol 8:277–280, 1982
167. Haim N, Epelbaum R, Cohen Y et al: Further studies on the treatment of advanced gastric cancer by 5-fluorouracil, Adriamycin, and mitomycin-C (modified FAM). Cancer 54:1999–2002, 1984
168. Panettiere F, Haas C, McDonald B et al: Drug combinations in the treatment of gastric adenocarcinoma. J Clin Oncol 2:420–424, 1984
169. Wils J, Bleiberg H, Dalesio O et al: An EORTC Gastrointestinal Group evaluation of the combination of sequential methotrexate and 5-fluorouracil, combined with Adriamycin in advanced measurable gastric cancer. J Clin Oncol 4:1799–1803, 1986
170. Klein H, Wickramanayake P, Farrokh G: 5-FU, adriamycin, and methotrexate: A combination protocol (FAMTX) for treatment of metastasized stomach cancer. Proc Am Soc Clin Oncol 5:84, 1986
171. Cazap E, Gisselbrecht C, Smith F et al: Phase II trials of 5-FU, doxorubicin, and cisplatin in advanced, measurable adenocarcinoma of the lung and stomach. Cancer Treat Rep 70:781–783, 1986
172. Wagener D, Burghouts J, van Dam F et al: A Phase II trial of 5-fluorouracil, Adriamycin, and cisplatin (FAP) in advanced gastric cancer. Proc Am Soc Clin Oncol 115, 1983
173. Moertel C, Rubin J, O'Connel M et al: A phase II study of combined 5-fluorouracil, doxorubicin, and cisplatin in the treatment of advanced upper gastrointestinal adenocarcinomas. J Clin Oncol 4:1053–1057, 1986
174. Robinson E, Haim N, Eppelbaum R et al: Phase II trials in the treatment of advanced gastric cancer. Proc Am Soc Clin Oncol 4:77, 1985
175. Levi J, Dalley D, Aroney R: Improved combination chemotherapy in advanced gastric cancer. Br Med J 2:1471–1473, 1979
176. Levi J, Fox R, Tattersall M et al: Analysis of a prospectively randomized comparison of doxorubicin versus 5-fluorouracil, doxorubicin, and BCNU in advanced gastric cancer: Implications for future studies. J Clin Oncol 4:1348–1355, 1986
177. Ahlgren J, Smith F, Harvey J et al: A phase II study of FAM plus triazinate for advanced measurable gastric carcinoma. Proc Am Soc Clin Oncol 3:145, 1984
178. De Lisi V, Cocconi G, Tonato M et al: Randomized comparison of 5-FU alone or combined with carmustine, doxorubicin, and mitomycin (BAFMi) in the treatment of advanced gastric cancer. Cancer Treat Rep 70:481–485, 1986
179. Bunn P, Nugent J, Ihde D et al: 5-Fluorouracil, methyl-CCNU, Adriamycin, and mitomycin C in the treatment of advanced gastric cancer. Cancer Treat Rep 62:1287–1293, 1978
180. Karlin D, Stroehlein J, Bennetts R et al: Phase I–II study of the combination of 5-FU, doxorubicin, mitomycin, and semustine (FAMMe) in the treatment of adenocarcinoma of the stomach, gastroesophageal junction, and pancreas. Cancer Treat Rep 66:1613–1617, 1982
181. Woolley PV, Macdonald JS, Smythe I et al: A phase II trial of Ftorafur, Adriamycin, and mitomycin-C (FAM II) in advanced gastric adenocarcinoma. Cancer 44:1211, 1979
182. Macdonald JS, Gohmann J: Chemotherapy of gastric cancer. Semin Oncol 15(suppl 4):42–49, 1988
183. Lokich J, Ahlgren J, Gullo J, Mid-Atlantic Oncology Program: A randomized trial of standard bolus 5-FU vs. protracted infusional 5-FU in advanced colon cancer. Proc Am Soc Clin Oncol 6:81, 1987
184. Nakajima T, Harashima S, Hirata M et al: Prognostic and therapeutic values of peritoneal cytology in gastric cancer. Acta Cytol 22:225–229, 1978

MURRAY F. BRENNAN
TIMOTHY KINSELLA
MICHAEL FRIEDMAN

CHAPTER 26 *Cancer of the Pancreas*

Pancreatic cancer is the fourth largest cancer killer in adults in the United States. The incidence of new cases of the disease and the death rate each year remain very close. In 1988, approximately 27,000 new cases will be seen in the United States, and 24,500 deaths will eventually result. The incidence is exceeded only by lung, colon and rectum, prostate, and breast cancer(s).

EPIDEMIOLOGIC CONSIDERATIONS

Because most patients with pancreatic cancer die of the disease, mortality data can be a good indicator of incidence provided that diagnostic accuracy is high.[1] Diagnostic accuracy can be checked by comparing the number of cases histologically confirmed at operation, biopsy, or autopsy with the number of cases diagnosed. For cancer of the pancreas, this varies from 75% to 95%.[1]

Cancer of the pancreas is increasing, and age-specific death rates increase with age (Fig. 26-1). The median age of presentation in national surveys is 69.2 years for men and 69.5 years for women from 1973 through 1977.[2] The overall male–female ratio of patients suspected of having peripancreatic cancer, presenting to Memorial Sloan-Kettering Cancer Center from October 1983 to October 1986, was 1.2:1. This differs from the male–female ratio of 1.7:1.0 for pancreatic cancer deaths in other series.[3] The male–female ratio differs according to age and has been previously reported for pancreatic cancer deaths varying from 2:1 for patients younger than age 40 to 1:1 for patients older than age 80. Our present data suggest that the male–female ratios for age at presentation younger than 40 are 3:1, 1.8:1 for 41 to 50 years; 1.2:1 for 51 to 80 years; and 1.1:1 for patients older than 80. The overall persistent male preponderance is completely reversed, however, in the Native Indian population in New Mexico (Fig. 26-2).[4]

The incidence of pancreatic cancer in several predominantly Spanish populations varies from 3.0 per 100,000 women in Puerto Rico to 11.7 per 100,000 Spanish men in New Mexico (Table 26-1). These racial differences are emphasized by the incidence in black men in Los Angeles (9.5 per 100,000) compared with the rate in Chinese men in the same city of 2.0 per 100,000 (Fig. 26-3). Intermediate rates are seen for the United States white population, the Spanish population, and the Japanese population.

The incidence in countries of origin and in first-generation and second-generation immigrants has been examined (Fig. 26-4). The rate in the first generation rapidly increases to the rate of U.S. whites. This is not solely due to smoking, although it may account for the effect in Japanese and Chinese populations.[5]

The influence of birthplace has been examined in Israel, and the incidence of carcinoma of the pancreas varies from 10.4 per 100,000 men born in Europe or America to 5.6 per

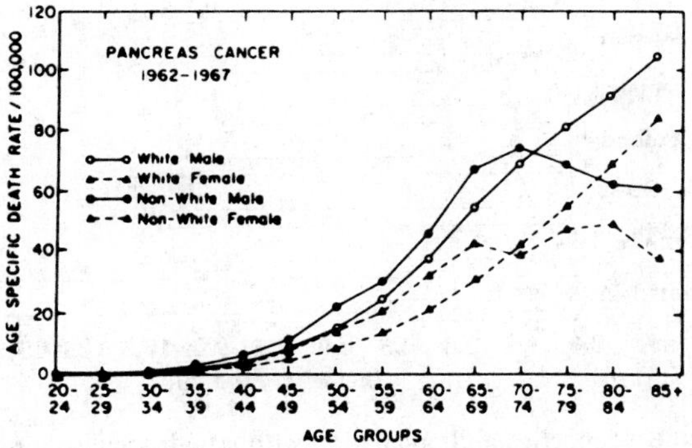

FIG. 26-1. Increasing U.S. age-specific mortality rates for cancer of the pancreas, by race and sex. (Levin DL, Connelly RR: Cancer of the pancreas. Available epidemiologic information and its implications. Cancer 31:1231–1236, 1973)

TABLE 26-1. Incidence of Pancreatic Cancer in Selected Areas by Sex

Location	*Men**	*Women**
New Mexico		
Spanish	11.7	9.2
Other white	10.1	6.6
American Indian	5.2	10.4
Cuba	4.9	3.2
Puerto Rico	4.9	3.0
Los Angeles		
Spanish	7.5	5.0
Other white	8.1	5.0
Cali, Colombia	5.0	3.2
Spain		
Navarra	4.0	2.6
Zaragoza	4.9	1.8

World Health Organization: Cancer Incidence in Five Continents, vol IV. IARC Sci Publ 42, 1982.
*Per 100,000 population.

100,000 men born in Israel. In non-Jewish residents, the incidence is 3.3 per 100,000 (Fig. 26-5).

Similar wide variations can be demonstrated in male incidence at various sites within different countries. For example, incidences vary from 11.0 per 100,000 in Ontario, Canada, to 3.7 in the Northwestern Territory of Canada. Countries with a high incidence are illustrated in Figure 26-6. There has been a progressive international increase in the incidence of pancreatic cancer. In England and Wales, from 1911 to 1971, the mortality from cancer of the pancreas in both men and women has increased at least fivefold.[6]

ETIOLOGY

Several environmental factors have been associated with an increased risk of pancreatic carcinoma, although the exact cause remains unclear. Pancreatic carcinoma, like several other common malignancies, appears to be more prevalent among persons in lower socioeconomic groups.[7] Close scrutiny of the available epidemiologic studies shows that pancreatic carcinoma has less of a demographic association with social class than do other common malignancies such as breast and lung carcinoma.[3,7]

Several dietary factors have been implicated. At least one study showed a positive correlation between coffee consumption and pancreatic carcinoma.[8] In this case-control study, patients with carcinoma of the pancreas were found to have a history of greater coffee consumption than the control group of patients with benign gastrointestinal disorders. Because the control group contained patients with peptic ulcer disease and had an overall average coffee intake below the level of consumption for the general population, it is difficult to confirm whether patients with cancer of the pancreas actually consumed more coffee than would be considered average. There have been at least two other studies that have not confirmed the association of coffee intake and pancreatic carcinoma.[9,10]

One study suggested an association between alcohol consumption and an increased risk of carcinoma of the pancreas.[11] In this study of Finnish men with a history of alcohol abuse, an excess of pancreatic carcinoma was found, compared with the overall Finnish male population. At least three other studies have shown little or no correlation between alcohol consumption and pancreatic carcinoma.[12–14]

FIG. 26-2. Male-to-female ratio for varying populations with pancreatic cancer. Note the major difference in the American Indian population in New Mexico. (World Health Organization: Cancer Incidence in Five Continents, vol IV. IARC Sci Publ 42, 1982)

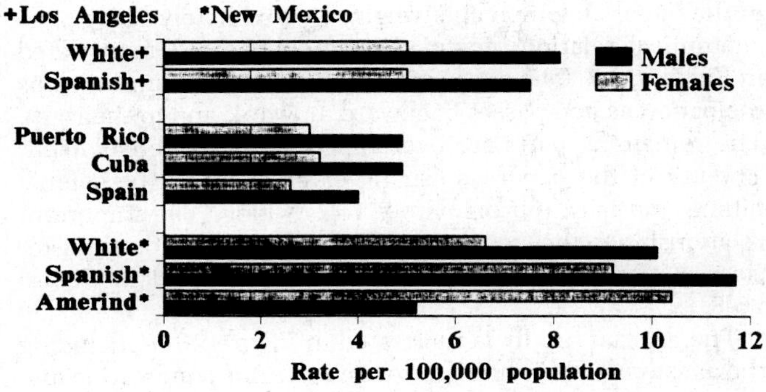

FIG. 26-3. Incidence of pancreatic cancer. Influence of race in a single geographic area: Los Angeles. (World Health Organization: Cancer Incidence in Five Continents, vol IV. IARC Sci Publ 42, 1982)

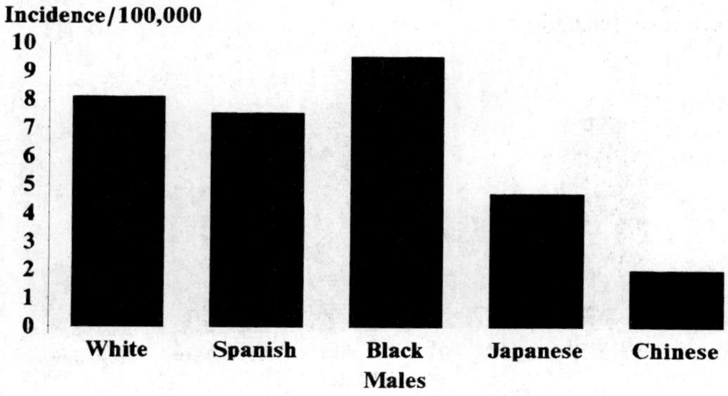

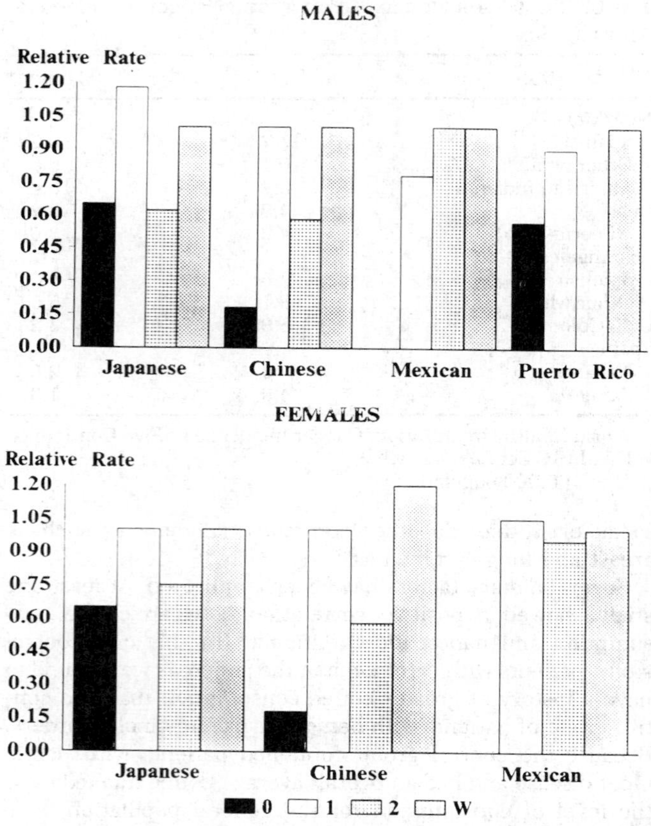

FIG. 26-4. Rates of pancreatic cancer in countries of origin and in first and second generation migrants relative to rates in white Americans. 0, country of origin; 1, first generation; 2, second generation; W, United States whites. (Thomas DB, Karagas MR: Cancer in first and second generation Americans. Cancer Res 47:5771, 1987)

Cigarette smoking has also been associated with an increased risk of pancreatic carcinoma.[1,15,16] In heavy cigarette smokers (at least two packs daily), a study from Veterans Administration hospitals showed almost twice the rate of pancreatic carcinoma compared with nonsmokers.[17] Cigarette smoke contains carcinogens, including the nitrosoamines that have induced pancreatic malignancies in laboratory animals.[18,19]

FIG. 26-5. Incidence of pancreatic cancer in Israel: effect of birthplace. Eur, Europe; Amer, North America; Afr, Africa. (World Health Organization: Cancer Incidence in Five Continents, vol IV. IARC Sci Publ 42, 1982)

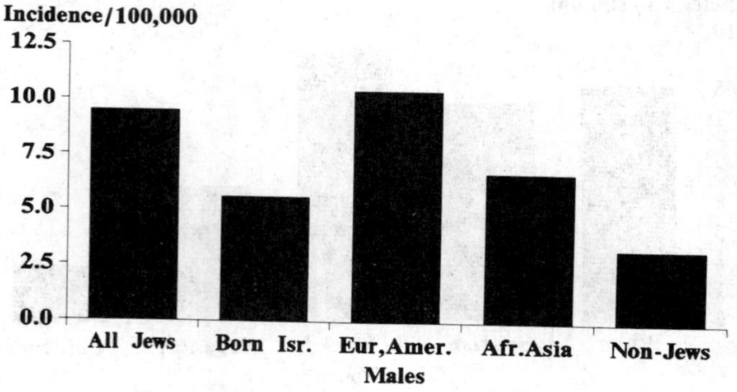

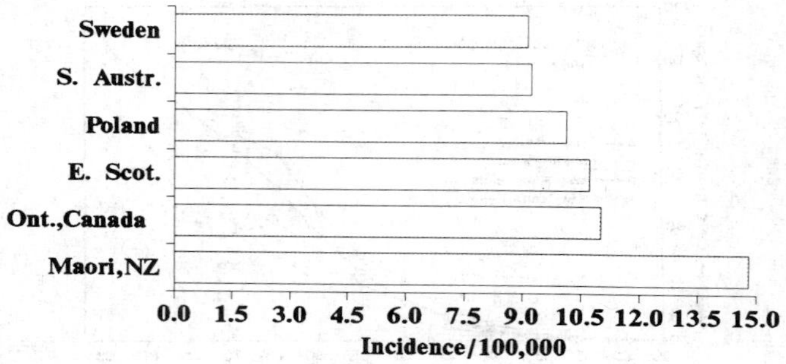

FIG. 26-6. Countries and population with a high incidence of pancreatic cancer. (World Health Organization: Cancer Incidence in Five Continents, vol IV. IARC Sci Publ 42, 1982)

An increased incidence of pancreatic carcinoma is present in patients with chronic pancreatitis.[20,21] Calcifications associated with chronic pancreatitis have been found in 3% of patients with documented pancreatic carcinoma.[22,23] However, there appears to be no association between biliary calcifications and carcinoma of the pancreas.[24] Epidemiologic studies of patients have also shown that almost 15% have a history of diabetes mellitus, which appears to be higher than expected.[25,26] However, in more than half of the patients with diabetes and pancreatic carcinoma, the onset of clinical diabetes preceded the diagnosis of pancreatic carcinoma by no longer than 3 months.[24,26] This suggests that the carcinoma may cause pancreatic endocrine insufficiency. Diabetes mellitus, presenting many months to years before the development of pancreatic carcinomas, would be better evidence for an etiologic correlation, but this type of temporal relationship is not commonly found.[25]

Long-term exposures to solvents and petroleum compounds appear to increase the risk of pancreatic carcinoma.[24] A prospective study of workers exposed to benzidine and beta-naphthylamine showed a higher incidence.[27] The nitrosoamines are recognized as potent pancreatic carcinogens in hamsters.[28] Azaserine has also been shown to produce pancreatic tumors in rats.[29] Exposure for 10 years or longer to these industrial chemicals may increase the risk of pancreatic carcinoma by a factor of five.[24]

ANATOMICAL CONSIDERATIONS

The pancreas lies transversely in the posterior peritoneum of the upper abdomen and weighs approximately 100 g. The anatomical relationships of the pancreas are demonstrated in Figure 26-7. The superior part of the duodenum overlaps the pancreas and passes backward, upward, and to the right. The remaining parts are overlapped by the pancreas itself. The tail of the pancreas usually extends out to the splenic hilum, and it is approximately 15 cm long. The important relationship to the transverse mesocolon and the deep posterior relationship of the pancreas are illustrated in Figure 26-8.

The arterial supply is illustrated in Figure 26-9, including the anastomoses of the superior and inferior pancreaticoduo-

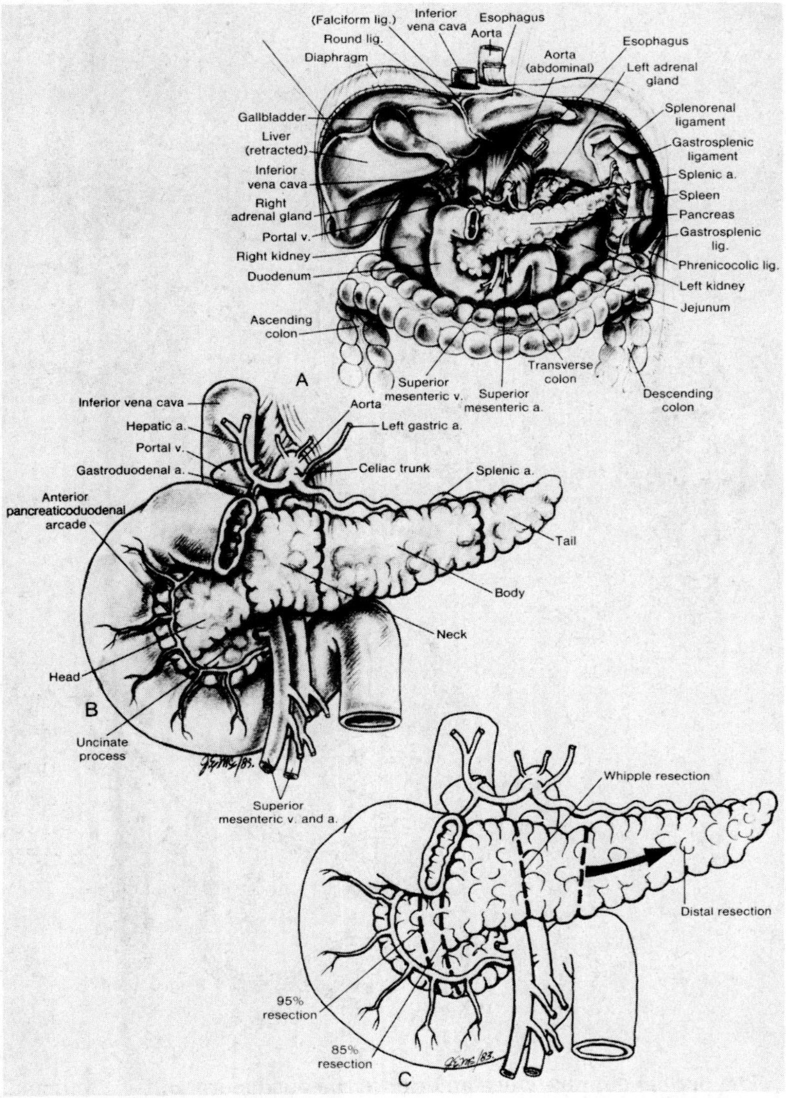

FIG. 26-7. Anatomical relationships of the pancreas. (Gray SW, Skandalakis JE, McCluskey DA: Atlas of Surgical Anatomy for General Surgeons. Baltimore, Williams & Wilkins, 1985)

denal arteries. The important venous drainage is illustrated in Figure 26-10. The surgically important lymphatic drainage is in intimate relationship with the surface and borders of the pancreas and indirectly with the celiac, preaortic, and superior mesenteric groups. Because of the diffuse, surrounding lymphatic drainage, it is thought that tumors in the pancreas can drain virtually to any of the surrounding nodal-bearing areas.

The diameter of the pancreatic duct varies: within the head, it is 3 to 4.8 mm; within the body, 2 to 3.5 mm; and within the tail, 0.9 to 2.4 mm.[30] Two milliliters to 3 ml of contrast material can fill the main pancreatic duct, and 7 to 10 ml can fill the smaller ducts.[31] The pancreatic duct variations have been widely described (Fig. 26-11). From the standard, both ducts open into the duodenum, with communication between the accessory and the main duct, to a blind accessory duct, an independent accessory duct, or missing accessory duct.

The extent of the uncinate process is variable: It can extend from just behind the vessels to the left of the superior mesenteric artery and is an important feature of transection during surgery. Failure to remove this portion of the uncinate process completely in a pancreatoduodenectomy can result in troublesome intraoperative and postoperative bleeding.

The most important anatomical abnormalities that influence pancreatic resection are those of vascular supply. There are usually variations in the hepatic artery, the most common abnormality being the right hepatic artery, arising from the superior mesenteric artery. The course is variable and usually proceeds behind the common duct and the portal vein. This can occur in as many as 25% of patients. The accessory left hepatic artery is rarely a problem because it tends to rise from the common hepatic or left gastric artery and passes in the left omentum. However, on rare occasions it may arise from the superior mesenteric or from the gastroduodenal artery. In 2% to 4% of patients the common hepatic artery arises from the superior mesenteric and occasionally passes through the head of the pancreas, which can be a major problem during resection.[32]

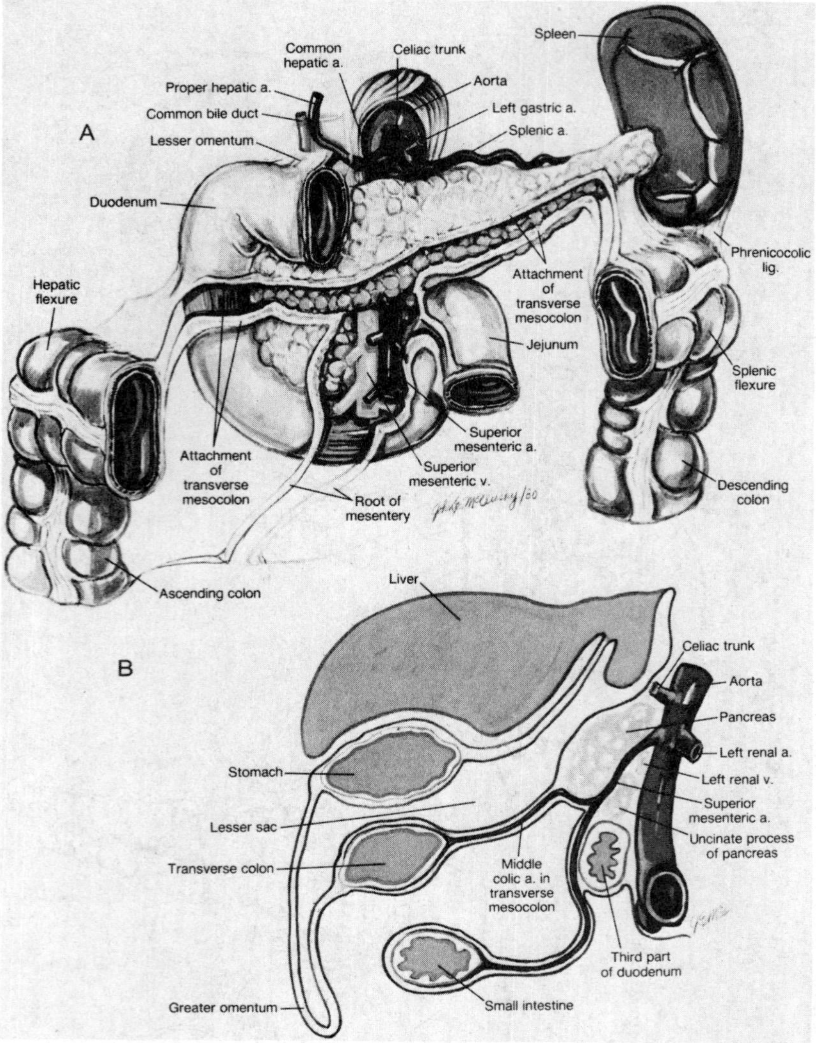

FIG. 26-8. Important relationship to the transverse mesocolon and the deep posterior relationship to the pancreas. (Gray SW, Skandalakis JE, McCluskey DA: Atlas of Surgical Anatomy for General Surgeons. Baltimore, Williams & Wilkins, 1985)

The portal vein rarely lies anterior to the duodenum. Biliary tract abnormalities usually accompany this vascular abnormality. The portal vein may communicate with the superior vena cava, and rarely, a pulmonary vein joins the portal vein. Congenital strictures in the portal vein can occur, and the preduodenal portal vein is often associated with other abnormalities of the pancreas, including malrotation.

PATHOLOGIC CLASSIFICATION

Pancreatic cancers arise from both the exocrine and endocrine parenchyma of the gland.[33,34] Approximately 95% occur within the exocrine portion of the pancreas and may arise from ductal epithelium, acinar cells, connective tissue, or lymphatic deposits. Only 2% of tumors of the exocrine pancreas are benign.[35] The less common tumors of the endocrine pancreas arise from islet of Langerhans cells, and most are benign. An overview of the classification of benign and malignant tumors of the pancreas is presented in Table 26-2. Tumors of endocrine origin are covered in Chapter 39.

The most common pancreatic cancer is a ductal adenocarcinoma, which accounts for about 80% of all pancreatic cancers.[36] In a recent analysis of patients presenting to the Memorial Sloan-Kettering Cancer Center, 79% of 575 admitted during 46 months with peripancreatic cancer had adenocarcinoma of the pancreas. Less common ductal cancers include squamous cell carcinomas, giant cell carcinomas, and carcinosarcomas. Carcinomas of the pancreas usually arise in the proximal gland, which includes the head, neck, and uncinate process.[37] Carcinomas arise in the distal gland less commonly, with 20% of all carcinomas occurring in the body and 5% to 10% occurring in the tail. Grossly, carcinomas appear hard and gritty and often are whitish. Microscopic changes of acute and, more commonly, chronic pancreatitis often surround a pancreatic carcinoma and can make the diagnosis difficult, especially when small amounts of tissue are obtained with a percutaneous biopsy.

Because most pancreatic tumors are ductal in origin, pancreatic ductal obstruction is a common finding. Cancers in the pancreatic head often produce obstruction of both the pancreatic and common bile ducts. Invasion of adjacent duodenum, with ulceration and partial or complete duodenal obstruction, occurs in as many as 25% of pancreatic head

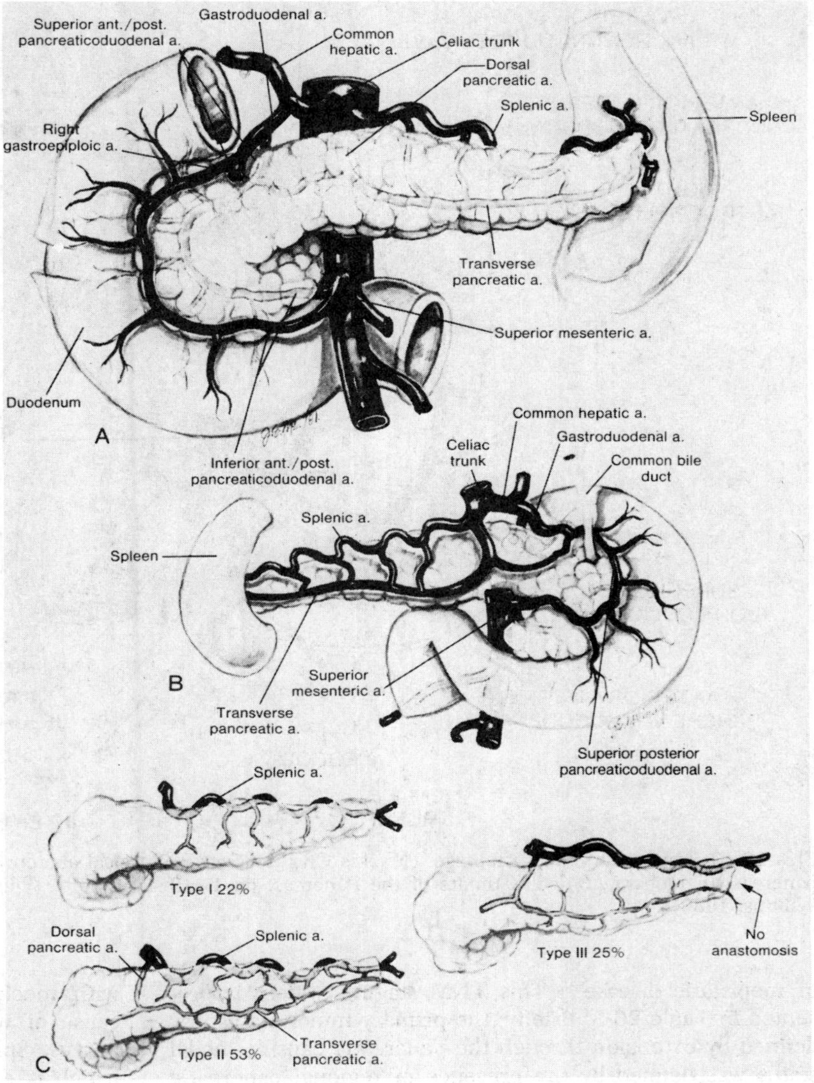

FIG. 26-9. Arterial drainage. (Gray SW, Skandalakis JE, McCluskey DA: Atlas of Surgical Anatomy for General Surgeons. Baltimore, Williams & Wilkins, 1985)

cancers.[37] Obstruction of the portal or superior mesenteric vein can result from local invasion of tumors of the proximal pancreas. Tumors of the distal gland are often larger at diagnosis (5–10 cm) than proximal gland tumors.[33,34] These distal tumors of the pancreatic body and tail can cause obstruction of the splenic vein.

A characteristic pathologic feature of pancreatic adenocarcinomas is the early development of subclinical metastases.[24,37] Fewer than 20% of patients have disease macroscopically confined to the pancreas at diagnosis; 40% of patients present with locally advanced disease, including involvement of regional lymph nodes and adjacent pancreatic tissue, and more than 40% have identifiable visceral metastases at presentation, usually involving the liver.[24] Peritoneal implants occur in 35% of patients at presentation. The natural history of pancreatic carcinomas is highlighted by widespread metastases to other abdominal viscera and extra-abdominal spread to lung, bone, and brain.

Cystic neoplasms of the pancreas are rare tumors that have characteristic pathologic features.[33,34] These tumors are usually large, filled with mucinous secretions, and may be multilocular. Microscopically, the cysts are lined with columnar epithelium alone (cystadenomas) or with a mixture of columnar epithelium and atypical malignant epithelial cells (cystadenocarcinomas). These carcinomas are usually localized, and approximately 50% of patients can be cured with surgery alone. Other rare (<1%) tumors of the nonendopancreas include acinar cell carcinomas, pancreatic sarcomas, and lymphomas. Islet cell tumors are covered in Chapter 39.

CLINICAL FEATURES

STAGING

In 1981, the American Joint Committee for Cancer Staging and End Results Reporting published a staging system for pancreatic carcinoma based on the extent of the primary tumor, the status of regional lymph nodes, and the presence

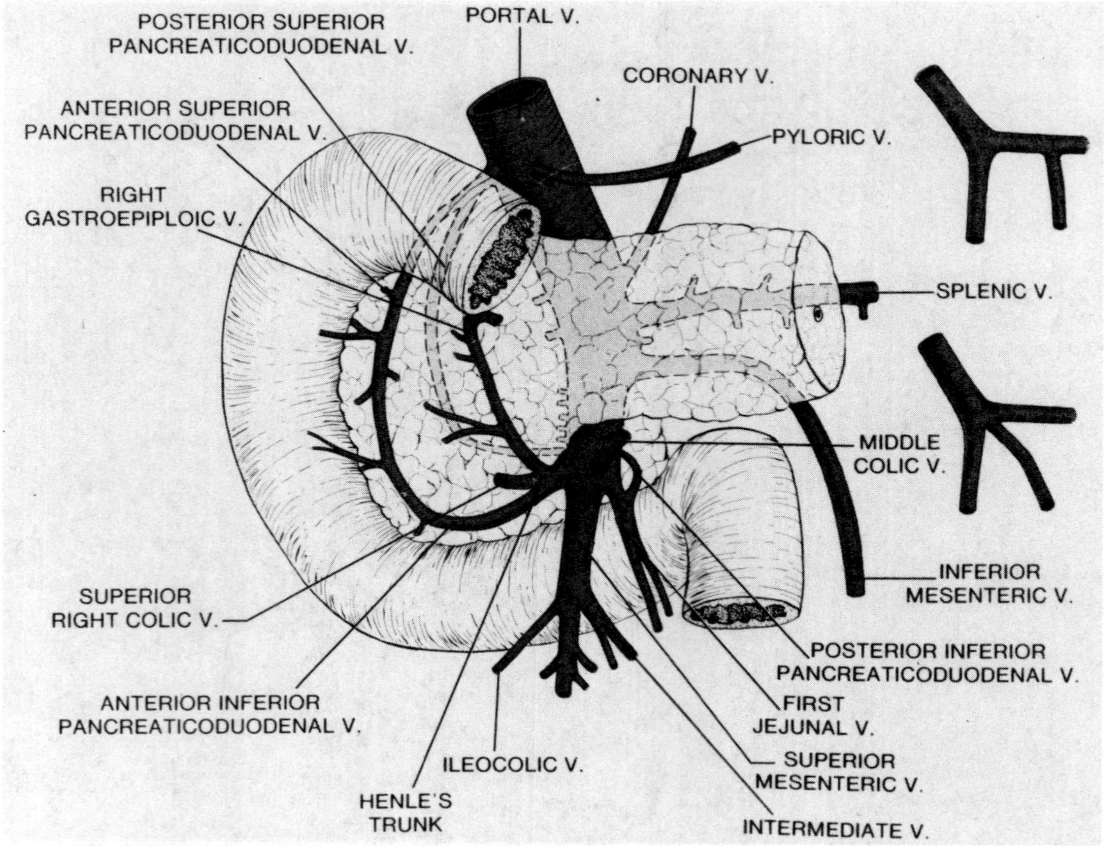

FIG. 26-10. Important venous drainage. (Mackie CR, Moossa AR: Surgical anatomy of the pancreas. In Moossa AR [ed]: Tumors of the Pancreas, pp 1–19. Baltimore, Williams & Wilkins, 1980)

of metastatic disease.[38] This TNM staging system is presented in Table 26-3. Briefly, the primary tumor status was defined by extension through the pancreatic capsule; nodal status was defined by the presence of regional pancreatic lymph node involvement; and metastatic disease status was defined by the presence of distal lymph node, peritoneal, or visceral metastatic disease. The surgical staging system based on the TNM system was defined as follows: Stage I disease is localized within the pancreatic capsule and amenable to surgical resection; Stage II disease is locally advanced with invasion of duodenum or peripancreatic soft tissues and not surgically resectable; Stage III disease has regional lymph node involvement; and Stage IV disease has distant metastases. The staging system used at Memorial Sloan-Kettering Cancer Center is illustrated in Table 26-4.[39]

SIGNS AND SYMPTOMS

Cancer of the pancreas is a highly malignant disease. The majority of patients present with disease advanced beyond the scope of potentially curative treatment. The hallmarks of pancreatic carcinoma are pain and clinical wasting. Tumors in the head of the pancreas often cause biliary obstruction. Patients also develop signs and symptoms of gastric outlet and duodenal obstruction because of local tumor invasion, with mechanical obstruction and motility problems, the cause of which is probably infiltration of the splanchnic nerves. Splanchnic nerve invasion results in severe pain, which is often difficult to eradicate by medication. Carcinoma of the body and tail rarely produces gastric obstruction because of local infiltration and is often asymptomatic until well advanced. Even in the absence of mechanical obstruction of the stomach and duodenum, marked loss of appetite is a common symptom. A typical patient with pancreatic carcinoma has lost more than 10% of his body weight at diagnosis, and wasting is progressive. Distant metastases, particularly to liver, occur early in the course of the disease.

The initial symptoms are nonspecific and insidious at onset. The typical patient reports a gradual onset of anorexia, nausea, upper abdominal to midabdominal pain, and weight loss. Because of the nonspecific nature of these symptoms, early diagnosis of pancreatic cancer is difficult and requires a high index of suspicion on the part of the physician initially involved in the patient's care. A delay in diagnosis of several months from the initiation of symptoms is common. In a report from the Cancer of the Pancreas Task Force, fewer than 33% of patients experienced symptoms for 2 months or less before diagnosis.[38] Delays in diagnoses are reported in other large reviews.[37,40]

Pain is the most common symptom in patients with pan-

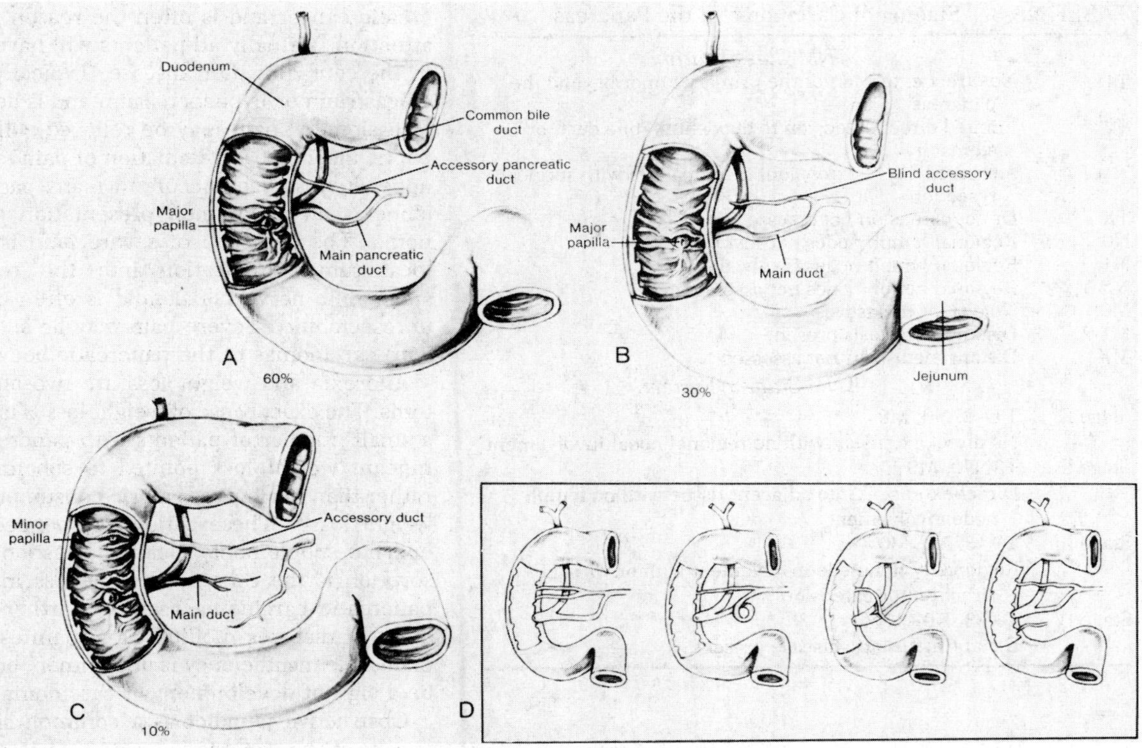

FIG. 26-11. Pancreatic duct variations. (Gray SW, Skandalakis JE, McCluskey DA: Atlas of Surgical Anatomy for General Surgeons. Baltimore, Williams & Wilkins, 1985)

TABLE 26-2. Histogenetic Classification of Pancreatic Neoplasms

Origin	*Benign*	*Malignant*
Duct Cell	Polyp	Duct cell carcinoma
	Papilloma	Giant cell carcinoma
	Adenoma	Adenosquamous carcinoma
	Cystadenoma	Microglandular adenocarcinoma
	Oncocytoma	Mucinous carcinoma
	Benign papillary cystic neoplasm	Cystadenocarcinoma
		Papillary cystic carcinoma
Acinar Cell	Acinar cell adenoma	Acinar cell carcinoma
	Acinar cell cystadenoma	Acinar cell cystadenocarcinoma
Connective Tissue	Lipoma	Malignant fibrous histiocytoma
	Leiomyoma	Fibrosarcoma
	Benign peripheral nerve tumor	Liposarcoma
	Hemangioma	Leiomyosarcoma
	Lymphangioma	Malignant peripheral nerve tumor
		Rhabdomyosarcoma
		Hemangiosarcoma
		Lymphangiosarcoma
		Hemangiopericytoma
		Malignant lymphoma
		Plasmacytoma
Islet Cell	Insulinoma	Malignant insulinoma
	Glucagonoma	Malignant glucagonoma
	Gastrinoma	Malignant gastrinoma
	Adenoma, functionally inactive	Islet cell carcinoma, functionally inactive
		Islet cell carcinoma carcinoid type
Uncertain	Fibroadenoma	Pancreaticoblastoma

Modified from Cubilla AL, Fitzgerald PJ: Tumors of the exocrine pancreas. Washington DC, Armed Forces Institute of Pathology, 1984, and from Legg MA: Pathology of the pancreas. In: Brooks JR (ed): Surgery of the Pancreas, pp 41–77. Philadelphia, WB Saunders, 1983.

TABLE 26-3. Staging of Carcinoma of the Pancreas

	TNM Classification
T1	No direct extension of the primary tumor beyond the pancreas
T2	Limited direct extension to duodenum, bile duct, or stomach
T3	Advanced direct extension, incompatible with surgical resection
TX	Direct extension not assessed
N0	Regional lymph nodes not involved
N1	Regional lymph nodes involved
NX	Regional lymph nodes not assessed
M0	No distant metastasis
M1	Distant metastasis present
MX	Distant metastasis not assessed
	TNM Staging System
Stage I	T1–2, N0, M0 No direct extension with no regional nodal involvement
Stage II	T3, N0, M0 Direct extension into adjacent tissue with no lymph node involvement
Stage III	T1–3, N1, M0 Regional lymph node involvement with or without direct tumor extension
Stage IV	T1–3, N0–1, M1 Distant metastatic disease present

creatic cancer and is often the reason for seeking medical attention. Virtually all patients will have pain at some point in the course of their disease. Typically, the pain is in the epigastrium or hypochondrium and is described as gnawing. Occasionally, pain may be relieved with meals, mimicking peptic ulcer disease. Radiation of pain to the low thoracic or upper lumbar back occurs in many patients, but back pain alone is an uncommon presentation of pancreatic carcinoma. The presence of severe pain is often indicative of local tumor infiltration into the retroperitoneum and splanchnic nerve plexus and is often considered a sign of unresectability. Severe pain may be slightly more common with carcinomas of the pancreatic body and tail.[37]

Anorexia and weight loss are two other common symptoms. The exact cause of weight loss is unknown. A report on a small number of patients with pancreatic cancer and significant weight loss pointed to subclinical malabsorption, rather than inadequate caloric consumption, as the source of weight loss.[41] These patients responded to oral pancreatic enzyme supplements, but the question of whether malabsorption is the cause of weight loss in most patients with pancreatic carcinoma requires further study. The sudden onset of diabetes mellitus as a manifestation of pancreatic endocrine insufficiency is uncommon, but is often thought to be a sign of development of carcinoma of the pancreas.[42]

Obstructive jaundice is a common sign, particularly for lesions of the pancreatic head. Associated symptoms of dark

TABLE 26-4. Postsurgical Staging for Cancer of the Pancreatic Region

Primary Tumor: T
- T1 2 cm or less in diameter
- T2 2 to 6 cm in diameter
- T3 Over 6 cm in diameter
- T4 Direct extension to contiguous structures
- TX Unknown or unrecorded

Nodes: N
- N0 None
- N1 Anterior, posterior, superior, inferior pancreatic nodes
  - a) Microscopic focus in one node
  - b) Solitary, macroscopic
  - c) Multiple nodes (microscopic or macroscopic)
- N2 Porta hepatic, common hepatic, celiac, proximal superior mesenteric lymph nodes
  - a) Microscopic focus in one node
  - b) Solitary, macroscopic
  - c) Multiple nodes (microscopic or macroscopic)
- N3 Periaortic, distal superior mesenteric, or other abdominal lymph nodes
- NX Unknown or unrecorded

Metastases Beyond Regional Nodes: M
- M0 None
- M1 Liver only
- M2 Other Intra-abdominal metastases
  - a) Without liver
  - b) With liver
- M3 Multiple peritoneal implants or malignant ascites
- M4 Extra-abdominal metastases
- MX Unknown or unrecorded

Clinical (cTNM) and Pathologic (pTNM) Staging

Stage I	T1–4,	N0,	M0
Stage II	T1–4,	N1–2,	M0
Stage III	T1–4,	N0–3,	M1–4

urine, light stools, and pruritus may proceed the clinical detection of jaundice. Totally painless jaundice is not common in pancreatic carcinoma and occurs more often in ampullary carcinoma or a primary bile duct carcinoma.[43] Although the gallbladder is commonly distended at exploration, fewer than 33% of patients will have a palpable gallbladder at presentation (Courvoisier's sign).[43] Splenomegaly, another uncommon physical finding, usually occurs with tumors of the distal gland involving splenic vein obstruction. Early spread of tumor to the liver and peritoneum may occur in 15% to 25% of patients and presents with the signs of a palpable liver or abdominal distension with ascites.[37]

Patients may have a higher risk of depression at diagnosis, compared with other abdominal tumors. One study reported depression in 67% of 46 patients with pancreatic carcinoma, compared with less than 10% of 64 patients with colon carcinoma.[44] Considering the delay in diagnosis of several months in most patients, a reactive depression may be expected. Patients with pancreatic carcinoma may have a higher frequency of venous thrombosis and migratory thrombophlebitis (Trousseau's sign).[45] Thrombophlebitis appears more commonly in patients with tumors of the distal pancreas, but there is no clear correlation between the development of thrombophlebitis with an underlying pancreatic carcinoma in an otherwise healthy patient.[43]

DIAGNOSIS

The algorithm for the diagnosis of adenocarcinoma of the pancreas is outlined in Figure 26-12. Once a suspicion of pancreatic cancer has been raised—because of nonspecific upper abdominal symptoms, weight loss, or jaundice—then clinical confirmation is required. This is usually obtained by physical examination to confirm jaundice, ascites, palpable mass, or metastatic disease. Chemical confirmation of the jaundice can be obtained by serum indices. Radiologic tests can also evaluate the extent of the disease. Radiologic confirmation requires ultrasonography to demonstrate a mass in the pancreas, dilated extrahepatic biliary ducts, or metastatic disease in the liver.

Computed tomography (CT) is the mainstay of both diagnostic confirmation and the evaluation of the extent of disease (Fig. 26-13). CT can demonstrate the mass in the pancreas, metastatic disease in the liver and the periaortic and retropancreatic lymph nodes, and ascites. Enormous masses arising from the pancreas suggest diagnoses such as lymphoma or sarcoma (Fig. 26-14). Clear identification of cystic changes, with or without calcification, suggests the possibility of cystadenoma or cystadenocarcinoma. Masses in young people suggest the possibility of pancreaticoblastoma.

Endoscopic retrograde cholangiopancreatography (ERCP) is a valuable tool in the diagnosis, or in the localization of the tumor to the ampulla or the demonstration of obstructed stenotic or sclerosed ducts (Fig. 26-15), all highly suggestive of adenocarcinoma. Conversely, the presence of a lesion on CT scans with a subsequently normal pancreatic duct (Figs. 26-13 and 26-14) may suggest an islet cell neoplasm or exclude pancreatic adenocarcinoma. Care must be taken, however, not to misinterpret a normal duct as an islet cell

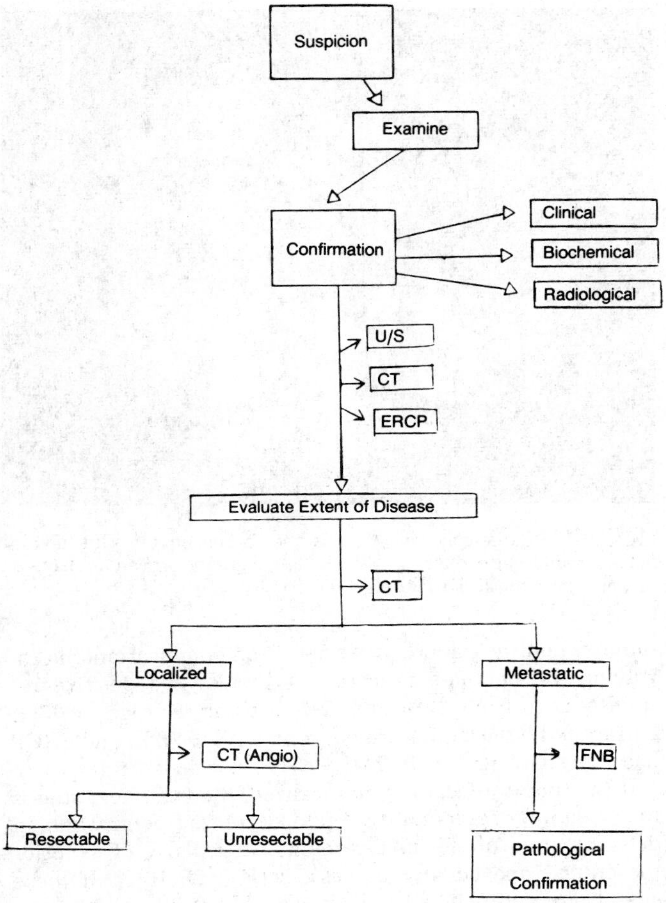

FIG. 26-12. Algorithm: diagnosis of pancreatic adenocarcinoma.

FIG. 26-13. Obvious mass on CT scan, shown to have normal pancreatic duct and benign minimal enlargement by operation and long-term follow-up.

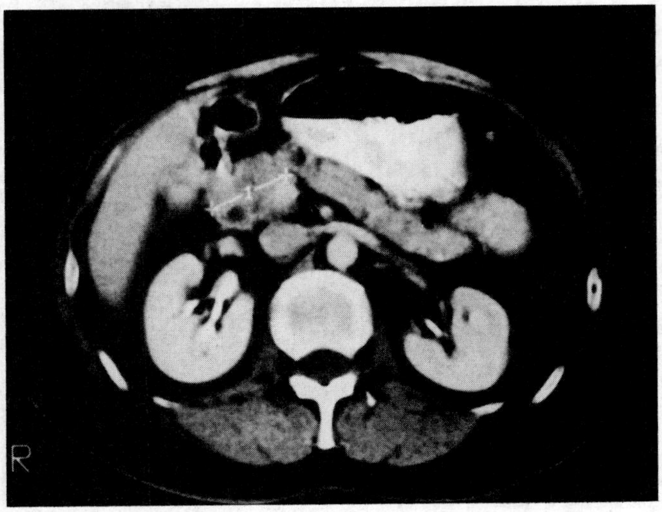

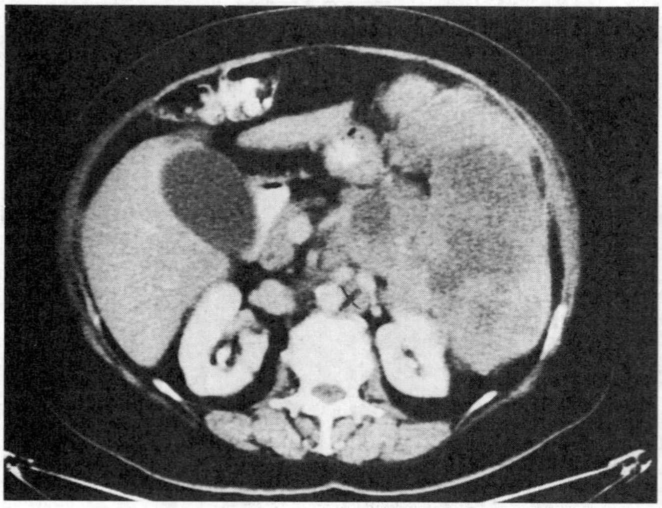

FIG. 26-14. Large pancreatic mass shown subsequently to have a normal pancreatic duct by ERCP. The patient proved to have a primary pancreatic lymphoma.

tumor when the pancreatic lesion is an adenocarcinoma involving the uncinate process. CT results had positive response rates from 63% to 100%, with an average of 65%. Ultrasound has a similar range, from 23% to 95%, and ERCP had a positive rate of 53% to 96%.[40]

If the tumor appears to be localized, then the next step is to evaluate for resectability. Again CT plays a central role in determination of the involvement, particularly of superior mesenteric and celiac axis vessels (Fig. 26-13).[40] If these vessels are not involved and a reasonable assessment can be made about obstruction of the portal vein on the basis of CT, then resection can be considered. If the tumor is clearly unresectable, or if metastatic disease is identified, based on the CT scan, we proceed to pathologic confirmation. However, if there is concern about resectability and if there are compelling reasons not to explore the patient, then we use angiography (Fig. 26-16).

FIG. 26-15. ERCP of patient with a localized mass in the head and body of the pancreas, confirmed as an unresectable adenocarcinoma.

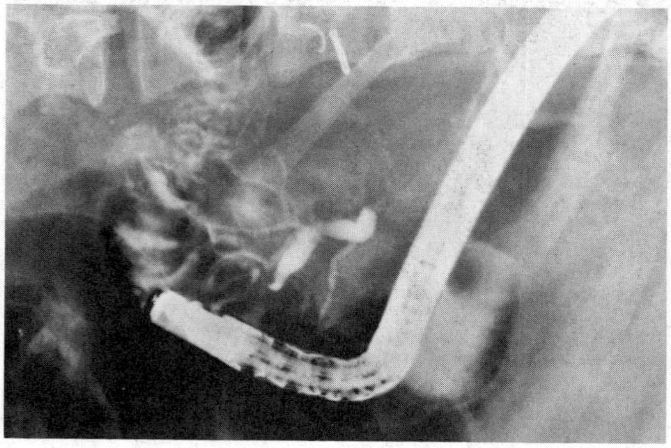

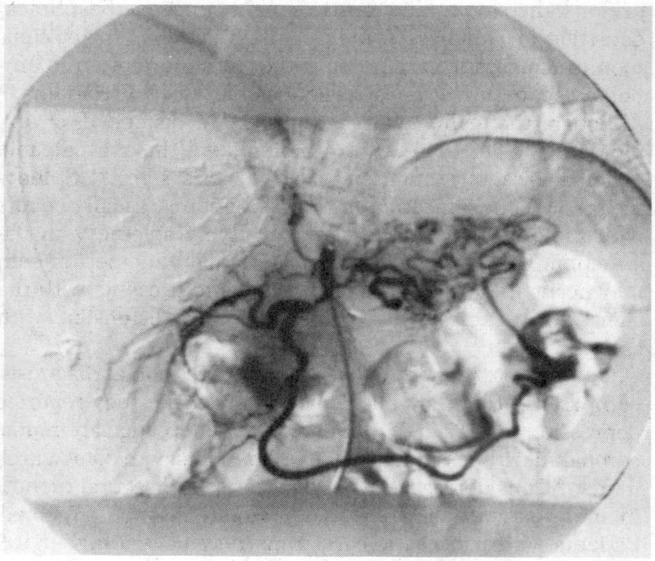

FIG. 26-16. Arteriogram demonstrating encasement of the common hepatic and splenic arteries, indicating unresectability.

Angiography is used to determine the presence of abnormal vasculature, such as a right hepatic artery arising from the superior mesenteric artery, and to determine unresectability based on encasement of the superior mesenteric or, rarely, hepatic or celiac axis arteries (Fig. 26-17). The abnormal vasculature does not warrant the uniform use of angiography before surgery. This vessel can usually be detected in the porta hepatis at the time of resection and often runs behind the pancreas, rather than directly through it. Conversely, the complete encasement of the superior mesenteric or celiac arteries is an absolute contraindication to resection.

If the tumor is deemed unresectable or metastatic disease is identified, then histopathologic confirmation should be

FIG. 26-17. Encasement of an abnormal right hepatic artery arising from the superior mesenteric artery.

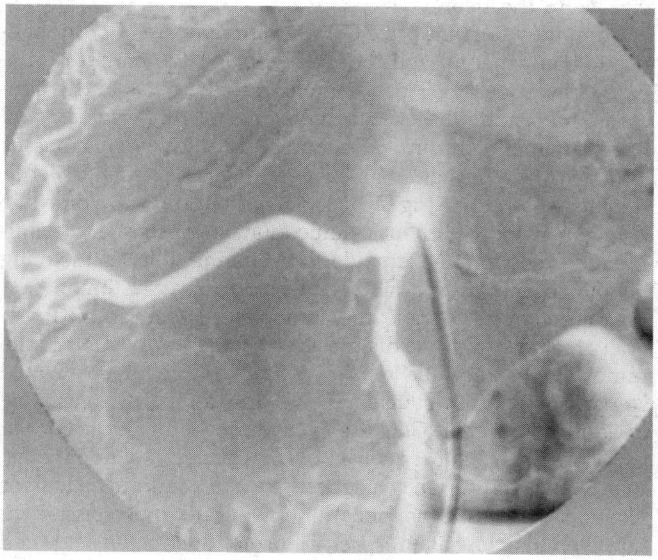

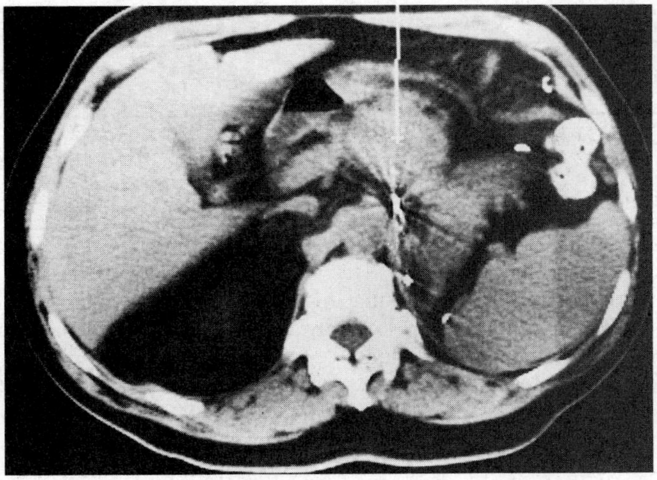

FIG. 26-18. Histopathologic confirmation obtained by "skinny" needle biopsy of the pancreas.

obtained, either by direct fine-needle biopsy of the pancreas (Fig. 26-18) or percutaneous biopsy of a liver metastasis.

Upper gastrointestinal (GI) contrast studies, which are rarely of value, are much less valuable than CT. This test is also redundant because most patients will have endoscopy as part of the ERCP. Magnetic resonance imaging (MRI) is only now undergoing serious evaluation in the pancreatic area. MRI may eventually displace CT, but for the present CT is the procedure of choice.

A new modality is endoscopic ultrasound. It is used mainly for staging gastric and esophageal cancer and can demonstrate local invasion by pancreatic neoplasms into the portal vein (Fig. 26-19).

Percutaneous transhepatic cholangiograms (PTHC) are indicated on limited occasions. They are primarily used if there is concern about a distal common bile duct lesion and the proximal extent of such a tumor is unclear. By use of ultrasound and CT, it is usually possible to determine the dilation of the extrahepatic biliary ducts and the proximal extent of any stenotic lesion of the common bile duct. It is appropriate at the time of ERCP, if the common bile duct can be entered, to place a stent or a nasobiliary catheter before considering further surgical intervention.

SEROLOGIC MARKERS

Serologic markers of pancreatic cancer are of interest for a variety of reasons. If sufficiently sensitive and specific, markers aid in the differential diagnosis of patients with abdominal or retroperitoneal disease. Markers can also identify a prognostically more favorable population of patients with resectable, curable disease. For postoperative and advanced pancreatic cancer patients with poorly measurable tumor, a convenient, reproducible, and accurate serologic test can assist in clinical follow-up.

The summarized results of four potential markers are shown in Table 26-5. One of the first markers to be investigated systematically was the carcinoembryonic antigen (CEA). CEA is a high-molecular-weight glycoprotein and the normal product of fetal gut tissue. This widely available test identifies about half of the pancreatic cancer patients and can discriminate malignant from benign pancreatic disease in over 90% of cases. However, CEA is not an efficient marker for either diagnosis or follow-up because it is elevated in many benign states, such as ulcerative colitis or biliary disease, and in many malignancies, such as colon or lung cancer.[53-56]

The CA 125 antigen is a well-recognized marker for epithelial ovarian neoplasms and has been screened in GI malignancies as well.[57-59] This large glycoprotein is identified by a murine monoclonal antibody raised against a human ovarian cell line.[60] In pancreatic cancer patients, CA 125 is detected less than 50% of the time. As a single test, CA 125

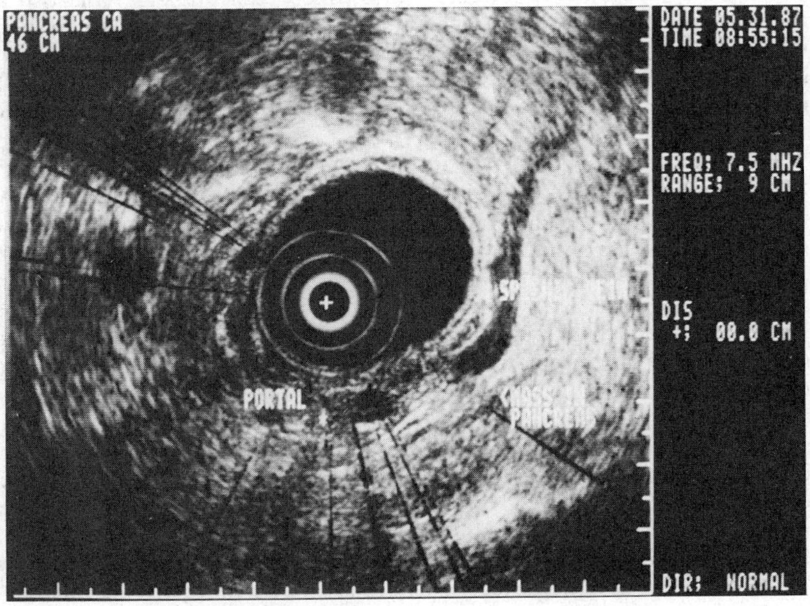

FIG. 26-19. Tissue to be removed. All of the finely shaded area, including distal stomach, duodenum, head of pancreas, gallbladder, and common bile duct, will be resected.

TABLE 26-5. Selected Tumor Markers in Pancreatic Cancer

Marker	*Reference*	*Serum Level*	*Pancreatic Cancer*	*Pancreatitis*	*Normal Levels*
CEA	46–49	2.5–50 ng/ml	114/231 (49%)	10/188 (5%)	0/34
CA 125	48–50	35 U/ml	55/132 (42%)	15/75 (20%)	0/38
CA 19-9	46–48, 50, 51	37 U/ml	255/319 (80%)	18/233 (8%)	1/72
DU-PAN-2	52	300 U/ml	31/33 (94%)		0/126

is not clinically satisfactory for pancreatic cancer and is probably more useful for ovarian cancer.

The tumor-associated carbohydrate antigen, CA 19-9, is detectable by a murine monoclonal antibody raised against a human colorectal adenocarcinoma cell line.[61] This mucin-like molecule is a sialated Lewis antigen, which has been associated more often with pancreatic than with other intra-abdominal malignancies.[62] The findings of five representative studies are summarized in Table 26-5. With this monoclonal antibody, approximately 80% of pancreatic cancer patients are correctly detected, compared with 8% of patients with pancreatitis and 1% of normal subjects incorrectly identified. Steinberg found CA 19-9 was statistically more specific than CEA (86.5% versus 48.4%) but only slightly more sensitive (92.5% versus 87.3%).[46] Data from Piantino demonstrated an identical superiority for CA 19-9.[47] Tempero suggests that CA 19-9 may provide a useful clinical marker for detecting pancreatic cancer progression in patients with recurrent or advanced disease.[63]

More recently, a murine monoclonal antibody directed against a pancreatic adenocarcinoma glycoprotein has been evaluated. The DU-PAN-2 antigen appears to be an oncofetal surface antigen that is quite specific for identifying and following pancreatic cancer.[52] DU-PAN-2 may be elevated in those with biliary cirrhosis, gastric cancer, and biliary cancer but seems to be sensitive and specific for pancreatic cancer and deserves further evaluation.

With the enthusiasm for and increasing sophistication of monoclonal antibody production, it is likely that new markers will be forthcoming. The simultaneous use of several species (*e.g.*, CA 19-9 and CA 125) may yield even more satisfactory discrimination between diseases and clinical results.[64,65]

SURGICAL TREATMENT

PREOPERATIVE BILIARY DECOMPRESSION FOR OBSTRUCTIVE JAUNDICE

Preoperative biliary drainage before surgery has been practiced for a number of years. Dr. Alan O. Whipple's early experience with a pancreaticoduodenectomy was preceded by relief of obstruction by bypass.[66] Retrospective studies suggested that preliminary decompression by cholecystectomy resulted in a decrease in operative mortality from 50% to 8%![67]

Percutaneous transhepatic biliary drainage (PTBD) resulted in a striking reduction in operative mortality to 8.2%, compared with 28% in historical controls.[68] Several other retrospective studies using historical controls and other trials, including concurrent nonrandomized controls and no controls, suggested benefit.[69–72] The combined results of these studies suggested an operative mortality of 13.7% among patients undergoing preoperative PTBD, compared with 26% among patients undergoing surgery without it (Table 26-6). Two of the five trials suggested a significant reduction in mortality and in morbidity. The apparent improvement associated with PTBD in these studies may be explained further by other factors, such as the exclusion of high-risk patients from subsequent operations or the use of PTBD as the definitive form of palliation. In fact, 98 (40%) of 246 of patients undergoing PTBD did not proceed to subsequent laparotomy.

More recent prospective randomized trials have challenged the value of PTBD. In 1982 the first prospective evaluation in a single-arm trial of 37 patients, 35 of whom had malignant obstruction, resulted in drainage-related morbidity of 54% and drainage-related mortality of 13.5%.[73] Postoperative mortality was 24%. In two well-controlled randomized trials, 127 patients, 94% of whom had malignant disease, showed no benefit in either morbidity or mortality by PTBD.[74,75] Overall mortality was 14% with or without preliminary drainage (Table 26-6). In-hospital mortality was 23% among patients drained and 16% among those not drained. In one of the trials, there was a 19% mortality among 31 patients not drained and 32% mortality among 34 patients drained, including five deaths before any operation and two additional deaths resulting from complications of drainage procedure. Five patients required early surgery for bile peritonitis.[75]

In all these trials, there have been many complications related to PTBD. A prospective controlled trial has been completed that showed no benefit in operative mortality and showed a prolongation of hospital stay with the drainage procedure for patients with both benign and malignant biliary obstruction.[76] Overall, no objective benefit other than decrease in bilirubin has been shown to result from preoperative drainage. The high complication rate with the percutaneous procedure has obscured any potential benefit from the biliary decompression.

The alternative is endoscopically placed biliary drainage, which has theoretical appeal in providing similar drainage with less risk of complication. In a comprehensive series of 595 cases collected from six centers in Japan and Europe, a 97.5% success rate has been claimed.[77] This is far in excess of any success rate that most North American centers have been able to provide. Complication rates are small (4%). The principal complication is cholangitis. Mortality is less than 2%. Current trials examine benefits of preoperative

TABLE 26-6. Postoperative Mortality in Obstructive Jaundice*: Results of Preoperative Drainage Studies

Author	Year	Method	Mortality	
			Drainage	No Drainage
Retrospective				
Whipple[66]	1983	Cholecystostomy	8% (2/25)	50% (16/32)
Nakayama[68]	1978	PTBD†	8% (4/49)	28% (36/148)
Dooley[72]	1979	PTBD	24% (5/21)	Not reported
Denning[69]	1981	PTBD	18% (4/22)	27% (7/26)
Norlander[20]	1982	PTBD	18% (8/44)	33% (14/42)
Gundry[71]	1984	PTBD	4% (1/25)	20% (5/25)‡
Total			14% (22/161)	26% (62/241)
Prospective, Nonrandom				
McPherson[73]	1982	PTBD	24% (8/33)	Not reported
Prospective, Random				
Hatfield[74]	1982	PTBD	5% (1/22)	8% (2/25)
McPherson[75]	1984	PTBD	22% (6/27)	19% (6/31)
Total			14% (7/49)	14% (8/56)

* Data presented for malignant causes only unless otherwise noted.
† PTBD = percutaneous transhepatic biliary drainage.
‡ Twenty-eight percent were benign.

nasobiliary drainage in alleviating the risks and complications of postoperative patients. In centers where the overall operative mortality is less than 5%, it is unlikely that any benefit in mortality can be shown by such studies without large numbers of patients. In a randomized trial comparing endoscopic and percutaneous stent insertion in 75 patients with malignant obstructive jaundice, the endoscopic route had a greater success rate in relieving jaundice and was associated with a significantly lower complication rate and 30-day mortality.[78] Proponents of the percutaneous route have challenged this study based on a too high percutaneous complication rate.[79]

RESECTION

Surgical resection remains the only possible chance for cure and allows confirmation of the histologic and site-specific subtypes. Candidates for resection can be carefully chosen by preoperative testing.

Incision and Evaluation

The bilateral subcostal incision with the extensive use of an upper-hand retractor to gain complete and adequate access to the upper abdomen is preferred. Rarely, an upper midline extension (Mercedes-Benz) is required.

Primary contraindications to resection are liver metastasis or extrapancreatic serosal implantation. It is important to examine the inferior surface of the mesocolon to be sure there is no tumor extending through the base. For many, this is an indication of unresectability. In essence, as resectability is evaluated, part of the dissection for the subsequent resection is completed. In most patients, evidence of obvious nodal involvement with cancer in the portal area precludes subsequent resection. If an ampullary or islet cell lesion is suspected, positive nodes are an absolute contraindication to further dissection.

Once it is clear that the tumor, duodenum, and the head of the pancreas are mobile, the histopathologic diagnosis is obtained, if it has not been obtained preoperatively. This is done by a single pass of a transduodenal tru-cut needle, holding the pancreas and tumor with the fingers and thumb of the left hand. Although difficulty may be encountered in obtaining a histologic diagnosis, most physicians have reported a very low false-negative rate, and a diagnosis was readily obtained.[37,80]

On rare occasions a decision has to be made to proceed with a pancreatic resection when no histologic diagnosis of carcinoma can be obtained. Some authors advocate this approach, but, whenever possible, a clear histologic diagnosis should be obtained. Conversely, repetitive transduodenal or open biopsies should be discouraged. Difficulties are encountered with persistent attempts at aggressive biopsy with no subsequent progression to resection than if the surgeon proceeds with conventional resection because of the very high likelihood that a pancreatic or periampullary carcinoma exists. Provided that this issue has been discussed preoperatively with the patient, the procedure can be continued.

If tumor invades or adheres to the celiac axis or origin of the common hepatic artery, it is a contraindication for further resection, and the procedure should be terminated. Once the hepatic vessels are free, the suprapancreatic portal vein is dissected just medial to the curve of the hepatic artery. This can be easily identified between common duct and hepatic artery, and its freedom from any local tumor invasion should be established. This exposure is limited, and the vein will be more easily demonstrated from the inferior approach.

The relationship of the tumor to the portal vein is then established inferiorly through the lesser sac. Gross and encompassing involvement and difficulty in obtaining dissection between vein and pancreas are limits to resection. Minimal adherence to the vein, however, does not prevent resection and can be dealt with by resection of the vein. The surgeon should assess whether the superior mesenteric artery is involved. It is rare that involvement of the origin of the superior mesenteric artery will exist without virtually complete encasement of the portal vein, often with obvious venous collaterals and varices. Once it has been established that the superior mesenteric artery is free and that the portal vein is free or only minimally involved, the decision to proceed is made.

Pancreaticoduodenectomy

The tissue to be resected includes the distal stomach, the gallbladder, the common bile duct, the head of the pancreas with the contained tumor, all four parts of the duodenum, and the first part of the small intestine (Fig. 26-20). The topography of the tumor in its relation to these tissues is illustrated in Figure 26-21. The common duct is commonly dilated and there may be some dilatation of the pancreatic duct. This may not be appreciated. Preoperative assessment can determine the degree of expected dilatation of the common hepatic duct, and the failure to find what was assessed preoperatively raises the question of an erroneous diagnosis.

The order in which dissection proceeds is a matter of personal preference. The continued mobilization of the third and fourth parts of the duodenum, at the ligament of Treitz, and the first part of the jejunum, early in the procedure rather than following the gastric dissection, is often appropriate. It may be easier to divide the stomach earlier in the procedure to gain access to the pancreas. Procedures reserving the pylorus can, on rare occasions, be done for very small lesions involving the ampulla.

FIG. 26-20. All tissues are now removed and the reconstruction can begin.

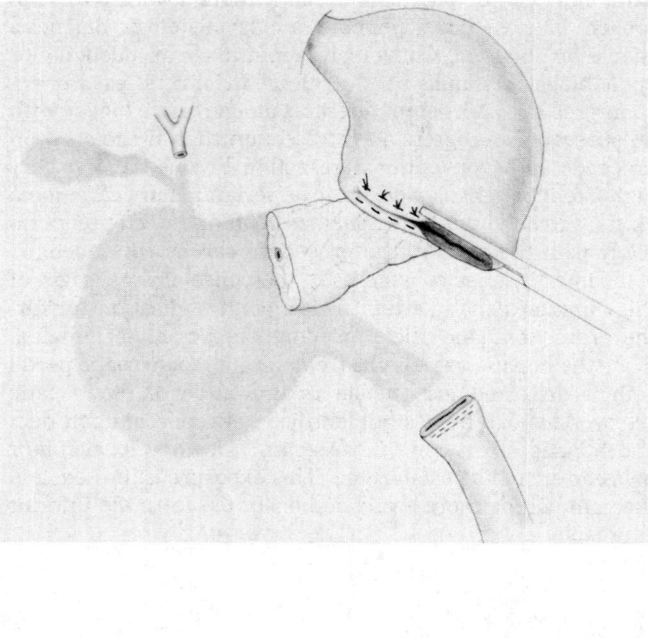

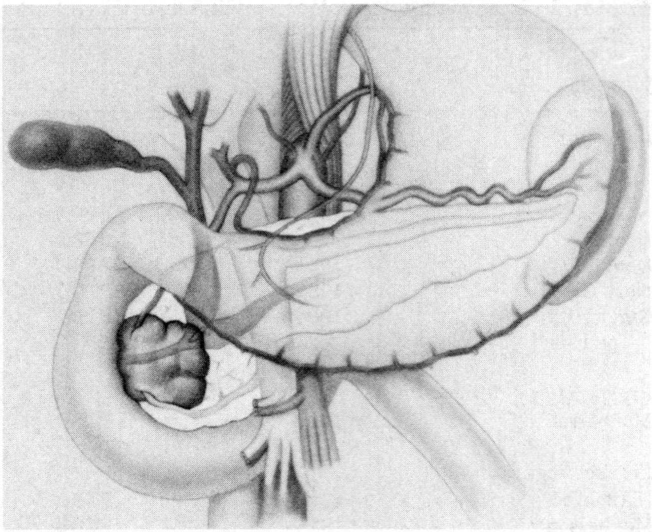

FIG. 26-21. Topography of the tumor, demonstrating both the dilatation of the common bile duct and pancreatic duct and the tissues that need to be exposed and resected.

Once the pancreas has been divided, then the final dissection of the porta hepatis is continued. The cholecystectomy is performed, and, when the duct enters low on the common duct, surgery can be done conventionally from fundus to duct such that the gallbladder will come with the specimen. If the entrance of the cystic duct is quite high on the common duct or into the right hepatic duct, then cholecystectomy is done in conventional fashion as an isolated procedure, ligating duct and artery and removing the gallbladder, discontinuous with the specimen.

Careful and diligent attention is then paid to the uncinate process. Many surgeons do not remove the uncinate process completely, but it is important to do so because it can be a worrisome site of subsequent bleeding. In uncinate process tumors, unresectability may be encountered quite late in the procedure. If that is suspected by the early assessment, then the uncinate process should be dissected before the small bowel is divided. If invasion of the portal vein is encountered, isolation above and below can be obtained and the vein transected if necessary. Conversely, a lateral sidebiting, vascular clamp can be placed along the pancreatic vein and a small portion of the vein taken. If the vein is taken, mobilization of the small intestine can easily make up several centimeters such that end-to-end approximation with vascular 4-0 sutures can be achieved. This allows the specimen to be removed, and the tissue remaining (see Fig. 26-20) is now ready for reconstruction.

Reconstruction

Choledochojejunostomy is performed first because it is the deepest anastomosis. A small longitudinal incision is made with a cautery over the serosa of the small bowel, and the serosa is gently teased from the mucosa to allow a greater entry site for mucosa than for serosa. The horizontal running everting mattress suture of 3-0 or 4-0 prolene is then used to

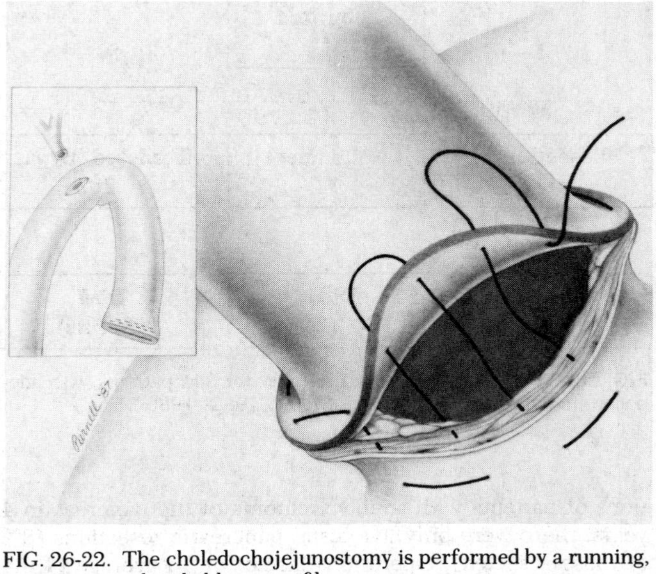

FIG. 26-22. The choledochojejunostomy is performed by a running, everting, nonabsorbable, monofilament suture.

settle the back wall and the anterior separate line suture (Fig. 26-22). This gives a comfortable, easy-to-place anastomosis that can slide down to approximate the tissues under direct vision. By taking a larger bite on the serosal site and a small bite on the mucosal site, a satisfactory mucosa-to-mucosa anastomosis can be obtained.

The pancreaticojejunostomy is performed next. A similar incision in the small intestine is made along the jejunal wall, and horizontal nonabsorbable mattress sutures are placed to attach the pancreas to the small bowel. A direct duct to the mucosal anastomosis is then performed with three interrupted 4-0 or 5-0 prolene sutures, bringing the duct directly to mucosa. A similar row of horizontal mattress sutures is then encompassed to place the remainder of the pancreas into the small intestine (Fig. 26-23). Once this has been completed the standard gastrojejunostomy is performed, usually with one absorbable and one nonabsorbable layer of sutures. The completed anastomoses appear as in Figure 26-24, although on occasion the gastrojejunostomy will be retrocolic. We prefer to use two Reliavac drains, one in the right upper quadrant and one from the left side of the pancreaticojejunostomy. The wound is closed in standard fashion with a running mass closure with nonabsorbable #1 suture material.

FIG. 26-23. The choledochojejunostomy is complete and the pancreaticojejunostomy is begun. The posterior layer of horizontal mattress sutures fixes the pancreas to the jejunum and two or three interrupted 5-0 nonabsorbable prolene complete a mucosa-to-mucosa anastomosis of the pancreatic duct to the jejunum.

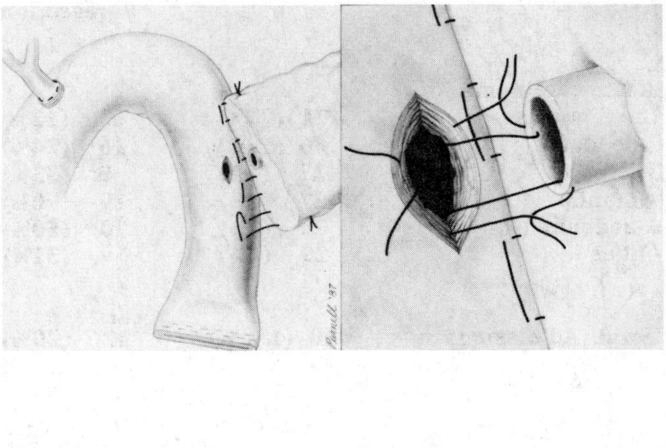

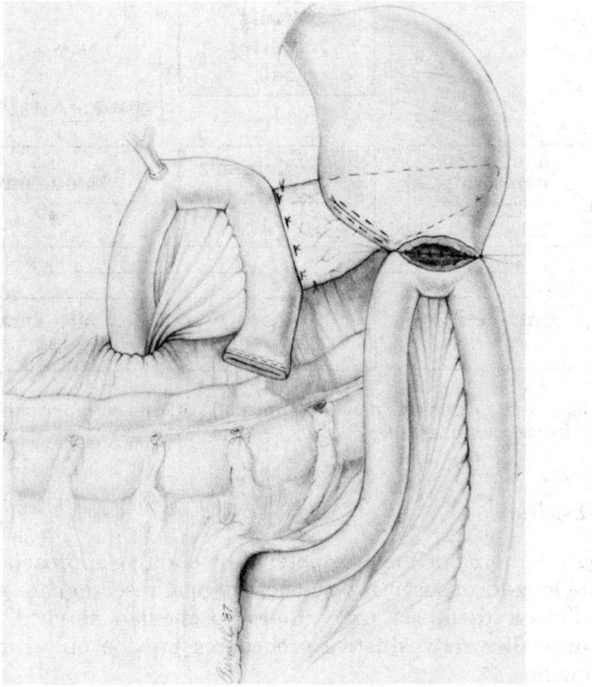

FIG. 26-24. The completed reconstruction, showing the pancreaticojejunostomy, the choledochojejunostomy, and gastrojejunostomy being performed. The pancreatic and jejunal anastomosis is usually done retrocholic and the gastrojejunostomy can be either retrocholic, as shown here, or anticholic.

Extended Resections

Extended pancreatic resections have been proposed to include resection of the portal vein, superior mesenteric artery, and celiac axis and an extended nodal dissection.[81] This "regional pancreatectomy" has undergone considerable evolution and refinement and has an improved operative morbidity and mortality.

Current approaches to pancreatic resection for adenocarcinoma have evolved from major arterial resection, but they have encompassed more extensive nodal dissection, liberal use of portal vein resection, and primary reanastomosis, if necessary.

The debate about total pancreatectomy as a preferred procedure over more limited resections continues. As operative morbidity from leakage from pancreaticojejunostomy has decreased, arguments for total pancreatectomy have become less forceful. Because the results in long-term survival do not clearly depend on the type of pancreatic resection, most experienced surgeons rely on the procedure that most easily and adequately removes the primary cancer.

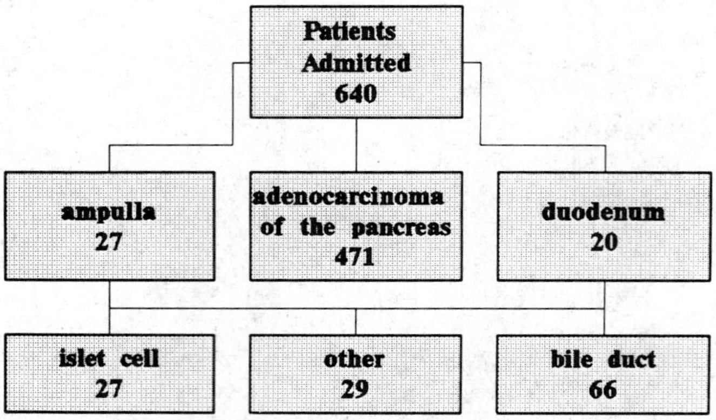

FIG. 26-25. Definitive diagnoses for 640 patients with peripancreatic cancer admitted to MSKCC, 1983–1987.

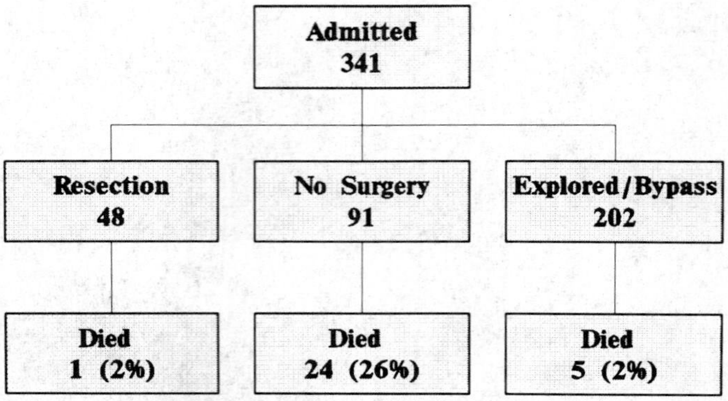

FIG. 26-27. In-hospital 30-day mortality for 341 patients with adenocarcinoma of the pancreas, MSKCC, 1983–1986.

Results

Surgery remains the only potentially curative approach, and the long-term survival results of surgical resection are poor. Adjuvant therapies have improved median survival only minimally, and palliative procedures provide only limited benefit.

The number of patients who present with suspected adenocarcinoma of the pancreas is clearly greater than the actual incidence. From 1983 through 1987, the Memorial Sloan-Kettering Cancer Center (MSKCC) admitted 640 adult patients suspected of having peripancreatic carcinoma. Of these, 471 (73%) had adenocarcinoma of the pancreas. The remainder had bile duct cancer (10%), islet cell cancer (4%), or ampullary or duodenal cancer (7%) (Fig. 26-25). Of 442 patients suspected of having a peripancreatic carcinoma admitted to the same institution between 1983 and 1986, 341 (77%) had adenocarcinoma of the pancreas. The age range for these patients was 31 to 90 years (Fig. 26-26).

OPERABILITY. Of 341 patients, 250 (73%) underwent exploration and 48 (19%) were resected (Fig. 26-27). Comparable figures for the resectability rate of other peripancreatic tumors are shown in Figure 26-28.

The majority of these patients require a pancreaticoduodenectomy or total pancreatectomy. In 63 successive resections of patients with adenocarcinoma of the pancreas in 4 years, there were only five distal pancreatic resections (8% of those resected). Operations lasted for an average of 6.4 hours (range, 2.2–14.5 hours), and the median intraoperative blood replacement was 1000 ml (0–6500 ml).

The results of resection, bypass, and pancreatic implantation have been previously reported from MSKCC.[82] Until 1980, operative and in-hospital mortality was between 16% and 20% for resection, biopsy, or bypass (Tables 26-7, 26-8, and 26-9). This was similar to the operative mortalities of 15% to 25% reported before 1982 (Table 26-8). In a recent report on 50 cases of adenocarcinoma, patients operated on between 1969 and 1980 were compared with those operated on between 1981 and 1986.[100] The operative mortality rate fell from 24% in the first period to 2% in the second, remarkably similar to the operative mortality of 18% until 1980 at MSKCC and of 2% between 1983 and 1986, with similar numbers of patients (Fig. 26-27). Age has not been a barrier to resection. Patients who are older than 70 years of age have no greater operative mortality and similar survival compared with younger patients (Fig. 26-29).

SURVIVAL. Operative morbidity and mortality have been markedly decreased. Long-term survival, however, is little changed (Table 26-8). The MSKCC experience is shown in Figure 26-30. The influence of brachytherapy on survival

FIG. 26-26. Age range of 341 patients with adenocarcinoma of the pancreas, MSKCC, 1983–1986.

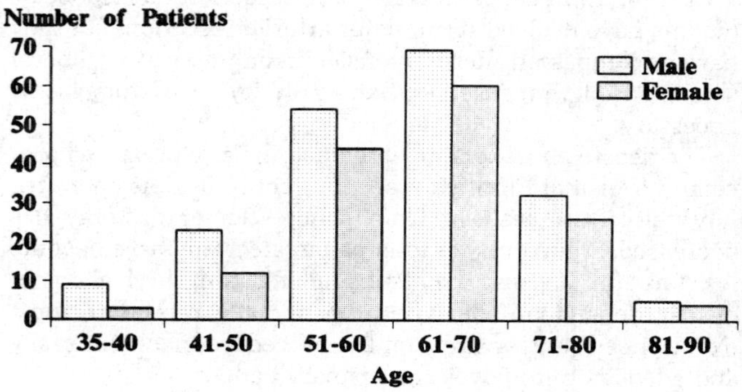

FIG. 26-28. Resectability rates of peripancreatic tumors, MSKCC, 1983–1987.

	n	# resections
Adenocarcinoma of the Pancreas	471 (74%)	63 (13%)
Bile duct	66 (10%)	16 (24%)
Islet cell	27 (4%)	9 (33%)
Ampulla	27 (4%)	19 (70%)
Duodenum	20 (3%)	10 (50%)
Other	29 (4%)	9 (31%)
Total Admissions	640 (100%)	126 (20%)

TABLE 26-7. In-Hospital and Long-Term Survival by Procedure

Procedure	*No. of Patients*	*Mortality (%)* 30-day	*Mortality (%)* In-Hospital	*Median Surviva (mo)*
Biopsy	80	15	16	4
Biopsy, alone	48	19	20	3
Biopsy, previous bypass	32	9	9	6
Bypass	76	12	14	4
Implant	33	0	3	8
All resection for cure	39	18	23	18
Conventional resection*	16	19	19	14
Resection	19	16	16	17

Morrow M, Hilaris B, Brennan MF: Comparison of conventional surgical resection, radioactive implantation, and bypass procedures for exocrine carcinoma of the pancreas, 1975–1980. Ann Surg 199:1–5, 1984.

*Figures exclude cystadenocarcinoma.

was shown to be a median of 8 months, with no in-hospital mortality (Table 26-7). Current experience is similar, with small improvement in those receiving brachytherapy (Fig. 26-31). Hospital stay was not affected by brachytherapy treatment (Table 26-10).

BYPASS PROCEDURES

Between 1970 and 1979, 34% of 46,888 patients in England and Wales had operations for pancreatic cancer, and 95% of these were biliary bypasses for relief of jaundice. Only 5% of the 34% underwent resection; between 1970 and 1979, fewer than 800 pancreatic resections were performed in all of England and Wales, despite their very high incidence of pancreatic cancer.[6] The hospital mortality for pancreatic bypass was 20%, compared with 14% mortality for resection in the same series.

Because more than 80% of the patients with carcinoma of the pancreas present with obstructive jaundice and resection is possible in only 25%, palliative bypass has received considerable attention.[98–100] In a collected series of more than 8000 patients with unresectable carcinoma of the pancreas, Sarr and Cameron showed that patients undergoing biliary bypass had a lower operative mortality rate (19%) than did patients subjected to diagnostic laparotomy only (26%).[101] The overall survival was longer (5.4 months) in the patients having bypass than for those patients subject to diagnostic laparotomy (3.5 months). For the 341 patients with adenocarcinoma of the pancreas admitted from 1983 through 1986, the operations performed are illustrated in Figures 26-32 and 26-33.

TABLE 26-8. Results of Pancreatic Resection for Cure of Exocrine Cancer

Author	*Year*	*Years of Treatment*	*No. of Patients*	*No. per Year*	*Operative Mortality (%)*	*Mean Survival (mo)*
Bowden[83]	1958	26	51	2	31	9
Portland Surg. Coop.[84]	1967	10	27	2	22	22
Crile[85]	1970	Selected	28		NS*	6
Feduska[86]	1971	11	16	1	44	7
Wilson[87]	1974	16	13	1	23	10
Brooks[88]	1975	10	16	1	13	23
Shapiro[89]	1975	Selected	24		8	11
Nakase[90]	1975	25	430	17	22 10 b + t 5 total	12 (head)
Tepper[91]	1976	10	31	3	16	11
Knight[92]	1978	10	16	1	14	16
Moosa[93]	1979	7	52	7	8	23
Longmire[94]	1980	21	50	2	NS	16†
Edis[95]	1980	25	162	6	16	10†
Fortner[96]	1981	9	36	4	15	NS
Herter[97]	1982	39	82	2	19	9
All patients			1034	4‡	18‡	12‡
Memorial Sloan-Kettering Cancer Center	1982	6	39	7	18%	18

Modified from Morrow M, Hilaris B, Brennan MF: Comparison of conventional surgical resection, radioactive implantation, and bypass procedures for exocrine carcinoma of the pancreas, 1975–1980. Ann Surg 199:1–5, 1984.

*NS = not stated; b + t = body and tail of pancreas.

†These figures are medians.

‡These figures are averages.

TABLE 26-9. Bypass Procedures

Author	*Year*	*No. of Patients*	*Mortality (%)*	*Mean Survival (mo)*
Bowden[83]	1958	114	57	5
Portland Coop.[84]	1967	248	18	5.4
Crile[85]	1970	28		8
Feduska[86]	1971	60	33	6
Wilson[87]	1974	80	14	6
Brooks[88]	1975	35	15	5.8
Shapiro[89]	1975	24	4	8
Nakase[90]	1975	1791	21	5 head 3 b + t* 3 total
Knight[92]	1978	155	22	7
Moosa[93]	1979	31	6	6
Longmire[94]	1980	103		6
Van Heerden[98]	1980	151	6	6†
Brooks[99]	1980	51	24	7
Herter[97]	1982	152	17	6
All patients		3023	18‡	6‡
Memorial Sloan-Kettering Cancer Center	1982	76	12	4

Modified from Morrow M, Hilaris B, Brennan MF: Comparison of conventional surgical resection, radioactive implantation, and bypass procedures for exocrine caracinoma of the pancreas, 1975–1980. Ann Surg 199:1–5, 1984.
*b + t = body and tail of pancreas.
†This is a median figure.
‡These figures are averages.

The question of the preferred biliary diversion—gallbladder to intestine or common bile duct to intestine—has been addressed.[101] The debate centers on the ease of doing cholecystojejunostomy versus the slower decline in bilirubin than in choledochal drainage. Other objections to the cholecystojejunostomy are that the cystic duct will become obstructed by the primary neoplasm and that the cystic duct must enter the common bile duct well above the malignant distal obstruction at the time of initial bypass.[102–104] Conversely, the choledochojejunal anastomosis is technically more difficult and requires greater exposure but has been favored by many.

There have been questions about the merits in terms of survival.[101] In a collected series of over 900 patients, the operative mortality was identical in patients undergoing biliary drainage through the common duct (20%) to those undergoing cholecystojejunostomy (16%). In addition, survival in more than 1600 patients was similar after biliary decompression using the common bile duct (6.5 months) to the gallbladder (5.3 months). These comparisons, although not addressing stage or extent of disease, suggest that either method is equally acceptable.

The problem of recurrent jaundice is poorly addressed. At worst, less than 5% to 10% of patients with obstructive jaundice in which the cholecystojejunostomy was used as the decompression route have recurrent jaundice, which can be resolved with an endoscopic procedure. The particular methods of diversion include not only simple cholecystojejunostomy with a loop but also other procedures such as Roux-en-Y cystojejunostomy, cholecystoduodenostomy, choledochoduodenostomy, and choledochojejunostomy by a loop or by the Roux-en-Y method. These have been looked at

FIG. 26-29. Age range of 48 patients resected for adenocarcinoma of the pancreas, MSKCC, 1983–1986.

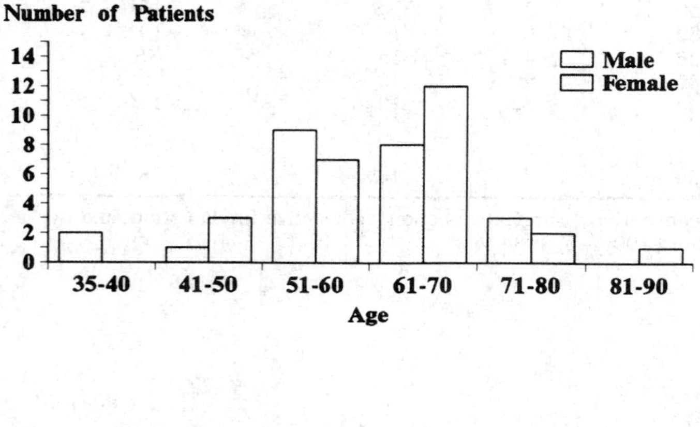

FIG. 26-30. Survival for adenocarcinoma of the pancreas, MSKCC, 1983–1987.

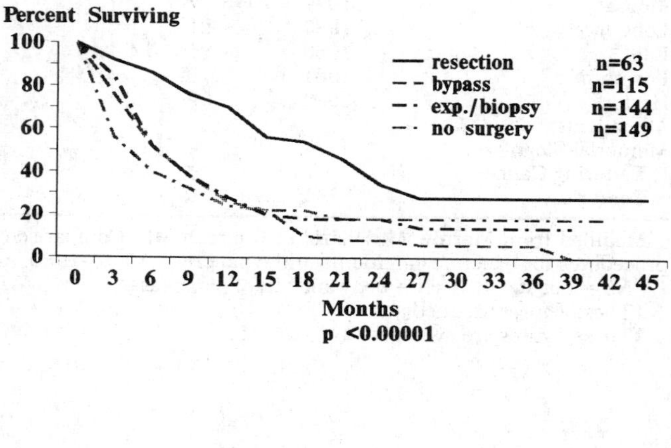

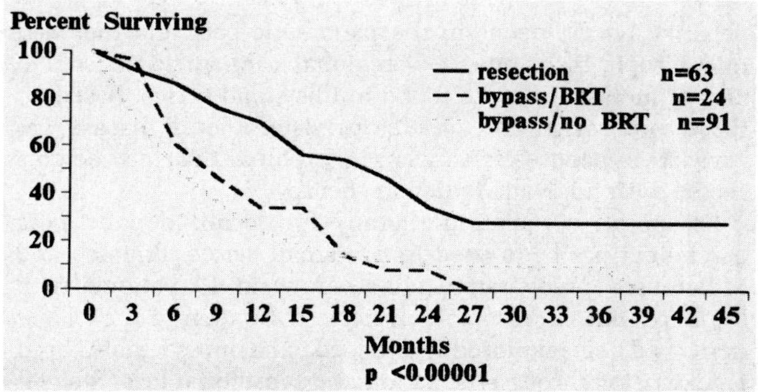

FIG. 26-31. Influence of brachytherapy on survival for adenocarcinoma of the pancreas, MSKCC, 1983–1987.

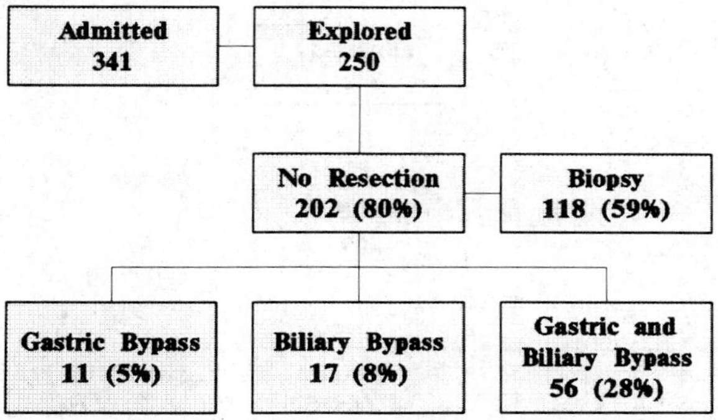

FIG. 26-32. Types of operations performed on 341 patients with adenocarcinoma of the pancreas, MSKCC, 1983–1986.

in terms of survival, and they do not seem to show any significant benefit. A review of 1114 patients shows all methods to give a range of survival between 4.8 and 7.8 months, with considerable overlap.[101]

Gastric Bypass for Obstructive Jaundice

Complete duodenal obstruction is an unusual presenting symptom of pancreatic cancer but is often a component of the disease. Many patients will have some abnormality of the duodenal outlet, detected either by endoscopy or by upper GI radiologic studies. Approximately 30% of patients will present with nausea and vomiting, some of which is associated with duodenal obstruction.[37,105] There has been considerable debate whether gastroenterostomy should be performed in all patients or only when apparently imminent obstruction is present. The objection to routine gastroenterostomy is based on the fact that most patients will not require it, that it increases morbidity due to increased operative time and additional anastomoses, and that some extrapolations have suggested increased mortality. The possibility of subsequent stomal ulceration or some contribution of the gastroenterostomy to functional gastric emptying delay has also been raised.

Reoperations for subsequent duodenal obstruction in patients who had not had previous gastroenterostomy appear to be quite high, ranging from 2% to 50% (Table 26-11). Sarr and Cameron suggest that 13% of patients not undergoing gastroenterostomy at the time of the initial operation subsequently required gastroenterostomy for development of duodenal obstruction.[101] One review reported that almost 50% of patients who did not have a gastric duodenal bypass initially and survived for 6 months or more were likely to develop duodenal obstruction and needed reoperation.[106] Others suggested a mortality of 10% to 20%.[107,112]

In a collected series of more than 500 patients, there was an average survival of 5.8 months for patients with gastroenterostomy and an average of 6.6 months for those not undergoing gastroenterostomy.[101] Similar figures for operative mortality are suggested in a review of 648 patients: 17% operative mortality with gastroenterostomy and 18% mortality without gastroenterostomy. We believe that gastroenterostomy should be routinely employed unless there is some circumstance specifically arguing against it.

RADIATION THERAPY

ADJUVANT RADIATION THERAPY FOR RESECTABLE DISEASE

Radiation therapy in combination with surgical resection has been used in an attempt to improve local disease control and survival. The pattern of failure after surgical resection by pancreaticoduodenectomy was analyzed for 31 patients from the Massachusetts General Hospital, in which survival (median, 10.5 months) and operative mortality (16%) were equivalent to other surgical series at that time (1963–1973).[91] Of 26 postoperative survivors, 22 patients died of recurrent (persistent) pancreatic carcinoma, 13 cases of which were confirmed by reexploration for suspected recurrence or by autopsy. When the clinical and pathologic findings were combined, 13 patients (50%) were believed to

TABLE 26-10. Hospital Stay for Patients with Pancreatic Adenocarcinoma*

Factors	*Resection*	*Explored Biopsy*	*Explored Bypass*	*Explored Brachytherapy*	*No Operation*
Number of patients	48	118	84	19	279
Median	26	17	19	18	14
Range	8–62	2–131	2–84	10–72	1–176
Estimated median survival (mo)	18	4	4	9	3
Hospital stay survival	5%	14%	16%	6%	16%

*Figures for Memorial Sloan-Kettering Cancer Center from October 15, 1983, to October 15, 1986.

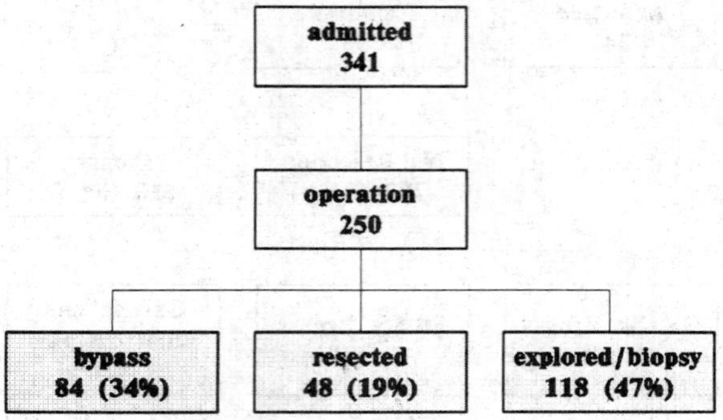

FIG. 26-33. Adenocarcinoma of the pancreas, Memorial Sloan-Kettering Cancer Center, 1983–1986.

have locoregional recurrence within the surgical bed. Only 4 (15%) of 26 patients demonstrated distant metastases without evidence of local failure.

The problem of persistent locoregional disease following surgical resection of Stage I disease was highlighted in a recent autopsy series from Japan.[127] Of eight patients with T1 and T2 tumors, six had microscopic metastases in grossly negative lymph nodes in the pancreatic bed, and four had microscopic involvement of regional para-aortic nodes. No distant metastases were found in this small series. Based on these two series and others, persistent local disease for early-stage pancreatic cancer is a problem that may be corrected with adjuvant radiation therapy.[82]

Preoperative radiation therapy for localized pancreatic carcinoma has been used in two small series. Pilepich and Miller used preoperative radiotherapy in 17 patients with localized, but unresectable, lesions.[128] Sixteen of the 17 patients had been explored and judged to be unresectable based on extension through the pancreatic capsule (at least Stage II disease). The primary tumor was less than 5 cm in 4 patients and 5 cm or larger in the remaining 13 patients. These patients then received conventionally fractionated 200 cGy/fraction) radiation therapy of 40 to 50 Gy in 4 to 5 weeks. Eleven of the 17 patients were reexplored, with 6 patients undergoing resection of tumors of the pancreatic head. Two patients remained disease-free at 5 years. The second series involved 7 patients with tumor of the pancreatic head or periampullary area who received a pancreaticoduodenectomy procedure and 45 Gy of radiation delivered preoperatively (5 patients) or postoperatively (2 patients).[129] Two

TABLE 26-11. Incidence of Duodenal Obstruction Requiring Gastroenterostomy (GE) After Initial Laparotomy or Biliary Bypass, 1965–1980

	Patients			
Author	*Total*	*% Undergoing GE at Initial Celiotomy*	*% Requiring GE in Future*	*Operative Mortality of Subsequent GE*
Glantz[107]	93	26	10*	40
Richards[108]	106	20	34	10
Webster[109]	74	4	26†	14
Pipes[110]	28	8	28‡	
Hertzberg[111]	169	3		
Collure[112]	79	37	20§	
Stuart[113]	48	0	20	
Elmslie[104]	27	20	23	
Douglass[114]	64	8	17	
Vijayanagar[115]	50	30	23	
Mendoza[116]	32	54	14	
Monge[117]	23	12	27	
Buckwalter[118]	296	69	6	
Winegarner[119]	112	29	6	
Williams[120]	135	10	8	
McDevitt[121]	13	46	15	
Howard[37]	81	15	2	
Brooks[88]	60		9	
Glassman[122]	20		20	
Blievernicht[103]	93	45	38	15
Linn[123]	43		16‖	
du Plessis[124]	4		50	
Reed[125]	56		11	
Forrest[126]	159	31	13	
Mean			13	16
Total	1865			

Sarr MG, Cameron JL: Surgical management of unresectable carcinoma of the pancreas. Surgery 91:123–133, 1982.

* Eleven additional patients died with duodenal obstruction.

† Six additional patients had symptoms of duodenal obstruction at death.

‡ One additional patient died with duodenal obstruction.

§ Two additional patients died with duodenal obstruction.

‖ Only 25% of these patients had abnormal UGI series findings originally.

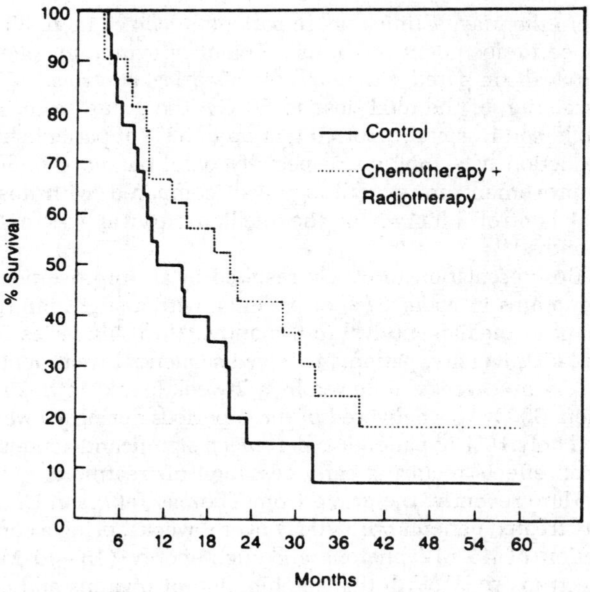

FIG. 26-34. GITSG: comparison of survival in treated with control group. Survival was greater in treated as compared with control groups throughout follow-up period (adjusted p = 0.03) (Kalser MH, Ellenberg SS: Pancreatic cancer: Adjuvant combined radiation and chemotherapy following curative resection. Arch Surg 120:901, 1985)

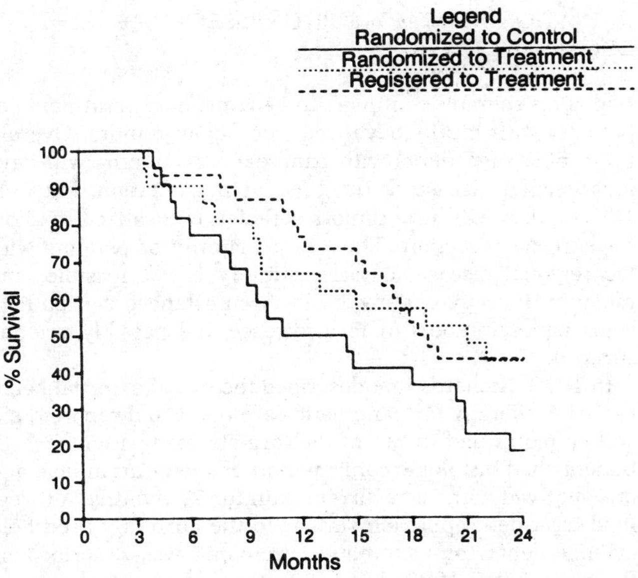

FIG. 26-35. GITSG: probability of survival by treatment. (Gastrointestinal Tumor Study Group [GITSG]: Further evidence of effective adjuvant combined radiation and chemotherapy following curative resection of pancreatic cancer. Cancer 59:2006–2010, 1987)

patients survived for 5 years, and there were no clinically detected local recurrences.

More recently, two groups have performed randomized prospective trials of postoperative radiation therapy in patients with resected carcinoma of the pancreas. In a study at the National Cancer Institute, 32 patients with locally confined pancreatic carcinoma underwent total or regional pancreatectomy and were randomly allocated to receive either intraoperative radiotherapy (IORT) as adjuvant treatment or conventional treatment.[130] The IORT group of 16 patients received 20 Gy, using 9 to 12 MeV electrons to the tumor bed and regional nodal basins immediately after resection. The surgical and radiotherapeutic details of IORT are described elsewhere.[131,132] The control group of 16 patients received surgery alone for Stage I disease and external-beam radiation therapy (50 Gy in 5–6 weeks) postoperatively for Stage II and Stage III disease. More than 90% of patients on both arms of this study were Stages II and III.

Operative mortality was high (9 of 32 patients) but was similar in both IORT and control groups, as was the incidence of complications in the postoperative period. When operative deaths were excluded from analysis, the disease-free survival was increased in the IORT patients (20 months) compared with the control group (12 months, p = 0.1), but overall survival was similar. Local disease control was significantly improved in the IORT group. Although the number of patients on this trial was modest, it appears that IORT can improve local disease control in locally advanced disease following pancreatectomy with acceptable morbidity.

The Gastrointestinal Tumor Study Group (GITSG) reported on a prospective randomized trial comparing surgery (usually a Whipple procedure) to postoperative adjuvant therapy with external-beam irradiation (40 Gy in 6 weeks) and 5-fluorouracil (500 mg/m² × 3 days, repeated monthly for 2 years).[133] Forty-three patients were randomized to surgery alone (22 patients) or postoperative adjuvant therapy (21 patients), with an equal distribution of patients with Stages I, II, and III disease. There was a significant improvement in median survival (21 months versus 11 months, p = 0.05) and 2-year survival (43% versus 18%, p = 0.05) in patients receiving postoperative combined modality therapy (Fig. 26-34). Median disease-free survival, however, was 9 months and 11 months in the control and treated groups, respectively, and the overall death rates were 86% and 71%, respectively. Subsequently, the GITSG entered an additional 30 patients with similar clinical and pathologic features into the postoperative combined modality treatment arm.[134] In this study (Fig. 26-35), results similar to the treated arm were obtained. However, the survival curves are carried to 60 months in the earlier study (see Fig. 26-34), whereas in the latter study results are only given for 24 months.

Although these reports from the National Cancer Institute and the GITSG support the use of postoperative adjuvant treatment, the routine use of external-beam irradiation with or without 5-fluorouracil (5-FU) cannot be recommended. Without studies of alternative therapies, postoperative radiation therapy with 5-FU appears to be the adjuvant therapy most likely to prolong survival, but the use of this therapy, given the limited survival prolongation, requires individualization. A series of resected pancreatic carcinoma shows considerable variation in the median survival of 10 to 23 months, with the upper limit similar to the results of the adjuvant therapy trials.[82,93–95,97]

RADIATION THERAPY FOR UNRESECTABLE LOCAL DISEASE

Radiation therapy continues to be a primary treatment for patients with locally advanced, resectable tumors. Overall, up to 50% of patients with pancreatic carcinoma will have locoregional disease at the time of presentation, but only 10% to 15% will have tumors sufficiently localized to allow for surgical resection. Thus, in a majority of patients with locoregional disease, curative surgery is not feasible, and radiation therapy under certain circumstances can palliate signs and symptoms of local disease and possibly prolong survival.

In 1922, Richards first described the use of external-beam radiation therapy for pancreatic carcinoma and reported excellent pain relief in two of the three treated patients.[135] All patients had histologic confirmation of adenocarcinoma, and one survived without recurrent pain for 27 months. A three-field treatment approach similar to the currently used field arrangements for pancreatic carcinoma was described by Richards. In the 1920s and 1930s, there were anecdotal case reports of effective palliation of pain in patients with pancreatic carcinoma by using external orthovoltage radiation.[136,137] Unfortunately, the limited tissue penetration of the available low-energy orthovoltage beams and the proximity of radiosensitive normal structures did not allow for delivery of homogeneously distributed, high doses of fractionated orthovoltage radiation, which we now recognize as being necessary for even a palliative tumor response.

The use of brachytherapy radiation for pancreatic carcinoma was initially described by Upcott in 1912, when he placed radium capsules in a cholecystostomy following resection of an ampullary carcinoma.[138] In 1934, Handley used multiple radium tubes to implant a patient with an unresectable pancreatic carcinoma.[137] The tubes contained up to 35 mg of radium and were removed through the operative wound 15 to 50 hours after implantation. Three of the seven patients treated in this fashion survived for more than 1 year. In the late 1930s, Pack and McNeer used a permanent radium implant in three patients with unresectable pancreatic carcinoma, one of whom survived pain-free for 16 months.[139]

In the 1950s and 1960s, the development of the betatron and the linear accelerator, which were capable of generating megavoltage x-rays, allowed the delivery of high doses of radiation to deep-seated tumors, such as pancreatic carcinoma, with relative sparing of adjacent normal tissues. Phillips from Memorial Hospital, reported the first series of megavoltage irradiation in unresectable pancreatic carcinoma and recorded the effective palliation of symptoms, particularly pain, in 25% of the patients treated to doses of 4400 to 5000 roentgens delivered during 4 weeks.[140] Shortly thereafter, Miller and Fuller from M.D. Anderson Hospital, reported an improvement in symptom palliation and in normal tissue tolerance, compared with orthovoltage radiation, in a series of patients with pancreatic carcinoma.[141]

A dose-response relationship for unresectable pancreatic carcinoma to megavoltage radiation therapy, at least in the palliation of symptoms, is suggested in a comparison of several radiation therapy series. Additionally, there may be a dose-response relationship for overall survival. Early reports from the Mayo Clinic, where patients received up to 35 Gy, failed to document any improvement of symptom relief or survival compared with untreated historical controls.[142] With escalation of the total dose to 50 Gy, the group from M.D. Anderson Hospital reported that up to 33% of patients had a reduction of symptoms, especially pain, but no significant improvement in overall survival compared with historical controls, for whom the median survival was only 6 months.[141]

Dose escalation to 60 Gy resulted in an improvement in symptoms in about 67% of patients, with a slight improvement in median survival to 8 months.[143] In this series from Duke University, patients received sequential treatments of 20 Gy in 2 weeks, followed by a 2-week break. In this regimen, 60 Gy was delivered in three periods during 10 weeks, and only 10% of patients experienced significant, acute radiation effects requiring early cessation of treatment.

More recently, the group from Thomas Jefferson University treated patients with 70 Gy over 9 weeks, using a combination of 45 MV photons and high-energy (15–40 MeV) electrons.[144,145] With this combination of photons and electrons, effective palliation was noted in 50% to 70% of patients, depending on the type and severity of symptoms. Thirty-six of 40 patients completed treatment, and there were only two cases of significant late radiation injury to bowel. A median survival of 10 months was observed, which is similar to some surgical series of resectable pancreatic carcinoma.[24,94]

Although it is difficult to compare retrospective treatment series because of varying and often unknown patient selection factors, as the total dose of external-beam radiation was increased from 35 to 70 Gy a trend of an increased tumor response, as measured by palliation of signs and symptoms and by increased overall survival, was evident. However, it is important to point out that even with doses as high as 70 Gy, local tumor control was achieved clinically in only 50% of patients.[144,145] Unfortunately, many patients who initially respond favorably to the external-beam irradiation of unresectable pancreatic carcinoma will later show evidence of tumor regrowth and the return of local signs and symptoms before death. Even with high-dose external-beam irradiation of 70 Gy, only a rare patient will be a long-term survivor of 5 years or more.[143,144] Because of these poor treatment results, experimental irradiation techniques have been used either alone or in combination with conventional external-beam photon irradiation in an attempt to improve local control and influence overall survival.

EXTERNAL-BEAM PHOTON IRRADIATION FOR UNRESECTABLE DISEASE

Selection of optimal treatment for a patient with a locally advanced unresectable pancreatic carcinoma poses a major problem to the radiation oncologist. Considerations in determining the radiation therapy technique include the extent of local tumor, the volume of normal tissues included within the radiation fields, and the baseline medical and nutritional status of the patient. Although the role of external-beam radiation therapy must be determined on an individual basis, certain guidelines should be followed.

Patients presenting with widespread metastatic disease are clearly not candidates for high-dose external-beam radiation. If local symptoms of pain and intestinal obstruction are the predominant symptoms in a patient presenting with metastasis, then lower doses of radiation (50 Gy) may be used in an attempt to provide temporary palliation. For the unresectable patient presenting with biliary obstruction and clinical jaundice, surgical bypass or endoscopic or percutaneous transhepatic biliary drainage is preferable to palliative external-beam radiation therapy. For a patient with no clinical evidence of visceral metastasis but with significant weight loss (> 10–15% of body weight) and locally advanced unresectable disease, high-dose external-beam irradiation again is not warranted because this type of radiation is typically complicated by acute symptoms of nausea, vomiting, anorexia, and diarrhea.[146] In the nutritionally depleted patient, the acute radiation symptoms are often severe enough to abort a planned course of high-dose radiation therapy. Even in selected patient series, at least 10% do not complete the planned course of high-dose radiation therapy.[143,144]

Patients with unresectable pancreatic carcinoma found suitable for aggressive external-beam radiation therapy should have locally advanced disease without evidence of dissemination and should demonstrate adequate nutritional status. In this patient group, the intent of external-beam radiation is to deliver a dose of at least 60 Gy to gross disease and 45 to 50 Gy to microscopic disease. The local tumor volume is determined by CT scanning with oral contrast

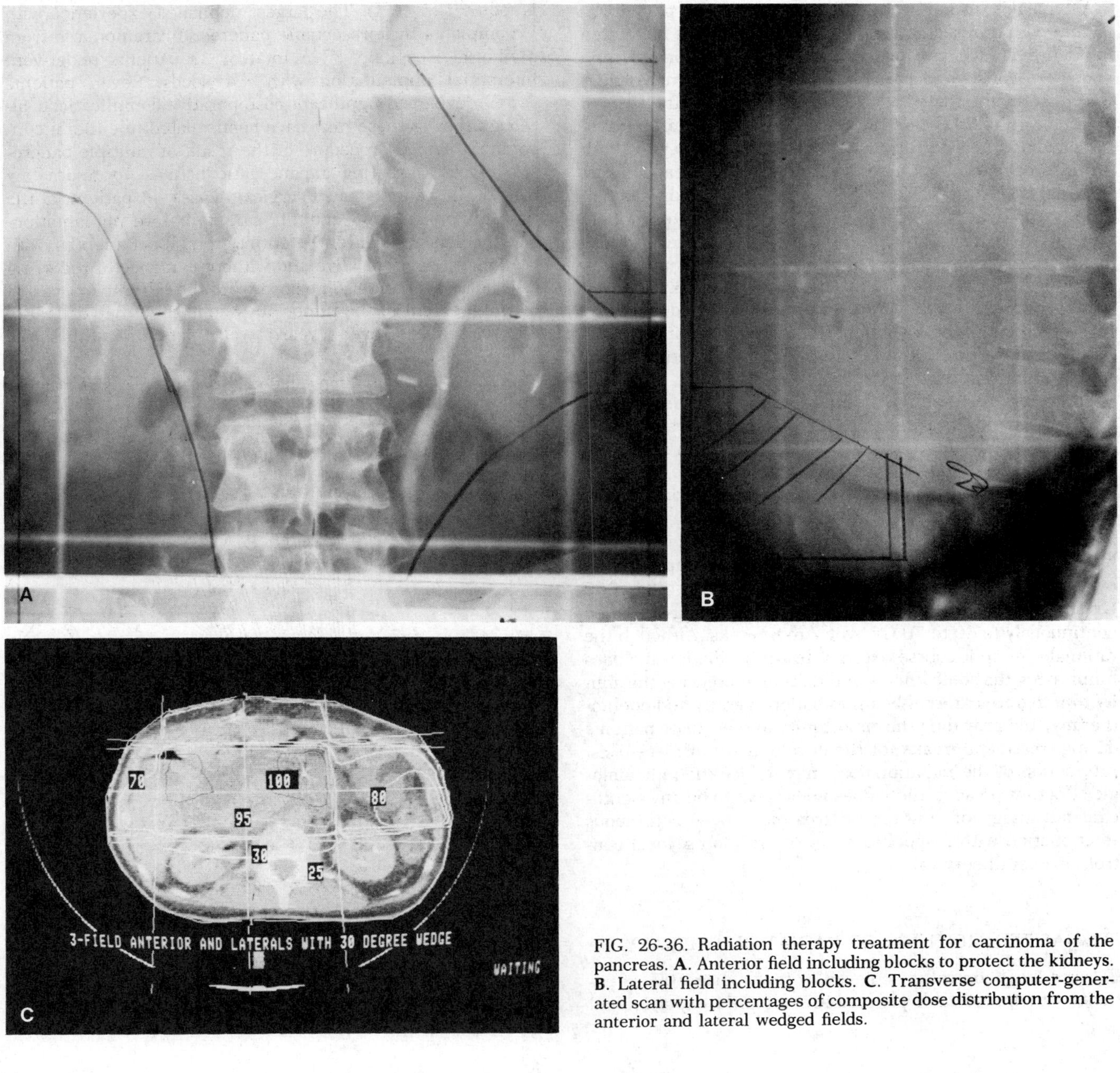

FIG. 26-36. Radiation therapy treatment for carcinoma of the pancreas. **A**. Anterior field including blocks to protect the kidneys. **B**. Lateral field including blocks. **C**. Transverse computer-generated scan with percentages of composite dose distribution from the anterior and lateral wedged fields.

material, by surgical clips placed at the time of exploration, and, if possible, by operative consultation with the radiation therapist or by a review of the surgical and pathology reports. The role of MRI scanning in defining the tumor volume for radiation therapy of unresectable pancreatic carcinoma has not been clearly defined at this time.

A major concern in radiation treatment planning for this patient group is the amount of normal tissues included within the high-dose volume. Organs that limit upper abdominal irradiation include stomach, small bowel, large bowel, liver, kidney, and spinal cord. Although the tolerance of each of these organs is reasonably well defined, when using conventionally fractionated irradiation (1.8–2.0 Gy daily), factors such as previous surgical procedures or the use of concomitant chemotherapy may lower the threshhold for acute and late radiation injury, particularly to the intestine.[146]

A typical external-beam radiation treatment plan for a patient with unresectable pancreatic carcinoma is illustrated in Figure 26-36. The primary tumor and regional lymph nodes are considered part of the initial treatment volume, which is usually treated at 1.8-Gy to 2.0-Gy daily fractions to a dose of 45 to 50 Gy. At the time of simulation, an intravenous pyelogram is performed to visualize the kidneys on both the anteroposterior and lateral radiation fields. Oral contrast material is used to visualize the stomach and proximal small bowel. Typically, a three-field plan, with an anterior field and two wedged lateral fields, usually results in the best dose distribution to cover the initial tumor volume and maximally spare normal tissues. Customized cerrobend blocks are used if appropriate to further protect normal tissue. Additionally, CT scanning in the radiation treatment position often is helpful to best direct the radiation dose distribution to the initial tumor volume.

Following treatment of the initial tumor volume by 45 to 50 Gy, a second simulation is done to plan an increase of the radiation dose to the primary gross disease by an additional 20 to 25 Gy. Although the "boost" field volume often requires a similar three-field or simple anteroposterior/posteroanterior field arrangement, rotational fields may be used for tumor volumes of 5 cm or smaller. Although some series have advocated the use of split-course radiotherapy (20 Gy over 2 weeks, followed by a 2-week break, with a total of 60 Gy administered over 10 weeks), other series have treated continuously to 60 to 70 Gy over 7 to 8 weeks. Although the rationale for split-course external-beam irradiation includes minimizing the acute effects of radiation, increasing the ability to integrate external-beam radiation therapy and chemotherapy, and providing the opportunity to reevaluate patients during treatment breaks for the development of metastasis, protraction of the radiation dose may reduce the radiobiologic effect. At present, there does not appear to be any significant advantage of split-course treatment over continuous fractionation with respect to relief of symptoms, local control, or overall survival.

SPECIALIZED METHODS OF RADIATION THERAPY

Because local control is achieved in fewer than 50% of patients with unresectable pancreatic carcinoma, experimental methods of radiation have been used, often in conjunction with external-beam therapy, to deliver higher effective tumor doses. These specialized experimental techniques include the use of interstitial implants, IORT, high linear energy transfer (high LET) or fast-neutron therapy, and charged-particle irradiation.

Interstitial Therapy

Interstitial irradiation involves implantation of radioactive sources into the pancreatic parenchyma (Fig. 26-37). The use of interstitial implants is attractive in theory because of the rapid falloff in dose from a radioactive source and because of the low dose rate delivered (< 1 Gy per hour), which can result in a greater biologic effectiveness.

The most commonly used isotope for pancreatic implants is iodine-125 (^{125}I). The largest published experience with ^{125}I implants in unresectable pancreatic carcinoma is from Memorial Hospital.[82,147] A total of 33 patients underwent interstitial implantation with ^{125}I seeds. Seven patients (21%) developed significant postoperative complications, although four of these may have been related to either a concomitant bypass procedure or the result of multiple pancreatic biopsies creating a pancreatic fistula. Approximately 67% of the patients had a surgical bypass, 11 patients at the time of implantation and 11 patients before implantation. The median survival for the entire group was 8 months, with the longest survivor alive and without evidence of recurring disease at 33 months. The dose from the ^{125}I implant varied with the extent of the tumor but was in the range of 160 to 200 Gy delivered over 1 year. Twelve patients in this series

FIG. 26-37. Interstitial implantation of the pancreas with radioactive sources for brachytherapy. (Shipley WU, Nardi GL, Cohen AM et al: Iodine-125 implant and external beam irradiation in patients with localized pancreatic carcinoma. A comparative study to surgical resection. Cancer 45:709–714, 1980)

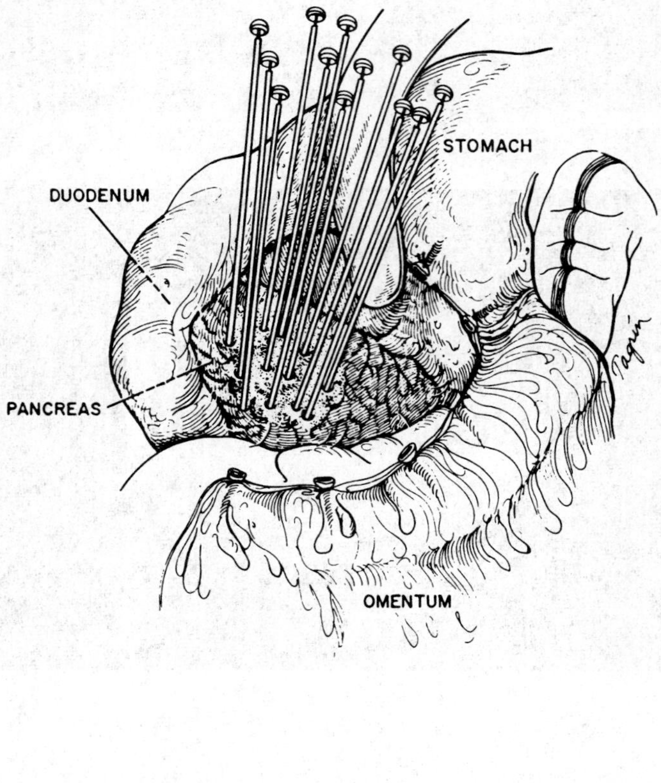

also received external-beam photon irradiation using conventional fractionation to a dose of 30 to 40 Gy.

There was no significant difference in overall survival in this series of 33 implanted patients (median, 8 months) compared with a separate group of 39 patients (median, 18 months) who underwent resection at Memorial Hospital during the same period (Table 26-8).[82] The recent experience with resection shows a highly significant improvement in survival between resection and no resection, with or without brachytherapy (Fig. 26-32).[148] Nine of 33 patients receiving the ^{125}I implant had documented liver metastasis at the time of implantation, and the other 24 patients had locally advanced unresectable disease. The 30-day mortality for this group was 0, compared with 18% for the surgically resected patients. Although showing improved survival, this does not demonstrate statistical significance for brachytherapy over bypass alone, but follow-up is short. Theoretically, significant complications can result from this therapy, but in the MSKCC experience hospital stay was not different for those patients receiving or not receiving brachytherapy (Table 26-10).

There are two other series using ^{125}I implants and external-beam irradiation for unresectable pancreatic carcinoma. At the Massachusetts General Hospital, Shipley and coworkers treated 12 patients with locally advanced pancreatic carcinoma with a combination of ^{125}I implantation (calculated dose of 160 Gy) and external-beam irradiation (45 Gy in 5 weeks), encompassing both the primary tumor and regional lymph nodes.[149] The median survival in this series was 11 months, with 30 months for the longest surviving patient. Clinical local tumor control was achieved in 9 of the 12 patients. Pancreatic fistulas developed in 2 patients, and both responded to conservative management. The group at Thomas Jefferson University also combined the ^{125}I implant with postoperative external-beam irradiation.[145] In this series, 18 patients received a ^{125}I implant (120 Gy) and external-beam radiation therapy (60 Gy); they had a median survival of 12 months, and only 1 patient was thought to have failed locally. Treatment complications included abscess formation in 3 patients, duodenal ulceration with perforation in 1 patient, and pancreatitis in 1 patient.

Intraoperative Radiotherapy

IORT involves the use of large single doses of radiation delivered directly to an exposed tumor and potential areas of regional spread at the time of surgical exploration. High-energy electrons have been used most frequently in Japan and in the United States. IORT has been used alone in patients with locally advanced unresectable pancreatic carcinoma with little obvious therapeutic gain.

In pilot studies from Howard University, the median survival of patients with unresectable pancreatic carcinoma treated with IORT was only 6 months, although 10 of the 19 treated patients had liver metastases documented at surgery and certainly represented a poor prognostic group.[150] The largest experience with IORT alone is from Kyoto University in Japan, where 108 patients were treated.[151] This study noted pain relief in patients receiving an IORT dose of greater than 20 Gy, although there was no documentation of the extent or duration of pain relief. The median survival was 6 months, and most patients died of progressive disease within 12 months. Ulceration and hemorrhage of the duodenum included within the IORT field occurred in 25% of the patients, but there were no treatment-related deaths. The investigators concluded that the IORT dose should be limited to less than 30 Gy if a significant segment of duodenum needs to be included within the IORT field. In a more recent study from two other Japanese centers, 33 patients received an IORT dose of 20 to 40 Gy, which gave prompt pain relief (within 1 week) in 50% of patients. There was a suggestion of an improved survival in IORT patients (median, 6 months) compared with patients treated with only surgical bypass (median, 2.5 months).[152]

A combination of intraoperative electron-beam irradiation and external-beam photon irradiation has been used in patients with unresectable pancreatic carcinoma at three major medical centers within the United States. A total of 63 patients with locally advanced disease were treated at the Massachusetts General Hospital between 1978 and 1985 on a single-arm pilot study.[153,154] All patients received preoperative external-beam radiation of 10 Gy delivered in five fractions during the week before exploration. At exploration, the patients received intraoperative electron-beam radiation of 15 to 20 Gy, with most receiving 20 Gy. Misonidazole, a hypoxic cell sensitizer, was given at a dose of 3.5 g/m^2 immediately before IORT in 41 of 63 patients. A surgical bypass of the bile duct or duodenum was performed as indicated. Postoperatively, the patients received an additional 39.6 Gy of external-beam radiation over 5 weeks. The median survival of the group was 14 months, with a 16.5-month median survival in patients receiving IORT without misonidazole and a 12-month median survival in patients receiving IORT with misonidazole. Approximately 60% of patients were alive at 1 year, and 25% were alive at 2 years. As determined clinically by follow-up CT scans, about 67% of patients had local control at 1 year, but only 40% continued to have local control at 2 years. The longest survival in the series was 52 months.

At the Mayo Clinic, a total of 44 patients with primary unresectable pancreatic carcinoma have been treated with a combination of IORT to 20 Gy and external-beam radiation therapy of 45 to 50 Gy, using conventional fractionation.[155] Some patients also received 5-FU given intravenously for three consecutive days at 500 mg/m^2 during weeks 1 and 5 of the external-beam irradiation. Median survival was in the range of 12 months, with only 10% of patients alive at 2 years. There was no significant difference in survival based on tumor size of less than or greater than 6 cm. Local tumor progression with the external-beam or IORT fields was uncommon and occurred in only 3 of 42 (7%) evaluable patients. Most patients died of metastatic disease. The most common postoperative problem was a periodic delay in gastric emptying. There were no major problems with duodenal hemorrhage.

At the National Cancer Institute there has been a randomized trial of IORT in patients with unresectable carcinoma of the pancreas.[130] In this study, 32 patients with unresectable Stage III disease or with limited Stage IV disease (liver and peritoneal metastases detected at exploration) were entered into a prospectively randomized trial. The patients in the treatment group received surgical biliary and gastric bypass followed by intraoperative radiation therapy to the primary tumor of 25 Gy using 18 to 22 MeV electrons. These patients then received postoperative external-beam radiation therapy of 50 Gy over 6 to 7 weeks. The control group received the biliary and gastric bypass and postoperative external beam radiation of 60 Gy delivered in split courses of 20 Gy over 2 weeks, with cycles separated by a 2-week break. Both the experimental and control groups received 5-FU begun concomitant with external-beam irradiation at 500 mg/m^2 for 3 days, repeated every 4 weeks for a year. In this study, in which a majority of patients had Stage IV disease, the median survival for both the IORT and control patients was 8 months. All patients on the control arm died within 18 months, and patients on the IORT arm died within 24 months. Time to local disease progression was longer in the IORT arm, but more than 50% of patients were judged to fail locally. Four patients had complete autopsies. Radiation-related changes were seen, with widespread necrosis and little or no viable tumor identified in two patients.[156] Although the treatment-related complication rates were similar for both the IORT and control groups, three patients receiving IORT developed severe, but not fatal, late duodenal hemorrhage.

Based on the published experience with IORT alone or with the combination of IORT and external-beam irradiation, there does not appear to be any major improvement in overall survival in patients with locally advanced unresectable pancreatic carcinoma. Although the initial experience on the contribution of misonidazole as a radiation sensitizer was positive, further follow-up at Massachusetts General Hospital and from the study at the National Cancer Institute suggests that there is no benefit from the addition of the sensitizer to IORT.[130,153,154] Some of these series suggest a decrease in local failure, but the development of widespread metastatic disease during or shortly after treatment continues to be the major problem.

High Linear Energy Transfer Radiation

The use of high LET radiation can theoretically improve tumor response because its ability to kill cells has little dependence on oxygen concentration. With photon irradiation, which is low linear energy radiation, cell kill can vary by a factor of 2.5 to 3.0, depending on the tissue concentration of oxygen. Fast-neutron irradiation is a type of high LET commonly used in the United States, although it is available only at a limited number of centers.

At the Fermi Laboratory in Illinois, 31 patients with unresectable pancreatic carcinoma received two or three treatments with fast neutrons weekly for up to 7 weeks.[157] These patients received approximately 1950 neutron cGy in 13 fractions, which is estimated to be biologically equivalent to 60 Gy of photon irradiation delivered in conventional fractionation. The median survival in this group was 9 months, with 25 of 31 patients showing clinical evidence of local failure. Additionally, almost 33% of the patients had severe late toxicity, with two treatment-related deaths from GI hemorrhage. At the Mid-Atlantic Neutron Therapy Facility outside Washington, D.C., 19 patients received 1750 neutron cGy in 24 fractions over 6 weeks.[158] Although local control was achieved in approximately 50% of the patients, median survival was only 6 months. There was an unacceptably high rate of late radiation complications, with seven patients experiencing significant GI injuries and one patient developing a transverse myelitis. At the M.D. Anderson Hospital, combined neutron and photon irradiation has been used in 13 patients, who received two neutron and three photon treatments weekly for up to 10 weeks.[159] Although acute and late radiation effects were minimal, median survival was 8 months.

Charged-Particle Irradiation

Both helium ions and negative pi mesons have been used to treat locally advanced pancreatic carcinoma. In contrast to photons or neutrons, for which the beam energy is attenuated continuously in tissue, the dose distribution of charged particles is characterized by a discrete stopping region called the Bragg peak, which is dependent on the initial beam energy. A relatively homogeneous dose distribution can be obtained for a tumor volume using beam modulators. These charged particles are biologically more effective than photons, with factors of relative biological effectiveness of 1.2 for helium ions and 1.5 for negative pi mesons, compared with 1.0 for photons. At the University of California at Berkeley, 34 patients with unresectable pancreatic carcinoma were treated with helium ions, receiving the equivalent of 50 to 60 Gy of photon irradiation over 8 weeks.[160] The median survival in this group was only 9 months, and 24 of the 34 patients had persistent local disease. Additionally, 4 patients developed late GI hemorrhage several months after treatment. At Los Alamos Laboratory, 10 patients received negative pi meson irradiation comparable to 45 to 55 Gy of photon irradiation; they had a survival of only 5 months.[161]

COMPLICATIONS OF TREATMENT

Many physicians have argued against pancreatic resection for adenocarcinoma of the pancreas because of operative mortality in the range of 20% to 30%. The operative mortality in our hands is less than 5%, similar to other reported series. Estimated median operative blood loss in the 48 resections performed at MSKCC for adenocarcinoma of the pancreas from 1983 to 1986 was 2200 ml, with a median replacement of 10,000 ml (0–6500 ml). Mortality is usually associated with a leak of the pancreaticojejunal anastomosis, with the second most common complication being postoperative hemorrhage. The high frequency of leakage from pancreaticojejunostomy has been used as an argument in favor of performing total pancreatectomy. We believe that these complications are small and uncommon, and with operative mortality less than 5%, they should not be used as an argument against resection.

One early postsurgical complication is delayed gastric emptying, which is usually self-limiting and requires agents such as Reglan. If drainage is adequate, pancreaticojejunal leaks and biliary leaks can usually be treated conservatively. On rare occasions, reexploration for such anastomotic difficulties is justified. Later technical complications include stenosis at the choledochojejunal anastomosis. Stenoses are often associated with the development of cholangitis and with progressive deterioration in liver function. The symptoms are intermittent fever and chills, accompanied by mildly elevated liver function test findings. Diagnosis can be confirmed by ultrasound or CT scanning, which can demonstrate a dilated duct and the presence of intraductal stones. If sufficient doubt exists, then transhepatic percutaneous cholangiography can clearly demonstrate the problem. This can be remedied by re-resection of the anastamosis, performed after all the biliary stones have been removed.

Metabolic complications include diabetes mellitus and pancreatic exocrine insufficiency. The development of insulin-dependent diabetes mellitus depends on the amount of normal pancreas left, and various tests of pancreatic reserve are being explored.[162] For most patients who do not have diabetes preoperatively and who require resection only of the head of the pancreas, no supplemental insulin is needed after the procedure.

Unless there was extensive antecedent pancreatitis or chronic obstruction and glandular obstruction, pancreatic insufficiency is usually mild. If there is significant diarrhea or fat malabsorption, then the addition of pancreatic enzyme supplementation before each meal is of significant benefit. Other complications are usually indicators of recurrent disease. Most commonly, the recurrence of pain, jaundice from obstruction or intrahepatic metastases, and the development of ascites are harbingers of relatively imminent demise and require only symptomatic or palliative treatment.

Complications of intraoperative radiation therapy can be significant, with pancreatic leak, the development of pancreatic ascites, and, occasionally, prolonged delays in return to normal GI function. Despite this, we were not able to demonstrate prolonged hospital stays because of brachytherapy (Table 26-10). In all of these situations, nutritional deficits are common, and perioperative use of nutritional support by the parenteral or enteral route is to be encouraged.

CHEMOTHERAPY

The overwhelming majority of pancreatic adenocarcinoma patients have unresectable, incurable disease. These patients have a predictably short survival, averaging only 14 weeks, and fewer than 10% are alive 1 year after diagnosis.[163] Moreover, they have severe, debilitating symptoms that require palliation. The typical patient has evidence of a poor performance status, malabsorption, weight loss, abdominal pain, bowel dysmotility, hepatic synthetic and detoxification derangement, obstructive jaundice, and effusions. Because of this constellation of symptoms, most patients cannot tolerate intensive chemotherapy. There are pharmacokinetic and pharmacodynamic reasons for intolerance of vigorous treatment, including hypoalbuminemia, ascites, anemia, and hepatic dysfunction. For these fragile patients, surviving so short a time, there is a thin therapeutic index and little opportunity for therapy to exert antitumor effects.

In addition to host disability and risk factors, the tumor itself has a virulently expressed biology. Arising within the retroperitoneum and involving deep abdominal structures, this cancer is usually detected in an advanced stage. These sites of original and metastatic disease have the two-fold effect of rarely providing easily measurable disease for judging objective antitumor effects and of presenting a complex picture of physiological derangement.

Pancreatic cancer cells are relatively resistant to conventional chemotherapy, but the reasons for this resistance have not been clearly defined. There has been no systemic evaluation of pancreatic adenocarcinoma cells to screen for the presence of the multiple-drug-resistant phenotype (*mdr*-1 gene or P-glycoprotein gene).[164,165] Nor has there been a full elucidation of possible intracellular mechanisms of biochemical resistance to nitrosoureas or fluoropyrimidines. A more thorough understanding of the cellular biology of this tumor is needed.

The general pessimism that accompanies chemotherapy for those with advanced disease is well founded but poorly understood. With more than 20,000 deaths in the United States each year, there are too few pancreatic cancer patients being treated in a formal research protocol manner and an insufficient effort to correlate laboratory insights with clinical outcome.

SINGLE-AGENT CHEMOTHERAPY

For more than three decades, efforts have been made to identify effective systemic agents.[163,166,167] Because pancreatic cancer is rarely a locoregional problem, systemic therapy has been the major clinical thrust. Unfortunately, many flaws have consistently characterized chemotherapy studies. Despite the number of new cases diagnosed each year, relatively small series of patients have usually been assembled and reported. Attempts to use objective response rate as a measure of effect have been confounded by interobserver variation or inaccuracy, and attempts to replicate clinical findings have often been frustrating. Differences in the mix of prognostic features of study populations seem to have more often accounted for a "therapeutic advance" than the new treatment itself. Comparisons of the survival of responders and nonresponders have inappropriately been used as prima facie evidence of the identification of new, effective treatments. These study design and analysis difficulties have limited the value of some clinical research efforts and should be considered in the design of future trials.

A therapy can be considered effective if it results in an appreciable number of complete tumor regressions; if it shifts the overall survival for a treated population, including both responders and nonresponders; or if it results in long-term survival for even a minority of patients, affecting the tail on the survival curve. By these criteria, there has been no satisfactory agent yet identified for patients with pancreatic adenocarcinoma.[167,168]

Table 26-12 provides an overview of many of the single agents that have been used in patients with advanced and metastatic pancreatic cancer. These data are a compilation of series reported to NCI Cancer Therapy Evaluation Program Information System (CTEP-IS) or found in the medical literature.[178] The objective response rates are displayed with 95% confidence intervals. The drugs most commonly used

TABLE 26-12. Single-Agent Chemotherapy in Pancreatic Cancer

Drug	*Author*	*Number of Patients*	*Response Rate ± 95% CI**
Commonly Used			
5-Fluorouracil	Carter[166]		
	Moertel[169]	251	26 ± 3%
Mitomycin C	Crooke[170]	53	21 ± 6%
Streptozotocin	Carter[166]	27	11 ± 6%
Doxorubicin	GITSG[171]		
	Carter[166]		
	Crooke[170]	28	7 ± 5%
Semustine (methyl-CCNU)	Moertel[169]	91	4 ± 2%
Nitrosoureas			
Carmustine (BCNU)	Moertel[169]	31	0
Lomustine (CCNU)	Carter[166]	19	16 ± 8%
Chlorozotocin	Moertel[169]		
	GITSG[172]	53	6 ± 3%
Intercalators			
Amsacrine	Inamasu[173]		
	Omura[174]		
	Sternberg[175]	109	0
Mitoxantrone (DHAD)	Bedikian[176]	14	0
4′DMDR	Mittleman[177]		
	CTEP-IS[178]	58	10 ± 7%
Epirubicin	Hochster[179]		
	Wils[180]	50	22 ± 6%
Esorubicin	Blayney[181]	16	0
Mitoxantrone	DeSimone[182]		
	CTEP-IS[178]	48	0
Aclacinomycin	CTEP-IS[178]	9	22 ± 14%
Alkylator			
Melphalan	Horton[183]		
	Smith[184]	58	5 ± 3%
Ifosfamide	Gad-El-Mawla[185]		
	Einhorn[186]		
	Bernard[187]	83	26 ± 5%
Miscellaneous			
AZQ	DeSimone[188]	17	0
BTGDR	GITSG[189]		
	CTEP-IS[178]	32	6 ± 4%
Cisplatin	CTEP-IS[178]	15	0
Dactinomycin	GITSG[171]	28	4 ± 4%
Dianhydrogalanul	CTEP-IS[178]	44	5 ± 3%
Etoposide	CTEP-IS[178]		
	Horton[183]	38	0
Hexamethylmelamine	CTEP-IS[178]	54	7 ± 3%
L-Asparaginase	Lessner[190]	10	0
Maytansine	GITSG[172]	33	0
Methotrexate	GITSG[171]	25	4 ± 4%
Metoprine	Sternberg[191]	27	0
MGBG	Inamasu[192]		
	Ravry[193]	66	6 ± 3%
Razoxane (ICRF159)	GITSG[189]	24	8 ± 6%
Tamoxifen	Crowson[194]	14	0
Vindesine	Smith[195]	15	7 ± 7%

*95% confidence interval for responses.

are 5-FU, mitomycin C, streptozotocin, doxorubicin, and methyl-CCNU. Of these agents, only 5-FU has been reported to have a minimum 95%-confidence-boundary response rate of greater than 20%. Whether administered in a bolus intravenous loading or by weekly schedule, there is not convincing evidence that any particular 5-FU regimen is superior.[196,197] As with other enteric adenocarcinomas, the response rates reported for 5-FU range from 0 to more than 50%.[198] Given the pharmacology of 5-FU, there is evidence that oral 5-FU is unpredictably and inconsistently absorbed and should never be used.[197]

Mitomycin C has become a very popular agent in combination therapy of pancreatic cancer patients. Because of delayed hematologic suppression, it has been used in an intermittent schedule of bolus dosing every 6 to 8 weeks. The chronic toxicities of cumulative marrow depletion, nephrotoxicity, and hemolytic-uremic syndrome are not commonly seen because pancreatic cancer patients rarely benefit sufficiently or live long enough to receive large total doses.[166,170]

The nitrosoureas have also been investigated. Streptozotocin has been the particular focus of study because it is toxic to both pancreatic islet and ductular epithelial cells.[199] Because the drug has relatively little bone marrow toxicity, it can be conveniently combined with other agents in combination programs. However, it does induce nausea, vomiting, anorexia, and renal tubular toxicity, which many patients find intolerable.[168,200,201] Other nitrosoureas, such as BCNU, CCNU, methyl-CCNU, and chlorozotocin, have also been screened, but they benefitted very few patients as single agents.[166,202]

The other interesting compounds are the anthracyclines. Doxorubicin has been evaluated in a small population of patients as a single agent.[203] Although the response rate is low, it has been incorporated in some combination programs.[170]

In recent years, many drugs have been used as first-line therapies. The attempt to study the best possible patient population is thought to aid the identification of potentially effective therapies. Anthracycline analogues, including epirubicin, 4′demethoxydoxorubicin (4′DMDR), and aclacinomycin A, have resulted in objective responses.[177–180] However, it is not clear whether they are superior to doxorubicin in terms of efficacy or toxicity. Responses have also been noted with the alkylators, melphalan and ifosfamide, but further evaluation is necessary.[183–187] There is no single agent of dramatic efficacy.

COMBINATION CHEMOTHERAPY

Attempts to improve on the unsatisfactory state of single-agent chemotherapy for pancreatic adenocarcinoma have led investigators to explore drug combinations. Clinical investigators recognized the variability and imprecision of small Phase II studies and began to perform larger, randomized studies to define activity more reliably. Table 26-13 summarizes selected randomized two-drug studies, based on 5-FU, which provided the therapeutic rationale for the subsequent three-drug combinations. Response rates for these two-drug regimens, including BCNU, streptozotocin, methyl-CCNU, and mitomycin C, are clustered between 5% and 33%, with 95% confidence limits of ± 3% to 9%. The median survival time for the entire treated population varies between 9 and 26 weeks. No two-drug combination provides satisfactory palliation or survival benefits.[169,208]

Some biologic similarities between gastric and pancreatic cancer have been noted, and similar therapeutic regimens have been applied. The most widely employed three-drug regimens derived from work begun at Georgetown University in the early 1970s. Patients with enteric adenocarcinoma were treated with, and responded to, combinations of 5-FU, mitomycin C, and either Adriamycin or streptozotocin, administered in a cyclic weekly program. In 1978, the SMF program was described.[209] All agents were administered by bolus or short-infusion IV injection: streptozotocin (1 gm/m²) and 5-FU (600 mg/m²) on days 1, 8, 29, and 36; mitomycin C (10 mg/m²) on day 1 of each 8-week treatment cycle. Of 23 patients treated with SMF, there were 10 (43%) objective responses, and there was an overall median survival of 24 weeks. Other investigators found a similar efficacy for the SMF program.[210,211]

In 1980, Smith and colleagues described their results with the FAM program: 5-FU (600 mg/m²) on day 1, 8, 29, 36; Adriamycin (30 mg/m²) on day 1 and 29; mitomycin C (10 mg/m²) on day 1, repeated every 8 weeks. An objective response rate of 37% in 27 patients was described.[212] Both SMF and FAM demonstrated increased survival times for responding patients compared with nonresponding patients; the toxicity proved tolerable, and some patients enjoyed meaningful palliation. However, these initial studies consisted of small numbers of patients, and the results of other Phase II attempts to confirm these FAM and SMF data were not entirely consistent. Response rates of as low as 13% were reported.[195,214–216] Table 26-14 lists some of the more popular three- or four-drug combinations tested. Where replica-

TABLE 26-13. Selected Two-Drug Combination Chemotherapy in Randomized Trials for Pancreatic Cancer

Author	*Treatment*	*Number*	*Objective Response Rate (±95% CI)**	*Median Survival (weeks)*
Kovach[204]	5-FU + BCNU†	30	10 (33 ± 9%)	24
	5-FU	31	5 (16 ± 7%)	26
	BCNU	21	0 (0%)	22
Moertel[205]	5-FU + streptozotocin	42	5 (12 ± 5%)	13
	Streptozotocin + cyclophosphamide	51	6 (12 ± 5%)	9
Moertel[206]	5-FU + spironolactone	89		18
	5-FU + streptozotocin ± spironolactone	87		16
Buroker[207]	5-FU + mitomycin C	45	10 (22 ± 6%)	19
	5-FU + methyl-CCNU	43	2 (5 ± 3%)	17

*95% confidence interval.
†5-FU = 5-fluorouracil; BCNU = carmustine; methyl-CCNU = semustine.

TABLE 26-14. Selected Combination Chemotherapy in Pancreatic Cancer

References	*Common Regimen Designations*	*Range of Response Rates*	*Range of Median Survival (weeks)*
195, 198, 212, 213	FAM*	13–40%	12–24
195, 209, 211, 214, 215	SMF	14–43%	13–24
216	FAC	21%	16
217	FAM-chlorozotocin	13%	25
218	FAM-streptozotocin	18–48%	18–22
219	FAMMe	22%	

*FAM = 5-fluorouracil, doxorubicin, mitomycin C; SMF = streptozotocin, mitomycin C, 5-fluorouracil; FAMMe = 5-fluorouracil, doxorubicin, mitomycin C, semustine; FAC = 5-fluorouracil, doxorubicin, cisplatin.

tion has been performed, the range of responses is given. With variable response rates and minimal impact on overall survival, no combination therapy demonstrates apparent superiority.

To define more precisely the efficacy of the competing FAM and SMF programs and to compare FAM with simpler, less-toxic regimens, three important randomized trials have been performed (Table 26-15). The Gastrointestinal Tumor Study Group (GITSG) compared several chemotherapy programs, including FAM and two SMF programs, in 1976. The FAM and SMF I regimens were modeled to conform exactly to the Georgetown University protocols, whereas SMF II was a modification, employing a 5-day loading course for 5-FU.[209,212,220] A total of 92 previously untreated patients were studied, 34 of whom had a performance status 0 or 1. The response rates were indistinguishable, and median survival very nearly so. The investigators concluded that SMF I "ranked first" among the regimens tested, but neither FAM nor SMF could be recommended for routine use.[220]

In 1986, Oster and colleagues described 184 patients treated with either FAM or SMF (as used by GITSG and Georgetown).[221] More than 70% of patients had a performance status 0 or 1 and had undergone a prior celiotomy. Objective responses were slightly more frequent for FAM (1 complete response and 8 partial responses in 90 patients) compared with SMF (3 partial responses in 94 patients), but there were no statistically significant differences in response or survival (medians, 18.3 for FAM versus 26.4 weeks for SMF). Reasonable levels of toxicity were produced, with 50% of FAM and 39% of SMF groups having severe or life-threatening toxicity. These investigators also concluded that neither regimen was truly satisfactory.

The third important study was reported by the North Central Cancer Treatment Group (NCCTG).[222] This was a Phase II comparison of 5-FU (500 mg/m² per day × 5, repeated at 4 weeks × 2, then at 5 weeks); 5-FU (400 mg/m² daily × 4) plus doxorubicin (40 mg/m² every 4 weeks × 2, then every 5 weeks); and FAM. A total of 144 cases were evaluated for survival, and 33 with measurable disease were evaluated for objective response. There was a nonsignificant greater number of responses for 5-FU and 5-FU plus doxorubicin than for FAM. The median survival times were clustered at 17 to 23 weeks. Although somewhat more marrow toxicity resulted with FAM, about 30% of the 5-FU and 5-FU plus doxorubicin groups had leukopenia (2000/mm³). Considering toxicity, cost, and survival, the authors concluded that neither drug combination was superior to 5-FU.[222]

Based on all the available data, it is difficult to recommend any particular combination program for patients outside a clinical trial setting. Simple attempts to combine the minimally effective agents in an empirical manner produce combinations of two to four drugs that more often yield toxicity rather than efficacy.[218,219,223–225] Trivial differences may exist between regimens, but the vast majority of patients are not benefitted.

CHEMOTHERAPY TRIALS

For patients with incurable disease, there is an ongoing effort to identify effective systematic chemotherapy drugs and

TABLE 26-15. Selected Combination Chemotherapy in Pancreatic Cancer: FAM and SMF Comparisons

Author	*Treatment*	*Number*	*Objective Response Rate (±95% CI)**	*Median Survival (weeks)*
GITSG[220]	FAM†	90	9 (14% ± 4%)	18.3
	SMF	94	3 (4% ± 2%)	26.4
Oster[221]	FAM	29	4 (14% ± 6%)	11.6
	SMF I	28	4 (14% ± 7%)	17.7
Cullinan[222]	5-FU	50	3/10 (30% ± 15%)	23
	5-FU + doxorubicin	44	3/10 (30% ± 15%)	23
	FAM	50	1/13 (8% ± 7%)	17

*95% confidence interval.
†FAM = 5-fluorouracil (5-FU), doxorubicin, mitomycin C; SMF = streptozotocin, mitomycin C, 5-fluorouracil.

biologicals. Formal disease-oriented Phase II screening efforts, sponsored by pharmaceutical companies or by the National Cancer Institute, are the focus of most clinical efforts. Additionally, there is a randomized trial being conducted by the NCCTG, which seeks to confirm the efficacy of a combination chemotherapy program described by Mallinson et al in 1980.[226] These authors randomized 40 patients either to supportive care only (no chemotherapy) or to a regimen consisting of 5-FU (270 mg/m^2 daily for 5 days), cyclophosphamide (160 mg/m^2 on day 1 and 5), methotrexate (11 mg/m^2 on day 1 and 4) and vincristine (0.7 mg/m^2 on day 2 and 5), followed in 5 weeks with 5-FU (350 mg/m^2) plus mitomycin C (3.5 mg/m^2), both daily for 5 days. The median survival of the control group was 9 weeks, compared with 44 weeks for those treated with chemotherapy ($p = 0.0006$). The toxicity was acceptable, and the treatment appeared to demonstrate substantial benefit. To assess this treatment, the NCCTG plans to randomize approximately 200 patients to one of three treatments: 5-FU (500 mg/m^2 daily for 5 days every 5 weeks); the Mallinson regimen; or 5-FU (300 mg/m^2, daily for 5 days, plus doxorubicin (40 mg/m^2 on day 1) plus cisplatin (60 mg/m^2, daily) repeated every 5 weeks.[216] This study should complete accrual in 1988 and should provide definitive confirmation or refutation of this therapy.

Studies based on laboratory information have produced Phase III trials comparing combinations of cisplatin, Ara-C, and caffeine to the more conventional SMF regimen.[227]

NEW DIRECTIONS

Several new themes in pancreatic adenocarcinoma clinical research are likely to develop in the near future. Formal clinical trials investigating biologic response modifiers (BRM) are anticipated. There are few data on the use of interferons in pancreatic cancer, and small studies with recombinant gamma-interferon and other products have neither been promising nor definitive.[228,229] There has been relatively little clinical exploration of interleukins, with or without activated lymphocytes, in these patients.[230,231]

There has been more, albeit incomplete, data on therapeutic monoclonal antibodies. Experience with the 17-1A antibody has been the best described. This is a murine-derived IgG2a monoclonal antibody generated against a human colorectal adenocarcinoma cell line. It binds to human enteric cancers in vitro and inhibits adenocarcinoma xenografts in athymic nude mice.[232–234] Preliminary studies in man demonstrated that 17-1A was tolerable, but antimouse antibodies were detected circulating in those treated.[235] Phase II studies in pancreatic cancer patients have used both 17-1A alone and 17-1A absorbed on autologous peripheral mononuclear white cells that are reinfused.[236,237]

Sindelar reported objective responses in 4 of 25 pancreatic cancer patients treated with 17-1A, but these benefits were brief, ranging from 6 to 40 weeks, with a median overall survival of 12 weeks.[236] Further analyses of these data suggest no significant objective response.[238] Patients have also been treated with 17-1A plus FAM chemotherapy.[239] Clinical responses have been noted, but the inclusion of conventional chemotherapy complicated the interpretation of the data. There are other monoclonal antibodies, such as DU-PAN-1 through DU-PAN-5 and ACI, that may prove to be of clinical relevance for pancreatic cancer patients.[240,241] This is a promising area of clinical investigation which is now only beginning to be explored.[66]

RELATIVE THERAPEUTIC EFFECTIVENESS

It is very difficult to evaluate cost effectiveness in the treatment of pancreatic adenocarcinoma. Length of hospital stay has been used as an indication of the effectiveness of treatment. Table 26-10 outlines the length of stay at the Memorial Sloan-Kettering Cancer Center in New York. It is clear that length of stay varies by only a small degree for patients undergoing major resection, those undergoing bypass procedures, with or without radiation therapy, or those being admitted and not undergoing surgery. Basing the length of subsequent survival on the length of stay, if the average survival for a bypass procedure is 4 months, the length of stay as a percentage of life expectancy is 14%. Conversely, if we do the same for resections, then the length of stay is 5% of mean estimated survival rates. This does not take into account perioperative or in-hospital mortality, and because mortality was greater in patients with advanced disease and shorter life expectancy, this only exaggerates these effects. In similar fashion, if conventional radiation therapy is delivered over 6 weeks for unresectable disease, patients will be in active daily treatment for 25% of their life expectancy. A clear indication of the costs or charges accrued by such a treatment has yet to be produced.

PAIN RELIEF

Epigastric pain is the most common symptom in patients with pancreatic carcinoma and often is the reason for seeking medical attention. Increase in the severity of epigastric pain, associated with radiation to the back or diffuse radiation in the abdomen, occurs in most patients during the course of their disease. Severe pain is the most incapacitating symptom of pancreatic cancer. In a study of pain prevalence in patients with lung, prostate, uterine, cervical, or pancreatic cancer that has recently been completed, 60% of patients with pancreatic cancer reported "moderate to bad" pain in the past week.[242] Patients (86%) were interviewed within 6 months of diagnosis and tended to be those who had survived after surgery. Daily "moderate to bad" pain occurred in 38% of these patients.

The cause of severe pain is believed to result from tumor infiltration into the retroperitoneum and splanchnic nerve plexus.[243] Treatment to palliate pain includes medical management with narcotic analgesics, surgical neurotomy, chemical neurolysis, and radiation therapy. Three treatment approaches are discussed here, and a discussion of the judicious use of narcotic analgesics in cancer patients is presented in Chapter 59. Medical management alone often is not successful in relieving pain in patients with pancreatic carcinoma.

Three types of surgical neurotomy have been used to ease pain in patients with pancreatic carcinoma, including a neurotomy of the preganglionic sympathetic plexus, a neurotomy of the celiac and superior mesenteric ganglions, and a neurotomy of the postganglionic plexus of the celiac ganglion.[244-246] Considerable expertise is required to perform these procedures, particularly in the patient with locally advanced or locally recurrent pancreatic carcinoma. Unfortunately, most patients will experience only partial and temporary pain relief following neurotomy, presumably resulting from inadequate surgical denervation or subsequent tumor infiltration of other nerve roots in the retroperitoneum.

Chemical neurolysis, using either an intraoperative or percutaneous approach, is used more often today than surgical neurotomy to relieve pain in patients with pancreatic carcinoma. The percutaneous injection of 50 ml of 50% alcohol after a diagnostic injection of pontocaine was described by Bridenbaugh and colleagues in 1964.[247] The efficacy of neurolytic block of the celiac plexus approaches 90%.[248,249] Needle verification by radiographic techniques, particularly CT scanning, appears to reduce morbidity and improve efficiency.[250,251] Serious complications of a percutaneous nerve block are rare (<1%) and result from inadvertent injection into the peritoneal cavity (causing peritonitis) or into the subarachnoid space (causing paralysis). Transient hypotension as a result of splanchnic pooling following injection occurs more commonly and responds to supportive care.

Chemical neurolysis may be more easily performed intraoperatively.[243] At laparotomy, both sides of the celiac axis are directly injected with 50% alcohol or 6% phenol. No increased morbidity or mortality, compared with laparotomy and surgical bypass alone, is reported by the University of Michigan.[243] Approximately 90% of their patients had effective and, occasionally, permanent pain relief.

External-beam radiation therapy is often effective in reducing pain associated with pancreatic carcinoma. Based on a comparison of retrospective series, doses of >50 Gy (usually > 60 Gy) are required.[143-145] Between 50% and 70% of patients will experience significant pain relief. Japanese investigators have used large, single doses of intraoperative electron-beam radiation.[151,152] Doses of 20 to 40 Gy delivered to unresectable pancreatic carcinoma results in effective and often prompt (within 1–2 weeks) pain relief in as many as 50% of patients. However, intraoperative radiation therapy remains an experimental approach available only in a limited number of medical centers within the United States.

REFERENCES

1. Levin DL, Connelly RR: Cancer of the pancreas: Available epidemiologic information and its implications. Cancer 31:1231, 1973
2. Pollack ES: The epidemiology of cancer and the delivery of medical care services. Public Health Rep 99:476, 1984
3. Buncher CR: Epidemiology of pancreatic cancer. In Moosa AR (ed): Tumors of the Pancreas, p 415. Baltimore, Williams & Wilkins, 1980
4. World Health Organization: Cancer Incidence in Five Continents, vol IV. IARC Sci Publ 42, 1982
5. Thomas DB, Karagas MR: Cancer in first and second generation Americans. Cancer Res 47:5771, 1987
6. Allen-Mersh TG, Earlam RJ: Pancreatic cancer in England and Wales: Surgeons look at epidemiology. Ann R Coll Surg Engl 68:154, 1986
7. Hoover R, Mason T, McKay F et al: Geographic patterns of cancer mortality in the United States. In Fraumeni JF (ed): Persons at High Risk of Cancer. An Approach to Cancer Etiology and Control, pp 343–360. New York, Academic Press, 1975
8. MacMahon B, Yen S, Trichopoulos D, et al: Coffee and cancer of the pancreas. N Engl J Med 304:630, 1981
9. Feinstein A, Horowitz R, Spitzer W et al: Coffee and pancreatic cancer: The problems of etiologic science and epidemiologic case-control research. JAMA 246:957, 1981
10. Wynder E, Hall N, Polansky M: Epidemiology of coffee and pancreatic cancer. Cancer Res 43:3900, 1983
11. Hakulinen T, Lehtimaki L, Lehtonen M et al: Cancer morbidity among two male cohorts with increased alcohol consumption in Finland. J Natl Cancer Inst 52:1711, 1974
12. Wynder E, Mabuchi K, Maruchi N et al: A case control study of cancer of the pancreas. Cancer 31:641, 1973
13. Wynder E, Mabuchi K, Maruchi N et al: Epidemiology of cancer of the pancreas. J Natl Cancer Inst 50:645, 1973
14. Monson R, Lyon J: Proportional mortality among alcoholics. Cancer 36:1077, 1975
15. Wynder E: An epidemiologic evaluation of the causes of cancer of the pancreas. Cancer Res 35:2228, 1975
16. Krain L: The rising incidence of carcinoma of the pancreas. An epidemiologic appraisal. Am J Gastroenterol 54:500, 1970
17. Kahn H: The Dorn study of smoking and mortality among U.S. veterans: Report on eight and one-half years of observation. Natl Cancer Inst Monogr 19:1, 1966
18. Pour P, Wilson R: Experimental tumors of the pancreas. In Moosa A (ed): Tumors of the Pancreas, p 37. Baltimore, Williams & Wilkins, 1980
19. Sindelar W, Kurman C: Nitrosamine-induced pancreatic carcinogenesis in outbred and inbred Syrian hamsters. Carcinogenesis 3:1021, 1982
20. Bartholomew L, Gross J: Carcinoma of the pancreas associated with chronic relapsing pancreatitis. Gastroenterology 35:473, 1958
21. Lundh G, Nordenstam H: Pancreas calcification and pancreas cancer. A discussion of two cases. Acta Chir Scand 136:493, 1970
22. Robin A, Scott J, Rosenfeld D: The occurrence of carcinoma of the pancreas in chronic pancreatitis. Radiology 94:289, 1970
23. Mainz D, Webster P: Pancreatic carcinoma. A review of etiologic considerations. Am J Dig Dis 19:459, 1974
24. Brooks J: Cancer of the pancreas. In Brooks JR (ed): Surgery of the Pancreas, p 263. Philadelphia, WB Saunders, 1983
25. Sasaki A, Kamado K, Horiuchi N: A changing pattern of causes of death in Japanese diabetics. Observations over fifteen years. J Chronic Dis 312:433, 1978
26. Karmody A, Kyle J: The association between carcinoma of the pancreas and diabetes mellitus. Br J Surg 56:362, 1969
27. Mancuso T, El-Attar A: Cohort study of workers exposed to betanaphythylamine and benzidine. J Occup Med 9:277, 1967
28. Pour P, Althoff J, Kruger F et al: The effect of N-Nitrosobis (2-oxopropyl)almine after oral administration to hamsters. Cancer Lett 2:323, 1977
29. Longnecker D, Curphey T: Adenocarcinoma of the pancreas in azaserine-treated rats. Cancer Res 35:2249, 1975
30. Skandalakis JE, Gray SW, Rower JS et al: Anatomical complication of pancreatic surgery. Contemp Surg 15:17, 1979
31. Kasugai T, Kuno N, Kobayashi S: Endoscopic pancreatocholangiography. Gastroenterology 63:217, 1972
32. Michels NA: The hepatic, cystic and retroduodenal arteries and their relations in the biliary ducts. Ann Surg 133:503, 1951
33. Cubilla AL, Fitzgerald PJ: Surgical pathology of tumors of the exocrine pancreas. In Moosa AR (ed): Tumors of the Pancreas, pp 159–193. Baltimore, Williams & Wilkins, 1980
34. Cello JP: Carcinoma of the pancreas. In Sleisenger MH, Fordtran JS (eds): Gastrointestinal Disease: Pathophysiology, Diagnosis, Management, 3rd ed, pp 1514–1527. Philadelphia, WB Saunders, 1983
35. Cubilla AL, Fitzgerald PJ: Tumors of the Exocrine Pancreas. Washington DC, Armed Forces Institute of Pathology, 1984
36. Legg MA: Pathology of the pancreas. In Brooks JR (ed): Surgery of the Pancreas, pp 41–77. Philadelphia, WB Saunders, 1983
37. Howard JM, Jordan GL: Cancer of the pancreas. Curr Probl Cancer 2:1, 1977
38. Cancer of the Pancreas Task Force: Staging of cancer of the pancreas. Cancer 47:1631, 1981
39. Fortner JG: Regional pancreatectomy for cancer of the pancreatic ampulla with other related sites: Tumor staging and results. Ann Surg 199:418, 1984
40. Gudjonsson B, Livestone EM, Spiro HM: Cancer of the pancreas. Diagnostic accuracy and survival statistics. Cancer 42:2494, 1978
41. Perez MM, Newcomer AD, Moertel CG et al: Assessment of weight loss, food intake, fat metabolism, malabsorption, and treatment of pancreatic insufficiency in pancreatic cancer. Cancer 52:346, 1983
42. Go VLW, Taylor WF, DiMagno EP: Efforts at early diagnosis of pancreatic cancer: The Mayo Clinic experience. Cancer 47:1698, 1981
43. Moertel CG: Exocrine pancreas. In Holland JF, Frei E (eds): Cancer Medicine, 2nd ed, pp 1792–1804. Philadelphia, Lea & Febiger, 1982
44. Fras I, Litin EM, Pearson JS: Comparison of psychiatric symptoms in carcinoma of the pancreas with those in some other intra-abdominal neoplasms. Am J Psychiatry 123:1553, 1967

45. Sack GH, Levin J, Bell WR: Trousseau's syndrome and other manifestations of chronic disseminated coagulapathy in patients with neoplasms: Clinical, pathophysiologic, and therapeutic features. Medicine 56:1, 1977
46. Steinberg WM, Gelfand R, Anderson KK et al: Comparison of the sensitivity and specificity of the CA 19-9 and carcinoembryonic antigen assays in detecting cancer of the pancreas. Gastroenterology 90:343, 1986
47. Piantino P, Andriulli A, Gindro T et al: CA 19-9 assay in differential diagnosis of pancreatic carcinoma from inflammatory pancreatic diseases. Am J Gastroenterol 81:436, 1986
48. Haglund C, Roberts PJ, Kuusela P et al: Gastrointestinal cancer associated antigen CA 19-9 in histological specimens of pancreatic tumors and pancreatitis. Br J Cancer 53:189, 1986
49. Haglund C: Tumour marker antigen CA 12-5 in pancreatic cancer: A comparison with CA 19-9 and CEA. Br J Cancer 54:897, 1986
50. Pasquali C, Sperti C, D'Andrea AA et al: Evaluation of carbohydrate antigens 19-9 and 12-5 in patients with pancreatic cancer. Pancreas 2:34, 1987
51. Sakahara H, Endo K, Nakajima K et al: Serum CA 19-9 concentrations and computed tomography findings in patients with pancreatic carcinoma. Cancer 57:1324, 1986
52. Mahvi DM, Meyers WC, Bast RC et al: Therapeutic efficacy as defined by a seriodiagnostic test utilizing a monoclonal antibody in carcinoma of the pancreas. Ann Surg 202:440, 1985
53. Moosa AR, Levin B: The diagnosis of "early" pancreatic cancer: The University of Chicago experience. Cancer 47:1688, 1981
54. Moosa AR, Mackie CR, Gelder FB et al: The value of tumor markers in the diagnosis and management of nonendocrine tumors of the pancreas. In Moosa AR (ed): Tumors of the Pancreas, pp 355–380. Baltimore, Williams & Wilkins, 1980
55. Holyoke ED, Evans JT, Mittleman A: Biochemical Markers for Cancer, pp 61–80. New York, Marcel Dekker, 1982
56. Cooper MJ, Mackie CR, Skinner DB et al: A reappraisal of the value of carcinoembryonic antigen in the management of patients with various neoplasms. Br J Surg 66:120, 1979
57. Van Nagell Jr: Tumor markers in ovarian cancer. Clin Obstet Gynecol 10:197, 1983
58. Pentti K, Keinonen KT, Koiwla T et al: Tumor associated antigen CA 12-5 in patients with ovarian cancer. Br J Obstet Gynaecol 92:528, 1985
59. Bast RC, Klug TL, St John E et al: A radioimmunoassay using a monoclonal antibody to monitor the course of epithelial ovarian cancer. N Engl J Med 309:883, 1983
60. Bast RC, Feeney M, Lazarus H et al: Reactivity of a monoclonal antibody with human ovarian carcinoma. J Clin Invest 68:1331, 1981
61. Koprowski H, Steplewski Z, Mitchell K et al: Colorectal carcinoma antigens detected by hybridoma antibodies. Somatic Cell Mul Genet 5:957, 1979
62. Ritts RE, Del Villano BC, Go VLM et al: Initial clinical evaluation of an immunoradiometric assay for CA 19-9 using the NCI serum bank. Int J Cancer 33:339, 1984
63. Tempero M, Uchida E, Takasaki H et al: Serial CA 19-9 levels and tumor response in pancreatic cancer (abstr). Proc Am Soc Clin Oncol 6:81, 1987
64. Benini L, Cavallini G, Zordan D et al: Prospective clinical evaluation of the diagnostic accuracy of monoclonal (CA 19-9, CA 50, CA 12-5) and polyclonal (CEA, TPA) antigens in respect to pancreatic cancer. Dig Dis Sci (66S) 31:254, 1986
65. Schlom J, Weeks MO: Potential clinical utility of monoclonal antibodies in the management of human carcinomas. In DeVita VT Jr, Hellman S, Rosenberg SA (eds): Important Advances in Oncology 1985, p 170. Philadelphia, JB Lippincott, 1985
66. Whipple AO, Parsons WB, Mullins CR: Treatment of carcinoma of the ampulla of Vater. Ann Surg 102:763, 1935
67. Maki T, Sato T, Kakizaki G: Pancreatoduodenectomy for periampullary carcinomas: Appraisal of a two-stage procedure. Arch Surg 92:825, 1966
68. Nakayama T, Ikeda A, Okuda K; Percutaneous transhepatic drainage of the biliary tract: Technique and results in 104 cases. Gastroenterology 74:554, 1978
69. Denning DA, Ellison EC, Carey LC: Preoperative percutaneous transhepatic biliary decompression lowers operative morbidity in patients with obstructive jaundice. Am J Surg 141:61, 1981
70. Norlander A, Kalin B, Sundblad R: Effect of percutaneous transhepatic drainage upon liver function and postoperative mortality. Surg Gynecol Obstet 155:161, 1982
71. Gundry SR, Strodel WE, Knol JA et al: Efficacy of preoperative biliary tract decompression in patients with obstructive jaundice. Arch Surg 119:703, 1984
72. Dooley JS, Dick R, Olney J et al: Non-surgical treatment of biliary obstruction. Lancet 2:1043, 1979
73. McPherson GAD, Benjamin IS, Habib NA et al: Percutaneous transhepatic drainage in obstructive jaundice: Advantages and problems. Br J Surg 62:261, 1982
74. Hatfield ARW, Tobias R, Terblanche J et al: Preoperative external biliary drainage in obstructive jaundice: A prospective controlled clinical trial. Lancet 2:896, 1982
75. McPherson GAD, Benjamin IS, Hodgson HJF et al: Preoperative percutaneous biliary drainage: The best results of a controlled trial. Br J Surg 71:371, 1984
76. Pitt HA, Cameron JL, Postier RG et al: Factors affecting mortality in biliary tract surgery. Am J Surg 141:66, 1981
77. Hagenmuller F, Classen M: Therapeutic endoscopic and percutaneous procedures for biliary disorders. Prog Liver Dis 7:299, 1982
78. Speer AG, Cotton PB, Russell RC et al: Randomised trial of endoscopic versus percutaneous stent insertion in malignant obstructive jaundice. Lancet 2:57, 1987
79. Bornman PC, Terblanche J, Harries-Jones EP et al: Endoscopic versus percutaneous stents for malignant jaundice. Lancet 2:689, 1987
80. Isaacson R, Weiland LH, McIlrath DC: Biopsy of the pancreas. Arch Surg 109:227, 1974
81. Fortner JG: Regional resection of the pancreas: A new surgical approach. Surgery 73:307, 1973
82. Morrow M, Hilaris B, Brennan MF: Comparison of conventional surgical resection, radioactive implantation, and bypass procedures for exocrine carcinoma of the pancreas, 1975–1980. Ann Surg 199:1, 1984
83. Bowden L, McNeer G, Pack G: Carcinoma of the head of pancreas—Five-year survival in four patients. Am J Surg 109:578, 1965
84. Portland Surgical Society Cooperative Study: A ten-year experience with carcinoma of the pancreas. Arch Surg 94:322, 1967
85. Crile G: The advantages of bypass operations over radical pancreaticoduodenectomy in the treatment of pancreatic carcinoma. Surg Gynecol Obstet 130:1049, 1970
86. Feduska N, Dent T, Lindenauer S: Results of palliative operations for carcinoma of the pancreas. Arch Surg 103:330, 1971
87. Wilson S, Block G: Periampullary carcinoma. Arch Surg 108:539, 1974
88. Brooks J, Culebras J: Cancer of the pancreas—palliative operation, Whipple procedure, or total pancreatectomy? Am J Surg 131:516, 1976
89. Shapiro T: Adenocarcinoma of the pancreas: A statistical analysis of biliary bypass vs. Whipple resection in good risk patients. Ann Surg 182:715, 1975
90. Nakase A, Matsumoto Y, Uchida K et al: Surgical treatment of cancer of the pancreas and the periampullary region: Cumulative results in 57 institutions in Japan. Ann Surg 185:52, 1977
91. Tepper J, Nardi G, Suit H: Carcinoma of the pancreas: Review of MGH experience from 1963 to 1973. Cancer 37:1519, 1976
92. Knight R, Scarborough J, Goss J: Adenocarcinoma of the pancreas—A ten-year experience. Arch Surg 113:1401, 1978
93. Moosa A, Lewis M, Mackie C: Surgical treatment of pancreatic cancer. Mayo Clin Proc 54:468, 1979
94. Longmire W, Transero L: The Whipple procedure and other standard operative approaches to pancreatic cancer. Cancer 47:1706, 1981
95. Edis A, Kiernan P, Taylor W: Attempted curative resection of ductal carcinoma of the pancreas. Review of Mayo Clinic experience: 1951–1975. Mayo Clin Proc 55:531, 1980
96. Fortner J: Surgical principles for pancreatic cancer: Regional total and subtotal pancreatectomy. Cancer 47:1712, 1981
97. Herter F, Cooperman A, Ahlborn T et al: Surgical experience with pancreatic and periampullary cancer. Ann Surg 195:274, 1982
98. Van Heerden J, Heath P, Alden C: Biliary bypass for ductal adenocarcinoma of the pancreas: Mayo Clinic experience, 1970–1975. Mayo Clin Proc 55:537, 1980
99. Brooks DC, Osteen R, Gray E et al: Evaluation of palliative procedures of pancreatic cancer. Am J Surg 141:430, 1981
100. Crist DW, Sitzmann JV, Cameron JL: Improved hospital morbidity, mortality, and survival after the Whipple procedure. Ann Surg 206:358, 1987
101. Sarr MG, Cameron JL: Surgical management of unresectable carcinoma of the pancreas. Surgery 91:123, 1982
102. Bufkin WJ, Smith PE, Krementz FT: Evaluation of palliative operations for carcinoma of the pancreas. Arch Surg 94:240, 1967
103. Blievernicht SW, Neifeld JP, Terz JJ et al: The role of prophylactic gastrojejunostomy for unresectable periampullary carcinoma. Surg Gynecol Obstet 151:794, 1980
104. Elmslie RG, Slovatinek AH: Surgical objectives in unresected cancer of the head of the pancreas. Br J Surg 59:500, 1972
105. Hart PF, Gillett DJ: Non-functioning palliative gastroenterostomy. Aust NZ J Surg 41:354, 1972
106. Gudjonsson B: Cancer of the pancreas: 50 years of surgery. Cancer 60:2284, 1987
107. Glantz G, Ozeran RS: Role of gastroenterostomy in management of pancreatic carcinoma. Am Surg 32:670, 1966
108. Richards AB, Chir M, Sosin H: Cancer of the pancreas: The value of radical and palliative surgery. Ann Surg 177:325, 1973
109. Webster DJT: Carcinoma of the pancreas and periampullary region: A clinical study in a district general hospital. Br J Surg 62:130, 1975
110. Pipes KE, Pareira MD: Duodenal obstruction appearing after palliative biliary diversion for pancreatic carcinoma. Surgery 44:636, 1958
111. Hertzberg J: Pancreatico-duodenal resection and bypass-operation in patients with carcinoma of the head of pancreas, ampulla, and distal end of the common duct. Acta Chir Scand 140:523, 1974
112. Collure DWD, Burns GP, Schenk WG Jr: Clinical, pathological, and therapeutic aspects of carcinoma of the pancreas. Am J Surg 128:683, 1974
113. Stuart M, Keo T, Hermann RE et al: Palliation of malignant obstruction of the common bile duct by side to side choledochoduodenostomy. Am J Surg 121:505, 1971
114. Douglass HO, Holyoke ED: Pancreatic cancer: Initial treatment as the determinant of survival. JAMA 229:793, 1974
115. Vijayanagar R, Tobins SH: Evaluation of palliative operations for carcinoma of the head of the pancreas: A ten-year study. Mt Sinai J Med (NY) 37:115, 1970
116. Mendoza CB, Easley GW: Bypass procedure for palliation in obstructive jaundice. W Va Med J 70:27, 1974
117. Monge JJ: Survival of patients with small carcinomas of the head of the pancreas: Biliary intestinal bypass vs pancreaticoduodenectomy. Ann Surg 166:908, 1967
118. Buckwalter JA, Lawton RL, Tidrick RT: Bypass operations for neoplastic biliary tract obstruction. Am J Surg 109:100, 1965
119. Winegarner FG, Haguea WH, Elliott DW: Tissue diagnosis and surgical management of malignant jaundice. Am J Surg 111:5, 1966
120. Williams RD, Elliott DW, Zollinger RM: Surgery for malignant jaundice. Arch Surg 80:992, 1960

121. McDevitt JB: Parenchymatous carcinoma of the head of the pancreas. J Ir Med Assoc 62:390, 1969
122. Glassman WS, Johnston PW: Palliative surgery in carcinoma of the pancreas. Geriatrics 10:456, 1955
123. Linn BS, Goldstein HS: Judgement in palliation of pancreatic carcinoma: With an assist by the computer. South Med J 62:116, 1969
124. du Plessis DJ: The palliative operation for obstructive jaundice due to carcinoma of the pancreas. S Afr J Surg 8:11, 1970
125. Reed K, Vose PC, Jarstfer BS: Pancreatic cancer: 30-year review (1947–77). Am J Surg 138:929, 1979
126. Forrest JF, Longmire WP Jr: Carcinoma of the pancreas and periampullary region: A study of 279 patients. Ann Surg 189:129, 1979
127. Nagai H, Kuroda A, Morioka Y: Lymphatic and local spread of T_1 and T_2 pancreatic cancer. Ann Surg 204:65–71, 1986
128. Pilepich MV, Miller HH: Pre-operative irradiation in carcinoma of the pancreas. Cancer 46:1945, 1980
129. Kopelson G: Curative surgery for adenocarcinoma of the pancreas/ampulla of Vater: The role of adjuvant pre- or post-operative radiation therapy. Int J Radiat Oncol Biol Phys 9:911, 1983
130. Sindelar WF, Kinsella TJ: Randomized trial of intraoperative radiotherapy in resected carcinoma of the pancreas. Int J Radiat Oncol Biol Phys (Suppl 1)12:148, 1986
131. Fraass BA, Miller RW, Kinsella TJ et al: Intraoperative radiation therapy at the National Cancer Institute: Technical innovations and dosimetry. Int J Radiat Oncol Biol Phys 11:1299, 1985
132. Sindelar WF, Hoekstra HJ, Kinsella TJ: Surgical approaches and techniques in intraoperative radiotherapy for intra-abdominal, retroperitoneal, and pelvic neoplasms. Surgery (in press)
133. Gastrointestinal Tumor Study Group: Pancreatic cancer: Adjuvant combined radiation and chemotherapy following curative resection. Arch Surg 120:899, 1985
134. Gastrointestinal Tumor Study Group: Further evidence of effective adjuvant combined radiation and chemotherapy following curative resection of pancreatic cancer. Cancer 59:2006, 1987
135. Richards GE: Possibilities of roentgen-ray treatment in cancer of the pancreas. Am J Roentgenol 9:150, 1922
136. Merritt EA, Rathbone RR: The diagnosis and roentgen treatment of carcinoma of the head of the pancreas. Radiology 26:459, 1936
137. Handley WS: Pancreatic cancer and its treatment by implanted radium. Ann Surg 100:215, 1934
138. Upcott H: Tumors of the ampulla of Vater. With a report of two cases. Ann Surg 56:710, 1912
139. Pack GT, McNeer G: Radiation treatment of pancreatic cancer. Am J Roentgenol Rad Ther Nucl Med 40:708, 1938
140. Phillips R: Principles and results of palliative radiotherapy in nonresectable cancer. Med Clin North Am 40:807, 1956
141. Miller TR, Fuller LM: Radiation therapy of carcinoma of the pancreas. Report on 91 cases. Am J Roentgenol Rad Ther Nucl Med 80:787, 1958
142. Billingsley JS, Bartholomew LG, Childs DS: A study of radiation therapy in carcinoma of the pancreas. Proc Staff Meet Mayo Clin 33:426, 1958
143. Haslam JB, Cavanaugh PJ, Stroup SL: Radiation therapy in the treatment of irresectable adenocarcinoma of the pancreas. Cancer 32:1341, 1973
144. Dobelbower RR, Borgelt BB, Strubler KA et al: Precision radiotherapy for cancer of the pancreas: Technique and results. Int J Radiat Oncol Biol Phys 6:1127, 1980
145. Whittington R, Dobelbower RR, Mohiuddin M et al: Radiotherapy of unresectable pancreatic carcinoma: A six-year experience with 104 patients. Int J Radiat Oncol Biol Phys 7:1639, 1981
146. Kinsella TJ, Sindelar WF, Bloomer WD: Radiation enteritis: Pathophysiology, clinical manifestations and management. In Nyhus LM, Nelson RL (eds): Surgery of the Small Intestine, pp 193–203. Norwalk, CT, Appleton-Century-Crofts, 1987
147. Hilaris B, Moorthy C, Kim J: Radiotherapeutic management of pancreatic cancer at Memorial Sloan-Kettering Cancer Center. In Conn I (ed): Pancreatic Cancer: New Directions in Therapeutic Management, pp 251–262. New York, Masson, 1980
148. Brennan MF, Hilaris B: Unpublished data
149. Shipley WU, Nardi GL, Cohen AM et al: Iodine-125 implant and external beam irradiation in patients with localized pancreatic carcinoma. A comparative study of surgical resection. Cancer 45:709, 1980
150. Goldson AL, Ashaveri E, Espinoza MC et al: Single high-dose intraoperative electrons for advanced stage pancreatic cancer: Phase I pilot study. Int J Radiat Oncol Biol Phys 7:869, 1981
151. Abe M, Takahashi M: Intraoperative radiotherapy: The Japanese experience. Int J Radiat Oncol Biol Phys 7:863, 1981
152. Nishamura A, Nakano M, Otsu H et al: Intraoperative radiotherapy for advanced carcinoma of the pancreas. Cancer 54:2375, 1984
153. Shipley WU, Wood WC, Tepper JE et al: Intraoperative electron beam irradiation for patients with unresectable pancreatic carcinoma. Ann Surg 200:289, 1984
154. Tepper JE, Shipley WU, Warshaw AL et al: The role of Misonidazole combined with intraoperative radiation therapy in the treatment of pancreatic carcinoma. J Clin Oncol 5:579, 1987
155. Gunderson LL, Martin JK, Kvols LT et al: Intraoperative and external beam irradiation ± 5-FU for locally advanced pancreatic cancer. Int J Radiat Oncol Biol Phys 13:319, 1987
156. Sindelar WF, Hoekstra H, Rstrepo C et al: Pathological tissue changes following intraoperative radiotherapy. Am J Clin Oncol 9:504, 1986
157. Kaul R, Cohen L, Hendrickson F et al: Pancreatic carcinoma: Results with fast neutron therapy. Int J Radiat Oncol Biol Phys 7:173, 1981
158. Smith FP, Schein PS, Macdonald JS et al: Fast neutron irradiation for locally advanced pancreatic cancer. Int J Radiat Oncol Biol Phys 7:1527, 1981
159. Al-Abdulla ASM, Hussey DH, Olson MH et al: Experience with fast neutron therapy for unresectable carcinoma of the pancreas. Int J Radiat Oncol Biol Phys 7:165, 1981
160. Castro JR, Quivey JM, Lyman JT et al: Current status of clinical particle radiotherapy at Lawrence Berkeley Laboratory. Cancer 46:633, 1980
161. Kligerman MM, Sala JM, Smith AR et al: Tissue reaction and tumor response with negative pi mesons. J Can Assoc Radiol 31:13, 1980
162. Bajorunas D, Horowitz DG, Dresler C et al: Amino acid kinetics under glucagon replacement in pancreatectomized patients (in preparation)
163. Moertel CG, Reitemeier RJ: Advanced Gastrointestinal Cancer: Clinical Management and Chemotherapy. New York, Harper & Row, 1969
164. Pastan I, Gottesman M: Multiple drug resistance in human cancer. N Engl J Med 316:1388, 1987
165. Myers C, Cowan K, Sinha B et al: The phenomenon of pleotropic drug resistance. In: DeVita VT Jr, Hellman S, Rosenberg SA (eds): Important Advances in Oncology 1987, pp 27–37. Philadelphia, JB Lippincott, 1987
166. Carter SK: The integration of chemotherapy into a combined modality approach for cancer treatment: VI. Pancreatic adenocarcinoma. Cancer Treat Rev 3:193, 1975
167. O'Connell MJ: Current status of chemotherapy for advanced pancreatic and gastric cancer. J Clin Oncol 3:1032, 1985
168. Schein PS: The role of chemotherapy in the management of gastric and pancreatic carcinoma. Semin Oncol 12:49, 1985
169. Moertel CG: Chemotherapy of gastrointestinal cancer. Clin Gastroenterol 5:777, 1976
170. Crooke ST, Bradner WT: Mitomycin C: A review. Cancer Treat Rev 3:121, 1976
171. Gastrointestinal Tumor Study Group: Randomized phase II clinical trial of adriamycin, methotrexate, and actinomycin D in advanced measurable pancreatic carcinoma. Cancer 42:19, 1978
172. Gastrointestinal Tumor Study Group: Phase II trials of maytansine, low-dose chlorozotocin, and high-dose chlorozotocin as single agents against advanced measurable adenocarcinoma of the pancreas. Cancer Treat Rep 69:417, 1985
173. Inamasu M, Oishi N, Chen T et al: Phase II trial of amsacrine in pancreatic carcinoma: A Southwest Oncology Group study. Cancer Treat Rep 68:1411, 1984
174. Omura GA, Bartolucci AA, Lessner HE et al: Phase II evaluation of amsacrine in colorectal, gastric, and pancreatic carcinomas: A Southeastern Cancer Study Group trial. Cancer Treat Rep 68:929, 1984
175. Sternberg CN, Magill GB, Sordillo PP et al: Phase II evaluation of m-AMSA (4′-(9-acridinylamino)-methane-sulfon-m-anisidide) in patients with adenocarcinoma of the pancreas. Am J Clin Oncol (CCT) 6:459, 1983
176. Bedikian AY, Stroehlein J, Korinek J et al: Phase II evaluation of dihydroxyanthracenedione (DHAD, NSC 301739) in patients with upper gastrointestinal tumors. A preliminary report. Am J Clin Oncol 6:473, 1983
177. Mittelman A, Magill GB, Raymond V et al: Phase II trial of Idarubicin in patients with pancreatic cancer. Cancer Treat Rep 712:657, 1987
178. National Cancer Institute: Cancer Therapy Evaluation Program Information System (CTEP-IS), 1987
179. Hochster H, Green MD, Speyer JL et al: Activity of epirubicin in pancreatic cancer. Cancer Treat Rep 70:299, 1986
180. Wils J, Bleiberg H, Blijham G et al: Phase II study of epirubicin in advanced adenocarcinoma of the pancreas. Eur J Cancer Clin Oncol 21:191, 1985
181. Blayney DW, Goldberg DA, Leong LA et al: Phase II trial of esorubicin in advanced pancreatic adenocarcinoma. Cancer Treat Rep 70:683, 1986
182. DeSimone PA, Gams R, Bartolucci A: Weekly mitoxantrone in the treatment of advanced pancreatic carcinoma: A Southeastern Cancer Study Group trial. Cancer Treat Rep 80:929, 1986
183. Horton J, Gelber R, Engstrom P et al: Trials of single agent and combination chemotherapy for advanced cancer of the pancreas. Cancer Treat Rep 65:65, 1981
184. Smith DB, Kenny JB, Scarffe JH et al: Phase II evaluation of melphalan in adenocarcinoma of the pancreas. Cancer Treat Rep 69:917, 1985
185. Gad-El-Mawla N: Ifosfamide in advanced pancreatic cancer. Cancer Chemother Pharmacol 18:555, 1986
186. Einhorn LH, Loehrer PJ: Ifosfamide chemotherapy for pancreatic carcinoma. Cancer Chemother Pharmacol 18:551, 1986
187. Bernard S, Noble S, Wilcosky T et al: A phase II study of ifosfamide (IFOS) plus N-acetyl cysteine (NAC) in metastatic measurable pancreatic adenocarcinoma (pc) (abstr). Proc Am Soc Clin Oncol 5:328, 1986
188. DeSimone P, Kramer B, Omura GA et al: Phase II evaluation of diaziquone in gastric and pancreatic cancers: A Southeastern Cancer Study Group trial. Am J Clin Oncol (CCT) 9:401, 1986
189. Gastrointestinal Tumor Study Group: Phase II trials of hexamethylmelamine, dianhydrogalactitol, razoxane, and beta-2′-deoxythioguanosine as single agents against advanced measurable tumors of the pancreas. Cancer Treat Rep 69:713, 1985
190. Lessner HE, Valenstein S, Kaplan R et al: Phase II study L-asparaginase in the treatment of pancreatic carcinoma. Cancer Treat Rep 64:1359, 1980
191. Sternberg CN, Magill GB, Sordillo PP et al: Phase II evaluation of metoprine in advanced pancreatic adenocarcinoma. Cancer Treat Rep 68:1053, 1984
192. Inamasu MS, Oishi N, Chen TT et al: Phase II study of mitoguazone in pancreatic cancer: A Southwest Oncology Group study. Cancer Treat Rep 70:531, 1986
193. Ravry MJR, Omura GA, Hill GJ et al: Phase II evaluation of mitoguazone in cancers of

the esophagus, stomach, and pancreas: A Southeastern Cancer Study Group trial. Cancer Treat Rep 70:533, 1986
194. Crowson MC, Dorrell A, Rolfe EB et al: A phase II study to evaluate tamoxifen in pancreatic adenocarcinoma. Eur J Surg Oncol 12:335, 1986
195. Smith FP, Stablein DM, Schein PS: Phase II combination chemotherapy trials in advanced measurable pancreatic cancer (abstr). Proc Am Soc Clin Oncol 3:150, 1984
196. Lokich J, Chawla PL, Brooks J et al: Chemotherapy in pancreatic carcinoma: 5-fluorouracil (5-FU) and 1,3, bis-(2 chlorethyl)-1-nitrosourea (BCNU). Ann Surg 179:450, 1974
197. Stolinsky DC, Pugh RP, Bateman JR: 5-fluorouracil (NSC-19383) therapy for pancreatic carcinoma: Comparison of oral and intravenous routes. Cancer Chemother Rep 59:1031, 1975
198. Mater MW, Theologides A, Cooper MR et al: Fluorouracil (F) + adriamycin (A) + mitomycin (M) (FAM) versus fluorouracil (F) + streptozotocin (S) + mitomycin (M) (FSM) in advanced pancreatic cancer (abstr). Proc Am Soc Clin Oncol 1:90, 1982
199. Schein PS, O'Connell MJ, Blom J et al: Clinical antitumor activity and toxicity of streptozotocin (NSC-85998). Cancer 34:993, 1974
200. Stolinsky DC, Sadoff L, Braunwald J et al: Streptozotocin in the treatment of cancer. Cancer 30:61, 1972
201. DuPriest RW, Huntington MC, Massey WH et al: Streptozotocin therapy in 22 patients. Cancer 25:358, 1975
202. Moertel CG, Doublass HO, Hanlet J et al: Phase II study of methyl-CCNU in the treatment of advanced pancreatic carcinoma. Cancer Treat Rep 60:1659, 1976
203. Schein PS, Lavin PT, Moertel CG et al: Randomized phase II clinical trial of adriamycin in advanced measurable pancreatic carcinoma: A Gastrointestinal Tumor Study Group report. Cancer 42:19, 1978
204. Kovach JS, Moertel CG, Schutt AJ et al: A controlled study of combined 1,3-bis-(2-chlorethyl)-1-nitrosorea and 5-fluorouracil therapy for advanced gastric and pancreatic cancer. Cancer 33:563, 1974
205. Moertel CG, Douglass HO Jr, Hanley J et al: Treatment of advanced adenocarcinoma of the pancreas with combinations of streptozotocin plus 5-fluorouracil and streptozotocin plus cyclophosphamide. Cancer 40:605, 1977
206. Moertel CG, Engstrom P, Lavin PT et al: Chemotherapy of gastric and pancreatic carcinoma. Surgery 85:509, 1979
207. Buroker T, Kim PN, Groppe C et al: 5-FU infusion with mitomycin C vs 5-FU infusion with methyl CCNU in the treatment of advanced upper gastrointestinal cancer. Cancer 44:1215, 1979
208. Stephens RL, Hoogstraten B, Haas C et al: Pancreatic cancer treated with carmustine, fluorouracil and spironolactone. A randomized study. Arch Intern Med 138:115, 1978
209. Wiggans RG, Wooley PV, MacDonald JS et al: Phase II trial of streptozotocin, mitomycin-C and 5-fluorouracil (SMF) in the treatment of advanced pancreatic cancer. Cancer 41:387, 1978
210. Aberhalden RT, Bukowski RM, Groppe CW et al: Streptozotocin (STZ) and 5-fluorouracil (5-FU) with and without mitomycin-C (Mito) in the treatment of pancreatic adenocarcinoma (abstr). Proc Am Soc Clin Oncol 18:301, 1977
211. Bukowski RM, Abderhalden RI, Hewlett JS et al: Phase II trial of streptogotocin, mitomycin-C, and 5-fluorouracil in adenocarcinoma of the pancreas. Cancer Clin Triasl 3:321, 1980
212. Smith FP, Hoth DF, Levin B et al: 5-fluorouracil in adenocarcinoma of the pancreas. Cancer Clin Trials 3:321, 1980
213. Bitran JD, Desser RK, Kozloff MF et al: Treatment of metastatic pancreatic and gastric adenocarcinoma with 5-fluorouracil, adriamycin, and mitomycin-C (FAM). Cancer Treat Rep 63:2049, 1979
214. Bukowski RM: Randomized comparison of 5-FU and mitomycin-C (MF) versis 5-FU, mitomycin-C and streptozotocin (SMF) in pancreatic adenocarcinoma. A Southwest Oncology Group study (abstr). Proc Am Soc Clin Oncol 22:543, 1981
215. Bukowski RM, Balcerzak ST, O'Bryan RM et al: Randomized trial of 5-fluorouracil and mitomycin-C with or without streptozotocin for advanced pancreatic cancer. A Southwest Oncology Group study. Cancer 52:1577, 1983
216. Moertel CG, Rubin J, O'Connell MJ et al: A phase II trial of combined 5-fluorouracil, doxorubicin and cisplatin in the treatment of advanced upper gastrointestinal adenocarcinoma. J Clin Oncol 4:1053, 1986
217. Smith FP, Rustgi VK, Schertz G et al: Phase II study of 5-FU, doxorubicin, and mitomycin (FAM) and chlorozotocin in advanced measurable pancratic cancer. Cancer Treat Rep 66:2095, 1982
218. Bukowski RM, Schacter LP, Groppe CT et al: Phase II trial of 5-fluorouracil, adriamycin, mitomycin-C and streptozotocin (FAM-S) in pancreatic cancer. Cancer 50:197, 1982
219. Karlin DA, Stroehlein JR, Bennetts RW et al: Phase I-II study of the combination of 5-FU, doxorubicin, mitomycin, and semustine (FAMMe) in the treatment of adenocarcinoma of the stomach, gastroesophageal junction, and pancreas. Cancer Treat Rep 66:1613, 1982
220. Gastrointestinal Tumor Study Group: Phase II studies of drug combination in advanced pancreatic carcinoma: Fluorouracil plus doxorubicin plus mitomycin-C plus fluorouracil. J Clin Oncol 4:1794, 1986
221. Oster MW, Gray R, Panasci L et al: Chemotherapy for advanced pancreatic cancer: A comparison of 5-fluorouracil, adriamycin, and mitomycin-C (FAM) with 5-fluorouracil, streptozotocin and mitomycin-C (FSM). Cancer 57:29, 1986
222. Cullinan SA, Moertel CG, Fleming TR et al: A comparison of chemotherapeutic regimens in the treatment of advanced pancreatic and gastric carcinoma. JAMA 253:2061, 1985
223. Bukowski RM, Inamasu M, Taylor S et al: Randomized trials of combination chemotherapy vs. a Phase II drug in metastatic adenocarcinoma of the pancreas. A Southwest Oncology Group Study (abstr). Proc Am Soc Clin Oncol 4:80, 1985
224. Magill GB, Jakubowski AA, Sternberg CN et al: Phase II trial of MIFA IV chemotherapy for advanced adenocarcinoma of the pancreas (abstr). Proc Am Soc Clin Oncol 6:88, 1987
225. Bukowski RM: Characteristics of long-term survivors receiving chemotherapy for pancreatic adenocarcinoma in Southwest Oncology Group studies (abstr). Proc Am Soc Clin Oncol 3:149, 1984
226. Mallinson CN, Rake MO, Cocking JB et al: Chemotherapy in pancreatic cancer: Results of a controlled, prospective, randomized, multicenter trial. Br Med J 281:1589, 1980
227. Kyriazis AP, Kyriazis AA, Yagoda AA: Enhanced therapeutic effect of cis-diamminodichloroplatinum against nude mouse grown human pancreatic adenocarcinoma when combined with I-B-D-arabionfuranosylcytosine and caffeine. Cancer Res 45:6083, 1985
228. Roh JK, Wooley PV, Reich SD et al: Phase II evaluation of recombinant interferon gamma (IF) in advanced pancreatic and gastric adenocarcinoma (abstr). Proc Am Soc Clin Oncol 5:85, 1986
229. Chachoua A, Green M, Muggia FM: Immune modulating therapy in gastrointestinal cancer. Am J Gastroenterol 81:623, 1986
230. Rosenberg SA, Lotze MT, Muul LM et al: A progress report on the treatment of 157 patients with advanced cancer using lymphokine-activated killer cells and interleukin-2 or high-dose interleukin-2 alone. N Engl J Med 316:889, 1987
231. West WH, Tauer KW, Yannelli JR et al: Constant-infusion recombinant interleukin-2 in adoptive immunotherapy of advanced cancer. N Engl J Med 316:898, 1987
232. Herlyn M, Steplewski Z, Herlyn D et al: Colorectal carcinoma-specific antigen: Detection by means of monoclonal antibodies. Proc Natl Acad Sci USA 76:1438, 1979
233. Herlyn DM, Steplewski Z, Herlyn MF et al: Inhibition of growth of colorectal carcinoma in nude mice by monoclonal antibody. Cancer Res 44:717, 1980
234. Herlyn DM, Koprowski H: IgG2a monoclonal antibodies inhibit human tumor growth through interaction with effector cells. Proc Natl Acad Sci USA 79:4761, 1982
235. Sears HF, Herlyn D, Steplewski Z et al: Effects of monoclonal antibody immunotherapy on patients with gastrointestinal adenocarcinoma. J Biol Response Mod 3:138, 1984
236. Sindelar WF, Maher MM, Herlyn D et al: Trial of therapy with monoclonal antibody 17-1A in pancreatic carcinoma: Preliminary results. Hybridoma 5:125, 1986
237. Tempero MA, Pour PM, Uchida E et al: Monoclonal antibody C017-1A and leukopheresis in immunotherapy of pancreatic cancer. Hybridoma 5:133, 1986
238. Glenn J, Steinberg WM, Kurtzman SH et al: Evaluation of the utility of a radioimmunoassay for serum CA 19-9 levels in patients before and after treatment of carcinoma of the pancreas. J Clin Oncol 6:462, 1988
239. Paul AR, Engstrom PD, Weiner LM et al: Treatment of advanced measurable evaluable pancreatic carcinoma with 17-1A murine monoclonal antibody alone or in combination with 5-fluorouracil, adriamycin and mitomycin (FAM). Hybridoma 5:171, 1986
240. Metzgar RS, Gaillard MT, Levine SJ et al: Antigens of human pancreatic adenocarcinoma cells defined by murine monoclonal antibodies. Cancer Res 42:601, 1982
241. Parsa I: Identification of human acinar cell carcinoma by monoclonal antibody and in vitro differentiation. Cancer Lett 15:115, 1982
242. Greenwald HP, Bonica JJ, Bergner M: The prevalence of pain in four cancers. Cancer 60:2563, 1987
243. Flanigan D, Kraft R: Continuing experience with palliative chemical splanchniectomy. Arch Surg 113:509, 1978
244. de Takats G, Walter L, Lasner J: Splanchnic nerve section for pancreatic pain. Ann Surg 131:44, 1949
245. Grimson K, Hesser F, Kitchin W: Early clinical results of transabdominal celiac and superior mesenteric ganglionectomy, vagotomy, or transthoracic splanchnioectomy in patients with chronic abdominal visceral pain. Surgery 22:230, 1947
246. Yoshioka H, Wakabavashi T: Therapeutic neurotomy on head of pancreas for relief of pain due to chronic pancreatitis. Arch Surg 76:546, 1958
247. Bridenbaugh L, Moore D, Campbell D: Management of upper abdominal cancer pain: Treatment with celiac plexus block with alcohol. JAMA 190:99, 1964
248. Jones J: Coeliac plexus block with alcohol for relief of upper abdominal pain due to cancer. Ann Coll Surg Engl 59:46, 1977
249. Thompson G, Moore D, Bridenbaugh L: Abdominal pain and alcohol celiac plexus nerve block. Anesth Analg 56:1, 1977
250. Hanowell S, Kennedy S, MacNamara T et al: Celiac plexus block. Diagnostic and therapeutic applications in abdominal pain. South Med J 73:1330, 1980
251. Buy JN, Moss A, Singler R: CT guided celiac plexus and splanchnic nerve neurolysis. J Comput Assist Tomogr 6:315, 1982

HAROLD J. WANEBO
GEOFFREY FALKSON
STANLEY E. ORDER

CHAPTER 27 *Cancer of the Hepatobiliary System*

Hepatobiliary cancer is relatively uncommon in the United States. In 1987, approximately 14,000 new cases were reported.[1] Worldwide, however, primary hepatocellular carcinoma may be the most common fatal cancer, having an estimated annual incidence between 300,000 and 1.2 million and a fatality ratio of 0.92.[2] In the United States primary cancers of the liver and biliary passages are considered collectively for incidence. It is estimated that gallbladder cancer is the most common, accounting for 4000 to 6000 deaths each year, followed by 4000 hepatocellular cancer deaths and a slightly smaller number of bile duct cancer deaths. In recent years, our understanding of the cause and distribution of hepatobiliary cancer has improved markedly, and newer technologies have become available for diagnosis and management. Therapeutic advances have been made through experimental approaches that combine the efforts of the radiation oncologist, the surgeon, and the medical oncologist.[3–6]

HEPATOCELLULAR CARCINOMA

EPIDEMIOLOGY

Primary hepatocellular carcinoma (HCC) or malignant hepatoma is one of the most common malignancies in the world, and it is estimated to be responsible for up to 1,250,000 deaths every year.[2,7,8] It occurs infrequently in the United States and North America, with fewer than 10,000 new patients annually, accounting for less than 2% of all malignancies.[1,7–9] The age-standardized annual incidence is 2.9 per 100,000 men and 1.2 per 100,000 women. A similar low incidence is found in Britain, Canada, Australia, and South America. In portions of Africa and Asia, HCC is the most common malignant tumor.[10–12] The incidence ranges from 34 per 100,000 men in Singapore of Chinese descent to 65 per 100,000 men in Zimbabwe to more than 100 per 100,000 men in Mozambique and Taiwan.[13] The incidence of HCC is so high in parts of China that population screening is advocated.[14] Worldwide, the disease occurs predominately in men over 30 years of age.[14,15] Five times more men have HCC than women in high-incidence regions, whereas in low-incidence areas the ratio is 2 : 1.[7] The fibrolamellar variant of HCC occurs in a younger population (mean, 23–26 years), occurs equally in both sexes, and has a relatively longer survival period (Table 27-1).[16–19]

Chinese immigrants to Singapore or low-risk areas, such as the United States, retain their high-risk rates for HCC, but this is not the case with black migrants. Blacks in South Africa have a higher incidence (28 per 100,000) than American blacks (8 per 100,000), in whom the rate is slightly higher than in American whites (2.4 per 100,000).[7,20] There is a close relationship between the distribution of hepatitis B virus (HBV) infections and HCC, and the carrier rate for HBV is high among native born and migrant Chinese and black Africans but low for blacks outside Africa and for whites in South Africa, Europe, and North America.[11,21,22–34]

TABLE 27-1. Incidence of Heptocellular Carcinoma

Country	*Incidence*	*Reference*
North America	10,000 cases per year	1–4, 7–9
Britain, Canada, Australia and South America	No figures cited	2, 4, 7
Mozambique and Taiwan	100 per 100,000	10, 11, 13
Singapore	34.2 per 100,000 Chinese men	14
Zimbabwe	65 per 100,000 men	14
South Africa	28 per 100,000 black men	7, 20
United States	8 per 100,000 black men	20
United States	2.4 per 100,000 white men	20

ETIOLOGY

There are many risk factors related to HCC, including malnutrition, dietary carcinogens, parasitic infections, cirrhosis from various causes (Tables 27-2 and 27-3), caval outflow obstruction, and hormone ingestion.[36–59] Although some of these factors may have a role in the disease, it appears that HBV plays a major role in the pathogenesis of most HCC.[23–34,50–54,60]

Although the association of HCC in West Africa with viral hepatitis was reported by Paget in 1956, it was not until the identification of HBV (Australian antigen) by Blumberg in 1967 and a marker for hepatitis A that the role of hepatitis could be defined.[7,25,27] Studies of the etiologic relationship between HBV and HCC were advanced by the demonstration of a human tumor cell line that has HBV DNA integrated into the cellular genome, which replicates HBsAg.[35] Integration of HBV DNA has been demonstrated both in hepatoma cell lines and in tumor samples from HCC patients.[24,34,35] The cirrhosis seen in HCC patients is usually the macronodular or postnecrotic type, which is caused by chronic HBV infection.[2,15,21,22] Prospective data from Taiwan strongly suggest a direct role for HBV in HCC.[26] Beasley's 4-year study of 3500 HBV carriers and 19,250 controls established a relative risk of 234, with HCC occurring in 40 carriers and 1 control subject.[28]

PATHOLOGY

About 90% of primary carcinomas of the liver are HCC, the remaining are cholangiocarcinomas (about 7%) and less common tumors such as hepatoblastomas, angiosarcomas, and sarcomas (Table 27-4).[60–73] The gross appearance varies from a single, large, dominant nodule or mass, which may be well-circumscribed or infiltrating, to a multicentric tumor. The tumor itself is characteristically soft, a factor that may lead to rupture and intraperitoneal hemorrhage. There may be areas of necrosis or hemorrhage, especially in large tumors. Intermediate forms of the large nodular tumor are often seen. Multicentric tumors frequently are found in cirrhotic livers, and in some cases, it may be difficult to distinguish neoplastic from regenerative nodules.[63–65] In livers with multiple small nodules, it is difficult to distinguish be-

TABLE 27-2. Risk Factors for Hepatocellular Carcinoma

Risk Factor	*Observation*	*Reference*
Chronic hepatic injury	Associated with HCC in North and South America in 22% to 60% of HCC patients	1, 7, 13, 14
Cirrhosis	Associated with HCC in Asia and Africa in 60% to 90% of HCC patients	7, 10–12, 23, 26, 37, 38, 51
Chronic hepatitis B infection	Increases the chance of developing HCC; persistent viral infection found in sera from 20% to 90% of HCC patients worldwide	7, 25, 34, 41, 42, 52
Aflatoxin	Implicated in etiology of HCC in Africa and Asia	7, 39, 41, 42
Alcoholism	Implicated in etiology of HCC, but association between alcoholism and HCC is less strong than between chronic alcohol intake and cancer of the mouth, larynx, and esophagus; possible promoter for hepatitis B virus	7, 29, 43, 44
Chronic hepatic outflow obstruction (CHOO)	Associated with HCC in 20% of South African cases and well documented in Japan; 61.6% of CHOO cases studied by Simson had HCC	45–49
Male sex	Most HCC occurs in men; suggested hormonal involvement	50, 53–59

TABLE 27-3. Clinical Features of Hepatocellular Carcinoma in High- and Low-Incidence Areas

Variables	*High Incidence*	*Low Incidence*
Geographic location	Asia, Africa	North America, Europe
Race	Asians, blacks	Mostly whites
Median age	Asians, 40–50 yr Blacks, 20–30 yr	50–60 yr
Duration of symptoms	Usually short, especially in young blacks	Can be indolent
Abdominal pain or discomfort	70–90%	50–70%
Anorexia and weight loss	Common	Common
Hemorrhage secondary to ruptured tumor	10–20%	$<$10%
Cirrhosis	60–80%	60–80%
Cirrhosis evolving to hepatocellular carcinoma	50% or more	5–10%
Type of cirrhosis	Mostly macronodular	Mostly micronodular
Etiology of cirrhosis	HBV probably most important	Often alcohol and HBV
Hepatocellular carcinoma associated with hepatitis B virus	80% or more	30–50%
Hepatitis B antigen	70–90%	15–40%
Possible exposure to aflatoxin	High	Most unlikely
AFP $>$ 400 ng/ml (radioimmunoassay)	70–85%	30–65%

tween a multicentric HCC or intrahepatic metastatic spread.[67] A high frequency of portal vein invasion may be responsible for retrograde tumor spread and multiple intrahepatic metastases.[65] Okuda and colleagues have drawn attention to an important encapsulated HCC.[66] This tumor is common in Japan but is less frequently seen in other areas.[63] Sclerotic tumors are uncommon and may be mistaken for carcinoma on gross examination.

Peters recognized six different histologic patterns of HCC: microtrabecular, macrotrabecular, acinar, pseudoglandular, cobblestone, and pelioid types.[63,67] Cytologically, HCC may range from a well-differentiated tumor that is difficult to distinguish from normal hepatocytes to a poorly differentiated neoplasm. Cells may be uniform or markedly pleomorphic or may form giant cells. Cell cytoplasm may be clear, containing large amounts of glycogen, or have large lipid-containing vacuoles. Hyland bodies and Mallory bodies may be present. The trabecular hepatic portal canaliculi are reproduced in well-differentiated tumors, and exaggerations of these histologic features are responsible for most of the microscopic subtypes. Well-differentiated carcinomas may secrete bile and formed bile plugs may be recognized in the canaliculi. Canaliculi lined by two or three hepatocytes may assume the appearance of rosettes, similar to those seen in non-neoplastic livers in chronic acute hepatitis—the pseudoglandular pattern.

Some have suggested that histologic classification of HCC should be simplified into two subtypes: trabecular or undifferentiated tumors. The macrotrabecular, microtrabecular, acinar, pseudoglandular, and adenomatous carcinomas are all considered trabecular. Other histologic variants of trabecular tumors are the carcinoid-like tumors and highly vascu-

TABLE 27-4. Classification of Hepatic Tumors

Epithelial		*Mesenchymal*		
Benign	*Malignant*	*Benign*	*Malignant*	*Others*
Focal nodular hyperplasia	Hepatoblastoma	Hemangioma	Mixed	Cysts
Adenoma Bile duct adenoma Bile duct cystadenoma	Hepatocellular carcinoma Cholangiocellular carcinoma	Hemangioendothelioma (types I and II) Mesenchymal hamartoma Peliosis hepatitis	Mesenchymal tumors Rhabdomyosarcoma Undifferentiated sarcoma Angiosarcoma Malignant histiosarcoma Neuroblastoma Germ cell tumor Endodermal sinus tumor Lymphoma Leiomyosarcoma Malignant tumor of bile duct origin, carcinomas, rhabdomyosarcoma	Metastasis
Adrenal rest Nodular hyperplasia				

Data from Rao BN, Green AA: Hepatic tumors in children and adolescents. In Wanebo HJ (ed): Hepatic and biliary cancer, pp 187–218. New York, Marcel Dekker, 1987.

larized types resembling peliosis hepatitis, called "peleoid" by Peters.[63,68]

Two histologic subsets of HCC can be classified separately because of their clinical and prognostic features. Fibrolamellar carcinoma occurs in younger patients of either sex and is associated with better resectability rates and survival than is the usual form of HCC.[67,69–72] Distinctive features include the marked fibrosis, which is arranged in a lamellar fashion around the neoplastic hepatocytes. These tumors have also been called "polygonal cell type" with fibrous stroma by Berman, Libbey, and Foster.[71] The more favorable prognosis of these patients, compared with those with other forms of HCC, has been disputed by Christopherson and his coworkers.[72]

Sclerosing HCCs (cholangiocarcinoma, carcinoma of bile duct) are adenocarcinomas that have a ductular arrangement.[73] They may secrete mucus but not bile. On gross examination they present as a solitary white mass containing more fibrous stoma than does HCC. It is histologically indistinguishable from the cholangiocarcinomas that arise in extrahepatic bile ducts. Sclerosing HCC is associated with hypercalcemia.[73]

Related Liver Tumors

Benign liver tumors include adenoma, focal nodular hyperplasia (FNH), hemangioma, and mesenchymal hamartoma.[61,62] In Christopherson's Liver Registry, FNH was the most common, diagnosed in 106 of the 201 cases. The median age was 31 years, compared with 30 years in the 83 patients with adenomas. Hemoperitoneum occurred in 9%, and 83% had a history of birth control pill use for an average of 71 months. FNH is usually described as having a large central scar from which radiates wide fibrous bands, somewhat resembling macronodular cirrhosis.

Of the patients with liver cell adenomas, 83% used oral contraceptives for an average of 80 months. In most cases, there was a single tumor, ranging in diameter from 1 to 22 cm. Adenomas were composed exclusively of hepatocytes, tended to be circumscribed, and were usually described as encapsulated.

Other malignant tumors include angiosarcoma of the liver which is related to ingestion or exposure to Thorotrast, an organic arsenical vinyl chloride, androgenic anabolic steroids, birth control pills, and diethylstilbestrol for prostatic cancer.[62] Patients usually die from liver destruction, even though at the time of diagnoses only a small number (12%) have distant metastases. The disease is multicentric and widespread throughout the liver, and there have been no survivors.

The ethnically global mixture of the American population and the infrequent incidence of HCC in North America limit the study of hepatoma. There is a diversity of underlying disease, including macronodular cirrhosis, primarily in Chinese men; diffuse cirrhosis, primarily in whites; and nodular and diffuse cirrhosis in patients with nonresectable HCC. The disease may be alpha-fetoprotein (AFP) positive or negative. This variable mixture must be analyzed in toto to develop realistic prognoses and therapeutic approaches.

Pathophysiologic Classification

HCC can be described morphologically by histologic characteristics, but a pathophysiologic classification that deals with underlying disease, as observed by CT scan and analyzed by biochemical markers, may be of more value in guiding chemical decisions than is the histologic description. One exception is the fibrolamellar form of HCC, which appears to be associated with prolonged survival.[66,67]

Underlying Disease

CHRONIC ACTIVE HEPATITIS. Patients with chronic active hepatitis present difficult management problems because most major cytotoxic agents adversely affect chronic active hepatitis and the damaged liver. The regenerative capacity of the normal liver decreases with relapsing viral infection. In addition, these patients are often managed with prednisone, Imuran, and other immunosuppressive agents that further complicate management. Even with reduced dosages of chemotherapy, a reactivation of hepatitis and further injury of tissue may occur.[74]

DIFFUSE CIRRHOSIS. Diffuse cirrhosis, common in the United States, is often associated with a loss of regenerative capacity in the normal liver. Experience suggests that if the liver involved by HCC is also small and cirrhotic, it is unlikely that it will be able to regenerate in response to tumor resection.[75] Depending on the degree of cirrhosis, sequelae such as modest liver failure and ascites may occur, and, in more marked circumstances, esophageal varices caused by portal hypertension and jaundice may occur. Each of these factors makes therapy more difficult and increases the complication rate, regardless of the treatment modality used.[76] A milder form of diffuse cirrhosis is one in which the regenerative capacity of the normal liver is suggested by increased liver size as detected by physical examination or CT scans. The expansion of the normal liver, in addition to the presence of the tumor, suggests to the oncologist a potential for liver regeneration after treatment of the tumor.

MACRONODULAR CIRRHOSIS. Macronodular cirrhosis is particularly prominent in Asians, in contrast to the more diffuse cirrhosis seen in North Americans. Hepatitis B has been commonly associated with macronodular cirrhosis.[77] The distinctive large and nodular liver is also associated with a poor regenerative capacity, as is the case with diffuse cirrhosis, and it severely limits the ability to resect. However, AFP screening has permitted identification of a large series of patients in China with early HCC. The majority of these patients underwent curative wedge resections of these early lesions.[77] Although this result has not been duplicated for diffuse cirrhosis, there are methods for converting nonresectable HCC to a resectable state through cytoreduction by means of isotopic labeled antibody therapy.[78] Furthermore, HCC that occurs in conjunction with macronodular cirrhosis is usually hypervascular, which enhances certain treatment methods, particularly radiolabeled antibodies.[78]

TUMOR MARKERS. AFP is the major tumor marker associated with HCC and is elevated in over 70% of patients with disease.[79–82] Correlations between tumor differentiation and the levels of AFP have been demonstrated.[69] Patients with high levels of the marker protein have short survival times and poorly differentiated carcinomas. Moderately differentiated tumors are associated with intermediate levels of AFP and intermediate survival times. Patients with low AFP levels fall into two groups. One group consists of long-term survivors with extremely well-differentiated tumors, and the second group with anaplastic carcinomas have ultrashort survival times.[69] Other series have shown that high AFP levels are associated with better survival rates than normal AFP levels, but these data may reflect a particular patient mix.[33]

Carcinoembryonic antigen (CEA) is elevated in more than 70% of patients with HCC, but it lacks specificity. There is no correlation between CEA and AFP concentrations: the CEA may rise when the AFP decreases. Alkaline phosphatase is invariably elevated, but it also lacks specificity.[83]

Other tumor markers have been found in patients with HCC, especially in low-incidence areas and usually in patients without HBV and without elevated AFP. Increased levels of chorionic gonadotropin, of chorionic somatotropin, and of calcitonin have been reported.[84,85] Elevated neurotensin levels have been found in patients with fibrolamellar carcinoma.[86]

In China, 70% to 75% of patients with HCC have positive AFP titers. Between 90% and 95% have either hepatitis B antigen or antibody. However, 25% to 30% of the patients with HCC are AFP negative.[87,88] These patients have not attracted general attention in Chinese medical practice.

In the randomized prospective study carried out through the Radiation Oncology Study Group (RTOG) in the eastern United States, 63% of the patients were AFP positive and 37% were AFP negative. Ten percent of the patients have HBV antigen, according to a study by DiBisceglie and coworkers.[25a] Twenty-one percent of 63 patients had positive anti-HBV antibody titers. This contrasts with no HBV-antigen positivity ($p < 0.004$) and 10% anti-HBV antibody positive titers ($p = 0.08$) in 98 consecutive cancer patients. In the western United States, however, the higher incidence of patients of Asian background leads to a higher incidence of AFP positivity, HBS antigenicity, and antibody levels. Finally, based on the original Phase I–II study with radiolabeled antibody, tumors that do not elevate AFP seem to grow slower than AFP-producing tumors.

CLINICAL PRESENTATION

Most patients complain of right upper quadrant pain or distention and weight loss. The pain is usually dull or aching, but it can be acute and frequently radiates to the right shoulder. Fatigue and loss of appetite are common, and unexplained fever may occur. Patients may present with hepatic decompensation and have ascites, variceal bleeding, jaundice, or encephalopathy.

The findings of firm nodular hepatomegaly and an arterial bruit, combined with a hepatic rub, strongly suggest HCC in an advanced stage. Earlier stages may have hepatomegaly only or have no specific findings. Among 569 patients referred to a hospital in South Africa as possible HCC cases based on hepatomegaly, more than 60% were confirmed to have HCC, 11% had cirrhosis only, 7.5% had tuberculosis, and 5% had amoebiasis.[81] Only 3.5% had metastatic cancer to the liver.

In high-risk patients having chronic HVB or cirrhosis, ultrasound and AFP monitoring may lead to earlier diagnoses. Metastases occur commonly in HCC, accounting for the variable modes of presentation. Lung metastases are found in approximately 20% of patients, and pulmonary or chest wall symptoms may be the first symptom. Occasionally, metastases to bone or other uncommon sites may draw attention to the disease. Although the liver disease dominates the clinical picture, more than half of the patients will have extrahepatic spread during the clinical course of the disease. Other modes of presentation include an acute abdomen from a spontaneous rupture of the tumor (more common in Asia), acute Budd-Chiari syndrome due to extension of the tumor into the inferior vena cava, and portal hypertension due to invasion of the portal venous system.[89,90] There are rare modes of presentation that receive undue attention, including endocrine and paraneoplastic complications. Erythrocytosis is the most common. Hypoglycemia occurs in the late stages of the disease but is very seldom the reason for suspecting HCC. Hypercalcemia, hyperthyroidism, and carcinoid syndrome are also described. Hypertrophic pulmonary osteoarthropathy is common in South African patients with HCC but is seldom symptomatic.[81]

METASTATIC DISEASE

HCC can invade the diaphragm and adjacent organs like the stomach, which may be related to the propensity for membranous obstruction of the inferior vena cava in patients with HCC.[90] HCC may also invade the portal vein and, less frequently, the hepatic veins. Bile duct obstruction and early jaundice can result, even in the setting of limited tumor burden.[91] Perineural metastases and intraperitoneal rupture of the hepatic tumor and hemorrhage can also occur.

Metastatic disease is present in a minority of patients at operation, but at the time of autopsy more than 50% of the patients have metastases. These occur most commonly in regional nodes, lung, bone, adrenal gland, and brain. Series by Simson, Peters, and Anthony show a distribution of metastases similar in African and non-African studies.[63,64,68] Approximately 40% of all patients have tumor in regional nodes. Other metastatic sites are very rare, with less than 10% involving bone, adrenal gland, heart, and central nervous system. Sternal metastases may be a specific type of spread in patients with membranous obstruction of the inferior vena cava.[90] Direct venous spread is an important factor in HCC. Invasion of the portal and hepatic vein is common, and tumor frequently involves the inferior vena cava. The gallbladder is invaded directly in approximately 6% of the cases, and the tumor obstructs large bile ducts in the porta hepatis or in the larger ducts within the liver.[91] The subsequent jaundice in these patients can falsely suggest a terminal status usually seen in patients with HCC who are jaundiced. Spontaneous hemoperitoneum caused by rupture, evident in 25% of Anthony's series, and hemorrhage from esophageal varices, evident in 19% of the same series, are serious complications of HCC.[68]

DIAGNOSIS

In areas of the world where HCC is common, chronic HBV infection, chronic membranous obstruction of the inferior vena cava, chronic hepatic outflow obstruction (CHOO), and male sex are factors that should draw attention to the possibility of developing HCC. These clear associations also apply to low-incidence areas of the world. HCC is insidious. If clinical signs and symptoms directly referable to HCC have developed, the prognosis is usually only a few months.

Tumor Markers

The presence of AFP in the serum of patients with HCC has led to its use as a screening method in high-risk populations. This has been effective in China, in patients with chronic hepatitis in Japan, and among Alaskan Eskimos, and it may have value in selected patients with HBV-positive hepatitis.[79,82,92–97] Elevated AFP, unfortunately, is not specific for the diagnosis of HCC, and histologic confirmation is essential. In a series of black South African patients suspected to have HCC and who had elevated levels of serum AFP, several nonhepatic malignancies of the gallbladder and the extrahepatic bile ducts and pancreas were demonstrated.[81]

Elevation of AFP levels is a well-recognized feature of metastatic liver cancer, endodermally derived tumors, and islet cell tumors.[80] Unlike germ cell tumors, in which the elevation of AFP may be related to the amount of tumor present, the levels vary in patients with HCC. The heterogeneity of AFP expression may relate to the cause of HCC, although in classic HCC, elevated AFP levels should raise concern about the diagnosis of HCC. Although AFP occurs in fetal blood in levels reaching 500 to 700 ng/ml, it decreases rapidly after birth.[92] Within the first year, infants achieve normal adult values of less than 10 ng/ml. The frequency of AFP elevation in HCC varies from 30% to 90%.[79–93] Although a normal AFP does not exclude HCC, very high values strongly suggest HCC.

A general diagnostic approach is outlined in Figure 27-1. The finding of an upper abdominal mass in a high-risk patient, who is HBV positive or who lives in an indigenous area for HCC, should prompt an AFP test, followed rapidly by an ultrasound and CT scan. If disease is extensive, a fine-needle biopsy may suffice. If liver resection is considered, an exploration with operative biopsy is preferred.

Radiologic Studies

Plain films of the chest and abdomen may provide some information.[98] An unusual hump or elevation of the diaphragm may correspond to an invasive liver tumor, pending exclusion of a primary nerve palsy or eventration. Abdominal films may show hepatomegaly and, occasionally, calcification is seen in primary hepatic tumors. An upper gastrointestinal (GI) series may show gross displacement of the stomach in patients with advanced disease. Some patients may present with hemothorax and corresponding ascites, along with metastases to the lung detected as large "cannonball lesions" or the rarer micronodule shadows.

Radionuclide-labeled colloids, in particular ^{99m}Tc-labeled sulfur colloid, are sensitive in evaluating space-occupying liver lesions. In a large Singapore study, ^{99}Tc-sulfur colloid detected HCC in 94% of the patients, ^{198}Au-colloid detected lesions in 81%, and gallium in 89%.[99] Gallium was more useful in distinguishing primary HCC from secondary lesions or abscesses. Most of the difficulties arose from background effects of a highly cirrhotic liver; here gallium may be more useful and provide better quality scanning, with improved specificity and sensitivity. A technetium scan would appear to be the preferred initial diagnostic examination, but gallium may be more useful if metastases are suspected.[100]

Ultrasound is a very versatile and inexpensive early diagnostic test. It is noninvasive, nontoxic, and rapidly used. It may be of equal or greater sensitivity than radionuclide scanning. Lesions less than 3 cm can be detected by ultrasound; for the small tumors, ultrasound is considered by some to be the most sensitive of imaging techniques, in which cases it is hypoechoic.[101] It also can guide an aspiration needle. Intraoperative ultrasound is useful in the detection of deep-seated small tumors.[102]

CT can detect and delineate the extent of hepatic tumors. The presence of isodense tumors or small lesions may lead to false-negative results, and occasionally false-positive results are also given. Magnetic resonance imaging (MRI) has been shown comparable to CT scanning and in some cases may be preferable. The degree of contrast between the

FIG. 27-1. Evaluation of hepatocellular cancer. A general guideline to the diagnostic workup of the patient at risk for hepatocellular carcinoma. An arteriogram is generally done if resection is planned. A biopsy could be done at that time, unless the patient is considered unresectable, at which time a percutaneous biopsy could be done. *Paraneoplastic syndrome may elevate or depress calcium or glucose. **Must indicate safety of biopsy or be corrected.

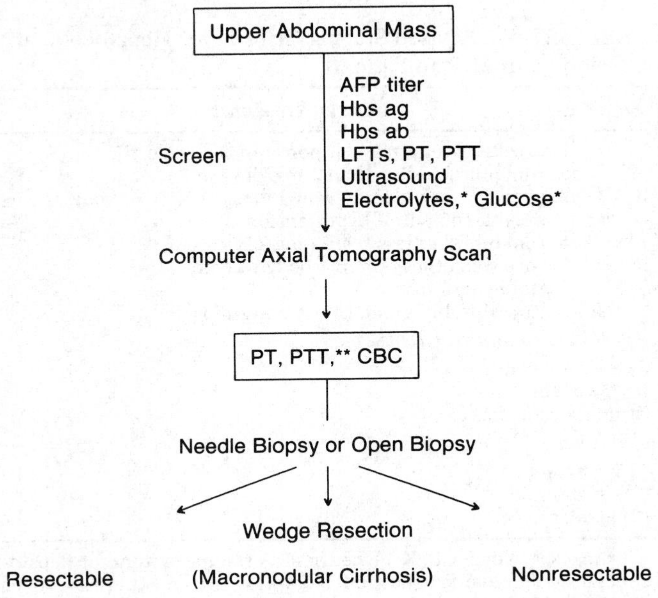

tumor and normal liver is better with MRI and distinguishes among HCC and angioma, cysts, and cirrhosis.

Comparisons of these methods suggest that scintography with technetium may be a good first choice, although if adequate ultrasound is available it is considered preferable by many. CT and technetium scanning are probably similar in sensitivity, but the CT scan better defines the anatomy of the disease and also shows the extrahepatic extent of tumor. Ultrasound in skilled hands is useful in distinguishing cysts and possible vascular lesions, as well as for detecting small HCC not visualized by the CT scan.[101]

Diagnosis by needle biopsy is frequently possible.[102] Caution is required because of the potential for hemorrhage from a hypervascular HCC or a misdiagnosed hemangioma. Peritoneoscopic visualization with biopsy is recommended by some.[103] This would allow direct assessment of the liver during the biopsy and minimize the potential for hemorrhage. In patients who are candidates for resection, a needle biopsy is not recommended in view of the risk for hemorrhage and tumor-cell contamination. Such patients are better explored and resected if curative surgery is undertaken.

Patients who are considered candidates for surgery (*i.e.*, localized lesion limited to one lobe or segment without extrahepatic spread) should have hepatic angiography.[104,105] This provides information about the tumor extent and an arterial and venous system road map essential for planned resection. These tumors are usually hypervascular, and, in some cases, the angiogram may demonstrate lesions in both lobes of the liver not detected by noninvasive techniques.[103–105] A late-phase angiogram can demonstrate the portal vein and its major branches, and a direct inferior vena cavogram may be useful in determining the metastasic or direct invasion. Angiography provides data for resection and for other surgical approaches, such as hepatic artery infusion therapy.

Although staging is essential to the primary management of all major cancers, an accepted system is not currently in use for HCC. One suggested system was based on risk factors in Ugandan patients (Table 27-5).[106] This system categorizes patients according to the presence or absence of ascites, weight loss, portal hypertension, or jaundice, and it further subdivides categories by the anatomical extent of tumor. In the Ugandan patients, the survival ranged from greater than 3 months in those with no ascites, weight loss <10%, no portal hypertension, and normal bilirubin to less than 2 months in those with all these factors present. Prognostic factors in advanced HCC are discussed in the section on chemotherapy.[107]

TABLE 27-5. Revised Staging Criteria for Hepatocellular Carcinoma in African Patients

Stage	*Cancer Presentation*
I	No ascites, weight loss or portal hypertension Serum bilirubin less than 2 mg/dl
II	Ascites and/or moderate weight loss (<25% of body weight), no portal hypertension Serum bilirubin less than 2 mg/dl
III	Severe weight loss (>25% body weight) Portal hypertension Serum bilirubin greater than 2 mg/dl
Anatomic Extent of Involvement	
A	One lobe only
B	Two lobes
C	Metastatic disease
Cirrhosis	
(+) = present	
(−) = absent	
(?) = uncertain	

Primack A, Vogel CL, Kyalwazi et al: A staging system for hepatocellular carcinoma: Prognostic factors in Ugandan patients. Cancer 35:1357–1364, 1975.

SURGERY

The preoperative assessment by the clinical and radiologic techniques described should provide the major determination of resectability.[103–105,108,109] During the laparotomy, the final decisions are made, based on the extent of tumor, the involvement of major vascular structures, lymph node metastases, or extrahepatic spread. Extension to the diaphragm or to the lateral parities under the rib cage requires a more extensive resection to insure adequate margins. In general, extension into the suprahepatic portion of the inferior vena cava or extension into the porta hepatis with involvement of the ducts or vessels on the contralateral major lobe precludes conventional resection.

In a jaundiced patient, a percutaneous cholangiogram or endoscopic cholangiopancreatiography (ERCP) may reveal a bile duct extension with contralateral hepatic duct involvement or common bile duct involvement, probably precluding resection except by very experienced surgeons or for patients selected for transplant surgery. Cirrhosis is also a major risk factor governing the extent of resection. Extensive cirrhosis, especially that associated with portal hypertension, precludes resection in most patients, except for very small tumors. Intraoperative ultrasound can determine the presence of small intrahepatic tumors, especially the presence of multicentric tumors, and can influence the plan for resection.

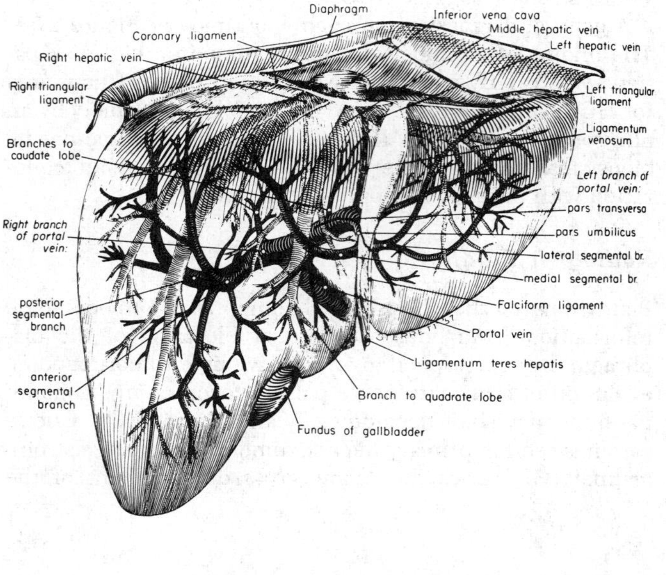

FIG. 27-2. The liver in transparency to show the branching and relative position of the parts of the portal and hepatic veins. (Goldsmith NA, Woodburne RT: The surgical anatomy pertaining to liver resection. Surg Gynecol Obstet 105:310, 1957. By permission of Surgery, Gynecology & Obstetrics)

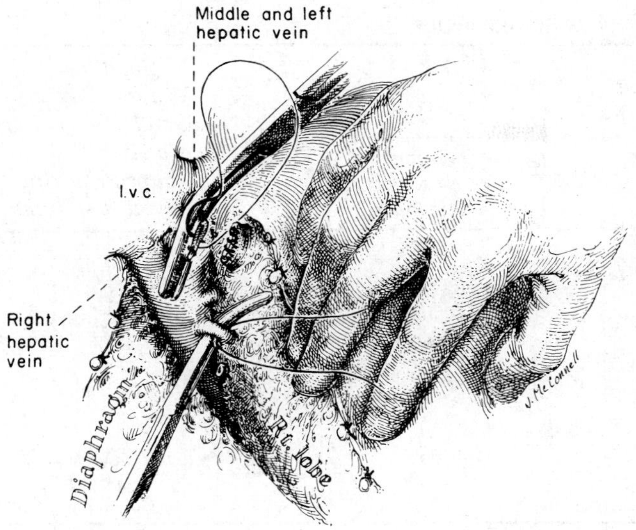

FIG. 27-3. Division of the right hepatic vein. With the right lobe of the liver retracted anteriorly and to the left, the vein is divided between Pott's clamps and oversewn with vascular sutures. Several smaller hepatic veins must be ligated as they enter the retrohepatic vena cava more inferiorly. (Starzl TE, Bell RH, Beart RW, et al: Hepatic trisegmentectomy and other liver resections. Surg Gynecol Obstet 141:429, 1974. By permission of Surgery, Gynecology & Obstetrics)

FIG. 27-4. Devascularization of the true right lobe. The cystic artery and cystic duct are ligated and divided to aid in the dissection. Of the structures of the portal triad, the bifurcation of the duct is almost always the most superior, that of the portal vein is intermediate, and that of the hepatic artery is most inferior. The lateral suture closure of the portal vein is at the site of detachment of the right portal branch. The tissue bridge conceals the umbilical fissure, behind which a finger can be inserted. The bridge is present in about half the patients. (Starzl TE, Bell RH, Beart RW, et al: Hepatic trisegmentectomy and other liver resections. Surg Gynecol Obstet 141:429, 1975. By permission of Surgery, Gynecology & Obstetrics)

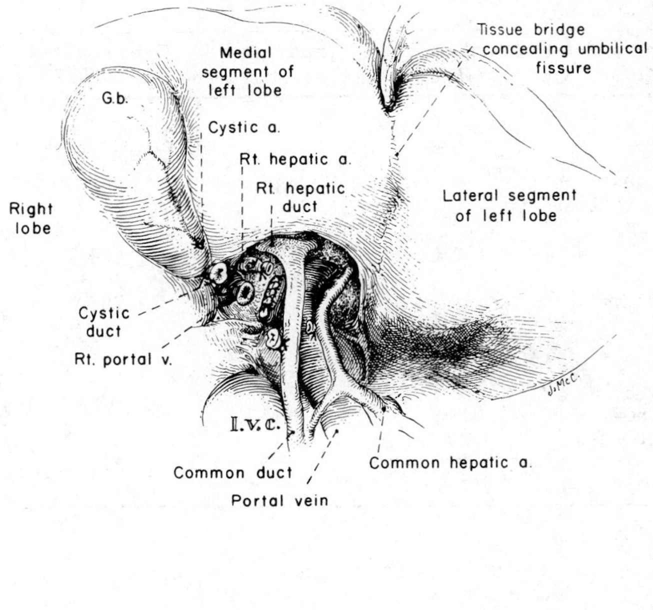

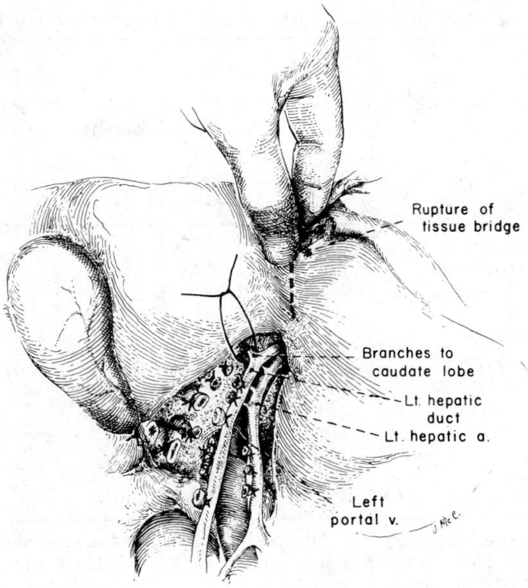

FIG. 27-5. Nearly completed mobilization of the left branches of the portal triad. The tissue bridge is being broken to permit access to the umbilical fissure. The final two branches before the main trunk reaches the umbilical fissure go to the left portion of the caudate lobe. These final branches (or at least the last one) should be preserved unless all of the caudate lobe is to be removed. Total caudate removal is not usually necessary. (Starzl TE, Bell RH, Beart RW, et al: Hepatic trisegmentectomy and other liver resections. Surg Gynecol Obstet 141:429, 1975. By permission of Surgery, Gynecology & Obstetrics)

FIG. 27-6. Liver transection nearly completed along the exact line of color change demarcated by viable and cyanotic liver tissue. Intersegmental veins are left attached to the lateral segment if possible. The last major structure to be encountered is the middle hepatic vein. (Starzl TE, Bell RH, Beart RW, et al: Hepatic trisegmentectomy and other liver resections. Surg Gynecol Obstet 141:429, 1975. By permission of Surgery, Gynecology & Obstetrics)

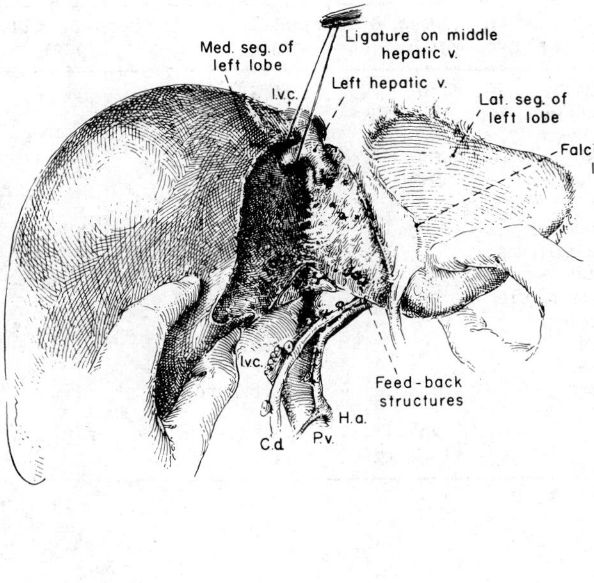

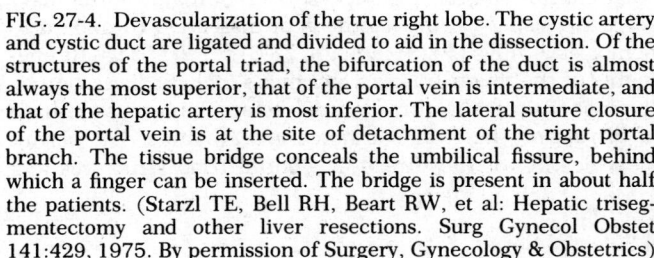

TABLE 27-6. Summary of Resection Experience with Primary Hepatic Malignancies

Resection Data	Clinical Cancers			Small or "Minute" Cancers Found by Screening in High-Risk Groups Requiring Limited Resections
	Western Experience	*Eastern Experience*	*Japan National Study*	
Total patients	~2000	4983	5496	147
No. of resections	482	969	1186	110
Resectability rate (range)	20–25%	19% (7–46%)	21.5%	73% (54–76%)
With cirrhosis, mean (range)	17% (0–43%)	68% (40–90%)	~80%	90%
Hospital mortality after resection	15%	18%		0–5%
Overall survival				
1 year	81%	48%	55%	73%
3 years	46%	24%	30%	66%
5 years	30%	14.5%		33–70%

Data from Nagorney DM, Adson MA: Major hepatic resections for hepatoma in the west. In Wanebo HJ (ed): Hepatic and biliary cancer, pp 167–185. New York, Marcel Dekker, 1987; Okuda K, Liver Cancer Study Group of Japan: Primary liver cancers in Japan. Cancer 45:2663–2669, 1980.

The operative exposure is important.[105,109–112] Some surgeons are comfortable with the bilateral subcostal incision with anterior traction on the costal border by a rigid retractor. Others may make liberal use of thoracoabdominal incisions, which afford improved exposure and may be necessary in patients having large lesions that involve the proximal portion of the inferior vena cava in the superior portion of the liver. This incision may also be necessary in patients in whom proximal control of the vena cava is required.

Anatomical Considerations

The liver substance is arranged segmentally. The classic descriptions of Goldsmith and Woodburne divide the liver into two major lobes, with the division line on a plane from the bed of the gallbladder to the inferior vena cava (Fig. 27-2).[113] Couinaud categorized eight hepatic subsegments.[114] The subsegments, based on the portobiliary drainage, have been more commonly used by European than North American surgeons, perhaps because of their greater familiarity with Couinaud's work.[115]

The classic approach consists of hilar dissection, with vascular control and subsequent resection of major portobiliary segments using various methods of dissection to maximize hemostasis (Figs. 27-3 through 27-6).[3,105,110,116,117] Refinements of the finger fracture technique include disruption by the sucker tip or the ultrasonic dissector. Numerous methods of disrupting the liver substance are available that permit identification of the thread-like portal triad structures and

TABLE 27-7. Resection of Hepatocellular Carcinoma: Results of Selected Series

	Western Series						
Author (Year)	*Adson (1986)*	*Lim and Bongard (1984)*	*Sorenson et al (1979)*	*Fortner et al (1981)*	*Bengmark et al (1982)*	*Iwatshi et al (1983)*	*Thompson et al (1983)*
Total study population	230	86					
% cirrhosis	50%	43%					
No resections	62	22	31	42	21	43	35
Resectability rate	27%	26%					
% resections with cirrhosis	3%	43%	16%		0%	12%	20%
Hospital mortality after resections		39%	26%	17%	14%	9%	20%
Survival							
1 year				85%		78%	
2 year	53%	Median 18.7 mo	62%	50% (3 yr)	38% (2 yr)	60%	
5 years	30%		16%	37%	20% (4 yr)	46%	31%

larger segmental vessels and ducts, which can be ligated, clipped, or in some cases, electrocoagulated. Larger vessels are easily identified within the liver substance and are formally ligated and bisected. Control of the hepatic veins is controversial and depends primarily on the experience of the individual surgeon rather than on any accepted surgical anatomical study. Although the right and left hepatic veins may be easily exposed in some patients, more commonly they are buried within the liver substance. Because of its position superior and posterior in the liver, the early exposure of this vein can be treacherous, and many prefer to expose and ligate it near the completion of the resection.[124] Many approaches have been described in the literature.[105,108–117]

The basic principles of safe hepatic resection require adequate exposure and complete mobilization of the liver, with division of ligamentous attachments (*i.e.*, the triangular ligament superiorly and the attachments of the right lobe posteriorly and laterally for right hepatic resections) and exposure of the superior hepatic cava. Isolation of the suprahepatic cava and vascular control with a looped umbilical tape may provide an additional safety measure for control of the suprahepatic cava in the event of a mishap. Although rarely necessary, use of a large-bore cardiac venous shunt, placed by means of the right atrium into the inferior vena cava using a large-bore shunt for very high-risk lesions, is possible.

Hilar dissection and vascular isolation of the major branches of hepatic artery and portal vein, encircling these with a vascular loop or an umbilical tape or ligating these structures directly, will markedly reduce the bleeding of both portal veins and arterial inflow to the segments. Some surgeons espouse total inflow occlusion by clamping the porta hepatis with a vascular clamp.[118] Occlusion times up to 1 hour have been reported, and blood loss and operative time have been markedly reduced from conventional approaches. If feasible, the numerous retrohepatic veins should be exposed and ligated. This may not be possible in all patients because of the extensive encircling of the cava by the liver. The same can be said for the hepatic veins, which may be located deep in liver. In some cases, however, the veins may be easily seen, mobilized, and ligated during the dissection.

Blood loss may be moderate or profound, depending on the extent of the resection and the presence of underlying cirrhosis or coagulopathy; it is imperative to minimize blood loss by all mechanical methods. Autotransfusions may be useful, although there are concerns about the potential for spreading cells unwittingly shed during the operative procedure. Adequate replacement with fresh-frozen plasma and platelets, if necessary, early in the dissection, especially in cirrhotic patients, may help reduce blood loss.

Lateral sublobar segmental resections (*i.e.*, tumors less than 5 cm in the lateral portion of the liver) may not require routine hilar vascular control. In contrast, even small tumors in the proximity of the hepatic vein on the posterior dome (segments 7 and 8) may preclude a safe resection for most surgeons. Intraoperative ultrasound can locate small nonpalpable HCC and major portal inflow to the subsegment, which allows for a more limited resection in cirrhotic patients.

After completion of the resection, the liver surface is irrigated copiously, small open ducts or vessels are ligated as necessary, and the open liver substance is covered with omentum. Most surgeons make use of a closed drainage system to provide egress of blood and bile during the immediate postoperative period. Antibiotics and adequate replacement of fluids and clotting factors are prerequisites to good clinical outcome.

Resectability

Twenty-five percent of patients with primary HCC seen at major centers have potentially resectable lesions (Tables 27-6 and 27-7).[119–128] Approximately 10% to 12% are actually resected.

Most surgeons consider severe cirrhosis to be a contraindication to major resection.[124–128] This is suggested from studies demonstrating retrospectively that cirrhosis and HCC

TABLE 27-7. Resection of Hepatocellular Carcinoma: Results of Selected Series *(continued)*

Eastern Series							
Honjo and Mizusoto (1974)	*Lin (1976)*	*Okuda et al (1980)*	*Wu et al (1980)*	*Lee et al (1982)*	*Okamato et al (1984)*	*Nagasue et al (1986)*	*Nagoa et al (1987)*
76	382	2411	748	935	266		
40%		83%			90%		
21	181	213	181	165	103	94	98
26%	31%	9%	24%	18%	46%		
48%	21%	71%	70%	85%		86%	75%
9%	12%	28%	9%	20%	13%	7.6%	19%
	35%	33%	56%	45%	65%	55%	73%
23%	20%	20%	29%	20%	27%		42%
(3 yr)	(3 yr)	(3 yr)	(3 yr)	(3 yr)			
14%	19%	12%	16%	18%	13%	3.5%	25%

coexisted in 81% of patients examined at autopsy, in only 35% of patients examined at laparotomy, and in only 21% of patients with resectable tumors.[124] Most experienced surgeons have recognized that the greater the extent of the liver resection, the more dangerous is the procedure in patients with cirrhosis.[123,126] This recognition has led to mass screenings of patients at risk for HCC, many of whom have cirrhosis, with the hope of finding small resectable tumors. Kanematsu and colleagues have explored the risk and the value of limited hepatic resection for smaller encapsulated hepatomas from cirrhotic livers.[129] They found operative mortality rates of 1% to 15% for limited resections in patients with severe hepatic impairment and for major resections in cirrhotic patients with better hepatic reserve.[129]

Patient selection remains a problem for cirrhotics. Lee and co-workers found that bromosulfaphthalein excretion greater than 10% at 45 minutes or serum albumin less than 3 g/dl contraindicated major resection.[130] Tobe observed that major resection was generally contraindicated in patients who were Child's C class and who had impaired clearance of indocyanine green.[131] Schemes to define liver reserve in cirrhotics and to determine safe hepatic resection limits have been offered by several clinicians.[131–133]

Table 27-6 presents an overview of the eastern and western experience.[119–135] In the western series fewer than 20% of patients have cirrhosis, and the overall resectability is about 20% to 25%, with a 15% operative mortality rate. The 5-year cure rate is approximately 30%. In the eastern series, the percentage of cirrhosis ranged between 40% and 90%. The overall resectability rate ranged from 7% to 46%. The overall hospital mortality after resection ranged from 9% to 33%; Okuda in Japan reports 28% and Okamoto reports 13%.[133,135] Among cirrhotics in the Japanese overview, the overall mortality was approximately 30%, but in other series it was less: 20% in Honjo and Mizsumoto's series and 12% in the Wu series.[123,127a] The 5-year survival rate in those resected ranged from 11% to 19%.

An update of the Japanese experience reviewed survival rates and the impact of cirrhosis in HCC patients undergoing surgery between 1980 and 1981.[135a] Cirrhosis had a significant, adverse impact on survival after resection (Fig. 27-7). In a review of the medical and surgical experience at the Chiba University Hospital, Okuda and Tobe reported HCC was resected in 64 (19.8%) of 324 patients, with an operative death rate of 9.9%; multiple resections were performed in 6 patients.[135a] The extent of resection in 71 patients included partial resection for 48, segmentectomies for 8, and lobectomy or trisegmentectomy in 15. The relationship of mortality to the extent of resection was 15% to 27% in the group having major resections and was only 5% (3 of 56) in those patients undergoing partial resections or segmentectomies. The operative mortality according to Child's class was 4% (47 cases) with Child A, 7% (18 cases) with Child B, and 50% (6 cases) with Child C.[135] This series also used intraoperative ultrasonography to detect nonpalpable or unrecognizable tumors smaller than 5 cm, of particular importance in cirrhotics.

The relationships of tumor size, AFP levels, and the diagnostic measures of ultrasound, CT, and angiography in this well-studied group of patients is shown in Table 27-8, and

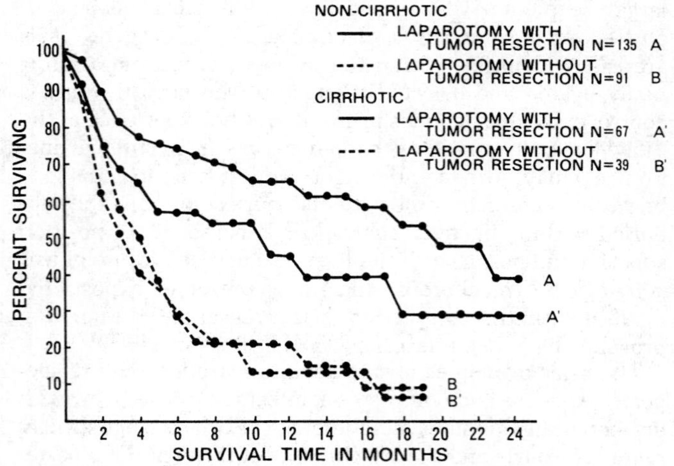

FIG. 27-7. Survival curves for the laparotomized cases in the latest National Study (1980–1981): (*A*) 135 noncirrhotic cases with resection; (*B*) 91 noncirrhotic cases without resection; (*A′*) 67 cirrhotic cases with resection; (*B′*) 39 cirrhotic cases without resection. There are significant differences between A and A′, between A and B, and between A′ and B′, but not between B and B′.

the surgical survival data relevant to Child's class and extent of resection are shown in Table 27-9. The survival rate at 3 years in this series was 80% for patients with small tumors (≥2 cm), compared with 20% for those with tumors larger than 5 cm. High rates of resectability and survival have been reported for other Japanese and Chinese series for small HCC lesions diagnosed at an early stage.[135a–135c] In patients with tumors larger than 5 cm, approximately half died from tumor recurrence and the remaining from hepatic failure. This selective series emphasizes the need for concentrated experience with the disease.

Pediatric Liver Tumors

HEPATOBLASTOMA. Hepatoblastoma is a distinctive tumor of the liver in infants and children, with the male-female ratio of 1.5 : 2.1.[136–141] It is usually diagnosed in the first 2 to 3 years of life and is rarely seen in children older than age 6. It may be associated with congenital anomalies, such as tetralogy of Fallot, persistent ductus arteriosis, or extrahepatic biliary atresia. The most common presentation is as an asymptomatic abdominal mass found by the parent or during a routine physical examination. Jaundice is rare. Abdominal roentgenographic examination usually shows a mass density in the upper abdomen, and liver scan usually shows decreased isotope uptake. About 67% of the tumors arise in the right lobe. The serum levels of AFP are elevated in 80% to 90% of all patients. Microscopically, hepatoblastoma is classified into the more common pure epithelial type and a mixed epithelial mesenchymal type.[136–142]

HCC is also seen in the pediatric population, but it is less frequent than hepatoblastoma, occurs in older children (median, 10–12 years), and has a male-female ratio of about 8 : 1. At the time of diagnosis most patients are symptomatic, with weight loss, abdominal pain, jaundice, and anemia, and serum AFP levels are elevated in 30% to 80%. Although it is

TABLE 27-8. Accuracy of Various Diagnostic Modalities for Hepatocellular Carcinoma (Chiba University Hospital Experience)

Size of Tumor (cm)	No. of Patients	*Alpha-Fetoprotein Levels (ng/ml)*			*Diagnosis Made by (%)*		
		<20	*20–499*	*>500*	*Ultrasound*	*CT*	*Angiography*
<2	12	5	7		75	92	67
<3	19	10	7	2	93	93	80
<5	23	5	13	5	100	94	95
<5.1	17	3	4	10	100	100	100
Total	71	23	31	17	94	95	89

From Okuda K, Ryu M, Tobe T: Surgical management of hepatoma. The Japanese experience. In Wanebo HJ (ed): Hepatic and biliary cancer, pp 219–238. New York, Marcel Dekker, 1987.

similar in its histologic pattern and clinical presentation to the adult form, the incidence of cirrhosis is only 5% in the children compared with about 75% in the adults.[136] In a review of pediatric hepatic tumors from St. Jude's Children's Research Hospital by Rao and Green, 29 of 7€ hepatic tumors were hepatoblastomas, 18 were HCC, 8 were sarcomas, 1 was neuroblastoma, 7 were hemangiomas or hemangioendotheliomas, 3 were visceral larval migrans, 2 were hepatic abscesses, and 8 were other miscellaneous non-neoplastic tumors (Table 27-10).[136]

Of 29 hepatoblastomas, 7 had associated congenital abnormalities (a major CNS defect in 4), and 10 were resectable by hepatic lobectomy.[136] Eight of ten patients survived 3 to 18 years after resection, and two patients developed intrahepatic recurrences resistant to chemotherapy and died after 17 and 31 months, respectively. Among the 18 patients with HCC, all but 2 had asymptomatic masses. Five had congenital abnormalities, and only three had complete tumor resection of their tumors. Two of these were alive 5 and 17 years after surgery, and one died with local tumor recurrence. Of the eight primary liver sarcomas, six were malignant mesenchymoma and two were intrahepatic rhabdomyosarcoma. Five patients were resected, and three were long-term survivors with adjuvant chemotherapy. Two patients not given adjuvant therapy developed metastases and died.[136]

Transplantation

PRIMARY LIVER CANCER. In view of the limited resectability rate of 15% to 30% in most of the series, the potential for retrieval by total hepatectomy and transplantation has intrigued and challenged surgeons for years. The largest experience has been reported by Starzl and his group, although other surgeons have participated.[142–146] In the Starzl experience, a total of 55 patients received orthotopic liver transplants who had primary hepatic malignancies. There were 32 women and 23 men, with ages between 2 and 68 years (Table 27-11). Malignancies included HCC in 38 patients (69%), of which 7 were the fibrolamellar variant; bile duct carcinoma (Klatskin's tumor) in 8 (14.5%); epithelioid hemangioendothelial sarcoma in 3 (5.5%); and cholangiocarcinoma in 2 (3.6%). Four additional tumors included hepatoblastoma, hemangiosarcoma, unclassified sarcoma, and adenocarcinoma from an unknown primary. Of 40 patients, 76% were thought to have unresectable lesions and received liver transplants as the primary method of therapy. In the first 20 of these the immune suppression regimen included azathioprine, prednisone, and antilymphocyte globulin; the other 19 were immunosuppressed with cyclosporin and prednisone.

Thirteen patients received transplants for non-neoplastic

TABLE 27-9. Hepatic Resection for Primary Liver Cancer: Relationship of Surgical Procedure, Child's Classification, and Operative Mortality (Chiba University Hospital Experience)

Child's Classification	*No. of Cases*	*Extent of Resection*		
		Partial	*1 Segment*	*2–3 Segments*
A	47	28	7	12
	(2)* (4.3%)	(1)†		(1)
B	18	16		2
	(2) (11.1%)			(2)
C	6	4	1	1
	(3) (50%)	(1)	(1)	(1)
Total	71	48	8	15
	(7) (9.9%)	(2) (4.1%)	(1) (12.5%)	(4) (26.7%)

Okuda K, Ryu M, Tobe T: Surgical management of hepatoma. The Japanese Experience. In Wanebo HJ (ed): Hepatic and Biliary Cancer, pp 219–238. New York, Marcel Dekker, 1987.

* Number in parentheses are operative deaths.

† Due to variceal bleeding.

TABLE 27-10. Therapy for Primary Malignant Liver Tumors (St. Jude Children's Research Hospital Experience)

Disease	*Total*	*Resected*	*AWD**	*DOD*	*DWD*	*NED*
Hepatoblastoma	29	10	1	14	3	11
Hepatocellular carcinoma	18	3	2	14	0	2
Sarcoma	8	5	0	5	0	3
Neuroblastoma	1	1				1

Rao BN, Green AA: Hepatic tumors in children and adolescents. In Wanebo HJ (ed): Hepatic and biliary cancer, pp 187–218. New York, Marcel Dekker, 1987.
*AWD = alive with disease; DOD = died of disease; DWD = died without disease; NED = no evidence of disease.

end-stage liver disease and were found to have coincidental primary liver malignancy. Hepatocellular carcinoma was found in 12 and hepatoblastoma in 1. Twelve of 13 patients are alive and free of disease from 10 months to more than 15 years. Among those operated for clinical HCC, the recurrence rate was 50%. All the HCCs recurred within 1 year (mean, 6 months; range, 4–12 months), but patients with the fibrolamellar type had recurrences after 1 year (mean, 20 months). There was a continued decline in survival because of recurrent malignancy. Of the 42 patients with unresectable malignancy, only 10 (24%) were alive and only 6 (14%) were free of tumor from 4 months to 9 years. In contrast, among the 13 patients who had liver replacements for non-neoplastic liver disease and were found to have incidental HCC, none had recurrence and 12 are living 10 months to 15 years after treatment. Thus, it appears that

TABLE 27-11. Liver Transplantation in Patients with Unresectable Liver Cancer (Starzl Group)

Histology	*Method of Immune Suppression**	*No. of Patients*	*Months Until Recurrence, (%)*	*Time of Survival (Mean)*	*No. of Survivors, (%)*
HCC	Az/ALG	8	5 (63)	2–13 mo 4 mo	0
	Cy/P	8	4 (50)	4–12 mo 6 mo	3 (38)
HCC fibrolamellar variant	Az/ALG	1	1 (10)	13 mo	0
	Cy/P	6	3 (50)	13–30 mo	4 (66)
Bile duct	Az/ALG	3	2 (66)	21–42 mo	0
(Klatskin) cholangiocarcinoma	Cy/P	2	2	6–10 mo	0
		1	1	15 mo	0
Sarcoma	Az/ALG	2	1 (50)		1 (50)
	Cy/P	2	1 (50)		1 (50)

TOTAL: Az/ALG, group (20) of 14 survivors:
6 postoperative deaths
9 (64%) died of recurrence
4 died NED; infection, 2, 2, 3, 6 mo
1 survival—9 yr

Cy/P group (22) of 21 survivors:
1 postoperative death
9 (41%) alive 4–48 mo (mean 23 mo)
4 died NED; infection, 1, 2, 2, 13 mo
8 DOD

Data from Esquirel CO, Iwatsuki S, Gordon RD et al: Transplantation for primary liver cancer. In Wanebo HJ (ed): Hepatic and biliary cancer, pp 477–486. New York, Marcel Dekker, 1987.
*Immunosuppression regimen: Az/ALG = azathioprine + antilymphocyte globulin; Cy/P = cyclosporine + prednisone.

Liver Transplantation in Patients with Incidental Primary Liver Cancer

Histology	*No. of Patients*	*Months Until Recurrence*	*No. of Survivors*
HCC	11	0	10 (10 mo–15 yr), 1 Postoperative death
Hepatoblastoma	1	0	1

HCC per se is not an absolute contraindication to total resection and transplantation. The extent of tumor in HCC appears to be the main determining factor, emphasizing the need for effective drug treatment.

CHEMOTHERAPY

Despite the poor prognosis of patients with inoperable HCC, there is sufficient prognostic diversity to confuse the analysis of the outcome of therapeutic trials, if known prognostic factors are not taken into account. Important factors of the natural history of the disease, such as sex, age, performance status, cirrhosis, race, and country of origin, should be considered in predicting survival in therapeutic trials. In many cases, these factors are more significant than the treatment used. Unique data are available in the analysis of 432 patients with advanced HCC prospectively studied by ECOG, in which eligibility and availability were standardized for all patients. Furthermore, the 301 North American patients and the 131 South African patients received similar treatment at the same time.[147]

Factors that had the most significant adverse effect on survival were impaired performance status, male sex, older age, and the presence of jaundice and reduced appetite. Cirrhosis by itself was associated with poorer survival but, viewed relative to sex and age, lost its statistical significance. Country of origin, but not race, was significant; North American patients had a longer survival. The importance can be seen in the following example: For patients with a good performance status, a South African man older than 45 years of age, with jaundice and reduced appetite, has a 5% probability of surviving 6 months, but a North American woman younger than 45 years of age, without jaundice or loss of appetite, has a 68% chance of surviving 6 months. The median survival time of the 432 ECOG patients was 14 weeks. Patients with a performance status of 4, with renal insufficiency or with any evidence of encephalopathy, were not entered into the study. The overall median survival time of all patients with advanced HCC was therefore even shorter.

In a French study, prognostic factors for 127 untreated patients were analyzed.[148] The median survival time was 73 days; four of these untreated patients survived longer than 1 year. A survival time longer than 60 days was seen in only 1 of 25 patients with evidence of encephalopathy. Predictive of very poor prognosis were encephalopathy, alcohol consumption, and elevated AFP, BUN, and bilirubin levels. The authors conclude that the natural history of patients with HCC in France shows no difference from those in Asia or Africa. Malaysian patients had a survival time between that of North American and South African patients.[160]

Although HBV infection has not been shown to have prognostic significance, a growing body of evidence suggests that North American and European patients without cirrhosis have a better prognosis than do patients in the high-incidence areas for cirrhosis of Africa and most of Asia.[33] In Pretoria, Simson's postmortem studies highlight the importance of membranous occlusion of the hepatic veins and demonstrate the paradoxical finding that survival is poorer for patients without cirrhosis than for those patients with cirrhosis.[90] It is important, therefore, to have ongoing Phase II trials in different parts of the world, in which standard eligibility criteria are used to compensate for known and unknown factors.

In evaluating clinical trials of HCC, certain rules must be observed: histologic confirmation of the diagnosis, proper stratification by important prognostic variables, and inclusion of all patients in the study for response and survival data. Early deaths should not be excluded.

Unfortunately, most of the literature on the treatment of HCC consists of uncontrolled trials with selected patients that do not take into account any of the above factors. Although important information can be gained from these trials, the results must be interpreted both in the light of selection factors, purposeful or not, and of exclusion factors.

Determination of Tumor Response

The criteria for objective response are as follows: *Complete response* is the absence of any clinically detectable tumor mass (*i.e.*, normal physical examination, liver chemistries, appropriate radiographic studies, and normal AFP if elevated before therapy); and a *partial response* is a reduction by at least 50% of the product of the largest perpendicular diameters of the most clearly measurable lesions, with no increase in any other indicator lesion, and the absence of new areas of malignant disease. If hepatomegaly is the primary indicator, there must be a reduction by at least 30% of the sum of liver measurements below each costal margin at the midclavicular line and xyphoid process. For complete and partial responses, there can be no significant deterioration in weight or performance status.

Survival time is the best objective measure of the effects of treatment in patients with HCC, but it is important to include patients who do not complete the prescribed program.

Single Agents

In controlled studies, no alkylating agent has been found to be of value in the treatment of patients with primary liver cancer. Response rates with these drugs are less than 10%, and median survival times are comparable to those achieved with placebos.[148–150] Various antimetabolites have been tested, and none have proved useful as single agents in the treatment of patients with HCC.[151–160,171] Data on single-agent results for 5-fluorouracil and dichloromethotrexate are given in Table 27-12. None of the plant alkaloids have been shown to be of value, nor has diaminodichloroplatinum (DDP).[161–168]

Various antibiotics and related substances have been tested, but none have been shown to be of definite value in controlled studies.[11,160,164,169–187] Data from the longer series of patients treated with doxorubicin, idarubicin, epirubicin, esorubicin, mitoxantrone, and neocarzinostatin are shown in Table 27-12.

Other diverse agents have been tested, including hormones, and biological response modifiers, but none have proved to be of clinical value.[162,170,188–201]

TABLE 27-12. Liver Cancer: Single-Agent Studies with ≥10 Patients

Agent	*No. of Patients*	*No. of Responses*	*Mean Survival (mo)*	*Author, Year*	*Reference*
5-Fluorouracil					
IV	19	2		Brennan, 1964	154
	16	0	2	Gailani, 1972	150
	10	1	5	Davis, 1974	153
Oral	9	0	2	Link, 1977	158
	12	6		Kennedy, 1977	159
	45	0	2	Falkson, 1978	172
Doxorubicin	13	2	3	Ihde, 1977	174
	41	7		Vogel, 1977	173
	44	14	3	Johnson, 1978	177
	74	22		Olweny, 1980	176
	31	8	4	Melia, 1983	164
	12	0	3	Barbare, 1984	179
	52	6	4	Chlebowski, 1984	175
	45	11	3	Choi, 1984	180
	63	6	3	Falkson, 1978–1984	170, 171
	109	1	4	Sciarrino, 1985	178
Idarubicin	15	0		Cheng, 1985	183
Epirubicin	18	3	3	Hochster, 1985	181
	17	0	4	Shiu, 1986	182
Esorubicin	35	3	3	Perry, 1987	167
Mitoxantrone	19	2	3	Falkson, 1984	185
	33	3	>4	Davis, 1986	184
	34	0	<3	Falkson, 1987	187
Neocarzinostatin	28	2	3	Falkson, 1980	169
	30	7	2	Falkson, 1984	170
m-AMSA	35	1	3	Falkson, 1981	189
	23	3	5	Bukowski, 1982	190
	16	0		Cheng, 1983	191
	20	1		Amrein, 1984	192
	24	0	3	Falkson, 1984	170
CDDP	13	1		Melia, 1981	166
	20	1	2	Ravry, 1986	168
	35	2	<3	Falkson, 1987	187
VP-16	25	3	<3	Cavalli, 1981	163
	24	3	2	Melia, 1983	164
DCMTX	17	1		Vogel, 1972	151

TABLE 27-13. Liver Cancer: Combination Chemotherapy in Series with ≥10 Patients

Agent	*No. of Patients*	*No. of Responses*	*Mean Survival (mo)*	*Author, Year*	*Reference*
5-FU + Ara C	22	1	2	Gailani, 1972	156
5-FU + BCNU	14	1		McIntire, 1976	202
5-FU PO + MeCCNU	44	2	<3	Falkson, 1978	172
5-FU PO + MeCCNU	20	4	4	Joishy, 1982	160
5-FU IV + MeCCNU	55	7	<3	Falkson, 1984	171
5-FU + MMC	13	5	2	Umsawasdi, 1978	203
5-FU + STZ	33	4	<3	Falkson, 1978	172
5-FU + STZ	49	4	<3	Falkson, 1984	171
5-FU + MTX, CYT, VCR	10	0	5	Cochrane, 1977	206
5-FU + MTX, CYT, VCR	19	0	1	Choi, 1984	180
DOX + 5-FU	38	5	3	Baker, 1977	207
DOX + DCMTX	12	1		Olweny, 1980	176
DOX + PRED	17	6	4	Oon, 1980	208
DOX + 5-FU, PRED, VCR	17	5	4	Oon, 1980	208
DOX + MeCCNU	21	3	3	Chlebowski, 1981	209
DOX + 5-FU, VM-26	36	16		Bezwoda, 1982	210
DOX + STZ	23	2	3	Morstyn, 1983	211
DOX + 5-FU, MeCCNU	38	8	3	Falkson, 1984	171
DOX + BLEO	49	8	2	Ravry, 1984	212
DOX + 5-FU, MMC	40	5	2	Al-Idrissi, 1985	213

*5-FU = 5-fluorouracil; Ara C = cytarabine; BCNU = carmustine; MeCCNU = methyl-lomustine; MMC = mitomycin-c; ST2 = streptozotocin; CYT = cyclophosphamide; VCR = vincristine; DOX = doxorubicin; PRED = prednisone; VM-26 = teniposide; BLEO = bleomycin.

TABLE 27-14. Liver Cancer: Chemotherapy Overview by Agent Class

Agent	*Response*	*Reference*
Alkylating Agents		
Cyclophosphamide, triethyleneglycol diglycidylether, alanine mustard, DL-serine bis (2-chloropropyl) carbamate ester, chlorethylcyclohexylnitrosourea, chloroethyl-methyl-cyclohexyl-nitrosourea	Response rates are less than 10% and median survival time is comparable to that achieved with placebo	149, 150
Antimetabolites		
Methotrexate Dichloromethotrexate 6-Mercaptopurine Hydroxyurea Cytosine-arabinoside 5-Fluorouracil	Various antimetabolites have been tested; none have proved of value as single agents	151–159, 196
Plant Alkaloids		
Vinblastine SPG 827 (podophyllin derivative) VP-16-213 (etoposide)	Vinblastine and SPG 827 of no therapeutic value; variable response for etoposide ranging from median survival of 22 weeks in one trial to no survival advantage in other trials;	161–165
Antibiotics and Related Substances		
Mitomycin-C Actinomycin-D Carzinophyllin Chromomycin-A_3 Neocarzinostatin	No value shown for mitomycin-C, actinomycin-D, carzinophyllin or chromomycin-A_3; neocarzinostatin showed response in 2/25 patients and median survival time of 11 weeks in one clinical trial	169–170
Doxorubicin		
Doxorubicin 4′-Epidoxorubicin Oral demethoxydaunorubicin Mitoxantrone Menogaril	For doxorubicin, clinical trials report response rates of 17%, 15%, 11%; for all patients in all trials median survival is less than 4 months; other analogues have been equally ineffective	171–186
Other Agents		
Dehydroemitine, Procarbazine, cobalt proporphyrin complex, Butyryloxyethylglyoxal Dithiosemicarbazone, [4′-(9-Acridinlyamino)-methanesulphon-m-anisidide] (m-AMSA) Acivin Alpha-interferon Gamma-interferon Beta-interferon	No therapeutic responses for all agents; minimal response rates for m-AMSA	166, 168, 170, 187–195
Cis-diamino-dichloroplatinum (DDP)	DDP shows little or no effect	166, 168, 187
Hormone Treatment		
Magesterol acetate Tamoxifen Cyproterone acetate Buserelin	No beneficial results for these agents, although the anti-androgen cyproterone acetate shows some promise in HCC patients with cirrhosis; the gonadotrophic agonist, Buserelin, is in clinical trials but is not yet evaluable	197–101
Combination Chemotherapies and Chemotherapy/Radiotherapy Combinations		
Vincristine (VCR) + methotrexate (MTX) + 6-mercaptopurine (6MP) + prednisone (Pred); BCNU + cytosine-arabinoside; 5-FU + thiotepa; 5-FU + mitomycin C (MMC); 5-FU + cyclophosphamide (CTX) + MTX + VCR; 5-FU + ara-C; 5-FU + MeCCNU; 5-FU + streptozotocin; Doxorubicin (ADM) + 5-FU; ADM + 5-FU + Pred + VCR; ADM + MeCCNU; ADM + 5-FU + VM26; ADM + STZ; ADM + bleomycin; ADM + 5-FU + MMC; radiotherapy (RT) + 5-FU + CTX + MTX + VCR; RT + intra-arterial 5-FU + ADM; RT + MTX or MMC + 5-FU + ADM.	No response or limited response in combination chemotherapies with high toxicity in 5-FU studies; chemoradiotherapies show no survival differences with combined chemotherapies	156, 171–172, 176, 180, 202–203, 206–213

Combination Chemotherapy

With few exceptions, it has been shown that nothing is gained by adding cytostatics that do not have single-agent activity to a drug combination regimen. This procedure leads to increased toxicity, necessitating a decrease in the amount of the therapeutically active agents that can be given at the same time. Various small series of uncontrolled trials of drug combinations in patients with primary liver cancer are reported in the literature, in which patient selection was ignored and the results can be explained by variations in the natural history of the disease.

None of the combination treatments have given results superior to single agents in clinical trials.[11,157,180,202–213] The response and the survival for larger series of patients treated with 5-fluorouracil (5-FU) or doxorubicin combinations are given in Table 27-13. An overview of the response to chemotherapy by agent class is shown in Table 27-14.

Chemoradiation Therapy

Combination treatment with chemotherapy and radiotherapy has been tried in various smaller series. Procarbazine and radiotherapy were randomly compared to other treatments and placebo and not found to be effective; nor was radiotherapy combined with 5-FU, cyclophosphamide (CTX), methotrexate (MTX), and vincristine (VCR).[11,206] Early trials of radiotherapy and intra-arterial (IA) 5-FU and doxorubicin (ADM) did give promising results, as did radiotherapy with MTX or mitomycin C in addition to 5-FU and ADM.[214–216] In a larger trial, no survival improvement was reported for patients given radiotherapy only or given radiotherapy with mitomycin C, ADM, and 5-FU given intra-arterially or intravenously.[215,225]

Status of Chemotherapy

Until better response rates can be documented for single agents or there is sufficient rationale for combination chemotherapy in patients with HCC, physicians cannot justify treating small groups of patients with combination of poorly active agents. The recommended approach is to have well-designed Phase II trials of new agents. The expanding knowledge about HCC as a disease may promote better clinical trials. Even in Phase II trials, patient discriminants such as age, sex, performance status, and country of origin are important. It may also be important to stratify patient categories according to type of HCC: normal and cirrhotic or precirrhotic patterns; encapsulated hepatocellular carcinomas (common in Japan), excluding the status of hepatitis B viral infection, and fibrosing varieties of expanding types of HCC, including fibrolamellar HCC. Although no cytostatic has shown reproducible response rates of 20% or more in patients with HCC, at least agents with occasional activity can be selected over others that are totally inactive.

Hepatic Artery Infusion

Although careful postmortem examination shows that metastases occur in the vast majority of patients with HCC, liver disease dominates the clinical picture in most of the patients, and only 25% of patients have extrahepatic metastases at the time of diagnosis. This has motivated attempts at regional chemotherapy. Results of treatment by hepatic artery infusion appear better than they are because of selection factors. In 1968, optimism was justified because early results seemed promising.[218] In 1970, continuous intra-arterial MTX was shown to be superior to intra-arterial 5-FU.[219] The median survival time of these selected patients was 375 days for the group treated intra-arterially with MTX, 118 days for 5-FU, and 55 days for the control group. The controls were patients who met the selection criteria for intraoperative placement of the catheter in the hepatic artery. Despite this survival difference, this form of treatment was not regarded as practical or advisable. No other controlled studies comparing intra-arterial to systemic chemotherapy or to no treatment have been done despite numerous publications on intra-arterial fluorinated pyrimidines and on intra-arterial doxorubicin in patients with HCC.[153,157,220–225]

No evidence from any of these studies supports the contention that intra-arterial treatment prolongs survival, nor is there evidence of a change in prognosis after intra-arterial HN_2, dichloromethotrexate, mitomycin C, or cisplatin.[226,227] Optimistic claims have been made and 50% response rates have been quoted for these therapies.[228–231] These series consist of selected patients with good pathologic discriminants. Most of the studies of intra-arterial chemotherapy require that the patients have adequate enough performance status to tolerate a laparotomy for placing the catheter, no distal metastases, and adequate liver function. With these preconditions, the median survival time should be good because these known prognostic factors give a 50% chance of surviving 1 year. The total number of patients with HCC seen was also not given.

Although adequate pharmacologic rationale for intra-arterial treatment is available, the clinical case remains to be proved. Intra-arterial chemotherapy is only indicated in a clinical trial setting if it is compared with systemic treatment and if *all* patients, including postoperative and early deaths, entered on the study are included in the denominator. These results of intra-arterial cytostatics in HCC are similar to those for patients with liver metastases from colon cancer. Local tumor shrinkage does occur, but considerable toxicity and morbidity and even mortality are associated with this approach, even in selected patients with good prognostic features.

In a randomized study comparing intra-arterial cytostatics and hepatic artery ligation with hepatic artery ligation and partial vein infusion with symptomatic treatment, no difference in survival between treated and untreated patients was observed.[232] Hepatic artery ligation was performed in a large series of patients with HCC in Mozambique before 1978, with disastrous results in this African population with advanced disease.[233] More recent experience has been more optimistic, with both simple ligation of the hepatic artery and selective arterial ligation to the specific lobe where the tumor is located and with total hepatic dearterialization.[176,231,232]

Hepatic arterial occlusion has been used with MTX, 5-FU, doxorubicin, and mitomycin C.[176,232,234–240] Causes of death included hepatic failure and hepatorenal syndrome. Various refinements in techniques, such as intermittent occlusion of the hepatic artery, selective transcatheter embolization, and introduction of Gelfoam or Ivalon particles have been introduced.[241–243]

Particles to which doxorubicin, mitomycin C, or a combination of mitomycin C, fluorodeoxyuridine (FudR), and doxorubicin have been added have been tried.[242,243] Neocarzinostatin suspended in a lipid lymphographic agent and injected into the arterial system has been tried in Japan.[245] Definite tumor necrosis can be produced by injecting ethiodol or lipiodol with doxorubicin, with or without nimustine hydrochloride (ACNU).[246,247] Intra-arterial BCNU has been given with starch microspheres.[248] In Japan, where resection is more often possible because of the nature of the disease, intra-arterial embolization and chemotherapy are being used as neoadjuvant therapy.[249–251]

Intra-arterial therapy by continuous infusion or by microspheres, with or without hepatic arterial occlusion, has many enthusiastic followers. In the absence of controlled clinical trials in which all patients entered on the study are evaluated, there can be no real assessment of its value.

A problem has already arisen in that intra-arterial doxorubicin is considered to be effective treatment. In a study on 64 patients with nonresectable HCC treated with intra-arterial epirubicin, tumor size was evaluated only in 53 patients, 8 of whom had objective improvement. The reported response rate was 15.1% but should have been 12.5%. The median survival time of 205 days was compared with the historic survival time obtained with intra-arterial doxorubicin. It was concluded that the epirubicin was more effective than doxorubicin in the intra-arterial treatment of nonresectable HCC.[252] As with systemic treatment, the results of the different intra-arterial treatments can be interpreted only in terms of the HCC subtype and the patient's prognostic factors.[253]

RADIATION

Evaluation for Radiotherapy

The distinctions between diffuse or nodular patterns of HCC are important for any review of the role of CT in hepatocellular cancer. A widely dispersed, nonmarginated, diffuse tumor is not only nonresectable, but also unlikely to have sufficient tumor remission to be resectable.[254] In contrast, nonresectable massive nodular disease with clear margins on CT scans can be converted to a resectable state by new techniques.[254,255] Similarly, multifocal, nodular, clearly demarcated patterns of HCC can be converted to a resectable state by new treatment modalities that include external radiation, sensitizing drugs, and radiolabeled antiferritin.[254]

In the past, a partial response of HCC was defined to be at least a 30% reduction in the sum of liver measurements below each costal margin at the midclavicular lines and the xyphoid process.[256] The dorsal to ventral dimension could not be obtained accurately by clinical measurement. CT scans in 8-mm sections now allow total reconstruction of the entire liver volume. Pixels may then be examined to determine density. Standardization of the pixels before scanning each patient provides uniform analysis and a more accurate comparison of results. When all pixels from the entire CT series are analyzed, a bimodal pattern of density is established for tumor and for normal tissue (Fig. 27-8). This more

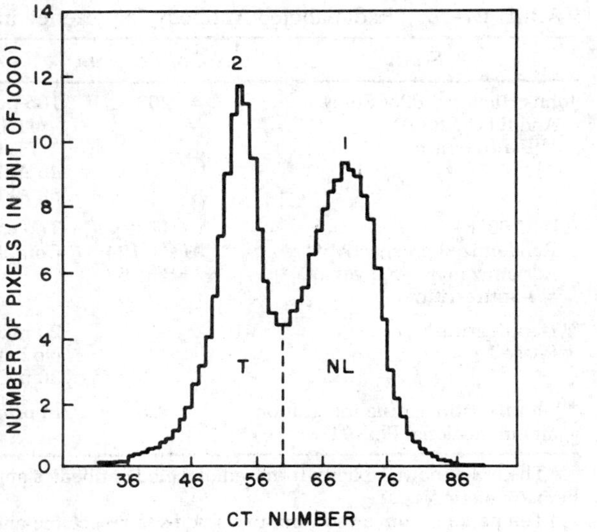

FIG. 27-8. When all of the pixels from the entire computerized axial tomographic series are analyzed, a bimodal pattern of density is established for tumor and another for normal tissue. This more accurate method to determine tumor volumetrics was originally designed from the dosimetry of radiolabeled antibody which requires tumor volumetrics. (Yang N-C, Leichner PK, Fishman EK et al: CT volumetrics of primary liver cancers. J Comput Assist Tomogr 10:621–628, 1986. Used with permission of Raven Press)

FIG. 27-9. Hepatocellular cancer with chronic active hepatitis. Note that with modest tumor reduction there is a greater normal liver reduction. The top line indicates the total liver volume, the intermediate line indicates normal liver volume, and the bottom line indicates the tumor volume. The reduced normal liver tolerance when chronic active hepatitis is an underlying disease is characteristic. See new methods of evaluation for tumor volumetrics and normal liver volumetrics. Compare normal liver volumetrics to Figure 27-10.

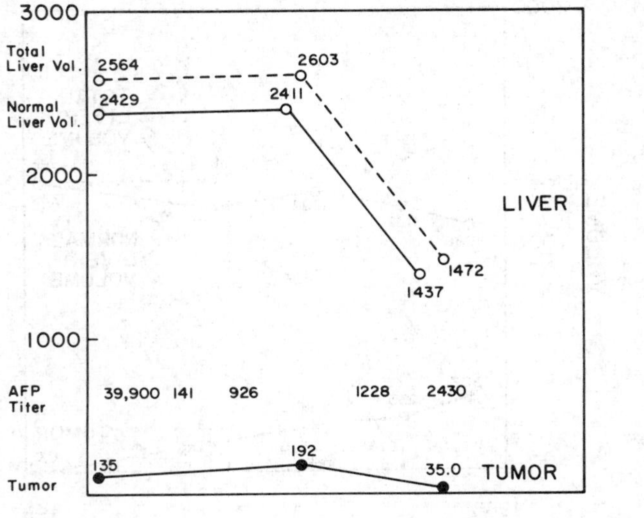

TABLE 27-15. Radiolabeled Antibody Experience in Hepatoma*

Study	*No. of Patients*	*Results*
Johns Hopkins' Pilot Study And RTOG 83-01 ^{131}I-antiferritin	263	105 patients reported 41% PR 7% CR 46 AFP+: 5 months median survival 59 AFP−: 10.5 month median survival
RTOG 83-19 Randomized prospective† Adriamycin + 5-FU versus ^{131}I-antiferritin	177 AFP+ 124 AFP− 53	Too early to evaluate Completion expected 1.5 years
^{90}Y-antiferritin* Phase I	15	20 mCi Yttrium No hematologic toxicity† 30 mCi grade 3
^{90}Y-antiferritin + drug integration and monoclonal Phase I	25	In progress

*The only known toxicity from radiolabeled antibodies applied to hepatocellular cancer has been hematopoietic.
†Ten patients converted from two studies to resectable and NED.

accurate method was originally designed for the dosimetry of radiolabeled antibody, which requires tumor volumetrics.[257]

The pragmatic application of tumor volumetrics for progression and remission analysis has become a valuable tool in determining patient response to therapy (Fig. 27-9).[258] Tumors of varying sizes cannot be quantitatively analyzed in terms of percentage of remission. If two tumors weighing 500 g and 2500 g regressed by 30%, the reduction would be 150 g and 750 g, respectively. From the viewpoint of applied cytotoxic therapy, more quantitative analyses offer better and more accurate appreciation of a given modality than does percent reduction. As use of the computer program becomes more pervasive in the major medical centers, a clearer understanding of the cytoreductive power of agents used to treat HCC will emerge.[257,258]

External Radiation

Radiation doses greater than 3000 rad within 3 weeks have caused radiation hepatitis.[259] In the treatment of metastatic lesions, 2100 rad was successful in achieving partial remission. This dose was later integrated with Adriamycin and 5-FU in the treatment of metastatic liver disease.[260–262] This same combination was then used as an induction therapy for a multimodality treatment program and achieved a 15% partial remission rate during the treatment course.[75] A variety of other radiation sources, including yttrium-90 microspheres and ^{131}ethiodol, have been proposed, but without meaningful dosimetry.[263–265]

FIG. 27-10. A 22-year-old woman, AFP negative, with no underlying pathology and with recurrent nonresectable nodular hepatocellular cancer. Volumetrics demonstrate total liver volume, normal liver volume, and tumor volume following radiolabeled antibody treatment.

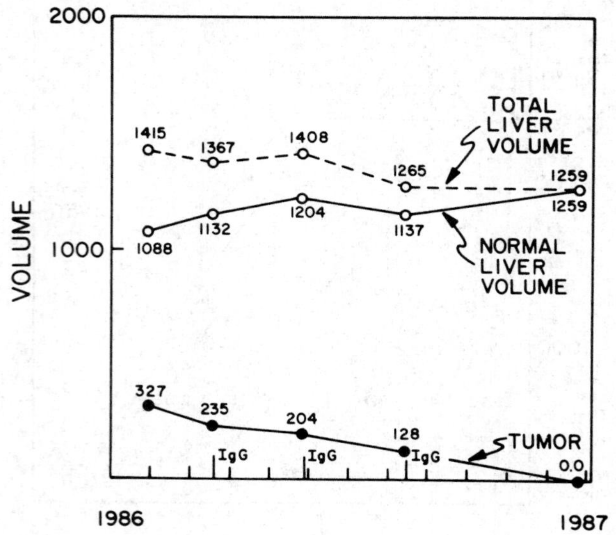

FIG. 27-11. An 83-year-old man with nodular massive nonresectable AFP negative hepatocellular cancer treated with multiple courses of ^{131}I-antiferritin radiolabeled antibodies.

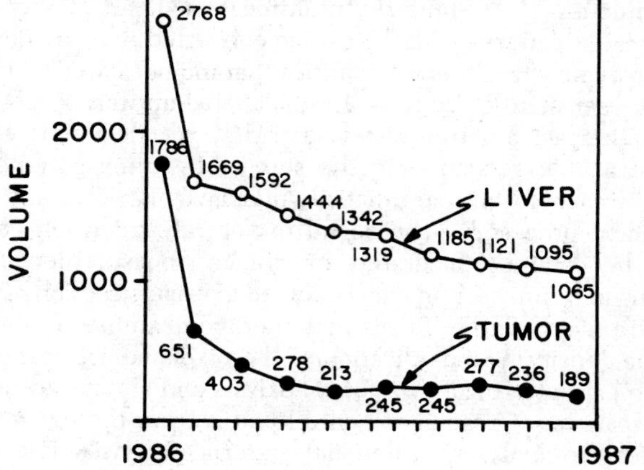

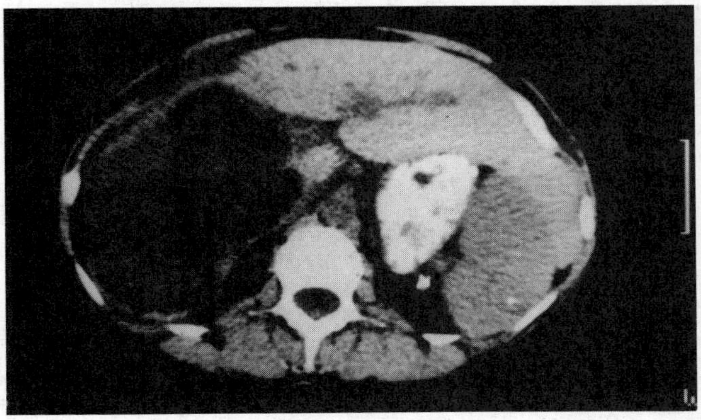

A

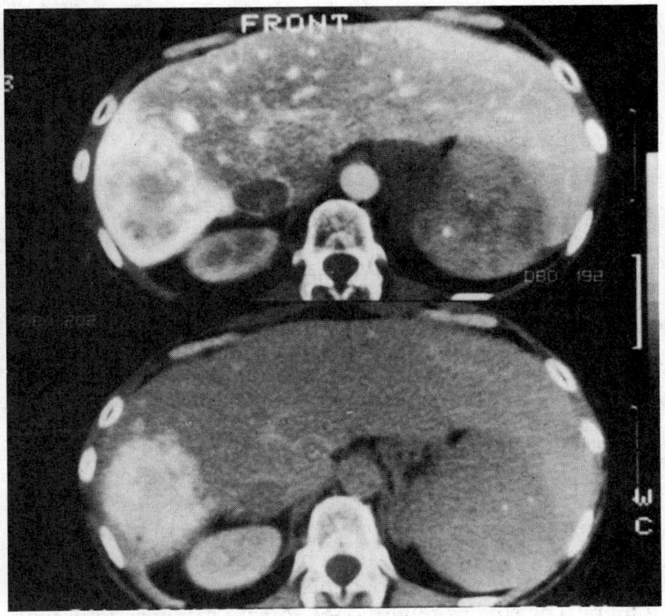

B

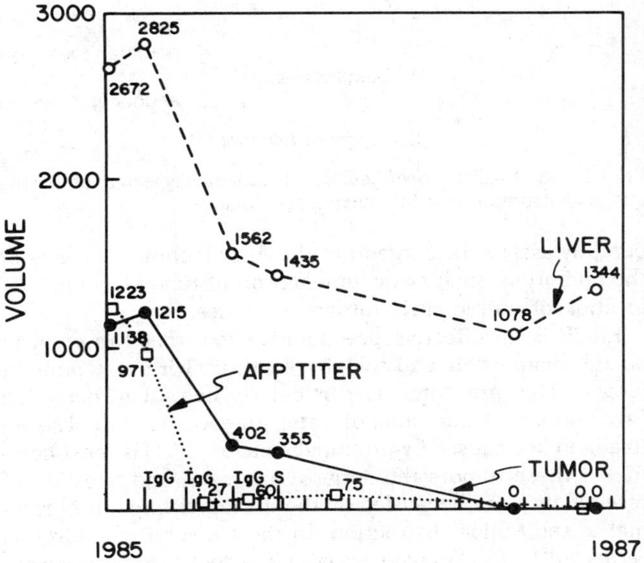

C

FIG. 27-12. **A**. A 56-year-old woman with nodular massive nonresectable AFP positive hepatocellular cancer with presenting computed tomogram. Bracket at right represents 5 cm. **B**. After treatment, the arteriographic computed tomographic arterial and venous phase before resection. Bracket at right represents 5 cm. **C**. Total liver, tumor volumetrics, and AFP titer of this patient converted from nonresectable to resectable. The patient remains disease-free. (Sitzman JV, Order SE, Klein JL et al: Conversion by new treatment modalities of nonresectable to resectable hepatocellular cancer. J Clin Oncol 5:1566–1578, 1987. Reproduced with permission of Grune & Stratton)

Radioactive Antibodies

HCC was known to produce ferritin.[266] This protein, normally associated with iron storage, is in the apoferritin form (*i.e.*, lacking iron) and is produced ubiquitously by a variety of malignancies.[266,267] The finding that selective tumor deposition of ^{131}I-antiferritin occurred due to increased tumor vascular permeability was described both in experimental models and in clinical investigation.[268–272] Tumor saturation, the dose of ^{131}I-antiferritin that binds accessible tumor ferritin, and the tumor effective half-life of 3 to 4 days led to the development of this new agent.[75] Two intravenous infusions led to a median dose of 1100 to 1200 rad and were later integrated with 15 mg of Adriamycin and 500 mg of 5-fluorouracil, which acted as potential sensitizers.[75] The newest laboratory information indicates that Adriamycin shifts the tumor cells into G2 and early M, both positions in the cell cycle in which increased radiosensitivity has been reported.[269]

The initial experience in 105 patients indicated an advantageous response in AFP-negative patients, who had a median survival of 10.5 months, and no significant difference from conventional therapy in AFP-positive patients, who had a median survival of 5 months.[75] The conversion from nonresectable to resectable disease in patients with nodular massive or nodular multifocal HCC has offered new treatment possibilities (Table 27-15; Figs. 27-10, 27-11, and 27-12).[254] The modification in China of the ^{131}I-antiferritin therapy by intra-arterial infusion was also followed by partial wedge resections in patients with macronodular HCC.[75] In both limited series of patients, an elevated serum AFP level was not a distinguishing factor because conversion to a resectable state occurred in patients with and without elevated AFP levels.[254,273]

Currently under investigation is the use of ^{90}Y, which is a more powerful beta-emitting isotope than ^{131}I (0.3 MeV versus 0.9 MeV).[271,272,274] Yttrium-90 has demonstrated remissions of metastatic lesions and primary HCC.[272,274]

The influence of radiolabeled antibody treatment on complete remissions, conversions to resectability, and remissions of metastasis indicate that more should be expected from further clinical research with them. Iodine-131-anti-

AFP has been reported by some investigators to have therapeutic activity, but others have not been able to document significant tumor deposition.[275,276] It would be reasonable to expect that Adriamycin, cis-platinum, and 5-FU may act as sensitizing agents for radiolabeled antibodies.[277,277a,278]

INTRAHEPATIC BILIARY CANCER

Intrahepatic biliary cancer occurs less frequently than extrahepatic Klatskin's tumor, and it represents about 0.5% of primary liver tumors in the United States. In contrast to extrahepatic bile duct cancer, this tumor has an associated significant neovasculature, produces CEA, and may be treated with ^{131}I-anti-CEA to achieve a partial remission. In 37 patients, a 25.9% partial remission and 7.4% complete remission rates were achieved.[279] These results took 8 years to accumulate, indicating the rarity of the disorder. It was also observed that elevated AFP levels do not distinguish hepatoma from intrahepatic cholangiocarcinoma because there are AFP-positive patients with intrahepatic biliary tumors. The studies reported 9% to 14% response rates with 14-day to 4-month median survivals. Overall, the median survival was 6.5 months, and the 33% of patients who responded to therapy demonstrated a median survival of 15.2 months.[279]

BILIARY TRACT CANCER

Primary malignancies of the biliary tract were first described by Fardel in 1890 with a subsequent description by Courvoisier in the last decade of the 19th century.[280,281] Baudoin performed the first biliary enteric bypass of a biliary malignancy in 1896, and in 1903 Mayo reported the first successful resection.[282,283]

The autopsy frequency of bile duct carcinoma is approximately 0.01 to 0.46%, and carcinoma is found in approximately 1 of every 200 operations involving the biliary tree.[284,285]

DIAGNOSIS

The clinical presentation of the patient with cancer of the bile duct is usually painless jaundice. Fatigue, pruritus, fever, and nonspecific abdominal pain are frequent accompanying findings.[286,287] Laboratory findings are often nonspecific. Hemoglobin, leukocyte counts, and serum electrolyte values are usually unaltered. Liver function tests reflect obstructive jaundice in more than 80% of cases.[286–288] A variety of diagnostic measures are available, and an orderly sequence is noted (Fig. 27-13).

Ultrasound is the simplest noninvasive test that can suggest extrahepatic biliary obstruction by confirming the presence of dilatation of intrahepatic biliary ducts.[289]

Cholangiography is the next consideration, and the options include endoscopic retrograde cholangiography (ERCP), percutaneous transhepatic cholangiography (PTC), or intraoperative cholangiography. Careful preoperative cholangiography is helpful in assessing the resectability of tumors and in planning the operative approach. Intraoperative cholangiography assists the surgeon in the finer technical aspects of the operation, such as documentation of tube placement or location of multicentric tumors or stones.

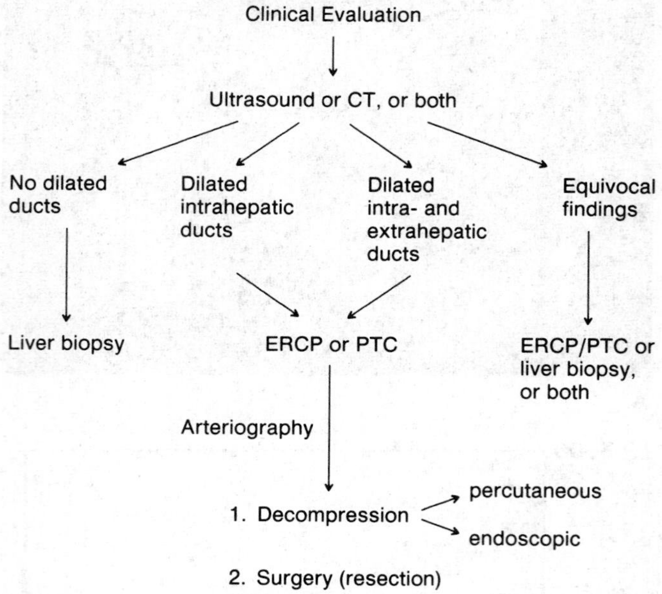

FIG. 27-13. Evaluation of jaundiced patient suspected of having cholangiocarcinoma or bile duct carcinoma.

ERCP is an effective preoperative tool that can confirm ductal anatomy and histologic diagnosis with concomitant biopsy. This procedure is particularly helpful in detecting carcinoma of the ampulla of Vater. In patients with obstructive jaundice caused by proximal cancers, PTC is most helpful. In these tumors the surgical approach and question of resectability can be settled by the ductal architecture proximal to the tumor obstruction. In the University of Virginia series, all 16 PTC in patients with bile duct carcinomas were interpreted as abnormal, and 15 (94%) were diagnosed as consistent with "malignancy." Although three patients (18%) had complications, none were fatal.[286] Elias and colleagues conducted a prospective randomized comparison of ERCP and PTC in jaundiced patients and concluded that both techniques had similar diagnostic accuracy.[291] PTC can also provide effective decompression of the biliary system and normalization of liver function test findings. PTC requires that any clotting abnormalities be corrected before the procedure.

Arteriography is not routinely used in the preoperative workup of obstructive jaundice but may be used for diagnosis in more difficult or confusing cases and in those cases in which resection is contemplated. The findings of neovascu-

TABLE 27-16A. Bile Duct Cancer (The UCLA Experience)

Laboratory Finding	*Mean*	*% Abnormal*
Alkaline phosphatase (U)	582	94
Total bilirubin (mg/dl)	17.4	84
SGOT (IU)	96	55
SGPT (IU)	121	50
Creatinine (mg/dl)	1.1	10
Albumin (g/dl)	3.3	52

TABLE 27-16B. Bile Duct Cancer (The UCLA Experience)

Test	1954–1978 No. Performed	1954–1978 Accuracy (%)	1979–1983 No. Performed	1979–1983 Accuracy (%)
Ultrasound	9	56	35	91
CT scan	0		19	95
Transhepatic cholangiogram	13	100	33	100
Transjugular cholangiogram	12	100	0	
ERCP	7	43	12	92

larity, major arterial encasement, or occlusion can lead to evaluation of nonresectability, particularly in tumors located in or near the hilum.[287] Late-phase arteriography allows visualization of the portal system and its relation to the neoplasm. Percutaneous transhepatic portography with direct cannulation of the portal system can also be done to evaluate tumor invasion.[292] The sensitivity of diagnostic measures is shown in Table 27-16, A and B.

Voyles and co-workers reported their experience with cholangiography and arteriography (with late-phase portography) in evaluation of the resectability of tumors of the proximal biliary tree.[293] All 37 patients in the study received PTC, and 20 received arteriography. Of the tumors, 32% were judged unresectable by cholangiography; 54% were judged unresectable by cholangiography and arteriography; and 65% were judged unresectable by cholangiography, arteriography, and "clinical considerations." Only 7 patients (18.9%) underwent resection. This represented 38.5% of those predicted to be unresectable and 8.3% of the patients whose tumors were predicted to be unresectable. The authors concluded that cholangiography with arteriography can predict resectability with a high degree of certainty and perhaps present laparotomy if cytological diagnosis can be confirmed by transcutaneous biopsy.

Although CT was not evaluated in the study, it can evaluate the hepatic parenchyma for other space-occupying lesions or metastases. In addition, CT allows a more precise evaluation of the head of the pancreas, which is important because carcinoma in this location is a common lesion.[287,294] Percutaneous needle aspiration for cytodiagnosis may also be done and may obviate laparotomy in those patients judged to be unresectable by preoperative studies. A fine needle can be advanced into the tumor under ultrasound or CT guidance. Evander and colleagues reported a 53% correct diagnosis in biliary tract and pancreatic carcinoma.[295] There were no false positives and no complications. This technique should probably not be performed in patients planned for resection because there is potential for tumor growth along the needle tract.[296]

Selected radiologic procedures in the patient with obstructive jaundice should allow a 90% to 95% accurate diagnosis of the malignancy of the biliary tract. Ultrasound is the first choice, and, if intrahepatic biliary dilatation is observed, PTC or fine-needle aspiration for cytodiagnosis can effectively be used for tissue evaluation and hepatic decompression. In some centers, ERCP has proved most useful in diagnosis of malignancy in the distal biliary tree. ERCP, CT, and arteriography can be used for evaluation of more confusing or difficult cases.

MANAGEMENT

Percutaneous Transhepatic Catheter

PTC drainage procedures can be effective diagnostic tools. In addition, PTC can provide internal or external drainage with biliary decompression of partial or complete obstructions. With proper hygiene and attention to catheter care, a patient can maintain a biliary catheter and provide decompression for many months.[287]

Resection of hilar tumors is often impossible. An alternative approach in such cases is to provide satisfactory drainage of bile through the occluding tumor.[308–311] In the past, this was accomplished by dilatation of the tumor and insertion of the proximal limb of a T tube through the tumor into the proximal duct so that the distal limb provided drainage into the common bile duct. Two additional techniques have been described and are probably superior to simple T tubes. Terblanche and colleagues suggested the use of the U tube for palliation of bile duct tumors.[311] The U tube is a Silastic tube passed into the distal common duct through the tumor and out the hepatic parencyhma proximally through the affected right or left hepatic duct. Each end of the tube is brought out through the abdominal wall. This apparatus can provide both internal and external drainage. An advantage of this tube is that it can be changed percutaneously as necessary.

Cameron and co-workers suggested stenting bile duct tumors and benign strictures with Silastic tubing introduced transhepatically into the common bile duct.[308–310] In addition to providing satisfactory splinting of the obstruction, only one tube remains external, and it can be easily changed over a guide wire. The rationale for employing stents is that primary bile duct carcinomas often do not metastasize to distant sites and the tumors may remain small for extended periods. Because the primary causes of death are the sequelae of obstructive jaundice, significant palliation may be achieved by biliary decompression, with prolongation of life and relief of the aggravating symptoms of obstructive jaundice. Stenting in particular is applicable for proximal bile duct cancers that are not resectable.[308–310]

In some cases, the bile ducts may be satisfactorily drained by hepaticojejunostomy using the approach to the left duct described by Blumgart or by intrahepatic cholangiojejunostomy.[312–316] For lesions in the common duct, resection should be employed.[317–322] The proximity of the hepatic artery and portal vein to these lesions, however, frequently limits the extent or possibility of resection because of direct invasion. If the lesion in the mid-duct is unresectable, palliation can be achieved by insertion of a stent or by performing a biliary enteric anastomosis. A Roux-en-Y jejunal anastomosis to the duct proximal to the tumor is the preferred approach.[308,309] For lesions of the distal duct that are resectable, pancreaticoduodenectomy is the preferred treatment.[317–322] For distal lesions that are not resectable, a bypass procedure, either cholecystojejunostomy or choledochojejunostomy, is preferable.

Preoperative decompression is a matter of debate. In 1978, Nakayama and co-workers suggested that a period of preoperative biliary decompression might improve liver function and the nutritional status, thereby decreasing morbidity and mortality of surgery for obstructive jaundice.[297] Although this view was held by many surgeons, Norlander and colleagues reported no significant difference in postoperative mortality patients with obstructive jaundice caused by benign or malignant processes.[298] Results continue to be mixed.[299] A recent report by Denning strongly suggests that preoperative decompression does lower surgical morbidity, but not mortality, for surgery for malignancies in the biliary tract.[300] MacPherson and co-workers reported a prospective randomized trial in Great Britain that entered 65 patients with obstructive jaundice.[301] Of these, 31 patients underwent exploration and were compared with 34 who received drainage for a mean duration of 18 days before exploration. Hospitalization was prolonged for the drainage group (40 versus 24 days). The mortality rate was 19% (6 of 31) for the laparotomy group and 32% (11 of 34) for the drainage group. The authors concluded that preoperative percutaneous biliary drainage fails to improve the mortality rate in patients treated surgically for obstructive jaundice.[301] More recently, Pitt and colleagues reported a prospective randomized trial that agrees with these results.[302]

Surgery

Traditional treatment for carcinoma of the bile duct has been surgical (Table 27-16C). The long-term results of surgery and other therapies have been exceedingly poor. Treatment has been palliative in most cases, although some patients with lesions detected early had fully resectable disease. Fortunately, today most patients operated on for bile duct cancer have the site of obstruction delineated preoperatively by PTC or ERCP, which optimizes treatment planning.

An important step in the intraoperative management of the patient suspected of having a bile duct tumor is a biopsy to establish the diagnosis. It is sometimes difficult to obtain biopsy specimens, particularly when the tumor is located in a relatively inaccessible area. Intraoperative choledoctoscopy permits direct visualization and biopsy of tumors and may aid in evaluating the extent of the tumor.[303]

The surgical approach to primary bile duct tumors depends on several factors, including the anatomical site of the tumor and the age and general condition of the patient. A localized intrahepatic cholangiocarcinoma can be resected in the patient in good general condition, ordinarily by lobectomy. A more difficult problem is presented by the tumor located at the ductal confluence (Klatskin's tumor), which may involve both right and left hepatic ducts and the common hepatic duct.[304] The preferred treatment is excision of the tumor and the involved ductal system, establishing enteric bile drainage by a Roux-en-Y hepaticojejunostomy. In a small number of cases, the tumor may involve only one hepatic duct, and the affected duct and its lobe can be removed by hepatic lobectomy, sparing the contralateral lobe. Biliary-enteric continuity is reestablished by a Roux-en-Y hepaticojejunostomy or hepaticocholedochostomy.[305–307]

PROGNOSIS

The overall results of treatment of primary biliary tract cancer have been poor. The strategic location of these tumors precludes excision in most cases.

In 1979, Akwari and Kelly reported 30 patients with cancers in the hilium.[305] Of 4 resected, 3 (75%) were alive at 1 year; 26% of 26 patients having drainage and none of the 8 who had laparotomies alone were alive at 1 year. In 1980, Evander and colleagues reported on 80 patients, of whom 27 (34%) were resected.[323] In that group there were 9 bile duct resections, 15 bile duct plus hepatic lobe resections, 2 pancreaticoduodenectomies with total pancreatectomy, and 1 local excision. The postoperative mortality was 11% after resection and 30% if the tumor was nonresectable. The median survival was 20 months after radical resection, 7.5 months after palliative resections, and 2.5 months for patients with unresectable tumors.[323]

In the UCLA series of 146 patients, the overall morbidity rate during the most recent 5 years was 67% and the overall mortality was 11%.[324] Complications were primarily wound

TABLE 27-16C. Bile Duct Cancer (The UCLA Experience)

	1954–1978		*1979–1983*	
Procedure	*No.*	*%*	*No.*	*%*
Resection	50	53	13	27
Palliation	45	47	33	73
PTD	0		5	10
Laparotomy, biopsy	23	24	8	11
Biliary-enteric bypass	21	22	23	50
Pancreatoduodenectomy	15	16	4	9
Cholangioscopy			25	54

Pitt H, Roslyn JJ, Tompkins R: Surgical resection of bile duct cancer. The UCLA Experience. In Wanebo HJ (ed): Hepatic and Biliary Cancer, pp 339–355. New York, Marcel Dekker, 1987.

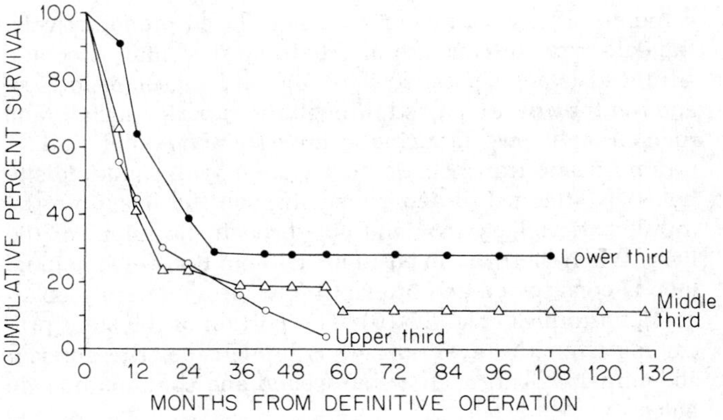

FIG. 27-14. Postoperative survival curves of 96 patients treated from 1954 to 1978 according to location of lesion within biliary system. Forty-seven were upper third, 24 were middle third and 18 were lower third. Six had diffuse lesions. (Tompkins RH, Thomas D, Longmire WP: Prognostic factors in bile duct carcinoma. Ann Surg 194:447–457, 1981)

and intra-abdominal infections. The mortality after resection was 13% in 63 patients, compared with 10% in 33 patients who underwent palliative procedures. The mortality after laparotomy alone, with or without chloecystectomy, was 2%, and it was 11% for choledochotomy with T tube or U tube insertion. For patients undergoing radical pancreatic resection or biliary enteric bypass, it was about 10%. The survival in this group was determined by the location, extent, and histology of the tumor and the operative procedure performed (Figs. 27-14 and 27-15).

Cumulative survival at 5 years was 8%. The rates were best for lower-third lesions (28%), which were commonly treated by Whipple procedure. For the upper-third lesions the 1- and 2-year survivals were 45% and 25%, respectively, but there were no 5-year survivors (Figs. 27-14 and 27-15). The total series of long-term survivors included one patient with a middle-third lesion who was alive at 11 years and another patient with a lower-third tumor who was alive with no recurrence at 9 years. There was no significant difference in mortality between biliary enteric anastomosis (9%) and intubation (7%). Survival was also related to microscopic pathology. Five-year survival was 31% in patients with papillary lesions, 20% in those with sclerosing cholangiocarcinomas, 8% in those with well-differentiated tumors, and 0 in patients with poorly differentiated bile duct cancers. Before 1979, 22 of 47 patients underwent resection of proximal lesions, and there were no 5-year survivors. Operative mortality was 23% in the resected patients and 19% for the entire group of 47 patients. Since 1979, only 7 (18%) of 40 patients with upper-third lesions have undergone resection with no mortality; the in-hospital mortality was 7.5% for the whole group. Thus, there has been a shift from resection to palliative bypass for proximal lesions.

FIG. 27-15. Postoperative survival curves of 96 patients treated from 1954 to 1978 according to type of operation performed. Results of pancreatic duodenectomy (Whipple procedure, 15 patients) for middle and lower third lesions were significantly better than biliary anterior bypass (21 patients) or intubation (45 patients). (Tompkins RH, Thomas D, Longmire WP: Prognostic factors in bile duct carcinoma. Ann Surg 194:447–457, 1981)

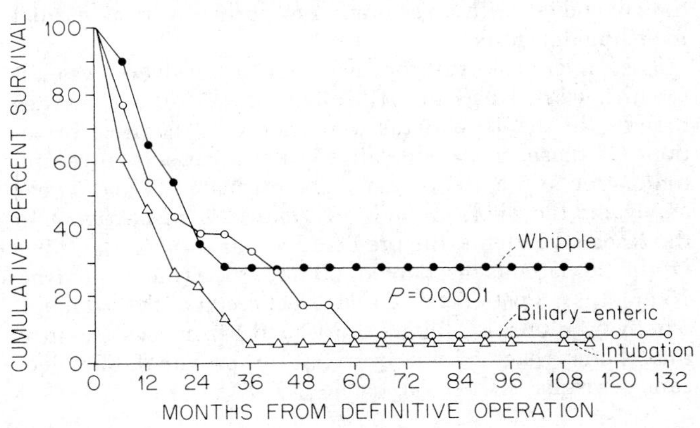

In a report by Blumgart's group, there were 94 patients with proximal lesions, of whom 19% underwent a resection.[307,325] Six had local resection with no mortality, and 12 had major resections with two 30-day mortalities and one delayed death. Of the 17 surgical survivors, 7 were alive and well at 2 years, with one surviving more than 70 months. The mean survival of this group was 36 months. Ten died of disease between 6 and 30 months (mean survival, 15.5 months), and two patients died of other causes at 7 and 9 months.[325] Of 57 treated by biliary enteric or intubational bypass, 19 died, primarily from infection. Previous surgery or biliary drainage appeared to complicate matters and increase morbidity and mortality rates. Of 24 patients previously manipulated, the mortality was 33%, compared with 18% in 22 patients palliated without previous interference. The long-term survival rate was not given.[325]

The Hopkins' approach has been to correct metabolic and septic problems by vitamin K administration and IV antibiotics. If a patient does not respond within 24 hours, percutaneous transhepatic cholangiographic decompression of the biliary tree is carried out with insertion of multiholed ring catheters, which are placed in a dilated hepatic duct and advanced through the tumor-constricted site into the duodenum.[308–310] If the catheter cannot be passed through the tumor at first attempt, external drainage for 2 to 3 days may reduce edema and allow a successful passage through the stricture in the duodenum. The side holes in the tube allow internal decompression. Decompressing the biliary tree reduces the need for urgent surgical intervention and may decrease operative morbidity and mortality. The ring catheter also assists in identifying the bile ducts during surgery. In the case of a Klatskin's tumor obstructing both the left and right hepatic ducts, it may be necessary to insert ring catheters into each side of the biliary tree. Biliary ring catheters were required in 6 of the 27 patients in the Hopkins' series, and preoperative internal drainage was maintained for a mean period of 7 days.[309] All patients received penicillin or ampicillin, gentamicin, and clindamycin or flagyl before surgery.

The surgical technique is shown in (Figs. 27-16 and 27-17). Preoperative insertion of the ring catheters allows easy identification of the ducts above the bifurcation. After the entire extrahepatic biliary tree has been removed, transhepatic stents are placed in both the right and left hepatic ducts. These stents can be placed by attaching them to their previously placed ring catheters and withdrawn by the ring

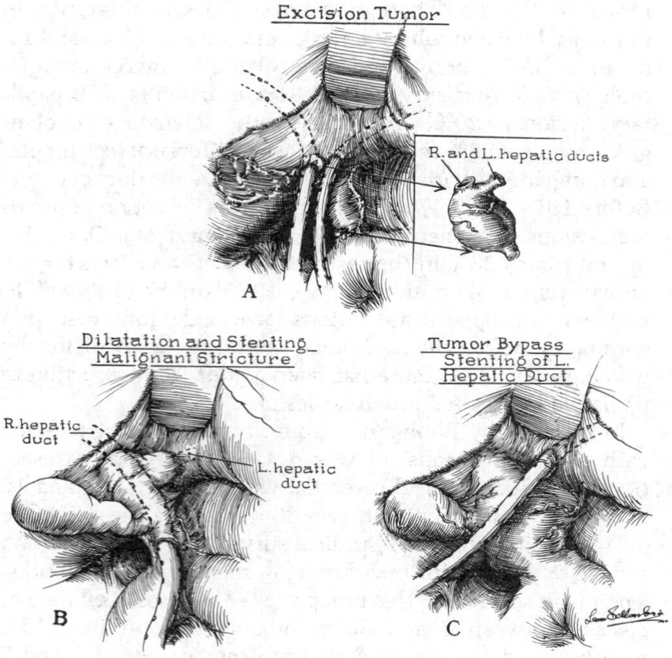

FIG. 27-16. Malignant biliary strictures can be resected (**A**), dilated from below (**B**), or bypassed by entubating the left hepatic duct above the tumor (**C**). A hepaticojejunostomy is then constructed over the stent. (Cameron JL, Gayler BW, Zuidema GD: The use of silastic transhepatic stents in benign malignant biliary strictures. Ann Surg 188:552–561, 1978)

FIG. 27-17. Procedure for replacing transhepatic biliary stents under fluoroscopic control. A stylet is threaded through the old silastic stent into the Roux-en-Y loop. The old stent is then removed, leaving the stylet in place, and the new stent is easily threaded back into place over the stylet. (Broe PJ, Cameron JL: Management of proximal biliary tract tumors. In Maclean LD (ed): Advances in Surgery, vol 15. Chicago, Year Book, 1981)

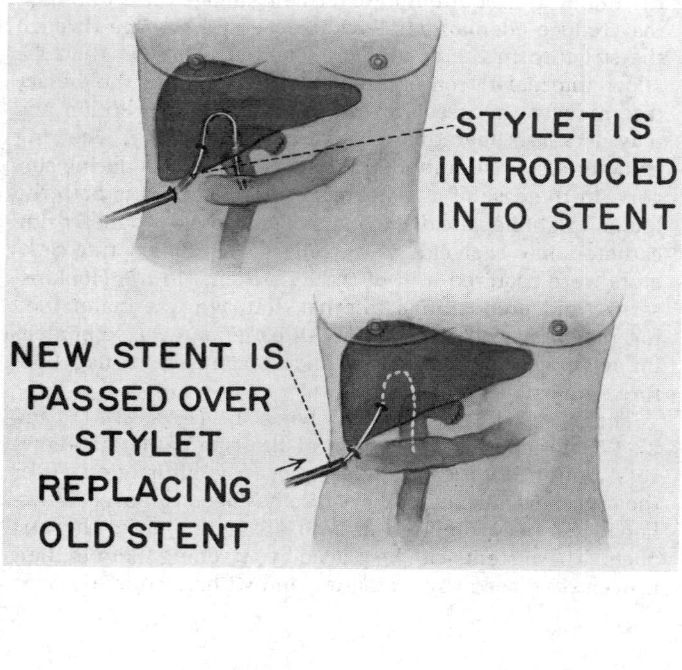

catheters. If ring catheters were not placed preoperatively, Randall-Stone forceps are inserted into the biliary tree and advanced as far as possible. The Glisson's capsule is incised, and the forceps are passed through the superior surface and then brought out through the anterior abdominal wall. A 6-mm Silastic transhepatic biliary stent (with multiple site holes) is attached to and pulled through the liver into the intrahepatic biliary tree and out through the hilum of the liver. When these are in position, a 60-cm Roux-en-Y jejunal loop is constructed and brought up to form bilateral hepaticojejunostomies (Fig. 27-16). The portion of the stent protruding from the liver surface is brought out the anterior abdominal wall through a stab wound and contains no side holes.

The stents are left in place permanently and are irrigated by the patient. They are replaced every 3 months as an outpatient procedure, using the guide wire technique (Fig. 27-17). If the tumor is resectable, that is the best option; if not, the tumor can be dilated and one or more intrahepatic ducts intubated with stents. It is advisable to place stents in both ducts if the lesion is not resected to reduce the risk of infection in the undrained duct. After palliative tumor dilatation and intubation, a Roux-en-Y jejunal loop is constructed and a hepaticojejunostomy performed. If it is not possible to dilate the stricture, the tumor is bypassed by inserting the stent into the left hepatic duct, proximal to the lesion. A hepaticojejunostomy is then fashioned over the distal end of the biliary stent.

In the Hopkins' series of 27 patients treated for proximal bile duct cancer, there was one postoperative death from sepsis secondary to cholangitis developing in an undrained left duct after an effort at dilatation and stent insertion in the right hepatic duct.[309] Thirteen patients had previous cholecystectomies or common duct explorations; 93% were jaundiced and had preoperative PTC placement of ring catheters as described. All gross tumor was removed in 10 of 13 patients in whom resection was attempted. Palliative dilatation and stenting was carried out in the remaining 14 patients. Hepaticojejunostomies were done in 25 patients and hepaticoduodenostomy in 1 patient.

Postoperative irradiation of the tumor bed was given to 20 patients, of whom 9 received a full course of 5000 rad and 5 received less than 3000 rad. Six patients who had undergone curative resection received 5000 rad externally and 2500 rad delivered by local radium-192 seeds placed in the Silastic stents for 24 to 48 hours (Fig. 27-18). All had a reduction of their jaundice, with a restoration to normal or near-normal liver function tests.

The mean survival for 26 surgical survivors was 22 months, with 6 patients still alive. Mean survival was 30 months for the 10 patients who underwent curative resection. Of these, 5 are still alive, with 2 patients alive and tumor-free at 5 and 7.5 years. The estimated 2- and 5-year survival in the whole group is 40% and 15%, respectively. In the resected patients, the predicted 5-year survival was 25%. Of the 26 patients discharged, 20 have died (mean survival, 15 months); 8 patients died as a direct result of their tumors, 5 of liver failure, 4 of biliary sepsis, and 1 from a gastrointestinal hemorrhage.[309] An overview of proximal bile duct cancer results is shown in Table 27-17.

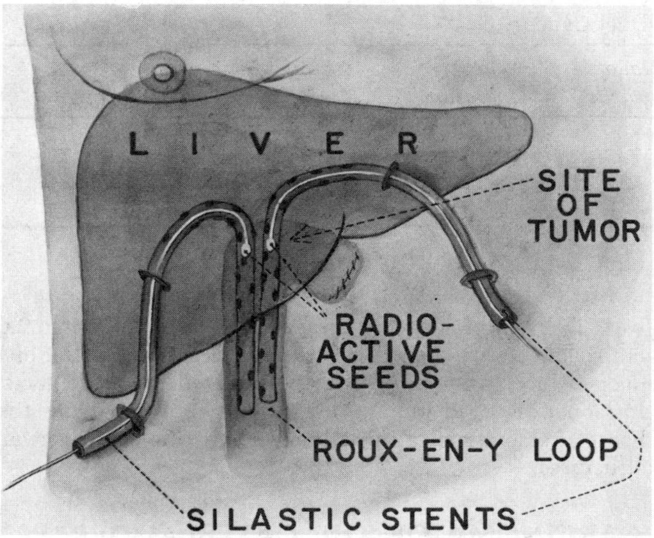

FIG. 27-18. The silastic transhepatic stents can be used as conduits for lowering radioactive ^{192}Ir seeds to the site of the tumor. These seeds are left in place for 24 to 48 hours and then removed. (Broe PJ, Cameron JL: Management of proximal biliary tract tumors. In Maclean LD (ed): Advances in Surgery, vol 15. Chicago, Year Book, 1981)

RESECTION OF MIDDLE AND DISTAL DUCT CANCERS. Cancer of the middle portion of the common bile duct is refractory to curative therapy. These tumors are within a few millimeters of the hepatic artery and portal vein. Of the 12 patients seen at the Lahey Clinic between 1965 and 1978, 4 were resected, and none survived beyond 2 years.[317–321]

Their most extensive experience has been with distal bile duct cancers. Between 1939 and 1978, the Lahey Clinic had experience with 282 patients with primary cancer of the bile duct, all but 6 of which were adenocarcinomas.[342–345] Of 173 patients treated between 1939 and 1965, most died of cancer 5 to 26 weeks after surgery, and only 25 survived more than 1 year.[319] Of 109 patients seen between 1965 and 1978, the median survival was 11 months. Of 41 patients with distal lesions resected by Whipple procedures (pyloris preserving), there were 10 (24%) postoperative deaths, and 8 (26%) of 31 survived free of disease beyond 5 years.[321]

Herter and colleagues also reported on pyloris-preserving Whipple procedures with pancreatic enteric anastomoses in 48 patients, of whom 33 had periampullary area neoplasms and 15 had pancreatitis without any postoperative deaths. Ten patients with distal bile duct cancers were alive 1 to 42 months after surgery (mean follow-up, 9 months).[322] A composite of experience with distal bile duct cancer is shown in Table 27-18.

Radiation Therapy

Although radiotherapy has a long history of use in treating patients with extrahepatic bile duct cancer, most of the published experiences have been anecdotal and retrospective and describe a variety of doses, fields, and delivery techniques.

Kopelson and co-workers reported on eight patients, of whom two were resected and six had palliative radiation only.[326] Doses ranged from 3800 to 7225 cGy in 25 to 29 treatments, using anterior and posterior fields. Obstructive jaundice was relieved. Palliation was achieved in seven of eight patients, with a mean survival of 7.4 months. In a Cleveland Clinic series of 79 bile duct cancer patients treated from 1958 to 1977, 16 were radiated postoperatively.[327] Intubation or bypass was done in 14; one was resected and one was biopsied only. The tumor was at the bifurcation in ten patients, in the common hepatic duct in four, and in the common bile duct in two. Cobalt irradiation of 2400 to 5000 rad was given. The proximal duct cancer patients survived an average of 1.7 years, and one patient was alive and tumor-free at 6 years. Nonirradiated patients survived an average of 6 months.

In a report by Wheeler, radiation was given to 9 of 21 patients with hepatic duct lesions in whom a T tube or U tube internal drain had been inserted.[328] Four patients received external radiation (4000–4500 rad), four had a radium wire passed through a T tube or U tube, delivering a dose of 4000 rad in 2 days, and one was treated by external and internal radiation. Actuarial survival appeared enhanced in those treated with radiation compared to patients treated with drainage only.[328] Fletcher and colleagues used internal radiation with iridium-192 wire to treat eight patients with proximal bile duct lesions.[329] A radiation dose of 4000 to 4800 rad at 0.5 cm from the wire was delivered over 48 hours. The median survival was 11 months, with two patients alive at 22

TABLE 27-17. Survival Data in Patients Undergoing Surgery for Proximal Biliary Tumors

Procedure	*No. of Patients*	*Postoperative Deaths (%)*	*Mean survival (mo)*
Laparotomy and biopsy	41	5 (12)	5.6 ± 4.2
Palliative Y- or T-tube stenting	251	44 (17)	9.9 ± 5.3
Intrahepatic cholangiojejunostomy	68	11 (16)	11.0 ± 7.6
Palliative transhepatic stenting	35	3 (9)	18.6 ± 15.3
Tumor resection	88	11 (12)	22.2 ± 16.7
Total	483	74 (15)	

Data from Cameron JL, Sanfey H: Surgical management of proximal cholangiocarcinomas. In Wanebo HJ (ed): Hepatic and Biliary Cancer, pp. 395–415, New York, Marcel Dekker, 1987.

TABLE 27-18. Survival After Surgical Resection of Distal Bile Duct Cancer

Author	*Institution*	*Series*	*Reference*	*No. of Patients*	*Whipple Operation*	*Postoperative Mortality (%)*	*5-Year Survival (%)*
Braasch	Lahey Clinic	1939–1965	319	62	27	26	30
		1965–1978	317	14	14	21	18
Herter	Cleveland Clinic	1940–1978	322	21	10	Not reported	33
Pitt	UCLA	1954–1983	324	22	15	13	30

and 23 months. An update of the experience to 18 patients continues to show a similar trend.

In the Johns Hopkins' experience with proximal bile duct cancers, 20 of 27 patients had postoperative radiation. Nine patients received 5000 rad externally and six patients received iridium-192 wire irradiation (2500 rad) and 5000 rad externally after tumor resection. The mean survival rate of the entire group was 18 months, with 11 patients remaining alive with the tumor controlled.[330] Between 1974 and 1981, Hashikawa treated 25 patients with hepatic duct lesions.[331] Most had percutaneous transhepatic drainage before irradiation, three had T tubes placed, and three had no surgical procedures. Survival appeared to be longer in patients treated with doses greater than 4000 rad. One of the 25 patients has survived disease-free for more than 6.5 years.

Intraoperative radiation has also been applied to bile duct cancers, primarily in Japan. Todoroki treated 25 patients with unresectable advanced cancer of the bile duct, using a single dose of 3000 rad with 11 to 20 MeV electrons.[332] Treatment was well-tolerated and palliation was effective, with recanalization of the obstructed ducts documented in all cases. Median survival was 13 months. Abe and Takahashi reviewed results of intraoperative therapy in Japan. A total of 59 patients with biliary cancer were treated in 12 institutions. Single doses of 2500 to 4000 rad were administered. Recanalization of the bile duct was demonstrated radiographically in 90% of the patients. Analysis of autopsied patients suggested that a single dose of 3500 rad was potentially curative.[333]

RADIOTHERAPEUTIC CONSIDERATIONS. A recent analysis of radiation for bile duct cancer by Pilepich suggested that radiation may have a potentially curative role in patients with local regional disease.[234] Because of slow growth, low propensity to metastasize, and small tumor bulk, the volume of normal tissues in irradiation treatment fields is generally small. External radiation doses of 6000 rad in 6 weeks, and preferably 7000 rad in 7 to 8 weeks, are suggested for consistent control of gross tumor. A dose of 4500 to 5000 rad is considered adequate for irradiation of microscopic disease.

The delivery of full tumoricidal doses of external-beam radiation is feasible for proximal bile duct lesions but difficult for distal duct cancers because of potential damage to the duodenum and stomach. In these cases, the best approach may be a combination of external-beam radiation of 5000 to 6000 rad and internal brachiotherapy as a boost. Internal radiation alone cannot be expected to provide adequate dosage to gross tumor unless the lesion is small and superficial. This is due to a rapid falloff of dosage around the wire. Delivery of adequate dosage for distances of 1.0 to 2.0 cm requires very high exposures at the surface of the bile ducts, which can produce scarring and stenosis of the ducts. Intraoperative radiation is another way of providing the boost after external irradiation while sparing some normal structures.

CARCINOMA OF THE GALLBLADDER

Carcinoma of the gallbladder is the fifth most common malignancy of the GI tract in the United States, after cancers of the colon, pancreas, stomach, and esophagus.[335] It occurs in about 1% of patients undergoing cholecystectomy for gallstones. It carries a grave prognosis, with most large series reporting 5-year survival rates of less than 5%. The disease is advanced and unresectable in most patients. A patient in whom the carcinoma was an incidental finding at the time of routine cholecystectomy may be cured by cholecystectomy alone. These are primarily patients with carcinoma in situ or with small cancers showing limited invasion of the gallbladder wall.[335–343] About 75% of the patients are women whose median age is in the seventh decade and in whom the diagnosis is made only on surgical exploration. More than 75% have associated cholelithiasis.[335,343]

PATHOLOGY

Cancer of the gallbladder usually presents as a locally extensive tumor.[335,337,343] The entire gallbladder may be involved, appearing thickened, contracted, and plastered into the liver, and it may be filled with purulent material, mucus, or stones.[343–345] Occasionally, extensive areas of hemorrhage and necrosis are present, even leading to perforation.[345] Frequently, one or more gallstones are present in the specimen, and about 85% of the cases have associated cholelithiasis. Carcinoma is most often present in the fundus and may present as a mucosal plaque, a polypoid or papillary excrescence, or discrete thickening of the wall, sometimes with an attached gallstone.[335,344,345] Papillary tumors are shaggy, friable lesions projecting into the lumina, and they may extend to and obstruct the cystic duct. A thickened gallbladder wall may exhibit diffuse calcification, a result of long-standing inflammation. A calcified or "porcelain gallbladder" is demonstrable radiographically and has about a 15% to 20% chance of containing cancer.[346,347] The series by Polk and colleagues included 22 cases of gallbladder cancer in approximately 100 porcelain gallbladders.[347]

Histologic types include adenocarcinoma in about 85% of patients and pure squamous cancers or mixed carcinomas with glandular and squamous elements in 10%.[345] About 5%

of the cases have neither squamous nor glandular differentiation and by light microscopy are found to be true sarcomas.

The adenocarcinomatous glands vary in size and may blend into the surrounding stoma and may be unrecognized. Occasionally, such cases are overlooked in the routine cholecystectomy but will be manifested subsequently by metastases; the occult cancer will be found frequently on reexamination of the original specimen.[345] Intramucosal lesions should be examined by multiple sections to determine the presence of invasion, which is frequently difficult if the tumor has grown into a Rokitansky-Aschoff sinus. Among the adenocarcinomas, 15% are predominantly papillary and about 9% are mucinous. The mucinous tumors contain large pools of mucin, with clusters of freely floating tumor cells, and such cases often have peritoneal implants and obstruction of the extrahepatic bile ducts.[344,345] Distant metastases are infrequent.[344]

Some adenocarcinomas may be poorly differentiated or anaplastic and are difficult to separate from sarcomas. Spindle-cell malignancies of the gallbladder are carcinomas, not sarcomas.[345,348,349] The distinction between carcinomas and rhabdomyosarcomas in children is important because of chemotherapeutic implications. Tumors with squamous components are observed commonly in North Americans, constituting almost 35% of gallbladder cancers in this population.[350] Mixed lesions with both glandular and squamous elements may occur. These have been called adenoacanthomas, but a better label may be adenosquamous carcinomas.[343–345]

Clear cell carcinomas of the gallbladder have been described by Albores-Saavedra and are historically identical to small cell undifferentiated cancers found in other sites.[351] Of 19 cases, all metastasized, and 9 patients were dead within 1 year.[351] Well-differentiated neuroendocrine tumors, such as carcinoids, have also been incidental findings at cholecystectomy.[345]

METASTATIC DISEASE

Modes of spread of carcinoma of the gallbladder have been examined in surgical cases and autopsy material. In a review by Fahim and co-workers, about 25% of 151 patients had nodal metastases at the time of surgery.[352] Most of the involved nodes were in the drainage of the cystic duct and the common hepatic and bile ducts. Vascular invasion was noticed in 14% and nerve invasion occurred in 24%. None of the patients had intraperitoneal tumor spread, but invasion of adjacent organs was common. Thirty-four percent had spread to the liver, and in 84% of these the involvement was restricted to the gallbladder bed. Satellite nodules surrounded the main hepatic extension in 8% and multiple distant nodules occurred in the right hepatic lobe in 8%.

At autopsy, carcinoma of the gallbladder involves the liver (90%) and bile ducts (60%) and extends to regional nodes in about 70% of the cases.[353] Over 60% had para-aortic nodal metastases and 33% had supraclavicular nodal disease. Approximately 33% had extension to the stomach, duodenum, pancreas, and peritoneum. The lung was involved in about 33%.[353] Most of the long-term survivors have had tumors that were unsuspected clinically at the time of surgery. In Piehler and Crichlow's review, survival was 14.9% among 15 patients whose tumors were detected by the pathologist after cholecystectomy and only 2.9% among 70 patients whose lesions were discovered by the surgeon and were resected completely.[335]

CLINICAL FEATURES

Common symptoms as noted in a representative series included pain (79%), nausea and vomiting (53%), weight loss (42%), jaundice (34%), anorexia (27%), abdominal distention (24%), pruritus (15%), and melena (3%). Most patients had multiple symptoms (Table 27-19A).[360] The major clinical findings included tenderness or a mass in the right upper quadrant or epigastrium in more than half the patients, hepatomegaly and jaundice in one third, and cachexia, fever, and ascites in about 10% to 15%. The duration of symptoms was variable, ranging from 1 month in 33% of the patients to 2 to 6 months in 50%, and 6 to 12 months in the remaining patients (Table 27-19).

Preoperative testing was distinctly inaccurate in most cases. The preoperative diagnosis based on both clinical and laboratory findings in one series was a benign process in 60% and a malignant process in 40% of the cases.[337] Acute or chronic cholecystitis and cholelithiasis were the most common of the preoperative benign diagnoses, considered in more than 60% of the patients; pancreatic cancer and biliary tract cancer were considered to be the most likely malignant diagnoses.[337] Liver function studies and radiologic tests failed to pinpoint the diagnosis in most cases. Percutaneous transhepatic cholangiography, although useful for showing obstruction and suggesting a possible cause, did not distinguish primary gallbladder cancer from other lesions in this region. Of the patients in the University of Virginia series, 75% had cholelithiasis, findings that are similar to those of most series.[337]

The diagnostic problems resulting in delayed diagnosis of gallbladder cancer have been confirmed by other studies. The University of Minnesota series listed a high percentage of abnormal oral or intravenous cholangiography, but other test findings, such as upper GI series, were abnormal in less than 50% of cases (Table 27-19B).[338] The Charity Hospital series reported by Hamrick and colleagues concluded that none of the preoperative tests were diagnostic.[354] Hyperbilirubinemia occurred in 44% of their patients, and anemia, leukocytosis, and hypoalbuminemia were frequent abnormalities, as were hepatic enzyme elevations in patients with more advanced disease. In most of their patients, the gallbladder was not visualized by oral cholecystogram, and intravenous cholangiography added no new information. The upper GI series was abnormal in 33% of the patients, and in half of these cases, there was gastric outlet obstruction. External duodenal compression was observed in about 33% of the cases. Percutaneous transhepatic cholangiograms helped to visualize the site of obstruction, but they were not diagnostic.

Although few of these patients had ultrasonography, it might be helpful in some patients to document a thickened wall or identify adenomata.[355–357] In addition, CT scans may assist in the earlier identification of a neoplastic process in the gallbladder fossa.

TABLE 27-19A. Symptoms in Patients with Carcinoma of the Gallbladder (University of Virginia Series, 1981)

*Symptom**	% Patients	Duration
Pain	79	<1 month, 30%
Nausea and vomiting	53	2–6 months, 50%
Weight loss	42	7–12 months, 20%
Jaundice	34	
Anorexia	27	
Abdominal distention	24	
Pruritus	15	
Melena	3	

Wanebo HJ, Costle WN, Fechner RE: Is carcinoma of the gallbladder a curable lesion? Ann Surg 195:624–631, 1982.
*Multiple symptoms in most patients.

SURGERY

Because of the variety of clinical presentations, ranging from occult malignancy to advanced diseases, surgical management has been quite varied in most series. In the University of Virginia series of 100 gallbladder cancer patients, surgical approaches consisted of cholecystectomy alone or with common duct drainage in 40 patients, cholecystectomy and partial liver resection in 8 patients, exploration with bypass or biopsy only in 44 patients, and autopsy only in 8 patients.[337] The median survival after cholecystectomy was 6 months, with two long-term survivals of 11 and 24 years. In many cases, the carcinoma was diagnosed postoperatively by the pathologist. The median survival after resection of the gallbladder and associated liver bed was 14 months, with one of seven long-term survivors (14%). Among 44 patients having miscellaneous procedures, the median survival time was 2 months with no long-term survivors.[337]

The impact of occult gallbladder cancer and the role of histopathologic stage has been addressed by many authors. In a Mayo Clinic report by Appleman, 21 of 166 patients who underwent definitive gallbladder surgery survived 5 years or longer.[340] None of the 21 involved adjacent structures, but 10 invaded the muscle of the gallbladder wall. Frank and Spjut described 16 patients whose tumors were first detected by the pathologist.[341] The cancer invaded the muscularis propria in 12 patients, the serosa in 3 patients, and the adjacent liver in 1 patient. The 5-year survival for the group was only 13%.[341]

Bergdahl reviewed 32 patients with clinically occult cancer whose gallbladders were removed for clinically benign disease. Among the 21 patients whose tumors involved all layers of the gallbladder, the longest survival was 2.5 years.[339] Among the 11 patients with tumors confined to the mucosa or submucosa, 7 were alive after 5 years.

TABLE 27-19B. Diagnostic Procedures Used in Primary Gallbladder Cancer*

Procedure	*% Abnormal Tests*
Oral cholecystogram, 42/47	89
Intravenous cholecystogram, 6/7	86
Upper gastrointestinal series, 24/53	45
Selective hepatic arteriogram, 1/3	33
Abdominal film, 7/109	6

Morrow CE, Sutherland DE, Florack G et al: Primary gallbladder carcinoma: Significance of suberosal lesions and results of aggressive surgical treatment and adjuvant chemotherapy. Surgery 94:709–714, 1983.
*University of Minnesota series, 1983.

Nevin and colleagues attempted to reconcile the prognostic heterogeneity of gallbladder cancer by formulating a staging system based on depth of invasion and spread of disease.[336] Five stages were delineated: Stage 1 (intramucosal); Stage 2 (mucosa and muscularis); Stage 3 (involvement of all three layers); Stage 4 (involvement of all three layers and cystic lymph nodes); and Stage 5 (involvement of liver by direct extension or metastases to distant organs). Of 17 patients with Stage 1 or Stage 2 disease, all survived. Of 23 patients with Stage 3, 2 survived 5 years, and of 5 with Stage 4 there was one 5-year survival. None of the 21 Stage 5 patients survived beyond 1 year.

In a similar study from the University of Virginia, microscopic staging failed to identify a favorable subgroup of patients.[337] Among 46 stageable patients, only two had Stage I and four had Stage II disease. Only 2 of these survived 5 years, and 1 had a carcinoid of the gallbladder. If the latter patient is excluded, there was a survival rate of 20% for lesions confined to the muscularis. This is not different from other studies with similarly staged patients.[337–339,357] The greatest number of cases was in the Stage III group, of whom only 3 of 21 survived 2 years and only 1 survived beyond 5 years. None of the Stage IV patients survived, and only 1 of 13 Stage V patients survived (a patient with extension to the liver). The disease was limited to the gallbladder in only 25% of the patients.

In most cases, extension was into the liver or metastasis to the common duct nodes, the ducts themselves, the pancreas, or the duodenum (Fig. 27-19). In some of the patients, the gallbladder and liver were not available for the definitive study that would have allowed those patients to be included in the staging system. Liver metastases alone occurred in 19 patients, and secondary GI tract carcinomas accompanied the primary disease in 13 patients.

Somewhat similar results occurred in the University of Minnesota series. Of 11 patients with invasive cancer of the muscular wall that did not extend through the serosa, 1 (20%) of 5 patients survived after cholecystectomy alone, and 4 of 6 survived after more radical resection: cholecystectomy and lymphadenectomy (with three hepatic wedge re-

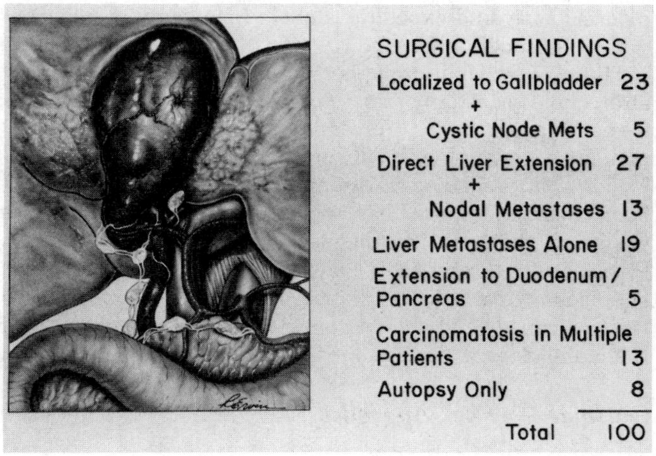

SURGICAL FINDINGS
Localized to Gallbladder 23
+
Cystic Node Mets 5
Direct Liver Extension 27
+
Nodal Metastases 13
Liver Metastases Alone 19
Extension to Duodenum / Pancreas 5
Carcinomatosis in Multiple Patients 13
Autopsy Only 8
Total 100

FIG. 27-19. Locoregional extent of disease in the University of Virginia series is enumerated above. Primary sites of extension are liver nodes, with occasional patients having extension to duodenum and pancreas.

sections and one pancreatic duodenectomy).[338] The three patients treated by cholecystectomy alone died of recurrent cancer at 18, 48, and 60 months, respectively. The overall survival rate in 11 patients with cancer confined to the wall was 46% (5 of 11). Of the 13 patients with cystic node metastases (Stage IV), 9 had cholecystectomy alone, 3 had lymphadenectomy, and 1 had pancreaticoduodenectomy. The cumulative survival was only 37% at 6 months, and all patients were dead within 18 months. Of 14 patients with advanced disease treated by aggressive surgery (lymphadenectomy in 6, hepatic wedge resection in 6, and right hepatic lobectomy in 2), the mean survival time was only 3 months.

The surgical results of four microstaged Western series are shown in Table 27-20 and emphasize the need to standardize the staging and reporting for surgical outcome. It would appear from the surgical series that the patient most likely to benefit from a cholecystectomy alone would be one with intramucosal disease only, but a composite resection (cholecystectomy with removal of the gallbladder bed by hepatic wedge resection and lymphadenectomy) would be required for those with invasive cancer confined to the wall (muscular coat or subserosal).

Among the Stage IV and V patients in the Minnesota series were 38 patients who were treated with either chemotherapy (35 patients) or radiation (3 patients) and who had a mean survival time of 4.5 months, compared with 3 months for the group of 14 patients receiving surgery only ($p = 0.0001$).[338] Although this series was not randomized, it suggests a rationale for pursuing adjuvant therapy in these patients.

The treatment is probably valid for early gallbladder cancer in which disease is limited to the gallbladder. In a report by Adson of 112 patients, 16 had carcinoma extending just beyond the gallbladder or regional nodes, which was theoretically resectable.[358] Of these, 12 had cholecystectomy, all but 1 died within 15 months. Four patients had a cholecystectomy plus wedge resection of the liver and lymphadectomy; all remained free of disease, but 3 died without cancer (3.5, 6, and 14 years), and 1 is alive at 9 years. This suggests the need for a more aggressive approach in the Stage III patients.

In the Scandinavian series by Bergdahl, 32 of 120 patients had a cholecystectomy performed for benign disease, whereupon cancer was found by the pathologist.[339] The survival was poor (longest, 2.5 years) in the 21 patients with cancer involving all layers of the wall, but it was 64% in the 11 patients with mucosal or submucosal cancers. Of the group having cholecystectomies, only 5 died of recurrence, suggesting the need for radical cholecystectomy (wedge resection of the liver and lymph node dissection). It also suggested a rationale for adjuvant therapy in patients with disease involving the entire wall.

In a review of 2567 patients with gallbladder cancer from

TABLE 27-20. Five-Year Survival After Resection of Gallbladder Cancer in Staged Series

		Surviving/Total				
Stage	*Extent of Invasion*	*Nevin (336)*	*Wanebo (337)*	*Morrow (338)*	*Bergdahl (339)*	*Composite Survival*
I	Mucosa	6/10	1/2	NS/4* 2/26 (8%)	6/11 (64%)	(Stage 1-II) 18/33 (55%)
II	Muscularis	5/7 [13/40 (33%)]	0/3	NS/4 7/8 (88%) at 3 yr		(Stage 1-III) 27/106 (26%)
III	Subserosal	2/23	1/21	NS/3 5/8 (63%) at 5 yr	0/21 (0)	
IV	Cystic LN+	1/5	0/6	0/13	NS	1/24 (4.2%)
Va	Extension to liver or adjacent organ (resectable)	0/21	1/3	0/14	NS/88 = 0? (presumed, not stated)	1/123 (8%)
Vb	Regionally advanced or metastatic (unresectable)			0/74		
Total series	(microstaged)	14/66 (21%)	3/46 (65%) 3/100 total series	5/112 (4.5%)	6/120 (5%) (calculated, not stated)	28/398 (7%)

Data from Wanebo HJ: Carcinoma of the gallbladder. In Wanebo HJ (ed): Hepatic and biliary cancer, pp 431–445. New York, Marcel Dekker, 1987.
*NS = not stated.

Japan, Tashiro and colleagues found 467 patients (20.6%) who were treated by radical resection.[359] Those with Stages I and II lesions had good survival times, but those with more extensive disease did poorly. As in the Western series, most patients (59%) had associated gallstones, and only a small percentage (1.6%) were diagnosed preoperatively. These authors recommend that patients with cancer extending through the wall should have an extended cholecystectomy, a right hepatic lobectomy, and pancreaticoduodenectomy.[359]

A surprisingly high survival rate was obtained in the 467 patients who had radical resections of various types. The 5-year survival by stage ranged from 97% to 58% for Stages I and II to 25% to 20% for Stages III and IV. Even Stage V had an 11% survival rate. These Japanese survival rates are quite superior to any of the American or European series. The reasons for these differences are not clear, but possible racial, cultural (nutritional), and pathobiologic differences should be studied. It is unlikely that the extent of surgery or basic treatment differences would explain these survival results. An international symposium to compare differences may be of value.

Most of the series from the United States and Europe are in agreement that a more extended cholecystectomy (including the gallbladder bed and a regional node dissection) should be done. Although there are reported 5-year survivors after hepatic lobectomy, most investigators believe that formal lobectomies or other organ resections are probably not indicated and that a wedge resection or subsegmental resection should suffice.[360–363]

Related Epithelial Abnormalities

Other epithelial abnormalities should be pointed out in addition to carcinoma. Benign tumors, such as papillomas, adenomas, lipomas, and hemangiomas, may occur.[364–367] Noncarcinomatous malignancies may also occur, such as melanoma, carcinosarcoma, and malignant mixed tumors.[345] For the most part, the epithelial abnormalities are generally related to chronic cholecystitis and are probably precursor lesions to cancer. The relationship of cholecystitis to epithelial abnormalities has been examined by Albores-Saavedra and colleagues.[366] In a report from Mexico, 13.5% of patients with cholecystitis had atypical hyperplasia, and 3.5% had what was thought to be carcinoma in situ.[366] Carcinoma in situ is very common in surgical cases of gallbladder cancer, suggesting that this epithelial abnormality is probably a precursor of invasive cancer. Removal of this level of disease should result in improved survival. The presence of polyps is also a consideration for surgery.

A series reported by Kozuka and colleagues of 1605 cholecystectomies included 11 benign adenomas (all <12 mm), 9 adenomas with malignant change (all >12 mm), and 79 patients with invasive cancer (most >30 mm).[367] Of the 79 patients, 15 had adenomatous residues. The average ages were 50 years in the adenoma group, 58 years in the patients with in situ cancer, and 64 years in the invasive cancer patients. Some of the long-term survivors of cholecystectomy alone may be patients with relatively benign lesions such as adenomas or in situ cancers. It also suggests a rationale for early and expeditious cholecystectomy in older patients with cholelithiasis.

There is evidence that the retained diseased gallbladder after cholecystostomy is at increased risk for the development of cancer. In the University of Virginia series, 8 of 100 patients presented with cancer developing in retained gallbladders after cholecystostomy.[368] These patients had all been observed for a median of 8 years before developing the symptoms that led to the diagnosis of the gallbladder cancer. Physicians can reasonably consider patients with a diseased gallbladder retained after cholecystostomy to be at increased risk for cancer and should consider expeditious removal of the gallbladder if the patient is fit medically.

Optimal Surgical Approach

The optimal surgical approach has not been defined from any published clinical trial data. Considering the infrequency of the cancer, it is unlikely that the answer will be available soon, but recommendations can be made on the basis of some of the findings of the larger clinical series, in particular the studies performed at the Mayo Clinic.[352] This group described a major route of spread of gallbladder cancer, which appears to be locoregional rather than distant. Direct extension to the liver is common, with frequent spread to cystic, common duct, and peripancreatic nodes. Further direct extension along the nodal pathways may also involve the pancreas and duodenum. Similar findings have been reported from several of the recent larger series.[337,338,343] Liver metastasis or direct liver extension occurs in about 30% to 40% of the cases.

A logical surgical approach is total removal of the organ and the gallbladder bed, with a wedge of 3 to 4 cm of underlying liver, and a node dissection of the draining lymphatics. A right hepatic lobectomy is probably unnecessary. The lymph node dissection should include the nodal drainage of the entire bile duct, including the superior and inferior peripancreatic nodes, the common duct nodes, nodes in the porta hepatis (the common hepatic duct), and periportal vein and perihepatic artery nodes.

Biopsies should be taken from strategic areas of the resection site to ensure that the margins are clear. If all margins are clear, the nodes are negative, and the lesions seem confined to the gallbladder only, then the physician may observe the patient, obtaining frequent CT scans. If the nodes are positive, the margins are positive, or the disease extends into the liver, then postoperative radiation and chemotherapy are indicated.

The surgeon should be suspicious of gallbladder cancer in the high-risk patient who is older, has stones, has a very thick-walled gallbladder, or has a calcified gallbladder that is not completely compatible with the expected findings of chronic cholecystitis. If cancer is suspected, a small biopsy should be obtained before the dissection of the gallbladder. This prevents the unnecessary spillage of tumor cells that invariably occurs if a cholecystectomy is done and the carcinomatous communication between gallbladder and liver is disrupted. Tumor spillage may account for the frequent rapid dissemination of this disease in many patients after cholecystectomy. If a cancer is recognized early, then the operative procedures outlined could be carried out at that time or delayed if the patient and family are not prepared for a more extended resection. If there are questions about the diagnosis (infection and inflammation versus tumor), a fine-needle aspiration of the gallbladder fluid for cytology and bacteriology could be done to assess drainage or malignancy.

In the event that a cholecystectomy was done for a clinically occult lesion, the physician should consider reexploration with resection of the gallbladder bed and lymph node dissection. In the medically high-risk patient, observation only should be considered for cancer limited to mucosa or submucosa, and radiation plus chemotherapy should be given for lesions invading beyond these layers.

RADIATION

The pattern of failure after resection clearly points to the limitation of surgical procedures for most patients.[326,369] Local recurrence is a common cause of death in patients who relapse after cholecystectomy.[326] In Kopelson's review, local recurrence was present or was a cause of death in 86% of 110 patients who died within 5 years after simple cholecystectomy.[326]

Radiation data for gallbladder cancer are sparse. Hanna and Rider reviewed data on 51 patients treated at the Princess Margaret Hospital in Toronto.[370] Radiation doses ranged from an average of 2600 rad in those treated for palliation to 4000 rad in 4 weeks in those treated with curative intent.[370] Two-thirds of the patients had disease confined to the right upper quadrant. Although all the patients eventually died of disease, survival was stated to be significantly longer for those who received postoperative radiotherapy than for those who had surgery only.[393] Similar impressions of the survival benefit of irradiation were recorded by other researchers, but patient numbers were very small.[326,334,371] In a retrospective review by Vaittinen, the median survival was 29 months with surgery alone and 63 months for patients who were irradiated postoperatively.[343] These data may reflect case selection bias, and more data on external-beam therapy are needed to evaluate the role of irradiation for these tumors.

Several preliminary reports on the use of intraoperative radiotherapy indicate that this technique may play a part in the palliative and curative management of biliary tract malignancies.[372]

Effective radiation for gallbladder carcinoma depends on the volume of the treatment fields necessary to encompass the tumor, the residual tumor burden, and the total dose and fractionation. The relationship between tumor bulk and tumor control is well established. A dose of 4500 to 5000 rad, using conventional 175 to 200 rad/day fractionation, is required to eradicate microscopic disease but will not control gross tumor.

The ideal candidates for adjuvant, postoperative radiotherapy are patients who have had resection of all gross disease and are at high risk of harboring microscopic, residual tumor. A dose of 4500 to 5000 rad in approximately 5 weeks delivered to the gallbladder bed and regional lymphatics is likely to provide permanent local-regional control and, in a subset of patients, cure. For patients who have gross residual disease after resection or who had unresectable disease, consistent locoregional control will require higher doses, in the range of 7000 rad in 7 to 8 weeks. Such doses cannot be delivered safely to intra-abdominal sites unless the treated volume is small and removed from vulnerable structures, such as small bowel, or unless such procedures as a radioactive implant or intraoperative radiotherapy are used in conjunction with external-beam radiotherapy.

Combined radiotherapy and chemotherapy have a potential for improving locoregional control. 5-FU has been used as a radiation potentiator in the treatment of other GI malignancies and appears to have improved locoregional control with radiotherapy in several trials.[373] Similar trials should be conducted in patients with carcinoma of the gallbladder, particularly in those with gross residual tumor after surgery.

CHEMOTHERAPY

Single-Agent Chemotherapy

The infrequent occurrence of biliary cancer has limited the evaluation of its response to chemotherapeutic agents (Table 27-21).[374] Because many reports have included data on hepatic and pancreatic cancer under hepatobiliary malignan-

TABLE 27-21. Chemotherapeutic Responses of Biliary Cancer

Drugs	*Response (%)*	*References*
5-Fluorouracil	4/17 (24)	Haskell (1980) [375]
	3/23 (13)	Davis et al (1980) [376]
Mitomycin C	7/15 (42)	Crooke and Bradner (1976) [377]
	0/10 (0)	Von Eyben et al (1980) [378]
BCNU	2/2 (100)	Haskell (1980) [375]
Adriamycin	1 (anecdotal)	Adolphson and Carpenter (1981) [379]
Neocarzinostatin	Anecdotal response	Bodey et al (1981) [380]
m-AMSA	2/23 (9)	Bukowski et al (1983) [381]
FAM	4/14 (31)	Harvey et al (1984) [382]
Ftorafur, Adriamycin, and BCNU	3/7 (43)	Hall et al (1979) [383]
Adriamycin and bleomycin	1/5	Ravey and Hester (1979) [384]
5-FU and mitomycin C via hepatic artery	9/13 (69)	Misra et al (1977) [385]

Andrews W, Smith F: Chemotherapy for cholangiocarcinoma and gallbladder cancer. In Wanebo HJ (ed): Hepatic and biliary cancer, pp 453–457. New York, Marcel Dekker, 1987.

cies, information on chemotherapy for these tumors lags behind that of the more common GI malignancies.

Several drugs beneficial in other upper GI malignancies have apparent single-agent activity in biliary cancer. In all of these single-agent trials, however, durations of response have been very short, on the order of weeks. This paucity of single-agent therapy needs to be remedied before combination chemotherapy or combined modality therapy for biliary cancer can be developed. The most commonly reported drug has been 5-FU. Haskell reported responses in 4 of 17 patients (24%).[375] Davis and co-workers reported three responses in 23 patients (13%).[376] Mitomycin C was effective in 7 of 15 patients (42%) in a study by Crooke and Bradner, but Von Eyben and colleagues noted no responses in 10 patients given mitomycin C.[377,378] Anecdotal reports of responses to BCNU, Adriamycin, and neocarzinostatin have also been published.[379–380]

Bukowski and colleagues reported on 23 cases of gallbladder carcinoma and cholangiocarcinoma treated with m-AMSA.[381] Doses of 60 to 120 mg/m², given IV at 4-week intervals, produced partial responses in 1 of 12 patients with gallbladder cancer and 1 of 11 patients with cholangiocarcinoma.

Combination Chemotherapy

Several combination chemotherapy regimens have been studied in biliary tract carcinomas. One used the FAM protocol developed for gastric carcinomas. This consisted of treatment in 8-week cycles, giving 5-FU at a dose of 600 mg/m² on days 1, 8, 29, and 36; Adriamycin at 30 mg/m² on days 1 and 29; and mitomycin C at 10 mg/m² only on day 1 of each cycle. Harvey and co-workers reported on 17 consecutive patients with metastatic disease treated with FAM, of whom 14 had objectively measurable disease.[382] Partial responses were noted in 4 patients (31%), with a median duration of 8.5 months and a median survival of 11.5 months. Seven patients had disease stabilization for a median of 6.7 months (range, 3–18 months) and a median survival of 8.4 months. Progressive disease was seen during the first cycle of FAM in 4 patients, with this group surviving from 2 to 5 months.

Hall and colleagues evaluated a combination chemotherapy (FAB) using 4 mg/m² of Ftorafur given IV on days 1 and 22 and 2 mg/m² on days 4 and 26; 60 mg/m² of Adriamycin given IV on day 1 and 45 mg/m² on day 22; and 150 mg/m² of BCNU given IV on day 1. This regimen was given on a 6- to 8-week cycle in a mixed population of seven patients with gallbladder and bile duct cancer.[383] They reported three responders (43%), with two complete responses. Responders had an 11-month median survival. Ravey and Hester used a combination of 60 mg/m² of Adriamycin given IV every 3 weeks, combined with 10 U/m² of bleomycin every 2 weeks. They reported one partial remission among five patients.[384]

Mirsa and co-workers reported the use of chemotherapy given directly into the hepatic artery.[385] This seemed to be more effective than intravenous therapy. By delivering 5-FU plus mitomycin C directly into the hepatic artery in patients with gallbladder carcinoma metastatic to the liver, they noted 9 responses in 13 treated patients (69%).[385]

Adjuvant chemotherapy was explored in a nonrandomized trial using 5-FU with and without other drugs as adjuvant therapy in 13 patients with gallbladder cancer.[386] Treated patients had a median survival of 20 weeks, compared with 8 weeks for untreated patients. Of these, 1 treated patient with gross disease remaining after surgery was alive at 6 years.

The paucity of chemotherapy and combined modality data in the treatment of biliary cancer and cancer of the gallbladder delineates the need for clinical trials to address these issues.[373,387] Intergroup studies are probably needed to provide adequate patient numbers.

REFERENCES

1. Silverberg E: Cancer statistics 1987. CA 38:5–22, 1988
2. Cook GG, Moosa B: Hepatocellular carcinoma: One of the world's most common malignancies. Am J Med 233:705–708, 1985
3. Cady B, MacDonald JS, Sunderson LL: Cancer of the hepatobiliary system. In DeVita VT Jr, Hellman S, Rosenberg SA (eds): Cancer: Principles and Practice of Oncology, 2nd ed, pp 741–770. Philadelphia, JB Lippincott, 1985
4. Knop R, Berg CD, Ihde D: Primary liver cancer in the adult. In Moossa AR, Robson MC, Schimpff SC (eds): Comprehensive Textbook of Oncology, pp 1087–1096, Baltimore, Williams & Wilkins, 1986
5. Herfarth C, Schlag P, Hohenberger P (eds): Therapeutic Strategies in Primary and Metastatic Liver Cancer, Berlin, Springer-Verlag, 1986.
6. Wanebo HJ (ed): Hepatic and Biliary Cancer. New York, Marcel Dekker, 1987

EPIDEMIOLOGY

7. Linsell A: Primary liver cancer: Epidemiology and etiology. In Wanebo HJ (ed): Hepatic and Biliary Cancer, pp 3–15. New York, Marcel Dekker, 1987
8. Chlebowski R, Tong M, Weissman J et al: Hepatocellular carcinoma–diagnostic and prognostic features in North American patients. Cancer 53:2701–2706, 1984
9. Lopez-Corella E, Ridaura-Sanz C, Albores-Saavedra J: Primary carcinoma of the liver in Mexican adults. Cancer 22:678–684, 1968
10. Sung J, Wang T, Yu J: Clinical study of primary carcinoma of the liver inTaiwan. Am J Dig Dis 12:1036–1049, 1967
11. Geddes EW, Falkson G: Malignant hepatoma in the Bantu. Cancer (Suppl 6) 25:1271–1278, 1970
12. Okuda K, Liver Cancer Study Group of Japan: Primary liver cancers in Japan. Cancer 45:2663–2669
13. Falk H: Liver. In Schottenfeld J, Fraumeni J (eds): Cancer Epidemiology and Prevention, pp 668–682. Philadelphia, WB Saunders, 1982
14. Tang Z-Y, Yank B-I: Early detection of subclinical hepatocellular carcinoma. In Tang Z-Y (ed): Subclinical Hepatocellular Carcinoma, pp 12–21. Berlin, Springer-Verlag, 1985
15. Cook GG, Mozaffari P, Van Rensberg S: Cancer of the liver. Br Med Bull 40:342–345, 1984
16. Berman M, Libbey P, Foster J: Hepatocellular carcinoma: Polygonal cell type with fibrous stroma—an atypical variant with a favorable prognosis. Cancer 46:1448–1455, 1980
17. Craig J, Peters R, Edmondson H et al: Fibrolamellar carcinoma of the liver: A tumor of adolescents and young adults with distinctive clinicopathologic features. Cancer 46:372–379, 1980
18. Lack E, Neave C, Vawter G: Hepatocellular carcinoma—Review of 32 cases in childhood and adolescence. Cancer 52:1510–1515, 1983
19. Ihde D, Matthews M, Makuch R et al: Prognostic factors in patients with hepatocellular carcinoma receiving systemic chemotherapy—Identification of two groups of patients with prospects for prolonged survival. Am J Med 78:399–406, 1985
20. Dunham LJ, Bailar JC III: World maps of cancer mortality rates and frequency ratios. JNCI 41:155–203, 1968
21. Omato M, Ashcavaii M, Liew CT et al: HCC in USA; etiologic consideration. Localization of hepatitis B antigen. Gastroenterology 76:279–287, 1979
22. Trichopolous D, Tabor E, Goetz RJ et al: Hepatitis B and primary hepatocellular carcinoma in European population. Lancet 2:1217–1219, 1978
23. Liver Cancer Study Group of Japan: Primary liver cancer in Japan. Cancer 54:1747–1755, 1984
24. Lin D, Liaw Y, Chu C et al: Hepatocellular carcinoma in noncirrhotic patients—A laparoscopic study of 92 cases in Taiwan. Cancer 54:1466–1468, 1984
25. DiBisceglie AM, Hoofnagle JH: Hepatitis B virus infection and hepatocellular carcinoma: Etiologic relationships and clinical implications. In Updates: Cancer: Principles and Practice of Oncology, vol 10, pp 1–10. Philadelphia, JB Lippincott, 1987

25a. DiBisceglie AM, Sjogren M, Klein J et al: Role of hepatitis B virus infection in hepatocellular carcinoma in the United States. Presented at International Sympo-

sium on Molecular Probes: Technology Medical Applications, Florence, Italy, April 11–13, 1988
26. Lai C, Lam K, Wong K et al: Clinical features of hepatocellular carcinoma: Review of 211 patients in Hong Kong. Cancer 47:2746–2755, 1981
27. Hall AJ, Winter PD, Wright R: Mortality of hepatitis B positive blood donors in England and Wales. Lancet 1:91–93, 1985
28. Beasley RP, Linn CC, Hwang LY et al: Hepatocellular carcinoma and hepatitis B virus: A prospective study of 22,707 men in Taiwan. Lancet 2:1129–1132, 1981
29. Bassendine MF, Della Seta L, Salmeron J et al: Incidence of hepatitis B virus infection in alcoholic liver disease, HBsAg negative chronic active liver disease and primary liver cell cancer in Britain. Liver 3:65–70, 1983
30. Yeh FS, Mo CC, Luo S et al: A serological case control study of primary hepatocellular carcinoma in Los Angeles. Cancer Res 43:6077–6079, 1983
31. Lohija G, Pirkle H, Hoefs J et al: Hepatocellular carcinoma in young mentally retarded HBsAg carriers without cirrhosis. Hepatology 5:824–826, 1985
32. Van den Heever A, Pretorius FJ, Falkson G et al: Hepatitis B surface antigen and primary liver cancer. S Afr Med J 54:359–361, 1978
33. Falkson G, Bohmer RH, Adam M et al: Hepatitis-B as a prognostic discriminant in patients with primary liver cancer. Cancer 57:812–815, 1986
34. Wen Y: Hepatitis B virus and hepatocellular carcinoma—cellular and molecular aspects. In Tang Z-Y (ed): Subclinical Hepatocellular Carcinoma, pp 218–231. Berlin, Springer-Verlag, 1985
35. MacNab GM, Alexander JJ, Lecatsas G et al: Hepatitis B surface antigen produced by a human hepatoma cell line. Br J Cancer 34:509–515, 1976
36. Smalley SR, Moertel CG, Hilton JF et al: Hepatoma in the noncirrhotic liver (in press)
37. Hislop W, Masterson N, Bouchier I et al: Cirrhosis and primary liver cell carcinoma in Tayside—A five year study. Scott-Med J 27:29–36, 1982
38. Fisher RL, Schauer PS, Sherlock S: Primary liver cancer in the presence or absence of hepatitis B-antigen. Cancer 38:901–905, 1976
39. Linsell CA, Peers FG: Aflatoxin and liver cell cancer. Trans R Soc Trop Med Hyg 71:471–473, 1977
40. Yaobin W, Lizun L, Benfa Y et al: Relationship between geographical distribution of liver cancer and climate—aflatoxin B_1 in China. Sci Sin [B] 26:1166–1175, 1983
41. Troillais P: Evidence that hepatitis B virus has a role in liver cell carcinoma in alcoholic liver disease. N Engl J Med 306:1384–1387, 1982
42. Kew MC, Roussow E, Paterson A et al: Hepatitis B virus status of black women with hepatocellular carcinoma. Gastroenterology 84:693–696, 1983
43. McSween RNM: Alcohol and cancer. Br Med Bull 38:31–33, 1982
44. Nakanuma J, Ohta G: Morphology of cirrhosis and occurrence of hepatocellular carcinoma in alcoholics with and without HBsAg and in nonalcoholic HBsAg positive patients. A comparative study. Liver 3:231–237, 1983
45. Simson IW: Budd Chiari syndrome and veno-occlusive disease in contemporary issues in surgical pathology. In Peters RL and Craig JR (eds): Liver Pathology, pp 299–314. Edinburgh, Churchill Livingstone, 1986
46. Simson IW: Membranous obstruction of the inferior vena cava and hepatocellular carcinoma in South Africa. Gastroenterology 82:171–178, 1982
47. Rector WG, Xu Y, Goldstein L et al: Membranous obstruction of the inferior vena cava in the United States. Medicine 64:134–143, 1985
48. Simson IW: The causes and consequences of chronic hepatic venous outflow obstruction. S Afr Med J 72:11–14, 1987
49. Nakamura S, Takezawa Y: Obstruction of the inferior vena cava in the hepatic portion and hepatocellular carcinoma. Tohoku J Exp Med 138:119–120, 1982
50. Johnson PJ, Krasner N, Portman B et al: Hepatocellular carcinoma in Great Britain: Influence of age, sex, HBsAg status and etiology of underlying cirrhosis. Gut 19:1022–1026, 1978
51. Melia WM, Wilkinson ML, Portman BC et al: Hepatocellular carcinoma in the non-cirrhotic liver: A comparison with that complicating cirrhosis. Q J Med (211)53:391–400, 1984
52. Cobden I, Bassendine MF, James OFW: Hepatocellular carcinoma in North East England: Importance of hepatitis B infection and extropical military service. Q J Med (233)60:855–863, 1986
53. Schonland MM, Millward-Sadler GH, Wright DH et al: Hepatocellular carcinoma. In Wright R, Millward-Sadler GH, Alberti KGMM et al (eds): Liver and Biliary Disease, 2nd ed, pp 1138–1184. London, Balliere Tindall, 1985
54. Iqbal MJ, Wilkinson ML, Forbes A et al: Preponderance of serum and intrahepatic 5-alpha-dihydrotestosterone in males with hepatocellular carcinoma despite low circulating androgen levels. J Hepatol 3:304–309, 1986
55. Iqbal MJ, Wilkinson ML, Johnson PJ et al: Sex steroid receptor proteins in foetal adult and malignant human liver tissue. Br J Cancer (Suppl 6)48:791–796, 1983
56. Wilkinson ML, Iqbal MJ, Williams R: Characterisation of high affinity binding sites of androgens in primary hepatocellular carcinoma. Clin Chim Acta 152:105–113, 1985
57. Nagasue N, Ito A, Yukaga H et al: Androgen receptors in hepatocellular carcinoma and surrounding parenchyma. Gastroenterology 89:643–647, 1985
58. Ohnishi S, Murakami T, Moriyama T et al: Androgen and estrogen receptors in hepatocellular carcinoma and in the surrounding non-cancerous liver tissue. Hepatology 6:440–443, 1986
59. Nagasue N, Yukaya H, Chang Y-C et al: Active uptake of testosterone by androgen receptors of hepatocellular carcinoma in humans. Cancer 57:2162–2167, 1986
60. Edmondson HA, Steiner PE: Primary carcinoma of the liver: An autopsy study of 100 cases among 48,900 necropsies. Cancer 7:462–502, 1954
61. Christopherson WM, Mays ET, Barrows GH: Liver tumors in young women: A clinical pathologic study of 201 cases in the Louisville registry. In Fenoglio CM, Wolff M (eds): Progress in Surgical Pathology, vol II, pp 187–205. New York, Masson Publishing USA, 1980
62. Christopherson WM, Mays ET: Risk factors, pathology and pathogenesis of selected benign and malignant liver neoplasms. In Wanebo HJ (ed): Hepatic and Biliary Cancer, pp 17–43. New York, Marcel Dekker, 1987

PATHOLOGY

63. Peters RL: Pathology of hepatocellular carcinoma. In Okuda K, Peters RL (eds): Hepatocellular Carcinoma, pp 107–168. New York, John Wiley & Sons, 1976
64. Simson IW: Personal communication, 1987
65. Steiner PE: Cancer of the liver and cirrhosis in Trans-Saharan Africa and the United States of America. Cancer 13:1085–1166, 1960
66. Okuda K, Musha H, Nakajima Y et al: Clinicopathologic features of encapsulated hepatocellular carcinoma. A study of 26 cases. Cancer 40:1240–1245, 1977
67. Nakashima T, Sakamoto K: A study of hepatocellular carcinoma among Japanese from the point of veiw of morpho-developmental pathology—gross anatomical types classified in its relation to capsule formation. Kurume Med J 24:S43–62, 1977
68. Anthony PP: Primary carcinoma of the liver: A study of 282 cases in Ugandan Africans. J Pathol 110:37–48, 1973
69. Matsumoto Y, Suzuki T, Asada I et al: Clinical classification of hepatoma in Japan according to serial changes in serum alpha-fetoprotein levels. Cancer 49:354–360, 1982
70. Craig JR, Peters RL, Edmondson HA et al: Fibrolamellar carcinoma of the liver. A tumor of adolescents and young adults with distinctive clinico-pathologic features. Cancer 46:372–379, 1980
71. Berman MM, Libbey NP, Foster JH: Hepatocellular carcinoma. Polygonal cell type with fibrous stroma—an atypical variant with a favorable prognosis. Cancer 46:1448–1455, 1980
72. Christopherson WM, Mays ET, Barrows GH: Liver tumors in young women: A clinical pathologic study of 201 cases in the Louisville registry. In Fenoglio CM, Wolff M (eds): Progress in Surgical Pathology, vol II, pp 187–205. New York, Masson Publishing USA, 1980
73. Omata M, Peters RL, Tatter D: Sclerosing hepatic carcinoma: Relationship to hypercalcemia. Liver 1:33–49, 1981
74. Rizzo PA, Young RC: Infections in the cancer patient. In DeVita VT Jr, Hellman S, Rosenberg SA (eds): Cancer: Principles and Practice of Oncology, 2nd ed. p 1963, Philadelphia, JB Lippincott, 1985
75. Order SE, Stillwagon GB, Klein JL et al: Iodine 131 antiferritin, a new treatment modality in hepatoma: A Radiation Therapy Oncology Group study. J Clin Oncol 3:1573, 1985
76. Tommasini M, Colombo M, Sangiovanni A et al: Intrahepatic doxorubicin in unresectable hepatocellular carcinoma: The unfavorable role of cirrhosis. Am J Clin Oncol 9:8, 1986
77. Tang Z-Y, Yu Y, Linz Zhou Y et al: Small hepatocellular carcinoma: Clinical analysis of 30 cases. Chin Med J [Engl] 92:455, 1979
78. Rostock RA, Klein JL, Leichner PK et al: Distribution of physiologic factors that affect 131-I antiferritin tumor localization in experimental hepatoma. Int J Radiat Oncol Biol Phys 10:1135, 1984
79. Okuda K, Kotoda K, Obata H et al: Clinical observations during a relatively early stage of hepatocellular carcinoma with special reference to serum alpha-fetoprotein levels. Gastroenterology 69:226–234, 1975
80. McIntyre KR, Waldmann TA, Moertel CG et al: Serum alpha-fetoprotein in patients with neoplasms of the gastrointestinal tract. Cancer Res 35:991–996, 1975
81. Geddes EW, Falkson G: Differential diagnosis of primary malignant hepatoma in 569 Bantu mineworkers. Cancer (Suppl 5)31:1216–1221, 1973
82. Waldmann TA, McIntire KR: The use of radioimmunoassay for alpha-fetoprotein in the diagnosis of malignancy. Cancer 34:1510–15, 1974
83. Melia WM, Johnson PJ, Carter S et al: Plasma carcinoembryonic antigen in the diagnosis and management of patients with hepatocellular carcinoma. Cancer 48:1004–1008, 1981
84. Nakagawara A, Ikeda K, Tsuneyoshi M et al: Hepatoblastoma producing both alpha-fetoprotein and human chorionic gonadotropin. Clinicopathologic analysis of four cases and a review of the literature. Cancer 56:1636–1642, 1985
85. Conte N, Ceccettin PM, Manente P et al: Calcitonin in hepatoma and cirrhosis. Acta Endocrinol (Copenh) 106:109–111, 1984
86. Collier NA, Weinbren K, Bloom SR et al: Neurotension secretion by fibrolamellar carcinoma of the liver. Lancet 1:538–540, 1984
87. Anderson JR, Cain KC, Gelber RD et al: Analysis and interpretation of the comparison of survival by treatment outcome variables in cancer clinical trials. Cancer Treat Rep (Suppl 10)69:1139–1144, 1985
88. Falkson G: Personal communication
89. Ong GB, Taw JL: Spontaneous rupture of hepatocellular carcinoma. Br Med J 4:146–149, 1972
90. Simson IW: Membranous obstruction of the inferior vena cava and hepatocellular carcinoma in South Africa. Gastroenterology 82:171–178, 1982
91. van Sonnenberg E, Ferrucci JT: Bile duct obstruction in hepatocellular carcinoma (hepatoma)—clinical and cholangiographic characteristics. Report of 6 cases and review of the literature. Radiology 130:7–13, 1979

92. Alpert E: Human alpha-fetoprotein (AFP): Developmental biology and clinical significance. In Popper H, Schaffner E (eds): Progress in Liver Diseases, vol V, pp 337–349. New York, Grune and Stratton, 1976
93. McIntire KR, Vogel CL, Primack A: Effect of surgical and chemotherapeutic treatment on alpha-fetoprotein levels in patients with hepatocellular carcinoma. Cancer 37:677–683, 1976
94. The Co-ordinating Group for the Research of Liver Cancer, People's Republic of China: Application of serum alpha-fetoprotein assay in mass survey of primary carcinoma of liver. Am J Clin Med 241:241–245, 1974
95. Heyward WL, Bender TR, Lanier AP et al: Serological markers of heptatitis B virus and alpha-fetoprotein levels preceding primary hepatocellular carcinoma in Alaskan eskimos. Lancet 2:889–891, 1982
96. Dodd RY, Vyas GN, Dienstag VL et al: HbsAg as a risk factor for hepatocellular carcinoma among Americans In Viral Hepatitis and Liver Disease, p 638. Orlando, Grune & Stratton, 1984
97. Lotze MT, Wanebo HJ: Current and future research directions in management of hepatic cancer. In Wanebo HJ (ed): Hepatic and Biliary Cancer, pp 501–534. New York, Marcel Dekker, 1987
98. Teates CD: Radiological techniques in the diagnoses and treatment of liver tumors. In Wanebo HJ (ed): Hepatic and Biliary Cancer, pp 57–95. New York, Marcel Dekker, 1987
99. Oon CJ, Yo SL, Chio LF et al: The evaluation of tumour marker proteins in the diagnosis of primary hepatocellular carcinoma. Ann Acad Med Singapore, (Suppl 2) 9:228–233, 1980
100. Ihde DC, Sherlock P, Winawer SJ et al: Clinical manifestations of hepatoma: A review of 6 years' experience at a cancer hospital. Am J Med 56:83, 1974
101. Ohto M et al: Detection of minute hepatocellular carcinoma for early diagnosis of real-time ultrasonography (abstr). Gastroenterology 79:1117, 1980
102. Ohto M, Karasawa E, Tsuchiya et al: Ultrasonically guided percutaneous contrast medicine injection and aspiration biopsy using a real time puncture transducer. Radiology 136:171–176, 1980
103. Cheng W-KE, Lightdale CJ: Primary liver cancer: Diagnosis and laboratory findings. In Wanebo HJ (ed): Hepatic and Biliary Cancer, pp 45–55. New York, Marcel Dekker, 1987
104. Fortner JG, Kim DK, McSweeney J et al: Tumors of the liver as demonstrated by angiography, scan and laparotomy. Surg Gynecol Obstet 141:409–411, 1975
105. Fortner JG: Current management of tumors of the liver. Surg Clin North Am 57:465–472, 1977
106. Primack A, Vogel CL, Kyalwazi SK et al: A staging system for hepatocellular carcinoma: Prognostic factors in Ugandan patients. Cancer 35:1357–1364, 1975
107. Falkson G, Moertel CG, Lavin P et al: Chemotherapy studies in primary liver cancer. Cancer 42:2149–2156, 1978
108. Adson NA, Beart RW: Elective hepatic resections. Surg Clin North Am 57:339, 1977
109. Adson MA: Diagnosis and surgical treatment of primary and secondary solid hepatic tumors in the adult. Surg Clin North Am 61:181–196, 1981
110. Adson MA: Hepatic resections: Technical considerations—One surgeons view. In Wanebo HJ (ed): Hepatic and Biliary Cancer, pp 487–499. New York, Marcel Dekker, 1987
111. Fortner JG, Maclean BA, Kim DK et al: The seventies' evolution in liver surgery for cancer. Cancer 47:2162–2166, 1981
112. Tobe T: Hepatectomy in patients—cirrhotic liver: Clinical and basic observations. In Nyhus LM (ed): Surgery Annual, pp 177–202. Norwalk, Appleton, 1984
113. Goldsmith NA, Woodburne RT: The surgical anatomy pertaining to liver resection. Surg Gynecol Obstet 105:310, 1957
114. LeFoie CC: Etudes anatomiques et chirurgicales. Paris, Masson, 1957
115. Bismuth H: Surgical anatomy and anatomical surgery of the liver. World J Surg 6:3–9, 1982
116. Starzl TE, Bell RH, Beart RW et al: Hepatic trisegmentectomy and other liver resections. Surg Gynecol Obstet 141:429, 1975
117. Foster JH, Berman MM: Solid liver tumors. Major Probl Clin Surg 22:1, 1977
118. Huguet C, Gallot D, Offenstadt G: Normothermine complete hepatic vascular exclusion for extensive resection of the liver. N Engl J Med 294:51, 1976
119. Nagorney DM, Adson MA: Major hepatic resections for hepatoma in the west. In Wanebo HJ (ed): Hepatic and Biliary Cancer, pp 167–185. New York, Marcel Dekker, 1987
120. Inouye AA, Whelan TJ Jr: Primary liver cancer: A review of 205 cases in Hawaii. Am J Surg 138:53, 1979
121. Harrison NW, Dhru D, Primack A et al: The surgical management of primary hepatocellular carcinoma in Uganda. Br J Surg 60:565, 1973
122. Lee NW, Wong J, Ong GB: The surgical management of primary carcinoma of the liver. World J Surg 6:66, 1982
123. Wu M, Chen H, Zhang X et al: Primary hepatic carcinoma resection over 18 years. Chin Med J [Engl] 93:723, 1980
124. Lin T-Y: Recent advances in technique of hepatic lobectomy and results of surgical treatment for primary carcinoma of the liver. Prog Liver Dis 4:668, 1976
125. Okuda K: Liver Cancer Study Group of Japan: Primary liver cancers in Japan. Cancer 45:2663, 1980
126. Tobe T: Current status of surgical therapy for primary liver cancer in Japan. Jpn J Surg 13:86, 1983
126a. Nagasue N, Yukaya H, Ogawa Y et al: Clinical experience with 118 hepatic resections for hepatocellular carcinoma. Surgery 99:694–701, 1986
126b. Nagao T, Inoue S, Goto S et al: Hepatic resection for hepatocellular carcinoma. Clinical features and long-term prognosis. Ann Surg 205:33–40, 1987
127. Okuda K, Musha H, Nakajima Y et al: Clinicopathologic features of encapsulated hepatocellular carcinoma. A study of 26 cases. Cancer 40:1240, 1977
127a. Honjo I, Mitzumoto R: Primary carcinoma of the liver. Am J Surg 128:31, 1974
128. Balasegram M, Joishy SK: Hepatic resection. The logical approach to surgical management of major trauma to the liver. Am J Surg (Suppl 5)142:580–583, 1981
129. Kanematsu T, Takenatio K, Matsumata T et al: Limited hepatic resection effective for selected cirrhotic pts with primary liver cancer. Ann Surg 199:51, 1984
130. Lee Y-T N: Primary carcinoma of the liver: Diagnosis, prognosis, and management. J Surg Oncol 22:17, 1983
131. Tobe T: Hepatectomy in patients with cirrhotic livers: Clinical and basic observations. Surg Annu 16:177 1984
132. Gill RA, Goodman MW, Golfus GE et al: Aminopyrine breath test predicts surgical risk for patients with liver disease. Ann Surg 198:701, 1983
133. Okamoto E, Kyo A, Yamanaka N et al: Prediction of the safe limits of hepatectomy by combined volumetric and functional measurements in patients with impaired hepatic function. Surgery 95:586, 1984
134. Tsuzuki T, Ogata Y, Iida S et al: Hepatic resection in 125 patients. Arch Surg 119:1025, 1984
135. Okuda K, Ryu M, Tobe T: Surgical management of hepatoma. The Japanese experience. In Wanebo HJ (ed): Hepatic and Biliary Cancer, pp 219–238. New York, Marcel Dekker, 1987
135a. Chen D, Sung J, Shev J et al: Serum AFP in early stage of human hepatocellular carcinoma. Gastroenterology 86:1404, 1984
135b. Shinagawa T, Ohto M, Kimura K et al: Diagnosis and clinical features of small hepatocellular carcinoma with emphasis on the utility of real-time ultrasonography. A study in 51 patients. Gastroenterology 86:495, 1984
135c. Ebara M, Ohto M, Shingawa T et al: Natural history of minute HCC smaller than 3 cm complicating cirrhosis. A study in 22 patients. Gastroenterology 90:289, 1986
136. Rao BN, Green AA: Hepatic tumors in children and adolescents. In Wanebo HJ (ed): Hepatic and Biliary Cancer, pp 187–218. New York, Marcel Dekker, 1987
137. Weinberg AG, Finegold MJ: Primary hepatic tumors of childhood. Hum Pathol 14:512–537, 1983
138. Edmondson HA: Differential diagnosis of tumors and tumor-like lesions of the liver in infancy and childhood. Am J Dis Child 91:168, 1956
139. Ishak KG: Primary hepatic tumors in childhood. In Popper H, Schafner R (eds): Progress in Liver Disease, Vol 5, pp 636–667. New York, Grune & Stratton, 1976
140. Lack EE, Neave C, Vawter GF: Hepatoblastoma: A clinical and pathological study of 54 cases. Am J Surg Pathol 6:693–702, 1982
141. Gonzales-Crussi F, Upton MP, Maurer HS: Hepatoblastoma: Attempt at characterization of histologic subtypes. Am J Surg Pathol (Suppl 7)6:599–612, 1982
142. Esquivel CO, Iwatsuki S, Gordon RD et al: Transplantation for primary liver cancer. Wanebo HJ (ed): Hepatic and Biliary Cancer, pp 477–486. New York, Marcel Dekker, 1987
143. Starzl TE, Putnam CW: Experiences in Hepatic Transplantation. Philadelphia, WB Saunders, 1969
144. Calne RY: Liver transplantation. In Calne RY (ed): The Cambridge and King's College Hospital Experience, pp 306–311. London, Grune & Stratton, 1983
145. Iwatsuki S, Gordon RD, Shaw BW Jr et al: Role of liver transplantation in cancer therapy. Ann Surg (Suppl 4)202:401–407, 1985
146. Starzl TE, Iwatsuki S, Shaw BW Jr et al: Treatment of fibrolamellar hepatoma with partial or total hepatectomy and transplantation of the liver. Surg Gynecol Obstet 162:145–148, 1986
147. Falkson G, Cnaan A: Prognostic factors in hepatocellular cancer (in press)
148. Attali P, Prod'Homme S, Pelletier G et al: Prognostic factors in patients with hepatocellular carcinoma. Attempts for the selection of patients with prolonged survival. Cancer 59:2108–2111, 1987
149. Falkson G, Snyman HJ: Experience with chemotherapy of cancer at the University of Pretoria. Acta Union Internationale Contre le Cancer (Suppl 1–2)20:439–446, 1964
150. South African Primary Liver Cancer Research Group: Malignant hepatoma—controlled therapeutic trials. S Afr Med J 41:309–314, 1967
151. Vogel C, Adamson R, DeVita V et al: Preliminary clinical trials of dichloromethotrexate (NSC-29630) in hepatocellular carcinoma. Cancer Chemother Rep 56:249–258, 1972
152. Tester W, Donhower R, Eddy J et al: Evaluation of weekly escalating doses of dichloromethotrexate in patients with hepatocellular carcinoma and other solid tumors. Cancer Chemother Pharmacol 8:305–310, 1982
153. Davis H, Ramirez G, Ansfield F: Adenocarcinomas of stomach, pancreas, liver and biliary tracts: Survival of 328 patients treated with fluoropyrimidine therapy. Cancer 33:193–197, 1974
154. Brennan M, Talley R et al: Critical analysis of 594 cancer patients treated with 5-fluorouracil. In Plattner A (ed): Proceedings of the International Symposium on Chemotherapy of Cancer, pp 118–149. New York, Elsevier North-Holland, 1964
155. Ramierz G, Ansfield F, Curreri A: Hepatoma: Long-term survival with disseminated tumor treated with 5-fluorouracil. Am J Surg 120:400–403, 1970
156. Gailani S, Holland JF, Falkson G et al: Comparison of treatment of metastatic gastrointestinal cancer with 5-fluorouracil (5-FU) to a combination of 5-FU with cytosine arabinoside. Cancer 29:1308–1313, 1972
157. Al-Sarraf M, Go T, Kithier K et al: Primary liver cancer. A review of the clinical features, blood groups, serum enzymes, therapy, and survival of 65 cases. Cancer 33:574–582, 1974
158. Link J, Bateman J, Paroly W et al: 5-Fluorouracil in hepatocellular carcinoma—Report of twenty-one cases. Cancer 39:1936–1939, 1977

159. Kennedy P, Lahane D, Smith F et al: Oral fluorouracil therapy of hepatoma. Cancer 39:1930–1935, 1977
160. Joishy SK, Bennett JM, Balasegaram M et al: Clinical and chemotherapeutic study of hepatocellular carcinoma in Malaysia—A comparison with African and American patients. Cancer 50:1065–1069, 1982
161. Damrongsak C, Viranuvatti V, Chearanai O et al: Vinblastine in the treatment of carcinoma of the liver. J Med Assoc Thai 56:370–372, 1973
162. Falkson G: The treatment of liver cell cancer. In Cameron HM, Linsell DA, Warwick GP (eds): Liver Cell Cancer, pp 81–92. Amsterdam, Elsevier Scientific Publishing, 1976
163. Cavalli F, Rozencweig M, Renard J et al: Phase II study of oral VP-16-213 in hepatocellular carcinoma. Eur J Cancer Clin Oncol (Suppl 10)17:1079–1082, 1981
164. Melia WM, Johnson PJ, Williams R: Induction of remission in hepatocellular carcinoma: A comparison of VP-16 with adriamycin. Cancer 51:206–210, 1983
165. Domingo GO, Lingao AL, Lao JY et al: Therapeutic activity and efficiency of etoposide in hepatocellular carcinoma. Phil J Intern Med 20:106–112, 1982
166. Melia WM, Westaby D, Williams R: Iamminodichloride platinum (cisplatinum) in the treatment of hepatocellular carcinoma. Clin Oncol 7:275–280, 1981
167. Perry DJ, Van Ecco DA, Mick R: A Phase II study of deoxydoxorubicin in patients with advanced liver cancer. Cancer Treat Rep 71:1117–1118, 1987
168. Ravery MJR, Omura GA, Bartolucci AA et al: Phase II evaluation of cisplatin in advanced hepatocellular carcinoma and cholangiosarcoma: A Southwestern Cancer Study Group trial. Cancer Treat Rep (Suppl 2)70:311–312, 1986
169. Falkson G, Von Hoff D, Klaassen D et al: A phase II study of neocarzinostatin (NSC 157365) in malignant hepatoma. An Eastern Cooperative Oncology Group pilot study. Cancer Chemother Pharamcol 4:33–36, 1980
170. Falkson G, MacIntyre J, Coetzer B et al: Phase II-III trial of neocarzinostatin versus m-AMSA adriamycin in hepatocellular carcinoma. J Clin Oncol (Suppl 6)2:581–584, 1984
171. Falkson G, Coetzer BJ, Terblance APS: Phase II trial of mitoxantrone in patients with primary liver cancer. Cancer Treat Rep (Suppl 10)68:1311–1312, 1984
172. Falkson G, Moertel C, Lavin P et al: Chemotherapy studies in primary liver cancer a prospective randomized clinical trial. Cancer 42:2149–56, 1978
173. Vogel CL, Bayley AC, Rocker RJ et al: A phase II study of adriamycin (NSC 123127) in patients with hepatocellular carcinoma from Zambia and the United States. Cancer 39:1923–1929, 1977
174. Ihde D, Kane R, Cohen M et al: Adriamycin therapy in American patients with hepatocellular carcinoma. Cancer Treat Rep 61:1385–1387, 1977
175. Chlebowski R, Brzechwa-Adjunkiewicz A, Cowden A et al: Doxorubicin (75 mg/m²) for hepatocellular carcinoma: Clinical and pharmacokinetic results. Cancer Treat Rep 68:487–491, 1984
176. Olweny CL, Katongole-Mbidde E, Bahendeka S et al: Further experience in treating patients with hepatocellular carcinoma in Uganda. Cancer 46:2717–2722, 1980
177. Johnson P, Thomas H, Williams R et al: Induction of remission in HCC with doxorubicin. Lancet 1:1006–1009, 1978
178. Sciarrino E, Simonetti R, LeMoli S et al: Adriamycin treatment for hepatocellular carcinoma—Experience with 109 patients. Cancer 56:2751–2755, 1985
179. Barbare J, Ballet F, Petit J et al: Carcinoma hepatocellulaire sur cirrhose: Traitment par la doxorbuicine. Essaie phase II. Bull Cancer (Paris) 71:442–445, 1984
180. Choi T, Lee N, Wong J: Chemotherapy for advanced hepatocellular carcinoma. Adriamycin versus quadruple chemotherapy. Cancer 53:401–405, 1984
181. Hochster HS, Green MD, Speyer S et al: 4′-Epidoxorubicin (epirubicin): Activity in hepatocellular carcinoma. J Clin Oncol (Suppl 3)3:1535–1540, 1985
182. Shiu W, Mok S, Tsao S et al: Phase II trial of epirubicin in hepatoma. Cancer Treat Rep 70:1035–1036, 1986
183. Cheng E, Chun H, Schiff C et al: Phase II trial of oral 4′demethoxydaunorubicin (DMDR) in patients (pts) with primary liver carcinoma (PLC) (abstr). Proc Am Soc Clin Oncol 4:88, 1985
184. Davis RB, Van Ecco DA, Leone LA et al: Phase II trial of mitoxantrone in advanced primary liver cancer: A cancer and leukemia group B study. Cancer Treat Rep 70:1125–1126, 1986
185. Falkson G, Coetzer BJ, Terblanche APS. Phase II trial of mitoxantrone in patients with primary liver cancer. Cancer Treat Rep (Suppl 10)68:1311–1312, 1984
186. Falkson G, Coetzer B: Phase II studies of mitoxantrone in patients with liver cancer. Invest New Drugs 3:187–189, 1985
187. Falkson G, Ryan LM, Johnson LA et al: Randomized phase II study of mitoxantrone and cis-platinum in patients with HCC. An ECOG study. Cancer 60:2141–2145, 1987
188. Falkson G: Therapeutic approaches to hepatoma. Cancer Treat Rev 2:73–76, 1975
189. Falkson G, Coetzer B, Klaassen DJ: A phase II study of m-AMSA in patients with primary liver cancer. Cancer Chemother Pharmacol 6:127–129, 1981
190. Bukowski RM, Legha S, Saiki J et al: Phase II trial of m-AMSA in hepatocellular carcinoma. A Southwest Oncology Group study. Cancer Treat Rep 66:1651–1652, 1982
191. Cheng E, Lightdale C, Young C et al: Phase II trial of (m-AMSA) 4′-9-(acridinlyamino)-methanesulfon-m-anisidide in primary liver cancer. Am J Clin Oncol 6:211–213, 1983
192. Amrein P, Richards F, Coleman M et al: Phase II trial of amsacrine in patients with hepatoma: A Cancer and Leukemia Group study. Cancer Treat Rep 68:923–924, 1984
193. Nair PV, Tong MJ, Kemp F et al: Clinical, serological and immunological effects of human leukocyte interferon in HBsAg positive hepatocellular carcinoma. Cancer 56:1018–1022, 1985
194. Sachs E, Bisceglie AM, Dusheiko GM et al: Treatment of hepatocellular carcinoma with recombinant leukocyte interferon. A pilot study. Br J Cancer 52:105–109, 1985
195. Forbes A, Johnson PJ, Williams R: Recombinant human gamma interferon in primary hepatocellular carcinoma. J R Soc Med 78:826–829, 1985
196. Falkson G: Chemoterapie van primere lewerkarsinoom. Spekulum 3:5–11, 1954
197. Gillman T, Hathorn M, Lamont NME: Alloxan as a possible therapeutic agent for primary carcinoma of the liver. Lancet 2:687–688, 1957
198. Friedman MA, Demanes DJ, Hoffman PG Jr: Hepatomas: Hormone receptors and therapy. Am J Med 73:362–366, 1982
199. Paliard R, Clement G, Saez S et al: Traitment du carcinome hepatocellulaire par le tamoxifene. Gastroenterol Clin Biol 8:680–681, 1984
200. Trinchet J-C, Roudil F, Vayasse J et al: Effects d'une association tamoxifene—norethisterone chez 16 malades de carcinome hepatocellulaire. Gastroenterol Clin Biol 9:455, 1985
201. Forbes A, Wilkinson ML, Iqbal MJ et al: Possible role of antiandrogens in treatment of hepatocellular carcinoma. Gut 27:A596, 1986
202. McIntyre K, Vogel C, Primack A et al: Effect of surgical and chemotherapeutic treatment on alpha fetoprotein levels in patients with hepatocellular carcinoma. Cancer 37:677–683, 1976
203. Umsawasdi T, Chainuvati T, Viranuvatti V: Combination chemotherapy of hepatocellular carcinoma (HC) with 5-fluorouracil (5-FU) and mitomycin-C (MMC) (abstr). Proc Am Assoc Cancer Res 19:193, 1978
204. Lee Y-TM: Systemic and regional treatment of primary carcinoma of the liver. Cancer Treat Rev 4:195–212, 1977
205. Falkson G: The management of tumors of the liver and biliary tract. In Carter SK, Glatstein E, Livingston RB (eds): Principles of Cancer Treatment, pp 426–433. New York, McGraw-Hill, 1982
206. Cochrane A, Muray-Lyon I, Brinkly D et al: Quadruple chemotherapy versus radiotherapy in treatment of primary hepatocellular carcinoma. Cancer 40:609–614, 1977
207. Baker LH, Saiki JH, Jones SE et al: Adriamycin and 5-fluorouracil in the treatment of advanced hepatoma. A Southwest Oncology Group study. Cancer Treat Rep 61:1595–1597, 1977
208. Oon CJ, Chua EJ, Foong WC et al: Adriamycin in the treatment of resectable and intersectible primary hepatocellular carcinoma. Ann Acad Med Singapore 9:256–259, 1980
209. Chlebowski R, Chan K, Tong M et al: Adriamycin and methyl-CCNU. Combination therapy in hepatocellular carcinoma: Clinical and pharmacokinetic aspects. Cancer 48:1088–1095, 1981
210. Bezwoda W, Derman D: Treatment of advanced malignant hepatoma with adriamycin or AMSA in combination with VM-26 plus 5-FU (abstr). Proc Am Soc Clin Oncol 1:91, 1982
211. Morstyn G, Ihde D, Eddy J et al: Combination chemotherapy of hepatocellular carcinoma with doxorubicin and streptozotocin. Am J Clin Oncol 6:547–551, 1983
212. Ravery MJR, Omura GA, Bartolucci AA: Phase II evaluation of epidoxorubicin plus bleomycin in hepatocellular carcinoma. A Southeastern Cancer Group trial. Cancer Treat Rep 68:1517–1518, 1984
213. Al-Idrissi H, Ibrahim E, Satir A et al: Primary hepatocellular carcinoma in the Eastern Province of Saudi Arabia: Treatment with combination chemotherapy using 5-fluorouracil, Adriamycin and mitomycin-C. Hepatogastroenterology 32:8–10, 1985
214. Friedman MA, Volberding P, Cassidy M et al: Therapy for hepatocellular cancer with intrahepatic arterial adriamycin and 5-fluorouracil combined with whole-liver irradiation: A Northern California Oncology Group study. Cancer Treat Rep 63:1885–1888, 1979
215. South African Primary Liver Cancer Research Group. Malignant hepatoma—Controlled therapeutic trials. S Afr Med J 41:309–314, 1967
216. Volberding P, Friedman M, Phillips T: Hepatoma treated with intraarterial (IA) polychemotherapy plus whole liver radiation (abstr). Proc Am Soc Clin Oncol 21:418, 1980
217. Okuda K, Peters RL, Simson IW: Gross anatomic features of hepatocellular carcinoma from three disparate geographic areas. Proposal of new classification. Cancer 54:2165–2173, 1984
218. Falkson G, Geddes EW: Infusion of liver tumours. Br Med J 4:454, 1968
219. Lange M, Falkson G, Geddes E: Intra-arterial chemotherapy in the treatment of primary liver cancer. S Afr J Surg (Suppl 4)12:245, 1974
220. Watkins E, Khazei A, Nahara K: Surgical basis for arterial infusion chemotherapy of disseminated carcinomas of the liver. Surg Gynecol Obstet 130:581–605, 1970
221. Cady B, Oberfield R: Arterial infusion chemotherapy of hepatoma. Surg Gynecol Obstet 138:381–4, 1974
222. Sullivan RD: Systematic and arterial infusion chemotherapy for metastatic liver cancer. Int J Radiat Oncol Biol Phys 1:973–976, 1976
223. Pettavel J, Morgenthaler F: Protracted arterial chemotherapy of liver tumors: An experience of 107 cases over a 12-year period. Prog Clin Cancer 7:217–233, 1978
224. Urist M, Balch C: Intra-arterial chemotherapy for hepatoma using adriamycin administered via an implantable infusion pump (abstr). Proc Am Soc Clin Oncol 3:148, 1984
225. Friedman MA, Volberding PA, Cassidy MJ: Therapy of hepatocellular cancer with combined intra hepatic arterial chemotherapy and whole liver irradiation. Ann Acad Med Singapore 9:260–268, 1980
226. Chearanai O, Plengvanit U, Tuchinda S et al: Treatment of advanced primary liver

carcinoma using intermittent intraarterial nitrogen mustard. Southeast Asian J Trop Med Public Health 5:96–104, 1974
227. Cheng E, Watson R, Fortner J et al: Regional intraarterial infusion of cisplatin in primary liver cancer: A phase II trial (abstr). Proc Am Soc Clin Oncol 22:179, 1982
228. Misra N, Jaiswal M, Singh R et al: Intrahepatic arterial infusion of the combination of mitomycin-C and 5-fluorouracil in treatment of primary and metastatic liver carcinoma. Cancer 39:1425–1429, 1977
229. Shildt R, Baker L, Stuckey W: Hepatic artery infusion (HAI) with 5-FUDR (F), Adriamycin (A) and streptozotocin (St) in unresectable hepatoma. A Southwest Oncology Group study (abstr). Proc Am Soc Clin Oncol 3:150, 1984
230. Douglass H: Prolongation of survival with periodic percutaneous multidrug arterial infusions in patients with primary and metastatic gastrointestinal carcinoma to liver (abstr). Proc Am Soc Clin Oncol 21:416, 1980
231. Patt Y, Charnsangavej C, Saski M: Hepatic arterial infusion of floxuridine, adriamycin, and mitomycin C for primary liver neoplasms. Dev Oncol 26:125–140, 1984
232. Lai EC, Choi TK, Tong SW et al: Treatment of unresectable hepatocellular carcinoma: Results of a randomized controlled trial. World J Surg 10:501–509, 1986
233. Coccia-Portugal MA: Personal communication
234. Almersjo O, Bengmark S, Rudenstam C et al: Evaluation of hepatic dearterialization in primary and secondary cancer of the liver. Am J Surg 124:5–9, 1972
235. Balasegaram M: Complete hepatic dearterialization for primary carcinoma of the liver—Report of twenty-four patients. Am J Surg 124:340–345, 1972
236. Fortner J, Mulcare R, Solis A et al: Treatment of primary and secondary liver cancer by hepatic artery ligation and infusion chemotherapy. Ann Surg 178:162–172, 1973
237. Al-Jurf A, Jochimsen P, Shirazi S et al: Hepatic artery ligation and chemotherapeutic infusion in the treatment of hepatic malignancy. J Surg Oncol 27:119–123, 1984
238. Almersjo O, Bengmark S, Hafstrom L et al: Results of liver dearterialization combined with regional infusion of 5-fluorouracil for liver cancer. Acta Chir Scand 142:131–138, 1976
239. Takagi H, Morimoto R, Yasue M et al: Ligation and catheterization of the hepatic artery for palliative treatment of malignant hepatic tumors. J Surg Oncol 23:219–222, 1983
240. Nagasue N, Inokuchi K, Kobayashi M et al: Hepatic dearterialization for nonresectable primary and secondary tumors of the liver. Cancer 38:2593–2603, 1978
241. El-Domeiri A, Mojab K: Intermittent occlusion of the hepatic artery and infusion chemotherapy for carcinoma of the liver. Am J Surg 135:771–775, 1978
242. Yamada R, Sato M, Kawabata M et al: Hepatic artery embolization in 120 patients with unresectable hepatoma. Radiology 148:397–401, 1983
243. Charnsangavej C, Chuang V, Wallace S et al: Work in progress: Transcatheter management of primary carcinoma of the liver. Radiology 147:51–55, 1983
244. Kinami Y, Miyazaki I: The superselective and the selective one shot methods for treating inoperable cancer of the liver. Cancer 41:1720–1727, 1978
245. Konno K, Maeda H, Iwai K et al: Effect of arterial administration of high-molecular-weight anticancer agents SMANCS with lipid lymphographic agent on hepatoma: A preliminary report. Eur J Cancer Clin Oncol 19:1053–1065, 1983
246. Tashiro S, Maeda H: Clinical evaluation of artyerial administration of SMANCS in oily contrast medium for liver cancer. Jpn J Med 2479–80, 1985
247. Kanematsu T, Inokuchi K, Sugimachi K et al: Selective effects of lipiodolized antitumor agents. J Surg Oncol 25:218–226, 1984
248. Dakhil S, Ensminger W, Cho K et al: Improved regional selectivity of hepatic arterial BCNU with degradable microspheres. Cancer 50:631–635, 1982
249. Nakamura H, Tanaka T, Hori S et al: Transcatheter embolization of hepatocellular carcinoma: Assessment of efficacy in cases of resection following emoblization. Radiology 147:401–405, 1983
250. Okamura J, Monden M, Kambayashi J et al: Experience of the multidisciplinary treatment of hepatocellular carcinoma. Follow-up studies on chemoembolization with surgical excision. Excerpta Med Int Cong Ser 629:400–417, 1984
251. Sakurai M, Okamura J, Kuroda C: Transcatheter chemo-embolization effective for treating hepatocellular carcinoma—A histopathologic study. Cancer 54:387–392, 1984
252. Epirubicin Study Group for Hepatocellular Carcinoma: Intra-arterial administration of epirubicin in the treatment of nonresectable hepatocellular carcinoma. Cancer Chemother Pharmacol 19:183–189, 1987
253. Ihde DC, Matthews MJ, Makuch RW et al: Prognostic factors in patients with hepatocellular carcinoma receiving systemic chemotherapy. Am J Med 78:399, 1985
254. Sitzmann JV, Order SE, Klein JL et al: Conversion by new treatment modalities of nonresectable to resectable hepatocellular cancer. J Clin Oncol 5:1566, 1987
255. Liu TF: Distribution of malignancies in China. Proceedings of the First International Radiation Therapy Congress, Shanghai, 1986
256. Falkson G, Lavin P, Moertel CG et al: Chemotherapy studies in primary liver cancer: A prospective randomized clinical trial. Cancer 42:2149, 1978
256a. Yang N-C, Leichner PK, Fishman EK et al: CT volumetrics of primary liver cancers. J Comput Assist Tomogr 10:621–628, 1986
257. Leichner PK, Klein JL, Siegelman SS et al: Dosimetry of 131-I labeled antiferritin in hepatoma: Specific activities in the tumor and liver. Cancer Treat Rep 66:647, 1983
258. Ettinger DS, Leichner PK, Siegelman SS et al: Computed tomography assisted volumetric analysis of primary liver tumors as a measure of response to therapy. Am J Clin Oncol 8:413, 1985
259. Kaplan HS, Bagshaw MA: Radiation hepatitis possible prevention by combined isotopic and external radiation therapy. Radiology 91:12, 1968
260. Sherman DM, Weichselbaum R, Order SE et al: Palliation of hepatic metastasis. Cancer 41:2013, 1978
261. Friedman MA, Volberding PA, Cassidy MJ et al: Therapy in hepatocellular cancer with intrahepatic arterial Adriamycin and 5-fluorouracil combined with whole liver irradiation. A Northern California Group study. Cancer Treat Rep 63:1885, 1979
262. Friedman MA: Primary hepatocellular cancer—present results and future prospects. Int J Radiat Oncol Biol Phys 9:1841, 1983
263. Grady ED, Nolan TR, Crumbley AJ et al: Internal radiation therapy of liver cancer. J Med Assoc Ga 66:625, 1977
264. Ohishi H, Uchida H, Yoshimura H et al: Hepatocellular carcinoma detected by iodized oil: Use of anticancer agents. Radiology 154:25, 1985
265. Park CH, Suh JH, Yoo HS et al: Evaluation of intrahepatic I-131 Ethiodol on a patient with hepatocellular cancer. Clin Nucl Med 11:514, 1986
266. Richter GW: Comparison of ferritin from neoplastic and nonneoplastic human cells. Nature 207:616, 1965
267. Lenhard RE, Order SE, Spunberg JJ et al: Isotopic immunoglobulin: A new systemic therapy for advanced Hodgkin's disease. J Clin Oncol 3:1296, 1985
268. Rostock RA, Klein JL, Leichner PK et al: Selective tumor localization in experimental hepatoma by radiolabeled antiferritin antibody. Int J Radiat Oncol Biol Phys 9:1345, 1983
269. Rostock RA, Klein JL, Kopher KA et al: Variables affecting the tumor localization of 131-I antiferritin in experimental hepatoma. Am J Clin Oncol 6:9, 1984
270. Rostock RA, Kopher KA, Bauer TW et al: Factors that affect antiferritin localization in four rat hepatoma models. In Freeman AI (ed): Cancer Drug Delivery, vol 2, p 139. New York, Mary Ann Liebert, 1985
271. Leichner PK, Yang NC, Frenkel TL et al: Dosimetry and treatment planning for ^{90}Y-labeled antiferritin in hepatoma. Int J Radiat Oncol Biol Phys 14:2775, 1988
272. Williams J: Personal communication, 1987
273. Tang ZY, Liu KD, Guo YD et al: Tumor imaging and targeting therapy for hepatocellular carcinoma: Preliminary results of experimental and clinical studies: Chung Hua I Hsueh Tsa Chih 99:855, 1986
274. Order SE, Klein JL, Leichner PK et al: 90-Yttrium antiferritin: A new therapeutic radiolabeled antibody. Int J Radiat Oncol Biol Phys 12:277, 1986
275. Kusumoto Y, Nakata K, Muro T et al: Serotherapy of AFP producing tumors with the purified antibody to AFP. Oncoder Bio-Med 4:95, 1983
276. Koji T, Ishi N, Munehisa T et al: Localization of radioiodinated antibody to alpha fetoprotein in hepatoma transplanted in rats and a case report of alpha fetoprotein antibody treatment of a hepatoma patient. Cancer Res 40:3013, 1980
277. Matsumoto Y, Suzuki T, Asada I et al: Clinical classification of hepatoma in Japan according to serial changes in serum alpha fetoprotein levels. Cancer 49:354, 1982
277a. Fu KK, Lam KN, Rayner PA: The influence of time sequence of Cisplatin administration and continuous low dose rate irradiation (CLDRI) on their combined effects on a murine squamous cell carcinoma. J Radiat Oncol Biol Phys 11:2119, 1985
278. Johnson PJ, Williams R: Serum alpha fetoprotein estimations and doubling time in hepatocellular carcinoma. Influence of therapy and possible value in early detection. JNCI 64:1329, 1980
279. Stillwagon GB, Order SE, Klein JL et al: Multi-modality treatment of primary nonresectable intrahepatic cholangiocarcinoma with 131-I anti-CEA—A Radiation Therapy Oncology Group study 13:687, 1987
280. Fardel D: Malignant neoplasms of the extrahepatic biliary ducts. Ann Surg 76:205, 1922
281. Courvoisier LG: Casuistisch-Statistische Beitrage zur Pathologie und Chirurgie der Gallenwege. Leipzig, Vogel, 1890
282. Baudoin CE: Surgery of the upper abdomen: II. Surgery of the Gallbladder, Liver, Pancreas and Spleen, vol 24, p 409. Philadelphia, Blakiston, 1913
283. Mayo WJ: Malignant disease of the common bile duct. In Mayo WJ, Mayo CH (eds): Collection of Papers Published Previous to 1909, p 401. Philadelphia, Saunders, 1912
284. Sako K, Seitzinger GL, Garside E: Carcinoma of the extrahepatic bile ducts: Review of the literature and report of six cases. Surgery 41:416, 1957
285. Neibling HH, Dockerty MB, Waugh JM: Carcinoma of the extrahepatic bile ducts. Surg Gynecol Obstet 89:429, 1949
286. Gibby DG, Hanks JB, Wanebo HJ et al: Bile duct carcinoma: Diagnosis and treatment. Ann Surg 202:139, 1985
287. Jones RS, Hanks J: Overview of Cancer of Bile Duct. In Wanebo HJ (ed): Hepatic and Biliary Cancer, pp 329–338. New York, Marcel Dekker, 1987
288. Faintuck J and Levin B: Diagnosis of Bile Duct Cancer. In Wanebo HJ (ed): Hepatic and Biliary Cancer, pp 299–338. New York, Marcel Dekker, 1982
289. McKay AJ, Duncan JG, Lau P et al: The role of gray scale ultrasonography in the investigation of jaundice. Br J Surg 66:162, 1979
290. Broughton NS, Evensen A, Osnes M: Endoscopic retrograde cholangiography in primary biliary tract carcinoma. Clin Radiol 29:647, 1978
291. Elias E, Hamlyn AN, Jain S et al: A randomized trial of percutaneous transhepatic cholangiography with the Chiba needle versus ERCP for bile duct visualization in jaundice. Gastroenterology 71:439, 1976
292. Hoevels J, Ihse I: Percutaneous transhepatic portography in bile duct carcinoma. Correlation with percutaneous transhepatic cholangiography and angiography. ROFO 131:140, 1979
293. Voyles CR, Bowley NJ, Allison DJ et al: Carcinoma of the proximal extrahepatic biliary tree: Radiologic assessment and therapeutic alternatives. Ann Surg 197:188, 1983
294. Goldberg HI, Filly RA, Korobkin M et al: Capability of CT body scanning and ultrasonography to demonstrate the status of the biliary ductal system in patients with jaundice. Radiology 129:713, 1978

295. Evander A, Ihse I, Lunderquist A et al: Percutaneous cytodiagnosis of carcinoma of the pancreas and bile duct. Ann Surg 188:90, 1978
296. Cutherell L, Wanebo HJ, Tegtmeyer CJ: Catheter tract seeding after percutaneous biliary drainage for pancreatic cancer. Cancer 57:2057–2060, 1986
297. Nakayama T, Ikeda A, Okuda K et al: Percutaneous transhepatic drainage of the biliary tract. Technique and results in 104 cases. Gastroenterology 74:554, 1978
298. Norlander A, Kalin B, Sunblad R: Effect of percutaneous transhepatic drainage upon liver function and post-operative mortality. Surg Gynecol Obstet 155:161, 1982
299. Ferrucci JY, Mueller PR: Interventional radiology of the biliary tract. Gastroenterology 82:974, 1982
300. Denning DA, Ellison EC, Carey LC: Pre-operative percutaneous transhepatic biliary decompression lowers operative morbidity in patients with obstructive jaundice. Am J Surg 141:61, 1981
301. MacPherson GAD, Benjamin IS, Hodgson HJF et al: Pre-operative percutaneous transphepatic biliary drainage: The results of a controlled trial. Br J Surg 71:371, 1984
302. Pitt HA, Gomes AS, Lois JF et al: Does pre-operative percutaneous biliary drainage reduce operative risk or increase hospital cost? Ann Surg 201:545, 1985
303. Tompkins RK, Johnson J, Storm FK et al: Operative encoscopy in the management of biliary tract neoplasms. Am Surg 132:174, 1976
304. Klatskin G: Adenocarcinoma of the hepatic duct with distinctive clinical and pathological features. Am J Med 38:241, 1965
305. Akwari OE, Kelly KA: Surgical treatment of adenocarcinoma. Location: Junction of the right, left and common biliary ducts. Arch Surg 114:22, 1979
306. Tompkins RK, Thomas D, Wile A et al: Prognostic factors in bile duct carcinoma. Analysis of 96 cases. Ann Surg 4:447–457, 1981
307. Beazley RM, Hadjis NS, Benjamin IS et al: Clinicopathological aspects of high bile duct cancer. Experience with resection and bypass surgical treatments. Ann Surg 199:623–636, 1984
308. Cameron JL, Gayler BW, Zuidema GD: The use of silastic transhepatic stents in benign and malignant biliary strictures. Ann Surg 188:552, 1978
309. Cameron JL, Sanfey H: Surgical management of proximal cholangiocarcinomas. In Wanebo HJ (ed): Hepatic and Biliary Cancer, pp 395–416. New York, Marcel Dekker, 1987
310. Broe PJ, Cameron JL: The management of proximal biliary tract tumors. Adv Surg 15:47–91, 1981
311. Terblanche J, Saunders SJ, Louw JH: Prolonged palliation in carcinoma of the main hepatic duct junction. Surgery 71:720, 1972
312. Blumgart LH, Kelley CJ: Hepaticojejunostomy in benign and malignant high bile duct strictures: Approaches to the left hepatic ducts. Br J Surg 71:257–261, 1984
313. Longmire WP Jr, Sanford MD: Intrahepatic cholangiojejunostomy with partial hepatectomy for biliary obstruction. Surgery 24:264, 1948
314. Longmire WP Jr, Lippman HN: Intrahepatic cholangiojejunostomy: An operation for biliary obstruction. Surg Clin North Am 36:849, 1956
315. Smith R: Hepaticojejunostomy with transhepatic intubation. A technique for very high strictures of the hepatic ducts. Br J Surg 51:186, 1964
316. Bismuth H, Corlette MB: Intrahepatic cholangioenteric anastimosis in carcinoma of the hilus of the liver. Surg Gynecol Obstet 140:170–178, 1975
317. Alexander F, Rossi RL, O'Bryan M et al: Biliary carcinoma: A review of 109 cases. Am J Surg 147:503–509, 1984
318. Braasch JW: Surgical resection of cancer of the mid-duct and distal common bile duct in hepatic and biliary cancer. In Wanebo HJ (ed): Hepatic and Biliary Cancer, pp 357–373. New York, Marcel Dekker, 1987
319. Braasch JW, Warren KW, Kune GA: Malignant neoplasms of the bile ducts. Surg Clin North Am 47:627–638, 1967
320. Braasch JW: Carcinoma of the bile duct. Surg Clin North Am 53:1217–1227, 1973
321. Braasch JW, Jin G, Rossi RL: Pancreatoduodenectomy with preservation of the pylorus. World J Surg 8:900–905, 1984
322. Herter FP, Cooperman AM, Ahlborn TN et al: Surgical experience with pancreatic and periampullary cancer. Ann Surg 195:274–281, 1982
323. Evander A, Fredlund P, Hoevels J et al: Evaluation of aggressive surgery in carcinoma of the extrahepatic bile ducts. Ann Surg 191:23, 1980
324. Pitt HA, Roslyn JJ, Tompkins RK: Surgical resection of bile duct cancer: The UCLA experience. In Wanebo HJ (ed): Hepatic and Biliary Cancer, pp 339–355. New York, Marcel Dekker, 1987
325. Blumgart LH, Hadjis NS: Proximal bile duct cancer: Curative resection or palliative bypass. In Wanebo HJ (ed): Hepatic and Biliary Cancer, pp 375–394. New York, Marcel Dekker, 1987
326. Kopelson G, Harisiadis L, Tretter P et al: The role of radiation therapy in cancer of the extra-hepatic biliary system: An analysis of thirteen patients and a review of the literature of the effectiveness of surgery, chemotherapy and radiotherapy. Int J Radiat Oncol Biol Phys 2:883–894, 1977
327. Lees CD, Zapolanski A, Cooperman AM et al: Carcinoma of the bile ducts. Surg Gynecol Obstet 151:193–198, 1980
328. Wheeler PG, Dawson JL, Nunnerley H et al: Newer techniques in the diagnosis and treatment of proximal bile duct carcinoma—an analysis of 41 consecutive patients. Q J Med 199:247–258, 1981
329. Fletcher MS, Brinkley D, Dawson JL et al: Treatment of hilar carcinoma by bile drainage combined with internal radiotherapy using 192-iridium wire. Br J Surg 70:733–735, 1983
330. Cameron JL, Broe P, Zuidema GD: Proximal bile duct tumors. Surgical management with silastic transhepatic biliary stents. Ann Surg 196:412–419, 1982
331. Hashikawa Y, Shimada T, Miura T et al: Radiation therapy of carcinoma of the extrahepatic bile ducts. Radiology 146:787–789, 1983
332. Todoroki T, Iwasaki Y, Okamura T et al: Intraoperative radiotherapy for advanced carcinoma of the biliary system. Cancer 46:2179–2184, 1980
333. Abe M, Takahashi M: Intraoperative radiotherapy: The Japanese experience. Int J Radiat Oncol Biol Phys 7:863–868, 1981
334. Pilepich MV: Radiation for carcinoma of the extrahepatic bile duct and Radiotherapy in carcinoma of gallbladder. In Wanebo HJ (ed): Hepatic and Biliary Cancer, pp 417–427, 447–452. New York, Marcel Dekker, 1987
335. Piehler JM, Crichlow RW: Primary carcinoma of the gallbladder. Surg Gynecol Obstet 147:929–942, 1978
336. Nevin JE, Moran TJ, Kay S et al: Carcinoma of the gallbladder. Cancer 37:141–148, 1976
337. Wanebo HJ, Castle WN, Fechner RE: Is carcinoma of the gallbladder a curable lesion? Ann Surg 195:624–631, 1982
338. Morrow CE, Sutherland DE, Florack G et al: Primary gallbladder carcinoma: Significance of suberosal lesions and results of aggressive surgical treatment and adjuvant chemotherapy. Surgery 94:709–714, 1983
339. Bergdahl L: Gallbladder carcinoma first diagnosed at microscopic examination of gallbladders removed for presumed benign disease. Ann Surg 191:19–22, 1980
340. Appleman RM, Morlock CG, Dahlin DC et al: Long-term survival in carcinoma of the gallbladder. Surg Gynecol Obstet 17:459–464, 1963
341. Frank SA, Spjut HJ: Inapparent carcinoma of the gallbladder. Am Surg 33:367–372, 1967
342. Jones CJ: Carcinoma of the gallbladder. A clinical and pathological analysis of fifty cases. Ann Surg 132:110–120, 1950
343. Vaittinen E: Carcinoma of the gallbladder: A study of 390 cases diagnosed in Finland 1953–1967. Ann Chir Gynaecol [Suppl] 168:7–81, 1970
344. Edmonsdon HA: Tumors of the Gallbladder and Extrahepatic Bile Ducts, Section VII, Fascicle 26. Washington DC, Armed Forces Institute of Pathology, 1967
345. Frierson HF, Fechner RE: Pathology of malignant neoplasms of the gallbladder and extrahepatic bile ducts. In Wanebo HJ (ed): Hepatic and Biliary Cancer, pp 281–297. New York, Marcel Dekker, 1987
346. Berk RN, Armbuster TG, Saltzstein SL: Carcinoma in the porcelain gallbladder. Radiology 106:29–31, 1973
347. Polk HC Jr: Carcinoma and the calcified gall bladder. Gastroenterology 50:582–585, 1966
348. Alpers CE, Smuckler EA: Pleomorphic carcinoma of the gallbladder. Case report and ultrastructural study. Ultrastruct Pathol 6:29–38, 1984
349. Appleman HD, Coopersmith N: Pleomorphic spindle-cell carcinoma of the gallbladder. Relation to sarcoma of the gallbladder. Cancer 25:535–541, 1970
350. Black WC, Key CR, Carmany TB et al: Carcinoma of the gallbladder in a population of Southwestern American Indians. Cancer 39:1269–1279, 1977
351. Albores-Saavedra J, Soriano J, Larraza-Hernandez O et al: Oak cell carcinoma of the gallbladder. Hum Pathol 15:639–646, 1984
352. Fahim RB, McDonald JR, Richards JC et al: Carcinoma of the gallbladder: A study of its modes of spread. Ann Surg 156:114–124, 1962
353. Ohlsson EG, Aronsen KF: Carcinoma of the gallbladder. A study of 181 cases. Acta Chir Scand 140:475–480, 1974
354. Hamrick RE Jr, Liner FJ, Hastings PR et al: Primary carcinoma of the gallbladder. Ann Surg 195:270–273, 1982
355. Detweiler DG, Biddinger P, Staab EV et al: The appearance of adenomyomatosis with the newer imaging modalities: A case with pathologic correlation. J Ultrasound Med 1:295–298, 1982
356. Lampman LE, Meijer JG, Stroucken AA: Sonographic detection of early gallbladder cancer. Diagn Imag Clin Med 53:99–103, 1984
357. Sato T, Koyama K, Yamauchi H et al: Early carcinoma of the gallbladder. Gastroenterol Jpn 16:459–464, 1981
358. Adson MA: Carcinoma of the gallbladder. In Moody F (ed): Advances in Diagnosis and Treatment of Biliary Tract Disease, Ch 12. New York, Masson, 1983
359. Tashiro S, Konno T, Mochinaga M et al: Treatment of carcinoma of the gallbladder in Japan. Jpn J Surg 12:98–104, 1982
360. Pack GT, Miller TR, Brasfield RD: Total right hepatic lobectomy for cancer of the gallbladder: Report of three cases. Ann Surg 142:6–16, 1955
361. Brasfield RD: Right hepatic lobectomy for carcinoma of the gallbladder: A five-year cure. Ann Surg 153:563–566, 1961
362. Pemberton LB, Diffenbaugh WF, Strohl EL: The surgical significance of carcinoma of the gallbladder. Am J Surg 122:381–383, 1971
363. Burdette WJ: Carcinoma of the gallbladder. Ann Surg 145:832, 1957
364. Shepard VD, Walters W, Dockerty MD: Benign neoplasms of the gallbladder. Arch Surg 45:1, 1942
365. Arbab A, Brasfield R: Benign tumors of the gallbladder. Surgery 61:535–540, 1967
366. Albores-Saavedra J, Alcantra-Vazquez A, Cruz-Ortiz H et al: The precursor lesions of invasive gallbladder carcinoma: Hyperplasia, atypical hyperplasia and carcinoma in situ. Cancer 45:919–927, 1980
367. Kozuka S, Tsubone N, Yasui A et al: Relation of adenoma to carcinoma in the gallbladder. Cancer 50:2226–2234, 1982
368. Castle WN, Wanebo HJ, Fechner RE: Carcinoma of the gallbladder and cholecystectomy. Arch Surg 117:946–948, 1982
369. Nagashima H, Watanabe A, Hayashi S et al: Primary carcinoma of the gallbladder and the extrahepatic bile duct. Gastroenterology 17:246–253, 1982
370. Hanna SS, Rider WD: Carcinoma of the gallbladder or extrahepatic bile ducts: The role of radiotherapy. Can Med Assoc J 118:59–61, 1978

371. Treadwell TA, Harding WJ: Primary carcinoma of the gallbladder. The role of adjunctive therapy in its treatment. Am J Surg: 703–706, 1976
372. Abe M, Takahashi M: Intraoperative radiotherapy: The Japanese experience. Int J Radiat Oncol Biol Phys 7:863–868, 1981
373. Schein DS, Stablein DM, Novah JW et al: A comparison of combination chemotherapy and combined modality therapy for locally adrenal gastric cancer. Cancer 49:1771–1777, 1982
374. Andrews W, Smith F: Chemotherapy for cholangiocarcinoma and gallbladder cancer. In Wanebo HJ (ed): Hepatic and Biliary Cancer, pp 453–457. New York, Marcel Dekker, 1987
375. Haskell CM: Cancer of the liver. In Haskell CM (ed): Cancer Treatment, pp 319–357. Philadelphia, WB Saunders, 1980
376. Davis HL Jr, Ramirez G, Ansfield FJ: Adenocarcinoma of stomach, pancreas, liver, and biliary tracts: Survival of 328 patients treated with fluoropyrimidine therapy. Cancer 33:193–197, 1974
377. Crooke ST, Bradner WT: Mitomycin-C: A review. Cancer Treat Rev 3:121–139, 1976
378. Von Eyben F, Hellekant C, Mattson M et al: Mitomycin-C in advanced gallbladder carcinoma. Acta Radiol [Diagn] (Stockh) 19:81–84, 1980
379. Adolphson CC, Carpenter JT Jr: Response to doxorubicin and mitomycin in cholangiocarcinoma: A case report. Cancer Treat Rep 66:209–210, 1982
380. Bodey GP, Bedikian AY, Valdivieso M et al: Chemotherapeutic management of hepatobiliary and pancreatic cancer. In Stroehlein JR, Romsdahl MM (eds): Gastrointestinal Cancer, pp 279–292. New York, Raven Press, 1981
381. Bukowski RM, Leichman LP, Rivkin SE: Phase II trial of m-AMSA in gallbladder and cholangiocarcinoma: A Southwest Oncology Group study. Eur J Cancer Clin Oncol 6:721–723, 1983
382. Harvey JH, Smith FP, Schein PS: 5-Fluorouracil, mitomycin, and doxorubicin (FAM) in carcinoma of the biliary tract. J Clin Oncol (Suppl 11)2:1245–1248, 1984
383. Hall SH, Benjamin RS, Murphy WK et al: Adriamycin, BCNU, Ftorafur chemotherapy of pancreatic and biliary tract cancer. Cancer 44:2008–2013, 1974
384. Ravey M Jr, Hester M: Phase II study of adriamycin plus bleomycin for the treatment of hepatocellular and biliary tract carcinoma. Proc Am Soc Clin Oncol 20:415, 1979
385. Misra NC, Jaiswal MSD, Singh RV et al: Intrahepatic arterial infusion of combination of mytomycin-C and 5-fluorouracil in treatment of primary and metastatic liver carcinoma. Cancer 39:1425–1429, 1977
386. Oswalt CE, Cruz AB: Effectiveness of chemotherapy in addition to surgery in treating carcinoma of the gallbladder. Rev Surg 34:436–438, 1977
387. Pilepich MV, Lambert PM: Radiotherapy of carcinomas of the extrahepatic biliary system. Radiology 127:767–770, 1978
388. Wanebo HJ: Carcinoma of the gallbladder. In Wanebo HJ (ed): Hepatic and Biliary Cancer, pp 431–445. New York, Marcel Dekker, 1987

WILLIAM F. SINDELAR

CHAPTER 28 *Cancer of the Small Intestine*

Neoplasms are uncommon in the duodenum and small intestine. The small bowel accounts for more than 75% of the length and more than 90% of the mucosal absorptive surface of the entire gastrointestinal (GI) tract; however, fewer than 5% of all GI neoplasms arise in the small intestine.[1,2] Cancers of the duodenum and small intestine constitute about 1% of all gastrointestinal tract malignancies.[3–5]

The diagnosis of neoplasms of the duodenum or small intestine can be difficult to establish because symptoms may be vague and nonspecific.[6,7] Metastatic disease is frequently present at the time of diagnosis of malignant tumors, and the prognosis is not favorable for small bowel cancers.[7,8] Surgical resection can cure some patients with small intestinal malignancies.[7–10] However, radiotherapy, chemotherapy, and other treatment modalities have been of little benefit in managing malignant diseases of the small intestine.[7,8,11–15]

HISTORY

Neoplasms occurring in the small intestine were first recognized in 1655.[16] The first clinically reported small bowel tumor was a duodenal carcinoma described in 1746.[17] Wesner discovered a leiomyosarcoma of the small intestine in 1883.[18] The first successful surgical resection of a small intestinal tumor was reported by Fleiner in 1885.[19]

Early reviews of small intestinal neoplasms were compiled by Heurtaux in 1899 and by King in 1917.[20,21] Modern reviews have examined benign or malignant tumors of the duodenum and small intestine.[1,3,4,6–10,14–16,22–32]

EPIDEMIOLOGY

Duodenal and small intestinal tumors have been reported in patients whose ages range from 1 year to 84 years, with a mean age of 59 years.[1,7,8,23] The average age at presentation of patients with benign neoplasms is 62 years, whereas patients with intestinal malignancies present at a mean age of 57 years.[33] The annual incidence of clinically diagnosed small bowel neoplasms in the United States is approximately 1200 cases.[5,34] The age-adjusted incidence in the United States for clinically diagnosed small intestinal neoplasms in the white population is 1.2 per 100,000 for men and 0.8 per 100,000 for women.[34] The incidence per 100,000 blacks is 1.6 for men and 0.7 for women.[34] The incidence and distribution of small intestinal tumors appears to be uniform worldwide.[5,8]

The autopsy incidence of small intestinal tumors is 0.2%, but the operative incidence of neoplasms of the small bowel is less than 0.01%.[35] Most benign tumors are asymptomatic and clinically innocent, but most malignancies become symptomatic and require surgical intervention.[8,36–39] Clinical series of symptomatic patients have revealed symmetric distribution of benign and malignant small intestinal tumors.[7–10,24,33–43] Table 28-1 summarizes the distribution of benign and malignant neoplasms of the duodenum and small intestine in various clinical series.[7–10,24,33,36–43]

Duodenal and small intestinal neoplasms are associated with certain inherited disorders of the GI tract, including familial polyposis, Gardner's syndrome, Peutz–Jeghers syndrome, Crohn's disease, celiac disease, and neurofibromatosis.

TABLE 28-1. Benign and Malignant Neoplasms of the Duodenum and Small Intestine

Author	Year	Number of Neoplasms		
		Benign	Malignant	Total
Darling et al[24]	1959	46	86	132
Krouse et al[36]	1961	24	12	36
Botsford et al[33]	1962	71	44	115
Skandalakis et al[9]	1962	340	257	597
Sawyer et al[37]	1963	23	27	50
Schmutzer et al[38]	1964	59	41	100
Ebert et al[10]	1965	48	29	77
Ostermiller et al[39]	1966	77	122	199
Spratt[40]	1966	11	19	30
Freund et al[41]	1978	37	79	116
Miles et al[42]	1979	11	31	42
Herbsman et al[8]	1980	20	54	74
Mittal et al[7]	1980	15	39	54
Giuliani et al[43]	1985	5	43	48
TOTAL		787 (47%)	883 (53%)	1670

ETIOLOGY

There have been no factors identified as having a definite role in the etiology of duodenal and small intestinal neoplasms. Because of the rarity of small bowel tumors compared with neoplasms occurring in the large bowel, stomach, or esophagus, there have been proposals that local factors in the small intestine may function in the prevention of neoplasia or in the deactivation of possible carcinogens.

The lack of acid in the small intestinal lumen has been suggested to be protective against tumorigenesis.[8,9] Neoplasms frequently are encountered in areas of GI tract acidity, such as the stomach and colon. Nitrosamines, which are potent experimental GI carcinogens, are formed only in acid environments.[44]

The rapid peristalsis of the small bowel has been suggested to protect against neoplasia in the duodenum and small bowel, possibly by minimizing the time of mucosal exposure to carcinogenic agents.[45] It has been proposed that the liquid small bowel content may be less abrasive or irritating to the mucosa than are particulates in the esophagus, chyme in the stomach, or fecal matter in the colon.[46]

Benzopyrene hydroxylase is present in large amounts in the mucosa of the small intestine and may detoxify carcinogens.[8,47] A large concentration of secretory immunoglobulin in the small intestine has been considered protective against the development of tumors, possibly by neutralizing oncogenic viruses.[28]

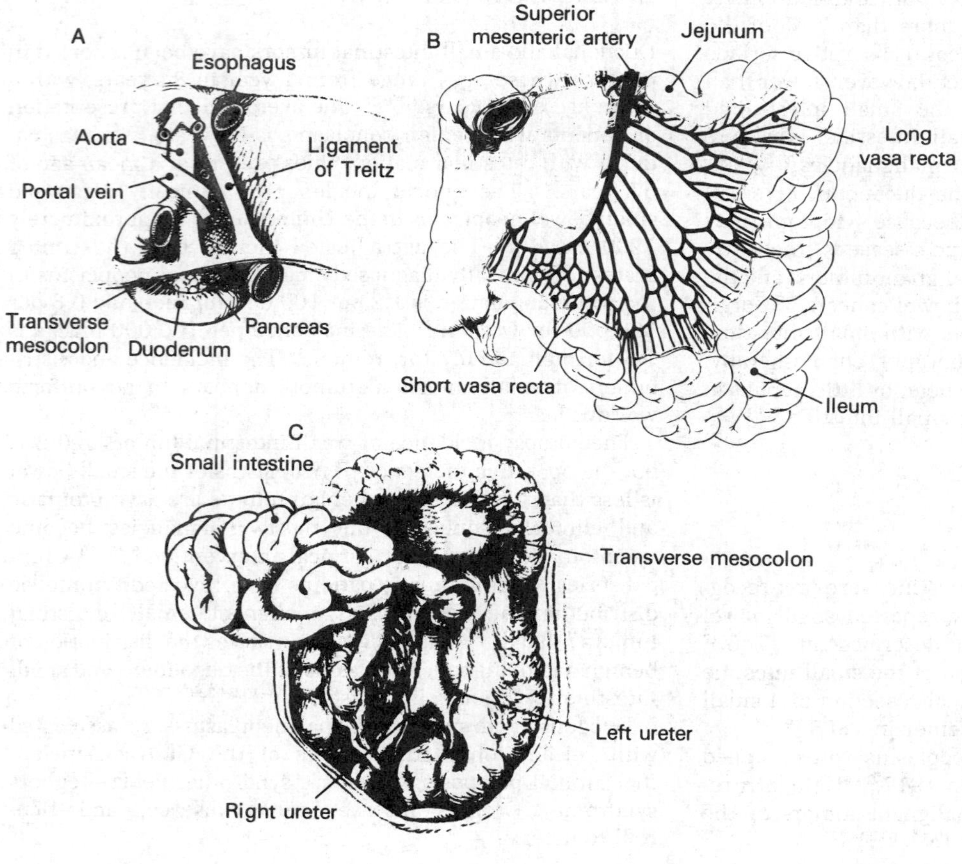

FIG. 28-1. Anatomy of the small intestine. **A.** Relationships of the duodenum. **B.** Vascular supply of the small intestine. **C.** Mesentery of the small intestine. (Adapted from Healey JE: A Synopsis of Clinical Anatomy, p 179. Philadelphia, WB Saunders, 1969)

The relative absence of bacteria in the duodenum and small intestine, compared with the esophagus or colon, may protect against neoplastic transformation resulting from bacterially produced carcinogens.[28]

ANATOMY

ANATOMIC RELATIONSHIPS

The small bowel is more than 600 cm long, extending from the gastric pyloric ring to the colonic ileocecal valve. The small bowel comprises the duodenum, jejunum, and ileum (Fig. 28-1).

The duodenum extends horizontally to the right from the pyloric ring as an intraperitoneal structure and then turns caudally to become retroperitoneal, surrounding the head of the pancreas and receiving openings from the biliary and pancreatic ducts. The duodenum then extends horizontally to the left, passing dorsally to the superior mesenteric vessels before turning superiorly and emerging as an intraperitoneal segment at the ligament of Treitz. The duodenum derives its arterial supply from the gastroduodenal branches of both the celiac axis and superior mesenteric artery. Duodenal venous drainage is into the portal system. Figure 28-2 illustrates the vascular anatomy in the region of the duodenum. Duodenal lymphatics drain behind the head of the pancreas into the pancreaticoduodenal group and into the celiac nodes.

The jejunum begins at the ligament of Treitz, situated to the left of the second lumbar vertebra, and extends caudally from the free border of the mesentery. The arterial supply is derived from branches of the superior mesenteric artery. Venous drainage is through mesenteric tributaries that terminate in the portal vein through the superior mesenteric vein. Lymphatic drainage flows through the mesentery, with nodes located within the mesenteric leaflets.

The ileum is located distal to and is continuous with the jejunum, with an indistinct division between the distal jejunum and proximal ileum. Arterial branches supply the ileum from the ileocolic artery, which arises as a branch of the superior mesenteric artery. Venous drainage into the portal system is through the superior mesenteric vein. Numerous lymph nodes occur along lymphatic channels that pass through the mesentery.

The mesentery attaches obliquely to the dorsal abdominal wall in a line extending from the left of the second lumbar vertebra to the right iliac fossa. The free mesenteric border fans out to allow convolutions within the abdominal cavity of the small intestine, which attaches to the edge of the mesentery. The small intestinal arterial supply, venous drainage, and lymphatic channels are supported within the mesentery. Blood vessels anastomose freely in the mesentery through arcades that supply the intestine through segmental branches.

MICROSCOPIC ANATOMY

The small intestine is a tubular organ containing an inner mucosal layer, a middle muscular layer composed of an inner circular and outer longitudinal array of smooth muscle, and an outer serosal layer of peritoneum and connective tissue.

The lining of the small intestine is arranged into circular folds, the valvulae conniventes, which increase the surface area of the mucosa. Valvulae are prominent in the duodenum, well developed in the jejunum, and poorly developed in the ileum. Mucosal villi are formed by epithelial foldings and provide a large absorptive surface area. The lining epithelium comprises columnar epithelial cells, goblet cells, and enterochromaffin cells.

The submucosa contains supportive connective tissue and carries the intestinal blood supply in both longitudinal and circular directions through a submucosal plexus. The submucosa contains considerable amounts of connective tissue throughout the small intestine, with increasing concentrations distally in the bowel.

The muscular portion of the small intestinal wall is formed of smooth muscle with small amounts of connective tissue, as well as blood vessels and lymphatics. The inner, circular muscular layer is thick. The thin, outer muscular layer is longitudinally oriented. The myenteric nerve plexus is con-

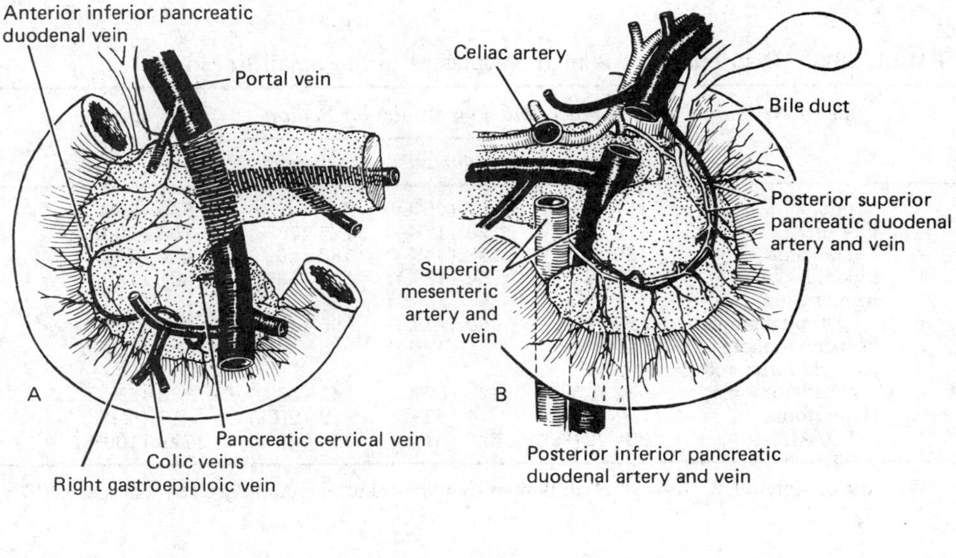

FIG. 28-2. Anatomy of the duodenum. **A**. Anterior view with pancreatic and duodenal vessels. **B**. Posterior view with posterior vascular arcades. (Edwards EA, Malone PD, MacArthur JD: Operative Anatomy of Abdomen and Pelvis, p 127. Philadelphia, Lea & Febiger, 1975)

TABLE 28-2. Classification of Neoplasms of the Duodenum and Small Intestine

Tissue of Origin	*Benign*	*Malignant*
Epithelium	Adenoma	Adenocarcinoma
Connective tissue	Fibroma	Fibrosarcoma
Smooth muscle	Leiomyoma	Leiomyosarcoma
Fat	Lipoma	Liposarcoma
Vascular tissue	Hemangioma	Angiosarcoma
	Lymphangioma	
Lymphoid tissue	Pseudolymphoma	Lymphoma
Nerve	Neurofibroma	Neurofibrosarcoma
	Neurilemmoma	Malignant schwannoma
Argentaffin	—	Carcinoid

tained in the connective tissue that separates the circular and longitudinal muscular layers.

The serosa is composed of epithelium that forms a peritoneal surface over a subserosa of loose connective tissue. The serosa covers the intestinal tube, except at the point of mesenteric attachment, where the intestinal serosa is continuous with the peritoneal epithelium of the mesentery.

PATHOLOGY

Benign or malignant intestinal neoplasms can arise from any portion of the duodenum, jejunum, or ileum.[48,49] Small intestinal tumors are classified in Table 28-2.

The most frequently encountered benign tumors of the small intestine are adenomas, leiomyomas, and lipomas.[48–51] Fibromas and neurofibromas are uncommon small bowel neoplasms.[50–52] Intestinal neurofibromas are sometimes seen in patients with neurofibromatosis. Vascular tumors, such as hemangiomas and lymphangiomas, are unusual. Hamartomas of the small intestine are associated with the Peutz–Jeghers syndrome. Lymphoid hyperplasia in the small intestine can lead to the formation of polypoid masses, and small intestinal pseudolymphoma can occur.[5,53,54] The distribution of benign neoplasms in the duodenum, jejunum, and ileum is given in Table 28-3.[29]

Adenocarcinomas make up about half of the malignancies involving the small intestine, and carcinoid tumors account for about 35% of malignant lesions.[3,8] Leiomyosarcomas are among the most common of the small intestine sarcomas which develop in the small intestine, and angiosarcomas and liposarcomas are seen rarely.[50] Neurofibrosarcomas occur in the small bowel and occasionally are associated with neurofibromatosis. Although secondary lymphomatous involvement of the small bowel regularly is seen in disseminated lymphomas, malignant lymphomas occur rarely as primary tumors. The distribution of malignant neoplasms in the duodenum, jejunum, and ileum is given in Table 28-4.[28,30,54]

CLINICAL FEATURES

SYMPTOMS

Benign small bowel tumors may remain occult and cause no symptoms, being found incidentally at autopsy.[24,33] The lack of symptoms may be due to the distensibility of the small intestine and the low viscosity of bowel fluid, which allow the passage of small bowel content in spite of partial occlusion of the intestinal lumen.[8] Approximately half of all patients with benign small bowel tumors eventually become symptomatic, usually presenting with abdominal pain.[2,24] The pain may be related to partial or complete intestinal obstruction, which is present in more than 50% of symptomatic cases. Intussusception is often the cause of intestinal obstruction, with the tumor acting as a lead point. Benign small bowel neoplasm is the most frequent cause of adult intussusception.[24] Intestinal obstruction often is chronic and intermittent, probably because of the distensibility of the small bowel, allowing the passage of bowel content around lesions of substantial size.[1,2,8,13–15] The symptoms produced by a proximal obstruction in the duodenum or jejunum usually are unrelenting nausea and vomiting with cramping epigastric pain. Distal obstructing lesions in the ileum typically result in intermittent vomiting, abdominal distension, and cramping periumbilical pain.

Hemorrhage may occur from benign tumors resulting from mucosal involvement by the neoplastic process, which becomes manifest in approximately 25% of symptomatic

TABLE 28-3. Distribution of Benign Neoplasms in the Small Intestine

Type of Neoplasm	*Number and Percentage by Region*			*Total*
	Duodenum	*Jejunum*	*Ileum*	
Adenoma	167 (33%)	127 (25%)	211 (42%)	505 (29%)
Fibroma	12 (7%)	28 (17%)	125 (76%)	165 (10%)
Leiomyoma	86 (19%)	188 (41%)	180 (40%)	454 (26%)
Lipoma	72 (24%)	54 (18%)	175 (58%)	301 (18%)
Hemangioma and lymphangioma	18 (8%)	99 (47%)	95 (45%)	212 (12%)
Pseudolymphoma	0	1 (17%)	5 (83%)	6 (<1%)
Neurofibroma and neurilemmoma	12 (15%)	25 (32%)	41 (53%)	78 (5%)
Hamartoma	1 (14%)	4 (57%)	2 (29%)	7 (<1%)
TOTAL	368 (21%)	526 (31%)	834 (48%)	1728 (100%)

Wilson JM, Melvin DB, Gray GF et al: Benign small bowel tumor. Ann Surg 181:247–250, 1975.

TABLE 28-4. Distribution of Malignant Neoplasms in the Small Intestine

Type of Neoplasm	*Number and Percentage by Region*			*Total*
	Duodenum	*Jejunum*	*Ileum*	
Adenocarcinoma	427 (40%)	408 (38%)	241 (22%)	1076 (46%)
Sarcoma	46 (10%)	162 (36%)	239 (54%)	447 (19%)
Lymphoma	4 (16%)	9 (36%)	12 (48%)	25 (1%)
Carcinoid	48 (6%)	78 (10%)	682 (84%)	808 (34%)
TOTAL	525 (22%)	660 (28%)	1171 (50%)	2356 (100%)

Loehr WH, Mujahed Z, Zahn FD, et al: Primary lymphoma of the gastrointestinal tract: A review of 100 cases. Ann Surg 170:232–238, 1969; Wilson JM, Melvin DB, Gray GF, et al: Primary malignancies of the small bowel: A report of 96 cases and review of the literature. Ann Surg 180:175–179, 1974; Barclay THC, Schapira DV: Malignant tumors of the small intestine. Cancer 51:878–881, 1983.

patients.[9,10,38] Hemorrhage is usually slow and chronic, resulting in anemia, weakness, and debilitation.[39] Severe intestinal bleeding sufficient to warrant surgical intervention is unusual in benign small bowel tumors.[24]

Malignant tumors of the small intestine produce symptoms in more than 75% of patients.[7–9,14,15,21,24–28,50,51] Pain is the most common presenting symptom, occurring in more than 65% of cases of malignant small bowel tumors.[8,14,24,37,51] The pain may occur intermittently as cramps or as diffuse, dull aches that may radiate through the abdomen or to the back. Weight loss occurs in more than half of the patients.[28,37,51] The most profound weight loss occurs in intestinal lymphomas. Symptoms of partial intestinal obstruction develop in approximately 35% of patients with malignant lesions.[8,15] Obstruction is usually due to malignant invasion of the intestinal wall, unlike benign intestinal tumors that frequently result in intussusception.

Hemorrhage may occur with small bowel malignancies.[10,39] Bleeding is often chronic and occult, leading to anemia. Rarely, massive hemorrhage may be the presenting complaint. Approximately 10% of patients with malignant small bowel tumors present with an acute abdomen resulting from bowel perforation and peritonitis.[24] Frequently the symptoms resulting from small intestinal malignancies may be vague and nonspecific, leading to difficulties in diagnosis.[52,54] Diarrhea or steatorrhea may occur, particularly with lymphomas involving the duodenum or jejunum.[53] Carcinoids can produce the carcinoid syndrome, characterized by cutaneous flushing, cyanosis, chronic diarrhea, and intermittent respiratory distress.[55,56] The carcinoid syndrome is manifest only in the presence of metastatic disease.

SIGNS

The clinical examination in patients with benign small intestinal tumors may be unrewarding, with many patients presenting with no abnormal findings.[57] Benign tumors are not palpable unless they are very large. If palpable, benign neoplasms typically are freely moveable.[5,10] Distension and visible peristaltic waves may be present in intestinal obstruction. Intussusception may cause the appearance of a tender, palpable mass, and melanotic stool may be present. Benign tumors may cause intestinal bleeding, which produces anemia and stools positive for gross or occult blood.

Malignancies of the small intestine often present without specific clinical findings but with indications of intestinal dysfunction or obstruction. Signs of weight loss are common as presenting findings, and cachexia may be present if the disease is advanced.[33] An abdominal mass is palpable in approximately 25% of cases.[4,8,33] Intestinal obstruction develops in about 25% of patients, with abdominal distension a frequent finding.[57,58] Gross or occult blood may be present in the stool if there has been hemorrhage from the tumor, and anemia frequently is present. Clinical jaundice is seen routinely with duodenal malignancies. Peritonitis can occur with tumors that have perforated the intestinal wall. Steatorrhea and malabsorption can be present with small intestinal malignancies, especially with lymphomas, in which villous atrophy of the intestinal mucosa occurs.[54,58–61] Peripheral lymphadenopathy may be present in disseminated lymphomas. Hypertension and cutaneous hyperemia may be present as a consequence of advanced carcinoid tumor.

DIAGNOSIS

GENERAL CONSIDERATIONS

The diagnosis of benign or malignant small intestinal tumors is difficult before surgical exploration because clinical symptoms and signs may be nonspecific and because diagnostic efforts may not confirm neoplasms. A correct preoperative diagnosis can be expected in less than half of the symptomatic patients.[39,50]

LABORATORY STUDIES

Laboratory studies rarely reveal specific abnormalities in patients with small intestinal neoplasms. A hypochromic, microcytic anemia may result from chronic blood loss from tumor ulceration. Elevations of bilirubin and hepatic enzymes routinely result from duodenal neoplasms that obstruct the bile duct. Hyperamylasemia can evolve following obstruction of the pancreatic duct by duodenal tumors. Tumor markers, such as carcinoembryonic antigen, are rarely elevated in small intestinal tumors unless metastatic disease is present in the liver. Carcinoid tumors frequently cause elevated levels of 5-hydroxyindoleacetic acid in the urine.

RADIOLOGIC STUDIES

Roentgenographic examinations are useful in the diagnosis of small intestinal neoplasms. Abdominal films are generally nonspecific in asymptomatic patients. If intestinal obstruction is present, air–fluid levels and intestinal dilatation can be observed. In bulky intestinal tumors, a mass may be visible on routine abdominal roentgenography.

Contrast radiography is the most valuable roentgenographic modality for diagnosing small intestinal tumors. Upper GI series with small bowel follow-through have been successful in demonstrating tumors of the small intestine, particularly in obstructing malignant lesions, for which the diagnostic accuracy can be as high as 50%.[27] The GI series can sometimes distinguish among various types of small bowel lesions.[8] Intraluminal masses typically represent benign intestinal lesions such as polyps or leiomyomas. Intramural masses that thicken the intestinal wall but cause little or no mucosal changes suggest mural sarcomas or malignant lymphomas. Ulcerative mucosal lesions generally result from carcinomas. GI series may demonstrate intussusception. Through the administration of glucagon or anticholinergic agents, hypotonic duodenography may improve the visualization of the duodenum and small bowel by arresting intestinal motility at the time of contrast roentgenography.[62] Selective intubation of the small intestine may be possible using Miller-Abbott or Cantor tubes, allowing detailed study of isolated intestinal segments through the direct instillation of contrast material and air. The distal ileum usually is poorly visualized in upper GI contrast studies, but it may be demonstrated through barium enemas in which contrast material from the colon is refluxed into the distal small intestine.

Angiography may be of benefit in the diagnosis and localization of small intestinal neoplasms. A tumor blush may be present on angiogram in vascular neoplasms such as carcinoids or hemangiomas. Displacement of normal bowel vascular architecture can occur with hypovascular tumors such as carcinomas. Vascular malformations of the small intestine are often demonstrated angiographically by the appearance of abnormal concentrations of blood vessels or arteriovenous shunting. Actively bleeding intestinal neoplasms may be localized by angiographic examination.

Chest roentgenography should be performed in the evaluation of patients for small intestinal tumors to examine for possible metastatic tumor deposits. Lung tomography should be performed to evaluate any questionable pulmonary metastatic lesions.[63]

Computed tomographic (CT) body scans have improved roentgenographic sensitivity and accuracy over conventional x-rays in diagnosing intra-abdominal neoplasms. However, body scans are rarely helpful in the detection of small intestinal tumors. The presence of fluid and gas within the small bowel can obscure masses within the intestinal wall or obscure projections into the bowel lumen. CT scans may benefit the definition of large tumors extending beyond the intestinal wall and may assist in the demonstration of advanced metastatic disease by resolving hepatic metastases or by revealing mesenteric lymphadenopathy or peritoneal tumor implants.

Magnetic resonance imaging (MRI) demonstrates neoplasms of the small intestine as intra-abdominal masses with signal intensities varying from the characteristics and configuration of normal bowel. Metastatic deposits may be detected by MRI in the mesentery, retroperitoneum, or liver.

Diagnostic ultrasonography is useful in evaluating intra-abdominal masses, particularly in distinguishing solid from cystic lesions. Ultrasonography has little role, however, in the diagnosis of small intestinal neoplasms because the fluid content of the bowel assumes a sonic density similar to the density of the intestinal wall and of intestinal tumors, obscuring the ultrasonic detection of small bowel masses. The presence of gas in the small bowel blocks the ultrasonic transmission and thereby eliminates the possibility of detection of masses in regions of gaseous bowel distension. Large tumors extending outside the intestine can be visualized, and ultrasound can reveal disseminated disease, particularly liver metastases.

RADIOISOTOPIC SCANS

Radionuclide scans have little role in diagnosing small bowel neoplasms because intestinal tumors rarely take up imaging agents selectively. Nonspecific intestinal incorporation of imaging material may obscure the visualization of bowel tumors in gallium scans. However, radioisotopic scans may be of benefit in detecting small bowel neoplasms that have metastasized. Liver scans show metastatic foci as hepatic filling defects, and bone scans demonstrate radionuclide uptake by osseous metastases.

ENDOSCOPIC EXAMINATIONS

Endoscopy can be used to examine the duodenum. Using flexible fiberscopes, the entire duodenum and portions of the proximal jejunum can be visualized. Direct biopsies or cytologic samples can be obtained. Periampullary lesions can be evaluated directly by endoscopic cannulation of the biliary and pancreatic ducts through the papilla of Vater and by directly injecting contrast material for roentgenographic visualization. The distal ileum occasionally can be examined by fiberoptic colonoscopy by passing the endoscope through the ileocecal valve and viewing the ileum retrograde. Experimental endoscopes capable of visualizing the entire small intestine are being developed.

TREATMENT

Therapy depends on the histologic type of small intestinal tumor and upon the malignant potential of the neoplasm. General principles can be followed in treating tumors of the duodenum and small intestine.

Surgery is the indicated treatment for virtually all symptomatic tumors of the small intestine. Benign tumors can be removed by local excision. Small tumors, particularly pedunculated neoplasms, can be removed adequately by enterotomy and simple excision of the lesion. Large sessile tumors may require segmental resection of the involved portion of intestine, with reestablishment of bowel continuity by end-to-end intestinal anastomosis. Malignant tumors require extensive surgical excision, which includes segmental resection of the involved bowel with wide margins around the neoplasm, including the mesentery with the vascular and lymphatic pedicle. Lesions in the jejunum and ileum are amenable to radical segmental resection. However, anatomic difficulties are encountered in attempts to radically extirpate tumors in the duodenum because of the retroperitoneal location of the duodenum and its proximity to the pancreas, biliary system, portal venous system, and stomach. Duodenotomy and local excision of benign tumors are possible. Segmental resection can be performed only in the distal free portion of the duodenum. Adequate resection of malignant duodenal lesions in the proximal portion or in the C-loop usually requires pancreaticoduodenectomy (Whipple's operation).

For nonresectable small intestinal tumors, surgical palliation is indicated if intestinal obstruction is present. Usually an obstruction is palliated through bypass, anastomosing unobstructed intestine proximal to the lesion to bowel located distal to the site of obstruction.

Radiation therapy has little role in the treatment of primary small intestinal neoplasms, although it sometimes palliates advanced disseminated disease by relieving pain in areas of metastatic deposits, such as the liver or bone. Chemotherapy has little impact on primary small intestinal neoplasms and is used only for the treatment of metastatic bowel malignancies. Adjuvant radiotherapy and chemotherapy are controversial treatment modalities in small bowel tumors and are subjects of current clinical investigations.

BENIGN NEOPLASMS

ADENOMAS

Adenomas are benign proliferations of epithelium arising from the mucosa or glandular elements. They comprise approximately 30% of all benign small intestinal neoplasms.[8,27,37,64,65] Adenomas can occur as adenomatous polyps, villous adenomas, and Brunner's gland adenomas.

Adenomatous polyps are found throughout the small intestine. They are located commonly in the ileum and in the duodenum but are also found in the jejunum.[8,23,24,27,51] Adenomatous polyps are usually solitary, but multiple polyps may occur within the small bowel. Rarely, the entire GI tract is involved in a polyposis syndrome.[23,37,66] Adenomatous polyps typically are pedunculated, but sessile polyps sometimes can be found. Adenomatous polyps often are asymptomatic and are identified incidentally at autopsy.[24,33] Symptomatic polyps usually present with intermittent intestinal obstruction caused by intussusception, with the polyp acting as the lead point.[2,13–15] Polyps frequently produce chronic, slow intestinal hemorrhage, leading to anemia.[10] Rarely, small intestinal adenomatous polyps result in profuse bleeding.[39]

Indications for the treatment of small intestinal adenomatous polyps include obstruction and hemorrhage. Pedunculated polyps may be excised at the base of the stalk by enterotomy. Some duodenal polyps may be removed endoscopically. For sessile polyps, complete excision of the base is required. Segmental intestinal resection may be necessary to prevent luminal narrowing after the removal of large polyps. Intussuscepted bowel segments must be reduced in all cases of intestinal obstruction, and segmental resection should be performed on any portion of the intestine suspected of vascular compromise. If no ischemic or damaged bowel results after intussusception reduction, simple enterotomy and polyp excision are sufficient treatment.

Villous adenomas are sessile polyps that form exuberant fronds.[67–69] They occur rarely in the small bowel. They are found most often in the duodenum but occasionally occur in the jejunum and ileum.[70,71] Most villous adenomas are smaller than 5 cm in diameter, but some may attain large sizes before becoming symptomatic.[72–74] Malignant degeneration has been reported in almost half of the villous adenomas exceeding 5 cm.[74,75] Malignancy is rare in small villous adenomas. Typical symptoms produced by villous adenomas are intestinal bleeding and intermittent cramping pain.[76] Bouts of intermittent partial intestinal obstruction develop in approximately 35% of patients.[74] Intestinal hemorrhage is seen in about half of the symptomatic patients and is usually associated with malignant degeneration.[74] Bleeding is usually occult or mild; however, massive bleeding from villous adenomas has been reported.[66] Villous adenomas in the small intestine are not heavily secretory and do not produce diarrhea and electrolyte loss as can villous adenomas located in the colon.[8] The diagnosis of intestinal villous adenomas can be established by contrast radiography in approximately 75% of cases.[71,77,78] Villous adenomas characteristically produce filling defects with striated patterns on roentgenographs, indicating where the contrast material infiltrates among the villous fronds.

The treatment of villous adenomas of the small intestine is surgical excision. Lesions should be removed because of the possibility of hemorrhage and malignant transformation. Although some small duodenal lesions may be amenable to endoscopic resection, the majority of villous adenomas require laparotomy for removal. Small lesions can be excised locally through enterotomy, but large lesions may require segmental bowel resection. For villous adenomas with evidence of malignant transformation, resection with wide margins of bowel and mesentery should be performed.

Adenomas of Brunner's glands are rare, pedunculated, solitary neoplasms found in the duodenum, which arise from the submucosal Brunner's glands that produce alkaline duodenal mucus.[26,79–81] Usually Brunner's gland adenomas are less than 1 cm in diameter. Malignant transformation has not been recognized, but adenomas of Brunner's glands can cause duodenal obstructive and hemorrhagic symptoms.[79] Clinically, they may mimic peptic ulcer disease, with epigastric pain, vomiting, and bleeding.[8] The diagnosis of Brunner's gland adenoma may be made by contrast roentgenography, which may show a duodenal polypoid lesion. Endoscopy and biopsy may establish the diagnosis. Symptomatic Brunner's gland adenomas should be surgically excised. Large tumors that are not amenable to local excision should be bypassed by gastroenterostomy, rather than performing a potentially hazardous pancreaticoduodenectomy for a benign neoplasm with no recognized potential for malignant transformation.

BENIGN TUMORS OF CONNECTIVE TISSUE

Benign tumors involving the small intestine can arise from connective tissues and include fibromas, lipomas, and tumors of vascular tissues.

Fibromas are rare benign neoplasms of connective tissue that typically are located within the intestinal wall.[82] Usually fibromas are smaller than 2 cm in diameter, although large tumors have been reported.[83] Fibromas can be pedunculated lesions, but most are sessile.[82,83] Most are asymptomatic and are discovered incidentally. Occasionally, intestinal fibromas can cause symptoms, including hemorrhage from mucosal ulceration and intestinal obstruction, chiefly intussusception. Symptomatic fibromas should be treated by surgical excision. Simple local excision suffices for small tumors, but large lesions may require segmental bowel resection.

Lipomas are neoplasms of mature adipose tissue that can be found throughout the GI tract as well-circumscribed tumors within the intestinal submucosa. More than 50% of all GI lipomas are found in the small intestine, accounting for approximately 20% of all benign small bowel neoplasms.[82] The incidence of lipomas increases distally in the small intestine, with 60% of lipomatous lesions in the ileum, 20% in the jejunum, and 20% in the duodenum.[24,29,84] Lipomas are usually solitary but can occur as multiple lesions. Their frequency increases with advancing age, and they are slightly more common in men than in women.[8] Lipomas of the small intestine remain asymptomatic in at least 35% of cases, being discovered incidentally.[83] Symptomatic lipomas usually cause cramping pain and intestinal obstruction, with intussusception occurring frequently.[29] Hemorrhage from intestinal lipomas is not common. The diagnosis of intestinal lipoma occasionally can be made on the basis of a GI series detecting the presence of a small bowel filling defect. Lipomas frequently occur at the ileocecal valve, where a filling defect may be demonstrated during a barium enema that refluxes into the small bowel. The treatment of symptomatic intestinal lipomas is surgical excision. Local excision is sufficient for small lesions, but for large or obstructing tumors, segmental intestinal resection is recommended.

Benign tumors of vascular tissue can occur in the duodenum and small intestine. Vascular neoplasms are considered to represent proliferative developmental malformations of vascular or lymphatic channels.[82,85]

Intestinal *hemangiomas* are rare benign tumors arising from a proliferation of vascular channels within the submucosal vascular plexus.[86-89] They account for approximately 10% of all benign tumors in the small bowel.[23,83] Hemangiomas are polypoid lesions that usually extend intraluminally. Large tumors may become annular, causing bowel constriction and mucosal ulceration.[86] Approximately 40% of intestinal hemangiomas are solitary. Single hemangiomas can be small and isolated or can involve long segments of the bowel.[82,86] Multiple lesions occur in 60% of patients with intestinal hemangiomas, with lesions found throughout the GI tract.[82,84,87,88] Hemangiomas are slightly more common in the jejunum than in the ileum, and they are unusual in the duodenum.[82,89] Hemangiomas appear grossly as congested small submucosal nodules. Multiple hemangiomas occurring in the GI tract are commonly designated as multiple phlebectasia. Although most cases of GI multiple phlebectasia are sporadic, a hereditary form exists, called the Osler–Weber–Rendu syndrome, in which telangiectatic lesions involve long segments of the small intestine.[85]

Most patients with intestinal hemangiomas develop clinical manifestations, especially diffuse intestinal bleeding.[8,82,87-90] Rarely, vague abdominal pain, intestinal obstructive symptoms, or intussusception characterize the clinical presentation. The diagnosis of intestinal hemangioma is difficult but should be suspected if hemangiomatous lesions are present in the skin or are detected on endoscopic examination of the esophagus, stomach, or colorectum. Hemangiomas of the small intestine may be revealed on contrast roentgenographic studies. Occasionally, they may be thrombosed and calcified, a condition that may be apparent on abdominal x-ray film.[91] Visceral angiography can detect arteriovenous malformations in hemangiomas and is often successful in confirming and locating intestinal hemangiomas when active hemorrhage is present.[92]

The treatment of symptomatic hemangiomas of the small intestine is surgical excision. Generally, the entire involved segment of bowel must be removed to ensure complete extirpation of the abnormal blood vessels giving rise to the tumor. Obstructing lesions should be removed by segmental bowel resection. Most instances of surgical intervention are for intestinal hemorrhage. Unless preoperative angiography can localize the point of hemorrhage, operative identification of the site of bleeding can be challenging. If a single lesion is present in the intestine, it may be identified by palpation or by inspection for fullness in the bowel wall. However, when multiple hemangiomas are present, localization of the bleeding can be difficult. Transillumination of the intestinal wall for hemorrhagic lesions, examination for engorgement of mesenteric vessels in the region of bleeding, division of the intestine and examination for bleeding in the lumen to determine whether hemorrhage is proximal or distal to the point of division, and multiple enterotomies to examine possible bleeding sources have been used to operatively localize bleeding hemangiomas in the small intestine.[86-89,92] Even if the bleeding site can be identified and resected, the patient may suffer future hemorrhage from unresected lesions if multiple phlebectasia is present.[8,87-90,93]

Lymphangiomas of the small intestine are rare tumors that arise from masses of dilated lymphatic vessels within the submucosa.[82,94] Lymphangiomas occur throughout the GI tract, usually as solitary intramural lesions, but occasionally as multiple lymphangiomas.[95] Most intestinal lymphangiomas are asymptomatic and are discovered incidentally. Rarely, lymphangiomas produce intussusception and intestinal obstruction. Symptomatic lymphangiomas should be treated by segmental resection of the involved bowel segment.

BENIGN TUMORS OF SMOOTH MUSCLE

Leiomyomas of the small intestine are benign neoplasms of smooth muscle. They are relatively common small bowel tumors, comprising about 25% of all benign intestinal tumors.[9,29,96] Leiomyomas are found throughout the small intestine, occurring equally in the jejunum and ileum and less commonly in the duodenum.[9,29,82] The benign tumors can occur in patients of any age, but the frequency increases with advancing age.[23,81,96] They typically occur with equal frequency in males and females.[9,23,96]

Leiomyomas grow as intramural masses that expand the intestinal wall. Tumor growth usually causes compression of the lumen and subserosal bulging.[29] A characteristic growth feature of leiomyomas involves central ulceration, probably from the compression of feeding blood vessels and resultant necrosis. The tumors typically are well-circumscribed but lack a true capsule. Leiomyomas frequently erode the overlying bowel mucosa. Leiomyomas produce clinical symptoms in more than 70% of patients.[9,23,29,82] Cramping, intermittent abdominal pain is a presenting symptom in at least 65% of patients.[29] Chronic intestinal obstructive symptoms are present in about 30% of cases.[29] Intussusception develops in about 15% of patients.[9,29] A palpable mass is present in up to 25% of patients with symptomatic leiomyomas.[9] Intestinal bleeding is a common clinical feature, often intermittent and frequently manifested as melena. Hematemesis can occur with lesions in the duodenum. Massive hemorrhage from intestinal leiomyomas is rare.[82] Patients with leiomyomas of the small bowel usually complain of fatigue, and many patients experience weight loss. The diagnosis of small intestinal leiomyoma sometimes can be established clinically. Detection of occult blood in the stool is possible in more than 50% of the symptomatic patients, and anemia usually is present.[8,16,23] Contrast radiography may identify an intestinal neoplasm, and ulcerations in the bowel mucosa sometimes are present at the site of the lesion. Leiomyomas of the small intestine should be treated surgically. Lesions should be removed by segmental bowel resection with margins of surrounding normal tissue.

OTHER BENIGN TUMORS OF THE SMALL INTESTINE

A variety of benign neoplasms can occur within the small intestine, including pseudolymphomas, neurogenic tumors, and hamartomas.

Pseudolymphoma of the small intestine presents as hyperplasia of lymphoid tissue in the bowel wall, which can occur with infectious stimuli such as viral illnesses or bacterial enteritis. Lymphoid hyperplasia has been reported with hypoglobulinemia, and lymphoid polyposis has been noted occasionally to precede the development of lymphoma or leukemia.[97,98] Enlarged lymphoid aggregates may cause abdominal pain or symptoms of intestinal obstruction. Usually, the enlarged lymphoid tissue collections are located in the ileum, but significant hypertrophy of lymphoid patches can occur in the jejunum. The duodenum rarely develops pseudolymphoma. Contrast radiologic studies may demonstrate enlarged lymphoid aggregates. Pseudolymphoma is a benign condition that resolves after treatment or removal of the infectious stimulus.

Benign tumors of neuroectodermal origin occur with low frequency in the small intestine, accounting for about 5% of all benign small bowel neoplasms.[23,29] *Neurofibromas* are composed of nerve elements and appear in the small intestine as nonencapsulated, intramural tumors. They can occur at any age as single, isolated lesions or as multiple neoplasms. Intestinal neurofibromas are found in von Recklinghausen's disease.[23,99–101] Neurofibromas usually occur in the ileum, but they also have been reported in the jejunum and duodenum.

Neurofibromas can remain asymptomatic, but an estimated 70% of patients eventually develop symptoms.[101] Pain occurs as the presenting symptom in approximately 40% of patients, and intestinal bleeding develops in 35%.[29] Intermittent intestinal obstruction can occur, often from intussusception.[82] The diagnosis of neurofibroma of the small intestine should be suspected in patients with the clinical manifestations of neurofibromatosis, including cutaneous neurofibromas, axillary freckling, and patchy skin pigmentation. The stool is usually positive for occult blood. Abdominal x-ray films may show signs of intestinal obstruction, and contrast roentgenography may demonstrate small bowel filling defects. Symptomatic intestinal neurofibromas are treated by surgical excision. Segmental intestinal resections are often necessary for bleeding lesions or obstruction. Small pedunculated tumors can be removed by local excision.

Neurilemmomas are benign tumors of nerve sheaths that are rare in the small intestine.[102] The tumors are small, encapsulated lesions that can occur in all areas of the small intestine, causing pain, hemorrhage, and intestinal obstruction. Symptomatic neurilemmomas should be excised.

Hamartomas are polyps containing myoepithelial elements and are formed from developmental overgrown portions of the bowel wall.[5,8,51] Hamartomatous polyps can cause pain, intussusception, intestinal obstruction, or bleeding. Occasionally, hamartomas may remain asymptomatic. Small intestinal hamartomatous polyps can occur as manifestations of various clinical syndromes. Multiple hamartomas have been identified in adenomatosis of the entire GI tract. A well-recognized clinical entity associated with multiple small intestinal hamartomas is the Peutz–Jeghers syndrome.[103–105] The disease is a hereditary condition carried as a simple mendelian dominant trait characterized by multiple polyps of the small intestine, circumoral pigmentation, and perianal mucosal melanosis. Polyps in the Peutz–Jeghers syndrome are hamartomatous. The polyps are concentrated in the jejunum but also occur in the ileum, duodenum, stomach, and occasionally the colon.

Most cases of Peutz–Jeghers polyps can be managed conservatively. However, symptomatic polyps may require surgical exploration and excision. Because polyps are multiple, it can be a difficult problem to distinguish the area of intestine that is responsible for clinical symptoms. Preoperative localization of obstructed intestinal segments or areas of bleeding by roentgenographic studies may be helpful. Frequently, patients with symptomatic Peutz–Jeghers intestinal polyps require multiple operations for recurrent obstruction or GI hemorrhage. Simple excision of symptomatic polyps is sufficient. If polyp removal compromises the bowel wall, lumen size, or vascular supply, segmental bowel resection must be performed. Although GI malignancies have been reported in the presence of the Peutz–Jeghers syndrome, malignant transformation of the hamartomatous polyps is unlikely.[2,105–107]

MALIGNANT NEOPLASMS

ADENOCARCINOMA

General Considerations

Adenocarcinomas are the most common small intestinal malignancies, accounting for approximately 50% of all cancers of the small bowel.[3,24,27,28,41,42,108–114] Adenocarcinomas increase in frequency with advancing age, with a peak incidence after age 70.[29] Small intestinal adenocarcinomas are slightly more frequent in males than females.

The distribution of adenocarcinomas tends to be greatest proximally in the duodenum, with reduced frequency in the jejunum, and with the lowest incidence distally in the ileum.[8,15,24,30,37,38,108–114] The duodenum is the site of approximately 40% of small bowel carcinomas, the jejunum 35%, and the ileum 25%. Considering the average length of the duodenum as 10% of the length of either the jejunum or the ileum, the frequency of occurrence of small bowel carcinomas in relation to intestinal length is lowest in the ileum, higher in the jejunum by a factor of approximately twofold, and highest in the duodenum by a factor of 20-fold. In the duodenum, approximately 65% of carcinomas occur in the periampullary region, 20% occur proximal to the ampulla, and 15% occur distal to the ampulla.[82] Carcinomas of the jejunum tend to develop proximally, with 70% of jejunal cancers located within 100 cm of the ligament of Treitz.[82] Ileal carcinomas are chiefly distal, with 70% of ileal cancers located within 100 cm of the ileocecal valve.[82]

Adenocarcinomas of the small intestine are derived from the glandular epithelium. Carcinomas tend to grow through the intestinal mucosa to form ulcerative lesions and tend to infiltrate the bowel wall and penetrate through the serosa. Adenocarcinomas can metastasize through lymphatics to the regional lymph nodes, locally to the peritoneal cavity and serosal surfaces, and hematogenously to the liver, lungs, bone, and other sites.

Clinical Features

The clinical manifestations of carcinoma of the small intestine depend upon the size and location of the neoplasm. They include abdominal pain, nausea and vomiting, weakness, weight loss, anemia, GI hemorrhage, bowel obstruction, or intestinal perforation.[5,8,35]

Duodenal carcinomas produce jaundice in more than half of the patients.[82] Periampullary lesions result in biliary obstruction in more than 75% of cases.[8,115] Hemorrhage is common with duodenal carcinomas, resulting in anemia and the presence of occult blood in the stool in more than 75% of patients.[34] Pain, usually epigastric, is often present, with a burning quality that often mimics an ulcer diathesis.[8] Obstruction is unusual in duodenal carcinomas. A palpable mass is present in 25% of cases and usually represents a dilated gall bladder rather than a neoplastic mass.[8]

Carcinomas of the jejunum produce complaints of vague, cramping abdominal pain, weight loss, and weakness. Hemorrhage is common and is usually chronic. Intestinal obstruction occurs in approximately 25% of patients.[28] A mass is palpable in about 30% of cases.[8,82]

Ileal carcinomas present clinically as cramping pain, chiefly in the lower abdomen. Weakness and weight loss are common. Chronic hemorrhage frequently occurs in carcinomas of the ileum. Obstructive symptoms can develop in 35% of patients. Tumors usually occur distally in the ileum and frequently grow circumferentially around the bowel. Approximately 35% of patients present with a palpable abdominal mass.[8,82] Some association between Crohn's disease and ileal carcinomas has been reported.[116–118]

Diagnosis

Duodenal carcinomas can be diagnosed by upper GI series, which may demonstrate filling defects, mucosal ulcerations, or visceral displacement suggestive of neoplasm (Fig. 28-3). In cases of jaundice, transhepatic cholangiography may reveal a malignant obstruction in the ampullary area. CT of the abdomen may reveal a duodenal or peripancreatic mass. Diagnostic ultrasonography can demonstrate a duodenal mass or confirm biliary obstruction and dilatation. Endoscopy allows duodenal carcinomas to be visualized and directly biopsied. Endoscopic retrograde cholangiopancreatography, with endoscopic cannulation of the pancreatic and biliary ducts for the injection of radiographic contrast material, can help in differentiating obstructive jaundice caused by neoplasm from jaundice resulting from biliary lithiasis or inflammatory pancreatic masses. Occasionally, duodenal carcinomas can be diagnosed from cytologic specimens obtained from the duodenum by intubation and aspiration or by endoscopic brushings.[8] Percutaneous needle aspiration has routinely enabled the diagnosis of malignancies in the region of the duodenum and head of pancreas.[119,120]

Carcinomas of the jejunum can be diagnosed by contrast radiography. GI series with small bowel follow-through can demonstrate filling defects, intramural lesions, mucosal abnormalities, or intestinal displacement suggestive of neoplasm. Arteriography can delineate jejunal neoplasms suspected of hemorrhage. CT body scans of the small intestine resolve poorly owing to shadow artifacts caused by intraluminal air and fluid. However, body scans can visualize large tumors and enlarged regional metastatic lymph nodes or metastatic disease in the liver. Ultrasonography resolution of jejunal cancers is limited by the inability of sound waves to pass through intestinal gas. Metastatic deposits, particularly in the liver, can be detected by ultrasonic examination. Endoscopy is not routinely possible beyond the ligament of Treitz and is not helpful in diagnosing carcinoma of the jejunum.

Carcinomas of the ileum generally can be diagnosed roentgenographically. GI series can show filling defects, ulcerations, or bowel loop displacements. Barium enemas with reflux of contrast material through the ileocecal valve into the terminal ileum can identify distal ileal lesions. Arteriography can detect carcinomas presenting with intestinal bleeding. Carcinomas occurring in the distal ileum and ileocecal valve areas occasionally can be visualized endoscopically by using colonoscopy and retrograde examination through the ileocecal valve. Usually, body scans and diagnostic ultrasonography are not helpful in diagnosing tumors of

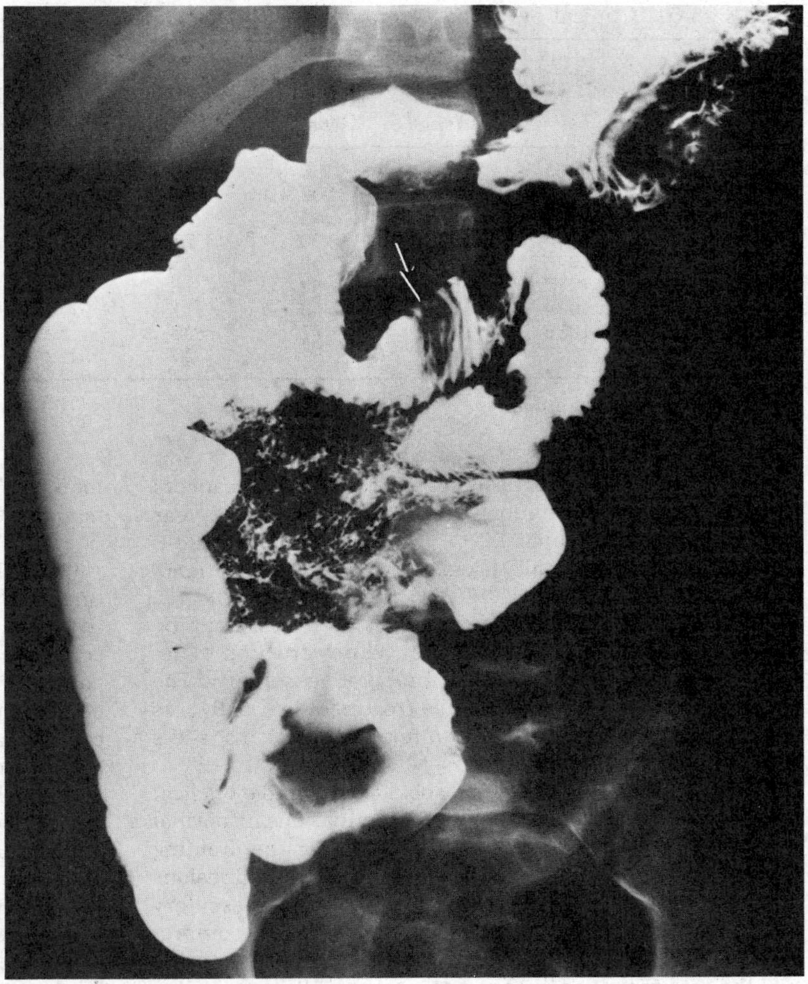

FIG. 28-3. Adenocarcinoma of the duodenum. A filling defect (*arrow*) is present in the duodenum proximal to the ligament of Treitz.

the ileum, except in detecting metastatic deposits in lymph nodes or in the liver.

Treatment and Prognosis

SURGERY. Carcinomas of the small intestine are treated by surgical resection, which should be radical to ensure complete excision of the tumor and the surrounding tissue. The resection should include the segment of bowel containing the tumor, the lymphovascular mesenteric pedicle, and the regional draining lymph nodes. In advanced nonresectable or metastatic disease, local resection or bypass of the tumor may be necessary to palliate obstructive symptoms.

Localized duodenal carcinomas should be treated by radical resection. Although segmental resections are sometimes possible for tumors occurring proximally or distally in the duodenum away from the pancreas, most duodenal carcinomas require extirpation of the entire duodenum and the head of the pancreas. Duodenal carcinomas are usually treated by pancreaticoduodenal resection, which includes duodenectomy, antrectomy, resection of the head of the pancreas, and resection of the distal common bile duct.[121–123] GI tract reconstruction after pancreaticoduodenectomy requires pancreaticojejunostomy, choledochojejunostomy, and gastrojejunostomy.[121–123] Radical resection for duodenal carcinomas has resulted in 5-year survival rates in most series averaging 20%.[43,114,115,123–129] Table 28-5 summarizes the clinical results for patients surgically treated for carcinoma of the duodenum.[43,114,115,125–129]

Patients with metastatic duodenal cancers or with malignant duodenal lesions not amenable to radical surgical resection should undergo palliative surgical bypass to correct or prevent biliary and gastric obstruction.[129,130] Survival after palliative treatment for duodenal cancers is usually short, averaging 4 months.[129] The survival in patients with untreated duodenal carcinomas is typically less than 3 months from diagnosis.[82]

Carcinoma occurring in the jejunum should be treated by radical surgical resection that includes the segment of intestine containing the neoplasm, wide margins of normal bowel around the tumor, and resection of the mesentery supporting the involved intestine, including all draining lymph nodes down to the mesenteric root. Tumor involvement of mesenteric blood vessels may limit radical resection if the sacrifice of most of the small intestine or its blood supply is not

TABLE 28-5. Clinical Series of Carcinoma of the Duodenum

Author	Year	Number of Patients	Resection Rate (%)	Operative Mortality (%)	Mean Survival (months)*	5-Year Survival* (%)
Spinazzola et al[125]	1963	12	50	0	16	0
Mongé et al[126]	1964	25	100	24	10	37
Cortese et al[127]	1972	32	44	29	46	30
Warren et al[128]	1975	39	100	21	31	23
Shulka et al[115]	1976	8	50	25	9	0
Nakase et al[129]	1977	50	62	16	19	8
Ouriel et al[114]	1984	34	56	11	28	29
Giuliani et al[43]	1985	13	77	40	36	17
TOTAL		213	69	20	24	22

* Survival of resected group.

feasible. The overall prognosis for resected jejunal cancers is not favorable, with tumor recurrence likely. The 5-year survival rate is less than 20%.[8,14,25,28,106–114,131,132] Table 28-6 summarizes the results of various surgical series of patients with jejunal carcinomas.[3,15,24,27,28,43,114]

Palliative segmental bowel resection or bypass may be necessary to relieve or prevent intestinal obstruction by jejunal carcinomas too extensive for curative surgery. The survival of patients given palliative treatment is usually less than 6 months, and the survival of untreated patients is less than 4 months.[8,82]

Adenocarcinomas of the ileum should be treated by radical resection of the involved intestine, wide margins of normal surrounding tissue, and mesentery containing the draining lymph nodes. Frequently, radical resections for ileal lesions require right colectomy because resection of the mesentery containing the lymph nodes that drain the ileum compromises the blood supply to the right colon. Tumor extension into the root of the mesentery may not permit wide excision. For patients with carcinomas of the ileum who can undergo surgical resection, 5-year survival rates average 20%.[8,14,28,43,109–114] Results of patients treated surgically for carcinoma of the ileum are given in Table 28-7.[3,15,24,27,28,43,114]

Palliative segmental intestinal resection or bypass may be required to relieve or to prevent obstruction in patients with carcinoma of the ileum that are metastatic or which are too extensive to cure by resection. The survival following palliative treatment of cancers of the ileum usually is less than 6 months.[8,82] The survival of untreated patients with carcinoma of the ileum is typically less than 4 months.[8,82]

RADIATION THERAPY. Carcinomas of the small intestine may be treated with radiation therapy if curative surgical resection is not possible. Radiotherapy has been reported occasionally to produce remissions and to prolong survival in patients with advanced disease. Palliative radiotherapy may decrease pain and relieve obstructive symptoms.[5,8,133] Many carcinomas are radioresistant, and the overall results of the role of radiation therapy in promoting survival in patients with small intestinal cancers are discouraging.[8] Radiotherapy to the intestinal tract is poorly tolerated, resulting in malaise, nausea, vomiting, and enteritis. Often, radiation toxicity prevents the delivery of sufficient tumoricidal dosage. A combination of radiation therapy and surgery may benefit situations in which the surgical resection is likely to leave behind microscopic residual tumor that can be sterilized subsequently by radiotherapy. The use of intraoperative radiation therapy may prove useful when, at the time of surgery, a single large dose of radiation can be given to the tumor or resected tumor bed and to areas at risk for residual tumor contamination and possible recurrence.[134–136] Normal tissues not at risk for tumor contamination may be moved operatively from the radiation beam path or may be shielded to prevent exposure to radiosensitive normal tissues.[134–139]

CHEMOTHERAPY. Chemotherapy may be used in the treatment of disseminated small intestinal carcinomas or in

TABLE 28-6. Clinical Series of Carcinoma of the Jejunum

Author	Year	Number of Patients	Resection Rate (%)	5-Year Survival (Resected Group) (%)
Darling et al[24]	1959	16	44	14
Rochlin et al[3]	1961	9	67	17
McPeak[15]	1967	17	100	6
Silberman et al[27]	1974	5	80	50
Wilson et al[28]	1974	16	88	21
Ouriel et al[114]	1984	21	76	50
Giuliani et al[43]	1985	16	81	38
TOTAL		100	77	27

TABLE 28-7. Clinical Series of Carcinoma of the Ileum

Author	*Year*	*Number of Patients*	*Resection Rate (%)*	*5-Year Survival (Resected Group) (%)*
Darling et al[24]	1959	4	75	0
Rochlin et al[3]	1961	4	75	33
McPeak[15]	1967	3	100	0
Silberman et al[27]	1974	4	75	33
Wilson et al[28]	1974	13	85	0
Ouriel et al[114]	1984	10	70	14
Giuliani et at[43]	1985	19	68	38
TOTAL		57	75	19

the treatment of small bowel cancers that are not amenable to curative surgical resection. Chemotherapy occasionally has been useful in advanced intestinal cancers, resulting in tumor regressions and improved survival in some patients.[13–15,26,28,132] The usual chemotherapeutic agents used in carcinomas of the small intestine are 5-fluorouracil and the nitrosoureas. Combination chemotherapy regimens have improved response rates in various GI cancers compared with single agents.[140,141] The roles of chemotherapy following surgical resection and in combination with radiotherapy in the treatment of small intestinal malignancies are under investigation.

SARCOMA

General Considerations

Sarcomas are malignant tumors that arise in tissues derived from embryonic mesoderm. Sarcomas can develop in all organs and may occur as neoplasms of the small intestine. The many types of sarcomas originate in connective tissue, muscle, fat, vascular tissue, neural elements, and other tissues. Despite a broad spectrum of histogenesis, all sarcomas have similar clinical behaviors and can be considered as a single class of malignant neoplasms for the purposes of diagnosis and management.

Sarcomas account for approximately 20% of all malignant small bowel tumors.[9,17,24,28,38,39,108] Sarcomas of the small intestine have been reported at all ages, with a general increase in frequency with advancing age and with most tumors presenting after the age of 50.[8] The frequency of small bowel sarcomas is approximately equal in men and women. Sarcomas may develop in all regions of the small intestine, but they are least common in the duodenum, which harbors approximately 10% of small intestinal sarcomas.[9,24,28,36] The jejunum is the site of about 35% of intestinal sarcomas, and the ileum is the site of 55% of the sarcomas of the small intestine.[9,24,28,36]

Small intestinal sarcomas usually develop in intramural locations and grow predominantly toward serosal surfaces, so that the tumors often extend outside the bowel wall where they may invade surrounding structures. The growth of intramural sarcomas toward intestinal mucosa can take place, producing ulceration. Intestinal sarcomas frequently develop into neoplasms of large size, with more than 75% being larger than 5 cm in diameter.[108] Because of their large sizes, sarcomas frequently outgrow their vascular supplies and develop ischemic central necrosis.

Sarcomas of the small intestine typically spread by direct extension into tissues that surround the bowel, such as mesentery, abdominal wall, retroperitoneum, and adjacent intestine or other viscera. Intestinal sarcomas disseminate chiefly by the hematogenous route, with the most frequent sites of metastases being the lungs and liver.[9,24,28,38,39] Lymphatic metastases are unusual in sarcomas.[8,82]

Histologic Types

Fibrosarcomas are derived from malignant connective tissue elements. Fibrosarcomas occurring in the small intestine are rare, accounting for less than 10% of small intestinal sarcomas.[24] Fibrosarcomas have been reported in both men and women, chiefly in persons over the age of 50. Fibrosarcomas are reported most frequently in the ileum, with moderate distribution in the jejunum and rare occurrence in the duodenum. The average 5-year survival is 35%.[82]

Leiomyosarcomas arise from malignant smooth muscle elements. Leiomyosarcomas are the most common small intestinal sarcomas, comprising more than 75% of GI sarcomas and accounting for approximately 15% of all malignant small bowel tumors.[8,9,16,38,39] Leiomyosarcomas have been reported at all ages, with a general increase in frequency with advancing age.[8] There is a slight male predominance over females in incidence in most series.[8,9,38,39] Intestinal leiomyosarcomas occur most often in the ileum, with a moderate incidence in the jejunum and least often in the duodenum. Leiomyosarcomas usually grow in an intramural location with serosal extension, and the neoplasms often become large masses that invade outside the intestine. The tumors often develop necrotic centers, which can lead to fistula or abscess formation. Leiomyosarcomas often exhibit protracted, slow growth, with approximately 50% of patients surviving 5 years or longer after diagnosis.[8,108]

Liposarcomas are malignant neoplasms derived from lipoblasts. Liposarcomas are found frequently in the retroperitoneum and abdominal wall but are quite rare as tumors arising within the small bowel. Intestinal liposarcomas typically occur in the serosa and develop into masses that result in extrinsic compression and intestinal obstruction, often growing slowly and achieving large sizes before causing clinical symptoms.[8] Intestinal liposarcomas are found chiefly in the ileum but can occur in the jejunum. Liposarcomas are extremely rare in the duodenum.

Angiosarcomas develop from vascular elements and are rare in the small intestine.[82] Angiosarcomas typically are aggressive, rapidly growing lesions with a poor clinical prognosis. They have been reported in all areas of the small intestine in both men and women. The lesions are intramural, with mucosal extension and ulceration. Angiosarcomas are highly vascular, often presenting with GI hemorrhage.

Neural sarcomas can occur in the small intestine and are derived from neural elements. Intestinal neural sarcomas include *neurofibrosarcomas* and *malignant schwannomas.* Neurofibrosarcomas are malignant tumors arising from neural elements and occur only rarely in the small intestine. Neurofibrosarcomas tend to be aggressive neoplasms that exhibit rapid growth and early dissemination.[82] The tumors develop intramurally and extend toward both the serosa and mucosa. Neurofibrosarcomas occur in all regions of the small bowel and develop equally in men and women. There is an increased incidence of intestinal neurofibrosarcomas in patients with von Recklinghausen's disease.[82]

Malignant schwannomas are sarcomas derived from nerve sheath cells. Schwannomas of the intestinal tract are rare.[82] Schwannomas generally develop in the intestinal wall and extend in subserosal directions, although mucosal invasion and ulceration can occur. Schwannomas are found most often in the ileum, less in the jejunum, and least in the duodenum. Most schwannomas grow slowly, and patient survivals of over 2 years are common even with metastatic disease.

Clinical Features

Patients with sarcomas of the small intestine often complain of cramping abdominal pain that is intermittent. Occasionally, the pain may be a steady discomfort or feeling of fullness. Pain is a feature at clinical presentation in more than 65% of patients.[4,16,24,28,108] Weight loss is seen in 30% of patients. Nausea and vomiting, although typically intermittent, are part of the clinical presentation in approximately 40% of cases.[24,28] An abdominal mass is palpable in more than 50% of patients at the time of presentation.[8,9,28] GI hemorrhage develops in about 50% of patients with sarcomas of the small intestine, usually with leiomyosarcomas.[8,9,24,28] Bleeding is usually chronic, resulting in melena and anemia. Hematemesis is occasionally present with tumors of the proximal intestine, and profuse hemorrhage can occur in some cases.[8] Intestinal obstruction develops in approximately 20% of patients from direct tumor occlusion of the bowel lumen, from intestinal kinking around a tumor mass, or from intussusception.[9,28,39]

Diagnosis

The diagnosis of sarcoma of the small intestine frequently depends on surgical exploration. However, intestinal sarcoma is suggested by the presence of an abdominal mass on radiographs. If extensive necrosis is present, a fluid level may be visible within the mass. Radiographic contrast studies can show intestinal filling defects, ulcerative lesions, or displacement of bowel loops. A barium enema can show colonic displacement by a large abdominal mass, and the reflux of contrast through the ileocecal valve can demonstrate neoplasms in the distal small bowel. Arteriography can show a mass or tumor blush.

CT can delineate the extent of an abdominal mass and identify areas where the tumor has invaded surrounding structures. Ultrasonography can show cystic or necrotic areas within a tumor mass. Metastatic disease in the liver, peritoneum, or retroperitoneum may be revealed by body scans or ultrasonography. Radionuclide liver scans can show hepatic metastatic disease, and gallium scintigraphy occasionally reveals the extent of a primary intestinal tumor or metastatic deposits, particularly if areas of necrosis are present within the neoplasm.

Endoscopy can provide a diagnosis of sarcoma located proximally in the intestine located within the reach of the fiberoptic gastroduodenoscope or distally within the viewing distance of the colonoscope passed retrograde through the ileocecal valve. Because many sarcomas grow subserosally and spare the mucosa, endoscopic biopsies may be negative for tumor unless mucosal invasion has taken place.

Treatment and Prognosis

SURGERY. Surgical excision should be performed whenever possible in sarcomas of the small intestine. Resection should include the intestinal segment giving rise to the tumor, along with surrounding normal tissues in areas of potential tumor spread. In addition, wide resection for intestinal sarcoma may require sacrifice of portions of tissues adjacent to the intestine, such as liver, retroperitoneum, or abdominal wall. Because lymphatic metastases are unusual in sarcomas, extensive dissections of the nodal drainage beds usually are not performed. Five-year survivals as high as 50% have been reported following resection.[8,108]

In nonresectable tumors, palliative segmental bowel excision or bypass of the tumor should be performed to relieve or prevent obstruction. Nearly all patients treated palliatively for unresected tumors succumb to their disease within 12 months of diagnosis.[108]

Pulmonary metastases should be treated by thoracotomy and wedge excision if all metastatic disease is removable from the lung and if no extrapulmonary dissemination is present. In many sarcomas, salvage rates as high as 25% are seen following aggressive surgical excision of pulmonary metastatic disease.[142–144]

If isolated hepatic metastases are present, surgical excision of the metastatic deposits should be considered. Hepatic metastases should be removed by wedge excision or by hepatic lobectomy if the deposits can be approached and extirpated with reasonable morbidity. Although the overall survival of patients with hepatic metastases is poor, some patients may derive long-term benefit from the surgical excision of metastatic deposits within the liver.[145] Patients with solitary hepatic metastases are likely to have longer survival after resection than patients with multiple or bilobar metastases.

RADIATION THERAPY. Radiotherapy may be of benefit in the palliation of patients with nonresectable intestinal sarcomas.[8,24,146] Sarcomas may respond to high-dose radiation, occasionally with long-term survivals resulting even in the presence of gross residual tumor.[147]

Radiation therapy should be considered as an adjunct following surgical resection of intestinal sarcoma, particularly if extraintestinal tissue invasion by microscopic residual disease remaining at the surgical margin is possible. Surgical resection combined with radiation therapy has achieved satisfactory disease control in some intra-abdominal sarcomas, even when incompletely resected.[148,149]

CHEMOTHERAPY. Chemotherapy can be of benefit in the palliation of advanced sarcomas.[150,151] Doxorubicin has broad activity against sarcomas. In metastatic sarcoma, objective response rates in excess of 65% have been reported using combination chemotherapy including doxorubicin, cyclophosphamide, vincristine, and imidazole carboxamide.

Adjuvant chemotherapy following surgical resection of sarcomas has been suggested to reduce the chance of local recurrence and of disease dissemination.[148,149] Adjuvant chemotherapy following surgery or given in combination with radiation therapy is being evaluated for possible benefit in the treatment of various sarcomas.

LYMPHOMA

Lymphoid elements are found throughout the small intestine, and the small bowel can become involved in lymphoid malignancies. Lymphoma can originate in the small bowel as a primary neoplasm, or the small intestine can become involved secondarily as a manifestation of systemic lymphoid malignancy.

Primary lymphoma of the small intestine typically is localized to a single segment of bowel, although multiple separate lesions may be present in up to 20% of cases.[152] All anatomic regions of the small intestine may develop lymphoma. The frequency of lymphoma is lowest in the duodenum, moderate in the jejunum, and highest in the ileum, a pattern consistent with the relative increase in the concentration of lymphatic tissue from the lymphatic-poor duodenum through the jejunum to the lymphatic-rich ileum.[152,153] Primary GI lymphoma constitutes approximately 5% of all lymphoid malignancies and accounts for about 1% of small bowel neoplasms.[8,53,152,153] There appears to be an epidemiologic association between intestinal lymphoma and chronic celiac disease, with chronic immunodeficiency diseases, and with ethnic origins from the Middle East.[154-157] Intestinal lymphomas occur in increased frequency below the age of 10, in low incidence between ages 10 and 50, and in dramatically increased incidence above 50 years of age.[158,159] Intestinal lymphoma shows a slight male predominance, with the male : female incidence ratio being approximately 1.5 : 1. In areas of the Middle East, the incidence of intestinal lymphoma is high, men and women are affected equally, and the disease tends to be manifested before the age of 30.[155]

Intestinal lymphoma arises in the lymphoid tissue of the submucosa. The tumor expands the bowel wall, invades and ulcerates the mucosa, and penetrates the intestinal wall into the serosa. The histologic architecture of the neoplasm can be nodular, with aggregations of lymphoid cells, or diffuse, with a uniform infiltration of malignant lymphoid elements. Involvement of the mesentery and regional lymph nodes in areas of small bowel lymphoma is common. Bowel involvement may be limited or may extend for considerable distances. Most intestinal lymphomas are large in size, with 70% of the lesions exceeding 5 cm in diameter.[108]

Lymphomas of the small intestine manifest clinical signs and symptoms attributable to the presence of a mass that may be ulcerated or obstructing.[159] Cramping abdominal pain is common and often associated with nausea and vomiting. Frequently, lymphoma causes partial intermittent intestinal obstruction. Complete obstruction can occur but is unusual. GI hemorrhage is frequent and usually chronic, leading to anemia. Rarely, massive intestinal bleeding can occur with acute ulceration of the tumor. Fever may be present, usually indicating systemic lymphoma. Occasionally, intestinal lymphomas cause perforation, with the clinical presentation of an acute abdomen. A palpable abdominal mass frequently is present. Diffuse lymphadenopathy or organomegaly suggests advanced systemic disease. Ascites can be present if there is extensive intra-abdominal or retroperitoneal lymphoma. The ascites may represent a malignant effusion or may be a chylous accumulation of intestinal lymph resulting from lymphomatous disruption of mesenteric and retroperitoneal lymphatic channels.

In many instances, the diagnosis of intestinal lymphoma can be made roentgenographically. GI contrast studies may show infiltration of the bowel wall with ulceration or thickening of the mucosa. Segmental intestinal constriction may be present. Displacement of bowel loops can occur with extensive bulky disease. A barium enema can show colonic displacement by large tumors or reveal abnormalities in the distal ileum by retrograde filling of the small intestine. Lymphangiography can determine lymphomatous involvement of intra-abdominal and retroperitoneal nodes. CT and MRI body scans can delineate large masses.

The treatment of lymphoma isolated to the small intestine should be surgical and should involve wide resection of the involved bowel segment, the surrounding tissues, and the regional mesenteric lymph nodes. Extensive disease or intestinal lymphoma presenting together with systemic disease may require palliative resection or bypass to relieve or prevent intestinal obstruction or hemorrhage. Many series report 5-year survival rates of patients with resected intestinal lymphoma averaging 40%.[108,153,159] Patients with nonresectable disease have an overall 5-year survival of 25%.[8] Radiotherapy is of benefit in the palliation of extensive, nonresectable intestinal lymphomas, and chemotherapy is indicated for the treatment of intestinal lymphoma patients unable to undergo curative resections.[8,159,160] Chemotherapy is universally administered for disseminated lymphoma. Chemotherapeutic agents with activity against malignant lymphomas include methotrexate, vincristine, cyclophosphamide, and 6-mercaptopurine.[159]

There is considerable debate over the possible roles of adjuvant radiation therapy and adjuvant chemotherapy following complete surgical excision of lymphoma isolated to the small intestine. Many centers advocate systemic treatment whenever lymphomatous involvement of the GI tract is diagnosed.[12] Although resection of isolated lymphoma of the small bowel can be curative in some patients, studies currently are being performed to evaluate whether adjuvant radiotherapy and chemotherapy after surgery can result in prolonged patient survival.[159]

CARCINOID

Carcinoids are malignant neoplasms that arise from argentaffin cells.[161] Carcinoids represent unusual tumors that can develop throughout the GI tract, in the respiratory tract, and in the gonads.[162,163] The appendix and the small intestine are the sites most frequently affected by carcinoid tumors. Carcinoids account for more than 30% of all small intestinal malignancies, and they typically occur in the intestine as small submucosal nodules.[164,165] Carcinoids are usually solitary, although multiple tumors can be seen in approximately 30% of cases.[166] Carcinoids are rarely located in the duodenum, are infrequent in the jejunum, and are most frequently located in the ileum.[163–168]

Small intestinal carcinoids typically exhibit a slow growth rate. As many as 70% of lesions may remain clinically asymptomatic and are discovered incidentally at autopsy or at laparotomy performed for reasons unrelated to small intestinal neoplasms.[39,163,164] When carcinoids of the small intestine produce symptoms, the clinical features can be vague and nonspecific. Abdominal pain is the chief symptom, although nausea and vomiting may be prominent features of the clinical presentation.[167,168] Intestinal obstruction may occur from fibrosis around the neoplasm or from intussusception. Occasionally, an abdominal mass is palpable. By the time patients present with clinical symptoms, metastatic disease has developed in as many as 90%.[164,169] Despite the high incidence of disseminated disease at the time of diagnosis, the overall 5-year survival rate of patients with carcinoid of the small intestine averages over 20%.[163]

The carcinoid syndrome is an infrequently occurring but well recognized clinical constellation of symptoms that develops in fewer than 10% of patients with carcinoid tumors of the small bowel.[167,170] Because of their derivation from argentaffin cells, which can produce various kinins, carcinoid tumors produce 5-hydroxytryptamine (serotonin) in large amounts, along with histamine, catecholamines, and kinins that are released into the circulation to produce vasoactive manifestations.[163,170,171] The clinical features of the carcinoid syndrome include cutaneous flushing, episodic watery diarrhea, and paroxysmal dyspnea or asthma. The carcinoid syndrome is clinically manifested only with advanced cases of carcinoid tumor when liver metastases are present. Circulating 5-hydroxytryptamine is metabolized and excreted in the urine as 5-hydroxyindoleacetic acid, which serves as a chemical marker for the carcinoid syndrome.

The diagnosis of carcinoid tumor of the small intestine can be difficult to establish before surgical exploration. Contrast roentgenography may reveal small bowel filling defects, obstructing lesions, or mural thickening. Carcinoids in the ileum occasionally can be demonstrated retrograde by a barium enema that is refluxed through the ileocecal valve. Arteriography often reveals a tumor blush because carcinoids typically are highly vascular. Urinary excretion of 5-hydroxyindoleacetic acid may be elevated particularly in patients with advanced disease.

The treatment of carcinoid tumor of the small intestine depends upon the extent of the disease. Curative surgical removal is possible for localized tumors. Carcinoids of the jejunum should be treated by wide segmental bowel resection. Carcinoids in the ileum should be segmentally resected and may require right hemicolectomy if the blood supply to the right colon is compromised by resection of the tumor. Duodenal carcinoids often require pancreaticoduodenectomy. The surgical treatment of advanced cases of carcinoid is indicated if the patient can clinically tolerate surgical intervention, because reducing primary tumor bulk and metastatic deposits can prolong survival.[25,163,172] The treatment of advanced cases demonstrating the carcinoid syndrome should consist of the pharmacological management of the symptoms of flushing, diarrhea, and dyspnea with antiserotonin and antibradykinin agents.[173,174] Although radiation therapy is of limited benefit in carcinoids, palliative liver irradiation has been successful in improving symptoms in some patients with extensive hepatic metastatic disease.[163,175] Chemotherapy has been of limited success. Streptozotocin has shown some efficacy against carcinoid tumors.[176] Intra-arterial chemotherapy for hepatic metastatic disease has palliative benefit in some patients.[177]

METASTATIC TUMORS

Nonintestinal malignancies may metastasize to the small bowel, involving the intestine by direct invasion or by spread to the bowel wall through peritoneal seeding, lymphatic spread, or hematogenous dissemination.

The small intestine may be involved by tumors that originate outside the bowel and invade the intestine secondarily. The duodenum can be involved by tumor extension from cancers of the colon, stomach, pancreas, biliary system, or kidney.[178–181] Metastatic tumors involving retroperitoneal lymph nodes may enlarge, spread, and invade intestine.[182] The jejunum can be invaded directly by malignancies of the colon, stomach, pancreas, kidney, or retroperitoneum.[8,183] The ileum may be affected by cancers arising in the colon or pelvis.[8,183]

Direct tumor extension into the small intestine produces clinical symptoms and signs of intestinal obstruction or of hemorrhage if the tumor ulcerates. The diagnosis of small bowel involvement by direct neoplastic extension may be made by radiologic contrast studies, which can demonstrate compression, displacement, or ulceration of the intestine. However, the diagnosis of a primary extraintestinal tumor must be established to distinguish secondary intestinal involvement from tumors arising primarily within the small bowel. GI series may demonstrate gastric or pancreatic malignancies. Barium enemas can show colonic tumors, and pyelography can reveal renal neoplasms. Lymphangiography localizes malignant retroperitoneal lymphadenopathy. CT or

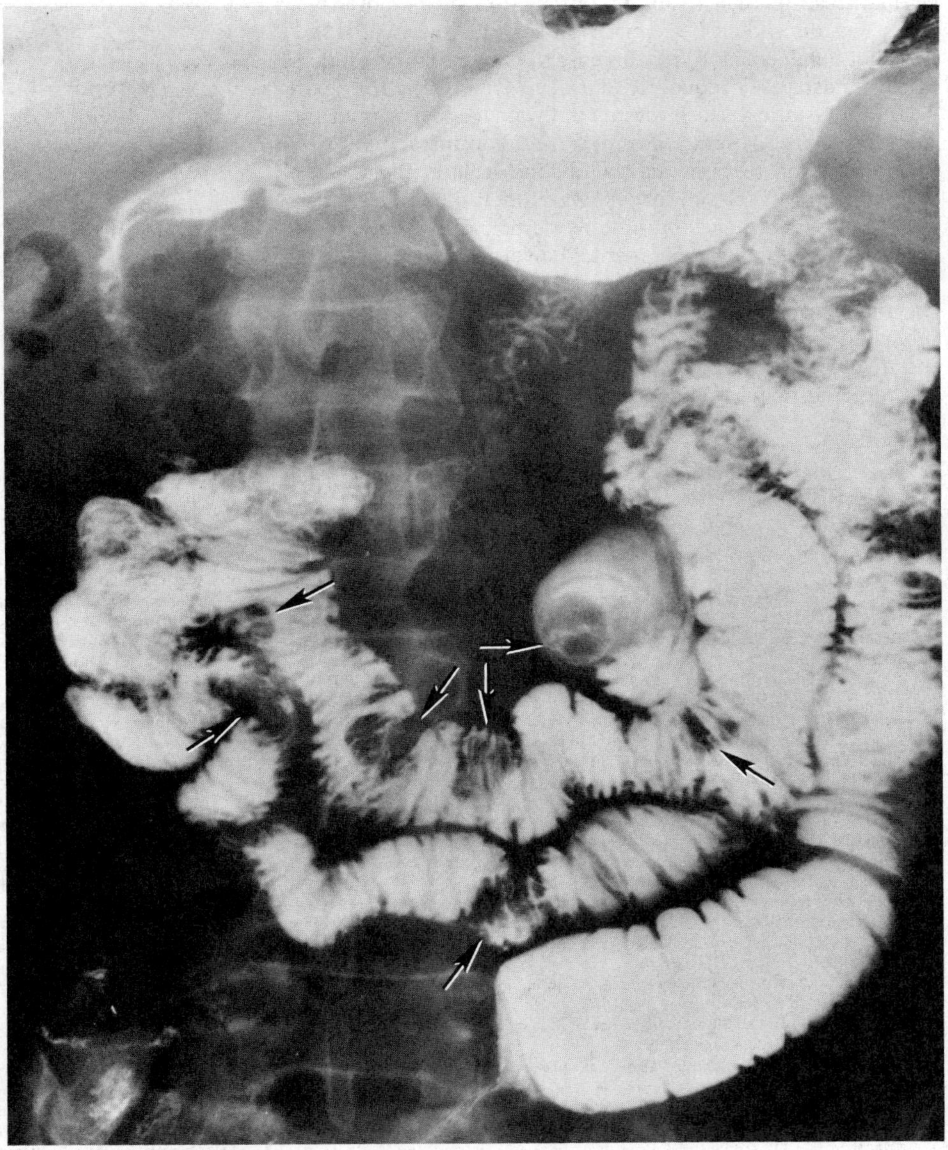

FIG. 28-4. Metastatic melanoma in the small intestine. Multiple filling defects (*arrows*) are present in the small bowel.

MRI body scans can demonstrate intra-abdominal tumor masses and indicate areas of small bowel invasion.

The treatment of tumors invading the small bowel should include surgical excision of the primary tumor, including the segment of bowel invaded. Resection may be quite extensive to include all areas at risk for tumor extension.[181,183,184]

The small intestine may be the site of metastatic deposits from malignancies arising outside the small bowel that involve the intestine by hematogenous, lymphatic, or transperitoneal spread.[185,186] Although the incidence of metastatic involvement of the small bowel is low, tumors that give rise to small intestinal metastases include carcinoma of the cervix, malignant melanoma, carcinoma of the lung, carcinoma of the esophagus, and carcinoma of the ovary.[181,182,185–189] Small intestinal metastatic deposits typically develop in the submucosa and produce intramural lesions. Metastases to the small intestine may form expansile segments within the bowel wall that lead to obstruction, ulcerated mucosal lesions that produce intestinal hemorrhage, or submucosal polypoid masses that result in intussusception. The most common presenting clinical complaint of patients with metastatic lesions to the small bowel is partial intestinal obstruction.[185] Chronic intestinal hemorrhage may be present, resulting in anemia and possibly intermittent melena.[185,186]

The diagnosis of metastatic involvement of the small intestine may be difficult. Roentgenographic contrast studies may reveal masses or filling defects in the small intestine (Fig. 28-4); however, in approximately 50% of cases of small bowel metastases no radiographic abnormalities can be demonstrated.[8]

Surgical resection should be used to treat metastases to the small intestine that result in obstruction or hemorrhage. Large lesions should be excised by segmental bowel resection, but local excision may be possible in small or pedunculated metastases. Frequently, surgical exploration for small bowel metastatic disease reveals multiple lesions. If multiple metastases are present, care must be taken intraoperatively to identify and to treat adequately the lesions causing the symptoms for which the surgery was undertaken. If a solitary small bowel metastasis is the only demonstrable site of disseminated malignancy, segmental bowel resection should be performed, because there is a small chance that resection of the metastatic deposit will be curative.[186] In resections of metastatic melanoma, the mesenteric lymph nodes draining the involved intestinal segment should be removed because the regional nodes frequently contain tumor.[186]

REFERENCES

1. Braasch JW, Denbo HF: Tumors of the small intestine. Surg Clin North Am 44:791–809, 1964
2. Schier J: Diagnostic and therapeutic aspects of tumors of the small bowel. Int Surg 57:789–792, 1972
3. Rochlin DB, Longmire WP: Primary tumors of the small intestine. Surgery 50:586–592, 1961
4. Good CA: Tumors of the small intestine. Am J Roentgenol 89:685–705, 1963
5. Moertel CG: Small intestine. In Holland JF, Frei E (eds): Cancer Medicine, 2nd ed, pp 1808–1818. Philadelphia, Lea & Febiger, 1982
6. Croom RD, Newsome JF: Tumors of the small intestine. Am Surg 41:160–167, 1975
7. Mittal VK, Bodzin JH: Primary malignant tumors of the small bowel. Am J Surg 140:396–399, 1980
8. Herbsman H, Wetstein L, Rosen Y et al: Tumors of the small intestine. Curr Probl Surg 17:121–184, 1980
9. Skandalakis JE, Gray SW, Shepard D et al: Smooth Muscle Tumors of the Alimentary Tract. Leiomyomas and Leiomyosarcomas—A Review of 2525 Cases, pp 1–468. Springfield, Charles C Thomas, 1962
10. Ebert PA, Zuidema GD: Primary tumors of the small intestine. Arch Surg 91:452–455, 1965
11. Sternlieb P, Mills M, Bellamy J: Hodgkin's disease of the small bowel. Am J Med 31:304–309, 1961
12. Weaver DK, Batsakis JG: Primary lymphomas of the small intestine. Am J Gastroenterol 42:620–625, 1964
13. Rochlin DB, Smart CR, Silva A: Chemotherapy of malignancies of the gastrointestinal tract. Am J Surg 109:43–46, 1965
14. Dorman JE, Floyd CE, Cohn I: Malignant neoplasms of the small bowel. Am J Surg 113:131–136, 1967
15. McPeak CJ: Malignant tumors of the small intestine. Am J Surg 114:402–411, 1967
16. Sarr GF, Dockerty MB: Leiomyomas and leiomyosarcomas of the small intestine. Cancer 8:101–111, 1955
17. Hamberger GE: Propempticum Auspicale quo Dissertationem Solemnen: Indicit et de Ruptura Intestini Duodeni Disserit, pp 1–8. Jena, Litteris Ritterianis, 1746
18. Wesner F: Beiträge zur Casuistik der Geschwülste: I. Ueber ein Telangiectatisches Myom des Duodenum von Ungewöhnlicher grösse. Virchows Arch [Pathol Anat] 93:377–386, 1883
19. Fleiner W: Zwei Fälle von Darmgeschwülsten mit Invagination. Virchows Arch [Pathol Anat] 101:484–523, 1885
20. Heurtaux A: Nôte sur les temeurs bénignes de l'intestin. Arch Prov Chir 8:701–712, 1899
21. King EL: Benign tumors of the intestines with special reference to fibroma. Surg Gynecol Obstet 25:54–71, 1917
22. Shallow TA, Eger SA, Carty JB: Primary malignant disease of the small intestine. Am J Surg 69:372–383, 1945
23. River L, Silverstein J, Tope JW: Benign neoplasms of the small intestine. A critical comprehensive review with reports of 20 new cases. Int Abstr Surg 102:1–38, 1956
24. Darling RC, Welch CE: Tumors of the small intestine. N Engl J Med 260:397–408, 1959
25. Brookes VS, Waterhouse JAH, Powell DJ: Malignant lesions of the small intestine: A ten-year survey. Br J Surg 55:405–410, 1968
26. Reyes L, Talley RW: Primary malignant tumors of the small intestine. Am J Gastroenterol 54:30–43, 1970
27. Silberman H, Crichlow RW, Caplan HS: Neoplasms of the small bowel. Ann Surg 180:157–161, 1974
28. Wilson JM, Melvin DB, Gray GF et al: Primary malignancies of the small bowel: A report of 96 cases and review of the literature. Ann Surg 180:175–179, 1974
29. Wilson JM, Melvin DB, Gray G et al: Benign small bowel tumor. Ann Surg 181:247–250, 1975
30. Barclay THC, Schapira DV: Malignant tumors of the small intestine. Cancer 51:878–881, 1983
31. Johnson AM, Harman PK, Hanks JB: Primary small bowel malignancies. Am J Surg 51:31–36, 1985
32. Ciccarelli O, Welch JP, Kent GG: Primary malignant tumors of the small bowel. The Hartford Hospital experience, 1969–1983. Am J Surg 153:350–354, 1987
33. Botsford TW, Crowe P, Crocker DW: Tumors of the small intestine: A review of experience with 115 cases including a report of a rare case of malignant hemangio-endothelioma. Am J Surg 103:358–365, 1962
34. Cutler SJ, Young JL: Third National Cancer Survey: Incidence data. Natl Cancer Inst Monogr 41:1–454, 1975
35. Spiro HM: Clinical Gastroenterology, 3rd ed, pp 643–666. New York, Macmillan, 1983
36. Krouse JM, Eyerly RC, Babcock JR: Tumors of the small bowel. Am J Surg 101:121–127, 1961
37. Sawyer RB, Sawyer KC, Sawyer KC et al: Benign and malignant tumors of the small intestine. Am Surg 29:268–272, 1963
38. Schmutzer KJ, Holleran WM, Regan JF: Tumors of the small bowel. Am J Surg 108:270–276, 1964
39. Ostermiller W, Joergenson EJ, Weibel L: A clinical review of tumors of the small bowel. Am J Surg 111:403–409, 1966
40. Spratt JS: Prevalence of neoplastic and pseudoneoplastic lesions of the small intestine. Geriatrics 21:231–238, 1966
41. Freund H, Lavi A, Pfeffermann R et al: Primary neoplasms of the small bowel. Am J Surg 135:757–759, 1978
42. Miles RM, Crawford D, Duras S: The small bowel tumor problem: An assessment based on a 20-year experience with 116 cases. Ann Surg 189:732–740, 1979
43. Giuliani A, Caporale A, Teneriello F et al: Primary tumors of the small intestine. Int Surg 70:331–334, 1985
44. Schmahl D: Carcinogenic substances and carcinogens: Their clinical significance. In Herfarth C, Schlag P (eds): Gastric Cancer, pp 15–18. New York, Springer-Verlag, 1979
45. Wattenberg LW: Carcinogen-detoxifying mechanisms in the gastrointestinal tract. Gastroenterology 51:932–935, 1966
46. Lowenfels AB: Why are small bowel tumors so rare? Lancet 1:24–25, 1973
47. Wattenberg LW: Studies of polycyclic hydrocarbon hydroxylases of the intestine possibly related to cancer: Effect of diet on benzopyrene hydroxylase activity. Cancer 28:99–102, 1971
48. Barnett WO: Benign tumors of the duodenum. Am Pract 13:625–632, 1962
49. Stassa G, Klingensmith WC: Primary tumors of the duodenal bulb. Am J Roentgenol 107:105–110, 1969
50. Everson TC: Carcinoma of the small intestine. In Everson TC, Cole WH (eds): Cancer of the Digestive Tract. Clinical Management, pp 75–85. New York, Appleton–Century–Crofts, 1969
51. Lowe WC: Neoplasms of the Gastrointestinal Tract, pp 125–144. Flushing, Medical Examination Publishing, 1972
52. Hancock RJ: An 11-year review of primary tumours of the small bowel including the duodenum. Can Med Assoc J 103:1177–1179, 1970
53. Loehr WJ, Mujahed Z, Zahn FD et al: Primary lymphoma of the gastrointestinal tract: A review of 100 cases. Ann Surg 170:232–238, 1969
54. Haghighi P, Nasr K: Primary upper small intestine lymphoma (so-called Mediterranean lymphoma). Pathol Annu 8:231–255, 1973
55. Cassidy M: Abdominal carcinomatosis associated with vasomotor disturbances. Proc R Soc Med 27:220–221, 1934
56. Thorson A, Biörck G, Björkman G, Waldenström J: Malignant carcinoid of the small intestine with metastases to the liver, valvular disease of the right side of the heart (pulmonary stenosis and tricuspid regurgitation without septal defects), peripheral vasomotor symptoms, bronchoconstriction, and an unusual type of cyanosis: A clinical and pathologic syndrome. Am Heart J 47:795–817, 1954
57. Montgomery GE, Liechty RD: Malignant small-bowel tumors. J Iowa Med Soc 56:249–251, 1966
58. Lee FD: Nature of the mucosal changes associated with malignant neoplasms in the small intestine. Gut 7:361–367, 1966
59. Brzechwa-Ajdukiewicz A, McCarthy CF, Austad W et al: Carcinoma, villous atrophy, and steatorrhea. Gut 7:572–577, 1966
60. Jinich H, Rojas E, Webb JA et al: Lymphoma presenting as malabsorption. Gastroenterology 54:421–425, 1968
61. Brunt PW, Sircus W, Maclean N: Neoplasia and the coeliac syndrome in adults. Lancet 1:180–184, 1969
62. Chernish SM, Miller RE, Rosenak BD et al: Hypotonic duodenography with the use of glucagon. Gastroenterology 63:392–398, 1972
63. Sindelar WF, Bagley DH, Felix EL et al: Lung tomography in cancer patients: Full-lung tomography in screening for pulmonary metastases. JAMA 240:2060–2063, 1978
64. Morson BC, Dawson IMP: Gastrointestinal Pathology, pp 352–377. London, Blackwell Scientific Publications, 1972
65. Muto T, Bussey HJR, Morson BC: The evolution of cancer of the colon and rectum. Cancer 376:2251–2270, 1975
66. Ravitch MM: Polypoid adenomatosis of the entire gastro-intestinal tract. Ann Surg 128:283–298, 1948

67. Perry EC: Papilloma of the duodenum. Trans Pathol Soc London 44:84–85, 1893
68. Wechselmann L: Polyp und Carcinom in Magen-darmkanal. Beitr Klin Chir 70:855–904, 1910
69. Joyeux R: Tumeur adenomato-villeuse du duodenum. J Chir (Paris) 66:437–448, 1950
70. Steinberg LS, Sheiber W: Villous adenomas of the small intestine. Surgery 71:423–428, 1972
71. Kutin ND, Ranson JHC, Gouge TH et al: Villous tumors of the duodenum. Ann Surg 181:164–168, 1975
72. Golden R: Non-malignant tumors of the duodenum: Report of two cases. Am J Roentgenol 20:405–413, 1928
73. Hoffman BP, Grayzel DM: Benign tumors of the duodenum. Am J Surg 70:394–400, 1945
74. Shulten MF, Dyasu R, Beal JM: Villous adenoma of the duodenum: A case report and review of the literature. Am J Surg 132:90–96, 1976
75. Bremer EH, Battaile WG, Bulle PH: Villous tumors of the upper gastrointestinal tract: Clinical review and report of a case. Am J Gastroenterol 50:135–143, 1968
76. Meltzer AD, Ostrum BJ, Isard HJ: Villous tumors of the stomach and duodenum. Radiology 87:511–513, 1966
77. Waters CA: The roentgenologic diagnosis of papilloma of the duodenum. Am J Roentgenol 24:544–557, 1930
78. Ring EJ, Ferrucci JT, Eaton SB et al: Villous adenomas of the duodenum. Radiology 104:45–48, 1972
79. Silverman L, Waugh JM, Huizenga KA et al: Large adenomatous polyp of Brunner's glands. Am J Clin Pathol 36:438–443, 1961
80. Deutschberger O, Tchertkoff V, Daino J et al: Benign duodenal polyp: Review of the literature and report of a giant adenomatous polyp of the duodenal bulb. Am J Gastroenterol 38:75–84, 1962
81. de Silva S, Chandrasoma P: Giant duodenal hamartoma consisting mainly of Brunner's glands. Am J Surg 133:240–243, 1977
82. Wood DA: Atlas of Tumor Pathology. Tumors of the Intestines, section VI, fascicle 22, pp 19–120. Washington, Armed Forces Institute of Pathology, 1967
83. Rankin FW, Newell CE: Benign tumors of the small intestine. Report of twenty-four cases. Surg Gynecol Obstet 57:501–507, 1933
84. Smith FR, Mayo CW: Submucous lipomas of the small intestine. Am J Surg 80:922–928, 1950
85. Gentry RW, Dockerty MB, Clagett OT: Vascular malformations and vascular tumors of the gastrointestinal tract. Int Abstr Surg 88:281–323, 1949
86. Moore RM, Schmeisser HC: Benign tumors of the small intestine. South Med J 27:386–393, 1934
87. Sivula A: Intestinal haemangioma: Observation on two cases treated surgically. Acta Chir Scand 131:485–491, 1966
88. Bilton JL, Riahi M: Hemangioma of the small intestine. Am J Gastroenterol 48:120–124, 1967
89. Hyun BH, Palumbo VN, Null RH: Hemangioma of the small intestine with gastrointestinal bleeding. JAMA 208:1903–1905, 1969
90. Brown AJ: Vascular tumors of the intestine. Surg Gynecol Obstet 39:191–199, 1924
91. Nys A, Buyssens N: Diffuse cavernous hemangiomatosis of the small intestine. Gastroenterology 45:663–666, 1963
92. Alfidi RJ, Esselstyn CD, Tarar R et al: Recognition and angio-surgical detection of arteriovenous malformations of the bowel. Ann Surg 174:573–582, 1971
93. Calem WS, Jimenez FA: Vascular malformations of the intestine. Their role as a source of hemorrhage. Arch Surg 86:571–579, 1963
94. Arnett NL, Friedman PS: Lymphangioma of the colon: Roentgen aspects. A case report. Radiology 67:882–885, 1956
95. Puppel ID, Morris LE: Lymphangioma of the jejunum. Arch Pathol 38:410–412, 1944
96. Golden T, Stout AP: Smooth muscle tumors of the gastrointestinal tract and retroperitoneal tissues. Surg Gynecol Obstet 73:784–810, 1941
97. Hermans PE: Nodular lymphoid hyperplasia of the small intestine and hypogammaglobulinemia: Theoretical and practical considerations. Fed Proc 26:1066–1611, 1967
98. Shaw EB, Hennigar GR: Intestinal lymphoid polyposis. Am J Clin Pathol 61:417–422, 1974
99. Shaw RC: Von Recklinghausen's disease of the small intestine associated with skin lesions. Am J Surg 80:360–363, 1950
100. Brasfield RD, Das Gupta TK: Von Recklinghausen's disease: A clinicopathological study. Ann Surg 175:86–104, 1972
101. Hochberg FH, DaSilva AB, Galdabini J et al: Gastrointestinal involvement in von Recklinghausen's neurofibromatosis. Neurology (Minneap) 24:1144–1151, 1974
102. Cedermark J: Neurinomas of the gastrointestinal tract. J Int Coll Surg 12:5–11, 1949
103. Jeghers H, McKusick VA, Katz KH: Generalized intestinal polyposis and melanin spots of the oral mucosa, lips and digits: A syndrome of diagnostic significance. N Engl J Med 241:993–1005, 1949
104. Dormandy TL: Gastrointestinal polyposis with mucocutaneous pigmentation (Peutz-Jeghers syndrome). N Engl J Med 256:1093–1102, 1141–1146, 1186–1190, 1957
105. Reid JD: Duodenal carcinoma in the Peutz-Jeghers syndrome: Report of a case. Cancer 18:970–977, 1965
106. Williams JP, Knudsen A: Peutz-Jeghers syndrome with metastasizing duodenal carcinoma. Gut 6:179–184, 1965
107. Humphries AL, Shepherd MH, Peters HF: Peutz-Jeghers syndrome with colonic adenocarcinoma and ovarian tumor. JAMA 197:296–298, 1966
108. Pagtalunan RJG, Mayo CW, Dockerty MB: Primary malignant tumors of the small intestine. Am J Surg 108:13–18, 1964
109. Goel IP, Didolkar MS, Elias EG: Primary malignant tumors of the small intestine. Surg Gynecol Obstet 143:717–719, 1976
110. Rich JD: Malignant tumors of the intestine: A review of 37 cases. Am Surg 43:445–454, 1977
111. Sager GF: Primary malignant tumors of the small intestine. A twenty-two-year experience with thirty patients. Am J Surg 135:601–603, 1978
112. Coutsoftides T, Shibata HR: Primary malignant tumors of the small intestine. Dis Colon Rectum 22:24–26, 1979
113. Williamson RC, Welch CE, Malt RA: Adenocarcinoma and lymphoma of the small intestine: Distribution and etiologic associations. Ann Surg 197:172–178, 1983
114. Ouriel K, Adams JT: Adenocarcinoma of the small intestine. Am J Surg 147:66–71,1984
115. Shukla SK, Elias EG: Primary neoplasms of the duodenum. Surg Gynecol Obstet 142:858–860, 1976
116. Morowitz DA, Block GE, Kirsner JB: Adenocarcinoma of the ileum complicating chronic regional enteritis. Gastroenterology 55:397–402, 1968
117. Tyers GFO, Steiger E, Dudrick SJ: Adenocarcinoma of the small intestine and other malignant tumors complicating regional enteritis: Case report and review of the literature. Ann Surg 169:510–518, 1969
118. Frank JD, Shorey BA: Adenocarcinoma of the small bowel as a complication of Crohn's disease. Gut 14:120–124, 1973
119. Smith EH, Bartrum RJ, Chang YC et al: Percutaneous aspiration biopsy of the pancreas under ultrasonic guidance. N Engl J Med 292:825–828, 1975
120. Goldman ML, Naib ZM, Galambos JT et al: Preoperative diagnosis of pancreatic carcinoma by percutaneous aspiration biopsy. Am J Dig Dis 22:1076–1082, 1977
121. Howard JM: Pancreatico-duodenectomy: Forty-one consecutive Whipple resections without an operative mortality. Ann Surg 168:692–640, 1968
122. Gilsdorf RB, Spanos P: Factors influencing morbidity and mortality in pancreaticoduodenectomy. Ann Surg 177:332–337, 1973
123. Howard JM, Jordan GL: Cancer of the pancreas. Curr Probl Cancer 2:1–52, 1977
124. Brunschwig A, Tiholiz IC: Surgical treatment of malignant tumors of the duodenum exclusive of those arising from the papilla of Vater. Surg Clin North Am 26:163–175, 1946
125. Spinazzola AJ, Gillesby WJ: Primary malignant neoplasms of the duodenum: Report of twelve cases. Am Surg 29:405–412, 1963
126. Mongé JJ, Judd ES, Gage RP: Radical pancreatoduodenectomy: A 22-year experience with the complications, mortality rate, and survival rate. Ann Surg 160:711–722, 1964
127. Cortese AF, Cornell GN: Carcinoma of the duodenum. Cancer 29:1010–1015, 1972
128. Warren KW, Choe DS, Plaza J et al: Results of radical resection for periampullary cancer. Ann Surg 181:534–540, 1975
129. Nakase A, Matsumoto Y, Uchida K et al: Surgical treatment of cancer of the pancreas and the periampullary region: Cumulative results in 57 institutions in Japan. Ann Surg 185:52–57, 1977
130. Coutsoftides T, MacDonald J, Shibata HR: Carcinoma of the pancreas and periampullary region: A 41-year experience. Ann Surg 186:730–733, 1977
131. Vuori JVA: Primary malignant tumors of the small intestine. Analysis of cases diagnosed in Finland, 1953–1962. Acta Chir Scand 137:555–561, 1971
132. Morgan DF, Busuttil RW: Primary adenocarcinoma of the small intestine. Am J Surg 134:331–333, 1977
133. Cavanaugh PJ: Considerations appropriate to a clinical trial of definitive radiation therapy in adenocarcinoma of the pancreas. J Surg Oncol 7:135–137, 1975
134. Abe M, Takahashi M, Yabumoto E et al: Techniques, indications and results of intraoperative radiotherapy of advanced cancers. Radiology 116:693–702, 1975
135. Abe M, Takahashi M, Yabumoto E et al: Clinical experiences with intraoperative radiotherapy of locally advanced cancers. Cancer 45:40–48, 1980
136. Gunderson LL, Tepper JE, Biggs PJ et al: Intraoperative ± external beam irradiation. Curr Probl Cancer 7:1–69, 1983
137. Sindelar WF, Kinsella T, Tepper J et al: Experimental and clinical studies with intraoperative radiotherapy. Surg Gynecol Obstet 157:205–219, 1983
138. Kinsella TJ, Glatstein E, Sindelar WF: Intraoperative radiotherapy. Hosp Pract 20:125–127, 130–131, 137–138, 140–141, 1985
139. Kinsella TJ, Sindelar WF, Tepper JE et al: Intraoperative radiotherapy. In Withers HR, Peters LJ (eds): Innovation in Radiation Oncology, pp 143–153. New York, Springer-Verlag, 1988
140. Bunn PA, Nugent JL, Ihde DC et al: 5-Fluorouracil, methyl-CCNU, adriamycin, and mitomycin-C in the treatment of advanced gastric cancer. Cancer Treat Rep 62:1287–1293, 1978
141. Higgins GA: Chemotherapy in advanced gastric cancer. In Herfarth C, Schlag P (eds): Gastric Cancer, pp 361–366. New York, Springer-Verlag, 1979
142. Thomford NR, Woolner LB, Clagett OT: The surgical treatment of metastatic tumors in the lungs. J Thorac Cardiovasc Surg 49:357–363, 1965
143. Ochsner A, Rush V: Treatment of pulmonary metastatic disease. Surg Clin North Am 46:1469–1473, 1966
144. Fallon RH, Roper CL: Operative treatment of metastatic pulmonary cancer. Ann Surg 166:263–265, 1967
145. Foster JH, Berman MH: Solid Liver Tumors, pp 209–234. Philadelphia, WB Saunders, 1977
146. McNeer GP, Cantin J, Chu F et al: Effectiveness of radiation therapy in the management of sarcoma of the soft somatic tissues. Cancer 22:391–397, 1968

147. Suit HD, Russell WO, Martin RG: Management of patients with sarcoma of soft tissue in an extremity. Cancer 31:1247–1255, 1973
148. Rosenberg SA, Kent H, Costa J et al: Prospective randomized evaluation of the role of limb-sparing surgery, radiation therapy, and adjuvant chemoimmunotherapy in the treatment of adult soft-tissue sarcomas. Surgery 84:62–69,1978
149. Rosenberg SA, Sindelar WF: Surgery and adjuvant radiation-chemoimmunotherapy in soft tissue sarcomas: Result of treatment at the National Cancer Institute. In van Oosterom AT, Muggia FM, Cleton FJ (eds): Therapeutic Progress in Ovarian Cancer, Testicular Cancer and the Sarcomas, pp 397–412. Boston, Martinus Nijhoff, 1980
150. Jacobs EM: Combination chemotherapy of metastatic testicular germinal cell tumors and soft part sarcomas. Cancer 25:324–332, 1970
151. Gottlieb JA: Combination chemotherapy for metastatic sarcoma. Cancer Chemother Rep 58:265–270, 1974
152. Rosenberg SA, Diamond HD, Jaslowitz B et al: Lymphosarcoma: A review of 1269 cases. Medicine (Baltimore) 40:31–84, 1961
153. Naqvi MS, Burrows L, Kark AE: Lymphoma of the gastrointestinal tract: Prognostic guides based on 162 cases. Ann Surg 170:221–231, 1969
154. Eidelman S, Parkins RA, Rubin CE: Abdominal lymphoma presenting as malabsorption: A clinico-pathologic study of nine cases in Israel and a review of the literature. Medicine (Baltimore) 45:111–137, 1966
155. Harris OD, Cooke WT, Thompson H et al: Malignancy in adult coeliac disease and idiopathic steatorrhoea. Am J Med 42:899–912, 1967
156. Whitehead R: Primary lymphadenopathy complicating idiopathic steatorrhoea. Gut 9:569–575, 1968
157. Dutz W, Asvadi S, Sadri S et al: Intestinal lymphoma and sprue: A systematic approach. Gut 12:804–810, 1971
158. Mestel AL: Lymphosarcoma of the small intestine in infancy and childhood. Ann Surg 149:87–94, 1959
159. McGovern VT: Lymphomas of the gastrointestinal tract. In Yardley JH, Morson BC, Abell MR (eds): The Gastrointestinal Tract, pp 184–205. Baltimore, Williams & Wilkins, 1977
160. Treadwell TA, White RR: Primary tumors of the small bowel. Am J Surg 130:749–755, 1975
161. Pearse AGE: The APUD cell concept and its implications in pathology. Pathol Annu 9:27–41, 1974
162. Ritchie AC: Carcinoid tumors. Am J Med Sci 232:311–328, 1956
163. Marks C: Carcinoid Tumors. A Clinicopathologic Study, pp 1–154. Boston, GK Hall, 1979
164. Moertel CG, Sauer WG, Dockerty MB et al: Life history of the carcinoid tumor of the small intestine. Cancer 14:901–912, 1961
165. Horsley BL, Baker RR: Fibroplastic response to intestinal carcinoid. Am Surg 36:676–680, 1970
166. Cunningham PJ, Norman J, Cleveland BR: Malignant carcinoid associated with thoraco-abdominal aneurysm and analysis of thirty-one cases of gastrointestinal carcinoid tumors. Ann Surg 176:613–619, 1972
167. Ostermiller WE, Joergenson EJ: Carcinoid tumors of the small bowel. Arch Surg 93:616–619, 1966
168. Sterling JA, Jayasanker MR, Galvez M: Carcinoids of the gastrointestinal tract. Am J Gastroenterol 47:373–378, 1967
169. Dockerty MB: Carcinoids of the gastrointestinal tract. Am J Clin Pathol 25:794–796, 1955
170. Diffenbaugh WG, Anderson RE: Carcinoid (argentaffin) tumors of the gastrointestinal tract. Arch Surg 73:21–37, 1956
171. Sjoerdsma A, Weissbach H, Udenfriend S: A clinical, physiologic and biochemical study of patients with malignant carcinoid (argentaffinoma). Am J Med 20:520–532, 1956
172. Chandler JJ, Foster JH: Malignant carcinoid syndrome treated by resection of hepatic metastases. Am J Surg 109:221–222, 1965
173. Melmon KL, Sjoerdsma A, Oates JA et al: Treatment of malabsorption and diarrhea of the carcinoid syndrome with methysergide. Gastroenterology 48:18–24, 1965
174. Tilson MD: Carcinoid syndrome. Surg Clin North Am 54:409–423, 1974
175. Herbsman H, Hassan A, Gardner B et al: Treatment of hepatic metastases with a combination of hepatic artery infusion chemotherapy and external radiotherapy. Surg Gynecol Obstet 147:13–17, 1978
176. Schein P, Kahn R, Gorden P et al: Streptozotocin for malignant insulinomas and carcinoid tumor. Report of eight cases and review of the literature. Arch Intern Med 132:555–561, 1973
177. Sparks FC,Mosher MB, Hallauer WC et al: Hepatic artery ligation and postoperative chemotherapy for hepatic metastases: Clinical and pathological results. Cancer 35:1074–1082, 1975
178. Grinnell RS: Lymphatic metastases of carcinoma of the colon and rectum. Ann Surg 131:494–506, 1950
179. Lawson LJ, Holt LP, Rooke HWP: Recurrent duodenal haemorrhage from renal carcinoma. Br J Urol 38:133–137, 1966
180. Treitel H, Meyers MA, Maza V: Changes in the duodenal loop secondary to carcinoma of the hepatic flexure of the colon. Br J Radiol 43:209–213, 1970
181. Veen HF, Oscarson JEA, Malt RA: Alien cancers of the duodenum. Surg Gynecol Obstet 143:39–42, 1976
182. Ngan H: Involvement of the duodenum by metastases from tumours of the genital tract. Br J Radiol 43:701–705, 1970
183. Van Prohaska J, Govostis MC, Wasick M: Multiple organ resection for advanced carcinoma of the colon and rectum. Surg Gynecol Obstet 97:177–182, 1953
184. Ellis H, Morgan MN, Wastell C: "Curative" surgery in carcinoma of the colon involving duodenum: A report of 6 cases. Br J Surg 59:932–935, 1972
185. de Castro CA, Dockerty MB, Mays CW: Metastatic tumors of the small intestines. Surg Gynecol Obstet 105:159–165, 1957
186. Das Gupta TK, Brasfield RD: Metastatic melanoma of the gastrointestinal tract. Arch Surg 88:969–973, 1964
187. Farmer RG, Hawk WA: Metastatic tumors of the small bowel. Gastroenterology 47:496–504, 1964
188. Beckly DE: Alimentary tract metastases from malignant melanoma. Clin Radiol 25:385–389, 1974
189. McNeill PM, Wagman LD, Neifeld JP: Small bowel metastases from primary carcinoma of the lung. Cancer 59:1486–1489, 1987

ALFRED M. COHEN

BRENDA SHANK

MICHAEL A. FRIEDMAN

CHAPTER 29 *Colorectal Cancer*

Adenocarcinoma of the large bowel affects approximately one person in 20 in the United States and in most Westernized countries. With more than 140,000 new cases diagnosed in the Unites States each year, representing 15% of all cancers, this disease constitutes a major public health problem. However, when diagnosed in its early stages, this common malignancy is highly curable by surgical treatment, with minimal morbidity and mortality. Because of the high potential cure rate, defining populations at risk and screening asymptomatic patients are important considerations. The presence of a number of "biomarkers" associated with colorectal cancer, such as adenomatous polyps and abnormal mucosal cell proliferation, will allow clinicians to test the efficacy of a number of preventive strategies in the next decade.[1]

This chapter reviews recent advances in the multidisciplinary treatment of primary colorectal cancer. Incremental benefits, risks, and toxic effects of these combined modality approaches are defined, and recent developments in chemotherapeutic protocols for metastatic disease are examined. Much of the discussion will consider *colon* cancer separately from *rectal* cancer. Although certain features of their biology and natural history are similar, patterns of tumor recurrence, surgical treatment, and adjuvant treatment programs are so disparate as to warrant the distinction. Treatment of patients with potentially curable cancers will be discussed separately from treatment of patients with unresectable, recurrent, or metastatic disease.

Figure 29-1 provides an overview of the end results of treatment of patients with colorectal adenocarcinoma. It demonstrates the need for improved earlier diagnosis and control of micrometastatic disease. Figure 29-2 suggests that efforts in these directions have reduced the overall death rate from this cancer. The 5-year relative survival rate from colon cancer increased from 41% in the 1950s to 54% in the 1980s; that for rectal cancer increased from 40% to 51.5% in the same period.[2]

ANATOMY

GROSS ANATOMY OF THE LARGE BOWEL

The large bowel is divided into the colon and rectum. However, for treatment purposes, it is also important to consider the large bowel in terms of free intraperitoneal location versus extraperitoneal location. Treatment failure of intraperitoneal tumors is more likely to be expressed as peritoneal seeding, whereas treatment failure of extraperitoneal tumors manifests as local recurrence. Extraperitoneal sites of tumor include the pelvis and the abdominal retroperitoneum.

The cecum, transverse colon, and sigmoid loop are mobile structures that lie free in the peritoneal cavity and are completely covered with serosa (visceral peritoneum). The dorsal or posterior aspect of the ascending and descending colon, and both flexures frequently lack serosa. Tumor spread from these segments may involve the retroperitoneal soft tissues, kidney, ureter, and pancreas. Although the rectum is frequently considered to be extraperitoneal, the anterior surface of the upper rectum is covered with serosa and is therefore intraperitoneal. Patterns of recurrence of high rectal cancer may depend on whether the location of the tumor is anterior or posterior.

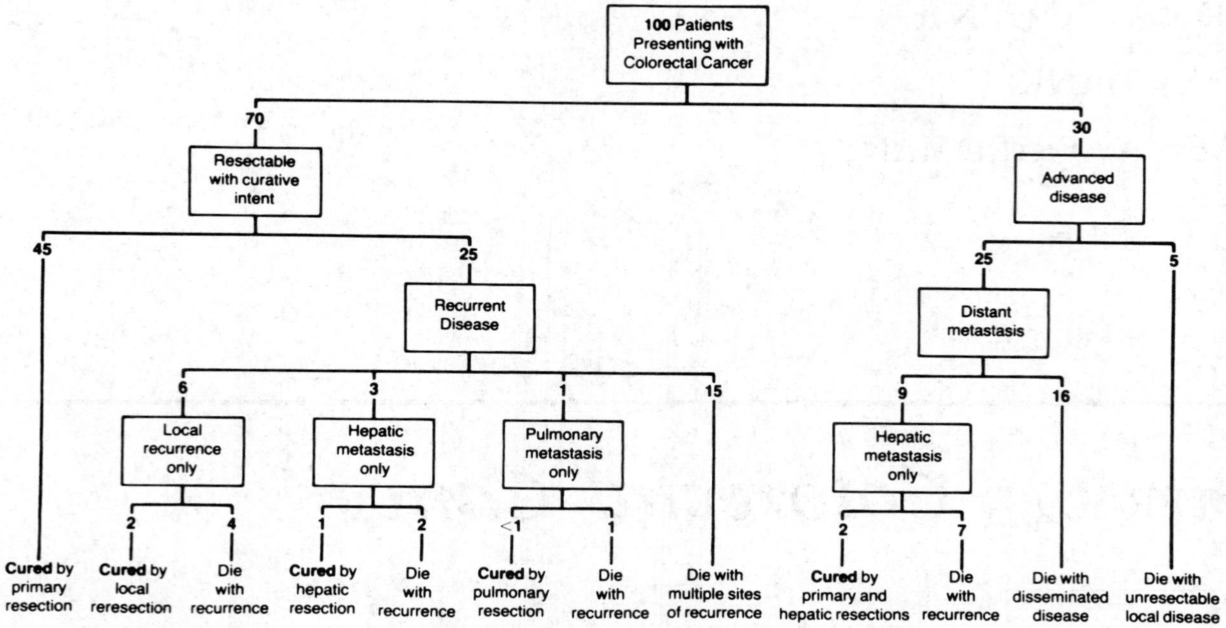

FIG. 29-1. Patterns of failure in 100 patients presenting with large bowel cancer. (August DA, Ottow RT, Sugarbaker PH: Clinical perspectives on human colorectal cancer metastases. Cancer Metastasis Rev 3:303–324, 1984)

RECTUM

The rectum in the adult is about 15 cm long; for treatment purposes it is divided into 5-cm segments. However, actual rectal length and division into surgical segments reflect several patient features, such as height, body habitus, pelvic width (gynecoid versus android), and curve of the sacral hollow, within which the rectum resides. The backward displacement of the rectum onto the sacrum is important in fecal continence, to be discussed later.

Frequently the lowermost location of a rectal cancer is defined in terms of distance from the anus. It should be stated whether the determination is made with a rigid or flexible endoscope, and whether the reference point is the anal verge (the lowermost portion of the anal canal) or the dentate line. Once the rectum is surgically mobilized from the sacral hollow, a posteriorly based tumor easily palpable on digital rectal examination may be well out of the pelvis.

About 1 to 2 cm above the dendate line is the posteriorly palpable muscular anorectal ring, or puborectalis sling. The dentate line is well defined visually, and the distance above this demarcation as determined with a rigid proctoscope is the most reliable way of defining the lowest extent of a rectal cancer (Fig. 29.3).

The rectal diameter, particularly 5 to 12 cm from the anal verge, is two to three times the diameter of the sigmoid and left colon, which allows the rectum to serve as a reservoir. Although rectal resection with anastomosis establishes intestinal continuity, the reservoir function of the rectum is abolished. This may lead to urgency and frequency in defecation, which usually improves with time and with dilation of the neorectum.

FIG. 29-2. Improvement in 5-year relative survival rates from colorectal cancer (white men and women).[2]

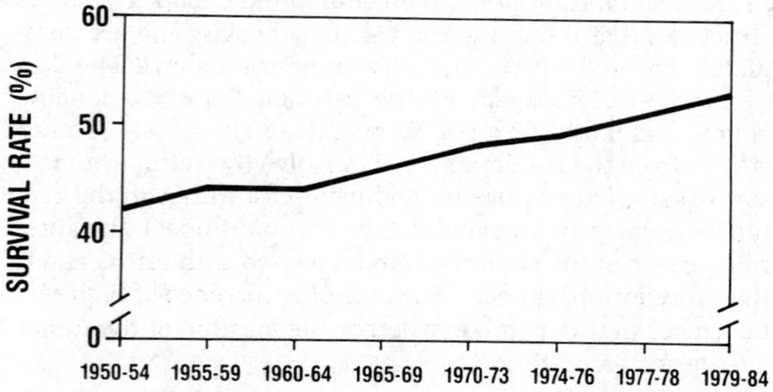

NORMAL HISTOLOGY

The histology of the large bowel directly reflects its functions of water absorption and mucus secretion. Water is absorbed primarily in the proximal half, with storage in the distal bowel. Mucus facilitates evacuation of the partially desiccated feces. The bowel wall consists of mucosa, lamina propria, muscularis mucosa, submucosa, muscularis propria, and, when present, visceral peritoneum (serosa). A layer of fat (subserosa) is present between the muscularis propria and the serosa. The serosa wraps around the colon to envelop the vascular/lymphatic structures and form the mesentery. This explains why tumors that grow completely through the muscularis are not necessarily "transmural" (see section on Surgical-Pathologic Staging, below).

The inside of the colon is relatively smooth, lacking the plicae of the small intestine. Only large folds (haustrations) are present. Microscopically, the entire thickness of the mucosa is composed of rather straight glands between which are

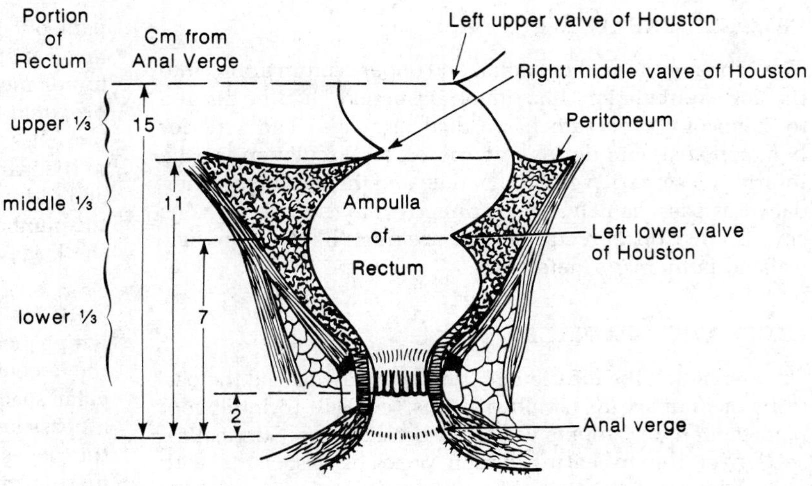

FIG. 29-3. Division of the rectum into upper, middle, and lower thirds. (Goligher JC [ed]: Surgical anatomy. In Surgery of the Anus, Rectum and Colon, 3rd ed. London, Bailliere Tindal, 1975) Diseases of the Colon and Anal Rectum. Philadelphia, WB Saunders, 1959)

the crypts of Lieberkühn. Goblet cells are interspersed with tall columnar cells. Mitoses are present primarily in the base of the crypts, and new cells move up the glands with continuous exfoliation into the bowel lumen.

ARTERIAL SUPPLY TO THE LARGE BOWEL

Although standard surgical treatment of large bowel cancer includes resection of the potentially involved node-bearing mesentery, the extent of mesenteric resection frequently depends on arterial supply (Fig. 29-4).

The cecum and the ascending and transverse colon are nourished by branches from the superior mesenteric artery. The ileocolic artery is quite constant, feeding the distal ileum as well as the proximal colon. When a right colectomy is performed, at least 15 cm of ileum is included to ensure adequate blood supply to the distal small bowel. The right colic artery is quite variable: it may be a branch of the superior mesenteric artery or a subdivision of the ileocolic artery. It is usually diminutive, which precludes a cecectomy and necessitates a full right hemicolectomy, even for early lesions in the cecum. The middle colic artery routinely divides proximally into a left and right branch.

The descending colon, the sigmoid, and the upper rectum are supplied by branches of the inferior mesenteric artery. Approximately 4 cm below the origin of the inferior mesenteric artery is the takeoff of the left colic artery. This ascending branch connects via the marginal artery of Drummond with the left branch of the middle colic artery. If there is significant stenosis of the origin of the superior mesenteric artery, the left colic artery may provide the major blood supply to the transverse and right colon, as well as to the entire small bowel. Pulses in the superior mesenteric artery and middle colic artery should always be felt before dividing the inferior mesenteric or left colic artery to prevent this potentially catastrophic complication. The collateral blood supply to the left colon from the middle colic artery must also be examined whenever the inferior mesenteric artery is ligated, as the marginal arterial arcade may be incomplete.

The upper rectum receives its blood supply from the superior hemorrhoidal artery, the continuation of the inferior mesenteric artery. The diminutive middle hemorrhoidal and the inferior hemorrhoidal arteries are branches of the internal iliac artery. In addition, blood is supplied to the anus and lower rectum via pudendal branches of the internal iliac artery. The blood supply to the distal 5 cm of rectum comprises a rich network of multiple small branches, which allows surgical clearance of all perirectal tissue down to the level of the levator muscles without producing an ischemic rectal remnant.

FIG. 29-4. Anatomical segments and vascular supply to the colon and rectum. (Jones T, Shepard WC: A Manual of Surgical Anatomy. Philadelphia, WB Saunders, 1945)

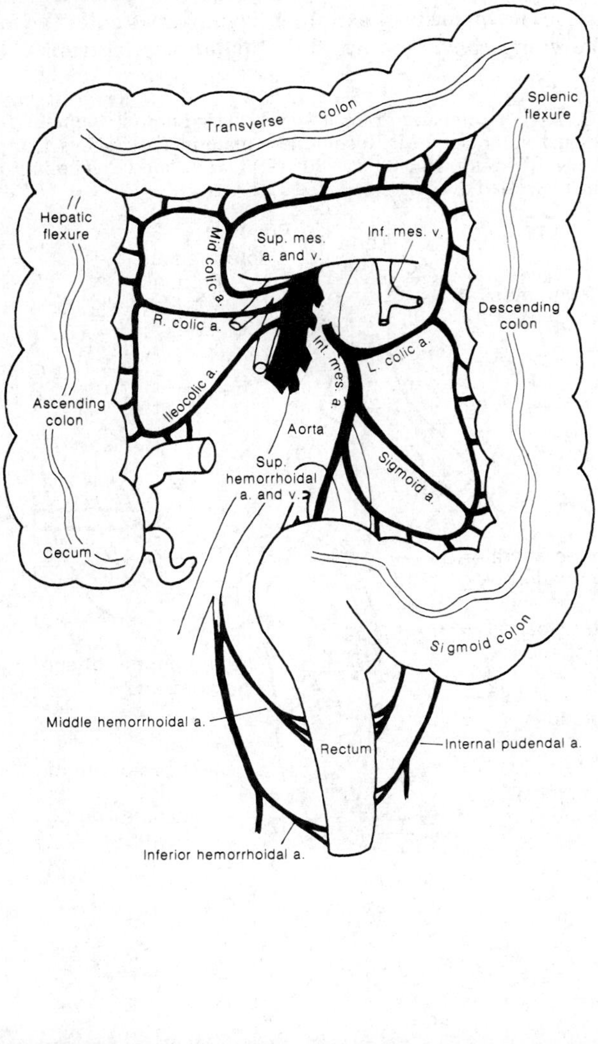

VENOUS DRAINAGE

The venous system of the colon and upper rectum drains into the portal circulation. It is important to note that the distal 5 to 7 cm of the rectum has a dual drainage. The superior hemorrhoidal vein drains into the portal circulation via the inferior mesenteric vein; the middle and inferior hemorrhoidal veins pass via pelvic veins directly into the inferior vena cava. Hence, distal rectal cancers are more likely to produce isolated pulmonary metastases.

LYMPHATIC DRAINAGE

Understanding the location of lymphatic vessels and the patterns of drainage to lymph nodes is requisite to intelligent management of patients with colorectal cancer. Surgical resection of tumor-bearing lymph nodes is associated with cure, albeit in a minority of patients. Hence, surgical lymphadenectomy should be considered a therapeutic procedure as well as a staging procedure.

The intramural lymphatics of the large bowel begin as a plexus beneath the lamina propria, superficial to the muscularis mucosa. This anatomical relationship explains the absence of lymph node metastases associated with in situ tumors. The lymphatics pass into the submucosa, where they follow blood capillaries. Efferent lymphatic vessels proceed radially outward through the circular and longitudinal muscle layers to communicate with an intramuscular and subserosal lymphatic plexus (Fig. 29-5).

Some lymphatics drain into subserosal epicolic lymph nodes. The majority of extramural lymphatics enter the mesentery and converge toward the major arterial trunks. The paracolic groups of lymph nodes along the marginal vascular arcades are the most numerous and are important sites of tumor metastases. The intermediate nodal groups are more proximal, involving the bifurcation of major arterial branches. Central or principal nodes are present contiguous to the inferior mesenteric and superior mesenteric arteries, and ultimately the entire para-aortic chain. Table 29-1 lists the numbers of lymph nodes in surgically cleared specimens; the largest number of nodes are in the paracolic group.[3]

RIGHT COLON. The cecal paracolic area is rich with lymph nodes. The dominant intermediate nodes are along the ileocolic artery. Medial to the ileocolic artery is the avascular space of Treves. Lateral to this space, the lymphatics all pass centrally and proximally, without any connection to the nodes of the small intestine. Anterior to the superior mesenteric vein, a continuous series of nodes follows the ileocolic artery, extending to the superior mesenteric artery. Some lymphatics pass up the superior mesenteric vein, which accounts for the portal lymph node metastases from right colon cancer.

TRANSVERSE COLON. The hepatic flexure and proximal two thirds of the transverse colon drain into the middle colic intermediate lymph nodes. The midcolic lymphatics pass directly into the superior mesenteric nodes. There are occasional connections from the transverse paracolic lymphatics to the omental and splenic hilar nodes.

SPLENIC FLEXURE AND DESCENDING COLON. The lymphatics of the splenic flexure and upper descending

FIG. 29-5. Lymphatic drainage of the large bowel, including the colon wall. (Villemin F, Huard P, Montague M: Recherches Anatomiques Sur les Lymphatiques du Rectum, et De l'Anus. Rev Surg Chir 63:39–80, 1925, and Cole PP: The intramural spread of rectal carcinoma. Br Med J 1:431–433, 1913)

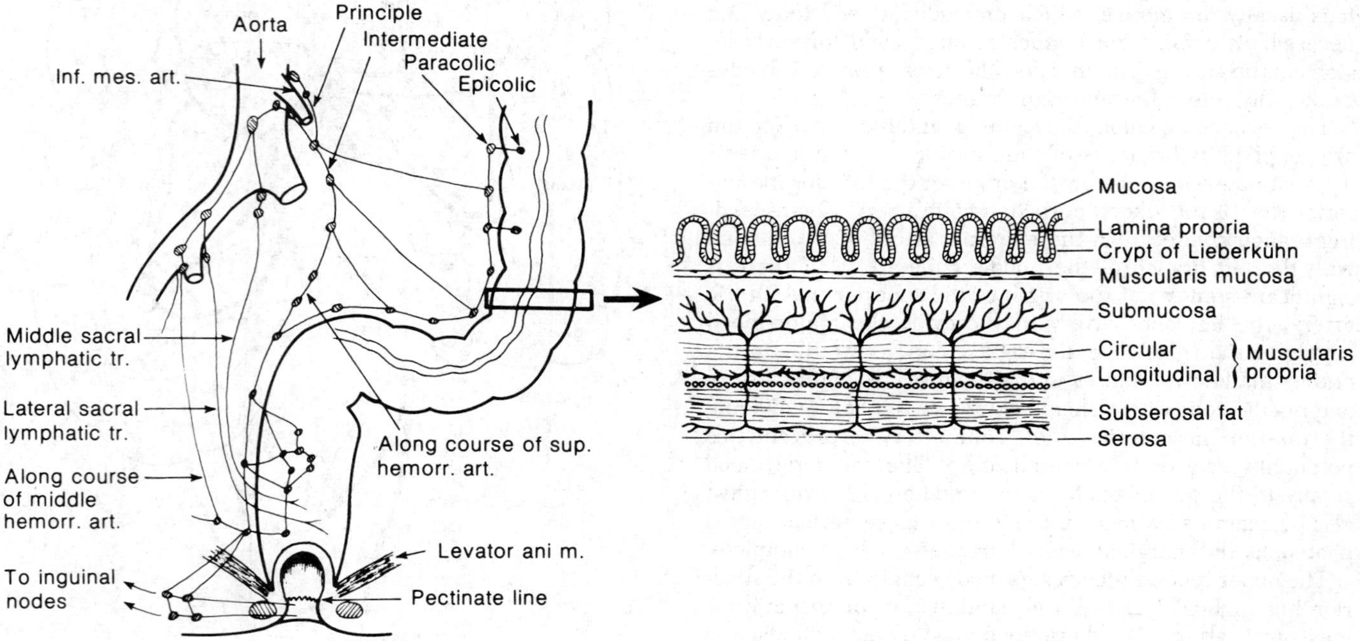

TABLE 29-1. Lymph Nodes in Various Nodal Groups

Regional Lymphatic Chain	*Average No. of Nodes*		
	Paracolic	*Intermediate*	*Central*
Ileocolic	19.0	6.7	3.3
Right colic	7.3	2.3	1.5
Middle colic	16.2	3.7	2.5
Left colic	19.5	4.6	1.3

Data modified from Slanetz CA Jr, Herter FP: The large intestine. In Haagensen CD, Feind CR, Harter FP et al (eds): The Lymphatics in Cancer, pp 489–564. Philadelphia, WB Saunders, 1972.

colon follow the course of the marginal vascular arcade and the left colic artery to reach the inferior mesenteric artery.

SIGMOID AND RECTOSIGMOID. The paracolic nodes in this area are numerous. Some intramural lymphatics bypass these nodes, passing directly to intermediate or central nodes, which explains the occasional finding of a skip metastasis. Approximately 20% of patients have predominantly paracolic and central lymph nodes, with few intermediate nodes. Even in this group, only an average of 4.3 lymph nodes can be obtained from along the inferior mesenteric artery proximal to the origin of the left colic artery.

RECTUM. The major portion of the lymphatic drainage of the rectum passes along the superior hemorrhoidal arterial trunk toward the inferior mesenteric artery. Only a few lymphatics pass along the inferior mesenteric vein. The pararectal nodes above the level of the middle rectal valve drain exclusively along the superior hemorrhoidal lymphatic chain. Below this level (approximately 7–8 cm above the anal verge), some lymphatics pass to the lateral rectal pedicle. These lymphatics are associated with nodes along the middle hemorrhoidal artery, obturator fossa, hypogastric, and common iliac arteries. In addition, extensive lymphatics are present in women contiguous with the rectovaginal septum, and in men along Denonvilliers' fascia.[4,5] The entire extraperitoneal soft tissue (mesorectum) is permeated with lymphatics.

NORMAL PHYSIOLOGY

The function of the large bowel is to absorb water from the small bowel contents and to act as a reservoir for fecal material. The right colon is primarily responsible for the solidification of ileal contents by the absorption of water. The left colon and the rectum are fecal storage sites. Mucus secretion by colonic goblet cells facilitates passage of the more solidified stool.

Two muscular mechanisms are involved in maintaining fecal continence. The internal and external sphincter muscles control the anal canal lumen. The puborectalis sling system elevates the distal rectum when intra-abdominal pressure increases, leading to kinking at the anorectal angle and enhanced continence, despite sneezing or coughing. This is the "flap-valve" theory of continence.[6] The intrarectal balloon proctogram defines the anorectal angle at rest and with straining.[7,8] Anorectal manometry and electromyography can be used to study subtle functional differences.[9]

Sphincter-saving treatment of rectal cancer may result in impaired function. Frequency and urgency occur when the normal rectal reservoir is replaced with the less capacious proximal colon. Poor control of gas and fecal soilage, particularly with coughing, may lead to considerable embarrassment. Besides impairing motor function of the sphincter systems, surgery can cause sensory changes. Normal innervation is sensitive enough to distinguish gas, liquid, and solid feces, resulting in controlled differential release of these substances.

EPIDEMIOLOGY

Worldwide, the incidence rates of colorectal cancer vary widely, from 3.4 cases per 100,000 population in Nigeria to 35.8 cases per 100,000 population in Connecticut.[10] In addition to North America, both Australia and New Zealand, as well as portions of northern and western Europe, have a relatively high incidence of the disease.[11,12] In the United States, the Northeast has had a particularly high mortality from bowel cancer, with a marked clustering of cases in more densely populated areas. These trends are gradually becoming less apparent but still exist.[11] Also, American immigrants from Germany, Ireland, Czechoslovakia, and Greece have a higher incidence of disease than immigrants from other nations.[13,14]

The age-specific incidence of disease in the United States appears to rise steadily from the second to the ninth decade. Men have proportionately more rectal cancer than women, but both sexes are relatively equally represented.[15]

In the United States two religious groups have a diminished risk of large bowel cancer. Seventh-Day Adventists and Mormons have a standardized mortality ratio of 0.52 to 0.81 for bowel cancer at all sites, compared to geographic cohorts of other religions. Both groups refrain from using alcohol and tobacco and practice some form of dietary moderation.[16–19] The reasons for the 20% to 50% risk reduction are not clear; these populations continue to be the subjects of careful scrutiny.

Colorectal cancer is a dynamically changing disease entity.[11] There has been a progressive trend toward disease of the more proximal colon and away from disease of the rectosigmoid bowel.[10,20-22] Less than 60% of cases are currently diagnosable with only rigid proctosigmoidoscopy.

ETIOLOGY

It has long been postulated that colorectal cancer is caused or promoted by environmental factors, and especially by dietary factors that affect the enteric milieu.[23,24] It is suspected that carcinogens are present and identifiable in feces.[25,26] Although it is not possible to identify a specific cause of colon cancer, epidemiologic studies of nutritional habits and migration patterns are revealing. Both national and international studies point to a clear association of colorectal cancer with certain diets (such as those rich in animal fats and meat and poor in fiber) and certain high-risk populations.[11,14,27,28]

Japanese in their native country have a low incidence of colorectal cancer, approximately 6 to 8 cases per 100,000 population.[10] However, first-generation Japanese emigrants to Hawaii have a 2.5-fold greater rate of large bowel cancer, similar to that of caucasians living in Hawaii.[29,30] Exposure to the typical American diet, rich in cholesterol and fat and low in fiber, appears to affect the risk even in first-generation immigrants.[31] Moreover, since 1945, the incidence of colorectal cancer has increased in Japan, perhaps related to a more American-style diet there.[32] Immigrants to Puerto Rico, Europe, Israel, Australia, and Poland assume the risk of these host countries.[33-38] Studies that relate cultural, dietary, and genetic factors with colorectal cancer incidence offer important insights into disease etiology and identify the test populations for intervention efforts. A variety of possibilities are being considered in order to identify the causative factors more precisely. Currently at least six etiologic hypotheses are being tested preclinically, epidemiologically, or with clinical intervention, as described below.

1. FECAPENTAENES. These potent mutagenic compounds, found in human feces and thought to be produced by gut microflora, were active in the Ames *Salmonella* assay[39] and mammalian cell systems.[40] Moreover, there is a correlation between the level of stool fecapentaenes and tumor incidence in select high- and low-risk populations in South Africa.[41] Bruce[42] and Correa et al[43] have suggested a positive association between fecapentaene levels and the incidence of colonic polyps. Intraluminal levels of fecapentaenes can be lowered by fiber, vitamin C, and vitamin E intake.[44,45]

2. 3-KETOSTEROIDS. These are potential tumor promoters or initiators, presumed to be derived from metabolic products of cholesterol. They induce genetic damage in cell cultures and rodent bowel.[46,47] At least two have been identified in human feces, and they may be present in higher concentrations in persons at higher risk for colon cancer.[48-50]

3. PYROLYSIS PRODUCTS. Compounds such as benzo [*a*] pyrene, which result from the broiling or frying of meat at high temperatures, have proved carcinogenic in rodents[51,52] and are suspected of contributing to gastric and esophageal cancers.[24]

4. NORMAL BILE ACIDS. Directly related to the intake of fat, bile acids such as deoxycholic and cholic acid are thought to induce gut lumen proliferation.[53,54] Populations that consume more fat have more bile acid secretion and an associated increased incidence of colonic cancer. Removing the gallbladder results in high levels of bile acids in the cecum, ascending colon, and stool[55,56] and may be associated with a greater frequency of right-sided colon cancer.[57] It is the free, not total, bile acid concentration that is most critical.[58,59]

5. INSUFFICIENT DIETARY CALCIUM. Calcium salts appear to modulate the damage described above by reducing the concentration of free bile acids by forming insoluble bile salt complexes.[58] At least one cohort study found that individuals with colon cancer tend to have a lower intake of calcium.[60]

6. FECAL PH. Alkaline environments support higher concentrations of free bile acids and other potential carcinogens.[61,62] In such an environment, bile acids are more soluble and carcinogens more damaging in animal model systems.[62,63] Epidemiologic studies from South Africa and the United States reveal a higher incidence of colon cancer in subjects with a higher stool *p*H.[60,64,65]

PRIMARY PREVENTION

Despite the inability to precisely identify the factor or factors responsible for colon cancer, a variety of dietary interventions have been considered and are being tested. Painter and Burkitt, observing dietary patterns in different African groups, postulated that those who ingested large volumes of fiber and consequently had high stool bulk had a lower incidence of many types of bowel disease, including colorectal cancer.[66,67] They suggested that high bulk stools promote faster colonic transit time, and thus intraluminal carcinogens have less opportunity to be formed or to interact with the epithelium at risk. However, this explanation is incomplete, since in some normal individuals fiber can slow fecal transit time. In addition to simple dilution, fiber may directly bind carcinogens, may favorably change the fecal *p*H, or may participate in other complex interactions.[68-70] Case–control and population studies in Scandinavia, Israel, and the United States support the contention that increased dietary fiber is of value.[25,71,72] Of the many types of fiber, cellulose and bran fiber may be more effective in reducing carcinogenesis than other fiber types.[73-75]

Limitation of total dietary fat and cholesterol has been proposed.[24] Studies of immigrant populations to Hawaii, populations in Nebraska,[14] and Seventh-Day Adventists[76] confirm that increased fat and cholesterol ingestion can be associated with increased risk of colorectal cancer. The use of *oral calcium* to potentially counteract bile acid effects has been suggested.[77] The use of *antioxidants* is also being evaluated. Vitamin C, tocopherol, and selenium are micronutrients that have many diverse biochemical effects but which also serve to protect gut epithelium from fecapentaene and other carcinogen (oxidative) damage.[78-80] However, simple dietary supplementation with these agents has not proved to be of dramatic benefit.[81,82]

With the identification of a number of phenotypic "intermediate biomarkers" associated with colorectal cancer, clinical prevention trials may generate useful insights without having to wait decades for the end results.[1]

SECONDARY PREVENTION. It is possible, in part, to identify patients at high risk for developing colorectal cancer. So-called secondary prevention strategies in these patients may include removal of precancerous lesions (neoplastic polyps), or excising the entire end-organ at risk. Management of patients with precancerous diseases will be discussed in a later section.

CLINICAL RISK FACTORS FOR COLORECTAL CANCER (TABLE 29-2)

GENETIC

FAMILIAL POLYPOSIS SYNDROMES. Several heritable syndromes are associated with adenomatous polyposis and a high risk of large bowel cancer.[83] The most important of these is the familial adenomatosis syndrome. Numerically, few colon cancer patients have this condition, since its incidence in the United States is between 1:6850 and 1:8300.[84] However, without intervention, virtually all affected individuals will develop colorectal cancer. The disease is inherited as an autosomal dominant trait, with greater than 90% penetrance. Affected persons develop pancolonic adenomatous polyposis. The polyps are not present at birth, but by late adolescence more than 1000 may be visualized. If the polyposis is untreated, the risk of cancer rises progressively with age so that by 40 years, nearly 80% of affected persons will have at least one adenocarcinoma. New mutations may arise in 20% to 30% of these cases of polyposis, and a careful evaluation of family members is necessary.[85-88]

Gardner's syndrome, also inherited as an autosomal dominant trait, occurs with half the frequency of familial adenomatosis syndrome. The entire large and small bowel may be affected by adenoma.[83] Other mesenchymal abnormalities that may coexist include desmoid tumors of the mesentery and abdominal wall, lipomas, sebaceous cysts, osteomas, and fibromas. Because the full clinical spectrum may not be expressed in a given patient, an evaluation of family members is warranted.[89,90] Related to this clinical entity may be the Oldfield syndrome of multiple sebaceous cysts associated with polyposis and adenocarcinoma.[91] It is likely that all of these syndromes are variations of the same genetic defect. Familial adenomatous polyposis is the generic appellation most recently selected to identify these groups. Less common is the Turcot syndrome, probably an autosomal recessive condition, which is associated with malignant central nervous system tumors in addition to bowel polyposis.[92]

Bodmer and co-workers have putatively identified one locus for the familial adenomatous polyposis gene on chromosome 5 near the fq21–22 bands.[93] Such molecular landmarks would permit screening in utero or before the development of signs or symptoms of disease. Moreover, the same researchers have identified a chromosome 5 allele loss in sporadic, noninherited colon cancer. Such molecular probes offer unprecedented opportunities for improved understanding of disease biology, diagnosis, prevention, and therapy.

TABLE 29-2. Clinical Risk Factors for Colorectal Cancer

Genetic
Familial adenomatous polyposis syndrome
Gardner, Oldfield, or Turcot syndrome
Peutz-Jegher syndrome
Familial
Familial colorectal cancer syndrome
Hereditary adenocarcinomatosis syndrome
Family history of colorectal cancer
Preexisting disease
Inflammatory bowel disease
Colorectal cancer
Pelvic cancer post irradiation
Neoplastic colorectal polyps
General
All men and women over age 40

HEREDITABLE SYNDROMES NOT PARTICULARLY ASSOCIATED WITH COLON CANCER. Both the Peutz-Jeghers syndrome and generalized juvenile polyposis are characterized by hamartomatous polyps of the bowel. The patient with Peutz-Jeghers syndrome has multiple tumors, usually clustered more in the small bowel (duodenum) than in the large intestine, and mucocutaneous pigmented lesions.[94] There is a small chance (2%–3%) of malignant degeneration.[95] The juvenile polyposis syndrome also is characterized by multiple hamartomas of the entire bowel. The chance of malignancy is considered to be quite small.[95,96]

FAMILIAL CANCER SYNDROMES. Certain families appear to have a high frequency of colon cancer without adenomatous polyposis of the bowel. A clinical condition described by Lynch and Lynch is inherited as an autosomal dominant trait with greater than 90% penetrance.[97] It has several unusual clinical features, including the development of multiple colon cancers at a relatively early age in several generations. The majority of these cancers are located in the proximal colon. A more generalized condition, also inherited as an autosomal dominant trait, has been described by Lynch et al and Law et al for some families with multiple colonic and extracolonic adenocarcinomas (familial adenocarcinomatosis).[97-99] This syndrome is characterized by the relatively early onset of colon, endometrial, breast, or gastric adenocarcinomas.[98]

For the majority of colorectal cancer patients, those with so-called sporadic disease, there is also evidence of an increased incidence in family members. Macklin has demonstrated that the relatives of individuals with sporadic colon cancer have a twofold to threefold greater chance of developing large bowel cancer than the general population.[100] The clustering of colon and rectal cancer in those with a positive family history but without an excess number of polyps has not been characterized as a specific genetic disorder.[83] Rather, environmental and dietary factors may be of greater importance—or, more likely, the etiology lies in a subtle interplay of heredity and environmental factors.[101] Burt et al analyzed a large family with multiple colon cancer cases but without a precisely definable pattern of inheritance and noted adenomatous polyps in 21% of 191 family members but in only 9% of 132 controls.[102] They proposed that this excess of polyps and colon cancer was the result of an unspecified autosomal dominant gene for susceptibility rather than chance occurrence. This group of patients is also the subject of investigation as to genotypic changes.[103]

INFLAMMATORY BOWEL DISEASE

There is a well-recognized increased risk (up to 30-fold) of colonic cancer in patients with inflammatory bowel disease. For patients with ulcerative colitis the incidence of malignancy increases with the extent of bowel involvement, age at onset, severity, and duration of the disease.[104-107] Patients who have had pancolitis for 30 years have a greater than 35% chance of developing bowel cancer.[108-111] At even greater risk are those in whom severe pancolitis began in childhood. Other atypical aspects of malignancy include multifocal disease (10%–20% of cases) and proximal colon primary sites (40%–50%).[106,112,113]

GRANULOMATOUS COLITIS

Crohn's disease also carries an increased risk of large as well as small bowel cancer.[114] Although granulomatous colitis is not as frequently associated with cancer as is ulcerative colitis, bowel adenocarcinomas with atypical presentations at younger ages are often noted.[113,115,116] Tumors usually arise in affected portions of the bowel, but they may also be metachronous and may occur in sites of prior surgery.[117]

PREVIOUS MALIGNANT DISEASE

Patients who have undergone treatment for a large bowel adenocarcinoma are at greater risk for developing a second colorectal tumor. There is at least a threefold greater likelihood that a second primary bowel cancer will develop either coincident with the index lesion or at a later time.[118-120] The implications for the follow-up of patients after definitive resection are obvious: regular reevaluation is required. Clustering of breast, ovarian, and colon cancer in the same patients has also been demonstrated. The aggregation of multiple adenocarcinomas is similar to the pattern described for familial adenocarcinoma syndrome.[121]

Irradiation of the pelvis also seems to enhance the risk of developing sigmoid cancer. Patients who have undergone radiation therapy for cervical, endometrial, or bladder cancer may be at enhanced risk of developing large bowel cancer, possibly related to irradiation-induced carcinogenesis.[122,123]

PRIOR NONCANCER SURGERY

Patients who have undergone cholecystectomy or ureterosigmoidostomy have a higher incidence of large bowel cancer. It is postulated that the high concentration of inciting or promoting compounds in the secretions accounts for the increased risk of neoplasia.[124-126]

POLYPS

Neoplastic and inflammatory polyps occur in the large bowel. Adenomatous polyps may be tubular or villous. The tubular adenomas are four times more common than the villous adenomas and are usually smaller. In general, large polyps are more likely to contain a malignant focus than the smaller ones; nearly half of polyps larger than 2 cm in diameter will contain malignancy.

Approximately 25% of patients with one tubular polyp will have others. Tubular adenomas are relatively more evenly distributed throughout the large bowel, while villous tumors are more frequently found in the rectum.[127] Villous adenomas are reported to have eight to ten times the probability of cancer than tubular polyps.[127-130]

Predictably, the larger the number of these adenomas, the greater the chance that cancer will develop.[131] Although it is not necessary to have a polyp prior to or coincident with a cancer, this sequence occurs five times more frequently than cancer alone.[10]

GENERAL POPULATION

By far the largest population at risk for colorectal cancer are men and women over the age of 40. Although colorectal cancer is sometimes found in children, the incidence of disease increases steadily up to the eighth decade.[132,133]

DIAGNOSIS

Colorectal cancer may be diagnosed when a patient presents with symptoms or as the result of a screening program. Except for patients with obstructing or perforating cancers, the duration of symptoms does not correlate with prognosis.[134-136] However, since early colorectal cancer produces no symptoms, and since many of the symptoms of colorectal cancer are nonspecific, aggressive efforts at detection through screening programs are essential.

We cannot adequately stress the vagueness of abdominal symptoms in colorectal cancer. Twelve percent of otherwise healthy patients without colorectal cancer complain of a change in bowel habits in the recent past, and 11% report abdominal pain.[137] Even rectal bleeding has a very low predictive value in the diagnosis of colorectal cancer.[138] Screening strategies will be discussed in subsequent sections.

EVALUATION OF THE SYMPTOMATIC PATIENT

COLON CANCER. Symptoms of colon cancer—intermittent abdominal pain, nausea, or vomiting—are secondary to bleeding, obstruction, or perforation. A palpable mass is common with right colon cancer. Bleeding may be acute and most commonly appears as red blood mixed with stool. Dark blood is most commonly secondary to diverticular bleeding. Occasionally, melena may be associated with a right colon cancer. Chronic blood loss with iron deficiency anemia can occur. Such patients may present with weakness and high output congestive heart failure. Lesser degrees of bleeding may be detected as part of a fecal occult blood test (discussed below under screening). Rectal bleeding associated with warfarin use should be investigated to rule out a colon cancer.

Malignant obstruction of the large bowel is most commonly associated with cancer of the sigmoid. If the ileocecal valve is competent, such obstructions manifest as acute abdominal illness. If the ileocecal valve is incompetent, the illness is more insidious, with increasing constipation and abdominal distention noted over many days. The major differential diagnosis in such cases includes cancer and diverticulitis. A limited barium enema examination may yield only suggestive data, and even fiberoptic endoscopy may not be diagnostic if associated edema precludes reaching the cancer with the endoscope. Cytology of a brush biopsy specimen obtained through the fiberoptic endoscope may be diagnostic.

TABLE 29-3. Qualitative Analysis of Screening Options for Colorectal Cancer

Technique	*Sensitivity for Cancer*	*Sensitivity for Polyps*	*Cost*	*Patient Discomfort*
Digital rectal examination	+	½+	½+	+
Fecal occult blood	++	+	½+	½+
Rigid sigmoidoscopy	++	++	++	++
Flexible sigmoidoscopy (60–65 cm)	+++	+++	++	+
Single column barium enema	++	+	++	++
Air contrast barium enema	+++	+++	++	+++
Colonoscopy	++++	++++	++++	+++

The perforation of colon cancer may be acute or chronic. The clinical picture of acute perforation may be identical to that of appendicitis or diverticulitis, with pain, fever, and a palpable mass. In the presence of obstruction, there may be a perforation either through the tumor or through proximal nontumorous colon (cecum). The distinction is important from a prognostic viewpoint. Chronic perforation with fistula formation into the bladder from sigmoid colon cancer is similar to diverticulitis. Gross pneumaturia may occur, or the patient may present only with recurrent urinary tract infections. The continued presence of multiple enteric organisms despite repeated treatment mandates diagnostic studies. Bladder cytologies, cystoscopy, brushings, and biopsies may not lead to the correct diagnosis. Fiberoptic endoscopy of the colon is the most valuable diagnostic procedure.

RECTAL CANCER. Rectal and rectosigmoid cancer is much more likely to be symptomatic prior to diagnosis. Gross red blood (mixed or covering stool, or by itself) is frequent. Hemorrhoidal bleeding should always be a diagnosis of exclusion. All patients with rectal bleeding should be evaluated. If the blood is minimal and bright red in appearance, is located only on the toilet paper, and is associated with normal-colored stool, a sigmoidoscopy (preferably fiberoptic sigmoidoscopy with a 60- to 65-cm instrument) may suffice. All other patients should undergo sigmoidoscopy and barium enema examination, or colonoscopy. Since a rectal cancer may be missed on barium enema examination, proctosigmoidoscopy complements the radiologic study.

With compromise of the rectal reservoir by tumor, a change in bowel activity may occur. Unexplained constipation or reduction in stool caliber should lead to evaluation. Obstructing rectal cancers frequently cause diarrhea rather than constipation. Rigid sigmoidoscopy and barium enema examination or colonoscopy are the appropriate studies.

In cases of locally advanced rectal cancer with circumferential growth and extensive transmural penetration, urgency and inadequate emptying lead to tenesmus. This is usually a grave sign. Some degree of tenesmus may occur with less extensive distal rectal cancer as part of the normal rectal reflex. Urinary symptoms may occur with compression of the bladder, invasion of the prostate, or destruction of the high sacral nerve roots. Buttock or perineal pain from posterior extension also is a grave sign.

METASTATIC DISEASE. Synchronous liver metastases occur in 5% to 10% of patients and occasionally are the presenting manifestation of colorectal cancer. The patient may complain of pain in the right upper quadrant, right hypochondrium, right posterior chest, or right shoulder. The pain may be a continuous ache, or it may be experienced as an acute episode related to hemorrhage or necrosis of a metastasis. Hepatomegaly may be detected on routine physical examination of an otherwise asymptomatic patient. It is important to evaluate the gastrointestinal (GI) tract in such patients, even if the fecal occult blood test is negative, before proceeding with a premature liver biopsy.

SCREENING

The early detection of colorectal cancer is potentially associated with a dramatic reduction in disease-related mortality. The relatively slow growth of most colorectal cancers and the high diagnostic sensitivity of colonoscopy and air contrast barium enema examination justify aggressive screening strategies. In addition, some screening approaches may detect not only early cancers, but benign neoplastic polyps as well. Endoscopic removal of such polyps may, to some extent, prevent subsequent colorectal cancer. Screening strategies must take into account the risk of the population being screened, the segments of the large bowel at greatest risk, the cost-effectiveness of screening, the availability of various technologies, and patient compliance.[139]

A qualitative assessment of the various screening options is outlined in Table 29-3. The reader should keep in mind that there has been a proximal shift in the location of many colorectal cancers, leading to a considerable increase in right colon cancers, particularly in women.[140-142] Predictive values for the various screening methods have not been included in Table 29-3, since they are prevalence dependent. For example, the predictive value of a positive fecal occult blood test in an otherwise healthy 40-year-old person will be much lower than in a 65-year-old person with a strong family history of colorectal cancer. The incidence of colorectal cancer in the 65-year-old population is 10 times as great as in the 40-year-old population.

HIGH-RISK FACTORS

FAMILY HISTORY. In persons with a family history of colorectal cancer, screening should begin at age 35 to 40 years with a yearly fecal occult blood test and probably some type of endoscopic surveillance.[143] Flexible sigmoidoscopy (with the 60- to 65-cm instrument) every 3 to 5 years should be considered, with full colonoscopy if an adenomatous polyp is identified.[144] Autosomal dominant cancer families require frequent invasive screening with colonoscopy or sigmoidoscopy combined with air contrast barium enema examinations every 3 to 5 years beginning at age 40.[139]

FAMILIAL ADENOMATOUS POLYPOSIS. Once the diagnosis of familial adenomatous polyposis is made, many patients will undergo either a total colectomy with ileorectal anastomosis, or total proctocolectomy with ileostomy or ileal pouch–anal anastomosis. Those with retained rectum should undergo rigid proctoscopy with fulguration of polyps every 6 months for the rest of their lives.

PERSONAL HISTORY OF CANCER OR POLYP. Endoscopic surveillance of the entire remaining bowel is appropriate every 1 to 3 years.[145] An air contrast barium enema examination combined with limited endoscopy is also reasonable. The National Polyp Study is prospectively gathering data on the frequency and type of follow-up appropriate for these patients.[146] Preliminary data indicate that patients with multiple polyps, particularly villous lesions, are at a greater risk for subsequent polyp formation.

ULCERATIVE COLITIS. Patients with a history of extensive ulcerative colitis (except patients with isolated ulcerative proctitis) present for at least 10 years and not treated by proctocolectomy, require colonoscopic surveillance every 1 to 2 years. Any worrisome area is biopsied, and multiple blind biopsies of "normal" mucosa are performed to detect dysplasia.[147,148] A recent review questions the efficacy of endoscopic screening in this population.[149]

SCREENING STRATEGIES FOR THE GENERAL POPULATION

DIGITAL RECTAL EXAMINATION. The digital rectal examination is a traditional part of the annual physical examination. In addition to low rectal cancers, anal and prostatic cancers may also be detected; and a stool specimen is obtained for occult blood determination. The sensitivity of the digital rectal examination has decreased with the more proximal shift in the location of colorectal cancer. Although it is difficult to demonstrate a reduction in cancer mortality from periodic rectal digital examinations, the procedure should remain part of any regular physical examination.[150]

RIGID SIGMOIDOSCOPY. Rigid sigmoidoscopy is comparatively inexpensive, but its usefulness is restricted by the length of bowel that can be examined and by patients' unwillingness to undergo the procedure. In a series of 26,000 patients over the age of 45 studied at the Strang Clinic, asymptomatic cancer was detected in 58 patients.[151] The cure rate in these patients was 90%. Gilbertsen et al studied 18,000 patients with serial sigmoidoscopies and polypectomies.[152] Although the variable length of follow-up makes accurate analysis difficult, their data indicate a substantial reduction in the incidence of subsequent rectal cancer in patients from whom premalignant polyps were removed.

FLEXIBLE SIGMOIDOSCOPY. Flexible proctosigmoidoscopes are available in 25 to 35 cm lengths and 60 to 65 cm lengths. The light source is provided by fiberoptic technology. Viewing may use fiberoptics or direct videoendoscopic technology. The shorter scopes are relatively easy to learn to use, more comfortable for the patient, and more applicable for screening programs using nonphysician personnel.[153,154] The longer flexible sigmoidoscopes reach on the average 45 cm proximal to the anus (the junction of the descending colon and sigmoid) and allow detection of approximately two thirds of colorectal cancers and polyps.[144,154-160] Any patient found to have a neoplastic polyp on screening endoscopy should be considered at high risk and should undergo complete examination of the remaining colon and more intense surveillance.

BARIUM ENEMA AND COLONOSCOPY. Because most studies compare these two procedures, a joint discussion follows. The standard barium enema examination is unsatisfactory for the detection of early cancers or polyps, missing one third of early cancers in a study by Gilbertsen et al.[152] Colonoscopy is the most accurate way of diagnosing early colorectal cancers and allows resection of premalignant polyps at the same time. However, the air contrast barium enema examination may be almost as accurate, except for diminutive polyps, and has the advantage of routine visualization of the ascending colon, not possible in 5% to 10% of colonoscopies.[161-164] Endoscopy is not completely accurate: polyps may not be visualized because of blind corners and mucosal folds, and the cecum may not be reached in every case.[165] The prospective data from the National Polyp Study will more clearly define the efficacy of these two modalities.

TABLE 29-4. Screening Programs for Colorectal Cancer Using Fecal Occult Blood Tests

Study	*No. of Patients*	*Compliance*	*Positive Tests (%)*	*No. of Cancers Detected*	*Predictive Value (%)*
Gilbertsen et al[152]	23,000	72	2.3	54	11.3
Winawer et al[177]	13,127	74	2.5	59	17.7
Winchester et al[184]	54,101	26	4.4	29	4.7
Sontag et al[185]	13,522	22	4.6	14	10.3
Cummings et al[178]	58,934	20	2.3	17	6.4
Hardcastle et al[176]	10,253	39	2.4	17	13.7

EXFOLIATIVE CYTOLOGY. Lavage-induced exfoliative cytology and brush biopsies can be used as an adjunct to endoscopic examination. Lavage cytology does not appear to improve the diagnostic yield, although brush techniques may be helpful.[166]

FECAL CARCINOEMBRYONIC ANTIGEN. This approach is at the earliest stages of investigation.[167] The concept of detecting shed tumor antigens in the feces needs to be explored in additional studies.

FECAL OCCULT BLOOD TESTING. Guaiac-impregnated paper slide tests for fecal occult blood have been available for 20 years. The relatively low cost and the potential for patient testing at home have generated considerable interest in this approach. All guaiac tests measure hemoglobin indirectly by the determination of its peroxidase activity. Two other approaches are being studied. The HemoQuant test, a quantitative assay for fecal hemoglobin, is based on the conversion of heme to fluorescent porphyrins.[168,169] The test is more costly and requires more complicated testing support. Data are not yet available comparing this test with existing guaiac-based systems in a large screening program. An immunochemical approach to the detection of human fecal hemoglobin is possible, which would obviate false positive test results associated with dietary hemoglobin and ingestion of peroxidase-containing foods.[170,171]

In considering the overall impact of fecal occult blood screening programs, a number of features must be stressed. False positive tests are extremely expensive and at best inconvenient for the patient. Patients with positive test results undergo extensive diagnostic testing, which may include sigmoidoscopy, barium enema, colonoscopy, and upper GI endoscopy.[172] Patients with false negative results may be inappropriately reassured, and may disregard subsequent symptoms.

All guaiac-based fecal occult blood tests are unreliable to some degree. Ahlquist and Beart[173] reported positive Hemoccult test results with as little as 0.04 mg hemoglobin per gram of stool (normal, $<$2 mg/g) and negative results with as much as 42.5 mg/g. Fecal occult blood testing as a screening technique assumes that colorectal cancers (many of which are ulcerated) are associated with detectable intraluminal blood loss. However, some colorectal cancers bleed intermittently, and others not at all. In several studies of patients with known colorectal cancer, 20% to 30% of patients had negative fecal occult blood tests.[174-176] Less than one third of patients with polyps have stools positive for occult blood.[176]

Several factors affect the accuracy of fecal occult blood tests.[169,178,179] The initial studies by Greegor suggested that dietary restriction was important in order to minimize peroxidase from red meat, fresh fruit, and raw vegetables. Macrae and associates did not find this to be very important, as long as the slides were not dehydrated.[180] This issue has yet to be completely resolved. The number of stool specimens tested will influence the reliability of the technique.[181] Separate specimens taken on three consecutive days is the usual recommendation. Slide hydration before testing reactivates the fecal peroxidase activity. Although this maneuver decreases the false negative rate, it dramatically increases the false positive rate.[177] Certain medications, including iron, cimetidine, antacids, and particularly large amounts of ascorbic acid, may interfere with the peroxidase reaction, leading to an increased false negative rate.[182]

Evaluation of the Positive Fecal Occult Blood Test. Because the predictive value of a positive test is less than 20%, the few dollars spent for the fecal occult blood test leads to a great expenditure of funds to identify patients with true positive results.[172] Although a complete colonoscopy is probably the most direct way to exclude cancer and polyps, an air contrast barium enema examination may be the most cost-effective approach to the evaluation of the patient with a positive test result.[183] Rigid or flexible sigmoidoscopy should complement the barium study.

Screening Programs. Data from selected large series are presented in Table 29-4.[152,176-178,184,185] Approximately 2.5% of tested patients are Hemoccult (or Hemoccult II) positive, with compliance rates ranging from 20% to 97%.

Three large-scale prospective population-based programs are attempting to demonstrate a reduction in colorectal cancer mortality with fecal occult blood test-screening, and to define compliance and cost issues associated with this test. These studies are taking place at the University of Minnesota; New York; Nottingham, England; and Goteborg, Sweden.[176,184]

SCREENING RECOMMENDATIONS FOR THE GENERAL POPULATION. We recommend yearly fecal occult blood tests and sigmoidoscopy every 3 to 5 years beginning at age 40. We would encourage the greater use of flexible sigmoidoscopy as part of a screening strategy.

PATHOLOGY

GROSS APPEARANCE

Tumor configuration may be divided into fungating (exophytic), ulcerating, stenosing, or constricting (annular, circumferential). Approximately two thirds of all tumors are ulcerating and one third are fungating.[186] These configurations do not represent different kinds of tumors but different phases of an orderly progression. Most malignant bowel tumors start out as a small polypoid lesions. These lesions may grow into the lumen, or into the bowel wall itself. As they grow laterally or circumferentially, they are termed *infiltrating.* Right-sided cancers, usually fungating in nature, tend to grow more into the lumen and extend along one wall, especially in the capacious cecum. Left-sided cancers tend to grow more into the bowel wall and circumferentially, having a typical "napkin ring" configuration on barium enema examination. These cancers are thought to start as sessile masses that gradually span the circumference over a 1- to 2-year period. Growth along circumferential lymphatics may account for much of this behavior. As tumors grow into the bowel, they eventually interfere with the blood supply, occasionally leading to necrosis, ulceration, and perforation.[187,188]

HISTOLOGIC TYPES

The major histologic type of large bowel cancer is adenocarcinoma, which accounts for 90% to 95% of all large bowel tumors.[189,190] It is the only histologic type further classified by grade. Adenocarcinoma consists of columnar or cuboidal epithelium with varying degrees of loss of the normal differentiation pattern.

A number of histologic types of large bowel cancer have been identified. The World Health Organization (WHO) has developed a classification of both benign and malignant tumors.[191] The classification of malignant tumors is given in Table 29-5. Descriptions of most of these pathologic types may be found in the Armed Forces Institute of Pathology Series[192]; illustrations of each may be found in that series and in the WHO series.[191]

Mucinous or "colloid" adenocarcinoma represents approximately 10% of large bowel tumors.[193] These adenocarcinomas are defined by large amounts of *extracellular* mucin retained within the tumor. A separate WHO classification is the rare (4% of mucinous carcinomas) *signet-ring cell* carcinoma, which contains intracellular mucin, which pushes the nucleus to one side. Some signet-ring tumors appear to form a linitis plastica type of tumor by spreading intramurally, usually not involving the mucosa.[194] Other rare variants of epithelial tumors include squamous cell carcinomas, of which about 40 cases have been reported in the literature.[195] Another rare variant is the adenosquamous carcinoma, sometimes called adenoacanthoma. This tumor has elements of both adenocarcinoma and squamous carcinoma and usually manifests as an ulcerated tumor. About 50 cases have been reported in the literature.[190]

Finally, there are the undifferentiated carcinomas, which contain no glandular structures or other features such as mucus secretions. Other designations for undifferentiated carcinoma include carcinoma simplex, medullary carcinoma, and trabecular carcinoma. Gibbs has emphasized that undifferentiated carcinomas are not necessarily anaplastic.[196] He describes undifferentiated carcinoma as a malignant epithelial neoplasm that does not differentiate into formed tubules, but exhibits little nuclear pleomorphism and few bizarre mitoses.

TABLE 29-5. World Health Organization Classification of Malignant Primary Tumors of the Large Intestine

Epithelial tumors
Adenocarcinoma
Mucinous adenocarcinoma
Signet-ring cell adenocarcinoma
Squamous cell carcinoma
Adenosquamous carcinoma
Undifferentiated carcinoma
Unclassified carcinoma
Carcinoid tumors
Argentaffin
Nonargentaffin
Composite
Nonepithelial tumors
Leiomyosarcoma
Others
Hematopoietic and lymphoid neoplasms
Unclassified

About 4% to 17% of carcinoids may appear in the rectum, and 2% to 7% may appear in the colon.[197-199] These small, firm, polypoid nodules are covered by an intact mucosa and rarely produce the carcinoid syndrome. The nonepithelial tumors include a variety of sarcomas, all rare; leiomyosarcomas appear to predominate. In one report of intestinal leiomyosarcoma, 4 of 41 cases were in the rectum and none were in the colon.[199] Primary malignant lymphomas that occur in the colon and rectum are usually of a diffuse histiocytic (large cell) type.[190]

DEGREE OF DIFFERENTIATION

Broders was a pioneer in classifying the adenocarcinomas by their degree of differentiation.[200] He designated four grades, based on the percentage of differentiated tumor cells. "Well differentiated" in Broders' system meant well-formed glands, resembling an adenoma. Broders included the mucinous carcinomas in his system. Dukes considered mucinous carcinomas separately.[201] Because of their poor prognosis, others group them with the most undifferentiated tumors.

Dukes' grading system considered the arrangement of cells rather than the percentage of differentiated cells. Dukes' initial approach evolved into a three-grade system, now most widely used. Grade 1 is the most differentiated, with well-formed tubules and the least nuclear polymorphism and fewest mitoses. Grade 3 is the least differentiated, having only occasional glandular structures, pleomorphic cells, and a high incidence of mitoses. Grade 2 is intermediate between Grades 1 and 3.[189,202]

Jass and colleagues use seven parameters in their grading criteria: histologic type, overall differentiation, nuclear polarity, tubule configuration, pattern of growth, lymphocytic infiltration, and amount of fibrosis.[203] It is clear that not everybody agrees on the grading criteria, but most agree on the use of a three-grade system, similar to that described in this section.

SPREAD OF COLORECTAL CANCER

Much of what we know about the local and distant spread of colorectal cancer is due to the meticulous and elegant studies of Cuthbert Dukes, a pathologist at St. Mark's Hospital in London, who did extensive studies on the local invasion of rectal cancer and on lymphatic involvement by this disease. In 1930, Dukes and his colleague Gordon-Watson described the spread of rectal cancer,[187] which Dukes amplified in later papers.[188,201,204]

LOCAL INVASION. After the initial mucosal growth, there are several directions in which a tumor may progress, but usually it protrudes first into the lumen. Dukes found that subsequent lateral invasion was greater in the transverse rather than the longitudinal direction, leading to circumferential growth.[201,205] Black and Waugh found that the same growth pattern occurred in colon cancer.[206]

In addition to intramural and circumferential spread, the growth of rectal cancer proceeds cephalad and caudad (longitudinally). Dukes described the growth as more extensive in the submucosa.[201] However, Miles in 1920 concluded that submucosal intramural spread was comparatively trivial.[207] In a 1966 study of curative resections, Grinnell found no retrograde submucosal spread in 67 of 76 cases.[208]

As the tumor traverses the muscularis mucosa and infiltrates the submucosa, it is termed *invasive*. As it reaches the muscle and blood supply becomes inadequate, ulceration may occur. As the tumor penetrates the rectal wall and extrarectal tissues, it directly invades neighboring structures.[204] Dukes and Bussey defined various degrees of local spread: slight local spread denotes invasion only of the extrarectal tissues; moderate spread refers to tumor well established in the mesentery; and extensive spread refers to deeply invasive carcinoma, possibly extending into neighboring organs.[204] They also found that the extent of spread increases with the grade of the tumor.

One of the more interesting ways of looking at histologic sections is with whole mounts of the cross-section of the bowel.[209,210] This histologic procedure allows one to define the invasion profile of lateral transmural penetration. This has not been used extensively yet, but it may prove to be of great use in future studies.

An additional pattern of local spread is perineural invasion, or spread along the perineural spaces, which may reach as far as 10 cm from the primary tumor.[211] Perineural invasion increases with the degree of local extension. In one study, no patient with Dukes' A tumors had perineural invasion, whereas 24% of those with Dukes' B and 69% with Dukes' C tumors did have perineural invasion, as did 23% of patients with Broders Grade 2 lesions and 58% with Grade 3 lesions.[212] Too few patients had Broders Grade 1 or 4 lesions to evaluate.

LYMPHATIC EXTENSION. In 1930 Dukes concluded, incorrectly, that lymph node metastases occurred only after local tumor spread into the perirectal tissues.[187] The exceptions were generally high-grade tumors. More recent studies have demonstrated a 10% to 20% incidence of nodal metastases from rectal cancer limited to the bowel wall.[213-225]

In 1935 Gabriel et al described the orderly and predictable course of spread of lymphatic disease in rectal cancer.[226] First, disease metastasizes to the perirectal nodes at the level of the primary tumor or immediately above it. Then the chain accompanying the superior hemorrhoidal vessels is involved. Very rarely are there discontinuous or skip metastases.[226-229] The pericolic lymph nodes along the mesenteric border of the pelvis usually are not involved by these rectal tumors unless there is extensive tumor with lymphatic blockage. Gabriel et al pointed out that in late stages of the disease, when the hemorrhoidal lymphatics are blocked, there is lateral or downward spread.[226] Grinnell also noted such retrograde flow in 34 (3.7%) of 913 cases of colon and rectum tumors.[230]

In colon carcinoma, the normal lymphatic flow is through the lymphatic channels along the major arteries, with three echelons of lymph nodes: pericolic, intermediate, and principal lymph nodes. If tumors lie between two major vascular pedicles, lymphatic flow may drain in either or both directions, as shown in Figure 29-6. If the central lymph nodes

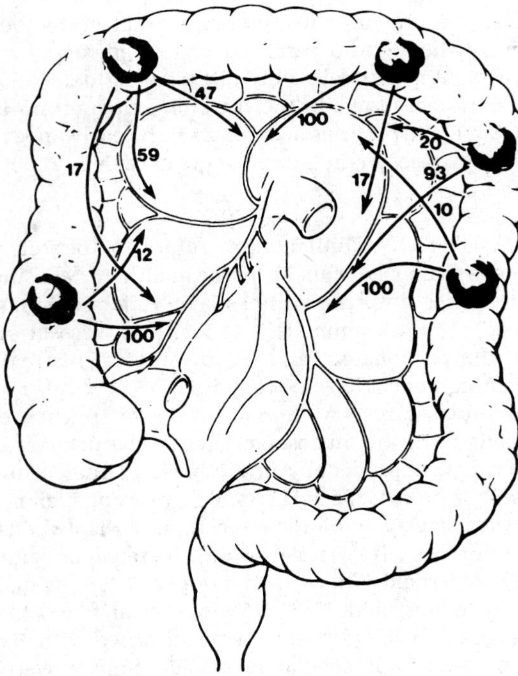

FIG. 29-6. For tumors that lie between two pedicles, lymphatic flow may drain in either or both directions. From a study of cleared specimens, it was possible to determine the preferential route by the location of lymphatic metastases. The numbers above signify the percentage of metastasizing carcinomas in the above locations that have demonstrated positive nodes along a given vascular route. For example, tumors lying between the ileocolic and right colic arcades metastasize along the ileocolic pedicle in 100% and along the right colin in 12%. (Hertzer FP, Slanetz CA: Patterns and significance of lymphatic spread from cancer of the colon and rectum. In Weiss L, Gilbert HA, Ballon SC (eds): Lymphatic System Metastasis. Boston, GK Hall, 1980)

are blocked by tumor, lymphatic flow can become retrograde along the marginal arcades, both proximally and distally.[231]

The risk of lymph node metastases increases with increasing tumor grade.[204] Dukes found that 30% of low-grade tumors were associated with positive lymph nodes, compared to 81% of high-grade tumors. The number of lymph nodes involved also increased with grade: an average of 3.2 nodes were involved for low-grade tumors and 6.8 for high-grade tumors.

HEMATOGENOUS SPREAD. The liver is the primary site of hematogenous metastases, followed by the lung. In approximately 40% of autopsy studies the liver is the only site involved.[232-234] Involvement of other sites in the absence of liver or lung involvement is rare.

The major venous drainage of the lower rectum is by a dual system: drainage from the superior hemorrhoidal veins enters the portal system to the liver, drainage from the middle and inferior hemorrhoidal veins eventually reaches the vena cava to get to the lungs. Bone metastases in the sacrum and the vertebral bodies may occur through the vertebral venous plexus, as originally described by Batson.[235] In 1977 Vider et al proposed that this system represented another mechanism of metastatic spread.[236] The portal mesenteric and caval systems offer low-pressure drainage to the liver and lungs, whereas the vertebral venous plexus is a high-pressure system that may only open during defecation, allowing metastases to go to the skeleton and central nervous system. Such a hypothesis accords with the early appearance of bone metastases in the sacrum, coccyx, pelvis, and lumbar vertebrae.

IMPLANTATION. Implantation refers to the release of tumor cells from the primary tumor and their deposition on another surface. Implantation has been reported with tumor cells shed (1) intraluminally, (2) from the serosal surface through the peritoneum, and (3) by surgical manipulation and resulting deposition on wound surfaces.[237]

Intraluminal spread of tumor occurs by release of the tumor cells from the mucosal surface of the primary tumor and their deposition distally in the bowel, either in fistulas, abscesses, or hemorrhoids. The mechanism of such implantation is considered to be the deposition of viable cells onto the raw surface of a fistula or an ulcerated or surgically treated hemorrhoid. There are a number of reports of tumor growth in hemorrhoids.[238-240] McGrew et al found that the percentage of positive cytologic smears varied with distance from the tumor in 50 specimens studied. Smears were positive in 42% at the proximal ends of resected specimens (average length, 21 cm) and in 65% at the distal ends (average length, 10 cm).[241]

Transcoelomic spread accounts for intraperitoneal seeding and carcinomatosis seen, even in the absence of nodal or hematogenous spread.

Other forms of implantation may be related to surgery. The incidence of disease recurrence at suture lines is about 10%.[242,243] At least half of these recurrences might be explained by implantation of cells from the stump.[242]

Tumor can also be implanted into the abdominal surgical scar,[244-246] into the perineal scar after an abdominoperineal resection,[247-249] or even into the mucocutaneous margin of a colostomy.[242,250] Pomeranz and Garlock performed studies to ascertain how easily cells might be dislodged from the serosal surface during surgery.[246] They looked at cells obtained by gently rubbing the serosal surface with a slide or cotton tip. Tumor cells were found in 2 of 20 cases. Boreham tried such studies in 52 patients and could not easily dislodge cells from the serosa.[245] However, in 4 of 16 samples, sections through areas of serosal puckering or ulceration opposite the growth revealed malignant cells on the peritoneal surface.

A concern is that surgical manipulation could also release cells into the venous circulation. Cole et al found malignant cells in the veins when isotonic saline was perfused from the artery to the vein when the vein and artery had been tied off before any colonic manipulation.[243] Fisher and Turnbull found tumor cells in the mesenteric veins in 32% of 25 consecutive bowel resections.[251]

STAGING AND PROGNOSTIC FEATURES

The staging of colorectal carcinoma has been complicated by the fact that it has evolved over half a century, and various authors have developed systems that use the same descriptors to represent different stages. Even one common and simple staging system, the Dukes classification for cancer of the rectum, has been misinterpreted by various authors.[252] This is perhaps not surprising, since the definitions changed even in Dukes' personal series of publications.[187,201] Because of these discrepancies in coding for the same stages, comparison of clinical studies reported in the literature is often impossible.

The ultimate value of any staging system lies not only in treatment planning but in comparing results of different studies and predicting recurrence patterns and survival.[253] Many pathologic features of colorectal carcinoma influence predictions of recurrence and survival. Independent pathologic variables include the depth of penetration through the bowel wall, whether lymph nodes are involved, and the number of involved lymph nodes. Nonindependent features that have been incorporated into a few staging systems include extent of local invasion,[214,254] level of lymph node involvement,[226] blood vessel invasion, lymphatic invasion, histologic grade,[255] and carcinoembryonic antigen (CEA) level.[256,257]

SURGICAL–PATHOLOGIC STAGING

This section describes various pathologic staging systems. Operative findings of liver metastases, peritoneal seeding, and adherence to or invasion of contiguous organs must be combined with the histologic findings.

Dukes' Classification and Its Modifications

The first practical staging system was Dukes' classification,[201] which classified rectal tumors from A to C, with stage A indicating penetration into but not through the bowel wall, stage B representing penetration through the bowel wall, and stage C representing involvement of lymph nodes, regardless of the extent of bowel wall penetration. This system, developed from an earlier clinical grouping by Lockhart-Mummery,[258] had the virtue of being simple and predictive of prognosis. However, it has since been modified by many authors, including Dukes,[226] to reflect finer levels of penetration and nodal metastases, and has been extended to include the colon as well as the rectum.

The most important of the staging systems that utilize the A, B, C terminology are shown in Figure 29-7. Kirklin and colleagues split Dukes' stage A into a new A (mucosa only) and B1 (into but not through the muscularis propria), and changed Dukes' stage B to B2.[259] The Astler–Coller staging system[213] allowed separation of wall penetration and nodal status.

A recent analysis of clinical trials in the National Surgical Adjuvant Breast and Bowel Project (NSABP) compared the prognostic abilities of various modifications of the original Dukes classification.[260] In Dukes' stage C the level of positive node involvement, defined as either less than 2 cm or 2 cm or more beyond the bowel wall, was not very predictive of ultimate survival. Researchers analyzing the clinical trial results found that depth of penetration and the number of positive nodes were significant predictors of survival, and the number of positive nodes was the strongest factor in this

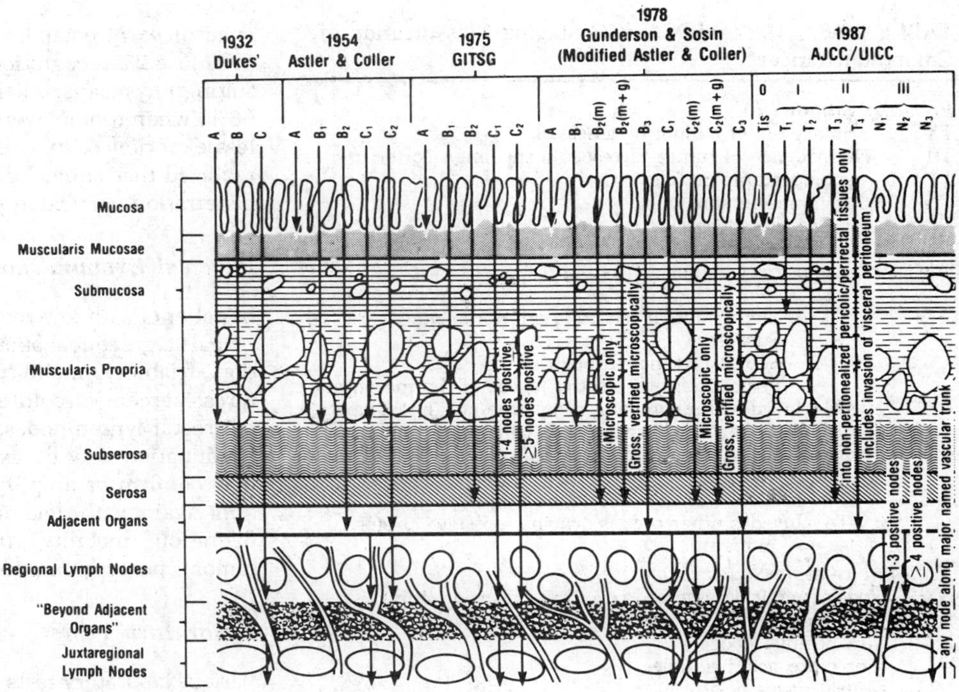

FIG. 29-7. Schematic comparison of the various pathological staging systems.

analysis. The number of positive nodes was also independently prognostic in the multivariate analysis from the Large Bowel Cancer Project in London.[261] Until now, the number of positive nodes has been included only in the Gastrointestinal Tumor Study Group (GITSG) classification.[262] The data suggest that any classification or staging system devised in the future should certainly consider the number of positive nodes as a predictive discriminant.

The TNM Classification

Both the American Joint Committee on Cancer (AJCC)[263] and the International Union Against Cancer (UICC)[264] have proposed staging systems utilizing the TNM classification. There was not, however, total agreement between the staging systems, and neither system specifically considered the number of positive nodes. In studies which looked at the prognostic ability of pathologic TNM staging,[265-267] survival was identical or even reversed for Stages II and III.

A revised, 1987 joint AJCC/UICC TNM staging system unified the two systems. The revised system is simpler and considers the important prognostic factor, the number of positive nodes.[268-270] Free mesothelial penetration is also considered.[271] We strongly recommend the universal use of the new TNM system for reporting end results. Table 29-6 defines the three most widely used systems: Dukes, Astler–Coller, and the 1987 TNM.

CLINICAL STAGING SYSTEMS

Pretreatment Evaluation

Because all three systems described above involve postsurgical pathologic staging, they cannot be used for making treatment decisions, and they are not applicable when sphincter-conserving procedures are used, such as fulguration, local excision, or contact radiation therapy. Therefore, clinical staging systems have been considered. Abrams tried to correlate the size of the tumor, the presence or absence of ulceration, and the degree of differentiation with the final Dukes' stage.[272] Ulceration was the principal feature, with 63% of nonulcerated cancers classified as Dukes' A, compared with only 28% of ulcerated lesions. Another clinical staging system, devised by a group from the Princess Margaret Hospital in Toronto,[273] was based on several prognostic variables: the presence or absence of metastases, whether the rectal tumor was fixed or mobile, whether it was annular, and whether the clinical symptoms of weight loss, anorexia, weakness, and anemia were present. These variables were grouped into four clinical classes. In Class I none of the variables were present; Class II was characterized by annular rectal tumor or the systemic symptoms; Class III denoted a fixed rectal tumor; and in Class IV metastases were present. Patient survival correlated well with breakdown into these classes and with breakdown by Dukes' stages, but the correlation between clinical classes and Dukes' stages was not good. Recently, univariate and multivariate analyses of prognostic features were done on 824 rectal cancer patients in the Medical Research Council's preoperative radiation therapy trial in the United Kingdom.[274,275] Mobility of the tumor was the most important preoperative assessment related to curative resection.

An Australian Clinicopathological Staging System combines features of both a pathologic staging system and a clinical system, based on local tumor characteristics alone.[276,277]

York Mason has also suggested the use of a clinical staging system based on mobility of the primary tumor. Clinical

TABLE 29-6. 1987 AJCC/UICC Staging Classification of Colorectal Cancer*

Primary Tumor (T)

TX	Primary tumor cannot be assessed
T0	No evidence of tumor in resected specimen (prior —polypectomy or fulguration)
Tis	Carcinoma in situ
T1	Invades submucosa
T2	Invades into muscularis propria
T3/T4	Depends on whether serosa is present
	Serosa present:
	T3 Invades through muscularis propria into
	Subserosa
	Serosa (but not through)
	Pericolic fat within the leaves of the mesentery
	T4 Invades through serosa into free peritoneal cavity, —or through serosa into a contiguous organ
	No serosa (distal two thirds rectum, posterior left of right —colon)
	T3 Invades through muscularis propria
	T4 Invades other organs (vagina, prostate, ureter, —kidney)

Regional Lymph Nodes (N)

NX	Nodes cannot be assessed (*e.g.,* local excision only)
N0	No regional node metastases
N1	1–3 positive nodes
N2	4 or more positive nodes
(N3	central nodes positive)

Distant Metastases (M)

MX	Presence of distant metastases cannot be assessed
M0	No distant metastases
M1	Distant metastases present

Dukes' staging system correlated with TNM

Dukes' A =	T1N0M0
	T2N0M0
Dukes' B =	T3N0M0
	T4N0M0
Dukes' C =	T(any)N1M0, T(any)N2M0
Dukes' D =	T(any)N(any)M1

Modified Astler–Coller (MAC) system correlated with TNM

MAC A =	T1N0M0
MAC B1 =	T2N0M0
MAC B2 =	T3N0M0, T4N0M0
MAC B3 =	T4N0M0
MAC C1 =	T2N1M0, T2N2M0
MAC C2 =	T3N1M0, T3N2M0
	T4N1M0, T4N2M0
MAC C3 =	T4N1M0, T4N2M0

Note: In all pathologic staging systems, particularly those applied to rectal cancer, the abbreviations (m) and (g) may be used: (m) denotes microscopic transmural penetration; (g) or (m + g) denotes transmural penetration visible on gross inspection and confirmed microscopically.

* Modified from American Joint Committee on Cancer: Manual for Staging of Cancer, 3rd ed. Philadelphia, JB Lippincott, 1987; and Union Internationale Contre le Cancer: TNM Classification of Malignant Tumors, 4th ed. Geneva, UICC, 1987; by permission.

Stage I represents a freely mobile tumor; Stage II, a mobile tumor; Stage III, tethered mobility; and Stage IV, fixed tumor.[278] Clinical Stages I and II should comprise cases in which local curative excision may be possible. Nicholls et al tested the accuracy of the digital examination by comparing it with the final pathologic stage.[279] They assessed the morphology, number of quadrants involved, fixation, and presence of extrarectal involvement. In 70 tumors, there was 67% to 83% recognition of the final pathology by the consulting physicians, whereas the correlation was less (44%–68%) when tumors were assessed by the registrars, who had less experience. In a subsequent publication, Nicholls et al reported that clinical determination of the local extent and penetration correlated positively with survival.[280]

Physical Examination

In patients with low rectal cancer, digital examination often reveals a great deal about the primary tumor size, configuration, friability, mobility, involvement of contiguous structures, percent circumference, and possibly involvement of perirectal lymph nodes. With rigid endoscopy, the physical examination may be extended to higher rectal tumors and may confirm or amplify the results of the digital examination. Again, with rigid endoscopy one may assess tumor configuration, mobility (using the endoscope to move the tumor), percent circumference, and size.

Laboratory Tests

Various laboratory tests such as standard liver function tests, 5′-nucleotidase, and γ-glutamyl transpeptidase (GGTP) may be useful in suggesting liver metastases. However, the results are not specific, and a liver imaging study is necessary, and sometimes even a biopsy, to verify metastases. Although it was hoped that the CEA level would be useful for staging, Moertel et al reported that whereas CEA levels usually increase with increasing stage of colorectal cancer, a large proportion of patients with tumors of all stages have no increase in CEA levels.[257]

Imaging Studies

Many imaging modalities have been used to rule out distant metastases in patients preoperatively. Chest radiography is performed to rule out lung metastases and to assess the patient's ability to tolerate surgery. Intravenous pyelography (IVP) has usually been done to look for ureteral deviation or hydronephrosis. However, computed tomography (CT) is making IVP obsolete.[281,282]

PRIMARY TUMOR AND NODES. Imaging studies for staging of the primary tumor must be capable of revealing the extent of penetration through the bowel wall. A barium enema or air contrast barium enema study is inadequate for this purpose, since either study offers only intraluminal images. Several authors report that intrarectal ultrasound (US) is extremely sensitive, as good as or better than CT for assessing extent of bowel wall penetration.[283-286] For example, Hildebrandt and Feifel compared the rectal US findings with pathologic findings in 25 patients.[283] The findings on digital examination correlated with pathologic findings in 15 of 17 patients and overestimated disease in 2 patients. Sonography correlated with the pathologic assessment in 23 of 25 patients; the other 2 were overstaged. These authors proposed a US staging category, uTNM. Nyberg et al have suggested a potential application for intraluminal US in assessing colon tumors as well.[287] In an in vitro study, they compared US examinations of colon specimens with the histopathology and found a good correlation. It has even been suggested that US may be useful in detecting metastases in lymph nodes. In a study by Rifkin and Marks,[285] CT demonstrated only 2 of 7 positive lymph nodes, with no false positives, whereas sonography demonstrated 6 of 7 positive nodes, with 2 false positives. The positive nodes were 0.5 to 1.0 cm in size. The single positive case not detectable with US had normal-sized nodes with only microscopic invasion. Neither CT nor US could detect such nodal disease.

Mayes and Zornoza reviewed 80 CT examinations done for colon and rectal carcinoma and concluded that CT was useful in assessing pelvic masses, para-aortic nodes, adrenals, and liver.[288] Nicholls et al[279] found that CT correctly demonstrated extensive local spread in rectal carcinoma in 89% of patients but was no better than the digital examination in cases of lesser spread or lymph node involvement.

Several investigators have indicated that CT staging is quite accurate,[282,289-292] with one study offering a CT staging system.[289] Staging was based on bowel wall thickness and penetration into surrounding fat, any positive lymph nodes, or distant disease in the liver. Other authors have indicated that CT staging is not accurate, primarily because of inability to assess the depth of invasion accurately from CT scans, or to detect positive lymph nodes.[293-299] Grabbe et al[294] indicated that CT staging was better than the clinical staging system of York Mason, but the problem of assessing slight perirectal spread and tumor in lymph nodes made CT staging inaccurate. On the other hand, Netri et al[296] indicated that CT staging was less accurate than the rectal examination in assessing extraparietal invasion but had a 77% accuracy for detecting positive lymph nodes.

Magnetic resonance (MR) imaging has been compared with CT in several studies[300-302]; the two modalities have been found to be roughly equivalent in demonstrating positive lymph nodes. CT affords better spatial resolution but MR imaging affords better contrast resolution.[301] Butch et al thought that CT and MR imaging were equally effective in staging but that neither modality could demonstrate the extent of bowel wall infiltration or tumor spread to normal-sized perirectal nodes.[302]

Other methods of assessing lymph node involvement include lymphangiography and lymphoscintigraphy. The lymphangiogram "inconstantly" demonstrated nodes associated with internal iliac vessels.[303] Ege and Cummings found pelvic lymphoscintigraphy feasible,[304] but Reasbeck et al found it of no use.[305] Some of the newer radiolabeled monoclonal antibodies may be of use in the future in assessing the presence of tumor in lymph nodes, as well as distant disease.[306,307]

LIVER. Radionuclide scintigraphy, once the prominent method for imaging the liver, has a low spatial resolution and does not demonstrate metastases less than 2 cm in size.[308-310] Although US is of low cost and widely available, it is less accurate than CT for imaging of hepatic disease.[296] The best modality for detecting small metastases at this time is CT.[311,312] MR imaging has generally proved not as useful as CT,[313] although in one study in which two very specific MR techniques were used,[314] MR imaging was better than conventional CT and comparable to CT enhanced with ethiodized oral emulsion-13.

STAGING OF ADVANCED DISEASE

As newer, more aggressive approaches are adopted for metastatic disease, particularly to the liver, a classification of the extent of metastatic disease becomes more pressing. There have been attempts to define classifications[312,314] based on extent of hepatic replacement, symptoms, extrahepatic disease, resectability, or liver function test results, but the definitive system has not yet evolved. An International Staging System has been proposed that is simple and logical.[314] It has four stages: O = curatively resected; I = <25% hepatic replacement (HR) with no extrahepatic disease (E) or symptoms attributable to liver metastases (S); II = 25% to 75% HR with no E and no S; III = >75% HR with no E and no S, or any HR with E and/or S. If this system is adopted, its utility will only be determined by prospective analyses of its predictive value.

ADDITIONAL PROGNOSTIC VARIABLES

Although operative findings and pathologic stage are the major determinants of prognosis, many clinical and pathologic features may be prognostic for ultimate survival. Many of these factors are interrelated and merely reflections of the same overall characteristic of the cancer. Very few multivariate analyses have been performed.[253,271]

Clinical Features

AGE. Ever since Hoerner in 1958 reported the poor prognosis for colorectal cancer in the very young,[315] numerous articles have supported this conclusion in patients less than 40 years old. Various explanations have been offered, including delay in diagnosis of the disease and the large number of mucoid adenocarcinomas in this group. Dukes and Bussey suggested that the much higher rate of lymphatic metastases in patients less than 40 years old was due to a delay in receiving treatment or to more rapid progression of the disease in young patients; they favored the latter explanation.[204] Their data indicated that the average age (62 years) of patients with low-grade malignancies was considerably higher than those with high-grade malignancies (55 years).[204] Recio and Bussey[316] found that 53% of tumors in young patients were high grade, versus only 20% of tumors in the older age groups where colorectal carcinoma is more common. They also noted an increased number of mucoid tumors in younger patients. Many other authors have supported these findings.[317-319] Adolescent patients less than 20 years old have presented with high-stage, mucin-producing, high-grade tumors and have had a poor survival as a result.[320]

When stage-adjusted survival has been analyzed, in almost all reports there is no difference in relative prognosis for the younger age group.[320-324] In one study, only Dukes' Stage C patients less than 30 years old had a worse outcome than older patients.[325]

GENDER. Women do better than men in terms of survival from colorectal cancer, just as they often survive better with other malignancies.[326,327] In the randomized preoperative radiation therapy study for rectal cancer at Memorial Sloan-Kettering Cancer Center,[328] the only variable besides stage that was predictive of prolonged survival was female gender. Four large analyses showed an improved survival for females.[329-332] However, other studies have not shown a difference in prognosis by gender.[323,325,333,334] Since women generally live longer than men, studies should address the causes of death to ascertain whether the improved long-term survival merely reflects fewer non-cancer-related deaths. Koch analyzed relative survival, independent of deaths from other causes, and still found a higher survival rate for women.[335]

SYMPTOMS. Beahrs and Sanfelippo[336] reported that symptomatic colorectal cancer patients had a 5-year survival rate of 49%, compared with 71% for asymptomatic patients. It is logical to assume that patients in whom colorectal cancer is detected by a screening technique such as fecal occult blood testing or sigmoidoscopy might be treated at an earlier stage and therefore might have a greater chance for cure. Several reports note high survival rates in patients in whom colorectal cancer was detected by screening. In these studies, the number of patients with positive lymph nodes has been small and the survival rates high.

DURATION OF SYMPTOMS. It appears that patients with symptoms lasting longer than 6 months have an increased 5-year survival rate. This improved survival may reflect the slow growth rate of tumors in these patients. In a study of 1084 patients reported by Copeland and colleagues, the 5-year disease-free survival rate for patients with symptoms of 6 months' duration or less was 31%, compared to 37% for patients who had had symptoms longer than 6 months.[337] In a study of 161 patients, Pescatori et al found that patients with symptoms for more than 6 months had a significantly higher rate of radical operations, a lower postoperative mortality, and a higher 5-year survival rate—43%, versus only 32% for patients with symptoms of less than 6 months' duration.[338] Pescatori et al found no correlation between the duration of symptoms and pathologic stage.[338] In a recent multivariate analysis, there was no effect of duration of symptoms on survival when stage was controlled.[332]

OBSTRUCTION OR PERFORATION. Obstruction and perforation appear to reduce survival.[223,332,339-348] One reason for the poor prognosis in this group of patients is the high operative mortality.[349] In one study, after resection performed with curative intent, patients whose lesions had obstructed or invaded other organs had the same 5-year survival rate as the curative resection group as a whole.[349] However, patients with perforating lesions had only half this life expectancy. A study of 2524 patients in the Large Bowel Cancer Project in the United Kingdom confirmed that obstruction was an important contributor to mortality during the initial in-patient period.[334] Obstruction was the only symptom that had an independent effect in the multivariate analysis of 709 patients in Sydney.[332]

A Danish study compared outcome in 219 patients who had obstruction and perforation and 732 patients who did not have these complications.[323] The 5-year survival rate was 23% for patients with either or both of these complications and 35% for patients without them. In the NSABP clinical trial, data from 1021 patients were analyzed.[347] The presence of bowel obstruction strongly influenced the prognostic outcome. Of interest, bowel obstruction in the right colon was associated with a significantly diminished disease-free survival, whereas obstruction in the left colon was not associated with a similar diminution in survival. Obstruction and circumferential growth were separate prognostic factors; neither one completely explained the effects of the other. The relative risk for patients with tumors that were both obstructing and encircling compared to patients with tumors that were neither obstructing nor encircling was 3.27. The GITSG used multivariate analysis to examine prognostic features in 572 patients.[348] Obstruction was an important indicator of prognosis, completely independent of Dukes' stage. Bowel perforation was important as a prognostic feature only for disease-free survival. In light of the findings of the NSABP study, it is of interest that the GITSG found no differences in the relative failure risks for obstruction in different sites in the bowel. A study reported from Massachusetts General Hospital indicated that both local failure and intra-abdominal metastatic failure were increased in patients with obstruction or perforation, compared with a control group of patients without these symptoms.[223] In regard to perforating cancers, one should distinguish between perforation through the tumor and perforation proximal to an obstructing cancer.

HEMORRHAGE OR RECTAL BLEEDING. Hemorrhage or rectal bleeding has been associated with an improved prognosis, perhaps because it is related to a surface erosion that can manifest early and lead to early intervention, and not a symptom reflective of tumor penetration.[350] In the GITSG experience, the presence of melena or rectal bleeding marginally prolonged survival ($p = 0.08$) even after the effects of Dukes' stage were accounted for.[348] In another study, symptomatic or asymptomatic anemia had no effect on prognosis.[337] In the analysis of the Sydney Hospital experience, patients with rectal bleeding had a significantly longer survival on univariate analysis; however, the significance of bleeding disappeared on multivariate analysis.[332]

LOCATION OF THE PRIMARY TUMOR. It has generally been found that the 5-year survival rate is less for patients with cancer of the rectosigmoid and rectum than for patients with cancer elsewhere in the colon.[329,330,333,337,347,351] In regard to colon primaries, some authors suggest a worse prognosis for patients with lesions in the right colon.[329,347] Others find no difference[323,331]; still others report a worse prognosis for patients with disease in the left colon.[338] For rectal disease, a decreased survival has been noted for patients with lesions below the peritoneal reflection, compared with patients with lesions above the peritoneal reflection.[352] These data are supported by the Medical Research Council's preoperative radiation therapy trial for rectal cancer.[275]

PRIMARY TUMOR SIZE. Colorectal cancer is unusual in that the majority of studies report no adverse relationship of tumor size to survival.[202,219,221,224,329,330,332,353,354] A few studies have shown improved survival with smaller tumors.[217] A recent study found that colon tumors 6 to 10 cm in size were associated with an improved survival, compared to lesions larger than 11 cm.[225] The relationship of size to survival did not hold for rectal tumors.[224] Of interest, some studies have shown increased tumor penetration through the bowel wall with larger tumors,[221,355] but not an increase in lymph node metastases.[221] The GITSG analysis of 572 colon patients in a randomized chemoimmunotherapy trial found that although tumor size was unimportant when analyzed as a single factor, when the effects of other factors were adjusted for, increasing size had a negative effect on survival and disease-free survival.[348]

PRIMARY TUMOR CONFIGURATION. As early as 1939 Grinnell reported that survival was higher in patients with tumors projecting into the lumen (83%) than in patients whose tumors were either intermediate (45% survival) or infiltrating (38%).[228] The reasons for such differences in survival include the lower frequency of penetration of the bowel wall by exophytic tumors compared with ulcerating tumors (24% versus 39%),[355] less frequent nodal metastases with exophytic tumors than with ulcerating lesions,[355–357] and fewer hematogenous metastases (23% versus 31%).[185] Overall, exophytic tumors are more frequently limited to the bowel wall (46%) than are ulcerating tumors (24%).[355] One recent study that has looked at exophytic versus nonexophytic tumors is the GITSG colon adjuvant study.[348] This study found that the presence of an exophytic lesion had a significantly beneficial effect on survival.

BLOOD TRANSFUSION. Several authors have suggested that perioperative blood transfusions have a negative effect on disease-free interval in patients with colorectal or colonic cancer.[358,359] Other prognostic variables were not considered in these studies. Foster et al did consider other variables and claimed a worse survival for patients with colonic cancers, regardless of stage, receiving perioperative transfusions but no adverse effects of transfusion for rectal cancers.[360] After adjusting for stage, age, and gender by Cox regression analysis, Nathanson et al found that blood transfusions were not detrimental.[361] Weiden and associates, in a retrospective multivariate analysis of 171 patients with colorectal cancer, found no relationship between perioperative blood transfusion and survival or disease recurrence.[362] Corman and associates also were unable to show an adverse effect after a multivariate analysis.[333] However, when they considered the number of units transfused, both as a single variable and in the multivariate analysis, this feature had a very strong prognostic value for colorectal cancer, and in particular for colon cancer ($p = 0.005$). It was not prognostic when patients with rectal cancer were analyzed separately, but there were only 74 patients in this group. In addition to perioperative blood transfusion, other surgical complications such as fever and sepsis may play a role.[365]

TABLE 29-7. Percent Survival as a Function of Histologic Tumor Grade

Study	(No. of Patients)	% Survival by Grade: 1	2	3	4
Broders[200]	Rectum (598)	56	38	25	15
Grinnell[228]	Colon/rectum (204)	66	48	25	*
Sunderland[378]	Rectum/sigmoid (210)	75	76	58	*
Dukes and Bussey[204]	Rectum (2097)	77	61	29	*
Copeland et al[337]	Colon/rectum (654)	58	42	21	*
Rao et al[219]	Rectum/sigmoid (107)	59	38	11	*
Riboli et al[366]	Colon/rectum (90)	65	33	25	*
Minsky et al[373]	Colon (158)	100	80	56	*
Minsky et al[373]	Rectum (82)	86	71	55	*

* No Grade 4 in system employed.

Pathologic Features

ADJACENT ORGAN INVOLVEMENT. Adjacent organs are involved in about 10% of colorectal cancer cases. Spratt and Spjut found that removal of a contiguous pathologically invaded organ did not alter 5- and 10-year survival rates.[329] To address this issue, Gunderson and Sosin devised a modification of the Astler–Coller staging system which added B3 and C3 stages, denoting adjacent organ involvement for node-negative or node-positive disease, respectively.[214] Several studies have analyzed both locoregional recurrence and 5-year survival rates by this modified Astler–Coller staging system.[227,363,364] The additional B3 and C3 staging predicted increased local recurrence, as well as decreased 5-year survival. Nathanson et al, in a multivariate analysis of prognostic factors, indicated that the second most important factor was involvement of adjacent organs, which increased the relative risk of dying of colorectal cancer to 2.6.[361] Minsky and colleagues analyzed patients with colon or rectal cancer according to whether they had stage B3 or C3 disease clinically or verified microscopically.[224,225] Patients with Stage B3 colon cancer verified pathologically had a 27% 5-year actuarial survival rate, significantly lower than the 88% survival in patients with B3 disease who were thought to have only clinical adjacent organ involvement.[225]

DEGREE OF DIFFERENTIATION. Dukes and others pointed out a correlation of grade with lymph nodal and distant metastases found at operation.[188,204,215] Disease grade has also been correlated with the likelihood of venous spread,[184,204] the risk of lymphatic penetration,[184] extent of local spread,[204] average number of lymphatic metastases,[355] and increasing wall penetration.[355] In another study, grade was not associated with the extent of local invasion.[366]

Univariate analysis has shown a definite relationship between survival and histologic grade in both colon and rectal cancer (Table 29-7). The relationship was significant in node-negative patients,[366] but too few patients with positive nodes were available to assess the influence of grade in this group. In several recent multivariate analyses, grade was independently prognostic of survival.[261,275,331,332,348,367]

The trend of the data indicates that grade should be consid-

TABLE 29-8. Scoring System for Prognostic Model Based on Grade- and Stage-Related Parameters*

Parameter	Score
Lymphocytic infiltration	
Marked	0
Moderate	3
Little or none	6
No. of Nodes involved	
0	0
—1–4	4
—≥5	8
Spread through bowel wall	
None	0
Slight to moderate	3
Extensive	6

* Grinnell RS: The grading and prognosis of carcinoma of the colon and rectum. Ann Surg 109:500–533, 1939.

Range of possible total scores: 0–20. A set of five prognostic categories (I to V) based on the model was highly predictive of survival. Scores of 0 are assigned to category I, scores of 1 to 6 to category II, scores of 7 to 11 to category III, scores of 12 to 16 to category IV, and scores of 17 to 20 to category V.

ered an independent prognostic factor; however, several problems are associated with its use, including the nonuniformity of grading systems, the designation of the majority of tumors as "intermediate" in grade, variability of grade in different parts of the tumor,[369] and concern as to pathologists' agreement on grading of the same tumor. The question of the adequacy of biopsies has been addressed.[228,281,370] Agreement between the grade of a resected rectal cancer specimen and the grade of the original biopsy specimen obtained at proctosigmoidoscopy varied from 56% to 78%. It was worse for poorly differentiated tumors, 38% to 52%, and somewhat better for moderately well differentiated tumors, 64%.[281,370] The proctosigmoidoscopy biopsy specimen was usually assigned a lower grade than the surgical specimen.[228] Complete agreement among three pathologists with respect to multiple biopsy specimens obtained under anesthesia and the resected specimens was only 44%.[281]

An interesting study from St. Mark's Hospital and St. Bartholomew's Hospital in London has addressed the problem of subjectivity in grading by defining the parameters of grading and then determining those most predictive of survival with a multivariate analysis.[203] The best-fitting parsimonious model comprised the grading variables of lymphocytic infiltration, tubular configuration, and pattern of growth (expanding versus infiltrating). A four-grade system was devised that proved to be reproducible and predictive of survival. The investigators took this one step further, allowing grade-related parameters to compete with stage-related parameters in an overall model of pathologic prognostic categories. The best model consisted of the number of affected lymph nodes, the presence of lymphocytic infiltration, and the extent of spread through the bowel wall (Table 29-8).[234] A set of five prognostic categories based on the model was highly predictive of survival.

COLLOID CARCINOMA (MUCINOUS CARCINOMA). Colloid or mucinous adenocarcinomas have a poor prognosis and frequently are grouped with high-grade carcinomas since their prognosis is quite similar. The percentage of regional or synchronous distant metastases is higher than in noncolloid carcinomas; Trimpi and Bacon reported a 70% incidence of regional or distant metastases.[371] Sundblad and Paz reported 43% Stage C or D carcinomas in patients with colloid carcinomas, compared with only 15% for patients with noncolloid carcinomas.[372] Cohen et al reported an 83% frequency of positive nodes and an increased incidence of gross transmural penetration in patients with colloid carcinomas, findings similar to those in patients with poorly differentiated adenocarcinomas.[355] Minsky et al noted that local recurrence and abdominal failure were higher.[373]

Many authors have reported a poorer survival rate in patients with colloid carcinomas—less than half in some series.[374,375] Symonds and Vickery reported a 34% survival in all patients with colloid colorectal carcinomas, compared to 53% for patients with other adenocarcinomas. The survival rate for patients with colloid rectal carcinoma was only 18%,[376] versus 49% for those with noncolloid rectal carcinoma. Others have found less dramatic differences.[373,377]

Signet-ring cell carcinoma is rarely cured. All four cases reported by Symonds and Vickery were fatal within 1 year of diagnosis.[376]

BLOOD VESSEL INVASION. It would be logical to assume that blood vessel invasion might signify dissemination to distant organs. However, as pointed out by Dukes, emboli within a vein may not mean dissemination but only spread along a path of least resistance.[188] Furthermore, failure to find emboli within a vein does not preclude earlier dissemination. Brown and Warren reported increased blood vessel invasion with higher grade of disease, increased bowel wall penetration, and increased visceral metastases.[232] The frequency of visceral metastases was reduced in the absence of blood vessel invasion: only 1 of 70 patients without blood vessel invasion had visceral metastases.[232] In a 1983 study, Knudsen et al found that liver metastases were three times as frequent in patients with venous invasion than in patients without it.[212] All seven patients with synchronous metastases studied by Madison and associates had blood vessel invasion, whereas only 31% of those patients without metastases had this finding.[368] Dukes and Bussey noted an increase in blood vessel invasion with both increasing grade and increasing local spread,[204] and verified an earlier study showing an increase in blood vessel invasion with positive lymph nodes.[188]

Blood vessel invasion is detected in 17% to 50% of cases.[202,211,221,251,368,378-380] This feature may predict decreased survival.[329,337,348,378,379,381-384] However, because blood vessel invasion is related to many other factors, whether it is an independent variable remains unclear. Blood vessel invasion is associated with a poor prognosis in Dukes' B and C patients, independent of lymph node status[378,381,382] and of Dukes' stage.[378,382] In the colon, a survival difference has been reported only for patients with Stage C2 disease.[383] In the rectum and sigmoid, a survival difference has been noted only for patients with Dukes' C disease.[378]

In multivariate analyses, vascular invasion was not an independent variable in one study,[384] but it was in five other large studies.[212,261,275,332,367]

LYMPHATIC VESSEL INVASION. Grinnell was one of the first to look at lymphatic vessel invasion.[233] Spratt and Spjut noted decreased survival at 5 and 10 years when lymphatic vessel invasion was present.[329] From their data it appears that once lymphatic vessel invasion was present, neither venous invasion nor perineural invasion decreased the survival rate much further. Khankanian et al grouped lymphatic vessel invasion with blood vessel invasion and designated the combined entity "vascular invasion."[385] They studied this phenomenon within the bowel wall only and noted no difference in disease-free interval with vascular invasion. Analysis of the GITSG data indicated that lymphatic invasion was "potentially harmful" ($p = 0.08$ in their analysis).[348] A recent multivariate study of rectal and rectosigmoid cancer considered stage, blood vessel invasion, and lymphatic vessel invasion.[384] Lymphatic vessel invasion was an independent prognostic feature ($p = 0.04$).

PERINEURAL INVASION. The classic study of perineural invasion was reported by Seefeld and Bargen,[211] who noted that malignant spread by growth along perineural spaces occurred as far as 10 cm from the primary tumor. The incidence of perineural invasion was 30% in 100 cases, increasing with grade and Dukes' stage. Patients with perineural invasion had more local recurrences in the scar or anastomotic site than those free of perineural invasion (81% versus 30%). The 5-year survival rate was also lower in the former group (7% versus 35%). Spratt and Spjut confirmed this survival difference.[329] One multivariate analysis included nerve invasion and found it to be an independent prognostic variable.[212]

IMMUNE RESPONSE TO THE PRIMARY TUMOR. Crude indicators of patients' general immune response have been analyzed for prognostic usefulness. Two studies of peripheral blood lymphocyte counts are contradictory. Kim and associates noted that when the peripheral blood lymphocyte count was less than 1000/mm^3, survival was 30%, compared to about 60% survival in patients with higher counts.[386] Corman et al, in a multivariate analysis, found no difference in survival by preoperative lymphocyte counts.[333] In a study of lymphocyte subsets, T-lymphocytes were depressed in 57% of preoperative and postoperative patients with colorectal carcinoma; B-lymphocyte counts were normal.[387] The impact of T-cell depression on prognosis was not evaluated.

A recent Southwestern Oncology Group (SWOG) study that analyzed humoral immunity reported no survival difference as a function of serum IgM concentration but prolonged survival with higher levels of IgA and IgG.[388] Baseler and associates noted that circulating IgA immune complexes were increased in patients with various carcinomas compared with healthy subjects or patients undergoing surgery for benign disease.[389] The highest levels of circulating IgA immune complexes were found in patients with colon carcinoma.

Considerable interest has been expressed in the prognostic value of local inflammatory reactions at the primary tumor site. Spratt and Spjut noted a decrease in survival with a lack of inflammatory response around the tumor periphery.[329] Murray et al reported an increased 5-year survival rate for patients with Dukes' B and C colon cancer when local inflammation was present (89% versus 46%).[390] Local inflammation has been found in approximately 50% to 75% of tumors.[202,390] Jass et al demonstrated that lymphocytic infiltration was the most important factor in their grading model (Cox regression analysis) and was also important in their "best" model with grade- and stage-related parameters.[203] Carlon et al similarly noted that lymphocytic infiltration around the primary and the pattern of growth were the most significant prognostic features.[391] Svennevig and associates reported a higher number of mononuclear cells in both the peritumoral stroma and within the tumor parenchyma from those patients cured by surgery.[392]

REACTIVE LYMPH NODES. Multiple investigators have shown that an apparent immunologic response in regional lymph nodes correlates with improved survival.[390,393–395] In sigmoid colon cancer, Patt and associates noted that sinus histiocytosis and paracortical immunoblastic activity individually correlated with an increased survival.[393] When both features were present, survival was even better. There was no benefit from increased germinal center activity in this study. Murray et al also reported an increased survival with sinus histiocytosis of the draining lymph nodes, and an even greater increase in survival when this feature was present with a local inflammatory reaction to the primary.[390] Pihl and colleagues observed that paracortical lymph node hyperplasia occupying more than 15% of the lymph node section was favorably associated with survival.[395]

CARCINOEMBRYONIC ANTIGEN AND OTHER BIOMARKERS. The value of the preoperative CEA level as an independent prognostic indicator is unclear. The preoperative CEA level does reflect tumor burden.[396–398] Many authors have reported that an increased level (5 ng/ml) indicates an increased risk of recurrence,[398–405] but others have not found it to be a good prognostic variable.[406-409] Steele et al reported that an increased CEA level was prognostic for colon cancer but not for rectal cancer.[410] Recently, a group from the Mayo Clinic reported that the CEA level was strongly associated with survival, but within stages, it was only independently prognostic for Dukes' C patients with four or more positive lymph nodes.[257]

The CEA level not only correlates with the extent of the tumor burden, it also correlates highly with venous invasion.[411] Tabuchi et al looked at peripheral as well as portal vein CEA levels immediately after laparotomy. In peripheral blood, increased CEA levels correlated only with venous invasion. In portal venous blood, CEA elevation correlated with venous invasion, tumor size, lymphatic invasion, Dukes' stage, and depth of invasion.[411]

De Mello et al looked at a large number of factors as potential prognostic variables.[331] They found that the CEA level was prognostic as a single variable, but not if age, stage, and sex were included in the model. Similarly, the possible tumor markers of γ-glutamyl transpeptidase and pseudouridine were found to be prognostic only as single variables. Phosphohexoseisomerase and three acute phase reactant proteins (APRP), α_1-antichymotrypsin, C-reactive protein, and α_1-acid glycoprotein, were found to be prognostic. When α_1-antichymotrypsin was included in the model, the other markers were no longer significant, although phosphohexoseisomerase was of borderline significance. Ward et al in 1977 found other APRP to be prognostic.[412] Durdey and colleagues demonstrated that APRP combined with CEA level were most useful in determining fixed versus mobile tumors, and whether tumors were fixed because of inflammation or invasion.[413] By using the criteria of increased APRP and CEA (>45 ng/ml) levels, Williams and coworkers were able to identify 10 of 11 tumors with extensive or moderate malignant spread, 4 of 5 with inflammatory spread, and 21 of 23 with no spread.[281] These were not very good criteria for determining minimal malignant spread, but for moderate and extensive spread, the sensitivity, specificity, and accuracy were 91%, 96%, and 94%, respectively. Others have found that preresection APRP levels are of no value in predicting who will develop metastases, or the site of metastases.[414]

CELL CYCLE PARAMETERS AND PLOIDY. In 100 patients, Meyer and Prioleau found no relationship between the fraction of cells in S-phase and histologic grade or other clinicopathologic features, such as age, sex, site of tumor, size, Dukes' stage, number of positive lymph nodes, presence of adenomas, or even relapse-free survival.[415] The question of alteration of prognosis was also considered by Blijham et al who noted an increased rate of recurrences with a high percentage of S-phase cells in Dukes' C colorectal cancer.[416] On the other hand, Bleiberg et al found no correlation between the mean labeling index and age, sex, tumor localization, Dukes' classification, or disease-free survival at 5 years.[417]

Some authors have found a relationship between aneuploidy and Dukes' stage[418-420]; others have not.[421-423] No significant relationship of aneuploidy to grade has been established.[416,421] Ota et al looked at primary colorectal cancer specimens for labeling index, flow cytometry parameters, and primer-available DNA-dependent polymerase index (PDPI), all of which bore no relation to Dukes' stage, tumor location, tumor size, or frequency of nodal metastases.[423]

Flow cytometry parameters may bear a relation to recurrence or survival. Streffer et al reported a high incidence of local recurrence in patients with rectal carcinoma who had a high ratio of S-phase cells.[424] For rectal carcinoma, the incidence of either lymph node metastases or distant metastases increased with an increased percentage of S-phase cells in the tumor. For tumors with more than 19.7% cells in S-phase, the incidence of lymph node or distant metastases was 82%. For tumors with less than 19.7% cells in S-phase, the incidence of positive lymph nodes or distant metastases was only 14%.

Several authors have found an increase in survival with diploid tumors and a worse survival with aneuploid tumors.[419,424-427] Scott et al found significantly better survival in patients with diploid tumors than in patients with aneuploid or tetraploid tumors.[427] Local recurrence was twice as common in patients with nondiploid tumors as in patients with diploid tumors. Using a Cox multivariate analysis that included multiple clinical and pathologic factors, Scott et al found that DNA ploidy and the operative assessment of tumor spread were the most important prognostic variables. Nondiploid tumors also were associated with an increased incidence of vascular invasion, tumor fibrosis, and high Dukes' stage. In a series of 33 patients with at least a 3-year follow-up, Melamed and associates were unable to document a poorer prognosis for patients with aneuploid tumors when ploidy was corrected for stage.[428] The potential for cell cycle analysis and its use in prognosis is only beginning to be realized.

SUMMARY OF STAGING AND PROGNOSTIC VARIABLES

Although the presence of hematogenous or nodal metastases are major determinants of curability, recent analyses utilize multivariate regression models to provide sophisticated outcome projections. These data have been applied toward unifying end-results reporting.[428d,428e]

ADDITIONAL TUMOR BIOLOGIC FEATURES

Oncogenes

The *ras* and *myc* oncogenes have been implicated in colorectal carcinoma. Der et al initially reported that carcinoma of the colon was associated with the activated oncogene (c-Ki-*ras*-2-gene).[429] Elevated expression of the *ras* oncogene family was also found in premalignant and malignant tumors of the colorectum by Spandidos and Kerr.[430] The *ras* oncogene protein product (p21) was detected by Gallick et al in 9 of 17 colon cancers.[431] However, in 4 of 5 patients with distant metastases this protein product was not elevated, suggesting that *ras* oncogene activation is an early phenomenon in carcinogenesis. Thor and associates demonstrated a correlation of p21 expression with the depth of invasion.[432] Overall, the protein was found to be increased in 22 of 47 malignant colon carcinomas but not in benign colon conditions or normal colon. Recently, two groups (the State University of New York at Stony Brook, and the University of Leiden with Johns Hopkins University) have detected specific mutations to the *ras* oncogene from the normal counterpart in about 40% of colon cancers.[433-435] These mutations were often present in villous adenomas as well, indicating strongly that *ras* oncogene activation is a relatively early event.

The c-*myc* oncogene has also been found in polyps and colon cancer.[436,437] In one study of 15 patients, tumors and adjacent normal tissues were examined for expression of c-*myc*.[437] The authors found no gene amplification or rearrangement of c-*myc*. However, the c-*myc* mRNA transcripts were elevated in 12 of 15 tumors and the protein product, p62 c-*myc*, was elevated in 8 of 15 tumors. In both cases the transcript elevation and protein product elevation were greatest in the well-differentiated tumors and lowest in the poorly differentiated tumors. Since there was no gene amplification, it was proposed that the increased transcripts were due to enhanced transcription or to an increase in mRNA stability.

Growth Factors and Receptors

Tumor growth is a function of the fraction of cells actively in cycle (growth fraction), the cell cycle time, and the amount of cell loss. Primary colon cancers have been radiologically observed to double in size in 138 to 1155 days.[438] Doubling times of human colon carcinoma in cell culture are from 16 to 36 hours. These rates of growth are exceedingly rapid compared with the observed doubling times of such cancers in situ, probably reflecting both a low growth fraction and a large cell loss to desquamation or necrosis.

Colorectal cancer cells have been found to secrete transforming growth factors (TGF) and tumor inhibitory factors (TIF).[439,440] Gastrin receptors have been found in cultured cells.[441,442] Androgen receptors at low levels have been detected.[443] Alford and colleagues studied hormone receptors in 23 primary tumors and found estrogen receptors in 30% and glucocorticoid receptors in 23%; in six patients, there were receptors for the three hormones estrogen, progesterone, and dihydrotesterone.[444] In that study, at least 70% of the tumors had at least one positive receptor. McClendon et al also found estrogen-binding activity in 5 of 21 human colon carcinomas.[445] Additional data have substantiated the presence of multiple hormone receptors.[446]

Ornithine Decarboxylase

The enzyme ornithine decarboxylase (ODC) has been implicated in both tumor promotion and proliferation by increasing polyamine synthesis.[447] It is the rate-limiting enzyme that is essential for mucosal proliferation in the colon.[448] A group at Johns Hopkins has shown that ODC activity increases from normal mucosa, through normal-appearing mucosa in patients with familial polyposis, to nondysplastic polyps in such patients, to dysplastic polyps.[448] Porter and associates found ODC levels eight times greater in cancer specimens than in normal adjacent mucosa; adenomatous polyps were intermediate, although there was a considerable overlap.[449]

Immunology and Markers

A large group of biologically interesting antigens has been detected in association with colorectal cancer cells. The CEA level was discussed earlier as a preoperative prognostic factor. Monoclonal antibody technology will allow identification of multiple additional antigens in the coming years. An overview of various antigens follows.

CARCINOEMBRYONIC ANTIGEN. CEA was referred to as an "Oncofetal protein" after Gold and Freeman isolated it in 1965 from human adult colon cancer and fetal colon epithelium using adsorption and tolerance techniques.[450] It is a heavily glycosylated, single chain peptide of 200,000 daltons molecular weight. Electron microscopic immunochemical techniques demonstrate the protein in normal colonic columnar and goblet cells.[451] Monoclonal antibody technology has indicated a large number of epitopes.[452,453] Studies with these epitopes are under way with the hope of improving the specificity of this antigen in the detection and treatment of colorectal cancer.

BLOOD GROUP ANTIGENS. Multiple investigators have confirmed the lack of expression of normal blood group ABH antigens in the distal colon and rectal mucosa and the presence of such antigens on cancers in these locations.[454-457] A recent report suggests that ABH antigens appear in neoplastic (adenomatous) polyps but not in hyperplastic polyps.[458] Many of the tumor-associated antigens detected with monoclonal antibodies are modified blood group glycolipids.[459] The modified Lewis antigens represent another group of oncofetal antigens[460-462]; variations in their expression are currently of great interest.

CA 19-9. Of the large number of antigens defined on colorectal cancers (albeit not exclusively), one of the most widely studied has been the carbohydrate cell surface antigen, designated 19-9, which was identified by Koprowski and associates.[463] This antigen is a sialylated lacto-*N*-fucopentose that is related to the Lewis blood group substance.[464] CA 19-9 is released into the blood of cancer-bearing patients and is detected with the CA 19-9 assay system. The antigen recognized by this antibody appears to be a class 3 differentiation antigen.[465]

ADDITIONAL MONOCLONAL ANTIBODY-DEFINED ANTIGENS. Koprowski's group defined another antigen identified with monoclonal antibody 17-1A.[466,467] This system has been of particular interest because immunologic inhibition of growth can result with infusion of this antibody. Johnson, Schlom, and associates defined a high molecular weight glycoprotein (referred to as TAG-72) using monoclonal antibody B72.3.[468] Although this antigen is present in 85% of colorectal cancers, there is considerable heterogeneity in its expression in the primary tumor, lymph nodes, and distant metastases.[469]

HUMAN CHORIONIC GONADOTROPIN. Human chorionic gonadotropin (hCG) has been found in approximately 50% of colorectal carcinomas, although increased serum levels are found considerably less often.[470,471] In an immunohistochemical study of 50 colorectal carcinomas, 20 adenomas, 8 ulcerative colitis specimens, and 10 normal mucosa specimens, Campo et al found hCG-producing cells in 52% of the carcinomas but in none of the normal mucosa or benign lesions.[471] They suggest that hCG may be a marker of prognostic significance: hCG was detected in the primary tumor in 15 of 19 patients with lymph node or hepatic metastases, but in only 9 of 23 patients without metastases.

TREATMENT OF PRECANCEROUS COLORECTAL DISEASE

NEOPLASTIC POLYPS (ADENOMAS)

Histologically, neoplastic polyps are tubular, villous, or a combination of both. Villous tumors have a higher propensity to be associated with cancer in the polyp. In addition, patients with multiple villous polyps are more likely to develop additional polyps following removal of the initial lesions. Since the finding of a polypoid mass on endoscopy or barium enema examination does not connote benignity, such lesions should be removed except in the most infirm patients. Almost all pedunculated polyps can be removed by endoscopic snare polpectomy. Sessile lesions can frequently be removed piecemeal, but with an increased risk of perforation. Several sessions may be necessary. Large villous lesions in the cecum and ascending colon may require colectomy.

Data accruing from the National Polyp Study will define more precisely the appropriate follow-up strategies for patients with polyps. Current data from several sources allow us to endorse the follow-up algorithms in Figures 29-8 and 29-9 as general guidelines.[472-475]

The large villous adenoma of the rectum can pose a difficult management problem. Transanal local excision at the level of the submucosa allows complete histologic examination. Some 75% of soft, nonulcerated tumors will prove benign on subsequent examination, 15% will contain superficial cancer, and 10% will contain invasive cancer.[476] Random biopsies of grossly benign-appearing lesions are unreliable and make subsequent surgical excision more difficult.[477] Electrocoagulation with cautery, piecemeal snare excision, and neodymium/yttrium-aluminum-garnet (Nd-YAG) laser ablation have all been used, but preclude complete histologic assessment. Very large tumors can be excised and the mucosa closed by muscle plication and mucosal advancement.[478,479] Low anterior resection, coloanal procedures, and abdominoperineal resection all play a role in the management of extensive benign rectal polyps.

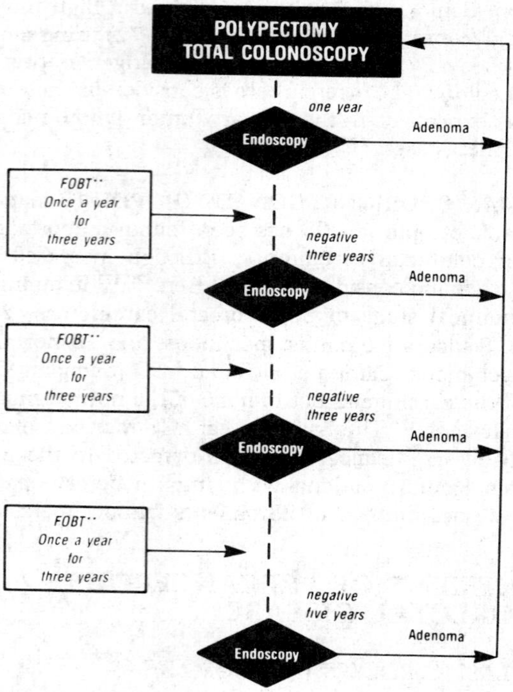

FIG. 29-8. Management of the minimal-risk patient with colorectal adenomas, defined as the patient with a solitary adenoma less than 2 cm, pedunculated, if sessile then having tubular histology, with only mild or moderate dysplasia.[472]

FAMILIAL ADENOMATOUS POLYPOSIS

There is continued controversy as to the appropriate surgical management of patients with familial adenomatous polyposis. Because almost all untreated patients develop colorectal cancer by age 40, prophylactic surgery is warranted. Total abdominal colectomy with ileorectal anastomosis is usually the procedure of choice if the rectum is relatively free of polyps. Bowel function is acceptable, and bladder and sexual function are preserved. The rectal stump must be examined frequently (as often as every 6 months) for signs of cancer. Polyps must be regularly removed or fulgurated. Cancer has been reported to develop in the retained rectal stump in 5% to 60% of patients. The results from the major centers are summarized in Table 29-9. Unquestionably, there is increased risk with increased duration of follow-up. The risk is considerably less if the rectum is not involved by the polyposis (20% of polyposis patients).[480] In patients not willing to risk developing cancer in the retained rectum, or in patients with a carpet of polyps in the rectum, total proctocolectomy is appropriate. In most younger patients, restorative proctocolectomy with a distal mucosal proctectomy and an ileal pouch–anal anastomosis will enhance the quality of life.[485] Multiple aspects of the management of these patients are described in a recent monograph.[486]

ULCERATIVE COLITIS

As described in the section on screening, many patients with ulcerative colitis can be followed endoscopically, with selective surgery performed in those who develop high-grade dys-

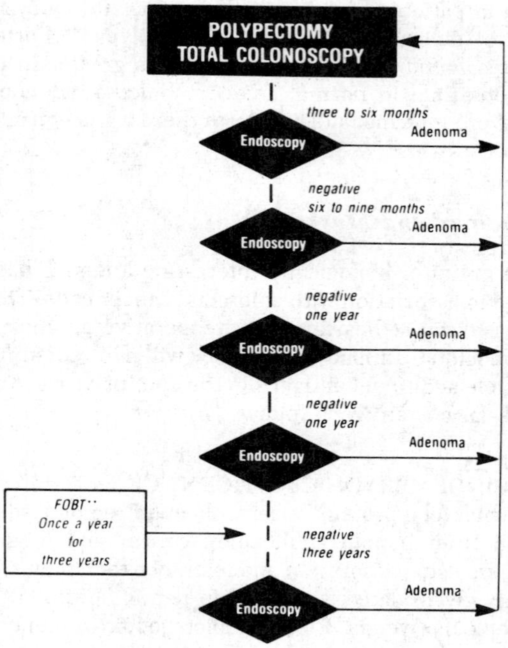

FIG. 29-9. Management of the high-risk patient with colorectal adenomas, defined as multiple adenomas, ≥2 cm, sessile, villous, or tubulovillous, with severe dysplasia, carcinoma in situ, or invasive cancer.[472]

TABLE 29-9. Risk of Rectal Cancer After Abdominal Colectomy for Polyposis

Center	No. of Patients	Subsequent Rectal Cancer
St. Marks Hosp.[481]	174	13% (at 25 yr)
Mayo Clinic[482]	178	59% (at 23 yr)
Memorial Hospital[483]	27	10%
Cleveland Clinic[484]	133	7.5%

plasia or cancer.[487-491] Restorative total proctocolectomy with distal submucosal proctectomy and ileal pouch–anal anastomosis should be considered in the younger patient undergoing elective surgery.[492,493]

TREATMENT OF POTENTIALLY CURABLE COLORECTAL CANCER

The remainder of this chapter describes multimodality treatment strategies for colorectal cancer, cure rates, and patterns of recurrence. Treatment strategies and end results are presented separately for four major disease groups: (1) resectable colon cancer (including cancer of the rectosigmoid), (2) resectable rectal cancers, (3) potentially curable but primarily surgically unresectable colorectal cancers, and (4) recurrent or metastatic disease.

PRETREATMENT EVALUATION

The following are general guidelines for the pretreatment evaluation of potentially curable colorectal disease:

History: In addition to the personal medical history, the family history of colorectal cancer, polyps, and other cancers should be obtained.

Physical Examination: Check for hepatomegaly, ascites, and lymphadenopathy. If rectal cancer is present, determine its distance from the anal verge and dentate line, distance from levators, configuration, mobility, involvement of contiguous organs or the pelvis, and involvement of pararectal nodes. In women, rule out synchronous ovarian pathology and breast cancer.

Laboratory Data: Blood count, CEA, liver chemistries.

GI: Full colonoscopy or proctosigmoidoscopy and air contrast barium enema (in the absence of obstruction or perforation).

Imaging: A preoperative chest radiograph is appropriate. Rectal cancer patients should undergo CT of the abdomen and pelvis, particularly if preoperative radiation therapy is planned. If available, intrarectal US may be helpful. Colon cancer patients need a perioperative CT or US study of their liver as a baseline. This study need not be performed preoperatively if liver chemistries are normal and hepatomegaly is not present.

Surgical: Examination under anesthesia and cystoscopy may be helpful in selected cancer cases.

TREATMENT OF RESECTABLE COLON CANCER, AND END RESULTS

Treatment strategies for potentially curable colon and intraperitoneal rectal cancer remain primarily surgical. However, preliminary data indicate that postoperative chemotherapy may improve the disease-free survival rate in patients who have undergone potentially curative surgery. Results from recent adjuvant systemic and regional portal vein chemotherapy studies supporting this statement will be presented. The rationale for adjuvant radiation in selected patients will be discussed.

GENERAL SURGICAL PRINCIPLES

The morbidity of elective colon surgery is directly related to mechanical and oral antibiotic bowel preparation, the use of perioperative systemic antibiotics, and the skill of the surgical and anesthesia team.

Extent of Bowel Resection

Except for the occasional minimally invasive polypoid cancer, which can frequently be cured by endoscopic polypectomy, en bloc surgical resection is the primary treatment approach in patients with colon cancer. Fortunately, almost all of these cancers can be treated without a permanent or even temporary colostomy. This should be explained to the patient and family at an early point in the consultation, since concern about a colostomy frequently supersedes all other considerations of the patient.

Surgical treatment of colon cancer requires excision of an adequate amount of normal colon proximal and distal to the tumor, adequate lateral margins if the tumor is adherent to a contiguous structure, and removal of the regional lymph nodes. Pathologic studies indicate that tumor rarely spreads more than 1.2 cm longitudinally beyond the area of gross involvement, and a 5-cm margin is more than adequate.[206] However, removal of intermediate and more central (principal) lymph nodes requires ligation and division of multiple main vascular trunks. Hence, the extent of the colonic resection for potentially curable colon cancer is determined by the biology of local tumor growth and by the associated lymphadenectomy.

Extent of Lymph Node Dissection

Patients with colon cancer metastatic to regional lymph nodes may still be cured with surgery. Hence, lymphadenectomy is not only necessary for staging, it is also therapeutic. The paracolic and intermediate lymph nodes are routinely resected, but it is not clear to what extent removal of more central or principal lymph nodes is therapeutic. Enker, Laffer, and Block described excellent results in the treatment of colon cancer which they believed were due in part to an extensive lymphadenectomy.[494] However, Grinnell reported that all 17 patients with carcinoma of the descending colon, sigmoid, or rectum and positive nodes around the origin of the inferior mesenteric artery died of cancer.[495]

Adequate regional lymph node dissection is therefore part of effective therapy for colon cancer. Small segmental resections with removal of only the paracolic lymph nodes are suitable only in the presence of liver metastases or peritoneal seeding, or in medically poor-risk patients. Relevant intermediate nodes should be routinely removed. The extent of resection of central nodes will depend on the patient's age, body habitus, overall medical condition, and the operative findings.

"No Touch" Technique

The discovery of large numbers of tumor cells within the portal vein associated with intraoperative manipulation of the tumor led to the suggestion that the lymphovascular pedicle be ligated prior to mobilization of the primary tumor.[496–498] Current concepts of tumor biology suggest that in the large majority of patients with subsequent liver metastases, micrometastases are already established before the primary tumor is resected. Thus, intraoperative vascular dissemination may play only a small role in the metastatic process. From a practical surgical viewpoint, it can be very difficult and potentially dangerous to isolate vascular structures prematurely. A randomized prospective trial of the "no touch" technique is underway in the Netherlands.[499] Preliminary results suggest a small benefit with preliminary vascular ligation only in the subset of patients with sigmoid colon cancer and histologic evidence of venous invasion. A complete analysis of mature data will be of interest in resolving this controversial issue.

Prevention of Intraluminal Spread

There appears to be little doubt that tumor cells are exfoliated into the intestinal lumen. It is likely that some of these cells are alive and capable of implanting on exposed cut surfaces of the bowel.[237,500] Isolated suture line recurrences are very rare after right colectomy, occurring more often after left-sided colectomies and in rectal operations. The greater longitudinal bowel margins with right-sided colon cancers, and the presence of active digestive enzymes and cytotoxic bile, may explain some of this discrepancy. Stapled anastomoses do not seem to be any more susceptible to tumor implantation than those that are hand-sewn. Precautions to minimize the implantation of cancer cells have been advised[501–503]; those that have shown efficacy in animal studies include isolation of the tumor with ligatures proximal and distal, irrigation of the lumen, Formalin or electrocautery treatment of bowel edges, and use of iodized suture material. No randomized clinical trial has ever tested these hypotheses.

Prophylactic Oophorectomy

Since 2% to 8% of women with colorectal cancer will have synchronous ovarian metastases,[504–506] and 1% to 7% of those who undergo potentially curative resections will develop subsequent ovarian metastases, prophylactic oophorectomy appears to be useful in the overall management of such patients. In addition, such an approach would reduce or eliminate the risk of primary ovarian cancer, which is approximately 1% for women over age 40, and is perhaps higher in colorectal cancer patients.[507] Extensive ovarian metastases are almost always part of widespread recurrent tumor, but it remains unclear as to whether prophylactic removal of grossly normal ovaries containing micrometastatic colonic cancer will actually increase the cure rate.

The mechanism of spread to ovaries remains unclear. It does not appear to be by peritoneal seeding, but more likely by lymphatic or hematogenous pathways. Most authors report that node-positive patients are at greater risk.[505,507,508] However, others are unable to show a predominance of ovarian metastases in node-positive patients.[509,510] Premenopausal women are at greater risk.[504,507] Whether this is related to the presence of steroid receptors in colon cancer cells is unknown.[444]

When nonrandomized patient groups that underwent prophylactic oophorectomy have been compared with appropriate matched controls, no survival benefit has been demonstrated.[505,511] It is likely that a 5% survival benefit is the maximum to be gained from prophylactic oophorectomy.

We recommend that women with colorectal cancer be asked preoperatively for permission to perform a bilateral oophorectomy. If the ovaries are grossly abnormal they should be removed. A hysterectomy is not required in the treatment of ovarian metastases. If a premenopausal woman is considering childbirth, prophylactic oophorectomy is not warranted. However, in the large majority of perimenopausal and postmenopausal women with potentially curable colorectal cancer, consideration should be given to removal of grossly normal ovaries.

SITE-SPECIFIC SURGERY

General guidelines for appropriate operative resection for colon cancers involving the major locations follow. The exact anastomotic technique (*e.g.*, hand-sewn versus stapled anastomoses, use of different suture materials, one or two layers) is not important for the purposes of this chapter; in general, all of these issues are a function of the surgeon's preference.[512]

CECUM/ASCENDING COLON. Tumors in the cecum or ascending colon are treated by right hemicolectomy. The ileocolic and right colic arteries are divided, and usually the right branch of the middle colic (Fig. 29-10). The right ureter, spermatic or ovarian veins, inferior vena cava, superior mesenteric vein, and duodenum are at risk during this procedure. In the obese patient, overly aggressive lymphadenectomy along the superior mesenteric artery can cause catastrophic damage to the superior mesenteric vein, which lies adjacent.

HEPATIC FLEXURE. An extended right hemicolectomy is necessary for tumors in the hepatic flexure. This procedure is identical to that for cancer in the ascending colon, except that the middle colic artery is resected at its origin (Fig. 29-11). The splenic flexure may be mobilized to facilitate anastomosis as well as subsequent endoscopy.

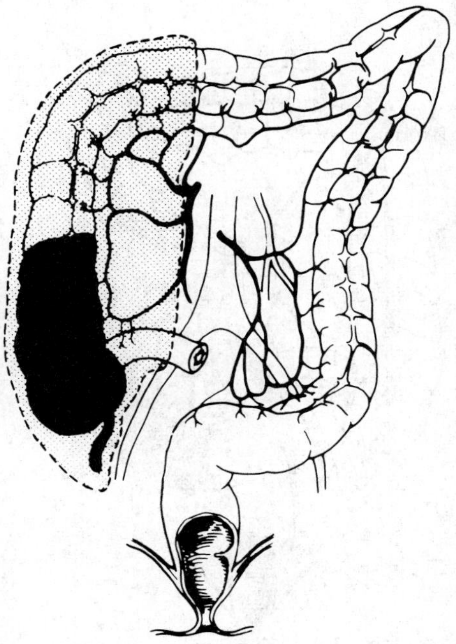

FIG. 29-10. Surgical resection for a cecal or ascending colon cancer.

TRANSVERSE COLON. Lesions of the middle and left transverse colon usually require resection of all colon proximal to the descending colon (Fig. 29-12). The right colon is removed for technical surgical reasons, and not to enhance cancer treatment. A more limited transverse colectomy is also acceptable, particularly with a lengthy ascending colon.

SPLENIC FLEXURE. As described for transverse colon lesions, an extensive resection of all proximal colon gener-

FIG. 29-11. Surgical resection for a cancer at the hepatic flexure.

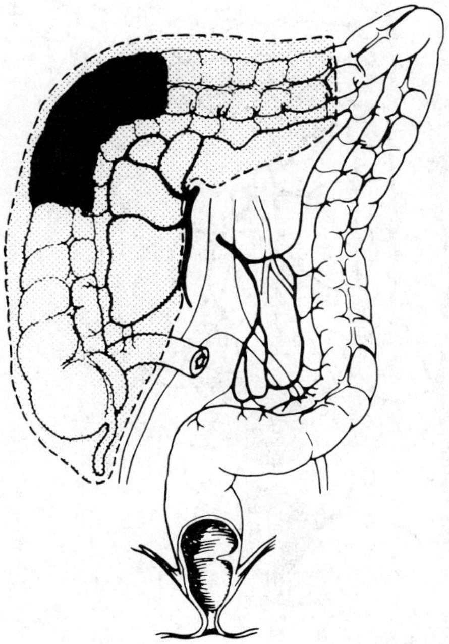

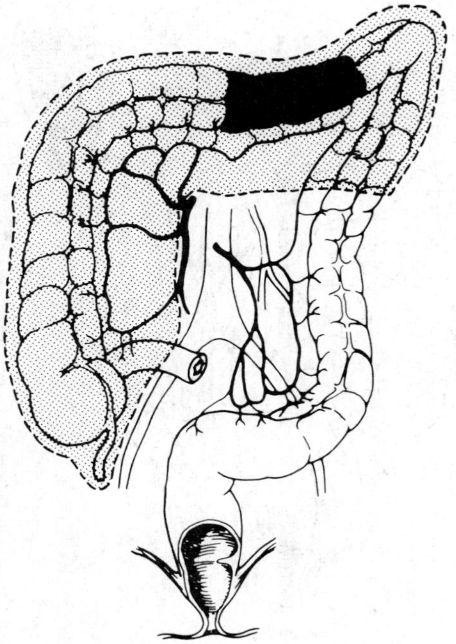

FIG. 29-12. Preferable surgical resection for cancer for the transverse colon. A segmental resection may be appropriate in poor-risk patients.

ally is preferred. The inferior mesenteric artery is preserved but cleared of contiguous nodes (Fig. 29-13). It is also acceptable to preserve the right branch of the middle colic artery and all proximal colon, with the mid-transverse colon anastomosed to the mid-descending colon (Fig. 29-14). Care must always be taken to avoid an unnecessary splenectomy, which may adversely affect survival.[513]

FIG. 29-13. Preferred extensive resection for cancer at the splenic flexure.

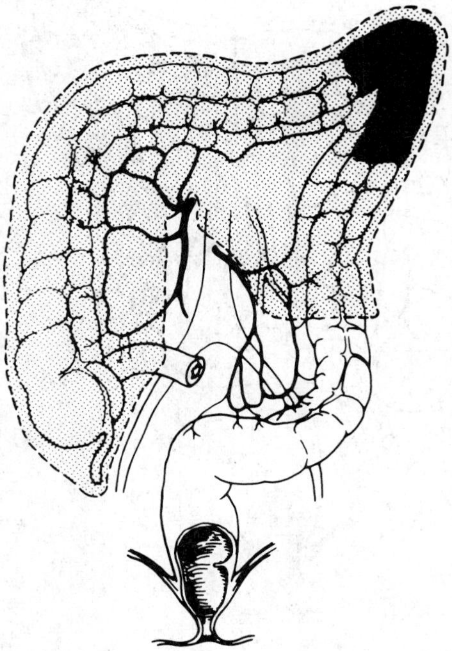

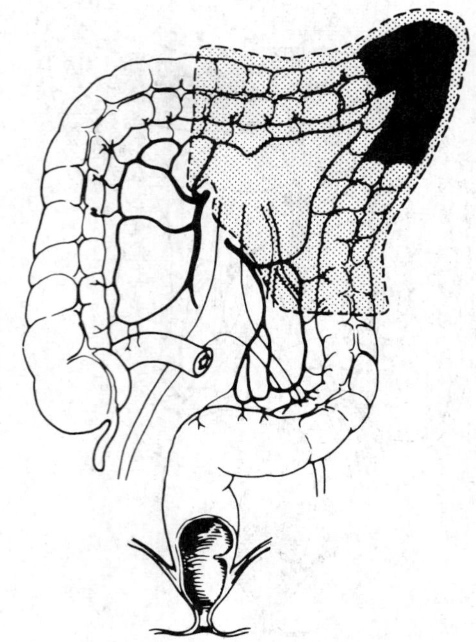

FIG. 29-14. A more limited resection for cancer of the splenic flexure in poor risk patients.

DESCENDING COLON. A left hemicolectomy with high ligation of the inferior mesenteric artery and vein is necessary for cancers of the descending colon. The transverse colon is brought to the distal sigmoid colon at the level of the pelvic brim (Fig. 29-15). The ureters, spermatic or ovarian veins, spleen, and pancreas are all at risk.

FIG. 29-15. Surgical resection for a descending colon cancer.

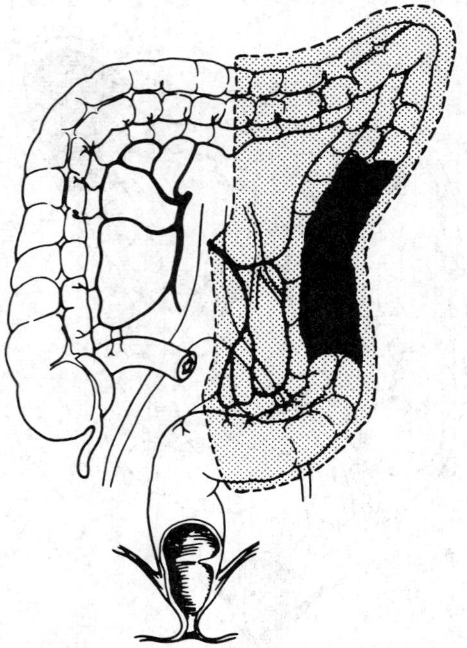

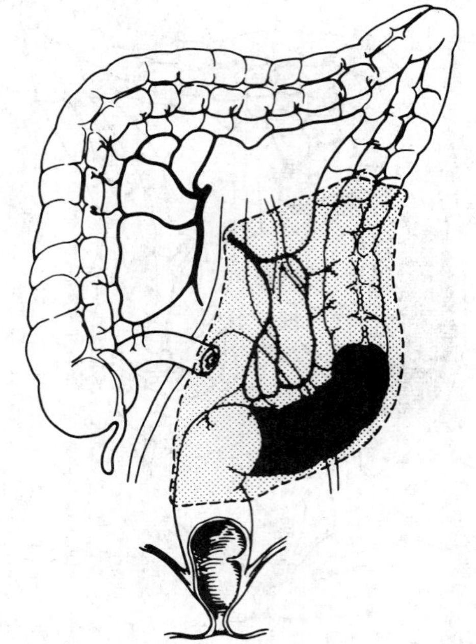

FIG. 29-16. Preferred surgical procedure for cancer of the mid and proximal sigmoid colon. In poor-risk patients, the inferior mesenteric artery and the left colic artery may be preserved.

SIGMOID COLON. Tumors in the sigmoid colon may be resected by wide sigmoid resection, with the superior hemorrhoidal artery ligated just distal to the origin of the left colic artery; or by a complete left hemicolectomy (Fig. 29-16). Both ureters must be identified and the presacral space entered.

FIG. 29-17. Surgical resection for cancer of the rectosigmoid.

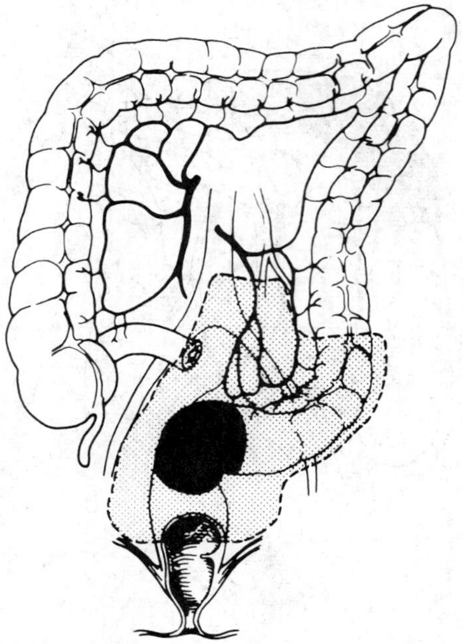

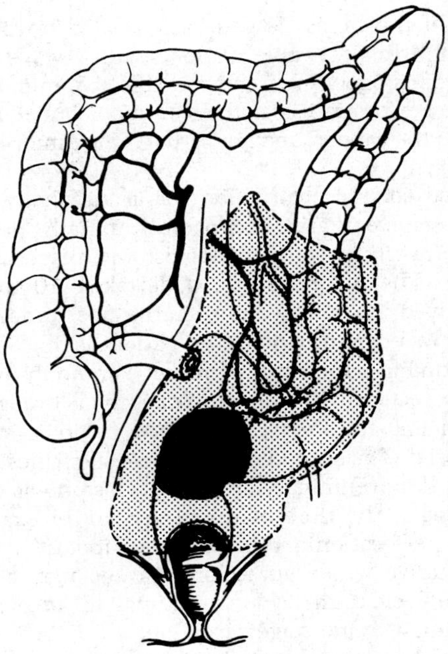

FIG. 29-18. A more radical surgical resection for cancer of the rectosigmoid.

RECTOSIGMOID (INTRAPERITONEAL RECTUM). Tumors of the distal sigmoid and intraperitoneal rectum are treated by "anterior" resection. Both ureters must be identified. The rectum is mobilized from the presacral space. The pelvic peritoneum is incised completely. The anterior prerectal plane along the prostate or vagina is opened. The lateral attachments of the rectum may be preserved. The middle sacral vessels are ligated. The proximal vessels may be ligated just distal to the left colic artery origin (Fig. 29-17) or at the level of the origin of the inferior mesenteric artery (Fig. 29-18). The higher ligation may be necessary to allow mobilization of the splenic flexure and adequate length of the proximal bowel to allow a tension-free anastomosis.

TREATMENT RESULTS

Many variables affect the curability of colorectal cancer. Multivariate analysis indicates that the surgical–pathologic stage is the most important. This section examines expected end results after surgery for potentially curable colon cancer as a function of stage. The impact of the many other prognostic variables on outcome was discussed earlier in the chapter. The management of patients with unresectable primary cancer or synchronous hematogenous metastases is discussed later.

Data appear to suggest that the 5-year survival rates after surgical resection have improved somewhat in recent years. Although such results may indicate the widespread application of appropriate surgical techniques in resecting these cancers, the use of perioperative CT may increase our ability to detect early liver metastases, and therefore to define more accurately the patient population selected for potentially curative surgery. However, whether one looks at a very large experience of a single surgeon (such as that of E. S. R. Hughes in Australia)[327] or the multicenter experience of the United Kingdom Large Bowel Cancer Project,[261] it appears that the majority of patients with colon cancer resectable at the time of laparotomy are cured by surgical extirpation.

TABLE 29-10. Five-Year Survival Rates in Node-Negative Colon Cancer

Study	*Stage*	*Survival (%)*
Willet et al[363]	T1N0M0	97
	T2N0M0	90
	T3N0M0	78
	T4N0M0	63
Eisenberg et al[325]	Dukes' A	82
	Dukes' B	73
GITSG[560,561]	T3N0M0	80

CURE RATES FOR NODE-NEGATIVE PATIENTS. The 5-year survival rate for patients with tumors involving the mucosa or submucosa is in excess of 90%. Muscle wall invasion decreases the 5-year survival rate slightly, to 80%. Transmural penetration is still associated with cure in the majority of patients, with survival in the 60% to 80% range. Data from selected series are listed in Table 29-10.

CURE RATES FOR NODE-POSITIVE PATIENTS. The overall 5-year cure rate for patients with regional lymph node metastases is approximately one third. However, recent data are consistent with a relatively good prognosis in patients with four or fewer lymph nodes involved. The end results reported by the GITSG indicate a survival of 56% in patients with one to four positive nodes. Results from the National Surgical Adjuvant Breast and Bowel Project (NSABP)[514] and the United Kingdom Large Bowel Cancer Project[261] support this distinction. Data from selected series are listed in Table 29-11.

PATTERNS OF RECURRENCE. We will examine local (direct extension), regional (lymphatic/nodal), and peritoneal seeding recurrence patterns.

The major risk of recurrence in patients with colon cancer remains disseminated disease. The liver is involved in as many as two thirds of patients who die of colon cancer.[363] Ovarian metastases develop in up to 7% of women with colon cancer and are a symptomatic problem in approximately half of those patients.

The risk of locoregional failure varies with the pathologic

TABLE 29-11. Five-Year Survival Rates in Node-Positive Colon Cancer

Study	*Stage*	*Survival (%)*
Willet et al[363]	T2N1M0	74
	T3N1M0	48
	T4N1M0	38
Eisenberg et al[325]	Dukes' C	40
GITSG[560,561]	Dukes' C (1–4 nodes)	56
	Dukes' C (>4 nodes)	26

stage of the primary tumor. In addition, posterior penetration in a portion of the colon devoid of serosa may increase the local recurrence rate. In an autopsy series reported from the University of Florida, the local recurrence rate (in patients who died of cancer) was 27% in those with T3N0M0 disease, 21% in those with T2N1M0 disease, and 52% in those with T3N1M0 disease.[515] A similar analysis from the University of Washington identified a 27% recurrence rate in patients with transmural tumor, but 69% if the tumor adhered to or invaded adjacent structures.[516] However, only 19% of the 53 patients autopsied had isolated locoregional recurrences. The rate of disease recurrence in retroperitoneal lymph nodes was 64% in that report, and included some patients with negative nodes in the originally resected specimen.

Recurrence patterns have been analyzed in a group of 533 patients with colon cancer treated at the Massachusetts General Hospital.[363,364] The overall locoregional failure rate was 19%, with only 6% isolated local failures. However, two thirds of the patients with disease recurrence at any site had some component of locoregional failure. The local recurrences correlated with gross transmural penetration of the primary, and particularly with adherence to or invasion of surrounding organs. The local failure rate approached 50% in patients with five or more positive lymph nodes. These findings are supported by a report from the Peter Bent Brigham Hospital, in which patients with sigmoid colon cancer had an overall regional recurrence rate of 18%.[217] However, this represented a two-thirds failure rate in patients with disease recurrence at any site. In half of these patients, failure was expressed as isolated regional recurrence.

In a clinical analysis of node-positive patients at Memorial Hospital, local recurrence was documented in only 6% of 148 patients, representing only 13% of those patients with overall tumor recurrence (Enker WE: Personal communication, 1988).

The incidence of peritoneal seeding has not been well documented. In the autopsy series reported from the University of Washington, treatment failure manifested as peritoneal seeding was identified in 36% of patients who died of colon cancer. Of note, peritoneal seeding occurred in the absence of locoregional recurrence in 58% of those cases.[516] The Massachusetts General Hospital autopsy series has yielded comparable data, a 32% failure rate by peritoneal seeding.[515a]

SPECIFIC MANAGEMENT PROBLEMS IN COLON CANCER

SYNCHRONOUS CANCERS. Synchronous colorectal cancers occur in 3% to 5% of patients.[517,518] In addition, approximately one third of cancer-bearing patients will have associated benign neoplastic polyps. These data suggest that preoperative clearance of the remaining colon is required, either by air contrast barium enema examination or, preferably, by colonoscopy.[519]

OBSTRUCTING CANCERS. Circumferential cancers of the colon may manifest as large bowel obstruction. The acuteness of the illness is generally related to the competence of the ileocecal valve. Patients with a valve that does not allow reflux experience considerable abdominal pain and distention. Perforation is not uncommon, but it is usually proximal to the cancer, and not through the tumor itself (see next section).

Left-sided colonic obstruction was traditionally managed by a three-stage operative approach.[345] Initially, patients underwent a diverting transverse colostomy, or occasionally a cecostomy. The second stage, undertaken 10 to 14 days later, involved tumor resection. As the final procedure, the colostomy was closed. Unless the patient is quite ill, a two-stage Hartmann procedure is more commonly used. The tumor is resected, with the proximal colon brought to the skin as an end-colostomy. The distal colon is sutured or stapled closed. The second operation reestablishes intestinal continuity. If a preliminary diverting colostomy is chosen, it is important at the time of initial surgery to examine the cecum for perforation and the liver for metastases.

Intraoperative whole gut colonic lavage may be used to mechanically clear the colon proximal to an obstruction. This may allow a one-stage resection.

The patient with an obstructing cancer of the ascending or transverse colon can usually be treated with a single-stage resection (Fig. 29-12). An ileal–colon anastomosis is performed, which even in the absence of bowel preparation usually heals without complication. Perioperative systemic antibiotics are essential.

PERFORATING CANCERS. Perforation of the colon can occur proximal to an obstructing cancer. Recognition of this catastrophe and the timely performance of radical surgical resection, peritoneal cavity irrigation, drainage, and antibiotic administration have lessened the morbidity and mortality. Chronic perforations into a contiguous organ with or without fistula formation will be discussed subsequently. Acute free perforations into the peritoneal cavity leading to generalized peritonitis or localized abscess formation can be catastrophic. The differential diagnosis primarily includes appendicitis, diverticulitis, or perforated gastroduodenal ulcer.

CONTIGUOUS ORGAN INVOLVEMENT. Direct involvement of adjacent organs occurs in approximately 10% of patients. Extended surgery in such patients is associated with cure rates of 20% to 50%.[346,520,521] The tumor-bearing colon may be adherent due to inflammatory adhesions, or may be attached by direct penetration of tumor. Penetration into an adjacent hollow organ such as bladder or small bowel may lead to a fistula. Almost one half of clinically adherent or invaded viscera are attached by inflammatory adhesions only.[521] All such attachments should be presumed to be due to direct tumor penetration and should not be divided and biopsied. If such attachments are inadvertently torn, the survival (albeit by retrospective analysis) is half that associated with direct multivisceral resection.[521,522]

CANCER IN POLYPS. Cancer is present in approximately 5% of adenomatous polyps.[523] Cancers invasive to the level of the muscularis mucosa do not have access to the lym-

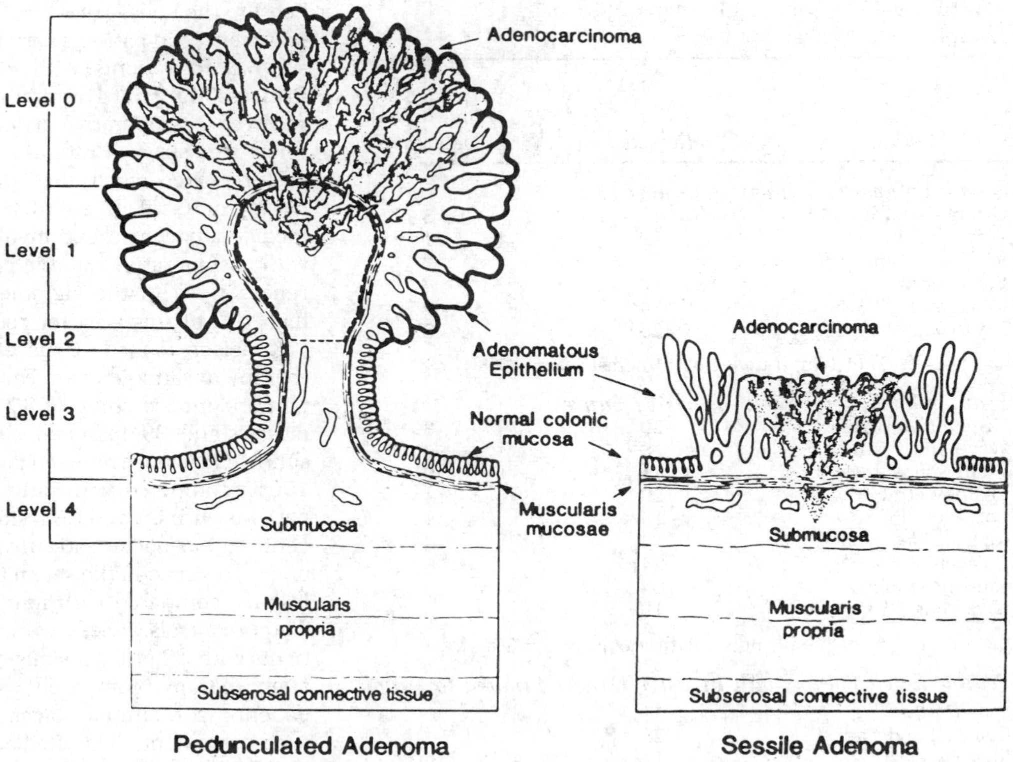

FIG. 29-19. Levels of invasion in a pedunculated adenoma (*left*) and a sessile adenoma (*right*). The stippled areas represent zones of carcinoma. Note that any invasion below the muscularis mucosae in a sessile lesion represents Level 4 invasion (submucosa). In contrast, invasive carcinoma in a pedunculated adenoma must traverse a considerable distance before it reaches the submucosa of the underlying bowel wall. However, any cancer that penetrates the muscularis mucosae is at risk for dissemination. (Haggitt RC, Glotzbach RE, Soffer EE, et al: Prognostic factors in colorectal carcinomas arising in adenomas: Implications for lesions removed by endoscopic polypectomy. Gastroenterology 89:328–336, 1985)

phatic pathways and can be cured by endoscopic or surgical polypectomy. This section considers the treatment of cancer invasive at least through the muscularis mucosa in an otherwise benign adenomatous or villous polyp. The extent of invasion must be considered, and whether the polyp is pedunculated or sessile. After endoscopic polypectomy of such lesions, one must address the risk of residual localized or nodal cancer versus the risk of definitive colectomy. Decision analysis theory can be applied for more elegant help with this troublesome problem.[524]

Figure 29-19 defines the various levels of invasion and helps in conceptualizing the problem. In addition to the level of invasion, histopathologic features to be taken into account include the degree of differentiation (grade), the presence of lymphatic or blood vessel invasion, and the adequacy of endoscopic resection (margin). Patients at high risk for local residual or nodal metastatic cancer have polyps containing one or several of the following features: poorly differentiated cancer, lymphatic vessel invasion, tumor invasive to level 3 or 4, or a positive or close polypectomy margin.[525–528]

The major issue is the risk of lymph node metastases. Colacchio and colleagues have documented what they feel is an unacceptable risk associated with conservative (nonresective) management of most of these patients.[529] The overall risk of nodal metastases is reported by these authors to be 10%. Nivatongs looked only at patients who subsequently underwent surgical resection and defined subsets based on polyp configuration and gross extent of invasion. His data and review of the literature provide the most realistic appraisal of the risk of lymph node metastases (Table 29-12). Since approximately half of patients with lymph node metastases die of cancer, the incremental survival benefit from surgery for cancer limited to the head of a polyp is only 1.5%.

In summary, polypectomy alone can cure almost all patients with a moderately or well-differentiated cancer limited to the head of a pedunculated adenomatous polyp, with clear margins on the stalk, and no histopathologic evidence of lymphatic vessel invasion. The polypectomy site should be examined endoscopically in 4 to 6 months to confirm the absence of mucosal recurrence.

Not all polyps can be removed endoscopically. Large sessile lesions, particularly of the thin-walled ascending colon, pose a major therapeutic challenge. Large villous tumors have a high likelihood (up to 40%) of containing carcinoma in the polyp. Hence, limited biopsies are subject to extensive sampling error false negatives. If endoscopic removal is attempted, piecemeal removal with the snare cautery over several sessions is required. Such patients should be observed as inpatients for 1 to 2 days to rule out a perforation. Large benign sessile adenomas may require surgical resection as the least morbid approach to removal.

ADJUVANT THERAPIES FOR COLON CANCER

Adjuvant Radiation Therapy

Adjuvant radiation therapy for colon carcinoma has been approached with two different philosophies, which we will consider separately: (1) localized irradiation to the tumor bed and potentially positive nodal sites, and (2) whole abdominal irradiation.

TABLE 29-12. Cancer in Polyps: Risk of Lymph Node Metastases

Study	No. Resected	No. of Lymph Node Metastases
Sessile Polyps with Invasive Cancer		
Grinnell and Lane[531]	13	3
Waye and Frankel[532]	9	1
Wolff and Shinya[523]	5	2
Locke et al[533]	12	4
Kodaira et al[534]	34	2
Nivatvongs[530]	25	3
% of lymph nodes with metastases = 15%		
Pedunculated Polyps with Invasive Cancer		
Grinnell and Lane[531]	39	3
Waye and Frankel[532]	8	0
Wolff and Shinya[523]	11	0
Shatney et al[535]	23	1
Locke et al[533]	15	1
Coutsoftides et al[536]	13	0
Colacchio et al[529]	24	6
Kodaira et al[534]	64	3
Nivatvongs[530]	16	3
% of lymph nodes with metastases = 8%		
Pedunculated Polyps with Invasive Cancer Limited to Head of Polyp		
Grinnell and Lane[531]	28	0
Shatney et al[535]	14	0
Nivatvongs[530]	12	0
Colacchio et al[529]	11	2
% of lymph nodes with metastases = 3%		

Nivatongs S: Management of polyps containing invasive carcinoma. In Codner IJ, Fry RD, Roe JP (eds): Colon, Rectal, and Anal Surgery 1985, pp 183–188. St. Louis, CV Mosby, 1985.

Adjuvant radiation therapy for colon carcinoma is associated with special problems of toxicity because of the large amount of small bowel that may lie in the treatment field. Radiologic imaging with contrast materials can be used to determine the location and mobility of small bowel while planning the treatment. A good shift of the small bowel can be achieved by placing the patient in the lateral decubitus position, allowing the target area to be treated with a minimum of bowel present.[537] Other techniques to reduce radiation toxicity will be discussed later.

Locoregional Adjuvant Irradiation

Several nonrandomized reports indicate that locoregional adjuvant irradiation improves local control of cancer of the cecum, a site at high risk for local recurrence. Doses of 4000 to 6000 cGy plus boost treatment have been used on primary and nodal drainage sites.[538–541] Shehata et al used postoperative radiation therapy on 40 patients and found that after a median follow-up of 4 years, 21 of the 31 living patients had had no recurrences. There were four local failures, one being an isolated local recurrence.[540]

In a study of 80 patients with Stages B2(g) to C3 colon tumors at various sites, Duttenhaver and associates gave 4500 cGy to the tumor bed, occasionally with a 540-cGy boost to the nodal areas.[542] Radiation therapy decreased local recurrences in patients with B3 and C2 disease and improved survival in patients with B3, C2, and C3 disease. At the Princess Margaret Hospital in Toronto, 82 patients who had received postoperative irradiation had a 67% local recurrence-free survival rate at 5 years.[541] Patients in whom disease recurred locally had primarily Stage B2 (3 of 18 patients) or C (9 of 24) disease. Duttenhaver et al did not include adjacent organ involvement in their analysis. Even with postoperative radiation therapy, 8 of the 25 local recurrences were in the sigmoid colon, which emphasizes the high risk of this area for recurrent disease.

Kopelson looked at the effect of postoperative radiation therapy in sigmoid colon cancer after curative resection in a nonrandomized study of 17 patients with Stages B2 to C3 disease and 39 matched controls.[543] The 5-year actuarial survival rate for irradiated patients with B2 or B3 disease was 100%, compared with only 64% in the control group. For patients with C2 and C3 lesions, the survival difference from controls was not statistically significant. At 3 years there was one recurrence in the seven irradiated patients with B2 or B3 lesions, compared with four recurrences in the 17 nonirradiated controls. There were no recurrences in the five patients with C2 or C3 lesions who received postoperative radiation therapy, compared with three recurrences in eight patients with similar stages of disease who did not receive such treatment. The Radiation Therapy Oncology Group (RTOG) and Eastern Cooperative Oncology Group (ECOG) are cooperating in a randomized study to compare the effects of "sandwich" radiation therapy versus postoperative radiation therapy alone. Patients are randomly assigned to receive preoperative low-dose radiation therapy for tumors in fixed portions of the large bowel and rectum. After surgery, patients with Stage B2, B3, or C tumors receive radiation therapy.[544] The ECOG also has a study in progress involving adjuvant large-field radiation therapy with low dose per fraction irradiation to the tumor bed, draining nodes, and liver for C1 and C2 colon tumors that have been completely excised.

Whole Abdomen Adjuvant Irradiation

Whole abdominal radiation therapy for patients with colon carcinoma has been explored by several investigators. In a series of papers from the Albert Einstein Medical Center, Turner, Ghossein, and their colleagues have described results in patients who received approximately 2100 cGy to the whole abdomen by a moving strip technique.[545–547] The right lobe of the liver received a dose of 1500 cGy. Seventeen of 31 patients were alive after a minimum follow-up of 1 year (mean follow-up, 2 years).[546] In five patients disease recurred locally with or without distant metastases; eight had distant metastases only. One patient died of radiation enteritis. Other studies of whole abdominal radiation therapy suggest a benefit.[548,549]

The Princess Margaret Hospital is conducting a randomized trial in patients with completely resected B2 and C colon carcinoma. Patients are randomly assigned to surgery alone, or 2200 cGy delivered over 4½ weeks to the whole abdomen.[549]

Abdominal Irradiation and Chemotherapy

Intraperitoneal 5-fluorouracil (5-FU) combined with local–regional radiation therapy may enhance local, peritoneal cavity, and hepatic control.[544] The SWOG has completed a Phase I–II trial of concomitant bolus 5-FU and whole abdominal irradiation, with modest toxicity.[550] The same group has recently activated a program of concomitant continuous infusion of 5-FU with whole abdominal irradiation.

Adjuvant Systemic Therapy for Colon Cancer

As the natural history of colon cancer has been better defined, patient populations at increased risk for overall recurrence after surgery have been identified. Systemic chemotherapy has been administered after primary resection for those with poor prognoses. The first generation of adjuvant trials was initiated in the late 1950s and is summarized in Table 29-13.[351,551–554] These were studies of heterogeneous patient groups, often including patients with colonic and rectal primaries, patients who had undergone curative and palliative resections, and all Dukes' stages. Only thiotepa and the fluoropyrimidines, 5-FU and floxuridine (FUDR), were available, and were usually employed with suboptimal intensity.

Despite these flaws in study design and conduct, relatively large patient cohorts were accrued and studied, establishing the clinical and scientific basis for subsequent adjuvant efforts. The trials listed in Table 29-13 are conventionally considered "negative studies," since dramatic benefits were not elicited. However, the third and fourth Veterans Administration Surgical Oncology Group (VASOG)[553] and the Central Oncology Group (COG)[554] studies demonstrated a 5% to 10% benefit in 5-year survival. For Dukes' C colon cancer, a significant disease-free survival benefit was noted ($p = 0.026$): 40% of adjuvantly treated patients had recurrences at 5 years, versus 52% of patients not given systemic adjuvant treatment.[554] Moreover, an overall analysis of the fluoropyrimidine trials indicates a relatively consistent therapeutic effect, confirmed by statistical pooling methodology.[555,556] Given the available drugs, existing pharmacologic understanding, size of patient groups studied, and dose intensity of therapy offered, it is not surprising that a major therapeutic impact was not observed. Rather, it is interesting that benefits were noted for any of the trials.

TABLE 29-13. First-Generation Randomized Trials of Adjuvant Therapy for Large Bowel Cancer*

Study	*Study Period*	*Treatment*		*Total Accrual*
		Regimen	*Duration*	
Dixon et al,[551]	1957–60	Thiotepa	2 days	695
Dwight et al,[351]	1957–61	Thiotepa	2 days	1064
Dwight et al,[552]	1961–64	FUDR	7 wk	548
Higgins et al,[553]	1965–69	5-FU	6 wk	308
	1969–73	5-FU	18 mo	518
Grage and Moss,[554]	1971–76	5-FU	12 mo	233

*All studies had a surgery-only control group.
FUDR = floxuridine; 5-FU = 5-fluorouracil.

The second generation of studies focused on combinations of agents and included both chemotherapy and immunotherapy. Table 29-14 describes six major trials initiated in the 1970s.[557–561] Five of the six studies employed a surgery-only control group (the exception was the ECOG 2276 study). Five utilized a combination of 5-FU + methyl-CCNU, with (MOF) or without (MF) vincristine. Combination chemotherapy—MF or MOF—was presumed to be more active than 5-FU alone in advanced disease. The empirical application of nonspecific immunotherapy with bacillus Calmette-Gúerin (BCG), BCG-MER (BCG with methanol extraction residue of BCG), or levamisole was studied. More than 4000 patients were evaluated; a trend favoring chemotherapy was noted in several studies, but statistically significant benefit was detected only in the NSABP C01 and the North Central Cancer Treatment Group (NCCTG) 78-48-52 studies.

In the NSABP C01 study, conducted from 1977 to 1983, 1116 patients were randomly assigned to observation, chemotherapy, or immunotherapy. There was a statistically significant superiority in both disease-free survival ($p = 0.05$) and overall survival ($p = 0.04$) for the MOF chemotherapy group compared to the control group. A patient not receiving adjuvant chemotherapy had a 1.34 greater likelihood of dying than his counterpart who did, a 5% to 8% survival improvement at the interim analysis.[559] Patients with right-sided colonic tumors appeared to derive the most salutary benefits. BCG treatment had no discernible impact on overall survival.

Based on preliminary data reported by Verhaegen et al,[562] the NCCTG assigned 408 patients to receive either the presumed immunomodulatory agent levamisole, 5-FU + levamisole, or observation only (see Table 29-14). With a median follow-up of 56 months, the levamisole and 5-FU + levamisole regimens improved disease-free survival ($p = 0.02$ to 0.04), especially for patients with Dukes' C lesions. Toxic effects were generally mild and reversible. These beneficial effects formed the rationale for the large intergroup study (INT 0035) described in Table 29-15.

Several preliminary conclusions were drawn from these second-generation studies. The benefits of adjuvant therapy were confidently observed only in large-scale clinical trials. No single therapeutic program could be recommended for all patients, but several attractive options existed. Another lesson learned was that methyl-CCNU had unexpected chronic bone marrow toxicity; acute nonlymphocytic leukemia was noted in 14 of 2067 adjuvantly treated patients. The excess risk to those receiving large doses of methyl-CCNU as an adjuvant was estimated to be 2.3 : 1000 persons per year. The promising leads developed in the second-generation trials are being pursued in the currently active group studies (see Table 29-15).

The NSABP in protocol C03 plans to utilize MOF as its standard control regimen. However, the total amount of therapy is decreased to 46 weeks (five cycles) to attempt to reduce the chance of nitrosourea-associated leukemia. A program of 5-FU biochemical modulation by folinic acid (leucovorin) will be compared to MOF (see Chemotherapy for Metastatic Colorectal Disease). Of interest will also be the results of a National Cancer Institute of Canada (NCIC) adjuvant study of 5-FU + folinic acid, initiated in 1987. This

TABLE 29-14. Second-Generation Colon Cancer Adjuvant Trials

Study	*Total Accrual*	*Chemotherapy*	*Immunotherapy*	*Chemoimmunotherapy*	*Results*
VASOG 5[557]	654	5-FU, 9 mg/kg on d 1, + methyl-CCNU, 120 mg/m² on d 1, every 7 wk for 12 cycles			MF results in survival benefit for Dukes' C1
GITSG 6175[558]	621	5-FU, 325 mg/m² on d 1–5, 375 mg/m² on d 36–40, + methyl-CCNU, 130 mg/m² on d 1, every 10 wk for 7 cycles	BCG-MER, 1 mg intradermally (ID) on d 1 and 0.5 mg ID once weekly at wk 1, 5, 10, 15, 20, 25, 40, 55, 70	MF + BCG-MER	Apparent overall improved survival compared to historical controls
ECOG 2276 —(unpublished)	866	5-FU + methyl-CCNU, same as GITSG 6175, for 8 cycles or 5-FU, 450 mg/m²/d × 5 d, every 5 wk for 15 cycles			
NSABP C01[559]	1166	MF, same as in GITSG 6175 protocol, + VCR, 1 mg/m² on d 1 every 10 wk for 8 cycles	BCG, 6 × 10⁸ organisms by scarification weekly for 12 wk, then every other week for 33 wk		MOF results in 67% 5-year survival, vs. 58% for control
SWOG 7510[560]	626	5-FU, 400 mg/m² on d 1, 8, 15, + methyl-CCNU, 175 mg/m² on d 1, every 8 wk for 7 cycles		MF + BCG (6 × 10⁸ organisms PO) every other wk for 26 wk	Superior disease-free survival benefit for MF ± BCG
NCCTG 78-48-52[561]	398		Levamisole, 150 mg on d 1, 2, 3 every 3 wk	Levamisole + 5-FU, 450 mg/m², weekly for 52 wk	5-FU ± levamisole results in superior disease-free survival

MF = methyl-CCNU + 5-FU; VCR = vincristine; BCG = bacillus Calmette-Guérin; MER = methanol extraction residue of BCG; VASOC = Veterans Administration Surgical Oncology Group; GITSG = Gastrointestinal Tumor Study Group; ECOG = Eastern Cooperative Oncology Group; NSABP = National Surgical Adjuvant Breast and Bowel Project; SW = Southwest Oncology Group; NCCTG = North Central Cancer Treatment Group.

TABLE 29-15. Currently Active Cooperative Group Trials of Adjuvant Systemic Therapy for Colon Cancer

Study	*Projected Accrual*	*Treatment/Arm*	*Comments*
INT 0035	300	Control 5-FU + levamisole	Dukes' B
	900	Control Levamisole 5-FU + levamisole	Dukes' C (Study duplicates and attempts to confirm NCCTG 78-48-52)
NSABP C03	855	MOF	Similar to NSABP C01, but only 5 —courses
		5-FU + folinic acid	Similar to regimen of Petrelli et al[817]
NCIC C03	400	Control 5-FU + folinic acid MOF	Similar to regimen of Ehrlichman et al[825]; high-dose FA
NCCTG 87-46-51	450	Control 5-FU + folinic acid. γ-interferon	Low-dose FA

INT = Intergroup; NSABP = National Surgical Adjuvant Breast and Bowel Project; NCIC = National Cancer Institute of Canada; NCCTG = North Central Cancer Treatment Group.

study has a surgery-alone control arm. The intergroup study (INT 0035) is attempting to confirm the NCCTG levamisole ± 5-FU experience. Begun in 1985, NCCTG, SWOG, and ECOG plan to accrue 1200 Dukes' B and C patients by late 1987.

There has never before been so much documentation to support the contention that adjuvant systemic therapy is of value for Dukes' B and C colon cancer patients. It is not possible to specify precisely which regimen is optimal for each patient subgroup at this time. Nonetheless, the current generation of national trials presents an ideal opportunity to confirm the magnitude and character of the impact of adjuvant therapy, and patients and physicians should be encouraged to participate. However, it is important to note that four of five major trials continue to use a surgery only control.

Adjuvant Portal Vein Chemotherapy

The rationale for adjuvant perioperative infusion of chemotherapy into the portal vein is based on the observation that, at the time of surgery, tumor cells embolize the portal venous system, seeding the liver.[337,563] Fisher and Turnbull in 1955 demonstrated tumor cells in the portal circulation in 32% of patients at the time of colonic carcinoma resection.[251] Moreover, there is considerable clinical and autopsy evidence that the liver may be the most frequent, and sometimes the only, site of metastasis.[337,563] Although established metastases are fed primarily by the hepatic artery, micrometastases are likely to still be dependent on the portal venous blood.

In 1975 Taylor et al began a randomized study of intraportal 5-FU, 700 mg/m²/d, with heparin, infused continuously for 7 days immediately postoperatively for patients with Dukes' A, B, and C lesions. Approximately 250 patients were studied; by 1985, with a greater than 50-month median follow-up, 80 deaths had occurred. Patients with Dukes' B colon cancer appeared to have a substantial survival benefit ($p = 0.002$) with intraportal venous 5-FU.[564] This preliminary study stimulated several randomized trials of generally similar design.

The Australia and New Zealand Trial evaluated 372 patients with colon cancer randomly allocated to observation alone or immediate postoperative chemotherapy with 5-FU, 600 mg/m²/d for 7 days given intravenously or intraportally. Compared to the other two groups, portal vein 5-FU infusion resulted in a highly significant superior disease-free and overall survival in Dukes' C patients.[565] These data are not fully mature and require further follow-up in order to determine the magnitude and duration of benefits.

A second study of similar design was conducted by the Swiss Group for Clinical Cancer Research (SAKK).[566] From 1981 to 1986, 378 evaluable patients who had undergone resection for Dukes' A, B, or C lesions were allocated to a control or a chemotherapy group; the chemotherapy group received immediate postoperative intraportal 5-FU, 500 mg/m²/d, with 5,000 units of heparin, given by continuous infusion for 7 days. On the first day of therapy, a 10 mg/m² bolus of mitomycin C was also administered. After a median follow-up of 24 months, recurrences were detected in 43 of 187 control patients, compared with 34 of 191 infused patients ($p < 0.05$). Too few deaths have occurred to establish a significant observable difference in survival, and a longer follow-up period is required before definitive conclusions can be drawn.

TABLE 29-16. Currently Active U.S. Studies of Adjuvant Portal Vein Chemotherapy

Study	*Projected Accrual*	*Treatment/Arm*
NCCTG 69-46-04	220	Control 5-FU, 500 mg/m²/d × 7 d, + heparin
NSABP C02	1334	Control 5-FU, 600 mg/m²/d × 7 d, + heparin

In the United States there are currently two active Phase III trials evaluating perioperative portal venous chemotherapy. Described in Table 29-16, these two studies should provide considerable information. Of special importance is the NSABP C02 study, since, with 1,334 patients, it will be the largest single trial of portal venous chemotherapy. It is anticipated that both studies will complete accrual by 1988 and that preliminary survival data will be available 1 to 3 years thereafter.

Use of a chemotherapy program such as that described by Taylor et al[564] in the immediate postoperative recovery period is attractive because of its convenience, modest toxicity, and relative lack of added expense. The clinical results reported to date are promising, but the impact of adjuvant portal venous chemotherapy on overall survival is not yet sufficiently clear that this therapy can be routinely recommended at this time. If ongoing trials confirm efficacy, subsequent programs will have to integrate systemic and portal venous chemotherapy.

Summary of Adjuvant Treatment for Colon Cancer

Less than 1% of all patients with colorectal cancer are entered into randomized trials. In order to help define further benefits of adjuvant treatment, patient participation in randomized trials is strongly encouraged. Preliminary data suggest a potential survival benefit with adjuvant chemotherapy. Pending maturation of recently initiated studies, high-risk patients should be considered for treatment. Adjuvant irradiation may also play a role in highly selected patients.

TREATMENT OF RESECTABLE RECTAL CANCER, AND END RESULTS

In the patient's mind, the treatment of rectal cancer is frequently associated with a colostomy. In some patients such concern may lead to a delay in seeking medical care. Fortunately, at most only one third of patients with rectal cancer require a permanent colostomy. For most patients, the primary treatment modality is radical surgical resection. As described in this section, the results of these primarily surgical approaches can be improved with adjuvant therapy, and several techniques can be utilized to maximize both local and overall cure rates of resectable colon cancers.

TABLE 29-17. Treatment of Cancers of the Extraperitoneal Rectum (<11 cm from Anal Verge)*

Abdominoperineal resection
Low anterior resection
End-to-end versus side-to-end
Sutures versus staples
Abdominosacral resection
Coloanal resection
Endoanal versus pull-through
Staples versus sutures
Localized procedures
Local excision
Fulguration
Endocavitary radiation/brachytherapy

*Exclusive of adjuvant therapies.

SITE-SPECIFIC TREATMENT OPTIONS

For surgical resections, the rectum is generally considered in three distinct sections in relation to the anal verge: the upper third, middle third, and lower third. These sections roughly correlate with 5-cm intervals. Treatment options for cancers of the lower two thirds of the rectum (extraperitoneal rectum) are outlined in Table 29-17.

UPPER THIRD. Treatment of cancers in the distal sigmoid or intra-abdominal rectum (rectosigmoid), cure rates, and patterns of recurrent cancer are similar to those of the more proximal colon. Tumors in the upper third of the rectum have their lowermost edge 11 to 12 cm from the anal verge. Extirpation is primarily surgical, by anterior or low anterior resection. In an anterior resection of the rectosigmoid, the rectum is mobilized from the sacral hollow. However, with a low anterior resection, the lateral rectal attachments (middle hemorrhoidal arteries) are divided. Bowel continuity is always restorable, either end to end or side to end. Single- or double-layer sutures or staples are suitable.

MIDDLE THIRD. Cancers in the middle third of the rectum are quite problematic to treat, because abdominoperineal resection with permanent colostomy does *not* yield superior results to those achieved with sphincter-saving surgical treatment.[567] Hence, every effort should be made to restore intestinal continuity in patients with cancers 6 to 11 cm from the anal verge. Overall surgical success depends not only on surgical expertise but also on patient body habitus, pelvic width, and the presence of associated colonic disease such as diverticulosis.

LOWER THIRD. Almost all cancers in the lower 5 cm of the rectum require an abdominoperineal resection. The abdominosacral resection or stapled low anterior resection may be feasible with early tumors if small margins are accepted. The restorative proctectomy with a coloanal anastomosis can be used in selected patients. Local procedures may also be appropriate for selected patients with low rectal cancers (see below).

EXTENT OF SURGERY ISSUES

Prior to describing the essential features of the various approaches outlined in Table 29-17, we will address a number of issues relevant to radical extirpative surgery.

DISTAL MUCOSAL MARGIN. One of the pivotal aspects of sphincter-saving surgery for patients with distal rectal cancers is the requirement to obtain an "adequate distal margin." A 5-cm distal margin is traditionally cited in surgical texts. The data do not support this rule. Distal spread may be via submucosal direct extension or intramural lymphatics. The spread may be continuous or discontinuous (satellites). Histologic examination of the bowel wall distal to the gross tumor reveals a predominance of tumors without any distal spread, and only 2.5% with spread greater than 2 cm.[567] The few patients with extensive distal spread usually have poorly differentiated, node-positive rectal cancers that disseminate rapidly.[568] A recent report from Copenhagen confirmed that a margin of 1.5 cm is adequate for potentially curable tumors.[569] There is no correlation between the risk of suture line or local recurrence and the extent of distal margin in excess of 2 cm.[570,571]

Measured operative surgical margins always exceed pathologically measured margins, because of shrinkage of the specimen. Because of the potential for miscalculation during the operative procedure, we recommend a surgical margin of 3 cm. If the transanal intraluminal circular stapler is used, margins of 2 cm plus the additional distal "donut" specimen are adequate. Exceptions are bulky, poorly differentiated or anaplastic carcinomas, which may require a longer distal margin to maximize local control. It is unacceptable to intraoperatively surgically transect a rectal cancer in a desperate attempt to avoid a permanent colostomy.

EXTENT OF PROXIMAL LYMPH NODE DISSECTION. In patients with rectal cancer the mesorectum should be removed to the level of the aortic bifurcation. This will include all nodes just distal to the origin of the left colic artery, but not the periaortic nodes or those along the inferior mesenteric artery. A nonrandomized comparison of "high ligation" of the inferior mesenteric artery and resection distal to the left colic artery, reported by the St. Mark's Hospital group, did not elicit any survival benefit for the higher lymphadenectomy group.[572] The results in patients from whom pathologically positive nodes along the inferior mesenteric artery were surgically removed justify limiting routine resection to below the left colic origin: Hojo et al had only one 5-year survivor,[573] and Grinnell none.[574] However, technically it is frequently necessary to divide the inferior mesenteric artery and vein in order to mobilize an adequate length of proximal colon to reach the rectal or anal remnant in sphincter-saving surgical procedures.

EXTENT OF PELVIC (DISTAL AND LATERAL) DISSECTION. Although the studies reviewed above justify a more limited mucosal distal margin than was recommended in the past, the extent of surgical excision of distal lymphatics or lymph nodes has not been discussed. These structures reside within the mesorectum. In a report by Williams and colleagues, only 3 of 50 patients who underwent abdominoperineal resection had positive lymph nodes caudad to the tumor within the mesorectum;[568] these cases were poorly differentiated cancers. Heald et al have strongly advocated complete excision of the mesorectum for distal rectal cancers, reporting an astonishing local recurrence rate of only 3.7% with such an approach.[575,576]

The appropriate extent of the lateral dissection for rectal cancer remains controversial. A formal pelvic lymphadenectomy is feasible in young slender patients. Not only does the procedure remove iliac and obturator lymph nodes, it may remove pararectal tissue more effectively. An adequate lateral dissection is crucial to effective local control.[576a] Such surgery may be associated with greater blood loss, a greater overall complication rate, more bladder dysfunction, and uniform erectile impotency in males.

Interest in formal pelvic lymph node dissection has been limited to a number of centers: Memorial Sloan–Kettering Cancer Center, the University of Chicago, St. Mark's Hospital, and the National Cancer Center Hospital in Tokyo. Elegant studies by Hojo et al have defined the incidence of metastasis to the various nodal groups.[573] These data were presented earlier in this chapter. An approximate 10% improvement in 5-year survival has been reported by a number of authors from these centers.[577–580] The survival benefit was most notable in patients who underwent a sphincter-saving procedure.[581] In a nonrandomized comparative report from St. Mark's Hospital, no survival advantage could be demonstrated with extended abdominopelvic nodal dissection.[582]

In summary, although a limited (2–3 cm) distal mucosal margin is adequate, local cure of rectal cancer requires maximum extirpation of mesorectal and lateral pararectal tissues. The role of formal pelvic lymphadenectomy is not defined.

RADICAL TREATMENT OPTIONS

ABDOMINOPERINEAL RESECTION. Abdominoperineal resection can be performed as a synchronous transabdominal/perineal procedure with two operative teams, or sequentially. Surgery is greatly facilitated by placing the patient in the modified lithotomy position with a single skin preparation and draping.

The abdomen is explored for nodal metastases, other primary cancers, and liver metastases. The superior hemorrhoidal vessels are ligated just caudad to the origin of the left colic artery (Fig. 29-20). If extensive nodal disease is present, higher arterial ligation may be appropriate (Fig. 29-21). The mid-sacral vessels are ligated. The rectum is mobilized from the sacral hollow beneath Waldeyer's fascia. The rectosacral fascia is incised to mobilize the rectum to beyond the coccyx. The peritoneum at the base of the bladder or posterior vagina is incised, and the rectum separated from the prostate or posterior vagina. If there is any suggestion of involvement of the rectovaginal septum, a hysterectomy with posterior vaginectomy will facilitate adequate tumor clearance. The "lateral ligaments" are divided, and the anus with pelvic floor muscles is excised.

An end sigmoid colostomy is brought out through the rectus sheath to minimize subsequent hernia. If postoperative radiation therapy is a possibility, clips should be placed around the tumor area to facilitate delivering the boost dose. Efforts to exclude the small bowel from the radiation field using the uterus, omentum, peritoneum, or absorbable mesh should be considered. The perineum was traditionally left open to heal by granulation, but in most patients the pelvic fat and skin can be closed primarily, with greatly improved recovery.

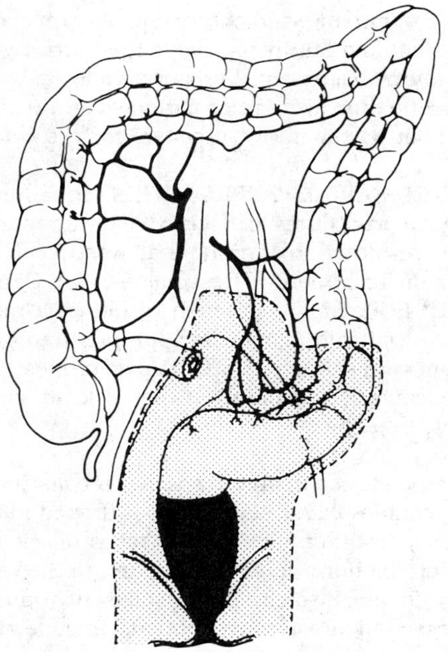

FIG. 29-20. Preferred extent of surgery in an abdominoperineal resection.

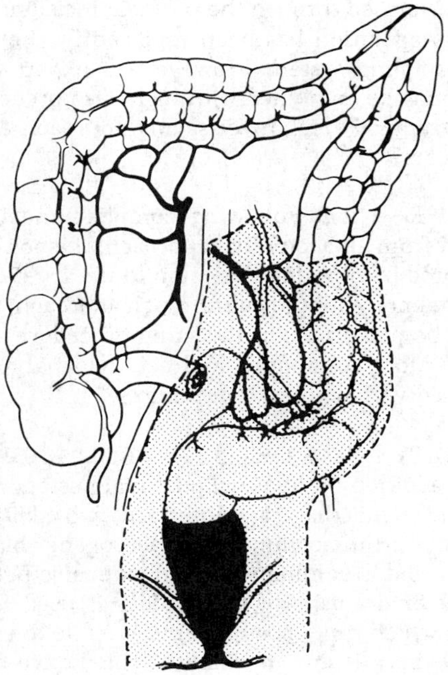

FIG. 29-21. Extended proximal lymphadenectomy in selected patients having abdominoperineal resection.

The surgical, nursing, and enterostomal team should work with the patient and family to relieve their anxiety concerning colostomy management. Preoperative visits by specially trained personnel or even other patients can greatly reduce concerns about postoperative life-style for the colostomate.

SPHINCTER-SAVING APPROACHES. In all sphincter-saving surgical procedures, considerable tumor manipulation is required, resulting in intraluminal tumor cell shedding (see section on Treatment of Resectable Colon Cancer: General Surgical Principles). Although results of a randomized study are not available, it appears appropriate to irrigate the distal rectum with saline or water as part of most sphincter-saving procedures to minimize the risk of suture line recurrences.

Low Anterior Resection. If a transanal reconstruction with a stapler is contemplated, the patient is draped in the modified lithotomy position. The initial stages of the operation with complete mobilization of the rectum to the level of the levators are identical to the initial stages of the abdominoperineal resection. Restorative options include end-to-end and side-to-end anastomoses constructed with sutures or staples. The most widely used approach utilizes the intraluminal circular stapler placed via a transanal approach. This approach allows the creation of very low anastomoses in the pelvis,[583] but the leak rate may be slightly higher.[584] Temporary protective transverse colostomy is no longer a routine adjunct with low anterior resection.

Abdominosacral Resection. An operation pioneered by D'Allaines in the 1940s has been modified by a number of surgeons to allow direct anastomosis through a perineal incision.[585,586] The rectum is mobilized to the pelvic floor, as in the operations described above. A second incision is made just above the anus, the coccyx is removed, and the pelvis is entered through the posterior fascia. An end-to-end anastomosis is performed through the perineal incision. To a great extent, this operation has been replaced by the use of the transanal stapling system. However, in expert hands, the operation may be combined with high-dose preoperative radiation therapy as a sphincter-saving approach to very low rectal cancers.[587,588]

Coloanal Resection. Following complete mobilization of the rectum from an abdominal approach, the bowel continuity is restored by bringing the colon to the level of the anus and dentate line. With the pull-through approach, the anastomosis can be performed at the same procedure, or delayed 10 days.[580] More commonly, a direct endoanal anastomosis is performed with staples[590] or sutures.[591]

MORBIDITY AND MORTALITY FROM RADICAL SURGERY. In addition to the usual potential postoperative complications of hemorrhage and infection, two additional areas of concern warrant comment. A neurogenic bladder with inability to void is common after an extensive pelvic dissection. Catheter drainage of the bladder is used for 7 to 10 days, after which time most patients are able to void spontaneously. If there is any mechanical obstructive component from urethral stricture or prostate enlargement, transurethral surgery may be required before voiding is possible. Bethanechol chloride may be useful in improving bladder emptying. Intermittent or continuous catheterization for months may be necessary in some patients.

Sexual dysfunction, particularly in males, is the rule. Retrograde ejaculation despite normal orgasm is the most common complaint. Erectile impotency is very common after abdominoperineal resection.

The mortality from radical surgery for rectal cancer is 2% to 6%, with no difference between abdominoperineal resection or sphincter-saving procedures.[592–594]

LOCAL TREATMENT OPTIONS FOR RECTAL CANCER

PATIENT SELECTION. Local treatment alone for rectal cancer was first applied to patients with medical contraindications to radical surgery. Severe cardiopulmonary disease may preclude extensive surgery because of high surgical mortality. Patient blindness has always been a concern if a colostomy is required, which makes subsequent self-care difficult. However, a small subset of patients with early rectal cancers may be treated preferentially by one of a number of more limited approaches. Exophytic, small (<3 cm), well-differentiated tumors, clinically limited to the submucosa, are ideal for a limited approach. However, tumors invasive into the muscle wall have also been treated in limited fashion, with good results. Improved clinical staging systems, combined with careful histologic and biologic analyses of various phenotypic markers, may enable us to define appropriate subsets of rectal cancer patients for these treatment strategies.[280] A detailed analysis of these considerations is outside the scope of this book, but the various approaches will be described to familiarize the reader with these therapeutic options. The results are presented in subsequent sections.

TRANSANAL LOCAL EXCISION. A transanal local excision is the most straightforward approach to removing rectal cancers. The deep plane of dissection can be submucosal or full-thickness, generally the latter. Adequate dilation of the anus and the use of special retractors, fiberoptic light, and traction sutures facilitate the procedure. Primary closure of the defect minimizes subsequent scarring, which is important in follow-up of these patients.

POSTERIOR PROCTOTOMY. For lesions too large or too proximal for transanal local excision, two other surgical approaches are available—the posterior proctotomy (Kraske procedure) and transsphincteric excision. In the posterior proctotomy, a perineal incision is made just above the anus, the coccyx is removed, and the fascia divided. The rectum is mobilized and a wide local excision is performed, or even a sleeve resection.[595]

TRANSSPHINCTERIC PROCEDURE. Also known as the Bevan or York Mason procedure, the transsphincteric approach is identical to the posterior proctotomy, except that the entire anal sphincter is divided posteriorly in the midline. As long as each portion of the sphincter mechanism is identified and marked, the anus can be reconstructed at the completion of the operation with minimal risk of functional impairment.[596]

FULGURATION. Fulguration or cauterization has been used as an alternative to abdominoperineal resection by Madden, Crile, Turnbull and others.[597,598] The procedure is done in multiple stages under general or regional anesthesia. Tumor is charred, then scraped with a curette. This approach is not without risk, primarily a delayed hemorrhage (in 10%–20% of cases) from the slough of the scar at 7 to 10 days.

ENDOCAVITARY IRRADIATION. Radiation has been used as a single modality approach to early rectal cancer with curative intent. External beam x-rays alone have been used,[599] but most investigators have used intracavitary irradiation, either alone or combined with temporary isotope implants.[600] The anus is dilated and a 4-cm proctoscope is introduced. A low-energy x-ray unit is placed through the scope almost against the tumor. Generally, 50-kV x-rays, in doses of 3000 cGy per treatment, are given using this "contact" approach. Three or four such sessions are required. Bulky tumors may require additional irradiation with iridium implants or external beam therapy to reach the deeper pararectal tissues.

OTHER LOCAL OPTIONS. Multiple other local treatment strategies have been used. Cryosurgery and Nd-YAG laser ablation may play a role in future years.

Treatment Results in Rectal Cancer

This section presents the end results after surgery for rectal cancer. Overall, cure rates for cancers in the lowermost third of the rectum are less than those for cancers in the upper two thirds.[601,602] In the discussion of patterns of recurrence, pelvic failure will be explored in detail.

CURE RATES FOR NODE-NEGATIVE RECTAL CANCER. Three fourths of patients with node-negative rectal cancer will be cured by radical surgical resection.[261,592] The 5-year survival figures from several major centers are listed in Table 29-18.

CURE RATES FOR NODE-POSITIVE RECTAL CANCER. Only a minority of patients whose rectal cancers have spread to regional lymph nodes are cured by surgery.

TABLE 29-18. Cure Rates in Node-Negative Rectal Cancer

Study	*Stage*	*5-Year Survival (%)*
Wilson and Beahrs[594]	Dukes' A, B	79
Eisenberg et al[325]	Dukes' A	88
McDermott et al[136]	Dukes' A	93
Eisenberg et al[325]	Dukes' B	79
McDermott et al[136]	Dukes' B	71

TABLE 29-19. Cure Rates in Node-Positive Rectal Cancer

Study	*Stage*	*5-Year Survival (%)*
Wilson and Beahrs[594]	Dukes' C	41
Eisenberg et al[325]	Dukes' C	29
McDermott et al[136]	Dukes' C	41

About one third of such patients achieve a 5-year disease-free survival (Table 29-19).

RESULTS WITH LOCAL TREATMENT OPTIONS. In analyzing the long-term results achieved with the various limited treatment options, it is important to appreciate that case selection favors excellent results.[602b] When in situ cancers were excluded, a local control rate of 82% was obtained in a total of 378 patients with invasive cancer treated by local excision.[602c–602g] In the most recent report from St. Marks Hospital, treatment failed locally in 4 of 39 patients.[602h] Hager and associates from Erlangen reported that 3 of 36 patients with T_1 cancers and 3 of 18 with T_2 cancers had local recurrences.[602i] The largest series has been reported from the Mayo Clinic, with a local failure rate of 27% (38 of 141 patients).[603]

Local failure after *fulguration* occurs in 10% to 50%.[602d,602e,604] Multiple sessions (average of 3.5) may be required to maximize local control.[602d,604] A subset of patients with recurrence are cured by subsequent radical surgery.[602d,602e,604–606]

Papillon and colleagues in Lyon, France, pioneered the treatment of selected patients with rectal cancers using *endocavitary irradiation.* Exophytic superficial cancers exclusive of poorly differentiated or colloid histology and less than 4.5 cm in diameter were treated. If the tumor was felt to invade muscle, interstitial iridium-192 was added. In 245 patients, the 5-year disease-free survival rate was 76%. The local failure rate was only 5.3%.[602g] Sischy and associates have reported equally good results.[607] The local failure rate in 94 patients treated with endocavitary irradiation alone was 5%.

Five-year survival rates with local treatment options vary from 50% to 90%, with many deaths secondary to medical illnesses and unrelated to cancer. In selected patients, a 10% cancer-related 5-year mortality can be expected with local excision, fulguration, or primary irradiation.

PATTERNS OF RECURRENCE AFTER RADICAL SURGERY. Despite radical surgery, local–regional failure occurs in 20% to 50% of patients with transmural or node-positive rectal cancers. Pelvic recurrence can be secondary to suture line tumor, retained lymph nodes, intralymphatic tumor, or shed tumor cells. The incidence of treatment failure in the pelvis is directly related to the extent of transmural penetration (microscopic versus gross) and the additive risks of lymph node metastases. Pelvic failure rates as a function of various pathologic parameters are listed in Tables 29-20 and 29-21.

Failure patterns determined at autopsy provide the most accurate insight into the relative risks of local and distant recurrence. In the series reported from the Massachusetts

TABLE 29-20. Pelvic Recurrence Rates After Surgery for Node-Negative Rectal Cancer

Study	*Stage*	*Locoregional Recurrence*
McDermott et al[610]	Dukes' B	15
Phillips et al[609]	Dukes' B	15
Pilipshen et al[608]	Dukes' B	30
Pilipshen et al[608]	T2N0M0	14
Pilipshen et al[608]	T3N0M0	30
Rich et al[221]	T3(m)N0M0*	17
Rich et al[221]	T3(g)N0M0*	25
Rich et al[221]	T4N0M0	53

*(m) denotes microscopic transmural extension; (g) denotes gross transmural extension.

General Hospital, isolated pelvic recurrences were documented in 25% of patients, but a total of 75% of cancer-related deaths were associated with tumor in the pelvis. These data suggest that improved local control through multimodality treatment of the primary cancer not only will dramatically reduce cancer-related morbidity, but also may improve survival, particularly in node-negative patients.

SPECIFIC MANAGEMENT PROBLEMS IN RECTAL CANCER

OBSTRUCTION. Subtotal obstruction from rectal cancers may manifest as increasing constipation or frank obstipation, more commonly as diarrhea and tenesmus. If dietary management with a minimal residue regimen is not effective in allowing an elective operation (perhaps including preoperative irradiation), a preliminary colostomy should be considered.

CONTIGUOUS ORGAN INVOLVEMENT. In patients with rectal cancer, contiguous organ involvement usually entails direct invasion of the prostate and base of the bladder in men, and of the vagina in women. In women who have previously undergone a hysterectomy, a cancer of the upper third of the rectum may invade the base of the bladder. Management issues are discussed in a later section on unresectable, recurrent cancer—locally advanced rectal cancer.

TABLE 29-21. Pelvic Recurrence Rates After Surgery for Node-Positive Rectal Cancer

Study	*Stage*	*Locoregional Recurrence (%)*
McDermott et al[610]	Dukes' C	32
Phillips et al[609]	Dukes' C	21
Pilipshen et al[608]	Dukes' C	39
Pilipshen et al[608]	T2 N1 M0	22
Pilipshen et al[608]	T3 N1 M0	49
Rich et al[221]	T3(m)N1M0*	28
Rich et al[221]	T3(g)N1M0*	52
Rich et al[221]	T4N1M0	67

*(m) denotes microscopic transmural extension; (g) denotes gross transmural extension.

ADJUVANT THERAPIES FOR RECTAL CANCER

Limited Local Surgery and Adjuvant Irradiation

As described previously, limited local treatment strategies such as local excision, fulguration, and intracavitary irradiation may be selected as palliative approaches, and, with appropriate case selection, as curative approaches. It is reasonable to postulate that locoregional failure secondary to microscopic residual primary tumor or pelvic lymph node metastases may be reduced with adjuvant radiation. Relatively little data are available in this regard, and none of it is randomized.

Some investigators have used supplementary radiation therapy in a subset of patients who were treated with electrocoagulation.[598,606,611–613] Wittoesch and Jackman reported a 47% 5-year survival rate in their poor-risk patients, of whom 62% had received some form of adjuvant irradiation.[614] Preoperative irradiation to about 2000 cGy was used in a local excision series at Memorial Hospital, in which many patients had undergone reexcision for recurrent disease.[615] The 5-year survival rate was 83%, similar to the 84% survival rate reported by that institution for primary local excisions without irradiation, with only 6% dead of disease during the 5-year interval.[616]

Rich et al described 17 patients with adenocarcinoma in the lower two thirds of the rectum who underwent a local procedure to remove gross tumor, either a local excision (in 16 patients) or fulguration (1), and who received adjuvant irradiation. There was only one local failure (6%) despite positive margins in 11 of the 17 patients.[617]

Radical Surgery and Adjuvant Irradiation

The multimodality management of patients with rectal cancer is directed toward maximizing local control, as well as increasing overall survival. The following discussion addresses the complex issues of radiation dose, sequencing, and toxicity prior to analyzing the end results of adjuvant radiation therapy.

Until recently, analyses of adjuvant irradiation for rectal carcinoma were nonrandomized, retrospective studies that compared results in patients who had received adjuvant radiation therapy as a complement to a radical surgical procedure with results in historical or, at best, concurrent controls. In the discussion of adjuvant radiation therapy, we will distinguish nonrandomized from randomized studies.

DOSE CONSIDERATIONS. If one looks at the series of preoperative radiation therapy studies done in the past, there appears to be a trend toward increasing local control as the preoperative dose of radiation therapy increased.[618] In a recent preoperative radiation therapy study, the local control rate was 67% with 4000 cGy, increasing to 91% with 5000 cGy.[619] A study of patients with gross residual cancer demonstrated a local control rate of 67% with doses between 5000 and 5499 cGy, increasing to 89% with doses above 6000 cGy.[620] In the randomized GITSG postoperative radiation therapy study, the local control rate was 76% without pelvic irradiation in the control group but increased only to 80% in the radiation therapy alone group, which had received only 4400 to 4800 cGy.[262] It seems apparent that doses of 5000 cGy or higher are needed to control microscopic disease.

SEQUENCING CONSIDERATIONS. *Preoperative Radiation.* The rationale for using preoperative radiation therapy is (1) to increase resectability, (2) to abrogate potential seeding of tumor during surgery, and (3) to destroy microscopic foci of tumor that may lie beyond the surgical margins or in lymph nodes outside the operative field.[621]

The potential advantages of delivering radiation therapy preoperatively are several. (1) The radiation is delivered under well-vascularized and well-oxygenated conditions, so that the cells are maximally radiosensitive. (2) One can avoid implantation of viable cells, either locally or through vascular channels, as the tumor is manipulated during surgery. (3) The radiation is delivered with a freely mobile small bowel (*i.e.,* without any adhesions resulting from a surgical procedure), so that any given portion of the small bowel lies within the radiation fields only part of the time during irradiation. (4) If there is a question regarding fixation, preoperative irradiation increases the chance of resectability. A decrease in the number of positive nodes has also been noted after preoperative radiation therapy,[622–624] but the ultimate effect of such a downstaging on survival is unclear.

Postoperative Radiation. A major reason for choosing postoperative irradiation is that the stage and extent of disease are known, and one may select the patients most likely to benefit from adjuvant therapy on the basis of these prognostic features. Other advantages include the following: (1) The extent of disease is determined at surgery, so that the radiation therapy field, including boost fields, may be more carefully defined. (2) Sphincter-preserving procedures can be done without (unfounded?) fear of healing of irradiated tissue. (3) Surgery is not delayed. (4) Patients with distant metastases found at surgery may be excluded from the treatment program or may be placed on a combined radiation-chemotherapy regimen. Potential disadvantages include the loss of the advantages that preoperative radiation therapy offers: (1) after surgery tumor cells may be in a hypoxic state because vascularity is compromised, and therefore the cells may be less radiosensitive; (2) the small bowel may be fixed within the radiation fields; and (3) the potential advantage of preventing seeding of viable cells at surgery cannot exist.

"Sandwich" Radiation Therapy. This technique entails a combination of preoperative radiation therapy, usually with relatively small doses (500–2000 cGy), and postoperative radiation therapy, to a high total dose only in high stage cases. The technique may offer the advantages of both preoperative and postoperative radiation therapy.

TECHNIQUES TO MINIMIZE TOXICITY. At the doses necessary to control microscopic disease before or after surgery for rectal carcinoma, the major organ of concern for tolerance is the small bowel.[625] If a large portion of the small bowel receives more than 5000 cGy, the risk of treatment-associated complications increases. These complications include obstruction, perforation, and fistula. The risk of complications may also be increased with other patient-related factors, such as hypertension or diabetes,[626] or a history of multiple surgical procedures in the abdomen. Many techniques have been developed to prevent such toxic effects (Table 29-22). These may be divided into surgical and radiation therapy techniques.

Surgical techniques include pelvic reconstruction to exclude small bowel from the pelvis.[537] An omental transposition flap[627] or retroverted uterus may be used, or an absorbable synthetic polyglycolic mesh pelvic sling.[628–631] Insertion of a tissue expander has also been described.[632]

During radiation therapy planning, small bowel radiographs with contrast material in the small bowel to determine its location and mobility are essential.[537,633–635] The severity of acute GI effects has been correlated with the small bowel volume included in the radiotherapy fields.[635] There was no diarrhea when the average volume of small bowel included in the fields was 58 cm^3, whereas when this volume was increased to 485 cm^3, unresponsive diarrhea developed. Late GI effects correlated with prior pelvic surgery and with the volume of small bowel that received more than 4500 cGy.

A three- or four-field technique with careful blocking is used for the large pelvic portion of treatment, with AP/PA and two lateral fields, to a dose of 4600 to 5000 cGy. After this, a carefully planned boost dose (1000–1500 cGy) is given to the tumor bed area, guided by the location of the original tumor as defined by various imaging methods and by clips placed at surgery. The boost field may be planned most effectively in this era with the aid of CT (Fig. 29-22).

During treatment of the prone patient, the bladder may be distended, which will push small bowel superiorly out of the pelvic fields.[537] External compression with the patient in the

TABLE 29-22. Techniques to Minimize Toxic Effects in Small Bowel with Pelvic Radiation Therapy

Surgical Techniques:
Pelvic reconstruction to exclude small bowel from pelvis:
Reperitonealize pelvic floor
Retrovert the uterus
Construct omental sling
Use temporary prosthesis
Place clips to delineate high-risk areas
Perform temporary colostomy
Radiation Therapy Techniques:
During planning:
Small bowel radiographs during simulation
Liberal use of other diagnostic tools such as US, CT, or MR imaging to delineate tumor–small bowel relationship
Place patient prone
Use multiple fields for pelvic treatment, with judicious blocking
Use carefully planned boost fields
During treatment:
Bladder distention (with patient prone)
Use external compression
Use "false tabletop"
Use small doses per fraction (180 cGy) or hyperfractionation (b.i.d.)
Diet regulation
Potential: use of radioprotectors

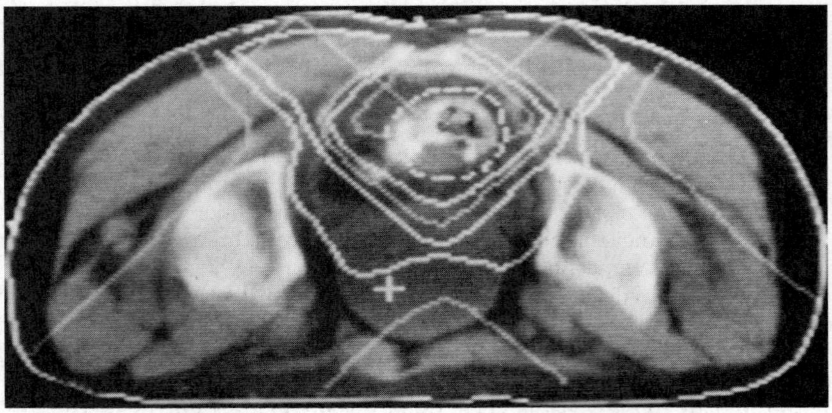

FIG. 29-22. Planning "boost" treatment for a rectal primary in an inoperable patient utilizing a computerized tomography treatment planning system. Dashed inner line = biological target volume. Other lines are isodoses from two wedged posterior oblique fields.

prone position has also been used. Gallagher et al demonstrated a reduction of small bowel within the fields when they combined the prone position, bladder distention, and external compression, in comparison with the supine position.[635]

It has been suggested that the use of special diets during a course of radiation therapy may be an advantage in preventing acute radiation effects.[636] Diets have included (1) a powdered elemental diet, (2) a lactose-restricted diet, and (3) a combination low-fat, low-residue, low-lactose diet. The elemental diet was of value in animal studies,[637] and preliminary results suggest benefit in clinical trials.[638] A lactose-restricted diet has not been shown to be of value in patients undergoing whole pelvis irradiation.[639] A randomized trial with a low-fat, low-residue, low-lactose diet is in progress at Memorial Sloan-Kettering Cancer Center for gynecologic patients receiving pelvic radiation therapy; the trial has been expanded to patients with other carcinomas receiving pelvic radiation therapy.[640]

Some pharmaceutical agents may possibly protect the small bowel while not jeopardizing the radiation effect on the tumor. The radioprotector, WR-2721, has been studied in mice.[641,642] A Phase II trial was initiated in April 1987 by the RTOG in which WR-2721 was administered before protracted fractionated radiation therapy for carcinoma of the rectum, cervix, or bladder. Other analogues may prove to be of more use in the future. A study in mice has shown that prostaglandin E_2 protected against acute toxicity, as measured by jejunal cell survival, when given 1 hour before radiation therapy.[643] At present, the best protection against toxic effects in the small bowel is careful coordination from the outset by the surgeon and radiation therapist.

Results of Preoperative Radiation Therapy

NONRANDOMIZED STUDIES. Seminal studies from Memorial Hospital[644,645] suggested a survival benefit at doses approximating 1500 to 2000 cGy. A variety of radiation techniques were used (radon seeds, orthovoltage, etc.) The overall 5-year survival rate was 55% in irradiated patients versus 45% in those treated by surgery alone. In subsequent studies doses have ranged from 2000 to 6000 cGy. In all of these studies, the local recurrence rates have been low (5%–15%),[587,646–651] considerably lower than in patients treated with surgery alone at the same institution.[647,649,650] The results with high-dose preoperative therapy are summarized in Table 29-23.

High-dose preoperative radiation therapy has also allowed downstaging of disease in some cases. In most series, the percentage of patients with positive lymph nodes is reduced from 30% to 40% without radiation therapy to a level of 20% to 25%.[647–649] In a few studies, no microscopic tumor was

TABLE 29-23. Nonrandomized Studies of High-Dose Preoperative Radiation Therapy

			Local Recurrence		*Survival*		
Study	*Date*	*Dose (cGy)*	*S*	*RT*	*S*		*RT*
Jewish Hospital of St. Louis and Mallinckrodt Institute of Radiology	1982	2000 *or* 4500	14%	2000 cGy: 8%	. . .		. . .
				4500 cGy: 4%			
University of Florida	1985	3000–4500	29%	8%	41%	5-yr NED	71%
Baystate Medical Center	1985	4000–4500	15%	6%	48%	5-yr adjusted overall	74%
					52%	Adjusted NED	79%
Thomas Jefferson Hospital	1987	4000–5000		All: 14%	. . .	4-yr all	66%
			Low lesions:	11%	41%	Low lesions (Memorial Hosp. comparison)	72%

S = surgery; RT = radiation therapy.

TABLE 29-24. Randomized Studies of Preoperative Radiation Therapy

			No. of Patients		*LR*		*5-Year Survival*	
Study	*Date*	*Dose (cGy)*	*S*	*RT*	*S*	*RT*	*S*	*RT*
Princess Margaret Hosp., Toronto[655]	1977	500	56	55	. . .	. . .	35% Overall	35%
							17% Stage C	35%
Medical Research Council[274,655a]	1982	500	275	277	57%	55%	38% Overall	42%
	1984	2000		272		53%		40%
Memorial Hosp.[328]	1974	2000	414	376	23%† Stage C	13%†	65% Overall	67%
					From autopsy:			
VASOG I[622,657]	1975	2000–2500	353	347	36% All	29%	32% Overall	40%
					40% APR	29%*	28% APR	41%
							32% Stage C	54%
Stockholm Rectal Group, Stockholm[656]	1987	2500	274	271	20 (p < .01)	8%	. . .	. . .
VASOG II[658]	1986	3150	180	181	. . .	. . .	50% APR	50%
Mainz[663,664]	1977, 1984	3450	106	64	20%	12.5%	64% (p < .05)	80%
EORTC[654,665]	1985, 1987	3450	166	152	35% (p = 0.002)	15%	60% (p = .08)	70%

LR = local recurrence; S = surgery alone; RT = adjuvant preoperative radiation therapy; APR = abdominoperineal resection.
* Statistically significant.
† Unpublished data (Shank et al).

found in 3% to 17% of the operative specimens.[651–653] A recent study stressed the safety and ability of preoperative radiation therapy to complement sphincter-saving procedures in low rectal cancer.[587] Complications have tended to be minimal, similar to the complications of surgery alone, although an increase in wound sepsis in one series was reported.[647] Friedmann et al noted an increase in bowel obstruction and organ injury during surgery to 5% with radiation therapy, compared with 1% without.[649]

RANDOMIZED STUDIES. Many randomized studies have used relatively low doses of preoperative irradiation, ranging from 500 cGy to 3450 cGy. Although large numbers of patients were treated in several of these studies, the lower doses produced little benefit in local recurrence rates. The major preoperative studies are summarized in Table 29-24.[654–665] The most impressive results are reported by the European Organization for Research on Treatment of Cancer (EORTC).[654] At 5 years, the actuarial local control rate was 85% in the group treated with preoperative radiation therapy group (3450 cGy in 230 cGy per day fractions) compared with 65% for the surgery-alone group (p = 0.001). Similar data have been reported by the group in Mainz, Federal Republic of Germany,[664] and the Stockholm Rectal Cancer Study Group.[656]

In the studies with doses less than 3000 cGy, there has been no improvement in overall survival. An exception is the VASOG I study in which patients who received preoperative irradiation (2500 cGy) before abdominoperineal resection had a 41% 5-year survival rate, compared with a 28% survival rate for those treated by surgery alone. Of the studies utilizing doses higher than 3000 cGy, the EORTC and the Mainz group report a difference in disease-free survival with preoperative irradiation.[664,665] A small study from Yale randomizing patients to 4500 cGY noted an improved 5-year survival, from 25% to 41%. Two studies from the Soviet Union have shown statistically significant increases in survival, but it is not clear whether they were truly randomized.[659,660]

In terms of complications with low-dose radiation therapy, the most complete observations have been done in the Medical Research Council study.[661] In this study, the complications were essentially identical between the two radiation therapy groups and the surgery-alone group, except for a significant decrease in anastomotic leaks in the radiation therapy groups compared with the surgery-alone group. In addition, there were no increases in long-term complications.[661] In the VASOG II study, most complications were similar in the two groups, except for an increase in moderate to severe complications, especially perineal infections, in the group treated with preoperative radiation therapy.[658]

SUMMARY OF PREOPERATIVE IRRADIATION. Adjuvant preoperative irradiation in sufficiently high doses likely improves the local control rate and may increase survival. To confirm these conclusions, the United Kingdom Medical Research Council (MRC) has begun trial II, randomizing patients with "tethered" cancers to receive 4,000 cGY preoperatively.

Results of Postoperative Radiation Therapy

NONRANDOMIZED STUDIES. The largest nonrandomized studies (Table 29-25) have been reported from the M. D. Anderson Hospital[666] and from the Massachusetts General Hospital.[662] In both studies, high doses were delivered to the pelvis (4000–5000 cGy at M. D. Anderson Hospital and 4500 cGy at Massachusetts General Hospital), with additional boost doses to high-risk areas in some cases. The results show a reduction in the local recurrence rate for patients with B2 and C2 lesions (the stages for which sufficient patients were available to draw valid comparisons with historical controls). In the Massachusetts General Hospital series, 5-year survival was higher with radiation therapy. The

TABLE 29-25. Nonrandomized Studies of Postoperative Radiation Therapy

Study	Year	Dose (cGy)	Total No. of Patients		Local Recurrence			5-Year Actuarial Survival	
			S	RT	Stage	S	RT	S	RT
M.D. Anderson Hosp.[666] (Follow-up range, 24–138 mo)	1987	4000–5000 to pelvis, + 600–1000 boost	?	105	B2	13%	4%	. . .	65%
					B3	26%	31%	. . .	48%
					C2	30%	18%	. . .	48%
					C3	49%	1/5		3/5
Mass. General Hosp.[662] (Median follow-up, 56 mo)	1987	4500 to pelvis, ± ≥540 boost	142	165 (79)*	B2	23%	9%	. . . (47%)	71% (76%)†
					B3	53%	0/7	. . . (27%)	67% (69%)
					C2	47%	21%	. . . (27%)	39% (34%)
					C3	4/6	53%	. . . (0/6)	17% (13%)
Thomas Jefferson Univ. Hosp.[668] (Follow-up range, 2–9 yr)	1985	4500 to pelvis	88	26	B2	26%	11%	34%	32%
					C1				
					C2				

S = surgery only; RT = adjuvant postoperative radiation therapy.
*Surgery done at the same institution
†( ) = NED survival; patients dying of intercurrent disease were excluded from analysis at time of death.

M. D. Anderson Hospital report does not include historical surgery-only controls in the survival analysis. The incidence of small bowel obstruction requiring surgery was higher at M. D. Anderson Hospital (13%) than at Massachusetts General Hospital (6%). However, the former group used larger parallel opposed anteroposterior pelvic fields for most of their patients, whereas the group at Massachusetts General Hospital used a four-field technique for the pelvic portion of the radiation therapy. A report from Thomas Jefferson University Hospital also suggests an advantage for postoperative radiation therapy (4500 cGy) in preventing local recurrences, but not in improving overall survival.[668]

RANDOMIZED STUDIES. Three major randomized studies of postoperative radiation therapy have included a surgery-only arm for comparison: a GITSG study, an NSABP study, and a study from multiple institutions in Denmark (Table 29-26).[262,669–671] In all three studies a slightly lower dose of radiation was used than in the nonrandomized stud-

TABLE 29-26. Randomized Studies of Postoperative Radiation Therapy for Rectal Carcinoma

Study	Year	Dose (cGy)	No. of Patients		Stage	Local Recurrence		Survival		
			S	RT		S	RT	S		RT
									At 5 yr:	
GITSG[262,669]	1985, 1986	4000–4800	58	50	B2–C:	24%	20%	43%		52%
									At 5 yr:	
NSABP[670]	1987	4600–4700 ≥ perineal boost	184	184	B2–C:	25%	16%	43%	Overall	41%
								30%	DFS	34%
									At 2 yr:	
Denmark[671]	1986	5000 (split course: 3000 —2 wk→ 2000)	250	244	B:	12%	12%	67%	LRF	82%
					C:	25%	21%			
					If > 4500 cGy delivered:					
					B:		9%			
					C:		16%			

S = surgery only; RT = adjuvant postoperative radiation therapy; DFS = disease-free survival; LRF = local recurrence free.

ies, and there were frequently many protocol violations with respect to the actual dose of radiation delivered. Nevertheless, all of the studies show some advantage for postoperative radiation therapy in terms of decreasing local recurrences. No survival difference has been seen at 5 years in any of these studies, although the study from Denmark is not yet mature.

These studies have shown disparate results in terms of complications. In the GITSG trial there was an 18% rate of severe or life-threatening toxicity(4% life-threatening) due to enteritis.[672] This was not a function of radiation dose. However, in the combined therapy arm, there was a 61% incidence of severe, life-threatening, or fatal toxic effects. In contrast, in the NSABP study, no severe complications were associated with radiation therapy. The Denmark study indicated a higher rate of severe complications in the radiation therapy group, 21%, versus only 8% in the surgery-only group.

SUMMARY OF POSTOPERATIVE IRRADIATION. A decreased local recurrence rate in nonrandomized studies of postoperative radiation therapy for rectal carcinoma has been confirmed in randomized studies. However, this has not yet been translated into any increase in overall 5-year survival. The studies are still maturing, and one must bear in mind that the doses of radiation used were somewhat lower than in the nonrandomized studies, or were given as a split course, as in the Denmark study.

A Swedish trial is comparing moderate dose/high fraction (2500–500 rad/day) preoperatively versus postoperative treatment of B2/C patients with >5000–200 rad/day.[667]

"Sandwich" Radiation Therapy

In nonrandomized studies, many authors have explored the use of combined preoperative and postoperative radiation therapy, or "sandwich" radiation therapy (Table 29-27). Preoperative doses have varied from 500 cGy as a single fraction[668,673] to as high as 2000 cGy.[674] In all trials, the preoperative portion of radiation therapy has been well tolerated. Mohiuddin et al reported the Thomas Jefferson University results in Stage B2 to C rectal cancer, comparing (1) combined preoperative and postoperative radiation therapy, (2) the preoperative portion of treatment only, (3) surgery alone, and (4) surgery plus postoperative radiation therapy (4500 cGy).[668] Local control was improved in the groups that had received high total doses of radiation therapy, namely the sandwich radiation therapy group and the postoperative radiation therapy group. Distant metastases were fewer in the patients who received 500 cGy preoperatively, either alone or with postoperative treatment, than in the surgery-alone group (24%, 13%, and 57% rate of distant metastases for the respective groups). The only significantly improved 5-year survival rate was in the group given sandwich radiation therapy—78%, compared with only 34% in the surgery-alone group.

In a study from the Massachusetts General Hospital,[673] in which patients were selected to receive postoperative irradiation based on pathologic criteria (C, B2(m+g), B2(m) with poor margins), the 4-year survival rate was 79% in the sandwich arm, similar to the results reported from Thomas Jefferson University. In a study reported by Brenner et al[674] in which 2000 cGy was given preoperatively and 2600 cGy postoperatively, there were no local recurrences in 26 patients with Dukes' B and C lesions after a follow-up of 14 to 42 months. In another nonrandomized study, reported by Shank et al,[675] about equal numbers of patients were assigned to receive either 1500 cGy in five fractions preoperatively or sandwich radiation therapy, consisting of 1500 cGy preoperatively and 4140 cGy postoperatively. There was only one local recurrence, in the group given preoperative radiation therapy only.

The RTOG and the ECOG have joined in a randomized study of patients with rectal lesions less than 12 cm from the anal verge. Patients were randomly assigned to receive 500 cGy preoperative radiation therapy or no preoperative radiation therapy. All patients with B2 to C disease received 4500 rad postoperatively. Results of this study are not yet available.

TABLE 29-27. Results of "Sandwich" Radiation Therapy for Rectal Cancer: Nonrandomized Studies

Study	*Date*	*No. of Patients* S	P	C	*Dose (cGy)* *Preop.*	*Postop.*	*Local Recurrence* S	P	C	*% Survival* S	P	C
										At 5 years		
Thomas Jefferson Univ. Hosp.[668]	1985	88	29	31	500	4500	26%	34%	7%	34	52	78
										At 4 years:		
Mass. General Hosp.[673]	1983	. . .	16	15	500	4500–5000 (6000–6500 for gross disease)	. . .	13%	29%	. . .	93	79
										At 3 years:		
Memorial Hosp.[675]	1987	. . .	24	23	1500	4140	. . .	4%	0%	. . .	92	82

S = surgery only; P = preoperative radiation therapy only; C = combined preoperative and postoperative radiation therapy.

Radical Surgery and Adjuvant Chemotherapy or Chemotherapy–Radiation Therapy Combinations for Rectal Cancer

The local anatomy and natural history of rectal adenocarcinoma require clinical attention to issues of both regional and systemic control of tumor. Three recently completed randomized studies are of particular relevance. As summarized in Table 29-28, these studies evaluated postoperative pelvic radiation therapy; two had surgery-only control groups and two had combined radiation therapy and chemotherapy arms.[262,669,670,676]

The GITSG[262,669] Study 7175, initiated in 1975, allocated patients with completely resected Dukes' B2 and C lesions to one of four treatment groups: (1) surgical control; (2) methyl-CCNU (130 mg/m² on day 1) and 5-FU (325 mg/m² on days 1–5, and 375 mg/m² on days 36–40), repeated every 10 weeks for 18 months; (3) radiation therapy, 4000 to 4800 cGy to the pelvis; or (4) radiation therapy, 4000 to 4400 cGy, plus 5-FU and methyl-CCNU as in (2). Although initially projected to accrue more than 500 patients, this trial was terminated after the entry of only 227 patients because of observed outcome differences between the regimens. At an 80-month median follow-up time, the control population had a 55% recurrence rate as compared to a 33% rate for the combination radiation therapy plus chemotherapy group ($p < 0.009$). There were 14 local recurrences in the 32 control patients and 5 local recurrences in the 46 patients treated by combination therapy. A subsequent analysis at 94 months' median follow-up showed an even larger margin of benefit for the combination therapy. In addition to a disease-free survival advantage, combination chemotherapy–radiation therapy was associated with a statistically significant overall survival benefit ($p = 0.005$). There was an approximate 20 percentage point superiority in survival at 6 years for the 96 patients at risk.[669] Although these data support an aggressive multimodality approach to patients with rectal cancer, the morbidity of combined radiation therapy plus 5-FU and methyl-CCNU must be considered.[672] Severe or life-threatening acute toxic effects occurred in 18% of patients in the radiation therapy arm and in 61% of those in the combined radiation therapy–chemotherapy arm. Three late deaths occurred, two from enteritis in the combined treatment group and one from nonlymphocytic leukemia in a chemotherapy-alone patient.

The second major trial of adjuvant therapy for rectal cancer was initiated by the NCCTG (study 79-47-51) in 1979.[676] A total of 200 patients with Dukes' B2 and C rectal cancer were randomly assigned to either postoperative radiation therapy only (4500 cGy with a 500-cGy boost) or to an integrated program of methyl-CCNU (130 mg/m² on day 1) plus 5-FU (350 mg/m²/d on days 1–5; 400 mg/m²/d on days 36–40), radiation therapy beginning on day 64, followed by one additional cycle of methyl-CCNU + 5-FU (sandwich therapy). The radiation therapy dose was 4500 to 5000 cGy. At a median follow-up time of 29 months, there were 38 recurrences in the group treated with radiation therapy alone, compared with only 23 recurrences in those treated with combination therapy. The disease-free survival doubled in patients who underwent sphincter-saving surgery followed by the combination treatment, compared with postoperative radiation therapy alone. The local failure rate in the combination treatment group was 11%, versus 20% in those treated with postoperative irradiation only. The overall disease-free survival was superior with combined treatment ($p = 0.001$). The time interval to tumor recurrence was statistically superior for the combination therapy group ($p = 0.025$). Overall survival differences could not be reported since the data were not sufficiently mature.

The largest study was performed by NSABP (R01) and required a decade (1977–1987) to complete accrual.[670] A total of 528 patients with Dukes' B2 and C lesions were randomized to (1) postoperative observation; (2) postoperative pelvic radiation therapy, 4700 cGy with a boost to 5300 cGy maximum; or (3) MOF chemotherapy (methyl-CCNU, vincristine, 5-FU) as utilized in the NSABP C01 study. After a 54-month mean follow-up time, there was a statistically significant disease-free survival advantage for MOF chemotherapy ($p = 0.05$) and an overall survival improvement for selected subsets of patients receiving MOF (particularly males and those less than 65 years old). Patients given only postoperative irradiation had no statistically demonstrable

TABLE 29-28. Recently Completed U.S. Trials of Adjuvant Therapy for Rectal Cancer

Study	*Total Accrual*	*Treatment* (Arms)*	*Results*
GITSG 7175[669]	227	Control MF Pelvic RT RT + 5-FU, then MF	RT + CT resulted in 59% 5-year survival versus 43% in controls ($p < 0.01$)
NCCTG 79-47-51[676]	200	Pelvic RT Sandwich MF + RT + MF	RT + MF resulted in 55% 5-year survival versus 49% for RT alone
NSABP R01[670]	551	Control Pelvic RT MOF	MOF resulted in 52% 5-year survival versus 42% in controls

MF = methyl-CCNU + 5-FU; MOF = methyl-CCNU + vincristine (Oncovin) + 5-FU.
*All patients underwent complete surgical resection.

improvement in overall or relapse-free survival. There was, however, a reduction in the locoregional recurrence rate from 25% without radiation therapy to 16% with radiation therapy. Despite the 80 weeks of MOF chemotherapy, no leukemias had yet been observed; other toxic effects were predictable and tolerated.[670]

In contrast to the above studies, the EORTC was unable to show a benefit with combined treatment.[677] This study of preoperative adjuvant therapies compared irradiation (3450 cGy in 230-cGy fractions) with the same radiation regimen combined with only an intravenous bolus of 5-FU (375 mg/m^2) on the first four days of irradiation. In the 247 patients followed up, overall survival was better with radiation therapy only. However, the incidence of liver metastases was reduced ($p = 0.07$) in the combined radiation therapy + 5-FU group.

As an integrated experience, the three recent U. S. studies summarized in Table 29-28 indicate that meaningful survival benefits can be achieved with programs utilizing postoperative chemotherapy. These data are supported by two earlier trials of adjuvant single-agent 5-FU in colorectal cancer patients; the results in the rectal cancer patients were reported separately. Survival benefits with intensive 5-FU regimens have been reported by Grage et al[554] for the Central Oncology Group and by Higgins et al for the VA group.[553]

Although radiation therapy alone has had little apparent impact on survival, the combination of radiation therapy and chemotherapy may offer the greatest survival advantage.[556] Several issues remain unclear: the exact choice of chemotherapy agent(s) that will provide the most benefit at the least toxicity, the duration of chemotherapy, the scheduling and dosage of radiation therapy, and the integration of all three modalities (surgery, radiation therapy, and chemotherapy). In an attempt to address some of the therapeutic issues, new studies have been initiated.

Currently, two large cooperative group randomized efforts are ongoing in the United States (Table 29-29). The NCCTG Study 864751 is using a 2 × 2 factorial statistical design and attempting to quantify the relative benefits of continuous infusion versus bolus 5-FU, as well as the value of including methyl-CCNU in the chemotherapy regimen. All patients receive pelvic radiation therapy and concomitant 5-FU in the sandwich sequence of chemotherapy–radiation–chemotherapy. Half the patients receive MF chemotherapy as in the previous NCCTG trial (79-4751), the other half receive 5-FU, 500 mg/m^2 on days 1 to 5 and days 36 to 40 before radiation therapy, and 450 mg/m^2 on days 1 to 5 and days 36 to 40 1 month after the completion of radiation therapy. During the irradiation interval patients receive either standard 5-FU, 500 mg/m^2 on days 1 to 3 and days 36 to 39 as an IV bolus, or 225 mg/m^2/d as a continuous IV infusion for 5 weeks. The planned pelvic radiation therapy dose is 4500 cGy, with a boost to a total of 5400 to 5900 cGy.

The recently activated NSABP R02 study is also summarized in Table 29-29. This protocol compares the standard NSABP MOF chemotherapy regimen with a 5-FU + folinic acid program and is complementary to NSABP Study C03 for patients with colon cancer. Half the patients will receive radiation therapy in conjunction with chemotherapy. Because of preliminary evidence of qualitative therapy interactions in specific subgroups, women will receive 5-FU + folinic acid, with or without radiation therapy; men will be randomly assigned to the four therapy options. The chemotherapy doses are identical to those used in NSABP Study C03.

These two active studies address some of the most demanding questions in the treatment of rectal cancer. Programs entailing pelvic irradiation and 5-FU + methyl-CCNU have demonstrated both benefits and toxicities. The new NSABP and NCCTG studies will help redefine the therapeutic ratio, and in addition will evaluate promising new ways of using 5-FU, by infusion or with folinic acid modulation.

Summary of Adjuvant Treatment for Rectal Cancer

Until a complete analysis of the above studies becomes available, some form of adjuvant therapy is recommended for most patients with T3 or T4 and/or N1 rectal cancer. Whenever possible, participation in a formal clinical trial is to be encouraged. However, for those not entering a clinical study, the choice of adjuvant therapy is contingent on many medical, psychological, and financial factors, which must be considered by the patient and physician. For many patients the use of high-dose preoperative or postoperative radiation therapy with postoperative 5-FU chemotherapy is entirely reasonable and justifiable.

TABLE 29-29. Currently Active U.S. Trials of Adjuvant Therapy for Rectal Cancer

Study	*Total Accrual*		*Treatment (Arms)*	
NCCTG 86-47-51	450		MF/RT + 5-FU/MF (5-FU infusion)	
			MF/RT + 5-FU/MF (5-FU bolus)	
			5-FU/RT + 5-FU/5-FU (5-FU infusion)	
			5-FU/RT + 5-FU/5-FU (5-FU bolus)	
NSABP R02	800	Men	MOF	
		Men	MOF + RT	
		Men	5-FU/FA	Women
		Men	5-FU/FA + RT	Women

FA = folinic acid; MF = methyl-CCNU + 5-FU.

MANAGEMENT OF UNRESECTABLE, RECURRENT, AND METASTATIC DISEASE

TREATMENT OF INITIALLY ADVANCED COLON CANCER

Synchronous Metastatic Cancer

Approximately 10% to 15% of patients with primary colon cancers will present with synchronous metastatic cancer. The treatment of patients with synchronous liver metastases is discussed under Treatment of Recurrent and Metastatic Cancer. The operative finding of peritoneal seeding or extensive unresectable intra-abdominal nodal metastases beyond the central nodal drainage should not deter surgical resection. An extended surgical lymphadenectomy in selected younger patients may be curative in a small subset despite gross involvement of high nodes, albeit probably at most 10% to 15%.

Locally Unresectable Colon Cancer

Such tumors may be unresectable for cure, whether or not distant metastases are present. Extensive direct extension into the retroperitoneum, pelvic side wall, or duodenum or pancreas may be found. In the presence of concomitant metastatic disease, a bypass enteroenterostomy is usually appropriate. In the absence of distant disease, an aggressive local surgical approach to these "unresectable" tumors should be taken in otherwise healthy patients.

TREATMENT OF INITIALLY ADVANCED RECTAL CANCER

Synchronous Metastatic Cancer

Synchronous metastatic cancer, particularly to the liver, is not a contraindication to resection of the rectal primary. Maximum surgical effort should be made to avoid a permanent colostomy if the surgery is considered palliative. However, a palliative abdominoperineal resection is appropriate in the presence of minimal distant disease, in order to prevent or treat bleeding, obstruction, or diarrhea. However, if massive liver metastases are present, palliation may be achieved with dietary restriction, radiation therapy, fulguration, or laser therapy. A diverting colostomy alone is to be avoided if at all possible.

Locally Advanced and Unresectable Rectal Cancer

Such cancers are adherent to or directly invade contiguous organs or structures. Many are *curable* with radical surgery and high-dose radiation therapy. Anterior exenteration in women with vaginal involvement is appropriate. The rectal tumor is resected in continuity with a hysterectomy and a posterior vaginectomy. Anterior extension of rectal cancer into the prostate or base of the bladder in men, or into the bladder in women who have had a hysterectomy, is surgically curable in one third of cases by pelvic exenteration.[678-680] Posterior extension into bone can be surgically treated by including the sacrum in the rectal resection.[681]

In the absence of distant disease, locally advanced rectal cancer that invades contiguous organs or pelvic structures is best treated locally with a combination of surgery and radiation therapy.[681]

PREOPERATIVE IRRADIATION. For unresectable or marginally resectable rectal cancer, the goal of preoperative irradiation is to increase the likelihood of pathologically negative margins at surgery. Such an approach would potentially lead to an increased local control rate as well as (one hopes) survival. The problem in evaluating any series involving preoperative irradiation is the use of variable subjective criteria for resectability. The doses needed to increase resectability must be high, 4500 cGy or above.

The results of preoperative radiation therapy in lesions that were considered marginally resectable or unresectable are shown in Table 29-30. Resectability and the complete resection rate are seen to be highly variable, as are the local failure rate and the survival rate.[619,652,682-685] The data in Table 29-30 suggest that if a sufficiently high dose of preoperative irradiation is given, a large percentage of tumors may become resectable, and many patients in this group may have a long survival. However, since the local failure rate remains high, with survival of only 25% to 50% of patients on average, better local and systemic control is needed. As a result, there have been attempts to add intraoperative therapy in the form of radioactive implants or electron beam irradiation to these preoperative irradiation regimens for enhanced local control, or to provide chemotherapy concurrently with radiation therapy for better systemic control.

Several studies of combined chemotherapy and irradiation have included small numbers of patients with advanced rectal carcinoma.[686-689] The definition of advanced disease has varied from study to study, but in general the tumors have been circumferential, fixed or partially mobile, large (≥4 cm), involving adjacent structures, and/or deeply ulcerated. Chemotherapy has consisted of 5-FU alone[686,689] or combined 5-FU and mitomycin C.[686-688] After the combined treatment, 71% to 98% of the patients underwent surgical resection. In two of the studies[686,687] no tumor was found in 13% to 20% of the operative specimens. Local failure rates varied from 7% to 22%, and the rate of distant metastases from 23% to 39%. Overall survival rates varied from 59% to 86%, with disease-free survival rates of 48% to 64%. The data of Taylor et al did not suggest any additive benefit to the 5-FU.[689] Because the follow-up time in these studies has been relatively short and no randomized studies have been done, it is difficult to ascertain whether the addition of chemotherapy will affect the long-term survival in patients with marginally resectable or unresectable disease.

INTRAOPERATIVE IRRADIATION. Intraoperative radiation therapy may be defined as the use of some form of irradiation during a surgical procedure. Low-energy photon beams, electron beams, and interstitial radioactive implants have been used.[690] The value of intraoperative radiation therapy is that the field of a boost dose may be reduced by directly visualizing the target volume. In addition, one may minimize the dose received by normal tissues by physically moving normal tissues out of the way of an external beam or

TABLE 29-30. Preoperative Radiation Therapy for Marginally Resectable or Unresectable Rectal Cancer

Study	*No. of Patients*	*Dose (cGy)*	*Follow-up*	*Resectability (%)**	*Complete Resection (%)**	*Local Failure (%)†*	*Survival (%)**
Netherlands Cancer Inst.[682]	21	3500 (marginally resectable)	$2\frac{1}{2}$–$6\frac{1}{2}$ yr	95	95	15	48
	38	6400 (unresectable)	$\frac{1}{2}$–$2\frac{1}{2}$ yr	0	0	. . .	18
Univ. of Oregon[652]	58	5000	≥4 yr	41	24	. . .	9
Univ. Hosp. of Bergen[683]	24	3150	4 mo to $3\frac{1}{2}$ yr	67	46	6	33
Tufts–New Engl. Med. Ctr.[684]	44	4500–5000‡	>3 yr	75	59	36	41
Mass. Genl. Hosp.[685]	25	4000–5200	2–6 yr	80	64	43	28
Univ. of Virginia[619]	60	4000–6000	>$3\frac{1}{2}$ yr (mean)	. . .	87	12	45
Thomas Jefferson Univ. Hosp.[588]	45	4500 (partially fixed)	≥3 yr	100	. . .	2	79
	19	5500 (totally fixed)	≥3 yr	84	. . .	29	52
	12	6500 (unresectable)	≥3 yr	58	. . .	43	24

* Original number of patients used as a denominator.
† Local failure as a percentage of patients resected.
‡ Two patients received higher doses (5400 and 6000 cGy).

by using rapid dose decrements at the periphery of the target volume with radioactive implants. As a result, a better therapeutic ratio may ensue. In this situation one may use a relatively high boost dose given in minutes as intraoperative beam therapy, or a relatively high localized dose given over a few days by means of an interstitial implant.

Pilot studies combining external irradiation and intraoperative electron beam therapy have been done by Gunderson et al at both Massachusetts General Hospital and the Mayo Clinic on patients with residual, unresectable, or recurrent disease of the colon or rectum.[691–693] At both institutions, preoperative external radiation therapy was given in doses of 4500 to 5000 cGy, with electron beam boosts of 1000 to 1500 cGy, usually with 6- to 18-MeV electrons. In both studies, the local recurrence rate has been low (6%–15%), and the survival rate without evidence of disease has been about 60%. In an analysis of unresectable rectal carcinoma cases at the Massachusetts General Hospital, Tepper et al reported a 92% actuarial local control rate at 3 years in patients with completely resected disease.[694] In patients with residual disease the actuarial local control rate at 3 years was 67%. Survival overall was 60% at 3 years, with 70% actuarial survival for those with completely resected disease and 30% for those with gross residual tumor. In an update from the Mayo Clinic, the disease-free survival rate was 53% after a follow-up of 10 to 64 months.[693] In an RTOG Phase I/II study of intraoperative radiation therapy for unresectable or recurrent carcinoma of the rectum, no toxic effects have been observed other than minor bladder problems. The RTOG is now planning to proceed with Phase III trials.[695]

Interstitial implants have been used for advanced and recurrent carcinoma of the colon and rectum.[696–698] A study reported from the University of Southern California involved locally extensive carcinoma of the anorectum.[697] Forty patients were treated, although only 32 had adenocarcinomas of the rectum. A preoperative radiation dose of 4000 to 5000 cGy was given to the pelvis, followed by insertion of an iridium-192 afterloading implant, either once to a dose of 3500 to 4000 cGy (in four patients treated early in the program) or twice to a dose of 1500 to 2000 cGy for each implant, spaced 2 to 3 weeks apart (for the remainder of the patients). With a 3-year average follow-up, the local recurrence rate was 30%.

In summary, combined preoperative external radiation therapy and intraoperative irradiation techniques may improve local control and survival rates in some patients. Complications with intraoperative electron beam therapy have been relatively few (ureteral obstruction, healing problems, or infectious complications), while complications with interstitial implants have been relatively serious, although it is reported that when implants are fractionated (*i.e.*, two separate implantations), complications are fewer.[697]

POSTOPERATIVE IRRADIATION. Wang and Schulz reported a few "cures" in patients treated with postoperative radiation therapy who had residual disease after surgery for initially advanced lesions.[699] In a series of papers from the Albert Einstein College of Medicine, the disease-free survival rate was about 67% after an average follow-up of about 3 years in patients with advanced rectal and rectosigmoid cancer treated postoperatively with 4600 cGy to the pelvis followed by a 1000 to 2000 cGy boost to areas of residual disease.[545,547,700] Allee et al differentiated between patients with gross residual and microscopic residual disease.[620] Those with gross residual disease had a local failure rate of 52% and an actuarial 3-year survival rate of only 6%, whereas those with microscopic residual disease had a local failure rate of 26% and an actuarial 3-year survival rate of 59%. These patients were treated with relatively high doses, initially to 4500 cGy, to pelvic fields, followed by a boost to 6000 to 7000 cGy if small bowel could be excluded.

Patients with advanced or residual local disease who have not received any preoperative or intraoperative irradiation should be considered for high-dose postoperative irradiation, although no randomized studies have been done to show a survival benefit in these patients.

FOLLOW-UP AFTER POTENTIALLY CURATIVE TREATMENT

PURPOSES OF REGULAR FOLLOW-UP

The detection of asymptomatic recurrence, discussed below, is only one facet of patient follow-up. Maximizing the quality of life by management of treatment-related problems is extremely important in patients with colorectal disease.

Management of Treatment-Related Problems

DISTURBANCES IN BOWEL FUNCTION. Dietary modifications and medications may be necessary for control of bowel function, in the short or long term. Severe diarrhea secondary to loss of the ileocecal valve and bile salt intolerance can occur after a right-sided colectomy. Many patients are chronically constipated before colorectal surgery and may need to continue increased intake of dietary roughage and the use of stool softeners. After sphincter-saving rectal surgery, fecal urgency and frequency may be ameliorated with stool bulking agents.

SMALL BOWEL OBSTRUCTION. This late-occurring problem, related to surgical scarring or radiation enteritis, necessitates surgery in 5% of patients.

COLOSTOMY-ASSOCIATED PROBLEMS. The need for continued advice about colostomy management, irrigation techniques, prevention of skin irritation, and so forth may necessitate consultation with an enterostomal therapist.

DISTURBANCES IN SEXUAL FUNCTION. Surgery or pelvic irradiation in females may lead to menopause and vaginal dryness with dyspareunia. Male impotence due to both psychological and organic factors may require intervention. Implants can improve erectile impotence. Retrograde ejaculation is the rule after pelvic surgery in males.

Detection of New Primary Colorectal Cancers

Since approximately 5% of patients will develop a metachronous large bowel cancer, the detection of new primary colorectal cancers is one of the more important aspects of follow-up. If colonoscopy was not performed preoperatively, it should be performed 4 to 6 months after surgery.

Detection of Other Primary Cancers

Patients who have had primary colorectal cancer may be at high risk for the development of other cancers, particularly of the female breast, ovary, and cervix. Coordinated screening for these potentially curable cancers is important.

DETECTION OF RECURRENT COLORECTAL CANCER

A subset of patients with recurrent colorectal cancer can be cured[702]; hence, a nihilistic approach to follow-up is not appropriate. Local failure in the pelvis and limited distant metastases to the liver or lung may be curable if detected at an asymptomatic stage.

Follow-up strategies directed toward the detection of recurrent cancer in asymptomatic patients will vary, based on the risks of such recurrence and the likelihood that such detection would lead to early intervention. The availability of multiple expensive tests has led to some uncertainty as to appropriate follow-up strategies. A recent prospective study from the National Institutes of Health provides common-sense guidelines for the follow-up of high-risk patients.[703] Interval history and physical examination were combined with serial abdominal CT, chest radiography, lung tomography, liver–spleen radionuclide scintigraphy, intravenous pyelography, bone scans, and barium studies. CEA levels were monitored monthly for 3 years, then every 3 months for an additional 2 years. Serial CEA testing combined with regular physician visits was the most useful approach to the detection of recurrent colorectal cancer. The controversial issue of CEA determinations is addressed below.[704,705]

General guidelines for the follow-up of patients after potentially curative treatment for colorectal cancer are outlined in Table 29-31. A more detailed discussion of various tests follows.

Blood Tests in the Detection of Recurrent Cancer

CARCINOEMBRYONIC ANTIGEN. Studies from a number of groups have confirmed that serial CEA assays do detect recurrent colorectal cancer in asymptomatic patients.[706–713] In approximately two thirds of patients with recurrent disease, an increased CEA level will be the first indicator of the tumor. The pattern of recurrence influences the likelihood of CEA elevation: 25% to 50% of patients with local or regional recurrences and 95% of those with liver metastases have increased CEA levels.[714] Primary anaplastic tumors that do not stain positively with immunohistochemical stains for CEA frequently are not associated with an elevated CEA level despite the presence of metastatic disease.[715]

The sensitivity and specificity of the CEA assay will depend to a great degree on the definition of an "elevated" CEA level. Minimal transient CEA elevations are common after surgery, and can be influenced not only by smoking history, chronic bronchitis, hepatitis, and colitis, but also simple factors such as the time of day the blood sample was drawn. A diurnal variation in CEA levels in normal people has been documented.[714,716] Minton and associates have developed a nomogram to identify pathologic elevations for an individual patient that may still fall within the normal range for large populations.[708] The rate of CEA elevation (the slope) may be a more accurate indicator, with a more rapid rise suggestive of liver metastases.[717] Denstman and colleagues have looked at decision matrices for various CEA levels, as well as rate of CEA elevation. Receiver-operating characteristic curve analysis has been used to define 6.0 ng/ml as the ideal upper limit of normal.[718] However, despite this analysis, Denstman et al point out that with this value the data indicate only a sensitivity of 62% and specificity of 83%.

In using the CEA test, it is important to consider the prognostic group (pathologic stage) and the interval between

TABLE 29-31. General Guidelines for Follow-up of Patients After Potentially Curative Surgery

Procedure/Test	*Frequency*	*Comment*
History/examination	Every 3–4 mo for 3 yr, then every 6 mo for 2 yr	Detects $\frac{1}{3}$ of recurrences
Fecal occult blood	Same	
Sigmoidoscopy	Same	Only if anastomosis in pelvis
Colonoscopy	Preoperatively or 4–6 mo postoperatively, then every 6–36 mo	Every 3 yr once free of polyps
Chest x-ray	Yearly	
CEA	Every 2–4 mo	
Liver chemistries Chest CT Abdominal CT Pelvic CT Liver–spleen scan Liver US IVP Bone scan	As indicated by findings on history, examination, or elevated CEA levels	

tests. Even if we accept a 95% sensitivity and 95% specificity, the predictive value will vary greatly based on the likely prevalence of recurrent cancer.[718] If an early node-negative cancer patient undergoes CEA testing monthly, the prevalence of interval disease may only be 1%. The predictive value of a positive test will be only 16%, with a 99.9% predictive value for a negative CEA test. At the other extreme, if a multiple node-positive patient undergoes CEA testing every 4 months, a tumor recurrence prevalence of 20% may be estimated. Under these circumstances, a positive CEA test will have a predictive value of 82.6% and a negative test will have a predictive value of 98.7%.[719]

Considering the speculative benefit of early detection of asymptomatic recurrent colorectal cancer, a number of oncologists have suggested that CEA assays should not be performed at all outside of clinical trials. By contrast, a group at Ohio State University recommends testing every 4 to 6 weeks to maximize the efficacy of second-look surgery.[720] The IUCC Workshop on the Immunodiagnosis of Cancer recommended that CEA assays be performed every 6 to 12 weeks.[721]

LIVER FUNCTION TESTS. Because the CEA level is elevated in 95% of patients with liver metastases, the CEA assay may be the most sensitive "liver function test" for the diagnosis of this condition. The following is limited to the various biochemical tests normally performed when liver disease is suspected. Unfortunately, published reports do not focus on the detection of early or minimal metastatic disease, but include in the analyses patients with gross metastatic cancer.

Lind and Singer, using Bayesian analysis, analyzed the predictive value of bilirubin, alkaline phosphatase (AP), lactic dehydrogenase (LDH), and SGOT values in the diagnosis of liver metastases.[722] Interested readers are encouraged to study this report. The accuracy of such tests is the highest when the prevalence of liver metastases is low. With a prevalence of 5% (in the range for screening purposes), accuracies are as follows: AP, 76%; SGOT, 86%; bilirubin, 90%; and LDH, 71%.

A prospective analysis of both single and multiple blood chemistries in the detection of liver metastases was reported by Kemeny, Sugarbaker, and colleagues.[311] CEA and γ-glutamyl transpeptidase (GGTP) were the most sensitive, while SGOT and 5′-nucleotidase were the most specific. The sensitivity of the CEA assay as a single test was 86%, the specificity was 60%, and the accuracy was 79%. Combinations of liver chemistries with and without CEA assay yielded accuracies only in the range of 60%. Tartter et al also found the combination of CEA and AP to be the most useful screening test for liver metastases.[723] With CEA values above 10 ng/ml and AP values above 135 IU/ml, the combination had a sensitivity of 88%, with a false negative rate of only 2%. In another prospective study of liver metastases, Kemeny et al looked at the subset of patients with resectable (minimal) liver metastases. Only 40% had an elevated AP level, and only 30% an elevated LDH level.[724]

ADDITIONAL BLOOD TESTS. Podolsky and associates reported results with galactosyl transferase isoenzyme II (GT II) in patients with colorectal cancer. The isoenzyme was elevated in 75% of patients with metastatic cancer; in three patients, increased levels preceded clinical recurrence by 3 to 7 months.[725]

The cancer-associated carbohydrate antigen 19-9 (CA 19-9), detected by monoclonal antibody, is present in the serum of patients with a diversity of cancers. Reports from a number of authors indicate that it is not as useful as the CEA assay.[726–728]

Diagnostic Imaging in the Detection of Recurrent Cancer

Chest radiographs are useful for the early detection of asymptomatic *lung metastases.* Before a major liver resection is undertaken, lung tomography or chest CT is appropriate.

For the detection of recurrent disease in the *pelvis and abdomen,* CT is the imaging modality of choice after a complete physical examination. It remains unclear whether magnetic resonance (MR) imaging will be superior to CT in this anatomical area or even complementary.

A variety of imaging techniques are available for the detection of *liver metastases.* The sensitivity of the modality is important, but specificity must also be considered because hepatic cysts and hemangiomas are common. The type of patient being studied is important in the selection of an imaging technique. For patients with symptomatic hepatomegaly, radionuclide scintigraphy of the liver allows excellent visualization of multifocal metastases.

The evaluation of patients with one or a few space-occupying lesions less than 3 cm in diameter is a more difficult problem. Kemeny and associates, reporting on 60 patients, noted that CT correctly demonstrated the size and location of the lesions in only 43%.[724] In 40% of patients lesions found at surgery were not visualized on CT. In a similar study reported by Sugarbaker's group, CT, radionuclide scintigraphy, and US all were unreliable for lesions less than 3 cm in diameter.[311,729] Overall, CT had the highest accuracy at 84%.

Gunven and colleagues in Tokyo studied CT and US preoperatively.[730] For lesions under 1 cm, CT was the most accurate, but still detected less than 50% of the lesions. Even with 1- to 2-cm lesions, the sensitivity of CT was only 50%, and that of US was only 40%.

The three-dimensional imaging capabilities of MR imaging have yet to be fully explored in characterizing liver metastases. Stark and associates found MR imaging to be superior to CT, and MR displayed definitive diagnostic features in small hemangiomas.[731] At present, MR imaging should not supplant CT in the search for minimal intra-abdominal and hepatic metastatic cancer.

TREATMENT OF RECURRENT AND METASTATIC CANCER

SPECIFIC MANAGEMENT PROBLEMS

Liver Metastases

Surgical excision of liver metastases is discussed in depth in Chapter 62, Section 3. It is important to stress that surgical resection of liver metastases is the only curative option and should be considered in most patients in otherwise good general health and lacking evidence of any tumor outside the liver. Overall, surgical resection is associated with a 25% to 30% 5-year disease-free survival rate. Results are better if the primary was node negative. Wedge resection with a 2-cm margin is adequate, unless size or location requires anatomical lobectomy. Although the presence of a single metastatic focus is ideal for treatment purposes, excision of as many as four lesions is associated with cure, particularly if the lesions are all greater than 4 cm or are unilobar.

Since hamartomas, bile duct cysts, hemangiomas, and granulomas are common in the liver, every attempt should be made to biopsy suspicious liver nodules found during surgery for the primary tumor. If an incisional biopsy is not feasible, flexible needle aspiration may be used to obtain material for cytological analysis.[732] A limited wedge resection of a single liver metastasis is reasonable at the time of surgery for the primary. More extensive resections should be delayed 4 to 6 weeks after surgery for the primary, particularly if a preoperative CT scan is not available.

Lung Metastases

Lung metastases are usually associated with widespread metastatic disease. However, isolated lung metastases may occur, and if they are single, resection should be considered. Lung metastases occur most commonly with cancers of the distal 5 cm of the rectum because of the dual venous drainage. In highly selected patients with isolated single lung lesions, resection results in a 20% 5-year survival rate.[733]

Local Failure in Rectal Cancer

Local or regional failure may occur after treatment of the primary cancer by local measures, sphincter-saving surgery, or abdominoperineal resection. Because recurrent pelvic cancer is frequently symptomatic and difficult to eradicate when it occurs, efforts should be directed toward maximizing the local cure at the time of the original treatment. Unexplained perineal or buttock pain that develops a few months to a few years after treatment of rectal cancer should be considered to indicate recurrence until proven otherwise. Most apparently localized pelvic recurrences are associated with more extensive diffuse pelvic cancer, which makes cure difficult. Some 25% to 50% of patients with rectal cancer have isolated locoregional recurrences, so aggressive treatment may lead to cure. Since management differs greatly, depending on the initial surgical treatment, the following discussion is organized according to the original approach to the primary tumor. In addition, aggressive multimodality locoregional treatment options are more limited in patients in whom disease recurs despite full-dose adjuvant radiation therapy.

RECURRENCE AFTER LIMITED LOCAL TREATMENT. After treatment of rectal cancer by local excision, intracavitary radiation, or fulguration, some patients with limited local recurrences can be cured by radical surgery, perhaps combined with radiation therapy. Selected patients with very superficial recurrences can be given additional local treatment prior to radical extirpative surgery, particularly if their medical condition would render radical surgery excessively risky. Although the data are scant, low anterior resection or abdominoperineal resection can often be performed (in the absence of distant disease), with 25% to 50% salvage rates.

RECURRENCE AFTER RADICAL SURGERY. Although isolated resectable local recurrences occur, most patients with pelvic failure have diffuse locoregional recurrences. In addition, many of these patients will also have distant metastatic disease. Patients with asymptomatic or minimally symptomatic pelvic recurrences and tumor outside the pelvis are usually treated with systemic chemotherapy. Regional chemotherapy of the pelvis is an experimental approach, with an encouraging initial report on the use of 5-FU and mitomycin C given by internal iliac artery infusion.[734] Results may be enhanced with hyperthermia.[735]

Irradiation is the most useful palliative technique in patients with symptomatic pelvic recurrence. Although 80% to 90% of patients will obtain initial pain relief, long-term symptom-free survival is uncommon with external beam irradiation alone.[736,737] If disease recurs in the pelvis despite adjuvant high-dose irradiation, additional palliative irradiation is frequently not feasible. In patients with uncontrolled pelvic pain despite irradiation, symptomatic relief must be sought with pain control measures, not cancer treatment.

Localized pelvic recurrences should be resected if feasible. These include instances of limited presacral tumor, vaginal apex masses, and isolated suture line and perineal recurrences. The useful surgical procedures include wide local excision, abdominoperineal resection, resection of pelvic tumors with en bloc partial sacrectomy, and total pelvic exenteration. Resection may be combined with external beam irradiation, intraoperative brachytherapy with iodine-125, intraoperative electron beam or photon radiation, or afterloading isotope catheter systems.

Surgical resection of highly selected patients with pelvic recurrence can be curative.[738] Exenteration can result in a 20% to 30% 5-year survival rate.[739] Posterior fixation to the lower sacrum may necessitate en bloc excision. As long as the S3 nerve roots are left intact, bladder function will be acceptable. Composite resection has been reported by Wanebo and associates, with 6 of 24 patients surviving 4 years.[740]

Patients with localized pelvic recurrences without prior irradiation have been treated at the Massachusetts General Hospital and Mayo Clinic with an aggressive multimodality approach. Patients undergo high-dose external beam irradiation and radical surgical resection with an intraoperative electron beam boost. In the Massachusetts General Hospital series of 22 patients, an actuarial local control rate of 56% was obtained at 4 years in the subset of patients with tumors amenable to complete resection.[690] Thirty-six patients have been treated at the Mayo Clinic, with only a 17% local failure rate after a short median follow-up.[741] Intraoperative brachytherapy has yielded comparable results at Memorial Hospital.[698]

SUTURE LINE RECURRENCE AFTER LOW ANTERIOR RESECTION. Limited suture line recurrence in a patient with metastatic cancer may not require treatment. Radiation therapy may be useful for more advanced disease, and to control bleeding. Prophylactic colostomy should be avoided if at all possible, with partial obstruction managed by diet restriction and stool softeners. The Nd-YAG laser may play a role in keeping the lumen patent. In patients without distant metastases, long-term disease-free survival can be achieved with abdominoperineal resection, although cures are infrequent.[742-744]

PERINEAL RECURRENCE AFTER ABDOMINOPERINEAL RESECTION. It is important to distinguish between pelvic and perineal recurrences after abdominoperineal resection.[745] Isolated perineal recurrences can be palliated by wide local excision, but the disease is rarely cured.[746,747]

Treatment Initiated on the Basis of CEA Assay

The definition of an elevated CEA level and the evaluation of patients with elevated levels were discussed earlier. After transient CEA elevations, associated benign disorders, and laboratory error have been ruled out, asymptomatic patients will fall into one of three groups: they will have a new primary cancer; they will have a recurrent colorectal cancer, which can be ascertained by a more complete history, physical examination, or a panoply of tests and scans; or they will have an entirely negative evaluation. This section discusses the management of the latter group.

Options in managing asymptomatic patients with elevated CEA levels and negative evaluations include (1) continued observation and repeat examinations and tests, (2) chemotherapy, and (3) surgical exploration (second-look surgery).

CHEMOTHERAPY. Because of the relative inefficacy of systemic chemotherapy, it is difficult to use this modality in asymptomatic patients without some way to monitor response to treatment. In a randomized trial of 5-FU and methyl-CCNU, a survival benefit could not be demonstrated in patients receiving early cytotoxic therapy rather than continued observation.[748]

SURGERY. In analyzing data on the usefulness of CEA-directed second-look surgery, a number of issues are important (Table 29-32).

The frequency with which CEA assays should be performed was discussed earlier in the section on Detection of Recurrent Colorectal Cancer. However, if second-look surgery is shown to be efficacious, it is likely that CEA assays will need to be done every 1 to 2 months to maximize this benefit. The Ohio State University group has strongly endorsed monthly CEA assays, followed by early reoperation if necessary (see below).[749] Currently, a prospective randomized trial is underway at the Memorial Sloan–Kettering Cancer Center comparing CEA assays performed monthly versus every 4 months.

Sites Most Amenable to Curative Resection. In the various studies of CEA-directed second-look operations, the term curative resection is used. This term is loosely applied to tumors amenable to complete surgical resection. It is unlikely that resection of para-aortic nodes, omental tumor, or other peritoneal nodules is truly curative. However, selected liver or lung metastases and some locally recurrent cancer may be resected for cure in a subset of patients.

Negative Exploration. Most groups have documented tumor recurrence in over 90% of patients selected for second-look surgery. At Ohio State University, tumor was confirmed in 139 of 146 surgical explorations.[720,749,750] The Memorial Hospital group found recurrence in 33 of 37 patients explored.[751] Staab and associates reported tumor confirmation in 29 of 32 patients.[752] However, most of the patients in whom surgical exploration is negative will likely develop clinical signs of recurrent cancer in the future.

Surgical Resections. There has been great variability in the reports of second-look operations in regard to the frequency of potentially curative resections. In a series of four reports from the Ohio State University group, a total of 146 patients underwent surgical exploration; 58% subsequently underwent resection with curative intent.[708,720,749,750] This high re-

TABLE 29-32. CEA-Initiated Second-Look Surgery Issues

Is overall survival, as well as symptom-free survival, prolonged compared to that achieved with regular interval history and physical examination?
Optimum CEA assay frequency
Optimum definition of abnormal CEA
Optimum timing of second-look surgery in patients with elevated CEA levels and negative evaluation for recurrent cancer
Value of adjuvant chemotherapy after second-look surgery
Cost–benefit analysis

sectability rate was ascribed to a policy of frequent CEA determinations (every 4–6 weeks), and early operation with CEA values less than 10 ng/ml. At Memorial Hospital, 43% of patients had resectable tumors.[751] However, Steele et al at Harvard University could resect only 27%,[753] Wilking et al at Roswell Park Memorial Cancer Institute only 15%,[754] and Staab et al in the Federal Republic of Germany only 12%.[752]

Cures. Despite considerable variability in long-term survival data, some patients who undergo second-look operations based on CEA assay results will have tumor resected and will be alive and free of cancer at 5 years. Most reports refer to actuarial 5-year survival rates. However, in a recent publication from the Ohio State University group, the 5-year survival rate in the 45 patients who underwent curative resection and were at risk for 5 years was 31%.[720]

Cost. The cost of CEA follow-up programs is considerable. When the expenses of the assays, additional laboratory tests and scans, and exploratory surgery are tabulated, such programs cost $25,000 per patient found to have resectable cancer.[755] If 25% of such patients are actually cured, then the true cost is $100,000 per patient cured.

Overall Impact on Survival. August, Ottow, and Sugarbaker have analyzed colorectal cancer from the perspective of the potential for surgical cure of recurrent cancer.[702] They estimate that 15% of patients have isolated local recurrence, with a cure rate of 20%. This results in a 3% incremental survival. Approximately 25% of patients appear to have isolated hepatic metastases, with one fourth of these appropriate for resection. With a 30% cure rate following liver resection, the overall incremental survival will be an additional 2%. Hence, it is likely that surgery, either based on clinical criteria or on a CEA blood test, can improve overall survival only by 5% (3% + 2%) of the entire patient population undergoing potentially curative resection of colorectal cancer.

Current Studies. The National Institutes of Health and the Medical Research Council are sponsoring a large cooperative trial in the United Kingdom to answer the following question: Does monthly CEA monitoring, added to quarterly routine histories and physical examinations, actually reduce the morbidity and mortality of colorectal cancer?[756] Following resection of B2 or C colon or rectal cancer, patients undergo monthly CEA assays. The results of the tests are unknown to the patient and the physician. If recurrence is detected because of symptoms or physical examination, appropriate treatment is instituted. If the patient remains asymptomatic but has a rising CEA level (>10 ng/ml), the patient is randomized. In the standard follow-up arm, again the physician and patient are not notified. In the intensive follow-up arm, the physician is notified, additional tests and scans are obtained, and second-look surgery is performed, if appropriate, based on the complete evaluation.

At this time, no groups are studying the issue of the optimum timing of second-look surgery in asymptomatic patients with a negative evaluation. Since most patients have no benefit from these explorations, a strategy of delayed surgery until tumor is detectable on a radiograph, scan, or examination or until symptoms develop may maximize symptom-free survival for the entire group.

One approach to focusing second-look surgery despite normal routine radiographs and scans is the use of isotope-labeled monoclonal antibodies to define recurrent tumor, both with external scanning and with intraoperative gamma detection. Iodine-131, iodine-125, and indium-111 isotopes with CEA antibody and monoclonal B72.3 have been studied.[757–760] The exact usefulness of these techniques is not yet known.

CHEMOTHERAPY FOR METASTATIC COLORECTAL CANCER

Single-Agent Chemotherapy

The fluoropyrimidines remain the most widely employed single chemotherapeutic agents for patients with colorectal cancer. Since the introduction of 5-FU in 1957,[761] tens of thousands of patients have been treated, and objective response rates of 8% to 85% have been reported.[701,762] The reasons for the wide range of response rates include various patient selection factors, such as performance status and co-morbid conditions; disease factors, such as sites of metastases and prior therapy; and treatment-related factors. A particularly important treatment-related variable seems to be the intensity of 5-FU administration. Moertel found a 9% response rate for 5-FU therapy that induced no leukopenia, compared with a 30% response rate for 5-FU therapy that reduced the white blood cell count to 4500 to 1500 cells/mm^3.[763] The Central Oncology Group compared four programs with different schedules, routes, and intensities of 5-FU.[764] They found that IV 5-FU, 12 mg/kg/d for 5 days, followed by 6 mg/kg every other day for 11 days, followed by 15 mg/kg/wk resulted in a superior response rate (35%) and response duration ($p < 0.001$). Associated with this benefit was a higher incidence of drug toxicity, with 18% of patients experiencing severe or life-threatening leukopenia. This loading course schedule of 5-FU did not, however, result in a significantly longer survival. It has been asserted that an objective response rate of about 20% is generally achievable with the fluoropyrimidines.[701,763] Overall, 5-FU does not demonstrably affect survival for all patients treated; it is associated with a median survival of 6 or 8 months. However, for the minority of patients who do evidence an objective response, the median survival may be in the 12- to 18-month range.[762] If 5-FU is administered with proper vigor, most patients experience mucositis, diarrhea, or leukopenia as dose-limiting effects of therapy.[762,765] Even after three decades of use, no single schedule or dose scheme has yet been shown to be ideal, but administration with proper intensity (to the point of definite but acceptable toxic effects) is appropriate.

Attempts to improve upon the therapeutic benefit of 5-FU have included modifications of route and schedule. Administering 5-FU by the oral rather than parenteral route has been abandoned because of erratic GI absorption and poor response rates.[765–768] However, the use of prolonged or nearly continuous IV infusions of 5-FU has gained in popularity. The advantages of ambulatory infusion 5-FU given over

TABLE 29-33. Hepatic Intra-arterial Floxuridine Therapy for Liver Metastases in Colorectal Cancer

Study	Mode	No. of Patients	Dose (mg/kg/d × 14 d q 28 d)	Objective Response Rate (%)
Kemeny et al, 1986[783]	IV	49	0.125	20
	IA	45	0.3	50
Hohn et al, 1987[784]	IV	46	0.075	10
	IA	67	0.20	37

IV = intravenous; IA = intra-arterial.

several days to months include the ability to deliver a relatively higher dose per unit time and the lack of myelotoxicity.[769-771] In order for continuous IV infusion to be practical and economically feasible, dependable and affordable infusion devices had to be developed. The current pump technology makes these devices easily available. Lokich et al[772] have demonstrated that for 5-FU the major toxic effect of 300 mg/m²/d given by continuous IV infusion for weeks to months is mucositis; an additional 5% to 25% of patients experience a hand-foot syndrome of painful erythroderma.[773] The relative lack of hematologic toxicity makes this regimen attractive for combinations with myelotoxic drugs. Response rates ranging from 25% to 50% have been reported,[774-779] and some comparative studies suggest that infusion is more efficacious than bolus therapy.[770] Prospective randomized trials comparing conventional with continuous infusion 5-FU are ongoing.[772,780] Because of the added expense and bother of this mode of therapy, it is hoped that substantial clinical advantages will be demonstrated.[781] Preliminary data indicate a 29% response rate with continuous IV infusion of 5-FU, compared to a 9% response rate with bolus administration.

Another special mode of administration of a fluoropyrimidine is hepatic intra-arterial (IA) therapy for those with liver metastases. Because of the favorable pharmacodynamics of fluorodeoxyuridine (FUDR), there is high hepatic extraction and drug concentration with relatively little systemic exposure. Moreover, preliminary Phase II studies with continuous intrahepatic arterial infusion of FUDR at 0.2 to 0.4 mg/kg/d for 14 days out of 28 have reported 80% objective response rates.[781,782] In order to confirm these findings, two randomized studies have been completed comparing IV with IA FUDR (Table 29-33). Although two to three times higher response rates can be obtained with IA therapy, the impact on disease-free and overall survival is unclear.[783,784]

Historically, the next most important family of compounds for colorectal cancer patients has been the nitrosoureas. Response rates of 10% to 15% have been reported for BCNU, CCNU, chlorozotocin, and methyl-CCNU.[701,785,786] Because of the convenience of oral administration and of single-agent activity equivalent to that of 5-FU demonstrated in one randomized trial, methyl-CCNU has probably been the most frequently employed.[785] There are, however, no firm data to support the contention of superiority for any particular nitrosourea.[787] The chloroethyl nitrosoureas have characteristic delayed and cumulative toxic effects on bone marrow, which often limits the ability to administer therapy for prolonged periods. In addition, patients receiving methyl-CCNU are at greater risk for myelodysplasia, preleukemia, and acute nonlymphatic leukemia. For 2067 patients retrospectively evaluated, the relative risk of such a hematologic syndrome was estimated to be 12.4 times greater than in those treated with other forms of chemotherapy. The chance of a leukemic syndrome was greater for those receiving higher total doses and living for a longer time. Obviously, patients receiving large total doses of methyl-CCNU as part of an adjuvant program are at the greatest risk.[788] Mitomycin C has produced the same general quantitative and qualitative responses as the nitrosoureas.[765,787,789] Since both mitomycin C and methyl-CCNU have potential for substantial chronic hematologic and renal toxicity and yield median response durations of approximately 3 months, there is little to recommend one agent over the other.

Unfortunately, although dozens of new drugs are being screened there is no convincing evidence of meaningful efficacy for any of them. Table 29-34 lists the other agents, which have produced a total response rate of 4% in almost 4000 patients studied.

The modest responsiveness of colon adenocarcinoma to currently available chemotherapy has been the subject of intense basic science investigation. Adenocarcinoma of cer-

TABLE 29-34. Single Chemotherapeutic Agents Examined in Phase II Studies

Acivicin	Ftorafur
Aclacinomycin A	F3TDR
Alanosine	Hexamethylmelamine
Aminothiadiazole	Ifosfamide
AMSA	Indicine-*n*-oxide
Anguidine	Maytansine
5-Azacytidine	Methyl-CCNU
B-TGDR	MGBG
Bisantrene	Mitoxantrone
Bleomycin	PALA
Chlorozotocin	PCNU
Cisplatin	Piperazinedione
Cyclocytidine	Razoxane
3-Deazauridine	Rubidazone
4-Deoxydoxorubicin	Streptonigrin
Dianhydrogalactidol	Streptozotocin
Diaziquone	Teniposide
Dibromodulcitol	TMCA
Dichloromethotrexate	Triazinate
Diglycoaldehyde	Tubercidin
4-DMDR	Vindesine
DON	Yoshi-864
Doxorubicin	Zinostatin
Etoposide	

tain other organs (breast, ovary, stomach) is initially responsive to a wide variety of alkylating and anthracycline agents, so histopathology is not an adequate explanation. One possible explanation for the poor response of colon adenocarcinoma to chemotherapy may lie in the observation of high expression of the *mdr* 1 gene in colon cancer cells de novo. This gene encodes a drug transport protein that modulates the access of cytotoxics to the interior of the cell. Other mechanisms of drug resistance, both acquired and arising de novo, are being explored.[790] Colon carcinoma cells also evidence other aspects of the pleotropic drug resistance phenomenon,[791] and characterization of the p170 glycoprotein, glutathione transferase and other biochemical marker activity is being pursued.

Combination Chemotherapy

Because of the limited number of chemotherapeutic options available, most attempts to improve systemic treatment have consisted of empirically adding drugs to 5-FU.[701,787] One such popular regimen is based on the addition of methyl-CCNU to 5-FU. Enthusiasm for this combination arose from a small randomized comparison of methyl-CCNU + Oncovin + 5-FU (MOF) versus 5-FU in metastatic bowel cancer patients at the Mayo Clinic. As initially reported, the objective response rate for MOF was twice that for 5-FU (43% versus 19%), but no significant survival advantage was observed.[792] Subsequent attempts to confirm this superiority have not been uniformly successful, and response rates for MOF or MF type regimens have ranged from 4% to 40%.[787,793-799] This observed heterogeneity should not be surprising, since the reported response rate for 5-FU alone varies tenfold. Perhaps MF combinations result in higher response rates than 5-FU alone, but most of the responses are partial and last less than 6 months. Nonetheless, the initial activity of MOF or MF combinations has influenced the design of adjuvant trials in both colon and rectum cancer for more than a decade.

Simple attempts to substitute or add another alkylating-type agent such as mitomycin C, for the nitrosourea have not generally resulted in clinically meaningful differences.[800,801] There have been attempts to combine multiple alkylating-type agents, such as 5-FU + methyl-CCNU + mitomycin C or MOF + streptozotocin. Randomized trials with appropriate control groups have failed to demonstrate a significant survival superiority for any such combination despite considerable increases in response rates.[799,802]

Loehrer and colleagues combined bolus IV 5-FU, 15 mg/kg/wk, with cisplatin, 60 mg/m^2 every 3 weeks, and noted a 32% response rate in 38 patients.[803] They presumed that this combination represents a special synergy, since at this dose cisplatin alone is nearly inactive in colon cancer.[804] This combination has been evaluated not only with bolus 5-FU[803,805] but also with infusion 5-FU, resulting in 21 responses in 30 patients.[806] As was noted for methyl-CCNU + 5-FU combinations, provocative preliminary results require confirmation in larger series. At least one trial comparing bolus 5-FU with 5-FU + cisplatin (as utilized by Loehrer[803]) has shown equivalent response and survival results.[807] Bolus

TABLE 29-35. Selected Randomized Trials of Chemotherapy for Patients with Metastatic Large Bowel Cancer

Study	*Treatment/Arms (mg/m^2)*
GITSG	5-FU, 500/d × 5 d q 4 wk
	FA, 500/wk, + 5-FU, 600/wk
	FA, 25/wk, + 5-FU, 600/wk
NCOG	5-FU, 440/d × 5 d, then 550/wk
	FA, 200/d × 5 d, + 5-FU, 400/d × 5 d q 28 d
	MTX, 50/6 h × 5 followed in 24 h by 5-FU, 500, and FA 10/6 h × 8 (rescue)
NCCTG	5-FU, 500/d × 5 d
	FA, 20/d × 5 d, + 5-FU, 425/d × 5 d
	FA, 200/d × 5 d, + 5-FU, 370/d × 5 d
	MTX, 200, followed in 7 h by 5-FU, 1000, and FA 15/6 h × 8 (rescue)
	MTX, 40, followed in 24 h by 5-FU, 700
	5-FU, 300/d × 5 d, + CDDP, 20/d × 5 d
ECOG	5-FU, 500/d × 5 d, then 600/wk
	5-FU, 500/d × 5 d, + CDDP, 20/d × 5 d
	5-FU, 300/d by continuous infusion
	5-FU, 300/d by continuous infusion, + CDDP, 20/d × 5 d

FA = folinic acid; CDDP = cisplatin.

and infusion 5-FU + cisplatin combinations are being evaluated in large-scale randomized trials (Table 29-35), with the appropriate comparison to 5-FU alone.

Fluorouracil Modulation

Another scientific theme currently being explored is the attempt to increase the effectiveness of the 5-FU. Efforts to biochemically modulate fluoropyrimidine cytotoxicity have recognized the crucial and complex interactions of fluoropyrimidine and folate molecular species. These studies have concentrated on altering folate metabolism with either methotrexate (MTX) or folinic acid (FA, leucovorin). The sequential use of MTX followed by 5-FU results in enhanced cell kill in various cell culture and animal tumor model systems.[808-810] This effect is assumed to result from MTX inhibition of purine metabolism causing more PRPP production or increasing dTMP synthetase binding, resulting in more 5-FU effect on RNA.[809,810] Many MTX dosages (ranging from 200–800 mg/m^2), intervals (1–24 hours before 5-FU), and schedules (bolus to infusion, weekly to monthly) have been reported. Mucositis and leukopenia have been the most notable toxic effects. Responses have been observed in untreated patients as well as patients who have failed 5-FU regimens, but currently there is no single regimen of proven superior therapeutic index.[806,811-816] Moreover, there is no convincing evidence that MTX/5-FU is better than 5-FU alone.[817]

Another and potentially more promising avenue of research is the modulation of 5-FU by folinic acid. Considerable preclinical evidence indicates that intracellular reduced folate cofactor enhances cytotoxicity by stabilizing the covalent ternary complex of thymidylate synthetase and

FdUMP.[818-820] Folinic acid effectively provides the pool of required reduced folates and is clinically available. Numerous Phase II studies have been performed with varying doses of folinic acid (25 to 250 mg/m² per course) and 5-FU (150–200 mg/m² per course). Response rates of 10% to 60% have been noted both in those with and without prior 5-FU exposure.[821-824] At least three randomized studies have suggested superiority for 5-FU + FA combinations. Ehrlichman and colleagues[825] concluded that the combination of FA in a dosage of 200 mg/m²/d for 5 days and 5-FU in a dosage of 370 mg/m²/d for 5 days every 28 days produces more objective responses than the single-agent schedule of 5-FU, 370 mg/m²/d for 5 days. Doroshow et al, using the same 5-FU dose with 500 mg/m² FA, demonstrated similar benefits.[826] Petrelli et al[817] suggested that weekly FA, 500 mg/m², plus 5-FU, 600 mg/m², produced a higher response rate than 5-FU, 450 mg/m²/d for 5 days, followed by 200 mg/m² every other day for 6 days. The toxicity of FA-modulated 5-FU therapy is noteworthy. When administered weekly, the combination results in relatively mild leukopenia in approximately 10% of patients. The dose-limiting toxic effects are enteritis and diarrhea, which can be life-threatening. In contrast, daily administration of the combination for 5 days produce oral mucositis in approximately 33% of all patients. In addition to these medical side-effects, the cost of administering high doses of folinic acid can exceed several thousand dollars for a treatment course.

In order to resolve the unanswered questions concerning efficacy and therapeutic index of 5-FU–modulating combination chemotherapy schedules, several major randomized trials have been initiated (see Table 29-35). With so many variables in dose intensity, schedule, and frequency of administration, it would be impossible to test all possible permutations. Nonetheless, those regimens which in Phase II testing appear to be the most promising candidates are being directly compared with 5-FU alone. The implications for adjuvant programs are obvious, since more active regimens could translate into greater therapeutic impact on Dukes' B and C patients. There are already two ongoing adjuvant studies of 5-FU + FA, the NSABP C03 and NCIC C02 studies.

Chemotherapy for Patients Not Benefiting from 5-FU Therapy

The majority of patients who receive 5-FU as a single agent will not benefit, and many are candidates for subsequent systemic therapy. Outside of a formal research program, the options available for such patients are limited. Occasional responses to nitrosoureas have been observed in those not benefiting from 5-FU. Moertel et al noted a 10% response rate in 112 patients treated with a chlorethyl nitrosourea as second-line therapy.[792] Likewise, two-drug combinations containing methyl-CCNU have proved to be effective in less than 10% of patients.[797] Some patients have been reported to respond to 5-FU + FA or 5-FU + MTX as subsequent therapy,[821,823,824] and to high-dose alkylators with autologous bone marrow support, but lasting benefits are not observed. However, in no situation have better response rates to such programs been demonstrated in those who failed prior 5-FU therapy than in previously untreated patients.

INNOVATIVE THERAPIES FOR COLORECTAL CANCER

BIOLOGICAL RESPONSE MODIFIERS

There has been a dramatic expansion in the understanding and synthesis of biological response modifiers. Historically, nonspecific immunostimulants such as BCG or MER-BCG were widely studied. Several adjuvant protocols tested BCG alone or in conjunction with conventional chemotherapy.[670,827,828] Hoover and colleagues have combined BCG with an autologous tumor cell vaccine.[829] None of these studies has demonstrated that a BCG product increases overall survival. Another nonspecific immunostimulant is the phenyl midazothiazole, levamisole. As described in the section on Adjuvant Therapies for Colon Cancer, levamisole, either alone or with 5-FU, appears to increase disease-free time.[561]

More intensive activity has centered on testing of the interferons (IFN) (Table 29-36).[830-845] At least three studies of an α-IFN preparation in patients with advanced colon cancer patients have been reported. A total of 45 patients were treated with various doses or schedules (up to 50×10^6 U/d for 5 days every 14–21 days), but no objective responses were noted.[830-832] α-IFN has been combined with 5-FU in Phase II studies and responses have been observed.[833,834] It is not yet known whether IFN adds to 5-FU efficacy in any way. Multiple other IFN species are being evaluated.[835-838]

Interleukin-2, either alone or with specific activated killer lymphocytes, is being tested, and some responses have been noted.[839,840]

Monoclonal antibodies directed against colon cancer are also being investigated.[841,842] The 17-1A antibody has been the most widely tested, and objective responses have been noted.[843,845] Although preliminary data do not permit any

TABLE 29-36. Selected Biological Response Modifiers

Class	*Biological Response Modifier*	*Reference*
Interferon (IFN)	Leukocyte IFN	830, 838
	Lymphoblastoid IFN	
	RIFN-α_2	
	RIFN leukocyte A	
	RIFN-β	
	RIFN-γ	
	RIFN-γ + 5-FU	
	RIFN-α + 5-FU	
Interleukins (IL)	IL-2 + LAK cells	839
	IL-2	839
	IL-2	840
Monoclonal antibodies	17-1A	841, 843
	44 × 14	845
	B 72.3	842
Autologous tumor vaccine	Antigen + BCG	844

From the Cancer Therapy Evaluation Program Information System.

definite conclusion of activity, the potential for this approach seems bright.[846]

BONE MARROW TRANSPLANTATIONS

Based on the responses noted in leukemias and lymphomas with very high dose chemotherapy accompanied by autologous bone marrow reconstitution, colon cancer patients have recently been treated with similar regimens. Leff et al treated 20 patients with IV bolus L-PAM at 180 mg/m² plus bone marrow transfusion and observed three complete and six partial responses.[847] In a similar program the same workers obtained 9 responses in 19 patients.[848] Responses have also been seen with combinations of very high dose alkylating agents, such as cyclophosphamide + cisplatin + BCNU.[829] Unfortunately, despite the impressive objective response rates, the duration of regression has been only 1 to 3 months and the toxicity is truly formidable. Attempts to evaluate high-dose chemotherapy and bone marrow reconstitution are continuing, and methods of integrating this approach with conventional therapies are being explored.

MISCELLANEOUS COLORECTAL TUMORS

CARCINOID TUMORS

Most alimentary tract carcinoids occur in the ileum and the appendix. The rectum is the next most common site, with occasional tumors in the colon.[849] Almost all rectal carcinoids present as asymptomatic submucosal nodules less than 2 cm in size. In contrast to other sites, hematogenous and lymph node metastases are rare (<15%).[850] Malignant potential is seen almost exclusively in patients with tumors larger than 2 cm.[851] Transanal local excision suffices for tumors less than 2 cm, with radical surgery reserved only for larger tumors and those with histologic evidence of invasion of the muscularis propria.[852]

SARCOMA

Almost all smooth muscle tumors in the bowel occur in the stomach and small bowel. A few cases of rectal leiomyosarcoma have been reported.[853-855] The tumors may be small and asymptomatic, or greater than 10 cm with typical rectal cancer symptomatology. The smaller, submucosal tumors arise from the muscularis mucosa. Most are low grade, and almost all are curable by local excision. Tumors arising in the muscularis propria are frequently high grade. Local recurrence is common with limited surgical approaches.[853,855] With high-grade tumors, metastases to liver and lung occur in almost all patients despite radical surgery.[854,855]

LYMPHOMA

Primary rectal lymphoma is rare; it can be cured by surgery and postoperative irradiation.[856]

This Chapter was critically reviewed and edited by Ms. Milicent Cranor, whose efforts are gratefully recognized.

REFERENCES

1. Lipkin M: Biomarkers of increased susceptibility to gastrointestinal cancer. Gastroenterology 92:1083–1086, 1987
2. National Institutes of Health: Annual Cancer Statistics Review, Including Cancer Trends; 1950–1985. NIH publication No. 88–2789, Bethesda, Md, February 1988
3. Slanetz CA Jr, Herter FP: The large intestine. In Lymphatics in Cancer pp 489–564. Haagensen CD, Feind CR, Herter FP et al (eds): Philadelphia, WB Saunders, 1972
4. Enquist IF, Block IR: Rectal cancer in females: Selection of proper operation based upon anatomic studies of rectal lymphatics. Prog Clin Cancer 2:73–85, 1966
5. Reinhold P: Contribution a l'Etude des Facteurs de Recidives Postoperatoire du Cancer Rectal. These, Paris, 1924
6. Bartolo DCC, Row AM, Locke-Edmunds JC et al: Flap-valve theory of anorectal continence. Br J Surg 73:1012–1014, 1986
7. Preston DM, Lennard-Jones JE, Thomas BM: The balloon proctogram. Br J Surg 71:29–32, 1984
8. Lahr CJ, Rothenberger DA, Jensen LL et al: Balloon topography. Dis Colon Rectum 29:1–5, 1986
9. Read NW, Bartolo DCC, Read MG: Differences in anal function in patients with incontinence to solids and in patients with incontinence to liquids. Br J Surg 71:39–42, 1984
10. Schottenfeld D, Winawer SJ: Large intestine. In Schottenfeld D, Fraumeni JF Jr (eds): Cancer: Epidemiology and Prevention, pp 703–709. Philadelphia, WB Saunders, 1982
11. Ziegler RG, Devesa SS, Fraumeni JF Jr: Epidemiology pattern of colorectal cancer. In Devita VT Jr, Hellman S, Rosenberg SA (eds): Important Advances in Oncology 1986, pp 209–232. Philadelphia, JB Lippincott, 1986
12. Waterhouse J, Muir C, Correa P et al: Cancer Incidence in Five Continents, Vol III. Lyon, International Agency for Research on Cancer, 1976
13. Blot WJ, Fraumeni JF, Stone BJ et al: Geographic patterns of large bowel cancer in the United States. JNCI 57:1225–1231, 1976
14. Pickle LW, Greene MH, Ziegler RG et al: Colorectal cancer in rural Nebraska. Cancer RES 44:363–369, 1984
15. Burdette WJ (ed): Carcinoma of the Colon and Antecedent Epithelium. Springfield, Ill, Charles C Thomas, 1970
16. Phillips RL, Kuzma JW, Lotz TM: Cancer mortality among comparable members versus non-members of the Seventh Day Adventist Church. In Cairns J, Lyon JL, Skolnick M (eds): Cancer Incidence in Defined Populations, pp 83–102. Banbury Report No. 4, Cold Spring Harbor, New York, Cold Spring Harbor Laboratory, 1980
17. Phillips RL, Garfinkel L, Kuzma JW et al: Mortality among California Seventh-Day Adventists for selected cancer sites. JNCI 65:1097–1107, 1980
18. Enstrom JE: Health and dietary practices and cancer mortality among California Mormons. In Cairns J, Lyon JL, Skolnick M (eds): Cancer Incidence in Defined Populations, pp 69–90. Banbury Report No. 4, Cold Spring Harbor, New York, Cold Spring Harbor Laboratory, 1980
19. Lyon JL, Sorenson AW: Colon cancer in a low-risk population. Am J Clin Nutr 31:227–230, 1978
20. Cady B, Persson AV, Monson DO et al: Changing patterns of colorectal cancer. Cancer 33:433–436, 1974
21. Axtell LM, Chiazze L: Changing relative frequency of cancers of the colon and rectum in the United States. Cancer 19:750–754, 1966
22. Rhodes JB, Holmes FF, Clarke GM: Changing distribution of primary cancers in the large bowel. JAMA 235:1641–1643, 1977
23. Bruce WR, Dion PW: Studies relating to a fecal mutagen. Am J Clin Nutr 33:2511–2512, 1980
24. Weisburger JH, Wynder EL: Etiology of colorectal cancer with emphasis on mechanism of action and prevention. In Devita VT, Hellman S, Rosenberg SA (eds): Important Advances in Oncology 1987, pp 197–221. Philadelphia, JB Lippincott, 1987
25. Modan B: Dietary role in cancer etiology. Cancer 40:1887–1891, 1977
26. Willett NC, MacMahon B: Diet and cancer—an overview. N Engl J Med 310:697–703, 1984
27. Palmer S, Bakshi K: Diet, nutrition, and cancer: I. Interim dietary guidelines. JNCI 70:1151–1170, 1983
28. Jain M, Cook GM, Davis FG et al: A case–control study of diet and colorectal cancer. Int J Cancer 26:757–768, 1980
29. Haenszel WM, Kurihara M: Studies of Japanese immigrants: I. Mortality from cancer and other diseases among Japanese in the United States. JNCI 40:43–47, 1968
30. Correa P, Haenszel W: The epidemiology of large-bowel cancer. Adv Cancer Res 26:1–141, 1978
31. Armstrong B, Doll R: Environmental factors and cancer incidence and mortality in different countries with special reference to dietary practices. Int J Cancer 15:617–631, 1975
32. Lee JAH: Recent trends of large bowel cancer in Japan compared to United States and England and Wales. Int J Epidemiol 5:187–194, 1976
33. Waterhouse J, Shanmugaratnam K, Mair C et al: (eds): Cancer Incidence in Five Continents, Vol IV. IARC Scientific Publication No. 42, Lyon, International Agency for Research on Cancer, 1982
34. Waterhouse J, Carrea P, Muir et al (eds): Cancer Incidence in Five Continents, Vol III. IARC Scientific Publication No. 15, Lyon, International Agency for Research on Cancer, 1976

35. McMichael AJ, McCall MG, Hartshorne JM et al: Patterns of gastrointestinal cancer in European migrants to Australia: The role of dietary change. Int J Cancer 25:431–437, 1980
36. Monk M, Warshauer ME: Stomach and colon cancer mortality among Puerto Ricans in New York City and Puerto Rico. J Chronic Dis 28:349–358, 1975
37. Martinez I, Torres R, Frias Z et al: Factors associated with adenocarcinoma of the large bowel in Puerto Rico. In Birch JM (ed): Advances in Medical Oncology Research and Education, Vol 3, pp 45–52. New York, Pergamon Press, 1979
38. Zhang YQ, MacLennan R, Berry G: Mortality of Chinese in New South Wales, 1969–1978. Int J Epidemiol 13:188–192, 1984
39. Ames BN, McCann J, Yamasaki E: Methods for detecting carcinogens and mutagens with the *Salmonella* mammalian microsome test. Mutat Res 31:347–364, 1975
40. Curren RD, Putman DL, Yang LL et al: Genotoxicity of fecapentaene-12 in bacterial and mammalian cell assay systems. Carcinogenesis 8:349–353, 1987
41. Ehrich M, Aswell JE, Van Tassell RL et al: Mutagens in the feces of three South African populations at different levels of risk for colon cancer. Mutat Res 64:231–240, 1979
42. Bruce WR: Recent hypotheses for the origin of colon cancer. Cancer Res 47:4237–4242, 1987
43. Correa P, Paschal J, Pizzolato P et al: Fecal mutagens and colorectal polyps: Preliminary report of an autopsy study. In Bruce WR, Correa P, Lipkin M et al (eds): Gastrointentinal Cancer: Endogenous Factors, pp. 119–123. Cold Spring Harbor, New York, Cold Spring Harbor Laboratory, 1981
44. Dion PW, Bright-See EB, Smith CC et al: The effect of dietary ascorbic acid and α-tocopherol on fecal mutagenicity. Mutat Res 102:27–37, 1982
45. Reddy BS, Sharma C, Simi B et al: Metabolic epidemiology of colon cancer: Effect of dietary fiber on fecal mutagens and bile acids in healthy subjects. Cancer Res 47:644–648, 1987
46. Susuki K, Bruce WR, Baptista J et al: Characterization of cytotoxic steroids in human feces and their putative role in the etiology of human colon cancer. Cancer Lett 33:307–317, 1986
47. Smith LL: Carcinogenic cholesterol products. In Cholesterol Autoxidation, pp 432–446. New York, Plenum Press, 1981
48. Lipkin M, Reddy BS, Weisburger J et al: Non-degradation of fecal cholesterol in subjects at high risk for cancer of the large intestine. J Clin Invest 67:304–307, 1981
49. Bird RP, Bruce WR: Toxicity of dietary components to colonic mucosa in vivo. Proc Am Assoc Cancer Res 24:89, 1983
50. Bird RP: Effect of dietary components on the pathobiology of colonic epithelium: Possible relationship with colon tumorigenesis. Lipids 21:289–291, 1986
51. Sugimura T: Carcinogenicity of mutagenic heterocyclic amines formed during the cooking process. Mutat Res 150:33–42, 1985
52. Tanaka T, Barnes WS, Weisburger JH et al: Multipotential carcinogenicity of the fried food mutagen 2-amino-3-methylimidazo[4,b-f]quinoline (IQ) in rats. Jpn J Cancer Res (Gann) 76:570–576, 1985
53. Suzuki K, Bruce WR: Increase by deoxycholic acid of the colonic nuclear damage induced by known carcinogens in C57B1/6J mice. JNCI 76:1129–1132, 1986
54. Hill MJ, Drasar BS, Williams RED et al: Faecal bile-acid and clostridia in patients with cancer of the large bowel. Lancet 1:535–539, 1975
55. Linos DA, Beard CM, O'Fallon et al: Cholecystectomy and carcinoma of the colon. Lancet 2:379–381, 1981
56. Vernick LF, Kuller LH: Cholecystectomy and right-sided colon cancer; An epidemiological study. Lancet 2:381–383, 1981
57. Vernick LJ, Kuller LH, Lohsoonthorn P et al: Relationship between cholecystectomy and ascending colon cancer. Cancer 45:392–395, 1980
58. Bird RP, Medline A, Furrer et al: Toxicity of orally administerd fat to the colonic epithelium of mice. Carcinogenesis 6:1063–1066, 1985
59. Caderni G, Stuart E, Bruce WR: Dietary factors affecting the proliferation of epithelial cells in the colon of the mouse. Gastroenterology 92:1336, 1987
60. Garland C, Shekelle RB, Barrett-Connor E et al: Dietary vitamin D and calcium and risk of colorectal cancer: A 19-year prospective study in men. Lancet 1:307–309, 1985
61. Thornton JR: High colonic pH promotes colorectal cancer. Lancet 1:1081–1082, 1981
62. Van Dokkum W, de Boer BCJ, van Faassen A et al: Diet, faecal pH and colorectal cancer. Br J Cancer 48:109–110, 1983
63. Samelson SL, Nelson RL, Nyhus LM: Protective role of faecal pH in experimental colon carcinogenesis. JR Soc Med 78:230–233, 1984
64. Walker ARP, Walker AJ: Faecal pH, dietary fibre intake, and proneness to colon cancer in four South African populations. Br J Cancer 53:489–495, 1986
65. Pietroiusti A, Guliano M, Vita S et al: Faecal pH and cancer of the large bowel. Gastroenterology 84:1273, 1983
66. Painter NS, Burkitt DP: Diverticular disease of the colon: A deficiency disease of Western civilization. Br Med J 12:450–454, 1971
67. Burkitt DP, Walker ARP, Painter NS: Dietary fiber and disease. JAMA 229:1063–1074, 1974
68. Doll R, Peto R: The causes of cancer: Quantitative estimates of avoidable risks of cancer in the United States today. JNCI 66:1193–1308, 1981
69. Reddy BS: Dietary fiber and colon carcinogenesis: A critical review. In Vahouny GV, Kritchevsky D (eds): Dietary Fiber in Health and Disease, pp 265–285. New York, Plenum Press, 1982
70. Kritchevsky D: Diet, nutrition and cancer. Cancer 58:1830–1836, 1986
71. Jensen OM, Mosbech J, Salaspuro M et al: A comparative study of the diagnostic basis for cancer of the colon and cancer of the rectum in Denmark and Finland. Int J Epidemiol 3:183–186, 1974
72. Modan B, Barell V, Lubin F et al: Low fiber intake as an etiologic factor in cancer of the colon. JNCI 55:15–18, 1975
73. Greenwald P, Lanza E: Role of dietary fiber in the prev of cancer. In DeVita VT Jr, Hellman S, Rosenberg SA (eds): Important Advances in Oncology 1986, pp 37–54. Philadelphia, JB Lippincott, 1986
74. Glauert HP, Bennick MR, Sander CH: Enhanced 1,2-dimethylhydrazine-induced colon carcinogenesis in mice by dietary agar. Food Cosmet Toxicol 19:281–286, 1981
75. Freeman HJ, Spiller GA, Kim YS: A double blind study of the effect of purified cellulose dietary fiber on 1,2-dimethylhydrazine-induced rat colonic neoplasia. Cancer Res 38:2912–2917, 1978
76. Reddy BS, Ekelund G, Bohe M et al: Metabolic epidemiology of colon cancer: Dietary pattern and fectal sterol concentrations of three populations. Nutr Cancer 5:a34–40, 1978
77. Lipkin M, Newmark H: Effect of added dietary calcium on colonic epithelial cell proliferation in subjects at high risk for familial colon cancer. N Engl J Med 313:1381–1384, 1985
78. Clark LC: The epidemiology of selenium and cancer. Fed Proc 44:2584–2589, 1985
79. Shamberger RJ: Nutrition and Cancer. New York, Plenum Press, 1984
80. Banner WP, DeCosse JJ, Tan QH et al: Selective distribution of selenium in colon parallels its antitumor activity. Carcinogenesis 5:1543–1546, 1984
81. Bussey HJ, DeCosse JJ, Deschner EE: A randomized trial of ascorbic acid in polyposis coli. Cancer 50:1434–1439, 1982
82. McKeown-Eyssen GE, Bright-See E: Dietary prevention of recurrences of adenomatous polyps in the colon and rectum. In: UICC Cancer Congress, Budapest, 1986. Geneva, International Union Against Cancer, 1986
83. McKusick VA: Genetics and large-bowel cancer. Am J Dig Dis 19:954–957, 1974
84. Lipkin M, Sherlock P, DeCosse JJ: Risk factors and preventative measures in the control of cancer of the large intestine. Curr Probl Cancer 4:1057, 1980
85. Bussey HJR: Gastrointestinal polyposis. Gut 11:970–978, 1970
86. Bussey AJR: Familial Polyposis Coli. Baltimore, Johns Hopkins University Press, 1975
87. Erbe RW: Inherited gastrointestinal polyposis syndromes. N Engl J Med 294:1101–1104, 1976
88. DeCosse JJ, Adaurs MB, Condon RF: Familial polyposis. Cancer 39:267–273, 1977
89. Kelly PB, McKinnon DA: Familial multiple polyposis of the colon: Review and description of a large kindred. McGill Med J 30:67–85, 1961
90. Gardner EJ: Follow-up study of a family group exhibiting dominant inheritance for a syndrome including intestinal polyps, osteomas, fibromas and epidermal cysts. Am J Hum Genet 14:376–390, 1962
91. Oldfield MC: The association of familial polyposis of the colon with multiple sebaceous cysts. Br J Surg 41:534–541, 1954
92. Turcot J, Despres JP, St. Pierre F: Malignant tumors of the central nervous system associated with familial polyposis of the colon: Report of two cases. Dis Colon Rectum 2:465–68, 1959
93. Bodmer WF, Bailey CJ, Bodmer J et al: Localization of the gene for familial adenomatous polyposis on chromosome 5. Nature 328:2–4, 1987
94. Jeghers H, McKusick VA, Katz KH: Generalized intestinal polyposis and melanin spots of the oral mucosa, lips and digits. N Engl J Med 241:993–1005, 1949
95. Reid JD: Intestinal carcinoma in the Peutz-Jeghers syndrome. JAMA 229:833–834, 1974
96. Kussin SZ, Lipkin M, Winawer SJ: Inherited colon cancer: Clinical implications. Am J Gastroenterol 72:443–457, 1979
97. Lynch HT, Lynch PM: Heredity and gastrointestinal tract cancer. In Lipkin M, Good RA (eds): Gastrointestinal Tract Cancer. New York, Plenum Press, 1978
98. Lynch HT, Albano WA, Lynch JF et al: Recognition of the cancer family syndrome. Gastroenterology 84:672–673, 1983
99. Law JP, Herberman RB, Oldham RL: Familial occurrence of colon, uterine and of lymphoproliferative malignancies: Clinical description. Cancer 39:1224–1228, 1977
100. Macklin MT: Inheritance of cancer of the stomach and large intestine in man. JNCI 24L:551–557, 1960
101. Sherlock P: Heredity versus environment in colorectal cancer. In Winawer S, Schottenfeld D, Sherlock P (eds): Colorectal Cancer: Prevention, Epidemiology and Screening, pp 65–66. New York, Raven Press, 1980
102. Burt RW, Bishop DT, Cannon LA et al: Dominant inheritance of adenomatous colonic polyps and colorectal cancer. N Engl J Med 12:1540–1544, 1985
103. Mulvihill JJ: Clinical ecogenetics: Cancer in families. N Engl J Med 312:1569–1570, 1985
104. Edwards FC, Truelove SC: The course and prognosis of ulcerative colitis. Gut 5:1–22, 1964
105. Morson BC: Cancer and ulcerative colitis. Gut 7:425–426, 1966
106. Mir-Modjlessi SH, Farmer RG, Easley KA et al: Colorectal and extracolonic malignancy in ulcerative colitis. Cancer 58:1569–74, 1986
107. MacDougall PM: The cancer risk in ulcerative colitis. Lancet 2:655–658, 1966
108. Ohman U: Colorectal carcinoma in patients with ulcerative colitis. Am J Surg 144:344–349, 1982
109. Kewenter J, Ahlman H, Hulten L: Cancer risk in extensive ulcerative colitis. Ann Surg 188:824–828, 1978

110. Katzka I, Body RS, Morris E et al: Assessment of colorectal cancer risk in patients with ulcerative colitis. Experience from a private practice. Gastroenterology 85:22–29, 1983
111. Prior P, Gyde SN, Macartney JC et al: Cancer morbidity in ulcerative colitis. Gut 23:490–497, 1982
112. Devroede GJ, Taylor WF, Sauer WG: Cancer risk and life expectancy of children with ulcerative colitis. N Engl J Med 285:17–21, 1971
113. Kirsner JB, Shorter RG: Inflammatory bowel disease of the large bowel and anal canal. In Kirsner JB, Shorter RG (eds); Diseases of the Colon, Rectum and Anal Canal, chap 17. Baltimore, Williams & Wilkins, 1987
114. Hamilton SR: Colorectal carcinoma in patients with Crohn's disease. Gastroenterology 89:398–407, 1985
115. Heaton K: Crohn's disease and ulcerative colitis. In Trowell H, Burkitt D, Heaton K et al (eds): Dietary Fibre, Fibre-Depleted Foods and Disease, pp 205–216. New York, Academic Press, 1985
116. Greenstein AJ, Sachar DB, Smith H et al: Patterns of neoplasia in Crohn's disease and ulcerative colitis. Cancer 46:403–407, 1980
117. Weedon DD, Shorter RG, Ilstrup DM et al: Crohn's disease and cancer. N Engl J Med 289:1099–1104, 1973
118. Morson BC: Genesis of colorectal cancer. Clin Gastroenterol 5(3): 505–525, 1976
119. Heald RJ, Bussey HJR: Clinical experience at St. Mark's Hospital with multiple synchronous cancers of the colon and rectum. Dis Colon Rectum 18:6, 1975
120. Schottenfeld D, Berg JW, Vitsky B: Incidence of multiple primary cancers: II. Index cancers arising in the stomach and lower digestive system. JNCI 43:77–86, 1969
121. Burbank F: Patterns in cancer mortality in the United States: 1950–1967. Natl Cancer Inst Monogr 33, 1971
122. MacMahon CE, Rowe JW: Rectal reaction following radiation therapy of cervical carcinoma: Particular reference to subsequent occurrence of rectal carcinoma. Ann Surg 173:264–269, 1971
123. Castro EB, Rosen PP, Quan SH; Carcinoma of large intestine in patients irradiated for carcinoma of cervix and uterus. Cancer 31:45–52, 1973
124. McMichael AJ, Potter JD: Host factors in carcinogenesis: Certain bile-acid metabolic profiles that selectively increase the risk of proximal colon cancer. JNCI 75:185–191, 1985
125. Lowenfels AB, Domellof L, Lindstrom CG et al: Cholelithiasis, cholecystectomy, and cancer: A case–control study in Sweden. Gastroenterology 83:672–676, 1982
126. Bristol JB, Williamson RCN: Ureterosigmoidostomy and colon carcinogenesis. Science 214:351, 1981
127. Appel MF, Spjut HJ, Estroda RG: The significance of villous component in colonic polyps. Am J Surg 134:770–771, 1977
128. Morson BC: Evolution of cancer of the colon and rectum. Cancer 34:845–849, 1974
129. Lipkin M: Phase 1 and phase 2 proliferative lesions of colonic epithelial cells in diseases leading to colonic cancer. Cancer 34:878–888, 1974
130. Muto T, Bussey HJR, Morson BC: The evolution of cancer of the colon and rectum. Cancer 36:2251–2270, 1975
131. Ekelund GR: Cancer risk with single and multiple adenomas, synchronous and metachronous tumors. In Winawer SJ, Schottenfeld D, Sherlock P (eds): Progress in Cancer Research and Therapy, Vol 13, Colorectal Cancer: Prevention, Epidemiology and Screening, pp 151–155. New York, Raven Press, 1980
132. Sherlock P, Lipkin M, Winawer SJ: The prevention of colon cancer. Am J Med 68:917–931, 1980
133. Winawer SJ, Miller DG, Sherlock P: Risk and screening for colorectal cancer. Adv Intern Med 30: 471–496, 1984
134. Devlin HB, Plant JA, Morris D: The significance of symptoms of carcinoma of the rectum. Surg Gynecol Obstet 137:399–402, 1973
135. Irvin TT, Greaney MG: Duration of symptoms and prognosis of carcinoma of the colon and rectum. Surg Gynecol Obstet 144:883–886, 1977
136. McDermott FT, Hughes ESR, Paihl E et al: Prognosis in relation to symptom duration in colon cancer. Br J Surg 68:846–849, 1981
137. Farrands PA, Hardcastle JD: Colorectal cancer by self completion questionnaire. Gut 25:4445–4447, 1984
138. Chapuis PH, Goulston KJ, Dent OF et al: Predictive value of rectal bleeding in screening for rectal and sigmoid polyps. Br Med J Clin Res 290:1546–1548, 1985
139. Eddy DM, Nugent FW, Eddy JF et al: Screening for colorectal cancer in a high-risk population: Results of a mathematical model. Gastroenterology 92:682–692, 1987
140. Snyder DN, Heston JF, Meigs JW et al: Changes in site distribution of colorectal carcinoma in Connecticut, 1940–1973. Dig Dis 22:791–797, 1977
141. Stewart RJ, Stewart AW, Turnbull PRG et al: Sex differences in subsite incidence of large bowel cancer. Dis Colon Rectum 26:658–660, 1983
142. Butcher D, Hassanein K, Dudgeon M et al: Female gender as a major determinant of changing subsite distribution of colorectal cancer with age. Cancer 56:714–716, 1985
143. Rozen P, Fireman Z, Figer A et al: Family history of colorectal cancer as a marker of potential malignancy within a screening program. Cancer 60:248–254, 1987
144. Gryska PV, Cohen AM: Screening asymptomatic patients at high risk for colon cancer with full colonoscopy. Dis Colon Rectum 30:18–20, 1987
145. Nava H, Pagana TJ: Postoperative surveillance of colorectal carcinoma. Cancer 49:1043–1047, 1982
146. Winawer SJ, Ritchie M, Diaz B et al: The National Polyp Study: Aims and Organization. In Rozen P, Winawer SJ (eds): Frontiers of Gastrointestinal Research, Vol 10, Secondary Prevention of Colorectal Cancer: An International Perspective, pp 216–225. Basel, Karger, 1986
147. Morson BC: Use of dysplasia as an indicator of risk for malignancy in patients with ulcerative colitis. In Winawer SJ, Schottenfeld D, Sherlock P (eds): Colorectal Cancer: Prevention, Epidemiology and Screening, pp 347–354. New York, Raven Press, 1980
148. Dobbins WO, Stock M, Ginsberg AL: Early detection and prevention of carcinoma of the colon in patients with ulcerative colitis. Cancer 40:25–48, 1977
149. Collins RH, Geldman M, Fordtran JS: Colon cancer, dysplasia, and surveillance in patients with ulcerative colitis. N Engl J Med 316:1654–1658, 1987
150. Dales LG, Friedman GD, Collen MF: Evaluating periodic multiphase health checkups: A controlled trial. J Chronic Dis 32:385–404, 1979
151. Hertz RE, Deddish MR, Day E: Value of periodic examination in detecting cancer of the rectum and colon. Postgrad Med 27:290, 1960
152. Gilbertsen VA, Williams SE, Schuman L et al: Colonoscopy in the detection of carcinoma of the intestine. Surg Gynecol Obstet 149:877–878, 1979
153. Winawer SJ, Cummins R, Baldwin NP et al: A new flexible sigmoidoscope for the generalist. Gastrointest Endosc 28:233–236, 1982
154. Dubow RA, Katon RM, Benner KG et al: Short (36 cm) versus long (60 cm) flexible sigmoidoscopy: A comparison of findings and tolerance in asymptomatic patients screened for colorectal neoplasia. Gastrointest Endosc 31:305–308, 1985
155. Wilking N, Petrelli NJ, Herrera L et al: A comparison of the 25 cm rigid proctosigmoidoscope with the 65 cm flexible endoscope in the screening of patients for colorectal carcinoma. Cancer 57:669–671, 1986
156. Winnon G, Beri G, Parnish J: Superiority of the flexible to the rigid sigmoidoscope in routine proctosigmoidoscopy. N Engl J Med 302:1011–1012, 1980
157. Marks G, Boggs HW, Castro AF et al: Sigmoidoscopic examinations with rigid and flexible fiberoptic sigmoidoscopes in the surgeon's office: A comparative prospective study of effectiveness in 1,012 cases. Dis Colon Rectum 22:162–168, 1979
158. Lipshutz GR, Katon RM, McCool MF et al: Flexible sigmoidoscopy as a screening procedure for neoplasia of the colon. Surg Gynecol Obstet 148:19–22, 1979
159. Marks G, Gathright JB, Boggs W et al: Guidelines for use of the flexible sigmoidoscope in the management of the surgical patient. Dis Colon Rectum 25:187–190, 1982
160. Wherry DC: Screening for colorectal neoplasia in asymptomatic patients using flexible fiberoptic sigmoidoscopy. Dis Colon Rectum 24:521–522, 1981
161. Rex DK, Rehman GA, Coppas JC et al: Sensitivity of double contrast barium study for left colon polyps. Radiology 158:69–72, 1986
162. Fork FT, Lindstrom C, Ekelund GR: Reliability of double contrast examination of the large bowel in polyp detection: A prospective clinical study. Gastrointest Radiol 8:163–172, 1983
163. Ott DJ, Albin OS, Gelfand GW et al: Predictive value of a diagnosis of colonic polyp on the double contrast barium enema. Gastrointest Radiol 8:75–80, 1983
164. Thoeni RF, Petras A: Double contrast barium enema and endoscopy in the detection of polypoid lesions in the cecum and ascending colon. Radiology 144:257–260, 1982
165. Miller RE, Lehman G; Polypoid colonic lesions undetected by endoscopy. Radiology 129:295–297, 1978
166. Winawer SJ, Leidner SD, Hajdu SI, et al: Colonoscopic biopsy and cytology in the diagnosis of colon cancer. Cancer 42:2849–2853, 1978
167. Shimano T, Okuda H, Mondes T et al: Usefulness of carcinoembryonic antigen measurement in feces of patients with colorectal cancer. Dis Colon Rectum 30:607–10, 1987
168. Ahlquist DA, McGill DB, Schwartz S et al: Hemoquant, a new quantitative assay for fecal hemoglobin. Ann Intern Med 101:297–302, 1984
169. Ahlquist DA, McGill DB, Schwartz S et al: Fecal blood levels in health and disease. N Engl J Med 312:22–1428, 1985
170. Songster CL, Barrows GH, Jarrett DD: Immumochemical detection of fecal blood—the fecal smear pinch disc test. A new non-invasive screening test for colorectal cancer. Cancer 45:1099–1102, 1980
171. Saito H, Tsuchida S, Nakaji S et al: An immunological test for fecal occult blood by counter immunoelectrophoresis. Cancer 56:1549–1552, 1985
172. Barry MJ, Mulley AG, Richter JM: Effect of workup strategy of the cost-effectiveness of fecal occult blood screening for colorectal cancer. Gastroenterology 93:301–310, 1987
173. Ahlquist DA, Beart RW Jr: Use of fecal occult blood test in the detection of colorectal neoplasia. Curr Probl Gen Surg 2:200–210, 1985
174. Winawer SJ, Fleisher M: Sensitivity and specificity of the fecal occult blood test for colorectal neoplasia. Gastroenterology 82:986–991, 1982
175. Griffith CDM, Turner DJ, Saunders JH: False-negative results of hemoccult test in colorectal cancer. Br J Med 283:472, 1981
176. Hardcastle JD, Armitage NC, Chamberlin J et al: Fecal occult blood screening for colorectal cancer in the general population. Cancer 58:397–403, 1986
177. Winawer SJ, Andrews M, Flehinger B et al: Progress report on controlled trial of fecal occult blood testing for the detection of colorectal neoplasia. Cancer 45:2959–2964, 1980
178. Cummings KM, Michalek AJ, Tidings J et al: Results of a public screening program for colorectal cancer. NY State Med 86:68–72, 1986
179. Simon JB: Occult blood screening for colorectal carcinoma: A critical review. Gastroenterology 88:820–837, 1985
180. Macrae FA, St. John DJ, Couligiore P et al: Optimal dietary conditions for hemoccult testing. Gastroenterology 82:889–903, 1982
181. Gnauck R, Macrae FA, Fleisher M: How to perform the occult blood test. CA 34:134–147, 1984
182. Jaffe RM, Kasten B, Young DS et al: False negative stool occult blood test caused by the ingestion of ascorbic acid. Ann Intern Med 83:824–826, 1975

183. Feczko PJ, Halpert RD: Reassessing the role of radiology and hemoccult screening. AJR 146:697–701, 1986
184. Winchester DP, Shull JH, Scanlon EF et al: A mass screening program for colorectal cancer using chemical testing for occult blood in the stool. Cancer 45:2955–2958, 1980
185. Sontag SJ, Durczak C, Aranha GV et al: Fecal occult blood screening for colorectal cancer in a Veteran's Administration hospital. Am J Surg 145:89–93, 1983
186. Jackman RJ, Beahrs OH: Tumors of the Large Bowel. Philadelphia, WB Saunders, 1969
187. Gordon-Watson C, Dukes C: The radium problem: III. The treatment of carcinoma of the rectum with radium. With an introduction on the spread of cancer of the rectum. Br J Surg 17:643–669, 1930
188. Dukes CE: Cancer of the rectum: An analysis of 1000 cases. J Pathol Bacteriol 50:527–539, 1940
189. Hermanek P: Evolution and pathology of rectal cancer. World J Surg 6:502–509, 1982
190. Spjut HJ: Pathology of neoplasms. In Spratt JS (ed): Neoplasms of the Colon, Rectum, and Anus: Mucosal and Epithelial. Philadelphia, WB Saunders, 1984
191. Morson BC, Sobin LH: Histological typing of intestinal tumours. Technical report No. 15, Geneva, World Health Organization, 1976
192. Wood DA: Tumors of the intestines. In: Atlas of Tumor Pathology, Section VI, Fascicle 22. Washington, DC, Armed Forces Institute of Pathology, 1967
193. Bonello JC, Sternberg SS, Quan SHQ: The significance of the signet-cell variety of adenocarcinoma of the rectum. Dis Colon Rectum 23:180–183, 1980
194. Mathews JL, Coyle D Jr, Little WP: Primary linitis plastica of the rectum: Report of a case. Dis Colon Rectum 25:488–490, 1982
195. Cooper HS: Carcinoma of the colon and rectum. In Norris HT (ed): Pathology of the Colon, Small Intestine, and Anus. New York, Churchill Livingstone, 1983
196. Gibbs NM: Undifferentiated carcinoma of the large intestine. Histopathology 1:77–84, 1977
197. MacDonald RA: A study of 356 carcinoids of the gastrointestinal tract: Report of four new cases of the carcinoid syndrome. Am J Med 21:867–878, 1956
198. Orloff MJ: Carcinoid tumors of the rectum. Cancer 28:175–180, 1971
199. Evans HL: Smooth muscle tumors of the gastrointestinal tract: A study of 56 cases followed for a minimum of 10 years. Cancer 56:2242–2250, 1985
200. Broders AC: The grading of carcinoma. Minn Med 8:726–730, 1925
201. Dukes CE: The classification of cancer of the rectum. J Pathol 35:323–332, 1932
202. Qizilbash AH: Pathologic studies in colorectal cancer: A guide to the surgical pathology examination of colorectal specimens and review of features of prognostic significance. Pathol Annu 17(part 1):1–46, 1982
203. Jass JR, Atkin WS, Cuzick I et al: The grading of rectal cancer: Historical perspectives and a multivariate analysis of 447 cases. Histopathology 10:437–459, 1986
204. Dukes CE, Bussey HJR: The spread of rectal cancer and its effect on prognosis. Br J Cancer 12:309–320, 1958
205. Cole PP: The intramural spread of rectal carcinoma. Br Med J 1:431–433, 1913
206. Black WA, Waugh JM: The intramural extension of carcinoma of the descending colon, sigmoid, and rectosigmoid: A pathologic study. Surg Gynecol Obstet 87:457–464, 1948
207. Miles WE: Discussion on the surgical treatment of cancer of the rectum. Br Med J 2:730–742, 1920
208. Grinnell RS: Lymphatic block with atypical and retrograde lymphatic metastasis and spread in carcinoma of the colon and rectum. Ann Surg 163:272–280, 1966
209. Montessori GA, Donald JC, Invasion profile of colorectal carcinoma. Dis Colon Rectum 21:26–28, 1978
210. Templeton A: The value of whole mount sections in determining adequacy of surgical margins and in staging carcinoma of the colorectum. Presented at the 24th annual meeting of the American Society of Therapeutic Radiology and Oncology, Oct 28, 1982
211. Seefeld PH, Bargen JA: The spread of carcinoma of the rectum: Invasion of lymphatics, veins and nerves. Ann Surg 118:76–90, 1943
212. Knudsen JB, Nilsson T, Sprechler M et al: Venous and nerve invasion as prognostic factors in postoperative survival of patients with resectable cancer of the rectum. Dis Colon Rectum 26:613–617, 1983
213. Astler VB, Coller FA: The prognostic significance of direct extension of carcinoma of the colon and rectum. Ann Surg 139:846–851, 1954
214. Gunderson LL, Sosin H: Areas of failure found at reoperation (second or symptomatic look) following "curative surgery" for adenocarcinoma of the rectum: Clinicopathologic correlation and implications for adjuvant therapy. Cancer 34:1278–1292, 1974
215. Gilbert SG: Symptomatic local tumor failure following abdomino-perineal resection. Int J Radiat Oncol Biol Phys 4:801–807, 1978
216. Cass AW, Million RR, Pfaff WW: Patterns of recurrence following surgery alone for adenocarcinoma of the colon and rectum. Cancer 37:2861–2865, 1976
217. Olson RM, Perencevich NP, Malcolm AW et al: Patterns of recurrence following curative resection of adenocarcinoma of the colon and rectum. Cancer 45:2969–2974, 1980
218. Malcolm AW, Perencevich NP, Olson RM et al: Analysis of recurrence patterns following curative resection for carcinoma of the colon and rectum. Surg Gynecol Obstet 152:131–136, 1981
219. Rao AR, Kagan AR, Chan PM et al: Patterns of recurrence following curative resection alone for adenocarcinoma of the rectum and sigmoid colon. Cancer 48:1492–1495, 1981
220. Mendenhall WM, Million RR, Pfaff WW: Patterns of recurrence in adenocarcinoma of the rectum and rectosigmoid treated with surgery alone: Implications in treatment planning with adjuvant radiation therapy. Int J Radiat Oncol Biol Phys 9:977–985, 1983
221. Rich T, Gunderson LL, Lew R et al: Patterns of recurrence of rectal cancer after potentially curative surgery. Cancer 52:1317–1329, 1983
222. Pilipshen SJ, Heilweil M, Quan SHQ et al: Patterns of pelvic recurrence following definitive resections of rectal cancer. Cancer 53:1354–1362, 1984
223. Willett C, Tepper JE, Cohen A et al: Obstructive and perforative colonic carcinoma: Patterns of failure. J Clin Oncol 3:379–384, 1985
224. Minsky BD, Mies C, Recht A et al: Resectable adenocarcinoma of the rectosigmoid and rectum: 1. Patterns of failure and survival. Cancer (in press)
225. Minsky BD, Mies C, Rich TA et al: Potentially curative surgery of colon cancer: 1. Patterns of failure and survival. J Clin Oncol 6:106–118, 1988
226. Gabriel WB, Dukes C, Bussey HJR: Lymphatic spread in cancer of the rectum. Br J Surg 23:395–413, 1935
227. Wood WQ, Wilkie DPD: Carcinoma of the rectum: An anatomico-pathologic study. Edinburgh Med J 40:321–331, 1933
228. Grinnell RS: The grading and prognosis of carcinoma of the colon and rectum. Ann Surg 109:500–503, 1939
229. Villemin F, Huard P, Montague M: Récherches anatomiques sur les lymphatiques du rectum et de l'anus. Rev Chir 63:39–80, 1925
230. Grinnell RS: Lymphatic block with atypical and retrograde lymphatic metastasis and spread in carcinoma of the colon and rectum. Ann Surg 108:621–642, 1938
231. Herter FP, Slanetz CA: Patterns and significance of lymphatic spread from cancer of the colan and rectum. In Weiss L, Gilbert HA, Ballon SC (eds); Lymphatic System Metastasis. Boston, GK Hall, 1980
232. Brown CE, Warren S: Visceral metastases from rectal carcinoma. Surg Gynecol Obstet 66:611–621, 1938
233. Grinnell RS: The lymphatic and venous spread of carcinoma of the rectum. Ann Surg 116:200–215, 1942
234. Weiss L, Grundmann E, Torhorst J et al: Haematogenous metastatic patterns in colonic carcinoma: An analysis of 1541 necropsies. J Pathol 150:195–203, 1986
235. Batson OV: The function of the vertebral veins and their role in the spread of metastases. Ann Surg 112:138–149, 1940
236. Vider M, Maruyama Y, Narvaez R: Significance of the vertebral venous (Batson's) plexus in metastatic spread in colorectal carcinoma. Cancer 40:67–71, 1977
237. Umpleby HC, Williamson RCN: Anastomotic recurrence in large bowel cancer. Br J Surg 74:873–878, 1987
238. Beahrs OH, Phillips JW, Dockerty MB: Implantation of tumor cells as a factor in recurrence of carcinoma of the rectosigmoid: Report of four cases with implantation at dentate line. Cancer 8:831–838, 1955
239. LeQuesne LP, Thompson AD: Implantation recurrence of carcinoma of rectum and colon. N Engl J Med 258:578–582, 1958
240. Boreham P: Implantation metastases from cancer of the large bowel. Br J Surg 46:103–108, 1958
241. McGrew EA, Laws JF, Cole WH: Free malignant cells in relation to recurrence of carcinoma of the colon. JAMA 154:1251–1254, 1954
242. Goligher JC, Dukes CE, Bussey HJR: Local recurrences after sphincter-saving excisions for carcinoma of the rectum and rectosigmoid. Br J Surg 39:199–211, 1951
243. Cole WH, Packard D, Southwick HW: Carcinoma of the colon with special reference to prevention of recurrence. JAMA 155:1549–1553, 1954
244. Lawrie H: Letter: Cancer contagion and inoculation. Br Med J 1:198–199, 1906
245. Ryall C; Cancer infection and cancer recurrence: A danger to avoid in cancer operations. Lancet 2:1311–1316, 1907
246. Pomeranz AA, Garlock JH: Postoperative recurrence of cancer of colon due to desquamated malignant cells. JAMA 158:1434–1436, 1955
247. Moossa AR, Ree PC, Marks JE et al: Factors influencing local recurrence after abdominoperineal resection for cancer of the rectum and rectosigmoid. Br J Surg 62:727–730, 1975
248. Walz BJ, Green MR, Lindstron BJ et al: Anatomical prognostic factors after abdominooperineal resection. Int J Radiat Oncol Biol Phys 7:477–484, 1981
249. Thomas PRM, Stablein DM, Kinzie JJ et al: Perineal effects of postoperative treatment for adenocarcinoma of the rectum. Int J Radiat Oncol Biol Phys 12:167–171, 1986
250. Mayo WJ: Grafting and traumatic dissemination of carcinoma in the course of operations for malignant disease. JAMA 60:512–513, 1913
251. Fisher ER, Turnbull RB Jr: The cytologic demonstration and significance of tumor cells in the mesenteric venous blood in patients with colorectal carcinoma. Surg Gynecol Obstet 100:102–108, 1955
252. Goligher JC: The Dukes' A, B and C categorization of the extent of spread of carcinomas of the rectum. Surg Gynecol Obstet 143:793–794, 1976
253. Wiggers T, Arends JW, Volovics A: Regression analysis of prognostic factors in colorectal cancer after curative resections. Dis Colon Rectum 31:33–41, 1988
254. Wood CB, Gillis CR, Hole D et al: Local tumour invasion as a prognostic factor in colorectal cancer. Br J Surg 68:326–328, 1981
255. Davis NC, Evans EB, Cohen JR et al: Staging of colorectal cancer: The Australian Clinico-Pathological Staging (ACPS) System compared with the Dukes' system. Dis Colon Rectum 27:707–713, 1984
256. Midiri G, Amanti C, Consorti F et al: Usefulness of preoperative CEA levels in the assessment of colorectal cancer patient stage. J Surg Oncol 22:257–260, 1983

257. Moertel CG, OFallon JR, Go VL et al: The preoperative carcinoembryonic antigen test in the diagnosis, staging, and prognosis of colorectal cancer. Cancer 58:603–610, 1986
258. Lockhart-Mummery JP: Two hundred cases of cancer of the rectum treated by perineal excision. Br J Surg 14:110–124, 1927
259. Kirklin JW, Dockerty MB, Waugh JM: The role of the peritoneal reflection in the prognosis of carcinoma of the rectum and sigmoid colon. Surg Gynecol Obstet 88:326–331, 1949
260. Wolmark N, Fisher B, Wieand HS: The prognostic value of the modifications of the Dukes' C class of colorectal cancer. Ann Surg 203:115–122, 1986
261. Phillips RKS, Hittinger R, Blesovsky L et al: Large bowel cancer: Surgical pathology and its relationship to survival. Br J Surg 71:604–610, 1984
262. Gastrointestinal Tumor Study Group: Prolongation of the disease-free interval in surgically treated rectal carcinoma. N Engl J Med 312:1465–1472, 1985
263. American Joint Committee on Cancer: Manual for Staging of Cancer, 2nd ed. Philadelphia, JB Lippincott, 1983
264. Harmer MH (ed): TNM Classification of Malignant Tumours, pp 69–76. Geneva, International Union Against Cancer [Union Internationale Contre le Cancer], 1978
265. Chapuis PH, Dent OF, Newland RC et al: An evaluation of the American Joint Committee (pTNM) staging method for cancer of the colon and rectum. Dis Colon Rectum 29:6–10, 1986
266. Enderlin F, Gloor F: Colorectal cancer: The relationship of staging to survival. A cancer registry study of 800 cases in St. Gallen-Appenzell. Soz Praventivmed 31:85–88, 1986
267. Hermanek P: Problems of pTNM classification of carcinoma of the stomach, colorectum and anal margin. Pathol Res Pract 181:296–300, 1986
268. American Joint Committee on Cancer: Manual for Staging of Cancer, 3rd ed. Philadelphia, JB Lippincott, 1987
269. Hermanek P, Sobin LH (eds): TNM Classification of Malignant Tumours (International Union Against Cancer), 4th ed. Berlin, Springer-Verlag, 1987
270. Nathanson SD, Schultz L, Tilley B et al: Carcinoma of the colon and rectum: A comparison of staging classifications. Am Surg 52:428–433, 1986
271. Newland RC, Chapuis PH, Smyth EJ: The prognostic value of substaging colorectal carcinoma: A prognostic study of 1117 cases with standardized pathology. Cancer 60:852–857, 1987
272. Abrams JS: Clinical staging of rectal cancer. Am J Surg 139:539–543, 1980
273. Zorzitto M, Germanson T, Cummings B et al: A method of clinical prognostic staging for patients with rectal cancer. Dis Colon Rectum 25:759–765, 1982
274. Duncan W, Smith AN, Freedman LF et al: Clinico-pathological features of prognostic significance in operable rectal cancer in 17 centres in the U.K. Br J Cancer 50:435–442, 1984
275. Freedman LS, Macaskill P, Smith AN: Multivariate analysis of prognostic factors for operable rectal cancer. Lancet 2:733–736, 1984
276. Davis NC, Newland RC: The reporting of colorectal cancer: The Australian clinicopathological staging system. Aust NZ J Surg 52:395–397, 1982
277. Davis NC, Evans EB, Cohen JR et al: Clinicopathological staging of colorectal cancer: Has the time arrived? Br J Surg 72 (suppl):S47–S52, 1985
278. York Mason A: Rectal cancer: The spectrum of selective surgery. Proc R Soc Med 69:237–244, 1976
279. Nicholls RJ, York Mason A, Borson BC et al: The clinical staging of rectal cancer. Br J Surg 69:404–409, 1982
280. Nicholls RJ, Galloway DJ, Mason AY et al: Clinical local staging of rectal cancer. Br J Surg 72 (suppl):S51–S52, 1985
281. Williams NS, Durdey P, Quirke P et al: Pre-operative staging of rectal neoplasm and its impact on clinical management. Br J Surg 72:868–874, 1985
282. Clark J, Bankoff M, Carter B et al: The use of computerized tomography scan in the staging and follow-up study of carcinoma of the rectum. Surg Gynecol Obstet 159:335–342, 1984
283. Hildebrandt U, Feifel G: Preoperative staging of rectal cancer by intrarectal ultrasound. Dis Colon Rectum 28:42–46, 1985
284. Romano G, de Rosa P, Vallone G et al: Intrarectal ultrasound and computed tomography in the pre- and postoperative assessment of patients with rectal cancer. Br J Surg [Suppl]:S117–S119, 1985
285. Rifkin MD, Marks GJ: Transrectal US as an adjunct in the diagnosis of rectal and extrarectal tumors. Radiology 157:499–502, 1985
286. Beynon J, Mortensen NJ, Foy DM et al: Endorectal sonography: Laboratory and clinical experience in Bristol. Int J Colorect Dis 1:212–215, 1986
287. Nyberg DA, Kimmey MB, Wang K et al: Sonographic staging of colon neoplasms: Accuracy in determining depth of spread (abst). Radiology 154: 1986
288. Mayes GB, Zornoza J: Computed tomography of colon carcinoma. AJR 135:43–46, 1980
289. Thoeni RF, Moss AA, Schnyder P, Margulis AR: Detection and staging of primary rectal and rectosigmoid cancer by computed tomography. Radiology 141:135–138, 1981
290. Hamlin DJ, Burgener FA, Sischy B: New technique to stage early rectal carcinoma by computed tomography. Radiology 141:539–540, 1981
291. Zaunbauer W, Haertel M, Fuchs WA: Computed tomography in carcinoma of the rectum. Gastrointest Radiol 6:79–84, 1981
292. van Waes PFGM, Koehler PR, Feldberg MAM: Management of rectal carcinoma: Impact of computed tomography. AJR 140:1137–1142, 1983
293. Dixon AK, Fry IK, Morson BC et al: Pre-operative computed tomography of carcinoma of the rectum. Br J Radiol 54:655–659, 1981
294. Grabbe E, Lierse W, Winkler R: The perirectal fascia: Morphology and use in staging of rectal carcinoma. Radiology 149:241–246, 1983
295. Adalsteinsson B, Glimelius B, Graffman S et al: Computed tomography in staging of rectal carcinoma. Acta Radiol Diagn 26:45–55, 1985
296. Netri G, Coco C, Valentine V et al: Clinical staging of rectal cancer: Results of a prospective continuing study. Ital J Surg Sci 15:169–174, 1985
297. Freeny PC, Marks WM, Ryan JA, Bolen JW: Colorectal carcinoma evaluation with CT: Preoperative staging and detection of postoperative recurrence. Radiology 158:347–353, 1986
298. Thompson WM, Halvorsen RA, Foster WL Jr et al: Preoperative and postoperative CT staging of rectosigmoid carcinoma. AJR 146:703–710, 1986
299. Shank B, Dershaw D, Caravelli J et al: A prospective, blinded trial of CT staging for rectal carcinoma (unpublished data)
300. Lee JKT, Heiken JP, Ling D et al: Magnetic resonance imaging of abdominal and pelvic lymphadenopathy. Radiology 153:181–188, 1984
301. Dooms GC, Hricak H, Crooks LE, Higgins CB: Magnetic resonance imaging of the lymph nodes: Comparison with CT. Radiology 153:719–728, 1984
302. Butch RJ, Stark DD, Wittenberg J et al: Staging rectal cancer by MR and CT. AJR 146:1155–1160, 1986
303. Fuchs WA: Normal anatomy. In Fuchs WA, Davidson JW, Fisher HW (eds): Lymphography in Cancer. Recent Results Cancer Res 23: 42–86, 1969
304. Ege GN, Cummings BJ: Interstitial radiocolloid ilio-pelvic lymphoscintigraphy: Technique, anatomy and clinical application. Int J Radiat Oncol Biol Phys 6:1483–1490, 1980
305. Reasbeck PG, Manktelow A, McArthur AM et al: An evaluation of pelvic lymphoscintigraphy in the staging of colorectal carcinoma. Br J Surg 71:936–940, 1984
306. Moldofsky PJ, Powe J, Mulhern CB Jr et al: Metastatic colon carcinoma detected with radiolabeled $F(ab')_2$ monoclonal antibody fragments. Radiology 149:549–555, 1983
307. Mach J–P, Chatal J–F, Lumbroso J–D et al: Tumor localization in patients by radiolabeled monoclonal antibodies against colon carcinoma. Cancer Res 43:5593–5600, 1983
308. Alderson PO, Adams DF, McNeil BJ et al: Computed tomography, ultrasound, and scintigraphy of the liver in patients with colon or breast carcinoma: A prospective comparison. Radiology 149:225–230, 1983
309. Zeman RK, Paushter DM, Schiebler ML et al: Hepatic imaging: Current status. Radiol Clin North Am 23:473–487, 1985
310. Thompson WM: Imaging strategies for tumors of the gastrointestinal system. CA 37:165–185, 1987
311. Kemeny NM, Sugarbaker PH, Smith TJ et al: A prospective analysis of laboratory tests and imaging studies to detect hepatic lesions. Ann Surg 195:163–167, 1982
312. Gennari L, Doci R, Bozzetti F et al: Surgical treatment of hepatic metastases from colorectal cancer. Ann Surg 203:49–54, 1986
313. Reinig JW, Dwyer AJ, Miller DL et al: Liver metastasis detection: Comparative sensitivities of MR imaging and CT scanning. Radiology 162:43–47, 1987
314. van de Velde CJH: The staging of hepatic metastases arising from colorectal cancer. Recent Results Cancer Res 100:85–90, 1986
315. Hoerner MT: Carcinoma of the colon and rectum in persons under twenty years of age. Am J Surg 96:47–53, 1958
316. Recio P, Bussey HJR: The pathology and prognosis of carcinoma of the rectum in the young. Proc R Soc Lond 58:789–790, 1965
317. Mayo CW, Pagtalunan JG: Malignancy of the colon and rectum in patients under 30 years of age. Surgery 53:711–718, 1963
318. Coffey RJ, Cardenas F: Cancer of the bowel in the young adult. Dis Colon Rectum 7:491–492, 1964
319. van Langenberg AV, Ong GB: Carcinoma of large bowel in the young. Br Med J 3:374–376, 1972
320. Odone V, Chang L, Caces J et al: The natural history of colorectal carcinoma in adolescents. Cancer 49:1716–1720, 1982
321. Safford KL, Spebar MJ, Rosenthal D: Review of colorectal cancer in patients under age 40 years. Am J Surg 142:767–769, 1981
322. Simstein NL, Kovalcik PJ, Cross GH: Colorectal carcinoma in patients less than 40 years old. Dis Colon Rectum 2:169–171, 1978
323. Bülow S: Colorectal cancer in patients less than 40 years of age in Denmark, 1943–1967. Dis Colon Rectum 23:327–336, 1980
324. Umpleby HC, Williamson RCN: Carcinoma of the large bowel in the first four decades. Br J Surg 71:272–277, 1984
325. Eisenberg B, DeCosse JJ, Harford F et al: Carcinoma of the colon and rectum: The natural history reviewed in 1704 patients. Cancer 49:1131–1134, 1982
326. Welch CE, Burke JF: Carcinoma of the colon and rectum. N Engl J Med 266:211–219, 1962
327. McDermott FT, Hughes ESR, Pihl E et al: Comparative results of surgical management of single carcinomas of the colon and rectum: A series of 1939 patients managed by one surgeon. Br J Surg 68:850–855, 1981
328. Stearns MW, Deddish MR, Quan SHQ et al: Preoperative reontgen therapy for cancer of the rectum and rectosigmoid. Surg Gynecol Obstet 138:584–586, 1974
329. Spratt JS Jr, Spjut HJ: Prevalence and prognosis of individual clinical and pathologic variables associated with colorectal carcinoma. Cancer 20:1976–1985, 1967
330. Godwin JD, Brown CC: Some prognostic factors in survival of patients with cancer of the colon and rectum. J Chronic Dis 28:441–454, 1975
331. deMello J, Struthers L, Turner R et al: Multivariate analysis as aides to diagnosis and assessment of prognosis in gastrointestinal cancer. Br J Cancer 48:341–348, 1983

332. Chapuis PH, Dent OF, Fisher R et al: A multivariate analysis of clinical and pathological variables in prognosis after resection of large bowel cancer. Br J Surg 72:698–702, 1985
333. Corman J, Arnoux R, Peloquin A et al: Blood transfusions and survival after colectomy for colorectal cancer. Can J Surg 29:325–329, 1986
334. Fielding LP, Phillips RKS, Fry JS et al: Prediction of outcome after curative resection for large bowel cancer. Lancet 2:904–907, 1986
335. Koch M, McPherson TA, Egedahl RD: Effect of sex and reproductive history on the survival of patients with colorectal cancer. J Chronic Dis 35:69–72, 1982
336. Beahrs OH, Sanfelippo PM: Factors in the prognosis of colon and rectal cancer. Cancer 28:213–217, 1971
337. Copeland EM, Miller LD, Jones RS: Prognostic factors in carcinoma of the colon and rectum. Am J Surg 116:875–881, 1968
338. Pescatori M, Maria G, Beltrani B et al: Site, emergency, and duration of symptoms in the prognosis of colorectal cancer. Dis Colon Rectum 25:33–40, 1982
339. Ulin AW, Ehrlich EW: Current views related to management of large bowel obstruction caused by carcinoma of the colon. Am J Surg 104:463–467, 1962
340. Chang WYM, Burnett WE: Complete colonic obstruction due to adenocarcinoma. Surg Gynecol Obstet 114:353–356, 1962
341. Miller LD, Boruchow IB, Fitts WT: An analysis of 284 patients with perforative carcinoma of the colon. Surg Gynecol Obstet 123:1212–1218, 1966
342. Floyd CE, Cohn I: Obstruction in cancer of the colon. Ann Surg 165:721–731, 1967
343. Crowder VH, Cohn I: Perforation in cancer of the colon and rectum. Dis Colon Rectum 10:415–420, 1967
344. Glenn F, McSherry CK: Obstruction and perforation in colorectal cancer. Ann Surg 173:983–992, 1971
345. Welch JP, Donaldson GA: Management of severe obstruction of the large bowel due to malignant disease. Am J Surg 127:492–499, 1974
346. Welch JP, Donaldson GA: Perforative carcinoma of colon and rectum. Ann Surg 180:734–740, 1974
347. Wolmark N, Wieand HS, Rockette HE et al: The prognostic significance of tumor location and bowel obstruction in Dukes B and C colorectal cancer: Findings from the NSABP clinical trials. Ann Surg 198:743–752, 1983
348. Steinberg SM, Barkin JS, Kaplan RS et al: Prognostic indicators of colon tumors: The Gastrointestinal Tumor Study Group experience. Cancer 57:1866–1870, 1986
349. Kelley WE Jr, Brown PW, Lawrence W Jr et al: Penetrating, obstructing, and perforating carcinomas of the colon and rectum. Arch Surg 116:381–384, 1981
350. Thomas WH, Larson, RA, Wright HK et al: An analysis of patients with carcinoma of the right colon. Surg Gynecol Obstet 127:313–318, 1968
351. Dwight RW, Higgins GA, Keehn RJ: Factors influencing survival after resection in cancer of the colon and rectum. Am J Surg 117:512–522, 1969
352. Gilchrist RK, David VC: A consideration of pathological factors influencing five year survival in radical resection of the large bowel and rectum for carcinoma. Ann Surg 126:421–438, 1947
353. Osnes S: Carcinoma of the colon and rectum: A study of 353 cases with special reference to prognosis. Acta Chir Scand 110:378–388, 1956
354. McSherry CK, Cornell GN, Glen F: Carcinoma of the colon and rectum. Ann Surg 169:502–512, 1969
355. Cohen AM, Wood WC, Gunderson LL et al: Pathological studies in rectal cancer. Cancer 45:2965–2968, 1980
356. Wolmark N, Fisher ER, Wieand HS et al: The relationship of depth of penetration and tumor size to the number of positive nodes in Dukes C colorectal cancer. Cancer 53:2707–2712, 1984
357. Coller FA, Kay EB, MacIntyre RS: Regional lymphatic metastasis in carcinoma of the colon. Ann Surg 114:56–63, 1941
358. Burrows L, Tartter P: Effect of blood transfusions on colonic malignancy recurrence rate. Lancet 2:662, 1982
359. Agarwal M, Blumberg N: Colon cancer patients transfused perioperatively have an increased incidence of recurrence (abst) Transfusion 23:421, 1983
360. Foster RS Jr, Costanza MC, Foster JC: Adverse relationship between blood transfusions and survival after colectomy for colon cancer. Cancer 55:1195–1201, 1985
361. Nathanson SD, Tilley BC, Schultz L et al: Perioperative allogeneic blood transfusions: Survival in patients with resected carcinomas of the colon and rectum. Arch Surg 120:734–738, 1985
362. Weiden PL, Bean MA, Schultz P: Perioperative blood transfusion does not increase the risk of colorectal cancer. Cancer 60:870–874, 1987
363. Willett CG, Tepper JE, Cohen AM et al: Failure patterns following curative resection of colonic carcinoma. Ann Surg 200:685–690, 1984
364. Willett C, Tepper JE, Cohen AM et al: Local failure following curative resection of colonic adenocarcinoma. Int J Radiat Oncol Biol Phys 10:645–651, 1984
365. Fucini C, Bandettini L, Dlia M et al: Are postoperative fever and/or septic complications prognostic factors in colorectal cancer resected for cure? Dis Colon Rectum 28:94–95, 1985
366. Riboli EB, Secco GB, Lapertosa G et al: Colorectal cancer: Relationship of histologic grading to disease prognosis. Tumori 69:581–584, 1983
367. Godwin JD II: Carcinoid tumors: An analysis of 2837 cases. Cancer 36:560–569, 1975
368. Madison MS, Dockerty MB, Waugh JM: Venous invasion in carcinoma of the rectum as evidenced by venous radiography. Surg Gynecol Obstet 99:170–178, 1954
369. Qualheim RE, Gall EA: Is histopathologic grading of colon carcinoma a valid procedure? Arch Pathol 56:466–472, 1953
370. Thomas GDH, Dixon MF, Smeeton NC et al: Observer variation in the histological grading of rectal carcinoma. J Clin Pathol [Suppl] 36:385–391, 1983
371. Trimpi HD, Bacon HE: Mucoid carcinoma of the rectum. Cancer 4:597–609, 1951
372. Sundblad AS, Paz RA: Mucinous carcinomas of the colon and rectum and their relation to polyps. Cancer 50:2504–2509, 1982
373. Minsky BD, Mies C, Rich TA et al: Colloid carcinoma of the colon and rectum. Cancer 60:3103–3112, 1987
374. DeMascarel A, Coindre JM, DeMascarel I et al: The prognostic significance of specific histologic features of carcinoma of the colon and rectum. Surg Gynecol Obstet 153:511–514, 1981
375. Walton WW, Hagihara PF, Griffen WO: Colorectal adenocarcinoma in patients less than 40 years old. Dis Colon Rectum 19:529–534, 1976
376. Symonds DA, Vickery AL Jr: Mucinous carcinoma of the colon and rectum. Cancer 37:1891–1900, 1976
377. Umpleby HC, Ranson DL, Williamson HC: Peculiarities of mucinous colorectal carcinoma. Br J Surg 72:715–718, 1985
378. Sunderland DA: The significance of vein invasion by cancer of the rectum and sigmoid: A microscopic study of 210 cases. Cancer 2:429–437, 1949
379. Grinnell RS: Lymphatic metastases of carcinoma of the colon and rectum. Ann Surg 131:494–506, 1950
380. Burns FJ, Pfaff J Jr: Vascular invasion in carcinoma of the colon and rectum. Am J Surg 92:704–709, 1956
381. Swinton NW: Cancer of the colon and rectum: A statistical study of 608 patients. Surg Clin North Am 39:745–753, 1959
382. Talbot IC, Ritchie S, Leighton MH et al: Spread of rectal cancer within veins: Histologic features and clinical significance. Am J Surg 141:15–17, 1981
383. Minsky BD, Mies C, Rich TA et al: Potentially curative surgery of colon cancer: 2. The influence of blood vessel invasion. J Clin Oncol 6:119–127, 1988
384. Minsky BD, Mies C, Recht A et al: Resectable adenocarcinoma of the rectosigmoid and rectum: 2. The influence of blood vessel invasion. Cancer 61:1408–1416, 1988
385. Khankanian N, Mavligit GM, Russell WO et al: Prognostic significance of vascular invasion in colorectal cancer of Dukes' B class. Cancer 39:1195–1200, 1977
386. Kim US, Papatestas AE, Aufses AH Jr: Prognostic significance of peripheral lymphocytic counts and carcinoembryonic antigens in colorectal carcinoma. J Surg Oncol 8:257–262, 1976
387. Shafir M, Bekesi JG, Papatestas A et al: Preoperative and postoperative immunological evaluation of patients with colorectal cancer. Cancer 46:700–705, 1980
388. Panettiere FJ, Chen TT: Prognostic significance of serum immunoglobulin levels in colorectal adenocarcinoma: Data from a SWOG study. Proc Am Soc Clin Oncol 6:73, 1987
389. Baseler MW, Maxim PE, Veltri RW: Circulating IgA immune complexes in head and neck cancer, nasopharyngeal carcinoma, lung cancer, and colon cancer. Cancer 59:1727–1731, 1987
390. Murray D, Hreno A, Dutton J et al: Prognosis in colon cancer: A pathologic reassessment. Arch Surg 110:908–913, 1975
391. Carlon CA, Fabris G, Arslan-Pagnini C et al: Prognostic correlations of operable carcinoma of the rectum. Dis Colon Rectum 28:47–50, 1985
392. Svennevig JL, Lunde OC, Holter J et al: Lymphoid infiltration and prognosis in colorectal carcinoma. Br J Cancer 49:375–377, 1984
393. Patt DJ, Byrnes RK, Vardiman JW et al: Mesocolic lymph node histology is an important prognostic indicator for patients with carcinoma of the sigmoid colon: An immunomorphologic study. Cancer 35:1388–1397, 1975
394. Tsakraklides V, Wanebo HJ, Sternberg SS et al: Prognostic evaluation of regional lymph node morphology in colorectal cancer. Am J Surg 129:174–180, 1975
395. Pihl E, Malahy MA, Khankanian N et al: Immunomorphological features of prognostic significance in Dukes' class B colorectal carcinoma. Cancer Res 37:4145–4149, 1977
396. LoGerfo P, Herter FP: Carcinoembryonic antigen and prognosis in patients with colon cancer. Ann Surg 181:81–84, 1975
397. Herrera MA, Chu TM, Holyoke ED; Carcinoembryonic antigen (CEA) as a prognostic and monitoring test in clinically complete resection of colorectal carcinoma. Ann Surg 183:5–9, 1976
398. Wanebo HJ, Rao B, Pinsky CM et al: Pre-operative carcinoembryonic antigen level as a prognostic indicator in colorectal cancer. N Eng J Med 299:448–451, 1978
399. Band PR, Beck IT, Dinner PJ et al: Two year follow-up study of patients with known serum concentrations of carcinoembryonic antigen. Can Med Assoc J 117:657–659, 1977
400. Evans JT, Mittleman A, Chu M et al: Pre- and post-operative uses of CEA. Cancer 42:1419–1421, 1978
401. Kohler JP, Simonowitz D, Paloyan D: Pre-operative CEA level: A prognostic test in patients with colorectal carcinoma. Am Surg 46:449–452, 1980
402. Staab HJ, Anderer FA, Brummendorf T et al: Prognostic value of pre-operative serum CEA level compared to clinical staging: I. Colorectal carcinoma. Br J Cancer 44:652–662, 1981
403. Szymendera J, Nowacki MP, Szalowski AW et al: Predictive value of plasma CEA levels: Preoperative prognosis and postoperative monitoring of patients with colorectal carcinoma. Dis Colon Rectum 25:46–52, 1982
404. Onetto M, Paganuzzi M, Secco GB et al: Preoperative carcinoembryonic antigen and prognosis in patients with colorectal cancer. Biomed Pharmacother 39:392–395, 1985
405. Aabo K, Pedersen H, Kjaer M: Carcinoembryonic antigen (CEA) and alkaline phos-

phatase in progressive colorectal cancer with special reference to patient survival. Eur J Cancer Clin Oncol 22:211–217, 1986
406. Goslin R, Steele G, MacIntyre J et al: The use of pre-operative plasma CEA levels for the stratification of patients after curative resection of colorectal cancer. Ann Surg 192:747–751, 1980
407. Chapuis PH, Newland RC, Payne JE et al: Preoperative carcinoembryonic antigen level and prognosis in colorectal cancer. Med J Aust 2:140–143, 1980
408. Blake KE, Dalbow MH, Concannon JP et al: Clinical significance of preoperative plasma carcinoembryonic antigen (CEA) level in patients with carcinoma of the large bowel. Dis Colon Rectum 25:24–32, 1982
409. Lewi H, Blumgart LH, Carter DC et al: Pre-operative carcinoembryonic antigen and survival in patients with colorectal cancer. Br J Surg 71:206—208, 1984
410. Steele G Jr, Ellenberg S, Ramming K et al: CEA monitoring among patients in multi-institutional adjuvant G.I. therapy protocols. Ann Surg 196:162–169, 1982
411. Tabuchi Y, Deguchi H, Imanishi K et al: Comparison of carcinoembryonic antigen levels between portal and peripheral blood in patients with colorectal cancer: Correlation with histopathologic variables. Cancer 59:1283–1288, 1987
412. Ward AM, Cooper EH, Turner R et al: Acute-phase reactant protein profiles: An aid to monitoring large bowel cancer by CEA and serum enzymes. Br J Cancer 35:170–178, 1977
413. Durdey P, Williams NS, Brown DA: Serum carcinoembryonic antigen and acute phase reactant proteins in the pre-operative detection of fixation of colorectal tumours. Br J Surg 71:881–884, 1984
414. Walker C, Grace BN: Acute-phase reactant proteins and carcinoembryonic antigen in cancer of the colon and rectum. Cancer 52:150–154, 1983
415. Meyer JS, Prioleau PG: S-phase fractions of colorectal carcinomas related to pathological and clinical features. Cancer 48:1221–1228, 1981
416. Blijham G, Schutte B, Reynders M et al: Flow cytometric (FCM) determination of ploidy level and life cycle analysis on 297 paraffin embedded colorectal carcinoma specimens. Proc Am Soc Clin Oncol 4:22, 1985
417. Bleiberg H, Buyse M, van den Heule B et al: Cell cycle parameters and prognosis of colorectal cancer. Eur J Cancer Clin Oncol 20:391–396, 1984
418. Mauro F, Teodori L, Schumann J, Gohde W: Flow cytometry as a tool for the prognostic assessment of human neoplasia. Int J Radiat Oncol Biol Phys 12:625–636, 1986
419. Wolley RC, Schreiber K, Koss LG et al: DNA distribution in human colon carcinomas and its relationship to clinical behavior. JNCI 69:15–22, 1982
420. Tribukait B, Hammarberg C, Rubio C: Ploidy and proliferation patterns in colorectal adenocarcinomas related to Dukes' classification and to histopathological differentiation. Acta Pathol Microbiol Immunol Scand [A] 91:89–95, 1983
421. Hiddemann W, von Bassewitz DB, Kleinemeier H–J et al: DNA stemline heterogeneity in colorectal cancer. Cancer 58:258–263, 1986
422. Frankfurt OS, Slocum HK, Rustum Ym et al: Flow cytometric analysis of DNA aneuploidy in primary and metastatic human solid tumors. Cytometry 5:71–80, 1984
423. Ota D, Johnston D, Drewinko B: Colorectal carcinoma (CA) cell kinetics: Need for new therapeutic strategies. Proc Am Soc Clin Oncol 6:13, 1987
424. Streffer C, van Beuningen D, Gross E et al: Predictive assays for the therapy of rectum carcinoma. Radiother Oncol 5:303–310, 1986
425. Armitage NC, Robins RA, Evans DF et al: Tumour cell DNA content in colorectal cancer and its relationship to survival. Br J Surg 72:828–830, 1985
426. Kokal W, Sheibani K, Terz J et al: Tumor DNA content in the prognosis of colorectal carcinoma JAMA 255:3123–3127, 1986
427. Scott NA, Rainwater LM, Wieand HS et al: The relative prognostic value of flow cytometric DNA analysis and conventional clinicopathologic criteria in patients with operable rectal carcinoma. Dis Colon Rectum 30:513–520, 1987
428. Melamed MR, Enker WE, Banner P et al: Flow cytometry of colorectal carcinoma with three-year followup. Dis Colon Rectum 29:184–186, 1986
428a. Chapuis PH, Dent OF, Fisher R et al: A multivariate analysis of clinical and pathological variables in prognosis after resection of large bowel cancer. Br J Surg 72:698–702, 1985
428b. Fielding LP, Phillips RK, Frey JS et al: The prediction of outcome after curative resection for large bowel cancer. Lancet 2:904–907, 1986
428c. Jass JR, Love SB, Northover JM: A new prognostic classification of rectal cancer. Lancet 1:1303–1306, 1987
428d. Fielding LP: Clinical-pathologic staging of large-bowel cancer: A report of the ASCRS committee. Dis Colon Rectum 31:204–209, 1988
428e. Williams NS, Jass JR, Hardcastle JD: Clinicopathological assessment and staging of colorectal cancer. Br J Surg 75:649–652, 1988
429. Der CJ, Cooper GM: Altered gene products are associated with activation of cellular *ras* genes in human lung and colon carcinomas. Cell 32:201–208, 1983
430. Spandidos DA, Kerr IB: Elevated expression of the human *ras* oncogene family in premalignant and malignant tumours of the colorectum. Br J Cancer 49:681–688, 1984
431. Gallick GE, Kurzrock R, Kloetzer WS et al: Expression of p21*ras* in fresh primary and metastatic human colorectal tumors. Proc Natl Acad Sci USA 82:1795–1799, 1985
432. Thar A, Hand PH, Wunderlich D et al: Monoclonal antibodies define differential *ras* gene expression in malignant and benign colonic diseases. Nature 311:562–565, 1984
433. Marx JL: Research news: *ras* oncogene activated in human colon cancers. Science 237:603, 1987
434. Bos JL, Fearon ER, Hamilton SR et al: Prevalence of *ras* gene mutations in human colorectal cancers. Nature 327:293–297, 1987
435. Forrester K, Almoguera C, Han K et al: Detection of high incidence of K-*ras* ongogenes during human colon tumorigenesis. Nature 327:298–303, 1987
436. Stewart J, Evan G, Watson JV, Sikora K: Detection of the c-*myc* oncogene product in colonic polyps and carcinomas. Br J Cancer 53:1–6, 1986
437. Sikora K, Chan S, Evan G et al: c-*myc* oncogene expression in colorectal cancer. Cancer 59:1289–1295, 1987
438. Welin S, Youker J, Spratt JS Jr et al: The rates and patterns of growth of 375 tumors of the large intestine and rectum observed serially by double contrast enema study (Malmo technique). AJR 90:673–687, 1963
439. Hanauske AR, Buchok J, Scheithauer W, Von Hoff DD: Human colon cancer cell lines secrete alpha TGF-like activity. BR J Cancer 55:57–59, 1987
440. Coffey RJ Jr, Shipley GD, Moses HL: Production of transforming growth factors by human colon cancer lines. Cancer Res 46:1164–1169, 1986
441. Beauchamp RD, Townsend CM Jr, Singh P et al: Proglumide, a gastrin receptor antagonist, inhibits growth of colon cancer and enhances survival in mice. Ann Surg 202:303–309, 1985
442. Singh P, Walker JP, Townsend CM Jr et al: Role of gastrin and gastrin receptors on the growth of a transplantable mouse colon carcinoma (MC-26) in BALB/c mice. Cancer Res 46:1612–1616, 1986
443. Stebbings WS, Farthing MJ, Vinson GP et al: Androgen receptors in rectal and colonic cancer. Dis Colon Rectum 29:95–98, 1986
444. Alford TC, Do HM, Geelhoed GW et al: Steroid hormone receptors in human colon cancers. Cancer 43:980–984, 1979
445. McClendon JE, Appleby D, Claudon DB et al: Colonic neoplasms: Tissue estrogen receptor and carcinoembryonic antigen. Arch Surg 112:240–241, 1977
446. Geelhoed GW, Crandall A, Lippman ME: Biologic implications of steroid hormone receptors in cancers of the colon. South Med J 78:252–254, 1985
447. Tempero M: Bile acids, ornithine decarboxylase, and cell proliferation in colon cancer: A review. Dig Dis 4:49–56, 1986
448. Luk GD, Baylin SB: Ornithine decarboxylase as a biologic marker in familial polyposis. N Engl J Med 311:80–83, 1984
449. Porter CW, Herrera-Ornelas L, Pera P et al: Polyamine biosynthetic activity in normal and neoplastic human colorectal tissues. Cancer 60:1275–1281, 1987
450. Gold P, Freeman SO: Specific carcinoembryonic antigens of the human digestive system. J Exp Med 122:467–481, 1965
451. Ahnen DJ, Nakane PK, Brown WR: Ultrastructural localization of carcinoembryonic antigen in normal intestine and colon cancer. Cancer 49:2077–2090, 1982
452. Primus FJ, Kuhns WJ, Goldenberg DM; Immunological heterogeneity of carcinoembryonic antigen: Immunohistochemical detection of carcinoembryonic determinants in colonic tumors with monoclonal antibodies. Cancer Res 43:693–701, 1983
453. Herlyn M, Blaszczyk M, Sears HF et al: Detection of carcinoembryonic antigen and related antigens in sera of patients with gastrointentinal tumors using monoclonal antibodies in double-determinant radioimmunoassays. Hybridoma 2:329–339, 1983
454. Wiley EL, Murphy P, Mendelson G, Eggleston JC: Distribution of blood group substances in normal human colon. Am J Clin Pathol 76:806–809, 1981
455. Ernst C, Thurin J, Atkinson B: Monoclonal antibody localization of A and B isoantigens in normal and malignant fixed human tissues. Am J Pathol 117:451–461, 1984
456. Schoentag R, Primus FJ, Kuhns W: ABH and Lewis blood group expression in colorectal carcinoma. Cancer Res 47:1695–1700, 1987
457. Compton C, Wyatt R, Konugres A et al: Immunohistochemical studies of blood group substance H in colorectal tumors using a monoclonal antibody. Cancer 59:118–127, 1987
458. Itzkowitz SH, Yuan M, Ferrell LD et al: Cancer-associated alterations of blood group antigen expression in human colorectal polyps. Cancer Res 46:5976–5984, 1986
459. Hakomori S: Blood group glycolipid antigens and their modifications as human cancer antigens. Am J Clin Pathol 82:635–648, 1984
460. Abe K, Hakomori S, Ohshiba S: Differential expression of difucosyl type II chain (Eey) defined by monoclonal antibody AH6 in different locations of colonic epithelia, various histological types of colonic polyps and adenocarcinomas. Cancer Res 46:2639–2644, 1986
461. Sakamoto J, Furukawa K, Cordon-Cardo C et al: Expression of Lewis A, Lewis B, X, Y blood group antigens in human colonic tumors and normal tissue in human tumor-derived cell lines. Cancer Res 46:1553–1561, 1986
462. Itzkowitz SH, Yuan M, Fukushi Y et al: Lewis X- and sialylated Lewis X-related antigen expression in human malignant and non-malignant colonic tissues. Cancer Res 46:2627–2632, 1986
463. Koprowski H, Steplewski Z, Mitchell K et al: Colorectal carcinoma antigens detected by hybridoma antibodies. Somatic Cell Mol Genet 5:957–972, 1979
464. Magnani JL, Nilsson B, Brockhaus M et al: A monoclonal antibody–defined antigen associated with gastrointestinal cancer is a ganglioside containing sialylated lacto-*N*-fucopentose. J Biol Chem 257:14365–14369, 1982
465. Atkinson BF, Ernst CS, Herlyn M et al: Gastrointenstinal cancer-associated antigen in immunoperoxidase assay. Cancer Res 42:4820–4823, 1982
466. Herlyn D, Herlyn M, Steplewski Z, Koprowski H: Monoclonal antibodies in cell mediated cytotoxicity against human melanoma and colorectal carcinoma. Eur J Immunol 9:657–659, 1979
467. Herlyn D, Steplewski Z, Herlyn M, Koprowski H: Inhibition of growth of colorectal carcinoma in nude mice by monoclonal antibody. Cancer Res 40:717–721, 1980

468. Johnson VG, Schlom J, Patterson AJ et al: Analysis of a human tumor associated glycoprotein (TAG-72) identified by monoclonal antibody B72-3. Cancer Res 46:850-857, 1986
469. Lottich SC, Szpak CA, Johnston WW et al: Phenotypic heterogeneity of a tumor-associated antigen in adenocarcinomas of the colon and their metastases as demonstrated by monoclonal antibody B72.3. Cancer Invest 4:387-395, 1986
470. Skinner JM, Whitehead R: Tumor-associated antigens in polyps and carcinoma of the large bowel. Cancer 47:1241-1245, 1981
471. Campo E, Palacin A, Benasco C et al: Human chorionic gonadotropin in colorectal carcinoma. Cancer 49:1611-1616, 1987
472. Lambert R, Sobin LH, Waye JD et al: The management of patients with colorectal adenomas. CA 34:167-176, 1984
473. Wegener M, Borsch G, Schmidt G: Colorectal adenomas: Distribution, incidence of malignant transformation, and rate of recurrence. Dis Colon Rectum 29:383-387, 1986
474. Neugut AI, Johnsen CM, Forde KA et al: Recurrence rates for colorectal polyps. Cancer 55:1586-1589, 1985
475. Nava H, Carlsson G, Petrelli NJ et al: Followup colonoscopy in patients with colorectal adenomatous polyps. Dis Colon Rectum 30:465-468, 1987
476. Nivatvongs S, Nicholson JD, Rothenberger DA et al: Villous adenomas of the rectum: The accuracy of clinical assessment. Surgery 87:549-551, 1980
477. Taylor EW, Thompson H, Oates GD et al: Limitations of biopsy in reoperative assessment of villous papilloma. Dis Colon Rectum 24:259-262, 1981
478. Groff W, Rubin RJ, Salvati EP et al: A method of management of a circumferential villous tumor of the rectum. Dis Colon Rectum 24:151-154, 1981
479. Pello MJ: Transanal excision of large sessile villous adenomas using an endorectal traction flap. Surg Gynecol Obstet 164:281-279, 1987
480. Bess MA, Adson MA, Elveback LR, Moertel CG: Rectal cancer following colectomy for polyposis. Arch Surg 115:460-467, 1980
481. Bussey HJR, Eyers AA, Ritchie SM et al: The rectum in adenomatous polyposis: The St. Mark's policy. Br J Surg 72:S29-S35, 1985
482. Moertel CG, Hill JR, Adson MA: Management of multiple polyposis of the large bowel. Cancer 28:160-164, 1971
483. Harvey JC, Quan SHQ, Stearns MW: Management of familial polyposis with preservation of the rectum. Surgery 84:476-482, 1978
484. Sarre RG, Jagelman DG, Beck GJ et al: Colectomy with ileorectal anastomosis for familial adenomatous polyposis: The risk of rectal cancer. Surgery 101:20-26, 1986
485. Heimann TM, Gelernt I, Salky B et al: Familial polyposis coli: Results of mucosal proctectomy with ileoanal anastomosis. Dis Colon Rectum 30:424-427, 1987
486. Herrera-Irbelas L (ed): Familial polyposis coli. Semin Surg Oncol 3:66-139, 1987
487. Kewenter J, Hulten L, Ahren C: The occurrence of severe epithelial dysplasia and its bearing on treatment of longstanding ulcerative colitis. Ann Surg 195:209-213, 1982
488. Nugent FW, Haggitt RC, Colcher H et al: Malignant potential of chronic ulcerative colitis. Gastroenterology 76:1-5, 1979
489. Lennard-Jones JE, Morson BC, Ritchie JK et al: Cancer and colitis—assessment of the individual risk by clinical and histological criteria. Gastroenterology 73:1280-1289, 1977
490. Lennard-Jones JE; Cancer risk in ulcerative colitis—surveillance or surgery? Br J Surg 72(suppl):S84-S86, 1985
491. Rosenstock E, Farmer RG, Petras R et al: Surveillance for colonic carcinoma in ulcerative colitis. Gastroenterology 89:1342-1346, 1985
492. Wong WD, Rothenberger DA, Goldberg SA: Ileoanal pouch procedures. Curr Probl Surg 22:1-78, 1985
493. Taylor BA, Dozois RR: The J ileal pouch-anal anastomosis. World J Surg 11:727-734, 1987
494. Enker WE, Laffer UT, Block GE: Enhanced survival of patients with colon and rectal cancer is based upon wide anatomic resection. Ann Surg 190:350-360, 1979
495. Grinnell RS: Results of ligation of inferior mesenteric artery at the aorta in resections of carcinoma of the descending and sigmoid colon and rectum. Surg Gynecol Obstet 120:1031-1036, 1965
496. Ault GW: A technique for cancer isolation and extended dissection for cancer of the distal colon and rectum. Surg Gynecol Obstet 106:467-477, 1958
497. Cole WH, Roberts SS, Strehl FW: Modern concepts of cancer of the colon and rectum. Cancer 19:1347-1358, 1966
498. Turnbull RB Jr, Kyle K, Watson FR, Spratt J: Cancer of the colon: The influence of the no-touch isolation technique on survival rates. Ann Surg 166:420-427, 1967
499. Wiggers T, Jeekel J, Arends JW et al: The no-touch isolation technique in colon cancer: A prospective controlled multi-center trial. Proc Am Soc Clin Oncol 5:269, 1986
500. Cohn I Jr, Gonzalez EA Jr, Atik M: Spillage and recurrence of colonic carcinoma. Surg Forum 12:153-155, 1961
501. Cohn I Jr, Floyd CE, Atik M: Control of tumor implantation during operations on the colon. Ann Surg 157:825-838, 1963
502. Cohn I Jr, Corley RG, Floyd CE: Iodized suture for control of tumor implantation in a colon anastomosis. Surg Gynecol Obstet 116:366-370, 1963
503. Douglass HO Jr, LeVeen HH: Tumor recurrence in colon anastomoses: Prevention by coagulation and fixation with formalin. Ann Surg 173:201-205, 1971
504. MacKeigan JM, Ferguson JA: Prophylactic oophorectomy in colorectal cancer in premenopausal patients. Dis Colon Rectum 22:401-405, 1979
505. Cutait R, Lesser ML, Enker WE: Prophylactic oophorectomy in surgery for large bowel cancer. Dis Colon Rectum 26:6-11, 1983
506. Graffner HOL, Alm POA, Oscarson JEA: Prophylactic oophorectomy in colorectal carcinoma. Am J Surg 146:233-235, 1983
507. O'Brien PH, Newton BB, Metcalf JS et al: Oophorectomy in women with carcinoma of the colon and rectum. Surg Gynecol Obstet 153:827-830, 1981
508. Blamey S, McDermott F, Pihl E et al: Ovarian involvement in adenocarcinoma of the colon and rectum. Surg Gynecol Obstet 153:42-44, 1981
509. Herrerra LO, Ledesma E, Natarajan N et al: Metachronous ovarian metastases from adenocarcinoma of the colon and rectum. Surg Gynecol Obstet 154:531-534, 1982
510. Morrow M, Enker WE: Late ovarian metastases in carcinoma of the colon and rectum. Arch Surg 119:1385-1388, 1984
511. Ballantyne GH, Raigel MM, Wolff BG et al: Oophorectomy in colon cancer: Impact on survival. Ann Surg 202:209-214, 1985
512. Wolmark N, Gordon PH, Fisher B et al: A comparison of stapled and hand-sewn anastomoses in patients undergoing resection of Duke's B and C colorectal cancer: An analysis of disease-free survival and survival from the NSABP prospective trials. Dis Colon Rectum 29:344-350, 1986
513. Davis CJ, Ilstrup DM, Pemberton JH: Influence of splenectomy on survival rate of patients with colorectal cancer. Am J Surg 155:173-179, 1988
514. Wolmark N, Fisher B, Wieand HS: The prognostic value of modifications of the Duke's C class of colorectal cancer: An analysis of the NSABP clinical trials. Ann Surg 203:115-122, 1986
515. Cass AW, Million RR, Pfaff WW: Patterns of recurrence following surgery alone for adenocarcinoma of the colon and rectum. Cancer 37:2861-2865, 1976
515a. Welch JP, Donaldson GA: The clinical correlation of an autopsy study of recurrent colorectal cancer. Ann Surg 189:496-502, 1979
516. Russell AH, Pelton J, Reheis CE et al: Adenocarcinoma of the colon: An autopsy study with implications for new therapeutic strategies. Cancer 56:1446-1451, 1985
517. Enker WE, Dragacevic S: Multiple carcinomas of the large bowel. Ann Surg 187:8-11, 1978
518. Langevin JM, Nivatvongs S: The true incidence of synchronous cancer of the large bowel. Am J Surg 147:330-333, 1984
519. Isler JJm Brown PC, Lewis FG et al: The role of preoperative colonoscopy in colorectal cancer. Dis Colon Rectum 30:435-439, 1987
520. Kelly WE Jr, Brown PW, Lawrence W, Tertz JJ: Penetrating, obstructing, and perforating carcinomas of the colon and rectum. Arch Surg 116:381-384, 1985
521. Gall FP, Tonak J, Altendorf A: Multivisceral resections in colorectal cancer. Dis Colon Rectum 30:337-341, 1987
522. Hunter JA, Ryan JA Jr, Schultz P: En bloc resection of colon cancer adherent to other organs. Am J Surg 154:67-71, 1987
523. Wolff WI, Shinya H: Definitive treatment of "malignant" polyps of the colon. Ann Surg 182:516-524, 1975
524. Wilcox GM, Beck JR: Early invasive cancer in adenomatous colonic polyps: Valuation of the therapeutic options by decision analysis. Gastroenterology 92:1159-1168, 1987
525. Cranley JP, Petras RE, Carey WD et al: When is endoscopic polypectomy adequate therapy for colonic polyps containing invasive carcinoma? Gastroenterology 91:419-427, 1987
526. Wilcox JM, Anderson PB, Colacchio TA: Early invasive carcinoma in colonic polyps: A review of the literature with emphasis on the assessment of the risk of metastasis. Cancer 57:160-171, 1986
527. Haggitt RC, Glotzbach RE, Soffer EE et al: Prognostic factors in colorectal carcinomas arising in adenomas: Implications for lesions removed by endoscopic polypectomy. Gastroenterology 89:328-336, 1985
528. Bartnik W, Butruk E, Orlowska J: A conservative approach to adenomas containing invasive carcinoma removed colonoscopically. Dis Colon Rectum 28:673-675, 1985
529. Colacchio TA, Forde KA, Scantlebury VP: Endoscopic polypectomy: Inadequate treatment for invasive colorectal carcinoma. Ann Surg 194:704-707, 1981
530. Nivatvongs S: Management of polyps containing invasive carcinoma. In Codner IJ, Fry RD, Roe JP (eds): Colon, Rectal, and Anal Surgery 1985, pp 183-188. St Louis, CV Mosby, 1985
531. Grinnell RS, Lane N: Benign and malignant adenomatous polyps and papillary adenomas of the colon and rectum: An analysis of 1,856 tumors in 1,335 patients. Int Abstr Surg 106:519, 1958
532. Waye JD, Frankel A: Treatment of early colon cancer. Gastroenterology 66:796, 1974
533. Locke MR, Cairns DW, Ritchie JK, Lockhart-Mummery HE: The treatment of early colorectal cancer by local excision. Br J Surg 65:346-349, 1978
534. Kodaira S, Teramoto T, Oro S et al: Lymph node metastases from carcinomas developing in pedunculated and semi-pedunculated colorectal adenomas. Aust NZ J Surg 51:429-433, 1981
535. Shatney CH, Lober PH, Gilbertsen VA, Sosin H: The treatment of pedunculated adenomatous colorectal polyps with focal cancer. Surg Gynecol Obstet 139:845-850, 1974
536. Coutsoftides T, Lavery I, Benjamin SP, Sivak MV Jr: Malignant polyps of the colon and rectum: A clinical pathological study. Dis Colon Rectum 22:82-86, 1979
537. Gunderson LL, Russell AH, Llewellyn HJ et al: Treatment planning for colorectal cancer: Radiation and surgical techniques and value of small-bowel films. Int J Radiat Oncol Biol Phys 11:1379-1393, 1985
538. Kopelson G: Adjuvant postoperative radiation therapy for colorectal carcinoma

above the peritoneal reflection: II. Antimesenteric wall ascending and descending colon and cecum. Cancer 52:633–636, 1983
539. Loeffler RK: Postoperative radiation therapy for adenocarcinoma of the cecum using two fractions/day. Int J Radiat Oncol Biol Phys 10:1881–1883, 1984
540. Shehata WM, Meyer RL, Jazy FK et al: Regional adjuvant irradiation for adenocarcinoma of the cecum. Int J Radiat Oncol Biol Phys 13:843–846, 1987
541. Wong CS, Harwood AR, Cummings BJ et al: Postoperative local abdominal irradiation for cancer of the colon above the peritoneal reflection. Int J Radiat Oncol Biol Phys 11:2067–2071, 1985
542. Duttenhaver JR, Hoskins RB, Gunderson LL et al: Adjuvant postoperative radiation therapy in the management of adenocarcinoma of the colon. Cancer 57:955–963, 1986
543. Kopelson G: Adjuvant postoperative radiation therapy for colorectal carcinoma above the peritoneal reflection: I. Sigmoid colon. Cancer 51:1593–1598, 1983
544. Richards F II, Atkins JN, Scarantino C et al: Phase I study of intraperitoneal 5-fluorouracil (IP-5FU) with local radiation therapy (RT) as adjuvant therapy in stage B3 and C1, 2, 3 colon cancer (abst). Proc Am Soc Clin Oncol 5:80, 1986
545. Turner SS, Vieira EF, Ager PJ et al: Elective postoperative radiotherapy for locally advanced colorectal cancer: A preliminary report. Cancer 140:105–108, 1977
546. Ghossein NA, Ager PJ, Ragins H et al: The treatment of locally advanced carcinoma of the colon and rectum by a surgical procedure and radiotherapy postoperatively. Surg Gynecol Obstet 148:917–920, 1979
547. Ghossein NA, Samala EC, Alpert S et al: Elective postoperative radiotherapy after incomplete resection of colorectal cancer. Dis Colon Rectum 24:252–256, 1981
548. Meek AG, Lam WC, Order SE: Carcinoma of the colon: Irradiation by delayed split whole-abdominal technique. Radiology 148:845–849, 1983
549. Wong CS, Harwood AR, Cummings BJ et al: Total abdominal irradiation for cancer of the colon. Radiother Oncol 2:209–214, 1984
550. Fabian CJ, Reddy E, Jewell et al: Phase I–II pilot of whole abdominal radiation and concomitant 5-FU as an adjuvant in colon cancer. A Southwest Oncology Group Study (unpublished manuscript)
551. Dixon WJ, Longmire WP Jr, Holden WD: Use of triethylenethiophosphomamide as adjuvant to the surgical treatment of gastric and colorectal cancer: Ten year follow-up. Ann Surg 173:26–39, 1971
552. Dwight RW, Humphrey EW, Higgins GA et al: FUDR as an adjuvant to surgery in cancer of the large bowel. J Surg Oncol 5:243–249, 1973
553. Higgins GA, Lee LE, Dwight RW et al: The case for adjuvant 5-fluorouracil in colorectal cancer. Cancer Clin Trials 1:35–41, 1978
554. Grage TB, Moss SE: Adjuvant chemotherapy in cancer of the colon and rectum: Demonstration of effectiveness of prolonged 5-FU chemotherapy in a prospectively controlled randomized trial. Surg Clin North Am 61:1321–1329, 1981
555. Buysce ME, Zeleniuch-Jacquotte A, Chalmers TC: Adjuvant therapy of colorectal cancer: Why we still don't know (unpublished manuscript)
556. Macdonald JS: Adjuvant therapy of gastrointestinal cancer. In Salmon SE (ed): Adjuvant Therapy of Cancer V, pp 479–496. New York, Grune & Stratton, 1987
557. Higgins GA, Amadeo JH, McElhinney J et al: Efficacy of prolonged intermittent therapy with combined 5-fluorouracil and me-CCNU following resection for carcinoma of the large bowel. Cancer 53:1–8, 1984
558. Gastrointestinal Tumor Study Group: Adjuvant therapy of colon cancer: Results of a prospectively randomized trial. N Engl J Med 310:737–743, 1984
559. Wolmark N, Fisher B, Rockette H: Adjuvant therapy in carcinoma of the colon: Five year results of NSABP protocol C-01. In Salmon SE (ed): Adjuvant Therapy of Cancer V, pp 531–536. New York, Grune & Stratton, 1987
560. Panettiere FJ, Chen TT: The SWOG large bowel study benefits from therapy (abst). Proc Am Soc Clin Oncol 4:76, 1985
561. Laurie J, Moertel C, Flemming T et al: Surgical adjuvant therapy of poor prognosis colorectal cancer with levamisole alone or combined levamisole and 5-fluorouracil: A North Central Cancer Treatment Group and Mayo Clinic Study (abst). Proc Am Soc Clin Oncol 5:81, 1986
562. Verhaegen H, DeCree J, DeCock W et al: Levamisole therapy in patients with colorectal cancer. In Terry WD, Rosenberg SA (eds): Immunotherapy of Human Cancer, pp 225–230. New York, Excerpta Medica, 1982
563. Pestana C, Reitemeyer RJ, Moertel CG et al: The natural history of carcinoma of the colon and rectum. Am J Surg 108:826–829, 1964
564. Taylor I, Machin D, Mullee M et al: A randomized controlled trial of adjuvant portal vein cytotoxic perfusion in colorectal cancer. Br J Surg 72:359–362, 1985
565. Gray BN, deZwart J, Fisher R et al: The Australia and New Zealand Trial of Adjuvant Chemotherapy in Colon Cancer. In Salmon SE (ed): Adjuvant Therapy of Cancer V, pp 537–554. New York, Grune & Stratton, 1987
566. Metzger U, Mermillod B, Aeberhard P et al: Intraportal chemotherapy in colorectal carcinoma as an adjuvant modality. World J Surg 11:452–458, 1987
567. Williams NS: The rationale for preservation of the anal sphincter in patients with low rectal cancer. Br J Surg 71:575–518, 1984
568. Williams NS, Dixon MF, Johnston D: Reappraisal of the 5 centimetre rule of distal excision for carcinoma of the rectum: A study of distal intramural spread and of patients' survival. Br J Surg 70:150–154, 1983
569. Madsen PM, Christiansen J: Distal intramural spread of rectal carcinomas. Dis Colon Rectum 29:279–282, 1986
570. Hojo K: Anastomotic recurrence after sphincter-saving resection for rectal cancer: Length of distal clearance of the bowel. Dis Colon Rectum 29:11–14, 1986
571. Pollett WG, Nicholls RJ: The relationship between the extent of distal clearance and survival and local recurrence rates after curative anterior resection for carcinoma of the rectum. Ann Surg 198:159–163, 1984
572. Pezim ME, Nicholls RJ: Survival after high or low ligation of the inferior mesenteric artery during curative surgery for rectal cancer. Ann Surg 200:729–733, 1984
573. Hojo K, Koyama Y, Moriya Y: Lymphatic spread and its prognostic value in patients with rectal cancer. Am J Surg 144:350–354, 1982
574. Grinnell RS: Results of ligation of inferior mesenteric artery at the aorta in resections of carcinoma of the descending and sigmoid colon and rectum. Surg Gynecol Obstet 120:1031–1036, 1965
575. Heald RJ, Husband EM, Ryall RDH: The meso-rectum in rectal cancer surgery: The clue to pelvic recurrence? Br J Surg 69:613–616, 1982
576. Heald RJ, Ryall RDH: Recurrence and survival after total meso-rectal excision for rectal cancer. Lancet 1:1479–1482, 1986
576a. Quirke P, Durdey P, Dixon MF et al: Local recurrence of rectal adenocarcinoma due to inadequate surgical resection. Histopathological study of lateral tumor spread and surgical excision. Lancet 1:996–999, 1986
577. Deddish MR: Surgical procedures for carcinoma of the left colon and rectum with five year end results following abdomino-pelvic dissection of lymph nodes. Am J Surg 99:188–191, 1960
578. Enker WE, Laffer UT, Block GE: Enhanced survival of patients with colon and rectal cancer is based upon wide anatomic resection. Ann Surg 190:350–360, 1979
579. Hojo K, Koyama Y: The effectiveness of wide anatomical resection and radical lymphadenectomy for patients with rectal cancer. Jpn J Surg 12:111–116, 1982
580. Koyama Y, Moriya Y, Hojo K: Effects of extended systemic lymphadenectomy for adenocarcinoma of the rectum: Significant improvement of survival rate and decrease of local recurrence. Jpn J Clin Oncol 14:623–632, 1984
581. Enker E, Heilweil ML, Hertz REL et al: En bloc pelvic lymphadenopathy and sphincter preservation in the surgical management of rectal cancer. Ann Surg 203:426–433, 1986
582. Glass RE, Ritchie JK, Thompson HR et al: The results of surgical treatment of cancer of the rectum by radical resection and extended abdomino-iliac lymphadenectomy. Br J Surg 72:599–601, 1985
583. Beart RW Jr, Kelly KA: Randomized prospective evaluation of the EEA stapler for colorectal anastomoses. Am J Surg 141:143–147, 1981
584. McGinn FP, Gartell PC, Clifford PC et al: Staples or sutures for low colorectal anastomoses: A prospective randomized trial. Br J Surg 72:603–605, 1985
585. Donaldson GA, Rodkey GV, Behringer GE: Resection of the rectum with anal preservation. Surg Gynecol Obstet 123:571–580, 1966
586. Localio SA, Eng K, Coppa GF: Abdominosacral resection for mid-rectal cancer. Ann Surg 198:320–324, 1983
587. Higgins GA, Humphrey EW, Dwight RW et al: Preoperative radiation and surgery for cancer of the rectum: Veterans Administration Surgical Oncology Group trial II. Cancer 58:352–359, 1986
588. Mohiuddin M, Yelovich RM, Komarnicky LT et al: Preoperative radiation and surgery in unfavorable cancers of the rectum (abst). Proc Am Soc Clin Oncol 6:97, 1987
589. Cutait DE, Cutait R, Ioshimoto M et al: Abdominoperineal endoanal pull-through resection: A comparative study between immediate and delayed colorectal anastomosis. Dis Colon Rectum 28:294–299, 1985
590. Enker WE, Stearns MW Jr, Janov AJ: Peranal coloanal anastomosis following low anterior resection for rectal carcinoma. Dis Colon Rectum 28:576–581, 1985
591. Parks AG, Percy JP: Resection and sutured colo-anal anastomosis for rectal carcinoma. Br J Surg 69:301–304, 1982
592. Welch JP, Donaldson GA: Recent experience in the management of cancer of the colon and rectum. Am J Surg 127:258–266, 1974
593. McDermott FT, Hughes ESR, Pihl EA et al: Changing survival prospects in rectal carcinoma: A series of 1,306 patients managed by one surgeon. Dis Colon Rectum 29:798–803, 1986
594. Slanetz CA Jr, Herter FP, Grinnell RS: Anterior resection versus abdominoperineal resection for cancer of the rectum and rectosigmoid. Am J Surg 123:110–117, 1972
595. Hargrove WC III, Gertner MH, Fitts WT Jr: The Kraske operation for carcinoma of the rectum. Surg Gynecol Obstet 148:931–933, 1979
596. Bevan AD: Carcinoma of the rectum: Treatment by local excision. Dis Colon Rectum 29:906–910, 1986
597. Madden JL, Kandalaft SI: Electrocoagulation as a primary curative method in the treatment of carcinoma of the rectum. Surg Gynecol Obstet 157:164–179, 1983
598. Crile G, Turnbull RB: Role of electrocoagulation in the treatment of carcinoma of the rectum. Surg Gynecol Obstet 135:391–396, 1972
599. Cummings BJ Jr, Rider WD, Harwood AR et al: Radical external beam radiation therapy for adenocarcinoma of the rectum. Dis Colon Rectum 26:30–36, 1983
600. Papillon J: New prospects in the conservative treatment of rectal cancer. Dis Colon Rectum 27:695–700, 1984
601. Lockhart-Mummery HE, Ritchie JK et al: The results of surgical treatment for carcinoma of the rectum at St. Marks Hospital from 1948 to 1972. Br J Surg 63:673–677, 1976
602. Whittaker M, Goligher JC: The prognosis after surgical treatment for carcinoma of the rectum. Br J Surg 63:384–388, 1976
602a. Wilson SM, Beahrs OH: A curative treatment of carcinoma of the sigmoid, recto-sigmoid and rectum. Ann Surg 183:556–565, 1976
602b. Accarpio G, Scopinaro G, Claudiani F et al: Experience with local rectal excision in light of two recent preoperative diagnostic methods. Dis Colon Rectum 30:296–298, 1987
602c. Allgower M, Durig M, Hochstetter A et al: The parasacral sphincter-splitting approach to the rectum. World J Surg 6:539–548, 1982

602d. Killingback MJ: Indications for local excision of rectal cancer. Br J Surg 2S:54–56, 1985
602e. Wilson E: Local treatment of cancer of the rectum. Dis Colon Rectum 16:194–199, 1973
602f. Mason AY: Transsphincteric approach to rectal lesions. Surg Ann 9:171–194, 1977
602g. Grigg M, McDermott FT, Pihl EA et al: Curative local excision in the treatment of carcinoma of the rectum. Dis Colon Rectum 27:81–83, 1984
602h. Whiteway J, Nicholls RJ, Morson BC: The role of surgical local excision in the treatment of rectal cancer. Br J Surg 72:694–697, 1985
602i. Hager T, Gall FP, Hermanek P: Local excision of cancer of the rectum. Dis Colon Rectum 26:149–151, 1983
603. Biggers OR, Beart RW Jr, Ilstrup DM: Local excision of rectal cancer. Dis Colon Rectum 29:374–377, 1986
604. Salvati EP, Rubin RJ: Electrocoagulation as primary therapy for rectal carcinoma. Am J Surg 132:583–586, 1976
605. Wanebo HJ, Quan SHQ: Failures of electrocoagulation of primary carcinoma of the rectum. Surg Gynecol Obstet 138:174–176, 1974
606. Eisenstat TE, Duke ST, Rubin RJ et al: Five year survival in patients with carcinoma of the rectum treated by electrocoagulation. Am J Surg 143:127–131, 1982
607. Sischy B, Granez MJ, Hinson EJ: Endocavitary irradiation for adenocarcinoma of the rectum. Cancer 34:333–339, 1984
608. Pilipshen SJ, Heilweil M, Quan SHQ et al: Patterns of pelvic recurrence following definitive resections of rectal cancer. Cancer 53:1354–1362, 1984
609. Phillips RKS, Hittinger R, Blesovsky L et al: Local recurrence following curative surgery for large bowel cancer. Br J Surg 71:17–20, 1984
610. McDermott FT, Hughes ESR, Pihl E et al: Local recurrence after potentially curative resection for rectal cancer in a series of 1,008 patients. Br J Surg 72:34–37, 1985
611. Jackman RJ: Conservative management of selected patients with carcinoma of the rectum. Dis Colon Rectum 4:429–434, 1961
612. Culp CE: Conservative management of certain selected cancers of the lower rectum: In Controversies in Surgery, pp 407–414. Philadelphia, WB Saunders, 1976
613. Gingold BS, Mitty WF Jr, Tadros M: Importance of patient selection in local treatment of carcinoma of the rectum. Am J Surg 145:293–296, 1983
614. Wittoesch JH, Jackman RS: Results of conservative management of cancer of the rectum in poor risk patients. Surg Gynecol Obstet 107:618, 1958
615. Deddish MR: Local excision. Surg Clin North Am 54:877–880, 1974
616. Stearns MW Jr, Sternberg SS, DeCosse JJ: Treatment alternatives: Localized rectal cancer. Cancer 54:2691–2694, 1984
617. Rich TA, Weiss DR, Mies C et al: Sphincter preservation in patients with low rectal cancer treated with radiation therapy with or without local excision or fulguration. Radiology 156:527–531, 1985
618. Enker WE, Kemeny N, Shank B et al: Defining the needs for adjuvant therapy of rectal and colonic cancer. Surg Clin North Am 61:1295–1310, 1981
619. Fortier GA, Krochak RJ, Kim JA et al: Dose response to preoperative irradiation in rectal cancer: Implications for local control and complications associated with sphincter sparing surgery and abdominal resection. Int J Radiat Oncol Biol Phys 12:1559–1563, 1986
620. Allee PE, Gunderson LL, Munzenrider JE: Postoperative radiation therapy for residual colorectal carcinoma (abst). Int J Radiat Oncol Biol Phys 7:1208, 1981
621. Powers WE, Tolmach LJ: Preoperative radiation therapy: Biological basis and experimental investigation. Nature 201:172–204, 1964
622. Higgins GA Jr, Conn JH, Jordan PH et al: Preoperative radiotherapy for colorectal cancer. Ann Surg 181:624–631, 1975
623. Boulis Wassif S, Langenhorst BL, Hop WCJ: The contribution of preoperative radiotherapy in the management of borderline operability rectal cancer. In: Jones SE, Salmon SE (eds): Adjuvant Therapy of Cancer II, pp 613–620. New York, Grune & Stratton, 1979
624. Kligerman MM, Urdanetta N, Knowlton A et al: Preoperative irradiation of rectosigmoid carcinoma including its regional lymph nodes. Am J Roentgenol Radium Ther Nucl Med 114:498–503, 1972
625. Kinsella TJ, Bloomer WD: Tolerance of the intestine to radiation therapy. Surg Gynecol Obstet 151:273–284, 1980
626. Maruyama Y, Van Nagell JR Jr, Utley J et al: Radiation and small bowel complications in cervical carcinoma. Radiology 112:699–703, 1974
627. Russ JE, Smoron GL, Gagnon JD: Omental transposition flap in colorectal carcinoma: Adjunctive use in prevention and treatment of radiation complications. Int J Radiat Oncol Biol Phys 10:55–62, 1984
628. Sugarbaker PH: Pelvic displacement prosthesis to prevent small bowel damage with pelvic irradiation. Surg Gynecol Obstet 157:269–271, 1983
629. Devereux DF, Kavanah MT, Feldman MI et al: Small bowel exclusion from the pelvis by a polyglycolic acid mesh sling. Surg Oncol 26:107–112, 1984
630. Kavanah MT, Feldman MI, Devereux DF et al: New surgical approach to minimize radiation-associated small bowel injury in patients with pelvic malignancies requiring surgery and high-dose irradiation: A preliminary report. Cancer 56:1300–1304, 1985
631. Devereux DF, Chandler JJ, Eisenstat T et al: Efficacy of an absorbable mesh in keeping the small bowel out of the human pelvis following surgery. Dis Colon Rectum 31:17–21, 1988
632. Dische S, Dowdell JW: A method to reduce radiation injury to intestine—a preliminary report. Radiother Oncol 1:277–279, 1984
633. Green N, Iba G, Smith WR: Measures to minimize small intestine injury in the irradiated pelvis. Cancer 35:1633–1640, 1975
634. Green N: The avoidance of small intestine injury in gynecologic cancer. Int J Rad Oncol Biol Phys 9:1385–1390, 1983
635. Gallagher MJ, Brereton HD, Rostock RA et al: A prospective study of treatment techniques to minimize the volume of pelvic small bowel with reduction of acute and late effects associated with pelvic irradiation. Int J Rad Oncol Biol Phys 12:1565–1573, 1986
636. Pezner R, Archambeau JO: Critical evaluation of the role of nutritional support for radiation therapy patients. Cancer 55:263–267, 1985
637. McArdle AH, Wittnich C, Duguid W, Freeman CR: The use of an elemental diet as prophylaxis in radiation enteropathy. [Works-in-Progress]. Am Soc Ther Radiol Mtg., September, 1981
638. McArdle AH, Reid EC, Laplante HP et al: Prophylaxis against radiation injury: The use of elemental diet prior and during radiotherapy for invasive bladder cancer and in early postoperative feeding following radical cystectomy and ileal conduit. Arch Surg 121:879–885, 1986
639. Stryker JA, Bartholomew M: Failure of lactose-restricted diets to prevent radiation-induced diarrhea in patients undergoing whole pelvic irradiation. Int J Radiat Oncol Biol Phys 12:789–792, 1986
640. Shike M: Personal communication, 1987
641. Ito H, Meistrich ML, Barkley HT Jr et al: Protection of acute and late radiation damage of the gastrointestinal tract by WR-2721. Int J Radiat Oncol Biol Phys 12:211–219, 1986
642. Travis EL, Thames HD Jr, Tucker SL et al: Protection of mouse jejunal crypt cells by WR-2721 after small doses of radiation. Int J Radiat Oncol Biol Phys 12:807–814, 1986
643. Hanson WR, Thomas C: 16,16-dimethyl prostaglandin E_2 increases survival of murine intestinal stem cells when given before photon radiation. Radiat Res 96:393–398, 1983
644. Stearns MW Jr, Deddish MR, Quan SH et al: Preoperative roentgen therapy for cancer of the rectum. Surg Gynecol Obstet 109:285–289, 1959
645. Quan SHQ, Deddish MR, Stearns MW: The effect of preoperative roentgen therapy upon the 10- and 5-year results of the surgical treatment of cancer of the rectum. Surg Gynecol Obstet 111:507–508, 1960
646. Gary-Bobo J, Pujol H, Solassol CI et al: L'irradiation préoperatoire du cancer rectal: résultats a 5 ans de 116 cas. Bull Cancer [Paris] 66:491–496, 1979
647. Glimelius B, Graffman S, Pahlman et al: Preoperative irradiation with high-dose fractionation in adenocarcinoma of the rectum and rectosigmoid. Acta Radiol Oncol 21:373–379, 1982
648. Mendenhall WM, Million RR, Bland KI et al: Preoperative radiation therapy for clinically resectable adenocarcinoma of the rectum. Ann Surg 202:215–222, 1985
649. Friedmann P, Garb JL, Park WC et al: Survival following moderate-dose preoperative radiation therapy for carcinoma of the rectum. Cancer 55:967–973, 1985
650. Roe JP, Kodner IH, Walz B et al: Preoperative radiation therapy for rectal carcinoma. Dis Colon Rectum 25:471–473, 1982
651. Papillon J: The future of external beam irradiation as initial treatment of rectal cancer. Br J Surg 74:449–454, 1987
652. Stevens KR Jr, Fletcher WS, Allen CV: A review of the value of radiation therapy for adenocarcinoma of the rectum and sigmoid. Front Gastrointest Res 5:93–101, 1979
653. Sischy B: The place of radiotherapy in the management of rectal adenocarcinoma. Cancer 50:2631–2637, 1982
654 Gerard A, Berrod J-L, Pene F et al: Interim analysis of a phase III study on preoperative radiation therapy in resectable rectal carcinoma: Trial of the Gastrointestinal Tract Cancer Cooperative Group of the European Organization for Research on Treatment of Cancer (EORTC). Cancer 55:2373–2379, 1985
655. Rider WD, Palmer JA, Mahoney LJ et al: Preoperative irradiation in operable cancer of the rectum: Report of the Toronto Trial. Can J Surg 20:335–338, 1977
655a. Duncan W: Adjuvant radiotherapy in rectal cancer: The MRC trials. Br J Surg 72 (suppl):S59–S62, 1985
656. Stockholm Rectal Cancer Study Group: Short-term preoperative radiotherapy for adenocarcinoma of the rectum. Am J Clin Oncol 10:369–375, 1987
657. Roswit B, Higgins GA Jr, Keehn R: Preoperative irradiation for carcinoma of the rectum and rectosigmoid colon: Report of a national Veterans Administration randomized study. Cancer 35:1597–1602, 1975
658. Higgins GA, Humphrey EW, Dwight RW et al: Preoperative radiation and surgery for cancer of the rectum: Veterans Administration Surgical Oncology Group trial II. Cancer 58:352–359, 1986
659. Dedkov IP, Zibina MA: Intensive preoperative gammatherapy in combined treatment of cancer of the rectum. Am J Proctol 27:43–47, 1976
660. Simbirtseva LP, Sneshko LI, Smirnov NM: Results of intensive combined therapy for carcinoma of the rectum. Vopr Oncol 21:7–12, 1975
661. Duncan W, Smith AN, Freedman LS et al: A trial of preoperative radiotherapy in the management of operable rectal cancer: First report of an MRC working party. Br J Surg 69:513–519, 1982
662. Tepper JE, Cohen AM, Wood WC et al: Postoperative radiation therapy of rectal cancer. Int J Radiat Oncol Biol Phys 13:5–10, 1987
663. Bruckner R, Kempf P, Kutzner J, Brunner H: Preliminary results of preoperative radiotherapy in carcinoma of the rectum. Dtsch Med Wochenschr 102:195–198, 1977
664. Kutzner J, Bruckner R, Kempf P: Präoperative Strahlentherapie beim Rektum Karzinomen. Strahlenther 160:236–238, 1984
665. Gerard A: Personal communication, 1988
666. Vigliotti A, Rich TA, Romsdahl MM et al: Postoperative adjuvant radiotherapy for

adenocarcinoma of the rectum and rectosigmoid. Int J Radiat Oncol Biol Phys 13:999–1006, 1987
667. Pahlman L, Glimelius B, Graffman S: Pre- versus postoperative radiotherapy in rectal carcinoma: An interim report from a randomized multicentre trial. Br J Surg 72:961–966, 1985
668. Mohiuddin M, Derdel J, Marks G et al: Results of adjuvant radiation therapy in cancer of the rectum: Thomas Jefferson University Hospital experience. Cancer 55:350–353, 1985
669. Douglass HO, Moertel CG, Mayer RJ et al: Survival after postoperative combination treatment of rectal cancer. N Engl J Med 315:1294–1295, 1986
670. Fisher B, Wolmark N, Rockette HE et al: Adjuvant chemotherapy or postoperative radiation for rectal cancer: Five year results of NSABP R01. In Salmon SE (ed): Adjuvant Therapy of Cancer V, pp 547–554. New York, Grune & Stratton, 1987
671. Balslev I, Pedersen M, Teglbjaerg PS et al: Postoperative radiotherapy in Dukes' B and C carcinoma of the rectum and rectosigmoid: A randomized multicenter study. Cancer 58:22–28, 1986
672. Thomas PRM, Lindblad AS, Stablein DM et al: Toxicity associated with adjuvant postoperative therapy for adenocarcinoma of the rectum. Cancer 57:1130–1134, 1986
673. Gunderson LL, Dosoretz DE, Hedberg SE et al: Low-dose preoperative irradiation, surgery, and elective postoperative radiation therapy for resectable rectum and rectosigmoid carcinoma. Cancer 52:446–451, 1983
674. Brenner S, Lanter BH, Seligman BR: Adjuvant therapy in treatment of rectal carcinoma (abst). Int J Radiat Oncol Biol Phys 6:1378, 1980
675. Shank B, Enker W, Santana J et al: Local control with pre-operative radiotherapy alone versus "sandwich" radiotherapy for rectal carcinoma. Int J Radiat Oncol Biol Phys 13:111–115, 1987
676. Krook J, Moertel C, Wieand H et al: Radiation vs. sequential chemotherapy–radiation–chemotherapy: A study of the North Central Cancer Treatment Group, Duke University and the Mayo Clinic. Proc Am Soc Clin Oncol 5:82, 1986
677. Boulis-Wassif S, Gerard A, Loygue J et al: Final results of a randomized trial on the treatment of rectal cancer with preoperative radiotherapy alone or in combination with 5-fluorouracil, followed by radical surgery. Cancer 53:1811–1818, 1984
678. Boey J, Wong J, Ong GB: Pelvic exenteration for locally advanced colorectal carcinoma. Ann Surg 195:513–518, 1982
679. Ledesma EJ, Bruno S, Mittelman A: Total pelvic exenteration in colorectal disease. Ann Surg 194:701–703, 1981
680. Bricker EM, Kraybill WG, Lopez MJ et al: The current role of ultraradical surgery in the treatment of pelvic cancer. Curr Probl Surg 23:871–953, 1986
681. Sugarbaker PH: Partial sacrectomy for en bloc excision of rectal cancer with posterior fixation. Dis Colon Rectum 25:708–711, 1982
682. Tierie AH: Radiotherapy in marginal resectable and non-resectable rectum cancer. Radiol Clin 47:222–227, 1978
683. Bjerkeset T, Dahl O: Irradiation and surgery for primarily inoperable rectal and adenocarcinoma. Dis Colon Rectum 23:298–303, 1980
684. Emami B, Pilepich M, Willett C et al: Effect of preoperative irradiation on resectability of colorectal carcinomas. Int J Radiat Oncol Biol Phys 8:1295–1299, 1982
685. Dosoretz DE, Gunderson LL, Hedberg S et al: Preoperative irradiation for unresectable rectal and rectosigmoid carcinomas. Cancer 52:814–818, 1983
686. Schnetzer G, Brickner T, Stone W et al: Adjuvant preoperative chemotherapy and radiation therapy in moderately advanced adenocarcinoma of rectum (abst). Proc Am Soc Clin Oncol 3:133, 1984
687. Haghbin M, Sischy B, Hinson J: Adjuvant preoperative irradiation and chemotherapy for primary large rectal carcinoma: nine-year follow-up (abst). Proc Am Soc Clin Oncol 5:80, 1986
688. Sedlacek S, Pearlman N: Locally advanced adenocarcinoma of the rectum (ACR): Concurrent preoperative chemotherapy (CT) and radiation therapy (RT) (abst). Proc Am Soc Clin Oncol 6:93, 1987
689. Taylor RE, Karr GR, Arnott SJ: External beam radiotherapy for rectal adenocarcinoma. Br J Surg 74:455–459, 1987
690. Cohen AM: Intraoperative radiation therapy for colorectal cancer. Probl Gen Surg 4:76–82, 1987
691. Gunderson LL, Cohen AC, Dosoretz DD et al: Residual, unresectable, or recurrent colorectal cancer: External beam irradiation and intraoperative electron beam boost ± resection. Int J Radiat Oncol Biol Phys 9:1597–1606, 1983
692. Gunderson LL, Martin JK Jr, Earle JD et al: Intraoperative and external beam irradiation with or without resection: Mayo pilot experience. Mayo Clin Proc 59:691–699, 1984
693. Gunderson LL, Martin JK, Beart RW et al: Intraoperative and external beam irradiation ± 5-FU for locally advanced colorectal cancer. Ann Surg (in press)
694. Tepper JE, Cohen AM, Wood WC et al: Intraoperative electron beam radiotherapy in the treatment of unresectable rectal cancer. Arch Surg 121:421–423, 1986
695. Calkins AR: Personal communication, 1987
696. Syed AMN, Puthawala A, Neblett D et al: Primary treatment of carcinoma of the lower rectum and anal canal by a combination of external irradiation and interstitial implant. Radiology 128:199–203, 1978
697. Puthawala AA, Syed AMN, Gates C et al: Definitive treatment of extensive anorectal carcinoma by external and interstitial irradiation. Cancer 50:1746–1750, 1982
698. Fourquet A, Enker WE, Shank B et al: The value of interstitial radiation in advanced and recurrent colorectal cancer. Endocr Hypertherm Oncol 1:113–117, 1985
699. Wang CC, Schulz MD: The role of radiation therapy in the management of carcinoma of the sigmoid, rectosigmoid and rectum. Radiology 79:1–5, 1962
700. Ghossein NA, Ager PJ, Ragins H et al: The treatment of locally advanced carcinoma of the colon and rectum by a surgical procedure and radiotherapy postoperatively. Surg Gynecol Obstet 148:917–920, 1979
701. Carter SK: Large bowel cancer: The current status of treatment. JNCI 56:3–10, 1976
702. August DA, Ottow RT, Sugarbaker PH: Clinical perspective of human colorectal cancer metastasis. Cancer Metastasis Rev 3:303–324, 1984
703. Sugarbaker PH, Gianola FJ, Dwyer A et al: A simplified plan for follow-up of patients with colon and rectal cancer supported by prospective studies of laboratory and radiologic test results. Surgery 102:79–87, 1987
704. Fletcher RH: Carcinoembryonic antigen. Ann Intern Med 104:66–73, 1986
705. Northover J: Carcinoembryonic antigen and recurrent colorectal cancer. Gut 27:117–122, 1986
706. Beart RW, Metzger PP, O'Connor MJ et al: Postoperative screening of patients with carcinoma of the colon. Dis Colon Rectum 24:585–589, 1981
707. Boey J, Cheung HC, Lai CK et al: A prospective evaluation of serum carcinoembryonic antigen levels in the management of colorectal carcinoma. World J Surg 8:279–286, 1984
708. Minton JP, James KK, Hurtubise PE et al: The use of serial carcinoembryonic antigen determinations to predict recurrence of carcinoma of the colon and the time for a second-look operation. Surg Gynecol Obstet 147:208–210, 1978
709. Smith AN, Gordon A, Browning GCP et al: Postoperative monitoring of CEA in the prediction of surgical outcome in colorectal cancer. J R Coll Surg Edinb 30:294–298, 1985
710. Sorokin JJ, Sugarbaker PH, Zamcheck N et al: Serial carcinoembryonic antigen assays: Use in detection of cancer recurrence. JAMA 228:49–53, 1974
711. Wanebo HJ: Are carcinoembryonic antigen levels of value in the curative management of colorectal cancer? Surgery 89:290–295, 1981
712. Sugarbaker PH, Zamcheck N, Moore FD: Assessment of serial carcinoembryonic antigen assays in postoperative detection of recurrent colorectal cancer. Cancer 38:2310–2315, 1976
713. Wedell J, Eisen PM, Luu TH et al: A retrospective study of serial CEA determinations in the early detection of recurrent colorectal cancer. Dis Colon Rectum 24:618–621, 1981
714. Moertel CG, Schutt AJ, Go LW: Carcinoembryonic antigen test for recurrent colorectal cancer. JAMA 239:1065–1066, 1978
715. Midiri G, Amanti C, Benedetti M et al: CEA tissue staining in colorectal cancer patients. Cancer 55:2624–2629, 1985
716. Focan C: Circadian CEA variability: When to sample. J Clin Oncol 3:607, 1985
717. Staab HJ, Anderer FA, Hornung A et al: Doubling time of circulating CEA and its relation to survival of patients with recurrent colorectal cancer. Br J Cancer 46:773–781, 1982
718. Denstman F, Rosen L, Khubchandani IT et al: Comparing predictive decision rules in postoperative CEA monitoring. Cancer 58:2089–2095, 1986
719. Vecchio TJ: Predictive value of a single diagnostic test in unselected populations. N Engl J Med 274:1171–1173, 1966
720. Martin EW Jr, Minton JP, Carey LC: CEA-directed second-look surgery in the asymptomatic patient after primary resection of colorectal cancer. Ann Surg 202:310–317, 1985
721. Neville AM: International Union Against Cancer Workshop on Immunodiagnosis. Cancer Res 46:3744–3746, 1986
722. Lind SE, Singer DE: Diagnosing liver metastases: A Bayesian analysis. J Clin Oncol 4:379–388, 1986
723. Tartter PI, Slater G, Gelernt I et al: Screening for liver metastases from colorectal cancer with carcinoembryonic antigen and alkaline phosphatase. Ann Surg 193:357–360, 1981
724. Kemeny NM, Ganteaume L, Goldberg DA et al: Preoperative staging with computerized axial tomography and biochemical laboratory tests in patients with hepatic metastases. Ann Surg 303:169–172, 1986
725. Podolsky DK, Weiser MM, Isselbacher KJ et al: A cancer-associated galactosyltransferase isoenzyme. N Engl J Med 299:703–705, 1978
726. Putzki H, Student A, Jablonski M et al: Comparison of the tumor marker CEA, TPA, and CA 19-9 in colorectal carcinoma. Cancer 59:223–226, 1987
727. Szymendera JJ, Nowacki MP, Kozlowicz-Gudzinska I et al: The value of serum levels of carcinoembryonic antigen, CEA, and gastrointestinal cancer antigen, GICA or CA 19-9, for preoperative staging and postoperative monitoring of patients with colorectal carcinoma. Dis Col Rectum 28:895–899, 1985
728. Novis BH, Gluck E, Thomas P et al: Serial levels of CA 19-9 and CEA in colonic cancer. J Clin Oncol 4:987–993, 1986
729. Smith TJ, Kemeny NM, Sugarbaker PH et al: A prospective study of hepatic imaging in the detection of metastatic disease. Ann Surg 195:486–491, 1982
730. Gunven P, Makuchi MM, Takayasu K et al: Preoperative imaging of liver metastases: Comparison of angiography, CT scan, and ultrasonography. Ann Surg 202:573–579, 1985
731. Stark DD, Felder RC, Wittenberg et al: Magnetic resonance imaging of cavernous hemangioma of the liver: Tissue specific characterization. Am J Radiol 145:213–222, 1985
732. Cohen AM: Needle biopsy technique to confirm suspected liver metastases at laparotomy. Surg Gynecol Obstet (in press)
733. McCormack PM, Attiyeh FF: Resected pulmonary metastases from colorectal cancer. Dis Colon Rectum 22:553–556, 1979
734. Patt YZ, Peters RE, Chuang VP et al: Palliation of pelvic recurrence of colorectal

cancer with intra-arterial 5-fluorouracil and mitomycin. Cancer 56:2175–2180, 1985
735. Estes NC, Morphis JG, Hornback NB, Jewell WR: Intraarterial chemotherapy and hyperthermia for pain control in patients with recurrent rectal cancer. Am J Surg 152:597–601, 1986
736. Dobrowsky W, Schmid AP: Radiotherapy of presacral recurrence following radical surgery for rectal carcinoma. Dis Colon Rectum 28:917–919, 1985
737. Pacini P, Cionini L, Pirtoll L et al: Symptomatic recurrence of carcinoma of the rectum and sigmoid: The influence of radiotherapy on the quality of life. Dis Colon Rectum 29:865–868, 1986
738. Benotti PN, Bothe A, Eyre RC et al: Management of recurrent pelvic tumor. Arch Surg 122:457–460, 1987
739. Pearlman NW, Donohue RE, Stiegmann GV et al: Pelvic and sacropelvic exenteration for locally advanced or recurrent anorectal cancer. Arch Surg 122:537–541, 1987
740. Wanebo HJ, Gaker DL, Whitehill R et al: Pelvic recurrence of rectal cancer: Options for curative resection. Presented at the 98th annual meeting of the Southern Surgical Association, Palm Beach, Fla, November–December, 1986
741. Beart RW Jr, Martin JK Jr, Gunderson LL: Management of recurrent rectal cancer. Mayo Clin Proc 61:448–450, 1986
742. Sannella NA: Abdominoperineal resection following anterior resection. Cancer 38:378–381, 1976
743. Vassilopoulos PP, Yoon JM, Ledesma EJ et al: Treatment of recurrence of adenocarcinoma of the colon and rectum at the anastomotic site. Surg Gynecol Obstet 152:777–780, 1981
744. Pihl E, Hughes ESR, McDermott FT et al: Recurrence of carcinoma of the colon and rectum at the anastomotic suture line. Surg Gynecol Obstet 153:495–496, 1981
745. Stearns MW Jr: Diagnosis and management of recurrent pelvic malignancy following combined abdominoperineal resection. Dis Colon Rectum 23:359–361, 1980
746. Polk HC Jr, Spratt JS Jr: The results of treatment of perineal recurrence of cancer of the rectum. Cancer 43:952–955, 1979
747. Wilking N, Herrera L, Petrelli NJ, Mittelman A: Pelvic and perineal recurrences after abdominoperineal resection for adenocarcinoma of the rectum. Am J Surg 150:561–563, 1985
748. Hine KR, Dykes PW: Prospective randomized trial of early cytotoxic therapy for recurrent colorectal carcinoma detected by serum CEA. Gut 25:682–688, 1984
749. Martin EW Jr, Cooperman M, King G et al: A retrospective and prospective study of serial CEA determinations in the early detection of recurrent colorectal cancer. Am J Surg 137:167–169, 1979
750. Martin EW Jr, Cooperman M, Carey LC, Minton JP: Sixty second-look procedures indicated primarily by rise in serial carcinoembryonic antigen. J Surg Res 28:389–394, 1980
751. Attiyeh FF, Stearns MW: Second-look laparotomy based on CEA elevations in colorectal cancer. Cancer 47:2119–2125, 1981
752. Staab HJ, Anderer FA, Stumpf E et al: Eighty-four second look operations based on sequential carcinoembryonic antigen determinations and clinical investigations in patients with recurrent gastrointestinal cancer. Am J Surg 179:198–204, 1985
753. Steele G Jr, Zamcheck N, Mayer R et al: Results of CEA-initiated second-look surgery for recurrent colorectal cancer. Am J Surg 139:544–548, 1980
754. Wilking N, Petrelli NJ, Derrera L et al: Abdominal exploration for suspected recurrent carcinoma of the colon and rectum based upon elevated carcinoembryonic antigen alone or in combination with other methods. Surg Gynecol Obstet 162:465–468, 1986
755. Sandler RS, Freund DA, Herbst CA et al: Cost effectiveness of postoperative carcinoembryonic antigen monitoring in colorectal cancer. Cancer 53:193–198, 1984
756. Northover J, Slack WW: A randomized controlled trial of CEA-prompted second look surgery in recurrent colorectal cancer: A preliminary report. Dis Colon Rectum 27:576, 1984
757. Beatty JD, Duda RB, Williams LE et al: Preoperative imaging of colorectal carcinoma with indium 111-labelled anticarcinoembryonic antigen monoclonal antibody. Cancer Res 46:6494–6502, 1986
758. Martin DT, Hinkel GH, Tuttle S et al: Intraoperative radio immunodetection of colorectal tumor with a hand-held radiation detector. Am J Surg 150:671–674, 1985
759. Lyden MJ, Thompson CH, Liechtenstein M et al: Visualization of metastases from colon carcinoma using an iodine 131-radio-labeled monoclonal antibody. Cancer 57:1135–1139, 1986
760. Begent RHJ, Keep PA, Searle F et al: Radioimmunolocalization and selection for surgery in recurrent colorectal cancer. Br J Surg 73:64–67, 1986
761. Heidelberger C, Chandhari NK, Dannenberg P et al: Fluorinated pyrimidines: A new class of tumor inhibitory compounds. Nature 179:665–666, 1957
762. Moertel CG, Reitemeyer RJ: Advanced Gastrointestinal Cancer: Clinical Management and Chemotherapy. New York, Harper & Row, 1969
763. Moertel CG: Large bowel. In Holland JF, Frei E (eds): Cancer Medicine, pp 1497–1626. Philadelphia, Lea & Febiger, 1973
764. Ansfield F, Klotz J, Nealor T et al: A phase III study comparing the clinical utility of four regimens of 5-fluorouracil. Cancer 39:34–40, 1977
765. Moertel CG: Clinical management of advanced gastrointestinal cancer. Cancer 36:675, 1975
766. Christophidis N, Vajda FJE, Lucas I et al: Fluorouracil therapy in patients with carcinoma of the large bowel: A pharmacokinetic comparison of various rates and routes of administration. Clin Pharmacokinet 3:330–336, 1978
767. Bateman J, Irwin L, Pugh R et al: Comparison of intravenous and oral administration of 5-fluorouracil for colorectal carcinoma. Proc Am Assoc Cancer Res 16:242, 1975
768. Hahn RG, Moertel CG, Shutt AJ et al: A double-blind comparison of intensive course 5-FU by oral vs. intravenous route in the treatment of colon carcinoma. Cancer 35:1031–1036, 1975
769. Lokich J, Bothe A, Fine N et al: Phase I study of protracted venous infusion of 5-fluorouracil. Cancer 48:2565–2568, 1981
770. Seifert P, Baker LH, Reed MD et al: Comparison of continuously infused 5-fluorouracil with bolus injection in treatment of patients with colorectal adenocarcinoma. Cancer 36:123–128, 1975
771. Caballero GA, Ausman RK, Quebbeman EJ: Long-term, ambulatory, continuous intravenous infusion of 5-fluorouracil for treatment of advanced adenocarcinoma. Cancer Treat Rep 69:13–15, 1985
772. Lokich J, Gillings D, Gallo J et al: Bolus versus infusion 5-fluorouracil (5-FU): A randomized clinical trial in advanced measurable colorectal cancer. Proc Am Soc Clin Oncol 5:83, 1986
773. Lokich JJ, Moor C: Chemotherapy associated palmar-plantar erythrodysesthesia syndrome. Ann Intern Med 101:798–800, 1984
774. Quebbeman E, Ausman R, Hansen R et al: Long-term ambulatory treatment of metastatic colorectal adenocarcinoma by continuous intravenous infusion of 5-fluorouracil. J Surg Oncol 30:60–65, 1985
775. Wade JL, Herbst S, Greenburg A: Prolonged venous infusion (PVI) of 5-fluorouracil (5-FU) for metastatic colon cancer. Proc Am Soc Clin Oncol 5:88, 1986
776. Benedetto P, Davila E, Solomon J: Chronic continuous systemic infusion of 5-fluorouracil (CCI-5-FU) in the treatment of metastatic colorectal carcinoma (CCA). Proc Am Soc Clin Oncol 3:142, 1984
777. Hansen E, Quebbeman R, Ausman R et al: Continuous 5-fluorouracil (5-FU) infusion in colorectal cancer: Update of the MCW experience. Proc Am Soc Clin Oncol 6:80, 1987
778. Belt RJ, Davidner ML, Myron MC et al: Continuous low dose 5-fluorouracil (5-FU) for adenocarcinoma: Confirmation of activity. Proc Am Soc Clin Oncol 4:90, 1985
779. Leichman L, Seichman CG, Kinzie J et al: Long term low dose 5-fluorouracil (5-FU) in advanced measurable colon cancer: No correlation between toxicity and efficacy. Proc Am Soc Clin Oncol 4:86, 1985
780. NCIC Ongoing Clinical Trial, initiated 1986
781. Lokich J: Optimal schedule for 5-fluorouracil chemotherapy: Intermittent bolus or continuous infusion? Am J Clin Oncol 8:445–448, 1985
782. Niederhuber JE, Ensminger W, Gyves J et al: Regional chemotherapy of colorectal cancer metastatic to the liver. Cancer 53:1336–1343, 1984
783. Kemeny N, Reichman B, Oderman P et al: Update of randomized study of intrahepatic (H) vs systemic (S) infusion of fluorodeoxyuridine (FUdR) in patients with liver metastases from colorectal carcinoma (CR). Proc Am Soc Clin Oncol 5:86, 1986
784. Hohn D, Stagg R, Friedman M et al: The NCOG randomized trial of intravenous (IV) vs. hepatic arterial (IA) FUDR for colorectal cancer metastatic to the liver. Proc Am Soc Clin Oncol 6:85, 1987
785. Moertel CG: Therapy of advanced gastrointestinal cancer with the nitrosoureas. Cancer Chemother Rep 3/4:27, 1973
786. Macdonald JS, Neefe J: Chemotherapy in the management of gastrointestinal cancer. Abdom Surg 21:126–131, 1979
787. Moertel CG: Chemotherapy of gastrointestinal cancer. N Engl J Med 299:1049–1052, 1978
788. Boice JD, Greene MH, Killen JY et al: Leukemia and pre-leukemia after adjuvant treatment of gastrointestinal cancer with semustine (methyl-CCNU). N Engl J Med 309:1079–1083, 1983
789. Wasserman TH, Comis RL, Goldsmith M et al: Tabular analysis of clinical chemotherapy of solid tumors. Cancer Chemother Rep 6:399, 1975
790. Pastan I, Gottesman M: Multiple-drug resistance in human cancer. N Engl J Med 316:1388–1393, 1987
791. Myers C, Cowan K, Sinha B et al: The phenomenon of pleiotropic drug resistance. In DeVita VT, Hellman S, Rosenberg SA (eds): Important Advances in Oncology 1987, pp 27–37. Philadelphia, JB Lippincott, 1987
792. Moertel CG, Schutt AJ, Hahn RG et al: Therapy of advanced colorectal cancer with a combination of 5-fluorouracil, methyl 3-cis-(2-chlorethyl)-1-nitrosourea and vincristine. JNCI 54:69, 1975
793. Posey L, Morgan LR: Methyl CCNU versus methyl CCNU and 5-fluorouracil in carcinoma of the large bowel. Cancer Treat Rep 61:1453–1458, 1977
794. Baker LH, Talley RW, Matter R et al: Phase III comparison of the treatment of advanced gastrointestinal cancer with bolus weekly 5-FU vs. methyl-CCNU plus bolus weekly 5-FU: A Southwest Oncology Group study. Cancer 38:1–7, 1976
795. Falkson G, Falkson HC: Fluorouracil, methyl-CCNU, and vincristine in cancer of the colon. Cancer 38:1468–1470, 1976
796. Macdonald JS, Kisner DF, Smythe T et al: 5-Fluorouracil (5-FU), methyl-CCNU and vincristine in the treatment of advanced colorectal cancer: Phase II study utilizing weekly 5FU. Cancer Treat Rep 60:1597, 1976
797. Kemeny N, Yagoda A, Braun D et al: Randomized study of 2 different schedules of methyl CCNU, 5-FU, and vincristine for metastatic colorectal carcinoma. Cancer 43:78–82, 1979
798. Engstrom P, MacIntyre J, Douglass H Jr et al: Combination chemotherapy of advanced bowel cancer. Proc AACR-ASCO 19:384, 1978
799. Kemeny N, Yagoda A, Braun J: Metastatic colorectal carcinoma: A prospective trial of methyl CCNU, 5-fluorouracil (5FU) and vincristine (MOF) versus MOF plus streptozotocin (MOF-Strep). Cancer 51:20–25, 1983

800. Buroker T, Kim PN, Groppe C et al: 5FU infusion with mitomycin C vs. 5FU infusion with methyl CCNU in the treatment of advanced colon cancer. Cancer 42:1228–1233, 1978
801. Ramming KP, Tesler AS, Haskell CM: Gastrointestinal tract neoplasms. In Haskell CM (ed): Cancer Treatment, pp 300–301. Philadelphia, WB Saunders, 1980
802. Richards FD, Case LD, White DR et al: Combination chemotherapy (5-fluorouracil, methyl-CCNU, mitomycin C) versus 5-fluorouracil alone for advanced previously untreated colorectal carcinoma: A phase III study of the Piedmont Oncology Association. J Clin Oncol 4:565–570, 1986
803. Loehrer PJ, Einhorn LH, Williams JD et al: Cisplatin plus 5-FU for the treatment of adenocarcinoma of the colon. Cancer Treat Rep 69:1359–1363, 1985
804. Kovach JS, Moertel CG, Shutt AS et al: Phase II study of cis-diamminedichloroplatin (NSC-119875) in advanced carcinoma of the large bowel. Cancer Chemother Rep 57:357–358, 1973
805. O'Connell MJ, Moertel CG, Kvols LK et al: Clinical trial of cisplatin and intensive 5-fluorouracil for the treatment of advanced colo-rectal cancer. Am J Clin Oncol 9:192–195, 1986
806. Cantrell J, Hart R, Taylor R et al: A Phase II trial of continuous infusion (CI) 5-FU and weekly low dose cis-platin (DDP) in colorectal carcinoma. Proc Am Soc Clin Oncol 5:84, 1986
807. Loehrer PJ, Turner S, Kubilis P et al: A prospective randomized study of 5-fluorouracil (5FU) alone or with cisplatin (P) in the treatment of metastatic colorectal cancer: A Hoosier Oncology Group trial. Proc Am Soc Clin Oncol 6:297, 1987
808. Bertino JR, Sawicki WL, Lindquist A et al: Schedule dependent autitumor effects of methotrexate and 5-fluorouracil. Cancer Rev 37:327–328, 1977
809. Cadman E, Heimer R, Davis L: Enhanced 5-fluorouracil nucleotide formation after methotrexate adminstration: Explanation for drug synergism. Science 205:1135–1137, 1979
810. Benz C, Cadman E: Modulation of 5-fluorouracil metabolism and cytotoxicity by antimetabolite pretreatment in human colorectal adenocarcinoma HCT-8. Cancer Rev 41:994–999, 1981
811. Mehrotra S, Rosenthal CJ, Gardner B: Biochemical modulation of antineoplastic response in colorectal carcinoma: 5-fluorouracil (F), high dose methotrexate (M) with calcium leukovorin (L) rescue (FML) in two sequences of administration. Proc Am Soc Clin Oncol 1:95, 1982
812. Kemeny N, Michaelson R: Phase II trial of low dose methotrexate and sequential 5-fluorouracil in the treatment of metastatic colorectal carcinoma. Proc Am Soc Clin Oncol 1:95, 1982
813. Mahajan SL, Ajan JA, Kanoj A et al: Comparison of two schedules of sequential high-dose methotrexate (MTX) and 5-fluorouracil (5-FU) for metastatic colorectal carcinoma. Proc Am Soc Clin Oncol 2:122, 1983
814. Rangineni RR, Ajani JA, Bedikian AY et al: Sequential conventional dose methotrexate (MTX) and 5-fluorouracil (5-FU) in the primary therapy of metastatic colorectal carcinoma. Proc Am Soc Clin Oncol 2:125, 1983
815. Hansen R, Ritch P, Anderson T: Sequential methotrexate (MTX), 5-fluorouracil (5-FU), and leukovorin (LCV) in colorectal cancer. Proc Am Soc Clin Oncol 2:117, 1983
816. Drapkin R, McAloon E, Lyman G: Sequential methotrexate (MTX) and 5-fluorouracil in advanced measurable colorectal cancer. Proc Am Soc Clin Oncol 2:118, 1983
817. Petrelli N, Herrera L, Stulc J et al: A phase III study of 5FU versus 5FU + methotrexate versus 5FU + high-dose leucovorin in metastatic colorectal adenocarcinoma. Proc Am Soc Clin Oncol 6:286, 1987
818. Ullman B, Lee M, Martin DW et al: Cytotoxicity of 5-fluoro-2′-deoxyuridine: Requirement for reduced folate cofactors and antagonism of methotrexate. Proc Natl Acad Sci USA 75:980–983, 1978
819. Evans RM, Laskin JD, Hakala MT: Effect of excess folates and deoxyinosine on the activity and site of action of 5-fluorouracil. Cancer Res 41:3283–3295, 1981
820. Houghton JA,Maroda SJ Jr, Philips JO et al: Biochemical determinants of responsiveness to 5-fluorouracil and its derivatives in xenografts of human colorectal adenocarcinomas in mice. Cancer Res 41:144–149, 1981
821. Machover D, Schwarzenberg L, Goldschmidt E et al: Treatment of advanced colorectal and gastric adenocarcinomas with 5-FU combined with high-dose folinic acid: A pilot study. Cancer Treat Rep 66:1803–1807, 1982
822. Greene H, Desai A, Levick S et al: Combined 5-fluorouracil infusion and high dose folinic acid in the treatment of metastatic gastrointestinal cancer. Proc Am Soc Clin Oncol 5:89, 1986
823. Lopez AR, Van Tilburg A, Bradley T et al: Treatment of advanced malignancy with 5-fluorouracil combined with folinic acid. Proc Am Assoc Cancer Res 25:178, 1984
824. Schmoll HJ, LeBlanc S: Sequential high dose folinic acid and 5-fluorouracil in advanced colorectal cancer with measurable, progressive disease. Proc Am Soc Clin Oncol 4:94, 1985
825. Ehrlichman C, Fine S, Wong A et al: A comparison of 5-fluorouracil and folinic acid versus 5FU in metastatic colorectal cancer. Proc Am Soc Clin Oncol 5:82, 1986
826. Doroshow JH, Bertrand M, Multhauf P et al: Prospective randomized trial comparing 5FU versus 5FU and high dose folinic acid (hdfa) for treatment of advanced colorectal cancer. Proc Am Soc Clin Oncol 6:374, 1987
827. Mavligit GM, Burgess MA, Seibert GB et al: Adjuvant immunotherapy and chemoimmunotherapy in colorectal cancer of the Dukes C classification. Cancer 36:2421–2427, 1975
828. Higgins GA, Donaldson R, Rogers L et al: Efficacy of MER immunotherapy when added to a regimen of 5-fluorouracil and methyl-CCNU following resection for carcinoma of large bowel. Cancer 54:193–198, 1984
829. Antman K, Eder JP, Schryber et al: Fifty-eight solid tumor patients treated with a high dose combination alkylating agent preparative regimen with autologous bone marrow support: The DFCI/BIH experience (abst). Proc Am Soc Clin Oncol 5:40, 1986
830. Silgals RM, Ahern JD, Neefe JR et al: A phase II trial of high dose intravenous interferon alpha 2 in advanced colorectal cancer. Cancer 54:2257–2261, 1984
831. Figlin RA, Callaghan N, Sarna G: Phase II trial of interferon administered daily in adenocarcinoma of the colon/rectum. Cancer Treat Rep 67:493–494, 1983
832. Niederle N, Kurschel E, Schmidt CG: Biologic effect of recombinant leukocyte 2 interferon in metastatic colorectal carcinomas. Dtsch Med Wochenschr 109:779–782, 1984
833. Wrigley PFM, Slevin ML, Clark P et al: Alpha-2 interferon in combination with 5-fluorouracil for advanced colorectal carcinoma. Proc Am Soc Clin Oncol 3:14, 1984
834. Kreuser ED, Porzsolt F, Digel W et al: Interferon alpha-2C in combination with 5-fluorouracil for refractory colorectal carcinoma (abst 611). Presented at the Fifth NCI–EORTC Symposium on New Drugs and Cancer Therapy, Amsterdam, 1986
835. Lillis PK, Brown T, Beougher K et al: Phase II trial of recombinant beta interferon (beta-seron) in advanced colorectal cancer. Proc Am Soc Clin Oncol 6:A336, 1987
836. O'Connell MJ, Moertel CG, Shutt AJ et al: Phase II clinical trial of human recombinant gamma interferon (RIFN-gamma) in patients (Pts) with advanced colorectal cancer. Proc Assoc Cancer Res 27:181, 1986
837. Rios A, Levin B, Ajani J et al: Combination of recombinant human interferon gamma (RIFN gamma) and 5-fluorouracil in the treatment of patients with advanced colorectal carcinoma (CRC). Proc Am Soc Clin Oncol 6:A328, 1987
838. Crown SE, Mintzer D, Cunningham-Rundles S et al: High-dose human lymphoblastoid interferon in metastatic colorectal cancer: Clinical results and modification of biological responses. Cancer Treat Rep 71:39–45, 1987
839. Rosenberg SA, Lotze MT, Muul LM et al: A progress report on the treatment of 157 patients with advanced cancer using lymphokine-activated killer cells and interleukin-2 alone. N Engl J Med 316:889–897, 1987
840. West WH, Tauer KW, Yannelli JR et al: Constant-infusion recombinant interleukin-2 in adoptive immunotherapy of advanced cancer. N Engl J Med 316:898–905, 1987
841. Sears H, Herlyn D, Steplewski Z, Koprowski H: Effects of monoclonal antibody immunotherapy on patients with gastrointestinal adenocarcinoma. J Biol Res Mod 3:138–150, 1984
842. Gallagher WJ, Burk MW: Monoclonal antibody ricin A chain conjugates (immunotoxins): Potential therapeutic agents for human colon carcinoma. J Surg Res 40:159–166, 1986
843. Douillard JY, LeMevel B, Curtet et al: Immunotherapy of gastrointestinal cancer with monoclonal antibodies. Med Oncol Tumor Pharmacother 3:141–146, 1986
844. Hoover HC Jr, Surdyke M, Dangel RB et al: Prospectively randomized trial of adjuvant active specific immunotherapy for human colorectal cancer. Cancer 55:1236–1243, 1985
845. Mellstedt H, Frodin JE, Christensson B et al: Application of monoclonal antibodies (Mab 17-1A) in the treatment of colo-rectal carcinomas. In Carrano RA, Douillard JY (eds): Monoclonal Antibodies in Clinical Oncology. New York, Marcel Dekker, 1988
846. Schlom J, Weeks MO: Potential clinical utility of monoclonal antibodies in the management of human carcinomas. In DeVita VT, Hellman S, Rosenberg SA (eds): Important Advances in Oncology, 1985, pp 170–192. Philadelphia, JB Lippincott, 1985
847. Leff RS, Thompson JM, Johnson DB et al: Phase II trial of high-dose melphalan and autologous bone marrow transplantation for metastatic colon carcinoma. J Clin Oncol 4(11):1586–1591, 1986
848. Leff RS, Johnson DB, Daly MB et al: High response rate with minimal toxicity in the treatment of metastatic colon carcinoma with high dose melphalan and autologous bone marrow transplantation (ABMT). (abst). Proc Soc Clin Oncol 5:88, 1986
849. Orloff MJ: Carcinoid tumors of the rectum. Cancer 28:175–180, 1971
850. Naunheim KS, Zeitels J, Kaplan EL et al: Rectal carcinoid tumors: Treatment and prognosis. Surgery 94:670–675, 1983
851. Quan SHQ, Bader G, Berg JW: Carcinoid tumors of the rectum. Dis Colon Rectum 7:197–206, 1964
852. Morgan JG, Marks C, Hearn D: Carcinoid tumors of the gastrointestinal tract. Ann Surg 180:720–727, 1974
853. Khalifa AA, Bong WL, Rao VK et al: Leiomyosarcoma of the rectum: Report of a case and review of the literature. Dis Colon Rectum 29:427–432, 1986
854. Walsh TH, Mann CV: Smooth muscle neoplasms of the rectum and anal canal. Br J Surg 71:597–599, 1984
855. Evans HL: Smooth muscle tumors of the gastrointestinal tract. Cancer 56:2242–2250, 1985
856. Devine RM, Beart RW Jr, Wolff BG: Malignant lymphoma of the rectum. Dis Colon Rectum 29:821–824, 1986

BRENDA SHANK
ALFRED M. COHEN
DAVID KELSEN

CHAPTER 30 *Cancer of the Anal Region*

The treatment of epidermoid cancer of the anal region has undergone a major change over the past decade. From radical surgery only—abdominoperineal resection—treatment has evolved to entail radiation therapy, either alone or combined with chemotherapy, with sphincter-sparing surgery.[1-3] This combined modality approach is now regarded as the model for successful combined modality therapy of cancer.

EPIDEMIOLOGY AND ETIOLOGY

INCIDENCE, AGE, AND SEX

In the United States, cancer of the anal region accounts for 1% to 2% of all large bowel cancers[4-6] and 3.9% of all anorectal carcinomas.[7] The figures are similar in the United Kingdom, where cancer of the anal region constitutes 3% to 3.5% of all anorectal tumors.[8,9] Most of these tumors are epidermoid carcinoma (Table 30-1).[10]

Epidermoid carcinoma of the anal region most commonly occurs between age 30 years and the late 80s, with the preponderance of cases occurring in persons aged 58 to 64 years.[4,5,7,11-13] McConnell correlated the site with age and found that 80% of *anal canal* carcinomas occurred in people over the age of 60, whereas more than 50% of the *anal margin* carcinomas occurred in people younger than 60 years old.[9] However, Stearns et al reported no age differences for patients with carcinomas in these two sites.[7]

In the United States, anal carcinoma occurs more frequently in females than in males (Table 30-2).[4,5,7,10,14] This is generally true for anal *canal* cancers in the Western world.[8,9,15-18] Anal *margin* cancers, however, are more frequent in males. In contrast, Kapur et al noted a strong male preponderance for anal cancer in New Delhi, India.[19]

Several recent studies have implicated male homosexuality in anal canal carcinoma, presumably from anal intercourse.[10,13,20-24] A case-control study reported by Daling et al compared potential risk factors in 148 patients with anal cancer and 166 controls with colon cancer.[24] A history of anal-receptive intercourse in men (but not in women) was strongly associated with anal cancer (relative risk [RR] = 33.1).

In a study by Peters and Mack of 970 Los Angeles County residents, the incidence of anal carcinoma was 6.1 times greater in single men than in married men ($p < 0.001$).[10] The increased incidence was limited to squamous and transitional cell carcinomas in the anus and did not apply to adenocarcinoma; single women were not at an increased risk. In the age group less than 35 years old, anal carcinoma was more common in men, the reverse of the sex ratio for patients over 35 years old, where again there was a substantial female predominance. Peters and Mack regarded these findings as consistent with the hypothesis that anal sexual activity is related to anal cancer. They also noted an increase in the incidence of anal carcinoma in 1980–1981 to twice that expected for men less than 45 years old (18 cases versus 8.3 expected). An increased incidence was not seen in women of any age or in men more than 45 years old. The investigators

TABLE 30-1. Anal Carcinoma: Distribution of Histologic Types in 970 Patients*

Type	*% of Patients*
Squamous cell carcinoma	63
Transitional (cloacogenic) carcinoma	23
Adenocarcinoma	7
Paget's disease	2
Basal cell carcinoma	2
Melanoma	2

* Modified from Peters RK, Mack TM: Patterns of anal carcinoma by gender and marital status in Los Angeles County. Br J Cancer 48:629–636, 1983.

could not rule out the possibility that the increased incidence in young single men may have been related to acquired immune deficiency syndrome (AIDS), which was also occurring in the same population. Mechanisms postulated were physical irritation of the anal canal, genital carcinogens (*e.g.*, lubricants), or the transmission of oncogenic viruses by sexual contact.

VIRUSES AND OTHER INFECTIOUS AGENTS

There appears to be a relationship between papillomaviruses and the development of genital warts (condylomata acuminata), which can convert to squamous cell carcinomas after a long latent period of 5 to 40 years.[25] Anal canal carcinoma has been associated with condylomata[26–29] in the general population and in male homosexuals.[30] In the case-control study reported by Daling et al,[24] squamous cell carcinoma (but not transitional cell carcinoma) was strongly associated with a history of genital warts (RR = 26.9 in males and 32.5 in females). Nine (64%) of 14 patients with tumors positive for human papillomavirus by in situ hybridization techniques had a history of warts.

In women without a history of genital warts, anal cancer was associated with seropositivity for herpes simplex virus type 2 (RR = 4.1) and *Chlamydia trachomatis* (RR = 2.3). In men without a history of warts, there was an association with gonorrhea (RR = 17.2).

OTHER ASSOCIATED CONDITIONS

Anal canal carcinomas, in particular mucinous adenocarcinomas, have been associated with anal fistulas[4,31–34] and other benign conditions such as lymphogranuloma venereum[35,36] and leukoplakia.[16] Brennan and Stewart reported the relationship with condylomata acuminata and fistulas as well as fissures, abscesses, and hemorrhoids.[37] In one study, 41% of anal canal carcinomas were preceded by benign anorectal disease for at least 5 years.[38] There is a sexual difference in susceptibility to development of anogenital malignancies in the presence of condylomata: in a study reported by Chuang et al that spanned 28 years, 41 of 500 women with condylomata acuminata developed anogenital malignancies, while only one of 246 men developed anogenital malignancies.[39]

TABLE 30-2. Anal Carcinoma: Geographic Variability in Male : Female Ratios

Geographic Area	*Male : Female Ratio* All	*Anal Canal*	*Anal Margin*
United States[4,5,7,10,14]	1 : 2	3 : 7	2 : 1
United Kingdom[8,9,15–17]	1 : 1	3 : 4	3–4 : 1
France[18]	. . .	1 : 3	. . .
India (New Delhi)[19]	3 : 1	. . .	. . .

Ellipses indicate data not reported or not subdivided by location.

Prior radiation therapy may play a role in the development of anal carcinoma,[16,40,41] as may immunosuppression. Immunosuppressed renal transplant patients have a 100-fold increase in anogenital tumors compared with the rest of the population.[42] Many of these patients have a history of condylomata acuminata (29%) or herpes genitalis. In the case-control study reported by Daling et al, current cigarette smoking was a major risk factor in both sexes (RR = 7.7 in women and 9.4 in men).[24] This substantiates the report by Daniell, who noted that 54% of 13 women with anal cancer were current smokers, in comparison to only 26% of 202 age-matched patients with colon cancer.[43]

Several general conclusions with regard to etiology can be made. Anal canal carcinoma appears to be related to immunosuppression and correlates highly with preexisting condylomata acuminata, which are probably caused by viruses. There is a clear-cut relationship with male homosexuality, which may relate both to the presence of other viral diseases in these individuals and to immunosuppression. The relationship between anal cancer and AIDS is unclear,[44] but numerous and diverse gastrointestinal tract disorders are associated with AIDS, and an increase in anal cancer incidence has been seen recently in the AIDS-prone population in Los Angeles County.

ANIMAL STUDIES

Animal studies offer some clues to the genesis of anal tumors. In mice, anal carcinomas may be induced by chemical carcinogens.[45,46] In a study by Kingsnorth et al, the induction of anal squamous cell carcinomas was promoted by epidermal growth factor (EGF).[46] The frequency of anal squamous cell carcinomas induced by dimethylhydrazine (DMH) alone was only 10%, whereas in mice treated with both DMH and EGF, the frequency was 33% ($p < 0.05$). Kingsnorth et al postulated that this potentiation was a result of EGF-stimulated squamous cell hyperplasia, with the EGF thus acting as a co-carcinogen. It is of particular interest that EGF did not promote the development of DMH-induced tumors in the rest of the colon, which occur at a high rate (approximately 75%) with DMH alone.

ANATOMIC CONSIDERATIONS

Squamous cell cancer of the anus can occur in the anal canal proper, the lowermost rectum, or the perianal skin.[47,48] Important gross anatomic landmarks associated with these lo-

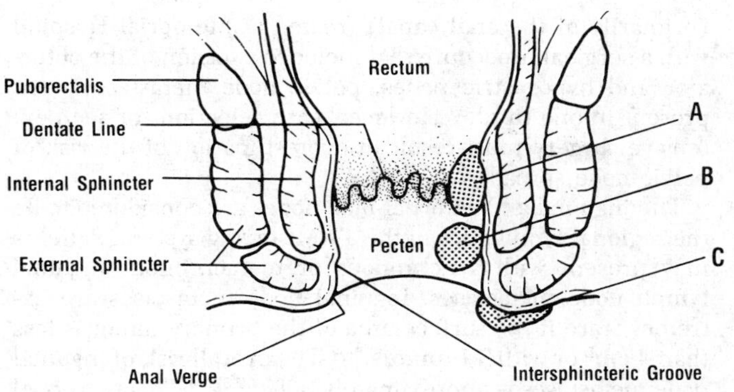

FIG. 30-1. Gross anatomy of the anal canal. A tumor in location *A* is always considered anal *canal* cancer; in location *C* it is anal *margin* cancer; in location *B* it is anal canal *or* margin, depending on institutional preference.

cations are illustrated in Figure 30-1. Each level is associated with histologically distinct epithelium.

The lowermost region lies caudad to the anal verge and is covered with keratinized stratified squamous epithelium. Pigmentation and hair follicles are present. Anal cancers are defined distally as those that are within 5 cm of the anal verge, and are referred to as *perianal* or *anal margin* cancers. Extending proximally from the anal verge to the pectinate or dentate line is the hairless stratified squamous epithelium of the anal canal. The rectal columns (columns of Morgagni) extend for 1.0 to 1.5 cm proximal to the level of the anorectal ring. Proximal to the ring the mucosa is columnar. The mucosa over the rectal columns is cuboidal, giving rise to the transitional cell or cloacogenic anal cancers. Squamous epithelium can extend proximally to the pectinate line, which explains the finding of squamous cell cancers in the distal rectum proper. The anal crypts are located in the distal columns of Morgagni. From microscopic glandular components within these crypts the rare mucoepidermoid cancers arise.

The definition of the proximal extent of tumors referred to as *anal margin* varies. The St. Marks Hospital, London, Memorial Hospital, New York (part of Memorial Sloan-Kettering Cancer Center), and Melbourne, Australia, groups consider all tumors below the dentate line as anal margin.[49–51] All tumors involving the dentate line are then considered *anal canal* cancers. The Mayo Clinic and other groups define anal margin tumors as those below the anal verge.[52] Figure 30-1 shows the various potential tumor sites within the anal region.

The *intersphincteric groove* is easily palpable on rectal examination. It represents the potential plane between the internal and external sphincter mechanism. The external sphincter surrounds the internal sphincter circumferentially and extends more caudad than the internal sphincter. Hence, the most superficial muscle beneath the anal verge is the superficial *external sphincter.* This is an important anatomic consideration when local excision is attempted. The superficial external and internal sphincter muscles can be resected without loss of continence in most patients. The entire sphincter mechanism caudad to the puborectalis sling can be resected over a partial circumference with acceptable continence (compared to a permanent colostomy).

The anal region is extremely well vascularized and has an extensive lymphatic system (Fig. 30-2). The lymphatics drain into the inguinal nodes, the lateral pelvic nodes, and the mesorectal nodes.[7] Tumors below the anal verge drain primarily into the inguinal nodal system. The distal 5 cm of rectum and the anal canal to the anal verge drain into the inguinal nodes, as well as along the middle hemorrhoidal vessels to the pelvic side walls, and into the inferior mesenteric system. Lymph node metastases are the rule with advanced anal cancer.

PATHOLOGY

HISTOLOGY

Many different histologic cell types may occur in the anal area.[53] In addition to the more common types (see Table 30-1), other rare histologic entities can arise, such as small cell carcinomas similar to oat cell carcinoma of the lung,[54] lymphoma, basal cell carcinoma, and Paget's disease.[55] Melanomas constitute 1% to 2% of all anal cancers, and anal melanoma constitutes only 1.6% of all melanomas.[56] The importance of anal melanoma lies in its poor prognosis, with a 5-year survival rate of only 8% to 12%[57,58]; survival is associated with tumors less than 2 mm in diameter.[57]

Some pathologists divide anal canal tumors into those that exhibit keratinization and those that do not,[49] and further subdivide nonkeratinizing tumors into basosquamous, basaloid, and cloacogenic carcinomas. Other investigators have found no difference in clinical outcome with such subdivisions and believe that all histologic varieties are subsets of squamous cell carcinoma.[59,60]

FIG. 30-2. Lymphatic drainage of the anus. Drainage is through three pathways: (1) inferiorly, from the *margin* and *canal*, across the perineum to the superficial inguinal lymph nodes; (2) from the upper canal and just superior to the dentate line, along the inferior and middle hemorrhoidal vessels to the hypogastric nodes; and (3) superiorly, from the rectum, along the superior hemorrhoidal vessels to the inferior mesenteric nodes.

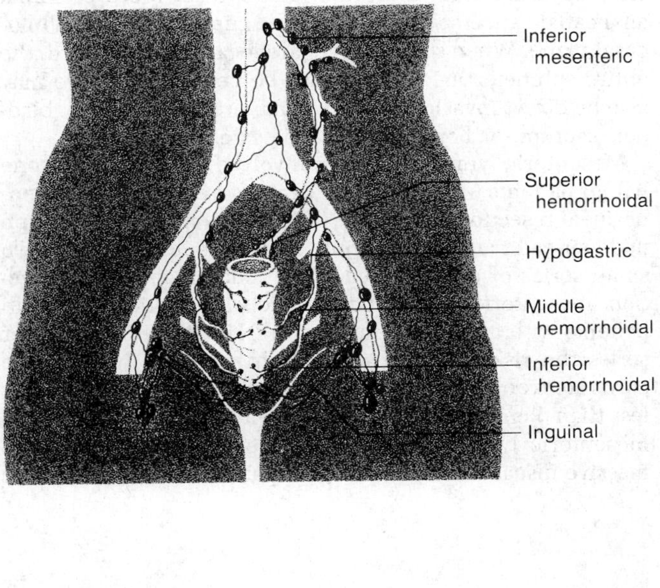

PRECANCEROUS CHANGES

Precancerous changes seen histologically in the anal canal, such as intraepidermal carcinoma of the Bowenoid type,[51] have been studied by a number of investigators. Fenger and Nielsen studied the incidence of precancerous changes in the anal canal epithelium.[61,62] Of 306 specimens, obtained at minor surgery, that included at least 1 cm of the anal transition zone (ATZ), seven (2.3%) showed squamous cell dysplasia, although the dysplasia was severe in only one. With an average follow-up of 27 months, no case of dysplasia had progressed to carcinoma. In a group of 139 patients who underwent abdominoperineal resections (most with carcinomas of the rectum, but some with anal canal tumors), 15 (10.8%) had dysplasia that was thought to be precancerous or to represent carcinoma in situ. Of the 16 patients with squamous cell carcinoma of the anal canal, severe dysplasia or carcinoma in situ was seen in 13 (81%). Fenger and Nielsen concluded that most anal canal tumors arising in the ATZ are preceded by multicentric areas of dysplasia.

Flow cytometric analysis of normal epithelium along the ATZ and, in smaller groups of patients, of anal canal tumors has been performed in fresh specimens by Fenger and Bichel.[63] A normal diploid population was seen in normal squamous epithelium in the ATZ, along with a small hyperdiploid peak, the relevance of which was unclear. Three patients with squamous cell carcinoma of the anal canal had a high proliferative index but near-diploid peaks. In contrast, Goldman et al found that most anal tumors had an aneuploid pattern.[64] Additional studies in larger numbers of patients are needed to clarify these findings.

NATURAL HISTORY

Squamous cell cancer of the anus and its variants spread by direct extension into contiguous soft tissues, with early dissemination via the lymphatics. Hematogenous spread is less common. The basaloid or cloacogenic subtypes have less biologic relevance than tumor location in a consideration of the natural history of anal cancer.[65,66]

Anal margin cancers invade local tissues and cause clinically apparent local ulceration and spread. More proximal anal canal cancers frequently spread cephalad in the submucosal plane. When such cancers are locally far advanced, the entire sphincter mechanism may be penetrated; there may also be direct invasion of the vagina, urethra, prostate, bladder, sacrum, or bone of the pelvic side walls.

Mesenteric lymph nodes are involved in one third to one half of patients with anal *canal* cancers treated by abdominoperineal resection,[6,16,51,59,67,68] The risk of mesenteric lymph node spread from anal *margin* cancers is less clear. In two small series of patients treated by abdominoperineal resection, mesenteric lymph node spread was identical to that in patients with anal canal cancers.[51,67] However, in two other series the risk was almost nil.[6,69] In addition, because the cure rate from local excision alone with anal margin cancers less than 5 cm in diameter is 90%,[50] it appears that spread to mesenteric lymph nodes is infrequent, except in cases of massive disease. In a series of 45 patients with anal cancer (primarily of the anal canal) treated at Memorial Hospital with a surgical procedure that included excision of the obturator and hypogastric nodes, pelvic node metastases were present in one third.[59] However, case selection for such extensive surgery must result in overestimation of the risk of pelvic node spread.

The inguinal and external iliac nodes are considered to be the regional lymphatics in the TNM staging system. Patients may present with synchronous or metachronous inguinal lymph node metastases. Inguinal node metastases are extremely rare if the surface area of the primary tumor is less than 4 cm^2 or with T1 tumors.[5,67] The overall risk of inguinal node metastases is approximately 30%.[59,67,70] This was equal to the incidence of pelvic node metastases in the Memorial Hospital series.[7] If inguinal nodes originally negative on physical examination are destined to become clinically positive, they usually do so within 18 months of treatment of the primary tumor.[67]

Hematogenous metastases occur in a minority of patients. Because of the dual venous drainage of the area, metastases occur equally to the liver and lung.[71]

Despite radical surgery, almost all recurrences of disease after surgery alone represent locoregional treatment failure. Most cancer-related deaths are secondary to uncontrolled pelvic and perineal disease.[52,54,68,72,73]

DIAGNOSIS

Because the initial symptoms of anal cancer are similar to those of common benign conditions, patient-related delay in diagnosis is very frequent. Because anal cancer is rare and examination may be painful and difficult if spasm is present, physician-related delay also occurs. Almost one third of the patients at Memorial Hospital with squamous cell cancer of the anorectum were thought to have had benign disease until a biopsy proved otherwise.[59] More than half of the patients in the Mayo Clinic study had associated benign anal pathology such as fistula-in-ano, fissure, or hemorrhoids.[52]

Bleeding, pain, and a sensation of a mass are the most common symptoms. Pruritus is less frequent, except in patients with perianal cancer.[52] Physical examination should include digital anorectal examination, anoscopy and proctoscopy, and palpation of the inguinal lymph nodes. Associated Bowen's or Paget's disease of the perianal skin increases the index of suspicion for anal carcinoma. The differential diagnosis of bleeding, pain, and/or a mass sensation includes thrombosed hemorrhoids, fissures, fistula, perianal or crypt abscess, benign anal papilloma, and adenocarcinoma of the rectum. Patients with severe pain and spasm may be treated empirically with analgesics, stool softeners, warm baths, and topical ointments for 1 to 2 weeks. Persistent symptoms may require examination under sedation or general anesthesia to avoid missing the diagnosis of cancer or an inadequately treated infection.

An incisional biopsy is necessary to confirm the diagnosis. Excision should not be attempted, except for superficial lesions detected very early. In general, suspicious inguinal lymph nodes should be biopsied to distinguish inflammatory from metastatic lymphadenopathy. Formal groin dissection should be avoided. Needle aspiration of the groin nodes for cytology may be attempted first. If the results are negative, surgical biopsy should follow. In addition to physical examination and surgical staging of a suspicious inguinal node site, an extent-of-disease staging includes chest radiography, liver function tests, and computed tomography of the abdomen and pelvis.

STAGING

An early attempt at staging was made at the Mayo Clinic in 1962.[5] This staging was similar to the Dukes' staging of rectal cancer, with Stage A representing invasion into sphincter muscle, Stage B, invasion through the sphincter muscle, and Stage C, lymph node involvement. They also graded the tumors by Broders' system. This simple system was found to be prognostic for 5-year survival. Because the sphincter muscle is thick, Stage B was later subclassified further and Stage D was added, representing unresectable regional tumor or distant metastases.[54] This classification was found to be prognostic for local and distant recurrence and for survival. Both of these classifications developed at the Mayo Clinic were pathologic classifications and applicable solely to anal canal carcinomas.

A similar surgical-pathologic staging classification was developed at the Roswell Park Memorial Institute[74] for application to the perianal area as well as the anal canal. A Stage O was introduced for carcinoma in situ, and perirectal and inguinal nodes were subclassified. That system was found to be prognostic, but the major decrements in survival came from sphincter muscle or inguinal node involvement. Involvement of perirectal nodes only was not particularly detrimental to survival compared with sphincter muscle involvement.[74]

The International Union Against Cancer (UICC) established a dual staging system with a clinical staging and a pathologic staging post-surgery,[75] to be used only for carcinoma in the anal region. Separate classifications were developed for the anal canal and for the anal margin, the anal margin staging system being analogous to that for other skin tumors. There were criticisms[76]; suggestions were incorporated into an illustrated guide of the UICC staging system.[77] A 1987 edition of the UICC staging system has now been published.[78] The American Joint Committee on Cancer (AJCC) adopted the same staging system for anal carcinoma.[79] This unified AJCC/UICC system (Table 30-3) takes into account the fact that anal canal carcinoma is increasingly treated by nonsurgical methods, such as radiation therapy alone or multimodality therapy.

Regardless of treatment, this standard clinical TNM staging system should be used to facilitate comparison of results. T staging is by size and invasion into other organs or tissues. The N classification for the anal canal subdivides the regional nodes, recognizing the poor prognosis of inguinal node involvement. Anal margin tumors are staged as for skin cancers, the T staging being almost the same as for the anal canal (see Table 30-3). Grading is also stipulated, with Grade 1 representing well-differentiated disease; Grade 2, moderately differentiated disease; Grade 3, poorly differentiated disease; and Grade 4, undifferentiated disease. Other variations of a TNM system have been used.[18,80]

In devising a staging system it is important to ascertain which clinical features are the most prognostic. Many studies have shown that survival correlates with size of the anal lesion (see section on Prognostic Factors). In one study survival correlated with the 1978 UICC clinical staging (circumferential invasion or invasion of adjacent organs) and with grade.[64] However, size, which may be more objectively assessed, also correlates with circumferential invasion. Therefore, any staging system should logically be based on tumor size and invasion into adjacent organs, and should also consider grade, as does the new AJCC/UICC system. We recommend that this system be used routinely so that results between institutions may be compared.

TABLE 30-3. AJCC/UICC Staging for Anal Canal and Anal Margin Cancer*

Primary tumor (T)	
TX	Primary tumor cannot be assessed
T0	No evidence of primary tumor
Tis	Carcinoma in situ
T1	≤2 cm in greatest dimension
T2	>2 cm but ≤5 cm in greatest dimension
T3	>5 cm in greatest dimension
Anal canal:	
T4	Any size, invading adjacent organ(s): vagina, urethra, bladder
Anal margin:	
T4	Invading deep extradermal structures: skeletal muscle, bone
Regional Lymph Node Involvement (N)	
NX	Regional lymph nodes cannot be assessed
N0	No regional lymph node involvement
Anal canal:	
N1	Metastasis to perirectal lymph nodes
N2	Metastasis to unilateral internal iliac and/or unilateral inguinal lymph nodes
N3	Metastasis to perirectal and inguinal lymph nodes and/or bilateral internal iliac and/or bilateral inguinal lymph nodes
Anal margin:	
N1	Ipsilateral inguinal lymph node metastasis
Distant Metastasis (M)	
MX	Distant metastasis cannot be assessed
M0	No distant metastasis
M1	Distant metastasis

Stage Grouping				
	Stage 0	Tis	N0	M0
	Stage I	T1	N0	M0
	Stage II	T2	N0	M0
		T3	N0	M0
Anal canal:				
	Stage IIIA	T4	N0	M0
		T1–3	N1	M0
	Stage IIIB	T4	N1	M0
		Any T	N2, 3	M0
Anal margin:				
	Stage III	T4	N0	M0
		Any T	N1	M0
Both:				
	Stage IV	Any T	Any N	M1

* Postsurgical histopathologic staging is the same, except determined by the pathologic examination (pT and pN).

PROGNOSTIC FACTORS

STAGE

Clinical stage (as measured by 1978 UICC T stage) has been correlated with prognostic outcome. Goldman and co-workers retrospectively analyzed findings in a group of 43 patients from Sweden with anal canal cancers.[64] Clinical stage was highly statistically correlated with outcome: patients with T1 and T2 cancers had a greater than 80% 5-year survival rate, while those with T3 and T4 disease had survival rates in the range of 0 to <20%; however, very few patients had T3 or T4 disease. This relationship is probably not an independent relationship, as T stage is related to size.

Metastasis to inguinal lymph nodes is also an indicator of a poor prognosis.[66,81] However, Greenall and co-workers found a 55% 5-year survival rate despite the presence of inguinal lymph node metastases, if lymphadenectomy could be performed.[81] It is not yet clear how the use of multimodality therapy will alter the historically poor prognosis associated with positive inguinal nodes. Treatment failure carries a poor prognosis, as might be expected. In one series patients in whom disease recurred despite treatment with chemotherapy and radiation, or radiation alone, had a median survival of 7 to 14 months.

SIZE

Tumor size (related to T stage) is of prognostic importance. A number of investigators have found that patients with lesions less than 2 cm in diameter have a markedly better prognosis than those with larger lesions.[54,67] Dillard et al found a 75% 5-year survival rate in a group of 12 patients with tumors less than 8 cm^2; only 47% of patients with tumors larger than 8 cm^2 survived.[67] Boman et al reported that of a total of 108 patients with anal canal tumors, 13 had small (<2 cm in diameter), superficially invasive lesions.[54] All were treated with local excision, and although one later required abdominoperineal resection, all were cured. Kuehn et al[82] reported no survivors with tumors >6 cm in diameter; and even with aggressive therapy, Wanebo et al found very poor survival in patients with lesions more than 10 cm in diameter.[83] Salmon et al also found that size was significantly related to survival in a study in which radiation therapy alone was the primary treatment.[66] In another radiation therapy series, size (≤4 cm or >4 cm in diameter) was prognostic for 5-year survival but not for tumor control.[84]

OTHER PROGNOSTIC FEATURES

Histologic cell type for squamous cancers of the anal canal (epidermoid versus cloacogenic) has not been found to be of major prognostic relevance. The cloacogenic carcinomas have been considered to have a slightly better prognosis in some series[66,85]; however, in 243 patients with resectable anal canal tumors, Papillon and Montbarbon found a worse prognosis for patients with nonkeratinizing and basaloid carcinoma than for patients with keratinizing lesions.[84] Small cell carcinomas of the anus, like extrapulmonary small cell cancers in other parts of the body, appear to have a worse prognosis, with a high propensity for systemic dissemination.[54]

Asymptomatic patients do better than symptomatic patients, but this may be directly related to the size of the tumor.[86] *Location* may be of slight prognostic importance, with anal margin tumors having a better outcome than those in the anal canal. On the other hand, Paradis et al found no difference in survival rates between patients with tumors within the anal canal and those with tumors in the perianal region.[74] No difference in survival according to *sex* was observed by Papillon and Montbarbon.[84]

Goldman et al looked at *DNA content, (i.e.,* whether tumors were diploid or greater than diploid) and found no correlation of survival with this factor.[64]

TREATMENT

ANAL MARGIN

Local Surgery

Superficial perianal skin carcinomas outside the anal verge may be treated with wide local excision with good results. A skin graft can be placed if the surgical defect is large. Rarely are formal skin flaps necessary or desirable. A split-thickness skin graft will shrink with time, leaving a relatively small defect that will not interfere with the detection of local recurrence. Primary abdominoperineal resection is almost never indicated as the initial treatment of these lesions. As with squamous cell cancer elsewhere on the integument, the cure rate after local excision for superficial tumors exceeds 80%.[49,50,52,70,87] Local failure rates are higher if the anal margin includes cancers in the anal canal distal to (not involving) the dentate line.[50] In the Memorial Hospital experience disease recurred locally in nine of 31 patients treated with local excision for such anal margin cancers.[50] Eight of these cases were amenable to a second local excision. In four patients, disease recurred in the inguinal nodes. There were only three cancer-related deaths in the 31 patients initially treated by local excision, and only one patient ultimately required abdominoperineal resection.

Deeply infiltrative anal margin lesions have been treated with abdominoperineal resection.[50,67] Although most patients are cured, the small number of reported cases of disease defined as anal margin cancers precludes detailed analysis of end results and patterns of failure.

External Irradiation

Epidermoid carcinoma of the anal margin tends to be early or only moderately advanced at the time of diagnosis,[88,89] with lymph nodes only rarely involved (0–15%),[88,90] usually in larger tumors (≥5 cm in diameter).[91] Although these early cancers of the anal margin are very successfully treated by local excision, radiation therapy should be considered in some patients. Papillon suggested that radiation therapy should be used in patients with anal margin carcinoma that is considered unresectable, or in patients who have extensive or recurrent lesions[80]; in addition, patients who are medically inoperable may have radiation therapy to this area.

Although some early studies of anal margin irradiation were done with interstitial radium needle implants,[80,88] the high incidence of radionecrosis and the relatively poor geometry indicate that external-beam radiation therapy is the radiation modality of choice.[80] Although photons are most frequently used for such treatments, electron-beam therapy may also be successfully utilized for early perineal epidermoid carcinomas.[92] Results in perineal anal canal lesions, stage for stage, are similar to results in anal canal lesions[89,93]; more extensive lesions therefore require more aggressive therapy. Although some authors have recommended abdominoperineal resections for extensive lesions,[89] from reported results radiation therapy appears to be an excellent alternative that yields a good cure rate with sphincter preservation.

Most studies group together patients with anal margin and anal canal carcinomas. Recently two groups reported on the results in anal margin carcinomas alone.[91,94] Neither study was a pure radiation therapy study, as chemotherapy with mitomycin C and 5-FU was given concurrently with radiation therapy in a large proportion of the patients. The study from the Centre Leon Berard used direct perineal fields and cobalt-60 as the source to deliver a surface dose of 4000 cGy in ten fractions. In a few patients with residual disease, iridium-192 implants were also used.[94] In the study from Princess Margaret Hospital, external-beam radiation therapy was used in most of the patients, who received a dose of 5000 cGy in 4 weeks, or in 8 weeks as a split course.[91] In both studies, local control was similar (80%–85%). In the Centre Leon Berard study, the 5-year disease-free survival rate was 50%, and only half of the deaths were secondary to cancer.[94] Treatment failed locally in five of 35 patients, but two patients were salvaged. Lymph node failures tended to occur later and were fatal in three patients. In the Princess Margaret Hospital study, local control was achieved in all 13 patients with a primary lesion less than 5 cm in diameter but in only two of five patients with a primary lesion larger than 10 cm.[91] Four patients had positive lymph nodes in this study, and disease in two was controlled by treatment. The investigators noted that local necrosis developed in three of 11 patients treated with radiation therapy alone.

In a study of both perianal and anal canal tumors, five patients with perianal tumors without nodal involvement were treated with radiation therapy (4000–6000 cGy) plus bleomycin; two of these patients with advanced disease (T4NO) also underwent abdominoperineal resection after chemotherapy and radiation therapy.[95] All five patients were alive and disease-free on follow-up of 16 to 84 months.

ANAL CANAL

Local Disease

LOCAL EXCISION. In a small series reported from the Cleveland Clinic, none of ten patients treated initially by local excision experienced recurrence of the disease.[96] Included were cancers of the anal margin and anal canal that extended less than one-half the circumference; cancers involving the dentate line were excluded. Internal or full-thickness sphincter excision with skin-graft coverage resulted in acceptable continence. In a review from the Connecticut Cancer Registry reported by Kuehn et al, 26 patients with anal cancer including distal anal canal cancers were treated by local excision, and 76% were cured.[47]

The Mayo Clinic experience[54] with anal cancers between the dentate line and the anal verge includes 19 patients treated by local excision. Treatment failed locally in one of 12 superficial tumors, which was subsequently cured with abdominoperineal resection. Seven patients with underlying sphincter muscle invasion refused radical surgery and were treated by wide local excision, some with adjuvant irradiation. Disease recurred locally in three.[54] In a group of five patients (four with T1 disease) treated at the Lahey Clinic by local excision, none had disease recurrence.[12] Of 144 patients treated at Memorial Hospital for anal canal cancers (dentate line involvement), only 11 were suitable candidates for local excision. The 5-year survival rate was only 45%, and the majority had local recurrence.[97] Less than 10% of the 91 anal canal tumors treated at St. Mark's Hospital with curative intent (dentate line involvement) were amenable to local excision; of these, 75% were cured.[70] Klotz et al compiled reports of anal canal "basaloid" cancers, 33 of which had been treated by local excision.[11] Most of the tumors had been found incidentally in hemorrhoidectomy specimens. The 5-year cure rate was 60%. Local excision should be considered only for small (T1) tumors with no evidence of nodal involvement, and in patients who can be followed up closely.

Locoregional Disease

MULTIMODALITY THERAPY. *Diagnostic Surgery.* Because integrated multimodality therapy not only improves overall survival but also allows radical surgery to be avoided in the majority of patients, the scope of initial diagnostic surgery should be limited to maximize the final functional result.

For anal margin cancers distal to the anal verge, a punch or surgical incisional biopsy performed in the office will suffice. For patients with considerable spasm and pain, examination and incisional biopsy under general anesthesia is appropriate. If a decision is made to proceed with local excision only (small anal margin or T1 anal canal lesion), the bowel is prepared and elective surgery is done.

Grossly positive inguinal lymph nodes are studied initially by needle aspiration cytology; open biopsy is performed if the result is benign. Minimally suspicious nodes warrant an excisional biopsy of one or two lymph nodes, with great care to avoid a hematoma or lymphatic leak. A superficial groin dissection is not necessary or useful as part of the initial treatment strategy, will delay definitive chemotherapy and radiation treatment, and may increase the risk of leg edema following combined treatment.

Combined Chemotherapy and Irradiation. In the past 10 to 15 years, increasing evidence amassed from single-arm Phase II studies has indicated that initial chemotherapy plus radiation therapy yields a very high rate of tumor regression

TABLE 30-4. Epidermoid Anal Canal Carcinoma: Treatment Plans and Results, by Institution

Treatment and Results	*Wayne State University, Detroit*	*Memorial Hospital, New York*	*Highland Hospital, Rochester, NY*	*Princess Margaret Hospital, Toronto*	*Fresno Community Hospital, Fresno, CA*
5-FU	1000 mg/m² × 4 d × 2 cycles	750 mg/m² × 5 d	1000 mg/m² × 4 d × 2 cycles from d 2	1000 mg/m² × 4 d	1000 mg/m² × 4 d × 2 cycles
Mitomycin C	15 mg/m², d 1	15 mg/m², d 1	10 mg/m², d 2	10 mg/m², d 1	10–15 mg/m², on d 1, × 2 cycles
RT	30 Gy/15 fx from d 1	30 Gy/15 fx starting d 6–9	50–57.5 Gy/25–32 fx from d 1 with boost	50 Gy/20 fx from d 1†	41–50 Gy/23–28 fx from d 1 with boost
Surgery	APR or LE 4–6 wk after RT	APR or LE 2–4 wk after RT	APR in 4 patients; no surgery in others; ¹⁹²Ir implant for residual disease	None	None
Maintenance Chemotherapy	None	For gross or microscopic residual disease*	None	None	None, but additional chemotherapy for residual disease
Total cases	45	44	33	30	30
Primary cases	45	44	33	30	27
Measurable response to chemotherapy and RT:					
CR	38	26	30	28	26
PR	7	. . .	3	2	4
No. having surgery	45	44	4	2‡	22
No. with sphincter preservation	27	20	29	30	30
No. with histologically neg. specimens	38	26	4	0	21
No. continuously NED	34	32	24	24§	27
5-Year Actuarial Survival	. . .	78%	. . .	72%	. . .
Median follow-up, mo (range)	50 (18–124)	39 (1–89)	51 (12–108)	25 (8–50)	? (9–76)

5-FU = 5-fluorouracil, RT = radiation therapy, CR = complete response, PR = partial response, APR = abdominoperineal resection, LE = local excision, fx = fraction(s), d = day, NED = no evidence of disease.
*Most patients did not receive maintenance chemotherapy.[106]
†Continuous radiation therapy in 16 patients and split course in 14.
‡Surgery for known residual disease only.
§One half of patients with local failure were salvaged with local resection.

(including a high complete remission rate) and that further surgery, if needed, can be limited to an excisional biopsy of residual scar. Thus, for many patients with relatively large anal epidermoid tumors, a colostomy can be avoided with an excellent survival expectation.

Table 30-4 summarizes the results of therapy in a number of large series.[98-103] Because anal canal tumors are rare, there are no prospective controlled randomized trials comparing chemotherapy plus irradiation with irradiation alone or surgery alone. However, because the combined approach yields comparable or superior results with modest morbidity and a high rate of sphincter preservation, a prospective controlled study does not seem to be required to accept multimodality therapy as conventional treatment for the majority of patients with anal canal disease. One retrospective study that compared multimodality therapy with surgery or radiation therapy alone suggested a higher cure rate with multimodality therapy in patients with higher stage disease (sphincter muscle and/or perirectal node involvement).[104]

All of the larger series have followed a chemotherapy protocol similar to that pioneered by Nigro and co-workers[105]: 5-FU given by continuous 24-hour infusion for 4 to 5 days, plus a single bolus dose of mitomycin C. Combined therapy has been given concurrently or sequentially. In the concurrent regimen, radiation therapy and chemotherapy are initiated on the same day. In the sequential regimen, chemotherapy is given before radiation therapy. In addition to differences in timing of administration, the dose of radiation therapy has also varied (see Table 30-4). Furthermore, in centers such as Wayne State University and the Memorial Sloan-Kettering Cancer Center, chemotherapy plus radiation therapy has been given prior to a planned surgical procedure—initially abdominoperineal resection, later local excision. At Highland Hospital in Rochester, New York, and the Princess Margaret Hospital, radiation therapy to higher total doses was definitive treatment; surgery was not part of the treatment plan. Despite these differences between trials, there is little evidence from these four studies, all of which were conducted on relatively small groups of patients, that one schedule or dose level is markedly superior to another. Response and survival rates are similar, although fewer patients may require an abdominoperineal resection after concurrent chemotherapy and radiation therapy to higher doses.

Some investigators have found that any patient with a positive biopsy result after completion of the initial treatment was certain to have recurrence of disease. All seven patients at Wayne State University with positive biopsy findings at that point had recurrent disease, despite salvage abdominoperineal resection performed in six patients.[98] However, this is not the experience of others.[99,106]

Combined therapy can be given in a community setting,[107] but because this approach involves careful interdigitation of several disciplines, it should be initiated only if there is a sufficient patient load to make such interactions workable (*e.g.*, more than ten patients per year). Results in 30 patients with anal canal tumors treated at a community hospital[102,103] in California (see Table 30-4) were similar to results achieved at the larger centers, with no patient experiencing more than group II toxicity on a modified scale.[108]

The best chemotherapy–radiation therapy regimen and the most appropriate radiation dose to use for patients with anal canal tumors limited to the primary site have not yet been defined. Distant recurrence is not the major problem in these patients. Local recurrence is more common, especially if the radiation dose is low (3000 cGy). 5-FU probably acts as a radiosensitizer,[109] while mitomycin is probably not synergistic.[110] Byfield and co-workers treated 11 patients with a 120-hour infusion of 5-FU at 25 mg/kg/24 h and concurrent irradiation, and omitted mitomycin.[111] Radiation therapy was given in 4-day cycles (1000 cGy/cycle) separated by at least 9 days, to a total dose of 3000 to 4750 cGy. All patients had complete clinical regressions; only one had active disease histologically. There was only one local recurrence.

The chemotherapy regimen of mitomycin C and 5-FU is quite active against anal canal tumors, with major response rates in the 50% to 60% range when used in chemotherapy alone trials. However, some patients do not respond or have less than a complete remission with this combination. It may be possible to identify subsets of patients at greater risk for failure who would be candidates for aggressive investigational chemotherapy–radiation therapy regimens.

RADICAL SURGERY. Before the widespread use of multimodality therapy, more than 90% of patients with potentially curable anal canal cancers required abdominoperineal resection. A wide perineal dissection in association with a posterior vaginectomy in women was recommended.[14,68] Despite initial enthusiasm from the group at Memorial Hospital in regard to vaginectomy, a more recent analysis discounted its routine application.[7] Lateral pelvic lymphadenectomy was initially advocated by the same group on the basis of a 24% incidence of pathologically positive nodes.[59] Subsequent analysis could not define any therapeutic benefit for this extended abdominoperineal resection.[7] The overall cure rate with abdominoperineal resection is approximately 50%.[112]

The Mayo Clinic experience initially reported in 1976 by Beahrs and Wilson[52] has been updated by Boman et al.[54] Disease recurred in 40% of the 114 patients, with subsequent treatment resulting in a 71% 5-year survival rate. At the Ellis Fischel State Cancer Hospital in Columbia, Missouri, the 5-year survival rate in 46 patients was 58%.[67] The M. D. Anderson Hospital group reported a 62% 5-year survival rate in 109 patients treated with only abdominoperineal resection.[90] One sixth of the cases were anal margin cancers. The most recent Memorial Hospital update includes 103 patients treated by radical surgery, with a 55% 5-year survival rate.[97] All of these tumors involved the dentate line. The 5-year survival in patients with tumors larger than 5 cm was only 40%. At St. Mark's Hospital, the 5-year survival rate in 83 patients with anal cancers involving the dentate line treated by radical surgery was 48%.[70]

Treatment failure despite radical surgery is both locoregional and distant. In the Mayo Clinic experience, 84% of initial sites of failure included local and regional disease.[54] The majority of cancer-related deaths are secondary to uncontrolled locoregional tumor. One third to one half of patients with locally advanced anal cancers treated by abdominoperineal resection at the major centers known for their expertise in this disease still had local recurrence in the pelvis or perineum.[54,68,70,90,97]

Today, with the success of combined modality therapy, an abdominoperineal resection should be reserved for salvage of the few patients in whom multimodality treatment fails.

INTERSTITIAL RADIATION THERAPY. Interstitial radiation therapy was originally used because of the limitations of orthovoltage irradiation. It had the potential of curing only early lesions that were unlikely to spread to the lymph nodes. Radium needles have been used primarily, although interstitial implants with ^{192}Ir have also been used. Radium needles were used for several years at the Christie Hospital in Manchester, England,[88,93] and are still used there for early anal lesions. In a recent update from that institution, radium needles were the exclusive treatment modality in 74 patients, 43 with anal canal lesions and 31 with anal margin lesions.[93] The minimum follow-up period was 5 years. Of the 68 evaluable patients, 33 (49%) were disease-free at 5-year follow-up or at death and were considered to have been cured. Of the 35 locoregional failures, 7 were salvaged by a surgical procedure. Local control was achieved in 64% of tumors less than 5 cm in diameter but in only 23% of tumors 5 cm or larger. The investigators recommend only local excision or an implant for tumors less than 5 cm in diameter with clinically negative nodes, and close follow-up and surgical resection for any recurrence.

Radium implantation has also been used extensively by Papillon,[80] but he has abandoned this technique because of painful local reactions and inability to achieve nodal control because of the small target volume.[84] Early studies with radium needles yielded a severe necrosis rate of about 25%.[88,113,114] Utilizing ^{192}Ir to a dose of 6000 cGy, Keiling and co-workers observed no local failures in 12 patients but a 16% local necrosis rate, although all healed with conservative treatment.[115] In two patients disease recurred in regional lymph nodes, again emphasizing the lack of control outside the very small target volume.

Combined multimodality techniques are yielding better

local control, sphincter preservation, and survival rates and should be considered for locoregional anal canal disease.

EXTERNAL IRRADIATION. External irradiation may be used with fields designed to cover the pelvic and inguinal node areas, which are at risk in anal canal cancer. In the modern megavoltage era, there is less morbidity from external irradiation than there was in the orthovoltage era. Computed tomography (CT) may aid in the planning of treatment. For example, boost doses, whether given by external irradiation or by interstitial implant, may be better designed with the use of CT. A study reported from Duke University Medical Center found excellent definition of tumor extent (local spread, lymph node involvement, and distant metastases) with CT of the pelvis, and CT was also useful for follow-up for potential recurrence.[116]

The results of major studies using external irradiation alone are given in Table 30-5. Local control overall ranges from 60% to 80%, while overall survival ranges from 50% to 80%. Two French studies, from the Institut Curie[108] and the Institut Gustave Roussy,[117] show that 5-year survival is related to the extent of the primary tumor as determined from either tumor size or the 1978 UICC T staging. A study from San Francisco found that survival is better in tumors less than 5 cm in diameter with negative nodes.[13,118] Of interest, in an update of the Institut Curie external irradiation data, the investigators expressed the belief that multimodality therapy is now the best approach for curative therapy.[119] Investigators at the Princess Margaret Hospital, who compared multimodality therapy with external irradiation, also concluded that multimodality therapy affords better local control and therefore a better colostomy-free survival.[100] In a study from Russia, in which the length of follow-up is unclear, similar results were obtained for 5-year survivals by T stage.[120]

In all of the studies listed in Table 30-5, the rate of complications requiring surgery remains around 5% to 15%, probably reflecting the high doses (6000–7000 cGy) that must be delivered to the primary site to control this disease when radiation therapy is the sole treatment modality. The addition of bleomycin to external irradiation in ten patients has not offered any added benefit in terms of decreased recurrence.[121]

COMBINED INTERSTITIAL AND EXTERNAL IRRADIATION. Several studies on small numbers of patients have been done with external irradiation combined with implants (^{137}Cs, ^{192}Ir, radium needles).[90,92,122,123] Good local control was achieved, but there was still a relatively high rate of complications requiring surgery or leading to death. Delouche et al reporting on 22 patients followed up for 5 to 13 years, noted a 32% rate of moderate to severe complications with 3000 to 4000 cGy external radiation therapy and 3500 to 4000 cGy ^{192}Ir implant.[122] However, a 78% local control rate was achieved, with an overall survival of 45%.

The most extensive series is that from the Centre Leon Berard in which 222 patients were treated over a 15-year period with external radiation therapy (^{60}Co) to a dose of 3000 to 4200 cGy across the target volume, followed by an ^{192}Ir implant 2 months later to a dose of 1500 to 2000 cGy.[84] The investigators reported only a 3% rate of serious complications, 65% 5-year disease-free survival, and 79% locoregional control. Combined brachytherapy and external irradiation may also be useful in very extensive lesions,[124,125] described below in the section on Locally Advanced and Recurrent Cancer.

In summary, combined interstitial and external radiation therapy may yield high local control rates but a significant complication rate. However, a 5-year disease-free survival rate of 65%, as reported by Papillon,[84] is excellent and compares favorably with results in surgically treated patients.

Locally Advanced and Recurrent Cancer

Recurrent *anal margin* cancer, after local excision, may require only further local excision for salvage. In a study from Memorial Sloan-Kettering Cancer Center, 16 patients in whom disease recurred underwent additional surgical procedures; of these, 12 were alive at 5 years and only two had died of disease.[81] One patient was unavailable for follow-up. Eleven of the 12 patients with local failure underwent local excision only for salvage. More advanced primary or recur-

TABLE 30-5. Anal Canal Carcinoma: Treatment with External Radiation Therapy Alone

Study	*No. of Patients*	*Primary Site Dose (cGy)*	*Follow-up (Yr)*	*Complications Requiring Surgery*	*5-Year Survival*		*Local Control*
Institut Curie[108]	158	6500–7000	3–14	8%	T ≤ 4 cm:	70%	
					>4 cm T≤6 cm:	57%	
					T > 6 cm:	33%	
					All:	51%	67%
					UICC 1978 stage		
Inst. Gustave Roussy[117]	64	6000–6500	2–13	14%	T1, T2:	72%	91%
					T3, T4:	35%	T3: 76%
							T4: 4/6
					All:	50%	81%
St Francis Hosp. et al[13,118]	39[13]	6500	0.5–8.5	13%	All:	79%	80%
	35[118]	4525–7550		6%	N0, <5 cm:	92%	77%
Princess Margaret Hosp.[100]	25	4500–6000	5–25	12%	All:	72%	60%

rent anal margin lesions may be salvaged by external radiation therapy.[80]

Patients with recurrent *anal canal* cancer after surgery should be considered for multimodality therapy (described in section on Multimodality Therapy for locoregional disease of the anal canal). Locoregional failures after initial multimodality therapy have been successfully treated with abdominoperineal resection[2] or with additional radiation and chemotherapy.[103]

Multimodality therapy for locally advanced primary anal canal tumors may yield good palliation and, in some cases, even cure. In a study reported from the University of Virginia, major regressions were observed in six of seven patients, three of whom were treated with chemotherapy alone and three with chemotherapy plus irradiation.[58] An abdominoperineal resection was performed on all patients, and all had delayed wound healing. Three of the seven patients remained disease-free for 24 to 26 months and four died, two of cancer and two of other causes. Another form of multimodality therapy, mitomycin C and 5-FU with external irradiation and interstitial ^{192}Ir implant, has been tried in 29 patients with advanced local disease.[126] With a follow-up of 5 to 54 months, 25 of 29 patients were alive and disease-free, only two of these having required radical salvage surgery with loss of sphincter function.

Brachytherapy combined with external irradiation has been used for advanced disease.[124,125] In a study from the University of California,[125] among 40 patients with anorectal cancer, eight had squamous cell or cloacogenic carcinoma and received combined external and interstitial ^{192}Ir irradiation. With a 2 to 6 year follow-up, there was a 10% rate of complications requiring surgery or leading to death. Although one cannot separate out the patients with epidermoid carcinomas in this study, there was a 70% local control rate and a 3-year disease-free survival rate of 60% in the entire group of 40 patients.

Inguinal Node Involvement

The initial experience from Memorial Hospital suggested that patients with grossly positive inguinal lymph nodes *synchronous* with the primary tumor were incurable.[127] A subsequent report indicated that two of 13 patients survived 5 years after abdominoperineal resection followed 6 weeks later by inguinal lymphadenectomy.[72] Other studies have confirmed a small cure rate for surgical treatment of patients with synchronous unilateral inguinal nodes.[52,67] Current recommendations are for limited surgical sampling, combined chemotherapy and radiation therapy with boost doses to the involved groin, and surgical salvage for isolated inguinal recurrence.

The development of unilateral *metachronous* inguinal lymph nodes does not carry such an ominous prognosis. After therapeutic groin dissection, the 5-7 year survival rate as reported from Memorial Hospital and St. Mark's Hospital exceeded 50%,[69,81] but it was nil in a small series reported from the Mayo Clinic.[52] Current strategies in patients with metachronous isolated inguinal node metastases after multimodality therapy include a formal groin dissection followed by chemotherapy. The use of radiation under these circumstances would depend on prior dose and fields.

Metastatic Disease

Because of its rarity and because many patients with anal canal tumors have locoregional disease that has been successfully treated by surgery alone, radiation therapy alone, or multimodality therapy, data on the use of chemotherapy as a single modality in the treatment of advanced disease are scanty. A number of anecdotal reports are available, however. Single-agent trials of Adriamycin and of cisplatin have been reported by several investigators. Fisher et al reported response to both Adriamycin as a single agent and cisplatin at a dosage of 2 mg/kg in an elderly man with advanced disease.[128] Salem et al studied cisplatin as a single agent in three patients: one achieved complete remission and the other two had partial regressions.[129] Earlier trials with 5-FU and vinblastine in small groups of patients were ineffective. Bleomycin and vincristine were used by Livingston et al in a single patient and a partial regression was observed.[130] Combination chemotherapy with cisplatin plus 5-FU has now been reported in two patients, again with major objective responses, one of which was a complete remission.[131]

One of the larger series of patients with advanced anal canal tumors treated with chemotherapy as primary management has been reported by Wilkin et al.[132] They treated a group of 15 patients with advanced disease with a non-cisplatin-containing combination of bleomycin, vincristine and high-dose methotrexate, with leucovorin rescue (BOM). Major objective regressions were seen in three (25%) of 12 patients with measurable disease, but the duration of response ranged from only 1 to 5 months. Toxicity was severe in one third of the patients, and four patients probably died as a result of toxicity. Wilkin et al concluded that although one fourth of the patients had responses, these were of short duration and associated with severe toxicity.

Magill et al treated a group of 19 patients (11 of whom had had prior chemotherapy) with a combination of cisplatin, bleomycin, and a vinca alkaloid (either vinblastine or vindesine). Six of 15 evaluable patients responded.[133]

In summary, anal canal tumors are sensitive to several chemotherapeutic agents, including cisplatin and mitomycin–5-FU. The optimal regimen remains to be defined. Complete remissions are possible, but relapse of distant metastases has always been seen.

FOLLOW-UP

Patients with squamous cell cancer of the anus require careful follow-up. Those with local or regional recurrence can be treated curatively, and those with systemic disease are eligible for effective chemotherapy. Follow-up should include interval history, physical examination, and liver function tests every 2 to 3 months for the first 3 years, then semiannually for another several years. The detection of local and inguinal node recurrence requires follow-up by the same physicians in order to differentiate post-treatment scar and inflammatory lymphadenitis from progressive recurrent tumor. Regular chest radiography and abdominal or pelvic CT at least yearly for the first 3 years is appropriate.

Management of patients with residual or recurrent local disease, as well as those with metachronous regional lymph nodes, was discussed earlier. The most recent report from the Memorial Hospital group documents the efficacy of surgical treatment of such patients.[81] Additional chemotherapy as definitive treatment or as a surgical adjuvant will likely improve these results further.[103]

ANORECTAL MELANOMA

Anorectal melanomas are rarely diagnosed at a curable stage, and most patients die within a year of diagnosis from systemic metastases. Fortunately, such tumors are rare, accounting for approximately 1% of anal cancers. Ultraradical surgery involving an abdominoperineal resection with inguinal and pelvic lymphadenectomy was the recommended approach for many years.[134] The end results with such approaches are poor, and current recommendations encourage a sphincter-saving local treatment if at all feasible.

Clinical and Pathologic Features

The diagnosis of anorectal melanoma is frequently delayed because the tumor is located deep within the anal canal and because symptoms are typically nonspecific "hemorrhoidal" complaints. Anal burning, pruritus, and minor intermittent blood on the toilet paper are usual. A mass, frequently nonpigmented, is seen at the dentate line, consistent with a thrombosed internal hemorrhoid. With progression, a prolapsing mass with increasing hemorrhage occurs, perhaps with palpable inguinal adenopathy. However, primary tumor progression is almost always cephalad. Although the majority of anal melanomas are pigmented on microscopic examination, only a small minority are grossly melanotic.[135] Asymptomatic anal melanoma is diagnosed as an incidental finding in hemorrhoidectomy specimens.

Patterns of Spread

Extensive proximal submucosal spread into the rectum occurs. Lymph node metastases are found in the mesorectal nodes in 50% of patients treated by radical surgery, and in the inguinal nodes in 20%.[134-136] Hematogenous metastases occur early and widely, primarily to the liver and lungs.

Treatment and End Results

The Memorial Hospital,[58,136-138] St. Mark's Hospital,[139] and Mayo Clinic[140] groups report the largest experience with these tumors, in addition to a composite experience from Israel.[141] In the initial reports from Memorial Hospital, abdominoperineal resection, alone or combined with pelvic and inguinal lymphadenectomy, was recommended for all patients without distant disease, but there were only three 5-year survivors of 50 patients so treated. In a smaller experience at St. Mark's Hospital, there were no 5-year survivors. In the few patients treated by wide local excision (2-cm margins), all patients died of distant disease without local recurrence. The Mayo Clinic experience with abdominoperineal resection is equally grim. In a report from Israel, only two of 30 patients survived 5 years, both after local excision.

A more recent analysis of the Memorial Hospital experience includes some patients treated by local measures, such as local excision, fulguration, and cryosurgery.[58] The end results as a function of tumor thickness provided the greatest insight into the far-advanced nature of these cancers when treatment is undertaken. All three patients with melanomas less than 2.0 mm thick were cured with abdominoperineal resection. No patient with a tumor thicker than 2.0 mm survived longer than 5 years, and 85% were dead in 2 years. Hence, it appears that only patients with "incidentally diagnosed" melanomas, usually as part of a hemorrhoidectomy specimen, are likely to be cured by surgery. Although the long-term survivors at Memorial Hospital were treated with radical surgery, that does not preclude cure with a more limited approach.[142] More advanced lesions may be treated by local excision combined with external-beam radiation therapy, at doses of at least 400 cGy per fraction.[143]

Summary

Patients with incidental anal melanomas less than 2 mm thick detected in hemorrhoidectomy specimens should undergo wide local excision. If the location of the tumor is unknown (multiple unmarked specimens sent to pathology), the patient may either be observed closely for signs of local recurrence or may undergo abdominoperineal resection.

Intermediate tumors, those more than 2 mm thick but not overly bulky, may be palliated with a local procedure — wide local excision, fulguration, laser vaporization, or cryosurgery. External-beam or implant radiation therapy may play an adjuvant role.

Despite the incurability of bulky anal melanoma, if the lesion cannot be controlled with a local approach, abdominoperineal resection or radiation therapy may still be necessary to palliate symptoms of bleeding, tenesmus, or obstruction.

Patients with systemic disease should be considered for chemotherapy and immunotherapy regimens appropriate for skin melanoma.

FUTURE DIRECTIONS

PREVENTION AND EARLY DETECTION. Prevention of epidermoid carcinoma of the anal canal will require better knowledge of etiologic factors. Meanwhile, because accumulating evidence implicates papillomaviruses as causative factors, and because the incidence of anal cancer appears to be increasing in the male homosexual community, it would be wise to direct further epidemiologic and virologic studies along these lines. Increasing use of measures for "safe sex" initiated to stem the spread of AIDS may also affect the incidence of anal cancer. Early detection could result from increased awareness in high-risk individuals; both male homosexuals and immunosuppressed renal transplant patients should be educated about anal cancer. Basic studies, such as the search for tumor markers or flow cytometric analyses for possible premalignant or diagnostic changes, may aid in detection as well as follow-up. Animal studies, such as those with epidermal growth factor, may offer insights into etiology and potentially lead to means of prevention.

THERAPY. Multimodality therapy has made great inroads in the sphincter-saving cure of anal cancer. Studies are now addressing issues such as the following: (1) decreasing thrombocytopenia during treatment by omitting mitomycin C from the regimen; (2) optimizing the treatment of patients with positive inguinal lymph nodes by limiting surgical excision to clinically grossly positive nodes and relying increasingly on high-dose nodal irradiation in combination with chemotherapy; (3) investigating more aggressive multimodality regimens for advanced local disease (*i.e.*, chemotherapy plus external-beam irradiation plus radioactive implants); and (4) exploring new aggressive chemotherapy regimens for patients with metastatic disease.

REFERENCES

1. Cummings BJ: The place of radiation therapy in the treatment of carcinoma of the anal canal. Cancer Treat Rev 9:125–147, 1982
2. Shank B: Treatment of anal canal carcinoma. Cancer 55:2156–2162, 1985
3. Papillon J: The responsibility of radiologists in the preservation of breast and rectum in cancer treatment. Clin Radiol 37:303–309, 1986
4. Grinnell RS: An analysis of forty-nine cases of squamous cell carcinoma of the anus. Surg Gynecol Obstet 98:29–39, 1954
5. Richards JC, Beahrs OH, Woolner LB: Squamous cell carcinoma of the anus, anal canal, and rectum in 109 patients. Surg Gynecol Obstet 114:475–482, 1962
6. Sawyers JL, Herrington JL Jr, Main FB: Surgical considerations in the treatment of epidermoid carcinoma of the anus. Ann Surg 157:817–824, 1963
7. Stearns MW Jr, Urmacher C, Sternberg SS et al: Cancer of the anal canal. Curr Probl Cancer 4:1–44, 1980
8. Morson BC, Volkstadt H: Malignant melanoma of the anal canal. J Clin Pathol 16:126–132, 1963
9. McConnell EM: Squamous cell carcinoma of the anus: A review of 96 cases. Br J Surg 57:89–92, 1970
10. Peters RK, Mack TM: Patterns of anal carcinoma by gender and marital status in Los Angeles County. Br J Cancer 48:629–636, 1983
11. Klotz RG, Pamukcoglu T, Souilliard DH: Transitional cloacogenic carcinoma of the anal canal. Cancer 20:1727–1745, 1967
12. Corman ML, Haggitt RC: Carcinoma of the anal canal. Surg Gynecol Obstet 145:674–676, 1977
13. Cantril ST, Green JP, Schall GL et al: Primary radiation therapy in the treatment of anal carcinoma. Int J Radiat Oncol Biol Phys 9:1271–1278, 1983
14. Welch JP, Malt RA: Appraisal of treatment of carcinoma of the anus and anal canal. Surg Gynecol Obstet 145:837–841, 1977
15. Gabriel WB: Discussion on squamous cell carcinoma of the anus and anal canal. Proc R Soc Med 53:403–409, 1960
16. Wolfe HRI, Bussey HJR: Squamous cell carcinoma of the anus. Br J Surg 55:295–301, 1968
17. Morson BC, Pang LSC: Pathology of anal cancer. Proc R Soc Med 61:623–624, 1968
18. Rousseau J, Mathieu G, Fenton J et al: La télécobaltothérapie des cancers du canal anal. J Radiol Electrol Med Nucl 54:622–626, 1973
19. Kapur BML, Dhawan IK, Singhal KK: Epidermoid carcinoma of the anorectum: Review of 31 cases. Dis Colon Rectum 20:252–254, 1977
20. Cooper HS, Patchefsky AS, Marks G: Cloacogenic carcinoma of the anorectum in homosexual men: An observation of four cases. Dis Colon Rectum 22:557–558, 1979
21. Li FP, Osborn D, Cronin CM: Anorectal squamous carcinoma in two homosexual men. Lancet 2:391, 1982
22. Austin DF: Etiologic clues from descriptive epidemiology: Squamous carcinoma of the rectum or anus. Natl Cancer Inst Monogr 62:89–90, 1982
23. Daling JR, Weiss NS, Klopfenstein LL et al: Correlates of homosexual behavior and the incidence of anal cancer. JAMA 247:1988–1990, 1982
24. Daling JR, Weiss NS, Hislop G et al: Sexual practices, sexually transmitted diseases, and the incidence of anal cancer. N Engl J Med 317:973–977, 1987
25. zur Hausen H: Human papillomaviruses and their possible role in squamous cell carcinomas. Curr Top Microbiol Immunol 78:1–30, 1977
26. Siegel A: Malignant transformation of condyloma acuminatum: Review of the literature and case report. Am J Surg 103:613–617, 1962
27. Friedberg MJ, Serlin O: Condyloma acuminatum: Its association with malignancy. Dis Colon Rectum 6:352–355, 1963
28. Oriel JD, Whimster IW: Carcinoma in situ associated with virus-containing anal warts. Br J Dermatol 84:71–73, 1971
29. Prasad ML, Abcarian H: Malignant potential of perianal condyloma acuminatum. Dis Colon Rectum 23:191–197, 1980
30. Croxson T, Chabon AB, Rorat E et al: Intraepithelial carcinoma of the anus in homosexual men. Dis Colon Rectum 27:325–330, 1984
31. McAnally AK, Dockerty MB: Carcinoma developing in chronic draining cutaneous sinuses and fistulas. Surg Gynecol Obstet 88:87–96, 1949
32. Winkelman J, Grosfeld J, Bigelow B: Colloid carcinoma of anal-gland origin: Report of a case and review of the literature. Am J Clin Pathol 42:395–401, 1964
33. Bretlau P: Carcinoma arising in anal fistula. Acta Chir Scand 133:496–500, 1967
34. Chaos A, Garrido H, Fernandez-Villoria JM: Carcinoma associated with fistula in ano. Int Surg 58:497–499, 1973
35. Binkley GE, Derrick WA: The association of squamous cancer with anal manifestations of lymphogranuloma venereum. Am J Dig Dis 12:46–47, 1945
36. Rainey R: The association of lymphogranuloma inguinale and cancer. Surgery 35:221–235, 1954
37. Brennan JT, Stewart CF: Epidermoid carcinoma of the anus. Ann Surg 176:787–790, 1972
38. Buckwalter JA, Jurayj MN: Relationship of chronic anorectal disease to carcinoma. Arch Surg 75:352–361, 1957
39. Chuang TY, Perry HO, Kurland LT et al: Condyloma acuminatum in Rochester, Minnesota, 1950–1978: II. Anaplasias and unfavorable outcomes. Arch Dermatol 120:476–483, 1984
40. Cabrera A, Tsukada Y, Pickren JW et al: Development of lower genital carcinomas in patients with anal carcinoma: A more than casual relationship. Cancer 19:470–480, 1966
41. Goligher JC: Surgery of the Anus, Rectum and Colon, 3rd ed, p 815. London, Bailere, Tindell and Cassell Ltd, 1975
42. Penn I: Cancers of the anogenital region in renal transplant recipients: Analysis of 65 cases. Cancer 58:611–616, 1986
43. Daniell HW: Re: causes of anal carcinoma. JAMA 254:358, 1985
44. Cone LA, Woodard DR, Potts BE et al: An update on the acquired immunodeficiency syndrome (AIDS): Associated disorders of the alimentary tract. Dis Colon Rectum 29:60–64, 1986
45. Kawaura A, Kumagai H, Shibata M et al: Tumors of the anal region induced in mice painted with methylazoxymethanol acetate. Gann 72:886–890, 1981
46. Kingsnorth AN, Abu-Khalaf M, Ross JS et al: Potentiation of 1,2-dimethylhydrazine-induced anal carcinoma by epidermal growth factor in mice. Surgery 97:696–700, 1985
47. Kuehn PG, Beckett R, Eisenberg H et al: Epidermoid carcinoma of the perianal skin and anal canal. N Engl J Med 270:614–617, 1964
48. Adam YG, Efron G: Current concepts and controversies concerning the etiology, pathogenesis, diagnosis and treatment of malignant tumors of the anus. Surgery 101:253–266, 1987
49. Morson BC: The pathology and results of treatment of squamous cell carcinoma of the anal canal and anal margin. Proc R Soc Med 53:414–420, 1960
50. Greenall MJ, Quan SHQ, Stearns MW et al: Epidermoid cancer of the anal margin. Am J Surg 149:95–101, 1985
51. Hardy KJ, Hughes ESR, Cuthbertson AM: Squamous cell carcinoma of the anal canal and anal margin. Aust NZ J Surg 38:301–305, 1969
52. Beahrs OH, Wilson SM: Carcinoma of the anus. Ann Surg 184:422–428, 1976
53. Wood DA: Tumors of the intestines. In: Atlas of Tumor Pathology, pp 200–223. Washington, DC, Armed Forces Institute of Pathology, 1967
54. Boman BM, Moertel CG, O Connell MJ et al: Carcinoma of the anal canal: A clinical and pathologic study of 188 cases. Cancer 54:114–125, 1984
55. Ordonez NG, Awalt H, Mackay B: Mammary and extramammary Paget's disease: An immunocytochemical and ultrastructural study. Cancer 59:1173–1183, 1987
56. Remigio PA, Der BK, Forsberg RT: Anorectal melanoma: Report of two cases. Dis Colon Rectum 19:350–356, 1976
57. Quinn D, Selah C: Malignant melanoma of the anus in a Negro: Report of a case and review of the literature. Dis Colon Rectum 20:627–631, 1977
58. Wanebo HJ, Woodruff JM, Farr GH et al: Anorectal melanoma. Cancer 47:1891–1900, 1981
59. Stearns MW, Quan SH: Epidermoid carcinoma of the anorectum. Surg Gynecol Obstet 191:953–957, 1970
60. Dougherty B, Evans H: Carcinoma of the anal canal: A study of 79 cases. Am J Clin Pathol 83:159–164, 1985
61. Fenger C, Nielsen VT: Precancerous changes in the anal canal epithelium in resection specimens. Acta Pathol Microbiol Immunol Scand [A] 94:63–69, 1986
62. Fenger C, Nielsen VT: Dysplastic changes in the anal canal epithelium in minor surgical specimens. Acta Pathol Microbiol Immunol Scand [A] 89:463–465, 1981
63. Fenger C, Bichel P: Flow cytometric DNA analysis of anal canal epithelium and ano-rectal tumours. Acta Pathol Microbiol Scand [A] 89:351–355, 1981
64. Goldman S, Auer G, Erhardt K et al: Prognostic significance of clinical stage, histologic grade, and nuclear DNA content in squamous-cell carcinoma of the anus. Dis Colon Rectum 30:444–448, 1987
65. Singh R, Nime F, Mittelman A: Malignant epithelial tumors of the anal canal. Cancer 48:411–415, 1981
66. Salmon RJ, Zafrani B, Habib A et al: Prognosis of cloacogenic and squamous cancers of the anal canal. Dis Colon Rectum 29:336–340, 1986
67. Dillard BM, Spratt JS Jr, Ackerman LV et al: Epidermoid cancer of anal margin and canal. Arch Surg 86:772–777, 1963
68. Clark J. Petrelli N, Herrera L et al: Epidermoid carcinoma of the anal canal. Cancer 57:400–406, 1986
69. Wolfe HRI: The management of metastatic inguinal adenitis in epidermoid cancer of the anus. Proc R Soc Med 61:626–629, 1961
70. Hardcastle JD, Bussey HJR: Results of surgical treatment of squamous cell carcinoma of the anal canal and anal margin seen at St. Mark's Hospital 1928–66. Proc R Soc Med 61:629–630, 1968
71. Kuehn PG, Beckett R, Eisenberg H et al: Hematogenous metastases from epidermoid carcinoma of the anal canal. Am J Surg 109:445–449, 1965

72. Greenall MJ, Quan SHQ, DeCosse J: Epidermoid cancer of the anus. Br J Surg 72:S97–S103, 1985
73. Pyper PC, Parks TG: The results of surgery for epidermoid carcinoma of the anus. Br J Surg 72:712–714, 1985
74. Paradis P, Douglass HO Jr, Holyoke ED: The clinical implications of a staging system for carcinoma of the anus. Surg Gynecol Obstet 141:411–416, 1975
75. Harmer MH (ed.): TNM Classification of Malignant Tumors, 3rd ed, pp 77–81. Geneva, International Union Against Cancer (Union Internationale Contre le Cancer), 1978
76. Hermanek P: Problems of pTNM classification of carcinoma of the stomach, colorectum and anal margin. Pathol Res Pract 181:296–300, 1986
77. Spiessl B, Hermanek P, Scheibe O et al (ed): TNM-Atlas: Illustrated Guide to the TNM/pTNM Classification of Malignant Tumours, 2nd ed, pp 114–123. New York, Springer-Verlag, 1982
78. Hermanek P, Sobin LH (eds): TNM Classification of Malignant Tumours, 4th ed, pp 50–52, 83–88. New York, Springer-Verlag, 1987
79. American Joint Committee on Cancer: Manual for Staging of Cancer, 3rd ed. Philadelphia, JB Lippincott Co, 1987
80. Papillon J: Rectal and Anal Cancers, pp 124–125. New York, Springer-Verlag, 1982
81. Greenall M, Magill G, Quan S et al: Recurrent epidermoid cancer of the anus. Cancer 57:1437–1441, 1986
82. Kuehn PG, Eisenberg H, Reed JF: Epidermoid carcinoma of the perianal skin and anal canal. Cancer 22:932–938, 1968
83. Wanebo H, Futrell W, Constable W: Multimodality approach to surgical management of locally advanced epidermoid carcinoma of the anorectum. Cancer 47:2817–2826, 1981
84. Papillon J, Montbarbon JF: Epidermoid carcinoma of the anal canal: A series of 276 cases. Dis Colon Rectum 30:324–333, 1987
85. Serota AI, Weil M, Williams RA et al: Anal cloacogenic carcinoma. Arch Surg 116:456–459, 1981
86. Grodsky L: Unsuspected anal cancer discovered after minor anorectal surgery. Dis Colon Rectum 10:471–478, 1967
87. Turell R: Epidermoid squamous cell cancer of the perianus and anal canal. Surg Clin North Am 42:1235–1241, 1962
88. Dalby JF, Pointon RS: The treatment of anal carcinoma by interstitial irradiation. AJR 85:515–520, 1961
89. Schraut WH, Wang C-H, Dawson PJ et al: Depth of invasion, location, and size of cancer of the anus dictate operative treatment. Cancer 51:1291–1296, 1983
90. Frost DB, Richards PC, Montague ED et al: Epidermoid cancer of the anorectum. Cancer 53:1285–1293, 1984
91. Cummings BJ, Keane TJ, Hawkins NV et al: Treatment of perianal carcinoma by radiation (RT) or radiation plus chemotherapy (RTCT) (abstr). Int J Radiat Oncol Biol Phys 12:170, 1986
92. Hintz BL, Charyulu KKN, Sudarsanam A: Anal carcinoma: Basic concepts and management. J Surg Oncol 10:141–150, 1978
93. James RD, Pointon RS, Martin S: Local radiotherapy in the management of squamous carcinoma of the anus. Br J Surg 72:282–285, 1985
94. Papillon J, Renard L, Pipard G: Le cancer de la marge de l'anus: Experience du Centre Leon Berard. J Eur Radiother 6:29–34, 1985
95. Glimelius B, Påhlman L: Recurrent epidermoid cancer of the anus. Cancer 57:1437–1441, 1986
96. Al-Jurf AS, Turnbull RB, Fazio VW: Local treatment of squamous cell carcinoma of the anus. Surg Gynecol Obstet 148:576–578, 1979
97. Greenall MJ, Quan SHQ, Urmacher C et al: Treatment of epidermoid carcinoma of the anal canal. Surg Gynecol Obstet 161:509–517, 1985
98. Leichman L, Nigro N, Vaitkevicius VK et al: Cancer of the anal canal: Model for preoperative adjuvant combined modality therapy. Am J Med 78:211–216, 1985
99. Enker WE, Heilweil M, Janov AJ et al: Improved survival in epidermoid carcinoma of the anus in association with pre-operative multi-disciplinary therapy. Arch Surg 121:1386–1390, 1986
100. Cummings B, Keane T, Thomas G et al: Results and toxicity of the treatment of anal canal carcinoma by radiation therapy or radiation therapy and chemotherapy. Cancer 54:2062–2068, 1984
101. Sischy B: The use of radiation therapy combined with chemotherapy in the management of squamous cell carcinoma of the anus and marginally resectable adenocarcinoma of the rectum. Int J Radiat Oncol Biol Phys 11:1587–1593, 1985
102. John MJ, Flam M, Lovalvo L et al: Feasibility of non-surgical definitive management of anal canal carcinoma. Int J Radiat Oncol Biol Phys 13:299–303, 1987
103. Flam MS, John M, Mowry P et al: Definitive combined modality therapy of carcinoma of the anus: A report of 30 cases including results of salvage therapy in patients with residual disease. Dis Colon Rectum 30:495–502, 1987
104. Ajlouni M, Mahrt D, Milad MP: Review of recent experience in the treatment of carcinoma of the anal canal. Am J Clin Oncol 7:687–691, 1984
105. Nigro ND, Vaitkevicius VK, Considine B Jr: Combined therapy for cancer of the anal canal: A preliminary report. Dis Colon Rectum 17:354–356, 1974
106. Michaelson RA, Magill GB, Quan SHQ et al: Pre-operative chemotherapy and radiation therapy in the management of anal epidermoid carcinoma. Cancer 51:390–395, 1983
107. Nigro ND: Multi-disciplinary management of cancer of the anus. World J Surg 11:446–451, 1987
108. Salmon RJ, Fenton J, Asselain B et al: Treatment of epidermoid anal canal cancer. Am J Surg 147:43–48, 1984
109. Byfield JE, Calabro-Jones P, Klisak I et al: Pharmacologic requirements for obtaining sensitization of human tumor cells *in vitro* to combined 5-fluorouracil or ftorafur and x rays. Int J Radiat Oncol Biol Phys 8:1923–1933, 1982
110. Rockwell S: Cytotoxicities of mitomycin C and X rays to aerobic and hypoxic cells *in vitro*. Int J Radiat Oncol Biol Phys 8:1035–1039, 1982
111. Byfield JE, Barone RM, Sharp TR et al: Conservative management without alkylating agents of squamous cell anal cancer using cyclical 5-FU alone and X-ray therapy. Cancer Treat Rep 67:709–712, 1985
112. Golden GT, Horsley JS III: Surgical management of epidermoid carcinoma of the anus. Am J Surg 131:275–280, 1976
113. Bond WH: Proc R Soc Med 53:411–414, 1960
114. Devois A, Decker R: La curiepuncture du cancer de l'anus. Arch Fr Mal Appar Dig Mal Nutr 49(suppl):54–67, 1960
115. Keiling R, Grunewald JM, Achille E: Radiothérapie des cancers malpighiens de l'anus: La curiethérapie interstitielle à l'iridium 192 des epitheliomas du canal anal. J Radiol Electrol Med Nucl 54:634–635, 1973
116. Cohan RH, Silverman PM, Thompson WM et al: Computed tomography of epithelial neoplasms of the anal canal. AJR 145:569–573, 1985
117. Eschwege F, Lasser P, Chavy A et al: Squamous cell carcinoma of the anal canal: Treatment by external beam irradiation. Radiother Oncol 3:145–150, 1985
118. Doggett SW, Green JP, Cantril ST: Efficacy of radiation alone for limited squamous cell carcinoma of the anal canal. Int J Radiat Oncol Biol Phys 12(suppl):170–171, 1986
119. Fenton J, Cutuli B, Rousseau J et al: Anal canal carcinoma: Survival and sphincter preservation after radiotherapy (195 cases) (abstr). Presented at the fifth annual meeting of the European Society of Radiologic Therapy and Oncology, 1986
120. Chruscov MM, Semakina EP, Raifel BA: Die Strahlentherapie des rektalen Epidermoidkarzinoms. Radiobiol Radiother (Berlin) 19:683–689, 1978
121. Glimelius B, Påhlman L: Radiation therapy of anal epidermoid carcinoma. Int J Radiat Oncol Biol Phys 13:305–312, 1987
122. Delouche G, Bachelot F, Cohen M et al: La radiothérapie des cancers malpighiens de l'anus. J Radiol Electrol Med Nucl 54:642–646, 1973
123. Ager P, Samala E, Bosworth J et al: The conservative management of anorectal cancer by radiotherapy. Am J Surg 137:228–230, 1979
124. Martinez A, Edmundson GK, Cox RS et al: Combination of external beam irradiation and multiple-site perineal applicator (MUPIT) for treatment of locally advanced or recurrent prostatic, anorectal, and gynecologic malignancies. Int J Radiat Oncol Biol Phys 11:391–398, 1985
125. Puthawala AA, Syed N, Gates TC et al: Definitive treatment of extensive anorectal carcinoma by external and interstitial irradiation. Cancer 50:1746–1750, 1982
126. Pipard G, Peytremann R, Marti MC: Conservative multidisciplinary treatment of locally advanced epidermoid and cloacogenic cancer of the anal canal (abst). Proc Am Soc Clin Oncol 5:268, 1986
127. Stearns MW Jr: Epidermoid carcinoma of the anal region. Surg Gynecol Obstet 106:92–96, 1958
128. Fisher W, Herbst K, Sims J et al: Metastatic cloacogenic carcinoma of the anus: Sequential responses to Adriamycin and cis-dichlorodiamineplatinum (II). Cancer Treat Rep 62:91–97, 1978
129. Salem P, Habboubi N, Naanasissie E et al: Effectiveness of cisplatin in the treatment of anal squamous cell carcinoma. Cancer Treat Rep 69:891–893, 1985
130. Livingston R, Bodey G, Gottlieb J et al: Kinetic scheduling of vincristine and bleomycin in patients with lung cancer and other malignant tumors. Cancer Chemother Rep 57:219–224, 1973
131. Khatr R, Frenay M, Bourry J et al: Cisplatin plus 5-fluorouracil in the treatment of metastatic anal squamous cell carinoma: A report of two cases. Cancer Treat Rep 70:1345–1346, 1986
132. Wilkin N, Petrelli N, Herrera L et al: Phase II study of combination of bleomycin, vincristine and high-dose methotrexate (BOM) with leucovorin rescue in advanced squamous cell carcinoma of the anal canal. Cancer Chemother Pharmacol 15:300–302, 1985
133. Magill GB: Personal communication, 1987
134. Pack GT, Martins FG: Treatment of anorectal malignant melanoma. Dis Colon Rectum 3:15–24, 1960
135. Morson BC, Volkstadt H: Malignant melanoma of the anal canal. J Clin Pathol 16:126–132, 1963
136. Quan SH, Deddish MR: Noncutaneous melanoma. CA 16:111–114, 1966
137. Quan SHQ, White JE, Deddish MR: Malignant melanoma of the anorectum. Dis Colon Rectum 2:275–283, 1959
138. Pack GT, Oropeza R: A comparative study of melanoma and epidermoid carcinoma of the anal canal: A review of 20 melanomas and 29 epidermoid carcinomas. Dis Colon Rectum 10:161–176, 1967
139. Ward MW, Romano G, Nicholls RJ. The surgical treatment of anorectal malignant melanoma. Br J Surg 73:68–69, 1986
140. Chiu YS, Unni KK, Beart RW: Malignant melanoma of the anorectum. Dis Colon Rectum 23:122–124, 1980
141. Siegel B, Cohen D, Jacob ET: Surgical treatment of anorectal melanomas. Am J Surg 146:336–338, 1983
142. Garnick M, Lokich JJ: Primary malignant melanoma of the rectum: Rationale for conservative surgical management. J Surg Oncol 10:529–531, 1978
143. Harwood AR, Cummings BJ: Radiotherapy for mucosal melanomas. Int J Radiat Oncol Biol Phys 8:1121–1126, 1982

W. MARSTON LINEHAN
WILLIAM U. SHIPLEY
DAN L. LONGO

CHAPTER 31 *Cancer of the Kidney and Ureter*

RENAL CELL CARCINOMA

Each year in the United States there are approximately 18,000 cases of renal cell carcinoma, resulting in more than 9,000 deaths. This tumor accounts for approximately 3% of adult malignancies and occurs in a male–female ratio of 2:1. It is more common among urban than rural residents. Although most cases of renal cell carcinoma occur in persons aged 50 to 70 years, it has been observed in children as young as 6 months of age. Between 1975 and 1984 there was a modest increase in the incidence of renal cell carcinoma, about 2% per year.[1–7]

Renal cell carcinoma was first described by Konig in 1826. As early as 1855 Robin concluded that the renal tubular epithelium was the most probable tissue of origin of the cancer, an observation that was confirmed by Waldeyer in 1867. In 1883 Grawitz, noting that the fatty content of the cancer cells was similar to that of adrenal cells, concluded that the tumors arose from adrenal rests within the kidney and introduced the term "stroma lipomatodes aberrata renis" for these clear cell tumors. The term "hypernephroid tumors" was introduced in 1894 by Birch-Hirschfeld. Since then the conceptually incorrect term "hypernephroma" has frequently been applied to renal tumors.[8–11]

Rarely, renal cell carcinoma occurs in a familial form. There is an increased incidence of renal cell carcinoma with von Hippel–Lindau syndrome: up to 35% of patients with von Hippel–Lindau syndrome will develop renal cell carcinoma. In both familial syndromes the renal cancer is often bilateral and tends to occur in a younger age group.[12–15] An increased incidence of renal cell carcinoma has also been observed in patients with autosomal dominant polycystic kidney disease.[16]

ETIOLOGY

A number of environmental, hormonal, cellular, and genetic factors have been studied as possible causal factors in the development of renal cell carcinoma. Cigarette smoking is a definite risk factor for the development of kidney cancer. It has been estimated that 30% of renal cell carcinomas in men and 24% in women may be directly due to smoking.[17–19] Obesity is associated with an increased risk of development of renal cell carcinoma, particularly in women.[18–20] Analgesic abuse, which is known to be associated with renal pelvis cancer, is also associated with an increased incidence of kidney cancer. The increased risk for the development of renal cell carcinoma is observed primarily in patients who abuse phenacetin-containing analgesics and develop analgesic nephropathy.[18,21]

A number of environmental and occupational factors have been associated with the development of kidney cancer. There is an increased incidence of renal cell carcinoma among leather tanners, shoe workers, and workers exposed to asbestos.[22,23] Exposure to cadmium is associated with an increased incidence of kidney cancer, particularly in men who smoke.[24] Patients exposed to thorotrast, a 2.5% solution of thorium dioxide used in the 1920s as a contrast medium for renal and hepatic visualization, have an increased incidence of kidney cancer. Thorium dioxide is a radioactive agent that produces α-rays, β-rays, and γ-rays; it is thought that chronic exposure to radiation emitted by this agent is responsible for the development of renal cancer.[25] An association between gasoline exposure and kidney cancer has been observed in animal studies. Although there is an increased incidence of renal cell carcinoma reported with exposure to petroleum, tar, and pitch products, studies of oil refinery workers and petroleum products distribution workers do not identify a definite relationship between gasoline exposure and renal cancer. There may be an increased risk of kidney cancer in older workers or in workers exposed to gasoline for prolonged periods of time.[26,27]

There is an increased incidence of renal cell carcinoma in patients who develop acquired cystic disease while on long-term hemodialysis.[28-31] Acquired cystic disease is a recently described phenomenon in which patients on long-term dialysis for renal failure develop cysts in their native kidneys. Renal cell carcinoma has been found in association with the papillary hyperplasia observed in the cyst epithelium of these kidneys. It is estimated that 35% to 47% of patients on long-term dialysis will develop acquired cystic disease, and about 5.8% of the patients with acquired cystic disease will develop renal cell cancer. Although most of these cancers are clinically insignificant and are found incidentally in autopsy or after bilateral nephrectomy, some will have an aggressive course.[28-30]

A hormonal etiology for renal cell carcinoma was suggested in 1947 based on a series of animal studies by Matthews and co-workers, who reported the induction of kidney tumors in male Syrian golden hamsters by prolonged administration of estrogen.[32,33] In a subsequent study published in 1952, Kirkman and Bacon reported treatment with estrogen of 100 male hamsters for 250 days; 97 developed renal tumors.[34] Bloom et al demonstrated that cortisone plus medroxyprogesterone acetate (Provera) could inhibit the growth of estrogen-induced, transplantable renal tumors, and that an estrogen antagonist could inhibit the growth of these tumors in the hamster.[35,36] The current role of hormonal therapy in the management of patients with metastatic renal cell carcinoma will be discussed.

GROWTH FACTORS

The role of tumor-produced growth factors in the initiation or progression of genitourinary malignancies is currently under study. In many patients with renal cell carcinoma there is evidence of tumor-produced factors that have systemic effects. Pyrexia, cachexia, abnormal liver function, increased alkaline phosphatase levels, hypercalcemia, polycythemia, neuromyopathy, and amyloidosis have all been reported in association with renal cell carcinoma.[37] Humoral hypercalcemia of malignancy, frequently observed in patients with renal cell carcinoma, is thought to be caused by a tumor-produced, systemically active bone-resorbing factor. Some studies suggest that this tumor-produced factor is parathyroid hormone (PTH)-like, others suggest that it is more transforming growth factor (TGF)-like.[38] A PTH-related protein that has been implicated in malignant hypercalcemia has been cloned from a human lung cancer cell line and expressed in mammalian cells.[39] Whether or not this PTH-like factor induces paracrine or endocrine effects such as bone resorption or hypercalcemia of malignancy in patients with renal cell carcinoma is currently under study.

It has been suggested that the bone-resorbing factor produced by human tumors may have TGF-like bioactivity. Derynck et al[40] have shown that renal cell carcinoma and renal cell carcinoma cell lines have increased expression of TGF-α, TGF-β, and epidermal growth factor (EGF) receptor.[40,41] Gomella and co-workers found greater expression of TGF-α and TGF-β in renal cell carcinoma than in normal renal tissue from the same patient.[42] TGF-α is known to bind to the EGF receptor and can induce reversible transformation of nontransformed cell lines.[43,44] TGF-β has been shown to inhibit both the growth of lymphokine-mediated stimulation of peripheral blood lymphocytes[45] and the lytic activity of lymphokine-activated killer cells.[46,47] These and other studies suggest the possibility that tumor-produced growth factors could have a number of roles in renal cell carcinoma. TGF-α, for example, could have an autocrine role in either initiation or progression of renal cell carcinoma by stimulation through the EGF-receptor and induction of unregulated cell growth. Bone resorption induced by TGF-α[48] or a PTH-like factor could release TGF-β from the bone (one of the largest reservoirs of TGF-β in the body), which could inhibit the host's immune response to the tumor.[45-47] It is hoped that an understanding of the role of soluble factors involved in regulation of growth of renal cell carcinoma will lead to new strategies for treatment of this disease. Studies of peptides that block growth factor receptor activation, antibodies that block growth factor receptors, and other agents that affect growth factor production and action are in progress.

MOLECULAR GENETICS

In the past ten years much information on the genetics of renal cell carcinoma has become available. In 1979 Cohen and co-workers described a pedigree with familial renal cell carcinoma in which the pattern of inheritance was consistent with an autosomal dominant gene.[49] Of particular interest was the association of renal cell carcinoma with a karyotypic abnormality, a balanced reciprocal translocation between the short arm of chromosome 3 and the long arm of chromosome 8. This abnormality was present in constitutional tissue and, therefore, presumably in tumor tissue of affected family members. All members of the family who developed renal cell carcinoma had a 3;8 translocation; no family member without a 3;8 translocation developed renal cell carcinoma. It has since been shown that in this kindred the cellular oncogene *c-myc* is translocated from chromosome 8 to chromosome 3 and the cellular oncogene *c-raf* is translocated from chromosome 3 to chromosome 8.[50] A second pedigree with renal cell carcinoma was described in 1982 by Pathak and co-workers.[51] In the propositus, the major karyotypic abnormality was a chromosome 3 to chromosome 11 translocation. This pedigree differed from the one described by Cohen et al. in that the karyotypic abnormality was limited to the tumor. Recently, chromosomal analysis performed on tumor cells from a patient with von Hippel–Lindau disease revealed a proximal deletion in the short arm of chromosome 3 in the 3p14 region.[52]

The studies of chromosomal abnormalities in familial renal cell carcinoma focused attention on the possible role of alterations in the short arm of chromosome 3 in the genesis of nonfamilial renal cell carcinoma. Chromosomal analysis by Yoshida et al,[53,54] Szucs et al,[55] and Carroll et al[56] suggested that a structural change in chromosome 3 is linked to sporadic as well as hereditary renal cell carcinoma. This information led to the use of restriction length fragment polymorphism (RFLP) analysis of chromosome 3 in constitutional and tumor tissue in patients with sporadic renal cell carcinoma.[57] The technique of RFLP analysis for detection of DNA sequence deletions in tumors, described by Cavanee et al in 1983, is more sensitive than karyotype analysis for detecting DNA sequence deletions.[58] RFLP analysis has been used to detect DNA sequence deletions in a number of human tumors, including Wilms' tumor,[59-62] retinoblastoma,[63] bladder cancer,[64] small cell lung carcinoma,[65] and colorectal carcinoma.[66] The use of RFLP analysis to define the somatic mechanisms involved in tumor development relies on the variability of DNA recognition sequences of bacterial restriction endonucleases.[63,67] Study of these RFLPs permits comparison of normal and tumor tissue for the presence or absence of DNA sequences. For example, the RFLP obtained with a particular probe for chromosome 3, pH3H2 (DNF15S2), detects a polymorphic locus at the 3p21 region.[68]

Zbar and co-workers performed RFLP analysis on normal and tumor tissue from 18 patients with renal cell carcinoma using three recombinant probes that have been mapped to the short arm of chromosome 3.[57] These investigators found evidence for a DNA sequence deletion (see Fig. 31-1) in 11 of 11 evaluable patients with renal cell carcinoma. The frequency of loss of 3p sequences in renal cell carcinoma is greater than that observed at other chromosomal loci in bladder carcinoma (42%), Wilms' tumor (55%), and colorectal carcinoma (20%) and suggests that loss of heterozygosity in this region is a nonrandom alteration and that a functioning gene located on 3p may be involved in the origin or evolution of renal cell carcinoma.[57,64,66]

Many of the biologic and genetic alterations in renal cell carcinoma are similar to those in retinoblastoma. Both neoplasms exist in hereditary and sporadic forms, and the hereditary form is associated with an earlier age at onset than is the sporadic form. The conceptual basis that seems to fit the current genetic data on retinoblastoma is consistent with the current molecular genetic data on renal cell carcinoma. The two-mutation theory of Knudson postulates that at least two mutations are necessary for the development of cancer (Fig. 31-2).[69,70] The data generated by chromosomal and RFLP analysis of renal cell carcinoma suggest that a somatic mutation is a chromosomal event that may involve the loss of the wild-type allele of a particular gene. In Wilms' tumor, which is associated with a DNA sequence deletion in the 13p region of chromosome 11, the introduction of a normal human chromosome 11 suppresses the tumorigenicity of Wilms' tumor cell lines.[71] Analogously, the introduction of a normal chromosome 3 back into a renal cell carcinoma cell line may be used to assess its effect on tumorigenesis.

FIG. 31-1. Chromosome 3 showing the area of interstitial deletion in renal cell carcinoma at 3p14-21 locus. * denotes the site of the c-erb a-2 oncogene; ** the c-raf-1 locus.

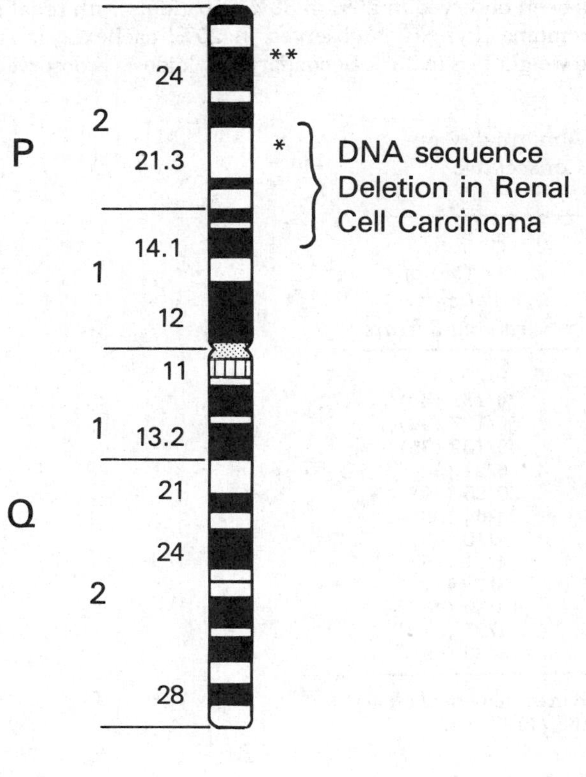

FIG. 31-2. Knudsen's hypothesis[69,70] as applied to renal cell carcinoma would suggest that RFLP analysis uncovers a DNA sequence deletion in allele A with a coexistent mutation at the same locus on allele A. In this region could be a gene that codes for a protein that regulates or suppresses growth factor or oncogene expression. (Comings, 1973).

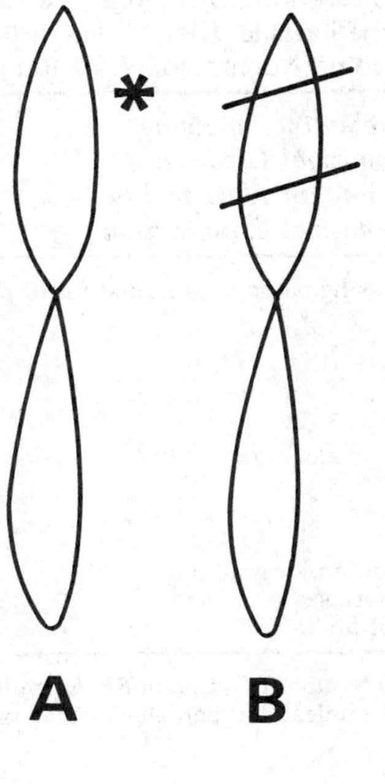

PATHOLOGY

For a number of years it was thought that renal cell carcinoma originated in adrenal rests within the kidney; immunohistologic and ultrastructural analysis has now established that the proximal renal tubular epithelium is the true tissue of origin.[1,72] Renal cell tumors tend to be round, but may vary widely in size. The average diameter is approximately 7 cm; however, renal tumors can often grow to fill the entire retroperitoneum. Previously, renal lesions 2 cm or less in diameter were considered to be renal adenomas, while lesions 2 cm or more in diameter were considered to be carcinomas. The distinction between benign and malignant tumors is no longer made on the basis of size but on the basis of classic histologic criteria.[72,73] Although renal cell carcinoma tends to arise in the cortex of the kidney, it can originate in the interior of the kidney. There is often a pseudocapsule formed around the tumor by compression of surrounding tissue. Hemorrhage and necrosis may be present, and frequently large areas of sclerosis and fibrosis are found within the tumor. Calcification and single or multiple fluid-filled cysts may be seen within the tumor. Sporadic renal cell carcinoma appears in either kidney with equal frequency; it is most often solitary and unilateral.

Renal cell carcinoma can occur in three different cellular types: clear cell, granular cell, and spindle or sarcomatoid variant. Clear cell carcinomas contain lightly staining cells with vacuolated cytoplasm containing cholesterol-like substances, neutral lipids, phospholipids, and glycogen.[1,74] Granular cell carcinomas contain cells that have a ground-glass–appearing, eosinophilic-staining cytoplasm with abundant mitochondria. The large nuclei of granular cells stain darker than the nuclei of clear cells. In sarcomatoid renal cell carcinoma there are spindle type cells which may resemble fibroblasts, rhabdomyoblasts, lipoblasts, or pleomorphic mesenchymal cells.[1,74–76] Few tumors are purely clear or granular cell type; most are mixtures of clear and granular cells. Depending on the series, 1% to 6% of renal cell carcinomas are sarcomatoid variant.[77,78]

Some studies suggest that there is slightly better prognosis with clear cell variant than with granular or mixed renal cell carcinomas.[79] The sarcomatoid variant is associated with a significantly poorer prognosis than are carcinomas of the clear, granular, or mixed cell type.[78,80–82] Sella and coworkers recently reported a median survival of only 6.6 months in 44 patients with sarcomatoid-type renal cell carcinoma, versus a 19.0-month median survival in 814 patients with nonsarcomatous renal cell carcinoma.[82] Although infrequently used in renal cell carcinoma, tumor grading may correlate with survival, particularly in patients with nonmetastatic cancer.[79,80,83]

CLINICAL PRESENTATION

Renal cell carcinoma may remain clinically occult for most of its course. The classic presentation of pain, hematuria, and flank mass occurs in only about 19% of patients and often is indicative of advanced disease.[1] A tumor in the kidney can progress unnoticed to a large size in the retroperitoneum until a metastasis appears. Approximately 30% of patients with renal cell carcinoma present with metastatic disease, 25% with locally advanced renal cell carcinoma, and 45% with localized disease (Table 31-1).[7,84] Some 75% of patients with metastatic renal cell carcinoma have metastases to the lung, 36% to soft tissues, 20% to bone, 18% to liver, 8% to cutaneous sites, and 8% to the central nervous system.[85]

A considerable number of patients with renal cell carcinoma develop systemic symptoms of this disease.[86–89] Hypochromic anemia, due to either hematuria or hemolysis, has been observed in 29% to 88% of patients with renal cell carcinoma. Pyrexia is observed in 20%; cachexia, fatigue, and weight loss in 33%. Secondary amyloidosis is observed in

TABLE 31-1. Presenting Symptoms, Laboratory Abnormality, or Abnormality on Physical Examination and Their Relation to Survival Rate in 309 Consecutive Patients Undergoing Nephrectomy for Renal Cell Carcinoma*

Presenting Symptom, Abnormal Laboratory Finding, or Abnormality on Physical Examination	*No. of Patients (% of total) (n = 309)*	*No. (%) of Patients Surviving 5 Years*
Classic triad (gross hematuria, abnormal mass, pain)	29 (9)	9/29 (31)
Hematuria	183 (59)	74/183 (40)
Pain	127 (41)	56/127 (44)
Abdominal mass	139 (45)	49/139 (35)
Fever	21 (7)	8/21 (38)
Weight loss	85 (28)	29/85 (39)
Anemia	64 (21)	24/64 (38)
Erythrocytosis	10 (3)	4/10 (40)
Hypercalcemia	11 (3)	4/11 (35)
Acute varicocele	7 (2)	3/7 (43)
Tumor calcification on x-ray film	39 (13)	18/39 (46)
Symptoms of metastases	31 (10)	1/31 (3)
Cancer, incidental finding	20 (7)	13/20 (65)

* Modified from Skinner DG, Colvin RB, Vermillion CD et al: Diagnosis and management of renal cell carcinoma: A clinical and pathologic study of 309 cases. Cancer 28:1165–1177, 1971.

3% to 5%.[37] Nonmetastatic hepatic dysfunction, initially described by Stauffer in 1961, is a reversible syndrome associated with renal carcinoma that tends to occur in association with fever, fatigue, and weight loss and resolves when the primary tumor is removed. Nonmetastatic hepatic dysfunction, which is usually associated with poor long-term prognosis, occurs in up to 7% of patients with renal cell carcinoma. Abnormal hepatic function is observed in up to 40%.[81,90–92]

Renin levels are often elevated in patients with renal cell carcinoma, but tend to return to normal after the kidney is removed. Whether the tumor itself produces renin or whether it induces renin production by compression of adjacent tissue is unclear. Immunocytochemical studies suggest that renal cell carcinoma may produce renin, which, however, may be biologically inactive.[89,93,94] Plasma fibrinogen levels are elevated in patients with renal cell carcinoma and may correlate with tumor stage, disease activity, and response to therapy.[95] Acquired dysfibrinogenemia has also been reported in association with renal cell carcinoma and can be a sensitive plasma marker for the disease and for tumor progression.[96]

RADIOGRAPHIC EVALUATION

It is often difficult to determine whether a space-occupying renal mass lesion is benign or malignant. In a series of 940 asymptomatic space-occupying renal mass lesions reported by Lang, 515 (55%) were benign renal cysts, and only 52 (5.5%) were malignant neoplasms (Table 31-2).[97] A number of diagnostic modalities are used to evaluate and stage renal mass lesions (Fig. 31-3), including excretory urography, computed tomography (CT), arteriography, venography, ultrasound, and magnetic resonance imaging (MRI). Excretory urography is commonly used in the initial evaluation of renal mass lesions, but because it is neither sensitive nor specific in renal cell carcinoma, a small to medium-sized tumor may be present when the excretory urogram appears normal. Excretory urography does provide important information about the location and function of the contralateral kidney, and this is particularly useful when surgery is being considered.

TABLE 31-2. Underlying Pathologic Conditions in 940 Asymptomatic Space-Occupying Lesions of the Kidney*

Type of Lesion	*No. of Lesions*	*% of Total No. of Lesions*
Cystic lesions		58
Benign cysts	515	
Benign hemorrhagic cysts	4	
Hydronephrosis	8	
Cystic dysplastic kidney	3	
Polycystic kidney	17	
Malignant neoplasms		5.5
Hypernephromas	21	
Other malignant neoplasms	31	
Benign neoplasms	40	4.2
Inflammatory lesions (pyelonephritis, abscess)	213	23
Intrarenal hematoma	7	0.7
Pseudotumors	81	8.6

* Modified from Lang EK: Diagnosis of renal and parenchymal tumors. In Skinner DG, deKernion JB (eds): Genitourinary Cancer, p 42. Philadelphia, WB Saunders, 1978.

Ultrasound examination provides excellent staging and diagnostic information and can provide accurate anatomic detail of extrarenal extension of tumor, adrenal involvement, involvement of lymph nodes, and infiltration of adjacent viscera.[1,98–100] It can also aid in the detection and delineation of renal vein or inferior vena caval involvement. Ultrasound examination is frequently used in the evaluation of renal cystic lesions that are detected on excretory urography or CT. If a cystic renal mass lesion appears potentially malignant on excretory urography, ultrasound, or CT, further evaluation by percutaneous cyst puncture under ultrasound or CT guidance may be performed. This procedure has two components: evaluation of cyst fluid and radiographic examination of the interior of the cyst. Cyst fluid aspirate is assessed for color, turbidity, and the presence of blood; and fat, protein, lactic acid dehydrogenase (LDH), and glucose content is measured. If the cyst is benign, there is typically a clear, straw-colored fluid that is low in fat, protein, and LDH content. When a cystic or necrotic tumor is aspirated, the fluid may be bloody and may have a high fat, protein, or LDH content. After the fluid is removed, the cyst is filled with contrast medium and air and imaged radiographically. A benign cyst should appear as a homogeneous sphere with a regular border; a tumor may show up as a nodule or mass protruding into the cyst.[98] The combination of ultrasound and cyst puncture enables the clinician to make the correct diagnosis in a very high percentage of suspicious renal mass lesions.[1]

Renal arteriography (see Figs. 31-4B, 31-4C) has historically been a standard part of the evaluation of patients with a suspicious renal mass. In a renal cell carcinoma the arteriogram will often show neovascularity, arteriovenous fistulas, pooling of contrast medium, and accentuation of capsular vessels. Epinephrine may be used as an aid in the diagnosis of an equivocal renal mass lesion. When epinephrine is infused into a normal kidney during arteriography the renal vessels constrict; the vessels in a renal cell carcinoma do not constrict owing to lack of musculature in the tumor vessels.[1] A renal arteriogram is particularly useful in evaluating an indeterminant small renal mass lesion and as an aid to the surgeon in defining the vasculature during the surgical removal of a large tumor.[101,102] Although renal arteriography can be performed with minimal risk, false aneurysms, arterial emboli, hemorrhage, and decreased renal function secondary to contrast agent injection have been reported.[1] Digital subtraction arteriography can define the tumor vasculature without the morbidity associated with standard arteriography and adequately demonstrates the main renal arterial anatomy in more than 80% of cases. The combination of CT and digital subtraction angiography yields satisfactory diagnostic and anatomic detail in most cases of renal cell carcinoma.[103]

CT is a useful imaging technique for renal cell carcinoma (see Fig. 31-5A).[5,100,101,104–109] In a study in which CT results were correlated with pathologic findings in 111 patients, perirenal extension was correctly identified in 79% of cases, lymph node involvement in 87%, renal vein involvement in

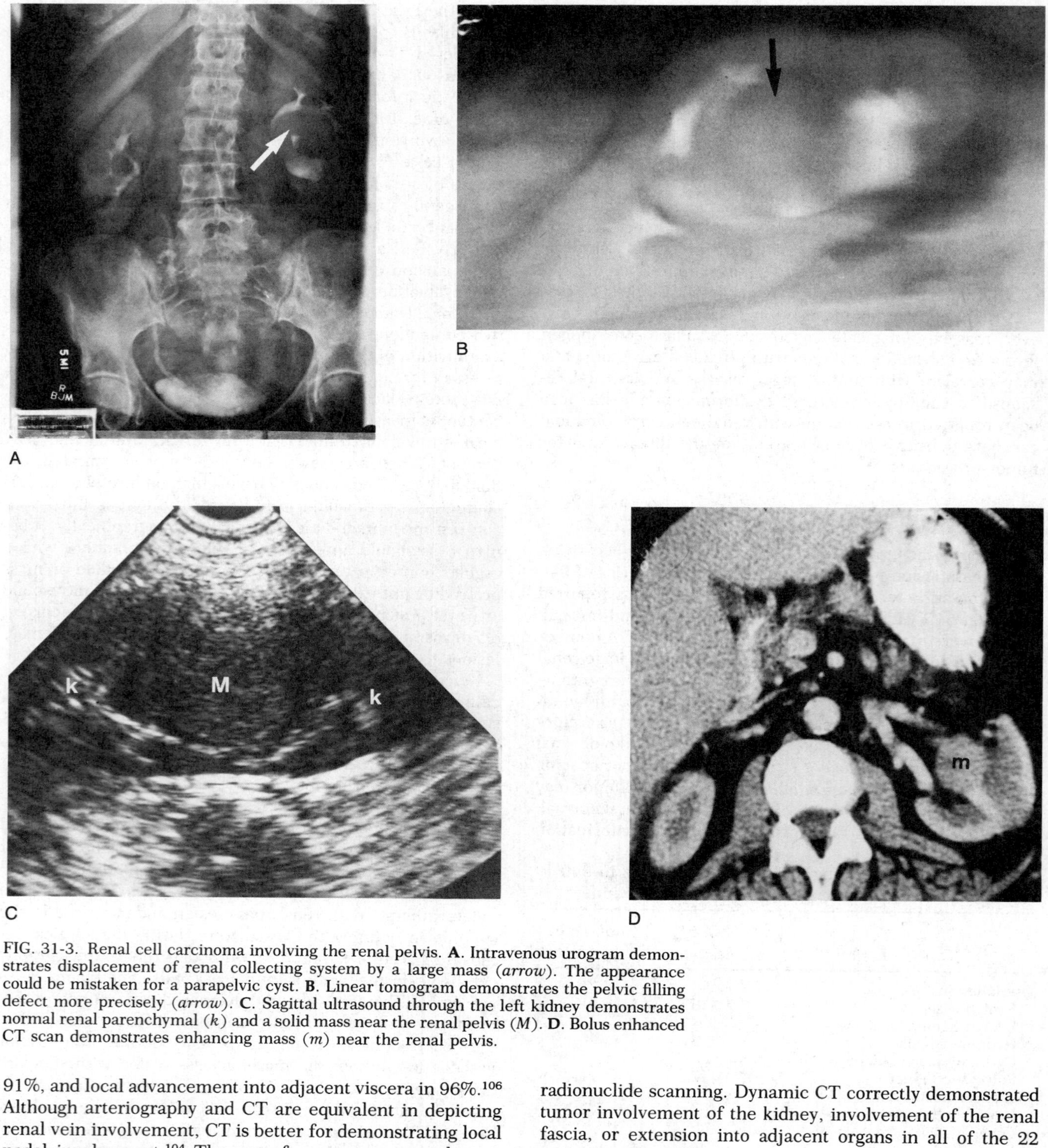

FIG. 31-3. Renal cell carcinoma involving the renal pelvis. **A**. Intravenous urogram demonstrates displacement of renal collecting system by a large mass (*arrow*). The appearance could be mistaken for a parapelvic cyst. **B**. Linear tomogram demonstrates the pelvic filling defect more precisely (*arrow*). **C**. Sagittal ultrasound through the left kidney demonstrates normal renal parenchymal (*k*) and a solid mass near the renal pelvis (*M*). **D**. Bolus enhanced CT scan demonstrates enhancing mass (*m*) near the renal pelvis.

91%, and local advancement into adjacent viscera in 96%.[106] Although arteriography and CT are equivalent in depicting renal vein involvement, CT is better for demonstrating local nodal involvement.[104] The use of contrast agent enhancement has greatly increased the sensitivity of CT for abnormal renal mass lesions.[107,108] Contrast-enhanced CT allows the clinician to detect very small changes in the density of a renal lesion that might indicate the presence of an early neoplastic lesion. In a comparison study, dynamic CT was superior to standard CT arteriography, ultrasonography, and radionuclide scanning. Dynamic CT correctly demonstrated tumor involvement of the kidney, involvement of the renal fascia, or extension into adjacent organs in all of the 22 patients studied.[100]

Inferior venacavography is performed when there is a large renal tumor or when there is uncertainty about tumor involvement of the vena cava. Ultrasound, CT, and MRI (Fig. 31-6) can provide information about tumor involvement of the vena cava; however, the inferior venacavogram is the most reliable means of accurately determining the precise

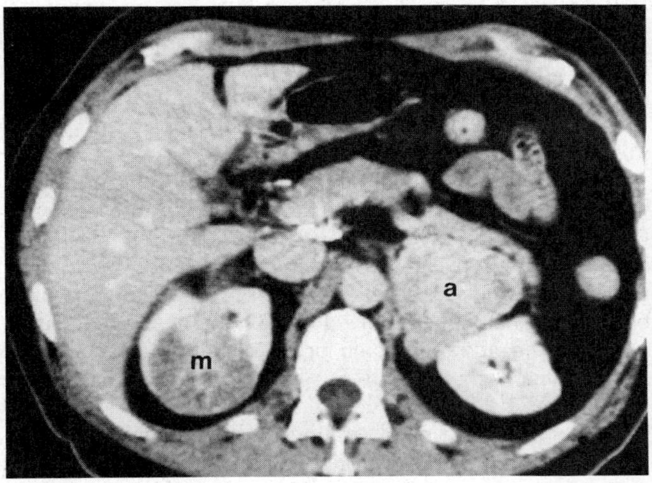

A

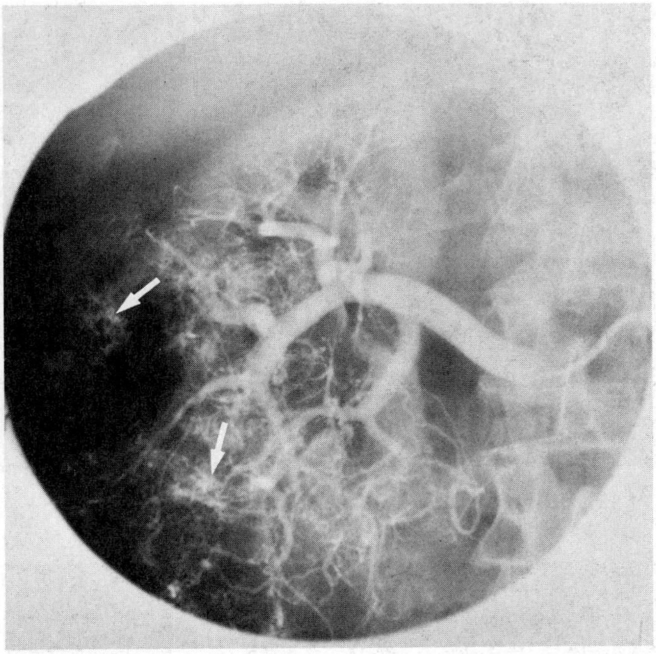

B

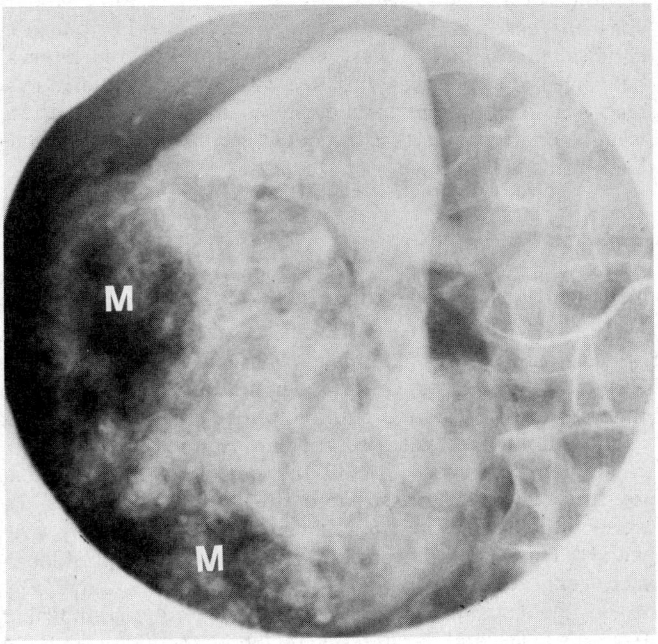

C

FIG. 31-4. Angiographic appearance of a renal cell carcinoma. **A.** CT demonstrates a right renal carcinoma (*m*) with a large contralateral adrenal metastasis (*a*). **B.** Early phase of arteriogram demonstrates vascular changes indicative of a malignancy with puddling and tortuosity (*arrows*). **C.** Late phase of the arteriogram demonstrates that the tumor (*M*) is relatively avascular despite its early appearance.

extent of vena caval involvement by tumor. This information is important to the surgeon in planning the vascular aspect of the operative procedure.

MRI is very useful for staging renal cell carcinoma.[110] MRI can produce a unique three-dimensional picture of the tumor which, in the case of a large tumor, may be an invaluable aid to the surgeon in planning the operative approach.

There is no single imaging technique that is best for all patients with renal cell carcinoma. Depending on the size of the primary tumor and the extent of extrarenal disease, excretory urography, CT, ultrasound, arteriography, venography, and MRI each can provide unique information in an individual case. Because CT, MRI, and ultrasound are outpatient procedures and are less invasive than arteriography, arteriography is now less frequently used. Multiple imaging modalities are often used to provide the most complete information, particularly when surgical removal of a large tumor is being considered.

STAGING AND PROGNOSIS

The staging system (Fig. 31-7) currently in use by most physicians in the United States is the Robson modification of the system of Flocks and Kadesky (Table 31-3).[111] In the Robson classification, Stage I renal cell carcinoma is confined to the kidney, Stage II carcinoma extends through the renal capsule but is confined to Gerota's fascia, and Stage III carcinoma involves the renal vein or inferior vena cava (III-

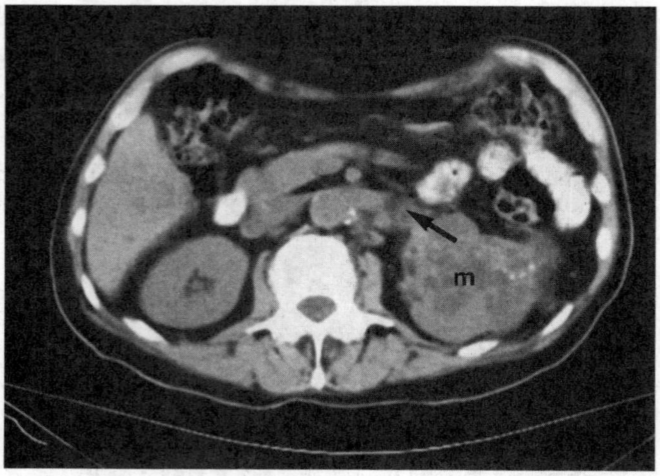

A

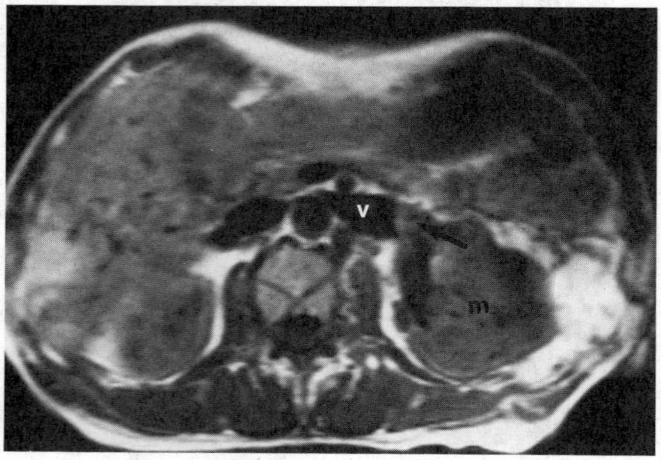

B

FIG. 31-5. Renal vein invasion by a renal carcinoma as shown by CT and MRI. **A**. Nonenhanced CT shows large left renal mass with calcification (*m*) invading the left renal vein (*arrow*). **B**. T1-weighted MRI demonstrates tumor (*m*) and vascular invasion (*arrow*). Flowing blood (*v*) in the left renal vein is black on this scan.

A) or the local hilar lymph nodes (III-B). In Stage IV renal cell carcinoma the tumor has spread to local, adjacent organs (other than the adrenal gland) or to distant sites. The Robson staging system is uncomplicated and widely used. A disadvantage of this system is that it combines stages that may have significantly different survival prognoses. In this classification system renal vein or inferior vena caval involvement (III-A) is the same stage as local lymph node metastasis (III-B). Although patients with Stage III-B renal cell carcinoma have a greatly decreased survival,[112,113] the prognosis for patients with Stage III-A renal cell carcinoma is not particularly different from that for patients with Stage I or Stage II renal cell carcinoma.

The TNM classification provides a more accurate method for classifying extent of tumor involvement. In the TNM classification, T1 denotes a small tumor confined to the kidney, T2 denotes a large tumor that deforms the kidney or collecting system but is still confined to the kidney, T3 denotes tumor with perinephric or hilar extension, and T4 denotes tumor that has extended to neighboring organs (Table 31-4). N+ indicates local nodal involvement, and in M+ disease there are metastases.

The 5-year survival initially reported by Robson and coworkers in 1969 was 66% for Stage I renal cell carcinoma, 64% for Stage II, 42% for Stage III, and only 11% for Stage IV.[111] These survival statistics remained essentially the same for a number of years (Table 31-5).[79,90] However, it has since been noted that while renal vein involvement does not have a markedly negative effect on prognosis, the 5-year survival for patients with Stage III-B renal cell carcinoma is only 18%.[7,79,80,90,114] Recent studies have reported better survival for patients with tumor confined to the kidney: approximately 95% 5-year survival for T1 renal cell carcinoma and 92% 5-year survival for Stage T2 disease.[80,106] The 5-year survival for patients with metastatic renal cell carcinoma continues to be low, from 0 to 20%.[7,80,85,115] Most studies show increased survival in patients in whom the following conditions obtain: (1) there is a long disease-free interval between initial nephrectomy and the appearance of metastases, (2) only pulmonary metastases are present, (3) there is a good performance status, and (4) the primary tumor has been removed.[85]

SURGICAL TREATMENT

Surgery is the only known effective therapy for localized renal cell carcinoma. The first nephrectomy was performed by Erastus B. Walcott in Milwaukee on June 4, 1861, on a 58-year-old man with a kidney tumor who died 15 days after surgery.[116] Professor Gustave Simon, after completing a number of experimental nephrectomies on dogs, undertook the first deliberate, planned and successful nephrectomy in Heidelberg on August 2, 1869, in a patient with a persistent ureteral fistula. The first successful nephrectomy in a patient with kidney cancer was performed in 1883 by Grawitz.[116] The standard procedure today for treatment of localized renal cell carcinoma is radical nephrectomy (Fig. 31-8).[117] Radical nephrectomy includes complete removal of Gerota's fascia and its contents, including the kidney and the adrenal gland, and provides a better surgical margin than simple removal of the kidney.

There are a number of different surgical approaches to removal of a kidney cancer. Common approaches are the anterior transperitoneal approach, the flank approach, and the thoracoabdominal approach. The choice of surgical approach depends on the location and size of the tumor and the body habitus of the patient. The type of incision is chosen to ensure that the tumor may safely be removed. A flank incision, with or without removal of a portion of the 10th or 11th rib, is often used for small tumors without venous involvement. A subcostal transabdominal incision may be used when there is a large tumor in the middle or lower aspect of the kidney or when vascular involvement is anticipated and access to the major vessels is essential. A thoracoabdominal incision is often required when there is a large middle or upper pole tumor. In a thoracoabdominal incision a rib is

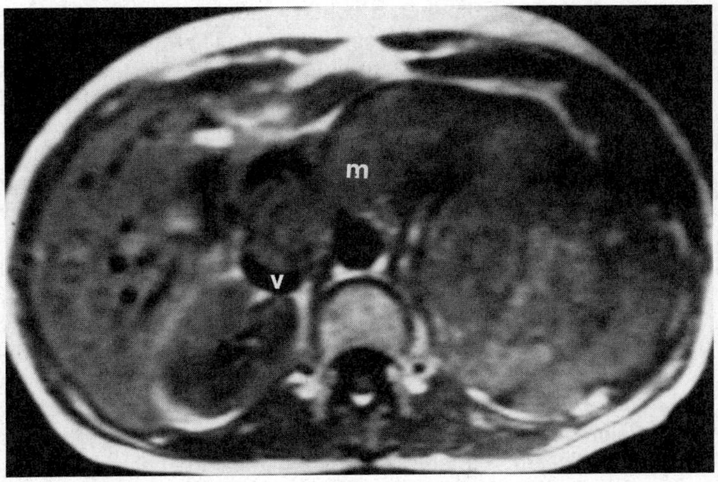

A

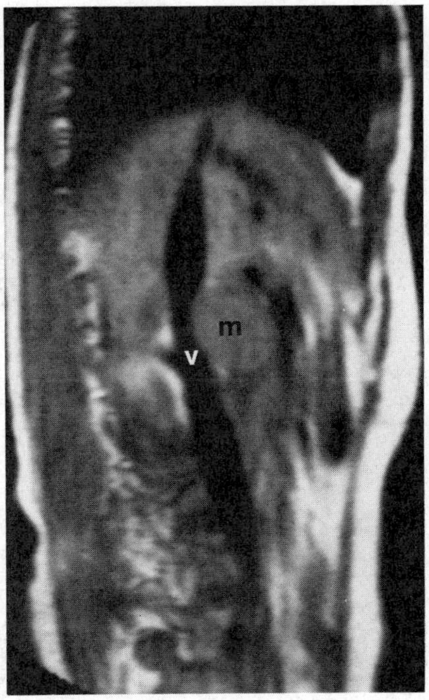

B

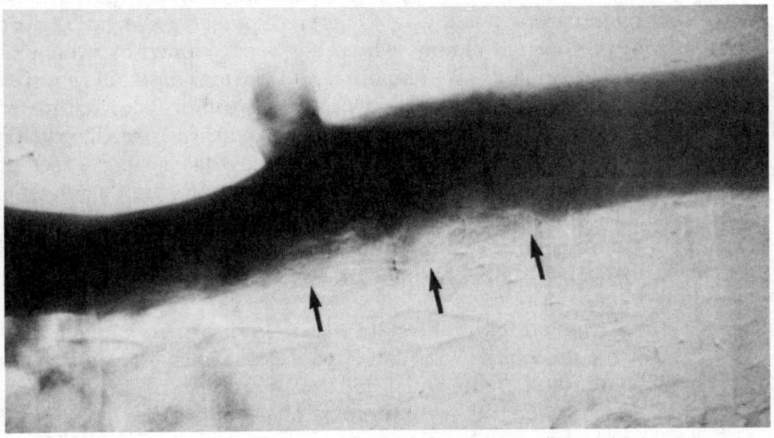

C

FIG. 31-6. Invasion of IVC by renal carcinoma demonstrated by MRI and venography. **A**. Axial T1-weighted image demonstrates a large left renal carcinoma with extension into the left renal vein (*m*) with protrusion into the IVC (*v*). **B**. Sagittal T1-weighted image shows the relation of the tumor thrombus (*m*) to the IVC (*v*) in the lateral projection. **C**. An AP image of the interior cavagram demonstrates tumor in the medial aspect of the inferior vena cava.

removed, the thoracic cavity is opened, and the diaphragm is incised. The incision is then carried down transabdominally to allow maximal exposure of the upper abdominal region and the great vessels. In removal of a right-sided tumor, the hepatic flexure of the colon is mobilized toward the midline away from the kidney and duodenum. The duodenum is also dissected up anteriorly and medially to the great vessels, and the renal artery and vein are identified. The renal vessels are divided and ligated early in the surgical procedure to decrease the vascularity of the tumor so that it may be removed with a minimum of blood loss. Following ligation of the vessels, Gerota's fascia is incised away from the posterior abdominal wall, diaphragm, and liver (pancreas and spleen on a left-sided tumor) (see Fig. 31-9). Once Gerota's fascia and its contents have been dissected away from the surrounding structures and the vasculature has been ligated with nonabsorbable suture, the specimen can be lifted out of the retroperitoneum. When there is tumor in the renal vein, the renal vein can be ligated distal to the tumor thrombus. If there is tumor extension into the vena cava, the vena cava may need to be partially resected. If the tumor has grown into the side wall of the vena cava or if the vena caval involvement is too extensive for a simple partial wall resection, a portion of the vena cava itself may be resected. When the tumor is in the right kidney, the adjacent vena cava can often be resected safely. If, however, the tumor in the left kidney and the adjacent vena cava are resected, vascular reconstruction of the right renal vein may be needed to establish adequate venous drainage.[114,118,119] If the suprahepatic caval extension of a renal tumor thrombus extends up to the right atrium, cardiopulmonary bypass may be required for tumor removal.[119,120]

Regional lymphadenectomy is often performed at the time of radical nephrectomy, although its role in prolonging survival has not been demonstrated. In a regional lymphadenectomy, ipsilateral nodal tissue from the diaphragm to the bifurcation of the aorta as well as nodal tissue in the interaortocaval region at the hilum of the kidney is removed. Proponents of regional lymphadenectomy point out that 5-year survival in patients with N+ renal cell carcinoma is greatly decreased, and there is no known effective therapy for metastatic renal cell carcinoma. If local nodes were the first site of metastasis, resection of microscopic disease might be of benefit. Long-term survival in patients with N+ disease who underwent lymphadenectomy has been reported. The ultimate role of regional lymphadenectomy remains to be determined in further randomized trials.[79,111–113,121–123]

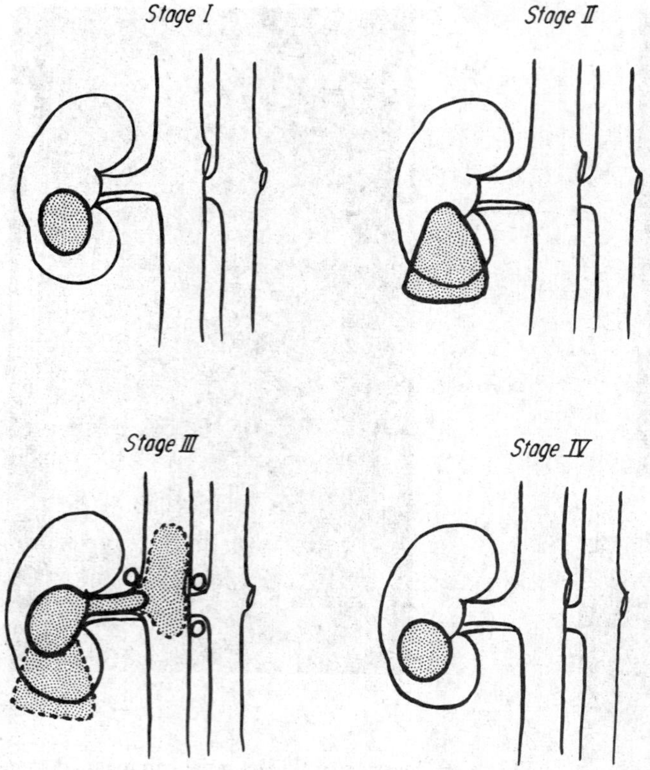

FIG. 31-7. Staging system for renal adenocarcinoma. (Modified from Skinner DG, Vermillion CD, Colvin RB: The surgical management of renal cell carcinoma. J Urol 107:705–716, 1972)

BILATERAL RENAL CELL CARCINOMA OR TUMORS IN SOLITARY KIDNEYS

The treatment of patients who present with either bilateral renal cell carcinoma or renal cell carcinoma in a solitary kidney is challenging. Patients with tumor in a solitary kidney may be treated by either partial nephrectomy or nephrectomy followed by dialysis and/or transplantation.[124–127] A 5-year survival of 60% in patients with bilateral renal cell carcinoma or tumor in a solitary kidney treated by partial nephrectomy has been reported.[128] Some surgeons advocate surgical enucleation of a tumor in a patient with a solitary kidney. In one series patients with either bilateral renal cell carcinoma or tumor in a solitary kidney treated with enucleation had a 90% 3-year survival. There was excellent renal function in all patients; none required dialysis.[129] Others advocate caution in using surgical enucleation and favor partial nephrectomy instead. Marshall and co-workers evaluated standard nephrectomy specimens that were enucleated ex vivo and found positive margins, satellite tumor nodules, and occult metastatic disease in lymph nodes in a number of cases that were not appreciated fully in the operating room.[130] Most surgeons favor resection of a narrow rim of normal tissue around the tumor in the kidney instead of simple enucleation.[131] Extracorporeal partial nephrectomy plus autotransplantation is a technique that allows the surgeon to accurately remove large tumors in the center of a solitary kidney.[128] This ex vivo procedure entails radical excision of the kidney and division of the ureter. The kidney is then placed on a table and is intermittently perfused with a chilled solution to enhance viability. Under optical magnification the tumor is carefully dissected from the surrounding renal parenchyma. Care is taken to preserve the vasculature of the normal kidney, which has been defined by preoperative arteriography. A small rim of normal tissue is removed along with the tumor to provide a tumor-free margin of resection. After the kidney has been surgically reconstructed it is autotransplanted back into the iliac space. Vascular anastomosis of the renal artery and vein to the iliac vessels and ureteroureterostomy are performed. If multiple tumors are encountered in which small tumors are distributed throughout the parenchyma, autotransplantation is not indicated.[124]

TABLE 31-3. Comparison of the Two Classification Systems for Staging of Renal Cell Carcinoma*

	TNM (1978)	*Robson*
Small tumor, no enlargement of kidney	T1	A
Large tumor, cortex not broken	T2	A
Perinephric or hilar extension	T3	B
Extension to neighboring organs	T4	D
Nodal invasion	N+	C
Renal vein involved	V1	C
Vena cava involved	V2	C
Distant metastases	M+	D

* Selli C, Hinshaw WM, Woodard BH, Paulson DF: Stratification of risk factors in renal cell carcinoma. Cancer 52:899, 1983.

Although familial renal cell carcinoma or renal cell carcinoma associated with von Hippel–Lindau syndrome is often bilateral, sporadic renal cell carcinoma is only rarely bilateral.[132] Bilateral (synchronous or asynchronous) renal cell carcinoma has been reported to occur in 1.8% to 3.8% of cases.[117] Patients with synchronous bilateral renal cell carcinoma have a better prognosis than patients with asynchronous disease. Zincke and co-workers reported a 78% 5-year survival for patients seen initially with bilateral renal cell carcinoma versus only a 38% 5-year survival for patients whose metastases in the contralateral kidney appeared after the primary had been removed.[132]

RADIATION THERAPY AS AN ADJUVANT TO NEPHRECTOMY

The cure rates for patients with high pathologic stage renal cell carcinoma (N+, M+) treated by nephrectomy are only fair and have improved little in the last two decades. However, because patients with renal cell carcinoma can have variable and protracted courses, the benefit in survival from any adjunctive therapy to nephrectomy is difficult to demonstrate. Currently no data clearly indicate that radical nephrectomy plus lymph node dissection provides enhanced cure rate over treatment by nephrectomy alone.[115] In addition, studies looking at the possible benefit of adjuvant irradiation combined with nephrectomy are few and inconclusive (Table 31-6). Reports of benefit with radiation therapy come from only one nonrandomized trial.[133] Two randomized studies found no benefit from postoperative irradia-

TABLE 31-4. TNM Classification — Kidney

Primary Tumor (T)

TX Minimum requirements cannot be met
T0 No evidence of primary tumor
T1 Small tumor, minimal renal and calyceal distortion or deformity. Circumscribed neovasculature surrounded by normal parenchyma
T2 Large tumor with deformity or enlargement of kidney or collecting system
T3a Tumor involving perinephric tissues
T3b Tumor involving renal vein
T3c Tumor involving renal vein and infradiaphragmatic vena cava
Note: Under T3, tumor may extend into perinephric tissues, into renal vein, and into vena cava as shown on cavography. In these instances, the T classification may be shown as T3a, b, and c, or some appropriate combination, depending on extension, e.g., T3a,b is tumor in perinephric fat and extending into renal vein.
T4a Tumor invasion of neighboring structures (e.g., muscle, bowel)
T4b Tumor involving supradiaphragmatic vena cava

Nodal Involvement (N)

The regional lymph nodes are the para-aortic and paracaval nodes. The juxtaregional lymph nodes are the pelvic nodes and the mediastinal nodes.
NX Minimum requirements cannot be met
N0 No evidence of involvement of regional nodes
N1 Single, homolateral regional nodal involvement
N2 Involvement of multiple regional or contralateral or bilateral nodes
N3 Fixed regional nodes (assessable only at surgical exploration)
N4 Involvement of juxtaregional nodes
Note: If lymphography is source of staging, add "1" between "N" and designator number; if histologic proof is provided "+" if positive, and "−" if negative. Thus N1+ indicates multiple positive nodes seen on lymphography and proved at operation by biopsy.

Distant Metastasis (M)

MX Not assessed
M0 No (known) distant metastasis
M1 Distant metastasis present
Specify
Specify sites according to the following notations

Pulmonary — PUL	Bone Marrow — MAR
Osseous — OSS	Pleura — PLE
Hepatic — HEP	Skin — SKI
Brain — BRA	Eye — EYE
Lymph Nodes — LYM	Other — OTH

Note: Add "+" to the abbreviated notation to indicate that the pathology (p) is proved.

TABLE 31-5. Summary of Published Survival Rates in Renal Cell Carcinoma

Study, Year	*Length of Survival (yr)*	*Survival (%) by Stage* I	II	III	IV
Robson et al, 1969[111]	5	66	64	42	11
	10	60	67	38	0
Skinner et al, 1971[79]	5	65	47	51	8
	10	56	20	37	7
Boxer et al, 1979[81]	5	56	100	50	8
	10	20	66	25	0
McNichols et al, 1981[83]	5	67	51	34	14
	10	56	28	20	3
Cherrie et al, 1982[114]	5	. . .	. . .	0–53	0
	10	. . .	. . .	. . .	. . .
Selli et al, 1983[80]	5	93	63	80	13
	10	. . .	. . .	. . .	. . .
Bassil et al, 1985[115]	5	91–100	. . .	. . .	18
	10	. . .	. . .	. . .	. . .
Golimbu et al, 1986[7]	5	88	67	40	2
	10	66	35	15	. . .

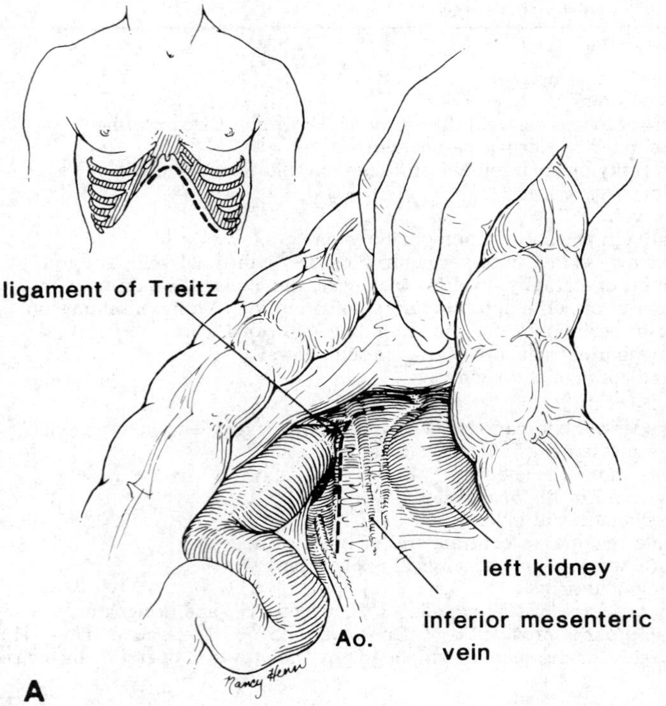

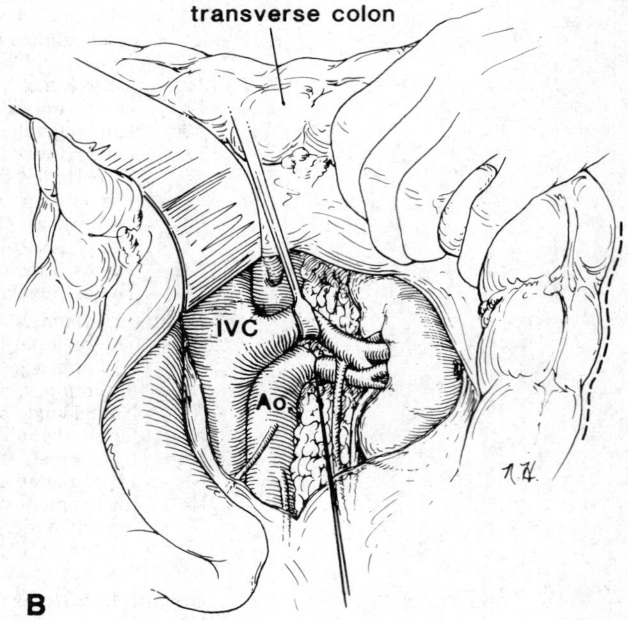

FIG. 31-8. Area of dissection for lymph node dissection for radical nephroureterectomy should be from the superior mesenteric artery to the level of the inferior mesenteric artery with the anatomic structures identified. The dotted line to the right of the descending colon indicates a line of incision on the left pericolic gutter that should extend superiorly to include division of the splenocolic attachments. (Paulson DF, Perez CA, Anderson T: Cancer of the kidney and ureter. In DeVita VT Jr, Hellman S, Rosenberg SA (eds): Cancer: Principles and Practice of Oncology, 2nd ed, p 898. Philadelphia, JB Lippincott, 1985)

FIG. 31-9. The left colon can be reflected from the anterior surface of Gerota's fascia with exposure of the renal artery before ligation and division. (Paulson DF, Perez CA, Anderson T: Cancer of the kidney and ureter. In DeVita VT Jr, Hellman S, Rosenberg SA (eds): Cancer: Principles and Practice of Oncology, 2nd ed, p 900. Philadelphia, JB Lippincott, 1985)

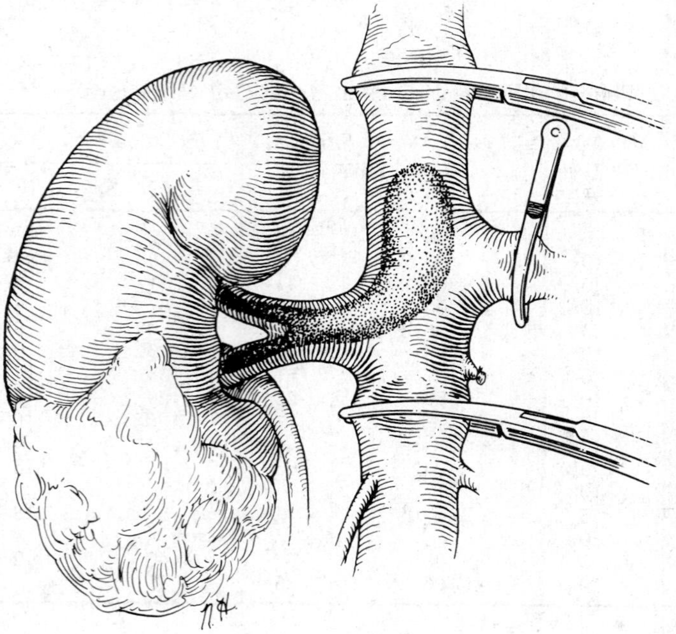

tion.[134,135] However, any possible benefit from radiation therapy in the latter two studies was likely compromised by either the radiation technique or the radiation dose. Four fatal liver complications occurred after postoperative irradiation of up to 5500 cGy in the 1973 study reported by Finney.[134] In a study in Denmark, reported in 1987, a high complication rate was noted.[135] In this series the dose per fraction was 250 cGy, for a total dose of 5000 cGy delivered over approximately 4 weeks. Because of complications (44% severe, 19% fatal), mainly gastrointestinal, this trial was stopped.[135]

Two studies of preoperative radiation therapy given before partial nephrectomy have been reported. The first, reported by van der Werf-Messing,[136] found no benefit with a dose of 3000 cGy given prior to nephrectomy. However, 37% of the patients had tumors of low pathologic stage and thus would have been unlikely to benefit from the adjuvant treatment. Likewise, in the Phase III trial reported from Finland of 3600 cGy given preoperatively, 70% of patients had tumors of low pathologic stage (pT1 and pT2). Thus, to date there are no wholly satisfactory analyses of the efficacy of well-tolerated modern megavoltage preoperative or postoperative radiation therapy as an adjunct to radical nephrectomy in patients judged to be at high risk for locoregional failure—those with high pathologic stage tumors.

Present information indicates that patients with pathologic stage T1 or T2 tumors without lymph node metastases are not good candidates for adjunctive therapy as they are likely

TABLE 31-6. Renal Cell Carcinoma: Treatment Results with and Without Adjuvant Radiation Therapy

Study, Year	No. of Patients	Local Treatment	5-Year Survival (%)	Local Recurrences (%)	Comments
Peeling et al, 1969[294]	96	Nephrectomy	52	. . .	Not randomized; ? RT dose
	68	Nephrectomy + RT	25	. . .	
Rafla, 1970[133]	96	Nephrectomy	37	25	Not randomized; ? RT dose
	94	Nephrectomy + RT	56	7	
Finney, 1973[134]	49	Nephrectomy	44	. . .	Randomized; RT dose to 5500 cGY
	51	Nephrectomy + RT	36	. . .	
van der Werf-Messing, 1973[136]	85	Nephrectomy	50	. . .	Randomized; 37% of patients had small tumors (pT1–2)
	89	RT (3000 cGy) + nephrectomy	45	. . .	
Juusela et al, 1977[295]	44	Nephrectomy	63	. . .	Randomized; 70% of patients had small tumors (pT1–2)
	38	RT (3600 cGy) + nephrectomy	47		
Kjaer et al, 1987[296]	33	Nephrectomy	62	3	Randomized; RT group with high complication rate—44% serious, 19% lethal
	32	Nephrectomy + RT (5000 cGy; 20 fractions)	38	0	

RT = radiation therapy.

to have an 80% or greater 5- to 10-year survival after radical nephrectomy alone.[113,115] Candidates for possible postoperative adjunctive radiation therapy include those with pathologic evidence of deep invasion of Gerota's fascia, adjacent organs, or regional lymph nodes and who have no known metastatic disease. Such patients are probably best treated by daily fractions of 180 to 200 cGy with 10- to 25-MV beams from linear accelerators to fields that include the renal fossa and tumor bed as well as the para-aortic and paracaval lymph nodes, to a total dose of 4500 cGy in 5 weeks. The usual parallel-opposed anterior-posterior isocentric fields are secondarily shaped with individual corner blocks. For right-sided tumors there is often a need for field reduction at the 3600 to 4600 cGy level to include only the tumor bed and the retroperitoneal lymph node regions, so that not more than 30% of the liver parenchyma receives a high dose. A post-nephrectomy, preirradiation CT scan is very useful as a baseline for subsequent comparison. Unless there is clear evidence of wound contamination by tumor spill at the time of nephrectomy, usually no effort is made to include the entire surgical incision in the treatment fields.

METASTATIC RENAL CELL CARCINOMA

NEPHRECTOMY AND RESECTION OF METASTASES

Adjuvant or palliative nephrectomy is not infrequently performed in patients with metastatic renal cell carcinoma, particularly those with pain, hemorrhage, malaise, hypercalcemia, erythrocytosis, or hypertension. Removal of the primary tumor may alleviate some or all of these abnormalities.[137,138] Although there are isolated reports of regression of metastatic renal cell carcinoma following removal of the primary tumor, only four (0.8%) of 474 patients in nine series who underwent nephrectomy experienced "regression" of metastatic foci.[139] DeKernion and co-workers reported results in 26 patients with metastatic renal cell carcinoma who underwent palliative or adjuvant nephrectomy and found no increase in survival, compared with survival in the entire group of 79 patients with metastatic renal cell carcinoma.[140] Middleton reported on 141 patients with metastatic renal cell carcinomas; 33 underwent adjuvant nephrectomy, however, none of the 141 patients survived more than 24 months.[141] Adjuvant nephrectomy is not recommended for the purpose of inducing spontaneous regression; rather, it is performed to decrease symptoms or to decrease tumor burden in preparation for subsequent therapy in carefully controlled environments.

Of the approximately 30% of patients with renal cell carcinoma who present with metastases, only 1.5% to 3.5% have solitary metastasis.[141–143] Patients with a solitary metastasis synchronous with a primary lesion have decreased survival when compared with patients who develop metastasis after the primary tumor is removed.[133,140,142] Surgical resection is appropriate in selected patients with metastatic renal cell carcinoma. In one study, 59 patients with renal cell carcinoma who underwent surgical resection for a solitary metastasis had a 45% 3-year survival and a 34% 5-year survival.[141] O'Dea et al reported on patients who presented with primary tumor in place and a solitary metastasis. Of the patients who underwent nephrectomy and who later developed metastasis, 23% lived more than 5 years after removal of the metastatic lesions. Three of the 26 patients were alive 58, 94, and 245 months after resection of the metastatic lesion.[142] Nephrectomy and resection of metastases will render few cures but will frequently produce some long-term survivors.

ANGIOINFARCTION

Angioinfarction of the kidney is used both with and without nephrectomy in the treatment of metastatic renal cell carcinoma. A number of techniques have been developed to occlude the renal artery for this purpose. Short-term embolization can be accomplished with alcohol, autologous blood clot, or gelatin sponge pads (Gelfoam). Other inert substances such as Silastic spheres, stainless steel pellets, or Gianturco steel coils are also used to embolize the renal artery.[144] Most patients develop a postinfarction syndrome consisting of pain, fever, and gastrointestinal complaints almost immediately after infarction.[137] Transcatheter arterial occlusion may decrease vascularity prior to nephrectomy in patients with large, locally advanced renal cell carcinoma or may lessen tumor bleeding, pain, or other systemic symptoms in patients with unresectable tumors.[144] Angioinfarction has not been demonstrated to be an effective method for inducing regression in patients with metastatic renal cell carcinoma. In a study by Swanson et al of patients with metastatic renal cell carcinoma who underwent angioinfarction followed by nephrectomy, a small number experienced complete or partial response of the metastatic disease to this therapy; however, there was no difference in survival between these patients (n = 100) and the patients who were treated with nephrectomy alone (n = 43).[145]

ROLE OF RADIATION THERAPY

The major sites of hematogenous metastases from renal cell carcinoma are bone, lung, and brain. Treatment in virtually all instances is noncurative, and thus the role of radiation therapy, neurosurgery, orthopedic surgery, or thoracic surgery in the local management of these metastases is nearly always palliative. However, patients presenting with an initially solitary metastatic lesion have a 30% to 40% chance of surviving for 5 years. Thus, in these patients it is important to ensure as durable a palliative response as possible. In patients presenting with a solitary metastasis to the lung, spine, or brain, initial or de novo surgery should be considered, usually followed by postoperative irradiation. For a solitary metastasis to the spine, vertebral body resection by the anterior approach has proved satisfactory in carefully selected patients.[146,147] External-beam radiation therapy, the usual initial palliative approach for patients with symptomatic metastases, has been reported to yield a subjective or objective response in one half to two thirds of patients.[148–150] In a selected and carefully reviewed subset of patients irradiated for metastatic renal carcinoma, subjective improvement was noted in 16 of 19 analyzed patients, whereas objective evidence of regression, usually radiographic, was documented in only 13 of 26 treated patients. The external-beam radiation doses were most commonly in the range of 4000 cGy.[148] Doses the equivalent of at least 5000 cGy in 5½ weeks are necessary to achieve a durable palliative response.[149] To deliver such high doses, multiple-field techniques are often necessary. Palliation of large renal bed recurrences by external-beam irradiation has been unsatisfactory. Some relief of pain has been achieved in about 50% of the patients, but it is usually of very short duration.[150]

SYSTEMIC THERAPY

The treatment of patients with metastatic renal cell carcinoma has been one of the most frustrating endeavors of medical oncology. A huge number of chemotherapeutic agents, hormones, and combinations have been tested, but none has yielded reproducible therapeutic effects. The history of the therapy of metastatic renal cell carcinoma is dotted with positive pilot studies that fail to remain positive when tested in another institution or in another group of patients. Recently it has been found that renal tubular epithelium, the tissue of origin of renal cell carcinoma, constitutively expresses the multidrug resistance gene, *mdr,* which encodes a transport protein called p170.[151] Whether this gene is responsible for the de novo drug resistance seen in nearly all renal cell carcinomas has not been examined.

In contrast to the results with chemotherapeutic agents and hormones, several biologic approaches to renal cell carcinoma have produced response rates so encouraging that many oncologists feel justified in offering biologic agents as primary treatment. When response rates in patients with metastatic disease approach 30%, it is probably reasonable to begin to apply the therapy in the adjuvant setting to patients with locally advanced disease with a high probability of relapse after surgery. Such studies are being planned for at least two biological therapies.

CHEMOTHERAPY

The conventional treatment for metastatic renal cell carcinoma is vinblastine, 0.2 or 0.3 mg/kg/wk. Hrushesky and Murphy found that the response rate among 39 patients receiving weekly doses of vinblastine of 0.2 mg/kg was 31%, but the response rate among 96 patients receiving less vinblastine was only 15%.[152] Responders have markedly prolonged survival. Dose-related variables and dose intensity have not been carefully evaluated prospectively in renal cell carcinoma. Most workers administer lower doses because of concern about toxic effects, and most agree that the response rate is closer to 15% than 30%.

Efforts to improve the response rate to vinblastine by adding other agents have been largely unsuccessful.[32] Usually the agents added to vinblastine are not active in renal cell carcinoma as single agents (a violation of one of the cardinal rules for building a more effective combination regimen), and often the dose of vinblastine is lowered or the frequency of administration decreased because of toxic effects produced by the less effective agents in the combination. A recent report of a 30% response rate to vinblastine (4 mg/m^2), bleomycin (30 mg), and methotrexate (500 mg/m^2 with leucovorin rescue) may represent a possible exception to this bleak picture.[153] However, it must be remembered that other initial reports of high response rates with combination therapy have uniformly failed to be confirmed.

An innovative approach to the use of chemotherapy in the treatment of metastatic renal cell carcinoma has been taken by Hrushesky and his colleagues.[154] Using programmable Medtronic pumps for automatic drug delivery, they found that the maximum tolerated dose of fluorodeoxyuridine (FUDR) infusions was more than twice that of conventional infusions if the FUDR infusion rate was sinusoidal, with the peak centered around 6 PM. Among 18 evaluable patients, five achieved partial responses and one a complete response. This small study suggests that a clever treatment design takes into account circadian influences on the therapeutic ratio and may allow augmentation of dose intensity to a clinically significant degree.

A complete response to neocarzinostatin has been reported, but the denominator is unknown.[155] A series of patients with primarily pulmonary disease were treated with chemotherapy infusions into the bronchial arteries.[156] Five of 12 patients were said to have responded, but the results are not evaluable because of extreme heterogeneity in agent, dose, and timing of administration.

CHEMOTHERAPY FOR LOCALLY ADVANCED RENAL CELL CARCINOMA

There are very few studies of adjuvant chemotherapy in renal cell cancer, and those few are not prospective and randomized.[157] However, one small study reported that the adjuvant use of bleomycin and lomustine (CCNU) was associated with fewer relapses and longer survival than in historical controls.[158] The intra-arterial administration of chemotherapeutic agents has been tried as a means of controlling locally advanced disease in single-arm studies that are difficult to interpret. Although tumors resected after intra-arterial chemotherapy with 5-FU[159] or mitomycin C in liposomes[160] are commonly found to be necrotic, it is not clear that this method prevents local or distant recurrences. This field of inquiry has been hampered by the paucity of active chemotherapeutic agents. It is hoped that the development of new approaches will allow a more careful assessment of the impact of treatment on locally advanced disease.

HORMONAL THERAPY

The possibility that hormonal therapy might be useful in renal cell cancer was briefly addressed earlier. Because prolonged estrogen administration induces renal tumors in male Syrian golden hamsters, it was reasoned that human renal cell cancer might be responsive to hormonal manipulation. Experimental studies showed that renal tumors in animals could be modulated by hormonal influences, and the findings were extrapolated to men on the basis of the more frequent occurrence of the tumor in men than in women. Human renal cancer was not evaluated for the presence of hormone receptors, but it was felt that there was little other effective therapy to offer and that the toxic effects of hormonal manipulation were less than those of experimental chemotherapy. Patients received progestogens (chiefly medroxyprogesterone acetate), testosterone, or antiestrogens, alone, in combination, or together with corticosteroids, chemotherapy, or immunotherapy.[32] Objective response rates in the compiled data range from 5% to 9%, with nearly all responses being partial and short-lived and affecting mainly pulmonary metastatic disease. In fact, one analysis suggested that as stricter response criteria are applied, the response rate to hormonal manipulation falls to less than 2%.[152] One study from Japan attempted to evaluate the role of medroxyprogesterone acetate given after definitive surgery in patients with Stages I to III disease.[161] Although a difference that was not statistically significant was seen between the treated and control groups, the study was not prospective and randomized, and it is not clear that both groups underwent similar surgical-pathologic staging. Recent work has documented the presence of receptors for some sex steroids on some human renal cell carcinomas, but efforts to correlate the presence of progesterone receptors, estrogen receptors, and androgen receptors with response have usually been fruitless.[162] Careful study of bona fide human cell lines of renal cell carcinoma is in the initial stages, but it appears that sex steroid hormones exert little trophic effect on human renal cell carcinoma. Any effect of hormonal manipulation could be due more to immune stimulation by the progestogen than to direct effects on the tumor. Although the side-effects of hormonal therapy are not life-threatening, they can be unpleasant. The recent development of biologic treatments with measurable response rates has relegated hormonal therapy to the third line of treatment approaches for metastatic renal cell carcinoma.

BIOLOGIC THERAPY

Several exciting developments in biologic therapy have altered substantially the prospects for the treatment of renal cell carcinoma. The development by Rosenberg and colleagues at the Surgery Branch of the National Cancer Institute (NCI) of adoptive cellular therapy with lymphokine-activated (LAK) cells plus interleukin-2 (IL-2) has changed our view of this resistant disease.[163,164] These investigators have obtained objective response rates of over 30%, and 10% of patients with metastatic disease achieve complete remissions that appear to have affected survival. Other biologic agents such as interferon, tumor necrosis factor, and monoclonal antibodies are being tested that may be effective alone or may have additive therapeutic effect when administered in combination with IL-2–based immunotherapy. Various interferons have been tested and have been found to be effective in 15% to 20% of patients, most of whom had had disease progression on chemotherapy.[165–167] A pilot study of cimetidine plus coumarin, two biologic response modifiers whose immune effects are not well characterized, has also demonstrated objective responses.[168] Active specific and nonspecific approaches have been explored, and monoclonal antibodies are just beginning to be characterized.

The new approach to the treatment of patients with metastatic renal cell carcinoma with adoptive immunotherapy developed by Rosenberg et al involves two elements, IL-2 and LAK cells. This therapy begins with 4 to 5 days of intravenous IL-2 every 8 hours. Patients are then given a 2-day rest, and those scheduled to receive LAK cells undergo four or five daily leukophoreses to harvest lymphocytes. The lymphocytes are cultured in medium containing IL-2 to generate LAK cells, which are then reinfused along with intravenous IL-2. Patients who receive intravenous IL-2 alone receive a second cycle of IL-2 beginning approximately 1 week after the last dose of IL-2 given in the first cycle. (Further details on the basic and clinical aspects of this therapy are given in Chapter 17, Principles and Applications of Biologic Therapy.) Because there were no responses in nine patients with metastatic renal cell carcinoma with the primary tumor in place who were treated in the Surgery Branch of the NCI with either IL-2 or IL-2 plus LAK cells, most patients who present with a kidney tumor in place undergo nephrectomy before receiving adoptive immunotherapy. The nephrectomy decreases the tumor bulk and provides tissue for possible subsequent use for therapy with tumor-infiltrating lymphocytes (discussed below). It is important that immunotherapy in patients with metastatic renal cell carcinoma not be instituted until the patient has fully recovered from surgery and renal function is normal. One of the toxic effects of IL-2 therapy involves the development of renal insufficiency. Although the renal insufficiency resolves quickly after IL-2 is withdrawn, patients with one kidney who have recently had surgery must be evaluated and monitored carefully.

Currently, 124 patients with metastatic renal cell carcinoma have been treated in the Surgery Branch of the NCI. Most of the patients underwent nephrectomy prior to treatment, and many had had chemotherapy, radiation, hormone, or other therapies previously. Seventy-two evaluable patients with metastatic renal cell carcinoma received IL-2 plus LAK cell therapy, 52 received IL-2 alone. Some received lower-dose IL-2 (30,000 U/kg every 8 hours), most received higher-dose IL-2 (100,000 U/kg every 8 hours).

Of the 72 evaluable patients who received LAK cells plus IL-2, 8 had complete responses and 17 had partial responses, for a 35% complete or partial response rate. Of the 52 evaluable patients who received IL-2 alone, 4 had complete responses and 7 had partial responses. Durations of responses to the two different regimens are given in Table 31-7. There were responses at a number of different sites, including lung, liver, soft tissue, subcutaneous tissue, and bone (Figs. 31-10, 31-11, 31-12, 31-13, 31-14).

A randomized trial is currently under way at the NCI comparing response to therapy with IL-2 plus LAK cells to IL-2 alone. Currently 48 patients with advanced renal cell carcinoma have been randomized to receive IL-2 plus LAK cells and 48 to receive IL-2 alone. Among the 46 evaluable patients who have received IL-2 plus LAK cells, 7 have achieved a complete response and 8 have had partial responses. Among the 42 evaluable patients who received IL-2 alone, so far 3 patients have achieved a complete response and 7 have achieved a partial response. (Inevaluable patients are those who for some reason did not receive IL-2; also, two patients in the LAK/IL-2 group, one with a complete response and one with no response, did not receive LAK cells. [Rosenberg SA et al: Submitted for publication].)

Other groups have also reported responses in metastatic renal cell carcinoma with adoptive immunotherapy with IL-2 plus LAK cells.[165] The NCI IL-2/LAK Extramural Working Group reported two complete and three partial responses in 32 evaluable patients treated with IL-2 plus LAK cells, for a 16% response rate.[169] The difference in response rate seems to be accounted for by the greater tumor burden present in the patients treated at the extramural centers. In the extramural trial there were more patients with bulky abdominal disease than in the NCI series, and 9 of 35 patients treated had not undergone nephrectomy before receiving adoptive immunotherapy. It has been reported that patients with renal cell cancer may have defects in their immune systems that correct with the excision of the primary tumor.[170] It seems likely that overcoming the immunosuppressive effects of factors produced by solid tumors would be easier at lower tumor burdens. Perhaps these further arguments support performing nephrectomy in the setting of metastatic disease. The success in treating metastatic disease has stimulated interest in performing adoptive cellular therapy with LAK cells plus IL-2 in a surgical adjuvant setting. A prospective randomized study in patients with N+ or T4A renal cell carcinoma is currently being conducted by Linehan, Rosenberg, and their colleagues.

Other recent *in vivo* and *in vitro* preclinical studies suggest that major improvements in adoptive immunotherapy are likely to occur. In an attempt to identify more potent cells for use in adoptive transfer, Rosenberg et al have performed murine studies in which lymphocytes grown from the tumor, tumor-infiltrating lymphocytes (TIL), have proved much more potent than LAK cells in mediating regression of established metastases.[171] It has been demonstrated recently that TIL from a number of human tumors, including renal cell carcinoma, can be isolated and expanded.[172–175] Based on these studies and on clinical experience demonstrating that selected patients who have recently undergone nephrectomy can safely undergo adoptive immunotherapy with IL-2 or IL-2 plus LAK cells, a clinical trial has been initiated in which the primary kidney tumor or accessible metastatic tissue is resected, the lymphocytes from the tumor are expanded in media containing IL-2, and the TIL cells plus intravenous IL-2 and cyclophosphamide are administered back into the patient.[176] A pilot trial has demonstrated that this therapeutic strategy is practical and that in carefully selected patients with renal cell carcinoma, IL-2 plus TIL cell therapy can safely be administered. Currently, after the renal tumor is removed, the enzyme-dispersed cells (containing tumor cells and lymphocytes) are cryopreserved and stored. After the patient has fully recovered from surgery and renal function is normal, the cells are thawed and the TIL cells are expanded for therapy.

The potential for improved outcome by combining adop-

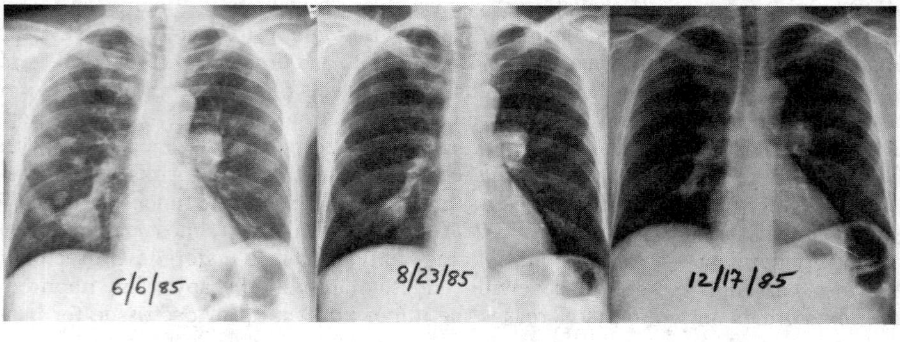

FIG. 31-10. Chest radiographs of multiple pulmonary nodules in a patient with metastatic renal cell cancer before (*left panel*) and after (*middle and right panels*) treatment with IL-2 and LAK cells. All of the nodules underwent a marked regression; most resolved completely.

TABLE 31-7. Results of Immunotherapy for Renal Cell Carcinoma, Surgery Branch, National Cancer Institute

	LAK Cells + IL-2		*IL-2*	
Total Evaluable Patients	*No. of Patients*	*Response Duration (mo)*	*No. of Patients*	*Response Duration (mo)*
	72		52	
No. with CR	8	20+, 17+, 15, 13+, 13, 11, 9, 6	4	24+, 18+, 17+, 15+
No. with PR	17	26+, 17+, 13, 11, 10+, 10+, 10, 9, 7, 7, 6, 6, 6, 6, 3, 1, 1	7	17+, 17+, 15+, 11+, 11, 9+, 5+
Total no. of CR + PR	25	(35%)	11	(21%)

tive cellular therapy with chemotherapy has been demonstrated in other animal experiments. Salup, Back, and Wiltrout found, in a murine renal cell carcinoma model, that neither LAK cells plus IL-2 nor single-agent doxorubicin were very effective therapy in advanced stage renal cancer. However, when doxorubicin and LAK cells plus IL-2 were combined and administered both systemically and intraperitoneally, 80% of animals with locally advanced and metastatic disease were cured of renal cell carcinoma.[177] A clinical trial applying the principles learned from these experiments is under way. Among the effects demonstrated for doxorubicin is that on the trafficking of adoptively transferred cells. When doxorubicin is administered with the cells, nearly twice as many cells home to a tumor-bearing kidney than to a normal kidney. Another drug, flavone-8-acetic acid (FAA), has been demonstrated to be a potent inducer of interferon. When used together with IL-2 in a murine model, FAA cured 80% or more of animals with advanced renal cell carcinoma.[178] Thus, the exploration of combined modality therapy may improve on the advances made to date.

FIG. 31-11. Lung tomograms of a patient with metastatic renal cell carcinoma with a right hilar mass, before treatment with IL-2 and LAK cells (*lower panels*) and afterward (*upper panels*). The tumor regresses almost completely.

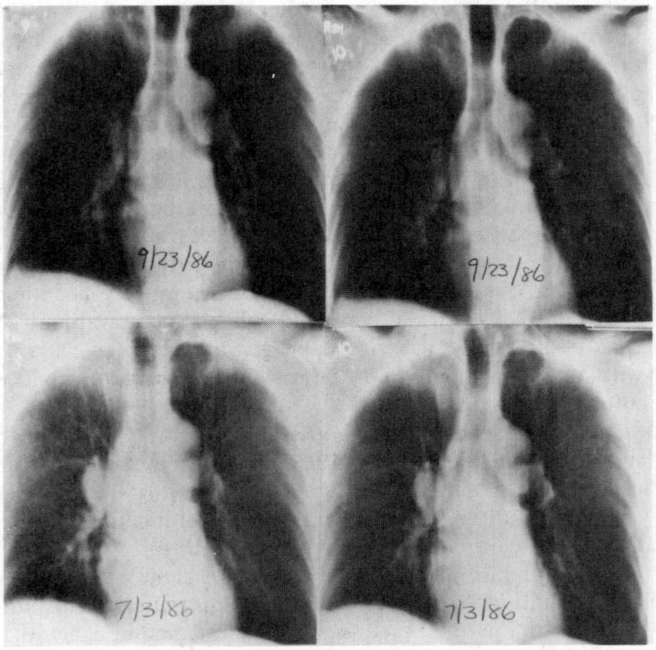

Interferon is perhaps the most extensively evaluated biologic agent in renal cell cancer treatment.[167,168] A large number of patients have been treated with purified and recombinant interferon-α, interferon-β, and interferon-γ; the results of such studies are summarized in Table 31-8.[179-198] The data suggest that the best response rates occur when interferon is administered daily at close to the maximum tolerated dose, rather than intermittently at high doses. The response rate for daily doses of interferon-α between 10 and 20 megaunits/m^2 is around 25%, and about 5% of the responses are complete. Responses last a median of 8 months. It would be expected that interferon might act additively or synergistically with certain other biologic agents like LAK cells plus IL-2, IL-2, other interferons, tumor necrosis factor, and other cytokines. Interferon should also potentiate the effects of antitumor monoclonal antibodies. A number of clinical trials employing combinations of biologic agents are under way. Substantial preclinical data support the use of interferon in combination with chemotherapeutic agents.[199] Clinical trials of interferon plus vinblastine[200-202] and interferon plus BCNU[203] have not shown dramatic enhancement or antitumor responses. A study conducted at the Mayo Clinic appears to show nearly a doubling of the response rate in patients with renal cell carcinoma treated with interferon (20 megaunits/m^2 three times weekly) with the addition of aspirin (2 tablets orally four times a day) to the therapeutic regimen.[204] Ten (34%) of 29 patients achieved objective responses lasting a median of over 10 months. This observation is being tested in a prospective randomized study by the North Central Oncology Group. The mechanism by which aspirin enhances the antitumor effects of interferon is unknown but could relate to the inhibition of lipoxygenase or the induction by aspirin of a protein that blocks phospholipase C, which is involved in cell proliferation through phosphoinositol turnover. Certainly the single-agent activity of interferon-α is at least comparable to that of the best chemotherapeutic agents. Interferon may form a building block for a combined modality regimen that includes chemotherapeutic agents and LAK cells plus IL-2. The M. D. Anderson group has suggested that tumors that progress after an interferon-induced partial or complete remission may be more

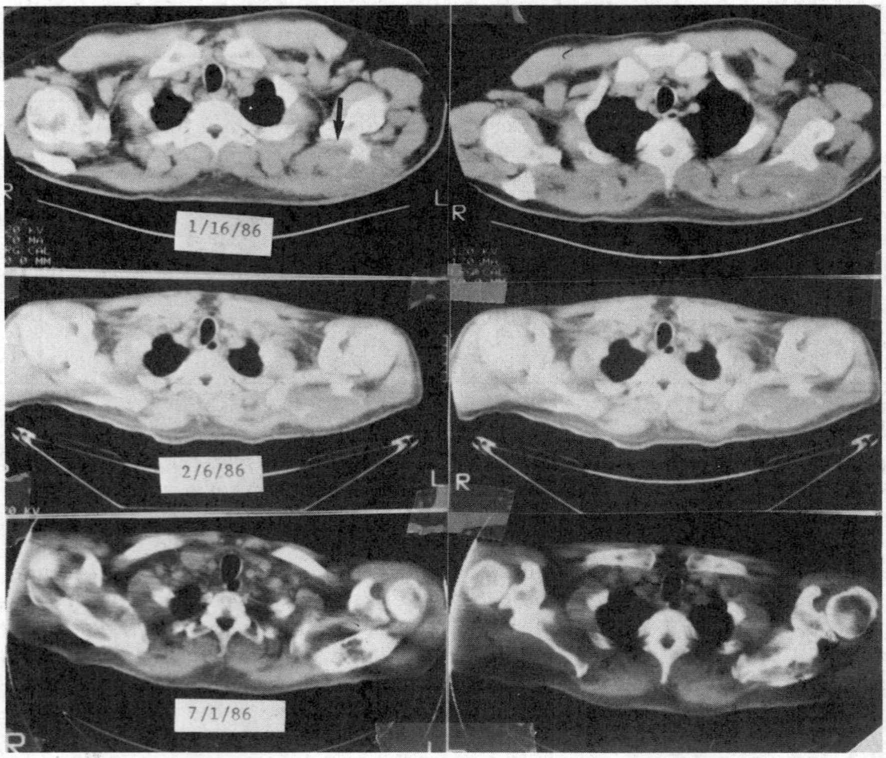

FIG. 31-12. CT scan of a patient with renal cell carcinoma with a metastasis in the scapula before treatment with IL-2 and LAK cells (*upper panels*) and afterward (*middle and lower panels*). All tumors regressed completely.

FIG. 31-13. Radiograph of the pelvis of a patient with metastatic renal cell carcinoma who had a large osseous metastasis before treatment with IL-2 and LAK cells (*upper panel*) and afterward (*lower panel*). The osseous lesion regressed completely and the bone recalcified.

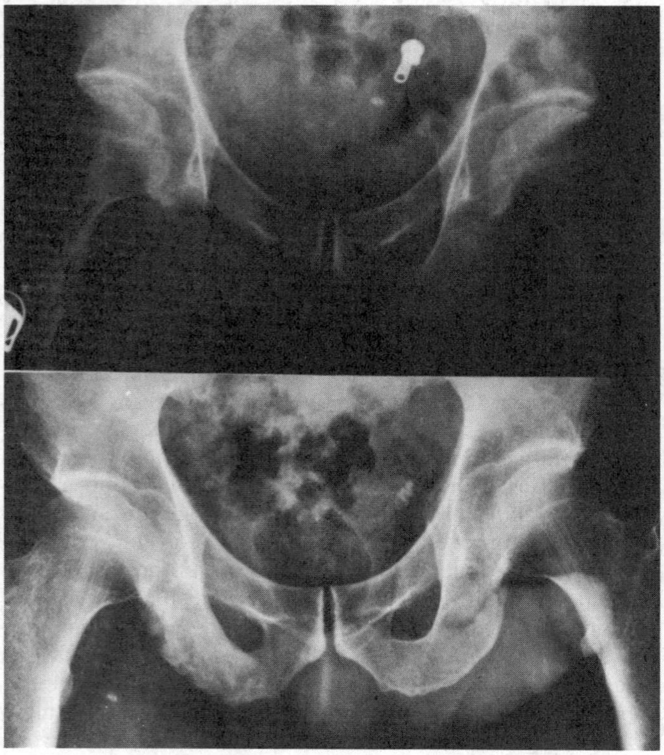

responsive to subsequent treatment with chemotherapeutic agents.[205] Sequential therapy also needs to be evaluated.

Ribonucleic acid (RNA) has been used in the treatment of patients with renal cell carcinoma, in the form of synthetic double-stranded polymer, polyinosinic-polycytidylic acid (poly IC), which induces interferon,[206] and in the form of xenogeneic immune RNA, RNA extracted from the lymphoid cells of animals immunized with human renal cell carcinoma cells.[207,208] Poly IC did not produce responses at the maximum tolerated dose.[206] The incubation of patient lymphocytes with immune RNA extracted from the lymphocytes of guinea pigs that had been immunized with the patient's tumor results in the development of tumor-specific cellular immunity by a mechanism that is not yet established. When such cells were reinfused into the patient, most patients had measurable changes in immune function, and complete or partial responses were obtained in 6 (22%) of 27 patients.[207] Patients with pulmonary metastases were the most likely to respond to this form of passive immunotherapy. Xenogeneic immune RNA from the lymphoid cells of sheep immunized with renal cancer has also been given directly to patients with renal carcinoma, but has not been shown to produce tumor regression.[208]

Active nonspecific immunotherapy has recently produced responses in a pilot study of 42 patients with metastatic renal cell cancer.[168] The use of two orally administered agents, coumarin (100 mg/d) and cimetidine (300 mg/four times a day), produced complete responses in three patients and partial responses in 11 (overall response rate, 33%). Response durations are not yet available for complete responders, but the partial responses lasted a median of 5 months. All the responses occurred in patients who had undergone

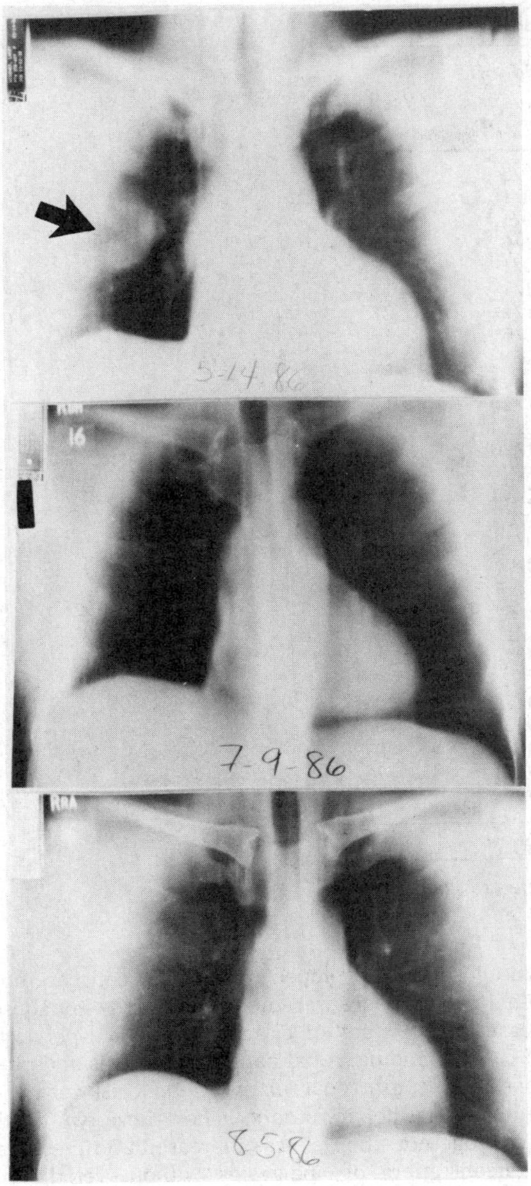

FIG. 31-14. Lung tomograms of a patient with renal cell carcinoma who had a large pulmonary metastasis before IL-2 treatment (*upper panel*) and afterward (*middle and lower panels*). The pulmonary nodule regressed completely.

nephrectomy (14 of 31, or 45%). Although cimetidine has been thought to modulate suppressor cells, the effects of coumarin on the immune system are unclear. These results need to be confirmed and extended. In contrast, the use of bacillus Calmette-Guérin (BCG) has not been associated with convincing therapeutic results in patients with metastatic disease. Pulmonary lesions may regress, but it is not known if such responses prolong survival. In one study of BCG given in the adjuvant setting after nephrectomy, survival did not appear to be improved.[209] However, if BCG and its related nonspecific immunostimulants are to be successfully applied to the treatment of cancer, one would expect their greatest effect to be seen in locally advanced disease when administered in the adjuvant setting. BCG has been given as a component of a multimodality treatment program that included combination chemotherapy and hormonal manipulation, but the response rate was not higher than that obtained with interferon or vinblastine as single agents.[210] In another study of vincristine, doxorubicin, medroxyprogesterone, and BCG, patients whose primary tumors were resected had a higher probability of responding than those in whom the primary tumor was left in place.[211] Thymosin fraction V appears to have no antitumor effects in renal cancer,[212] but an acid mucopolysaccharide called catrix-s, extracted from bovine tracheal cartilage, produced a dramatic complete remission in one of two patients with renal cell carcinoma who were treated with it.[213]

A variety of approaches to inducing tumor-specific immunity have been taken. Treatment with autologous cells modified by dimethyldioctadecyl ammonium bromide,[214] or with autologous cells irradiated and given with adjuvants like *Corynebacterium parvum* with[215] and without[216] cyclophosphamide to eliminate suppressor cells, is associated with response rates of 10% to 20%.[217] Antigens have been extracted from tumors, polymerized, and administered together with immune stimulants like BCG,[218,219] and attenuated vaccinia virus[220] has been given in an effort to elicit a tumor-specific immune response. Such approaches have been minimally effective at eliciting appropriate immune responses, and antitumor responses in vivo have been rare. However, the success that has been demonstrated in colorectal cancer using an autologous tumor vaccine plus BCG, and the availability of recombinant molecules such as IL-2 that may be superior at boosting cell-mediated immunity, make this approach to treatment worthy of further exploration.

An early attempt at using an immunologic approach to the treatment of renal cell cancer was reported in 1971. Horn and Horn infused plasma from a patient previously cured of renal cell carcinoma into a family member who had diffusely metastatic renal cell carcinoma, and produced a complete remission that lasted almost 2 years.[221] The patient relapsed with metastases to the cerebrum, a site that might be considered a sanctuary from the effects of antibodies. Investigators have been slow to apply the field of serotherapy to renal cell carcinoma. Only very recently have efforts been made to characterize the cell surface of renal cell cancers and the polyclonal and monoclonal antibodies that recognize the cell surface antigens.[222,223] Antibodies directed against renal cell cancer are expected to be useful adjuncts to therapy with interferons and LAK cells plus IL-2.

CARCINOMA OF THE RENAL PELVIS

Carcinoma of the renal pelvis is a relatively rare tumor that accounts for 5% of all renal tumors. It occurs more frequently in men than in women (2–3 : 1). Upper urinary tract carcinoma is a multifocal process; patients with cancer at one site in the upper urinary tract are at greater risk of developing tumors elsewhere. The probability of multifocal occurrence is greater in patients with larger lesions and in those with carcinoma in situ. A patient with one upper tract urothelial tumor has a 30% to 50% chance of developing a bladder tumor as well. Some 2% to 4% of patients with an

TABLE 31-8. Response Rate of Renal Cell Carcinoma to Various Interferons

Interferon Type and Source	*Dose (megaunits/m²), Route, and Schedule*	*No. of Evaluable Patients*	*No. of Responses (CR/PR)*	*Response Rate (%)*
HuIFN(Le)[179,180]	3 IM daily	19	0/5	26
	3 IM daily	50	3/10	26
HuIFN(Le)[181]	6 IM daily × 3 d, for 4 wk	4	0/1	25
HuIFN(Le)[182]	3 IM daily × 5 d, for 12 wk	43	1/6	16
HuIFN(Le)[183]	1 IM daily × 28 d	14	0/1	7
	10 IM daily × 28 d	16	1/1	12.5
HuIFN(Le)[184]	3 IM daily	11	1/2	27
HuIFN(Ly)[185]	5 IM 3 times a wk × 24 wk	33	0/5	15
HuIFN(Ly)[186]	3 IM on d 1, 5 on d 2, 10 on d 3, 20 on d 4–10	39	0/5	13
HuIFN(Ly)[187]	3 IM daily	18	1/2	17
HuIFN(Ly)[188]	3 IM 3 times a wk × 6 wk	21	0/1	5
HuIFN(Ly)[189]	5 IM daily	73	1/16	23
αA	3–36 IM daily	45	1/7	18
rIFN-α2	6–10 IM daily	108	2/13	14
rIFN-α2[190]	2 SC 3 times a wk,	10	0/0	0
	30 IV daily × 5 d, for 2–3 wk	10	0/1	10
rIFN-α2[191]	2 IM daily	15	0/0	0
	20 IM daily	41	1/11	29
rIFN-α2[192]	3–36 IM daily × 5 d × 14 wk	19	1/4	26
rIFN-α2[193]	10 IM daily × 3 mo	8	1/1	25
rIFN-α2[194]	2 SC 3 times a wk,	51	1/4	10
	30 IV daily × 5 d, for 3 wk	46	1/2	7
rIFN-α2[195]	3–36 IM daily × 10 wk	22	0/5	23
rIFN-β[196]	150 IV twice a wk × 4 wk	15	0/2	13
rIFN-γ[197]	Up to 75 IV twice a week	13	0/0	0
rIFN-γ[198]	Varying doses IM	14	0/1	7
	Varying doses IV	16	0/1	6
Total		747	16/107	16.5

IM = intramuscular, SC = subcutaneous, IV = intravenous, CR = complete response, PR = partial response.

upper tract urothelial tumor develop bilateral renal pelvic tumors. If a patient has both a renal pelvic tumor and a ureteral tumor at the same time, there is a 75% chance that a bladder tumor will develop. Alternatively, a patient with a bladder tumor initially has a 2% to 3% chance of developing an upper tract tumor.[224–228]

ETIOLOGY

In 1965 Hultengren et al first identified a connection between epithelial tumors of the renal pelvis and abuse of compound analgesics.[229,230] Since then a number of other reports from Sweden,[231,232] Australia,[233–235] the Netherlands,[236] Denmark,[237] Italy,[238] and Germany[239] have demonstrated an association between analgesic abuse and renal pelvic tumors. Most of the patients ingested a significant amount (5 kg) of compound analgesics, usually containing phenacetin, phenazone, and caffeine.[228,234] Typically, upper genitourinary (GU) tract tumors occur in patients in whom prolonged and heavy analgesic ingestion is followed by renal papillary necrosis.[234] Although the precise mechanism is not completely understood, studies have suggested a possible etiologic role of orthoaminophenols, the major phenacetin metabolites, in the development of renal pelvic tumors.[228] In a study of 192 patients with chronic pyelonephritis, 104 had pyelonephritis secondary to analgesic abuse. Of the 104 analgesic abusers, 8 developed transitional cell carcinoma of the renal pelvis. There were no tumors in the nonabusers.[231] In a case-control study of patients with renal pelvic transitional cell carcinoma, renal papillary necrosis and phenacetin abuse both conferred a relatively equal risk for the development of renal pelvic tumors. When these two conditions occurred together, the risk was increased 20 times over that for nonconsumers of analgesics without renal papillary necrosis.[235]

There is also an association between cancer of the renal pelvis and Danubian endemic familial nephropathy (Balkan nephropathy). Balkan nephropathy is a slowly progressive inflammation of the interstitium of the kidney that ultimately results in renal failure. This disorder, which is prevalent in the Balkan countries (Yugoslavia, Rumania, Bulgaria, and Greece), is associated with multifocal, slow-growing, superficial, low-grade tumors of the renal pelvis.[228] The cause of Balkan nephropathy is unclear; however, a number of potential etiologic agents such as fungal toxins, viruses, silicates, and heavy metals have been studied.[224]

An association has been observed between renal pelvic tumors and urban residence as well as occupation in the aniline dye, textile, plastics, and rubber industries.[228,240] There is a significant increase in risk for upper genitourinary tract urothelial cancer in smokers; the risk is highest among the heaviest smokers.[228] Chronic inflammation and irritation are associated with the development of renal pelvic tumors, particularly in patients who have upper urinary tract stones.

There are in-depth studies of the molecular genetics of transitional cell carcinoma. DNA sequence deletions have been detected by RFLP analysis at the *c-H-ras* locus in 42% of patients with bladder carcinoma, suggesting the possibility of a recessive or activated oncogene at this site.[64] There are reports of nine kindreds exhibiting a familial pattern in the development of transitional cell carcinoma of the urinary tract.[241,242] Of the affected family members, 22% had upper tract tumors, 59% had bladder cancer, and 18% had both upper and lower tract tumors.[241] One member of another cancer-prone family (Li-Fraumeni syndrome) developed bilateral upper tract urothelial carcinoma. A molecular defect, an activated *c-raf*-1 gene, has been isolated from noncancerous cells from members of a family with Li-Fraumeni syndrome; however, material from affected family members with bladder or upper tract transitional cell carcinoma has not yet been analyzed.[243] Studies of the molecular and cellular aspects of urothelial transformation should provide further insight into the etiology and mechanisms of progression and metastasis of this disease.

PATHOLOGY

Transitional cell carcinoma accounts for 90% of the tumors of the renal pelvis and can be in situ, papillary, or planar. Squamous cell carcinoma, which is usually associated with chronic inflammation or infection of the renal pelvis, accounts for 7% of renal pelvic tumors. Squamous cell cancer of the renal pelvis is often deeply invasive and is associated with a worse prognosis than is transitional cell carcinoma. Adenocarcinoma of the renal pelvis has been reported in few patients and occurs in association with inflammation, infection, or calculi.[224,228,240,244]

DIAGNOSTIC AND STAGING TECHNIQUES

The differential diagnosis of renal pelvic carcinoma is given in Table 31-9. Hematuria is the initial presenting symptom in the majority of patients. Gross hematuria is present in 62% to 75%, microscopic hematuria in 10%. The triad of flank mass, pain, and hematuria is encountered frequently, in 20% or less, and often is associated with advanced disease.[228,240,245–248]

Excretory urography is frequently used to evaluate patients with renal pelvic tumors and will often reveal a filling defect in the collecting system. There may also be either a hydronephrotic or a nonfunctional kidney due to obstruction by a blood clot or mass.[224,227] Retrograde pyelography (in which contrast medium is injected into the ureter through an endoscope) accurately delineates upper tract filling defects. If there is uncertainty about the nature of a renal pelvic lesion, CT performed before and after administration of intravenous contrast material will differentiate a tumor from another radiolucent mass such as a stone. Angiography is not often used in the diagnostic evaluation of a suspected renal pelvic tumor. However, a renal mass lesion that lacks the characteristic neovascularity of a renal cell carcinoma may be the first indication of a renal pelvic tumor invading the renal parenchyma.[249–251]

Urine cytology is useful in evaluating a renal pelvis mass, and endoscopically obtained barbotage specimens allow an accurate diagnosis to be made in about 80% of cases.[252,253] Tissue can also be obtained by introducing a biopsy brush into the ureter and removing a specimen for cytologic or histologic examination. Brush biopsy increases diagnostic accuracy to between 80% and 90%. Endoscopic ureteroscopy and percutaneous nephroscopy are recently developed clinical techniques that have improved the diagnosis of upper tract tumors. With currently available flexible endoscopic instruments, the renal pelvis can be inspected visually in almost 90% of patients.[240,246,254,255]

TABLE 31-9. Differential Diagnosis of Cancer of the Renal Pelvis*

Intrinsic Lesions
Calculus
Blood clot
Cholesteatoma
Malakoplakia
Inflammatory lesions of urothelium (pyelitis cystica, etc.)
Benign ureteropelvic junction obstruction
Benign (connective tissue) tumors of renal pelvis
Renal cell carcinoma
Suburothelial hemorrhage
Extrinsic Lesions
Vascular impressions
Parapelvic cyst

*Modified from Fraly EE: Cancer of the renal pelvis. In Skinner DG, de Kernion JB (eds): Genitourinary Cancer, p 141. Philadelphia, WB Saunders, 1978.

STAGE AND GRADE

The most significant prognostic factors for survival of patients with renal pelvic carcinoma are stage and grade of tumor.[246,256] Renal pelvic cancer is divided into four stages. Stage I is papillary carcinoma without evidence of invasion, Stage II denotes tumor that is superficially invasive but limited to the lamina propria, Stage III denotes involvement of the muscularis, Stage III denotes involvement of the muscularis, and stage IV denotes extent to adjacent structures or metastatic disease (Table 31-10). Renal pelvic tumors are graded from I to III. The 5-year survival for patients with

TABLE 31-10. Renal Pelvic Cancer*

Stage I	Papillary or planar (nonpapillary) carcinoma with no evidence of invasion.
Stage II	Papillary or planar carcinoma. Superficially invasive but with invasion limited to the lamina propria.
Stage III	Papillary or planar carcinoma, extending to the level of the muscularis (may extend beyond the muscularis in intrarenal portions of the renal pelvis if confined to the kidney.)
Stage IV	Papillary or planar carcinoma extending to the adventitial surface and either involving adjuvant structures or metastatic or both.

*Modified from Bennington JL, Beckwith JB: Armed Forces Institute of Pathology, 2nd ed, Fasc 12, 1975.

Grade I transitional cell carcinoma of the renal pelvis approaches 100%; for Grade II, it is 60% to 70%; and for Grade III, it is 5%. Invasion of the renal hilum occurs in 95% of patients who ultimately develop metastases.[246,256,257]

TREATMENT

Carcinoma of the renal pelvis may be treated with a radical nephrectomy that includes removal of Gerota's fascia and its contents, total removal of the ipsilateral ureter, and removal of a cuff of bladder.[224,228,246,248,258–260] Simple intrafascial nephrectomy is associated with a decreased 5-year survival rate compared to that for radical nephrectomy, particularly in patients with Stage III or IV tumors.[259] When transitional cell carcinoma of the renal pelvis invades the renal vein or vena cava, an extensive surgical procedure including thrombus extraction and/or partial vena cava resection may be required.[224,228,240,246,248,258–262]

A more conservative surgical excision is advocated by some who note that renal pelvic carcinoma can be bilateral and that survival of patients with low-stage, low-grade renal pelvic carcinoma treated with a conservative surgical procedure is approximately the same as in patients treated with more radical surgery.[263–265] The incidence of low-grade, low-stage renal pelvic carcinoma is approximately 8% and that of bilateral disease is 2%. There is also often a long latent period prior to recurrence.[240,247,260] In most studies reporting a low recurrence rate after local excision, the follow-up period is short. When even low-stage, low-grade tumors were resected from the renal pelvis, a 29% to 30% incidence of recurrence in the ipsilateral ureter was found during a 10-year follow-up.[240] Although the availability of new techniques such as intraoperative nephroscopy and brush cytology have made staging much more accurate, intraoperative pyeloscopy is not without risk. In a recent series of 18 patients with renal pelvic carcinoma who underwent intraoperative pyeloscopy for evaluation and staging, two experienced disease recurrence in the renal fossa.[266] Currently, most clinicians consider that local, partial excision is most appropriate for patients with a solitary kidney, with bilateral renal pelvic carcinoma, or with renal insufficiency. New treatment strategies involving percutaneous resection of renal pelvic tumors followed by either laser irradiation or supplemental intracavitary therapy with mitomycin C or BCG are currently being evaluated.[255]

FOLLOW-UP

Conscientious follow-up after surgery for renal pelvic carcinoma is essential. Urinalysis, urine cytology, and cystourethroscopy are performed every 3 months for 2 to 3 years, then less frequently. For patients who undergo a conservative upper tract procedure, periodic retrograde pyelography is also performed.[240]

URETERAL CARCINOMA

Ureteral carcinoma is an uncommon neoplasm that accounts for only 1% of all malignancies of the upper GU tract. Ureteral carcinoma was first described by the French pathologist Rayer in 1841; the first ureteral carcinoma to be removed by nephroureterectomy was reported by Vorphl in 1905. Ureteral carcinoma tends to occur in the older age groups, predominantly in the sixth, seventh, and eighth decades of life. The male–female ratio is 2:1. The most common site for the occurrence of a ureteral tumor is in the lower third of the ureter, with a lesser incidence higher up.[267–272]

TABLE 31-11. Classification of Tumors of the Ureter*

Primary Tumors
Epithelial
Malignant
Transitional cell carcinoma (71%)
Transitional cell carcinoma with differentiation (20%)
Squamous differentiation
Glandular differentiation
Mixed
Squamous cell carcinoma (pure) (8%)
Adenocarcinoma (1%)
Undifferentiated carcinoma (1%)
Benign
Papilloma
Mesodermal
Malignant
Leiomyosarcoma
Benign
Fibroepithelial polyp
Leiomyoma
Neurilemmoma
Angioma
Secondary Tumors (All Malignant)
Drop metastases
Metastases via blood or lymph
Direct extension

*Modified from Bennington JL, Beckwith JB: Armed Forces Institute of Pathology, 2nd ed, Fasc 12, 1975.

HISTOLOGY AND ETIOLOGY

Ninety percent of malignant tumors of the ureter are transitional cell carcinomas; 20% have squamous or glandular differentiation. Eight percent of the tumors are pure squamous cell carcinomas and 1% are adenocarcinomas (Table 31-11). Tumors of the ureter share embryologic, morphologic, and etiologic characteristics with renal pelvic tumors. As with renal pelvic tumors, there is an increased incidence of ureteral carcinoma associated with Balkan nephropathy, prolonged exposure to phenacetin, or prolonged exposure to environmental agents such as aniline dyes.[273]

CLINICAL PRESENTATION

Hematuria is the most common presenting symptom and is present in 75% of patients with ureteral carcinoma. The hematuria is usually painless; however, colicky pain due to obstruction by clot or by tumor occurs in up to 35%. Urinary frequency or dysuria, present in only 10% of patients with renal pelvic carcinoma, occurs in up to 50% of patients with ureteral carcinoma.[269,273]

Ureteral carcinoma is divided into five stages (Table 31-12). Stage 0 ureteral carcinoma is confined to the mucosa of the ureter; Stage A disease involves the lamina propria. In Stage B the tumor involves the muscularis of the ureter; in Stage C the tumor extends through the muscularis to the

TABLE 31-12. Staging of Ureteral Carcinoma

Stage 0	Limited to mucosa
Stage A	Lamina propria invasion
Stage B	Confined to muscularis
Stage C	Invasion through muscularis with involvement of adjacent structures or metastases
Stage D	Metastatic

adventitia. Stage D is metastatic disease. Although up to 100% of Grade I tumors and 85% of Grade II tumors may be noninvasive, only 30% of Grade III and 8% of Grade IV tumors are noninvasive.[273]

DIAGNOSIS

Excretory urography is an initial part of the evaluation of a suspected ureteral mass lesion. On excretory urography the upper tract above the tumor may be completely normal or there may be hydronephrosis or complete nonfunction. Retrograde pyelography is performed to delineate accurately the precise location of the ureteral lesion.[273,274] Urine is collected for cytologic examination, and brush biopsy may be performed to obtain tissue for histologic examination. The availability of flexible endoscopy has greatly improved the surgeon's ability to visualize and biopsy ureteral lesions.[255] Abdominal CT also provides useful staging information, particularly with regard to extension of the tumor outside the ureter.

TREATMENT

Carcinoma of the ureter is treated by either nephroureterectomy (Fig. 31-15) or partial ureterectomy.[227,268,269,275] The advantage of a partial ureterectomy is that the more conservative procedure preserves the kidney. However, mapping studies of the urothelium have demonstrated that carcinoma of the upper urinary tract is a multifocal disease. There is often atypia and carcinoma in situ in multiple areas of the urothelium, particularly in high-grade, high-stage carcinomas. Ureteral carcinoma treated by partial ureterectomy or by nephrectomy plus partial ureterectomy is associated with a 12% to 40% recurrence rate.[269,275] Those who advocate more conservative management of ureteral carcinoma note that recent studies demonstrate that in low-stage, low-grade carcinomas, distal ureterectomy with reimplantation of the distal ureter is associated with excellent survival,[227,264] and that survival is more dependent on grade and stage of disease (Table 31-13) than on the type of operation performed.[247,276] In a study reported by Babain and Johnson there was a 100% 5-year survival rate in patients with Stage 0 or A distal ureteral carcinoma who were treated with distal ureterectomy plus reimplantation.[227] Currently, distal ureterectomy plus reimplantation is recommended for patients with low-stage, low-grade disease that occurs in the distal third of the ureter. Nephroureterectomy is recommended for patients with high-grade or high-stage tumor and for those with disease at a location other than the distal third of the ureter.

The surgical procedure of radical nephrectomy plus ureterectomy entails removal of the kidney and the entire con-

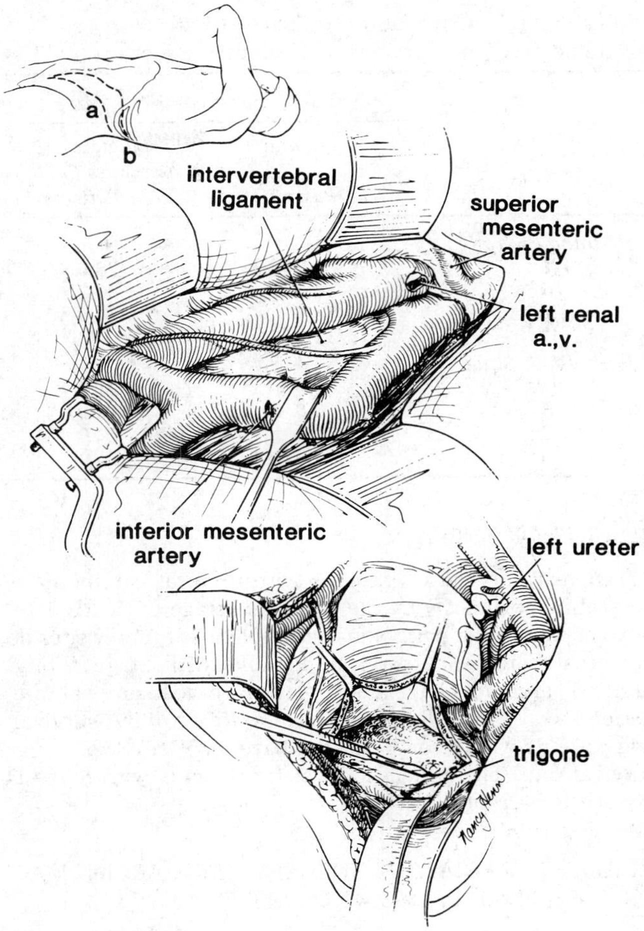

FIG. 31-15. The patient for a nephroureterectomy with lymph node dissection should be placed in a modified flank position and an incision made either through line a or line b. The area of dissection is as indicated in the middle panel, being divested from the superior mesenteric artery to the bifurcation. The ureter is removed by opening the bladder, circumscribing the orifice, and sharply dissecting the ureter from the surrounding detrusor muscle. The defect in the bladder is then closed appropriately. (Paulson DF, Perez CA, Anderson T: Cancer of the kidney and ureter. In DeVita VT Jr, Hellman S, Rosenberg SA (eds): Cancer: Principles and Practice of Oncology, 2nd ed, p 907. Philadelphia, JB Lippincott, 1985)

tents of Gerota's fascia, the ureter, and a cuff of bladder including the ureteral orifice and intramural ureter. Regional lymph nodes may be removed, particularly if there is indication of involvement. This surgical procedure may be performed using one or two incisions, depending on the patient's body habitus and the surgeon's preference. When partial ureterectomy is performed, urinary tract continuity is reestablished with either ureteroureterostomy or ureteroneocystostomy.

New strategies involving endoscopic fulguration and laser photocoagulation have been developed for treatment of patients with ureteral carcinoma. Carcinoma in situ of the distal ureter has been treated with endoscopic fulguration, with encouraging preliminary results.[277] These new therapeutic strategies will be important in the future evaluation of the role of radical versus local surgery for treatment of this disease.

TABLE 31-13. Correlation of Survival Rate with Pathologic Characteristics of Ureteral Cancer

	5-Year Survival Rate (%)	
	Bloom and Associates (1970) (54 Patients)	*Batata and Associates (1975) (41 Patients)*
Histologic Grade		
I	83.0	78.0
II	52.0	50.0
III	18.0	0
IV	12.0	0
Pathologic Stage		
0,A	62.0	91.0
B	50.0	43.0
C	33.3	23.0
D	0	0

RESULTS OF THERAPY

The 5-year survival of patients with ureteral carcinoma is determined primarily by the grade and stage of the disease. Sex and age of the patient and multiplicity of tumor sites do not greatly influence survival. Patients with Stage A or 0 ureteral carcinoma have a 90% to 100% 5-year survival rate. Patients with Stage B disease have a 45% to 85% survival, and patients with Stage C disease have a 25% to 30% 5-year survival rate. The 5-year survival for patients with Stage D disease is currently 0 to 5%.

ADJUVANT RADIATION THERAPY FOR CARCINOMA OF THE RENAL PELVIS AND URETER

There would seem to be no role for adjuvant therapy for low-stage upper tract transitional cell tumors; most series report less than 20% of the patients failing treatment or dying within 5 years after surgical resection.[270,245] Moreover, the results of surgical resection for patients with high-stage tumors—those with pathologic evidence of periurethral, peripelvic, or perirenal extension, or those with regional lymph node metastases—are also poor; less than 30% of the patients are cured by surgery alone.[278–280] Autopsy studies indicate that lymph node involvement occurs in 37% to 82% of patients with pelvic tumors.[245,281] In patients with ureteral tumors, lymph node involvement occurs in 22% to 41% of cases.[271] Local recurrence rate has been reported to be higher after surgical resection for invasive pelvic tumors (43%) than for invasive tumors of the ureter (14%).[269,244] A recent retrospective review of patients with poor-risk (high-stage or high-grade) transitional cell carcinoma of the renal pelvis and ureter found that patients treated with postoperative irradiation of 4000 to 5000 cGy had a lower incidence of local recurrence (1% versus 46%) and a higher 5-year survival (27% versus 17%) than patients treated with surgery alone.[280] Also, 45% of the patients in the poor prognosis group developed distant metastases.

A study of the best available information suggests that postoperative radiation therapy following radical surgical resection should be considered only for patients with locally advanced disease—those with pathologically confirmed periureteral, perirenal, or peripelvic extension of tumor, or those with proven regional lymph node metastases. Some centers are embarking on Phase I or II studies or pilot studies combining such local radiation therapy with adjuvant cisplatin-based chemotherapy regimens.[282] The dose of radiation therapy if no adjuvant chemotherapy is given would be in the range of 4500 cGy delivered in 180-cGy fractions over 5 weeks to the tumor bed, and to the regional lymph nodes with a boost to the tumor bed of up to 5000 cGy. However, if adjuvant chemotherapy is given, these doses should be decreased by 10% to 15%.

CHEMOTHERAPY FOR CARCINOMAS OF THE RENAL PELVIS AND URETER

Carcinomas arising in the ureters and renal pelvis are mainly transitional cell carcinomas,[227] can be multiple (either metachronously or synchronously),[283] occur with increased frequency in Balkan nephropathy (a toxic nephropathy indigenous to the Danube basin),[284] and give rise to metastases in about 40% of patients.[227] The histology, biology, and natural history make it senseless for the medical oncologist to consider transitional cell carcinomas of the ureter and renal pelvis as pathologic entities distinct from transitional cell carcinoma of the bladder. There are certainly distinctive features to the surgical management of ureteral and renal pelvis tumors based on anatomic differences; however, the patterns of local recurrence and systemic spread and response to treatment are very similar to histologically identical tumors arising in the bladder.[285]

In light of the frequent epithelial atypia in a normal-appearing ureter adjacent to primary tumors and the high incidence of local recurrence (up to 64%) and subsequent development of bladder tumors (21%),[286] it is surprising that adjuvant chemotherapy has been reported only anecdotally.[287] Topical thiotepa has been employed, but it is not possible to discern whether it exerts beneficial effects. A systematic study of postoperative or preoperative chemotherapy or immunotherapy is indicated.

The treatment of metastatic disease is the treatment for metastatic bladder cancer. At the moment, the most active regimen is M-VAC, a four-drug regimen consisting of methotrexate, vincristine, doxorubicin, and cisplatin, developed by Yagoda and colleagues at Memorial Sloan-Kettering Cancer Center.[288] M-VAC produces objective responses (complete and partial) in 69% of patients with metastatic transitional cell carcinoma of bladder, ureter, and renal pelvis.[288] The use of cyclophosphamide, doxorubicin, and cisplatin in varying doses, routes (intravenous, intra-arterial), and schedules has produced a similar response rate.[289] Both regimens are being tested in neoadjuvant trials. The administration of doxorubicin followed by cyclophosphamide 12 hours later allowed nearly 100% of the projected doses of the two drugs to be given, with a 57% overall response rate and a 23% complete response rate.[290] The capacity of WR-2721 to enhance the antitumor effects of cisplatin in patients with melanoma[291] makes it important to test its use in transitional cell tumors, which are also highly responsive to cisplatin-containing regimens. The apparent superiority of BCG over thiotepa in superficial bladder cancer[292] has suggested that immunotherapy approaches may also be useful. In addition to the active nonspecific approaches (BCG, interferon) and passive nonspecific approaches, there is a burgeoning preclinical literature on monoclonal antibodies that alone or conjugated to a drug or toxin or used in combination with other treatment modalities may prove useful in treating transitional cell tumors.[293] The reader is referred to Chapter 32 for a more complete discussion of treatment options and the direction of current treatment approaches.

REFERENCES

1. DeKernion JB: Renal tumors. In Walsh PC, Gittes RF, Perlmutter AD et al (eds): Campbell's Urology, 5th ed, pp 1294–1342. Philadelphia, WB Saunders, 1986
2. Goodman MT, Morgenstern H, Wynder EL: A case-control study of factors affecting the development of renal cell carcinoma. Am J Epidemiol 124:926–941, 1986
3. Lack EE, Cassady R, Sallan SE: Renal cell carcinoma in childhood and adolescence: A clinical and pathological study of 17 cases. J Urol 133:822–828, 1985
4. Lieber MM, Tomera FM, Taylor WF et al: Renal adenocarcinoma in young adults: Survival and variables affecting prognosis. J Urol 125:164–168, 1981
5. Castellanos RD, Aron BS, Evans AT: Renal adenocarcinoma in children: Incidence, therapy and prognosis. J Urol 111:534–537, 1974
6. National Institutes of Health: 1986 Annual Cancer Statistics Review. NIH publication No. 87–2789, Washington, DC, 1986
7. Golimbu M, Joshi P, Sperber A et al: Renal cell carcinoma: Survival and prognostic factors. Urology 27:291–301, 1986
8. Carson WJ: Tumors of the kidney: Histologic study. In: Transactions of the Section on Urology, American Medical Association, 1928
9. Glenn JF: Renal tumors. In Harrison JH, Gittes RF, Perlmutter AD et al (eds): Campbell's Urology, 4th ed, pp 967–1009. Philadelphia, WB Saunders, 1979
10. Grawitz P: Die sogenannten Lipome der Niere. Virchows Arch Pathol Anat 93:39–63, 1883
11. Doderlein A, Birch-Hirschfeld FV: Embryonale Drusengeschwulst der Nierengegend im Kindesalter. Sex Organe 3:88–99, 1984
12. Outzen HC, Maguire HC Jr: The etiology of renal-cell carcinoma. Semin Oncol 10:378–384, 1983
13. Lauritsen JG: Lindau's disease: A study of one family through six generations. Acta Chir Scand 139:482–486, 1973
14. Green JS, Bowmer MI, Johnson GJ: Von-Hippel-Lindau disease in a Newfoundland kindred. Can Med Assoc J 134:133–146, 1986
15. Malek RS, Omess PJ, Benson RC Jr et al: Renal cell carcinoma in von Hippel–Lindau syndrome. Am J Med 82:236–238, 1987
16. Gregoire JR, Torres VE, Holley KE et al: Renal epithelial hyperplastic and neoplastic proliferation in autosomal dominant polycystic kidney disease. Am J Kidney Dis 9:27–38, 1987
17. Kantor AF: Current concepts in the epidemiology and etiology of primary renal cell carcinoma. J Urol 117:415–417, 1977
18. McLaughlin JK, Mandel JS, Blot WJ et al: A population-based case-control study of renal cell carcinoma. J Natl Cancer Inst 72:275–284, 1984
19. Yu MC, Mack TM, Hanisch R et al: Cigarette smoking, obesity, diuretic use, and coffee consumption as risk factors for renal cell carcinoma. J Natl Cancer Inst 77:351–356, 1986
20. Whittemore AS, Paffenbarger RS Jr, Anderson K et al: Early precursors of urogenital cancers in former college men. J Urol 132:1256–1261, 1984
21. Lornoy W, Becaus I, de Vleeschouwer M et al: Renal cell carcinoma, a new complication of analgesic nephropathy. Lancet 1:1271–1272, 1986
22. Malker HR, Malker BK, McLaughlin JK et al: Kidney cancer among leather workers. Lancet 1:56, 1984
23. Maclure M: Asbestos and renal adenocarcinoma: A case-control study. Environ Res 42:353–361, 1987
24. DeKernion JB, Smith RB: The kidney and adrenal glands. In Paulson DF (ed): Genitourinary Surgery, pp 1–153. New York, Churchill-Livingstone, 1984
25. Kauzlaric D, Barmeir E, Luscieti P et al: Renal carcinoma after retrograde pyelography with thorotrast. AJR 148:897–898, 1987
26. Enterline PE, Viren J: Epidemiologic evidence for an association between gasoline and kidney cancer. Environ Health Perspect 62:303–312, 1985
27. McLaughlin JK, Blot WJ, Mehl ES et al: Petroleum-related employment and renal cell cancer. J Occup Med 27:672–674, 1985
28. Grantham JJ, Levine E: Acquired cystic disease: Replacing one kidney disease with another. Kid Int 28:99–105, 1985
29. Hughson MD, Buchwald D, Fox M: Renal neoplasia and acquired cystic kidney disease in patients receiving long-term dialysis. Arch Pathol Lab Med 110:592–601, 1986
30. MacDougall ML, Welling LW, Wiegmann TB: Renal adenocarcinoma and acquired cystic disease in chronic hemodialysis patients. Am J Kidney Dis 9:166–171, 1987
31. Bretan PN, Busch MP, Hricak H et al: Development of acquired renal cysts and renal cell carcinoma: Case reports and review of the literature. Cancer 57:1871–1879, 1986
32. Harris DT: Hormonal therapy and chemotherapy of renal-cell carcinoma. Semin Oncol 10:422–430, 1983
33. Matthews VS, Kirkman H, Bacon RL: Kidney damage in the golden hamster following chronic administration of diethylstilbestrol and sesame oil. Proc Soc Exp Biol Med 66:195–196, 1947
34. Kirkman H, Bacon RL: Estrogen-induced tumors of the kidney: I. Incidence of renal tumors in intact and gonadectomized male golden hamsters treated with diethylstilbestrol. J Natl Cancer Inst 13:745–755, 1952
35. Bloom HJG, Dukes CE, Mitchley BCV: Hormone-dependent tumours of the kidney: I. The oestrogen-induced renal tumour of the syrian hamster. Hormone treatment and possible relationship to carcinoma of the kidney in man. Br J Cancer 17:611–646, 1963
36. Bloom HJG, Roe FJC, Mitchley BCV: Sex hormones and renal neoplasia: Inhibition of tumor in hamster kidney by an estrogen antagonist, an agent of possible therapeutic value in man. Cancer 20:2118–2124, 1967
37. Chisholm GD: Nephrogenic ridge tumors and their syndromes. Ann NY Acad Sci 230:403–423, 1974
38. Strewler GJ, Williams RD, Nissenson RA: Human renal carcinoma cells produce hypercalcemia in the nude mouse and a novel protein recognized by parathyroid hormone receptors. J Clin Invest 71:769–774, 1983
39. Suva LJ, Winslow GA, Wettenhall EH et al: A parathyroid hormone-related protein implicated in malignant hypercalcemia: Cloning and expression. Science 237:893–895, 1987
40. Derynck R, Goeddel DV, Ullrich A et al: Synthesis of messenger RNAs for transforming growth factors alpha and beta and the epidermal growth factor receptor by human tumors. Cancer Res 47:707–712, 1987
41. Derynck R, Roberts AB, Winkler ME et al: Human transforming growth factor-alpha: Precursor structure and expression in E. coli. Cell 38:287–297, 1984
42. Gomella LG, Sargent ER, Wade TP et al: Expression of transforming growth factor alpha in normal adult kidney and enhanced expression of transforming growth factor alpha and beta in renal cell carcinoma (submitted for publication)
43. Rosenthal A, Lindquist PB, Bringman TS et al: Expression in rat fibroblasts of a human transforming growth factor-alpha cDNA results in transformation. Cell 46:301–309, 1986
44. Coffey RJ Jr, Derynck R, Wilcox JN et al: Production and autoinduction of transforming growth factor-alpha in human keratinocytes. Nature 328:817–820, 1987
45. Kehrl JH, Wakefield LM, Roberts AB et al: Production of transforming growth factor beta by human T lymphocytes and its potential role in the regulation of T cell growth. J Exp Med 163:1037–1050, 1986
46. Mule JJ, Schwarz SL, Roberts AB et al: Transforming growth factor-beta inhibits the in vitro generation of lymphokine-activated killer cells and cytotoxic T cells (unpublished manuscript)
47. Kasid A, Director EP, Bell GI: Effects of TGF-beta on human lymphokine activated killer cell precursors: Autocrine inhibition of cellular proliferation and differentiation to immune killer cells (unpublished manuscript)
48. Ibbotson KJ, Harrod J, Gowen M et al: Human recombinant transforming growth factor alpha stimulates bone resorption and inhibits formation in vitro. Proc Natl Acad Sci USA 87:2228–2232, 1986
49. Cohen AJ, Li FP, Berg S et al: Hereditary renal-cell carcinoma associated with a chromosomal translocation. N Engl J Med 301:592–595, 1979
50. Drabkin HA, Bradley C, Hart I et al: Translocation of c-myc in the hereditary renal cell carcinoma associated with a t(3:8) (p14.2;q24.13) chromosomal translocation. Proc Natl Acad Sci USA 82:6980–6984, 1985
51. Pathak S, Strong LC, Ferrell RE et al: Familial renal cell carcinoma with a 3;11 chromosome translocation limited to tumor cells. Science 217:939–941, 1982
52. King CR, Schimke RN, Arthur T et al: Proximal 3p deletion in renal cell carcinoma cells from a patient with von Hippel–Lindau disease. Cancer Genet Cytogenet 27:345–348, 1987
53. Yoshida HA, Ohyashiki K, Ochi H et al: Cytogenetic studies of tumor tissue from patients with nonfamilial renal cell carcinoma. Cancer Res 46:2139–2147, 1986
54. Yoshida HA, Ohyashiki K, Ochi H et al: Rearrangement of chromosome 3 in renal cell carcinoma. Cancer Genet Cytogenet 19:351–354, 1986
55. Szucs S, Muller-Brechlin R, DeRiese W et al: Deletion 3p: The only chromosome loss in a primary renal cell carcinoma. Cancer Genet Cytogenet 26:369–373, 1987
56. Carroll PR, Murty VVS, Reuter V et al: Abnormalities at chromosome region 3p 12-14 characterize clear cell renal carcinoma. Cancer Genet Cytogenet 26:253–259, 1987
57. Zbar B, Brauch H, Talmadge C et al: Loss of alleles of loci on the short arm of chromosome 3 in renal cell carcinoma. Nature 327:721–727, 1987
58. Cavenee WK, Dryja TP, Phillips RA et al: Expression of recessive alleles by chromosomal mechanisms in retinoblastoma. Nature 305:779–784, 1983
59. Koufos A, Hansen MFM, Lampkin BC et al: Loss of alleles at loci on human chromosome 11 during genesis of Wilms' tumour. Nature 309:170–172, 1984
60. Orkin SH, Goldman DS, Sallan SE: Development of homozygosity for chromosome 11p markers in Wilms' tumour. Nature 309:172–174, 1984
61. Reeve AE, Hiusiaux PJ, Gardner RJM et al: Loss of a Harvey ras allele in sporadic Wilms' tumour. Nature 309:174–176, 1984

62. Fearon ER, Vogelstein B, Feinberg AP: Somatic deletion and duplication of genes on chromosome 11 in Wilms' tumours. Nature 309:175–177, 1984
63. Cavenee WK, Murphree AL, Shull MM et al: Prediction of familial predisposition to retinoblastoma. N Engl J Med 314:1201–1207, 1986
64. Fearon ER, Feinberg AP, Hamilton SH et al: Loss of genes on the short arm of chromosome 11 in bladder cancer. Nature 318:377–380, 1985
65. Brauch H, Johnson B, Hovis J et al: Molecular analysis of the short arm of chromosome 3 in small-cell and non-small-cell carcinoma of the lung. N Engl J Med 317:1109–1113, 1987
66. Solomon E, Voss R, Hall V et al: Chromosome 5 allele loss in human colorectal carcinomas. Nature 328:616–619, 1987
67. White R, Leppert M, Bishop T et al: Construction of linkage maps with DNA markers for human chromosomes. Nature 313:101–105, 1985
68. Carritt B, Welch HM, Parry-Jones NJ: Sequences homologous to the human D1S1 locus present on human chromosome 3. Am J Hum Genet 38:428–436, 1986
69. Knudson AG Jr: Genetics of human cancer. Annu Rev Genet 20:231–251, 1986
70. Moolgavkar SH, Knudson AG Jr: Mutation and cancer: A model for human carcinogenesis. J Natl Cancer Inst 66:1037–1051, 1981
71. Weissman BE, Saxon PJ, Pasquale SR et al: Introduction of a normal human chromosome 11 into a Wilms' tumor cell line controls its tumorigenic expression. Science 236:175–180, 1987
72. Tannenbaum M: Ultrastructural pathology of human renal cell tumors. Pathol Annu 6:249–277, 1971
73. Fisher ER, Horvat B: Comparative ultrastructural study of so-called renal adenoma and carcinoma. J Urol 108:382–386, 1972
74. Mostofi FK, Davis CJ Jr: Pathology of urologic cancer. In Javadpour N (ed): Principles and Management of Urologic Cancer, 2nd ed, pp 54–126. Baltimore, Williams & Wilkins, 1983
75. Thoenes W, Storkel ST, Rumpelt HJ: Histopathology and classification of renal cell tumors (adenomas, oncocytomas and carcinomas): The basic cytological and histopathologoical elements and their use for diagnostics. Pathol Res Pract 181:125–143, 1986
76. Bonsib SM, Fischer J, Plattner S et al: Sarcomatoid renal tumors: Clinicopathologic correlation of three cases. Cancer 59:527–532, 1987
77. Bertoni F, Ferri C, Bacchini BP et al: Sarcomatoid carcinoma of the kidney. J Urol 137:25–28, 1987
78. Ro JY, Ayala AG, Sella A et al: Sarcomatoid renal cell carcinoma: Clinicopathologic. A study of 42 cases. Cancer 59:519–526, 1987
79. Skinner DG, Colvin RB, Vermillion CD et al: Diagnosis and management of renal cell carcinoma: A clinical and pathologic study of 309 cases. Cancer 28:1165–1177, 1971
80. Selli C, Hinshaw WM, Woodard BH et al: Stratification of risk factors in renal cell carcinoma. Cancer 52:899–903, 1983
81. Boxer RJ, Waisman J, Lieber MM et al: Renal carcinoma: Computer analysis of 96 patients treated by nephrectomy. J Urol 122:598–601, 1979
82. Sella A, Logothetis CJ, Ro JY et al: Sarcomatoid renal cell carcinoma: A treatable entity. Cancer 60:1313–1318, 1987
83. McNichols DW, Segura JW, DeWeerd JH: Renal cell carcinoma: Long-term survival and late recurrence. J Urol 126:17–23, 1981
84. Silverberg E: Cancer statistics. CA 31:13–28, 1981
85. Maldazys JD, deKernion JB: Prognostic factors in metastatic renal carcinoma. J Urol 136:376–379, 1986
86. Samaan NA: Paraneoplastic syndromes associated with renal carcinoma: A pilot study. J Clin Oncol 6:862, 1987
87. Pinals RS, Krane SM: Medical aspects of renal carcinoma. Postgrad Med J 38:507–519, 1962
88. Cherukuri SV, Johenning PW, Ram MD: Systemic effects of hypernephroma. Urology 10:93–97, 1977
89. Sufrin G, Mirand EA, Moore RH et al: Hormones in renal cancer. J Urol 117:433–438, 1977
90. Utz DW, Warren MM, Gregg JA et al: Reversible hepatic dysfunction associated with hypernephroma. Mayo Clin Proc 45:161, 1970
91. Boxer RJ, Waisman J, Lieber MM et al: Non-metastatic hepatic dysfunction associated with renal carcinoma. J Urol 119:468–471, 1978
92. Hanash KA, Utz DC, Khalil L et al: Syndrome of reversible hepatic dysfunction associated with hypernephroma: An experimental study. Invest Urol 8:399–404, 1971
93. Lindop GB, Fleming S: Renin in renal cell carcinoma: An immunocytochemical study using an antibody to pure human renin. J Clin Pathol 37:27–31, 1984
94. Lindop GB, Leckie B, Winearls CG: Malignant hypertension due to renin-secreting renal cell carcinoma: An ultrastructural and immunocytochemical study. Histopathology 10:1077–1088, 1986
95. Sufrin G, Mink I, Moore FR et al: Coagulation factors in renal adenocarcinoma. J Urol 119:727–730, 1978
96. Dawson NA, Barr CF, Alving BM: Acquired dysfibrinogenemia: Paraneoplastic syndrome in renal cell carcinoma. Am J Med 78:682–686, 1985
97. Lang EK: Asymptomatic space-occupying lesions of the kidney: A programmed sequential approach and its impact on quality and cost of health care. South Med J 70:277–285, 1977
98. Frohmuller HGW, Grups JW, Heller V: Comparative value of ultrasonography, computerized tomography, angiography and excretory urography in the staging of renal cell carcinoma. J Urol 138:482–484, 1987
99. Juul N, Torp-Pedersen S, Gronvall S et al: Ultrasonically guided fine needle aspiration biopsy of renal masses. J Urol 133:579–581, 1985
100. Lang EK: Comparison of dynamic and conventional computed tomography, angiography, and ultrasonography in the staging of renal cell carcinoma. Cancer 54:2205–2214, 1984
101. Karp W, Ekelund L, Olafsson G et al: Computed tomography, angiography and ultrasound in staging of renal carcinoma. Acta Radiol 22:625–632, 1981
102. Mauro MA, Wadsworth DE, Stanley RJ et al: Renal cell carcinoma: Angiography in the CT era. AJR 139:1135–1138, 1982
103. Zabbo A, Novick AC, Risius B et al: Digital subtraction angiography for evaluating patients with renal carcinoma. J Urol 134:252–255, 1985
104. Richie JP, Garnick MC, Seltzer S et al: Computerized tomography scan for diagnosis and staging of renal cell carcinoma. J Urol 129:1114–1116, 1983
105. Stephenson TF, Tyengar S, Rashid HA: Comparison of computerized tomography and excretory urography in detection and evaluation of renal masses. J Urol 131:11–13, 1984
106. Jashke W, Kaick GV, Peter S et al: Accuracy of computed tomography in staging of kidney tumors. Acta Radiol (Stockh) 23:593–598, 1982
107. Kothari K, Segal AJ, Spitzer RM et al: Preoperative radiographic evaluation of hypernephroma. J Comput Assist Tomogr 5:702–704, 1981
108. Yokoyama M, Watanabe K, Inatsuki S et al: Computerized tomography of the kidney: Tissue-plasma ratio of contrast enhancement with bolus injection and renal function. J Urol 127:721–723, 1982
109. Lang EK: Angio-computed tomography and dynamic computed tomography in staging of renal cell carcinoma. Radiology 151:149–155, 1984
110. Karstaedt N, McCullough DL, Wolfman NT et al: Magnetic resonance imaging of the renal mass. J Urol 136:566–570, 1986
111. Robson CJ, Churchill BM, Anderson W: The results of radical nephrectomy for renal cell carcinoma. J Urol 101:297–301, 1969
112. Peters PC, Brown GL: The role of lymphadenectomy in the management of renal cell carcinoma. Urol Clin North Am 7:705–709, 1980
113. Siminovitch JMP, Montie JE, Straffon RA: Prognostic indicators in renal adenocarcinoma. J Urol 130:20–23, 1983
114. Cherrie RJ, Goldman DG, Lindner A et al: Prognostic implications of vena caval extension of renal cell carcinoma. J Urol 128:910–912, 1982
115. Bassil B, Dosoretz DE, Prout GR Jr: Validation of the tumor, nodes and metastasis classification of renal cell carcinoma. J Urol 134:450–454, 1985
116. Gilbert JB: Diagnosis and treatment of malignant renal tumors. J Urol 39:223–237, 1938
117. McDonald MW: Current therapy for renal cell carcinoma. J Urol 127:211–217, 1982
118. Kearney GP, Waters WB, Klein LA et al: Results of inferior vena cava resection for renal cell carcinoma. J Urol 125:769–773, 1981
119. Sogani PC, Herr HW, Bains MS et al: Renal cell carcinoma extending into the inferior vena cava. J Urol 130:660–663, 1983
120. Marshall FF, Reitz BA, Diamond DA: A new technique for management of renal cell carcinoma involving the right atrium: Hypothermia and cardiac arrest. J Urol 131:103–107, 1984
121. deKernion JB, Berry D: The diagnosis and treatment of renal cell carcinoma. Cancer 45:1947–1956, 1980
122. deKernion JB: Lymphadenectomy for renal cell carcinoma. Urol Clin North Am 7:697–703, 1980
123. Marshall FF, Powell KC: Lymphadenectomy for renal cell carcinoma: Anatomical and therapeutic considerations. J Urol 128:677–681, 1982
124. Zincke H, Engen DE, Henning KM et al: Treatment of renal cell carcinoma by in situ partial nephrectomy and extracorporeal operation with autotransplantation. Mayo Clin Proc 60:651–662, 1985
125. Mandel J, Kjellstrand CM: Long-term results of dialysis and transplantation in patients with end-stage renal failure from hypernephroma. Nephron 44:111–114, 1986
126. Smith RB, deKernion JB, Ehrlich RM et al: Bilateral renal cell carcinoma and renal cell carcinoma in the solitary kidney. J Urol 132:450–454, 1984
127. Jacobs SC, Berg SI, Lawson RK: Synchronous bilateral renal cell carcinoma: Total surgical excision. Cancer 46:2341–2345, 1980
128. Topley M, Novick AC, Montie JE: Long-term results following partial nephrectomy for localized renal adenocarcinoma. J Urol 131:1050–1052, 1984
129. Novick AC, Zincke H, Neves RJ et al: Surgical enucleation for renal cell carcinoma. J Urol 135:235–238, 1986
130. Marshall FF, Taxy JB, Fishman EK et al: The feasibility of surgical enucleation for renal cell carcinoma. J Urol 135:231–234, 1986
131. deKernion JB, Mukamel E: Selection of initial therapy for renal cell carcinoma. Cancer 60:539–546, 1987
132. Zincke H, Swanson SK: Bilateral renal cell carcinoma: Influence of synchronous and asynchronous occurrence on patient survival. J Urol 128:913–915, 1982
133. Rafla S: Renal cell carcinoma: Natural history and results of treatment. Cancer 25:26–40, 1970
134. Finney R: Radiotherapy in the treatment of hypernephroma: A clinical trial. Br J Urol 45:258–269, 1973
135. Kjaer M, Frederiksen PL, Engelholm SA: Postoperative radiotherapy in stage II and III renal adenocarcinoma: A randomized trial by the Copenhagen renal cancer study group. Int J Radiat Oncol Biol Phys 13:665–672, 1987
136. van der Werf-Messing B: Carcinoma of the kidney. Cancer 32:1056–1062, 1973
137. deKernion JB: Treatment of advanced renal cell carcinoma: Traditional methods and innovative approaches. J Urol 130:2–7, 1983
138. Freed SZ: Nephrectomy for renal cell carcinoma with metastases. Urology 9:613–615, 1977

139. Montie JE, Stewart BH, Straffon RA et al: The role of adjunctive nephrectomy in patients with metastatic renal cell carcinoma. J Urol 117:272–275, 1977
140. deKernion JB, Ramming KP, Smith RB: The natural history of metastatic renal cell carcinoma: A computer analysis. J Urol 120:148–151, 1978
141. Middleton RG: Surgery for metastatic renal cell carcinoma. J Urol 97:973–977, 1967
142. O'Dea MJ, Zincke H, Utz DC et al: The treatment of renal cell carcinoma with solitary metastasis. J Urol 120:540–542, 1978
143. Tolia BM, Whitmore WF Jr: Solitary metastasis from renal cell carcinoma. J Urol 114:836–838, 1975
144. Swanson DA, Wallace S, Johnson DE: The role of embolization and nephrectomy in the treatment of metastatic renal carcinoma. Urol Clin North Am 7:719–730, 1980
145. Swanson DA, Johnson DE, von Eschenbach AC et al: Angioinfarction plus nephrectomy for metastatic renal cell carcinoma: An update. J Urol 130:449-452, 1983
146. Sundaresan N, Galicich JH, Baines MS et al: Vertebral body resection in the treatment of cancer involving the spine. Cancer 53:1393–1396, 1984
147. Sundaresan N, Scher H, Whitmore WF Jr: Spinal cord compression in kidney cancer (abstr). Proceedings of the American Society of Clinical Oncology, March 1986, p 267
148. Fossa SD, Kjolseth I, Lund G: Radiotherapy of metastasis from renal cancer. Eur Urol 8:340–342, 1982
149. Onufrey V, Mohiuddin M: Radiation therapy in the treatment of metastatic renal cell carcinoma. Int J Radiat Oncol Biol Phys 11:2007–2009, 1985
150. Halperin EC, Harisiadis L: The role of radiation therapy in the management of metastatic renal cell carcinoma. Cancer 51:614–617, 1983
151. Fojo AT, Ueda K, Slamon DJ et al: Expression of a multidrug-resistance gene in human tumors and tissues. Proc Natl Acad Sci USA 84:265, 1987
152. Hrushesky WJ, Murphy GP: Current status of the therapy of advanced renal carcinoma. J Surg Oncol 9:277, 1977
153. Bell DR, Aroney RS, Fisher RJ et al: High-dose methotrexate with leucovorin resue, vinblastine, and bleomycin with or without tamoxifen in metastatic renal cell carcinoma. Cancer Treat Rep 68:587, 1984
154. Hrushesky WJM, Roemeling R, Rabatin J et al: Continuous FUDR infusion is effective in progressive renal cell cancer. Proc Am Soc Clin Oncol 6:108, 1987
155. Satake I, Tari K, Yamamoto M et al: Neocarzinostatin-induced complete regression of metastatic renal cell carcinoma. J Urol 133:87, 1985
156. Kakizoe T, Matsumoto K, Nishio Y et al: Chemotherapy by bronchial arterial infusion for pulmonary metastases of renal cell carcinoma. J Urol 131:1053, 1984
157. Poster DS, Pinna K, Bruno S et al: Current status of chemotherapy, hormonal therapy, and immunotherapy in the treatment of renal cell carcinoma. Am J Clin Oncol 5:53, 1982
158. Miller CF: Adjuvant chemotherapy of renal cell carcinoma using a combination of bleomycin and lomustine. Proc Am Soc Clin Oncol 21:C-171, 1980
159. Leiter E, Edelman S, Brendler H: Continuous preoperative intraarterial perfusion of renal tumors with chemotherapeutic agents. J Urol 95:169, 1966
160. Kato T, Nemoto R, Mori H et al: Transcatheter arterial chemoembolization of renal cell carcinoma with microencapsulated mitomycin C. J Urol 125:19, 1981
161. Satomi Y, Takai S, Kondo I et al: Postoperative prophylactic use of progesterone in renal cell carcinoma. J Urol 127:919, 1982
162. Ronchi E, Pizzocaro G, Miodini P et al: Steroid hormone receptors in normal and malignant human renal tissue: Relationship with progestin therapy. J Steroid Biochem 21:329, 1984
163. Rosenberg SA, Lotze MT, Muul LM et al: Observations on the systemic administration of autologous lymphokine-activated killer cells and recombinant interleukin-2 to patients with metastatic cancer. N Engl J Med 313:1485, 1985
164. Rosenberg SA, Lotze MT, Muul LM et al: A progress report on the treatment of 157 patients with advanced cancer using lymphokine-activated killer cells and interleukin-2 or high dose interleukin-2 alone. N Engl J Med 316:889, 1987
165. West WH, Tauer KW, Yannelli JR et al: Constant infusion recombinant interleukin-2 in adoptive immunotherapy of advanced cancer. N Engl J Med 316:898–905, 1987
166. Krown SE: Interferon treatment of renal cell carcinoma: Current status and future prospects. Cancer 59:647, 1987
167. Goldstein D, Laszlo J: Interferon therapy in cancer: From imaginon to interferon. Cancer Res 46:4315, 1986
168. Marshall ME, Mendelsohn L, Butler K et al: Treatment of metastatic renal cell carcinoma with coumarin (1,2-benzopyrone) and cimetidine: A pilot study. J Clin Oncol 6:682, 1987
169. Fisher RI, Coltman CA, Doroshow JH et al: Phase II clinical trial of interleukin-2 plus lymphokine activated killer cells in metastatic renal cancer. Proc Am Soc Clin Oncol 6:244, 1987
170. Krishnan EC, Mebust WK, Weigel JW et al: Culture of peripheral monocytes in vitro in patients with renal cell carcinoma: A possible prognostic indicator. J Urol 130:597, 1983
171. Rosenberg SA, Spiess P, Lafreniere R: A new approach to the adoptive immunotherapy of cancer with tumor-infiltrating lymphocytes. Science 233:1318, 1986
172. Belldegrun A, Linehan WM, Robertson CN et al: Isolation and characterization of lymphocytes infiltrating human renal cell cancer: Possible application for therapeutic adoptive immunotherapy. Surg Forum 37:671, 1986
173. Belldegrun A, Muul LM, Rosenberg SA: Interleukin-2 expanded tumor infiltrating lymphocytes in human renal cell cancer: Isolation, characterization and antitumor activity. Cancer Res 48:206–214, 1988
174. Topalian SL, Muul LM, Solomon D et al: Expansion of human tumor infiltrating lymphocytes for use in immunotherapy trials. J Immunol Methods 102:127–141, 1987
175. Muul LM, Spiess PJ, Director EP et al: Identification of specific cytolytic immune responses against autologous tumor in humans bearing malignant melanoma. J Immunol 138:989–995, 1987
176. Topalian SL, Solomon D, Avis FP et al: Immunotherapy of patients with advanced cancer using tumor infiltrating lymphocytes and recombinant interleukin-2: A pilot study. J Clin Oncol 6:839–853, 1988
177. Salup RR, Back TC, Wiltrout RH: Successful treatment of advanced murine renal cell cancer by bicompartmental adoptive chemoimmunotherapy. J Immunol 138:641, 1987
178. Wiltrout RH, Boyd MR, Back TT et al: Flavone-8-acetic acid augments systemic natural killer cell activity and synergizes with interleukin-2 for treatment of murine renal cancer. J Immunol 140:3261–3265, 1988
179. Quesada JR, Swanson DA, Trindade A et al: Renal cell carcinoma: Antitumor effects of leukocyte interferon. Cancer Res 43:940, 1983
180. Quesada JR, Swanson DA, Gutterman JU: Phase II study of interferon alpha in metastatic renal-cell carcinoma: A progress report. J Clin Oncol 3:1086, 1985
181. Medenica R, Slack N: Clinical results of leukocyte interferon-induced tumor regression in resistant human metastatic cancer resistant to chemotherapy and/or radiotherapy—pulse therapy schedule. Cancer Drug Deliv 2:53, 1985
182. deKernion JB, Sarna G, Figlin R et al: The treatment of renal cell carcinoma with human leukocyte alpha-interferon. J Urol 130:1063, 1983
183. Kirkwood JM, Harris JE, Vera P et al: A randomized study of low and high doses of leukocyte alpha interferon in metastatic renal cell carcinoma: The American Cancer Society collaborative trial. Cancer Res 45:863, 1985
184. Edsmyr F, Eposti PL, Andersson L et al: Interferon therapy in disseminated renal cell carcinoma. Radiother Oncol 4:21, 1985
185. Neidhart JA, Gagen MM, Yound D et al: Interferon-alpha therapy of renal cancer. Cancer Res 44:4140, 1984
186. Trump DL, Elson PJ, Borden EC et al: High-dose lymphoblastoid interferon in advanced renal cell carcinoma: An Eastern Cooperative Oncology Group study. Cancer Treat Rep 71:165, 1987
187. Marumo K, Murai M, Hayakawa M et al: Human lymphoblastoid interferon therapy for advanced renal cell carcinoma. Urology 24:567, 1984
188. Vugrin D, Hood L, Taylor W et al: Phase II study of human lymphoblastoid interferon in patients with advanced renal carcinoma. Cancer Treat Rep 69:817, 1985
189. Umeda T, Niijima T: Phase II study of alpha interferon on renal cell carcinoma: Summary of three collaborative trials. Cancer 58:1231, 1986
190. Kempf RA, Grunberg SM, Daniels JR et al: Recombinant interferon alpha-2 (Intron A) in a phase II study of renal cell carcinoma. J Biol Response Mod 5:27, 1986
191. Quesada JR, Rios A, Swanson D et al: Antitumor activity of recombinant-derived interferon alpha in metastatic renal cell carcinoma. J Clin Oncol 3:1522, 1985
192. Sarna G, Figlin R, deKernion J: Interferon in renal cell carcinoma: The UCLA experience. Cancer 59:610, 1987
193. Kuzmits R, Kokoschka EM, Micksche M et al: Phase II results with recombinant interferons: Renal cell carcinoma and malignant melanoma. Oncology 42 (suppl):26, 1985
194. Muss HB, Costanzi JJ, Leavitt R et al: Recombinant alpha interferon in renal cell carcinoma: A randomized trial of two routes of administration. J Clin Oncol 5:286, 1987
195. Buzaid AC, Robertone A, Kisals C et al: Phase II study of interferon alpha-2a, recombinant (Roferon-A) in metastatic renal cell carcinoma. J Clin Oncol 5:1083, 1987
196. Rinehart J, Malspeis L, Young D, Neidhart J: Phase I/II trial of human recombinant beta-interferon serine in patients with renal cell carcinoma. Cancer Res 46:5364, 1986
197. Rinehart J, Malspeis L, Young D et al: Phase I/II trial of human recombinant interferon gamma in renal cell carcinoma. J Biol Response Mod 5:300, 1986
198. Quesada JR, Kurzrock R, Sherwin SA et al: Phase II studies of recombinant human interferon gamma in metastatic renal cell carcinoma. J Biol Response Mod 6:20, 1987
199. Trotta PP: Preclinical biology of alpha interferons. Semin Oncol 13 (suppl 2):3, 1986
200. Figlin RA, deKernion JB, Maldazys J et al: Treatment of renal cell carcinoma with alpha (human leukocyte) interferon and vinblastine in combination: A phase I-II trial. Cancer Treat Rep 69:263, 1985
201. Fossa SD, DeGaris ST, Heier MS et al: Recombinant interferon alpha-2a with or without vinblastine in metastatic renal cell carcinoma. Cancer 57:1700, 1986
202. Schnornagel J, Verwey J, tenBokkel Huinink W et al: Phase II study of recombinant interferon alpha-2 and vinblastine in advanced renal carcinoma. Proc Am Soc Clin Oncol 6:106, 1987
203. Creagan ET, Kovach JS, Long HJ et al: Phase I study of recombinant leukocyte A human interferon combined with BCNU in selected patients with advanced cancer. J Clin Oncol 4:408, 1986
204. Creagan ET, Kovach JS, O'Connell MJ et al: Improved response of renal cell carcinoma to alpha interferon by the addition of aspirin. Cancer (in press)
205. Dexeus FH, Logothetis CJ, Quesada J et al: Potential increase in efficacy of chemotherapy after treatment of patients with metastatic renal cell carcinoma with interferon. Proc Am Soc Clin Oncol 6:100, 1987
206. Droller MJ: Immunotherapy of metastatic renal cell carcinoma with polyinosinic-polysytidylic acid. J Urol 137:202, 1987
207. deKernion JB, Ramming KP: The therapy of renal adenocarcinoma with immune RNA. Invest Urol 17:378, 1980
208. Richie JP, Steele GD Jr, Wilson RE et al: Current treatment of metastatic renal cell carcinoma with xenogeneic immune ribonucleic acid. J Urol 131:236, 1984
209. Morales A, Wilson JL, Pater JL Loeb M: Cytoreductive surgery and systemic bacillus

Calmette-Guerin therapy in metastatic renal cancer: A phase II trial. J Urol 127:230, 1982
210. Stanisic TH: Renal cell carcinoma (hypernephroma). Ariz Med 37:164, 1980
211. Ishmael DR, Burpo LJ, Bottomley RH: Combined therapy of advanced hypernephroma with medroxyprogesterone, BCG, Adriamycin, and vincristine. Proc Am Soc Clin Oncol 19:407, 1978
212. Dimitrov NV, Arnols D, Munson J et al: Phase II study of thymosin fraction 5 in the treatment of metastatic renal cell carcinoma. Cancer Treat Rep 69:137, 1985
213. Romano CF, Lipton A, Harvey HA et al: A phase II study of catrix-s in solid tumors. J Biol Response Mod 4:585, 1985
214. Prager MD, Baechtel FS, Peters PC et al: Specific immunotherapy of human metastatic renal cell carcinoma. Proc Am Assoc Cancer Res 22:163, 1981
215. Sahasrabudhe DM, deKernion JB, Pontes JE et al: Specific immunotherapy with suppressor function inhibition for metastatic renal cell carcinoma. J Biol Response Mod 5:581, 1986
216. McCune CS, Patterson WB, Henshaw EC: Active specific immunotherapy with tumor cells and *Corynebacterium parvum*. Cancer 43:1619, 1979
217. McCune CS: Immunologic therapies of kidney carcinoma. Semin Oncol 10:431, 1983
218. Tallberg T, Tykka H, Mahlberg K et al: Active specific immunotherapy with supportive measures in the treatment of palliatively nephrectomized, renal adenocarcinoma patients: A thirteen-year follow-up study. Eur Urol 11:233, 1985
219. Neidhart JA, Murphy SG, Hennick LA et al: Active specific immunotherapy of stage IV renal carcinoma with aggregated tumor antigen adjuvant. Cancer 46:1128, 1980
220. Arakawa S Jr, Hamami G, Umezu K et al: Clinical trial of attenuated vaccinia virus AS strain in the treatment of advanced adenocarcinoma: Report on two cases. J Cancer Res Clin Oncol 113:95, 1987
221. Horn L, Horn JL: An immunological approach to the therapy of cancer? Lancet 2:466, 1971
222. Yoshida SO, Imam A, Olson CA et al: Proximal renal tubule surface membrane antigens identified in primary and metastatic renal cell carcinoma. Arch Pathol Lab Med 110:825, 1986
223. Iizumi Y, Yazaki T, Kanoh S et al: Fluorescence study of renal cell carcinoma with antibodies to renal tubular antigens, intermediated filaments, and lectins. Urol Int 41:57, 1986
224. Fraley EE: Cancer of the renal pelvis. In Skinner DG, deKernion JB (eds): Genitourinary Cancer, pp 134–149. Philadelphia, WB Saunders, 1978
225. Mahadevia PA, Larwa GL, Koss LG: Mapping of urothelium in carcinomas of the renal pelvis and ureter: A report of nine cases. Cancer 51:890–897, 1983
226. McCarron JP Jr, Chasko SB, Gray GF Jr: Systemic mapping of nephroureterectomy specimens removed for urothelial cancer: Pathological findings and clinical correlations. J Urol 128:243–246, 1982
227. Babaian RJ, Johnson DE: Primary carcinoma of the ureter. J Urol 123:357–359, 1980
228. Droller MJ: Transitional cell cancer: Upper tracts and bladder. In Walsh PC, Gittes RE, Perlmutter AD et al (eds): Campbell's Urology, pp 1343–1440. Philadelphia, WB Saunders, 1986
229. Hultengren N, Lagergren C, Ljungqvist A: Carcinoma of the renal pelvis in renal papillary necrosis. Acta Chir Scand 130:314–320, 1965
230. Palvio DHB, Andersen JC, Falk E: Transitional cell tumors of the renal pelvis and ureter associated with capillarosclerosis indicating analgesic abuse. Cancer 59:972–976, 1987
231. Bengtsson U, Angervall L, Ekman H et al: Transitional cell tumors of the renal pelvis in analgesic abusers. Scand J Urol Nephrol 2:145–150, 1968
232. Bengtsson U, Johansson S, Angervall L: Malignancies of the urinary tract and their relation to analgesic abuse. Kidney Int 13:107–113, 1978
233. Adam WR, Dawborn JK, Price CG et al: Anaplastic transitional-cell carcinoma of the renal pelvis in association with analgesic abuse. Med J Aust 1:1108–1109, 1970
234. Mahony JF, Storey BG, Ibanez RC et al: Analgesic abuse, renal parenchymal disease and carcinoma of the kidney or ureter. Aust NZ J Med 7:463–469, 1977
235. McCredie M, Stewart JH, Carter JJ et al: Phenacetin and papillary necrosis: Independent risk factors for renal pelvic cancer. Kidney Int 30:81–84, 1986
236. Gaakeer HA, De Ruiter HJ: Carcinoma of the renal pelvis following the abuse of phenacetin–containing analgesic drugs. Br J Urol 51:188–192, 1979
237. Hoybye G, Nielsen OE: Renal pelvic carcinoma in phenacetin abusers. Scand J Urol Nephrol 5:190–192, 1971
238. Campo B, Zanitzer L, Torelli T et al: Renal cell carcinoma and transitional cell carcinomas of the pelvis and bladder in a patient affected by chronic renal failure due to abuse of phenacetin. Tumori 72:215–217, 1986
239. Rathert P, Melchior H, Lutzeyer W: Phenacetin: A carcinogen for the urinary tract. J Urol 113:653–657, 1975
240. Clayman RV, Lange PH, Fraley EE: Cancer of the upper urinary tract. In Javadpour N (ed): Principles and Management of Urologic Cancer, pp 544–559. Baltimore, Williams & Wilkins, 1983
241. Orphali SLJ, Shols GW, Hagewood J et al: Familial transitional cell carcinoma of renal pelvis and upper ureter. Urology 27:394–396, 1986
242. Frischer Z, Waltzer WC, Gonder MJ: Bilateral transitional cell carcinoma of the renal pelvis in the cancer family syndrome. J Urol 134:1197–1198, 1985
243. Cahng EH, Pirollo KF, Zou ZQ et al: Oncogenes in radioresistant, noncancerous skin fibroblasts from a cancer-prone family. Science 237:1036–1041, 1987
244. Blacher EJ, Johnson DE, Abdul-Karim FW et al: Squamous cell carcinoma of the renal pelvis. Urology 25:124–126, 1985
245. Johansson S, Angervall L, Bengtsson U et al: A clinicopathologic and prognostic study of epithelial tumors of the renal pelvis. Cancer 37:1376–1383, 1976
246. Grabstald H, Whitmore WF, Melamed MR: Renal pelvic tumors. JAMA 218:845–854, 1971
247. Murphy DM, Zincke H, Furlow WL: Management of high grade transitional cell cancer of the upper urinary tract. J Urol 125:25–29, 1981
248. Wagle DG, Moore RH, Murphy GP: Primary carcinoma of the renal pelvis. Cancer 33:1642–1648, 1974
249. Lang EK: The arteriographic diagnosis of primary and secondary tumors of the ureter or ureter and renal pelvis. Radiology 93:799–805, 1969
250. Pontes JE, Christensen LC, Pierce JM Jr: Angiographic aspects of tumors of renal pelvis and ureter. Urology 7:334–336, 1976
251. Gatewood OMB, Goldman SM, Marshall FF et al: Computerized tomography in the diagnosis of transitional cell carcinoma of the kidney. J Urol 127:876–887, 1982
252. Cullen TH, Pophom RR, Vos HJ: Urine cytology and primary carcinoma of the renal pelvis and ureter. Aust NZ J Surg 41:230–236, 1972
253. Highman WJ: Transitional carcinoma of the upper urinary tract: A histological and cytopathological study. J Clin Pathol 39:297–305, 1986
254. Smith AD, Orihuela E, Crowley AR: Percutaneous management of renal pelvic tumors: A treatment option in selected cases. J Urol 137:852–856, 1987
255. Bagley DH, Huffman JL, Lyon ES: Flexible ureteropyeloscopy: Diagnosis and treatment in the upper urinary tract. J Urol 138:280–285, 1987
256. Davis BW, Hough AJ, Gardner WA: Renal pelvic carcinoma: Morphological correlates of metastatic behavior. J Urol 137:857–861, 1987
257. Tumors of the renal pelvis and ureter. In Bennington JL, Beckwith JB (eds): Tumors of the Kidney, Renal Pelvis, and Ureter, pp 243–310. Washington, DC, Armed Forces Institute of Pathology, 1975
258. Cummings KB: Nephroureterectomy: Rationale in the management of transitional cell carcinoma of the upper urinary tract. Urol Clin North Am 7:569–578, 1980
259. Johansson S, Wahlqvist L: A prognostic study of urothelial renal pelvic tumors. Cancer 43:2525–2531, 1979
260. Johnson DE, deBerardinis M, Ayala AG: Transitional cell carcinoma of the renal pelvis: Radical or conservative surgical treatment? South Med J 67:1183–1186, 1974
261. Geiger J, Fong O, Fay R: Transitional cell carcinoma of renal pelvis with invasion of renal vein and thrombosis of subhepatic inferior vena cava. Urology 28:52–54, 1986
262. Jitsukawa S, Nakamura K, Nakayama M et al: Transitional cell carcinoma of kidney extending into renal vein and inferior vena cava. Urology 25:310–312, 1985
263. Gittes RF: Management of transitional cell carcinoma of the upper tract: Case for conservative local excision. Urol Clin North Am 7:559–568, 1980
264. Bazeed MA, Scherge T, Becht E et al: Local excision of urothelial cancer of the upper urinary tract. Eur Urol 12:89–95, 1986
265. Wallace DMA, Wallace DM, Whitfield HN et al: The late results of conservative surgery for upper tract urothelial carcinomas. Br J Urol 53:537–541, 1981
266. Tomera KM, Leary FJ, Zincke H: Pyeloscopy in urothelial tumors. J Urol 127:1088–1089, 1982
267. McIntyre D, Pyrah LN, Raper FP: Primary ureteric neoplasms with a report of forty cases. Br J Urol 37:160–191, 1965
268. Foord AG, Ferrier PA: Primary carcinoma of the ureter with report of seven cases. JAMA 112:596–601, 1939
269. Abeshouse BS: Primary benign and malignant tumors of the ureter: A review of the literature and report of one benign and twelve malignant tumors. Am J Surg 91:237–271, 1956
270. Heney NM, Nocks BN, Daly JJ et al: Prognostic factors in carcinoma of the ureter. J Urol 125:632–636, 1981
271. Hawtrey CE: Fifty-two cases of primary ureteral carcinoma: A clinical-pathologic study. J Urol 105:188–193, 1971
272. Batata MA, Whitmore WF Jr, Hilaris BS et al: Primary carcinoma of the ureter: A prognostic study. Cancer 35:1626–1632, 1975
273. Richie JP: Management of ureteral tumors. In Skinner DG, deKernion JB (eds): Genitourinary Cancer, pp 150–165. Philadelphia, WB Saunders, 1978
274. Bergman H, Friedenberg RM, Sayegh V: New roentgenologic signs of carcinoma of the ureter. Am Roentgen Ray Soc 86:707–717, 1961
275. Strong DW, Pearse HD: Recurrent urothelial tumors following surgery for transitional cell carcinoma of the upper urinary tract. Cancer 38:2178–2183, 1976
276. Bloom NA, Vidone RA, Lytton B: Primary carcinoma of the ureter: A report of 102 new cases. J Urol 103:590–598, 1970
277. Herr HW, Whitmore WF Jr: Ureteral carcinoma in situ after successful intravesical therapy for superficial bladder tumors: Incidence, possible pathogenesis and management. J Urol 138:292–294, 1987
278. Heney NM, Nocks BN, Daly JJ et al: Prognostic factors in carcinoma of the ureter. J Urol 125:632–636, 1981
279. Johannson A, Angerval L, Benstsson U et al: A clinicopathologic and prognostic study of epithelial tumors of the renal pelvis. Cancer 37:1376–1381, 1976
280. Brookland RK, Richter MP: Postoperative irradiation of transitional cell carcinoma of the renal pelvis and ureter. J Urol 133:952–955, 1985
281. Saitoh H, Hida N, Nakamura K et al: Distant metastases urothelial tumors of the renal pelvis and ureter. Tokai J Exp Clin Med 7:355–361, 1982
282. Shipley WU: Radiation therapy in the management of patients with genitourinary malignancies. In Wang CC (ed): Clinical Radiation Oncology: Indications, Techniques, and Results. Boston, PSG, 1987
283. Maruf NJ, Godec CJ, Kahn A et al: Synchronous tumors in both ureters and left renal pelvis. Urology 21:305, 1983
284. Hall P, Dammin G: Balkan nephropathy. Nephron 22:281, 1968
285. Trindade A, Samuels ML, Logothetis CJ: Chemotherapy of carcinoma of renal pelvis: Preliminary report. Urology 18:54, 1981

286. Nocks BN, Heney NM, Daly JJ et al: Transitional cell carcinoma of renal pelvis. Urology 19:472, 1982
287. DeKock MLS, Breytenbach IH: Local excision and topical thiotepa in the treatment of transitional cell carcinoma of the renal pelvis: A case report. J Urol 135:566, 1986
288. Sternberg C, Scher H: Current status of chemotherapy for urothelial tract tumors. Oncology 1:41, 1987
289. Logothetis CJ, Samuels ML, Selig DE et al: Combined intravenous and intraarterial cyclophosphamide, doxorubicin, and cis-platin (CISCA) in the management of select patients with invasive urothelial tumors. Cancer Treat Rep 69:33, 1985
290. Hrushesky WJM, Roemeling RV, Wood PA et al: High-dose intensive systemic therapy of metastatic bladder cancer. J Clin Oncol 5:450, 1987
291. Glover D, Glick JH, Weiler C et al: WR-2721 and high-dose cisplatin: An active combination in the treatment of metastatic melanoma. J Clin Oncol 5:574, 1987
292. Pinsky CM, Camacho FJ, Kerr D et al: Intravesical administration of bacillus Calmette-Guerin in patients with recurrent superficial carcinoma of the urinary bladder: Report of a prospective, randomized trial. Cancer Treat Rep 69:47, 1985
293. Bander NH: Monoclonal antibodies in the diagnosis and treatment of bladder cancer. In Yagoda A (ed): Bladder Cancer: Future Directions for Treatment, p 75. New York, John Wiley & Sons, 1986
294. Peeling WB, Mantell BS, Shepheard BGF: Post-operative irradiation in the treatment of renal cell carcinoma. Br J Urol 41:23–31, 1969
295. Juusela H, Malmio K, Alfthan D et al: Preoperative irradiation in the treatment of renal adenocarcinoma. Scand J Urol Nephrol 11:277–281, 1977
296. Kjaer M, Frederiksen PL, Engelholm SA: Postoperative radiotherapy in stage II and III renal adenocarcinoma. A randomized trial by the Copenhagen Renal Cancer Study Group. Int J Radiat Oncol Biol Phy 13:665–772, 1987

JEROME P. RICHIE
WILLIAM U. SHIPLEY
ALAN YAGODA

CHAPTER 32 *Cancer of the Bladder*

Carcinoma of the urinary bladder accounts for approximately 2% of all malignant tumors. The American Cancer Society has estimated that there will be 46,400 new cases of bladder cancer in 1988, with an estimated 10,400 deaths.[1] Although the disease is localized at the time of initial diagnosis in 90% of patients, as many as 80% will subsequently develop recurrent tumors. Close follow-up is mandatory because of both the potential for recurrence and the potential change in the biologic behavior of recurrent tumors. Indeed, patients with recurrent superficial bladder tumors give a glimpse of the process of carcinogenesis in vivo, with polychronotopism and subsequent invasion of the muscle wall and metastases.

Traditionally, management of the patient with carcinoma of the bladder has been the responsibility of the urologic surgeon. Currently, however, proper management requires the concerted effort of a team approach, with involvement from the radiotherapist and medical oncologist as well as the urologist. The increased incidence of bladder cancer and the rising mortality from bladder cancer underscore the need for effective combination treatment programs for all stages of disease in order to reduce recurrences and improve survival rates.

EPIDEMIOLOGY

The incidence of carcinoma of the bladder is higher in industrialized countries than in underdeveloped regions such as Asia and Africa. Bladder cancer is more prevalent in urban than in rural areas, giving credence to the effects of industrial carcinogens on the development of bladder cancer. The incidence of bladder cancer increases with age, with a peak incidence in the seventh decade of life. The male to female ratio is 3:1.

The association of occupational factors with the development of bladder malignancies was first suggested by Rehn[2] in 1895, who observed an increased risk of bladder cancer in aniline dye workers. Subsequent studies over the next 50 years have identified benzidine, 1 naphthylamine, and 2 naphthylamine as the primary agents. The average latency between exposure and development of bladder cancer is between 16 and 22 years. Other occupational categories associated with bladder cancer have been the dye, rubber, leather, paint, and organic chemical industries.

A consistent relationship has been demonstrated between cigarette smoking and bladder cancer. The rate of development of bladder cancer is about twice as high in smokers as in nonsmokers.[3] Winder and Goldsmith[4] reported a consistent relationship between the amount and duration of smoking and the incidence of bladder cancer in both men and women. The disparity in habits of cigarette smoking may account for the male to female ratio in bladder cancer of 3:1, which seems to be decreasing as more women have smoked for longer periods of time. A Canadian study[5] showed that the risk ratio of bladder cancer in men who smoked 10 cigarettes a day, between 10 and 20, and more than 20 cigarettes a day was 1.0, 3.8, and 5.1 respectively. The relationship of artificial sweeteners to bladder cancer was highlighted by the Food and Drug Administration. Some pioneering work by Hicks and associates[6] has shown that both cyclamate and saccharine function as potent promoting agents in the rat model in which a single subthreshold initiating dose of methyl-nitrosourea (MNU) is followed by oral saccharine or cyclamates. These promoters increase the rate of tumors from 2% to 50% and telescope the time of induction from 2 years to 8 weeks. These findings were explained by the subthreshold dose of MNU serving as an initiator, with cyclamate or saccharine serving as a promoter. Although epidemiologic studies have suggested that artificial sweeteners are only weak human carcinogens,[7] these studies would be expected to show only an increased risk of 30% or more. Although the studies did not reach statistical significance, in the small group of nonsmoking females who represent the lowest risk the relative risk ratio for development of bladder cancers with cyclamates was 2.9.

A close relationship exists between bilharziasis and squamous cell carcinoma of the bladder. A recent review has focused on the presence of urinary nitrite in association with squamous cell carcinoma secondary to bilharziasis. Urinary tract infection associated with urinary nitrites and the production of nitrosourea may act as a proximate carcinogen for the production of squamous cell cancer of the bladder.[8]

PATHOLOGY

Ninety percent of urothelial bladder tumors are of the transitional cell variety. These tumors are usually papillary and often multicentric, reflecting the field change phenomena so often observed in transitional cell malignancies. Squamous cell carcinoma accounts for 6% to 8% of bladder tumors, and 2% are adenocarcinomas, usually arising in the dome of the bladder from the urachus. Tumors in association with exstrophy of the bladder are often adenocarcinomas.

Tumors are graded by the degree of cellular atypia and nuclear abnormalities as well as the number of mitotic figures. Broder's classification segregates tumors on a scale of I to IV, based on the degree of anaplasia. Some pathologists prefer to use a three grade system because the behaviors of grades III and IV are so similar that combining these two into a single grade seems justified.[9]

Mostofi and the World Health Organization (WHO) have called attention to the importance of recognizing and recording the growth pattern of bladder cancer (papillary or infiltrating, or both, or nonpapillary and noninfiltrating). Papillary tumors seem to have pushing borders that do not invade the muscularis on a broad front and therefore have a relatively better prognosis. Nonpapillary lesions, however, tend to invade on a broader front and hence have a more ominous prognosis.[10] A major problem in treating patients with bladder cancer has been in distinguishing the benign "papilloma" from malignant epithelial tumors. For many years, the variable nature of the benign-appearing papilloma has caused most pathologists to classify this lesion as a low grade carcinoma. Based on studies by Lerman et al and Koss,[11,12] it would appear that sufficient data exist to justify the separation of papilloma from carcinoma. The WHO has defined a papilloma as a papillary tumor with a delicate fibrovascular core covered by normal transitional cell epithelium that is less than six layers thick.[10] These benign transitional cell lesions have a recurrence rate of up to 50%; hence, semiannual surveillance is required for patients with this diagnosis.

Carcinoma in situ is defined as diffuse presence of highly anaplastic malignant cells within the confines of the urothelial lining. This term is used to designate a flat intraurothelial cancer with crowding of the larger nuclei and numerous mitoses. The lamina propria reveals no specific abnormalities. A lesion may appear cystoscopically as normal bladder mucosa or as a red velvety area related to vascular proliferation and dilatation. Carcinoma in situ, in association with overt bladder tumors, signifies a field change and indicates the need for more aggressive therapy.

CLINICAL PRESENTATION

There are no pathognomonic signs or symptoms of bladder cancer. Hematuria, with or without irritative symptoms, occurs in 75% of patients with bladder cancer. Vesical irritability alone is the persisting symptom in 30% of patients and often signifies the presence of carcinoma in situ. Advanced cases may present with rectal obstruction, pelvic pain, or lower extremity edema secondary to lymphatic or venous occlusion. Urinary cytology or flow cytometry may lead to a presumptive diagnosis of bladder cancer, especially in patients with higher grade lesions. Many patients will have an excretory urogram, which often suggests an intraluminal filling defect in the bladder.[13] The diagnosis of bladder cancer is confirmed by cystoscopic examination and transurethral biopsy of the suspected area. At the time of biopsy, bimanual examination is conducted to ascertain the extent of tumor and the presence or absence of fixation to adjacent pelvic structures. The biopsy should be adequate to determine the presence or absence of muscle invasion. Random biopsies at sites adjacent to and distant from the tumor should be evaluated for carcinoma in situ. A cold cup or punch biopsy forceps is useful for obtaining tissue without cautery artifact.

STAGING

Bladder carcinoma that has invaded the muscular wall or deeper is a potentially lethal disease, often metastasizing before major urinary symptoms appear in the patient. Once a diagnosis has been ascertained by biopsy, a chest roentgenogram, radionuclide bone scan, and liver and renal function studies should be performed. The first site of failure in patients with invasive bladder cancer is usually in the bones or the lungs; therefore these areas should be evaluated carefully.[14] Computed tomography scans or magnetic resonance imaging have gained increasing popularity as an adjunct to staging. Ultrasonography of the bladder has been evaluated but has yet to be very helpful in delineating the extent of local involvement.

Modern-day staging began with the observations of Jewett and Strong[15] in 1946, in a study that related the depth of penetration of the bladder wall to the incidence of local extension in metastases. This staging system was modified by Marshall into an O, A, B, C, D system that was based on the bimanual examination under anesthesia and the histologic evaluation of the tumor resected transurethrally.[16] The Jewett, Strong, Marshall staging system and its counterpart in the UICC and the American Joint Committee tumor,

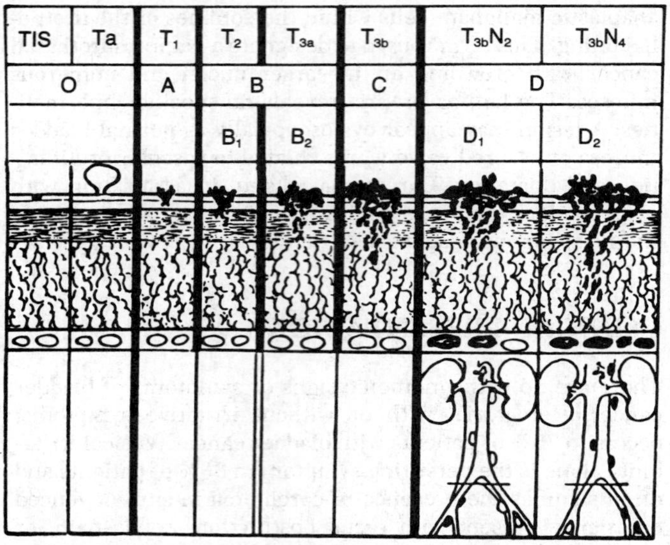

FIG. 32-1. Comparison of TNM system and Jewett, Marshall, Strong (O, A, B, C, D) system for staging of transitional cell carcinoma of the bladder. (Prout GR Jr: Bladder carcinoma. In Pilch YH [ed]: Surgical Oncology, p 683. New York, McGraw-Hill, 1984)

nodes, and metastases (TNM) system are illustrated in Figure 32-1.[18] The stage O lesion indicated tumor that is limited to the mucosa, which includes both a visible papillary carcinoma (T_a) and carcinoma in situ (TIS). Clinical stage T1 (A) lesions have invaded into the lamina propria but not beyond. Clinical T2–T4 (B,C) are tumors that invade at least into muscle. Clinical T2 (B1) tumors infiltrate muscle but have no palpable mass or induration on bimanual examination after transurethral resection. A stage T3 (B2-C) tumor infiltrates muscle and has a palpable mass or induration present on bimanual examination after transurethral resection. (T3A or B2 tumors do not have evidence of invading beyond the bladder muscle; stage T3B or C tumors have invasion documented into perivesical fat.) The clinical T4 tumors are those that extend into neighboring structures (T4A invasion into vagina, uterus, or prostate with histologic confirmation; T4B tumors are fixed to the bony pelvis or abdominal wall or invade rectum). The staging criteria for lymph nodal involvement are based on the surgical and pathologic staging of the lymph nodes. In the absence of any histologic confirmation of nodal metastasis, the disease is staged as Nx. Patients with biopsy-proven metastatic lymph nodes limited to the pelvis have either stage D_1 or N_{1-3}. N_1 is involvement of a single homolateral node; N_2 is involvement of contralateral or multiple pelvic lymph nodes; N_3 is involvement of fixed pelvic lymph node(s). Patients with involvement of lymph nodes outside the pelvis are classified either D_2 or N_4. Among the muscle-invading tumors the prognostic difference between clinical stage T2 (B1) and clinical T3 (B2-C) is significant in some series,[15,16,40–42,54,56,59] but in others no difference was noted.[17,39,57]

One difficulty with clinical staging systems is that they are only as good as the techniques available to assess the extent of disease. Many American urologists continue to use the Jewett, Strong, Marshall system of classification, but there is a growing trend in the United States to join international colleagues in using the TNM system. The National Surgical Adjuvant Group and the Memorial Sloan-Kettering Cancer Center have documented an error rate as high as 50% between clinical and pathologic stages for patients with muscle-invading tumors.[54,64] Skinner and associates,[19] in a review of 130 patients, found that clinical and pathologic stages were concordant in 53% of patients with Stage T1 tumors, in only 13% of patients with clinical Stage T2 tumors, and in 50% of patients with Stage T3 tumors. The overall rate of agreement was only 36%, with 41% of patients understaged and 23% overstaged. Refinements in the clinical staging system with more emphasis on histopathologic information of the biopsy such as degree of invasion, grade of tumor, configuration of tumor, and the presence or absence of carcinoma in situ are in order. It is hoped that many of these factors can be consistently shown independently to influence prognosis following treatment for patients with muscle-invading tumors. The TNM pathologic staging criteria by microscopic evaluation of the tumor in the radical cystectomy specimen are quite accurate for predicting prognosis (Table 32-1). A refined clinical staging system that would correlate well with the TNM pathologic staging will be quite useful if and when such refinements can be developed and tested prospectively.

TREATMENT

PHILOSOPHIC CONSIDERATIONS

Treatment of the patient with bladder carcinoma should be selected so as to prevent death from the malignancy and to do so with as little treatment-related morbidity as possible. In

TABLE 32-1. Therapeutic Results for Radical Cystectomy for Invasive Bladder Cancer (Patients Grouped by Pathologic Stage)

Series (Year)	*No. of Patients*	*5-Year Survival Rate (%) for Pathologic Stage*				
		P0/P1/Pcis	*P2*	*P3a*	*P3b*	*P4 or N+*
Bowles and Cordonier,[4] 1963	50		63	50	20	0
Jewett, King, Shelley,[45] 1964	61		50	16	12	
Pearse, Reed, Hodges,[46] 1978	52		50	16	12	
Mathur, Krahn, Ramsey,[47] 1981	58	71	88	57	40	29
Skinner, Lieskovsky,[48] 1984	197	75	64		44	36
Skinner, Lieskovsky,[49] 1988	189	83	83	69	29	27

patients with superficial tumors, recurrences are likely and increase with the size and the multiplicity of the tumor and the association of carcinoma in situ. Treatment directed toward recurrent superficial bladder tumors is mainly for patient convenience and the reduction of the need for resection; fewer than 25% of these patients will progress to invasive disease. In patients with muscle-invading tumors, surgical extirpation remains as the gold standard for long-term tumor-survival. However, innovative approaches for patients with muscle-invading tumors that incorporate more extensive transurethral surgery with chemotherapy or radiation therapy, or both, and selective bladder preservation are now being studied in careful prospective protocols.[119,120]

SUPERFICIAL BLADDER CANCER

Stage O (in situ) tumors are frequently treated with transurethral resections or fulguration. Many of these lesions are papillary and can be controlled locally with conservative therapy in more than 80% of the cases. However, some lesions are more infiltrating and less differentiated, and recurrences in more than 50% of the patients have been reported. It is important for the urologist to remove the base of the lesion with an adequate margin.

Intravesical Chemotherapy

Postoperative intravesical chemotherapy has been used to reduce recurrence rates. Agents such as doxorubicin have been used in a cyclic fashion, beginning on the day of surgery, with good success.[20] Randomized trials have been undertaken specifically to destroy existing tumors or tumor implants that could occur during local resection or fulguration, and to prevent recurrence of resected primary tumors or development of new cancers.[21,22] Ideally, agents for intravesical administration should be poorly absorbed through the bladder mucosa, thereby preventing systemic toxicity and exposing local lesions to a high drug concentration.

Thiotepa, which has been studied extensively in the carcinogen-induced FANFT murine bladder cancer model, has little effect on normal murine urothelium, destroys established cancers, inhibits tumor reimplantation, and retards development of new lesions.[21,22] The usual dose is 30 to 60 mg/30 to 60 ml given intravesically for 1 to 2 hours weekly for 4 weeks and thereafter monthly. When given to patients with established tumors, approximately 30% achieve complete and 30% achieve partial remissions. In a randomized trial using 90 mg for 30 minutes given immediately after complete resection of all tumors versus no therapy, tumor recurrence (or implants) decreased by 40%.[23] In a study in patients with no visible tumor, 66% of the thiotepa group versus 40% of the control group remained tumor free at 1 year.[24] Because of its low molecular weight, 189, thiotepa is absorbed and myelosuppression can be seen in 18% to 40% of cases; pancytopenia is uncommon.[25]

Mitomycin-C in doses of 20 to 60 mg/20 to 40 ml weekly for eight doses produces complete response in approximately half and partial response in one third of the cases.[26] Higher response rates are noted with doses greater than 40 mg/40 ml. The drug seems to be as effective as thiotepa as primary therapy and can induce complete remission in patients failing thiotepa therapy. Myelosuppression is rare because the molecular weight, 334, is too large for absorption through the bladder mucosa. Bladder irritation and genital and palmar rashes secondary to direct contact with the drug have been described.[21] Doxorubicin, epodyl, and tenoposide (VM-26) have been used extensively in Europe and Japan. In two randomized studies, doxorubicin, given three times per week in doses of 20 mg to 30 mg, 50 mg, and 60 mg, produced responses in 31% to 56%, 69% to 72%, and 59% to 74% of cases, respectively.[27] Other studies have described complete remission with negative cytologic and endoscopic findings in two thirds of the cases.[21] However, bladder irritation is frequent, 27% to 44%, and severe when given immediately after fulguration. Of note, cisplatin, intravesically as well as intravenously, is ineffective and can induce severe hypersensitivity reactions.[28]

Bacillus Calmette-Guerin (BCG) in doses of 120 mg/50 ml of normal saline intravesically with weekly intradermal administration for 6 weeks has also proved extremely effective. Prospective randomized trials by Lamm et al[29] and Pinsky et al[30] have shown a 50% prophylaxis versus untreated cases. In a study of 86 cases, half of whom served as controls, the number of recurrent tumors was reduced, and the disease-free interval, including negative cytology, and the time to progression locally and to cystectomy (BCG 3 of 43 cases versus control 15 of 43 cases) was significantly ($p = 0.001$) prolonged.[31] Conversion to a negative cytology was frequently observed ($p = 0.05$).[32] A few patients who after achieving complete remission eventually required surgery for recurrent, abnormal cytology showed new tumors only in the renal pelvis, ureter, or urethra; areas that had direct contact with BCG remained free of disease. Present data suggest that intradermal administration can be omitted.[32]

Lamm[32] reported his experience in patients with superficial bladder cancer receiving intravesical BCG (Pasteur) strain (120 mg/50 ml saline weekly for 6 weeks). A highly significant reduction recurrence rate was noted: 20% versus 52% in controls. Brosman[33] reported 35 patients treated with TICE strain of BCG for carcinoma in situ. By 24 weeks, all 27 patients who tolerated BCG were rendered tumor free and placed on maintenance regimen. Six patients did not receive full treatment; thus, 31 of 33 patients (94%) were rendered free of disease.

CARCINOMA IN SITU

Management of carcinoma in situ may present specific problems in patients with transitional cell carcinoma. Carcinoma in situ is noninvasive but has a high potential for subsequent invasion. Carcinoma in situ is multifocal and diffuse and reflects the potential for the entire urothelial surface to undergo exposure to potential carcinogens.

If the lesion involves only a small portion of the bladder (<5 cm), is reasonably well delineated, does not involve the prostatic urethra, vesical neck, or either ureteral orifice, and there is no evidence of positive cytologic findings from the upper urinary tract, thorough electrofulguration of the involved areas is indicated followed by a course of intravesical thiotepa or doxorubicin for 6 months. Another alternative is

BCG weekly for 6 to 12 weeks. The patient should be followed post-treatment with cystoscopic and urinary cytologic studies at 2- to 3-month intervals for the first year, at 4-month intervals for the second year, and at 6-month intervals thereafter. If the lesion does not respond, if cytologic findings do not convert to negative, and if the irritative bladder symptoms remain after treatment, cystoprostatectomy with urinary diversion is recommended. In patients who have diffuse lesions, involvement of the prostatic urethra, or severe irritative bladder symptomatology, radical cystectomy is warranted.

Involvement of the prostatic urethra with carcinoma in situ should prompt in-continuity urethrectomy.

The initiation of aggressive treatment of carcinoma in situ is prompted by the previous experience of Utz and co-workers.[34] In their initial series in which carcinoma in situ was treated primarily by transurethral electroresection and fulguration, subsequent invasion developed in 73% of patients, with 57% of these patients dying of their disease in 5 years. The more aggressive approach of cystectomy after diagnosis of carcinoma in situ demonstrated no deaths in 15 subsequent patients. Three of these patients had microinvasion with more than 80% of the bladder replaced by in situ cancer at the time of pathologic examination.

In a more recent series, however, Utz and co-workers[35] have identified a subset of patients with positive cytologic findings in whom carcinoma in situ has been found without associated irritative symptoms or overt bladder tumors. These patients seem to represent an earlier state along the road to invasion and metastases, and some have been followed for longer than 10 years without progression. Thus, management of the patient with carcinoma in situ should be individualized, with more conservative treatment such as intravesical chemotherapy used for those patients at lower risk of progression.

INVASIVE DISEASE

PARTIAL CYSTECTOMY

The role of segmental resection in the management of transitional cell carcinoma of the bladder remains controversial. However, this operative option presents an attractive alternative for carefully selected patients. Selection of patients for partial cystectomy is complicated by the tendency of the entire vesical urothelium to be unstable in the presence of an isolated and well-defined lesion, and because of the probability of undetected microinvasion and carcinoma in situ in remote areas of the bladder. The additional problem of wound seeding at the time of partial cystectomy must not be underemphasized.

A series of specific criteria must be established in order to select the appropriate patient for surgery. The tumor should be invasive. The tumor should be less than 6 cm to 8 cm in size to permit resection with sufficient tumor-free margins for acceptable functional bladder capacity. The lesion should be solitary and primary and, ideally, located in the upper part of the bladder or on the posterior wall. Invasion of the vesical neck or the prostate is a contraindication. Transitional cell carcinomas have a better response to partial cystectomy than do squamous cell carcinomas owing to the tendency of the latter to extend intramurally via lymphatics and venous plexus of the bladder wall. The appearance of carcinoma in situ adjacent or distant to the lesion itself indicates urothelial instability and is a contraindication to partial cystectomy.

Before partial cystectomy, preoperative radiotherapy in the form of a minimum dose of 1000 to 2000 rad should be established to devitalize the tumor cells and prevent wound seeding. Before opening the bladder, the bladder should be irrigated with sterile water. When laterality of the lesion can be established, a unilateral pelvic node dissection should be established in continuity.

The necessity for rigid patient selection makes segmental resection appropriate for only 5% of patients with bladder cancer. Five-year survival rates in patients with Stage O, A, or B bladder cancer carefully selected for treatment by partial cystectomy range from 65% to 81%.[36,37]

RADICAL CYSTECTOMY: TREATMENT RESULTS

For most patients whose tumor demonstrates invasion of the muscle wall, more aggressive treatment is clearly indicated. Once the urothelial malignancy has penetrated into the muscularis, radical cystoprostatectomy in men or anterior exenteration in women has been the treatment of choice. This operation satisfies the treatment of field changes that are common in urothelial malignancy and results in reasonable potential for cure if the cancer is still confined within the bladder wall. Unfortunately, many tumors have progressed beyond the point of curability by means of local therapy with radical cystectomy alone. Failures in patients managed by radical cystectomy are usually due to distant metastases, with fewer than 10% of patients failing locally.

Prognosis in patients with carcinoma of the bladder who have undergone cystectomy has traditionally been reported on the basis of 5-year survival rates. Originally, this was based on observed survival data, with all patients followed at least 5 years. Beginning in the 1970s, however, actuarial survival rates using statistical correlation such as Kaplan Meyer curves have been used to present projected 5-year survival rates (Table 32-1). This technique allows the incorporation of patients followed for less than 5 years but considered at risk for the interval over which they have been followed. One problem with reports of survival is that most 5-year survivals have been based on pathologic stage (Table 32-1), which may be at some variance from the clinical stage (Table 32-2).

Up until the 1950s, survival rates had little meaning since the operative mortality varied from 25% to 60%. In 1966, Glantz[50] reported a mortality rate of 20% in patients who underwent total cystectomy in the 1950s and early 1960s. Whitmore and Marshall[51] reported a mortality rate of 14% in radical cystectomies done between 1945 and 1955. Richie and associates[17] reported a 15% overall operative mortality from 1955 to 1971 but a 2% operative mortality in the most recent 50 patients done in the early 1970s. Johnson and Lamy[52] reported a 3.3% mortality rate in 214 radical cystec-

TABLE 32-2. Therapeutic Results for Radiation Therapy and Radical Cystectomy for Invasion Bladder Cancer

Series and Year	*No. of Patients*	*Clinical Stage*	*Total Dose (cGY)*	*Maintained Local Control (%)*	*5-Year Survival Rate (%)*
Radiation Therapy					
Miller and Johnson,[38] 1973	263	T2,T3	5800–6500	56	22
Shipley et al,[40] 1985	37	T2,T3	6400–6840	49	39
Timmer et al,[41] 1985	76	T2,T3	6000–6500	41	38
Quilty and Duncan,[42] 1986	333	T3	5000–5750	24	26
Blandy,[43] 1988	138	T2,T3	6000	40	
Preoperative Radiation and Surgery			*Preoperative XRT*		
Boileau and Johnson et al,[39] 1980	112	T2,T3	5000	90	50
Batata et al,[117] (1981)	133	T3,T4	2000	88	35
van der Werf-Messing et al,[58] 1982	183	T3	4000	100	52
National Bladder Cancer Group[59]	175	T2–T4	4000	92	52

tomies done from 1969 to 1975. More recently, Skinner[53] reported a less than 1% operative mortality in 128 radical cystectomies from 1971 to 1977.

With the improvement in postoperative mortality rate, survival data have become more meaningful (see Table 32-1). Before 1975, most survival rates were broken down into patients with superficial (O,A and B1; T-O,TA, T1) and deep (B2, C or T3A, T3B) pathologically staged lesions. Whitmore and associates[54] reported a 63% 5-year survival rate for superficial tumors by pathologic stage and a 20% 5-year survival rate for deep lesions by pathologic stage in 137 patients who underwent radical cystectomy alone from 1949 to 1958. With preoperative radiation therapy of 4500 rad and improved surgical techniques, 5-year survival rates for 119 patients operated on from 1959 to 1966 were 58% for the superficial group and 48% for the deep group. Eighty-six patients who received a short course (2000 rad) to the bladder and true pelvis and then radical cystectomy from 1966 to 1970 had a 5-year survival rate of 56% for the superficial lesions and 58% for the deep lesions. Although this series suggests improvement in survival rate related to preoperative radiation, an equally plausible alternative explanation relates to improved survival rates from improved techniques of surgical approach, anesthetic management, and patient monitoring.

In an effort to improve patient survival, various combinations of radiation therapy along with radical cystectomy have been advocated. Randomized trials of radiation therapy prior to radical cystectomy have shown a trend in improvement in survival but not one that is statistically significant when compared with surgery alone.[62,64] Nonrandomized concurrent studies have not shown any survival advantage to preoperative radiation therapy versus current surgical cystectomy.[48,55] At present, one has the clear impression that for patients with tumors that minimally invade muscle (clinical and pathologic stage T2 or B_1), there seems to be no benefit from radiation therapy in addition to immediate radical cystectomy. Such opinion is supported by the fact that the 5-year survival rates with radical cystectomy alone for patients with pathologic stage T1 or T2 are 80% or more in recent series (see Table 32-1).

FULL-DOSE RADIATION THERAPY: TREATMENT RESULTS

External Beam Irradiation

Full-dose radiation therapy as definitive treatment has yielded 5-year survival rates of 22% to 39% for patients presenting with clinical stage T2 and T3 (B1, B2-C) tumors (see Table 32-1).[38,40–43] The major clinical problem in such patients is that permanent eradication of the cancer in the bladder occurs in only 30% to 50% of the patients (see Table 32-2) compared to more than 85% in patients treated by cystectomy following preoperative radiation therapy.[39,58,59,117] However, patients who do have an excellent response to radiation therapy have an excellent survival probability. In the retrospective review from the Massachusetts General Hospital, the survival of patients with clinical stage T2 and T3 tumors from their bladder cancer was 79% in patients who had local control of their cancer compared to only 11% for patients who developed a local recurrence.[40] In these retrospective series, several clinically useful observations can be made: fewer than half of the treated patients will have a complete response to conventional external beam radiation therapy, and only one third to two fifths of the whole group will have permanent control of their local bladder tumor; radical cystectomy may be deferred in the completely responding patients, most of whom will not require this operation; patients needing salvage cystectomy have been, during the most recent decade, better able to tolerate that operation, perhaps because of improvements in surgery, radiation therapy, and perioperative care; and, finally, the radiation response rate has not changed over the past two decades, and thus expecting further progress with conventional radiation therapy alone and prompt salvage cystectomy seems unrealistic. Salvage cystectomy still carries significant risks, with mortality rates from 2% to 19%.[41,52]

Tumor-related prognostic factors that contribute to an improved treatment outcome by full-dose radiation therapy in patients with muscle-invading tumors include the clinical stage of the tumor, the accomplishment of a visibly complete transurethral resection of the tumor, the histologic characteristic of a papillary tumor surface, and the absence of

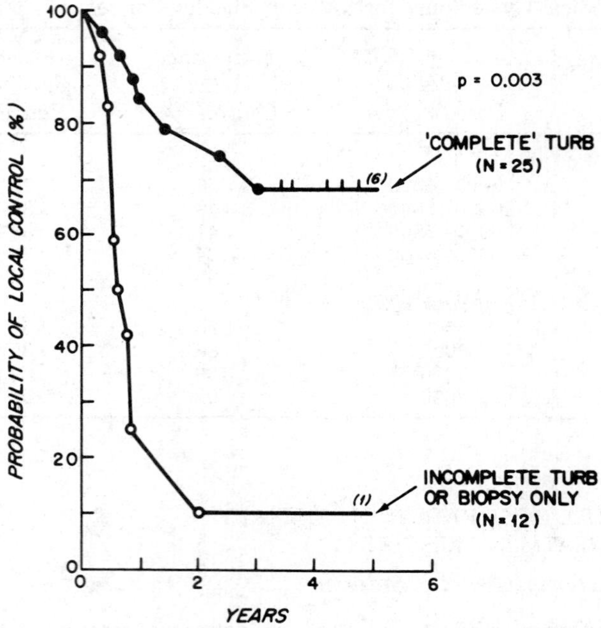

FIG. 32-2. Probability of local control by full-dose radiation therapy in patients with Stages T2 and T3 bladder cancer in whom a "visibly complete" transurethral resection of the bladder tumor (TURB) was possible, and in patients in whom only an incomplete resection or biopsy was done. The numbers in parentheses indicate the number of patients followed up more than 5 years. (Shipley WV, Prout GE Jr, Kaufman SD et al: Full-dose irradiation for patients with invasive bladder carcinoma: Clinical and histological factors prognostic of improved survival. Cancer 60:511, 1987)

ureteral obstruction by tumor. In patients with clinical stage T2 and T3 tumors, the local control rate at 5 years in 25 patients in whom the urologist judged that a visibly complete transurethral resection had been accomplished was 68% versus 10% for those patients who had undergone a biopsy only or incomplete resection ($p = 0.003$).[40] The 5-year survival rate from bladder cancer in the group who underwent a complete resection was 54% versus 17% in the group who did not (Figure 32-2). There are almost certainly some inaccuracies in the endoscopic estimate of the extent of tumor debulking. Nevertheless, this is a favorable prognostic factor and very likely correlates both with initial tumor size and with the number of remaining tumor cells that must be inactivated by irradiation.

Many reports have documented that papillary tumors are of less malignant potential than are solid tumors.[60-63] Muscle invading papillary tumors are more effectively treated by radiation therapy than are solid tumors.[40,62,64,65] For tumors of the same clinical stage, radiation therapy has led to both better local tumor control and patient survival in those tumors of papillary histology, as compared to the solid tumors for patients treated with external beam radiation therapy[40] and by combined external beam and interstitial radiation therapy.[65]

Intraoperative Radiation Therapy

The ability to deliver selectively more radiation therapy directly to the tumor and less to the uninvolved portion of the bladder can be provided in appropriate patients by open surgery. Brachytherapy using radium-226 (^{226}Ra) needle implantation has been used with great success over the past 25 years by van der Werf-Messing and colleagues at the Rotterdam Radiotherapy Institute for patients with solitary tumors of less than 5 cm in greatest diameter. Intraoperatively, the radium needles are inserted into and immediately adjacent to the tumor at the time of open cystotomy. Recently, however, the radioactive source has been changed to cesium-137 (^{137}Cs).[66] Sutures that are attached to the needles are brought out through a separate track from the incision and are used to remove the needles in 3 to 6 days, or following the delivery of 3,250 to 6,500 cGy of radiation. Problems of wound seeding by tumor resulting from the open cystotomy have been solved by the use of preoperative radiation therapy with doses of 1,050 cGy over 3 elapsed days in 3 fractions. The largest number of patients (328) who have been treated by this approach have had clinical stage T2 tumors, although not all of these patients have had proof of muscle invasion. Seventy-seven percent have remained free of recurrence of tumor in their bladder for at least 5 years (Table 32-3), for an overall survival of 56%.[66] For patients with clinical stage T2 tumors a similarly high 5-year local tumor control rate as well as survival rate is seen by groups from Amsterdam and Creteil.[67,68]

Intraoperative radiation therapy by electron beam has been used with similar success in Japan.[69] The treatment was also done at the time of open cystotomy but without tumor resection or fulguration. The electron beam dose of 2,500 to 3,000 cGy by 3.5 to 7.5 MeV electrons was delivered via cylinders of 4, 5, or 6 cm in internal diameter. Three thousand to 4,000 cGy of external beam irradiation was given postoperatively to the whole bladder in 15 to 20 treatments. In 28 patients treated for stage T2 tumors there was freedom from local recurrence in 82%, with an overall 62% 5-year survival rate.

RECENT MODIFICATIONS IN TREATMENT TECHNIQUES

Surgical Techniques

POTENCY PRESERVING TECHNIQUE FOR RADICAL CYSTECTOMY. Before the early 1980s, virtually all patients who had undergone radical cystectomy were impotent postoperatively. Following the pioneering work by Walsh and associates of delineation of the anatomy of Santorini's plexus[70] and the description of the anatomic relationships between the nerves supplying the corpora cavernosum and the apex of the prostate,[71] anatomical approaches have been described for radical prostatectomy and radical cystectomy that can preserve potency in a high percentage of patients. Radical cystectomy proceeds in standard fashion, including bilateral pelvic lymph node dissection and division of the lateral pedicles to the prostate. A plane is developed between the bladder and rectum by incising the peritoneum and using gentle blunt dissection to free the rectum from the prostate at Denonvilliers' fascia. Dissection is stopped before encountering lateral pedicles of the bladder near the pelvic fascia. Attention is then turned to the dorsal-venous complex and plexus of Santorini as for radical retropubic prostatec-

TABLE 32-3. Intraoperative Radiation Therapy: Clinical Stage T2 Bladder Cancer

Series	*No. of Patients*	*Treatment*	*5-Year Local Control (%)*	*5-Year Survival (%)*
van der Werf-Messing et al[66]	328	XRT, ^{226}Ra	77	56
Batterman et al[67]	85	XRT, ^{226}RA	74	55
Mazeron et al[68]	24	Resection, ^{192}Ir, XRT	92	58
Matsumoto et al[69]	28	IORT, XRT	82	62

XRT, external Beam irradiation; ^{226}Ra, brachytherapy by radium needles; ^{192}Ir, brachytherapy by after-loading iridium in catheters; IORT, single dose electron beam irradiation.

tomy. Isolation of the dorsal-venous complex is achieved and the membranous urethra transected with division of the lateral pelvic fascia and pedicles to the prostate. The seminal vesicles are then dissected away from the neurovascular bundle on each side and the remainder of the lateral bladder pedicles ligated.

Using these principles, radical removal of bladder cancer can be performed with preservation of the neurovascular bundles and therefore preservation of potency. Indeed, approximately two thirds of the patients who were potent preoperatively will recover potency from 3 months to 1 year after radical cystectomy using this modified technique.

URINARY DIVERSION. The standard method of urinary diversion following cystectomy in 1988 remains the ileal conduit. However, newer techniques have been described to include continent forms of urinary diversion such as the Kock pouch, Camey procedure, or ileocecal segment. These techniques involve innovative use of bowel segments either brought to the skin or sutured to the urethra, allowing the patient to void in a normal fashion or be catheterized intermittently rather than wearing an external collecting device. The Kock pouch involves use of a long segment of ileum and creation of an internal pouch with antirefluxing intussuscepted nipple connected to both ureters and a second nipple to preserve continence. The pouch is usually brought to the abdominal wall but may, on rare occasions, be placed down to the urethra.[72] The Camey procedure involves use of a long segment of ileum hooked to the end of the urethra in an end-to-side anastomotic fashion.[73] Each ureter is implanted into one end of the upper portion of the U using an antirefluxing ureteroileal anastomosis. The patients void normally during the daytime but have problems with nocturnal enuresis. The ileocecal segment can be used with the ileocecal valve as an antireflux mechanism and the cecum brought to the skin for intermittent catheterization or a cecoileal segment anastomosed directly to the urethra for normal voiding.[74,75] All of these techniques are somewhat experimental and should be used only in selected patients. Urinary diversion continues to evolve through a variety of new techniques, all of which will require long-term follow-up to be certain that complications not yet suspected do not arise.

NORMAL TISSUE-SPARING TECHNIQUES WITH IRRADIATION. Over the past decade improvements in the use of higher energy megavoltage irradiation (XRT) primarily from linear accelerator beams have been used for full-dose or definitive treatment of patients with bladder cancer. These have been well tolerated by the pelvic soft tissues and likely represent a clinically significant reduction in late radiation sequelae in the pelvic tissues without compromising bladder and bowel function. The four-field box technique has become the accepted method of treating the bladder tumor volume and the pelvic lymph nodes.[38] These fields are based inferiorly 1.0 cm below the lower border of the obturator foramena so as to include adequate urethral tissue distally. (The fields may have to be even lower in women with cystoceles.) The width is 1 to 1.5 cm lateral to the bony pelvis at its widest point to cover adequately the external iliac lymph nodal tissues. For conventional radiation fractionation, daily doses (5 sessions per week) in the 180 to 200 cGy range were judged to offer an optimal therapeutic index. For instance, when 180 cGy per fraction doses were used with full-dose radiation therapy, only 4 of 35 patients developed severe frequency or hematuria, or both, either causing incontinence or requiring surgery.[40] In a series in which high radiation doses per fraction (240–275 cGy) were delivered to the whole bladder and to some surrounding nodal tissues in patients with T3 tumors to total doses of 4,750 to 5,500 cGy, the incidence of severe bladder damage was 45% in patients who lived 3 years or more after treatment.[76]

The technique of administering the boost to the tumor volume depends on the equipment available and the size of the patient. The goal is to exclude as much uninvolved normal tissue as possible from the region that receives the total dose (6,000–7,000 cGy in 7–8 weeks). Ideally the technique should limit the total dose to less than 6,000 cGy to the uninvolved section of the bladder and the posterior half of the rectosigmoid, and to less than 4,500 to 5,000 cGy to the anus and the head and neck regions of the femorae. The information allowing the boost dose to be only to the bladder tumor volume and not the whole bladder requires close coordination between the urologist and radiation oncologist. A diagram of the bladder tumor, the extent of transurethral resection, the bimanual examination, and the selected mucosal biopsies are all helpful in planning the cone-down boost field to the tumor volume. The boost can be optimally given with treatment beams of 10 MV x-rays or greater by paired lateral fields that maximally exclude the rectum. However, if the beam of a 4 or 6 MV accelerator is to be used, the 120 degree arc rotation is usually the most desirable boost technique (Fig. 32-3).

CHEMOTHERAPY FOR ADVANCED DISEASE

Transitional cell carcinoma of the urothelium (renal pelvis, ureter, urinary bladder, urethra, and prostatic ducts) is a chemotherapeutically responsive tumor, evidenced by com-

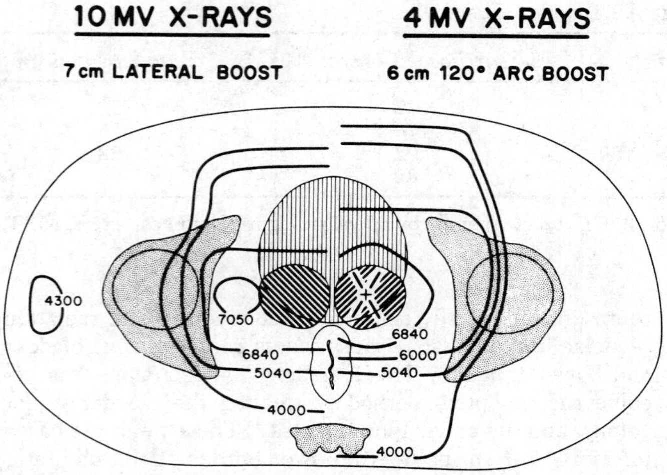

FIG. 32-3. A comparison for full-dose radiation therapy (XRT) of invasive T2–T3 bladder tumor by 10 MV x-rays or 4 MV x-rays. The XRT dose to the whole pelvis is 5040 cGy; the XRT boost dose to the bladder tumor volume is 1800 cGy.

plete and partial remissions observed in 45% to 70% of selected cases with some combination regimens.[77,78] Single agents can produce objective tumor regression in 10% to 30% of cases; only with multidrug regimens have a significant number of complete remissions been reported. Of cardinal importance, such combinations still need to be proved in prospective randomized Phase III studies against active single agents such as cisplatin or methotrexate.

The major problem in evaluating therapy in this tumor is patient selection bias owing to different patient populations, sites of metastases being evaluated, extent of prior therapies, and response criteria.[79–81] The last-mentioned problem has come under scrutiny in a Consensus Development Conference on Guidelines for Clinical Research in Bladder Cancer.[80,81]

Single Agents

The most active single agents are cisplatin and methotrexate (Table 32-4).[77,78] Cisplatin has been evaluated in more than 320 cases, generally in a dose of 70 mg/m² IV every 3 to 4 weeks. Response is observed within 3 to 6 weeks and persists for 3 to 5 months; complete remission is uncommon. No evidence exists to suggest that higher cisplatin doses will induce a better or a more prolonged response. In randomized Phase III studies, cisplatin singly has produced response in 17% to 20% of cases.[82–84] Although some data suggest that cisplatin may be more effective against soft tissue metastases than against primary intravesical disease,[84] two studies[85,86] using cisplatin alone neoadjuvantly described significant efficacy. Methotrexate produces remission in 30% of cases.[77,78] The optimum dose is still unknown, but the schedule most frequently used is 40 mg/m² IV weekly. Tumor regression occurs within 2 to 4 weeks and persists for 3 to 4 months. Complete remission is infrequent. No randomized trial has evaluated high- versus low-dose methotrexate, but in 57 cases culled from the literature giving high dose with citrovorum favor rescue, the response rate was 45% (95% confidence intervals, 32–50%).

Doxorubicin and the vinca alkaloids have also shown moderate antitumor activity. Doxorubicin, 45, 60, and 75 mg/m² IV every 3 weeks, produces response in 17% of cases. Complete remission for 17 to 48 months has been reported; most responses are partial and persist a median of 3 months. A possible dose response relationship has been suggested. Vin-

TABLE 32-4. Single-Agent Trials in Previously Treated and Untreated Patients with Advanced Urothelial Tract Tumors[77,78]

Drugs	*No. of Patients*	*% Complete and Partial Remission*
Amsacrine (AMSA)	61	12 (4–20)*
Bisantrene	13	0 (0–23)
Bleomycin	79	5 (0–10)
Carboplatin	80	11 (7–15)
Cisplatin	**320**	**30 (25–35)**
Cyclophosphamide	26	7 (0–17)
10-Deazaaminopterin	15	20 (0–40)
Diaziquone (AZQ)	16	0 (0–17)
Doxorubicin	**248**	**17 (12–23)**
Etoposide (VP-16-213)	47	2 (0–4)
5-Fluorouracil	105	15 (18–22)
Gallium nitrate	26	27 (11–48)
Hexamethylmelamine	24	13 (0–31)
Methotrexate	**236**	**29 (23–35)**
(high dose)	57	45 (32–50)
Mitomycin-C	42	13 (3–23)
Mitoxantrone	28	0 (0–10)
Neocarcinostatin	19	5 (0–19)
PALA	18	0 (0–16)
Teniposide (VM-26)	64	11 (3–19)
(intravesical)	148	13 (8–18)
Vinblastine	**38**	**16 (4–28)**
Vincristine	42	14 (3–25)

* Numbers in parentheses indicate range of 95% confidence intervals.

blastine sulfate and vincristine in limited trials were observed to induce remission in 16% and 14% of cases, respectively.[77,78] Both agents are now being used only in combination regimens.

Few trials have investigated lymphokines or immunologic agents. Interferon exhibited significant antiproliferative activity against five human bladder lines,[87] and interleukin-2 has induced tumor regression of T2–T4 primary bladder lesions with intralesional administration.[88] Of note, three of six patients were observed to have had complete tumor regression, and two additional patients obtained a partial remission.[88] Both agents have not yet been investigated in a systematic disease-site trial for bladder cancer.

Combination Regimens

Cisplatin has been combined with various drugs; the most common are doxorubicin and cyclophosphamide. In most Phase II studies, significantly higher response rates have been observed only with cisplatin and doxorubicin combinations, with or without cyclophosphamide (Table 32-5).[77,78] However, randomized Phase III trials have generally been unable to find a statistically significant prolongation in survival for such combinations compared to a single drug therapy.[82,84,89] Many Phase II studies of cisplatin plus doxorubicin have noted an increased number of complete responses, with some patients living 2 to 8 years. In a trial by the Eastern Cooperative Oncology Group,[84] 33% of 45 patients responded to cisplatin, adriamycin, and cyclophosphamide (CAP) combination compared to 17% of 48 patients given cisplatin alone. However, in another Phase III randomized trial in 46 cases, response rates were similar, 20% and 16%, respectively.[77,78] This CAP combination has also been given intra-arterially to patients with advanced local disease.[78] In contrast, the doxorubicin non-cisplatin non-methotrexate-containing regimen and the methotrexate non-cisplatin-containing regimen have generally shown no enhanced antitumor activity greater than that which could be achieved with doxorubicin or with methotrexate alone.[78]

The most efficacious new regimens combine cisplatin and methotrexate.[77,78,90,91] The European Organization for Research on Treatment of Cancer (EORTC)[90] has had the most experience, using a schedule of cisplatin, 70 mg/m² administered on day 1, and methotrexate, 40 mg/m² administered on days 8 and 15, IV, every 3 weeks. In 43 evaluable cases, 23% achieved complete and 23% partial remissions (95% confidence intervals, 31–61%).[90] Median remission duration was 54 and 24 weeks, respectively; survival had not been reached at 26 months for those achieving complete remission compared to 9 months for partial responders and stable disease cases. Toxicity was significant, with more than 50% having severe mucositis, resulting in 83% of cases never receiving the protocol as planned. Other investigators have used this two-drug combination in various schedules and dosages and have reported a significant response rate in the primary bladder lesion as well as in metastatic sites.[77,78] In a randomized trial[83] comparing the two-drug combination against cisplatin alone, the response rate was 45% in 49

TABLE 32-5. Combination Agent Trials in Previously Treated and Untreated Patients with Advanced Urothelial Tract Tumors[77,78]

Drugs	*No. of Patients*	*% Complete and Partial Remission*
Cisplatin	**320**	**30 (25–35)**
+Cyclophosphamide	113	25 (17–33)
+Doxorubicin +	142	51 (43–59)
cyclophosphamide	351	46 (41–51)
5-fluorouracil	44	44 (29–59)
5-fluorouracil + teniposide	12	58 (29–82)
+Teniposide (VM-26)	41	51 (36–67)
+Vinca + bleomycin	18	50 (24–76)
Cistaplatin + Dichloromethotrexate	49	47 (33–61)
Cisplatin + Methotrexate +	**160**	**46 (38–54)**
cyclophosphamide + doxorubicin	13	38 (17–67)
vinblastine (CMV)	**50**	**56 (42–70)**
vinblastine + doxorubicin (M-VAC)	**83**	**67 (55–76)**
Doxorubicin	**248**	**17 (12–23)**
+Cyclophosphamide +	56	23 (12–34)
5-fluorouracil	58	19 (9–29)
bleomycin	23	35 (15–55)
+5-Fluorouracil +	103	39 (29–48)
teniposide + mitomycin-C	29	48 (30–66)
+Teniposide (VM-26)	27	19 (8–36)
+Bleomycin	7	0 (0–96)
Methotrexate	**236**	**29 (23–35)**
+Cyclophosphamide + doxorubicin +	38	39 (27–52)
bleomycin + vinicristine + mitomycin-C	22	32 (13–58)
+Mitomycin-C	16	31 (9–54)
+Vinblastine	47	40 (22–55)

* Numbers in parentheses indicate range of 95% confidence limits.

cases (95% confidence intervals, 31–59%) compared with 33% in 51 cases (95% confidence intervals, 20–46%), respectively. In more than 160 patients given this two-drug combination, the response rate was 46% (95% confidence limits, 38–54%), with a 14% (95% confidence intervals, 9–19%) complete remission rate.[77,78] At this time, the cisplatin, methotrexate, vinblastine (CMV) and the methotrexate, vinblastine, Adriamycin (doxorubicin), cisplatin (M-VAC) regimens have not been evaluated against cisplatin plus methotrexate, and these three- and four-drug regimens may be no more active than the two-drug combination. Dichloromethotrexate, a drug excreted by way of the biliary system, thereby avoiding additive toxicity with cisplatin, in a weekly dosage schedule of 300 to 400 mg/m² was combined with cisplatin 50 to 70 mg/m² on days 1, 28, and thereafter every 6 weeks.[92] Remission rates were similar to those achieved with methotrexate and cisplatin combinations. This antifol analogue is potentially a useful agent in such combinations because of its mode of excretion, and future trials are planned.

Harker et al[93] using the CMV regimen (Table 32-6) achieved a 28% complete (95% confidence intervals, 16–41%) and 28% partial remission rate in 50 adequately treated patients: overall response rate was 56% ± 14%. Dose modifications were made for myelosuppression, changes in creatinine clearance, nausea and vomiting, and age. Approximately 31% of cases required a dose modification. Six patients (12%) experienced nadir sepsis, and 2 (4%) died secondary to chemotherapy. Median duration of complete remission was 9 months, with 6 patients in remission for 6 to 35 months. Median survival for complete remission was 44 weeks compared to 29 weeks for partial remission and 25 weeks for nonresponders. Four additional patients who had significant tumor regression with CMV plus irradiation had all disease surgically removed (CR_s). In 17 patients who still had an intact bladder, 11 had complete tumor regression: 6 given CMV alone and 5 given CMV plus irradiation.[94] Of these 11 patients, 10 clinical complete responses ($_cCR$) and 1 pathologic complete response ($_pCR$), 5 had no evidence of disease for 4 to 41 months.

Using the M-VAC regimen (Table 32-7), Sternberg et al[95] reported complete remission in 37% (95% confidence intervals, 21–41%). Of 92 patients entered, 83 were adequately treated and had transitional cell carcinoma: 19 with N_{3-4} M_o and 64 with M + disease. $_cCR$ was achieved in 13%, $_pCR$ in 12%, and CR_s in 12%. Median survival for the whole CR group has not yet been reached and will exceed 30 months: median survival for $_cCR$ and $_pCR$ will exceed 28 and 33 months, respectively; median survival has been reached for CR_s at 27 months. Considering only the N + cases, 53% achieved complete remission versus 33% for the M + cases. Liver and bone metastases were not as responsive as nodal, soft tissue, and pulmonary lesions. Patients who achieved a partial or minor remission survived a median of 11 months and nonresponders only 7 months. There were no 2-year survivors for partial or minor responders and nonresponders, whereas 71% of complete responders survived 2 years and 55% were projected to survive 3 years. Brain metastases have been noted in 18% of responders beginning 6 to 42 months after remission, half of whom never experienced systemic relapse. Nontransitional cell histologies (two cases) and carcinoma in situ lesions did not respond. Toxicity was moderately severe, with nadir sepsis in 20% of cases and 4% having a drug-related death. Renal toxicity greater than + 1 was noted in 31% and mucositis in 41%. Of note, in 25 patients who underwent surgical restaging, 24% were clinically understaged, confirming the inaccuracy of $_cCR$ status.

TABLE 32-6. CMV Regimen* [93]

Drugs†	*Days*		
	1	*2*	*8¶*
Cisplatin‡		100	
Vinblastine	40		40
Methotrexate§	4		4

* All doses in mg/m² with cycles repeated on day 22.

† Patients > 70 years old receive 80% of all doses; if vomiting persists to day 8, no drug is given.

‡ For each cycle adjust cisplatin to 100% for Ccr > 60 ml/min; 50% of dose for Ccr 50–60 ml/min; none for Ccr < 50 ml/min.

§ No drug for a decrease on day 8 of > 30 ml/min compared to day 1 or Ccr < 50 ml/min or Cr > 1.8 mg/dl.

¶ Major dose modifications for both drugs depending on myelosuppression.

TABLE 32-7. M-VAC Regimen* [95]

Drugs	*Days*			
	1	*2*	*15*	*22‡*
Methotrexate	30		30	30
Vinblastine		3†	3	3
Doxorubicin		30		
Cisplatin		70		

* All doses are in mg/m² and cycles are repeated every 28–32 days (see text).

† For patients having prior pelvic irradiation equivalent to > 2500 rad in 5 days, reduce the dose of doxorubicin 15 mg/m².

‡ No doses given when the WBC < 2500 cells/mm³, platelets > 100,000 cells/mm³, or mucositis present.

Although preliminary data from other M-VAC trials have found similar efficacy,[96–98] others have described significantly less responsiveness and considerably more toxicity.[99–101] In one study,[99] only three patients (15%) achieved complete remission and four (20%) had a partial response; two complete responders are alive without evidence of disease for 2 to 3.5 years. These data suggest that M-VAC may be beneficial only for low volume metastatic disease. In other trials, 1 of 12 (8%)[100] and 10 of 23 (43%)[101] patients responded. M-VAC is now being evaluated in two randomized series against methotrexate and cisplatin, each used singly; results of these Phase III studies should define more clearly the role for this regimen.

Adjuvant Neoadjuvant

Increasing efficacy of combination regimens in treatment of patients with advanced disease has led to many pilot Phase II trials employing chemotherapy adjuvantly and neoadjuvantly. Since clinically staged high-grade, high-stage (T_{3B-4}) bladder lesions are frequently (40–60%) found at radical cystectomy to have lymph node involvement ($_pN+$) and such metastases denote a poor prognosis (17%, 2-year survival, and less than 7%, 5-year survival) because of eventual tumor dissemination,[102] the rationale for systemic therapy is obvious. Additionally, if primary bladder lesions can be significantly downstaged, further therapy with irradiation or other modalities may permit surgical resection or even bladder preservation.[107–110,119,120]

While nonrandomized Phase II trials[85,86] have described significant clinical (pretherapy T versus post-therapy T stage) and, in some series, pathologic ($P < T$) downstaging with chemotherapy and radiation therapy, used singly or together, these positive results still need prospective randomized Phase III trials to confirm such efficacy. Many cooperative groups recently have undertaken such prospective studies; until results become available, investigators in this area need not feel compelled to institute adjuvant or neoadjuvant therapies because published randomized neoadjuvant and adjuvant studies,[103–105] generally with less than 50 cases in each arm, have yet to demonstrate benefit with chemotherapy.

These pilot trials, however, have delineated future difficulties in interpreting results from neoadjuvant therapy, suggesting that disease-free survival with or without bladder preservation at designated intervals may be the only appropriate end-point. Generally, significant clinical downstaging can be observed cystoscopically in 50% to 70% of cases,[85,106–110] cystoscopically in 60%, and pathologically in 30% to 40%.[106,111–115] The more noninvasive diagnostic T procedures used (CT and MRI scan, transrectal or abdominal sonography, urine cytology and flow cytometry, and transurethral resection with biopsy) in one series[106] decreased the clinical T remission rate to 24%. Using T staging by cystoscopic examination alone leads to significant clinical understaging ($T < P$), whereas noninvasive procedures can also be confusing and lead to clinical overstaging ($T > P$).[106] Most regimens seem to be ineffective against mixed histologies (transitional cell carcinoma plus squamous cell carcinoma or adenocarcinoma) and carcinoma in situ. Definitions of response and time to clinical and pathologic restaging vary, thereby leading to confusion in the interpretation of results. In some series, disappearance of a T_{3-4} lesion with persistence of carcinoma in situ has been interpreted as a complete response; in others, response is downgraded to a partial remission—yet both may be correct and simply represent different response criteria. Additionally, small lesions, T_2, may have been completely removed after an aggressive surgical transurethral resection, thereby rendering the patient disease-free (T_0) at the next cystoscopy[106,109–110]; chemotherapy, in this instance, actually was administered adjuvantly rather than neoadjuvantly since response may have been secondary to surgery alone. Aggressive surgical transurethral resection of tumor may explain the favorable reports of neoadjuvant chemotherapy for T_2 lesions. However, so-called radical transurethral resection of 5 to 7 cm lesions described by Hall et al[109,110] prior to initiating chemotherapy may be an important factor in increasing survival and in maintaining bladder preservation. Of 60 patients subjected to radical transurethral resection followed by 2 g IV of methotrexate every 3 weeks for 8 doses, 57% were tumor-free at 3 years, 12% experienced a recurrent T_{1-2} lesion, 12% had progressive disease and died, and 20% still had muscle invasive tumors. The 1-, 2-, and 3-year survival rates were 81%, 60%, and 52%, respectively, a rate believed to be similar to that of historical controls with irradiation and surgery alone; however, bladder preservation was possible. Preliminary results using cisplatin plus methotrexate suggested even better control (11 of 14 patients tumor-free), and this combination is now being evaluated in a prospective trial.[110] Thus, the benefit of complete endoscopic resection at the onset of treatment for removal of tumor bulk is difficult to ignore, and randomized phase III studies will need to stratify such patients, based on surgical resection, before randomization.

Adjuvant trials, which define more precisely tumor stage prior to chemotherapy, should require fewer patient entries because there is less need to compensate for the 30% to 50% error in clinical staging. Patient selection can be minimized but still may be a major factor in the interpretation of results, as illustrated in one series in which 475 patients were considered for therapy, 220 were entered onto the study, 180 completed radiation and radical cystectomy, and only 83 were able to be randomized to cisplatin versus no therapy. Of note, of the 43 patients randomized to cisplatin, only 9 received the planned 8 doses.[103] It is not surprising that there was no major improvement in the disease-free survival for the cisplatin-treated group.

The roles for combined cisplatin and radiation therapy for selected patients in whom medical indications precluded radical cystectomy[98,107,115] and for a sandwich technique of chemotherapy and radiation therapy are also under investigation, with interesting preliminary results.

The National Bladder Cancer Group treated patients with muscle-invading bladder cancer (clinical stages T2–T4) who were *not* candidates for cystectomy. The initial complete response rate was high (77%), however, among the 57 patients who had gross residual disease and who were evaluated cystoscopically, 23% of the completely responding tumors have recurred to date, mostly in patients with large tumors.[115] The actuarial 4-year survival rate for the entire group, whether or not they completed the planned treatment, is 35% and is significantly better for patients with clinical stage T2 tumors (64%) than those with clinical stage T3 or T4 cancers (Fig. 32-4). Jakse and colleagues[116] from Innsbruck report a similar experience in 44 patients, with a complete response rate of 75% and with local relapse in only 15% of the completely responding group. The actuarial 5-year survival for all patients in this series is 46% and is 66% for the completely responding patients. Currently, many institutions and multidisciplinary groups are using combinations of chemotherapy and radiation therapy.[119,120] both together and alone, as "upfront" or neoadjuvant treatment in patients with invasive bladder carcinoma to evaluate the possibility of selecting for treatment with bladder preservation only patients who have a complete response to this regimen following chemotherapy and 4000 cGy of irradiation, and thus who have a high probability of having had, without cystectomy, the local cure of their bladder cancer. The complete responding patients undergo consolidation with irradia-

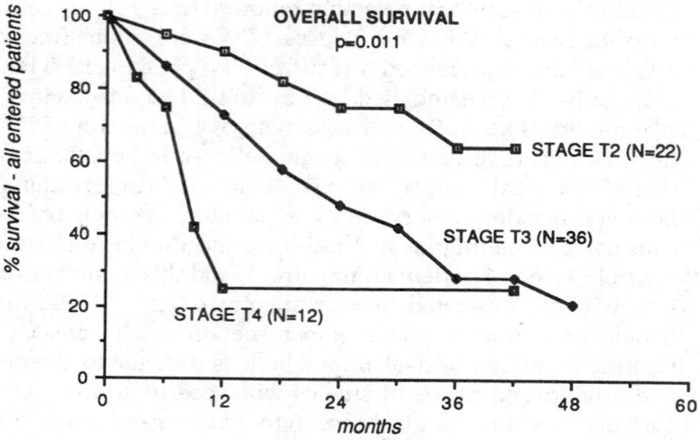

FIG. 32-4. Actuarial survival by clinical stage for all 70 patients entered on the National Bladder Cancer Group protocol of cisplatin and full-dose radiation therapy.[115]

tion to 6000 to 6500 cGy plus cisplatin. The patients whose tumors do not respond completely to chemotherapy plus 4000 cGy are recommended to undergo immediate cystectomy.

In the final analysis, however, we must await the data from investigative prospectively randomized trials before accepting adjuvant or neadjuvant treatment modalities.

FUTURE CONSIDERATIONS

Improvement in survival rates must rely on earlier detection and development of new therapeutic strategies to combat unrecognized micrometastases. Flow cytomtery holds promise as an automated technique to identify changes in DNA/RNA ratio and, when further refined, may serve an important screening function. Identification of oncogenes related to cellular transformation should open exciting new pathways for diagnosis and treatment. Although surgical extirpation has been the mainstay of treatment, therapy combining local–regional control with systemic control, with agents such as cisplatin in combination with other chemotherapeutic agents, may help to reduce the overall mortality from distant metastases and result in improved long-term disease-free survival rate. Phase III trials randomized with or without adjuvant cisplatin-and-methotrexate-containing regimens are underway to evaluate this hopeful possibility. Innovative selective bladder-sparing approaches await confirmation of efficacy by prospective multi-institutional trials.

REFERENCES

1. Silverberg E: Cancer Statistics, 1988. CA 38:14, 1988
2. Rehn L: Blasen Geschwulste Bei Fuchsin—Arbeitern. Arch Klin Chir 50:588, 1895
3. Clayson DB: Epidemiology of Bladder Cancer. In Cooper EH, Williams RE, (eds): The Biology and Clinical Management of Bladder Cancer p, 65. Oxford, England, Blackwell Scientific Publications, 1975
4. Winder EL, Goldsmith R: The Epidemiology of Bladder Cancer: The Second Look. Cancer 40:1246, 1977
5. Miller AB: Bladder Cancer—Epidemiology. In Wilkinson PM (ed): Advances in Medical Oncology, Research and Education; Vol XI, Clinical Cancer—Principal Sites II, p 201. Elmsford, New York, Pergamon Press, 1979
6. Hicks RM, Chowaniec J: Experimental induction, histology and ultrastructure of hyperplasia and neoplasia in the urinary bladder epithelium. International Review Experimental Pathology 18:199, 1978
7. Morrison AS, Buring JE: Artificial sweeteners in cancer of the lower urinary tract. N Eng J Med 302:537, 1980
8. El-Asar AA, et al: Study of the etiological factor of bilharzial bladder cancer in Egypt: Five-urinary nitrite in a rural population. Tumori 66:409, 1980
9. Collan Y, Makinen J, Heikkenen A: Histologic grading of transitional cell tumors of the bladder: Value of histologic grading (WHO) in prognosis. Eur Urol 5:311, 1979
10. Mostofi FK: Pathology in staging of bladder cancer. In Wilkinson PM (ed): Advances in Medical Oncology Research and Education, Vol XI, Clinical Cancer—Principal Site II, p 213. Elmsford, New York, Pergamon Press, 1979
11. Lerman RI, Hutter RVP, Whitmore WF Jr: Papilloma of the urinary bladder. Cancer 25:333, 1970
12. Koss LG: Mapping of the urinary bladder: Its impact on the concepts of bladder cancer. Hum Pathol 10:533, 1979
13. DeFelippo N, Fortunato R, Mellins HZ, et al: Intravenous urogram: Important adjunct for the diagnosis of bladder tumors. Br J Urol 56:502, 1984
14. Prout GR Jr, Griffin PP, Shipley WU: Bladder carcinoma as a systemic disease. Cancer 43:2532, 1979
15. Jewett HJ, Strong GH: Infiltrating carcinoma of the bladder: Relation of depth of penetration of the bladder wall to incidence of local extension in metastases. J Urol 55:366, 1946
16. Marshall VF: The relation of the preoperative estimate to the pathologic demonstration of the extent of vesical neoplasms. J Urol 68:714, 1952
17. Richie JP, Skinner DG, Kaufman JJ: Radical cystectomy for carcinoma of the bladder: 16 years of experience. J Urol 113:186, 1975
18. American Joint Committee for Cancer Staging, Beahrs OH, Myers MH (eds): Manual for Staging of Cancer, 2nd ed, p 171. Philadelphia, JB Lippincott, 1983
19. Skinner DG, Tift JP, Kaufman JJ: High-dose, short-course preoperative radiation therapy and immediate single stage radical cystectomy with pelvic node dissection in the management of bladder cancer. J Urol 127:671, 1982
20. Garnick MB, Schade D, Israel M, et al: Intravesical doxorubicin for prophylaxis in the management of recurrent superficial bladder carcinoma. J Urol 131:43, 1984
21. Soloway MS: Surgery and intravesical chemotherapy in the management of superficial bladder cancer. Semin Urol 1:23, 1983
22. Soloway MS, Murphy WM: Experimental chemotherapy of bladder cancer systemic and intravesical. Semin Oncol 6:168, 1979
23. Burnand KG, Boyd PJR, Mayo ME, et al: Single dose intravesical thiotepa as an adjuvant to cystodiathermy in the treatment of transitional cell bladder carcinoma. Br J Urol 50:237, 1978
24. Koontz WW Jr, Prout GR Jr, Smith W, et al: The use of intravesical thio-tepa in the management of non-invasive carcinoma of the bladder. J Urol 125:307, 1981
25. Hollister D, Coleman M: Hematologic effects of intravesicular thiotepa therapy for bladder cancer. JAMA 244:2065, 1980
26. Bracken RB, Johnson DE, von Eschenbach AC, et al: Role of intravesical mitomycin-C in management of superficial bladder tumors. Urology 16:11, 1980
27. Niijima T: Intravesical therapy with adriamycin and new trends in the diagnostics and therapy of superficial urinary bladder tumors. In Montedison Laekermedol AB (ed): Diagnostics and Treatment of Superficial Urinary Bladder Tumours, p 37. Stockholm, WHO Collaborating Centre for Research and Treatment of Urinary Bladder Cancer, 1979
28. Blumenreich MS, Needles B, Yagoda A, et al: Intravesical cisplatin for superficial bladder tumors. Cancer 50:863, 1982
29. Lamm DL, Thor DE, Winters WD, et al: BCG immunotherapy of bladder cancer: Inhibition of tumor recurrence and associated immune response. Cancer 48:82, 1981
30. Pinsky C, Camacho F, Kerr D, et al: Treatment of superficial bladder cancer with intravesical BCG. Proc Am Soc Clin Oncol (abstract C-223). 2:57, 1983
31. Herr HW: Carcinoma in situ of the bladder. Semin Urol 1:15–22, 1983
32. Lamm DL: Bacillus Calmette-Guerin immunotherapy for bladder cancer. J Urol 134:40, 1985
33. Brosman SA: The use of Bacillus Calmette-Guerin in the therapy of bladder carcinoma in situ. J Urol 134:36, 1985
34. Utz DC, Hanash KA, Farrow GM: The plight of the patient with carcinoma in situ of the bladder. J Urol 103:160, 1970
35. Utz DC, Farrow GM, Rife CC, et al: Carcinoma in situ of the bladder. Cancer 45:1842, 1980
36. Marshall VF, Holden J, Ma KT, et al: Survival of patients with bladder carcinoma treated by simple segmental resection. Cancer 9:568, 1956
37. Masina F: Segmental resection for tumors of the urinary bladder: Ten-year follow-up. Br J Surg 52:279, 1965
38. Miller LS, Johnson DE: Megavoltage radiation for bladder carcinoma: Alone, post-operative, or pre-operative, p 771. Seventh National Cancer Conference Proceedings, 1973
39. Boileau MA, Johnson ED, Chan RC, et al: Bladder carcinoma: Results with preoperative radiation therapy and radical cystectomy. Urology 16: 569–576, 1980
40. Shipley WU, Rose MA, Perrone TL, et al: Full-dose irradiation for patients with invasive bladder carcinoma: Clinical and histological factors prognostic of improved survival. J Urol 134:679–683, 1985
41. Timmer PR, Hartlief HA, Hoojikaas JA: Bladder cancer: Pattern of recurrence in 142 patients. Int J Radiat Oncol Biol Phys 11:899–905, 1985
42. Quilty PM, Duncan W: Primary radical radiotherapy for T3 transitional cell cancer of

the bladder: An analysis of survival and control. Int J Radiat Oncol Biol Phys 12:853–860, 1986
43. Blandy JP, Jenkins BJ, Fowler CG, et al: Radical radiotherapy and salvage cystectomy for T2 and T3 cancer of the bladder. In Smith PM, Pavone-Macaluso MM (eds): The Treatment of Advanced Bladder Cancer. New York, AR Liss (in press)
44. Bowles WT, Cordonnier JJ: Total cystectomy for carcinoma of the bladder. J Urol 90:731, 1963
45. Jewett HJ, King LR, Shelley WM: A study of 365 cases of infiltrating bladder cancer: Relation of certain pathological characteristics to prognosis after extirpation. J Urol 92:668, 1964
46. Pearse HD, Reed RR, Hodges CV: Radical cystectomy for bladder cancer. J Urol 119:216, 1978
47. Mathur VK, Krahn HP, Ramsey EW: Total cystectomy for bladder cancer. J Urol 125:784, 1981
48. Skinner DG, Lieskovsky G: Contemporary cystectomy with pelvic node dissection compared to preoperative radiation therapy plus cystectomy in management of invasive bladder cancer. J Urol 131:1069, 1984
49. Skinner DG, Lieskovsky G: Management of invasive and high-grade bladder cancer. In Skinner DG, Lieskovsky G (eds): Diagnosis and Management of Genitourinary Cancer pp 295–312. Philadelphia, WB Saunders, 1988
50. Glantz GN: Cystectomy and urinary diversion. J Urol 96:714, 1966
51. Whitmore WF Jr, Marshall VF: Radical total cystectomy for cancer of the bladder: 230 consecutive cases five years later. J Urol 87:853, 1962
52. Johnson DE, Lamy SM: Complications of a single stage radical cystectomy and ileal conduit diversion: review of 214 cases. J Urol 117:171, 1977
53. Skinner DG: Current perspectives in the management of high-grade invasive bladder cancer. Cancer 45:1866–1874, 1980
54. Whitmore WF Jr, Batata MA, Ghoneim MA, et al: Radical cystectomy with or without prior radiation in the treatment of bladder cancer. J Urol 118:184, 1977
55. Montie JE, Straffon RA, Stewart BH: Radical cystectomy without radiation therapy for carcinoma of the bladder. J Urol 131:477, 1984
56. Goffinet DR, Schneider NJ, Glatstein EJ, et al: Bladder cancer: Results of radiation therapy in 384 patients. Radiology 117:149, 1975
57. Blandy JP, England HR, Evans SJW, et al: T3 bladder cancer—the case for salvage cystectomy. Br J Urol 52:506, 1980
58. van der Werf-Messing B: Carcinoma of the urinary bladder T3 NX MO treated by preoperative radiation followed by simple cystectomy. Int J Radiat Oncol Biol Phys 8:1849–1855, 1982
59. Shipley WU, Coombs LJ, Prout GR Jr: Preoperative irradiation and radical cystectomy for invasive cancer—patterns of failure and prognostic factors associated with patient survival and disease progression. J Urol 135:222A, 1986
60. Jewett HJ, King LR, Shelley WJ: A study of 365 cases of infiltration bladder cancer: Relation of certain pathologic characteristics to prognosis after extirpation. J Urol 92:668, 1964
61. Soto EA, Friedell GH, Tiltman AJ: Bladder cancer as seen in giant histologic sections. Cancer 39:447, 1977
62. Slack NH, Prout GR Jr: The heterogeneity of invasive bladder carcinoma and different responses to treatment. J Urol 123:644, 1980
63. Heney NM, Proppe K, Prout GR Jr, et al: Invasive bladder cancer: Tumor configuration, lymphatic invasion and survival. J Urol 130:895, 1983
64. Prout GR Jr: Radiation therapy and cystectomy. Urol 23(Suppl 4):104, 1984
65. van der Werf-Messing B, Menon RS, Hop WCJ: Carcinoma of the urinary bladder category T2, T3, Nx, MO, treated by interstitial radium implant. In Smith PH, Pavone-Macaluso MM (eds): The Treatment of Advanced Bladder Cancer. New York, AR Liss, (in press)
66. van der Werf-Messing B, Menon RS, Hop WL: Cancer of the urinary bladder T2, T3 (NXMO) treated by interstitial radium implant: Second report. Int J Radiat Oncol Biol Phys 7:481–485, 1983
67. Battermann JJ, Tierie AH: Results of implantation for T1 and T2 bladder tumors. Radiother Oncol 5:85–90, 1986
68. Mazeron JJ, Marinello G, Pierquin B, et al: Treatment of bladder tumors by iridium-192 implantation: The Creteil technique. Radiother Oncol 4:111–119, 1985
69. Matsumoto L, Kakizoe T, Mikuriya S, et al: Clinical evaluation of intraoperative radiotherapy for carcinoma of the urinary bladder. Cancer 47:509–513, 1981
70. Reiner WG, Walsh PC: An anatomical approach to the surgical management of the dorsal vein and Santorini's plexus during radical retropublic surgery. J Urol 121:998, 1978
71. Walsh PC, Donker PJ: Impotence following radical prostatectomy: Insight into etiology and prevention. J Urol 128:492, 1982
72. Kock NG, Nilson AE, Nilsson LO, et al: Urinary diversion via a continent ileal reservoir: Clinical results in 12 patients. J Urol 128:469, 1982
73. Lilien OM, Camey M: 25-year experience with replacement of the human bladder (Camey procedure). J Urol 132:886, 1984
74. Rowland RG, Mitchell ME, Bihrle R, et al: Indiana continent urinary reservoir. J Urol 137:1136, 1987
75. Thuroff JW, Alken P, Riedmiller H, et al: The Mainz pouch (mixed augmentation ileum and cecum) for bladder augmentation and continent diversion. J Urol 136:17, 1986
76. Duncan W, Williams JR, et al: An analysis of the radiation related morbidity observed in a randomized trial of neutron therapy for bladder cancer. Int J Radiat Oncol Biol Phys 12:2085–2092, 1986
77. Yagoda A: Chemotherapy of urothelial tract tumors. Cancer 60:1879, 1987
78. Yagoda A: Chemotherapy for advanced bladder cancer. In Yagoda A (ed): Bladder Cancer: Future Directions for Treatment, p 87. New York, John Wiley & Sons, 1986
79. Yagoda A: Future implications of phase II chemotherapy trials in 95 patients with measurable advanced bladder cancer. Cancer Res 37:2775–2780, 1977
80. Yagoda A: Progress in treatment of advanced urothelial tract cancer tumors. J Clin Oncol 3:1448, 1985
81. Van Oosterom AT, Akaza H, Hall R, et al: Response criteria phase II/phase III invasive bladder cancer. In Denis L, Niijima A, Prout GR Jr, et al (eds): Developments in Bladder Cancer, p 301. New York, Alan R Liss, 1986
82. Soloway MS, Einstein A, Corder MP, et al: A comparison of cisplatin and the combination of cisplatin and cyclophosphamide in advanced urothelial cancer. Cancer 52:767, 1983
83. Hillcoat BL, Raghavan D: A randomized comparison of cisplatin (C) versus cisplatinum and methotrexate (C + M) in advanced bladder cancer. Proc Am Soc Clin Oncol 5(Abstr 426):110, 1986
84. Khandekar JD, Elson PJ, DeWys WD, et al: Comparative activity and toxicity of cis-diamminedichloroplatinum (DDP) and a combination of doxorubicin, cyclophosphamide, and DDP in disseminated transitional cell carcinoma of the urinary tract. J Clin Oncol 3:539, 1985
85. Ragahavan D, Pearson B, Duval P, et al: Initial intravenous cisplatin therapy: Improved management for invasive high risk bladder cancer. J Urol 133:399, 1985
86. Fagg SL, Dawson-Edwards P, Hughes MA, et al: Cis-diamminedichloroplatinum (DDP) as initial treatment of invasive bladder cancer. Br J Urol 56:296, 1984
87. Borden EC, Groveman DS, Nasu T, et al: Antiproliferative activities of interferons against human bladder carcinoma cell lines in vitro. Int J Cancer 34:359, 1984
88. Pizza G, Severni G, Menniti D, et al: Tumor regression after intralesional injection of interleukin 2 (IL-2) in bladder cancer: preliminary report. Int J Cancer 34:359, 1984
89. Al-Sarraf M, Frank J, Smith J Jr, et al: Phase II trial of cyclophosphamide, doxorubicin and cisplatin (CAP) versus amsacrine in patients with transitional cell carcinoma of the urinary bladder: A southwest oncology group study. Cancer Treat Rep 69:189, 1985
90. Stoter G, Splinter TAW, Child JA, et al: Combination chemotherapy with cisplatin and methotrexate in advanced transitional cell cancer of the bladder. J Urol 137:663, 1987
91. Carmichael J, Cornbleet MA, MacDougall RH, et al: Cis-platin and methotrexate in treatment of transitional cell carcinoma of the urinary tract. Br J Urol 57:299, 1985
92. Natale RB, Wheeler RH, Ensminger W, et al: Cisplatin and dichloromethotrexate (DCM): A pharmacologically rational combination with high activity. Proc Am Assoc Cancer Res 24:166(Abstr. 659), 1983
93. Harker WG, Meyers FJ, Freiha FS, et al: Cisplatin, methotrexate and vinblastine (CMV): An effective chemotherapy regimen for metastatic transitional cell carcinoma of the urinary tract. A Northern California oncology group study. J Clin Oncol 134:1118, 1985
94. Meyers FJ, Palmer JM, Freiha FS, et al: The fate of the bladder in patients with metastatic bladder cancer treated with cisplatin, methotrexate, and vinblastine: A Northern California Oncology group study. J Urol 134:118, 1985
95. Sternberg CN, Yagoda A, Scher HI, et al: M-VAC (methotrexate, vinblastine, adriamycin, and cisplatin) for advanced transitional cell carcinoma of the urothelium. J Urol 139:461, 1988
96. Hasun R, Pont J, Marberger M, et al: M-VAC for recurrent urothelial tumor after radical surgery. 10th International Symposium on the Chemotherapy of Bladder Cancer, Abstr 149. Vienna, Austria, February 18–21, 1987
97. Chong C, Logothetis CJ, Dexus FH, et al: M-VAC as salvage chemotherapy in transitional cell carcinoma (TCC) of the urothelium previously treated with cisplatin combination chemotherapy. Proc Am Assoc Cancer Res 28(Abstr 810):204, 1987
98. Srougi M: Estrategia de tratamento do cander de bexiga. J Brasil Urol (in press)
99. Tannock I: Chemotherapy with M-VAC at the Princess Margaret Hospital (Abstr 9). Acta Urol Ital 1(Suppl 1):7, 1987
100. Droz JP, Lupera H, Gliosen M, et al: Phase I trial of methotrexate (M), vinblastine (V), adriamycin (A), and cisplatin (C) (M-VAC regimen) in advanced stage bladder cancer (Abstr 11). Acta Urol Ital 1(Suppl 1):8, 1987
101. de La Pena J, Martinez-Peneiro JM, Cisneros J, et al: M-VAC chemotherapy in disseminated bladder cancer (Abstr 10). Acta Urol Ital 1(Suppl 1):7, 1987
102. Smith JA, Whitmore WF: Regional lymph node metastases from bladder cancer. J Urol 126:591, 1981
103. Einstein A, Coombs J, Pearse H, et al: Cisplatin (CP) adjuvant therapy following pre-operative radiotherapy plus radical cystectomy (RT + RCy) for invasive bladder carcinoma: A randomized trial of the National Bladder Cancer group (NBCP). Am Urol Assoc 133(Abstr 433):222, 1985
104. de La Pena J, Martinez-Pineiro JA, Leon JJ, et al: Cisplatinum plus cystectomy vs. cystectomy alone in invasive bladder cancer: Preliminary results of a randomized multicentre study (Abstr 19). Acta Urol Ital 1(Suppl 1):10, 1987
105. Daniels JR, Skinner DG, Lieskovsky G: Chemotherapy of carcinoma of the bladder. In Skinner DG, Lieskovsky G: Diagnosis and Management of Genitourinary Cancer, pp 313–322. Philadelphia, WB Saunders, 1988
106. Scher HI, Yagoda A, Herr H, et al: Neoadjuvant M-VAC (methotrexate, vinblastine, adriamycin, and cisplatin): The effect on the primary bladder lesion. J Urol (in press)
107. Shipley WU, Coombs LJ, Einstein AB, et al: Cisplatin and full dose irradiation for patients with invasive bladder cancer: A preliminary report of tolerance and local response. J Urol 132:899, 1984
108. Jaske G, Frommhold H, Nedden DZ: Combined radiation and chemotherapy for

locally advanced transitional cell carcinoma of the urinary bladder. Cancer 52:767, 1983
109. Hall RR, Newling DWW, Ramsden PD, et al: Treatment of invasive bladder cancer by local resection and high dose methotrexate. Br J Urol 56:668, 1984
110. Hall RR: Transurethral resection and systemic chemotherapy as primary treatment for T_3 bladder cancer. In Yagoda A (ed): Bladder Cancer: Future Directions for Treatment, p 111. New York, John Wiley & Sons, 1986
111. Scher HI, Yagoda A, Herr H, et al: Neoadjuvant M-VAC (methotrexate, vinblastine, adriamycin and cisplatin) for extravesical urinary tract tumors. J Urol (in press)
112. Simon SD, Srougi M: Systemic M-VAC chemotherapy for primary treatment of locally invasive transitional cell carcinoma of the bladder (TCCB): A pilot study. Pro Am Soc Clin Oncol 5(Abstr 432):11, 1987
113. Bukowski RM, Montie JE, Lee M, et al: Neoadjuvant M-VAC with intraarterial (i.a.) cisplatin in locally advanced transitional cell carcinoma of the bladder. J Urol 137(Abstr 211):156A, 1987
114. Sabri SE, Zincke H, Keating JP, et al: Neoadjuvant chemotherapy (M-VAC) prior to cystectomy for high stage (T2-4NxMo) bladder cancer: Do local pathological findings suggest a potential for bladder salvage. J Urol 137(Abstr 212):156A, 1987
115. Shipley WU, Prout GR Jr, Einstein AB Jr, et al: Treatment of invasive bladder cancer by cisplatin and radiation in patients unsuited for surgery. JAMA 258:931–935, 1987
116. Jakse G, Frommhold H, Nedden DZ: Combined radiation and chemotherapy for locally advanced transitional cell carcinoma of the urinary bladder. Cancer 55:1659–1664, 1985
117. Batata MA, Chu FCH, Hilaris BS, et al: Preoperative whole pelvis versus through pelvis irradiation and cystectomy for bladder cancer. Int J Radiat Oncol Biol Phys 7:1349–1355, 1981
118. Bloom HCG, Hendry WR, Wallace DM, et al: Treatment of T3 Bladder Cancer: A controlled trial of preoperative radiotherapy and radical cystectomy versus radical radiotherapy, 2nd report and review. Br J Urol 54:136, 1982
119. Prout GR Jr, Kaufman SD, Shipley WU, et al: Combined therapy in the treatment of patients with muscle-invading bladder cancer: A preliminary report of a bladder-sparing effort. J Urol 139:268A, 1988
120. Wajsman Z, Klimberg IW, Parsons JJ, et al: Bladder sparing treatment for muscle invasive transitional cell carcinoma: Cystemic chemotherapy followed by radiation therapy with adjunctive cysplatin. J Urol 139:268A, 1988

CARLOS A. PEREZ
WILLIAM R. FAIR
DANIEL C. IHDE

CHAPTER 33 *Carcinoma of the Prostate*

Adenocarcinoma of the prostate is a common tumor in man. In 1987 it was estimated that in the United States 90,000 new cases were clinically diagnosed and 26,000 patients died of the disease.[1]

The prostatic cell is the target for many hormonal and chemical substances that control the gland's proliferative rate and biologic behavior[2]; this influence stems from organs as close as the testicle or the adrenal cortex and as far away as the pituitary and the hypothalamus.[3] Recently tissue- and tumor-specific antigens and associated antigens have been identified in several animal tumor systems.[4,5]

The role of the prostate in causing bladder outlet obstruction was first defined by Ferri of Naples in 1530.[6] The earliest anatomical illustration depicting the prostate was published in the Tabulae Anatomicae by Vesalius in 1538. The first known reference to a prostatic tumor causing obstruction of the bladder neck was by Riolan in 1649,[7] but the earliest specific reference to carcinoma of the prostate was made by Baillie in 1794.[8]

In 1786 John Hunter, the great English anatomist, demonstrated that removing the testicles from young male animals prevented the growth of the prostate; in a mature animal orchiectomy was followed by prostatic atrophy.[9] Some 150 years later Huggins and Hodge demonstrated that regression of carcinoma of the prostate could be induced by endocrine manipulation.

EPIDEMIOLOGY AND GENETICS

The annual incidence of prostatic cancer in the United States is approximately 58 per 100,000 white men and 95 per 100,000 black men. Although some reports indicate that the incidence of prostatic cancer is rising,[10] the overall incidence from 1940 to 1980 remained unchanged. The 5-year survival rate in white men increased to 63% for those diagnosed between 1970 and 1973, compared with 50% for those diagnosed a decade earlier. For blacks, the 5-year survival rate for those diagnosed between 1970 and 1973 was 55%, a 20% increase over the survival rate for those diagnosed in the period 1960 to 1963.[11]

There is a 40-fold difference in incidence of prostatic cancer between U.S. blacks, who have one of the highest rates in the world, and residents of Japan, who have one of the lowest rates.[12] Breslow and co-workers found significant differences between the low rate of latent carcinoma in Chinese populations from Hong Kong and Singapore compared with the high rate in men in Sweden, the Federal Republic of Germany, and blacks from Jamaica; an intermediate frequency was found for Israelis and black Ugandans.[13] The prevalence of small latent carcinomas was about 12% in all areas studied, and they occurred at a constant frequency in all age groups. Support for the concept that these differences may be related to environmental factors stems from the observation that persons emigrating from low-risk countries to the United States have rates of clinical disease intermediate between those of their country of origin and the United States.[14,15]

No particular influence of urban or rural residence on the subsequent development of prostatic cancer has been demonstrated; this is inconsistent with the hypothesis that environmental factors may play a major role in causing the disease.[10,16–20] The prostate is one of the major cancer sites in man for which an association with smoking has not been demonstrated.[21] An intensive study of the incidence of prostatic cancer in Japanese men found no relationship between residence in the Hiroshima and Nagasaki areas at the time of the atomic bomb explosions and the subsequent development of prostatic carcinoma.[22] A familial association has been reported in several studies.[17,18,23,24]

Steele and co-workers identified an increased number of sexual partners and a higher occurrence of venereal disease in a patient group compared with controls, suggesting a possible viral-venereal relationship to prostatic cancer.[24] Although there is little agreement in the literature as to the possible roles of coital frequency or numbers of sexual partners, some studies confirm a higher frequency of previous venereal disease in patients with prostatic cancer.[25,26] The role of circumcision in the development of prostatic cancer was studied by Wynder et al[18] and Rotkin[27]; no significant correlations were found. Despite long debate, the role of hormones in the etiology of carcinoma of the prostate is obscure, for the following reasons: (1) prostatic cancer does not develop in eunuchs; (2) many cases of metastatic disease of the prostate appear to be hormonally dependent; and (3) latent prostatic cancer is lower than expected in cirrhotic men who have elevated blood levels of endogenous estrogens.[28,29] Despite the decrease in latent carcinoma of the prostate in patients with cirrhosis, when worldwide mortality rates for patients with cirrhosis are correlated with the rate of prostatic cancer, the presence or absence of cirrhosis appears entirely unrelated to death from prostatic cancer.[30]

Prostatic cancer and benign prostatic hyperplasia are often found concurrently in older men. Greenwald and co-workers observed 838 patients with benign prostatic hyperplasia and 802 age-matched controls for an average of 10 years and found no difference in the prevalence of prostatic cancer between the two groups[31] Armenian et al,[32] in a study of 296 patients with benign prostatic hyperplasia diagnosed either histologically or clinically and 299 age-matched controls followed up for 7 to 27 years, found the incidence of prostatic cancer to be 3.7 times higher in men with benign prostatic hyperplasia than in the controls. This issue is still unsettled.

ANATOMICAL CONSIDERATIONS

The prostate gland is a solid organ that surrounds the urethra between the base of the bladder and the urogenital diaphragm. It has a walnut-shaped, somewhat pyramidal configuration and is situated just distal to the bladder neck, its apex resting against the urogenital diaphragm (Fig. 33-1). The normal prostate has a consistency similar to that of the tip of the nose, carcinoma characteristically having a firmer consistency.[33] The normal prostate weighs about 20 g. The lateral margins of the prostate are delineated usually against the levator ani muscles forming the lateral prostatic sulci. Often there is a midline furrow that demarcates the left and right lobes of the prostate. These anatomical structures may be lost when there is extensive involvement of the gland by tumor or periprostatic extension. The prostate consists of fibrous acinar, glandular, muscular, and vascular elements.

Anteriorly the prostate is attached to the pubic symphysis by the puboprostatic ligaments; posteriorly it is separated from the rectum by Denonvilliers' fascia. In the fetus the peritoneum of the pelvic floor extends down as a continuation of the pouch of Douglas behind the prostate gland. In later life the two layers are fused, with a potential space between them. Denonvilliers' fascia is attached above to the peritoneum and below to the urogenital diaphragm; it limits the posterior extension of prostatic carcinoma into the rectum. Attached to the posterior superior aspect of the prostate are the seminal vesicles and the vas deferens, which pierce the gland to enter the urethra at the verumontanum.

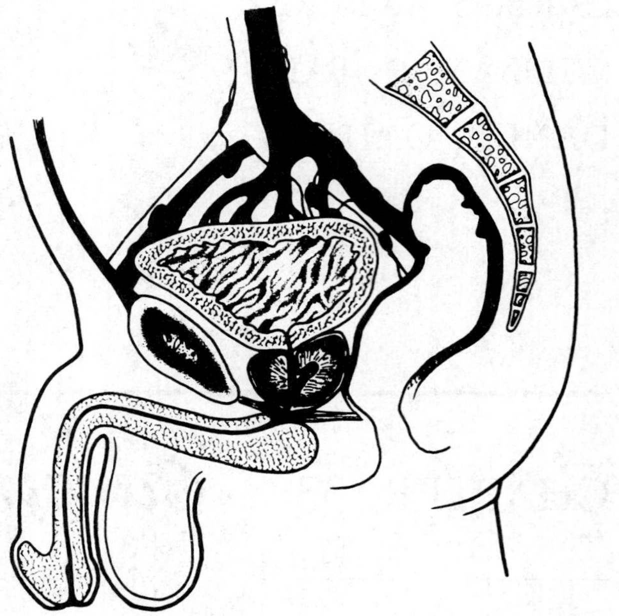

FIG. 33-1. Anatomy of male urogenital system (sagittal section).

Classically the prostate has been described as consisting of five lobes: anterior, posterior, median, and two lateral lobes. The posterior lobe extends across the entire posterior surface of the gland and is the portion of the gland felt by the examining rectal finger. McNeal, in an elegant study of the morphological anatomy of the prostate, defined four basic anatomical areas[34]:

1. The peripheral zone, constituting 70% of the glandular prostate. Almost all carcinomas of the prostate arise in this gland.
2. The central zone, constituting 25% of the glandular prostate. The central zone is markedly different histologically from the peripheral zone.
3. The preprostatic region, the urethral segment proximal to the verumontanum. The preprostatic region is the exclusive site of benign prostatic hyperplasia.
4. The anterior fibromuscular stroma, which forms the anterior surface of the prostate.

The prostatic acini are lined with a columnar epithelium with two cell layers (basal and principal cells); the peripheral ducts are lined by a single layer of glandular epithelium that merges with the transitional epithelium of the central prostatic ducts and urethra.

NATURAL HISTORY AND ROUTES OF SPREAD

More than 95% of prostatic carcinomas arise in the glandular epithelium of the peripheral glands of the prostate,[35-37] in contrast to benign prostatic hyperplasia, which originates from the central or periurethral portions of the gland. These observations led McNeal to conclude that "evidence from volume distribution data suggests that there are not two types of prostatic carcinoma with different biologic potential, but a single species having slow growth rate with a logarithmic growth curve. The development of carcinoma in the gland follows predictable patterns, including early involvement of the capsule and perineural spaces. The later course of tumor growth is characterized by a loss of differentiation and the ability to penetrate the capsule and periurethral stroma."[35]

Breslow et al demonstrated that carcinoma is more common in the apex (caudal portion) of the prostate; 64% of 350 carcinomas were detected in a section taken 5 mm from the distal end of the prostate.[13] Thus, unless the urethra is transected distal to the prostate, the likelihood of leaving prostatic cancer behind is extremely high; this is a further argument against the common practice of leaving a "button" of distal prostate to facilitate the urethrovesical anastomosis.[35,38-40]

An increased incidence of Stage A lesions has been found in older patients.[41-44] As stated by Whitmore, "although it is reasonable to assume that the stage A prostatic lesion is the source of all clinically evident prostatic cancers, it is also apparent that most stage A tumors never become clinically manifest."[41] The clinical incidence of Stage A tumors is about half of that predicted by autopsy studies, strongly suggesting that these lesions do not become clinically manifest within the lifetime of the host.

The tumor may form one or more nodules involving one or more lobes; in 77% of pathologic specimens of radical prostatectomies resected by Jewett, multiple tumor foci were found throughout the gland.[45] Because of the peripheral location of the lesions, tumor later extends into and through the capsule of the gland, and invades periprostatic tissues. It may extend into the seminal vesicles, and later involve the bladder neck or the rectum. Tumor invasion of the perineural spaces and the lymphatics as well as the blood vessels explains the tendency of the tumor to produce lymphatic or distant metastases.

LYMPH NODE METASTASES

Depending on the extent of the tumor and the degree of differentiation, the tumor may metastasize to the regional lymphatics. Flocks et al in a study of 411 patients were among the first to correlate the size of the gland and the probability of lymphatic metastases.[46] Table 33-1 shows the relationship of clinical stage and degree of differentiation of the tumor with the frequency of nodal metastases.[47]

McLaughlin et al found that multiple lymph nodes were frequently affected in patients with well-differentiated tumors, not only those with poorly differentiated tumors.[48] The lymph nodes most commonly involved were the obturator and hypogastric, followed by the external iliac group.

The earliest lymph nodes to be involved are those in the periprostatic and obturator area (Fig. 33-2). The tumor subsequently involves the external iliac and hypogastric lymph nodes, and later the common iliac and periaortic nodes. Approximately 7% of patients have involvement of the presacral and presciatic lymph nodes (including promontorial and middle hemorrhoidal group) without evidence of metastases to the external iliac or hypogastric lymph nodes.[49]

Pistenma et al reported findings in 93 patients in whom lymphangiography and pelvic and retroperitoneal lymph node dissections were carried out.[50] Table 33-2 lists the frequency of lymph node involvement by anatomical site in these 93 patients.

Prout et al reported similar findings in 92 patients with various stages of prostatic carcinoma who underwent pelvic lymphadenectomy.[51] More patients with extracapsular extension had pelvic nodal metastases. Solitary lymph node metastases were noted in 11 of 32 patients with positive nodes. Bilateral pelvic lymph node involvement was present in 14 of 24 patients with more than one metastatic lymph node.

Prognosis is closely related to the presence or absence of lymph node metastases (Fig. 33-3).[51] Prout et al found that

TABLE 33-1. Frequency of Pelvic Node Metastasis by Histologic Grade and Clinical Stage*

	Grade			
	Well Differentiated	*Moderately Differentiated*	*Poorly Differentiated*	
Stage	*No./Total (%)*	*No./Total (%)*	*No./Total (%)*	*Total (%)*
A1	0/28	0/12	0/1	0/41
A2	0/7	5/19 (26)	3/7 (43)	8/33 (24)
B1	2/53 (4)	13/94 (14)	3/9 (33)	18/156 (12)
B2	5/27 (18)	29/106 (27)	9/21 (43)	43/154 (28)
C	5/10 (50)	18/44 (41)	13/14 (93)	36/68 (53)
Total	12/125 (10)	65/275 (24)	28/52 (54)	105/452 (23)

*Middleton RG: Value of and indications for staging pelvic lymph node dissection. Presented at the NIH Consensus Development Conference, Management of Clinically Localized Prostate Cancer, Bethesda, MD, June 15–17, 1987.

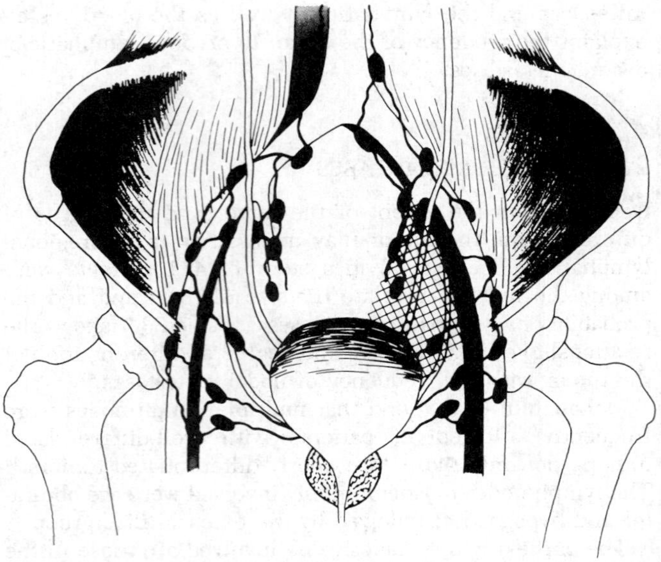

FIG. 33-2. Anatomy of prostate and lymphatic drainage. Shaded area depicts boundaries of limited staging lymphadenectomy.

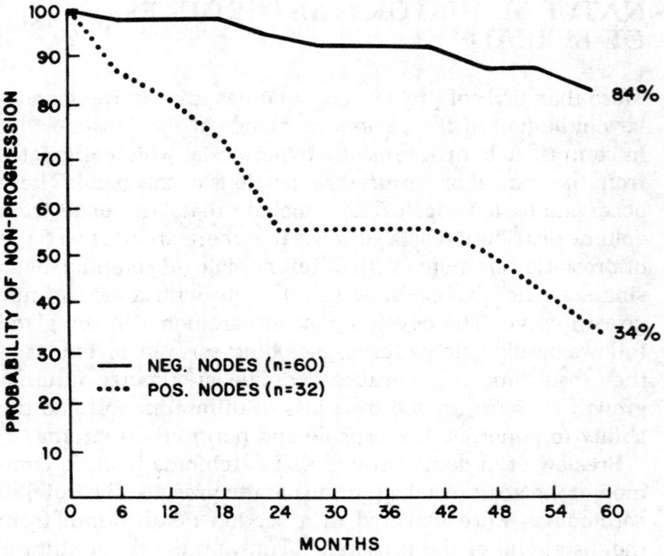

FIG. 33-3. Probability of survival without progression of clinical prostatic adenocarcinoma related to presence of pelvic lymph node metastases. (Prout GR et al: Nodal involvement as a prognostic indicator in patients with prostatic carcinoma. J Urol 124:226–231, 1980)

the presence of a single nodal metastasis was not an unfavorable prognostic sign: only 2 (18%) of 11 patients experienced tumor progression, in comparison to 16 (76%) of 21 with multiple lymph node involvement.

DISTANT METASTASES

Distant metastases usually occur to the skeleton, liver, and lungs, and less frequently to the brain or other sites. It is generally accepted that prostatic carcinoma metastasizes preferentially to the bones of the pelvis and the spine by way of the vertebral veins, a concept popularized by Batson.[52] However, Dodds et al found that the distribution of skeletal metastases is comparable in patients with prostatic or other primary tumors,[53] thus not confirming Batson's hypothesis. The preponderance of metastases to the axial skeleton and proximate long bones may be a function of regional arterial blood flow and not of any specific venous drainage.

PATHOLOGY

The most common tumor arising in the prostate is adenocarcinoma, which originates from the peripheral acinar glands. Adenocarcinomas are classified by some pathologists as well, moderately, and poorly differentiated, according to cellular characteristics, nuclear content, number of nuclei, pleomorphism, invasion of the stroma, and so forth.

Mostofi has used the following criteria for defining the various histological grades.[54] Well-differentiated tumors form glands that may be large, intermediate, or small, and have a papillary configuration. Of the moderately differentiated tumors, only 50% to 75% form glands, and there may be a cribriform, less papillary pattern. In poorly differentiated tumors, cells are arranged in rows, columns, or sheets; 25% or less of the tumors will form glands. Poorly differentiated tumors carry a much worse prognosis than the better

TABLE 33-2. Frequency of Lymph Node Involvement by Tumor in Adenocarcinoma of the Prostate (93 Patients)*

Lymph Node Group	*No. of Patients Undergoing Biopsy*	*No. (%) with Tumor*	*% Opacified†*
Para-aortic	74	13 (18)	93
Common iliac	76	13 (17)	95
External iliac	74	16 (22)	94
Internal iliac	63	15 (24)	87
Obturator	51	16 (31)	94

*Pistenma DA, Bagshaw MA, Freiha FS: Extended-field radiation therapy for prostatic adenocarcinoma: Status report of a limited prospective trial. In Johnson DE, Samuels ML (eds): Cancer of the Genitourinary Tract, pp 229–247. New York, Raven Press, 1979.

†Refers to histologic evidence of retained contrast material within the lymph node specimen.

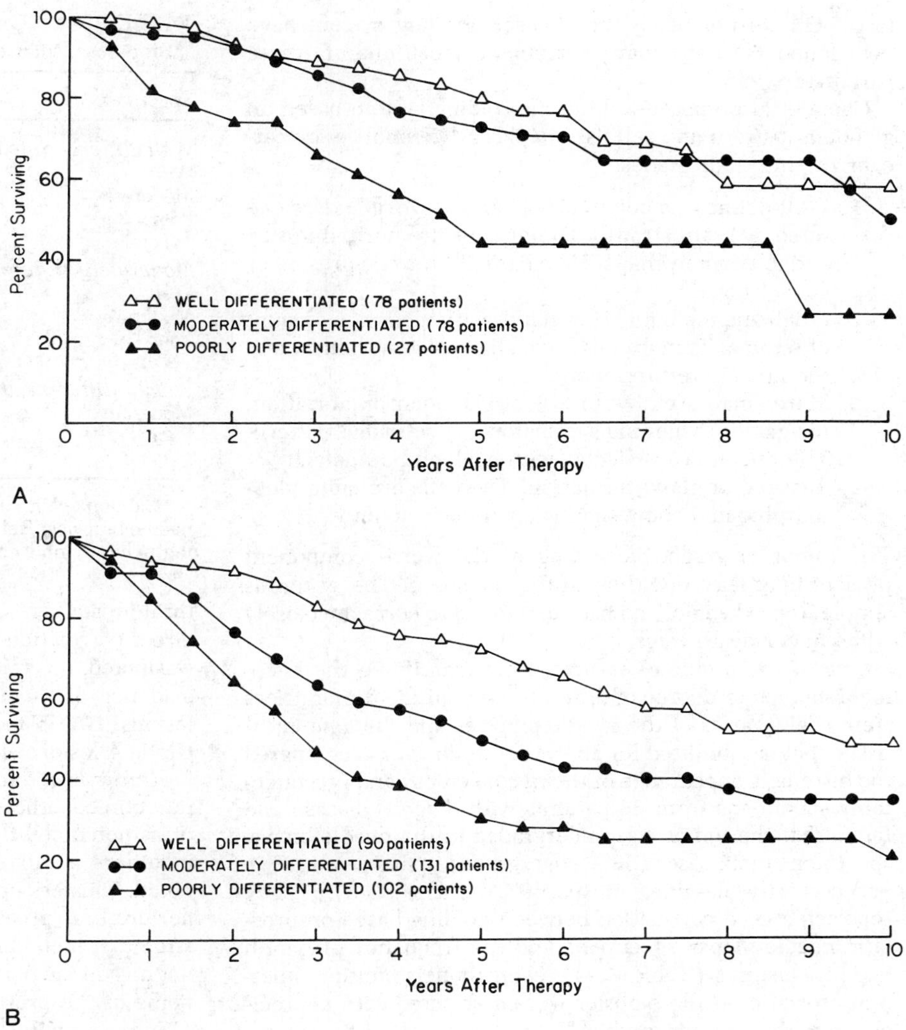

FIG. 33-4. Tumor-free survival according to histologic degree of differentiation of the tumor in patients with carcinoma of the prostate treated at Washington University from 1967 to 1983. **A**. Stage B. **B**. Stage C. (Perez CA et al: Definitive radiation therapy in carcinoma of the prostate localized to the pelvis: Experience at the Mallinckrodt Institute of Radiology. Natl Cancer Inst Monogr [in press])

differentiated lesions (Fig. 33-4). The poorer prognosis is closely related to the tendency of such tumors to metastasize to regional lymph nodes and distant sites (Fig. 33-5).[55]

Gleason and associates proposed a prognostic classification system based on the clinical stage and the degree of differentiation of primary and secondary patterns of the tumor.[56] Patients with tumors with a Gleason score of less than 5 have relatively early stage disease and well-differentiated lesions, with excellent prognosis. Patients with scores of 6 through 10 usually have Stage B or C tumors, with moderate differentiation and an intermediate prognosis. Scores higher than 10 in general correspond to anaplastic lesions and are associated with a poor prognosis. As Gleason pointed out, the degree of histologic differentiation of prostatic adenocarcinoma is the simplest, strongest, and most readily available measure of the biologic malignancy of this tumor.[57]

Paulson and the Uro-Oncology Research Group[58] and Kramer et al[59] have concluded that the Gleason grade of prostatic carcinoma as determined from needle biopsy specimens is an accurate predictor of pelvic lymph node metas-

FIG. 33-5. Anatomical sites of failure in patients with carcinoma of the prostate according to pathologic degree of tumor differentiation (1967–1983). (Perez CA et al: Definitive radiation therapy in carcinoma of the prostate localized to the pelvis: Experience at the Mallinckrodt Institute of Radiology. Natl Cancer Inst Monogr [in press])

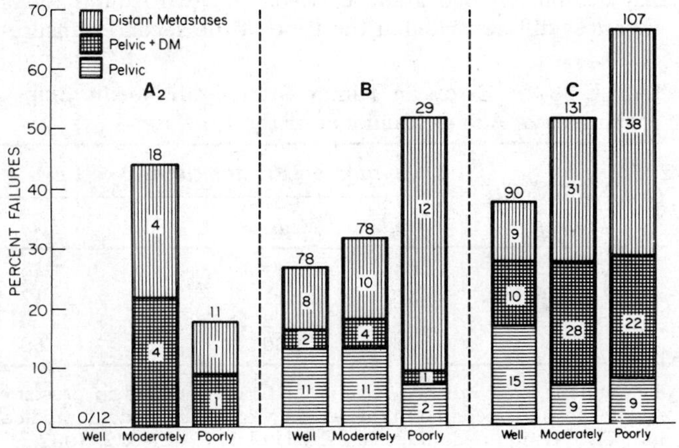

tases. Others not using the Gleason grading system have not found a particularly strong correlation of these parameters.[51,60]

Gaeta et al proposed a different grading system based on glandular pattern and cellular anaplasia.[61] Tumors were categorized into four grades:

1. Well-defined, medium-sized, and large glands separated by scant stroma. Tumor cells are normal in size and uniform in shape. No clear light may be present or conspicuous.
2. Small and medium-sized glands with moderate amount of stroma. Tumor cells have slight pleomorphism and the nuclei are prominent.
3. More small ascini with loss of glandular organization, the glands exhibiting a cribriform or scirrhous pattern. The nuclei are vesicular with acidophilic nuclei.
4. Absence of gland formation. The cells are quite pleomorphic and show significant mitotic activity.

The tumor is graded according to the worse component present in at least one third of the specimen. The system is simple, reproducible, and has been found to correlate closely with cancer death rates.

One of the problems in accurately identifying the histologic subtype or degree of differentiation of the tumor arises from the vagaries of the needle biopsies and the amount of tissue that is submitted for analysis. Catalona et al compared the histologic appearance of the needle biopsy and prostatectomy specimens from 66 patients with Stage B disease and found that the tumor was undergraded in the needle biopsy specimens in 22 cases (33%), overgraded in five cases (8%), and correctly classified in 39 (59%) (Table 33-3).[62] They reported a good correlation between grading based on prostatic needle biopsy specimens and the frequency of lymph node metastases (Table 33-4), even though multiple bilateral prostatic needle biopsies were associated with appreciable errors in tumor grading.

Brawn reported on 54 patients with prostatic carcinoma who underwent two transurethral resections of the prostate separated by 3 to 11 years.[63] He observed significant dedifferentiation of the tumors, going into higher grades, in 19 (73%) of 26 initially Grade 1 tumors, 9 (75%) of 12 Grade 2 tumors, and 7 (88%) of 8 Grade 3 tumors. Even the tumors that did not change grade between the two examinations were less differentiated at the time of the second transurethral prostatic resection when compared with the first one. A direct correlation between dedifferentiation and metastases was noted: no Grade 1 lesions in the second analysis showed evidence of metastases, whereas 4 (19%) of 21 Grade 2 lesions, 10 (55%) of 18 Grade 3 lesions, and 28 (80%) of 35 Grade 4 lesions showed evidence of metastases at the time.

TABLE 33-3. Errors in Tumor Grading on Needle Biopsy Specimens of Adenocarcinoma of the Prostate*

Grade on Needle Biopsy	Grade on Prostatectomy Specimen: Well	Moderate	Poor	Totals
Well	21	17	2	40
Moderate	3	11	3	17
Poor	0	2	7	9
Total	24	30	12	66

*Catalona WJ, Stein AJ, Fair WR: Grading errors in prostatic needle biopsies: Relation to the accuracy of tumor grade in predicting pelvic lymph node metastases. J Urol 127:919–922, 1982.

Well, poor, and moderate refer to degree of tumor differentiation.

TABLE 33-4. Grading Errors in Prostatic Needle Biopsies: Relation to Lymph Node Metastases*

Specimen	*Positive Nodes/Total*	*%*
Well differentiated on needle biopsy, 40 cases		
Well	0/21	0
Moderate	1/17	6
Poor	0/2	0
Total	1/40	3
Moderately differentiated on needle biopsy, 17 cases		
Well	1/3	33
Moderate	4/11	36
Poor	1/3	33
Total	6/17	35
Poorly differentiated on needle biopsy, 9 cases		
Moderate	0/2	0
Poor	5/7	71
Total	5/9	56

*Catalona WJ, Stein AJ, Fair WR: Grading errors in prostatic needle biopsies: Relation to the accuracy of tumor grade in predicting pelvic lymph node metastases. J Urol 127:919–922, 1982.

Periurethral duct carcinoma has been described as a separate clinicopathologic entity.[64–69] Histologic sections show a transitional cell type of carcinoma in most instances, while in others a mixture of glandular and transitional cells is noted. Clusters of large anaplastic tumor cells often fill the periurethral prostatic ducts and spread into the prostatic stroma. A high number of mitoses is seen.[70] This tumor does not invade the perineural spaces as commonly as adenocarcinoma of the prostate for localized tumors.

Some authors believe periurethral duct carcinomas are relatively benign,[71] yet most reports indicate aggressive behavior, with invasion of the prostatic stroma and the bladder neck and metastases to the lymph nodes, bone, and lung. In most series the majority of patients died of the tumor within 4 years.[68,72]

The treatment of choice is radical cystoprostatectomy.[73] Kopelson et al reported a good prognosis in patients with early stage disease; however, in patients with Stage C disease the 5-year survival rate was only 34.5%.[69] It is important to recognize this tumor, since it is not hormonally responsive but is moderately sensitive to radiation therapy. Kopelson et al reported a 76% local tumor control and a 58% 5-year survival rate in patients treated with irradiation, in contrast to 14% local tumor control and 24% 5-year survival rate in patients not receiving this treatment.

Another rare type of epithelial tumor in the prostate is the *adenoid cystic carcinoma* (representing less than 0.01% of all tumors of the prostate). Its histologic appearance is similar to that of the salivary gland counterpart, with a cribriform pattern and cystic structures associated with gland formation.

Endometrioid tumors occasionally arise from the verumontanum. These tumors may have an exophytic configuration in the prostatic urethra or may infiltrate the adjacent tissues. Endometrial glands and cells with numerous mitotic figures may be seen. Melicow and Pachter postulated that this tumor originates in müllerian duct tissue of the prostatic utricle.[74]

Carcinosarcoma of the prostate represents 0.1% of prostatic neoplasias. As in the endometrial counterpart, there is a mixed pattern of adenocarcinoma invading the stroma and sarcomatous elements. Smooth or striated muscle, fibroblasts, or other mesenchymal malignant cells may be identified.

Sarcomas constitute about 0.1% of all primary neoplasias of the prostate gland[70] and may be characterized histologically as leiomyosarcoma, rhabdomyosarcoma, or fibrosarcoma. These tumors have the propensity to develop early lymphatic and vascular invasion with widespread regional lymphatic and distant metastases.

Primary *malignant lymphomas* of the prostate are rare. The tumors may be of the lymphocytic, histiocytic, or mixed cell type.[75] These tumors behave similarly to extranodal malignant lymphomas in other sites and should be treated accordingly.

CLINICAL FEATURES

SYMPTOMS

Patients with localized prostatic carcinoma frequently are asymptomatic and the diagnosis is suspected during a routine rectal examination. Patients with Stage A disease may have symptoms of bladder outlet obstruction and rectal findings compatible with benign prostatic hyperplasia. Larger tumors may produce symptoms of urethral obstruction with resulting frequency, nocturia, hesitancy, and narrow stream. Occasional patients have severe irritative bladder symptoms in the absence of clinical evidence of infection. Isolated hematuria or hematospermia is rare.

In advanced disease the majority of patients present with symptoms of bony metastases manifested by back pain or stiffness; occasionally the disease is erroneously treated as degenerative arthritis. Pathologic fractures are occasionally seen, with lytic metastases in the subtrochanteric areas of the femur.

SCREENING STUDIES

Mass screening for prostate cancer is somewhat difficult, because rectal examination still remains the most effective means of detecting early carcinoma of the prostate, other tests not being particularly sensitive or specific for this malignancy.[76,77] The efficacy of a screening test is a function of three factors: (1) the sensitivity of the test, (*i.e.*, the proportion of true positive tests), (2) the specificity of the test (*i.e.*, the proportion of true negative tests), and (3) the prevalence of prostatic carcinoma in the population being screened. Digital rectal examination has about 80% sensitivity and 50% specificity. Radioimmunoassays for prostatic acid phosphatase (PAP) have a sensitivity of only 10% and a specificity of 90% for tumors.

Recently, clinical application of prostate-specific antigen (PSA) has come under investigation. This antigen, initially identified and purified by Wang et al in 1979 from prostatic tissue,[78] is a protein with a molecular weight of 33,000 in about 7% carbohydrate. PSA is detected not only in prostatic tissue (normal, benign hyperplasia, malignant tumors) and seminal fluid but also in the sera of patients with prostatic cancer. PSA is localized within the cytoplasm ductal epithelial cells and in secretory materials in ductal lamina.[79,80] Seamonds et al reported a specificity of PSA assay of 95% in 40 patients with newly diagnosed carcinomas of the prostate and 97.1% in 35 patients with recurrent tumors.[81] The corresponding values for PAP were 24 of 40 (60%) and 23 of 35 (65.7%), respectively. The overall sensitivity of PSA was 96% compared with 62.7% for PAP. The specificity of PSA and PAP assays is comparable in their experience (96.8% and 98.9%, respectively). Seamonds et al believe that the PSA assay is more sensitive for monitoring therapy, since the PSA titer usually rises before the PAP level and always precedes clinical signs of relapse. Although there may be some false positive tests, since PSA titers may be elevated more frequently than PAP levels in selected patients with benign prostatic hypertrophy or prostatitis, Seamonds et al postulate that these patients may fall into a high-risk population that may have early undetected carcinoma of the prostate or precancerous conditions, and they recommend close follow-up. The PSA titer used at our institution is 0.4 to 4 ng/ml. Elevated titers have been found to be associated with a greater probability of lymph node metastases or distant dissemination.

Recently Stamey et al reported a comparison of PSA and PAP as measured by radioimmunoassay in 2200 serum samples from 699 patients, 378 known to have prostatic carcinoma.[82] The PSA titer was elevated in 122 of 127 patients with newly diagnosed and treated prostatic carcinoma. The antigen titer increased with advancing clinical stage and was proportional to estimated volume of the tumor. On the other hand, the PAP concentration was elevated in only 57 of the patients with cancer and correlated less closely with tumor volume. However, the PSA titer was increased in 86% and the PAP concentration in 14% of the patients with benign prostatic hyperplasia. After radical prostatectomy for cancer, PSA titers routinely fell to undetectable ranges with a half-life of 2.2 days. PAP concentration, if initially elevated, fell to normal levels within 24 hours but always remained detectable. PSA but not PAP appeared to be useful in detecting residual and early recurrence of tumor and in monitoring response to radiation therapy. Stamey et al concluded that the PSA titer is more sensitive than the PAP level in the detection of prostatic carcinoma and probably will be more useful in monitoring response and recurrence after therapy. However, a caveat is that both PSA and PAP levels may be elevated in benign prostatic hyperplasia.

DIAGNOSTIC STUDIES

Rectal examination of the prostate is critical. The examination is best performed with a well-lubricated glove and with the patient standing, bent over at the waist with his elbows resting comfortably on a firm surface. The examiner notes

TABLE 33-5. Results of Screening Tests for Prostate Cancer*

Test	No. of Patients	Sensitivity	Specificity	Predictive Value: Positive Test	Predictive Value: Negative Test	Efficiency
Rectal examination	300	0.69	0.89	67	91	85
Acid phosphatase—enzyme	300	0.56	0.94	72	88	84
Acid phosphatase—RIA	100	0.20	0.85	29	78	70
Acid phosphatase—CIEP	100	0.20	0.95	56	80	78
Urine cytology before massage	202	0.17	0.98	67	80	79
Prostatic secretion cytology after massage	211	0.29	0.98	78	82	81
Urine cytology after massage	209	0.22	0.98	71	81	80
Aspiration cytology	200	0.55	0.91	65	88	83
Lactic dehydrogenase V/I ratio	132	0.47	0.82	44	83	73
Leukocyte adherence inhibition	113	0.50	0.79	43	83	72

*Guinan P, Bush I, Ray V et al: The accuracy of the rectal examination in the diagnosis of prostate carcinoma. N Engl J Med 303:499–503, 1980.

the size of the gland, its overall consistency, and the presence of any firm areas. A typical neoplastic nodule of prostatic carcinoma is extremely firm, often not elevated above the surface of the gland, but surrounded by compressible prostatic tissue. The examiner should determine whether or not the lateral sulcus is involved by the tumor and also the degree of spread superiorly. In most patients the seminal vesicles cannot be palpated as discrete structures, and the finding of a firm area extending above the prostate suggests involvement of the seminal vesicles by malignancy. After palpating the prostate the physician should always examine the posterior aspect of the rectum as well. Not all areas of induration felt on prostatic examination represent carcinoma. Other causes of induration are prostatic calculi, infections, granulomatous prostatitis, prostatic infarction, and firm nodules of benign prostatic hyperplasia. Approximately 50% of prostatic nodules found on rectal examination are confirmed to be malignant on biopsy.[83–85]

In a study by Guinan and associates,[86] the digital rectal examination had the highest overall efficacy of ten screening tests for prostatic cancer (Table 33-5).

Although the rectal examination remains the keystone for early detection, the actual diagnosis of carcinoma of the prostate can be made only with histologic or cytologic evaluation. Needle biopsy is the standard method of diagnosing this tumor in the United States. Closed needle biopsy of the prostate can be performed via either the perineal or the transrectal route. The transperineal route minimizes the risk of infection because the needle is not placed through the rectum. Proponents of the transrectal route (Fig. 33-6) believe that this approach allows the surgeon to guide the point of the biopsy needle into the suspect area more accurately.

Currently there is little enthusiasm for routine transurethral biopsy of the prostate. Although by definition, this is the only method of diagnosing Stage A cancer of the prostate, it is of no value in determining the nature of a solitary nodule felt on rectal examination and may miss even larger tumors that have not extended to the periurethral area.

In Europe and especially Scandinavia, aspiration biopsy has been utilized for many years with impressive results; it is a relatively simple procedure and permits the physician to make the diagnosis in an outpatient procedure with a minimum of expense and patient morbidity. The most commonly used instrument is the needle described by Franzen et al,[87] which is guided by the rectal examining finger to the nodule; an aspirate is obtained directly from the suspect area. No anesthesia is required. With sufficient experience in obtaining a specimen and interpreting the cytology, the results of cytologic aspiration compare favorably with histologic results in material obtained by needle biopsy. With adequate examiner skills, unsatisfactory cell samples resulting from faulty biopsy technique are found in fewer than 1% of all specimens.[88,89] False negative diagnoses range from less than 5% to 30%. False positive diagnoses are relatively rare,

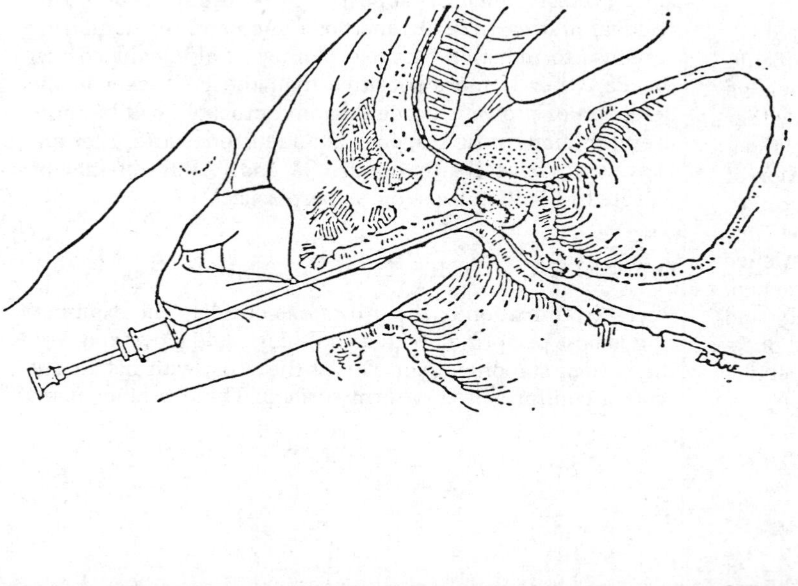

FIG. 33-6. Transrectal needle biopsy of the prostate.

TABLE 33-6. Transrectal Aspiration Biopsy for Clinical Staging and Cytologic Grade in Carcinoma of the Prostate*

Cytologic Grade	*No. of Patients*	*Stage (%)*		
		B	*C*	*D*
High	131	62 (47.3)	56 (42.8)	13 (9.9)
Moderate	265	65 (24.5)	172 (64.9)	28 (10.6)
Poor	73	7 (9.6)	42 (57.5)	24 (32.9)
Total	469	134 (28.6)	270 (57.5)	65 (13.9)

*Esposti PL: Cytologic malignancy grading of prostatic carcinoma by transrectal aspiration biopsy. Scand J Urol Nephrol 5:199–209, 1971.

but granulomatous prostatitis or aspiration of cells from the seminal vesicle can confuse the cytopathologist.

Esposti found a significant correlation between the cytologic grade of the specimen and the clinical stage of disease (Table 33-6).[90]

STANDARD WORKUP

The standard tests currently required in the evaluation of patients with prostatic carcinoma are listed below.

Standard Workup for Prostatic Carcinoma

- Physical examination
- Rectal examination
- Serum acid phosphatase
- Serum alkaline phosphatase
- Prostate-specific antigen (PSA)
- Chest radiograph
- Radioisotope bone scan
- Needle biopsy (or TURP)

Other Tests as Indicated

- Pelvic CT
- Ultrasonography
- Bipedal lymphangiography
- Pelvic lymphadenectomy
- Radiographic bone survey

The value of serum acid phosphatase in the detection or staging of prostatic cancer is limited.[91-93] Neither radioimmunoassay nor conventional enzymatic methods are accurate enough to use as routine screening tests for the detection of carcinoma of the prostate.[92,93] In patients with surgical Stage D disease the acid phosphatase level may be in the normal range.[94] There is little evidence to warrant the routine use of bone marrow acid phosphatase assays in staging carcinoma of the prostate.[95]

In a large-scale study conducted by the Uro-Oncology Research Group (UROG), 509 men with newly diagnosed prostatic adenocarcinoma were assigned a preliminary clinical stage based on the results of physical examination, routine bone survey, and serum phosphatase levels.[96] Patients underwent, in sequence, a radioisotope bone scan, lymphangiography, and a staging pelvic lymph node dissection before being assigned a final clinical stage. Technetium-99 medronate bone scanning demonstrated bony metastases in approximately 25% of all patients judged free of disease from a routine bone survey, the incidence being related to the stage of the disease (Table 33-7). Lund et al[97] and Merrick et al[98] have stressed the value of bone scanning in the staging of patients with clinically localized carcinoma of the prostate in whom radiation therapy or a surgical procedure is planned. Abnormalities in the bone scan coupled with elevation of either the PAP level or PSA titer are strongly suggestive of clinically inapparent metastatic disease. Merrick et al noted that repeated follow-up bone scans may be of value in detecting post-treatment metastases, since patients with normal bone scans will live longer than those with abnormal scans.[98] However, from a clinical standpoint, this procedure in follow-up is of questionable value since treatment of symptomatic bone metastases may not be justifiable. Of course, bone scans will be of substantial diagnostic help in patients with bone pain and normal radiographs. Roentgenograms may sometimes be necessary to better evaluate areas of increased uptake on the radioisotope bone scan, but routine radiographic bone surveys are of little value and add unnecessary expense to the evaluation of the patient, even though occasionally a lesion seen on radiographs may not appear on the bone scan.[99]

Lymphangiography has shown an overall accuracy of 75% in several studies.[100,101] Pistenma et al described a true negative rate of 88% (52/59) but a true positive rate of only 50% (15/30).[101] The lymphangiogram cannot demonstrate microscopic metastases, or lymph nodes that are totally replaced by metastatic tumor. On bipedal lymphangiography the internal iliac and obturator nodes, frequently involved in early nodal tumor extension, do not opacify. This accounts

TABLE 33-7. Adenocarcinoma of the Prostate: Incidence of Positive Bone Scans as a Function of Preliminary Clinical Stage*

Preliminary Stage	*No. of Patients*	*Bone Scan Positive, No. (%)*
IA	31	3 (10)
IB	51	4 (8)
II	101	20 (20)
III	79	19 (24)
IVA	94	33 (35)
IVC	69	65 (94)

*Paulson DF, Uro-Oncology Research Group: The impact of current staging procedures in assessing disease extent of prostatic adenocarcinoma. J Urol 121:300–302, 1979.

TABLE 33-8. Adenocarcinoma of the Prostate: Impact of Radioisotope Bone Scan and Staging Pelvic Node Dissection on Change in Assigned Clinical Stage*

		Final Stage													
	No. of														
Preliminary	*Patients*	*IA*		*IB*		*II*		*III*		*IVA*		*IVB*		*IVC*	
Stage	*(N = 452)*	No.	(%)	No.	(%)	No.	(%)	No.	(%)	No.	(%)	No.	(%)	No.	(%)
IA	70	67	(95)	1										2	
IB	41	1		22	(53)	4		1		1		10	(24)	2	(5)
II	83	1		1		45	(54)	5		6		17	(20)	8	(10)
III	73	0		0		0		42	(57)	4		12	(16)	15	(20)
IVA	82	3		1		1		6		22	(26)	14	(16)	35	(42)
IVC	103	0		0		0		0		0		0		103	

* Paulson DF, Uro-Oncology Research Group: The impact of current staging procedures in assessing disease extent of prostatic adenocarcinoma. J Urol 121:300–302, 1979.

for the relatively high incidence—22% to 40%—of false negative results with routine lymphangiography.[60,96,100,102]

Computed tomography (CT) also has problems in detecting positive pelvic lymph nodes in patients with cancer of the prostate. CT does not accurately demonstrate intranodal metastasis unless the nodes are enlarged more than 2 cm.[103] Large lymph nodes in a patient with prostatic cancer do not necessarily indicate metastatic tumor in the nodes, because they may be enlarged for other reasons (*e.g.*, hyperplasia). In a study by Golimbu et al, the accuracy of CT was only 70% for assessing the lymph node status and 47% for determining the tumor extent.[104]

In the UROG study, almost 50% of patients with Stages IB, II, and III disease were shifted to a more advanced disease category as a result of radioisotope bone scans and lymph node biopsy. The impact was greatest in those patients originally thought to have disease confined to the prostate (Table 33-8.)[96] Failure to determine the presence of bone or nodal extension with these studies would have resulted in inappropriate treatment selection.

Several reports have described the technique of transrectal ultrasound (US) as well as the anatomy of the prostate and preliminary US findings in benign hyperplasia or carcinoma of the prostate.[105,106] In a study of 443 men who underwent transrectal endosonography of the prostate, Rifkin found 130 pathologically proven cancers and 313 cases of benign prostatic disease.[105] Cancers were hyperechoic in 69% of cases and had poorly defined margins, whereas benign lesions were hyperechoic in only 46% of cases and tended to be more accurately measured because of their sharper borders. However, Rifkin concluded that there are no specific characteristics on transrectal US that differentiate among many cases of benign prostatic disease and malignancy, and therefore biopsy is always required.[105] Rectal US may assist in determining the location of the areas to be biopsied, and a needle inserted through the perineum or the rectum can be guided to the suspect nodule by means of US.

Chodak et al, in a prospective randomized study of transrectal US in 216 men, reported a sensitivity of 86% but a specificity of only 41%.[107] Tumors less than 1 cm in diameter were the most difficult to detect. To date, the use of transrectal US remains a controversial issue: in our experience at the Memorial Sloan-Kettering Cancer Center, only 5% of patients with positive findings on transrectal US will have carcinoma confirmed on subsequent biopsy.[108] Further evaluation of this procedure will be required before more definite conclusions can be made regarding its usefulness in the early detection of carcinoma of the prostate.

STAGING AND PROGNOSIS

LYMPHADENECTOMY

Because of increased morbidity associated with pelvic lymph node dissection extending from the common iliac artery superiorly to the genitofemoral nerve laterally and the obturator fossa medially, a number of surgeons recommend a more limited dissection.[109,110] The incidence of identified nodal spread by clinical stage is similar whether the dissection is limited or more extensive. The limited dissection outlined by Paulson et al is the procedure of choice (see Fig. 33-2).[58] Dissection is begun at the bifurcation of the common iliac vessels and carried down the medial inferior margin of the external iliac artery to the pelvic floor, medially across the pelvic floor to the inferior border of the prostate, and then superiorly along the hypogastric vessels back to the bifurcation of the common iliacs. The tissue surrounding the obturator nerve should be included in the specimen. The obturator artery and vein may be sacrificed if necessary. The UROG failed to find a single case of positive periaortic nodes among 54 patients with negative pelvic nodes,[111] confirming similar observations by Flocks et al[46] and Arduino and Glucksman.[112]

Is a staging pelvic lymphadenectomy of prognostic value in patients with prostatic cancer? The answer is clearly yes. Whitmore et al found that 40% of patients with positive lymph nodes after a pelvic lymph node dissection and ^{125}I prostate implantation had recurrent disease within 24 months.[113] Furthermore, more than 75% of the patients with positive pelvic nodes had evidence of distant metastases within 60 months after treatment. Cline and co-workers, in a series of patients treated with pelvic lymph node dissection and radical perineal prostatectomy, found that 50% of patients with positive lymph nodes had recurrent disease within 24 months after treatment.[114]

Is pelvic lymph node dissection of value in planning radiation therapy? The rationale is that if the nodes are negative, irradiation should be confined to the prostate, whereas if the nodes are positive, irradiation should be extended to pelvic and/or periaortic lymph nodes. Freiha et al have questioned whether radiation therapy can sterilize metastatic pelvic lymph nodes.[115] Paulson studied 90 patients with surgical Stage D1 carcinoma.[116] The mean time to failure was 23 months in a group of patients who received extended field radiation therapy (inverted T field extending from the diaphragm to the prostate with lateral extension to the pelvic side walls, with a total of 7000 cGy delivered to the prostate and 5000 cGy to the periaortic and pelvic nodes). The mean relapse-free survival period was 12 months in patients receiving delayed hormonal treatment ($p = 0.02$). Although radiation therapy might delay the onset of recurrent or metastatic disease, it may have little impact on prolonging overall survival in these patients.

Is pelvic node dissection curative? Controversy still exists over the curative value of pelvic lymph node dissection. Barzell et al[117] in a study of patients treated with interstitial radiation and pelvic node dissection, reported that when the total tumor volume in the lymph nodes was less than 3 cc there was some therapeutic benefit from the lymph node dissection. However, a more recent study at the same institution[118] and one by Kramer et al[119] do not confirm these findings and provide convincing evidence that in most patients, staging lymphadenectomy is not a curative procedure. In the series reported by Kramer et al, of 11 patients with Stage D1 carcinoma of the prostate who were treated with radical perineal prostatectomy plus pelvic lymph node dissection, 50% had recurrent disease within 18.3 months. In 33 other patients with Stage D1 disease who were treated with either radiation therapy or delayed hormonal therapy, the time to 50% patient failure was 19.2 months. The same authors found no notable difference between the mean time to treatment failure in 17 patients with one positive node and in 10 patients with multiple positive nodes. It appears that either surgery or radiation therapy is rarely curative in the presence of positive lymph nodes. Hence, staging lymph node dissection should be considered only if the physician has predetermined that if positive nodes are found, no attempt at curative therapy will be made.

DIGITAL EXAMINATION

Experienced digital examination of the prostate yields relatively accurate information about tumor volume. Byar and Mostofi noted that 85% of the nodules in 208 patients treated with radical prostatectomy were multifocal or extensive[2]; 17% of the patients with Stage A2 and B tumors had extracapsular tumor extension in the specimen. Jewett reported that after radical prostatectomy, 25% of patients with Stage A and B disease had seminal vesicle involvement in the operative findings.[85]

CLINICAL STAGING SYSTEMS

The American Joint Committee schema for staging carcinoma of prostate is shown in Table 33-9 and Figure

TABLE 33-9. TNM Classification—Prostate*

Primary Tumor (T)

- TX Minimum requirement to assess the primary tumor cannot be met.
- T0 No tumor present
  - T1a No palpable tumor; on histologic sections no more than three high-power fields of carcinoma found
  - T1b No palpable tumor; histologic sections revealing more than three high-power fields of prostatic carcinoma
  - T2a Palpable nodule less than 1.5 cm in diameter with compressible, normal-feeling tissue on at least three sides
  - T2b Palpable nodule more than 1.5 cm in diameter or nodule or induration in both lobes
- T3 Palpable tumor extending into or beyond the prostatic capsule
  - T3a Palpable tumor extending into the periprostatic tissues, or involving one seminal vesicle
  - T3b Palpable tumor extending into the periprostatic tissues, involving one or both seminal vesicles; tumor size more than 6 cm in diameter
- T4 Tumor fixed or involving neighboring structures

Nodal Involvement (N)

The regional nodes are those within the true pelvis; all others are distant nodes. Histologic examination is required for stages N0 through N3, except for subset "c."

- NX Minimum requirements to assess the regional nodes cannot be met.
- N0 No involvement of regional lymph nodes
- N1 Involvement of a single homolateral regional lymph node
- N2 Involvement of contralateral, bilateral, or multiple regional lymph nodes
- N3 A fixed mass present on the pelvic wall with a free space between this and the tumor

Distant Metastasis (M)

- MX Minimum requirements to assess the presence of distant metastasis cannot be met
- M0 No (known) distant metastasis
- M1 Distant metastasis present

Specify____________________

Specify sites according to the following notations:

Distant lymph nodes	LYM	Pleura	PLE
Pulmonary	PUL	Skin	SKI
Osseous	OSS	Eye	EYE
Hepatic	HEP	Other	OTH
Brain	BRA		

*Beahrs OH, Myers MH (eds): Manual for Staging Cancer, American Joint Committee on Cancer. Philadelphia, JB Lippincott, 1983.

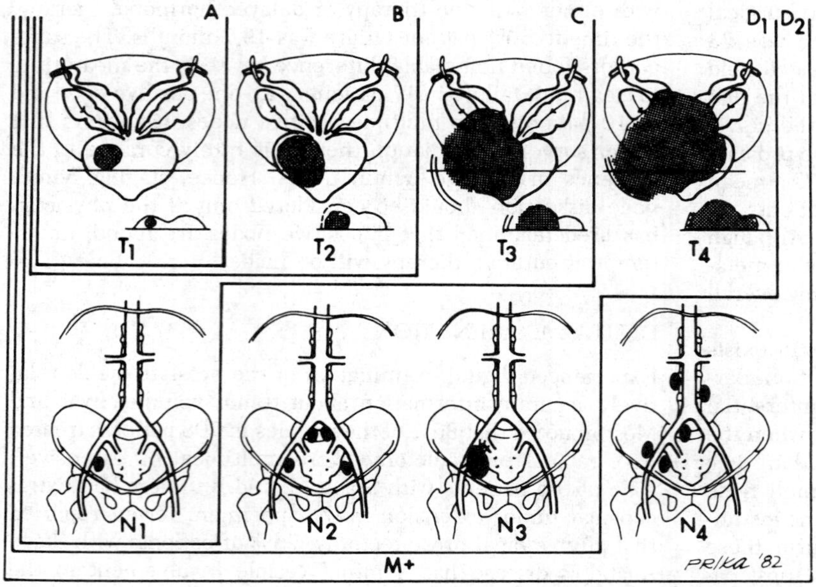

FIG. 33-7. Anatomic staging for carcinoma of the prostate. Stage groupings follow the T categories and are incorporated into the American Urologic System of Stage A1, B1, C1, D1, and D2. The AJC and UICC do not stage group. Regional nodes are N1 = T3 and D1 and juxtaregional nodes are considered metastatic; therefore, T4–N1 equivalence, same as D2. The AJC and UICC classification systems are identical. The American (Jewett-Marshall) system utilizes A, B, C, D designations that are translated to correspond to TNM categories. Modified from AJC. (Frank IN et al: Urologic and male genital cancers. In Rubin P [ed]: Clinical Oncology. American Cancer Society, 1983)

33-7.[120,121] Other systems such as the American Urological Society system are used to express the clinical extent of this tumor (Table 33-10). *Stage A1* lesions are well-differentiated local adenocarcinomas that are not clinically apparent but are found incidentally during transurethral prostatic resection or needle biopsy of the prostate.[122] *Stage A2* tumors also are not clinically apparent, but they have a more diffuse pattern or larger volume, frequently with multifocal involvement of the prostate, and are not well differentiated histologically.

McMillen and Wettlaufer[123] repeated transurethral resection 3 months after the first procedure in 27 patients with an initial diagnosis of Stage A adenocarcinoma of the prostate; 7 (26%) of the 27 patients were found to have substantial residual tumor at the time of repeat resection and were reclassified as having Stage A2 disease. Parfitt et al in similar studies found that only 7% to 9% of patients originally diagnosed as having focal carcinoma of the prostate had more extensive disease on repeat transurethral resection or radical prostatectomy.[124]

Golimbu and Morales analyzed findings in 24 patients with clinical Stage A2 tumors and concluded that such tumors are more aggressive biologically than Stage B1 lesions.[125] Review of several papers in the literature disclosed a 24% incidence of lymph node metastases in this group of patients. Bauer and associates analyzed the 10-year survival of 24 patients with clinically unsuspected prostatic carcinoma (Stages A1 and A2) and noted that 50% of those with moderately and poorly differentiated lesions (Stage A2) died of the disease.[126] Furthermore, if the lesion was diffusely infiltrating the gland, the deaths from or with cancer rose to 80%. Similar findings have been reported by Heaney et al,[127] Barnes et al,[128] and DeVere White et al.[129]

Stage B represents palpable tumor confined within the capsule of the prostate gland. It has been divided into B1, in which the nodule involves a single lobe and is less than 1.5 cm in diameter, and B2, in which there is more extensive intraglandular palpable tumor.

Stage C denotes lesions with extracapsular extension. These lesions have been subclassified as C1, when there is involvement of the periprostatic tissues, and C2, when the tumor involves the seminal vesicles. Neglia et al also include in the C2 subgroup tumors that extend into the bladder neck, rectum, or pelvic wall.[130]

Stage D tumors can be subclassified as D1 when there is metastatic disease to the regional lymph nodes or when, as

TABLE 33-10. Preliminary Stage Classification—Prostate

AUS Stage	*Stage*	*AJC-UICC Classification*	*Local Lesion*	*Prostatic Acid Phosphatase*	*Bone Metastases By Bone Roentgenogram*
A1—focal	IA	T0NxM0	Not palpable, focal	Not elevated	No
A2—diffuse	IB	T0NxM0	Not palpable, diffuse	Not elevated	No
B	II	T1T2NxM0	Confined to prostate	Not elevated	No
C	III	T3NxM0	Local extension	Not elevated	No
D1	IVA	TanyNxM0	Any	Elevated	No
D1	IVB	*TanyN1-4M0	Any	Any	No
D2	IVC	TanyNanyM1	Any	Any	Yes

*IVB patients cannot be assigned a stage classification until after node dissection as this category is reserved for patients with lymph node extension.

used by Perez et al,[131] there is extensive involvement of the bladder, rectum, or pelvic tissues extending to the pelvic wall (by clinical examination). Stage D2 denotes clinically evident metastatic carcinoma when the patient is first seen, as evidenced by abnormal radionuclide bone scans, liver and spleen scans, skeletal radiographs, or surgically proved extrapelvic soft tissue or lymph node metastases.

In general, 10% of newly diagnosed cases of prostatic adenocarcinoma belong to Stage A, 15% to 20% to Stage B, 40% to stage C, and the remaining to Stage D. The proportion of patients with Stage D2 lesions has decreased from about 40% 20 years ago to 25% at the present time, a reflection of professional and public education that has increased the awareness of the disease.

It should be kept in mind that the accuracy of clinical staging is not optimal. In 175 prostatectomy specimens thought to be clinical Stage I or II, Byar and Mostofi reported definite histologic evidence of seminal vesicle involvement in 37 (21%).[2] Furthermore, the presence of metastatic lymph nodes in the pelvis, which significantly alters the prognosis, frequently correlates with clinical stage as well as with histologic differentiation of the tumor.

PROGNOSTIC FACTORS

There is a striking correlation between clinical stage, degree of differentiation of the tumor, and biologic behavior and prognosis. Secondary prognostic factors, which are closely dependent on the former, include (1) extent (size) of the tumor within each clinical stage, (2) plasma acid phosphatase levels, (3) regional lymph node involvement by tumor, (4) findings on radionuclide bone scan, and (5) response to therapy.

McNeal noted that 80% of the tumors less than 10 mm in diameter were focal, whereas 78% of those larger than 10 mm were diffuse, and 84% of the latter had penetrated and spread outside the capsule.[35] This work was confirmed by Scott et al.[132] Byar and Mostofi have shown that the depth of penetration of the tumor in the capsule before there is periprostatic involvement has prognostic implications.[2]

Of the diagnostic tests used to determine tumor extent, the plasma acid phosphatase levels have been shown to correlate closely with tumor dissemination and prognosis,[93,94] with elevations over 25% of maximum normal values carrying a poorer prognosis.

Oesterling et al reported on 275 patients with clinically localized carcinoma of the prostate treated surgically.[133] They noted that the serum prostatic acid phosphatase and Gleason degree of tumor differentiation correlated very well with prognostic factors such as capsular penetration, seminal vesical involvement, and lymph node involvement (Fig. 33-8).

Hilaris et al[100] noted very few distant metastases in patients with Stage T1 and T2 disease and negative pelvic lymph nodes; of those with T3–T4 disease and negative nodes, about 50% have distant metastases after 5 years. Patients with positive lymph nodes, regardless of the initial stage of the primary tumor, have a 75% to 80% rate of distant metastases during the same period of observation.

The location of the metastatic lymph nodes has great prog-

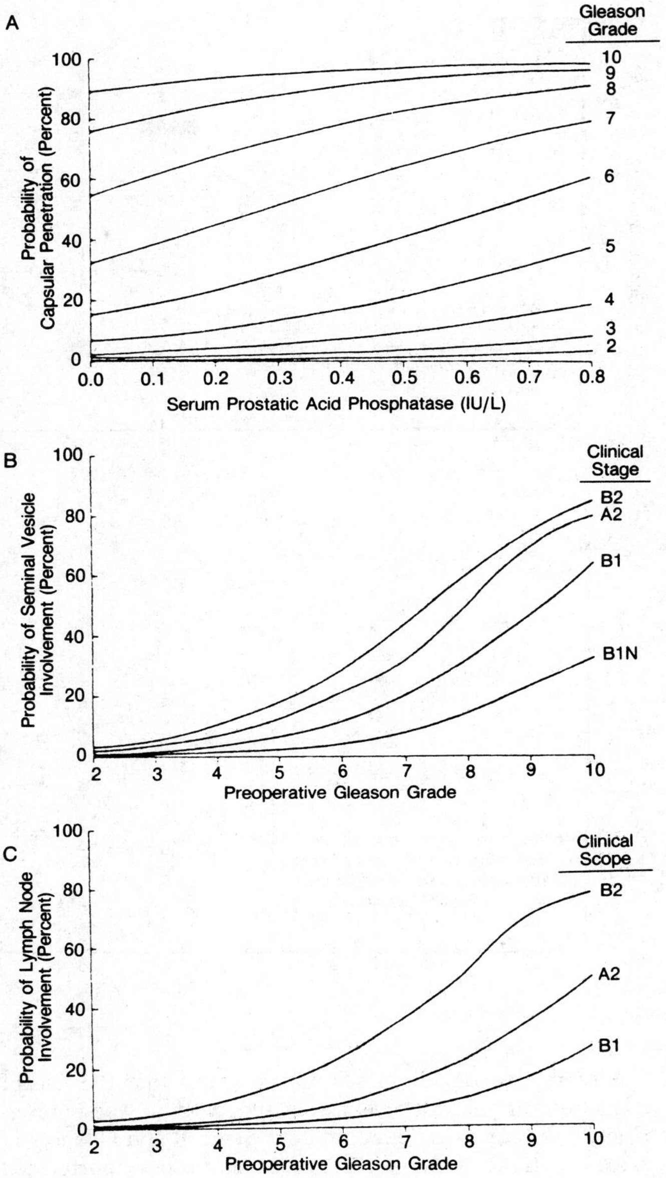

FIG. 33-8. **A**. Probability of capsular penetration as a function of serum prostatic acid phosphatase level and preoperative Gleason grade. **B**. Probability of seminal vesicle involvement as a function of preoperative Gleason grade and clinical stage. There is no curve for A1 disease because no patient in this series with that clinical stage cancer had seminal vesicle involvement. **C**. Probability of lymph node involvement as a function of preoperative Gleason grade and clinical stage. There are no curves for A1 and B1N disease because no patient with either of these clinical stages had positive lymph nodes. (Oesterling JE et al: Correlation of clinical stage, serum prostatic acid phosphatase and preoperative Gleason grade with final pathological stage in 175 patients with clinically localized adenocarcinoma of the prostate. J Urol 138:92–98, 1982)

nostic importance. Bagshaw et al reported that the disease-free survival rate in patients with negative lymph nodes was 86%, in those with positive pelvic lymph nodes it was 71%, while in those with positive periaortic lymph nodes it was only 30%.[134]

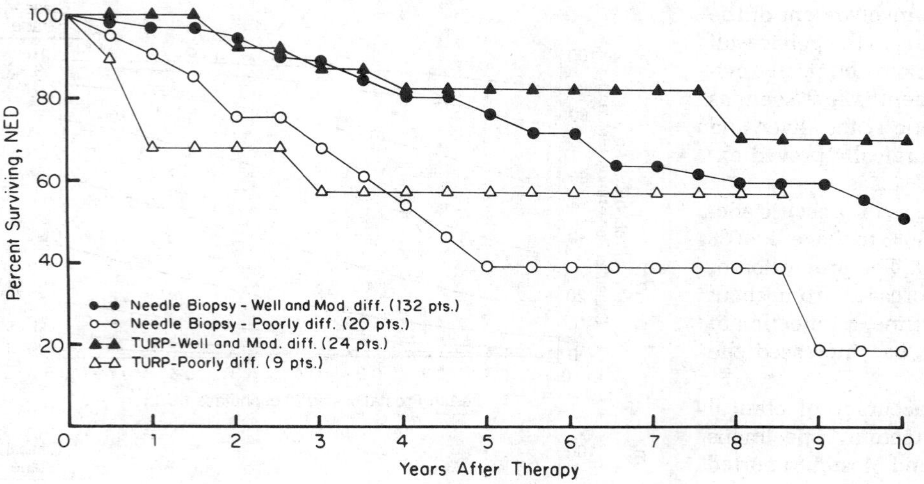

A

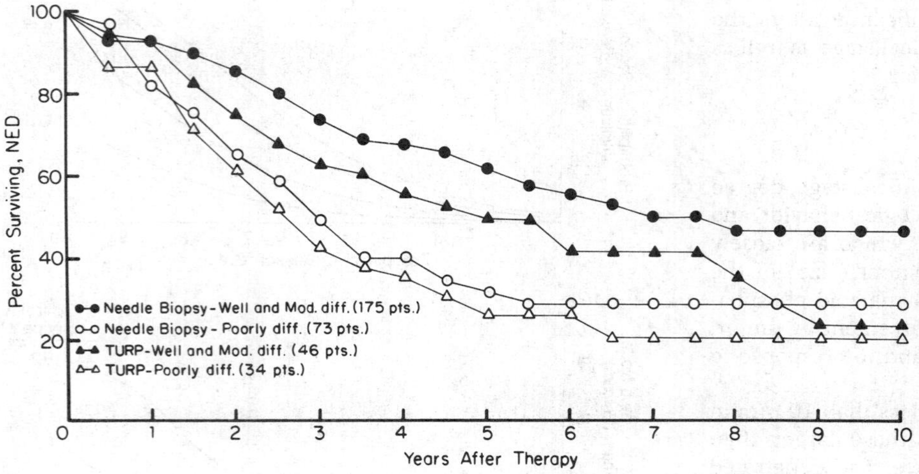

B

FIG. 33-9. NED survival of patients with carcinoma of the prostate correlated with method of diagnosis (needle biopsy or transurethral prostatic resection) and histologic grade. **A**. Stage B. **B**. Stage C. (Perez CA et al: Definitive radiation therapy in carcinoma of the prostate localized to the pelvis: Experience at the Mallinckrodt Institute of Radiology. Natl Cancer Inst Monogr [in press])

A report by McGowan strongly suggests that the use of transurethral resection is associated with a worse prognosis.[135] In our experience, in both Stage B and C, survival rates in patients in whom this procedure has been performed are comparable to survival rates in those with disease diagnosed by needle biopsy, if the patients are grouped according to tumor differentiation (Fig. 33-9). It is likely that the bulk of tumor, which presumably will be greater in patients requiring transurethral resection of the prostate because of urethral obstruction, and the lesser differentiation may account for the worse prognosis. Similar conclusions were reached by Kuban et al[136] but not by Hanks et al.[137] These observations need to be further investigated.

Hormonal Receptors

In 75% to 80% of cases, tumors of the prostate respond to hormonal therapy. Huggins et al in 1939 and subsequently others demonstrated experimentally the dependency of prostatic enlargement on circulating androgens.[138] Animal studies have confirmed the correlation between prostatic tumor growth and hormonal stimulation by androgens, and between tumor depression and androgen deprivation or estrogen administration. Huggins and Hodges in 1941 reported historical observations on the treatment of carcinoma of the prostate with hormonal manipulation.[139]

There are some technical difficulties to the characterization of hormonal receptors in human prostatic tissues,[140] which are related to the following factors:

1. The composition of the prostate, with intermixed epithelial and stromal cells; 17β-estradiol receptors are present in both epithelial and stromal tissues from normal, benign prostatic hyperplasic, and adenocarcinoma prostatic specimens.
2. Cellular heterogeneity in prostatic carcinoma.
3. Contamination of tissue with serum testosterone-estradiol binding globulin.
4. High endogenous content of dihydroxytestosterone in human prostate, with near saturation of receptor protein.
5. High content of proteolytic enzymes, difficult to homogenize, which leads to receptor inactivation.

6. The presence of a protein in cytosol of human prostate that binds with high affinity to methyltrienolone (R1881), but has the features of a progesterone receptor.

Nevertheless, Ekman et al in a study of 23 patients reported a significant correlation between the presence of steroid receptors and response to hormonal therapy.[141] Fifteen (83%) of 18 patients with "positive" receptors experienced clinical tumor regression, in contrast to only one response (20%) in 5 patients with "negative" receptors.

TREATMENT

At present, several therapeutic options are available:

1. Observation (in patients with Stage A1 disease), although Walsh[142] believes radical prostatectomy is justified in selected cases.
2. Radical prostatectomy, including the nerve-sparing operation (limited to selected patients with Stage A2 or B disease).
3. Interstitial irradiation combined with staging lymphadenectomy (for selected patients with Stage A2 or B disease).
4. External irradiation (for patients with Stage A2, B, C, or D1 disease).
5. Hormonal manipulation (for various stages).
6. Chemotherapy.

Patients with Stage A1 disease found incidentally on transurethral resection require no treatment because the disease has many years of natural evolution before it becomes a clinical problem.[143] Byar et al reported on 148 patients with Stage A focal carcinoma treated conservatively or not at all.[144] Only 6.8% of these patients experienced disease progression. A literature review disclosed a death rate of only 1.9% in 262 patients with stage A1 cancer.

Barnes and Ninan demonstrated comparable survival for patients with Stage A and B lesions treated with either radical prostatectomy or endocrine therapy.[145] On the other hand, the survivals reported by Thompson[146] from the Mayo Clinic in patients treated with transurethral resection before 1940 are well below those reported with more aggressive therapy. Hanash et al reviewed findings in 200 patients with histologically proven carcinoma of the prostate treated with only transurethral resection between 1934 and 1942 (probably the same population studied by Thompson).[44] Patients were not clinically staged. In those with clinically latent (occult) tumors, the 5-year survival rate was about 50%; the 10-year survival rate for all histologic grades was 30%. This was similar to the expected survival for a comparable normal population. In contrast, patients with clinically manifest tumors had a 5-year survival rate of 20% for those with Grade 1, 2 or 3 disease and less than 5% for those with Grade 4 disease. The 10-year survival rate was below 10% for all grades, significantly below the expected normal survival rate (about 40%). Patients with Stage A2 or B tumors may be treated with a radical prostatectomy, external irradiation, or interstitial ^{125}I implants combined with a staging pelvic lymphadenectomy.

Today many urologists agree that patients with Stage C tumors may be treated with definitive external irradiation, or in some instances palliatively with hormonal manipulation. Patients with distant metastases should be initially treated with hormonal therapy or chemotherapy; irradiation may be useful in controlling local or metastatic tumor growth.

RADICAL PROSTATECTOMY

Radical prostatectomy, initially described by Young in 1905,[147] was popularized by Jewett.[45] Radical prostatectomy is a therapeutic option only when the tumor is confined to the prostate; it has no role in the management of extracapsular disease or in the presence of positive lymph nodes. Freiha reviewed specimens obtained at autopsy or during radical prostatectomy in more than 300 patients and concluded that the largest optimal volume amenable to cure by radical prostatectomy is 1 to 4 cc (1.4-cm nodule), if capsular penetration is considered a proved prognostic sign.[148]

Radical prostatectomy should not be performed for at least 6 to 8 weeks after transurethral resection or open prostatectomy, to minimize technical difficulties. The obliteration of tissue planes during open surgery or a particularly aggressive transurethral resection may make radical prostatectomy difficult to perform, and other therapeutic modalities may have to be considered.

The anatomical location of the prostate makes successful removal of the organ technically difficult and has led to the development of several approaches for radical prostatovesiculectomy, whether by a retropubic or a perineal approach.[149–151] The procedure consists of radical in-continuity removal of the prostate and its investing capsule, together with the seminal vesicles, the ampulla, and the vas deferens (Fig. 33-10). The prostate should be completely removed by excision of the urethra at the prostatomembranous junction; no residual "button" of prostatic tissue should be left at the apex. The fascia extending between the bladder and seminal vesicles should be removed with the specimen despite the potential danger of damage to the posterior bladder wall and ureters. These two fascia layers do provide an area for containment of local tumor growth.

The vascular supply to the prostate arises from the inferior vesical artery, and both veins and arteries course together with their fascia at the vesicoprostatic junction in a posterior lateral direction. The vascular supply of the seminal vesicles also arises from the inferior vesical plexus and is routinely controlled during division and ligation of the vascular pedicles of the prostate.

Arterial bleeding during a radical prostatectomy will often cease spontaneously; however, bleeding from branches of the internal pudendal artery adjacent to the prostate may be difficult to control as these vessels retract into the fat surrounding the rectum. Venous bleeding usually causes the major blood loss during the performance of radical prostatectomy, particularly when the dorsal vein of the penis is divided as it courses under the symphysis pubis. At this point, the vein courses over the anterior surface of the prostate and forms free anastomoses with the veins from Santorini's

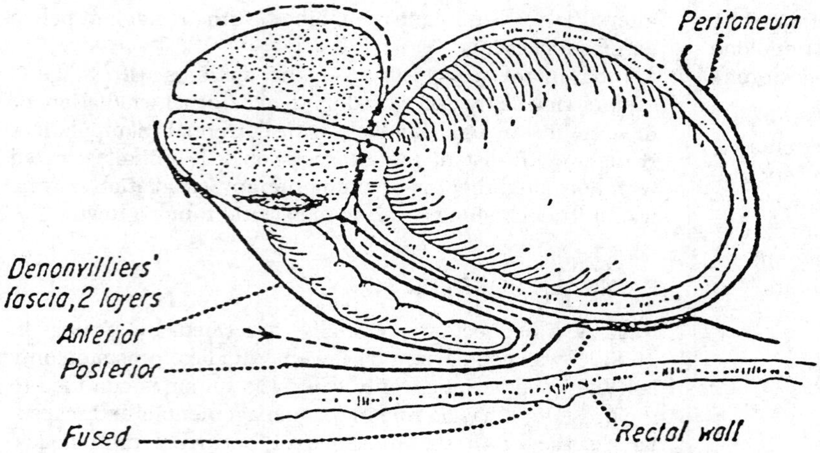

FIG. 33-10. Limits of dissection for radical prostatectomy.

plexus. Any laceration of these friable structures can lead to considerable blood loss that is often difficult to control.

The retropubic approach to radical prostatectomy is preferred by many surgeons. As a rule, urologic oncologists are more familiar with the pelvic anatomy than with the perineal approach. The retropubic prostatectomy also allows the simultaneous performance of a bilateral pelvic lymph node dissection. The use of nerve-sparing techniques to avoid impotence following radical prostatectomy[152] has led to renewed enthusiasm among surgeons for the retropubic approach.

The disadvantages of the retropubic approach to the prostate are the vascularity of the field and the difficulty in establishing a direct vesicourethral anastomosis beneath the pubis, particularly in obese patients. Removal of the pubic symphysis has been advocated. This does not decrease stability of the pelvis postsurgically, but may enhance the degree of postoperative incontinence. Additionally, a nerve-sparing prostatectomy may be more difficult to perform from the perineal approach. The primary contraindications to a surgical procedure are ankylosis of the hips and previous prostatic surgery, which may fix the prostate and bladder in the pelvis and make reconstruction of the vesicourethral junction difficult.

Perineal prostatoseminovesiculectomy has the advantage of providing a relatively avascular field for dissection, good exposure for reconstruction of the vesicourethral anastomosis, and postoperative drainage. The procedure is well tolerated by elderly patients, in whom an intra-abdominal approach may compromise pulmonary function. The principal disadvantage is that it does not afford simultaneous exposure of the pelvic lymphatic drainage and thus a second operative procedure is required.

NERVE-SPARING RADICAL RETROPUBIC PROSTATECTOMY

The successful performance of a nerve-sparing radical prostatectomy is based on attention to important recent observations concerning the prostatic and pelvic anatomy. The first of these, which described the anatomy of the dorsal vein complex and Santorini's plexus, led to modifications in the surgical procedure that reduced blood loss and improved surgical exposure, thereby facilitating the ease of identification and preservation of the nerves.[153] The second observation delineated the location of the autonomic nerves that innervate the corpora cavernosa and modified the operative approach to avoid damaging these structures, thereby retaining potency in many patients.[154] Additionally, improved visualization of the anatomy of the urethrovesical function has led to improvements in the technique of performing the anastomosis between the urethra and the bladder neck, with a resulting decrease in the frequency of postoperative incontinence.[155,156]

The improvement in the rate of impotence and incontinence associated with radical surgery for carcinoma of the prostate has led to a renewed enthusiasm for total prostatectomy to control localized prostatic cancer. The details of the operative technique should be familiar to all urologic oncologists.

The operation is best performed under regional anesthesia. An epidural anesthetic has the advantage of allowing excellent anesthetic control during the surgery, and the resulting peripheral vasodilation appears to greatly reduce blood loss during pelvic surgery. The epidural catheter also allows additional anesthetic agents to be administered in the immediate postoperative period and obviates the need for injectable narcotic medication in many patients.

Before the prostatectomy is begun, a bilateral pelvic lymph node dissection is performed. In the presence of metastatic disease in the lymph nodes, there are no data to support the position that total prostatectomy is a curative procedure, and our policy is not to proceed with the prostatectomy if positive nodes are found.

If the frozen section samples of the lymph nodes are negative for metastatic cancer, the operative procedure is carried out as described by Walsh.[157] After the endopelvic fascia has been incised bilaterally and the puboprostatic ligaments cut to allow the prostate to drop dorsally, the dorsal vein complex is ligated and divided. This maneuver allows direct visualization of the urethroprostatic junction. The neurovascular bundles run parallel and in close proximity to the prostatic capsule and the lateral walls of the proximal urethra.

An important step at this juncture is to spread the tips of

the dissecting scissors just adjacent to the lateral walls of the urethroprostatic junction. This maneuver separates the neurovascular bundles laterally from the urethra and allows passage of a right angle clamp under the urethra. This in turn makes possible the division of the urethra under direct vision and enables the surgeon to cut only the urethra and avoid transecting the neurovascular bundles at the apex of the prostate. Once the urethra is transected, the prostate is separated from the rectum in the midline. This maneuver is facilitated by upward traction on the cut end of the Foley catheter, the balloon of which is still inflated in the bladder. The surgeon can now visualize the relationship of the neurovascular bundles to the tumor and decide whether they must be excised or can be safely preserved. If the decision is made to excise the neurovascular bundle on the side of the tumor, the neurovascular bundle on the contralateral side can usually be preserved. With wide excision of the neurovascular bundle, it is now possible to obtain wider soft tissue margins than were previously attainable with standard radical prostatectomy.[158] The specific operative steps in the surgical procedure have been detailed elsewhere.[159,160]

If a bilateral nerve-sparing technique is appropriate, the lateral pelvic fascia is then divided between fine silk ligatures close to the prostatic capsule. Proceeding in a cephalad direction will bring the seminal vesicles into view, and these structures are excised in their entirety with the prostate.

The bladder neck is then transected at its junction with the prostatic urethra. In performing this maneuver it is important to define a plane between the prostate and the bladder that will allow a relatively small bladder neck opening when the junction between the prostate and bladder is cut.

To ensure coaptation of the bladder mucosa to the proximal urethra, the bladder mucosa is exteriorized by a series of 0000 chromic catgut sutures everting the mucosa over the cut bladder neck. The anastomosis between the bladder and urethra is also done under direct vision using five or six 00 chromic catgut sutures. A Foley catheter is left in place for 3 weeks before removal.

PRESERVATION OF SEXUAL FUNCTION. Walsh recently described the results in 320 men who had undergone a nerve-sparing prostatectomy and were followed up for 1 year or longer.[158] Of the 320 men, 259 were potent preoperatively and had sexual partners. Postoperatively, 192 (74%) were potent.

Potency, which was defined as the ability to achieve an erection sufficient for vaginal penetration and orgasm, returned gradually over the first 2 years following surgery. Potency correlated with both the age of the patient and the stage of the disease (Table 33-11). Thus, potency returned in 93% of patients with Stage A1 disease, 72% with Stage A2 disease, 92% with Stage B1N disease, 72% with Stage B1 disease, and 56% with Stage B2 disease. Of note, in those patients in whom it was necessary to sacrifice the neurovascular bundle on one side, 69% were potent postoperatively.[161]

Of concern has been the possibility that preservation of the neurovascular bundle might compromise the adequacy of the surgical margins obtained. In a recent analysis of 414 patients treated by Walsh and colleagues (Table 33-12), 10% of patients had disease in the surgical margin, a frequency similar to that reported with the older techniques of radical prostatectomy.[158]

IRRADIATION

Interstitial Irradiation

Starting with Pasteau in 1911,[162] radium was used in the treatment of patients with prostatic carcinoma, either by implanting needles through a perineal route or by inserting special applicators through the rectum or the prostatic urethra.[163-166] Bumpus[167] and Nitch[168] utilized rectal, urethral, or external applicators or interstitial implantation into the prostate gland through a suprapubic cystostomy; Caulk[169] combined brachytherapy with supplemental external x-ray therapy. Flocks[170] used interstitial injection of radioactive

TABLE 33-11. Influence of Age and Clinical Stage on Postoperative Potency in 320 Men Followed for at Least 1 Year

Clinical Stage	*Age (years)* 30–39	40–49	50–59	60–69	70–75	*Total*
A1		100% (2/2)	90% (9/10)	100% (3/3)		93% (14/15)
A2			90% (9/10)	57% (4/7)	0% (0/1)	72% (13/18)
B1N	100% (2/2)	80% (4/5)	97% (30/31)	92% (11/12)	0% (0/1)	92% (47/51)
B1		79% (11/14)	82% (42/51)	65% (39/60)	20% (1/5)	72% (93/130)
B2		67% (2/3)	68% (15/22)	40% (8/20)		56% (25/45)
Total	100% (2/2)	79% (19/24)	85% (105/124)	64% (65/102)	14% (1/7)	74% (192/259)

Walsh PC: Preservation of sexual function in the surgical treatment of prostatic cancer—an anatomic surgical approach. In DeVita VT Jr, Hellman S, Rosenberg SA (eds): Important Advances in Oncology 1988, p 165. Philadelphia, JB Lippincott, 1988.

TABLE 33-12. Pathologic Findings in 414 Consecutive Radical Prostatectomies (in %)

		Pathologic Findings (%)				
Clinical Stage	*No. of Patients*	*Organ Confined*	*Capsular Penetration*	*Seminal Vesicle Involvement*	*Positive Surgical Margin*	*Positive Lymph Nodes*
A1	16	94	6	0	0	0
A2	40	83	17	15	15	10
B1N	78	82	18	3	3	0
B1	196	65	35	10	9	3
B2	84	29	71	31	19	23
Total	414	64	36	13	10	7

Walsh PC: Preservation of sexual function in the surgical treatment of prostatic cancer—an anatomic surgical approach. In DeVita VT Jr, Hellman S, Rosenberg SA (eds): Important Advances in Oncology 1988, p 167. Philadelphia, JB Lippincott, 1988.

colloidal gold into the prostate gland. A local control of over 50% was achieved, with few complications.

In the early 1970s Whitmore et al popularized the retropubic implantation of ^{125}I for clinical Stage A2, B, and selected C cases.[171] A limited staging lymphadenectomy is always performed, and in general, only patients with negative lymph nodes are treated with radioactive implants. The prostate is freed from the endopelvic fascia and the puboprostatic ligament is partially sectioned for better exposure; metallic stylettes are placed in the prostate gland, about 1 cm apart, and not too close to the rectum or the bladder neck (Fig. 33-11A). ^{125}I seeds, usually 0.4 to 0.5 mCi strength, are inserted at various intervals. In general, an adequate seed implant will deliver 7000 to 8000 cGy to the tumor, with higher doses to the central portion of the gland. The rectum and bladder receive 5000 to 6000 cGy (Fig. 33-11B). Patients who have undergone a complete transurethral prostatic resection have insufficient tissue left to support the ^{125}I seeds.

Charyulu et al[172] and Syed et al[173] described a peritoneal approach with afterloading techniques for implantation of radon or ^{125}I seeds or removable ^{192}Ir implants.

Carlton et al have used radioactive gold (^{198}Au) grains combined with external irradiation in the treatment of carcinoma of the prostate.[174] After staging pelvic lymphadenectomy, gold grains are implanted into the prostate gland through a suprapubic incision to deliver 3000 to 3500 cGy, followed by external pelvic irradiation to the pelvis (approximately 4000 cGy).

External Irradiation

With the advent of megavoltage equipment, irradiation has been increasingly used for the treatment of prostatic carcinoma.[175,176] A variety of techniques have been used, varying from parallel anterioposterior (AP) ports with a perineal appositional field, to lateral ports (box technique), or rotational fields to supplement the dose to the prostate. At present, it is not known whether pelvic and periaortic lymph node irradiation may improve survival.[177,178] In patients with obstructive lower urinary tract symptoms who have undergone transurethral resection, 4 weeks should elapse before radiation therapy is initiated, in order to decrease sequelae (urinary incontinence, urethral strictures).

Hormonal manipulation concurrent with irradiation has not been shown to improve survival or tumor control.[131,166,179] Therefore, it is strongly recommended that hormonal therapy be withheld until there is evidence of tumor progression after initial therapy.

PORTALS, BEAM ENERGY, AND TUMOR DOSES. If it is decided to treat the pelvic lymph nodes, as is customarily done at Washington University, the field size for Stage A2 and B lesions is 15 × 15 cm at the patient surface (16.5 cm at isocenter). For Stages C and D1 tumors, the field size is increased to 15 × 18 cm at the patient surface (16.5 × 20.5 cm at isocenter) to cover the common iliac lymph nodes (Fig. 33-12A)

The reduced field for treatment of the prostatic volume can be about 7 × 9 cm to 10 × 12 cm, depending on the size of the gland and periprostatic extensions (Fig. 33-12B). Pilepich et al have issued practical guidelines on the size of the gland as determined by CT in 100 patients and have recommended specific landmarks for use in determining field sizes.[180]

The periaortic lymph nodes can be treated through a separate periaortic port placed above the pelvic fields, in which case an appropriate gap should be calculated. If large-field linear accelerator beams are available, it is more convenient to use a single port that includes both the pelvic and periaortic lymph nodes.

The use of high-energy photon beams (above 10 MV) will simplify the technique and decrease morbidity. Up to 5000 cGy total dose can be delivered through AP and PA ports; the additional dose is administered through rotational ports. Although anterior arc rotation has been employed, a better distribution is obtained with bilateral 120-degree arc rotations that skip the midline anteriorly and posteriorly (Fig. 33-13). With lower energy photon beams (4–10 MV), lateral ports are necessary to deliver part of the dose (box technique) (Fig. 33-14). Posterior oblique fields are occasionally used for the same purpose.

The usual dose of irradiation is 4500 to 5000 cGy to the pelvic and periaortic lymph nodes (when the latter are to be irradiated), with a boost to the prostate. The minimal total tumor dose to the prostate in Stage A2 or B tumor is 6500 cGy, and for Stage C, 7000 cGy. For Stage D1 lesions,

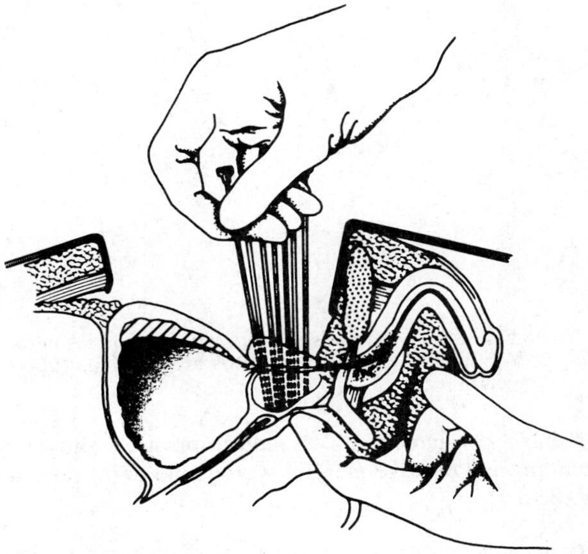

A

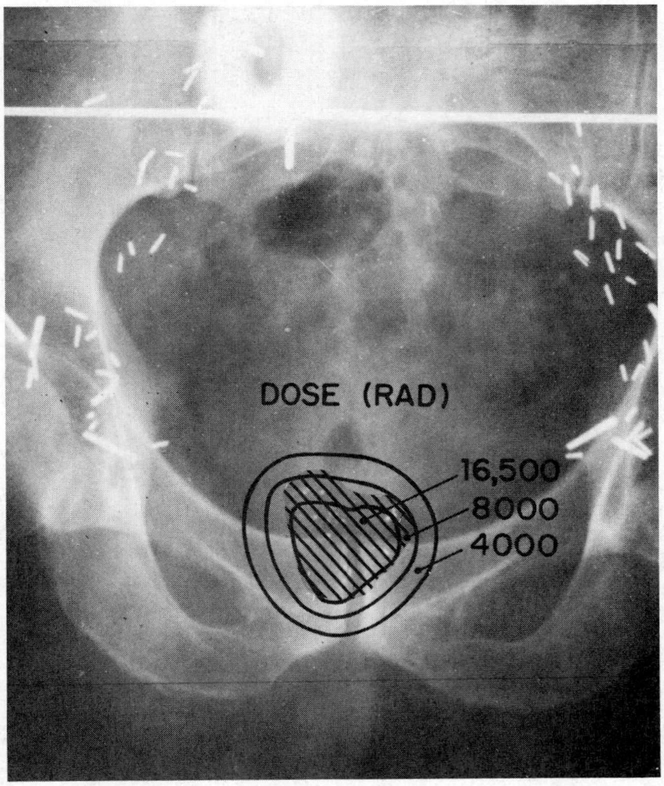

B

FIG. 33-11. **A**. Suprapubic interstitial implantation in the prostate. **B**. Anteroposterior radiograph of pelvis showing iridium-192 seed implant in the prostate and isodose curves.

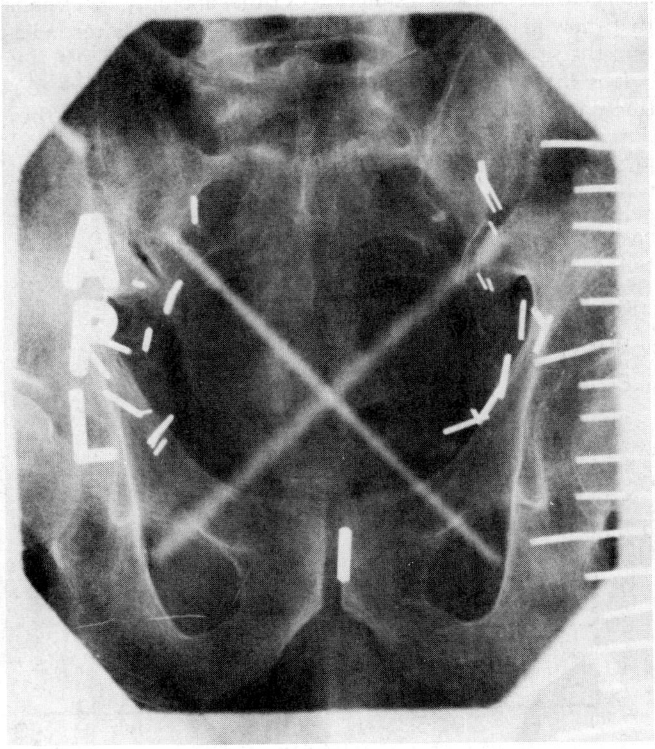

A

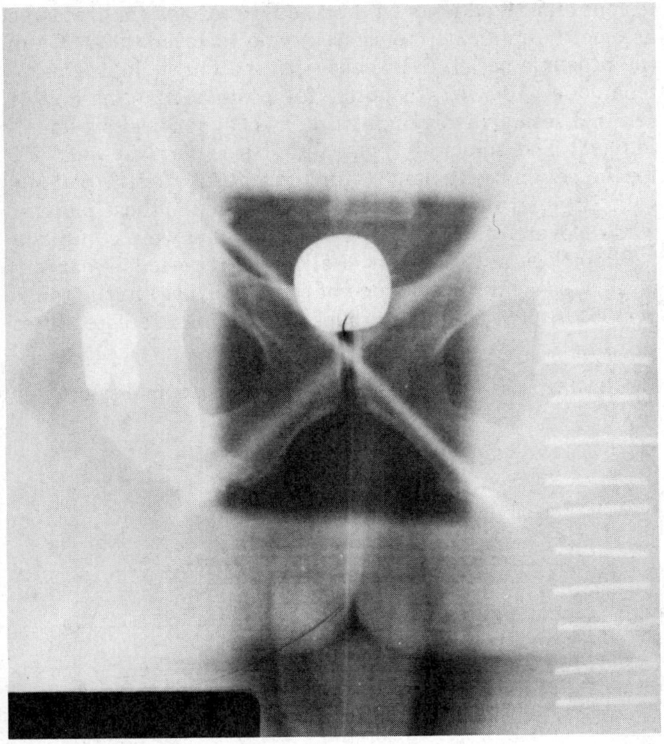

B

FIG. 33-12. **A**, **B**. Ports for pelvic lymph nodes and prostate boost.

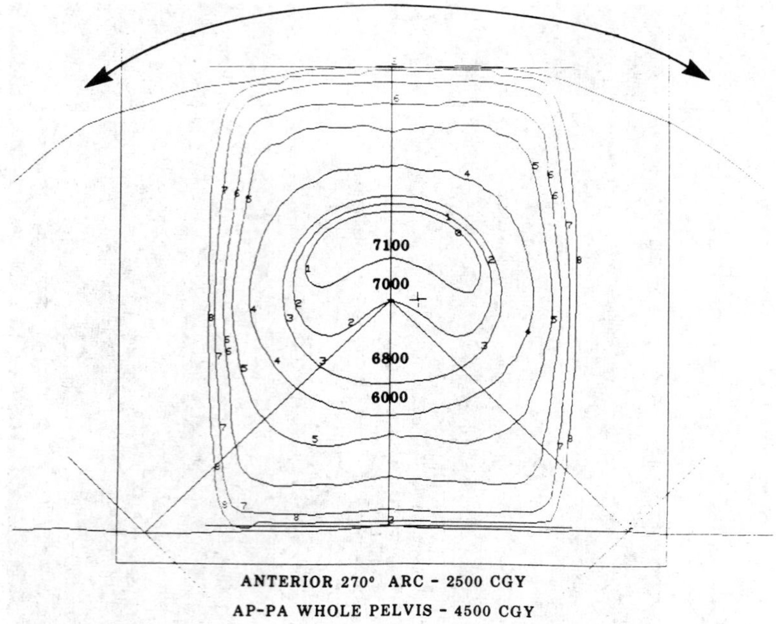

FIG. 33-13. Dose distribution with AP and PA ports (4500 cGy) and bilateral 120° arc rotations (2500 cGy).

because this treatment is palliative, the minimal tumor dose can be held at 6500 cGy to decrease morbidity.

Most institutions treat with daily fractions of 180 to 200 cGy, five fractions per week.

Irradiation After Prostatectomy

Lang reported treatment results in 30 patients with Stage C lesions and 26 patients with Stage D1a lesions (microscopic areas of lymph node metastases) who received 6000 cGy to the prostatic bed in 6½ weeks with the four-field isocentric technique (10 × 10 cm ports) for positive margins and/or seminal vesical involvement after radical perineal prostatectomy.[181] The actuarial 5-year tumor-free survival was 72% for the patients with Stage C tumors and 70% for the patients with Stage D1 tumors. Therapy was limited to those patients who recovered fully from the operation and were continent.

Pilepich et al[182] and Ray et al[183] also reported 5-year survival rates (without evidence of tumor relapse) in the range of 50% to 60% in small groups of patients irradiated after suprapubic prostatectomy or radical prostatectomy when carcinoma and positive margins were found in the specimen (Fig. 33-15).

FIG. 33-14. Dose distribution with box technique, 6-MV photons.

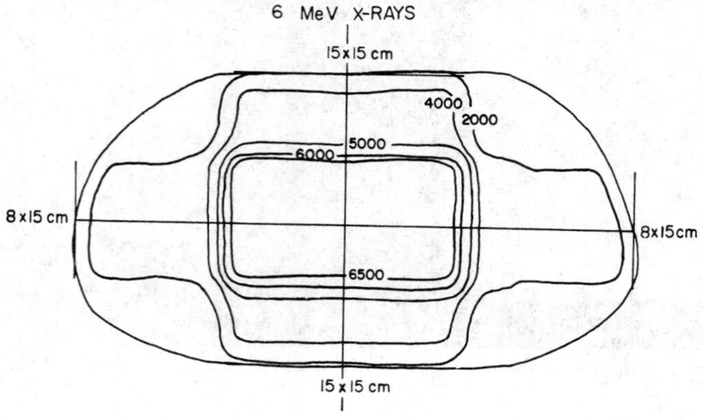

PROSTATE BIOPSIES AFTER DEFINITIVE IRRADIATION. Numerous reports describe the microscopic disappearance of tumor, fibrosis, obliteration of glandular structure, and occasionally calcifications in the prostate after definitive radiation therapy.[184-188] The number of positive biopsies decreases as a function of time, and only specimens that show persistent tumor more than 18 months after radiation therapy may have clinical import.

It is important to determine whether biopsies were routinely done regardless of clinical findings or whether they

FIG. 33-15. Disease-free survival (actuarial life-table method) for patients with carcinoma of the prostate treated with postoperative radiotherapy. (Pilepich MV et al: Postoperative irradiation in carcinoma of the prostate. Int J Radiat Oncol Biol Phys 10:1869–1873, 1984)

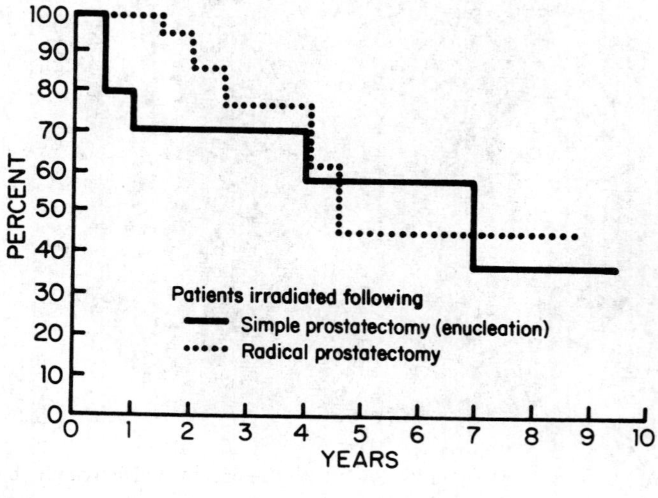

were indicated because of clinical suspicion of tumor progression. In a report by Freiha and Bagshaw on biopsies performed in 64 of 146 patients 2 or more years after completion of irradiation, only 29% of the prostates normal on digital rectal examination contained cancer, in contrast to 85% of those that seemed abnormal.[115]

Cox and Kline recently reported on 46 consecutive patients, many of whom underwent serial transperineal needle biopsies of the prostate following definitive radiation therapy (7000 cGy in 30 to 37 fractions); a decreased incidence of positive specimens was noted, with 19% showing persistent tumor after 24 months and 15% after 42 months.[184] Perez et al recorded the time at which complete tumor regression took place after definitive radiation therapy in patients with Stage B or C carcinoma of the prostate.[55] Figure 33-16 superimposes Perez's clinical findings on the pathologic observations of Cox and Kline. There is a similar pattern of clinical and histologic tumor regression, with about 20% of the cases showing persistent tumor by either method. Therefore, careful periodic digital examination is adequate for evaluating the effects of irradiation on local control of prostatic carcinoma, and biopsies are required only when the gland remains persistently indurated after 18 months or there is evidence of tumor regrowth.

Another important issue discussed in many of the reports is the import of positive biopsy specimens. In general, if the biopsies are done routinely, there is no significant correlation between the positive needle biopsy findings and the clinical course of the patients.[55,184–188] However, Freiha et al[115] and Carlton et al[189] noted that residual viable prostatic carcinoma in needle biopsy specimens more than 2 years after external irradiation is associated with a high rate of local recurrence and distant metastases.

Scardino reported on 475 patients with clinical Stage A2, B, or C1 prostatic carcinoma treated with radioactive gold seed implantation and external beam irradiation.[190] In 124 patients, one or more needle biopsies of the prostate were performed 6 to 36 months after completion of the radiation therapy. Biopsy results were consistently negative in 81 (65%) of the 124 patients and were positive for cancer on one or more occasions in 43 (35%). The rate of local recurrence was 14% in patients with negative biopsy results and 47% in those with positive biopsy results. Distant metastases were noted in 30% of those with negative biopsies and in 51% of those with positive biopsies.

Palliative Irradiation

Patients with massive pelvic extensions of prostatic carcinoma or with lymph node involvement may complain of pelvic pain or hematuria, or may develop urethral obstruction or leg edema due to lymphatic obstruction. Radiation therapy in the range of 5000 cGy may be quite efficacious in the treatment of these symptoms. Carlton et al reported relief of bladder neck obstruction in 20 (50%) of 40 patients treated palliatively, improvement of hydronephrosis in 8 (73%) of 11 patients, and disappearance of intractable hematuria in 7 (100%) of 7 patients who had either failed to respond to estrogen therapy or had been treated with hormones after irradiation.[189]

Kraus et al reported satisfactory results in the palliative treatment of locally advanced prostatic cancer with doses ranging from 2250 to 6600 cGy; most patients received between 4000 and 5000 cGy.[191] Disappearance of gross hematuria was noted in 13 (100%) of 13 patients, and a definitive decrease in the size and induration of the gland was observed in 19 (82%) of 23 patients. Marked improvement in rectal symptoms (pain, constipation, tenesmus) was reported in 5 (100%) of 5 patients after irradiation, and severe rectal bleeding due to tumor invasion was controlled in one patient. Symptoms of lower urinary tract obstruction showed improvement after irradiation in 14 patients; 4 of 5 patients treated for urethral obstruction had a favorable response. Severe edema of the lower extremities improved in 3 patients, and perineal and inguinal pain was relieved in 3 patients.

Increasing urinary difficulty may develop in patients with partial urethral obstruction because of swelling during the initial phase of irradiation. An indwelling catheter may avert a complete blockage, but this should not be used for more than 2 or 3 weeks because of irritation and the danger of superimposed infection. A transurethral resection may be performed occasionally if the obstruction does not improve during the initial course of irradiation.

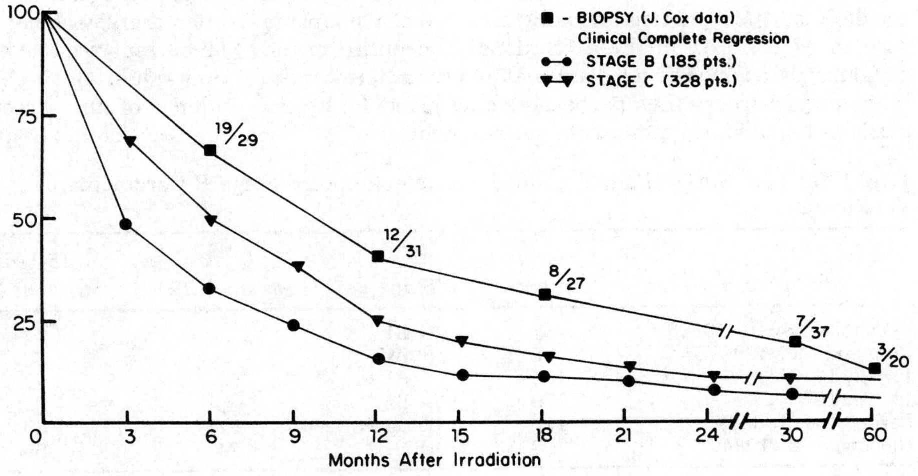

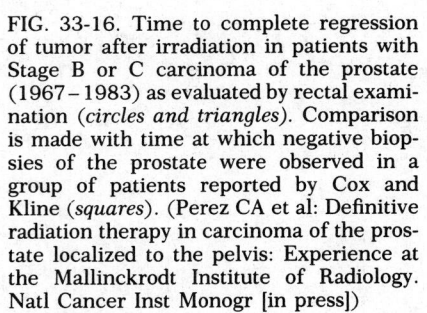

FIG. 33-16. Time to complete regression of tumor after irradiation in patients with Stage B or C carcinoma of the prostate (1967–1983) as evaluated by rectal examination (*circles and triangles*). Comparison is made with time at which negative biopsies of the prostate were observed in a group of patients reported by Cox and Kline (*squares*). (Perez CA et al: Definitive radiation therapy in carcinoma of the prostate localized to the pelvis: Experience at the Mallinckrodt Institute of Radiology. Natl Cancer Inst Monogr [in press])

Radiation therapy is also used in the treatment of *distant metastases* from prostatic carcinoma. Marked symptomatic relief is noted in over 80% of the patients treated with doses of 3000 to 3500 cGy in 2 to 3 weeks. Large ports to include the entire bone, such as in the extremities of the pelvis, must be used. Also, portals encompassing the entire thoracic or lumbar spine, as the case may be, will decrease the need for retreatment. Brain metastases may be successfully treated with doses in the range of 3000 to 3500 cGy delivered over 2 or 3 weeks to the entire cranial contents (75% of the patients have multiple lesions).

When practically all the bones of the body are involved by tumor, several investigators have advocated systemic administration of radioactive phosphorus (^{32}P) after priming with testosterone[192–194] or parathormone.[195,196] Testosterone cyprionate, 100 mg, is given intramuscularly each day for 7 to 15 days. After the first 5 or 6 days, ^{32}P (sodium phosphate) administration is begun, either orally or intravenously (1.5 mCi for 6–7 days). Others advocate administration of a single dose of 5 to 7 mCi. Edland reported good to excellent relief of pain in 86% of 42 patients treated.[197]

Pinck and Alexander treated 32 patients with parathormone prior to ^{32}P administration and noted acute pain relief in 22 (69%) and extended (1 year or longer) pain relief in 14 (44%).[198] In these patients, the usual acute gastrointestinal symptoms secondary to irradiation may appear, and there is a certain degree of bone marrow depression.

Straffon et al reported the use of yttrium-90 hypophysectomy in the palliative treatment of patients with painful widespread bony metastases.[199] About half of 13 patients had good response, including 7 that had not responded to orchiectomy or estrogen therapy.

Prophylactic Breast Irradiation Before Hormonal Therapy

Gynecomastia is a common and unwanted side-effect of estrogen therapy that may cause pain, discomfort, and embarrassment. The prevention of gynecomastia and related symptoms has been reported in approximately 80% of patients treated with irradiation in the range of 1000 cGy delivered as a single dose through small appositional ports with superficial x-rays.[200–202] We employ tangential ports with a cobalt-60 or 4-MV photons and deliver a 1200 cGy midplane dose to each breast in three fractions. The entire breast glandular tissue must be irradiated before orchiectomy or the initiation of estrogen therapy, because once glandular hyperplasia is initiated, the process is not reversible.

RESULTS OF THERAPY

SURVIVAL

Radical Prostatectomy

Table 33-13 gives the 10- and 15-year survival rates after radical prostatectomy for Stage B carcinoma of the prostate.[85,203–207] The major difficulties in accurately assessing the impact of treatment on disease that is presumably localized to the prostate are as follows.

1. Patients treated in the past, included to allow an adequate follow-up period, were not staged by modern techniques, such as radioisotope bone scanning, CT, and sensitive tumor biomarkers.
2. None of the studies included bilateral pelvic lymphadenectomy to determine the presence of lymph node metastases at the time of surgery.
3. In many older series, patients with Stage A and B disease were grouped together. Some patients received empirical hormonal therapy in addition to surgery, making it impossible to assess the effect of surgery alone.

In 1970 Jewett described the results of prostatectomy in 111 consecutive patients with tumors less than 1.5 cm in diameter.[205] Ten-year tumor-free survival was 41%. Overall tumor-free survival was 27%. Of the 38 patients who died with disease, 17 had microscopic invasion of the seminal vesicles at the time of prostatectomy; in the remaining 21 the disease was histologically limited to the prostate. In Jewett's series, of 79 patients with Stage B2 disease, 18% survived 15 years, 50% had invasion of the seminal vesicles, and only 5% lived without evidence of tumor for 15 years.

In 1987 Lepor et al updated the results of radical perineal prostatectomy performed at Johns Hopkins University between 1951 and 1963.[208] Seventy patients with clinical Stage I disease, 57 of whom were followed up, had a 5-year survival rate of 83%, a 10-year survival rate of 63%, and a 15-year survival rate of 52%. Survival in these patients was virtually identical to the projected life expectancy of age-matched men in the general population. These results are similar to those reported by Bagshaw in 491 patients with clinical Stage A2 and B carcinoma of the prostate treated with radiation therapy alone, 60% of whom survived 15 years.[209] Gibbons reported that 46 (84%) of 55 patients followed up for a minimum of 15 years were alive or had died without evidence of tumor recurrence.[210]

The Veterans Administration Cooperative Urological Re-

TABLE 33-13. Survival After Radical Prostatectomy for Stage B Carcinoma of the Prostate

Study, Year	*No. of Patients*	*Stage*	*10-Year Survival (%)*	*15-Year Survival (%)*
Walsh and Jewett, 1980[203]	57	B1	. . .	51
Culp and Meyer, 1973[204]	86	B1	. . .	33
Jewett, 1970[205]	103	B1	50	27
Jewett, 1956[84]	79	B2		33
Berlin et al, 1968[206]	116	Localized	57	39
Gibbons et al, 1984[207]	54	B1/B2	74	55

search Group reported a randomized trial of radical prostatectomy plus placebo (37 patients) versus placebo alone (29 patients) in patients with Stage A and B tumors.[211] Nine of the placebo-treated patients and seven of the prostatectomy patients were omitted from analysis for various reasons. The results were comparable at a median 7.7-year follow-up of all survivors. Madsen et al noted that six patients in the prostatectomy group had Gleason scores of 8 to 10, in contrast to none in the placebo group. Of the patients treated with radical prostatectomy plus placebo, 45% were alive at 8.5 years, compared to 62% of those treated with placebo alone. The differences were not statistically significant. Also, there was no significant difference in the rate of progression of Stage B prostatic carcinoma after either therapy, only two patients dying with tumor.[212]

Long-term results with the nerve-sparing radical prostatectomy are awaited with high expectation. Unfortunately, patients have not been followed up for a long enough time, and survival results are not yet available.

Direct randomized comparison of radiation therapy versus radical prostatectomy for early prostatic carcinoma was reported by Paulson et al in 97 patients with clinical Stage A2 or B disease.[213] Fifty-six patients received radiation therapy and 41 were treated with radical prostatectomy. The authors did not specify the stratification criteria used or why, in a randomized study, 59 patients were assigned to radiation and 47 to radical prostatectomy. Also, 7 patients in the radiation treatment group and 9 patients in the surgical group did not receive the prescribed treatment. The actuarial disease-free survival was 85% for the surgical patients and 60% for the radiation therapy group. Most treatment failures occurred because of metastases to bone (as evidenced by a positive bone scan) or other distant sites. This certainly should not have been the direct effect of the local irradiation and may be related to the initial distribution of the patients in the two study groups. Furthermore, serious reservations regarding the statistical processing of the data have been raised.[214]

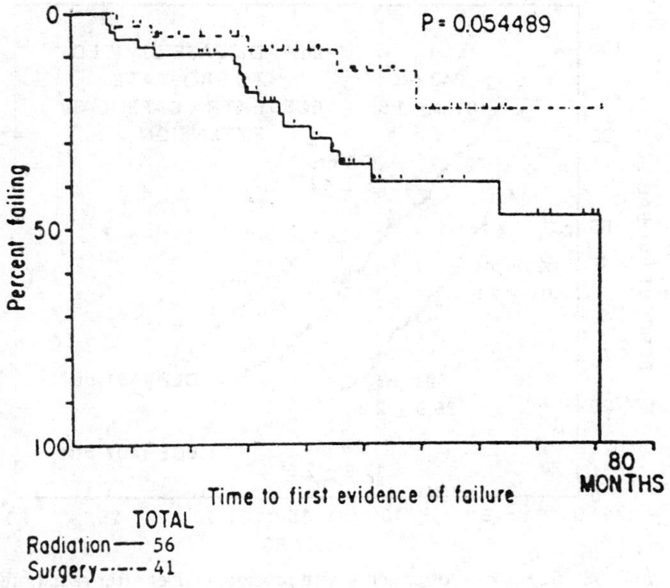

FIG. 33-17. Disease-free survival after additional 20 months of follow-up. (Paulson DF: Randomized series of surgery versus radiation therapy. Presented at the NIH Consensus Development Conference, Management of Clinically Localized Prostate Cancer, Bethesda, MD, June 15–17, 1987).

In 1987 Paulson updated the results in these patients and again noted better survival in the prostatectomy patients (Fig. 33-17).[215] However, the results obtained with radiation therapy in this series are inferior to those reported by other authors.[216] Figure 33-18 illustrates a comparison of survival in patients with similar surgical stage treated with radiation therapy alone by Bagshaw.[209] Therefore, a properly designed prospective clinical trial to compare these two modalities is warranted.

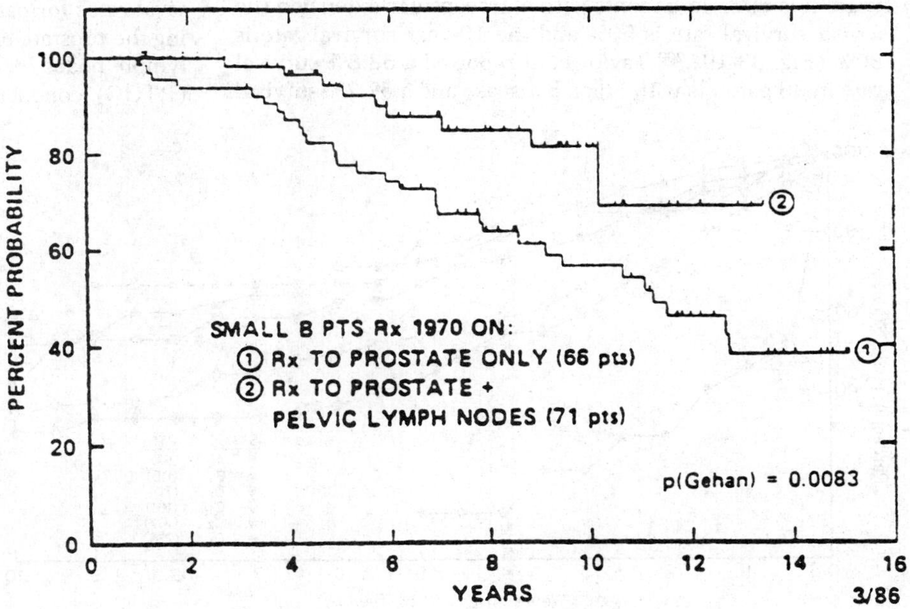

FIG. 33-18. Survival in patients with B_2 disease, limited to the prostate, according to extent of irradiation. This stage was selected for study because the probability of lymph node metastases is high but the metastases may be microscopic or less well developed than in Stage C. There was a highly significant survival advantage for patients who received radiation to the pelvic nodes and the prostate. (Bagshaw MA: Status of the radiation treatment of prostatic cancer at Stanford. Presented at the NIH Consensus Development Conference, Management of Clinically Localized Prostate Cancer, Bethesda, MD, June 15–17, 1987)

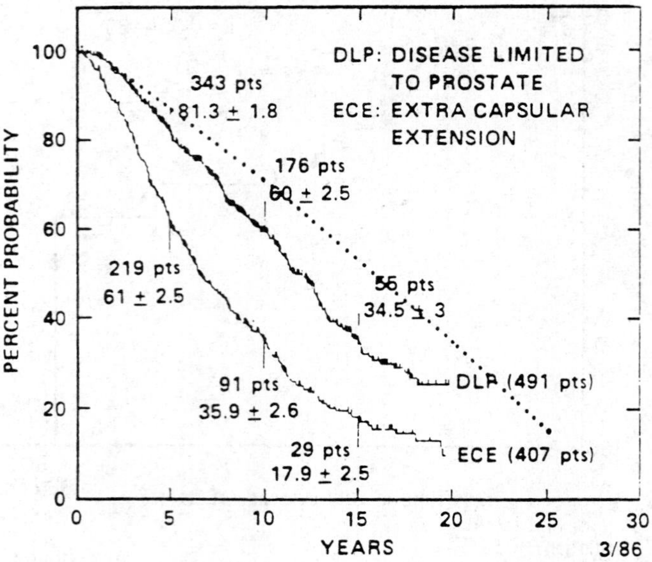

FIG. 33-19. Survival of patients with prostate cancer after radiation therapy, Stanford University. Each upward tick indicates the length of survival for each survivor and that the patient was alive at the time of the last follow-up notation. A downward step indicates the death of one or more patients. The curves are uncorrected, and deaths due to all causes are counted. The expected survival of an age-adjusted cohort of American men is plotted as a separate curve. Percentage survival ±SD at 5-year intervals is annotated to 15 years. (Bagshaw MA: Status of the radiation treatment of prostatic cancer. Presented at the NIH Consensus Development Conference, Management of Clinically Localized Prostate Cancer, Bethesda, MD, June 15–17, 1987)

Irradiation

The largest experience with the use of external irradiation in the treatment of prostatic carcinoma localized to the pelvis has been reported by Stanford University. Their results indicate that at 5 years the disease-free survival rate for patients with tumors localized to the prostate is about 75%, and at 10 years it is 60%. In patients with extracapsular extension the 5-year survival rate is 50% and the 10-year survival rate is 30% (Fig. 33-19).[209] Taylor et al reported a 58.8% survival rate in 36 patients with Stage B disease and a 57.7% survival rate in 221 patients with Stage C disease with a minimum follow-up of 2 to 3 years.[217] Perez et al recently reported results in 577 patients with various stages of prostatic carcinoma who were followed up for a minimum of 3 years after therapy (median follow-up, 6.5 years).[55] The actuarial disease-free 5-year survival rate was 78% for patients with Stages A2 and B disease, 60% for those with Stage C disease, and 15% for those with Stage D1 disease (Fig. 33-20). The 10-year tumor-free survival rate was 60% for patients with Stages A2 and B disease and 40% for those with Stage C disease (Table 33-14). The local failure rate was about 12% ($9/41$) in patients with Stage A2 tumors and 17% ($31/185$) in those with Stage B tumors; no particular difference was noted with doses ranging from 6000 to 7000 cGy. A significantly higher failure rate was noted in patients with Stage C disease treated with doses below 7000 cGy than in those treated with higher doses (Fig. 33-21). Approximately half of the pelvic failures were also associated with distant metastases. The overall rate of distant metastases was 20% in Stage B, 40% in Stage C, and 65% in Stage D1. Others have reported similar results.[130,135,218–221]

Hanks et al reported the results of definitive radiation therapy (6000–7000 cGy) in 619 patients treated throughout the United States and reported in the Patterns of Care Study.[222] The 5-year survival rate was 75% for Stage A, 85% for Stage B, and 58% for Stage C. The 10-year survival rate was 50% for Stage A2, 61% for Stage B, and 38% for Stage C. These figures are comparable to those reported by single institutions. Furthermore, Hanks et al noted a greater probability of in-field recurrences in patients treated with less than 6500 cGy for Stage T3 or T4 tumors. The complication rate was 6.9% in 174 patients treated with doses above 7000 cGy and 3.5% in those treated with doses below this level ($p = 0.03$).

McGowan reported that patients with Stage B2 and C tumors in whom the pelvic lymph nodes were treated had a better survival than those who underwent irradiation to the prostate only.[135] By contrast, Neglia et al noted similar survival rates for patients treated either with fields encompassing the prostate only or with larger ports including the pelvic lymph nodes.[130] The Radiation Therapy Oncology Group (RTOG) conducted two randomized studies assessing the

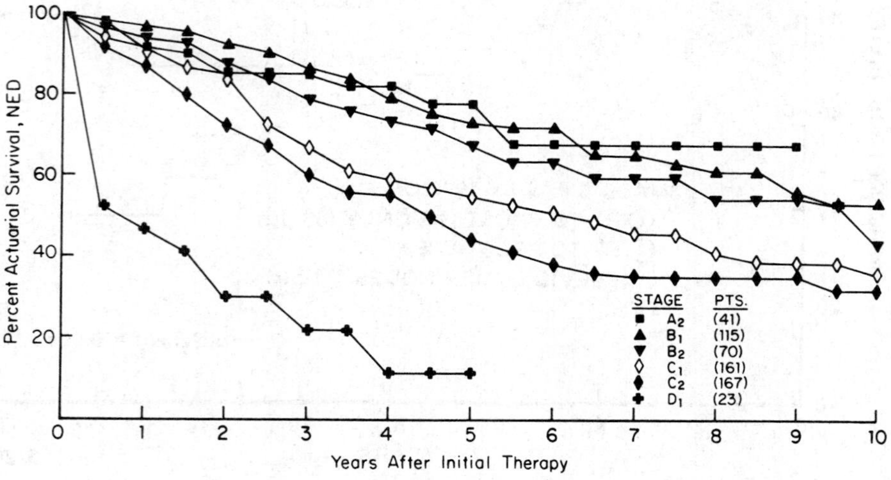

FIG. 33-20. NED survival by stage for 577 patients with carcinoma of the prostate localized to the pelvis treated with definitive irradiation at Mallinckrodt Institute of Radiology (1967–1983). (Perez CA et al: Definitive radiation therapy in carcinoma of the prostate localized to the pelvis: Experience at Mallinckrodt Institute of Radiology. Natl Cancer Inst Monogr [in press])

TABLE 33-14. Carcinoma of the Prostate, 1967–1983: 10-Year Survival

Clinical Stage	*No. of Patients at Risk*	*10-Year Direct Survival*		*Death—ICD*	*Adjusted Survival (%)*
		No.	*(%)*		
A2	3	2	(66.7)	1	100
B1	30	21	(70)	2	75
B2	16	10	(62.5)	4	83.3
C1	76	30	(39.5)	16	50
C2	61	20	(32.8)	10	39.2
D1	12	2	(16.7)	2	20

value of irradiation to the pelvic nodes in Stage B disease or the periaortic nodes in Stage C disease.[223,224] Preliminary data reported by Asbell et al[225] and Pilepich et al[177,178] show similar survival, whether or not the pelvic lymph nodes are electively irradiated, in Stage A2 or B tumors. Elective irradiation of the periaortic lymph nodes in patients with Stage C disease or with Stage A2–B disease and positive pelvic nodes failed to improve survival. However, a slightly higher survival rate has been reported by Pistenma et al for patients with positive nodes when the pelvic and periaortic lymph nodes were irradiated.[50]

Hilaris et al[100,226] and Sogani et al[227] reported 5-year survival rates of 80% or higher for patients with T1 and T2 tumors and 55% to 60% for those with T3 tumors treated with ^{125}I implants and staging lymph node dissection. The local failure rate was approximately 15%. Local recurrence was 10% or less with doses over 15,000 cGy and 30% or greater with lower doses.

FIG. 33-21. Correlation of pelvic recurrences and dose of irradiation for patients with Stage B carcinoma of the prostate (1967–1983). (Perez CA et al: Definitive radiation therapy in carcinoma of the prostate localized to the pelvis: Experience at Mallinckrodt Institute of Radiology. Natl Cancer Inst Monogr [in press])

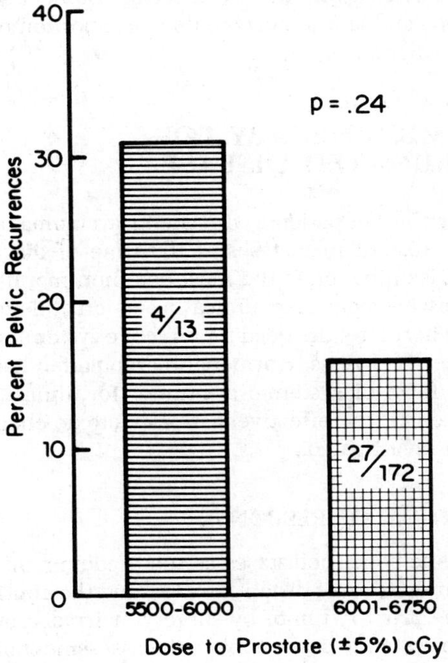

Carlton et al reported results in 542 patients treated with ^{198}Au grains and external irradiation, with a minimum follow-up of 1 year.[174,189] The survival rates are comparable to those reported after radical prostatectomy or other radiation therapy techniques. Approximately 65% of the patients with Stage A, B, or C1 disease had negative biopsies 1 year or longer after therapy. Exact patterns of failure were not reported.

Batata et al reported on 28 patients who had positive nodes at the time of interstitial therapy and pelvic lymphadenectomy and who then received irradiation to the whole pelvis alone or to the pelvis and the periaortic lymph nodes; they were compared with a group of 24 patients not given external irradiation. The determinate 5-year survival rate was 54% in both groups; the tumor-free 5-year survival rate was 15% (2/13) with and 21% (5/24) without external irradiation.[228] Similar results were reported by Prout et al, who compared results in 16 patients given external irradiation and 16 patients who received no additional therapy after ^{125}I implantation in the prostate.[51] Nodal external irradiation is probably not effective because 75% to 80% of these patients develop distant metastases and few survive more than 5 years.

TREATMENT SEQUELAE

Surgery

The major objection to the routine use of radical prostatectomy to control localized prostatic carcinoma has been the nearly 100% rate of impotence. However, after the nerve-sparing radical retropubic prostatectomy described by Walsh, 83% of his patients retained potency,[152] whereas Catalona et al observed preservation of potency in only 22 (52%) of 42 sexually potent patients treated with this procedure.[229] From 3% to 7% of the patients will experience urinary incontinence of varying degrees; in a small percentage it can be permanent and disabling.

Other complications of radical prostatectomy include excessive blood loss and fistula formation between the bladder and rectum due to injury to the rectum when the prostate is freed off this structure. The ureters may be damaged if the surgeon dissects within layers of the trigone while attempting to define a cleavage plane between the bladder and seminal vesicles. Fortunately, injuries to the surrounding structures are relatively rare. They occur most commonly in patients who have had previous prostatic surgery or pelvic irradiation.

Thrombophlebitis may occur in a small percentage of patients following bilateral pelvic lymphadenectomy. The incidence does not appear to be appreciably reduced by the routine use of preoperative minidose heparin.[230] Modification of the limits of the node dissection may minimize this problem.

Irradiation

Acute side-effects of irradiation include diarrhea, abdominal cramping, rectal discomfort, and occasionally rectal bleeding, which may be related to a transient enteroproctitis. Patients with hemorrhoids may experience discomfort earlier than other patients, and aggressive symptomatic treatment should be instituted promptly. The symptoms can be controlled with the administration of diphenoxylate hydrochloride with atropine sulfate (Lomotil), opium preparations such as paregoric, Imodium, and emollients such as kaolin and pectin. The local symptoms of proctitis and rectal discomfort can be relieved by administration of small enemas with cod liver oil, and suppositories containing bismuth, benzyl benzoate, zinc oxide, or Peruvian balsam (Anusol, Wyanoids, Medicone, etc.). Some of the suppositories may contain cortisone. Other preparations that can be quite effective are small enemas with hydrocortisone (Proctofoam, Cortifoam). An adequate diet with low residue and no grease or spices usually helps to decrease gastrointestinal symptoms.

Genitourinary symptoms are secondary to cystourethritis and are characterized by dysuria, frequency, and nocturia. The urine is usually clear, although occasionally it may show microscopic or even gross hematuria. Preparations such as mandelamine and antispasmodics, phenazopyridine HCl (Pyridium), or a smooth muscle antispasmodic such as flavoxate HCl (Urispas, Cistopaz) can be effective in relieving symptoms. An adequate fluid intake is extremely important (at least 2000–2500 ml daily). Superimposed infections of the urinary tract may occur and should be diagnosed with appropriate urine culture studies, including tests of sensitivity to sulfonamides and antibiotics. Therapy should be promptly instituted.

Erythema and dry or moist desquamation may develop in the perineum or intergluteal fold. Good skin hygiene and topical application of Vaseline, Aquaphor, or lanolin should suffice. However, if more severe reactions develop, use of zinc oxide ointment or Desitin and intensive skin care are necessary.

More severe late sequelae of treatment include persistent proctitis or proctosigmoiditis, with an occasional patient requiring a colostomy. This complication was noted in 1% of 577 patients. The incidence of rectal ulcers is 2% to 3%, and that of persistent proctitis is about 6%.[55]

Hazra and Giri noted a 43% incidence of proctitis, with 2% of the patients requiring colostomy, in a group of 32 patients with localized prostatic carcinoma treated with 5000 cGy to the pelvic lymph nodes and 1000 cGy to the prostate and adjacent tissues with conventional fractionation, and an additional 800 cGy single-dose exposure to the pelvic girdle.[231] This is not usual and customary therapy.

Chronic cystitis is observed in less than 5% of the patients; with doses of more than 7500 cGy to the bladder hemorrhagic cystitis may occasionally develop, requiring a cystectomy (less than 1% of the patients). Urethral stricture has been reported in approximately 5% of patients,[128,232,233] most frequently in patients who underwent transurethral prostatic resection before or during radiation therapy.

A complete tabulation of the reported incidence of severe intestinal or urinary complications was published by Dewit et al.[234]

One of the most vexing sequelae of irradiation is sexual impotence, which has been reported in about 40% of initially potent patients treated with external radiation therapy, but in only 15% of those treated with interstitial ^{125}I. Age may be a factor in this difference, since implants tend to be used in younger patients and external beam irradiation in older patients. Possible causes of sexual impotence include decreased testosterone and dihydroxytestosterone levels, fibrosis or decreased external glandular secretions, pudendal or sympathetic nerve injury, and anxiety or depression.

Serial determinations of plasma dihydroxytestosterone and testosterone levels in patients treated with external irradiation showed no notable changes in hormone levels.[235]

Combined Surgery and Irradiation

The combination of a surgical procedure and definitive radiation therapy is associated with a higher complication rate. Pilepich et al described no excessive edema of the lower extremities in 236 patients treated with definitive radiation therapy alone, in contrast to 15.5% (18/116) of patients who had undergone limited pelvic lymph node dissection and 66% (4/6) of patients who had undergone extended lymphadenectomy.[236]

Pistenma et al reported a high frequency of small bowel complications in patients in whom a transperitoneal periaortic lymph node dissection was performed and 5500 cGy was delivered through AP and PA ports.[50] The frequency was greatly decreased with the use of retroperitoneal lymph node dissections and lateral ports to deliver a portion of the periaortic irradiation.

SYSTEMIC THERAPY FOR DISSEMINATED DISEASE

Up to one third of patients with adenocarcinoma of the prostate have distant metastases at the time of diagnosis, and distant dissemination is the most common manifestation of disease progression after surgical resection or definitive irradiation. Therefore, the need for effective systemic therapy of this cancer is obvious. Hormonal manipulation has been the standard form of systemic treatment for almost 50 years. More recently, the effectiveness of cytotoxic chemotherapy has been investigated.

EVALUATION OF RESPONSE

Osteoblastic bone metastases as the predominant and often sole manifestation of distant disease, and the continued control of the primary tumor by surgery or irradiation in many men with systemic cancer, make the assessment of response to chemotherapy in prostatic carcinoma especially difficult. Because of this, response in therapeutic trials reported in the literature has been determined by variable and often subjective methods. The need for reproducible and standardized response definitions in prostatic cancer is emphasized by the observation that the "objective" response to cisplatin in one chemotherapy trial ranged from 4% to 23%, depending on which of several published systems of response determination was employed.[237] Methods frequently employed to monitor tumor response are listed in Table 33-15.

Since most patients receiving systemic therapy will have bone metastases, reliable response assessment with radionuclide bone scintigraphy and bone radiography would be of great value. Improvement on serial bone scans and radiographs provides specific evidence of tumor response and is associated with improved survival,[97,238] but radiographic resolution of osteoblastic lesions is rare, scan improvement often lags behind other evidence of response, and the detection of scintigraphic changes requires careful attention to technical details of scanning. Findings on both examinations often worsen with tumor progression, but worsening on either, especially radiography, can also occur with osteoblastic activity associated with bone healing in responding patients[239] and cannot be relied on as the sole evidence of disease progression.

Some investigators do not find primary tumor assessment to be helpful,[240] but the National Prostatic Cancer Project (NPCP) found that regression of the primary tumor correlates with favorable response at 12 weeks of therapy and with normalization of acid phosphatase levels.[241,242] Recent experience suggests that rectal US improves the ability to detect changes in the primary tumor volume during therapy.[243,244]

Substantial declines in elevated values of serum acid phosphatase, which are present in most men with disseminated prostatic cancer, correlate with improved survival on both hormonal therapy[245] and chemotherapy,[246] pain relief, and reduction in size of the primary tumor.[242] Furthermore, elevated values normalize significantly more often in patients with stable disease than in those with progressive disease by NPCP criteria.[247] Radioimmunoassays for acid phosphatase appear no more useful than enzymatic assays for monitoring tumor status on systemic treatment.[248] Because of fluctuation in results of repeated measurements of acid phosphatase,[249] reliance should be placed only on confirmed, substantial (twofold or greater) changes in values that persist for at least a month, preferably longer.[248,249] Recent studies of a newly characterized prostate-specific antigen indicate that this test could prove useful in evaluating tumor response.[250]

TABLE 33-15. Methods for Monitoring of Tumor Response in Patients with Metastatic Prostatic Cancer Given Systemic Therapy

Assessment of primary prostatic tumor:
Physical examination
Ultrasound examination
Radionuclide bone scans and bone radiographs
Measurement of serum acid phosphatase levels
Determination of serum specific prostatic antigen
Nonspecific indicators of disease status:
Performance status
Bone pain
Weight
Hemoglobin level
Measurable or evaluable tumor masses:
Physical examination
Chest radiographs and/or other radiographs or radionuclide studies
Computed tomography

Until recently, the nonspecific indicators of performance status, bone pain, weight, and hemoglobin level have been the most commonly utilized end points for the evaluation of response in metastatic prostate cancer. Although these parameters frequently worsen with tumor progression and improve with response, especially response to hormonal therapy, 23% to 63% of improvements can occur in patients who experience tumor progression within 12 weeks of initiation of therapy.[241]

Sites of clearly measurable or evaluable masses in metastatic prostatic cancer are infrequently documented with routine tests. Pulmonary metastases are found in 10% to 20% of patients, liver metastases in 10% to 15%, and peripheral lymph node metastases in 10%,[246,251–253] but these patients probably have a worse prognosis than men without such measurable lesions.[246,254] Abnormally enlarged pelvic and abdominal lymph nodes can be detected in 30% to 35% of patients with bone metastases if CT is performed.[252] Objective responses in these more "measurable" sites are associated with improved survival[237,246,251,255] and in one series with improvement in a mean of 4.6 other objective and subjective indicators of response.[252]

Currently, the most widely used response criteria are those of the NPCP, which require normalization of acid phosphatase level, improvement in some evaluable tumor lesion if present, and no new tumor lesions or symptomatic deterioration for 12 weeks in order to declare a partial response.[256] If only the last two criteria plus the failure of any evaluable lesion to worsen are observed, the patient is declared to have stable disease. These criteria may fail to identify some objective tumor regressions. More importantly, studies that utilize NPCP response criteria often report results in terms of "objective response rate," which includes both partial response and stable disease categories.

When NPCP criteria are applied, survival and response duration are similar for patients with partial response or stable disease on both hormonal therapy and chemotherapy.[256] This is also true when other response criteria emphasizing measurable disease are utilized.[255] Criteria that emphasize disease stability are clearly inadequate to document antitumor activity in nonrandomized Phase II trials. A simple, reproducible, universally applicable system for unequivocally and objectively demonstrating tumor response in prostatic cancer remains elusive. This enhances the importance of survival as a measure of therapeutic efficacy in this disease. Response criteria and prognostic factors in prostatic cancer have been reviewed.[257]

HORMONAL THERAPY OF PROSTATIC CARCINOMA

Multiple types of hormonal therapy have been employed since 1941 when Huggins and colleagues demonstrated

TABLE 33-16. Effect of Endocrine Therapy on Hormonal Levels in Prostatic Cancer Patients*

Therapy	*Testosterone Levels*			*Luteinizing Hormone Levels*	*Estradiol Levels*
	First Week	*Long-term*	*Duration*		
Orchiectomy	Castrate	Castrate	Indefinite	Increased	Decreased
Estrogens	Decreased	Castrate	Reversible	Decreased	Increased
LHRH Agonists	Increased	Castrate	Reversible	Increased, then decreased	Decreased
Progestational agents	Decreased	May rebound	Reversible	Decreased	Unknown
Pure antiandrogens	Increased	Increased	Reversible	Increased	Increased
Inhibitors of steroid synthesis	Castrate	Unknown	Reversible	Increased	Decreased

*Modified from Grayhack JT, Keeler TC, Kozlowski JM: Carcinoma of the prostate: Hormonal therapy. Cancer 60:589–601, 1987.

tumor regression and diminution of serum acid phosphatase levels after orchiectomy or estrogen administration in patients with prostatic cancer.[139,258] All protocols seek to reduce androgenic stimulation of the carcinoma by one or more of four mechanisms: ablation of androgen-producing tissue, suppression of pituitary gonadotropin release, inhibition of androgen synthesis, or interference with androgen action in target tissues.[259] Changes in hormone levels induced by, and side-effects of various types of endocrine treatments are summarized in Tables 33-16 and 33-17.

Orchiectomy removes the source of 95% of circulating testosterone and is followed by a prompt, long-lasting decline in serum testosterone levels. Elevated levels of this hormone are not routinely observed with tumor recurrence after orchiectomy.[260] Adrenalectomy reduces extratesticular sources of androgen production in castrated patients, but is now infrequently performed.

The principal action of estrogens in prostatic cancer is thought to be suppression of pituitary gonadotropin release with consequent reduced stimulus for testicular testosterone synthesis, although direct interference with hormonal synthesis or a direct effect on the prostatic cancer cell may also be contributory.[259,260] The nonsteroidal estrogen diethylstilbestrol (DES) suppresses serum testosterone to castrate levels in a dosage of 3 mg/day, while higher dosages have no additional effect.[261] Testosterone is not uniformly suppressed by a 1 mg/day dosage, which nonetheless appears to have similar antitumor effects. Progestational agents suppress gonadotropin release[262] and may also directly interfere with hormonal synthesis or, in some cases, act as antiandrogens in target tissues.[259,260] With prolonged use of progestins, however, suppressed testosterone levels may rise in some patients.[259] The newly introduced leutinizing hormone–releasing hormone (LHRH) agonists such as leuprolide and buserelin induce an initial rise in gonadotropin levels followed by a sharp decline associated with castrate levels of testosterone within 2 to 3 weeks.[263] Hypophysectomy eliminates gonadotropin and adrenocorticotropic hormone stimulation of testicular and adrenal androgen secretion.

Androgen production in the adrenal gland and the testicle may be inhibited at several points in the synthetic pathway. Aminoglutethimide, which is administered with a glucocorticoid, inhibits the synthesis of all adrenal steroids and leads to further reduction of serum testosterone in castrate patients that may correlate with tumor regression.[264,265] Ketoconazole, an antifungal agent, impairs steroid synthesis, including testicular and adrenal androgens, and can often be administered without supplemental glucocorticoids.[266] Spironolactone, which also has some direct antiandrogenic effects, inhibits male sex hormone production further down the synthetic pathway,[267] and estrogens and progestational agents exert such effects even more distally.[260]

Cyproterone acetate is the most potent of the progestational antiandrogens, which are thought to act by inhibiting formation of the dihydrotestosterone–receptor complex in prostatic nuclei.[259,260] Flutamide is a nonsteroidal antiandrogen that does not suppress gonadotropin or testosterone levels but does have estrogenic side-effects.[268] In contrast to

TABLE 33-17. Morbidity of Endocrine Therapy in Prostatic Cancer Patients*

Effect	*Orchiectomy*	*Estrogens*	*LHRH Agonists*	*Antiandrogens*
Cardiovascular	−	+†	−	−
Tumor flare	−	−	++	−
Gastrointestinal distress	−	+	−	+
Impotence	++	++	+++	−
Gynecomastia	−	+++	−	++
Hot flashes	+	±	+	−

*Modified from Grayhack JT, Keeler TC, Kozlowski JM: Carcinoma of the prostate: Hormonal therapy. Cancer 60:589–601, 1987.
†Dose dependent.

other forms of hormonal manipulation, it infrequently induces impotence.[259,268] Tamoxifen is a nonsteroidal antiestrogen that has been studied in prostatic cancer because of some evidence of estrogen receptors in neoplastic cells, but it appears to have minimal or no antitumor effects.[269]

Orchiectomy, DES, or LHRH agonists (especially leuprolide) are the most common initial hormonal treatments for metastatic prostate cancer in the United States. When NPCP objective response criteria are applied to patients with disseminated cancer, 37% to 46% of patients have complete or partial responses to any of these maneuvers, and in an additional 39% to 48% the disease stabilizes for 12 weeks or more.[270-272] Pain and impaired ambulatory status improve in 40% to 70% of cases.[271,272] In a large randomized study by the Veterans Administration Cooperative Urologic Research Group (VACURG), DES in a dosage of 5 mg/day, orchiectomy, or the combination was markedly superior to placebo after 6 months in terms of pain relief, improved ambulation, and reduction in primary tumor size, soft tissue metastases, and ureteral dilation. All hormonal therapies delayed the development of distant metastases compared with placebo,[273] and none of the three treatments was superior to another by any parameter.

In contrast to breast cancer, objective response with a second endocrine manipulation is only infrequently observed (5%–15% of cases) in carcinoma of the prostate after termination of response to initial hormonal therapy. Subjective improvement of short duration, however, is not uncommon. DES or orchiectomy,[274] adrenalectomy,[275] hypophysectomy,[276] high-dose DES-diphosphate,[277] progestins,[262] LHRH agonists,[278] aminoglutethimide,[265,279] ketoconazole,[266] antiandrogens,[259] and antiestrogens[280] have been employed in this setting. For most patients their value is undefined. In an early randomized study,[281] DES was not superior to a placebo in orchiectomized patients with progressive tumor.

There is no doubt of the palliative efficacy, both subjective and objective, of hormonal therapy in prostatic cancer, and survival beyond 10 years can occur in up to 10% of patients with bony metastases on such treatment.[282] The influential study of Nesbit and Baum,[274] published in 1950, compared the survival of men given hormonal treatment with survival in a control group treated from 1925 to 1940, before the introduction of endocrine therapy (and of antibiotics), and concluded that orchiectomy, DES, or the combination improved survival in locally advanced or metastatic tumor. A more recent study employing multivariate analysis, however, found that improvement in survival after 1940 in prostatic cancer patients could potentially be explained by a trend toward lower mortality which was occurring from 1937 to 1944 independently of treatment.[283]

The principal prospectively collected data addressing the impact of hormonal therapy on survival was generated by the VACURG in a series of randomized trials. In men with Stage A cancer who did not receive any locoregional therapy, hormone treatment had no impact on survival,[284] and DES in a dosage of 5 mg/day given as an adjuvant after radical prostatectomy to men with Stages A and B disease significantly shortened survival.[285] Adjuvant therapy with DES in patients treated with prostatic or pelvic irradiation confers no survival advantage in randomized studies.[130] Therefore, hormonal treatment should not be administered to any patient with localized or locally advanced cancer unless it is the most feasible method of relieving tumor-related symptoms.

The first large VACURG study randomized patients with locally advanced or metastatic cancer to receive DES (5 mg/day), orchiectomy, both treatments simultaneously, or placebo. In patients with Stage III (locally advanced) disease, estrogen-containing treatments actually shortened survival because of the increased risk of death from cardiovascular causes, while patients with Stage IV disease (distant metastases or elevated serum acid phosphatase levels) had a similar survival rate regardless of treatment.[273] Since changes in treatment were allowed in this study for patients with worsening symptoms, and since almost half the patients with Stage IV disease who were initially given placebo received some form of active treatment within the first year, this trial actually evaluated the merits of immediate hormonal treatment versus withholding such therapy until symptoms worsen.[273] The results imply that hormonal treatment can be withheld in symptomatic patients without compromising survival, provided that therapy is later given when needed. This concept has recently been questioned on theoretical grounds, but no conclusive data that mandate immediate therapy in asymptomatic patients have been forthcoming.[259]

In the second VACURG study in advanced disease, placebo was compared with DES in dosages of 5, 1, or 0.2 mg/day. Excessive cardiovascular deaths in patients with Stage III disease were again noted with the 5-mg dose of DES, but with the 1-mg dose cardiovascular deaths were no greater than with placebo. The 1- and 5-mg doses of DES were similar in retarding progression from Stage III to IV and in reducing overall cancer deaths.[286] Despite the ability of DES to retard development of metastases in Stage III disease, initial therapy with placebo yielded better survival than DES 5 mg/day in Stage III disease and was no worse than the 1-mg dose regimen,[287] once again confirming that withholding hormonal treatment in less advanced disease is not deleterious provided that it is administered when metastases develop. Later analysis of this randomized trial[288] revealed that survival is modestly but significantly better with DES, 1 or 5 mg/day, than with DES, 0.2 mg/day, or placebo in men less than 75 years old (those with the least cardiovascular risk from estrogens) with Stage IV or high-grade tumor, the subgroup most in need of effective anticancer therapy. Recent mature results of this study are said to demonstrate superior survival with DES, 1 mg/day, as initial therapy for men with Stages III and IV disease combined. Nonetheless, proof that hormonal therapy prolongs survival in metastatic prostatic cancer cannot be considered to be established.

A few large trials have compared different forms of hormonal manipulation as initial systemic therapy for prostate cancer. Recent studies have shown that LHRH agonists produce antitumor effects and survival rates similar to those seen with DES and orchiectomy.[272,289] The initial increase in levels of circulating androgens induced by LHRH agonists is not of clinical import in most patients, but in less than 10% worsening pain or urinary symptoms can occur.[272] Some investigators do not advise use of LHRH agonists as sole treatment in patients with impending neurologic compromise.[290] In a European trial in men with locally advanced and metastatic disease, DES, 3 mg/day, and the progestational antiandrogen cyproterone acetate were both superior to medroxyprogesterone acetate in terms of time to tumor progression and survival. Antitumor effects of the former two agents were not significantly different.[291] When a lower dose of medroxyprogesterone acetate was compared with DES, 1 mg/day, in a VACURG study, the progestational agent was again inferior to DES in retardation of tumor progression, though not in overall survival.[292] Some of these randomized trials have established that the 3 mg/day dosage of DES, which currently is often utilized, is associated with more frequent fluid retention and cardiovascular toxicity than the LHRH agonist[272] or antiandrogen[293] to which DES was compared.

Recently the concept of "total blockade" of the effects of both testicular and adrenal androgen production has aroused renewed interest because of the availability of pharmacologic means of achieving this effect with an LHRH agonist and an antiandrogen. Whether adrenal androgens contribute to the growth of prostatic cancer, either supplementary to the testicular hormonal source or after castration, is controversial, but elevated levels of dihydrotestosterone, the active metabolite of testosterone, have been demonstrated in prostatic cancer tissue after orchiectomy.[290,294] The lowest concentration of androgen that is capable of stimulating prostatic cancer growth is unknown, however.[290]

Early promising results with the combination of an LHRH agonist or orchiectomy and an antiandrogen as initial treatment for Stage D2 prostate cancer were obtained by Labrie and colleagues. Recently published data in 131 such patients indicate complete or partial response rates by NPCP criteria of 61%, disease stability in another 34%, actuarial 2-year freedom from tumor progression of 61%, and actuarial 2-year survival of 89%.[295] These results, if reproducible, appear superior to those achieved with previous forms of endocrine therapy. Preliminary results of a randomized study of leuprolide alone versus leuprolide plus flutamide in more than 600 patients with Stage D2 cancer indicate improvement in time to tumor progression with the combination regimen, but the magnitude of this difference is quite modest, with an increase from 13.8 to 16.5 months at the median point. The frequency of improvement in pain and serum acid phosphatase levels after 12 weeks of therapy also favors the two-drug regimen, but there is no significant difference in overall response to therapy or survival with the addition of flutamide to leuprolide, compared to results with leuprolide alone.[296]

Orchiectomy, an LHRH agonist (currently leuprolide in the U.S.), or DES in a dosage of 1 mg/day is presently the recommended standard therapy when hormonal therapy is required in prostatic cancer. Orchiectomy is preferred in men with cardiovascular disease or those who do not wish to take daily medication. LHRH agonists avert some of the psychological effects of orchiectomy, but leuprolide requires daily parenteral administration. Currently there is no proof that any form of hormonal therapy is superior to orchiectomy,[259,290] and initial therapy can be selected based on patient preference, consideration of side-effects, and expense.

The presence of elevated levels of nuclear androgen receptor proteins in prostatic tumor specimens is associated with improved response and survival on initial hormonal manipulation in most[297,298] but not all[299] studies. Heterogeneity of receptor content among tumor cells, sampling problems with small tissue specimens, and technical complexities of current assay systems limit widespread application of these tests. After patients fail initial treatment, a receptor assay would have major clinical utility if it could identify the small minority of patients with a high likelihood of response to a second endocrine therapy.

CYTOTOXIC CHEMOTHERAPY

In addition to major difficulties in objectively documenting tumor response, there are several other reasons for the modest utilization of chemotherapeutic agents in this disease. Prostatic cancer is a disease of older men, many of whom will die of intercurrent illness rather than of the tumor. Even in men with osseous metastases, the course of the disease varies markedly, making survival a poor criterion of treatment efficacy except in prospective randomized clinical trials. Customarily employed endocrine therapies are relatively nontoxic compared with chemotherapy. Finally, and perhaps most important, there are major limitations to the effectiveness of currently available drugs. The present status of chemotherapy in this tumor has been the subject of several reviews.[300-302]

Table 33-18 summarizes results of single-agent chemotherapy in hormone-resistant metastatic prostate cancer. Only drugs administered to at least 40 patients in Phase II or randomized NPCP trials that report "objective" response rates are included.[300] Although response criteria are variable, no chemotherapeutic agent has reproducibly yielded even a 20% complete plus partial remission rate in this setting. Despite its failure to produce tumor regression in all reported studies, doxorubicin had a superior response rate and was associated with better survival (after adjustment for prognostic factors) in a randomized comparison with 5-fluorouracil.[246] Estramustine phosphate, a nitrogen mustard covalently bound to estradiol, produces a high response rate in patients who have not had previous hormone therapy.[303] However, castrate levels of testosterone result from administration of the drug,[304] and the therapeutic contribution of the alkylating moiety is uncertain. As shown in Table 33-18, objective antitumor effects are minimal in men failing hormonal manipulation.

The initial prospective randomized trials of the NPCP compared single-agent cytotoxic chemotherapy in men with Stage D cancer who had failed endocrine treatment with "standard therapy," which included continued administration of other hormonal treatments and palliative irradiation. Of those who had not had major previous irradiation, 41% and 36% of men given cyclophosphamide and 5-fluorouracil, respectively, had *not* developed tumor progression after 12 weeks of treatment, compared with 19% given standard therapy. The difference in freedom from progressive disease between the cyclophosphamide and standard therapy treatment groups was statistically significant[305] and provided an impetus for further evaluation of chemotherapy in prostatic cancer. There was no significant difference in survival

TABLE 33-18. Single-Agent Chemotherapy in Hormone-Resistant Metastatic Prostatic Cancer*

Drug	*No. of Evaluable Patients*	*CR + PR (%)*	*Stable Disease (%)*
Doxorubicin	88	15	20
Cyclophosphamide	119†	6	34
Cisplatin	117	20	7
	92†	2	27
Estramustine phosphate	86	17	20
	163	3	25
5-Fluorouracil	14	29	21
	33†	12	42
Hydroxyurea	30	50	13
	28†	7	7
Prednimustine	23	0	0
	62†	0	13
Dacarbazine	55†	4	24
Methotrexate	58†	5	36
Amsacrine	40	0	25

*Modified from Eisenberger MA, Simon R, O'Dwyer PJ et al: A reevaluation of nonhormonal cytotoxic chemotherapy in the treatment of prostatic carcinoma. J Clin Oncol 3:827–841, 1985.
†NPCP trial.
CR = complete response, PR = partial response.

among the treatment arms, however.[300] In men who had had prior irradiation, the less myelosuppressive agents estramustine phosphate and streptozocin were compared with standard therapy. There were no significant differences in response rates or survival.[300,306] No other randomized trials of cytotoxic chemotherapy versus further endocrine management or supportive care in hormone-resistant prostate cancer have been reported to date.

Given the very modest efficacy of the available individual drugs, it is perhaps not surprising that randomized trials have failed to demonstrate any superiority of combination chemotherapy to single agent treatment (Table 33-19). In these studies, the intensity of drug administration was less than in some Phase II studies that were able to demonstrate objective response rates over 20% in good-prognosis patients who were extensively evaluated to document sites of measurable or evaluable tumor.[251,255] A two-drug combination that included doxorubicin produced a significantly higher response rate than hydroxyurea alone, although the survival rate was unaffected.[307]

Cytotoxic chemotherapy has also been administered to prostatic cancer patients without prior hormonal therapy, either in addition to or instead of an endocrine manipulation. The NPCP reported two prospective randomized trials in men with newly diagnosed Stage D2 disease who had not received prior systemic therapy; control patients received

TABLE 33-19. Randomized Trials of Combination Chemotherapy Versus Single-Agent Chemotherapy in Prostatic Cancer*

Study, Treatment	*No. of Evaluable Patients*	*CR + PR*	*Stable Disease*	*Median Survival*
Smalley et al[308]				
5-FU	32	2	5	34 wk
CTX + DXR + 5-FU	39	2	4	25 wk
Chlebowski et al[309]				
CTX	15	0	8	7.2 mo
CTX + DXR + 5-FU	12	0	6	8.9 mo
Muss et al[310]				
CTX	17	0	9	8 mo
CTX + MTX + 5-FU	15	1	7	5 mo
Herr[311]				
CCNU	20	0	6	24 wk
CTX + MTX + 5-FU	20	3	4	26 wk
Stephens et al[307]				
HU	69	1/24†	9	28 wk
CTX + DXR	68	6/19†	18	27 wk

*Modified from Eisenberger MA, Simon R, O'Dwyer PJ et al: A reevaluation of nonhormonal cytotoxic chemotherapy in the treatment of prostatic carcinoma. J Clin Oncol 3:827–841, 1985.
†Patients with measurable disease only.
5-FU = 5-fluorouracil, CTX = cyclophosphamide, DXR = doxorubicin, MTX = methotrexate, CCNU = lomustine, HU = hydroxyurea, CR = complete response, PR = partial response.

DES or orchiectomy. DES plus cyclophosphamide or estramustine phosphate plus cyclophosphamide were compared with standard therapy in the first study; DES plus cyclophosphamide plus 5-fluorouracil and estramustine phosphate were evaluated in the second study. There were no significant differences in response rate, time to tumor progression, or survival rate among treatment groups in either study.[259,260] Other studies have also confirmed that estramustine is not superior to DES as initial hormonal therapy in terms of time to tumor progression[303] or survival rate.[303,312]

Combination chemotherapy followed by hormone manipulation only after tumor progression has been given as initial treatment for good-risk patients presenting with distant metastases. Although the anticipated high response to subsequent endocrine treatment did occur, the response rate to chemotherapy alone was not remarkably higher than in the authors' experience with similar chemotherapy given after development of hormone resistance.[313]

Because male hormones are trophic for the malignant tissue in most prostatic cancer patients, an enhanced sensitivity to chemotherapy after stimulation of tumor growth by androgen administration has been postulated. Both early[314] and more recent[315,316] experience, however, suggests that even in men who have failed standard hormone treatment, androgens can produce subjective, objective, and possibly fatal tumor stimulation. A recent randomized study in hormone-refractory patients showed no benefit to "androgen priming" prior to administration of combination chemotherapy.[316]

Tumor regressions with cytotoxic chemotherapy do occur in patients with prostatic cancer resistant to hormonal therapy. Chemotherapy may be modestly better than continued hormone manipulation in delaying further tumor progression in this setting. Its impact is still marginal, however, and no drugs or regimens can be recommended as "standard treatment." Research to identify more drugs with greater antitumor activity is needed.

REFERENCES

1. American Cancer Society 1987 Cancer Facts & Figures. New York, American Cancer Society, 1986
2. Byar DP, Mostofi FK, Veterans Administration Cooperative Urological Research Group: Carcinoma of the prostate: Prognostic evaluation of certain pathologic features in 208 radical prostatectomies examined by the step-section technique. Cancer 30:5–13, 1972
3. Catalona WJ, Chretien P, Trahan EE: Abnormalities of cell-mediated immunocompetence in genitourinary cancer. J Urol 111:229–237, 1974
4. Wang MC, Papsidero LD, Valenzuela LA et al: Prostate antigen: A new potential marker for prostatic cancer. Prostate 2:89–96, 1981
5. Coffey DS, Isaacs JT: Requirements for an idealized animal model of prostatic cancer. In Murphy GP (ed): Models for Prostate Cancer pp 379–391. New York, Alan R Liss, 1980
6. Ferri A: Decaruncla Cusive callo quae cervici vesicae innascitur. Naples, 1553
7. Riolan J: Encheiridium Anatomicum et Pathologicum. Lugd Batav, 1649
8. Baillie M: The morbid anatomy of the human body. London, Longmans, 1794
9. Hunter J: Treatise on the Venereal Disease. London, 1788
10. Winkelstein W Jr, Ernster FL: Epidemiology and etiology of prostatic cancer. In Murphy GP (ed): Prostatic Cancer, pp 1–18. Littleton, Mass, PSG Publishing, 1979
11. Rotkin ID: Distribution and risk of prostatic cancer. In: Cancer Epidemiology in the USA and USSR, pp 111–123. NIH publication AD-2044, Washington, DC, US Government Printing Office, 1980
12. Doll R: Geographic variation in cancer incidence: A clue to causation. World J Surg 2:595–602, 1978
13. Breslow N, Chan CW, Dhom G et al: Latent carcinoma of prostate at autopsy in seven areas. Int J Cancer 20:680–688, 1977
14. Staszewshi J, Haenszel W: Cancer mortality among the Polish-born in the U.S. JNCI 35:291–297, 1965
15. Haenszel W, Kurihara M: Studies of Japanese migrants: I. Mortality from cancer and other disease among Japanese in the United States. JNCI 40:43–68, 1968
16. Malcolm D: Potential carcinogenic effect of cadmium in animals and man. Ann Occup Hyg 15:33–36, 1972
17. Krain LS: Epidemiologic variables in prostatic cancer. Geriatrics 2:93–97, 1973
18. Wynder EL, Mabushi K, Whitmore WJ Jr: Epidemiology of cancer of the prostate. Cancer 18:344–360, 1971
19. Haenszel WM, Marcus SC, Zimmerer EG: Cancer morbidity in urban and rural Iowa. Public Health Service monograph 37, Bethesda, Md, US Department of Health, Education and Welfare, 1957
20. Akazaki K, Stemmermann GN: Comparative study of latent carcinoma of the prostate among Japanese in Japan and Hawaii. JNCI 50:1137–1144, 1973
21. Hammond EC: Tobacco in persons at high risk of cancer. In Fraumani JF (ed): Persons at High Risk of Cancer: An Approach to Epidemiology and Control, pp 131–138. New York, Academic Press, 1975
22. Bean MA, Yatani R, Liu PI et al: Prostatic carcinoma at autopsy in Hiroshima and Nagasaki Japanese. Cancer 32:498–506, 1973
23. Woolf CM: An investigation of the familial aspects of carcinoma of the prostate. Cancer 13:739–744, 1960
24. Steele R, Lees REM, Kraus AS et al: Sexual factors in the epidemiology of cancer of the prostate. J Chronic Dis 24:29–37, 1971
25. Krain LS: Some epidemiologic variables in prostatic carcinoma in California. Prev Med 3:154–159, 1974
26. Schumman LM, Mandel J, Blackard C et al: Epidemiologic study of prostatic cancer: Preliminary report. Cancer Treat Rep 61:181–186, 1977
27. Rotkin ID: Studies in the epidemiology of prostatic cancer: Expanded sampling. Cancer Treat Rep 61:173–179, 1977
28. Glantz GM: Cirrhosis and carcinoma of the prostate gland. J Urol 91:291–293, 1964
29. Robson MC: Cirrhosis and prostatic neoplasms. Geriatrics 21:150–154, 1966
30. Rotkin ID: Epidemiologic clues to increase risk of prostatic cancer. In Spring-Mills E, Hafez ESE (eds): Male Accessory Sex Glands: Biology and Pathology, pp 289–309. New York, Elsevier/North-Holland, 1980
31. Greenwald PKV, Polan AK et al: Cancer of the prostate among men with benign prostatic hyperplasia. JNCI 53:335–340, 1974
32. Armenian HK, Lilienfeld AM, Diamond EL et al: Relationship between benign prostatic hyperplasia and cancer of the prostate. Lancet 2:115–117, 1974
33. Catalona WJ: Prostate Cancer. Orlando, Fla, Grune & Stratton, 1984
34. McNeal JE: Zonal anatomy of the prostate. Prostate 2:35–49, 1981
35. McNeal JE: Origin and development of carcinoma in the prostate. Cancer 23:24–34, 1969
36. McNeal JE: Morphogenesis of prostatic carcinoma. Cancer 18:1659–1666, 1965
37. McNeal JE: Regional morphology and pathology of the prostate. Am J Clin Pathol 49:347–356, 1968
38. Franks LM: Benign nodular hyperplasia of the prostate: A review. Ann R Coll Surg Engl 14:92–106, 1954
39. McNeal JE: Anatomy of the prostate: An historical survey of divergent views. Prostate 1:3–13, 1980
40. Blennerhassett JB, Vickery AL: Carcinoma of the prostate gland: An anatomical study of tumor location. Cancer 19:980–984, 1966
41. Whitmore WF Jr: The natural history of prostatic cancer. Cancer 32:1104–1112, 1973
42. Halpert B, Sheehan EE, Schmalhorst WR et al: Carcinoma of the prostate: A survey of 5,000 autopsies. Cancer 16:737–742, 1963
43. Halpert B, Schmalhorst WR: Carcinoma of the prostate in patients 70 to 79 years old. Cancer 19:695–698, 1966
44. Hanash KA, Utz DC, Cook EN et al: Carcinoma of the prostate: A 15-year follow up. J Urol 107:450–453, 1972
45. Jewett HJ: Radical perineal prostatectomy for palpable, clinically localized, non-obstructive cancer: Experience at the Johns Hopkins Hospital 1909–1963. J Urol 124:492–494, 1980
46. Flocks RH, Culp D, Porto R: Lymphatic spread from prostatic cancer. J Urol 81:194–196, 1959
47. Middleton RG: Value of and indications for staging pelvic lymph node dissection. Presented at the NIH Consensus Development Conference, Management of Clinically Localized Prostate Cancer, Bethesda, Md, June 15–17, 1987
48. McLaughlin AP, Saltzstein SL, McCullough DL et al: Prostatic carcinoma: Incidence and location of unsuspected lymphatic metastases. J Urol 115:89–94, 1976
49. Golimbu M, Morales P, Al-Askari S et al: Extended pelvic lymphadenectomy for prostatic cancer. J Urol 121:617–619, 1979
50. Pistenma DA, Bagshaw MA, Freiha FS: Extended-field radiation therapy for prostatic adenocarcinoma: Status report of a limited prospective trial. In Johnson DE, Samuels ML (eds): Cancer of the Genitourinary Tract, pp 229–247. New York, Raven Press, 1979
51. Prout GR Jr, Heaney JA, Griffin P et al: Nodal involvement as a prognostic indicator in patients with prostatic carcinoma. J Urol 124:226–231, 1980
52. Batson OV: The role of the vertebral veins in metastatic processes. Ann Intern Med 16:38–45, 1942

53. Dodds PR, Caride VJ, Lytton B: The role of vertebral veins in the dissemination of prostatic carcinoma. J Urol 126:753–755, 1981
54. Mostofi FK: Grading of prostatic carcinoma. Cancer Chemother Rep 59:111–117, 1975
55. Perez CA, Pilepich MV, Garcia D et al: Definitive radiation therapy in carcinoma of the prostate localized to the pelvis: Experience at the Mallinckrodt Institute of Radiology. Natl Cancer Inst Monogr (in press)
56. Gleason DF, Mellinger GT, Veterans Administration Cooperative Urological Research Group: Prediction of prognosis for prostatic adenocarcinoma by combined histological grading and clinical staging. J Urol 111:58–64, 1974
57. Gleason DF, Veterans Administration Cooperative Urological Research Group: Histologic grading and clinical staging of prostatic carcinoma. In Tannenbaum M (ed): Urologic Pathology: The Prostate, pp 171–198. Philadelphia, Lea & Febiger, 1977
58. Paulson DF, Uro-Oncology Research Group: The impact of current staging procedures in assessing disease extent of prostatic adenocarcinoma. J Urol 121:300–302, 1979
59. Kramer SA, Spahr J, Brendler CB et al: Experience with Gleason's histopathologic grading in prostatic cancer. J Urol 124:223–224, 1980
60. Freiha FS, Pistenma DA, Bagshaw MA: Pelvic lymphadenectomy for staging prostatic carcinoma: Is it always necessary? J Urol 122:176–177, 1979
61. Gaeta JF, Asirwatham JE, Miller G et al: Histologic grading of primary prostatic cancer: A new approach to an old problem. J Urol 123:689–693, 1980
62. Catalona WJ, Stein AJ, Fair WR: Grading errors in prostatic needle biopsies: Relation to the accuracy of tumor grade in predicting pelvic lymph node metastases. J Urol 127:919–922, 1982
63. Brawn N: The dedifferentation of prostate carcinoma. Cancer 52:246–251, 1983
64. Albert PS, Mallouh C, Nagamatsu GR: Transitional-cell carcinoma of the prostate. Urology 2:128–130, 1973
65. Bates RH Jr: Transitional cell carcinoma of the prostate. J Urol 101:206–207, 1969
66. Dube VE, Farrow GM, Greene LF: Prostatic adenocarcinoma of ductal origin. Cancer 32:402–409, 1973
67. Greene LF, O'Dea MJ, Dockery MD: Primary transitional cell carcinoma of the prostate. J Urol 116:761–763, 1976
68. Johnson DE, Hogan JM, Ayala AG: Transitional-cell carcinoma of the prostate: A clinical morphological study. Cancer 29:287–293, 1972
69. Kopelson G, Harisiadis L, Romas NA et al: Periurethral prostatic duct carcinoma: Clinical features and treatment results. Cancer 42:2894–2902, 1978
70. Tannenbaum, M: Histology of the prostate gland. In Tannenbaum M (ed): Urologic Pathology: The Prostate, pp 312–315. Philadelphia, Lea & Febiger, 1977
71. Bates HR: Transitional cell carcinoma of the prostate. J Urol 101:206–207, 1969
72. Greene LF, Mulcahy JJ, Warren MM et al: Primary transitional cell carcinoma of the prostate. J Urol 110:235–237, 1973
73. Wolfe JHN, Lloyd-Davis RW: The management of transitional cell carcinoma in the prostate. Br J Urol 53:253–257, 1981
74. Melicow MM, Pachter MR: Endometrial carcinoma of prostatic utricle (uterus masculinua). Cancer 20:1715–1722, 1967
75. Mostofi FK, Price EB Jr: Malignant tumors of the prostate. In: Atlas of Tumor Pathology: Tumors of the Male Genital System, 2nd series, fascicle 8, p 253. Washington, DC, Armed Forces Institute of Pathology, 1973
76. Galen RS, Gambino SR: Beyond Normality: The Predictive Value and Efficiency of Medical Diagnosis. New York, John Wiley & Sons, 1978
77. Watson RA, Tang DB: The predictive value of prostatic acid phosphatase as a screening test for prostatic cancer. N Engl J Med 303:497–499, 1980
78. Wang MC, Valenzuela LA, Murphy GP et al: Purification of a human prostatic specific antigen. Invest Urol 17:159–163, 1979
79. Papsidero LD, Kuriyama M, Wang MC et al: Prostate antigen: A marker for human prostate epithelial cells. JNCI 66:37–42, 1981
80. Papsidero LD, Wang MC, Valenzuela LA et al: A prostate antigen in sera of prostatic cancer patients. Cancer Res 40:2428–2432, 1980
81. Seamonds B, Yang N, Anderson K et al: Evaluation of prostate-specific antigen and prostatic acid phosphatase as prostate cancer markers. Urology 28:472–479, 1986
82. Stamey TA, Yang N, Hay AR et al: Prostate-specific antigen as a serum marker for adenocarcinoma of the prostate. N Engl J Med 317:909–916, 1987
83. Emmett JL, Barber KW Jr, Jackman RJ: Transrectal biopsy to detect prostatic carcinoma: A review and report of cases. J Urol 87:460–474, 1962
84. Jewett HJ: Significance of a palpable prostatic nodule. JAMA 160:838–839, 1956
85. Jewett HJ: The present status of radical prostatectomy for stages A and B prostatic cancer. Urol Clin North Am 2:105–124, 1975
86. Guinan P, Bush I, Ray V et al: The accuracy of the rectal examination in the diagnosis of prostate carcinoma. N Engl J Med 303:499–503, 1980
87. Franzen S, Giertz G, Zajicek J; Cytological diagnosis of prostatic tumor by transrectal aspiration biopsy: A preliminary report. Br J Urol 32:193–196, 1960
88. Andersson L, Jonsson G, Brunk U: Puncture biopsy of the prostate in the diagnosis of prostatic cancer. Scand J Urol Nephrol 1:227–234, 1967
89. Willems JS, Lowhage T: Transrectal fine needle aspiration biopsy for cytologic diagnosis in grading of prostatic carcinoma. Prostate 2:381–395, 1981
90. Esposti PL: Cytologic malignancy grading of prostatic carcinoma by transrectal aspiration biopsy. Scand J Urol Nephrol 5:199–209, 1971
91. Foti AG, Cooper JF, Herschman H et al: Detection of prostatic cancer by solid phase radio-immunoassay of serum prostatic acid phosphatase. N Engl J Med 297:1357–1361, 1977
92. Fair WR, Heston WDW, Kadmon D et al: Prostatic cancer, acid phosphatase, creatinine kinase-BB and race: A prospective study. J Urol 128:735–738, 1982
93. Yam LT: Clinical significance of the human acid phosphatase: A review. Am J Med 56:604–616, 1974
94. Whitesel JA, Donohue RE, Mani JH et al: Acid phosphatase-its influence on pelvic lymph node dissection (abstr 236). Presented at the annual meeting of the American Urologic Association, Kansas City, MO, May 1982
95. Belleville WD, Mahan DE, Sepulveda RA et al: Bone marrow acid phosphatase by radio-immuno assay: Three years of experience. J Urol 125:809–811, 1981
96. Paulson DF, Uro-Oncology Research Group: The impact of current staging procedures in assessing disease extent of prostatic adenocarcinoma. J Urol 121:300–302, 1979
97. Lund F, Smith PH, Suciu S, EORTC Urological Group: Do bone scans predict prognosis in prostatic cancer? A report of the EORTC protocol 3762. Br J Urol 56:58–63, 1984
98. Merrick MV, Ding CL, Chisholm GD et al: Prognostic significance of alkaline and acid phosphatase and skeletal scintigraphy in carcinoma of the prostate. Br J Urol 57:715–720, 1985
99. Murphy GP, Natarajan N, Pontes JE et al: The national survey of prostate cancer in the United States by the American College of Surgeons. J Urol 127:928–934, 1982
100. Hilaris BS, Whitmore WF, Batata MA et al: Behavioral patterns of prostate adenocarcinoma following an I-125 implant and pelvic node dissection. Int J Radiat Oncol Biol Phys 2:631–637, 1977
101. Pistenma DA, Bagshaw MA, Freiha FS: Extended-field radiation therapy for prostate adenocarcinoma: Status report of a limited prospective trial. In Johnson DE, Samuels ML (eds): Cancer of the Genitourinary Tract, pp 229–247. New York, Raven Press, 1979
102. Ray GR, Pistenma DA, Castellino RA et al: Operative staging of apparently localized adenocarcinoma of the prostate: Results in 50 unselected patients. I. Experimental design and preliminary results. Cancer 38:73–83, 1976
103. Gore RM, Moss AA: Value of computed tomography in interstitial ^{125}I brachytherapy of prostatic carcinoma. Radiology 146:453–458, 1983
104. Golimbu M, Morales P, Al-Askari S et al: CAT scanning in staging of prostatic cancer. Urology 18:305–308, 1981
105. Rifkin MD: Endorectal sonography of the prostate: Clinical implications. AJR 148:1137–1142, 1987
106. Lee F, Gray JM, McLeary RD et al: Prostatic evaluation of transrectal sonography: Criteria for diagnosis of early carcinoma. Radiology 158:91–95, 1986
107. Chodak GW, Wald V, Parmer E et al: Comparison of digital examination and transrectal ultrasonography for the diagnosis of prostate cancer. J Urol 135:951–954, 1986
108. Stone NN, Sogani PC, Rosenberg SM et al: Screening of ambulatory patients for prostate cancer by transrectal ultrasonography (unpublished manuscript)
109. Fisher H, Herr H, Sogani P et al: Modified pelvic lymph node dissection in patients undergoing I-125 implantation for carcinoma of the prostate (abstr). Presented at a conference on Prostate and Bladder Cancer, San Francisco, Oct 9–10, 1981
110. Paulson DF: The prognostic role of lymphadenectomy in adenocarcinoma of the prostate. Urol Clin North Am 7:615–622, 1980
111. Paulson DF, Perez CA, Anderson T: Genitourinary malignancies in cancer. In DeVita VT, Hellman S, Rosenberg SA (eds): Cancer: Principles and Practice of Oncology, ed 1, pp 732–785. Philadelphia, JB Lippincott, 1982
112. Arduino LJ, Glucksman MA: Lymph node metastases in early carcinoma of the prostate. J Urol 8:91–93, 1962
113. Whitmore WF Jr, Batata MA, Hilaris BS: Prostate irradiation: Iodine-125 implementation. In Johnson DE, Samuels ML (eds): Cancer of the Genitourinary Tract. New York, Raven Press, 1979
114. Cline WA, Kramer SA, Farnham R et al: Impact of pelvic lymphadenectomy in patients with prostatic adenocarcinoma. Urology 17:129–131, 1981
115. Freiha FS, Bagshaw MA: Carcinoma of the prostate: Results of post-irradiation biopsy. Prostate 5:19–25, 1984
116. Paulson DF, Cline WA, Hinshaw W, Uro-Oncology Research Group: Extended field radiation therapy vs delayed hormonal therapy in node positive prostatic adenocarcinoma. J Urol 127:935–937, 1982
117. Barzell W, Bean MA, Hilaris BS et al: Prostatic adenocarcinoma: Relationship of grade and local extent to pattern of metastases. J Urol 118:278–282, 1977
118. Grossman HB, Batata M, Hilaris D et al: I-125 implantation for carcinoma of prostate: Further follow-up of first 100 cases. Urology 20:591–598, 1982
119. Kramer SA, Cline WA Jr, Farnham R et al: Prognosis of patients with stage D-1 prostatic adenocarcinoma. J Urol 125:817–819, 1981
120. American Joint Committee on Cancer: Manual for Staging of Cancer. Beahrs OH, Myers MH (eds): Philadelphia, JB Lippincott, 1983
121. Rubin P (ed): Clinical Oncology. New York, American Cancer Society, 1983
122. Sheldon CA, Williams RD, Fraley EE: Incidental carcinoma of the prostate: A review of the literature and critical appraisal of classification. J Urol 124:626–631, 1980
123. McMillen SM, Wettlaufer JN: The role of repeat transurethral biopsy in stage A carcinoma of the prostate. J Urol 116:759–760, 1976
124. Parfitt HE, Smith JA, Gliedman JB et al: Accuracy of staging in A1 carcinoma of the prostate. Cancer 51:2346–2350, 1983
125. Golimbu M, Morales P: Stage A2 prostatic carcinoma: Should staging system be reclassified? Urology 13:592–596, 1979
126. Bauer WC, McGavran MH, Carlin MR: Unsuspected carcinoma of the prostate in

suprapubic prostatectomy specimens: A clinico-pathological study of 55 consecutive cases. Cancer 13:370–378, 1960
127. Heaney JA, Chang HC, Daly JJ et al: Prognosis of clinically undiagnosed prostatic carcinoma and the influence of endocrine therapy. J Urol 118:283–287, 1977
128. Barnes R, Hirst A, Rosenquist R: Early carcinoma of the prostate: Comparison of stages A and B. J Urol 115:404–405, 1976
129. DeVere White R, Paulson DF, Glenn JF: The clinical spectrum of prostate cancer. J Urol 117:323–327, 1977
130. Neglia WJ, Hussey DH, Johnson DE: Megavoltage radiation therapy for carcinoma of the prostate. Int J Radiat Oncol Biol Phys 2:873–882, 1977
131. Perez CA, Walz BJ, Zivnuska FR et al: Irradiation of carcinoma of the prostate localized to the pelvis: Analysis of tumor response and prognosis. Int J Radiat Oncol Biol Phys 6:555–563, 1980
132. Scott R Jr, Mutchnik DL, Laskowski TZ et al: Carcinoma of the prostate in elderly men: Incidence, growth characteristics and clinical significance. J Urol 101:602–607, 1969
133. Oesterling JE, Brendler CB, Epstein JI et al: Correlation of clinical stage, serum prostatic acid phosphatase and preoperative Gleason grade with final pathological stage in 175 patients with clinically localized adenocarcinoma of the prostate. J Urol 138:92–98, 1987
134. Bagshaw MA, Pistenma DA, Ray GR et al: Evaluation of extended-field radiotherapy for prostatic neoplasm: 1976 progress report. Cancer Treat Rep 61:297–306, 1977
135. McGowan DG: The value of extended field radiation therapy in carcinoma of the prostate. Int J Radiat Oncol Biol Phys 7:1333–1339, 1981
136. Kuban DA, El-Mahdi AM, Schellhammer PF: The effect of TURP on prognosis in prostatic carcinoma. Int J Radiat Oncol Biol Phys 13:1653–1659, 1987
137. Hanks GE: Optimizing the radiation treatment and outcome of prostate cancer. Int J Radiat Oncol Biol Phys 11:1235–1246, 1985
138. Huggins C, Masino MH, Eichelberger L et al: Quantitative studies of prostatic secretion. Characteristics of the normal secretion: The influence of thyroid suprarenal and testis extirpation and androgen substitution on the prostatic output. J Exp Med 70:543–556, 1939
139. Huggins C, Hodges CV: Studies on prostatic cancer: I. The effect of castration of estrogen and of androgen injection on serum phosphatases in metastatic carcinoma of the prostate. Cancer Research 1:293–297, 1941
140. Murphy GP, Sandberg AA (eds): Progress in Clinical and Biological Research, Vol 23, Prostate Cancer and Hormone Receptors. New York, Alan R Liss, 1979
141. Ekman P, Snochowski M, Zetterberg A et al: Steroid receptor content in human prostatic carcinoma and response to endocrine therapy. Cancer 44:1173–1181, 1979
142. Walsh PC: Radical prostatectomy with preservation of sexual function. Presented at the NIH Consensus Development Conference, Management of Clinically Localized Prostate Cancer, Bethesda, Md, June 15–17, 1987
143. Stamey TA: Cancer of the prostate: An analysis of some important contributions and dilemmas. Monogr Urol 67–94, 1982
144. Byar DP, Veterans Administration Cooperative Urological Research Group: Survival of patients with incidentally found microscopic cancer of the prostate: Results of a clinical trial of conservative treatment. J Urol 108:908–913, 1972
145. Barnes RW, Ninan CA: Carcinoma of the prostate: Biopsy and conservative therapy. J Urol 108:897–900, 1972
146. Thompson GJ: Transurethral resection of malignant lesions of the prostate gland. JAMA 120:1105–1109, 1942
147. Young YH: Early diagnosis and radical cure of carcinoma of the prostate: Being a study of 40 cases and presentations of radical operation. Bull Johns Hopkins Hosp 16:315–321, 1905
148. Freiha FS: Selection criteria for radical prostatectomy based on morphometric studies. Presented at the NIH Consensus Development Conference, Management of Clinically Localized Prostate Cancer, Bethesda, Md, June 15–17, 1987
149. Hutch JA: A new theory of anatomy of the internal urinary sphincter and the physiology of micturition: IV. the urinary sphinteric mechanism. J Urol 97:705–712, 1967
150. Vickery AL Jr, Kerr WS Jr: Carcinoma of the prostate treated by radical prostatectomy: A clinical pathological survey of 187 cases followed for five years and 148 cases followed for ten years. Cancer 16:1598–1608, 1983
151. Weyrauch HM: Surgery of the Prostate. Philadelphia, WB Saunders, 1959
152. Walsh PC: Radical prostatectomy with preservation of sexual function. Urologist Letter Club, March 24, 1983
153. Reiner WG, Walsh PC: An anatomical approach to the surgical management of a dorsal vein and Santorini's plexus during radical retropubic surgery. J Urol 121:198–200, 1979
154. Walsh PC, Donker PJ: Impotence following radical prostatectomy: Insight into etiology and prevention. J Urol 128:492–497, 1982
155. Fowler JE Jr, Clayton M, Roohallah S et al: Early experience with Walsh technique of radical retropubic prostatectomy. Urology 29:242–246, 1987
156. O'Donnell PD, Finan B: Urinary continence following nerve sparing radical prostatectomy. J Urol 137:225A, 1987
157. Walsh PC: Radical retropubic prostatectomy with preservation of sexual function: Evolution of a surgical procedure. AUA Update Series, vol 5, lesson 5, American Urological Association, 1985
158. Walsh PC: Preservation of sexual function and the surgical treatment of prostatic cancer: An anatomic surgical approach. In DeVita VT Jr, Hellman S, Rosenberg SA (eds): Important Advances in Oncology 1988. Philadelphia, JB Lippincott, 1988
159. Walsh PC: Radical retropubic prostatectomy and cystoprostatectomy: Surgical technique for preservation of sexual function. Film produced by Aegis Productions, distributed by Norwich Eaton Pharmaceuticals, 1984
160. Walsh PC: Radical retropubic prostatectomy. In Walsh PC, Gittes RF, Perlmutter AD et al (eds): Campbell's Textbook of Urology, 5th ed, vol 3, pp 2754–2775. Philadelphia, WB Saunders, 1986
161. Walsh PC, Epstein JI, Lowe FC: Potency following radical prostatectomy with wide unilateral excision of the neurovascular bundle. J Urol 138:823–827, 1987
162. Pasteau O: Traitement du cancer de la prostate par le radium. Rev Mal Nutr 1911, p 363
163. Young YH: Use of radium in cancer of the prostate and bladder. JAMA 68:1174–1177, 1917
164. Manon G: D'un moyen simple et facile d'applique le radium dans le cancer de la prostate. J Urol (Paris) 7:335, 1918
165. Deming CL: Results of 100 cases of cancer of the prostate and seminal vesicles treated with radium. Surg Gynecol Obstet 34:99–118, 1922
166. Barringer BS: Radium in the treatment of prostatic carcinoma. Ann Surg 80:881–884, 1924
167. Bumpus HC Jr: Radium in cancer of the prostate: Report of 217 cases. JAMA 78:1374–1376, 1922
168. Nitch CAR: The conservative treatment of carcinoma of the prostate. Br J Urol 8:329–336, 1936
169. Caulk JR: Carcinoma of the prostate. J Urol 37:832–839, 1937
170. Flocks RH: Interstitial irradiation therapy with a solution of Au198 as part of combination therapy for prostatic carcinoma. J Nucl Med 5:691–705, 1964
171. Whitmore WF Jr, Hilaris B, Grabstald H: Retropubic implantation of Iodine 125 in the treatment of prostatic cancer. J Urol 108:918–920,1972
172. Charyulu K, Block N, Sudarsanam A: Preoperative extended field radiation with I-125 seed implant in prostatic cancer: A preliminary report of a randomized study. Int J Radiat Oncol Biol Phys 5:1957–1961, 1979
173. Syed AMN, Puthwala AA, Tansey LA et al: Management of prostate carcinoma: Combination of pelvic lymphadenectomy, temporary IR-192 implantation and external irradiation. Radiology 19:829–833, 1983
174. Carlton CE Jr, Hudgins PT, Guerriero WG et al: Radiotherapy in the management of stage C carcinoma of the prostate. Trans Am Assoc Genitourinary Surg 67:70–74, 1975
175. Cosgrove MD, George FW III, Terry R: The effects of treatment on the local lesion of carcinoma of the prostate. J Urol 109:861–865, 1973
176. DelRegato JA: Long term curative results of radiotherapy of patients with inoperable prostatic carcinoma. Radiology 131:291–297, 1979
177. Pilepich MV, Krall JM, Sause WT et al: Prognostic factors in carcinoma of the prostate: Analysis of RTOG Study 75-06. Int J Radiat Oncol Biol Phys 13:339–349, 1987
178. Pilepich MV, Asbell SO, Krall JM et al: Correlation of radiotherapeutic parameters and treatment related morbidity: Analysis of RTOG Study 77-06. Int J Radiat Oncol Biol Phys 13:1007–1012, 1987
179. van der Werf-Messing D, Sourek-Zikova V, Blonk DI: Localized advanced carcinoma of the prostate: Radiation therapy vs hormonal therapy. Int J Radiat Oncol Biol Phys 1:1043–1048, 1976
180. Pilepich MV, Prasad SC, Perez CA: Computed tomography in definitive radiotherapy of prostatic carcinoma: Part 2. Definition of target volume. Int J Radiat Oncol Biol Phys 8:235–240, 1982
181. Lang PH: Adjuvant postoperative radiation therapy following radical prostatectomy. Presented at the NIH Consensus Development Conference, Management of Clinically Localized Prostate Cancer, Bethesda, Md, June 15–17, 1987
182. Pilepich MV, Walz BJ, Baglan RJ: Postoperative irradiation in carcinoma of the prostate. Int J Radiat Oncol Biol Phys 10:1869–1873, 1984
183. Ray GR, Cassady JR, Bagshaw MA: External beam megavoltage radiation treatment of post-radical prostatectomy residual or recurrent tumor: Preliminary results. J Urol 114:98–101, 1975
184. Cox JD, Kline RW: Do prostate biopsies 12 months or more after external irradiation for adenocarcinoma stage III, predict long-term survival? Int J Radiat Oncol Biol Phys 9:299–303, 1983
185. Leach GE, Cooper JF, Kagan AR et al: Radiotherapy for prostatic carcinoma: Postirradiation prostatic biopsy and recurrent patterns with long term followup. J Urol 128:505–509, 1982
186. Kiesling VJ, McAninch JW, Goebel JL et al: External beam radiotherapy for adenocarcinoma of the prostate: A clinical followup. J Urol 124:851–854, 1980
187. Kagan AR, Gordon J, Cooper JF et al: A clinical appraisal of post-irradiation biopsy in prostatic cancer. Cancer 39:637–641, 1977
188. van der Werf-Messing B: Prostatic cancer treated at the Rotterdam Radiotherapy Institute. Strahlentherapie 154:537–541, 1978
189. Carlton CE Jr, Dawoud F, Hudgins P et al: Irradiation treatment of carcinoma of the prostate: A preliminary report based on 8 years of experience. J Urol 108:924–927, 1972
190. Scardino PT: Local control of prostate cancer with radiation therapy: Frequency and significance of positive postirradiation prostatic biopsy results. Presented at the NIH Consensus Development Conference, Management of Clinically Localized Prostate Cancer, Bethesda, Md, June 15–17, 1987
191. Kraus PA, Lytton B, Weiss RM et al: Radiation therapy for local palliative treatment of prostatic cancer. J Urol 108:612–614, 1972
192. Joshi DP, Seery WH, Goldberg LG et al: Evaluation of phosphorus 32 for intractable pain secondary to prostatic carcinoma metastases. JAMA 193:621–623, 1965

193. Kaplan E, Fels IG, Kotlowski BR et al: Therapy of carcinoma of the prostate metastatic to bone with P32 labeled condensed phosphate. J Nucl Med 1:1, 1960
194. Smart JG: The use of P32 in the treatment of severe pain from bone metastases of carcinoma of the prostate. Br J Urol 37:139–147, 1965
195. Tong ECK, Finkelstein P: The treatment of prostatic bone metastases with parathormone and radioactive phosphorus. J Urol 109:71–75, 1973
196. Rubenfeld S: Treatment of bone metastases from carcinoma of the prostate with parathyroid hormone and radioactive phosphorus. Urology 1:268–269, 1973
197. Edland RW: Testosterone potentiated radiophosphorus therapy of osseous metastases in prostatic cancer. AJR 120:678–683, 1974
198. Pinck BD, Alexander S: Parathormone potentiated radiophosphorus therapy in prostatic carcinoma. Urology 1:201–204, 1972
199. Straffon RA, Kiser WS, Robitaille M et al: Yttrium hypophysectomy in the management of metastatic carcinoma of the prostate gland in 13 patients. J Urol 99:102–105, 1968
200. Larsson L-G, Sundbom C-M: Roentgen irradiation of the male breast. Acta Radiol Ther Phys Biol 58:253–256, 1962
201. Corvalan JG, Gill WM, Egleston TA et al: Irradiation of the male breast to prevent hormone produced gynecomastia. Am J Roentgenol Radiat Ther Nucl Med 106:839–840, 1969
202. Rodriguez-Antunez A, Cook SA, Jelden GL et al: Management of primary and metastatic carcinoma of the prostate by the radiotherapist. AJR 118:876–880, 1973
203. Walsh PC, Jewett HJ: Radical surgery for prostatic cancer. Cancer 45:1906–1908, 1980
204. Culp OS, Meyer JJ: Radical prostatectomy in the treatment of prostatic cancer. Cancer 32:1113–1118, 1973
205. Jewett HJ: The case for radical perineal prostatectomy. J Urol 103:195–199, 1970
206. Berlin BB, Cornwell PM, Connelly RR et al: Radical perineal prostatectomy for carcinoma of the prostate survival in 143 cases treated from 1935-1958. J Urol 99:97–101, 1968
207. Gibbons RP, Korrea RJ, Brannen GE et al: Total prostatectomy for localized prostatic cancer. J Urol 131:73–76, 1984
208. Lepor H, Kimball AW, Walsh PC: Cause-specific survival analysis following radical prostatectomy: The Johns Hopkins Experience. Presented at the NIH Consensus Development Conference, Management of Clinically Localized Prostate Cancer, Bethesda, Md, June 15–17, 1987
209. Bagshaw MA: Status of the radiation treatment of prostatic cancer at Stanford. Presented at the NIH Consensus Development Conference, Management of Clinically Localized Prostate Cancer, Bethesda, Md, June 15–17, 1987
210. Gibbons RP: Total prostatectomy for localized prostatic cancer: Long-term surgical results and current morbidity. The Virginia Mason Clinic experience. Presented at the NIH Consensus Development Conference, Management of Clinically Localized Prostate Cancer, Bethesda, Md, June 15–17, 1987
211. Byar DP, Corle DK: VACURG randomized trial of radical prostatectomy for stages I and II prostate cancer. Urology 17(suppl):7–11, 1981
212. Madsen PO, Corle DK, Byar DP: Radical prostatectomy for carcinoma of the prostate: Stages I and II. In Rost A, Fielder U (eds): Proceedings, International Symposium on the Treatment of Carcinoma of the Prostate, p 46. Berlin, Berlin Urologische Klinik, Klinikum Steglitz, Freie Universität, 1980
213. Paulson DF, Lin GH, Hinshaw W, Stephani S, Uro-Oncology Research Group: Radical surgery versus radiotherapy for adenocarcinoma of the prostate. J Urol 128:502–504, 1982
214. Hanks GE: National practice results of external beam radiation for prostate cancer. Presented at the NIH Consensus Development Conference, Management of Clinically Localized Prostate Cancer, Bethesda, Md, June 15–17, 1987
215. Paulson DF: Randomized series of surgery versus radiation therapy. Presented at the NIH Consensus Development Conference, Management of Clinically Localized Prostate Cancer, Bethesda, Md, June 15–17, 1987
216. Pilepich MV, Bagshaw MA, Asbell SO et al: Definitive radiotherapy in resectable (stage A2 and B) carcinoma of the prostate: Results of a nationwide overview. Int J Radiat Oncol Biol Phys 13:659–663, 1987
217. Taylor WJ, Richardson RG, Hafermann MD: Radiation therapy for localized prostate cancer. Cancer 43:1123–1127, 1979
218. Gibbons RP, Mason JT, Correa RJ Jr et al: Carcinoma of the prostate: Local control with external beam radiation therapy. J Urol 121:310–312, 1979
219. Hussey DH, Chan R, Delclos L et al: Radiotherapy for carcinoma of the prostate. Cancer Bull 30:131–134, 1978
220. Harisiadis L, Veenema RJ, Senyszyn JJ et al: Carcinoma of the prostate: Treatment with external radiotherapy. Cancer 41:2131–2152, 1978
221. Lipsett JA, Cosgrove MD, Green N et al: Factors influencing prognosis in the radiotherapeutic management of carcinoma of the prostate. Int J Radiat Oncol Biol Phys 1:1049–1058, 1976
222. Hanks GE, Leibel SA, Krall JM et al: Patterns of care studies: Dose-response observations for local control of adenocarcinoma of the prostate. Int J Radiat Oncol Biol Phys 11:153–157, 1985
223. Radiation Therapy Oncology Group: Protocol 75-06 randomized radiation therapy for adenocarcinoma of the prostate, stage C or stage B, with positive pelvic nodes. Philadelphia, Radiation Therapy Oncology Group, 1975
224. Radiation Therapy Oncology Group: Protocol 77-06 randomized radiation therapy for adenocarcinoma of the prostate, stage B or A2. Philadelphia, Radiation Therapy Oncology Group, 1977
225. Asbell SO, Krall JM, Pilepich MV et al: Elective pelvic irradiation in stage A_2, B carcinoma of the prostate: Analysis of RTOG 77-06. Int J Radiat Oncol Biol Phys (in press)
226. Hilaris BS, Whitmore WF, Batata MA et al: ^{125}I implantation of the prostate: Dose-response considerations. Front Radiat Ther Oncol 12:82–90, 1978
227. Sogani PC, DeCosse JJ Jr, Montie J et al: Carcinoma of the prostate: Treatment with pelvic lymphadenectomy and 125 iodine implants. Clin Bull 9:24–31, 1979
228. Batata MA, Hilaris BS, Chu FCH et al: Radiation therapy in adenocarcinoma of the prostate with pelvic lymph node involvement on lymphadenectomy. Int J Radiat Oncol Biol Phys 6:149–153, 1980
229. Catalona WJ, Dresner SM: Nerve-sparing radical prostatectomy: Extraprostatic tumor extension and preservation of erectile function. J Urol 134:1149–1151, 1985
230. Hindsley JP Jr, Sanfelippo CJ, Fowler JE Jr et al: Mini dose heparin therapy in pelvic lymphadenectomy and ^{125}I implantation for localized prostatic cancer. Urology 15:272–274, 1980
231. Hazra TA, Giri S: Prophylactic pelvic girdle irradiation in the treatment of prostatic carcinoma. Int J Radiat Oncol Biol Phys 7:817–819, 1981
232. Pilepich MV, Perez CA, Walz BJ et al: Complications of definitive radiotherapy for carcinoma of the prostate. Int J Radiat Oncol Biol Phys 7:1341–1348, 1981
233. Ray GR, Cassady R, Bagshaw MA: Definitive radiation therapy of carcinoma of the prostate: A report on 15 years of experience. Radiology 106:407–418, 1973
234. Dewit L, Ang KK, van der Schueren E: Acute side effects and late complications after radiotherapy of localized carcinoma of the prostate. Cancer Treat Rev 10:79–89, 1983
235. Perez CA: Carcinoma of the prostate, a vexing biological and clinical enigma. Int J Radiat Oncol Biol Phys 9:1427–1438, 1983
236. Pilepich MV, Pajak T, George FW et al: Preliminary report on phase III RTOG studies on extended-field irradiation in carcinoma of the prostate. Am J Clin Oncol 6:485–491, 1983
237. Yagoda A, Watson RC, Natale RB et al: A critical analysis of response criteria in patients with prostatic cancer treated with cis-diamminedichloride platinum: II. Cancer 44:1553–1562, 1979
238. Pollen JJ, Gerber K, Ashburn WL et al: Nuclear bone imaging in metastatic cancer of the prostate. Cancer 47:2585–2594, 1981
239. Levenson RM, Sauerbrunn BJL, Bates HR et al: Comparative value of bone scintigraphy and radiography in monitoring tumor response in systemically treated prostatic carcinoma. Radiology 146:513–518, 1983
240. Paulson DF, Berry WR, Cox EB et al: Treatment of metastatic endocrine-unresponsive carcinoma of the prostate gland with multiagent chemotherapy: Indicators of response to therapy. JNCI 63:615–622, 1979
241. Schmidt JD, Johnson DE, Scott WW et al: Chemotherapy of advanced prostatic cancer: Evaluation of response parameters. Urology 7:602–610, 1976
242. Johnson DE, Scott WW, Gibbons RP et al: Clinical significance of serum acid phosphatase levels in advanced prostatic carcinoma. Urology 8:123–126, 1976
243. Fujino A, Scardino PT: Transrectal ultrasonography for prostate cancer: II. The response of the prostate to definitive radiotherapy. Cancer 57:935–940, 1986
244. Kojima M, Watanabe H, Ohe H et al: Kinetic evaluation of the effect of LHRH analog on prostatic cancer using transrectal ultrasonography. Prostate 10:11–17, 1987
245. Byar DP: VACURG studies on prostatic cancer and its treatment. In Tannenbaum M (ed): Urologic Pathology: The Prostate, pp 241–267. Philadelphia, Lea & Febiger, 1977
246. DeWys WD, Begg CB, Brodovsky H et al: A comparative clinical trial of Adriamycin and 5-fluorouracil in advanced prostatic cancer: Prognostic factors and response. Prostate 4:1–11, 1983
247. Slack NH, Mittelman A, Brady MF et al: The importance of the stable category for chemotherapy treated patients with advancing and relapsing prostate cancer. Cancer 46:2393–2402, 1980
248. Zweig MH, Ihde DC: Assessment of serum radioimmune and enzymatic prostatic acid phosphatase and radioimmune creatine kinase BB for monitoring response to therapy in metastatic prostate cancer. Cancer Res 45:3945–3950, 1985
249. Brenckman WD, Lastinger LB, Sedor F: Unpredictable fluctuations in serum acid phosphatase activity in prostatic cancer. JAMA 245:2501–2504, 1981
250. Killian CS, Yang N, Emrich LJ et al: Prognostic importance of prostate specific antigen for monitoring patients with stages B2 to D1 prostate cancer. Cancer Res 45:886–891, 1985
251. Logothetis CJ, Samuels MJ, von Eschenbach AC et al: Doxorubicin, mitomycin-C, and 5-fluorouracil (DMF) in the treatment of metastatic hormonal refractory adenocarcinoma of the prostate, with a note on the staging of metastatic prostate cancer. J Clin Oncol 1:368–379, 1983
252. Winkler CF, Dunnick NR, Eddy J et al: Computed tomography of the abdomen and pelvis: Documentation of tumor response and progression in disseminated prostate cancer. Med Pediatr Oncol 4:20–25, 1986
253. Torti FM, Aston D, Lum BL et al: Weekly doxorubicin in endocrine-refractory carcinoma of the prostate. J Clin Oncol 1:477–482, 1983
254. Berry WR, Laszlo J, Cox E et al: Prognostic factors in metastatic and hormonally unresponsive carcinoma of the prostate. Cancer 44:763–775, 1979
255. Ihde DC, Bunn PA, Cohen MH et al: Effective treatment of hormonally-unresponsive metastatic carcinoma of the prostate with Adriamycin and cyclophosphamide: Methods of documenting tumor response and progression. Cancer 45:1300–1310, 1980
256. Slack NH, Brady MF, Murphy GP et al: A reexamination of the stable category for evaluating response in patients with advanced prostate cancer. Cancer 54:564–574, 1984

257. Torti FM: Response criteria in urologic malignancies: Recent results. Cancer Res 85:50–57, 1983
258. Huggins C, Stevens RE, Hodges CV: Studies on prostatic cancer: II. The effects of castration on advanced carcinoma of the prostate gland. Arch Surg 43:209–223, 1941
259. Grayhack JT, Keeler TC, Kozlowski JM: Carcinoma of the prostate: Hormonal therapy. Cancer 60:589–601, 1987
260. Menon M, Walsh PC: Hormonal therapy for prostatic cancer. In Murphy GP (ed): Prostatic Cancer, pp 175–200. Littleton, Ma, PSG Publishing, 1979
261. Shearer RJ, Hendry WF, Sommerville IF et al: Plasma testosterone: An accurate monitor of hormone treatment of prostatic cancer. Br J Urol 45:668–677, 1973
262. Geller J, Albert J, Yen SSC: Treatment of advanced cancer of prostate with megestrol acetate. Urology 12:537–541, 1978
263. Warren B, Worgul TJ, Drago J et al: Effect of very high dose D-leucine-6-gonadotropin-releasing hormone proethylamide on the hypothalamic-pituitary testicular axis in patients with prostatic cancer. J Clin Invest 71:1842–1853, 1983
264. Worgul TJ, Santen RJ, Samojlik E et al: Clinical and biochemical effect of aminoglutethimide in the treatment of advanced prostatic carcinoma. J Urol 129:51–55, 1983
265. Ahmann FR, Crawford ED, Kreis W et al: Adrenal steroid levels in castrated men with prostatic carcinoma treated with aminoglutethimide plus hydrocortisone. Cancer Res 47:4736–4739, 1987
266. Tapazoglou E, Subramanian MG, Al-Sarraf M et al: High-dose ketoconazole therapy in patients with metastatic prostate cancer. Am J Clin Oncol 9:369–375, 1986
267. Walsh PC, Siiteri PK: Suppression of plasma androgens by spironolactone in castrated men with carcinoma of the prostate. J Urol 114:254–256, 1975
268. Sogani PC, Vagaiwala MR, Whitmore WF: Experience with flutamide in patients with advanced prostatic cancer without prior endocrine therapy. Cancer 54:744–750, 1984
269. Torti FM, Lum BL, Lo R et al: Tamoxifen in advanced prostatic carcinoma: A dose escalation study. Cancer 54:739–743, 1984
270. Murphy GP, Huben RP, Priore R: Results of another trial of chemotherapy with and without hormones in patients with newly diagnosed metastatic prostatic cancer. Urology 28:36–40, 1986
271. Murphy GP, Beckley S, Brady MR et al: Treatment of newly diagnosed metastatic prostate cancer patients with chemotherapy agents in combination with hormones versus hormones alone. Cancer 51:1264–1272, 1983
272. Leuprolide Study Group: Leuprolide versus diethylstilbestrol for metastatic prostatic cancer. N Engl J Med 311:1281–1286, 1984
273. Blackard CE, Byar DP, Jordan WP: Orchiectomy for advanced prostatic carcinoma: A reevaluation. Urology 1:553–560, 1973
274. Nesbit RM, Baum WC: Endocrine control of prostatic carcinoma: Clinical and statistical survey of 1,818 cases. JAMA 143:1317–1320, 1950
275. Bhanalaph T, Varkarakis MJ, Murphy GP: Current status of bilateral adrenalectomy for advanced prostatic carcinoma. Ann Surg 179:17–23, 1974
276. Silverberg GD: Hypophysectomy in the treatment of disseminated prostatic carcinoma. Cancer 39:1727–1731, 1977
277. Citrin DL, Kies MS, Wallemark C-B et al: A phase II study of high dose estrogens (diethylstilbestrol diphosphate) in prostate cancer. Cancer 56:457–460, 1985
278. Eisenberger MA, O'Dwyer PJ, Friedman MA: Gonadotropin hormone-releasing hormone analogues: A new therapeutic approach for prostatic cancer. J Clin Oncol 4:414–424, 1986
279. Drago JR, Santen RJ, Liptonk A et al: Clinical effect of aminoglutethimide, medical adrenalectomy, in treatment of 43 patients with advanced prostatic carcinoma. Cancer 53:1447–1450, 1984
280. Glick JH, Wein A, Padavic K et al: Phase II trial of tamoxifen in metastatic carcinoma of the prostate. Cancer 49:1367–1372, 1982
281. Brendler H, Prout G: A cooperative group study of prostatic cancer: Stilbestrol versus placebo in advanced progressive disease. Cancer Chemother Rep 16:323–328, 1962
282. Reiner WG, Scott WW, Eggleston JC et al: Long-term survival after hormonal therapy for stage D prostatic cancer. J Urol 122:183–184, 1979
283. Lepor H, Ross A, Walsh PC: The influence of hormonal therapy on survival of men with advanced prostatic cancer. J Urol 128:335–340, 1982
284. Byar DP: Survival of patients with incidentally found microscopic cancer of the prostate: Results of a clinical trial of conservative treatment. J Urol 108:908–913, 1972
285. Arduino LJ, Bailar JC, Becker LE et al: Carcinoma of the prostate: Treatment comparisons. J Urol 98:516–522, 1967
286. Byar DP: The Veterans Administration Cooperative Urologic Research Group's studies of cancer of the prostate. Cancer 32:1126–1130, 1973
287. Bailar JC, Byar DP: Estrogen treatment for cancer of the prostate: Early results with 3 doses of diethylstilbestrol and placebo. Cancer 26:257–261, 1970
288. Byar DP, Green SB: The choice of treatment for cancer patients based on covariate information. Bull Cancer 67:477–490, 1980
289. Parmer H, Edwards L, Phillips RH et al: Orchiectomy versus long-acting D-trp-6-LHRH in advanced prostatic cancer. Br J Urol 59:249–254, 1987
290. Smith JA: New methods of endocrine management of prostatic cancer. J Urol 137:1–10, 1987
291. Pavone-Macaluso M, de Voogt HJ, Viggiano G et al: Comparison of diethylstilbestrol, cyproterone acetate, and medroxyprogesterone acetate in the treatment of advanced prostatic cancer: Final analysis of a randomized phase III trial of the EORTC urological group. J Urol 136:624–631, 1986
292. Byar DP: Hormone therapy: Results of the VACURG studies. In: Management of Clinically Localized Prostate Cancer: NIH Consensus Development Conference, pp 117–119. Bethesda, MD, National Cancer Institute, 1987
293. de Voogt HJ, Smith PH, Pavone-Macaluso M et al: Cardiovascular side effects of diethylstilbestrol, cyproterone acetate, medroxyprogesterone acetate, and estramustine phosphate used for the treatment of advanced prostatic cancer: Results from EORTC trials 30761 and 30762. J Urol 135:303–307, 1986
294. Geller J: Rationale for blockade of adrenal as well as testicular androgens in the treatment of advanced prostate cancer. Semin Oncol 12(suppl 1):28–35, 1985
295. Labrie F, Dupont A, Giguere M et al: Advantages of the combination therapy in previously untreated and treated patients with advanced prostate cancer. J Steroid Biochem 25:877–883, 1986
296. Crawford ED, McLeod D, Dorr A et al: A comparison of leuprolide with flutamide and leuprolide in previously untreated patients with clinical stage D2 cancer of the prostate. J Urol 137:256A, 1987
297. Trachtenberg J, Walsh PC: Correlation of prostatic nuclear androgen receptor content with duration of response and survival following hormonal therapy in advanced prostatic cancer. J Urol 127:466–471, 1982
298. Benson RC, Gorman PA, O'Brien PC et al: Relationship between androgen receptor binding activity in human prostate cancer and clinical response to endocrine therapy. Cancer 59:1599–1606, 1987
299. Gorelic LS, Lamm DL, Ramzy I et al: Androgen receptors in biopsy specimens of prostate adenocarcinoma: Heterogeneity of distribution and relation to prognostic significance of receptor measurements for survival of advanced cancer patients. Cancer 60:211–219, 1987
300. Eisenberger MA, Simon R, O'Dwyer PJ et al: A reevaluation of nonhormonal cytotoxic chemotherapy in the treatment of prostatic carcinoma. J Clin Oncol 3:827–841, 1985
301. Tannock IF: Is there evidence that chemotherapy is of benefit to patients with carcinoma of the prostate? J Clin Oncol 3:1013–1021, 1985
302. Torti FM: Prostatic cancer chemotherapy: Recent results. Cancer Res 85:58–69, 1983
303. Smith PH, Suciu S, Robinson RG et al: A comparison of the effect of diethylstilbestrol with low dose estramustine phosphate in the treatment of advanced prostate cancer: Final analysis of a phase III trial of the EORTC. J Urol 136:619–623, 1986
304. Nickel CJ, Morales A: Estramustine phosphate versus stilbestrol as primary treatment for metastatic cancer of the prostate. Can J Surg 26:434–438, 1983
305. Scott WW, Johnson DE, Schmidt JE et al: Chemotherapy of advanced prostatic carcinoma with cyclophosphamide or 5-fluorouracil: Results of first national randomized study. J Urol 114:909–911, 1975
306. Murphy GP, Gibbons RP, Johnson DE et al: A comparison of estramustine phosphate and streptozotocin in patients with advanced prostatic carcinoma who have had extensive irradiation. J Urol 118:288–291, 1977
307. Stephens RL, Vaughn C, Lane M et al: Adriamycin and cyclophosphamide versus hydroxyurea in advanced prostatic cancer: A randomized Southwest Oncology Group study. Cancer 53:406–410, 1984
308. Smalley RV, Bartolucci AA, Hemstreet G et al: A phase II evaluation of a 3-drug combination of cyclophosphamide, doxorubicin, and 5-fluorouracil in patients with advanced bladder carcinoma or stage D prostatic carcinoma. J Urol 125:191–195, 1981
309. Chlebowski RT, Hestorff R, Sardoff L et al: Cyclophosphamide versus the combination of Adriamycin, 5-fluorouracil, and cyclophosphamide in the treatment of metastatic prostatic cancer: A randomized trial. Cancer 42:2546–2552, 1978
310. Muss HB, Howard V, Richards F et al: Cyclophosphamide versus cyclophosphamide, methotrexate, and 5-fluorouracil in advanced prostatic cancer: A randomized trial. Cancer 47:1949–1953, 1981
311. Herr HW: Cyclophosphamide, methotrexate, and 5-fluorouracil combination chemotherapy versus chlorethyl-cyclohexyl-nitrosourea in the treatment of metastatic prostatic cancer. J Urol 127:4620–4625, 1982
312. Benson RC, Gill GM: Estramustine phosphate compared with diethylstilbestrol: A randomized, double-blind, crossover trial for stage D prostate cancer. Am J Clin Oncol 9:341–351, 1986
313. Seifter EJ, Bunn PA, Cohen MH et al: A trial of combination chemotherapy followed by hormonal therapy for previously untreated metastatic carcinoma of the prostate. J Clin Oncol 4:1365–1373, 1986
314. Fowler JE, Whitmore WF: Considerations for the use of testosterone with systemic chemotherapy in prostatic cancer. Cancer 49:1373–1377, 1982
315. Suarez AJ, Lamm DL, Radwin HM et al: Androgen priming and cytotoxic chemotherapy in advanced prostatic cancer. Cancer Chemother Pharmacol 8:261–265, 1982
316. Manni A, Santen RJ, Boucher AE et al: Androgen priming and response to chemotherapy in advanced prostatic cancer. J Urol 136:1242–1256, 1986

WILLIAM R. FAIR
CARLOS A. PEREZ
TOM ANDERSON

CHAPTER 34 *Cancer of the Urethra and Penis*

Malignant lesions of the urethra and penis are uncommon tumors. This fact has contributed somewhat to the controversy regarding their treatment, in that no single institution has sufficient patients to define the natural history and proper therapy. Treatment has often been empiric and published reports anecdotal.

Squamous cell carcinoma is the most common cancer in the penis and urethra. The pattern of spread is primarily a reflection of the area of the organ affected. Likewise, the treatment approach, and in large measure the overall prognosis, is directly related to the region of the urethra or penis involved.

CARCINOMA OF THE MALE URETHRA

Carcinoma of the male urethra is extremely rare, with only approximately 600 cases reported in the world literature.[1] Such carcinomas have been reported in boys as young as 13 years and in men as old as 91, although most patients are over 50 years of age with a peak incidence at 58 years.[2] Significant etiologic factors have not been identified, but chronic inflammation is thought to play a role in the initiation of the disease on the basis of the observation that many patients give a history of prior venereal disease, urethritis, or urethral stricture. The incidence of urethral stricture in men with carcinoma of the male urethra is reported to range from 24% to 76%, with the most frequent site also being the most frequent site of malignancy.[3–6] No racial predisposition has been recorded.

As in bladder cancer, a high percentage of males with carcinoma of the urethra give a history of smoking or occupational exposure to known carcinogens. However, no epidemiologic studies have unequivocally linked these factors to the development of urethral carcinoma.

SYMPTOMS

The lesion is often insidious at onset, with the symptoms being attributed primarily to benign stricture disease rather than to malignancy. Urethral stricture or bleeding in a patient without a history of trauma or venereal disease, or the onset of a perineal abscess or fistula in an elderly man, should suggest the possibility of urethral carcinoma. Because of the nonspecific nature of the symptoms, the interval between the initiation of symptoms and the diagnosis is as long as 15 years with an average of 5 months.[7] The most common presenting symptoms are listed in Table 34-1; most reflect local involvement by the lesion.

PATHOLOGY

Tumors of the male urethra may be categorized according to the histology of the cells lining the anatomic region of origin (Fig. 34-1). The transitional epithelium of the prostatic urethra gives rise to transitional cell malignancy that is histologically and clinically distinct from the adenocarcinoma commonly associated with prostatic malignancy. Benign lesions of condyloma acuminatum, benign papillomas, and urethral caruncles are found within the distal penile urethra and

TABLE 34-1. Presenting Symptoms of Carcinoma of the Male Urethra in 47 Cases

Symptoms	*Number*	*(%)*
Palpable urethral mass	34	(72)
Obstructive symptoms (with or without retention)	32	(65)
Pain	12	(26)
Urethral fistula/periurethral abscess	10	(21)
Hematuria	10	(21)
Palpable inguinal mass	9	(19)

meatus. In published reports, 59% of tumors occurred in the bulbomembranous urethra, 34% in the penile urethra, and 7% in the prostatic urethra. Histologically, 78% of male urethral carcinomas were squamous cell carcinoma, 15% transitional carcinoma, 6% adenocarcinoma, and 1% undifferentiated carcinoma.

Male urethral carcinoma tends to spread by direct extension to adjacent structures and usually involves the vascular spaces of the corpus spongiosum and the periurethral tissues. Carcinoma of the bulbomembranous urethra often extends to the urogenital diaphragm, prostate, perineum, and scrotal skin. Hematogenous spread is uncommon except in advanced disease. Metastasis occurs by lymphatic embolization to regional lymph nodes. The lymphatics from the anterior urethra drain into the superficial and deep inguinal nodes and occasionally to the external iliac nodes, whereas the lymphatics from the posterior urethra drain into the external iliac, obturator, and hypogastric nodes. Tumors of the anterior urethra generally metastasize to the inguinal nodes and tumors of the posterior metastasize to pelvic nodes; however, there are some exceptions.[8]

FIG. 34-1. Anatomy and pathology of urethral carcinoma.

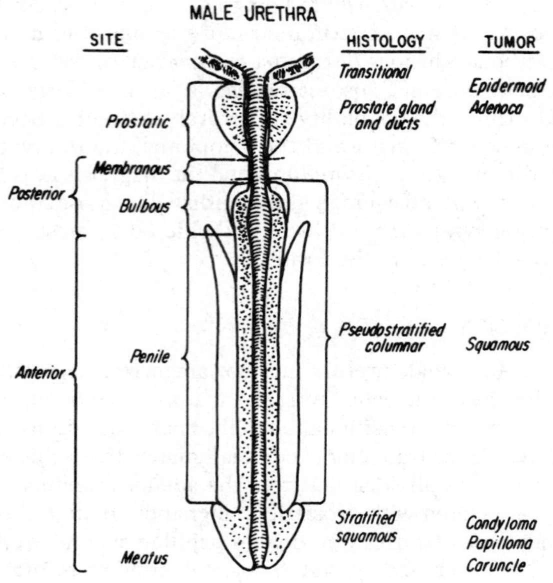

TABLE 34-2. Staging System for Carcinoma of the Male Urethra

Stage	*Criteria*
O	Confined to mucosa only (in situ)
A	Into but not beyond lamina propria
B	Into but not beyond substance of corpus spongiosum or into but not beyond prostate
C	Direct extension into tissues beyond corpus spongiosum (corpora cavernosa, muscle, fat, fascia, skin, direct skeletal involvement), or beyond prostatic capsule
D_1	Regional metastasis including inguinal and/or pelvic lymph nodes (with any primary tumor)
D_2	Distant metastasis (with any primary tumor)

Modified from Ray B, Canto AR, Whitmore W: Experience with primary carcinoma of the male urethra. J Urol 117:591–594, 1977.

EVALUATION AND STAGING

The diagnosis is made by transurethral or needle biopsy. The extent of local involvement can be determined by careful inspection and palpation of the external genitalia and perineum at the time of cystourethroscopy and by bimanual examination with the patient under anesthesia. Cytologic studies of voided urine may be helpful for the diagnosis in some patients.[1] A CT scan or MRI is helpful in evaluating the pelvic and para-aortic nodes. A lymphangiogram may be of value in selected cases but is not required routinely.

The most common staging system currently is that proposed by Ray and associates (Table 34-2). A system proposed by the American Joint Committee (AJC) based on the extent of the primary tumor and the presence or absence of regional lymph node involvement or distant metastases is given in Table 34-3.

TABLE 34-3. Staging System for Urethral Cancer (American Joint Committee)

T–Primary Tumor (Male)	
Tx	Primary tumor cannot be assessed
T0	No evidence of primary tumor
Tis	Carcinoma in situ
Ta	Noninvasive papillary, polypoid, or verrucous carcinoma
T1	Tumor invades subepithelial connective tissue
T2	Tumor invades corpus spongiosum or prostate or periurethral muscle
T3	Tumor invades corpus cavernosum or beyond prostatic capsule or bladder neck
T4	Tumor invades other adjacent organs
N–Regional Lymph Nodes	
Nx	Regional lymph nodes cannot be assessed
N0	No regional lymph node metastasis
N1	Metastasis in a single lymph node, 2 cm or less in greatest dimension
N2	Metastasis in a single lymph node, more than 2 cm but no more than 5 cm in greatest dimension, or multiple lymph nodes, none more than 5 cm in greatest dimension
N3	Metastasis in a lymph node(s) more than 5 cm in greatest dimension
M–Distant Metastasis	
Mx	Presence of distant metastasis cannot be assessed
M0	No distant metastasis
M1	Distant metastasis

TREATMENT

General Philosophy

The primary mode of therapy for carcinoma of the male urethra is surgical excision of the lesion. The extent of surgery depends on the location and stage of the tumor. In general, anterior urethral carcinoma seems more amenable to surgical control than does posterior urethral carcinoma; perhaps as a consequence, the prognosis for patients with lesions originating in the anterior urethra is better than that of those with tumors situated posteriorly.

A comparison of the results of surgical excision and radiation therapy is difficult because of the low incidence of the disease. As with surgery, the results of radiation therapy are very much dependent on the site of the tumor, with anterior urethral lesions responding better than posterior ones.[2]

Modern combinations of chemotherapy are capable of producing meaningful objective regression of regionally advanced or metastatic urothelial carcinomas. The MVAC regimen (methotrexate, vinblastine, doxorubicin, and cisplatin) has produced significant tumor regression in a majority of patients with transitional cell carcinoma of the urinary tract.[9–11] Of note is that tumors of nontransitional histology appear to be resistant to this combination. The MVAC regimen causes significant myelosuppression, and the potential for nephrotoxicity and cardiotoxicity necessitate careful attention to detail in drug administration. However, on the basis of the response to MVAC chemotherapy in bladder and upper tract urothelial tumors, investigation into its use in transitional cell carcinoma of the urethra is warranted.

Untreated patients with carcinoma of the urethra can anticipate a median survival of 3 months, with a range of 1 week to 15 months. Only 16% of these patients will survive more than 5 years.[12]

Carcinoma of the Distal Urethra

Carcinoma of the penile urethra may be treated by transurethral resection, local excision, partial amputation, or radical amputation with or without emasculation. For superficial, papillary, or in situ tumor, transurethral resection may be sufficient. For tumor infiltrating the corpus and localized to the distal half of the penis, a partial amputation with a 2-cm margin proximal to any visible or palpable lesion is the generally accepted treatment. If the infiltrating tumor is located in the proximal penile urethra or involves the entire penile urethra, radical amputation should be done. Emasculation is indicated only when the scrotal skin is involved.

Unlike the situation in carcinoma of the penis, clinically palpable adenopathy in the groin of patients with urethral carcinoma usually represents metastases and is not often the result of reactive inflammation. Ilioinguinal node dissection is indicated only if the inguinal nodes are palpable; there is no evidence of benefit from prophylactic groin dissection. After excision of the primary tumor, the patient should be followed with careful examination of the inguinal areas for evidence of lymphadenopathy, and a groin dissection should be done on the finding of metastatic disease.[1,3,5,7,13] In general, the survival rates correlate with the location and type of lesion and overall are poor (Table 34-4).

Carcinoma of the Bulbomembranous Urethra

Early lesions of the bulbomembranous urethra have been treated successfully by transurethral resection or by resection of the involved urethral segment with end-to-end anastomosis, but cases appropriate for such limited resection are rare.[13,14] Poor survival figures have been recorded with all forms of treatment; however, it appears that radical excision offers the best opportunity for long-term disease control with the lowest incidence of local recurrence. Unfortunately, most patients with bulbomembranous urethral carcinoma present with locally advanced disease.

In-continuity resection of the pubic rami has been suggested as a means of improving local control,[15] but the small number of patients thus treated prevents definitive conclusions. Patients with carcinoma of the posterior urethra should have simultaneous deep pelvic node dissection to determine the presence of nodal metastatic disease. There is no evidence that cure can be effected in patients with gross pelvic disease by either surgical excision or radiation therapy alone.

Carcinoma of the Prostatic Urethra

Carcinoma arising from the prostatic urethra is rare. There are no characteristic symptoms of this lesion, and the serum acid phosphatase concentration is not elevated. Superficial lesions of the prostatic urethra have been managed successfully by transurethral resection in some patients;[1] however, such tumors are uncommon. In the majority of instances, the tumor involves the bulk of the prostate with variable exten-

TABLE 34-4. Five-Year Survival in Carcinoma of Male Urethra

Histologic Type	*No. of Cases (%)*			
	Penile	*Bulbomembranous*	*Prostatic*	*Total*
Squamous	12/27 (44)	4/40 (10)	0/1 (0)	
Transitional	1/3 (33)	0/4 (0)	4/13 (31)	
Adenocarcinoma	–	1/4 (25)	–	
Undifferentiated	–	0/1 (0)	–	
Total	13/30 (43)	5/49 (10)	4/14 (29)	

Modified from Ray B, Canto AR, Whitmore WF: Experience with primary carcinoma of the male urethra. J Urol 117:591–594, 1977.

sion to the bulbomembranous urethra or the bladder neck and trigone. In this situation, radical prostatectomy alone may not provide a tumor-free margin, and anterior exenteration is the treatment of choice. As with other carcinomas in the posterior urethra, the overall 5-year survival rates for invasive prostatic urethral carcinoma are poor.[5]

The results of radiation therapy for carcinoma of the male urethra are difficult to evaluate because the incidence of the tumor is so low and few cases have been treated. In lesions of the distal urethra, the response to either penectomy or radiation therapy is similar.[16] Aggressive external radiation to the prostate (6000–7000 cGy) in combination with transurethral resection has produced an occasional long-term survivor.

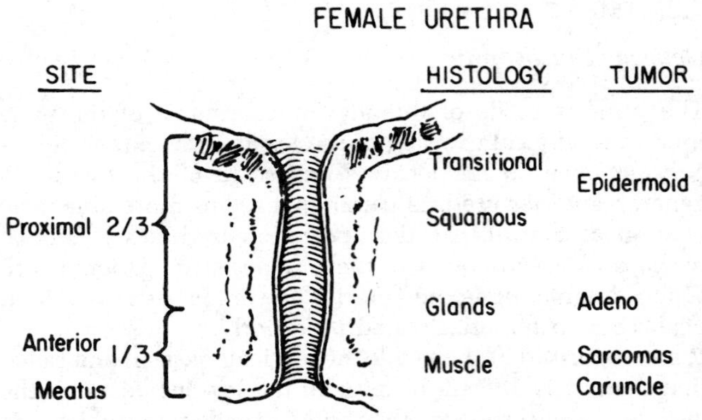

FIG. 34-2. Anatomy and pathology of the female urethra.

CARCINOMA OF THE FEMALE URETHRA

Carcinoma of the urethra is unusual among genitourinary tract neoplasms in occurring more often in females than in males. The tumors most commonly present in older, postmenopausal women, with 75% of patients being over 50 years of age. The disease is more prevalent in whites than in other races.

ETIOLOGY

The etiology of urethral carcinoma in females has not been established, although a causal relation is reported between chronic irritation and malignancy. Proliferative lesions such as caruncles, papillomas, adenomas, and polyps have been reported to be associated with subsequent malignancy. Leukoplakia of the urethra should be considered a premalignant lesion and treated accordingly.

SYMPTOMS

The tumor usually presents as a papillary growth and later becomes a soft, fungating mass that bleeds easily. Ulcerative lesions may produce a foul-smelling discharge. Spread from the primary lesion is by local extension and infiltration with subsequent involvement of the bladder neck and vulva. It may be difficult on initial physical examination to differentiate malignant tumors of the urethra from those of the vulva.

The lymphatic drainage of the various segments of the female urethra is poorly defined. However, it is generally accepted that the lymphatics of the distal urethra drain into the inguinal region, whereas the drainage from the more proximal urethra is to the obturator and iliac nodes. Between 25% and 50% of patients will have inguinal node involvement at the time of initial diagnosis[2,17–19]; an additional 15% of patients will develop tumorous nodes during follow-up. As with urethral carcinoma in males, inguinal lymphadenopathy usually indicates malignant involvement.

PATHOLOGY

Stratified squamous epithelium lines the distal two thirds of the female urethra, whereas transitional epithelium lines the proximal one third (Fig. 34-2). Tumor histology is a reflection of the site, with the predominant tumor being squamous cell carcinoma, usually presenting in the proximal two thirds. In general, carcinomas of the anterior urethra are low grade, whereas carcinomas of the proximal or entire urethra are of higher grade. However, histologic characteristics do not significantly affect the prognosis; thus, for practical purposes, transitional cell carcinoma, squamous cell carcinoma, and adenocarcinoma are treated in a similar fashion, although for metastatic transitional cell carcinoma, combination chemotherapy may be considered.[9,10]

TREATMENT

The most significant prognostic factor is the anatomical location of the tumor. For example, meatal tumors, when diagnosed early, are associated with an excellent 5-year survival rate.[20,21] The treatment is based primarily on the tumor stage at the time of presentation. Local excision is often sufficient in selected patients with carcinoma of the distal urethra, as the incidence of lymph node metastasis with distal urethral carcinoma is low.

For tumors involving the proximal urethra or with extension beyond the urethra into the adjacent structures, more extensive surgical resection is necessary, including total urethrectomy, cystectomy with pelvic node dissection, and, in cases of palpable inguinal lymph nodes, inguinal lymphadenectomy. Removal of the vulva and vagina have also been advocated as part of an anterior exenteration.[13,22]

Bracken and co-workers reported on 81 cases of carcinoma of the female urethra,[21] with the overall 5-year survival rate of the entire group being 32%. There is a high incidence of local recurrence for all forms of single-modality therapy ranging from 46% to 64%, suggesting the need to explore combination treatment.

Radiation Therapy

In carcinoma of the urethral meatus, irradiation can control the tumor and preserve the function of the urethra. Meatal carcinomas are usually treated with interstitial implants; large tumors that extend into the labia, vagina, or urinary bladder require the addition of external beam therapy. The combination of surgery and brachytherapy irradiation[23] or external beam irradiation[15] has been advocated to improve the results in advanced urethral tumors.

RADIATION THERAPY TECHNIQUES. Declois[24] thoroughly described the techniques for interstitial irradiation of the female urethra. Single- or double-plane or a volume implant is performed, depending on the volume of tumor to be treated. With the advent of ^{192}Ir, after-loading implants utilizing this material have largely replaced radium or ^{60}Co. Pierquin et al[25] described the use of "directional gutters" through which ^{192}Ir pins are inserted. Should the tumor involve the inferior aspect of the urethral meatus, care must be exercised to encompass this part of the lesion adequately, sometimes utilizing "crossing" needles. In this case, it is advisable to use a vaginal cylinder that will extend the periphery of the implant into the labia minora.

Radiographs are obtained to verify the insertion of the sources, and computer calculation displays the dose distributions in multiple planes. An estimated dose of 6000 to 7000 cGy is given, depending on tumor extent.

For larger tumors involving the labia, vagina, or the base of the urinary bladder, an implant technique alone will be inadequate to control the disease. For these patients, a combination of external beam radiotherapy with an interstitial implant is recommended.

Tumors involving the posterior urethra should be treated in a manner similar to those of the urinary bladder.[26]

RESULTS. Small meatal tumors show 5-year cure rates in the range of 70% to 90%.[20,26–28] Neoplasms involving the proximal urethra or the entire urethra are more difficult to treat, and the overall control rate for these tumors is only 20% to 30%. In some studies, the combination of preoperative radiotherapy and radical cystourethrectomy appeared to increase the survival rate in patients with advanced disease.[29,30]

SEQUELAE. Urethral strictures will develop in some patients, necessitating dilatation. More severe complications are necrosis secondary to overdosage and, occasionally, fistula, primarily vesicovaginal or urethrovaginal.[21,26] In the case of advanced neoplasms, fistula formation is unavoidable because of tumor erosion of the organ and subsequent tumor necrosis.[30] Other less common complications include osteomyelitis of the symphysis pubis, radiation cystitis and urinary incontinence or stress incontinence, radiation enteritis, and small-bowel obstruction. Johnson and O'Connell[29] encountered a 42% complication rate in patients treated by radiotherapy, whereas in the series by Prempree et al,[28] two of ten patients treated definitively by means of radiotherapy developed strictures. Bracken et al[21] reported a complication rate of 45% among their patients who were treated with radiation, whereas Taggart et al[26] encountered severe complications in 5 of 37 patients.

CANCER OF THE PENIS

INCIDENCE

Carcinoma of the penis represents 2% to 5% of all urogenital cancers.[31] Although rare in North America, tumors of the penis are a significant clinical problem in populations where circumcision is not a common practice and proper hygiene is lacking. Indeed, in some populations, squamous cell carcinoma of the penis accounts for 10% to 12% of all malignancies in males. Although malignant penile lesions have been found in young men, most patients are more than 50 years of age.

ETIOLOGY

The occurrence of penile carcinoma correlates strongly with the presence of a foreskin and the irritative effects of smegma combined with the products of poor hygiene within the preputial sac. Carcinoma is rare among men who were circumcised in the neonatal period,[32] but circumcision performed at puberty or in adulthood does not have the same

TABLE 34-5. Malignant Lesions of the Penis

Lesions	*Characteristics*	*Treatment*
Squamous carcinoma	Mass of foreskin or glans; phimosis often	Partial penectomy ± lymph node dissection; local excision or radiation therapy in appropriate, localized lesions
Malignant melanoma	Mass of foreskin or glans; phimosis often	Excision with wide margins; partial/total penectomy may be required. Lymph node dissection
Basal cell carcinoma	Extremely rare. Rolled, well-defined edges	Local excision with adequate margins.
Carcinoma in situ	Red or scaly plaque, no deep invasion	Local excision
Mesenchymal tumors	From stromal/connective tissue of penis. Approximately 50% are malignant. Sarcomas (Kaposi's and fibrosarcoma) most common malignant lesions	Partial/total penectomy
Metastatic tumors	Usually from genitourinary tract	Local control only
Leukemic or lymphomatous infiltrate	Rare	Treatment of systemic disorder

TABLE 34-6. Premalignant Lesions of the Penis

Lesion	*Characteristics*	*Treatment*
Leukoplakia	White plaque	Local excision
Erythroplasia of Queyrat	Raised, red, velvet lesion; cellular disorientation with multiple mitoses; identical to carcinoma in situ of skin; 10%–20% may develop areas of squamous cell carcinoma. May be painful	Local excision; topical 5-fluorouracil; radiation
Bowen's disease	Red plaque	Local excision
Balanitis xerotica obliterans	Scaly, atrophic with fissure or ulceration; meatus often involved	Local excision; topical steroids (?)
Buschke–Lowenstein tumor	Large verrucous lesion, histologically benign; may undergo malignant degeneration	Local excision with negative margins. Topical therapy doubtful; radiation therapy has limited effectiveness

protective potential as does neonatal circumcision.[33–35] Although the annual age-adjusted incidence of carcinoma of the penis for males in the United States is only 1.0 per 100,000, the incidence in uncircumcised males is approximately 1 in 600.[36] Smegma, the product of bacterial action or desquamated epithelial cells, has been identified as carcinogenic in animal systems, although the specific component responsible for malignant degeneration in human males has not been identified.

Conflicting reports both support and deny the association of penile carcinoma with the presence of cervical carcinoma in sexual partners as well as a possible relation to herpetic infection.[37,38] No persistent etiologic relation has been documented between carcinoma of the penis and the venereal diseases of syphilis, granuloma inguinale, and chancroid.

SYMPTOMS

The most common presenting clinical manifestation of penile cancer is a mass or a persistent sore or ulcer of the glans or foreskin.[31,39] Most penile carcinomas are painless, and there may be significant ulceration and bleeding without patient concern. Less commonly, the initial symptoms are related to inguinal lymphadenopathy.

It has been estimated that more than one-half of patients will delay more than a year in seeking treatment after the appearance of the lesion.[12,35,39–41]

TABLE 34-7. Minimal Diagnostic Criteria for Carcinoma of the Penis

T = primary tumor
Clinical examination
Incisional/excisional biopsy
N = Regional lymph nodes
Clinical examination
CT/MRI
Intravenous urography (optional)
Lymphangiography (optional)
Superficial femoral node biopsy (optional but recommended)
M = Distant Metastases
Clinical examination
Chest radiography
CT/MRI
Biochemical determinations (liver function, calcium)
Liver scan, bone scan (optional)

PATHOLOGY

Penile carcinoma is most often squamous cell in origin, although a variety of other malignancies may also involve the penis (Table 34-5). In addition, a number of premalignant lesions have been identified (Table 34-6).

STAGING

The initial diagnosis must be made by incisional or, preferably, excisional biopsy. Careful physical examination to determine the extent of local invasion and the status of the inguinal lymph nodes is essential to proper staging. A CT scan or MRI to evaluate the pelvic or abdominal lymph nodes or both is also required. A lymphangiogram appears to be optional (Table 34-7).

Table 34-8 shows the Jackson staging system for penile carcinoma.[42] Although widely used, this system suffers to the extent that inguinal nodal involvement is not subcategorized; all patients with tumorous nodes are grouped together.[43] The tumor–node–metastasis (TNM) classification, outlined in

TABLE 34-8. Jackson Classification for Penile Cancer

Stage	*Criteria*
I	Tumor confined to glans or prepuce
II	Invasion into shaft or corpora; no nodal or distant metastases
III	Tumor confined to penis; inguinal metastases that are operable
IV	Tumor involves adjacent structures; inoperable and/or distant metastases

TABLE 34-9. TNM Classification of Squamous Carcinoma of Penis*

T		N		M	
TX	Minimum requirements cannot be met	NX	Minimum requirements cannot be met	MX	Minimum requirements cannot be met
T0	No evidence of primary tumor	N0	No evidence of involvement of regional lymph nodes	M0	No evidence of distant metastases
TIS	Carcinoma *in situ* (Bowen's disease, erythroplasia of Queyrat)	N1	Involvement of a single regional node	M1	Distant metastases present
T1	Tumor not more than 1 cm in largest dimension and clearly superficial	N2	Involvement of single bilateral inguinal nodes or multiple unilateral nodes	M1a	Evidence of occult metastases based on biochemical and/or other tests
T2	Tumor 1 cm in any dimension and clearly superficial	N3	Fixation of regional nodes or ulceration of skin over involved regional nodes	M1b	Single metastasis in a single organ site
T3	Tumor of any size invading underlying tissues	N4	Involvement of juxtaregional lymph nodes	M1c	Multiple metastases in a single site
T4	Tumor invading adjacent structures, that is, corpus, urethra, symphysis, perineum			M1d	Metastases in multiple organ sites

* Minimal requirements for tumor (*T*) include clinical examination with biopsy; for nodes (*N*) clinical examination, lymphography, or urography; for distant metastasis (*M*) clinical examination, chest x-ray film, lymphography or metastatic bone studies. The regional nodes are those of the superficial inguinal region. Juxtaregional nodes are those of the external iliac chain below the bifurcation of the common iliac artery and those of the hypogastric region.

Table 34-9, is an attempt to quantify more precisely the nodal and metastatic disease.

TREATMENT PRINCIPLES

Adequate therapy of patients with penile cancer implies an accurate assessment of the extent of the disease with particular reference to the status of the regional lymph nodes. Surgery, in the form of partial or total penectomy with or without inguinal and pelvic lymph node dissection is the most commonly accepted treatment. Radiation therapy as external irradiation, penile brachytherapy, or both, also have been given in an attempt to lessen the functional sacrifice associated with ablation of the primary tumor.

Paramount in any treatment philosophy is a consideration of the lymphatic drainage of the penis as a prelude to rational therapeutic planning (Fig. 34-3). The skin of the penis and the lymphatics of the prepuce drain primarily into the superficial inguinal nodes. As a result of a freely anastomosing system and crossover at the base of the penis, bilateral drainage occurs.[44] The glans is likewise drained by the superficial inguinal nodes, but, along with those of the corpora, the glans lymphatics also empty into the deep inguinal and iliac nodes. The superficial nodes are located in the deep portion of Camper's fascia superficial to the deep fascia of the thigh, the fascia lata. Subsequently, the superficial lymphatics drain into the deep inguinal lymphatics surrounding the femoral vessels and thence to the external iliac, common iliac, and periaortic lymphatic channels. Tumor invasion of the corpora cavernosa or the posterior urethra also is consistent with involvement of the deep pelvic lymphatic structures of the internal iliac and obturator regions.

Surgical Treatment

Two areas of surgical concern in disease management are the selection of the appropriate treatment for the primary lesion and the role of surgery in the evaluation and therapy of nodal disease.

TREATMENT OF PRIMARY LESION. Adequate control of the primary tumor must be accomplished for a cure to be expected. Surgical therapy involves removal of the lesion with adequate margins to minimize the risk of local recur-

FIG. 34-3. Lymphatic drainage of penis.

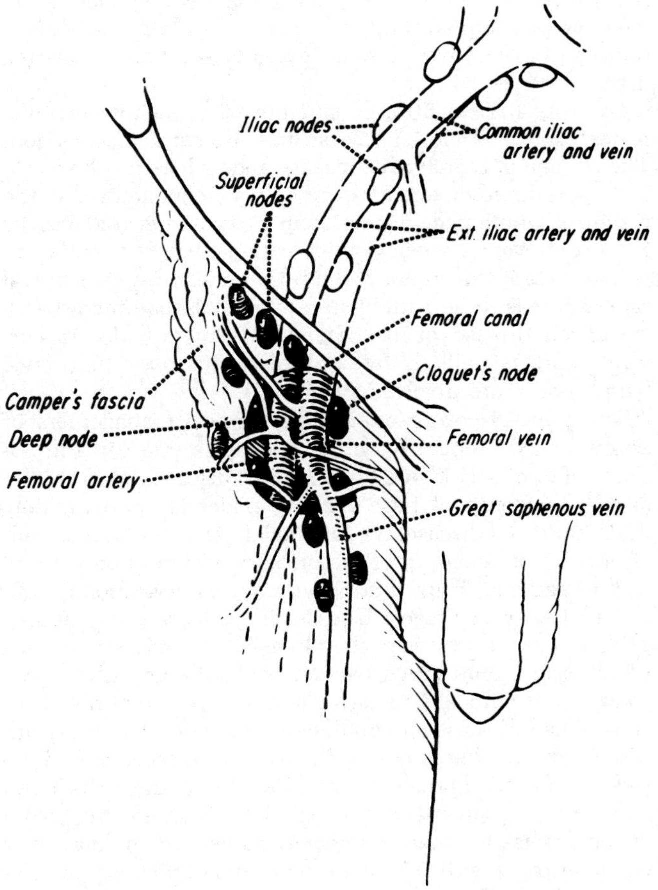

rence. Small tumors that are limited to the prepuce are treated by circumcision alone. Lesions that on physical examination involve only the skin, not the underlying structures, may be controllable by excisional biopsy. Penectomy, either partial or total, is indicated for lesions that, because of their size, invasiveness, or location on the shaft, are not amenable to more conservative treatment. Partial penectomy requires that a 2-cm margin of grossly normal shaft be available proximal to the primary lesion. For lesions that approach the base of the shaft or that are extensive, total penectomy should be accomplished with excision of both corpora and creation of a perineal urethrostomy.[45]

MANAGEMENT OF REGIONAL LYMPH NODES. Several important facts should be kept in mind concerning the role of regional lymphadectomy in patients with penile cancer. First, between 35% and 60% of patients with squamous cell penile cancer will present with palpable inguinal lymph nodes.[46,47] Second, the incidence of false-positive lymph nodes on clinical examination averages 40%, with various series reporting figures between 13% and 82%,[12,43,45] because of the well-known association of inflammatory inguinal lymphadenopathy with ulcerated or infected penile lesions. Clinical assessment of the lymph nodes thus should be delayed until after a 4- to 6-week course of antibiotic therapy, especially in patients with obviously infected or inflamed penile lesions. Third, approximately 20% of patients with clinically tumor-free inguinal lymph nodes in fact have lymphatic metastases.[45,46] Fourth, lymph node dissection can be curative in some patients with tumor-bearing inguinal nodes.

Overall, 40% to 50% of patients with positive inguinal nodes can be rendered disease free by surgical resection. The volume of lymph node disease and its location appear to be important predictors of success. In a recent analysis of the results of lymph node dissection in 119 patients at Memorial Sloan-Kettering Cancer Center, patients with unilateral inguinal-node involvement had a 56% median 5-year survival rate, whereas those with bilateral inguinal-node metastases, extranodal disease, or iliac node involvement had a 9% survival. Cure is unlikely by surgical means once the pelvic lymph nodes are involved.[44]

The primary controversy in the surgical management of penile cancer concerns lymph node dissection in the absence of clinically identifiable inguinal disease. Whereas the overall incidence of false-negative nodes is approximately 20%, in Stage I disease, the late nodal extension to the groin after adequate excision of the primary occurs in only 5% to 11% of patients, Thus, routine lymph node dissection is difficult to justify in Stage I disease. In patients with invasive primary tumors, however, the likelihood of nodal metastases increases; in some series, two-thirds of patients with Stage II disease and clinically negative nodes were found histologically to have disease on lymph node dissection.[48] The significant morbidity that may accompany groin dissection and the lack of controlled prospective studies to document the benefit of early "prophylactic" versus late "therapeutic" groin dissection has led many surgeons and centers to delay lymphadenectomy until clinical evidence of lymph node involvement exists.[37,47]

Ekstrom and Edsmyr identified a 50% disease control rate in patients who had node dissection delayed until adenopathy was evident.[49] Frew et al[50] could identify no cancer deaths in patients in whom lymph node excision was deferred until clinical node disease was present. Beggs and Spratt reported no significant adverse effect on survival in patients with delayed groin dissection; the 1% mortality rate from lymphadenectomy was essentially the same as the percentage of patients who died from cancer as a result of therapeutic delay.[47] More recently, others have reported a significant decrease in 5-year survival rates in patients with therapeutic as opposed to prophylactic groin dissection[48,51] and have suggested that delayed surgery is inappropriate.

Cabanas[52] has described a technique of "sentinel node" biopsy followed by a formal node dissection if metastatic disease is found. The sentinel lymph node is found radiographically, on the anteroposterior view, at the junction of the femoral head and the ascending pubic ramus. Anatomically, the sentinel node is part of the lymphatic system around the superficial epigastric vein located medial to and above the superficial epigastric–saphenous junction. In Cabanas' series, inguinel–femoral–iliac node involvement was not demonstrated in the absence of a positive sentinel node biopsy. However, subsequently, Perinetti et al[53] reported a case of a patient with a negative sentinel-node biopsy who had unresectable bilateral groin disease 3 months later.

It thus seems appropriate that patients with noninvasive tumor and clinically negative nodes (Stage I) be followed carefully and groin dissection considered only if lymphadenopathy occurs. In patients with Stage II disease, the sentinel node biopsy is appealing as a means of increasing diagnostic and prognostic accuracy without significant morbidity, although proponents of both prophylactic and therapeutic groin dissection exist. In patients with clinically positive nodes (Stage II), initial bilateral dissection should be performed because of the high incidence (60%) of bilateral inguinal node involvement.[49] Unilateral node dissection in patients managed by delayed lymphadenectomy is reasonable because the incidence of contralateral involvement in these patients is less than 10%.[12] Controversy also exists over the benefit obtained by pelvic node dissection in the presence of pelvic nodal metastatic disease. Although positive pelvic nodes appear to be an indicator of incurable disease, some authors report a 20% to 29% cure rate with surgery in these patients. Whether this apparent long-term survival reflects a beneficial impact of surgery or represents a subset of patients with apparently indolent disease is undetermined.[52]

Technical Aspects of Lymphadenectomy. The operation is performed essentially as described by Whitmore and Vagaiwala.[54] The patient is placed in the supine position with the thighs slightly flexed, abducted, and externally rotated with support under the knees. The incision for the bilateral pelvic node dissection, which may be performed before (usually) or after the inguinal dissection, is a midline incision from the umbilicus to the pubis. The dissection limits are defined by the genitofemoral nerve laterally, the bladder medially, the bifurcation of the common iliac artery superiorly, and the fascia covering the obturator internus and levator ani mus-

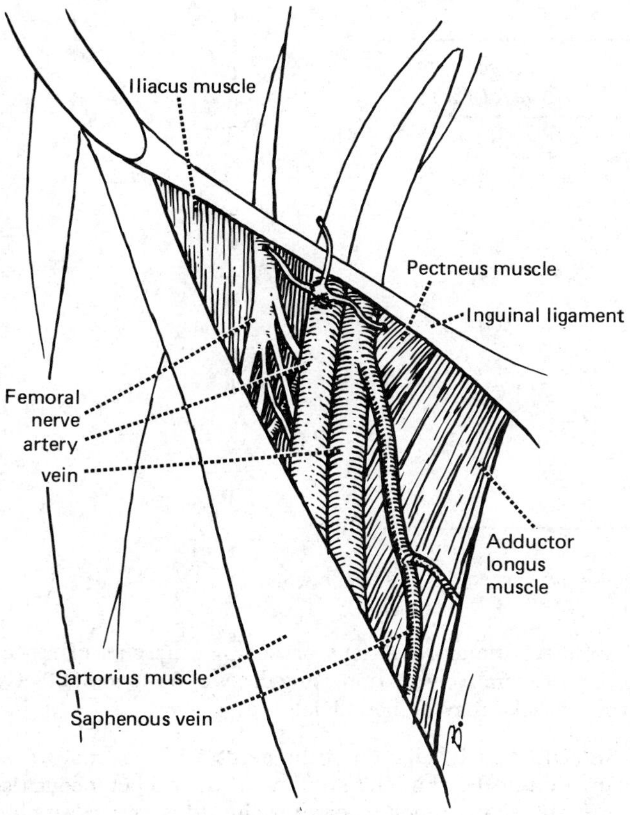

FIG. 34-4. Anatomical limits of deep groin dissection.

cles inferiorly (Fig. 34-4). Cloquet's node can usually be removed through the pelvic incision as the vessels are cleaned as they enter the femoral canal. The inguinal incision is planned to provide adequate margins surrounding lymph nodes containing obvious tumor and simultaneously to remove the area of skin at greatest risk of devitalization and necrosis. An elliptical incision is made over the inguinal ligament from the anterosuperior iliac spine toward, but lateral to, the pubic tubercle. The borders of the ellipse parallel the inguinal ligament and extend 4 to 6 cm in a vertical diameter at the widest point. The incision is bevelled outward from the skin down so as to describe a pyramidal wedge of tissue, truncated by the skin surface. Because penile cancers appear to involve the inguinal lymph nodes by tumor embolization rather than through permeation of lymphatic channels, wide, thin skin flaps and a thorough dissection, such as is required for malignant melanoma, are not indicated. The surgeon's goal should be to remove completely the nodes in the superficial and deep inguinal areas; this can be done without widely undermining the skin flaps.

Complications. The most common complication is skin flap necrosis. Particular attention to operative detail, especially with regard to skin flap thickness, infection control, protection of femoral vessels by sartorius transfer, appropriate drainage, and postoperative immobilization appears to lessen this most disturbing complication. Other problems include lymphedema (19%–45%), wound infection (10%), and, rarely, hemorrhage, hernia, or death. The presence of persistent lymphedema can be a particular problem. Meticulous ligation of lymphatic channels during the dissection by cautery, metal clips, or fine ligatures appears to reduce the likelihood of severe, persistent lymphedema. The use of preoperatively fitted compression stockings, elevation, and immobilization also appears to be important in reducing the incidence of this problem.

Radiation Therapy

As with surgery, radiation therapy has been used in treatment of both the primary lesion and nodal disease.

RADIATION OF THE PRIMARY LESION. The principal advantage of irradiation in treating the primary lesion is preservation of the penis. Irradiation alone will control the tumor in a significant number of patients, thus avoiding anatomic and functional deficits that may produce devastating psychological effects. In addition, if radiation therapy fails, a surgical procedure may control the recurrent disease if it is not too extensive and metastases are not present.

Before initiation of radiotherapy for carcinoma of the penis, routine circumcision must be performed. This procedure will minimize the radiotherapy-associated morbidity, swelling and irritation of the skin, moist desquamation, and secondary infection.[55]

RADIATION THERAPY. A wide variation of techniques, doses, and fractionation schemes have been employed.[56–60] Implants, molds, contact therapy, orthovoltage therapy, and megavoltage therapy are used. The most commonly employed techniques are as follows.

Low-energy orthovoltage (60–150 kVp) has been used for the treatment of relatively superficial invasive carcinoma or for carcinoma in situ (including the erythroplasia of Queyrat). The lesion is treated with a margin of 1 to 2 cm beyond visible or palpable tumor. Doses in the range of 6000 cGy in 5 to 6 weeks will produce local control in most instances.

Megavoltage irradiation is necessary for infiltrating tumors with thickness greater than 0.5 cm. It also is required for the inguinal lymph nodes. When the tumor in the lymph nodes is infiltrating the skin, bolus therapy should be used to avoid skin-sparing effect. For the treatment of the primary lesion, the entire penis should be included in the irradiated volume. This can be done with appositional portals using special positioning devices. The doses of irradiation should be 6500 to 7000 cGy, in five-weekly fractions, for 5 to 7 weeks, depending on the volume treated.

External beam radiotherapy requires specially designed accessories to achieve adequate bolus over the organ and homogeneous dose distribution. The device usually consists of a plastic box with a central opening that can be fitted over the organ; the space between the skin and the box must be filled with tissue-equivalent material. This box can then be treated with a parallel opposed megavoltage beam.

Although external beam radiotherapy has become a prevalent modality in the treatment of the primary lesion in carci-

TABLE 34-10. Control of Primary Lesion with Radiotherapy

Author	*No. of Patients*	*Treatment Method*	*Dosage*	*Local Control (%)*
Engelstad[58]	72	Mold, teleradium	3500–3700 R 500–700 R/day	50
Jackson[42]	39	Mold (most cases), external beam (some cases)	?	49
Murrell & Williams[59]	108	External beam	3000–6700 cGy 200 cGy/day	52
Kelley et al.	10	External beam (electrons)	5100–5400 cGy 300 cGy/day	100
Haile & Delclos	20	Mold, implant, external beam	?	90
Pointon[61]	32	External beam	5250–5500 cGy in 16 Rx/22 days	84
Salverria	41	Iridium mold	6000 cGy/several days	84

noma of the penis, molds are still used. The mold is usually built as a box with a central opening, and radioactive sources should be sufficiently long to prevent underdosage at the tip of the penis. A dose of 6500 cGy at the surface and approximately 6000 cGy at the center of the organ is delivered over 6 to 7 days.

Control rates of the primary lesions with radiation therapy achieved by several authors are summarized in Table 34-10.

RADIATION OF REGIONAL LYMPHATICS. Irradiation of the involved regional lymph nodes in patients with carcinoma of the penis may result in permanent control and cure of a substantial percentage of patients.[60]

In cases in which irradiation is used to treat lymph nodes, both inguinal and pelvic nodes as far as the common iliac bifurcation should be irradiated with paralleled anteroposterior and posteroanterior portals. Beçause of the anterior position of the lymph nodes, an unequal loading favoring the anterior portals can be used. For elective treatment (without clinical evidence of metastatic tumor), doses of approximately 5000 cGy in 5 weeks are adequate. In those patients with palpable lymph nodes, doses on the order of 7000 to 8000 cGy over 7 to 8 weeks (180–200 cGy per day) are indicated.

Special skin care must be instituted to prevent moist epidermitis and serious discomfort. The prevention of infection is critical to the satisfactory completion of the radiation therapy.

PALLIATION. Good palliative effects can be achieved in patients with extensive, advanced, infiltrating, or ulcerated tumors. A direct appositional port may be adequate, and doses in the range of 4000 to 6000 cGy may cause temporary tumor regression with decreased pain and bleeding and healing of neoplastic ulceration.

POSTOPERATIVE IRRADIATION. In those patients with incomplete tumor resections or positive margins of resection, postoperative radiation using doses of 5000 to 6000 cGy over 6 weeks may be beneficial.

SEQUELAE. Irradiation of the penis produces moist desquamation of the skin and swelling of the subcutaneous tissue of the shaft. Albeit uncomfortable, this is a reversible reaction that subsides within a few weeks. Telangiectasia is a common late consequence of radiation therapy and is usually asymptomatic (Fig. 34-5).

Ulceration, necrosis of the glans, or necrosis of the skin of the shaft area are rare. Lymphedema of the legs has been reported following inguinal and pelvic radiotherapy, but the role of radiotherapy in the development of this complication remains controversial; the majority of the patients with this symptom have disease in the lymphatics that may be responsible for lymphatic blockage.

In the reported series, meatal–urethral strictures occur with a frequency ranging from 0 to 40%.[7,14–17] This incidence compares favorably with the incidence of urethral stricture following penectomy. Most of the strictures after radiotherapy are at the meatus.

Chemotherapy

Primarily because of the rarity of penile cancer in those countries that have the most experience in doing controlled clinical trials, optimal chemotherapy for this lesion has not yet been defined. Bleomycin is the most active drug tested to date, with rates of objective response ranging from 21% to 60%.[62,63] Methotrexate in doses necessitating leucovorin rescue has produced objective responses in 61% of patients,[62] including an occasional complete remission.[64] Cisplatin has produced responses in 21% of patients.[62]

As yet, no meaningful combination regimens have been tested. The drugs with demonstrable activity could be judiciously combined. However, current chemotherapy must be considered primarily palliative.

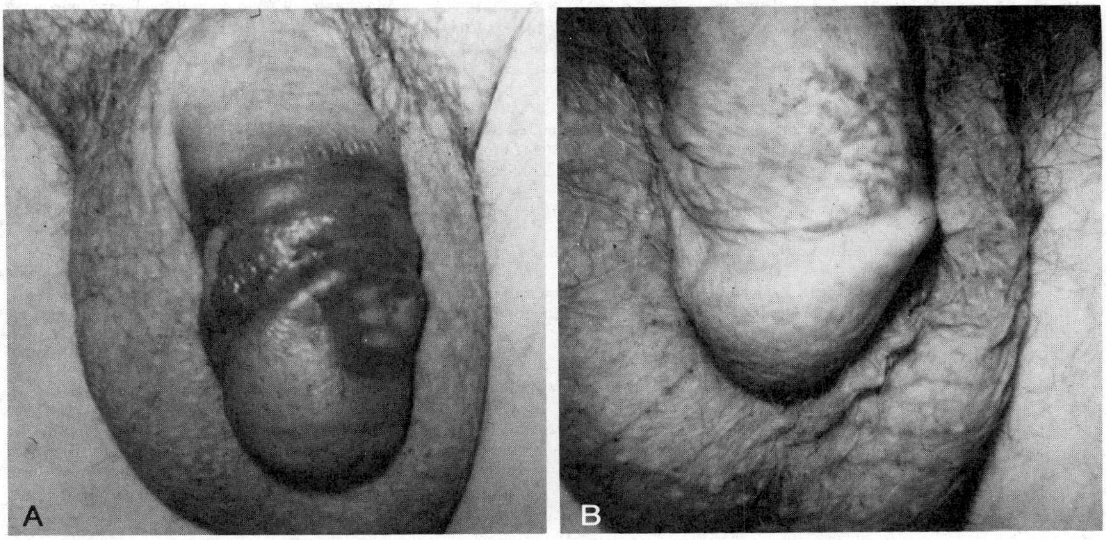

FIG. 34-5. Squamous-cell carcinoma of balanopreputial region with extension into glans (Stage I). Patient was treated with 120 kVp x-rays, 0.3 mm^3 HVL, receiving 6000 cGY skin dose in 5 weeks. **A**. Before treatment. **B**. Same patient 4 years later; no evidence of disease. Telangiectasia is present. (Reproduced with permission from Pilepich MV: Carcinoma of the penis and male urethra. In Perez CA, Brady LW [eds]: Principles and Practice of Radiation Oncology, pp 912–918. Philadelphia, JB Lippincott, 1987)

REFERENCES

1. Fair WR, Yang CR: Urethral carcinoma in males. In Resnick M, Kursh E (eds): Current Therapy in Surgery. Toronto, BC Decker, 1987
2. Grabstald H: Tumors of the urethra in men and women. Cancer 32:1236–1255, 1973
3. Kaplan GW, Bulkey GJ, Grayhack JT: Carcinoma of the male urethra. J Urol 96:365–371, 1967
4. King LR: Carcinoma of the urethra in male patients. J Urol 92:555–559, 1964
5. Ray B, Canto AK, Whitmore WF Jr: Experience with primary carcinoma of the male urethra. J Urol 117:591–594, 1977
6. Zaslow J, Priestly JT: Primary carcinoma of the male urethra. J Urol 58:207–211, 1947
7. Mandler JT, Pool TL: Primary carcinoma of the male urethra. J Urol 96:67–72, 1966
8. Yang CR, Fair WR, Whitmore WF Jr: Urethral carcinoma in males (submitted for publication)
9. Sternberg CN, Yagoda A, Scher HI, et al: Preliminary results of M-VAC (methotrexate, vinblastine, Adriamycin and cisplatin) for transitional cell carcinoma of the urothelium. J Urol 33:403–407, 1985
10. Scher HI, Yagoda A, Herr HW, et al: Neoadjuvant M-VAC (methotrexate, vinblastine, Adriamycin and cisplatin) for extravesical urinary tract tumors. J Urol (in press)
11. Scher HI, Yagoda A, Herr HW, et al: Neoadjuvant M-VAC (methotrexate, vinblastine, Adriamycin and cisplatin): Effect on the primary bladder lesion (submitted for publication)
12. Paulson DF, Perez CA, Anderson T: Cancer of the urethra and penis, In Devita VT Jr, Hellman S, Rosenberg SA (eds): Principles and Practice of Oncology, vol 1, pp 965–977. Philadelphia, JB Lippincott, 1985
13. Pointon RCS, Poole-Wilson DS: Primary carcinoma of the urethra. Br J Urol 40:682–685, 1968
14. Lower WE, Hausfeld KF: Primary carcinoma of the male urethra: Report of 10 cases. J Urol 58:192–206, 1947
15. Klein FA, Whitmore WF Jr, Herr HW, et al: Inferior pubic rami resection with en bloc radical excision for invasive proximal urethral carcinoma. Cancer 51:1238–1242, 1983
16. Raghavaiah NV: Radiotherapy in the treatment of carcinoma of the male urethra. Cancer 41:1313–1316, 1978
17. Desai S, Libertino JA, Zinman L: Primary carcinoma of the female urethra. J Urol 110:693–695, 1973
18. Staubitz WJ, Carden LM, Oberkircher OJ, et al: Management of urethral carcinoma in the female. J Urol 73:1045–1053, 1955
19. Ritter DW: Primary malignancy of the female urethra. West J Surg Obstet Gynecol 51:420–429, 1953
20. Antioniades J: Radiation therapy in carcinoma of the female urethra. Cancer 24:70–76, 1969
21. Bracken RB, Johnson DE, Miller LS, et al: Primary carcinoma of the female urethra. J Urol 116:188–192, 1976
22. Grabstald H, Hilaris B, Henschike U, Whitmore WF Jr: Cancer of the female urethra. JAMA 197:835–837, 1966
23. Hopkins SC, Vider M, Nag SK, et al: Carcinoma of the female urethra: Reassessment of the modes of therapy. J Urol 129:958–961, 1983
24. Declois L: Carcinoma of the female urethra: Interstitial irradiation in genitourinary tumors, In Johnson DE, Boileau MA (eds): Fundamental Principles and Surgical Techniques, pp 275–286. New York, Grune & Stratton, 1982
25. Pierquin B, Chassange D, Cox JD: Toward consistent local control of certain malignant tumors: Endoradiotherapy with iridium 192. Radiology 99:661–667, 1971
26. Taggart CG, Castro JR, Rutledge FN: Carcinoma of the female urethra. Am J Roentgenol 114:145–151, 1972
27. Prempree T, Amoremarn R, Patanaphan V: Radiation therapy in primary carcinoma of the female urethra. Cancer 54:729–733, 1984
28. Prempree T, Wizenberg MJ, Scott RM: Radiation treatment of primary carcinoma of the female urethra. Cancer 42:1177–1184, 1978
29. Johnson DE, O'Connell JR: Primary carcinoma of the female urethra. Urology 21:42–45, 1983
30. Antoniades J, Pilepich MV: Carcinoma of the female urethra, In Perez CA, Brady LW (eds): Principles and Practice of Radiation Oncology, pp 863–866. Philadelphia, JB Lippincott, 1987
31. Hanash K, Furlow W, Utz D, et al: Carcinoma of the penis: A clinicopathologic study. J Urol 104:291–297, 1970
32. Jackson SM: The treatment of carcinoma of the penis. Br J Surg 53:33–35, 1966
33. Kuruvilla JT, Garlic RH, Mamnen KE: Results of surgical treatment of carcinoma of the penis. Aust NZ J Urol 41:157–159, 1971
34. Schellhammer PF, Spaulding JP: Carcinoma of the penis, In Paulson DF (ed): Genitourinary Surgery, p 629. New York, Churchill Livingstone, 1983
35. Thomas JA, Small CS: Carcinoma of the penis in southern India. J Urol 160:520–524, 1963
36. Paymaster JC, Gangadharin P: Cancer of the penis in India. J Urol 97:110–113, 1967
37. Gursel EO, Georgountzod C, Uson AC, et al: Penile cancer. Urology 1:569–578, 1973
38. Schrek L, Lenowitz H: Etiologic factors in carcinoma of the penis. Cancer Res 7:180–184, 1947
39. Hardner GJ, Bhanalaph T, Murphy GP, et al: Carcinoma of the penis: Analysis of therapy in 100 consecutive cases. J Urol 108:428–430, 1972
40. Buddington WT, Kickham CJ, Smithy WE: An assessment of malignant disease of the penis. J Urol 89:442–446, 1963
41. Dean AL: Epithelioma of the penis. J Urol 33:252–254, 1935
42. Jackson SM: The treatment of carcinoma of the penis. Br J Surg 53:33–35, 1966
43. Srinivas V, Morse MJ, Herr HW, et al: Penile cancer: Relation of extent of nodal metastasis to survival. J Urol 137:880–882, 1987
44. Skinner DG, Leadbetter WR, Kelley SP: The surgical management of squamous cell carcinoma of the penis. J Urol 107:273–277, 1972
45. Persky L, deKernion JB: Carcinoma of the penis. CA 36:258–272, 1986
46. deKernion JB, Tynberg P, Persky L, et al: Carcinoma of the penis. Cancer 32:1256–1262, 1973

47. Beggs JH, Spratt JS Jr: Epidermoid carcinoma of the penis. J Urol 91:166–172, 1964
48. McDougal WS, Kirchner FK Jr, Edwards RH, et al: Treatment of carcinoma of the penis: The case for primary lymphadenectomy. J Urol 136:38–41, 1986
49. Ekstrom T, Edsmyr F: Cancer of the penis: A clinical study of 29 cases. Acta Chir Scand 115:25–45, 1958
50. Frew ID, Jefferies JD, Swinney J: Carcinoma of the penis. Br J Urol 39:398–401, 1967
51. Johnson DE, Lo RK: Management of regional lymph nodes in penile carcinoma: Five-year results following therapeutic groin dissections. Urology 24:308–311, 1984
52. Cabanas RM: An approach for the treatment of penile carcinoma. Cancer 39:456–466, 1977
53. Perinetti EP, Crane DD, Catalona WJ: Unreliability of sentinel lymph node biopsy for staging penile carcinoma. J Urol 124:734–735, 1980
54. Whitmore WF Jr, Vagaiwala MR: A technique of ilioinguinal lymph-node dissection of carcinoma of the penis. Surg Gynecol Obstet 159:573–578, 1984
55. Pilepich MV: Carcinoma of the penis and male urethra, In Perez CA, Brady LW (eds): Principles and Practice of Radiation Oncology, pp 912–918. Philadelphia, JB Lippincott, 1987
56. Almgard LE, Edsmyr F: Radiotherapy in treatment of patients with carcinoma of the penis. Scand J Urol Nephrol 7:1–5, 1973
57. Engelstad RB: Treatment of cancer of the penis at the Norwegian Radium Hospital. Radiology 60:801–806, 1948
58. Murrell DS, Williams JL: Radiotherapy in the treatment of carcinoma of the penis. Br J Urol 37:211–222, 1965
59. Newaisy GA, Deeley TG: Radiotherapy in the treatment of carcinoma of the penis. Br J Urol 41:519–521, 1968
60. Pointon RCS: External beam therapy. Proc R Soc Med 68:779–781, 1975
61. Narayana AS, Olney LE, Loening SA, et al: Carcinoma of the penis: Analysis of 219 cases. CA 49:2185–2191, 1982
62. Ahmed T, Sklaroff R, Yagoda A: Sequential trials of methotrexate, cisplatin, bleomycin. J Urol 132:465–468, 1984
63. Kyalwazi SK, Bhana D, Harrison NW: Carcinoma of the penis and bleomycin chemotherapy in Uganda. Br J Urol 46:689–696, 1974
64. Garnick MB, Szkarin AT, Ceele GD Jr: Metastatic carcinoma of the penis: Complete remission after high dose methotrexate chemotherapy. J Urol 122:265–266, 1979

LAWRENCE H. EINHORN
E. DAVID CRAWFORD
WILLIAM U. SHIPLEY
PATRICK J. LOEHRER
STEPHEN D. WILLIAMS

CHAPTER 35 *Cancer of the Testes*

Although testicular cancer is a relatively uncommon disease, accounting for only 1% of all male malignancy,[1] it is important for several reasons. Because testis cancer is the most common carcinoma in the 15- to 35-year-old age group, it has the potential for reducing productive years of life in this young patient population. Moreover, testicular cancer is one of the few neoplasms associated with accurate serum markers: human chorionic gonadotropin (hCG) and alphafetoprotein (AFP). Also, whereas in most disseminated cancers, if a complete remission is not attained with chemotherapy, the patient ultimately dies of the disease, in testicular cancer, it is possible to resect residual disease surgically, changing a partial remission (PR) to a surgical complete remission (CR) and curing the patient. Finally, testicular cancer has become a model for a curable neoplasm.[2]

ANATOMY AND HISTOLOGY OF THE TESTIS

The normal testis measures about 4 × 3 × 2.5 cm. The testes acquire various tunics or coverings during their descent from the area of the genital ridge in the retroperitoneum through the inguinal canal into the scrotum. These tunics are the tunica vaginalis, the internal spermatic fascia, the cremasteric fascia, the external spermatic fascia, and the scrotum, which consists of skin and the dartos tunic. The testicular tubules themselves have a dense fascial covering called the tunica albuginea, which posteriorly is invaginated into the body of the testis to form the mediastinum testis. This mediastinum sends fibrous septae into the testis, thus separating it into several hundred lobules. The upper pole of the testis has a vestigial structure, the appendix testis. Posteriorly, the adnexal structures associated with the testis are the epididymis, the vas deferens, and the spermatic cord.

Histologically, each lobule of the testis contains convoluted seminiferous tubules, which are freely anastomotic. An estimated 250 to 400 lobular ducts converge at the mediastinum testis, where they connect with 12 to 20 efferent ducts that drain into the globus major of the epididymis.[3] The testicular seminiferous tubule is surrounded by a basement membrane of connective and elastic tissue. The basement membrane encloses the seminiferous cells, which are of two types: the supporting, or Sertoli, cells and the spermatogenic cells, called spermatogonia. The stroma between the seminiferous tubules is connective tissue in which the interstitial (Leydig) cells are located.

The blood supply to the testes is derived from their site of origin at the genital ridges. The arteries to the testes are the internal spermatic arteries arising from the aorta just below the renal arteries. They course through the spermatic cords directly to the testes, where they anastomose with the vas deferential arteries, which are branches of the hypogastric artery. The venous return from the testis begins as a pampiniform plexus of the spermatic cord. At the internal ring, this plexus joins to form the common spermatic vein. The right spermatic vein enters the vena cava anteriorly, usually several centimeters below the right renal vein. The left spermatic vein empties directly into the left renal vein, usually at a right angle. The lymphatics of the testis pass up the cord to the lumbar lymph nodes, the distribution of which is discussed in a separate section of this chapter.

The appendages of the testis and epididymis are embryologic remnants. The appendix testis is a remnant of the müllerian duct, whereas the remaining appendages (epididymis, superior and inferior vas aberrans, and paradidymis) arise from the mesonephric (wolffian) duct and are attached to the globus major, the upper and lower epididymis, and the junction of the epididymis and vas deferens, respectively. The appendage most commonly present is the appendix testis, found in 90% of autopsies. The appendix epididymis is present in one-third of patients, and the remaining appendages are found in only 1% to 3% of patients.

ETIOLOGY OF TESTICULAR TUMORS

The etiology of germinal cell tumors is unknown. There is an increased frequency in patients with abnormal testicular development and descent.[4,5] For example, in atrophic cryptorchid (undescended) testes, tumors are much more frequent even after orchiopexy. Gilber and Hamilton report that 12% of all testicular neoplasms arise in cryptorchid testes, and the chance of a tumor developing in an undescended testis is more than 40 times greater than in a normally descended scrotal testis.[6]

HISTOLOGY

The classification of malignant tumors for practical clinical purposes in this country is based on the classification of Dixon and Moore as reported in the Armed Forces Institute of Pathology fascicles (Table 35-1).[7] Ninety-six percent of all primary tumors are malignant and arise from germinal cells. They are either seminomas or nonseminomatous tumors.

TABLE 35-1. Pathologic Classification of Testicular Neoplasms

Primary Neoplasms
- Germinal neoplasms (may demonstrate any one or more of the following components):
  1. Seminoma
     a. Classic (typical)
     b. Anaplastic
     c. Spermatocytic
  2. Embryonal carcinoma
  3. Teratoma
     a. Mature
     b. Immature
  4. Chloriocarcinoma
  5. Yolk sac tumor (endodermal sinus tumor; embryonal adenocarcinoma of the prepubertal testis)
- Nongerminal neoplasms
  1. Specialized gonadal stromal neoplasms
     a. Leydig cell tumors
     b. Other gonadal stromal tumors
  2. Gonadoblastomas*
  3. Miscellaneous neoplasms
     a. Adenocarcinoma of the rete testis
     b. Neoplasms of mesenchymal origin
     c. Adrenal rest "tumors"
     d. Adenomatoid tumor

Secondary neoplasms
- Reticuloendothelial neoplasms
- Metastatic carcinomas

* Gonadoblastomas show both germ-cell and gonadal stromal elements and, strictly speaking, should not be considered nongerminal. They are included under this heading for convenience, as they differ clinically from germ-cell tumors.

There have been at least six major attempts since 1940 to classify germinal tumors along clinically meaningful lines. Beginning with the work of Freedman and Moore in 1946,[8] Dixon and Moore in 1952,[7] and Mostofi and Price in 1973,[9] this nomenclature is now incorporated in a classification proposed by the World Health Organization International Reference Center.[10] In Table 35-2, it can be noted that the British refer to all nonseminomatous germ-cell tumors as "malignant teratomas" of one type or another. American pathologists prefer the term "embryonal carcinoma" to signify a tumor that appears as the most undifferentiated form of teratoma. Despite these differences in language, the classifications are easily correlated (Table 35-2).

CLASSIC SEMINOMA

Classic seminoma usually presents in the fourth or fifth decade of life and accounts for about 40% of testicular tumors. The most common presenting symptom is gradual, painless testicular enlargement. The tumor is homogeneous on cut section and tan to pink with areas of infarct-like granular necrosis. Microscopically, it forms sheets of uniform cells segregated into compartments by slender fibrous septae containing a lymphocytic infiltrate that may vary in density. The nuclei are large, central, and hyperchromatic; the cytoplasm is clear or granular; and the cell borders are well defined. Occasional giant cells may occur in seminoma in the form of a Langerhans' giant cell and also a multinucleated giant cell, which may resemble that of a syncytiotrophoblast. Of course, when the seminoma is combined with other teratomatous or embryonal elements, it is not considered a pure or classic seminoma.

Whether anaplastic seminoma is truly intrinsically distinct from typical seminoma is doubted seriously. Consequently, a panel of pathologists at a 1980 international symposium on testicular cancer suggested the deletion of this term from the literature.[11] Until recently, the histologic diagnosis of anaplastic seminoma was made on the basis of the following microscopic features: (1) a large number of mitotic figures (an average count exceeding five per high-power field); (2) tumor cell anaplasia; and (3) a low-power impression of a solid neoplasm that does not appear as well nested and organized as the classic counterpart. In one report, 55% of a series of primary "anaplastic seminomas" contained multinucleated giant cells with positive histochemical staging for intracytoplasmic hCG, yet the clinical behavior of these tumors of low clinical stage was favorable when patients were treated with radiotherapy in the conventional manner.[12,13]

Approximately 10% of seminomas will be associated with an elevated serum hCG concentration. An elevated AFP concentration is never seen in pure seminoma.

SPERMATOCYTIC SEMINOMA

Spermatocytic seminoma accounts for about 7% of all seminomas and carries a good prognosis. It occurs in older patients, with an average age of 65 years. It is slow growing and

TABLE 35-2. Comparison of Classifications of Testicular Germ-Cell Tumors*

Dixon and Moore	*Mostofi and Price*	*WHO*	*British Testicular Tumour Panel*
	Tumors of one histologic type	*Tumors of one histologic type*	
Seminoma	Seminoma (typical) Spermatocytic seminoma Anaplastic seminoma†	Seminoma Spermatocytic seminoma	Seminoma Spermatocytic seminoma
Embryonal carcinoma	Embryonal carcinoma Polyembryoma Adult	Embryonal carcinoma Polyembryoma	Malignant teratoma, undifferentiated (MTU)
Teratoma, adult	Teratoma Mature Immature With malignant change‡	Teratoma Mature Immature With malignant transformation	Teratoma, differentiated
	Embryonal carcinoma juvenile	Yolk sac tumor (embryonal carcinoma, juvenile type; endodermal sinus tumor)	Yolk sac tumor
Choriocarcinoma	Choriocarcinoma	Choriocarcinoma	
	Tumors of more than one histologic type	*Tumors of more than one histologic type*	
Teratoma with embryonal carcinoma ("teratocarcinoma")	Embryonal carcinoma with teratoma ("teratocarcinoma")	Embryonal carcinoma with teratoma ("teratocarcinoma")	Malignant teratoma, intermediate (MTI)
	Specify types	Choriocarcinoma and any other types (specify)	Malignant teratoma trophoblastic (MTT)
	Specify types	Other combinations (specify)	"Combined tumor" when seminoma present

* Excluding intratubular germ-cell neoplasia.
† This term has been discarded in a more recent formulation.
‡ Refers to malignant areas independent of seminoma, embryonal carcinoma, or choriocarcinoma.

rarely metastasizes. The cut surface is pale gray, soft, and friable with a gelatinous or mucoid appearance. The tumor cells form solid sheets with poor segregation by fibrous septae, in contrast to its classic counterpart, which is well segregated by septae. A marked variation in the size of the tumor cells is a classical confirming histologic feature. Cells range from giant cells (50–100 μm) to many small cells (6–8 μm). There is no lymphocytic infiltration or granuloma formation, as would be seen in the classic seminoma.

EMBRYONAL CARCINOMA

Embryonal carcinoma is a highly malignant tumor with a cellular structure that is anaplastic with embryoid features such as immature tubular, papillary, or reticular appearance. The adult type has a variable histologic pattern. The polyembryonic type contains embryonal bodies that resemble those in its ovarian counterpart. Infantile embryonal carcinoma usually occurs as endodermal sinus (yolk sac) tumors. It varies in its size grossly, and cut surfaces show a varied appearance, with hemorrhagic necrosis often interspersed among yellow or gray bulging soft tissue. Its microscopic appearance is of characteristic primitive epithelial cells that are distinctly malignant in appearance. There is great variation in their size and arrangement, including some with very large pleomorphic nuclei and without distinct cell borders and others that are small with obvious borders. Mitotic figures and multinucleation are common. Acinar and papillary structures are noted frequently. The stroma is variable; it may be loose or quite thick and fibrous. Some tumors contain trophoblastic cells. These tumors generally are more aggressive and have a high metastatic potential compared with seminoma. Embryonal cells can secrete hCG, AFP, or both.

TERATOCARCINOMA

"Teratocarcinoma" describes a germinal tumor with elements of histologically mature teratoma. Behaviorally, it lies somewhere between the mature teratoma and the highly anaplastic and malignant embryonal carcinoma. On cut surface, it has a mixture of solid and cystic spaces, the solid spaces often containing hemorrhagic or necrotic material. Histologically, there is a mixture of frankly malignant tissue, as in embryonal carcinoma, and fully differentiated cartilage, muscle, or epithelial tissue. Trophoblastic cells may also be found. The British would classify this as malignant teratoma, intermediate.

ADULT (MATURE) TERATOMA

Adult teratoma has elements of one or more of the three germinal layers showing evidence of complete histologic maturity. It is necessary to sample such a tumor thoroughly to exclude undifferentiated foci. Although this type is the least aggressive of the nonseminomatous tumors, it can metastasize in the adult and so cannot be regarded as biologically benign. In fact, only 75% of patients with mature teratoma survived when treated with orchiectomy alone; the remaining 25% died of metastatic disease. Therefore, appropriate pathologic staging is indicated in adults. However, this is not the case in children, particularly newborn infants and those under the age of 2. When an adult teratoma has cellular and active stroma with mitotic figures, it is referred to as immature teratoma.

YOLK SAC TUMOR

Yolk sac (endodermal sinus) tumor presents more commonly in infants and young children but also can present in its histologically distinct form in adults. It is an aggressive tumor in the adult, with early hematogenous dissemination. It is especially virulent when it presents as a primary in the mediastinum. In contrast, its clinical behavior is considerably less aggressive in infants and young children.[14,15] Pure yolk sac tumors routinely are associated with an elevated AFP and a normal hCG.

CHORIOCARCINOMA

Choriocarcinoma is the most aggressive of the nonseminomatous tumors and is rare in its pure form. More frequently, it is seen mixed with other germ cell elements such as embryonal carcinoma and teratocarcinoma. It is recognized grossly by focal hemorrhages on the cut surface. The microscopic diagnosis requires definition of syncytiotrophoblastic cells, which are giant cells with multiple hyperchromatic nuclei and abundant eosinophilic cytoplasm, in relation to cytotrophoblasts, which are sheets of cells with single nuclei, abundant clear cytoplasms, and well-defined borders. HCG has long been used as a diagnostic marker of trophoblastic neoplasia. Beta subunits of hCG (β-hCG) have been identified, and accurate radioimmunoassays have been developed. Monitoring of this diagnostic marker now forms an indispensable part of the management and follow-up of patients with germ-cell tumors of the testis.[16]

BENIGN TUMORS

Tumors of stromal cell origin represent about 3% to 4% of primary testicular tumors. They are grouped as tumors of the specialized gonadal stroma and are called interstitial (Leydig) cell tumors, Sertoli cell tumors, granulosa cell tumors, androblastomas, testicular tubular adenomas, and so on.[17] Histologically, they have the appearance of the supporting tissues of the gonads of either sex and therefore may resemble Sertoli cells, granulosa cells, or theca cells. They constitute almost 20% of childhood testicular tumors.[18] Their behavior usually is benign; no more than 10% are reported to have malignant potential.[19,20] Gynecomastia occurs in about 15% of adults having interstitial cell tumors and in about one-third of adults with Sertoli cell tumors.[20] Management is accomplished with orchiectomy alone and clinical staging with CT scan and lymphangiography. Routine lymphadenectomy is not considered necessary if these studies are negative.

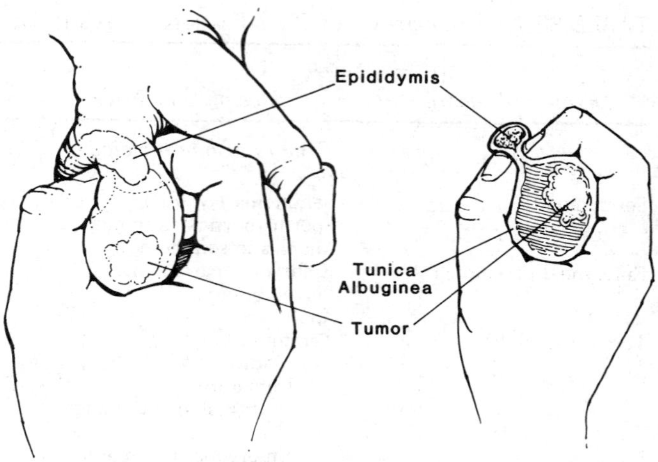

FIG. 35-1. Male scrotal examination. (Einhorn LH, Donohue JP, Peckham MJ, et al: Cancer of the testis. In DeVita VT Jr, Hellman S, Rosenberg SA [ed]: Cancer: Principles and Practice of Oncology, 2nd ed, p 985. Philadelphia, JB Lippincott, 1985)

SIGNS AND SYMPTOMS

The usual presentation of a testicular cancer is a painless enlargement of one gonad with the patient seeking medical evaluation of a lump, swelling, or hardness of the testis. In our experience, approximately 40% of patients also complain of a dull ache or heavy sensation in the scrotum, inguinal area, or lower abdomen. Acute onset of pain is rare unless the patient has concomitant epididymitis or develops bleeding within the testis, as expansion of the tunica albuginea produces pain.

Physical examination of the testis is performed by carefully palpating the organ between the thumb and first two fingers. The normal testis is homogeneous in consistency and freely movable (Fig. 35-1). Any nodular, hard, or fixed area discovered within the substance must be considered neoplastic until proved otherwise. The contralateral testis provides a comparative model for the examiner.

Simple palpation of a testis mass may give some clue as to its pathology. For example, seminomas tend to expand through the entire testicular substance, whereas teratomas and embryonal cell tumors tend to produce discrete nodular masses within the substance of the testis. Evaluation of the epididymis and cord structure is recommended.

DIFFERENTIAL DIAGNOSIS

The differential diagnosis of a testicular mass includes torsion, epididymitis, and tumor. Ancillary studies, including ultrasonography, are helpful in establishing a diagnosis, but suspicion is raised by the physical examination alone. In a retrospective review of our testicular cancer population, 55% of patients were initially treated for presumed epididymitis, resulting in a delay of definitive therapy from several weeks to 9 months or longer.

LABORATORY INVESTIGATION

Along with the blood cell count and urinalysis, the basic laboratory studies for patients suspected of having testicular tumors are specified radiologic studies and measurement of serum markers. HCG and AFP have become the ultimate tumor markers, and their use is routine in all stages of germ-cell tumors. In disseminated nonseminomatous germ-cell tumors, approximately 40% of all patients will have an elevated AFP and 75% an elevated hCG, and 85% will have one or both markers elevated. A marker that fails to return to normal or rises after a chemotherapy-induced CR almost invariably implies persistent or recurrent disease. The half-life of hCG is 18 to 24 hours and that of AFP, 5 days. Marked elevations of AFP may take several months to normalize after a curative treatment, either surgery (retroperitoneal lymphadenectomy; RPLND) or chemotherapy.

Occasionally, elevated hCG or AFP levels are found in the absence of active germ-cell tumors. The most obvious cause of such a result is a laboratory error. No patient should be treated as having a relapse purely on the basis of a single elevation of hCG. Although there is a sense of urgency to treat patients immediately with chemotherapy for a post-RPLND or first-line chemotherapy relapse, in reality, there is no necessity for prompt institution of chemotherapy as long as there is no obvious hematogenous spread (normal chest radiograph) or extensive nodal disease (on physical examination, abdominal CT, or both). For example, if a patient achieves a CR with cisplatin combination chemotherapy and subsequently has an hCG of 18 mIU/ml (normal less than 1.50-mIU/ml) while all other studies are normal, the worst error an oncologist can make is to start salvage chemotherapy; in reality, there may not be a relapse at all. Initially, we would repeat the hCG assay with another laboratory if appropriate. We also would query the patient about recent marijuana abuse, as this can cause gynecomastia and modest elevations of hCG. Finally, some patients will have cisplatin-induced atrophy in the remaining normal testis, with resultant low serum testosterone levels. The pituitary gland, by normal feedback mechanisms, will secrete large quantities of luteinizing hormone (LH) to stimulate the Leydig cells of the testis to secrete more testosterone. The beta subunit of hCG is not supposed to have cross-reactivity with LH; however, there is always some degree of interference even in the best radioimmunoassays. A simple test in this clinical situation is to give a patient a single injection of 300 mg of depotestosterone and repeat the hCG assay in 2 weeks. If hCG has been suppressed, the cause of the apparent elevation is cross-reactivity of the assay with LH.

Only rarely is a false-positive AFP elevation observed. This marker can be elevated in other tumors, especially hepatoma. Also, regenerating hepatitis or cirrhotic nodules can cause a false-positive elevation of AFP, but this is usually obvious clinically.

Markers are also of value in seminoma. HCG is elevated in only 10% of seminoma; however, 50% of patients Stage III seminomas will have elevated hCG. Moreover, AFP is never elevated in pure seminoma, so if an orchiectomy reveals pure seminoma, but the AFP is elevated, the patient should be managed as having nonseminomatous disease,[13]

Lactic dehydrogenase (LDH) is a nonspecific marker akin to the erythrocyte sedimentation rate in Hodgkin's disease. Most patients with bulky metastases of germ-cell tumor will have an elevated LDH.

A potential new marker has recently been described for metastatic seminoma. Kuzmits and colleagues measured serum neuron-specific enolase (NSE) in 11 patients with metastatic seminoma, and eight had elevated levels.[21] Only 3 of 11 had elevated hCG, and all 11 had normal AFP levels. The NSE levels fell to normal with cisplatin combination chemotherapy. These authors also documented the localization of NSE in seminoma cells immunohistochemically. NSE assays may be of particular value in bulky Stage II–III seminoma with persistent radiographic abnormalities after cisplatin-based chemotherapy in helping to determine the need for subsequent laparotomy or radiotherapy.

RADIOGRAPHIC STUDIES AND STAGING

In nonseminomatous disease, Stage I (or A) refers to tumor confined to the testis; this implies tumor-free lymph nodes and a clear chest. Stage II (or B) indicates metastatic disease in the node-bearing area of the periaortic or vena caval zone but with no demonstrable metastases above the diaphragm or in visceral organs. Stage III (C) designates clinical or radiographic evidence of metastases above the diaphragm or in other viscera. Stages IIA (B_1) and IIB (B_2) refer to microscopic (IIA with fewer than five positive nodes) and grossly positive nodes or more than 5 positive nodes, respectively.

Radiographic studies are designed to rule out Stage III disease (pulmonary metastases) and retroperitoneal nodal metastases (Stage II disease). Useful in this regard are chest CT, which we consider essential before embarking on lymphadenectomy. Of less value are lymphangiography and intravenous urography. The possible error in pedal lymphangiography is roughly 25% false negative and 5% to 10% false positive.[22] With such overall inaccuracy, lymphangiography is no longer needed for staging purposes in our view. We have been impressed with the value of CT as a staging mechanism for the retroperitoneal space. Gross nodal metastases usually are detected by this method, although microscopic metastases are not, and our overall accuracy rate with CT is 70% to 80%.[23,24] Independent clinical studies in the United States reveal at least a 20% understaging rate when combining all diagnostic tests such as CT scan and serum markers.[22–24]

SEMINOMA

Seminoma is the most common histologic subtype of testis tumors in adults, accounting for about 60% of all germ-cell tumors. Its treatment is one of the most gratifying endeavors in all of oncologic clinical practice: with the advent of multidrug chemotherapy that allows the cure of men with disseminated disease, the overall cure rate for all stages is now at or above 90% in most treatment centers. Because these tumors occur in a young population, and because surgical resection, external-beam radiation, and multidrug chemotherapy are

TABLE 35-3. Staging of Seminoma

Stage I	Tumor confined to the testis
Stage II	Nodal metastases (usually based on radiologic studies) but limited to the infradiaphragmatic lymphatics
	A. Minimal retroperitoneal disease
	B. Bulky metastases
Stage III	Tumor involving lymphatics above the diaphragm
Stage IV	Extranodal metastases

all effective (either alone or in combinations) in treating patients with metastatic deposits, consideration of cure *with* maintenance of fertility *and* avoidance of potential harmful sequelae is very important.

Seminoma is exquisitely sensitive to radiation and usually presents at an early stage. Postorchiectomy external-beam radiation therapy to the retroperitoneal lymph nodes achieves very high cure rates for patients with low-stage tumors. The optimum treatment of patients presenting with distant metastases is chemotherapy initially. The role, if any, of consolidation surgery or radiotherapy in clinical scenarios in which there are persistent radiographic abnormalities remains controversial. Likewise, the optimal treatment of bulky Stage II disease is uncertain.

After radical orchiectomy (see below) that reveals seminoma, the clinical evaluation for possible extragonadal metastatic disease should always include postorchiectomy serum radioimmunoassays for hCG and AFP, tomography, a retroperitoneal CT scan, and a bipedal lymphangiogram if the retroperitoneal CT scan is negative. Because the AFP concentration is never elevated with pure seminoma and the serum hCG rarely is, these markers contribute nothing to the clinical staging of patients with seminoma (Table 35-3). The absolute incidence of occult retroperitoneal lymph node metastases in Stage I seminoma (CT and lymphangiograms are normal) is not known because for the last three decades, patients have been treated by regional radiation after noninvasive staging. The accepted incidence of occult metastases is 10% to 25% [22,25,26]

Recently, several specific histopathologic characteristics of the primary tumor have been evaluated with regard to their influence on metastatic spread in men with pure seminoma.[27,28] Unfortunately, no significant predictors have been identified, although because all patients evaluated had retroperitoneal irradiation, the false-negative rate of noninvasive staging has not truly been tested. In preliminary data from the Massachusetts General Hospital, no difference has been found in the incidence of either vascular invasion or invasion of the epididymis or spermatic cord in patients clinically staged as I compared with those in Stage II.

POSTORCHIECTOMY RADIATION TECHNIQUE (STAGES I AND IIA)

The retroperitoneal lymph nodal groups usually included in the radiation treatment fields are the ipsilateral external iliac, the bilateral common iliac, the paracaval, and the para-aortic nodes superiorly including coverage of the cisterna cyli. Lymphangiographic study of the retroperitoneal lymph nodes is very useful in the design of the treatment fields at the time of simulation. An excretory urogram or an abdominal CT scan must be carefully evaluated prior to or at the time of simulation with the patient in the treatment position to assure the exact localization of the kidneys with respect to the treatment fields. When such care is taken to localize the kidneys properly, the risk of radiation-induced damage is essentially eliminated.

The exact definition of the fields depends on the unique characteristics of the individual patients and the type of megavoltage equipment available. The boundaries of the fields usually are *superiorly* to the origin of the thoracic duct or to include the entire anterior surface of the T11 vertebral body; *inferiorly* to the internal inguinal ring and the inguinal excision; and *laterally* to include the ipsilateral renal hilum, usually more generously on the left than on the right. The contralateral para-aortic or paracaval and common iliac lymph node groups are contoured with individually cut Cerrobend blocking and treated with 4 to 12 MeV linear accelerator beams.

These fields should be expanded to include additional areas in the following not-uncommon situations. First, in patients who have a history of herniorrhapy or orchiopexy, which may predispose to atypical lymphatic drainage, the inferior portion of the field should be extended to include the contralateral inguinal region. Second, in patients with histo-

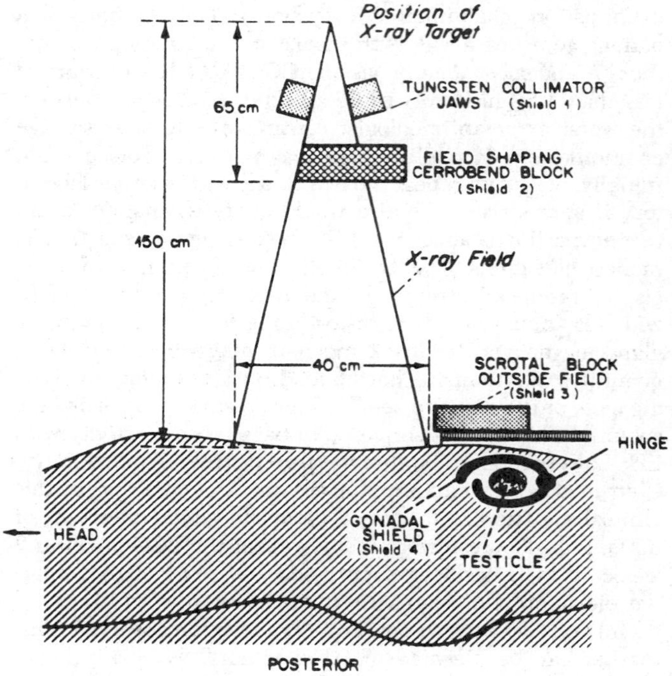

FIG. 35-2. A schematic sagittal diagram of the treatment set-up and shielding for the treatment of a patient with a testicular seminoma following radical orchiectomy. Patient is supine and the contralateral testis is shown diagrammatically. Field size is 40 cm in the longitudinal direction, and the treatment distance from source to skin is 150 cm. Four shielding devices are illustrated: the collimator jaws of the linear accelerator, cerrobend field shaping blocks, a lead scrotal block, and a gonadal shield whose front or cephalad wall separates the testicle from the horizontal internal scatter. (Kubo HD, Shipley WU: Int J Radiat Oncol Biol Phys 8:1741–1745, 1982)

logic evidence of epididymal or spermatic cord invasion, the field should be enlarged to include the ipsilateral hypogastric lymph nodes as potential site of metastases.

Recent improvements in shielding the contralateral testis include using three additional shields outside the primary beam. A system that has proved convenient, effective, and useful at the Massachusetts General Hospital is shown in Figure 35-2 and includes a 10-cm lead shield immediately above the contralateral testis; an extension of Cerrobend block for an additional 5 cm below the inferior border of the field at the level of the blocking tray; and a more comprehensive gonadal shielding, preventing the majority of internally scattered photons from hitting the remaining testis. This combination has lowered the dose received by the contralateral testis to approximately 0.1% of the treatment dose.[29]

The fields are treated with conventional fractionations (150 cGy per day, five sessions per week) using 10-MeV linear accelerator beam. Both the anterior and the posterior fields are treated each day. If the patient has had a huge primary tumor invading part of the scrotum but not requiring a hemiscrotectomy, or if the tumor has been removed through a scrotal incision, the ipsilateral hemiscrotum is treated by a 12 to 15 MeV electron-beam field that is matched to the lower border of the photon field. The ipsilateral hemiscrotum is held to the involved side with a soft clamp while the patient places and holds his remaining testis high in the inguinal canal and under a 2-cm-thick lead cup. With this technique, the contralateral testis can usually be moved more than 4 cm from the electron beam edge and has been consistently found to receive 3% or less of the given electron dose by scatter.

TREATMENT RESULTS: STAGE I

The results from many major centers in clinical Stage I seminoma treated with postorchiectomy radiation therapy are all outstanding (for examples, see Table 35-4). The 3- to 5-year disease-free survival rates are very near the absolute cure rates in patients with testicular seminoma in that there are very few late relapses with death in these series. Now, with the advent of chemotherapy effective against disseminated disease, we would anticipate being able to cure nearly all of these few patients who will relapse with distant disease.

The outstanding 3- to 5-year survival rates (all above 95%) seem not to be influenced by whether the reporting institution did or did not use prophylactic mediastinal irradiation. In the absence of any data to support its usefulness,[36,37] prophylactic mediastinal irradiation has been discontinued by most treatment centers for at least 5 years. Moreover, supradiaphragmatic irradiation will certainly compromise a patient's ability to receive and tolerate multidrug chemotherapy should it be necessary.[38] Thus, this practice seems further contraindicated.

TABLE 35-4. Results of Postorchiectomy Radiation Therapy in Stage I Seminoma

Treatment Center	*Total Patients*	*5-Year Survival (%)*
Walter Reed Army Hosp.[30]	284	97
Royal Marsden Hosp.[31]	232	98
M.D. Anderson Hosp.[28]	161	95
Stanford Univ. Hosp.[32]	71	100
Massachusetts General Hosp.[33]	135	98
U.S Patterns of Care Study[34]	229	98
Cross Cancer Institute[35]	139	98
Total	1151	98

Patients treated with postorchiectomy radiation therapy for Stage I seminoma have only a 2% probability of developing metastatic disease, a 2% incidence of a second testis tumor, and a less than 0.5% incidence of leukemia.[28,31,33] The incidence of second tumors has been no higher than the age-standardized national incidence rates.[31]

TABLE 35-5. Results of Postorchiectomy Radiation Therapy in Stage II Seminoma

Treatment Center	*Total Patients*	*5-Year Survival (%)*
Walter Reed Army Hosp.[30]	34	76
Royal Marsden Hosp.[36]	63	79
M.D. Anderson Hosp.[39]	48	88
Ontario Cancer Institute[37]	86	74
Massachusetts General Hosp.[33]	25	92
Cross Cancer Institute[35]	32	70
Total	288	79

TREATMENT RESULTS: STAGE II

Postorchiectomy radiation therapy for patients with Stage II seminoma has been reported to yield a 70% to 88% survival rate (Table 35-5). The "correct" management of these patients has become increasingly controversial over the last 5 years with the demonstrated effectiveness of multidrug chemotherapy against advanced or disseminated seminoma. Several not completely satisfactory staging systems for the size of the metastatic deposits in retroperitoneal lymph nodes exist. However, it is clear from all series that those patients with bulky retroperitoneal metastases (Stage IIB) have had, with radiation alone before the cisplatin and chemotherapy era, survival or cure rates in the 60% range, compared with rates above 90% in those with minimal disease (Stage IIA), which statistically is not significantly lower than for Stage I. Patterns of failure following radiation for Stage IIB seminoma by wide-field or extended-field radiation therapy alone in the 1960s and 1970s suggest, in most[33,36,39] (Tables 35-6 and 35-7), but not all,[40] series, that 30% or more of the patients so treated will develop metastatic disease outside the treated volume. In contrast, those patients with Stage IIA disease have a very low incidence of distant metastases whether or not they are given prophylactic mediastinal irradiation.[37,39]

Observations 15 to 20 years ago in patients with testicular seminoma suggested that those with anaplastic tumor histology or an elevated urinary gonadotropin titer did uniquely poorly. However, recent reviews by several large institutions, including the Walter Reed Army Hospital[41] and the

TABLE 35-6. Results of Treatment in Stage II Seminoma: Royal Marsden Hospital 1962–1979

Stage	*Size of Retroperitoneal Node Metastases (cm)*	*No. of Patients*	*Total Relapsing (%)*	*Died of Seminoma*	*Died of Intercurrent Disease*
IIA	<2	31	3 (9.7)	2	5
IIB	<5	11	2 (18)	1 0	
IIC	>5	21	tap(38)	6	3
Total		63	13 (21)	9 (14%)	8 (13%)

Memorial Sloan-Kettering Cancer Center,[42] documented that patients with Stages I and IIA disease and anaplastic histology have, when treated with conventional radiation therapy, as high an overall success rate as do patients with well-differentiated seminoma. Also, in recent reviews, all patients with Stage I or Stage IIA disease who had an elevated serum hCG by radioimmunoassay have remained in complete remission after conventional radiation therapy.[43,44] Thus, patients with Stages I and IIA pure seminoma with elevated serum hCG, as well as those with anaplastic seminoma, should be treated by radiation therapy with doses that are usual for the patient's clinical stage.

TREATMENT OF ADVANCED SEMINOMA

Radiation therapy was the treatment of choice for Stage IIB, III, or IV seminoma before the advent of cisplatin combination chemotherapy. The cure rate for Stage IIB was about 60%, and the cure rate for Stages III and IV ranged from 20% to 60%.[33,36,45] Extended radiation therapy to both infradiaphragmatic and supradiaphragmatic fields often precludes the administration of effective doses of chemotherapy to control any later failure.[38]

Alkylating agents were used against metastatic seminoma in the 1970s. However, beginning in 1974, the combination of cisplatin, vinblastine, and bleomycin (PVB) was instituted as first-line chemotherapy in disseminated testicular seminoma at Indiana University. Seminoma was judged at least as chemosensitive as any other germ-cell type to cisplatin-based chemotherapy, and even as a single agent, cisplatin has produced excellent results. For example, Oliver at the Institute of Urology in London utilized cisplatin 50 mg/m^2 on days one and two every 3 weeks for four courses and achieved a CR in 13 of 14 patients.[46] The response rates are high whether cisplatin-based chemotherapy is given as the first treatment with no prior radiation (Table 35-8) or as salvage treatment for relapse after initial radiation (Table 35-9). Although most authors have not reported separately the maintained CR rate with and without prior radiation therapy, it seems clear that extensive prior radiation is a significant negative influence on both the chemotherapy tolerance and the CR rate. The Southeastern Cancer Study Group has recently published the largest experience in the treatment of patients with advanced seminoma with and without prior radiation therapy.[38] In their series, 43 of 62 patients treated by PVB with or without VP-16 or doxorubicin have achieved and maintained CR. However, in 13 of these 43 patients the response was "consolidated" by surgery, radiation therapy, or both to the site of original tumor bulk. There were six drug-related fatalities and 12 patients dying of progressive disease, 11 of whom were never disease-free.

In patients treated with cisplatin-containing chemotherapy regimens, one difficulty has been that 50% or more will not have a radiographic CR. The need for further treatment versus observation in these patients is still unclear. Surgical resection following such chemotherapy is difficult because of the severe fibrotic reaction frequently noted in the retroperitoneum. Friedman and associates reported two perioperative deaths in three patients who underwent surgery to remove residual disease.[48] In a recent Memorial Sloan-Kettering Cancer Center review of patients with bulky Stage II or Stage III seminoma, residual viable tumor was found only when the residual mass was 3 cm or greater radiologically and clear rather than desmoplastic.[49]

In summary, advanced seminoma is a rare disease and one that is chemosensitive and has a cure potential with chemotherapy competitive with that seen in nonseminomatous germ-cell tumors: 93 of 111 (84%) patients achieved a continuous disease-free status with cisplatin combination chemotherapy. A reasonable approach, shared by many

TABLE 35-7. Sites of Initial Relapse After Radiotherapy for Stage II Seminoma: Royal Marsden Hospital, 1962–1979

Stage	*Size of Retroperitoneal Node Metastases (cm)*	*No. of Patients*	*Lung± Mediastinum*	*Cervical*	*Scrotum or Groin Nodes**	*Liver*	*Extradural*	*Multiple Sites*
IIA	2	31	1	0	2	0	0	0
IIB	2–4.9	11	0	0	1	0	1	0
IIC	5–9.9	9	2	0	0	1	0	0
IID	10	12	1	2	0	0	0	2
Total		63	4	2	3	1	1	2

* Two of three patients who had scrotal interference prior to orchiectomy and who did not receive scrotal and groin-node irradiation suffered relapses.

TABLE 35-8. Results of Postorchiectomy Initial Chemotherapy in Stages IIB, III, and IV Seminoma

Treatment Center	*Chemotherapy*	*No. of Patients*	*Maintained CR**
London Inst. Urology[46]	Cisplatin	10	9
M.D. Anderson Hosp.[39]	Cisplatin ± cyclophosphamide	10	8
University of Munich[47]	VIP	6	5
Southeastern Cancer Study Group[38]	PVB ± doxorubicin or PVP-16B	27	21
Norwegian Random Hosp.[51]	PVB or PVP-16B	39	33
National Cancer Inst., Milan[52]	PVB or PVP-16B	19	17
Total		111	93(84%)

* Includes some patients receiving postchemotherapy surgery or radiation to remove residual disease.

treatment centers, is to use multidrug cisplatin-based chemotherapy initially and to use no further treatment in the patients with a radiographic CR. In those with residual masses, either careful close observation or consolidation by radiation therapy or surgery is appropriate.[50,51] Possibly the recent identification of two potentially useful serum markers for seminoma, placental alkaline phosphatase[52] and neuron-specific enolase[21] will aid in the difficult decision concerning appropriate management of patients with persistent radiographic abnormalities.

ORCHIECTOMY

Removal of the testis through an inguinal approach is the definitive procedure for both pathologic diagnosis and local control of the primary tumor. The inguinal approach is preferred as it permits early control of both the vascular and lymphatic supply of the testis as well as the en bloc removal of the paratesticular fascial layers. Scrotal orchiectomy and biopsy are to be condemned and have been associated with a 24% incidence of local recurrence or spread to inguinal lymph node areas.[53] Although (β-hCG and AFP) are sensitive markers germ-cell tumors, 30% of patients with nonseminomatous germ-cell tumor and 92% of those with seminomas will have normal marker levels. Therefore, a decision against surgical exploration of a testicular mass should not be based on negative results of tumor markers.

The management of the patient who has undergone a scrotal orchiectomy is predicated on whether a testicular biopsy was performed prior to the orchiectomy. If the operating surgeon recognized the presence of a tumor and did not biopsy the testis, then the inguinal portion of the spermatic cord can be removed through a metachronous inguinal incision or at the time of an RPLND. If a biopsy was performed and a nonseminomatous germ-cell tumor identified, a hemiscrotectomy should be done; an inguinal lymphadenectomy is performed only in the unusual case where palpable nodes are identified. In patients who have a seminoma, the groin and lateral scrotum should be included within the irradiated field.

The surgical procedure for orchiectomy is as follows. The patient is placed supine on the operative table, and adequate anesthesia is attained. The inguinal area is prepared and draped, and an incision is made 2 cm superior and parallel to the inguinal ligament. The incision is carried through the subcutaneous tissue, and the several large veins encountered are identified and ligated. The aponeurosis of the external oblique and the external inguinal ring are identified, and an incision is made in the external fascia. Care is taken to dissect bluntly the underlying medial muscle and nerve from the fascia. The medial and inferior aspects of the spermatic cord are dissected free from the external fascia, exposing the pubic tubercle. At this point, a Penrose drain is placed around the spermatic cord at the level of the pubic tubercle. After the cremasteric vessels have been divided, the drain is doubled around the spermatic cord and clamped securely 1 inch from the internal ring. By both blunt and sharp dissection, the testis is delivered from the scrotum to the operative field. With large tumors, it is often necessary to extend the incision down to the upper aspects of the scrotum.

If a tumor appears obvious, then the surgeon should proceed with division of the spermatic cord at the internal ring. If the existence of a neoplasm is questionable, a frozen section may be performed by isolating the testis away from the operative field, covering the incision, and performing the biopsy with the testis encircled by towels or sponges. In order

TABLE 35-9. Results of Chemotherapy After Orchiectomy and Radiation Therapy for Disseminated Relapse of Seminoma Salvage (Chemotherapy)

Treatment Center	*Chemotherapy*	*No. of Patients*	*Maintained CR**
London Inst. Urology[46]	Cisplatin, etoposide	4	4
University of Munich[47]	VIP	7	5
Southeastern Cancer Study Group[38]	PVB ± doxorubicin or PVP-16B	33	20
Norwegian Radium Hosp.[50]	PVB or PVP-16	15	9
National Cancer Institute, Milan[51]	PVB or PVP-16B	13	6
Total		72	44(61%)

* Includes some patients receiving postchemotherapy surgery for residual disease.

to remove the testis, the structures of the spermatic cord should be identified and divided. It is necessary to identify and ligate the vas separately from the spermatic vessels. The cord stump is placed in the retroperitoneum so that the distal aspects of the cord can be removed without difficulty in the event a RPLND is performed.

RADICAL RETROPERITONEAL LYMPH NODE DISSECTION

Retroperitoneal lymphadenectomy remains the mainstay of surgical therapy for nonseminomatous germ-cell tumors. In patients with low-volume disease, including Stages I, IIA, and IIB, RPLND permits accurate staging, minimizes the risk of retroperitoneal recurrence, and cures a substantial number of patients without chemotherapy. Controversies surrounding management by observation for clinical Stage I disease as well as the role of primary and adjuvant chemotherapy for early Stage II are discussed elsewhere in this chapter. RPLND is also performed to remove residual disease after chemotherapy and to define further therapy in this subset of patients.

HISTORICAL PERSPECTIVES

Jamieson and Dobson in 1910 described the lymphatic drainage of the testis, establishing the primary echelon of drainage for right-sided tumors to the interaortocaval, preaortic, and precaval nodes and for left-sided tumors to the left periaortic and preaortic nodes.[54] There exists some crossover, especially from right to left, of these lymphatics. Their anatomical study was the basis for lymph node dissection in the management of these tumors. The first site of metastases is the retroperitoneal lymph nodes in nearly 90% of patients who have nonseminomatous tumors; in only 7% to 15% of patients will the site of first metastasis be outside the surgical margins of the lymph node dissection.

The first successful retroperitoneal lymph node dissection was reported by Cuneo and Marcille.[55] Other investigators soon described performing lymph node dissections in an attempt to cure testicular tumors.[56,57] The classic report by Lewis in 1948 was the first to establish RPLND as a primary therapy for nonseminomatous germ-cell tumors.[58] He reported a 46% 5-year survival rate among 28 patients who were treated with combined retroperitoneal lymphadenectomy and radiation after orchiectomy.

Various surgical approaches have been advocated for the removal of the retroperitoneal lymph nodes. Cooper and associates were among the first to popularize the transthoracic approach[59] based on Sweet's gastroesophageal procedures. The transabdominal approach was popularized by Staubitz, Whitmore, and others.[60,61] Donohue and his coworkers later modified this dissection by including an extended bilateral suprahilar removal using a transabdominal midline incision with mobilization of the pancreas and surrounding structures.[62] In addition, Donohue's group depicted the distribution of retroperitoneal lymph node metastases in patients who had Stages IIA, IIB, and IIC disease.[62] This significant, meticulously performed study provides the rationale for tailoring the surgical procedure to the amount of disease present. Furthermore, it serves as a rationale for modifying RPLND in order to preserve ejaculatory function in patients with clinical Stage I disease.

There is minimal morbidity and virtually no mortality associated with RPLND.[62,63] The principal long-term complication remains loss of ejaculation. However, recent reports by Lange and colleagues reveal that fertility can be preserved in selected patients undergoing radical retroperitoneal dissection,[64] and this subject will be discussed later in this chapter.

Radiologic tests to detect lymph node metastases, including magnetic resonance imaging (MRI), CT scanning, and lymphangiography, have false-positive and false-negative rates that range from 15% to 25%.[65] Therefore, RPLND is the most accurate way to detect retroperitoneal metastases. Moreover, it is therapeutic in the majority of patients with Stages I through IIB disease, being associated with a recurrence rate of less than 2% in the retroperitoneum.[66]

Adequate preoperative preparation of the patient undergoing an RPLND is imperative. Vigorous preoperative overnight hydration with 5% dextrose in 0.45% saline at a rate of 150 ml per hour is instituted; in combination with intravenous mannitol at the time of dissection of the renal hilum, this fluid reduces the risk of arterial thrombosis and renal ischemia. Broad-spectrum antimicrobials are administered preoperatively. General anesthesia is routine. Occasionally, in patients with residual disease after chemotherapy, sodium nitroprusside-induced hypotension is employed to reduce blood loss when resecting bulky retroperitoneal disease associated with a dense desmoplastic reaction around the vessels and other retroperitoneal structures. Central venous lines and arterial lines are helpful in monitoring hemodynamic status in patients judged to be at high risk for bleeding or other complications.

SURGICAL PROCEDURE: THORACOABDOMINAL LYMPH NODE DISSECTION

Patient position for thoracoabdominal RPLND is of paramount importance. The patient is placed on the ipsilateral side of the operating table with the break located just above the iliac crest (Fig. 35-3). The ipsilateral shoulder is positioned 30° off the horizontal, and the arm is extended across the chest and placed on a Mayo stand or a Kraus armrest. The hips are nearly flat. Once the incision is made, this position results in an uncoiling phenomenon similar to that observed when opening an empty paper towel roll.

The incision is made over an appropriately selected rib so that the medial aspect of the incision lies halfway between the xiphoid process and the umbilicus. The lateral extent of the incision is the posterior axillary line. The costochondral junction is crossed, and a gentle curve like that of a hockey stick is made so that the incision becomes either a left paramedian or a midline. In general, the thoracic and abdominal limbs of the incision should be of equal length.

With the electrocautery device, the subcutaneous tissues and latissimus dorsi muscle are divided. The distal two-thirds of the selected rib is identified and resected. At this point, the surgeon can proceed either in an extraperitoneal or in-

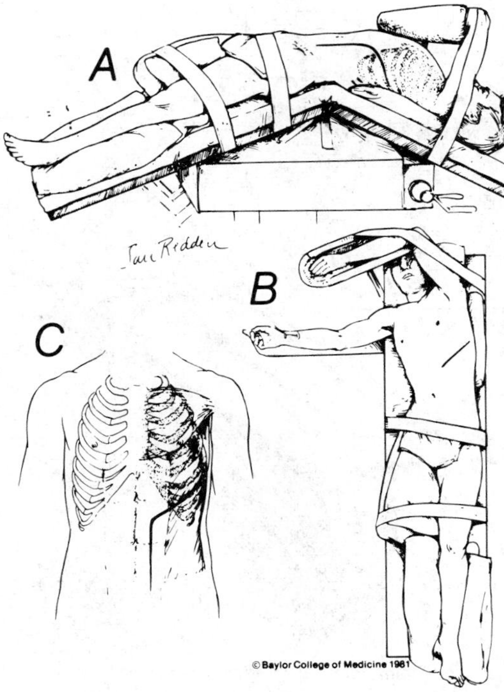

FIG. 35-3. Position and incision for left thoracoabdominal retroperitoneal lymphadenectomy. **A**. The soft tissue of the flank is placed directly over the break in the table, with the contralateral leg triangulated and the ipsilateral leg straight. The table is maximally hyperextended. **B**. The right arm rests on an arm board; the left arm is elevated on a well-padded Kraus support. **C**. The incision begins over the rib at the left posterior axillary line, is directed toward a point midway between the xiphoid and the umbilicus, and then turns over the abdomen to become a paramedian incision. (Scardino PT: Thoracoabdominal retroperitoneal lymphadenectomy for testicular cancer. In Crawford ED, Borden TA [eds]: Genitourinary Cancer Surgery. Philadelphia, Lea & Febiger, 1982)

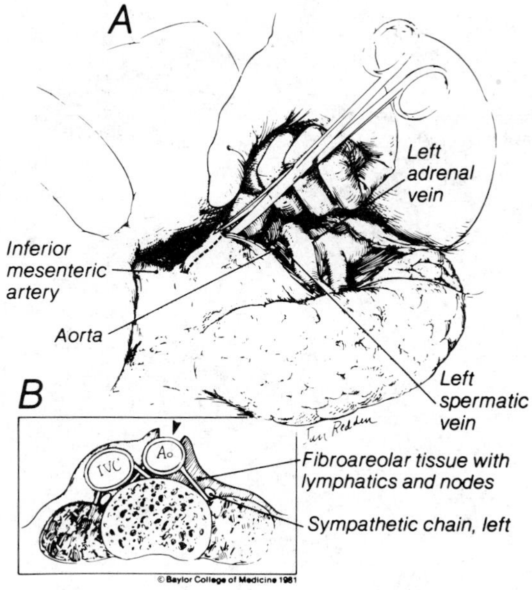

FIG. 35-4. **A**. The left renal vein is mobilized by dividing the adrenal and spermatic veins. The plane between the aorta and the retroperitoneal tissue to be dissected can be established bluntly as illustrated. **B**. The dissection is viewed in cross-section to illustrate the tissue to be dissected from the great vessels. (Scardino PT: Thoracoabdominal retroperitoneal lymphadenectomy for testicular cancer. In Crawford ED, Borden TA [eds]: Genitourinary Cancer Surgery. Philadelphia, Lea & Febiger, 1982)

traperitoneal fashion after division of the costochondral junction. In general, an extraperitoneal approach is indicated in patients who have not had chemotherapy or who have small amounts of retroperitoneal disease. In patients undergoing RPLND after chemotherapy, it is difficult to proceed extraretroperitoneally, and the peritoneum should be opened to expose the retroperitoneal structures.

With both sharp and blunt dissection, the diaphragm and peritoneum are dissected from the posterior sheath medially to the linea alba. Once the peritoneal envelope is retracted, a plane must be developed between the Gerota's fascia and the posterior peritoneum. After the peritoneal envelope is freed from the retroperitoneal structures, a Finochietto retractor is placed in the wound in such a fashion as to allow the costochondral margins to protrude through its open blades. For a left-sided dissection, the left renal vein represents the center of the anatomic dissection. Located immediately above the left renal vein is the superior mesenteric artery; laterally is the kidney, posteriorly and laterally is the left renal artery, posteriorly are the aorta and right renal artery, inferiorly are the aorta and inferior mesenteric artery, and medially is the inferior vena cava.

The initial dissection proceeds along the root of the superior mesenteric artery. This artery is an important landmark, and great care must be observed so that the vessel is not injured. There are numerous lymphatics that circumscribe the superior mesenteric artery, and these must be clipped and divided carefully. The dissection is carried laterally to the crus of the left hemidiaphragm and then continued medially and superiorly to the adrenal gland (Fig. 35-4).

Once this is accomplished, the dissection is carried over to the inferior vena cava, further delineating the upper limits of the dissection. The areolar tissues surrounding the left renal vein are divided and ligaclipped. The dissection then proceeds to the superior aspect of this vein, where the adrenal vein is identified and ligated. As the dissection is carried posteriorly, the lumbar vein will be encountered and should be identified and ligated, as it can be the source of troublesome bleeding (Fig. 35-5). In general, with anterior and superior traction, the aorta and root of the left renal artery are identified. A plane is located and developed between the adventitia of the aorta and the anteriorly located areolar and nodal tissues. Dissection is carried inferiorly on the aorta, identifying the inferior mesenteric artery. This artery may be divided; however, in older patients and in patients in whom ejaculatory function is to be preserved, this artery is not divided.

Both the renal artery and renal vein can now be dissected from proximal to distal or from the hilum to the root. Bivalving Gerota's fascia provides safe access to the renal hilar area and easy identification of aberrant renal arteries and veins (Fig. 35-5). Prior to dissection of the renal vessels, administration of 12.5 g of mannitol intravenously is recom-

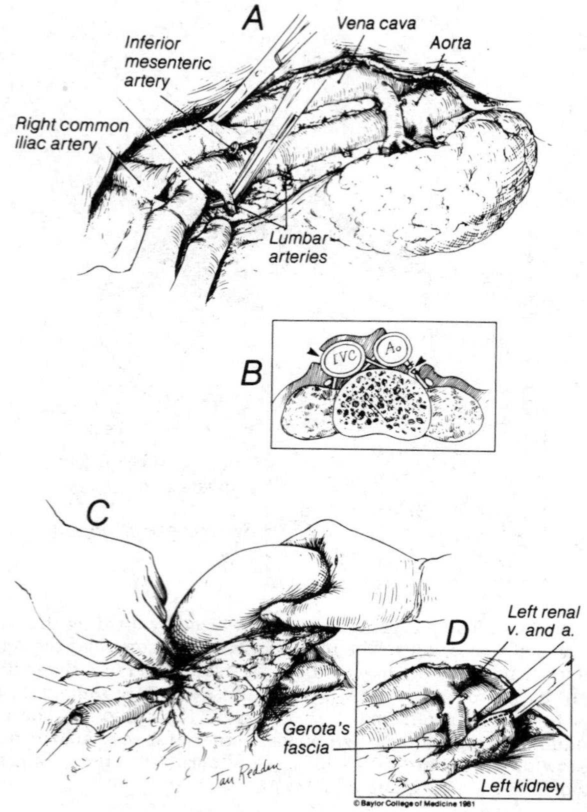

FIG. 35-5. **A**. The lateral border of the dissection is the lateral aspect of the inferior vena cava. Hemoclips must be applied along this margin. The lumbar arteries are identified, ligated, and divided. **B**. Cross-sectional view. **C**. Gerota's fascia is divided over the lateral border of the kidney and split into an anterior and posterior bundle. **D**. The ring of perirenal fat can be divided at the renal hilum while the renal vessels are directly visible. (Scardino PT: Thoracoabdominal retroperitoneal lymphadenectomy for testicular cancer. In Crawford ED, Borden TA [eds]: Genitourinary Cancer Surgery. Philadelphia, Lea & Febiger, 1982)

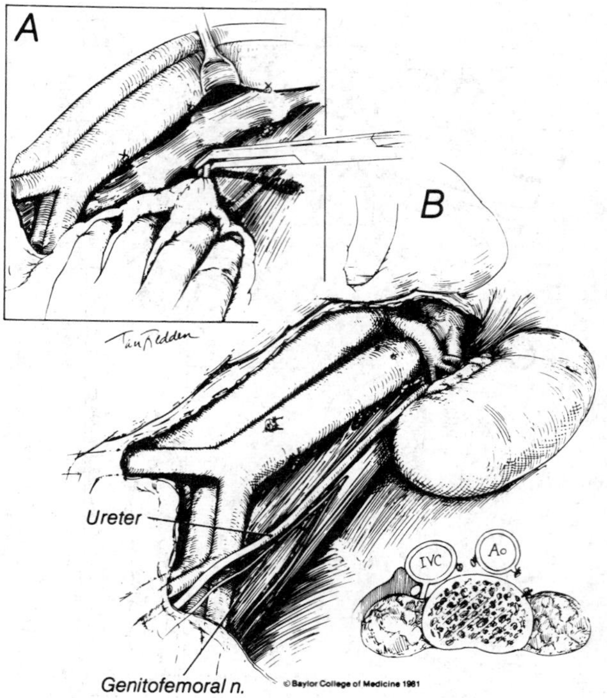

FIG. 35-6. **A**. Clips are applied to the vessels along the left aortic groove in the area of the sympathetic chain. **B**. The completed dissection is illustrated both as an overview and as a cross-section. The left common iliac artery and vein are dissected to a point just beyond their bifurcation. (Scardino PT: Thoracoabdominal retroperitoneal lymphadenectomy for testicular cancer. In Crawford ED, Borden TA [eds]: Genitourinary Cancer Surgery. Philadelphia, Lea & Febiger, 1982)

mended. In patients requiring extensive dissection after chemotherapy, intravenous mannitol is again administered 20 minutes after vessel manipulation.

With both blunt and sharp dissection, Gerota's fascia is freed from the anterior and posterior surface of the kidney. This maneuver allows for the removal of node-bearing hilar tissue en bloc with the surgical specimen. We routinely remove the adrenal gland with the specimen.

Once this tissue is freed, attention is directed to the inferior margins of the great vessels. Areolar and nodal tissues are divided in and around the aorta and vena cava, and the lumbar arteries and veins are isolated and divided. A right-angle clamp is passed around each vessel prior to ligation with 4-0 silk suture. The left renal vein is retracted to expose the origin of the right renal artery. The areolar tissue cephalad to the right renal artery is mobilized, clipped, and divided. Dissection continues behind the vena cava, exposing the prevertebral ligaments. On the ipsilateral side, the dissection should be carried down to the great vessels to just below the bifurcation of the external and internal common iliac arteries. Dissection on the ipsilateral side includes all tissue lateral to the aorta and medial to the ureter (Fig. 35-6).

In patients who have lymph node involvement clinically judged as IIB or IIC, a similar margin is obtained on the contralateral side. Modification of the lymph node dissection to preserve ejaculatory function can be performed by preserving the sympathetic supply roots and postganglionic fibers (Fig. 35-7). All remnants of the spermatic cord are removed with the surgical specimen by tracing the testicular vessels to the internal ring, palpating the ligature on the stump, and dissecting the vas from the vessels. The margins of the dissection have now been outlined, and attention is directed to removing the remaining retroperitoneal node tissue.

Modification of the operation is necessary in patients who have residual disease after chemotherapy, as it is frequently impossible to remove all tumor en bloc, because the normal anatomic cleavage plane between the nodal tissue and the great vessels may be obliterated. Sharp dissection with a No. 10 knife blade on a scalpel may be necessary for removal of tumor, as may ligation and resection of the inferior vena cava. Rarely, aortic resection with graft placement is required. Nephrectomy and bowel resection may be performed in order to remove all gross tumor. Cytoreductive surgical procedures of this nature may require 12 to 15 hours of operating time and should be performed only by surgeons

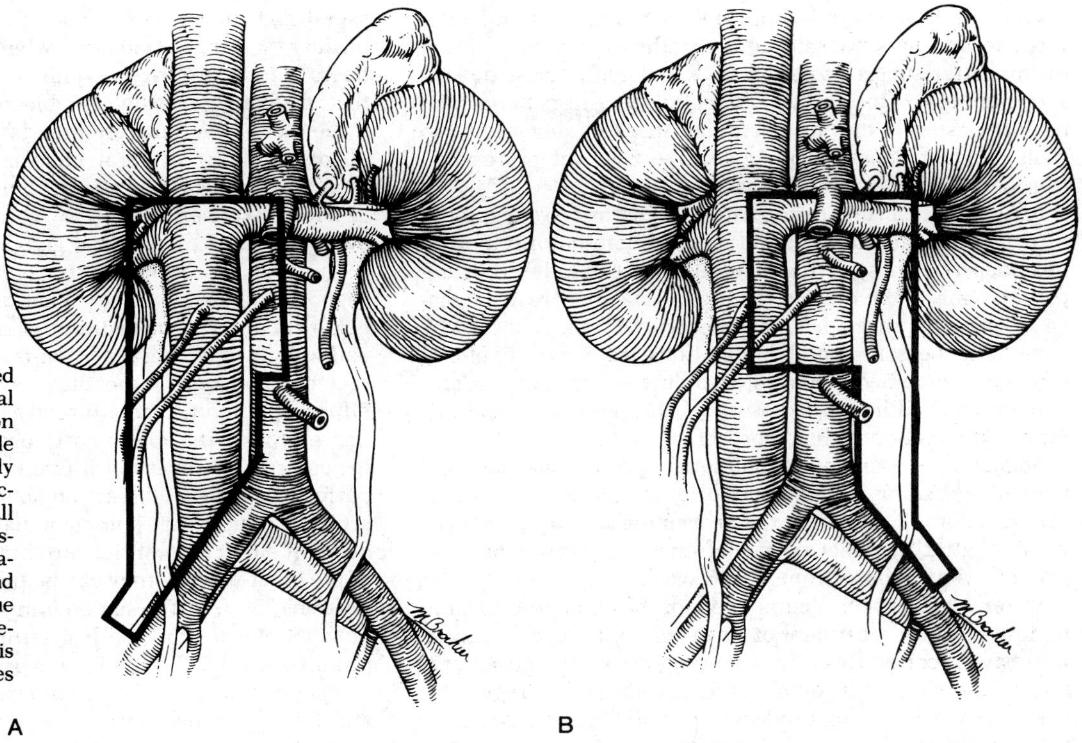

FIG. 35-7. Limits of modified nerve sparing retroperitoneal lymph node dissection on right side (**A**) and left side (**B**) for patients with grossly negative nodes. The dissection is designed to remove all nodes likely to contain metastases yet preserve the contralateral sympathetic chain and hypogastric plexus. (Donohue JP: Options in the management of low stage testis cancer. AUA Update Series 6:27, 1987)

well versed in retroperitoneal anatomy and surgery. After properly administered and effective chemotherapy, this operation is indicated in patients with partial resolution of retroperitoneal or thoracic disease as demonstrated on CT scan or other radiographic studies. Patients who have persistently elevated serum markers are, in general, not candidates for this surgical procedure. In patients who have both abdominal and thoracic disease, we have modified the incision to include a median sternotomy coupled with a midline abdominal incision. A complete bilateral dissection, including the suprahilar areas, is indicated in all postchemotherapeutic node dissections.

As Donohue has pointed out, the "heterogenicity of the tissue in the retroperitoneum makes it visually impossible to distinguish between necrotic changes, teratoma, and carcinoma" (cited by Einhorn and associates).[67] The surgeon must be cognizant of the existence of the lymph nodes in the retrocrual space, especially in patients with lower abdominal lymphadenopathy. CT scans may demonstrate lymph node enlargement in this area.[68]

RADIATION THERAPY FOR PATIENTS WITH NONSEMINOMATOUS GERM-CELL TUMORS

Because of the very high success rate with first-line chemotherapy, the quite satisfactory response rates with secondline chemotherapeutic regimens, and the excellent results using surgical resection of residual disease, many clinicians do not appreciate the marked sensitivity of embryonal carcinoma and teratocarcinoma to local radiation — about that of non-Hodgkin's lymphoma. The best of the documentation of the efficacy of external-beam radiation with conventional fractionation in doses of 4500 to 5000 cGy comes from the Royal Marsden Hospital experience. In that series, only 2 of 84 patients with clinical Stage I disease developed a retroperitoneal recurrence, 1 each in 44 patients with primary teratocarcinoma and 40 patients with primary embryonal carcinoma. In patients with clinical Stage II tumors with metastases that were 2 cm or smaller by lymphangiography, radiation therapy sterilized these deposits in 93%. However, radiation was effective in permanently sterilizing the retroperitoneum in only 31% of the patients with bulky retroperitoneal metastases.[69] Radiation in nonseminomatous germcell tumors is reserved for those patients with incompletely responding (radiographically) metastases that are not amenable to postchemotherapy surgical resection, such as metastases in the central mediastinum, the bone, and the brain when there is clinical or pathologic evidence of persistent carcinoma. Doses with conventional fractionation are used in this setting, usually approximately 3600 cGy over 4 weeks. In sites in which the heart and central nervous system can be completely excluded, boosts to higher doses should be considered.

SURGICAL RESECTION OF RESIDUAL DISEASE

The incidence of demonstrable residual disease in the retroperitoneum, chest, or both after combination chemotherapy is between 30% and 60%.[53,63,70] Patients who achieve a PR to chemotherapy are considered candidates for resection of the residual disease providing they do not have persistently elevated serum markers; salvage chemotherapy should be used in this latter subset of patients. Occasionally, urologic surgeons are asked to remove residual disease in patients who have persistently elevated or rising markers, but rarely do such patients benefit from extensive removal of residual retroperitoneal or chest disease.

Patients harboring retroperitoneal disease are explored through either a midline or a thoracoabdominal intraperitoneal incision. Those with unilateral disease in either the lung parenchyma or the mediastinum can have their residual disease removed through thoracotomy incision. Those who have both thoracic and abdominal disease can be explored through a combined median sternotomy and midline abdominal incision, although exposure of the posterior mediastinum is difficult with this approach.

Adequate assessment of pulmonary, cardiovascular, and hematologic status is mandatory prior to this extensive surgical procedure. We attempt to perform the surgery as soon as possible after the final course of chemotherapy, which, in general, is anywhere from 4 to 6 weeks.

Bleomycin has been a component of the chemotherapeutic regimens for the treatment of germ-cell tumors, and patients who have received this drug are at high risk for a postoperative pulmonary catastrophe, as discussed by Goldinger and colleagues.[71] This drug produces chronic fibrotic changes in the lung leading to restrictive pulmonary disease and impaired carbon monoxide diffusion. These changes are subtle and require pulmonary function testing to be appreciated. Patients who are overhydrated during surgery and who have a fixed pulmonary arterial resistance can develop interstitial edema, enhancing the diffusion defect caused by bleomycin. Elevated FiO_2 concentrations can lead to destruction of Type I and Type II pneumocytes, producing an adult respiratory distress syndrome (ARDS). In order to avert this complication, the patient should be maintained at a relative hypovolemic state, being carefully monitored by a Swan-Ganz catheter to assess central and pulmonary pressures. In addition, there should be judicious use of crystalloids in fluid replacement. Colloids are preferable. Inspired FiO_2 concentration should not exceed 25% both intraoperatively and postoperatively.

FERTILITY ISSUES AFTER RPLND

The majority of patients undergoing a bilateral radical RPLND will be rendered infertile by virtue of the development of retrograde ejaculation or ejaculatory failure. This complication has surfaced as an important issue that often determines the type of therapy for a patient. There are several reasons for the contemporary interest in this complication, including the fact that the majority of patients with germ-cell tumors can expect to be cured of their cancer.

The neuroanatomy of ejaculation is not completely understood. The efferent impulses are mediated by sympathetic fibers from the thoracolumbar outflow at T12 to L3 and travel by the paravertebral ganglia and hypogastric neuroplexus.[72] Efferent impulses that mediate ejaculation are carried by autonomic and somatic nerves originating in the sacral and lumbar cord areas. Sympathetic fibers augment bladder and neck closure, whereas the parasympathetic fibers relax the internal sphincter. The sympathetic fibers that mediate emission and bladder neck closure traverse three paths: the paravertebral ganglia, the aortomesenteric plexus, and the ureteral plexus. Preservation of many of these sympathetic paths is possible by modifying the extent of node dissection and also by carefully dissecting the tissue overlying the paravertebral ganglia.

Lange and associates at the University of Minnesota have supported changing from a bilateral to a unilateral dissection below the inferior mesenteric artery in order to preserve the pathway of these nerves.[72] On the ipsilateral side, they dissect only on top of the iliac vessels and avoid the aortic bifurcation and the area directly below it. The sympathetic fibers around the lower aorta are thus preserved, and the hypogastric plexus is not injured. Those authors continue to perform a bilateral dissection above the inferior mesenteric artery. Because the thoracolumbar sympathetic ganglia are deep on either side of the vertebral column under the edges of the great vessels, they can be preserved. With these modifications, 51% of the patients in the Minnesota series with Stages I and IIA disease had return of ejaculatory function postoperatively. Fossa and co-workers have reported return of ejaculation in 100% of patients with right-sided tumors and 56% with left-sided tumors with a limited dissection above the inferior mesenteric artery.[73]

The majority of patients with testicular cancer can expect to achieve a long-term disease-free status. Because this population is sexually active and frequently concerned about fathering children, both the short-term and the long-term effects of treatment on their reproductive system is of concern. Lange and co-workers stated that 25% of patients with testis cancer are permanently infertile before any therapy is instituted, 35% are temporarily infertile, and 40% are fertile.[64] Therefore, approximately 75% of the patients are at risk for loss of fertility from either lymph node dissection, chemotherapy, or both. The exact reasons for the impaired fertility at the time of diagnosis remain poorly understood. Berthelsen and Skakkeback evaluated 218 patients with testicular cancer and found 9% had a history of cryptochidism.[74] When the contralateral testes were biopsied, irreversible changes were noted in 24%, and carcinoma in situ was found in 5%. Fifteen percent had lowered serum testosterone, and LH was elevated in 12%.

CHEMOTHERAPY FOR DISSEMINATED TESTIS CANCER

HISTORICAL PERSPECTIVES: PRE-CISPLATIN ERA

Even in the 1950s and 1960s, disseminated testicular cancer was considered a chemosensitive tumor, with a respectable 50% objective response rate and a modest 5% to 10% cure rate with dactinomycin-based chemotherapy.[75,76] During the 1960s, several other single agents such as mithramycin, vinblastine, and bleomycin demonstrated similar activity.[77–79] These early chemotherapy studies achieved a 10% to 20% CR rate, and approximately half of these patients relapsed,

TABLE 35-10. VAB-VI Chemotherapy Regimen

Drug	*Dose*	*Day*
Vinblastine	4 mg/m^2	
Cyclophosphamide	600 mg/m^2	1
Dactinomycin	1 mg/m^2	1
Bleomycin	30 units by IV push	1
	20 $units/m^2$ by continuous IV infusion	1–3
Cisplatin	120 mg/m^2	4

usually within 1 year. With modern cisplatin combination chemotherapy, patients achieving a CR have only a 10% relapse rate owing to the more effective induction therapy and the availability of tumor markers and CT scans to define CR more accurately.

Combination chemotherapy with vinblastine plus bleomycin was first described by Samuels and colleagues at M.D. Anderson Hospital and Tumor Institute.[80] In 1973, these authors switched from intermittent therapy to continuous infusion bleomycin in combination with vinblastine.[81]

The discovery of cisplatin was a major advance in the field of medical oncology. Cisplatin is one of a group of coordination compounds of platinum identified by Rosenberg, Van Camp, and Krigas that strongly inhibits bacterial replication.[82] Cisplatin as a single agent had significant activity in refractory advanced testicular cancer.[83] Indeed, it is the single most active agent in the treatment of testicular cancer and has become an integral part of combination chemotherapy programs for disseminated disease.

VAB PROGRAMS: MEMORIAL SLOAN-KETTERING CANCER CENTER

The Memorial group evaluated combination chemotherapy with vinblastine plus actinomycin D (dactinomycin) plus bleomycin (VAB-1) from June 1972 to April 1974.[84] This regimen was utilized in 71 evaluable patients and produced 14% CR and 22% PR rates. From June 1974 to January 1976, cisplatin administered every 3 to 4 months plus continuous-infusion bleomycin was added to the VAB regimen (VAB-II).[85] There was a 50% CR rate in 50 evaluable patients, and 12 (24%) remained alive and disease-free.[84] Slight modifications were made in the protocol from July 1975 through September 1976, creating VAB-III. Forty-four per cent of these 80 patients were disease free with follow-up 17 to 31 months.[86] In September 1976, another slight modification resulted in VAB-IV, with 50% of 48 patients disease free with shorter follow-up than for VAB-III.[86]

Between January 1979 and November 1982, 166 patients were treated with VAB-VI. This regimen represented a major departure from the prior VAB programs in that cisplatin (120 mg/m^2) was given monthly for three courses (Table 35-10). Therapy was repeated every 4 weeks for three courses. Bleomycin was not given on the third cycle. The complete response rate was 78%, with 67% of patients disease free with chemotherapy alone and 11% after chemotherapy plus resection of viable residual carcinoma.[87] The overall relapse rate was 12% and was greater in tumors of extragonadal origin (21%) than for testis primary (11%).

The Memorial group has recently completed a randomized prospective study comparing VAB-VI with the two-drug regimen of cisplatin plus VP-16 in good-risk disseminated testicular cancer.[88] The therapeutic results were identical, but there was a highly statistically significant reduction in toxicity with the two-drug regimen.

PVB STUDIES AT INDIANA UNIVERSITY

In August 1974, we began studies at Indiana University in disseminated testicular cancer with the already-established two-drug regimen of vinblastine plus bleomycin and adding to this the then-experimental drug, cisplatin.[89] The original regimen is depicted in Table 35-11. The cisplatin was dissolved in 50 ml of normal saline and given at a rate of 1 mg/min. Saline hydration at a rate of 100 ml/hour was given continuously during all 5 days of cisplatin administration. Mannitol diuresis was not employed and has never been felt to be necessary in any of our subsequent studies. In this trial, 33 of 47 patients (70%) achieved a CR, and an additional five patients (11%) were rendered disease free by post-PVB resection of teratoma or carcinoma. Thirty patients (64%) survived 5 years and 28 (60%) 10 years.

Today, after four courses of PVB, if the markers are normal and there are persistent radiographic abnormalities, we resect residual disease 4 to 6 weeks after the final cisplatin chemotherapy if anatomically feasible. Surgery consists of RPLND, lateral thoracotomy, median sternotomy with wedge resection of bilateral pulmonary metastases, or a combined thoracoabdominal procedure.[93] If carcinoma is found in the completely resected specimen and the markers remain normal, two postoperative courses of the original induction regimen (fifth and sixth courses of cisplatin combination chemotherapy) are given. This strategy will result in a 67% long-term disease-free survival rate in such patients.[90] Similar results have been obtained with post-VAB-VI resection at Memorial.[87]

The principal serious toxicity of the original PVB protocol was related to the high-dose (0.4 mg/kg) vinblastine. Myalgias, constipation, neuropathy, and paralytic ileus all were troublesome, but severe granulocytopenia and potential

TABLE 35-11. Original PVB Regimen

Cisplatin	20 mg/m^2 every 3 weeks × 4
Vinblastine	0.2 mg/kg day 1 and 2 every 3 weeks × 4
Bleomycin	30 units IV push weekly × 12

Maintenance vinblastine 0.3 mg/kg monthly × 21 months

TABLE 35-12. Three Treatment Arms of PVB Study No. 2

Cisplatin 20 mg/m² × 5 every 3 weeks × 4 Vinblastine 0.4 mg/kg Bleomycin 30 units IV weekly × 12
Cisplatin 20 mg/m² × 5 every 3 weeks × 4 Vinblastine 0.3 mg/kg Bleomycin 30 units weekly × 12
Cisplatin 20 mg/m² × 5 every 3 weeks × 4 Vinblastine 0.2 mg/kg every 3 weeks × 4 Doxorubicin 50 mg/m² every 3 weeks × 4 Bleomycin 30 units weekly × 12

sepsis was the most worrisome toxicity. Therefore, in 1976, we started a randomized prospective trial comparing our original PVB with the same regimen but with a 25% reduction in the vinblastine dosage (to 0.3 mg/kg). A third arm adding doxorubicin to PVB with vinblastine at 0.2 mg/kg was also studied (Table 35-12). Once again, maintenance vinblastine was employed for a total of 2 years.

Seventy-eight patients were entered on this study. The 25% reduction in the vinblastine dosage resulted in the expected decrease in hematologic and neuromuscular toxicity. There was no significant difference in the efficacy of the three induction arms (Table 35-13).[91] Fifty-eight patients (73%) are currently alive and disease free for 9^+ years.

On the basis of the results of this study, we abandoned our original PVB regimen in 1978 in favor of the equally effective but less toxic regimen involving the reduced dosage of vinblastine. A similar but larger study was conducted by the EORTC in 214 patients randomized to vinblastine 0.4 or 0.3 mg/kg in combination with cisplatin and bleomycin.[92] This study also showed no benefit for the higher dose of vinblastine: the CR rates were 68% for the regimen using vinblastine at 0.4 mg/kg versus 71% with 0.3 mg/kg. There was no significant difference in the disease-free or overall survival rates, but there was a significant increase in both hematologic ($p = 0.01$) and nonhematologic toxicity with the higher dose of vinblastine.

We began a third-generation study in 1978 in conjunction with the Southeastern Cancer Study Group. This study randomized patients achieving CR or disease-free status after resection of teratoma to maintenance vinblastine, as in our first two studies, versus no maintenance therapy (just four courses of PVB over 12 weeks). This study confirmed the fact that optimal cure rates were achieved with induction PVB and that maintenance vinblastine was unnecessary.[93] One hundred forty-seven patients from Indiana University entered this study, and 117 (80%) are alive and disease free with a minimum follow-up of 5 years. The Memorial group has also evaluated maintenance therapy (vinblastine plus dactinomycin) with VAB-VI and likewise found no value.[87]

The results of these three PVB studies are depicted in Table 35-14. Overall, with follow-up of 6 to 13 years, 201 of 272 (74%) patients with disseminated testicular cancer are alive and presumably cured of their disease. Similar results with PVB have been published by numerous other investigators and cooperative groups around the world.

PVB VERSUS CISPLATIN PLUS VP-16 PLUS BLEOMYCIN (PVP-16B)

Etoposide (VP-16) is an epipodophyllotoxin derivative with definite single-agent activity in refractory testicular cancer.[94] In preclinical systems, there is marked synergy with VP-16 plus cisplatin.[95] In 1978, we began our initial salvage chemotherapy studies with cisplatin plus VP-16 in patients who were not cured with PVB or similar induction therapy (vide infra). VP-16, unlike vinblastine, is essentially devoid of neuromuscular toxicity.

The three-drug combination of cisplatin, VP-16, and bleomycin was initially used as first-line induction chemotherapy at the Royal Marsden Hospital.[96] Thirty-seven of 43 patients (86%) achieved disease free status.

From 1981 through 1984, the Southeastern Cancer Study Group conducted a randomized prospective study comparing PVB and PVP-16B as initial induction chemotherapy (Table 35-15).[97] Once again, no maintenance therapy was given in either arm, and if the markers were normal postchemotherapy but there was persistent radiographic abnormalities, appropriate surgery was done. If carcinoma was found, two more courses of the original induction regimen were given.

A total of 244 patients from 24 institutions entered this trial. Of 121 patients treated with PVB, 74 (61%) had a CR, and another 15 (13%) became disease free after resection of teratoma (10 patients) or carcinoma (5 patients). Among the 123 patients given PVP-16B, 74 (60%) had a CR, and 28 (23%) became free of disease after resection of teratoma (22 patients) or carcinoma (6 patients). Thus, 74% became disease free after treatment with PVB and 83% after PVP-16B. Nine patients on PVB and six receiving PVP-16B subsequently had recurrences. The 2-year survival rate was approximately 80% in both arms, with a slight but not statistically significant survival advantage for PVP-16B. However, in the subgroup of advanced disseminated disease, there was a clear survival advantage for this combination ($p = 0.02$).

Granulocytopenic toxicity, including granulocytopenic fever, was similar in the two arms. Severe thrombocytopenia

TABLE 35-13. Results of PVB Study No. 2

	PVB (0.4 mg/kg) (*n* = 26)	*PVB (0.3 mg/kg)* (*n* = 27)	*PVB + Doxorubicin* (*n* = 25)
NED*	23 (88%)	21 (78%)	20 (80%)
Relapses	5 (19%)	2 (10%)	3 (15%)
Currently NED	20 (77%)	19 (70%)	18 (72%)

* No evidence of disease.

TABLE 35-14. Summary of PVB Studies at Indiana University

Study No.	*Time*	*No. of Patients*	*CR (%)*	*NED with Surgery (%)*	*Currently NED (%)*
1	1974–76	47	33 (70)	5 (11)	27 (57)
2	1976–78	78	53 (68)	13 (17)	57 (73)
3	1978–81	147	92 (63)	31 (21)	117 (80)

was more common with PVP-16B, as 14% had a platelet count below 50,000/mm³ at some time during treatment compared with 5% of the patients given PVB. However, hemorrhage was seen in two patients given PVB but in none given PVP-16B. There was a major reduction in neuromuscular toxicity, as manifested by paresthesia, abdominal cramps and ileus, and myalgias. This was significant not only statistically but also clinically (Table 35-16). On the basis of this study, which demonstrated a reduction in morbidity and equivalent, if not superior, survival, we now utilize PVP-16B as first-line therapy for disseminated testicular cancer.

EXTRAGONADAL GERM-CELL TUMORS

Primary extragonadal germ-cell tumors may arise in midline structures such as the mediastinum and retroperitoneum or in the pineal gland, prostate, stomach, or thymus. During early embryogenesis, germinal epithelium arises in the yolk sac and undergoes a midline migration (from the sixth cervical vertebra to the second sacral vertebra) down the dorsal mesentery of the hindgut to the urogenital ridge and eventually forms aggregrates of testicular tissue in the scrotum. During the migration, germinal epithelium may be sequestered along the route and ultimately undergo malignant transformation.

Patients with presumed primary retroperitoneal germ-cell tumors must have a careful search for an occult testicular primary. This is critically important, because the testis is a relative sanctuary site from the effects of chemotherapy, and a missed small primary there will not necessarily be eradicated with chemotherapy.[98] Patients with a normal testis on palpation should have bilateral testicular ultrasound performed. If physical examination or ultrasound is abnormal, an orchiectomy should be performed, usually after completion of chemotherapy. Also, a primary retroperitoneal germ-cell tumor should be a midline mass: if the abdominal CT scan reveals predominantly right- or left-sided adenopathy, this is compatible with an occult primary site of origin in the ipsilateral testis, and strong consideration should be given to removal of the suspected testis.

TABLE 35-15. Treatment Arms of Southeastern Cancer Study Group Comparison of PVB and PVP-16B

Cisplatin 20 mg/m² × 5 every 3 weeks × 4
Vinblastine 0.15 mg/kg days 1 and 2 every 3 weeks × 4
Bleomycin 30 units weekly × 12
Cisplatin 20 mg/m² × 5 every 3 weeks × 4
VP-16 100 mg/m² × 5 every 3 weeks × 4
Bleomycin 30 units weekly × 12

The treatment philosophy for a primary retroperitoneal germ-cell tumor should parallel that for the testicular tumors in general, and the prognosis for cure is similar to that of testicular primaries with similar amounts of disease and marker elevation.

There is a paucity of literature guidelines for the management of suprasellar germ-cell tumors (pinealomas). Most of these are seminoma, but anatomical location often precludes accurate histologic diagnosis. An area of significant controversy is whether cranial irradiation alone is adequate or whether the entire neuroaxis should be radiated. The incidence of positive spinal-fluid cytology ranges from 6% to 55% in various series, and about 35% of patients relapse in the spine. However, the routine use of craniospinal radiotherapy makes the subsequent delivery of myelosuppressive chemotherapy very difficult should the patient relapse. The Harvard Joint Center for Radiotherapy recently detailed their results in 25 suprasellar germ-cell tumors.[99] Nineteen of the patients (76%) are continuously disease free, and most of these received radiation to the entire neuroaxis.

Primary mediastinal germ-cell tumors are fascinating biologic entities and therapeutically challenging disorders. The curve rate with cisplatin combination chemotherapy for nonseminomatous tumors is well below 50% and that for endodermal sinus (yolk sac) tumors below 25%. However, primary mediastinal seminomas have an extremely high cure rate with either radiotherapy or chemotherapy. There are a variety of known, suspected, and unknown reasons for the poor prognosis of primary mediastinal nonseminomatous tumors. One obvious reason is the initial presence of teratoma, which is often unresectable after chemotherapy because of anatomical constraints that do not exist in the retroperitoneum. However, even when a CR is achieved with resection of just necrotic fibrous tissue after cisplatin combination chemotherapy, there is a higher than expected relapse rate.

Primary mediastinal nonseminomatous germ-cell tumors have recently been associated with hematologic disorders and Klinefelter's syndrome. Nichols and coworkers described three patients with such tumors and hematologic malignancy (two cases of megakaryocytic leukemia and one myelodysplastic syndrome). These authors reviewed the case records of 688 patients with germ-cell tumors treated at Indiana University and the Dana Farber Cancer Institute.[100] Thirty-four (4.9%) of these tumors arose in the mediastinum, and three of these patients had hematologic malignancies. By contrast, there were no hematologic malignancies in the 654 patients with primary testicular or retroperitoneal germ-cell tumors. Subsequent to this report, we have seen six additional cases of hematologic malignancies associated with primary mediastinal germ-cell tumors.

TABLE 35-16. Neuromuscular Toxicity (% of Patients)

	PVB (N = 114)		*PVP-16B (N = 110)*
Paresthesias		p = 0.0003	
None	62		77
Mild	27		19
Moderate	11		4
Abdominal Cramps		p = 0.0008	
None	80		95
Mild	12		3
Moderate	8		2
Myalgias		p = 0.00002	
None	81		99
Mild	5		1
Moderate	14		0

The Indiana group has also prospectively performed chromosomal studies on 22 consecutive patients with mediastinal germ-cell tumors.[101] Five (22%) had karyotypic or pathologic evidence of Klinefelter's syndrome. All five had tumors with nonseminomatous histology and were relatively young (median age 15).

Extragonadal germ-cell tumors must always be considered in the diagnosis of "carcinoma, primary unknown," especially in young patients with mediastinal or retroperitoneal masses. Assays for hCG and AFP should be performed. The investigators at Vanderbilt accumulated data on 119 patients with poorly differentiated carcinoma, primary unknown.[102] Reviewing pathologists found features suggestive of germinal neoplasm in only six cases, and only two of these achieved CR with cisplatin combination chemotherapy. Overall, 27 of 96 patients (28%) who received at least one course of chemotherapy attained a CR and an additional 42 (44%) a PR. Sixteen patients (17%) are currently without evidence of disease 16 to 133 months (median 65 months) after completion of chemotherapy. Only three of the 27 achieving a CR were hCG or AFP positive. This article points out that neither light microscopy nor marker elevation can differentiate curable and incurable patients.

The results of PVB in extragonadal germ-cell tumors at Indiana and Vanderbilt have been published.[103] Eighteen of 32 (56%) patients had no evidence of disease for 1 to 5^+ years at the time of publication. Identical chemotherapy was employed by the Southeastern Cancer Study Group with similar results.[104] VAB-VI gave similar results at Memorial Sloan-Kettering Cancer Center.[105] All eight patients with extragonadal seminomas achieved a CR compared with 6 of 11 whose tumors had nonseminomatous elements. Twelve of nineteen (63%) were continuously disease free at the time of publication. Investigators at M.D. Anderson used a complicated five-drug regimen and, again, achieved similar results, with 16 of 19 patients with seminomas and 12 of 30 with nonseminomatous tumors without evidence of disease.[106]

CENTRAL NERVOUS SYSTEM METASTASES

Metastasis in the central nervous system (CNS) is an uncommon initial presentation, occurring in less than 5% of all patients with Stage III disease. Most of these patients have concomitant advanced pulmonary metastases with testicular-tumor histology mainly of choriocarcinoma or yolk sac elements. The presence of CNS metastases does not preclude cure, and such patients should be treated aggressively.

At M.D. Anderson Hospital and Tumor Institute, 12 patients with disseminated testicular cancer and CNS metastases were treated from 1977 to 1979 with chemotherapy plus whole-brain radiotherapy.[107] Although none of the six patients with multiple CNS metastases were cured, four of the six with single CNS metastases were disease free at 13^+ to 41^+ months.

A unique approach for CNS metastases has been advocated by investigators at Charing Cross Hospital in London, England.[108] Ten patients with germ-cell tumors and CNS metastases were treated from 1977 to 1984 with no CNS irradiation. A complicated chemotherapy regimen (POMB/ACE or EP/OMB) was employed in conjunction with high-dose (1 g/m^2) methotrexate and intrathecal methotrexate. Eight patients were disease free at 3^+ to 54^+ months.

At Indiana University, five patients presented with CNS metastases, and four are without evidence of disease at 2^+ to 8^+ years with cisplatin combination chemotherapy plus simultaneous cranial irradiation (5000 rad in 5 weeks). In addition, five patients had the termination of a chemotherapy CR with the development of CNS metastases, and three of these are disease free 2^+ to 8^+ years. We have not seen any acute or delayed neuropsychological sequelae from this combined-modality approach.[109]

Our current recommendation at Indiana University for CNS metastases at the time of diagnosis is to initiate full-dose cisplatin combination chemotherapy plus 5000 rad of whole-brain irradiation in 5 weeks with both modalities starting on day 1. If a patient with a chemotherapy CR relapses with only CNS metastases, we employ identical CNS irradiation plus two courses of cisplatin combination chemotherapy, because we feel that a CNS relapse can herald a systemic relapse, similar to meningeal relapse of childhood acute lymphoblastic leukemia.

THE TESTIS AS A SANCTUARY SITE

Testicular relapse can terminate a CR in childhood acute lymphoblastic leukemia in the absence of marrow or meningeal relapse, implying that the testis is a sanctuary site. In germ-cell tumors, the testis is affected by chemotherapy, with resultant testicular atrophy and impaired spermatogenesis. Nevertheless, the primary tumor in the testis is not always eradicated by systemic chemotherapy. Greist and coworkers described 20 patients with occult testicular primaries who underwent a delayed orchiectomy after cisplatin combination chemotherapy.[110] These patients were initially believed to have a primary retroperitoneal germ-cell tumor but subsequently were found to have a testicular primary upon careful palpation or bilateral testicular ultrasound demonstrating a characteristic hypoechogenic mass. Three of these patients had embryonal cell carcinoma in the testis after cisplatin chemotherapy, and an additional six had teratoma. None of the 20 patients had persistent carcinoma in the original areas of bulky retroperitoneal disease. Similar results have been reported by others.[111,112]

An orchiectomy therefore must be performed initially or after chemotherapy in any patient with a known or suspected testicular primary, as it is erroneous to assume that the chemotherapy will eradicate the primary. If carcinoma is found in the orchiectomy specimen, we recommend two postoperative courses of cisplatin combination induction chemotherapy, as we do if carcinoma is found in the retroperitoneum or chest after chemotherapy. However, this view is controversial,[111] and there is not enough information to permit a firm recommendation based on hard data.

SALVAGE CHEMOTHERAPY

First-line cisplatin combination chemotherapy will cure 70% of patients with disseminated germ-cell tumors. By definition, then, 30% become candidates for salvage chemotherapy.

It is our philosophy to resect residual disease after a maximum of four courses of induction therapy if the serum markers are normal and if it is anatomically feasible to extirpate the persistent disease. We traditionally do not give more than four courses of induction therapy even if there is continued serologic and radiographic regression. Most patients with persistently elevated markers at this time demonstrate a plateau in their marker decline, allowing the physician to realize that a fifth or sixth course will be incapable of normalizing the markers. Furthermore, by continuing the same "ineffective" induction regimen beyond four courses, there is a risk that the disease will worsen, thereby depriving the patient of the opportunity to enroll on a potentially curative cisplatin salvage regimen. A patient who progresses *during* cisplatin combination chemotherapy is not a candidate for a cisplatin salvage chemotherapy regimen, whereas a patient progressing while no longer receiving cisplatin is still potentially curable with agents to which his tumor has not been exposed.

The marker results of a hypothetical patient of this type are shown in Table 35-17. This patient had his maximal marker regression with his first course of chemotherapy. He still had a greater than 1 log reduction with his second course; however, he subsequently had a clear plateau in his hCG decline. It should be obvious that giving a fifth and sixth course of the identical induction regimen would never normalize his hCG. Instead, because of continuation of a noncurative regimen, he eventually develops marker-evidenced progression and is no longer a candidate for a cisplatin-based salvage regimen, as his disease has progressed during cisplatin chemotherapy.

TABLE 35-17. Hypothetical Example of Disease Progression During Cisplatin Combination Chemotherapy (see text for discussion)

Chemotherapy Course	*hCG*
1	100,000
2	5000
3	450
4	300
5	240
6	220
7	2000

If a patient has a PR with anatomically unresectable disease but has normal serum markers, he is observed monthly (on no therapy) until he develops serologic or radiographic evidence of progressive disease. This practice is followed because some patients with an "unresectable PR" have no remaining tumor; that is, they have persistent necrotic fibrous tissue with or without teratoma. Some of these patients will become radiographically free of disease with the passage of time as their necrotic fibrous deposits spontaneously dissipate.

The two-drug combination of cisplatin and VP-16 is highly synergistic in preclinical systems.[113] Single-agent VP-16 is an active, albeit noncurative, drug in refractory testicular cancer. We first began PVP-16 salvage chemotherapy in 1978 and documented a 30% cure rate.[114] These results have subsequently been confirmed by other single institutions as well as by the Southeastern Cancer Study Group.[115] This represented the first curative salvage regimen for an adult solid tumor.

Another active drug in refractory testicular cancer is ifosfamide, with a 22% single-agent response rate after PVB and PVP-16.[116] We have evaluated cisplatin plus ifosfamide in refractory testicular cancer.[117] Perhaps the most impressive results are with this therapy as a third-line or later regimen in patients previously given PVB or PVP-16 combinations: 16 of 54 patients (30%) achieved disease-free status, and 10 (18%) are 18^+ months continuously disease free, including seven who are 2^+ years free of disease with this third-line regimen.[118] Our current first-line regimen is PVP-16B. Therefore, our present initial salvage regimen is cisplatin plus vinblastine plus ifosfamide (Table 35-18). The uroprotector mesna, in a dosage of 120 mg/m^2 by intravenous push, is given just prior to starting ifosfamide and then by continuous infusion 1200 mg/m^2 per day for all 5 days of each ifosfamide course.

The second course of salvage chemotherapy always begins

TABLE 35-18. Initial Salvage Chemotherapy at Indiana University

Cisplatin 20 mg/m^2 × 5
Vinblastine 0.22 mg/kg on day 1
Ifosfamide 1.2 g/m^2 × 5
Drugs are given every 3 weeks for four courses.

on day 22, regardless of the blood count. We try to give courses three and four on time also, and if we do delay therapy, we never delay by more than 7 days. If, on day 5 of a course of salvage chemotherapy, there is no obvious hematologic recovery, we delete the fifth day of ifosfamide. We do not ever lower drug dosages based on nadir blood counts or day-of-treatment counts. However, if granulocytopenic fever or thrombocytopenic bleeding occurs, we reduce subsequent ifosfamide and vinblastine 25%. We never reduce cisplatin dosages. If the serum creatinine exceeds 2 mg/dl, we reduce ifosfamide (alone) 25%, and if hematuria (more than 10 erythrocytes per high-power field) is found, during daily urinalysis, we hold ifosfamide that particular day and resume regular dose after hematuria clears.

We are now evaluating high-dose chemotherapy with autologous bone-marrow transplantation in patients who are otherwise incurable (progression during cisplatin or prior PVB, VP-16, and ifosfamide). Results with this approach in the past have been disappointing, with virtually no 1^+-year remissions. However, most preparative regimens used chemotherapy regimens without cisplatin (*e.g.*, cyclophosphamide, VP-16, BCNU). Carboplatin (CBDCA) is as active as cisplatin, with myelosuppression as its dose-limiting toxicity, making it ideal for high-dose therapy with bone-marrow transplantation in refractory testicular cancer. Furthermore, in preclinical systems, the drug is highly synergistic with VP-16. We are currently evaluating very high-dose CBDCA plus VP-16 with marrow transplantation in this setting, with very encouraging (albeit early) results.

MANAGEMENT OF POOR-PROGNOSIS TESTICULAR CANCER

The first important issue is determining which patients with germ-cell tumors have advanced disease and would be candidates for more aggressive (and therefore, by definition, more toxic) chemotherapy. No author disputes the fact that patients with advanced disease have a relatively poor prognosis with standard-dose cisplatin plus vinblastine (or VP-16) plus bleomycin; however, not all authors agree on the criteria for advanced disease. Tumor volume, variously defined, is important prognostically in all series. Serum markers, especially hCG, are independently important in most, but not all, series.[119]

TABLE 35-19. Indiana University Staging System for Disseminated Testicular Cancer

Minimal Extent
1. Elevated markers only
2. Cervical nodes (±nonpalpable retroperitoneal nodes)
3. Unresectable nonpalpable retroperitoneal disease
4. Fewer than five pulmonary metastases per lung field AND largest <2 cm (±nonpalpable retroperitoneal nodes)

Moderate Extent
1. Palpable abdominal mass only (no supradiaphragmatic disease)
2. Moderate pulmonary metastases: 5–10 metastases per lung field and largest <3 cm OR solitary pulmonary metastasis of any size >2 cm (±nonpalpable retroperitoneal disease)

Advanced Extent
1. Advanced pulmonary metastases: primary mediastinal nonseminomatous germ-cell tumor OR >10 pulmonary metastases per lung field, OR multiple pulmonary metastases with largest >3 cm (±nonpalpable retroperitoneal disease)
2. Palpable abdominal mass plus supradiaphragmatic disease
3. Liver, bone, or CNS metastases

TABLE 35-20. Therapeutic Results in Advanced Testicular Cancer According to Indiana Staging System, 1978–1983*

Minimal	*Moderate*	*Advanced*
102/103 (99%)	50/55 (91%)	43/81 (53%)

* Numerator is all patients who became disease free with PVB or PVP-16B with or without surgery for residual disease.

At Indiana University, we have developed a staging system that places patients with disseminated germ-cell tumors into three separate categories: minimal, moderate, or advanced disease (Table 35-19).[119] Table 35-20 demonstrates the therapeutic outcome of these patients. It should be noted that our "moderate disease" category included patients who did extremely well with standard chemotherapy, with 50 of 55 (91%) achieving disease-free status. These patients would have been classified as having advanced disease in many other staging systems and would have been inappropriately subjected to a newer, more aggressive chemotherapy regimen instead of standard chemotherapy.

A recent British study from six medical centers treating patients from 1976 to 1982 also identified three separate prognostic categories with 3-year survival rates of 91%, 72%, and 47% and overall a 75% 3-year survival rate.[120] Therapeutic results improved with the passage of time, presumably because of greater familiarity of cisplatin combination chemotherapy regimens and surgical resection of residual disease (Table 35-21). If the 1981–1982 regimen had been a newer, more aggressive regimen, the authors might have erroneously believed a therapeutic advance had been made when comparing the results with those of the 1976–1978 regimens. This table demonstrates the hazard of historical control analysis in documenting superiority of a new regimen. The improved results with time were seen in both advanced and less advanced disease.

A similar demonstration of the importance of experience with chemotherapy was also observed in patients with disseminated germ-cell tumors treated at Indiana University (Table 35-22). As discussed in detail earlier, our original regimen (1976–1976) consisted of cisplatin plus vinblastine plus bleomycin (PVB). Our second study demonstrated that we could achieve identical therapeutic results with less hematologic and neuromuscular toxicity by reducing the vin-

TABLE 35-21. Improvement of Outcome in Advanced Disease with Time (Multicenter British Study)

Year(s)	*No. of Patients*	*3-Year Survival Rate (%)*
1976–78	110	68
1979	102	72
1980	101	81
1981–82	145	89

TABLE 35-22. Comparison of Results of Sequential PVB Studies at Indiana University

Study No. (Year)	*No. of Patients*	*No. with CR (%)*	*NED with Surgery (%)*	*Now NED (%)*
1 (1974–76)	47	33 (70)	5 (11)	27 (57)
2 (1976–78)	78	51 (65)	13 (17)	57 (73)
3 (1978–81)	147	92 (63)	31 (21)	117 (80)

blastine dosage from 0.4 to 0.3 mg/kg, and our third study documented that optimal cure rates could be achieved with 12 weeks (four courses of PVB) and that maintenance vinblastine was unnecessary. In these studies, our cure rate increased from 57% to 80% with the identical chemotherapy regimens except for the reduction in the vinblastine dosage and the elimination of maintenance vinblastine. Unfortunately, many descriptions of "new improved" regimens compare the results in a small number of patients with brief follow-up with our original regimen despite the fact that their new, more aggressive regimens were all given in the 1980s. Such claims of superiority obviously must be viewed with caution, if not skepticism.

Cisplatin plus VP-16 plus bleomycin has been recently utilized as initial chemotherapy in both Europe and the United States. Peckham and associates treated 43 patients, with 37 (86%) becoming disease-free. Cisplatin was given in a dosage of 20 mg/m² five times a week, bleomycin at 30 mg weekly, and VP-16 at 120 mg/m² on one through three days. Fourteen of these patients had advanced disease, and 12 (86%) were continuously disease free at the time of the publication.[96]

From 1981 to 1984, the Southeastern Cancer Study Group randomized patients with disseminated germ-cell tumors to 12 weeks of PVB or 12 weeks of PVP-16B.[97] The cisplatin and bleomycin in both regimens were the same (20 mg/m² five times weekly every 3 weeks for four courses and 30 units weekly for 12 weeks); the vinblastine dosage was 0.15 mg/kg on days one and two and the VP-16 dosage was 100 mg/m² five times a week every 3 weeks for four courses. In the subgroup of patients with advanced disease, 48% are continuously disease-free with PVP-16B and 33% with PVB, and there is a statistically significant survival advantage ($p = 0.02$) for the PVP-16B arm in these patients with advanced disseminated disease (Table 35-23).

Pizzocaro and colleagues recently published their results with PVP-16B in advanced germ-cell cancer.[121] The cisplatin dosage was 20 mg/m² for five consecutive days, the VP-16 dosage was 100 mg/m² for three consecutive days, and the bleomycin dosage 30 units weekly. Forty patients were treated from August 1981 through November 1983. Any patient with a larger than 10-cm abdominal mass, a larger than 5-cm pulmonary nodule, metastases outside the nodes and lung (*e.g.*, liver, bone, CNS), a serum AFP exceeding 1000 ng/ml, or a serum hCG exceeding 50,000 mIU/ml was eligible. All but three patients (92%) achieved disease-free status, and with a median follow-up of 24 months (range 13–40 months), 34 (85%) remain free of disease.

TABLE 35-23. Randomized Southeastern Cooperative Group Comparison of PVB and PVP-16B: Number (%) of Patients Achieving CR

Initial Extent of Disease	*PVB*	*PVP-16B*
Minimal	52/54 (96)	54/56 (97)
Moderate	22/26 (85)	23/30 (77)
Advanced	12/36 (33)	17/35 (48)
Total	116	121

An innovative aggressive regimen for advanced testicular cancer was devised by Ozols and colleagues at the U.S. National Cancer Institute (NCI). This pilot regimen tested double-dose cisplatin (40 mg/m² five times weekly) combined with vinblastine, VP-16, and bleomycin (PVeBV). Starting in May 1981, the NCI performed a randomized study comparing the new regimen with standard PVB. Of 30 patients, 26 (87%) achieved a CR with PVeBV, and 21 of the 30 (70%) are continuously free of disease. There were two deaths secondary to bleomycin and one death from recurrent embryonal carcinoma (malignant teratoma, undifferentiated), and two patients had recurrent teratoma (teratoma, differentiated). In this randomized study, 10 of 16 (62%) achieved a CR on standard dose PVB; however, only 5 of 16 (31%) are continuously free of disease (one death from bleomycin pulmonary fibrosis; two patients with recurrent teratoma). Although there is a trend favoring PVeBV, after 4 years, the only parameter that has achieved statistical significance is the number of patients who are alive and without recurrent embryonal carcinoma or teratoma ($p = 0.027$).

High-dose cisplatin plus high-dose VP-16 in 22 poor-prognosis patients was reported by Daugaard and Rørth.[122] Their criteria for advanced disease included greater than 10-cm abdominal nodes, liver metastases, greater than 5-cm supradiaphragmatic metastases, multiple pulmonary metastases with at least one larger than 5 cm, extragonadal primary tumor with elevated marker(s), or hCG greater than 100,000 mIU/ml. Drug dosages were cisplatin 40 mg/m² five times weekly, plus VP-16 200 mg/m² five times weekly, plus bleomycin 15 mg/m² weekly, with courses repeated every 3 weeks. Nineteen patients (86%) achieved a CR, and 17 (77%) had no evidence of disease with a median follow-up of 11 months (range $1^+–19^+$ months). However, toxicity was severe, with five drug-related deaths and 20 of 22 patients having at least one episode of granulocytopenic fever and 15 having two to five episodes of granulocytopenic fever, including four cases of documented bacteria.

A present national intergroup study of two cisplatin doses (20mg/m² $\times$ 5 versus 40 mg/m² $\times$ 5) in combination with VP-16 and bleomycin in advanced disseminated germ cell tumors (Table 35-24) will clarify the role of high-dose cisplatin in this patient population.

TABLE 35-24. Protocol for Randomized High-Dose Cisplatin Trial in Advanced Disease

*Cisplatin Dose**	*Other Drugs (Both Arms)*
20 mg/m^2 OR 40 mg/m^2	VP-16 100 mg/m^2 × 5 q 3 weeks × 4 Bleomycin 30 units weekly × 12

* Dose given five times weekly every 3 weeks for four courses.

The principal reason for chemotherapy failure and subsequent death from disseminated testicular cancer is bulky advanced diseases, but it must be remembered that another cause of treatment failure is moderate-size or bulky teratoma that persists after chemotherapy and is unresectable.[123] Alternatively, teratoma may be associated with non-germ-cell elements that are as chemoresistant as is teratoma.[124] More aggressive chemotherapy will not solve either of these latter two problems.

SURVEILLANCE VERSUS RPLND FOR CLINICAL STAGE I DISEASE

Retroperitoneal lymph dissection remains the only modality that can prove that clinical Stage I nonseminomatous germ-cell tumor is in fact pathologic Stage I. (Even in the most experienced of hands, clinical understaging of the disease occurs in approximately 25% of patients and overstaging in 20%). Nevertheless, approximately 70% of patients undergoing RPLND will receive no definitive therapeutic benefit from the operation. Additionally, 10% to 13% of patients undergoing the procedure will nevertheless experience relapse, usually outside of the operative field. Moreover, in the past, loss of ejaculation and sterility occurred in most patients who underwent RPLND. Because of these drawbacks of surgery, and in view of the development of sensitive tumor markers and effective chemotherapeutic agents, postorchiectomy observation or surveillance is appealing. As previously discussed, the overall survival rate for patients with pathologic Stage I disease who undergo a RPLND should approach 100%, so the standard by which surveillance programs must be judged is formidable.

The results of several large surveillance programs throughout the world consistently show a disease progression rate of approximately 30%,[72] and unfortunately, there have been several deaths in these programs, although, as expected, the majority of patients do well. Recent reports suggest that, even with monitoring, 80% of relapses are of a more advanced stage,[65,72] compared to those patients undergoing RPLND who tend to relapse in the chest with a lower volume of disease.

As more experience is generated, it becomes clear that patient selection for surveillance protocols requires individualization. A meticulous work-up should be performed and interpreted by a multidisciplinary team consisting of urologists, medical oncologists, radiologists, and pathologists experienced in evaluating these patients and tests. As a minimum for consideration of entry into an observation protocol, the patient should have undergone a radical inguinal orchiectomy with negative surgical margins. Postorchiectomy, the tumor markers β-hCG, AFP, and LDH should fall to normal within their expected metabolic half-lives. Both CT scan of the abdomen and chest or whole-lung tomograms should show no suspicious nodes or evidence of pulmonary parenchymal metastases. Finally, a lymphangiogram should be unequivocally negative.

If all these criteria are met, known prognostic factors are analyzed. Patients who have an embryonal carcinoma are felt to be at high risk of relapse, as are patients having vascular, lymphatic, or cord invasion by tumor. Finally, a judgment must be made about the reliability of the patient in returning for rigorous follow-up examination. Because, in effect, surveillance is a form of treatment, the physician also maintains a degree of responsibility for ensuring the follow-up. It should be emphasized to the patient that surveillance is an as yet-unproven method of therapy, whereas RPLND has been performed in many large centers with few complications and no deaths. The principal criticism is the ejaculatory dysfunction that occurs, but with the modifications in the operation recently described by Lange and others, this argument no longer seems important. Thus, patients with a grossly normal retroperitoneum can be offered a modified nerve-sparing lymphadenectomy, which will maintain antegrade ejaculation and subsequent fertility in approximately 90% of cases. In our experience, once these matters are discussed with the patient, the majority opt for surgical staging and therapy by RPLND.

Regardless of the initial form of therapy, careful follow-up during the perioperative period is mandatory. Physical examination, chest radiography, and serum marker assays are performed monthly during the first year, every 2 months during the second year, and every 6 months thereafter. Patients who elect surveillance should have a CT scan approximately every 2 to 3 months for the first 2 years.

LATE CONSEQUENCES OF CISPLATIN COMBINATION CHEMOTHERAPY

Approximately 80% of patients with disseminated cancer are cured with initial cisplatin combination chemotherapy or salvage chemotherapy. At Indiana University, we recently reviewed 207 patients with a minimum follow-up of 5$^+$ years.[125] The overwhelming majority of these patients have returned to a productive life with few, if any, long-term toxicities other than sterility and Raynaud's phenomenon. In our experience, only rarely is the Raynaud's condition of sufficient severity to impair health.

FERTILITY

Drasga and associates have evaluated with serial semen analyses 69 patients with disseminated germ-cell tumors who did not undergo an RPLND.[126] Before any chemotherapy was administered, 77% of patients were severely oligospermic and 17% azoospermic. After four courses of PVB, 96% were azoospermic. However, 2 years after initiation of chemotherapy, 50% had recovered a normal sperm count and motility, and approximately half of the patients who had attempted to impregnate their wives had been successful, with the infants having no congenital abnormalities. Fossa and colleagues at the Norwegian Radium Hospital in Oslo reported similar results,[127] with 50% to 60% of patients having active spermatogenesis 1 to 3 years after PVB. In contrast, Nijman and associates recently reported that 2 years after PVB, only 28% of patients had greater than 60,000,000 spermatozoa/ml; however, unlike the previous two studies, these patients all received maintenance cisplatin for 12 months.[128]

RAYNAUD'S PHENOMENON

Vogelzang and colleagues were among the first to observe the relation of Raynaud's phenomenon to testicular cancer chemotherapy.[129] In their series, 22 of 60 men (37%) treated with vinblastine plus bleomycin with or without cisplatin developed Raynaud's. Digital ischemia occurred in 21% of patients treated with vinblastine plus bleomycin and in 41% treated with PVB. This complication began a median of 10 months after chemotherapy was instituted (range 2–28 months). Other authors have reported on Raynaud's phenomenon with vinblastine plus bleomycin.[130]

VASCULAR COMPLICATIONS

The incidence of Raynaud's phenomenon with distal arteriolar narrowing raises the specter of generalized vascular disease with acute myocardial infarction secondary to coronary artery disease, deep venous thrombosis, and cerebrovascular accident. Bleomycin and vinca alkaloids such as vinblastine have been anecdotally associated with myocardial ischemia.[131,132] In 1979, Edwards and associates reported two patients in their 20s treated with PVB for eight courses who died of far-advanced testicular cancer and at autopsy had clinically unsuspected severe arteriosclerosis of the coronary arteries.

Two recent reports have increased concern about vascular complications of cisplatin combination chemotherapy. Samuels and colleagues described five patients with both acute and long-term vascular toxicity,[134] and three of these patients had no evidence of cancer at autopsy (Table 35-25). These cases were culled from 65 patients treated at the University of Minnesota from 1978 to 1982. However, one of these patients came from the University of Chicago, and the denominator at that institution is unknown. Thus, the frequency of these problems cannot be determined at present.

These five cases are not proof of PVB-based toxicity. Patient 1 may have had clostridial sepsis as the causative agent of rectal infarction. Patient 3 had sepsis and hypotension during high-dose ara-C and a questionable myocardial infarction. Patient 4 received doxorubicin, a known cardiotoxic drug, as well as other agents. Finally, in patient 5, Koch's postulates were not fulfilled, as rechallenge with five more courses of PVB produced no immediate further problems.

Doll and associates described four additional cases of vascular complications after cisplatin combination chemotherapy in 23 patients treated from 1983 to 1985 (Table 35-26).[135] None of these patients had known risk factors

TABLE 35-25. Vascular Complications Associated with Cisplatin Combination Chemotherapy[134]

Age	*Vascular Event*	*Timing Postchemotherapy (mo)*	*Comments*
23	Rectal infarction	Course 4 PVB	Rectal pain and bleeding with blood cultures positive for *Clostridia*
24	Myocardial infarction	18	Obese; sudden death with 75% occlusion left anterior descending coronary artery
33	Myocardial infarction	6	PVB, then cisplatin+ VP-16, then high-dose ara-C; developed sepsis, hypotension, and questionable MI.
42	Myocardial infarction	46	Prior radiotherapy to abdomen + cyclophosphamide, bleomycin, and doxorubicin; subsequent PVB
58	Cerebrovascular accident	Course 1 PVB	CVA resolved; received 5 further cycles of PVB without problems. Subsequent cyclophosphamide + dactinomycin + methotrexate with worsening left hemiparesis and subsequent death

TABLE 35-26. Vascular Complications Associated with Cisplatin Combination Chemotherapy

Age	*Vascular Event*	*Timing Postchemotherapy (mo)*	*Comments*
21	Cerebrovascular accident	7	Double-dose cisplatin + VP-16 + bleomycin; developed headaches, slurred speech, and right hemiparesis with normal head CT, MR, and cerebral arteriogram
24	Myocardial infarction	18	No risk factors
25	Cerebrovascular accident	course 3	No risk factors
27	Myocardial infarction	course 2	Double-dose cisplatin + VP-16 + bleomycin; PVB 5 years previously; patient completed 3 additional courses without further problems

such as prior mediastinal radiotherapy, family history of cardiac disease, heavy smoking, hypertension, diabetes, or hyperlipedemia.

There are several plausible explanations for vascular toxicity, including the previously mentioned Raynaud's phenomenon progressing to generalized vascular disease. Also, bleomycin can cause endothelial changes cumulatively in capillaries and arterioles.[136] Cisplatin-induced hypomagnesemia can cause ventricular irritability and coronary artery spasm. High levels of circulating von Willebrand's factor antigen have been associated with Raynaud's, may be a marker for endothelial damage,[137] and may lead to thrombosis.[138]

There are several conclusions and statements that can be made:

1. The incidence of vascular complications is low (less than 5%).
2. Vascular complications are various.
3. Some patients with complications can be retreated with the same chemotherapy without apparent problems.
4. It is not possible to know whether these vascular complications are secondary to treatment or to the disease process (*e.g.*, tumor emboli, deep venous thrombosis in association with large pelvic mass). If treatment is implicated, which drug or drug combination is the culprit remains unknown.

The recently completed adjuvant intergroup Stage I–II study provides a unique forum to address these important concerns. Questionnaires concerning deep venous thrombosis, pulmonary embolus, myocardial infarction, and cerebrovascular accident have been sent to several hundred patients. It will be of great interest to see if there is an increase in vascular complication in patients who received cisplatin combination chemotherapy versus those patients who were cured with surgery alone.

BLEOMYCIN-RELATED COMPLICATIONS

Barneveld and colleagues evaluated 93 patients treated with PVB, of whom eight had clinical evidence of bleomycin pneumonitis.[139] One of these patients died from bleomycin toxicity; the other seven were fully recovered with a minimum follow-up of 2 years. Chest films normalized at a median of 9 months (range 6–13 months), and all symptoms abated in 4 to 5 months.

A different bleomycin-related complication relates to radiographic abnormalities that can simulate metastatic pulmonary nodules.[140,141] Subclinical bleomycin pulmonary fibrosis can produce a coalescence of fibrous tissue that on chest roentgenography or, especially, CT has the appearance of metastatic nodules. If such nodules are seen after chemotherapy in areas different from those of the original pulmonary metastases, they are assumed to be secondary to bleomycin, and it is not necessary to biopsy these areas by fine-needle aspiration or thoracotomy.

LEUKEMIA

Testicular cancer patients are immunologically intact and receive short-duration chemotherapy, and there is no appreciable risk of secondary leukemia. However, if alkylating agents are used long term, secondary leukemia can be a late consequence of curative therapy.[142] The Memorial Sloan-Kettering Cancer Center group retrospectively evaluated patients treated from 1950 through 1979 and found four cases of acute myeloblastic leukemia and one of chronic myelomonocytic leukemia, with a relative risk estimate of 13.7 in the total patient population and 50.1 in the group receiving chemotherapy. Two of these patients were treated with VAB-III (2 years of chlorambucil), two with radiotherapy alone, and one with radiotherapy plus 18 months of chemotherapy.

TABLE 35-27. Characteristics of Late Relapses at Walter Reed Army Medical Center[143]

Patient	Timing of Relapse (mo)	Initial Chemotherapy	Comments
1	45	VAB-III	Large abdominal mass ? CR; late relapse in abdomen with elevated AFP
2	54	VAB-III	Large abdominal mass with abdominal recurrence
3	76	Adjuvant dactinomycin	CR with PVB for 65+ months
4	87	Mithramycin	Initial pulmonary metastases, recurred in lungs
5	56	PVB	Recurred with solitary pulmonary metastases
6	51	Adjuvant VAB-III	Pelvic recurrence of teratocarcinoma with elevated AFP
7	86	VAB-III	Late abdominal and pelvic recurrence with elevated AFP

LATE RELAPSES

Perhaps the most ominous late consequence is a relapse. In our experience at Indiana University, we see occasional late (more than 2 years) relapses after chemotherapy. The usual scenario is a patient presenting with bulky teratocarcinoma who has normalization of markers with chemotherapy and undergoes an RPLND with resection of large-volume teratoma. Theoretically, microscopic teratoma may have been left behind; it can be biologically inert, grow slowly as teratoma, or, possibly, transform as teratocarcinoma with the preponderant mass consisting of mature and immature teratoma with small components of embryonal cell carcinoma. Such patients relapse in the original area of bulk teratoma, frequently with elevated AFP concentrations. Our present recommendations for patients with postchemotherapy resection of teratoma that is larger than 5 cm is to obtain abdominal CT scans every 3 to 4 months for 2 years and then one or two times per year for an additional 2 to 3 years.

The Walter Reed group has reported seven patients with late relapse (45–87 months after chemotherapy).[143] These patients are detailed in Table 35-27.

Another issue of "late relapse" is a second primary germ-cell tumor, which will occur in 1% to 3% of all cured patients. Instruction in testicular self-examination as well as physician palpation of the testis is part of our routine follow-up in all patients.

ADJUVANT CHEMOTHERAPY

The criteria for successful application of adjuvant chemotherapy are (1) poor prognosis for cure with primary therapy alone, and (2) evidence that the proposed adjuvant therapy is effective in metastatic disease. However, in nonseminomatous germ-cell tumors, there is a third consideration, namely, whether similar cure rates can be achieved by using chemotherapy when a patient relapses after an RPLND; adjuvant chemotherapy may be unnecessary.

A national intergroup study has been recently completed in patients with pathologic Stage II nonseminomatous germ-cell tumors. Patient entry was from 1979 to 1987, and there were 197 evaluable patients.[144] Median time on study is in excess of 4 years. Patients were randomized to two postoperative courses of cisplatin combination chemotherapy versus observation, which consisted of history and physical examination, and hCG and AFP assays, and posteroanterior and lateral chest films monthly the first postoperative year, every 2 months during the second year, and subsequently every 6 months. Ninety-seven patients entered the adjuvant arm, and only one patient has relapsed. This patient subsequently died of metastatic testicular cancer. Forty-eight of 98 patients on the observation arm have relapsed. However, with this close follow-up, relapse was detected in a favorable setting: only three of these patients have died from recurrent testicular cancer, and the remaining 95 remain disease free. There was no independent risk factor for relapse that would mandate adjuvant chemotherapy in any subtype (*e.g.*, marker-negative patients, vascular invasion). Two courses of cisplatin-based adjuvant chemotherapy will almost always prevent relapse. However, when surgery, follow-up, and chemotherapy are optimal, either approach produces excellent cure rates.

NEW STUDIES

In addition to the studies already mentioned in this chapter, there are other important studies that are still awaiting final analysis (Table 35-28). In the Memorial study, the results with the two-drug regimen of cisplatin and VP-16 produced therapeutic results equivalent to those of the five-drug regimen of VAB-VI with considerably less treatment-related morbidity. In the Southeastern Cancer Study Group protocol,

TABLE 35-28. New Studies

Institution	Patient Population	Study Design
Memorial Sloan-Kettering	Favorable prognosis	VAB-VI versus PVP-16
Southeastern Cancer Study Group	Minimal and moderate disseminated disease	PVP-16B × 4 courses versus PVP-16B × 3 courses
EORTC	Favorable prognosis	PVP-16B versus PVP-16
ECOG	Advanced disseminated disease	PVP-16B versus cisplatin + VP-16 + ifosfamide

approximately 200 patients were randomized, and at present, it appears that three courses of PVP-16B over 9 weeks gives results identical to those of four courses over 12 weeks. The EORTC study is still too early for any conclusions, and the ECOG study has just recently begun patient accrual.

REFERENCES

1. Drain LS: Testicular cancer in California from 1942–1969: The California Tumor Registry experience. Oncology 27:45–51, 1973
2. Einhorn LH: Testicular cancer: A model for a curable neoplasm. Cancer Res 41:3275–3280, 1981
3. Strecker JF, Floyd JW III: The testis. In Devine CJ, Stecker JF (eds): Urology in Practice, pp 73–79. Boston, Little, Brown, 1978
4. Hausfeld KF, Schrandt D: Malignancy of testis following atrophy: Report of three cases. J Urol 94:69–72, 1965
5. Herr HW, Silber I, Martin DC: Management of inguinal lymph nodes in patients with testicular tumors following orchiopexy, inguinal, or scrotal operation. J Urol 110:223–224, 1973
6. Gilbert JB, Hamilton JB: Incidence and nature of tumors in ectopic testes. Surg Gynecol Obstet 71:731–743, 1940
7. Dixon FJ, Moore RA (eds): Atlas of Tumor Pathology, Fascicle 31B, section 8, p 32. Washington, DC, Armed Forces Institute of Pathology, 1952
8. Friedman NB, Moore RA: Tumors of the testis: A report on 922 cases. Milit Surgeon 99:573–593, 1946
9. Mostofi FK, Price EB (eds): Tumors of the Male Genital System Atlas of Tumor Pathology, Second Series, Fascicle 8, p 7. Washington, DC, Armed Forces Institute of Pathology, 1973
10. Mostofi FK, Sobin LH: Histological Typing of Testis Tumors. International Histological Classification of Tumors, No. 16. Geneva, World Health Organization, 1977
11. Rosai J, Heyderman E, Kurman RJ, Mostofi FK, Nochomovitz LE, Scully RA: Report of the Pathology Review Committee. International Symposium on Human Testis Cancer, Mouse Teratocarcinoma and Oncofetal Proteins. Minneapolis, 1980
12. Rosen SW, Weintraub BD, Vaitukaitis JL et al: Placental proteins and their subunits as tumor markers. Ann Intern Med 82:71–83, 1975
13. Lange PH, Nochomovitz LE, Rosai J, et al: Serum alpha-fetoprotein and human chorionic gonadotropin in patients with seminoma. J Urol 124:472–478, 1980
14. Drago JR, Nelson RP, Palmer JM: Childhood embryonal carcinoma of the testis. Urology 12:499–503, 1978
15. Duckett J: Panel on testis tumors, American Cancer Society. Atlanta, October, 1980
16. Lange PH, Fraley EE: Serum alpha-fetoprotein and human chorionic gonadotropin in the treatment of patients with testicular tumors. Urol Clin North Am 4:393–406, 1977
17. Mostofi FK, Theiss EA, Ashley DJB: Tumors of specialized gonadal stroma in human male patients: Androblastoma, Sertoli cell tumor, granulosa-theca cell tumor of the testis, and gonadal stromal tumor. Cancer 12:944–957, 1959
18. Holtz F, Abell MR: Testicular neoplasms in infants and children I: Tumors of non-germ cell origin. Cancer 16:982–986, 1963
19. Silverberg SG, Thompson JW, Higashi G, Baskin AM: Malignant interstitial cell tumor of the testis: Case report and review. J Urol 96:356–363, 1966
20. Hopkins GB: Interstitial cell tumor of the testis: Case report and review of the literature. J Urol 103:449–451, 1970
21. Kuzmits R, Schernthaner G, Krisch K: Serum neuron-specific enolase: A marker for response to therapy in seminoma. Cancer 60:1017–1021, 1987
22. Barzell W, Whitmore WF: Neoplasms of the testis. In Harrison JH, Gittes RF, Perlmutter AD et al (eds): Campbell's Urology, 4th Ed, p 1141. Philadelphia, WB Saunders, 1979
23. Richie JP, Garnick MB, Finberg H: Computerized tomography: How accurate for abdominal staging of testis tumors? J Urol 127:715–717, 1982
24. Rowland RG, Weisman D, Williams S, Einhorn L, Donohue, JP: Accuracy of preoperative staging in Stage A and B non-seminomatous germ cell testis tumors. J Urol 127:718–720, 1982
25. Maier JG, Sulak MH, Mittemeyer BT: Seminoma of the testis: Analysis of treatment success and failure. 102:596–602, 1968
26. Heiken JP, Balfe DM, McClennan BL: Testicular tumors: Oncologic imaging and diagnosis. Int J Radiat Oncol Biol Phys 10:275–287, 1984
27. Hoeltl W, Kosak D, Pont J et al: Testicular cancer: Prognostic implications of vascular invasion. J Urol 137:683–685, 1987
28. Zagars GK, Babaian RJ: Stage I testicular seminoma: Rationale for post-orchiectomy radiation therapy. Int J Radiat Oncol Biol Phys 13:155–162, 1987
29. Kubo HD, Shipley WU: Reduction of the scatter dose to the testicle outside the radiation treatment fields. Int J Radiat Oncol Biol Phys 8:1741–1745, 1982
30. Maier JG, Sulak MH: Radiation therapy in malignant testis tumors seminoma. Cancer 32:1212–1216, 1973
31. Hamilton C, Horwich A, Peckham MJ et al: Radiotherapy for Stage I seminoma testis: Results of treatment and complications. Radiat Ther Oncol 6:115–120, 1986
32. Earle JD, Bagshaw MA, Kaplan HS: Supervoltage radiation therapy of testicular tumors. Am J Roentgenol 117:653–661, 1973
33. Dosoretz DE, Shipley WU, Blitzer PH et al: Megavoltage irradiation for pure testicular seminoma: Results and patterns of failure. Cancer 48:2184–2190, 1981
34. Hanks GE, Herring DF, Kramer S: Patterns of care outcome studies: Results of the National Practice in Seminoma of the Testis. Int J Radiat Oncol Biol Phys 7:1413–1417, 1981
35. Willan BD, McGowan DG: Seminoma of the testis: A 22 year experience with radiation therapy. Int J Radiat Oncol Biol Phys 11:1769–1775, 1985
36. Peckham MJ: Testicular tumors: Investigation and staging. In The Management of Testicular Tumors, pp 89–101. London, Edwin Arnold, 1981
37. Thomas GM, Rider WD, Dembo AJ et al: Seminoma of the testis: Results of treatment and patterns of failure after radiation therapy. Int J Radiat Oncol Biol Phys 8:165–174, 1982
38. Loehrer PJ, Birch R, Williams SD et al: Chemotherapy of metastatic seminoma: The Southeastern Cancer Study Group experience. J Clin Oncol 5:1212–1220, 1987
39. Zagars GK, Babian RJ: The role of radiation therapy in Stage II testicular seminoma. Int J Radiat Oncol Biol Phys 13:163–170, 1987
40. Smalley SR, Evans RG, Richardson RL et al: Radiotherapy as initial treatment for bulky Stage II seminoma. J Clin Oncol 3:1333–1338, 1985
41. Percarpio B, Clements JC, McLeod DG et al: Anaplastic seminoma: An analysis of 77 patients. Cancer 43:2510–2513, 1979
42. Cockburn AG, Vugrin D, Batata M et al: Poorly differentiated (anaplastic) seminoma of the testis. Cancer 53:1991–1994, 1984
43. Mauch P, Weichselbaum R, Botnick L: The significance of positive chorionic gonadotropins in apparently pure seminoma of the testis. Int J Radiat Oncol Biol Phys 5:887–889, 1979
44. Mirimanoff RO, Shipley WU, Dosoretz DE et al: Pure seminoma of the testis: The results of radiation therapy in patients with elevated human chorionic gonadotropin titers. J Urol 134:1124–1126, 1985
45. Quivey JM, Fu KK, Herzog KA et al: Malignant tumors of the testis: Analysis of treatment results and sites and causes of failure. Cancer 39:1247–1253, 1977
46. Oliver RTD: Surveillance for Stage I seminoma in single agent cisplatinum for metastatic seminoma (abstr). Proc Am Soc Clin Oncol 3:162, 1984
47. Clemm C, Hartenstein R, Willich N et al: Vinblastine–ifosfamide–cisplatinum treatment of bulky seminoma. Cancer 58:2203–2207, 1986
48. Friedman EL, Garnick MB, Stomper PC et al: Therapeutic guidelines and results in advanced seminoma. J Clin Oncol 3:1325–1332, 1985
49. Motzer R, Bosl G, Heelan R et al: Residual mass: An indication for surgery in patients with advanced seminoma following systemic chemotherapy. J Clin Oncol 5:1064–1070, 1987
50. Fossa S, Borge L, Aass N et al: The treatment of advanced metastatic seminoma: Experience in 55 cases. J Clin Oncol 5:1071–1077, 1987
51. Pizzocaro G, Salvioni R, Piva L et al: Cisplatin combination chemotherapy in advanced seminoma. Cancer 58:1625–1629, 1986
52. Horwich A, Tucker DF, Peckham MJ: Placenta alkaline phosphatase as a tumor marker in seminoma using the H17E2 monoclonal antibody assay. Br J Cancer 51:625–629, 1985
53. Crawford ED, Scardino PT: Testicular carcinoma: An overview. In Crawford ED, Borden TA (eds): Genitourinary Cancer Surgery, pp 249–261. Philadelphia, Lea & Febiger, 1982
54. Jamieson JK, Dobson JF: The lymphatics of the testicle. Lancet 1:493–495, 1910
55. Cuneo B, Marcille M: Topographie des ganglions iliopelviens. Bull Soc Anat [Paris], 6s(III):653, 1901
56. Howard RJ: Malignant disease of the testis. Practitioner 79:794–810, 1907
57. Hinman F: The operative treatment of tumor of the testicle. JAMA 63:2009–2015, 1914
58. Lewis LG: Radioresistant testis tumors: Results in 133 cases—Five-year followup. J Urol 69:841–844, 1953
59. Cooper JF, Leadbetter WF, Chute R: The thoracoabdominal approach for retroperitoneal gland dissection: Its application to testis tumors. Surg Gynecol Obstet 90:486–496, 1950
60. Staubitz WJ, Early KS, Magoss IV, Murphy GP: Surgical management of testis tumors. J Urol 111:205–209, 1974
61. Whitmore WF: Surgical treatment of adult germinal testis tumors. Semin Oncol 6:55–68, 1979
62. Donohue JP, Zachary JM, Maynard BR: Distribution of nodal metastases in non-seminomatous testis cancer. J Urol 128:315–320, 1982
63. Donohue JP: Surgical management of testicular cancer. In LH Einhorn (ed): Testicular Tumors: Management and Treatment, pp 29–46. New York, Masson Publishing, 1980
64. Lange P, Narayan P, Fraley E: Fertility issues following therapy for testicular cancer. Semin Urol 4:264, 1985
65. Rowland RG, Weisman D, Williams S et al: Accuracy of preoperative staging in Stage A and B non-seminomatous germ cell testis tumors. J Urol 127:718–720, 1982
66. Pizzocaro G, Musumeci R: The relative value of lymphangiograph (LAG) and computed tomography (CT) in diagnosing small retroperitoneal metastases. In S Khoury (ed): Testicular Cancer, p 261. New York, 1985
67. Einhorn LH, Donohue JP, Peckham MJ et al: Cancer of the testes. In DeVita VT, Hellman S, Rosenberg SA (eds): Cancer: Principles and Practice of Oncology, pp 979–1011. Philadelphia, JB Lippincott, 1985

68. Crawford ED, Mettler FA, Duncan PR: Retrocrural lymphadenopathy in testicular cancer. J Urol 131:343–345, 1984
69. Tyrell CJ, Peckham MJ: The response of lymph node metastases of testicular teratoma to radiation therapy. Br J Urol 48:363–370, 1976
70. Skinner DG: Surgical management of germ cell tumors of the testis. In DG Skinner (ed): Urological Cancer, pp 301–304 Grune & Stratton, 1983
71. Goldinger PL, Scheweizer O: The hazards of anesthesia and surgery in bleomycin-treated patients. Semin Oncol 6:121–124, 1979
72. Lange PH, Narayan P, Vogelzang NJ et al: Return of fertility after treatment for non-seminomatous testicular cancer: Changing concepts. J Urol 129:1131–1135, 1983
73. Fossa SD, Klepp O, Molne K et al: Testicular function after unilateral orchiectomy for cancer and before further treatment. Int J Androl 5:179–184, 1982
74. Berthelsen JG, Skakkeback NE: Gonadal function in men with testis cancer. Fertil Steril 39:68–75, 1983
75. Li MC, Whitmore WF, Golbey R et al: Effects of combined drug therapy on metastatic cancer of the testis. JAMA 174:145–153, 1960
76. MacKenzie AR: Chemotherapy of metastatic testis cancer: Results in 154 patients. Cancer 19:1369–1376, 1966
77. Kennedy BJ: Mithramycin therapy in advanced testicular neoplasms. Cancer 26:755–766, 1970
78. Blum RH, Carter S, Agre K: A clinical review of bleomycin: A new anti-neoplastic agent. Cancer 31:903–914, 1973
79. Samuels ML, Howe CD: Vinblastine in the management of testicular cancer. Cancer 25:1009–1017, 1970
80. Samuels ML, Johnson DE, Holoye PY: Continuous intravenous bleomycin therapy with vinblastine in Stage III testicular neoplasia. Cancer Chemother Rep 59:563–570, 1975
81. Samuels ML, Lanzotti VJ, Holoye PY et al: Combination chemotherapy in germinal cell tumors. Cancer Treat Rev 3:185–204, 1976
82. Rosenberg B, VanCamp L, Krigas T: Inhibition of cell division in *E. coli* by electrolysis products from a platinum electrode. Nature 205:678–699, 1965
83. Higby DJ, Wallace HJ, Albert DJ et al: Diamminedichloroplatinum: A Phase I study showing responses in testicular and other tumors. Cancer 33:1219–1225, 1974
84. Wittes RE, Yagoda A, Silvay O et al: Chemotherapy of germ cell tumors of the testis. Cancer 37:637–645, 1976
85. Cheng E, Cvitkovic E, Wittes RE et al: Germ cell tumor: VAB II in metastatic testicular cancer. Cancer 42:2162–2168, 1978
86. Cvitkovic E, Wittes R, Golbey R et al: Primary combination chemotherapy for metastatic or unresectable germ cell tumors (abstract). Proc Am Assoc Cancer Res 19:174, 1978
87. Bosl GJ, Gluckman R, Geller NL et al: VAB-6: An effective chemotherapy regimen for patients with germ cell tumors. J Clin Oncol 4:1493–1499, 1986
88. Bosl GJ, Geller NL, Cirrincione CC et al: Multivariate analysis of prognostic variables in patients with metastatic testicular cancer. Cancer Res 43:3403–3407, 1983
89. Einhorn LH, Donohue JP: Cis-diamminedichloroplatinum, vinblastine, and bleomycin combination chemotherapy in disseminated testicular cancer. Ann Intern Med 87:293–298, 1977
90. Nichols C, Gupta S, Loehrer P et al: Outcome in patients with residual germ cell cancer after post-chemotherapy surgery (abstr). Proc Am Soc Clin Oncol 6:100, 1987
91. Einhorn LH, Williams SD: Chemotherapy of disseminated testicular cancer. Cancer 46:1339–1344, 1980
92. Stoter G, Sleyfer DT, Bokkel Huinink WW et al: High-dose versus low-dose vinblastine in cisplatin–vinblastine–bleomycin combination chemotherapy of non-seminomatous testicular cancer: A randomized study of the EORTC Genitouurinary Tract Cancer Cooperative Group. J Clin Oncol 4:1199–1206, 1986
93. Einhorn LH, Williams SD, Troner M et al: The role of maintenance therapy in disseminated testicular cancer. N Engl J Med 305:727–731, 1981
94. Fitzharris BM, Kaye SB, Saverymuttu S et al: VP-16-213 as single agent in advanced testicular tumors. Eur J Cancer 16:1193–1197, 1980
95. Schabel FM Jr, Trader MW, Laster WR Jr et al: Cis-dichlorodiammineplatinum: Combination chemotherapy and cross-resistance studies with tumors of mice. Cancer Treat Rep 63:1459–1473, 1979
96. Peckham MJ, Barrett A, Liew KH et al: The treatment of metastatic germ cell testicular tumors with bleomycin, etoposide, and cisplatin (BEP). Br J Cancer 47:613–619, 1983
97. Williams SD, Birch R, Einhorn LH et al: Treatment of disseminated germ-cell tumors with cisplatin, bleomycin, and either vinblastine and etoposide. N Engl J Med 316:1435–1440, 1987
98. Greist A, Einhorn LH, Williams SD et al: Pathologic findings at orchiectomy following chemotherapy for disseminated testicular cancer. J Clin Oncol 2:1025–1027, 1984
99. Rich TA, Cassady JR, Strand RD et al: Radiotherapy for pineal and suprasellar germ cell tumors. Cancer 55:932–940, 1985
100. Nichols CR, Hoffman R, Einhorn LH, et al: Hematologic malignancies associated with primary mediastinal germ cell tumors. Ann Intern Med 102:603–609, 1985
101. Nichols CR, Heerema NA, Palmer C et al: Klinefelter's syndrome associated with mediastinal germ cell neoplasms. J Clin Oncol 5:1290–1294, 1987
102. Hainsworth JD, Wright EP, Gray GF, Greco FA: Poorly differentiated carcinoma of unknown primary: Correlation of light microscopic findings with response to cisplatin-based combination chemotherapy. J Clin Oncol 5:1275–1280, 1987
103. Hainsworth JD, Einhorn LH, Williams SD et al: Advanced extragonadal germ cell tumors. Ann Intern Med 97:7–11, 1982
104. Vugrin D, Einhorn LH, Williams SD et al: A multi-institutional experience in extragonadal germ cell tumors: An SECSG study (abstr). Proc Am Assoc Cancer Res 26:172, 1985
105. Israel A, Bosl GJ, Golbey RB et al: The results of chemotherapy for extragonadal germ-cell tumors in the cisplatin era: The MSKCC experience (1975–1982). J Clin Oncol 3:1073–1078, 1985
106. Logothetis CJ, Samuels ML, Selig DE et al: Chemotherapy of extragonadal germ cell tumors. J Clin Oncol 3:316–325, 1985
107. Logothetis CJ, Samuels ML, Trindode A: The management of brain metastases in germ cell tumors. Cancer 49:1278–1281, 1982
108. Rustin GJS, Newlands ES, Bagshawe KD et al: Successful management of metastatic and primary germ cell tumors in the brain. Cancer 57:2108–2113, 1986
109. Lester SG, Morphis JG, Hornback NB et al: Brain metastases and testicular tumors: Need for aggressive treatment. J Clin Oncol 2:1397–1403, 1984
110. Greist A, Einhorn LH, Williams SD et al: Pathologic findings at orchiectomy following chemotherapy for disseminated testicular cancer. J Clin Oncol 2:1025–1027, 1984
111. Chong C, Logothetis CJ, von Eschenbach A et al: Orchiectomy in advanced germ cell carcinoma following intensive chemotherapy: A comparison of systemic to testicular response. J Urol 136:1221–1223, 1986
112. Fowler JE Jr, Whitmore WF Jr: Intratesticular germ cell tumors: Observations on the effect of chemotherapy J Urol 126:412–415, 1981
113. Schabel FM Jr, Trader MW, Laster WR Jr et al: Cis-dichlorodiammineplatinum: Combination chemotherapy and cross-resistance studies with tumors of mice. Cancer Treat Rep 63:1459–1573, 1979
114. Williams SD, Einhorn LH, Greco FA et al: VP-16-213 salvage therapy for refractory germinal neoplasms. Cancer 46:2154–2158, 1980
115. Hainsworth JD, Williams SD, Einhorn LH et al: Successful treatment of resistant germinal neoplasms with VP-16 and cisplatin: Results of a Southeastern Cancer Study Group trial. J Clin Oncol 3:666–671, 1985
116. Wheeler BM, Loehrer PJ, Williams SD, Einhorn LH: Ifosfamide in refractory germ cell tumors. J Clin Oncol 4:28–34, 1986
117. Loehrer PJ, Einhorn LH, Williams SD: Salvage therapy for refractory germ cell tumors with VP-16 + ifosfamide + cisplatin. J Clin Oncol 4:528–536, 1986
118. Lauer RL, Roth B, Loehrer PJ et al: Cisplatin + ifosfamide + either VP-16 or vinblastine as third-line therapy for metastatic testicular cancer (abstr). Proc Am Soc Clin Oncol 6:99, 1987
119. Birch R, Williams SD, Cone A et al: Prognostic factors for favorable outcome in disseminated germ cell tumors. J Clin Oncol 4:400–407, 1986
120. Peckham MJ, Oliver RTD, Bagshawe KD et al: Prognostic factors in advanced non-seminomatous germ-cell testicular tumors: Results of a multicentre study. Lancet 1:8–11, 1985
121. Pizzocaro G, Piva L, Salvioni R et al: Cisplatin, etoposide, bleomycin as first-line therapy and early resection of residual tumor in far-advanced germinal testis cancer. Cancer 56:2411–2415, 1985
122. Daugaard G, Rorth M: High-dose cisplatin and VP-16 with bleomycin in the management of advanced metastatic germ cell tumors. Eur J Cancer Clin Oncol 22:477–485, 1986
123. Loehrer PJ, Sledge GW, Einhorn LH: Heterogeneity among germ-cell tumors of the testis. Semin Oncol 12:304–316, 1985
124. Ulbright TM, Loehrer PJ, Roth LM et al: The development of non-germ cell malignancies within germ cell tumors. Cancer 54:1824–1833, 1984
125. Greist A, Roth B, Einhorn LH et al: Cisplatin-combination chemotherapy for disseminated germ cell tumors: Long-term followup (abstr). Proc Am Soc Clin Oncol 4:98, 1985
126. Drasga RE, Einhorn LH, Williams SD et al: Fertility after chemotherapy for testicular cancer. J Clin Oncol 1:179–183, 1983
127. Fossa SD, Ous S, Abyholm T et al: Post-treatment fertility in patients with testicular cancer. Br J Urol 57:210–214, 1985
128. Nijman JM, Koops HS, Kremer J et al: Gonadal function after surgery and chemotherapy in men with Stages II and III non-seminomatous testicular tumors. J Clin Oncol 5:651–656, 1987
129. Vogelzang NJ, Bosl GJ, Johnson K et al: Raynaud's phenomenon: A common toxicity after combination chemotherapy for testicular cancer. Ann Intern Med 95:288–292, 1981
130. Teutsch C, Lipton A, Harvey HA: Raynaud's phenomenon as a side effect of chemotherapy with vinblastine plus bleomycin for testicular cancer. Cancer Treat Rep 61:925–926, 1977
131. Subar M, Muggia FM: Apparent myocardial ischemia associated with vinblastine administration. Cancer Treat Rep 70:690–691, 1986
132. Vogelzang NJ, Freming DH, Kennedy BJ: Coronary artery disease after treatment with bleomycin and vinblastine. Cancer Treat Rep 64:1159–1160, 1980
133. Edwards GS, Lane M, Smith FE: Long-term treatment with PVB: Possible association with severe coronary artery disease. Cancer Treat Rep 63:551–552, 1979
134. Samuels BL, Vogelzang NJ, Kennedy BJ: Severe vascular toxicity associated with vinblastine, bleomycin, and cisplatin chemotherapy. Cancer Chemother Pharmacol 19:253–256, 1987
135. Doll DC, List AF, Greco FA et al: Acute vascular ischemic events after cisplatin-based combination chemotherapy for germ cell tumors of the testis. Ann Intern Med 105:48–51, 1986
136. Burkhardt A, Haltje WJ, Gebbens JO et al: Vascular lesions following perfusion with bleomycin: Electron microscopic observations. Virchows Arch [Pathol Anat] 372:227–236, 1976

137. Kahaleh MD, Osborn I, LeRoy EC: Increased Factor VIII antigen in scleroderma and Raynaud's phenomenon. Ann Intern Med 94:842–845, 1981
138. Pui CH, Chesney CM, Weed J et al: Altered von Willebrand factor molecule in children with thrombus following asparaginase–prednisone–vincristine therapy for leukemia. J Clin Oncol 3:1266–1271, 1985
139. Barneveld PW, Sleijfer DT, van der Mark TW et al: Natural course of bleomycin induced pneumonitis. Am Rev Resp Dis 135:48–51, 1987
140. Nachman JB, Baum ES, White H et al: Bleomycin-induced pulmonary fibrosis mimicking recurrent metastatic disease in a patient with testicular cancer. Cancer 47:236–239, 1981
141. McCrea ES, Diaconis JN, Wade JC et al: Bleomycin toxicity simulating metastatic nodules to the lungs. Cancer 48:1096–1100, 1981
142. Redman JR, Vugrin D, Arlin ZA et al: Leukemia following treatment of germ cell tumors in men. J Clin Oncol 2:1080–1087, 1984
143. Terebelo HR, Taylor HG, Brown A et al: Late relapse of testicular cancer. J Clin Oncol 1:566–571, 1983
144. Williams SD, Stablein DM, Einhorn LH et al: Pathologic Stage II testis cancer: Immediate adjuvant chemotherapy versus observation with treatment relapse: A report from the Testicular Cancer Intergroup Study. N Engl J Med 317:1433–1438, 1987

WILLIAM J. HOSKINS
CARLOS PEREZ
ROBERT C. YOUNG

CHAPTER 36 *Gynecologic Tumors*

Gynecologic cancer represents 14.9% of all cancers in women and accounts for 10% of all cancer deaths.[1] Table 36-1 lists the estimated number of new cases and deaths of the female genital cancers for 1987. For the physician called on to diagnose and treat patients with female genital cancer, it is important to have a thorough understanding of the pathophysiology of the disease as well as an understanding of the various therapeutic options available. In this chapter we present current information on all of the female genital cancers except ovarian cancer, which is covered separately in Chapter 37. Epidemiology, natural history, and routes of spread are presented as well as the essential pathologic characteristics necessary for planning therapy. Major emphasis is placed on methods of diagnosis and current therapeutic options.

CARCINOMA OF THE VULVA

Carcinoma of the vulva accounts for approximately 3% of all female genital cancers.[1] Squamous cancer accounts for 90% of these cancers. Other cell types encountered are malignant melanoma, basal cell carcinoma, and adenocarcinoma of the Bartholin's and Skene's glands. Occasionally, primary vulvar sarcoma and verrucous carcinoma are seen. Paget's disease, which is discussed under the section on preinvasive cancer, may be associated with invasive adenocarcinoma of the sweat glands.

Usually vulvar cancers tend to develop slowly and spread by direct continuity to adjacent tissues or via the lymphatics to the inguinal lymph nodes. Treatment is most often surgical and results in physical disfigurement and sexual dysfunction.[2] Ongoing clinical protocols in this disease are evaluating alternative methods of therapy that researchers hope will allow modifications of treatment so as to reduce disfigurement and improve survival.

EPIDEMIOLOGY

The median age for patients with carcinoma in situ of the vulva is 44[3–9] and for those with microinvasive carcinoma it is 58.[8,10,11] Patients with frankly invasive carcinoma have a median age of 61.[12–14] Some authors have suggested that carcinoma in situ and microinvasive carcinoma are being seen more frequently and are occurring in younger women, but there are too few large series to document that impression. There does not appear to have been any change in the age incidence of invasive cancer.

Japaze et al[6] reported no increased incidence of vulvar cancer in any ethnic group, but Mack and Casagrande[15] reported an incidence in women of the lowest socioeconomic class that was three times the incidence in women of the highest socioeconomic class. Medical illnesses associated with vulvar cancer are hypertension, cardiovascular disease, obesity, and diabetes.[5,11,16–18] A variety of sexually transmitted diseases have been found in association with vulvar carcinoma including granulomatous venereal disease, syphilis, herpes hominis type II, and condylomata acuminata.[9,19] An increased incidence of anogenital carcinoma, especially cervical cancer, has been reported in patients with vulvar cancer.[20,21]

NATURAL HISTORY AND PATTERNS OF SPREAD

The association of carcinoma in situ, microinvasive carcinoma, and invasive vulvar carcinoma indicates that there is a

TABLE 36-1. Estimated New Cases and Deaths from Female Genital Cancer in 1988

Site	*Estimated New Cases*	*Estimated Deaths*
Corpus	34,000	3,000
Ovary	19,000	12,000
Cervix	12,900	7,000
Other	4,800	1,100
Total	70,700	23,100

Adapted from Silverberg E, Lubera J: Cancer statistics, 1988. CA 38:5, 1988.

continuum from preinvasive to invasive disease. There seems little doubt, however, that this process is much slower in the vulva than in the vagina or cervix, with almost two decades separating the peak incidence of vulvar carcinoma in situ and invasive carcinoma. Some authors have suggested that the multifocal carcinoma in situ of women in their 30s or 40s may not be as likely to progress to invasive cancer as the localized carcinoma in situ of the older woman. Although this may be true, there is no definite proof of this theory, and certainly one should not delay therapy in young women on this basis.

Plentl and Friedman[22] reported that primary vulvar lesions are most common in the labia and next most common on the clitoris. Labial lesions occurred three times more frequently on the labia majora as on the labia minora. These same authors pointed out the predictable spread of metastatic lesions to the inguinal lymph nodes followed by spread to the pelvic nodes. With the possible exception of vulvar melanoma, it is unusual for vulvar cancer to spread via the bloodstream.

The embryologic derivation of the lymphatics of the vulvar skin is similar to that of the abdominal skin,[22] and it is logical that primary drainage would be to the superficial and deep inguinal lymph nodes. Direct drainage to the pelvic lymph nodes occurs infrequently. The labia minora are characterized by a fine network of lymphatics that extend to the folds between the labia minora and labia majora. At these folds the lymphatic vessels become more coarse and extend cephalad. The lymphatics of the labia majora are more coarse than those of the labia minora and run laterally to the crural fold where they turn cephalad. Both of these lymphatic channels drain to the inguinal nodes. The clitoral vessels drain into the connecting trunks of the labia minora. All of these channels eventually drain into the superficial inguinal nodes that lie beneath Camper's fascia and anterior to the cribriform fascia. Connecting lymphatics lead to the deep inguinal nodes that surround the femoral vessels and drain into the iliac nodal system. Although it appears that clitoral lymphatics also drain directly into the pelvic lymphatics,[22] metastases to pelvic nodes without inguinal involvement are rare. Way[23] found involvement of the pelvic lymph nodes in the absence of inguinal lymph nodes in only 3% of his cases.

The overall incidence of positive lymph nodes (both inguinal and pelvic) in vulvar cancer was found to be 46% in a literature review of more than 1,100 patients by Plentl and Friedman.[22] Since the incidence of pelvic node metastases is 5% to 10%, one can expect inguinal node metastases to occur in 35% to 40% of cases. These same authors reported a 62% incidence of metastases in clinically palpable lymph nodes and a 35% incidence of metastases in nonpalpable lymph nodes. The incidence of positive lymph nodes increases with the size of the lesion, with the depth of invasion, and by location, with midline lesions having a higher incidence of bilateral positive lymph nodes.

PATHOLOGY

Intraepithelial neoplasia of the vulva exhibits a variety of gross and microscopic patterns. Grossly, the lesions may be flat and raised (maculopapular) or verrucous. They may be brown (hyperpigmented), red (erythroplastic) or white (leukoplakia). The various gross and microscopic patterns led to these lesions being termed Bowen's disease, erythroplasia of Queyrat, carcinoma simplex, and Paget's disease.[24] In order to standardize nomenclature, the International Society for the Study of Vulvar Disease published a classification in 1976 that is widely accepted throughout the world.[26] A summary of that classification is shown in Table 36-2. In this classification system only two types of true intraepithelial neoplasia are accepted: carcinoma in situ and Paget's disease. Histologically, carcinoma in situ is characterized by disordered orientation and maturation of the epithelial cells that extend the full thickness of the epithelium. Giant cells, multinucleated cells, dyskeratosis, parakeratosis, and increased density of cells are seen as well as abnormal nuclear morphology with irregular nuclear borders and clumped chromatin.[26] Paget's disease is characterized microscopically by the Paget's cells, which are large and round or oval with pale, vacuolated cytoplasm. These cells appear singly and in nests surrounded by small hyperchromatic basaloid cells. Helwig and Graham[27] reported that one third of their cases of Paget's disease of the vulva were associated with underlying adenocarcinomas of an adnexal structure. Associated carcinomas of the breast[28] and of Bartholin's gland[29] and squamous carcinoma of the cervix[30] have been reported.

Invasive squamous cancer is the most common vulvar malignancy and accounts for more than 90% of all cases. Grossly, the lesions will be ulcerated and endophytic in one third of cases and exophytic in the remainder.[26] Histologically, squamous cancers are usually well differentiated with whorls and nests of keratin. Gosling et al[31] and Way[32] have reported that 5% to 10% of these cancers will be anaplastic.

TABLE 36-2. International Society for the Study of Vulvar Disease: Classification of Vulvar Diseases*

A. Hyperplastic dystrophy
   1. Without atypia
   2. With atypia
B. Lichen sclerosis
C. Mixed dystrophy
   1. Without atypia
   2. With atypia
D. Paget's disease of the vulva
E. Carcinoma in situ

* Abbreviated classification.

Squamous cancers that are less than 2 cm in diameter and invade less than 5 mm are often termed microinvasive carcinoma.[33,34] The actual metastatic potential and the proper management of such patients are currently being evaluated. Two varieties of squamous cancer that occur rarely are adenoid squamous cancer described by Lasser et al[35] and verrucous carcinoma.[36] Verrucous carcinoma resembles extensive condylomata acuminata and is very well differentiated. It invades locally but rarely metastasizes.[37]

Melanoma accounts for 2% to 9% of vulvar cancers.[26] Two varieties of melanoma are described: the nodular melanoma and the superficial spreading melanoma.[26] Depth of invasion is directly related to the incidence of nodal metastases and survival.[38] Although a common finding in other parts of the body, basal cell carcinomas of the vulva occur infrequently.[39] Sarcomas may rarely arise in the vulvar connective tissue and, although leiomyosarcoma is the most common, neurofibrosarcomas, rhabdomyosarcomas, fibrosarcomas, and angiosarcomas have been reported.[40] Adenocarcinomas may occasionally arise from the periurethral Skene's glands, but most adenocarcinomas are either of the Bartholin's gland or from vulvar adnexal structures associated with Paget's disease.

Bartholin's carcinomas can be squamous if they originate near the orifice of the duct, papillary if they arise from the transitional epithelium of the duct, and adenocarcinoma if they arise from the gland itself. The adenoid cystic variety of Bartholin's gland carcinoma is similar to the adenoid cystic tumor of the salivary gland and tends to invade locally with metastases occurring late, if at all.[26]

CLINICAL PRESENTATION AND STAGING

The most common complaint of the patient with vulvar cancer is of a growth or mass of the vulva.[18] Pruritus vulvae, bleeding, and pain are also seen, and up to 20% of patients will be asymptomatic.[16,41] Although both physician and patient delay have been attributed to delays in diagnosis, better education appears to have had an influence since most recent series report smaller lesions and there is a growing body of literature on microinvasive cancer.

The best method of diagnosis of vulvar cancer is a high index of suspicion and early biopsy. Either a wedge biopsy with a knife or a circular biopsy with a Keye's dermal punch under local infiltration anesthesia will provide an excellent specimen and early diagnosis. The Keye's punch is especially good since hemostasis can usually be obtained with silver nitrate application without need for suture. Colposcopy will often be of use in defining the limits of the lesion, but it is too time-consuming to be significantly useful as a screening procedure. Toluidine blue staining of the vulva has been advocated as a method of identifying areas for biopsy but has a 20% false positive rate.

If invasive carcinoma is found on biopsy, the patient should undergo a metastatic evaluation. The vagina and cervix should be carefully inspected and a Papanicolaou smear of the cervix obtained. A careful bimanual examination, cystoscopy, proctoscopy, barium enema, intravenous pyelogram, chest radiograph, and biochemical profile are required. Computed tomography or nuclear magnetic resonance imaging (MRI) of the pelvis may be helpful in evaluating retroperitoneal nodal areas. Since most of these patients will be elderly, a thorough medical evaluation is often indicated before treatment.

The International Federation of Gynecology and Obstetrics classification for vulvar cancer is based on the tumor, nodes, and metastases (TNM) classifications with descriptive phraseology. Both the TNM classifications and the descriptions for each stage are listed in Table 36-3. For malignant melanoma, either the Clark[42] or Breslow[43] classifications of depth of invasion should also be provided. Bartholin's gland carcinomas are staged by the International Federation of Gynecology and Obstetrics (FIGO) system and

TABLE 36-3. Carcinoma of the Vulva: FIGO Method of Staging (TNM Classification)

T Primary tumor	
T1	Tumor confined to the vulva—2 cm or less in larger diameter
T2	Tumor confined to the vulva—more than 2 cm in diameter
T3	Tumor of any size with adjacent spread to the urethra or vagina or perineum or anus
T4	Tumor of any size infiltrating the bladder mucosa or the rectal mucosa or both, including the upper part of the urethral mucosa, or fixed to the bone
N Regional lymph nodes	
N0	No nodes palpable
N1	Nodes palpable in either groin, not enlarged, mobile (not clinically suspicious of neoplasm)
N2	Nodes palpable in either one or both groins, enlarged, firm and mobile (clinically suspicious of neoplasm)
N3	Fixed or ulcerated nodes
M Distant Metastases	
M10	No clinical metastases
M1a	Palpable deep pelvic lymph nodes
M1b	Other distant metastases
Definitions of the different clinical stages in carcinoma of the vulva (FIGO)	
Stage I	
T1 N0 M0	Tumor confined to the vulva—2 cm or less in the larger diameter. Nodes are not palpable, or are palpable in either groin, not enlarged, mobile (not clinically suspicious of neoplasm)
Stage II	
T2 N0 M0	Tumor confined to the vulva—more than 2 cm in diameter. Nodes are not palpable, or are palpable in either groin, not enlarged, mobile (not clinically suspicious of neoplasm)
Stage III	
T3 N0 M0 T3 N1 M0 T3 N2 M0 T1 N2 M0 T2 N2 M0	Tumor of any size with adjacent spread to the lower urethra or the vagina, perineum, or anus, or nodes palpable in either one or both groins, enlarged, firm and mobile, not fixed (but clinically suspicious of neoplasm)
Stage IV	
T4 N0 M0 T4 N1 M0 T4 N2 M0 T1 N3 M0 T2 N3 M0 T3 N3 M0 T4 N3 M0	Tumor of any size infiltrating the bladder mucosa or the rectal mucosa or both, including the upper part of the urethral mucosa, or fixed to the bone or other distant metastases. Fixed or ulcerated nodes in either one or both groins
All other conditions containing M1 or M1b	

metastatic tumors are not staged. It must be realized that the above staging system does not include a subdivision for microinvasive vulvar cancer. It is thus important to describe accurately the depth of invasion for Stage I tumors. For future prognostic evaluation, the presence or absence of lymphovascular invasion should also be noted.

TREATMENT

Historically, vulvar carcinoma has been considered to be effectively managed only by radical surgery with little place for radiation therapy, chemotherapy, or conservative surgery. The slow growth of the disease with its orderly progression of metastases to regional lymph nodes lends itself to en bloc surgical resection, and survival rates of 80% to 85% for patients with negative lymph nodes and 40% to 50% for those with positive inguinal nodes have been consistently reported. Table 36-3A shows 5-year survival rates in patients with carcinoma of the vulva. Unfortunately, the operation of radical vulvectomy and inguinal or inguinal and pelvic node dissection results in significant disruption of normal anatomy and is complicated by wound breakdown, lymphedema, and sexual dysfunction. Because of the above, several innovative approaches are being evaluated to decrease the short- and long-term morbidity of treatment of this disease. It is quite possible that the next decade will see rapid changes in the therapy of vulvar cancer.

STAGE 0

In the 1960s, Collins et al[44] advocated radical vulvectomy for carcinoma in situ of the vulva, pointing out that 4 of their 41 patients had unsuspected invasive cancer in the final specimen. Boutselis[4] reported survival rates approaching 100% with simple vulvectomy, and Rutledge and Sinclair[45] described the skinning vulvectomy that removed the skin of the vulva but preserved the fat, muscular, and glandular structures. When covered with a split-thickness skin graft from the thigh or buttocks, better cosmesis was obtained. Forney et al[7] used this procedure in 8 patients and noted only 1 recurrence. In 1983, Barnhill et al[46] described the rhomboid flap technique for vulvar reconstruction following wide local excision of carcinoma in situ.

Current management of carcinoma in situ of the vulva is wide local excision using either primary closure, skin flaps, or skin graft for restoration of normal anatomy. Many authors[7,9,47,48] have reported successful control of the disease with recurrence rates of 9% to 12%. Given the improved function and cosmesis with wide local excision, there is little doubt that optimal management consists of this method of therapy and close follow-up. Most patients, even if they require repeat excisions for recurrence, can be managed by wide local excision providing they adhere to a schedule of frequent follow-up examinations. Other methods of treating carcinoma in situ of the vulva include topical 5-fluorouracil, cryosurgery, dinitrochlorobenzene-induced hypersensitivity, and laser vaporization. Of these methods, only laser vaporization has proved significantly useful, and none provide a pathologic specimen for histologic review.

Paget's disease of the vulva extends subepithelially and requires wide excision in order to achieve free margins. Frozen section of the margins in the operating room may assist the surgeon in ensuring complete removal. Although some authorities recommend simple vulvectomy, this lesion, like carcinoma in situ, can usually be managed by less radical excision so that sexual function is maintained. A slightly deeper excision to remove the epidermis and corium down to the level of the underlying fat is indicated to ensure removal of the adnexal skin structures. Breen et al[49] reported a 12.4% recurrence rate after surgical excision, many of these patients having undergone simple vulvectomy initially. Some authors[50] have reported success with topical chemotherapy for recurrent Paget's disease, but such treatment should not be used as primary therapy because of the possibility of missing an underlying adenocarcinoma. If an invasive adenocarcinoma is found, the patient should be managed according to the extent of the invasive disease.

TABLE 36-3A. Survival Rates for Carcinoma of the Vulva

Stage	*Five-Year Survival Rate (%)*
Stage I	70
Stage II	50
Stage III	30
Stage IV	10

STAGE I

Stage I vulvar cancer encompasses all tumors that show any invasion (of any depth) as long as the tumor is less than 2 cm in diameter, does not involve the anus, vagina, or urethra, and there are no palpably enlarged lymph nodes. There is a growing body of literature, however, that indicates that certain early lesions should be separated into a category called microinvasive vulvar carcinoma. Wharton et al[33] in 1974 described a series of patients with vulvar cancers that were less than 2 cm in diameter and exhibited less than 5 mm of stromal invasion. They performed lymphadenectomies in 10 of 25 such patients and found no positive lymph nodes. Parker et al,[34] using the same definition of microinvasion, found inguinal metastases in 3 of 37 patients. Since those reports, several authors have reported small series of patients with an average incidence of inguinal node metastases of 5% to 10%.[8,11,51,52] Factors that may influence the incidence of nodal metastases are invasion greater than 2 mm,[52] anaplastic tumors,[11,34,52] confluency of invading foci,[11] and lymphovascular invasion.[34]

At present, there is no consensus as to how patients with microinvasive carcinoma should be managed. Nor is there clear-cut evidence in the literature that enables us to establish firm guidelines. DiSaia et al[53] have recommended an operative procedure in which the superficial inguinal lymph nodes are removed and sent for frozen section. If positive nodes are found, bilateral complete groin dissections and radical vulvectomy are performed; but if the nodes are negative, wide local excision of the primary cancer is performed and the procedure terminated. This therapeutic option appears to offer the best treatment plan to date, based on the meager information available. However, no large prospective trial of this method of therapy has been conducted to date. The Gynecologic Oncology Group (GOG) is currently evaluating prospectively all patients with tumor diameter of less than 2 cm and tumor invasion of less than 5 mm. In this protocol, patients are being managed by modified radical hemivulvectomy and ipsilateral node dissection. Perhaps a large number of patients, followed prospectively, will allow us to set reasonable treatment guidelines.

All other Stage I carcinomas of the vulva (those with invasion greater than 5 mm) should be managed by radical vulvectomy and bilateral inguinal lymphadenectomy. The therapeutic options for these patients are the same as those for Stage II carcinoma discussed below.

STAGES II AND III

Stage II vulvar carcinoma is a cancer that is greater than 2 cm in diameter, does not involve the anus, vagina, or urethra, and in which there are no palpable suspicious inguinal lymph nodes. The treatment of Stage II carcinoma of the vulva is radical vulvectomy and bilateral inguinal lymphadenectomy. There are three basic surgical approaches. The so-called butterfly incision removes the skin over the mons from the level of the iliac crest, the vulva, and a wedge of skin over the inguinal dissection. An alternative to this is to mobilize a skin flap over the inguinal dissection without excision of this skin. Finally, some authors have advocated separate groin incisions for the inguinal dissections coupled with a radical excision of the vulva. The incidence of local recurrence is similar in each type, and the choice of incision is primarily a matter of preference. Although some authors still recommend routine performance of pelvic lymphadenectomy as part of this operation,[54] most surgeons who perform pelvic lymphadenectomy do so only if the inguinal lymph nodes are positive. Green[16] found no patients with pelvic nodal metastases in patients with negative inguinal nodes. Recently, the GOG completed a randomized trial of pelvic irradiation or pelvic lymphadenectomy in patients with positive inguinal nodes and demonstrated statistically significant improved survival and no increased morbidity in the group receiving pelvic irradiation.[55] They have since begun a randomized trial of pelvic and inguinal irradiation versus inguinal lymphadenectomy in patients with Stages I and II vulvar cancer.

STAGES III AND IV CARCINOMA OF THE VULVA

Stage III vulvar carcinoma is a tumor of any size with spread to the urethra, vagina, or anus, or with clinically suspicious nodes in the inguinal area. In these patients, radical vulvectomy often requires removal of a portion of the distal urethra or vagina and may require excision of a portion of the anus. Exenteration is rarely required. Based on the GOG study cited earlier, these patients should undergo postoperative pelvic irradiation if the inguinal lymph nodes contain cancer.

Stage IV vulvar cancer involves the upper one third of the urethra or involves the bladder or rectum. Patients will also be considered Stage IV if they have fixed inguinal lymph nodes, fixation of tumor to bone, or distant metastases. Treatment of tumors involving the bladder or upper urethra is best managed by the addition of anterior exenteration to the radical vulvectomy and inguinal node dissections. Posterior exenteration is used when the lesion involves the rectum. When the tumor is fixed to bone or there are distant metastases, treatment is usually palliative and consists of combinations of irradiation and chemotherapy.

MALIGNANT MELANOMA OF THE VULVA

Chung et al[38] found no lymph node metastases in patients with Clark's level I or II malignant melanoma. Positive lymph nodes were present in deeper levels. Current recommendations for treatment are radical vulvectomy and bilateral inguinal node dissection for levels of invasion greater than Clark's level II and wide local excision for Clark's level I and II. Some authorities recommend wide local excision and ipsilateral inguinal node dissection for all cases of vulvar melanoma. The GOG is prospectively evaluating wide local excision and inguinal lymphadenectomy for all cases of vulvar melanoma.

BARTHOLIN'S GLAND CARCINOMA

Bartholin's gland carcinoma is managed by radical vulvectomy and bilateral inguinal node dissection. Resection of the local tumor must be extensive because of its deep location. Although some authors recommend pelvic node dissection in all Bartholin's gland carcinoma, current evidence would suggest that pelvic irradiation may be an acceptable treatment option. Adenoid cystic carcinoma of the Bartholin's gland usually requires only wide local excision because lymph node metastases are rare.

OTHER VULVAR TUMORS

Basal cell carcinoma and verrucous carcinoma are managed by wide local excision. Lymph node dissection is not indicated in these patients. Metastatic tumors of the vulva should usually be excised, if possible, to control local symptoms. Further treatment will depend on the site of the primary cancer. All soft tissue sarcomas should be locally excised, if possible. After excision, treatment should include combinations of systemic chemotherapy and local and regional irradiation.

SURGICAL TREATMENT OF VULVAR CARCINOMA

Radical vulvectomy was first described in 1912 by Basset.[56] The classical operation as practiced until the mid-1960s included both bilateral inguinal and pelvic lymph node dissection. In the middle to late 1960s, many surgeons began to perform pelvic lymph node dissections only if the inguinal lymph nodes contained metastatic cancer. The validity of this approach has been clearly documented by several authors who have shown that pelvic node metastases rarely occur in patients with negative inguinal lymph nodes.[57–59] Additionally, the literature indicates that survival in patients with positive pelvic lymph nodes is very poor.

For many years, most surgeons utilized some form of en bloc dissection of the vulva and inguinal lymph nodes with

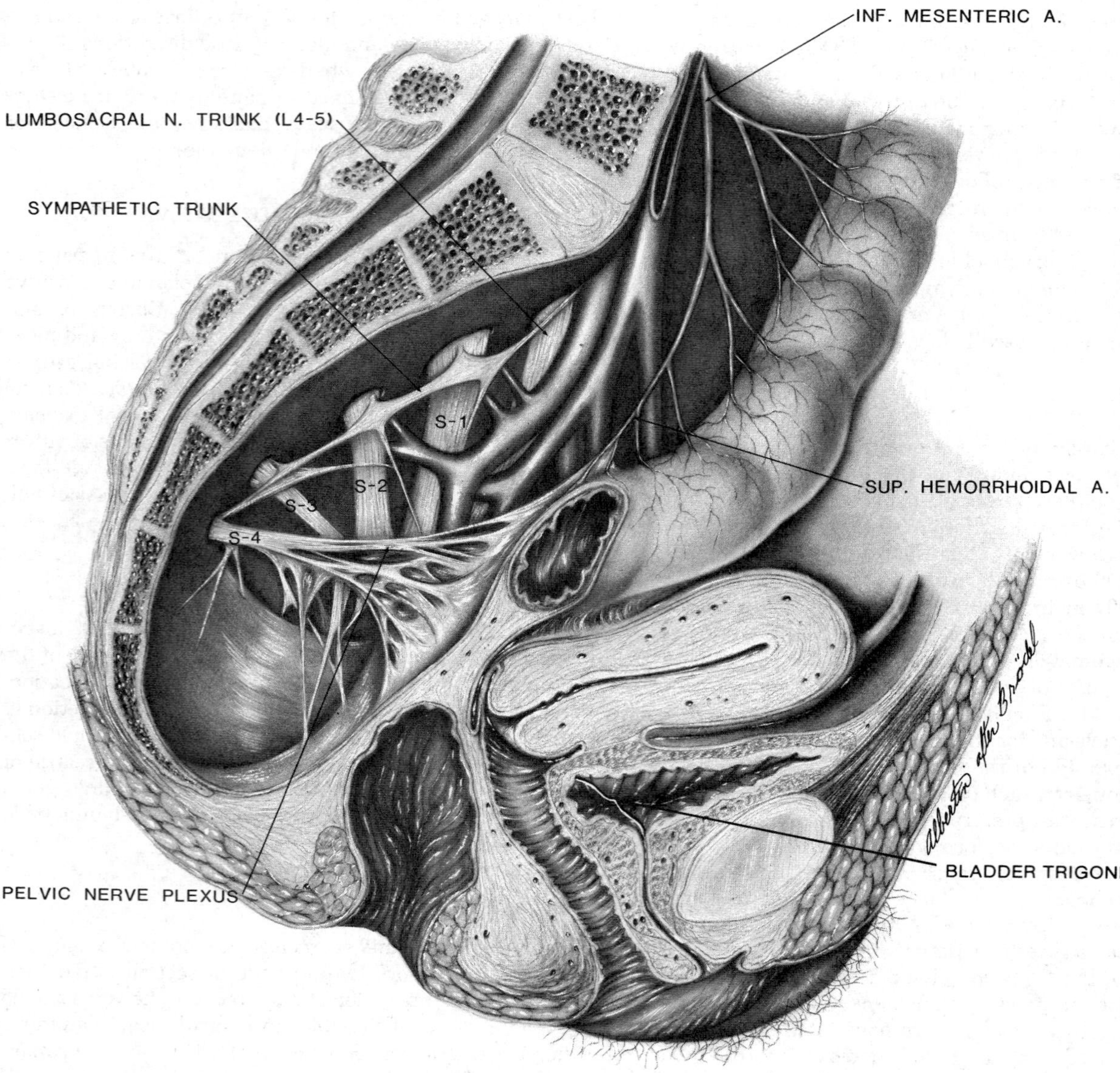

FIG. 36-1**A**. Sagittal view of female pelvis, including relationships of pelvic viscera, vasculature, and nerve plexuses. (*Figure continues on facing page.*)

the overlying skin as illustrated in Figure 36-1C. In recent years, many surgeons have used separate inguinal incisions without removal of the skin overlying the nodal areas. When combined with a radical vulvectomy, this procedure leaves a "bridge" of skin between the vulvectomy and the inguinal incision. Hacker et al[60] reviewed 100 cases and reported no recurrence of tumor in this skin bridge; they found a 14% incidence of wound breakdown compared to more than 40% wound breakdown in patients managed by a classical type of en bloc dissection. Figure 36-1D illustrates the lines of incision for a radical vulvectomy with separate inguinal incisions.

The necessity of performing a bilateral inguinal lymph node dissection in all patients was first questioned by Morris in 1977.[61] A review of Way's total experience indicates that only 5% of patients with negative ipsilateral inguinal lymph nodes had contralateral nodal involvement.[62] Recent prospective series by the GOG also indicate a low incidence of contralateral positive lymph nodes in patients with negative ipsilateral nodes.[63]

Iversen et al[64] have recommended hemivulvectomy and ipsilateral inguinal dissection for lesions of less than 1 cm with no vascular invasion and the GOG is currently evaluating hemivulvectomy for lesions of less than 2 cm with invasion of less than 5 mm. Figure 36-1E illustrates this procedure. Although there is currently no consensus about the necessary radicality of the approach to vulvar cancer, it is apparent that many investigators are questioning the uniform practice of the classical radical vulvectomy and bilateral inguinal node dissection. Further investigations into the results of less radical approaches are necessary before definite recommendations can be made.

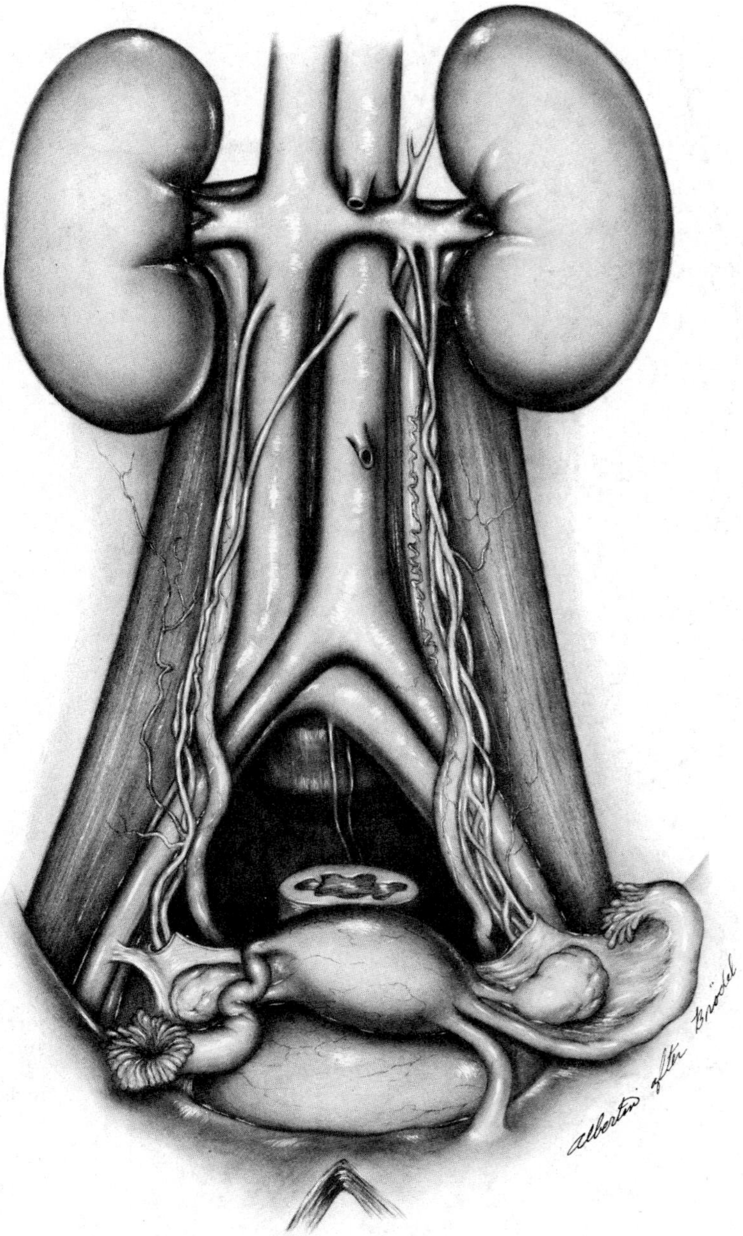

FIG. 36-1**B**. Abdominal and pelvic anatomy of the female reproductive tract. (*Figure continues on next page.*)

The major surgical complication associated with radical vulvectomy is wound breakdown with rates of 30% to 80% depending on the definition used. The use of perioperative antibiotics, separate inguinal incisions, and careful attention to a lack of tension on the wound edges will help minimize this complication. The formation of lymphocysts and chronic lymphedema can be minimized by use of suction drains but still remains a significant problem in patients who undergo surgical therapy of vulvar carcinoma. Catastrophic hemorrhage from the denuded femoral vessels is a rare complication if the sartorius muscle is transposed to cover the inguinal dissection. Introital stenosis can be minimized by use of skin flaps and avoidance of excessive tension at the time of closure of the surgical incision.

Despite better patient and physician education, one occasionally sees patients with vulvar cancers that involve the rectum or bladder. In such cases, anterior or posterior exenteration must be combined with radical vulvectomy and inguinal node dissection. It is possible that continued development of radiation therapy techniques will make possible combined therapy that can spare these organs.

RADIATION THERAPY IN VULVAR CANCER

The role of radiotherapy in the management of carcinoma of the vulva remains a controversial issue, primarily because of the lack of data on the results of treatment with modern techniques. The traditional belief that vulvar tissues cannot tolerate therapeutic doses of radiation has limited the role of

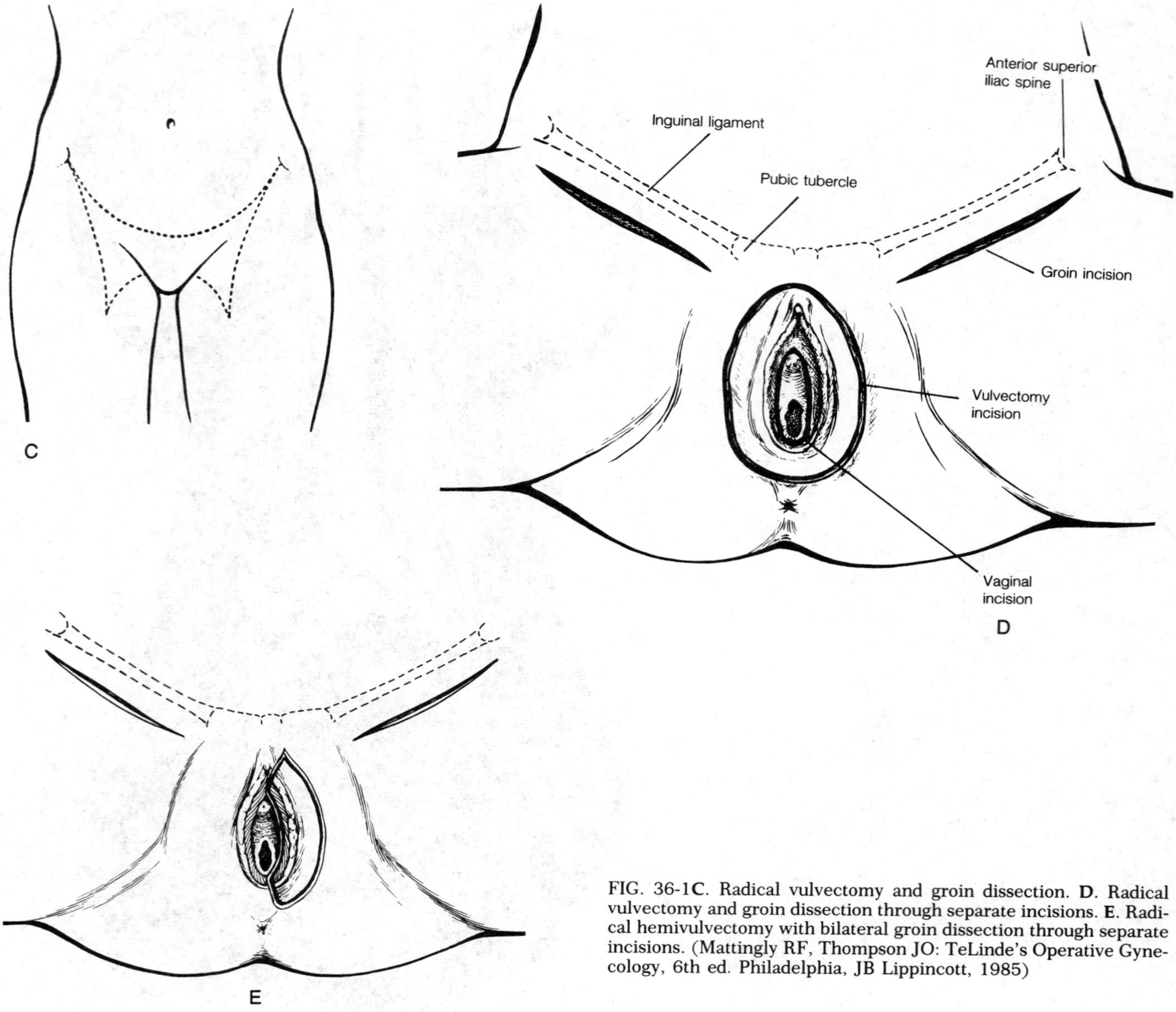

FIG. 36-1**C**. Radical vulvectomy and groin dissection. **D**. Radical vulvectomy and groin dissection through separate incisions. **E**. Radical hemivulvectomy with bilateral groin dissection through separate incisions. (Mattingly RF, Thompson JO: TeLinde's Operative Gynecology, 6th ed. Philadelphia, JB Lippincott, 1985)

radiotherapy to palliation or for treatment of patients who are not amenable to surgical resection.

Radiation Therapy Techniques for the Primary Site (Vulva)

In patients who are not candidates for surgical resection, the primary tumor site needs to be irradiated to the customary tumoricidal dose of approximately 7000 cGy in 35 to 40 treatments. Very small lesions may be controlled with somewhat lower doses (6000–6500 cGy). It is important to use a daily fraction size of 180 cGy or less. Usually, parallel opposed AP-PA portals are used, preferentially loaded anteriorly (or using a high energy single anterior beam), that cover the vulva and the regional lymphatics. An electron beam or low energy photon beam supplement aimed directly at the vulva is needed at the end of the course to bring doses to full tumoricidal level. An implant may also be considered as a means of providing a boost to the primary tumor site. Use of appropriate bolus material over the areas of the skin (vulva) at risk for tumor involvement is essential. Interruption of the course is often necessary in the third or fourth week of treatment to prevent severe moist desquamation and maceration of tissues.

Radiation Therapy Techniques for the Regional Lymphatics

In patients with no clinical indications of regional lymphatic involvement, the inguinal lymph nodes are treated electively (prophylactically) to a dose of 5000 cGy (180–200 cGy per day). Depending on the available equipment, either an anteroposterior beam or a differentially loaded parallel opposed beam or an electron beam (for part of the treatment) can be used. Care should be taken to deliver adequate doses not only to the superficial inguinal nodes but also to the femoral nodes and the first echelon of deep pelvic nodes (Figs. 36-1 and 36-2).

In patients with findings indicative of regional lymph node involvement, the doses to the involved lymph nodes need to be in the range of 6500 to 7000 cGy, depending on the size of the involved nodes. In patients with evidence of involvement of the inguinal lymph nodes, the pelvis should be treated with prophylactic irradiation of 4500 to 5000 cGy. In patients with evidence of spread to the pelvic nodes, these fields may be boosted to 5500 to 6000 cGy (Fig. 36-3). Because some of the patients with involved pelvic lymph nodes remain curable, irradiation of the lower para-aortic chain in the presence of pelvic lymph node involvement might be appropriate.

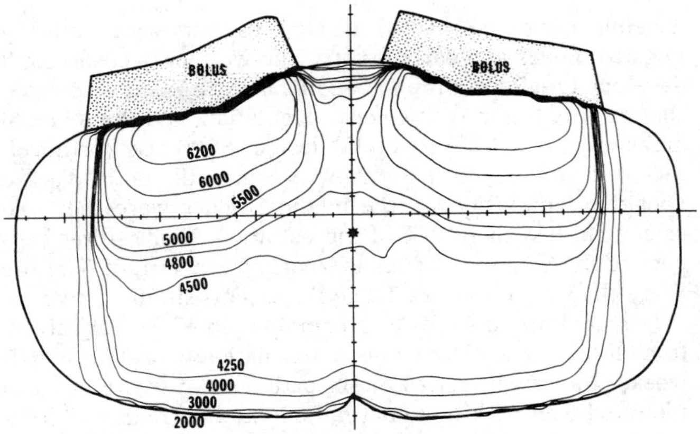

FIG. 36-3. Representative treatment plans for irradiation of regional lymphatics. Parallel opposed 18 MV photon beams are preferentially loaded anteriorly (2700 cGy anteriorly, 1800 cGy posteriorly), and a bolus is added over the inguinal areas to improve dose distribution in subcutaneous tissues in that area. A boost of 1500 cGy using 16 MeV electrons (without bolus) is added to the groin. (Pilepich MV: Carcinoma of the vulva. In Perez CA, Brady LW [eds]: Principles and Practice of Radiation Oncology, pp 1036–1043. Philadelphia, JB Lippincott, 1987)

Postoperative Radiotherapy

Radiotherapy is used increasingly in combination with surgery. In patients who have undergone a resection of the primary lesion and are considered at high risk for recurrence because of inadequate resection margins, postoperative irradiation is well indicated and should consist of at least 4500 cGy, preferably 5000 cGy, (175–200 cGy per day). If the resection margins are clearly involved or there is known gross residual tumor, higher doses of irradiation (6000–7000 cGy) are required.

FIG. 36-2. Set-up for patients with positive inguinal lymph nodes. The entire pelvis is treated to a dose of 4500 to 5000 cGy. This is followed by a boost to the inguinal-femoral areas and distal iliac chain to bring the total dose to that area to 5500 to 6000 cGy and a final boost to the positive inguinal lymph nodes consisting of 500 to 1000 cGy, bringing the total dose to that area to approximately 6500 cGy (calculated at 3–4 cm). (Pilepich MV: Carcinoma of the vulva. In Perez CA, Brady LW [eds]: Principles and Practice of Radiation Oncology, pp 1036–1043. Philadelphia, JB Lippincott, 1987)

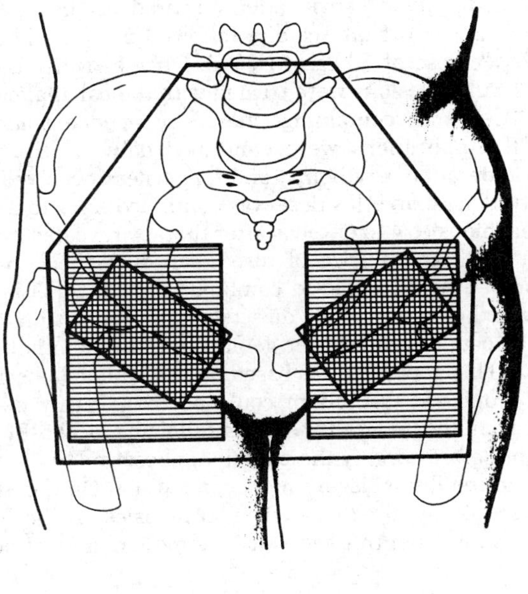

Preoperative Radiotherapy

Patients with advanced primary lesions involving surrounding structures that are either of questionable resectability or are clearly unresectable can be treated with preoperative intent. By delivering moderately high doses of 4500 to 5500 cGy preoperatively, one can expect an increase in the resectability rate and also avoid mutilating procedures such as exenteration.

Irradiation of Recurrent Lesions

Recurrences following surgical resection remain potentially curable and need to be treated aggressively in the manner described above, with doses in the range of 6500 to 7000 cGy, and daily fractions of 180 cGy.

RESULTS OF RADIATION THERAPY IN VULVAR CANCER

There have been numerous attempts to combine radiotherapy and surgery in order to improve the therapeutic results.[65–72] Frankendal et al[65] reported on 55 patients of whom 22 had palpable lymph nodes considered tumerous; in 19 of these there was histologic confirmation of nodal involvement. Primary lesions were either electrocoagulated, resected, or irradiated. The regional nodes were dissected if clinically involved. Clinically negative nodes were observed without treatment unless the primary tumor was quite large or poorly differentiated. In such a situation, the groins were irradiated to a dose of 3000 to 6000 cGy in 15 to 55 days. Of the 12 patients who were irradiated prophylactically to the inguinal areas because of unfavorable primary lesions, none developed inguinal metastasis. Of 7 patients with clinically negative nodes and early lesions who were only observed, 3 developed regional lymph node metastases. Kucera[71] treated the primary lesion with electrocoagulation, and the inguinal areas were irradiated to a total dose of 6000 cGy (orthovoltage or cobalt-60). In patients with Stages III and IV disease (positive lymph nodes), the inguinal nodes were then dissected (in less than 20% of the patients). Eighty-three percent of the Stage I patients, 69% of the Stage II, 58% of the Stage III, and 10% of the Stage IV patients survived 5 years.

Daly and Million[69] tested a combination of radical vulvectomy followed by elective nodal irradiation to 4500 cGy in 5 weeks. In a small series of six patients the treatment was tolerated well with no nodal failures and no radiation complications. No delay in healing of the surgical site was recorded. Homesley et al[55] reported on 114 patients with invasive carcinoma of the vulva and positive inguinal nodes randomized (after radical vulvectomy and bilateral groin lymphadenectomy) to receive postoperative radiation therapy to the pelvic and groin lymph nodes (4500–5000 cGy in 5–6 weeks). The irradiated patients had a recurrence rate of 32.3% and a 68% 2-year survival rate in contrast to a recurrence rate of 45.5% and a 2-year survival rate of 54% in the nonirradiated group. The incidence of recurrence at the primary site was similar in both groups (8.5% in the irradiated and 9.1% in the pelvic lymph node dissection groups). Surgical morbidity and late side effects of irradiation and surgery were similar in both groups.

The rationale for a combination of radiotherapy and conservative surgery in advanced tumors that would ordinarily require exenteration has been discussed by Boronow.[68] In a series of nine cases, only one local recurrence was observed. The incidence of operative morbidity was minimal, and five patients remained disease-free for a period ranging from 11 months to 4.5 years. This experience has recently been updated,[67] indicating a 75% to 80% 5-year salvage probability in advanced primary and recurrent cancer. Hacker et al[70] treated eight patients with locally advanced vulvar cancer, who would ordinarily require an exenteration, with 4400 to 5400 cGy prior to resection (vulvectomy). Significant tumor regression was observed in seven and there was no viable tumor in the surgical specimen in four patients. Five of eight patients (62.5%) remained alive without evidence of disease from 15 months to 10 years.

Pao et al[74] reported the results on 40 patients with histologically confirmed primary or recurrent vulvar carcinoma treated with radiation therapy for locoregional disease at Washington University Medical Center. Nineteen of the patients with primary tumors received postoperative radiotherapy (5000 cGy in 6 weeks) after wide local excision or simple vulvectomy (9 patients) or radical vulvectomy (10 patients). Fifteen of the 19 exhibited local tumor control. Five patients with Stage III or IV disease were managed with radiotherapy alone. Four had a complete response with two currently with no evidence of disease (NED). Two patients who received preoperative radiotherapy with local excision are also currently free of disease. The 4-year NED survival rate for the study population is 100%, 28%, 50%, 0% and 10% for Stages I, II, III, IV and recurrent tumors, respectively. The poor results obtained in Stage II tumors are probably due to selection because 4 of 7 patients developed distant metastases. Two of 14 patients treated for recurrent disease remain NED after local excision of their tumors and irradiation. No dose response for subclinical disease could be found between 4500 and 7000 cGy. Treatment morbidity was acceptable with 2 patients developing severe long-term complications requiring surgical intervention.

The wide range of techniques, doses, and fractionation patterns makes it difficult to evaluate accurately the side effects of radiotherapy using modern techniques and treatment schemes. When dealing with a tumor at the skin or mucosal surface, which requires that the peak dose be at the surface, it is to be expected that all patients will have a significant acute (cutaneous and mucosal) irritation. Of more concern, however, is the incidence of late sequelae, some of which can be attributed to the fractionation schemes. Schulz et al,[75] for example, reported a very high incidence in patients who were treated with 500 cGy fractions. The complication rate has been consistently low in patients who were treated with the conventional 200 cGy per day or similar fractionation schemes. Prospective, large scale, multidimensional studies are needed to define the optimal indications for radiotherapy in vulvar carcinoma and its efficacy using modern techniques.

CHEMOTHERAPY OF CARCINOMA OF THE VULVA

Topical chemotherapy has been used for treatment of selected patients with vulvar or vaginal intraepithelial neoplasia. Topical 5-fluorouracil (5-FU) has been the most commonly used agent.[76] Often, three 7-day courses of 5% 5-FU cream are given 2 weeks apart. A study of 27 patients treated in this manner demonstrated that although 3 patients required retreatment at 3, 9, and 11 months, all 25 evaluable patients were free of disease for 3+ to 40+ months after treatment.[77]

Foster and Woodruff[73] treated six patients with histologically documented atypical vulvar dystrophy with topical dinitrochlorobenzene (DNCB) after surgery and topical 5-FU had failed. Contact sensitization was produced using 2000 μg of DNCB per 0.1 ml acetone followed 2 weeks later by a challenge dose of 50 μg of DNCB. Once sensitized, the patients' vulvar lesions were treated with topical application of DNCB cream containing increasing concentrations of DNCB. Applications were continued daily by the patient until induration, erythema, and tenderness occurred in the involved area, and this dose was continued for 1 to 2 weeks. Repeat biopsies 4 to 6 weeks after therapy revealed improvement or disappearance of disease in 5 of the 6 patients. Stillman et al[78] have used combined topical 5-FU pretreatment and colposcopically directed surgical excision to manage 16 patients with lower genital tract intraepithelial neoplasia. This approach was based on the authors' observation that neoplastic epithelium could be more easily dissected away from the underlying stroma following local 5-FU application. Before surgery the patient applies 4 ml of 5% topical 5-FU to the lesions every night for 1 week. On the 8th day, colposcopically directed excisional biopsies are performed. All 16 patients in this series had remission, and, although 2 have required retreatment, no patient has had a recurrence of severe dysplasia.

Levin et al[79] have used preoperative chemotherapy (mitomycin C and 5-FU) followed by pelvic irradiation prior to surgery for advanced carcinoma of the vulva. On day 1, mitomycin C (10 mg/m^2) is given intravenously followed 30 minutes later by a 24-hour infusion of 5-FU (1000 mg/m^2). 5-FU is repeated for 3 additional days at a similar dose and schedule followed by 10 days of equal fractions of radiation therapy. Courses of chemotherapy and radiation therapy last 2 weeks. Once adequate response was achieved (usually 1–2 cycles), surgery was performed. The researchers observed marked local tumor shrinkage in six patients that allowed more definitive surgery following the chemotherapy.

FUTURE CONSIDERATIONS IN CARCINOMA OF THE VULVA

Future studies in vulvar cancer should be directed toward defining microinvasive carcinoma and continuing the search for methods to reduce the radicality of the surgical therapy. Further investigations of plastic surgical reconstruction of the vulva should be directed at restoring normal anatomy and function, especially for the young patient.[80,81]

If the ongoing GOG study shows inguinal and pelvic irradiation to be as good as or better than bilateral inguinal node dissection, attention should next be turned to combining local excision with vulvar irradiation in an attempt to improve functional and cosmetic results.

From our limited experience as well as the reports in the literature, it is possible that radiation therapy may play a significant role in the management of patients with carcinoma of the vulva:

1. Radical vulvectomy could, in selected patients (those with tumors less than 2 cm and clinically negative nodes), be replaced by a wide local excision of the tumor to be followed by irradiation of the vulvar region as well as elective irradiation of the regional lymphatics in patients with clinically negative inguinal-femoral lymph nodes (5000 cGy). The margins of the primary tumor specimen should be microscopically negative (no residual tumor).
2. In patients with lesions smaller than 2 cm and clinically positive regional lymph nodes, the primary tumor could be removed by wide local excision, a superficial inguinal lymph node dissection carried out, and postoperative irradiation delivered (5000 cGy to the primary tumor area and 6000 cGy to the inguinal-femoral and pelvic lymph nodes).
3. Patients on whom a radical vulvectomy is carried out when the surgical margins at the primary site are negative and the regional lymph nodes have no evidence of metastatic tumor should not require postoperative radiation therapy. However, in patients with positive lymph nodes, postoperative irradiation has been shown to improve the probability of tumor control and survival. Frankendal et al[65] reported on 19 of 55 patients on whom there was histologic evidence of lymph node metastases and who received postoperative radiation therapy (3000–6000 cGy in 15–55 days). Of 12 patients given elective irradiation because of unfavorable primary tumors, none developed inguinal lymph node recurrences. Seven patients who were observed developed regional lymph node metastases.
4. In patients with advanced inoperable carcinoma of the vulva, radiation therapy combined with chemotherapy (cisplatin and 5-FU) is beginning to be used with encouraging preliminary results.[82] Continued research into combinations of chemotherapy and irradiation may make even large tumors curable.

None of these approaches to therapy of vulvar cancer have been widely used, and careful, prospective trials of patients treated by these methods are necessary. The prospect of irradiation playing a major role in the management of carcinoma of the vulva is very promising.

CARCINOMA OF THE VAGINA

Carcinoma of the vagina is defined as a primary carcinoma arising in the vagina that does not involve the cervix or vulva. As a primary carcinoma, it is not a common cancer and accounts for about 2% of all gynecologic cancers.[83–85] The most common carcinomas of the vagina are actually tumors that involve the vagina by direct extension or are metastases from other genital areas, particularly the cervix. The vagina is also frequently involved by tumors of the rectum. With the exception of diethylstilbestrol (DES)-related clear cell carcinomas, primary carcinomas of the vagina are squamous cell cancers. Primary sarcomas occur but are rare.

EPIDEMIOLOGY

The median age for patients with carcinoma in situ of the vagina is the early fifth decade,[86–88] whereas the median age for patients with invasive cancer is the mid-sixth decade.[83–85,89] One percent to 3% of patients who develop squamous carcinoma of the vagina will have had squamous neoplasia of the cervix.[87] Hummer et al[88] reported that carcinoma in situ of the vagina followed carcinoma in situ of the cervix within up to 17 years, but that one third of the cases were diagnosed within 2 years. Prior radiation therapy may be a predisposing factor in primary vaginal carcinoma.[83,89,90] Pride et al[89] noted that 9 of 43 patients (20.9%) with invasive cancer of the vagina had a history of radiation therapy. The interval from previous irradiation to development of the primary squamous cancer was 7 to 20 years. Other authors[83,90] have noted intervals from 10 to 15 years.

In 1971 Herbst et al[91] related an increase in the number of clear cell carcinomas of the vagina to maternal ingestion of DES during pregnancy. The youngest DES exposed patient to develop clear cell adenocarcinoma was 7 years old and the peak incidence occurred at age 19.[92,93] The actual risk of an exposed female developing clear cell adenocarcinoma is 0.14 to 1.4 per 1,000 through age 24.[92] A plateau of cases was reached in the mid-1970s with a gradual decline in the number of cases each year since that time. It is not known whether these women will be at risk for the development of other cancers of the genital tract as they become older.

Primary sarcomas of the vagina account for about 2% of all vaginal cancer.[94,95] Leiomyosarcoma is the most frequent, but reticulum cell and stromal sarcomas have been reported. Age at diagnosis is in the fifth and sixth decades.[94] Sarcoma botryoides, although rare, is the most common tumor of the genital tract in female children.[96] The mean age for the appearance of these tumors is between 2 and 3 years.

Malignant melanomas occur in the vagina infrequently as a primary neoplasm. As in other parts of the genital tract, they spread locally by direct extension as well as by lymphatics and via the bloodstream.[97,98]

NATURAL HISTORY AND PATTERNS OF SPREAD

The location of primary vaginal carcinoma was evaluated in an extensive literature review of more than 1,200 cases by Plentl and Friedman.[85] They found that 26.9% occurred on the anterior wall, 57.2% on the posterior wall, and 15.9% on the lateral walls. Of 743 cases reviewed for axial location, they found that 50.7% occurred in the upper third of the vagina, 18.8% in the middle third, and 30.4% in the lower third. Clear cell adenocarcinomas of the vagina associated with maternal DES ingestion occur more commonly on the anterior vagina and are more frequently seen in the upper third of the vaginal canal.

Vaginal carcinomas spread to adjacent structures by direct extension or via lymphatics. By convention, tumors that involve the cervix or vulva are considered as primary in those sites because they are more common. The proximity of the urethra, bladder, and rectum results in early involvement of those structures and has a major effect on treatment planning. When spreading laterally, the tumor may invade the paracolpial, parametrial, and pararectal tissues, with extension to the pelvic side walls.

The lymphatic drainage of the vagina begins with the fine capillary meshwork in the mucosa and submucosa.[85] Both of these systems flow into collecting trunks near the lateral aspect of the vagina. The ventral portion of the vagina drains primarily to lateral pelvic lymph nodes while the posterior portion drains into the rectal and para-aortic lymph nodes. There is significant overlap in these patterns of drainage. The upper third of the vagina drains primarily like the cervix, whereas the middle third tends to spread both into the pelvic nodes and into the inferior gluteal nodes in the area of the ischial spine. The lower third of the vagina drains laterally, posteriorly, and to the femoral nodes.

In addition to the above distribution of lymphatics, there is a rich interconnection between the lymphatics of the vagina and those of the bladder and rectum. In their review of the literature, Plentl and Friedman[85] reported an overall positive node rate of 20.8% for vaginal carcinoma. These results were obtained both from surgical series and autopsy reports. Patients with clear cell carcinoma have distant spread (supraclavicular nodes or lungs) more frequently than would be expected for a similar group of patients with squamous cell carcinoma of the vagina or cervix.[93]

Pathology

Squamous carcinomas of the vagina may appear grossly as either ulcerated and endophytic tumors or they may be exophytic and protrude into the vaginal canal. Microscopically, they are epidermoid carcinomas with pleomorphic squamous cells that display a lack of organization and loss of cellular cohesion.[99] The lesions may exhibit patterns of dysplasia, carcinoma in situ, and invasion. Premalignant lesions may be multifocal.

Most clear cell adenocarcinomas of the vagina are polyploid or nodular with a reddish color. Some, however, are flat with a granular surface. Microscopically, three histologic patterns have been described: a tubulocystic pattern, a solid pattern, and a papillary pattern.[100]

Leiomyosarcoma of the vagina has a similar gross and microscopic appearance to leiomyosarcoma of other sites. Tavassoli and Norris[101] reviewed smooth muscle tumors of the vagina and concluded that tumors with moderate to marked atypia and greater than 5 mitoses per 10 high power fields should be considered leiomyosarcomas. The sarcoma botyroides of infancy is characterized by friable polypoid growths that appear like a bunch of grapes. Microscopically, these tumors comprise poorly differentiated spindle cells and a myxoid stroma and tend to grow around blood vessels.[99]

CLINICAL PRESENTATION, DIAGNOSIS, AND STAGING

Preinvasive lesions of the vagina are asymptomatic, and diagnosis is usually made during the evaluation of an abnormal Pap smear. Examination of the vagina by colposcopy should be conducted in all patients with abnormal cytology, even if there is a lesion of the cervix that appears to explain the cytology. Although not totally painless, vaginal biopsies do not usually require local anesthesia. A skin hook used to tent up the vaginal mucosa and stabilize it is often helpful in obtaining an adequate biopsy.

Abnormal vaginal bleeding is the most common symptom of invasive vaginal carcinoma.[94,102] The bleeding is often postmenopausal because that is the most common age group to develop the disease, but may also be postcoital or, in younger patients, intermenstrual. Vaginal discharge is also common. Pain or symptoms referable to the bladder or rectum usually occur with more advanced disease.[103] Brady[104] has reported that the average duration of symptoms before diagnosis is up to 7.4 months.

Detection of invasive vaginal carcinoma is made by inspection, palpation, and biopsy. In performing a speculum examination, it is important to either rotate the speculum or remove it slowly so as to visualize the entire vagina. Lesions arising on the posterior vaginal wall are particularly likely to be missed because they can be obscured by the posterior blade of the speculum. Any lesions noted during examination should be biopsied. Wharton et al[102] published data from M.D. Anderson Hospital that showed that 67.5% of patients seen at that institution had lesions larger than 2 cm when initial diagnosis was made.

The staging workup of the patient with vaginal cancer includes careful inspection of the vagina and cervix with biopsies as needed and a careful bimanual examination. Chest radiograph, biochemical profile, intravenous pyelogram, barium enema, cystoscopy, and proctoscopy are necessary. CT, MRI, and lymphangiography may be helpful in

TABLE 36-4. International Federation of Gynecology and Obstetrics Classification for Carcinoma of the Vagina

Stage 0	Carcinoma in situ: intraepithelial carcinoma
Stage I	Carcinoma limited to the vaginal wall
Stage II	Carcinoma has invaded the subvaginal tissue but has not extended to the pelvic wall
Stage III	Carcinoma has extended to the pelvic wall
Stage IV	Carcinoma has extended beyond the true pelvis or has involved the mucosa of the bladder or rectum. Bullous edema as such does not permit a case to be alloted to Stage IV
Stage IVA	Spread of the growth to adjacent organs
Stage IVB	Spread to distant organs

certain situations. The FIGO classification of vaginal carcinoma is listed in Table 36-4.

TREATMENT OF VAGINAL CANCER

The anatomical position of the vagina, lying between the urethra and bladder anteriorly and the rectum posteriorly, has been the predominant factor in treatment planning. The vaginal tube is thin walled, and the thickness of the vesicovaginal and rectovaginal septa is usually measured in millimeters.

Surgical extirpation of carcinoma of the vagina is often not feasible because the proximity of the bladder and rectum requires exenterative procedures to achieve adequate surgical margins. Therefore, with the exception of clear cell adenocarcinoma of the vagina occurring in young women and localized to the upper third of the vaginal canal, the primary treatment of vaginal carcinoma, especially squamous cell carcinoma, has been radiotherapy. Chau[105] pointed out the complexity of management of these patients and the need for careful radiotherapeutic techniques, which has resulted in survival similar to that for carcinoma of the uterine cervix. Perez et al[106] suggested that a correlation can be drawn between the doses of irradiation given to various tumor stages and the probability of local tumor control.

Carcinoma in situ

A wide range of therapeutic options are available for carcinoma in situ of the vagina and the choice of the correct option depends on the location of the lesion, the size of the lesion, and whether it is a single focus or multiple foci. Local excision is ideal therapy for patients with either single lesions or several lesions located in a single portion of the vagina, especially patients who develop recurrence in the vaginal cuff following hysterectomy. Total vaginectomy, on the other hand, is a difficult procedure and requires split thickness grafts for repair. Multiple lesions may often be treated in stages, with multiple excisions and primary closure. Cryotherapy has limited usefulness in the treatment of vaginal carcinoma in situ as it usually must be performed under anesthesia, requires multiple applications, and can easily damage the urethra, bladder, or rectum because of the difficulty in controlling the depth of the freeze. CO_2 laser has become very popular recently and has the advantage of being able to be tailored to rather exact depth and extent of disease. Further studies with long-term follow-up are needed to define the extent of its usefulness in this disease. Woodruff et al[107] reported the use of topical 5-FU in preinvasive vaginal carcinoma and noted complete eradication of lesions in 8 of 9 patients. Townsend[108] recommends 5 g of 5-FU cream instilled in the vagina every night for 5 days. He repeats these courses of therapy every 6 to 12 weeks until eradication of the lesion is documented. Contamination of the vulva must be prevented because 5-FU cream can produce an intense chemical reaction on the vulva. Radiation therapy of carcinoma in situ is rarely indicated; however, in selected cases in which the patient is a poor operative risk, irradiation of the vagina has been reported to afford excellent cure rates using intracavitary and interstitial sources alone.[109,110] Radiation therapy may also be considered in cases in which extensive surgical resection is necessary because of multifocal involvement of the entire vagina.

Stage I

Stage I lesions of the vagina that are located in the upper one third of the vagina can be managed by either radical hysterectomy, partial vaginectomy and pelvic lymphadenectomy, or standard radiotherapy. Some authors[110–113] have recommended a surgical approach in most of these cases. Lesions of the middle or lower vagina, unless they are very superficial and do not lie in the rectovaginal or vesicovaginal septa, often require either anterior or posterior exenteration for primary surgical therapy. Frick et al[111] have considered low and middle vaginal posterior lesions similar to rectal carcinoma and thus justified posterior exenteration as a logical choice of therapy. Although there is little doubt that individualization of therapy may often be best for any given patient, the difficulties encountered in surgical therapy of vaginal carcinoma because of the proximity of the bladder and rectum have resulted in most of these cancers being managed by irradiation. Irradiation appears to allow considerably more flexibility than does surgery, and good functional results are obtained with adequate radiation therapy. Surgical procedures may be reserved for the treatment of irradiation failures.

Brown et al[109] and Perez and Camel[110] have reported excellent tumor control and survival in patients with Stage I vaginal carcinoma. These authors have cautioned against an overly aggressive therapy in these early lesions because of the possibility of producing mucosal injury and interference with sexual function. Most patients with Stage I superficial tumors can be treated adequately with intracavitary and interstitial sources alone. If the carcinoma is less than 0.5 cm thick, intracavitary irradiation with a vaginal cylinder to deliver 8000 cGy to the mucosa will yield excellent results (over 90% tumor control). If the lesion is thicker or localized to one of the walls of the vagina, the addition of an interstitial single plane implant will deliver an adequate dose of irradiation to the tumor, limiting the exposure to the uninvolved normal tissues.

In patients with more extensive Stage I lesions, external irradiation should be administered to treat the paravaginal tissues and the regional lymph nodes, in addition to intracavitary and interstitial therapy.

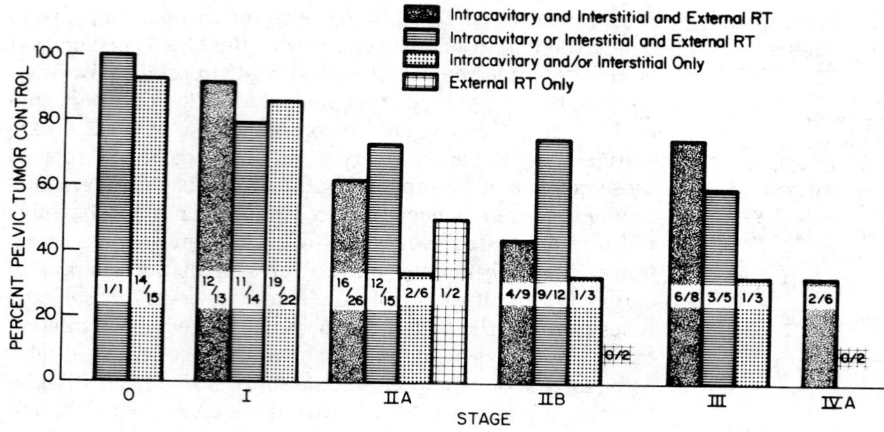

FIG. 36-4. Tumor control in the vagina and the pelvis (MIR 1950–1984) as a function of the type of treatment used and the anatomical stage of the disease. In patients with tumor beyond Stage I there is a critical need for the addition of external beam irradiation in order to improve tumor control. (Perez CA, Camel HM, Galakatos AE, et al: Definitive irradiation in carcinoma of the vagina. Long-term evaluation. Personal communication, 1987)

Stage II

Patients with Stage II carcinoma of the vagina require a more comprehensive approach that should include external beam irradiation and brachytherapy. Better survival has been observed by Perez et al[106] in Stage II carcinomas with the addition of external irradiation in comparison to brachytherapy alone (Fig. 36-4). They reported 65% survival with brachytherapy plus external irradiation and 40% survival with brachytherapy alone. In general, doses of 2000 cGy to the whole pelvis are delivered followed by a supplemental dose (3000 cGy) to the parametria with a midline shielding block. This is combined with interstitial and intracavitary therapy to deliver a minimum of 6500 to 7000 cGy to the base of the tumor and 5000 cGy to the pelvic lymph nodes.

Stages III and IV

In the more advanced lesions (Stages III and IVA) the results with irradiation have been less than satisfactory, with only 25% to 30% pelvic tumor control and survival. Therefore, higher irradiation doses with a greater contribution from the external irradiation are used. Table 36-5 summarizes the results in 165 patients with carcinoma of the vagina treated at the Mallinckrodt Institute of Radiology, Washington University School of Medicine Center.[106] Several authors have suggested a combination of irradiation and surgery in an effort to improve therapeutic results.

TECHNIQUES OF RADIATION IN VAGINAL CARCINOMA

The pelvic portals should encompass the entire vagina down to the introitus and the pelvic lymph nodes to the upper portion of the common iliac chain. Portals of 15 × 15 cm or 15 × 18 cm are usually adequate. In lesions of the lower two thirds of the vagina, it is necessary to electively include the inguinal lymph nodes in the irradiated field even when no palpable lymph nodes are present.

Intracavitary therapy is carried out with varying diameter vaginal cylinders, such as the Burnett, Bloedorn, or Delclos applicators. The largest possible diameter should be used to improve the ratio of mucosa/tumor dose (Fig. 36-5).[114,115] A new afterloading vaginal applicator retaining the characteristics of the Bloedorn applicator has recently been designed at Washington University Medical Center by Perez et al.[116] Interstitial therapy with ^{137}Cs, ^{226}Ra needles or afterloading ^{192}Ir needles have been employed. Single plane, double plane, or volume implants should be planned depending on the extent and thickness of the tumor.

When the lesion is in the upper third, it is the authors' practice to treat the upper vagina with the same intracavitary arrangement as in carcinoma of the uterine cervix, including an intrauterine tandem and vaginal colpostats. The middle and distal vagina are treated with a vaginal cylinder. For smaller lesions (carcinoma in situ and Stage I), a dose of 6000 cGy at 0.5 cm under the mucosa is adequate. For larger lesions, doses in the range of 7000 to 8000 cGy are neces-

TABLE 36-5. Carcinoma of the Vagina, Mallinckrodt Institute of Radiology: Anatomical Sites of Failure

Stage	*No. of Patients*	*Local/Parametrial Only*	*Local/Parametrial + Distant Metastases*	*Distant Metastases Only*	*Dead of Intercurrent Disease*
0	16	1 (6.3%)	0	0	6 (37.5%)
I	50	4 (8%)	3 (6%)	5 (10%)	20 (40%)
IIA	49	10 (20.4%)	9 (18.4%)	6 (12.2%)	15 (30.6%)
IIB	26	5 (19.2%)	7 (26.9%)	5 (19.2%)	6 (23.1%)
III	16	0	6 (37.5%)	4 (25%)	1 (6.3%)
IVA	8	2 (25%)	4 (50%)	0	1 (12.5%)

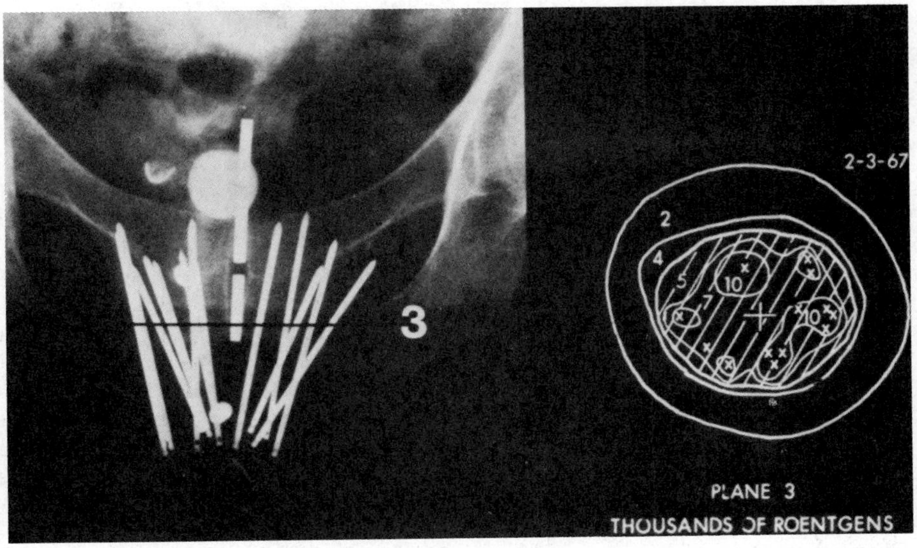

A

FIG. 36-5. **A**. Example of an intracavitary and double plane interstitial implant used to treat an extensive carcinoma of the vagina. This was combined with external beam 22 MV photon irradiation (4000 cGy whole pelvis and additional 2000 cGy parametrial dose). **B**. Distribution of radioactive sources and minimal tumor doses around primary tumor. **C**. Dose profile for patients with advanced vaginal carcinoma, using a combination of whole pelvic (WP) and parametrial external irradiation (SF), and intracavitary and double plane interstitial implant. (Perez CA, Korma A, Sharma S: Dosimetric considerations in irradiation of carcinoma of the vagina. Int J Radiat Oncol Biol Phys 2:639, 1977)

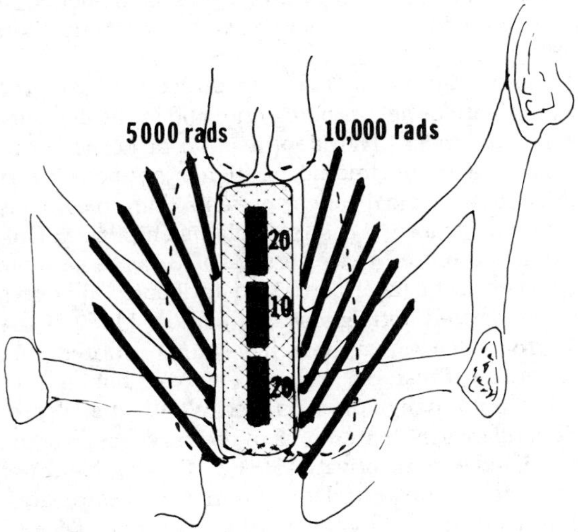

B

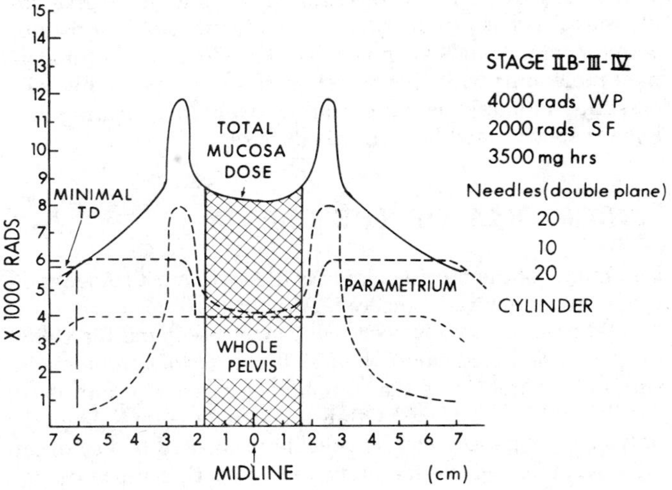

C

sary. In general, the vaginal mucosa receives an estimated 9000 to 10,000 cGy, which usually is well tolerated. The pelvic lymph nodes usually receive 5000 to 6000 cGy with whole pelvis and split fields.

TREATMENT OF CLEAR CELL CARCINOMA OF THE VAGINA

Stage I lesions of the cervix or vagina can be treated with either surgery or radiation therapy.[93,117] All other stages should be treated with radiation therapy.

Surgery for Stage I clear cell carcinoma may have the advantage of ovarian preservation and better vaginal function following skin graft although Wharton et al[117] have advocated intracavitary or transvaginal irradiation for the treatment of small tumors. They describe excellent tumor control with a functional vagina and preservation of ovarian function.

A radical hysterectomy and vaginectomy with radical lymph node dissection are necessary for vaginal clear cell carcinoma. Para-aortic nodes should be sampled before the procedure to determine whether there is lymphatic disease beyond the pelvis.

Fletcher[118] reported the results in 19 young women treated with irradiation alone (2 treated with irradiation combined with surgery), 15 of them followed for more than 2 years. Eighteen of the patients are surviving, 17 of them tumor free. One patient with an extensive lesion has a vaginal recurrence, and 1 patient died of a pulmonary embolus after removal of radium needles.

TREATMENT OF NONEPITHELIAL TUMORS OF THE VAGINA

The treatment of embryonal rhabdomyosarcoma of the vagina has undergone significant change in the past few years.

Combined treatment with chemotherapy, irradiation, and surgery has allowed many children to be treated without performing pelvic exenteration.[119,120] Survival rates of 46% to 63% have been reported using such combinations of therapy.[120,121] Sordillo et al[122] and Kinsella and Glatstein[123] have reported on the use of combinations of chemotherapy or radiation sensitizer and irradiation in adult soft tissue sarcomas. These same principles may be applicable to adult sarcomas of the vagina.

The results of surgical or irradiation therapy or both for vaginal melanoma are poor. Morrow and DiSaia[124] reported only 21% survival following radical surgery. These authors reported an 80% recurrence rate in cases managed by excisions with or without irradiation. Further studies of these patients are needed to determine optimal methods of therapy.

CHEMOTHERAPY OF VAGINAL CARCINOMA

Chemotherapy for squamous carcinoma of the vagina is no different from that outlined later in this chapter for cervical squamous carcinoma. The treatment of embryonal rhabdomyosarcoma has primarily used combinations of vincristine, actinomycin D, and cyclophosphamide. Treatment of malignant melanoma with chemotherapy has not been highly successful, and many institutions are actively investigating biologic response modifiers in this disease.

CARCINOMA OF THE CERVIX

Carcinoma of the uterine cervix is the third most frequent of the female genital cancers.[1] Although there were only 12,900 cases of invasive cervical cancer predicted for 1988, this does not include more than 50,000 cases of carcinoma in situ and several times that number of cases of preinvasive dysplasias of the cervix.[1] Of all the female genital cancers, only cervical cancer can be reliably prevented by use of an effective, inexpensive screening technique that allows detection of precancerous conditions that can be treated effectively so as to prevent the development of invasive cancer. Thus, the vast majority of deaths due to cervical cancer each year can be said to be preventable if women avail themselves of routine screening with cervical cytology.

EPIDEMIOLOGY

The peak age incidence for carcinoma of the cervix is between 48 and 55 years with the mean age 53.8 years and the median age 51.5 years.[125,126] This compares to a peak age incidence between the ages of 25 and 40 for carcinoma in situ.[126] Barber[127] reviewed data from the state of Connecticut and the Third National Cancer Survey and found that only 9% of women with invasive cancer were under age 35 whereas 53% of women with carcinoma in situ were under age 35.

Cervical cancer is more frequent in women of low socioeconomic status, women who begin sexual intercourse at a young age, women with a larger number of sexual partners, women who become pregnant at a young age, multiparous women, and prostitutes.[127–131] In contrast, carcinoma of the cervix is infrequent in nulliparous women, in those with inactive sexual lives, such as nuns, and in women married to one husband without children.[127,131,132] Cancer of the cervix is infrequent in Jewish and Moslem women, and circumcision of Jewish and Moslem men has been postulated as a cause.[133] Abou-Daoud[134] questioned the role of circumcision as a protective factor when he found an equal incidence of cervical cancer in Lebanese Moslems and Christians. Ackerman and del Regato[135] postulated genetic factors as a cause of the low incidence of cervical cancer in Jewish women. Kessler[136] has shown that the risk of cervical cancer may be increased in the wives of men who have been previously married to women who developed cervical cancer.

Chemical irritants have not been demonstrated to increase the incidence of cervical carcinoma in women, although cervical carcinoma has been induced in animals by direct application of chemical carcinogens.[137] Hormonal compounds in the form of oral contraceptives cannot be linked to an increased incidence of cervical cancer, but use of DES by pregnant women has resulted in an increased incidence of clear cell carcinoma of the cervix and vagina in their offspring.[138–140]

Recently, major attention has been directed toward the possibility of infectious agents being etiologic in the development of cervical cancer. The identification of herpes virus type 2 (HSV-2) and the finding of higher antibody titers against the virus in cervical cancer patients than in controls are suggestive of a cause and effect relationship.[141,142] Hollinshead et al[143] reported that the sera of 88% of patients with invasive cervical cancer contained antibodies to herpes virus tumor-associated antigens as compared to 11% of the sera of controls. Several authors have demonstrated that HSV-2 viruses can transform animal cells[144] or human embryonic cells[145] into malignant cells, and Wentz et al[146] produced in situ and invasive carcinoma of the cervix and vagina of mice inoculated with inactivated HSV-2. Finally, Notter et al[147] were able to demonstrate HSV-2 tumor-associated antigens in biopsies of cervical cancer using a peroxidase-antiperoxidase stain.

Meisels and Fortin[148] first demonstrated the high frequency of human papillomavirus (HPV) infection in 1976 and noted its association with dysplasias of the cervix. Kurman et al[149] studied 322 cases of cervical dysplasia and carcinoma in situ for the presence of papilloma antigen and found these proteins in over 20% of cases. Current studies would indicate that almost 50% of intraepithelial neoplasia will show evidence of HPV infection,[150,151] and viral particles have been demonstrated in invasive cervical cancer.[151] HPV types 6 and 11 are common in non-neoplastic condylomata acuminata, and HPV types 16 and 18 (and less often types 31, and 33–35) are common in cervical intraepithelial neoplasia and invasive cervical cancer. Several authors have recently found HPV infections of the penis in sexual partners of women with cervical intraepithelial neoplasia.[152,153] Krebs and Schneider[154] examined 127 male partners of women with cervical intraepithelial neoplasia and found 83 men (65%) with penile HPV lesions of which 3 had penile dysplasia.

Although definitive answers as to the exact mechanism for

the development of cervical cancer are not available, considerable insight has been obtained during the past few years. High-risk populations can be identified, and it would appear that viral infection may play an important role in the development of the disease process.

NATURAL HISTORY AND PATTERNS OF SPREAD

Squamous cell carcinoma usually arises from the squamocolumnar junction of the cervix and is preceded by cervical dysplasia and carcinoma in situ.[155,156] Petersen[154a] reported 127 patients with untreated carcinoma in situ of the cervix and described invasive carcinoma in 30% of cases by the 10th year. Clemmesen and Poulsen[157] reported a progression rate of 40% from carcinoma in situ to invasive cancer, whereas Kottmeier[157a] reported that of 31 patients with carcinoma in situ 71% developed invasive cancer within 12 years and 80% within 30 years. Although most authorities agree that dysplasias and carcinoma in situ do proceed to invasive cancer, there is less agreement on the time scale of this progression. The Walton report[158] described intervals of 1 to 20 years.

Invasive carcinoma occurs when the malignant epithelial cells break through the basement membrane and enter the stroma. Continued growth results in a visible lesion that involves progressively more of the cervical tissue. Cervical cancer spreads by direct extension into the paracervical tissue, the vagina, or the endometrium. Continued local growth will involve the pelvic side walls laterally, the bladder anteriorly, or the rectum posteriorly. Metastases occur primarily by means of the lymphatics, although blood-borne metastases do occur.

The cervix has a rich lymphatic network. Microscopic lymphatics lie beneath the squamous mucosa and surround the endocervical glands.[159] In the outer third of the cervix the lymphatics turn cephalad. In these lateral channels the cervical lymphatics are joined by vaginal lymphatics. Plentl and Friedman[159] comment on the interconnection of all of the lymphatics from the various levels of the cervix with those of the uterus and upper vagina. The lateral collecting trunks are relatively large and leave the cervix with the uterine artery and veins. The upper branches of these collecting lymphatics drain into the interiliac lymph nodes, whereas the middle branches drain into the obturator and deep hypogastric lymph nodes. The lower branches drain into the inferior gluteal and sacral lymph nodes and then into the lower aortic nodes. The interiliac, obturator, and hypogastric nodes drain into the common iliac and aortic lymph nodes.

In a review of 31 reports (more than 6,000 patients), Plentl and Friedman[159] found that the average incidence of positive lymph nodes was 15.4% in Stage I and 28.6% in Stage II. A recent series from Memorial Sloan-Kettering Cancer Center evaluated 431 patients and reported 15% positive lymph nodes in Stage IB and 22% in Stage IIA cervical cancer.[160] Table 36-6 shows the distribution of para-aortic nodal metastases reported by several authors.[161–169] As can be seen, the incidence of positive para-aortic nodes is 6% in Stage IB, 12% in Stage IIA, 19% in Stage IIB, and 29% in Stage IIIB.

Spread by hematogenous dissemination is relatively unusual in early stages of cervical cancer but increases with more advanced stages. Carlson et al[170] reported distant metastases in 4.7% of patients with Stage IB and 9.2% in Stage IIA. In Stage IIB through Stage IV the average incidence of distant metastases was 20.4%, ranging from 16.2% in Stage IIB to 24% of Stage IV.

PATHOLOGIC CHARACTERISTICS

Gross Characteristics

In situ and microinvasive cervical cancers are, in general, diagnosed by exfoliative cytology and colposcopy and do not present with gross abnormalities. The term "occult" carcinoma refers to an invasive cancer that is not clinically apparent and usually is the result of an endophytic carcinoma that develops high in the endocervix. Visible lesions are usually divided into endophytic and exophytic lesions. A variant of the endophytic type of tumor extends into and expands the endocervix so that the diameter of the corpus and cervix appear to be equal, resembling a barrel. These so-called barrel-shaped carcinomas are usually described as having transverse diameters of 6 cm or more and present special treatment problems.[171] Just as endophytic tumors can have a misleading appearance and be more extensive than they appear at first examination, exophytic tumors may appear more extensive than they actually are when examined more

TABLE 36-6. Metastases to Para-Aortic Lymph Nodes in Carcinoma of the Cervix

	Stage					
	IB	*IIA*	*IIB*	*IIIA*	*IIIB*	*IV*
Sudarsanam et al[161]	11/53 (7%)	3/31 (14%)	4/22 (18%)	2/3 (66%)	3/16 (19%)	0/3 (0)
Nelson et al[162]			5/31 (16%)		13/28 (46%)	
Piver et al[163]			6/46 (13%)		18/49 (36%)	4/7 (57%)
Wharton et al[164]	0/21 (0)	0/10 (0)	10/47 (21%)		14/42 (33%)	
Lagasse et al[165]	8/143 (5%)	4/22 (18%)	19/58 (33%)	0/3 (0)	19/61 (31%)	1/4 (25%)
Buchsbaum[166]	0/23 (0)	1/12 (7%)			7/20 (35%)	1/2 (50%)
Averette et al[167]	3/40 (8%)	1/12 (7%)	2/9 (22%)		2/20 (10%)	1/2 (50%)
Welander et al[168]			8/41 (20%)	2/6 (33%)	8/32 (25%)	4/12 (33%)
Berman et al[169]	8/158 (5%)	3/25 (12%)	40/240 (17%)	1/3 (33%)	44/177 (25%)	3/17 (18%)
Total	30/438 (6%)	13/109 (12%)	94/494 (19%)	5/15 (33%)	128/445 (29%)	14/47 (30%)

carefully. Often an exophytic tumor appears to fill the upper vagina and be connected to the cervix by a relatively small stalk with only moderate invasion into, or enlargement of, the cervix.

Microscopic Characteristics

Preinvasive cervical carcinoma is usually described by one of two different classifications, both of which are common usage. The first system divides lesions into dysplasias (mild, moderate, and severe) and carcinoma in situ. The second system uses three divisions of the term cervical intraepithelial neoplasia (CIN-1, CIN-2, and CIN-3). This precursor stage of cervical carcinoma begins with minimal morphologic changes (CIN-1 or mild dysplasia) and progresses to the point that the entire epithelium from the basement membrane to the surface is composed of malignant cells (CIN-3 or carcinoma in situ).

The vast majority of invasive carcinomas of the cervix are squamous cell carcinomas. Although many authors state that these carcinomas represent 90% or more of all cervical cancer, Regan and Ng[172] have pointed out that when rigid histologic criteria are used, only 75% to 80% are of the squamous cell type. Regan and Ng[172] have proposed that squamous carcinomas be classified as large-cell nonkeratinizing, large-cell keratinizing, and small-cell nonkeratinizing. They reported survival by cell type of 68.3% with large-cell nonkeratinizing carcinomas, 41.7% with large-cell keratinizing carcinomas, and 20% with small-cell nonkeratinizing carcinomas. Other authors have used different types of histologic grading. Wentz[173] divided these cancers into well-differentiated, moderately differentiated, and poorly differentiated carcinomas and reported differences in survival by grade. Many other terms have been used including high grade and low grade, anaplastic, and grades 1 through 4. This lack of uniformity has often made comparison of results difficult and often prohibits rational clinical protocol development that might be based on differentiation of the carcinomas.

Adenocarcinomas of the cervix arise from the endocervical columnar cells.[174] They account for 10% to 15% of cervical carcinomas,[172,174] although some authors have recently reported incidences of 16% to 34%.[175,176] This relative increase in incidence has been postulated to be due to improved detection and treatment of squamous cancers during their relatively prolonged preinvasive stage.[176] Histologically, endocervical adenocarcinoma is composed of glands formed of malignant columnar cells with enlarged, bizarre nuclei and increased mitoses. As these adenocarcinomas become less differentiated, they may lose their glandular appearance and become more solid.

Adenosquamous carcinomas of the cervix represent 2% to 5% of all cervical carcinomas[172,177] and are a mixture of malignant adenocarcinoma and malignant squamous cell carcinoma. These tumors are poorly differentiated and associated with decreased survival.[172,178] Clear cell carcinoma[178,179] glassy cell carcinoma,[180] adenoid cystic carcinoma[181] and mucoepidermoid carcinoma[182] are seen infrequently, but in general behave as poorly differentiated carcinomas. Also reported rarely as primary carcinomas arising in the cervix are malignant melanoma,[183] carcinoid,[184] sarcomas,[185] malignant lymphoma and Hodgkin's disease,[186,187] and verrucous carcinoma.[188] The last carcinoma mentioned, verrucous carcinoma, is a very well-differentiated squamous cell carcinoma that invades locally but rarely metastasizes.

CLINICAL MANIFESTATIONS

Preinvasive cervical carcinoma is detected by the Papanicolaou smear at the time of routine periodic examination and is not associated with symptoms. Any symptoms the patient might have, such as vaginal discharge, represent coexisting problems. Early invasive carcinoma can produce a vaginal discharge or vaginal bleeding (the most common type of vaginal bleeding being postcoital spotting). As the tumor of the cervix becomes more extensive, a serosanguinous or prurulent discharge is more pronounced and bleeding may become intermenstrual and more copious in quantity.

Pain is a late symptom in cervical carcinomas as are symptoms relative to the urinary tract or rectum. Dull aching pain low in the pelvis may be associated with chronic inflammation, tumor necrosis, or a combination of these factors. Low back pain or leg pain may be due to compression of lumbosacral nerves, direct involvement of lumbosacral nerve roots, pressure from a large tumor mass, or, on occasion, ureteral obstruction. Urinary frequency or urgency, hematuria, rectal tenesmus, and rectal bleeding result from direct invasion of the bladder or rectum from advanced disease.

DIAGNOSIS, CLINICAL EVALUATION, AND STAGING

Diagnosis

The purpose of periodic cytologic screening by means of the Papanicolaou smear is to prevent invasive cervical cancer. Although microinvasive and early invasive cervical cancers will be detected and this early detection is valuable in decreasing the death rate from cervical cancer, the ideal is to detect all cervical abnormalities in the premalignant stage and thus prevent invasive cervical cancer.

Papanicolaou smears are performed at the time of routine pelvic examination, and there appears to be little doubt that this technique has resulted in a decline in the mortality from cervical cancer.[189,190] The frequency with which this routine screening examination should be performed, however, is the subject of considerable debate. In 1976, the task force appointed by the Conference of Deputy Ministers of Health of Canada was reported (The Walton Report).[158] They identified two major categories of risk. The "low risk" group is made up of women who have never had a period of sexual activity during their lives, who have had a hysterectomy for nonmalignant disease, or who have reached the age of 60 after regular participation in a screening program never having had an abnormal cytologic smear. The "at risk" group is made up of women who have reached the age of 18, who are sexually active, and who do not otherwise fall into the low risk group. Within the "at risk" group is a "high risk" subgroup made up of women who have had an early onset of sexual activity with multiple partners. Largely as a result of this report, the American Cancer Society recommended that asymptomatic women 20 years of age and older and those under 20 years of age who are sexually active have cytologic screening for 2 consecutive years and at least one screening every 3 years until age 65. They further recommended that women at high risk of developing cervical carcinoma because of early age at first coitus, multiple sexual partners, and multiparity should have a yearly cytologic screening. A complete gynecologic examination should be performed when the vaginal smears are obtained.[191] The American College of Obstetricians and Gynecologists refused to accept this recommendation, however, and still recommends that cervical cytologic screening take place at the time of an annual gynecologic examination.[192]

To date, there is no clear and unified recommendation concerning periodic screening of women by cervical cytology in the United States. Although the distribution of women into risk groups seems reasonable, that distribution in practice is quite difficult. To effectively establish risk categories, one must have a detailed and reliable sexual history, and even then there is the question of whether the woman's risk status is also influenced by the sexual history of her partner (which may be even more difficult to determine accurately). Also unanswered is whether the value of annual screening is influenced by the bimanual examination and the breast examination and whether that annual examination by the gynecologist is the only periodic health screening that the woman receives.

If the cytologic smear reveals dysplastic or malignant cells, the patient should be evaluated by colposcopy and biopsy. Atypical smears due to inflammation should be managed by treating the inflammation and repeating the Papanicolaou smear. Persistent atypical smears that do not clear with treatment of infection require colposcopic evaluation and biopsy.

Colposcopy is the recommended method of evaluating an abnormal Papanicolaou smear. Using a bright light with a green filter to enhance vascular patterns and 10 to 15 power magnification, abnormal areas can be visualized and identified for biopsy with considerable accuracy. Most obstetrics and gynecology programs in the United States provide a thorough experience in this technique, and colposcopes are a relatively inexpensive piece of office equipment. Colposcopy is designed to allow properly directed biopsies; it is not a substitute for cervical biopsy and endocervical curettage. When colposcopy is inadequate in the patient with dysplastic or malignant cells on a Papanicolaou smear, cervical conization is mandatory.

Cervical conization is the removal of a cone shaped portion of tissue from the cervix that includes most or all of the transformation zone. This procedure is indicated in any patient who has dysplastic or malignant cells on cervical cytology, inadequate colposcopy, and no grossly visible lesion on the cervix. It is also indicated in patients with microinvasive cancer and in patients where the depth of invasion cannot be determined by biopsy. A cone biopsy should not be performed on a patient with a visible lesion of the cervix unless a cervical biopsy of the area fails to make the diagnosis of invasive cancer.

As mentioned above, any grossly visible cervical lesion should be biopsied. The performance of a Papanicolaou smear or colposcopy, or both, does not substitute for cervical biopsy. The inflammation that accompanies many cervical carcinomas can be misleading on both colposcopic examination and on the Papanicolaou smear, resulting in false negative evaluation.

Clinical Evaluation

The standard clinical evaluation for patients with cervical carcinoma includes examination by inspection and palpation (under anesthesia, if necessary), biochemical profile to include evaluation of liver and renal functions, chest radiograph, cytoscopy, proctosigmoidoscopy, and intravenous pyelography. In patients with advanced stage or in all patients over age 40, a barium enema should be obtained. CT scan can be helpful in evaluating retroperitoneal lymph nodes or in treatment planning of bulky lesions for irradiation. The reliability of this method of evaluation of lymph nodes has been reported in nonsurgically staged patients[193] and is currently under investigation in patients who are undergoing surgical staging by the GOG. Lymphangiograms have been used in the nonsurgical evaluation of cervical cancer and may be helpful when clearly positive. Piver and Chung[194] reported 98% accuracy by biopsy or laparotomy in patients with a positive lymphangiogram but a 20% false negative rate in those studies reported as negative. MRI is being evaluated and may prove to be helpful. Other symptoms may also require evaluation with appropriate studies.

Clinical Staging of Cervical Carcinoma

The staging of cervical carcinoma is a clinical staging classification that consists of physical examination (inspection, palpation, and biopsy), laboratory studies, and roentgenographic evaluation as outlined above. Surgical staging, if performed, does not alter the official stage of the patient for the purpose of reporting treatment results. Whenever possible, cervical cancer should be staged as part of a multidisciplinary effort involving the gynecologist, radiation therapist, and medical oncologist. The staging examination can usually be performed adequately in the outpatient setting, but if there is significant question about the adequacy of the examination or the examination is perceived not to be adequate, examination under anesthesia should be performed.

In 1985 the Oncology Committee of the FIGO made changes in the FIGO classification of cervical carcinoma. Although these changes will not officially be published until the 20th annual report in 1988, FIGO allowed publication of the changes in early 1987.[195] The new FIGO classification is listed in Table 36-7. As can be seen, the changes in the staging system are limited to Stage I. Stage IA, which in the 19th report published in 1985 was described as "microinvasive carcinoma (early stromal invasion)," is now divided into two categories. Stage IA_1 is defined as "preclinical carcinomas of the cervix, that is, those diagnosed only by microscopy," and should be limited to the very earliest forms of microinvasion, including cases in which invasion can be seen but the area of invasion is too small for measurement. Stage IA_2 are "lesions detected microscopically that can be mea-

TABLE 36-7. Staging of Invasive Carcinoma of the Uterine Cervix Adopted in 1987 by the International Federation of Gynecology and Obstetrics (FIGO)

Stage 0	Carcinoma in situ, intraepithelial carcinoma Cases of Stage 0 should not be included in any therapeutic statistics for invasive carcinoma
Stage I	The carcinoma is strictly confined to the cervix (extension to the corpus should be disregarded)
Stage IA1	Preclinical carcinomas of the cervix, that is, those diagnosed only by microscopy
Stage IA2	Lesions detected microscopically that can be measured. The upper limit of the measurement should not show a depth of invasion of more than 5 mm taken from the base of the epithelium, either surface or glandular, from which it originates, and a second dimension, the horizontal spread, must not exceed 7 mm. Larger lesions should be staged as IB
Stage IB	Lesions of greater dimensions than Stage IA2 whether seen clinically or not. Preformed space involvement should not alter the staging but should be specifically recorded so as to determine whether it should affect treatment decisions in the future
Stage II	The carcinoma extends beyond the cervix, but has not extended on to the pelvic wall. The carcinoma involves the vagina but not the lower third
Stage IIA	No obvious parametrial involvement
Stage IIB	Obvious parametrial involvement
Stage III	The carcinoma has extended to the pelvic wall. On rectal examination there is no cancer-free space between the tumor and the pelvic wall The tumor involves the lower third of the vagina All cases with a hydronephrosis or nonfunctioning kidney should be included, unless they are known to be due to other cause
Stage IIIA	Extension on to the pelvic wall
Stage IIIB	Extension on to the pelvic wall and hydronephrosis or nonfunctioning kidney
Stage IV	The carcinoma has extended beyond the true pelvis or has clinically involved the mucosa of the bladder or rectum. A bullous edema as such does not permit a case to be allotted to Stage IV
Stage IVA	Spread of the growth to adjacent organs
Stage IVB	Spread to distant organs

sured." The upper limit of the measurement should not show a depth of invasion of more than 5 mm taken from the base of the epithelium (either surface or glandular) from which it originates, and a second dimension, the horizontal spread, should not exceed 7 mm. Larger lesions should be staged as IB. Stage IB is now defined as "lesions of greater dimensions than Stage IA_2 whether seen clinically or not." Performed space involvement should not alter the staging but should be specifically recorded to determine whether it might affect treatment decisions in the future. The remainder of the staging classification is unchanged.

The impact of these changes on the staging system is not clear at this time since most authorities in the United States use "less than 3 mm of invasion without lymphovascular invasion" as the definition of Stage IA cervical carcinoma. It appears doubtful at this time that clinical practice patterns will be changed by this new classification, and its effect on reporting of results cannot be defined.

Surgical Staging of Cervical Carcinoma

In the early 1970s, Averette et al[167,196] and Nelson et al[162] introduced the concept of pretreatment surgical staging of cervical carcinoma. Averette et al[167] reported a high lack of correlation between clinical staging and the results of surgical exploration with reported errors of 26% in Stage IB, 45% in Stage IIA, 60% in Stage IIB, 66% in Stage IIIA, and 95% in Stage IIIB. Both authors demonstrated the relatively high frequency of para-aortic nodal metastases in cervical carcinoma, particularly in more advanced stages. Table 36-6 summarizes the results of several reports of positive para-aortic lymph nodes in cervical cancer.

Wharton et al[164] and Piver and Barlow[163] reported on the treatment of patients with positive para-aortic nodes with extended field radiotherapy. Wharton et al[164] gave 5500 cGy to the para-aortic area and noted a 27% serious complication rate with a 13% treatment related mortality rate. Piver and Barlow[163] used 6000 cGy and noted a similar high complication rate. Berman et al[197] reported fewer intestinal complications using a retroperitonial approach to the para-aortic lymph nodes, and Welander et al,[168] using a transperitoneal approach to the para-aortic lymph nodes, reported that a 4400 cGy dose to the para-aortics was not associated with a high complication rate.

Survival in patients with positive para-aortic lymph nodes has been addressed by several authors and is summarized in Table 36-8. The average disease-free survival is approximately 18%. Welander et al[168] pointed out that because the maximum tolerated para-aortic irradiation appears to be in the range of 4400 to 4500 cGy, it is unlikely that patients with more than microscopic disease will be cured by extended field irradiation. They also pointed out that because many patients with positive para-aortic lymph nodes have bulky local disease, control of para-aortic disease may not benefit survival because of inability to control the local disease. Also, spread to para-aortic lymph nodes may be a sign only of systemic disease. Buchsbaum[166] reported that 34.8% of patients with positive para-aortic lymph nodes had metastatic cancer in the scalene lymph nodes, and Welander et al[168] found that 54.8% of patients with positive para-aortic lymph nodes developed distant metastases as compared to 25% of a similar group of patients with negative para-aortic lymph nodes.

The place of pretreatment surgical staging in cervical carcinoma of the cervix remains unclear. Several large institutions across the United States routinely perform such procedures as prospective protocols and the GOG has used pretreatment laparotomy as an integral part of many of their advanced cervix protocols. Certainly the operation has a place in a research setting. Whether data being accumulated

TABLE 36-8. Survival in Cervical Carcinoma Patients with Positive Para-Aortic Lymph Nodes

Author	*Year Published*	*Survival (%)*	*Duration of Survival Analysis (yr)*
Wharton et al[164]	1977	14.2	2
Piver and Barlow[163]	1977	12.5	
Nelson et al[162]	1977	13	4
Buchsbaum[166]	1979	18.8	2
Welander et al[168]	1981	25.8	2+
Berman et al[169]	1984	25	3
Mean		18.2	

in these studies will show enough survival benefit to recommend the procedure routinely remains to be elucidated.

PROGNOSTIC FACTORS IN CERVICAL CANCER

Prognosis in cervical cancer is worse with advancing stage of disease, which in general represents increasing tumor bulk or increasing extent of tumor involvement of adjacent or distant organs. In early stage disease, however, survival appears to be influenced by multiple factors. The accurate identification of these risk factors has been addressed by several authors. Patients with Stages IB and IIA carcinoma treated by radical hysterectomy and pelvic lymphadenectomy have survival rates of 82% to 92% when there are no metastases to pelvic lymph nodes, compared to survival rates of 45% to 61% in patients with positive lymph nodes (Table 36-9). The incidence of positive lymph nodes in these patients has, in turn, been related to tumor diameter greater than 4 cm,[194,198,208] lymphovascular invasion,[198,208,209] deep invasion into the cervical stroma,[198,210,211] and histologic grade.[198,211] At least two of these authors also looked at recurrence in patients who had negative lymph nodes.[198,211] Fuller et al[198] found that after stratifying for nodal metastases, size of the primary tumor, depth of invasion into the cervix, and histologic grade were associated with an increased incidence of recurrence. They also noted an increased incidence of recurrence in patients who had adenocarcinoma as compared to squamous histology, even though patients with adenocarcinoma did not have an increased incidence of positive lymph nodes. Burke et al[211] found adenomatous cell type and lymphovascular invasion to place patients with negative lymph nodes at increased risk. Figge and Tamimi[212] noted an increased recurrence rate in patients with adenocarcinoma, but in their series this was only in association with lymphovascular space involvement and positive lymph nodes. Several authors have reported increased recurrence rates and decreased survival as the number of metastatic lymph nodes or the number of metastases in lymph node groups increase.[194,199,213]

In patients managed by radiotherapy, several authors have reported lower survival and an increased incidence of pelvic recurrences in patients with anemia.[214,215] Jenkin and Stryker[216] found more pelvic recurrences and complications in patients with hypertension, whereas Van Herik[217] found decreased survival when patients had oral temperatures over 100° F. Although some patients with elevated temperatures had pelvic infection, over half of them had no specific etiologic factor for the temperature elevation.

Prempree et al[218] reported an increased incidence of poorly differentiated tumors and decreased survival in patients with cervical cancer who were younger than 35 years of age. Other authors, however, have not found age at onset of the disease to affect survival.[219,220]

TREATMENT OF CERVICAL CARCINOMA

General Principles of Management

The primary method of therapy for preinvasive (Stage 0) and microinvasive (Stages IA_1 and IA_2) carcinoma of the cervix is surgery. Only rarely is there a place for radiation therapy in the management of such early disease. Stages IB and IIA carcinoma of the cervix can be managed equally effectively by either radical surgery or irradiation therapy.[221] There is no purpose in comparing the efficacy of these two treatment modalities because there has been, and should be, definite selection of patients in that some patients are better managed surgically whereas others will benefit most from primary therapy with irradiation. The optimum approach is that all patients be treated in institutions that have personnel

TABLE 36-9. Influence of Positive Pelvic Lymph Nodes on Survival in Stages IB and IIA Carcinoma of the Cervix

	Percent Survival	
	Positive Lymph Nodes	*Negative Lymph Nodes*
Piver and Chung (1975)[194]	45	82
Fuller et al (1987)[198]	50	85
Burghardt et al (1987)[199]	60.9	88.1
Martimbeau et al (1982)[200]	53	92
Mean	52.2	86.8

and equipment suitable for either type of therapy and that selection of therapy be a joint decision among the surgeon, the radiation oncologist, and the patient. Only in this setting will the very best results be obtained for all patients.

Patients with Stage IIB through Stage IVA are usually managed by radiotherapy. Although the rare patient with IVA carcinoma of the cervix may be a candidate for primary pelvic exenteration, such patients are usually managed by radiotherapy. Patients with IVB cervical carcinoma are usually managed by combinations of chemotherapy and irradiation. Recently, there have been reports of Phases I and II trials of concomitant chemotherapy and irradiation in patients with locally advanced disease. Although this is an intriguing concept, its usefulness is uncertain as yet.

Selected types of cervical carcinoma may be managed by combinations of surgery and irradiation. Those specific areas will be discussed later in this chapter.

Stage 0 (Carcinoma in situ)

Although the standard therapy for cervical intraepithelial neoplasia (CIN), grade 3 (severe dysplasia and carcinoma in situ) is conization of the cervix, selected patients can be managed by outpatient therapy using either cryotherapy or laser ablation. For these patients to be candidates for such therapy, their lesions should be entirely visible by colposcopy, the squamocolumnar junction must be visible, the endocervical curettage must be negative, and the colposcopically directed biopsy must be at least as severe as the cytologic smear. Some authorities also require that the lesion occupy no more than one quadrant of the cervix and there be no gland involvement. To be a candidate for outpatient therapy, the patient must be reliable and agree to long-term follow-up. Townsend et al[222] reviewed cases of invasive carcinoma following outpatient therapy and found that in most cases in which invasive cancer developed, there had been obvious deviation from above criteria. Similar findings were reported by Sevin et al.[223]

In the past, abdominal or vaginal hysterectomy has been considered the treatment of choice for CIN-3. Based on the evidence now available in the literature, this is no longer justified. In an extensive review of the literature, Coppleson[224] found that only 18 of 5,442 women (0.3%) treated for carcinoma in situ by conization of the cervix subsequently developed overt invasive cancer. This compared to 38 of 8,995 women (0.4%) who developed invasive carcinoma of the vagina after hysterectomy for carcinoma in situ. Based on these results, routine hysterectomy for CIN-3 cannot be recommended. Patients who do not desire further childbearing and have intraepithelial neoplasia that involves the margins of the cone biopsy may be treated by hysterectomy. Hysterectomy can also be indicated in patients with other gynecologic disorders that require removal of the uterus. It is the rare patient desirous of further childbearing who will ever require hysterectomy for preinvasive cancer.

Stage IA Carcinoma of the Cervix

In the 1987 classification of cervical carcinoma by FIGO, microinvasive carcinoma is divided into IA_1 and IA_2 (see Table 36-7). Stage IA_1 (microinvasive carcinoma that is so small it cannot be measured) should be treated by abdominal or vaginal hysterectomy in the healthy patient who is not desirous of further childbearing. Women who desire preservation of fertility or who are poor surgical risks can be managed by conization and followed closely, providing the cone margins are free of disease.

The proper management of Stage IA_2 is less clear. Averette et al[225] found no cases with positive lymph nodes if invasion was less than 1 mm without lymphovascular invasion but reported a 3.5% incidence of positive nodes in the literature if invasion extended to 5 mm. Simon et al[226] found no metastases to lymph nodes in 43 patients with invasion less than 3 mm and 3.9% positive lymph nodes in 26 patients with invasion of 3.1 to 5 mm. These same authors reviewed the literature and reported 8% nodal metastases in patients with invasion of 3 to 5 mm. In addition to depth of invasion, several authors have reported an increased incidence of nodal metastases if there was lymphovascular space invasion.[227,228] Based on these results, most authorities in the United States recommend abdominal or vaginal hysterectomy for Stage IA cervical cancer if invasion is less than 3 mm and there is no lymphovascular space involvement. Cervical carcinoma with invasion of more than 3 mm or in which there is lymphovascular invasion is managed in the same way as Stage IB. The influence of volume of invasive cancer as a criteria for planning therapy has been recommended by Burghardt.[227,232] Because such measurements are now part of the new FIGO classification, further data may be available in the future.

Patients with Stage IA may also be treated with intracavitary irradiation. In 32 patients with microinvasive carcinoma treated at Washington University, 18 of whom received intracavitary therapy alone, no local or regional failures occurred, and the corrected 5-year survival (for intercurrent disease) was 100%.

Hamberger et al[229] reported on 151 patients with Stage IA or IB lesions less than 1 cm in diameter treated with intracavitary therapy alone. No failures were noted in 41 patients with Stage IA, and only 4 failures in 93 (4%) were seen in patients with small volume Stage IB carcinoma. However, of 17 patients with more advanced Stage IB lesions, 3 patients (18%) treated with intracavitary therapy alone had regional failures.

Stages IB and IIA Carcinoma of the Cervix

Stages IB and IIA cervical carcinoma can be managed equally effectively by either radical hysterectomy and pelvic lymphadenectomy or full pelvic irradiation.[221] Surgical therapy is preferred by some because ovarian function is preserved in young women, the vagina is usually more pliable than when irradiation is used, overall treatment time is shorter, and long-term radiation complications in pelvic tissues are avoided. Other reasons for selection of surgery are concomitant inflammatory gastrointestinal disease, pelvic inflammatory disease, presence of an adnexal mass, and pregnancy. Radiation therapy has the advantages that it avoids major intraoperative and postoperative surgical complications, the patient can receive most of the therapy as an outpatient, and

TABLE 36-10. Survival Rates for Stages I and II Carcinoma of the Cervix Treated by Radical Hysterectomy and Pelvic Lymphadenectomy

Author	*Stage*	*No. of Patients*	*Survivors**	*Survival (%)*
Blaikley et al[201]	IB	98	64	65.5
	IB and IIA	161	96	50.8
Brunschwig and Barber[202]	IB (A)	173	141	81.5
	IB and IIA (B)†	308	231	76.0
Christensen et al[203]	IB	168	137	82.7
	IB and IIA	219	168	77.0
Ketcham et al[204]	IB	28	Actuarial	86.0
	IB and IIA	42		87.0
Liu and Meigs[205]	IB	116	91	78.4
	IB and IIA	165	119	72.1
Masterson[206]	IB	120	105	87.5
	IB and IIA	150	124	82.5
Park et al[207]	IB	126	Actuarial	91.0
Average	IB			81.9
	IB and IIA			74.2

Modified from Hoskins WJ, Ford JH Jr, Lutz MH, et al: Radical hysterectomy and pelvic lymphadenectomy for the management of early invasive carcinoma of the cervix. Gynecol Oncol 4:278, 1976.

* Patients dead of intercurrent disease were included with survivors when data were available.

† Surgical and pathologic classification.

it is suitable for virtually any patient. Several authors[207,230,231] have reported noncontrolled studies that demonstrate that both methods are equally effective therapy for Stages IB and IIA cervical cancer. Newton[233] and Roddick and Greenlow[234] have reported similar survival and complication rates in Stages IB and IIA cervical cancer when patients were prospectively randomized to either radiation therapy or radical hysterectomy. The results of a literature review that compared the two modalities were reported by Hoskins et al[221] and are presented in Tables 36-10 and 36-11.

Volterrani and Lombari[242] reported a 5-year survival rate of 82.6% in 23 patients with occult Stage IB carcinoma of the cervix treated with intracavitary radium only (^{226}Ra application using a derivation from the Paris method to deliver 7500 mgh). However, in Stage IB the 5-year survival rate was only 65.8%, in Stage II 50%, and in Stage III 29.8%. The results are substantially inferior to those obtained with a combination of intracavitary and external irradiation. It is obvious that intracavitary therapy alone is grossly inadequate to effectively irradiate the larger primary tumors, including the

TABLE 36-11. Five-Year Survival Rates of Patients with Stages I and II Carcinoma of the Cervix Treated by Radiotherapy

Author	*Stage*	*No. of Patients*	*Survivors**	*Survival (%)*
Blaikley et al[201]	I	183	123	67.2
	I and II	551	296	53.7
Dickson[235]	IB	348	249	71.6
	IB and IIA	983	598	60.0
Fletcher[236]	IB	549	Actuarial	91.5
	IB and IIA	973		83.5
Kline et al[237]	IB	45	37	81.4
	IB and IIA	64	47	70.5
Kottmeier[238]	IB	611	547	89.5
	IB and IIA	1576	1244	78.9
Muirhead and Green[239]	I	194	152	78.0
	I and II	306	208	68.0
Perez et al[240]	IB	312	Actuarial	87.0
	IIA	98	NED	73.0
Wall et al[241]	I	101	87	86.4
	I and II	208	153	73.5
Average	I			83.5
	I and II			75.6

Modified from Hoskins WJ, Ford JH Jr, Lutz MH, et al: Radical hysterectomy and pelvic lymphadenectomy for the management of early invasive carcinoma of the cervix. Gynecol Oncol 4:278, 1976.

* Patients dead of intercurrent disease were included with survivors when data were available.

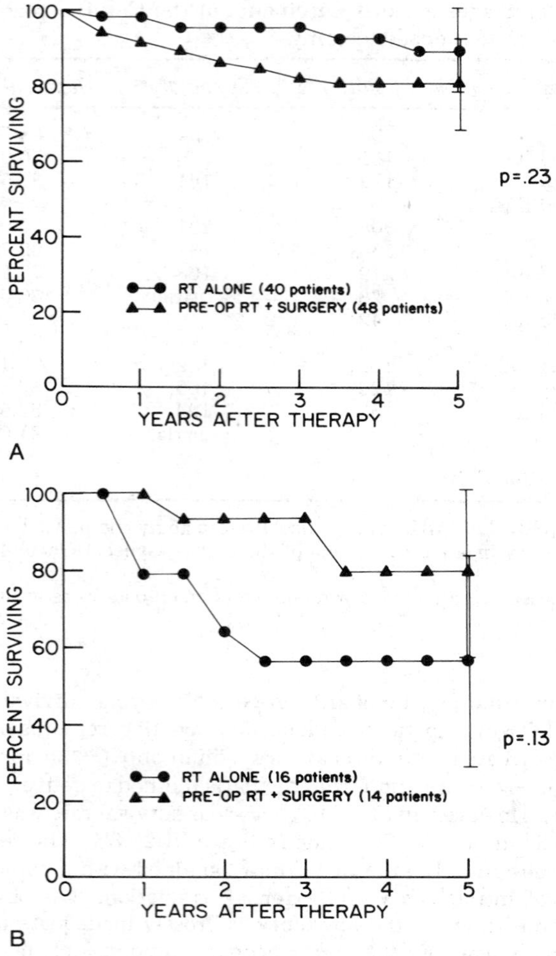

FIG. 36-6. **A**, **B**. NED actuarial survival in patients with Stage IB (**A**) or IIA (**B**) carcinoma of the uterine cervix treated with either irradiation alone (*solid circles*) or a combination of low dose preoperative irradiation and surgery (*solid triangles*). Randomized study, 1966–1979. Difference in survival is not statistically significant. (Perez CA, Camel HM, Kao MS, et al: Randomized study of preoperative radiation and surgery or irradiation alone in the treatment of stage IB and IIA carcinoma of the uterine cervix: Final report. Gynecol Oncol 27:129, 1987)

barrel-shaped lesions as well as any parametrial extension. Unfortunately, the authors did not report the exact location of the failures.

Van Nagell et al,[243] after radical hysterectomy or irradiation for Stage IB disease, found that the recurrence rate was 5% for tumors less than 2 cm in diameter treated with either modality. In lesions 2 to 5 cm in diameter, the failure rate was 24% for surgery but only 11% for radiation. Kielbinska et al,[244] in a long-term follow-up of 792 women treated by irradiation and 789 women treated with hysterectomy and irradiation for Stage I cervical carcinoma, found no difference in survival, general health, incidence of recurrent carcinoma, or appearances of second primary malignancies. Perez et al[245] have recently reported a randomized trial of preoperative irradiation and radical hysterectomy versus irradiation alone in Stage IB and Stage IIA cervical cancer (Fig. 36-6).

Bulky endocervical carcinoma (barrel-shaped cervix) has been reported to have a higher incidence of central recurrence, pelvic and para-aortic node metastases, and distant metastases.[246] Because of the difficulty of obtaining central control of these large lesions, higher doses of irradiation to the central pelvis or a surgical procedure to remove the uterus or both have been advocated.[247] Currently, the GOG is evaluating the benefit of postirradiation hysterectomy in such patients in a prospective, randomized trial.

The use of irradiation for patients with positive lymph nodes following radical hysterectomy is controversial. In a panel report summarizing the experience at several institutions in the United States, Morrow[248] reported no consistent practice and no evidence of benefit from such therapy. Recently, investigators from the Memorial Sloan-Kettering Cancer Center reported improved survival in patients with nodal metastases at radical hysterectomy when they were treated postoperatively with a combination of whole pelvis irradiation and chemotherapy.[249]

Stages IIB, III, and IV Carcinoma of the Cervix

The treatment of cervical cancer more advanced than Stage IIA is irradiation. Isolated cases of Stage IVA cervical cancer with involvement of the bladder or rectum without pelvic sidewall involvement can be treated by primary pelvic exenteration, but the better choice of therapy, even in these patients, is primary irradiation.

In Stage IIB the 5-year survival rate is 60% to 65% and practically all patients are treated with irradiation alone. Occasionally a conservative hysterectomy is performed after high-dose preoperative irradiation in patients with a barrel-shaped cervix and limited medial parametrial infiltration that regresses completely 4 to 6 weeks after completion of irradiation.

In Stage IIIB, the 5-year survival rates range from 25% to 48%. This may be related to the socioeconomic status of the patients, extent of the disease, technique of irradiation, and dose delivered to the parametrium. Johns[250] reported better pelvic tumor control and survival and fewer complications in a group of 65 patients with Stages IIB and III cervical carcinoma treated with 23 MV photons in comparison with 61 patients treated with ^{60}Co external irradiation and intracavitary insertions (Fig. 36-7).

Interstitial parametrial implants have been used to supplement standard external and intracavitary techniques. Prempree[251] reported a 96% local tumor control rate and a 61% 5-year disease-free survival rate in 23 patients with an intact uterus and Stage IIIB carcinoma of the cervix treated with a combination of external irradiation and intracavitary and interstitial implants to the parametrium. Likewise, he described a 23% local failure rate and a 69% 5-year survival rate in 26 patients with similar stage carcinoma of the cervix treated in the same manner but on whom the uterine cavity could not be probed or was absent.

Aristizabel et al[252] described the treatment of 21 patients with locally advanced invasive carcinoma of the uterine cervix treated with transperineal interstitial implants using a

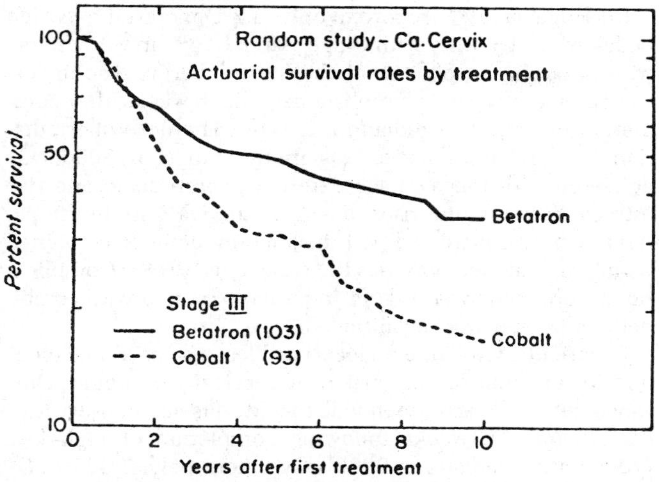

FIG. 36-7. Survival curves for patients with Stage III carcinoma of the uterine cervix on a randomized treatment study with either betatron or cobalt-60 external beams in addition to intracavitary insertion (unpublished data). (Johns HE: Optimization of energy and equipment. In Kramer S, Suntharalingam N, Zinniger GF [eds]: High Energy Photons and Electronics: Clinical Applications in Cancer Management, p 333. New York, John Wiley and Sons, 1976)

specially designed plastic template. With a mean follow-up of 26 months, local tumor control was reported in 18 of the patients (85%). Seven patients (33%) developed grade 2 or 3 complications, which included vesicovaginal (1 patient), rectovaginal (1 patient), or both fistulae (1 patient). Three patients developed severe radiation proctitis or cystitis, or both (one each).

Martinez et al,[253] using a special applicator consisting of two acrylic cylinders, a template with an array of holes that serve as guides to localize the trocars, and a cover plate, treated 37 patients with advanced or recurrent carcinoma of the cervix and 26 with vaginal-urethral tumors. They reported six local failures in the patients with cervical lesions and five in the group with vaginal-urethral tumors. The overall complication rate was 5.1%.

Maruyama and Muir[254] have used Californium-252 (^{252}Cf) neutron brachytherapy in conjunction with fractionated external irradiation to treat carcinoma of the uterine cervix. They reported on 41 patients with Stage IB treated with 4000 to 5000 cGy to the whole pelvis followed by 500 to 1500 cGy boost dose to the lateral pelvic wall. Cs neutron-252 therapy was usually delivered in a single intracavitary insertion in about 8 hours. Nearly total tumor clearance was achieved in more than 90% of the patients by the completion of therapy, only a small group exhibiting a slow clearance pattern.

When brachytherapy procedures cannot be performed because of medical reasons or unusual anatomical configuration of the pelvis or the tumor (*i.e.,* extensive lesion and inability to identify the cervical canal), higher doses of external irradiation alone may be used. Castro et al[255] reported results in 118 patients with invasive cervical carcinoma treated with 5000 to 6000 cGy to the whole pelvis (four-field box technique) and additional doses to residual tumor with reduced AP-PA portals to complete 7000 cGy tumor dose. With doses below 5000 cGy, no pelvic tumor control was obtained in 32 patients, but disease control and survival were significantly enhanced with higher doses. Complications increased with higher doses.

Combinations of Irradiation and Surgery in Carcinoma of the Cervix

The results of several series are similar to those obtained with irradiation alone. Perez et al[245] reported on a prospectively randomized study of 118 selected patients with Stages IB and IIA carcinoma of the uterine cervix. All patients were followed for a minimum of 5 years or until death. Patients were randomly assigned to be treated with irradiation alone (as described previously) or with irradiation and surgery (2000 cGy to the whole pelvis and one intracavitary insertion for 5000–6000 mgh followed by a radical hysterectomy with pelvic lymphadenectomy 26 weeks later). The tumor-free actuarial 5-year survival rate for 40 Stage IB patients treated with irradiation alone was 80% and for 48 patients treated with preoperative irradiation and surgery was 82%

TABLE 36-12. Carcinoma of the Uterine Cervix, Stages IB and IIA: Percentage of Metastatic Pelvic Lymph Nodes and Dose of Irradiation Delivered to Lymph Nodes

	Stage IB		*Stage IIA*		
Author	*Surgery Alone*	*Preoperative XRT*	*Surgery Alone*	*Preoperative XRT*	*Estimated Dose (cGy) to Nodes*
Christensen[203]	29/167 (17.4%)		27/104 (26%)		0
Morley[257]	18/143 (12.6%)				0
Morton[258]	9/38 (23.7%)	4/32 (12.5%)			1800
Sweeney and Douglas[259]		5/39 (13%)		9/54 (17%)	3500
Rampone[260]		81/137 (15%)			2000
Decker[261]		5/38 (13.2%)		11/45 (24.4%)	4000
Quigley[262]		13/136 (9.6%)			1800
Parker[263]	15/95 (16%)	6/73 (8%)	7/16 (44%)	20/71 (28%)	Not stated
Gray[264]	5/44 (11.4%)	3/58 (5.2%)	6/17 (35.3%)	Inc. with I	4500
Perez[265]		2/43 (4.6%)		2/24 (8.3%)	3000–4000
Perez[265]	0/32 (0)				4001–5000
Rutledge[266]		1/30 (3.3%)		4/39 (10.3%)	5000

Modified from Perez CA, Breaux S, Askin F, et al: Irradiation alone or in combination with surgery in Stage IB and IIA carcinoma of the uterine cervix. A non-randomized comparison. Cancer 43:1062, 1979.

(p = 0.23). In 16 patients with Stage IIA, actuarial tumor-free survival was 56% with irradiation alone and 79% in 14 patients treated with irradiation and surgery (p = 0.13). In the patients with Stage IB treated with irradiation alone, the pelvic failure rate was 2.5% and distant metastases 7.5%. In the preoperative irradiation-surgery group, the pelvic failure rate was 12.5% and distant metastases 4.2%. In Stage IIA, patients receiving radiotherapy alone had a pelvic failure rate of 6.3%, combined pelvic recurrence with distant metastases of 18.8%, and distant metastases alone of 12.5%. The incidence of grade 2 to 3 complications in the patients receiving radiation therapy alone was 13.8% (two vesicovaginal fistulae, one rectovaginal fistula, and one rectal stricture). In the patients treated with preoperative irradiation and surgery, 11% developed grade 2 to 3 complications (one rectal stricture, one severe proctitis, one small bowel obstruction, and three ureteral strictures).

Einhorn et al[256] in a nonrandomized study reported better survival in 49 patients with Stage IB using a combination of surgery and irradiation (100% at 5 years) in comparison with 64 patients treated with irradiation alone (81% at 5 years). No difference was observed in 25 patients with Stage IIA treated with combined therapy and 40 treated with irradiation alone (about 75% 5-year survival rate). Patients with metastatic lymph nodes have survival rates that are approximately 50% of those with negative nodes.

The dose of irradiation delivered to the lymph nodes, the time of the operation, and the pathologic examination of the specimens are critical in determining the presence of postirradiation residual tumor (Table 36-12). Rampone et al[260] reported a 15% incidence of metastatic lymph nodes in a group of 537 patients with Stage IB treated with two preoperative intracavitary insertions (total of 6000 mgh), which delivered 1500 cGy to the pelvic lymph nodes. All patients with positive nodes in the operative specimen were given postoperative external radiation to the pelvis. The 5-year survival rate was 92.9% for 456 patients with negative nodes in contrast to 52% in 81 patients with positive nodes.

Rutledge et al[266] reported only 3.3% metastatic lymph nodes in 30 patients with Stage I and 10.3% in 39 patients with Stage IIA carcinoma of the uterine cervix who underwent a bilateral pelvic lymphadenectomy 6 weeks after completion of definitive radiation therapy. The dose of irradiation to the lymph nodes was in the range of 5000 cGy delivered with megavoltage external photon beam and two intracavitary radium insertions. The survival rate in the patients who were treated with irradiation alone or combined with lymphadenectomy was the same (Fig. 36-8). Complications were somewhat higher in patients treated with combinations of the two modalities.

In patients with large endocervical lesions (barrel-shaped) or with endometrial extension of cervical carcinoma, Durrance et al[267] recommended an extrafascial conservative hysterectomy 6 weeks following completion of high-dose preoperative radiation (2000 cGy whole pelvis, 3000 cGy split fields, and one intracavitary insertion of 6000 mgh). Perez et al[268] reported that in patients with primary carcinoma of the uterine cervix who have endometrial stromal invasion of tumor only in the curettings, the addition of a hysterectomy did not improve the survival since most of the patients failed because of distant dissemination. Stage IVB cancer is managed by combinations of irradiation and chemotherapy.

RADIATION THERAPY TECHNIQUES

The application of radium therapy in the treatment of carcinoma of the cervix was first presented in 1913 at the Congress at Halle. Despite a slower regression after irradiation, reflecting cellular kinetics and slow growth, no difference in tumor control or survival has been observed in adenocarcinomas when compared with epidermoid carcinoma.[268,269] Because of the predilection for endocervical involvement in adenocarcinoma, a combination of irradiation and conservative hysterectomy has been advocated.[231,271]

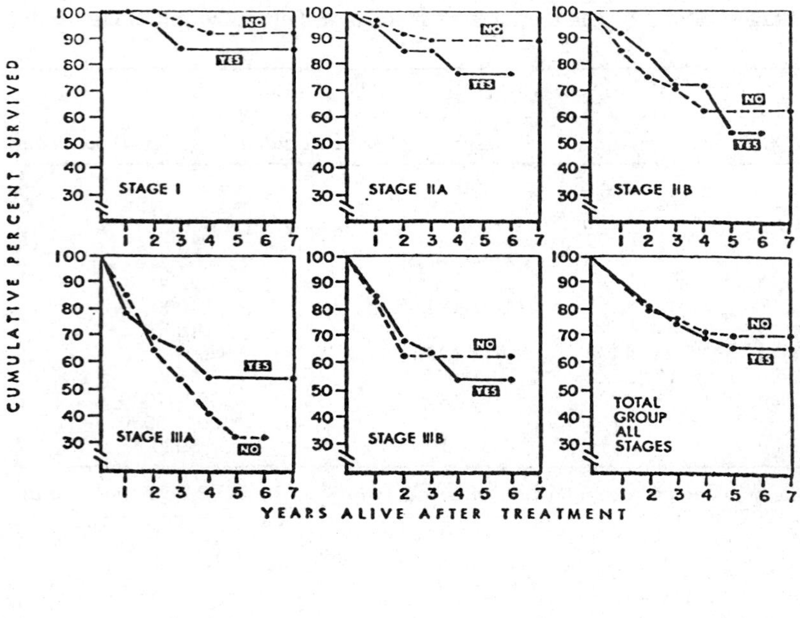

FIG. 36-8. Survival curves of patients treated for squamous cell carcinoma of the cervix, Stages I, IIA, IIB, IIIA, IIIB, and all stages combined. Patients who had lymphadenectomy after definitive irradiation to their treatment are represented by solid line curves. The broken line curves are for patients who had radiation treatment only. (Rutledge FM, Fletcher GM, Macdonald EJ: Pelvic lymphadenectomy as an adjunct to radiation therapy in treatment for cancer of the cervix. Am J Roentgenol Radium Ther Nucl Med 106:831, 1969)

External Irradiation

External irradiation is used to treat the whole pelvis and the parametria including the common iliac lymph nodes, whereas the central disease (cervix, vagina, and medial parametria) is primarily irradiated with intracavitary sources. External pelvic irradiation is delivered before intracavitary insertions in patients with the following:

1. Bulky cervical lesions, to improve the geometry of the intracavitary application
2. Exophytic easily bleeding tumors
3. Tumors with necrosis or infection.

Volume

In the treatment of invasive carcinoma of the uterine cervix, it is critical to deliver adequate doses of irradiation to the pelvic lymph nodes. For Stage IB carcinoma, 15 × 15 cm portals (at the surface of the patient) are sufficient. For patients with IIA-B, III, and IVA carcinoma, somewhat larger portals, 18 × 15 cm, are required to cover all of the common iliac nodes in addition to the cephalad half of the vagina (Fig. 36-9). A 2 cm margin lateral to the bony pelvis is sufficient. If there is no vaginal extension, the lower margin of the port is at the inferior border of the obturator foramen. When there is vaginal involvement, the entire length of this organ should be treated down to the introitus.

If metastatic periaortic lymph nodes are suspected or confirmed, the retroperitoneal tissues need to be irradiated either through a separate portal or with a field that includes both the periaortic nodes and the pelvic tissues (anterior and posterior, occasionally lateral portals).

FIG. 36-9. Simulation AP film of pelvis showing volume treated with external irradiation that includes uterus, upper vagina, parametria, and pelvic lymph nodes.

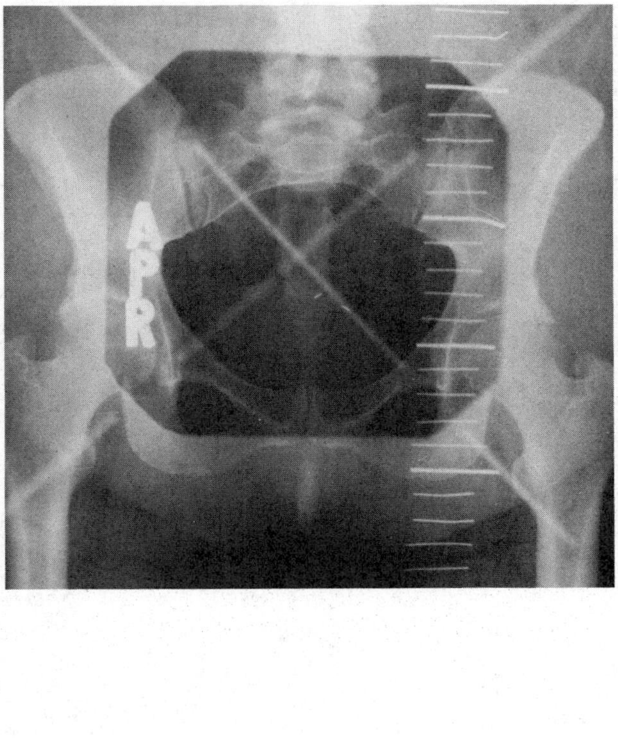

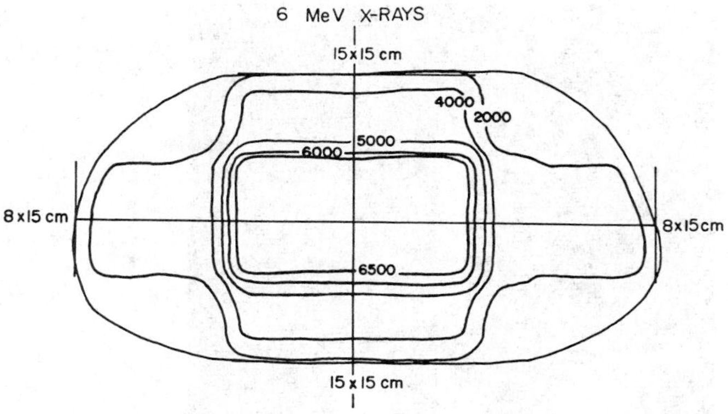

FIG. 36-10. Example of "box technique" with anterior/posterior and lateral portals used for the treatment of pelvic tumors.

Beam Energies

Because of the thickness of the pelvis, high-energy beams are especially suited for this treatment. They decrease the dose of radiation delivered to the peripheral normal tissues and provide a more homogeneous dose distribution in the central pelvis. With lower-energy megavoltage beams (^{60}Co, 4–6 MV photons), higher maximum doses must be given and there is a need to use more complex portal arrangements (three fields or pelvic box technique) to minimize the dose to the bladder and the rectum while delivering an adequate dose in the cervix and the parametria (Fig. 36-10).

Brachytherapy

Brachytherapy can be delivered with intracavitary techniques using applicators consisting of an intrauterine tandem and vaginal colpostats or, when necessary, with vaginal cylinders. Also, intersititial implants with needles in limited tumor volumes are helpful in specific clinical situations (*i.e.*, localized residual tumor).

The intracavitary therapy, with its rapid dose fall-off as a function of distance, yields a high dose to the uterus and paracervical tissues, but as the only modality it is inadequate to treat the pelvic lymph nodes (Fig. 36-11). Several isotopes are available, such as ^{226}Ra and ^{60}Co, although currently ^{137}Cs is the most popular. Various applicators are used for intracavitary therapy, most at present being afterloading. Afterloading applicators allow a better application because the operators are not concerned with radiation exposure; also, the technique can be exploited to achieve more optimal dose distribution with replacement or removal of sources in the tandem or the vaginal ovoids at different times. Radiographs of the application can be obtained using dummy sources; the active sources will be inserted only after the films have been reviewed and the position of the applicators is believed to be satisfactory.

In general, the first intracavitary insertion is scheduled after 1000 to 2000 cGy of external irradiation if an adequate geometry exists in the pelvis. Otherwise, 2000 to 4000 cGy are delivered before the first application to decrease the size of the lesion and improve the relationship of the applicators

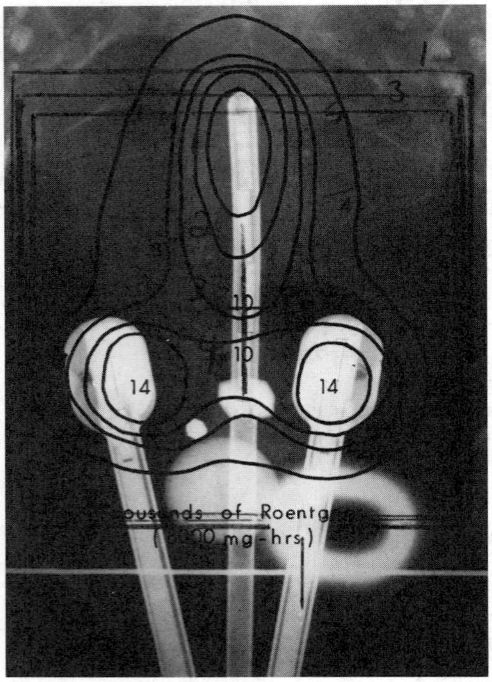

A

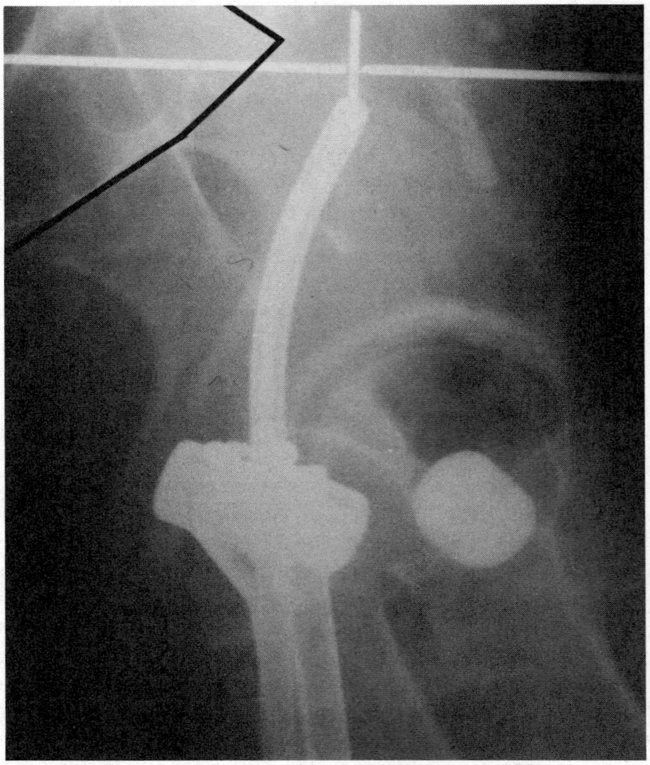

B

FIG. 36-11. AP (**A**) and lateral (**B**) radiographs of the pelvis showing an intracavitary application with interuterine tandem and vaginal colpostats. Isodose dose curves on a coronal plane are superimposed on AP port.

to the cervix and vagina. The second application is performed 1 to 3 weeks after the first insertion.

Doses of Irradiation

Optimal dose for invasive carcinoma of the cervix is delivered with a combination of whole pelvis, intracavitary, and, at times, interstitial therapy. Some institutions use lower doses of whole pelvis, external irradiation (1000 cGy for Stage IB and 2000 cGy for Stages IIA–B, III, and IVA) in addition to parametrial doses to complete 5000 cGy in Stages IB and IIA–B and 6000 cGy for more advanced stages. An assortment of step wedges designed in accordance with the isodose curves of the intracavitary applications or a 3 cm wide rectangular 5 half value lead block are used to shield the midline. This is combined with two intracavitary insertions that deliver 7000 to 8000 mgh (6500–7200 cGy to point A).

This technique affords a high central dose to the cervix, paracervical tissues, and parametria and a moderate homogeneous dose to the external iliac lymph nodes without exceeding the bladder and rectal tolerance doses (Fig. 36-12). Other institutions prefer higher doses of whole pelvic external irradiation (usually 4000 cGy) with an additional parametrial dose to complete 5000 cGy in patients with Stages IB and IIA and 6000 cGy for patients with IIB, III, or IVA tumors. This is usually combined with one or two intracavitary insertions for approximately 5000 to 6000 mgh (4500–5500 cGy to point A). When residual tumor is palpated at the completion of the prescribed course of therapy, an additional 1000 cGy through a small 8 × 12 cm field to one parametrium or 12 × 12 cm to both parametria may be used to deliver an additional 1000 cGy. The midline block is left in place.

FIG. 36-12. Isodose distribution in the pelvis with combined external and intracavitary irradiation showing doses to be delivered to the cervix and parametria without exceeding irradiation of bladder and rectum.

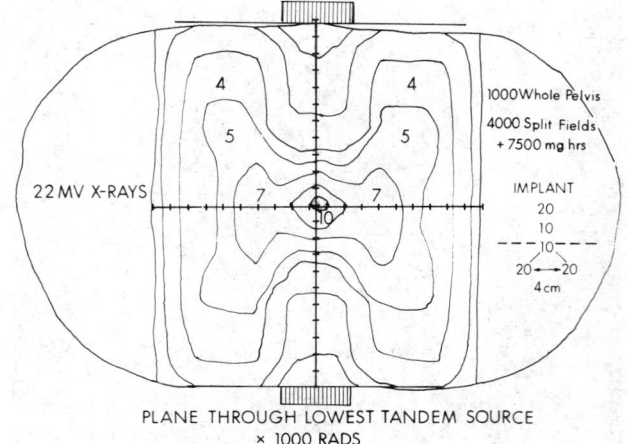

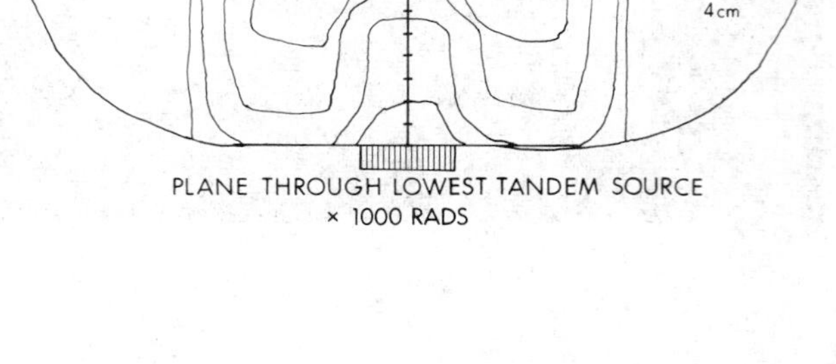

Techniques for Combination of Irradiation and Surgery

PREOPERATINE IRRADIATION. At some institutions the combination of preoperative irradiation and a hysterectomy has been used to treat patients with Stages IB and IIA.[272,273] Sometimes an intracavitary insertion alone is used (5000–6000 mgh) before radical hysterectomy with pelvic lymphadenectomy. At some institutions this brachytherapy is combined with external irradiation (2000 cGy to the whole pelvis in which case a radical hysterectomy and pelvic lymphadenectomy is performed). In other patients 2000 cGy to the whole pelvis plus 3000 cGy to the parametria and an intracavitary insertion (5000–6000 cGy to point A) are delivered, to be followed 4 to 6 weeks later by a conservative extrafascial hysterectomy.[272,273] The rationale for the use of an operation in addition to irradiation has been the alleged inability of irradiation to eradicate completely the tumor at bulky primary sites or in the pelvic lymph nodes[274,275] and the belief of some gynecologists that a more functional vagina in sexually active patients will be left after the surgical procedure.[276]

POSTOPERATIVE IRRADIATION. When metastatic pelvic lymph nodes or positive surgical margins are found after a hysterectomy, postoperative irradiation is delivered. If only intracavitary therapy was given preoperatively, 2000 cGy whole pelvis and 3000 cGy to the parametrial are administered, shielding the midline. If some external therapy is delivered preoperatively, an additional parametrial dose to complete 5500 cGy should be given again, shielding the midline with an appropriate block.

In patients not irradiated preoperatively on whom postoperative irradiation is indicated because of positive (central) surgical margins, we administer a combination of external irradiation (2000 cGy whole pelvis and 3000 cGy to the parametria with a small midline block) combined with an intracavitary insertion for 6000 cGy to the vaginal mucosa (1800 mgh) with two colpostats. In patients with metastatic pelvic lymph nodes external irradiation alone (5000 cGy to the midplane of the pelvis) has been administered.

In patients receiving postoperative irradiation, extreme care should be exercised in designing treatment techniques that include intracavitary insertions; because of the surgical extirpation of the uterus, the bladder and the rectosigmoid may be closer to the radioactive sources than in the patient with an intact uterus.[277] Furthermore, vascular supply may be affected by the surgical procedure and adhesions can prevent mobilization of the small bowel loops that occasionally may be fixed in the pelvis, which increases the risk of complications.

Hyperbaric Oxygen, Hypoxic Sensitizer, and Hyperthermia Combined with Irradiation

Several reports have been published on clinical trials evaluating the efficacy of hyperbaric oxygen (HBO)[278] combined with irradiation in the treatment of a variety of human tumors, one of them carcinoma of the uterine cervix. Watson and co-workers,[279] in a randomized clinical trial involving 320 patients (Stages III and IVA) treated at four institutions, reported a 5-year survival rate of 33% in the oxygen-treated group in contrast to 27% in the control patient group treated in air ($p = 0.08$). The greatest improvement in survival was observed in women below the age of 55, in whom the 5-year survival rate for those treated with oxygen was 50% in contrast to 30% for the control group treated in air. The local recurrence rate was 33% in the 161 patients treated with oxygen and 53% in 159 patients treated in air. The difference is statistically significant ($p = 0.001$). The morbidity in the patients treated with oxygen was greater (20 severe and 13 moderate) than in those treated in air (6 severe and 8 moderate). The difference was particularly striking in the bowel (13 versus 2 severe complications, respectively).

On the other hand, an extensive trial of carcinoma of the cervix reported by Fletcher et al[280] in 233 patients with Stages IIB, III, and IV randomized to be treated with conventional irradiation in air or with hyperbaric oxygen demonstrated no significant benefit in survival or tumor control (20 of 109 patients treated with oxygen failing in the pelvis in contrast to 29 of 124 treated in air). Further, the morbidity was greater (26 complications) in patients treated with hyperbaric oxygen compared with the control group (15 complications). A smaller series reported by Glassburn and colleagues[281] showed no benefit in survival but increased morbidity with hyperbaric oxygen in carcinoma of the cervix. It is possible that hyperbaric oxygen administered with fewer high-dose fractions may be more efficacious than when combined with conventional dose and fractionation schemes.[282] The trials reported have not shown an increased incidence of distant metastasis, which has been reported in a clinical study and in some animal experiments.[283]

Thomas and co-workers[284] described a Phase I study of metronidazole carried out on 80 patients with various stages of carcinoma of the uterine cervix. The authors suggested that a daily dose of 1.3 g/m^2 was well-tolerated but no tumor response data were reported; Phase III clinical trials were recommended.

Dische[285] reported preliminary observations on the use of misonidazole in the treatment of advanced carcinoma of the cervix in 10 patients. The morbidity of this therapy is similar to that observed with irradiation alone, except for some misonidazole neurotoxicity. All 10 patients had more than 50% tumor regression, results believed to be very promising. A randomized study was recently carried out by the Radiation Therapy Oncology Group to evaluate the sensitizing effects of misonidazole in Stages III and IVA carcinoma of the cervix (daily dose of 400 mg/m^2 for a total of 12 g/m^2) treated with conventional fractionation. Preliminary results show no significant differences in survival, tumor control, or morbidity. The GOG has developed a protocol to compare misonidazole or hydroxyurea in combination with definitive irradiation in patients with Stages IIB, III, or IV carcinoma of the uterine cervix.

Because of technological limitations to deliver adequate heat to large parts of the body such as the pelvis, the evaluation of hyperthermia in the treatment of carcinoma of the uterine cervix has been sparse. Hornback and co-workers[286] recently reported on a nonrandomized study stating that the combination of microwave hyperthermia and irradiation

TABLE 36-13. Carcinoma of the Uterine Cervix, MIR 1959–1977, Irradiation Alone: Type of Grade III Severe Treatment Sequelae

	Stage						
	IA	*IB*	*IIA*	*IIB*	*IIIA*	*IIIB*	*IVA*
Total no. of patients treated	26	277	86	215	10	183	14
Number of complications (%)	1 (3.8)	22 (7.9)	7 (8.1)	32 (14.9)		13 (7.1)	2 (14.3)
Intestinal							
Rectovaginal fistula		2		5			
Sigmoid perforation		1		3			
Small bowel perforation			1				
Proctitis		2		2		2	
Rectal ulcer			3				
Sigmoid stricture		3	1	3		1	
Small bowel obstruction		1		4		4	
Other GI	1	1		2			
Urinary							
Cystitis		1					
Bladder ulcer		2		1			
Vesicovaginal fistula		3		2		3	1
Ureteral stricture		4	2	4		2	
Other GU							1
Other							
Pulmonary embolus						1	
Pelvic hemorrhage				1			
Pelvic abscess		1		1			
Arteriosclerosis				2			
Other		1		2			

Perez CA, Breaux S, Madoc-Jones H, et al: Radiation therapy alone in treatment of carcinoma of the uterine cervix: II. Analysis of complications. Cancer 54:235, 1984.

TABLE 36-14. Carcinoma of the Uterine Cervix, MIR 1966–1979, Stages IB and IIA: Major Complications of Treatment

	Stage IB				*Stage IIA*			
	Radiation Therapy Alone (40 Patients)		*Preoperative Radiation Therapy + Surgery (48 Patients)*		*Radiation Therapy Alone (16 Patients)*		*Preoperative Radiation Therapy + Surgery (14 patients)*	
	Grade 2	*Grade 3*	*Grade 2*	*Grade 3*	*Grade 2*	*Grade 3*	*Grade 2*	*Grade 3*
Rectovaginal fistula		1 (2.5%)						
Vesicovaginal fistula		2 (5%)						
Ureteral stricture		1 (2.5%)		1 (2.1%)				2 (14.3%)
Wound infection			1 (2.1%)					
Subcutaneous fibrosis	1 (2.5%)							
Vault necrosis	1 (2.5%)		1 (2.1%)		1 (6.3%)		1 (7.1%)	
Pelvic infection		1 (2.5%)						
Vaginal stenosis	6 (15%)		1 (2.1%)		2 (12.5%)			
Thrombophlebitis			2 (4.2%)					
Pelvic arteriosclerosis	1 (2.5%)							
Proctitis								1 (7.1%)
Rectal stricture						1 (6.3%)		1 (7.1%)
Acute pelvic cellulitis							1 (7.1%)	
Small bowel stricture								1 (7.1%)
Lymphocyst							1 (7.1%)	

Perez CA, Camel HM, Kao MS, et al: Randomized study of preoperative radiation and surgery or irradiation alone in the treatment of Stage IB and IIA carcinoma of the uterine cervix: Final report. Gynecol Oncol 27:129, 1987.

(433 mgh) resulted in improved tumor control in a group of 79 patients with Stage IIIB (72% local tumor control) in comparison with previously irradiated controls (35% and 53% tumor control). However, 5-year survival rates were similar in all groups (22–30%).

COMPLICATIONS OF IRRADIATION

Major complications of radiation therapy for Stages I and IIA carcinoma of the cervix range from 3% to 5% and for Stages IIB and III, between 10% and 15%. The most frequent major complications for the various stages are listed in Tables 36-13 and 36-14. Perez et al,[287] Kottmeier,[288] Pourquier et al,[289] and others have demonstrated a greater incidence of complications with higher doses of irradiation. Higher doses of external irradiation to the whole pelvis have also been associated with a greater number of complications (Fig. 36–13)[287] Injury to the gastrointestinal tract usually appears within the first 2 years after radiotherapy, whereas complications of the urinary tract are seen more frequently 3 to 4 years after treatment.[290] When preoperative radiation is combined with surgery, the complication rate tends to be somewhat higher (5–10%), particularly because of injury to the ureter or the bladder (ureteral stricture or uretero–vaginal or vesicovaginal fistula).

The dose and techniques of irradiation and the type of surgical procedures performed are important in determining the morbidity of combined therapy. Nelson et al[272] reported an incidence of severe complications of 17.5% in a group of 80 patients treated with radiation and radical hysterectomy in contrast to 7.4% major complications in a group of 95 patients treated with high-dose preoperative radiation and a conservative extrafascial hysterectomy.

The pretherapy staging laparotomy is fraught with a significant number of complications, particularly if irradiation is given (over 5000–5500 cGy) when metastatic para-aortic lymph nodes are found. The usual operative complications may be noted, such as pneumonia, thrombophlebitis, cardiovascular accident, hepatitis, or evisceration. Late complications include those of combined surgery and irradiation in the abdomen and pelvis, such as small bowel obstruction, stricture and fibrosis of the intestine or rectosigmoid, and rectovaginal or vesicovaginal fistula. With improving anesthesia, surgical techniques, and antibiotic therapy, the mortality for radical hysterectomy with pelvic lymphadenectomy has decreased to 1% or less.[221] Other complications include ureterovaginal fistula, the incidence of which has decreased to less than 3%.

FIG. 36-13. Major treatment sequelae (grades 2 and 3), radiation only, carcinoma of the uterine cervix. MIR, 1959–1977. (Perez CA, Breaux S, Mudoc-Jones H, et al: Radiation therapy alone in treatment of carcinoma of the uterine cervix. II. Analysis of complications. Cancer 54:235, 1984)

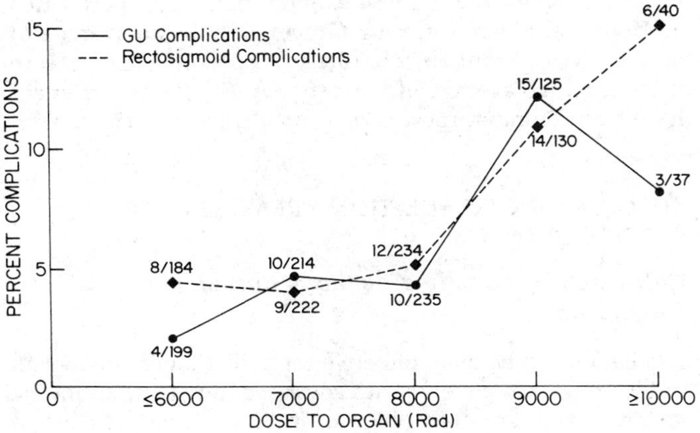

The incidence of complications has been listed between 5% and 20%, depending on the extent of the periaortic lymph node dissection, the transperitoneal or retroperitoneal approach for the operation, and the dose of irradiation given.[291,292] Tewfik et al[293] reported 27.8% complications in a group of 23 patients mostly with Stage IIIB carcinoma of the cervix treated with laparotomy and pelvic/periaortic nodal irradiation. Komaki et al[292] observed 3 small bowel obstructions in 22 patients (14%) receiving 5000 to 5500 cGy to the periaortic areas for histologically proven nodal metastases from carcinoma of the cervix or endometrium. In contrast, Potish et al[294] described only 2 patients with small bowel obstructions and 3 with large bowel complications in 81 patients (6%) with cervical carcinoma treated with radiotherapy alone (including periaortic lymph nodes) and not undergoing a surgical exploration. The risk of para-aortic nodal irradiation, when indicated, must be evaluated with respect to survival. Several authors[292,293,295] have reported survival rates of 30% to 40%, but, as previously noted in Table 36-9, other authors have reported lower survival rates.[292,293,295]

SURGICAL TECHNIQUES FOR CARCINOMA OF THE CERVIX

From the first hysterectomy for cervical cancer in 1878 by Freund[296] until the description of total pelvic exenteration by Brunschwig in 1948,[297] surgical treatment has played a vital role in the management of cervical cancer. In the following sections, the major surgical procedures are discussed briefly. No attempt has been made to describe the procedures in detail or to show drawings of the operations more suitable to a surgical text. The interested reader is referred to *Telinde's Operative Gynecology*.[298]

Cervical Conization

Conization of the cervix may be either diagnostic or therapeutic. It is indicated for the diagnostic evaluation of patients with cervical intraepithelial neoplasia or microinvasive carcinoma and is the standard therapeutic option for patients with CIN-3. Complications associated with cervical conization are hemorrhage, cervical stenosis, and uterine perforation.

Total Extrafascial Abdominal Hysterectomy

Total abdominal hysterectomy for the treatment of cervical carcinoma includes the removal of the uterus and the cervix.

The plane of excision lies just outside the pubocervical fascia and does not require unroofing of the ureters as they pass through the cardinal ligaments. A small vaginal cuff can easily be excised. Hysterectomy is indicated in selected cases for CIN-3 and for microinvasive cervical carcinoma when invasion is less than 3 mm and there is no lymphovascular invasion. Extrafascial hysterectomy is also used by some authorities after irradiation for barrel-shaped Stages IA and IB cervical carcinoma and after irradiation in early stage disease if the endometrium is involved.

Modified Radical Hysterectomy

In the modified radical hysterectomy, the ureter is unroofed from its canal, but the lateral attachments with their blood supply are preserved. Parametrial and paracervical tissue medial to the ureter is removed and a larger vaginal cuff is taken. Some authorities have recommended this operation for carcinoma in situ or microinvasive carcinoma of the cervix, but it is rarely used today.

Radical Abdominal Hysterectomy with Bilateral Pelvic Lymphadenectomy

In the radical hysterectomy, the ureters are dissected completely free from their tunnels through the paracervical tissues and the bladder is dissected free of the upper one third of the vagina. The uterosacral ligaments are severed near their point of origin posteriorly and the cardinal ligaments are severed at the lateral pelvic sidewall. This allows complete removal of the parametrial, paracervical, and upper paravaginal tissues as well as removal of the upper one fourth to one third of the vagina. The lymphadenectomy begins at the middle of the common iliac vessels and consists of removal of the distal one half of the common iliac and complete removal of the external iliac, hypogastric, obturator, and presacral lymph nodes. Many surgeons combine this operation with a selective para-aortic lymphadenectomy and begin the pelvic dissection at the bifurcation of the aorta.[221]

Average blood loss from radical hysterectomy and pelvic lymphadenectomy for cervical cancer is 1,500 to 1,800 ml, and most patients will require blood transfusions.[176,221] Aside from minor postoperative infections, the most common complication is neurogenic bladder dysfunction, and Webb and Symmonds[299] have reported poor bladder sensation in 31.5% of patients who required catheter drainage more than 14 days after surgery. Urinary tract fistulae are the most common serious complications of radical hysterectomy, but most modern series report the incidence to be less than 2%.[176,221,300] Pelvic lymphocysts and pelvic abscess are infrequent problems resulting from the use of closed suction drainage of the pelvis by most surgeons.

Radical hysterectomy is used for Stages IB and IIA cervical carcinoma. Its advantages and disadvantages have been cited previously. In the hands of well-trained, experienced surgeons it has an acceptable complication rate that is similar to that for full pelvic irradiation. Symmonds[300] has pointed out that the complications of radical hysterectomy are more often amenable to correction than the late complications of irradiation.

Selective Para-Aortic Lymphadenectomy

Selective para-aortic lymphadenectomy or para-aortic lymph node biopsy is an integral part of the management of patients with cervical carcinoma. Its use in pretreatment surgical staging has already been discussed. Many surgeons perform this procedure prior to radical hysterectomy, believing that if these lymph nodes contain metastatic cancer, the patient is better treated by extended field irradiation. Enlarged or suspicious lymph nodes seen on CT scan or lymphangiography can sometimes be sampled by fine needle aspiration guided by CT scan or fluoroscopy. If this sampling procedure is inadequate, para-aortic node biopsy is indicated.

Pelvic Exenteration

The use of pelvic exenteration for recurrent cervical cancer after irradiation therapy was introduced at Memorial Sloan-Kettering Cancer Center by Brunschwig in 1948.[297] In 1960 Brunschwig and Daniel[301] reported on 592 exenterations with a 5-year survival rate of 17% and an operative mortality of 23%. In 1987, Lawhead et al[302] reviewed the Memorial Sloan-Kettering Cancer Center experience with pelvic exenteration for the years 1972 through 1981 and reported an operative mortality of 9.8% and a 5-year survival rate of 23%. As of December 1981, 1,129 pelvic exenterations had been performed on the Gynecology Service at Memorial Sloan-Kettering Cancer Center.

Total pelvic exenteration consists of removal of the bladder, urethra, uterus, cervix, vagina, and rectum along with all lateral supporting tissues. Most surgeons differentiate between supralevator exenterations which stop at the floor of the pelvis and infralevator exenterations which excise part or all of the pelvic floor and include removal of the vulva. Posterior exenteration allows preservation of the urinary tract and anterior exenteration preserves the rectum. The urinary conduit can be constructed from the ileum, sigmoid, or transverse colon. On occasion, in a supralevator exenteration, the continuity of the large intestine can be maintained by low rectal anastomosis.

In recent years, improved radiation therapy equipment, improved training of radiotherapists, and better techniques for administration of irradiation have made central recurrence alone an unusual finding in cervical carcinoma. Between 1948 and 1971, 1,064 exenterations were performed at Memorial Sloan-Kettering Cancer Center, an average of 46.3 per year. From 1972 until 1981, 65 exenterations were performed, an average of 6.5 per year. Similar experiences have been found at most centers that treat cervical cancer.

SURGICAL OR IRRADIATION TREATMENT OF SPECIAL PROBLEMS

Palliation of Locally Advanced Carcinoma of the Cervix

Irradiation can be quite effective for palliation of pelvic pain or bleeding or in patients with advanced tumors in whom the general condition does not warrant a prolonged course of external irradiation with conventional fractionation. If vaginal bleeding is the main concern, a single intracavitary insertion with tandem and colpostats for about 6000 mgh (5500 cGy to point A) will suffice. If previous irradiation was delivered, lower intracavitary doses should be prescribed (4500–5000 mgh).

Several high dose fractionation schedules have been used, and Meoz et al[303] described satisfactory palliation with single doses of 1000 cGy combined with misonidazole, delivered every 3 to 6 weeks for a total 3000 cGy. Complications in the long-term survivors were relatively high (15%). The Radiation Therapy Oncology Group is conducting a Phase I/II trial using multiple (twice daily) fractions of 370 cGy each to deliver 740 cGy on two consecutive days, repeating every 3 to 6 weeks for a total of 4400 cGy.

Treatment of Recurrent Carcinoma of the Cervix

AFTER DEFINITIVE IRRADIATION. The irradiation of previously irradiated patients must be undertaken with extreme caution. It is very important to analyze the techniques used in the initial treatment (beam energy, volume, doses delivered with external or intracavitary irradiation) and the period of time between the two treatments. In general, we give external irradiation to limited volumes (4000–4500 cGy, 180 cGy total dose per fraction preferentially using lateral portals). Occasionally, intracavitary or interstitial irradiation can be used to treat relatively circumscribed recurrences.

Puthawala et al[304] treated 14 patients with interstitial implants who had received definitive radiotherapy at the time of initial treatment for carcinoma of the uterine cervix that recurred in the pelvis. Seven of them exhibited tumor control (50%). Palliation of symptoms after reirradiation was obtained in about 80% of the patients. The authors described no postoperative mortality. Severe complications occurred in 15% of the patients (soft tissue necrosis and one instance each of rectovaginal fistula, vesicovaginal fistula, enterovaginal fistula, and rectal stricture).

Prasavinichai et al[305] noted a 17.6% 5-year survival rate in 51 patients with recurrent tumors limited to the pelvis, treated with irradiation alone, pelvic exenteration (10 patients), or combination of exploratory laparatomy, debulking, and irradiation (10 patients). Prempree et al[306] treated 8 patients with late invasive cervical carcinoma recurrent after primary irradiation. Three survived tumor free more than 5 years after retreatment.

AFTER PREVIOUS SURGERY. It is easier to treat surgical recurrences with irradiation. We believe that a combination of external irradiation (2000–4000 cGy total dose) depending on volume of tumor and an additional parametrial dose with midline shielding for a total of 5000 to 6000 cGy is needed. In addition, an intracavitary insertion that may cover the vaginal vault or the entire vagina depending on tumor volume should be delivered. The total mucosal dose from the external and intracavitary therapy can approach 12,000 cGy without a high risk. It is extremely useful to combine these techniques with interstitial irradiation to boost the dose to the vaginal vault or the parametrium or paravaginal tissues when the volume of disease requires it. Doses in the range of 2000 to 3000 cGy are administered with single, double, or volume implants, depending on the extent of the tumor.

Friedman and Pearlman[307] reported a 42% tumor-free survival rate in 38 patients treated with irradiation after primary surgical therapy (7 were irradiated electively for close or positive margins, lymphatic permeation, or pelvic lymph node involvement). Six of the 7 patients were tumor free for 2 to 5 years. Of 14 patients with limited central recurrence, 8 were tumor free from 3.5 to 9 years. The worst results were noted with persistent or recurrent peripheral pelvic tumor (3 of 11 patients survived tumor free more than 5 years) or with massive pelvic recurrences (in 6 patients only palliation was achieved). Evans et al[308] reported on 114 patients found to have unresectable recurrent carcinoma of the cervix after primary irradiation or surgical treatment. Seventy patients were treated with irradiation (external, interstitial, or combination). Ten percent of the patients lived 15 months or longer and 5% survived 5 or more years (Fig. 36-14). Satisfactory palliation was observed in a large proportion of the patients.

FIG. 36-14. Survival of 70 patients in nonrandomized study with recurrent carcinoma of the uterine cervix treated with radiation therapy (external, brachytherapy, or a combination). (Evans SR Jr, Hilaris BS, Borber HRK: External vs. interstitial irradiation in unresectable recurrent cancer of the cervix. Cancer 28:1284, 1971)

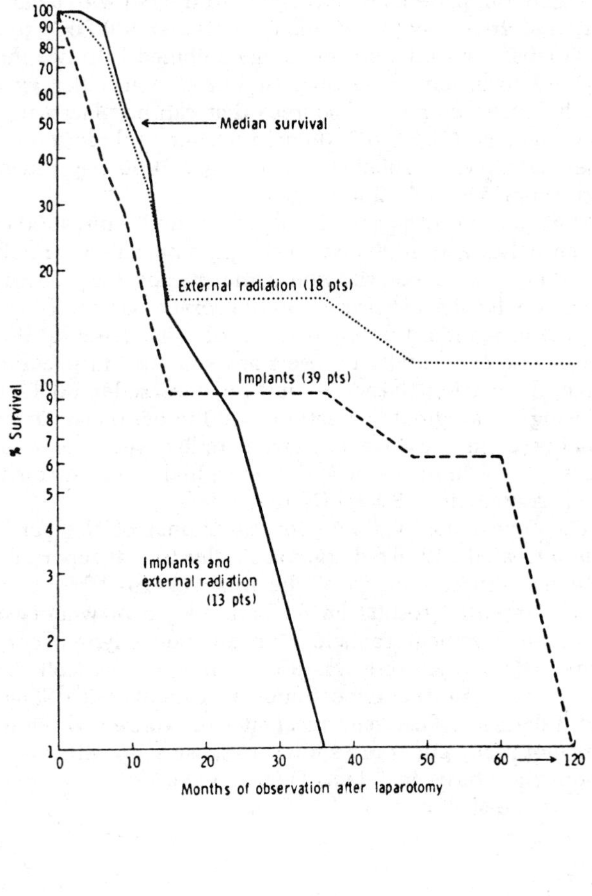

Carcinoma of the Cervical Stump

Subtotal hysterectomy, a relatively popular procedure for benign conditions of the uterus in past years, is performed rarely today. These patients are, of course, at risk to develop carcinoma of the uterine cervix. It is important to divide patients with carcinoma of the cervical stump into the following groups: *true,* when the first symptom occurs 3 or more years after subtotal hysterectomy, or *coincidental,* when the symptoms are noticed before the third postoperative year.[309] Moss et al[310] recommend two elapsed years after hysterectomy as the time for the classification of these lesions. This distribution is important because the prognosis for carcinoma of the true stump is significantly better than for coincidental lesions, which probably means that carcinoma was present at the time the hysterectomy was performed. The natural history and patterns of spread of carcinoma of the cervical stump are similar to those for the cervix in the intact uterus. The diagnostic workup, clinical staging, and basic principles of therapy are the same. When surgery is performed for Stage I tumors, it is somewhat more difficult because of the previous surgical procedures and the presence of adhesions in the pelvis.

When irradiation is administered, the lack of a uterine cavity into which to insert a tandem containing three or more sources makes intracavitary therapy more difficult. Whenever possible, sources should be inserted in the remaining cervical canal. Occasionally, transvaginal irradiation may be used to boost the dose delivered to central disease in the stump. It is important to deliver more whole pelvis irradiation.

In general, patients with Stage I are treated with a combination of 2000 cGy to the whole pelvis and 3000 cGy to the parametria with midline shielding combined with two intracavitary insertions. The dose of intracavitary therapy depends on the number of sources that can be placed in the cervical canal (1000 to 3000 mgh for one to three sources). The vaginal vault should receive about 7000 cGy mucosal dose (approximately 2000 mgh).

More advanced stages should be treated with 4000 cGy whole pelvis and 2000 cGy to the parametria with midline shielding, combined with the same intracavitary doses. If there is bulky disease present in the cervix, parametrium, or vagina, interstitial therapy with needles is advisable. When there is no opportunity to insert any sources in the cervical canal, the whole pelvis dose must be increased to 6000 cGy. In using intravaginal irradiation, 3000 to 5000 cGy air dose is delivered in 2 to 4 weeks in three to five weekly fractions. Moss et al[310] limit the dose to the vaginal vault for transvaginal irradiation to 3000 cGy in 10 days.

The 5-year survival rate for carcinoma of the cervical stump treated with irradiation is similar to that reported for patients with carcinoma of the intact uterus.[309,311] Creadnick[312] reported results on 83 patients, 25 of whom were treated with radical trachelectomy and pelvic lymphadenectomy. The salvage rate was 85.7% in squamous cell carcinoma and 50% in adenocarcinoma (patients with Stages I and II disease). The anatomical sites of failure and the incidence of recurrences are similar to those seen with cases in whom the uterus in intact. Distant metastasis also follows the same distribution.

Because of the proximity of the bladder, rectum, and small intestine to the intracavitary sources and the often higher doses of whole pelvis external beam irradiation given, complications are somewhat more frequent than in the carcinoma of the cervix with intact uterus. Wimbush and Fletcher[311] reported 5 fistulas, 6 cases of severe proctosigmoiditis, and 12 cases of vault necrosis in 238 patients treated with definitive radiotherapy.

Carcinoma of the Cervix During Pregnancy

Preinvasive and invasive cervical carcinoma that occurs during pregnancy requires the combined expertise of the gynecologic oncologist, maternal-fetal medicine specialist, and on occasion, the radiation oncologist. An abnormal Papanicolaou smear in the pregnant patient should be evaluated by colposcopy and biopsy.[313] Although an endocervical curettage should not be performed, the physiologic eversion of the cervix in pregnancy usually allows easy visualization of the squamocolumnar junction. Biopsy of the cervix requires a well-equipped treatment room because of the likelihood of profuse bleeding. Although conization of the cervix should be performed in patients with biopsies or Papanicolaou smears suspicious for invasion, less severe lesions can usually be followed by colposcopy and Papanicolaou smears with biopsy as necessary until the postpartem period. Several authors have reported the use of cervical conization in pregnancy with small to significant increases in morbidity and pregnancy wastage.[314,315]

When invasive cancer of the cervix is encountered, it is imperative that the patient be evaluated by the oncologist and the specialist in maternal-fetal medicine. The patient must be informed of all therapeutic options and their possible effects on both her fetus and her. In 1988, a tertiary level intensive care nursery can reliably obtain survival rates of about 80% for fetuses delivered at 28 weeks of gestation (1000-g fetus).[316] For patients less than 24 weeks gestation the pregnancy should be disregarded, whereas patients who are 28 weeks pregnant or more should have delivery of the fetus by cesarean section. Between 24 and 28 weeks, the patient and her physician must weigh the advantages and disadvantages of all courses of action because even though fetal survival rates at 28 weeks' gestation may be excellent, there is significant morbidity associated with the small birth weight infant.

The actual treatment of the cancer depends on the stage of disease and the usual considerations for selecting therapy. Radical hysterectomy can be performed either with the fetus in situ or in the case of a viable fetus immediately after delivery by cesarean section. If radiation is to be used, the patient will usually abort during the course of whole pelvis irradiation. If this does not occur, the uterus must be evacuated before insertion of intracavitary irradiation.[317,318] Survival has been reported to be similar in pregnant and nonpregnant patients matched by stage of disease regardless of the gestational age of the pregnancy.[317,319] Common practice is to avoid vaginal delivery in pregnancy because of the fear that delivery through a cervix involved with carcinoma will result in more rapid spread of the disease. However, Creasman et al[317] were not able to document decreased survival in

Stage I patients who had vaginal delivery before definitive treatment.

CHEMOTHERAPY OF CARCINOMA OF THE CERVIX

Because effective initial therapy with surgery and irradiation is available for most patients with cervical carcinoma, chemotherapy has been studied less completely.[320,321] Nevertheless, there are circumstances in which chemotherapy would play an important role, if effective regimens were identified. Groups of patients who are candidates for chemotherapy include those with advanced (Stages III and IV) disease, patients who have recurrent disease after surgery and radiation therapy, and patients who present with pelvic and periaortic nodal metastasis and therefore have a low potential for cure with standard treatment modalities.

In addition, chemotherapy could play a role as a radiation sensitizer, enhancing conventional irradiation. Finally, the location of cervical carcinoma and the regional localization in the pelvis have provided a rationale for the study of regional perfusion of the chemotherapy using intra-arterial infusion.

Factors that complicate the effective use of chemotherapy in cervical carcinoma include decreased pelvic vascular perfusion, limited bone marrow reserve, and poor renal function related to ureteral obstruction from tumor or fibrosis.

Single-Agent Chemotherapy

Table 36-15 lists the single agents that have some activity in cervical carcinoma. These data can be used only to suggest activity because, for the most part, they represent collected information from the literature in which variable criteria for response were used. Significant activity in well-designed studies with adequate patient numbers has been documented only for 5-FU and cisplatin,[322,323] although activity for dibromoducitol,[324] dianhydrogalactitol,[325] ifosfamide[325] and the platinum derivatives CHIP,[326] and carboplatin[327] has recently been documented.

Cisplatin remains the single agent with the best-documented activity.[323] The GOG evaluated 497 patients on three separate dose schedules: 50 mg/m^2 every 3 weeks; 100 mg/m^2 every 3 weeks; or 20 mg/m$^2 \times 5$ every 21 days. Responses were seen in 20%, 31%, and 25%, with complete responses in 10%, 13%, and 9%, respectively. The median duration of response was 4 months and the median survival 6.5 months. Significant nephrotoxicity and myelosuppression were seen with all regimens. Although there was a statistically significant difference in response rates favoring the high dose schedule, there were no differences in complete response rates or survival.

Combination Chemotherapy

Because there are several classes of cytotoxic agents with different mechanisms of action that have activity in carcinoma of the cervix, a number of combinations have been used. None of these combinations has been definitely shown to be more effective than single agents. Recently, however, several studies show 10% to 29% complete remission rates, suggesting some enhancement of effect. Table 36-16 lists combination chemotherapy studies in which reasonable numbers of evaluable patients have been studied, and the response rates appear to exceed those of single agents. However, the majority of the studies have not compared combination chemotherapy regimens to standard single agents, and the toxicity of these combinations is substantial. Although some of these combinations produce higher response rates, none has been definitely shown to be superior to single agent cisplatin in either duration of response or survival, particularly in patients who have recurrent disease after primary therapy.

Intra-arterial Chemotherapy

Intra-arterial infusions of chemotherapeutic agents in cervical carcinoma have been of considerable theoretical interest for some years based on the distinct arterial supply to the

TABLE 36-15. Single-Agent Chemotherapy in Cervical Cancer

Drugs	*Responders/Total Treated*	*Overall Response (%)*
Alkylating Agents		
Cyclophosphamide	31/228	14
Chlorambucil	11/44	25
Dibromodulcitol	4/15	27
Dianhydrogalactitol	7/36	17
Ifosfamide	10/30	30
Antimetabolites		
5-Fluorouracil	68/348	20
Methotrexate	12/77	16
Mitotic Inhibiters		
Vincristine	10/44	23
Antitumor Antibiotics		
Doxorubicin (Adriamycin)	8/78	10
Bleomycin	17/172	10
Other Agents		
Cisplatin	21/52	40
CHIP	7/36	21
Carboplatin	11/39	28
Piprazinedione	5/38	13

TABLE 36-16. Combination Chemotherapy in Cervical Carcinoma

Regimen	*Evaluable Patients*	*Number of Responses (%)*	*Complete Responses (%)*
Doxorubicin (Adriamycin) and methotrexate	59	39 (66)	13 (22)
	24	7 (28)	0 (0)
Doxorubicin and methyl-CCNU	13	14 (45)	9 (29)
Doxorubicin and cisplatin	19	6 (31)	2 (10)
Mitomycin C and bleomycin	33	12 (36)	5 (15)
Mitomycin C, vincristine and bleomycin	91	46 (51)	14 (15)
Mitomycin C, vincristine, bleomycin and cisplatin	14	6 (43)	4 (29)
Cisplatin, bleomycin and velban	33	22 (66)	6 (18)
Cisplatin, bleomycin, vincristine and methotrexate	15	10 (66)	3 (20)

tumor-bearing area. Unfortunately, the responses have been limited and the toxicity significant. Morrow et al[328] and Swenerton et al[329] each studied 20 patients using bleomycin or a combination of bleomycin and mitomycin-C and vincristine. Morrow et al[328] observed only 2 of 26 objective regressions; Swenerton et al[329] reported 3 of 20. The approach continues to be evaluated, using injections of either single drugs or combinations into the internal iliac arteries, and some studies report a reduction in complications related to the procedure and some responses.[330-333] However, randomized comparisons will be required to establish the benefits, if any, of intra-arterial chemotherapy infusions.

Chemotherapy as a Radiosensitizer

Continued interest in the use of chemotherapeutic agents as radiation sensitizers has been stimulated by the initial positive results with hydroxyurea. Piver et al[334] studied 130 patients with Stages IIB–IIIB cervical carcinoma in a prospective double-blind randomized study in which patients received split-course radiation therapy with or without hydroxyurea. In clinical Stage IIB patients, a significant improvement in 2-year survival was achieved for the group receiving hydroxyurea (74%) in comparison to the control group treated with radiotherapy and a placebo (43.5%). In clinically staged IIIB patients, 52% of those receiving hydroxyurea were alive at 2 years compared with 33% of those receiving a placebo with radiation ($p = 0.22$). Increased toxicity was noted in the hydroxyurea arm.[335,336]

Hreshchyshyn et al[337] and Piver[338] compared hydroxyurea or placebo combined with irradiation in Stages IIIB and IV cervical cancer. In 104 evaluable patients randomized to two treatment regimens, the complete response rate was 68% for the hydroxyurea-treated group and 48% for the placebo group ($p < 0.05$).[337] Duration of progression-free intervals and survival were also significantly better in the patients receiving hydroxyurea. Hematologic toxicity was more common and more severe in those patients receiving hydroxyurea. However, the results are less secure because the patients were not all surgically staged and substantial numbers of randomized patients were inevaluable. With effective radiotherapy alone, Fletcher[339] and Perez et al[340] demonstrated survival and tumor control similar to those observed with the addition of hydroxyurea in the two series described. Nevertheless, the two studies do suggest a potential role for radiation sensitizers in cervical carcinoma. Recently, cisplatin has been used as a radiation sensitizer in cervix carcinoma. Studies by Choo et al[341] randomized 45 Stage I and II patients to receive either radiation alone or radiation therapy with cisplatin 25 mg/m^2 intravenously weekly. Significantly higher complete response rates were noted in the radiotherapy and chemotherapy group (55%) compared with radiation alone (20%), but no differences in local recurrence rates or survival were reported. Two other studies have demonstrated that weekly low-dose cisplatin with irradiation is feasible and not associated with significant increases in toxicity but may be associated with a modest improvement in disease-free survival (54% versus 45%).[342,342a]

FUTURE DIRECTIONS

Conservative therapy (less than hysterectomy) is well established for Stage 0 (CIN-3) of the cervix. Prospective studies may show that conization of the cervix with negative margins and close follow-up may be sufficient for some patients with microinvasive cervical cancer. For patients with Stages IB and IIA cervical cancer, identifications of high risk subgroups may allow early use of adjunctive therapy with further improvements in survival. Combination therapy using irradiation and chemotherapy may be able to improve survival in advanced disease. Most important, every effort should be expended to develop chemotherapeutic agents effective in the therapy of squamous cell and adenocarcinoma of the cervix. All patients with advanced and recurrent cervical cancer should be considered for entry in clinical trials.

CARCINOMA OF THE ENDOMETRIUM

Carcinoma of the endometrium is the most common of the female genital cancers. It is estimated that there will be 34,000 new cases in 1988, which represents 48% of all female genital cancers and 6.9% of all malignancies occurring in women.[1] Although carcinoma of the endometrium accounts for 48% of all new cases of female genital cancer, it will cause only 13% of all gynecologic cancer deaths.[1] The low death rate in this disease is primarily due to early diagnosis. Approximately 78% of all uterine cancer is diagnosed while it is still confined to the uterus.[1]

EPIDEMIOLOGY

The largest number of cases of endometrial cancer occurs between the ages of 55 and 60, although 75% to 80% of cases occur after menopause and a significant number of cases are reported in each decade after age 50. The median age is 61.1 years.[343] Obesity,[344–346] nulliparity,[346,347] late menopause,[343] polycystic ovarian disease,[343,348] estrogen secreting tumors of the ovary,[348,349] and exogenous estrogen[350,351] are associated with an increased incidence of endometrial cancer. Nachtigall et al[352] and Gambrel[353] have shown that when progesterone is given with exogenous estrogen, there is no increased risk of endometrial cancer. Medical disorders associated with the development of endometrial cancer include diabetes, hypertension, arthritis, and hypothyroidism. Of these, hypertension and diabetes mellitus are most frequently observed.[343,354,355]

Carcinoma of the endometrium has been observed more frequently in Jewish women and is rare among Japanese women.[355] Sommers et al[356] have reported an increased susceptibility to endometrial cancer in some families, but in general the familial association does not appear to be strong.[357]

NATURAL HISTORY, ROUTES OF SPREAD, AND CLINICAL MANIFESTATIONS

The association of hyperplasia of the endometrium with endometrial carcinoma is well documented.[358] Cystic and adenomatous hyperplasias may be physiologic when they occur in an anovulatory hormonal environment before menopause but must be of more concern in a postmenopausal woman. Atypical adenomatous hyperplasia is a cause of concern in any woman, regardless of menstrual status.

Carcinoma of the endometrium may spread along the uterine cavity to the cervix, penetrate the uterine wall, or spread through the fallopian tubes. The carcinoma can spread by local extension to the ovary, broad ligament, vagina, or other pelvic organs. Malignant cells may spread by way of the lymphatics or less frequently through the bloodstream. The endometrial lymphatics begin beneath the glandular lining cells of the endometrium and drain into lymphatic vessels in the myometrium. Myometrial lymphatics, in turn, drain into the subserosal network which coalesces into larger channels before exiting the uterus. Lymph flow from the fundus travels toward the adnexa and infundibulopelvic ligaments, whereas flow from the lower and middle thirds tends to spread in the base of the broad ligament toward the lateral pelvic sidewall.[359] There are four drainage channels from the uterus according to Plentl and Friedman[359]: (1) from the fundus with the ovarian vessels, (2) in the folds of the broad ligament, (3) along the mesosalpinx and fallopian tubes, and (4) along the round ligaments to the femoral nodes.

In a review of the literature, Plentl and Friedman[359] found nodal metastases in 202 of 1,978 cases (10%) undergoing lymphadenectomy at the time of surgical therapy for endometrial carcinoma. In autopsy series, these same authors reported an incidence of 65%. Creasman et al,[360] reporting on a pilot study of the GOG in which patients with Stage I adenocarcinoma had selective pelvic and para-aortic lymph node sampling, reported an incidence of positive pelvic lymph nodes of 11.4% and of aortic nodes of 5.7%.

Metastases or extension of endometrial cancer to the fallopian tubes or the ovaries has been reported to occur in 5% to 10% of patients.[361] Cervical involvement has been found to occur with the same frequency.[362] Extension to the vagina occurs in about 7% of cases.[359] Metastases to the peritoneal cavity and the omentum are occasionally seen. Creasman et al[363] reported a recurrence rate of 34% in patients wtih positive peritoneal cytology as compared to a 10% recurrence rate in patients with negative peritoneal cytology. However, other authors have not confirmed this high recurrence rate.[364]

Almost all women with endometrial cancer report abnormal vaginal bleeding. Since 70% to 75% of women who develop the disease are postmenopausal, this symptom should be easily identified. The character of the abnormal bleeding varies from a serosanguinous discharge to frank bleeding. Pyometria and hematometria may be seen in patients with stenosis of the cervical canal. The finding of a pyometria in a postmenstrual woman should be considered highly suggestive of endometrial cancer. Pain is usually a symptom of advanced disease.

PATHOLOGY

Grossly, endometrial carcinoma is a polypoid growth that arises most often in the fundus of the uterus. The tumor may be small and focal or diffusely involve the uterine cavity. The diffuse lesions often show extensive hemorrhage and necrosis. The posterior wall is more likely to be involved than the anterior wall.

Histologically, most endometrial carcinomas are adenocarcinomas.[365] There is no evidence that adenoacanthoma behaves differently from pure adenocarcinoma. Recently several pathologists have begun using the term "adenocarcinoma with squamous metaplasia" to describe an adenocanthoma. Adenosquamous carcinoma of the endometrium contains malignant adenocarcinoma and malignant squamous carcinoma. Ng et al[366] and Silverberg[367] have described these lesions in detail, and both have reported a worse prognosis for them compared to pure adenocarcinomas. Both Silverberg et al[367] and Salazar et al[368] have related prognosis in these tumors to the differentiation of the adenocarcinoma portion of the tumor.

Infrequently seen carcinomas of the endometrium include clear cell carcinoma,[369] secretory carcinoma,[370] and squamous carcinoma.[371] Recently attention has been directed toward the papillary variety of endometrial carcinoma. Two varieties are recognized: an endometrioid papillary carcinoma and a serous papillary carcinoma. Although both have been reported to behave as poorly differentiated tumors, the serous papillary variety appears to carry the worse prognosis.[372,373]

The histologic grading of endometrial carcinoma is divided by FIGO into well differentiated (Grade 1), moderately differentiated (Grade 2), and poorly differentiated (Grade 3). In a GOG pilot study of 222 patients, Boronow et al[374] found the distribution of cases to be 42% Grade 1, 40% Grade 2, and 18% Grade 3. These authors were able to correlate increasing grade with an increased frequency of nodal metastases.

DIAGNOSIS, CLINICAL EVALUATION, AND STAGING

The diagnosis of endometrial carcinoma is made on the basis of a fractional dilation and curettage. The endocervical curettage should be performed before sounding or dilating the cervix to prevent contamination of the cervical sample by endometrial tissue that may be dislodged by the sound or dilator. If there is a visible lesion or a suspicious area on the cervix, biopsies should be obtained. If the diagnosis was made by office biopsy, a separate endocervical curettage should be obtained. Some authorities recommend that a formal dilatation and curettage be performed if carcinoma is diagnosed on office biopsy to be sure that the worst lesion is sampled. The Papanicolaou smear is not a reliable method of detecting endometrial cancer, even though occasionally malignant endometrial cells may be found in the Papanicolaou smears of asymptomatic patients with endometrial cancer. In such cases, a dilatation and curettage is indicated.

Patients diagnosed as having endometrial carcinoma should undergo a thorough history and physical examination, a careful pelvic examination, a chest radiograph, an intravenous pyelogram, a barium enema, cystoscopy, and proctosigmoidoscopy. Laboratory studies should include a complete blood count and biochemical profile to include renal and liver function tests. Other diagnostic studies such as CT, MRI, and lymphangiography may occasionally be helpful. Additional tests should be performed if warranted by symptoms.

The FIGO staging classification is listed in Table 36-17. As with other gynecologic cancers, staging should be performed jointly by the gynecologic oncologist, radiation oncologist, and medical oncologist. Stage I tumors are subclassified according to the grade of the tumor.

TABLE 36-17. FIGO Classification of Endometrial Carcinoma

Stage I	The carcinoma is confined to the corpus
Stage Ia	The length of the uterine cavity is 8 cm or less
Stage Ib	The length of the uterine cavity is 8 cm or more Stage I cases should be subgrouped with regard to the histologic type of the adenocarcinoma as follows: G1—Highly differentiated carcinoma G2—Differentiated adenocarcinomas with partly solid areas G3—Predominantly solid or entirely undifferentiated carcinomas
Stage II	The carcinoma involves the corpus and the cervix
Stage III	The carcinoma extends outside the corpus, but not outside the true pelvis (it may involve the vaginal wall or the parametrium but not the bladder or rectum)
Stage IV	The carcinoma involves the bladder or rectum or extends outside the pelvis

PROGNOSTIC FACTORS IN CARCINOMA OF THE ENDOMETRIUM

Age at time of diagnosis of endometrial carcinoma has long been known to be a prognostic factor. Frick et al[354] reported improved survival in patients under age 59 with Stage I disease even after correcting for deaths from intercurrent disease. Other authors[375a,376] have reported similar findings. Jones[376] attributed the improved survival to an increased incidence of less extensive, better differentiated lesions in younger women. Stage at diagnosis is directly related to survival. Creasman and Weed[343] reviewed three large series and reported average survivals of 79% for Stage I, 50% for Stage II, 27% for Stage III, and 9% for Stage IV. Cervical involvement has been associated with a worse prognosis in most series. Surwit et al[377] reviewed 117 patients with histologic involvement of the cervix. Overall survival for the entire group was 58%. However, when divided into those with stromal invasion and those with only involvement of endocervical glands, the survival rates were 47% and 74%, respectively. Uterine size in Stage I disease appears to be a less reliable indicator of prognosis. Lutz et al[378] state that uterine size does not always reflect actual tumor volume because of the association of benign uterine disease such as leiomyomata. Creasman et al,[360] however, noted an increased incidence of both pelvic and para-aortic lymph node metastases in stage IB as compared to Stage IA.

Perhaps the most significant prognostic factors for planning therapy in patients with early disease are histologic grade, depth of myometrial penetration, and lymph node metastases. Lewis et al[375] in 1970 reported an 11.2% incidence of nodal metastases in Stage I endometrial cancer, and in a literature review Morrow et al[360] reported that 10.6% of 369 patients with Stage I and 36.5% of 85 patients with Stage II disease had positive lymph nodes. Creasman et al[360] and Boronow et al,[375] reporting on a GOG pilot study, found that the incidence of both pelvic and para-aortic nodal metastases was related to increasing histologic grade, increasing depth of myometrial invasion, and, to a lesser extent, uterine size. DiSaia et al[379] evaluated recurrence and survival in that same group of patients and found those risk factors to be related to both increased rates of recurrence and decreased survival. Plentl and Friedman,[359] in an extensive review of the literature, found decreased survival in endometrial cancer to be directly related to both histologic grade and depth of tumor penetration of the myometrium. These same authors found that vaginal recurrence was also directly related to histologic grade. They reported 4.3% vaginal recurrence with Grade 1 tumors, 9.2% with Grade 2, and 24.4% with Grade 3.

TREATMENT OF CARCINOMA OF THE ENDOMETRIUM

Although the numbers of deaths from endometrial carcinoma are low in relation to cervical carcinoma and ovarian carcinoma, this is due to the large percentage of patients diagnosed in Stage I rather than the survival rates per stage. In a literature review, Morrow et al[380] reported survival rates of 76% for Stage I, 51% for Stage II, 26% for State III, and 9% for Stage IV. Boronow[381] found that survival in endometrial cancer was very similar to cervical cancer when corrected for stage distribution. In other series, the 5-year survival rate of surgery alone or combined with preoperative or postoperative radiation therapy has varied from 80% to 95%.[382-385]

The therapeutic approach for endometrial cancer is determined by FIGO stage, histologic type and grade, depth of myometrial penetration, and the medical condition of the patient.[386,387] Hysterectomy is the central feature of the management of most cases. The place of radiation therapy is in the adjunctive therapy of high-risk early-stage disease, in the management of advanced disease, and for those patients with early disease who are medically unsuitable for hysterectomy.[388,389]

Stages IA and IB Carcinoma of the Endometrium

Patients with Stages IA and IB endometrial carcinoma whose tumor is grade 1 can be managed by total abdominal hysterectomy and bilateral salpingo-oophorectomy. Removal of pelvic or para-aortic lymph nodes is not indicated as the incidence of nodal metastases is less than 5%.[360,374] If pathologic analysis of the uterus reveals invasion of greater than 50%, whole pelvic irradiation should be added even though the major effect of this irradiation may be to decrease the incidence of central recurrence rather than improve survival.[379,390] DiSaia et al[379] found that only 4% of grade 1 patients had deep myometrial invasion. Whether postoperative vaginal irradiation should be added in grade 1 patients with minimal myometrial invasion is controversial. The incidence of vaginal metastases is reported to be less than 5%[359,391] in grade 1 carcinomas.

Patients with histologic grade 2 or grade 3 carcinomas have a 15% and 39% incidence, respectively, of deep myometrial invasion.[374] The incidence of metastases to pelvic lymph nodes is 10% for grade 2 and 36% for grade 3, and aortic lymph nodes are involved in 4% of grade 2 tumors and 28% of grade 3 tumors.[360] Because of these factors, preoperative whole pelvis irradiation is used at Memorial Sloan-Kettering Cancer Center and para-aortic nodal sampling is performed at the time of hysterectomy. Vaginal irradiation is added postoperatively.

In preoperative insertions (^{137}Cs) for Stage I tumors, Perez at Washington University has used 3500 to 4000 mgh in the endometrial cavity. A surface dose of 6000 to 6500 cGy is also delivered to the surface of the vaginal fornices (1800–2000 mgh). Surgery is usually scheduled 3 days to 1 week after removal of the brachytherapy insertion to ensure that the true pathologic extent of the tumor can be adequately evaluated histologically. Although a higher degree of tumor sterilization is observed when surgery is performed 4 to 6 weeks after the brachytherapy placement, the pathologic features that can be helpful in determining whether further treatment is necessary, such as depth of myometrial invasion, are more difficult to evaluate.[392-394] Preoperative brachytherapy has the disadvantage that inadequate radiation dose is delivered to the pelvic lymph nodes. If tumor extension greater than 50% thickness of the myometrium or tumor extension beyond the uterus is demonstrated at the time of surgery, external beam irradiation should be added postoperatively.

In patients treated after total abdominal hysterectomy and bilateral salpingo-oophorectomy, the irradiation fields are the same as those used for preoperative irradiation. Whole pelvis fields are used for this boost, using a midline shield at some point during the treatment course as determined by calculating the bladder and rectal doses from the intracavitary insertion. Usually, 2000 cGy are delivered to the whole pelvis and 3000 cGy to the parametria with a midline block. If the patient has residual tumor left in the pelvis, a boost to the area of residual tumor is indicated. The indications for postoperative radiation therapy are deep myometrial invasion, transection of tumor, unsuspected advanced stage (ovary/tube/node involvement), and unsuspected poorly differentiated tumors.

Creasman and Weed[343] have recommended initial total abdominal hysterectomy with selective pelvic and para-aortic lymph node sampling in all Stage IA and IB grade 2 and 3 patients. These authors would then add postoperative pelvic or vaginal irradiation based on findings at surgery.

Stage II Carcinoma of the Endometrium

In Stage II endometrial carcinoma, the cancer has involved the cervix *(corpus et collum)*. There appears to be little doubt that survival is significantly lower in these patients.[359,367,377,395] Surwit et al[377] reported survival rates of 74% if only the endocervical glands were involved. Homesley et al[345] in a review from Memorial Sloan-Kettering Cancer Center reported survival rates of 61% if cervical involvement was occult and 48% if there was gross involvement of the cervix. Recently, however, Larson et al[396] from M.D. Anderson Hospital divided patients into three groups: gross cervical involvement, occult stromal invasion, and no evidence of stromal invasion. They reported survival rates of 70%, 65%, and 67% in each group respectively and concluded that there is no prognostic significance in the extent of cervical involvement.

Most authorities use a combination of whole pelvis irradiation and a single intracavitary application of cesium followed by total abdominal hysterectomy and bilateral salpingo-oophorectomy for Stage II carcinoma of the endometrium.[396,397] At Washington University, based on previous experience recently reported by Grigsby et al,[398] patients with Stage II endometrial carcinoma who have only microscopic involvement of the endocervix are treated with a preoperative intracavitary insertion followed by an extrafascial hysterectomy and bilateral salpingo-oophorectomy. In general, the dose delivered is 3500 to 4000 mgh to the body of the uterus and 6000 cGy to the vaginal vault (1800 to 2000 mgh) with 2 cm colpostats. If there is gross or multiple quadrant microscopic involvement of the exocervix, in addition to the intracavitary insertion, the patient receives external irradiation (2000 cGy whole pelvis and 3000 cGy additional dose to the parametria with midline shield) followed by an extrafascial hysterectomy approximately 4 weeks later. For the inoperable patient, or in the case in which surgery is refused, radiation alone is used. At Memorial Sloan-Kettering Cancer Center, whole pelvis irradiation followed in 3 to 4 weeks by modified radical hysterectomy with para-aortic nodal sampling is used for Stage II endometrial carcinoma.

Although some series have reported the use of radical hysterectomy and bilateral pelvic lymphadenectomy in these patients, Rutledge[399] has pointed out that therapy with irradiation followed by hysterectomy has greater usefulness for most patients and the cure rate is comparable.

Stages III and IV Carcinoma of the Endometrium

Most patients with advanced endometrial cancer will not be candidates for operation. Because the distribution of tumor within the pelvis may vary, no single technique is applicable to all patients. External beam therapy is the mainstay of treatment; whole pelvis irradiation is given for 2000 to 4000 cGy, with an additional boost to the parametria given with midline shield to complete 5000 to 6000 cGy in 5 to 7 weeks. The central dose is supplemented with at least two brachytherapy applications for approximately 8000 mgh. Afterloading Simon-Heyman capsules and the Fletcher-Suit applicators lend themselves best to the differential loading necessary to achieve the best possible dose distribution. If lower third vaginal extension is present, volume interstitial implantation with brachytherapy sources is indicated.

Endometrial carcinoma that is Stage III based on involvement of the upper vagina may be managed by preoperative whole pelvis and intracavitary irradiation and total abdominal or modified radical hysterectomy and a wide vaginal cuff.

RESULTS OF TREATMENT USING RADIATION THERAPY IN CARCINOMA OF THE ENDOMETRIUM

Statistically valid data are not available to support the impact of adjuvant radiotherapy on survival. However, in a randomized study, Graham[400] reported better 5-year survival rates with combination therapy as opposed to hysterectomy alone, although the differences between the preoperative and postoperative irradiation groups were not statistically significant. Nolan et al[384] in a nonrandomized study also demonstrated improved survival with combined therapy in patients with Stage I in high risk groups (large uterus or less differentiated lesions).

Nevertheless, there has been a significantly decreased incidence of vaginal recurrences in patients treated with irradiation (1–3%) in contrast to those treated with hysterectomy alone (15%). A review of 304 patients treated at the Mallinckrodt Institute of Radiology, using preoperative intracavitary therapy alone in 199 patients, in addition to 43 patients on whom additional external irradiation was given (usually 2000–3000 cGy whole pelvis), demonstrated an overall pelvic recurrence rate of 4% for grade 1, 3% for grade 2, and 9% for grade 3 lesions.[401] Survival is shown in Figure 36-15. Table 36-18 shows 5-year survival figures for patients with Stage I disease, as reported in the literature.

Several authors have reported a greater incidence of vaginal pelvic recurrences and distant metastases in patients with poorly differentiated (grade 3 tumors) or in those with advanced stage. However, radiation therapy has been shown to decrease the incidence of pelvic recurrences. Bedwinek et al[407] reported a 71% overall 5-year disease-free survival,

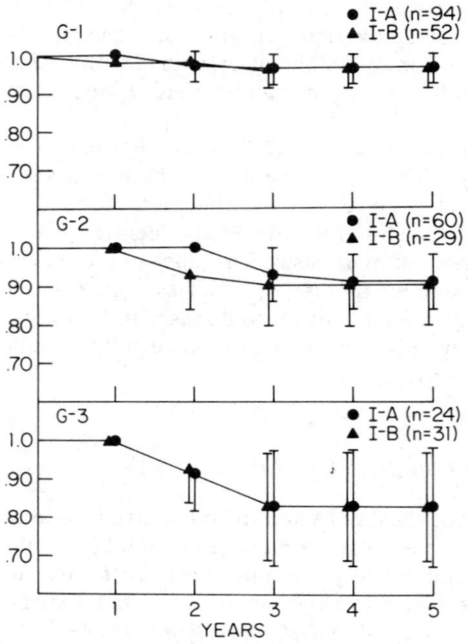

FIG. 36-15. Disease-free survival by grade and stage. (Stokes S, Bedwinek JM, Kao M-S, et al: Treatment of Stage I adenocarcinoma of the endometrium by hysterectomy and adjuvant irradiation: A retrospective analysis of 304 patients. Int J Radiat Oncol Biol Phys 12:339, 1986)

9.6% incidence of pelvic recurrences, and 15.6% distant failures in 83 patients with Stage I grade 3 endometrial carcinoma treated with either intracavitary irradiation alone or combined with pelvic external radiotherapy.

Uterine size in Stage I has been found to correlate with prognosis only if the enlargement is related to tumor infiltration in the myometrium (Table 36-19). Wade et al[415] and Javert[416] noted that often benign conditions such as myomata and adenomyosis may contribute to uterine enlargement and have no significant impact on prognosis. Stokes et al[401] observed similar survival rates in Stages IA and IB patients regardless of the tumor differentiation. Myometrial invasion decreases the 5-year survival rate from 85% to 90% when it is absent to 60% to 79% when involvement is more

TABLE 36-18. Stage I Endometrial Carcinoma Survival at 5 Years

Author	*No. of Patients*	*% Survival at 5 Years*
Bleiler et al[402]	282	64 crude
Wharam et al[403]	269	81 NED
Graham[400]	123	74 crude
Malkasian et al[404]	409	82 actuarial
Underwood et al[385]	220	91 actuarial
Frick et al[354]	239	78 crude
Salazar et al[405]	307	84 actuarial
Brady et al[406]	99	88 crude
Stokes et al[401]	304	

Modified from Glassburn JR, Brady LW: Carcinoma of the endometrium. In Perez CA, Brady LW (eds): Principles and Practice of Radiation Oncology, pp 966–987. Philadelphia, JB Lippincott, 1987.

TABLE 36-19. Five-Year Survival Rates Correlated with Depth of Myometrial Invasion

	No Invasion		*Superficial Invasion*		*Deep Invasion*	
	No. of Patients	*5-Year Survival Rate (%)*	*No. of Patients*	*5-Year Survival Rate (%)*	*No. of Patients*	*5-Year Survival Rate (%)*
Author						
Anderson[408]	12	100	22	86	7	42
Gusberg[409]	245	67	96	70	94	34
Climie[335]	56	87	20	80	23	56
Austin[336]	133	91	239	95	163	81
Cheon[410]	181	81	91	77	73	42
Nilson[411]			205	89	131	76
Lewis[375]	16	93	41	88	22	54
Ng[412]	129	88	48	72	22	27
Sall[413]			75	92	16	75
Nahhas[414]	75	85	33	82	28	56
Frick[354]	63	79	101	77	42	45
Total patients	910		971		621	
Total survivors	736		827		376	
Average 5-year survival rate		80		85		50

Adapted from Jones HW III: Treatment of adenocarcinoma of the endometrium. Obstet Gynecol Surv 30:147, 1975.

than half way through the myometrium (Fig. 36-16).[376,379] Similar results are correlated with the degree of differentiation of the tumor (Table 36-20).

A few reports have compared the effectiveness of external irradiation or intracavitary radium without conclusive results. Sala and del Regato[422] compared the survival after 4000 cGy external irradiation to the pelvis (70 patients) or a radium implant for 6000 cGy (48 patients). The 3-year survival rate was 87% and 77%, respectively. No vaginal recurrences were noted in either group. The survival rate was similar whether residual tumor was present in the surgical specimen or not. Similar findings were reported by Silverberg and DeGeorgi[423] in 76 patients treated with preoperative irradiation and hysterectomy. Weigensberg[424] in a randomized study involving small groups of patients in two community hospitals observed a 5-year actuarial disease-free survival rate of 75% in 53 patients treated with intracavitary irradiation and hysterectomy and of 48% in 38 patients treated with external beam irradiation. Patients treated with intracavitary radium received 5400 cGy and with external beam irradiation, 4000 cGy. Only 2 of the intracavitary therapy patients had pelvic recurrences in contrast to 9 in the external beam group. Uterine size and degree of tumor differentiation were similar in both groups. Aalders et al[390] in a randomized trial, and Bedwinek et al[407] in a nonrandomized retrospective review, reported similar survival rates with intracavitary therapy alone or combined with external irradiation. However, pelvic recurrences can be decreased with external irradiation in patients with less differentiated tumors from about 20% to 5%.

FIG. 36-16. NED survival by depth of myometrial invasion (quick or postoperative radiotherapy) for endometrial carcinoma patients. (Stokes S, Bedwinek JM, Kao M-S, et al: Treatment of Stage I adenocarcinoma of the endometrium by hysterectomy and adjuvant irradiation: A retrospective analysis of 304 patients. Int J Radiat Oncol Biol Phys 12:339, 1986)

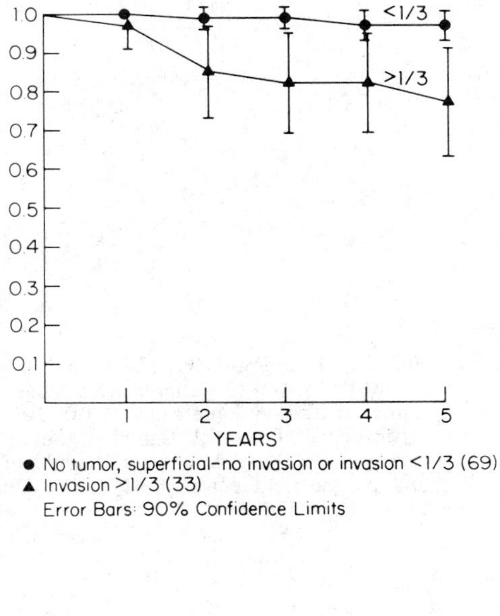

In 19 patients with Stage II endometrial carcinoma treated by an intracavitary insertion and external beam radiation to the whole pelvis, a 63% 5-year survival rate was obtained.[425] A report by Grigsby et al[398] from the Mallinkrodt Institute of Radiology disclosed 8 pelvic recurrences in 79 patients (10%) with stage II endometrial carcinoma treated by a combination of preoperative or postoperative intracavitary insertion and external irradiation. Eleven patients with microscopic endocervical involvement treated only with a preoperative intracavitary insertion had no pelvic or vaginal recurrence. In a small group of 26 patients with Stage II endometrial carcinoma treated with irradiation alone, the overall incidence of pelvic failure was 34.6%, in contrast to only 8.9% in those treated with a combination of irradiation and surgery. The survival and NED survival rates are illustrated in Figure 36-17.

It is known that gross involvement of the cervix carries a

TABLE 36-20. Relationship Between Tumor Differentiation and 5-Year Survival Rates in Patients with Endometrial Carcinoma

	Grade I		*Grade II*		*Grade III*	
	No. of Patients	*5-Year Survival Rate (%)*	*No. of Patients*	*5-Year Survival Rate (%)*	*No. of Patients*	*5-Year Survival Rate (%)*
Author						
Webb[417]	32	84	155	52	37	30
Lindgren[418]	120	88	153	82	56	80
Gusberg[409]	204	62	85	53	65	32
Boutselis[419]	81	75	42	64	49	14
Anderson[408]	14	100	51	82	26	65
Climie[335]	56	93	24	75	18	44
Dobbie[420]	147	81	74	78	45	73
Roman[421]	47	87	105	78	113	51
Wade[415]	65	84	150	78	50	42
Austin[336]	126	96	239	96	163	75
Cheon[410]	196	81	72	78	77	44
Ng[412]	91	86	101	75	62	37
Nahhas[414]	106	84	57	75	35	48
Beiler[402]	54	83	130	65	67	40
Frick[354]	218	79	76	54	54	30
Total patients	1558		1515		917	
Total survivors	1267		1124		462	
Average 5-year survival rate		81		74		50

Adapted from Jones HW III: Treatment of adenocarcinoma of the endometrium. Obstet Gynecol Surv 30:147, 1975.

worse prognosis than microscopic involvement. Noteably, Grigsby et al[398] reported lower survival in patients with ectocervical tumor invasion, even if it was microscopic only. Patterns of failure reported by various authors in patients with Stage II endometrial carcinoma are summarized in Table 36-21.

Unfortunately the results of treatment for Stage III disease are poor. A 25% 5-year survival is to be expected with aggressive therapy, with somewhat better results being obtained in patients who had ovarian involvement only (Table 36-22). Patients with Stage IV disease are rarely cured, and most authors report 5% of the patients alive at 5 years.

SURGERY FOR CARCINOMA OF THE ENDOMETRIUM

The usual surgical procedure for adenocarcinoma of the endometrium is abdominal hysterectomy and bilateral salpingo-oophorectomy. On occasion, some authorities will recommend modified radical hysterectomy or radical hysterectomy for Stage II disease. The techniques for these procedures are identical to those described under the section on cervical cancer and need not be repeated here. Most surgeons do not recommend that the cervix be sutured closed before abdominal hysterectomy for endometrial carcinoma although this was common practice in the past. Nei-

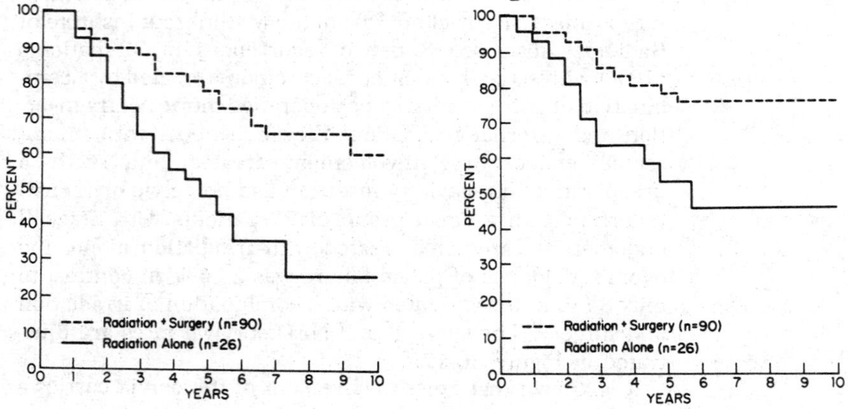

FIG. 36-17. Overall survival (**A**) and disease-free survival (**B**) in 116 patients with Stage II carcinoma of the endometrium. MIR, 1960–1981. (Grigsby PW, Perez CA, Camel HM, et al: Stage II carcinoma of the endometrium: Results of therapy and prognostic factors. Int J Radiat Oncol Biol Phys 11:1915, 1985)

TABLE 36-21. Carcinoma of the Endometrium: Treatment Outcome of Stage II Disease

Investigator	No. of Patients	Survival (%)	No. of Recurrences (%): Vagina	Pelvis	Vagina + Pelvis	Pelvis + DM	DM
		Stage II—Radiation Therapy and Surgery					
Gagnon et al[426]	20	44.8*		1 (5)			2 (10)
Onsrud et al[427]	44†	85			1 (2.3)		4 (9.1)
	40‡	85	2 (5)	2 (5)	3 (7.5)		4 (10)
Salazar et al[405]	20			1 (5)			3 (15)
Spanos et al[428]	61				12 (19.7)§		Not reported
Total‖	124		2 (1.6)	4 (3.2)	4 (3.2)	0	13 (10.5)
				Total pelvis 8%			Total DM 10.5%
		Stage II—Radiation Therapy Alone					
Landgren et al[429]	38	65**		3 (7.9)		4 (10.5)	9 (23.7)
Salazar et al[405]	8			3 (37.5)			2 (25)
Spanos et al[428]	21				4 (19)††		Not reported
Total‖	46			6 (13)		4 (8.7)	11 (23.9)
					Total pelvis 21.7%		Total DM 32.6%

Perez CA, Bedwinek JM, Breaux SR: Patterns of failure after treatment of gynecological tumors. Cancer Treat Symp 2-217, 1983.
* Five years.
† Radium only.
‡ Radium + external.
§ Value = combined total or recurrences in pelvis, vagina and pelvis, and pelvis + DM in study by Spanos et al.
‖ Excluding Spanos et al.
** Actuarial, 5 years.
†† Value = combined total of recurrences in pelvis and pelvis + DM in study by Spanos et al.

ther do most surgeons tie the fimbriated ends of the fallopian tubes upon opening the abdomen, although most do recommend placing clamps across the cornual region to occlude the fallopian tubes and provide traction during the procedure. Pelvic exenteration has been used for central recurrence after irradiation, but the utility of this procedure in endometrial carcinoma is limited.[437]

TECHNIQUES OF IRRADIATION FOR CARCINOMA OF THE ENDOMETRIUM

Combinations of Irradiation and Surgery

A variety of techniques have been used combining irradiation and surgery in the treatment of Stage I endometrial cancer, including external beam, brachytherapy, or combinations of

TABLE 36-22. Stage III Endometrial Carcinoma: Survival Rates at 5 Years

Author	No. of Patients	Survival at 5 Years (%)
Antoniades et al[430]	37	25
Rutledge and Ehrlich[431]		21
Buchler et al[357]	32	22
Kottmeier[432]	136	30
Homesley et al[433]	23	4
Boronow[434]	49	18
Geisler and Gibbs[435]	19	5.3
Ng and Reagan[412]	14	13.6
Danoff et al[436]	17	11.7

Danoff BF, McDay J, Louka M, et al: Stage III endometrial carcinoma: Analysis of patterns of failure and therapeutic implications. Int J Radiat Oncol Biol Phys 6:1491, 1980.

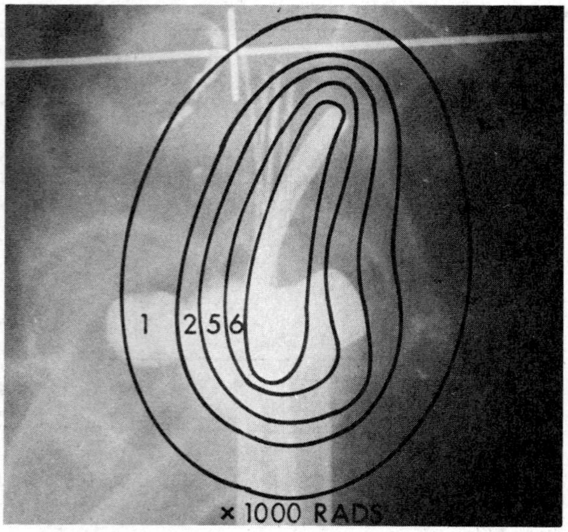

A

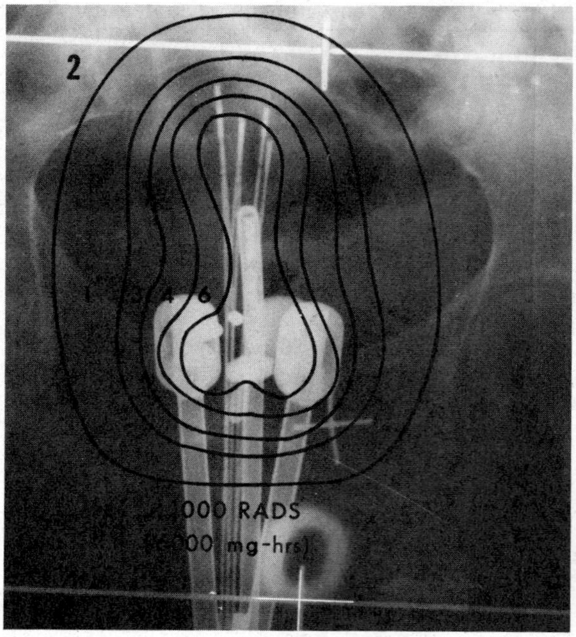

B

FIG. 36-18. Frontal (**A**) and lateral (**B**) radiographs of intracavitary insertion in patient with carcinoma of the endometrium showing Heyman-Simon afterloading capsule in the uterine fundus, tandem in the lower uterine segment, and ovoids in the vaginal vault. (Perez CA, DiSaia PJ, Knapp RC: Gynecologic tumors. In DeVita VT Jr, Hellman S, Rosenberg SA [eds]: Cancer: Principles and Practice of Oncology, 2nd ed, pp 1013–1081. Philadelphia, JB Lippincott, 1985)

both. Irradiation has been administered preoperatively or postoperatively or as a combination of both.

Preoperative irradiation has several aims: to decrease the opportunity of viable tumor cells seeded in the operative field to develop into a local recurrence, to render the tumor cells nonviable and decrease the possibility of distant dissemination of the tumor, and to irradiate the areas of frequent nodal involvement that are not removed at the time of surgery. The techniques of external beam irradiation, volume to be treated, and portals used are similar to those used in the treatment of carcinoma of the uterine cervix.

For the intracavitary insertions, in addition to afterloading tandem and vaginal ovoids, it is common practice to pack the uterine cavity with Heyman or afterloading Heyman-Simon capsules (Fig. 36-18). This technique allows the placement of sources in the body of the uterus around the tumor and, at the same time, some pressure can be exerted on the uterine wall, it is hoped with some reduction in its thickness. These two effects may result in higher doses of irradiation delivered to the serosa of the uterus and immediately adjacent paracervical tissues. The lower segment of the uterus and the endocervical canal can be treated with capsules or with a tandem. The vaginal vault is always irradiated with vaginal colpostats. If there is tumor extension into the vagina, the entire length of this organ should be treated with a cylinder or special applicator (*i.e.*, Burnett, Bloedorn, Delclos) to include the suburethral regions and introitus because of the propensity of advanced endometrial adenocarcinoma to metastasize to this site through submucosal venous and lympathatic plexuses.

Radiation Therapy Alone

Medically inoperable patients with Stage I or II disease in a significant percentage of cases can be cured with a combination of external beam therapy and brachytherapy. Usually two intracavitary insertions are carried out, 2 weeks apart, to deliver 4500 to 5000 mgh to the uterine cavity and an additional 3000 mgh to the vaginal vault. This is combined with external beam therapy for an additional 2000 to 4000 cGy to the whole pelvis, and subsequent boosting of the lateral pelvic dose to a total of 5000 cGy with a midline pelvic shield to protect the bladder and bowel. Survival rates of 74% to 78% at 5 years have been reported.[389,438]

COMPLICATIONS OF THERAPY

Surgical or combined treatment by surgery and adjuvant irradiation in endometrial carcinoma is well tolerated. Major complications, as reported by Stokes et al,[439] with a preoperative implant and hysterectomy, were noted in 1% of 199 patients. However, if the intracavitary insertion was given postoperatively, 12% of the patients (3 of 26) had significant complications. When external irradiation was given—the dose to the whole pelvis combined with an intracavitary insertion—the complication rate was 2% (5 in 264 patients) but increased to 18% (7 in 40 patients) when the whole pelvis dose exceeded 3000 cGy. A total of 8 major gastrointestinal and 4 urinary complications were noted in 304 patients, the most frequent being bowel obstruction, ureterovaginal fistula, uretheral stricture, hemorrhagic cystitis, and rectal ulcer.

CHEMOTHERAPY OF CARCINOMA OF THE ENDOMETRIUM

Hormonal Therapy

The most commonly used systemic treatment in recurrent endometrial carcinoma has been synthetic progestational agents. The response rates range from 30% to 37%.[440] Responses are associated with prolonged survival; median survival for patients responding to progesterone therapy has been 23 to 29 months compared to 6 months for patients without an objective response.[440] Response to hormonal therapy is related to the histologic grade of the tumor, and well-differentiated tumors respond more frequently than do those with poorly differentiated histologies. Other factors that influence response to hormonal therapy include disease-free interval, age, and presence of areas of squamous metaplasia within the tumor. Responses are more likely in vaginal or lung metastases and lymph nodes and less likely in pelvic recurrences.

The progesterone receptor content of endometrial tumors correlates well with subsequent response to progesterone therapy.[441,442,443] Even though well-differentiated tumors tend to have the highest progesterone receptor positivity, the receptor positivity appears to be a better correlate than grade.

In studies on 114 endometrial adenocarcinomas, the mean progesterone-binding capacity was inversely related to tumor grade.[441] Although more data are needed to firmly establish the value of progesterone receptor (PR) analysis, it is noteworthy that this study reported that 88% (30 of 34) of progesterone-responsive lesions were PR(+) and 94% (34 of 36) of unresponsive lesions were PR(−).

Systemic hormonal therapy with progestogens has been well established as first-line systemic therapy for patients with recurrent or disseminated disease. The most commonly used progestogens have been hydroxyprogesterone (Delalutin) or medroxyprogesterone (Depo-Provera, 400 mg intramuscularly weekly). Oral megastrol acetate (Megase), 160 mg/day, produces similar results. These progestogens should be continued indefinitely until recurrence or distant metastases develop.

Studies using alternative endocrine therapy for advanced endometrial cancer, including the antiestrogen tamoxifen[444,445] and the synthetic 17-ethinyl testosterone derivative danazol, have suggested some activity. Data from several studies with tamoxifen[446-449] suggest an overall response rate of approximately 39% with well-differentiated tumors being more likely to respond. Recently, attempts have been made to enhance the activity of hormonal therapy by sequential therapy with tamoxifen that induces progesterone receptors.[450] Although an increase in progesterone receptors was documented, the overall response rate was 33%, not significantly different from progesterone alone. However, further studies to study the modulation of progesterone receptors in endometrial cancer are warranted.

The use of progestogen therapy as prophylaxis in early-stage endometrial carcinoma remains controversial. In one large adjuvant trial, Stage I patients received either adjuvant Depo-Provera or a placebo.[451] Despite unbalanced stratification with regard to prognostic factors and frequent unevaluability, there was no difference in 5-year survival rates. Another study of 35 Stage IA and Stage IB patients treated with surgery with or without subsequent treatment with 6-methyl-17-hydroxyprogesterone reported no benefit.[452] Despite this, several investigators have advocated the use of prophylactic progestational agents in high risk patients.[453-457] However, the worth, if any, of adjuvant progesterone therapy in early-stage endometrial carcinoma must be considered unproven. Two ongoing trials, one in Australia[440] and one in Italy[458] that include only high risk patients, suggest some beneficial effect, but further follow-up is needed in this important subgroup of patients.

Single-Agent Chemotherapy

Nonhormonal chemotherapy has been studied to a limited degree. Table 36-23 lists the single agents that appear to have some activity in advanced endometrial cancer.[459-462] These data can be used only to suggest activity because of the small numbers of patients studied and the variability of prognostic factors. Of these agents, only doxorubicin, hexamethylmelamine, and cisplatin appear to have clearly established

TABLE 36-23. Single Agent Chemotherapy in Endometrial Carcinoma

Drugs	*Patients Responding/Total Treated*	*Response Rate (%)*
Alkylating agents		
Cyclophosphamide	7/33	21
Nitrogen mustard	3/11	27
Antimetabolites		
5-Fluorouracil	10/43	23
Antitumor Antibiotics		
Doxorubicin (Adriamycin)	33/92	36
Bleomycin	3/8	37
Miscellaneous Agents		
Hexamethylmelamine	6/29	30
Cisplatin	11/26	42
Cisplatin	4/13	31

activity[463,464] with response rates in the 30% to 40% range.

Of all the single agents, doxorubicin has been most extensively evaluated and appears to be the standard single agent to which new agents or combinations should be compared. Thigpen et al[465] treated 43 patients with advanced or recurrent disease using 60 mg/m^2 intravenous doxorubicin every 3 weeks. They reported a 37% response rate (16 of 43), and 26% (11 of 43) had clinical complete regression of disease. Median survival was 14 months for patients achieving a complete response, 6.8 months for those with a partial regression, and 3.5 months for patients with progressive disease. Age, time to first recurrence, histologic grade of primary site of metastasis, and previous therapy had no effect on probability of response. Toxicity was similar to other studies in which doxorubicin was used as a single agent.

Conflicting reports on the activity of cisplatin in this disease may relate to its low activity (1 of 25, 4%) when used as second-line treatment[460] and its reasonable response rate (46%) when used at higher doses (100 mg/m^2) in patients who had not been previously treated with chemotherapy.[461]

Combination Therapy

Combination chemotherapy for advanced endometrial carcinoma has not been studied extensively. The relatively few studies that have been published generally include small patient numbers.[463,464] Recent studies employing doxorubicin and cisplatin[466,467] report higher response rates (30–90%) but with only a few patients treated. Comparison of this two-drug regimen with doxorubicin alone[468] demonstrates a 45% response rate for the combination compared to 20% for the single agent. Cisplatin, doxorubicin (Adriamycin), and cyclophosphamide (PAC) demonstrated a 45% overall response rate in 209 patients at a cost of moderate to severe toxicity.[469] Another study of the three-drug regimen CAP, including cisplatin 50 mg/m^2, cyclophosphamide 500 mg/m^2, and doxorubicin 50 mg/m^2 intravenously every 4 weeks, produced a 58% response rate, including 28% complete remissions in 18 patients with advanced disease.[470] Both the AP and CAP combinations appear to have some enhanced activity and should be compared to doxorubicin alone in larger trials. Other studies have added combination chemotherapy and progestogens, but the independent contribution of the drugs and the hormone cannot be assessed in these single-arm studies.[471-474]

The combination of megestrol, cyclophosphamide, and doxorubicin with or without 5-FU was given to 126 patients in a cooperative group study.[475] The response rate (22%) and the median survival (27 weeks) were the same in both arms and represent only a marginal improvement over the 19% response rate achieved by the same group with doxorubicin alone.

Whether the use of combinations of hormones with single agent chemotherapy or combinations enhances the antitumor effect substantially remains unresolved and should be subjected to well-controlled clinical trials.

FUTURE DIRECTIONS

Major efforts should be made to better define the relative risk groups in early-stage endometrial cancer. The GOG has closed its surgical staging protocol in which more than 1,000 cases of patients have undergone rigidly controlled surgical staging. When these data are available, a great deal of information will be gleaned from careful analysis of those cases. Prospective studies should then be undertaken to improve therapeutic results in high risk groups.

It is imperative that chemotherapeutic agents useful in endometrial cancer be developed. Not only will this provide hope for recurrent disease, but also it will allow the development of useful neoadjuvant regimens. At this time, all patients with advanced and recurrent disease should be considered candidates for investigational protocols.

UTERINE SARCOMAS

Uterine sarcomas account for 1% to 6% of all cancers of the corpus uteri.[476-484] These variations in reported incidence depend on the criteria used to classify these cancers as well as the nature of the series on which the reports are based. Table 36-24 lists a classification of uterine sarcomas. It is based on Kempson's[479] simplification of the classification by Ober.[479a] For practical purposes, however, there are three main histologic types of uterine sarcomas that are of clinical significance: (1) malignant mixed mullerian tumors, (2) leiomyosarcomas, and (3) stromal sarcomas. Although there is no FIGO staging classification for uterine sarcomas, most authors utilize a modification of the FIGO classification for endometrial carcinoma. This classification is listed in Table 36-25. As has been pointed out by Lewis et al,[476] this classification is a surgical classification based on the findings at initial surgical treatment of the sarcoma.

TABLE 36-24. Classification of Uterine Sarcomas

I. Pure sarcomas
A. Pure homologous
1. Leiomyosarcoma
2. Stromal sarcoma
3. Angiosarcoma
4. Fibrosarcoma
B. Pure heterologous
1. Rhabdomyosarcoma
2. Chondrosarcoma
3. Osteogenic sarcoma
4. Liposarcoma
II. Mixed sarcomas
A. Mixed homologous
B. Mixed heterologous
C. Mixed homologous and heterologous
III. Malignant mixed mullerian tumors
A. Malignant mixed mullerian tumor, homologous type; carcinoma plus one or more of the homologous sarcomas listed under IA above
B. Malignant mixed mullerian tumor, heterologous type; carcinoma plus one or more of the heterologous sarcomas listed under IB; homologous sarcoma(s) may also be present
IV. Sarcoma, unclassified
V. Malignant lymphoma

TABLE 36-25. Staging Classification of Uterine Sarcomas

Stage I	Sarcoma is confined to the corpus
Stage II	Sarcoma is confined to the corpus and cervix
Stage III	Sarcoma has spread outside the uterus but is confined to the true pelvis
Stage IV	Sarcoma has spread outside the true pelvis

MALIGNANT MIXED MULLERIAN TUMORS

Malignant mixed mullerian tumors or mesodermal mixed tumors are composed of two types of cells: an adenocarcinoma of the endometrium and a sarcomatous element. They are termed homologous if the sarcomatous element is from a cell type found in the uterus and referred to as heterologous if the sarcomatous element is from cell types not found in the uterus (rhabdomyosarcoma, chondrosarcoma, osteosarcoma, or liposarcoma). The reported peak age incidence for malignant mixed mullerian tumors is between 55 and 65 years.[476,477] Vaginal bleeding is the most common presenting symptom.[480,481] Prior irradiation is reported in 5% to 30% of patients.[480,481] Diagnosis is made by dilatation and curettage. Spread of disease is usually by local extension in the pelvis, to lymph nodes, and to the lungs similar to endometrial adenocarcinoma, although these tumors are more aggressive than most endometrial adenocarcinomas. Major et al[482] reported at 15.5% incidence of positive lymph nodes in 174 cases of malignant mixed mullerian tumors and correlated these metastases with depth of myometrial penetration, lymphovascular invasion, and cervical involvement.

The primary treatment for malignant mixed mullerian tumors is surgical removal of the uterus, fallopian tubes, and ovaries. Adjunctive radiotherapy has been reported to decrease the incidence of local recurrence but not to enhance survival.[477]

Perez et al[483] reported on a group of 54 patients with mixed mesodermal sarcomas of the uterus who received combined radiation therapy and surgery as their treatment. In Stage I disease, a preoperative uterine packing for 6000 mgh was recommended. Treatment for patients with Stage II disease consisted of an intracavitary insertion for 5000 to 6000 mgh, combined with external beam whole pelvis irradiation for 2000 cGy and a 3000 cGy boost to the parametrium with a midline shield. They found that local failures were decreased, as compared with other series in which surgery alone was the only local treatment.[484] This increase in local control with radiation has been confirmed by others, and there is a tendency in the combined radiation and surgery group toward improved survival.[485–487] However, numbers in most series are quite small, the reports are unrandomized, and it is quite difficult to make a definite statement about treatment efficacy.

Belgrad et al,[487] in reviewing patients treated at four institutions, also found improved 2-year survival rates in patients treated by combined radiation and surgery for both endometrial stromal sarcomas and mixed mesodermal sarcomas. In the mixed mesodermal category, 35% survived 2 years with combined modality therapy, whereas 20% survived with surgery only. Salazar et al[488] found that in patients who received local radiotherapy as part of their program of management, local failures decreased but survival was not changed.

In a GOG randomized trial of chemotherapy in advanced uterine sarcomas, responses to Adriamycin alone or Adriamycin plus DTIC were noted in 10% to 23% of patients.[489] This same group was unable to demonstrate a statistically significant survival advantage with the adjunctive use of Adriamycin in early (Stages I and II) disease.[490]

Prognosis of malignant mixed mullerian tumors is directly related to the extent of disease at the time of diagnosis. Kempson and Bari[479] reported that all of their patients with disease extending into the outer half of the myometrium died. Piver and Lurain[491] reviewed 610 cases and reported an overall survival rate of 21%. Most reports in their review indicated survival rates of 15% to 30%.

LEIOMYOSARCOMA

Leiomyosarcomas are tumors of the smooth muscle and arise in the myometrium. The exact dividing line between cellular leiomyomata and leiomyosarcoma is not clear. Taylor and Norris[492] found that tumors of less than 10 mitoses per 10 high power fields did not recur or metastasize and called these tumors cellular leiomyomata. Kempson and Bari[479] reported death from tumor or metastases in all of their patients if the tumors had 5 to 9 mitoses per 10 high power fields. Silverberg[493] reported death or metastases in one-half of his patients if the tumor had 5 to 9 mitoses per 10 high power fields. Other factors that seem to influence prognosis are cellular atypia, vascular invasion, and infiltrating tumor margins.[493] It thus appears clear that most, if not all, tumors with less than 5 mitoses per high power field are benign, all with greater than 10 mitoses per 10 high power fields are malignant, and those with 5 to 9 mitoses per 10 high power fields are of uncertain malignant potential. Piver and Lurain[491] in a literature review of 265 cases reported 99% survival for 0 to 4 mitoses per 10 high power fields, 30% survival for 5 to 9 mitoses per 10 high power fields, and 16% survival for tumors with 7 to 10 mitoses per 10 high power fields.

The median age for patients who develop leiomyosarcoma is between 43 and 56 years.[494,495] The presenting symptoms are abnormal vaginal bleeding, an enlarging pelvic mass, and pain or pressure in the pelvis. Dilatation and curettage will result in a correct diagnosis in fewer than one third of cases.[496] Spread of disease is by direct extension to other pelvic viscera, through the lymphatics, and by invasion of blood vessels and hematogenous spread, especially to the lung. Treatment consists of removal of the uterus and adnexa. Adjuvant radiotherapy has not been found to be of benefit in patients with leiomyosarcoma.[447,448] Adjuvant chemotherapy with Adriamycin in Stages I and II disease was evaluated by the GOG.[490] The recurrence rate was 40% in patients receiving Adriamycin and 57% in the no therapy group. The difference was not significant. Responses of 25% and 30% were seen in advanced disease by the GOG using Adriamycin alone versus Adriamycin and DTIC.[489] Prognosis for uterine leiomyosarcoma varies from essentially nil in advanced disease to 20% to 30% for disease confined to the uterus at initial diagnosis.[478]

ENDOMETRIAL STROMAL SARCOMA

Two varieties of this tumor are recognized: endometrial stromal sarcoma and endolymphatic stromal myosis. A third type of this tumor is referred to as stromal nodule, but this is a universally benign tumor. Stromal sarcomas arise from the endometrial stroma, and the distinction between stromal sarcoma and endolymphatic stromal myosis is on the basis of mitotic count. Tumors with 10 or more mitoses per 10 high power fields are stromal sarcomas, and those with fewer mitoses are endolymphatic stromal myosis.[476,492]

Stromal tumors are seen most frequently between the ages of 45 and 50 years, and the most common symptoms are vaginal bleeding and an enlarged, boggy uterus. Diagnosis is made by dilatation and curettage or as an unexpected finding at hysterectomy for leiomyomata. Endolymphatic stromal myosis spreads by direct extension and via the lymphatics. It has extended beyond the uterus by the time of diagnosis in 40% of cases, although two thirds of cases will have the disease confined to the pelvis.[491] Recurrence rates of 50% are reported, but spread outside of the pelvis is not usually seen.[497] Endometrial stromal sarcomas are highly malignant neoplasias with tumor-free survival rates of 0 to 33% being reported.[479,490,498] Distant metastases are more frequent in this group of patients.

The treatment of endolymphatic stromal myosis and endometrial stromal sarcoma is removal of the uterus and adnexa. More radical local resection has been recommended for endolymphatic stromal myosis, but no large series supports this recommendation. Adjunctive irradiation for stromal sarcoma is probably effective in obtaining local control and preventing pelvic recurrences, and Belgrad et al[487] have reported modest improvements in survival. In their report, the 2-year survival rate in patients with endometrial stromal sarcoma treated by radiation therapy and surgery was 57% while in those treated by surgery alone it was 37%.

Norris and Taylor[498] reported a beneficial effect of irradiation on residual disease with endolymphatic stromal myosis, and Koss et al[499] recommended pelvic irradiation for recurrences as well as postsurgical residual disease. There are very few data on chemotherapy for stromal sarcomas, although Baggish and Woodruff[500] have reported responses with high-dose progestins.

CONCLUSIONS AND FUTURE DIRECTIONS

Surgery remains the treatment of choice for all sarcomas arising from the uterus. A total abdominal hysterectomy and bilateral salpingo-oophorectomy are the preferred treatment, although there are advocates of a more radical surgical approach for endolymphatic stromal myosis. In general, lymph node dissections or lymph node sampling, although adding information with regard to prognosis, have not improved survival. Although local failures are unfortunately quite common, the vast majority of patients will fail because of hematogenous dissemination of their tumor. The role of radiation therapy in the treatment of uterine sarcomas remains controversial, with no clear evidence at present that its use, either preoperatively or postoperatively, improves survival. In patients with Stages III and IV disease who are not operative candidates, some palliation and control of local symptoms can be achieved by the judicious use of both external beam therapy and brachytherapy placements.

Since the major pattern of failure is that of disseminated tumor, either alone or in combination with local failure, an effective systemic means of therapy must be devised if a significant improvement in survival is to be obtained. Because of the rarity of sarcomas arising from the uterus, multi-institutional studies are necessary to evaluate new treatment approaches.

CARCINOMA OF THE FALLOPIAN TUBE

Of all the organs of the female genital tract, the fallopian tube gives rise to the smallest number of primary malignant tumors. Such tumors comprise between 0.5% and 1.1% of all gynecologic malignancies.[501–504] Because of its anatomical location in association with the uterus and ovary (the two most common sites of gynecologic cancers), rigid criteria have been recommended to label a tumor as being a primary cancer of the fallopian tube.[503,504] To be considered a primary carcinoma of the fallopian tube, the tumor must be located grossly within the fallopian tube, the uterus and ovary must either not contain carcinoma or, if they contain carcinoma, it must be clearly different from the fallopian tube carcinoma, and the tubal carcinoma must involve the tubal mucosa with transition from benign to malignant epithelium (except in the case of sarcomas arising from nonmucosal structures). By far the most common malignant tumors involving the fallopian tube are metastatic from other genital organs.[505]

EPIDEMIOLOGY

Benedet and White[506] reviewed eight reports of fallopian tube carcinomas reported between 1961 and 1979 (393 cases) and found a mean age incidence of 55 years. They stated that although the disease had been reported to occur between 18 and 87 years, the vast majority of cases occurred between the ages of 40 and 65. The most commonly associated conditions are infertility and chronic salpingitis. However, the common association of infertility and salpingitis and the high frequency in which salpingitis is found, compared to the rarity of fallopian tube carcinoma, renders chronic infection as an etiologic factor unlikely. Some authors have also found an increased incidence of tuberculous salpingitis in association with tubal carcinoma, but again no definite etiologic link has been proved.

PATHOLOGY

The most common malignant tumors of the fallopian tube are adenocarcinomas. Grossly, adenocarcinoma of the fallopian tube presents as a swollen, dilated fallopian tube that, when opened, is filled with papillary and solid tumor. Areas of degeneration with hemorrhage and necrosis are commonly seen.[504] The fimbriated end of the tube is closed in approximately one half of cases, and, prior to opening the tube, it is difficult to differentiate tubal carcinoma from a hydrosalpinx or tubo-ovarian abscess.[507] Microscopically, alveolar, papillary, and medullary patterns of tumor growth have been described with abrupt transitions from normal to neoplastic epithelium.[508] Mixtures of the above patterns are common. Grading of fallopian tube carcinomas has not been proved to be of prognostic significance by some authors,[509] but this may be due to the relatively small numbers in most series. Hu et al[503] did relate survival to histologic grade and found that grade was important in those cases in which the serosa was not involved but that after involvement of the serosa, metastases developed irrespective of grade.

Pure sarcomas of the fallopian tube such as leiomyosarcoma and chondrosarcomas have been reported but are exceedingly rare.[510] Mixed mesodermal tumors of the fallopian tube contain mixtures of adenocarcinoma and sarcoma and are either homologous, when they contain sarcomas of tubal elements such as smooth muscle, or heterologous, when they contain tissues not found in the tube such as cartilage or bone.[511]

Other rare tumors that may be seen in the fallopian tube are lymphomas,[512] hydatidiform moles,[513] and choriocarcinoma.[512] The last two types are probably associated with tubal pregnancies. A primary adenosquamous carcinoma has recently been reported.[514]

PATTERNS OF SPREAD, CLINICAL MANIFESTATION, AND STAGING

Malignant tumors of the fallopian tube spread by exfoliation of clonogenic cells into the lumen of the fallopian tube that then migrate into the pelvic and abdominal cavity, or in the case of tumors that penetrate the serosa, shed cells directly into the pelvic and abdominal cavity. Although a large percentage of tubal carcinomas exhibit occlusion of the fimbriated end of the tube, one must assume that the potential for transtubal migration may have existed earlier in the course of the disease. Following entry of cells into the abdominal cavity, spread is similar to that of ovarian carcinoma. Fallopian tube cancer also spreads by contiguous invasion of adjacent structures and via the lymphatics. Hematogenous spread appears to occur less frequently. Commonly involved organs are the pelvic peritoneum, broad ligament, omentum, diaphragm, and surfaces of the intestines.[501,515] Plentl and Friedman[515] described the lymphatics of the fallopian tube. Efferent lymphatics travel in the mesosalpinx to join efferent channels from the ovary and uterus and follow the ovarian vessels to para-aortic lymph nodes. Lymphatics also course within the broad ligament to the iliac lymph nodes and superior gluteal lymph nodes. Metastatic disease to pelvic and para-aortic nodes is most common, although inguinal node metastases are occasionally seen.[515]

Bilateral tubal involvement was reported in one half of their cases by Novak and Woodruff.[516] Benedet and White[506] in their review of more than 400 cases from the literature reported the incidence of tumors to be roughly equal in the right and left fallopian tubes and found bilaterality in 21%. Whether bilaterality is due to multicentric involvement of paired organs or due to metastases is not clear.

Frick[517] has stated that the diagnosis of fallopian tube cancer is made preoperatively in only 5% of cases. The most common symptoms are abnormal vaginal bleeding and abdominal pain. Benedet and White[506] reviewed 8 series of cases and found that of 203 patients, 101 (50%) reported abnormal vaginal bleeding or discharge, 62 (30%) described abdominal pain, and in 25 (12%) a mass was the presenting symptom. Pain may be intermittent and colicky or dull and aching in nature and probably results from tubal distension similar to that seen with a tubal pregnancy. On rare occasions, an asymptomatic patient may present with adenocarcinoma cells on a Papanicolaou smear.[504] The symptoms complex of hydrops tubae profluens consists of the triad of a profuse vaginal discharge, abdominal pain, and an adnexal mass. This triad is said to be pathognomonic for tubal carcinoma but is uncommon in most series.

Staging of carcinoma of the fallopian tube is determined at surgical exploration, as in ovarian carcinoma. The preoperative diagnostic evaluation is also the same as for ovarian carcinoma since most patients undergoing surgery will do so with the diagnosis of a pelvic mass. Only rarely will fallopian tube cancer be high on the list of differential diagnoses. There is no FIGO staging classification for fallopian tube carcinoma. Dodson et al[518] in 1970 modified the staging for ovarian carcinoma and adapted it to tubal carcinoma by substituting fallopian tube for ovary, and vice versa. Shiller and Silverberg[519] in 1971 developed a different system that is more like the Dukes' classification for colon cancer. Benedet and White[506] modified the staging system reported by Erez et al[520] in 1967 and reported survival in 142 patients staged by their "modified Erez" classification. They found 5-year survival rates of 60% in Stage I, 30% in Stage II, 16% in Stage III, and 19% in Stage IV. Table 36-26 lists and compares the three staging systems mentioned above.

TREATMENT OF CARCINOMA OF THE FALLOPIAN TUBE

General Principles

Because of the relative rarity of fallopian tube carcinoma and because its histology and patterns of spread are so similar to carcinoma of the ovary, most authors have recommended treatment plans of surgery, radiation therapy, and chemotherapy similar to carcinoma of the ovary.

Surgery

The recommended surgical approach for tubal carcinoma is total abdominal hysterectomy, bilateral salpingo-oophorectomy, omentectomy, and resection of as much gross disease as possible. If the disease is limited to the pelvis or if all gross disease is resectable, a full surgical staging operation to include multiple peritoneal biopsies, diaphragmatic biopsy, and sampling of the pelvic and para-aortic nodes is required. Because of the potential early exfoliation of malignant cells via the tubal lumen, no recommendation for conservative surgery in the young patient can be made. This same potential for early dissemination of malignant cells has led most authorities to recommend that all patients with tubal cancer be treated adjunctively with either irradiation or chemother-

TABLE 36-26. Three Suggested Classifications for Fallopian Tube Carcinoma

Stage		*FIGO Type**	*Dukes' Type†*	*Modified Erez‡*
0			Carcinoma in situ	
I		Growth limited to tube	Tumor extends into submucosa or muscularis, not serosa	Tumor limited to the tube (mucosa or muscularis)
	IA	One tube, no ascites		
	IB	Both tubes, no ascites		
	IC	One or both tubes with ascites with malignant cells		
II		Growth limited to the true pelvis	Tumor extends to serosa	
	IIA	Extension to uterus or ovary		Tumor has extended through the serosa but not to contiguous organs
	IIB	Extension to other pelvic tissues		Tumor directly invading surrounding organs in pelvis or abdomen or metastases to pelvic organs
III		Growth involving one or both ovaries with intraperitoneal metastases	Tumor extends to ovary or endometrium	True metastatic lesions outside the pelvis but confined to the abdomen
IV		Growth involving one or both tubes with distant metastases outside the peritoneal cavity	Tumor extends beyond reproductive organs	Metastatic disease outside the abdomen

* Modified from Dodson MG, Ford JH Jr, Averette HE: Clinical aspects of fallopian tube carcinoma. Obstet Gynecol 36:935, 1970.
† Modified from Shiller HM, Silverberg SG: Staging and prognosis in primary carcinoma of the fallopian tube. Cancer 28:389, 1971.
‡ Modified from Benedet JL, White GW: Malignant tumors of fallopian tube. In Coppleson M (ed): Gynecologic Oncology: Fundamental Principles and Clinical Practice, pp 621–629. New York, Churchill Livingstone, 1981.

apy. McMurray et al[521] suggested that all patients with disease greater than Stage I be treated with aggressive postoperative therapy. They state that in their series of 30 patients, 50% of failures were in the upper abdomen and 44% failed in extraperitoneal sites. As with ovarian cancer, there does not seem to be any place for radical hysterectomy, complete lymphadenectomy, or pelvic exenteration in this disease.

Radiation Therapy for Carcinoma of the Fallopian Tube

Postoperative radiotherapy in patients with fallopian tube carcinoma has been recommended by some investigators and questioned by others.[502,509,522,523] Radiotherapy techniques currently used include 5000 cGy whole pelvis external beam irradiation for the more aggressive Stages I and II tumors. For Stage III disease, whole pelvic and abdominal radiation is required. Techniques resemble those used for ovarian tumors.[524] Instillation of radioactive colloidal gold (^{198}Au) and chromic phosphate (^{32}P) has been recommended in cases in which no macroscopic disease is present in the peritoneal cavity.

Several studies have suggested benefits from postoperative radiotherapy. In 1957 Engstrom[525] reported significant improvement in his cases of fallopian tube carcinoma treated with postoperative radium and deep external beam radiation (patients treated with postoperative radiotherapy showed a 38% 5-year survival rate versus a 15% 5-year survival rate in patients treated with surgery only). Greene and Scully[526] reported an average survival of 2 years with postoperative radiation and no survivors 1 year after surgery without radiotherapy.

Boutselis and Thompson[522] reported an increased 5-year survival rate in 7 of 8 patients treated with postoperative radiotherapy. Phelps and Chapman[527] reported good results for patients with Stages I and II disease treated with megavoltage irradiation. Nine patients with Stage I or II disease received 2500 to 5000 cGy to the pelvis or abdomen. Six also received intraperitoneal radioactive colloidal gold or phosphate. Eight of the 9 patients were alive at the time of publication of the study, with 6 patients being 5-year survivors. Six patients with Stage III disease were treated with postoperative radiotherapy; none survived. In a study of 34 patients, Amendola et al[528] reported 1 of 4 patients alive 5 years after therapy consisting of less than 3000 to 5000 cGy. However, 5 of 14 patients who received more than 5000 cGy were alive and disease free.

McMurray et al[521] reported on 30 patients with adenocarcinoma of the fallopian tube treated at Washington University. Nine had Stage I disease, 11 had Stage II, 7 had Stage III, and 3 had Stage IV. Primary surgical treatment consisted of total abdominal hysterectomy and bilateral salpingo-oophor-

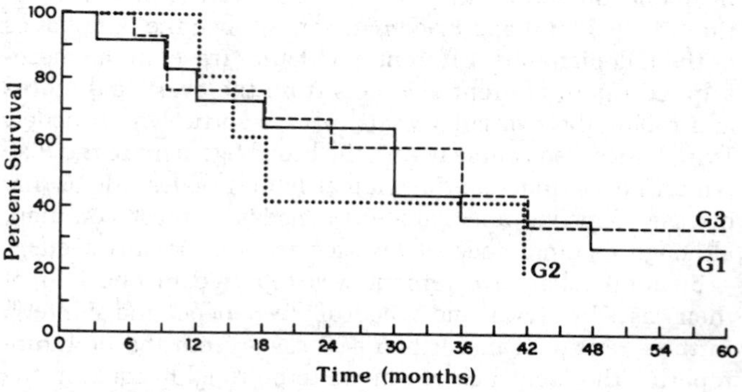

FIG. 36-19. Grade versus survival in fallopian tube carcinoma according to histologic differentiation, Washington University, 1950–1981.

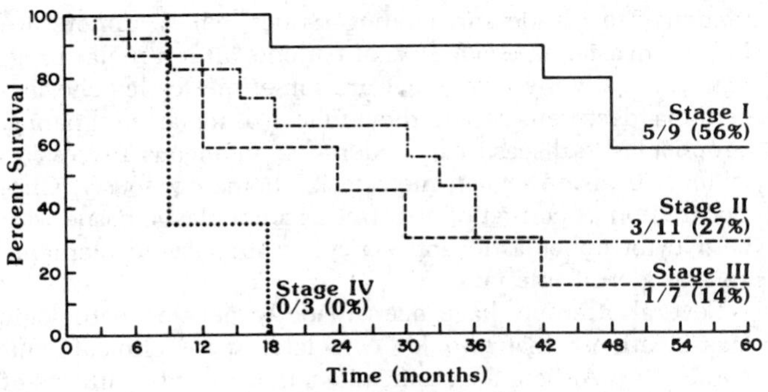

FIG. 36-20. Stage versus survival in fallopian tube carcinoma according to surgical stage, Washington University, 1950–1981.

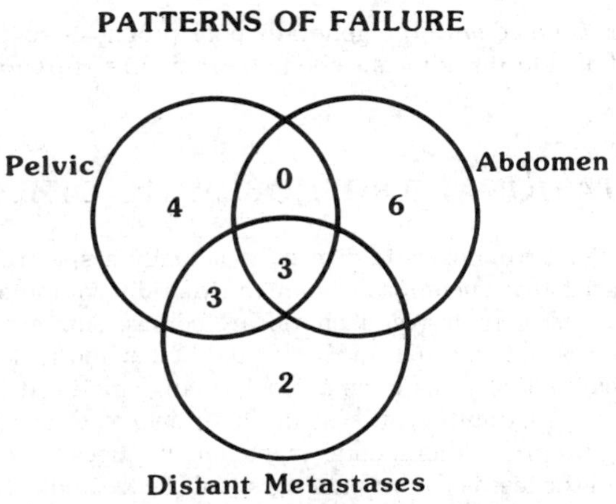

FIG. 36-21. Site of recurrence in fallopian tube carcinoma, Washington University, 1950–1981.

ectomy in 70% of patients; 23% had more extensive surgery than this, whereas 13% had incomplete extirpation of the female genitalia. Three patients with Stage I tumors were treated with surgery alone, and the remainder received postoperative radiation, chemotherapy, or both. Survival was unrelated to grade (Fig. 36-19), but highly dependent upon stage. Disease-free survival at 3 years was 86% for Stage I, 27% for Stage II, 29% for Stage III, and 0% for Stage IV (Fig. 36-20). Four of 5 patients treated after surgery with a combination of cisplatin, doxorubicin, and cyclophosphamide survived at least 3 years. Patterns of initial treatment failure showed 56% with a component of pelvic failure, 50% with a component of upper abdominal failure, and 44% with extraperitoneal metastases as a component of failure (Fig. 36-21). The results according to method of treatment (Table 36-27) suggest that aggressive postoperative adjuvant therapy targeted at upper abdominal and distant sites for metastases in all lesions beyond Stage I will improve survival and tumor control.

Chemotherapy of Carcinoma of the Fallopian Tube

Because it is a rare tumor, data on the chemosensitivity of tubal carcinoma must be obtained from individual case reports and small series. There are anecdotal reports of responses to triple drug therapy with cyclophosphamide, dactinomycin, and 5-FU[529] and to cyclophosphamide, doxorubicin, and progestogens.[530] Adjuvant chlorambucil has been used with pelvic irradiation with some long-term survivors.[531] Raju et al[523] reported experience with 22 cases of tubal carcinoma collected from 1955 to 1980. Six patients had been treated with chemotherapy, and only 1 showed an objective regression following treatment with cisplatin (100 mg/m^2 every 4 weeks).

A recent experience with chemotherapy for recurrent disease documented complete responses in one of six patients treated with oral alkylating agents and two of three patients treated with intravenous cisplatin.[532] Recently, the CAP (cyclophosphamide, Adriamycin, and cisplatin) regimen has been used in nine patients. Four complete remissions were seen; three of the four were without evidence of disease at 18 to 56 months.[532] This small study suggests significant activity for this combination, and it should be further investigated.

Because of the paucity of specific data about the chemosensitivity of this tumor and because its histology and pattern of spread resemble that of epithelial ovarian tumors, it has been common practice to treat these rare carcinomas with chemotherapeutic regimens active in epithelial ovarian cancer. However, a recent review of 30 patients[521] suggests that although the tumors behave similarly to ovarian cancer, they present at earlier stages and there is an increased frequency of failure due to distant metastases. Both these obser-

TABLE 36-27. Survival According to Treatment and Stage (Treatment of Patients Surviving 3 Years or More)

Stage	*S*	*S + RT*	*S + CT*	*S + PAC*	*S + CT + RT*	*Total*
I	3/3	1/2	3/3*		1/1	8/9
II		2/5	0/2	3/3†	0/1	5/11
III			0/3	1/2	1/2*	2/7
IV			0/1		0/2	0/3

Jacob AJ, Perez CA, et al: Carcinoma of the fallopian tube: Management and sites of failure. Cancer 58:2070, 1986.

* Two patients received RT.

† One patient alive with disease.

S, surgery; RT, radiotherapy; CT, chemotherapy; PAC, cisplatin, Adriamycin (doxorubicin), and Cytoxan (cyclophosphamide).

vations coupled with the generally poor prognosis suggest a potential role for adjuvant chemotherapy after surgery.

GESTATIONAL TROPHOBLASTIC DISEASE

Gestational trophoblastic disease is actually a spectrum of neoplasias that encompasses benign hydatidiform moles, locally invasive moles, and choriocarcinomas. Although the disorder is not common in the United States and makes up less than 1% of female gynecologic malignancies, it is extremely important because of the high degree of curability with appropriate therapeutic management. Because of the rarity of the disease, most patients should be treated at trophoblastic disease centers where sufficient expertise exists to deal with the complex and life-threatening nature of this disorder. Because of adherence to these principles, death from this disease is now rare, and in 1983 there were only 24 deaths reported in the United States from choriocarcinoma.[533]

EPIDEMIOLOGY

Although rare in the United States, the disease is much more common in other areas of the world, particularly in Asia and in South America, where incidences as high as 1 : 120 pregnancies have been reported. Although the precise explanation for this increase is unknown, many investigators have suggested nutritional or dietary factors. Studies in Philippine populations[534] revealed a lower incidence in the meat-eating, wealthy populations than in the poorer populations whose diets were heavily based on fish and rice and whose incidence of molar pregnancy was as high as 1 in 200. This contrasts to the incidence of approximately 1 in 1,200 pregnancies in the United States. In most series, increasing age, particularly above the age of 40, increases the risk. This is true in all countries but is most dramatic in countries in which a high baseline risk is already existent. Studies in Singapore demonstrate a 12-fold increase in risk for women above the age of 45.[535] Although risk increases with pregnancies over age 40, there appears to be no increasing risk with advancing parity. Furthermore, the patient's age or the parity does not affect the outcome of a molar pregnancy.

CLASSIFICATION AND PATHOLOGY

Approximately half of all trophoblastic tumors develop after a molar pregnancy, but they can develop after an abortion, an ectopic pregnancy, or after an apparently normal term pregnancy. If the disease occurs after a molar pregnancy, the tumor can be either a hydatidiform mole or a choriocarcinoma. However, if the disease develops in any of the other settings, virtually all the tumors are choriocarcinoma. Generally, the trophoblastic neoplasias can be classified morphologically as hydatidiform mole, invasive mole, and choriocarcinoma.

Hydatidiform moles have clusters of hydropic villi, absence of fetal vessels, and trophoblastic hyperplasia. Invasive moles have similar histologic findings but display a greater tendency to invade surrounding tissues. These tumors are locally invasive in about 15% of patients after a molar pregnancy. Locally invasive moles are sometimes called chorioadenoma destruens when they follow a molar pregnancy. Trophoblastic disease can undergo spontaneous regression or local invasion or can metastasize hematogenously. Choriocarcinomas consist of anaplastic trophoblastic tissue with both cytotrophoblastic and syncytiotrophoblastic elements and no identifiable villi.

Several attempts have been made to develop pathologic classifications that would correlate wtih clinical outcome.[536,537] Although classifications that include patterns of growth, extent of stromal invasion, nuclear grade, and lymphocytic infiltration have broadly correlated, the management and outcome generally have been based on staging and clinical definition of low, moderate, and high risk patients.

TUMOR MARKERS (HUMAN CHORIONIC GONADOTROPIN [HCG])

A major reason for the successful management of this tumor has been the availability of this marker substance that is invariably present with the disease. All types of trophoblastic disease produce hCG, and the quantity produced is proportional to the volume of the disease.[538] As a result, one can use hCG titers as an accurate monitor of disease response to therapy. Both diagnosis and management depend on careful radioimmunoassay of this substance. Pregnancy tests or biological assays have no place in the management of the disease. hCG consists of an alpha and beta chain. Because the alpha chain is cross-reactive with leutinizing hormone (LH), it has been the source of some confusion in diagnosis and subsequent management. As a result, a specific assay for the beta subunit was developed[539] and will selectively assay hCG in the presence of normal LH. Use of this specific radioimmunoassay is required for monitoring all patients with trophoblastic disease. Generally, after evacuation of a molar pregnancy, the elevated hCG titers disappear in 8 to 10 weeks, although in about 25% of patients clearance may be delayed as long as 14 to 16 weeks.[540]

CLINICAL EVALUATION AND STAGING

Generally, molar pregnancies are associated with first trimester bleeding, ectopic pregnancies, or threatened abortions. Often, the uterus is large for the estimated length of the gestation and the hCG titers are elevated in excess of a normal pregnancy. Fetal heart sounds are absent and obviously fetal parts are not palpable. Early toxemia of pregnancy may be present. Expulsion of grape-like villi will often provide the diagnosis of hydatidiform mole although vaginal bleeding is the most common presenting finding with invasive mole or choriocarcinoma. Occasionally patients will present with metastatic disease as their first manifestation of the illness.

Ultrasound evaluation is increasingly used to diagnose molar pregnancies, and the characteristic findings can be diagnostic. These techniques may also define extrauterine extension but are not always diagnostic.[541] Amniography also produces a typical moth-eaten appearance that is also characteristic. Neither amniography or angiography is frequently used because of the current sophistication of ultrasonography. The diagnosis is generally based on the clinical findings, hCG titer, ultrasound, and pathological confirmation. Patients with molar pregnancy should be evaluated further with chest radiographs, careful pelvic examinations, and weekly serial monitoring of the hCG titers. Patients who have evidence of persistent disease and those found to have choriocarcinoma should have chest radiographs and brain and liver scans to define the extent of metastatic spread.

Distant metastases are noted in about 5% of those patients who have molar pregnancies. Choriocarcinoma spreads hematogenously, and the common metastatic sites are lungs (80%), vagina (30%), pelvis (20%), liver (10%), brain (10%), bowel, kidney and spleen (5%).[542]

Unfortunately, no uniform staging classification has received widespread adoption. Many investigators classify patients according to whether disease is metastatic or nonmetastatic and then, among those with metastatic disease, further divide patients into those with low risk and high risk.[543] Several staging schemes have been used, including those of Bagshawe,[543] the Dutch Working Group for trophoblastic tumors,[544] and the New England Trophoblastic Disease Center.[543] Comparisons of all three staging classifications generally documented similar degrees of specificity and prognostic value.[544] The last two classifications are easier to apply because they are based on data readily available and do not require information about the husband's blood group, lymphocytic infiltration of the tumor, or the patient's immune status. Unfortunately, none of these retrospective comparisons identify a particular staging classification as superior. Nevertheless, the staging classification used by the New England Trophoblastic Disease Center is straightforward and useful as outlined in Table 36-28. Patients are divided into high risk and low risk molar pregnancies, patients with disease confined to the corpus of the uterus (Stage I), patients wtih local pelvic spread (Stage II), and patients with more advanced disease (Stages III and IV). Patients believed to have low risk molar pregnancies include those with hCG titers less than 100,000 IU/ml, small uterine size, ovarian enlargement less than 6 cm, and no other poor-prognosis metabolic or epidemiologic factors.[545] Patients at high risk include those with hCG titers greater than 100,000 IU/ml, uterine size greater than normal for date of gestation, enlarged ovaries, and any of the poor-prognosis metabolic or epidemiologic factors, including maternal age over 40, toxemia, coagulopathy, trophoblastic tumor with or without embolization, and hyperthyroidism.

TABLE 36-28. Staging of Gestational Trophoblastic Neoplasms

Stage 0	Molar pregnancy A. Low risk B. High risk
Stage I	Confined to uterine corpus
Stage II	Metastases to pelvis and vagina
Stage III	Metastasis to lung
Stage IV	Distant metastases

Goldstein DP, Berkowitz RS: The management of gestational trophoblastic neoplasms. Curr Prob Obstet Gynecol 4:1, 1980.

The majority of patients with Stage I disease (75%) have classical invasive mole, and the remaining 25% have locally invasive choriocarcinoma. Stages 0 to 3 all have good prognoses when treated with currently available therapies. Stage IV patients include those with poor prognostic findings. All have choriocarcinoma and include those with initial hCG titers of greater than 100,000 IU/ml, persistence of disease longer than 4 months after initial therapy, and those with brain or liver metastasis.

TREATMENT

Patients with hydatidiform mole require evacuation of the uterus by suction curettage and oxytocin. After evacuation, patients generally have a dilatation and curettage. In 80% of patients, no further therapy will be needed. Subsequent follow-up requires weekly hCG assay until the titer returns to normal.

The mainstay of treatment for the other gestational trophoblastic neoplasias is chemotherapy. Before chemotherapy, only 40% of patients could be cured with hysterectomy alone even when the disease appeared localized. In the presence of any evidence of metastatic spread, fewer than 10% of those patients survived despite aggressive surgery and irradiation. The classical reports of Li and colleagues[546] of the activity of methotrexate in the 1950s and the subsequent documentation of the curative capacity of chemotherapy by Hertz et al[547] represent milestones in cancer treatment and ushered in the era of modern chemotherapy.

Chemotherapy is now commonly used to manage patients with gestational trophoblastic neoplasia. Patients with hydatidiform mole receive chemotherapy if there is a persistent plateau in the weekly β-hCG level, a rise in the β-hCG titer, or the development of metastases. Patients with invasive mole or choriocarcinoma or those who present with metastatic disease require immediate chemotherapy.

Generally, patients requiring chemotherapy are divided into good risk patients who can be cured with single-agent chemotherapy and poor risk patients who generally require initial combination chemotherapy for best results. Poor-risk features include Stage IV disease, cerebral or hepatic metastases, β-hCG levels of greater than 100,000 IU/ml, previous unsuccessful treatment, persistence of symptoms for greater than 4 months, or disease after a full-term pregnancy. Using these criteria, treatment selection can be based on risk factors and stage.

Treatment of Low Risk Patients (Stages I and II and Low Risk Metastatic Disease)

Historically, single-agent chemotherapy is most commonly used for these patients. Intramuscular methotrexate (Mtx) or actinomycin D (Act D) have been the standard single-agent therapies with Mtx given intramuscularly 0.4 mg/kg/day × 5 days every 2 weeks or Act D 10 to 12 μg/kg/day × 5 days every 2 weeks. Although this therapy is extremely effective for low risk trophoblastic disease, both regimens have significant toxicity, and more recently moderate dose Mtx with leucovorin rescue has achieved similar results wtih less toxicity. The New England Trophoblastic Disease Center has recently summarized its 10-year experience with this regimen.[548] One hundred eighty-five patients were treated. Complete remissions were achieved in 88% of patients, including 90% of the 163 patients with nonmetastatic disease and 68% of those with low risk metastatic disease. In 82% of these patients, complete remission was achieved with a single course of methotrexate and leucovorin. The regimen includes Mtx 1 mg/kg intramuscularly every other day for 4 doses, followed by leucovorin intramuscularly 0.1 mg/kg 24 hours after each Mtx dose.

After the initial course of chemotherapy, the response to therapy is monitored by β-hCG regression curves.[549] One log or greater fall in hCG titer over the subsequent 18 days allows the physician to withhold further therapy. If the βhCG titer does not fall to this degree, reaches a plateau, or begins rising, a second course of therapy is administered. Therapy continues until the βhCG titer has normalized for 3 weeks. Patients are subsequently monitored at monthly intervals for 1 year. If βhCG titers remain normal for a year, pregnancy may be allowed.

Toxicity was modest. Granulocytopenia occurred in 6% of patients and thrombocytopenia in less than 2%. There was no alopecia, and nausea and vomiting were rare. Although 14% of patients developed enzyme evidence of hepatic toxicity, this resolved within 2 weeks of completing therapy. All of the patients in this series, who failed initial induction therapy with Mtx-leucovorin, achieved a complete remission with subsequent combination chemotherapy. On the basis of this extensive experience, this regimen appears to be the treatment of choice for low risk gestational trophoblastic disease.

Treatment of High Risk Patients

All high risk patients should receive initial combination chemotherapy. The most common regimen used contains methotrexate 0.3 mg/kg intramuscularly, actinomycin D 10 μg/kg intravenously, and chlorambucil 10 mg orally daily $\times$ 5 days with courses repeated as required until 3 successive weeks of normal β-hCG levels are achieved.[550] Other effective regimens include the CHAMOCA regimen of Bagshawe,[551,552] MAC,[553,554] or PVB (cisplatin, vinblastine, bleomycin).[554] Using these regimens, complete responses are generally achieved in approximately 80% of patients, although generally lower responses (60–70%) are seen in patients with hepatic or cerebral metastases.[555]

Salvage chemotherapy for patients failing initial induction therapy for high risk disease has generally employed six to seven drug combinations.[556,557] Although many of these early trials achieved some salvage, small numbers of patients were included. One salvage regimen using high-dose cisplatin, vincristine, and methotrexate with leucovorin achieved durable complete remissions in 35% of previous failures.[558] With the identification of VP-16[497,559] and cisplatin[560] as active agents in a salvage setting, several investigators have used these drugs in new regimens.

PVB, after failure of conventional triple therapy, achieved a complete remission in 50% of patients, although only 20% (2 of 11) had a sustained complete remission. More recently, high dose Mtx (1 g/m^2) with leucovorin rescue, VP-16, and bleomycin were used in 9 patients failing initial therapy with the modified Bagshawe regimen. Eight of the 9 (89%) achieved a sustained remission for more than 2 years. Bone marrow toxicity was universal and substantial.[498]

Patients with brain or liver metastasis are generally treated with local irradiation to the sites. Patients with proven brain metastasis or elevations of cerebrospinal fluid hCG are treated with 3000 cGy whole brain irradiation. Surgery is rarely required. Patients with hepatic metastasis are often treated with 2500 cGy before the start of chemotherapy to reduce the risk of intrahepatic hemorrhage during chemotherapy.

Long-Term Complications of Chemotherapy

Several studies of the long-term consequences of successful therapy for this disease have been published, and as yet there is no evidence of increased risk of maternal complications or fetal abnormalities associated with these treatments.[562,563]

POSTIRRADIATION GYNECOLOGIC MALIGNANCIES

Several reports have been published on the incidence of malignant tumors of the endometrium or other pelvic organs in patients treated with irradiation for benign or malignant pelvic conditions. Smith and Doll[564] reported an increased incidence of leukemia (7 deaths observed against 2.3 expected) and cancers of the heavily irradiated sites (59 observed versus 40.1 expected) 5 years or more after irradiation to the pelvis for benign metropathia haemorrhagica. The mean dose of radiation to the bone marrow was extimated to correlate with the projected excess rate of leukemia, which is about 1.1 case/woman/cGy/year. However, other authors such as Hutchinson[565] have not observed this increased incidence (3 cases observed versus 16 expected). Dickson[566] reported 2 deaths from leukemia whereas only 1.1 were expected. Wagoner[507] observed no excess of leukemia among 7,835 women treated with radium and roentgen rays for primary uterine cancer. Arneson and Schellhas[568] and Spratt and Hoag[569] observed no significant increase of malignancy in patients treated with irradiation for carcinoma of the uterine cervix.

Lee et al[570] reviewed 1,150 patients treated with irradiation for carcinoma of the uterine cervix at Washington University. Table 36-29 shows the observed and expected incidence of malignancy in several series. Thus, the current data fail to support the suggestion that irradiation may increase the incidence of malignancy in patients irradiated for gynecologic cancer.

Wagoner[567] also studied 1,803 patients treated for benign gynecologic disorders with radium and observed 10 deaths from leukemia against 3.6 expected; in a similar series in Connecticut, 9 cases of leukemia were seen against 2.8 expected. A decreased death rate from carcinoma of the breast has been observed by Smith and Doll[564] and others[571,572] with an artificial inducement of menopause. In the patients treated for carcinoma of the cervix at Washington University, a similar lower mortality from breast cancer was noted. It is possible that the castration induced by irradiation in younger women may influence the subsequent development

TABLE 36-29. Incidence of Postirradiation Gynecologic Malignancy

	Average Age (yr)	*No. of Patients*	*No. 2 NDI*	*Human Years Observed*	*CA per Human Year*	*Rate per 100,000*
Lee et al[570]	52	1053	49	6244	0.00785	785
Arneson and Schellhas[567]	49	874	36	6142	0.00586	586
Spratt and Hoag[569]	54	1853	36	6264	0.00574	574

Lee JY, Perez CA, Ettinger N, et al: The risk of second primaries subject to irradiation for cervix cancer. Int J Radiat Oncol Biol Phys 8:207, 1982.

of carcinoma of the breast. Villasanta and Rubel[573] reported 15 cases of pelvic malignancy in 174 patients irradiated for benign uterine bleeding in contrast to only 3 malignant tumors in 147 nonrandomized control patients who were not irradiated. Most of the tumors developed in the endometrium or the ovary. The dose of irradiation was relatively small (2000–2400 mgh). In contradistinction, the same authors observed only 19 patients developing a second pelvic malignancy in 569 women with malignant tumors of the gynecologic tract treated wtih doses of irradiation above 5000 cGy and followed for 4 years or longer. Dickson[566] pointed out that the incidence for malignancy after irradiation for benign uterine bleeding was significantly less in patients treated with external irradiation than in those treated with intracavitary radium. As reported by Thomas et al[574] most postirradiation malignancies of the uterus are adenocarcinomas of the endometrium, followed by mixed mullerian tumors and sarcomas of the uterine cervix. The prognosis of these patients after treatment was similar to that of patients who had not had irradiation.[574]

The principles of management for these patients are similar to those patients who receive no previous irradiation. Most authors agree that the primary treatment of these patients is surgical. There is some controversy whether preoperative or postoperative irradiation should be delivered. However, the number of patients is small, and no definite conclusions can be drawn.

REFERENCES

1. Silverberg E, Lubera J: Cancer statistics, 1988. CA 38:5, 1988
2. Anderson BL, Hacker NF: Psychosexual adjustment after vulvar surgery. Obstet Gynecol 62:457, 1983
3. Collins CG, Roman-Lopez JJ, Lee FYL: Intraepithelial carcinoma of the vulva. Am J Obstet Gynecol 108:1187, 1987
4. Boutselis JG: Intraepithelial carcinoma of the vulva. Am J Obstet Gynecol 113:733, 1972
5. Franklin EW, Rutledge FD: Epidemiology of epidermoid carcinoma of the vulva. Obstet Gynecol 39:165, 1972
6. Japaze H, Garcia-Buneul R, Woodruff JD: Primary vulvar neoplasia. Obstet Gynecol 49:404, 1977
7. Forney JP, Morrow CP, Townsend DE, et al: Management of carcinoma in situ of the vulva. Am J Obstet Gynecol 127:801, 1977
8. Kunschner A, Kanbour AI, David B: Early vulvar carcinoma. Am J Obstet Gynecol 132:599, 1978
9. Friedrich EG, Wilkinson EJ, Fu YS: Carcinoma in situ of the vulva: A continuing challenge. Am J Obstet Gynecol 136:880, 1980
10. Parker RT, Duncan I, Rampone J, et al: Operative management of early invasive epidermoid carcinoma of the vulva. Am J Obstet Gynecol 123:349, 1975
11. Magrina JF, Webb MJ, Gaffey TA, et al: Stage I squamous cell cancer of the vulva. Am J Obstet Gynecol 134:453, 1975
12. Podratz KC, Symmonds RE, Taylor WF, et al: Carcinoma of the vulva: Analysis of treatment and survival. Obstet Gynecol 61:63, 1983
13. Rutledge F, Smith JP, Franklin EW: Carcinoma of the vulva. Am J Obstet Gynecol 106:1117, 1970
14. Hacker NF, Leuchter RS, Berek JS, et al: Radical vulvectomy and bilateral inguinal lymphadenectomy through separate groin incisions. Obstet Gynecol 58:574, 1981
15. Mack T, Casagrande JT: Epidemiology of gynecologic cancer: II. Endometrium, ovary, vagina, vulva. In Coppleson M (ed): Gynecologic Oncology: Fundamental Principles and Clinical Practice, pp 28–30. New York, Churchill Livingstone, 1981
16. Green TH: Carcinoma of the vulva: A reassessment. Obstet Gynecol 52:462, 1978
17. Collins CG, Lee FYL, Ramon-Lopez JJ: Invasive carcinoma of the vulva with lymph node metastases. Am J Obstet Gynecol 109:446, 1971
18. Morley GW: Infiltrative carcinoma of the vulva: Results of surgical treatment. Am J Obstet Gynecol 124:874, 1976
19. Josey WE, Nahmais AJ, Naib ZM: Viruses and cancer of the lower genital tract. Cancer 38:526, 1976
20. Deligdisch L, Szulman AE: Multiple and multifocal carcinoma in female genital organs and breast. Gynecol Oncol 3:181, 1975
21. Stern BD, Kaplan L: Multicentric foci of carcinoma arising in structures of cloacal origin. Am J Obstet Gynecol 104:255, 1969
22. Plentl AA, Friedman EA: Lymphatic System of the Female Genitalia: The Morphologic Basis of Oncologic Diagnosis and Therapy, pp 15–50. Philadelphia, WB Saunders, 1971
23. Way S: Carcinoma of the vulva. In Meigs JV, Sturgis SH (eds): Progress in Gynecology, vol 3. New York, Grune & Stratton, 1957
24. Kaufman RH, Gardner HL: Intraepithelial carcinoma of the vulva. Clin Obstet Gynecol 8:1035, 1965
25. International Society for the Study of Vulvar Disease. New nomenclature for vulvar disease: I. Obstet Gynecol 47:122, 1976
26. Friedrich EG Jr, Wilkinson EJ: The vulva. In Blaustein A (ed): Pathology of the Female Genital Tract, pp 13–58. New York, Springer-Verlag, 1977
27. Helwig EB, Graham JH: Anogenital (extramammary) Paget's disease. Cancer 16:387, 1963
28. Friedrich EG Jr, Wilkinson EJ, Steingraeber PH, et al: Paget's disease of the vulva and carcinoma of the breast. Obstet Gynecol 46:130, 1975
29. Tchang F, Okagaki T, Richart R: Adenocarcinoma of Bartholin's gland associated with Paget's disease of vulvar area. Cancer 31:221, 1973
30. Woodruff JD, Richardson EH: Malignant vulvar Paget's disease. Obstet Gynecol 10:10, 1957
31. Gosling JRG, Abell MR, Drolette BM, et al: Infiltrative squamous cell carcinoma of the vulva. Cancer 14:330, 1961
32. Way S: Carcinoma of the vulva. Am J Obstet Gynecol 79:692, 1960
33. Wharton JT, Gallagher S, Rutledge FN: Microinvasive carcinoma of the vulva. Am J Obstet Gynecol 118:159, 1974
34. Parker RT, Duncan I, Rampone J, et al: Operative management of early invasive epidermoid carcinoma of the vulva. Am J Obstet Gynecol 123:349, 1975
35. Lasser A, Cornorg JT, Morris JM: Adenoid squamous carcinoma of the vulva. Cancer 33:224, 1974
36. Gallousis S: Verrucous carcinoma. Obstet Gynecol 40:502, 1972
37. Lucas WE, Bernischke K, Lebherz TB: Verrucous carcinoma of the female genital tract. Am J Obstet Gynecol 119:435, 1974
38. Chung AF, Woodruff JM, Lewis JL Jr: Malignant melanoma of the vulva. Obstet Gynecol 45:638, 1975
39. Breen JL, Neubecker RD, Greenwald E, et al: Basal cell carcinomas of the vulva. Obstet Gynecol 46:122, 1975
40. Tavassoli FA, Norris HJ: Smooth muscle tumors of the vulva. Obstet Gynecol 53:213, 1979
41. Buscema J, Woodruff JD, Parmley TH, et al: Carcinoma in situ of the vulva. Obstet Gynecol 55:225, 1980
42. Clark WH Jr: A classification of malignant melanoma in man correlated with histiogenesis and biologic behavior. In Montagna W, Hu F (eds): Advances in Biology of Skin and Pigmentary System, pp 621–647. London, Pergamon Press, 1967
43. Breslow A: Thickness, cross-sectional areas and depth of invasion in the prognosis of cutaneous melanoma. Ann Surg 172:902, 1970
44. Collins CG, Ramon-Lopez JJ, Lee FYL: Intraepithelial carcinoma of the vulva. Am J Obstet Gynecol 18:1187, 1970
45. Rutledge FN, Sinclair M: Treatment of intraepithelial carcinoma of the vulva by skin excision and graft. Am J Obstet Gynecol 102:806, 1986

46. Barnhill DR, Hoskins WJ, Metz P: Use of the rhomboid flap after partial vulvectomy. Obstet Gynecol 62:444, 1983
47. Woodruff JD, Julian C, Puray T, et al: The contemporary challenge of carcinoma in situ of the vulva. Am J Obstet Gynecol 115:677, 1973
48. Dean RE, Taylor ES, Weisbrod DM, et al: The treatment of premalignant and malignant lesions of the vulva. Am J Obstet Gynecol 119:59, 1974
49. Breen JL, Smith CI, Gregori CA: Extramammary Paget's disease. Clin Obstet Gynecol 21:1107, 1978
50. Watring WG, Roberts JA, Lagasse LD, et al: Treatment of recurrent Paget's disease of the vulva with topical bleomycin. Cancer 41:10, 1978
51. DiPaola GR, Gomez-Rueda N, Arrighi L: Relevance of microinvasion in carcinoma of the vulva. Obstet Gynecol 45:647, 1975
52. Kneale BLG, Elliott PM, McDonald IA: Microinvasive carcinoma of the vulva: Clinical features and management. In Coppleson M (ed): Gynecologic Oncology: Fundamental Principles and Clinical Practice, pp 320–328. New York, Churchill Livingstone, 1981
53. DiSaia PJ, Creasman WT, Rich WM: An alternate approach to early cancer of the vulva. Am J Obstet Gynecol 133:825, 1979
54. Krupp PJ: Invasive tumors of vulva: clinical features and management. In Coppleson M (ed): Gynecologic Oncology: Fundamental Principles and Clinical Practice, pp 329–338. New York, Churchill Livingstone, 1981
55. Homesley HD, Bundy BN, Sedlis A, et al: Radiation therapy versus pelvic node resection for carcinoma of the vulva with positive groin nodes. Obstet Gynecol 68:733, 1986
56. Basset A: Traitement chirurgical operatoire de l'epithelioma primitf du clitoris. Rev Chir 46:546, 1912
57. Krupp PJ, Bohm JW: Lymph node metastases in invasive squamous cell cancer of the vulva. Am J Obstet Gynecol 130:943, 1978
58. Hacker NF, Berek JS, Lagasse LD: Management of regional lymph nodes and their prognostic influence in vulvar cancer. Obstet Gynecol 61:408, 1983
59. Podratz KC, Symmonds RE, Taylor WF, et al: Carcinoma of the vulva: Analysis of treatment and survival. Obstet Gynecol 61:63, 1983
60. Hacker NF, Leuchter RS, Berek JS, et al: Radical vulvectomy and bilateral inguinal lymphadenectomy through separate groin incisions. Obstet Gynecol 58:574, 1981
61. Morris JM: A formula for selective lymphadenectomy: Its application to cancer of the vulva. Obstet Gynecol 50:152, 1977
62. Mattingley RF, Thompson JD: Surgical conditions of the vulva. In Mattingley RF, Thompson JD (eds): Telinde's Operative Gynecology, p 720. Philadelphia, JB Lippincott, 1985
63. Sedlis A, Marshall R, Homesley H, et al: Positive groin lymph nodes in vulvar cancer with superficial penetration. Gynecol Oncol 17:259, 1984
64. Iversen T, Abeler D, Aalders J: Individualized treatment of Stage I carcinoma of the vulva. Obstet Gynecol 57:158, 1976
65. Frankendal B, Larsson LG, Westing P: Carcinoma of the vulva. Acta Radiol [Ther] (Stockh) 12:165, 1973
66. Acosta AA, Given FT, Frazier AB, et al: Preoperative radiation therapy in the management of squamous cell carcinoma of the vulva: Preliminary report. Am J Obstet Gynecol 132:198, 1978
67. Boronow RC: Combined therapy or an alternative to exenteration for locally advanced vulvovaginal cancer. Cancer 49:1085, 1982
68. Boronow RC: Therapeutic alternative to primary exenteration for advanced vulvovaginal cancer. Gynecol Oncol 1:233, 1973
69. Daly JW, Million RR: Radical vulvectomy combined with elective node irradiation to TxNO squamous carcinoma of the vulva. Cancer 34:161, 1974
70. Hacker NF, Berek JS, Juillard GJF, et al: Preoperative radiation therapy for locally advanced vulvar cancer. Cancer 54:2056, 1984
71. Kucera H: Die Behandlung des Vulvakzinoms an der I. Universitats-Frauenklinik Wien (386 Falle). Strahlentherapie 156:598, 1980
72. Simonsen E, Nordberg UB, Johnson JE, et al: Radiation therapy and surgery in the treatment of regional lymph nodes in squamous cell carcinoma of the vulva. Acta Radiol Oncol 23:433, 1984
73. Foster DC, Woodruff JD: The use of dinitrochlorobenzene in the treatment of vulvar carcinoma in situ. Gynecol Oncol 11:330, 1981
74. Pao WM, Perez CA, Kuske RR, et al: Radiation therapy and conservation surgery for primary and recurrent carcinoma of the vulva: Report of 40 patients and a review of the literature. Int J Radiat Oncol Biol Phys (in press)
75. Schulz U, Callies R, Kruger KG: Effizienz der postoperativen electronentherapie des lekalisierten vulvarkarzinoms. Strahtertherapie 156:326, 1980
76. Stillman FH, Sedlis A, Boyce JG: A review of lower genital intraepithelial neoplasia and the use of topical 5-fluorouracil. Obstet Gynecol Surf 40:190, 1985
77. Calgar H, Hertzog AW, Hreschyshyn MM: Topical 5-fluorouracil treatment of vaginal intraepithelial neoplasia. Obstet Gynecol 5:580, 1981
78. Stillman FH, Boyce JG, Macasaet MA, et al: 5-Fluorouracil/chemosurgery for intraepithelial neoplasia of the lower genital tract. Obstet Gynecol 58:356, 1981
79. Levin W, Rad FF, Goldberg G, et al: The use of concomitant chemotherapy and radiotherapy prior to surgery in advanced stage carcinoma of the vulva. Gynecol Oncol 25:20, 1986
80. Hoskins WJ, Burke TW, Weiser EB, et al: The use of rotation flaps in vulvar surgery. Contemp Ob/Gyn 28:159, 1986
81. Julian CG, Callison J, Woodruff JD: Plastic management of extensive vulvar defects. Obstet Gynecol 38:193, 1971
82. Lovett RD, Kuske RR, Perez CA, et al: Preliminary evaluation of toxicity and tumor response to radiotherapy with cis-platinum and 5-fluorouracil for advanced or recurrent gynecologic malignancies. Presented at the 29th Annual Meeting of American Society for Therapeutic Radiology and Oncology, October 1987
83. Rutledge F: Cancer of the vagina. Am J Obstet Gynecol 97:635, 1967
84. Herbst AL, Green TH Jr, Ulfelder H: Primary carcinoma of the vagina. Am J Obstet Gynecol 106:210, 1970
85. Plentl AA, Friedman EA: Lymphatic System of the Female Genitalia: The Morphologic Basis of Oncologic Diagnosis and Therapy, pp 51–74. Philadelphia, WB Saunders, 1971
86. Gallup DG, Morley GW: Carcinoma in situ of the vagina. Obstet Gynecol 46:334, 1975
87. Graham JB, Meigs JV: Recurrence of tumor after total hysterectomy for carcinoma in situ. Am J Obstet Gynecol 64:1159, 1952
88. Hummer WK, Massey E, Decker DG, et al: Primary invasive squamous carcinoma of the vagina. Obstet Gynecol 53:218, 1959
89. Pride GL, Schultz AE, Chuprevich TW, et al: Primary invasive squamous carcinoma of the vagina. Obstet Gynecol 53:218, 1979
90. Novak ER, Woodruff JD: Postirradiation malignancies of the pelvic organs. Am J Obstet Gynecol 77:667, 1959
91. Herbst AL, Ulfelder H, Poskanzer DC: Adenocarcinoma of the vagina: Association of maternal stilbestrol therapy with tumor appearance in young women. N Engl J Med 11:284, 1971
92. Herbst AL, Cole P, Colton T, et al: Age-incidence and risk of diethylstilbestrol-related clear cell adenocarcinoma of the vagina and cervix. Am J Obstet Gynecol 128:48, 1977
93. Herbst AL, Robboy SJ, Scully RE, et al: Clear cell adenocarcinoma of the vagina in girls: Analysis of 170 registry cases. Am J Obstet Gynecol 119:713, 1974
94. Park RC, Parmley TH: Vaginal cancer. In McGowan L (ed): Gynecologic Oncology, pp 174–184. New York, Appleton-Century-Crofts, 1978
95. Perez C, Arneson AN, Galakatos A, et al: Malignant tumors of the vagina. Cancer 31:36, 1973
96. Smith J: Malignant gynecologic tumors in children. Am J Obstet Gynecol 116:201, 1973
97. Norris HJ, Taylor HB: Melanomas of the vagina. Am J Clin Pathol 46:420, 1966
98. Ragiri MV, Tobon H: Primary malignant melanoma of the vagina and vulva. Obstet Gynecol 43:658, 1974
99. Blaustein A: Diseases of the vagina. In Blaustein A (ed): Pathology of the Female Genital Tract, pp 59–86. New York, Springer-Verlag, 1977
100. Scully RE, Robboy SJ, Welch WR: Pathology and pathogenesis of diethylstilbestrol-related disorders of the female genital tract. In Herbst AL (ed): Intrauterine Exposure to Diethylstilbestrol in the Human. Chicago, The American College of Obstetricians and Gynecologists, 1978
101. Tavassoli FA, Norris HJ: Smooth muscle tumors of the vagina. Obstet Gynecol 53:689, 1979
102. Wharton JT, Fletcher GH, Declos L: Invasive tumors of vagina: Clinical features and management. In Coppleson M (ed): Gynecologic Oncology: Fundamental Principles and Clinical Practice, pp 345–359. New York, Churchill Livingstone, 1981
103. Livingstone RC: Primary carcinoma of the vagina. Springfield, IL, Charles C Thomas, 1950
104. Brady LW: Radiation therapy for carcinoma of the vagina. In McGowan L (ed): Gynecologic Oncology, pp 185–190. New York, Appleton-Century-Crofts, 1978
105. Chau PM: Radiotherapeutic management of malignant tumors of the vagina. Am J Roentgenol Radium Ther Nucl Med 89:502, 1963
106. Perez CA, Camel HM, Galakatos AE, et al: Definitive irradiation in carcinoma of the vagina. Long-term evaluation (personal communication)
107. Woodruff JD, Parmley TH, Julian CG: Topical 5-flourouracil in the treatment of vaginal carcinoma in situ. Gynecol Oncol 3:124, 1975
108. Townsend DE: Intraepithelial neoplasia of the vagina. In Coppleson M (ed): Gynecologic Oncology: Fundamental Principles and Clinical Practice, pp 339–344. New York, Churchill Livingstone, 1981
109. Brown GR, Fletcher GH, Rutledge FN: Irradiation of 'in situ' and invasive squamous cell carcinomas of the vagina. Cancer 28:1278, 1971
110. Perez CA, Camel HM: Longterm followup in radiation therapy of carcinoma of the vagina. Cancer 49:1308, 1982
111. Frick HC, Jacox HW, Taylor HC Jr: Primary carcinoma of the vagina. Am J Obstet Gynecol 101:695, 1968
112. Herbst AL, Green TH, Ulfelder H: Primary carcinoma of the vagina. Am J Obstet Gynecol 106:210, 1970
113. Underwood PB, Smith RT: Carcinoma of the vagina. JAMA 217:46, 1971
114. Perez CA, Korba A, Sharma S: Dosimetric considerations in irradiation of carcinoma of the vagina. Int J Radiat Oncol Biol Phys 2:639, 1977
115. Perez CA, DiSaia PJ, Knapp RC: Gynecologic tumors. In DeVita VT Jr, Hellman S, Rosenberg SA (eds): Cancer: Principles and Practice of Oncology, 2nd ed, pp 1013–1081. Philadelphia, JB Lippincott, 1985
116. Perez CA, Grigsby DW, Slessinger E: A new afterloading vaginal applicator (personal communication) 1987
117. Wharton JT, Rutledge FN, Gallagher HS, et al: Treatment of clear cell adenocarcinoma in young females. Obstet Gynecol 45:365, 1975
118. Fletcher GH (ed): Textbook of Radiotherapy, 3rd ed, pp 821–824. Philadelphia, Lea & Febiger, 1980
119. Piver MS, Barlow JJ, Wang JJ, et al: Combined radical surgery, radiation therapy and

chemotherapy in infants with vulvo-vaginal embryonal rhabdomyosarcoma. Obstet Gynecol 42:522, 1973
120. Grosfeld JL, Smith JP, Clatworthy JR: Pelvic rhabdomyosarcoma in infants and children. J Urol 107:673, 1973
121. Ghavimi F, Exelby PR, D'Angio GJ, et al: Combination therapy of urogenital embryonal rhabdomyosarcoma in children. Cancer 32:1178, 1973
122. Sordillo P, Magill GB, Shauer PK, et al: Preliminary trial of combination therapy with Adriamycin and radiation therapy in sarcomas and other malignant tumors. J Surg Oncol 21:23, 1982
123. Kinsella TJ, Glatstein E: Clinical experience with intravenous radiosensitizers in unresectable sarcoma. Cancer 59:908, 1987
124. Morrow CP, DiSaia PJ: Malignant melanoma of the female genitalia: A clinical analysis. Obstet Gynecol Surv 31:233, 1976
125. Barber HRK: Incidence, prevalence and median survival rates of gynecologic cancer. In van Nagell JR Jr, Barber HRK (eds): Modern Concepts of Gynecologic Oncology, pp 1–19. Boston, John Wright PSG Inc, 1982
126. Cramer D, Cutler SJ: Incidence and histopathology of malignancies of the female genital organs in the United States. Am J Obstet Gynecol 118:443, 1974
127. Barber HRK: Cervical Cancer. In McGowan L (ed): Gynecologic Oncology, pp 206–216. New York, Appleton-Century-Crofts, 1975
128. Christopherson WM, Parker JE: Relation of cervical cancer to early marriage and childbearing. N Engl J Med 273:235, 1965
129. Keighley E: Carcinoma of the cervix among prostitutes in a women's prison. Br J Vener Dis 44:254, 1968
130. Rotkin ID: Adolescent coitus and cervical cancer associations of related events with increased risk. Cancer Res 27:603, 1967
131. Rotkin ID: Sexual characteristics of a cervical cancer population. Am J Public Health 57:815, 1967
132. Taylor RS, Carroll BE, Lloyd JW: Mortality among women in 3 Catholic religious orders with special references to cancer. Cancer 12:1207, 1959
133. Terris M, Wilson F, Nelson JH Jr: Relation of circumcision to cancer of the cervix. Am J Obstet Gynecol 117:1056, 1973
134. Abou-Daoud KT: Epidemiology of cancers of the cervix in Lebanese Christians and Moslems. Cancer 20:1706, 1967
135. Ackerman LV, del Regato JA (eds): Cancer. Diagnosis, Treatment and Prognosis. St. Louis, CV Mosby, 1977
136. Kessler I: Human cervical cancer as a venereal disease. Cancer Res 36:783, 1976
137. Joneja MG, Coulson DB: Histopathology and cytogenetics of tumors induced by application of 7,12-dimethyl-benz (a) centhracene (DMBA) in mouse cervix. Eur J Cancer 9:367, 1973
138. Herbst AL, Cole P, Norusis MJ, et al: Epidemiologic aspects and factors related to survival in 384 registry cases of clear cell adenocarcinoma of the vagina and cervix. Am J Obstet Gynecol 135:876, 1979
139. Boyce JG, Lu T, Nelson JH Jr: Cervical carcinoma and oral contraceptives. Gynecol Obstet Invest 40:139, 1972
140. Drill VA: Oral contraceptives: Relation to mammary cancer, benign breast lesions and cervical cancer. Am Rev Pharmacol 15:367, 1975
141. Melnick JL, Adams E, Rawls WE: The causative role of herpes virus 2 in cervical cancer. Cancer 34:1375, 1974
142. Nahmias AJ, Naib ZM, Josey WE, et al: Prospective studies of the association of genital herpes simplex infection and cervical anaplasia. Cancer Res 33:1491, 1973
143. Hollinshead AC, Chretien PB, O'bong L, et al: In vivo and in vitro measurements of the relationship of human squamous carcinoma to herpes simplex virus tumor-associated antigen. Cancer Res 36:821, 1976
144. Rapp F, Duff R: Oncogenic conversion of normal cells by inactivated herpes simplex virus. Cancer 34:1353, 1974
145. Darai G, Munk K: Human embryonic lung cells abortively infected with herpes hominus Type 2 show properties of cell transformation. Nature New Biol 241:268, 1973
146. Wentz WB, Reagan JW, Heggie AD: Cervical carcinogenesis with herpes simplex virus, Type 2. Obstet Gynecol 46:117, 1975
147. Notter MFD, Docherty JJ, Martel R, et al: Detection of herpes simplex virus tumor associated antigen in uterine cervical tissue: Five case studies. Gynecol Oncol 6:574, 1978
148. Meisels A, Fortin R: Condylomatous lesions of the cervix and vagina I. Cytologic patterns. Acta Cytol 20:505, 1976
149. Kurman RJ, Jenson AB, Lancaster WD: Papillomavirus infections of the cervix: Relationship to intraepithelial neoplasia based on the presence of specific viral structural proteins. Am J Surg Pathol 7:39, 1983
150. Reid R, Crum CP, Herschman BR, et al: Genital warts and cervical cancer. III Subclinical papillomaviral infection and cervical neoplasia are linked by a spectrum of continuous morphologic and biologic change. Cancer 53:943, 1984
151. Crum CP, Levine RU: Human papillomavirus infection and cervical neoplasia: New perspectives. Int J Gynecol Pathol 3:376, 1984
152. Durst M, Gissman L, Ikenberg H, et al: A papillomavirus DNA from a cervical cancer and its prevalence in cancer biopsies from different geographical regions. Proc Natl Acad Sci USA 80:3812, 1983
153. Levine RU, Crum CP, Herman E, et al: Cervical papillomavirus infection and intraepithelial neoplasia: A study of male sexual partners. Obstet Gynecol 64:16, 1984
154. Krebs HB, Schneider V: Human Papillomavirus-associated lesions of the penis: colposcopy, cytology and histology. Obstet Gynecol 70:299, 1987
154a. Petersen O: Spontaneous course of cervical pre-cancerous conditions. Am J Obstet Gynecol 72:1063, 1956
155. Richart RM: Natural history of cervical intraepithelial neoplasia. Clin Obstet Gynecol 110:748, 1967
156. Reagan JW, Wentz WB: Genesis of carcinoma of the uterine cervix. Clin Obstet Gynecol 10:883, 1967
157. Clemmesen J, Poulsen H: Report of the Ministry of the Interior. Document 3, Copenhagen, 1971
157a. Kottmeier HL: Evolution et traitment des epitheliomas. Rev Fr Gynec Obstet 56:821, 1961
158. Walton Report: Cervical cancer screening program, epidemiological and natural history of cancer of the cervix. Can Med Assoc J 114:1003, 1976
159. Plentl AA, Friedman EA: Lymphatic system of the female genitalia: The morphologic basis of oncologic diagnosis and therapy, pp 75–115. Philadelphia, WB Saunders, 1971
160. Fuller AF, Elliott N, Kosloff C, et al: Lymph node metastases from carcinoma of the cervix, Stages IB and IIA: Implications for progress and treatment. Gynecol Oncol 13:165, 1982
161. Sudarsanam A, Komanduri C, Belinson J, et al: Influence of exploratory celiotomy on the management of carcinoma of the cervix. A preliminary report. Cancer 41:1049, 1978
162. Nelson JH Jr, Macasaet MN, Lu T, et al: The incidence and significance of para-aortic lymph node metastases in late invasive carcinoma of the cervix. Amer J Obstet Gynecol 118:749, 1974
163. Piver MS, Barlow JJ: High dose irradiation to biopsy confirmed aortic node metastases from carcinoma of the cervix. Cancer 39:1243, 1977
164. Wharton JT, Jones HW III, Day TG, et al: Preirradiation celiotomy and extended field irradiation for invasive carcinoma of the cervix. Obstet Gynecol 49:333, 1977
165. Lagasse LD, Creasnan WT, Singleton HM, et al: Results and complications of operative staging in cervical cancer: Experience of the Gynecologic Oncology Group. Gynecol Oncol 9:90, 1980
166. Buschbaum HJ: Extrapelvic lymph node metastases in cervical carcinoma. Am J Obstet Gynecol 133:814, 1979
167. Averette HE, Ford JH Jr, Dudan RC, et al: Staging of cervical cancer. Clin Obstet Gynecol 18:215, 1975
168. Welander CE, Pierce VK, Nori D, et al: Pretreatment laparatomy in carcinoma of the cervix. Gynecol Oncol 12:336, 1981
169. Berman ML, Keys H, Creasman W, et al: Survival and patterns of recurrence in cervical cancer metastatic to periaortic lymph nodes: A Gynecologic Group Study. Gynecol Oncol 19:8, 1984
170. Carlson V, Delclos L, Fletcher GH: Distant metastases in squamous-cell carcinoma of the uterine cervix. Radiology 88:961, 1987
171. Rutledge FN, Warton JT, Fletcher GH: Clinical studies with adjunctive surgery and irradiation therapy in the treatment of carcinoma of the cervix. Cancer 38:596, 1976
172. Regan JW, Ng ABP: The cellular manifestations of uterine carcinomas. In Norris HJ, Hertig AT, Abell MR (eds): The Uterus. International Academy of Pathology, Monographs in Pathology. Baltimore, Williams & Wilkins, 1973
173. Wentz WB: Histological grade and survival in cervical cancer with respect to cell type. Cancer 18:412, 1961
174. Abell MR, Gosling JRG: Gland cell carcinoma (adenocarcinoma) of the uterine cervix. Am J Obstet Gynecol 83:729, 1962
175. Davis JR, Moon LB: Increased incidence of adenocarcinoma of uterine cervix. Obstet Gynecol 45:79, 1975
176. Artman LE, Hoskins WJ, Bibro MC, et al: Radical hysterectomy and pelvic lymphadenectomy for stage IB carcinoma of the cervix: 21 years experience. Gynecol Oncol 28:8, 1987
177. Dougherty CM, Cottin N: Mixed squamous cell and adenocarcinoma of the cervix: Combined adenosquamous and mucoepidermoid types. Cancer 17:1132, 1964
178. Noller KL, Decker DG, Dockerty MD, et al: Mesonephric (clear cell) carcinoma of the vagina and cervix. Obstet Gynecol 43:640, 1974
179. Hart WR, Norris HJ: Mesonephric adenocarcinoma of the cervix. Cancer 29:106, 1972
180. Ulbright TM, Gersell DJ: Glassey cell carcinoma of the uterine cervix. A light and electron microscopic study of five cases. Cancer 51:2255, 1983
181. Hoskins WJ, Ng APB, Averette HE, et al: Cylindroma of the cervix uteri: Report of six cases and review of the literature. Gynecol Oncol 7:371, 1979
182. Dougherty CM, Cotten N: Mixed squamous cell and adenocarcinoma of the cervix: Combined, adenosquamous and mucoepidermoid types. Cancer 17:1132, 1964
183. Abell MR: Primary melanoblastoma of the uterine cervix. Am J Clin Pathol 36:248, 1961
184. Warner TFCS: Carcinoid tumor of the uterine cervix. J Clin Pathol 31:990, 1978
185. Abell MR, Ramirez JA: Sarcomas and carcinosarcomas of the uterine cervix. Cancer 31:1176, 1973
186. Charlton I, Karnei RF, King FM, et al: Primary malignant reticuloendothelial disease involving the vagina, cervix and corpus uteri. Obstet Gynecol 44:735, 1974
187. Retikas DG: Hodgkin's sarcoma of the cervix. Report of a case. Am J Obstet Gynecol 80:1104, 1960
188. Jennings RH, Barclay DI: Verrucous carcinoma of the cervix. Cancer 30:430, 1972
189. Breslow L: Cytology and the decline in uterine cervix mortality in California. In Clark RL, Cumley RW, McCoy JE, et al (eds): Oncology 1970. Proceedings of the

Tenth International Cancer Congress, vol IV. Diagnosis and Management of Cancer: Specific sites. Chicago, Year Book, 1971
190. Fidler HK, Boyes DA, Worth AJ: Cervical cancer detection in British Columbia. J Obstet Gynecol Br Comm 75:392, 1968
191. American Cancer Society: ACS report on the cancer-related health check-up. Cancer 30:194, 1980
192. The American College of Obstetricians and Gynecologists Statement of Policy. Periodic cancer screening for women. American College of Obstetricians and Gynecologists, June 1980
193. Walsh JW, Amendola MA, Konerding KF, et al: Computed tomographic detection of pelvic and inguinal lymph node metastases from primary and recurrent pelvic malignant disease. Radiology 137:157, 1980
194. Piver MS, Chung WS: Prognostic significance of cervical lesion size and pelvic node metastases in cervical carcinoma. Obstet Gynecol 46:507, 1975
195. Changes in definitions of clinical staging for carcinoma of the cervix and ovary: International Federation of Gynecology and Obstetrics. Am J Obstet Gynecol 156:263, 1987
196. Averette HE, Dudan RC, Ford JH: Exploratory celiotomy for surgical staging in cervical cancer. Am J Obstet Gynecol 113:1090, 1972
197. Berman ML, Lagasse LD, Watring WG, et al: The operative evaluation of patients with cervical carcinoma by an extraperitoneal approach. Obstet Gynecol 50:658, 1977
198. Fuller AF, Elliott N, Kosloff C, et al: Determinants of increased risk for recurrence in patients undergoing radical hysterectomy for stage IB and IIA carcinoma of the cervix. Gynecol Oncol (in press)
199. Burghardt E, Pickel H, Haas J, et al: Prognostic factors and operative treatment of stages IB to IIB cervical cancer. Am J Obstet Gynecol 156:988, 1987
200. Martimbeau PW, Kjorstad KE, Jenson T: Stage IB carcinoma of the cervix, the Norwegian Radium Hospital. II Results when pelvic nodes are involved. Obstet Gynecol 60:215, 1982
201. Blaikley JB, Lederman M, Pollard W: Carcinoma of the cervix at Chelsea Hospital for Women, 1935–1965. Five-year and 10-year results of treatment. J Obstet Gynecol Brit Commonw 76:729, 1969
202. Brunschwig A, Barber HRK: Surgical treatment of carcinoma of the cervix. Obstet Gynecol 27:21, 1966
203. Christensen A, Lange P, Neilsen E: Surgery and radiotherapy for invasive cancer of the cervix: Surgical treatment. Acta Obstet Gynecol 43:59, 1964
204. Ketcham AS, Hoye RC, Taylor PT: Radical hysterectomy and lymphadenectomy for carcinoma of the uterine cervix. Cancer 28:1272, 1971
205. Liu W, Meigs JV: Radical hysterectomy and pelvic lymphadenectomy: A review of 473 cases including 244 for primary invasive carcinoma of the cervix. Am J Obstet Gynecol 69:1, 1955
206. Masterson JG: The role of surgery in the treatment of early carcinoma of the cervix. Clin Obstet Gynecol 10:922, 1967
207. Park RC, Patow WE, Rogers RR, et al: Treatment for stage I carcinoma of the cervix. Obstet Gynecol 41:117, 1973
208. Chung CK, Nahlas WA, Stryker JA, et al: Analysis of factors contributing to treatment failures in stages IB and IIA carcinoma of the cervix. Am J Obstet Gynecol 138:550, 1980
209. van Nagell JR, Donaldson ES, Wood EG, et al: The significance of vascular invasion and lymphocytic infiltration in invasive cervical cancer. Cancer 41:228, 1978
210. Boyce J, Fruckter RC, Nicastri A, et al: Prognostic factors in stage I carcinoma of the cervix. Gynecol Oncol 12:154, 1981
211. Burke TW, Hoskins WJ, Heller PB, et al: Prognostic factors associated with radical hysterectomy failures. Gynecol Oncol 26:153, 1987
212. Figge DC, Tamimi HK: Patterns of recurrence of carcinoma following radical hysterectomy. Am J Obstet Gynecol 140:213, 1981
213. Fuller AF, Elliott N, Kosloff C, et al: Lymph node metastases from carcinoma of the cervix, stages IB and IIA. Implications for prognosis and treatment. Gynecol Oncol 13:165, 1982
214. Bush RS, Jenkin RDT, Alet WEC, et al: Definitive evidence for hypoxic cells influencing cure in cancer therapy. Br J Cancer 37:302, 1978
215. Vigario G, Kurohara SS, George FW III: Association of hemoglobin levels before and during radiotherapy with prognosis in uterine cervix cancer. Radiology 106:649, 1973
216. Jenkin RDT, Stryker JA: The influence of the blood pressure on survival in cancer of the cervix. Br J Radiol 41:913, 1968
217. Van Herik M: Fever as a complication of radiation therapy for carcinoma of the cervix. Am J Roentgenol Radium Ther Nuc Med 43:104, 1965
218. Prempree T, Patanaphan V, Sewchanel W, et al: The influence of patient's age and tumor grade on the prognosis of carcinoma of the cervix. Cancer 51:1764, 1983
219. Berkowitz RS, Ehrmann RL, Lavizzo-Mourey R, et al: Invasive cervical carcinoma in young women. Gynecol Oncol 8:311, 1979
220. Kyriakos M, Kempson RL, Perez CA: Carcinoma of the cervix in young women. Obstet Gynecol 8:311, 1979
221. Hoskins WJ, Ford JH Jr, Lutz MH, et al: Radical hysterectomy and pelvic lymphadenectomy for the management of early invasive carcinoma of the cervix. Gynecol Oncol 4:278, 1976
222. Townsend DE, Richart RM, Marks E, et al: Invasive carcinoma following outpatient evaluation and therapy for cervical disease. Obstet Gynecol 57:145, 1971
223. Sevin B, Ford JH, Girtanner RD, et al: Invasive cancer of the cervix after cryosurgery. Pitfalls of conservative management. Obstet Gynecol 53:465, 1979
224. Coppleson M: Cervical intraepithelial neoplasia: Clinical features and management. In Coppleson M (ed): Gynecologic Oncology: Fundamental Principles and Clinical Practice, pp 451–464. New York, Churchill Livingstone, 1981
225. Averette HE, Nelson JH, Ng ABP, et al: Diagnosis and management of microinvasive (stage IA) carcinoma of the uterine cervix. Cancer 38:414, 1976
226. Simon NL, Gore H, Shingleton HM, et al: Study of superficially invasive carcinoma of the cervix. Obstet Gynecol 69:19, 1986
227. Burghardt E: Microinvasive carcinoma. Obstet Gynecol Surv 34:836, 1979
228. van Nagell JR, Greenwell N, Powell DF, et al: Microinvasive cancer of the cervix. Am J Obstet Gynecol 145:981, 1983
229. Hamberger AD, Fletcher GH, Wharton JT: Results of treatment of early stage I carcinoma of the uterine cervix with intracavitary radium alone. Cancer 41:980, 1978
230. Pilleron JP, Durand JC, Lenoble JC: Carcinoma of the uterine cervix stages I and II, treated by radiation therapy and extensive surgery (1,000 cases). Cancer 29:593, 1972
231. Sall S, Pineda AA, Cananoq A, et al: Surgical treatment of stages IB and IIA invasive carcinoma of the cervix by radical abdominal hysterectomy. Am J Obstet Gynecol 135:422, 1979
232. Burghardt E: Early Histological Diagnosis of Cervical Cancer. Philadelphia, WB Saunders, 1973
233. Newton M: Radical hysterectomy or radiotherapy for stage I cervical cancer. Am J Obstet Gynecol 123:535, 1975
234. Roddick JW Jr, Greenlow RH: Treatment of cervical cancer. Am J Obstet Gynecol 19:754, 1971
235. Dickson RJ: Late results of radium treatment of carcinoma of the cervix. Clin Radiol 23:528, 1972
236. Fletcher GH: Cancer of the uterine cervix. Janeway Lecture. Am J Roentgenol Radium Ther Nucl Med 111:225, 1971
237. Kline JC, Schultz AE, Vermund H: High dose radiotherapy for carcinoma of the cervix. Method and results. Am J Obstet Gynecol 104:479, 1969
238. Kottmeier HL (ed): Annual Report on the Results of Treatment in Carcinoma of the Uterus, Vagina and Ovary, vol 15. Stockholm, International Federation of Gynecology and Obstetrics, 1973
239. Muirhead W, Green LS: Carcinoma of the cervix. Five-year results sequelae of treatment. Am J Obstet Gynecol 101:744, 1968
240. Perez CA, Camel HM, Kuske RR, et al: Radiation therapy alone in the treatment of carcinoma of the uterine cervix: A 20-year experience. Gynecol Oncol 23:127, 1986
241. Wall JA, Collins VP, Hudgins PT: Carcinoma of the cervix. Review of clinical experience during a 20-year period. Am J Obstet Gynecol 96:57, 1966
242. Volterrani F, Lombardi F: Long term results of radium therapy in cervical cancer. Int J Radiat Oncol Biol Phys 6:565, 1980
243. van Nagell JR, Rayburn W, Donaldson ES: Therapeutic implications of patterns of recurrence in cancer of the uterine cervix. Cancer 44:2354, 1979
244. Kielbinska S, Ludwika T, Fraczek O: Studies of mortality and health status in women cured of cancer of the cervix uteri: Comparison of long-term results of radiotherapy and combined surgery and radiotherapy. Cancer 32:245, 1973
245. Perez CA, Camel HM, Kao MS, et al: Randomized study of preoperative radiation and surgery or irradiation alone in the treatment of stage IB and IIA carcinoma of the uterine cervix. Final report. Gynecol Oncol 27:129, 1987
246. Lu T, Macasaet M, Nelson JH Jr: The barrel shape cervix. Am J Obstet Gynecol 124:596, 1976
247. O'Guinn AG, Fletcher GH, Wharton JT: Guidelines for conservative hysterectomy after irradiation. Gynecol Oncol 9:68, 1980
248. Morrow CP: Panel report: Is pelvic radiation beneficial in the postoperative management of stage IB squamous cell carcinoma of the cervix with pelvic node metastases managed by radical hysterectomy and pelvic lymphadenectomy? Gynecol Oncol 10:105, 1980
249. Wertheim MS, Hakes TB, Doghestani AN, et al: A pilot study of adjuvant therapy in patients with cervical cancer at high risk of recurrence after radical hysterectomy and pelvic lymphadenectomy. J Clin Oncol 3:912, 1985
250. Johns HE: Optimization of energy and equipment. In Kramer S, Suntharalingam N, Zinniger GF (eds): High Energy Photons and Electrons: Clinical Applications in Cancer Management, p 333. New York, John Wiley & Sons, 1976
251. Prempree T: Parametrial implant in stage IIIB cancer of the cervix. III. A five-year study. Cancer 52:748, 1983
252. Aristazabel SA, Surwit EA, Hevezi JM, et al: Treatment of advanced cancer of the cervix with transperineal interstitial irradiation. Int J Radiat Oncol Biol Phys 9:1013, 1983
253. Martinez A, Edmundson GK, Cox RS, et al: Combination of external beam irradiation and multiple-site perineal applicator (Mupit) for treatment of locally advanced or recurrent prostatic, anorectal, and gynecologic malignancies. Int J Radiat Oncol Biol Phys 11:391, 1985
254. Maruyuma Y, Muir W: Human cervical cancer clearance after ^{252}Cf neutron brachytherapy versus conventional photon brachytherapy. Am J Clin Oncol 7:347, 1984
255. Castro JR, Issa P, Fletcher GH: Carcinoma of the cervix treated by external irradiation alone. Radiology 95:163, 1970
256. Einhorn N, Bygdeman M, Sjoberg B: Combined radiation and surgical treatment for carcinoma of the uterine cervix. Cancer 45:720, 1980
257. Morley GW, Seski JC: Radical pelvic surgery versus radiation therapy for stage I carcinoma of the cervix (exclusive of microinvasion). Am J Obstet Gynecol 1126:785, 1976

258. Morton DG, Lagasse LD, Moore JG: Pelvic lymphadenectomy following radiation in cervical carcinoma. Am J Obstet Gynecol 88:932, 1964
259. Sweeney WJ III, Douglas RG: Treatment of carcinoma of the cervix with combined radiation and extensive surgery. Am J Obstet Gynecol 84:981, 1962
260. Rampone JF, Klem V, Kolstad P: Combined treatment of stage IB carcinoma of the cervix. Obstet Gynecol 41:163, 1973
261. Decker DG, Aaro LA, Hunt AB, et al: Sequential radiation and operation in carcinoma of the uterine cervix. Am J Obstet Gynecol 92:35, 1965
262. Quigley MM, Knab DR, McMahan ER: Carcinoma of the cervix. A third treatment. Obstet Gynecol 45:650, 1975
263. Parker RT, Wilbanks GD, Yowell RK: Radical hysterectomy with and without preoperative radiotherapy for cervical cancer. Am J Obstet Gynecol 99:993, 1967
264. Gray MJ, Gusberg SB, Guttman R: Pelvic lymph node dissection following radiotherapy. Am J Obstet Gynecol 76:629, 1958
265. Perez CA, Camel HM, Kao MS, et al: Randomized study of preoperative radiation and surgery or irradiation alone in the treatment of stage IB and IIA carcinoma of the uterine cervix. Preliminary analysis of failures and complications. Cancer 45:2759, 1980
266. Rutledge FN, Fletcher GH, Macdonald EJ: Pelvic lymphadenectomy as an adjunct to radiation therapy in treatment for cancer of the cervix. Am J Roentgenol Radium Ther Nucl Med 93:607, 1965
267. Durrance FY, Fletcher GH, Rutledge FN: Analysis of central recurrent disease in stage I and II squamous cell carcinomas of the cervix on intact uterus. Am J Roentgenol Radium Ther Nucl Med 106:831, 1969
268. Perez CA, Breaux S, Askin F, et al: Irradiation alone or in combination with surgery in stage IB and IIA carcinoma of the uterine cervix. A non-randomized comparison. Cancer 43:1062, 1979
269. Cuccia AA, Blodorn FG: Treatment of primary adenocarcinoma of the cervix. Am J Roentgenol Radium Ther Nucl Med 99:371, 1967
270. Rutledge FN, Galakatos AE, Wharton JT, et al: Adenocarcinoma of the uterine cervix. Am J Obstet Gynecol 122:236, 1975
271. Nelson AJ, Fletcher GH, Wharton T: Indications for adjunctive conservative extrafascial hysterectomy in selected cases of carcinoma of the uterine cervix. Am J Roentgenol Radium Ther Nucl Med 123:91, 1975
273. Perez CA, Kao M-S: Radiation therapy alone or combined with surgery in the treatment of barrel-shaped carcinoma of the uterine cervix (stages IB, IIA, IIB). Int J Radiat Oncol Biol Phys 11:1903, 1985
274. Leveuf J, Godord H: Le'exerese chirugicale des ganglions pelviens complement de la curtherapie des cancers du col de 'uterus. J Chir 43:177, 1934
275. Taussig FJ: Iliac lymphadenectomy with irradiation in the treatment of cancer of the cervix. Am J Obstet Gynecol 28:650, 1934
276. Abitol NM, Davenport JH: Sexual dysfunction after therapy for cervical carcinoma. Am J Obstet Gynecol 119:181, 1974
277. Perez CA: Carcinoma of the uterine cervix. In Perez CA, Brady LW (eds): Principles and Practice of Radiation Oncology, pp 919. Philadelphia, JB Lippincott, 1987
278. Fowler JF: Radiobiological considerations from the hyperbaric oxygen trials. A personal view. Br J Radiol 51:68, 1978
279. Watson ER, Halnan KE, Dische C, et al: Hyperbaric oxygen and radiotherapy: A Medical Research Council trial in carcinoma of the cervix. Br J Radiol 51:879, 1978
280. Fletcher GH, Lindberg RD, Caderao JB, et al: Hyperbaric oxygen as a radiotherapeutic adjuvant in advanced carcinoma of the uterine cervix. Preliminary results of a randomized trial. Cancer 39:617, 1977
281. Glassburn JR, Damsker JI, Brady LW, et al: Hyperbaric oxygen and radiation in the treatment of advanced cervical carcinoma. In Fifth International Hyperbaric Congress Proceedings, II, p 813, Simon Fraser University
282. Dische S: Hyperbaric oxygen: The Medical Research Council trials and their clinical significance. Br J Radiol 51:888, 1979
283. Johnson RJR, Walton RF: Sequential study on the effect of the addition of hyperbaric oxygen on the 5-year survival rates of carcinoma of the cervix treated with conventional fractional irradiations. Am J Roentgenol Radium Ther Nucl Med 120:111, 1974
284. Thomas GM, Rauth AM, Bush RS, et al: A toxicity study of daily dose metronidazole with pelvic irradiation. Cancer Clin Trials 3:223, 1980
285. Dische S: Misonidazole in the clinic at Mount Vernon. Cancer Clin Trials 3:175, 1980
286. Hornback HB, Shupe RE, Shidnia H, et al: Advanced stage IIIB cancer of the cervix treatment by hyperthermia and radiation. Gynecol Oncol 23:160, 1986
287. Perez CA, Breaux S, Madoc-Jones H, et al: Radiation therapy alone in treatment of carcinoma of the uterine cervix. II. Analysis of complications. Cancer 54:235, 1984
288. Kottmeier HL: Complications following radiation therapy in carcinoma of the cervix and their treatment. Am J Obstet Gynecol 88:854, 1964
289. Pourquier H, Dubois JB, Deland R: Cancer of the uterine cervix. Dosimetric guidelines for prevention of late rectal and rectosigmoid complications as a result of radiotherapeutic treatment. Int J Radiat Oncol Biol Phys 8:1887, 1982
290. Strockbine MJ, Hancock JE, Fletcher GH: Complications in 831 patients with squamous cell carcinoma of the intact uterine cervix treated with 3000 cGy or more whole pelvis irradiation. Am J Roentgenol Radium Ther Nucl Med 108:293, 1970
291. Piver MS, Vongtama V, Barlow JJ: Para-aortic lymph node irradiation for carcinoma of the uterine cervix using split-course technique. Gynecol Oncol 3:168, 1975
292. Komaki R, Mattingly RF, Hoffman RG, et al: Irradiation of para-aortic lymph node metastases from carcinoma of the cervix or endometrium. Radiology 147:245, 1983
293. Twefik HH, Buschbaum HJ, Latourette HB, et al: Para-aortic lymph node irradiation in carcinoma of the cervix after exploratory laparotomy and biopsy-proven positive aortic nodes. Int J Radiat Biol Phys 8:13, 1982
294. Potish R, Adcock L, Jones T, et al: The morbidity and utility of periaortic radiotherapy in cervical carcinoma. Gynecol Oncol 15:1, 1983
295. Rotman M, John M: Para-aortic irradiation in cervical carcinoma. Int J Radiat Oncol Biol Phys 5:2139, 1979
296. Freund AW: Zu meiner methods des totalen uterus-exstripation. Zentralbl Gynak 2:265, 1878
297. Brunschwig A: Complete excision of pelvic viscera for advanced carcinoma: A one-step abdominoperineal operation with end colostomy and bilateral ureteral implantation into the colon above the colostomy. Cancer 1:177, 1948
298. Mattingly RF, Thompson JD (eds): Telinde's Operative Gynecology, 6th ed. Philadelphia, JB Lippincott, 1985
299. Webb MJ, Symmonds RE: Wertheim hysterectomy: A reappraisal. Obstet Gynecol 54:140, 1979
300. Symmonds RE: Morbidity and complications of radical hysterectomy with pelvic lymph node dissection. Am J Obstet Gynecol 94:663, 1966
301. Brunschwig A, Daniel WW: Pelvic exenteration operations. Ann Surg 151:571, 1960
302. Lawhead RA, Clark DGC, Smith DH, et al: Pelvic exenteration for recurrent or persistent gynecologic malignancies: A ten-year review of the Memorial Sloan-Kettering Cancer Center experience (1972–1981). Gynecol Oncol (in press)
303. Meoz RT, Spanos WJ, Doss L, et al: Misonidazole combined with large-fraction pelvic irradiation in the treatment of patients with advanced pelvic malignancies. Preliminary report of an ongoing RTOG phase I–II study. Am J Clin Oncol 6:417, 1983
304. Puthawala AA, Syed AM, Fleming PA, et al: Re-irradiation with interstitial implant for recurrent pelvic malignancies. Cancer 50:2810, 1982
305. Prasavinichai S, Glassburn JR, Brady LW: Treatment of recurrent carcinoma of the cervix. Int J Radiat Oncol Biol Phys 4:957, 1978
306. Prempree T, Kwon T, VillaSanta U, et al: Management of late second or late recurrent squamous cell carcinoma of the cervix uteri after successful initial radiation treatment. Int J Radiat Oncol Biol Phys 5:2053, 1979
307. Friedman M, Pearlman AW: Carcinoma of the cervix; radiation salvage of surgical failures. Radiology 84:801, 1965
308. Evans SR Jr, Hilaris BS, Barber HRK: External vs. interstitial irradiation in unresectable recurrent cancer of the cervix. Cancer 28:1284, 1971
309. Sala JM, deLeon AD: Treatment of carcinoma of the cervical stump. Radiology 81:300, 1963
310. Moss WT, Brand WN, Battifor H (eds): Radiation Oncology. Rational, Technique, Results, p 408. St. Louis, CV Mosby, 1973
311. Wimbush PR, Fletcher GH: Radiation therapy of carcinoma of the cervical stump. Radiology 93:655, 1969
312. Creadnick RN: Carcinoma of the cervical stump. Am J Obstet Gynecol 75:5465, 1958
313. DePetrillo AD, Townsend DE, Morrow CP, et al: Colposcopic evaluation of the abnormal Papanicoloau test in pregnancy. Am J Obstet Gynecol 121:441, 1975
314. Averette HE, Nasser N, Yankow SL, et al: Cervical conization in pregnancy. Analysis of 180 operations. Am J Obstet Gynecol 106:543, 1970
315. Miluta JH, Enterline HT, Braun TE Jr: Carcinoma in situ of the cervix and pregnancy associated with pregnancy. JAMA 204:763, 1968
316. Boyle MH, Torrance GW, Sinclair JC, et al: Economic evaluation of neonatal intensive care of very low-birth-weight infants. N Engl J Med 308:1330, 1983
317. Creasman WT, Rutledge FN, Fletcher GH: Carcinoma of the cervix associated with pregnancy. Obstet Gynecol 36:495, 1970
318. Sablinska R, Tarlowska L, Stelmachar J: Invasive carcinoma of the cervix associated with pregnancy: Correlation between age advancement of cancer and gestation, and result of treatment. Gynecol Oncol 5:383, 1979
319. Kinch RAH: Factors affecting the prognosis of carcinoma of the cervix in pregnancy. Am J Obstet Gynecol 82:45, 1961
320. Bonomi PD, Yordan EL: Chemotherapy of cervical carcinoma. In Deppe G (ed): Chemotherapy of Gynecologic Cancer, p 103. New York, Alan R Liss, 1984
321. Wasserman TH, Carter SKL: The integration of chemotherapy into combined modality treatment of solid tumors: VIII. Cervical cancer. Cancer Treat Rep 4:25, 1977
322. Malkasian GD, Decker DG, Jorgensen EP: Chemotherapy of carcinoma of the cervix. Gynecol Oncol 5:109, 1976
323. Thigpen T, Shingleton H, Homsley H, et al: Cis-platinum in treatment of advanced or recurrent squamous cell carcinoma of the cervix: A phase II study of the Gynecologic Oncology Group. Cancer 48:899, 1981
324. Lira-Puerta V, Tenovio F, Wernz J, et al: Phase II study of cisplatin or dibromoducitol for carcinoma of the cervix. Proc Am Soc Clin Oncol 1:111, 1982
325. Stehman FB, Blom J, Blessing J, et al: Phase II trial of galactitol 1,2:5,6-dianhydro (NSC 132313) in the treatment of advanced gynecologic malignancies: a Gynecologic Oncology Group study. Gynecol Oncol 15:381, 1983
326. McGuire WP, Blessing JA, Hatch K, et al: A Phase II study of CHIP in advanced squamous cell carcinoma of the cervix (a Gynecologic Oncology Group study). Invest New Drugs 4:181, 1986
327. Arseneau J, Blessing JS, Stehman FB, et al: A Phase II study of carboplatin in advanced squamous cell carcinoma of the cervix (a Gynecologic Oncology Group study). Invest New Drugs 4:187, 1986
328. Morrow CP, DiSaia PJ, Mangan CF, et al: Continuous pelvic arterial infusion with bleomycin for squamous carcinoma of the cervix recurrent after irradiation therapy. Cancer Treat Rep 61:1403, 1977

329. Swenerton KD, Evers JA, White GW, et al: Intermittent pelvic infusion with vincristine, bleomycin and mytomycin C for advanced recurrent carcinoma of the cervix. Cancer Treat Rep 63:1379, 1979
330. Ohta A: Basic and clinical studies on the simultaneous combination treatment of cervical cancer (especially advanced cases) with a carcino-static agent and radiation. J Tokyo Med Coll 36:529, 1978
331. Oku T, Iwaskaki M, Tojo S: Study on surgical chemotherapy for advanced cancer of the uterine cervix—Particularly on the problem of clinical effect and drug concentration. Acta Obstet Gynaecol Jpn 31:1833, 1979
332. Kavanagh JJ, Rutledge F, Wharton JT, et al: Palliation of advanced recurrent pelvic malignancies by selective intra-arterial combination chemotherapy. Proc Am Soc Clin Oncol 1:109, 1982
333. Carlson JA, Freedman RS, Wallace S, et al: Intraarterial cis-platinum in the management of squamous cell carcinoma of the uterine cervix. Gynecol Oncol 12:92, 1981
334. Piver MS, Varlow JJ, Vongtama V, et al: Hydroxyurea and radiation therapy in advanced cervical cancer. Am J Obstet Gynecol 120:969, 1974
335. Climie ARW, Rachmaninoff N: A ten-year experience with endometrial carcinoma. Surg Gynecol Obstet 120:73, 1965
336. Austin JH, MacMahon B: Indicators of prognosis in carcinoma of the corpus uteri. Surg Gynecol Obstet 128:1247, 1969
337. Hreshchyshyn MM, Aron BS, Boronow RC, et al: Hydroxyurea or placebo combined with radiation to treat stages IIIB and IV cervical cancer confined to the pelvis. Int J Radiat Oncol Biol Phys 5:317, 1979
338. Piver MS, Barlow JJ, Vongtama V, et al: Hydroxyurea as a radiation sensitizer in women with carcinoma of the uterine cervix. Am J Obstet Gynecol 129:379, 1977
339. Fletcher GH: Cancer of the uterine cervix. Janeway Lecture. Am J Roentgenol Radium Ther Nucl Med 111:225, 1971
340. Perez CA, Breaux S, Madoc-Jones H, et al: Radiation therapy alone in the treatment of carcinoma of the uterine cervix: I. Analysis of tumor recurrence. Cancer 51:1393, 1983
341. Choo YC, Choy TK, Wong LC: Potentiation of radiotherapy by cis-dichlorodiammine platinum (II) in advanced cervical carcinoma. Gynecol Oncol 23:94, 1986
342. Twiggs LB, Potish RA, McIntyre S, et al: Concurrent weekly cis-platinum and radiotherapy in advanced cervical cancer: a preliminary dose escalating toxicity study. Gynecol Oncol 24:143, 1986
342a. Potish RA, Twiggs LB, Adcock LL, et al: Effect of cis-platinum on tolerance to radiation therapy in advanced cervical cancer. Am J Clin Oncol 9:387, 1986
343. Creasman WT, Weed JC Jr: Carcinoma of the endometrium (FIGO Stages I and II): Clinical features and management. In Coppleson M (ed): Gynecologic Oncology: Fundamental Principles and Clinical Practice, pp 562–574. New York, Churchill Livingstone, 1985
344. Damon A: Host factors in cancer of the breast and uterine cervix and corpus. J Natl Cancer Inst 24:485, 1960
345. Wynder EL, Escher GC, Montel N: An epidemiological investigation of cancer of the endometrium. Cancer 19:489, 1966
346. MacMahon B: Risk factors for endometrial cancer. Gynecol Oncol 2:122, 1974
347. Masubuchi K, Nemoto H: Epidemiologic studies on uterine cancer at Cancer Institute Hospital, Tokyo, Japan. Cancer 30:208, 1972
348. McDonald TW, Malkasian GD, Gaffney TA: Endometrial cancer associated with feminizing ovarian tumor and polycystic ovarian disease. Obstet Gynecol 49:654, 1977
349. Gusberg SB, Kardon P: Proliferative endometrial response to theca-granulosa cell tumors. Am J Obstet Gynecol 3:633, 1971
350. Smith DC, Prentice R, Thompson DJ, et al: Association of exogenous estrogen and endometrial carcinoma. N Engl J Med 293:1164, 1975
351. Amtunes CMF, Stolley PD, Rosensheim NB, et al: Endometrial cancer and estrogen use (Report of a large case-control study). N Engl J Med 300:9, 1979
352. Nachtigall LE, Nachtigall RH, Nachtigall RD, et al: Estrogen replacement therapy II: A prospective study in the relationship to carcinoma and cardiovascular metabolic problems. Obstet Gynecol 54:74, 1979
353. Gambrel DR Jr: Role of hormones in the etiology and prevention of endometrial and breast cancer. Acta Obstet Gynecol Scand [Suppl] 106:337, 1982
354. Frick HC, Munnell EW, Richart RM, et al: Carcinoma of the endometrium. Am J Obstet Gynecol 115:663, 1973
355. Moss WT: Common peculiarities of patients with adenocarcinoma of the endometrium, with special reference to obesity, body build, diabetes and hypertension. Am J Roentgenol Radium Ther Nucl Med 58:203, 1947
356. Sommers SC, Hertig AT, Beugloff H: Genesis of endometrial carcinoma. 11 cases 19 to 35 years old. Cancer 2:957, 1949
357. Buchler DA, Peckham BM, Carr WF: Treatment and results of endometrial carcinoma from 1956–1974. In Gray LA Sr (ed): Endometrial Carcinoma and Its Treatment: The Role of Irradiation, Extent of Surgery, and Approach to Chemotherapy, pp 146–150. Springfield, IL, Charles C Thomas, 1977
358. Gore H, Hertig AT: Premalignant lesions of the endometrium. Clin Obstet Gynecol 5:1148, 1962
359. Plentl AA, Friedman EA: Lymphatic system of the female genitalia: The morphologic basis of oncologic diagnosis and therapy, pp 116–152. Philadelphia, WB Saunders, 1971
360. Creasman WT, Boronow RC, Morrow CP, et al: Adenocarcinoma of the endometrium: Its metastatic lymph node potential. Gynecol Oncol 4:239, 1976
361. Berman ML, Ballon SC, Lagasse LD, et al: Prognosis and treatment of endometrial cancer. Am J Obstet Gynecol 136:679, 1980
362. Tak WK: Carcinoma of the endometrium, with cervical involvement (Stage II). Cancer 43:2504, 1979
363. Creasman WT, DiSaia PJ, Blessing J, et al: Prognostic significance of peritoneal cytology in patients with endometrial cancer and preliminary data concerning therapy and intraperitoneal pharmaceuticals. Am J Obstet Gynecol 141:931, 1981
364. Kennedy AW, Peterson FL, Becker SN, et al: Experience with pelvic washings in Stage I and II endometrial carcinoma. Gynecol Oncol 28:50, 1987
365. Reagan JW, Fu YS: Pathology of endometrial carcinoma. In Coppleson M (ed): Gynecologic Oncology: Fundamental Principles and Clinical Practice, pp 546–561. New York, Churchill Livingstone, 1981
366. Ng ABP, Reagan JW, Storaasli JP, et al: Mixed adenosquamous carcinoma of the endometrium. Am J Clin Pathol 59:765, 1973
367. Silverberg SG, Bolin MG, DeGiorgio LS: Adenoacanthoma and mixed adenosquamous carcinoma of the endometrium. A clinico-pathologic study. Cancer 30:1307, 1972
368. Salazar VM, DePapp EW, Bonifiglio TA, et al: Adenosquamous carcinoma of the endometrium: An entity with an inherent poor prognosis? Cancer 40:119, 1977
369. Kurman RJ, Scully RE: Clear cell carcinoma of the endometrium: an analysis of 21 cases. Cancer 37:872, 1976
370. Hertig AT, Gore H: Tumors of the female sex organs: Part 2. Tumors of the vulva, vagina and uterus. In Atlas of Tumor Pathology, Series 1, Fascicle 33. Washington, DC, Armed Forces Institute of Pathology, 1960
371. Fluhman CF: Squamous epithelium in benign and malignant conditions. Surg Gynecol Obstet 46:309, 1928
372. Hendrickson M, Ross J, Eifel P, et al: Uterine papillary serous carcinoma: A highly malignant form of endometrial adenocarcinoma. Am J Surg Pathol 6:93, 1982
373. Ramirez-Gonzalez CE, Adams K, Mangual-Vazquez TY, et al: Papillary Adenocarcinoma in the Endometrium. Obstet Gynecol 70:212, 1987
374. Boronow RC, Morrow CP, Creasman WT, et al: Surgical staging in endometrial cancer: Clinical-pathologic findings of a prospective study. Obstet Gynecol 63:825, 1984
375. Lewis BW, Stallworthy JA, Cowdell R: Adenocarcinoma of the body of the uterus. J Obstet Gynecol Br Commonw 77:343, 1970
376. Jones HW: Treatment of adenocarcinoma of the endometrium. Obstet Gynecol Surv 30:147, 1975
377. Surwit EA, Fowler WC Jr, Rogoff EE, et al: Stage II carcinoma of the endometrium. Int J Radiat Oncol Biol Phys 5:323, 1979
378. Lutz MH, Underwood PB, Kreutner A, et al: Endometrial carcinoma: A new method of classification of therapeutic and prognostic significance. Gynecol Oncol 6:83, 1978
379. DiSaia PJ, Creasman WT, Boronow RC, et al: Risk factors and recurrent patterns in Stage I endometrial cancer. Am J Obstet Gynecol 151:1009, 1985
380. Morrow CP, DiSaia PJ, Townsend DE: Current management of endometrial carcinoma. Obstet Gynecol 42:399, 1973
381. Boronow RC: Endometrial cancer: Not a benign disease. Obstet Gynecol 47:630, 1976
382. Arneson A: Clinical results and histologic changes following the radiation treatment of cancer of the corpus uteri. Am J Roentgenol Radium Ther Med 36:461, 1936
383. Kempson RL, Pokorny GE: Adenocarcinoma of the endometrium in women 40 years of age and younger. Cancer 21:650, 1968
384. Nolan JF, Dorough ME, Anson JH: The value of preoperative radiation therapy in Stage I carcinoma of the uterine corpus. Am J Obstet Gynecol 98:663, 1967
385. Underwood PB, Lutz MH, Kreutner A, et al: Carcinoma of the endometrium: Radiation followed immediately by operation. Am J Obstet Gynecol 128:86, 1977
386. Gusberg SB, Chen SY, Cohen CJ: Endometrial cancer: Factors influencing the choice of treatment. Gynecol Oncol 2:308, 1974
387. Malkasian GD Jr: Carcinoma of the endometrium: Effect of stage and grade on survival. Cancer 41:996, 1978
388. Kottmeier HL: Individualization of therapy in carcinoma of the corpus. In Cancer of the Uterus and Ovary. MD Anderson Hospital, pp 102–108. Chicago, Year Book, 1969
389. Landgren RD, Fletcher GH, Deldos L, et al: Irradiation of endometrial cancer in patients with medical contraindication to surgery or with unresectable lesions. Am J Roentgenol Radium Ther Nucl Med 126:148, 1976
390. Aalders H, Abler Z, Kolstad P, et al: Postoperative external irradiation and prognostic parameters in stage I endometrial carcinoma. Clinical and histopathologic study of 540 patients. Obstet Gynecol 56:419, 1980
391. Wharam MO, Phillips TL, Bagshaw MA: The role of radiation therapy in clinical stage I carcinoma of the endometrium. Int J Radiat Oncol Biol Phys 1:1081, 1976
393. Landgren RC, Fletcher GH, Delclos L, et al: Irradiation of endometrial cancer in patients with medical contraindications to surgery or with unresectable lesions. Am J Roentgenol Rad Ther Nucl Med 126:148, 1976
394. Strickland PL: Carcinoma corpus uteri: A radical intracavitary treatment. Br J Radiol 16:112, 1965
395. Homesley HD, Boronow RC, Lewis JL: Stage II Endometrial Adenocarcinoma: Memorial Hospital for Cancer, 1949–1965. Obstet Gynecol 49:604, 1977
396. Larson DM, Copeland LJ, Gallager HS, et al: Nature of cervical involvement in endometrial carcinoma. Cancer 59:959, 1987
397. Kinsella TJ, Bloomer WD, Lavin PT, et al: Stage II endometrial carcinoma: Ten-year followup of combined radiation and surgical treatment. Gynecol Oncol 10:290, 1980
398. Grigsby PW, Perez CA, Camel HM, et al: Stage II carcinoma of the endometrium:

Results of therapy and prognostic factors. Int J Radiat Oncol Biol Phys 11:1915, 1985
399. Rutledge F: The role of radical hysterectomy in adenocarcinoma of the endometrium. Gynecol Oncol 2:331, 1974
400. Graham H: The value of preoperative or postoperative treatment by radium for carcinoma of the uterine body. Surg Gynecol Obstet 1323:855, 1971
401. Stokes S, Bedwinek JM, Kao M-S, et al: Treatment of stage I adenocarcinoma of the endometrium by hysterectomy and adjuvant irradiation: A retrospective analysis of 304 patients. Int J Radiat Oncol Biol Phys 12:339, 1986
402. Beiler DD, Schmitz DA, O'Rourke TL: Carcinoma of the endometrium: Radiation and surgery versus surgery alone. Radiology 102:159, 1972
403. Wharam MO, Phillips TL, Bagshaw MA: The role of radiation therapy in clinical stage I carcinoma of the endometrium. Int J Radiat Oncol Biol Phys 1:1081, 1976
404. Malkasian GD Jr, McDonald TW, Pratt JH: Carcinoma of the endometrium. Mayo Clinic Experience. Mayo Clinic Proc 51:175, 1977
405. Salazar OM, Feldstein ML, DePapp EW, et al: Endometrial carcinoma: Analysis of failures with special emphasis on the use of initial preoperative external pelvic radiation. Int J Radiat Oncol Biol Phys 2:1101, 1977
406. Brady LW, Lewis GC, Antoniades J, et al: Evolution of therapeutic techniques. Gynecol Oncol 2:253, 1974
407. Bedwinek JM, Galakatos A, Camel HM, et al: Stage I, grade III adenocarcinoma of the endometrium treated with surgery and irradiation: Sites of failure and correlation of failure rate with irradiation technique. Cancer 54:40, 1984
408. Anderson JC, Meltzer HD, Scarborough JE, et al: Adenocarcinoma of the endometrium. Cancer 18:955, 1965
409. Gusberg SB, Yannopoulos D: Therapeutic decisions in corpus cancer. Am J Obstet Gynecol 120:73, 1964
410. Cheon HK: Prognosis of endometrial carcinoma. Obstet Gynecol 34:680, 1969
411. Nilson PA, Koller O: Carcinoma of the endometrium in Norway 1957–1960 with special reference to treatment results. Am J Obstet Gynecol 105:1099, 1969
412. Ng ABP, Reagan JW: Incidence and prognosis of endometrial carcinoma by histologic grade and extent. Obstet Gynecol 35:437, 1970
413. Sall S, Sonneblick B, Stone ML: Factors affecting survival of patients with endometrial adenocarcinoma. Am J Obstet Gynecol 107:116, 1970
414. Nahhas WA: Prognostic factors in endometrial carcinoma (personal communication, 1971)
415. Wade E, Kohorn EI, Morris JM: Adenocarcinoma of the endometrium. Evaluation of preoperative irradiation and factors influencing prognosis. Am J Obstet Gynecol 99:869, 1967
416. Javert CT: The spread of benign and malignant endometrium in the lymphatic system with a note on coexisting vascular involvement. Am J Obstet Gynecol 64:780, 1952
417. Webb GA, Margolis AJ, Traut HF: Adenocarcinoma of the endometrium: An evaluation of factors influencing prognosis and an outline of a plan of therapy based on these factors. West J Surg Obstet Gynecol 63:407, 1955
418. Lindgren L: The prognosis of carcinoma of the endometrium in its different stages treated by surgery combined with postoperative radiotherapy. Acta Obstet Gynecol Scand 36:426, 1957
419. Boutselis JG, Bair JR, Nichols V, et al: Carcinoma of the uterine corpus: A study of 269 cases, 1947–1959. Am J Obstet Gynecol 85:994, 1963
420. Dobbie BMW, Taylor CW, Waterhouse JAH: A study of carcinoma of the endometrium. J Obstet Gynaecol Br Commonw 72:659, 1965
421. Roman R, Beck R, Latour J: Correlation of histologic grading with 5-year survival rates in endometrial carcinoma. Am J Obstet Gynecol 97:117, 1967
422. Sala JM, del Regato JA: The treatment of carcinoma of the endometrium. Radiology 79:12, 1969
423. Silverberg SG, DeGiorgi LS: Histopathologic analysis of preoperative radiation therapy in endometrial carcinoma. Am J Obstet Gynecol 119:698, 1974
424. Weigensberg IJ: Preoperative radiation therapy in endometrial carcinoma: Preliminary report of a clinical trial. Am J Roentgenol Radium Ther Nucl Med 127:391, 1976
425. Greenberg SB, Glassburn JR, Antoniades J, et al: Management of carcinoma of the uterus stage II. Cancer Clin Trials 4:183, 1981
426. Gagnon JD, Moss WT, Gabourel LS, et al: External irradiation in the management of stage II endometrial carcinoma. A logical approach. Cancer 44:1247, 1979
427. Onsrud M, Aalders J, Abeler V, et al: Endometrial carcinoma with cervical involvement (stage II): Prognostic factors and value of combined radiological-surgical treatment. Gynecol Oncol 13:76, 1982
428. Spanos WJ, Fletcher GH, Wharton JT, et al: Patterns of pelvic recurrence in endometrial carcinoma. Gynecol Oncol 6:495, 1978
429. Landgren RC, Fletcher GH, Delclos L, et al: Irradiation of endometrial cancer in patients with medical contraindication to surgery or with unresectable lesions. Am J Roentgenol Radium Ther Nucl Med 126:148, 1976
430. Antoniades J, Brady LW, Lewis GC: The management of stage III carcinoma of the endometrium. Cancer 38:1838, 1967
431. Rutledge F, Ehrlich C: Adenocarcinoma of the endometrium. In Gray LA Sr (ed): Endometrial Carcinoma and Its Treatment: The Role of Irradiation, Extent of Surgery, and Approach to Chemotherapy, pp 128–137. Springfield, IL, Charles C Thomas, 1977
432. Kottmeier HL: Endometrial carcinoma and its treatment: Recent experience of the Radiumhemmet, Stockholm. In Gray LA Sr (ed): Endometrium Carcinoma and Its Treatment: The Role of Irradiation, Extent of Surgery and Approach to Chemotherapy, pp 118–126. Springfield, IL, Charles C Thomas, 1977
433. Homesley HD, Lewis JL Jr: Treatment of endometrial adenocarcinoma at Memorial Hospital, New York, 1884–1976. In Gray LA Sr (ed): Endometrial Carcinoma and Its Treatment: The Role of Irradiation, Extent of Surgery and Approach to Chemotherapy, pp 99–17. Springfield, IL, Charles C Thomas, 1977
434. Boronow RC: Endometrial cancers: Staging, pretreatment evaluation and factors in outcome. In Gray LA Sr (ed): Endometrial Carcinoma and Its Treatment: The Role of Irradiation, Extent of Surgery and Approach to Chemotherapy, pp 38–57. Springfield, IL, Charles C Thomas, 1977
435. Geisler HE, Gibbs CP: Invasive carcinoma of the endometrium. A 5 to 16 year followup of 183 patients. Am J Obstet Gynecol 102:516, 1968
436. Danoff BF, McDay J, Louka M, et al: Stage III endometrial carcinoma: Analysis of patterns of failure and therapeutic implications. Int J Radiat Oncol Biol Phys 6:1491, 1980
437. Barber HRK, Brunschwig A: Treatment and results of recurrent cancer of the corpus uteri in patients receiving anterior and posterior pelvic exenteration (1947–1963). Cancer 22:949, 1968
438. Stander RW: Vaginal metastases following treatment of endometrial carcinoma. Am J Obstet Gynecol 71:776, 1956
439. Stokes S, Bedwinek J, Breaux S, et al: Treatment of stage I adenocarcinoma of the endometrium by hysterectomy and adjuvant irradiation: Analysis of complications. Obstet Gynecol 65:86, 1985
440. Kneale BLG: Adjunctive and therapeutic progestins in endometrial cancer. Clin Obstet Gynecol 13:789, 1986
441. Ehrlich CE, Young PCM, Cleary RE: Cytoplasmic progesterone and estradiol receptors in normal, hyperplastic and carcinomatous endometria: Therapeutic implications. Am J Obstet Gynecol 141:539, 1981
442. Podratz KC, O'Brien PC, Malkasian GD Jr: Effects of progestational agents in treatment of endometrial carcinoma. Obstet Gynecol 66:106, 1985
443. Quinn MA, Cauchi M, Fortuna D: Endometrial carcinoma: Steroid receptors and response to medroxyprogesterone acetate. Gynecol Oncol 21:314, 1985
444. Swenerton KD: Treatment of advanced endometrial adenocarcinoma with tamoxifen. Cancer Treat Rep 64:805, 1980
445. Bonte J: Recente aanwinsten in de behandeling van endometriaal adenocarcinoma. Tijdschm. Voor Geneeskind 37:1377, 1981
446. Rendina GM, Donadio C, Saccucci P, et al: La nostra esperienza sulla terapia endocriva del carcinoma endometriale in fase avanzata (studio comparativo SW 269 casi). G Ital Oncol 3:153, 1983
447. Rendina GM, Donadio C, Fabri M, et al: Tamoxifen and medroxyprogesterone therapy for advanced endometrial carcinoma. Eur J Obstet Gynecol Reprod Biol 17:285, 1984
448. Slavik M, Petty WM, Blessing JA, et al: Phase II clinical study of tamoxifen in advanced endometrial adenocarcinoma. A Gynecology Oncology Group Study. Cancer Treat Rep 68:809, 1984
449. Hald I, Salimschick M, Mouridsen HT: Tamoxifen treatment of advanced endometrial carcinoma a phase II study. Eur J Gynecol Oncol 4:83, 1983
450. Carlson JA, Allegra JC, Day TG, et al: Tamoxifen and endometrial carcinoma: Alterations in estrogen and progesterone receptors in untreated patients and combination hormonal therapy in advanced neoplasia. Am J Obstet Gynecol 149:149, 1984
451. Lewis GC Jr, Slack NH, Mortel R, et al: Adjuvant progestogen therapy in the primary definitive treatment of endometrial cancer. Gynecol Oncol 2:368, 1974
452. Malkasian GD Jr, Decker DG: Adjuvant progesterone therapy for stage I endometrial carcinoma. Int J Gynecol Obstet 16:48, 1978
453. Beck RP: Experience in treating two hundred and eighty-eight patients with endometrial carcinoma from 1968 to 1972. Am J Obstet Gynecol 133:260, 1979
454. Gusberg SB: Current concepts in cancer: The changing nature of endometrial cancer. N Engl J Med 302:729, 1980
455. Kucera VH, Gerstner G, Michalica W, et al: Hormonprophylaxe bel der strahlenbehandlung des korpuskarzinomas mit hochdosierten gestagenen. Wien Med Wochenschr 129:395, 1979
456. Fournier D, Kubli F, Bauer M, et al: Hochdosierte gestagenlaznzeittherapie biem korpuskarizon, einflub aut uberlebenzeit. Geburtsh Frauenheilk 41:266, 1981
457. Bochman YV, Chepik OF, Volkova AT, et al: Can primary endometrial carcinoma stage I be cured without surgery and radiation therapy? Vopr Onkol 28:42, 1982
458. De Palo G, Spatti GB, Luciani L: Pilot study with adjuvant hormone therapy in FIGO Stage I endometrial carcinoma with myometrial invasion. Tumori 69:65, 1983
459. Lagasse L, Thigpen T, Morrison F: Phase II trial of piperazinedione in treatment of advanced endometrial carcinoma, uterine sarcoma, and vulvar carcinoma. Proc Am Assoc Cancer Res 20:388, 1970
460. Thigpen T, Blessing J, DiSaia P, et al: Phase II trial of cisplatinum in the management of advanced or recurrent endometrial carcinoma. Proc Am Soc Clin Oncol 22:469, 1981
461. Seski JC, Edwards CL, Herson J, et al: Cisplatin chemotherapy for disseminated endometrial cancer. Obstet Gynecol 59:225, 1982
462. Seski JC, Edwards CL, Copeland LG, et al: Hexamethylmelamine chemotherapy for disseminated endometrial cancer. Obstet Gynecol 58:361, 1981
463. Depe G, Malviya VK, Zbella E: Non-hormonal chemotherapy in endometrial cancer —a review. Wien Klin Wochenschr 96:747, 1984
464. Cohen CJ: Cytotoxic chemotherapy for patients with endometrial carcinoma. Clin Obstet Gynecol 13:811, 1986

465. Thigpen JT, Buschbaum HJ, Mangan C, et al: Phase II trial of adriamycin in the treatment of advanced or recurrent endometrial carcinoma. A Gynecologic Oncology Group Study. Cancer Treat Rep 63:21, 1979
466. Pasmantier MW, Coleman M, Silver RT, et al: Treatment of advanced endometrial carcinoma with doxorubicin and cisplatin: Effects on both untreated and previously treated patients. Cancer Treat Rep 69:539, 1985
467. Seltzer V, Vogl SE, Kaplan BH: Adriamycin and cisdiaminedichloroplatinum in the treatment of endometrial adenocarcinoma. Gynecol Oncol 19:308, 1984
468. Chauvergne J, Granger C, Mage PH, et al: Chimiotherapie palliative des cancers de l'endometre. Rev Fr Gynecol Obstet 81:547, 1986
469. Turbow MM, Thornton J, Ballon S, et al: Chemotherapy of advanced endometrial carcinoma with platinum, adriamycin, and cyclophosphamide. Proc Am Soc Clin Oncol 1:108, 1982
470. Hancock KC, Freedman RS, Edwards CL, et al: Use of cisplatin, doxorubicin, and cyclophosphamide to treat advanced and recurrent adenocarcinoma of the endometrium. Cancer Treat Rep 70:789, 1986
471. Bruckner HW, Deppe G: Combination chemotherapy of advanced endometrial adenocarcinoma with adriamycin, cyclophosphamide, 5-fluorouracil and medroxyprogesterone acetate. Obstet Gynecol 50:415, 1977
472. Cohen CJ, Deppe G, Bruckner HW: Treatment of advanced adenocarcinoma of the endometrium with melphalan, 5-fluorouracil and medroxyprogesterone acetate. A preliminary study. Obstet Gynecol 50:415, 1977
473. Lovecchio JL, Averette HE, Lichtinger M, et al: Treatment of advanced or recurrent endometrial adenocarcinoma with cyclophosphamide, doxorubicin, cis-platinum and megestrol-acetate. Obstet Gynecol 63:557, 1984
474. Piver MS, Lele SB, Patsner B, et al: Melphalan, 5-fluorouracil, and medroxyprogesterone acetate in metastatic endometrial carcinoma. Obstet Gynecol 67:261, 1986
475. Horton J, Elson P, Jordan P, et al: Combination chemotherapy for advanced endometrial cancer: An evaluation of three regimens. Cancer 49:2441, 1982
476. Lewis JL Jr, Berchuck A, Rubin SC, et al: Uterine Sarcomas in Shu MH, Brennan M (eds): Surgical Management of Soft Tissue Sarcoma. Philadelphia, Lea & Febiger (in press)
477. DiSaia PJ, Castro JR, Rutledge FN: Mixed mesodermal sarcoma of the uterus. Am J Roentgenol Rad Ther Nucl Med 117:632, 1973
478. Berchuck A, Rubin SC, Hoskins WJ, et al: Treatment of uterine leiomyosarcoma. Obstet Gynecol (in press)
479. Kempson RL, Bari W: Uterine sarcomas: Classification, diagnosis and prognosis. Hum Pathol 1:331, 1970
479a. Ober WB: Uterine sarcomas. Histogenesis and taxonomy. Ann NY Acad Sci 75:568, 1959
480. Norris HJ, Roth E, Taylor HB: Mesenchymal tumors of the uterus. II. A clinical and pathological study of 31 mixed mesodermal tumors. Obstet Gynecol 28:57, 1966
481. Salazar OM, Bonfiglio TA, Patten SF, et al: Uterine sarcomas. Natural history, treatment and prognosis. Cancer 42:1152, 1978
482. Major F, Silverberg S, Morrow P, et al: A preliminary analysis of prognostic factors in uterine sarcomas. A Gynecologic Oncology Group Study. Gynecol Oncol 26:411, 1987
483. Perez CA, Askin F, Baglan RJ, et al: Effect of irradiation on mixed mullerian tumors of the uterus. Cancer 43:1274, 1979
484. Edwards CL: Undifferentiated tumors. In Cancer of the Uterus and Ovary, pp 84–94. Chicago, Year Book, 1969
485. DiSaia PJ, Castro JR, Rutledge FN: Mixed mesodermal sarcoma of the uterus. Am J Roentgenol Radium Ther Nucl Med 117:632, 1973
486. Vongtama V, Karlen JR, Piver SM, et al: Treatment, results and prognostic factors in stage I and II sarcomas of the corpus uteri. Am J Roentgenol 126:139, 1976
487. Belgrad R, Elbadaw N, Rubin P: Uterine sarcoma. Radiology 114:181, 1975
488. Salazar OM, Bonfiglio TA, Patten SF, et al: Uterine sarcomas. Analysis of failures with special emphasis on the use of adjuvant radiation therapy. Cancer 42:1161, 1978
489. Omura GA, Major FJ, Blessing JA, et al: A randomized study of Adriamycin with and without Dimethyltriazenomidazole Carboxamide in advanced uterine sarcomas. Cancer 52:626, 1983
490. Omura GA, Blessing JA, Lifshitz S, et al: A randomized trial of adjacent Adriamycin in uterine sarcomas: A Gynecologic Oncology Group study. J Clin Oncol 3:1240, 1985
491. Piver MS, Lurain JR: Uterine sarcomas: Clinical features and management. In Coppleson M (ed): Gynecologic Oncology: Fundamental Principles and Clinical Practice, pp 608–618. New York, Churchill Livingstone, 1981
492. Taylor HB, Norris HJ: Mesenchymal tumors of the uterus. IV. Diagnosis and Prognosis of leiomyosarcomas. Arch Pathol 82:40, 1966
493. Silverberg SC: Leiomyosarcoma of the uterus: A clinicopathologic study. Obstet Gynecol 38:613, 1971
494. Bartsich EG, Bowe ET, Moore JG: Leiomyosarcoma of the uterus: A 50 year review of 42 cases. Obstet Gynecol 32:101, 1968
495. Christopherson WM, Williamson EO, Gray LA: Leiomyosarcoma of the uterus. Cancer 29:1512, 1972
496. Giarratano RC, Slate TA: Sarcoma of the uterus. Obstet Gynecol 38:472, 1971
497. Newlands ES: New chemotherapeutic agents in the management of gestational trophoblastic disease. Semin Oncol 9:239, 1982
497a. Hart WR, Yoonessi M: Endometrial stromatosis of the uterus. Obstet Gynecol 49:393, 1977
498. Wong LC, Choo YC, Ma HK: Etoposide, methotrexate, and bleomycin in drug-resistant gestational trophoblastic disease. Gynecol Oncol 24:51, 1986
498a. Norris HJ, Taylor HB: Mesenchymal tumors of the uterus. I. A clinical and pathologic study of 53 endometrial stromal tumors. Cancer 19:755, 1966
499. Koss LG, Spiro RH, Brunschwig A: Endometrial stromal sarcoma. Surg Gynecol Obstet 121:531, 1965
500. Baggish MS, Woodruff JD: Uterine stromatosis: Clinicopathologic features and hormone dependency. Obstet Gynecol 40:487, 1972
501. Sedlis A: Primary carcinoma of the fallopian tube. Obstet Gynecol 16:209, 1961
502. Roberts JA, Lifshitz S: Primary adenocarcinoma of the fallopian tube. Gynecol Oncol 13:301, 1982
503. Hu CY, Taymor ML, Hertig AT: Primary carcinoma of the fallopian tube. Am J Obstet Gynecol 59:58, 1950
504. Green TH, Scully RE: Tumors of the fallopian tube. Clin Obstet Gynecol 5:886, 1962
505. Woodruff JD, Julian CG: Multiple malignancy in the upper genital canal. Am J Obstet Gynecol 103:810, 1969
506. Benedet JL, White GW: Malignant tumors of fallopian tube. In Coppleson M (ed): Gynecologic Oncology: Fundamental Principles and Clinical Practice, pp 621–629. New York, Churchill Livingstone, 1981
507. Woodruff JD, Pauerstein CJ: The Fallopian Tube. Baltimore, Williams & Wilkins, 1969
508. Wheeler JE, Mastroianni L Jr: Pathology of the fallopian tube. In Blaustein A (ed): Pathology of the Female Genital Tract, pp 359–362. New York, Springer-Verlag, 1977
509. Hanton EM, Malkasian GD Jr, Dahlin DC, et al: Primary carcinoma of the fallopian tube. Am J Obstet Gynecol 94:832, 1966
510. Scheffey LC, Lang WR, Nugent FB: Clinical and pathologic aspects of primary sarcoma of the uterine tube. Am J Obstet Gynecol 52:904, 1941
511. Wu JP, Tanner WS, Fardal PM: Malignant mixed Mullerian tumor of the uterine tube. Obstet Gynecol 41:707, 1973
512. Hertig AT, Gore H: Tumors of the female sex organs: Part 3. Tumors of the ovary and fallopian tube. In Atlas of Tumor Pathology Series 1, fasc 33. Washington, DC, Armed Forces Institute of Pathology, 1961
513. Patton GWJ, Goldstein DP: Gestational choriocarcinoma of the tube and ovary. Surg Gynecol Obstet 137:608, 1973
514. Weiss PD, MacDougall MK, Regan JW, et al: Primary adenosquamous carcinoma of the fallopian tube. Obstet Gynecol 55:885, 1980
515. Plentl AA, Friedman EA: Lymphatic system of the female genitalia: The morphologic basis of oncologic diagnosis and therapy, pp 153–157. Philadelphia, WB Saunders, 1971
516. Novak ER, Woodruff JD: Novak's Gynecologic and Obstetric Pathology. Philadelphia, WB Saunders, 1971
517. Frick MC: Cancer of the fallopian tube. In Gusberg SG, Frick MC (eds): Corscaden's Gynecologic Cancer. Baltimore, Williams & Wilkins, 1978
518. Dodson MG, Ford JH Jr, Averette HE: Clinical aspects of fallopian tube carcinoma. Obstet Gynecol 36:935, 1970
519. Shiller HM, Silverberg SG: Staging and prognosis in primary carcinoma of the fallopian tube. Cancer 28:389, 1971
520. Erez S, Kaplan AL, Wall JA: Clinical staging of the uterine tube. Obstet Gynecol 30:547, 1967
521. McMurray EH, Jacob AJ, Perez CA, et al: Carcinoma of the fallopian tube: Management and sites of failure. Cancer 58:2070, 1986
522. Boutselis JG, Thompson JN: Clinical aspects of primary carcinoma of the fallopian tube. Am J Obstet Gynecol 111:98, 1971
523. Raju KS, Barker GH, Wiltshaw E: Primary carcinoma of the fallopian tube: Report of 22 cases. Br J Obstet Gynaecol 88:1124, 1981
524. Pauerstein CJ: The Fallopian Tube: A Reappraisal. Philadelphia, Lea & Febiger, 1974
525. Engstrom L: Primary carcinoma of the fallopian tube. Acta Obstet Gynecol Scand 36:289, 1957
526. Greene TH Jr, Scully RE: Tumors of the fallopian tube. Clin Obstet Gynecol 5:886, 1962
527. Phelps MH, Chapman EK: Role of radiotherapy in treatment of primary carcinoma of the uterine tube. Obstet Gynecol 43:669, 1974
528. Amendola BE, LaRouere J, Amendola MA, et al: Adenocarcinoma of the fallopian tube. Surg Gynecol Obstet 158:223, 1983
529. Henderson SR, Harper RC, Salazar OM, et al: Primary carcinoma of the fallopian tube. Difficulties of diagnosis and treatment. Gynecol Oncol 5:168, 1977
530. Guthrie D, Cohen S: Carcinoma of the fallopian tube treated with a combination of surgery and cytotoxic chemotherapy. Br J Obstet Gynaecol 88:1051, 1981
531. Griffiths CT: Ovary and the fallopian tube. In Holland JF, Frei E III (eds): Cancer Medicine, p 1718. Philadelphia, Lea & Febiger, 1972
532. Jacobs AJ, McMurray EH, Parham J, et al: Treatment of carcinoma of the fallopian tube using cisplatin, doxorubicin, and cyclophosphamide. Am J Clin Oncol 9:436, 1986
533. U.S. Public Health Service, National Vital Statistics Division Vital Statistics of the United States, Annual 1930–1983, Washington, U.S. Government Printing Office, 1934–1985
534. Acosta-Sison H: Statistical study of chorionephithelioma in the Phillipine General Hospital. Am J Obstet Gynecol 58:125, 1949
535. Teoh ES, Dawood MY, Ratnam SS: Epidemiology of hydatidiform mole in Singapore. Am J Obstet Gynecol 110:53, 1947
536. Hertig AT, Sheldon WH: Hydatidiform mole—A pathologicoclinical correlation of 200 cases. Am J Obstet Gynecol 53:1, 1947

537. Deligdisch L, Driscoll SG, Goldstein DP: Gestational trophoblastic neoplasms: Morphologic correlates of therapeutic response. Am J Obstet Gynecol 130:801, 1978
538. Goldstein DP: Endocrine assay in chorionic tumors. Clin Obstet Gynecol 18:41, 1978
539. Vaitukaitis JL, Braunstein GD, Ross GT: A radioimmunoassay which specifically measures human chorionic gonadotropin in the presence of human luteinizing hormone. Am J Obstet Gynecol 38:453, 1976
540. Goldstein DP: Chorionic gonadotropin. Cancer 38:453, 1976
541. Woo JSK, Ngan HYS, Ma HK: Non-resolution of pelvic sonographic abnormality after chemotherapy for persistent trophoblastic disease—A word of caution. Eur J Obstet Gynecol Reprod Biol 22:153, 1983
542. Goldstein DP, Berkowitz RS: The management of gestational trophoblastic neoplasms. Curr Prob Obstet Gynecol 4:1, 1980
543. Bagshawe DK: Risk and prognostic factors in trophoblastic neoplasia. Cancer 38:1373, 1976
544. Dijkema HE, Aalders JG, DeBruijn HWA, et al: Risk factors in gestational trophoblastic disease, and consequences for primary treatment. Eur J Obstet Gynecol Reprod Biol 22:145, 1986
545. Goldstein DP, Berkowitz RS, Cohen SM: The current management of molar pregnancy. Curr Prob Obstet Gynecol 3:1, 1978
546. Li MC, Hertz R, Spence DB: Effect of methotrexate therapy upon choriocarcinoma and chorioadenoma. Proc Soc Exp Biol Med 93:361, 1956
547. Hertz R, Lewis JL Jr, Lipsett MB: Five years experience with the chemotherapy of metastatic choriocarcinoma and related trophoblastic disease. Gynecol Oncol 23:111, 1986
548. Berkowitz RS, Goldstein DP, Bernstein MR: Ten years experience with methotrexate and folinic acid as primary therapy for gestational trophoblastic disease. Gynecol Oncol 23:111, 1986
549. Berkowitz RS, Goldstein DP: Methotrexate with citrovorum factor rescue for nonmetastatic gestational neoplasms. Obstet Gynecol 54:725, 1979
550. Surwit EA, Hammond CB: Treatment of metastatic trophoblastic disease with poor prognosis. Obstet Gynecol 53:207, 1979
551. Bagshawe KD: Treatment of trophoblastic tumors. Ann Acad Med 5:273, 1976
552. Weed JC, Barnard DE, Currie JL, et al: Chemotherapy with the modified Bagshawe protocol for poor prognosis metastatic trophoblastic disease. Obstet Gynecol 59:377, 1982
553. Berkowitz RS, Goldstein D, Bernstein M: Modified triple chemotherapy in the management of high risk metastatic gestational trophoblastic tumors. Gynecol Oncol 19:173, 1984
554. Hansen LA, Clayton BD: Treatment of gestational trophoblastic tumors. Drug Intell Clin Pharm 18:569, 1984
555. Ballon SC, Berman ML, Lagasse LD, et al: The unique aspects of gestational trophoblastic disease. Obstet Gynecol Surv 32:405, 1977
556. Bagshawe KD: Treatment of trophoblastic tumors. Ann Acad Med 5:273, 1976
557. Surwit EA, Suciu TN, Schmidt HJ, et al: A new combination chemotherapy for resistant trophoblastic disease. Gynecol Oncol 8:110, 1979
558. Newlands ES, Bagshawe KD: Activity of high dose cis-platinum (NCI 119875) in combination with vincristine and methotrexate in drug resistant gestational choriocarcinoma. A report of 17 cases. Br J Cancer 40:943, 1979
559. Newlands ES, Bagshawe KD: The role of BP16-213 (Etoposide) in gestational choriocarcinoma. Cancer Chemother Pharmacol 7:211, 1982
560. Amiel JL, Droz JP, Tursz T: Placental tumors resistant to usual chemotherapy: Treatment using cis-diaminedichloroplatinum. Two cases. Nouv Presse Med 7:1933, 1978
561. Gordan AN, Lavanagh JJ, Gershenson DM, et al: Cisplatin, vinblastine, and bleomycin combination therapy in resistant gestational trophoblastic disease. Cancer 58:1407, 1986
562. Ross GT: Congenital anomalies among children born to mothers receiving chemotherapy for gestational trophoblastic neoplasms. Cancer 37:1043, 1976
563. Kuten A, Cohen Y, Thatcher M, et al: Pregnancy and delivery after successful treatment of epidural metastatic choriocarcinoma. Gynecol Oncol 6:464, 1978
564. Smith PG, Doll R: Late effects of X irradiation in patients treated for metropathia haemorrhagica. Br J Radiol 49:224, 1976
565. Hutchinson GB: Leukemia in patients with cancer of the cervix uteri treated with radiation. A report covering the first five years of an international study. J Natl Cancer Inst 40:9591, 1968
566. Dickson RJ: The late results of radium treatment for benign uterine haemorrhage. Br J Radiol 42:582, 1969
567. Wagoner JK: Leukemia and other malignancies following radiation therapy for gynecological disorders. Boice, Fraumeni (eds): Radiation Carcinogenesis: Epidemiology and Biological Significance, pp 153–159. New York, Raven Press, 1984
568. Arneson AN, Schellhas HF: Multiple primary cancers in patients treated for carcinoma of the cervix. Am J Obstet Gynecol 106:1155, 1970
569. Spratt JS, Hoag MG: Incidence of multiple primary cancers per man years of follow-up: Twenty-year review from Ellis Fischel State Cancer Hospital. Ann Surg 164:775, 1966
570. Lee JY, Perez CA, Ettinger N, et al: The risk of second primaries subsequent to irradiation for cervix cancer. Int J Radiat Oncol Biol Phys 8:207, 1982
571. Wagoner JK: Presented at the 1969 meeting of the American Public Health Association
572. Feinleib M: Breast cancer and artificial menopause: A cohort study. J Natl Cancer Inst 41:315, 1968
573. Villasanta U, Rubel H: Radium treatment of benign uterine bleeding. Long-term follow-up. Obstet Gynecol 33:813, 1969
574. Thomas WO Jr, Harris HH, Enden JA: Postirradiation malignant neoplasms of the uterine fundus. Am J Obstet Gynecol 104:209, 1969

ROBERT C. YOUNG
ZVI FUKS
WILLIAM J. HOSKINS

CHAPTER 37 *Cancer of the Ovary*

Ovarian cancer is the fourth most frequent cause of cancer death in women and the leading cause of gynecologic cancer death in the United States. More women die of ovarian cancer yearly than from cervical and endometrial carcinoma combined. Incidence and mortality estimates for 1986 indicate that 19,000 new cases are diagnosed yearly and 11,600 women die.[1] A steady increase in the age-adjusted ovarian cancer death rates has been observed over the past 25 years, with similar increases in other industrialized nations as well.[2] Approximately 1 woman in 70 will develop the disease, and about 1% of all female deaths are due to ovarian cancer.

EPIDEMIOLOGY

The highest ovarian cancer rates are reported from highly industrialized countries, with age-adjusted mortality rates that range from 3.02 : 100,000 in Italy to 7.04 : 100,000 in the United States and 11.02 : 100,000 in Denmark. The notable exception is Japan, where rates of death from ovarian cancer are 1.69:100,000, among the lowest in the world. Studies of migrant populations suggest significant environmental influences. Japanese migrants to Hawaii and their first-generation offspring in the United States have an incidence significantly higher than women in Japan but lower that that in the indigenous white population of the United States.[3,4]

In the United States, the common epithelial ovarian neoplasms are most frequent in adult white populations. They are rarely seen before menarche but tend to increase significantly thereafter, with peak incidence in the 40- to 70-year-old group. In contrast, germ-cell ovarian tumors are seen primarily in children and young women and are more frequent in nonwhite populations.

Several epidemiologic studies suggest that disordered endocrine function may contribute to the development of ovarian cancer. For example, a higher incidence of epithelial tumors is seen in women with lower mean number of pregnancies, in those never pregnant, and in those with a history of infertility.[5–7] No clear-cut association between ovarian cancer and the administration of synthetic estrogens has been established,[8] but oral contraceptives appear to reduce the risk.[9] Also, cancer of the ovary and cancer of the breast appear to share some etiologic factors. For example, women with breast cancer have twice the expected risk of ovarian carcinoma, and women with ovarian cancer have a threefold to fourfold increase in the frequency of subsequent breast cancer.

No association with viral infections has been identified. Paradoxically, a lower-than-expected frequency of mumps and other viral exanthems is reported for women with ovarian cancer.[10]

Familial and genetic associations have been reported but are rare. Ovarian cancer has been reported in multiple members of the same or succeeding generations.[11] Several unusual genetic disorders seem to predispose to ovarian neoplasms, although the tumors are usually benign and stromal in origin. Females with Peutz–Jeghers syndrome (mucocutaneous pigmentation and intestinal polyps) have a 5% to 14% chance of developing ovarian tumors, and women with inherited basal-cell nevus syndrome develop benign fibromas or, rarely, other tumors. Patients with gonadal dysgenesis (46XY genotype or mosaic) are prone to gonadoblastomas, but, interestingly, patients with Turner's syndrome (45X0) and undeveloped gonads have no such tendency. An increased frequency of ovarian thecomas has been described in patients on long-term anticonvulsant therapy and is believed to be related to variations in the ability to metabolize these drugs.[12]

Although epidemiologic evidence strongly suggests environmental causes, few, if any, associations have been firmly established. There is no good evidence that either diagnostic or therapeutic irradiation increases the frequency of this malignancy. Likewise, there is no established association with known chemical carcinogens. Ovarian cancer has not been seen among women with industrial exposure to dyes, tars, or anthracene-containing compounds.[13] However, exposure to asbestos or talc is associated with an increased risk of ovarian carcinoma in humans. Studies indicate a higher-than-expected frequency of ovarian and peritoneal neoplasms in asbestos workers. Passage of such materials through the bowel wall or retrograde through the female reproductive tract has been described and could explain how such agents arrive at the ovarian epithelium.[14,15]

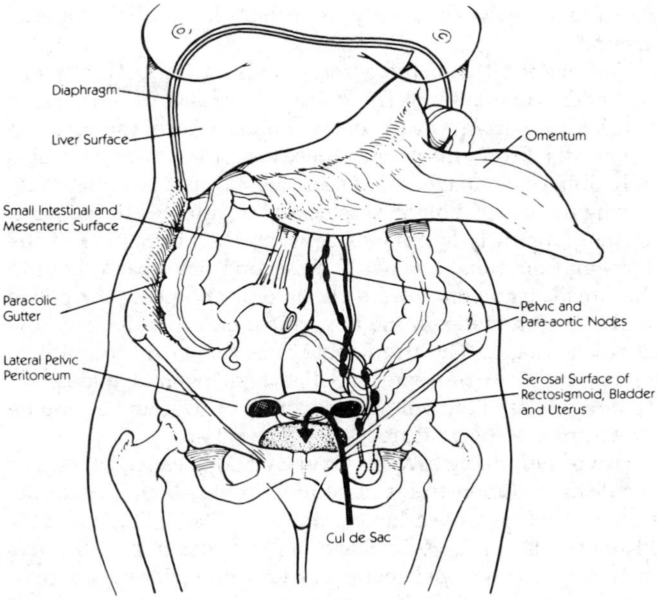

FIG. 37-1. Spread of disease in ovarian cancer.

PATHOGENESIS AND BEHAVIOR

Epithelial carcinomas account for 80% to 90% of ovarian malignancies; the remaining ovarian tumors arise from the germ or stromal cells. Epithelial tumors arise from the serosal mesothelial layer of the gonads. In the embryo, the ovary develops from the genital ridge of thickened coelomic epithelium. The germ cells originate in the primitive streak and migrate to the gonad, where they proliferate to form the bulk of the cortex. The mesenchyma of the medulla gives rise to the ovarian stroma. All three of these cell types (coelomic epithelial cells, germ cells, and stromal cells) can give rise to malignant neoplasms.[16] Because the coelomic epithelium has the multipotential capability to differentiate into endometroid, mucinous, or serous epithelium, the common epithelial tumors of the ovary have these characteristic cell types.[17]

Epithelial tumors disseminate primarily by surface shedding, lymphatic spread, or, rarely, metastasizing hematogenously. Most of the errors committed by surgeons in the operative management of this disease can be directly related to a lack of understanding of the patterns of spread. Figure 37–1 illustrates the typical spread of the disease. Commonly, these tumors spread by continuity and intraperitoneal dissemination.[18] Spread to the opposite ovary occurs in 6% to 13% of patients with otherwise Stage IA disease,[19,20] and transperitoneal tumor implantation or lymphatic spread to the uterus and fallopian tubes occurs in approximately 5% of patients otherwise thought to be Stage IA (see below for discussion of staging system).[19] However, with more advanced stages of disease, the uterus is involved in 25%,[18] sometimes with demonstrable retrograde lymphatic tumor emboli. Direct spread may also involve the peritoneal surfaces of the bladder, the rectosigmoid, or the pelvic peritoneum.

The most common type of extraovarian spread is transperitoneal dissemination of cells shed from gross or microscopic excrescences on the surface of the primary tumor. The presence of malignant cells in the peritoneal cavity in spite of an apparently intact capsule indicates that some cancers exfoliate cells even before there is disruption of the capsule.[21] The exfoliated clonogenic cells attach to the peritoneal surfaces and form micrometastases, which continue to exfoliate clonogenic cells. These free-floating cells are removed from the peritoneal cavity through lymphatic channels located in the diaphragm.[22,23] Clearance does not take place evenly over the whole diaphragmatic surface, being more extensive on the right side overlying the liver[24] because respiratory movements create a flow of peritoneal fluid along the abdominal gutters that ultimately flows predominantly to the right hemidiaphragm.[25] Drainage then occurs into the submesothelial lymphatic capillaries of the diaphragm, which intercommunicate with the pleural surface and subsequently with the anterior mediastinal lymph nodes.[22,26,27] This pathway quantitatively accounts for 80% of the peritoneal clearance. Peritoneoscopic studies have shown that a significant fraction of patients otherwise thought to have Stage I or Stage II disease have involvement of the undersurface of the diaphragm,[28–30] and this fact accounts for the failure to cure some patients with "Stage I–II" disease. Partial or complete obstruction of the diaphragmatic lymphatics by tumor cells allows implantation on the omentum and at various other sites on the serosal surface of the peritoneum. It also causes accumulation of carcinomatous ascites.[31] The force of gravity in the upright patient leads to early implantation in the cul-de-sac and along the surface of the rectum.

Autopsy studies have demonstrated virtual 100% involvement of the omenta of patients dying of ovarian carcinoma. Occult omental metastases have been found in 3% to 11% of untreated patients who were thought to have Stage I or II disease at initial surgical exploration.[30,32] Steinberg and associates[33] reported that 22% of 55 grossly negative omenta had histologically proven tumor. In one-half of these patients, the omentum was the only demonstrable site of Stage III disease.

The ovarian lymphatic system is also an important pathway of dissemination.[34] The lymphatic vessels of the ovarian parenchyma drain into the ovarian hilus to form the subovarian plexus. From this plexus, there are three different routes of lymphatic drainage. The main pathway ascends bilaterally among the ovarian blood vessels and terminates in the para-aortic group of lymph nodes between the bifurcation of the aorta and the renal arteries. The second route passes within the broad ligaments toward the lateral and posterior pelvic wall and terminates in the uppermost external iliac and hypogastric nodes. The third route runs along the round ligaments and into the external iliac and inguinal nodes, accounting for the uncommon instances of ovarian carcinoma spread to the inguinal nodes.

Use of lymphangiography in early and advanced stages of the disease demonstrates dissemination in about 15% of patients with Stage I ovarian carcinoma, 17% in Stage II, 31% in Stage III, and 64% in Stage IV.[35-37] At autopsy, the frequency of involved pelvic and aortic lymph nodes is approximately equal, with 80% of patients showing metastases.[38] Burghardt and associates[39] performed complete pelvic and para-aortic lymphadenectomies in 48 patients with untreated ovarian cancer and found that 14% had positive lymph nodes in Stages I and II and 63% in Stages III and IV. Pelvic nodes were involved more frequently than para-aortic nodes, which were never involved unless pelvic nodes were involved. Preliminary data from a Gynecologic Oncology Group (GOG) surgical staging study indicate that in patients with disease in Stage I, Stage II, or optimal Stage III (defined in this study as less than 3 cm of abdominal disease prior to debulking), the incidence of positive pelvic lymph nodes is 11% and the incidence of positive para-aortic lymph nodes is 8%[40].

Although peritoneum, omentum, bowel surfaces, and retroperitoneal lymph nodes are the most frequent sites of spread, other organs are also at risk for metastasis. Among the distant organs that may be involved are (in order of decreasing frequency) liver, lung, pleura, kidney, bone, adrenal gland, bladder, and spleen.[18] Recent studies of recurrence after negative second-look laparotomy have found disease outside the abdominal cavity in as many as 50% of patients.[41,42]

PATHOLOGY

Several comprehensive reviews of the pathology of ovarian cancer have been published that provide detailed descriptions for each of the individual tumor types.[43-47] The World Health Organization (WHO) and the International Federation of Gynecology and Obstetrics (FIGO) have adopted a unified classification of the common epithelial tumors, the sex cord-stromal tumors, and the germ-cell tumors (Table 37-1). The vast majority (85%-90%) of malignant ovarian tumors seen in the United States are of the epithelial type, and their approximate overall frequency is as follows: serous cystadenocarcinoma, 42%; mucinous cystadenocarcinoma, 12%; endometrioid carcinoma, 15%; undifferentiated carci-

37-1. World Health Organization Classification of Malignant Ovarian Tumors

Common Epithelial Tumors
- Malignant serous tumors
  - Adenocarcinoma, papillary adenocarcinoma, papillary cystadenocarcinoma
  - Surface papillary carcinoma
  - Malignant adenofibroma, cystadenofibroma
- Malignant mucinous tumors
  - Adenocarcinoma, cystadenocarcinoma
  - Malignant adenofibroma, cystadenofibroma
- Malignant endometroid tumors
  - Carcinoma
    - Adenocarcinoma
    - Adenoacanthoma
    - Malignant adenofibroma, cystadenofibroma
  - Endometroid stromal sarcomas
  - Mesodermal (müllerian) mixed tumors: homologous and heterologous
- Clear-cell (mesonephroid) tumors, malignant
  - Carcinoma and adenocarcinoma
- Brenner tumors, malignant
- Mixed epithelial tumors, malignant
- Undifferentiated carcinoma
- Unclassified

Sex Cord-Stromal Tumors
- Granulosa-stromal cell tumors
  - Granulosa-cell tumor
  - Tumors in the thecoma-fibroma group
  - Fibroma
  - Unclassified
- Androblastomas: Sertoli-Leydig cell tumors
  - Well-differentiated
    - Tubular androblastoma, Sertoli cell tumor (tubular adenoma of Pick)
    - Tubular androblastoma with lipid storage, Sertoli cell tumor with lipid storage (folliculome lipidique of Lecene)
    - Sertoli-Leydig cell tumor (tubular adenoma with Leydig cells)
  - Leydig cell tumor, hilus cell tumor
    - Of intermediate differentiation
    - Poorly differentiated (sarcomatoid)
    - With heterologous elements
- Gynandroblastoma
- Unclassified

Lipid (Lipoid) Cell Tumors
- Germ-Cell Tumors
  - Dysgerminoma
  - Endodermal sinus tumor
  - Embryonal carcinoma
  - Polyembryoma
  - Choriocarcinoma
  - Teratomas
    - Immature
    - Mature dermoid cyst with malignant transformation
    - Monodermal and highly specialized
      - Struma ovarii
      - Carcinoid
      - Struma ovarii and carcinoid
      - Others
  - Mixed forms
- Gonadoblastoma
  - Pure
  - Mixed with dysgerminoma or other form of germ cell tumor

Modified from Serov SF, Scully RE, Solvin LH: International Histological Classification of Tumors, No. 9. Histological Typing of Ovarian Tumors. Geneva, World Health Organization, 1973.

noma, 17%; and clear-cell carcinoma, 6%. The remaining 8% of primary tumors are the sex cord–stromal and germ-cell tumors.

EPITHELIAL OVARIAN CARCINOMA

Tumors of Low Malignant Potential (Borderline Tumors)

Epithelial tumors are generally classified as benign, malignant (invasive), or carcinomas of low malignant potential (tumors of borderline malignancy). The latter group has neoplastic epithelial cells, cellular clusters detached from sites of origin, increased mitotic activity, and nuclear abnormalities. However, they lack obvious invasion of the supporting stroma. The incidence of these borderline epithelial tumors is variable but may approach 15% of all epithelial tumors.

These tumors clearly possess a different natural history; they grow and metastasize slowly. Five-year survival rates for patients with serous and mucinous low-malignant-potential epithelial tumors range from 74% to 98%.[48] In another study, the 5- and 10-year survival rates of patients with low-malignant-potential tumors were 93% and 91%, respectively, compared with 34% and 29% for patients with invasive epithelial carcinomas.[49] It is therefore important to identify patients with tumors of low malignant potential and to distinguish them from the patients with invasive ovarian carcinoma when planning treatment or analyzing results and survival.

The optimal treatment for borderline tumors is unclear. In early-stage (I and II) disease, surgical resection alone usually produces excellent results. However, in the more advanced stages, some investigators advocate therapeutic approaches similar to those used for more invasive tumors, for despite the fact that these tumors grow more slowly, approximately 10% to 15% of patients will die of their disease within the first 5 to 10 years.

Histology: Importance of Type and Grade

For the invasive epithelial carcinomas, an independent correlation of survival with histologic type has not been found consistently.[50–54] The current consensus is that there is limited prognostic significance to the histologic type of these cancers independent of clinical stage, extent of residual disease, and histologic grade.

In contrast to histologic type, the degree of cellular differentiation of epithelial cancers (histologic grade) is an important independent predictor of response to treatment and survival.[55–58] For example, studies from the Mayo Clinic of Stage II serous cystadenocarcinoma demonstrate an 80% survival for patients with Broder's Grade 1 tumors, 47% for Grade 2, and 10% for Grade 3 and 4 tumors.[56] Day and colleagues have made similar observations using the pattern system of grading.[57] In Stages I and II serous carcinoma of the ovary, patients with Grade 1 tumors had a 78% 7-year survival rate compared with 35% for Grade 2 and 0 for Grade 3. Although initial studies emphasized the effect of grade on prognosis in early-stage disease, subsequent studies suggest it is important even in more advanced disease. Using grading systems based on cytologic detail (Broder's) or the pattern-grading classification based on the degree to which the tumor forms papillary structures or glands rather than solid sheets, several investigators have shown survival significance to grading systems for patients with advanced disease treated with chemotherapy.[58,59]

A study by Dembo and Bush suggests a more complex interaction of grade and histologic type.[60] In patients with serous tumors, the effect of grade was highly significant, whereas grade was not of prognostic significance in patients with mucinous, endometrioid, or clear-cell tumors. When the two variables of grade and histologic type were combined, it was possible to show significant survival differences between patients with "favorable" pathologies (serous well-differentiated and mucinous, endometrioid, and clear-cell types of all grades), in whom the 5-year survival rate was 59%, and patients with "unfavorable" pathologies (serous, moderately, and poorly differentiated and the unclassified type), in whom the 5-year survival rate was 19%.

Histologic grading of ovarian tumors has not been accepted enthusiastically by pathologists, primarily because no standardized and easily reproducible objective classification exists. Nevertheless, in spite of the different classifications used, virtually every published study thus far indicates an important survival impact of tumor grade, and grading is now a requirement in every carefully designed clinical study.

STROMAL AND GERM-CELL TUMORS

Stromal Tumors

Fewer than 10% of all ovarian tumors are of stromal origin. These include tumors containing granulosa, theca, Sertoli, Leydig, and collagen-producing stromal cells or their embryonic precursors.[47,61] Only the granulosa-cell tumor, of the many stromal tumors listed in Table 37–1, is seen with significant frequency. This tumor is composed of granulosa cells with or without an admixture of theca cells and may contain folliculoid structures known as Call–Exner bodies. These tumors can be associated with feminizing effects and precocious puberty secondary to tumor-related estrogen secretion. Presenting signs and symptoms are similar to those of epithelial ovarian tumors with the exception of those related to hyperestrogenism. These tumors tend to be discovered at earlier stages and to have a more indolent course than the epithelial tumors. Late recurrences sometimes can be treated effectively with repeated cytoreductive surgery. There is no convincing evidence that the tumor is particularly responsive to radiation therapy or chemotherapy, but responses to alkylating agents and Adriamycin (doxorubicin) have been described. Recently, 6 of 11 patients treated with a combination of cisplatin, vinblastine, and bleomycin (PVB) achieved pathologically documented complete remission (CR),[62] but follow-up is short and toxicity significant.

Sertoli–Leydig cell tumors are characterized by differentiation toward testicular structures. These contain various mixtures of Sertoli and Leydig cells and tissues similar to those of the fetal testis.

Gonadal stromal tumors occasionally contain granulosa-cell elements combined with tubules and Leydig cells characteristic of the arrhenoblastoma. Such tumors are called gynandroblastomas.

Germ-Cell Tumors

Although germ-cell tumors constitute less than 5% of all ovarian malignancies, they are important because they occur in young women, display a vastly different natural history than epithelial tumors, and require different treatment. Nearly all of these patients can be cured using combination chemotherapy and limited surgery. Irradiation is now used only for the dysgerminomas.

Of these tumors, dysgerminoma, endodermal sinus tumor, and embryonal carcinoma are most often encountered. The dysgerminomas comprise less than 2% of all ovarian malignancies, are cytologically similar to seminoma of the testis, and display a very similar natural history. These tumors are frequently (90%) unilateral and tend to be localized, with secondary spread by way of the lymphatics to the para-aortic nodes. The tumor is highly radiosensitive, and primary management is with surgery and radiation. Five-year survival rates with effective conventional therapy approach 80% to 90%.

The terms "endodermal sinus tumor" and "embryonal carcinoma" have, in the past, often been used interchangeably to describe highly malignant germ-cell tumors of the ovary. However, there is now convincing evidence that the two disorders are different.[61] Embryonal carcinoma, with patterns typical of embryonal carcinoma of the testis and associated with elevations of serum human chorionic gonadotropin (hCG) or alpha-fetoprotein (α-FP), is rarely seen in the ovary. Endodermal sinus tumors are more common and are similar morphologically to the infantile orchioblastoma. The endodermal sinus tumor, also called yolk sac tumor, is characterized by reticular patterns, papillary formations known as Schiller–Duval bodies, and both intracellular and extracellular hyaline droplets. This tumor is derived from extraembryonic rather than embryonic tissues. Both tumors are highly aggressive, metastasize hematogenously, and are poorly controlled even with radical surgery and irradiation. Chemotherapy is highly effective however and will be discussed in a later section.

DIAGNOSIS AND STAGING

There are no specific symptoms or signs of ovarian cancer, particularly in early stages, and as a result, when symptoms and signs appear, they are usually manifestations of advanced disease. Early on, ovarian cancer is often asymptomatic; symptoms of nausea, dyspepsia, and vague lower abdominal discomfort are frequently ignored by the patient or the doctor. Seventy-five percent of patients will have spread beyond the ovary at diagnosis, and 60% will have spread beyond the pelvis.[63,64] Sall and Stone[65] found that 37% of patients had abdominal discomfort or pain, 35% had abdominal swelling or masses, and 15% experienced vaginal bleeding. Gastrointestinal symptoms were present in 10% and urinary tract symptoms in 1.5% In two other large series, the presenting symptoms were pain (57%), abdominal distention (51%), and vaginal bleeding (25%).[66,67]

Because the ovary lies in the rather spacious pelvic cavity and is suspended loosely by the ovarian and infundibulopelvic ligaments, a mass may become quite large without producing symptoms of either pain or pressure. When pain does occur, it is probably caused by stretching of the supporting ligaments and may be both nonspecific and intermittent. Discomfort from compression of the bladder or rectum is also nonspecific. It is therefore essential that all women, particularly perimenopausal or postmenopausal women, with pelvic or abdominal symptoms have a thorough physical and pelvic examination with careful evaluation of the adnexal area. All too often, women are subjected to several weeks or months of expensive diagnostic radiographic studies when a pelvic examination in the office would have revealed the large pelvic mass that was finally discovered on computed tomography (CT) scan or magnetic resonance imaging (MRI). Of even more concern is the delay in diagnosis that results from trying various symptomatic therapies without having performed a pelvic examination.

Palpation of an adnexal mass in a premenarchal or postmenopausal female is one indication for exploratory laparotomy. Functional ovarian cysts should not occur in these age groups, and a palpable mass usually indicates neoplastic growth. The incidence of malignancy in such patients is difficult to determine, but the high mortality rate of ovarian cancer that has spread beyond the ovary mandates early surgical exploration. Barber and Graber[68] have pointed out that the normal ovary during the reproductive years is approximately 3.5 × 2.0 × 1.5 cm but that in the postmenopausal patient it should be 2.0 × 1.0 × 0.5 cm or less. As a result, palpation of an ovary in a postmenopausal woman indicates ovarian enlargement, and surgical exploration should be considered. However, Flynt and Gallup[69] performed exploratory laparotomy on 11 patients with a palpable postmenopausal ovary and found only one malignancy: a colon carcinoma. A larger series of patients is needed to clarify whether all such patients should undergo surgical exploration.

Ovarian enlargement in a woman during the reproductive years is more often benign. Most of these enlargements are attributable to either follicular or corpus luteum cysts (functional cysts), and the vast majority will regress in one to three menstrual cycles. Such patients should be followed by repeat pelvic examination at 4- to 6-week intervals. Some gynecologists recommend oral contraceptives to increase the speed of spontaneous resolution by preventing stimulation of the ovary by pituitary hormones. Table 37-2 outlines the suggested management of patients with an adnexal mass. Although still in the reproductive age group, patients who are over age 40 are at greater risk for ovarian cancer. Fortunately, retention of reproductive function is usually of less concern in these patients.

Conventional Papanicolaou smears offer little diagnostically because they are rarely positive and then only in advanced disease. However, any patient with adenocarcinoma cells on a Pap smear and a negative evaluation of the vulva, vagina, cervix, and endometrium should be considered to have carcinoma of the ovary, fallopian tubes, or other intra-

TABLE 37-2. Management of the Patient with an Adnexal Mass

Observe and Repeat Examination in 4–6 Weeks	*Surgical Exploration*
Reproductive age	Premenarchal Post-menopausal
Less than 8 cm	Greater than 8 cm
Decreasing size	Increase in size or persistence through 2–3 menstrual cycles
Cystic and smooth	Solid and irregular
Mobile	Fixed
Unilateral	Bilateral
Asymptomatic	Pain or other symptoms of acute intra-abdominal process
No ascites	Ascites

TABLE 37-3. Evaluation of Patients with Suspected Ovarian Carcinoma

Careful history and physical examination to include breast and pelvic examination and Papanicolaou smear
Complete blood count, biochemical profile, and CA-125 assay
Chest radiograph
Intravenous urogram
Cystoscopy
Proctoscopy
Barium enema
CT, MRI, or ultrasound*
Upper-gastrointestinal series with small-bowel follow-through in patients with upper gastrointestinal symptoms or symptoms of partial bowel obstruction

* As indicated by clinical evaluation.

abdominal organs. If a metastatic evaluation is negative, the patient should be considered for surgical exploration.

Some investigators have attempted mass screening of asymptomatic patients by peritoneal lavage with culdocentesis,[70–72] but poor patient acceptance and low positive yield make this an ineffective method of diagnosing ovarian cancer. Moreover, Rubin and associates[73] have recently shown that peritoneal washings were negative in more than 50% of patients with gross intraperitoneal disease at second-look surgical exploration.

Laparoscopy as a diagnostic tool for ovarian carcinoma should, in general, be discouraged. Although it may occasionally be useful in differentiating uterine leiomyomata or endometriosis from ovarian cancer, such cases are infrequent. Laparoscopic biopsy or needle aspiration of an unruptured ovarian mass should not be performed because malignant cells may be spilled into the peritoneal cavity.

Ultrasound is a safe, noninvasive procedure that may be used to define intra-abdominal disease. Solid elements and prominent papillary projections with involvement of adjacent viscera suggest a malignant neoplasm. Ultrasound can also be used to distinguish ascites from a large ovarian cyst. A mass separate from the uterus associated with internal echoes of normal sensitivity suggests ovarian cancer. Ultrasound can also be used to guide direct percutaneous needle aspiration of suspected metastasis or aspiration biopsies of aortic nodes.[74,75]

Lymphangiography is useful in the evaluation of patients with ovarian carcinoma[35–37,76] and detects nodal involvement in 30%. In those positive, 32% had disease in the pelvic nodes only, and in 46%, there was diffuse retroperitoneal involvement of both pelvic and para-aortic nodes.[19] Lymphangiography is accurate when the aortic lymph nodes are enlarged by tumor and the radiologist has sufficient expertise. In one study of 33 patients with positive preoperative lymphangiograms, histologic confirmation was obtained in 100%. In 63 patients with negative preoperative lymphangiograms, the lymphographic–histologic correlation was 87.3%. Eight of these 63 patients (12.7%) had microscopic nodal involvement at surgery. The overall accuracy of bipedal lymphangiography in this study thus was 91.7%.[37]

CT adds useful diagnostic and staging information to that obtained by ultrasound, lymphangiography, and surgery. CT may clearly delineate liver and pulmonary nodules, abdominal and pelvic masses, and retroperitoneal nodal involvement. However, it is costly and still cannot reliably detect masses smaller than 2 cm in diameter. The technique has been particularly useful in ovarian carcinoma when bowel ileus makes an ultrasonogram difficult to interpret.[77] CT has also been used to detect subcutaneous metastases in patients with ovarian cancer.[78]

Preoperative evaluation of a patient with suspected ovarian cancer is outlined in Table 37–3. The extent of such an evaluation requires that the physician use clinical judgment: a young woman with a persistent unilateral cystic mass may require only basic biochemical evaluation and an intravenous urogram, whereas a postmenopausal woman with a large, irregular mass should undergo a more extensive evaluation.

TUMOR MARKERS

Tumor markers that can detect early ovarian cancer would be valuable because most disease currently is diagnosed only when it is already advanced. Whereas markers have often been helpful in monitoring the rare germ-cell malignancies, they have not been very helpful thus far in detecting early epithelial ovarian malignancies.

The serial measurement of α-FP has facilitated the postsurgical evaluation of therapy for patients with endodermal sinus tumors.[79] After surgical resection, serum α-FP levels progressively decline and, with recurrence, become elevated prior to clinically palpable disease. Assays for α-FP are also helpful in diagnosing an endodermal sinus tumor in a woman with a rapidly enlarging, solid ovarian mass. Human chorionic gonadotropin or its beta subunit has been a valuable tumor marker in the postsurgical evaluation of patients with ovarian choriocarcinoma and embryonal carcinoma or in evaluating germ-cell tumors with choriocarcinomatous elements.[80]

Carcinoembryonic antigen (CEA) is elevated in approximately 58% of patients with Stage III epithelial ovarian cancer.[81] The frequency of elevated CEA levels increases progressively with advancing stage and bulk of tumor. However, because serum CEA levels have also been elevated in patients with cirrhosis, chronic pulmonary disease, inflammatory bowel disease, or a history of heavy cigarette smoking, CEA is of limited diagnostic use in ovarian cancer. Nevertheless, in patients who do have elevated CEA levels before therapy, serial measurements may be valuable in monitoring subclinical disease.

Numerous investigators have attempted to isolate tumor-specific antigens that could be used for both serologic diagnosis and monitoring of patients during therapy.[82–85] Of all of these, the monoclonal antibody OC-125 directed against the antigen CA-125 common to most nonmucinous epithelial ovarian tumors appears to be the most useful.[86] The OC-125 antibody recognizes multiple antigen determinants on a high-molecular-weight (> 500,000 daltons) glycoprotein. These determinants are found in coelomic epithelium during embryonic development and can be detected on fetal tissues, müllerian duct remnants, amnion, and amnionic fluid. The antigen is not found in normal ovarian tissue but is found in nonmucinous epithelial ovarian carcinomas. Eighty-two percent of ovarian cancer patients react positively, and rising or falling titers correlate with disease in 93% of patients. Approximately 25% of patients with nongynecologic malignancies, 5% of patients with benign disease, and 1% of apparently healthy persons have elevated antigen levels (> 35 units of CA-125 per ml of serum).

Recently, several studies have explored CA-125 use in the detection of ovarian carcinoma. Zurawski and colleagues[87] studied 915 nonhospitalized Roman Catholic nuns, in whom CA-125 levels ranged from 0 to 574 U/ml. Thirty-six women (3.9%) had CA-125 levels greater than 35 U/ml, and 7 had levels greater than 65 U/ml. Of the latter 7 women, 5 were found to have benign or malignant neoplasms, including one colon carcinoma, one uterine leiomyoma, one endometrioma, one fibroadenoma of the breast, and one sclerosing adenosis of the breast. None of the 36 patients with levels of greater than 35 U/ml was found to have an ovarian cancer. Einhorn and associates[88] measured CA-125 levels in 100 women undergoing diagnostic laparotomy for a palpable adnexal mass. Levels were greater than 35 U/ml in 11 of 18 patients (61%) with some form of ovarian cancer and were greater than 65 U/ml in 9 of these 11 patients. Malkasian and co-workers[89] studied 64 women with benign ovarian lesions and found 13 of 31 (42%) with endometriosis to have levels greater than 35 U/ml. Other authors[90] have also found elevated levels in patients with endometriosis or hepatitis,[91] during menses in women with and without endometriosis,[92,93] and in patients with pelvic inflammatory diseases or pregnancy.[94]

From these studies, it is clear that CA-125 is not at present specific enough to be an accurate diagnostic test for ovarian cancer. There are insufficient data to determine its sensitivity in an asymptomatic population. Continued evaluation of the test in patients at high risk because of either the presence of an adnexal mass or a family history of ovarian carcinoma is warranted.

On the other hand, a persistent elevation of CA-125 in patients with a history of ovarian cancer has invariably been associated with the finding of residual disease at second-look surgery. Unfortunately, the level may fall into the normal range even though disease remains. Bast and coworkers performed second-look surgery on 15 women whose OC-125 levels had fallen into the normal range, and in 11 of the women residual disease was detected.[86]

The elevation of CA-125 levels may antedate the appearance of detectable disease or recurrence. Levels are often elevated 2 to 7 months before clinical detection of recurrent disease, and, in one unusual patient, elevated levels of CA-125 were present up to a year before the initial diagnosis of ovarian cancer. Unfortunately, the large amount of circulating antigen in most patients prevents the monoclonal antibody from being used effectively in its present form for either imaging or therapeutic purposes.

TREATMENT METHODS

SURGERY

Initial Surgical Staging

Unlike most gynecologic cancers, in which clinical evaluation is used to stage the diseases, ovarian cancer is staged surgically. The FIGO classification was revised in 1985, and although the official report has not been published, FIGO allowed publication of the changes in early 1987[95] (Table 37-4).

Major changes have been made in Stages I, II, and III. In Stages I and II, the former subdivisions "Ai and Aii" and "Bi and Bii" that identified tumor rupture or surface spread have been made part of subdivision C. It is required that malignant cells be identified in either washings or ascites to assign a patient to Stages IC or IIC; the presence of ascites alone without malignant cells is insufficient. In Stage III, subdivisions A, B, and C designate the size of the tumor found at surgical exploration. Inguinal node metastases are included in Stage IIIC. Of particular importance, this staging classification is based on the findings on opening the abdomen and *not* following surgical debulking: (i.e. a patient with disease larger than 2 cm confined to the omentum who has cytoreduction such that no residual tumor is apparent still has Stage IIIC disease). It is essential for the surgeon to define clearly the amount of disease found upon opening the abdomen.

Although only a few patients with ovarian cancer can be managed by surgery alone, the success of subsequent therapy is in large part determined by the accuracy and comprehensiveness of the initial surgical procedure. Proper selection of appropriate adjunctive therapy requires accurate assessment of the extent of residual disease at the conclusion of the initial operation, and the chance of achieving a complete pathologic response (negative second-look operation) is directly related to residual disease volume.

For best results, the surgeon must have a thorough understanding of the pathogenesis of the disease, be thorough in both preoperative preparation and postoperative care, and be appropriately aggressive intraoperatively. Most surgeons prefer a vertical midline incision for patients with suspected ovarian cancer because it provides excellent access to the pelvis and can be extended as far as proves necessary into the upper abdomen. Moreover, patients with apparent early-

TABLE 37-4. FIGO Stage Grouping for Primary Carcinoma of the Ovary (1987)

Stage I	Growth limited to the ovaries	
	IA	Growth limited to one ovary; no ascites. No tumor on the external surface, capsule intact
	IB	Growth limited to both ovaries; no ascites. No tumor on the external surfaces; capsules intact
	IC*	Tumor either Stage IA or IB but with tumor on the surface of one or both ovaries, or with capsule ruptured, or with ascites present containing malignant cells, or with positive peritoneal washings
Stage II	Growth involving one or both ovaries with pelvic extension	
	IIA	Growth involving one or both ovaries with pelvic extension
	IIB	Extension and/or metastases to the uterus and/or tubes
	IIC*	Tumor either Stage IIA or IIB but with tumor on the surface of one or both ovaries, or with capsule(s) ruptured, or with ascites present containing malignant cells, or with positive peritoneal washings
Stage III	Tumor involving one or both ovaries with peritoneal implants outside the pelvis and/or positive retroperitoneal or inguinal nodes. Superficial liver metastases equal Stage III. Tumor is limited to the true pelvis but with histologically verified malignant extension to small bowel or omentum	
	IIIA	Tumor grossly limited to the true pelvis with negative nodes but with histologically confirmed microscopic seeding of abdominal peritoneal surfaces
	IIIB	Tumor of one or both ovaries with histologically confirmed implants of abdominal peritoneal surfaces, none exceeding 2 cm in diameter. Nodes negative
	IIIC	Abdominal implants greater than 2 cm in diameter and/or positive retroperitoneal or inguinal nodes
Stage IV	Growth involving one or both ovaries with distant metastasis. If pleural effusion is present, there must be positive cytologic test results to allot a case to Stage IV. Parenchymal liver metastasis equals Stage IV.	

* To evaluate the impact on prognosis of the different criteria for alloting cases to Stage IC or IIC, it would be of value to know if rupture of the capsule was (1) spontaneous or (2) caused by the surgeon, and if the source of malignant cells detected was (1) peritoneal washings or (2) ascites.

stage disease may require different therapy than those found to have microscopic metastases to the upper abdomen, and proper evaluation of the upper abdomen is rarely possible through a lower-abdominal incision. When gross disease is present in the upper abdomen, proper resection requires adequate exposure. Unfortunately, it is still common to see patients who have had two or more operations for ovarian cancer yet no abdominal scar that extends above the umbilicus.

In a young patient with a nonsuspicious pelvic mass, a low transverse incision may be quite appropriate but must be large enough to remove the mass without danger of rupture. It is never appropriate to aspirate an ovarian mass to reduce its size to fit the incision. In instances in which carcinoma is found and a Pfannenstiel's incision has been used, the incision should be converted to a true transverse incision by dividing the rectus muscles and a second, upper-abdominal midline, incision made to explore the upper abdomen adequately. The patient should be made aware of this possibility preoperatively.

Initial exploration of the abdomen must be thorough and methodical. Figure 37-2 illustrates the essentials. The presence, amount, and character of any ascitic fluid should be noted and the fluid submitted in toto for cytology study. In the absence of ascitic fluid, washings should be obtained from the pelvis, each abdominal gutter, and each subdiaphragmatic surface.

If a unilateral mass is found, the surgeon must decide whether simply to remove it or to remove the tube and ovary. Generally, a cystectomy would be indicated only in a young (less than age 40) patient. If cystectomy is to be performed, the abdomen should be protected by the use of laparotomy tapes from spillage secondary to inadvertent rupture. If frozen-section study indicates a malignant neoplasm, a full metastatic search is mandated. In a patient not concerned about future childbearing, a total abdominal hysterectomy and bilateral salpingo-oophorectomy are indicated. Unilateral salpingo-oophorectomy is indicated only in the young patient desirous of further childbearing in whom careful inspection reveals no evidence of disease other than in one ovary. If careful and methodical inspection of the entire abdomen is negative, biopsies, as outlined in Table 37-5, are performed. In general, it is best to establish a set sequence for inspecting the abdomen and obtaining biopsies so that nothing will be omitted; Table 37-5 outlines the recommended exploration and biopsy procedure. It is not unreasonable to maintain the written protocol in the operating room to ensure accuracy.

Cytoreductive Surgery

Cytoreductive surgery is an integral part of initial patient management and demands substantial skill and judgment. Technically difficult cytoreductive surgery requires not only detailed knowledge of gynecologic surgery but also readiness for complicated abdominal and urologic surgery. Formal residency programs in obstetrics and gynecology and in general surgery do not usually provide the depth of knowledge and experience necessary for the surgical management of ovarian cancer. Whenever possible, therefore, patients with ovarian cancer should be referred to individuals with special training in surgical or gynecologic oncology.

The surgeon faces a formidable task when ovarian carcinoma has spread throughout the abdomen and pelvis. Often, the tumor fills the pelvis, and there is little room for examination of vital structures such as the iliac vessels and ureter. All peritoneal surfaces may be involved, including the lateral pelvic sidewalls, the bladder peritoneum, and the serosa of the rectosigmoid. The optimal approach to the pelvis is via the retroperitoneum. By opening the peritoneum lateral to the iliac vessels (and, if necessary, the colon), the surgeon gains access to the pararectal and paravesical spaces, allowing identification of the major blood vessels, ureter, and

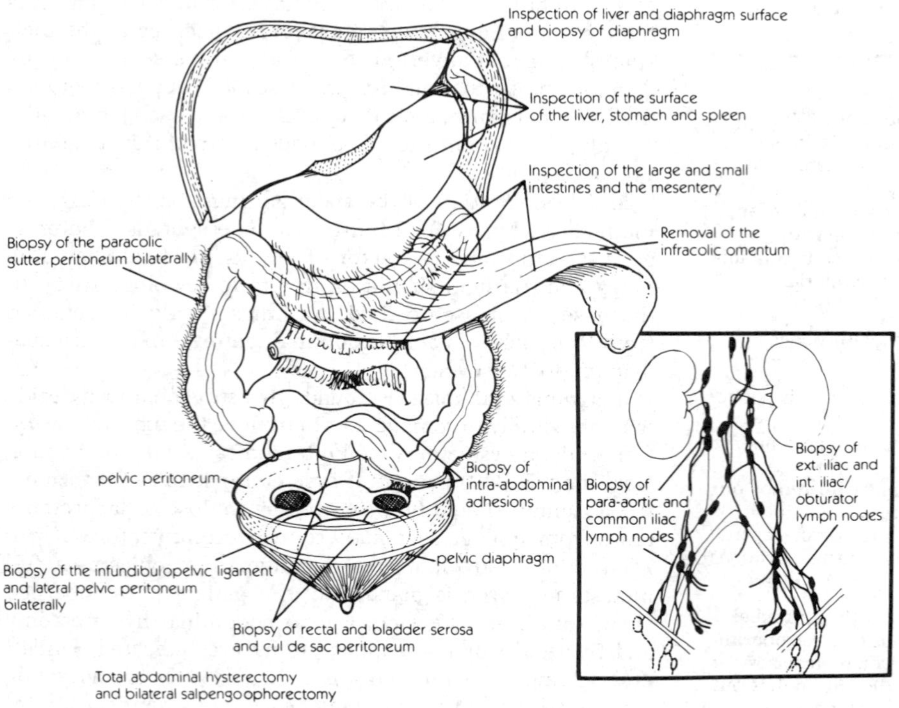

FIG. 37-2. Staging laparotomy for the patient with ovarian cancer. (Hoskins WJ: The role of cytoreductive surgery in ovarian cancer. PPO Update 1(2), February 1987)

infundibulopelvic ligament. Ligation of this ligament and of the round ligament allows the surgeon to mobilize the pelvic viscera and tumor masses. The ureter can be dissected free of the medial flap of peritoneum, and the uterine artery can be identified and ligated. If the tumor is large or has extended into the obturator foramen, the obturator nerve should be identified and preserved. With the ureter, obturator nerve, and major blood vessels identified and the uterine artery and infundibulopelvic ligament ligated, the surgeon can remove the uterus, adnexa, and pelvic tumor. In some cases, the tumor will peel away from the peritoneum, whereas in other cases the peritoneum must be removed with the tumor. On occasion, it is necessary to remove a portion of the bladder or rectosigmoid colon. Primary reanastomosis of the rectum is usually feasible, although on occasion a colostomy will be necessary. In some patients, pelvic involvement of the cecum or terminal ileum necessitates resection of these structures with reconstruction of intestinal continuity by ileoascending or ileotransverse colostomy. Although the ureter can usually be separated from the pelvic tumor, resection and reimplantation into the bladder may be necessary to achieve complete cytoreduction.

Resection of disease in the abdominal cavity should be as complete as possible. If disease involves the infracolic omentum, it can be removed below the transverse colon. If disease involves the supracolic omentum, it should be detached from the transverse colon and resected along the greater curvature of the stomach, as shown in Figure 37-3. Particular attention should be given to carrying the dissection up toward the spleen in order to remove all gross tumor. On occasion, it is necessary to remove the spleen. Tumor implants in the paracolic gutters and on the surface of the intestine can usually be separated from the underlying structures, although it is sometimes necessary to resect portions of the intestine. Disease on the liver surface and undersurface of the diaphragm can often be partially debulked, and venous oozing can usually be controlled with pressure from a laparotomy pack.

The surgeon must often make difficult decisions as to how extensive the resection of gross tumor should be in relation to possible benefit. There is probably little benefit in leaving a patient with a colostomy or resecting large segments of small intestine if bulk disease cannot be removed from other sites. On the other hand, such resection may be quite feasible in order to leave the patient with minimal residual disease.

Impact of Primary Cytoreductive Surgery

In 1968, Munnel[96] reported improved survival in Stages III and IV ovarian carcinoma if omentectomy was performed. He further demonstrated improved survival in patients undergoing definitive operation rather than "partial removal" or "laparotomy and biopsy." A year later, Delcos and Quinlan[97] reported that patients with "nonpalpable" disease survived longer than patients with "palpable" ovarian cancer when treated with radiotherapy. For nonpalpable disease, the 4-year survival rates for Stages II and III were 72% and 25%, respectively, and for palpable disease, the rates were 33% and 9%, respectively.

In the mid-1970s, Griffiths[98] used chemotherapy after cytoreductive surgery and compared the survival of patients grouped by the amount of residual disease. He demonstrated

TABLE 37-5. Operative Procedure for Proper Surgical Staging of the Patient with Ovarian Cancer

Step 1. If ascites is present, remove as much as possible for cytology. If no ascites is present, obtain cell washings from the pelvis, both abdominal gutters, and both subdiaphragmatic areas.

Step 2. Determine whether the mass is malignant; if malignant, perform appropriate pelvic procedure (total abdominal hysterectomy and bilateral salpingo-oophorectomy unless patient desires further childbearing and there is no evidence of spread beyond the ovary).

Step 3. Carefully examine pelvic peritoneum; if lesions are present, remove as much as possible and biopsy any lesion that cannot be removed. If no lesions are seen, sample at a minimum the peritoneum of the lateral pelvic sidewalls, the bladder, the rectosigmoid, and the cul-de-sac.

Step 4. Examine the paracolic gutters, and remove any lesions seen. If no lesions are seen, obtain a 1 × 3-cm strip of peritoneum on either side.

Step 5. Examine the omentum, and remove any that contains visible tumor (including the supracolic omentum if involved by tumor). If no lesions are seen, remove the infracolic omentum.

Step 6. Examine and palpate both diaphragms and the surface of the spleen and liver. If lesions are present, remove as much as possible; biopsy if they cannot be removed. If no lesions are seen, a strip of peritoneum 1 × 2 cm should be carefully excised from the right hemidiaphragm. (*Note:* only peritoneum is needed, and care should be taken not to create a pneumothorax.)

Step 7. Beginning at either the rectum or cecum, carefully inspect the entire large colon and remove and/or biopsy any suspicious lesion of the intestine or mesentery.*

Step 8. Beginning at either the ileocecal valve or ligament of Treitz, carefully inspect the entire small bowel and mesentery, removing and/or biopsing any lesions.*

Step 9. If, after all of the above procedures, no gross disease larger than 1 or 2 cm is left, the pelvic and para-aortic lymph nodes should be sampled.

* If resection of intestine is necessary to cytoreduce the tumor optimally or to relieve obstruction, this should be performed.

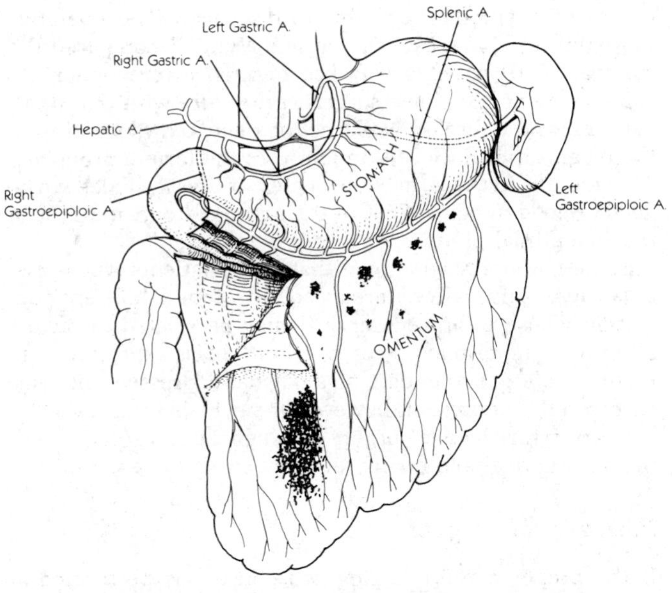

FIG. 37-3. Omentectomy in patients with metastatic ovarian cancer. (Hoskins WJ: The role of cytoreductive surgery in ovarian cancer. PPO Update 1(2), February 1987)

that the duration of survival was directly related to the amount of residual disease after initial cytoreductive surgery: patients with no residual disease had a mean survival of 39 months compared with 29 months for those with residual disease of no more than 0.5 cm and 18 months for those with residual disease of 0.6 cm to 1.5 cm. Patients with larger volumes of disease had a mean survival of 11 months, and none of these suboptimally cytoreduced patients survived beyond 26 months.

Table 37-6 summarizes four reports in which the median length of survival is reported based on primary cytoreductive surgery to less than, or greater than, 2 cm of residual disease. Most of these patients received postoperative multidrug chemotherapy. The mean survival was 29.4 months in the optimally cytoreduced group and 13.4 months in the group in whom cytoreductive surgery was suboptimal. A recent study of the GOG,[103] which compared two cisplatin-based regimens, showed a significant difference in both the progression-free interval and the survival rate for patients with no residual disease compared with those with residual masses as large as 1 cm. Fuks and associates[104] described two radiotherapy series in which the median survival was 24 months for "small residual" or "no residual" disease compared with 6 to 11 months for "large residual" disease. Dembo[105] reported a 43% 5-year survival rate in Stage III with less than 2 cm of residual disease in patients treated with whole-abdominal irradiation compared with an 18% 5-year survival rate for patients with greater than 2 cm of disease.

To evaluate the operative morbidity and quality of life of primary cytoreductive surgery. Chen and co-workers[106] reviewed 60 patients who underwent optimal primary cytoreductive surgery. They reported a mean operating time of 3.6 hours, a mean blood loss of 1644 ml, and a mean hospital stay of 16 days, with most patients receiving their first

TABLE 37-6. Effect of Volume of Residual Disease on Survival in Patients with Stage III Epithelial Ovarian Carcinoma Given Postcytoreduction Chemotherapy

	Survival (mo)		
	<2 cm	*>2 cm*	*Reference*
	44.5	15.9	99
	25+	13.5	100
	30+	18	101
	18*	6*	102
Mean	29.4	13.4	

* 0.5–1.5 cm.

course of chemotherapy prior to discharge. The operative morbidity rate was 5%. Blythe and Wahl[107] compared the survival of 19 patients who had optimal cytoreduction (to <2 cm) by an extensive surgical procedure with that of 17 patients whose disease could not be debulked (suboptimal); the mean survival was 14.3 months in the former group and 10.2 months in the latter. The quality of life was judged to be good or good to fair in 75% of the optimal group and 18% of the suboptimal group.

Some authors have argued that these patients whose disease can be optimally cytoreduced represent a different population whose improved survival may be related to factors other than the primary cytoreduction. This is a difficult argument to refute, and to date no study has addressed this issue successfully. At present, however, the evidence suggests that primary cytoreductive surgery is beneficial in terms of both median survival and quality of life.

Postsurgical Staging

If the proper careful staging procedure was performed at initial surgery, then little additional evaluation is ordinarily required postoperatively. However, if the upper abdomen was not properly evaluated during the initial operation, postoperative reevaluation by either laparotomy or laparoscopy may be necessary even before other treatment is begun. Unfortunately, understaging as a result of inadequate initial surgery is common: several laparoscopy studies have documented unappreciated intra-abdominal spread in 30% to 40% of patients with early (FIGO Stages I and II) disease explored through lower-abdominal incisions.[28,29] Piver and co-workers found diaphragmatic metastases in 11% and aortic lymph node metastases in 13% of patients otherwise felt to have Stage I disease.[30]

The use of laparoscopy in patients with ovarian carcinoma is of value both for initial staging and as a means of surveillance to assess therapeutic response.[28,29] In the U.S. National Cancer Institute (NCI) experience, laparoscopy documented involved sites that had gone undetected during conventional radiologic and isotopic procedures in 42% of patients.[108] In addition, this technique provided the only evidence of disease in 38%. Twenty percent to 30% of patients referred with presumed Stage I or II disease were reclassified as having Stage III disease on the basis of diaphragmatic metastases detected at laparoscopy.

Laparoscopy was found to be safe and feasible even in patients who had had prior laparotomies.[108] In 6% of patients, technical problems occurred that precluded complete evaluation. Of 159 procedures performed, there were few serious complications; only 2.5% of the patients required medical therapy to manage a complication. Complications included pneumothorax (one case), bleeding necessitating transfusion (one), wound infection (one), and hypotension (two). Other complications not requiring therapy were pneumomediastinum and subcutaneous or mesenteric emphysema. There were no deaths or viscus perforations, and no patient required surgical exploration because of a complication.

Other institutions have had similar experiences. Berek, Griffiths, and Leventhal reviewed 112 laparoscopies performed in 57 patients without clinical evidence of disease.[109] In 80 (71%) of the procedures, the entire peritoneal cavity was examined; visibility was totally inadequate in only 16 procedures. Similar complications occurred in this series, but none was serious.

Second-Look Surgical Reassessment

The term "second-look surgical reassessment" should be restricted to a systematic surgical reexploration of patients who have completed a planned course of treatment after initial surgical staging and cytoreductive surgery. Such patients should be clinically without evidence of disease by physical examination and routine diagnostic studies such as chest film, liver function tests, CA-125 assay, intravenous urogram, barium enema, and CT scan. The fact that approximately 50% of patients so evaluated will be found to have residual disease illustrates the difficulty of nonsurgical evaluation in this disease.

Wangenstein and associates introduced the concept of second-look surgery,[110] and a series of studies from the M.D. Anderson Hospital and Tumor Institute defined its application to ovarian cancer.[111–113] The technique of second-look reassessment requires considerable care because most patients with negative second-look operations do not receive further therapy. The abdomen should be entered through a generous midline incision extending from the symphysis pubis to at least 6 cm above the umbilicus. If no disease is found or if upper-abdominal disease is to be cytoreduced, the incision will probably need to be extended further toward the xyphoid. All adhesions in the abdomen and pelvis should be lysed, and portions of these adhesions should be submitted for pathologic analysis. A thorough examination of the abdomen and pelvis is then done. In general, the same procedures are followed as for the primary staging of ovarian cancer (see Table 37-5). Washings of the pelvis, paracolic gutters, and subdiaphragmatic areas are essential. If no gross disease is found, pelvic and para-aortic lymph nodes should be biopsied. Usually, a second-look operation results in 20 to 40 pathologic specimens. Residual disease should be resected whenever possible, and any disease that cannot be resected should be noted in the operative report.

Table 37-7 summarizes the effect of initial residual disease on the outcome of second-look surgical reassessment in epithelial ovarian cancer. The likelihood of a complete pathologic response (negative second-look reassessment) is 82% if no apparent residual disease remained after the initial surgery, 53% if minimal residual disease remained, and 23% if only suboptimal resection was possible.

The timing of second-look surgical reassessment has varied since the concept was introduced. Patients treated with single alkylating agents were usually treated for 12 to 18 months, and Smith and associates[113] indicated that patients given at least 10 courses of melphalan had a better survival rate than those who had shorter courses of therapy prior to the second look. With the introduction of multidrug regimens, toxicity was greater and 10 to 12 months of such chemotherapy was difficult to administer without significant dose reduction or prolongation of chemotherapy intervals. Greco and Berek and their co-workers[114,115] have used sec-

TABLE 37-7. Effect of Residual Disease at End of Initial Cytoreductive Operation on Presence of Disease at Second-Look Surgical Reassessment

	Percentage with Negative Second Look			
	No Residual	*Optimal Residual*	*Suboptimal Residual*	*Reference*
	67	61	14	41
	76	50	28	118
	–	40	11	119
	75	–	25	120
	95	36	20	121
	82	44	33	122
	–	49	13	123
	79	45	22	124
	100	100	40	125
Mean	82	53	23	

ond-look laparotomy after six courses of therapy. In a prospective randomized trial under way at Memorial Sloan-Kettering Cancer Center, five courses of cyclophosphamide, Adriamycin, and cisplatin (CAP) are being compared with 10 courses of the same regimen. It is too early to provide final results, but a preliminary review[116] has indicated no difference in the frequency of negative second-look surgical reassessment in the two arms. Although the optimal timing for second-look surgery has not been established, the use of multiagent chemotherapy has decreased the interval from the onset of chemotherapy to the surgical reassessment.

Unfortunately, Rubin and co-workers[42] reported that shorter courses of cisplatin-based chemotherapy produce a higher complete response rate but a higher recurrence rate after negative second-look surgical reassessment. They suggest that the longer intervals of therapy with earlier regimens allowed a longer time for patients whose tumors had developed drug resistance to have recurrences and thus not have second-look surgery.

Second-look surgical reassessment has recently been reviewed by Rubin and Lewis,[117] and the results are summarized in Table 37-8. The chance of a patient having a negative second-look surgical reassessment is directly related to the stage of disease, the grade of tumor, and the amount of residual disease at the conclusion of the initial cytoreductive operation. Of 1255 patients included in the 16 reports reviewed by Rubin and Lewis, 53.9% had residual disease detected at second-look surgery.

Persistent disease at second-look reassessment has been described in the pelvis, on the surfaces of the intestine, on the diaphragm, in the omentum, and retroperitoneal lymph nodes.[120,122,126,127] Both Berek and colleagues[119] and Creasman and associates[128] have reported retroperitoneal lymph node spread as the sole positive finding at second-look surgery.

Second-look surgical reassessment is a significantly invasive procedure that involves the expense and discomfort of a major abdominal operation and disrupts the patient's normal activities. Nevertheless, published reports have documented acceptable morbidity. In the excellent review by Rubin and Lewis, there were no deaths in 682 operations, and the overall morbidity rate (including minor complications) was 19%. Most of these complications were infections involving the incision, the urinary tract, or the lungs.

Recurrent ovarian carcinoma after negative second-look surgery occurred in 15% to 20% of all cases in the many references previously cited. However, in certain groups of patients, the recurrence rate is much higher. Barnhill and co-workers[41] and Rubin et al[42] have reported recurrence rates of approximately 50% in patients with Stages III and IV, Grade 2 and 3 tumors after treatment with cisplatin-based chemotherapy. It is possible that patients in these high-risk categories should receive additional therapy after negative second-look surgical reassessment.

Several authors have questioned the value of second-look surgery because of the poor survival of patients with positive findings and the high recurrence rates of patients with negative ones. However, new second-line experimental therapeutic options are available and should encourage further use of the second-look reevaluation technique. In areas in which such second-line therapeutic options are not available, the patient should be referred to centers where investigational treatment is being used.

TABLE 37-8. Results (as %) of Second-Look Surgery in Ovarian Carcinoma (Collected Series)*

	Negative
Stage	
I	80
II	68
III	35
Grade	
1	61
2	50
3	41
Residual disease after cytoreductive operation	
None	77
"Optimal"	45
"Suboptimal"	25

* Adapted from Rubin and Lewis.[117]

Other techniques for monitoring the response to therapy short of second-look laparotomy can be used under some circumstances. For example, the NCI group has utilized peritoneoscopy.[108] In 66 restaging peritoneoscopies, residual disease was found in 33 patients; peritoneoscopic findings provided the only evidence of disease in 24 patients (36%). These patients were spared an unnecessary second-look laparotomy, whereas those patients with negative results on peritoneoscopy underwent laparotomy. Residual ovarian cancer was found in 55%, mainly in the pelvis and mesentery. Therefore, a negative peritoneoscopy must be followed by laparotomy before a patient with ovarian cancer can be considered disease free. However, in patients undergoing therapy, laparoscopy proved a useful tool for monitoring subclinical disease.

Secondary Cytoreductive Surgery

Although the worth of primary cytoreductive surgery is clear, the value of secondary cytoreduction is controversial. The recent availability of cisplatin analogues, intraperitoneal chemotherapy, and a new generation of biologic response modifiers has expanded our second-line treatment capabilities, and because these agents are most effective against minimal residual disease, secondary cytoreduction may be important.

Table 37-9 summarizes the frequency with which secondary cytoreduction can be accomplished. Berek and coworkers[129] performed secondary cytoreduction on 32 patients and found that in 12 (38%), residual disease could be reduced to optimal (less than 1.5 cm). Median survival for that group was 20 months compared with 5 months for the 20 patients whose disease could not be optimally cytoreduced. Factors that were associated with a greater likelihood of optimal secondary cytoreduction were previous optimal primary cytoreduction, less than 1000 ml of ascites, tumor size less than 5 cm at second operation, and interval from primary to secondary surgery of greater than 12 months. Age, tumor grade, type of subsequent chemotherapy, and the presence or absence of bowel obstruction did not influence survival following secondary cytoreductive surgery.

Griffiths and associates[130] compared the incidence of successful cytoreduction and survival in patients undergoing primary versus secondary operations. Although effective cytoreduction was equally possible in both types of patients, survival was significantly less in those undergoing secondary cytoreduction. Wiltshaw et al[131] showed that partial responders to chemotherapy had improved survival if they underwent secondary cytoreductive surgery. Copeland and co-workers[132] evaluated nine patients who had undergone secondary cytoreduction and concluded that such surgery could contribute to long term survival. Several other groups also have reported successful secondary cytoreduction.[113,133–135]

Although the role of secondary cytoreduction surgery remains controversial, the increased availability of second-line therapy may increase the importance of such surgical procedures.

TABLE 37-9. Frequency of Successful Secondary Cytoreductive Operations in Patients with Advanced or Recurrent Epithelial Ovarian Cancer

	No. of Patients	*Patients Optimally Cytoreduced (%)*	*Reference*
	32	12 (37.5)	129
	13	11 (84.6)	130
	29	13 (44.7)	133
	26	15 (57.7)	134
	69	29 (42.0)	113
	38	9 (24.0)	135
Total	207	89 (43.0%)	

RADIATION THERAPY

Historical Considerations

The first report of radiation therapy for ovarian carcinoma was published in 1912 by Eymer,[136] who described long-term remissions in eight patients treated with low-dose whole-abdominal irradiation. The low-energy radiation beams available with the early orthovoltage machines had poor penetration and produced high skin doses and significant skin toxicity, which prevented the delivery of high-dose radiation to peritoneal tumors. Therefore, although radiation was shown to have significant palliative effects, its curative value was justifiably questioned.

The introduction of megavoltage radiotherapy in the early 1950s allowed more penetrating and skin-sparing radiation and made possible the application of large and shaped fields carried to high doses. However, the extreme radiation sensitivities of some of the normal abdominal contents have limited the use of radiotherapy as a curative modality in many patients, especially those with advanced disease. Nonetheless, when appropriate precautions are taken, radiotherapy does represent an effective curative modality for certain patients with ovarian carcinoma.

Tumoricidal Radiation Doses

The shape and distribution of the radiation fields as well as the dose and fractionation schemes employed in the treatment of ovarian carcinoma represent a compromise between the need to employ tumoricidal doses to eradicate tumor deposits and the desire to avoid injury to normal tissues included in the treatment fields. Although the tumoricidal dose levels for ovarian tumors have not been determined with great accuracy, there is ample evidence that radiation can permanently eradicate tumor deposits in patients with residual ovarian cancer. Fuks and Bagshaw[137] reported an actuarial 5-year disease-free survival rate of 46% in 16 Stage IIB patients with residual pelvic disease treated with 5000 to 6000 cGy. Schray and associates[138] treated 26 patients with small residual tumors (less than 2 cm in diameter) with similar radiation doses. Only four relapsed in the pelvis compared with 9 of 20 (45%) who had larger residual tumors. Dembo[139,140] treated patients with Stage I, II, or IIIA tumors with 4500 cGy to the pelvis and 2250 cGy to the upper abdomen. The 5-year survival rate in 50 patients with small or no residual tumors was 78% compared with 19% in 26 patients with larger residua. These data suggest that tumoricidal doses are tumor size dependent. For large tumors, this dose probably exceeds 5000 to 6000 cGy, whereas for small (< 2 cm) tumors it is probably 4500 to 5000 cGy, and for microscopic tumor deposits, the existing data suggest that the tumoricidal dose levels may be even lower. The Princess Margaret Group randomized patients with no residual tumors after surgery to receive either 4500 cGy to the pelvis or the same dose to the pelvis and 2250 cGy to the upper abdomen.[140–142] The 5-year survival rate for the patients receiving abdominopelvic radiotherapy was 78% compared with 51% in the patients treated to the pelvis only, the survival difference resulting from a 30% higher control rate of occult upper-abdominal metastases in the group that received abdominopelvic radiation. These data suggest that the 2250 cGy given was tumoricidal to microscopic upper-abdominal tumor deposits. These observations are supported by data of Delclos and Smith,[143] who showed that patients with Stage II disease treated with 5000 cGy to the pelvis and 2600 to 2800 cGy to the upper abdomen by the moving-strip technique had an improved survival rate at 5 years (57%) compared with the patients treated to the pelvis only (17%). Similarly, Perez et al[144,145] report a 5-year survival rate of 57% in patients with Stage II disease treated with a similar technique to the whole abdomen and of 16% in patients receiving pelvic irradiation only. It is therefore generally accepted that a dose of 2500 to 3000 cGy given in daily fractions of 150 to 200 cGy is probably tumoricidal for microscopic ovarian carcinoma.

Design of Treatment Fields, Total Dose, and Fractionation

In carcinoma of the ovary, the entire peritoneal cavity is at risk. However, the doses that would be required to eradicate large tumors in the upper abdomen cannot be administered because of the limited tolerance of some abdominal organs, such as the liver, kidneys, spinal cord, stomach, and intestines. Therefore, restrictions of the dose and special shielding for vital viscera are necessary to ensure that normal-tissue tolerance is not exceeded.

Two radiotherapy techniques have been employed routinely in patients with ovarian carcinoma: the open-field technique[146] and the moving-strip technique.[147,148] The open field employs irradiation through two large fixed portals (anterior and posterior) shaped to encompass the entire peritoneal cavity (Fig. 37-7). In some patients with Stage I or Stage II disease, radiation portals have been restricted to the lower half of the peritoneal cavity. However, in view of the frequent involvement of the retroperitoneal para-aortic group of lymph nodes in early-stage ovarian carcinoma, Hanks and Bagshaw[146] suggested that treatment should include the para-aortic region. Further, because many of these patients also have metastatic deposits on the undersurface of the diaphragms,[28] Glatstein and colleagues[149] suggested further modifications to encompass, in addition to the para-aortic region, large portions of the diaphragms (Fig. 37-4).

Using the open-field techniques, radiation is delivered at a rate of 800 to 1000 cGy per week. The total dose to the lower abdomen usually is 5500 cGy delivered in 27 fractions over 37 days. When calculated by the Ellis nominal standard dose (NSD) method,[150,151] the total dose to the pelvis is 1646 rets, and the corresponding tumor dose fractionation (TDF) value[152] is 89. When treating the upper abdomen, the dose usually is 4000 cGy delivered in 20 fractions over 33 days (1325 rets; TDF value 64), but shielding provided to the kidneys and liver (including the right hemidiaphragm) to protect these organs from radiation damage limits the effective dose to the underlying organs to approximately 2000 cGy.

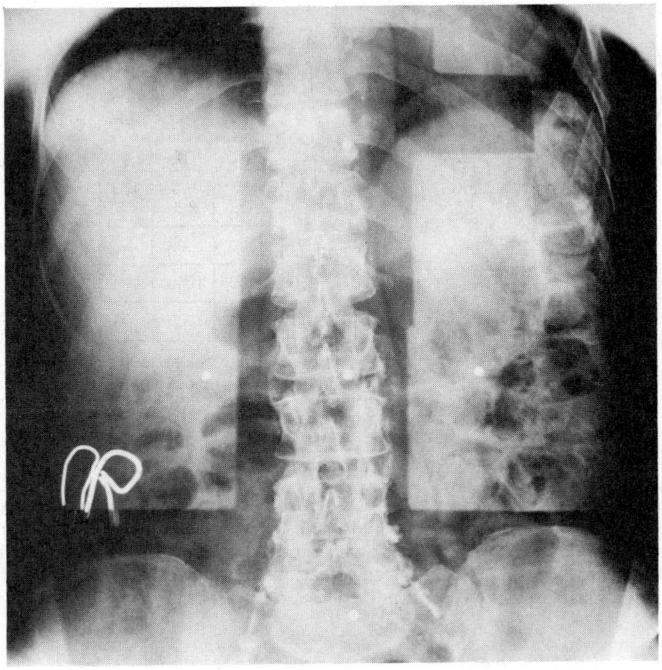

FIG. 37-4. Simulator portal film (Fuks Z, Bagshaw MA: The rationale for curative radiotherapy for ovarian carcinoma. Int J Radiat Oncol Biol Phys 1:21–32, 1975) demonstrating the anterior-posterior T-shaped field designed for the treatment of the para-aortic lymph nodes, the medial two thirds of the diaphragms, and the subpleural diaphragmatic lymph nodes. The technique, which is a four-field technique, also involves two opposed cross-table lateral fields. Its posterior margin is placed at the midplane of the lumbar vertebral bodies, providing protection to both kidneys from radiation damage. Its anterior margin is placed at the anterior periperitoneal fat line to encompass the total peritoneal cavity and the diaphragms. (Glatstein E, Fuks Z, Bagshaw MA: Diaphragmatic treatment in ovarian carcinoma: A new radiotherapeutic technique. Int J Radiat Oncol Biol Phys 2:357–362, 1977)

A further modification of the open-field technique has recently been suggested by Martinez and associates[153,154] (Fig. 37-5). This modification involves a special field design and dose fractionation scheme designed to improve the tolerance of the open-field technique. Briefly, treatment is delivered by a series of anteroposterior–posteroanterior opposed fields. Beginning with radiation to the true pelvis, the field extends from the lower borders of the obturator foramina up to the level of L5. Five fractions of 180 cGy each are given in 1 week. The field is then opened to include the entire ab-

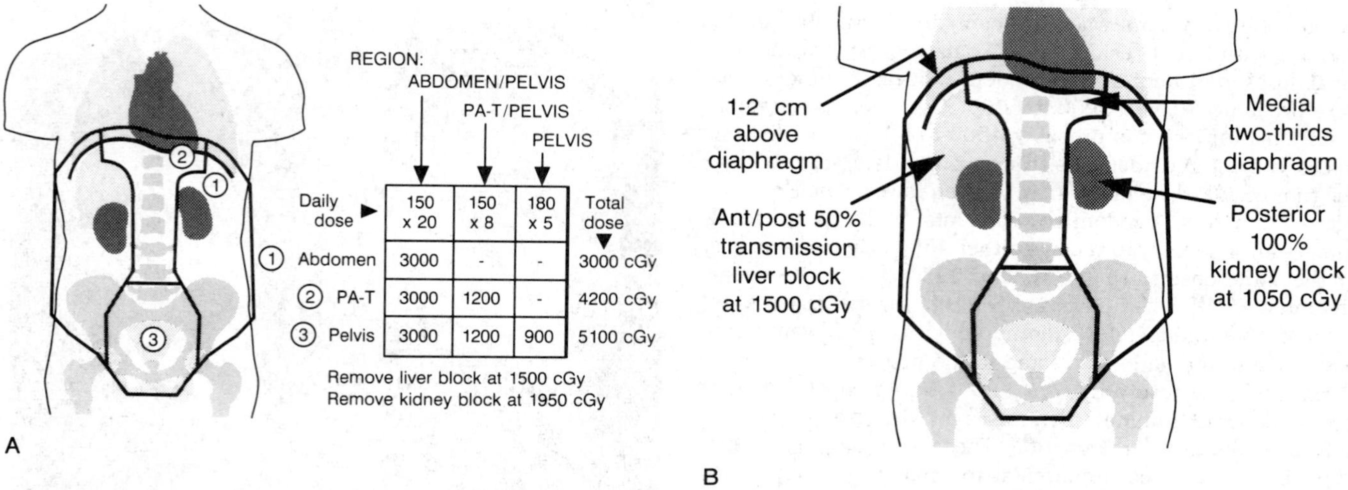

FIG. 37-5. Martinez technique and dose schedule. Field boundaries and blocks for treatment of gynecologic malignancies by whole-abdomen irradiation with diaphragmatic, para-aortic, and pelvic boost. PA'N, para-aortic nodes; DIAPH, diaphragm. (Martinez A, Schray MF, Howes AE, et al: Postoperative radiation therapy for epithelial ovarian cancer: The curative role based on a 24-year experience. J Clin Oncol 3:901–922, 1985)

dominal and pelvic peritoneum, extending up to 1 cm above the diaphragms. Twenty fractions of 150 cGy each are given to this volume in 4 weeks. A full-thickness posterior block is introduced after 1000 cGy to shield the kidneys, and a 50% transmission block is introduced anteriorly and posteriorly to shield the liver after 1500 cGy. The third and last field is a continuous pelvic, para-aortic, and partial diaphragmatic T-shaped field. Eight fractions of 150 cGy each are given in 10 days. In summary, the whole peritoneal cavity receives 3000 cGy in 20 fractions in 4 weeks, the pelvis receives 5100 cGy in 33 fractions in 6 to 7 weeks, and the para-aortic region, together with the medial part of the diaphragm, receives 4200 cGy in 28 fractions in 5 to 6 weeks. The total dose to the liver is 2250 cGy and to the kidneys 2000 cGy in 20 fractions in 4 weeks. This technique appears to be well tolerated.[154,155]

The moving-strip technique[147] involves the division of the peritoneal cavity into equal horizontal segments (strips) (Fig. 37-6). Treatment begins with irradiation to the lowest segments of the pelvis. At each radiotherapy session, a fixed number of adjacent segments are treated simultaneously. On consecutive days, the irradiated volume is moved cephalad from one segment to the adjacent segment in an orderly fashion until the entire abdomen has been treated. The dose to each point in the abdominal cavity usually is 3000 cGy delivered in 10 fractions over 12 days (1313 rets; TDF value 62). The kidneys and liver are usually shielded by partial-thickness lead blocks designed to allow the delivery of 50% of this dose. An additional dose of 2000 cGy in 10 fractions over 12 days usually is delivered to the pelvis by an open-field technique to increase the pelvic dose. When calculated by the NSD method, the total dose to the pelvis is 1713 rets (TDF value 95).

The moving-strip technique was designed to decrease the morbidity of whole-abdominal irradiation observed with the open-field technique.[143,147] However, when the NSD doses and the TDF values for the two techniques are compared, they prove similar. The NSD doses and the TDF values provide an estimate of normal tissue tolerance for fractionated radiation programs, and identical values imply biologically equivalent programs.[150–152] Indeed, studies comparing the open-field and moving-strip techniques[139,156] have shown that the rates of acute morbidity, chronic complications, and survival are similar.

FIG. 37-6. Total abdominal irradiation approach using the moving strip technique. Volume covered with the megavoltage moving strip technique. Kidneys are shielded from the posterior beam by two half-value layers of lead. The liver is shielded from the anterior beam by two half-value layers of lead. To compensate for the lower dose at both ends of the irradiated volume, treatment is started one strip below the lower margin of the pelvic field and completed one strip above the diaphragm.

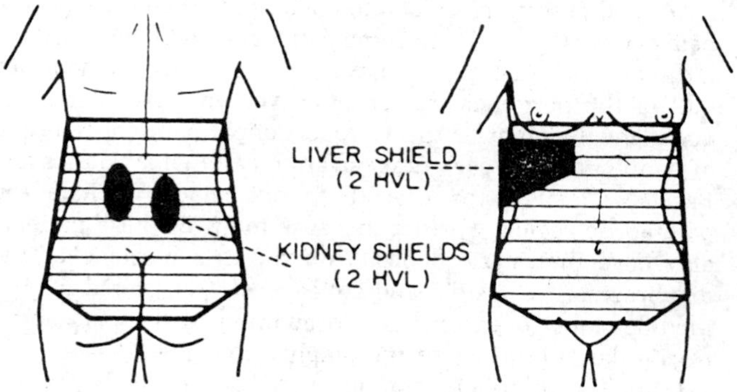

Acute Morbidity and Long-term Complications

The most common complication of radiation therapy for ovarian carcinoma is radiation-induced enteritis.[35,52,156] Its incidence and severity are directly related to the radiation dose. Acute morbidity, including diarrhea, nausea, vomiting, and weight loss, was seen in 78% of 167 patients treated with high-dose radiotherapy (4500 to 6000 cGy) to the lower abdomen.[157] In most of the patients, the gastrointestinal symptoms subsided within a few weeks after completion of treatment, although in 29% of the patients, diarrhea with or without gastrointestinal bleeding persisted for months to years. In 24 of the 167 patients (14%), severe bowel stenosis and bleeding developed, necessitating surgical intervention. Similar rates of acute and chronic radiation-induced enteritis have been reported by other investigators using the moving-strip technique.[158,159] Although still within acceptable limits, these rates of morbidity and complications are regarded as very high, despite the fact that they result from a treatment that is considered potentially curative for a malignant disease.

Some reduction in the peripheral blood counts almost always accompanies radiation.[35] Counts usually return to normal shortly after cessation of the treatment, but there is evidence that the activity of irradiated bone marrow remains impaired to a certain degree for extended periods.[160]

Radiation-induced hepatitis and nephritis are well-known hazards of doses exceeding 2500 cGy.[161,162] When careful port design and shielding are not performed, these syndromes are not uncommon in patients treated for ovarian carcinoma.[52,147,163] More recently, however, symptoms of hepatitis and nephritis have not been as common because of careful application of appropriate shielding of the liver and kidneys.

Preoperative Radiation

Preoperative radiation has been used sporadically.[164] Kottmeier reported a 40% (34/86) 3-year survival rate with preoperative radiation and total hysterectomy with bilateral salpingo-oophorectomy.[165] However, further information on these patients is not available. Kjorstad and co-workers[166] studied 145 patients with Stage III disease, 96 of whom had unresectable disease at initial surgery. Following a dose of 3000 cGy in 4 weeks to the whole abdomen, resection of the primary tumor, uterus, and omentum was possible in 38%. However, the operative mortality rate was 9% and the 5-year survival rate only 16%. The authors concluded that they achieved only a small increase in the salvage rate. Preoperative irradiation has not been popular for several reasons. One is the lack of histologic confirmation of malignancy without a laparotomy. Furthermore, after irradiation, the full extent of the disease is not known. Finally, there may be technical difficulties in carrying out surgery in the wake of high doses of preoperative irradiation.

Radioisotopes

The intraperitoneal instillation of radioactive colloidal gold (^{196}Au) or phosphorus (^{32}p) to irradiate the peritoneal cavity was popular in the past.[167,168] Colloidal ^{196}Au is no longer available for therapy. The colloidal particles increase isotope uptake by the mesothelial peritoneal cells and lymph nodes and decrease systemic radioisotope elution. Radioactive phosphorus (chromic phosphate) has a half-life of 14.2 days and emits only beta particles (1.7 MeV maximum energy). The range of beta particles in tissue is only 3 to 5 mm; thus, radioisotopes such as ^{32}p may sterilize microscopic peritoneal implants, but they are inadequate to treat large masses because of the short range of the beta particle. Also, because of adhesions or loculation, poor distribution in the peritoneal cavity may occur. This can be defined by injecting dilute Hypaque or by instilling technetium into the peritoneal cavity and scanning the patient before the therapeutic isotope is administered.

After radioisotope therapy, surgical management may be more difficult because of reactive fibrosis, although with ^{32}p, this problem has been infrequent. The usual dose of intraperitoneal radiophosphorus (as chromic phosphate) is 20 to 25 mCi diluted with sterile saline (1000–1500 ml) and properly distributed throughout the entire peritoneal cavity. If the average peritoneal surface is estimated at 30,000 cm^2, the dose of radiation delivered to the peritoneum is 6000 cGy and the dose delivered to the omentum is 7000 cGy.[168] Various methods for the administration of isotopes and verification of adequate distribution in the peritoneal cavity have been published.

The most common complication of intraperitoneal colloidal radioisotopes is small-bowel obstruction and stenosis. Pezner and co-workers[169] reviewing 104 patients treated intraperitoneally with radioisotopes, found that 11 required surgery for adhesions or fibrosis of the small intestine with severe chronic diarrhea; 1 patient with partial small-bowel obstruction was treated conservatively. In the patients receiving radioactive colloidal gold, only 1 of 45 (2.2%) developed small-bowel complications, in contrast to 12 of 50 (24%) treated with this technique in addition to pelvic external radiotherapy (about 4000 cGy in 4 weeks with ^{60}Co or 2-MeV photons). The frequency of small-bowel complications appears to be lower with ^{32}P than with ^{196}Au. Complications tend to be slightly more common in patients who have uneven distribution of the radioactive material in the peritoneal cavity.

CHEMOTHERAPY

Single Agents

Chemotherapy has ordinarily been used as the initial treatment in patients with advanced disease (FIGO Stages III and IV) and, in the past, for patients who were not considered appropriate candidates for radiation therapy.[170] Recently, with the discovery of more active agents, chemotherapy has become the most common form of therapy for patients with advanced disease.

Alkylating agents have been used more extensively than any other class of chemotherapeutic drugs. Melphalan, chlorambucil, cyclophosphamide, and thiotepa have produced similar objective response rates (33%–65%).[53] The median survival of treated patients is approximately 10 to 14 months; the median survival of those responding to chemotherapy is 17 to 20 months, and that for those not responding, 6 to 13 months. The 5-year survival rate of patients treated with alkylating agents ranges from 0 to 9% (mean 7%). The 5-year survival rate of the largest single series of patients treated with melphalan was 9%; approximately 20% of the responders in that series were alive at 5 years, with some patients alive and free of disease for periods in excess of 10 years. Second-look studies indicate that patients with no residual tumor at that time have a 5-year survival rate of 60% to 80% without further therapy.[171,172] It is therefore clear that some women with advanced ovarian cancer can be cured with single alkylating-agent therapy alone, although the number is small (5%–10%).

In addition to the alkylating agents, three other drugs—hexamethylmelamine,[173,174] Adriamycin, and cisplatin—have been fairly extensively studied and have response rates in the 20% to 35% range.[175] Cisplatin is one of the most active agents in ovarian cancer; overall response rates of 25% to 40% have been reported in single-agent trials.[176] In a randomized trial of cisplatin versus cyclophosphamide, a longer duration of response (18 versus 8 months) and significantly better survival (19 versus 12 months; $p = 0.009$) was seen with cisplatin.[177] Toxicities include nausea and vomiting, ototoxicity, peripheral neuropathy, nephrotoxicity, and bone-marrow suppression. Techniques are now available using hydration and chloruresis that markedly reduce the nephrotoxicity of the agent.[178–180] However, bone-marrow toxicity, peripheral neuropathy, and ototoxicity remain significant problems.

Several studies have demonstrated a clinically important dose–response relation with cisplatin.[181,182] Recently, Levin and Hryniuk[183] demonstrated a relation between dose intensity and outcome in 33 chemotherapy trials in ovarian cancer. The overall response rate and median survival correlated with the dose intensity (measured as mg/m² per week) for combinations of drugs, particularly those containing cisplatin. When analyzed as single drugs, the dose intensity relation was seen primarily for cisplatin. Because of the importance of dose intensity in cisplatin therapy, studies of high-dose (40 mg/m² daily for 5 days) cisplatin have been performed, demonstrating 32% response rates in refractory cases.[178]

Adriamycin is an active first-line agent in advanced ovarian cancer: collected experience indicates a response rate of approximately 30%.[175] Unfortunately, several studies indicate that the drug has very little activity when used as a second- or third-line agent, with only 3 of 56 patients (5%) responding to the drug after failing initial chemotherapy.[184,185]

One study of hexamethylmelamine in 54 previously untreated patients documented an overall response rate of 32%.[186] The drug was given orally continuously in this study, and there was significant gastrointestinal, hematologic, and neurologic toxicity. Recent studies suggest reduced toxicity with intermittent 14-day per month schedules. A recent update of information on hexamethylmelamine indicates definite single-agent activity.[187]

The cisplatin derivatives carboplatin (CBDCA) and CHIP have been studied extensively in ovarian cancer, and both have significant activity.[188–190] Carboplatin (400 mg/m²) appears to be roughly equivalent to 100 mg/m² of cisplatin.[188] The toxicity of carboplatin is primarily bone-marrow suppression with little or no nephrotoxicity, ototoxicity, or peripheral neuropathy. Preliminary evidence suggests that carboplatin has less cumulative toxicity than CHIP. Other single agents that appear to have some activity in advanced ovarian cancer after adequate testing include ifosfamide,[189–191] AZQ,[190] VP-16 (etoposide),[192,193] Peptichemio,[194] and low-dose mitomycin C.[195] Table 37-10 summarizes the activity of potentially important single agents in ovarian cancer.

Hormone Therapy

Although the ovary is the principal source of estrogen in women, the extent to which hormones regulate the ovarian epithelium is unclear. With the demonstration of the presence of both estrogen and progesterone receptors in approximately half of all ovarian carcinomas,[196–198] hormone treatment of the disease has been actively investigated. Initial reports of activity for megestrol (Megase),[199] medroxyprogesterone (MPA),[200,201] and tamoxifen[202,203] have been followed by larger studies with less-impressive results. One recent trial of MPA in 41 patients resulted in one partial response,[204] and two recent trials of tamoxifen have demonstrated no responses in 22[205] and 23[206] patients.

One recent study attempted to induce progesterone receptors by sequencing estradiol with MPA. Sixty-five patients were treated in two different dose schedules, and the overall response rate was 14%.[207] Although the toxicity of these agents is low, the activity appears to be extremely modest.

In Vitro Clonogenic Assays in Ovarian Cancer

For many years, attempts have been made to define the activity of potentially useful chemotherapeutic agents using a variety of in vitro screening techniques. These have not been particularly successful. An in vitro tumor colony assay that evaluates clonogenic potential after exposure to chemotherapy has been used in a variety of tumors and has received considerable study in ovarian carcinoma.[208] Unfortunately, subsequent larger studies with ovarian cancer, as well as other solid tumors, have highlighted serious shortcomings of the human tumor clonogenic assay.[209] The technical limitations of the assay include difficulty in preparation of single-cell suspensions, lack of optimum growth conditions for specific tumor types, and persistence of nonclonogenic clumps of tumor cells. In addition, it is unclear whether the assay is predictive for a specific drug or merely identifies those patients whose tumors are more generally responsive to chemotherapy. These technical limitations, coupled with the absence of sufficient numbers of active drugs for relapsed ovarian cancer patients and the short duration of response in relapsed patients, make the assay an experimental tool, not a clinically proven means for selection of chemotherapy.

Combination Chemotherapy

Combination chemotherapy in advanced ovarian cancer has been extensively studied over the past decade. From these

TABLE 37-10. Single Agents Active in Advanced Ovarian Adenocarcinoma

Drugs	*No. of Patients*	*Percent Response (% CR)*
Alkylating agents		
Melphalan	494	47 (20)
Chlorambucil	280	50
Thiotepa	144	65
Cyclophosphamide	126	49
Mechlorethamine	81	35
Ifosfamide	61	78
AZQ	26	15
Antimetabolites		
5-Fluorouracil	81	32 (18–20)
	21	33
Methotrexate	16	25
	23	13
Antitumor antibiotics		
Doxorubicin (Adriamycin)	18	28
	33	36
Mitomycin C	43	23
Plant Alkaloids		
Vinblastine	16	13
VP-16	22	32
Miscellaneous		
Hexamethylmelamine	53	41
Cisplatin	34	27
Carboplatin	22	50 (17)
Dianhydrogalacticol	39	15
Peptichemio	47	24 (14)

studies, important prognostic factors such as stage, histologic grade, and extent of residual disease have been well defined; the majority of trials now either stratify for important prognostic factors or at least analyze trials by these factors.[175] Nevertheless, response rates have varied from 20% to 90%, with CR rates ranging from 10% to 65% depending on the types of patients included and the criteria used for assessing response. The great variation in patient selection, prognostic factors, and response criteria makes it difficult, if not impossible, to compare many of these studies. Furthermore, in many of the studies, the differences in patient characteristics may have a more important influence on survival than the therapies being reported. In general, the recently published studies can be divided into three major groups: those comparing single agents with combinations, salvage chemotherapy studies on patients who have failed previous therapy, and studies on previously untreated patients.

SINGLE AGENTS VERSUS COMBINATION CHEMOTHERAPY. The first study to demonstrate significantly improved survival with any combination in a prospective comparison with a standard alkylating agent was published in 1978.[210] Eighty previously untreated patients were randomized to receive either melphalan in conventional doses, or Hexa-CAF (hexamethylmelamine, cyclophosphamide, methotrexate, and 5-fluorouracil [5-FU]). Treatment with the four-drug combination achieved a significantly higher overall response rate (75% versus 54%; $p < 0.05$), more complete remissions (33% versus 16%; $p = 0.06$), and significantly longer median survival (29 months versus 17 months; $p < 0.02$). However, Hexa-CAF was most effective in patients with small amounts of residual disease, in whom a higher overall response rate was achieved than in patients with extensive residual disease (84% versus 53%; $p < 0.05$). Important stratification factors, such as the extent of residual disease and histologic grade, as well as age, stage, and histologic type, were well balanced in the two groups. Careful definition of CR using peritoneoscopy or second-look laparotomy was utilized. Patients achieving CR, documented by restaging, had a long survival: 60% of these women were alive more than 4 years later. The toxicity of the combination was greater than that of the single agent, primarily because of greater hematologic toxicity, along with nausea, vomiting, and alopecia.

Dutch investigators confirmed the activity of the Hexa-CAF combination in previously untreated patients (overall response rate 57% with 30% CR)[211] but also demonstrated that in previously treated patients, Hexa-CAF has a much lower overall response rate (3 of 13 with no CR) and increased toxicity. Their study emphasizes the marked reduction of activity of any regimen used as second-line therapy in advanced ovarian cancer and, in addition, illustrates the futility of beginning therapy with an alkylating agent, then later attempting to salvage relapsing patients with more aggressive combination chemotherapy.

Subsequently, a series of randomized trials comparing single-agent chemotherapy (generally alkylating agents) with combination chemotherapy have been published. Generally, these trials either show improved response rates, improved disease-free or overall survival, or all three (Table 37–11).[212–218] In addition to the Hexa-CAF study, two other prospective randomized trials have demonstrated better survival. The first was a multi-institutional Swedish study. Trope and co-workers compared melphalan plus Adriamycin

TABLE 37-11. Combination Chemotherapy Versus Single Agents in Advanced Previously Untreated Ovarian Carcinoma

*Regimen**	*Results*	*Reference*
Clinical Trials Demonstrating Increased CR Rates and/or Disease-Free Survival		
CHAD vs. LPAM	38% CR vs. 21% CR: progression-free survival increased for CHAD	212
CHF vs. LPAM	85% RR vs. 57% RR; 50% CR vs. 17% CR	213
AC vs. C	Improved progression-free survival with AC in patients with minimal residual disease	214
PAC vs. CLB	RR: 68% vs. 26%, p = 0.0004 PCR: 26% vs. 15%	215
Clinical Trials Demonstrating Improved Survival		
Hexa-CAF vs. LPAM	75% RR vs. 43%; 33% CR vs. 16%; median survival, 29 mo. vs. 17 mo.	210
A + LPAM vs. LPAM	67% RR vs. 40%; 23+ mo. vs. 8.1 mo. for duration of response; median survival, 17 mo. vs. 11 mo.	217
CP vs. C	2-year disease-free interval: 52% vs. 10%; 2-year survival: 62% vs. 19%	218

*CHAD = cyclophosphamide, hexamethylmelamine, Adriamycin, cisplatin; LPAM = melphalan; CHF = cyclophosphamide, hexamethylmelamine, 5-fluorouracil; AC = Adriamycin, cyclophosphamide; C = cyclophosphamide; PAC = cisplatin, Adriamycin, cyclophosphamide; CLB = chlorambucil; Hexa-CAF = hexamethylmelamine, cyclophosphamide, methotrexate, 5-fluorouracil; CP = cyclophosphamide, cisplatin.

with melphalan alone in 142 patients with bulky Stage III or Stage IV disease.[217] The combination was superior to the single agent in overall response rate (63% versus 40%; $p < 0.01$), duration of response (23^+ months versus 8.1 months; $p < 0.001$), and overall median survival (16.8^+ months versus 10.7 months; $p < 0.03$). The second study was a Mayo Clinic trial[218] of 41 patients and showed a 2-year survival rate of 52% for cyclophosphamide and cisplatin compared with 19% for cyclophosphamide alone. The projected median survivals were 40 months and 16 months, respectively.

These trials provide substantial evidence for the increased effectiveness of combinations compared with single agents in this disease. Other studies have not shown such benefit,[216,219,220] but patient compliance and substantial dose modifications may have played a significant role in the results of these negative studies. One recent example is a large cooperative trial in Australia and New Zealand that compared oral chlorambucil with cisplatin at relapse with the combination of chlorambucil and cisplatin.[215] Response rates (53% versus 51%) and median survival (16 versus 17 months) were similar. However, only 57% of patients on combination chemotherapy had any significant myelosuppression, and even fewer (25%) did on the sequential treatment, yet the authors demonstrated that myelosuppression had an important favorable effect on survival. The relatively poor survival for both arms of the trial (similar to that achieved with single alkylating agents alone) and the authors' demonstrated positive effect of myelosuppression on subsequent survival illustrate the problem with this and similar trials. One is likely to demonstrate equivalence of single agents and combinations if the trial is designed with insufficient dose intensity of the drugs used in combination.

Several recent trials have also utilized maintenance alkylating agent therapy for several years.[215,221] These trials have failed to show a benefit for such maintenance and have reported leukemias in long-term survivors. In light of the dangers of long-term alkylating agent therapy[222,223] and in the absence of demonstrated benefit, this approach should be abandoned.

Several general conclusions emerge from these prospective randomized trials. Combination chemotherapy continues to provide higher overall response rates and higher CR rates than single agents, although in some studies survival time is not altered significantly. Nevertheless, long-term disease-free survivors, although uncommon, are more frequent with combinations, particularly when the dose intensity is adequate. Several newer combinations may be more effective than those originally used in the prospective comparisons with single alkylating agents.

At present, it would appear that the best chance for achieving a complete remission in advanced ovarian carcinoma exists when the initial therapy is an effective combination used in full therapeutic doses.

COMBINATION CHEMOTHERAPY AFTER ALKYLATING AGENT FAILURE. Many investigators have used combination chemotherapy after the tumor has failed to respond to initial single-agent therapy. Details of these regimens are presented in the original publications, in recent reviews,[224–227] and in Table 37-12. Unfortunately, none of these trials really established any regimen as particularly successful in managing chemotherapy failures. In spite of the high overall response reported for many of these combinations, the number of patients in the studies is small, and the majority of the responses are partial and of short duration (4–6 months). Moreover, the toxicity, when reported, appears to be substantial. Very few of these patients, regardless of the regimen, are alive at 1 year.

Two recent studies suggest some activity for VP-16 and

TABLE 37-12. Combination Chemotherapy After Alkylating Agent Failure

Regimen*	No. of Patients	CR + Pr (%)	Survival of Responders (mo)	Reference
ADR/CDDP	20	42	NS	228
	43	36	7	229
	20	25	7.2	230
ADR/CDDP/5-FU	103	48	12	231
CTX/HEX/ADR/CDDP	35	49	NS	232
	21	49	15	233
HEX/ADR/CDDP	27	41	7.5	234
	21	19	5.3	230
CTX/MTX/CF ± VCR	55	30	7.5	235
HEX/CDDP	38	55	10.8	236
	10	20	NS	237
VP-16/CDDP	10	50	NS	238
	25	40	NS	239

* ADR = Adriamycin; CDDP = cisplatin; 5-FU = 5-fluorouracil; HEX = hexamethylmelamine; CTX = cyclophosphamide; VCR = vincristine; MTX = methotrexate; CF = citrovorum factor; NS = not stated.

cisplatin regimens, although only a small number of patients were treated.[238,239] With the currently available drugs and regimens, combination chemotherapy used after the initial treatment fails is not likely to improve the cure rate in this disease but can, at present, be thought of as a way to identify interesting regimens for primary therapy of the untreated patient.

COMBINATION CHEMOTHERAPY AS INITIAL TREATMENT. Many studies have now been published of combination chemotherapy as the initial treatment in advanced disease. These studies have either been single-arm studies or randomized trials in which two or more combinations have been compared. A summary of a representative group of the single-arm trials is shown in Table 37-13. Most of these

TABLE 37-13. Combination Chemotherapy in Advanced Ovarian Carcinoma

Regimen	Schedule	No. of Evaluable Patients	Complete and Partial Remissions (%)	No. of Clinical CR (%)	No. of Pathologic CR (%)
PAC[240]		56	44/56 (79)	23/56 (41)	10/56 (18)
Cisplatin	20 mg/m² IV day × 5 q 4 wk				
Adriamycin	50 mg/m² IV day 1 q 4 wk				
Cyclophosphamide	750 mg/m² IV day 1 q 4 wk				
A-C (Dana Farber)[241]		41	35/41 (83)	20/41 (48)	12/41 (29)
Cyclophosphamide	500 mg/m² IV				
Adriamycin	40 mg/m²				
Hexa-CAF (NCI)[210]		40	30/40 (75)		13/40 (33)
Hexamethylmelamine	150 mg/m² PO qd × 14				
Cyclophosphamide	150 mg/m² PO qd × 14				
Methotrexate	40 mg/m² IV days 1,8				
5-Fluorouracil	600 mg/m² IV days 1,8				
CHAD[114]		46	45/46 (98)	35/46 (76)	14/46 (30)
Cyclophosphamide	600 mg/m² IV day 1				
Hexamethylmelamine	200 mg/m² PO days 8–22				
Adriamycin	25 mg/m² IV day 1				
Cisplatin	50 mg/m² IV day 1				
CHEX-UP[171]		62	43/62 (69)	29/62 (47)	12/62 (19)
Cyclophosphamide	150 mg/m² PO days 2–8 and 2–16				
Hexamethylmelamine	150 mg/m² PO days 2–8 and 9–16				
5-Fluorouracil	600 mg/m² IV days 1 and 8				
Cisplatin	30 mg/m² IV days 1 and 8				
CHAP-5[244]		84	66/84 (79)	Not Stated	25/84 (30)
Cyclophosphamide	100 mg/m² PO days 15–29				
Hexamethylmelamine	150 mg/m² PO days 15–29				
Adriamycin	35 mg/m² IV day 1				
Cisplatin	20 mg/m² IV days 1–5				
PC[243]		52	Not Stated	Not Stated	12/52 (23)
Cisplatin	20 mg/m² IV days 1–5				
Cyclophosphamide	600 mg/m² IV day 4				

studies now contain sufficient information about prognostic factors, response duration, and survival to allow realistic comparisons with currently established combination chemotherapy regimens or single agents.

Several groups have reported results of two-, three-, and four-drug combinations in nonrandomized studies in previously untreated Stage III and Stage IV disease. Most of these trials have used combinations of cisplatin, Adriamycin, cyclophosphamide, hexamethylmelamine, methotrexate, or 5-FU.[114,171,210,240–245] The overall response rates have been 60% to 80%, with clinical CR in approximately 40% to 50% of patients. Approximately half of those clinically free of disease actually have residual disease at second-look laparotomy. As a result, about 25% to 30% of all patients treated with combination chemotherapy will be free of disease at restaging, and it is this subset of patients who experience long-term disease-free survival. At present, there does not seem to be a striking difference between combinations, although the addition of cisplatin appears beneficial. Randomized trials between platinum-containing combinations have generally demonstrated equivalent results in terms of survival (see Table 37-14).

Recently, several well-designed trials have been performed of various combination regimens in an attempt to define the relative contributions of individual drugs as well as the combinations themselves. Several of the more significant studies are summarized in Table 37-14.

Dutch investigators compared CHAP-5 (cyclophosphamide, hexamethylmelamine, Adriamycin, and cisplatin) with Hexa-CAF and demonstrated a statistically greater response rate (79% versus 50%) and CR rate (30% versus 17%) as well as an improved disease-free survival (19.5 versus 6.8 months) and improved overall survival (30.7 versus 19.6 months) for the CHAP-5 combination.[244] The GOG compared Adriamycin and cyclophosphamide (AC) with cisplatin, Adriamycin, and cyclophosphamide (PAC) in 227 patients with measurable disease.[246] The CR rate was 51% for CAP and 26% for AC ($p < 0.0001$). The progression-free interval (13 versus 7.7 months) and overall survival (19.7 versus 15.7 months) were also statistically better with the cisplatin-containing combination.

These trials provide substantial evidence of the importance of platinum in any ovarian cancer regimen. Indeed, it is not clear whether the addition of other agents to regimens that include full-dose intensities of cyclophosphamide and cisplatin is necessary or beneficial. The Netherlands Cancer Institute recently completed a large trial comparing CHAP-5 with cyclophosphamide and cisplatin (CP). The overall response rate (78% versus 76%) and the pathologically documented CR rate (34% versus 37%) were similar for the two regimens.[246] A study from the Mayo Clinic compared CP with hexamethylmelamine, cyclophosphamide, Adriamycin, and cisplatin (HCAP) in 181 patients.[247] At a median follow-up of 30 months, the regimens produced identical survivals (24.6 months). A similar experience was seen in the preliminary analysis of a GOG trial comparing CAP with CP.[248] In this trial, the numbers of negative second looks (39% versus 38%) were similar, as were the times to disease progression and survival for the two arms.

Two studies comparing CP with CAP have come to somewhat different conclusions. A study by Conte et al[249] compared CP and PAC in 125 patients, including some with localized as well as those with advanced disease. The objective response rates were similar for the two groups (54% versus 56%), but the PAC regimen induced a higher percentage of CRs (41% versus 20%) in patients with measurable disease and there were more surgically documented CRs (62% versus 40%). However, progression-free interval and survival were not statistically different. The second trial[250] compared CP and PAC in 154 patients with advanced disease. The CR rate favored PAC (24% versus 11%), and at 3 years' follow-up there was a better survival rate in the PAC-treated group (48% versus 20%).

On the basis of the available data, there is very little evidence that any combination regimen produces better results than the two-drug CP regimen used in full therapeutic doses.

Late Complications of Chemotherapy

As therapy for advanced ovarian cancer improves, a variety of late complications are being observed that are related either to the treatment or to the altered natural history of the disease. Late relapses with unusual lesions such as bone metastases or central nervous system involvement have now

TABLE 37-14. Randomized Comparisons of Combination Chemotherapy in Advanced Ovarian Adenocarcinoma

Study	*Results*	*Reference*
CHAP-5 vs. Hexa-CAF	79% RR vs. 50%; 30% CR vs. 17%; median survival, 31 mo. vs. 20 mo.	244
PAC vs. AC	51% CR vs. 26% in patients with measurable disease. Response duration (15 mo. vs. 19 mo.), progression-free interval (13 mo. vs. 7 mo.), and overall survival (20 mo. vs. 16 mo.) all statistically significant	245
CHAP-5 vs. CP	78% RR vs. 76%. PCR 34% vs. 37% and no differences in survival	246
HCAP vs. CP	Survival at 30 months equivalent for the two regimens (24.6 mo.)	247
PAC vs. PC	41% clinical CR vs. 20% CR; in those patients going to second-look, significant increase in PCR for PAC (62% vs. 40%, $p < 0.05$). No difference in overall survival	249
PAC vs. CP	CR 24% vs. 11% ($p < 0.05$); at 3 yrs more PAC survivors (48% vs. 20%)	250

been reported.[251] Acute leukemia as a late complication of therapy has been reported in several studies. A published survey of 70 institutions with 5455 patients revealed 13 patients who developed leukemia, representing a 21-fold increase in risk.[222] Risks were highest in patients who had chemotherapy in excess of 2 years, and approximately two-thirds of the patients with leukemia had received radiation as well. Often, a long period of pancytopenia preceded frank leukemic transformation. Two-thirds of the leukemic patients who died had no evidence of ovarian cancer at autopsy. Similar results have been published in an analysis of 1399 women in five randomized trials in which the cumulative risk of acute nonlymphocytic leukemia was 9.6% at 7 years.[223] Nevertheless, it is important to emphasize that the overall risk of acute leukemia is small (0.3%).[222] However, techniques for minimizing the risk, such as cyclic intermittent chemotherapy rather than continuous daily treatment, avoidance of combined radiation–chemotherapy treatments, no maintenance alkylating-agent therapy, and better techniques for defining the CRs so that therapy can be discontinued, will undoubtedly be helpful.

Experimental Approaches

IMMUNOTHERAPY. Immunotherapy has been investigated in only a few studies, although a good theoretical basis for immunotherapy exists, including (1) the existence of tumor-associated antigens in ovarian cancer; (2) circulating lymphocytes that are reactive to the patient's tumor cells; (3) defects in B-cell function in patients with advanced ovarian cancer, although T-cell function appears intact; and (4) animal models of ovarian cancer that demonstrate enhanced tumor killing with chemotherapy and either nonspecific immunotherapy or specific antibodies generated against ovarian tumor cells.[252,253] Most studies have used nonspecific immunotherapy with chemotherapy. However, trials with intraperitoneal *Corynebacterium parvum*[255,256] interferon,[254] and melphalan–levamisole[257] have been reported.

Nonspecific immunotherapy in conjunction with chemotherapy has shown activity in two randomized studies in ovarian carcinoma,[258,259] and, although the independent contribution of immunotherapy to the therapeutic result is not completely clear, these studies are provocative. Further prospective studies with careful stratification of known prognostic factors will be required to define the role, if any, of this modality in advanced ovarian cancer.

Recently, studies have been done utilizing intraperitoneal IL-2 with or without lymphokine-activated killer (LAK) cells.[253,260] Some reduction in the systemic toxicity of this therapy is achieved when the biologicals are administered intraperitoneally, and objective regressions in ovarian cancer patients have been seen.[260] Unfortunately, at present, the therapy is associated with abdominal pseudocyst formation, which limits its effectiveness.

Several murine monoclonal antibodies have been generated against ovarian cancer specifically or are cross-reactive with ovarian cancer cell lines. Because for the most part these murine antibodies lack intrinsic cytotoxicity, they have been coupled to toxic moieties such as radioisotopes, chemotherapeutic agents, or natural toxins such as ricin or *Pseudomonas* exotoxin.[261,262] Preliminary results in cell lines in vitro and in a nude mouse model of human ovarian cancer[256] are encouraging, and these and other monoclonal antibodies are now entering clinical trial.[253]

DRUG RESISTANCE. The effectiveness of drug therapy in this disease is limited by the development of drug resistance. This resistance not only is drug–specific but also is frequently associated with a broad cross-resistance to structurally dissimilar drugs. Such pleiotropic resistance may be the result of presence of the *MDR*-1 gene with its protein product, the P-170 glycoprotein,[263,264] which enables the drug-resistant tumor to limit accumulation of structurally unrelated agents.[265–268] This cross-resistance is most frequently seen with natural products such as the vinca alkaloids, Adriamycin, and VP-16. Although this mechanism appears to be important in certain other tumors, it does not seem to be the primary mechanism of broad cross-resistance in ovarian cancer. Other mechanisms of resistance include the elevation of intracellular glutathione (GSH)[269] and increased DNA repair.[270]

Potential approaches to overcoming these mechanisms of drug resistance are now being explored. Certain calcium-channel blockers can overcome resistance associated with decreased drug accumulation. For example, verapamil reverses Adriamycin resistance in ovarian carcinoma cell lines[271] by blocking drug efflux. A pilot clinical trial has been completed;[272] levels of verapamil adequate for clinical effect could not be reached without unacceptable cardiac toxicity. Other calcium-channel blockers are now under study.

GSH is a tripeptide thiol found ubiquitously in human cells. Drug resistance in ovarian cancer cells is associated with a marked increase in intracellular GSH.[273,274] Buthionine sulfoximine (BSO), a synthetic amino acid analogue, inhibits the synthesis of GSH and markedly reduces intracellular GSH in vitro and in vivo.[277,278] This change is associated with a restoration of drug sensitivity in cell lines and a prolongation of survival in the in vivo nude mouse model of ovarian cancer. BSO has recently been approved for clinical trials in the salvage therapy of ovarian cancer.

It has also been demonstrated that drug resistance in ovarian cancer is associated with increased DNA repair after both chemotherapeutic or radiotherapeutic injury.[277] Aphidicolin, a potent inhibitor of α and β polymerase, can block this DNA repair and thus partially restore drug sensitivity in these resistant cell lines.[270] This approach may be applicable clinically.

These studies, taken as a whole, indicate that drug resistance in ovarian cancer is an interaction of multiple factors and that a single explanation of drug resistance is not likely. Nevertheless, there are now clinical trials under way to test a variety of ways in which resistance can be overcome.

RESULTS OF TREATMENT

Historically, the treatment of ovarian cancer has been discussed in the context of FIGO stage; that is, separating early disease (FIGO Stage I and Stage II) from advanced disease (FIGO Stage III and Stage IV). However, recent analyses of long-term survival results from several major institutions indicate that other patient- and tumor-related characteristics are extremely important. In addition to FIGO stage, the most important prognostic variables are tumor residuum, grade, histologic subtype, and the age of the patient at diagnosis.[49,60,154,278–281] A multivariate analysis of these variables in 430 ovarian carcinoma patients demonstrates that residual disease and tumor grade are the most important ($p < 0.001$) followed by stage ($p = 0.002$), age ($p = 0.004$), and histologic type ($p = 0.058$).[60] Thus, it appears that tumor residuum and stage are independent variables and that tumor residuum is significantly more powerful in predicting the therapeutic outcome than is the FIGO stage. This finding is now reflected in the change in the FIGO stage classification for advanced disease, as discussed earlier in this chapter.

That the amount of tumor remaining after initial surgery affects the final results of treatment has been known for years.[60,98,278] It is now common to describe three prognostically distinct subgroups based on early disease (Stages I and II) and the presence or absence of large postsurgical residual disease (usually > 2 cm). Patients with small amounts of residual disease stand a good chance of disease eradication by postoperative therapy and have the highest probability of long-term survival. For these reasons, it seems justified to discuss the treatment of three groups of patients separately: (1) those with early (FIGO Stages I and II) cancer and microscopic or no residual disease; (2) those with advanced disease but minimal residua (< 2 cm) after initial surgery; and (3) those more-frequent patients with bulky residual tumor and advanced (Stage III or IV) disease.

EARLY OVARIAN CANCER (FIGO STAGES I AND II) WITH MICROSCOPIC OR NO RESIDUAL DISEASE

The surgical management of Stage I ovarian cancer is influenced by the histologic type and grade of the tumor as well as by the reproductive desires of the patient. Although certain types of epithelial ovarian cancer are more likely than others to present at an early stage, there is probably little difference in either survival or recommended surgical management of these carcinomas when matched for stage and grade. Scully[43,47] summarized three series in which cancer was confined to a single ovary and reported a 78% survival rate with conservative surgical treatment and a 79% rate with radical therapy. Munnell[20] reported a 75% survival rate in two similar groups of patients, and Webb et al[283] reported 90% survival in patients with Stage I tumors with intact capsules and 57% survival when the tumor had penetrated the capsule or ruptured.

From these studies, it would appear that patients with epithelial cancer confined to one ovary with an otherwise-negative comprehensive surgical exploration can be managed by unilateral salpingo-oophorectomy and no further therapy providing the tumor is Grade 1 or 2 and the patient wants to have children. In patients who undergo conservative (unilateral salpingo-oophorectomy) therapy, the opposite ovary should be biopsied. In patients with Grade 3 tumors or those who do not desire to have children, a total abdominal hysterectomy and bilateral salpingo-oophorectomy should be performed.

A series of studies have attempted to define whether well-staged patients with IA and IB, well- or moderately well-differentiated tumors require further therapy. Dembo and associates[59] studied a group of 54 patients with Stage IA disease who were randomized between observation or pelvic radiotherapy after initial surgery. There were nine relapses among 30 patients with moderately or poorly differentiated tumors compared with none among 24 patients with well-differentiated tumors regardless of whether pelvic radiation was given. Similarly, the GOG[284,285] reported only one relapse among 56 patients with Stage IA–IB well- or moderately differentiated tumors randomized to receive either melphalan or no treatment postoperatively. On the basis of these observations, it has been suggested that patients with well-differentiated Stage I tumors who are without positive peritoneal cytology, densely adherent tumors, or cyst rupture do not require postoperative therapy.[142,284,285]

For patients with Stage II disease or with Stage I disease with incomplete surgical staging or poor prognostic findings, more aggressive management is required. Stage II epithelial ovarian carcinoma requires total abdominal hysterectomy, bilateral salpingo-oophorectomy, and a full staging operation in all cases. Particular care must be exercised to ensure that the carcinoma has not spread to the upper abdomen. Every effort should be made to remove all visible tumor in the pelvis utilizing techniques involving retroperitoneal approaches if necessary. If microscopic or small macroscopic residual disease remains, then adjuvant therapy is generally employed, and the management is similar to that used for patients with advanced stages and small residua.

The GOG, in an early trial, studied patients with Stage IA and IB epithelial ovarian cancer (staged in a conventional manner) and compared no additional therapy, pelvic irradiation, or intermittent oral melphalan.[284] Forty-nine percent of patients were not evaluable, and the three treatment arms were not well balanced for prognostic variables. The frequency of relapse was greatest after pelvic irradiation: 7 of 23 (30%) compared with observation (5 of 29; 17%) and intermittent oral melphalan (2 of 34; 6%), although there were no significant differences in overall survival. In subsequent trials that required careful surgical staging prior to entry, the Ovarian Cancer Study Group–GOG studied two groups of patients with early disease. The first, which was mentioned earlier, studied patients with good-prognosis Stage I disease; the second included patients with IC, IIA,B,C, and poor-prognosis Stage I disease and compared melphalan with intraperitoneal ^{32}p. Follow-up on this study is not complete, but the 5-year disease-free survival rate of both treatment approaches is good (≅ 80%).[285] A replacement trial has been initiated in the same patient population comparing intraperitoneal ^{32}p with three courses of cyclophosphamide–cisplatin. Because radiocolloids are transported to the diaphragm and concentrated there,[167,286] this treatment technique delivers high-dose radiation to the diaphragm, perhaps explaining the improved survival rate observed in patients receiving intraperitoneal radioactive colloids.

PATIENTS WITH POOR-PROGNOSIS STAGE I AND STAGES II–IV WITH LITTLE OR NO RESIDUAL DISEASE POSTOPERATIVELY

Patients in this category include most of those with poor-prognosis Stage I or II disease and 20% to 30% of those with Stage III disease who are left without gross tumor after initial surgery. Current evidence indicates that these patients require postoperative therapy, although it is not clear what form of therapy is optimal.

One approach has been to use postoperative irradiation, with doses of 4500 to 5000 cGy given to the pelvis and 2250 to 3000 cGy to the upper abdomen. Previous studies indicate that whole-abdominal radiation is necessary. Bush[287] showed that 4500 cGy given to the pelvis reduced the number of pelvic recurrences in Stage I disease, but the overall risk of relapse did not decrease, as most of the irradiated patients relapsed in the upper abdomen. Similarly, Schray and associates[138] reported that 14 of 19 Stage I and II patients treated with high-dose lower-abdominal irradiation relapsed in the upper abdomen. Irradiation of the upper abdomen will decrease the risk of relapse there and improve survival. The Princess Margaret Group studied patients with Stage IB, II, or IIIA ovarian carcinoma who were randomized to receive pelvic radiation, pelvic radiation plus oral chlorambucil for 2 years, or pelvic and upper-abdominal radiation.[140,141] In 8 of 31 patients treated with radiation to the pelvis only, upper-abdominal relapses without concomitant pelvic relapses were observed, compared with none in patients receiving whole-abdominal irradiation.[141] The 5-year survival rate for patients with whole-abdominal irradiation was 78% compared with 51% in the patients receiving pelvic radiation with or without chlorambucil.[287] Similarly, Delclos and Smith[143] reported that only 17% of 18 Stage II patients irradiated to the pelvis alone survived at 5 years compared with 49% of 71 patients treated with whole-abdominal irradiation. From these data, it is generally accepted that whole-abdominal radiotherapy is the optimal technique for this group of patients.

Chemotherapy has also been used in this group of patients, and the data suggest that results are similar to those observed with external-beam radiotherapy. The M.D. Anderson group studied patients with Stages I–IIIA and small amounts of residual disease, comparing single-agent melphalan with total-abdominal irradiation by moving strip in a slightly different dose and schedule than that used by the Princess Margaret group.[288,289] The 2- and 5-year survival rates for the groups were 86.5% and 71.5% for radiation and 90% and 78% for melphalan. Furthermore, now with 10 years' follow-up, there are still no differences in survival rates in the two groups.[290] The M.D. Anderson group concluded that chemotherapy is as effective as irradiation, has fewer serious side-effects, and is less expensive.

In contrast, the Radiumhemmet Group randomized patients with Stage I or Stage IIA seropapillary ovarian carcinoma to adjuvant postsurgical treatment with either lower-abdominal radiation, single alkylating-agent chemotherapy, or radiotherapy followed by chemotherapy.[291] The lowest 5-year survival rate was observed in patients treated with chemotherapy alone (68%) compared with 88% in the radiation alone group and 91% in the combined radiation–chemotherapy group.

Many of these early studies did not require comprehensive surgical staging before therapy. When systematic restaging is performed prospectively in such patients, 31% are found to have a more advanced stage, and 77% actually have Stage III disease.[282] Thus, it is clear that a significant reason why local treatment fails in many patients with apparently localized disease is that they have unsuspected extrapelvic metastases that are not being treated by surgery or pelvic irradiation.

Although both radiation and chemotherapy are effective against small (< 2 cm) ovarian tumors, resulting in high rates of clinical and pathologic CR, the cure rates for patients with residual tumor after initial surgery have been less favorable than those in patients with no residual tumor.[142,154] Whole-abdominal irradiation has frequently been employed in such patients with doses of 5000 to 6000 cGy to the lower abdomen and 3000 to 4000 cGy to the upper abdomen. Using radiotherapy, Dembo[142] reported a 58% 5-year survival rate in 36 patients with Stage II disease and a 43% rate in 55 patients with Stage III disease left with small residual tumors after initial surgery. Martinez et al[154] reported a 54% 5-year survival rate in 42 similar patients with Stage II or III disease.

Combination chemotherapy has been used in similar groups of patients. The initial response rates are high, and the pathologically confirmed complete remission rates are about 56% (Table 37-15). These patients generally experience long survival. The M.D. Anderson Group reported 34% 4-year survival rate in 83 patients treated with a variety of single-agent chemotherapies (melphalan, 5-FU, Adriamycin, cisplatin, hexamethylmelamine) and 51% in 66 patients treated with various combinations (HAC, HMM-CYT, MEL-DDP).[293,294] Lambert and Berry[177] reported a 35% 4-year survival rate in 42 patients treated with high-dose cyclophosphamide or high-dose cisplatin, and Belinson and associates[293] reported a 53% survival rate in 21 patients treated with CAP. These survival rates are generally similar to those observed with total-abdominal radiation.

The frequency of surgically confirmed CRs is approximately half the clinical CR rate but is heavily dependent on the volume of disease at initial therapy. The effect of extent of residual disease on the frequency of a pathologic CR is shown in Table 37-15.

Generally, patients who have negative second-look laparotomies after combination chemotherapy experience long survival, although this varies from institution to institution.[295] Greco et al[296,297] reported a 74% 4-year disease-free survival rate in patients with negative second-look operations postchemotherapy. The NCI experience is similar: among patients treated with CHEX-UP, 63% of the patients with pathologically documented CR are alive without relapse

TABLE 37-15. Effect of Residual Disease on Pathologic Complete Remission Rate

	Surgically Confirmed Complete Remissions (%)	
Chemotherapy	*<3 cm Residua*	*>3 cm Residua*
Hexa-CAF[210]	8/8 (100)	5/32 (16)
CHEX-UP[242]	5/14 (36)	5/37 (14)
H-CAP[247]	18/21 (86)	3/29 (11)
A-C[241]	11/12 (92)	1/24 (4)
PAC[240]	5/17 (30)	5/39 (13)
PAC/Hexa-CAF[292]	6/22 (27)	1/17 (6)
Total	53/94 (56)	20/178 (11)

at 5 years.[242] In contrast, studies from Memorial Hospital on survival of patients with negative second-look operations project a 65% relapse rate by 48 months.[298] In a 7-year follow-up of patients treated with PAC, only three of eight were alive without recurrence 7 to 8 years after treatment.[240] It is not clear why there are significant differences from institution to institution in the survival of patients with negative second-look operations postchemotherapy.

PATIENTS WITH STAGES II–IV AND BULKY RESIDUAL DISEASE

Unfortunately, most patients with Stage III disease and some with Stage II disease are left with extensive residual disease after initial surgery. These patients respond poorly to conventional therapies of all types, and the major challenge for the future lies in the development of successful management approaches for this large group of women.

In recent years, the mainstay of therapy for this group has been systemic chemotherapy; however, some patients with unique presentations may be appropriately treated with radiation. It is worthwhile to separate patients with gross abdominal tumor from those with only retroperitoneal lymph node metastases, because the latter group may have a different prognosis when given appropriate irradiation. Hintz and colleagues noted that patients with retroperitoneal lymph nodes as the only site of extrapelvic disease have a survival rate of about 55% at 5 years, in contrast to 10% for patients with peritoneal spread.[299]

In contrast, the prognosis of patients with gross abdominal tumors exceeding 2 cm in diameter has been poor with whole-abdominal irradiation. Even when aggressive radiotherapeutic approaches were used, with radiation to the whole peritoneal cavity at maximal tolerable doses, the 5-year survival rates were only 9% to 12%.[96,301,302] Further, the tolerance of treatment in these patients generally has been extremely poor. Additional treatment with single alkylating-agent chemotherapy, given either before or after radiotherapy,[300,303–306] usually failed to improve survival and was even less well tolerated. Therefore, it has been generally accepted that postoperative whole-abdominal irradiation given as the primary modality with curative intent is not indicated for patients with large (> 2 cm) abdominal tumors unless effective cytoreductive surgery can be performed before radiotherapy, leaving the peritoneal cavity either without gross disease or with little (< 2 cm) residual disease.

The lack of satisfactory cure rates with either radiation or combination chemotherapy in patients with bulky disease, and the frequent inability to cytoreduce the tumors at the initial laparotomy, have led to the introduction of combined-modality therapy. Combination chemotherapy is highly effective in debulking such tumors, resulting in 80% to 90% significant clinical responses. If second-look surgery is performed, the residual tumors are often small, and their complete or nearly complete resection can frequently be achieved. The elimination of this minimal residual disease after induction therapy has been under intensive study.[307]

Fuks et al[308] gave 38 patients initial induction therapy using 3 to 14 courses of the CHAD combination for tumor mass reduction and a second laparotomy for resection of residual tumors, followed by a consolidation phase with curative doses of whole-abdominal irradiation. The initial clinical response (CR and partial response) to CHAD was 91%. After second-look surgery, 76% of patients were without residual disease. Whole-abdominal irradiation using the Martinez technique was then given. The actuarial 5-year survival and disease-free survival rates for the whole group were 27% and 17%, respectively. These survival data are similar to those of patients treated with CHAP-5 combination chemotherapy without subsequent whole-abdominal irradiation,[246,309] suggesting that the consolidation radiotherapy had little if any effect on the survival probability already achieved by chemotherapy.

This observation is consistent with other recent reports. Hacker et al[292] treated 30 patients with a variety of combination-chemotherapy protocols, followed by a second surgical tumor reduction and whole-abdominal radiotherapy. Only 4 of 16 patients with completely resected tumors during the second laparotomy survived 22 to 41 months after radiotherapy. Hainsworth and associates,[297] using a similar approach after H-CHAP or H-FAP combination chemotherapy, found that 14 of 17 patients relapsed between 2 and 20 months after completion of radiotherapy. Coltart et al[310] reported 30% 3-year survival rate in 10 Stage III patients treated with cisplatin–cyclophosphamide chemotherapy, second debulking surgery, and whole-abdominal radiation. Not only was survival poor, but also the authors reported poor tolerance to radiation, including early discontinuation of the radiation in

TABLE 37-16. Survival for ≥2 Years After Salvage Abdominal Irradiation Following Positive Second-Look Surgery

		Residual Disease		
	Microscopic	*< 1 cm*	*> 1 cm*	*Reference*
	1/4	0/3	0/1	311
	3/11	0/5	0/1	297
	2/10	0/4	0/2	312
	4/16	2/6	0/18	292
	0/1	0/6	0/1	313
	2/9	0/7	0/6	314
	0/4		0/4	315
Total	12/55 (22%)	2/31 (7%)	0/33 (0%)	

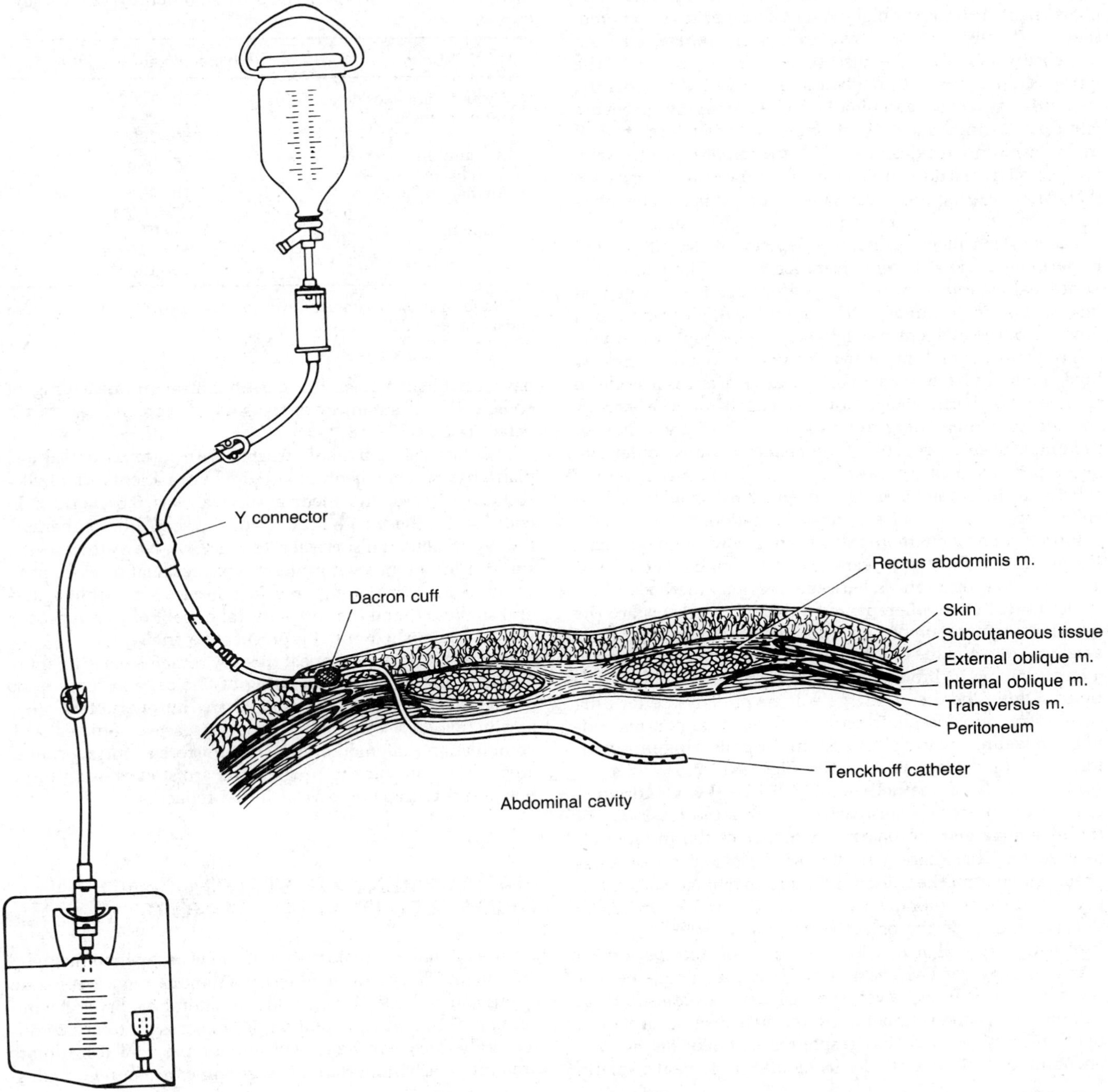

FIG. 37-7. Tenckhoff dialysis catheter system for the delivery of intraperitoneal chemotherapy in ovarian cancer.

30% to 53% of patients because of marrow toxicity and radiation enteritis necessitating surgery in 27% to 63% of the patients. Indeed, the probability of achieving a long (> 2-year) disease-free survival using postchemotherapy total-abdominal irradiation is low in general and a function of the extent of residual disease (Table 37-16). Other attempts to control small amounts of residual disease remaining after initial induction chemotherapy have included intraperitoneal radioisotopes (primarily ^{32}p) or chemotherapy.

Intraperitoneal Chemotherapy

Techniques for delivering chemotherapy to the patient with small amounts of peritoneally dispersed residual disease have been extensively studied. The clinical rationale and pharmacologic basis for high-volume intraperitoneal chemotherapy ("belly bath") in ovarian cancer are derived from the observation that the disease remains confined to the intraperitoneal space throughout most of its natural history; currently available combination chemotherapy produces clinical CRs in about 40% of patients, but at least half of these have some residual disease. Furthermore, in vitro studies demonstrate a dose–response effect for some drugs, such that cytotoxic drug concentrations may be achieved by intraperitoneal, but not by intravenous, administration.

The pharmacologic principles depend on the differences in peritoneal and systemic clearance.[317–319] The slower the peritoneal clearance of a drug, the greater is the potential pharmacologic advantage. The peritoneal clearance is a function of the molecular weight and the hydrophilic properties of the drug: high-molecular-weight compounds with low lipid solubility have a slow peritoneal clearance, leading to an increased pharmacologic advantage. Two other properties are necessary for a drug to be useful in the intraperitoneal treatment of ovarian cancer: the concentrations achievable in the peritoneal cavity must be cytotoxic to ovarian cancer cells, and the cytotoxic drug concentration should produce an acceptable degree of peritoneal irritation.

Intraperitoneal chemotherapy is not a new technique, having been used for many years to control malignant ascites. The principal differences between previous methods of intraperitoneal chemotherapy and current techniques are the use of a semipermanent Tenckhoff dialysis catheter or Port-a-cath system and the delivery of the antineoplastic agents in a large volume (2 liters of dialysate) instead of in 50 to 100 ml of saline. The use of a large volume of dialysate for drug administration is based, in part, on theoretical pharmacokinetic modeling studies.[317] A system for delivering intraperitoneal chemotherapy is shown in Figure 37-7.

Initial trials of methotrexate,[320] 5-FU,[321] and Adriamycin[322] were performed primarily to define the feasibility of the technique and the pharmacokinetics of the intraperitoneal route. The Phase I studies of these and other drugs documented a marked pharmacologic advantage with intraperitoneal chemotherapy (Table 37-17), and most of the Phase I trials reported objective responses.[319,320]

Although the pharmacologic success of intraperitoneal chemotherapy has been established, the therapeutic benefit remains less clear. However, the early trials established that patients with small amounts of residual disease are most likely to respond and that responses of bulky disease are uncommon.[331,332] Two studies using intraperitoneal cisplatin have established it as the current intraperitoneal drug of choice.[333,334] A summary of the study design and results are listed in Table 37-18.

TABLE 37-17. Intraperitoneal Chemotherapy in Ovarian Cancer

Drug	*Pharmacologic Advantage**
Cytosine arabinoside	300–1000[323]
5-Fluorouracil	111–898[321]
	550–7852[324]
Adriamycin	474[322]
Melphalan	63–93[325]
Methotrexate	18–36[320]
	7–303[326]
Cisplatin	21[327]
	47–72[328]
	50–100[329]

* Ratio of peak peritoneal level to plasma level or ratio of area under curve (AUC).

The survival of patients treated with intraperitoneal cisplatin has recently been reported.[335] For patients with bulky residual disease, the median survival was 6.5 months. In contrast, for those with little residual disease before therapy, the 2-year actuarial survival rate was 74%. Nevertheless, the survival of patients with microscopic residual disease, positive washings, or minimal residual disease is variable in several studies,[246] and the true survival benefit of this approach will be established only by prospective trials.

At present, intraperitoneal therapy remains experimental. Cisplatin appears to be the drug of choice, and there is no evidence of substantial activity of any intraperitoneal therapy in patients with bulky residual disease. Studies with combination chemotherapy administered intraperitoneally[332,336,337] are now in progress, as are studies using intraperitoneal therapy as part of initial induction.

MANAGEMENT OF STROMAL AND GERM-CELL OVARIAN TUMORS

Germ-cell and stromal tumors of the ovary, which make up only about 5% to 10% of all ovarian tumors, require separate discussion because of their unusual natural history and clinical manifestations. In addition, it is necessary to utilize different therapies for the various tumor types.[338] These tumors are particularly important because some of the most aggres-

TABLE 37-18. Intraperitoneal Cisplatin in Small Volume Residual Disease Ovarian Cancer After Induction Chemotherapy

	Mt Sinai[334]	*Netherlands Cancer Institute*[333]
No. of patients	23	21
Cisplatin dose	50 mg/m² in 2 liters every 3 wk	60–150 mg/m² in 2 liters every 2–3 wk
No. of cycles	6	6–10
Sodium thiosulfate	Not used	If toxicity developed in previous cycle
Catheter	Temporary in 75% of patients	Tenckhoff
Results	6/19 (32%) negative laparotomy	7/21 (33%) negative laparatomy

sive ones are now curable with combination chemotherapy and conservative surgery.

These tumors can be separated into three groups:

1. Those with ovarian stromal components, such as the granulosa-cell and Sertoli–Leydig cell tumors;
2. Those derived from germ-cell elements, such as malignant teratoma, embryonal carcinoma, endodermal sinus tumor, and dysgerminoma; and
3. Choriocarcinoma.

OVARIAN STROMAL TUMORS

Ovarian stromal tumors account for approximately 1% to 3% of all ovarian tumors, generally have an indolent natural history, and sometimes recur many years after initial therapy. They are sometimes associated with precocious feminization, and their association with unopposed estrogen secretion and an increased incidence of concomitant endometrial carcinoma (7.8%) has been well documented.[339] In a review of 51 patients, 43% of the tumors were theca-cell tumors, 24% were pure granulosa-cell tumors, and 33% were mixed granulosa–theca-cell tumors.[340] None of the patients with thecomas died as a result of their disease; deaths occurred only in patients having the granulosa cell-containing tumors with metastases.

Stromal tumors can be managed by unilateral salpingo-oophorectomy in young patients and rarely required adjunctive therapy. The incidence of bilaterality is very low. There are too few reported cases of Stage II stromal tumors to make definitive recommendations, but the lack of proven adjunctive therapy does not permit recommending conservative surgery in such patients. Factors such as tumor size, degree of differentiation, histologic patterns, and tumor spillage are of prognostic importance. Because of their protracted natural history, it is difficult to document the value of postoperative radiation. However, in tumors that are not completely resected, a dose of 5000 to 6000 cGy to the pelvis has been advocated. Such treatment of 37 patients at M.D. Anderson Hospital resulted in a 5-year survival rate of 75% for Stage I and 50% to 60% for Stages II and III.[338]

The role of chemotherapy in treating the granulosa–theca cell tumors has been poorly defined because so few patients have been studied. There are anecdotal reports of responses to alkylating agents[338,341] and Adriamycin.[342]

Experience with nine patients with Sertoli–Leydig cell tumors has been reported from the M.D. Anderson Hospital, five seen for initial therapy, and four with recurrent tumor. Two patients with recurrent lesions had a complete response after administration of a combination of vincristine, dactinomycin, and cyclophosphamide.[338] There is a report of partial regressions using CAP in two patients.[343] The largest recent study described 11 patients with granulosa-cell tumors who were treated with PVB.[62] Six of the 11 had surgically confirmed CRs. Substantial drug toxicity was seen, but this combination merits further study in stromal tumors in light of the paucity of activity with other regimens and with radiation therapy.

Recurrent stromal tumors are treated by resection and postoperative irradiation, if the residual tumor can be encompassed by external irradiation, or with chemotherapy, if the disease is extensive.

OVARIAN GERM-CELL TUMORS

Ovarian germ-cell tumors are rare, accounting for about 2% to 3% of all ovarian cancers. These tumors may have a mixed histologic pattern, and treatment should be designed to deal with the most malignant component. Historically, embryonal carcinoma, endodermal sinus tumors, and malignant teratomas had an extremely poor prognosis with surgery alone, and long-term survival was achieved only in a small percentage of patients even with Stage I disease.[344] For example, the Ovarian Tumor Registry of the American Gynecological Society reported in 1977 that 31 of 34 patients with endodermal sinus tumor were dead of disease after surgery alone; the three survivors, all with Stage IA disease, were living 2.5, 9, and 12 years after surgery.[345] Gallion and co-workers have reviewed the published literature on 150 cases of pure endodermal sinus tumors.[346] Before the use of chemotherapy, the overall 2-year survival rate of patients with Stage I disease was 27%, which did not differ from that of patients presenting with more advanced disease. Surgery alone was ineffective, producing only a 16% 2-year survival rate. Even total abdominal hysterectomy and bilateral salpingo-oophorectomy for Stage IA disease in one study produced only a 13% 2-year survival rate. Pelvic or total-abdominal radiation added little to these 2-year survival figures.

Improved cure rates for these tumors have followed the observation that germ-cell tumors are highly curable with combination chemotherapy. Surgery can now be more limited.

For germ-cell tumors confined to one ovary, unilateral salpingo-oophorectomy is the operation of choice for the young patient. For tumors that have spread to pelvic structures other than the opposite ovary, fallopian tube, or uterus, complete tumor removal without total abdominal hysterectomy or removal of the uninvolved adnexa is indicated. These patients can usually be cured with adjunctive chemotherapy and retain reproductive function.

Endodermal Sinus Tumors

Endodermal sinus tumors are unusual and aggressive tumors of germ-cell origin that reproduce the extraembryonic structures of the early embryo. The tumor is rarely bilateral. Before the use of combination chemotherapy, the tumor was almost invariably fatal.

The consensus at present is that all patients, regardless of stage, should receive chemotherapy. The earliest effective regimen reported was the VAC (vincristine, actinomycin D, cyclophosphamide) program. Two studies have summarized the results with VAC in a variety of more aggressive germ-cell tumors. Cangir and co-workers described 21 patients (8 with malignant teratomas, 6 with endodermal sinus tumors, 6 with mixed germ-cell tumors, and 1 with Sertoli–Leydig tumor),[347] 14 of whom showed no evidence of malignancy at a second-look operation after chemotherapy. These authors concluded that maximal surgical removal followed by adjuvant VAC was appropriate and that irradiation had no role in the initial management of these patients. Slayton and colleagues have recently summarized the experience of the GOG with VAC in aggressive germ-cell tumors.[348] Seventy-six patients were treated with VAC postoperatively, including 54 who were believed disease free after surgery, and 39 of these 54 (72%) remain disease free. The best results were seen in patients with immature (Grades II and III) teratoma, where 19 of 20 remained disease free. Results were not nearly as good in patients with significant residual disease after surgery; in this group, only 7 of 22 were disease free after VAC chemotherapy.

Although the largest experience has been with the VAC combination, recent reports indicate that PVB is at least as good as and may be better than VAC. Collected experience from published series[349–351] shows 53 of 61 (87%) of PVB-treated patients alive without evidence of disease. Recently, platinum, VP-16, and bleomycin (PVP-16B) has been used by the Royal Marsden group in nine patients (six with Stages III and IV disease), eight of whom are disease free at 6 to 62$^+$ months.[350] Although no randomized trials exist comparing VAC with PVB or P-VP-16B, it is likely that the last two regimens will become the therapy of choice for endodermal sinus tumors.

Malignant Teratoma

Malignant teratoma of the ovary is a rare, lethal germ-cell tumor. More than half of the patients present before the age of 20. The tumor is rarely bilateral. Prognosis seems to be related to the histologic grade of the tumor, according to the M.D. Anderson experience with 25 patients.[352]

Before the use of combination chemotherapy, patients were managed with aggressive surgery followed by irradiation or single-agent chemotherapy. Of eight patients managed in this manner, none survived, although all different grades of tumor were represented. In contrast, using the VAC combination without irradiation, 10 of 12 patients are surviving at a median of 43 months. A combination-chemotherapy approach with VAC or one of the other regimens mentioned in the previous section is now the therapy of choice for these tumors. Of all the germ-cell tumors, the Grade II and III immature teratomas appear to respond best to VAC.

Dysgerminoma

Dysgerminomas constitute only about 2% of all ovarian malignancies, and they are unique among the germ-cell tumors because of the high cure rate and sensitivity to radiation. They are the only ovarian germ-cell malignancy that occurs bilaterally with significant frequency (10% to 15%). Although these tumors are the counterpart of testicular seminoma in males, they are rarer. The tumor metastasizes to the regional lymph nodes in about 20% of the patients and can be cured with limited surgical procedures and low-dose radiation therapy.

Any other malignant germ-cell tumor components should be identified because they influence the prognosis. Asadourian and Taylor reported an admixture of germinal elements in 12 of 117 patients with dysgerminoma reviewed at the Armed Forces Institute of Pathology.[353] Several studies indicate that extension through the capsule of the tumor, extraovarian spread, large tumor size, or bilateral lesions are poor prognostic findings.[354,355]

At initial surgery, the contralateral ovary should be carefully examined. If there is any question of involvement, it should be bivalved, and wedge biopsies should be obtained for frozen section. If the tumor is localized to one ovary, a unilateral salpingo-oophorectomy should be performed. Also, the pelvic and periaortic nodes should be evaluated carefully by palpation; biopsies should be taken of any suspicious areas. If the tumor is localized inside the capsule of one ovary, no postoperative irradiation is indicated. Otherwise, a dose of 2000 to 2500 cGy should be delivered to the midplane of the hemipelvis on the side of the lesion, in addition to the pelvic and periaortic nodes.[355,356] If there is bilateral disease, bilateral salpingo-oophorectomy should be carried out and irradiation given to the pelvis and iliac and para-aortic nodes. If grossly metastatic nodes are present, a boost of 500 to 1000 cGy should be delivered with reduced fields. High-energy linear accelerator beams should be used to decrease the scatter dose to the contralateral ovary.

The group from the M.D. Anderson Hospital has reported results on 36 patients with pure dysgerminoma.[356] Sixty-one percent of the patients were in Stage I, and 34% had advanced disease (FIGO Stages III and IV). In 5 patients with Stage IA disease treated only with unilateral salpingo-oophorectomy, no recurrences were noted. All patients are alive 3 to 20 years after initial treatment, and 3 of these patients have had children. Management of the other patients was generally with aggressive debulking surgery followed by total-abdominal irradiation. Lymphangiography was used to assess disease in the para-aortic nodes. The overall survival for their group of patients was 86%. Similar results have been reported from the Radiumhemmet Institute.[355] Of 56 patients treated with radiation therapy, the overall 5-year survival rate was 75%, with 36% of the patients developing recurrences. The extent of the tumor was a critical factor in determining survival and recurrences. In 40 patients treated initially at the Radiumhemmet, 13 recurrences were noted, and of these patients 8 survived for 5 years or more after the beginning of therapy. Asadourian and Taylor reported recurrences or metastases in 23 of 105 patients (24%); additional therapy resulted in the cure of 10 of these patients.[353] These authors also observed a 96% 5-year actuarial survival rate in 78 patients with tumor localized to one or both ovaries, in contrast to 63% in 17 patients with extraovarian extension. There were 18 pregnancies after treatment in 10 patients. Fifteen of the babies were normal, 1 was malformed, and there were two abortions, one therapeutic and 1 spontaneous.

Recurrent tumors, when extensive or with distant metastasis, have been treated with combination chemotherapy.[357] In light of the activity of PVB in the testicular counterpart of this tumor, seminoma, the ovarian tumor has recently been treated with PVB. The Royal Marsden group treated seven patients with Stage III or IV dysgerminoma, four of whom had not responded to radiation, with PVB.[350] All seven had a CR, and six have been free of disease for more than 1 year.

Choriocarcinoma

This tumor is extremely rare (less than 1% of ovarian tumors). Chemotherapy, as in trophoblastic lesions, has been the treatment of choice.[358] The prognosis, however, is extremely poor. Rutledge reported a few patients responding to a combination of methotrexate, dactinomycin, and cyclophosphamide (MAC).[338] Recently, Fanning et al[359] reported the successful treatment of a patient with Stage III mixed germ-cell tumor with pure choriocarcinoma in the para-aortic nodes. The patient was treated with alternating sequences of VAC and PVB and at 30 months is free of disease. The authors state that this is the first reported long-term survival of a patient with pure choriocarcinoma metastases.

TREATMENT OF OVARIAN CARCINOMA ASSOCIATED WITH PREGNANCY

Although unusual, ovarian carcinoma does occur during pregnancy.[360] Palpation of an adnexal mass during the first trimester without other evidence of malignancy should be managed by close follow-up with pelvic examinations and, if necessary, ultrasound. A persistent corpus luteum cyst will usually resolve spontaneously, and surgical exploration for an asymptomatic mass is best carried out during the second trimester. Although most adnexal masses in pregnancy will be benign, a persistent mass should be removed. Creasman et al[361] reported on 17 patients with ovarian carcinoma managed at M.D. Anderson Hospital who were either pregnant or within 6 months of delivery at the time of diagnosis. One-third of the tumors were diagnosed at delivery.

Unless there is spread outside the ovary, unilateral salpingo-oophorectomy and a full staging operation are the treatments of choice. If the carcinoma has spread beyond the ovary, a full staging and debulking operation should be performed, although hysterectomy with sacrifice of the fetus should be undertaken only if necessary to debulk the tumor properly. Postoperative chemotherapy should be administered as indicated by the stage, cell type, and grade of the tumor, because most chemotherapeutic agents useful in ovarian cancer can be administered during pregnancy without known adverse effects on the fetus.

REFERENCES

1. Cancer Facts and Figures 1986. New York, American Cancer Society, 1986
2. Doll R, Muir C, Waterhouse J (eds): International Union Against Cancer: Cancer Incidence in Five Continents, vol 2. Berlin, Springer-Verlag, 1970
3. Buell P, Dunn JE: Cancer mortality among Japanese Issei and Nisei of California. Cancer 18:656–664, 1965
4. Haenszel W, Kurihara M: Studies of Japanese migrants: I. Mortality from cancer and other disease among Japanese in the United States. J Natl Cancer Inst 40:43–48, 1968
5. Joly DJ, Lilienfield AM, Diamond EL et al: An epidemiologic study of the relationship of reproductive experience to cancer of the ovary. Am J Epidemiol 99:190–209, 1974
6. Beral V, Fraser P, Chilvers C: Does pregnancy protect against ovarian cancer? Lancet 2:1083–1086, 1978
7. Lingeman CH: Etiology of cancer of the human ovary: A review. J Natl Cancer Inst 53:1603–1618, 1974
8. Hoover R, Gray LA, Fraumeni JF: Stilbestrol and the risk of ovarian cancer. Lancet 2:533–534, 1977
9. The Cancer and Steroid Hormone Study of the Centers for Disease Control and The National Institute of Child Health and Development: The reduction in risk of ovarian cancer associated with oral contraceptive use. N Engl J Med 316:650–655, 1987
10. West BO: Epidemiologic study of malignancies of the ovaries. Cancer 19:1001–1007, 1966
11. Fraumeni JF, Grundy GW, Creagan ET: Six families prone to ovarian cancer. Cancer 36:364–369, 1975
12. Schweisguth O, Gerard-Marchant R, Plainfosse B et al: Bilateral nonfunctioning thecoma of the ovary in epileptic children under anticonvulsant therapy. Acta Paediatr Scand 60:6–10, 1971
13. Hueper WC, Conway WD: Chemical Carcinogenesis and Cancers. Springfield, IL, Charles C Thomas, 1964
14. Longo DL, Young RC: Cosmetic talc and ovarian carcinoma. Lancet 2:349–351, 1979
15. Cramer DW, Welch WR, Scully RE, Wojciechowski CA: Ovarian cancer and talc. Cancer 50:372–376, 1982
16. Scully RE: Tumors of the Ovary and Maldeveloped Gonads. Armed Forces Institute of Pathology, Second Series, Fascicle 16. Washington, DC, Armed Forces Institute of Pathology, 1979
17. Janovski NA, Paramandandhan, TL: Tumors and tumor-like conditions of the ovaries, fallopian tubes and ligaments of the uterus. In Friedman EA (ed): Major Problems in Obstetrics and Gynecology, vol 4, p 12. Philadelphia, WB Saunders, 1973
18. Plentl AA, Friedman EA: Lymphatic System of the Female Genitalia: The Morphologic Basis of Oncologic Diagnosis and Therapy, pp 168–180. Philadelphia, WB Saunders, 1973
19. Fuks Z: Patterns of spread of ovarian carcinoma: Relation to therapeutic strategies. Adv Biosci 26:39–51, 1980
20. Munnell EW: Is conservative therapy ever justified in Stage I (Ia) cancer of the ovary? Am J Obstet Gynecol 103:641–650, 1969
21. Keettel WC, Pixley E: Diagnostic value of peritoneal washings. Clin Obstet Gynecol 1:592, 1958
22. Joffey JM, Courtice FC: Lymphatics, Lymph and Lymphoid Complexes, pp 295–305. New York, Academic Press, 1970
23. Feldman GB, Knapp RC: Lymphatic drainage of the peritoneal cavity and its significance in ovarian cancer. Am J Obstet Gynecol 119:991–994, 1974
24. Meyers MA: The spread and localization of acute intraperitoneal effusions. Radiology 95:547–554, 1970
25. Dyre JC: Intraperitoneal pressure in the human. Surg Gynecol Obstet 87:472, 1948
26. French JE, Florey HW, Morris BL: The absorption of particles by the lymphatics of the diaphragm. Q J Exp Biol 45:88–103, 1960
27. Coates G, Bush RS, Aspin N: A study of ascites using lymphoscintigraphy with 99m Tc-sulfur colloid. Radiology 107:577–583, 1973
28. Bagley CM, Young RC, Schein PS, Chabner BA, DeVita VT: Ovarian carcinoma metastatic to the diaphragm: Frequently undiagnosed at laparotomy. Am J Obstet Gynecol 116:397–400, 1973
29. Rosenoff SH, DeVita VT, Hubbard S, Young RC: Peritoneoscopy in the staging and follow-up of ovarian cancer. Semin Oncol 2:223–228, 1975
30. Piver MS, Barlow JJ, Lele SB: Incidence of sub-clinical metastasis in Stage I and II ovarian carcinoma. Obstet Gynecol 52:100–104, 1978
31. Feldman GB, Knapp RC, Order SE, Hellman S: The role of lymphatic obstruction in the formation of ascites in a murine ovarian carcinoma. Cancer Res 32:1663–1666, 1972
32. Fisher RI, Young RC: Advances in the staging and treatment of ovarian cancer. Cancer 39:967, 1977
33. Steinberg JJ, Demopoulos RI, Bigelow B: The evaluation of the omentum in ovarian cancer. Gynecol Oncol 2:253, 1975
34. Eichner E, Bove ER: In vivo studies on the lymphatic drainage of the human ovary. Obstet Gynecol 3:287–297, 1954
35. Fuks Z: External radiotherapy of ovarian cancer: Standard approaches and new frontiers. Semin Oncol 2:253–266, 1975
36. Kwaney R, Fuchs WA: Die Lymphographie bei malignen ovarial Tumoren. Fortschr Geb Röntgenstr Nuklearmed 126:564–566, 1977
37. Musumeci R, DePalo G, Kenda R, Tesoro-Tess JD et al: Retroperitoneal metastases from ovarian carcinoma: Reassessment of 365 patients studied with lymphography. AJR 134:449–452, 1980
38. Fuks Z: Patterns of spread of ovarian carcinoma: Relation to therapeutic strategies. In Newman CE, Ford CH, Jordan JA (eds): Ovarian Cancer. Oxford, Pergamon Press, 1980
39. Burghardt E, Pickel H, Stettner H: Management of advanced ovarian cancer. Eur J Gynaecol Oncol 3:155, 1984
40. Buchsbaum HJ, Delgado G, Blessing J et al: Surgical staging of ovarian carcinoma (abstr). Gynecol Oncol 23:253, 1986
41. Barnhill DR, Hoskins WJ, Heller PB et al: The second look surgical reassessment of epithelial ovarian carcinoma. Gynecol Oncol 19:148, 1984
42. Rubin SC, Hoskins WJ, Hakes TB et al: Recurrence after negative second-look laparotomy for ovarian cancer: Analysis of risk factors. Am J Obstet Gynecol 159:1094, 1988
43. Scully RE: Recent progress in ovarian cancer. Hum Pathol 1:73–98, 1970
44. Novak ER, Woodruff JD: Novak's Gynecologic and Obstetric Pathology, p 389. Philadelphia, WB Saunders, 1974
45. Serov SF, Scully RE, Solvin LH: International Histological Classification of Tumors, No. 9: Histological Typing of Ovarian Tumors. Geneva, World Health Organization, 1973

46. International Federation of Gynaecology and Obstetrics: Classification and staging of malignant tumors in the female pelvis. Acta Obstet Gynaecol Scand 50:1–7, 1971
47. Scully RE: Ovarian tumors. Am J Pathol 87:686–720, 1977
48. Nikrui N: Survey of clinical behavior of patients with borderline tumors of the ovary. Gynecol Oncol 12:107–119, 1981
49. Bjorkholm E, Pettersson F, Einhorn N et al: Long term follow-up and prognostic factors in ovarian carcinoma. The Radiumhemmet series 1953–1973. Acta Radiat Oncol 21:413–419, 1982
50. Kottmeier HL: Ovarian cancer with special regard to radiotherapy. Am J Roentgenol Rad Ther Nucl Med 111:417–421, 1971
51. Aure JC, Høeg K, Kolstad P: Clinical and histologic studies of ovarian carcinoma: Long-term follow-up of 900 cases. Obstet Gynecol 37:1–9, 1971
52. Perez CA, Walz BJ, Jacobson PL: Radiation therapy in the management of carcinoma of the ovary. Natl Cancer Inst Monogr 42:119–125, 1975
53. Young RC, Hubbard SP, DeVita VT: The chemotherapy of ovarian carcinoma. Cancer Treat Rev 1:99–110, 1974
54. Smith JP, Rutledge F, Wharton JT: Chemotherapy of ovarian cancer: New approaches to treatment. Cancer 30:1565–1571, 1972
55. Munnell EW, Taylor HC: Ovarian carcinoma: A review of 200 primary and 51 secondary cases. Am J Obstet 58:943, 1949
56. Decker DG, Mussey E, Williams TJ: Grading of gynecologic malignancy: Epithelial ovarian cancer. In Proceedings of the 7th National Cancer Congress, pp 223–231. Philadelphia, JB Lippincott, 1972
57. Day TG, Gallager HS, Rutledge F: Epithelial carcinoma of the ovary: Prognostic importance of histologic grade. Natl Cancer Inst Monogr 42:15–18, 1975
58. Ozols RF, Garvin AJ, Costa J et al: Advanced ovarian cancer: Correlation of histologic grade with response to therapy and survival. Cancer 45:572–581, 1980
59. Dembo AJ, Bush RS, Beale FA: Ovarian carcinoma: Improved survival following abdominopelvic irradiation in patients with a completed pelvic operation. Am J Obstet Gynecol 134:793–800, 1979
60. Dembo AJ, Bush RS: Choice of postoperative therapy based on prognostic factors. Int J Radiat Oncol Biol Phys 8:893–897, 1982
61. Scully RE: World Health Organization classification and nomenclature of ovarian cancer. Natl Cancer Inst Monogr 42:5–7, 1975
62. Colombo N, Sessa C, Landoni F et al: Cisplatin, vinblastine, and bleomycin combination chemotherapy in metastatic granulosa cell tumor of the ovary. Obstet Gynecol 67:265, 1986
63. Perez CA, Bradfield JS: Radiation therapy in the treatment of carcinoma of the ovary. Cancer 29:1027, 1972
64. Fisher RI, Young RC: Chemotherapy of ovarian cancer. Surg Clin North Am 58:143, 1978
65. Sall S, Stone ML: The treatment of ovarian cancer. Prog Clin Cancer 5:249, 1973
66. Kent SN, McKay DG: Primary cancer of the ovary. Am J Obstet Gynecol 80:430–438, 1960
67. Pearse WH, Behrman SJ: Carcinoma of the ovary. Obstet Gynecol 3:32–45, 1954
68. Barber HRK, Graber EA: The PMPO syndrome. Obstet Gynecol 38:921, 1971
69. Flynt JR, Gallup DG: The postmenopausal palpable ovary syndrome: A 14-year review. Milit Med 146:686, 1981
70. Bolandgray A, Mehellati KA, Ardekany MS: Early detection of ovarian malignancy by culdocentesis. J Reprod Med 9:32, 1971
71. Graham JB, Graham RM, Schueller DF: Preclinical detection of ovarian cancer. Cancer 17:414, 1964
72. McGowan L, Stein DB, Miller W: Cul-de-sac aspiration for diagnostic cytology study. Obstet Gynecol 96:413, 1966
73. Rubin SC, Dulaney ED, Markman M et al: Peritoneal cytology as an indicator of disease in patients with residual ovarian carcinoma. Obstet Gynecol 71:851, 1988
74. Samuels BI: Usefulness of ultrasound in patients with ovarian cancer. Semin Oncol 2:229–233, 1975
75. Berkowitz RS, Leavitt T Jr, Knapp RC: Ultrasound directed percutaneous aspiration biopsy of periaortic lymph nodes in cervical carcinoma recurrence. Am J Obstet Gynecol 131:906–908, 1978
76. Parker BR, Castellino RA, Fuks ZY, Bagshaw MA: The role of lymphography in patients with ovarian cancer. Cancer 34:100–105, 1974
77. Schaner EG, Head GL, Kalman MA et al: Whole body computed tomography in the diagnosis of abdominal and thoracic malignancy: Review of 600 cases. Cancer Treat Rep 61:1537–1560, 1977
78. Dunnick NR, Schaner EG, Doppman JL: Detection of subcutaneous metastasis by computed tomography. J Comp Assist Tomogr 2:275–279, 1978
79. Kurman RJ, Norris HJ: Endodermal sinus tumor of the ovary: A clinical and pathologic analysis of 71 cases. Cancer 38:2404–2419, 1976
80. Goldstein DP, Piro AJ: Combination chemotherapy in the treatment of germ cell tumors containing choriocarcinoma in males and females. Surg Gynecol Obstet 134:61–66, 1972
81. DiSaia PJ, Morrow CP, Haverback BJ, Dyce BJ: Carcinoembryonic antigen in cancer of the female reproductive system: Serial plasma values correlated with disease state. Cancer 39:2365–2370, 1977
82. Imamura N, Takahasi T, Lloyd KO et al: Analysis of human ovarian tumor antigens using heterologous antisera: Detection of new antigenic system. Int J Cancer 21:570–577, 1978
83. Dorsett BH, Ioachim HL, Stolbach L et al: Isolation of tumor-specific antibodies from effusions of ovarian carcinoma. Int J Cancer 16:779–786, 1975
84. Bhattacharya M, Barlow JJ: Ovarian Cancer. In Herberman RB, McIntyre KR (eds): Immunodiagnosis of Cancer, pp 632–643, New York, Marcel Dekker, 1979
85. Knauf S, Urbach GI: The development of a double-antibody radioimmunoassay for detecting ovarian tumor-associated antigen fraction OCA in plasma. Am J Obstet Gynecol 131:780–787, 1978
86. Bast RC, Klug TL, St John E et al: A radioimmunoassay using a monoclonal antibody to monitor the course of epithelial ovarian cancer. N Engl J Med 309:883–887, 1983
87. Zurawski VR, Broderick SF, Pickens P et al: Serum CA-125 levels in a group of nonhospitalized women: Relevance for the early detection of ovarian cancer. Obstet Gynecol 69:606, 1987
88. Einhorn N, Bast RC Jr, Knapp RC et al: Preoperative evaluation of serum CA-125 levels in patients with primary epithelial ovarian cancer. Obstet Gynecol 67:414, 1986
89. Malkasian GD Jr, Podratz KC, Stanhope RE et al: CA-125 in gynecologic practice. Am J Obstet 155:515, 1986
90. Barbieri RL, Niloff JM, Bast RC Jr et al: Elevated serum concentrations of CA-125 in patients with advanced endometriosis. Fertil Steril 45:630, 1986
91. Ruibol A, Encabo G, Martinez–Miralles E et al: CA-125 serum levels in non-malignant pathologies. Bull Cancer (Paris) 71:45, 1984
92. Pittaway DE, Foyez JA: Serum CA-125 antigen levels increase during menses. Am J Obstet Gynecol 156:75, 1987
93. Mastropaolo W, Fernandez Z, Miller EL: Pronounced increases in the concentration of an ovarian tumor marker, CA-125, in serum of a healthy subject during menstruation. Clin Chem 32:2110, 1986
94. Halila H, Stennan A, Seppala M: Ovarian cancer antigen CA-125 levels in pelvic inflammatory disease and pregnancy. Cancer 57:1327, 1986
95. International Federation of Gynecology and Obstetrics: Changes in definitions of clinical staging for carcinoma of the cervix and ovary: Am J Obstet Gynecol 156:236, 1987
96. Munnell EW: The changing prognosis and treatment in cancer of the ovary: A report of 235 patients with primary ovarian carcinoma 1952–1961. Am J Obstet Gynecol 100:790, 1968
97. Delclos L, Quinlan EJ: Malignant tumors of the ovary managed with postoperative megavoltage irradiation. Radiology 93:659, 1969
98. Griffiths CT: Surgical resection of tumor bulk in the primary treatment of ovarian carcinoma. Natl Cancer Inst Monogr 42:101, 1975
99. Delgado G, Oram DH, Petrilli EG: Stage III epithelial ovarian cancer: The role of maximal surgical reduction. Gynecol Oncol 18:293, 1984
100. Conte PF, Sertoli MR, Bruzzone M et al: Cisplatin, methotrexate and 5-fluorouracil regimen in the treatment of advanced and recurrent ovarian cancer. Gynecol Oncol 20:23, 1985
101. Posada JG Jr, Marantz AB, Yeung KY et al: The cyclophosphamide, hexamethylmelamine, 5-fluorouracil regimen in the treatment of advanced and recurrent ovarian cancer. Gynecol Oncol 20:23, 1985
102. Hacker NF, Berek JS, Lagasse LD et al: Primary cytoreductive surgery for epithelial ovarian cancer. Obstet Gynecol 61:424, 1983
103. Omura GA, Bundy B, Wilbanks G et al: A randomized trial of cyclophosphamide (C) plus cisplatin (P) with or without Adriamycin (A) in ovarian cancer (abstr). Proc Am Soc Clin Oncol 6:439, 1987
104. Fuks Z, Rizel S, Anteby SO et al: The multimodal approach to the treatment of Stage IV ovarian carcinoma. Rad Oncol Biol Physics 8:903, 1982
105. Dembo AJ: Radiotherapeutic management of ovarian cancer. Semin Oncol 11:238, 1984
106. Chen SS, Bochner R: Assessment of morbidity and mortality in primary cytoreductive surgery for advanced ovarian cancer. Gynecol Oncol 20:190, 1985
107. Blythe JG, Wahl TP: Debulking surgery: Does it increase the quality of survival? Gynecol Oncol 14:396, 1982
108. Ozols RF, Fisher RI, Anderson T, Makuch R, Young RC: Peritoneoscopy in the management of ovarian cancer. Am J Obstet Gynecol 140:611–619, 1981
109. Berek JS, Griffiths CT, Leventhal JM: Laparoscopy for second-look evaluation in ovarian cancer. Obstet Gynecol 58:192–198, 1981
110. Wangenstein OH, Lewis FJ, Tongen L: The "second look" in cancer surgery. Lancet 71:303, 1951
111. Rutledge FN, Burns BC: Chemotherapy for advanced ovarian cancer. Am J Obstet Gynecol 96:761, 1966
112. Smith JP, Rutledge F: Chemotherapy in the treatment of cancer of the ovary. Obstet Gynecol 107:691, 1970
113. Smith JP, Delgado G, Rutledge F: Second look operation in ovarian cancer. Cancer 38:1438, 1976
114. Greco FA, Julian CG, Richardson RL et al: Advanced ovarian cancer: Brief intensive combination chemotherapy and second look operation. Obstet Gynecol 58:199, 1981
115. Berek JS, Hocha NF, Lagasse LD et al: Second look laparotomy in Stage III epithelial ovarian cancer: Clinical variables associated with disease status. Obstet Gynecol 64:14, 1981
116. Hakes TB, Chalas E, Saigo P et al: Randomized trial of cyclophosphamide, doxorubicin and cisplatin (CAP) chemotherapy: 5 versus 10 cycles in Stage III and IV ovarian cancer (abstr). Proc Am Soc Clin Oncol 6:456, 1987
117. Rubin SC, Lewis JL, Jr: Second-look surgery in ovarian carcinoma. CRC Crit Rev Oncol Hematol 8:75, 1988
118. Cain JM, Saigo PE, Pierce VJ et al: A review of second look laparotomy for ovarian cancer. Gynecol Oncol 23:14, 1986
119. Berek JS, Hacker NF, Lagasse LD et al: Second look laparotomy in Stage III epithelial ovarian cancer: Clinical variables associated with disease status. Obstet Gynecol 64:207, 1984

120. Smirz LR, Stehman FB, Ulbright TM et al: Second look laparotomy after chemotherapy in the management of ovarian malignancy. Am J Obstet Gynecol 152:661, 1985
121. Webb MJ, Snyder JA, Williams TJ et al: Second look laparotomy in ovarian cancer. Gynecol Oncol 14:285, 1982
122. Podratz KC, Malkasian GD Jr, Hilton JF, et al: Second look laparotomy in ovarian cancer: Evaluation of pathologic variables. Am J Obstet Gynecol 152(2):230–238, 1985
123. Phibbs GC, Smith JP, Stanhope CR: An analysis of sites of persistent cancer at "second look" laparotomy in patients with ovarian cancer. Am J Obstet Gynecol 147:611, 1983
124. Curry SL, Zembo MM, Nahhas WA et al: Second look laparotomy for ovarian cancer. Gynecol Oncol 11:114, 1981
125. Dauplat J, Ferriere JP, Gorbinet M et al: Second look laparotomy in managing epithelial ovarian carcinoma. Cancer 57:1627, 1986
126. Ballon SC, Protnuf JC, Sikic BI et al: Second look laparotomy in ovarian carcinoma: Precise definition, sensitivity and specificity of the operative procedure. Gynecol Oncol 17:154, 1984
127. Schwartz PE, Smith JP: Second-look operations in ovarian cancer. Am J Obstet Gynecol 138:1124–1130, 1980
128. Creasman WT, Aba-Ghazaleh S, Schmidt HJ: Retroperitoneal metastatic spread of ovarian carcinoma. Gynecol Oncol 6:447, 1978
129. Berek JS, Hacker WF, Lagasse LD et al: Survival of patients following secondary cytoreductive surgery in ovarian cancer. Obstet Gynecol 61:189, 1983
130. Griffiths CT, Parker LM, Fuller AF Jr: Role of cytoreductive surgical treatment in the management of advanced ovarian cancer. Cancer Treat Rep 63:235, 1979
131. Wiltshaw E, Raju KS, Dawson I: The role of cytoreductive surgery in advanced carcinoma of the ovary: An analysis of primary and second surgery. Br J Obstet Gynaecol 92:522, 1985
132. Copeland LJ, Wharton JT, Rutledge FN et al: Role of "third look laparotomy" in the guidance of ovarian cancer treatment. Gynecol Oncol 15:149, 1983
133. Maggino T, Tredese F, Valente S et al: Role of second look laparotomy in multidisciplinary treatment and in the follow up of advanced ovarian cancer. Eur J Gynaecol Oncol 4:26, 1983
134. Luesley DM, Chan KK, Fielding WL et al: Second look laparotomy in the management of epithelial ovarian carcinoma: An evaluation of fifty cases. Obstet Gynecol 64:421, 1984
135. Raju KS, McKinna JA, Barker GH et al: Second look operations in the planned management of advanced ovarian carcinoma. Am J Obstet Gynecol 144:650, 1982
136. Eymer H: Beeinflussung von proliferenden Ovarialtumoren durch Rötgenstrahlen. Strahlen 1:358–361, 1912
137. Fuks Z, Bagshaw MA: The rationale for curative radiotherapy for ovarian carcinoma. Int J Radiat Oncol Biol Phys 1:21–32, 1975
138. Schray MF, Ox RS, Martinez A: Lower abdominal radiotherapy for Stages I, II and selected III epithelial ovarian cancer: 20 years' experience. Gynecol Oncol 15:78–87, 1983
139. Dembo AJ: Radiotherapeutic management of ovarian cancer. Semin Oncol 11:238–250, 1984
140. Dembo AJ: Abdominopelvic radiotherapy in ovarian cancer: A 10-year experience. Cancer 55:2285–2290, 1985
141. Dembo AJ, Bush RS, Beale FA et al: The Princess Margaret study of ovarian carcinoma Stages I, II, and asymptomatic III presentations. Cancer Treat Rep 63:249–254, 1979
142. Dembo AJ: The sequential multiple modality treatment of ovarian cancer. Radiol Oncol 3:187–192, 1985
143. Delclos L, Smith JP: Tumors of the ovary. In Fletcher G (ed): Textbook of Radiotherapy, 2nd Ed, pp 690–702. Philadelphia, Lea & Febiger
144. Perez CA, Korba A, Zivnusk F et al: Cobalt 60 moving strip technique in the management of carcinoma of the ovary: Analysis of tumor control and morbidity. Int J Radiat Oncol Biol Phys 4:379–388, 1978
145. Perez CA, Walz BZ, Jacobson PL: Radiation therapy in the management of carcinoma of the ovary. Natl Cancer Inst Monogr 42:119–125, 1975
146. Hanks G, Bagshaw MA: Megavoltage radiation therapy and lymphangiography in ovarian cancer. Radiology 93:649–654, 1969
147. Delclos L, Barun EJ, Herrera JR et al: Whole abdominal irradiation by cobalt-60 moving strip technique. Radiology 81:632–641, 1963
148. Perez CA, Korba A, Zivnuska F et al: ^{60}Co moving strip technique in the management of carcinoma of the ovary: Analysis of tumor control and morbidity. Int J Radiat Oncol Biol Phys 4:379–388, 1978
149. Glatstein E, Fuks Z, Bagshaw MA: Diaphragmatic treatment in ovarian carcinoma: A new radiotherapeutic technique. Int J Radiat Oncol Biol Phys 2:357–362, 1977
150. Ellis F: Dose–time fractionation: A clinical hypothesis. Clin Radiol 20:1–7, 1969
151. Dixon RL: General equation for the calculation of nominal standard dose. Acta Radiol [Ther] 11:305–311, 1972
152. Orton CG, Ellis F: A simplification in the use of the NSD concept in practical radiotherapy. Br J Radiol 46:529–537, 1973
153. Martinez A: Perspective: The role of radiation therapy in the treatment of epithelial ovarian cancer. In Ballon SC (ed): Gynecologic Oncology: Controversies in Cancer Treatment, pp 300–310. Boston, GK Hall, 1981
154. Martinez A, Schray MF, Hoes AE, Bagshaw MA: Postoperative radiation therapy for epithelial ovarian cancer: The curative role based on a 24-year experience. J Clin Oncol 3:901–922, 1985
155. Schray MF, Cox RS, Martinez A: Lower abdominal radiotherapy for Stages I, II and selected III epithelial ovarian cancer: 20 years' experience. Gynecol Oncol 15:78–87, 1983
156. Fazekas JT, Maier JF: Irradiation of ovarian carcinomas: A prospective comparison of the open-field and moving-strip techniques. Am J Roentgenol Rad Ther Nucl Med 120:118–123, 1974
157. Fuks Z: The role of radiation therapy in the management of ovarian carcinoma. Isr J Med Sci 8:815–828, 1977
158. Smith JP, Rutledge FN, Delclos L: Postoperative treatment of early cancer of the ovary: A random trial between postoperative irradiation and chemotherapy. Natl Cancer Inst Monogr 42:149–153, 1975
159. Brady LW: Advances in the management of gynecologic cancer: Radiation therapy. Cancer 36:661–668, 1975
160. Kjellgren O, Johnsson L: Bone marrow depression in the pelvis after megavoltage irradiation for ovarian carcinoma. Obstet Gynecol 105:849–855, 1969
161. Luxton R: Radiation nephritis. Q J Med 22:215–242, 1953
162. Ingold JA, Reed GB, Kaplan HS et al: Radiation hepatitis. Am J Roentgenol Rad Ther Nucl Med 93:200–205, 1965
163. Hintz BL, Fuks Z, Kempson RL et al: Results of postoperative megavoltage radiotherapy of malignant surface epithelial tumors of the ovary. Radiology 114:695–700, 1975
164. Long RT, Sala JM: Radical surgery combined with radiotherapy in the treatment of advanced ovarian carcinoma. Surg Gynecol Obstet 117:201–204, 1963
165. Kottmeier HL: Carcinoma of the uterine cervix, endometrium and ovary. In Year Book of Cancer, p 293. Chicago, Year Book Medical Publishers, 1962
166. Kjorstad KE, Welander G, Kolstad P: Preoperative irradiation in Stage III carcinoma of the ovary. Acta Obstet Gynecol Scand 56:449–452, 1977
167. Aure JC, Hoeg K, Kolstad P: Radioactive colloidal gold in the treatment of ovarian carcinoma. Acta Radiol [Ther] (Stockh) 10:399–407, 1971
168. Moore DW, Langley II: Routine use of radiogold following operation for ovarian cancer. Am J Obstet Gynecol 98:624–630, 1967
169. Pezner RD, Stevens KR Jr, Tong D, Allen CV: Limited epithelial carcinoma of the ovary treated with curative intent by intraperitoneal installation of radiocolloids. Cancer 42:2563–2671, 1978
170. Bagley CM Jr, Young RC, Canellos GP, DeVita VT: Treatment of ovarian carcinoma: Possibilities for progress, N Engl J Med 287:856–862, 1972
171. Louie KG, Ozols RF, Myers CE et al: Long-term results of a cisplatin-containing combination chemotherapy regimen for the treatment of advanced ovarian carcinoma. J Clin Oncol 4:1579, 1986
172. Schwartz PE, Smith JP: Second-look operations in ovarian cancer. Am J Obstet Gynecol 138:1124–1130, 1980
173. Johnson BL, Fisher RI, Bender RA et al: Hexamethylmelamine in alkylating agent resistant ovarian carcinoma. Cancer 42:2157, 1978
174. Bolis G, D'Incalci M, Belloni C et al: Hexamethylmelamine in ovarian cancer resistant to cyclophosphamide and Adriamycin. Cancer Treat Rep 63:1375, 1979
175. Ozols RF, Young RC: Chemotherapy of ovarian cancer. Semin Oncol 11:251–263, 1984
176. Young RC, Von Hoff DD, Gormley P et al: Cis-dichlorodiammineplatinum(II) for the treatment of advanced ovarian cancer. Cancer Treat Rep 63:1539–1544, 1979
177. Lambert HE, Berry RJ: High-dose cisplatin compared with high-dose cyclophosphamide in the management of advanced epithelial ovarian cancer (FIGO Stages III and IV): Report from the North Thames Cooperative Group. Br Med J 290:889–892, 1985
178. Ozols RF, Ostchega Y, Myers CE et al: High-dose cisplatin in hypertonic saline in refractory ovarian cancer. J Clin Oncol 3:1246–1250, 1985
179. Ozols RF, Corden BJ: High-dose cisplatin in hypertonic saline. Ann Intern Med 100:19–24, 1984
180. Ozols RF, Young RC: High-dose cisplatin therapy in ovarian cancer. Semin Oncol 12:21–30, 1985
181. Bruckner HW, Wallach R: High-dose cisplatinum for the treatment of refractory ovarian cancer. Gynecol Oncol 12:64–67, 1984
182. Barker GH, Wiltshaw E: Use of high dose cis-dichlorodiammine platinum-II following failure on previous chemotherapy for advanced carcinoma of the ovary. Br J Obstet Med 88:1192–1199, 1981
183. Levin L, Hryniuk WM: Dose intensity analysis of chemotherapy regimens in ovarian carcinoma. J Clin Oncol 5:756–767, 1987
184. Bolis G, D'Incalci M, Gramellini F et al: Adriamycin in ovarian cancer patients resistant to cyclophosphamide. Eur J Cancer 14:1401, 1978
185. Hubbard SM, Barkes P, Young RC: Adriamycin therapy for advanced ovarian carcinoma after chemotherapy. Cancer Treat Rep 62:1375, 1978
186. Wharton JT, Rutledge F, Smith JP et al: Hexamethylmelamine: An evaluation of its role in the treatment of ovarian cancer. Am J Obstet Gynecol 133:833, 1979
187. Foster BJ, Clagett–Carr K, Marsoni S et al: Role of hexamethylmelamine in the treatment of ovarian cancer: Where is the needle in the haystack? Cancer Treat Rep 70:1003, 1986
188. Wiltshaw E, Evans BD, Jones et al: JM8, successor to cisplatin in advanced ovarian carcinoma. Lancet 1:587, 1983
189. Canetta R, Carter SK: Developing new drugs for ovarian cancer: A challenging task in a changing reality. J Cancer Res Clin Oncol 107:111, 1984
190. Thigpen JT, Vance RB, Balducci L, Khansur T: New drugs and experimental approaches in ovarian cancer treatment. Semin Oncol 11:314, 1984
191. Bruhl P, Gunther V, Hoefer–Janker H et al: Results obtained with fractionated ifosfamide massive-dose treatment in generalized malignant tumors. Int J Clin Pharmacol Biopharmacol 14:29–39, 1976

192. Kuhnle H, Achterrath W, Frischkorn R: Krankheitsorientierte Phase II Studie mit Etoposid (NSC 141540) bei Cisplatin-refraktaren Ovarialkarzinomen. Tumor Diagn Ther 5:152, 1984
193. Hillcoat BL, Campbell JJ, Pepperell R et al: Phase II trail of VP-16-213 in advanced ovarian carcinoma. Gynecol Oncol 22:162, 1985
194. Paccagnella A, Tredese F, Salvagno L et al: Peptichemio in pretreated patients with ovarian cancer. Cancer Treat Rep 69:17, 1985
195. Creech RH, Shah MK, Catalano RB et al: Phase II study of low-dose mitomycin in patients with ovarian cancer previously treated with chemotherapy. Cancer Treat Rep 69:1271, 1985
196. Willocks D, Toppila M, Hudson CN et al: Estrogen and progesterone receptors in human ovarian tumors. Gynecol Oncol 16:246, 1983
197. Wurz H, Wussner E, Citoler P et al: Multiple cytoplasmic steroid hormone receptors in benign and malignant ovarian tumors and in disease-free ovaries. Tumor Diagn Ther 4:15, 1983
198. Ford LC, Berek JS, Lagasse LD et al: Estrogen and progesterone receptors in ovarian neoplasms. Gynecol Oncol 15:299, 1983
199. Geisler H: Megestrol acetate for the palliation of advanced ovarian carcinoma. Obstet Gynecol 61:95, 1983
200. Aabo K, Pedersen AG, Haid I et al: High-dose medroxyprogesterone acetate (MPA) in advanced chemotherapy-resistant ovarian carcinoma: A Phase II study. Cancer Treat Rep 66:407–408, 1982
201. Trope C, Johnsson JE, Sigurdsson K et al: High-dose medroxyprogesterone acetate for the treatment of advanced ovarian carcinoma. Cancer Treat Rep 66:1441–1443, 1982
202. Myers M, Moore GE, Major FJ: Advanced ovarian carcinoma: Response to antiestrogen therapy. Cancer 48:2368–2370, 1981
203. Schwartz P, Kenting G, Maclusky N et al: Tamoxifen therapy for advanced ovarian cancer. Obstet Gynecol 59:583–588, 1982
204. Hamerlynck JVTH, Maskens AP, Mangioni C et al: Phase II trial of medroxyprogesterone acetate in advanced ovarian cancer: An EORTC Gynecological Cancer Cooperative Group study. Gynecol Oncol 22:313, 1985
205. Slevin ML, Harvey VJ, Osborne RJ et al: A Phase II study of tamoxifen in ovarian cancer. Eur J Cancer Clin Oncol 22:309, 1986
206. Shirey DR, Kavanagh JJ, Gershenson DM et al: Tamoxifen therapy of epithelial ovarian cancer. Obstet Gynecol 66:575, 1985
207. Freedman RS, Saul PB, Edwards CL et al: Ethinylestradiol and medroxyprogesterone acetate in patients with epithelial ovarian carcinoma: A Phase II study. Cancer Treat Rep 70:369, 1986
208. Hamburger AW, Salmon SE, Kim MB et al: Direct cloning of human ovarian carcinoma cells in agar. Cancer Res 38:3438–3444, 1978
209. Hanauske AR, Von Hoff DD: The value of the human tumor cloning assay in ovarian cancer. Clin Obstet Gynecol 29:638, 1986
210. Young RC, Chabner BA, Hubbard SP et al: Prospective trial of melphalan (L-PAM) versus combination chemotherapy (Hexa-CAF) in ovarian adenocarcinoma. N Engl J Med 299:1261–1266, 1978
211. Neijt JP, Vanlindert ACM, Vendrijk CPJ et al: Hexa-CAF combination chemotherapy and other multiple drug regimens in advanced ovarian carcinoma: Present and future. Neth J Med 22:28, 1979
212. Vogl SE, Pagano M, Davis T et al: Platinum based combination chemotherapy versus melphalan for advanced ovarian carcinoma. Proc Int Congr Chemother 207:9–13, 1983
213. Delgado G, Smith FP, McLaughlin EF et al: Single agent vs. combination chemotherapy for ovarian cancer. Am J Clin Oncol 8:33–37, 1985
214. Edmonson JH, Fleming TR, Decker DG et al: Different chemotherapeutic sensitivities and host factors affecting prognosis in advanced ovarian carcinoma versus minimal residual disease. Cancer Treat Rep 63:241–247, 1979
215. Williams CJ, Mead GM, Macbeth FR et al: Cisplatin combination chemotherapy versus chlorambucil in advanced ovarian carcinoma: Mature results of a randomized trial. J Clin Oncol 3:1455–1462, 1985
216. Carmo–Pereria J, Costa FO, Henique E: Cis-platin, Adriamycin and hexamethylmelamine vs. cyclophosphamide in advanced ovarian cancer. Cancer Chemother Pharmacol 10:100, 1983
217. Trope C: A prospective randomized trial comparison of melphalan vs. melphalan–Adriamycin in advanced ovarian carcinoma (abstr). Proc Am Soc Clin Oncol 22:469, 1981
218. Decker DG, Fleming TR, Malkasian GD et al: Cyclophosphamide plus cisplatinum in combination: Treatment program for Stage III or IV ovarian carcinoma. Obstet Gynecol 60:481–486, 1982
219. MRC Working Party on Ovarian Cancer: Medical Research Council study on chemotherapy in advanced ovarian cancer. Br J Obstet Gynaecol 88:1174, 1981
220. Carmo–Pereira J, Costa FO, Henriques E et al: Advanced ovarian carcinoma: A prospective and randomized clinical trial of cyclophosphamide versus combination cytotoxic chemotherapy (Hexa-CAF). Cancer 48:1947–1951, 1981
221. Ludwig Institute for Cancer Research: Chemotherapy of advanced ovarian adenocarcinoma: A randomized comparison of combination versus sequential therapy using chlorambucil and cisplatin. Gynecol Oncol 23:1–13, 1986
222. Reimer RR, Hoover R, Fraumeni JF, Young RC: Acute leukemia after alkylating agent therapy in ovarian cancer. N Engl J Med 297:117, 1977
223. Greene MH, Boice JD, Greer BE et al: Acute non-lymphocytic leukemia after therapy with alkylating agents for ovarian cancer. N Engl J Med 307:1416, 1982
224. Weiss GR: Second-line chemotherapy for ovarian cancer. Clin Obstet Gynecol 29:665, 1986
225. Bruntsch U: Sekundare Chemotherapie beim fortgeschrittenen Ovarialkarzinoma: Neue Medikamente. Onkologie 8:410, 1985
226. Kardinal CG, Luce JK: Evaluation of a hexamethylmelamine and 5-fluorouracil combination in the treatment of advanced ovarian carcinoma. Cancer Treat Rep 61:1691, 1977
227. Barlow JJ, Piver MS: High-dose methotrexate plus Cytoxan in ovarian cancer (abstr). Proc Am Assoc Cancer Res 20:361, 1979
228. Briscoe KE, Pasmantier MW, Ohnuma T et al: Cis-dichlorodiammineplatinum (II) and Adriamycin treatment of advanced ovarian cancer. Cancer Treat Rep 62:2027, 1978
229. Bruckner HW, Cohen CJ, Kabakow B et al: Ovarian cancer: Secondary cisplatin regimens and prognostic factors (abstr). Proc Am Assoc Cancer Res 22:469, 1981
230. Neijt JP, ten Bokkel Huinink WW, Hamersma E et al: Combination chemotherapy including cisplatinum in previously treated patients with advanced ovarian carcinoma (abstr). Proc Am Soc Clin Oncol 1:108, 1982
231. Alberts DS, Hilgers RD, Moon TE et al: Combination chemotherapy for alkylator-resistant ovarian carcinoma: A preliminary report of a Southwest Oncology Group trial. Cancer Treat Rep 63:301, 1979
232. Kane R, Harvey H, Andrews T et al: Phase II trial of cyclophosphamide, hexamethylmelamine, Adriamycin and cis-dichlorodiammineplatinum(II) combination chemotherapy in advanced ovarian carcinoma. Cancer Treat Rep 63:307, 1979
233. Bruckner HW, Cohen CJ, Deppe G et al: Ovarian cancer schedule modification and dosage intensification of cyclophosphamide, hexamethylmelamine, adriamycin, cisplatin regimen (CHAP-II) (abstr). Proc Am Soc Clin Oncol 1:107, 1982
234. Bernath A, Andrews T, Dixon R et al: Long term follow-up of HAP vs. CAP in alkylating agent resistant advanced ovarian carcinoma (abstr). Proc Am Soc Clin Oncol 1:110, 1982
235. Barlow JJ, Piver MS: Second-line efficacy of intermediate high dose methotrexate with citrovorum factor rescue and cyclophosphamide in ovarian cancer. Gynecol Oncol 7:233, 1979
236. Vogl SE, Pagano M, Davis TE et al: Hexamethylmelamine and cisplatin in advanced ovarian cancer after failure of alkylating agent therapy. Cancer Treat Rep 66:1285, 1982
237. Lopez JA, Krikorian JG, Dias SF et al: Cisplatin–hexamethylmelamine therapy for advanced ovarian cancer. Gynecol Oncol 11:64, 1981
238. Barlow JJ, Lele SB: Etoposide (VP-16) plus cisplatin (DDP): A new active chemotherapeutic combination in patients with Stage III–IV ovarian adenocarcinoma. J Surg Oncol 32:43, 1986
239. De Lena M, Lorusso V, Romito S: Cisplatin plus etoposide as second-line treatment in advanced ovarian carcinoma. Cancer Treat Rep 70:893, 1986
240. Ehrlich CE, Einhorn L, Williams SD et al: Chemotherapy for Stage III–IV epithelial ovarian cancer with cis-dichlorodiammineplatinum(II), Adriamycin, and cyclophosphamide: A preliminary report. Cancer Treat Rep 63:281–288, 1979
241. Parker LM, Griffiths CT, Yankee RA et al: Combination chemotherapy with Adriamycin–cyclophosphamide for advanced ovarian carcinoma. Cancer 46:669–674, 1980
242. Wiltshaw E, Evans B, Rustin G et al: A prospective randomized trial comparing high-dose cisplatin with low-dose cisplatin and chlorambucil in advanced ovarian carcinoma. J Clin Oncol 4:722, 1986
243. Piccart M, Speyer J, Wernz J et al: Advanced epithelial ovarian cancer (OV-CA): Update with impressive survival utilizing cisplatin (DDP) (100 mg/m²/cycle) and cyclophosphamide (CTX) (abstr). Proc Am Soc Clin Oncol 4:117, 1985
244. Neijt JP van der Burg MEL, Vriesendorp R et al: Randomized trial comparing two combination chemotherapy regimens (Hexa-CAF vs. CHAP-5) in advanced ovarian carcinoma. Lancet 2:594–598, 1984
245. Omura G, Blessing JA, Ehrlich CE et al: A randomized trial of cyclophosphamide and doxorubicin with or without cisplatin in advanced ovarian carcinoma. Cancer 57:1725–1730, 1986
246. Neijt JP, ten Bokkel Huinink WW, van der Burg MEL: Randomized trial comparing two combination chemotherapy regimens (CHAP-5 v. CP) in advanced ovarian carcinoma. J Clin Oncol 5:1157–1168, 1987
247. Edmonson JH, McCormack GW, Fleming TR et al: Comparison of cyclophosphamide plus cisplatin versus hexamethylmelamine, cyclophosphamide, doxorubicin, and cisplatin in combination as initial chemotherapy for Stage III and IV ovarian carcinomas. Cancer Treat Rep 69:1243, 1985
248. Omura GA, Bundy B, Wilbanks G et al: A randomized trial of cyclophosphamide (C) plus cisplatin (P) with or without Adriamycin (A) in ovarian carcinoma. Proc Am Soc Clin Oncol 6:A439, 1987
249. Conte PF, Bruzzone M, Chiara S et al: A randomized trial comparing cisplatin plus cyclophosphamide versus cisplatin, doxorubicin, and cyclophosphamide in advanced ovarian cancer. J Clin Oncol 4:965–971, 1986
250. Jakobsen A, Bertelsen K, Sell A et al: Advantage of CAP over CP in terms of survival in advanced ovarian carcinoma (abstr). Proc Am Soc Clin Oncol 4:113, 1985
251. Mayer RJ, Berkowitz RS, Griffiths CT: Central nervous system involvement by ovarian carcinoma: A complication of prolonged survival with metastatic disease. Cancer 41:776, 1978
252. Bast RC, Knapp RC: Immunologic approaches to the management of ovarian carcinoma. Semin Oncol 11:264–274, 1984
253. Hamilton TC, Ozols RF, Longo DL: Biologic therapy for the treatment of malignant common epithelial tumors of the ovary. Cancer 60:2054–2063, 1987
254. Bast RC, Berek JS, Obrist R et al: Intraperitoneal immunotherapy of human ovarian carcinoma with *Corynebacterium parvum* (abstr). Proc Am Soc Clin Oncol 1:38, 1982
255. Mantovani A, Sessa C, Peri G et al: Intraperitoneal administration of *Corynebacterium*

parvum in patients with ascitic ovarian tumors resistant to chemotherapy: Effects on cytotoxicity of tumor-associated macrophages and NK cells. Int J Cancer 27:437–446, 1981
256. Hamilton TC, Young RC, McKoy WM et al: Characterization of a human ovarian carcinoma cell line (NIH:OVCAR-3) with androgen and estrogen receptors. Cancer Res 43:5379–5389, 1983
257. Gudson JP, Homesley HD, Muss HB et al: Chemotherapy of advanced ovarian epithelial carcinoma with melphalan and levamisole: A pilot study of the Gynecologic Oncology Group. Am J Obstet Gynecol 141:65–70, 1981
258. Creasman WT, Yale SA, Blessing JA et al: Chemoimmunotherapy in the management of primary Stage III ovarian cancer. Cancer Treat Rep 63:319, 1979
259. Alberts DS, Moon TE, Stephens RA et al: Randomized study of chemoimmunotherapy for advanced ovarian carcinoma. Cancer Treat Rep 63:325, 1982
260. Steis R, Bookman M, Clark J et al: Intraperitoneal lymphokine activated killer (LAK) cell and interleukin-2 (IL-2) therapy for peritoneal carcinomatosis: Toxicity, efficacy and laboratory results. Proc Am Soc Clin Oncol 6:A984, 1987
261. Pirker R, Fitzgerald DJP, Hamilton TC et al: Anti-transferrin receptor antibody linked to *Pseudomonas exotoxin* as a model immunotoxin in human ovarian carcinoma cell lines. Cancer Res 45:751–757, 1985
262. Pirker R, Fitzgerald DJP, Hamilton TC, et al: Characterization of immunotoxins active against ovarian cancer cell lines. J Clin Invest 76:1261–1267, 1985
263. Shen DW, Fojo A, Chin JE et al: Human multidrug-resistant cell lines: Increased *mdr*-1 expression can precede gene amplification. Science 232:643–645, 1986
264. Fojo A, Hamilton TC, Young RC et al: Multidrug resistance in ovarian cancer. Cancer 60:2075–2080, 1987
265. Juliano RL, Ling V: A surface glycoprotein modulating drug permeability in Chinese hamster ovary cell mutants. Biochim Biophys Acta 455:152–162, 1976
266. Debenham PG, Kartner N, Siminovitch L et al: DNA-mediated transfer of multiple drug resistance and plasma membrane glycoprotein expression. Mol Cell Biol 2:881–889, 1982
267. Roninson IB: Detection and mapping of homologous, repeated and amplified DNA sequences by DNA renaturation in agarose gels. Nucleic Acids Res 11:5413–5432, 1983
268. Riordan JR, Deuchars K, Kartner N et al: Amplification of P-glycoprotein genes in multidrug-resistant mammalian cell lines. Nature 316:817–819, 1985
269. Louie KG, Hamilton TC, Winker MA et al: Adriamycin accumulation and metabolism in Adriamycin-sensitive and resistant human ovarian cancer cell lines. Biochem Pharmacol 35:467–472, 1986
270. Hamilton TC, Masuda H, Young RC, Ozols RF: Modulation of cisplatin cytotoxicity by inhibition of DNA repair in a cisplatin resistant human ovarian cancer cell line 2780^{CP} (abstr). Proc Am Soc Cancer Res 28:291, 1987
271. Rogan AM, Hamilton TC, Young RC et al: Reversal of Adriamycin resistance by verapamil in human ovarian cancer. Science 224:994–998, 1984
272. Ozols RF, Cunnion RE, Klecker RW Jr et al: Verapamil and Adriamycin in the treatment of drug resistant ovarian cancer patients. J Clin Oncol 5:641–647, 1987
273. Meister A: Selective modification of glutathione metabolism. Science 20:472–477, 1983
274. Green JA, Vistica DT, Young RC et al: Potentiation of melphalan cytotoxicity in human ovarian cancer cell lines by glutathione depletion. Cancer Res 44:5427–5431, 1984
275. Ozols RF, Louis KG, Plowman J et al: Enhanced alkylating agent cytotoxicity in human ovarian cancer in vitro and in tumor bearing nude mice by buthionine sulfoximine depletion of glutathione. Biochem Pharmacol 36:147–153, 1987
276. Ozols RF, Hamilton TC, Masuda H, Young RC: The role of thiols in drug resistance. In Woolley PV III, Tew KD (eds): Mechanisms of Drug Resistance in Neoplastic Cells, 289–306 New York, Academic Press, 1988
277. Behrens BC, Hamilton TC, Masuda H et al: Characterization of a cis-diamminedichloroplatinum(II)-resistant human ovarian cancer cell line and its use in evaluation of platinum analogs. Cancer Res 47:414–418, 1987
278. Smith JP, Day TG: Review of ovarian cancer at the University of Texas Center, M.D. Anderson Hospital and Tumor Institute. Am J Obstet Gynecol 135:984–993, 1979
279. Einhorn L, Nilsson BO, Sjorall K: Factors influencing survival in carcinoma of the ovary: Study from a well-defined Swedish population. Cancer 55:2019–2025, 1985
280. Swenerton KD, Hislop TG, Spinelli J et al: Ovarian carcinoma: A multivariate analysis of prognostic factors. Obstet Gynecol 65:265–254, 1985
281. Redman JR, Petroni GR, Saigo PE et al: Prognostic factors in ovarian carcinoma. J Clin Oncol 4:515–523, 1986
282. Young RC, Decker DG, Wharton JT et al: Staging laparotomy in early ovarian cancer. JAMA 250:3072–3076, 1983
283. Webb MJ, Decker DG, Massey et al: Factors influencing survival in Stage I ovarian cancer. Am J Obstet Gynecol 166:222, 1973
284. Hreshchyshyn MW, Park RC, Blessing JA et al: The role of adjuvant therapy in Stage I ovarian cancer. Am J Obstet Gynecol 138:139–145, 1980
285. Young RC, Walton L, Decker D et al: Early stage ovarian cancer: Preliminary results of randomized trials after comprehensive initial staging (abstr). Proc Am Soc Clin Oncol 2:148, 1983
286. Piver SM: Radioactive colloids in the treatment of Stage IA ovarian cancer. Obstet Gynecol 40:42–44, 1972
287. Bush RS: Radiation therapy for patients with ovarian cancer. Strahlentherapie 159:131–137, 1983
288. Smith JP: Treatment of ovarian cancer. In Carter SK, Goldin A, Kuretroi K et al (eds): Advances in Cancer Chemotherapy, pp 493–503. Baltimore, University Park Press, 1978
289. Drouin P, Rutledge FN, Delclos L et al: Comparison of external radiotherapy and chemotherapy in ovarian cancer. Ann R Coll Phys Surg Can 12:61, 1979
290. Delclos L: International Symposium on Combined Modalities Approach on Gynecologic Cancer, Mexico City, May 1983, p 61
291. Einhorn N: The place of adjuvant chemotherapy in early stages. Int J Radiat Oncol Biol Phys 8:257–258, 1982
292. Hacker NF, Berek JS, Burnison CM et al: Whole abdominal radiation salvage therapy for epithelial ovarian cancer. Obstet Gynecol 65:619–623, 1985
293. Belinson JT, McClure M, Ashikaga T, Karakoff IH: Treatment of advanced and recurrent ovarian carcinoma with cyclophosphamide, doxorubicin and cisplatin. Cancer 54:1983–1990, 1984
294. Wharton JT, Edwards CL, Rutledge FN: Long term survival after chemotherapy for advanced epithelial ovarian carcinoma. Am J Obstet Gynecol 148:997–1005, 1984
295. Ozols RF, Young RC: Ovarian Cancer. In Haskell CM (ed): Current Problems in Cancer, Vol 11, pp 59–122. Chicago, Year Book Medical Publishers, 1987
296. Greco FA, Hande KR, Jones HW et al: Advanced ovarian cancer: Long-term follow-up after brief intensive chemotherapy (abstr). Proc Am Soc Clin Oncol 3:166, 1984
297. Hainsworth JD, Malcolm A, Johnson DH: Treatment of minimal residual advanced ovarian carcinoma: Abdominopelvic irradiation following incomplete response to combination chemotherapy. Obstet Gynecol 61:619–623, 1983
298. Dougherty J, Hakes T, Cain J et al: Recurrence pattern of advanced ovarian carcinoma after negative laparotomy (abstr). Proc Am Soc Clin Oncol 4:122, 1985
299. Hintz BL, Fuks Z, Kempson RL et al: Results of postoperative megavoltage radiotherapy of malignant surface epithelial tumors of the ovary. Radiology 114:695–700, 1975
300. Griffiths CT, Grogan RH, Hall TC: Advanced ovarian cancer: Primary treatment with surgery, radiotherapy, and chemotherapy. Cancer 29:1–7, 1972
301. Sigurdson K, Johnsson JE, Trope C: Carcinoma of the ovary in stage III: Effects of postoperative chemotherapy, radiation therapy and repeat laparotomy. Acta Radiat Oncol 21:181–189, 1982
302. Aure JC, Hoeg K, Kolstad P: Clinical and histologic studies of ovarian carcinoma: Long term follow-up of 990 cases. Obstet Gynecol 37:1–9, 1971
303. Delclos L, Quinlan EJ: Malignant tumor of the ovary managed with postoperative megavoltage irradiation. Radiology 93:659–663, 1969
304. Potish R, Adcock L, Brooker D et al: Sequential surgery, radiation therapy and Alkeran in the management of epithelial caricnoma of the ovary. Cancer 45:2754–2758, 1980
305. Nevin JE, Pinzon G, Baggerly TJ et al: The use of intravenous phenylalanine mustard followed by supervoltage irradiation in the treatment of carcinoma of the ovary. Cancer 51:1273–1283, 1984
306. Perez CA, Korba A, Zivnuska F et al: ^{60}Co moving strip technique in the management of carcinoma of the ovary: Analysis of tumor control and morbidity of carcinoma of the ovary: Analysis of tumor control and morbidity. Int J Radiat Oncol Biol Phys 4:379–388, 1978
307. Fuks Z, Rizel S, Anteby SO, Biran S: The multimodal approach to the treatment of stage III ovarian carcinoma. Int J Radiat Oncol Biol Phys 8:903–908, 1982
308. Fuks Z, Rizel S, Biran S: Chemotherapeutic and surgical induction of pathological complete remission and whole abdominal irradiation for consolidation does not enhance the cure of stage III ovarian carcinoma. J Clin Oncol 6:509–516, 1988
309. Neijt JP, ten Bokkel Huinink WW, van der Burg MEL et al: Complete remission at laparotomy: Still gold standard in ovarian cancer? Lancet 1:1028, 1986
310. Coltart RS, Nethersell BW, Brown CH: A pilot study of high dose abdominopelvic radiotherapy following surgery and chemotherapy for Stage III epithelial carcinoma of the ovary. Gynecol Oncol 23:105–110, 1986
311. Piver MS, Barlow JJ, Lee FT, Vongtama V: Sequential therapy for advanced ovarian adenocarcinoma: Operation, chemotherapy, second-look laparotomy and radiation therapy. Am J Obstet Gynecol 122:355–357, 1975
312. Kucera PR, Sheets EE, Micha JP et al: Whole abdominal radiotherapy for patients with minimal residual epithelial ovarian cancer. Presented at the Thirteenth Annual Meeting of the Western Association of Gynecologic Oncologist, San Diego, June 1985
313. Hoskins WJ, Lichter AS, Whittington R et al: Whole abdominal and pelvic irradiation in patients with minimal disease at second-look surgical reassessment for ovarian cancer. Gynecol Oncol 20:271–280, 1985
314. Peters WA, Blasko JC, Bagley CM et al: Salvage therapy with whole-abdominal irradiation in patients with advanced carcinoma of the ovary previously treated by combination chemotherapy. Cancer 58:880–882, 1986
315. Menczer J, Modan M, Brenner et al: Abdominopelvic irradiation for Stage II–IV ovarian carcinoma patients with limited or no residual disease at second-look laparotomy after completion of cisplatin-based combination chemotherpay. Gynecol Oncol 24:149, 1986
316. Young JA, Johnson A, Kroener J et al: Alternating combination chemotherapy for Stages III and IV ovarian carcinoma. J Clin Oncol 2:1317–1320, 1984
317. Dedrick RL, Myers CE, Bungay PM et al: Pharmacokinetic rationale for peritoneal drug administration in the treatment of ovarian cancer. Cancer Treat Rep 62:1, 1978
318. Dedrick RL: Theoretical and experimental bases of intraperitoneal chemotherapy. Semin Oncol 12:1–6, 1985
319. Myers C: The use of intraperitoneal chemotherapy in the treatment of ovarian cancer. Semin Oncol 11:275–284, 1984
320. Jones RB, Myers CE, Guarino AM et al: High volume intraperitoneal chemotherapy ("belly bath") for ovarian cancer. Cancer Chemother Pharmacol 1:161–166, 1978
321. Speyer JL, Collins JM, Dedrick RL et al: Phase I and pharmacologic studies of 5-fluorouracil administered intraperitoneally. Cancer Res 40:567, 1980
322. Ozols RF, Young RC, Speyer JL et al: Phase I and pharmacologic studies of Adriamy-

cin administered intraperitoneally to patients with ovarian cancer. Cancer Res 42:4265, 1982
323. Brenner DE: Intraperitoneal chemotherapy: A review. J Clin Oncol 4:1135–1147, 1986
324. Gyves JW, Ensminger WD, Stetson P et al: Constant intraperitoneal 5-fluorouracil infusion through a totally implanted system. Clin Pharmacol Ther 35:83–89, 1984
325. Howell SB, Pfeifle CL, Wung WE et al: Intraperitoneal chemotherapy with melphalan. Ann Intern Med 101:14–18, 1984
326. Howell SB, Chu BB, Wung WE et al: Long-duration intracavitary infusion of methotrexate with systemic leucovorin protection in patients with malignant effusions. J Clin Invest 67:1161–1170, 1981
327. Howell S, Pfeifle C, Wung W et al: Intraperitoneal cisplatin with systemic thiosulfate protection. Ann Intern Med 97:845–851, 1982
328. Pretorius RG, Hacker NF, Berek JS et al: Pharmacokinetics of IP cisplatin in refractory ovarian carcinoma. Cancer Treat Rep 67:1085–1092, 1983
329. Casper ES, Kelsen DP, Alcock NW et al: IP cisplatin in patients with malignant ascites: Pharmacokinetic evaluation and comparison with the IV route. Cancer Treat Rep 67:235–238, 1983
330. Ozols RF: Intraperitoneal chemotherapy in the management of ovarian cancer. Semin Oncol 12:75–80, 1985
331. Ozols RF, Speyer JL, Jenkins J et al: Phase II trial of 5-FU administered IP to patients with refractory ovarian cancer. Cancer Treat Rep 68:1229–1232, 1984
332. Markman M, Howell SB, Lucas WE et al: Combination intraperitoneal chemotherapy with cisplatin, cytarabine, and doxorubicin for refractory ovarian carcinoma and other malignancies principally confined to the peritoneal cavity. J Clin Oncol 2:1321–1326, 1984
333. ten Bokkel Huinink WW, Dubbelman R, Aartsen E et al: Experimental and clinical results with intraperitoneal cisplatin. Semin Oncol 12:43–46, 1985
334. Cohen CJ: Surgical considerations in ovarian cancer. Semin Oncol 12:53–56, 1985
335. Markman M, Howell S, Cleary S et al: Survival following cisplatin (DDP)-based intraperitoneal chemotherapy for refractory ovarian carcinoma (abstr). Proc Am Soc Clin Oncol 5:113, 1986
336. Markman M, Cleary S, Lucas WE, Howell SB: Intraperitoneal chemotherapy with high-dose cisplatin and cytosine arabinoside for refractory ovarian carcinoma and other malignancies principally involving the peritoneal cavity. J Clin Oncol 3(7):925–931, 1985
337. Zimm S, Cleary S, Lucas W et al: Phase I/pharmacokinetic study of intraperitoneal (IP) cisplatin (DDP) and etoposide (VP-16) (abstr). Proc Am Soc Clin Oncol 5:49, 1986
338. Rutledge FN, Fletcher GH, Smith JP et al: In Clark RL, Howe CD (eds): Cancer Patient Care at M.D. Anderson Hospital and tumor Institute, pp 263–308. Chicago, Year Book Medical Publishers, 1976
339. Stage AH, Grafton WD: Thecomas and granulosa–theca cell tumors of the ovary: An analysis of 51 tumors. Obstet Gynecol 50:21, 1977
340. Diddle AW: Granulosa and thecal-cell ovarian tumors: Prognosis. Cancer 5:215–228, 1952
341. Lusch CJ, Mercurio TM, Runyeon WK: Delayed recurrence and chemotherapy of a granulosa cell tumor. Obstet Gynecol 51:505–507, 1978
342. DiSaia PJ, Saltz A, Kagan AR et al: A temporary response of recurrent granulosa cell tumors to Adriamycin. Obstet Gynecol 52:355–358, 1978
343. Kaye SB, Davies E: Cyclophosphamide, Adriamycin, and cis-platinum for the treatment of advanced granulosa cell tumor, using serum estradiol. Gynecol Oncol 24:261–264, 1986
344. Woodruff JD, Protos P, Peterson WF: Ovarian teratomas. Am J Obstet Gynecol 102:702–715, 1968
345. Jimerson GK, Woodruff JD: Ovarian extraembryoneal teratoma I: Endodermal sinus tumor. Am J Obstet Gynecol 127:73–79, 1977
346. Gallion H, Van Nagell JR, Powell DR et al: Therapy of endodermal sinus tumor of the ovary. Am J Obstet Gynecol 135:447–451, 1979
347. Cangir A, Smith J, VanEys J: Improved prognosis in children with ovarian cancers following modified VAC (vincristine sulfate, dactinomycin and cyclophosphamide) chemotherapy. Cancer 42:1234–1238, 1978
348. Slayton RE, Park RC, Silverberg SG et al: VAC treatment of malignant germ cell tumors of the ovary. Cancer 56:243–248, 1985
349. Williams S, Blessing J, Adcock L, Homesley H: Treatment of ovarian germ cell tumors with cisplatin + vinblastine + bleomycin (PVB). Proc Am Soc Clin Oncol 3:175, 1984
350. Smales E, Peckham MJ: Chemotherapy of germ cell ovarian tumors. Eur J Cancer Clin Oncol 23:469–473, 1987
351. Carlson RW, Sikic BI, Turbow MM, Ballon SC: Combination PVB for malignant germ cell tumors of the ovary. J Clin Oncol 1:546–651, 1983
352. Curry SL, Smith JP, Gallagher HS: Malignant teratoma of the ovary: Prognostic factors and treatment. Am J Obstet Gynecol 131:845–849, 1978
353. Asadourian LA, Taylor HB: Dysgerminoma: An analysis of 105 cases. Obstet Gynecol 33:370–379, 1969
354. Pedowitz P, Felmus LB, Grayzel PM: Dysgerminoma of the ovary. Am J Obstet Gynecol 70:1282–1297, 1955
355. Brody S: Clinical aspects of dysgerminoma of the ovary. Acta Radiol [Ther]56:209–230, 1961
356. Krepart G, Smith JP, Rutledge F, Delclos L: The treatment for dysgerminoma of the ovary. Cancer 41:986–990, 1978
357. Cohen SM, Goldsmith MA: Prolonged chemotherapeutic remission of metastatic ovarian dysgerminoma: Report of a case. Gynecol Oncol 5:299, 1977
358. Goldstein DP, Piro AJ: Combination chemotherapy in the treatment of germ cell tumors containing choriocarcinoma in males and females. Surg Gynecol Obstet 134:61–66, 1972
359. Fanning J, Walker RLA, Shah NR: Mixed germ cell tumor of the ovary with pure choriocarcinoma metastasis. Obstet Gynecol 68:84S, 1986
360. Munnel EW: Primary ovarian cancer associated with pregnancy. Clin Obstet Gynecol 6:983–993, 1963
361. Creasman WT, Rutledge F, Smith JP: Carcinoma of the ovary associated with pregnancy. Obstet Gynecol 38:111, 1971

I. CRAIG HENDERSON
JAY R. HARRIS
DAVID W. KINNE
SAMUEL HELLMAN

CHAPTER 38 *Cancer of the Breast*

In North America, breast cancer is the most common malignancy among women and accounts for 27% of their cancers. Eighteen per cent of the cancer deaths in women are due to breast cancer, but since 1985, lung cancer has equalled or exceeded breast cancer as a cause of cancer death in women.[1] It was estimated that 130,900 new cases of breast cancer would be diagnosed in the United States in 1987 and that 41,300 women would die of breast cancer in that year.

The risk of an individual American woman developing breast cancer over a lifetime exceeds 10%, but this figure is somewhat misleading, because it represents the probability of developing breast cancer in the interval from birth to age 110. The greatest risk is expressed after the age of 65. The cumulative risk for an individual woman before age 70 is about 7%. The risk of dying of breast cancer is about one-third of this (Table 38-1). The relative risk of developing breast cancer for an individual woman in a defined risk group is usually multiplied by the probability of any woman developing breast cancer during a lifetime, and this figure is usually taken as the cumulative risk of that individual's developing breast cancer. However, the observed risk has rarely exceeded 30% in any study. Therefore, a more meaningful calculation to use in counseling women regarding their risk of breast cancer might be a 20-year interval. For example, if a 35-year-old woman with a strong family history of breast cancer is thought to have a relative risk of 2.0, her risk of developing breast cancer by the age of 55 is slightly under 5% and her risk of dying of breast cancer is slightly over 1% (Table 38-1).

ETIOLOGY AND RISK FACTORS

The cause of breast cancer is not known, but epidemiologic evidence points strongly toward three areas: endocrine factors, environment, and genetics (Table 38-2). Breast cancer may be induced by radiation, but this probably is not an important cause of breast cancer in the general population.

ENDOCRINE FACTORS

The age of menarche, menopause, and first pregnancy have been linked to the incidence of breast cancer in numerous studies. Although there is a direct relation between the total duration of menstrual life and the risk of developing breast cancer, the most important interval appears to be the time between menarche and first pregnancy. In one study, women with menarche before the age of 12 had almost a twofold higher incidence of breast cancer than women with menarche occurring after the age of 13.[2] The same investigators observed that a delay in the onset of regular menstrual cycles decreased the risk of breast cancer by one-third to one-half in both the women who had early onset of menarche and those with late onset.[3] Because starvation and strenuous physical activity delay menarche, it is tempting to correlate international differences in the incidence of breast cancer with differences in diet, physical activity, and the onset of menarche.[4] The relative risk of developing breast cancer in women with a natural menopause before age 45 is 0.73 compared with women whose natural menopause occurs be-

TABLE 38-1. Probability of Eventually Developing and Dying of Breast Cancer*

Age (yr)	*Risk of Developing Breast cancer (%)*	*Risk of Developing Invasive Breast Cancer (%)*	*Risk of Dying of Breast Cancer (%)*
Birth to 110	10.2	9.8	3.6
20 to 30	0.04	0.04	0.00
20 to 40	0.49	0.42	0.09
20 to 110	10.34	9.94	3.05
35 to 45	0.88	0.83	0.14
35 to 55	2.53	2.37	0.56
35 to 110	10.27	9.82	3.56
50 to 60	1.95	1.86	0.33
50 to 70	4.67	4.48	1.04
50 to 110	8.96	8.66	2.75
65 to 75	3.17	3.08	0.43
65 to 85	5.48	5.29	1.01
65 to 110	6.53	6.29	1.53

* Data from Surveillance, Epidemiology, and End Results (SEER): white females. Seidman H, Mushinski MH, Gelb SK et al: Probabilities of eventually developing or dying of cancer: United States, 1985. CA–A Cancer Journal for Clinicians 35:36–56, 1985.

tween the ages of 45 and 54.[5] The relative risk of breast cancer in women with a natural menopause after the age of 55 is 1.48. An artificial menopause before the age of 35 decreases the relative risk to 0.36. Oophorectomy performed between the ages of 35 and 44 reduces the relative risk to between 0.68 and 0.65, but the relative risk of breast cancer is not decreased when ovarian ablation is performed after the age of 50 or in women who have had an early natural menopause.

Nulliparous women have a higher incidence of breast cancer than women who have had one or more pregnancies, but the age of first pregnancy is an even more important determinant. In one study, the risk of developing breast cancer was increased fourfold to fivefold in women whose first pregnancy was after the age of 30 compared with those whose first pregnancy was before the age of 18.[6] It is possible that a first pregnancy after the age of 35 actually increases the risk of breast cancer.[7] It has been observed that prolactin levels in parous women are lower than in nulliparous women,[3] and the observations on the relations between a woman's menstrual history, pregnancy history, and risk of breast cancer suggest that high estrogen and high prolactin levels may promote the development of breast cancer.[3] The role of progesterone in inhibiting this process is less well understood.[3,8]

TABLE 38-2. Risk Factors Associated with Development of Breast Cancer

History of breast cancer
Family history of breast cancer, especially in first-degree relatives
Benign breast "cancer:" atypical hyperplasia
Early menarche, late menopause
Late first pregnancy > no pregnancy
Exogenous estrogens (postmenopausal, prior contraceptives)
Alcohol
Radiation
?Diet

The use of estrogens as postmenopausal replacement therapy or in oral contraceptives may be associated with a small increase in the risk of developing breast cancer, but this association is weak compared with the effect of estrogen in inducing or promoting endometrial cancer.[8] The use of small doses of estrogen for short periods as replacement therapy in postmenopausal women appears relatively safe. High daily doses and large cumulative doses of estrogens may result in higher risk, especially in patients who have had an oophorectomy or who have benign breast disease.[9,10] It has been estimated that the risk of developing breast cancer is increased twofold to threefold when estrogens are given for more than 10 years to women who have had an oophorectomy.[9]

There are more than 20 epidemiologic studies of the potential carcinogenic effect of oral contraceptives, and most of these have showed no relation between birth control pills and breast cancer incidence.[8,11] Nevertheless, it is not possible to rule out entirely a promotional effect in at least some patients. Assessment of these studies necessitates consideration of the composition of the oral contraceptive involved, the daily and cumulative doses of the hormone administered, and the latency for the development of breast cancer. The latency period for solid tumors is usually greater than 15 years, and the peak cancer incidence following exposure to a carcinogen occurs in the third decade. The time of exposure to a carcinogen may also be an important consideration in breast cancer epidemiology studies. For example, radiation appears to be carcinogenic for the breast only when exposure occurs at a relatively young age.[12] The only patient groups found to be at increased risk for the development of breast cancer from oral contraceptives are those with exposure prior to a first pregnancy or after the age of 45.[3] In one study, the relative risk of breast cancer was 2.25 after 4 years of oral contraceptive use and 3.52 after 8 years when oral contraceptives were administered prior to the first pregnancy ($p = 0.009$). These same durations of oral contraceptive use after the first pregnancy resulted in a relative risk of 1.31 and 1.74, respectively ($p > 0.30$).[2] Although the duration of exposure to oral contraceptives has been the single most important factor in some studies,[2,13] even exposure for more than 15 years did not increase the risk of breast cancer in other studies. Indeed, in one study, there was actually a significant decrease in the incidence of breast cancer with long-term oral contraceptive administration.[14]

ENVIRONMENTAL FACTORS AND DIET

The possibility that environmental factors are important in the etiology of breast cancer is suggested by observations on the incidence of breast cancer in Japanese women who migrate from Japan, where the incidence of breast cancer is low, to North America, where the incidence is high.[15] In a study performed in the San Francisco Bay area during 1969–1971, both Nisei (first-generation U.S. born) and Issei (immigrant) women were found to have an incidence of breast cancer nearly equal to that of the white population in the same area. These data suggest that environmental factors are as important as or more important than genetic considerations.

Diet is an obvious environmental factor, and possible relations between fat or cholesterol intake and steroid hormone metabolism have led to an emphasis on dietary fat as a possible etiologic agent. International studies relating age-adjusted cancer mortality rates and national per-capita fat intake demonstrate a direct correlation.[16] The correlation is stronger in postmenopausal women ($r = 0.81$) than in premenopausal women ($r = 0.66$). Laboratory studies provide further evidence of a possible relation between dietary fat and breast cancer.[17] The incidence of mammary cancer in DMBA-challenged rats is much higher among rats fed a diet with 10% to 20% corn oil than in those on a diet with no more than 5% corn oil.

Despite these compelling indirect data, epidemiologic studies correlating dietary fat and the incidence of breast cancer have been inconclusive. In the largest epidemiologic survey, 89,538 nurses between the ages of 34 and 59 were studied.[18] There was no relation between the relative risk of breast cancer and calorie-adjusted total fat, saturated fat, linoleic acid, or cholesterol intake. In fact, the relative risk of developing breast cancer among the women with the highest quintile of total fat intake was 0.85 compared with women in the lowest quintile. However, the difference in fat intake among women in these two extremes was only 25%. Practically, this suggests that women who reduce fat intake in the context of the usual American diet are not likely to reduce their breast cancer risk.

These epidemiologic studies do not rule out the possibility that a greater reduction in fat intake or a reduction in fat intake at an earlier age might have an important effect on breast cancer incidence. Cohort studies in countries where there has been a gradual increase in the incidence of breast cancer demonstrate that the risk is dependent on the year of birth.[19] In Iceland, the incidence of breast cancer increased steadily from 1911 to 1972, but the shape of the breast cancer incidence curves did not change during that period, suggesting that the etiologic or promotional factor important for the increasing incidence of breast cancer was operative well before the age at which the breast cancers were usually diagnosed.

Seventeen cohort or case-control studies on the relation between alcohol intake and breast cancer have been performed, and all but three show an increased risk with use of alcohol. This risk is dose related: a moderate alcohol intake is associated with a 40% to 60% increase in risk.[20,21]

FAMILY HISTORY

Women (and, to a much lesser extent, men) with any family history of breast cancer are at increased risk. However, the relative risk of developing breast cancer in women with a family history in second-degree relatives is about 1.5[22,23] compared with 1.7 to 2.5 among women with a history in first-degree relatives.[22] In some epidemiologic studies, the risk was even greater when two sisters or a mother and one or more sisters had breast cancer,[23,25] but in other studies, no association with the number of cancer-affected first-degree relatives was observed. It has been reported that breast cancer occurring in the premenopausal years or in younger women imparts a higher risk,[23] but this, too, is an inconsistent finding.[22,26] In one study, the risk was greatest in relatives of patients with bilateral breast cancer,[26] whereas in others, it was greatest in relatives of patients with unilateral breast cancer.[23] However, no risk group has been shown to have a lifetime risk in excess of 30%.[26] It is estimated that the probability of a 30-year-old woman developing breast cancer by the age of 70 is 28% if she has two sisters with breast cancer, one bilaterally, and 25% if her mother and sister have breast cancer, one bilaterally.[26]

RADIATION

Radiation is associated with an increased risk of breast cancer in survivors of the atomic bomb blast, in patients given radiation for postpartum mastitis, in women receiving multiple fluoroscopies during therapy for tuberculosis, and in animal models.[12,27] Radiation exposure results in an increased risk after a latency of 10 to 15 years, but there is very little increased risk in women exposed to radiation after the age of 40.[12]

BENIGN BREAST DISEASE

The risk of breast cancer in patients with a history of benign breast disease, especially "fibrocystic disease," has ranged from 1.86 to 2.13.[28] However, the incidence of fibrocystic disease diagnosed on the basis of histologic findings has ranged from 13% to 71% in various studies. "Lumpy breasts," which are often confused with fibrocystic disease, probably occur in more than 85% of patients. As a result, this term and the general category of "benign breast disease" have little practical significance in counseling women regarding their risk of breast cancer.

A retrospective review of more than 10,000 biopsies per-

TABLE 38-3. Patterns of Benign Breast Disease Associated with Increased Risk of Breast Cancer and Association with Family History

Histology	*Family History**	*No. of Patients*	*Relative Risk†*	*p*
All patients	—	3303	1.5	<0.0001
	No	2934	1.4	0.0007
	Yes	369	2.5	<0.0001
No proliferative disease	—	1378	0.89	0.51
Proliferative disease	—	1925	1.9	<0.0001
Atypical hyperplasia	—	232	4.4	<0.0001
	No	193	3.5	<0.0001
	Yes	39	8.9	<0.0001

Data from Dupont WD, Page DL: Risk factors for breast cancer in women with proliferative breast disease. N Engl J Med 312:146–151, 1985.

* Cancer in first-degree relative.

† Compared with age-matched population from Third National Cancer Survey.

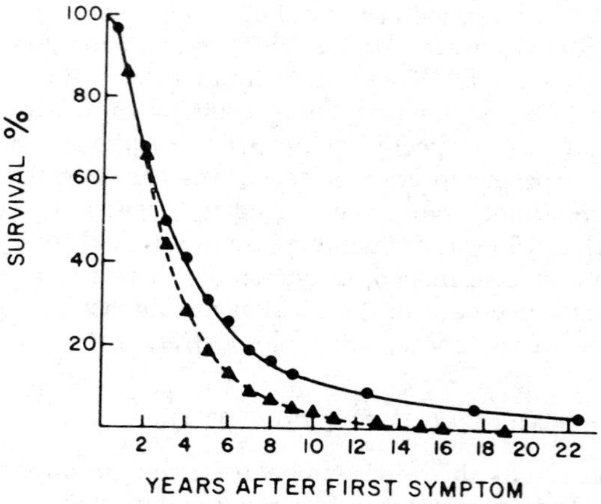

FIG. 38-1. Survival of untreated patients (*triangles*) seen at the Middlesex Hospital, England, between 1805 and 1933, juxtaposed with survival of patients treated with radical mastectomy (*circles*) at Johns Hopkins between 1889 and 1931 (Henderson IC, Canellos GP: Cancer of the breast: the past decade. Reprinted by permission of N Engl J Med 302:17–30, 1980)

formed at the Vanderbilt Hospital has led to the conclusion that most of the risk associated with benign breast disease is attributable to the small percentage of patients who have atypical hyperplasia or both atypical hyperplasia and a family history of breast cancer (Table 38-3). In this study, 3303 biopsies were reviewed among the total population. Patients with a family history of breast cancer had a higher incidence of subsequent invasive breast cancer. About one-third of the patients had no evidence of proliferative disease at all, and there was no evidence of an increased risk among this group. Atypical hyperplasia was observed in only 7% of the patients, but their risk of developing breast cancer was increased fourfold. For the 39 patients (about 1% of the total) who had both atypical hyperplasia and a history of breast cancer in a first-degree relative, the risk of subsequent breast cancer was increased ninefold. However, even in this very high-risk group, the observed incidence of breast cancer over 25 years was only about 40%, and less than one-third of these patients eventually died of breast cancer. These data suggest that benign breast disease is rarely an indication for special monitoring and may never be an indication for therapeutic intervention.

NATURAL HISTORY OF BREAST CANCER

The natural history of breast cancer is characterized by a long duration and marked heterogeneity within and between patients. Breast cancer is among the more slowly growing tumors, and as a result, both the preclinical period (before diagnosis) and the clinical phases after initial treatment and metastases are measured in years and decades. Nevertheless, some patients have a very aggressive form of the disease and do poorly. An equal number have such an indolent form of the disease that it is difficult to demonstrate that therapy has any effect at all on survival. During the long clinical phase, there is ample opportunity for clonal mutation and evolution, and it seems probable that almost all breast cancer patients have multiple tumor clones, each with its own unique growth requirements, growth rates, propensity to metastasize, and sensitivity to drugs.

The long natural history of breast cancer has been emphasized in about a half-dozen studies of patients with untreated breast cancer. Most of the patients in these studies were identified in the late nineteenth and early twentieth century, and then, as now, such patients were self-selected. It therefore cannot be assumed that they are truly representative of the full spectrum of breast cancer patients. All of these series, like the one shown in Figure 38-1, include some patients who lived for two to three decades without any treatment at all. Nevertheless, the median survival for the untreated patients in the Middlesex series was 2.7 years. The survival of patients treated with radical mastectomy by

FIG. 38-2. Relative mortality per year (±SE) of all stages of breast cancer diagnosed in the United States, 1950–1973. (Data from End Results Section, Biometry Branch, National Cancer Institute 1977; Fox M: On the diagnosis and treatment of breast cancer. JAMA 241:489–494, 1979)

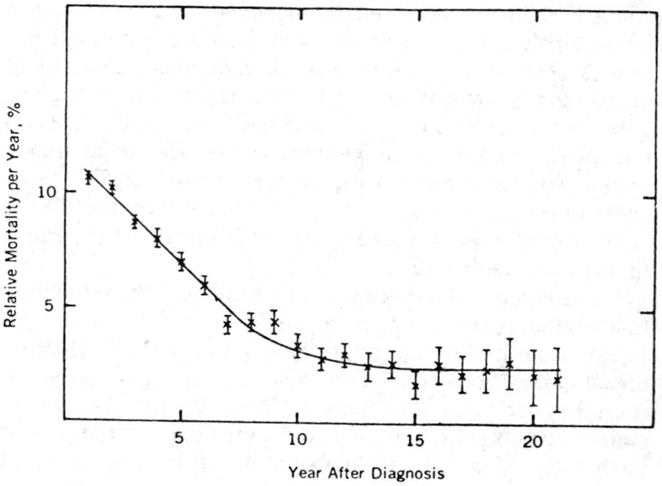

Halsted and his colleagues at Johns Hopkins, also shown in Figure 38-1, is not much different from that of untreated patients. The percentages of patients who ultimately died as a direct result of breast cancer are almost identical in the two series.[29] This comparison undermines the claim that the radical mastectomy is the "proven" therapy for breast cancer.

The heterogeneity of breast cancer is illustrated by an analysis of disease mortality rates in Connecticut between the years 1950 and 1973.[30] The highest mortality rate was observed immediately after diagnosis, and the rate gradually fell during the first decade of follow-up (Fig. 38-2). During the second decade of follow-up, the yearly relative mortality rate for breast cancer remained constant. Maurice Fox has suggested that this Connecticut mortality curve results from superimposition of at least two separate mortality curves from breast cancer populations with uniquely different natural histories (Fig. 38-3). One group, which constituted about 60% of all the patients in the series, had an annual mortality rate of approximately 2.5% per year. Half of these patients died in the first 15 years postmastectomy and the other half between years 15 and 30 (closed circles in Fig. 38-3). The remaining approximately 40% of the patient population had an annual mortality rate of about 25% per year. Most of these patients died within the first decade postmastectomy (open circles in Fig. 38-3). These observations are consistent with the concept that there is both an aggressive form of breast cancer, which contributes most of the observed morbidity and deaths, and an indolent form, which is compatible with long life regardless of the therapy given. Although intuitively one might anticipate that patients with a more indolent form of the disease would be disproportionately represented in an

FIG. 38-3. Relative survival of patients with a yearly mortality rate of ≤2.5% (*closed circles*) or >2.5% (*open circles*). (Fox M: On the diagnosis and treatment of breast cancer. JAMA 241:489–494, 1979)

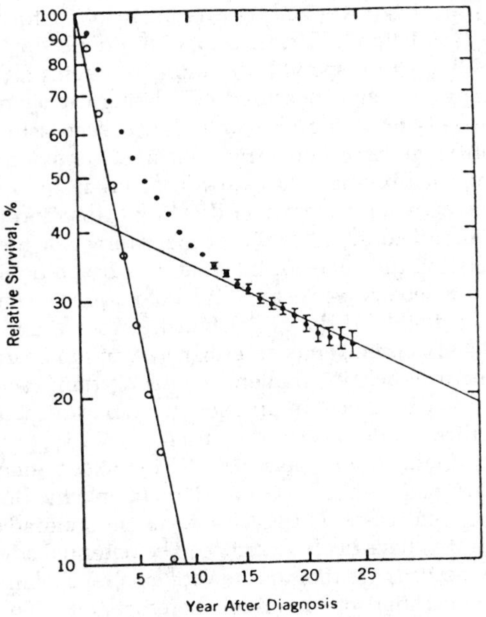

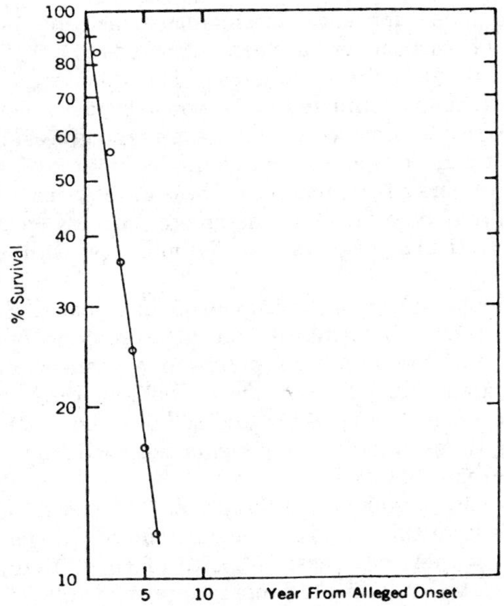

FIG. 38-4. Survival of the untreated patients shown in Fig. 38-1 replotted semilogarithmically.

untreated historical series, such as the one described in Figure 38-1, a semilogarithmic plot of the survival of these patients suggests that these untreated patients were primarily from the group with a mortality rate of about 25% per year (Fig. 38-4). It seems likely that many of the patients being identified in the current era are not represented among historical controls.

The heterogeneity of this disease can also be illustrated by the wide variability in growth rates as measured with labeling indices. The labeling index is a measure of the percentage of cells in a tumor that are undergoing cell division at a single point in time. Patients with high labeling indices are therefore more likely to have rapidly growing cancer than are those with low labeling indices. About 60% of patients have labeling indices less than 4%. The remaining 40% have indices that range from 4% to 41%.[31]

PRECLINICAL EVENTS

Our understanding of the preclinical behavior of breast cancer is dependent on either extrapolation backward from clinical observation or the use of tumor models. Both of these approaches have important limitations. Tumors large enough to be detected and measured in the clinic are likely to have a slower growth rate than microscopic preclinical lesions. Animal model tumors are usually selected because of a high growth fraction, which facilitates laboratory study. However, many human breast cancers have low growth fractions.

The *relative* growth rates of human tumors can be determined from clinical measurements, and these studies suggest that, on average, breast cancer has a lower labeling index, a longer doubling time, and a lower growth fraction than most other human tumors.[32] For example, the mean labeling index for adenocarcinomas consisting predominantly of breast cancer has been estimated to be 2.1%, compared with 29% for lymphomas. The doubling time for breast cancer is estimated to be about 83 days, compared with 27 days for embryonal tumors, and the growth fraction of breast cancer is about 6%, compared with 90% for embryonal tumors and lymphomas. These differences in growth fraction may be a factor in the greater success obtained in curing testicular cancers and lymphomas with chemotherapy.

The doubling time of breast cancer in its earliest clinical phases has been determined from measurements of lesions present but not initially appreciated as cancer in serial mammograms.[33-36] The observed doubling time in these studies averaged between 115 and 325 days, but the range of doubling times in individual patients extended from 23 days to more than 940 days.

It is usually assumed that the preclinical growth of breast cancer is logarithmic and continuous. Tumors can usually be palpated within the breast at a size of about 1 cm, and a sphere of this size could contain approximately 10^9 cells. Assuming origin of the cancer in a single-cell mutation, it would take 30 doublings for a malignant cell to produce 10^9 cells, assuming no cell loss during that interval. If all of these assumptions are true, and if one accepts a preclinical doubling time of about 100 days (a value substantially lower than all the mean values obtained in doubling-time measurements of clinically measurable lesions), then the preclinical phase of breast cancer should, on average, exceed 10 years. Even if breast cancer doubling times are actually one-half to one-fourth of that assumed in this illustration, the preclinical phase of breast cancer would still range from 2.5 to 5 years. Of course, these assumptions are all subject to challenge and may seriously underestimate differences in the growth rate of preclinical lesions growing logarithmically compared with clinically detectable lesions in a plateau phase of growth (*i.e.*, Gompertzian growth). It is also possible that the preclinical growth of breast cancer is less than logarithmic or even discontinuous, in which case the preclinical phase would be even longer.

It has recently been suggested that the assumption that preclinical breast cancer growth is logarithmic is inconsistent with observations from large clinical studies. Utilizing data on the interval from initial diagnosis of breast cancer to the appearance of clinically detectable metastases, it has been concluded by mathematical modeling that preclinical breast cancer might be better characterized as having short spurts of logarithmic growth alternating with quiescent periods of little or no growth.[37] To further complicate the issue, it is plausible that growth at various metastatic sites within each patient is asynchronous.

DEFINING PATIENT SUBSETS

The recognition that patients at extremes of the disease spectrum are very different provides a basis for attempting to identify groups of patients likely to benefit uniquely from one or another treatment strategy. However, all such attempts share some limitations, the most important of which is that the spectrum of the disease is continuous. That is, there are no groups of patients uniquely different from all others, and most patients are somewhere in the middle between the two extremes. Well-differentiated tumors slowly merge into moderately well-differentiated tumors. Patients with no evidence of tumor hormone receptors have only a slightly worse prognosis or a slightly lower probability of responding to endocrine therapy than patients with a low-positive receptor value.

A second problem with the use of many subsets is the lack of reproducibility from one observer to the next. In one study, the concordance between two pathologists in defining the cell type (ductal carcinoma not otherwise specified versus nonductal carcinoma) or assigning one of three nuclear grades was little more than might be expected by chance.[38]

In considering the notion of patients "subsets," one must also consider that differences in prognosis between patients in different subsets may be not in the ultimate probability of relapse but rather in the probable time to relapse. This is illustrated in a comparison of the survival of patients without lymph node metastases with that of patients with one lymph node involved.[39] At the end of the first 5 years of observation, the disease-free survival of these two groups of patients was nearly identical, and this was initially taken as evidence that there was no difference in the propensity of these two patient groups to develop distant metastases. However, further follow-up over 12 years demonstrated that the two curves slowly diverged, so that by the end of the 12th year, patients with a single involved node had a significantly higher recurrence rate than those with no lymph node involvement. This observation, once again, underscores the long natural history of the disease.

HORMONE RECEPTORS

It has long been known that only a subset of all patients with breast cancer respond to endocrine therapy and that these patients are characterized by a more indolent form of the disease (see below). Early attempts to define the group of patients likely to respond to hormone therapies utilized endocrine profiles and measured circulating estrogens or androgen levels, or both. However, the most successful method of identifying these endocrine-sensitive tumors has come from the measurement of estrogen or progesterone receptors. The estrogen receptor (ERP) is a cytosol protein that can be identified in either the primary tumor or metastases by incubating the supernatant fluid of a tissue homogenate with a radiolabeled estrogen.[40] Receptors present in the supernatant fluid bind the radiolabeled estrogen, and the unbound label is then removed either by dextran-coated charcoal, sucrose density-gradient centrifugation, or one of several other methods. In practice, the dextran-coated charcoal method is the most widely used.

Newer methods of measuring ERP involve monoclonal antibodies made to the receptor. Both an enzyme-linked immunochemical assay (ERICA) and an immunoradiometric assay (IRMA) have been described. The potential advantages of these methods are their utility with smaller specimens and the demonstration of tumor-cell heterogeneity. The use of these staining techniques also permits an estimate of the percentage of cells with ERP and theoretically permits a better estimate of the maximum cell kill that might be achieved by the use of endocrine therapy. On the other hand, quantification of results is more difficult. At present, there is good correlation between the results of these methods and the bioassay, and it is likely that the techniques utilizing antibodies to ERP or progesterone receptors (PR) will find increasing use.

Approximately two-thirds of all patients have ERP present in their tumor, and about half of the receptor-positive tumors will respond to endocrine therapy. Postmenopausal patients and older patients more frequently have receptor-positive tumors than do younger and premenopausal patients.[40] In general, the incidence of receptor positivity decreases with time, and several studies suggest that a biopsy obtained just before treatment is more predictive of response than a biopsy obtained months or years before. However, receptor status should be measured on all biopsies or mastectomy specimens when feasible. This information has prognostic significance, may influence the selection of an adjuvant therapy, and may be of use in the selection of palliative therapy for metastatic disease in the event that the sites are not easily accessible for biopsy and measurement of receptors.

It is not understood why not all receptor-positive tumors respond to endocrine therapy. It is plausible that many patients have a sufficient number of cells to cause the assay result to be positive but an insufficient number of receptor-positive cells for their death to result in a measurable reduction in the tumor mass. It is also possible that the ER measured in many tumors is not truly functional. Therefore, measurement of the PR has been used as a means of identifying intact ERP. When cancer cells with intact and functioning ERP are exposed to estrogen, the estrogen is transported into the nucleus, where messenger RNA is formed. Among the products of this interaction are additional ERP, PR, and various growth factors[41,42] (Fig. 38-5). Clinical observations appear to confirm the hypothesis that PR are a marker of intact ERP, as tumors with both types of receptors are much more likely to respond to endocrine therapy than are those with ERP alone (see below, Table 38-33).

FIG. 38-5. Role of estrogen receptor (*ER*) in processing estrogens (*E*) resulting in production of progesterone receptor (*PgR*) and growth factors. (Osborne CK: Receptors. In Harris J, Hellman S, Henderson IC, Kinne DW: [eds]: Breast Diseases, pp 210–232. Philadelphia, JB Lippincott, 1987)

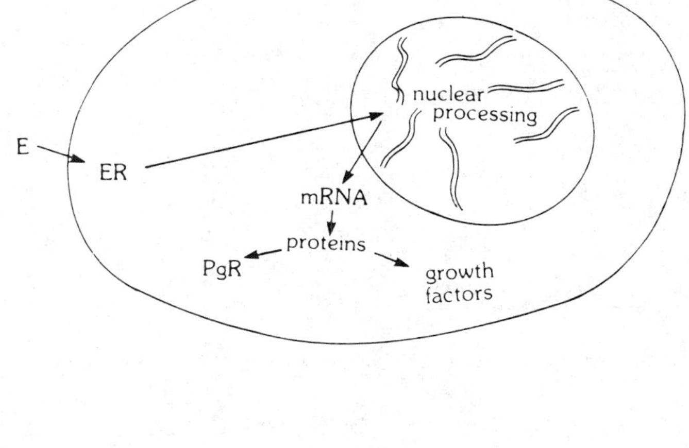

USE OF RECEPTORS TO DEFINE PROGNOSTIC SUBSETS

Because patients who respond to endocrine therapy are those with the longest disease-free intervals (see below), it is not surprising that patients with ERP or PR are also more likely to have a long disease-free interval. In fact, receptor-positive patients have a longer overall survival and a longer survival from evidence of first metastases than do receptor-negative patients.[43,44] Both ERP status and PR status are predictive of recurrence, and several studies suggest that the PR status has more prognostic value than the ERP status, especially in node-positive patients.[43,45] A multivariate analysis of 1529 patients with Stage II disease demonstrated that the PR had about the same prognostic value as did the presence of histologically involved nodes or tumor size (Table 38-4).

It is tempting to assume that the patient's receptor status is a reflection of the intrinsic growth rate of the tumor. In some studies, receptor-positive patients have had a better short-term prognosis or an improved short-term survival rate. However, the percentages of receptor-positive patients and receptor-negative patients who eventually relapse and die of breast cancer are identical.[46-51] Other investigators have concluded that receptor status is predictive only of the response to endocrine therapy and thus indirectly appears to predict growth rate.[52] In these studies, patients with receptor-positive tumors had an increased overall survival and an increased survival following the appearance of metastases but an insignificant prolongation of the disease-free interval. An improvement in survival was found only among those patients who were both receptor-positive and responsive to endocrine treatment.

Patients without histologically involved lymph nodes have better 10-year disease-free survival and overall survival rates than do node-positive patients. However, 15% to 30% of these patients will relapse, and 12% to 22% will die within 5 years of diagnosis.[53-58] If it were possible to identify those node-negative patients most likely to relapse and die of

TABLE 38-4. Prognostic Value of Receptors for Disease-Free Survival and Overall Survival in Patients with Stage II Breast Cancer (Multivariate Analysis of 1529 Patients)

	p Value	
Factor	*Disease-Free Survival*	*Overall Survival*
Positive nodes	<0.0001	<0.0001
Tumor size	<0.0001	0.0001
Progesterone receptor status	0.0001	0.0001
Endocrine therapy	0.0004	0.0017
Chemotherapy	0.0731	0.0191
Estrogen receptor status	0.1376	0.0017
Age	0.8990	0.0622

McGuire WL, Clark GM, Dressler LG et al: Role of steroid hormone receptors as prognostic factors in primary breast cancer. NCI Monogr 1:19–23, 1986.

breast cancer, they could be considered for treatment with adjuvant chemotherapy, sparing those with the best prognosis from the toxicities of this therapy. Many investigators have tried to use receptor status to identify this poor-prognosis group, but the results are contradictory (Table 38-5). In the Milan study, premenopausal patients without receptors had a significantly poorer survival rate than receptor-positive patients, but survival differences among postmenopausal patients were less obvious.[46] A study performed in the Cleveland area showed that receptor status was more predictive of relapse and death among postmenopausal than premenopausal patients.[47] In the largest of the studies shown in Table 38-5, there was no difference in the relapse rate or the length of survival by receptor status among either premenopausal or postmenopausal women.[59] A similar result has been found by investigators in England, who have demonstrated that the presence of receptors is highly predictive of relapse and survival among node-positive patients but not among node-negative patients.[60] In all of these studies, a substantial portion of the ERP-positive patients relapsed even though the relapse rate among ERP-negative patients was somewhat higher. Collecting these data led to the conclusion that patients who are receptor-negative have a small but significant increase in the risk of early relapse and early death from breast cancer, but that receptor status alone is insufficient to identify the 20% to 30% of node-negative patients at risk of eventually dying of breast cancer.

CLASSIFICATION OF TUMOR TYPES

Histopathologic examination of breast cancer makes available information that establishes the diagnosis of the lesion, aids in determining patient prognosis, and leads to a better understanding of the biology of the disease. This section presents a general overview of the subject, with emphasis on recent contributions that have enhanced our understanding of the nature of breast cancer or that have raised important questions that require resolution.

A number of pathologic classifications of mammary carcinomas are in use. The most commonly used are those presented by the Armed Forces Institute of Pathology (AFIP)[61] and the World Health Organization (WHO).[62] Breast carcinomas are classified as either ductal or lobular, corresponding to the ducts and lobules of the normal breast. However, there is evidence that most tumors arise in the terminal duct section of the breast, regardless of pathologic type.[63]

The frequency of the various histologic types of breast cancer in 1000 cases from NSABP Protocol B-04 is presented in Table 38-6. More than half (52.6%) are pure infiltrating duct lesions, not otherwise specified (NOS).

CARCINOMA IN SITU

Tumors arising from duct epithelium that are confined within the lumen of the ducts or lobules of the breast are

TABLE 38-5. Comparison of Disease-Free and Overall Survival of Patients Without Histologic Node Involvement Who Have Received No Adjuvant Therapy and Are Either Estrogen-Receptor Positive (ER^+) or Negative (ER^-)

Study	*Patient Population*	*Total No. of Patients*	*4–6-Year Disease-Free (%)* ER^+	ER^-	*p Value*
Milan (46)	Premenopausal	464	88	59	<0.0001
	Postmenopausal		75	70	0.22
Memorial (59)	Premenopausal	1034	88	83	NS*
	Postmenopausal		84	84	NS
Cleveland (47)	Premenopausal	510	72	72	0.65
	Postmenopausal		80	65	<0.06
			4–6-Year Survival (%)		
Milan (46)	Premenopausal	464	95	77	0.0001
	Postmenopausal		88	79	0.02
Memorial (59)	Premenopausal	1034	92	89	NS
	Postmenopausal		94	92	NS
Cleveland (47)	All Patients	510	87	74	<0.003

* NS = not significant.

TABLE 38-6. Incidence of Histologic Types of Breast Cancer (%)

Pure Tumor Groups	
Infiltrating duct NOS	52.6
Medullary	6.2
Lobular invasive	4.9
Mucinous	2.4
Tubular	1.2
Adenocystic	0.4
Papillary	0.3
Carcinosarcoma	0.1
Paget's Disease	2.3
With intraductal carcinoma	0.2
Infiltrating duct NOS	1.6
Infiltrating duct NOS + tubular	0.4
Infiltrating duct NOS + mucinous	0.1
Combinations with Infiltrating Duct NOS	28.0
+ Tubular	16.5
+ Lobular invasive	3.3
+ Mucinous	1.6
+ Lobular invasive + tubular	1.6
+ Papillary	1.2
+ Adenocystic	1.0
+ Tubular + adenocystic	0.8
+ Tubular + papillary	0.8
+ Mucinous + papillary	0.4
+ Adenocystic + mucinous	0.2
+ Lobular invasive + adenocystic	0.1
+ Lobular invasive + mucinous	0.1
+ Lobular invasive + papillary	0.1
+ Tubular + mucinous	0.1
+ Adenocystic + papillary	0.1
+ Lobular invasive + tubular + adenocystic + mucinous	0.1
Other Combinations of Tumor Types Exclusive of NOS	1.6
Tubular + papillary	0.5
Lobular invasive + tubular	0.4
Tubular + mucinous	0.2
Lobular invasive + mucinous	0.1
Tubular + adenocystic	0.1
Adenocystic + mucinous	0.1
Mucinous + papillary	0.1
Lobular invasive + tubular + adenocystic + papillary	0.1

generally referred to as carcinoma in situ. Carcinoma in situ has been classified as either ductal or lobular, depending on the cytologic features and pattern of growth. Both ductal carcinoma in situ (DCIS), also known as intraductal carcinoma or noninvasive ductal carcinoma, and lobular carcinoma in situ (LCIS) are characterized by a proliferation of malignant epithelial cells confined to the mammary ducts or lobules, without light-microscopic evidence of invasion through the basement membrane into the surrounding stroma. The distinction between DCIS and LCIS is usually not difficult, but overlaps exist. The natural history and management of these lesions will be discussed later in this chapter.

INFILTRATING CARCINOMA, NOS

A variety of histologic types of invasive (infiltrating) carcinomas of the breast have been described. Infiltrating ductal carcinomas in which no special histologic features are recognized are designated NOS and are by far the most common ductal tumors, accounting for almost 70% of breast cancers. They are characterized by their stony hardness to palpation. When transected, a gritty resistance is typically encountered, and the tumor retracts below the cut surface. Histologically, various degrees of fibrotic response and associated DCIS are present. These tumors commonly metastasize to the axillary lymph nodes, and their prognosis is the poorest of the various ductal types.

MEDULLARY CARCINOMA

Medullary carcinomas are circumscribed lesions that can attain large dimensions but demonstrate only low-grade infiltrative properties. They constitute 5% to 7% of all mammary carcinomas and are characterized by poorly differentiated nuclei and infiltration with small lymphocytes and plasma cells. The 5-year survival rate following treatment for medullary carcinoma is better than for NOS ductal carcinomas.

TUBULAR CARCINOMA

A tumor in which tubule formation is conspicuous is known as tubular or well-differentiated carcinoma. Generally, this diagnosis is made only when 75% or more of the tumor is composed of these elements. Axillary metastases are uncommon, and the prognosis is considerably better than for ductal carcinoma, NOS.

MUCINOUS CARCINOMA

Another ductal type, the mucinous or colloid carcinoma, comprises about 3% of all mammary carcinomas and is characterized microscopically by nests and strands of epithelial cells floating in a mucinous matrix. It usually is slow growing and can reach bulky proportions. When the tumor is predominantly mucinous, the prognosis tends to be good.

Other, rarer, types of ductal carcinomas include papillary, adenocystic, and carcinosarcoma or metaplastic duct carcinoma. Of note, in many cases, NOS ductal carcinomas contain small areas of these special types.

INFILTRATING LOBULAR CARCINOMA

Another histologic type of breast cancer is infiltrating lobular carcinoma. It is relatively uncommon, accounting for only 5% to 10% of breast tumors in most series. The clinical presentation is more often an area of ill-defined thickening in the breast, in contrast to the dominant lump characteristic of ductal carcinoma. Microscopically, lobular carcinomas typically are composed of small cells in a linear arrangement ("Indian-filing") with a tendency to grow around ducts and lobules (targetoid growth). Lobular carcinomas are also characterized by a greater proportion of multicentric tumors, either in the same or the opposite breast, when compared with NOS ductal carcinoma. Overall, infiltrating lobular carcinoma has a similar likelihood of axillary nodal involvement and prognosis as infiltrating duct carcinoma. However, the sites of metastases for these two types tend to differ. Ductal carcinomas more characteristically metastasize to bone or to intraparenchymal sites within lung, liver, or brain, whereas lobular carcinomas more often show a predilection for meningeal and serosal surfaces.

PAGET'S DISEASE

Paget's disease of the breast occurs in 1% to 4% of all patients with breast cancer. Clinically, the patient presents with a relatively long history of eczematous changes in the nipple with itching, burning, oozing, bleeding, or some combination of these. The nipple changes are associated with an underlying carcinoma in the breast that can be palpated in about two-thirds of the patients. The subadjacent tumor may be either intraductal or of the invasive duct type. The prognosis is related to the histologic type of the associated tumor. Histologically, the nipple epidermis contains tumor cells singly and in nests. Treatment of Paget's disease is discussed in the section on special problems later in this chapter.

INFLAMMATORY BREAST CARCINOMA

Inflammatory breast cancer is characterized clinically by prominent skin edema, redness and warmth, a visible erysipeloid margin, and induration of the underlying tissue. These criteria in the past were sufficient for the diagnosis. Currently, pathologic corroboration must be obtained. Biopsies of the involved skin reveal cancer cells in the dermal lymphatics. Inflammatory cells rarely are present. The prognosis of patients with inflammatory breast cancer is poor, even if the disease is apparently localized. The management of inflammatory cancer is discussed later in this chapter.

EVALUATION OF BREAST SPECIMENS

In the past, when mastectomy was the standard treatment for breast cancer, it was sufficient for the pathologist to diagnose the disease. Now that breast-conserving treatment is commonly employed, a more extensive evaluation of the resected specimen is critical. The exterior surface of the specimen should be inked to facilitate the assessment of the margins of resection for microscopic tumor involvement. The pathologist should describe the gross appearance of the resected specimen and, after inking, should describe the specimen on cut section, particularly in regard to the greatest dimension of the tumor and the distance from the periphery of the tumor to the closest margin of resection. A tissue sample for measurement of ERP and PR proteins should be obtained in a way that interferes as little as possible with the later evaluation of the margins of resection for tumor involvement. It is important to determine if there is microscopic tumor involvement at the margins of resection. This is best achieved by careful evaluation of permanent sections. One feature of the tumor that should be routinely noted, because it may influence the need for further resection of the primary tumor, is the extent of associated intraductal carcinoma, both in the primary tumor and in the grossly normal adjacent breast tissue.[64]

TUMOR CHARACTERISTICS

A number of morphologic aspects of breast tumors have been evaluated in terms of their relation to prognosis. The most important of these are histologic grade and the presence of lymphatic invasion. Other morphologic features that correlate less consistently with the prognosis include nuclear grade, the presence of necrosis, the frequency of mitoses, and the nature and extent of the cellular reaction of the tumor.

Tumor grading describes the degree of differentiation. The histologic grade of duct carcinoma can be scored by the degree of tubule formation, the size of the nuclei, the degree of nuclear hyperchromatism, and the number of mitoses. Tumors of low-grade malignancy have been designated Grade I and are believed to have the best prognosis. Tumors of high-grade malignancy have been designated Grade III and have the worst prognosis.

Lymphatic invasion refers to the presence of tumor emboli in breast lymphatics. Because tumor cells within an invasive cancer commonly grow in clumps, it is generally best to judge lymphatic invasion in breast tissue adjacent to the tumor. Such invasion is observed in approximately 25% of breast tumors and is associated with a lower likelihood of survival.

The prognostic importance of these morphologic features must be evaluated in relation to stage (the clinical extent of the cancer) and the number of involved axillary nodes, features with well-known prognostic value. It is also important to note that these morphologic features might predict the *pace* of the disease rather than the likelihood of long-term survival. This point is illustrated in the experience of Bloom, Richardson, and Field from the Middlesex and Royal Marsden Hospitals in London.[65] They examined the 20-year results in 1411 patients treated with modified radical mastectomy between 1936 and 1949. Table 38-7 shows the 5- and 15-year survival rates in relation to axillary node involvement and histologic grade, which suggest that histologic grade is a more useful indicator of prognosis at 5 years than it is at 15 years. The likelihood of long-term survival in patients with positive axillary nodes is low regardless of histologic grade. These results suggest that histologic grade is an indicator of the pace of the disease in patients with positive nodes and may be a good indicator of long-term prog-

TABLE 38-7. Corrected 5- and 15-year Survival by Axillary Nodal Involvement and Tumor Grade

	Nodal Involvement (%)		
	Grade	*Negative*	*Positive*
5 Years	1	86	68
	2	68	33
	3	64	19
15 Years	1	49	15
	2	29	11
	3	25	7

Bloom HJG, Field JR: Impact of tumor grade and host resistance on survival of women with breast cancer. Cancer 28:1580–1589, 1971.

nosis in patients with negative axillary nodes. Similar results have been noted by others in regard to histologic and nuclear grade.[66,67]

The level of concordance between different observers in assessing these histologic features can be low. This has been demonstrated in studies by the Eastern Cooperative Oncology Group (ECOG) in the evaluation of specimens for nuclear grade and lymphatic invasion. For example, among three reviewers of nuclear grade, there was complete agreement in only 34% of cases; among five reviewers, there was complete agreement in only 17% of cases.[38] This difficulty in assigning reproducible scores poses a significant practical problem to the use of these histologic features in estimating prognosis.

More recently, investigators have attempted to evaluate biologic aspects of breast tumors in a more quantitative fashion in order to estimate prognosis. These aspects include the determination of ER and PR proteins (ERP, PRP), measurements of tumor-cell kinetics, measurements of DNA content, and the determination of oncogene expression. The ERP and PRP determination has been described earlier in this chapter. The parameter of tumor-cell kinetics that has been studied most extensively is the labeling index, which can be determined by incubating tumor cells with ^{3}H-thymidine and counting the percentage of cells that take up the isotope by autoradiography. Because thymidine is primarily taken up by cells in the DNA synthetic or S phase of the cycle, the labeling index is a measure of the percentage of the cells in this phase and thus a reflection of tumor proliferative activity. More recently, the labeling index has been determined by the use of DNA flow cytometry, which identifies the percentage of cells in each phase of the cell cycle using DNA-specific fluorescent stains. In addition, flow cytometry can determine the degree of abnormality of DNA content (aneuploidy) in the tumor cells.

The labeling index is an important prognostic factor. This is illustrated by the data of Tubiana and colleagues from the Institut Gustave-Roussy.[68] They studied tumor samples from 128 breast cancer patients seen at that institution between 1972 and 1973, 96 of whom had diagnostic axillary dissections. The likelihood of relapse and death was analyzed by the labeling index for the 125 patients evaluable at 10 years. Their results indicate that the index is highly predictive of both relapse and death. Similar findings have been described by Meyer[69] and Silvestrini[70] and their co-workers.

The relation between the labeling index and other prognostic factors was also investigated by Meyer and associates.[69] They found that the index correlated significantly with the histologic features of the tumor but not with tumor size or the number of positive axillary nodes. Tubiana et al. similarly found that the labeling index is not correlated with nodal involvement and that the index was an important prognostic factor independent of clinical and pathologic staging.[68] They found in a multivariate analysis of their results that the index, tumor size, and tumor grade (and not axillary node involvement) were the main independent prognostic factors. Silvestrini and coworkers also did not find any correlation between the labeling index and tumor size or nodal involvement.[70] The index was found to be a highly significant prognostic factor for patients with negative nodes. All these results indicate that the labeling index correlates with histologic grade and appears to be an important prognostic factor independent of clinical or pathologic staging.

The index is inversely related to the level of steroid hormone receptors (ERP and PRP). At present, the relative prognostic importance of the index and receptors has not been clearly delineated. It is also important to note that the labeling index is not readily obtainable in most institutions. Its determination by autoradiography is tedious, and flow cytometry is not generally available at this time. This limits its utility as a prognostic factor in clinical practice.

More recently, flow cytometry has been used to investigate the relation between aneuploidy and prognosis. Patients with aneuploid tumors have been found to have a worse short-term prognosis than patients with diploid tumors.[71,72] The relation between DNA content, labeling index, and steroid hormone receptors as independent prognostic factors remains to be elucidated. McDivitt and co-workers found that DNA content, S-phase fraction (SPF) as measured by flow cytometry, and ERP were all correlated.[73] It should also be noted that flow cytometry offers the possibility of even more sophisticated characterization of a tumor by the use of monoclonal antibody probes. At present, there are not enough long-term data to support the routine use of these measures of proliferative activity to guide the clinical care of patients.

The most recent attempt to estimate prognosis involves the determination of oncogene expression in breast tumors. The most notable of these studies is by Slamon and colleagues, in which the amplification of the *HER-2/neu* oncogene was correlated with prognosis in 189 patients.[74] Amplification was seen in 35% of cases and was not correlated with ERP, PRP, tumor size, or number of positive axillary nodes. In a multivariate analysis for relapse-free survival, which included the number of positive nodes, *HER-2/neu* amplification, ERP, PRP, tumor size, and patient age, only the number of positive nodes and *HER-2/neu* amplification were statistically significant (both p values = 0.001). Additional studies will be required with more patients and longer follow-up to confirm the results. It is likely, however, that these newer determinations of the biologic aspects of breast tumors will emerge as important predictors of prognosis.

LOCAL SPREAD OF BREAST CANCER

The primary site of breast cancer is described by the quadrant of the breast in which it is found. In one series of 696 cases, 48% of the tumors were located in the upper outer quadrant, 15% in the upper inner quadrant, 11% in the lower outer quadrant, 6% in the lower inner quadrant, and 17% in the central region (designated as within 1 cm of the areola).[75] An additional 3% were termed diffuse because of multifocal origin or involvement of the entire breast. The higher frequency of breast cancer in the upper outer quadrant is thought to be attributable simply to the greater amount of breast tissue in that quadrant. In this series of patients, no differences in survival based on quadrant location were noted. The relation between the location of the primary tumor and prognosis also was examined in another

TABLE 38-8. Five-Year Relapse Rate (%) According to the Location of the Primary and Nodal Status (NSABP)

Location	*Negative Nodes*	*Positive Nodes*
UOQ	17 (208)*	63 (239)
UIQ	25 (75)	59 (37)
LIQ	22 (23)	55 (22)
LOQ	26 (46)	70 (44)

* Number of patients in subgroup.

large series from the National Surgical Adjuvant Breast Project (NSABP). Relapse and ultimate survival were related to the pathologic status of the axillary nodes, and there were no significant differences in prognosis by primary tumor location (Table 38-8).[76]

The spread of cancer through the breast has been summarized by Haagensen.[77] This spread occurs by direct infiltration into the breast parenchyma, along mammary ducts, and via breast lymphatics. Direct infiltration tends to occur by ramifying projections that have a characteristic stellate appearance on gross examination. If untreated, direct involvement of overlying skin or deep pectoral fascia is common. Involvement along ducts is observed frequently and may include wide segments of the breast. It is unclear, however, whether this intraductal involvement represents true spread of a primary cancer along previously uninvolved ducts or a "field cancerization" that results in simultaneous transformation along entire lengths of ducts. Spread can also occur by the extensive network of breast lymphatics. Investigators have emphasized lymphatic spread vertically down to the lymphatic plexus in the deep pectoral fascia underlying the breast. In addition, spread to the central subareolar region has been described. These multiple mechanisms of spread emphasize the likelihood of cancer being present in the breast well beyond the palpable primary mass.

A detailed study of the sites of cancer in a breast containing a primary tumor has been performed by Holland et al.[78] They examined 264 mastectomy specimens from patients with clinically unifocal breast cancer measuring 4 cm or less. In only 40% of cases was the cancer in the breast restricted to the primary tumor (Fig. 38-6). The probability of finding additional foci of cancer decreased as a function of distance from the primary tumor: 41% of the specimens had additional foci of cancer 2 cm or more from the primary tumor, whereas only 11% had additional foci 4 cm or more from the primary tumor. Of the cases with additional foci beyond 2 cm, the additional foci were intraductal in approximately two-thirds of cases.

FIG. 38-6. Distribution of tumor foci at different distances from reference tumor and proportions of cases with and without tumor foci around reference tumor. The pathologic size served as reference size.[78]

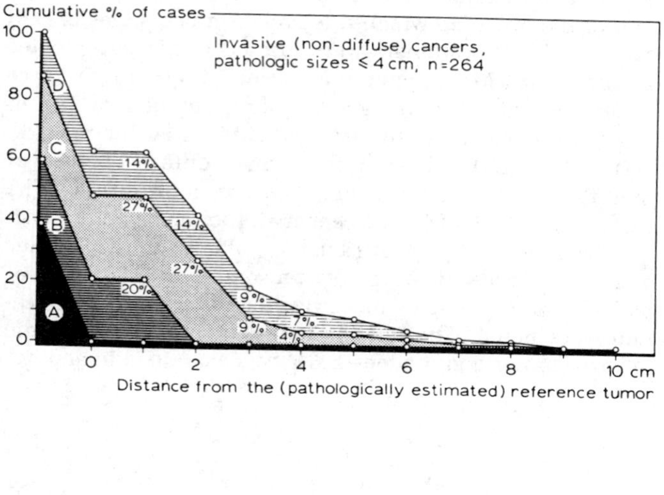

REGIONAL SPREAD

The most common routes of spread of breast cancer to regional lymph nodes are to the axillary, internal mammary, and supraclavicular lymph node regions. A knowledge of the likelihood of spread to these areas and their significance is critical for planning treatment.

AXILLARY NODE INVOLVEMENT

The axillary lymph node region is the principal site of regional metastases from carcinoma of the breast, and approximately 40% to 50% of patients have evidence of spread to the axillary nodes. The likelihood of axillary nodal involvement appears to be related directly to the size of the primary tumor, as shown in Figure 38-7. Also, although the evidence for this is not clear-cut, most data suggest, that axillary node positivity is slightly more common with tumors located in the lateral portion of the breast than with those in the medial or central portion.

To some extent, the incidence of histologic involvement of axillary nodes is dependent on the extent of the pathologic analysis of the specimen. Pickren was the first to show that a more thorough clearing and sectioning of the axillary specimen resulted in a greater yield of positive nodes.[79] Of 51 specimens analyzed in routine fashion and found to be negative, 11 (22%) showed evidence of involvement on more careful analysis in that study.

Detection of axillary involvement by physical examination has both a high false-positive and a high false-negative rate (Table 38-9). When axillary lymph nodes are palpable, histologic evidence of metastatic disease is not found in approx-

FIG. 38-7. Relation between tumor size and axillary node involvement and recurrence and mortality rates. (Fisher B, Slack NH, Bross ID et al: Cancer of the breast: Size of neoplasm and prognosis. Cancer 24:1071–1080, 1969)

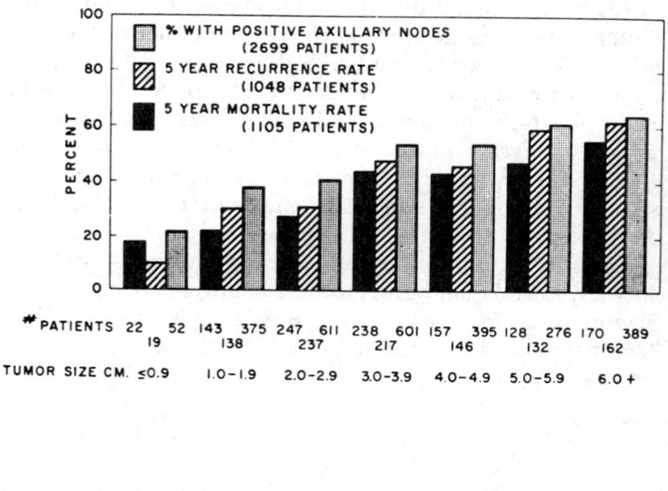

TABLE 38-9. Accuracy of Physical Examination in Predicting Histologic Involvement of Axillary Nodes

	*Series 1**	*Series 2†*	*Series 3‡*	*Series 4§*
False-positive (%)	25	24	26	29
False-negative (%)	32	32	27	29

* Butcher H: Radical mastectomy for mammary carcinoma. Ann Surg 170:883–884, 1969.
† Haagensen CD, Cooky E, Miller E et al: Treatment of early mammary carcinoma: A cooperative international study. Ann Surg 170:875–879, 1969.
‡ Schottenfeld D, Nash A, Robbins G, Beattie E: Ten-year results of the treatment of primary operable breast cancer. Cancer 38:1001–1007, 1976.
§ Bucalossi P, Veronesi U, Zingo L, Conti C: Enlarged mastectomy for breast cancer: Review of 1,213 cases. Am J Roentgenol Rad Ther Nucl Med 111:119–122, 1971.

TABLE 38-11. Ten-Year Survival (%) Related to Primary Tumor Size (cm) and Level of Axillary Involvement*

	Size of Primary (cm)			
Axillary Status	<2	2–5	>5	*Total*
Negative	82	65	44	72
Positive				
Proximal only	73	74	39	65
Middle or distal	–†	28	37	31
All	68	51	37	

* Schottenfeld D, Nash AG, Robbins GF et al: Ten-year results of the treatment of primary operable breast carcinoma. Cancer 38:1001–1007, 1976.
† Insufficient data.

imately 25% of cases. Conversely, when axillary nodes are not palpable, histologic involvement is detected in approximately 30% of cases. These shortcomings of clinical evaluation are of particular importance because histologic involvement of axillary nodes has a high correlation with prognosis. Table 38-10 shows 10-year survival figures according to axillary involvement from six separate series of patients treated with radical mastectomy. Patients with histologically negative axillary nodes have a markedly greater likelihood of survival than patients with histologic involvement. Furthermore, the prognosis is inversely related to the number of involved nodes.[80] At the current level of understanding, the presence and extent of metastases to the axilla represents the single most important prognostic factor for patients with breast cancer.

For the purposes of analysis, the axilla is commonly divided into three levels: proximal—tissue inferior to the lower border of the pectoralis minor muscle (I); middle—tissue directly beneath the pectoralis minor (II); and distal—tissue superior to the pectoralis minor (III). Prognosis is related to the level of axillary involvement (Table 38-11). Involvement of the upper level nodes carries a worse prognosis than involvement of proximal level nodes alone. In a series of 182 mastectomy specimens examined by clearing, involvement of nodes at the apex of the axilla was found in 15, and all 15 patients relapsed,[77] indicating the grave prognosis associated with involvement high in the axilla. Also, in general, involvement of upper-level nodes is associated with a high total number of lymph nodes involved; in this group of 15 patients, the mean number of involved nodes was 16.2 (range 4–37). In another study, axillary node involvement and survival were examined in 385 patients to determine whether the total number of involved nodes or the level of axillary involvement was the better indicator of prognosis.[81] For any given number of involved nodes, survival was independent of the level of involvement, and those investigators concluded that prognosis was related more directly to the total number of nodes involved than to the level of involvement.

The distribution of axillary node involvement by level has

TABLE 38-10. Percent Overall Survival (OS) and Disease-Free Survival (DFS) at 10 Years in Relation to Histologic Involvement of Axillary Lymph Nodes for Patients Treated by Radical Mastectomy

	*Series 1 DFS**	*Series 2 OS†*	*Series 3 OS‡*	*Series 4 DFS§*	*Series 5 OS¶*	*Series 6 OS‖*
Histologically negative	72	76	72	76	68	76
Histologically positive	25	48	43	24	27	35
1–3 nodes	34	63		36		
≥4 nodes	16	27		14		

* Valagussa P, Bonadonna G, Veronesi U: Patterns of relapse and survival following radical mastectomy. Cancer 41:1170–1178, 1978.
† Haagensen CD: Treatment of curable carcinoma of the breast. Int J Radiat Oncol Biol Phys 2:975–980, 1977.
‡ Schottenfeld D, Nash A, Robbins G, Beattie E: Ten-year results of the treatment of primary operable breast carcinoma. Cancer 38:1001–1007, 1976. *(A significant number of patients received postoperative irradiation.)*
§ Fisher B, Slack N, Katrych D: Ten-year followup results of patients with carcinoma of the breast in a cooperative clinical trial evaluating surgical adjuvant chemotherapy. Surg Gynecol Obstet 140:528–534, 1975.
¶ Spratt JS, Donegan WL: Cancer of the Breast. Philadelphia, WB Saunders, 1967.
‖ Payne WS, Taylor WF, Khonsari S: Surgical treatment of breast cancer: Trends and factors affecting survival. Arch Surg 101:105–113, 1970.

TABLE 38-12. Five-Year Relapse Rate (%) According to Size of Primary and Axillary Node Involvement

Axillary Status	Size of Primary (cm) <2	2–5	>5
Axillary Nodes Negative			
Fisher et al[84]	12	24	27
Nemoto et al[80]	13	19	25
Valagussa et al[53]	8	24	19
Axillary Nodes Positive			
Fisher et al[84]	50	60	79
Nemoto et al[80]	39	50	65
Valagussa et al[53]	37	64	74

been studied in two large series, with nearly identical results.[82,83] Involvement of level I alone was seen in 54% to 58% of cases; levels I and II in 20% to 22% of cases; and levels I, II, and III in 16% to 22% of cases. Involvement of levels II or III in the absence of involvement of level I ("skip metastases") was seen in only 2% to 4% of cases with nodal involvement. These results indicate that involvement of the axilla is by and large sequential. A level I dissection is therefore highly effective at determining the presence of nodal involvement but will frequently underestimate the extent of involvement.

Prognosis thus is related both to the size of the primary tumor and to axillary node involvement. Whether these two factors independently predict the outcome is addressed in Table 38-12. When axillary nodes are involved, the size of the tumor is still of prognostic value. For example, in the data from Valagussa and colleagues, the 5-year relapse rate was 37% for patients with positive nodes and small (≤2 cm) tumors and 79% for patients with positive nodes and large (>5 cm) tumors.[53] In the data from Fisher and coworkers, this correlation was analyzed further according to the number of positive axillary nodes (1 to 3 or 4 or more).[84] Within each subgroup with positive axillary nodes, the size of the primary tumor was still an independent prognostic factor. When axillary nodes are negative, however, the relation is less clear. The prognosis for patients with small (≤2 cm) tumors and negative nodes is exceptionally good, with a 5-year relapse rate of approximately 10%. For tumors larger than 2 cm, the prognosis is not as good. However, the prognosis for patients with large (>5 cm) tumors and negative nodes is not significantly worse than that of patients with 2- to 5-cm tumors and negative nodes. These data imply that the results of an axillary sampling are of value for prognostic purposes in patients with large primary tumors, because patients with histologically negative axillary nodes do relatively well even without adjuvant therapy. The 30-year results from Adair and associates support these observations: for patients with negative nodes, the 30-year survival rate was 61% when the primary tumor was no larger than 2 cm, 46% when it was 2 cm to 5 cm, and 50% when it was larger than 5 cm.[85] In contrast, for patients with involvement of level I axillary nodes, the 30-year survival rate was 40% when the tumor was no larger than 2 cm, 31% when it was 2 cm to 5 cm, and only 14% when it was larger than 5 cm.

In summary, the axillary nodal region is the principal drainage site for carcinoma of the breast, and a histologic analysis of the axilla provides a useful guide to prognosis. The more practical issue of what, if any, treatment is required for the axillary region will be addressed in later sections.

INTERNAL MAMMARY NODE INVOLVEMENT

The second major site of regional metastases for carcinoma of the breast is in the internal mammary lymph node (IMN) chain, which lies at the anterior ends of the intercostal spaces by the side of the internal thoracic artery. Because of their intrathoracic location and their uncommon clinical presentation, the frequency of internal mammary node involvement was not appreciated as early as was axillary node involvement. One of the first to document this second route of spread was Sampson Handley, who reported his results of internal mammary node biopsy in 1000 patients in 1975 (Table 38-13).[86] These results illustrate the following two points: (1) internal mammary node involvement is more common for inner quadrant or central tumors than for outer quadrant tumors; and (2) axillary lymph node involvement is more likely than is IMN involvement.

In the Handley study, even in patients with inner or central tumors, axillary involvement was more common than IMN involvement (42% versus 28%). Furthermore, if the axillary nodes were uninvolved, IMN involvement was uncommon (8%). Another larger series of patients reported from Italy has confirmed the Handley results.[87] In addition, these authors stressed the importance of primary tumor size in relation to IMN involvement: IMN involvement was seen in 19% of patients with tumors smaller than 5 cm, compared with 37% of patients with tumors larger than 5 cm.

The significance of IMN involvement is similar to that of axillary node involvement. In a large series reported by Veronesi and co-workers, the 10-year rate of disease-free survival was 73% when both the axillary nodes and the IMN were negative, 47% when axillary nodes alone were positive, 52% when the IMN alone were positive, and only 25% when both areas were positive.[88] In practice, however, biopsy of the IMN is associated with greater morbidity than biopsy of axillary nodes and is rarely performed.

SUPRACLAVICULAR NODE INVOLVEMENT

The principal route of spread to the supraclavicular lymph node areas is through the axillary node chain. In one series of

TABLE 38-13. Internal Mammary Node Involvement (%) in Relation to Location of the Primary and Axillary Node Involvement

	Primary Site UIQ	LIQ	Central	UOQ	LOQ
Total	27	33	32	14	13
	67/248	20/61	70/216	54/382	12/93
Axilla not involved	14	6	7	4	5
	20/143	2/36	5/76	7/170	2/40
Axilla involved	45	72	46	22	19
	47/105	18/25	65/140	47/212	10/53

Handley RS: Carcinoma of the breast. Ann R Coll Surg 57:59–66, 1975.

TABLE 38-14. Percentage of Patients with Metastases from Breast Cancer at Various Sites in Three Collected Series

	Series 1 (*n* = 160)*	*Series 2* (*n* = 43)†	*Series 3* (*n* = 100)‡
Lung	59	65	69
Liver	58	56	65
Bone	44	–	71
Pleura	37	23	51
Adrenals	31	41	49
Kidneys	NR§	14	17
Spleen	14	23	17
Pancreas	–	11	17
Ovaries	9	16	20
Brain	–	9	22
Thyroid	–	–	24
Heart	–	–	11
Diaphragm	–	–	11
Pericardium	5	21	19
Intestine	–	–	18
Peritoneum	12	9	13
Uterus	–	–	15
Lymph nodes	72	–	76
Skin	34	7	30

* Warren S, Witman EM: Studies on tumor metastases: The distribution of metastases in cancer of the breast. Surg Gynecol Obstet 57:81–1018, 1937.

† Saphillo O, Parker ML: Metastases from primary carcinoma of the breast with special reference to spleen, adrenal glands and ovaries. Arch Surg 42:1003, 1941.

‡ Haagensen CD: Diseases of the Breast. Philadelphia, WB Saunders, 1971.

§ NR = not recorded.

patients undergoing routine supraclavicular dissection, involvement of the region was found in 23 (18%) of the 125 patients who had involvement of axillary nodes but in none of the 149 patients who did not have involvement of axillary nodes.[89] The significance of supraclavicular node involvement was first shown by Halsted, who performed a supraclavicular dissection in 119 patients. Forty-four women (37%) were found to have involvement of these nodes, and only two were free of cancer at 5 years.[90] Supraclavicular node involvement represents a late stage of axillary nodal involvement and carries a grave prognosis.

DISTANT METASTASES

Metastatic spread from carcinoma of the breast can be present in a variety of organs. The likelihood of organ involvement has been studied in a number of autopsy series (Table 38-14).

STAGING

Staging refers to the grouping of patients according to the extent of their disease. It is useful in choosing treatment for individual patients, estimating their prognosis, and comparing the results of different treatment programs. Staging of breast cancer is performed initially on a clinical basis, according to the physical examination as well as laboratory and radiologic evaluation.

The most widely used clinical staging system is the one adopted by both the International Union against Cancer (UICC) and the American Joint Commission on Cancer Staging and End Results Reporting (AJC). It is based on the tumor–nodes–metastases (TNM) system as detailed in the *Manual for Staging of Cancer* (2nd edition, 1983):

T	Primary tumors
T1	Tumor 2 cm or less in its greatest dimension a. No fixation to underlying pectoral fascia or muscle b. Fixation to underlying pectoral fascia or muscle
T2	Tumor more than 2 cm but not more than 5 cm in its greatest dimension
T3	Tumor more than 5 cm in its greatest dimension a. No fixation to underlying pectoral fascia or muscle b. Fixation to underlying pectoral fascia or muscle
T4	Tumor of any size with direct extension to chest wall or skin. *Note:* Chest wall includes ribs, intercostal muscles, and serratus anterior muscle, but not pectoral muscle. a. Fixation to chest wall b. Edema (including peau d'orange), ulceration of the skin of the breast, or satellite skin nodules confined to the same breast c. Both of the above d. Inflammatory carcinoma

Dimpling of the skin, nipple retraction, or any other skin changes except those in T4b may occur in T1, T2, or T3 without affecting the classification.

N	Regional lymph nodes
N0	No palpable homolateral axillary nodes
N1	Movable homolateral axillary nodes a. Nodes not considered to contain growth b. Nodes considered to contain growth
N2	Homolateral axillary nodes containing growth and fixed to one another or to other structures
N3	Homolateral supraclavicular or infraclavicular nodes containing growth or edema of the arm.

M	Distant metastasis
M0	No evidence of distant metastasis
M1	Distant metastasis present, including skin involvement beyond the breast area.

Clinical stage grouping

Stage I	T1a or T1b,	N0 or N1a,	M0
Stage II	T0,	N1b,	M0
	T1a or T1b,	N1b,	M0
	T2a or T2b,	N0, N1a, or N1b,	M0
Stage III	T1a or T1b,	N2,	M0
	T2a or T2b,	N2,	M0
	T3a or T3b,	N0, N1 or N2,	M0

Stage IV	T4,	any N,	any M
	any T,	N3,	any M
	any T,	any N,	M1

Another clinical staging system, the Columbia Clinical Classification, (CCC), is at present less widely used but is of historical importance. Like the UICC–AJC system, patients are grouped according to the extent of disease in the primary tumor site, nodal areas, and distant metastases:

Stage A: No skin edema, ulceration, or solid fixation of the tumor to the chest wall. Axillary nodes are not involved clinically.

Stage B: No skin edema, ulceration, or solid fixation of the tumor to the chest wall. Clinically involved nodes, but less than 2.5 cm in transverse diameter and not fixed to overlying skin or deeper structures of the axilla.

Stage C: Any one of the five grave signs of advanced breast carcinoma:
- (1) Edema of the skin of limited extent (involving less than one-third of the skin over the breast)
- (2) Skin ulceration
- (3) Solid fixation of the tumor to the chest wall
- (4) Extensive involvement of axillary lymph nodes (measuring 2.5 cm or more in transverse diameter)
- (5) Fixation of the axillary nodes to overlying skin or deeper structures of the axilla.

Stage D: All other patients with more advanced breast carcinoma, including:
- (1) A combination of any two or more of the five grave signs listed under Stage C
- (2) Extensive edema of the skin (involving more than one-third of the skin over the breast)
- (3) Satellite skin nodules
- (4) Inflammatory type of carcinoma
- (5) Clinically involved supraclavicular lymph nodes
- (6) Internal mammary metastases as evidenced by a parasternal tumor
- (7) Edema of the arm
- (8) Distant metastases.

Both clinical systems are based on the results of surgery in treating breast cancer. The principal points of discrepancy between the UICC–AJC system and the CCC system are the recognition by the UICC–AJC that primary tumor size by itself is of prognostic importance, and the recognition by the CCC that axillary metastases larger than 2.5 cm usually indicate extension beyond the lymph node capsule and therefore a high risk of local recurrence.

As noted before, clinical evaluation of spread to the axilla has a high false-positive and false-negative rate. For this reason, pathologic staging based on histologic study of the axillary specimen is preferable. For the individual patient, prognosis is better determined by pathologic staging than by clinical staging (Table 38-15). For patients who have clinical indications of spread of tumor but negative histologic evaluations, the survival rate (72%) is similar to that of the entire group of patients with histologically negative nodes (76%), not to that of the group with histologically positive nodes (48%).[91] Similarly, if a patient does not have clinical evidence of axillary involvement but microscopic involvement is detected pathologically, the survival rate (57%) is similar to that of the entire group of patients with microscopic involvement (48%).

TABLE 38-15. Ten-Year Survival (%) According to Clinical and Pathologic Assessment of Axillary Nodes*

	Pathologic Assessment		
Clinical Assessment	*N–*	*N+*	*All*
N0	77	57	71
N1	72	34	44
All	76	48	

* Haagensen CD: Treatment of curable carcinoma of the breast. Int J Radiat Oncol Biol Phys 2:975–980, 1977.

Pathologic stage is commonly given as Stage I (axillary nodes not involved) or Stage II (axillary nodes involved). Refinements of this simple staging format have been made, such as subdividing Stage II according to the number of positive axillary nodes. Because prognosis is clearly related to the extent of axillary involvement (see Table 38-10), it has become convention to subdivide axillary involvement into one to three nodes positive or more than four nodes positive. Another refinement is based on the recognition that micrometastatic involvement of axillary lymph nodes is not associated with the poor prognosis seen with macrometastatic involvement. A comparison of the significance of these two types of axillary metastases has been the object of recent pathologic study. In one study, occult metastases were demonstrated in the regional lymph nodes by an extended histopathologic technique in 24% of 78 cases of invasive breast cancer that would have been regarded as pathologic Stage I (no nodal metastases) after "routine" pathologic examination.[92] Patients in whom the largest nodal metastases measured 2 mm or less in greatest diameter (micrometastases) were compared with those in whom the lesions were larger than 2 mm (macrometastases). Life-table analysis revealed no significant difference in survival rates of patients with micrometastases and those without nodal metastases, and both of these groups exhibited a significantly greater likelihood of survival than patients with macrometastases. In another study, by Huvos and coworkers from Memorial Hospital in New York City, prognosis also was related to the pathologic extent of axillary nodal involvement.[93] For the 62 patients with no involvement of the axillary nodes, the 8-year survival rate was 82% (51 of 62). When micrometastatic involvement (defined as less than 2 mm) of level I axillary nodes was found, the 8-year survival rate was 94% (17 of 18). In comparison, the survival rate was 62% (28 of 45) for patients with macrometastatic involvement of level I axillary nodes.

Other refinements of the pathologic staging scheme are based on the recognition that extension of metastatic disease beyond the lymph node capsule or involvement of an axillary node larger than 2 cm have been associated with a worse prognosis, independent of the number of nodes involved. These refinements have been included in the Postsurgical Treatment Pathological Classification given by the UICC–AJC in 1977:

Primary tumor (T)
- T0 No evidence of primary tumor
- T1–4 Same as UICC–AJC classification except for subdivision of T1 into
  - i: Tumor less than 0.5 cm
  - ii: Tumor 0.5 cm–0.9 cm
  - iii: Tumor 1.0 cm–1.9 cm

Nodal involvement (N)
- N No metastatic homolateral axillary nodal involvement
- N1 Movable homolateral axillary metastatic nodes not fixed to one another or to other structures
- N1a Lymph nodes with only histologic evidence of metastatic growth
- N1b Gross metastatic carcinoma in lymph nodes
  - i: Micrometastatic (smaller than 0.2 cm)
  - ii: Metastasis (larger than 0.2 cm) in one to three lymph nodes
  - iii: Metastasis to four or more lymph nodes
  - iv: Extension of metastasis beyond the lymph node capsule
  - v: Any positive node greater than 2 cm in diameter
- N2–3 Same as clinical UICC–AJC classification.

SCREENING FOR BREAST CANCER

Screening for cancer represents an important advance in the management of the disease. Two randomized clinical trials have demonstrated a 25% to 30% reduction in breast cancer mortality rates in screened individuals.[94-97] These results are consistent with those obtained in nonrandomized studies.[98-100] The cost : benefit ratio for the use of mammography and its optimal frequency are still a matter of debate.[101-107] However, a randomized controlled clinical trial from Sweden has shown that single view mammography in women 40 years of age or older with repeat screening every 2 or 3 years resulted in an approximately 30% reduction in mortality (Fig. 38-8).[97] These issues are discussed in detail in Chapter 20, section 4.

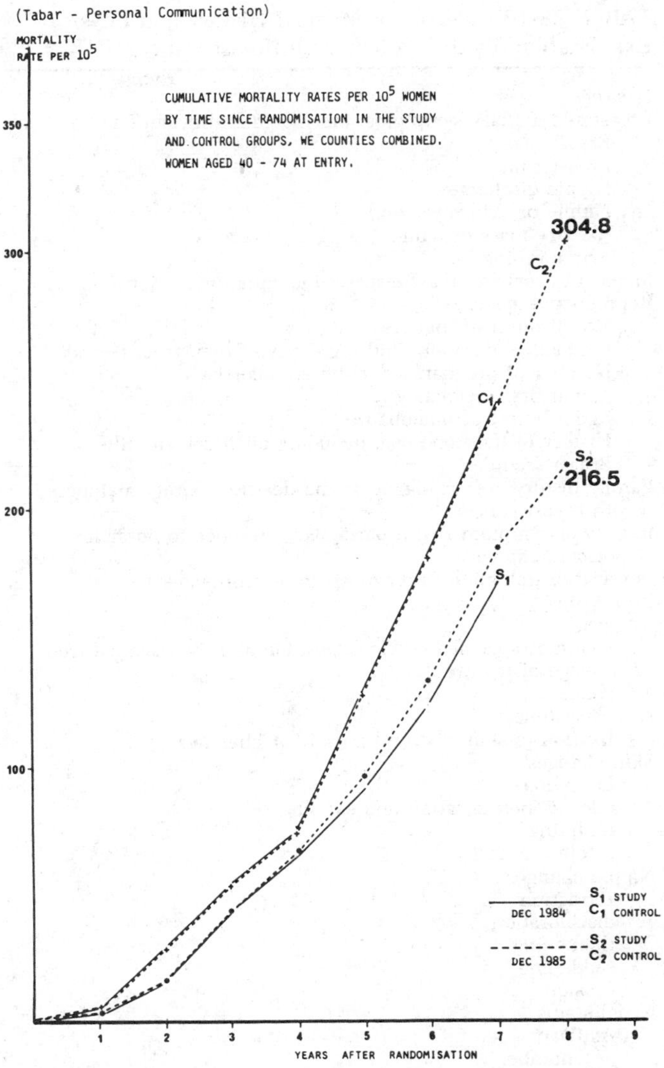

FIG. 38-8. Cumulative mortality rates for screened and control populations. (Tabar L: Unpublished data)

PRETREATMENT EVALUATION

There is general agreement that the pretreatment evaluation of a patient with breast cancer should include a thorough medical history and physical examination (Table 38-16), chest roentgenogram (postero-anterior and lateral views), complete bloodcount, and liver chemistries. The value of other tests (bone scan, liver scan, and mammogram) has been a matter of controversy.

Radionuclide scans are acknowledged to be a sensitive test for early bone metastases. However, the yield of bone scanning in asymptomatic patients with early breast cancer is small. For example, in one study from John Hopkins, only 1 of 64 patients with clinical Stage I or II breast cancer had a positive preoperative bone scan, whereas 25% of patients with Stage III disease had positive scans preoperatively.[108] In another study from the Peter Bent Brigham Hospital, the yield of bone scanning was 0 of 37 in clinical Stage I, 4% in Stage II, and 16% in Stage III.[109] In addition, bone scans can be positive in a number of benign bone conditions, and this can delay treatment and increase patient anxiety. These data suggest that a scan is warranted in Stage III breast cancer, but its usefulness in early stage disease is less certain. Some clinicians claim that a bone scan should be obtained in all patients as a baseline for future comparison, but this justification has not been established.

TABLE 38-16. Pertinent Medical History and Physical Examination for the Patient with Breast Cancer

History

- Breast and axillary symptoms: first noted and evolution
  - Breast mass
  - Breast pain
  - Nipple discharge
  - Nipple or skin retraction
  - Axillary mass or pain
  - Arm swelling
- Medical history of breast disease, including prior biopsies
- Reproductive history
  - Age of onset of menses
  - Frequency, duration, and regularity of menstrual periods
  - Number of pregnancies, children, abortions
  - Age at first pregnancy
  - Age of onset of menopause
  - History of hormone use, including birth control pills
  - Breast feeding
- Family history: age at diagnosis and death of family members with breast cancer
- Review of symptoms, with particular reference to possible metastatic spread
- Physical examination (a diagnosis is recommended)
- Breast Mass
  - size
  - location (specified by clock position and the distance from edge of the areola)
  - shape
  - consistency
  - fixation to skin, pectoral muscle or chest wall
- Skin changes
  - erythema
  - edema (note location and extent)
  - dimpling
  - satellite nodules
- Nipple changes
  - retraction
  - discoloration
  - thickening
  - reddening
  - erosion
- Nodal status
  - Axillary
    - number
    - location
    - size
    - fixation to other nodes or underlying structures
    - clinically suspicious or benign
  - Infraclavicular fullness
  - Supraclavicular nodes or area swelling

The yield of positive pretreatment liver scans is even smaller than that of bone scans. In a series of 234 patients studied with routine preoperative liver scans at the Mt. Sinai Hospital of Cleveland, only 12 (5%) had abnormal scans.[110] Of further interest, eight of these abnormal scans were established as false-positive by further evaluation, so that the ultimate result of the test was only 1% positivity. These findings are not surprising when one considers that metastases larger than 2 cm are required for visualization on liver scans.[111] It generally is recommended that liver scans be reserved for patients with abnormal liver chemistries or hepatomegaly.

It is worth emphasizing that a positive bone or liver scan does not necessarily establish metastatic disease. Both these tests commonly have significant false-positive rates, and the results of a positive scan must be viewed within the context of the total evaluation of the patient. In many cases, histologic confirmation should be obtained before definitive primary therapy is abandoned.

Bilateral mammograms are recommended before a biopsy of a suspicious breast mass to detect any occult lesion that also should be biopsied, either in the ipsilateral or the contralateral breast. The use of mammograms in this setting clearly improves the preoperative diagnostic accuracy, but a negative mammogram in the presence of a suspicious breast mass is not a justification to avoid biopsy. The use of mammography in patients with a positive biopsy is also important, especially in checking the contralateral breast. For patients who will be treated with mastectomy, the detection of additional lesions in the involved breast is of limited value. If a patient is to be treated with conservative surgery and radiation therapy, however, the detection of additional lesions is important, as discovery of multicentric lesions would influence a decision for additional surgery, an altered radiotherapeutic program, or possibly mastectomy. Occult, suspicious areas found on mammography should be removed after preoperative needle localization, which ensures excision of these areas with minimal deformity. When more than one lesion is to be excised, placement of the incisions should be planned to be most cosmetically acceptable if breast preservation is to be done yet without compromise of a possible mastectomy incision.

Newer diagnostic modalities, such as ultrasound, CT scan, and magnetic resonance imaging (MRI) of the breast, have been compared with mammography. None has proved more accurate, and they have the disadvantages of not detecting calcifications, delivering higher radiation doses (CT), and taking more patient time and costing more (CT and MRI).[112]

Radionuclide brain scans and CT scans of the head are both sensitive tests to detect early metastatic involvement. The yield of these studies in a pretreatment setting is very small, however, and they are not recommended in the absence of suspicious signs or symptoms.

An area of growing interest has been the use of biologic markers (see section on markers). A number of substances including carcinoembryonic antigen (CEA), ferritin, and human chorionic gonadotropin (hCG) have been suggested as possible markers. In patients with metastatic breast cancer, 70% have elevated CEA levels, 50% have elevated hCG levels, and 67% have elevated ferritin levels.[113-117] There is preliminary evidence that pretreatment marker concentrations can be a prognostic indicator. In one study, patients with postoperative CEA levels greater than 2.5 ng/ml had a 2-year recurrence rate of 65% compared with 20% for those with normal CEA levels ($p < 0.001$). The use of serial marker determination in the follow-up period also has been suggested as a means for the early detection of recurrence. This field is rapidly evolving, and firm recommendations are not possible at this time. Nevertheless, pretreatment measurements, particularly of CEA, are obtained easily and relatively inexpensively.

SURGICAL MANAGEMENT OF PRIMARY BREAST CANCER

HISTORICAL BACKGROUND

Surgical attempts to provide local–regional control of breast cancer through the end of the 19th century failed uniformly. Patients generally presented with advanced, bulky disease, and various surgeons reported local recurrence rates of 60% to 80%.

In 1894, Halsted published a description of his technique of radical mastectomy, which included excision of a wide margin of skin around the tumor, dissection of thin skin flaps, and en bloc removal of the breast, axillary lymph nodes, and pectoralis major and minor muscles. The local recurrence rate with this technique was 6%.[118] Although most patients later died of distant metastases, the Halsted procedure was recognized as a significant advance and was widely practiced. Indeed, for the first three-quarters of the 20th century, it was the surgical procedure of choice for patients with operable breast carcinoma. Haagensen extended this approach, advocating a wider skin excision which required a skin graft for closure.[119] He also developed the CCC staging system to select patients with lesions more favorable for mastectomy and to classify those with more advanced stages ("grave signs") as inoperable (see section on staging).

The extended radical mastectomy, described by Urban and Baker,[120] added an en bloc dissection of the IMN chain to the radical mastectomy. This operation required an intrapleural dissection with removal of a portion of the sternum and rib cage and closure of the defect with fascia over a chest tube.

In the same time period, other surgeons explored the feasibility of preserving the pectoralis major muscle to improve the cosmetic results. This procedure, termed "modified radical mastectomy," included total mastectomy, axillary dissection, preservation of the pectoralis major muscle, and excision of the pectoralis minor muscle, as described by Patey or later, with preservation of this small muscle, as reported by Auchincloss.[121] This procedure has been the standard surgical approach since the 1970s because of the availability of long-term results showing its effectiveness both in treating multicentric disease in the breast and in treating the axilla. The factors underlying the use of modified radical mastectomy will be discussed below.

MULTICENTRICITY

The reported incidence of multicentric (or multifocal) breast cancer in areas away from the primary tumor in mastectomy specimens ranges from 9% to 75%.[122] This large discrepancy is caused by three factors: differences in the precision of the definition of multicentricity, different techniques of examination, and variations in the extent of the tissue sampling. When sections of breast tissue are taken from each of the three quadrants apart from that containing the primary tumor, high rates of multicentricity have been reported. This was true in a simulated partial mastectomy series of Rosen and colleagues,[123] who reported residual cancer in 56% of patients. In a more recent study of patients with clinically occult (nonpalpable) breast cancers detected by mammography, there was a 44% incidence of multicentricity.[124] When these tumors were microinvasive pathologically, 57% showed multicentricity. In another series of patients from Memorial Hospital who underwent mastectomy for in situ cancers, multicentric disease was present in 60%.[125] Thus, even in the earliest (or nonpalpable) breast cancers treated, occult multicentricity is frequently present.

Lagios and associates[126] examined mastectomy specimens for tumor foci outside a 5-cm radius of the reference tumor, the hypothetical border of a breast quadrant. Multicentricity was found in 20% of cases. This is similar to the findings of Rosen's group of residual tumor in 26% and 38% of cases with reference tumors smaller than and larger than 2 cm, respectively.[123] More recently, Holland and associates examined the mastectomy specimens of patients who would have been considered candidates for breast-sparing procedures and mapped cancer at various distances from the primary tumor.[127] As described elsewhere in this chapter, although most of the cancer was found within the quadrant containing the primary tumor, many patients also had evidence of cancer far from the primary tumor site. In all of these studies, the principal form of breast cancer found in other quadrants was in situ cancer.

The more important question is whether these histologic findings of breast cancer indicate clinical activity, or if they represent "anatomic cancers," with little or no biologic implication. There are few long-term studies of patients with in situ breast cancer treated with biopsy alone. However, the available data for both lobular carcinoma in situ and intraductal carcinoma indicate that over a long period, a significant percentage of these patients will develop invasive breast cancer (see section on in situ cancer).

Additional circumstantial evidence that untreated cancer will progress is that unsuspected cancer is rarely found on autopsies done on elderly women dying of causes other than breast cancer. In a series of 70 patients over the age of 70 years, only four patients (5.7%) had intraductal cancer, one of these with microinvasion.[128] This result contrasts with the much higher incidence of unsuspected prostate cancer found in men at autopsy[129] and suggests that breast cancer is more likely to express itself as a clinical entity during the patient's life.

AXILLARY NODE METASTASES

There are four potential advantages to axillary dissection. First, the procedure provides prognostic information and helps determine the treatment plan. Patients with histologically involved nodes are considered candidates for adjuvant systemic therapy. Accurate staging thus benefits the patient, her family, and physicians.

Second, such dissection is reliable treatment of the axilla: few local recurrences in this area are seen after such dissection in patients with histologically positive nodes.[85,130] If conservative surgery and radiotherapy is the treatment of choice, irradiation of the axilla is unnecessary if complete dissection has been done.

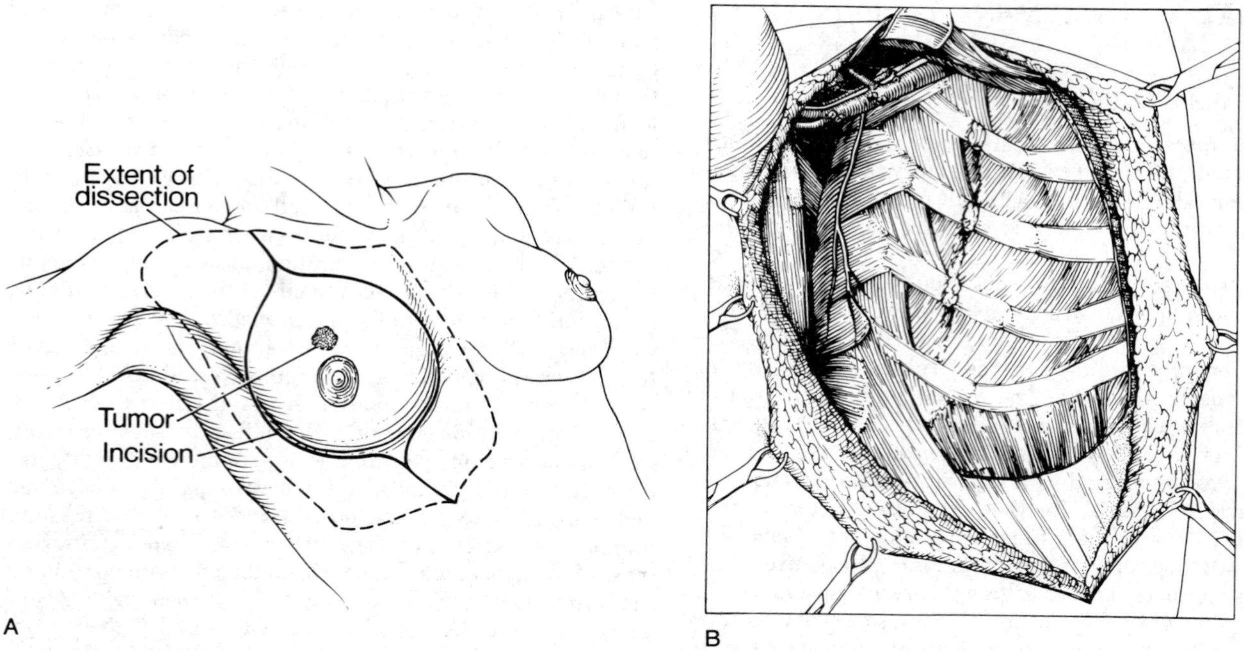

FIG. 38-9. Radical mastectomy. **A**. Outline of vertical incision (*solid lines*) widely encompassing a tumor at the 12:00 axis. Extent of underlying tissue removed is outlined by dotted lines. **B**. Operative field after removal of specimen, showing complete removal of breast, axillary nodes, and both pectoral muscles. Underlying chest wall is shown with intact long thoracic nerve laterally. (Kinne DW. In Harris JR, Hellman S, Henderson IC, Kinne DW [eds]: Breast Diseases, pp 267–268. Philadelphia, JB Lippincott, 1987)

Third, it is possible that axillary dissection improves overall survival. Long-term retrospective studies have shown that many patients with positive nodes are disease free many years after mastectomy, although their prognosis is certainly worse than that of patients with negative nodes.[85,131] However, modern studies suggest that axillary treatment does not greatly affect survival.[132] These studies will be discussed below.

A fourth potential benefit of axillary dissection is palliative. If bulky nodal disease can be excised, patients who eventually succumb to distant metastases may be spared painful lymphedematous extremities caused by tumor involvement of the neurovascular bundle.

LONG-TERM RESULTS WITH MASTECTOMY

Radical mastectomy was once the standard treatment for breast cancer in this country and, as a result, there are many studies using this procedure with long-term results. This en bloc dissection of the breast, all axillary nodes, and both pectoralis muscles is depicted in Figure 38-9. Haagensen reviewed his 50-year personal experience with 1036 patients treated by this procedure.[131] Results were given according to the CCC (see section on staging, above). Local recurrence rates 10 years after radical mastectomy were 3.7% in Stage A disease and 12% in Stage B. Pathologically involved nodes were recovered in 31% of patients with clinical Stage A and 72% of those with Stage B disease. The overall 10-year disease-free survival rate was 77% for patients with negative nodes and 49% for patients with positive nodes.

Robbins and Berg[133] reported 30-year follow-up on 1458 patients treated at Memorial Hospital with standard radical mastectomy. Thirteen percent of these women survived 30 years free of cancer, 57% died of breast cancer, 24% died of other causes, and 6% were lost to follow-up. As noted before, axillary nodal status was a more important determinant of prognosis than was the size of the primary tumor: patients with tumors smaller than 2 cm and involved nodes did worse than those with large tumors and negative nodes.

The 10-year follow-up of 304 patients treated at Memorial Hospital and classified by the TNM system is reported by Schottenfeld and associates.[130] Eighty-five percent of patients were treated with radical mastectomy and the rest with extended radical, modified radical, or total mastectomy. Thirty-six percent of patients with Stage II or III disease received postoperative radiotherapy. No patient received adjuvant systemic therapy. No local recurrences developed in patients with Stage I disease within 10 years, but recurrence was noted in 6% of those with clinical Stage II or III disease, which is similar to the local recurrence risks reported by Haagensen quoted above.[131] Overall 10-year survival rates were 91% for clinical Stage I, 57% for Stage II, and 34% for Stage III. Overall, patients with clinically negative nodes had a 71% survival rate compared with 48% in patients with positive nodes. As in the Robbins series, the level of axillary metastases was correlated with survival. If the highest axillary node involved was level I, the survival rate was 65%, with a decrease in survival to 30% if levels II and III had metastases. As noted earlier, there is a close correlation between the level of involvement and the total number of nodes harboring metastases.

AXILLARY NODE TREATMENT

The optimal extent of an axillary dissection is not clear. As noted in the section on local spread, skip metastases to the upper levels of axillary nodes are uncommon. The difficulty in interpreting these studies is that they are undertaken in the pathology laboratory on radical or modified radical mastectomy specimens. Although axillary levels were indicated by placement of tags in the operating room, the boundaries between levels are indistinct. Perhaps of more clinical importance is the study by Davies and colleagues at Guy's Hospital[134] comparing clinical examination with a simple axillary node biopsy done in the operating room, with axillary node sampling, and with the completed axillary dissection in the same patients. Axillary node biopsy failed to detect metastases in 42% of patients, and axillary node sampling or excision of nodes in the axillary tail missed 14% of patients with axillary metastases. Even if axillary dissection is considered only a staging procedure, it is apparent that a significant number of patients with involved nodes would not be identified by lesser sampling procedures.

One rationale for a complete dissection is that the upper levels of the axilla are commonly involved when the lower level nodes are involved. An incomplete dissection will therefore underestimate the extent of involvement and will commonly leave involved nodes behind. This is likely to influence the risk of axillary recurrence even if there is no association with an effect on survival. In an analysis of 539 patients with axillary metastases who underwent total axillary dissection, 40% of patients who had involved level I nodes also had positive nodes at higher levels.[82] If a level I and II dissection had been done, 20% would have had involved level III nodes left behind. In another study, 20% of patients with one to three positive lymph nodes in a sampling procedure were found to have four or more involved nodes by complete axillary dissection.[135] This result may have implications for the systemic therapy program undertaken. However, recent studies suggest that a level I and II dissection[136,137] or even a level I dissection alone[138] may adequately stage patients and control disease in the axilla.

The value of treating axillary nodes was examined in a trial performed by the NSABP. The NSABP B-04 trial, begun in 1971, randomized patients with clinically negative axillae to either radical mastectomy, total mastectomy and irradiation of the axillary nodes, or total mastectomy with delayed axillary dissection if nodes became clinically involved. The 10-year results showed no significant differences among the three groups of patients in disease-free or overall survival rates (57%).[132] Forty percent of patients with clinically negative axillary nodes who were treated with radical mastectomy had histologically positive nodes. Assuming that the same percentage of patients undergoing total mastectomy had microscopic involvement of these nodes, it is of interest that only 18% required delayed axillary dissection because of the development of clinically positive nodes. This finding has been interpreted to mean that not all histologically positive nodes will become biologically active. The results of the NSABP B-04 trial suggest that untreated positive nodes did not serve as a source of further dissemination, leading to a higher rate of distant metastases. There is no support in this study for the concept that nodal metastases in themselves instigate distant metastases. Also of importance is that in the group receiving irradiation to the axilla, these foci were well controlled, with only 3.1% presenting with axillary recurrence.

An analysis of NSABP B-04 trial by Harris and Osteen[139] points out that 35% of patients assigned to treatment by total mastectomy alone actually had a limited axillary dissection. This subgroup of patients required subsequent axillary dissection in fewer instances than did patients who had no nodes removed initially. Furthermore, many patients likely developed axillary metastases at the time of or subsequent to the appearance of distant metastases, thus making axillary dissection unnecessary, and some patients may have had unresectable axillary recurrences. Therefore, the true incidence of axillary failure is unknown. The impact of axillary treatment on survival is also unknown from this study. Because 60% of patients did not have axillary involvement and many of the 40% who did have also had occult distant metastases, the percentage of patients helped by axillary treatment can only be small. It is possible that the trial was simply not large enough to detect a small but clinically significant benefit.

Although providing interesting and important information on the biologic behavior of breast cancer, the NSABP study provides little practical guidance in the management of patients today. With the widespread use of adjuvant systemic therapy for patients with positive axillary nodes, most, if not all, breast cancer patients are advised to undergo axillary dissection as part of the staging. If patients are judged prior to treatment not to be candidates for any systemic therapy—for example, because of advanced age or severe medical illness—this study indicates that either irradiation of the nodes or observation with delayed dissection when they become clinically involved are reasonable options.

MODIFIED RADICAL MASTECTOMY

The modified radical mastectomy, also termed total mastectomy with axillary lymph node dissection and preservation of the pectoralis major muscle, is not as precisely defined or standardized as the radical mastectomy. The pectoralis minor muscle may be excised or divided or left intact, and, more importantly, there may be variation in the extent of axillary lymph node dissection ranging from sampling to full dissection.

One virtue of the modified radical mastectomy is that nearly all patients with operable breast cancers are unquestionable candidates for it. This includes patients with Stages I, II, and III breast cancer not fixed to the pectoralis major muscle or accompanied by bulky axillary lymph node involvement (the latter clinical settings suggesting the advis-

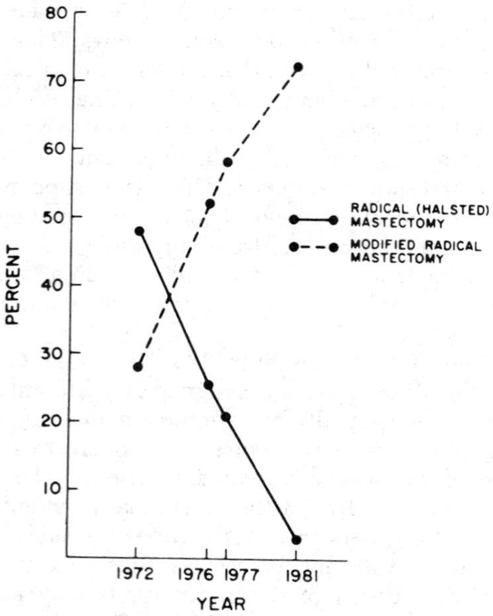

FIG. 38-10. Percentage of patients undergoing Halsted radical mastectomy and modified radical mastectomy in the 1982 National Survey of Cancer of the Breast in the United States. (Wilson RE et al: Trends in operative procedures in the United States, 1972–87, Surg Gynecol Obstet 159:309, 1984)

ability of radical mastectomy). The 1982 National Survey of Carcinoma of the Breast in the United States by the American College of Surgeons,[140] an aggregation of data from several hundred hospitals in the United States, encompassed about one-fifth of the incident cases of breast cancer for that year and is compared with similar surveys conducted in 1972 and 1977 in Figure 38-10. Although breast-sparing procedures were carried out in only 7.2% of cases in this survey, a lag time exists, and it is likely that a higher percentage of breast-conserving operations is being done today. At Memorial Sloan-Kettering Cancer Center, 824 patients with breast cancer were treated by members of the Breast Service in 1986. Sixty-six percent of patients underwent modified radical mastectomy compared with 3% having radical mastectomy. Breast preservation approaches (partial mastectomy, axillary dissection followed by radiation therapy) were performed in 215 patients, or 26%. This represents an increase from 8% of the total number of patients so treated in 1983 and 21% in 1985.

The procedure for modified radical mastectomy is shown in Figure 38-11. The cosmetic difference between this and radical mastectomy, shown in Figure 38-12, is apparent. With a low transverse scar, an intact pectoralis major muscle, and the use of an external prosthesis, more options for clothing are possible with the modified procedure. Also, the breast is easier to reconstruct with intact tissues whereas with a radical mastectomy, a myocutaneous flap is required to fill in the axillary hollow.

The change to modified radical mastectomy was brought about by several factors. Pathologic analysis of axillary nodes indicated that similar numbers were removed in the modified and the radical mastectomy procedures, and retrospective analysis showed similar overall survival rates for patients treated with either procedure.[141] Of note, a higher local recurrence rate was observed for patients with Stage III disease treated with modified radical mastectomy. This observation was corroborated in a prospective trial by Maddox and colleagues,[142] who noted no differences in overall or disease-free survival in patients undergoing radical or modified radical mastectomies but higher local recurrence rates for patients in the modified operation group who had Stage III lesions. Long follow-up of retrospective series, as reported by the Mayo Clinic,[143] shows nearly identical 10-year survival rates for patients treated by either procedure (approximately 74% for each). These data support the adoption of modified radical mastectomy as the procedure of choice.

Local recurrence after modified radical mastectomy is apparently not influenced by the proximity to the pectoralis major muscle. Patients with a deep margin of 1 mm or less have few local recurrences,[144] suggesting that an intact pectoral fascia is an effective tumor barrier. However, en bloc excision of a small portion of muscle beneath a deep tumor (or a biopsy site of uncertain depth) is useful to ensure an adequate deep margin.[145]

EXTENDED RADICAL MASTECTOMY

Extended radical mastectomy is defined as a standard radical mastectomy plus resection of the internal mammary nodes. Urban reported favorable results with this procedure for selected patients.[146] The survival rate of patients with involved IMN and uninvolved axillary nodes (54%) was identical to that of patients with a positive axilla and a negative internal mammary chain. A prospective randomized trial by Veronesi and Valagussa showed no survival differences between patients treated with radical or extended radical mastectomy.[147] The operation is seldom practiced in this country, accounting for about 1% of all procedures.[140]

However, Lacour and associates recently published 15-year results of patients treated at the Institut Gustave-Roussy with either radical or extended radical mastectomy.[148] For the subset of patients with medial lesions and positive nodes, the overall survival rate was 53% for extended radical mastectomy compared with 28% for radical mastectomy. The small numbers of patients in this subset cast doubt on the significance of this finding.

TOTAL MASTECTOMY

Sometimes referred to as simple mastectomy, this procedure removes the entire breast, including the nipple–areolar complex, but without axillary node dissection or removal of the pectoralis muscles. The operation has four principal indications:

1. Patients with in situ carcinoma (ductal or lobular) with no suspicious axillary lymphadenopathy, among whom metastatic disease to the axillary nodes occurs in less than 1%;
2. Carefully selected patients undergoing prophylactic mastectomy, often of the contralateral breast;

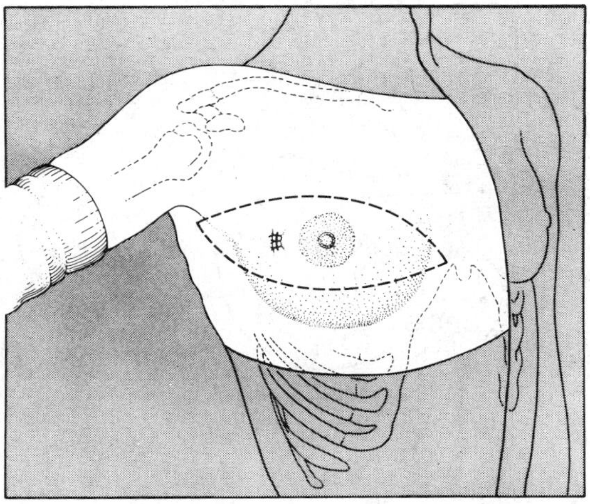

A

FIG. 38-11. Modified radical mastectomy. **A**. Skin incision, transversely placed. **B**. Pectoralis major muscle with intact neuromuscular bundle retracted medially. Pectoralis minor has been divided near coracoid process and will be excised. **C**. Completely dissected axilla, with intact pectoralis major muscle and long thoracic nerve and divided thoracoabdominal bundle (the latter may be preserved in a clinically negative axilla). (Kinne DW: In Harris JR, Hellman S, Henderson IC, Kinne DW [eds]: Breast Diseases, pp 263–266. Philadelphia, JB Lippincott, 1987)

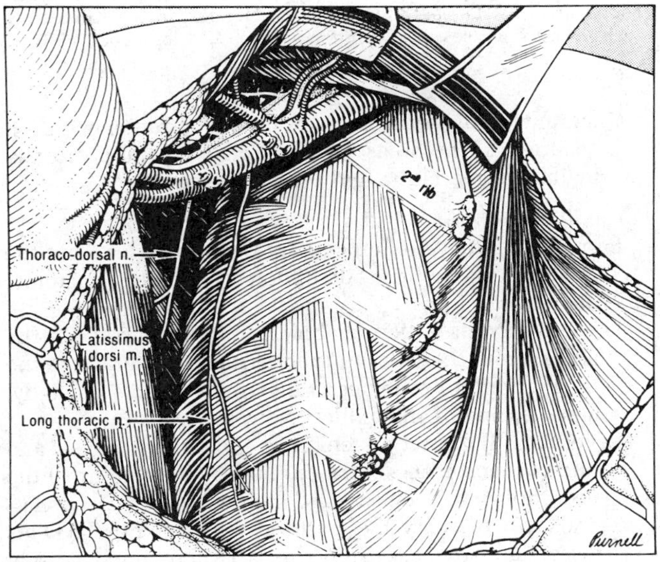

B

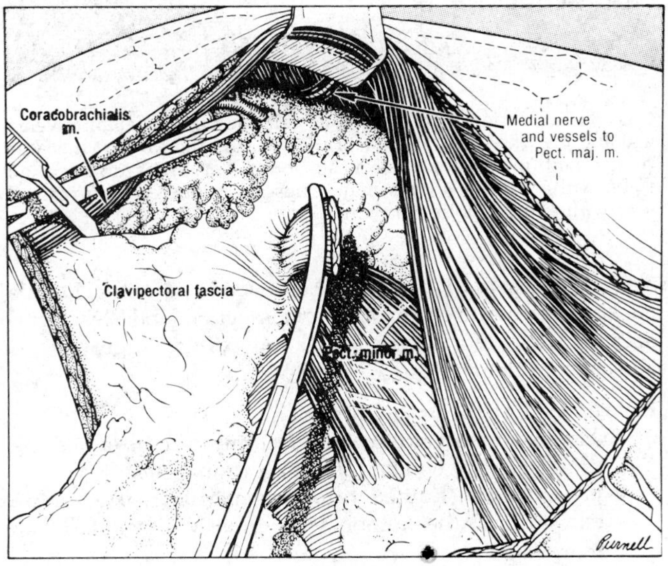

C

3. Patients who develop breast recurrence after partial mastectomy and axillary dissection (or axillary irradiation), with or without breast irradiation, and who remain free of distant disease ("salvage" mastectomy); and
4. As a palliative procedure in patients with bulky breast tumors and distant metastases in whom local control will be facilitated by removal of the breast.

SUBCUTANEOUS MASTECTOMY

Proposed as a prophylactic and cosmetic procedure, subcutaneous mastectomy involves the removal of the major portion of the breast but spares the nipple–areolar complex. It leaves 10% to 15% of breast tissue behind,[149] and carcinoma has developed in patients after this procedure.[150] Also, the cosmetic results are frequently unsatisfactory. There is thus very little, if any, indication for this procedure.

BREAST PRESERVATION PROCEDURES

Many attempts have been reported to treat infiltrating breast cancer by excision (partial mastectomy) alone, without treatment of the remaining breast tissue or axilla. As summarized in Table 38-17, the failure rate in the ipsilateral breast is significant, ranging from 25% to 37% within 5 years. These local failure rates are similar to that reported for a subgroup of the NSABP B-06 trial patients treated with segmental mastectomy, axillary dissection, and no further treatment to the breast. In a highly selected series reported by the Cleveland Clinic,[151] a 23% failure rate in the breast and axilla was reported with 15-year follow-up.

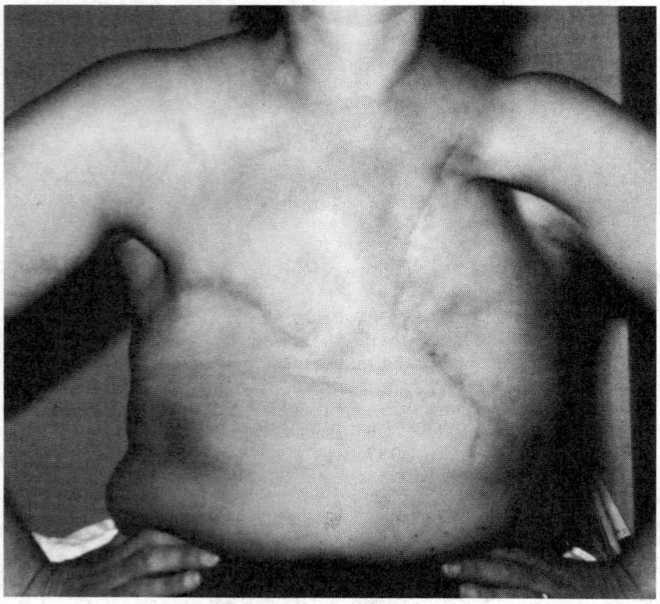

FIG. 38-12. Patient had undergone left radical mastectomy years ago and presented with a new primary in the right breast that was treated with modified radical mastectomy. Note transverse scar on right, with intact pectoralis major muscle, compared with vertical scar with axillary hollow on left.

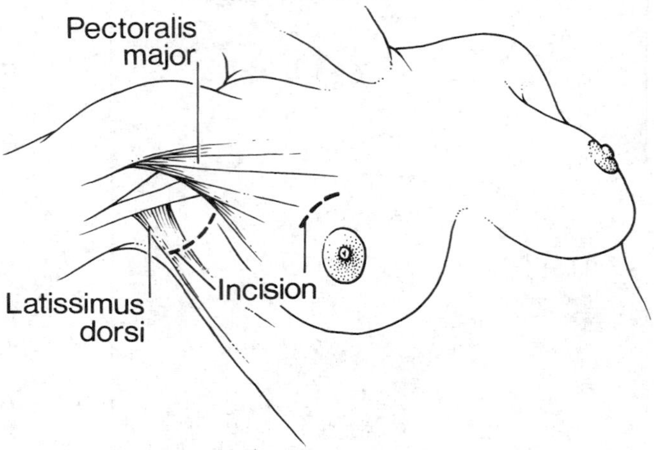

FIG. 38-13. Placement of incisions within skin lines for breast preservation cases. Two incisions are preferable to one when possible. (Kinne DW: In Harris JR, Hellman S, Henderson IC, Kinne DW [eds]: Breast Diseases, p 270. Philadelphia, JB Lippincott, 1987)

Breast preservation approaches outside of clinical trials consist of tumor excision, axillary dissection, and breast irradiation. The extent of both breast and axillary surgery varies and may be defined as follows:[152]

For removal of the breast tumor:

- Excision (tumorectomy, lumpectomy): removal of the tumor grossly without attention to margins;
- Wide excision (limited resection, partial mastectomy): excision of the tumor with grossly normal, clean margins;
- Quadrantectomy: en bloc excision of the tumor within a quadrant of the breast tissue along with the pectoralis major muscle fascia and overlying skin.

For axillary dissection:

- Sampling: removal of an axillary node or nodes from the lower axilla without definition of precise anatomic boundaries;
- Low axillary dissection: en bloc excision of level I of the axilla, from the latissimus dorsi muscle laterally to the lateral border of the pectoralis minor muscle medially, and clearing of the axillary vein superiorly;
- Level I and II dissection: en block excision of the low and mid portions of the axilla, facilitated by elevation of the pectoralis minor muscle and mobilization of the ipsilateral arm to relax the pectoralis major muscle. This dissection proceeds from the latissimus dorsi muscle

TABLE 38-17. Results of Partial Mastectomy Alone as Treatment for Early Breast Cancer

Institution	*Stage*	*Breast Relapse Rate (%)*	*Follow-up (yr)*
Princess Margaret*	T1–T2, N0	25	5
Royal Marsden†	T1–T2, N0	33	5
Suffolk‡	T1–T2, N0 or N1	37	3
McGill§	T1–T2, N0	28	5
Children's Hospital, San Francisco¶	T1–T2, N0 or N1	28	2

* Clark RM, Wilkinson RH, Mahoney LJ et al: Breast cancer: A 21 year experience with conservative surgery and radiation. Int J Radiat Oncol Biol Phys 8:967–975, 1982.

† Montgomery ACV, Greening WP, Levene AL: Clinical study of recurrence rate and survival time of patients with carcinoma of the breast treated by biopsy excision without any other therapy. J R Soc Med 71:339–342, 1978.

‡ Tagart REB: Partial mastectomy for breast cancer. Br Med J 2:1268, 1978.

§ Freeman CR, Belliveau NJ, Kim TH et al: Limited surgery with or without radiotherapy for early breast carcinoma. J Can Assoc Radiol 32:125–128, 1981.

¶ Lagios MD, Richards VE, Rose MR, Yee E: Segmental mastectomy without radiotherapy: Short-term follow-up. Cancer 52:2173–2179, 1983.

laterally to the medial border of the pectoralis minor muscle medially, with clearing of the axillary vein superiorly;

Full axillary dissection (levels I, II, and III): removal of the entire axillary contents, from the latissimus dorsi muscle laterally to the subclavius muscle (Halsted's ligament) medially, clearing the axillary vein, with preservation of or excision of the pectoralis minor muscle.

Ideal placement of the incisions is shown in Figure 38-13. Although controversy exists, present opinion favors wide excision of the breast tumor in order to achieve complete removal with clear margins, and either a level I and II or a full axillary dissection for adequate staging and axillary treatment.

BREAST RECONSTRUCTION AFTER MASTECTOMY

All women who undergo mastectomy for cancer should be made aware of the possibilities for breast reconstruction.[153-159] Although the attitudes of individual patients toward the psychological and cosmetic effects of the loss of the breast differ greatly, many patients find significant comfort in the possibility of future breast reconstruction.

Prior to undertaking surgery for breast reconstruction, the patient and physician should carefully discuss the expectations and motivation of the patient. It is essential that she have realistic expectations of the cosmetic and sensory differences that will exist in the reconstructed compared with the original breast. It is often helpful to show the prospective patient photographs of typical as well as good and poor results following breast reconstruction.

Considerable flexibility exists as to the timing of breast reconstruction. The breast can be reconstructed at the time of mastectomy, although there is considerably less experience with this technique, and the complication rates are higher.[154,156,160] Most plastic surgeons advocate a delay of 3 to 6 months before the reconstruction procedure. This provides adequate time for resolution of skin changes and contractures and is thought to lead to a more secure blood supply to the skin and soft tissue around any subsequent implants. Longer delays are possible, and many patients have had reconstruction as late as 10 years or more after mastectomy.

There is no evidence that reconstruction either increases the likelihood of local recurrence or makes its detection more difficult. In most cases, the prosthesis used in reconstruction is placed beneath the skin and the pectoralis major muscle, and local recurrence is most likely to develop superficial to this region. Also, in the absence of nodal disease, chest wall recurrence is so rare that most surgeons have abandoned it as an important factor in selecting such patients for breast reconstruction.

TYPES OF BREAST RECONSTRUCTION

Many techniques have been developed for reconstruction of the breast after mastectomy, and decisions for each patient must be made on an individual basis, taking into account the presence of adequate skin coverage, the laxity of the skin on the anterior chest wall, the presence and intact innervation of the pectoralis major muscle, and the contour of the opposite breast. When even slight laxity in the skin over the anterior chest exists, direct implants of inorganic material are the treatment of choice for recreating the breast contour.[153,161-164] Silicone gel implants are the most commonly used, and in a recent survey by Cocke, 310 of 419 patients had this type of prosthesis placed.[155] Also available are inflatable prostheses and polyurethane-coated prostheses with Dacron patches, although the latter are used infrequently.[153] Although contour-form types of prostheses are available, these tend not to be as satisfactory as round prostheses in the majority of patients. Prostheses come in a variety of sizes that can be individualized to the patient.

If the skin of the anterior chest wall is very tight, or if skin changes exist because of radiation, then it is necessary either to use available tissue and a tissue expander[166,167] or to advance both skin and subcutaneous tissue to the area of the breast using one of the various flaps.[154-159] Medially based transverse abdominal flaps can be used to replace or to add skin to the central or lower portion of the mastectomy defect. Perforating branches of the superior epigastric artery enter this flap near the medial aspect of the rectus abdominis sheath.

The latissimus dorsi myocutaneous flap is effective for replacing the bulk lost by removal of the pectoralis major muscle and brings a generous amount of skin to the reconstruction site. Skin in this flap is supplied by musculocutaneous perforating vessels from the latissimus dorsi muscle originating from the thoracodorsal artery. When adequate skin coverage exists and bulk tissue is required to fill the pectoralis major muscle defect, then latissimus dorsi muscle flaps supplied by the thoracodorsal branch of the subscapular artery are useful.

A variety of other types of flaps are possible, including local skin transfer from surrounding tissue, reconstructions that take part of the opposite breast, and the use of distant skin flaps such as elevation of abdominal tubes.[163-165] It is also possible to use a flap of greater omentum pedicled on a single gastroepiploic artery and vein covered with a skin graft.[168,169] Free flap reconstruction is also possible, involving the transfer of composite tissue from a distant area and microvascular anastomoses to nearby vessels, such as the internal mammary chain. The most common donor site is the gluteus maximus.[170,171] Although these flap procedures are more involved, sometimes they represent either the only or the best possible reconstructive approach and offer the additional benefit of obviating the need for a prosthesis. Usually, a satisfactory breast mound can be fashioned from the tissue brought into place. Choosing the exact type of reconstruction to be used requires judgment based on experience and must be determined individually for each patient. It is sometimes necessary to perform a plastic reconstructive procedure, such as reduction mammoplasty, on the remaining breast also because of significant asymmetry that may otherwise exist after reconstruction.

NIPPLE–AREOLAR RECONSTRUCTION

Although the procedures mentioned above can reconstruct the breast mound, reconstruction of the nipple–areolar complex is desired by many women for cosmetic reasons. Preservation of the patient's own nipple–areolar complex is cosmetically superior to other methods for substituting or reconstructing the areola.[153-155,172] However, this procedure has been associated with recurrent cancer in a number of cases[172-174] and should never be done. Another procedure for reconstructing the nipple–areolar complex involves the use of labia minora grafts or grafts of the upper inner thigh skin, where the pigment is darker.[175] A semicircle of these areas can be excised and transferred as full-thickness grafts to the de-epithelialized site on the breast eminence. Nipple prominence can be created by using pursestring sutures at the desired site. Techniques also have been devised for partitioning the nipple on the remaining breast and transplanting one section to the breast eminence on the opposite side.[153-155,176] This produces little cosmetic defect in the remaining breast. It also is possible to simulate the presence of an areola by tattooing the surface of the breast mound, and this method is often satisfactory in creating the appearance of a nipple.

COMPLICATIONS OF RECONSTRUCTIVE PROCEDURES

A variety of complications can attend breast reconstruction.[153-159] The presence of skin changes caused by previous radiation can substantially increase complication rates and may necessitate the use of a myocutaneous flap to provide adequate reconstruction. Other complications include hematoma, infections, soft-tissue ischemia, skin loss, and prosthesis extrusion, all of which are infrequent in experienced hands. A more common problem is capsule formation, in which tight or heavy fibrotic capsules form around breast implants. Secondary procedures may be required to release this capsule.

POSTOPERATIVE RADIOTHERAPY

The first major use of radiotherapy in the primary management of patients with breast cancer was not as definitive treatment but rather as an adjuvant to radical mastectomy. There were two rationales for such prophylactic radiotherapy. The first was that prophylactic radiotherapy could be used to reduce the risk of local–regional tumor recurrence. The risk of local recurrence after mastectomy is 10% to 15% and is related to whether axillary nodes are negative or positive (Table 38-18); it was hoped that postoperative radiotherapy would decrease this risk of local recurrence. This result seemed especially important because these recurrences are often very distressing for afflicted patients, and once clinically manifest, they can be treated effectively in only approximately 50% of patients. The second rationale for postoperative radiotherapy was to improve the likelihood of survival.[177]

It has been well established that radiotherapy after radical mastectomy markedly decreases the risk of local–regional recurrence. At the M. D. Anderson Hospital between 1963 and 1977, 920 patients underwent radiation after radical or modified radical mastectomy. Supraclavicular recurrence was minimal in irradiated patients, and chest wall recurrence was less common than in comparable patients who were not irradiated, particularly for high-risk patients (those with four or more positive nodes) (Table 38-19).

Despite this documented improvement in local–regional disease control, the effect of adjuvant radiation therapy on survival remains uncertain. The survival value of postoperative radiotherapy ideally would be determined by a large, properly conducted, prospective, randomized clinical trial. There are now four trials with published results in which patients have been randomized after radical or modified radical mastectomy to either postoperative radiotherapy or no further treatment (Table 38-20). As indicated in the "comments" column, there are methodologic problems in these trials, particularly the earlier ones. As a group, however, these trials indicate that postoperative radiotherapy decreases local–regional recurrence but does not significantly improve the likelihood of survival.

It is possible that postoperative irradiation is detrimental to survival. This possibility was suggested by Stjernsward, who hypothesized that postoperative radiation increased the mortality rate by suppressing host immunity.[178] More recently, an overview of postoperative radiotherapy has been published by Cuzick and associates.[179] Included in this study were the results from the Manchester trials, the Oslo trials, the Stockholm trial, and an unpublished small trial from Heidelberg. The results of these various trials were combined by the use of a summary logrank statistic (Mantel–Haenzel) obtained by adding together across trials the difference between observed and "expected" deaths. No difference was seen in the summary observed-minus-expected deaths comparing patients treated with and without radiotherapy over the first 10 years after surgery. After 10 years, however, there was a lower rate of survival associated with the use of radiotherapy ($p = 0.005$). Among patients followed longer than 10 years, 271 of the 683 (40%) who received radiotherapy died compared with 235 of the 691 patients (34%) who did not receive radiotherapy (Fig. 38-14). The overview analysis thus raises the possibility that postoperative irradiation is actually detrimental to survival, although it should be stressed that the technique of radiotherapy used in these older trials is considerably different from that currently used.

At this time, it is clear that postoperative radiation is not of

TABLE 38-18. Likelihood (%) and Site of First Relapse 5 to 10 Years After Radical Mastectomy According to Status of Axillary Nodes

	*Series 1**		*Series 2†*	
Site of Relapse	*Nodes+*	*Nodes–*	*Nodes+*	*Nodes–*
Local–regional only	18	6	25	4
Distant only	49	20	43	20
Local–regional and distant	9	2		

* Fisher B, Ravdin RG, Ausman RK et al: Surgical adjunct chemotherapy in cancer of the breast: results of a decade of cooperative investigation. Ann Surg 168:337–356, 1968.

† Valagussa P, Bonadonna G, Veronesi U: Patterns of relapse and survival following radical mastectomy. Cancer 41:1170–1178, 1978.

TABLE 38-19. Incidence of Local–Regional Recurrence After Radical Mastectomy and Postoperative Radiotherapy (M. D. Anderson Hospital)

		Recurrence (%)	
Site of Irradiation	*No. of Positive Axillary Nodes*	*Chest Wall*	*Supraclavicular Region*
Peripheral lymphatics	0	5	1
	1–3	9	2
	≥4	20	1
Peripheral lymphatics and chest wall	0	2	2
	1–3	8	1
	≥4	11	3

value in unselected patients. However, further study will be required to determine whether there are subsets of patients for whom postoperative therapy is beneficial. There is preliminary evidence that patients with inner or central primary tumors and positive axillary nodes are such a subset.[180] In addition, many physicians feel that for high-risk patients, the prevention of local–regional recurrence is sufficient reason to recommend this treatment. As noted above, local–regional recurrence can be highly distressing to a patient and, once manifest, is controlled in only 50% of cases.[181,182]

The above discussion applies to patients who do not receive adjuvant chemotherapy. The use of postoperative radiotherapy also must be considered in the light of adjuvant chemotherapy. It is possible that the chest wall and regional nodes are the site of greatest tumor burden after mastectomy in certain subgroups, such as patients with larger primary tumors or positive axillary nodes. According to the Goldie–Coldman hypothesis, spontaneous mutations of tumor cells to drug resistance may account for failures of chemotherapy. The greater the tumor burden, the more likely it is that drug-resistant cells will emerge.[183] Adjuvant radiation therapy, by decreasing the local tumor burden, therefore might decrease the probability of drug resistance and hence increase the probability of cure.

A few studies have addressed the value of adding radiation therapy to adjuvant chemotherapy.[184-187] Overall, no significant differences in survival rates were seen between those patients randomized to chemotherapy alone and those randomized to chemotherapy and radiotherapy. However, among all patients, local and regional control were significantly improved by the addition of radiation therapy. More recently, the results were published of a randomized trial examining the necessity and effectiveness of postoperative radiotherapy in 510 patients with T1–T2 tumors and pathologically positive nodes or T3 tumors and negative nodes who were treated with adjuvant chemotherapy at the Dana-Farber Cancer Institute in conjunction with the Joint Center for Radiation Therapy (DFCI/JCRT).[188] Patients with four or more positive nodes or at least one positive apical node were randomized to receive either five or ten cycles of cyclophosphamide/Adriamycin (doxorubicin) (CA). Patients with one to three positive nodes, or operable tumors larger than 5 cm and pathologically negative nodes, were randomized to receive eight cycles of either cyclophosphamide–methotrexate–5-fluorouracil (5-FU) (CMF) or methotrexate–5-FU (MF) chemotherapy. Two hundred and six of these patients were subsequently rerandomized to receive either no further treatment or adjuvant radiotherapy. Radiation therapy consisted of 4500 cGy in 5 weeks to the chest wall and appropriate draining lymph nodes. The median follow-up time from chemotherapy randomization was 45 months for patients in the CA arm and 53 months for those in the CMF/MF arm. The crude rate of local failure (chest wall or draining lymph node areas) as the first site of failure for patients randomized to receive chemotherapy only was 14%; for those randomized to receive both chemotherapy and ra-

TABLE 38-20. Results of Randomized Trials of Postoperative Radiotherapy After Radical Mastectomy

Study	*No. of Patients*	*Areas Treated*	*Follow-up (yr)*	*Local Control**	*Relapse-free Survival**	*Survival**	*Comments*
Manchester I	720	Chest wall + axilla	20–30	+		0	Randomization not strict; orthovoltage
Manchester II	741	Regional lymph nodes	20–30	+		0	
NSABP	RT = 91 control = 235	Regional lymph nodes	5	+	0	0	Randomization not strict; short follow-up
Oslo I	546	Chest wall + regional nodes	>11	+	0	0	Orthovoltage
Oslo II	542	Regional nodes	>11	++	+ Stage II	0	Supervoltage
Stockholm	644	Chest wall + regional nodes	8–14	++	+	0	

* 0 = no significant difference; + = improved with radiotherapy; ++ = greatly improved with radiotherapy.

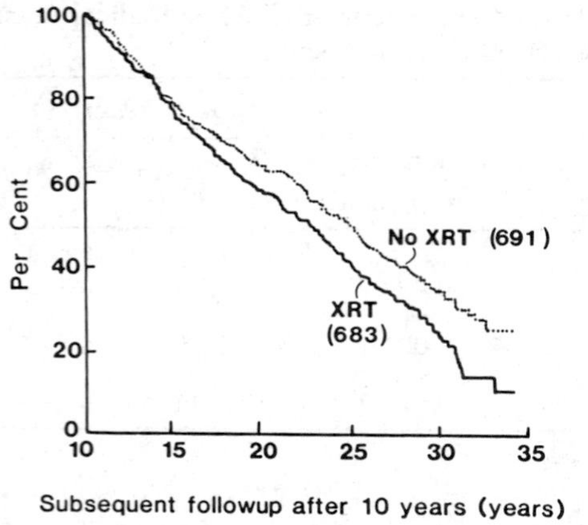

FIG. 38-14. Subsequent survival in patients surviving 10 years in a trial using radical mastectomy. There is a significant difference favoring patients treated with radical mastectomy alone ($p = 0.002$). Numbers in parentheses are total patients at risk in each arm of trial.[179]

diotherapy, it was 5% ($p = 0.03$). For patients in the CMF/MF arm, the rate of local failure as the first site of failure was nearly the same for patients randomized to chemotherapy only as for those randomized to adjuvant radiotherapy as well (5% and 2%). For patients in the CA arm, the crude rate of local failure was 20% for patients randomized to receive chemotherapy only and 6% for those randomized to both types of adjuvant treatment ($p = 0.03$). Moreover, some patients did not actually receive the treatments they were randomized to receive. Among the 43 patients treated with CA who actually received radiotherapy, there was only one local failure, compared with 12 local failures among the 59 patients (20%) who actually did not receive radiotherapy ($p = 0.007$). No significant difference was seen in disease-free survival or overall survival in either the CA or the CMF/MF arm between patients randomized to receive radiation therapy and those randomized to no further treatment (Fig. 38-15). Taken together, these results suggest that adjuvant chemotherapy alone is not highly effective at preventing local recurrence in patients with four or more positive axillary nodes and that radiation given after chemotherapy significantly reduces local failure as the first site of relapse in these patients. However, none of the available studies provides strong support for a survival benefit for radiotherapy in this setting.

At this time, the use of adjuvant radiotherapy in patients with four or more positive nodes who are treated by adjuvant chemotherapy is a matter of clinical judgment. Many clinicians will judge it useful to add radiotherapy in these patients in order to prevent local recurrence. The results of the DFCI/JCRT trial indicate that radiotherapy can be added at the completion of adjuvant chemotherapy, thus avoiding any possible interference with the administration of the chemotherapy.

CONSERVATIVE SURGERY AND RADIATION THERAPY FOR EARLY BREAST CANCER

The theoretical plan for the use of conservative surgery and radiation therapy is to preserve the breast by resecting only the tumor, leaving behind, in many cases, a subclinical burden of cancer cells. It has been well established that a resection of the tumor without subsequent irradiation results in a 15% to 40% risk of local recurrence.[189-193] Moderate doses of radiation are therefore used to eradicate this residual cancer while preserving an acceptable cosmetic appearance. It is critical to the success of this approach that the conservative resection not leave behind a tumor burden too large to be destroyed completely by the dose of radiation to be employed. Therefore, it is important to identify clinical or pathologic features that indicate when a conservative surgical resection is likely to be associated with a large residual tumor burden.

The recent pathologic study described above by Holland and colleagues from Nijmegen, The Netherlands,[78] is pertinent to the successful application of breast-conserving treatment. They found that 37% of cases showed no residual tumor foci in the breast beyond the primary tumor, 20% showed other tumor foci within 2 cm of the reference tumor, and 43% showed tumor foci further than 2 cm away from the reference tumor. The likelihood of residual tumor foci decreased with increasing distance from the reference tumor. For women with tumors 4 cm or smaller, 61% had tumor foci more than 1 cm away, 41% more than 2 cm away, 18% more than 3 cm away, and 11% more than 4 cm away. This study does not describe the bulk of the residual tumor or which patients are likely to have tumor foci at a great distance from the reference tumor, but it suggests that the residual tumor burden is greater in patients who have exci-

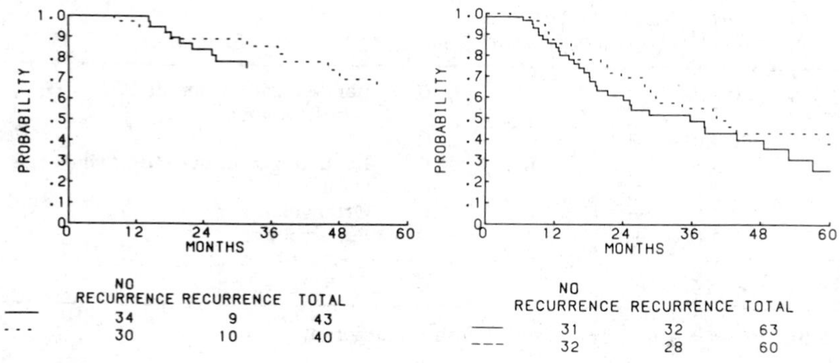

FIG. 38-15. Actuarial relapse-free survival in DFCI–JCRT trial testing value of postoperative radiotherapy (RT) after adjuvant chemotherapy (CT) for moderate-risk patients (*left*) and high-risk patients (*right*). Solid lines indicate patients treated with CT and RT; dotted lines indicate patients treated with CT alone.[188]

sion of the primary tumor with only narrow gross margins than in patients undergoing wider excision, such as quadrantectomy. It also implies that a cosmetically acceptable excision probably will leave behind microscopic disease near the biopsy site in many patients, thus explaining the high rate of local recurrence in the series testing excision only.

RETROSPECTIVE RESULTS

Ten-year results of retrospective studies of conservative surgery and radiotherapy are available from a number of institutions in the United States and Europe.[194-198] The results of the JCRT are representative of these studies and will be discussed in detail.

From July 1968 through December 1980, 525 patients with AJCC clinical Stage I or II carcinoma of the breast were treated at the JCRT. The follow-up was updated and the data were reanalyzed in August 1986. The median follow-up was 74 months, with a range of 33 to 185 months. All of the patients in this series had invasive carcinoma diagnosed by the original hospital pathologist and confirmed by the study pathologists. Nine of the patients had an opposite-breast cancer treated during this period, for a total of 534 breast cancers. The breakdown by TN stages was as follows: T1N0, 248; T1N1, 29; T2N0, 202; and T2N1, 55. The median age of the patients was 52 years, with a range from 25 to 93 years.

The treatment technique at the JCRT has been detailed previously.[199-201] There were some variations in treatment over the years of the study period, and the effect of these variations has been analyzed. Five hundred eight breasts were treated after excisional biopsy and 26 after incisional or needle biopsy. Of the patients treated after excisional biopsy, 411 received supplemental radiation (boost) to the primary site to 6000 cGy or greater. It is important to emphasize that an "excisional biopsy" in this series, for the most part, was simply a gross resection of the tumor without an attempt to obtain microscopically negative margins of resection.

Local recurrence was scored whenever tumor was noted in the treated breast or the skin overlying the breast. Fifty-seven patients had an isolated local recurrence, and two patients had simultaneous local and distant recurrence. The crude incidence of local recurrence thus was 11%. Eight patients had suspected or proven local recurrence after distant recurrence but were censored at the time of distant recurrence. By 10 years, the actuarial probability of local recurrence was 20%, with 23 patients still at risk past that point. The last breast failure was seen 109 months after the start of radiotherapy. When this curve is plotted semilogarithmically as local tumor control over time, a straight line is obtained, implying that the risk of local recurrence is fairly constant for the first 9 years after treatment.

The association between the type of biopsy and the probability of local recurrence was examined. The 10-year probability of local recurrence was 19% for patients treated with excisional biopsy and 43% for patients treated with incisional or needle biopsy ($p<0.0001$). For the 411 patients treated with excisional biopsy and a boost to the primary site to 6000 cGy or more (now considered optimal treatment) the 10-year probability of local recurrence was 15% (Fig. 38-16). The use of excisional biopsy facilitates the use of radiation therapy and is now routinely recommended for all patients treated at the JCRT. The optimal extent of the resection beyond the primary tumor into the adjacent grossly normal breast tissue is a more complicated matter (see below).

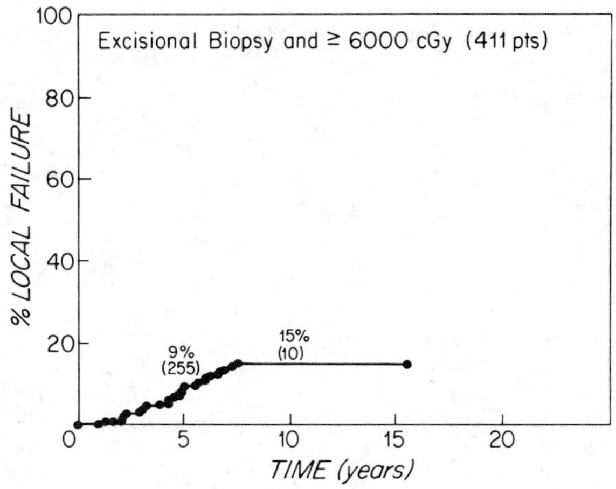

FIG. 38-16. Actuarial risk of breast (or local) failure among 411 patients treated with excisional biopsy and radiotherapy including a boost to the primary site of 6000 cGy or greater (JCRT).

Local recurrences after breast-conserving treatment can be classified on clinical and pathologic grounds as a true recurrence (TR), a marginal miss (MM), elsewhere in the breast (E), or in skin (S). A TR is one within the borders of the boost or at the site of the primary tumor in the absence of a boost. An MM is a recurrence near the site of the primary tumor but just outside the borders of the boost. An E is a recurrence at least several centimeters from the boosted volume and at a substantial distance from the primary tumor site. An S is a recurrence confined to the skin of the breast without evidence of parenchymal disease. Both TR and MM most likely represent a recurrence of the original cancer as opposed to a new primary tumor in the same breast.

The probability of a TR in the JCRT series for patients treated with radiation therapy after an excisional biopsy of the tumor was 4% at 5 years and 11% at 10 years. The probability of a TR in the 411 patients treated with a boost to the primary site to 6000 cGy or more was compared with that in the 97 patients treated without a boost, although the validity of this comparison is limited by selection bias, because patients thought to be at greater risk for local recurrence more often received a boost. Despite this, patients treated with a boost had a lower probability of a TR (7% at 10 years) than did patients treated without a boost (15% at 10 years; $p = 0.19$). This result suggests that a boost to the primary site may decrease the likelihood of a true recurrence. The probability of an MM in patients treated with excisional biopsy and radiation therapy including a boost to the primary site was 4% at both 5 and 10 years. The probability of developing either a TR or an MM (*i.e.*, a recurrence of the primary tumor) was 7% at 5 years and 11% at 10 years for patients treated with an excisional biopsy and a boost

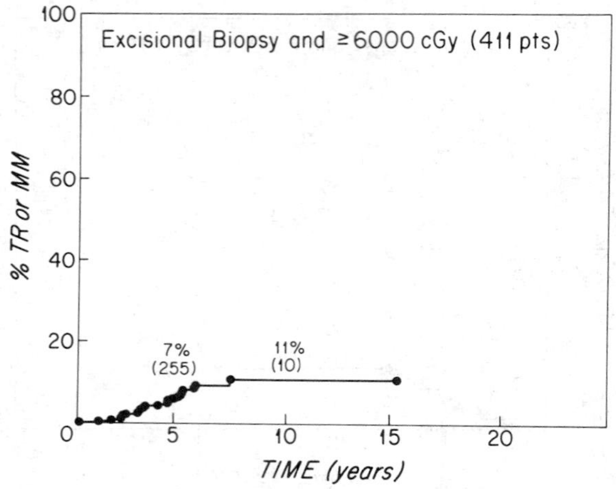

FIG. 38-17. Actuarial risk of a recurrence at (true recurrence, *TR*) or near (marginal miss, *MM*) primary tumor site among 411 patients treated with excisional biopsy and radiotherapy including a boost to the primary site of 6000 cGy or greater (JCRT).

(Fig. 38-17). No TRs or MMs occurred more than 8 years after treatment in the 30 patients followed at least that long.

The probability of a recurrence elsewhere in the treated breast was 1% at 5 years and 7% at 10 years. The time course to this type of recurrence is different from that to TR or MM. TRs and MMs are more common in the first 5 years and less common thereafter, whereas Es are less common in the first 5 years and more common thereafter. The probability of a recurrence elsewhere in the treated breast was greater for patients 49 years of age or younger at the time of diagnosis than in patients 50 or older, but this difference did not reach statistical significance (8% versus 5% at 10 years; $p = 0.08$).

Skin recurrence was an uncommon event in this series, being seen in only three patients. The 5- and 10-year probability of an S was 0.7%. All three Ss were seen in patients who had pathologically positive axillary nodes on initial presentation. The 5-year probability of an S was 2.5% for node-positive patients compared with 0 for node-negative patients ($p = 0.03$). These few patients had a rapid downhill course, with distant metastases appearing simultaneously with or soon after the local recurrence. This is very different from the usual course after local recurrence, which will be discussed in more detail below.

Nine women (2%) had bilateral tumors at the time of initial presentation. In the remaining patients, the probability of developing a metachronous opposite breast cancer was 4% at 5 years and 10% at 10 years, similar to that reported after mastectomy.

IMPLICATIONS OF THE JCRT RESULTS

The results obtained from the JCRT illustrate several common findings regarding the use of conservative surgery and radiation therapy. One observation is that the time to local recurrence is protracted: there was a fairly constant risk over a 9-year period. Of note, in a collaborative study of patients treated at the Princess Margaret Hospital, the Institut Curie, and the Marseilles Cancer Institute, a constant risk of local recurrence was observed over a 14-year period.[202] The time to local recurrence after breast-conserving treatment is different from that after mastectomy, in which the majority of recurrences appear within 3 years. In the JCRT series, the site of breast recurrence was different in the first 5 years (when nearly all recurrences were at or near the primary site) than in the second 5 years (when recurrences elsewhere in the treated breast were more common). These observations have implications for the follow-up observation of treated patients, which will be discussed below.

Another important observation is that most local recurrences are at or near the primary site (TR or MM) and likely represent a recurrence of the primary tumor. This observation has also been noted in the NSABP B-06 trial.[193,203,204] Pathologic studies of the primary tumor and the recurrences from both the JCRT[205] and the NSABP[204] indicate that the histologies are identical or similar in nearly all cases. This finding suggests that the techniques of surgery and radiation should emphasize adequate treatment of both the primary tumor and the surrounding area. This observation also provides a rationale for employing a boost to the primary site, a view which is reinforced by pathologic studies such as that of Holland and associates.[78] When patients are treated with excisional biopsy and radiotherapy including a boost to the primary site, recurrences of the primary tumor are rare after 8 years. There are at present very limited long-term data for patients routinely treated without a boost.

A related finding is that recurrences elsewhere in the treated breast are uncommon and are generally seen after a delay of several years. In the JCRT experience, whole-breast irradiation primarily appears to delay the appearance of second tumors in the treated breast. Whether failure elsewhere in the breast is due to multicentric carcinoma or represents a newly developed cancer is unknown. At the JCRT, recurrence elsewhere in the treated breast is viewed as a risk incurred by breast-conserving treatment, just as the appearance of an opposite-breast cancer is a risk incurred by unilateral treatment.

COSMETIC RESULTS

The cosmetic results of conservative surgery and radiotherapy have generally been good to excellent, and most patients have been very satisfied. The cosmetic results of patients treated at the JCRT are typical of other series using modern equipment and currently accepted doses. Measured features included breast edema, retraction, telangiectasia, arm edema, and overall cosmetic appearance as judged by the physician. A series of 239 patients was treated from 1976 to 1980. No patient in this series received chemotherapy. The overall cosmetic results fluctuated during the first 3 years after treatment but then stabilized.[206] At 5 years, the overall cosmetic results were judged excellent (little or no observable change) in 77% of patients, good (minimal but identifiable changes) in 9%, fair (significant results of radiation therapy noted) in 9%, and poor (severe normal-tissue sequelae) in 5% (Fig. 38-18). Moderate or severe retraction was the most common element of a fair or poor result, whereas telangiectasia, breast edema, and arm edema were rarely the cause of a fair or poor result. The cosmetic results were

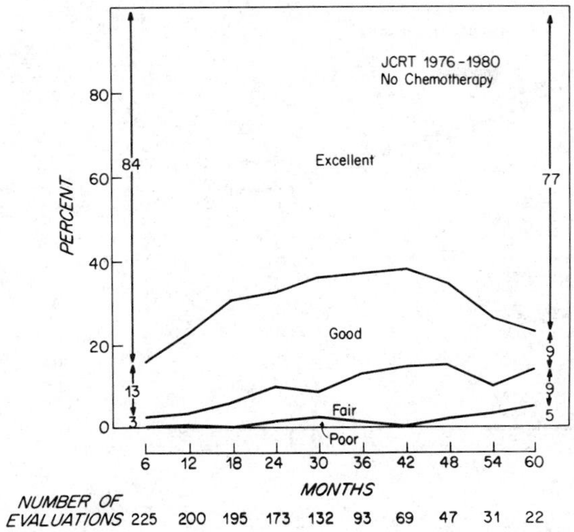

FIG. 38-18. Overall cosmetic results after completion of primary radiation treatment.

somewhat correlated with the dose and technique of radiotherapy, in that poorer cosmetic results were associated with very large implants (more than 100 seeds) and with implant doses exceeding 1800 cGy. Breast and arm edema were more common in patients who underwent axillary dissection.

RANDOMIZED PROSPECTIVE STUDIES OF CONSERVATIVE SURGERY AND RADIATION THERAPY VERSUS MASTECTOMY

The critical issue regarding primary radiation therapy is whether it yields survival rates equal to those achieved with mastectomy. This issue is best addressed by randomized prospective trials in which the treatment arms are well balanced in terms of prognostic features. Since 1970, there have been five prospective randomized trials using modern radiation therapy techniques. One such trial was performed at the National Cancer Institute of Italy in Milan.[207-209] From 1973 to 1980, 701 evaluable patients with primary tumors 2 cm or smaller and clinically uninvolved axillary nodes (T1N0) were entered. Patients were randomized to treatment with either conservative surgery and radiotherapy or radical mastectomy. Conservative surgery consisted of a resection of the entire involved quadrant of the breast (quadrantectomy) and a full axillary dissection. Radiotherapy was then administered to the breast alone through two opposing tangential fields, giving a dose of 5000 cGy in 5 weeks. Another 1000 cGy was then administered to the tumor site using orthovoltage radiation. From 1973 to 1975, patients with involved lymph nodes were further randomized to receive radiotherapy either to the breast alone or to the breast and to the draining lymph node areas as well. After 1975, all patients with involved lymph nodes were treated with 12 cycles of chemotherapy. The two arms of the trial were well balanced with regard to age, tumor size, and axillary nodal status. Microscopically involved axillary nodes were found in 25% of the radical mastectomy group and 27% of the conservatively treated group. Seven patients from the mastectomy group and seven in the quadrantectomy group had developed a local recurrence. Seven additional cases of a second primary cancer in the remnant ipsilateral breast were found in the group that was treated conservatively. The number of deaths in each treatment group since the start of treatment and the relapse-free and overall survival rates were similar between the two groups (Fig. 38-19). Patients with involved axillary nodes had a greater likelihood of relapse-free survival if treated with quadrantectomy and radiotherapy than with mastectomy (72% versus 59% at 10 years; $p = 0.03$).

The NSABP began a three-arm trial (Protocol B-06) in 1976 comparing mastectomy with segmental mastectomy with or without radiotherapy.[193,203] A total of 1843 evaluable patients with clinical Stage I or II carcinoma whose primary tumors clinically measured no more than 4 cm were entered. One hundred seventy-four patients refused their assigned treatment and were excluded from analysis. All patients underwent axillary dissection. Those with involved lymph nodes received adjuvant chemotherapy. Whereas in the Milan trial an entire quadrant of the breast was removed, segmental mastectomy as performed in the NSABP trial involved resection of the tumor with only enough normal tissue around it to attempt to ensure that the microscopic margins of the specimen were tumor free. It was considered impossible to obtain tumor-free margins in 10% of the patients randomly assigned to segmental mastectomy, and total mastectomy was carried out in these patients. Radiotherapy was delivered to the breast alone with supervoltage equipment using opposed tangential fields (often without wedge filters to compensate for the slope of the breast) to a dose of 5000 to 5300 cGy in 5 to 6 weeks. The regional lymph nodes were not treated, and no boost was given to the tumor site. For the patients who received radiotherapy, the 5-year actuarial incidence of recurrence in the breast was 7%, compared with 32% for patients who did not have radiotherapy ($p<0.001$).[203] This marked difference was seen both in patients with histologically involved and those with uninvolved lymph nodes. Of note, patients with positive lymph nodes who were treated with segmental mastectomy and adjuvant chemotherapy but without radiotherapy had a greater risk of breast recurrence (38%) than did patients with negative nodes who were treated only with segmental mastectomy (28%). However, patients with positive nodes treated with segmental mastectomy, radiotherapy, and adjuvant chemotherapy had a smaller risk of breast recurrence (4%) than did patients with negative nodes treated with segmental mastectomy and radiotherapy without chemotherapy (9%). This suggests that chemotherapy by itself does little to prevent breast recurrence but that radiotherapy and chemotherapy are additive or synergistic in reducing tumor recurrence in the breast.

Another trial was conducted from 1972 to 1979 at the Institut Gustave-Roussy in Villejuif, France, under the sponsorship of the WHO.[210] This trial included 179 patients with tumors pathologically 2 cm or smaller with either clinically involved or uninvolved lymph nodes. Patients were randomized to receive either modified radical mastectomy or conservative surgery, which consisted of removal of the tumor with a surrounding margin of 2 cm of grossly normal breast

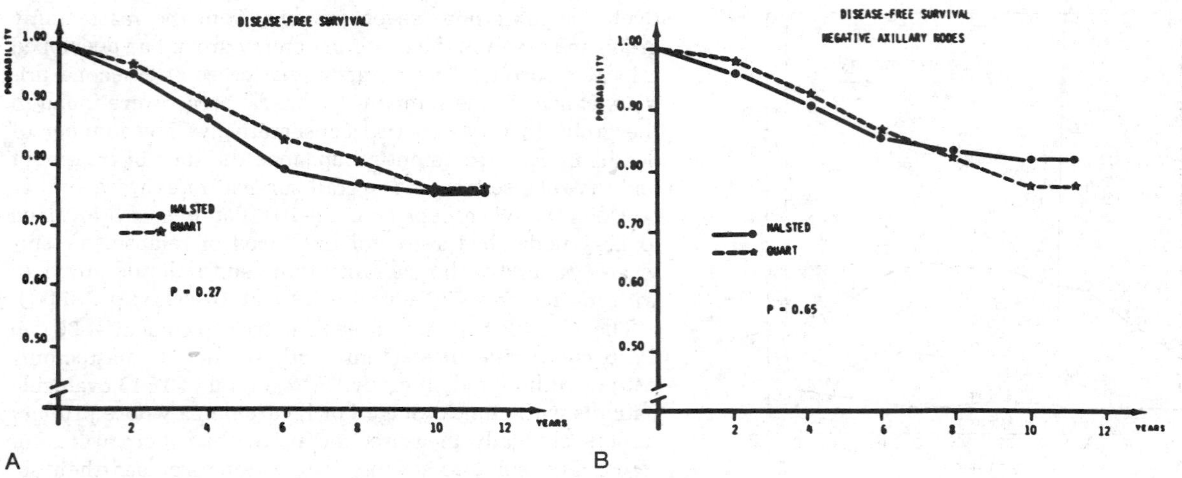

FIG. 38-19. Disease-free survival rates in Milan trial according to type of treatment. **A**. All patients. **B**. Patients with pathologically negative axillary nodes.

tissue ("tumorectomy"). All patients underwent low axillary dissection; if involved lymph nodes were detected, this was extended to a complete axillary dissection. All patients randomized to tumorectomy received breast irradiation. Patients randomized to either mastectomy or tumorectomy who had involved lymph nodes were further randomized to receive postoperative axillary, supraclavicular, and IMN irradiation or no further treatment. Adjuvant chemotherapy was not used. Radiotherapy was given with cobalt-60 to a dose of 4500 cGy in 18 fractions over 1 month, treating the breast four times weekly. A boost of 1500 cGy was given to the tumor bed in six fractions. The total length of irradiation was 6 weeks. With a median follow-up of approximately 10 years, there was no statistically significant difference in local recurrence, freedom from distant metastases, or overall survival rates in the two treatment groups.

The fourth recent prospective randomized trial was begun by the National Cancer Institute of the United States in 1979.[211] By September 1985, 197 patients with clinical Stage I or II cancers had been randomized to receive either modified radical mastectomy or conservative excision, full axillary dissection, and radiotherapy to the breast. Patients with histologically involved nodes also received doxorubicin and cyclophosphamide. With a median follow-up of 32 months, there was no significant difference in outcome between these two groups.

The fifth and most recent trial is one conducted from 1981 to 1986 at Guy's Hospital, London.[212] Patients with tumors smaller than 4 cm in diameter were randomized to treatment with modified radical mastectomy (185 patients) or conservative surgery, axillary clearance, and radiotherapy (214 patients). Patients with positive axillary nodes were subsequently randomized to be watched or to receive 12 cycles of CMF chemotherapy. So far, there are no differences in outcome between the two treatment arms, and the doses of chemotherapy delivered have been the same in both groups.

These randomized prospective trials demonstrate that when adequate treatment techniques are used, there is no significant difference in survival between patients treated with radical surgery and those treated with conservative surgery and radiotherapy. As such, they confirm the evidence of the retrospective trials as to the value of using conservative surgery and radiotherapy for patients with early breast cancer.

COMPLICATIONS

The complications associated with treatment have recently been reviewed elsewhere.[213] Acute complications of radiotherapy for early breast cancer include fatigue and erythema of the skin, occasionally with moist desquamation. However, these are self-limited and resolve within several weeks.

Significant long-term complications are uncommon when good technique is used. At the JCRT, transient or mild complications occurred in a small percentage of patients. The most common were rib fractures (5%), cosmetically (though rarely functionally) significant arm edema (4%),[214] radiation pneumonitis (2%), and, rarely, paresthesias or brachial plexus disorders.[215] Other rare complications were radiation pericarditis (one patient), soft-tissue necrosis (one patient), and occasionally fibrosis of the pectoral muscles.

RADIATION TECHNIQUE AND DOSES

The extent of surgery and the dose of radiation required for local tumor control are complementary: the more extensive the surgical procedure, the less radiation is required for tumor control. The entire breast should be treated with 180 to 200 cGy per day, for a total dose of 4500 to 5000 cGy. Doses exceeding 5000 cGy to the entire breast commonly result in an unacceptable degree of fibrosis and retraction and so should be avoided. It is important to maximize the homogeneity of the dose delivered to the breast. Inhomogeneities above 15% are not advisable, and it is preferable to maintain inhomogeneity below 10%. Bolus (material applied to the skin to circumvent the skin sparing of supervoltage radiation) is not required in the treatment of early breast cancer and should be avoided in most cases.

The question of whether to use a boost to the primary site is controversial. There are a number of reasons to justify routine use of a boost. First, in all reported series, most recurrences are seen at or near the primary site. Second, the data of Holland and colleagues indicate that most of the residual tumor burden after tumor excision is at or near the primary site.[78] Furthermore, excellent long-term local tumor control rates have been demonstrated from institutions in which a boost has been employed.

The principal justification for not using a boost is the report of the NSABP B-06 trial, which demonstrated excellent local tumor control in the absence of a boost.[193,203] However, the follow-up in this trial is still relatively short. In addition, because compensating wedges often were not employed, the actual dose to the site of the primary tumor may have been substantially greater in many cases than the nominal delivered dose of 5000 to 5300 cGy.

The need for a boost should also be considered in relation to the size of the tumor and the extent of the resection. For very small tumors treated with quadrantectomy, a boost is not likely to be of great importance, whereas for larger tumors treated with a gross excision, a boost is more likely to be important to maximize local tumor control. Given the multiplicity of clinical circumstances and the small differences in outcome, it is unlikely that a randomized trial will be useful in settling this issue.

The data from the JCRT have defined the volumes and doses of boost radiation consistent with preserving the cosmetic appearance of the breast. In most situations, this can be achieved using external-beam radiation (electron beam). Late failure at the primary site is rare when a boost is employed. It therefore seems prudent to deliver a modest boost dose (usually 1600 cGy or enough to bring the dose to the primary site to 6000 cGy or more) to the primary site following a local or wide excision of the tumor and 4600 to 5000 cGy to the whole breast.

It is also controversial whether radiation therapy should be delivered to the draining lymph node regions. The preponderance of evidence indicates that such nodal treatment does not have a detectable impact on survival. Nodal treatment will improve tumor control in these areas, but its use must be balanced against the risk of complications, which is related to the dose and techniques of radiotherapy used. It is important to stress that the results achieved in both the Milan and the NSABP trials involved irradiation to the breast alone. In light of their findings, treatment to the breast alone is reasonable in all situations. Treatment of high-risk nodal areas is also reasonable, provided it can be achieved without a significant risk of complications. It is well established that a fully dissected axilla should not be irradiated routinely because of the high risk of developing arm edema.[214,216,217]

FOLLOW-UP OF TREATED PATIENTS

Recurrence in the breast after conservative surgery and radiation therapy has a much better prognosis than a chest-wall recurrence after mastectomy, with approximately 50% of patients being alive and free of distant metastases 5 years later.[202,218] The time to local recurrence is protracted; therefore, treated patients require long-term follow-up to detect such a recurrence promptly. Both physical examination and mammography are critical. One reasonable follow-up program is to obtain mammograms 6 months and 1 year after treatment and then annually thereafter and to perform physical examinations every 4 to 6 months. It is not uncommon for changes in the texture and characteristics of the irradiated breast to continue to take place for 12 to 18 months after treatment, but changes after that time should be regarded with particular suspicion. When warranted, a small open biopsy (1–20 cc of tissue) can be performed safely, with little risk of wound nonhealing, infection, or worsening of the cosmetic outcome.

APPROACH TO THE PATIENT WITH EARLY BREAST CANCER

The preceding pages have discussed extensively the traditional treatment of breast cancer with mastectomy and the preservative approaches combining local excision and radiation therapy. How should one apply these discussions to the individual patient with early breast cancer? Any recommendations given must be considered conditional. The current data have been interpreted, but they are a portion of a continuum that includes both new studies and continued follow-up of earlier series, and it is important to consider the evolutionary nature of these data in the context of improving techniques and increased observation times. As the quality of these techniques improves and the length of follow-up increases, we can come to firmer conclusions as to the appropriate treatment for individual patients.

Analysis of treatment data must include a number of endpoints. The most obvious of these is survival; however, survival data alone do not reveal all the pertinent information. Because the purpose of both mastectomy and preservative management is to eradicate the primary tumor and regional disease, local control is an important endpoint in itself. Even this evaluation must be modified by understanding the consequences for the patient of having a recurrence. It appears that local recurrence after mastectomy has a different outcome than a recurrence following preservative treatment, with the former being more ominous than the latter. A third and very important endpoint is the quality of the functional and cosmetic result, because the purpose of either treatment is to eradicate the disease while allowing the patient to return as closely as possible to her predisease state. Finally, both short- and long-term undesirable consequences of treatment must be considered.

To determine the treatment for an individual patient, one must consider the age of the patient. Whereas younger patients are often more concerned with body image, they also have the longest life expectancy and therefore are potentially most exposed to the long-term complications of treatment. There are also important emotional and physiological considerations, including the woman's feelings about preserving the breast and her body image. Loss of the breast may have devastating psychological consequences; however, selection of breast preservation requires that the woman accept the presence of a potential site of residual or new disease. These considerations must be explored in helping the patient arrive at an appropriate decision. Other considerations that affect the selection of local treatment include breast size, tumor location, number of tumors, and the histologic character of the biopsy. There are no simple answers applicable for all patients. Today, both alternatives must be discussed with the patient; only through this discussion can an informed patient receive information and guidance sufficient to permit her to reach a reasonable decision.

From the available data, it seems clear that both mastectomy and breast preservation utilizing local excision and radiation therapy are acceptable alternatives for the treatment of early breast cancer. Although there are no simple rigid rules to determine which therapy is appropriate for an individual patient, there are some useful guidelines. First among the considerations favoring breast preservation procedures is the patient's desire for such treatment; in the absence of such a desire, there is no incentive. Second, the primary tumor should be small relative to the breast, so that local excision with a negative margin will result in an acceptable cosmetic appearance. Third, there should be a single lesion, as experience in treating patients with multiple lesions in one breast with breast-preserving techniques is limited. There should be no suspicious microcalcifications on the postexcision mammogram, and a review of the excision specimen using an appropriate method to ink the margins should show that these margins are clear of invasive or intraductal disease. Extensive diffuse intraductal disease in a specimen appears to increase the risk of local recurrence, although in studies showing this, resection margins were not always evaluated. It is uncertain whether the presence of extensive intraductal disease will continue to be a factor when carefully reviewed margins are found to be free of such disease. Finally, the patient should understand the requirements of the treatment course, as daily treatments for 5 to 8 weeks require a patient's commitment to such a program.

Considerations that favor mastectomy are in general the converse of those that favor preservative management. For example, some patients have no desire to preserve the affected breast; in fact, some may have a morbid fear of persistent disease lurking within the breast, and such patients are better served by mastectomy. If a cosmetically acceptable incision is not possible, then little is to be gained by preservative treatment. This may be the case when the primary tumor is large relative to the size of the breast and for tumors in certain locations, especially central lesions close to the areola. If there is multifocal disease extending beyond one quadrant, such disease usually cannot be encompassed in a cosmetically acceptable procedure, and the patient is better served by mastectomy. If the excision margins are positive and re-excision still shows disease at the resection margin, mastectomy is preferable. However, if the patient strongly desires preservative treatment, increasing the local radiation dose by means such as interstitial implantation of radioactive material can be considered.

Some women have had breast augmentation procedures with a prosthesis. Such appliances may cause unusual problems for the preservative technique. There is not a large experience in treating patients with a prosthesis, and thus it is difficult to make firm recommendations. A prudent recommendation is to remove the prosthesis, although for some women, this will negate the cosmetic advantage of a preservation technique. Such patients may be better served by mastectomy with appropriate reconstructive procedures.

For individual patients, there are often other considerations. Usually, a frank discussion with the patient and ample time for consideration of the alternatives allows an easy selection. These choices must be made by the patient with the advice, recommendation, and guidance of the physician. The relative importance of each of these considerations will change depending on the accumulated data and the physician's experience with the technical improvements of the various treatment techniques.

The use of adjuvant chemotherapy is discussed separately in this chapter. It may be combined with either mastectomy or preservative management with equal effectiveness and thus should not be a factor in the selection of the primary treatment modality. The timing of chemotherapy relative to the radiation treatment in preservative management is still unresolved. In general, we favor not administering them concomitantly, especially if doxorubicin is a part of the treatment regimen. There are strong reasons to consider giving the adjuvant chemotherapy first in patients at very high risk for distant metastases, the best indicator of which seems to be a large number of positive nodes. This is especially appropriate in patients who have had a good local excision. In patients with only a few positive nodes, the data support the use of chemotherapy following radiation, although some suggest that one cycle may precede the radiation. There are a number of studies in this area that require continued evaluation.

ADJUVANT THERAPY

Screening trials, especially the Health Insurance Plan of Greater New York (HIP) trial described above, have demonstrated conclusively that mastectomy or some other form of local therapy improves the likelihood of survival of some portion of breast cancer patients. Contrary to Halsted's expectations, however, improved local control with more extensive surgery or adjuvant radiotherapy has generally not improved survival. The effects of local therapy are "all or none": either the patient is cured by local treatment, or she dies of distant metastases at about the same time she would have died without local intervention because these metastases were established prior to the time of diagnosis and are outside the scope of even the most extensive local treatment.

These observations on the limitations of local therapy provided the initial rationale for the use of adjuvant systemic therapy (either chemotherapy or endocrine therapy) immediately following local treatment. In addition, it has been shown in animal models that tumors incurable by any form of therapy at a more advanced stage may be cured by surgical excision and adjuvant systemic therapy early after implantation.[219] Breast cancer was the first tumor in which adjuvant therapy was employed, and randomized trials evaluating adjuvant oophorectomy were begun as early as 1948.[220] Although success with adjuvant chemotherapy was first obtained in the treatment of pediatric tumors,[221] it is now firmly established that adjuvant chemotherapy will prolong the survival of premenopausal patients and adjuvant tamoxifen that of postmenopausal patients. These adjuvants to surgery and radiotherapy should now be considered standard treatment for node-positive patients.

ADJUVANT CHEMOTHERAPY

The chemotherapy trials that set today's standards were begun in 1972 and 1973. The first of these was conducted by the NSABP and used a single agent, L-phenylalanine mustard (L-PAM), 0.15 mg/kg orally for 5 days of each 6-week cycle for 2 years. Although less effective than some other agents then available for the treatment of metastatic breast cancer, L-PAM was associated with remarkably little acute toxicity and required no intravenous injections.[222] About 1 year later, the National Cancer Institute of Milan, Italy, initiated a similar trial of CMF. This regimen required intravenous injections on days 1 and 8 of each monthly cycle and oral administration of cyclophosphamide on days 1 through 14. The CMF was given for 1 year and had considerably more acute toxicity, including nausea, vomiting, mucositis, alopecia, leukopenia, and thrombocytopenia.[223] Similar patients were included in these two studies. All patients had operable cancers, including some T3 lesions, and axillary lymph node metastases and were stratified into two groups; those with one to three histologically involved nodes and those with more than four involved nodes. Patients were also stratified by menstrual status as premenopausal or postmenopausal (Milan) or by age (younger than 50 or 50 or older) (NSABP).

The 10-year results from these two trials are summarized in Table 38-21. All treated patients in both studies had a prolongation of disease-free survival, but this was statistically significant only for premenopausal women. Treated premenopausal women also had a statistically significant increase in overall survival. At 10 years, this was 24% for patients treated with L-PAM ($p = 0.02$) and 14% for patients given CMF ($p < 0.02$).

Subsequent published trials have more or less confirmed the results of these first studies.[224] In 11 such trials, premenopausal women were randomized to receive either chemotherapy (usually a combination of drugs for at least 6 months) or local therapy alone (mastectomy with or without adjuvant radiotherapy). In all of these trials, the patients who received adjuvant chemotherapy had better disease-free and overall survival rates, and improvement in disease-free survival reached levels of conventional statistical significance in five of the studies. The significant overall survival advantage observed for premenopausal women in the NSABP and Milan trials has now been confirmed in a third trial. In this study by the Danish national trials group, more than 1000 women were randomized to receive either cyclophosphamide as a single agent (130 mg/m² daily for 14 days of each monthly cycle) or CMF in about 75% to 80% of the doses given in the Milan trial. After more than 6 years of follow-up, there is a statistically significant survival advantage for those patients receiving adjuvant CMF and a trend toward improved survival for those receiving cyclophosphamide alone. The follow-up on all of the other published premenopausal studies is shorter than the follow-up of the studies from the NSABP, Milan, and Denmark, and it is reasonable to anticipate that a survival advantage for the treated patients will emerge with additional follow-up of the other trials.

There are also 11 published trials in which postmenopausal women were randomized to receive at least 4 months of adjuvant chemotherapy or local treatment only. In many cases, these were separate studies and not merely strata of larger trials that included both premenopausal and postmenopausal women. There is a trend toward improved disease-free survival in seven of the trials and a trend toward improved survival in three of the trials. However, the disease-free survival advantage reached conventional statistical significance in only three of the trials, and a significant survival advantage has never been observed.[224]

TABLE 38-21. Ten-Year Results of NSABP and Milan Trials in Which Patients with Histologically Involved Nodes Were Randomized to 1 to 2 Years of Adjuvant Chemotherapy or to Mastectomy Alone

	NSABP[222]			*Milan*[58,223]		
Patient Group	*Control*	*L-Pam*	*p*	*Control*	*CMF*	*p*
		Recurrence-Free at 10 Years (%)				
All patients	29	38	0.06	31	43	0.001
Premenopausal	29	46	0.02	31	48	0.0005
Postmenopausal	28	34	0.49	32	38	0.32
Premenopausal						
1–3 nodes	41	66	0.02	40	61	0.0002
>3 nodes	17	22	0.42	15	26	0.03
		Alive at 10 Years (%)				
All patients	41	48	0.30	47	55	0.10
Premenopausal	37	61	0.02	45	59	<0.02
Postmenopausal	43	41	0.80	50	52	0.89
Premenopausal						
1–3 nodes	48	81	0.01	51	68	0.025
>3 nodes	26	35	0.54	30	42	0.29

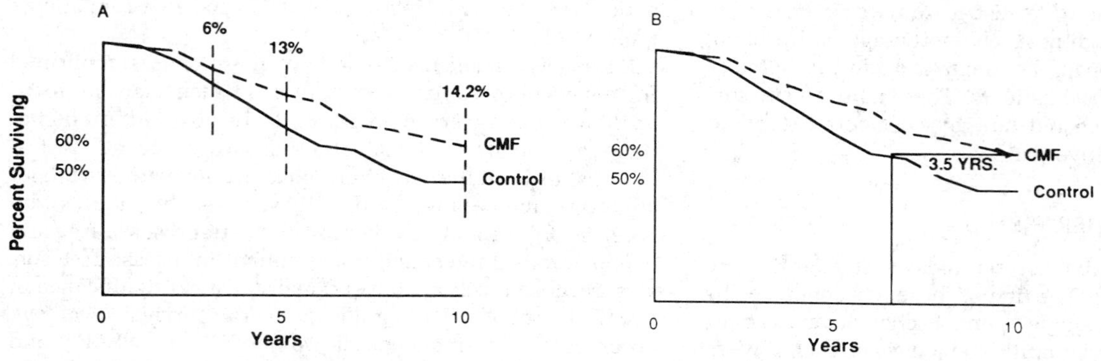

FIG. 38-20. Ten-year survival rate of all premenopausal patients treated in the Milan CMF trial. **A**. Usual way of interpreting survival curves by calculating vertical difference between curves at various time points after entry onto study. **B**. Estimating average survival benefit by calculating difference in the medians of the two curves. Because median has not yet been reached for the treated group in this study, a horizontal at the 60th percentile has been used. (Bonadonna G, Valagussa P, Rossi A et al: Ten-year experience with CMF-based adjuvant chemotherapy in resectable breast cancer. Breast Cancer Res Treat 5:95–115, 1985)

ESTIMATING THE SIZE OF THE BENEFIT

There are several ways in which the benefits of adjuvant chemotherapy in premenopausal women can be expressed. To some clinicians, the fact that the survival difference is statistically significant may be sufficient reason to utilize adjuvant chemotherapy in all node-positive premenopausal women. Others may wish to know the size of the benefit as well. The Kaplan-Meier survival plots for node-positive premenopausal women in the Milan trial are illustrated in Figure 38-20A. These demonstrate an absolute survival difference at 5 years (13%) and 10 years (14.2%) between treated patients and controls. However, it should not be erroneously assumed that only 14% of all treated patients benefited, and it is equally incorrect to conclude that 14% of all patients have been "cured" by adjuvant therapy.

Whereas the absolute survival differences shown in Figure 38-20A provide an estimate of treatment effect in the context of all patients given the treatment, a ratio reduction in mortality rate provides an estimate of benefit for the patients who would have died without therapy. If adjuvant therapy had no effect on patient survival, we would expect the number of deaths in each arm of a randomized study to occur in the same ratio as the number of patients originally randomized to each study arm. If, however, the number of deaths observed is smaller than that expected under the null hypothesis, the ratio of observed to expected deaths (O:E) will be less than 1.0 and will provide some measure of the reduction in mortality rate as a result of therapy. In the Milan trial, the O:E ratio for CMF-treated premenopausal patients was 0.78 and for control patients 1.31. This represents a 40% reduction in the mortality rate during the first 10 years of follow-up.[226]

A third way of expressing the size of the benefit from therapy requires longer follow-up but provides an estimate more consistent with the known biologic effect of systemic therapy. As noted, the effects from mastectomy and local radiotherapy are "all or none": either the patient's tumor is eradicated and the patient is cured, or the patient dies at approximately the time she would have died without treatment. In contrast, the effects of adjuvant systemic therapy are likely to be more variable: some patients may derive several months of additional life as a result of treatment, others may live several decades as a result of therapy, and a few may regain a normal life expectancy (*i.e.*, be "cured") as a result of the therapy. The Kaplan-Meier plots shown in Figure 38-20 are actually a summation of these variable effects. Conventionally, physicians calculate the vertical differences between the two curves (Fig. 38-20A). However, it may be more appropriate to evaluate horizontal differences between the curves, as shown in Figure 38-20B. If this horizontal difference is calculated at the point where 50% of the treated and control patients have died, it would represent a difference in medians. However, this set of data illustrates one of the significant limitations of this method: even after 10 years of follow-up, the median survival of the patients treated with CMF has not been reached. Ideally, the median follow-up of all patients in the study would exceed the median survival of the group with the best survival before a difference in medians is calculated. If the difference illustrated in Figure 38-22B, 3.5 years, were a true difference in medians, it could be interpreted as the average life gained by each treated patient over what she might have had with mastectomy only.

Recently published results from the Milan trial have been expressed as differences in medians. As shown in Table 38-22, the median disease-free survival of all patients randomized to the control arm of the study is 40 months, the median disease-free survival of all patients treated with CMF is 83 months, and the difference in the medians is 43 months. The difference in median disease-free survival for premenopausal women is in excess of 9 years, whereas postmenopausal women treated with one year of CMF had a median prolongation of disease-free survival of only 5 months. The longest benefits accrued to women with one to three positive nodes. Survival data are also shown in Table

TABLE 38-22. Differences in Median Disease-Free Survival and Overall Survival at 12 Years for Patients Randomized to 1 Year of Adjuvant Chemotherapy (CMF) or No Systemic Therapy (Control) in Milan Trial

	Disease-Free (mo)			*Survival (mo)*		
Patient Group	*Control*	*CMF*	*Difference*	*Control*	*CMF*	*Difference*
All	40	83	43	104	140	36
1–3 positive nodes	63	141	78	130	*	*
≥4 positive nodes	20	44	24	77	82	5
Premenopausal	32	141	109	96	*	*
Postmenopausal	59	64	5	128	113	−15

Modified from Bonadonna G, Valagussa P, Zambetti M et al: Milan adjuvant trials for stage I–II breast cancer. In Salmon SE (ed): Adjuvant Therapy of Cancer V, pp 211–222. New York, Grune & Stratton, 1987.

* Median survival not yet reached for CMF group, and difference in median cannot be calculated.

38-22. The difference in medians for all patients is 3 years; the difference in medians for premenopausal women has still not been reached, and the difference in medians for postmenopausal women is actually a negative value, suggesting a potential detrimental effect of therapy in this group.

ADJUVANT TAMOXIFEN

The first of the adjuvant tamoxifen trials was begun about 3 years after the adjuvant chemotherapy trials just described. Interest in the use of tamoxifen increased when a few studies demonstrated a benefit from adjuvant oophorectomy in premenopausal women and adjuvant chemotherapy failed to prolong the survival of postmenopausal women significantly.

The earliest trial to demonstrate that adjuvant tamoxifen could prolong the survival of patients with early breast cancer was the Nolvadex Adjuvant Therapy Organization (NATO) trial.[227,228] In this British study, node-positive and node-negative patients were randomized to receive either 2 years of tamoxifen following local therapy or local therapy only. At the end of 8 years, the survival advantage for the tamoxifen-treated groups exceeds 10%, and this difference is statistically significant. In this study, the O:E ratio of deaths is 0.86 for tamoxifen-treated patients and 1.14 for the control patients. The reduction of the mortality rate as a result of tamoxifen is estimated to be about 30%.[228] Although more than 1100 patients were enrolled in this trial, only 11% were premenopausal and 45% were node-positive. As a result, the power to detect even moderate to large differences in survival within patient subsets is not great. To circumvent this problem, these data have been analyzed using a Cox model, and in this model, the O:E ratio was similar for all subsets of the trial including premenopausal node-positive patients and postmenopausal patients with or without histologically involved nodes.

Results from nine additional trials in which patients were randomized to either tamoxifen or to no adjuvant systemic therapy have been published.[224] Most or all of the patients in each of these studies were postmenopausal. In each case, tamoxifen treatment resulted in a statistically significant improvement in disease-free survival. However, the overall survival advantage observed in the NATO trial has only recently been confirmed in a second study. In this trial, performed by the Scottish National Trial Group, more than 1300 women were randomized to receive either 5 years of adjuvant tamoxifen or no adjuvant systemic therapy. Unlike most other adjuvant trials, patients in the control group were scheduled to receive tamoxifen as their first systemic therapy after recurrence, and 93% of the patients in the control group were actually treated as planned. At the end of 8 years, there was a 15% survival advantage for the patients given adjuvant tamoxifen. The survival: hazard ratio of the tamoxifen patients was 0.71 compared with the control group ($p = 0.002$) (Table 38-23). This effect of tamoxifen was evident in all subgroups but was statistically significant only among postmenopausal women and among node-positive patients. All of the premenopausal women entered in this trial were node negative (in contrast to the NATO trial), and the number of deaths observed in the node-negative group, whether postmenopausal or premenopausal, is still considerably

TABLE 38-23. Eight-Year Results of Scottish Trial in which Patients with and without Histologically Involved Nodes Were Randomized to 5 Years of Adjuvant Tamoxifen (TAM) or Tamoxifen as First Systemic Therapy of Recurrence[243]

		Hazard Ratio
Patient Group	*No. of Patients*	*5-Year TAM (±95%CI)*
	Disease-Free Survival	
All patients	1312	0.57*(0.47–0.68)
	Survival	
All patients	1312	0.71†(0.58–0.89)
Node negative	751	0.73 (0.51–1.04)
Node positive	456	0.61 (0.46–0.81)
Premenopausal†	242	0.57 (0.27–1.19)
Postmenopausal‡	1070	0.73 (0.59–0.89)

* $p < 0.0001$.
† $p = 0.002$.
‡ All premenopausal patients had negative nodes; both node-negative and node-positive postmenopausal patients were included.

fewer than the number of deaths observed in the node-positive group.

A calculation of the differences in median disease-free survival and overall survival rates for patients randomized in the adjuvant tamoxifen trial are shown in Table 38-24. Because so many patients in this study were node negative, the median survivals have not been reached for the entire patient group. However, among the node-positive patients, there was a 53-month difference in the median disease-free survival period of the tamoxifen patients compared with the group who received no adjuvant systemic therapy. The overall survival advantage from adjuvant tamoxifen was 22 months. In this study, survival after recurrence was longer in the control group than in the tamoxifen group.

OVARIAN ABLATION

The first trial of ovarian ablation was begun in 1948, the last in 1965.[224] There were seven of these trials. Some used ovarian radiation and others oophorectomy. Some of the studies included both premenopausal and postmenopausal patients. None of the trials demonstrated a survival benefit from adjuvant oophorectomy at the end of the first 5 years of follow-up, and survival differences at 10 years were not large for most of the studies. As a result, adjuvant ovarian ablation had been abandoned by the time the first adjuvant chemotherapy trials utilizing long courses of chemotherapy were begun in 1972. In retrospect, it is plausible that adjuvant ovarian ablation was abandoned prematurely. The 10- and 15-year results from three of these trials now show larger survival advantages than anticipated. These observations, coupled with the fact that adjuvant chemotherapy appears to benefit premenopausal but not postmenopausal women, have been interpreted by some as evidence that adjuvant chemotherapy is really a form of chemical oophorectomy.[229]

The earliest and largest of the studies conducted in premenopausal women was initiated by the Christie Hospital in 1948. Women were randomized to receive either ovarian ablation or no further therapy after mastectomy.[220] At the end of 10 years, there was a 13% mortality reduction for all patients entered into the trial, a 37% mortality reduction for the node-negative patients, and an 11% mortality reduction for the node-positive patients. These differences were less evident after 15 years of follow-up (Table 38-25).

In a trial conducted in Toronto, Canada, patients under age 45 were randomized to receive ovarian ablation or no further systemic therapy. Those over age 45 were randomized to receive ovarian ablation alone, ovarian ablation plus at least 5 years of prednisone (7.5 mg daily), or no systemic therapy. There were only 150 patients in the group under age 45, and the small survival advantage for patients treated with ovarian ablation alone in this group did not reach statistical significance. However, premenopausal women over age 45 treated with both ovarian radiation and prednisone had a significant disease-free and overall survival advantage that persisted through year 15, at which time 72% of the patients in the treated group were alive compared with 44% in the control group ($p = 0.02$).[230]

Only one surgical oophorectomy trial has demonstrated a significant survival benefit for treated patients.[231] In this study, half of the patients were node negative, and some of the patients were postmenopausal. At 10 years, 71% of the patients treated with adjuvant oophorectomy were alive compared with 60% of the control group ($p < 0.05$). A similar trial from Malmö, Sweden, with 20 years of follow-up showed a trend toward improved survival with adjuvant oophorectomy, but this did not reach statistical significance.[232] The median survival of premenopausal women in the treated group was 62 months compared with 53 months in the control group, a difference that was not statistically significant.

OVERVIEW ANALYSIS

It is possible that a survival benefit of scientific or clinical importance may be overlooked even in randomized trials enrolling more than 1000 patients. For example, a mortality reduction of 20% could easily be missed in most of the randomized trials conducted thus far even though a statistically significant mortality reduction of this magnitude represents a large number of lives saved with a disease as common as breast cancer. A smaller but real benefit could also provide impetus for the design of additional clinical trials to develop an apparently promising idea further. However, there are limitations and potential pitfalls in the use of overviews.[233] For example, the greater statistical power may distort and exaggerate a very small benefit and so lead to inappropriate or excessive use of a therapy. The magnitude of a benefit determined in an overview may also be overestimated or

TABLE 38-24. Differences in Median Disease-Free Survival and Overall Survival for Patients Randomized to 5 Years of Adjuvant Tamoxifen (TAM) or No Systemic Therapy Control Group in Scottish National Trial (8-Year Follow-up Data)

	Disease-Free (mo)			*Survival (mo)*		
Patient Group	*Control*	*TAM*	*Difference*	*Control*	*TAM*	*Difference*
All	73	*	*	95	*	*
Node negative	*	*	*	*	*	*
Node positive	31	84	53	63	85	22

Modified from Scottish Cancer Trials Office: Adjuvant tamoxifen in the management of operable breast cancer: The Scottish trial. Lancet 2:171–175, 1987.

* Median survival not yet reached for tamoxifen or control group, and difference in medians cannot be calculated.

TABLE 38-25. Disease-Free Survival and Overall Survival Among Patients Randomized to Ovarian Irradiation or No Systemic Treatment in the Christie Hospital Trial*

		Disease-Free Survival (%)		*Overall Survival (%)*		
Patient Group	*Analysis Year*	*Control*	*Irradiation*	*Control*	*Irradiation*	*p*
All	10	44	53	48	55	0.07
	15			40	45	NS†
Node negative	10			69	80	0.06
	15	61	64	64	66	NS
Node positive	10			37	44	0.16
	15	24	34	29	36	NS

* Data from Cole MP: A clinical trial of an artificial menopause in carcinoma of the breast. In: Namer M, Lalanne CM (eds): Hormones and breast cancer. Paris: INSERM, 143–150, 1976, and Cole MP: Prophylactic compared with therapeutic x-ray artificial menopause. In Joslin CAF, Gleave EN (eds): The Clinical Management of Advanced Breast Cancer, pp 2–11. Cardiff, Alpha Omega Alpha Publishing, 1970.

† NS = Differences in survival figures not statistically significant.

underestimated. For example, an effect may be overestimated when one large trial with an inordinately large false-positive result contributes most of the weight to the overview estimate. Underestimation may occur when several trials with false-negative results (*e.g.*, from poor patient compliance in utilizing the treatment under study) are summated with the results from more positive trials. The main advantage of an overview thus can also be its weakness, and estimates of benefit obtained in an overview should never be accepted without a careful evaluation of the individual trials that have contributed to it.

Several overview analyses of adjuvant breast trials have now been published. One of these was limited to studies in the published literature.[234] A second attempted to include every trial, published and unpublished, that has been conducted throughout the world.[235] The latter study included patients randomized in trials comparing tamoxifen with no tamoxifen (*e.g.*, tamoxifen versus no systemic therapy, tamoxifen plus chemotherapy versus chemotherapy only) and trials that compared adjuvant chemotherapy with no adjuvant chemotherapy (*e.g.*, chemotherapy versus no systemic therapy, chemotherapy plus tamoxifen versus tamoxifen). This analysis included more than 9000 women randomized in chemotherapy trials and 16,000 women in tamoxifen trials. The estimated reduction in the mortality rate resulting from the use of adjuvant chemotherapy with combination agents was $26 \pm 7\%$ in women under the age of 50 and $8 \pm 6\%$ in those over the age of 50. The effects of adjuvant tamoxifen were $-2 \pm 8\%$ in women under age 50 and $20 \pm 3\%$ in women over the age of 50. No significant benefit accrued to patients treated with single-agent cytotoxic therapy.

The results of this overview analysis confirm the results of individual trials. Adjuvant chemotherapy is highly effective in premenopausal women and adjuvant tamoxifen in postmenopausal women. Also, adjuvant chemotherapy imparts no significant survival advantage to postmenopausal women, and adjuvant tamoxifen treatment has not yet been proved advantageous for premenopausal women.

NODE-NEGATIVE PATIENTS

Most of the chemotherapy trials just described involved primarily or exclusively patients with histologically involved nodes. In contrast, a large proportion of the patients in the endocrine therapy trials had no lymph node involvement. This is understandable in light of the relative toxicities of the two therapies. Even if the ratio reduction in mortality rate for node-negative and node-positive patients is the same, the absolute differences in mortality rates are likely to be different. Because node-negative patients generally have a better prognosis, the absolute differences in the survival of the treated and untreated patients may be quite small, and in this context, the toxicity of the therapy may easily outweigh the gain. Late toxicity, such as an increased incidence of second tumors, is also a more important consideration in a patient population more likely to live long enough to express the carcinogenic effect of the therapy (see below under toxicity). Because of this, many investigators have tried to identify a "bad prognostic group" among the node-negative patients, anticipating that adjuvant chemotherapy with its attendant toxicities might be more justified, as well as more effective, in patients with high-growth-fraction tumors. Until recently, the lack of ER or PR has been considered a marker of this poor prognosis group. However, a careful analysis of all studies on the prognosis of node-negative patients demonstrates that the 20% to 30% of node-negative patients likely to have recurrences and die of breast cancer in the first decade after diagnosis are not predominantly or exclusively ER-negative patients (see above).

Studies specifically designed to test the efficacy of adjuvant chemotherapy in node-negative patients are of recent vintage.[224] The largest of these trials randomized 457 patients to receive either adjuvant LMF (chlorambucil, methotrexate, and 5-FU) or no systemic treatment. At the end of 7 years, there was no significant difference in the disease-free survival rates of the two groups.[236] A Swiss study using a similar regimen demonstrated a transient effect but no significant long-term improvement in survival.[237] A small Austrian study using a slightly more intensive chemotherapy regimen demonstrated a significant survival benefit without an improvement in the recurrence-free survival rate.[238] This contradiction cannot be fully explained.

The study most frequently cited to support the use of chemotherapy in node-negative patients is the Milan trial in which patients who were both node-negative and ER-negative were randomized to receive either 12 courses of intravenous CMF over a period of 9 months or no systemic treatment.[239] Only 90 patients were enrolled in this trial, and the 5-year mortality rate for the control patients exceeded 35%. There was a significant survival advantage for the patients given adjuvant CMF ($p = 0.02$), and this was apparent in both premenopausal and postmenopausal women. The number of relapses in the control and treated populations, respectively, was 7 of 27 and 2 of 27 premenopausal patients, and 5 of 18 and 1 of 18 postmenopausal patients.

These results from Milan must be interpreted in the context of two other trials of node-negative patients, each of which has enrolled 500 to 1000 treated patients.[240–242] Although results from these studies have not been published, each has been monitored regularly for evidence of benefit. One of these trials is limited to node-negative, receptor-negative patients. The other stratified patients on the basis of receptor status. Because it is highly unlikely that a significant benefit anywhere near the magnitude of that described in the Milan trial has been observed but not reported, the dramatic results of the Milan trial must be accepted cautiously lest they prove to be an overestimate of the benefit.

Adjuvant systemic therapy is not recommended for node-negative patients at the present time and should not be considered for any patient until it has been reproducibly demonstrated that the survival benefits outweigh both the early and the delayed toxicities.

ENDOCRINE THERAPY IN RECEPTOR-NEGATIVE PATIENTS

In the NATO trial comparing 2 years of adjuvant tamoxifen with no systemic therapy, there was no evidence that the survival benefits for tamoxifen were greater or more significant among receptor-positive than receptor-negative patients.[227] The ratio of O:E deaths in patients with an ER concentration below and above 5 fmol/mg of cytosol protein was 0.63 and 0.82, respectively. The O:E ratio for patients with receptor levels below and above 30 fmol/mg was 0.76 and 0.71.

The data recently published from the Scottish National Trial appear to confirm the observations from the NATO study (Table 38-26). Patients were divided into groups based on receptor concentrations of 0 to 4, 5 to 19, 20 to 99, and 100 or more fmol/mg.[243] The 3-year disease-free survival rate was higher for the tamoxifen-treated group than for the control group within each subset. The survival: hazard ratio for the total follow-up period was also decreased as a result of tamoxifen treatment for each subgroup. However, this advantage for tamoxifen reached levels of statistical significance only in the group with the highest receptor level. Several other studies evaluating adjuvant tamoxifen have shown a nonsignificant trend toward better survival among ER-negative patients, but two large trials have shown a trend toward decreased survival among the tamoxifen-treated ER-negative patients.[242,244]

Until recently, it was difficult to accept the possibility that tamoxifen might have an effect in receptor-negative patients, as the response rate to endocrine therapy is less than 10% among receptor-negative patients with metastatic disease. However, recent laboratory investigations suggest that estrogen-dependent cells might produce paracrine growth factors that could support the growth of estrogen-independent cells[42] (see below). If so, the eradication of very few receptor-positive, tamoxifen-sensitive cells might affect the growth of a much larger mass of cells.

DURATION OF THERAPY

Perioperative adjuvant chemotherapy trials utilized one or a few doses of chemotherapy during the first week or two after diagnosis and mastectomy. One of these studies demonstrated a statistically significant survival advantage for patients treated with daily doses of intravenous cyclophosphamide.[245] However, the results of this trial have not been confirmed, and other perioperative studies of similar design have not shown such a significant survival benefit.[224]

TABLE 38-26. Correlation of ER Concentration and Disease-Free Survival Benefits from Adjuvant Tamoxifen in the Scottish National Trial (8-Year Report)

ER (fmol/mg)	*No. of Patients*	*Disease-Free (%) at 3 Years*		*Hazard Ratio Total Follow-up (95% CI)*
		Control	*Tamoxifen*	
All patients	1312	64	79	0.57 (0.47–0.68)
0–4	218	55	66	0.70 (0.47–1.05)
5–19	89	61	72	0.67 (0.36–1.28)
20–99	214	74	86	0.57 (0.33–1.00)
100+	221	61	86	0.35 (0.22–0.57)
Not tested	570	65	80	0.56 (0.43–0.47)

Modified from Scottish Cancer Trials Office. Adjuvant tamoxifen in the management of operable breast cancer: The Scottish trial. Lancet 2:171–175, 1987.

Large survival benefits from adjuvant chemotherapy were first demonstrated with regimens given for 1 to 2 years. A second generation of trials has now been completed in which patients were randomized to two durations of treatment. In the first of these studies, patients were randomized to receive either 15 or 30 weeks of a combination of cyclophosphamide and doxorubicin.[246] With a median follow-up in excess of 5 years and a maximum follow-up in excess of 10 years, there is no survival benefit for patients given the longer course of treatment, and there is a nonsignificant trend toward better survival for patients who received the short course. In Milan, patients were randomized to either 6 or 12 months of CMF,[223,247] and there was a nonsignificant trend toward improved survival with the shorter course of treatment in this study as well. This survival trend in favor of shorter therapy was most evident among the postmenopausal patients, for whom the value of chemotherapy is limited at best. Other studies addressing the issue of optimal therapy duration have randomized patients to intervals of 12 or 6 months, 24 or 6 months, and 2 years or 1 year.[246] None has demonstrated an advantage for the longer treatment.

There are no published results from randomized trials comparing different durations of tamoxifen treatment. Tamoxifen was given for 2 years in one and 5 years in the second trial in which an overall survival advantage was demonstrated. However, the duration of therapy was not the only distinguishing characteristic of these two trials, and it cannot yet be concluded that the optimal duration of adjuvant tamoxifen treatment is known. Until the results from randomized trials specifically designed to address this question are available, it is recommended that tamoxifen be given for at least 2 years and not more than 5 years.

OPTIMAL CHEMOTHERAPY

SINGLE AGENTS VERSUS COMBINATION CHEMOTHERAPY

The results of trials comparing the efficacy of combination chemotherapy with that of a single drug are contradictory.[224] Among premenopausal women, there is a statistically significant survival advantage for patients given combination chemotherapy in two of the studies, a nonsignificant but positive trend in two of the studies, and a nonsignificant negative survival trend in two more studies. The data from a similar number of studies in postmenopausal women are similarly contradictory.

DOXORUBICIN COMBINATIONS

Combination chemotherapy regimens that include doxorubicin have repeatedly induced a higher response in patients with metastatic breast cancer than regimens not including this drug (see below). Several recently reported trials suggest that this may be true in the adjuvant setting as well. In a French trial, patients were randomized to receive either 1 year of adjuvant CMF at conventional doses or one year of AVCF (doxorubicin, vincristine, cyclophosphamide, 5-FU).[249] In the seventh year of follow-up, 58% of the CMF patients and 75% of the AVCF patients were alive ($p = 0.015$). A trend toward improved disease-free survival rates among postmenopausal women was not statistically significant, but both the disease-free and the overall survival rates of premenopausal women randomized to AVCF were significantly better than those of patients randomized to CMF ($p = 0.001$). The NSABP randomized receptor-negative patients to receive either PF (L-PAM and 5-FU) or PAF (PF plus doxorubicin). Receptor-positive patients were randomized to the same two combinations with the addition of tamoxifen to each.[250] At the end of 5 years, there was a 20% decrease in the relapse rate and a 15% decrease in the mortality rate among patients receiving the combinations containing doxorubicin. The improvements in the disease-free survival rates were highly significant. The improvement in survival was marginally significant in postmenopausal women but not in premenopausal women.

The Cancer and Leukemia Group B (CALGB) has evaluated the possibility that the introduction of a doxorubicin-containing compound after induction with CMFVP might improve survival.[251] Patients were randomized to receive CMFVP for 14 months or CMFVP for 8 months followed by vinblastine, doxorubicin, thiotepa, and Halotestin (VATH). This trial showed an improvement in the disease-free survival rate that was statistically significant at the time of first analysis and a trend toward improved survival as well.

Conventional CMF has been compared with either CMFP or CMFVP in randomized trials. None of these studies has shown a statistically significant improvement in the overall survival rate, although the authors of these studies have concluded that there may be some advantage for the four- or five-drug regimen for some patient subsets. These conclusions must remain tentative until more data from mature trials are available.

DOSE

In a retrospective analysis of the Milan CMF trial, it was observed that the patients who received more than 85% of the planned dose of CMF had a statistically significant improvement in survival compared with patients who received reduced doses.[223,252] However, only 20% of the patients received full doses of therapy. The survival advantage for patients given the higher doses was seen among both premenopausal and postmenopausal women and has persisted through 10 years of follow-up. Other investigators have performed similar retrospective analyses correlating the dose of chemotherapy with either disease-free or overall survival, and none has found a statistically significant survival advantage for higher doses. Indeed, in some trials, there was not even a trend toward improved disease-free survival among patients who received the higher doses. A retrospective analysis of multiple trials has been reported that shows dose rate to be an important variable in disease-free survival.[253] However, this retrospective analysis is based on many assumptions inconsistent with the general principles of medical oncology practice. In addition, the statistical methodology is probably not appropriate to the data set selected.[254] This analysis therefore cannot be accepted as evidence that dose is an important variable in the use of adjuvant chemotherapy. On the basis of present knowledge, it seems unwise either to escalate or to decrease chemotherapy beyond the limits set by trials in which adjuvant chemotherapy resulted in a significant survival benefit.

CHEMOHORMONAL THERAPY

Many randomized trials have been conducted comparing either chemotherapy alone or endocrine therapy alone with a combination of chemotherapy and endocrine therapy.[224] In spite of this abundance of data, the critical questions regarding the appropriate use of these two modalities cannot yet be fully answered. These questions are:

1. Can all of the benefits of adjuvant chemotherapy be achieved by adjuvant oophorectomy? No published results are available from any trial evaluating the relative efficacy of chemotherapy and oophorectomy (or ovarian radiation) in premenopausal women, and very few randomized trials of this type have been initiated.
2. Is there a benefit from combining endocrine therapy (either tamoxifen or oophorectomy) with chemotherapy in premenopausal women? In one study, there was a nonsignificant trend toward improved survival when oophorectomy was added to CMFP,[242] and in another study, tamoxifen added very little to CMF or CMFP.[255] In NSABP trial B-09, patients who received a combination of PFT (L-PAM, 5-FU, and tamoxifen) had a shorter survival than patients treated with PF alone, but this trend was not statistically significant.
3. Do postmenopausal women who receive a combination of chemotherapy and tamoxifen live longer than those who receive tamoxifen alone? The definitive published trial addressing this issue is the Ludwig III trial.[256] Four hundred sixty-three patients were randomized to receive either daily oral prednisone plus tamoxifen for 12 months (pT), CMFpT for 12 months, or no systemic adjuvant therapy. At the end of 7 years, there is a statistically significant survival advantage for the patients treated with CMFpT compared with either those given pT alone or those randomized to observation (Fig. 38-21). Preliminary results from a somewhat smaller trial comparing 3 years of adjuvant tamoxifen alone with CMFP plus 3 years of tamoxifen has demonstrated a significant increase in the disease-free survival rate among those patients receiving both chemotherapy and endocrine therapy but no overall survival advantage.[257]
4. Is tamoxifen alone as effective as or more effective than chemotherapy in postmenopausal women? Although there are several such studies under way, results have been published from only one.[224,258] At the end of 5 years, the disease-free survival rate of women over age 50 who received tamoxifen was significantly better than that of patients randomized to CMF (p = 0.009), but a small trend in favor of improved survival with tamoxifen alone was not statistically significant. In contrast, women under age 49 who were treated with CMF had a marginally significant improvement in disease-free survival and a highly significant improvement in overall survival compared with women of the same age randomized to treatment with tamoxifen alone.

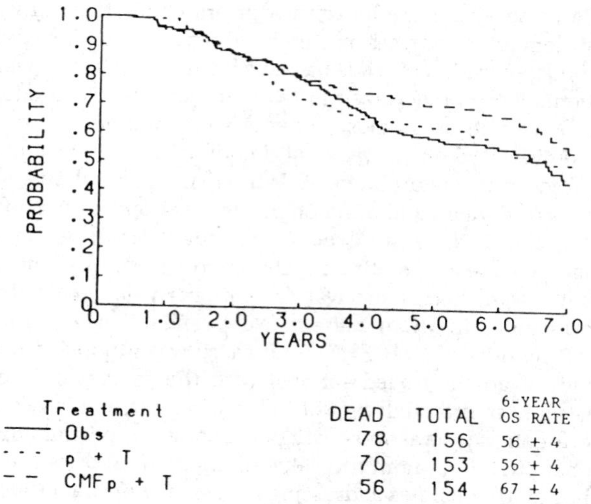

FIG. 38-21. Overall survival of postmenopausal patients in Ludwig III trial randomized to observation (*Obs*), prednisone plus tamoxifen (*p + T*), or CMFp + T. Three-way comparison, p = 0.12. CMFp + T vs Obs, p = 0.04; CMFp + T vs p + T, p = NS. (Goldhirsch A, Gelber RD: Adjuvant therapy for breast cancer: The Ludwig breast cancer trials 1987. In Salmon SE [ed]: Adjuvant Therapy of Cancer V, pp 297–309. Orlando, Grune & Stratton, 1987)

STANDARD REGIMEN

On the basis of the data currently available, 6 months of CMF should be considered standard adjuvant therapy for premenopausal node-positive patients. Regimens that contain doxorubicin appear to be as effective as CMF-type regimens, but it is plausible that mature data from ongoing trials will demonstrate the superiority of doxorubicin-containing combinations. Postmenopausal women should be treated with adjuvant tamoxifen, especially those who are node-positive and ER-positive. The value of chemotherapy in this group remains to be demonstrated, but the available evidence suggests that chemotherapy, when employed, should be given in combination with adjuvant tamoxifen.

INTEGRATION OF ADJUVANT THERAPY WITH OTHER MODALITIES

The optimal time to initiate adjuvant therapy is not known. It has been suggested that adjuvant chemotherapy be initiated as soon as possible after completion of primary therapy[259] or be given before treatment with mastectomy or radiotherapy.[260] This emphasis on timing is based on theoretical considerations and arises in part from a retrospective analysis of the Scandinavian trial in which patients were randomized to receive six daily doses of intravenous cyclophosphamide or no therapy.[259] The perioperative chemotherapy used in this trial resulted in a survival benefit in all but one of the hospitals contributing patients to the study. In that hospital, therapy was delayed for 2 to 4 weeks compared with the other hospitals, leading to the hypothesis that the time at which chemotherapy is started is important. However, similar retrospective analyses from other studies have not confirmed the observations of the Scandinavian trial. In addition, in a prospective randomized trial conducted to test this hypothesis,[256] in which patients were randomized to receive either no therapy immediately after mastectomy or CMF within 36 hours followed by 6 months of CMFPT or 6 months of CMFPT beginning 25 to 32 days after mastectomy, no significant advantage for early therapy has emerged with a median follow-up of 30 months. However, these results must be considered very preliminary.

Most adjuvant therapy trials have been performed in patients treated with mastectomy or mastectomy plus adjuvant radiotherapy. There are as yet no randomized controlled trials to determine the optimal integration of adjuvant chemotherapy and conservative surgery plus radiotherapy. Although chemotherapy and radiotherapy have been given sequentially and concomitantly, it has not been determined that the use of radiotherapy prior to chemotherapy will compromise the doses of chemotherapy that may be administered or that a compromise in dose is very important (see above). Because short courses of chemotherapy have proved as effective as longer courses, it is reasonable to consider administering all adjuvant chemotherapy after the surgical excision of the breast cancer and before the radiation therapy. However, it has not been shown that this can be done without compromising control of cancer within the breast itself. Uncontrolled trials have shown that chemotherapy may compromise the cosmetic results obtained when conservative surgery and primary radiation are used,[261] and preliminary results suggest that a sequential course of radiotherapy and chemotherapy is preferable to concomitant administration of these two modalities.[262]

TOXICITY

Although the acute toxicities of chemotherapy and the lack of acute toxicity from tamoxifen are well known, the possibility of a second tumor as a result of the therapy awaits further follow-up. The NSABP has reported an 11-fold increase in acute leukemia and a 24-fold increase in acute myelogenous leukemia ($p < 0.01$) within the first 10 years of follow-up after adjuvant therapy with L-PAM.[263] A similarly increased incidence of leukemia has not been observed after the administration of adjuvant CMF,[264] but the database from which this observation has been derived is probably too small to rule out any increased incidence of secondary cancers.[265] Firm evidence regarding the incidence of solid tumors resulting from either adjuvant chemotherapy or adjuvant tamoxifen will require two to three decades of follow-up. The very real possibility of inducing second tumors with adjuvant chemotherapy is readily apparent, as these agents are known to be carcinogens both in the laboratory and in the clinic. However, long-term administration of tamoxifen, a weak estrogen, may also be associated with an increased incidence of second tumors, especially adenocarcinoma. At present, this possibility must remain speculative, although endometrial carcinoma has been observed in patients treated with adjuvant chemotherapy plus tamoxifen.[266]

In spite of the toxicity associated with chemotherapy, the net benefits in overall survival or quality of disease-free survival outweigh the toxic costs. The Ludwig group has addressed this issue by calculation of the average time spent without symptoms or toxicity (TWiST) for postmenopausal women randomized on their trial comparing pT, CMFpT, and observation.[267] In this analysis, a month of TWiST was removed for any month in which a patient experienced even 1 day of subjective treatment toxicity, such as nausea, vomiting, or mucositis. Three months were removed beyond the end of therapy for patients who had alopecia, weight gain, or a local recurrence. The remainder of a patient's lifetime was removed from the analysis if the patient developed distant metastases or a second primary tumor other than a breast cancer. The net TWiST for patients on the three study arms is shown in Table 38-27. During the first years of life, patients under observation had a larger TWiST than patients

TABLE 38-27. Average Time Spent Without Symptoms (of Disease) or Toxicity (from Therapy) (TWiST) among Patients Randomized to Observation Only, Adjuvant Endocrine Therapy with Prednisone and Tamoxifen (p + T), or Adjuvant Chemohormonal Therapy with CMFp + T in Ludwig Breast Cancer Study III

	Months from Mastectomy					
Patient/Treatment Groups	*12*	*24*	*36*	*48*	*60*	*72*
All patients						
Observation	11	19	25	30	31	38*
p + T	9	18	25	31	37	42
CMFp + T	3	13	21	30	37	44*
Estrogen receptor-positive						
Observation	11	20	27	33	38	43
p + T	9	19	27	36	43	49
CMFp + T	3	13	22	30	38	45
Estrogen receptor-negative						
Observation	10	18	23	28	32	35
p + T	8	14	19	23	26	28
CMFp + T	2	11	19	27	34	41

Modified from Gelber RD, Goldhirsch A, Castiglione M et al: Time without Symptoms and Toxicity (TWiST): A quality-of-life-oriented endpoint to evaluate adjuvant therapy. In Salmon SE (ed): Adjuvant Therapy of Cancer, pp 455–465, Orlando, Grune & Stratton, 1987.

* Difference statistically significant. Other differences do not reach conventional levels of statistical significance.

under treatment because of the toxicities from treatment. However, as the disease-free survival benefits began to emerge for the patients receiving adjuvant therapy, these patients began to have a net increase in TWiST compared with the patients under observation. At 72 months of follow-up, the patients given CMFpT had a net TWiST advantage of 6 months compared with controls randomized to observation only. This advantage was statistically significant. Among patients who were ER-positive, however, the greatest TWiST was obtained by patients treated with endocrine therapy alone, whereas for those who were ER-negative, there was actually a loss of TWiST as a result of endocrine therapy. However, these differences among patient subsets defined by receptor status were not statistically significant.

VALUE OF FOLLOW-UP PHYSICAL EXAMINATIONS AND TESTS AFTER PRIMARY TREATMENT

Follow-up of patients with breast cancer is often carried out in an irregular and costly manner. For patients who have been treated for a potentially curable disease, the objectives of follow-up examinations should be oriented principally to the potentially curable diagnoses, that is, early detection of persistent or new breast cancers (in the contralateral breast and, in breast-preservation cases, the ipsilateral breast also) and early detection and treatment of other lesions, such as large-bowel and gynecologic cancers. Bone and other scans, as well as markers such as CEA, do not uniformly detect occult metastases and do not detect curable disease. They are useful in the evaluation of symptomatic patients, but their value in routine follow-up is uncertain.[268]

A considerable proportion of first metastases in breast cancer patients are in the skeletal system. Consequently, the NSABP protocols require radionuclide scans every 6 months for the first 3 postoperative years and yearly thereafter. Recent data from the NSABP indicate that routinely scheduled bone scans to detect metastases in asymptomatic breast cancer patients are relatively unrewarding,[269] as only 52 of 7984 scans (0.06%) detected asymptomatic bone lesions. The average charge for a bone scan is estimated to be $200. Based on a total expenditure of $1.5 million for all scans in this one NSABP clinical trial, the cost of each positive scan in asymptomatic patients thus was approximately $29,000. Pertinent to this issue also is the lack of evidence that the treatment of patients with asymptomatic skeletal metastases improves survival over that obtained when one waits for the appearance of symptoms. As a result of the minimal benefit from such routine scanning, it was recommended that only those asymptomatic patients in the NSABP studies who had positive axillary nodes receive scans at yearly intervals for the first 3 years. Many others, however, would advise these tests for symptomatic patients only.

Most recurrences after mastectomy are symptomatic; in approximately one-third of patients, asymptomatic recurrences are detected on routine follow-up physical examinations.[270,271] Nevertheless, management of chest wall or supraclavicular nodal disease (usually by excision and radiation therapy) may provide significant palliation. Although these patients are seldom curable, avoidance of chest wall ulceration or painful neurovascular involvement of the brachial plexus is of value.

SPECIAL PROBLEMS IN BREAST CANCER MANAGEMENT

DUCTAL CARCINOMA IN SITU

A review of this subject was recently published in the *New England Journal of Medicine* (Schnitt and associates, April 7, 1988), portions of which are abstracted here.

In 1932, Broders defined carcinoma in situ as "a condition in which malignant epithelial cells and their progeny are found in or near positions occupied by their ancestors before the ancestors underwent malignant transformation."[272] In the breast, carcinoma in situ has traditionally been categorized as either lobular or ductal, depending on the cytologic features and the pattern of growth. Ductal carcinoma in situ (DCIS, also known as intraductal carcinoma or noninvasive ductal carcinoma) is characterized by a proliferation of malignant epithelial cells confined to the mammary ducts, without light microscopic evidence of invasion through the basement membrane into the surrounding stroma.

The clinical spectrum of DCIS is broad and includes lesions discovered incidentally during microscopic examination of breast tissue removed because of another abnormality (*e.g.*, a fibroadenoma or an area of fibrocystic change), small foci detected by mammography, palpable but localized masses, and large palpable tumors or large areas of abnormality on mammography. The frequency with which these various patterns of presentation are observed depends on the population under study. In series reported prior to the advent of screening mammography, most patients with DCIS presented with a palpable mass, nipple discharge, or both.[273-275] In contrast, in a recent nationwide study of patients who underwent mammographic screening, 59% of the in situ cancers were detected exclusively by mammography.[99] Thus, small (often less than 1 cm), mammographically detected lesions currently comprise the majority of cases of DCIS at many institutions.

In the past, most patients with DCIS were treated with mastectomy, so the natural history of this lesion could not be studied. The available information on the risk of progression of DCIS to invasive cancer thus is extremely limited. The only studies that have addressed this issue are those in which patients with DCIS were treated with biopsy alone. There are two studies that identified patients with DCIS during histologic review of biopsies originally categorized as benign. One of these, by Page and colleagues, noted subsequent invasive carcinoma in the ipsilateral breast in 7 of 25 patients (28%) at intervals of 3 to 10 years (mean 6.1 years) after the initial biopsy.[276] In the other, by Betsill and colleagues, 8 of 30 patients (27%) developed an invasive carcinoma in the same breast an average of 9.7 years after the initial biopsy showing DCIS, and in nearly all of these patients, the invasive tumor occurred at or near the original biopsy site.[125,277] In both series, the cases of DCIS were all of the micropapillary or cribriform types; neither included examples of comedo-type

DCIS. These studies suggest that some, but not all, patients with DCIS treated with biopsy alone will develop an invasive cancer in the ipsilateral breast, usually in the region of the initial lesion. In these studies, the invasive carcinomas most commonly occurred within 10 years of the initial biopsy.

Insight into the biologic significance of DCIS can also be obtained from studies that indicate that foci of this lesion are frequently detected in the contralateral breast of women with invasive breast cancer. There is, however, a discrepancy between this incidence of contralateral DCIS and the risk of developing a subsequent, clinically evident, opposite-breast cancer. Alpers and Wellings found DCIS in 48% of breasts contralateral to cancer-containing breasts,[278] yet the cumulative risk of opposite-breast cancer has been reported to be only 12.5% at 20 years after diagnosis of the initial tumor.[279] These data also suggest that not all histologically detectable DCIS will progress to clinically significant cancer.

Mastectomy has been the standard form of treatment for DCIS. Although the multicentricity of DCIS and the occasional finding of foci of invasive cancer in breasts removed because of a biopsy diagnosis of DCIS have been used as arguments for mastectomy,[191] the principal rationale for this treatment of DCIS is its demonstrated efficacy: local tumor control and survival rates approaching 100% can be obtained.[273-275]

There are two other treatment options for patients with DCIS: excision combined with radiation therapy and excision alone.[280-284] Both options provide breast preservation, an important goal in terms of the quality of life. The available data indicate that breast-conserving treatment can be associated with reasonably high levels of local tumor control with a significant chance for salvage in the event of local recurrence. Experience with *invasive* breast cancers that have a prominent intraductal component and with pure DCIS has emphasized that the extent of intraductal involvement in the breast is typically not appreciated by palpation and may not even be recognizable at the time of surgery.[285] Therefore, there must be increased reliance on careful mammographic and pathologic evaluation to aid in defining the extent of the DCIS and ensuring that the lesion has been resected if breast-conserving treatment is being considered.

At many institutions, patients with DCIS in whom the lesion has been excised with clearly negative margins are considered candidates for excision and radiotherapy. At some institutions, selected patients with very limited disease are offered the option of treatment with wide excision alone. For example, Lagios and colleagues consider patients for treatment with excision alone if the DCIS is mammographically detected by the presence of microcalcifications, the lesion is 25 mm or smaller, an excision with pathologically negative margins of resection has been performed, a postoperative mammogram reveals no residual calcifications at the biopsy site, the breast is favorable for mammographic and clinical follow-up, and the patient agrees to undergo the careful follow-up required.[191] At the other extreme, in patients with extensive DCIS, mastectomy is recommended.

The need for axillary dissection in patients with DCIS is a matter of debate.[286] Because of the occasional difficulty in identifying foci of stromal invasion, there is a small likelihood of axillary lymph node involvement in patients having DCIS. This likelihood may be related to tumor size.[191] Therefore, in patients with extensive DCIS, it is generally recommended that a lower axillary dissection be performed. In patients with limited DCIS treated using a breast-preserving approach, an axillary dissection is typically not recommended because of the extremely low probability of nodal metastases and because of the desire to reserve this procedure in the event of a local recurrence.

An important consideration in the use of breast-conserving treatment for DCIS is the feasibility and efficacy of salvage in the event of local recurrence. Even with careful selection and treatment, the risk of local recurrence is likely to be greater with breast-conserving treatment than with mastectomy. Of note, approximately 50% of patients who develop a local recurrence after breast-conserving treatment for DCIS will have invasive cancer on relapse.[280-284] Nonetheless, preliminary data suggest that salvage after a local recurrence in patients with DCIS initially treated with excision with or without radiotherapy is highly effective. Salvage for patients initially treated with excision and radiotherapy generally consists of mastectomy, whereas salvage for patients initially treated with excision alone may consist of either excision and radiotherapy or mastectomy. The impact of a recurrence within the breast on survival is an unsettled issue.[132,287,288] In the absence of definitive information on this subject, we believe that the risk of local recurrence should be kept as low as possible, and that patients with DCIS treated with breast-conserving therapy should be monitored carefully to detect such local recurrences promptly. A reasonable follow-up program is physical examination every 4 months and mammograms every 6 months for the first 2 years and annually thereafter.

LOBULAR CARCINOMA IN SITU

In 1941, Foote and Stewart, as well as Muir, called attention to an in situ form of carcinoma of the female breast that apparently arises within the end parts of the lobule, a lesion they designated lobular carcinoma in situ or lobular CIS.[289,290] These in situ carcinomas may develop into, or at least be associated with, either infiltrating lobular or ductal carcinoma, although the frequency or even the absolute certainty of such a progression has been debated.[291-293]

It is virtually impossible to make a diagnosis of lobular carcinoma in situ by clinical examination.[275] In most instances, the signs and symptoms that lead to biopsy are related to benign lesions, such as fibrocystic mastopathy, that have no relation to the lobular carcinoma in situ. Roentgenologic methods (conventional mammography or xeroradiography) are likewise not usually helpful. Lobular carcinoma in situ also cannot be diagnosed by gross pathologic examination, although occasionally and retrospectively, one may gain the impression of an ill-defined area of induration within the breast substance.

The microscopic diagnosis of lobular carcinoma in situ is sometimes difficult because of its similarity to lobular hyperplasias.[294] This dilemma is analogous to that encountered in the differential diagnosis of proliferative or hyperplastic lesions and intraductal carcinomas. Such difficulty and uncertainty frequently are reflected by the designation "atypical" lobular hyperplasia.

In 1967, McDivitt and co-workers from Memorial Hospital (New York) published a report on the long-term follow-up of patients with lobular CIS.[293] Of 40 patients treated with biopsy alone, nine developed infiltrating carcinoma in the ipsilateral breast after 2 to 23 years. The cumulative risk of ipsilateral breast cancer was 10% at 5 years, 15% at 10 years, and 30% at 15 years. Of the 47 evaluable patients, seven subsequently developed contralateral breast cancer at intervals of 1 to 22 years. The cumulative risk of contralateral breast cancer was 5% at 5 years, 10% at 10 years, and 15% at 15 years. Of the subsequent breast cancers detected, approximately half were lobular and half ductal. In 1978, Rosen and associates updated the results at Memorial Hospital and found a similar risk of cancer.[295]

Subsequent reports of the risk of infiltrating cancer with lobular CIS have not indicated figures as high as those reported by McDivitt and colleagues. Wheeler and co-workers studied 25 women with lobular CIS treated with biopsy alone.[296] Only one of these women subsequently developed ipsilateral infiltrating cancer with a mean follow-up for the entire group of 17.5 years. Of this group, three developed contralateral infiltrating cancer. Haagensen and associates reported follow-up on 211 patients with lobular CIS.[297] The cumulative risk at 25 years for ipsilateral breast cancer was 22% and that for contralateral breast cancer was 15%.

The management of lobular CIS is controversial. Rosen and colleagues from Memorial Hospital have recommended ipsilateral mastectomy and generous biopsy of the opposite breast for this condition. In contrast, Haagensen and co-workers have recommended a more conservative approach of periodic follow-up. Those advocating the conservative approach point out that the considerations in the management of lobular CIS are, in effect, similar to those in the management of women at high risk because of family history or prior breast cancer: in all these groups, the risk of breast cancer approaches 1% per year and persists. As discussed above, it is reasonable to adopt a conservative viewpoint on the management of these other high-risk patients. As a result, many surgeons now favor a program of breast self-examination, periodic physician examinations, and mammograms as management of lobular CIS. In selected patients who are particularly anxious about the development of cancer, bilateral total mastectomies and prompt reconstruction is a reasonable approach.

Radiation therapy does not have a role in the management of lobular CIS.

TREATMENT OF LOCALLY ADVANCED BREAST CANCER (STAGE III)

"Locally advanced cancer of the breast" refers to breast carcinomas with significant primary or nodal disease but where distant metastases cannot be documented. This group of cancers has been shown to be poorly controlled by radical surgery alone and also to have a poor prognosis. Any T3b–T4, N2 or N3, M0 lesion now is regarded as locally advanced, inoperable breast cancer. T3a, N0 or N1, M0 cancers are included in the UICC Stage III because of their poor prognosis but generally are considered operable.

Following Halsted's popularization of the radical mastectomy at the turn of the century, the operation was performed without an understanding of which patients benefited from its use. Haagensen and Stout reviewed the records of patients undergoing radical mastectomy at the Presbyterian Hospital between 1915 and 1942 and identified various clinical features that were associated with high local recurrence rates and poor survival.[298] Table 38-28 lists the clinical features that marked a tumor as categorically inoperable by virtue of local recurrence rates greater than 50% and no 5-year clinical cures, and these features form the basis for classifying patients as CCC Class D or inoperable. In addition, those authors identified five "grave signs" that were associated with a somewhat increased likelihood of local recurrence and poor survival (Table 38-29). Although a single grave sign was not necessarily thought to indicate inoperability, in the presence of any two grave signs, 42% of patients developed local recurrence, and only one (2%) was free of disease at 5 years. The presence of a single grave sign forms the basis of CCC Class C, whereas patients with two or more grave signs are included in Class D.

Because of this high incidence of local–regional recurrence with surgical treatment, radiation therapy, either alone or in conjunction with surgery, has come to play a significant role in this stage of the disease. For radiation therapy to be effective in controlling these locally advanced cancers, however, doses greater than those used to treat

TABLE 38-28. Clinical Features of Breast Cancer Associated with Poor Results Following Radical Mastectomy

Clinical Feature	*No. of Patients*	*Local Recurrence (%)*	*5-Year Clinical Cure (%)*
Extensive edema of skin over breast	51	61	0
Satellite nodules	7	57	0
"Inflammatory" carcinoma of the breast	25	60	0
Distant metastases	10	20	0
Parasternal or supraclavicular node metastases	16	56	0
Edema of the arm	4	50	0

Haagensen CD: Diseases of the Breast, rev 2nd Ed., p. 623. Philadelphia, WB Saunders, 1971.

TABLE 38-29. Grave Signs of Breast Cancer

Clinical Feature	*No. of Patients*	*Local Recurrence (%)*	*5-Year Clinical Cure (%)*
Edema of the skin of the breast (less than one-third)	75	32	23
Skin ulceration	14	14	36
Solid fixation of the tumor to the chest wall	20	40	5
Axillary lymph node greater than 2.5 cm	24	13	38
Fixed axillary nodes	8	13	13

Haagensen CD: Diseases of the Breast, rev 2nd Ed., pp. 625–628. Philadelphia, WB Saunders, 1971.

early-stage tumors are required. Whereas 5000 cGy is effective in eradicating microscopic amounts of tumor, doses in excess of 6000 cGy are required for gross tumor. François Baclesse was one of the first to show that tumor control was achievable using sufficiently high radiation doses.[299] In a more recent study, Fletcher and Montague administered 6000 cGy in 8 weeks and obtained local control in 72% of patients with inoperable breast cancers.[300]

In a review from the JCRT, the results of primary radiation therapy in 192 patients with locally advanced cancers (five with bilateral disease) were analyzed.[301] Patients typically received 4500 to 5000 cGy in 5 weeks to the breast and draining lymph nodes. A local boost to areas of gross disease was delivered in 157 patients, using interstitial implantation (124 cases), electrons (6), or photons (27). Excisional biopsy (gross tumor removal) was performed in only 54 of the 197 breasts. Multiagent chemotherapy was given to 53 patients. The median follow-up was 65 months, with a range of 16 to 158 months. The actuarial probability of survival for the entire group was 41% at 5 years and 23% at 10 years. The probability of relapse-free survival was 30% at 5 years and 19% at 10 years. The addition of multiagent chemotherapy was associated with a significantly improved 5-year relapse-free survival (40% versus 26%, $p = 0.02$) (Fig. 38-22). The 5-year survival rate was 51% for patients who received adjuvant multiagent chemotherapy and 38% for patients who did not ($p = 0.16$). The actuarial rate of local–regional tumor control (not censored for distant failure) for all patients was 73% at 5 years and 68% at 10 years, and the crude incidence of local–regional control was 78% (153 of 197 breast and nodal groups treated). Local–regional tumor control was influenced principally by the radiation dose. Patients who received 6000 cGy or more to the primary site had a better 5-year rate of control in the breast than did patients who received less than 6000 cGy (83% versus 70%; $p = 0.06$). Significant complications were seen in 15 patients (8%), including moderate or severe arm edema in six patients and brachial plexopathy in four patients. Cosmetic results at last evaluation were excellent or good in 56% of evaluable patients, fair in 25%, and poor in 19%. These results indicate that high-dose radiation therapy without mastectomy is an effective means of achieving local–regional tumor control in patients with locally advanced breast cancer.

The results from the JCRT emphasize that a number of technical factors are important in achieving a good outcome. A dose to the primary site greater than 6000 cGy results in better local control. Furthermore, a dose in the range of 7500 cGy may be preferable for patients who have large tumors not amenable to resection.[302] For such patients, the JCRT recommends external-beam radiation to the breast at 180 cGy per day to a total dose of 4500 cGy in 5 weeks, followed by an interstitial implant of the primary site for an additional dose of 3000 cGy. An adequate dose to the axillary nodes is also important. Five thousand cGy in 5 weeks appears to be sufficient for patients without palpable disease in the axilla, whereas for patients with palpable disease, a total dose of 5600 cGy to the axilla is advised. Bolus is another important technical factor: the use of bolus over the entire breast for half or more of the external-beam treatment was associated with a greater degree of breast retraction and telangiectasia and poorer cosmetic results. For this reason, the use of bolus should be limited as much as possible in extent and frequency.

The results of the JCRT study also suggest an improvement in both relapse-free and total survival rates among patients who received multiagent chemotherapy, even though those patients had a worse T–N profile than did patients who were not treated with chemotherapy. These data support other retrospective studies that have shown

FIG. 38-22. Relapse-free survival for patients with Stage III breast cancer treated with conservative surgery and radiation therapy with (*open circles*) or without (*closed circles*) adjuvant CMF or Adriamycin.[298]

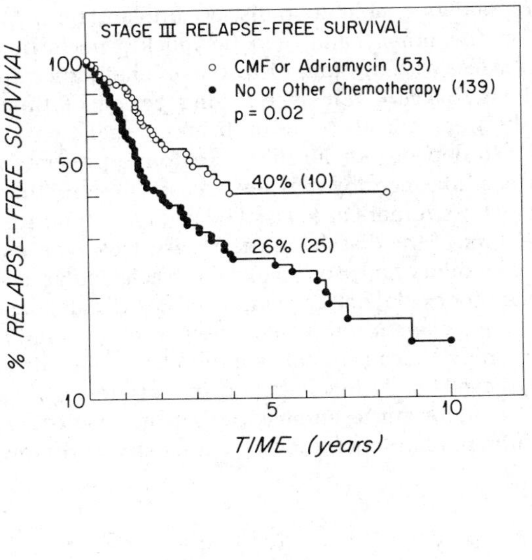

similar results.[303,304] However, in one prospective randomized trial comparing treatment with radiation therapy alone with radiation therapy plus adjuvant systemic therapy, no advantage to the use of adjuvant systemic therapy was noted.[305] This issue requires further prospective analysis.

The relative roles of primary radiation therapy and mastectomy in the treatment of locally advanced breast cancer have been addressed in prospective trials.[306,307] DeLena and colleagues reported rates of local tumor control at 5 years of 75% for patients treated with primary radiotherapy and 82% for patients undergoing mastectomy. No statistically significant differences were seen between the groups in the 5-year rates of either distant disease or overall survival. The probability of disease progression increased at a constant rate over time in both groups, which emphasizes the similarly poor results of both forms of local therapy, even when combined with vigorous systemic therapy. Similar results have been reported by the CALGB.[307] In their study, patients with locally advanced breast cancer were randomized after induction chemotherapy to either modified radical mastectomy or primary radiation therapy, both followed by 2 years of additional chemotherapy. The rates of local relapse, distant metastases, and overall survival were similar in the two groups. The results from these two randomized trials show no advantage for mastectomy over primary radiation therapy in patients with Stage III disease treated with initial chemotherapy.

The benefit of combining mastectomy and postoperative radiation for patients with locally advanced breast cancer has not yet been demonstrated in a prospective study. Retrospective studies of patients treated with a combination of mastectomy and radiation have shown excellent local tumor control at 5 years.[308] The addition of radiation to mastectomy to improve local tumor control must be balanced against a possible increase in the likelihood of complications, such as arm edema.

In considering the options for local treatment, there are a number of factors to be weighed. Primary radiation therapy, which involves 5 to 6 weeks of external-beam irradiation and interstitial implantation, is a time-consuming and technically demanding form of treatment. Furthermore, a breast that has undergone significant cosmetic alteration secondary to the cancer itself is not likely to have a good cosmetic result after treatment. Also, breast masses beyond a certain size are not amenable to radiation implantation. Mastectomy, on the other hand, can be quickly performed and interferes less with the administration of chemotherapy, particularly if this is given over a long period of time. The choice between mastectomy or primary radiation therapy should also depend on the initial anatomic presentation of the disease. Mastectomy may be a reasonable treatment for patients whose tumors are classified as Stage III on the basis of the extent of the disease in the breast. However, patients with fixed axillary nodes or involved infraclavicular or supraclavicular nodes do not appear to be good candidates for mastectomy, even after a good response to combination chemotherapy, because such surgery does not adequately address these sites of involvement. In considering these options, it is important to emphasize that the results achieved using combination chemotherapy and any form of local treatment are generally poor, with relatively few patients surviving free of systemic relapse beyond 5 years.[306,307] Although mastectomy may be more convenient than radiotherapy, consideration should be given to the psychological and physical effects of mastectomy and to the classic features of "inoperability" in a disease that carries a poor long-term prognosis.

In the absence of definitive data, a reasonable approach is to treat patients who have locally advanced breast cancer with initial combination chemotherapy for 4 to 8 months. If the cosmetic appearance is acceptable at that point, primary radiation therapy is given. However, if the breast tumor appears to be too large for interstitial implantation or the cosmetic appearance is already poor, and if N2 or N3 involvement was not present initially, the policy is to recommend mastectomy. As noted above, the use of postoperative radiation may be considered in this setting in order to optimize local tumor control.

The available data indicate that although locally advanced breast cancer can have a long natural history, systemic relapse and death from breast cancer are eventually observed in the large majority of patients. Substantial improvements in the treatment of locally advanced breast cancer will depend on new developments in systemic therapy.

PAGET'S DISEASE OF THE NIPPLE

Paget's disease of the nipple is characterized clinically by an itchy, eczematoid eruption involving the nipple and pathologically by large cells with pale cytoplasm and prominent irregular nuclei (Paget's cells) in the nipple epidermis. In approximately 60% of patients, an associated breast mass is present. In all cases, either invasive or noninvasive carcinoma is present in the involved breast, sometimes at a considerable distance from the nipple. The relation between the nipple involvement and the underlying malignancy is still a matter of controversy. It has been hypothesized that the nipple involvement represents migration of malignant cells from the underlying carcinoma, or alternatively, that it is an independent process.[309]

The prognosis is related to whether a mass is present. If a mass is present, the prognosis is similar to that in patients with similar masses but without Paget's disease. If a mass is absent, the prognosis is excellent. Nance and associates observed that none of 16 patients without a mass had axillary metastases, whereas axillary metastases were found in 50% when a mass was present.[310] Moreover, none of 21 patients without a mass died of cancer, whereas 18 of 32 with a mass died of cancer within 5 years. Consequently, these authors recommended radical mastectomy for patients with masses and total mastectomy for those without. On the other hand, Maier and coworkers reported that 8 of 56 patients without a mass had positive axillary nodes and advocated radical mastectomy in all patients.[311] At present, total mastectomy and axillary dissection is considered the surgical treatment of Paget's disease, particularly if a mass is present. Breast-preserving surgery, with or without radiotherapy, has been reported in 46 collected cases from the literature.[312] Three local recurrences were seen, indicating that this approach may be acceptable. However, follow-up is short, and the cosmetic results after nipple–areolar excision have not been evaluated.

CARCINOMA OF THE BREAST IN MEN

Carcinoma of the breast occurs infrequently in men, with an estimated incidence about 1% of that in women.[313,314] The average age at diagnosis appears to be about 10 years older for men than for women.[314–317] There have been fewer epidemiologic studies of male breast cancer, but there does appear to be some familial distribution, with very rare families having more than one male with breast cancer.[318,319] Some families with a high likelihood for breast cancer in the women have an occasional male with breast cancer. Male breast cancer appears to be associated with disease that causes hyperestrogenism. For example, bilharzias appear to be associated with the disease.[320] This infection damages the liver and causes hyperestrogenism, and in Egypt, where bilharzias is common, men constitute about 6% of all patients with breast cancer, as opposed to the 1% usually described. There is some evidence that gynecomastia also predisposes to breast cancer in men. There is a significant elevation of the incidence in patients with Klinefelter's syndrome.[321] Whereas earlier reports postulated that the incidence of breast cancer in men with Klinefelter's syndrome was about the same as in women, a recent analysis[322] of 27 reported cases suggested that males with Klinefelter's syndrome have a 3% increased risk of breast cancer.

On pathologic examination, male breast cancer resembles carcinoma of the breast in women with the exception that lobular carcinoma in situ is not seen. Estrogen receptors have been found in as many as 84% of the specimens.[323] Clinically, the disease presents as a unilateral mass, usually firm and painless. There may be abnormality of the nipple, including retraction, crusting or discharge, and ulceration. The tumor is frequently less well defined than in female breast cancer, and, because of the limited breast tissue in men without evidence of lobules, the tumor is frequently closely applied to the pectoral fascia and can involve the muscle itself. Male breast cancer usually presents in a more advanced stage.[315,316] Review of breast cancer cases at the Ellis Fischel State Cancer Hospital revealed a statistically significant difference in stage between male and female breast cancers.[324]

The method of treatment in most reported experience has been mastectomy, usually radical mastectomy because of frequent involvement of the pectoral muscle. Occasionally, if the muscle is not involved extensively, it can be spared. Use of radiation therapy alone for early carcinoma of the male breast has not been reported in significant numbers. It has been used as an adjuvant, both postoperatively following mastectomy, and in advanced cancer.[317] Some authors have advocated routine radiation after modified radical mastectomy except for patients with very small tumors.[325] Lymph node involvement has the same prognostic significance in men as it does in women.

There is some difference of opinion in the literature as to the prognosis. Most authors believe that, although male breast cancer presents in a more advanced stage, within each stage, the prognosis is similar to that in women.[315,316,328] The Memorial Hospital series, reporting follow-up of 97 male breast cancer patients, showed 80% free of disease 10 years after mastectomy when axillary nodes were histologically negative.[326] This was similar to the data in node-negative female patients. However, male patients with positive nodes had a prognosis much worse than that of women with positive nodes.

The pattern of metastases in men is similar to that in women, with bone (48%), soft-tissue (60%), and various visceral sites predominating.[320] The standard therapy for metastatic disease is orchidectomy, which produces an objective remission rate higher than that of female castration (50%–60%).[327,328] The high response rate most likely reflects the high incidence of ER protein. The responses last 3 to 40 months, with a median duration of 12 months. Further palliation may be obtained by adrenalectomy. A review of the literature by one author identified 17 cases, of which 12 were evaluable.[329] Nine patients objectively responded for 5 months to 5 years.

Hypophysectomy also may palliate advanced disease. A review of the experience with that operation confirmed objective responses in five of eight patients, including three complete remissions.[330] More recent studies report that comparable response rates may be achieved with antiestrogen and other hormonal agents, indicating a shift away from major surgical ablation.[331–333]

The experience with systemic adjuvant therapy in males with positive nodes is anecdotal. The regimen is generally the same combination chemotherapy used in women. In a recent report from the National Cancer Institute, 24 male patients were treated with adjuvant CMF. The 5-year survival rate exceeded 80%, a substantial improvement over that for historical controls.[334]

TREATMENT OF METASTASES

GENERAL PRINCIPLES

Recurrent breast cancer is incurable. This is true whether the site of recurrence is a solitary lesion on the chest wall or multiple foci within the liver and other viscera. The median length of survival after a diagnosis of recurrence is about 2 years, but this span may range from a few months to three decades.[335,336]

There is a role for all of the major modalities in the treatment of breast cancer metastases. Surgery is often used to excise local recurrences, to drain pleural effusions, or to ablate endocrine organs. Radiotherapy may be used alone or in conjunction with surgery to treat locally recurrent disease, and it is the treatment of choice for brain metastases. Radiotherapy is probably also the most effective method of relieving pain from bone lesions. However, when there are multiple sites of disease, and especially when disease involves visceral organs, some form of systemic therapy is usually employed. This may consist of relatively nontoxic endocrine therapies such as tamoxifen, aminoglutethimide, or progestins. Alternatively, symptoms may be relieved with chemotherapy, and most of the cytotoxic agents developed over the

TABLE 38-30. Factors of Importance in Determining When to Treat and Which Therapies to Use for Metastatic Breast Cancer

Patient symptoms
Disease-free interval
Sites of metastases
Menstrual status
Receptor status
Prior therapy
Response to prior therapy
Toxicities of therapy

last 30 years have at least some activity in breast cancer patients.

Patients seeking treatment for breast cancer metastases usually desire palliation of their symptoms, prolongation of survival, or both. The judicious use of the various treatment modalities in sequence may keep a patient symptom-free for many years. Unfortunately, the impact of these therapies on survival is limited. For this reason, this goal is usually of secondary importance in determining when a patient with breast cancer metastases should be treated or which modality to use (Table 38-30).

In making treatment decisions, the presence and nature of the patient's symptoms is the single most important consideration. Patients may live for months or even years with abnormalities on bone scan, elevated tumor markers, or small skin recurrences with almost no symptoms. There is no evidence that earlier treatment with an effective regimen will prolong survival. For example, when patients with metastatic disease are randomized to two regimens, one of which is associated with a significantly higher response rate than the other, and then crossed over to the opposite regimen at the time of progression, there is generally no survival advantage for the group of patients initially treated with the more effective program.[337,338]

The time from first diagnosis of breast cancer to documentation of metastatic disease is referred to as the disease-free interval, and few other pieces of clinical or laboratory data provide as much prognostic information as this figure (Table 38-31). For example, the median survival of patients who relapse in a single site less than 1 year after initial diagnosis is 11 months, whereas the median survival of a similar group of patients with a disease-free interval of more than 5 years is 40 months.[339] The disease-free interval is also an important predictor of the response to endocrine therapy. Patients with an interval in excess of 2 years have a significantly higher probability of responding to endocrine therapy than do those with an interval less than 2 years.[29] Patients who present with metastases but without a prior diagnosis of breast cancer (*i.e.*, with an interval of 0) have a better prognosis than those with a disease-free interval of less than 1 year, presumably because these patients represent a mixed group, some of whom have had long-standing disease that has been indolent and asymptomatic, whereas others have an unusually aggressive form of the disease that metastasizes early.

The number of sites of disease is also an important prognostic indicator, as shown in Table 38-31, and the number and specific sites of disease may strongly influence the type of therapy administered. For example, a patient with a single site of recurrence on the chest wall after a long disease-free interval might appropriately be treated with excision, or radiotherapy, or both. A patient with multiple sites of disease, including a local recurrence, should be treated with some form of systemic therapy. Patients with central nervous system (CNS) and liver metastases are thought to have a particularly dire prognosis. However, CNS metastases may respond dramatically to radiotherapy. Liver metastases are usually treated with chemotherapy, especially if the disease-free interval has been short.

Menstrual status is of help in determining whether the patient is likely to respond to endocrine therapy and if so, which endocrine therapy to use. Postmenopausal women rarely, if ever, respond to oophorectomy, and premenopausal women have not been shown to benefit from estrogens. Postmenopausal women less than 5 years from their last menstrual period are less likely to benefit from any form of endocrine therapy. The ER and PR determinations obtained at the time of the patient's original diagnosis have both prognostic and predictive value after the appearance of metastases: patients without these receptors have a poorer prognosis (see above) and a very low probability of responding to endocrine therapy. However, receptor status may change, and biopsy of a metastatic lesion should be performed for testing whenever possible.

Finally, the toxicity of the therapy must be balanced with a

TABLE 38-31. Effect of Disease-Free Interval and Number of Metastatic Sites on the Median Survival (Months) of Patients from First Recurrence of Breast Cancer

Disease-Free Interval (yr)	*Number of Metastatic Sites** 1	2	3	4	*Liver, CNS*
<1	11	7	5	5	5
1–2	16	13	7	6	8
2–5	20	14	12	5	7
>5	40	22	14	21	11

* Excluding patients with liver and central nervous system (CNS) metastases

Modified from Cutler S: Classification of extent of disease in breast cancer. Semin Oncol 1:91–96, 1974.

realistic estimate of the probability of a meaningful response. In controlled trials, even a toxic therapy that induces remission proved more likely to improve the overall quality of a patient's life than a nontoxic therapy that has a low probability of benefit. In one study, patients were randomized to receive either a nontoxic endocrine therapy or a toxic chemotherapy program without regard to usual selection factors such as receptor status or the patient's clinical characteristics.[340] The response rate to the chemotherapy was twice that to the endocrine therapy. Serial evaluation demonstrated that the quality of life associated with the more toxic but more effective chemotherapy was significantly greater than that achieved with the nontoxic but less effective endocrine therapy. Fortunately, there are many situations where the probability of response to two therapies is nearly identical, and in this setting, the less toxic should be used. For example, a 60 year-old postmenopausal woman with a 5-year disease-free interval and a receptor-positive tumor is as likely to respond to endocrine therapy as she is to chemotherapy, and in this circumstance, the nontoxic endocrine therapy is preferred. A patient with a local recurrence on the chest wall and no other site of distant disease 5 years after her mastectomy might more reasonably be treated with local excision alone or radiotherapy alone rather than the more toxic forms of systemic therapy. Similar considerations may be important in selecting radiotherapy fields, choosing among several different types of endocrine therapy, or utilizing a single cytotoxic agent rather than a combination of drugs.

The patient's long-term prognosis is a poor guide to the selection of therapy for patients with metastases. Many physicians feel compelled to treat a patient merely because metastases have been diagnosed and because the patient will eventually die of these metastases. Although it is not necessary to wait until the patient is bedridden to begin treatment, there is no evidence that earlier treatment is better. If the patient is desirous of treatment and is asymptomatic, the physician should consider recommending a new or experimental therapy. A second fallacy of clinical judgment is the use of a nontoxic therapy as a placebo in an asymptomatic patient. Endocrine therapy (*e.g.*, tamoxifen) or radiotherapy are often used in this way. However, the injudicious use of tamoxifen may limit its future value as palliation when a patient is symptomatic, and inappropriate use of radiotherapy may reduce bone marrow reserves and limit the future use of chemotherapy.

INITIAL EVALUATION OF METASTATIC DISEASE AND MONITORING RESPONSE TO THERAPY

Breast cancer may metastasize to almost any site in the body, as evidenced in the autopsy series cited above (see Table 38-14). The symptoms of metastases will usually direct the physician to one site, but a more thorough staging to detect metastases at other sites is recommended. There are several reasons for this. First, the presence of asymptomatic disease in multiple sites or in a visceral organ may suggest the use of systemic therapy rather than a more limited focus on the single symptomatic area. Second, patients frequently develop new symptoms shortly after the initiation of therapy; documenting these metastases before treatment is begun may discourage premature abandonment of a therapy because of a mistaken assessment that the disease is progressing during therapy. Third, the response to one therapy may influence the choice of future therapies. Finally, documentation of all sites of measurable disease may permit a more accurate assessment of the response to therapy at a later time.

The basic evaluation should encompass the most common sites of metastases. Physical examination should include a careful assessment of regional lymph nodes, the skin overlying the mastectomy site or the irradiated breast, the chest, and the abdomen. Signs of pleural effusions, ascites, and hepatomegaly should be specifically sought. Abnormalities in the blood count may suggest bone metastases. Liver function studies should be obtained for evaluation of potential liver metastases, but liver scans are not recommended as a routine because the frequency of false-positive results exceeds that of true-positive scans in patients without hepatomegaly or abnormal liver function studies.[341] Even though brain metastases are not uncommon in patients with metastatic breast cancer, there is no evidence that a radionuclide brain scan or a CT scan of the head is likely to reveal asymptomatic disease in other than a rare patient.[342]

Serial follow-up bone scans after treatment of the breast primary are no longer recommended in asymptomatic patients without evidence of extraosseous metastases because of the low yield observed in a number of recent studies[343] (see above). A baseline bone scan in a patient with documented metastases at other sites may be of help because of the frequency with which bone metastases appear soon after the initiation of therapy, but these scans must be interpreted very cautiously. Approximately 15% of patients with extraosseous metastases have solitary lesions on such baseline bone scans, and more than a third of these solitary lesions prove to be a benign process.[344] This is especially true when these solitary lesions are in the ribs; as many as 90% of these lesions may be benign.[345] Follow-up bone scans must also be interpreted cautiously, as patients may appear to have increased intensity of radionuclide uptake in responding lesions.[346] It has even been reported that some responding patients develop new abnormalities on bone scan after the initiation of therapy without these representing progressive disease.[347]

Between 50% and 80% of patients with metastatic breast cancer will have elevations of CEA, gross cystic disease protein (GCDP), CA 15-3, casein, ferritin, pregnancy-associated macroglobulin, beta-2-microglobulin, sialytransferase, tissue polypeptide antigen (TPA), or 5-nucleotide phosphodiesterase isoenzyme V (5′-NPD-V).[348,349]

CEA has been studied more extensively than any of the other markers. A serum CEA concentration of more than 3 ng/ml has been observed in 55%, and a CEA greater than 5 ng/ml in 40% to 45%, of patients with metastatic breast cancer.[350,351] Between 69% and 83% of patients who respond to therapy at other sites will also have a fall in CEA,[351,352] although approximately half of these will have a transient early rise in CEA level.[351] CEA is a useful tool for monitoring patients with metastatic breast cancer, although it is difficult to use. A CEA of more than 10 ng/ml almost always reflects metastases. In a rare patient, CEA elevations appear as long as 1.5 years prior to evidence of metastases at specific sites. A falling CEA almost always reflects a response to therapy, and this may be helpful in deciding to persist with therapy in a patient whose response in other sites is ambiguous. Because a rise in CEA may be transient, it cannot be taken as a sign of failure to respond and should not be an indication for discontinuing therapy unless the patient has other good evidence of progressive disease. Finally, a stable or falling CEA in a patient who is responding at other sites might be a basis for continuing therapy if the status of the patient's disease is ambiguous.

GCDP levels may also rise and fall with disease progression or regression, but this marker is abnormal in only 30% of patients with metastatic breast cancer.[353] CA 15-3 is a recently described marker for metastatic breast cancer. This antigen is measured in a bideterminant immunoradiometric assay utilizing two monoclonal antibodies, DF3 and 115 D8. CA 15-3 may be a more sensitive marker of metastatic breast cancer with only a small loss of specificity. A CA 15-3 value of 30 units/ml approximates a CEA of 5 ng/ml. Both CA 15-3 and CEA are abnormally high in most patients with liver metastases, but CA 15-3 is more likely to be abnormal in patients with local recurrences and bone metastases. Preliminary data suggest that changes in CA 15-3 levels accurately reflect disease progression and regression.[350]

USE OF ENDOCRINE THERAPY

Breast cancer is one of the few human tumors very responsive to endocrine therapy. The mechanism of this response is not fully understood. The simplest explanation is that breast cancer growth is directly dependent on a hormone, most likely estrogen.[354,355] However, human breast cancer cell lines have recently been shown to secrete growth factors, such as transforming growth factor (TGF). In estrogen-sensitive cell lines, such as the MCF-7, the secretion of growth factors appears to be controlled by estrogen and mediated through the estrogen receptor.[42] In cell lines without ER, secretion of growth factors appears to be independent of estrogen. These growth factors may stimulate the tumor cell from which they have been secreted (autocrine stimulation) or neighboring cells (paracrine stimulation). It is possible that estrogen may affect the growth of estrogen-independent cells through the release of paracrine growth factors from estrogen-dependent cells. In this way, the destruction of a very small number of estrogen-dependent cells could, theoretically, affect the growth of many estrogen-independent cells as well, and this might account for the apparent benefits from adjuvant tamoxifen given to patients whose tumors are ER-negative (see above).

Simple estrogen dependence does not fully explain the clinical phenomena observed during endocrine therapy. Patients who respond to one type of endocrine therapy are very likely to respond to a second, a third, and on occasion even to a fourth or fifth sequential endocrine maneuver. For example, a postmenopausal woman may respond to the administration of estrogens, have a secondary response to the discontinuance of the estrogen therapy when her tumor regrows after an initial response, and have a tertiary response to major ablative therapy, such as adrenalectomy, after the estrogen withdrawal response. It is difficult to understand why the same tumor responds to both the addition and the removal of estrogens. In addition, breast cancer is responsive to endocrine therapies such as progestins, androgens, and corticosteroids that do not involve estrogens. The "endocrine" therapy most widely used today, tamoxifen, has a cytotoxic effect independent of its ability to block estrogen uptake into tumor cells.[356]

The effects of all forms of endocrine therapy appear to be mediated through receptors, especially the ER. Although about one of three unselected patients will respond to endocrine therapy, the response rate among patients with ER is about twice that (Table 38-32). Patients whose tumors are without ER have a very low probability of responding, less than 10% in most series, whereas patients with a high receptor value have an even greater probability of responding (Table 38-33).[357,358] The receptor value likely reflects the total percentage of tumor cells that are ER positive, and cancer-cell death following endocrine therapy is likely to be greater in patients with higher receptor values. As a result, the durability of response among patients with high receptor values will also be greater.[357]

Patients whose tumors have both ER and PR have a higher response rate to a variety of endocrine therapies than do patients whose tumors have ER without PR (Table 38-33). Because the PR are produced only in cells with functional ER, very few tumors have been found to be ER negative and PR positive. In fact, these few patients may have a false-negative ER assay.[359] However, patients with high ER values are more likely to have PR than those with lower ER values. In one study 40% of tumors were PR positive if the ER was between 3 and 10 fmol/mg, 70% were PR positive if the ER level was 10 to 100 fmol/mg, and 77% were PR positive if the ER exceeded 100 fmol/mg.[496] There may be no advantage in determining both ER and PR values over careful quantification of ER alone.

Receptor information should be combined with other clinical characteristics to select those patients most likely to benefit from endocrine therapy. The clinical characteristics usually associated with endocrine response include a long disease-free interval, usually more than 2 years; disease localized to bone and soft tissues; late premenopausal or late postmenopausal status; and a prior response to endocrine therapy. In one study, 60% of patients with ER and a disease-free interval greater than 10 months responded to endocrine therapy, whereas only 25% of patients who were receptor-positive with a disease-free interval of less than 10 months responded.[360] The response to a second endocrine maneuver was 50% among ER-positive patients who had previously responded to another endocrine maneuver, whereas the response rate was only 30% among the ER-positive patients who had failed the first endocrine therapy.

Choice of Endocrine Therapy

In general, there is little evidence that the response rate or survival benefit from one endocrine therapy is superior to

TABLE 38-32. Endocrine Therapy for Metastatic Breast Cancer: Response (%) and Toxicity (Therapies Listed in Order of Increasing Toxicity)

Endocrine Therapy	*Patient Group*			*Major Toxicities*
	Unselected	*ERP+*	*ERP–*	
Tamoxifen*	32	54	9	Nausea, hot flashes, "flare," hypercalcemia, thrombocytopenia
Oophorectomy†	33	62	6	Surgical complications, hot flashes
Progestins*	31	(35)§	8	Weight gain, fluid retention, nausea, vaginal bleeding, hotflashes
Aminoglutethimide‡	31	54	6	Lethargy, dizziness/ataxia, rash, Cushingoid symptoms, nausea
LHRH analogues	42	–	–	Hot flashes, nausea, headache
Estrogens*	26	57	9	Nausea and vomiting, fluid retention, incontinence, vaginal bleeding, "flare," hypercalcemia
Androgens*	21	43	8	Masculinization, nausea, weight gain, "flare," hypercalcemia
Adrenalectomy*	32	46	10	Surgical mortality, Addisonian crises, Cushingoid symptoms
Hypophysectomy*	36	–	–	Surgical mortality, Addisonian crises, diabetes insipidus, anosmia

Modified from Henderson IC: Endocrine therapy in metastatic breast cancer. In Harris JR, Hellman S, Henderson IC, Kinne DW (eds): Breast Diseases, pp 398–428. Philadelphia, JB Lippincott, 1987.

* Primarily postmenopausal patients.
† Exclusively premenopausal patients.
‡ Exclusively postmenopausal patients.
§ See text commentary

that achieved with other such therapies.[361] Tamoxifen, oophorectomy, progestins, aminoglutethimide, estrogens, adrenalectomy, and hypophysectomy have been shown to be equivalent in many randomized trials. However, androgen therapy has a lower response rate than estrogens[362] or tamoxifen,[363] and corticosteroids, although they have not been compared with other endocrine therapies in randomized trials, are thought to be less effective on the basis of historical comparisons.

Because most endocrine therapies are equally effective, the choice of a particular one is based primarily on toxicity. The various endocrine therapies are listed in Table 38-32 in order of increasing toxicity, tamoxifen being associated with the least toxicity and adrenalectomy or hypophysectomy with the greatest. Luteinizing-hormone–releasing hormone (LHRH) analogues are still relatively untested forms of endocrine therapy and have not yet been evaluated in randomized trials. Thus, the full range of toxicity is unknown, as is their precise role relative to other forms of endocrine therapy. In premenopausal and postmenopausal patients, tamoxifen is the treatment of choice. Premenopausal patients who respond may later be treated with oophorectomy, then progestins, and finally aminoglutethimide as long as they respond before progression on the previous regimen. Second-

TABLE 38-33. Response to Endocrine Therapy Correlated with Either ER Value or ER and PR Status

ER Value (fmol/mg)	*Response Rate (%)**	*Frequency PR Positive (%)*†	*Combined ER/PR Status*	*Response Rate (%)*†
<3	6	9	ER – /PR –	9
3–10		40		
	46		ER + /PR –	32
10–100		70		
>100	81	77	ER + /PR +	71

* McGuire WL, Horwitz KB, Zava DT et al: Progress in endocrinology and metabolism: Hormones in breast cancer: Update 1978. Metabolism 27:487–501, 1978.

† Clark GM, McGuire WL: Progesterone receptors and human breast cancer. Breast Cancer Res Treat 3:157–163, 1983.

ary endocrine therapies in postmenopausal women could be administered in the sequence: progestins, aminoglutethimide, and estrogens.

Tamoxifen

Tamoxifen is usually administered in a dose of 10 mg twice daily. It has been shown in randomized trials that there is no advantage for higher doses of therapy.[364–367] Moreover, long-term administration of very high doses of tamoxifen (*e.g.*, 12 months of 60–100 mg/m^2 twice daily) has been associated with decreased visual acuity and a retinopathy.[368]

With a dose schedule of 10 mg twice daily, serum tamoxifen levels rise gradually to reach a steady state at about week 16.[369] The half-life of a single dose of tamoxifen is 9 to 12 hours, but the half-life of a chronic dose is 7 days. Circulating plasma levels can be detected 6 weeks after discontinuation of therapy.[369] As a result, the beneficial effects are not likely to be affected if patients miss one or even several doses. Because circulating tamoxifen may result in a false-negative ER determination, at least 6 weeks should elapse after discontinuing tamoxifen before performing a biopsy for receptor determination.

The effectiveness of tamoxifen in premenopausal women has been compared with oophorectomy in two randomized trials.[370,371] In the larger of these studies, there was no difference in the overall response rate to tamoxifen and oophorectomy.[371] The secondary response rate to oophorectomy after tamoxifen treatment was somewhat higher than that to tamoxifen ($p = 0.045$). The median time to treatment failure, response duration, and survival rate of patients randomized to oophorectomy or tamoxifen were nearly identical. The secondary response rate to oophorectomy following tamoxifen treatment was 33%; to tamoxifen following oophorectomy, 11%.[370] Although there are isolated case reports of patients responding to oophorectomy after tamoxifen failure, the probability of a secondary response to oophorectomy is much higher in patients who have an initial response to tamoxifen. In fact, the initial response to tamoxifen is a better predictor of the response to subsequent oophorectomy than is receptor status.[372]

Tamoxifen is remarkably nontoxic. Less than 10% of patients will experience mild and transient nausea that rarely requires discontinuation of therapy and can sometimes be alleviated if the patient takes tamoxifen before meals. Tamoxifen may cause a transient thrombocytopenia or leukopenia, but this rarely requires treatment or even careful monitoring. Thrombophlebitis has been observed to be increased in 1% to 3% of patients.[373] There is one report of an increased incidence of endometrial carcinoma in patients receiving tamoxifen, but this finding has not yet been confirmed by other observers.[266] A tumor "flare" or hypercalcemia occurs in 4% to 5% of patients (see below).

Ablation Therapy

Adrenalectomy and hypophysectomy are very effective endocrine therapy and were once commonly employed. More recently, these modalities have been abandoned because of the development of treatments with less toxicity. The overall operative mortality rate with these major forms of ablation was about 5%, but in the hands of inexperienced surgeons, it reached to 17% to 25%.[374] In addition, adrenalectomy and hypophysectomy cause permanent endocrine defects that necessitate life-long replacement, usually with corticosteroids.

Ovarian ablation is still commonly used and is considered by many specialists to be the endocrine therapy of choice for premenopausal women. Ablation of ovarian function may be obtained by either surgery or radiation. Although there are no randomized trials comparing these two methods, historical comparisons suggest that the response rates are equivalent.[361] However, the time to response after radiation ablation may be longer than that after surgical oophorectomy. Many patients undergo an inadvertent ovarian ablation when radiation therapy is administered to bone metastases in the pelvis or lumbosacral spine. When these areas are irradiated in a patient who is otherwise a good candidate for endocrine therapy, the patient should be evaluated initially for the response to ovarian ablation before another form of endocrine therapy is employed.

The best responses to ovarian ablation are seen in women over the age of 35 who are either still menstruating or within 1 year of the last menstrual period. Response rates to ovarian ablation in women younger than 35 are usually below 20%.[375,376] The response rate in postmenopausal women is less than 6%, and oophorectomy should never be employed in this group.[375,377,378] The operative mortality rate with surgical oophorectomy is low, usually less than 2% to 3%. In appropriately selected patients, the operative mortality rate is even lower. The principal side effects of this procedure are menopausal symptoms, especially hot flashes.

Aminoglutethimide and Corticosteroids

Corticosteroids are rarely used alone, because the response rate is thought to be lower than that to other forms of endocrine therapy. However, about 25% of patients will respond to corticosteroids.[379] Corticosteroids cause Cushingoid symptoms and osteoporosis when used for long periods of time. However, their value in palliating symptoms such as shortness of breath and bone pain, as well as their ability to improve the patient's overall sense of well-being, should not be overlooked, especially in the terminal phases of the disease.

Aminoglutethimide, given with corticosteroids, is among the more effective and less toxic forms of endocrine therapy. Aminoglutethimide blocks steroid hydroxylation and cleavage enzymes, including cholesterol sidechain cleavage in the initial step of steroidogenesis in the adrenal gland. However, aromatase reactions are more sensitive to the effects of aminoglutethimide.[380] For example, the concentration of aminoglutethimide required to block the conversion of androstenedione to estrone or the conversion of testosterone to estradiol is approximately one-tenth that required to block the cholesterol side chain cleavage. For this reason, it is thought that the principal site of aminoglutethimide action is outside the adrenal gland in fat tissue or within the breast itself.

The standard dose of aminoglutethimide is 250 mg orally

four times per day. Hydrocortisone, 40 mg per day divided into three or four doses, is usually administered with aminoglutethimide. Aminoglutethimide is effective at much lower doses and without hydrocortisone, but dose reduction does not decrease toxicity proportionately.[381] Aminoglutethimide at a dose of 250 mg twice daily will result in the same degree of estrogen suppression as 250 mg four times a day,[382] and this lower dose of aminoglutethimide might be considered an acceptable alternative to 250 mg four times daily. However, neither dose has been specifically approved by the Food and Drug Administration (FDA) for general use in the treatment of breast cancer in the United States.

Aminoglutethimide has been compared with tamoxifen, adrenalectomy, and hypophysectomy in randomized trials. In general, response rates are equivalent, but in several trials, aminoglutethimide plus hydrocortisone appeared to be more effective than tamoxifen in patients with bone metastases.[383,384]

Aminoglutethimide is somewhat more toxic than tamoxifen, oophorectomy, or progestins, although most of the toxicities disappear within 6 weeks of the initiation of therapy.[385] Aminoglutethimide is chemically related to the sedative glutethimide (Doriden), so it is not surprising that approximately one-third of the patients experience lethargy. However, this side-effect can be circumvented by the initial use of a dose of 250 mg twice daily. When this lower dose of aminoglutethimide is given with a full dose of corticosteroids, the patient is likely to experience euphoria, insomnia, and other signs of steroid excess. Approximately one of five patients will develop a rash during the first weeks of aminoglutethimide therapy. This is not an indication for discontinuation of aminoglutethimide, and it can be alleviated by a transient doubling of the steroid dose (*e.g.*, to 80 mg of hydrocortisone a day). Between 2% and 3% of the patients experience Cushingoid symptoms, which can be alleviated by a decrease in the hydrocortisone replacement dose. Addisonian crises are rare among patients who are given any steroid replacement. Patients may have a transient thrombocytopenia or, less commonly, leukopenia. On several occasions, this has been reported to be life threatening. However, in all instances, the thrombocytopenia and leukopenia appeared between weeks two and seven.[386] Monitoring platelet and leukocyte counts during this interval is therefore recommended.

Progestins

This group of compounds was once considered ineffective for the treatment of breast cancer, but more recent studies have shown that both medroxyprogesterone acetate and megestrol acetate are as active as any of the other endocrine therapies commonly used. Although there are no direct comparisons of these two forms of progestational therapy, they appear to be equally effective. Medroxyprogesterone acetate is more frequently used in Europe and megestrol acetate in the United States. Each has been compared in randomized trials with tamoxifen, and there are no differences in the response rates.[361] Although the summary response rate to progestins suggests that these agents are less effective than other endocrine therapies among ER-positive patients (see Table 38-32), this may reflect the fact that progestins were used as second- or third-line therapy in most of the studies used to calculate this summary response rate. It is premature to conclude that receptor status is unimportant in the selection of patients for the use of progestins.

Although uncontrolled early studies suggested that there might be an advantage to the use of high doses of medroxyprogesterone acetate, this has not been confirmed in randomized trials comparing two doses of this progestin.[361] Moreover, high doses of medroxyprogesterone acetate are associated with more side effects, including an increased incidence of gluteal abscesses, facies lunaris, increased sweating, and fine tremors. There are similar but more recent reports from uncontrolled trials that high doses of megestrol acetate increase the response rate.[387] This remains to be evaluated in controlled trials. In the absence of good evidence for a dose–response correlation, it is recommended that megestrol acetate be administered at a dose of 40 mg four times daily and that medroxyprogesterone acetate be limited to a total dose of 400 mg per day.

The principal toxicity of both of these progestational agents is weight gain, which may occur in 20% to 50% of patients and appears to be dose related.[388] Patients experiencing weight gain may have fluid retention, but it is not certain that fluid is responsible for all of the weight gain. Vaginal bleeding occurs in 5% to 10% of patients either while the patients are taking the progestational agent or when it is discontinued. Somewhat less than 10% of patients experience hot flashes.

Estrogens and Androgens

This group of compounds is rarely used today because estrogens and androgens are more toxic than the other drugs discussed thus far. For example, approximately one-third of patients placed on estrogens will discontinue them because of toxic side-effects, the most important of which are vomiting and fluid retention. Androgens may be associated with a marked improvement in the patient's sense of well-being but are also associated with masculinization, including hoarseness, hirsutism, and acne, in more than 50% of patients. Also, androgens are the endocrine therapy most often associated with "flare" (see below). However, both estrogens and androgens may be useful as third- or fourth-line treatment and are certainly preferable to the major ablative procedures. For example, estrogens might be used in an older patient who has previously responded to tamoxifen and progestational agents. Also, estrogen would be preferred to aminoglutethimide, especially in a patient over age 70, because of the increased frequency of lethargy and CNS effects associated with the latter drug. Androgens are occasionally useful in an older population with congestive heart failure, because androgen use is not accompanied by fluid retention, whereas both progestins and estrogens can exacerbate congestive heart failure.

The estrogens used most frequently are diethylstilbestrol (DES) (5 mg three times daily), ethinyl estradiol (1 mg three times daily), or Premarin (2.5 mg three times daily). The doses of estrogens used for palliation of metastatic breast cancer are usually higher than those commonly used to alleviate postmenopausal symptoms, but the evidence that higher doses of estrogens are more effective than lower doses is weak.[389] It is appropriate to use half doses of estrogen during the first month of therapy, with a gradual increase in dosage as the patient experiences fewer side-effects. There is no evidence that estrogens stimulate tumor growth in premenopausal patients with breast cancer, but estrogens are not effective in these patients.[390] About one-third of patients who respond to estrogens will have a withdrawal response if estrogens are discontinued at the first evidence of tumor regrowth.

Androgens have been shown in randomized trials to be less effective than estrogens.[361] All of the effective androgens tested have masculinizing effects. The androgen most commonly used today is fluoxymesterone (Halotestin) at a dose of 10 mg orally two to four times daily.

LHRH Analogues

The LHRH analogues have only recently been introduced and cannot be considered standard therapies for breast cancer at present. Both buserelin and leuprolide have been used in premenopausal and postmenopausal women.[391–393] Leuprolide has been more extensively tested, and in one study, 12 of 31 (39%) postmenopausal women and 11 of 25 (44%) premenopausal women responded.[392,394] These compounds are associated with minimal toxicity, but premenopausal women develop amenorrhea and postmenopausal symptoms. If further studies show similar response rates with low toxicity, it is possible that these compounds will soon become more widely used for breast cancer therapy, especially in premenopausal women.

Endocrine Therapy Combinations

A variety of endocrine therapies have been utilized in combination. This includes tamoxifen with fluoxymesterone, tamoxifen with DES, tamoxifen with aminoglutethimide, tamoxifen with medroxyprogesterone acetate, and tamoxifen with both aminoglutethimide and danazol. Although there is a trend in a few of these studies toward higher response rates among patients given two or more endocrine therapies, only one study has demonstrated an improvement in the overall survival rate.

Recently, randomized trials have been conducted comparing oophorectomy alone and oophorectomy plus prednisone in premenopausal women and tamoxifen alone versus tamoxifen plus prednisone in postmenopausal women. In both an initial study and a confirmatory study, there was a significant increase in the response rate when prednisone was added to either of the other two forms of endocrine therapy. In one of these two trials, there was a significant improvement in survival as well.[395,396]

Flare

Patients given almost any form of endocrine therapy may experience new symptoms or an exacerbation of old symptoms of their cancers beginning a few hours to a few days after initiation of therapy and subsiding spontaneously within a month. Most commonly, these symptoms consist of a diffuse achiness or increase in pain at sites of known metastases. There may be a transient erythema and slight swelling around skin or soft-tissue lesions. The serum CEA concentration may increase transiently. The most serious side-effect is hypercalcemia. The underlying mechanism for flare is not understood, but patients who experience these side-effects are as likely to go on to respond to endocrine therapy as are patients who do not have such side-effects. Flare has been most frequently observed in patients treated with androgens, tamoxifen, estrogens, and progestins. The incidence of this side-effect ranges from 3% to 9% in various studies.[361] Aminoglutethimide has not been reported to cause flare. However, rare instances of flare have been observed following oophorectomy and adrenalectomy.[397]

USE OF CHEMOTHERAPY

Combination chemotherapy will induce an objective response in approximately two-thirds of patients previously unexposed to chemotherapy, but complete eradication of disease at all sites will occur in less than 20%. The median duration of the response is usually less than 1 year (Table 38-34). The subjective response rate is higher than the objective response rate.[398] The median survival after the first course of chemotherapy is usually in excess of 3 years. However, these "average" figures mask the dramatic response that sometimes occurs: patients bedridden with bone pain not infrequently return to work for periods of several years. Although the numbers of patients with a long but unmaintained remission is small, there are reports of increasing numbers of such patients living almost symptom-free 5 to more than 10 years after completion of a course of chemotherapy.[399–402]

The time to the appearance of a response among breast cancer patients contrasts sharply with experience in patients with lymphomas, testicular cancers, and other tumors especially responsive to combination chemotherapy. The median time to response has ranged from 2 to 3 months in most studies, but this period is dependent in large part on the site of measurable disease. Thus, the median time to the appearance of a response is between 3 and 6 weeks in the skin and

TABLE 38-34. Response to and Survival after Treatment with Commonly Used Drug Combinations for Metastatic Breast Cancer

Percentage of patients with a response	43–82
Percentage with a complete response	4–27
Time to response (wk)	
Median	7–14
Maximum	72
Duration of response (mo)	
Median	5.3–13
Maximum	180+
Survival of responders (mo)	
Median	14.8–33
Maximum	180+

Modified from Henderson IC: Chemotherapy for advanced disease. In Harris JR, Hellman S, Henderson IC, Kinne DW (eds): Breast Diseases, pp 428–479. Philadelphia, JB Lippincott, 1987.

lymph nodes, 6 and 9 weeks in the lung, about 15 weeks in the liver, and nearly 18 weeks in the bones.[403,404] Practically, this means that a physician should not be discouraged if a response is not immediately apparent and should continue therapy until there is unequivocal evidence of progressive disease (see below regarding duration of chemotherapy). The possibility of disease progression during the first weeks of therapy may be suggested by new lesions on bone scans, increased intensity in old bone scan lesions, and transient elevations of CEA. The possibility of a "flare" following the administration of chemotherapy, similar to that described above for endocrine therapy, has not been carefully studied. However, it is known that some patients may have increased bone pain after chemotherapy begins before having a good response.

Identifying Chemotherapy-Responsive Patients

There are no well-defined clinical characteristics or established tests to identify patients likely to benefit from chemotherapy. This is in contrast to the situation described for endocrine therapy. Patients with metastatic breast cancer who should be treated with chemotherapy include all those who are symptomatic and who have either not responded or are very unlikely to respond to endocrine therapy based on the sites of metastases, disease-free interval, menstrual status, or ER status.

The profile of patients who have the highest response rates to chemotherapy is otherwise quite similar to the profile of patients who respond to endocrine therapy (Table 38-35). Responding patients with a long disease-free interval are more likely to have a durable response. Patients with only a few sites of metastatic disease are more likely to respond and to have a durable response to chemotherapy. Almost all studies have found that patients with a good performance status have a higher response rate than patients who are less than fully ambulatory, an important consideration in the use of historical controls in the evaluation of high- or low-dose chemotherapy regimens. Patients with a good performance status are more likely to tolerate high doses of chemotherapy, and this may erroneously lead to the conclusion that higher doses of drugs are more likely to induce a response.[398] Patients whose disease progresses during chemotherapy have a lower probability of response to a different type of chemotherapy. However, this is not necessarily true for patients who are given a chemotherapy combination after some interval during which they have received no chemotherapy of any type.

Twenty years ago, there were very few chemotherapy agents used routinely for the treatment of breast cancer, and new drugs were introduced earlier in the course of the patient's disease. Phase II studies of new agents are now performed in patients with more advanced disease who have had extensive prior chemotherapy and who have a poor performance status. A comparison of the response to a recently studied new agent with the response to an agent first studied 20 years ago thus may lead to the erroneous conclusion that the current drug is less effective.

Patients who do not respond to endocrine therapy are as likely to respond to chemotherapy as patients who are treated with chemotherapy as a primary modality. In a recent trial, patients were randomized to receive chemotherapy alone or tamoxifen alone. Patients who did not respond to the initial therapy were crossed over to the other therapy.[338] The primary response to chemotherapy in this study was 45%, and the secondary response to chemotherapy among those who did not respond to tamoxifen was 35%. The failure to respond to endocrine therapy appeared to have little or no effect on the subsequent response to chemotherapy.

On the basis of in vitro and animal models, one might anticipate that the most responsive patients would be those with the most rapidly growing tumors, possibly receptor-negative tumors. For example, the response to chemotherapy in vitro is twice as high in cell lines with a short doubling time and no ER as in receptor-positive cell lines with a long doubling time.[405] In clinical studies, however, ER status has not proved helpful in selecting chemoresponsive patients.[398] In five of seven studies performed to correlate response to chemotherapy and receptor status, the response rate among patients with receptor-positive tumors was higher than or equal to that in patients with receptor-negative tumors. Other potential markers of patients with high-growth-fraction tumors have been less extensively studied. In one small study, chemotherapy responders were found to have an average labeling index twice as high as that observed in patients who did not respond to chemotherapy.[406] The response rate

TABLE 38-35. Identifying Patients with Metastatic Breast Cancer Most Likely to Benefit from Chemotherapy

Factors Associated with:
Increased Probability of Response
Good performance status
Ambulatory status
Limited number (1–2) of disease sites
Prior hormone therapy
Metastases to lymph nodes
High labelling indices
High thymidine kinase levels
Increased Response Duration or Survival
Good performance status
Disease-free interval
Limited number of disease sites
Prior hormone therapy
Prior response to hormone therapy
Decreased Probability of Response
Bone metastases
Liver metastases
Prior chemotherapy
Prior radiotherapy
Decreased lymphocyte count
Decreased Response Duration or Survival
Prior radiotherapy
Decreased lymphocyte count
Factors Not Associated with Response Rate:
Age
Menopausal status
Dominant disease site
Carcinoembryonic antigen
Receptor status

Modified from Henderson IC: Chemotherapy for advanced disease. In Bonadonna G (ed): Breast Cancer: Diagnosis and Management, pp 274–280. New York, John Wiley & Sons, 1984.

to chemotherapy of tumors with a high thymidine kinase level was significantly greater than that of tumors with a low level of this enzyme (86% and 13%, respectively; $p < 0.001$).[407] Although promising, these data are too limited to recommend the use of labeling indices routinely to select patients for chemotherapy.

Active Drugs

Most chemotherapeutic agents active in the treatment of other cancers have at least some activity against breast cancer as well. However, the alkylating agents and the anthracyclines are the main components of most standard regimens. Cyclophosphamide is the most active of these agents, but thiotepa, L-PAM, and chlorambucil are also active. The relative effectiveness of these alkylating agents has never been determined in controlled trials. Cyclophosphamide may be given intravenously or orally. Chlorambucil and L-PAM have less acute toxicity but may be associated with a higher incidence of delayed toxicity, especially late leukemia.[263,408]

The anthracyclines are the most active drugs used as single agents, and doxorubicin has been shown effective against tumors resistant to cyclophosphamide.[409] In some studies, doxorubicin alone has been as active as the drug combinations CFP or CMFVP.[410,411] Although doxorubicin has conventionally been given as an intravenous bolus every 3 weeks, continuous administration over 48 to 96 hours and weekly administration schedules are less cardiotoxic.[412] Although both the continuous and weekly schedules are known to be effective for breast cancer, only the weekly schedule has been shown in a randomized trial to be as effective as a 3-weekly schedule.[413] 4′Epidoxorubicin has been as effective as doxorubicin in a number of randomized trials.[398] Although cardiotoxicity from 4′epidoxorubicin may be less than that from doxorubicin, it is not firmly established that the therapeutic index for 4′epidoxorubicin is really superior.

Although usually incorporated into second-line regimens, there is considerable evidence that mitomycin C and vinblastine are effective against tumors resistant to doxorubicin and cyclophosphamide. The response rate for mitomycin C, shown in Table 38-36, has been determined exclusively in patients refractory to other drugs. Although mitomycin C has recently been included in some first-line regimens, its principal use is still for the treatment of patients refractory to doxorubicin.

Vincristine is frequently used in combination programs for breast cancer, probably because it is not myelosuppressive and so does not compromise the doses of other drugs used in the combination. However, vincristine does cause neurotoxicity, and the incidence of severe neurotoxicity was high in the Phase II studies originally performed to demonstrate that it had any activity.[398] Five randomized trials have shown that vincristine adds nothing to combination chemotherapy. For example, when the regimen CMFP was compared with CMFVP in 427 patients,[414] there was no significant advantage in response rate or survival for patients given CMFVP. Also, doxorubicin alone was compared with the combination of doxorubicin and vincristine in randomized trials that enrolled 109 patients,[415] and the response rate was not significantly higher for the combination than for patients receiving doxorubicin alone. The use of vincristine for early or metastatic breast cancer is not recommended.

TABLE 38-36. Cytotoxic Drugs Active for Treating Breast Cancer

Drug	*Response Rate (%) in Phase II Trials*
4′-epidoxorubicin	34
Cyclophosphamide	33
Doxorubicin	32
Thiotepa	29
Methotrexate	28
Elliptinium	27
5-fluorouracil	27
Prednimustine	26
Vindesine	23
Mitomycin C	22
Vinblastine	21
L-Phenylalanine mustard	20
Mitoxantrone	20
Chlorambucil	17
Mitolactol	17

Modified from Henderson IC: Chemotherapy for advanced disease. In Harris JR, Hellman S, Henderson IC (eds): Breast Diseases, pp 428–479. Philadelphia, JB Lippincott, 1987.

Two other vinca alkaloids are effective. Vinblastine has recently been used as a 5-day continuous infusion, with a response rate of 37% in 106 patients, all of whom were considered refractory to doxorubicin.[416] Studies of bolus infusion of vinblastine are more limited, but the drug is active in this schedule as well. There are no randomized comparisons of the relative efficacy of bolus and continuous-infusion vinblastine. The other active vinca alkaloid, vindesine, has less neurotoxicity than vincristine and causes less myelosuppression than vinblastine. In randomized trials, vindesine has been as active as vinblastine and considerably more active than vincristine.[417,418] However, vindesine has not yet been approved by the FDA for general use in the treatment of metastatic breast cancer.

Other active drugs for breast cancer are listed in Table 38-36. Methotrexate and 5-FU are frequently used in combination, and methotrexate may be given intrathecally or orally to treat carcinomatous meningitis from metastatic breast cancer.[419] Methotrexate is also effective at moderate or high doses with leukovorin rescue, but it has not been demonstrated in controlled trials that there is any therapeutic advantage to the use of higher doses of methotrexate with leukovorin rescue instead of more conventional doses.[420,421] Mitoxantrone and prednimustine are much less toxic but also somewhat less effective than standard agents. Mitolactol has been used in a number of experimental combination programs but has not been shown to be superior to other alkylating agents in controlled trials and may have an unusual degree of tumorgenicity. Elliptinium appears to be very active for breast cancer and has a unique set of side-effects. However, it also does not have a place in the standard treatment of this disease. Several Phase II trials enrolling more than 100 patients failed to show much activity for cisplatin.[398] In one randomized trial, there was no advantage for CAP (49%) compared to CFP (46%).[422] However, two trials have used cisplatin in breast cancer patients not previously exposed to any form of chemotherapy, and in both studies, cisplatin appeared to be active. In one of these trials, cisplatin was used as a single agent,[423] and in the other, cisplatin was compared in a combination, CAP, with a more conventional CMVP.[424] Cisplatin appears to be cross-resistant with the agents most commonly used for breast cancer, and has no established role in the treatment of this disease, but may be an active drug nonetheless.

Drug Combinations

Several randomized trials have been performed to compare the relative efficacy of a single cytotoxic agent and a combination regimen.[398] In most of these studies, the response rate with the combination program was significantly higher, frequently twice as high, as that to the single agent. However, many of these studies were performed to determine if the additional toxicity associated with combination therapy resulted in sufficient benefit to justify its routine use, and the single agents may have been used at less-than-optimal doses. When a very intense program of cyclophosphamide was compared with the combination of CMF plus vinblastine, the efficacy of the two programs was nearly identical,[425] but a lower dose of cyclophosphamide was less effective than CMFVP.[426] Doxorubicin alone has been shown in several studies to be as effective as a combination program. Several randomized trials compared the strategy of sequential single agents with simultaneous use of all the same agents initially. Survival was marginally shorter and the total time spent in remission considerably less for patients treated with sequential single agents.[427,428] None of these studies systematically evaluated the quality of life. The duration of response and length of survival of responders to a single agent are nearly identical to those of responders to a combination. In some instances, the net quality of life may be better with a single agent rather than a combination.

The combinations most frequently utilized for the treatment of metastatic breast cancer are shown in Table 38-37. CMFP represents a truncation of the original Cooper regimen, which utilized CMFVP. As noted above, randomized trials have demonstrated that vincristine adds nothing to the regimen. However, two separate studies have demonstrated that the response rate to CMFP is higher than that to CMF alone. Prednisone may contribute to the efficacy of the regimen because of a direct antitumor effect. However, patients treated with CMFP have significantly less nausea and vomiting and have higher nadir leukocyte counts. As a result, patients treated with CMFP receive higher doses of cyclophosphamide, methotrexate, and 5-FU than patients treated with 5-FU alone.[429,430] The addition of prednisone may cause additional toxicity in some patients, including an increase in the incidence of infection, insomnia, or psychological sequelae. When these symptoms occur, it is advisable to discontinue the prednisone. In the standard CMFP program (Table 38-37), methotrexate and 5-FU are administered together. Attempts to increase the efficacy of CMFP by administering methotrexate and 5-FU sequentially with intervals of 1 to 24 hours have not been universally successful.[396] In conventional CMFP regimens, cyclophosphamide is given orally daily for 14 days. Because cyclophosphamide is effective when administered intravenously, CMF has also been given as an entirely intravenous regimen. However, a recently published randomized trial comparing intravenous CMF with conventional CMF demonstrated both a higher response rate to and a survival advantage for the conventional program.[431]

TABLE 38-37. Combination Chemotherapy Regimens Commonly Used to Treat Metastatic Breast Cancer

Regimen	*Dose (mg/m²)*	*Route*	*Day of Cycle Given*	*Cycle Length (wk)*
CMF (P)*†				
Cyclophosphamide	100	PO	1–14	
Methotrexate	40–60	IV	1 + 8	4
5-Fluorouracil	600–700	IV	1 + 8	
(Prednisone)	(40)	(PO)	(1–14)	
CA‡				
Cyclophosphamide	200	PO	3–6	3–4
Adriamycin	40	IV	1	
CAF§¶				
Cyclophosphamide	400–500	IV	1	
Adriamycin	40–50	IV	1	3
5-Fluorouracil	400–500	IV	1 + 8	

* Canellos GP, DeVita V, Gold GL et al: Cyclical combination chemotherapy for advanced breast cancer. Br Med J 1:218–220, 1974.

† Canellos GP, Pocock S, Taylor S et al: Combination chemotherapy for metastatic breast carcinoma. Cancer 38:1882–1886, 1976.

‡ Jones SE, Durie BGM, Salmon SE: Combination chemotherapy with Adriamycin and cyclophosphamide for advanced breast cancer. Cancer 36:90–97, 1975.

§ Bull J, Tormey D, Li SH, et al: A randomized comparative trial of Adriamycin versus methotrexate in combination drug therapy. Cancer 41:1649–1657, 1978.

¶ Smalley R, Carpenter J, Bartolucci A, Vogel C, Krauss S: A comparison of cyclophosphamide, Adriamycin, 5-fluorouracil (CAF) and cyclophosphamide, methotrexate, 5-fluorouracil, vincristine, prednisone (CMFVP) in patients with metastatic breast cancer. Cancer 40:625–632, 1977.

Combination programs that include doxorubicin produce a 15% to 20% higher response rate than identical regimens without doxorubicin.[398] The median duration of response and survival after treatment with a doxorubicin combination is 3 to 6 months longer, but in randomized trials, this difference usually has not been statistically significant. In the largest of these studies, patients were randomized to received CAF, CAFVP, or CMF.[432] Patients treated with CAF and CAFVP had a significantly higher response rate, and the median survival of patients treated with CAF was almost 11 months longer than that of patients treated with CMFVP. However, patients treated with CAFVP had only a 1.5-month prolongation of median survival, and this difference was not significant. In most studies, the doxorubicin combination has been associated with significantly more toxicity, and the rather dramatic alopecia that follows treatment with doxorubicin is unacceptable to many patients. The advantages of a doxorubicin-containing regimen as the initial treatment of patients with metastatic disease must be carefully weighed against the additional toxicity of these regimens and the fact that patients have fewer remaining alternative treatments for palliation at the time of further disease progression.

Secondary and Tertiary Treatments

The probability of a secondary response to chemotherapy among patients whose disease worsens while they are receiving a first combination regimen is between 20% and 35%, depending on whether the previous regimen included doxorubicin. Patients who have been treated with chemotherapy but whose disease progresses after an interval during which chemotherapy was not given (*e.g.*, 6 months or more) have a much higher probability of a secondary response, including a secondary response to the regimen to which they previously responded.

The response to secondary chemotherapy among patients without prior exposure to doxorubicin is approximately 35% (range 17%–54% in 17 separate studies). The median duration of response ranged from 4 to 11.5 months, and the median duration of survival ranged from 7 to 16 months.[398] The response rate to doxorubicin as a single agent in these patients was usually between 30% and 40%. Two combination programs have been reported to have relatively high response rates. One, VATH, has a reported response rate between 45% and 53%, a median duration of response of almost 1 year, and a median survival between 13 and 16 months.[433,434] The second program consists of 5-FU, vincristine (Oncovin), doxorubicin (Adriamycin), and mitomycin C (FOAM). The number of patients treated with this regimen is larger. The reported response rate is 35%, the median duration of response is 7 months, and the median survival is 9 months.[435]

Studies of patients already exposed to doxorubicin are more likely to include extensively treated patients with exposure to at least two separate combination programs. The overall response to chemotherapy in these patients is about 21% (range 0–40% in 11 separate studies), with a median survival of 4 to 6 months and a median duration of response of 2 to 8 months.[398] A particularly popular combination for this group of patients includes mitomycin C, 20 mg/m² intravenously on day one, and vinblastine, 0.5 mg/kg intravenously on days one and twenty-eight, administered on a 6- to 8-week cycle. This regimen is associated with severe myelosuppression, neurologic complications, and pulmonary toxicity.[436] The highest response rate observed in three trials evaluating the combination of mitomycin C and vinblastine was 40%, with a median duration of response of 4 months.[436–438]

No controlled studies have compared the relative efficacy of doxorubicin alone with that of a doxorubicin combination or of mitomycin C alone with that of the combination of mitomycin C and vinblastine as secondary or tertiary treatment. The only goal of therapy in these patients is palliation. The response rate to drug combinations administered in the setting of prior exposure to chemotherapy is unlikely to be much greater than the response to single agents, but the toxicity will almost certainly be greater. In light of this, CMF is recommended as first-line chemotherapy for patients with metastatic disease. Treatment at the time of disease progression should be single-agent doxorubicin, then single-agent mitomycin C, and finally single-agent vinblastine.

Optimal Duration of Therapy

There is no evidence that more than 6 months of chemotherapy is more beneficial than programs that end at about the sixth month. In one study, patients who were stable after 6 months of CMFVP therapy were randomized to continue CMFVP until evidence of disease progression or to stop CMFVP at 6 months.[427] Patients who stopped therapy were frequently retreated with CMFVP at the time of further disease progression, and many had a secondary response. There was a slight trend toward better survival among the patients who stopped CMFVP at the end of the first 6 months of treatment (Figure 38-23). Similar results have been ob-

FIG. 38-23. Effect of duration of therapy on survival. Patients treated with CMFVP who were stable beyond 6 months of therapy were randomized to continue CMFVP beyond 6 months or to discontinue therapy. (Smalley RV, Murphy S, Huguley CM et al: Combination versus sequential five-drug chemotherapy in metastatic carcinoma of the breast. Cancer Res 36:3911–3916, 1976)

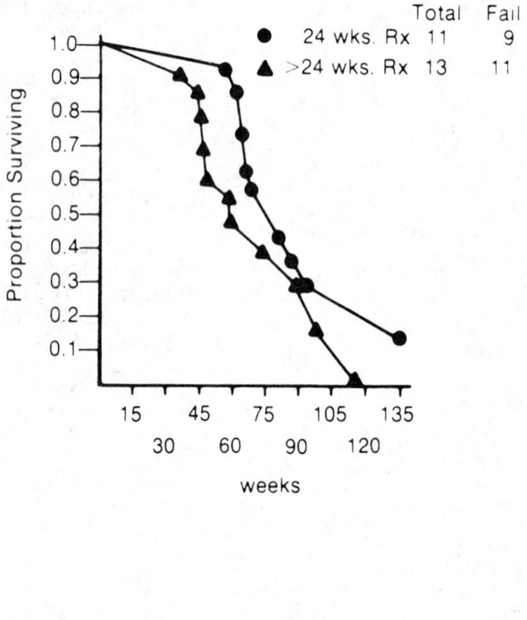

tained in a study of patients with locally advanced breast cancer.[439] In a more recent study, patients were randomized to receive either continuous chemotherapy (CA or CMF) until disease progression or three courses of chemotherapy and observation without treatment until evidence of disease progression.[440] Both objective response rates and quality of life, measured by a linear analogue self-assessment format, were significantly better among the patients randomized to receive chemotherapy continuously, and there was even a marginal survival advantage for the continuous-therapy program.

The optimal duration of chemotherapy is not known; it probably exceeds 3 months but might not exceed 6 months. On the basis of the evidence currently available, it is reasonable to discontinue therapy among patients whose disease is stable after 6 months of chemotherapy.

New Principles in the Use of Chemotherapy

Recent innovations designed to improve the efficacy of combination chemotherapy have included the use of high doses of drugs, alternating regimens, and continuous infusion.

There is undeniably a dose–response effect for most of the drugs used to treat breast cancer, but it has not been demonstrated that the therapeutic index of these agents is increased with higher doses. Most breast cancer dose studies are retrospective. Although patients receiving (or tolerating) a higher dose of drug had a higher response rate, patients with a higher performance status also had a higher response rate. It is likely that patients able to tolerate a higher dose of drug in these studies had a better initial performance status.[398,441,442] A retrospective analysis combining the results of many trials has been performed by Hryniuk and is frequently cited as evidence for a dose–response correlation in the use of chemotherapy for the treatment of breast cancer.[253,443] However, this analysis is based on numerous assumptions, many of which are inconsistent with the general principles of oncologic practice, and the conclusions from this oft-cited reference cannot be accepted as sound evidence of a dose response.[254]

Two randomized trials evaluating dose–response correlations have been performed. In one of these, patients were randomized to either a standard dose or a high dose of CMF.[444] There was no difference in the overall response rate, the median duration of response, or the survival of the two groups. A more recent and larger study randomized patients to standard-dose or low-dose CMF.[445] Patients receiving the standard doses of CMF had a significantly higher response rate and a marginal prolongation of survival.

Very high doses of single agents or drug combinations have been used with autologous bone-marrow transplantation to circumvent dose-limiting myelosuppression.[398] These trials involved from 1 to 16 patients, and the response rates have been as high as 100% with complete response rates between 30% and 100%. Because the number of patients entered in these trials is too small to permit meaningful interpretation, this approach must be considered entirely experimental.

Although dose may eventually be shown to be an important factor in determining the effectiveness of chemotherapy, it has not yet been shown that increasing the drug dose results in much added benefit, nor has it been demonstrated that drug doses can be safely reduced without compromising patient response, quality of life, and survival. Standard regimens are recommended until further evidence emerges from well-designed trials that specifically address these issues.

All tumors eventually develop resistance to these chemotherapeutic agents. Goldie, Coldman, and Gudauskas have hypothesized that the drugs induce resistance and that such resistance occurs very quickly after the first exposure to chemotherapy.[446] One strategy to circumvent this early resistance is the use of alternating, non-cross-resistant regimens. A large number of such trials have been performed,[447] none of which has shown a large advantage for the use of alternating regimens. In one study, more than 300 patients were randomized to receive either CMFP alternating every second cycle with two course of doxorubicin and vincristine.[448] Response to the two programs was almost identical, and both the duration of response and the duration of survival were slightly better for patients randomized to the nonalternating program.

More-frequent administration of drug in an intense dose schedule may result in higher overall response and complete response rates than administration of the same drugs at slightly higher doses intermittently.[411,427,449] In these studies, there was no significant survival advantage for the more intense program. The logical extension of these studies is the continuous administration of drug either for weeks via an implantable pump or for shorter courses using more conventional intravenous therapy in the hospital. Uncontrolled trials using continuous-infusion vinblastine, mitomycin C, doxorubicin, and 5-FU or FUDR suggest an improvement in the therapeutic index with more constant treatment, but none of these studies had appropriate control groups. The data thus are still inadequate to conclude that continuous-infusion therapy is more efficacious than intermittent bolus administration.[398]

Chemotherapy-Endocrine Therapy Combinations

The hypothesis that chemotherapy and endocrine (chemoendocrine) therapy are synergistic depends on the assumption that there are at least two distinctly different clones of cells, one clone responsive to chemotherapy but resistant to hormone therapy and the other resistant to chemotherapy but responsive to hormone therapy. There is abundant evidence that clones of the first type exist, but little evidence for the second.

The first generation of studies evaluating chemoendocrine therapy combinations demonstrated that the response rate to these combinations was consistantly and significantly higher than the response rate to endocrine therapy alone, but only 1 of 12 trials of this type showed a significant improvement in survival for patients receiving the chemoendocrine combination.[398] The response rate to chemoendocrine therapy is also usually higher than the response to chemotherapy alone, but this improvement reached levels of statistical significance in only 4 of 11 of trials designed to address this question. Improvement in the duration of response was marginal, and there was no significant improvement in survival for patients in these studies.[398]

The results from these studies can be illustrated and summarized by a recent large trial performed by the Australian–New Zealand Breast Cancer Trials Group.[338] Patients were randomized to receive either tamoxifen alone, combination chemotherapy with AC (doxorubicin plus cyclophosphamide), or a combination of tamoxifen plus AC (ACT). Patients whose tumors progressed on tamoxifen or AC were immediately crossed over to the other arm of the study. The initial response rates to tamoxifen, AC, and ACT were 22%, 45%, and 51%, respectively ($p = <0.001$). Because the secondary response to AC among tamoxifen failures is 35%, 43% of the patients randomized to tamoxifen eventually had a response either to tamoxifen alone or to subsequent chemotherapy. Only 6% of the patients whose tumors progressed on AC had a subsequent response to tamoxifen. As a result, the overall response rate of patients randomized to each of these three treatment arms was nearly the same. The median survival was not significantly different: 21 months, 18 months, and 20 months for patients randomized respectively to tamoxifen, AC, or ACT. This study not only failed to show any significant advantage for using chemoendocrine therapy but also suggested an advantage for the initial use of endocrine therapy alone, as more than 20% of the patients randomized to receive initial tamoxifen without chemotherapy had a period in which the symptoms of tumor were palliated without the toxicities of chemotherapy.

Several studies of chemoendocrine therapy have stratified patients by receptor status. In one study, patients were randomized to receive either CAF or CAF plus tamoxifen.[450] Among ER-positive patients, the response rate to CAF was 56% and to CAF plus tamoxifen, 67%. Among ER-negative patients, the response rates were 56% and 62%, respectively (not statistically significant). Receptor status thus does not identify patients more likely to benefit from chemoendocrine therapy.

Combinations of chemotherapy and endocrine therapy are not recommended for the treatment of metastatic breast cancer. Patients who are good candidates for endocrine therapy should be treated with endocrine therapy alone, as these patients may have long-term palliation without the side-effects of therapy. Patients who are not good candidates for endocrine therapy are not likely to derive much benefit from adding tamoxifen or other forms of endocrine therapy to an effective chemotherapy program.

TREATMENT OF SPECIFIC METASTATIC SITES

Breast cancer can, and usually does, metastasize to almost any organ site in the body (see Table 38-14). When multiple sites of disease are involved, systemic therapy should be used. However, in some situations, radiotherapy and, less often, surgery should be employed in addition to or instead of endocrine therapy or chemotherapy.

LOCAL RECURRENCE AFTER MASTECTOMY

Breast cancer recurrent in overlying skin and regional lymph nodes following a mastectomy must be distinguished from a recurrence entirely within breast parenchyma after primary radiation therapy. The natural history and prognosis of the latter is more like that of a new cancer in a contralateral breast and is discussed above in the section on conservative surgery and radiation therapy. Local recurrences after mastectomy are a common problem, occurring in 19% to 27% of patients with histologically involved nodes and in 3% to 8% of patients without node involvement.[218] These local recurrences have the same significance as metastases to distant organs: almost all of these patients will eventually die of breast cancer. Treatment of the isolated metastases will not be curative. On the other hand, many of these patients will live years after the appearance of a local recurrence. Factors predictive of survival are the same as those predictive of survival after recurrence at distant sites. The most important of these factors is the disease-free interval. The median survival of patients with locally recurrent disease is between 2 and 3 years, the 5-year survival rate being less than 35% and the 10-year survival rate less than 25%. The 10-year disease-free survival rate is usually less than 15%. In this context, it may be reasonable to treat some of these patients with local modalities without immediate systemic therapy.

Radiotherapy to the chest wall will result in an initial response rate of 63% to 79%,[218] but one-third to two-thirds of these patients will have a subsequent local recurrence. In a recent series from the JCRT, the actuarial local control rate at 5 years after local radiotherapy was 43%.[451] Local control following radiotherapy will be improved if prior surgery with excision of all apparent disease is possible, if higher doses of radiation therapy are used, or if a boost of radiotherapy is given to areas of gross residual disease.

Systemic therapy may also be useful in inducing regression of local disease. Overall response rates in several recent series are 62% to 85%.[452,453] Endocrine therapy may be as effective as or even more effective than chemotherapy in controlling a local recurrence.[453] This is consistent with the observation from postmastectomy adjuvant therapy trials in which adjuvant tamoxifen appears to be better in reducing local recurrence rates than is adjuvant chemotherapy.

Several other modalities available for the treatment of disease at specific sites include hyperthermia, photoradiation with hematoporphyrin photosensitization, and superficial laser therapy. Hyperthermia has been utilized alone, with radiotherapy, and with chemotherapy. Anecdotal reports concerning all three of these approaches are sometimes impressive and suggest the possibility of local control of disease refractory to more conventional forms of therapy. However, all of these approaches must be considered experimental at present.

When local recurrences accompany distant metastases, systemic therapy should be employed initially and radiotherapy added only if the locally recurrent disease is particularly symptomatic or fails to respond to systemic therapy. On the other hand, if an isolated local recurrence appears after a long disease-free interval and without evidence of distant metastases, initial therapy may consist of excision alone or of excision plus radiation therapy. Several recurrences of this type without evidence of distant metastases should preferentially be treated with radiation therapy.

METASTASES TO THE NERVOUS SYSTEM, SPINE, AND CHOROID

Between 20% and 25% of patients with metastatic breast cancer will eventually develop a problem related to the nervous system: brain metastases, epidural spinal cord compression, carcinomatous meningitis, brachial plexus syndrome, choroidal metastases, or a paraneoplastic syndrome. Breast cancer is one of the two or three most common tumors responsible for metastases at each of these sites. In autopsy series, CNS metastases are observed in 9% to 25% of all breast cancer patients.[349] However, antemortem diagnoses of brain metastases (about 10%) or carcinomatous meningitis (about 5%) are less frequent.[419,454,455]

Radiotherapy plays a central role in the treatment of all types of metastases to the nervous system, and dexamethasone should be administered promptly after the documentation of metastases on CT scan. (Dexamethasone administered prior to the CT scan obscures the diagnosis in occasional patients.) The optimal dose schedule of radiation is a point of some controversy. There is no evidence that either the response rate or the duration of response is significantly different when a high dose of radiation is delivered in multiple fractions over 4 weeks compared with low doses administered in two fractions over 3 to 7 days.[456] However, short high-dose courses of radiation may result in a higher complication rate.[457] Approximately 20% of patients with brain metastases deteriorate rapidly and are unable to complete the course of radiotherapy. However, 50% to 75% of patients who do complete the radiotherapy will have decreased neurologic symptoms, and some patients will remain free of symptoms for years. Dexamethasone should be tapered after the completion of radiation therapy and can be discontinued altogether in more than 50% of patients.

It has not been established that surgical excison of brain metastases has any advantage over radiation therapy alone, especially as radiation is usually administered after surgery. Moreover, brain metastases from breast cancer are often multicentric.[457] Surgery is indicated only when the diagnosis is in doubt or when patients have surgically accessible disease, persistent symptoms, and radioresistant tumors. Concomitant breast cancer metastases to the brain and a meningioma within the brain have been reported.[458] The possibility of meningioma in a breast cancer patient may be suspected on the basis of the CT finding and should lead to surgical exploration.

Until recently, systemic therapy has not been utilized for the treatment of brain metastases of breast cancer because it was assumed that these agents would not cross the blood–brain barrier. However, newer pharmacologic studies have demonstrated that many of the standard drugs utilized to treat breast cancer do indeed cross into the brain. These drugs include cyclophosphamide and 5-FU in conventional doses[459] and methotrexate in high doses.[460] Objective response was observed in 50% of a recent series of 66 patients treated for brain metastases with combination chemotherapy programs that included prednisone.[461] Even tamoxifen has been reported to induce remission of a brain metastasis.[462] However, until comparative studies on the relative efficacy of radiotherapy and systemic therapy have been performed, radiotherapy must be preferred for treatment of brain metastases because of both the high response rate and the very durable responses achieved in some patients.

Carcinomatous meningitis is generally thought to have a dire prognosis; the median survival is 7 months, and the 1-year survival rate is less than 10%.[419,463,464] Because of the diffuse nature of carcinomatous meningitis and the difficulties inherent in delivering radiotherapy to the entire cranial–spinal axis, intrathecal chemotherapy is almost always employed. Methotrexate, thiotepa, and cytosine arabinoside can be utilized; the first two of these agents are especially effective against breast cancer. Recommended regimens include methotrexate, 7 to 12 ml/m^2, twice weekly until neurologic symptoms have subsided. This may be optimally administered through an Ommaya reservoir. Systemic symptoms from methotrexate may be avoided if leukovorin rescue is given as well. When cerebrospinal fluid cytology becomes negative, the frequency of methotrexate administration may be gradually decreased, first to a weekly course and eventually to a single administration every 2 months.[464] Radiotherapy is reserved for symptomatic areas in the brain or spinal cord. However, when cranial nerve palsies are evident, radiation therapy is given to the whole brain because the tumor usually involves the entire subarachnoid space and extends over the convexities of the brain, brainstem, and even throughout the spinal cord. Because radiation therapy to the entire spine would involve more than 40% of bone marrow areas, this is generally not recommended.[464] When both radiotherapy to the CNS and methotrexate are administered, the possibility of a leukoencephalopathy increases.

Choroidal metastases may be the first sign of metastases, occur in 2% to 6% of all patients, and are bilateral in 20% to 50% of those patients who develop choroidal metastases.[465] Radiotherapy will improve visual acuity in 80% to 90% of patients, and complications, such as cataracts or radiation retinitis, are rare. Although there are anecdotal reports of chemotherapy being effective, there is generally no role for either chemotherapy or enucleation when radiation therapy is effective.

Epidural spinal-cord compression causing paralysis and sphincter dysfunction is among the most serious complications from breast metastases and is not an uncommon problem. Compression may occur either from direct encroachment on the spinal cord by expanding tumor or secondary to fractures of the vertebrae. The most common source of tumor growing to compress the spinal canal is metastases to the vertebrae. Because more than two-thirds of patients with breast cancer eventually develop bony metastases and the most common sites of bony metastases are the vertebrae, it is not surprising that this is a frequent problem in the differential diagnosis and management of patients with metastatic breast cancer.

Although radiotherapy remains the most important modality for the prevention of epidural spinal-cord compression, considerable clinical judgment is required to determine when to irradiate and which vertebrae to irradiate. Patients with metastatic breast cancer often have multiple painful areas and multiple abnormalities on bone scan. It is rarely necessary or appropriate to irradiate all of these, especially because large areas of bone marrow may be involved, and subsequent or concomitant chemotherapy will therefore be compromised. The precise nature of the underlying causes of spinal compression should be determined by the use of MRI, CT scans, and myelography. Soft-tissue masses likely to respond rapidly to radiotherapy should be distinguished from compression fractures, which may require surgical stabilization for adequate relief of symptoms or for prevention of paralysis.

When a diagnosis of impending or early epidural spinal-cord compression has been made, dexamethasone should be given first. Radiotherapy to the involved areas (which can be best defined by MRI in a sagittal plane or by myelography) will provide pain relief in two-thirds to three-fourths of patients and will maintain ambulation and sphincter function in more than half.[466] In general, the results of laminectomy plus radiotherapy are no better than the results of radiation therapy alone. However, surgery may be of value in patients with further deterioration after radiation therapy, recurrence in a previously irradiated area, or instability of the vertebral column.[466]

Bone pain in patients with multiple lesions and no evidence of epidural spinal-cord compression should be treated first with systemic therapy. Radiation can then be added to relieve symptoms when systemic therapy is not effective. Chemotherapy and endocrine therapy are not likely to relieve pain when radiation therapy has not been effective. Under these circumstances, other causes of pain or neurologic dysfunction should be sought. Often, compression fracture and other structural abnormalities will persist after treatment of the tumor, and antineoplastic therapy is not likely to provide further relief of these symptoms.

Brachial plexopathy in patients with breast cancer may occur because of tumor infiltration of the brachial plexus or because of radiation damage. A history of radiation treatment, the nature of the symptoms, and their distribution should provide some clues to distinguish between these two causes of plexopathy.[467] Early diagnosis of brachial plexopathy secondary to tumor and prompt administration of radiotherapy may alleviate symptoms before deafferentiation has occurred. When symptoms have advanced before diagnosis, the patient is usually left with permanent disability including permanent intractable pain.

BONE AND BONE MARROW METASTASES AND HYPERCALCEMIA

Because bone metastases are rarely isolated or rarely remain as a single focus for any length of time, the mainstay of treatment is systemic, namely, endocrine therapy or chemotherapy. The response rate of bone lesions in patients with ER-positive tumors or other clinical characteristics predictive of a response to endocrine therapy is nearly equal to the response to chemotherapy in patients refractory to endocrine therapy or with receptor-negative tumors. Intensive chemotherapy programs may induce some response in sites of bone disease in 80% to 90% of patients, with a complete response seen in 25% to 50% of patients.[421,468,469]

Radiotherapy is probably more effective than systemic therapy in relieving bone pain but can be applied to only one bone at a time.[470,471] However, the relative effectiveness of these two modalities has never been fully evaluated in randomized controlled trials. The value of radiotherapy or prophylactic surgical fixation in the prevention of fractures has likewise not been evaluated in controlled trials. By convention, prophylactic fixation has been recommended when lesions exceed 2.5 cm, involve 50% of the bone diameter, and invade the bone cortex.[472] Patients with persistent pain 6 to 8 weeks after the completion of radiotherapy should also be evaluated for a possible incomplete or nondisplaced fracture.

Bone-marrow metastases have been found in as many as 55% of patients with bone metastases diagnosed on bone scan or plain films.[473] Marrow metastases are seldom diagnosed by conventional means in patients without bone metastases[474] but may actually be found more frequently when extremely sensitive methods, such as immunocytochemical stains, are used. In one study, 28% of patients with operable breast lesions were found to have occult bone marrow metastases.[475] Bone marrow metastases from breast cancer should be treated with systemic therapy. The choice of endocrine therapy or chemotherapy is made utilizing the criteria described for the selection between these two modalities for other sites of metastases.

Between 5% and 10% of all patients with breast cancer will develop hypercalcemia at some time in the course of their metastatic disease.[476] Not infrequently, hypercalcemia occurs within a few hours to several weeks after the initiation of endocrine therapy. Its management in these patients is similar to the management of this condition in other patients with malignancy.[477] However, when hypercalcemia promptly follows the initiation of endocrine therapy, the endocrine therapy should be continued unless the hypercalcemia is life threatening or exceeds 14 mg/dl. Many of these patients will respond to endocrine therapy despite the hypercalcemia.[361]

PULMONARY METASTASES

Metastases to the lungs may appear as pulmonary nodules, lymphangetic spread, or pleural effusions. Pulmonary nodules are exquisitely sensitive to systemic therapy and may be completely eradicated with chemotherapy in 40% to 80% of patients.[421,468,469] Lymphangetic spread within the lungs has been found in 24% to 34% of patients at autopsy, but an unequivocal antemortem diagnosis is usually made in less than 20% of patients.[478] Although this diagnosis is considered dire, the 1-year survival rate is 80% and the 2-year survival rate is 30% when lymphangetic metastases are the first site of metastatic disease. Because this diagnosis is difficult to document, it is not surprising that it is also difficult to document objective responses to therapy. Systemic therapy is always indicated, and the criteria described above to choose between endocrine therapy and chemotherapy should be applied here as well.

More than 50% of patients with metastatic breast cancer are likely to develop malignant effusions.[479] Pleural effusion, especially when it is an isolated finding, does not carry a bad prognosis. In one series, the median survival of patients who presented with pleural effusion alone was 48 months.[480] Asymptomatic pleural effusions, especially if they are only one manifestation of systemic disease in a patient with multiple other sites, requires no specific therapy. Only 10% of pleural effusions are controlled by the first thoracentesis,[479] and repeated thoracenteses are likely to lead to loculation of fluid and increased difficulty in long-term control. Thoracostomy alone may lead to control of effusion in 20% to 50% of patients, but instillation of agents that induce sclerosis will lead to better control. Although a number of different agents have been shown to be effective, tetracycline is among those that are most readily available and have the least toxicity.[479] The best long-term control will be obtained with talc pleurodesis through a thoracostomy, and this treatment should be considered for patients with a good long-term prognosis who are able to withstand this procedure.[481]

REFERENCES

1. Silverberg E, Lubera J: Cancer Statistics, 1987. CA 37:2–19, 1987
2. Pike MC, Henderson BE, Casagrande JT, Rosario I, Gray GE: Oral contraceptive use and early abortion as risk factors for breast cancer in young women. Br J Cancer, 43:72–76, 1981
3. Henderson BE, Pike MC, Ross RK: Epidemiology and risk factors. In Bonadonna G (ed): Breast Cancer: Diagnosis and Management, pp 15–33. Chichester, John Wiley & Sons, 1984
4. Henderson BE, Ross RK, Judd HL, Krailo MD, Pike MC: Do regular ovulatory cycles increase breast cancer risk? Cancer 56:1206–1208, 1985
5. Thomas DB, Lilienfeld AM: Geographic, reproductive and sociobiological factors. In Stoll B (ed): Risk Factors in Breast Cancer, pp 25–53. Chicago, Wm Heinemann Medical Books, 1976
6. Brinton LA, Hoover R, Fraumeni JF: Reproductive factors in the aetiology of breast cancer. Br J Cancer 47:757–762, 1983
7. Trichopoulos D, Hsieh C, MacMahon B et al: Age at any birth and breast cancer risk. Int J Cancer 31:701–704, 1983
8. Thomas DB: Do hormones cause breast cancer? Cancer 53:595–604, 1984
9. Brinton LA, Hoover RN, Szklo M, Fraumeni JFJ: Menopausal estrogen use and risk of breast cancer. Cancer 47:2517–2522, 1981
10. Ross RK, Paganini-Hill A, Gerkins VR et al: A case-control study of menopausal estrogen therapy and breast cancer. JAMA 243:1635–1639, 1980
11. McPherson K, Drife JO: The pill and breast cancer: Why the uncertainty? Br Med J 293:709–710, 1986
12. Miller AB: Epidemiology and prevention. In Harris JR, Hellman S, Henderson IC, Kinne DW (eds): Breast Diseases, pp 87–102. Philadelphia, JB Lippincott, 1987
13. Meirik O, Adami HO, Christoffersen T, Lund E, Bergstrom R, Bergsho P: Oral contraceptive use and breast cancer in young women. Lancet 2:650–654, 1986
14. Cancer and Steroid Hormone Study of the Centers for Disease Control, the National Institute of Child Health and Human Development: Oral-contraceptive use and the risk of breast cancer. N Engl J Med 315:405–411, 1986
15. Buell P: Changing incidence of breast cancer in Japanese-American women. J Natl Cancer Inst 51:1479–1483, 1973
16. Wynder EL, Rose DP, Cohen LA: Diet and breast cancer in causation and therapy. Cancer 58:1804–1813, 1986
17. Mettlin C: Diet and the epidemiology of human breast cancer. Cancer 53:605–611, 1984
18. Willett WC, Stampfer MJ, Colditz GA, Rosner BA, Hennekens CH, Speizer FE: Dietary fat and risk of breast cancer. N Engl J Med 316:22–28, 1987
19. Bjarnason O, Day N, Snaedal G, Tulinius H: The effect of year of birth on the breast cancer age-incidence curve in Iceland. Int J Cancer 13:689–696, 1974
20. Willett WC, Stampfer MJ, Colditz GA, Rosner BA, Hennekens CH, Speizer FE: Moderate alcohol consumption and the risk of breast cancer. N Engl J Med 316:1174–1180, 1987
21. Schatzkin A, Jones Y, Hoover RN et al: Alcohol consumption and breast cancer in the epidemiologic follow-up study of the First National Health and Nutrition Examination Survey. N Engl J Med 316:1169–1173, 1987
22. Adami H, Hansen J, Jung B, Rimsten A: Characteristics of familial breast cancer in Sweden. Cancer 48:1688–1695, 1981
23. Sattin RW, Rubin GL, Webster LA et al: Family history and the risk of breast cancer. JAMA 253:1908–1913, 1985
24. Dupont WD, Page DL: Risk factors for breast cancer in women with proliferative breast disease. N Engl J Med 312:146–151, 1985
25. Baak JPA, Van Dop H, Kurver PHJ, Hermans J: The value of morphometry to classic prognosticators in breast cancer. Cancer 56:374–382, 1985
26. Anderson DE, Badzioch MD: Risk of familial breast cancer. Cancer 56:383–387, 1985
27. Bailar JC: Screening for early breast cancer: Pros and cons. Cancer 39:2783–2795, 1977
28. Love SM, Gelman RS, Silen W: Fibrocystic "disease" of the breast—A nondisease? N Engl J Med 307:1010–1014, 1982
29. Henderson IC, Canellos GP: Cancer of the breast: The past decade. N Engl J Med 302:17–30; 78–90, 1980
30. Fox MS: On the diagnosis and treatment of breast cancer. JAMA 241:489–494, 1979
31. Silvestrini R, Daidone MG, Gentili C: Biologic characteristics of breast cancer and their clinical relevance. In Bulbrook RD (ed): Commentaries on Research in Breast Disease, Vol 2, pp 1–40. New York, Alan R Liss, 1981
32. Malaise EP, Chavaudra N, Tubiana M: The relationship between growth rate, labelling index and histological type of human solid tumours. Eur J Cancer 9:305–312, 1973
33. von Fournier D, Weber E, Hoeffken W, Bauer M, Kubli F, Barth V: Growth rate of 147 mammary carcinomas. Cancer 45:2198–2207, 1980
34. Heuser L, Spratt JS, Polk HC: Growth rates of primary breast cancers. Cancer 43:1888–1894, 1979
35. Lundgren B: Observations on growth rate of breast carcinomas and its possible implications for lead time. Cancer 40:1722–1725, 1977
36. Gershon-Cohen J, Berger SM, Klickstein HS: Roentgenography of breast cancer moderating concept of "biologic predeterminism." Cancer 16:961–964, 1963
37. Speer JF, Petrosky VE, Retsky MW, Wardwell RH: A stochastic numerical model of breast cancer growth that simulates clinical data. Cancer Res 44:4124–4130, 1984
38. Gilchrist KW, Kalish L, Gould VE et al: Interobserver reproducibility of histopathological features in Stage II breast cancer: An ECOG study. Breast Cancer Res Treat 5:8–10, 1985
39. Rosen PP, Saigo PE, Braun DW et al: Axillary micro- and macrometastases in breast cancer. Ann Surg 194:585–591, 1981
40. Osborne CK: Receptors. In Harris JR, Hellman S, Henderson IC, Kinne DW (eds): Breast Diseases, pp 210–232. Philadelphia, JB Lippincott, 1987
41. Horwitz KB, McGuire WL: Estrogen control of progesterone receptor in human breast cancer: Correlation with nuclear processing of estrogen receptor. J Biol Chem 253:2223–2228, 1978
42. Lippman ME, Dickson RB, Bates S et al: Autocrine and paracrine growth regulation of human breast cancer. Breast Cancer Res Treat 7:59–70, 1986
43. McGuire WL, Clark GM, Dressler LG, Owens MA: Role of steroid hormone receptors as prognostic factors in primary breast cancer. NCI Monogr 1:19–23, 1986
44. Singhakowinta A, Potter H, Buroker T, Samal B, Brooks S, Vaitkevicius V: Estrogen receptor and natural course of breast cancer. Ann Surg 183:84–88, 1976
45. Thorpe SM, Rose C, Rasmussen BB, Mouridsen HT, Bayer T, Keiding N: Prognostic value of steroid hormone receptors: Multivariate analysis of systemically untreated patients with node negative primary breast cancer. Cancer Res 47:6126–6133, 1987
46. Valagussa P, Bignami P, Buzzoni R et al: Are estrogen receptors alone a reliable prognostic factor in node negative breast cancer? In Jones SE, Salmon SE (eds): Adjuvant Therapy of Cancer IV, pp 407–415. Orlando, Grune & Stratton, 1984
47. Crowe JP, Hubay CA, Pearson OH et al: Estrogen receptor status as a prognostic indicator for Stage I breast cancer patients. Breast Cancer Res Treat 2:171–176, 1982
48. Adams HO, Graffman S, Lindgren A, Sallstrom J: Prognostic implication of estrogen receptor content in breast cancer. Breast Cancer Res Treat 5:293–300, 1985
49. Blamey RW, Bishop HM, Blake JRS et al: Relationship between primary breast tumor receptor status and patient survival. Cancer 46:2765–2769, 1980
50. Raemaekers JMM, Beex LVAM, Koenders AJM et al: Disease-free interval and estrogen receptor activity in tumor tissue of patients with primary breast cancer: Analysis after long-term follow-up. Breast Cancer Res Treat 6:123–130, 1985
51. Hahnel R, Woodings T, Vivian AB: Prognostic value of estrogen receptors in primary breast cancer. Cancer 44:671–675, 1979
52. Howell A, Harland RNL, Bramwell VHC et al: Steroid-hormone receptors and survival after first relapse in breast cancer. Lancet 1:588–591, 1984
53. Valagussa P, Bonadonna G, Veronesi U: Patterns of relapse and survival in operable breast carcinoma with positive and negative axillary nodes. Tumori 64:241–258, 1978
54. Fisher B, Slack N, Katrych D, Wolmark N: Ten year follow-up results of patients with carcinoma of the breast in a co-operative clinical trial evaluating surgical adjuvant chemotherapy. Surg Gynecol Obstet 140:528–534, 1975
55. Donegan WL, Skibba JL: Patterns of survival and disease recurrence after mastectomy for carcinoma of the breast. Cancer Treat Symp 2:107–116, 1983
56. Fisher B, Bauer M, Wickerham DL, Redmond CK, Fisher ER: Relation of number of positive axillary nodes to the prognosis of patients with primary breast cancer. Cancer 52:1551–1557, 1983
57. Fisher ER, Sass R, Fisher B: Pathological Findings from the National Surgical Adjuvant Project for Breast Cancers (Protocol No. 4) X: Discriminants for tenth year treatment failure. Cancer 53:712–713, 1984
58. Bonadonna G, Rossi A, Valagusssa P: Adjuvant CMF chemotherapy in operable breast cancer: Ten years later. World J Surg 9:707–713, 1985
59. Butler JA, Bretsky S, Menendez-Botet C, Kinne DW: Estrogen receptor protein of breast cancer as a predictor of recurrence. Cancer 55:1178–1181, 1985

60. Williams MR, Todd JH, Ellis IO et al: Oestrogen receptors in primary and advanced breast cancer: An eight year review of 704 cases. Br J Cancer 55:67–73, 1987
61. McDivitt RW, Stewart FW, Berg JW: Tumors of the Breast. Washington, DC, Armed Forces Institute of Pathology, 1968
62. World Health Organization: Histologic typing of breast tumors. Tumori 68:181, 1982
63. Wellings SR, Jensen HM: On the origin and progression of ductal carcinoma in the human breast. J Natl Cancer Inst 50:1111–1118, 1973
64. Connolly J, Schnitt SJ: Evaluation of breast biopsy specimens in patients considered for treatment by conservative surgery and radiotherapy for early breast cancer. Pathol Annu 23:1–23, 1988
65. Bloom HJG, Field JR: Impact of tumor grade and host resistance on survival of women with breast cancer. Cancer 28:1580–1589, 1971
66. Parl FF, Dupont WD: A retrospective cohort study of histologic risk factors in breast cancer patients. Cancer 50:2410–2416, 1982
67. Rosen PP, Saigo PE, Braun DW Jr, Weathers E, DePalo A: Predictors of recurrence in Stage I (T1 N0 M0) breast carcinoma. Ann Surg 193:15–25, 1981
68. Tubiana M, Pejovic MH, Chavaudra N: Long term prognostic significance of the thymidine labeling index in breast cancer. Int J Cancer 33:441–445, 1984
69. Meyer JS, Freedman E, McCrate MM: Prediction of early course of breast carcinoma by thymidine labeling. Cancer 51:1879–1886, 1983
70. Silvestrini R, Daidone MG, Gasparini G: Cell kinetics as a prognostic marker in node-negative breast cancer. Cancer 56:1982–1987, 1985
71. Hedley DW, Rugg CA, Ng ABP: Influence of cellular DNA content on disease free survival of Stage II breast cancer patients. Cancer Res 44:5395–5398, 1984
72. Coulson PB, Thornthwaite JT, Woolley TW: Prognostic indicators including DNA histogram type, receptor content, and staging related to human breast cancer patient survival. Cancer Res 44:4187–4196, 1984
73. McDivitt RW, Stone KR, Craig B, Palmer JO, Meyer JS, Bauer WC: A proposed classification of breast cancer based on kinetic information. Cancer 57:269–276, 1986
74. Slamon DJ, Clark GM, Wong SG et al: Human breast cancer: Correlation of relapse and survival with amplification of *HER-2/neu* oncogene. Science 235:177–182, 1987
75. Spratt JS, Donegan WL: Cancer of the breast. Philadelphia, WB Saunders, 1967
76. Fisher B, Slack NH, Ausman RK: Location of breast carcinoma and prognosis. Surg Gynecol Obstet 129:705–716, 1969
77. Haagensen CD: Diseases of the Breast. Philadelphia, WB Saunders, 1971
78. Holland R, Velig SHJ, Mravunac M, Hendriks JHCL: Histologic multifocality of Tis, T1-2 breast carcinomas. Cancer 56:979–990, 1985
79. Pickren JW: Significance of occult metastases. Cancer 14:1266–1271, 1961
80. Nemoto T, Vana J, Bedwani RN et al: Management and survival of female breast cancer. Cancer 45:2917–2924, 1980
81. Smith JA, Gamez-Araujo JJ, Gallager HS, White EC, McBride CM: Carcinoma of the breast. Cancer 39:527–532, 1977
82. Veronesi U, Rilke F, Luini A: Distribution of axillary node metastases by level. Cancer 59:682–687, 1987
83. Rosen PP, Lesser ML, Kinne DW, Beattie EJ: Discontinuous or "skip" metastasis in breast carcinoma. Ann Surg 187:276–283, 1983
84. Fisher B, Slack NH, Bross IDJ: Cancer of the breast: Size of neoplasm and prognosis. Cancer 24:1071–1080, 1969
85. Adair F, Berg J, Joubert L, Robbins GF: Long-term followup of breast cancer patients: The 30-year report. Cancer 33:1145–1150, 1974
86. Handley RS: Carcinoma of the breast. Ann R Coll Surg 57:59–66, 1975
87. Bucalossi P, Veronesi U, Zingo L, Conti C: Enlarged mastectomy for breast cancer: Review of 1,213 cases. Am J Roentgenol Rad Ther Nucl Med 111:119–122, 1971
88. Veronesi U, Cascinelli N, Greco M et al: Prognosis of breast cancer patients after mastectomy and dissection of internal mammary nodes. Ann Surg 202:702–707, 1985
89. Dahl-Iversen E: Recherches sur les Métastases microscopiques des cancers du sein dans les ganglions lymphatiques parasternaux et susclaviculaires. Mem Acad Chin 78:651–652, 1952
90. Halsted WS: The results of radical operations for the cure of cancer of the breast. Ann Surg 46:1–19, 1907
91. Haagensen CD: Treatment of curable carcinoma of the breast. Int J Radiat Oncol Biol Phys 2:975–980, 1977
92. Fisher ER, Swamidoss S, Lee CH: Detection and significance of occult axillary lymph node metastases in patients with invasive breast cancer. Cancer 42:2025–2031, 1978
93. Huvos AG, Hutter RVP, Berg JW: Significance of axillary macrometastases and micrometastases in mammary cancer. Ann Surg 173:44–46, 1971
94. Shapiro S, Strax P, Venet L: Changes in 5 year breast cancer mortality in a breast cancer screening program. Proceedings of the Seventh National Cancer Conference, pp 663–678. Philadelphia, JB Lippincott, 1973
95. Shapiro S, Venet W, Strax P, Venet L, Roeser R: Ten- to fourteen-year effect of screening on breast cancer mortality. J Natl Cancer Inst 69:349–355, 1982
96. Habbema JPF, Van Oortmarssen GJ, VanPutten DJ, Lubbe JT, van der Maas PJ: Age specific reduction in breast cancer mortality for screening: An analysis of the results of the Health Insurance Plan of Greater New York Study. J Natl Cancer Inst 77:317–320, 1986
97. Tabar L, Fagerberg CJG, Gad A et al: Reduction in mortality from breast cancer after mass screening with mammography. Lancet 1:829–832, 1985
98. Verbeek ALM, Hendriks JH, Holland R, Mravunac M, Sturmans F, Day NE: Reduction of breast cancer mortality through mass screening with modern mammography. Lancet 1:1222–1224, 1984
99. Baker LH: Breast Cancer Detection Demonstration Project: Five-year summary report. CA 32:194–225, 1982
100. Seidman H, Gelb SK, Silverberg E, LaVerda N, Lubera JA: Survival experience in the Breast Cancer Detection Demonstration Project. Ca 37:258–290, 1987
101. Bailar JC III: Mammography: A contrary view. Ann Intern Med 84:77–84, 1976
102. Gohagan JK, Darby WP, Spitznagel EL, Monsees BS, Tome AE: Radiogenic breast cancer effects of mammographic screening. J Natl Cancer Inst 77:71–76, 1986
103. Case C: The Breast Cancer Digest, 2nd ed. Washington, DC, US Government Printing Office, 1984
104. Moskowitz M: Breast cancer: Age-specific growth rates and screening strategies. Radiology 161:37–41, 1986
105. Gisvold JJ, Martin JK: Prebiopsy localization of nonpalpable breast lesions. AJR 143:477–481, 1984
106. Meyer VE, Kopans DB, Stomper PC, Lindfors KK: Occult breast abnormalities: Percutaneous preoperative needle localization. Radiology 150:335–337, 1984
107. Poller SR, Mettle E, Bartow SA, Moradian G, Moscowitz M: Occult breast cancer: Prevalence and radiographic detectability. Radiology 163:459–462, 1987
108. Baker ER: The indications for bone scan in the pre-operative assessment of patients with operable breast cancer. Breast Dis 3:43–45, 1977
109. McNeil B, Pace PPD, Gray E: Pre-operative and follow-up bone scans in patients with primary carcinoma of the breast. Surg Gynecol Obstet 147:745–748, 1978
110. Wiener SN, Sachs SH: An assessment of positive liver scanning in patients with breast cancer. Arch Surg 113:126–127, 1970
111. Casta GNA, Benfield J Jr, Yamama H: The reliability of liver scans and function tests in detecting metastases. Surg Gynecol Obstet 124:463–469, 1972
112. Dash N, Lupetin AR, Daffner RH: Magnetic resonance imaging in the diagnosis of breast disease. AJR 146:119–125, 1986
113. Steward AM, Nixon D, Zamcheck N: Carcinoembryonic antigen in breast cancer patients. Cancer 33:1246–1252, 1979
114. Tormey DC, Wastros TT, Ahmann D: Biological markers in breast cancer I: Incidence of abnormalities of CEA, hCG, polyamines and three minor nucleosides. Cancer 35:1095–1100, 1975
115. Tormey DC, Waalkes TP, Semon RM: Biological markers in breast cancer II: Clinical correlation with chorionic gonadotropin. Cancer 39:2391–2396, 1976
116. Marcus DM, Zinbergt N: Measurement of serum ferritin by radioimmunoassay: Results in normal individuals and patients with breast cancer. J Natl Cancer Inst 55:791–795, 1975
117. Waalkes TP, Tormey DC: Biological markers and breast cancer. Semin Oncol 5:434–444, 1978
118. Halsted WS: The results of operations for the cure of cancer of the breast performed at Johns Hopkins Hospital from June, 1889 to January, 1894. Johns Hopkins Hosp Bull 4:497–555, 1894
119. Haagensen CD: Diseases of the Breast, 3rd Ed. Philadelphia, WB Saunders, 1986
120. Urban JA, Baker HW: Radical mastectomy in continuity with en bloc resection of the internal mammary lymph node chain. Cancer 5:992, 1952
121. Auchincloss H: Significance of location and number of axillary metastases in carcinoma of the breast: A justification for a conservative operation. Ann Surg 158:37, 1963
122. Lagios MD, Westdahl PR, Rose MR: The concept and implications of multicentricity in breast carcinoma. Pathol Annu 16:83–102, 1981
123. Rosen PP, Fracchia AA, Urban JA: "Residual" mammary carcinoma following simulated partial mastectomy. Cancer 35:739–747, 1975
124. Schwartz GF, Patchesfsky AS, Feig SA, Shaber GS, Schwartz AB: Multicentricity of non-palpable breast cancer. Cancer 45:2913–2916, 1980
125. Rosen PP, Braun DW, Kinne DW: The clinical significance of pre-invasive breast carcinoma. Cancer 46:919–925, 1980
126. Lagios MD, Richards VE, Rose MR, Yee E: Segmental mastectomy without radiotherapy: short-term follow-up. Cancer 52:2173–2179, 1983
127. Holland R, Solke HJV, Mravunac M: Histologic multifocality of Tis, T1-2 breast carcinomas. Cancer 56:979–990, 1985
128. Kramer WM, Ruch BF Jr: Mammary duct proliferation in the elderly. Cancer 31:130–137, 1973
129. Franks LM: Latent carcinoma of the prostate. J Pathol Bacteriol 68:603–616, 1954
130. Schottenfeld D, Nash A, Robbins G, Beattie E: Ten-year results of the treatment of primary operable breast carcinoma. Cancer 38:1001–1007, 1976
131. Haagensen CD, Bodian C: A personal experience with Halsted's radical mastectomy. Ann Surg 199:143–150, 1984
132. Fisher B, Redmond C, Fisher ER, Bauer M, Wolmark N et al: Ten-year results of a randomized clinical trial comparing radical mastectomy and total mastectomy with or without radiation. N Engl J Med 312:674–681, 1985
133. Robbins GF, Berg J: Curability of patients with invasive breast carcinoma based on a 30-year study. World J Surg 1:284–286, 1977
134. Davies GC, Millis RR, Hayward JL: Assessment of axillary lymph node status. Ann Surg 192:148–151, 1980
135. Danforth DN Jr, Findlay PA, McDonald HD et al: Complete axillary lymph node dissection for Stage I–II carcinoma of the breast. J Clin Oncol 4:655–662, 1986
136. Schwartz GF, Domenico M, D'Ugo MD: Extent of axillary dissection preceding irradiation for carcinoma of the breast. Arch Surg 121:1395–1398, 1986
137. Cady B: Usefulness and technique of axillary dissection in primary breast cancer. J Clin Oncol 4:623–624, 1986
138. Dewar JA, Sarrazin D, Benhamou E: Management of the axilla in conservatively

treated breast cancer: 592 patients treated at Institut Gustave-Roussy. Int J Radiat Oncol Biol Phys 13:475–481, 1987
139. Harris JR, Osteen RT: Patients with early breast cancer benefit from effective axillary treatment. Breast Cancer Res Treat 5:17–21, 1985
140. Wilson RE, Donegan WL, Mettlin C, Smart CR, Murphy GP: The 1982 National Survey of Carcinoma of the Breast in the United States by the American College of Surgeons. Surg Gynecol Obstet 159:309–318, 1984
141. Baker RR, Montague ACW, Childs NJ: A comparison of modified radical mastectomy to radical mastectomy in the treatment of operable breast cancer. Ann Surg 189:553–559, 1979
142. Maddox WA, Carpenter JT, Laws HL: A randomized prospective trial of radical (Halsted) mastectomy versus modified radical mastectomy in 311 breast cancer patients. Ann Surg 198:207–212, 1983
143. Martin JK Jr, van Heerden JA, Taylor W: Is modified radical mastectomy really equivalent to radical mastectomy in treatment of carcinoma of the breast? Cancer 57:510–518, 1986
144. Mentzer SJ, Osteen RT, Wilson RE: Local recurrence and the deep resection margin in carcinoma of the breast. Surg Gynecol Obstet 163:513–517, 1986
145. Kinne DW, DeCosse JJ: Modified radical mastectomy for carcinoma of the breast. Am Surg 48:543–556, 1982
146. Urban JA: Management of operable breast cancer: The surgeon's view. Cancer 42:2066–2077, 1978
147. Veronesi U, Valagussa P: Inefficacy of internal mammary nodes dissection in breast cancer surgery. Cancer 47:170–175, 1981
148. Lacour J, Le MG, Hill C: Is it useful to remove internal mammary nodes in operable breast cancer? Eur J Surg Oncol 13:309–314, 1987
149. Goldman LD, Goldwyn RM: Some anatomical considerations of subcutaneous mastectomy. Plast Reconstr Surg 51:501–505, 1973
150. Goodnought JE, Quagliana JM, Morton DL: Failure of subcutaneous mastectomy to prevent the development of breast cancer. J Surg Oncol 26:198–201, 1984
151. Hermann RE, Esselstyn CB Jr, Crile G Jr: Results of conservative operations for breast cancer. Arch Surg 120:746–751, 1985
152. Harris JR, Hellman S, Kinne DW: Limited surgery and radiotherapy for early breast cancer. N Engl J Med 313:1365–1368, 1985
153. Hohler H: Reconstruction of the female breast after radical mastectomy. In Converse JM (ed): Reconstructive Plastic Surgery, pp 3710–3726. Philadelphia, WB Saunders, 1977
154. Georgiade NG: Reconstructive Breast Surgery. St Louis, CV Mosby, 1976
155. Cocke WM Jr: Breast Reconstruction Following Mastectomy for Carcinoma. Boston, Little, Brown, 1977
156. Hartwell SW Jr, Anderson R, Hall MD: Reconstruction of the breast after mastectomy for cancer. Plast Reconstr Surg 57:152–157, 1976
157. Bostwick J III, Vasconez LO, Jurkiewicz MJ: Breast reconstruction after a radical mastectomy. Plast Reconstr Surg 61:682–693, 1978
158. Lewis JR Jr: Reconstruction of the breasts. Surg Clin North Am 51:429–440, 1971
159. Edgerton MT: Breast reconstruction after radical mastectomy for cancer. South Med J 60:719–723, 1967
160. Watts GT: Restorative prosthetic mammaplasty in mastectomy for carcinoma and benign lesions. Clin Plast Surg 3:177–191, 1976
161. Williams JE: Experience with a late series of Silastic breast implants. Plast Reconstr Surg 49:253–258, 1972
162. Synderman RK, Guthrie RH: Reconstruction of the female breast following radical mastectomy. Plast Reconstr Surg 47:565–567, 1971
163. Bradley SA: Acceptable Plastic Implants. In Simpson DC (ed): Modern Trends in Biomechanics, pp 25–51. London, Butterworths, 1970
164. Rees TD, Guy CL, Coburn RJ: The use of inflatable breast implants. Plast Reconstr Surg 52:609–615, 1973
165. Birnbaum L, Olsen JA: Breast reconstruction following radical mastectomy, using custom designed implants. Plast Reconstr Surg 61:355–363, 1978
166. Radovan C: Tissue expansion in soft-tissue reconstruction. Plast Reconstr Surg 74:482–490, 1984
167. Argenta LC: Reconstruction of the breast by tissue expansion. Clin Plast Surg 11:257–264, 1984
168. Phillips CM: Reconstructive surgery after classical radical mastectomies using omental pedicled grafts and fascia lata. Breast 4:10–18, 1978
169. Arnold PG, Hartrampf CR, Jurkiewicz MJ: One-stage reconstruction of the breast, using the transposed greater omentum (case report). Plast Reconstr Surg 57:520–522, 1976
170. Shaw WW: Breast reconstruction by superior gluteal microvascular free flaps without silicone implants. Plast Reconstr Surg 72:490–499, 1983
171. Bostwick J III: Breast reconstruction after mastectomy. In Harris JR, Hellman S, Henderson IC, Kinne DW (eds): Breast Diseases, pp 668–682. Philadelphia, JB Lippincott, 1987
172. Hohler H: Reconstruction after mastectomy. In Symposium on Neoplastic and Re constructive Problems of the Female Breast. St Louis, CV Mosby, 1973
173. Allison AB, Howorth MB Jr: Carcinoma in a nipple preserved by heterotopic auto-implantation. N Engl J Med 298:1132, 1978
174. Parry RG, Cochran TC Jr, Wolfort FG: When is there nipple involvement in carcinoma of the breast? Plast Reconstr Surg 59:535–537, 1977
175. Smith J, Payne WS, Carney JA: Involvement of the nipple and areola in carcinoma of the breast. Surg Gynecol Obstet 143:546–548, 1976
176. Adams WM: Labial transplant for correction of lesions of the nipple. Plast Reconstr Surg 4:295–299, 1949
177. Tapley N, Spanos WJ, Fletcher GH: Results in patients with breast cancer treated by radical mastectomy and post-operative irradiation with no adjuvant chemotherapy. Cancer 49:1316–1319, 1982
178. Stjernsward J: Decreased survival correlated to local irradiation in "early" operable breast cancer. Lancet 2:1285–1286, 1974
179. Cuzick J, Stewart H, Peto R et al: Overview of randomized trials comparing radical mastectomy without radiotherapy against simple mastectomy with radiotherapy in breast cancer. Cancer Treat Rep 71:7–14, 1987
180. Host H, Brennhovd IO: The effect of postoperative radiation therapy in breast cancer. Int J Radiat Oncol Biol Phys 2:1061–1067, 1977
181. Chu FCH, Lin FJ, Kim JH: Locally recurrent carcinoma of the breast: Results of radiation therapy. Cancer 37:2677–2681, 1976
182. Zimmerman KW, Montague ED, Fletcher GH: Frequency, anatomic distribution, and management of local recurrences after definite therapy for breast cancer. Cancer 19:67–74, 1966
183. Goldie JH, Coldman AJ: A mathematical model for relating the drug sensitivity of tumors to their spontaneous mutation rate. Cancer Treat Rep 63:1727–1731, 1979
184. Marcial VA, Velez-Garcia E, Moore M: Radiotherapy related adjuvant chemotherapy initiation delay in breast cancer with positive nodes: Does it affect prognosis?—A Southeastern Cancer Study Group Report. Proc ASTRO p 150, 1985
185. Cooper MR, Rhyne AL, Muss HB: A randomized comparative trial of chemotherapy and irradiation therapy for Stage II breast cancer. Cancer 47:2833–2839, 1981
186. Cooper MR, Muss H, Ferree C: A six and one half year follow-up of a randomized adjuvant study of chemotherapy with and without radiation therapy for Stage II breast cancer. Breast Cancer Res Treat 6:169, 1985
187. Ahmann D, O'Fallon J, Scanlon P et al: A preliminary assessment of factors associated with recurrent disease in a surgical adjuvant clinical trial for patients with breast cancer with special emphasis on the aggressiveness of therapy. Am J Clin Oncol 5:371–381, 1982
188. Griem KL, Henderson IC, Gelman R et al: The 5-year results of a randomized trial of adjuvant radiation therapy after chemotherapy in breast cancer treated with mastectomy. J Clin Oncol 5:1546–1555, 1987
189. Crile G: Multicentric breast cancer: The incidence of new cancers in the homolateral breast after partial mastectomy. Cancer 35:475–477, 1975
190. Peters MV: Wedge resection with or without radiation in early breast cancer. J Radiat Oncol Biol Phys 2:1151–1156, 1977
191. Lagios MD, Westdahl PR, Margolin FR, Rose MR: Duct carcinoma-in-situ. Cancer 50:1309–1314, 1982
192. Montgomery ACV, Greening WP, Levene AL: Clinical study of recurrence rate and survival time of patients with carcinoma of the breast treated by biopsy excision without any other therapy. J R Soc Med 71:339–342, 1978
193. Fisher B, Bauer M, Margolese R et al: Five-year results of a randomized clinical trial comparing total mastectomy and segmental mastectomy with or without radiation in the treatment of breast cancer. N Engl J Med 312:666–673, 1985
194. Calle R, Vilcoq JR, Zafrani B, Vielh P, Fourquet A: Local control and survival of breast cancer treated by limited surgery followed by irradiation. Cancer 12:873–878, 1986
195. Kurtz JM, Spitalier JM, Amalric R: Late breast recurrence after lumpectomy and irradiation. Int J Radiat Oncol Biol Phys 9:1191–1194, 1983
196. Clarke DH, Le MG, Sarrazin D et al: Analysis of local-regional relapses in patients with early breast cancers treated by excision and radiotherapy: Experience of the Institut Gustave-Roussy. Int J Radiat Oncol Biol Phys 11:137–145, 1985
197. Clark RM: Alternatives to mastectomy—The Princess Margaret Hospital experience. In Harris JR, Hellman S, Silen W (eds): Conservative Management of Breast Cancer, pp 35–46, Philadelphia, JB Lippincott, 1983
198. Spitalier JM, Gambarelli J, Brandone H: Breast-conserving surgery with radiation therapy for operable mammary carcinoma: A 25-year experience. World J Surg 10:1014–1020, 1986
199. Recht A, Silver B, Schnitt S, Connolly J, Hellman S, Harris JR: Breast relapse following primary radiation therapy for early breast cancer I: Classification, frequency, and salvage. Int J Radiat Oncol Biol Phys 11:1271–1276, 1985
200. Svensson GK, Bjarngard BE, Larson RD, Levene MB: A modified three-field technique for breast treatment. Int J Radiat Oncol Biol Phys 6:689–694, 1980
201. Siddon RL, Buck BA, Harris JR, Svensson GK: Three field corner technique for breast irradiation using tangential field corner blocks. Int J Radiat Oncol Biol Phys 9:583–588, 1983
202. Harris JR, Recht A, Amalric A et al: Time course and prognosis of local recurrence following primary radiation therapy for early breast cancer. J Clin Oncol 2:37–41, 1984
203. Fisher B, Wolmark N: Conservative surgery: The American experience. Semin Oncol 13:425–433, 1986
204. Fisher ER, Sass R, Fisher B, Gregorio R, Brown R, Wickerham L: Pathologic findings from the National Surgical Adjuvant Breast Project (Protocol 6). II: Relation of local breast recurrence to multicentricity. Cancer 57:1717–1724, 1986
205. Schnitt S, Connolly J, Recht A, Silver B, Harris JR: Breast relapse following primary radiation therapy for early breast cancer II: Detection, pathologic features, and prognostic significance. Int J Radiat Oncol Biol Phys 11:1277–1284, 1985
206. Beadle GF, Silver B, Botnick L, Hellman S, Harris JR: Cosmetic results following primary radiation therapy for early breast cancer. Cancer 54:2911–2918, 1984
207. Veronesi U, Saccozzi R, DelVecchio M et al: Comparing radical mastectomy with

quadrantectomy, axillary dissection and radiotherapy in patients with small cancers of the breast. N Engl J Med 305:6–11, 1981
208. Veronesi U: Randomized trials comparing conservation techniques with conventional surgery: An overview. In Tobias JS, Peckham MJ (eds): Primary Management of Breast Cancer: Alternatives to Mastectomy, pp 131–152. London, Edward Arnold Publishers, 1985
209. Veronesi U, Zucali R, Luini A: Local control and survival in early breast cancer: The Milan trial. Int J Radiat Oncol Biol Phys 12:717–720, 1986
210. Sarrazin D, Le M, Contesso G et al: Conservative treatment versus mastectomy in breast cancer: 10 year results of a randomized trial. Proc ESTRO p 249, 1987
211. Findlay P, Lippman M, Danforth D: A randomized trial comparing mastectomy to radiotherapy in the treatment of stage I–II breast cancer: A preliminary report. Proc Am Soc Clin Oncol 5:63, 1986
212. Habibollahi F, Fentiman IB, Chaudary MA: Conservation treatment of operable breast cancer. Proc Am Soc Clin Oncol 6:59, 1987
213. Recht A, Connolly JL, Schnitt SJ et al: Conservative surgery and radiation therapy for early breast cancer: Results, controversies, and unsolved problems. Semin Oncol 13:434–449, 1986
214. Larson D, Weinstein M, Goldberg I et al: Edema of the arm as a function of the extent of axillary surgery in patients with stage I–II carcinoma of the breast treated with primary radiotherapy. Int J Radiat Oncol Biol Phys 12:1575–1582, 1986
215. Salner AL, Botnick LE, Herzog AG et al: Reversible brachial plexopathy following primary radiation therapy for breast cancer. Cancer Treat Rep 65:797–802, 1981
216. Kissin MW, della Rovere GQ, Easton D, Westbury G: Risk of lymphoedema following treatment of breast cancer. Br J Surg 73:580–584, 1986
217. Mazeron JJ, Otmezguine Y, Huaro J, Pierquin B: Conservative treatment of breast cancer: Results of management of axillary lymph node area in 3353 patients. Lancet 1:1387, 1985
218. Recht A, Hayes DF: Specific sites and emergencies: Local recurrence. In: Harris JR, Hellman S, Henderson IC, Kinne DW (eds): Breast Diseases, pp 508–524. Philadelphia, JB Lippincott, 1987
219. Skipper HE: Kinetics of mammary tumor cell growth and implications for therapy. Cancer 28:1479–1499, 1971
220. Cole MP: A clinical trial of an artificial menopause in carcinoma of the breast. Inserm 55:143–150, 1975
221. Frei EF I: Selected considerations regarding chemotherapy as adjuvant in cancer treatment. Cancer Chemother Rep 50:1–8, 1966
222. Fisher B, Fisher ER, Redmond C: Ten year results from the NSABP clinical trial evaluating the use of L-phenylalanine mustard (L-PAM) in the management of primary breast cancer. J Clin Oncol 4:929–941, 1986
223. Bonadonna G, Valagussa P, Rossi A et al: Ten-year experience with CMF-based adjuvant chemotherapy in resectable breast cancer. Breast Cancer Res Treat 5:95–115, 1985
224. Henderson IC: Adjuvant systemic therapy for early breast cancer. Curr Probl Cancer 11:125–207, 1987
225. Brincker H, Rose C, Rank F et al: Evidence of a castration-mediated effect of adjuvant cytotoxic chemotherapy in premenopausal breast cancer. J Clin Oncol 5:1771–1778, 1987
226. Bonadonna G, Valagussa P, Tancini G et al: Current status of Milan adjuvant chemotherapy trials for node-positive and node-negative breast cancer. NCI Monogr 1:45–49, 1986
227. Nolvadex Adjuvant Trial Organisation: Controlled trial of tamoxifen as single adjuvant agent in management of early breast cancer: Analysis at six years. Lancet 1:836–839, 1985
228. Baum M, Wilson AJ, Ebbs SR: The role of adjuvant endocrine therapy in primary breast cancer. In Salmon SE (ed): Adjuvant Therapy of Cancer V, pp 377–390. Orlando, Grune & Stratton, 1987
229. Padmanabhan N, Howell A, Rubens RD: Mechanism of action of adjuvant chemotherapy in early breast cancer. Lancet 2:411–414, 1986
230. Meakin JW, Allt WEC, Beale FA et al: Ovarian irradiation and prednisone following surgery and radiotherapy for carcinoma of the breast. Breast Cancer Res Treat 3:s45–s48, 1983
231. Bryant AJ, Weir JA: Prophylactic oophorectomy in operable instances of carcinoma of the breast. Surg Gynecol Obstet 153:660–664, 1981
232. Tengrup I, Nittby LT, Landberg T: Prophylactic oophorectomy in the treatment of carcinoma of the breast. Surg Gynecol Obstet 162:209–214, 1986
233. Gelber RD, Goldhirsch A: The concept of an overview of cancer clinical trials with special emphasis on early breast cancer. J Clin Oncol 4:1696–1703, 1986
234. Himel HN, Liberati A, Gelber RD, Chalmers TC: Adjuvant chemotherapy for breast cancer: A pooled estimate based on published randomized control trials. JAMA 256:1148–1159, 1986
235. Early Breast Cancer Trialists Collaborative Group: The effects of adjuvant tamoxifen and of cytotoxic therapy on mortality in early breast cancer: An overview of 70 randomized trials among 30,000 women. N Engl J Med (in press)
236. Morrison JM, Howell A, Grieve RJ et al: The West Midlands Oncology Association Trials of adjuvant chemotherapy for operable breast cancer. In Jones SE, Salmon SE (eds): Adjuvant Therapy of Cancer IV, pp 253–259. Orlando, Grune & Stratton, 1984
237. Senn HJ, Barett–Mahler R: Update of Swiss adjuvant trials with LMF and CMF in operable breast cancer. In Salmon SE (ed): Adjuvant Therapy of Cancer V, pp 243–252. Orlando, Grune & Stratton, 1987
238. Jakesz R, Kolb R, Reiner G et al: Adjuvant chemotherapy in node-negative breast cancer patients. In Salmon SE (ed): Adjuvant Therapy of Cancer V, pp 223–231. Orlando, Grune & Stratton, 1987
239. Bonadonna G, Valagussa P, Zambetti M, Bozzoni R, Moliterni A: Milan adjuvant trials for stage I–II breast cancer. In Salmon SE (ed): Adjuvant Therapy of Cancer VI, pp 211–221. Orlando, Grune & Stratton, 1987
240. Fisher B, Redmond C, Fisher ER, Wolmark N: Systemic adjuvant therapy in treatment of primary operable breast cancer: National Surgical Adjuvant Breast and Bowel Project experience. NCI Monogr 1:35–43, 1986
241. Carbone PP: Multiple trials of adjuvant chemohormonal therapy in the treatment of breast cancer: Preliminary results—The ECOG experience. Breast Cancer Res Treat 3:35–38, 1983
242. Goldhirsch A, Gelber R: Adjuvant treatment for early breast cancer: The Ludwig Breast Cancer studies. NCI Monogr 1:55–70, 1986
243. Scottish Cancer Trials Office: Adjuvant tamoxifen in the management of operable breast cancer: The Scottish trial. Lancet 2:171–175, 1987
244. Pritchard KI, Meakin JW, Boyd NF et al: A randomized trial of adjuvant tamoxifen in postmenopausal women with axillary node positive breast cancer. In Jones SE, Salmon SE (eds): Adjuvant Therapy of Cancer IV, pp 339–347. Orlando, Grune & Stratton, 1984
245. Nissen–Meyer R, Host H, Kjellgren K, Mansson B, Norin T: Neoadjuvant chemotherapy in breast cancer: As single perioperative treatment and with supplementary long-term chemotherapy. In: Salmon SE (ed): Adjuvant Chemotherapy for Cancer V, pp 253–261. Orlando, Grune & Stratton, 1987
246. Henderson IC, Gelman RS, Harris JR, Canellos GP: Duration of therapy in adjuvant chemotherapy trials. NCI Monogr 1:95–98, 1986
247. Tancini G, Bonadonna G, Valagussa P, Marchini S, Veronesi U: Adjuvant CMF in breast cancer: Comparative 5-year results of 12 versus 6 cycles. J Clin Oncol 1:2–10, 1983
248. Osborne CK, Rivkin SE, McDivitt RW et al: Adjuvant therapy of breast cancer: Southwest Oncology Group studies. NCI Monogr 1:71–74, 1986
249. Mathe G, Plagne R, Morice V, Misset JL: Consistencies and variations of observations during serial analyses of a trial of adjuvant chemotherapy in breast cancer. In Salmon SE (ed): Adjuvant Chemotherapy for Cancer V, pp 271–280. Orlando, Grune & Stratton, 1987
250. Fisher B, Redmond CK, Wolmark N: Long term results from NSABP trials of adjuvant therapy for breast cancer. In Salmon SE (ed): Adjuvant Therapy of Cancer V, pp 283–295. Orlando, Grune & Stratton, 1987
251. Perloff M, Norton L, Korzun A et al: Advantage of an Adriamycin (A) combination plus Halotestin (H) after initial cyclophosphamide, methotrexate, 5-fluorouracil, vincristine and prednisone (CMFVP) for adjuvant therapy of node-positive Stage II breast cancer (abstract). Proc Am Soc Clin Oncol 5:70, 1986
252. Bonadonna G, Valagussa P: Dose–response effect of adjuvant chemotherapy in breast cancer. N Engl J Med 304:10–15, 1981
253. Hryniuk W, Levine MN: Analysis of dose intensity for adjuvant chemotherapy trials in Stage II breast cancer. J Clin Oncol 4:1162–1170, 1986
254. Henderson IC, Gelman RS: A reanalysis of dose intensity for adjuvant chemotherapy trials in Stage II breast cancer. SAKK Bull 1:10–12, 1987
255. Tormey DC, Gray R, Taylor IV SG, Knuiman M, Olson JE, Cummings FJ: Postoperative chemotherapy and chemohormonal therapy in women with node-positive breast cancer. NCI Monogr 1:75–80, 1986
256. Goldhirsch A, Gelber RD: Adjuvant therapy for breast cancer: The Ludwig Breast Cancer Trials 1987. In Salmon SE (ed): Adjuvant Therapy of Cancer V, pp 297–309. Orlando, Grune & Stratton, 1987
257. Hubay CA, Pearson OH, Gordon NH et al: Randomized trial of endocrine versus endocrine plus cytotoxic chemotherapy in women with Stage II, estrogen receptor positive breast cancer (abstract). Proc Am Soc Clin Oncol 5:63, 1986
258. Kaufmann M, Jonat W, Caffier H et al: Adjuvant systemic risk adapted cytotoxic plus/minus tamoxifen therapy in women with node positive breast cancer. In Salmon SE (ed): Adjuvant Therapy of Cancer V, pp 337–346. Orlando, Grune & Stratton, 1987
259. Nissen–Meyer R, Kjellgren K, Mansson B: Adjuvant chemotherapy in breast cancer. Recent Results Cancer Res 80:142–148, 1982
260. Ragaz J: Emerging modalities for adjuvant therapy of breast cancer: Neoadjuvant chemotherapy. NCI Monogr 1:145–152, 1986
261. Beadle G, Come S, Henderson IC et al: The effect of timing of primary breast irradiation and chemotherapy on the cosmetic results. Int J Radiat Oncol Biol Phys 10(suppl 2):77, 1984
262. Gore SM, Come SE, Griem K et al: Influence of the sequencing of chemotherapy and radiation therapy in node-negative breast cancer patients treated by conservative surgery and radiation therapy. In Salmon SE (ed): Adjuvant Therapy of Cancer V, pp 365–373. Orlando, Grune & Stratton, 1987
263. Fisher B, Rockette H, Fisher ER, Wickerham DL, Redmond C, Brown A: Leukemia in breast cancer patients following adjuvant chemotherapy or postoperative radiation: The NSABP experience. J Clin Oncol 3:1640–1658, 1985
264. Valagussa P, Tancini G, Bonadonna G: Second malignancies after CMF for resectable breast cancer. J Clin Oncol 5:1138–1142, 1987
265. Henderson IC, Gelman R: Second malignancies from adjuvant chemotherapy? Too soon to tell. J Clin Oncol 5:1135–1137, 1987
266. Killackey MA, Hakes TB, Pierce VK: Endometrial adenocarcinoma in breast cancer patients receiving antiestrogens. Cancer Treat Rep 69:237–238, 1985
267. Gelber RD, Goldhirsch A, Castiglione M, Price K, Isley M, Coates A: Time without Symptoms and Toxicity (TWiST): A quality-of-life-oriented endpoint to evaluate adjuvant therapy. In Salmon SE (ed): Adjuvant Therapy of Cancer V, pp 455–465. Orlando, Grune & Stratton, 1987
268. Horton J: Follow-up of breast cancer patients. Cancer 53:790–797, 1984

269. Wickerham L, Fisher B, Cronin W, Members of the NSABP Committee for Treatment Failure Criteria: The efficacy of bone scanning in the follow-up of patients with operable breast cancer. Breast Cancer Res Treat 1:24–84, 1983
270. Tomin R, Donegan WL: Screening for recurrent breast cancer—Its effectiveness and prognostic value. J Clin Oncol 5:62–67, 1987
271. Marrazzo A, Solina G, Puccia V: Evaluation of routine follow-up after surgery for breast carcinoma. J Surg Oncol 32:179–181, 1986
272. Broders AC: Carcinoma in situ contrasted with benign penetrating epithelium. JAMA 99:1670–1674, 1932
273. Ashikari R, Huvos AG, Snyder RE: Prospective study of noninfiltrating carcinoma of the breast. Cancer 39:435–439, 1977
274. Sunshine JA, Moseley HS, Fletcher WS, Krippaehne WW: Breast carcinoma in situ: A retrospective review of 112 cases with a minimum 10 year follow-up. Am J Surg 150:44–50, 1985
275. Farrow JH: The James Ewing Lecture: Current concepts in the detection and treatment of the earliest of the early breast cancers. Cancer 25:468–477, 1970
276. Page DL, Dupont WD, Rogers LW, Landenberger M: Intraductal carcinoma of the breast: Follow-up after biopsy only. Cancer 49:751–758, 1982
277. Betsill WL, Rosen PP, Lieberman PH, Robbins GF: Intraductal carcinoma: Long-term follow-up after treatment by biopsy alone. JAMA 239:1863–1867, 1978
278. Alpers CE, Wellings SR: The prevalence of carcinoma in situ in normal and cancer associated breasts. Hum Pathol 16:796–807, 1985
279. Robbins GF, Berg JW: Bilateral primary breast cancers: A prospective clinicopathological study. Cancer 17:1501–1527, 1964
280. Recht A, Danoff BS, Solin LJ: Intraductal carcinoma of the breast: Results of treatment with excisional biopsy and irradiation. J Clin Oncol 3:1339–1343, 1985
281. Zafrani B, Fourquet A, Vilcoq JR, Legal M, Calle R: Conservative management of intraductal breast carcinoma with tumorectomy and radiation therapy. Cancer 57:1299–1301, 1986
282. Montague ED: Conservation surgery and radiation therapy in the treatment of operable breast cancer. Cancer 53:700–704, 1984
283. Fisher ER, Saas R, Fisher B, Wickerham L, Paik SM: Pathologic findings from the National Surgical Adjuvant Breast Project (Protocol 6) I: Intraductal carcinoma (DCIS). Cancer 57:197–208, 1986
284. Lagios MD: Human breast precancer: Current status. Cancer Surv 2:383–402, 1983 (Updated by personal communication, 1987.)
285. Harris JR, Connolly JL, Schnitt SJ et al: The use of pathologic features in selecting the extent of surgical resection necessary for breast cancer patients treated by primary radiation therapy. Ann Surg 201:164–169, 1985
286. Silverstein MJ, Rosser RJ, Gierson ED: Axillary lymph node dissection for intraductal breast carcinoma: Is it indicated? Cancer 59:1819–1824, 1987
287. Fisher B: Breast cancer management: Alternatives to radical mastectomy. N Engl J Med 301:326–328, 1979
288. Hellman S, Harris JR: The appropriate breast cancer paradigm. Cancer Res 47:339–342, 1987
289. Foote FW Jr, Stewart FW: Lobular carcinoma in situ: A rare form of mammary cancer. Am J Pathol 17:491–496, 1941
290. Muir R: The evolution of carcinoma of the mamma. J Pathol Bacteriol 52:155, 1941
291. Benfield JR, Jacobson M, Warner NE: In situ lobular carcinoma of the breast. Arch Surg 91:130, 1965
292. Newman W: Lobular carcinoma of the female breast: Report of 73 cases. Ann Surg 164:305, 1966
293. McDivitt RW, Hutter RVP, Foote FW Jr: In situ lobular carcinoma: A prospective follow-up study indicating cumulative patient risks. JAMA 201:96–100, 1967
294. Stewart FW: Tumors of the Breast: Atlas of Tumor Pathology. Washington, DC, Armed Forces Institute of Pathology, 1950
295. Rosen P, Lieberman P, Braun D, Kosloff C, Adair F: Lobular carcinoma in situ of the breast. Am J Surg Pathol 2:225–251, 1978
296. Wheeler JE, Interline HT, Roseman JM: Lobular carcinoma-in situ of the breast: Long-term follow-up. Cancer 34:554–563, 1974
297. Haagensen C, Lane N, Lattes R, Bodian C: Lobular neoplasia (so-called lobular carcinoma in situ) of the breast. Cancer 42:737–769, 1978
298. Haagensen CD, Stout AP: Carcinoma of the breast: Criteria of operability. Ann Surg 118:859–870, 1932
299. Baclesse FL: Roentgen therapy as the sole method of treatment of cancer of the breast. Am J Roentgenol Rad Ther Nucl Med 62:311–319, 1949
300. Fletcher GH, Montague ED: Radical irradiation of advanced breast cancer. Am J Roentgenol Rad Ther Nucl Med 93:573–584, 1965
301. Sheldon T, Hayes DF, Cady B et al: Primary radiation therapy for locally advanced breast cancer. Cancer 60:1219–1225, 1987
302. Arriagada R, Mouriesse H, Sarrazin D, Clark RM, Doboer G: Radiotherapy alone in breast cancer I: Analysis of tumor parameters, tumor dose and local control: The experience of the Gustave-Roussy Institute and the Princess Margaret Hospital. Int J Radiat Oncol Biol Phys 11:1751–1757, 1985
303. De Lena M, Varini M, Zucali R et al: Multimodal treatment for locally advanced breast cancer: Results of chemotherapy-radiotherapy versus chemotherapy-surgery. Cancer Clin Trials 4:229–236, 1981
304. Rubens RD, Sexton S, Tong D, Winter PJ, Knight RK, Hayward JL: Combined chemotherapy and radiotherapy for locally advanced breast cancer. Eur J Cancer 16:351–356, 1980
305. Schaake-Koning C, van der Linden EH, Hart G, Engelsman E: Adjuvant chemo- and hormonal therapy in locally advanced breast cancer: A randomized clinical study. Int J Radiat Oncol Biol Phys 11:1759–1763, 1985
306. Valagussa P, Zambetti M, Bignami P et al: T3b–T4 breast cancer: Factors affecting results in combined modality treatments. Clin Exp Metastasis 1:191–202, 1983
307. Perloff M, Korzun A, Chu F, Lesnick G: Combination chemotherapy (CT) with surgery (S) or radiotherapy (RT) for Stage III breast carcinoma (abstract). Proc Am Soc Clin Oncol 4:60, 1985
308. Balawajder I, Antich PP, Boland J: An analysis of the role of radiotherapy alone and in combination with chemotherapy and surgery in the management of advanced breast carcinoma. Cancer 51:574–580, 1983
309. Paone JF, Baker RR: Pathogenesis and treatment of Paget's disease of the breast. Cancer 48:825–829, 1981
310. Nance FC, DeLoach DH, Welsh RA: Paget's disease of the breast. Ann Surg 171:864–874, 1970
311. Maier WP, Rosemond GP, Harasym EL: Paget's disease in the female breast. Surg Gynecol Obstet 128:1253–1263, 1969
312. Osteen RT: Paget's disease of the nipple. In Harris JR, Hellman S, Henderson IC, Linne DW (eds): Breast Diseases, pp 589–595. Philadelphia, JB Lippincott, 1987
313. Treves N, Holleb AI: Cancer of the male breast: A report of 146 cases. Cancer 8:1239–1250, 1955
314. Haagensen CD: Carcinoma of the male breast. In Diseases of the Breast, 2nd Ed, pp 779–792. Philadelphia, WB Saunders, 1971
315. Langlands AO, Maclean N, Ken GR: Carcinoma of the male breast: Report of a series of 88 cases. Clin Radiol 27:21–25, 1976
316. Donegan WL, Perez-Mesa C: Carcinoma of the male breast. Arch Surg 106:273–279, 1973
317. Roswit B, Edlis H: Carcinoma of the male breast: A thirty-year experience and literature review. Int J Radiat Oncol Biol Phys 4:711–715, 1978
318. Anderson DE: Genetic considerations in breast cancer. In Breast Cancer: Early and Late, pp 27–36. Chicago, Year Book Medical Publishers, 1970
319. Everson RB, Li FP, Fraumeni JF: Familial male breast cancer. Lancet 1:9–12, 1976
320. El-Gazayerli MM, Abel-Aziz AS: On biharziasis and male breast cancer in Egypt. Br J Cancer 17:566–571, 1963
321. Harnden DG, Maclean N, Langlands AO: Carcinoma of the male breast and Klinefelter's syndrome. J Med Genet 8:460–461, 1971
322. Evans DB, Crichlow RW: Carcinoma of the male breast and Klinefelter's syndrome: Is there an association? Cancer 37:246–251, 1987
323. Gupta N, Cohen JL, Rosenbaum C: Estrogen receptors in male breast cancer. Cancer 46:1781–1784, 1980
324. Yap HY, Tashima CK, Blumenschein GR: Male breast cancer: A natural history study. Cancer 44:748–754, 1979
325. Robinson R, Montague ED: Treatment results in males with breast cancer. Cancer 49:403–406, 1982
326. Heller KS, Rosen PP, Schottenfeld D: Male breast cancer: A clinicopathologic study of 97 cases. Ann Surg 188:60–65, 1978
327. Treves N: Treatment of cancer of the male breast by ablative surgery and hormonal therapy: An analysis of 42 patients. Cancer 12:820–832, 1959
328. Holleb A, Freeman HP, Farrow JH: Cancer of the male breast. NY State J Med 68:544–553, 1968
329. Li MC, Janelli DE, Kelly EJ: Metastatic carcinoma of the male breast treated with bilateral adrenalectomy and chemotherapy. Cancer 25:678–681, 1970
330. Kennedy BJ, Kiang DT: Hypophysectomy in the treatment of advanced cancer of the male breast. Cancer 29:1606–1612, 1972
331. Patterson JS, Battersby LA, Bach BK: Use of tamoxifen in advanced male breast cancer. Cancer Treat Rep 64:801–804, 1980
332. Lopez M, DiLauro L, Lazzaro B: Hormonal treatment of disseminated male breast cancer. Oncology 42:345–349, 1985
333. Bezwoda WR, Hesdorffer C, Dansey R: Breast cancer in men: Clinical features, hormone receptor status, and response to therapy. Cancer 60:1337–1340, 1987
334. Bagley CS, Wesley MN, Young RC, Lippman ME: Adjuvant chemotherapy in males with cancer of the breast. Am J Clin Oncol 10:55–60, 1987
335. Paterson AHG, Lees AW, Hanson J, Szafran O, Cornish F: Impact of chemotherapy on survival in metastatic breast cancer. Lancet 2:312, 1980
336. Fey MF, Brunner KW, Sonntag RW: Prognostic factors in metastatic breast cancer. Cancer Clin Trials 4:237–247, 1981
337. Cavilli F, Beer M, Martz G et al: Concurrent or sequential use of cytotoxic chemotherapy and hormone treatment in advanced breast cancer: Report of the Swiss Group for Clinical Cancer Research. Br Med J 286:5–8, 1983
338. Australian and New Zealand Breast Cancer Trials Group: A randomized trial in postmenopausal patients with advanced breast cancer comparing endocrine and cytotoxic therapy given sequentially or in combination. J Clin Oncol 4:186–193, 1986
339. Cutler S: Classification of extent of disease in breast cancer. Semin Oncol 1:91–96, 1974
340. Baum M, Priestman T, West RR, Jones EM: A comparison of subjective responses in a trial comparing endocrine with cytotoxic treatment in advanced carcinoma of the breast. In Mouridsen HT, Palshof T (eds): Breast Cancer—Experimental and Clinical Aspects, pp 223–226. Oxford, Pergamon Press, 1980
341. Sears HF, Gerber FH, Sturtz DL, Fouty WJ: Liver scan and carcinoma of the breast. Surg Gynecol Obstet 140:409–411, 1975
342. Muss HB, White DR, Cowan RJ: Brain scanning in patients with recurrent breast cancer. Cancer 38:1574–1576, 1976
343. Pedrazzini A, Gelber R, Isley M, Castiglione M, Goldhirsch A: First repeated bone scan in the observation of patients with operable breast cancer. J Clin Oncol 4:389–394, 1986
344. Corcoran RJ, Thrall JH, Kyle RW, Kaminski RJ, Johnson MC: Solitary abnormalities

in bone scans of patients with extraosseous malignancies. Radiology 121:663–667, 1976
345. Tumeh SS, Beadle G, Kaplan WD: Clinical significance of solitary rib lesions in patients with extraskeletal malignancy. J Nucl Med 26:1140–1143, 1985
346. Gillespie PJ, Alexander JL, Edelstyn GA: Changes in 87m-Sr concentrations in skeletal metastases in patients responding to cyclical combination chemotherapy for advanced breast cancer. J Nucl Med 16:191–193, 1975
347. Rossleigh MA, Lovegrove FTA, Reynolds PM, Byrne MJ: Serial bone scans in the assessment of response to therapy in advanced breast carcinoma. Clin Nucl Med 7:397–402, 1982
348. Buckman R, Coombes RC, Dearnaley DP, Gore M, Gusterson B, Neville AM: Some clinical uses of biological markers. In Bonadonna G (ed): Breast Cancer: Diagnosis and Management, pp 109–126. Chichester, Wiley & Sons, 1984
349. Smith IE: Recurrent disease. In Harris JR, Hellman S, Henderson IC, Kinne DW (eds): Breast Diseases, pp 369–384. Philadelphia, JB Lippincott Company, 1987
350. Hayes DF, Zurawski VR Jr, Kufe DW: Comparison of circulating CA 15-3 and carcinoembryonic antigen levels in patients with breast cancer. J Clin Oncol 4:1542–1550, 1986
351. Loprinzi CL, Tormey DC, Rasmussen P et al: Prospective evaluation of carcinoembryonic antigen levels and alternating chemotherapeutic regimens in metastatic breast cancer. J Clin Oncol 4:46–56, 1986
352. Mughal AW, Hortobagyi GN, Fritsche HA, Buzdar AU, Yap H, Blumenschein GR: Serial plasma carcinoembryonic antigen measurements during treatment of metastatic breast cancer. JAMA 249:1881–1886, 1983
353. Haagensen DE Jr, Mazoujian G, Holder WD Jr, Kister SJ, Wells SA Jr: Evaluation of a breast cyst fluid protein detectable in the plasma of breast carcinoma patients. Ann Surg 185:279–285, 1977
354. Welsch CW: Host factors affecting the growth in carcinogen-induced rat mammary carcinomas: A review and tribute to Charles Brenton Huggins. Cancer Res 45:3415–3443, 1985
355. Aitken SC, Lippman ME: Effect of estrogens and antiestrogens on growth-regulatory enzymes in human breast cancer cells in tissue culture. Cancer Res 45:1611–1620, 1985
356. Lippman M, Bolan G, Huff K: Interactions of antiestrogens with human breast cancer in long-term tissue culture. Cancer Treat 60:1421–1429, 1976
357. Campbell FC, Elston CW, Blamey RW et al: Quantitative oestradiol receptor values in primary breast cancer and response of metastases to endocrine therapy. Lancet 2:1317–1319, 1981
358. Allegra J, Lippman M, Thompson E et al: Estrogen receptor status: An important variable in predicting response to endocrine therapy in metastatic breast cancer. Eur J Cancer 16:323–331, 1980
359. Kiang DT, Kollander R: Breast cancers negative for estrogen receptor but positive for progesterone receptor: A true entity? J Clin Oncol 25:662–666, 1987
360. Byar D, Sears M, McGuire W: Relationship between estrogen receptor values and clinical data in predicting the response to endocrine therapy for patients with advanced breast cancer. Eur J Cancer 15:299–310, 1979
361. Henderson IC: Endocrine therapy of metastatic breast cancer. In Harris JR, Hellman S, Henderson IC, Kinne DW (eds): Breast Diseases, pp 398–428. Philadelphia, JB Lippincott, 1987
362. Cooperative Breast Cancer Group: Results of studies of the Cooperative Breast Cancer Group—1961–63. Cancer Chemother Rep 41:1–24, 1964
363. Westerberg H: Tamoxifen and fluoxymesterone in advanced breast cancer: A controlled clinical trial. Cancer Treat Rep 64:117–121, 1980
364. Ward HWC: Anti-oestrogen therapy for breast cancer: A trial of tamoxifen at two dose levels. Br Med J 1:13–14, 1973
365. Tormey DC, Lippman ME, Edwards BK, Cassidy JG: Evaluation of tamoxifen doses with and without fluoxymesterone in advanced breast cancer. Ann Intern Med 98:139–144, 1983
366. Rose C, Theilade K, Boesen E et al: Treatment of advanced breast cancer with tamoxifen. Breast Cancer Res Treat 2:395–400, 1982
367. Bratherton DG, Brown CH, Buchanan R et al: A comparison of two doses of tamoxifen (Nolvadex) in postmenopausal women with advanced breast cancer: 10 mg BD versus 20 mg BD. Br J Cancer 50:199–205, 1984
368. Kaiser-Kupfer MI, Lippman ME: Tamoxifen retinopathy. Cancer Treat Rep 62:315–320, 1978
369. Fabian C, Sternson L, El-Serafi M, Cain L, Hearne E: Clinical pharmacology of tamoxifen in patients with breast cancer: Correlation with clinical data. Cancer 48:876–882, 1981
370. Ingle JN, Krook JE, Green SJ et al: Randomized trial of bilateral oophorectomy versus tamoxifen in premenopausal women with metastatic breast cancer. J Clin Oncol 4:178–185, 1986
371. Buchanan RB, Blamey RW, Durrant KR et al: A randomized comparison of tamoxifen with surgical oophorectomy in premenopausal patients with advanced breast cancer. J Clin Oncol 4:1326–1330, 1986
372. Pritchard K, Meakin JW, Sawka C et al: The role and mechanism of action of tamoxifen in premenopausal women with metastatic carcinoma of the breast: An update (abstract). Proc Am Soc Clin Oncol 4:54, 1985
373. Lipton A, Harvey HA, Hamilton RW: Venous thrombosis as a side effect of tamoxifen treatment. Cancer Treat Rep 68:887–889, 1984
374. Robin PE, Dalton GA: The role of major endocrine ablation. In: Stoll BA (ed): Breast Cancer—Early & Late, pp 147–156. Chicago, Year Book Med Publishers, 1977
375. Dao TL: Ablation therapy for hormone-dependent tumors. Annu Rev Med 23:1–18, 1972
376. Fracchia AA, Farrow JH, DePalo AJ, Connolly DP, Huvos AG: Castration for primary inoperable or recurrent breast carcinoma. Surg Gynecol Obstet 128:1226–1234, 1969
377. Veronesi U, Pizzocaro G, Rossi A: Oophorectomy for advanced carcinoma of the breast. Surg Gynecol Obstet 141:569–570, 1975
378. Fitzpatrick PJ, Garrett PG: Metastatic breast cancer: Ovarian ablation with lower half-body irradiation. Int J Radiat Oncol Biol Phys 7:1523–1526, 1981
379. Stuart-Harris RC, Smith IE: Aminoglutethimide in the treatment of advanced breast cancer. Cancer Treat Rev 11:189–204, 1984
380. Santen RJ, Samojlik E, Worgul TJ: Aminoglutethimide. In Santen RJ, Henderson IC (eds): A Comprehensive Guide to the Therapeutic Use of Aminoglutethimide, pp 101–160, Basel, S Karger, 1982
381. Stuart-Harris R, Bozek T, Gazet JC et al: Low-dose aminoglutethimide in treatment of advanced breast cancer. Lancet 2:604–607, 1984
382. Santen RJ, Boucher AE, Santner SJ, Henderson IC, Harvey H, Lipton A: Inhibition of aromatase as treatment of breast carcinoma in postmenopausal women. J Lab Clin Med 109:278–289, 1987
383. Lipton A, Harvey HA, Santen RJ et al: Randomized trial of aminoglutethimide versus tamoxifen in metastatic breast cancer. Cancer Res 42:3434s–3436s, 1982
384. Smith IE, Harris AL, Morgan M, Gazet JC, McKinna JA: Tamoxifen versus aminoglutethimide versus combined tamoxifen and aminoglutethimide in the treatment of advanced breast carcinoma. Cancer Res 42:3430s–3433s, 1982
385. Santen RJ, Worgul TJ, Samojlik E et al: A randomized trial comparing surgical adrenalectomy with aminoglutethimide plus hydrocortisone in women with advanced breast cancer. N Engl J Med 305:545–551, 1981
386. Messeih AA, LiptonA, Santen RJ et al: Aminoglutethimide-induced hematologic toxicity: Worldwide experience. Cancer Treat Rep 69:1003–1004, 1985
387. Tchekmedyian NS, Tait N, Aisner J: Phase I/II trial of high-dose (HD) megestrol acetate (MA) in breast cancer (abstract). Proc Am Soc Clin Oncol 5:72, 1986
388. Hortobagyi GN, Buzdar AU, Frye D et al: Oral medroxyprogesterone acetate in the treatment of metastatic breast cancer. Breast Cancer Res Treat 5:321–326, 1985
389. Carter AC, Sedransk N, Kelley RM, Ansfield FJ, Ravdin RG, Potter NR: Diethylstilbestrol: Recommended dosages for different categories of breast cancer patients—Report of the Cooperative Breast Cancer Group. JAMA 237:2079–2085, 1977
390. Kennedy BJ: Massive estrogen administration in premenopausal women with metastatic breast cancer. Cancer 15:641–648, 1962
391. Klijn JGM, deJong FH: Treatment with a luteinising-hormone–releasing-hormone analogue. Lancet 1:1213–1216, 1982
392. Harvey HA, Lipton A, Santen RJ et al: Phase II study of a gonadotropin-releasing hormone analogue (leuprolide) in postmenopausal advanced breast cancer patients (abstract). Proc Am Soc Clin Oncol 22:444, 1981
393. Nagasawa H: Prolactin and human breast cancer: A review. Eur J Cancer 15:267–279, 1979
394. Harvey HA, Lipton A, Max DT et al: Medical castration produced by the GnRH analogue leuprolide to treat metastatic breast cancer. J Clin Oncol 3:1068–1072, 1985
395. Rubens RD, Knight RK: The contribution of prednisone (P) to primary endocrine therapy (PET) in advanced breast cancer (abstract). Proc Am Soc Clin Oncol 4:53, 1985
396. Stewart JF, Rubens RD, King RJB et al: Contribution of prednisolone to the primary endocrine treatment of advanced breast cancer. Eur J Cancer Clin Oncol 18:1307–1314, 1982
397. Wilson RE, Jessiman AG, Moore FD: Severe exacerbation of cancer of the breast after oophorectomy and adrenalectomy: Report of four cases. N Engl J Med 258:312–317, 1958
398. Henderson IC: Chemotherapy for advanced disease. In Harris JR, Hellman S, Henderson IC, Kinne DW (eds): Breast Diseases, pp 428–479. Philadelphia, JB Lippincott, 1987
399. Nemoto T: Metastatic breast cancer: Prolonged complete response or possible cure by chemotherapy (abstract). Proc Am Soc Clin Oncol 2:110, 1983
400. Legha SS, Buzdar AU, Smith TL et al: Complete remissions in metastatic breast cancer treated with combination drug therapy. Ann Intern Med 91:847–852, 1979
401. Decker DA, Ahmann DL, Bisel HF, Edmonson JH, Hahn RG, O'Fallon J: Complete responders to chemotherapy in metastatic breast cancer. JAMA 242:2075–2079, 1979
402. Abramowitz JW: Long term complete remissions from chemotherapy +/− hormonal therapy in breast cancer patients (abstract). Proc Am Soc Clin Oncol 1:76, 1982
403. Mattson W, Arwidi A, von Eyben F, Lindholm C: Phase II study of combined vincristine, Adriamycin, cyclophosphamide, and methotrexate with citrovorum factor rescue in metastatic breast cancer. Cancer Treat Rep 61:1527–1531, 1977
404. Henderson IC, Gelman RS, Canellos GP, Frei EI: Time to first response (IMP), partial response (PR), and complete response (CR) in breast cancer (BC) patients (PTS) treated with intensive chemotherapy (abstract). Proc Am Soc Clin Oncol 22:445, 1981
405. Franco LA, Shafie SM: Estrogen receptor status, doubling time and sensitivity of breast carcinoma cells to Adriamycin in tissue culture (abstract). Proc Am Assoc Cancer Res 22:5, 1981
406. Sulkes A, Livingston RB, Murphy WK: Tritiated thymidine labeling index and response in human breast cancer. J Natl Cancer Inst 62:513–515, 1979

407. Zhang HJ, Kennedy BJ, Kiang DT: Thymidine kinase as a predictor of response to chemotherapy in advanced breast cancer. Breast Cancer Res Treat 4:221–225, 1984
408. Lerner HJ: Acute myelogenous leukemia in patients receiving chlorambucil as long-term adjuvant chemotherapy for Stage II breast cancer. Cancer Treat Rep 62:1135–1138, 1978
409. Brambilla C, DeLena M, Rossi A, Valagussa P, Bonadonna G: Response and survival in advanced breast cancer after two non-cross-resistant combinations. Br Med J 1:801–804, 1976
410. Ahmann D, Bisel H, Eagan R, Edmonson J, Hahn R: Controlled evaluation of Adriamycin (NSC-123127) in patients with disseminated breast cancer. Cancer Chemother Rep 58:877–882, 1974
411. Hoogstraten B, George SL, Samal B et al: Combination chemotherapy and Adriamycin in patients with advanced breast cancer. Cancer 38:13–20, 1976
412. Legha SS, Benjamin RS, Mackay B et al: Adriamycin therapy by continuous intravenous infusion in patients with metastatic breast cancer. Cancer 49:1762–1766, 1982
413. Jain K, Wittes R, Benedetto P et al: A randomized comparison of weekly (arm I) vs. monthly (arm II) doxorubicin(DOX) in combination with mitomycin C (MMC) in advanced breast cancer (abstract). Proc Am Soc Clin Oncol 2:109, 1983
414. Segaloff A, Carter AC, Escher GC, Ansfield FJ, Talley RW: An evaluation of the effect of vincristine added to cyclosphosphamide, 5-fluorouracil, methotrexate, and prednisone in advanced breast cancer. Breast Cancer Res Treat 5:311–319, 1985
415. Steiner R, Stewart JF, Rubens RD: Results of endocrine therapy do not predict response to chemotherapy in advanced breast cancer. Eur J Cancer Clin Oncol 19:1559–1563, 1983
416. Fraschini G, Yap HY, Hortobagyi GN, Buzdar A, Blumenschein G: Five-day continuous-infusion vinblastine in the treatment of breast cancer. Cancer 56:225–229, 1985
417. Yap HY, Blumenschein GR, Hortobagyi GN, Buzdar A, Bodey GP: A randomized comparative study of vinblastine (VLB), vindesine (VDS) and vincristine (VCR) in patients (PTS) with refractory metastatic breast cancer (abstract). Proc Am Soc Clin Oncol 22:441, 1981
418. Smith IE, Powles TJ, Coombes RC et al: A control randomized trial comparing vindesine and Adriamycin with vincristine and Adriamycin in the treatment of advanced breast carcinoma. In Brade W, Nagel GA, Seeber S (eds): Proceedings of the International Vinca Alkaloid Symposium—Vindesine, pp 185–194. Karger Basel, Frankfurt, 1980
419. Yap HY, Yap BS, Rasmussen S, Levens ME, Hortobagyi GN, Blumenschein GR: Treatment for meningeal carcinomatosis in breast cancer. Cancer 49:219–222, 1982
420. Yap HY, Blumenschein GR, Yap BS et al: High-dose methotrexate for advanced breast cancer. Cancer Treat Rep 63:757–761, 1979
421. Henderson IC, Gelman R, Canellos GP, Frei E: Prolonged disease-free survival in advanced breast cancer treated with "super-CMF" Adriamycin: An alternating regimen employing high-dose methotrexate with citrovorum factor rescue. Cancer Treat Rep 65:67–75, 1981
422. Creagan ET, Green ST, Ahmann DL, Ingle JN, Edmonson JH, Marschke RF: A Phase III clinical trial comparing the combination cyclophosphamide, Adriamycin, cisplatin with cyclophosphamide, 5-fluorouracil, prednisone in patients with advanced breast cancer. J Clin Oncol 2:1260–1265, 1984
423. Sledge GW Jr, Loehrer PJ Sr, Roth BJ, Einhorn LH: Cisplatin as first-line therapy for metastatic breast cancer (abstract). Proc Am Soc Clin Oncol 6:53, 1987
424. Kolaric K, Roth A, Vukas D, Cervek J: CAP (cyclophosphamide, Adriamycin, platinum) vs CMFVP (cyclophosphamide, methotrexate, 5-fluorouracil, vincristine, prednisolone) combination chemotherapy in untreated metastatic breast cancer: A preliminary report of a controlled clinical study. Cancer Chemother Pharmacol 13:142–144, 1984
425. Rubens RD, Knight R, Hayward JL: Chemotherapy of advanced breast cancer: A controlled randomized trial of cyclophosphamide versus a four-drug combination. Br J Cancer 32:730–736, 1975
426. Mouridsen HT, Palshof T, Brahm M, Rahbek I: Evaluation of single-drug versus multiple-drug chemotherapy in the treatment of advanced breast cancer. Cancer Treat Rep 61:47–50, 1977
427. Smalley RV, Murphy S, Huguley CM, Bartolucci AA: Combination versus sequential five-drug chemotherapy in metastatic carcinoma of the breast. Cancer Res 36:3911–3916, 1976
428. Chlebowski R, Irwin LE, Pugh RP et al: Survival of patients with metastatic breast cancer treated with either combination or sequential chemotherapy. Cancer Res 39:4503–4506, 1979
429. Tormey DC, Gelman R, Band PR et al: Comparison of induction chemotherapies for metastatic breast cancer. Cancer 50:1235–1244, 1982
430. Ramirez G, Klotz J, Strawitz JG et al: Combination chemotherapy in breast cancer: A randomized study of 4 versus 5 drugs. Oncology 32:101–108, 1975
431. Englesman E, Rubens RD, Klijn JGM, Wildiers J, Rotmensz N, Sylvester R: Comparison of "classical CMF" with a three-weekly intravenous CMF schedule in postmenopausal patients with advanced breast cancer: An EORTC study (Trial 10808). Proc 4th EORTC Breast Cancer Working Conf 1987, p 1
432. Aisner J, Weinberg V, Perloff M et al: Chemotherapy versus chemoimmunotherapy (CAF v CAFVP v CMF each plus/minus MER) for metastatic carcinoma of the breast: A CALGB study. J Clin Oncol 5:1523–1533, 1987
433. Hart R, Perloff M, Holland J: One-day VATH (vinblastine, Adriamycin, thiotepa, and Halotestin) therapy for advanced breast cancer refractory to chemotherapy. Cancer 48:1522–1527, 1981
434. Perloff M, Hart R, Holland J: Vinblastine, Adriamycin, thiotepa, and Halotestin (VATH). Cancer 42:2534–2537, 1978
435. Friedman MA, Marcus FS, Cassidy MJ et al: 5-Fluorouracil + Oncovin + Adriamycin + mitomycin C (FOAM): An effective program for breast cancer, even for disease refractory to previous chemotherapy. Cancer 52:193–197, 1983
436. Konits P, Aisner J, VanEcho D, Lichtenfeld K, Wiernik P: Mitomycin C and vinblastine chemotherapy for advanced breast cancer. Cancer 48:1295–1298, 1981
437. Denefrio JM, East DR, Troner MB, Vogel CL: Phase II study of mitomycin C and vinblastine in women with advanced breast cancer refractory to standard cytotoxic therapy. Cancer Treat Rep 62:2113–2115, 1978
438. Garewal HS, Brooks RJ, Jones SE, Miller TP: Treatment of advanced breast cancer with mitomycin C combined with vinblastine or vindesine. J Clin Oncol 1:772–775, 1983
439. De Lena M, Zucali R, Viganotti G, Valagussa P, Bonadonna G: Combined chemotherapy–radiotherapy approach in locally advanced (T3b–T4) breast cancer. Cancer Chemother Pharmacol 1:53–59, 1978
440. Coates A, Gebski V, Bishop JF et al: Improving the quality of life during chemotherapy for advanced breast cancer. N Engl J Med 317:1490–1495, 1987
441. Bonadonna G, Valagussa P: Dose–response effect of CMF in breast cancer (abstract). Proc Am Soc Clin Oncol 21:413, 1980
442. Brufman G, Sulkes A, Fuks Z, Biran S: Cytoxan, methotrexate and 5-fluorouracil (CMF) chemotherapy (CHTX) in metastatic breast cancer (MBC): The influence of dose levels (DL) and performance status (PS) upon response rates and survival (abstract). Proc Am Soc Clin Oncol 2:103, 1983
443. Hryniuk W, Bush H: The importance of dose intensity in chemotherapy of metastatic breast cancer. J Clin Oncol 2:1281–1288, 1984
444. Hortobagyi GN, Buzdar AU, Bodey GP et al: High-dose induction chemotherapy of metastatic breast cancer in protected environment: A prospective randomized study. J Clin Oncol 5:178–184, 1987
445. Tannock IF, Boyd NF, Perrault DJ: Randomized trial of two doses of CMF chemotherapy for metastatic breast cancer (abstract). Proc Am Soc Clin Oncol 6:50, 1987
446. Goldie JH, Coldman AJ, Gudauskas GA: Rationale for the use of alternating non-cross-resistant chemotherapy. Cancer Treat Rep 66:439–449, 1982
447. Henderson IC, Hayes DF, Come S, Harris J,Canellos G: New agents and new medical treatments for advanced breast cancer. Semin Oncol 14:34–64, 1987
448. Tormey D, Gelman R, Falkson G: Prospective evaluation of rotating chemotherapy in advanced breast cancer. Am J Clin Oncol 6:1–18, 1983
449. Tormey DC, Weinberg VE, Leone LA et al: A comparison of intermittent vs. continuous and of Adriamycin vs. methotrexate 5-drug chemotherapy for advanced breast cancer. Am J Clin Oncol 7:231–239, 1984
450. Perry MC, Kardinal CG, Korzun AH et al: Chemohormonal therapy in advanced carcinoma of the breast: Cancer and Leukemia Group B protocol 8081. J Clin Oncol 5:1534–1545, 1987
451. Aberizk WJ, Silver B, Henderson IC, Cady B, Harris JR: The use of radiotherapy for treatment of isolated locroregional recurrence of breast carcinoma after mastectomy. Cancer 58:1214–1218, 1986
452. Hoogstraten B, Gad-El-Mawla N, Maloney TR et al: Combined modality therapy for first recurrence of breast cancer: A Southwest Oncology Group study. Cancer 54:2248–2256, 1984
453. Beck TM, Hart NE, Woodard DA, Smith CE: Local or regionally recurrent carcinoma of the breast: Results of therapy in 121 patients. J Clin Oncol 1:400–405, 1983
454. Tsukada Y, Fouad A, Pickren JW, Lane WW: Central nervous system metastasis from breast carcinoma. Autopsy study. Cancer 52:2349–2354, 1983
455. DiStefano A, Yap HY, Hortobagyi GN, Blumenschein GR: The natural history of breast cancer patients with brain metastases. Cancer 44:1913–1918, 1979
456. Borgelt B, Gelber R, Kramer S et al: The palliation of brain metastases: Final results of the first two studies by the Radiation Therapy Oncology Group. Int J Radiat Oncol Biol Phys 6:1–9, 1980
457. Glass JP, Foley KM: Specific sites of metastatic disease and emergencies: Brain metastases in patients with breast cancer. In Harris JR, Hellman S, Henderson IC, Kinne DW (eds): Breast Diseases, pp 480–487. Philadelphia, JB Lippincott, 1987
458. Burns PE, Jha N, Bain GO: Association of breast cancer with meningioma: A report of five cases. Cancer 58:1537–1539, 1986
459. Ushio Y, Posner JB, Sharpiro WR: Chemotherapy of experimental meningeal carcinomatosis. Cancer Res 37:1232–1237, 1977
460. Bertino JR: Toward improved selectivity in cancer chemotherapy: The Richard and Hinda Rosenthal Foundation Award Lecture. Cancer Res 39:293–304, 1979
461. Rosner D, Nemoto T, Lane WW: Chemotherapy induces regression of brain metastases in breast carcinoma. Cancer 58:832–839, 1986
462. Carey RW, Davis JM, Zervas NT: Tamoxifen-induced regression of cerebral metastases in breast carcinoma. Cancer Treat Rep 65:793–795, 1981
463. Smith DB, Howell A, Harris M, Bramwell VHC, Sellwood RA: Carcinomatous meningitis associated with infiltrating lobular carcinoma of the breast. Eur J Surg Oncol 11:33–36, 1985
464. Glass JP, Foley KM: Specific sites of metastatic disease and emergencies: Carcinomatous meningitis. In Harris JR, Hellman S, Henderson IC, Kinne DW (eds): Breast Diseases, pp 497–505. Philadelphia, JB Lippincott, 1987
465. Rose MA, Feldman EL: Specific sites of metastatic disease and emergencies: Choroidal metastases from breast cancer. In Harris JR, Hellman S, Henderson IC, Kinne DW (eds): Breast Diseases, pp 506–508. Philadelphia, JB Lippincott, 1987
466. Stillman M, Foley KM: Specific sites of metastatic disease and emergencies: Breast cancer and epidural spinal cord compression: Diagnostic and therapeutic strategies. In Harris JR, Hellman S, Henderson IC, Kinne DW (eds): Breast Diseases, pp 488–497. Philadelphia, JB Lippincott, 1987

467. Foley KM: Specific sites of metastatic disease and emergencies: Brachial plexopathy in patients with breast cancer. In Harris JR, Hellman S, Henderson IC, Kinne DW (eds): Breast Diseases, pp 532–538. Philadelphia, JB Lippincott, 1987
468. Israel L, Breau JL, Aguilera J: High-dose cyclosphosphamide and high-dose 5-fluorouracil: A new first-line regimen for advanced breast cancer. Cancer 53:1655–1659, 1984
469. Tormey DC, Kline JC, Palta M, Davis TE, Love RR, Carbone PP: Short term high density systemic therapy for metastatic breast cancer. Breast Cancer Res Treat 5:177–188, 1985
470. Cheng DS, Seitz CB, Eyre HJ: Nonoperative management of femoral, humeral, and acetabular metastases in patients with breast carcinoma. Cancer 45:1533–1537, 1980
471. Tong D, Gillick L, Hendrickson FR: The palliation of symptomatic osseous metastases: The final results of the study by the Radiation Therapy Oncology Group. Cancer 50:893–899, 1982
472. Cornell CN, Lane JM: Specific sites of metastatic disease and emergencies: Management of pathologic fractures. In Harris JR, Hellman S, Henderson IC, Kinne DW (eds): Breast Diseases, pp 525–532. Philadelphia, JB Lippincott, 1987
473. Ingle JN, Tormey DC, Tan HK: The bone marrow examination in breast cancer. Cancer 41:670–674, 1978
474. Come SE, Schnipper LE: Specific sites of metastatic disease and emergencies. In Harris JR, Hellman S, Henderson IC, Kinne DW (eds): Breast Diseases, pp 557–562. Philadelphia, JB Lippincott, 1987
475. Redding WH, Monaghan P, Imrie SF et al: Detection of micrometastases in patients with primary breast cancer. Lancet 2:1271–1273, 1983
476. Kennedy BJ, Tibbetts DM, Nathanson IT, Aub JC: Hypercalcemia: A complication of hormone therapy of advanced breast cancer. Cancer Res 13:445–459, 1953
477. Henderson IC: Hypercalcemia of malignant disease. In: Brain MC, Carbone PP (eds): Current Therapy in Hematology–Oncology 1985–86, pp 254–257. Philadelphia, BC Decker, 1985
478. Henner WD: Specific sites of metastatic disease and emergencies: Lymphangetic spread of carcinoma of the breast. In Harris JR, Hellman S, Henderson IC, Kinne DW (eds): Breast Diseases, pp 538–540. Philadelphia, JB Lippincott, 1987
479. Henner WD: Specific sites of metastatic disease and emergencies: Malignant effusions in breast cancer. In Harris JR, Hellman S, Henderson IC, Kinne DW (eds): Breast Diseases, pp 540–547. Philadelphia, JB Lippincott, 1987
480. Poe RH, Qazi R, Israel RH, Wicks CM, Rubins JM: Survival of patients with pleural involvement by breast carcinoma. Am J Clin Oncol 6:523–527, 1983
481. Fentiman IA, Rubens RD, Hayward JL: Control of pleural effusions in patients with breast cancer. Cancer 52:737–739, 1983
482. Butcher H: Radical mastectomy for mammary carcinoma. Ann Surg 170:883–884, 1969
483. Haagensen CD, Cooley E, Miller E et al: Treatment of early mammary carcinoma: A cooperative international study. Ann Surg 170:875–879, 1969
484. Valagussa P, Bonadonna G, Veronesi U: Patterns of relapse and survival following radical mastectomy. Cancer 41:1170–1178, 1978
485. Fisher B, Slack N, Katrych D: Ten-year followup results of patients with carcinoma of the breast in a cooperative clinical trial evaluating surgical adjuvant chemotherapy. Surg Gynecol Obstet 140:528–534, 1975
486. Payne WS, Taylor WF, Khonsari S: Surgical treatment of breast cancer: Trends and factors affecting survival. Arch Surg 101:105–113, 1970
487. Warren S, Witman EM: Studies on tumor metastases: The distribution of metastases in cancer of the breast. Surg Gynecol Obstet 57:81–85, 1937
488. Saphir O, Parker ML: Metastases of primary carcinoma of the breast with special reference to spleen, adrenal glands and ovaries. Arch Surg 42:1003–1018, 1941
489. Clark RM, Wilkinson RH, Mahoney LJ et al: Breast cancer: A 21 year experience with conservative surgery and radiation. Int J Radiat Oncol Biol Phys 8:967–975, 1982
490. Davis HL, Wiseley AN, Ramirez G, Ansfield FJ: Hypercalcemia complicating breast cancer. Oncology 28:126–137, 1973
491. Freeman CR, Belliveau NJ, Kim TH et al: Limited surgery with or without radiotherapy for early breast carcinoma. J Can Assoc Radiol 32:125–128, 1981
492. Fisher B, Ravdin RG, Ausman RK, Slack NH, Moore GE, Noer RJ: Surgical adjuvant chemotherapy in cancer of the breast: Results of a decade of cooperative investigation. Ann Surg 168:337–356, 1968
493. Baum M, Wilson AJ, Ebbs SR: The role of adjuvant endocrine therapy in primary breast cancer. In Salmon SE (ed): Adjuvant Therapy of Cancer V, pp 377–390. Orlando, Grune & Stratton, 1987
494. Cole MP: Prophylactic compared with therapeutic X-ray artificial menopause. In Joslin CAF, Gleave EN (eds): The Clinical Management of Advanced Breast Cancer: 2nd Tenovous Workshop, pp 2–11. Cardiff, Wales, Alpha Omega Alpha Publishing, 1970
495. McGuire WL, Horwitz KB, Zava DT, Garola RE, Chamness GC: Progress in endocrinology and metabolism: Hormones in breast cancer: Update 1978. Metabolism 27:487–501, 1978
496. Clark GM, McGuire WL: Progesterone receptors and human breast cancer. Breast Cancer Res Treat 3:157–163, 1983
497. Canellos GP, Devita V, Gold GL et al: Cyclical combination chemotherapy for advanced breast carcinoma. Br Med J 1:218–220, 1974
498. Canellos GP, Pocock S, Taylor S et al: Combination chemotherapy for metastatic breast carcinoma. Cancer 38:1882–1886, 1976
499. Jones SE, Durie BGM, Salmon SE: Combination chemotherapy with Adriamycin and cyclophosphamide for advanced breast cancer. Cancer 36:90–97, 1975
500. Bull J, Tormey D, Li SH et al: A randomized comparative trial of Adriamycin versus methotrexate in combination drug therapy. Cancer 41:1649–1657, 1978
501. Tranum B, Hoogstraten B, Kennedy A et al: Adriamycin in combination for the treatment of breast cancer. Cancer 41:2078–2083, 1978
502. Smalley R, Carpenter J, Bartolucci A, Vogel C, Krauss S: A comparison of cyclophosphamide, Adriamycin, 5-fluorouracil (CAF) and cyclophosphamide, methotrexate, 5-fluorouracil, vincristine, prednisone (CMFVP) in patients with metastatic breast cancer. Cancer 40:625–632, 1977

JEFFREY A. NORTON
JOHN L. DOPPMAN
ROBERT T. JENSEN

CHAPTER 39 *Cancer of the Endocrine System*

THE THYROID GLAND

Malignant disease of the thyroid gland is a heterogeneous disorder that affects all age groups, but is more serious in the elderly. No single treatment plan exists because of the high long-term survival of most patients with differentiated thyroid cancers, regardless of the type or extent of treatment.[1] Because some thyroid cancers are potentially lethal, a definitive diagnosis of all lesions of the thyroid gland is indicated, which will suggest appropriate therapy.

HISTORY

The name *thyroid* comes from the Greek word for shield. The gland was named by Wharton in 1646 either because of its shieldlike shape or because it shielded the larynx. Hyperthyroidism was described by Graves in 1835, and hypothyroidism or myxedema was described by Curling in 1850. In 1882, Reverdin produced experimental hypothyroidism by thyroidectomy. Hypothyroidism was successfully treated with thyroid extract in 1890.[2,3] In 1914, Kendall isolated the hormone thyroxine (T_4).

Theodor Kocher is the father of modern thyroid surgery. In 1878, he excised a thyroid to alleviate goiter, an operation he performed many times. Kocher also confirmed that total thyroidectomy in humans resulted in hypothyroidism, which he subsequently prevented by subtotal thyroidectomy. For these and other contributions, Kocher received the Nobel Prize in 1909. After consulting with Kocher, William Halsted at Johns Hopkins University developed his own technique of thyroidectomy.[4]

Thyroxine was first synthesized by Harrington and Barger in 1927. Thiouracil, the first antithyroid drug, was introduced in 1943 by McKenzie and Astwood.[4]

EPIDEMIOLOGY

The estimated number of new cases of thyroid cancer in the United States during 1986 was 10,600, with 7,700 cases in women (Table 39-1). Deaths from thyroid cancer in 1986 were about 1,100, approximately 10% the total new cases (Table 39-1). The incidence of thyroid cancer in women was 5.9/100,000 in 1984; the incidence in men was only 2.2/100,000 (Table 39-2). Thyroid neoplasms account for 90% of all endocrine malignancies (Table 39-3).

The majority of cases occur between 25 and 65 years of age, but thyroid cancer can occur in the very young and the elderly. For well-differentiated thyroid cancers, recent studies from several independent groups indicate that age at diagnosis is an important prognostic variable, and one report indicates that it is the *most* important prognostic variable.[5–9] The recurrence and survival rates of patients in the low-risk group (men younger than 40 years and women younger than 50 years) are strikingly different from patients in the high-risk group (all older patients). The high-risk age for differentiated thyroid cancer falls in the fourth or fifth decade.[5–9]

Although there appeared to be a definite increase in the

TABLE 39-1. Estimated New Cases of and Deaths from Thyroid Cancer

	Estimated New Cases			*Estimated Deaths*		
	Both Sexes	*Male*	*Female*	*Both Sexes*	*Male*	*Female*
Thyroid cancer	10,600	2,900	7,700	1,100	400	700

American Cancer Society 1986 Cancer Facts and Figures. Incidence estimates are based on rates from National Cancer Institute SEER Program 1977–1981.

incidence of thyroid cancer between the Second National Cancer Survey in 1947 and the Third National Cancer Survey during 1969–1971, and another increase between 1973 and 1977, the incidence between 1975 and 1984 appears to be stable (Table 39-2).

Following the report in 1969 by Sampson and associates on the prevalence of thyroid carcinoma in the autopsy population of Hiroshima and Nagasaki, there have been similar studies of the prevalence of thyroid cancer in patients dying of other diseases.[10,11] The more carefully the gland is examined, the more occult, often minute, cancers are found. Most series report a prevalence of thyroid cancer at autopsies between 5% and 10%, except in Japan and Hawaii, where the incidence is as high as 28%.[12,13] There is general agreement that these small, occult, and mostly papillary cancers are of small or no clinical significance even if lymph node spread is present. The prevalence of thyroid cancer in autopsy series does not correlate with increased clinical incidence, recurrence, or mortality from thyroid cancer.[14]

The prevalence of clinical thyroid cancer increases with either solitary nodular or multinodular thyroid disease, and therefore the evaluation of nodular thyroid disease is an integral part of the clinical evaluation of thyroid cancer. The prevalence of thyroid nodules depends on the population studied. In two large series of children not exposed to radiation, the rates were 0.22% and 1.5%.[15,16] Incidence increases linearly with age, with spontaneous nodules occurring at a rate of 0.08% per year through the eighth decade. In the U.S., clinical nodules are present in 4% to 7% of the adult population and are more common in women than men.[17] The absolute prevalence of thyroid cancer in solitary and multinodular glands is approximately 10% to 20%.[18–21]

PATHOLOGY

The majority of malignant tumors of the thyroid gland are of glandular–epithelial origin and are carcinomas (Table 39-4). Because some well-differentiated thyroid cancers grow very slowly, the diagnosis depends on blood vessel or capsular invasion rather than histopathologic appearance.[1,14] Because some lesions that have clear vascular invasion and distant spread may still have a benign clinical course, some physicians argue that aggressive therapy is not warranted.[1] The pathologist must receive adequate primary tissue, which includes the thyroid nodule and the adjacent ipsilateral thyroid lobe, in order to carefully evaluate the margins of the nodule and the thyroid. The junction of the neoplasm and the thyroid allows the pathologist to discern capsular invasion.

Often malignant papillary neoplasms of the thyroid are multifocal, which is indicative of an adverse prognosis (Table 39-5). Multifocality has been documented in up to 80% of patients with papillary cancer.[22] Another important prognostic feature is the age of the patient at diagnosis which is an important criterion in staging (Table 39-5).[9] An important clinicopathologic observation is the presence of direct extension into contiguous structures in the neck or extracapsular invasion, which affects subsequent recurrence rates.[7] Lymph node metastases do not have prognostic significance in papillary thyroid cancer (one group suggests that they are a good indication) but they have a negative prognostic value in medullary thyroid cancer.[23] The diagnosis of undifferentiated or anaplastic thyroid cancer has a uniformly poor prognosis.[24]

Because of the problems in staging thyroid carcinoma, a

TABLE 39-2. Age-Adjusted Cancer Incidence for Thyroid Cancer

	Year of Diagnosis									
Group	*1975*	*1976*	*1977*	*1978*	*1979*	*1980*	*1981*	*1982*	*1983*	*1984*
All races										
Men and Women	4.1*	4.1	4.6	4.3	3.8	3.6	3.8	3.9	4.0	4.1
All races										
Men	2.6	2.5	2.9	2.6	2.2	2.0	2.2	2.4	2.4	2.2
Women	5.5	5.7	6.2	5.9	5.2	5.1	5.3	5.2	5.6	5.9
White										
Men	2.3	2.4	2.8	2.5	2.1	1.9	2.2	2.3	2.2	2.1
Women	5.4	5.5	6.1	5.7	5.2	5.2	5.3	5.2	5.8	5.8
Black										
Men	1.4	1.2	1.5	1.2	1.6	1.0	1.1	1.7	1.5	1.4
Women	3.6	4.2	4.6	3.3	3.6	2.9	2.8	3.9	3.0	3.6

Data from SEER program NCI 1975–1984.
*Rates per 100,000 persons.

TABLE 39-3. Distribution of Endocrine Cancers at Presentation

	All Stages (no. of cases per year)	*Localized (% of cases)*	*Regional (% of cases)*	*Distant (% of cases)*	*Unstaged (% of cases)*
Thyroid gland	7975	61	28	7	3
Other endocrine	835	29	19	40	12
Total	8810	58	27	10	4

Data, for all races and both sexes, taken from the SEER program NCI 1975–1984.

uniform staging system has not been routinely applied. An acceptable staging system based on the TNM classification, the type of thyroid cancer, and the age of the patient is listed in Table 39-5.

Papillary Adenocarcinoma

In the United States and Sweden, papillary cancer is the most common type of thyroid malignancy (approximately 60%, Table 39-6). Viewed by electron microscopy, the papillary cancer cells are similar to hyperplastic cells except for nuclear inclusions and variations in size and shape.[25] The nuclear membrane of the papillary cancer cells is delicate, with an opaque, ground-glass appearance—the so-called "Orphan Annie" appearance.[26] Mixed papillary and follicular carcinomas are classified as papillary carcinomas, because they have similar biologic behavior and prognosis. Hawk and Hazard noted no difference in prognosis for papillary thyroid cancers that were principally papillary, principally follicular, or equally mixed.[27] Most papillary cancers are so slow growing that it would take many years' follow-up to distinguish differences, and even with good follow-up there have been no prognostic differences detected.

Papillary thyroid carcinoma varies in necrosis and gross appearance depending on size. Occult thyroid papillary cancers are usually small, less than 1.0 or 1.5 cm in diameter, often minute, sometimes multiple, and have no clinical significance. Most patients (517 of 518 in one study) have normal life spans without any awareness or clinical manifestation of tumor.[28] Even if occult papillary cancers metastasize to lymph nodes, the prognosis is still excellent, and it is important not to overtreat these occult tumors. Only a rare case of a metastasis to bone from an occult cancer has been reported.[29] The larger tumors usually are poorly defined, although some may be partially encapsulated.[30]

TABLE 39-4. Classification of Malignant Tumors of the Thyroid Gland

Well-Differentiated Carcinoma	
	Papillary or papillary-follicular adenocarcinoma
	Follicular carcinoma
	Hurthle cell carcinoma
	Medullary carcinoma
Undifferentiated (Anaplastic) Carcinoma	
Other Malignant Tumors	
	Sarcoma
	Lymphoma
	Metastatic tumor

Associated fibrosis is common, and calcium may be deposited in fibrotic areas. The classic appearance is one of papillary projections formed by a fibrovascular pedicle with its covering epithelium. Mitoses are uncommon. Squamous metaplasia, psammoma bodies, lymphatic invasion, and multifocality (30–40%) are common.[31] Multifocality may be multicentricity of primary papillary tumors or lymphatic spread throughout the thyroid. Extension of the tumor into adjacent neck structures worsens the prognosis, as does the presence of distant metastasis. Aggressive papillary thyroid carcinomas usually occur in patients over 45, with a greater risk in men (Table 39-5).

Follicular Carcinoma

Follicular carcinoma of the thyroid gland occurs less often than papillary carcinoma, except in iodine-deficient areas or in goiter areas like Switzerland (Table 39-6). Follicular adenomas and carcinomas usually have a relatively uniform, microfollicular pattern. Papillations and cytologic characteristics of papillary carcinoma (Orphan Annie nucleus, psammoma bodies) are not seen in follicular carcinoma. In contrast to follicular adenomas, follicular carcinomas show some degree of invasion of blood vessels or of the tumor capsule. An *atypical adenoma* is a follicular tumor without invasion but with sufficient cellular and nuclear atypia to suggest cancer. *Encapsulated follicular carcinoma* is a follicular tumor that appears to be encapsulated but shows microscopic invasion of the capsule, vessels, or both. Nineteen patients with this diagnosis treated with surgical resection and thyroid hormone replacement had a 10-year survival rate of 78%. Primary lesions larger than 3.5 cm were associated with recurrent or metastatic disease.[32]

The American Joint Committee on Cancer studies on staging emphasize the slow growth and good prognosis of follicular cancers if the tumor is small (≤3 cm) and localized (Table 39-5). Compared with papillary thyroid carcinomas, lymph node metastases are infrequent. The prognosis is poorer for patients over 45 years of age, for men in whom cancer extends into contiguous neck structures, and for patients with distant metastases.[33] The most important prognostic distinction is between minimally invasive (encapsulated) and extensively invasive carcinomas.[34] Growth rates of distant metastases may be very slow, and they often respond well, at least temporarily, to radioiodine therapy after ablation of the thyroid gland.

Hurthle cell or oxyphil cell tumors have been shown to be derived from the follicular cell by electron microscopy and

TABLE 39-5. Clinicopathologic Staging of Malignant Tumors of the Thyroid Gland

TNM Classification

Primary tumor (T)
- T_1 diameter ≤3 cm
- T_2 diameter >3 cm
- T_3 Multiple intraglandular tumor foci
- T_4 Fixation of thyroid, direct invasion through thyroid capsule

Nodal Involvement (N)
- N_x nodes cannot be assessed
- N_0 no clinically or pathologically positive nodes
- N_1 clinically positive or pathologically positive nodes

Metastases (M)
- M_x not assessed
- M_0 no known metastases
- M_1 distant metastases present

Stage Grouping

Cancer Type		*<45 yr*	*>45 yr*
Papillary:	Stage I	Any T Any N M_0	Any T N_0 M_0 T_1 N_1 M_0
	Stage II	Any T Any N M_1	T_{2-4} N_1 M_0
	Stage III	None	None
	Stage IV	None	Any T Any N M_1
Follicular	Stage I	Any T Any N M_0	T_1 N_0 M_0
	Stage II	Any T Any N M_1	T_{2-4} N_0 M_0
	Stage III	None	Any T N_1 M_0
	Stage IV	None	Any T Any N M_1
Medullary	Stage I	None	None
	Stage II	Any T Any N M_0	None
	Stage III	None	Any T Any N M_0
	Stage IV	Any T Any N M_1	Any T Any N M_1
Undifferentiated			
	Stage I	None	None
	Stage II	None	None
	Stage III	None	None
	Stage IV	Any T Any N Any M	Any T Any N Any M

10-year Survival

Stage I	>95%
Stage II	50–95%
Stage III	15–50%
Stage IV	<15%

From Staging of Cancer of Head and Neck Sites and of Melanoma. American Joint Committee on Cancer, 1980.

biochemical studies. Tumors show occasional formation of colloid and thyroglobulin and may synthesize thyroid hormone.[35,36] Hurthle cell neoplasms are usually composed of sheets of Hurthle cells. Criteria for malignancy of these tumors are similar to other follicular neoplasms, namely capsular or vascular invasion. Thompson and colleagues started a controversy in 1974, when they described 25 patients with Hurthle cell tumors. Most of the patients died, including 3 of 4 in whom the diagnosis of adenoma had been made.[37] They concluded that the diagnosis of oxyphil or Hurthle cell adenoma should not be used. A follow-up study from the same institution indicated that total thyroidectomy for malignant Hurthle cell neoplasms or benign neoplasms greater than 2 cm in diameter resulted in a lower recurrence rate than historical controls (21% versus 59%).[38] Recent studies indicated that Hurthle cell carcinomas can usually be distinguished pathologically from benign adenomas and that only 1.5% to 2.5% of benign Hurthle cell adenomas become malignant.[39,40] The pathologist's diagnosis of Hurthle cell adenoma or carcinoma usually corresponds to the clinical behavior, but an occasional adenoma may behave like carcinoma.

TABLE 39-6. Incidence (%) of Different Thyroid Cancer Types Based on Geographic Location

	Boston	*Stockholm*	*Basel*
Papillary	58	58	25
Follicular	24	19	39
Medullary	3	7	2
Anaplastic	15	16	26

Meissner WA: Tumors of the thyroid gland. In: Atlas of Pathology. Washington, DC, Armed Forces Institute of Pathology, 1984; Jereb B, Stjernsward J, Lowhagen T: Anaplastic giant-cell carcinoma of the thyroid gland. Cancer 35:1293, 1975, Heitz P, Moser H, Staub JJ: Thyroid cancer. Cancer 37:2329, 1976.

Medullary Carcinoma

Medullary carcinomas make up approximately 5% of all thyroid cancers (Table 39-6). They are slightly more common in women and occur at all ages, with the highest incidence in the fifth and sixth decades. A tumor of calcitonin-secreting C cells of the thyroid gland, this cancer represents an important potential model for the mechanisms of human epithelial cell transformation, because approximately 20% of these patients exhibit an autosomal dominant inheritance pattern.[41] Little is known about the specific genetic abnormalities associated with medullary carcinomas. Babu and colleagues proposed that a constitutional deletion of part of the short arm of chromosome 20 may be a predisposing factor in some families.[42] Other investigators have been unable to detect this deletion either in families with the tumor or in medullary carcinoma cells growing in tissue culture.[43-45]

In patients with multiple endocrine neoplasia-type 2a (MEN-2a), the earliest thyroid abnormality is referred to as C cell hyperplasia, which is characterized by multicentric patches of C cells. With time, these lesions progress to foci of microscopic carcinoma as the cells break out of the C cell hyperplasia cluster. Ultimately macroscopic foci of medullary thyroid carcinoma are evident. Hybridization histochemistry by Northern gel analysis of mRNA for calcitonin and calcitonin-gene-related peptide (CGRP) may be helpful in the future to diagnose specific C-cell hyperplasia and medullary carcinoma in situ.[46] This diagnosis is difficult to make pathologically. Some physicians have instead used preoperative specific elevations in calcitonin in response to calcium or pentagastrin stimulation, because they are especially useful in establishing an early diagnosis.[47]

In patients with familial medullary carcinoma or MEN-2a, the neoplasm is present in both thyroid lobes; in sporadic (nonfamilial) medullary carcinoma, the tumor occurs unilaterally.[48] The solid, firm tumor is usually gray-white. The cut surface shows areas of hemorrhage, necrosis, fibrosis, and calcification. The tumors are usually located at the junction of the upper and middle portion of each lobe, the area that has the highest concentration of C cells. The tumor cells are commonly arranged into solid, irregular groups. There is even an anaplastic variant recognized only by argyrophilia and by calcitonin immunoreactivity. The tumor stroma is hyaline and variable in size. Amyloid is often demonstrated by amyloid stains, such as congo red, or by electron microscopy. Calcitonin determination of the tumor by immunoperoxidase technique has been highly successful.

The tumor metastasizes both by lymphatics and blood stream. The growth rate, compared with anaplastic carcinoma, is relatively slow, yet the ultimate prognosis is not good, with only a 50% ten-year survival. Prognosis is worse for the older-age group, for patients with MEN-2b, for large tumor size, for lymph node metastases, and for distant metastases.[49,50] Lippman and others showed that patients having tumors with poor calcitonin-staining intensity and patchy calcitonin distribution (tumor-cell heterogeneity) had a higher risk for developing metastases and had a grave clinical course.[51] Recent experimental observations with human medullary thyroid carcinoma in tissue culture support this observation. Phorbol esters and cAMP induce growth inhibition, calcitonin secretion, and calcitonin gene transcription, and they decrease c-*myc* mRNA levels.[52,53] Therefore, phorbol esters in vitro reduce tumor-cell heterogeneity and increase more differentiated, homogeneous cells, which make calcitonin and are less likely to divide, reducing malignant potential. There is considerable evidence that hyperplasia of the C cells precedes neoplasia; if calcitonin levels are elevated in hyperplasia, thyroidectomy is recommended. In familial settings, the cure rate is high (95%) when calcitonin levels are elevated and the tumor is not palpable, but low (17%) if the tumor is palpable.[54]

Anaplastic Carcinoma

The relative frequency of undifferentiated or anaplastic thyroid carcinoma has been steadily decreasing for several decades. Currently it accounts for 18% of all thyroid cancers (Table 39-6).[59] The decreasing incidence of anaplastic thyroid tumors may mean that better diagnostic techniques are able to differentiate two confusing diagnoses, medullary thyroid carcinoma and lymphoma. In one study, 9 of 14 undifferentiated thyroid cancers reviewed with immunoperoxidase staining for calcitonin and with electron microscopy were found to be medullary carcinoma.[55] Monoclonal antibody methods specific for lymphoma are also detecting lymphomas masquerading as small cell anaplastic thyroid carcinoma.[56] There remain some anaplastic thyroid cancers with cells that are neither *spindle or giant cell carcinoma* nor demonstrate abortive follicle formation. Electron microscopy has shown that anaplastic cancer cells feature lysosomal bodies and microvilli, which resemble normal follicular cells.[57,58] Studies to determine the frequency of hormonal, epithelial, and sarcoma markers in anaplastic thyroid carcinoma indicate that 27% stain for thyroglobulin, 48% for alpha-antichymotrypsin, and 47% for vimentim, 30% were not positive for any marker, indicating a total lack of differentiation.[59]

The prognosis is dismal. All anaplastic thyroid tumors are placed in Stage IV (Table 39-5), regardless of the extent of disease. Most studies show a near zero 2-year survival. Aldinger found a 7% 5-year survival in 84 patients treated with combination therapy.[60] Often anaplastic thyroid cancers develop in pre-existing differentiated thyroid cancers in the elderly. There is a greater incidence in countries with endemic goiter (Table 39-6).[14,31]

ETIOLOGY

Radiation

The treatment of thymic enlargement in infancy with external radiation was first reported in 1907. Subsequently, x-irradiation was used to treat enlarged tonsils and adenoids, mastoiditis, sinusitis, hemangiomas, lymphadenopathy, and acne. Thousands of patients in the United States have received neck irradiation for these indications. In 1950, thyroid carcinoma was first reported in 9 of 28 children who had previously received thymic irradiation.[61] Subsequently, many studies have confirmed the association between therapeutic irradiation of the head and neck region and the development of thyroid carcinoma, salivary tumor, neural tumors, and parathyroid tumors 20 to 35 years later.[62]

The risk of developing thyroid cancer is radiation dose-dependent, increasing from as little as 6.5 rad to 1200 rad. Over 2000 rad the risk declines because the thyroid gland becomes sterilized. Treatment of Graves' disease with radioactive iodine does not cause thyroid cancer because the gland receives a dose in excess of 5000 rads.[63] Marshall Islanders, especially children, who received approximately 1200 rad as fallout from the nearby atomic bomb tests showed an increased incidence of thyroid neoplasia.[64] It seems likely that doses lower than 2000 rad damage thyroid tissue DNA, which leads to mutations. Thyroid neoplasia is a function of the radiation dose, described by a linear dose–response curve, starting at 3 per 200 person years at risk per 1000 rad.

Several factors elevate risk. Women have increased risk. The younger the patient at the time of irradiation, the greater the risk of subsequent cancer. The risk increases in proportion to time after exposure, and the risk is linear from 300 to 1200 rad. Increased secretion of thyroid-stimulating hormone (TSH) as a result of impaired thyroid hormone secretion may also play a role as a cancer-promoting agent after irradiation.[65]

Iodine

Papillary carcinoma of the thyroid may be more common in areas with iodination of salt (U.S.A.) or a high-iodine diet (Sweden).[66] Follicular carcinoma is much more common in iodine-deficient goiterous areas, such as Switzerland (Table 39-6). The high incidence of follicular neoplasia in goiterous areas may be related to the prolonged stimulatory effect of TSH.[67]

Goiters

In the rat, prolonged exposure of the thyroid gland to TSH stimulation induced by antithyroid drugs causes a high yield of malignant tumors, including rat medullary thyroid carcinoma. Some series have indicated a higher proportion of anaplastic and follicular carcinomas of the thyroid gland in endemic goiter regions.[31,68] A history of nodular goiter is obtained in approximately 80% of patients affected with anaplastic carcinoma.[59,68] The pre-existing abnormality may represent an adenomatous goiter, an adenoma, or a well-differentiated carcinoma. This striking association has led several investigators to infer transformation of a low-grade or benign lesion into a highly malignant one, and external radiation may enhance the potential for this transformation.[14,59,68,69] However, most radiation-induced thyroid cancers are well differentiated and behave biologically exactly like curable papillary cancers.[70,71]

Heredity

The thyroid carcinoma that is most influenced by genetic factors is medullary thyroid carcinoma, although the exact abnormality remains controversial.[42–45] This tumor is inherited by an autosomal dominant defect in 20% of the cases.[41] It occurs in three familial settings: familial medullary thyroid carcinoma, MEN-2a, and MEN-2b. Papillary thyroid carcinoma does not usually show a familial disposition, but there have been two studies suggesting that it occurs in families. One suggests that it is associated with familial polyposis of the colon and Gardner's syndrome (benign adenomatous colonic polyps, lipomas, fibromas, and mandibular osteomas).[73,74]

Other Risk Factors

Thyroiditis does not appear to predispose to carcinoma; however, there appears to be an increased incidence of lymphoma of the thyroid gland in patients with severe Hashimoto's thyroiditis.[75] The risk factors for thyroid malignancy are listed in Table 39-7.

DIAGNOSIS

Clinical Presentation

The manner of evaluating and treating a thyroid nodule is evolving. Thyroid nodules occur in 4% to 7% of the nonexposed adult population and in 20% to 30% of the radiation-exposed adult population, but only 10% to 20% of these nodules become malignant without radiation exposure and 30% to 50% become malignant after exposure.[17,76–78] Therefore, the work-up of a thyroid nodule should suggest surgical resection only for nodules that are malignant and avoid unnecessary surgery for nodules that are benign. The problem is that no preoperative test at present perfectly discriminates malignant from benign nodular disease.

History and Physical Examination

The patient's history may increase the suspicion of cancer in a thyroid nodule. Exposure to ionizing radiation is a well-documented risk factor for the subsequent development of thyroid cancer.[79] Whether patient age affects the likelihood of a nodule being cancerous is not clear.[80–82] Local symptoms like airway obstruction, hoarseness, and dysphagia may be associated with either extensive thyroid cancer or with goiter. Fewer than 5% of patients with thyroid cancer present with these symptoms.[82] This nonspecificity of symptoms has been emphasized in a report in which 40% of patients with benign goiter had vocal cord paralysis.[83] The appearance of a new nodule or rapid growth of a nodule are associated with malignancy but are also nonspecific. Because thyroid cancer usually grows slowly, a dominant nodule of long duration needs the same diagnostic attention as a new nodule. The risk of malignant disease in a multinodular

TABLE 39-7. Factors Predisposing to Thyroid Cancer

Factor	*Associated Malignancy*
TSH	Papillary
Low-dose radiation	Papillary
Iodine deficiency	Follicular
Iodine abundance	Papillary
Genetic	Medullary
Thyroiditis	Lymphoma
Preexisting goiter or neoplasia ± radiation	Anaplastic

Adapted from Jackson IMD, Cobb WE: Disorders of the thyroid. In Kohler PO (ed): Clinical Endocrinology. New York, John Wiley, 1986.

goiter is significantly lower than the risk in a solitary nodule.[17] It is important to examine the neck for enlarged jugular or central lymph nodes, which increase the likelihood of a thyroid nodule being malignant. Although physical characteristics of the nodule are poor predictors of a malignant lesion, it is important to palpate the thyroid nodule, because work-up and evaluation of a nodule is based on physical examination and not ultrasound or thyroid scanning.

Laboratory Tests

Laboratory tests are not helpful in the evaluation of a thyroid nodule. Serum levels of thyroglobulin are elevated in patients with differentiated thyroid tumors that arise from follicular epithelium, but levels are normal or low in patients with anaplastic or medullary tumors. The level of thyroglobulin cannot predict whether a given nodule is benign or malignant, nor can it predict whether a cancer is present in a multinodular goiter.[83] However, following total thyroidectomy for differentiated thyroid cancer with follicular elements, thyroglobulin levels return to normal and then may again become elevated with recurrent or metastatic disease.[84] Thyroglobulin levels have been used to follow patient populations at risk for developing thyroid cancer following irradiation in childhood. Increasing levels of thyroglobulin in serial determinations were found in individuals who subsequently developed thyroid nodules and cancer. The increment was 17 ± 8 ng/ml ($\bar{x} \pm$ SEM).[85] Thyroglobulin levels are also elevated in noncancerous thyroid diseases like Graves' disease, nontoxic goiter, and thyroiditis.[83] Because of the lack of specificity and sensitivity, thyroglobulin determinations are only useful in sequential determinations in an individual patient, for following patients with metastatic or recurrent thyroid disease and for following patients with a history of radiation exposure.

Carcinoembryonic antigen (CEA) is elevated in many patients with medullary thyroid carcinoma, but serum calcitonin elevations are specific for medullary cancer.[86] Combined with provocative agents like calcium or pentagastrin, calcitonin levels become the most sensitive marker available in clinical oncology.[87] Although medullary carcinoma is rare, these tests should be performed when there is a family history of this cancer.

Thyroid Gland Suppression

A thyroid nodule is suppressed by administering thyroid hormone exogenously for several months. Supposedly, benign nodules will shrink but maligant nodules will not. However, TSH receptors cause ligand binding on both normal and malignant thyroid tissue.[88,89] Indirect evidence for TSH dependence of thyroid cancer includes a report of lower recurrence rates for patients receiving thyroid hormone postoperatively than for those who did not receive it and one report of tumor regression in a patient treated with thyroid hormone alone.[90] The success rate of suppression therapy for solitary nodules ranged from 0 to 60%, with 0 to 38% having a complete response and 10% to 60% a partial response.[17] The incidence of malignant disease that it may suppress is completely unknown. Successful suppression of thyroid nodules does not exclude malignant disease; confirmed carcinomas have been reported that responded to suppression.[91,92] Also the lack of response to thyroid hormone is not specific for malignant disease; some benign nodules will not suppress. In two small studies in which nonresponders to suppression underwent thyroid resection, the incidence of thyroid cancer was 20% and 40%.[93,94] We employ suppression of selected small nodules that have a benign appearance on aspiration cytology. If an aspiration indicates malignancy, we operate without suppression. During hormonal treatment, the physician should measure TSH levels and ascertain that circulating levels are suppressed with a given thyroxine dose. The strategy should be altered to surgical resection if the nodule increases on suppression. At the end of 6 months, re-evaluation with another aspiration is necessary if the nodule is smaller but has not disappeared. If it remains unchanged, resection is necessary. With careful follow-up, delay in definitive treatment of well-differentiated thyroid cancer does not usually translate into increased morbidity or mortality.

Radionuclide Imaging

The three common isotopes used in thyroid scanning are ^{123}I, ^{131}I, and ^{99m}Tc-pertechnetate, which classify nodules by their ability to trap iodine. Iodine-123 has advantages over ^{131}I for imaging studies, because ^{123}I does not have the high beta-emission of ^{131}I. This particular emission, although it can be useful therapeutically, does not contribute diagnostic information and adds to the patient's dose of radiation.[95] A survey indicated that ^{99m}Tc and ^{123}I accounted for 54% and 35% respectively, of the thyroid imaging done in the United States.[96] Iodine 131 is indicated for uptake studies and for evaluation and treatment of metastatic thyroid carcinoma.

Because malignant thyroid tissue either does not trap or incorporate iodine or it incorporates less iodine than normal thyroid tissue, a malignant lesion appears as a "cold" area on a scan.[97] The main limitation of thyroid scanning is that it cannot distinguish benign from malignant nodules and can be used only to assign a probability of malignancy based on the functional status of a nodule. In Ashcraft and Van Herle's analysis of the literature in which radioiodine scans were obtained and all patients underwent surgery regardless of the functional status of a nodule, 84% were cold, 10.5% were warm (same as thyroid), and 5.5% of nodules were hot.[98,99] Malignant thyroid disease was documented in 16% of the cold nodules, in 9% of the warm nodules, and in 4% of the hot nodules. Their results indicate that thyroid scanning does not successfully discriminate between benign and malignant thyroid nodules. Cold nodules are more likely to be malignant but hot and warm nodules can also be malignant.[17] However, another group takes strong exception to the claim that hot nodules can be malignant, because they have found no clear evidence for any malignant hot nodules.[100,101] Whether hot thyroid nodules can be malignant or not is not critical, because hot nodules comprise 5.5% of all nodules and only 4% of these are malignant. The problem is that 10% to 20% of cold nodules, which compromise 85% of all nodules, may be malignant, and the nuclide scan can not reliably discriminate benign from malignant nodules in these cases.

Medullary thyroid carcinoma recurrent in the neck following thyroidectomy and in metastatic locations has been imaged using ^{201}Tl ^{99m}Tc scintigraphy.[102,103] This may be useful to image cross recurrent or metastatic disease in patients following thyroid resection who develop elevation of serum calcitonin levels.[102,103] Thallium is a blood pool marker. Because medullary carcinoma and the thyroid are very vascular, ^{201}Tl is concentrated in the tumor and thyroid, but the ^{99m}Tc is concentrated only in thyroid. A computer is used to subtract the technetium scan from the thallium scan to image medullary cancer. However, this same technique has also been used to image parathyroid adenomas, so it is not specific.[104] Metaiodobenzylguanidine (MIBG) labelled with ^{131}I has also successfully imaged primary and metastatic medullary carcinoma.[105,106] ^{131}I-MIBG has been used to image pheochromocytomas, and in one patient with MEN-2a, it also imaged both pheochromocytomas and medullary carcinoma.[105] Subsequently, it was used to image metastatic thyroid carcinoma to bone and liver. The isotope is taken up and incorporated into the medullary cancer cell, so it may be possible to treat metastatic disease with larger doses of ^{131}I-MIBG.[106]

Ultrasonography

Ultrasound examination of the thyroid gland accurately measures the size of a given nodule, whether it is solid or cystic, and the number of nodules.[107,108] Conventional B-mode ultrasound classifies nodules as solid, cystic, or mixed solid–cystic with an accuracy of more than 90%.[107,108] In one large review of 16 series in which conventional techniques were used, 21% of the solid lesions, 12% of the mixed lesions, and only 7% of the cystic lesions were malignant.[98] A solid mass within the thyroid is most often benign, but it also has the highest chance of being malignant. Conversely, a cystic mass is not always benign, but it is more likely to be benign than a solid mass. High-resolution real-time ultrasonography with near-field transducers is being used to image the thyroid gland with great detail, and it can discriminate nodules as small as 1 mm in diameter. The incidence of clinical cancer in these small nodules is not known, and the clinical significance of nodules detected by ultrasonography that are not palpable is unclear. In patients who are at risk for developing radiation-induced thyroid carcinoma, the results of two different groups support conservative management (close observation or aspiration and no resection) of small nodules that are not palpable or barely palpable, which are detected by ultrasonography. The chance of this type of nodule, even in patients with prior irradiation, becoming clinically significant thyroid cancer is very low.[109]

Currently, ultrasonography is not able to distinguish benign from malignant lesions. High-resolution real-time scanning depicts most malignant thyroid tumors as sonolucent, compared with the surrounding echogenic thyroid. Ultrasonography cannot distinguish between malignant and benign tumors. The "halo sign," a thin, sonolucent rim supposedly around a benign tumor, has been observed around both papillary and follicular carcinomas.[110,111] Lymph node metastases from a thyroid neoplasm can be detected and have the sonolucent characteristics of the primary tumor, but nonspecific lymph node enlargement may also appear sonolucent. A dedicated ultrasonographer who is committed to high-resolution thyroid imaging is necessary. The process is noninvasive, sensitive but not specific. It is the most accurate method to measure and follow the exact size of a lesion of a patient on thyroid suppression. Ultrasonography can be used to guide aspiration or biopsy of large lesions (1–3 cm) in the posterior part of the thyroid, which may be clinically significant but not readily palpable. It can detect small foci of medullary carcinoma that appear sonolucent in patients with a family history of MEN-2 or in patients with elevated calcitonin levels.[112] It is more sensitive than physical exam in detecting locally recurrent thyroid carcinoma in high-risk patients following thyroidectomy.[113] Because of its safety, flexibility, and sensitivity and because of its nature as a real-time extension of the physical examination, high-resolution ultrasonography has a role in the evaluation and follow-up of thyroid neoplasms, but information obtained is not specific for cancer.

Biopsy

Fine-needle aspiration biopsy has emerged as the most valuable aid in the diagnosis and management of thyroid nodular disease, because it is safe and inexpensive and has resulted in better selection of patients for surgery.[17] The diagnostic accuracy of cytologic analysis with aspiration biopsy has been low (50%) in some centers and very high (97%) in other centers.[99,114] The experience and technique of the physicians performing the biopsy and of the cytopathologists reading the slides appear to be the major factors influencing results. We use local anesthesia, a syringe holder, and a 25-gauge needle in most instances. The lesion should be fixed between two fingers and the needle placed in the center of the nodule for small (1–2 cm) lesions and at the periphery for larger (2–3 cm), often cystic lesions. We advocate at least six good samples. For a detailed description of the preferred method for aspiration cytology the reader should review Hamburger and Hamburger.[115] Most of the false negatives are caused by inadequate sampling. The problem of obtaining inadequate cytologic specimens decreases with physician experience and number of aspirations, such that satisfactory specimens can be obtained from approximately 95% of nodules.[94,114,116]

Large, rapidly growing lesions (>3 cm in diameter), which are suspected for lymphoma or anaplastic thyroid carcinoma, can be better assessed by cutting needle biopsy.[117,118] In lymphoma of the thyroid, fine-needle aspiration may give a diagnosis of thyroiditis, but a cutting needle biopsy usually provides the correct diagnosis.[118] This is important because surgery is not part of the usual treatment for lymphoma. The fine-needle aspiration and the large-needle biopsy are complementary. In studies analyzing both in the same patient, the biopsy was more reliable than aspiration in that it gave fewer false negative diagnoses.[117,119] Reported false-negative rates for fine-needle aspiration range from 2.2% to 10%.[120] The addition of large-needle biopsy can decrease the false negative rate to 1%.[121] The problem with large-needle cutting biopsy is that small nodules (<2 cm) are not amenable to this technique. Large-needle cutting biopsy has more side-effects than fine-needle aspiration, and in general, it has similar accuracy rates.[109,117] Nevertheless, large-needle cutting biopsy of lesions that are indeterminant on aspiration can result in a more definitive diagnosis.[117,122] We reserve cytologic examination by fine-needle aspiration for the majority of thyroid nodules, but we use large-needle biopsy for larger nodules (> 3 cm), which are more likely to be malignant carcinoma or lymphoma.

When a satisfactory fine-needle aspirate has been obtained, three cytologic results are possible: benign, suspicious, or malignant. Reviewing results from four recent series with a total of 848 patients, 78% of the patients had benign aspirates, 20% had suspicious aspirates, and 12% had malignant aspirates.[123–126] These data indicate improvement in fine-needle aspiration results with more experience, because previous studies included approximately 35% of patients in the suspicious or indeterminant group.[122,127,128] The incidence of thyroid cancer found in studies in which all patients with suspicious lesions underwent surgery ranged from 11% to 71% in different series (Table 39-8). The predictive value of fine-needle aspiration biopsy is affected by whether suspicious lesions are considered positive. If a suspicious nodule is not included in the positive group, then the procedure has few false-positive results, but it also misses many cancers in the suspicious group (22% chance of a suspicious aspirate having cancer). If the suspicious aspirate is included in the positive group, then the cytologic examination can diagnose approximately 97% of thyroid cancers, but the specificity decreases to approximately 70% (Table 39-8).

The difficulty in evaluating suspicious lesions reflects the inability to distinguish benign Hurthle cell and follicular tumors from their malignant counterparts.[127] Papillary carcinoma is less of an analytic problem, except when the sample is poor or diagnostic features of cancer-like psammoma bodies are not present. Repeat aspiration or large-needle biopsy may help. However, with follicular neoplasms, no preoperative evaluation has consistently been able to differentiate benign from malignant tumors. The actual diagnosis does not depend on cell pathology but on invasion of the capsule or blood vessels. This distinction is poorly evaluated by frozen section examination. Attempts have been made to use DNA content, nuclear size, and nuclear ploidy to distinguish malignant follicular neoplasms from benign neoplasms, but conflicting results have been reported.[133–135] In general, surgical excision of all suspicious thyroid nodules is recommended, because the complications of surgery are small (≤ 1%), the chance of malignancy is 20%, and no other method is currently available to identify malignant nodules.

The real benefit of fine-needle aspiration is for the benign aspiration group and the malignant aspiration group. Benign aspiration results were recorded for 78% of patients in four recent studies.[123–126] Only approximately 3% of patients with benign aspiration results will have thyroid cancer, and those cancers can be detected by subsequent aspirations.[123] Therefore, surgical resection is not necessary for patients with benign aspirations and these patients can undergo suppression and careful follow-up evaluations with repeat aspirations. Patients with malignant cytologic results should undergo immediate surgical resection, and they will have approximately an 84% chance of a true malignant lesion. Some researchers advocate surgical resection based solely upon the cytologic examination, rather than frozen section.[124] We do not advocate this strategy, because nearly 20% of aspiration-positive lesions will not be malignant on pathologic analysis.

Fine-needle aspiration has had a substantial impact on the management of thyroid nodules, and it provides far more diagnostic information than any other current diagnostic technique available. Work-up of nodules with history, physical exam, thyroid scan, and ultrasound yielded only 10% to

TABLE 39-8. Accuracy of Preoperative Fine-Needle Aspiration (FNA) Cytology in Six Recent Series

Author (Ref)	*Group*	*FNA (n)*	*Benign (n)*	*Malignant (n)*	*Malignant (%)*
Hawkins et al[128]	Benign	336	326	10	3
	Suspicious	28	13	15	54
	Malignant	51	3	47	92
Harsoulis et al[129]	Benign	150	146	4	3
	Suspicious	14	4	10	71
	Malignant	26	3	23	88
Abu-Nema et al[130]	Benign	89	88	1	1
	Suspicious	28	28	0	0
	Malignant	7	0	7	100
Ramacciotti et al[131]	Benign	87	79	8	9
	Suspicious	15	12	3	20
	Malignant	17	4	13	76
Hamburger et al[115]	Benign				
	Suspicious	149	133	16	11
	Malignant	284	66	218	77
Mayo[115]	Benign				
	Suspicious	233	173	60	26
	Malignant	98	0	98	100
Cumulative experience	Benign	662	639	23	3
	Suspicious	467	363	104	22
	Malignant	483	76	406	84

20% malignancy rates in surgically resected nodules. Fine-needle aspiration has halved the number of patients who undergo operations and has doubled the incidence (40%) of malignant disease confirmed at surgical resection.[17] If the results from two recent studies[123,124] can be reproduced at other institutions, only 20% of patients with nodules would require surgical excision, and if a nodule was excised it would have a 76% chance of being malignant. This increased efficiency would save the health care system about $400 to $750 per patient with a thyroid nodule.[125,126]

Standard Work-up

A careful history of childhood irradiation, the dose or reason for radiation treatment, and the interval from treatment to presentation is the first step in the evaluation of a thyroid nodule. Physical examination of the thyroid gland determines the size and location of any nodule or nodules. Carefully palpate for jugular, supraclavicular, and submandibular lymph nodes. Hoarseness, difficulty swallowing liquids, and dyspnea with exertion necessitate indirect laryngoscopy. Fine-needle aspiration, as previously described, is the initial diagnostic procedure for small lesions (<3 cm). If the cytologic specimens are suspicious or malignant, surgical resection is preferred. If the cytologic specimens are benign, thyroid suppression and follow-up is employed. Ultrasonography is used to measure the exact lesion size before suppression and to be certain no larger thyroid masses or suspicious lymph nodes have been missed. If the lesion appears to be totally cystic on ultrasound, aspiration should completely eliminate it. If the thyroid mass is large (> 3 cm) and there is a history of rapid recent growth plus symptoms related to recurrent laryngeal nerve function, large-needle biopsy is the preferred initial evaluation technique after physical examination. Therapeutic intervention is based on biopsy results.

If the cytologic specimen or the biopsy is benign, ultrasonography is used to measure the mass, and thyroid suppression is started. The responsible physician must be certain that TSH levels are suppressed by the dosage of thyroxine. If the nodule remains unchanged after 6 months, repeat aspirations are evaluated. If the nodule decreases in size, simple follow-up is continued while maintaining exogenous thyroxine. If the nodule increases in size, surgical resection is indicated. Nodule size can be accurately reevaluated by physical examination or ultrasound as necessary. The entire diagnostic approach is outlined in Fig. 39-1.

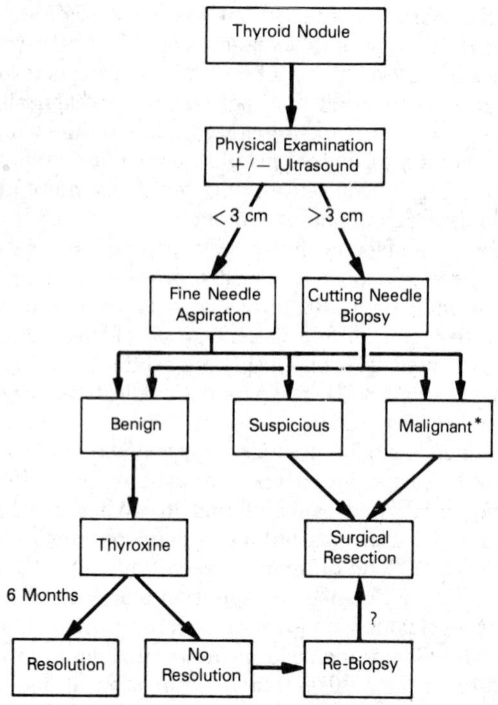

FIG. 39-1. Flow diagram for the evaluation of a thyroid nodule. *Anaplastic thyroid cancer and thyroid lymphoma may not require surgical resection.

TREATMENT

Surgery for Thyroid Nodules

Surgical resection is performed on the assumption that the nodule is a carcinoma. Nodule excision is not performed. Thyroid lobectomy of the ipsilateral thyroid lobe is the procedure of choice for the lobe with the nodule. For isthmus lesions, the isthmus is resected along with the lobe in closer propinquity to the nodule. The pathologist needs to know the relationship of the nodule to the adjacent normal thyroid tissue to make an adequate diagnosis. In the event that a given nodule is malignant and a simple nodulectomy is performed, any reoperation in the same lobe is technically difficult and increases the risk of recurrent laryngeal nerve injury sixfold.[136] The local recurrence rate after a simple nodulectomy, compared with a lobectomy, may be higher because 20% to 40% of well-differentiated carcinomas are multicentric.[127]

The patient is positioned so that the neck is extended by a longitudinal roll between the shoulders. The operating table is flexed, and the patient is in a sitting position. This reduces venous bleeding during the dissection. A horizontal incision is made 2 cm cephalad to the sternal notch in a skin crease. The incision is deepened through the subcutaneous tissue and the platysma muscle. Flaps are raised cephalad to the thyroid notch and caudad to the sternal notch.

The cervical fascia is divided at the midline and deepened to the level of the thyroid and trachea. The strap muscles are mobilized laterally around the thyroid lobe, and the thyroid lobe is mobilized upward and medially. If the strap muscles are densely adherent to the lobe because of tumor invasion (rate situation), the adjacent strap muscle can be removed en bloc with the lobe and tumor. It is imperative to meticulously dissect posterior to the thyroid gland. In this region are the major morbid structures, including the inferior thyroid artery, the recurrent laryngeal nerve, and two parathyroid glands (Fig. 39-2). Attempt to remove the lobe and save the parathyroid glands with intact blood supply, usually from the inferior thyroid artery. If the tumor extends into this area by either direct invasion or lymphatic metastases, then the parathyroid glands on the side of the advanced tumor can be sacrificed, but the recurrent laryngeal nerve should be preserved if possible. Remove any lymph nodes in the central

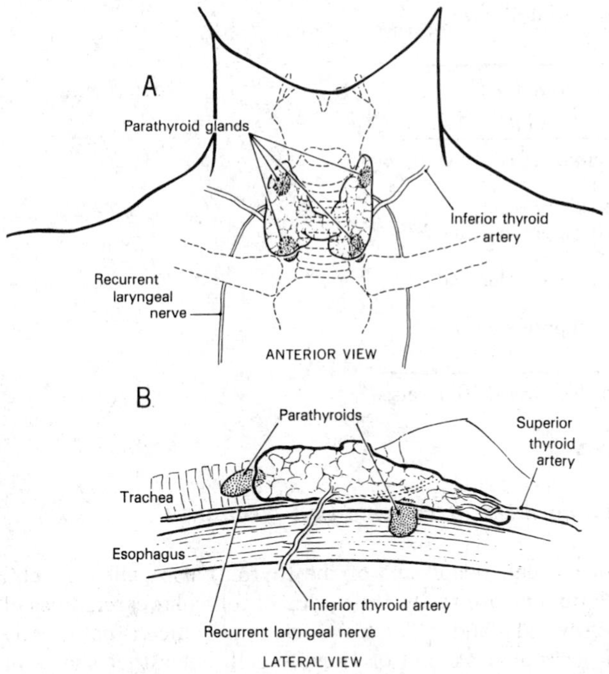

FIG. 39-2. Surgical anatomy of the thyroid and parathyroid gland. **A**. Anterior view. **B**. Lateral view. There are two major arteries to each thyroid lobe, the superior thyroid artery and the inferior thyroid artery. The superior parathyroid glands are superior and lateral to both the recurrent laryngeal nerve and the inferior thyroid artery. The inferior parathyroid glands are inferior and medial to both the recurrent laryngeal nerve and the inferior thyroid artery. The inferior thyroid artery is usually superficial to the recurrent laryngeal nerve, but this anatomical relationship may vary.

cervical neck area (medial to the jugular veins on each side) that are suspicious. If the nodes are unquestionably involved and bulky, removal of the nodes with the thyroid lobe en bloc is preferred.

Once the lobe is removed and the nodule is confirmed as well-differentiated carcinoma on frozen section, a total or near-total thyroidectomy is completed if the nodule is greater than 2 cm, leaving only a small portion of the thyroid gland on the contralateral side to preserve the recurrent laryngeal nerve and the parathyroid glands. If the parathyroid glands are either subcapsular or devascularized, the acceptable procedure is to autograft tissue into the sternocleidomastoid muscle of the contralateral side from the primary tumor.[137,138] Frozen section confirmation that the graft tissue is parathyroid is necessary.

Most studies that have considered the extent of thyroid resection for primary well-differential thyroid carcinoma have concluded that subtotal resection is preferred, especially in patients with small tumors and who are younger than 45 years of age.[139,140] There are no differences in survival or recurrence rates between the total and subtotal thyroidectomy groups, and greater morbidity associated with total thyroidectomy.[141,142] In older patients with larger, locally aggressive or metastatic well-differentiated tumors, near-total or total thyroidectomy is preferred because it lessens the dose and facilitates the administration of ^{131}I.[142] Prospective, randomized trials regarding the extent of resection for thyroid carcinoma have not been done; they may be impossible because of the slow-growing, "benign" nature of the neoplasm in the majority of patients. However, it is absolutely clear that thyroid carcinoma can behave in a very malignant manner in older patients with large tumors and extracapsular invasion.[5–9]

If the nodule is benign on frozen section, malignant and less than 2 cm in diameter, or the pathologist cannot be certain, only one lobe should be removed. The contralateral lobe is exposed and carefully palpated to be certain that no obvious tumors or suspicious nodules are present in it. If permanent pathology results indicate that the nodule removed is malignant, we use the same criteria to remove the contralateral lobe. Large lesions (>2 cm) in patients older than 45 years of age require near-total thyroidectomy. This point is controversial.[4] The risk of a reoperation on the contralateral lobe done approximately 1 week postoperatively is no greater than the same procedure performed at the initial operation.

Surgery for Well-Differentiated Thyroid Cancer

Surgical resection is the method of choice for exact diagnosis and initial treatment of well-differentiated thyroid and medullary thyroid carcinoma. Large-needle biopsy is the method of choice for diagnosis of thyroid lymphoma and anaplastic thyroid carcinoma. Resection may also be indicated for small (<3 cm) thyroid lymphomas and small anaplastic carcinomas, but the vast majority of these malignancies present with large bulky lesions and surgery has no role in treatment.[143,144] The extent of surgical resection and adjuvant treatment for well-differentiated thyroid carcinoma is given in Table 39-9. In general, the use of subtotal or total thyroidectomy is advocated, except in younger patients with nodules less than 2 cm in diameter. In patients undergoing subtotal or total thyroidectomy for well-differentiated thyroid carcinoma, the incidence of disease in the contralateral lobe is between 20% and 87%.[127,145,146] Disease recurs more than twice as often in patients who have had subtotal thyroidectomy than in patients who have had total thyroidectomy, although these local recurrences are not associated with decreased survival.[79] Another argument for total thyroidectomy is the ease of subsequent documentation of recurrent or metastatic disease by thyroglobulin determination or ^{131}I uptake. In addition, ^{131}I ablation dosage is reduced, allowing treatment doses to be administered within a safer range.

Two studies indicate that the postoperative mortality after total thyroidectomy for differentiated thyroid carcinomas is zero, with a 2% to 2.5% incidence of permanent recurrent laryngeal nerve damage and with a 1% to 2.7% incidence of permanent hypoparathyroidism.[147,148] Experienced surgeons can perform total thyroidectomy safely.

In patients with papillary and follicular thyroid carcinoma, TSH suppression of thyroid hormone and ^{131}I ablation following thyroidectomy have each decreased recurrence rates, but neither have improved survival.[79,149] Lymph node metastases at diagnosis are not associated with decreased survival rates, but they are associated with increased local recurrence rates. The correlation of young age with frequent nodal metastases and, conversely, of older age with less frequent nodal metastases supports the suggestion that there is a bio-

TABLE 39-9. Recommended Therapeutic Approach to Well-Differentiated Thyroid Cancer

Patient Age	*Size of Lesion*	*Extrathyroidal Disease*	*Recommended Therapy*
Any	≤2 cm	Absent	Thyroid lobectomy or NTT* with suppression
<45	2–4 cm	Absent	NTT/TT with suppression
≥45	2–4 cm	Absent	NTT/TT with suppression and ^{131}I ablation
Any	>4 cm	Present with direct invasion	NTT/TT with suppression and ^{131}I ablation†
Any	Any	Distant metastases (bone on lung)	NTT/TT with suppression and ^{131}I ablation

*NTT/TT = near total/total thyroidectomy; suppression = thyroxine to decrease TSH levels; ^{131}I = treatment with ^{131}I.
†One may consider additional local radiation therapy.

logic difference between risk groups with thyroid cancer. Even in poor-prognosis older patients with thyroid cancer, lymph node involvement does not influence survival.[9]

In general, the prognosis of well-differentiated thyroid cancer is excellent as long as some degree of thyroid resection is performed. Most groups add thyroxine to suppress TSH and use ^{131}I in certain risk groups. A suggested treatment strategy is listed in Table 39-9. Certain factors indicate more aggressive disease and may dictate more aggressive treatment. The higher risk groups include patients with distant metastases at presentation, older (>45 years) patients, males, patients whose disease has invaded adjacent structures from large primary lesions, and patients whose cancer is follicular.[5-7,150,151] Contrary to previous reports, radiation-induced thyroid carcinoma does not worsen prognosis.[71] It behaves the same as well-differentiated thyroid carcinoma. If surgical resection is performed, with or without thyroxine or ^{131}I, the survival of patients with papillary or follicular thyroid carcinoma is excellent (Table 39-10). The major morbidity and mortality occurs in the 5% minority of elderly patients who present with locally advanced or distant secondary disease. The use of more aggressive therapy may be indicated in this subgroup.

Management of Hurthle Cell Neoplasia

Hurthle cell neoplasms of the thyroid, also called oxyphil cell tumors, are really a subgroup of follicular carcinomas of the thyroid gland.[14] The histologic appearance is not merely an occasional oxyphil or Hurthle cell, but rather sheets of uniform Hurthle cells. The controversy regarding these tumors comes from a single institution's experience in which the authors state that Hurthle cell neoplasms larger than 2 cm, even without vascular or capsular invasion, can result in metastatic or locally recurrent disease and in the death of the patient.[37,38] They indicate that total thyroidectomy for all malignant tumors and for tumors greater than 2 cm in size results in a lower recurrence rate (21% versus 59%) than a historical control group.[38] In addition, Rosen and others indicate that, following total thyroidectomy, 9% of patients with Hurthle cell malignancies had carcinoma in the contralateral lobe, and following lobectomy, 12% of patients developed contralateral lobe tumors.[152] Therefore, the incidence of bilateral malignant Hurthle cell neoplasms was approximately 10%.[152]

Review of eight recent series indicate that the majority of Hurthle cell neoplasms appear benign pathologically; that is,

TABLE 39-10. Survival of Well-Differentiated Thyroid Carcinoma After Surgical Resection ± Ablation or Suppression, or Both

Group (Ref)	*n*	*5-Year Survival*	*10-Year Survival*	*20-Year Survival*
Papillary				
Schroder et al[142]	104	97%		
McConahey et al[127]	859			93%
Mazzaferri et al[79]	576		92.4%	
Joensuu et al[5]	121	92%	74%	
Radiation-Induced Papillary				
Schneider et al[62]	296		99%	
Follicular				
Schroder et al[142]	23	96%		
Lang et al[150]	170		94%	
Harness et al[151]	37		84%	
Crile et al[33]	84	73%	43%	
Joensuu et al[5]	46	87%	66%	

TABLE 39-11. Incidence, Recurrence Rates, and Late Metastases in Patients with Hurthle Cell Neoplasm of the Thyroid Gland

Author (Ref)	*Patients with Hurthle Cell Tumors (benign and malignant)*	*Patients with Benign Tumors (%)*	*% Recurrence Rate in Malignant Tumors*	*% Recurrence Rate in Benign Tumors*
Thompson[37] and Gundry[38]	62	26 (42)	29	12
Heppe[154]	20	10 (50)		0
Savino[155]	42	27 (64)	53	0
Rosen[152]	34	25 (73)		0
Bondeson[156]	42	34 (81)	25	0
Arganini[153]	47	40 (85)	43	2.5
Caplan[157]	27	24 (88)	33	0
Gosain[158]	75	71 (95)	25	0
Total	349		35	2

Adapted from Arganini M, Behar R, Wu TC et al: Hurthle cell tumors: a twenty-five-year experience. Surgery 100:1108, 1986.

they do not have vascular or capsular invasion (Table 39-11). The recurrence rate in tumors that are diagnosed as malignant is between 25% and 53%, with a mean rate of 35%. The recurrence rate in benign tumors is between 0 and 12%, with a mean rate of 2% (Table 39-11). The majority of Hurthle cell neoplasms are benign and act benign after thyroid lobectomy. If the pathologists diagnose a malignant Hurthle cell carcinoma, they are accurate because there is a higher incidence of recurrent disease; therefore, total or near-total thyroidectomy is advocated for selected Hurthle cell carcinomas proven pathologically malignant, but total thyroidectomy should not be performed for benign Hurthle cell neoplasms.

Radiation-Induced Thyroid Carcinoma

Considerable evidence exists that clinically inapparent thyroid cancer, even radiation-induced occult thyroid cancer, runs an indolent course and does not result in morbidity or mortality. There is evidence from autopsy studies of increased papillary cancer in patients exposed to prior radiation, but the clinical course of that cancer was benign and the patients died of other causes.[10,12] Stockwell and others advocated not scanning patients with a history of head and neck irradiation, but merely re-examining them at 2-year intervals for the development of thyroid nodules.[159] Schneider and others reviewed their experience with radiation-induced thyroid carcinoma, compared with thyroid carcinoma in patients with no history of head and neck irradiation, and found that patients with prior thyroid irradiation more often presented with bilateral thyroid lobe involvement and metastatic disease ($p < 0.005$).[160] However, the prognosis for well-differentiated thyroid cancer in patients with a history of irradiation was similar to patients with the same extent of disease but without such a history.[160] These data underline the importance of careful follow-up with physical examination and of serial serum thyroglobulin levels as a predictor of new malignancy.[85]

If a patient has a history of head and neck irradiation, other risk factors make certain subgroups more likely to develop cancer, including receiving higher doses, being female, and being young at the time of irradiation. Some groups recommend total thyroidectomy for all radiation-induced thyroid carcinomas because the incidence of bilaterality is high (54–75%).[161] However, a recent prospective study indicated that, although thyroid lobectomy may leave occult malignancies in unresected thyroid tissue, there was no significant difference in outcome between limited resection and total thyroidectomy after a 12-year follow-up.[162]

The administration of thyroid hormone to suppress TSH levels reduced the number of postresection recurrences in radiation-induced papillary and follicular carcinoma.[71] Reductions in recurrence rate could not be linked to the extent of surgical resection performed or the administration of postoperative radioactive iodine, which has been advocated in all radiation-induced carcinomas.[71,163] It appears that the clinical course of radiation-induced thyroid carcinomas is similar to other neoplasms without a history of radiation (Table 39-10) and that the therapy should be similar to that for other well-differentiated thyroid carcinomas (Table 39-9).

Postoperative Therapy and Follow-up

There is reasonably good evidence that all patients with well-differentiated thyroid cancer should take thyroid hormone postoperatively to suppress TSH levels.[79,149] This treatment is also able to decrease recurrence of radiation-induced thyroid carcinoma.[71] Reduced recurrence rates with the use of thyroxine postoperatively do not appear to translate into improved survival times, but studies have not demonstrated a negative impact of thyroxine on survival.[79,149,164] We recommend the postoperative administration of thyroxine to suppress TSH levels in all patients with thyroid carcinoma (Table 39-9).

The use of postoperative ^{131}I therapy has decreased recurrence rates but not prolonged survival.[88,156] Ablative doses of ^{131}I (30 mCi) should be administered postoperatively for both papillary and follicular primary lesions that occur in patients who are older than 45 years; whose lesions are multiple, locally invasive, and larger than 2.5 cm; and who have local or distant metastases, provided adequate uptake of the radionuclide can be demonstrated.[163]

Locally recurrent disease in the neck detected by physical examination or ultrasonography should be surgically excised if the procedure can be performed with low morbidity. Radical neck dissections are not indicated for differentiated thyroid carcinoma. Radiation therapy may be of help for less-differentiated recurrent or locally advanced lesions (see Treatment of Anaplastic Carcinoma).

Metastatic thyroid carcinoma confined to the lung has been successfully treated by ^{131}I, and 54% of patients were alive and without disease 20 years after ^{131}I treatment.[165] In contrast, no patient with bony involvement treated by ^{131}I has survived more than 10 years after treatment.[165] Following a successful ablation and failure to find extrathyroidal uptake, the patient is placed on thyroid hormone replacement and TSH levels are measured to ensure suppression. The patient is not rescanned again if the ablation was successful, unless serum thyroglobulin levels are persistently elevated or become elevated, suggesting recurrent or persistent disease.[166] The side effects of ^{131}I therapy, in order of frequency, include temporary bone marrow suppression, nausea, sialadenitis, pain in metastatic deposits, vomiting, pulmonary fibrosis, and leukemia.[166] Most authorities use a therapeutic dose of 100 to 200 mCi to treat recurrent or metastatic disease, which may be repeated several times.

A reasonable limiting factor is 200 rad to blood, and 1 mCi of ^{131}I gives 0.67 rad to blood, so 300 mCi would be the maximum tolerable dosage. When bulk disease or distant metastatic disease exists, dosimetry is required to allow maximal dose with minimal risk. In patients with metastatic disease that concentrates iodine, the mean radiation dose to metastases exceeds 100,000 rad.[167]

Hematologic complications, including hypoplasia and leukemia, may occur when the total dose exceeds 800 mCi.[165,168] Women have had normal pregnancies and deliveries following a total dosage between 500 and 600 mCi.

Survival rates from time of discovery of lung or bone metastases from differentiated thyroid carcinoma in a recent analysis of 283 patients indicate that 53% were alive at 5 years, 38% at 10 years, and 30% at 15 years.[168] Four variables had independent prognostic significance for survival: extensive metastases, older age at discovery of metastases, absence of ^{131}I uptake by metastases, and follicular cell type.[168] These variables were documented in another study, which also reported that pulmonary metastases occurred less often in patients treated initially by total thyroidectomy than in those treated with subtotal thyroidectomy.[169]

These results suggest that the aim of management of patients with differentiated thyroid carcinoma following surgery should be to detect and treat metastases as early as possible. The incidence of pulmonary metastases are lowest in patients with papillary carcinoma (9%), intermediate with follicular carcinoma (13%), and highest with Hurthle cell carcinoma (25%).[169] Surgical resection of distant metastases from differentiated thyroid carcinoma have been advocated by some.[170] Indications for resection included reduced administration of ^{131}I, pain, and pathologic fracture. Estimated cumulative survival rate (Kaplan-Meier) from resection was 45% for 5 years and 33% for 20 years after removal of a solitary metastasis.[170] This heroic treatment may be indicated for solitary metastasis to bone or lung that do not take up ^{131}I.

Management of Medullary Thyroid Carcinoma

In 1959, Hazard, Hawk, and Crile described medullary thyroid carcinoma as a distinct clinical and pathological entity. This neoplasm presents in sporadic form (nonfamilial) and is associated with three clinical syndromes: MEN-2a, MEN-2b, and familial non-MEN medullary thyroid carcinoma, a disease characterized by hereditary medullary cancer without associated endocrinopathies.[48,72] In the three familial presentations, the disease is nearly always bilateral and requires a total thyroidectomy and central lymph node dissection. When the disease presents sporadically, it is usually unilateral, but it still requires the same operation because the familial disease cannot be ruled out by history alone. In MEN-2a and MEN-2b, the medullary thyroid carcinoma is associated with pheochromocytoma, a potentially life-threatening situation if an unprepared patient undergoes anesthetic stress for thyroidectomy. For this reason, whenever the preoperative diagnosis of medullary cancer is indicated either by abnormal serum calcitonin levels or cutting needle biopsy, pheochromocytoma must be ruled out by measurement of 24 hour urine samples for VMA, metanephrines, and catecholamines or by serum norepinephrine and epinephrine levels.[48]

If suspected from the family history, the early diagnosis of C-cell hyperplasia, C-cell carcinoma in situ, or medullary carcinoma confined to the thyroid gland can be made by provocative testing with calcium and pentagastrin. An abnormal response is a rise in plasma calcitonin levels after administering these agents. Plasma calcitonin levels (basal and stimulated) increase as extent of disease increases. In 25 patients from kindreds with medullary carcinoma who had undetectable basal calcitonin levels and who had levels less than 1000 pg/ml following pentagastrin-calcium stimulation, 24 of 25 had disease localized to the thyroid gland and were cured following total thyroidectomy.[171] Telander and colleagues have demonstrated that medullary carcinoma is present in children from kindreds at a mean age of 7 years (range, 1.5–12 years). Total thyroidectomy in 17 children cured 14 of 17, the three with persistent disease had MEN-2b.[172] Provocative testing helps in kindreds with MEN-2a and familial non-MEN medullary carcinoma, but it is usually not helpful in patients with MEN-2b. In MEN-2b, the disease usually presents as a palpable neck mass in childhood, and carcinoma has spread outside the thyroid gland at presentation. These patients are seldom cured by surgery alone.[49]

Sporadic medullary carcinoma usually presents as a neck mass, and the diagnosis can be obtained by fine-needle aspiration, cutting needle biopsy, or measurement of serum calcitonin. Serum calcitonin is a specific, sensitive circulating marker for medullary carcinoma, but it is usually not measured as part of the work-up of a thyroid nodule. Patients with sporadic disease usually present with lymph node metastases or extrathyroidal disease, and they are not usually cured by surgery. High-resolution real-time ultrasonography can be used to accurately stage the extent of disease in the necks of these patients. The cancer appears bright and echogenic and is detectable within the thyroid or lymph nodes.[173]

The only significant predictor of survival following resection of primary medullary carcinoma is tumor invasion beyond the thyroid capsule or metastases to cervical lymph nodes.[174] The overall survival following surgical resection varies, but the ten-year survival is between 40% and 60%.[14,174]

Several studies have reported attempts to localize and resect lymph nodes containing micro- or macroscopic medullary carcinoma following thyroidectomy. One study described selective venous catheterization and pentagastrin stimulation to detect disease and regions draining calcitonin.[175] Another study used additional extensive neck dissections following thyroidectomy to remove tumor in lymph nodes.[176] Both studies were able to remove medullary carcinoma in clinically normal-appearing lymph nodes, and both were able to normalize postoperative basal calcitonin levels, but whether either method will influence subsequent survival is not yet proved.[175,176] Several groups have used thallium/technetium scanning to detect recurrent disease and to advocate resection of recurrent or persistent macroscopic disease.[102,103] Whether resection of local or distant metastases increases survival is not clear because of the indolent course of this neoplasm.

The tragedy of not detecting medullary carcinoma confined to the thyroid gland, when it is surgically curable, can be appreciated by considering the ineffectiveness of nonoperative treatment of recurrent or metastatic disease.[48] Chemotherapy has had little utility. Gottlieb and Hill reported remissions in 3 of 5 patients with metastatic disease, but these results have not been confirmed by others.[177,178] Cis-platinum, streptozotocin, BCNU, methotrexate, and 5-fluorouracil have all been used without benefit.[48]

Iodine-131 has been reported as an adjunct to surgery when postoperative plasma calcitonin levels remain elevated.[179,180] Iodine-131 is taken up by the remaining follicular cells, and the adjacent C cells are indirectly irradiated. Each of the above studies describe a case in which plasma calcitonin levels decreased following postoperative ^{131}I therapy. Another report documented a minimal response in one patient with metastatic medullary carcinoma treated with ^{131}I and lithium administration, which slowed whole-body turnover of iodine.[181] The physiology of C cells suggest that they would not transport iodine, so ^{131}I is a poor treatment for metastatic disease. If meticulous total thyroidectomy and central node dissection have been performed, minimal normal thyroid tissue will remain, therefore, radioiodine is seldom indicated. The fact that metastatic and recurrent medullary carcinoma takes up ^{131}I-MIBG indicates its potential for treating metastatic disease, but no studies have been reported.

Radiation therapy for localized, inaccessible tumors may be useful in patients with medullary cancer.[182,183] Steinfeld reported local control of disease in 3 of 5 patients with widespread metastases.[183] Sensitizers may increase radiation efficacy, but limited data are available. In general, medullary carcinoma is radioresistant and potential benefits from radiation therapy must be weighed against complications.

Patients with metastatic disease may be without symptoms, even with substantial tumor burdens. The most bothersome symptom that patients with metastatic medullary carcinoma develop is severe, voluminous secretory diarrhea, which generally develops when plasma calcitonin levels exceed 20 ng/ml. The cause of this diarrhea is unknown. It may be due to calcitonin or some other tumor-produced hormone because malignant C cells can secrete many different hormones.[48,184] This symptom is especially bothersome because it is not controlled by medical regimens. In some cases, debulking of grossly evident tumor will ameliorate the diarrhea. One patient with metastatic disease, elevated pancreatic polypeptide levels, and severe refractory diarrhea responded with complete resolution of the diarrhea to the long-acting somatostatin analog SMS-201-995.[185]

Management of Anaplastic Thyroid Carcinoma

Prognosis for anaplastic thyroid carcinoma is poor, and most patients with this diagnosis are dead within one year, with a median survival of 4 months.[186] Thyroid carcinoma has in its clinical manifestations a true paradox: it is a cancer that in its differentiated form may be one of the most benign types and in its undifferentiated form may be one of the most malignant forms.[1,186] Surgical resection is indicated for small tumors or tumors in which it is technically feasible; however, the majority of tumors are unresectable at presentation.[144] If the tumor is large and apparently unresectable, cutting-needle biopsy is recommended to establish the diagnosis. Radiotherapy alone has not been useful for anaplastic thyroid carcinoma; however, the combination of doxorubicin as a sensitizer and 5760 rad delivered in fractions over 40 days has had dramatic control rates for local anaplastic giant and spindle cell carcinoma of the thyroid gland.[187] The regimen consists of one weekly low dose of doxorubicin (10 mg/m^2) and hyperfractionated radiation therapy. The radiation therapy is carried out with fractional doses of 160 rad per treatment, twice a day for three days each week. Eight of nine patients achieved complete tumor regression in the primary area, and six remained disease free in the neck until death.[187] Of 8 patients with locally advanced differentiated thyroid carcinoma who were given the same treatment regimen, seven of eight achieved complete tumor regression.[188] The regimen produced no disproportionate morbidity of normal tissue. This regimen appears to be a real breakthrough for the treatment of locally advanced anaplastic or differentiated thyroid carcinoma. It remains to be seen whether other groups using the same regimen get similar results.

Drug therapy for advanced thyroid carcinoma or anaplastic thyroid carcinoma has been disappointing. Regimens with doxorubicin have shown the highest response rates, and doxorubicin is the best single agent (Table 39-12). Cisplatin and bleomycin have also had some activity. Two recent trials using these agents in advanced thyroid carcinoma had conflicting results. The combination of doxorubicin (60 mg/m^2) plus cisplatin (60 mg/m^2) had only 2 (9%) partial remissions in 22 evaluable patients with advanced thyroid cancer.[189] These results were inconsistent with a previous study, which showed that doxorubicin plus cisplatin was significantly better than doxorubicin alone in a similar group of patients with advanced thyroid carcinoma.[190] Eighty-four evaluable patients were stratified by histologic type and ran-

TABLE 39-12. Chemotherapy for Thyroid Carcinoma

Drugs	*First Author (ref)*	*Number of Evaluable Patients*	*Number of Responders (%)*	*Number of Complete Responders (%)*
Doxorubicin alone	Gottlieb[177]	43	15 (35)	
Doxorubicin alone	Shimaoka[190]	41	7 (17)	0
Doxorubicin plus cisplatin	Shimaoka[190]	43	11 (26)	5 (12)
Doxorubicin plus cisplatin	Williams[189]	22	2 (9)	0
Doxorubicin plus bleomycin plus vincristine plus melphalan	Bukowski[191]	11	4 (36)	1 (19)
Doxorubicin plus vincristine plus bleomycin	Sokal[194]	14	9 (64)	0

domized to doxorubicin alone (60 mg/m² IV every 3 weeks) or combination doxorubicin (60 mg/m²) and cisplatin (40 mg/m² IV every 3 weeks). The total dose of doxorubicin was 550 mg/m². Forty-one patients received doxorubicin alone and seven had partial responses (17%). Forty-three patients received the combination, and there were 5 complete and 6 partial responses (26%, NS). However, 5 complete responses in the combination group was significantly better than no complete responses in the doxorubicin alone group ($p = 0.03$), including 3 complete responders of 18 with anaplastic carcinoma, and an overall response rate in anaplastic carcinoma of 33%. Four of 5 complete responders survived for more than 2 years. The toxicity was similar in the two-drug regimens, and the results indicated that doxorubicin plus cisplatin was better than doxorubicin alone.[190] Bukowski and others treated 11 patients with advanced thyroid carcinoma with the combination of doxorubicin, bleomycin, vincristine, and melphalan.[191] They reported a response rate of 4 (36%) of 11, with one durable complete responder, a patient with anaplastic carcinoma.[191]

The findings of durable complete response in patients with anaplastic carcinoma are provocative. One worrisome potential diagnostic problem is thyroid lymphoma, which may mask as anaplastic carcinoma.[192,193] The differential diagnosis and treatment of thyroid lesions must include lymphoma, which is discussed in the chapter on lymphoma.[195–202] It is conceivable that there are subsets of patients with advanced or anaplastic thyroid carcinoma that will respond to combination chemotherapy. Patients with anaplastic thyroid carcinoma are rare, and it will take cooperative trials to answer questions about certain regimens.

THE PARATHYROID GLAND

One hundred years ago a Swedish student named Ivan Sandstrom discovered the parathyroid glands and described their macroscopic and microscopic characteristics in humans and in several animals.[203] Several decades passed before it was discovered that a hormone secreted by these glands controlled the level of blood calcium. Subsequently, it was discovered that calcitonin, vitamin D, and parathyroid hormone (PTH) all maintained calcium homeostasis. Diseases of parathyroid glands are usually manifested by hyperfunction, characterized by glandular enlargement, elevated serum PTH levels, and hypercalcemia.

Hyperparathyroidism is a common disease, the prevalence of which is between 1 and 5 per 1000 persons. An increased incidence of hyperparathyroidism has been reported in individuals who have been previously exposed to irradiation of the head and neck.[204] The parathyroid tumor associated with prior radiation is adenoma. Patients usually present with symptoms related to increased urinary excretion of calcium (urinary calculi and/or nephrocalcinosis) or demineralization of bony skeleton (bone pain or elevated serum alkaline phosphatase). The diagnosis of primary hyperparathyroidism is established biochemically by concomitant serial elevations of serum calcium levels and inappropriately elevated serum parathyroid hormone levels. Elevated urinary cyclic adenosine monophosphate (UcAMP) levels are also present in 92% of patients with primary hyperparathyroidism.[205] Once the diagnosis is established, surgical exploration is generally recommended and the extent of surgery depends on the cause of the hyperparathyroidism.

The three possible causes of primary hyperparathyroidism and their incidences are adenoma (83%), hyperplasia (15%), and carcinoma (1–2%). Parathyroid hyperplasia means multiple gland involvement, and it can be inherited as part of two familial syndromes (MEN-1, MEN-2a). Parathyroid adenomas are the most common cause of primary hyperparathyroidism, and they require identification and simple excision of the tumor. Parathyroid carcinomas are rare, and they require identification and resection of the tumor along with the ipsilateral lobe of the thyroid and abnormal central nodal tissue. The diagnosis of parathyroid carcinoma can be confusing.

Parathyroid carcinoma has been reported in three patients of several families with familial hyperparathyroidism. This is rare and implies transformation of hyperplastic parathyroid tissue into carcinoma.[206,207] Parathyroid carcinoma usually presents in the fourth decade. The hallmark preoperative signs are severe hypercalcemia (serum calcium >15 mg/dl), palpable neck mass, and bone and renal disease.[208] Parathyroid adenomas rarely present with palpable tumors, and calcium levels are usually significantly lower, although similar hypercalcemia can be seen with parathyroid adenomas.[209] The principal histologic features of parathyroid carcinoma that distinguish it from adenoma are a trabecular pattern, mitotic figures, thick fibrous bands, and capsular and blood vessel invasion.[208] The major problems with parathyroid carcinoma is intraoperative recognition of the pathology and performance of an appropriate resection procedure, including ipsilateral thyroid lobectomy and dissection of the central lymph node region.[210]

In two series of 28 patients and 70 patients, the 5-year survival was 44% and 29%, respectively, and the 10-year survival was 22% and 15%, respectively.[211,212] This is in marked distinction to another series of only 9 patients in which 8 of 9 patients were alive after a median follow-up period of 6 years.[210]

Distant metastases develop in lung, bone, and liver.[212,213] Radiation therapy has been unsuccessful at controlling primary and metastatic lesions.[212,213] Bukowski and colleagues reported a single patient with metastatic lesions who had a complete remission for 5 months after a combination of fluorouracil (500 mg/m^2), cyclophosphamide (500 mg/m^2), and dacarbazine (DTIC, 200 mg/m^2).[214] Another group also documented a dramatic response of metastatic parathyroid carcinoma to DTIC.[215]

The major morbidity factor of recurrent or metastatic parathyroid carcinoma is severe hypercalcemia, which is difficult to control medically and will eventually kill the patient. Aggressive surgical resection of bulk recurrent or metastatic disease has been advocated because of the indolent, slow-growing nature of the tumor and because of the potential to control hypercalcemia.[216] Unfortunately, surgery is not always possible or successful, especially if the carcinoma has metastasized widely. Attempts to inhibit the actions of parathyroid hormone with calcitonin, mithramycin, or diphosphonates have also been disappointing. The diphosphonates appear to be the most promising, but investigations in this area are preliminary.[212]

The crucial point in therapy of parathyroid carcinoma is proper intraoperative identification of malignancy and appropriate initial surgery. The characteristics that distinguish patients at risk preoperatively, as well as intraoperative malignant tumor characteristics which ensure a correct diagnosis, are listed in Table 39-13. If malignant parathyroid neoplasms are recognized and proper initial resections performed, a greater number of patients will be cured. The comments of Albright regarding surgery for hyperparathyroidism have held true for more than 50 years: "There is no time like the initial operation to find and remove the tumor."[217]

TABLE 39-13. Hyperparathyroidism: Etiology, Incidences, Diagnostic Features, and Long-Term Results

Diagnosis	*Etiology*	*Relative Frequency*	*Palpable Neck Mass and/or Vocal Cord Paralysis*	*Serum Calcium Level (mg/dl)*	*Parathyroid Hormone*	*Gross Pathology*	*Surgical Procedure*	*Microscopic Pathology*	*Recurrent* Hyperparathyroidism*
Hyperplasia	Familial pattern	14%	Absent	12	Elevated	Multiple gland enlargement, soft reddish brown appearance	Either 3.5 gland resection or 4 gland resection with autograft	Decreased fat content and increased gland cellularity in multiple glands	Intermediate (10%–30%)
Adenoma	Associated with prior irradiation	85%	Absent	12	Elevated	Single gland enlargement, soft reddish brown appearance	Excision of abnormal gland	Decreased fat content increased cellularity occasionally attached normal parathyroid gland	Low (<1%)
Carcinoma	? familial pattern	1%	Usually Present	>14	Elevated	Single enlarged gland that is firm, and whitish gray	Resection of abnormal gland in continuity with ipsilateral thyroid lobe and suspicious central lymph nodes	Trabecular pattern mitotic figures thick fibrous bands capsular and blood vessel invasion	High (>50%)

*Recurrent means that patient has normal serum calcium levels postoperatively and more than 6 months later develops recurrent hypercalcemia.

THE ADRENAL GLAND

HISTORY

Modern knowledge of adrenal physiology began in 1855 with Thomas Addison, who was the first to describe adrenal insufficiency in humans. The following year, Brown-Sequard demonstrated in animal experiments that the adrenals are essential for life. In 1896, Sir William Osler treated one patient with Addison's disease (adrenal insufficiency) with suprarenal extract and noted temporary benefit. Cushing's disease was first described in 1912, when Harvey Cushing wrote his monograph, *The Pituitary Body and its Disorders.* In 1933, both Kendall and Grollman independently obtained crystals from adrenal cortex extracts with adrenal cortical hormone-like activity. In 1949, the Mayo Clinic and Merck succeeded in producing "compound E" for the treatment of rheumatic fever. Thorn and Forsham used cortisone acetate to treat Addison's disease but noted salt-losing and supplemented it with sodium chloride. The naturally secreted hormone cortisol (hydrocortisone) was first synthesized in 1950 by Wendler.[218]

Aldosterone was isolated in 1952 from adrenal cortex by Grundy and colleagues. In 1955, Jerome Conn described a syndrome of primary aldosteronism, caused by excessive secretion of aldosterone by a benign cortical adenoma. In 1962, Bartter and colleagues described hyperplasia of the juxtaglomerular complex with secondary hyperaldosteronism.[218]

In 1805, Currier confirmed that the adrenal gland was composed of both medulla and cortex. Felix Fraenkel described a patient with an adrenal tumor and pressor attacks in 1886, and the first successful removal of a pheochromocytoma was done by Charles Mayo in 1927. Adrenaline was isolated from the adrenal medulla, and its structure determined and synthesized by three different groups in 1924. Ulf Swante von Euler won the Nobel Prize in 1970 for demonstrating that noradrenaline was the main transmitter of sympathetic nerve impulses. The association of medullary thyroid carcinoma with bilateral pheochromocytomas was first described in 1961 by John H. Sipple.[218]

PATHOLOGY OF THE ADRENAL CORTEX

Hyperplasia

Hyperplasia is defined as an increased number of cells in an organ.[219] It is a pathologic change associated with increased function or compensatory change. In pituitary-based hypercortisolism (Cushing's disease), which is the most common endogenous form of hypercortisolism, the gross adrenal enlargement is not impressive. The adrenal gland is approximately twice its normal size. The weight of each adrenal, normally between 3 and 6 g, may reach 6 to 8 g, and occasionally the weight reaches 12 g. Microscopically, there is a widened inner zone of the compact zona reticularis and a sharply demarcated outer zone of clear cells. The appearance of adrenal glands in ectopic ACTH syndrome is similar, except that the glands are usually larger, weighing at least 12 g, and maybe 30 g. Bilateral adrenal hyperplasia with increased aldosterone production must be ruled out in the search for an aldosteronoma because removal of one adrenal will not ameliorate the clinical situation.[220] Macronodular adrenal hyperplasia, consisting of 3-cm adrenal nodules weighing between 30 g and 100 g, usually is a secondary response of the adrenal to ACTH. Micronodular adrenal hyperplasia with 1- to 5-mm pigmented nodules, is more likely to be autonomous and occur in children, including infants. ACTH levels are low or undetectable. Although rare, this can occur in a familial pattern.[221,222]

Adrenal Cortical Adenoma

Adrenal adenoma is a benign neoplasm of adrenal cortical cells resembling normal adrenal cells histologically but possessing functional autonomy.[219] In general, an adenoma usually does not exceed 5 cm in its largest dimension, although benign tumors exceeding 10 cm have been reported. A 100-gram weight has been suggested as the upper limit for benign adenomas. Some cellular pleomorphism and tumor necrosis may be present but is rare. It is not possible to describe the exact functional neoplasm based solely on histology, although there are consistent indications. Adenomas produce syndromes of hypercortisolism and hyperaldosteronism, but seldom produce adrenogenital syndromes. Larger tumors producing adrenogenital syndromes are evidence for carcinoma, as are pleomorphism, tumor necrosis, and mitotic activity.[223] The prognosis of adrenal cortical adenomas producing Cushing's syndrome is excellent, and successful resection invariably produces a cure. The prognosis for adrenal cortical adenomas producing hyperaldosteronism is less favorable. Resection is followed by a response in blood pressure and correction of hypokalemia; however, 30% of patients with aldosteronomas resected develop recurrent hypertension, but not recurrent hypokalemia. Of course, if the preoperative diagnosis was incorrect and the patient had hyperaldosteronism secondary to hyperplasia, unilateral adrenalectomy will not improve the syndrome. Adenomas that produce the adrenogenital syndrome have the least favorable outcome, probably because many of these tumors are really misdiagnosed carcinomas, which will develop local recurrence or metastases.[223]

Adrenal Cortical Carcinoma

Adrenal cortical carcinoma is a malignant neoplasm of adrenal cortical cells demonstrating partial or complete histologic and functional differentiation.[219] Adrenal cortical carcinomas are rare. They only comprise between 0.05% and 0.2% of all cancers.[224,225] This translates to a rate of only 2 per million in the world population.[226] Women appear to develop functional adrenal cortical carcinomas more commonly than men, but men develop nonfunctioning malignant adrenal tumors more commonly than women.[224] There is a bimodal occurrence by age, with a peak incidence at less that 5 years and a second peak in the fourth and fifth decades. Adrenocortical carcinoma has been described as part of a complex hereditary syndrome that includes sarcoma, breast, and lung cancers.[227]

Cytogenetic analysis of primary adrenocortical carcinoma revealed clonal rearrangements of several autosomes and sex chromosomes. In all metaphases the following marker chromosomes were present: 4 pt, t(3;12) (p14;p13), 14q+, t(15;20)(p11;q11), t(5;18)(p13.3;p11.2), psu dic (18) t(18;3) (p11.39;p12), and psu dic (20) t(20;9) (q11.2;p11).[228]

Adrenal cortical carcinomas weigh between 100 and 5000 g. Areas of necrosis and hemorrhage are common and are consistent with malignancy. Invasion and metastases are also common. Microscopically, their appearance is variable, even within the same tumor. The presence of cells with big nuclei, hyperchromatism, and enlarged nucleoli are all consistent with malignancy.[219] Nuclear changes are more common in tumors larger than 500 g. Vascular invasion and clear mitoses are diagnostic of adrenocortical malignancy. Broad desmoplastic bands are associated with increased metastatic potential.

Twenty-one patients with adrenocortical carcinoma were separated by the extent of cellular pleomorphism into anaplastic and differentiated groups. Anaplastic tumors occurred more commonly in men, produced more frequent cutaneous metastases, and were more often associated with a lack of clinical or laboratory evidence of hormone production. In contrast, differentiated adrenal carcinoma usually occurred in women and produced clinical or laboratory evidence of hormonal excess. Median survival time of patients with anaplastic adrenal carcinoma was only 5 months, whereas median survival of patients with differentiated carcinoma was 40 months ($p = 0.005$). Patients with differentiated carcinoma lived for long periods with metastatic disease and more commonly had objective responses to mitotane (o,p-DDD) chemotherapy.[230]

The diagnosis of malignancy in adrenal cortical neoplasms is difficult, especially in tumors that weigh between 50 g and 100 g. In addition, the distinction between adrenal carcinoma and renal carcinoma can be difficult. However, immunostaining for vimentin, epithelial membrane antigen, cytokeratin, and blood group antigens can separate the two diagnoses. Adrenal carcinoma and adenoma stain positive for vimentin while renal carcinoma is negative for vimentin but positive for the others.[231] Table 39-14 attempts to differentiate between benign and malignant tumors based on criteria suggested by Page, DeLellis, and Hough of the Armed Forces Institute of Pathology.[219] Because the immunostaining profiles of adrenocortical carcinoma and adenoma are similar, the pathologist must still rely on clinical and morphological criteria.[231] Although the difference in natural history between benign and malignant adrenal cortical neoplasms is clear, it is not always possible to reliably separate them. The only reliable, single criterion is the presence of nodal or distant metastases. The data used to differentiate benign from malignant adrenocortical neoplasms include hormone production, amount of tumor necrosis, fibrosis, vascular invasion, mitoses, and tumor weight. In a series of 43 adrenocortical tumors analyzed using the histologic criteria outlined, mitotic activity and venous invasion correlated best with metastasizing or recurring (i.e., carcinoma) tumors.[232] In addition, cells from carcinomas produce abnormal amounts of androgens and 11-deoxysteroids and have a minimal response to ACTH compared with cells from benign adenomas.[233] Only 10% of malignant tumors are associated with masculinization and 12% with feminization, the rest usually produce a combination of hormones, including aldosterone.

Cushing's Syndrome or Hypercortisolism

Hypercortisolism results in the diverse signs and symptoms of Cushing's syndrome. Nearly every organ in the body is affected, and there is no single symptom or sign that is common to every patient with endogenous hypercortisolism.[234] Although hypercortisolism is the most common presentation for adrenal cortical neoplasms, Cushing's syndrome is rare, with an estimated incidence of only 10 per 1 million persons.[234]

The most common cause of hypercortisolism is iatrogenic administration of steroids to treat other diseases. Hypercortisolism is not usually associated with MEN-1, although it can be present in this familial syndrome.[235] It is present in 5% of patients with sporadic Zollinger-Ellison syndrome (ZES) and in 19% of patients with ZES and MEN-1.[234,236]

The clinical features of hypercortisolism are listed in Table 39-15. Progressive weight gain is the most universal symptom of patients with hypercortisolism. Obesity is usually truncal, and patients demonstrate thin extremities due to muscle wasting.[237] Increased fat in the dorsal neck region, combined with dorsal kyphosis as a result of osteoporosis,

TABLE 39-14. Diagnosis of Malignancy in Adrenal Cortical Neoplasms

Reliability	*Clinical Criteria*	*Pathologic Criteria*
Diagnostic malignancy	Weight loss, Feminization, Nodal or distant metastases	Tumor weight >100 g, tumor necrosis, fibrous bands, vascular invasion, mitoses
Consistent with malignancy	Virilism, Cushing's/virilism, No hormone production	Nuclear pleomorphism
Suggestive of malignancy	Elevated urinary 17-ketosteroids	Capsular invasion
Unreliable	Hypercortisolism Hyperaldosteronism	Tumor giant cells, cytoplasmic size variation, ratio between compact and clear cells

Adapted from Page DL, DeLellis RA, Hough AJ: Tumors of the adrenal. In: Atlas of Tumor Pathology, Washington, DC, AFIP, 1986.

TABLE 39-15. Signs and Symptoms of Endogenous Hypercortisolism

Sign or Symptom	*Incidence (%)*
Weight gain	88
Round face	75
Hypertension	74
Striae	66
Hirsutism	65
Glucose intolerance	65
Weakness	61
Amenorrhea	60
Plethora	60
Acne	45
Bruising	42
Mental changes	42
Osteoporosis	40
Edema	39
Pigmentation	21
Hypokalemia	17

Loriaux DL, Cutler GB: Diseases of the adrenal glands. In Kohler PO (ed): Clinical Endocrinology. New York, John Wiley and Sons, 1986.

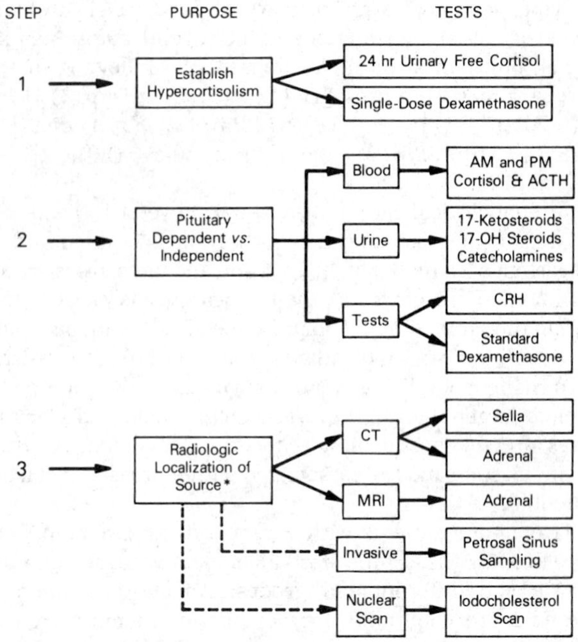

FIG. 39-3. Diagram for the work-up of a patient with suspected hypercortisolism or Cushing's syndrome. *In patients with ACTH-oma, additional studies are necessary (see text).

gives the appearance of a "buffalo hump." Serial photographs demonstrate a rounding of the face. Increased blood pressure in Cushing's syndrome is usually mild and is caused primarily by excess mineralocorticoid secretion.[238] Hypertension is less frequent in iatrogenic Cushing's syndrome because physicians prescribe pure glucocorticoids.[239] Striae are reliable clinical signs of Cushing's. Hirsutism consists of excessive fine hair on face, upper back, and arms. Virilization, including clitoromegaly, deep voice, and balding, suggest adrenocortical carcinoma. Glucose intolerance with hyperglycemia is common, and patients may present with diabetes mellitus.[240] Weakness because of muscle atrophy is a common complaint, and it is especially common in ectopic ACTH syndrome with hypokalemia. Menstrual irregularity or amenorrhea is common in women with Cushing's; men with Cushing's have loss of libido or impotency.[241] Dilatation of blood vessels and thinning of the subcutaneous tissue give the face a ruddy appearance.[242] Mental changes in Cushing's vary from mild depression to severe psychosis, correlating directly with cortisol and ACTH levels.[243,244] Hypokalemia worsens the weakness associated with Cushing's syndrome and suggests adrenocortical carcinoma or ectopic ACTH syndrome. Impaired immune surveillance is an important part of the morbidity associated with Cushing's syndrome. Opportunistic infections, including cryptococcosis, aspergillosis, nocardiosis, and pneumocystis carinii, are more common in patients with Cushing's syndrome and may be lethal.[245–247] In children with Cushing's syndrome, the most common presenting sign is obesity or short stature, an arrest of normal growth.[248] The early diagnosis of Cushing's syndrome depends primarily on a knowledge of the many different signs and symptoms of the disorder (Table 39-15) and a high clinical index of suspicion. Of 10 patients screened for presumptive hypercortisolism, one will have true Cushing's syndrome.[234]

The initial step in the work-up of a patient with presumptive hypercortisolism is to establish biochemically whether hypercortisolism is present. The second step is to determine whether the hypercortisolism is pituitary-dependent (Cushing's disease) or pituitary-independent, and the final step is to determine the exact cause of the hypercortisolism, (Fig. 39-3). Current laboratory testing allows the correct diagnosis of the hypercortisolism in nearly every case.[234]

Urinary excretion of unmetabolized or free cortisol is directly proportional to the amount of free cortisol in the plasma.[249] As the cortisol-binding globulin becomes saturated (plasma cortisol levels of 20 μg/dl), small increases in cortisol secretion produce exponential increases in urinary free cortisol.[238] This amplification makes 24-hour urinary free cortisol samples the single best measurement for discriminating normal from hypercortisolemic states (Fig. 39-3).[239] The single-dose dexamethasone test (Fig. 39-3) works because of the lack of normal feedback (Fig. 39-4) that occurs in all forms of hypercortisolism.[250] Normal subjects given 1 mg of dexamethasone orally at 11:00 PM have plasma cortisol levels less than 5 μg/dl at 8:00 AM the next day. Patients with endogenous hypercortisolism do not suppress and have cortisol levels greater than 5 μg/dl. The major advantage of this test is only a 3% incidence of false negatives, occurring in patients with Cushing's whose cortisol levels are suppressed. This test does have false positives (30%) caused by depression, alcoholism, stress, and primary cortisol resistance.[251–253] A normal single-dose dexamethasone test and a normal urinary free cortisol level (less than 100 μg/day) virtually exclude the diagnosis of hypercortisolism.[234]

The initial patient evaluation can further establish unequivocal proof of endogenous hypercortisolism and indicate the cause so that appropriate treatment can be initiated. In patients with depression or alcoholism, insulin-induced (0.15–0.3 U/kg) hypoglycemia (blood glucose < 40 mg/dl) can be used to distinguish these causes from endogenous

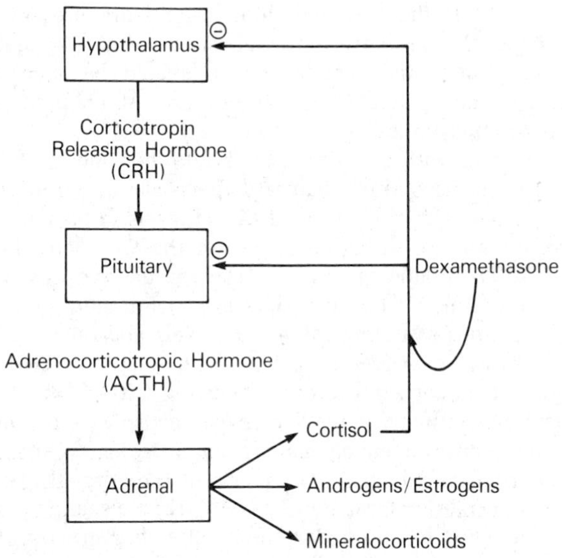

FIG. 39-4. Model of cortisol secretion indicating the mechanism of dexamethasone suppression of normal cortisol secretion.

hypercortisolism. Patients who have Cushing's do not increase plasma cortisol levels with hypoglycemia, but others will. Another method for discriminating is the corticotropin-releasing hormone (CRH) test. Patients with Cushing's disease (95%) respond to 1 μg/kg CRH by increasing plasma ACTH and cortisol levels, and patients with depression have a blunted ACTH response to CRH.[254] Twenty-nine of 33 patients with Cushing's disease increased plasma ACTH and cortisol levels following CRH, but none of 8 with ectopic ACTH responded. The CRH test worked as well as the standard dexamethasone test, and the diagnostic power was enhanced when the two tests were combined.[255]

Patients with Cushing's syndrome have abnormalities in the diurnal rhythm of plasma cortisol and ACTH levels. Serial samples over days are necessary because patients with Cushing's disease can have episodic secretion of cortisol. Nevertheless, a low midnight cortisol level (<2 μg/dl) excludes the diagnosis of endogenous hypercortisolism. Determination of simultaneous plasma ACTH levels are also helpful. Primary adrenal tumors or hyperplasia cause very low plasma ACTH levels; pituitary-dependent hypercortisolism has intermediate levels; and ectopic ACTH-producing tumors have very high levels, with approximately 60% of these patients having ACTH levels >300 pg/ml. Radioimmunoassays for ACTH in plasma have been difficult to perform reliably and interpret because of the platelet-associated proteases that degrade ACTH. Samples must be collected using recommended procedures, including prechilled tubes on ice. Urinary 17-ketosteroids can help the differential diagnosis of hypercortisolism. Low levels (<10 mg/day) suggest an adrenal adenoma, and very high levels (>60 mg/day) occur more commonly in patients with adrenal cancer and ectopic ACTH.[256,257] Hypokalemia is seen in most patients with ectopic ACTH (16 of 16 in one series) and in only 10% of patients with Cushing's disease.[258]

The standard dexamethasone suppression test is still one of the most useful tests in establishing the cause of hypercortisolism (Fig. 39-3).[255] The expected results are that urinary 17-hydroxysteroid levels will be less than 2.5 mg/day when normal subjects receive 2 mg of dexamethasone per day, a dose that has no effects on patients with endogenous hypercortisolism. High-dose dexamethasone (8 mg/day) will suppress urinary 17-hydroxysteroids to less than 50% of baseline levels in patients with pituitary-dependent hypercortisolism, but it has no effect on hypercortisolism from other causes. This single test has an accuracy rate of approximately 95%.[259]

CT scans (Fig. 39-3) detect abnormal sellar enlargement in up to 15% of patients with pituitary-dependent disease and detect more subtle abnormalities in 23% to 60% of patients.[260,261] Sellar CT scans can detect ACTH-secreting tumors whose greatest diameter is between 6 and 10 mm, but they cannot detect the more common microadenoma (<5 mm). In 10 patients with pituitary-dependent hypercortisolism, CT was normal, but simultaneous bilateral petrosal sinus sampling for ACTH concentrations produced a hormone gradient in each instance. Resection of the ipsilateral half of the pituitary with the ACTH gradient was followed by biochemical and clinical remission in each case, and pathologic analysis demonstrated microadenomas in 7 of 10 patients.[262] Petrosal sinus sampling for ACTH gradients may revolutionize the ability to correct hypercortisolism, eradicate tumor, and avoid hormonal deficiency for patients with Cushing's disease.[262]

Adrenal CT (Fig. 39-3) has been able to detect small adrenal abnormalities with certainty. CT can accurately detect normal adrenal glands in approximately 97% of the patients.[263] Although CT has great sensitivity ($>95\%$), it lacks specificity. Early detection of an adrenal neoplasm by CT greatly simplifies the work-up, and approximately 25% of patients with Cushing's syndrome will have a primary adrenal neoplasm as the source of the hypercortisolism. Unilateral adrenal tumors require the detection of a normal adrenal gland on the contralateral side (Fig. 39-5A). Adrenal hyperplasia can also be detected if both glands appear to be enlarged.

MRI is still experimental, but it may be able to add specificity to the sensitivity of CT.[264] MRI can distinguish adrenal adenoma (Fig. 39-5B) from carcinoma and from a pheochromocytoma by the brightness of the lesion on the T_2 weighted image.

Radioisotope imaging of adrenals with labeled iodocholesterol can be useful in distinguishing unilateral adrenal adenoma with suppression of the contralateral gland from bilateral hyperplasia.[265] It can differentiate a benign cortical adenoma, which usually takes up iodocholesterol, from a malignant cortical carcinoma, which usually does not take up the tracer.[266,267] In micronodular hyperplasia, uptake in both adrenal glands confirms the diagnosis. It can be useful in instances of recurrent hypercortisolism following bilateral adrenalectomy in which ectopic tissue enlarges with chronic ACTH stimulation. The limitations of radioiodocholesterol scans are the radiation dose, limited scanning and isotope availability, and poor imaging of malignant adrenal neoplasms (Fig. 39-3).

Once the laboratory tests confirm endogenous hypercortisolism, the work-up can pinpoint its cause. If an adrenal cortical neoplasm is the source of the hypercortisolism, the

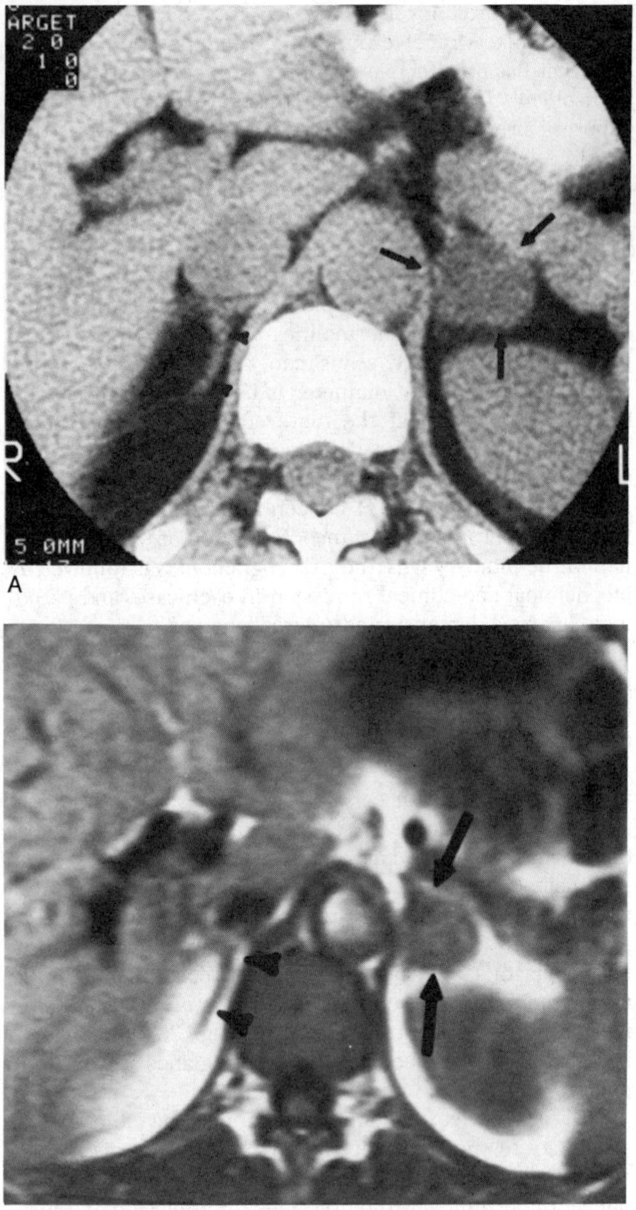

A

B

FIG. 39-5. Left adrenal adenoma in a patient with Cushing's syndrome. **A.** CT scan of the left adrenal (*arrows*) showing a mass and a normal contralateral adrenal gland (*arrowheads*). **B.** T_2 weighted magnetic resonance image of the same tumor (*arrows*) and normal contralateral adrenal gland (*arrowheads*). Because the tumor has a similar signal intensity to the liver on the T_2 image, the image indicates a benign adrenal adenoma, which was subsequently removed with resolution of the Cushing's syndrome.

work-up will produce the following results: (1) imaging of the tumor on CT and MRI (Fig. 39-5); (2) consistently low plasma ACTH levels when concomitant cortisol levels are elevated; (3) and no suppression of urinary 17-hydroxysteroids with high-dose dexamethasone. If the first criterion is absent, but the second and third are present, primary micronodular adrenal hyperplasia must be ruled out by an iodocholesterol scan or by pertrosal sinus sampling for ACTH levels, which should be low or undetectable (Fig. 39-3).[268,269] If the first and third criteria are present but ACTH levels are consistently elevated, urinary catecholamines, VMA, and metanephrines should be measured because the patient may have an ACTH-producing pheochromocytoma.[270]

In patients with ectopic ACTH syndrome, one would expect to find normal or bilateral hyperplasia of adrenals on CT, normal or greatly elevated ACTH levels in plasma, and no suppression with high-dose dexamethasone. Some bronchial ACTH-producing carcinoid tumors may suppress with dexamethasone.[234] If the results are inconsistent, rely on petrosal sinus sampling for ACTH levels and on the CRH test, in which over 95% of patients with ectopic ACTH have no ACTH or cortisol increase following CRH.[255,262] If the patient has pituitary-dependent hypercortisolism, the most common cause of endogenous hypercortisolism, expect to find normal or bilateral hyperplasia of the adrenal glands, normal or mildly elevated plasma ACTH levels, and no suppression with low-dose dexamethasone, but greater than 50% suppression with high-dose dexamethasone. With Cushing's disease, over 90% of individuals increased plasma ACTH and cortisol following CRH, and most patients will have a gradient on petrosal sinus sampling for ACTH.[255,262] In $<$5% of these tests, results will be confusing and ectopic ACTH syndrome will only be distinguishable from Cushing's disease at autopsy.[271]

Conn's Syndrome or Primary Aldosteronism

Aldosterone overproduction with elevated plasma levels is the cause of hypertension in patients with primary aldosteronism or Conn's syndrome.[272] Elevated urinary or serum levels of deoxycorticosterone, 18-hydroxycorticosterone, 18-hydroxydeoxycorticosterone, corticosterone, 18-hydroxycortisol, 18-oxocortisol, and other mineralocorticoids have also been detected in patients with primary aldosteronism.[273–276] These mineralocorticoid metabolites contribute to the hypertension.[277] The most common cause of primary aldosteronism is idiopathic adrenal hyperplasia, and the second most common cause is what Conn originally described, a solitary adenoma.[272] The third most common cause is adrenal cortical carcinoma, but it is rare for adrenal cancers to present solely with primary aldosteronism.[278] The cause of idiopathic adrenal hyperplasia is not clear, recent studies have suggested a pituitary factor that stimulates proliferation of the adrenal cortex.[279]

Hypertension, hypokalemia, hyperaldosteronism, and decreased plasma renin levels are essential for the diagnosis of primary aldosteronism. Secondary aldosteronism, which occurs with renal artery stenosis, cirrhosis, and conditions of decreased kidney perfusion, is diagnosed by an increase in plasma renin activity. Primary hyperaldosteronism is associated with weakness, muscle cramps, polyuria, and polydipsia, all of which are manifestations of the prominent hypokalemia.[277] The hypertension is usually mild to moderate.

The serum potassium level in primary aldosteronism is usually less than 3.9 mEq/liter.[280] Another possible explanation is essential hypertension that is being treated with diuretics, although these patients seldom have potassium levels less than 3.9 meq/liter. The diuretic should be withdrawn, and 24-hour urinary potassium excretion levels should be measured. In patients with primary aldosteronism, 24-hour urinary excretion of potassium will be greater than 30 mEq.[281] Patients who are taking antihypertensive medications, including diuretics and spironolactone, must stop all medications 1 month before measurements of plasma aldosterone levels and concomitant plasma renin activity. Patients with primary hyperaldosteronism should have elevated plasma aldosterone levels and low renin activity, with a plasma aldosterone/renin ratio that is usually greater than 30:1. The final proof of primary hyperaldosteronism relies on the inability to lower plasma aldosterone levels and a similar inability to raise plasma renin activity.

A new suppression test, which simplifies the evaluation of primary aldosteronism, uses captopril.[282,283] The patient takes 25 mg of captopril orally in the morning. Two hours later, plasma levels of aldosterone and renin activity are obtained. In normal subjects and patients with essential hypertension, the plasma aldosterone levels decrease and plasma renin activity increases. In patients with primary aldosteronism, plasma levels of aldosterone and renin activity do not change. A post-captopril plasma aldosterone level greater than 15 ng/dl and an aldosterone/renin ratio greater than 50 indicate primary aldosteronism (Table 39-16).

Once the diagnosis of primary aldosteronism has been established, it is important to establish whether the patient has idiopathic adrenal cortical hyperplasia (IAH) or a tumor that produces aldosterone (Table 39-16). The exact cause of primary aldosteronism is critical because treatment is primarily chemical for IAH and primarily surgical for a neoplasm. Patients with neoplasms generally have serum 18-hydroxycorticosterone levels greater than 100 ng/dl, while patients with IAH have levels less than 90 ng/dl; however, there is some overlap and these measurements don't totally discriminate between the two diagnoses.[274]

CT series indicate that approximately 75% to 90% of aldosteronomas can be accurately preoperatively imaged on CT, but tumors less than 7 to 10 mm may be missed.[284–288] CT does not accurately identify IAH because these glands appear normal, and small tumors may be missed on CT. CT evidence of a tumor does not predict the functional significance of the tumor.[284–287]

Iodocholesterol scans have improved with the availability of newer imaging agents. For example, ^{131}I-19-iodocholesterol is able to image 64% of aldosteronomas, but the newer agent, ^{131}I-6-beta-iodomethyl-19-norcholesterol, combined with adrenal suppression with dexamethasone, can image 88% of tumors, which is similar to CT (91%).[285] The advantage of these nuclear studies over CT is the functional information about the neoplasm. CT is more sensitive, more available, and uses less radiation per study than iodocholesterol scans, but in certain patients with equivocal studies, iodocholesterol scans can be very helpful. In patients with IAH, the adrenal scan shows symmetrical uptake in both adrenal glands; in patients with adrenal carcinoma, the study may show no uptake by the tumor; and in patients with adenomas, uptake is usually evident (88%).[285]

The single study of choice in hyperaldosteronism is sampling of the adrenal veins for aldosterone.[288] The procedure is performed by selective catheterization of the veins, and simultaneous blood samples for aldosterone and cortisol are collected from both adrenal veins and a peripheral vein. A unilateral elevation of the aldosterone level or of the aldosterone/cortisol ratio indicates the presence of an aldosterone-secreting adenoma. Bilateral levels of aldosterone that are similar and greater than peripheral levels are consistent

TABLE 39-16. Evaluation of Patient with Hyperaldosteronism

I. Diagnosis of Primary Aldosteronism

Measure	*Result*
Blood pressure	Hypertension
Serum K	Hypokalemia serum K < 3.9 mEq/liter
Urinary K	Elevated Urinary K Excretion (>25–30 mEq/day)
Plasma aldosterone and plasma renin activity	Ratio > 30:1 (elevated aldosterone and low renin)
Captopril suppression test (25 mg orally)	Post-captopril aldosterone > 15 ng/ml Aldosterone/renin ratio > 50

II. Etiology of Primary Aldosteronism: Idiopathic Adrenal Hyperplasia (IAH) Versus Neoplasm

IAH	*Measurement*	*Neoplasm*
<90 ng/dl	Serum 18-hydroxy-corticosterone	>100 ng/dl
Normal adrenals	High resolution CT	Tumor (<7–10-mm tumors can be missed)
Symmetrical uptake bilaterally	Iodocholesterol scan	Uptake of tracer by benign adenoma (malignant tumors may not take up tracer)
Fair response	Spironolactone	Good response
Aldosterone levels elevated from both adrenal veins and greater than simultaneous peripheral sample	Adrenal vein sampling	Aldosterone levels elevated on side with tumor, contralateral side equal to simultaneous peripheral samples

with IAH. Adrenal venous sampling for aldosterone (96%) was more sensitive than CT (75%) and adrenal venography (78%) in a prospective comparison.[288] Venous sampling is invasive and expensive, but it is the most reliable way to confirm a functioning aldosteroma.

The clinical response to spironolactone is useful in predicting the subsequent outcome of surgical resection of an adenoma. Before testing was done with spironolactone, only 66% of patients with adenoma were cured following surgical resection. After the guideline of a good response to spironolactone was used, the cure rate increased to 92%.[289]

The treatment of primary aldosteronism depends on the diagnosis. Idiopathic adrenal hyperplasia is best managed with spironolactone or amiloride, in conjunction with other antihypertensive drugs. This regimen usually allows effective blood pressure control.[277] There are subsets of patients with primary adrenal hyperplasia who responded favorably to subtotal (75%) adrenalectomy.[290] These patients may be easily identified because their hypertension responds to spironolactone. Following subtotal adrenalectomy, mineralocorticoid levels and renin–angiotensin levels return to normal despite the indicated hyperplasia. These results confirm a subset of patients with hyperplasia in whom 75% surgical resection may be helpful.[290] However, it is important to remember that the vast majority of patients with IAH should be treated with drugs.

Because of adrenal venous aldosterone levels and the ability to localize a small aldosteronoma to one adrenal gland, it is now preferable to use a posterior approach for unilateral adrenalectomy in patients with a localized adrenal cortical adenoma. Results for resection of an aldosteronoma have not been entirely satisfactory. A high percentage initially become normotensive and normokalemic postoperatively (approximately 95%), but 20% to 30% of these patients will develop recurrent hypertension within 2 to 3 years.[291] This hypertension is not usually associated with recurrent hypokalemia. Prolonged preoperative hypertension from an aldosteronoma may alter renal function, which leads to renal impairment, causing persistent hypertension despite successful resection of an adrenal cortical adenoma.[292]

A new drug with potential for managing the hypokalemia and hypertension associated with primary aldosteronism is the calcium channel blocker nifedipine. In a 4-week study of 10 patients (5 with aldosteroma and 5 with IAH), nifedipine controlled blood pressure and normalized potassium and aldosterone levels in every patient.[293]

Aldosterone-producing adrenocortical carcinomas are rare (2% of all carcinomas).[294] Patients with primary aldosteronism due to adrenocortical carcinoma usually have higher levels of deoxycorticosterone and aldosterone than patients with benign adenomas.[295] In addition, their hypokalemia and weakness is usually more severe than the typical patient with Conn's syndrome.[295] Their treatment is similar to other patients with adrenal carcinoma and will be discussed later.

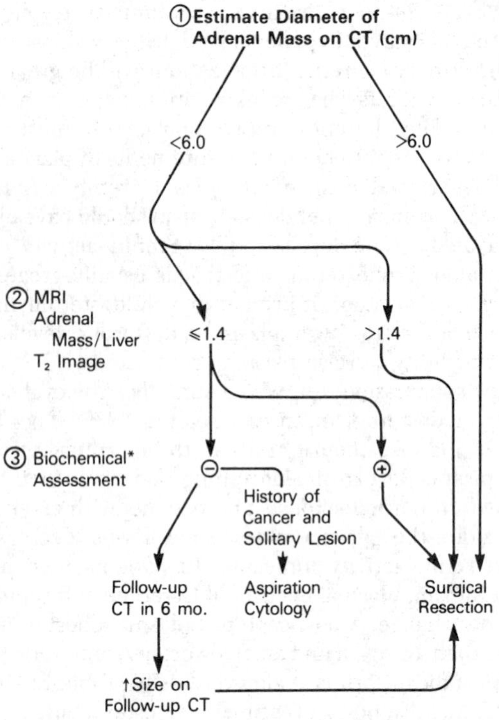

FIG. 39-6. Flow diagram for evaluation of an incidentally discovered adrenal mass. All three studies are performed on each patient. *Biochemical assessment includes 24-hour urine for 17-hydroxy, 17-ketosteroids, and catecholamines; low-dose dexamethasone test; and serum testosterone or estrogen, if suspicion.

Asymptomatic Adrenal Mass

With the availability of high-resolution CT scanners, a new diagnostic problem has arisen: the detection of an asymptomatic adrenal mass in patients with or without a history of cancer. Unexpected adrenal masses have been detected on 0.6% of abdominal CT scans.[296,297] The majority of adrenal masses detected in this manner will be benign, silent adrenal cortical adenomas, which occur in up to 8.7% of autopsy cases.[298] CT is not sufficient to differentiate metastases to the adrenal gland from a known or occult primary tumor, a pheochromocytoma, or an early, rare adrenal carcinoma.

When managing these masses, remember that the great majority are benign and nonfunctional. The work-up and therapy must not create an iatrogenic disease greater than the primary process. Percutaneous aspiration of occult pheochromocytomas has resulted in severe morbidity, including hypertensive crisis, hemorrhage, and even sudden death.[299,300] The suggested evaluation of an incidental adrenal mass (incidentaloma) detected by CT scan is given in Fig. 39-6.

When an adrenal mass is discovered in this manner, two questions arise: Does the adrenal mass produce hormones, and is it cancer?[298] A positive answer to either question indicates either surgery or some other therapy. It is possible to overlook a nonfunctioning adrenocortical carcinoma, which occurs in approximately 50% of patients in most series.[230,301] However, with earlier diagnosis and measurement of urinary 17-ketosteroids, the majority of nonfunctional adrenal cortical carcinomas actually do have increased secretions of steroids.[302,303]

The first step in evaluation of an asymptomatic adrenal mass is a careful history and physical examination. The clinician should note weight change, weakness, hypokalemia, Cushing's syndrome, hypertension, virilization, feminization, change in menstruation, and evidence of occult malignancy (stool guaic, Pap smear, anemia).

The laboratory evaluation of an asymptomatic adrenal mass should consist of a 24-hour urine test for 17-hydroxycorticosteroids and 17-ketosteroids. As previously mentioned, 17-ketosteroids may be elevated in patients with adrenal cortical cancer in the presence of normal 17-hydroxycorticosteroids.[302] Patients with carcinoma may have inactivity of the enzyme 11-beta-hydroxylase, which can cause elevated urinary levels of 17-hydroxycorticosteroids without Cushing's syndrome.[304] Single-dose dexamethasone (1 mg) suppression tests should be performed because patients with Cushing's syndrome caused by an adrenal neoplasm will not respond, but they may have normal basal steroid excretion.[302,305] Plasma testosterone levels should be measured if a woman or child has clinical evidence of hirsutism or virilization. Elevated testosterone levels are usually associated with elevated urinary 17-ketosteroids, but testosterone levels can be elevated in a patient with normal urinary 17-ketosteroids.[306] Serum estrogen levels should be measured if feminization is suspected. Again, 17-ketosteroids are usually elevated in patients with feminization, but they can also be normal, in which case, estrogen levels may be increased.[298] Aldosterone levels should be measured in any patient with hypertension, hypokalemia, and an adrenal mass. Twenty-four hour urine tests for catecholamines should be performed to rule out a pheochromocytoma.

The size of the adrenal mass on CT is probably the most helpful determinant of the nature of the biochemically silent lesion.[298] Most adrenal cortical carcinomas are greater than 6 cm in diameter, and most benign lesions are less than 6 cm. A small lesion cannot be totally ignored. Early diagnosis may lead to discovery of smaller adrenal cortical carcinomas, which may lead to better prognosis and survival. In three series, all five patients with nonmetastatic adrenocortical carcinoma and primary tumors less than 5 cm in diameter were alive 5 years postoperatively, but only approximately 10% of patients with larger tumors or metastases survived longer than 5 years.[307–309] CT can accurately image normal glands, hyperplastic adrenal glands, and adrenal neoplasms, but it cannot distinguish benign from malignant neoplasms by criteria other than size, direct invasion, or distant metastases.[310,311,312]

MRI of the adrenal is a relatively new modality, but already it has attained similar resolution to CT. Small tumors (< 1 cm) can be accurately imaged by MRI.[313] Studies indicate that MRI can reliably distinguish between adrenal metastases and nonfunctioning adenomas based on T_2-weighted spin echo scans.[313] Pheochromocytomas could also be clearly imaged and appeared bright on T_2-weighted spin echo scans.[314] These findings prompted a study of whether MRI could be used to differentiate masses indeterminate on CT. It was clear from this study that pheochromocytomas could be reliably diagnosed based on MR ratios between the adrenal mass and the adjacent liver on the T_2-weighted image.[315] Pheochromocytomas always had a ratio greater than 3 : 1, and this finding has been consistent for 21 patients (Table 39-17).[316] Patients with either benign nonfunctioning or hormone-producing adrenal adenomas had ratios between 0.7 and 1.4 (Fig. 39-5).[315] Patients with metastatic cancers

TABLE 39-17. Magnetic Resonance Imaging of the Adrenal: Ability to Predict Histology

	T_2 Image Adrenal Mass/Liver Ratio
Nonfunctioning or hyperfunctioning cortical adenomas	0.7–1.4
Metastases from other primary	1.2–2.8
Adrenal carcinoma	1.2–2.8
Pheochromocytoma	>3

Doppman JL, Reinig JW, Dwyer AJ et al: Differentiation of adrenal masses by magnetic resonance imaging. Surgery 102:1018, 1987.

or adrenocortical cancers (Fig. 39-7) had ratios between those measured for pheochromocytomas and those measured for adenomas (Table 39-17). Eight (21%) of 38 of these tumors could not be differentiated among adenomas, carcinoma, or metastases. Differentiation between incidental adenomas and metastases could be conclusively achieved if the primary neoplasm could be imaged and displayed by high signal intensity on T_2-weighted images.[315]

Fine-needle aspiration of an adrenal mass has a limited ability to differentiate benign from malignant adrenal lesions. Table 39-14 indicates how difficult it is to distinguish these tumors based on histopathologic or cytologic examinations. Fine-needle aspiration may be catastrophic if the patient has an unsuspected pheochromocytoma, so urinary catecholamines or MRI imaging are indicated before needle biopsy.[299,300] In patients with suspected metastatic disease and inconclusive MRI, needle aspiration may be helpful. In 16 patients with known primary cancers, 7 patients had adrenal metastases confirmed by cytologic examination.[317] Because it usually cannot distinguish between benign and malignant adrenal neoplasms and because the patient's life may be threatened by an unsuspected pheochromocytoma, fine-needle aspiration should not be routinely performed in the evaluation of asymptomatic adrenal masses.

The suggested approach to an asymptomatic adrenal mass is outlined in Fig. 39-6. All three suggested tests—CT, MRI, and biochemical assessment—should be performed on each patient, because each study can provide information important to the management. Initially the adrenal mass's diameter is carefully measured by CT. A size greater than 6 cm does play an important part in the differential diagnosis. It is also important to carefully examine the contralateral adrenal gland to be certain that the mass is only unilateral. Ultrasound can distinguish between solid and cystic large masses. Large adrenal masses (>6 cm) are probably malignant, and surgical resection is indicated.[318] MRI and biochemical assessment of such lesions are also important, because pheochromocytomas can be large and proper preoperative and intraoperative management is necessary to reduce the chance of intraoperative death. Small lesions (<3.5 cm) are usually benign adenomas, but functional adenomas, pheochromocytomas, and early carcinomas must be ruled out.[316] MRI is best for diagnosing pheochromocytomas because of the dramatically bright appearance on the T_2-weighted image (adrenal mass/liver ratio, >3 : 1), and it can also help with the diagnosis of a smaller malignant lesion,

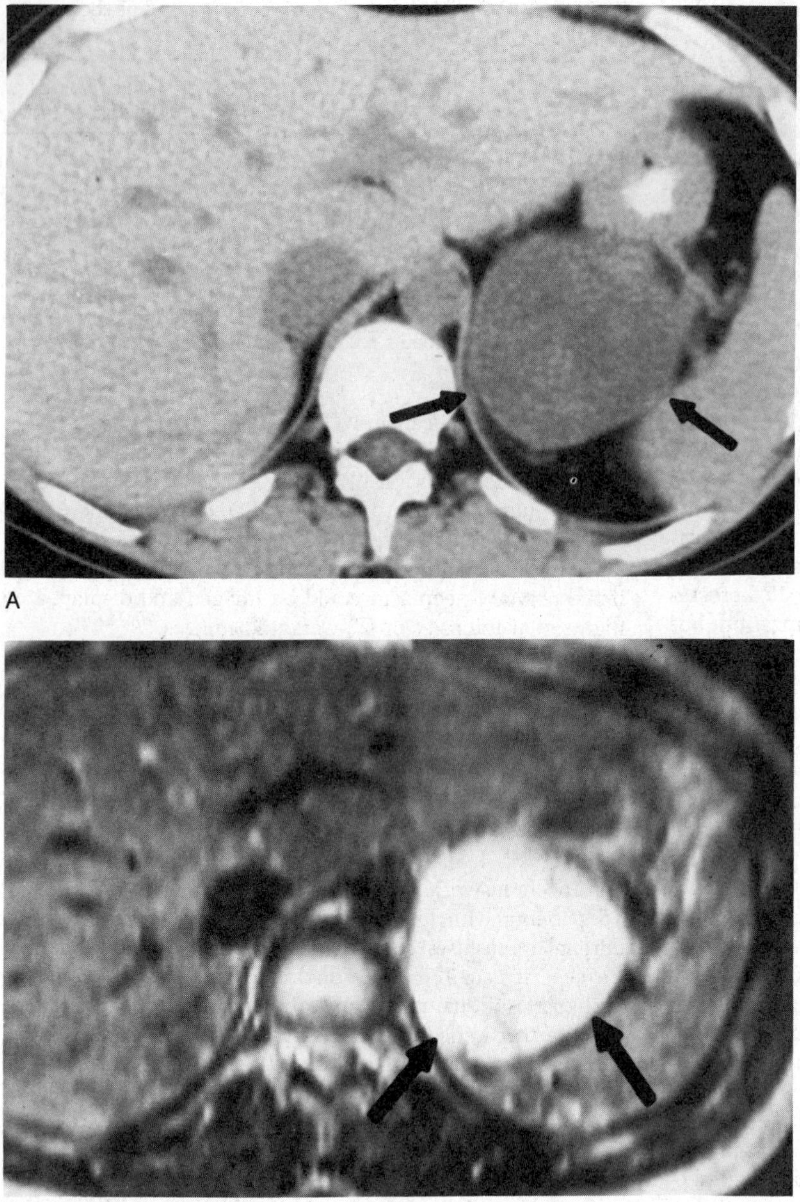

FIG. 39-7. Adrenocortical carcinoma of left adrenal. **A**. Computed tomography image of mass in left adrenal gland (*arrows*) in a patient with Cushing's syndrome. **B**. Magnetic resonance T_2 weighted image demonstrates that the mass (*arrows*) is brighter than the liver, consistent with adrenal cortical carcinoma. Surgical examination demonstrated an adrenal cortical carcinoma.

which has a ratio between 1.2 and 3.0. A ratio in this intermediate range and a nonfunctioning tumor (3.5–6.0 cm) suggest surgical resection, unless the patient has a history of a previous cancer and is at risk for adrenal metastases from a primary site. A positive biochemical assessment also mandates surgical resection. Follow-up CT is indicated for small nonfunctional adrenal masses with low intensity on MRI. If a mass of this type enlarges on subsequent CT, surgical resection is again indicated. This schema should provide early surgical intervention for functional or malignant adrenal masses and limit resection of adrenal metastases and nonfunctional benign adrenal adenomas.

Excess Sex Hormones

A patient with adrenocortical carcinoma may present with excessive sex hormone secretion. This may be combined with excessive cortisol or aldosterone, or the hormones may be primarily excessive estrogen or testosterone. In children, the clinical signs of increased androgen production include increased growth, premature development of pubic and facial hair, acne, genitalia enlargement, increased muscle mass, and deep voice. In women, the clinical signs of excess androgen include hirsutism, acne, amenorrhea, infertility, increased muscle mass, deep voice, and temporal balding. In children, the clinical signs of increased estrogen production include gynecomastia in boys and precocious breast enlargement or vaginal bleeding in girls. In adult men, hyperestrogenism presents with gynecomastia, decreased sexual drive, impotence, and infertility. In adult women, hyperestrogenism presents primarily with irregular menses in premenopausal women and with dysfunctional uterine bleeding or vaginal bleeding in postmenopausal women.[234] The work-up requires tests of 24-hour urinary 17-ketosteroids, 17-hydroxysteroids, urinary free cortisol, and depending on virilization or feminization, serum testosterone or estrogen determinations.

Virilization caused by an adrenal neoplasm may accompany Cushing's syndrome, and if it does occur, it usually indicates adrenal cortical carcinoma. Adrenal-induced virilization in the absence of Cushing's syndrome may be due to adrenal cortical adenoma or carcinoma.[319,320] There are many other disorders which cause virilization in women and children, but in working-up a patient with virilization, a CT or MRI study of both adrenals is indicated to rule out an adrenal neoplasm. Hyperestrogenism of adrenal origin is usually caused by an adrenal adenoma or carcinoma and may be associated with hypercortisolism. An imaging study of both adrenal glands should rule out a neoplasm before proceeding with the differential diagnosis of hyperestrogenism.

TREATMENT FOR ADRENAL CORTICAL NEOPLASMS

Adenomas of the Adrenal Cortex

The definitive treatment of benign adenomas is surgical resection of the adrenal gland with the adenoma. For tumors less than 6 cm in diameter, the posterior or lateral approach with resection of the 12th rib is recommended because of excellent exposure and less morbidity postoperatively (Fig. 39-8). For tumors greater than 6 cm, an anterior or flank approach is recommended because of malignant potential of larger tumors (Fig. 39-9). MRI can characterize a malignancy, because the adrenal mass–liver ratio is > 1.4 or < 3.0 on T_2 image.[264] Baker and colleagues reported two patients who had benign adrenal adenomas with increased adrenal mass–liver ratio on T_2-weighted MRI, but they agree with the ability of the MRI signal intensity to distinguish malignant neoplasms or pheochromocytomas.[321]

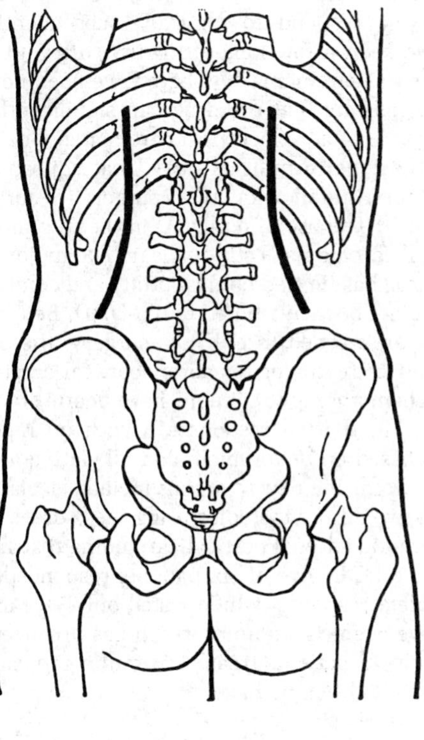

FIG. 39-8. Posterior approach to adrenalectomy. This method is recommended for small, benign tumors. Resection of the 12th rib is required.

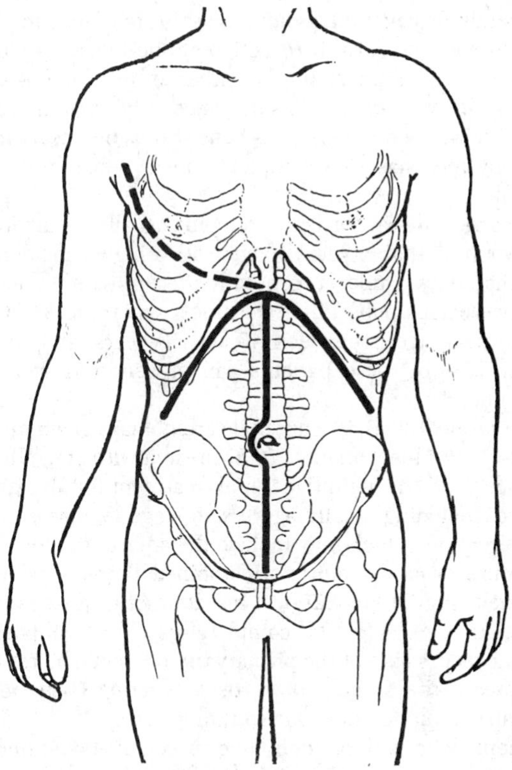

FIG. 39-9. Anterior approach to adrenalectomy. This method is recommended for large, malignant tumors or pheochromocytomas. Either a midline abdominal incision (thin patient with narrow costal margin) or a bilateral subcostal abdominal incision (obese patient with wide costal margin) is used. Extension into the right chest (*dotted line*) may be necessary to resect malignant tumors.

Steroid replacement before or during surgery is carried out as for bilateral adrenalectomy. Mineralocorticoid replacement is not required. Postoperative glucocorticoid replacement is necessary for 3 to 6 months to allow recovery of the hypothalamic–pituitary–adrenal axis. Surgical resection of an adenoma in this fashion is curative. Larger lesions weighing between 50 and 100 g, which exhibit no mitoses and no vascular invasion should be carefully followed. Long-term follow-up of patients has shown that resection of true adrenal adenomas is curative.[322]

Carcinoma of the Adrenal Cortex

The mainstay of treatment of adrenal cortical carcinoma is complete resection of all gross tumor. If the carcinoma is intimately associated with the kidney or liver or diaphragm on the right, or pancreas on the left, it may be necessary to resect part of or all of the contiguous structures at the time of definitive resection. The best chance for curative surgery is the initial operation. The surgeon needs adequate imaging of the mass by both CT and MRI. The CT and MRI scans should include the chest to rule out metastatic disease above the diaphragm. If the right adrenal is involved and the inferior vena cava is compressed, either an inferior vena cava contrast study or caval ultrasound is useful to determine blood flow through the cava. If resection of one kidney is planned along with the primary tumor, either an intravenous pyelogram or an IV contrast CT is indicated to be sure the contralateral kidney is functioning. A bone scan is necessary to rule out bony metastases. A complete bowel preparation is also helpful.

Pediatric adrenal cortical carcinoma usually occurs in children younger than 6 years of age, with a higher incidence in girls than boys. Children generally present with either virilism, precocious puberty, or Cushing's syndrome.[323–325] The second peak age is between 40 and 50 years, and approximately 70% of these patients will present with hormonal syndromes.[294]

The surgical staging of adrenal carcinoma is given in Table 39-18.[326–328] Most patients (70%) present with Stage III or IV disease.[294,328] The definitive initial treatment for all stages of disease, including locally aggressive stage IV disease, is en bloc resection, which may include the adjacent kidney. This procedure usually requires a combined thoraco-abdominal approach (Fig. 39-9). Surgical resection of localized disease can be curative.[294,327,328] If complete resection is impossible, as much as possible of the primary tumor should be removed to decrease the amount of cortisol-secreting tissue and to minimize complications due to tumor mass.

Patients who undergo definitive resection should undergo monthly monitoring of appropriate steroid secretion to detect a recurrence as early as possible. The steroid measured depends on the tumor secretion at the time of diagnosis. If hypercortisolism was present, urinary free cortisols should be measured. If urinary 17-ketosteroids were elevated preoperatively, their levels postoperatively should be tested. Plasma levels of 11-deoxycortisol, dehydroepiandrosterone, deoxycorticosterone, or other steroids may also signal recurrences in a patient.[234] CT and MRI can also disclose local recurrences or pulmonary metastases. If an apparently solitary recurrence is detected, it should be removed surgically if possible.

TABLE 39-18. Staging Criteria for Adrenal Cortical Carcinoma

Criteria	
T1	tumor ≤5 cm, invasion absent
T2	tumor >5 cm, invasion absent
T3	tumor outside adrenal in fat
T4	tumor invading adjacent organs
N0	no positive lymph nodes
N1	positive lymph nodes
M0	no distant metastases
M1	distant metastases
Stage	
I	T_1, N_0, M_0
II	T_2, N_0, M_0
III	T_1 or $T_2N_1M_0$, $T_3N_0M_0$
IV	any T, any NM_1, $T_3T_4N_1$

Macfarlane DA: Cancer of the adrenal cortex: The natural history, prognosis and treatment in a study of fifty-five cases. Ann R Coll Surg Engl 23:155, 1958; Sullivan M, Boileau M, Hodges CV: Adrenal cortical carcinoma. J Urol 120:660, 1978; Henley DJ, van Heerden JA, Grant CS et al: Adrenal cortical carcinoma—a continuing challenge. Surgery 94:926, 1983.

Prolonged remissions have been reported following resections of hepatic, pulmonary, and cerebral metastases from adrenal cortical carcinoma.[329–332] When complete resection of tumor metastases is not possible, near-total resection may still diminish the effects of some hormonally productive, slow-growing adrenal cortical cancers.[230] Palliation of bony metastases can be achieved by radiation therapy.[294] Percapto and Knowlton indicated that abdominal radiation therapy can be palliative in 67% of patients with local recurrences, and it even relieved one bowel obstruction.[332] However, it failed to improve the length of survival in two series.[294,332]

Once the patient has recurrent or metastatic adrenal cortical carcinoma, chemotherapy with o,p-DDD, is usually started.[333] Therapy is initiated at a dosage of 2 to 6 g daily, given in two or three divided doses and increased until adverse reactions occur. Adverse reactions include gastrointestinal toxicity (anorexia, nausea, vomiting, diarrhea), neuromuscular toxicity (depression, dizziness, tremors, headache, confusion, weakness), and skin rash. Of the patients treated, 79% experience some gastrointestinal toxicity, 50% develop neuromuscular toxicity, and 15% develop a skin rash.[333] A decrease in urinary 17-hydroxysteroids and 17-ketosteroids occurs in 67% of patients treated due to a direct effect on steroid metabolism,[334,335] and a partial response occurs in approximately a third of the patients treated. It is important to measure blood levels of o,p-DDD to ensure serum levels higher than 14 μg/ml. In one study, patients who had blood levels less than 10 μg/ml had no demonstrable therapeutic effects, while 7 of 8 patients who had levels greater than 14 μg/ml had objective responses and lived significantly longer.[336] Levels greater than 20 μg/ml are associated with symptoms of neuromuscular toxicity.[336]

Unfortunately, it can be an unpleasant drug, and when clinical toxicity is present, the dose must be adjusted to miminize side-effects. Tumor responses usually occur in the first 6 weeks after initiation of treatment. Although most patients who respond to o,p-DDD subsequently relapse, there have been a few long-term survivors with metastatic adrenocortical carcinoma.[337] There have been no controlled studies to indicate that the drug can significantly alter the natural course of adrenocortical carcinoma. One group suggests, without performing a study, that adjuvant o,p-DDD improves survival following initial surgery for adrenocortical carcinoma.[338] The use of o,p-DDD in the treatment of adrenal cortical carcinoma is still unclear. The major problem is that the drug has limited clinical utility and complete remissions have not been attributed to o,p-DDD. Better therapeutic agents are needed to enhance surgery, the only potentially curative treatment for adrenocortical carcinomas.

Other chemotherapy regimens have been very ineffective (Table 39-19). Partial responses have been reported with regimens based on doxorubicin and alkylating agents.[339,340] The most promising new regimens include cisplatin and etoposide. In two different studies using these drugs in patients with metastatic adrenal cortical carcinoma that failed to respond to o,p-DDD, five of six patients responded, including one complete response, which lasted only 1 year.[341,342] Another active agent is suramin, which has produced 5 partial responses in 12 patients treated. Suramin can cause thrombocytopenia and hemorrhage.[343]

TABLE 39-19. Chemotherapy for Adrenal Cortical Carcinoma

Drug	*Dose*	*Frequency*	*Number of Patients*	*Efficacy*	*Reference*
o,p-DDD	1–12 g/day	b.i.d. or t.i.d.		33% PR* 0 CR	(333–337)
Cisplatin + etoposide	40 mg/m²/day 100 mg/m²/day	Daily for 3 days	2	2 PR 0 CR	(341)
Cyclophosphamide + doxorubicin + cisplatin	600 mg/m² 40 mg/m² 50 mg/m²	Every 3 weeks	11	2 PR 0 CR	(339)
Cyclophosphamide + vincristine + methyl-CCNU + bleomycin	Not given		2	1 PR 0 CR	(340)
Doxorubicin alone	40 mg/m²	Every 4 weeks	8	1 PR 0 CR	(340)
Cyclophosphamide, melphalan, or peptichermio	Not given		12	2 PR 0 CR	(340)
Cisplatin	120 mg/m²	Every 4 weeks	5	0 PR 0 CR	(344)
Cisplatin + etoposide + bleomycin	40 mg/m² 100 mg/m² 30 U	Every 4 weeks	4	1 CR 2 PR	(342)

*PR = partial remission; CR = complete remission.

There is no consistently active cytotoxic drug or drug combination available for the treatment of adrenal cortical carcinoma. The activity of cisplatin in combination with bleomycin or doxorubicin suggests the continued evaluation of these compounds in the treatment of poor-risk or metastatic adrenal cortical carcinoma. Steroid hormone receptors have been detected *in vitro* in adrenal cortical carcinomas, indicating their dependence on progesterone and glucocorticoids.[345] However, *in vivo* studies of therapeutic manipulation of receptors have not been done.

Improved therapy is needed because adrenal cortical carcinoma is a very malignant tumor. One study categorized it into two subpopulations with different prognoses and different survival. The anaplastic variant occurred more commonly in males, produced more frequent cutaneous metastases, and was associated with a lack of clinical or laboratory evidence of hormone production. The median survival of patients with anaplastic adrenal cortical cancer was only 5 months. Differentiated adrenal cortical cancer usually occurred in women and produced clinical or laboratory evidence of hormonal excess. The median survival of patients with differentiated adrenal cortical cancer was 40 months.[230]

Most patients present with Stage III and Stage IV tumors (Table 39-18). Surgical cure is realistically only possible in Stage I or Stage II tumors, tumors confined to the adrenal gland.[346] In one large series from the Mayo Clinic, 39% of patients presented with Stage I or Stage II adrenal cortical carcinoma.[326] However, mean survival for patients presenting with Stage I and Stage II tumors was only 25 and 24 months, respectively, compared with 28 and 12 months for Stages III and IV. The only group with a significantly shortened survival was Stage IV patients.[328] These data indicate the poor prognosis for adrenal cortical carcinoma and support the use of adjuvant chemotherapy for resectable lesions (Stages I–III). Results from Vanderbilt, where physicians treated 21 patients with Cushing's syndrome and adrenal cortical cancer, demonstrated two subgroups of the 19 who died. Ten patients died in 12 to 24 months, while 9 patients died in 3 to 16 years. In the subgroup who had the longer survival, response to o,p-DDD and aggressive reoperations appeared to provide some benefit.[322]

A recent study indicated that most patients presented with functional tumors, an abdominal mass, and distant or nodal metastases (Stage IV). In patients with tumors confined to the adrenal gland, the mean survival was 5 years.[294] In patients with invasion of contiguous structures at presentation, mean survival was 2.3 years.[294] The metastatic sites of adrenal cancer are lymph nodes (68%), lung (71%), liver (42%), and bone (26%).[347]

Challenges for better treatment of adrenal cortical carcinoma include earlier diagnosis and better adjuvants than o,p-DDD. Earlier diagnosis can be facilitated by screening for symptoms or signs of hormonal excess during history and physical examinations. Changes in body appearance and menstrual history are important clues to earlier diagnosis. The use of MRI may help clinicians find early resectable adrenal cortical cancers. Drugs like cisplatin and etoposide, which appear to provide objective responses in patients with metastatic adrenal cortical cancer who have failed o,p-DDD, need to be tried as adjuvant therapy following resection of Stage II or III adrenal carcinomas.

Ectopic ACTH Syndrome

The first patient who exhibited features of Cushing's syndrome had an oat-cell carcinoma of the bronchus secreting a peptide now called corticotrophin or ACTH.[348] Similar patients who had adrenal hyperplasia without pituitary tumors were reported over the next 30 years, but it was Christy and Liddle who established the presence of ACTH-like material in the blood, and noted subnormal quantities of ACTH in the pituitary itself.[349,350] The name ectopic ACTH syndrome was introduced in 1962.[350]

The diagnosis of ectopic ACTH syndrome is based on the metabolic evaluation of the patient who presents with hypercortisolism. Early clues are Cushing's and severe hypokalemia (potassium < 3.3 meq/liter). The diagnosis is based primarily on very high plasma ACTH and cortisol levels, which don't change with high-dose dexamethasone or administration of CRH, and results of petrosal sinus sampling, which demonstrate low levels of ACTH draining from the pituitary gland.[255,262]

Once the diagnosis is established, the goal is to eradicate the neoplasm that is secreting ACTH. When this is accomplished either by surgery, chemotherapy, or radiation therapy, long-term cures can be achieved.[234] The main clinical problems have been finding the source of ectopic ACTH in some patients and treating the aggressive tumor in others.

The causative tumors, in approximate order of frequency, are oat-cell carcinoma of the bronchus, carcinoid tumor of the bronchus, epithelial carcinoma of the thymus or thymic carcinoids, islet-cell tumor of the pancreas, medullary carcinoma of the thyroid gland, pheochromocytoma, gut carcinoids, ovarian adenocarcinoma, pancreatic cystadenoma, and adenocarcinoma of unknown site.[351-353] Even if ectopic ACTH production is not a factor, all of these tumors can be malignant and can metastasize and kill the patient.

In many patients with ectopic ACTH production, the primary disease cannot be eradicated, and therapy is directed toward correcting the metabolic and hormonal abnormalities. Hypokalemia and excess mineralocorticoid activity may be managed with potassium supplementation and spironolactone. Hypercortisolism may be managed with metyrapone, aminoglutethimide, or new glucocorticoid receptor antagonist RU 486.[354-356] Bilateral adrenalectomy is recommended for patients who have ectopic ACTH caused by tumors that cannot be localized and do not appear immediately life threatening.[353]

Tumors may be elusive, and extensive localization procedures are indicated for the occult ACTH-producing neoplasm. One of the procedures is to sample various veins (e.g., thymic, inferior thyroid, inferior mesenteric) for ACTH in order to localize a tumor to a specific area or organ. The procedure has not been very successful for localizing occult tumors and is not recommended. The recommended procedures include chest CT and bronchoscopy, urinary catecholamines to screen for pheochromocytoma, plasma calcitonin or pentagastrin-calcium stimulation tests to rule out medullary thyroid carcinoma, CT scans to look for pancreatic neoplasms, and bone-marrow aspiration to rule out metastatic oat-cell carcinoma. Any suspicious finding in chest or abdomen can be unequivocally confirmed by fine-needle aspiration and radioimmunoassay for ACTH in the aspirate.[357] The proper therapy for ACTH-producing neoplasms depends on the exact tumor that produces ACTH and the extent of disease.

Pheochromocytoma

Pheochromocytomas, which arise from chromaffin cells in the adrenal medulla and elsewhere, secrete catecholamines and cause either intermittent, episodic, or sustained hypertension.[358] In autopsy series, only 0.005% to 0.1% of persons have unsuspected pheochromocytomas.[219] When urinary catecholamines are measured as a screening test for pheochromocytoma in hypertensive patient populations, the tumor is present in only 0.1% of the patients.[359,360] Although these tumors are rare, it is important to diagnose and localize pheochromocytomas for several reasons.[361] Sustained hypertension caused by a pheochromocytoma may be curable with tumor resection, and sudden death has occurred in patients with pheochromocytomas secondary to paroxysmal hypertensive crisis. Early diagnosis and therapy may lessen the probability of death from malignancy and improve the prognosis. Incidence of malignancy in pheochromocytomas is as low as 5% and as high as 46% in different series.[361,362] Extra-adrenal tumors are more commonly cancerous.[363]

Bilateral adrenal medullary pheochromocytomas are components of multiple endocrine neoplasias. MEN-2a includes medullary carcinoma of the thyroid gland, parathyroid hyperplasia, and pheochromocytomas. MEN-2b includes a characteristic body and facial appearance, bony abnormalities, medullary carcinoma of the thyroid gland, and pheochromocytomas. It is important to exclude pheochromocytoma before operating on medullary thyroid carcinomas, because unexpected pheochromocytomas during general anesthesia can result in hypertensive crisis and death. Familial pheochromocytoma has also been described. Affected individuals have bilateral adrenal pheochromocytomas and no other manifestation of MEN syndromes.[364] In other families without evidence of MEN, extra-adrenal pheochromocytomas have been reported, usually in the same extra-adrenal location (e.g., bladder) in all affected individuals from one kindred.[365] Pheochromocytomas also occur in approximately 25% of patients with Von Hippel-Lindau's disease,[366] and it has been reported in <1% of patients with neurofibromatosis and von Recklinghausen's disease.[366,367]

Pheochromocytomas typically produce catecholamines, which result in clinical symptoms of attacks of anxiety and marked hypertension or sustained hypertension. However, pheochromocytomas also produce other hormones, including ACTH, so patients may have concomitant Cushing's syndrome.[368] Pheochromocytomas also contain many other peptide hormones, including somatostatin, calcitonin, oxytocin, and vasopressin.[369-371] These hormones are seldom of clinical relevance.

PATHOLOGY. Pheochromocytomas arise from chromaffin cells.[361] Chromaffin cells are widespread and associated with sympathetic ganglia during fetal life. After birth, most chromaffin cells degenerate and the majority remain in the adrenal medulla.[361] This may explain why approximately 90% of pheochromocytomas are in the adrenal medulla. Extra-adrenal pheochromocytomas may arise anywhere, including the carotid body, in the heart, along the aorta, and within the urinary bladder.[372] The most common extra-adrenal location is the organ of Zuckerkandl, which is near the origin of the inferior mesenteric artery, to the left of the aortic bifurcation. Bilateral adrenal pheochromocytomas occur in MEN-2a and MEN-2b. Some believe that unilateral adrenal medullary tumor can occur in these patients, but in patients with MEN-2a who undergo unilateral adrenalectomy for pheochromocytoma, recurrent biochemical disease and/or imageable pheochromocytomas may develop in the contralateral adrenal gland with long follow-up.[373] Sturge-Weber syndrome is associated with cavernous hemangiomas of the trigeminal nerve and pheochromocytoma.

Data from series of patients with sporadic pheochromocytomas indicate that the right adrenal gland more commonly harbors a tumor than the left gland.[359,374] Pheochromocytomas resected from hypertensive patients usually measure between 3 and 5 cm in diameter and weigh approximately 100 g.[360] These tumors appear tan to gray and have a soft, smooth consistency. Larger tumors may be cystic, have necrotic areas, and often have calcification. Microscopically, pheochromocytomas resemble their cells of origin. They are usually arranged in cords or alveolar patterns.[219] Tumors may be composed of cords of cells lining vascular structures that have an angiomatous appearance.[375] Tumors are generally clearly separated from the adrenal cortex by a thin band of fibrous tissue. Extension of the pheochromocytoma into the cortex or vascular invasion may occur in benign neoplasms.[219]

The pathologic distinction between benign and malignant pheochromocytomas is not clear, and pathologists have relied on the reported benign natural history of most pheochromocytomas. However, recent reports indicate that more pheochromocytomas than expected may be malignant.[362] In one large series, the tumor recurrence rate was 10%, and most recurrences occurred within 5 years.[374] In two more recent series, the recurrence rates were 23% and 46% of the patients studied.[362,376] Although these rates partly reflect the referral pattern of tertiary institutions, they also reflect a higher malignancy rate than originally predicted.

Malignant tumors tend to be larger and weigh more than benign pheochromocytomas, although this is not an absolute criterion.[219] The only absolute criteria for malignancy are the presence of secondary tumors in sites where chromaffin cells are not usually present and visceral metastases.[377] Benign pheochromocytomas can demonstrate marked nuclear pleomorphism, and paradoxically, malignant ones demonstrate less.[219] Malignant pheochromocytomas usually have many more mitoses than benign tumors, but capsular and vascular invasion occurs with equal frequency in both.[219] Nuclear DNA ploidy may be an indicator of malignant potential.[378,379] Flow cytometry has been used recently to define a subgroup of patients with pheochromocytomas who have malignant tumors. Tumor DNA ploidy studies that showed tetra- or polyploidy and aneuploidy had a significantly higher chance of a malignant course than the majority of tumor cells that were normally diploid.[379] Studies by Medeiros and others indicate that the size (weight) of tumor and the degree of necrosis correlated best with malignant potential (Table 39-20).[380] The distinction between benign and malignant pheochromocytoma based on pathological criteria remains a challenge. Improved methods are vital because studies indicate that many more patients bear malignant, recurrent tumors than originally estimated.

DIAGNOSIS. Patients with pheochromocytomas can present with a range of symptoms from mild labile hypertension to sudden death secondary to a hypertensive crisis, myocardial infarction, or cerebral vascular accident. The classic patient describes "spells" of paroxysmal headaches, pallor, palpitation, hypertension, and diaphoresis. In 50% of patients the hypertension is intermittent; in the others it is sustained. In 90% of children with pheochromocytomas, the hypertension is sustained.[358] Patients may have signs of chronic hypovolemia, like orthostatic hypotension caused by excess alpha-catecholaminergic stimulation and vasoconstriction. The majority of patients have mild weight loss, but obesity does not rule out pheochromocytoma.

The diagnosis of pheochromocytoma is based on measuring catecholamines in the urine and blood and on the clonidine suppression test (Fig. 39-10). There is no single best screening test for pheochromocytoma. Some physicians prefer measurement of a spot urine for metanephrines. The false-negative rate is approximately 5%. A recent recommended screening method is the separate measurement of norepinephrine and epinephrine and their metabolites in the urine or serum.[381] Measuring urinary free catecholamines by ion-pair HPLC is another sensitive screening test.[382] If a

TABLE 39-20. Differentiation of Pheochromocytomas

Characteristics	*Benign*	*Malignant*	*Reference*
Metastases	—*	+	(377)
Weight (g)	156	759	(380)
Occurrence (%)	50–90	10–50	(374, 362)
Vascular invasion	+	+	(219)
Capsular invasion	+	+	(219)
Mitoses	±	++++	(219)
Nuclear pleomorphism	+	−	(219)
Ploidy	Diploid	Hyperdiploid triploid	(377, 378, 379)
Necrosis	±	++	(380)

*— does not occur; + occurs; ++ more prevalent; ++++ most prevalent.

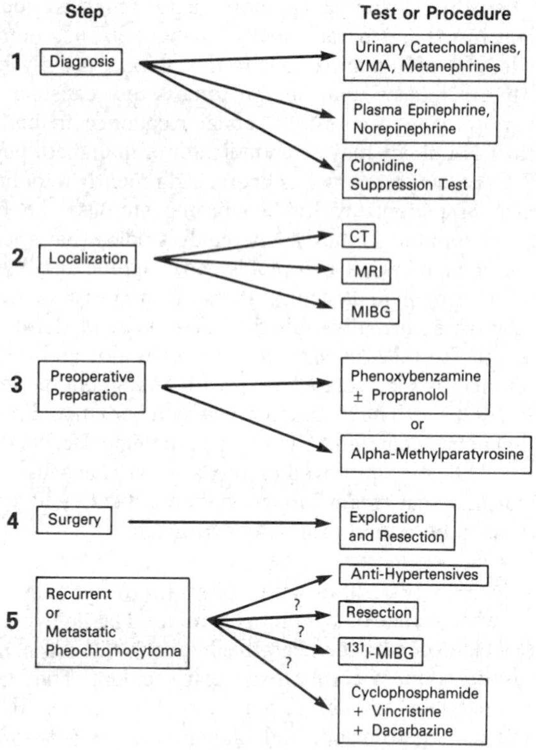

FIG. 39-10. Suggested flow diagram for the work-up, preparation, and treatment of a patient with a pheochromocytoma.

pheochromocytoma is suspected clinically or if a patient has a family history of MEN-2a or 2b, the next study is a 24-hour urine for catecholamines, metanephrines, and VMA. When patients with medullary thyroid carcinoma and MEN-2 family histories are screened for pheochromocytomas by these urinary studies, false negative results can occur.

Methods are now available to measure plasma catecholamines using a radioenzymatic assay.[383] This can provide a more direct measurement of catecholamine excess, but there have been conflicting reports comparing the value of urinary or plasma catecholamines in the diagnosis of pheochromocytoma.[384,385] As the plasma assays become more reliable, they offer a more sensitive and specific method than the urinary assays, especially when combined with clonidine.[381] The clonidine suppression test has become the test of choice to determine whether a patient with borderline urinary or plasma catecholamines has a pheochromocytoma.[386–389] While the patient rests supine in a quiet room, a venous catheter is inserted and blood samples are obtained and tested for plasma epinephrine, norepinephrine, and total catecholamines after 30 minutes. Then 300 μg of clonidine is administered orally, and 3 hours later, another blood sample is obtained. In normal patients with idiopathic hypertension, clonidine suppresses epinephrine and norepinephrine levels into the normal or less than normal range. In patients with pheochromocytomas, clonidine does not suppress plasma levels. In combining two studies from different groups, 14 normal persons suppressed, 51 essential hypertensive patients without pheochromocytomas suppressed, and 16 patients with proven pheochromocytomas did not suppress plasma epinephrine and norepinephrine levels following clonidine.[388,389] Only two incorrect diagnoses have been reported using the clonidine suppression test: one false positive and one false negative.[390] Autopsy of the patients with the false-positive test found diffuse infiltration of lymphoplasmacytic cells throughout the sympathetic ganglia and adrenal medulla. This finding suggested some unusual autoimmune disorder that resulted in excessive catecholamine production.[390] Despite the two unusual patients, the clonidine suppression test remains the best test for pheochromocytomas in patients with plasma catecholamine concentrations between 500 and 2000 pg/ml.[391]

LOCALIZATION STUDIES. CT and MRI are used to localize pheochromocytomas preoperatively.[311,316] Both are noninvasive, sensitive, and able to detect tumors approximately 1 cm in diameter. MRI is also specific because of the signal intensity on the T_2-weighted image. Pheochromocytomas appear more than three times as bright as liver, and few if any other adrenal tumors have a similar MRI appearance.[311] CT scanners have some advantages because of greater resolution and greater availability, but MRI scanners are rapidly improving in both areas. In a Mayo Clinic study of 52 patients with pheochromocytoma, CT detected 51 of 52 tumors, including 9 of 10 bilateral tumors.[392] In a more recent study, unenhanced, high-resolution CT detected pheochromocytomas in 6 of 6 patients who had tumors found at surgery, including 2 extra-adrenal retroperitoneal tumors.[393] In 7 patients with pheochromocytomas demonstrated on CT, MRI detected all primary lesions and metastases to the chest, retroperitoneum, and liver.[314] Because it has no radiation exposure, it has been used to successfully image a life-threatening pheochromocytoma during pregnancy in a patient with severe hypertension.[394] In addition, MRI successfully imaged an intrapericardial pheochromocytoma and distinguished it from the cardiac chambers and surrounding great vessels, which could not be determined by CT.[395] Adrenal arteriography and venography, which were formerly the best studies to localize pheochromocytomas, but were invasive and occasionally associated with hypertensive crises in unprepared patients, are no longer used to localize pheochromocytomas.

Another important new technique for the localization of functional pheochromocytomas is nuclear scanning following the administration of labelled MIBG. The compound is similar to norepinephrine and is taken up and concentrated in adrenergic tissue. ^{131}I-MIBG has been used in 400 patients to localize suspected pheochromocytoma.[396] The results were rated as true positive, false positive, true negative, or false negative, based on a combination of other imaging studies, venous sampling or pathologic results following surgical exploration. The sensitivity of MIBG scanning was 78% in sporadic pheochromocytoma, 91% in malignant pheochromocytoma, and 94% in familial pheochromocytoma. The overall sensitivity was 87%. The specificity was nearly 100% in all categories. MIBG scanning is safe, noninvasive, and efficacious for the localization of pheochromocytomas, including those that arise in nonadrenal sites and for malignant disease.[396] In addition, labelling MIBG with ^{123}I improves the quality of the images and allows detection of some pheochromocytomas not detectable with ^{131}I.[397] In a patient with extra-adrenal pheochromocytoma, ^{123}I-MIBG successfully imaged the tumor whereas ^{131}I-MIBG did not.[398] Metastatic bone involvement of pheochromocytoma can be imaged by ^{131}I-MIBG, but standard bone scintigraphy is more sensitive.[399,400] Iodine-131-MIBG used in 48 patients demonstrated a sensitivity of 77% and a specificity of 96%, and two other institutions had similar findings.[401–403] Whereas CT and MRI reflect changes in morphology, scintigraphic imaging relies on tissue function.[403] False-positive results with MIBG scintigraphy are rare, although tumors like medullary thyroid carcinoma and neuroblastoma can image. False-negative results (13%) are more common with multiple tumors and metastatic disease in the same patient.[397,404]

PREOPERATIVE PREPARATION. Once the diagnosis is established and the tumor localized, preoperative preparation includes alpha-adrenergic blockade. Phenoxybenzamine (10 mg) is taken orally two or three times a day (Fig. 39-10). If tachycardia develops (heart rate > 100 beats/min), beta-adrenergic blocking agents (propranolol) are added 1 week before surgery. Propranolol should never be started before alpha blockade, because unopposed vasoconstriction may worsen hypertension. One problem with intraoperative management of patients with pheochromocytomas is decreased blood volume and plasma volume because of tumor production of excess alpha-adrenergic hormones. Phenoxybenzamine blocks this excessive alpha-adrenergic activity, and after 14 days, the total blood volume and plasma volume increase to normal levels in patients with pheochromocytoma.[405] This standard regimen has been used by many institutions and has been a marked improvement over historical unprepared patients with pheochromocytomas.[406] In addition, lactic acidosis often results from the effect of catecholamines on intermediary metabolism and the peripheral circulation.[407] The measurement and correction of arterial blood pH should be performed in all patients before anesthesia and surgery.[407]

Alpha-methyltyrosine is a competitive inhibitor of tyrosine hydroxylase, the rate-limiting step in catecholamine biosynthesis. Treatment with alpha-methyltyrosine reduces catecholamine production by 50% to 80% in patients with pheochromocytoma. The usual dose is 250 mg twice daily, which may be increased to a maximum dosage of 3 to 4 g per day.[408] It has been used to prepare some patients with pheochromocytoma and unusual cardiac complications for surgery, and it can be used to treat hypertensive crisis in patients with pheochromocytoma.[409] The calcium-antagonist nifedipine is also used with phenoxybenzamine to control labile hypertensive episodes in patients with pheochromocytoma.[410]

INTRAOPERATIVE MANAGEMENT. If the patient is elderly or has had cardiac complications, the patient should be transferred to the intensive care unit 1 day before surgery. A Swan-Ganz catheter should be inserted, allowing correction of hemodynamic imbalances. The morning of the operation, an arterial catheter and peripheral intravenous catheters should be inserted. During surgery, especially during manipulation of the tumor, marked increases in blood pressure may occur, and hypertensive episodes should be controlled with either alpha-adrenergic blocking agents, like regitine, or with agents that directly relax arterial and venous smooth muscle, like sodium nitroprusside. Nitroprusside is the preferred drug because of its rapid onset and short duration. It is administered by a continuous intravenous infusion with a pump, and the blood pressure is continuously titrated to acceptable levels. Preoperative preparation with oral alpha-adrenergic blocking agents and intraoperative regulation of blood pressure with nitroprusside have greatly facilitated the surgical resection of pheochromocytomas.

The operation is performed using a transabdominal incision, either a bilateral subcostal or a long midline incision (Fig. 39-9). Preoperative localization studies guide the exploration, but the entire abdomen must be carefully viewed and palpated. Most pheochromocytomas will be well localized. However, some malignant pheochromocytomas or multiple pheochromocytomas in known or unsuspected MEN syndrome patients may be missed. Extra-adrenal pheochromocytomas may be difficult to find. The most common locations of intra-abdominal extra-adrenal pheochromocytoma are in the hilum of the kidneys and in the chromaffin tissue along the aorta from the celiac axis to the aortic bifurcation. The organ of Zuckerkandl at the aortic bifurcation is the most common extra-adrenal location, and pheochromocytomas have even been found within the bladder.[411] Multiple locations, metastatic potential, and multiple tumors all support the necessity for a thorough exploration of the entire abdominal cavity, which includes Kocherization of the duodenum and exploration of the lesser sac. The rule of ten should be considered in localizing pheochromocytomas: 10% malignant, 10% extra-adrenal, and 10% bilateral in the adrenal medulla.[387] This old rule may need to be modified. Recent results indicate that 26% to 47% of pheochromocytomas are malignant.[362,376] Almost 100% of patients with MEN-2 may have or develop bilateral benign adrenal medullary pheochromocytomas.[412]

MALIGNANT PHEOCHROMOCYTOMAS. Malignant pheochromocytomas are thought not to occur in MEN syndromes, but may account for almost half of the tumors in patients with pheochromocytomas.[362,376] In one study, 25 (36%) of 69 patients had malignant pheochromocytomas diagnosed by recurrent or metastatic disease, in another study using the same criteria, 81 (46%) of 176 patients with pheochromocytomas had malignant disease.[362,376] In the later study, the original histologic review failed to discriminate accurately between malignant and benign neoplasms. Pathologic analysis was not helpful in predicting which tumors were malignant.[362] Patients who developed metastases did not develop them until 0.2–28.7 years after their initial surgery. Incidence of detection for the first 9 years was 5% per year. Men were more likely to develop metastatic pheochromocytoma. Imaging with ^{131}I-MIBG was usually able to detect recurrent or metastatic pheochromocytoma, and yearly ^{131}I-MIBG scans are recommended for all patients following resection of pheochromocytoma.[362] Other groups also recommend lifetime follow-up.[376] The detection methods for primary, recurrent, or metastatic pheochromocytoma are the same: tests for urinary and serum catecholamines, clonidine suppression test, CT scan, MRI scan, and

^{131}I-MIBG scan. Careful follow-up requires some, but not necessarily all, of these studies annually. The incidence of malignant pheochromocytoma is greater than 10%, and careful follow-up may disclose a rate that approaches 50%.

TREATMENT. The basic principles in the treatment of malignant pheochromocytomas have been to surgically resect recurrences or metastases whenever possible and to treat hypertensive symptoms by catecholamine blockade.[413,414] Painful bony metastases, which can be diagnosed by either ^{131}I-MIBG scans or standard bone nuclide scans, respond well to radiotherapy.[400,415] Localized or solitary soft tissue masses can be successfully resected surgically.[416] Standard chemotherapy regimens including doxorubicin plus streptozotocin and BCNU plus doxorubicin have not had any efficacy in the treatment of malignant pheochromocytomas.[413]

Survival data of patients with malignant pheochromocytoma are difficult to obtain because of the rarity and indolence of the tumor.[416] In a large series from the Mayo clinic, the 5-year survival rate was 36%.[414] Patients who died did so within 3 years of the appearance of metastases.[417]

The early success with streptozotocin in the treatment of neuroendocrine tumors of the gastrointestinal tract suggested that it might also be useful in the treatment of malignant pheochromocytomas.[418] Initial work with streptozotocin was disappointing and suggested no role for it in the treatment of malignant pheochromocytoma.[413,417] However, Feldman suggested that the dosage schedule might be important in obtaining a beneficial result.[419] He provided an additional 3-year follow-up on a patient who responded well, noting that the patient maintained an 85% reduction in urinary homovanillic acid levels and a 73% reduction in urinary VMA levels, with normal renal function despite 66 g of streptozotocin.[420] Other investigators who have tried this high-dose streptozotocin regimen have seen no response and noticed a deterioration of renal function.[421] Although some patients with malignant pheochromocytoma may respond to streptozotocin chemotherapy, it does not appear to play a major role in the treatment of patients with these rare tumors.

Because of the high sensitivity (85%) and specificity (100%) of ^{131}I-MIBG for imaging pheochromocytomas, its use in higher doses to treat recurrent or metastatic pheochromocytomas is a logical progression. Current imaging modalities of pheochromocytoma permit relatively accurate dosimetry on the basis of the diagnostic dose of ^{131}I-MIBG administered. If uptake by primary or metastatic lesions is good, it is possible to deliver radiation doses of several thousand rad by increasing the administered activity. Specific activity of ^{131}I-MIBG of 200 mCi in 5 mg has now been achieved.[422] Unfortunately, treatment results have not been very dramatic. Treatment response in patients with pheochromocytomas can be measured by catecholamine secretion and standard tumor measurements. In 12 patients treated with ^{131}I-MIBG, only 5 had reduced catecholamine levels and 2 had decreased tumor size.[423] Vetter and colleagues reported two patients with malignant pheochromocytomas who had minor reduction in tumor size but no change in catecholamine secretion.[424] There have been no complete responses.[422]

In order for a malignant pheochromocytoma to concentrate and retain ^{131}I-MIBG the tumor must have an active neuronal pump mechanism.[424] Keiser and colleagues found that only one of five patients with metastatic pheochromocytoma had appreciable uptake of ^{131}I-MIBG into the tumor.[425] When ^{131}I-MIBG was administered to 9 patients with metastatic pheochromocytoma, 40% to 55% of the administered radioactivity appeared in the urine as ^{131}I-MIBG in 24 hours, and 70% to 90% appeared in the urine within 4 days.[426] The agent was rapidly excreted via the kidneys and was stable. This reduced ability of malignant pheochromocytomas to take up ^{131}I-MIBG may be partially explained by a recent study in which plasma levels of dopa and catecholamines from patients with benign pheochromocytomas were compared with levels from patients with malignant pheochromocytomas and neuroblastomas.[427] Neuroblastomas are aggressive tumors of neural-crest origin that occur in children and have no association with hypertension. All the patients with neuroblastoma had high plasma levels of dopa. Patients with benign pheochromocytomas had elevated plasma levels of norepinephrine or epinephrine, and none had elevated plasma levels of dopa. Sixty percent of patients with malignant pheochromocytomas had elevated plasma levels of dopa compared with benign pheochromocytomas. These observations suggest that patients with benign pheochromocytomas have well-differentiated tumor cells that function as normal chromaffin tissue. These cells synthesize and store norepinephrine and epinephrine, which lead to hypertension. Maligant pheochromocytomas, which are composed of less-differentiated cells, grow more rapidly and have relatively deficient mechanisms for catecholamine synthesis or storage, explaining why malignant tumors do not take up as much ^{131}I-MIBG and why dopa is detected in the plasma of 60% of patients with malignant pheochromocytoma, but not in patients with benign pheochromocytoma.[427] The similarity between malignant pheochromocytoma and neuroblastoma is further supported by the astonishing responsiveness of malignant pheochromocytomas to therapy that is effective in treating neuroblastomas.[425,428]

There are many similarities between pheochromocytoma and neuroblastoma: both arise from neuroectoderm, both contain neuron-specific enolase, and dopa circulates in the plasma of patients with both.[425,427] Because of these similarities and because a combination of cyclophosphamide, vincristine, and dacarbazine is 80% effective for metastatic neuroblastoma, this regimen was used in patients with metastatic pheochromocytoma.[425,429] The chemotherapy regimen consisted of cyclophosphamide (750 mg/m^2 IV on day 1), vincristine (1.4 mg/m^2 IV on day 1), and dacarbazine (600 mg/m^2 on days 1 and 2) in 21- to 28-day cycles. Doses of cyclophosphamide and dacarbazine were adjusted on the basis of neurotoxicity. Three patients were treated, and each had clear decreases in catecholamines and blood pressure and each had a documented partial response on imaging studies. Patients had either progressed on ^{131}I-MIBG therapy or failed to show tumors on ^{131}I-MIBG scan.[425]

This chemotherapy regimen has been used in 15 patients

TABLE 39-21. Treatment of Metastatic Malignant Pheochromocytoma

Year	*Compound*	*Number of Patients*	*Catecholamine Secretion (%)*	*Result of Imaging (%)*	*Reference*
1985	^{131}I-MIBG	12	5 PR (40%)	2 PR (16%)	(422)
1983	^{131}I-MIBG	3	NC*	±	(423)
1983	High-dose streptozotocin	1	PR	PR	(419)
1985	High-dose streptozotocin	1	NC	NC	(421)
1985	Cyclophosphamide + vincristine + dacarbazine	3	3 PR	3 PR	(425)
1987	Cyclophosphamide + vincristine + darcarbazine	15	13 PR (87%)	1 CR 7 PR (53%)	(428)

*NC = no change; ± = questionable decrease; PR = partial response; CR = complete remission.

with metastatic pheochromocytoma.[428] The ability to respond to the regimen correlated with the plasma norepinephrine level before therapy. One patient had a complete response and seven patients had partial responses, for an overall response rate of 53%. Decreased urinary catecholamine levels correlated well with the response evaluated by imaging studies. The median response lasted about 18 months. All responding patients have had dramatic improvement in hypertension control and performance status. The regimen has been well tolerated and toxicity has been mild.[428] Malaise, nausea, and vomiting have been limited to the initial 48 hours after therapy. Reversible granulocytopenia has been controlled by reductions of cyclophosphamide and dacarbazine. Hypertensive crisis following cytotoxic drug therapy in patients with unsuspected pheochromocytomas have been reported,[430] but this potentially life-threatening complication is not a problem as long as the patients have adequate alpha-adrenergic blockade.[425,430] Table 39-21 lists treatment regimens for metastatic pheochromocytoma.

CARCINOID TUMORS

In 1907, Oberndorfer described a group of intestinal tumors which grew slowly and appeared to be more benign than adenocarcinomas. He called these tumors "Karzinoide" or carcinoid.[431] Later it was recognized that carcinoid tumors were associated with an unusual syndrome that included flushing, wheezing, watery diarrhea, and valvular heart disease.[473] Carcinoid tumors arise from enterochromaffin (EC) cells, which are scattered throughout the body but occur primarily in the submucosa of the intestine and main bronchi. In the intestine, these cells are present at the base of the crypts and are sometimes called Kultschitzky cells.[432,433] Some EC cells, called argentaffin, can take up and reduce silver. Others, called argyrophilic, take up silver, but do not reduce it. EC cells contain peptides, such as substance P, enkephalins, or motilin.[434]

PATHOLOGY

According to Pearse, the EC cells are thought to migrate from the neural crest to their final adult location in a manner similar to C cells of the thyroid, melanocytes of the skin, and chromaffin cells of the adrenal medulla.[435,436] Tumors arising from these cells, such as carcinoid tumors, medullary carcinoma of the thyroid, melanomas, and pheochromocytomas, have been classified by Bolande and Pearse as APUDomas (*a*mine *p*recursor *u*ptake and *d*ecarboxylation).[435,436]

The APUDomas share a number of histological, ultrastructural, and biochemical features. Histologically, they are similar to islet cell tumors.[437] Both are composed of monotonous sheets of small round cells with uniform nuclei and cytoplasm. Mitotic figures are rare. Pathologists cannot differentiate benign from malignant carcinoids based on histology, nor can they differentiate islet cell tumors from carcinoids. Malignancy can only be unequivocally determined if there is documentation of lymph node or distant metastases. Ultrastructurally, they possess electron-dense neurosecretory granules.[438] It has been shown by immunoperoxidase staining that carcinoid tumors synthesize numerous peptides, including neuron-specific enolase, 5-hydroxytryptamine, 5-hydroxytryptophan, insulin, growth hormone, neurotensin, ACTH, beta-melanocyte stimulating hormone, gastrin, calcitonin, substance P, growth hormone-releasing hormone, and bombesin.[439–442] Shared biochemical characteristics include the presence of increased activity of various tissue enzymes, including diamine oxidase, L-dopa decarboxylase, cholinesterase, and nonspecific esterase.[436] Although recent evidence suggests that islet cell and parathyroid adenomas are not of neural crest origin, the similarity of these tumors to carcinoid tumors makes the concept of the APUDoma useful.[442]

Williams and Sanders originally proposed classifying carcinoids (Table 39-22) according to their site of origin: foregut carcinoids, including the respiratory tract, pancreas, stomach and duodenum; midgut carcinoids arising from the ileum and appendix; and hindgut carcinoids, arising from the left colon and rectum.[443] Foregut carcinoids generally have a

TABLE 39-22. Classification of Carcinoid Tumors

	Origin		
Characteristics	*Foregut*	*Midgut*	*Hindgut*
Organ	Respiratory tract pancreas, stomach, duodenum	Ileum, appendix	Rectum, left colon
Silver staining	Argentaffin negative, argyrophilic, or negative	Argentaffin positive	Argentaffin negative or occ. argyrophilic
Cytoplasmic granules	Round, variable density, 180 μm	Pleomorphilic, uniform density, 230 μm	Round, variable density, 190 μm
Tumor	Low 5-HT content, multihormonal*	High 5-HT content, multihormonal*	Rarely 5-HT, multihormonal*
Blood	5-HTP, histamine, multihormonal,* Occ. ACTH	5-HT, multihormonal,* rarely ACTH	Rarely release 5-HTP or ACTH
Urine	5-HTP, 5-HT, 5-HIAA, histamine and others	5-HT, 5-HIAA	Negative
Carcinoid syndrome	Yes	Frequently (with metastases)	Rarely
Metastasize to bone	Common	Rarely	Common

* Multihormonal products include tachykinins (substance P, substance K, neuropeptide K), neurotensin, pancreatic polypeptide, ACTH, or alpha subunit of human chorionic gonadotrophin.

low serotonin (5-HT) content, are argentaffin negative but argyrophilic, occasionally secrete 5-hydroxytryptophan (5-HTP) or ACTH, are often multihormonal, and may metastasize to bone. Although many of these foregut carcinoids contain peptides, clinical syndromes are rarely produced and elevated levels of hormones in the plasma are generally not detected. Gastric carcinoids in particular, although containing a variety of gastrointestinal hormones, are almost always asymptomatic.[447] Midgut carcinoids are argentaffin positive, have a high serotonin content, have a smaller number of endocrine cells than foregut tumors, release 5-HT and tachykinins (substance P, neuropeptide K, substance K), rarely secrete 5-HTP or ACTH, and rarely metastasize to bone. Hindgut carcinoid tumors are argentaffin negative, are often argyrophilic, rarely contain 5-HT, contain numerous gastrointestinal hormones, rarely secrete 5-HTP or ACTH, and may metastasize to bone.

Carcinoid tumors can be ubiquitous, but most will originate in four sites: bronchus, appendix, rectum, or small intestine (Table 39-23). Carcinoid tumors most frequently occur in the appendix (38%). The exact incidence of carcinoid tumors is not known, although an annual incidence has been reported in Ireland of 3.2 cases per million persons, making them four times as common as insulinomas and eight times as common as gastrinomas.[448] The clinical presentation of carcinoids far underestimates their occurrence because many are frequently asymptomatic. SEER data report an annual incidence of 2.8 per million persons for small intestinal carcinoids, but in an autopsy study at the Mayo Clinic the incidence was 6500 per million.[437,448]

Approximately 1 in every 200 to 300 appendectomies has a carcinoid tumor in the resected appendix.[437] Most of these neoplasms occur in the tip of the appendix, and 90% of these appendiceal carcinoids will be smaller than 1 cm in diameter and have no metastases.[437,451] However, approximately 50% of all appendiceal carcinoids between 1 and 2 cm will metastasize to lymph nodes.[452]

Small intestinal carcinoids may be multiple; 87% occur within the ileum and 40% within 2 feet of the ileocecal valve.[437] Primary tumors tend to remain small and extend outward into the lumen. They may spread to local lymph nodes, and a marked fibrotic reaction can occur, which distorts the gut or mesentery and presents as a small bowel obstruction or mesenteric infarction. Further spread invades the liver or bone. Approximately 20% to 35% of small intestinal carcinoid tumors are malignant and metastasize (Table 39-23). The incidence of metastases depends on the size of the primary lesion. Only 15% of the tumors less than 1 cm in diameter metastasize.[437] If the tumor is between 1 and 2 cm, metastases occur between 60% and 80% of the time.[437] If the tumor is greater than 2 cm in size, metastases nearly always occur.[437,452]

In approximately 1 in every 2500 proctoscopies, a small gray-yellow nodule will be seen, which on pathologic examination is diagnosed as a carcinoid tumor.[437] Nearly all rectal carcinoids occur submucosally on the anterior or lateral walls of the rectum between 4 and 13 cm above the dentate line.[437]

Bronchial carcinoids are rare and account for only 1% to 6% of all primary lung tumors.[453] Poor prognosis is indicated by high mitotic count, nuclear pleomorphism, vascular invasion, undifferentiated growth pattern, and lymphatic invasion. The bronchus is the site of the primary carcinoid tumor in about 12% of cases.[453,454]

Carcinoid tumors are classified based on their histologic growth pattern as either insular, trabecular, glandular, undif-

TABLE 39-23. Location, Incidence of Metastases, and Incidence of Carcinoid Syndrome by Location

Distribution	*Location of Tumors (%)*	*Incidence of Metastases (%)*	*Incidence of Carcinoid Syndrome (%)*
Foregut			
Esophagus	<1		
Stomach	2	22	9.5
Duodenum	2.6	20	3.4
Pancreas	<1	20	20
Gallbladder	<1	33	5
Bile Duct	<1		
Ampulla	<1	14	
Larynx	<1	50	
Bronchus	11.5	20	13
Thymus	2	25	
Midgut			
Jejunum	1.3	35	9
Ileum	23	35	9
Meckel's	1	18	13
Appendix	38	2	<1
Colon	2	60	5
Liver	<1		
Ovary	<1	6	50
Testis	<1		50
Cervix	<1	24	3
Hindgut			
Rectum	13	3	

Maton PN: The carcinoid tumor and the carcinoid syndrome. In Becker K (ed): Principles and Practice of Endocrinology and Metabolism. Philadelphia, JB Lippincott, 1987.

ferentiated, or mixed.[455] The histologic types have prognostic significance.[456,457] Glandular and undifferentiated carcinoids have the worst prognosis. Midgut carcinoids have a better prognosis than either foregut or hindgut carcinoids.[456] A study demonstrated that 27% of the midgut carcinoids that had the best prognosis were in the favorable histologic group (insular structure), whereas none of foregut carcinoids and none of hindgut carcinoids, which have a worse prognosis, were in the insular histologic group.[457] Multivariate analysis demonstrated that both histologic type and primary site have independent prognostic significance.[457]

Neither the stimulus for induction of malignant growth nor the factors that promote growth of carcinoid tumors are known. Recent data demonstrate that gastrin may be an important growth factor for gastric carcinoids. In pernicious anemia and atrophic gastritis, basal hypergastrinemia develops as achlorhydria develops, a disease state for which endocrine cell hyperplasia, nodules of mucosal argyrophilic cells, and carcinoid tumors have been reported.[439,458–461] Gastric carcinoids have also been reported in Zollinger-Ellison syndrome, which suggests that the hypergastrinemia may be the important factor.[439] Rats treated for prolonged periods of time with omeprazole, which is a potent long-acting inhibitor of the gastric H^+-K^+ ATPase, develop prolonged achlorhydria and basal hypergastrinemia, which results in EC hyperplasia and gastric carcinoids.[462] These experimental changes occur more frequently in female rats, suggesting that hormonal factors may also influence development of gastric carcinoids.[462]

CLINICAL FEATURES

Carcinoid Tumors Without Systemic Features

Some carcinoid tumors do not cause the carcinoid syndrome. In the most common site of occurrence the appendix (Table 39-23), carcinoid tumors are almost always found incidentally during surgery for appendicitis. Small intestinal carcinoids are the most common location for carcinoid tumors of clinical significance.[437] Most small intestinal carcinoids rarely cause symptoms, but these tumors can cause fibrosis of the mesentery, which results in kinking of the bowel, intestinal obstruction, obstruction of blood supply, and gut infarction or intussusception caused by the tumor itself or by spread of the tumor. The most common clinical presentation for small intestinal carcinoid is periodic abdominal pain that is consistent with a diagnosis of intermittent small bowel obstruction.[437] Gastrointestinal bleeding is uncommon and small intestinal carcinoids rarely ulcerate.[437] Because of the vagueness of the symptoms, the diagnosis of small intestinal carcinoid is frequently delayed by an average of 2 years.[437] Except for an abdominal mass with or without hepatomegaly, there are no physical signs to suggest small intestinal carcinoid tumors.[437]

Duodenal and gastric carcinoids are usually found incidentally during endoscopy. Rectal carcinoids are also found incidentally during endoscopy but can be quite large and cause obstruction. Rectal carcinoid tumors seldom cause bleeding because of their submucosal location, and they rarely ulcerate. Bronchial carcinoids are usually discovered as a coin lesion on x-ray films. Patients may present with cough, wheeze, hemoptysis, or with segmental obstruction and pneumonia. Thymic carcinoids present as anterior mediastinal masses usually on x-ray films or CT scans. Ovarian and testicular carcinoids may present as masses which can be reliably detected by physical examination or ultrasound. Most carcinoids present as an isolated disease, but there are associations between foregut carcinoids and multiple endocrine neoplasia type I, between gastric carcinoids and diseases causing hypergastrinemia, and between ampullary carcinoids and von Recklinghausen's disease.[439,458–461,463–466] Metastatic carcinoid tumors may frequently be found in patients with a grossly enlarged liver. These patients are fully active with minimal symptoms and have normal or near normal liver function tests.[437]

Carcinoid Tumors with Systemic Features

Carcinoid tumors contain and occasionally secrete a number of gastrointestinal peptides, which are thought to be involved in the pathogenesis of the carcinoid syndrome.[434,440,441,444,445,466–468] Because all APUDomas are carcinoid tumors and it cannot be determined which of the gastrointestinal hormones are released in sufficient amounts to cause symptoms, the carcinoid tumors that are found in a patient with a given clinical syndrome due to excess peptide are classified by that clinical syndrome, e.g., gastrinoma, insulinoma, somatostatinoma, GRFoma. Elevated serum concentrations of pancreatic polypeptide have been reported in 43% of patients with carcinoid tumors, motilin in 14%, somatostatin in 5%, calcitonin in 4%, alpha-subunit of HCG in 28%, beta-subunit of HCG in 12%, gastrin in 15%.[440,468] None had an elevated VIP or gastrin-releasing peptide serum concentration.[440] Even though these gastrointestinal peptides were present in the sera, it is not apparent that they contributed to any clinical symptoms.

Foregut carcinoids have been reported to be more likely to produce various gastrointestinal peptides than midgut carcinoids.[434] Foregut carcinoids have been reported to release ACTH, causing Cushing's syndrome, and release growth hormone, causing acromegaly.[434,472]

The Carcinoid Syndrome

MANIFESTATIONS. Even though carcinoid tumors have been known for 80 years, the endocrine manifestations of these tumors were not described until 1954.[473,474] The principal clinical manifestations are cutaneous flushing, diarrhea, valvular heart disease, asthma or wheezing, and facial telangectasia (Table 39-24).

Flushing attacks initially occur in 25% to 73% of patients and in 63% to 94% of patients at some time during the course of the disease. The typical flush is the sudden appearance of a deep red or violaceous erythema of the upper part of the body, primarily the face and neck. Flushes are associated with an unpleasant feeling of warmth, lacrimation, itching, palpitations, facial or conjunctival edema, and diarrhea. Flushes may be spontaneous or may be precipitated by stress, alcohol, certain foods (e.g., cheese), exercise, or injections of catecholamines (adrenaline, noradrenaline, isoproterenol), calcium, pentagastrin, or the COOH-terminal octapeptide of cholecystokinin.[467,475–481] Initial flushing attacks may last only 2 to 5 minutes; later attacks may last for hours. The most distinctive types of flushing are those associated with bronchial carcinoids or gastric carcinoids. With bronchial carcinoids the flushes are reported to be prolonged, reddish, and associated with salivation, lacrimation, diaphoresis, facial swelling, palpitations, diarrhea, and hypotension.[475] The flushing can cause diffuse body involvement, and after repeated flushing of this type, patients may develop a constant red or cyanotic coloration.[437] The flush associated with gastric carcinoids is also reddish but is distributed in patches over the neck and face. It is frequently provoked by food intake or pentagastrin. The erythema is associated with blotches and wheals with central clearing, and the lesions are frequently associated with pruritis.[437,475,476,481]

Diarrhea initially occurs in 32% to 78% of patients with

TABLE 39-24. Clinical Characteristics in Patients with Malignant Carcinoid Syndrome

Patients and Characteristics	*At Presentation*		*During Course of Disease*			
	1973[467]	*1987*[468]	*1961*[471]	*1958*[469]	*1987*[470]	*1987*[468]
Total patients	91	103	138	79	111	103
Symptom (%)						
Diarrhea	73	32	78	68	73	84
Flushing	65	23	94	74	63	75
Pain		10				
Asthma/wheezing	8	4	19	18	3	15
Pellagra	2		7	5		
None	12				22	
Carcinoid heart disease (%)	11		53	41	14	33
Sex (% males)	59	46		61		46
Mean age (yr)	57	59		52		
(range)	(25–79)			(18–80)		
Tumor location (%)						
Foregut	5	9		2		9
Midgut	78	87		75		87
Hindgut	5	1		8		1
Unknown	11	2		15		2

the carcinoid syndrome and is common in 68% to 84% at some time during the course of the disease. Diarrhea usually occurs with flushing (85% of cases), but it may occur alone (15% of cases).[470] Typically, the patient describes the stools as watery or less commonly as frothy or as the pale, bulky stool of steatorrhea, with the stool number ranging from 2 to 30 per day.[467,475] The diarrhea usually occurs independent of the flushing attacks.[467] Steatorrhea is much less common than diarrhea.[475,482] Abdominal pain may occur with or without diarrhea in 10% to 50% of patients.[469]

Cardiac manifestations have been reported in 11% to 53% of patients in different series. This cardiac disease is a unique form of fibrosis involving the endocardium, primarily of the right side of the heart, although left-side lesions can also occur.[475,483] The fibrous deposits are found most commonly on the ventricular aspect of the tricuspid valve and the associated chordae and less commonly on the pulmonary valve cusps. These fibrous deposits tend to cause constriction of both the tricuspid and pulmonic valves. At the pulmonic valve, stenosis is predominant, whereas at the tricuspid valve, the constriction results in the valve being fixed open, and tricuspid regurgitation is predominant, although some degree of clinical tricuspid stenosis can occur.[475,483,484] In two series, 80% of the patients with cardiac lesions had evidence of heart failure.[467,469]

Other clinical manifestations of carcinoid syndrome are wheezing or asthma-like symptoms in 8% to 25% of patients and pellagra-like skin lesions with hyperkeratosis and pigmentation in 2% to 6% of cases. Rarely reported to occur in carcinoid syndrome are rheumatoid arthritis, arthralgias, changes in mental state or confusion, ophthalmic changes during flushing leading to vessel occlusion, and retroperitoneal fibrosis leading to ureteral obstruction or Peyronie's disease of the penis.[469,485]

PATHOBIOLOGY. The carcinoid syndrome occurs only when the hormonal products released by the tumor reach the systemic circulation in sufficient concentration to result in clinical manifestations. The severity of the carcinoid syndrome is directly related to tumor size in an area that drains into the systemic circulation.[437] In almost all cases, especially with midgut carcinoids, this occurs after distant metastases, especially to the liver. With gastrointestinal carcinoids, the syndrome was associated with hepatic metastases in 95% of patients in one study and with distant metastases in 100% of patients in another study.[467,486] Rarely, primary gut tumors with nodal or extensive peritoneal metastases or peritoneal metastases with direct access to the ovarian veins or systemic circulation can produce the carcinoid syndrome without hepatic metastases.[467,487] Bronchial tumors can also give rise to the carcinoid syndrome without metastatic disease; however, in most cases metastases are present.[488–490] Rarely, tumors of thyroid C cells or oat cell tumors have been reported to cause the carcinoid syndrome.[475,489] All carcinoid tumors do not have the same propensity to metastasize and to produce the carcinoid syndrome (Table 39-23). Because midgut tumors are the most common and frequently metastasize in almost all series, midgut tumors account for 75% to 87% of the carcinoids causing the carcinoid syndrome. Foregut tumors account for 2% to 9%, hindgut for 1% to 8%, and unknown primary tumors for 2% to 15% (Table 39-24).

In the original description of the complete carcinoid syndrome, the dramatic symptom complex of valvular heart disease, peripheral vasomotor symptoms, bronchoconstriction, and cyanosis was attributed to secretion of 5-HT by the tumor.[473,474] In previous reports, the carcinoid syndrome with overproduction of 5-HT was estimated to occur in 6%, 10%, and 18% of patients.[467,491,492] These studies assumed that the patients with carcinoid syndrome had overproduction of 5-HT, but production was not systematically examined in all patients with carcinoid tumors.[470] About half of 220 patients with carcinoid tumor had evidence of 5-HT overproduction in one study.[470] In two other studies, 18% of 500 patients and 88% of 103 patients with carcinoid tumors had an elevated urinary 5-hydroxyindoleacetic acid (5-HIAA), the major metabolite of 5-HT.[467,468] In two of these studies, 12% to 22% of all patients with evidence of 5-HT overproduction had no symptoms, and in one study, only 58% of the patients having 5-HT overproduction had both flushing and diarrhea.[470] However, in patients without evidence of 5-HT overproduction, 5% had facial swelling or diarrhea.[470] Therefore, 5-HT overproduction cannot be equated with the symptoms of the carcinoid syndrome.[470]

Characteristically patients with carcinoid syndrome have expansion of the 5-HT pool size, increase in blood and platelet concentrations of 5-HT, and elevations of 5-HIAA in the urine.[493] In patients with the typical carcinoid syndrome, the conversion of tryptophan to 5-HTP is the rate limiting step. The 5-HTP is converted to 5-HT in the tumor and either stored in the tumor or released into vascular compartments. The majority is taken up by platelets, with a small amount remaining in the plasma (Fig. 39-11). Most of the 5-HT in the circulation is converted by monoamine oxidase and aldehyde dehydrogenase to 5-HIAA, which appears in large amounts in the urine.[470,493]

This is the typical pattern seen in midgut carcinoids, which characteristically secrete large amounts of 5-HIAA and 5-HT and which made up to 75% to 87% of all cases of carcinoid syndrome. Some carcinoid tumors cause an atypical carcinoid syndrome.[434,484,494,495] They are deficient in the enzyme dopa decarboxylase and they cannot convert 5-HTP to 5-HT, and 5-HTP is secreted into the blood stream (Fig. 39-11). Plasma levels of 5-HT are normal in patients with these tumors, but urinary levels are usually elevated because some of the 5-HTP is decarboxylated in the kidney and excreted as 5-HT. Patients with this type of carcinoid tumor may have a marked increase in urinary 5-HT and 5-HTP levels, but normal or only slightly elevated 5-HIAA levels.[470] Foregut carcinoid tumors are more likely to excrete high levels of 5-HT and 5-HTP in the urine and appear as the atypical carcinoid syndrome.

Flushing is not thought to be due to serotonin overproduction because serotonin antagonists such as methysergide, cyproheptadine, or ketanserin generally have no effect on the flushing. It has been proposed that 5-HT may play a role in provoking flushing attacks.[470,496–499] Early studies demonstrated that kinins, which are vasoactive substances, were released from carcinoids and that carcinoids contain kallikrein, an enzyme that can convert plasma kininogen to lysylbradykinin, which is converted to bradykinin.[500-502] However, not all patients have increase in bradykinin during flushing, and a study demonstrated that plasma kallikrein levels were not different in patients with carcinoids from those of normal controls and that levels did not increase in patients following alcohol administration despite the fact that some patients developed a flush.[480,500] This study suggested that circulating kallikrein levels were not a cause of the flush in these patients.[503]

The exact cause of the flushing in patients with carcinoid syndrome may differ according to tumor types and their secretory products. In patients with gastric carcinoids, the red, patchy, pruritic flush is thought to be mediated by histamine, because this type of flushing can be prevented by the use of H_1 and H_2 histamine receptor antagonists.[477,504,505] Candidates for mediators of flushing seen with midgut carcinoids include the tachykinins (substance P, neuropeptide K), various gastrointestinal peptides, and prostaglandins.[470,499,510] PGE, PGF, and other prostaglandins have been extracted from carcinoid tumors.[506] In one patient, plasma concentrations were correlated with the severity of flushing, but in other studies, no correlation existed between the clinical symptoms and prostaglandin levels.[506-508] Furthermore, a review of numerous reports of prostaglandin measurements in the carcinoid syndrome and of studies showing the ineffectiveness of prostaglandin synthesis inhibitors on flushing or diarrhea indicate that prostaglandins are unlikely to be the mediators.[470,509]

Recent studies demonstrated that substance P, neurokinin A (substance K), and neuropeptide K are stored in carcinoid tumor and released during flushing.[440,468,510-514] One study reported that plasma neuropeptide K increased during spontaneous and pentagastrin-stimulated flush.[515] Even though flushing can be produced by infusion of substance P, changes in plasma substance P or neuropeptide K does not always correlate with flushing, suggesting that circulating tachykinins have only a minor role, if any, in causing the flushing.[440,470,499,516] Even though various gastrointestinal peptides have been proposed, no changes in VIP, GIP, neurotensin, pancreatic polypeptide, motilin, insulin, glucagon, or enteroglucagon occurred with provocation of the flush.[503] Thus, the exact cause of flushing in the carcinoid syndrome remains unexplained.

5-HT is thought to be predominantly responsible for the diarrhea because of its effects on gut motility.[470,517,518] It also may cause fat malabsorption, and probably induces a secretory state in the small intestine.[470,519] Furthermore, 5-HT receptor antagonists (methylsergide, cyproheptadine, ketanserin) all relieve the diarrhea but not the flushing.[496-499] In combination with histamine, 5-HT may be responsible for producing asthma, and it is thought to be involved in the fibrotic reactions involved in causing heart disease, Peyronie's disease, and ureteral obstruction.[434,475,499,520]

DIAGNOSIS

Diagnosis of the carcinoid syndrome relies on the measurement of 5-HT or 5-HIAA in the urine, with the measurement of 5-HIAA in a 24-hour urine sample the most commonly used test. False positives may occur if the patient eats foods such as bananas, plantains, pineapple, kiwi fruit, walnuts, hickory nuts, pecans, and avocados, which would falsely elevate urinary levels.[521] Medications, including cough medicine containing guafanesin, acetaminophen, salicylates, and L-dopa, should also be avoided because they may affect urinary 5-HIAA levels.[522] Although a simple and inexpensive qualitative test can be used to measure increased excretion of 5-HIAA in the urine, the test is only positive when patients excrete more than 30 mg of 5-HIAA daily.[523] For properly controlled dietary and medicinal intake, the normal range for urinary 5-HIAA excretion is between 2 and 8 mg/24 hours. Many patients with 5-HT secreting carcinoid tumors have an increase in urinary 5-HIAA excretion, but in the range of 8 to 30 mg/24 hours; thus, the measurement of urinary 5-HIAA levels is the best method to diagnose the carcinoid syndrome.[524] 5-HIAA determinations alone have been shown to have a 73% sensitivity and a 100% specificity for the carcinoid syndrome.[470]

Although most physicians rely totally on the measurement of urinary 5-HIAA excretion to diagnose carcinoid tumors, measurements of urinary and platelet 5-HT may give additional information, and it is now recommended that these should also be measured.[470,524] Elevations of 5-HIAA can occur in malabsorption states, such as celiac disease, blind loop syndrome, chronic intestinal obstruction, and Whipple's syndrome.[475,496] Also, foregut carcinoids tend to produce the atypical carcinoid syndrome with increased 5-hydroxytryptophan but normal 5-HT. If there is a strong suspicion of the carcinoid syndrome in patients with a normal or minimally elevated 5-HIAA, they should be screened for other urinary metabolites of tryptophan.[524] This is usually not necessary because some of the 5-HTP is decarboxylated in the intestine and other tissues, and many of these patients have elevated urinary 5-HT or 5-HIAA.[481,524] In evaluating 75 patients with known carcinoid tumors, 15 patients had normal or slightly elevated urinary 5-HIAA levels, 11 of whom had elevated urinary 5-HT levels and 4 of whom had elevated platelet 5-HT levels.[524] The radioenzymatic assay for urinary or platelet serotonin levels is not readily available.[524,526]

Diagnostic difficulties may arise in patients who flush for reasons other than the carcinoid syndrome, in patients with the carcinoid syndrome in whom flushing is not apparent, in patients with carcinoid tumors in whom 5-HIAA may be normal or minimally elevated, or in the rare patient without metastatic disease who presents with flushing.[487,524,527] Other causes of flushing include menopausal flushing, reactions to alcohol and glutamate, side-effects from drugs like chlorpropamide, calcium channel blockers, or nicotinic acid, and other tumors, such as chronic myelogenous leukemia and systemic mastocytosis.[527] None of these conditions causes increased urinary 5-HIAA, and these tumors can be distinguished pathologically.

The diagnosis of a carcinoid tumor may be suggested by clinical symptoms or be made in relatively asymptomatic patients only after a histologic examination of a liver biopsy specimen or of a tumor specimen removed during endoscopy or surgery. In one study involving 154 consecutive patients with GI carcinoid tumors, 60% of those found at surgery were asymptomatic and 48% were symptomatic.[452] Radiographic studies were of limited value in detecting the carcinoids preoperatively, but endoscopy was valuable in that it detected all gastric carcinoids preoperatively and 45 of 46 rectal carcinoids preoperatively.[452] Positive barium studies usually showed dilated loops of small bowel or an extrinsic filling defect, but rarely showed a mucosal lesion in one study; ileal carcinoids were diagnosed or suggested in studies by others.[452,528,529] Although CT scan, ultrasonography, or arteriography will detect most hepatic metastases, the primary site is frequently not detected by these procedures.[468,528–534] One study demonstrated that ^{131}I-MIBG localized 71% of midgut carcinoids and 33% of foregut carcinoid tumors.[536] In patients with symptomatic carcinoid tumor, the time from the onset of symptoms until the diagnosis is frequently delayed by 1 to 2 years.[437,468]

Because metastatic carcinoid tumors can not be distinguished in many cases from metastatic islet cell tumors and because many metastatic carcinoids do not produce clinical symptoms of the carcinoid syndrome, recent studies have attempted to identify specific and sensitive serum markers for carcinoid tumors.[440,468,470] In one study, urinary 5-HIAA had a sensitivity of 73% and a specificity of 100%; plasma substance P had a sensitivity of 32% and a specificity of 85%; and plasma neurotensin had a sensitivity of 41% and a specificity of 60%.[440] In another study 88% of patients with carcinoid tumors (93% with hepatic metastases) had an elevated 5-HIAA, 66% had an elevated plasma neuropeptide K, and 43% had an elevated plasma pancreatic polypeptide concentration.[468]

PROGNOSIS

The occurrence and severity of the carcinoid syndrome are directly related to tumor bulk in an area that drains into the systemic circulation. This usually implies distant metastases, except in carcinoids of the bronchus, ovary, or testis. The carcinoid syndrome is a manifestation of advanced disease. Two of three patients with the carcinoid syndrome have physical signs of cancer, such as an abdominal mass or hepatomegaly.[437] In the remaining patients, the disease will be easy to identify on imaging studies. There is a direct correlation between tumor mass and urinary 5-HIAA levels.[437,456,467] Therefore, this laboratory test is a good marker for presence and extent of disease. Flushing does not indicate an extremely poor prognosis, nor does it require immediate or aggressive intervention. Patients with raised levels of urinary 5-HIAA may have only minimal symptoms, occasional flushing, or mild diarrhea for many years.

In patients with carcinoid tumors, survival rates depended on both the site and the extent of the tumors.[537] For all patients with local disease only, the 5-year survival was 94%, varying from 75% for tumors in the small intestine and ileum to 99% for tumors in the appendix (Table 39-25). In patients with regional involvement, 5-year survival was 64% overall, varying from 23% for the stomach to 100% for the appendix. For patients with distant metastases, the overall 5-year survival was 18%, varying from zero for stomach tumors to 19% for small intestinal carcinoid tumors. In different studies, 5-year survival was the highest for carcinoids of the appendix (92–99%), followed by lung (87%), rectum (76–100%), small intestine (42–71%), and colon and stomach (52%).[437,452,491,537–541] The chance of finding regional invasion or metastatic disease is directly proportional to the size of the primary tumors.[437] With carcinoid tumors <1 cm in diameter in the small bowel, less than 15% to 18% have metastatic disease; in the rectum, 0 to 20%; and in the appendix, 0 to 2%.[437,451,468,540,541] With carcinoid tumors >2 cm in diameter of the small bowel, 86% to 95% have metastases; in the rectum, almost all patients have metastatic diseases; and in the appendix, 33% have metastatic disease.[437,491,540,541] For all patients with carcinoid tumors, the 5-year survival rate varies from 65% to 82% in different studies.[468,537] Race, age, or sex had no influence on survival.[537]

The median survival from onset of symptoms of patients in three studies varied from 3.5 to 8.5 years.[467,468,542] The mean survival after recognition of abnormal excretion of 5-HIAA was 23 months, and the 5-year survivals after onset of symptoms in two studies were 30% and 67%.[467,468] An occasional patient lives for 30 years with carcinoid syndrome.[437] Some may live for many years excreting 300 to 400 mg of 5-HIAA per day, but the level of urinary 5-HIAA excretion usually correlates with survival.[467,475] In one study, patients who excreted 10 to 49 mg/day had a median survival of 29 months; those secreting 50 to 149 mg/day a survival of 24 months; those secreting >150 mg/day of 5-HIAA had a mean survival of 13 months.[467]

The most immediate life-threatening complication of the carcinoid syndrome, the carcinoid crisis, is observed in patients who have intense symptoms from foregut carcinoids

TABLE 39-25. Prognosis for Carcinoid Tumors

Site	*Number of Patients*	*% with Metastases*	*5-Year Survival (%)* Local	Regional Metastases	Distant Metastases	All Stages
Appendix	820	5	99	102	27	99
Rectum	295	15	92	44	7	83
Lung and bronchus	190	21	96	71	11	87
Small intestine and ileocecum	366	60	75	59	19	54
Colon	112	71	77	65	17	52
Stomach	41	54	93	23	0	52
All sites	1824	23	94	64	18	82

Modified from Godwin JD: Carcinoid tumors: an analysis of 2837 cases. Cancer 36:560, 1975.

or who have greatly elevated urinary 5-HIAA levels (>200 mg/24 hours). The carcinoid crisis may occur spontaneously or it may be associated with stress, anesthesia, or chemotherapy. Patients usually develop an intense flush, diarrhea, and abdominal pain. Mentation is altered ranging from lightheadedness to coma. Cardiac abnormalities also occur, including tachycardia, hypertension or profound hypotension. This crisis may be successfully treated, but in many patients, it may also be a terminal event.[544] Recent treatment strategies using the somatostatin analog, SMS-201-995, have greatly improved the treatment of carcinoid crises.

TREATMENT OF CARCINOID SYNDROME

Many patients have hepatic metastases from carcinoid tumor and remain active and well except for occasional episodes of flushing or diarrhea. Management of these patients includes avoiding stress and conditions or substances that precipitate flushing and dietary supplementation with nicotamide.[434] Heart failure may require diuretics; wheezing may require salbutamol, a bronchodilator that interacts with beta-adrenergic receptors and does not induce flushing, or aminophylline, and diarrhea may respond to loperamide. If patients still have carcinoid symptoms, various agents should be used on a trial-and-error basis to relieve the flushing, diarrhea, or wheezing (Table 39-26).

These agents act by inhibiting the synthesis of 5-HT, as 5-HT receptor antagonists, by blocking the action of 5-HT on target tissues, or by inhibiting the release of various vasoactive substances (Fig. 39-11). Parachlorophenylalanine, which blocks the hydroxylase enzyme that converts tryptophan to 5-HTP, has been shown to relieve diarrhea and improve flushing in some patients and to reduce urinary 5-HIAA.[543,544] However, the side-effects of this agent, including hypersensitivity reactions and psychiatric disturbances,

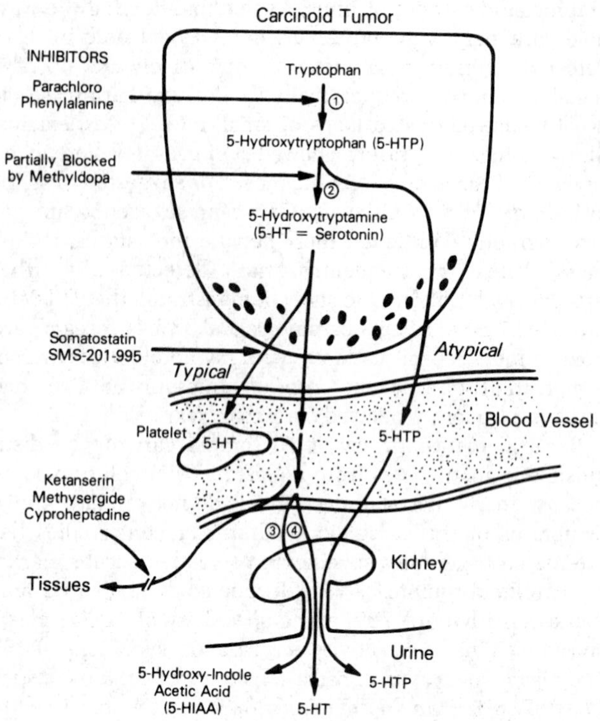

FIG. 39-11. Synthesis, secretion, and metabolism of serotonin (*5-HT*) and 5-hydroxytryptophan (*5-HTP*) in patients with typical and atypical carcinoid syndrome. (*1*) Tryptophan hydroxylase; (*2*) aromatic 1-amino acid decarboxylase (dopa decarboxylase); (*3*) monoamine oxidase; (*4*) aldehyde dehydrogenase. *Arrows* indicate the sites of action of therapeutic agents used in the treatment of carcinoid syndrome.

TABLE 39-26. Therapy of Carcinoid Syndrome

Group	*Drug*	*Dose*	*Flush*	*Diarrhea*	*Remarks*
Alpha-adrenergic blockers	Phenoxybenzamine	10–30 mg daily	Improves	No effect	May cause drowsiness, dry membranes
	Chlorpromazine	10–25 mg every 8 h	Improves if foregut tumor	No effect	Blocks acetylcholine, histamine, serotonin, and kinin
5-Hydroxytryptamine synthesis inhibitors	Methyldopa	4–6 g daily	May improve	No effect	Blocks tryptophan decarboxylase and alpha-adrenergic action
	Parachlorophenylalanine	0.5–1 g every 6 h	May improve	Improves	Blocks amino acid hydroxylase
5-Hydroxytryptamine receptor antagonists	Cyproheptadine	4–7 mg every 8 h	No effect	Improves	H_1-histamine antagonist
	Ketanserin	40–160 mg daily	May improve	Improves	Also H_1-histamine, alpha-adrenergic and dopamine antagonist
	Methysergide	3–8 mg daily	No effect	Improves	Anticholinergic, H_1-antagonist may cause retroperitoneal fibrosis
Somatostatin analogue	SMS-201-995	50–150 μg every 8–12 h	Improves	Improves	No oral preparation, antitumor effects in 14%

make it intolerable for long-term clinical use.[543,544] Alphamethyldopa partially blocks the conversion of 5-HTP to 5-HT, but its effect is partial.[481] It occasionally relieves flushing, but has little effect on GI symptoms.[434,475] Phenoxybenzamine, an alpha-adrenergic antagonist, and phenothiazines may block flushing provoked by alcohol or other agents, although patients frequently become refractory.[434,475,496,497] The 5-HT receptor antagonists methysergide, cyproheptadine, and ketanserin have all been used successfully to treat the GI symptoms without affecting the flushing.[496–498] Cyproheptadine (3–8 mg three times a day) reduced diarrhea in 50% of patients, with minimal effect on flushing or excretion of 5-HIAA.[437] Methysergide use is limited because it can cause or enhance retroperitoneal fibrosis. Cyprohepatidine can result in dry mouth or sedation, which are decreased by decreasing the dose. Ketanserin is a selective S_2-type 5-HT inhibitor, which is not effective in most patients.[434] A combination of histamine H_1- and H_2-receptor antagonists have been reported to be effective in carcinoid syndrome caused by gastric carcinoids.[504] Prednisone in doses of 20 mg/day has given occasional relief for severe flushing; however, it is ineffective in controlling the GI symptoms.[434,475] Tamoxifen was reported to cause symptomatic improvement in 2 patients with carcinoid syndrome, but 16 patients with malignant carcinoid tumors had no improvement or sustained reduction in 5-HIAA.[545–547]

Native somatostatin has been shown to inhibit flushing and increased pulse rate provoked by pentagastrin, food ingestion, or carcinoid syndrome.[476] Native somatostatin in patients with the carcinoid syndrome reversed the hypotension associated with surgical manipulation of a carcinoid tumor, inhibited the cutaneous vasodilation induced by ethanol or norepinephrine, inhibited the diarrhea and bronchoconstriction in one patient, and reversed intestinal chloride secretion in a patient with a carcinoid tumor and secretory diarrhea.[548–551] However, the natural form has a very short half-life (2.5–3 minutes) and has to be given by continuous intravenous infusion (Fig. 39-12).

A long-acting analog of somatostatin, SMS-201-995 (Sandostatin), has been synthesized which has a half-life of 90 min. It is 70 times as potent at inhibiting growth hormone release as somatostatin and can be given subcutaneously (50–150 mg) every 6 to 12 hours.[552–554] SMS-201-995 effectively relieves symptoms and decreases hormone levels when self-administered every 6 to 12 hours subcutaneously by patients with carcinoid syndrome, VIPomas, insulinomas, gastrinomas, glucagonomas, GRFoma, and glucagonomas.[437,555–560] In recent studies from the Mayo Clinic involving 53 patients with the carcinoid syndrome, SMS-201-995 completely improved flushing in 53% and caused a $\geq$ 50% decrease in an additional 32%. Diarrhea was completely improved in 25% and partially improved in an additional 49%.[437,559] 5-HIAA excretion was reduced to normal in 5% and partially decreased in an additional 63%.[437] Only 7% of patients failed to respond in some way.[437] Forty percent of patients ceased to respond after a median time of 4 months (range, 1 week to 12.5 months). The remaining patients sustained control for up to 2.5 years, with all of these responding for $>$1 year and 33% for $>$2 years).[437] The current dosage used in these studies was 150 mg given subcutaneously three times a day. Tolerance to SMS-201-995 was excellent. The only side-effects were transient hyperglycemia in 2 patients and mild to moderate steatorrhea in some patients.[437,559] Several patients developed decreased responsiveness to SMS-201-995 with time that was partially overcome by increasing the dose.[437]

SMS-201-995 has also been described to be effective in cases of carcinoid crises.[561] Carcinoid crises usually occur in patients with foregut carcinoids with $>$250 mg/day of 5-HIAA excretion, most frequently precipitated by stressful

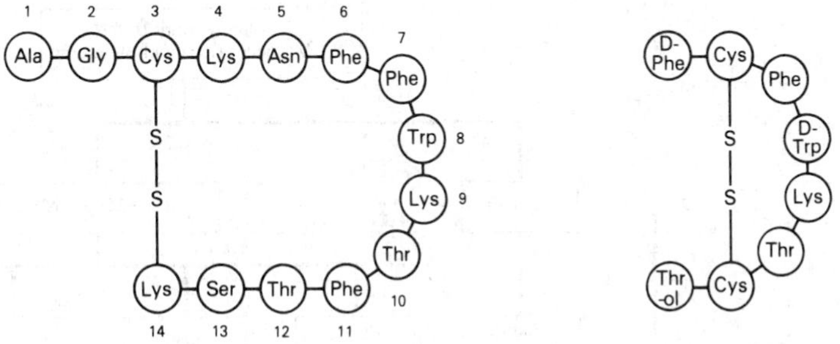

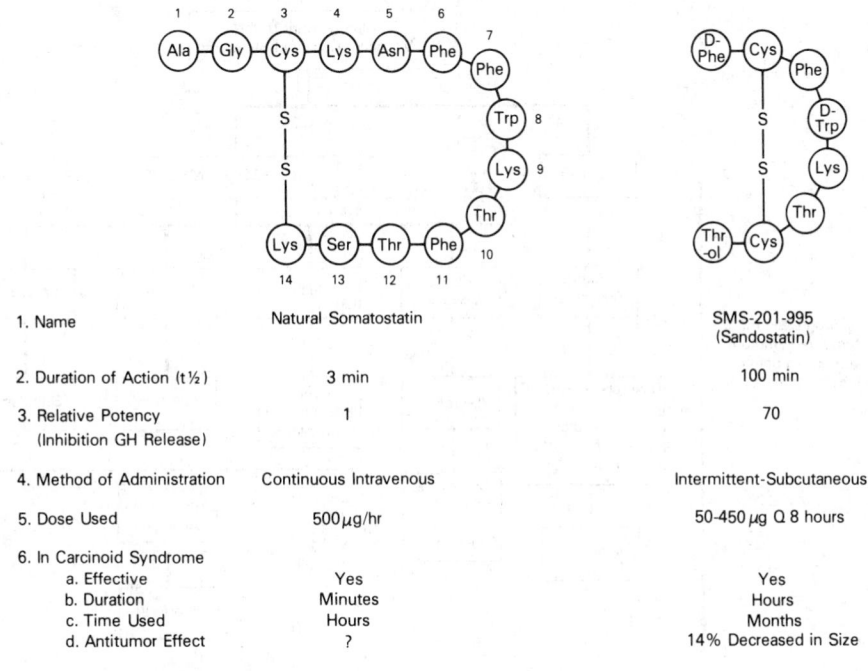

	Natural Somatostatin	SMS-201-995 (Sandostatin)
1. Name	Natural Somatostatin	SMS-201-995 (Sandostatin)
2. Duration of Action (t½)	3 min	100 min
3. Relative Potency (Inhibition GH Release)	1	70
4. Method of Administration	Continuous Intravenous	Intermittent-Subcutaneous
5. Dose Used	500 μg/hr	50-450 μg Q 8 hours
6. In Carcinoid Syndrome		
a. Effective	Yes	Yes
b. Duration	Minutes	Hours
c. Time Used	Hours	Months
d. Antitumor Effect	?	14% Decreased in Size

FIG. 39-12. Comparison of the structure and properties of native somatostatin and of a long-acting analogue of somatostatin, SMS-201-995.

situations such as chemotherapy or anesthesia, and may result in death. For these patients, SMS-201-995 may be life saving.[437,561]

For a patient with severe carcinoid syndrome not responsive to other measures, hepatic artery embolization or ligation may be effective.[437,562–567] In two studies of patients with carcinoid syndrome, hepatic artery ligation or embolization, resulted in symptomatic improvement of the carcinoid syndrome in 100% and 75%, respectively, of patients, with the response lasting from 1 to 18 months.[562,566] This procedure can have severe side-effects, including septicemia, and 5% of patients in one study died of a complication of hepatic artery occlusion.[567]

Interferon has recently been reported to be effective in relieving symptoms of the malignant carcinoid syndrome.[568] All six patients with the carcinoid syndrome had a decline in 5-HIAA excretion and significant symptomatic improvement.

The approach to treatment of the carcinoid syndrome is summarized in Figure 39-13. After symptomatic treatment, SMS-201-995 is the drug of choice. If tachyphylaxis develops, the dose can be increased. If symptoms recur, are severe, and do not respond to increased SMS-201-995, interferon should be considered.

TREATMENT OF CARCINOID TUMOR

Surgery should be considered as the only curative therapy for carcinoids. Resection of local disease or resection of local and regional nodal metastatic disease can result in cure in some patients. For most carcinoid tumors, the possibility of metastatic disease is directly related to the size of the primary lesion, the extent of surgical resection should be determined accordingly. In the case of appendiceal tumors ≤ 1 cm in diameter without gross metastases (over 98% of cases), a simple appendectomy is sufficient.[437] Of 110 such patients treated with simple appendectomy, of which 108 were followed for 5 years and 83 for 10 to 35 years, no patient developed a recurrence or metastatic carcinoid.[437,451] With rectal carcinoids <1 cm, local resection is adequate and will result in cure.[437] With small intestinal carcinoids ≤ 1 cm, there is not complete agreement; however, in two series, 15% and 18% of tumors <1 cm had metastases, leading one group to recommend a wide resection with en bloc resection of the adjacent lymph-node-bearing mesentery for all small intestinal carcinoids.[452] If the carcinoid tumor is ≥ 2 cm, a full-scale cancer operation should be done.[437] In the case of a ≥ 2-cm carcinoid tumor of the appendix, a right hemicolectomy is the operation of choice.[437,452,451] For a large tumor of the rectum, an abdominoperineal resection or a low anterior resection with primary anastomosis is recommended.[452] In the case of a $\geq$2-cm small intestinal carcinoid, a wide resection is recommended, with en bloc resection of the adjacent lymph-node-bearing mesentery.[452] For carcinoids of the appendix between 1 and 2 cm, simple appendectomy is recommended by some, but others favor partial cecectomy for those lesions located at the base of the appendix to ensure clear margins or formal right hemicolectomy.[437,451,452] For carcinoids of the rectum between 1 to 2 cm, tumors should be locally resected with a wide local full-thickness excision, and those tumors found to invade the muscularis propria should undergo abdominoperineal or low anterior resection.[437,452,570] Small gastric and duodenal carcinoids should be locally excised, but for larger, invasive tumors, subtotal gastrectomy with omentectomy or pancreatoduodenectomy should be performed.[452,570]

Resection of isolated hepatic metastases may also be markedly beneficial or curative in selected patients.[544] In one series, ten patients with hepatic metastases were chosen for possible resection who had apparently isolated areas of hepatic metastases in a surgically accessible region of the

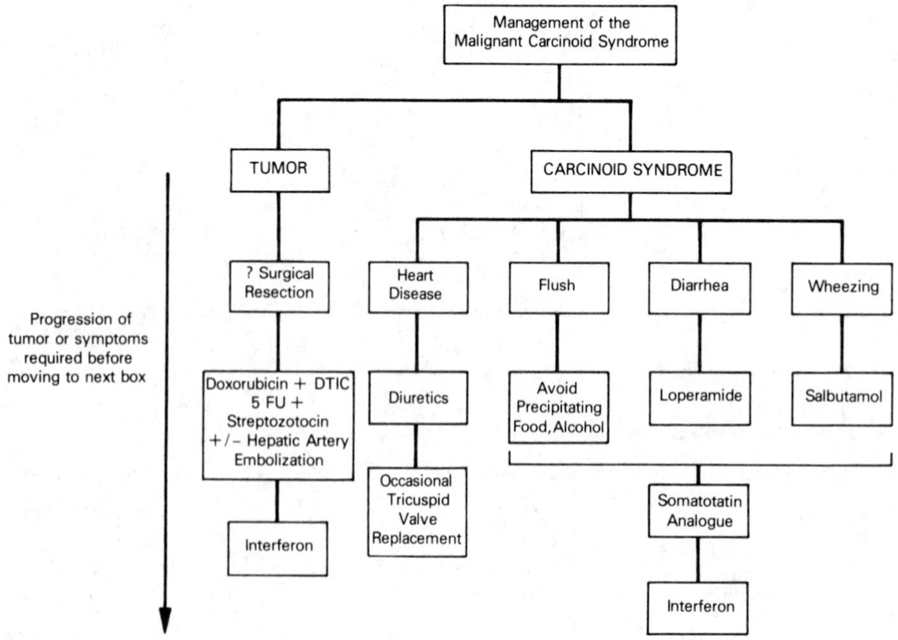

FIG. 39-13. Schematic diagram of the treatment of malignant carcinoid syndrome. † = control of the tumor will alleviate the carcinoid syndrome.

liver.[437,544] All patients with carcinoid syndrome had symptomatic relief, and 5-HIAA levels were reduced to normal. Although only one patient was cured, mean survival was 5 years and extended to 13.5 years for one patient.[437] In the presence of extensive metastases, partial hepatic resection is not indicated, nor is resection of the primary tumor unless it is causing obstruction or bleeding. Resection is helpful only when the operative procedure can remove all gross tumor.

Although a study reported that radiotherapy induced a prolonged disease-free remission for carcinoid tumors with metastases, a follow-up study showed no benefit.[571,572] Radiotherapy has not been useful in the treatment of metastatic carcinoid tumors, except for treatment of symptomatic bone and skin metastases.[434]

There is no general agreement on when chemotherapy should be started. One group with considerable experience suggests that only patients suffering significant symptoms or disability from malignant disease or who have a poor prognosis should undergo chemotherapy.[437] The signs of a poor prognosis include impaired liver function, very high levels of 5-HIAA (≥150 mg/day), or clinical evidence of carcinoid heart disease.[437] Chemotherapy for metastatic carcinoid tumors has been disappointing, with a response rate between 0 and 30% for single agents and between 22% and 40% for combined agents (Table 39-27). Remissions have been short-lived, averaging 4 to 7 months.[437,544] Given the indolent nature of the tumor, poor drug efficacy, undisputed toxicity of chemotherapy, and availability of excellent symptomatic therapy (somatostatin analog), chemotherapy is usually reserved for advanced tumors with radiologic evidence of progression. Active drugs include 5-fluorouracil, doxorubicin, cyclophosphamide, and streptozotocin, either alone or in combination.[544] Combination chemotherapy for metastatic carcinoid has not been clearly shown to have any major advantage compared with single-agent chemotherapy.[581]

Selective hepatic artery infusion of 5-fluorouracil had a similar response to rates reported for systemic 5-fluorouracil.[434] Hepatic artery ligation by surgery or embolization by interventional radiology have been reported to reduce hepatic tumor bulk.[437,564-566] After hepatic artery occlusion in 14 patients with metastatic carcinoid to the liver, 7% showed complete improvement, 43% showed 75% to 100% improvement, and 43% showed 50% to 75% improvement in both endocrine responses and in regression of hepatic metastases.[437] The response, however, was short, with a mean of 5 months.[437] The combination of hepatic artery ligation plus combination chemotherapy with dacarbazine, doxorubicin, 5-fluorouracil and streptozotocin has led to dramatic response rates in patients with carcinoid and hepatic metastases.[437,557,567] Of 21 patients with carcinoid tumors treated with sequential hepatic artery occlusion and cytotoxic drugs, 19% had complete improvement, 57% had 75% to 100% improvement, and 10% had 50% to 75% improvement, for an 80% overall response rate that lasted a median 24 months.[437]

The long-acting somatostatin analog, SMS-201-995, has had dramatic results in treating carcinoid syndrome, and thus researchers questioned its ability to reduce carcinoid mass. Carcinoid tumors and other neuroendocrine tumors have somatostatin receptors, which may mediate cellular antiproliferation.[582] In a recent study 29 patients with carcinoid syndrome were evaluated for the effects of SMS-201-995 on tumor size (usually hepatic metastases) by CT scan.[559] Tumor size increased in 3, remained unchanged in 22, and was reduced in 4 (14% response rate).[559] The antitumor effects of SMS-201-995 have not been impressive.

Human leukocyte interferon can cause a decrease in tumor size in a significant number of patients with metastatic carcinoid tumors.[577] In one study, 36 patients with malignant carcinoid tumors were treated with doses of 3 to 6 million units/day of interferon.[577,583] Nineteen of 36 patients

TABLE 39-27. Drug Therapy of Carcinoid Tumors

Strategy	*Agent*	*Patients*	*Number of Objective Responses (%)*	*Reference*
Single-Dose	DOX*	33	7 (21)	(544)
	5-FU	19	5 (26)	(544)
	DTIC	15	2 (13)	(574)
	ACT D	17	1 (6)	(574)
	CISPL	15	1 (6)	(575)
	Alkylating agents	39	9 (23)	(434)
	VP-16	17	0 (0)	(576)
	STZ	23	7 (30)	(434)
	Interferon	36	17 (47)	(577)
	SMS-201-995	29	4 (14)	(559)
Combination	STZ + 5-FU	43	14 (33)	(456)
	STZ + 5-FU	80	18 (22)	(578)
	STZ + CTX	47	12 (26)	(456)
	DOX + CTX + STZ	20	7 (35)	(579)
	STZ + DOX	10	4 (40)	(580)
	Hepatic artery			
	occlusion + DTIC	21	18 (86)	
	+ DOX + 5-FU + STZ	10	9 (90)	437

*DOX = doxorubicin; 5-FU = 5-fluorouracil; DTIC = dacarbazine; ACT D = actinomycin D (dactinomycin); CISPL = cisplatin; VP-16 = etoposide; STZ = streptozotocin; SMS-201-995 = somatostatin analog; Interferon = human leukocyte interferon.

had previously failed standard chemotherapy. With interferon, objective responses were seen in 17 of 36 patients (47%), stable disease in 39%, and progression in 14%. The median response lasted 34 months. Responders had a greater than 50% reduction in urinary 5-HIAA levels, and 4 patients (11%) had a significant reduction of tumor size on CT scan. Two patients achieved complete remission. Adverse side-effects were surmountable and less severe than with cytotoxic chemotherapy.[577,584] Using 12 to 24 million units three times weekly of recombinant alpha-interferon, 3 (20%) of 15 patients with metastatic carcinoid tumors had measurable regressions of tumor metastases, and a >50% reduction in 5-HIAA levels occurred in 6 (46%) of the 13.[437] Interferon used alone appears to be an active drug against carcinoid tumors, but its antitumor activity does not seem to be substantially greater than cytotoxic drug therapy.[437] No studies have combined interferon with cytotoxic drugs.

ZOLLINGER-ELLISON SYNDROME

In 1955, Zollinger and Ellison described two patients with severe peptic ulcer disease treatable only by total gastrectomy. It was characterized by extreme hypersecretion of gastric acid and a non-beta islet-cell tumor of the pancreas.[585] Zollinger and Ellison suggested that this syndrome was caused by the tumor releasing a humoral substance that caused the gastric hypersecretion.[585] Within 5 years, this prediction was confirmed when extracts of tumors from patients with Zollinger-Ellison syndrome (ZES) were found to contain a potent acid secretagogue that was "gastrin-like."[586] Amino acid analysis and enzymatic degradation of purified tumor extracts demonstrated that the secretagogue in the tumor was identical to human antral gastrin.[587,588] With the subsequent development of specific radioimmunoassays for gastrin, high concentrations of gastrin were identified both in the serum and in the tumors of patients with ZES.[589,590] Because these tumors synthesize and release large amounts of gastrin, they have been called gastrinomas.

Although the precise incidence of the disease is not known, recent studies estimate ZES to occur in 1 per 100,000 persons in Denmark and in approximately 0.1% of patients with duodenal ulcer disease in the United States.[591,592] It is the second most common islet cell tumor after insulinoma, occurring in 0.5 persons per million per year in Ireland.[593]

PATHOLOGY

Almost all of the clinical manifestations, except for those late in the course of the disease, are due to the gastric hypersecretion caused by hypergastrinemia. Effective control of the gastric hypersecretion abolishes all clinical manifestations (Table 39-28), such as peptic ulcer disease or diarrhea.[594–597,601] In patients with metastatic gastrinoma or large primaries, symptoms such as pain or cachexia can arise due to the tumor itself. Hypergastrinemia also causes trophic changes in the gastric mucosa, with the result that patients with ZES have increased numbers of parietal cells and an increased maximal acid secretory capacity.[594,602–604]

Many patients with ZES have diarrhea, and in some patients it is the sole presenting manifestation. The diarrhea is due to a number of consequences of gastric acid hypersecretion, including direct injury to the small intestinal mucosa, inactivation of pancreatic lipase at low pH levels, and precipitation of bile acids at low pH levels.[594] Although it has been proposed that hypergastrinemia itself, by increasing intestinal secretion, could contribute to the diarrhea, this hypothesis is not supported.[605] If the gastric acid hypersecretion is controlled in patients with diarrhea, even though the hypergastrinemia remains unchanged, the diarrhea disappears and the patients remain asymptomatic.[594]

Gastrin in both normal persons and in patients with ZES has been found in many different molecular sizes. In gastrinomas, gastrin-17 (G-17) is the major component, comprising 74% to 80% of the total immunoreactivity, with "big gastrin" or gastrin-34 (G-34) comprising most of the remainder.[594,606,607] In sera from normal persons and patients with gastrinoma, G-34 comprises more than 60% of the total gastrin immunoreactivity.[594,606,608] In addition to G-17 and G-34, smaller and larger forms of gastrin have been described in sera or gastrinomas from patients with ZES. These include a large-molecular-weight gastrin (big, big gastrin), and uncategorized gastrin slightly larger than G-34 (component I gastrin), and small amounts of amino-terminal, carboxyl-terminal, and carboxyl-terminal extended fragments of gastrin.[594,606–610] Each of the different gastrins can exist in either a sulfated or nonsulfated form, which are reported to

TABLE 39-28. Clinical Features of Patients with Zollinger-Ellison Syndrome

Patients and Features	*Year of Study (Ref)*				
	1964 (598)	*1978 (599)*	*1979 (600)*	*1986 (671)*	*1986*
Total patients	260	40	34	144	80
Multiple endocrine neophasia-type 1 (%)	21	23	24	24	21
Duration of symptoms before diagnosis (yr)		6.5	6.4		3.8
First symptoms (%)					
Abdominal pain	93	98	85	26	43
Pain and diarrhea	30	28	56	49	29
Diarrhea only	7	2	9	15	35
Dysphagia/pyrosis	0	0	6		13
Mean age at onset (yr)		50.5	50.4	47	45
Sex (% male)	60	60	62	68	64

TABLE 39-29. Pathology, Tumor Location, and Tumor Extent in Patients with Zollinger-Ellison Syndrome

Tumor Characteristics	*% of All Patients*	*Range (%)*
Extent of Tumor		
No tumor found	30	13–48
Localized tumor	36	23–51
Metastatic tumor	34	13–52
Tumor Location		
Pancreas	42	21–65
Duodenum	15	6–31
Other	11	1–26
Metastases only	2	0–11
Pathology		
Gastrinoma	90	87–94
Malignant		61–90
Benign		10–39
Islet cell hyperplasia	10	6–13

be equipotent.[594] In early studies, G-17 was reported to be five times more potent than G-34; however, in a study using synthetic peptides, G-34 and G-17 have been found to be equally potent.[611,612]

Gastrinomas most commonly occur in the pancreas with the exact percentage differing in different series (Table 39-29). In early studies, gastrinomas were reported to occur in a frequency of 4 : 1 : 4 for the pancreatic head : body : tail, and 14% of all gastrinomas were found in the duodenum.[595,621] Gastrinomas in the duodenum and in lymph nodes in the pancreatic head area have been increasingly reported, occurring in some studies in 40% of all cases in which tumor is found at surgery.[613–615,623] In recent studies, 65% to 90% of all gastrinomas found at surgery occur in the pancreatic head or duodenal area.[614,615] Gastrinomas have also occurred in other sites such as the liver, stomach, ovary, jejunum, mesentery, and spleen.

Because gastrin-containing cells (G cells) are not normally present in the adult human pancreas, pancreatic gastrinomas can be considered ectopic, but gastrinomas in areas that normally contain G cells (duodenum, stomach, jejunum) are considered entopic.[461,620–627] The incidence of malignant change is lower (38%) when gastrinomas occur in entopic locations and higher (60–70%) when they are ectopic.[624–626] In early studies, 60% to 90% of patients with ZES had metastatic gastrinoma at the time of diagnosis, whereas in recent studies, only 34% had metastatic disease at the time of diagnosis.[598,606,620,622] Metastases are usually to peripancreatic lymph nodes and to the liver, with pulmonary or bony metastases rarely reported. Gastrinomas are generally slow growing, and 42% of patients with metastatic gastrinoma survive for 5 years, and 30% survive for 10 years.[628]

The cell of origin of gastrinomas remains obscure. There is evidence that duodenal gastrinoma, which contain many well-differentiated antral G cells, originates from gastrin cells in the duodenal crypts and Brunner's glands.[461,626–627] Because G cells are not seen in the human pancreas, and because pancreatic gastrinomas are pleomorphic with heterogeneous cell types, it has been proposed that they originate from a multipotential, endocrine-programmed stem cell that undergoes somewhat inappropriate and incomplete differentiation toward the G cell.[461,626–627] An argyrophilic cell with atypical granules has been described in islet cell tumors, and it has been postulated that this cell may be the precursor or stem cell for both the normal islet-cell tumors.[606]

In early studies, gastrinomas were found at surgery in most patients (81–94%) with ZES.[598,606,620] In recent studies, gastrinomas have been found in only 70% of the patients with ZES. In half of the patients, the tumor is nonmetastatic, and in approximately half of these, the tumors are multiple.[587,620] Therefore, in only 20% of all patients with ZES is a single, nonmetastatic gastrinoma found. It has been suggested that islet cell hyperplasia or nesidioblastosis could be the cause of ZES in some of the cases in which no gastrinoma is found.[598,620,629] At present most authorities do not accept islet-cell hyperplasia or nesidioblastosis as a cause of ZES, because islet-cell hyperplasia is common in patients with ZES who have a gastrinoma; the hyperplastic islets do not contain gastrin; and the possibility that a small gastrinoma was not detected at surgery cannot be excluded. Islet-cell hyperplasia or nesidioblastosis is instead regarded as a consequence of the disease.[606,626,630]

The percentage of gastrinomas that are malignant is unclear. In early studies 60% to 90% of patients with ZES had a malignant gastrinoma, but in recent studies only half of patients have a malignant gastrinoma at the time of diagnosis.[588,606,620,622] This change may represent earlier diagnosis or inclusion of a spectrum of the disease not previously appreciated. The diagnosis of malignancy is complicated because no histologic crtieria predict malignancy. Malignancy can only be established by the presence of metastases. Even metastatic disease can be difficult to establish, because a number of cases of extrapancreatic gastrinoma localized in lymph nodes have been described with no evidence of primary tumor. Some of these cases have been cured by excision of the lymph nodes, which suggests that the gastrinoma was not metastatic, but originated in the lymph node.[613,614,631]

Approximately 25% of patients with ZES have a familial form with evidence of multiple endocrine neoplasia-type 1 (MEN-1), and the remaining 75% have a sporadic form with no evidence of MEN-1. MEN-1 is an autosomal dominant trait characterized by hyperplasia or tumors of multiple endocrine organs, with hyperparathyroidism the most common abnormality (97%).[463,632] Islet cell tumors of the pancreas occur in 82% of MEN-1 patients: 57% have ZES and 25% have insulinomas.[463] Pituitary and adrenal adenomas are less common. Patients with MEN-1 and ZES differ from sporadic ZES patients in that they frequently present at a younger age and their tumors are almost always small and multiple. Some studies report that patients with MEN-1 have an increased survival rate compared with sporadic cases.[613,618,619,633]

Immunocytochemical assays of tumors from patients with ZES have demonstrated gastrin in 90% to 100% of tumors in some studies and in 56% to 78% in others.[597] This difference may be due to differences in tissue fixation, in the type of gastrin antibody used, or in the small gastrin content in small tumors. More than 50% of tumors from patients with ZES also secreted other peptides, including pancreatic polypeptide (17–50%), insulin (20–33%), glucagon (0–33%), somatostatin (0–33%), and an ACTH-like protein (0–30%).[597,606,634-638] Only plasma levels of pancreatic polypeptide and motilin are elevated in more than 10% of the patients, suggesting that gastrinomas do not release any or release only small quantities of many of the peptides in the tumors.[597,639-644] Except for the occasional patient with Cushing's syndrome, patients with elevated levels of pancreatic polypeptide, motilin, or neurotensin do not vary clinically from those without elevations.[642,645]

Histologic studies have demonstrated that tumors from patients with ZES are similar to other carcinoid tumors.[597] Different histologic classifications have been proposed based on growth patterns, including classifying tumors into a glandular pattern, solid nests of cells (solid pattern), trabecular or ribbon like structure (gyriform pattern), and unclassified patterns.[597,626,634,637,646-648] Similar patterns have been demonstrated in tumors from patients with other endocrine tumors, and the type of histologic pattern does not correlate with the type of hormone produced, clinical symptoms, or malignancy. Ultrastructural classifications have all been proposed based on the type of granules seen, but this does not also correlate with malignancy or clinical features.[461,597,606,626,627,634,646]

CLINICAL FEATURES

The clinical features of ZES are summarized in Table 39-28. ZES is slightly more common in men (60%) than in women (40%); the mean age of patients is 45 to 50 years old. Approximately 25% of the patients have MEN-1. Abdominal pain is the most common initial symptom. Between 90% and 95% of patients develop peptic ulcer disease at some time during the course of the disease, and the abdominal pain cannot be distinguished from that which occurs with idiopathic peptic esophagitis or peptic ulcer disease. Diarrhea and esophageal disease are increasingly among the first symptoms.

The change in presenting symptoms is also reflected in changes in radiological and endoscopic findings. In early studies, up to 93% of patients had peptic ulcers, and in 36% of patients, the ulcers were multiple or in unusual locations.[598] Although atypical ulcers strongly suggest the diagnosis, today most patients with ZES have typical duodenal ulcers, and 18% to 25% of patients have no ulcer at the time of diagnosis.[594] This change is presenting symptoms and severity of peptic disease suggests that patients with ZES are being diagnosed earlier; nevertheless, there is still a delay of 3 to 6 years between the onset of symptoms and diagnosis.

In patients with MEN-1 and ZES, additional symptoms such as flank pain due to recurrent renal calculi secondary to the hyperparathyroidism, which is almost always present by the time the ZES presents, may also be apparent.[463,632]

DIAGNOSIS

None of the original triad described by Zollinger and Ellison is required for the diagnosis of ZES. At diagnosis, 38% to 68% of patients have a solitary peptic ulcer, and 14% to 25% have no peptic ulcer.[594] Although gastric hypersecretion remains an essential criterion of ZES, it may not be extreme, and in 13% to 48% of patients, gastrinomas are not located at the time of diagnosis (Table 39-29). ZES is suspected on the basis of the clinical presentation and established in almost all patients by demonstrating elevated basal acid output (BAO) and fasting hypergastrinemia.

ZES should be suspected in any patient who has an ulcer with diarrhea, a familial ulcer, an ulcer in an unusual location, or a recurrent or resistant ulcer. Because most patients present with symptoms that are similar to those in patients with idiopathic peptic disease, every patient who has peptic ulcer disease severe enough to require gastric surgery should have at least one preoperative fasting serum gastrin done.[594,600]

The diagnosis of ZES requires a fasting hypergastrinemia and an elevated BAO. The fasting gastrin concentration is usually done first and is usually elevated in more than 98% of all patients with ZES.[649] Disorders other than ZES that are known to elevate the fasting gastrin concentration fit into two categories: those associated with gastric acid hypersecretion (Table 39-30) and those associated with hypochlorhydria or achlorhydria, including chronic gastritis, gastric cancer, pernicious anemia, or postvagotomy.[594] No absolute level of serum gastrin distinguishes these two categories; they can only be distinguished by measuring BAO. If this is not possible, then a simple determination of the pH of the gastric contents while the patient is not taking antisecretory medications should be performed. A pH of 3 or higher virtually excludes the diagnosis of ZES.[650]

The most commonly used secretory criteria for diagnosing ZES are a BAO ≥ 15 mEq/h in patients without and ≥ 5 mEq/h in patients with previous acid-reducing operations.[594,651] The mean BAO in five series varied from 34 to 53 mEq/h in patients without previous gastric surgery and from 6 to 20 mEq/h for patients with previous acid-reducing surgery.[596,597,599,617,651] In early studies, 33% of patients with ZES without previous gastric surgery were reported to have a BAO < 15 mEq/h; however, in recent studies, only 1 of 77 patients without previous gastric surgery had a BAO less than 15 mEq/h.[596,597,599,617,651,652] Requiring a BAO of at least 15 mEq/h will include 66% to 99% of all patients with ZES and exclude 90% of patients with routine duodenal ulcer.[594] In most patients with previous acid-reducing surgery, the mean BAO exceeded 5 mEq/h, but in three studies, 10%, 33%, and 45% of patients had a BAO of less than 5 mEq/h.[597,641,653]

Patients with ZES also have an elevated maximal acid output (MAO) and an elevated BAO/MAO ratio that often exceeds 0.6; however, in a significant portion of patients, the BAO/MAO ratio is <0.6.[596,599,617,651,654] Criteria based on the MAO or BAO/MAO ratio have been shown to offer no advantage over the BAO alone.[594]

If a patient has a fasting gastrin concentration ≥ 1000 pg/ml and basal acid hypersecretion, then the diagnosis of ZES is generally established.[597,650] The only other disorder that can mimic ZES and cause similar elevations of both acid secretion and fasting gastrin is the retained gastric antrum syndrome, which is a rare condition that occurs in patients who have undergone a Billroth II gastroenterostomy, in which part of the antrum is left attached to the excluded proximal duodenal stump.[655,656] This diagnosis can be ex-

TABLE 39-30. Differential Diagnosis of Increased Fasting Gastrin and Basal Acid Output

Diagnosis	*Secretin Injection*	*Calcium Infusion*	*Meal Test*	*Other Discriminating Features*
Zollinger-Ellison syndrome	Increase >200 pg/ml over basal	Increase >395 pg/ml over basal	NC or increase <50% over basal*	Approximately 50% of patients have tumor
Retained gastric antrum	NC, or increase <200 pg/ml	NC or small increase	NC, decrease or increase <50% over basal	History of Billroth II operation. Positive ^{99m}Tc-pertech scan
Chronic gastric outlet obstruction	NC, or increase <200 pg/ml	NC or small increase	ND	Decreased gastric emptying: with nasogastric suction, serum gastrins return to normal
Antral G-cell hyperplasia	NC, decrease or increase <200 pg/ml	NC or small increase	Increase >100% over basal	Increased numbers of G cells may be seen by immunocytochemical staining
Antral G-cell hyperfunction	NC, decrease or increase <200 pg/ml	NC or small increase	Increase >100% over basal	Normal numbers of G cells Frequently familial. May be associated with hyperpepsinogenemia I
After small bowel resection	NC or increase <200 pg/ml	NC or small increase	ND	Hx of extensive small bowel resection

*NC = no change; ND = not determined.

cluded if there is no history of gastric surgery, or if there is a history, by the use of secretin test and by gastric ^{99m}Tc-pertechnetate scanning as outlined in Table 39-30.[656,657]

Approximately 40% of patients with ZES have a fasting gastrin concentration ≥ 1000 pg/ml. In the remaining 60%, the fasting gastrin concentration is elevated, but < 1000 pg/ml, a level which can be caused by other conditions (Table 39-30) that can cause similar elevations of fasting gastrin and BAO.[594] To distinguish them from ZES, various gastrin-provocative tests are necessary, including the secretin test, calcium infusion test, and meal test.[611,652,658–661] Because of its ease, lack of side-effects, high sensitivity, and very low occurrence of false positives, the secretin test is favored.[594,660] The calcium infusion test is cumbersome, there are frequent side-effects, and it has lower sensitivity and specificity for ZES than the secretin test. It is only used in the rare patient in whom ZES is strongly suspected but the secretin test is negative.[650,660] The meal test is used when the secretin test is negative and antral G cell hyperplasia or hyperfunction could explain the elevated fasting gastrin and BAO.[661]

Antral G-cell hyperplasia mimics ZES clinically with elevated fasting gastrins and BAO, frequently occurs in patients postvagotomy, is curable by antrectomy, and is differentiated from ZES by a negative secretin test and an exaggerated (≥ 100%) postmeal increase in serum gastrin.[594,662–666] Antral G-cell hyperfunction is similar to antral G-cell hyperplasia, except that there are normal numbers of G cells; the syndrome is frequently familial with autosomal dominant inheritance patterns; and it is associated with hyperpepsinogenemia I.[667,668] This syndrome is distinguished from ZES by having a negative secretin test and an exaggerated postmeal increase in serum gastrin.[594,667,668] Chronic gastric outlet obstruction can be difficult to distinguish from ZES because the obstruction can be caused by ZES, or it can mimic ZES and be caused by idiopathic duodenal ulcer, postbulbar peptic ulcer, or Crohn's disease, all of which can present with hypergastrinemia and elevated BAO.[594] ZES can be differentiated from the other causes of obstruction by a secretin test and prolonged gastric suction.[594,669] In ZES the secretin test will be positive (>200 pg/ml increase) and prolonged nasogastric suction will not change the serum gastrin concentrations; in the other conditions, the secretin test will be negative and serum gastrins will decrease with nasogastric suction. Massive small bowel resection can cause a transient hypergastrinemia and elevation of BAO, and it can be excluded from ZES by the patient's history and the secretin test.[594]

TUMOR LOCALIZATION

Precise localization of the gastrinoma has become increasingly important in evaluating patients with ZES. With the increased ability to control gastric acid hypersecretion with histamine H_2-receptor antagonists, emergency total gastrectomy is now rarely necessary, allowing time to determine the location and extent of the gastrinoma.[594] With the increased ability to control gastric acid hypersecretion, the growth and possible metastatic spread of the gastrinoma has become an increasingly important determinant of long-term survival.[595,597,622,670] As many as 52% of all patients at surgery have metastatic disease (usually to the liver), and by identifying these patients preoperatively unnecessary surgery can be prevented.[613,614,671] Gastrinomas are frequently multiple and extrapancreatic.[598,613,616,672] In up to 60% of patients in some series, no gastrinoma was found during surgery, and careful imaging could assist the surgeon in localizing the tumor.[616,673] One study identified by careful imaging 15% of the patients with metastatic disease to the liver in which the gastrinoma was resectable.[674]

A number of different techniques, including abdominal ultrasound, CT scanning, selective abdominal angiography,

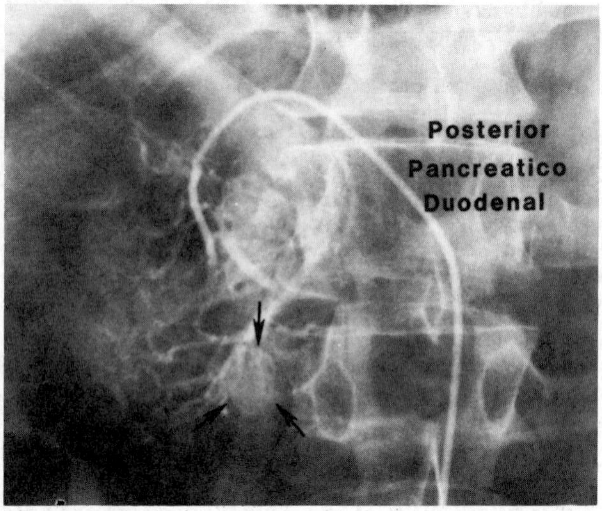

FIG. 39-14. Selective injection of the posterior pancreaticoduodenal artery showing a small gastrinoma in the posterior inferior portion of the pancreatic head in a patient with Zollinger-Ellison syndrome.

selective venous sampling for gastrin from portal venous tributaries, and intraoperative ultrasonography, have all been helpful in localizing gastrinomas.[615,675–690] Abdominal ultrasound in general has a sensitivity of 14% and a specificity of 100% for hepatic metastases and a sensitivity of 21% to 28% and a specificity of 92% to 93% for primary gastrinoma.[615,650,680] CT scanning performed with intravenous contrast agents had a sensitivity of 35% to 72% and a specificity of 98% to 100% for hepatic metastases and a sensitivity of 35% to 59% and a specificity of 83% to 100% for primary gastrinomas.[615,650,679,681,682]

Selective abdominal angiography was originally reported to give high false-positive and false-negative rates; however, in recent studies selective angiography has been shown to have improved (Fig. 39-14).[613,683] Angiography has a sensitivity of 33% to 86% and a specificity of 96% to 100% for hepatic metastases and a sensitivity of 35% to 68% and a specificity of 84% to 94% for primary gastrinomas.[615,650,682,684] In a comparison of CT and angiography, angiography identified 17% more hepatic metastases.[684] Angiography identified 13% more gastrinomas than CT, and a combination of techniques gave the same results as angiography alone.[684] In this study the specificity of CT was 98% and angiography was 100%.[684] CT scanning, because of its general availability, ease of performance, sensitivity, and specificity, should be the initial imaging procedure.[681] If the localization and extent of tumor are still in question, selective angiography should be performed.[684]

FIG. 39-15. Transhepatic portal venous sampling for gastrin concentration in the same patient with Zollinger-Ellison syndrome (see Fig. 39-14) demonstrates a marked increase in the inferior pancreaticoduodenal vein, localizing the gastrinoma to the head of the pancreas. Darkened circle represents the site of the gastrinoma at surgery.

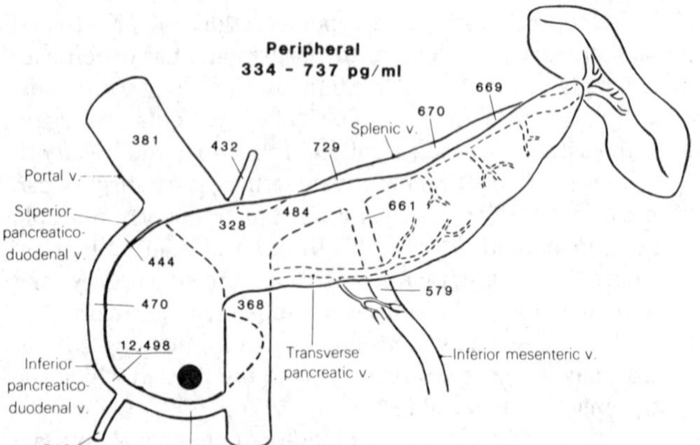

Two new techniques, selective venous sampling for gastrin from portal venous tributaries (Fig. 39-15) and intraoperative ultrasonography, have been used in localizing gastrinomas. A recent prospective study demonstrated that a combination of selective venous sampling and imaging yielded only marginally better results than imaging alone in identifying gastrinomas preoperatively.[683,685–687] Therefore, selective venous sampling for gastrin, although occasionally helpful, should not be used routinely.[650,687] Intraoperative ultrasonography has been demonstrated to change operative management in 10% of all ZES cases either by localizing additional gastrinomas or by determining that a gastrinoma was malignant.[688–690] Although this equipment is expensive and requires considerable experience, these results suggest that intraoperative ultrasonography will play an increasing role in the future.

TREATMENT

All patients with ZES have two problems. First, gastric acid hypersecretion must be controlled immediately and for the long-term, because most patients will not be cured by surgical excision. There are now effective drug and surgical means to accomplish this, and studies have shown that if acid hypersecretion is controlled, these patients have an excellent quality of life.[594,597] Second, long-term prognosis is increasingly determined by the natural history of the gastrinoma. The exact percentage is not clear, but as many as 60% to 90% of gastrinomas may be malignant (Table 39-29).[691] Therefore, it is important to consider therapy directed at the gastrinoma itself, including chemotherapy for metastatic disease and surgical excision of nonmetastatic gastrinoma.

Surgery for Gastric Hypersecretion

Until recently, all patients with ZES required total gastrectomy to control gastric acid hypersecretion. Patients were often debilitated by complicated ulcer disease, electrolyte abnormalities, and malnutrition. The operation frequently had to be done as an emergency, leading to a mortality of 15% in the postoperative period.[620] In these early studies, operative results were unsatisfactory for patients who had less than total gastrectomies. Most patients developed recurrent ulcer disease, often with lethal complications, within days of surgery. With the development of increasingly effective medical therapy, the mortality for patients with ZES undergoing total gastrectomy has decreased. In 10 series involving 248 ZES patients undergoing total gastrectomy, the operative mortality was 5.6%. If patients undergoing emergency procedures are excluded, the operative mortality was 2.4%.[613] However, the actual morbidity rate associated with total gastrectomy is not apparent from most published series, because adequate follow-up is not always apparent.[613] In at least one series of 18 patients undergoing total gastrectomy, all patients experienced one or several side-effects, including symptoms of esophageal reflux, early satiety, cramping, or diarrhea.[618] In 50% of the patients, these side-effects were moderate to severe, and in three (27%) patients, serious additional complications developed, including stenosis of the esophageal anastomosis in two patients and recurrent, severe vomiting in the third patient.[618]

It was once claimed that total gastrectomy could lead to regression of the gastrinoma in some patients, recent reports from several different centers have failed to substantiate this claim.[617,622,628,692] There is no evidence that either therapy for gastric hypersecretion or total gastrectomy affects the growth rate of the gastrinoma.

The development of better medical therapy has led to a considerable debate over the role of total gastrectomy in controlling gastric acid hypersecretion.[594,613,693] Some groups continue to advocate total gastrectomy as the treatment of choice for controlling gastric acid in all patients with ZES, citing high medical failure rates and improved morbidity and mortality now that total gastrectomy can be performed after correcting malnutrition.[601,613,693] However, many studies have demonstrated that gastric acid hypersecretion can be controlled medically using either cimetidine or ranitidine, if sufficiently high doses are used.[594,597] Furthermore, with the recent availability of even more potent histamine H_2-receptor antagonists, such as famotidine and the H^+K^+ ATPase inhibitor, omeprazole, medical therapy is becoming more effective.[696,697] Although drug therapy is not simple and may be costly, it is safe and effective if patients are followed closely. Therefore, we believe that total gastrectomy is only appropriate for patients who are unreliable or do not have access to routine medical follow-up. In all other patients, medical therapy is the treatment of choice, preferably by a group skilled in the medical management of this disease.

In patients who require high doses of histamine H_2-receptor antagonists, even when combined with an anticholinergic agent (*e.g.*, > 4.8 g of cimetidine or the equivalent per day), a parietal cell vagotomy should be considered if omeprazole is not available (Fig. 39-16). A combination of anticholinergic agents and H_2-receptor antagonists has a greater effect than either drug alone.[695,698–700] However, the use of anticholinergics is frequently associated with side-effects that limit patient acceptance. Richardson and colleagues reported that parietal cell vagotomy in patients with ZES in whom no tumor was found at surgery decreased the BAO by 66% and decreased the antisecretory-drug requirement by 95% in all patients.[673] It is likely that the need for antisecretory drug may increase slowly with time as the gastrinoma progresses, but it is evident that vagotomy will delay high-dose requirements for years in most patients. However, because of increasing availability of very potent antisecretory agents and limited long-term follow-up, parietal cell vagotomy should not be performed routinely.[650] It should be reserved for the occasional patient in whom high-dose antisecretory medication does not adequately control gastric acid hypersecretion and in whom at the time of the laparotomy no tumor or unresectable metastatic disease has been found.

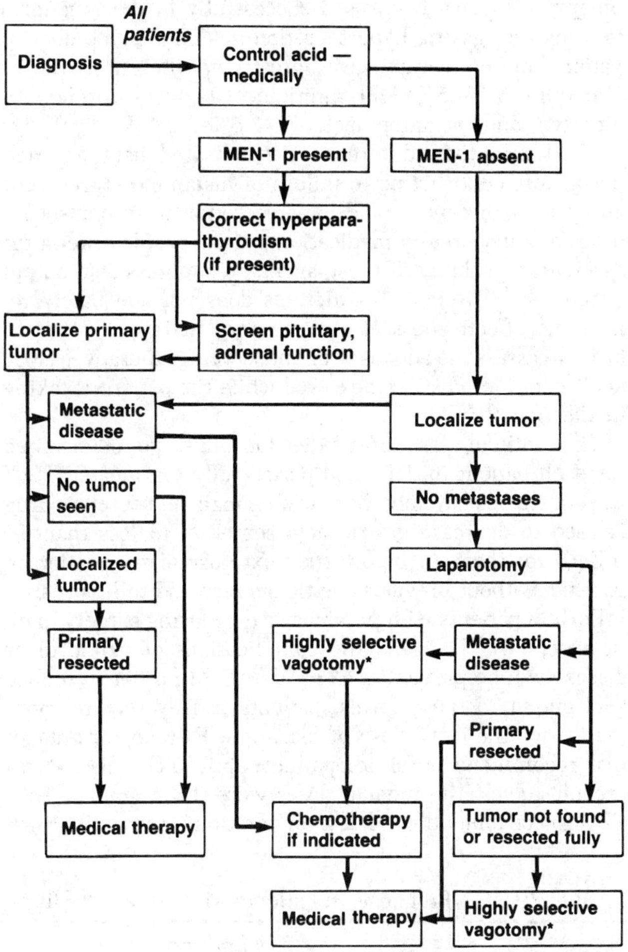

FIG. 39-16. Flow diagram for the management of patients with Zollinger-Ellison syndrome.* Consider highly selective vagotomy if high antisecretory drug requirement (i.e., >4.8 g cimetidine/day).

In patients with ZES and the MEN-1 syndrome, medical control of gastric hypersecretion can be greatly facilitated by correcting hyperparathyroidism.[632] Correction of hyperparathyroidism reduces the fasting serum gastrin concentration, increases the responsiveness to a given dose of antisecretory medication, and decreases the BAO.[701–703] Therefore, parathyroidectomy should be performed in these patients before any other surgical procedure to control gastric acid hypersecretion.

Medical Therapy of Gastric Hypersecretion

The results of medical treatment of gastric acid hypersecretion have been reviewed extensively recently.[594,597,650,704] Histamine H_2-receptor antagonists (cimetidine, ranitidine, famotidine), alone or in combination with anticholinergic agents (probanthine, isopropamide) and more recently with omeprazole, have been used successfully in the long-term treatment of gastric hypersecretion in ZES. The number of patients failing therapy varies greatly in different series for cimetidine (0–65%), for ranitidine (0–40%), for famotidine (0), and for omeprazole (0–7.5%).[594,597,618,694–697,705–713] Analysis of these different series indicated that the principal factors contributing to failure of histamine H_2-receptor antagonists to control acid hypersecretion were inadequate doses of antisecretory medication and unreliable criteria for assessing the ability of these agents to suppress acid output adequately.[704] Relief of symptoms does not adequately reflect the effectiveness of antisecretory therapy.[707,709,714] In order to assess the adequacy of antisecretory therapy, gastric acid secretion must be measured while the patient is taking medication.[594,597]

The optimal dose of medication must be determined for each patient initially and periodically reevaluated.[594,597] Recent studies have shown that if enough antisecretory drug is used to decrease gastric acid secretion to less than 10 mEq/h for the hour before the next dose of medication in patients without previous gastric surgery and to less than 5 mEq/h in patients with previous acid-reducing surgery, peptic ulcers will heal and the complications of peptic ulcer disease will be prevented.[596,696,711,714–716] In order to reduce acid output to these levels, patients usually require more than twice the usual dose of histamine H_2-receptor antagonist recommended for idiopathic peptic ulcer disease. In recent studies, the median doses were 3.6 g (range, 1.2–12.6 g) for cimetidine, 1.2 g for ranitidine (range, 0.45–6 g), and 0.25 g for famotidine (range, 0.05–0.8 g).[650,694,695,711] It is not completely clear why patients with ZES require more than the usual dose of histamine H_2-receptor antagonist to inhibit acid output adequately. Some patients have a decreased sensitivity to antisecretory drugs, or they have impaired or delayed absorption, but in 25% of patients no alteration in drug pharmacokinetics is found.[717,718]

Although relatively high doses of antisecretory agents are required initially and patients may require small dosage increases each year, the long-term use of H_2 antagonists and omeprazole has been proved effective and safe.[650] Except for antiandrogen side-effects (impotence, gynecomastia, breast tenderness) with high-dose cimetidine in up to 60% of male patients, long-term treatment with cimetidine in females or treatment with ranitidine, famotidine, or omeprazole in patients of either sex is safe.[597,650,719] Gastric carcinoids have been reported in rats receiving long-term omeprazole treatment, but no gastric carcinoids have been detected in clinical studies of patients with ZES treated with omeprazole up to 48 months.[462,696,697,712,713,720,721]

Most patients with ZES require histamine H_2-antagonists every 4 to 8 hours to inhibit adequately gastric secretion.[594,595] In contrast to optimally effective doses of cimetidine or ranitidine, which each are active for 6 to 8 hours, and of famotidine, which is active for 10 hours, the optimal dose of omeprazole is active for more than 48 hours, allowing most patients to use omeprazole only once or twice a day.[695–697]

TABLE 39-31. Prognosis in Patients with Zollinger-Ellison Syndrome

Prognosis	*Number of Patients*	*5-Year Survival (%)*	*10-Year Survival (%)*	*Year (Ref)*
All Patients				
	144	62	53	1986 (671)
	40	62	47	1984 (633)
	27	75	52	1983 (613)
Related to Tumor Resectability				
No tumor found	13	100	100	1983 (618)
	10	90	90	1985 (619)
	6	100		1984 (633)
Tumor resected	7	100	100	1983 (618)
	10	90	90	1985 (619)
	22	76		1984 (633)
Tumor incompletely resected or	10	75	20	1983 (618)
recurrence	7	14		1984 (633)
Unresectable	13	80		1983 (618)
	14	40	30	1985 (619)
	7	30		1984 (633)
	15	20		1986 (675)
*MEN-1 Status**				
With MEN-1	23	80	75	1985 (619)
	14		80	1983 (618)
	13	85	62	1984 (633)
	11	85	85	1983 (613)
Without MEN-1	42	70	65	1985 (619)
	36		64	1983 (618)
	27	52	40	1984 (633)
	26	70	50	1983 (613)

*MEN-1 = multiple endocrine neoplasia-type 1.

Treatment of Gastrinoma

The 5-year survival rate for all patients with ZES was 62% to 75% and the 10-year survival rate was 47% to 53% (Table 39-31). Although the growth of gastrinoma is slow, in long-term studies of patients originally treated by total gastrectomy, 57% died of tumor progression.[620,622] With the ability to control gastric acid hypersecretion, the malignant potential of the tumor is an increasingly important determinant of survival. A number of factors contribute to the long-term survival. The extent of the tumor and the effect of MEN-1 determine survival rates. In patients with no tumor found at laparotomy or in whom tumor is completely resectable, 5- and 10-year survival rates are 90% to 100%. In contrast, patients with tumor incompletely resected or unresectable, 5- and 10-year survival rates are 43% and 25%, respectively. Some patients with MEN-1 are reported to have better 5- and 10-year survival rates than patients without MEN-1, but in other studies, the difference was not significant.[608,613,619,633] However, these comparisons may not be valid because patients with both ZES and MEN-1 frequently present at an early age and may be in an earlier phase of their disease.

Therefore, because of the excellent prognosis of patients with resected gastrinoma and the evidence that the malignancy determines survival, surgical resection of the gastrinoma should be considered in all patients with ZES. The general approach to the gastrinoma is summarized in the flow diagram in Fig. 39-16. After gastric acid hypersecretion is adequately controlled medically, it must be determined whether the patient has ZES with or without MEN-1.[597] Pathology studies have demonstrated that patients with ZES and MEN-1 have many, small islet cell tumors.[722] In addition, surgical studies have demonstrated that none of 47 patients with ZES and MEN-1 were cured surgically without proximal pancreaticoduodenectomy.[613,615,616,618,633,686]

NONMETASTATIC GASTRINOMA. The role of surgery in the treatment of the gastrinoma is becoming better defined. All physicians agree that the ideal treatment of ZES is the surgical excision of the gastrinoma, but in early studies this was possible in only 8 (5%) of 157 patients.[594-596,600,617] Even this figure was probably an overestimation because often the follow-up period was less than 1 year and in no cases were multiple secretin tests performed postoperatively.[594]

Studies suggest a cure rate averaging 20% in series reported since 1981 (Table 39-32), and surgical cure rates may be even higher than 20% in the future. First, with the development of effective antisecretory agents, all patients can undergo extensive preoperative investigational studies, and surgery can be done electively. The surgery can be directed at gastrinoma localization and removal, without the emphasis on performing surgery to control gastric acid hypersecretion. Second, the preoperative localization and clinical distinction between patients with and without MEN-1 will identify groups of patients with different potentials for cure. Recent reports suggest more than 90% of patients with metastatic gastrinoma in the liver can be identified with either a CT scan or angiogram, obviating unnecessary attempts at curative surgery in these patients.[681,684] Third, in patients with nonmetastatic, sporadic gastrinoma, the cure rate may be much higher in patients with extrapancreatic gastrinoma (up to 66%) than in those with pancreatic gastrinomas.[613,615,616,618,621,623] However, preoperative localization studies frequently do not identify extrapancreatic gastrinomas, and even when the gastrinoma is localized, if hepatic metastases are not present, potential resectability cannot be predicted.[597,681,684]

It seems reasonable to recommend that all patients with sporadic gastrinoma (ZES not associated with MEN-1) and no serious contraindication to surgery undergo localization studies, preferably in a center with considerable experience with these diseases.[597,650] If no metastases are found, the patient should undergo surgical exploration (Fig. 39-20). In our experience, the single most important factor in achieving good surgical results, which is not emphasized in most studies, is the expertise of the surgeon. Even very experienced pancreatic surgeons have almost no experience with islet cell tumors and thus have no appreciation of the difficulty in identifying the extrapancreatic gastrinomas or of the

TABLE 39-32. Long-term Results of Surgical Resection of Gastrinoma

*Number of Patients Operated**	*Number with Normal Gastrin Postoperatively*	*% with Normal Gastrin Postoperatively*	*Year (Ref)*
25	1	4 (6 mo–4 yr)	1979 (600)
42	2	5	1980 (595)†
32	6	6.5	1981 (601)†
23	9	39	1982 (693)†
18	4	22	1982 (623)†
26	3	12	1983 (613)†
52	6	12	1983 (616)†
44	7	16	1983 (618)
45	5	11	1984 (614)†
22	4	18	1985 (673)
29	12	43 (postop) 30 (6 mo–4 yr)	1986 (615)
20	5	25	1987 (723)†

*Number of patients includes the patients reported to have undergone exploratory laparotomy in each series.

†Series in which total gastrectomy was performed in most cases.

technique of enucleating lesions within the pancreas. Because of limited experience with ZES, errors in judgment regarding the type and extent of surgical resection may often be made.

At surgery either a long midline or a bilateral subcostal incision is used. The liver, pelvis, small intestine, pancreas, stomach, duodenum, and mesenteric and retroperitoneal regions in the upper abdomen and the pelvis, particularly the ovaries in a female, are carefully explored and palpated. The pancreas should be examined visually and by careful palpation. The pancreatic head should be inspected after an extended Kocher maneuver.[615] The pancreatic body and tail are inspected by opening the lesser sac along the avascular plane of the transverse colon and the inferior border of the pancreas is freed so that the body and tail can be palpated between two fingers. The entire duodenum should be carefully palpated, and any suspicious nodule should be exposed by opening the duodenum. Any suspicious pancreatic, stomach, duodenal, bowel, or peripancreatic nodule or lymph node should be removed for pathologic examination. The same extensive search should be made regardless of the preoperative localization information. Even if one gastrinoma is found, the extensive search should still be completed because gastrinomas are frequently multiple or metastatic.

If a gastrinoma is found as a solitary lesion in the liver, it should be removed, provided the resection can be performed safely. If a gastrinoma is found in the pancreatic head, it should be enucleated.[615,650] If an unresectable gastrinoma is found in the pancreatic head area, a pancreaticoduodenectomy (Whipple's operation) is not indicated. No studies have demonstrated increased survival in patients with ZES after pancreaticoduodenectomy, and furthermore because of the marked morbidity and mortality associated with this operation (up to 37%) and the excellent long-term prognosis of these patients, the adverse consequences of a pancreaticoduodenectomy may outweigh the adverse consequences of an unresected solitary gastrinoma.[683] If no gastrinoma is found at surgery, as occurs in 30% to 60% of cases, a blind distal pancreatectomy should not be performed, because 65% to 90% of gastrinomas are found in the pancreatic head or duodenum (gastrinoma triangle) and because such an approach has not improved cure rates.[614,615,650,673] If no tumor is found or if the gastrinoma is unresectable or metastatic and the patient had a high antisecretory drug requirement (>4.8 g/day of cimetidine), then a highly selective vagotomy may be considered.

The role of surgery in the treatment of patients with ZES and MEN-1 is unclear.[635,724] Because of the low possibility of cure and because recent studies suggest that the gastrinoma in familial cases is less malignant, some groups recommend no explorative laparotomy, or a laparotomy only if a localized lesion is predicted by a localized gastrin gradient from selective venous sampling for gastrin or if the fasting serum pancreatic polypeptide concentration is more than three times normal.[614,620,725,726] It is not clearly established that familial gastrinoma has a less malignant course.[594] Also, too few patients have had exploratory laparotomies after measurement of pancreatic polypeptide concentrations or gastrin sampling studies to assess adequately their potential usefulness. Because many of these patients' parents died of metastatic gastrinoma and many of the patients present at relatively young ages with a large tumor, a surgical approach similar to the one used in patients with sporadic disease may be warranted for a particular kindred.[650] Therefore, we recommend that all patients with ZES and MEN-1 undergo extensive localization studies, but that only those patients with unequivocally positive imaging studies undergo surgical exploration (Fig. 39-18). This approach is suggested because these patients can not be cured without total pancreaticoduodenectomy and because the imaging studies detect most large tumors (> 3 cm) that may metastasize if left untreated.[681,684]

METASTATIC GASTRINOMA. Because patients with metastatic gastrinomas have markedly decreased survivals (Table 39-31) and because the malignant nature of the gastrinoma is an important determinant of survival, there is a need for improved treatment of metastatic gastrinoma (Table 39-33). Chemotherapy, hepatic embolization, systematic removal of all resectable tumor, hormonal therapy with a somatostatin analog, and treatment with interferon have all been advocated, but the role of each remains unclear.[427,428,437,595,674]

Chemotherapy using streptozotocin alone or in combination with 5-fluorouracil or 5-fluorouracil plus doxorubicin has been reported to be effective in reducing tumor size in 20% to 63% of patients with islet cell tumors (Table 39-33). In one study, the combination of streptozotocin plus 5-fluorouracil was more effective than streptozotocin alone.[728] DTIC and doxorubicin have given poor response rates alone (9–20%), and chlorozotocin has given approximately the same response rate (50%) as streptozotocin alone.

Almost all single studies that include significant numbers of patients and investigate the effects of chemotherapeutic agents on islet cell tumors have combined all islet cell tumors together. Whether these results apply to metastatic gastrinoma is unclear. Two studies have demonstrated no difference in the response rates of various islet cell tumors to streptozotocin, but there were only small numbers of patients with the different types of islet cell tumors for comparison.[728–730] Moreover, the chemotherapeutic responses have suggested differential responses by gastrinomas, glucagonomas and VIPomas to agents such as DTIC or streptozotocin.

When results are combined from a number of small series, streptozotocin alone appears to cause an objective response in 50% of patients with metastatic gastrinoma. Streptozotocin combined with 5-fluorouracil or 5-fluorouracil plus doxorubicin caused objective responses in 20% to 80% of patients with metastatic gastrinoma. For all islet tumors, the combination of streptozotocin plus 5-fluorouracil gave a response rate of 63%, which was significantly better than the 40% response rate with streptozotocin alone.[728] Whether similar results would be obtained for gastrinoma alone is unknown. Relatively few cases have been studied, cases that did not respond are generally not reported, different protocols are used in different studies, follow-up is incomplete, and different indications for treatment are frequently used. Furthermore, in a recent prospective study of 10 patients with metastatic gastrinomas to the liver that increased in size

TABLE 39-33. Drug Therapy for Islet Cell Tumors and Gastrinomas

Agent	*Patients (Number)*	*Objective Response (%)*	*Reference*
All Islet Tumors		*Number (Rate)*	
STZ	52	26 (50)	(729)
	17	7 (41)	(573)
	16	10 (62)	(730)
DOX	20	4 (20)	(731)
CZT	13	7 (53)	(732)
DTIC	11	1 (9)	(437)
Tubercidin	6	2 (33)	(437)
STZ + 5-FU	40	25 (63)	(728)
STZ + DOX	5	1 (20)	(580)
STZ + 5-FU + DOX	10	40 (40)	(727)
SMS-201-995	46	8 (17)	(558)
Interferon	22	6 (27)	(737)
Gastrinomas			
STZ	24	12 (50)	(594, 728, 729)
DTIC	5	0 (0)	(NIH 1987)
STZ + 5-FU	3	1 (33)	(728)
	10	8 (80)	(671)
	5	1 (20)	(621)
STZ + 5-FU	28	19 (42)	(733)
STZ	17		
STZ + 5-FU + DOX	10	4 (40)	(727)
SMS-201-995	10	3 (19)	(558)
Interferon	4	2 (50)	(737)

*STZ = streptozotocin; DOX = doxorubicin; CZT = chlorozotocin; 5-FU = 5-fluorouracil; DTIC = dacarbazine; Interferon = human leukocyte interferon.

over 6 months before entering the study, chemotherapy with streptozotocin, 5-fluorouracil, and doxorubicin resulted in only a 40% objective response rate, no complete remissions, and no statistical difference in survival between responders and nonresponders.[727] Therefore, the precise role and efficacy of chemotherapy in patients with metastatic gastrinoma have not been established.

Also not established is when chemotherapy should be considered in a given patient with metastatic disease. Some patients have had stable metastatic disease for 20 years, but most die within 5 years; the mean survival is 3 to 5 years.[595,601,613,617,622,674] Of the two groups of physicians with considerable experience with metastatic gastrinoma, one group proposes that patients be treated with chemotherapy when they become symptomatic.[728] However, if gastric acid hypersecretion is adequately controlled, symptoms that result only from the tumor arise very late in the course of the disease. Another group proposes that after the initial evaluation, patients be reassessed in 3 to 6 months, and those patients with increasing hepatic metastases should be treated with chemotherapy.[594,727] No studies have recommended chemotherapy in patients with metastases only to regional lymph nodes.

For metastatic liver tumors, hepatic arterial embolization has been of value in patients with gastrinoma and other GI endocrine tumors.[566,734] However, only small numbers of gastrinomas have been treated by this technique, and it is not possible to determine whether this procedure affects long-term survival. Distant metastases to bone occur in 12% of all patients with hepatic metastases, suggesting that procedures directed only at the disease in the liver may be of limited value in many patients with extensive disease.[738]

The data of Zollinger and colleagues suggest that removal of all resectable tumor or "debulking surgery" prolongs life expectancy.[595] There are no studies that have systematically evaluated debulking surgery. However, Norton and others reported the successful resection of all metastatic disease in 4 of 20 patients with extensive disease, 2 of whom have maintained normal gastrin levels postoperatively.[674] Although this requires systematic evaluation before it can be routinely recommended, these results raise the possibility that a small percentage of patients with extensive disease can be identified in whom removal of all resectible tumor may provide prolonged benefit.

Hormonal therapy with SMS-201-995 has been shown to be effective in controlling the symptoms due to a number of different islet cell or carcinoid-like tumors, including VIPomas, glucagonomas, GRFomas, insulinomas, gastrinomas, and carcinoids.[558,560] SMS-201-995 has decreased the size of metastases or tumor growth of islet cell tumors in animals and humans.[558,739] Studies have reported decreases in hepatic metastases in two patients with gastrinoma, but another study of nine patients with metastatic gastrinoma treated with SMS-201-995 for 1 to 11 months reported no effect.[560,735,736] Until controlled trials are done, treatment with SMS-201-995 can not be recommended for routine use in patients with metastatic gastrinoma.

Human leukocyte interferon may be helpful in patients with metastatic islet cell tumors including gastrinoma.[237] Seventeen of 22 patients, most of whom had previously failed chemotherapy, demonstrated an objective response with interferon treatment, defined as a decrease of more than 50% in tumor size or in tumor markers. Two of 4 patients with metastatic gastrinoma responded, but because of the small numbers of cases and limited follow-up, it is unclear whether interferon can provide long-term benefit for patients with metastatic gastrinoma.

INSULINOMA

Insulin-secreting islet cell tumors encompass a broad range of diagnostic and therapeutic features. The diagnosis of insulinomas relies on an interplay of clinical suspicion and careful laboratory analysis. Insulinomas were first recognized by Whipple, who had seen 30 patients with hypoglycemia and pancreatic adenomas by 1935.[740] Whipple's triad consisting of the characteristic symptoms of hypoglycemia associated with blood sugars below 50 mg/dl and immediate relief following ingestion of glucose remained the major criteria for many years for the diagnosis of insulinoma.[740]

Insulinomas usually occur in patients between the ages of 20 and 75 years. The average age of presentation is between 44 and 46 years.[691,741,742] There is a preponderance (60%) of women in most series.[691,743]

SYMPTOMS

The clinical symptoms of insulinomas are due to hypoglycemia in most instances. Greater than 80% of patients have intermittent, transient symptoms of central nervous system dysfunction from drowsiness to loss of consciousness and coma.[691,743] Many patients also report autonomic nervous system symptoms, such as palpitations or diaphoresis.[744] There are numerous reports of erroneous psychiatric or neurologic diagnoses for patients with insulinomas.[745] These reports highlight the need for blood glucose measurements during any transient neuropsychiatric incident, particularly if it is recurrent. Neuroglycopenic symptoms usually exist for more than 3 years before diagnosis. Some patients present with a history of self-treatment by consuming small frequent meals.[746] Most patients with insulinomas are clearly overweight, and many are obese.

DIAGNOSIS

Although there are useful clues to diagnosis of insulinoma, such as symptoms following a fast, often the symptoms are nonspecific and the diagnosis can be established only by fasting with concomitant laboratory examination (Fig. 39-17). Investigation of patients with neuroglycopenic episodes begins with the documentation of hypoglycemia during the symptoms provoked by a fast. Organic hypoglycemia is usually defined as a blood sugar less than 40 mg/dl in the fasting state. In normal women, blood values are frequently lower than men during fasting, and values may decrease below 40 mg/dl. Therefore, it is important that blood glucose and insulin concentrations be obtained during the fast.[691,743,747] It is necessary to reproduce hypoglycemia and desirable to reproduce mild neuroglycopenic symptoms during the fast and measure concomitant serum insulin levels. This is accomplished by obtaining baseline glucose and insulin levels and then fasting the patient (with free access to water) for 72 hours. More than 90% of the insulinomas are detected in this manner, most becoming symptomatic within 24 hours.[691,743] In the evaluation, the combination of an inappropriately elevated immunoreactive insulin (IRI > 6 μU/ml), a low level of blood glucose (<40 mg/dl), and a ratio of insulin to glucose <0.3 most clearly points to insulinoma. In addition, patients with insulinomas frequently have an elevated proinsulin component. Normal persons have less than 25% of the serum insulin as proinsulin and over 90% of patients with insulinomas have a proinsulin component greater than 25%, with mean levels of 50% (Fig. 39-17).[691]

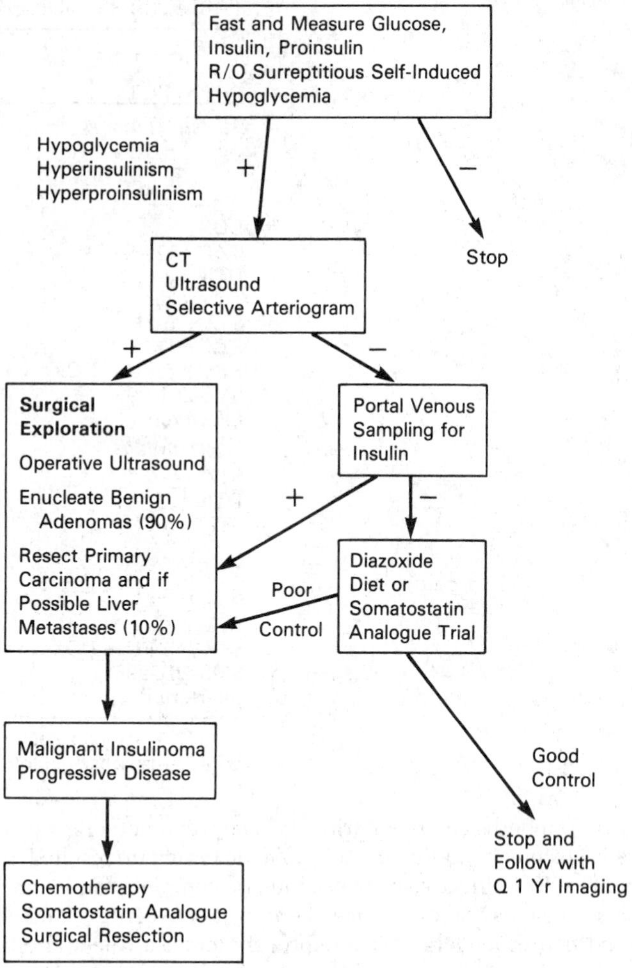

FIG. 39-17. Flow diagram for the management of patients with hypoglycemia.

PATHOLOGY

The distinction between benign and malignant insulinomas is of great clinical significance; however, as with other APUDomas it is not possible to distinguish these two types of tumor by pathological analysis alone. Malignancy is only defined by the presence of metastases at the time of surgery or metastases documented by other investigations.[748] Insulinomas are the opposite of gastrinomas: 60% to 90% of gastrinomas are malignant, but only 10% of insulinomas are malignant (Table 39-34).[691] In approximately 50% of malig-

TABLE 39-34. Incidence of Benign and Malignant Insulinomas

Category	*Incidence*	*Family History*
Single benign adenoma	80%	Negative
Multiple benign or malignant islet cell tumors (usually multiple endocrine neoplasia-type 1)	10%	Positive
Carcinoma, diagnosed by regional or hepatic metastases	10%	Usually negative but may be positive

nant islet cell tumors, human chorionic gonadotropin or its alpha-subunit may be elevated.[749] Other markers like chromogranin, neuron specific enolase, and synaptophysin are specific for neuroendocrine cells, such as pancreatic endocrine tumors, but these markers do not distinguish benign from malignant neoplasms.[750,751] The pattern of metastatic spread of insulinomas is limited to local invasion, peripancreatic and portal nodes, and the liver.

The majority of insulinomas are a solitary, benign pancreatic nodules that are often encapsulated. These tumors are uniformly distributed throughout the entire pancreas and are usually less than 2 cm in diameter. Ten percent of patients with insulinoma will have multiple islet cell tumors in the pancreas and will have MEN-1 (Table 39-34).[463]

LOCALIZATION

After a firm diagnosis of insulinoma is established, the next task is localization of the tumor (Table 39-35, Fig. 39-17). These radiographic investigations are concentrated on the pancreas because the vast majority of insulinomas are located there.[691,752–754] Preoperative localization is essential because insulinomas are frequently small (90% < 2 cm in diameter) and if metastatic spread is present, unnecessary surgery may be prevented.[743] Most insulinomas can be accurately localized preoperatively with either CT or selective arteriography.[691] Most large series report an even distribution of insulinomas within the pancreas, so that blind distal pancreatectomy would only have a one of three chance of finding a tumor.[755]

Selective venous sampling of the portal vein and its tributaries can accurately localize an insulinoma to the exact region of the pancreas in nearly all patients.[691] This finding is contrary to venous sampling results in patients with gastrinoma, in whom venous sampling was not as helpful.[687]

TABLE 39-35. Localization Procedures for Insulinoma

Procedure	*Successful Localization (%)*	*References*
Ultrasound	10–20	(755)
CT	20–40	(755)
Selective arteriogram	80–90	(755)
Transhepatic portal venous sampling	90–100	(756, 757, 758)
Operative ultrasound	90	(754, 759)

Insulinomas are almost always in the pancreas, but 50% of the gastrinomas are extrapancreatic.

In localization of insulinoma, rely on selective arteriography, which is positive in 80% to 90% of patients. If that study is negative, proceed with transhepatic portal venous sampling for insulin levels, which can localize the insulinoma to a region of the pancreas in almost every patient. Two groups have reported successful localizations by transhepatic sampling in the subgroup of patients not visualized by angiography, identifying 10 of 10 in one series and 6 of 7 in another.[691,755–758] If the arteriogram is positive, venous sampling is not necessary. Intraoperative ultrasonography has been useful in localizing insulinomas at the time of surgery.[689,754,759]

In our experience, more than 80% of insulinomas are visualized by arteriography, and most of the unidentified lesions are localized by venous sampling.[691] In cases where all the preoperative localization studies are negative, the decision for surgical exploration rests upon whether the patient's symptoms can be effectively controlled medically (Fig. 39-17). Such decisions should be made on an individual basis following adequate trials of suppression therapies and attempts to rule out malignancy.

TREATMENT

Surgery

All insulinomas without evidence of metastases and localized by angiography or transhepatic venous sampling should be surgically removed, regardless of the severity of symptoms. Of all insulinomas, 80% are benign isolated lesions whose surgical removal is curative (Table 39-34). The surgical approach itself is guided by the tumor's location and degree of encapsulation. The liver must always be explored for evidence of metastatic disease, and the entire abdomen should be explored to rule out rare extrapancreatic tumors. The entire pancreas must be explored for other tumors, since multifocal tumors occur in at least 10% of all cases.[691] Isolated lesions of the tail may be enucleated or removed en bloc by distal pancreatectomy. Body and head lesions require enucleation with careful dissection to avoid damage to the main pancreatic duct and its attendant morbidity. Division of the peritoneum lateral to the duodenum (Kocher maneuver) is necessary to palpate the pancreatic head, and division of the peritoneum along the inferior border of the pancreas is required to adequately palpate the body and the tail. Distal pancreatectomy usually requires concomitant splenectomy. Pneumococcal vaccine (Pneumovax) should be administered preoperatively to lower the risk of catastrophic postsplenectomy sepsis.

Anecdotal reports of hypoglycemia during manipulation of the pancreas have focused attention on glucose monitoring during surgery. Use of the artificial pancreas (Biostator) has documented an increased glucose requirement during removal of insulinomas.[691] A number of centers have made use of the artificial pancreas or frequent glucose measurement to monitor patients for hypoglycemia and to document successful removal of the tumor by noting a "rebound hyperglycemia" or suddenly decreased glucose requirement. However, a large retrospective study at the Mayo Clinic showed that the rebound hyperglycemia did not occur in 23% of patients who had successful extirpation of their insulinomas.[760] This technique may aid the localization of occult insulinomas. Kudlow and colleagues showed sensitive detection of an unlocalized tumor by using a noncrushing clamp to isolate regions of the pancreas from the circulation while monitoring blood glucose with an artificial pancreas programmed to amplify small increases in blood glucose concentrations.[761] Also germane to such cases are attempts to develop a rapid immunoassay for insulin, capable of detecting falls in insulin concentration within 20 minutes of removing a section of the pancreas. We do not currently use intraoperative monitoring of insulin or glucose to guide tumor localization or removal.

In nonlocalized insulinomas in which symptoms persist despite therapy to suppress insulin release, surgical exploration is indicated (Fig. 39-17).[691] Even in cases of documented metastatic disease, refractory debilitating symptoms may be an indication for debulking the pancreatic lesion. Metastases are not always secretory. Removal of peripancreatic lymph nodes may be curative for malignant insulinoma if no liver metastases are present.[691]

Nonsurgical Management

The simplest form of nonsurgical treatment for insulinoma is dietary management. Many insulinoma patients begin frequent small meals to alleviate symptoms before seeking medical evaluation, and a significant percentage report weight gain in the year before diagnosis. In unusually severe cases, intravenous glucose may be required to prevent neuroglycopenic attacks. Hypertonic solutions, such as 10% dextrose, should be avoided because of electrolyte imbalances generated by combining high levels of glucose and hyperinsulinemia simultaneously. We have used slowly absorbed oral nutrients, such as cornstarch, to provide stable euglycemia in preoperative patients. This may prove to be particularly useful in preventing sudden hypotension during anesthetic induction in patients requiring diazoxide treatment until just before surgery.[691]

The usual drug therapy for suppression of insulin secretion is diazoxide. Diazoxide suppresses insulin release through unknown mechanisms, in oral doses of 200 to 600 mg daily. The plasma half-life is approximately 28 hours, and peak hyperglycemia effect occurs about 12 hours after an oral dose and 4 hours after an intravenous dose.[691,743] The primary side-effects are nausea and salt and water retention. These effects can be minimized by administration of diazoxide with meals and by restriction of salt. The primary mode of clearance of diazoxide is renal, and diazoxide is known to displace protein-bound drugs and increase their free concentrations in serum. Therapy should be initiated at low doses and increased to a maximum of 600 mg in two or three divided doses, as tolerated or until symptoms are relieved. Clinical response to diazoxide may be related to the degree of differentiation of the tumor. Approximately 60% of insulinoma patients will respond to this medication.[691,743]

The long-acting SMS-201-995 is effective in controlling symptoms in 50% of patients with insulinoma.[558]

Malignant Insulinoma

The documentation of metastatic disease, either at the time of surgery or by imaging studies, is the only accurate means of diagnosing malignant insulinoma. Unlike all other islet cell tumors, malignant insulinomas are uncommon (10%). Malignant primary insulinomas are usually not occult and have a mean size of 6 cm, which is more than twice as large as benign insulinomas. The median disease-free survival following curative resection of malignant insulinomas was 5 years in one series.[748] The recurrence rate was 63%, with a median interval to recurrence of 2.8 years and a median survival after recurrent tumor of 19 months. Palliative re-resection was associated with a median survival of 4 years, and biopsy only, 11 months.[748] Insulin-secreting carcinomas are slow-growing tumors with significant metastatic potential. Surgical resection of primary and metastatic insulinomas is desirable when possible.[748] Malignant insulinomas, like other islet cell tumors, may respond to chemotherapy and treatment with SMS-201-995. The use of these agents for all malignant islet cell neoplasms will be described in the section on treatment.

OTHER ISLET CELL TUMORS

The remainder of the islet cell tumors, which occur infrequently, include nonfunctional islet cell tumors, vasoactive intestinal-peptide-producing tumors (VIPomas), glucagonomas, ACTHomas, somatostatinomas, and growth-hormone-stimulating pancreatic tumors (GRFomas). Each of these islet cell tumors can be malignant, but all are slow growing and indolent. Individual tumors and their syndromes are listed in Table 39-36.

Pathology of Nonfunctional Islet Cell Tumor

Nonfunctioning malignant islet cell tumors present in the fourth and fifth decades of life.[762,763] Because no active hormone is secreted by these tumors, symptoms arise from mechanical or crowding effects of the neoplasm. These tumors are usually quite large and locally invasive at diagnosis. Most patients present with abdominal pain, a palpable mass, or metastatic tumor in the liver. These tumors have a propensity to metastasize and are usually not cured by resection. Pancreatic polypeptide, neuron-specific enolase, and HCG may each function as a marker of the disease. Chemotherapy should be used for progressive disease and may be tried for known metastases after surgery. Mean survival from the time of diagnosis in one series was only 23 months (range, 4–72 months).[762]

VIPomas

Episodic and severe secretory diarrhea plus hypokalemia, hypochlorhydria, and metabolic acidosis (WDHA syndrome, pancreatic cholera syndrome, or Verner Morrison syndrome) are the classic findings associated with a pancreatic islet cell tumor producing vasoactive intestinal peptide (VIP). The diagnosis is established by an elevated VIP level, which can also serve as a marker for a malignant tumor.[764] It is now well-established that the VIP released by the VIPoma causes the symptoms.[765] Initial, preoperative supportive therapy includes intravenous fluids to correct the reduced volume, hypokalemia, and metabolic acidosis. Localization of the tumor in a manner similar to that for insulinoma should be followed by surgical resection and documentation of the extent of disease.[764] The long-acting SMS-201-995 frequently controls the secretory diarrhea and metabolic derangements in patients with pancreatic cholera.[555,558] Most VIPomas are responsive to chemotherapy with streptozotocin and 5-fluorouracil, and the use of these agents is discussed in the section on treatment.

Glucagonoma

The glucagonoma syndrome is characterized by a migratory necrolytic erythematous rash, mild diabetes mellitus, severe muscle wasting, and marked hypoaminoacidemia.[743,766] The diagnosis is established by a marked elevation in plasma glucagon concentration. Other causes of hyperglucagonemia, such as chronic pancreatitis, uremia, severe illness, trauma, or cirrhosis, should be excluded. Besides increased glucagon plasma levels, it is not clear what causes the rash. One group suggested that hypoaminoacidemia caused the rash in one patient with glucagonoma and reported that the rash cleared after parenteral normalization of plasma amino acid levels.[770] However, another group studying another patient noticed that the glucagonoma rash disappeared after surgical resection of the tumor, but not during dietary normalization of serum amino acids.[771] The role of prostaglandins in the rash is unclear, but Peterson recently demonstrated that glucagon increases epidermal arachidonic acid.[772] SMS-201-995 can induce remission of the rash and other components of the glucagonoma syndrome.[558,773] Treatment consists of tumor localization, resection, and chemotherapy.

Somatostatinoma

Somatostatin is a hormone that inhibits numerous endocrine and exocrine functions. Almost all gut hormones, including insulin, glucagon, gastrin, secretin, cholecystokinin, and motilin, are inhibited by somatostatin. In addition to the inhibition of endocrine secretions, somatostatin directly affects several target organs. It inhibits gastric acid secretion, and it increases intestinal motility and reduces the absorption of fat.[763] The somatostatinoma syndrome is caused by tumors that produce somatostatin. The clinical features include diabetes, diarrhea/steatorrhea, cholelithiasis, hypochlorhydria and weight loss.[774,775]

There have been 27 cases of pancreatic somatostatinoma and 21 cases of intestinal somatostatinomas reported in the world literature.[763] Most of the intestinal tumors arise in the duodenum, ampulla, or biliary ducts. Twenty-three of 27 pancreatic somatostatinomas and 11 of 21 intestinal somatostatinomas had evidence of metastatic disease at the time of diagnosis.[763] Diagnosis depends on the presence of an islet cell tumor with elevated circulating levels of somatostatin.

TREATMENT

Most islet cell tumors, including VIPomas, glucagonomas, nonfunctional tumors, and somatostatinomas, will be discovered to be malignant with diligent follow-up.[743,762,763,776] The exception is insulinoma, which has a low incidence of malignancy.[691] The malignant nature of these islet cell carcinomas cannot be accurately detected by pathology. They require careful follow-up with imaging studies and serum markers. The principles of treatment of malignant insulinomas, VIPomas, glucagonomas, somatostatinomas, and nonfunctioning islet cell tumors are similar to those discussed for gastrinomas. Although these tumors frequently metastasize, many patients will live comfortably and productively for many years with metastatic islet cell tumors if the symptoms can be controlled.

Chemotherapy alone has yielded few, if any prolonged complete remissions in patients with metastatic disease. Chemotherapy plus aggressive surgical resection of all visible disease has helped a few select patients; complete remission has lasted for 3 to 4 years in some.[674] Because of the indolent growth pattern of these tumors and the fact that chemotherapy has not cured any patients with metastatic islet cell carcinoma, chemotherapy has usually been withheld until a patient demonstrates refractory symptoms or progression of disease during carefully monitored follow-up. Progression usually means an increase in size or number of metastatic lesions on an imaging study, but it may mean increase in the serum hormone marker for a given tumor. Tumor size is generally more reliable.

Treatment of metastatic and primary islet cell carcinoma requires control of bulk disease and control of the symptoms caused by hormonal excess. Control of the tumor will usually control symptoms, but some tumors may not be treatable by surgery or chemotherapy, and control of symptoms will improve quality and may improve length of life. The initial consideration and the only potentially curative treatment of malignant islet cell carcinoma is surgical resection (Fig. 39-18). This is considered for any patient with a primary or metastatic islet cell tumor. The goal of surgery is to locate and remove all gross disease. Resection must be performed with acceptable morbidity and mortality, because often the disease is slow-growing. Patients may have lived for years with documented metastases.

Therapy for malignant islet cell tumors is currently divided between the new somatostatin analogue, SMS 201-995, to control symptoms by its antihormonal effects and chemotherapy to reduce tumor size and to control disease by its antitumor effects.[558]

Somatostatin Analogue

Recently, the development and availability of SMS 201-995 has enabled a new approach to the treatment of these islet cell tumors. The principal difference between SMS-201-995 and native somatostatin is that the analog is long-acting and allows a patient to self-administer the drug subcutaneously two to four times a day. SMS 201-995 (50–150 μg, two to three times daily) improved diarrhea in 14 of 17 patients (80%) with VIPomas, and plasma VIP levels decreased in 15

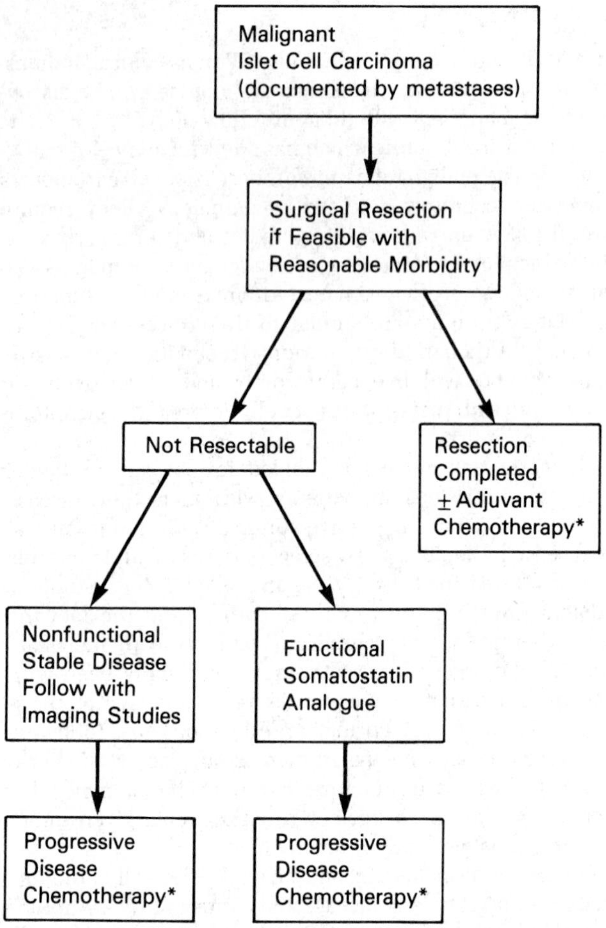

FIG. 39-18. Flow diagram for management of patients with malignant islet cell tumors. *Chemotherapy: DTIC for glucagonomas; streptozotocin or chlorozotocin + fluorouracil for others.

of 17 patients (Table 39-37).[558] Tumor size decreased in 4 of 10 patients. SMS-201-995 remained effective in 16 of 18 patients for more than 1 month and for more than 6 months in 50% of the patients.[558] Some patients became refractory and the dose had to be increased.[558]

SMS 201-995 improved symptoms in 83% of 12 patients with glucagonoma, with resolution of the rash in the 8 patients who had a rash at the start of treatment. The drug reduced the plasma glucagon level in 75%.[558] In 8 patients in whom tumor size was measured, none demonstrated any reduction on imaging study. In no patient did the diabetes improve. The rash responded quickly, and in some patients the response was independent of the effects on plasma glucagon levels. SMS-201-995 remained effective for more than 12 months in some patients.[558]

In 20 patients with insulinomas treated with SMS 201-995, hypoglycemic symptoms were improved in 40% and plasma insulin levels decreased in 65% (Table 39-37). However, 65% of the patients received SMS-201-995 for less than 1 week because most had curative surgery.[558] Only 1 patient with a somatostatinoma has been treated with SMS-201-995, and it was ineffective. Three patients with GRFomas have been treated, and in each case symptoms were controlled.[558]

Side-effects of the somatostatin analogue have been minimal. Patients with tumors that produce somatostatin develop constipation, malabsorption, gallstones and diabetes, but an SMS-201-995-induced form of this syndrome has not been described.[763,774,775] Steatorrhea has been described in some patients taking high doses, but in many cases the effect was transient.[558]

There is a role for SMS-201-995 in both the short-term and long-term management of the symptoms of VIPoma, glucagonoma, and GRFomas. SMS-201-995 may help some patients with metastatic insulinoma, but present results demonstrate only minimal antitumor action at the well-tolerated dosages administered.

Chemotherapy

Chemotherapy for insulinomas and the less common islet cell tumors is the same as that for gastrinomas (Table 39-33). Because of the rarity of these tumors, chemotherapy of all islet cell tumors is considered together. Although two series reported no difference in responsiveness to chemotherapeutic agents between these different tumors, the number of individual tumors used to make this comparison was small, and it is not established that each tumor type responds equally to chemotherapy.[728,729] As with gastrinomas, chemo-

TABLE 39-36. Less Frequent Islet Cell Tumors

Tumor	*Syndrome or Symptoms*	*Location*	*Marker Hormones*	*References*
Nonfunctional islet cell carcinoma	Weight loss, abdominal mass, pain	Pancreas	Pancreatic polypeptide, neuron-specific enolase, human chorionic gonadotrophin	(762)
VIPoma (pancreatic cholera) WDHA, Verner-Morrison syndrome	Severe watery diarrhea, hypokalemia, achlorhydria	Pancreas	VIP	(764)
Glucagonoma	Dermatitis, glucose intolerance, hypoaminoacidemia	Pancreas	Glucagon	(743, 766)
ACTHoma	Cushing's syndrome	Pancreas	ACTH	(645, 767)
Somatostatinoma	Diabetes mellitus, cholelithiasis, diarrhea and steatorrhea, hypochlorhydria	Pancreas Duodenum Jejunum	Somatostatin	(763, 774)
Pancreatic islet cell carcinoma and hypercalcemia	Increased calcium	Pancreas	Parathyroid hormone-like substance, urinary cyclic AMP	(768)
GRFoma	Acromegaly	Pancreas	Growth hormone-releasing factor	(769)

TABLE 39-37. Effect of SMS-201-995 in Patients with Islet Cell Tumors

	VIPoma	*Glucagonoma*	*Insulinoma*	*Nonfunctioning Islet Cell Tumor*
Patients treated	18	12	20	5
Symptoms improved (%)	83	83	40	60
Marker hormone level reduced (%)	89	75	65	
Dosage (μg/day)	300	100	600	450
Decrease in (%) tumor size	40	0	0	0

Abstracted from Maton PN, Gardner JD, Jensen RT: The use of long-acting analogue SMS-201-995 in patients with pancreatic islet cell tumors. Dig Dis Sci, in press.

therapy is reserved for patients with refractory symptoms or with metastatic disease shown to be increasing in size on imaging studies. These chemotherapeutic agents may have significant side-effects. It is possible that chemotherapy may have greater benefit in patients who have had metastatic disease resected or in patients with less extensive or aggressive metastatic disease, but this is not yet established.[674]

In several series, streptozotocin alone caused objective remissions in 41% to 60% of islet cell tumors, and the combination of tubercidin, doxorubicin, and DTIC caused remissions in 9% to 33% (Table 39-33). Streptozotocin with 5-fluorouracil, with or without doxorubicin, has caused objective responses in 20% to 63% of patients. The current agents of choice for these tumors are streptozotocin and 5-fluorouracil. Moertel and colleagues demonstrated that streptozotocin had a 40% response rate for treatment of metastatic islet cell carcinoma. This was significantly lower than the 63% partial response rate and the 33% complete response rate seen in patients treated with the combination of streptozotocin and 5-fluorouracil.[728] It appears that VIPomas are more sensitive to streptozotocin, with up to 90% responding; many patients show a complete remission.[764] Chlorozotocin is a drug similar to streptozotocin, with considerably less GI toxicity and nephrotoxicity, but increased myelosuppression. In one study, chlorozotocin had similar efficacy as a single agent to streptozotocin, and its improved tolerance may make it the nitrosourea of choice for treatment of metastatic islet cell carcinoma.[732] Because its mechanism of action is similar to streptozotocin, a patient will not respond to chlorozotocin if he fails streptozotocin therapy.

Kessinger and others identified DTIC as an effective agent in the treatment of malignant glucagonoma that is resistant to streptozotocin.[777–782] This high degree of responsiveness to DTIC (14 of 15 patients, including several complete remissions) make it the drug of choice for malignant glucagonoma.[573] In contrast, DTIC had no beneficial effect in metastatic gastrinoma that did not respond to streptozotocin.[594]

Experience with other chemotherapeutic agents, such as etoposide, actinomycin, or cisplatin, in islet cell tumors is limited, but in a few case reports they were ineffective.[573]

Human leukocyte interferon has been effective in controlling symptoms of hormonal excess in patients with islet cell tumors.[584,737,783] In one study, 17 of 22 patients with various islet cell tumors had a mean response of 8.5 months (range, 2–36 months).[737] With VIPomas 7 of 7 responded. With nonfunctioning tumors 6 (66%) of 9 patients had decreased serum levels or tumor size. The only patient with somatostatinoma responded. One insulinoma had no response. Six (27%) of the 22 patients demonstrated a decrease in tumor size.[737] Because each of the 22 patients had failed chemotherapy, these results suggest human leukocyte interferon may be of value for this subset of patients with islet cell tumors.[737] No response to recombinant alpha-interferon was seen in 2 patients with VIPoma.[784]

Hepatic artery occlusion with or without postocclusion chemotherapy has also been used successfully for islet cell tumors.[437,567] In 7 patients with various islet cell tumors, hepatic artery occlusion led to complete improvement in symptoms in 14%, a 75% to 99% improvement in 57%, and a 50% to 75% improvement in 14%.[437] Parallel regression of hepatic metastases was reported. In another study hepatic occlusion was combined with postocclusion chemotherapy, and 64% of 11 patients with islet cell tumors had complete improvement in symptoms; 18% had a 75% to 99% improvement; and 9% had a 50% to 75% improvement. The improvements lasted longer than with hepatic artery occlusion alone.[437,567]

It is critically important to ascertain the effects of any treatment in these rare patients with metastatic islet cell carcinomas. Active agents and partial objective responses may not truly benefit these patients. One study indicated that survival was not improved in the cohort of patients with metastatic gastrinoma who responded to chemotherapy compared with the group that showed no response.[727] Considering the toxic side-effects of chemotherapy and the less toxic alternate methods like SMS-201-995, the risks and benefits should be carefully evaluated before instituting any therapy. We believe that the great majority of islet cell tumors, except insulinoma, are malignant. Drugs like streptozotocin, chlorozotocin, fluorouracil, and doxorubicin have clear activity. With an early demonstration of recurrent or metastatic disease, the patient should be evaluated for the possibility of surgical resection of all tumor. If this is possible, it should be followed with a course of adjuvant chemotherapy.[674] Dramatic results have been demonstrated in some patients, and these complete remissions have been durable for over 3 years.[674]

MULTIPLE ENDOCRINE NEOPLASIAS

MULTIPLE ENDOCRINE NEOPLASIA TYPE 1

In 1954, Wermer described the familial occurrence of tumors involving the pituitary gland, parathyroid glands, and the endocrine pancreas.[785] Of the five affected patients, four had pituitary tumors, three had hyperparathyroidism, and three had pancreatic tumors. The syndrome initially called

Wermer's syndrome was once called multiple endocrine adenomatosis type 1, and is now called multiple endocrine neoplasia type 1 (MEN 1), because it is clear that some of the pancreatic islet cell tumors in affected individuals can be malignant.[786,787]

MEN-1 is inherited as an autosomal dominant trait.[786,787] The gene defect is unknown. It is also unknown whether a gene abnormality causes the pathology in all affected or one abnormal focus secretes substances that affect other sites. Recent work concerning the cause of primary hyperparathyroidism in patients with MEN-1 suggests that there is a circulating factor in the serum that stimulates bovine parathyroid cells to proliferate.[788] This parathyroid mitogenic factor may induce the parathyroid hyperplasia detected in these patients.[788]

Clinical Presentation

The peak incidence of symptoms in women with MEN-1 is during the third decade of life, and the peak incidence in men is during the fourth decade. More than half of patients with MEN-1 will have adenomas of more than one gland, and approximately 20% will have three affected glands. The frequency of glandular involvement, in descending order, is parathyroid, pancreatic islets, pituitary, adrenal cortex, and thyroid. The frequency of clinical symptoms, in descending order, is hypercalcemia, nephrolithiasis, peptic ulcer disease, hypoglycemia, headache, visual-field loss, hypopituitarism, acromegaly, galactorrhea-amenorrhea, and Cushing's syndrome.[786,787]

Parathyroid Gland Involvement

Hyperparathyroidism is the most common clinically detected abnormality in patients with MEN-1, occurring in 88% to 97% of all patients in different series.[786,789,790] The pathology associated with primary hyperparathyroidism is always hyperplasia or multiple gland disease (Table 39-38).[789,790] Surgical management requires removal of 3.5 or 4 parathyroid glands to control the hypercalcemia. If 4 glands are removed, immediate autograft of some of the parathyroid tissue into the musculature of the nondominant forearm is recommended.[791] Unfortunately, the incidence of recurrent or persistent hyperparathyroidism following surgery is between 16% and 54%, and the incidence of hypoparathyroidism is between 10% and 25%.[792,793] Proper surgical management requires a skilled, experienced surgeon who can find all 4 glands. Primary hyperparathyroidism adversely affects the medical management of the gastric acid hypersecretion in MEN-1 patients with hyperparathyroidism and ZES. Successful parathyroidectomy in these patients greatly facilitates the management of the gastric acid hypersecretion.[703]

Pancreatic Islet Cell Tumors

Pathologic examination of the resected pancreas in patients with MEN-1 demonstrates multiple islet cell tumors producing many different hormones.[794,795] In two large series, 81% to 82% of patients with MEN-1 developed islet cell tumors, of which 54% had multiple gastrinomas, 21% had insulinomas, 3% had glucagonomas, and 1% had VIPomas (Table 39-38).[786,790]

The ideal treatment of the ZES is usually surgical excision of the gastrinoma; however, in patients with MEN-1, excision of gastrinomas rarely results in normal serum gastrin levels. In six different surgical series, no patients with MEN-1 were cured by resection of their gastrinomas, indicating that the probability of curing these patients in this manner is remote.[650] However, many of these patients will develop islet cell carcinomas, which may metastasize. Therefore, we recommend that all patients with MEN-1 and ZES undergo extensive localization studies, but that only patients with positive imaging studies undergo surgical resection.[650]

Hypersecretion of insulin by islet cell tumors may produce clinical symptoms of hypoglycemia, and less commonly, hypersecretion of vasoactive intestinal peptide may produce secretory diarrhea and hypokalemia in patients with MEN-1. The management of these tumors is different from gastrin-

TABLE 39-38. Multiple Endocrine Neoplasia Syndromes and Familial Medullary Thyroid Cancer

	*MEN-1**	*MEN-2a*	*MEN-2b*	*Familial non-MEN MTC*
Medullary thyroid carcinoma	None	Bilateral	Bilateral	Bilateral
Course of medullary thyroid carcinoma	None	Variable, frequently indolent	Generally more virulent	Indolent
Pheochromocytoma	None	70% Bilateral	70% Bilateral	None
Parathyroid disease	Hyperplasia	Hyperplasia	Rare	None
Specific phenotype	None	None	Bony abnormalities, multiple mucosal neuromas, marfanoid habitus, bumpy lips	None
Familial, autosomal dominant trait	Yes	Yes	Yes, but may be nonfamilial	Yes
Islet cell tumors	Common (81–82%) Gastrinomas (54%) Insulinomas (21%) Glucagonomas (3%)	None	None	None

*MEN = multiple endocrine neoplasia; MTC = medullary thyroid carcinoma.

oma in patients with MEN-1. Medical management of hyperinsulinism and elevated VIP levels is not as reliable as medical management of gastric acid hypersecretion in ZES patients. Diazoxide and SMS-201-995 may be useful for short-term treatment, but they are not as reliable as surgical resection for long-term treatment. In patients with MEN-1, insulinomas or VIPomas are usually solitary tumors, resection of which manages symptoms and may result in cure.[683,725,794] Preoperative portal venous sampling for insulin or VIP can help to identify the tumor or region of the pancreas from which the abnormal hormone originates.[725]

Pituitary Tumors

Pituitary tumors occur in 54% to 65% of patients with MEN-1.[786,790] Symptoms, including headache and visual-field defects, caused by pituitary adenomas in MEN-1 are usually due to local encroachment of the tumor. The tumor is usually a chromophobe adenoma. The most common hormone secreted by pituitary adenomas is prolactin (70%), which may give rise to the galactorrhea-amenorrhea syndrome. The second most common hormone secreted is growth hormone (30%), which causes acromegaly. Cushing's syndrome rarely occurs in a patient with MEN-1 and is caused by excessive ACTH secretion from a pituitary adenoma; however, it can also be caused by a pancreatic islet cell tumors secreting ACTH.[645,795,796]

Adrenal and Thyroid Tumors

Adrenal abnormalities occur in 27% to 36% of the patients with MEN-1.[786,790] The most common abnormality is a benign, nonfunctional cortical adenoma, although adrenal cortical carcinomas and hyperplasia may occur.[786,790] Adrenal cortical hyperfunction may occur more frequently than thought previously.[786,790] It was recently reported in 15% of patients with MEN-1 and gastrinoma and in all MEN-1 patients with pituitary adenomas.[645] Adrenal cortical neoplasms usually are nonfunctional in patients with MEN-1.

Thyroid adenomas occur in approximately 5% to 30% of patients with MEN-1. They involve diffuse or nodular hyperplasia and have little clinical significance.

FAMILIAL MEDULLARY THYROID CARCINOMA AND MULTIPLE ENDOCRINE NEOPLASIA TYPE 2a AND 2b

History and Pathology

The coexistence of thyroid cancer and pheochromocytoma were first described in 1932 by Eisenberg and Wallerstein.[797] In 1959, Hazard and colleagues first described medullary thyroid carcinoma and its striking characteristics of cellular argentaffin staining and amyloid production.[798] Medullary thyroid carcinoma is associated with three distinct familial syndromes: MEN-2a, MEN-2b, and familial non-MEN medullary thyroid carcinoma, a disease characterized by hereditary thyroid cancer without associated endocrinopathies (Table 39-38).[799]

In 1962, a hypocalcemic factor was discovered in the thyroid and named calcitonin.[800] In 1968, a hypocalcemic substance was found in medullary carcinoma.[801] In 1970, a radioimmunoassay was developed for calcitonin, and a kindred with MEN-2a was described with elevated serum calcitonin levels.[802] Subsequently, patients with increased levels of serum calcitonin were identified whose resected thyroid glands were normal macroscopically but microscopically showed C-cell hyperplasia.[803,804]

In 1961, Sipple reported an unusually high incidence of bilateral pheochromocytomas in patients with thyroid malignancy.[805] These patients were later found to have medullary thyroid carcinoma, and the familial disease was inherited as a mendelian autosomal dominant trait with high gene penetrance.[806,807] Subsequently, hyperparathyroidism was also identified as part of the syndrome.[808] In 1968, this syndrome of medullary carcinoma of the thyroid gland, pheochromocytomas, and hyperparathyroidism was called multiple endocrine neoplasia type II.[801] Now it is called MEN-2a.

In the late sixties, Williams and Pollock and Gorlin and colleagues called attention to the finding that some patients had multiple mucosal neuromas, with or without marfanoid habitus, puffy lips, prominent jaw, pes cavus, and medullated corneal nerves with medullary carcinoma and pheochromocytomas (Fig. 39-19).[809,810] For this group of patients the term MEN-2b or MEN-3 was suggested.[811] Patients with MEN-2b seldom have parathyroid disease. Some have presented at a young age with constipation and toxic megacolon caused by intestinal ganglioneuromatosis. The disease usually occurs sporadically, but like MEN-2a, it may be inherited as an autosomal dominant trait. In patients with MEN-2b, the medullary carcinoma presents at an early age and appears to be more aggressive because few patients live beyond 30 years of age.[49] The characteristic appearance of these patients is often the first sign of disease and may suggest the diagnosis before other clinical abnormalities appear (Fig. 39-19). The medullary thyroid carcinoma is always present at the time of clinical recognition.

Histologically, the disease in patients with familial medullary carcinoma, MEN-2a, and MEN-2b appears identical to the medullary cancer occurring sporadically. In each syndrome there is bilateral involvement, and the medullary carcinoma usually occupies the superior-lateral part of the thyroid lobe(s) and may be multicentric. The neoplasm appears as a circumscribed, whitish-tan nodule, and it is composed of sheets or cords of round or spindle-shaped cells separated by a variable amount of amorphous stroma. It is a malignant tumor of the parafollicular cells or the calcitonin-secreting cells (C cells). Medullary carcinoma comprises 5% to 12% of all thyroid cancers, and only 10% is familial.[812]

The pheochromocytomas in patients with MEN-2a or MEN-2b usually present in the second or third decades of life and are usually (70%) bilateral.[812,813] Even in patients with unilateral pheochromocytomas, the contralateral adrenal gland almost always demonstrates medullary hyperplasia on pathologic analysis.[813] However, patients with medullary hyperplasia rarely have symptoms of pheochromocytoma. Pheochromocytomas in patients with MEN-2a or MEN-2b are seldom malignant and are usually contained within the adrenal gland. Histologically, these tumors are indistinguishable from those occurring sporadically in a nonfamilial setting.

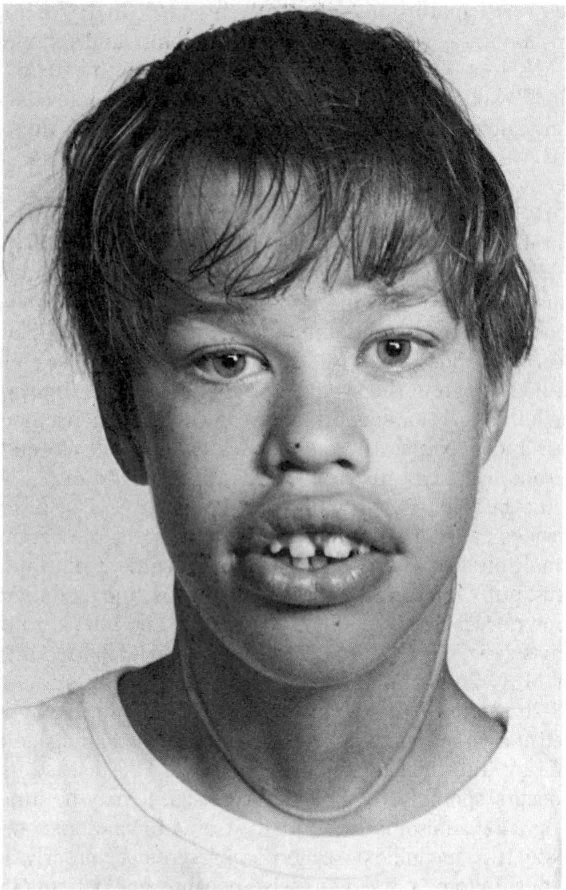

FIG. 39-19. Characteristic appearance of a patient with multiple endocrine neoplasia type 2b. Note the mucosal neuromas, pronounced lips, poor dentition, and prominent jaw. (Norton et al: Multiple endocrine neoplasia type 2b. Surg Clin North Am 59:109, 1979)

The parathyroid lesions in MEN-2a consist of generalized multiglandular hyperplasia, and they must be managed as the parathyroid disease is in MEN-1.[789,791]

Clinical Presentation

Any of the neoplasms that make up the syndromes of MEN-2a or MEN-2b may be the presenting problem; however, medullary thyroid carcinoma is a constant feature that affects 100% of these patients. Of 164 patients with MEN-2a, all had medullary cancer, 35 (21%) had pheochromocytomas, and 28 (17%) had hyperparathyroidism.[812] In another study of patients with MEN-2a, all had medullary carcinoma, 40% had pheochromocytomas, and 60% had parathyroid hyperplasia.[814]

Patients may initially seek medical advice because of episodic headaches, dizziness, or symptoms suggestive of hypertension. Patients with MEN-2a or MEN-2b should have a pheochromocytoma excluded before undergoing surgery for medullary carcinoma. Pheochromocytomas can usually be excluded by measuring urinary levels of epinephrine, norepinephrine, VMA, and metanephrines. If an elevated level is detected, abdominal CT or MRI and ^{131}I-MIBG scans are helpful in locating the lesion(s).[815] It is unusual for patients with MEN-2a to have symptoms related to parathyroid disease.[799]

Preoperative Evaluation

When a suspicion of MEN-2a or MEN-2b exists, precise diagnosis depends upon hormonal changes consistent with medullary carcinoma, hyperparathyroidism, and pheochromocytoma. The production of calcitonin by the tumor cells holds the key for diagnosis of medullary cancer. Most investigators believe that the upper normal limit of plasma calcitonin is 300 pg/ml. Virtually all patients with medullary cancer will have elevated basal or stimulated levels of calcitonin. Patients who present with clinically apparent disease will usually have basal plasma calcitonin levels exceeding 1 ng/ml.[816] Generally, there is a direct correlation between the tumor mass and plasma calcitonin levels.[816]

Radioimmunoassay for calcitonin has been especially helpful in evaluating family members from kindreds proven to have MEN-2a. Minimal elevations of plasma calcitonin are indicative of medullary carcinoma in patients who have no other clinical evidence of the neoplasm.[817] Some patients with normal basal levels of plasma calcitonin will have an increase to abnormal levels following calcium infusion (15 mg/kg over 4 hours) or pentagastrin injection.[818] Short-bolus calcium injection (2 mg calcium gluconate/kg over 1 minute) also provokes elevated plasma calcitonin levels in medullary carcinoma patients. Provocative tests for the diagnosis of medullary thyroid carcinoma were compared. The peak plasma calcitonin levels in patients with medullary cancer were higher with the combination test of calcium and pentagastrin injection than with calcium chloride alone, calcium gluconate alone, or pentagastrin alone. The patients with undetectable basal calcitonin levels (<300 pg/ml) had peak calcitonin responses above 300 pg/ml following pentagastrin and calcium injection. Three of 12 patients had peak calcitonin levels below 300 pg/ml with pentagastrin alone or with calcium gluconate alone, and they would not have been diagnosed if these two provocative agents had been used separately. The combination test of pentagastrin and calcium gluconate provides a higher diagnostic accuracy than any other provocative test, and it is the simplest, most effective method of screening for medullary thyroid carcinoma.[818]

In kindred members at risk who have borderline elevated plasma calcitonin levels (200–600 pg/ml), selective inferior thyroid venous catheterization and sampling during provocative testing is recommended.[819] Patients with medullary carcinoma have strikingly increased plasma calcitonin levels in the inferior thyroid vein effluent following provocative testing, but normal persons do not. Patients with minimally elevated plasma calcitonin levels following stimulation have minimal medullary carcinoma and are usually cured by thyroidectomy.[816]

Surgical Management

The ability to diagnose medullary thyroid carcinoma in patients at risk for the familial form allows the physician to diagnose and treat this malignancy in an early preclinical stage. If a patient from a MEN-2a kindred has medullary cancer, it is absolutely essential that the other family members at risk be screened. It is in this situation that calcium gluconate and pentagastrin provocative test has its greatest utility. Most patients diagnosed with only biochemically evident disease will have surgically curable C-cell hyperplasia or carcinoma confined to the thyroid gland.[820] Testing is usually done in family members at risk beginning at 5 years of age and continuing at yearly intervals through the fifth decade.

Patients with pheochromocytoma merit abdominal exploration and evaluation of both adrenal glands, the sympathetic chain, the organ of Zuckerkandl, and the bladder. If a solitary adrenal pheochromocytoma is present, it should be resected. Some advocate only resecting abnormal adrenal glands confirmed by palpation; others recommend routinely resecting both adrenal glands.[813,821] Bilateral adrenal resection is recommended because bilateral adrenal medullary pathology will be present in most patients.[813] However, some patients have only unilateral adrenalectomy and remain asymptomatic, with normal urinary catecholamines, for a mean follow-up period of 8 years.[821] Patients with MEN-2a undergoing unilateral adrenalectomy for pheochromocytoma should be followed carefully at 6-month or yearly intervals, because a second adrenal tumor may be diagnosed biochemically before it is clinically apparent.

The surgical management of familial medullary thyroid carcinoma is total thyroidectomy with a central lymph node dissection. It is essential that a total thyroidectomy be performed, because the disease is always bilateral.

Postoperative Follow-Up

In patients with MEN-2a and MEN-2b, the medullary thyroid carcinoma is the disease that is most frequently lethal. It seems to be more virulent in patients with MEN-2b than in patients with MEN-2a.[49] Survival of patients with MEN-2a is difficult to predict, because some patients die at a young age and others have a normal life expectancy. However, survival of patients with MEN-2a does depend on the extent of medullary carcinoma at initial surgical resection.[816]

In a familial setting it is imperative that the carcinoma be diagnosed at an early stage when it is confined to the thyroid gland.[820] The prognostic significance of the stimulated plasma calcitonin level was demonstrated in a study of 92 patients with hereditary medullary cancer.[820] The patients were divided into four groups according to their preoperative stimulated plasma calcitonin levels: Group 1, 250 to 1,000 pg/ml; Group 2, 1,000 to 5,000 pg/ml; Group 3, 5,000 to 10,000 pg/ml; and Group 4, above 10,000 pg/ml. In the 25 patients in Group 1, the carcinoma was clinically occult and only evident on biochemical testing. Only one of these patients had regional lymph node metastases, and only one had an elevated stimulated plasma calcitonin level postoperatively, indicating residual disease. None of the patients had distant metastases, and none died during the period of observation. In the Group 4 patients, 13 of the 23 had metastases to regional lymph nodes, and 14 had biochemical evidence of residual disease.[820] The only patients who had distant metastatic disease and succumbed to disease were in Group 4.[820]

With the widespread availability of reliable radioimmunoassays for calcitonin, an individual patient can be easily followed postoperatively. Detection of an elevated basal plasma calcitonin level or the finding of an abnormal response to calcium and pentagastrin indicates recurrent or persistent disease.

In patients with metastatic medullary thyroid carcinoma, the best strategy is unclear. Radioactive iodine ablation, thyroid suppression, and radiation therapy have not been helpful. The disease is relatively insensitive to chemotherapy. Because of the indolent nature of the tumor, most physicians have chosen not to aggressively treat metastatic disease.

The ten-year survival of medullary carcinoma is approximately 50%. Aggressive surgical resection has been used to control locally recurrent MTC because it is the only known effective therapy. However, it must be remembered that in patients with MEN-2a, the disease may be well tolerated. The average life expectancy of patients with medullary cancer and MEN-2a is 50 years.[822] The current best therapy for familial medullary thyroid carcinoma is early diagnosis and complete resection of intrathyroidal disease at the initial surgery. Ablation of extrathyroidal disease when detected as persistent or recurrent elevations of plasma calcitonin levels following total thyroidectomy requires the development of effective systemic adjuvant therapy.

REFERENCES

1. Schwartz TB: Benign metastases from thyroid malignancies. Lancet 1:733, 1986
2. Halsted WS: The operative story of goiter. Johns–Hopkins Hosp Rep 19:71,1929
3. Halsted WS: Surgical Papers, vol II, p 257. Baltimore, The Johns–Hopkins Press, 1924
4. Brennan MF: Cancer of the endocrine system. In DeVita VT, Hellman S, Rosenberg SA (eds): Cancer Principles and Practice of Oncology, 2nd ed, pp 1179–1241. Philadelphia, JB Lippincott, 1985
5. Joensuu H, Klemi PJ, Paul R et al: Survival and prognostic factors in thyroid carcinoma. Acta Radiol 25:243, 1986
6. Tubiana M, Schlumberger M, Rougier P et al: Long-term results and prognostic factors in patients with differentiated thyroid carcinoma. Cancer 55:794, 1985
7. Torres J, Volpato RD, Power EG et al: Thyroid cancer survival in 148 cases followed for 10 years or more. Cancer 56:2298, 1985
8. Hannequin P, Liehn JC, Delisle MJ: Multifactorial analysis of survival in thyroid cancer. Cancer 58:1749, 1986
9. Cady B, Rossi R, Silverman M et al: Further evidence of the validity of risk group definition in differentiated thyroid carcinoma. Surgery 98:1171, 1985
10. Sampson RJ, Key CF, Buncher CR et al: Thyroid carcinoma in Hiroshima and Nagasaki. Prevalence of thyroid carcinoma at autopsy. JAMA 209:65, 1969
11. Bondeson L, Ljungberg O: Occult thyroid carcinoma at autopsy in Malmo, Sweden. Cancer 47:319, 1981
12. Sampson RJ, Woolner LB, Bahn RC et al: Occult thyroid carcinoma in Olmsted County, Minnesota. Prevalence at autopsy compared with that in Hiroshima and Nagasaki. Cancer 34:2070, 1974
13. Fukunaga FH, Yatani R: Geographic pathology of occult thyroid carcinomas. Cancer 36:1095, 1975
14. Meissner WA: Tumors of the thyroid gland. In: Atlas of Tumor Pathology. Washington, DC, Armed Forces Institute of Pathology, 1984
15. Trowbridge FL, Matovinovic J, McLaren GD et al: Iodine and goiter in children. Pediatrics 56:82, 1975
16. Rallison ML, Dobyns BM, Keating FR et al: Thyroid nodularity in children. JAMA 233:1069, 1975
17. Rojeski MT, Gharib H: Nodular thyroid disease. N Engl J Med 313:428, 1985
18. Shimaoka K, Sokal JE: Differentiation of benign and malignant thyroid nodules by scnitiscan. Arch Intern Med 114:36, 1974
19. Groesbeck HP: Evaluation of routine scintiscanning of nontoxic thyroid nodules 1: the preoperative diagnosis of thyroid carcinoma. Cancer 12:1, 1959
20. Leichty RD, Stoffel PT, Zimmerman DE et al: Solitary thyroid nodules. Arch Surg 112:59, 1977
21. Messaris G, Kyriakou K, Vasilopoulos P et al: The single thyroid nodule and carcinoma. Br J Surg 61:943, 1974
22. Clark RL, White EC, Russell WO: Total thyroidectomy for cancer of the thyroid: significance of intraglandular dissemination. Ann Surg 149:858, 1959
23. Cady B, Sedgwick E, Meisner WA et al: Changing clinical pathologic therapeutic and surgical patterns indifferentiated thyroid carcinoma. Ann Surg 192:701, 1980

24. Nel CJC, van Heerden JA, Goellner JR et al: Anaplastic carcinoma of the thyroid: A clinicopathologic study of 82 cases. Mayo Clin Proc 60:51, 1985
25. Albores-Saavedra J, Altamirano-Dumas M, Alcorta-Anguizola B et al: Fine structure of human papillary thyroid carcinoma. Cancer 28:763, 1971
26. Lindsay S: Carcinoma of the Thyroid Gland, p 30. Springfield, IL, C Charles Thomas, 1960
27. Hawk WA, Hazard JB: The many appearances of papillary carcinoma of the thyroid. Cleve Clin Q 43:207, 1976
28. Sampson RJ: Thyroid carcinoma (letter). Arch Pathol Lab Med 102:270, 1978
29. Patchefsky AS, Keller IB, Mansfield CM: Solitary vertebral column metastasis from occult sclerosing carcinoma of the thyroid gland. Am J Clin Pathol 53:596, 1970
30. Jereb B, Stjernsward J, Lowhagen T: Anaplastic giant-cell carcinoma of the thyroid gland. Cancer 35:1293, 1975
31. Heitz P, Moser H, Staub JJ: Thyroid cancer. Cancer 37:2329, 1976
32. Schmidt RJ, Wang CA: Encapsulated follicular carcinoma of the thyroid: diagnosis, treatment and results. Surgery 100:1068, 1986
33. Crile G, Pontius KI, Hawk WA: Factors influencing the survival of patients with follicular carcinoma of the thyroid gland. Surg Gynecol Obstet 160:409, 1985
34. Lang W, Choritz H, Hundeshagen H: Risk factors in follicular thyroid carcinomas. Am J Surg Pathol 10:246, 1986
35. Roediger WEW: The oxyphil and C cells of the human thyroid gland. Cancer 36:1758, 1975
36. Valenta LJ, Michel-Bechet M: Electron microscopy of clear cell thyroid carcinoma. Arch Pathol Lab Med 101:140, 1977
37. Thompson NW, Dunn EL, Batsakis JG et al: Hurthle cell lesions of the thyroid gland. Surg Gynecol Obstet 139:555, 1974
38. Gundry SR, Burney RE, Thompson NW et al: Total thyroidectomy for Hurthle Cell Neoplasm of the thyroid. Arch Surg 118:529, 1983
39. Heppe H, Armin A, Calandra DB et al: Hurthle cell tumors of the thyroid gland. Surgery 98:1162, 1985
40. Arganini M, Behar R, Wu TC et al: Hurthle cell tumors: a twenty-five-year experience. Surgery 100:1108, 1986
41. Chong GC, Beahrs OH, Sizemore GW, et al: Medullary carcinoma of the thyroid gland. Cancer 35:695, 1975
42. Babu VR, Van Dyke DL, Jackson CE: Chromosome 20 deletion in human multiple endocrine neoplasias types 2A and 2B: a double blind study. Proc Natl Acad Sci USA 84:2525, 1985
43. Hsu TC, Pathak S, Samaan N et al: Chromosome instability in patients with medullary carcinoma of the thyroid. JAMA 246:2046, 1981
44. Emmertsen K, Lamm LU, Rasmussen KZ et al: Linkage and chromosome study of multiple endocrine neoplasia IIa. Cancer Genet Cytogenet 9:251, 1983
45. Tanaka K, Baylin SB, Nelkin BD et al: Cytogenetic studies of a human medullary thyroid carcinoma cell line. Cancer Genet Cytogenet 25:27, 1987
46. Zajac JD, Penschow J, Mason T et al: Identification of calcitonin and calcitonin gene-related peptide messenger ribonucleic acid in medullary thyroid carcinomas by hybridization histochemistry. J Clin Endocrinal Metab 62:1037, 1986
47. Wells SA Jr, Ontjes DA, Cooper CW et al: The early diagnosis of medullary carcinoma of the thyroid gland in patients with multiple endocrine neoplasia type II. Ann Surg 182:362, 1975
48. Cance WG, Wells SA Jr: Multiple endocrine neoplasia type IIa. Current Prob Surg 22:1, 1985
49. Norton JA, Fromme LC, Farrell RE et al: Multiple endocrine neoplasia type 2b: the most aggressive form of medullary thyroid carcinoma. Surg Clin North Am 59:109, 1979
50. Rossi R, Cady B, Meissner WA et al: Nonfamilial medullary thyroid carcinoma. Am J Surg 139:554, 1980
51. Lippman SM, Mendelsohn G, Trump DL et al: The prognostic and biological significance of cellular heterogeneity in medullary thyroid carcinoma: a study of calcitonin, L-dopa decarboxylase and histaminase. J Clin Endocrinol Metab 54:233, 1982
52. de Bustros A, Baylin SB, Levine MA et al: Cyclic AMP and phorbol esters separately induce growth inhibition, calcitonin secretion, and calcitonin gene transcription in cultured human medullary thyroid carcinoma. J Biol Chem 261:8036, 1986
53. de Bustros A, Baylin SB, Berger CL et al: Phorbol esters increase calcitonin gene transcription and decrease c-myc m-RNA levels in cultured human medullary thyroid carcinoma. J Biol Chem 260:98, 1985
54. Block MA, Jackson CE, Greenawald KA et al: Clinical characteristics distinguishing hereditary from sporadic medullary thyroid carcinoma. Arch Surg 115:142, 1980.
55. Kruseman ACN, Bosman FT, Henegouw JCV et al: Medullary differentiation of anaplastic thyroid carcinoma. Am J Clin Pathol 77:541, 1982
56. Carcangiu ML, Steeper T, Zampi G et al: Anaplastic thyroid carcinoma. Am J Clin Pathol 83:135, 1985
57. Gaal JM, Horvath E, Kovacs K: Ultrastructure of two cases of anaplastic giant cell tumor of human thyroid gland. Cancer 35:1273, 1975
58. Krisch K, Holzner JH, Kokoschkar et al: Hemangioendothelioma of the thyroid gland — true endothelioma or anaplastic carcinoma? Pathol Res Pract 170:230, 1980
59. LiVolsi VA, Brooks JJ, Arendash-Durand B: Anaplastic thyroid tumors immunohistology. Am J Clin Pathol 87:434, 1987
60. Aldinger KA, Samaan NA, Ibanez M et al: Anaplastic carcinoma of the thyroid. Cancer 41:2267, 1978
61. Duffy BJ Jr, Fitzgerald PJ: Cancer of the thyroid in children: a report of 28 cases. J Clin Endocrinol Metab 10:1296, 1950
62. Schneider AB, Shore-Freedman E, Ryo UY et al: Radiation-induced tumors of the head and neck following childhood irradiation. Medicine 64:1, 1985
63. Holm LE, Dahlquist I, Israelsson A et al: Malignant thyroid tumors after iodine 131 therapy. N Engl J Med 303:188, 1980
64. Conrad RA, Dobyns BM, Sutow WW: Thyroid neoplasia as a late effect of exposure to radioactive iodine in fallout. JAMA 214:316, 1970
65. Larsen PR, Conrad RA, Knudsen KD et al: Thyroid hypofunction after exposure to fallout from a hydrogen bomb explosion. JAMA 247:1571, 1982
66. Harach HR, Escalant DA, Onatavia A et al: Thyroid cancer and thyroiditis in an endemic goiter region before and after iodine prophylaxis. Acta Endocrinol 108:55, 1985
67. William ED: The aetiology of thyroid tumours. Clin Endocrinol Metab 8:193, 1979
68. Franssila K: Value of histologic classification of thyroid cancer. Acta Pathol Microbiol Scan Suppl 225:5, 1971
69. Kapp DS, Li Volsi VA, Sanders MM: Anaplastic carcinoma following well-differentiated thyroid cancer. Etiological considerations. Yale J Biol Med 55:521, 1982
70. Deaconson TF, Wilson SD, Cerletty JM et al: Total or near total thyroidectomy versus limited resection for radiation-associated thyroid nodules: A twelve-year follow-up of patients in a thyroid screening program. Surgery 100:1116, 1986
71. Schneider AB, Recant W, Pinsky SM et al: Radiation-induced thyroid cancer. Ann Intern Med 105:405, 1986
72. Farndon JR, Leight GS, Dilley WG et al: Familial medullary thyroid carcinoma without associated endocrinopathies: a distinct clinical entity. Br J Surg 73:278, 1986
73. Phade VR, Lawrence WR, Max MH: Familial papillary carcinoma of the thyroid. Arch Surg 116:836, 1981
74. Lote K, Andersen K, Nordal E et al: Familial occurrence of papillary thyroid carcinoma. Cancer 46:1291, 1980
75. Jackson IMD, Cobb WE: Disorders of the thyroid. In Kohler PO (ed): Clinical Endocrinology, pp 73–165. New York, John Wiley, 1986
76. Vander JB, Gaston EA, Dawber TR: Significance of solitary nontoxic thyroid nodules: preliminary report. N Engl J Med 251:970, 1954
77. De Groot LJ, Reilly M, Pinnameneni K et al: Retrospective and prospective study of radiation-induced thyroid disease. Am J Med 74:852, 1983
78. Rosen IB, Palmer JA, Bain J et al: Efficacy of needle biopsy in postradiation thyroid disease. Surgery 94:1002, 1983
79. Mazzaferri EL, Young RL, Oertel JE et al: Papillary thyroid carcinoma: the impact of therapy in 576 patients. Medicine 56:171, 1977
80. Thomas CG Jr, Buckwalter JA, Staab EV et al: Evaluation of dominant thyroid masses. Ann Surg 183:463, 1976
81. Messaris G, Evangelou GN, Tountas C: Incidence of carcinoma in cold nodules of the thyroid gland. Surgery 74:447, 1973
82. Hoffman GL, Thompson NW, Heffron C: The solitary thyroid nodule: a reassessment. Arch Surg 105:379, 1972
83. Baschieri L, Giani C, Taddei P et al: Serum thyroglobulin as a marker of thyroid carcinoma. In Andreoli M, Monaco F, Robbins J (eds): Advances of Thyroid Neoplasia, pp 189–201. Rome, 1981
84. Van Herle AJ, Uller RP: Elevated serum thyroglobulin: a marker of metastases in differentiated thyroid carcinoma. J Clin Invest 56:272, 1975
85. Schneider AB, Shore-Freedman E, Ryo UY et al: Prospective serum thyroglobulin measurements in assessing the risk of developing thyroid nodules in patients exposed to childhood neck irradiation. J Clin Endocrinol Metab 61:547, 1985
86. Wells SA Jr, Haagensen DE Jr, Linehan WM et al: The detection of elevated plasma levels of carcinoembryonic antigen in patients with suspected or established medullary thyroid carcinoma. Cancer 42:1498, 1978
87. Wells SA Jr, Dilley WG, Farndon JA et al: Early diagnosis and treatment of medullary thyroid carcinoma. Arch Intern Med 145:1248, 1985
88. Clark OH: TSH suppression in the management of thyroid nodules and thyroid cancer. World J Surg 5:39, 1981
89. Field JB, Bloom G, Chou MCY et al: Effects of thyroid-stimulating hormone on human thyroid carcinoma and adjacent normal tissue. J Clin Endocrinol Metab 47:1052, 1978
90. Balme HW: Metastatic carcinoma of the thyroid successfully treated with thyroxine. Lancet 1:812, 1954
91. Getaz EP, Shimaoka K, Razack M et al: Suppressive therapy for postirradiation thyroid nodules. Can J Surg 23:558, 1980
92. Hill LD, Beebe HG, Hipp R et al: Thyroid suppression. Arch Surg 108:403, 1974
93. Blum M, Rothschild M: Improved nonoperative diagnosis of the solitary "cold" thyroid nodule: surgical selection based on risk factors and three months of suppression. JAMA 243:242, 1980
94. Gershengorn MC, McClung MR, Chu EW et al: Fine-needle aspiration cytology in the preoperative diagnosis of thyroid nodules. Ann Intern Med 87:265, 1977
95. Schick RM: Thyroid nodules, letter to editor. N Engl J Med 314:452, 1986
96. Parker TW, Mettler FA Jr, Christie JH et al: Radionuclide thyroid studies: a survey of practice in the United States in 1981. Radiology 150:547, 1984
97. Dobyns BM, Maloof F: The study and treatment of 119 cases of carcinoma of thyroid with radioactive iodine. J Clin Endocrinol Metab 11:1323, 1951
98. Ashcraft MW, Van Herle AJ: Management of thyroid nodules I. History, Physical Examination, blood tests, x-ray tests and ultrasonograph. Head Neck Surg 3:216, 1981
99. Ashcraft MW, Van Herle AJ: Management of thyroid nodules II. Scanning techniques, thyroid suppressive therapy, and fine-needle aspiration. Head Neck Surg 3:297, 1981
100. Hamburger JI: Thyroid nodules, letter to the editor. N Engl J Med 314:452, 1986
101. Miller JM, Hamburger JI: The thyroid scintigram. I hot nodule. Radiology 84:66, 1965
102. Talpos GB, Jackson CB, Froelich JW et al: Localization of residual medullary thyroid cancer by thallium/technetium scintigraphy. Surgery 98:1189, 1985

103. Arnstein NB, Juni JE, Sisson JC et al: Recurrent medullary carcinoma of the thyroid demonstrated by thallium 201 scintigraphy. J Nucl Med 27:1564, 1986
104. Skibber JM, Reynolds JC, Spiegel AM, et al: Computerized technetium/thallium scan and parathyroid reoperation. Surgery 98:1077, 1985
105. Asari AN, Siegel ME, DeQuattro V et al: Imaging of medullary thyroid carcinoma and hyperfunctioning adrenal medulla using iodine-131 metaiodobenzylguanidine. J Nucl Med 27:1858, 1986
106. Sone T, Fukunaga M, Otsuka N et al: Metastatic medullary thyroid cancer: localization with iodine-131 metaiodobenzylguanidine. J Nucl Med 26:604, 1985
107. Thijs LG: Diagnostic ultrasound in clinical thyroid investigation. J Clin Endocrinol Metab 32:709, 1971
108. Simeone JF, Daniels GH, Mueller PR et al: High-resolution real-time sonography of the thyroid. Radiology 145:431, 1982
109. Stockwell R, Davidoff F: Radiation-induced thyroid carcinoma, letter to the editor. Ann Intern Med 106:637, 1987
110. Nassani SN, Bard R: Evaluation of solid thyroid neoplasms by gray scale and real-time ultrasonography: the halo sign. Ultrasound Med Biol 4:323, 1978
111. Propper RA, Skolnick ML, Weinstein BJ et al: The nonspecificity of the thyroid halo sign. JCU 8:129, 1980
112. Schwerk WB, Grun R, Wahl R: Ultrasound diagnosis of C-cell carcinoma of the thyroid. Cancer 55:624, 1985
113. Simeone JF, Daniels GH, Hall DA, et al: Sonography in the follow-up of 100 patients with thyroid carcinoma. AJR 148:45, 1987
114. Van Herle AJ, Rich P, Ljung BME et al: The thyroid nodule. Ann Intern Med 96:221, 1982
115. Hamburger JI, Hamburger SW: Fine-needle biopsy of thyroid nodules: avoiding the pitfalls. NY State J Med 86:241, 1986
116. Walfish PG, Hazani E, Strawbridge HTG et al: Combined ultrasound and needle aspiration cytology in the assessment and management of hypofunctioning thyroid nodule. Ann Intern Med 87:270, 1977
117. Nishiyama RH, Bigos ST, Goldfarb WB et al: The efficacy of simultaneous fine-needle aspiration and large-needle biopsy of the thyroid gland. Surgery 100:1133, 1986
118. Hamburger JI, Miller JM, Kini SR: Lymphoma of the thyroid. Ann Intern Med 99:685, 1983
119. Broughan TA, Esselstyn CB: Large-needle biopsy: still necessary. Surgery 100:1138, 1986
120. Schwartz AE, Nieburgs HE, Davies TF et al: The place of fine-needle biopsy in the diagnosis of nodules of the thyroid. Surg Gynecol Obstet 155:54, 1982
121. Boey J, Hsu C, Collins RJ: False-negative errors in fine-needle biopsy of dominant thyroid nodules: a prospective follow-up study. World J Surg 10:623, 1986
122. Block MA, Dailey GE, Robb JA: Thyroid nodules indeterminant by needle biopsy. Am J Surg 146:72, 1983
123. Hamburger JI: Consistency of sequential needle biopsy findings for thyroid nodules, management implications. Arch Intern Med 147:97, 1987
124. Hamburger JI, Hamburger SW: Declining role of frozen section in surgical planning for thyroid nodules. Surgery 98:307, 1985
125. Miller JM, Hamburger JI, Kini SR: The impact of needle biopsy on the preoperative diagnosis of thyroid nodules. Henry Ford Hosp Med J 28:145, 1980
126. Hamburger B, Gharib H, Melton LJ III et al: Fine-needle aspiration biopsy of thyroid nodules: Impact on thyroid practice and cost of care. Am J Med 73:381, 1982
127. McConahey WM, Hay ID, Woolner LB et al: Papillary thyroid cancer treated at the Mayo Clinic, 1946 through 1970: initial manifestations, pathologic findings, therapy and outcome. Mayo Clin Proc 61:978, 1986
128. Hawkins F, Bellido D, Bernal C et al: Fine-needle aspiration biopsy in the diagnosis of thyroid cancer and thyroid disease. Cancer 59:1206, 1987
129. Harsoulis P, Leontsini M, Economou A et al: Fine-needle aspiration biopsy cytology in the diagnosis of thyroid cancer: comparative study of 213 operated patients. Br J Surg 73:461, 1986
130. Abu-Nema T, Ayyash K, Tibblin S: Role of aspiration biopsy cytology in the diagnosis of cold solitary nodules. Br J Surg 74:203, 1987
131. Ramacciotti CE, Pretorius HT, Chu EW et al: Diagnostic accuracy and use of aspiration biopsy in the management of thyroid nodules. Arch Intern Med 144:1169, 1984
132. Gharib H, Boellner JR, Zinsmeister AR et al: Fine-needle aspiration biopsy of the thyroid: the problem of suspicious cytologic findings. Ann Intern Med 101:25, 1984
133. Boon ME, Lowhagen T, Cardozo PL et al: Computation of preoperative diagnosis probability for follicular adenoma and carcinoma of the thyroid on aspiration smears. Anal Quant Cytol Histol 4:1, 1982
134. Luck JB, Mumaw VR, Frable WJ: Fine-needle aspiration biopsy of the thyroid: differential diagnosis by videoplan image analysis. Acta Cytol 26:793, 1982
135. Sprenger E, Lawhagen T, Vogt-Schaden M: Differential diagnosis between follicular adenoma and follicular carcinoma of the thyroid by nuclear DNA determination. Acta Cytol 21:528, 1977
136. Patow CA, Norton JA, Brennan MF: Vocal cord paralysis and reoperative parathyroidectomy: A prospective study. Ann Surg 203:282, 1986
137. Brennan MF, Brown EM, Spiegel AM et al: Autotransplantation of cryopreserved parathyroid tissue in man. Ann Surg 189:139, 1979
138. Rossi R, Cady B, Silverman ML et al: Current results of conservative surgery for differentiated thyroid carcinoma. World J Surg 10:612, 1986
140. Cohn KH, Backdahl M, Forsslund G et al: Biologic considerations and operative strategy in papillary thyroid carcinoma: arguments against the routine performance of total thyroidectomy. Surgery 96:957, 1984
141. Crile G Jr, Antunez AR, Esselstyn CB Jr et al: The advantages of subtotal thyroidectomy and suppression of TSH in the primary treatment of papillary carcinoma of the thyroid. Cancer 55:2691, 1985
142. Schroder DM, Chambous A, France CJ: Operative strategy for thyroid cancer, is total thyroidectomy worth the price? Cancer 58:2320, 1986
143. Tupchong L, Phil D, Hughes F et al: Primary lymphoma of the thyroid: clinical features, prognostic factors and results of treatment. Int J Radiat Oncol Biol Phys 12:1813, 1986
144. Goldman JM, Goren EN, Cohen MH et al: Anaplastic thyroid carcinoma: long-term survival after radical surgery. J Surg Oncol 14:389, 1980
145. Tollefson HR, DeCosse JJ: Papillary carcinoma of the thyroid. Recurrence in the thyroid gland after initial treatment. Am J Surg 106:728, 1983
146. Clark RL, White EC, Russel WO: Total thyroidectomy for cancer of the thyroid: significance of intraglandular dissemination. Ann Surg 149:858, 1959
147. van Heerden JA, Groh MA, Grant CS: Early postoperative morbidity after surgical treatment of thyroid carcinoma. Surgery 101:224, 1986
148. Harness JK, Fung L, Thompson NW et al: Total thyroidectomy: complications and technique. World J Surg 10:781, 1986
149. Young RL, Mazzaferri EL, Rahe AJ et al: Pure follicular thyroid carcinoma: impact of therapy in 214 patients. J Nucl Med 21:735, 1980
150. Lang W, Choritz H, Hundeshagen H: Risk factors in follicular thyroid carcinomas. Am J Surg Pathol 10(4):246, 1986
151. Harness JK, Thompson NW, McLeod MK et al: Follicular carcinoma of the thyroid gland: trends and treatment. Surgery 96:972, 1984
152. Rosen IB, Luk S, Katz I: Hurthle cell tumor behavior: dilemma and resolution. Surgery 98:777, 1985
153. Arganini M, Behar R, Wu TC et al: Hurthle cell tumors: a twenty-five-year experience. Surgery 100:1108, 1986
154. Heppe H, Armin A, Calandra DB et al: Hurthle cell tumors of the thyroid gland. Surgery 98:1162, 1985
155. Savino D, Sibley RK, Sumner H: Significance of Hurthle cell in thyroid neoplasms: reexamination of an old but persistent problem. Lab Invest 44:59A, 1981
156. Bondeson L, Bondeson AG, Ljungberg O et al: Oxyphil tumors of the thyroid. Follow-up of 42 cases. Ann Surg 194:677, 1981
157. Caplan RH, Abellera RM, Kisken WA: Hurthle cell tumors of the thyroid gland, a clinicopathologic review and long-term follow-up. JAMA 251:3114, 1984
158. Gosain AK, Clark OH: Hurthle cell neoplasms. Arch Surg 119:515, 1984
159. Stockwell RM, Davidoff BM: Managing thyroid abnormalities in adults exposed to upper body irradiation in childhood: A decision analysis. J Clin Endocrinol Metab 58:804, 1984
160. Schneider AB, Shore-Freedman E, Weinstein RA: Radiation-induced thyroid and other head and neck tumors: occurrence of multiple tumors and analysis of risk factors. J Clin Endocrinol Metab 63:107, 1986
161. Calandra DB, Shah KH, Lawrence A et al: Total thyroidectomy in irradiated patients. Ann Surg 202:356, 1985
162. Deaconson TF, Wilson SD, Cerletty JM et al: Total or near total thyroidectomy versus limited resection for radiation-associated thyroid nodules: a twelve-year follow-up of patients in a thyroid screening program. Surgery 100:1116, 1986
163. DeGroot LJ, Reilly M: Comparison of 30- and 50-mCi doses of iodine-131 for thyroid ablation. Ann Intern Med 96:51, 1982
164. Cady B, Cohn K, Rossi RL et al: The effect of thyroid hormone administration upon survival in patients with differentiated thyroid carcinoma. Surgery 94:978, 1983
165. Brown AP, Greening WP, McCready VR et al: Radioiodine treatment of metastatic thyroid carcinoma: the Royal Marsden experience. Br J Radiol 57:323, 1984
166. Leeper RD: Thyroid cancer. Med Clin North Am 69:1079, 1985
167. Maxon HR, Thomas SR, Hertzburg VS et al: Relation between effective dose and outcome of radioiodine therapy for thyroid cancer. N Engl J Med 309:937, 1983
168. Schlumberger M, Tubiana M, De Vathaire F et al: Long-term results of treatment of 283 patients with lung and bone metastases from differentiated thyroid carcinoma. J Clin Endocrinol Metab 63:960, 1986
169. Samaan NA, Schultz PN, Haynie TP et al: Pulmonary metastasis of differentiated thyroid carcinoma: treatment results in 101 patients. J Clin Endocrinol Metab 65:376, 1985
170. Niederle B, Roka R, Schemper M et al: Surgical treatment of distant metastases in differentiated thyroid cancer: indication and results: Surgery 100:1088, 1986
171. Wells SA Jr, Dilley WG, Farndon JA: Early diagnosis and treatment of medullary thyroid carcinoma. Arch Intern Med 145:1248, 1985
172. Telander RL, Zimmerman D, van Heerden JA et al: Results of early thyroidectomy for medullary thyroid carcinoma in children with multiple endocrine neoplasia type 2. J Pediatr Surg 21:1190, 1986
173. Gorman B, Charboneau JW, James EM et al: Medullary thyroid carcinoma: role of high-resolution U.S. Radiology 162:147, 1987
174. Tennvall J, Biorklund A, Moller T et al: Prognostic factors of papillary, follicular and medullary carcinoma of the thyroid gland. Acta Radiol Oncol 24:17, 1985
175. Norton JA, Doppman JL, Brennan MF: Localization and resection of clinically inapparent medullary carcinoma of the thyroid. Surgery 87:616, 1980
176. Tisell LE, Hansson G, Jansson S et al: Reoperation in the treatment of asymptomatic metastasizing medullary thyroid carcinoma. Surgery 99:60, 1986
177. Gottlieb JA, Hill CS Jr: Chemotherapy of thyroid cancer with adriamycin: experience with 30 patients. N Engl J Med 290:193, 1974
178. Stepanas AV, Samaan NA, Hill CS Jr, et al: Medullary thyroid carcinoma: importance of serial serum calcitonin measurement. Cancer 43:825, 1979
179. Deftos LJ, Stein MF: Radioiodine as an adjunct to the surgical treatment of medullary thyroid carcinoma. J Clin Endocrinol Metab 50:967, 1980

180. Hellman DE, Kartchner M, Van Antwerp PJD et al: Radioiodine in the treatment of medullary carcinoma of the thyroid. J CLin Endocrinol Metab 48:451, 1979
181. Michael BE, Forouhar FA, Spencer RP: Medullary thyroid carcinoma with radioiodide transport. Clin Nucl Med 4:274, 1985
182. Tubiana M, Haddad E, Schlumberger M et al: External radiotherapy in thyroid cancers. Cancer 55:2062, 1985
183. Steinfeld AD: The role of radiation therapy in medullary carcinoma of the thyroid. Radiology 123:745, 1977
184. Cox TM, Fagan EA, Hillward CJ et al: Role of calcitonin in diarrhoea associated with medullary carcinoma of the thyroid. Gut 20:629, 1979
185. Jerkins TW, Sacks HS, O'Dorisio TM et al: Medullary carcinoma of the thyroid, pancreatic nesidioblastosis and microadenosis, and pancreatic polypeptide hypersecretion: a new association and clinical and hormonal responses to long-acting somatostatin analog SMS-201-995. J Clin Endocrinol Metab 64:1313, 1987
186. Nel CJC, van Heerden JA, Goellner JR et al: Anaplastic carcinoma of the thyroid: a clinicopathologic study of 82 cases. Mayo Clin Proc 60:51, 1985
187. Kim JH, Leeper RD: Treatment of anaplastic giant and spindle cell carcinoma of the thyroid gland with combination adriamycin and radiation therapy a new approach. Cancer 52:954, 1983
188. Kim JH, Leeper RD: Combination adriamycin and radiation therapy for locally advanced carcinoma of the thyroid gland. Int J Radiat Oncol 9:565, 1983
189. Williams SD, Birch R, Einhorn L: Phase II evaluation of doxorubicin plus cisplatin in advanced thyroid cancer: a southeastern cancer study group trial. Cancer Treat Rep 70:405, 1986
190. Shimaoka K, Schoenfeld DA, DeWys WD et al: A randomized trial of doxorubicin versus doxorubicin plus cisplatin in patients with advanced thyroid carcinoma. Cancer 56:2155, 1985
191. Bukowski RM, Brown L, Weick JK et al: Combination chemotherapy of metastatic thyroid cancer. Am J Clin Oncol 6:579, 1983
192. Heimann R, Vannineuse A, DeSloover C et al: Malignant lymphoma and undifferentiated small cell carcinoma of the thyroid: A clinicopathological review in light of the Kiel classification for malignant lymphomas. Histopathology 2:201, 1978
193. Rayfield Ed, Nishiyama RH, Sisson JC: Small cell tumors of the thyroid. Cancer 28:1023, 1971
194. Sokal M, Harmar GI: Chemotherapy for anaplastic carcinoma of the thyroid. Clin Oncol 4:3, 1978
195. Compagno J, Oertel JE: Malignant lymphoma and other lymphoproliferative disorders of the thyroid gland; a clinicopathologic study of 245 cases. Am J Clin Pathol 74:1, 1980
196. Devine RM, Edis AJ, Banks PM: Primary lymphoma of the thyroid: a review of the Mayo Clinic experience through 1978. World J Surg 5:33, 1981
197. Williams ED: Malignant lymphoma of the thyroid. Clin Endocrinol Metab 10:379, 1981
198. Hamburger JI, Miller JM, Kini SR: Lymphoma of the thyroid. Ann Intern Med 99:685, 1983
199. Aozasa K, Inoue A, Tajima K et al: Malignant lymphomas of the thyroid gland. Cancer 58:100, 1986
200. Rasbach DA, Mondschein MS, Harris NL et al: Malignant lymphoma of the thyroid gland: a clinical and pathological study of twenty cases. Surgery 98:1166, 1985
201. Tupchong L, Phil D, Hughes F et al: Primary lymphoma of the thyroid: clinical features, prognostic factors and results of treatment. Int J Radiat Oncol Biol Phys 12:1813, 1986
202. Vigliotti A, Kong JS, Fuller LM et al: Thyroid lymphomas stages 1E and 11E: comparative results for radiotherapy only, combination chemotherapy only and multimodality treatment. Int J Radiat Oncol Biol Phys 12:1807, 1986
203. Sandstrom I: Om en ny Kortel hos menniskan och atskilliga daggdjur. Ups J Med Sci 15:441, 1980
204. Christensson T: Hyperparathyroidism and radiation therapy. Ann Intern Med 89:216, 1978
205. Norton JA, Brennan MF, Saxe AW et al: Intraoperative urinary cyclic adenosine monophosphate as a guide to successful reoperative parathyroidectomy. Ann Surg 200:389, 1984
206. Mallette LE, Bilizikian JP, Ketcham AS et al: Parathyroid carcinoma in familial hyperparathyroidism. Am J Med 57:642, 1974
207. Dinnen JS, Greenwood RH, Jones JH et al: Parathyroid carcinoma in familial hyperparathyroidism. J Clin Pathol 30:966, 1977
208. Schantz A, Castleman B: Parathyroid carcinoma a study of 70 cases. Cancer 31:600, 1973
209. Levin KE, Galante M, Clark OH: Parathyroid carcinoma versus parathyroid adenoma in patients with profound hypercalcemia. Surgery 101:649, 1987
210. Cohn K, Silverman M, Corrado J et al: Parathyroid carcinoma: the Lahey Clinic experience. Surgery 98:1095, 1985
211. Wang CA, Gaz RD: Natural history of parathyroid carcinoma. Am J Surg 149:522, 1985
212. Shane E, Bilezikian JP: Parathyroid carcinoma: a review of 62 patients. Endocr Rev 3:218, 1982
213. Gutter RD, Maier H: Carcinoma of the parathyroid. Arch Intern Med 130:413, 1972
214. Bukowski RM, Sheeler L, Cunningham J et al: Successful combination chemotherapy for metastatic parathyroid carcinoma. Arch Intern Med 144:399, 1984
215. Calandra DB, Chejfec G, Foy BK et al: Parathyroid carcinoma: biochemical and pathologic response to DTIC. Surgery 96:1132, 1984
216. Flye MW, Brennan MF: Surgical resection of metastatic parathyroid carcinoma. Ann Surg 193:425, 1981
217. Albright F, Aub JC, Bauer W: Hyperparathyroidism. JAMA 102:1276, 1934
218. Medvei VC: A History of Endocrinology. Lancaster, England, MTP Press Limited, 1982
219. Page DL, DeLellis RA, Hough AJ: Tumors of the adrenal. In: Atlas of Tumor Pathology. Washington, DC, AFIP, 1986
220. Ferris JB, Brown JJ, Fraser R et al: Hypertension with aldosterone excess and low plasma-renin: Preoperative distinction between patients with and without adrenocortical tumour. Lancet 2:995, 1970
221. Arce B, Licea M, Hung S et al: Familial Cushing's syndrome. Acta Endocrinol 87:139, 1978
222. Schweizer-Cagrianut M, Salomon F, Hedinger E: Primary adrenocortical nodular dysplasia with cardiac myxomas. Virchow Arch 397:183, 1982
223. Hough AJ, Hollifield JW, Page DL et al: Diagnostic factors in adrenal cortical tumors. Am J Clin Pathol 72:390, 1979
224. Macfarlane DA: Cancer of the adrenal cortex. Ann R Coll Surg Engl 23:155, 1958
225. Hutter AM Jr, Kayhoe DE: Adrenal cortical carcinoma. Am J Med 41:572, 1966
226. DHEW Publication No. (NIH) 75-787. Third National Cancer Surgery: Incidence Data, Natl Cancer Inst Monogr 41, 1975
227. Lynch HT, Katz DA, Bogard JP et al: The sarcoma, breast cancer, lung cancer, and adrenocortical carcinoma syndrome revisited. Am J Dis Child 139:134, 1985
228. Limon J, Dal Cin P, Kakati S et al: Cytogenetic findings in a primary adrenocortical carcinoma. Cancer Genet Cytogenet 26:271, 1987
229. Schteingart DE, Seabold JE, Gross MD et al: Iodocholesterol adrenal tissue uptake and imaging in adrenal neoplasms. J Clin Endocrinol Metab 52:1156, 1981
230. Hogan TF, Gilchrist KW, Westring DW et al: A clinical and pathological study of adrenocortical carcinoma. Cancer 45:2880, 1980
231. Wick MR, Cherwitz DL, McGlennen RC et al: Adrenocortical carcinoma, an immunohistochemical comparison with renal cell carcinoma. Am J Pathol 122:343, 1986
232. Weiss LM: Comparative histologic study of 43 metastasizing and nonmetastasizing adrenocortical tumors. Am J Surg Pathol 8:163, 1984
233. O'Hare MJ, Monaghan P, Neville AM. The pathology of adrenocortical neoplasia: a correlated structural and functional approach to the diagnosis of malignant disease. Hum Pathol 10:137, 1979
234. Loriaux DL, Cutler GB: Diseases of the adrenal glands. In Kohler PO (ed): Clinical Endocrinology, pp 167–238. New York, John Wiley and Sons, 1986
235. Raker JW, Henneman PH, Graf WS: Coexisting primary hyperparathyroidism and Cushing's syndrome. J Clin Endocrinol Metab 22:273, 1962
236. Maton PN, Gardner JD, Jensen RT: Cushing's syndrome in patients with the Zollinger-Ellison Syndrome. N Engl J Med 315:1, 1986
237. Hiramatsu R, Yoshida K, Sato T: A body measurement to evaluate the pattern of fat distribution in central obesity: a screening and monitoring technique for Cushing's syndrome. JAMA 250:3174, 1983
238. Brown RD, Strott CA: Plasma deoxycorticosterone in man. J Clin Endocrinol Metab 32:744, 1971
239. Christy NP: Iatrogenic Cushing's syndrome. In Christy NP (ed): The Human Adrenal Cortex, p 95. New York, Harper & Row, 1971
240. McArthur RG, Cloutier MD, Hayes AB et al: Cushing's disease in children: findings in 13 cases. Mayo Clin Proc 47:318, 1972
241. McKenna TJ, Lorber D, LaCroix A et al: Testicular activity in Cushing's disease. Acta Endocrinol 91:501, 1979
242. Ferguson JK, Donald RA, Weston TS et al: Skin thickness in patients with acromegaly and Cushing's syndrome and response to treatment. Clin Endocrinol 18:347, 1983
243. Kelly WF, Chekcley SA, Bender DA et al: Cushing's syndrome and depression: a prospective study of 26 patients. Br J Psychiatr 142:16, 1983
244. Starkman MN, Schteingert DE, Schork MA: Depressed mood and other psychiatric manifestations of Cushing's syndrome: relationship to hormone levels. Psychosom Med 43:3, 1981
245. Kramer M, Corrado ML, Bacci V et al: Pulmonary cryptococcosis and Cushing's syndrome. Arch Intern Med 143:2179, 1983
246. Fulkerson WJ, Newman JH: Endogenous Cushing's syndrome complicated by pneumocystis carinii pneumonia. Am Rev Respir Dis 129:188, 1984
247. Graham BS, Tucker WS Jr: Opportunistic infections in endogenous Cushing's syndrome. Ann Intern Med 101:334, 1984
248. Thomas CG Jr, Smith AT, Griffith JM, et al: Hyperadrenalism in childhood and adolescence. Ann Surg 199:538, 1984
249. Beisel WR, Cos JJ, Horton R et al: Physiology of urinary cortisol excretion. J Clin Endocrinol Metab 24:884, 1964
250. Pavlatos FC, Smilo RP, Forsham PH: A rapid screening test for Cushing's syndrome. JAMA 193:720, 1965
251. Willenbring ML, Morley JE, Niewoeher CB et al: Adrenocortical hyperactivity in newly admitted alcoholics: prevalence, course and associated variables. Psychoneuroendorcinology 9:415, 1984
252. Chrousos GP, Vingerhoeds A, Brandon D et al: Primary cortisol resistance in man: a glucocorticoid receptor-mediated disease. J Clin Invest 69:1261, 1982
253. Chrousos GP, Vingerhoeds AC, Loriaux DL et al: Primary cortisol resistance: a family study. J Clin Endocrinol Metab 56:1243, 1983
254. Chrousos GP, Schuermeyer TH, Doppman J et al: Clinical applications of corticotropin-releasing factor. Ann Intern Med 102:344, 1985
255. Nieman LK, Chrousos GP, Oldfield EH et al: The ovine corticotropin-releasing hormone stimulation test and the dexamethasone suppression test in the differential diagnosis of Cushing's syndrome. Ann Intern Med 105:862, 1986
256. Ernest I: Steroid excretion and plasma cortisol in 41 cases of Cushing's syndrome. Acta Endocrinol 51:511, 1966

257. Nichols T, Nugent CA, Tyler FH: Steroid laboratory tests in the diagnosis of Cushing's syndrome. Am J Med 45:116, 1968
258. Howlett TA, Drury PL, Perry L et al: Diagnosis and management of ACTH-dependent Cushing's syndrome: comparison of the features in ectopic and pituitary ACTH production. Clin Endocrinol 24:699, 1986
259. Weiss ER, Rayjis SS, Nelson DH et al: Evaluation of stimulation and suppression tests in the etiological diagnosis of Cushing's syndrome. Ann Intern Med 71:941, 1969
260. Salassa RM, Laws ER Jr., Carpenter PC et al: Transsphenoidal removal of pituitary mucioadenoma in Cushing's disease. Mayo Clin Proc 53:24, 1978
261. Tyrrell JB, Brooks RM, Fitzgerald PA et al: Cushing's disease: selective transsphenoidal resection of pituitary microadenomas. N Engl J Med 298:753, 1978
262. Oldfield EH, Chrousos GP, Schulte HM et al: Preoperative lateralization of ACTH-secreting pituitary microadenomas by bilateral and simultaneous inferior petrosal venous sampling. N Engl J Med 312:100, 1985
263. Epstein AJ, Patel SK, Petasnick JP: Computerized tomography of the adrenal gland. JAMA 242:2791, 1979
264. Doppman JL, Reinig JW, Dwyer AJ et al: Differentiation of adrenal masses by magnetic resonance imaging. Surgery 102:1018, 1987
265. Bierwaltes WH, Sisson JC, Shapiro JC et al: Diagnosis of adrenal tumors with radionuclide imaging. Spec Top Endocrinol Metab 6:1, 1984
266. Schteingart DE, Seabold JE, Gross MD et al: Iodocholesterol adrenal tissue uptake and imaging in adrenal neoplasms. J Clin Endocrinol Metab 52:1156, 1981
267. Sarkar SD, Cofhen EL, Bierwaltes WH et al: A new and superior adrenal imaging agent, ^{131}I-6B-iodomethyl-19-nor-cholesterol (NP-59): evaluation in humans. J Clin Endocrinol Metab 45:353, 1977
268. McArthur RB, Bahn RC, Hayles AB: Primary adrenocortical nodular dysplasia as a cause of Cushing's syndrome in infants and children. Mayo Clin Proc 57:58, 1982
269. Donaldson MDC, Grant DB, O'Hare MJ et al: Familial congenital Cushing's syndrome due to bilateral nodular adrenal hyperplasia. Clin Endocrinol 14:519, 1981
270. Spark RF, Connolly PB, Gluckin DS et al: ACTH secretion from a functioning pheochromocytoma. N Engl J Med 301:416, 1979
271. Boggan JE, Tyrrell JB, Wilson CB: Transsphenoidal microsurgical management of Cushing's disease: report of 100 cases. J Neurosurg 59:195, 1983
272. Conn JW: Presidential address. Part I. Painting background. II. Primary aldosteronism, a new clinical syndrome. J Lab Clin Med 264:9, 1972
273. Biglieri EG, Schambelan M: The significance of elevated levels of plasma 18-hydroxycorticosterone in patients with primary aldosteronism. J Clin Endocrinol Metab 49:87, 1979
274. Kern DC, Tang K, Hanson CS et al: The prediction of anatomical morphology of primary aldosteronism using serum 18-hydroxycorticosterone levels. J Clin Endocrinol Metab 60:67, 1985
275. Gomez-Sanchez CE, Montgomery M, Ganguly A et al: Elevated urinary excretion of 18-oxocortisol in glucocorticoid-suppressible aldosteronism. J Clin Endocrinol Metab 59:1022, 1984
276. Chu MD, Ulick S: Isolation and purification of 18-hydroxycortisol from the urine of patients with primary aldosteronism. J Biol Chem 257:2218, 1982
277. Brown RD, Hollifield JW: Endocrine hypertension. In Kohler PO (ed): Clinical Endocrinology, p 239–262. New York, John Wiley & Sons, 1986
278. Tenschert W, Maurer R, Vetter H, Vetter W: Primary aldosteronism by carcinoma of the adrenal cortex. Klin Wochenschr 65:428, 1987
279. Carey RM, Sen S, Dolan LM et al: Idiopathic hyperaldosteronism: a possible role for aldosterone-stimulating factor. N Engl J Med 311:94, 1984
280. Weinberger MH, Grim CE, Hollifield JW et al: Primary aldosteronism: diagnosis, localization and treatment. Ann Intern Med 90:386, 1979
281. Kaplan NW: Commentary on incidence of primary aldosteronism: current estimations based on objective data. Arch Intern Med 123:152, 1969
282. Lyons DG, Kern DC, Brown RD et al: Single-dose captopril as a diagnostic test for primary aldosteronism. J Clin Endocrinol Metab 57:892, 1983
283. Thibonnier M, Sassano P, Joseph A et al: Diagnostic value of a single dose of captopril in renin- and aldosterone-dependent, surgically curable hypertension. Cardiovasc Rev Rep 3:1659, 1982
284. White EA, Schambelan M, Rost CR et al: Use of computed tomography in diagnosing the cause of primary aldosteronism. N Engl J Med 303:1503, 1980
285. Guerin CK, Wahner HW, Gorman CA et al: Computed tomographic scanning versus radioisotope imaging in adrenocortical diagnosis. Am J Med 75:653, 1980
286. Whaley D, Becker S, Presby T et al: Adrenal myelolipoma associated with Conn syndrome: CT evaluation. J Comput Assist Tomogr 9:959, 1985
287. Falke TH, Strake L, Shaff MI et al: MR imaging of the adrenals: correlation with computed tomography. J Comput Assist Tomogr 10:242, 1986
288. Geisinger MA, Zelch M, Bravo E et al: Primary hyperaldosteronism: comparison of CT, adrenal venography, and venous sampling. AJR 141:299, 1983
289. Auda SP, Brennan MF, Gill JR: Evolution of the surgical management of primary aldosteronism. Ann Surg 191:1, 1980
290. Banks WA, Kastin AJ, Biglieri EG, Ruiz AE: Primary adrenal hyperplasia: a new subset of primary hyperaldosteronism. J Clin Endocrinol Metab 58:783, 1984
291. Alder GK, Williams GH: Primary aldosteronism. In Krieger DT, Bardin CW (eds): Current Therapy in Endocrinology and Metabolism, pp 116–121. Toronto, BC Decker, 1985
292. Biglieri EG, Schambelan M, Slaton PE et al: The intercurrent hypertension of primary aldosteronism. Circ Res 26, 27(1):1, 1970
293. Nadler JL, Hsueh W, Horton R: Therapeutic effect of calcium channel blockade in primary aldosteronism. J Clin Endocrinol Metab 60:896, 1985
294. Cohn K, Gottesman L, Brennan MF: Adrenocortical carcinoma. Surgery 100:1170, 1986
295. Arteaga E, Biglieri EG, Kater C et al: Aldosterone-producing adrenocortical carcinoma, preoperative recognition and course in three cases. Ann Intern Med 101:316, 1984
296. Glazer HS, Weyman PJ, Sagel SS et al: Nonfunctioning adrenal masses: incidental discovery on computed tomography. Am J Roentgenol 139:81, 1982
297. Prinz RA, Brooks MH, Churchill R et al: Incidental asymptomatic adrenal masses detected by computed tomographic scanning: is operation required? JAMA 248:701, 1982
298. Copeland PM: The incidentally discovered adrenal mass, diagnosis and treatment. Ann Intern Med 98:940, 1983
299. McCorkell SJ, Miles NL: Fine-needle aspiration of catecholamine-producing adrenal masses; a possibly fatal mistake. AJR 145:113, 1985
300. Casola G, Nicolet V, Van Sonnenberg E et al: Unsuspected pheochromocytomas: risk of blood pressure alterations during percutaneous adrenal biopsy. Radiology 159:733, 1986
301. Didolkar MS, Bescher RA, Elias EG et al: Natural history of adrenal cortical carcinoma: a clinicopathologic study of 42 patients. Cancer 47:2153, 1981
302. Bertagna C, Orth DN: Clinical and laboratory findings and results of therapy in 58 patients with adrenocortical tumors admitted to a single medical center (1951 to 1978). Am J Med 71:855, 1981
303. Lewinsky BS, Grigor KM, Symington T et al: The clinical and pathologic features of "non-hormonal" adrenocortical tumors: report of twenty new cases and review of the literature. Cancer 33:778, 1974
304. Lipsett MB, Hertz R, Ross GT: Clinical and pathophysiologic aspects of adrenocortical carcinoma. Am J Med 35:374, 1963
305. Charbonnel B, Chatal JF, Ozanne P: Does the corticoadrenal adenoma with "pre-Cushing's syndrome" exist? J Nucl Med 22:1059, 1981
306. Gabrilove JL, Seman AT, Sabet R et al: Virilizing adrenal adenoma with studies on the steroid content of the adrenal venous effluent and a review of the literature. Endocr Rev 2:462, 1981
307. Tang CK, Gray GF: Adrenocortical neoplasms: prognosis and morphology. Urology 5:691, 1975
308. Sullivan M, Boileau M, Hodges CV: Adrenal cortical carcinoma. J Urol 120:660, 1978
309. Bradley E III: Primary and adjunctive therapy in carcinoma of the adrenal cortex. Surg Gynecol Obstet 141:507, 1975
310. Dunnick NR, Schaner EG, Doppman JL et al: Computed tomography in adrenal tumors. AJR 132:43, 1979
311. Dunnick NR, Doppman JL, Gill JR et al: Localization of functional adrenal tumors by computed tomography and venous sampling. Radiology 142:429, 1982
312. Hussain S, Belldegrun A, Seltzer SE et al: Differentiation of malignant from benign adrenal masses: Predictive indices on computed tomography. AJR 144:61, 1985
313. Reinig JW, Doppman JL, Dwyer AJ et al: Distinction between adrenal adenomas and metastases using MR imaging. J Comput Assist Tomogr 9:898, 1985
314. Fink IJ, Reinig JW, Dwyer AJ et al: MR imaging of pheochromocytomas. J Comput Assist Tomogr 9:454, 1985
315. Reinig JW, Doppman JR, Dwyer AJ et al: MRI of indeterminate adrenal masses. AJR 147:493, 1986
316. Reinig JW, Doppman JL: Magnetic resonance imaging of the adrenal. Radiologe 26:186, 1986
317. Katz RL, Shirkhoda A: Diagnostic approach to incidental adrenal nodules in the cancer patient. Cancer 55:1995, 1985
318. Belldegrun A, Hussain S, Seltzer SE et al: Incidentally discovered mass of the adrenal gland. Surg Gynecol Obstet 163:203, 1986
319. Gabrilove JL, Seman AT, Sabet R et al: Virilizing adrenal adenoma with studies on the steroid content of the adrenal venous effluent and review of the literature. Endocr Rev 2:462, 1981
320. Gabrilove JL, Frieberg EK, Nicolis GL: Peripheral blood steroid levels in Cushing's syndrome due to adrenocortical carcinoma or adenoma. Urology 22:576, 1983
321. Baker ME, Spritzer C, Blinder R et al: Benign adrenal lesions mimicking malignancy on MR imaging: report of two cases. Radiology 163:669, 1987
322. Scott HW, Abumrad NN, Orth DN: Tumors of the adrenal cortex and Cushing's syndrome. Ann Surg 201:586, 1985
323. Jones GS, Shah KJ, Mann JR: Adreno-cortical carcinoma in infancy and childhood: a radiological report of ten cases. Clin Radiol 36:257, 1985
324. Daneman A, Chan HSL, Martin J: Adrenalcarcinoma and adenoma in children: a review of 17 patients. Pediatr Radiol 13:11, 1983
325. Neblett W, Frexes-Steed M, Scott HW: Experience with adrenocortical neoplasms in childhood. Am Surg 53:117, 1987
326. Macfarlane DA: Cancer of the adrenal cortex: the natural history, prognosis and treatment in a study of fifty-five cases. Ann R Coll Surg Engl 23:155, 1958
327. Sullivan M, Boileau M, Hodges CV: Adrenal cortical carcinoma. J Urol 120:660, 1978
328. Henley DJ, van Heerden JA, Grant CS et al: Adrenal cortical carcinoma—a continuing challenge. Surgery 94:926, 1983
329. Hajjar RA, Hickey RC, Samaan NA: Adrenal cortical carcinoma: a study of 32 patients. Cancer 35:549, 1975
330. Appleqvist P, Kostianinen S: Multiple thoracotomy combined with chemotherapy in metastatic adrenal cortical carcinoma: a case report and review of the literature. J Surg Oncol 24:1, 1983
331. Potter DA, Strott CA, Javadpour N et al: Prolonged survival following six pulmonary resections for metastatic adrenal cortical carcinoma: a case report. J Surg Oncol 25:273, 1984

332. Percarpio B, Knowlton AH: Radiation therapy of adrenal cortical carcinoma. Acta Rad Ther Phys Biol 15:288, 1976
333. Gutierrez ML, Crooke ST: Mitotane (o,p-DDD). Cancer Treat Rev 7:49, 1980
334. Fukushima DK, Bradlow HL, Hellman L: Effects of o,p-DDD on cortisol and 6-B-hydroxycortisol secretion and metabolism in man. J Clin Endocrinol Metab 32:192, 1971
335. Hellman L, Bradlow HL, Zumoff B: Decreased conversion of androgens to normal 17-ketosteroid metabolites as a result of treatment with o,p-DDD. J Clin Endocrinol Metab 36:801, 1973
336. Van Slooten H, Moolenaar AJ, Van Seters AP et al: The treatment of adrenocortical carcinoma with o,p-DDD: prognostic simplications of serum levels monitoring. Eur J Clin Oncol 20:47, 1984
337. Jarabak J, Rice K: Metastatic adrenal cortical carcinoma, prolonged regression with mitotane therapy. JAMA 246:1706, 1981
338. Thompson NW: Adrenocortical carcinoma. In Thompson NW, Vinik AI (eds): Endocrine Surgery Update pp 119–128. New York, Grune & Stratton, 1983
339. van Slooten H, van Oosterom AT: CAP (cyclophosphamide, doxorubicin and cisplatin) regimen in adrenal cortical carcinoma. Cancer Treat Rep 67:377, 1983
340. Haq MM, Legha SS, Samaan NA et al: Cytotoxic chemotherapy in adrenal cortical carcinoma. Cancer Treat Rep 64:909, 1980
341. Johnson DH, Creco A: Treatment of metastatic adrenal cortical carcinoma with cisplatin and etoposide (VP-16). Cancer 58:2198, 1986
342. Hesketh PJ, McCaffrey RP, Finkel HE et al: Cisplatin-based treatment of adrenocortical carcinoma. Cancer Treat Rep 71:222, 1987
343. Stein CA, LaRocca R, Myers CE: A phase II trial of suramin in metastatic adrenocortical cancer (personnel communication)
344. Chun HG, Yagoda A, Kemeny N: Cisplatin for adrenal cortical carcinoma. Cancer Treat Rep 67:513, 1983
345. Sanfilippo JS, Wittliff JL: Steroid hormone receptors in adrenal cortical carcinoma. Am J Obstet Gynecol 150:326, 1984
346. Richie JP, Gittes RF: Carcinoma of the adrenal cortex. Cancer 45:1957, 1980
347. Didolkar MS, Bescher RA, Elias EG et al: Natural history of adrenal cortical carcinoma. Cancer 47:2153, 1981
348. Brown WH: A case of pluriglandular syndrome. Lancet 2:1022, 1928
349. Christy NP: Adrenocorticotrophic activity in plasma of patients with Cushing's syndrome associated with pulmonary neoplasms. Lancet 1:85, 1961
350. Liddle GW, Island D, Meador CK: Normal and abnormal regulation of corticotropin secretion in man. Recent Prog Horm Res 18:125, 1962
351. Imura H: Ectopic hormone syndrome. Clin Endocrinol Metab 9:235, 1980
352. Davies CJ, Hoplin GF, Welbourn RB: Surgical management of the ectopic ACTH syndrome. Ann Surg 196:246, 1982
353. Jex RK, van Heerden JA, Carpenter PC et al: Ectopic ACTH syndrome. Am J Surg 149:276, 1985
354. Liddle GW, Nicholson WE, Island DP et al: Clinical and laboratory studies of ectopic humoral syndromes. Rec Prog Horm Res 25:283, 1969
355. Misbin RI, Canary J, Williard D: Aminoglutethimide in the treatment of Cushing's syndrome. J Clin Pharmacol 16:645, 1976
356. Gaillard R, Poffet D, Riondel A et al: RU486 inhibits peripheral effects of glucorticoids in humans. J Clin Endocrinol Metab 61:1009, 1985
357. Doppman JL, Loughlin T, Miller DL et al: Identification of ACTH-producing intrathoracic tumors by measuring ACTH levels in aspirated specimens. Radiology, 163:501, 1987
358. Manger WM, Gifford RW Jr: Pheochromocytoma. New York, Springer-Verlag, 1977
359. Beard CM, Sheps SG, Kurland LT et al: Occurrence of pheochromocytoma in Rochester, Minnesota, 1950 through 1979. Mayo Clin Proc 58:802, 1983
360. Sutton MGS, Sheps SG, Lie JT: Prevalence of clinically unsuspected pheochromocytoma. Review of a 50-year autopsy series. Mayo Clin Proc 56:354, 1981
361. Cryer PE: Phaeochromocytoma. Clin Endocrinol Metab 14:203, 1985
362. Beierwaltes WH, Sisson JC, Shapiro B et al: Malignant potential of pheochromocytoma. Proc AACR 27:617, 1986
363. Melicow MM: One hundred cases of pheochromocytoma (107 tumors) at the Columbia Presbyterian Medical Center, 1926–1976. Cancer 40:1987, 1977
364. Irvin GL, Fishman LM, Sher JA: Familial pheochromocytoma. Surgery 94:938, 1983
365. Glowniak JV, Shapiro B, Sisson JC et al: Familial extra-adrenal pheochromocytoma a new syndrome. Arch Intern Med 145:257, 1985
366. Loughlin KR, Gittes RF: Urological management of patients with von Hippel-Lindau's disease. J Urol 136:789, 1986
367. Nakagawara A, Ikeda K, Tsuneyoshi M et al: Malignant pheochromocytoma with ganglioneuroblastomatous elements in a patient with von Recklinghausen's disease. Cancer 55:2794, 1985
368. Spark RF, Connolly PB, Gluckin DS et al: ACTH secretion from a functioning pheochromocytoma. N Engl J Med 301:416, 1979
369. Berelowitz M, Szabo M, Barowsky HW et al: Somatostatin-like immunoactivity and biological activity is present in huma pheochromocytoma. J Clin Endocrinol Metab 56:134, 1983
370. Weinstein RS, Ide LF: Immunoreactive calcitonin in pheochromocytomas. Proc Soc Exp Biol Med 165:215, 1980
371. Ang VTY, Jenkins JS: Neurohypophysical hormones in the adrenal medulla. J Clin Endocrinol Metab 58:688, 1984
372. Orringer MB, Sisson JC, Glazer G et al: Surgical treatment of cardiac pheochromocytomas. J Thorac Cardiovasc Surg 89:753, 1985
373. Lips KJM, Veer JVDS, Struyvenberg A et al: Bilateral occurrence of pheochromocytoma in patients with multiple endocrine neoplasia syndrome type 2a (Sipple's syndrome). Am J Med 70:1051, 1981
374. Remine WH, Chang GC, van Heerden JA et al: Current management of pheochromocytoma. Ann Surg 179:740, 1974
375. Shin WY, Groman CS, Berkman JI: Pheochromocytoma with angiomatous features. Cancer 40:275, 1977
376. Scott HW, Halter SA: Oncologic aspects of pheochromocytoma: the importance of follow-up. Surgery 96:1061, 1984
377. Sherwin RP: Present status of the pathology of the adrenal gland in hypertension. Am J Surg 107:136, 1964
378. Lewis PD: A cytophotometric study of benign and malignant pheochromocytomas. Virchows Arch 9:371, 1971
379. Hosaka Y, Rainwater LM, Grant CS et al: Pheochromocytoma: nuclear deoxyribonucleic acid patterns studied by flow cytometry. Surgery 100:1003, 1986
380. Medeiros LJ, Wolf BC, Balogh K et al: Adrenal pheochromocytoma. a clinicopathologic review of 60 cases. Hum Pathol 16:580, 1985
381. Hengstmann JH: Evaluation of screening tests for pheochromocytoma. Cardiology 72:153, 1985
382. Kremer R, Crawhall JC, Kolanitch R: Rapid and reliable estimation of urinary free catecholamines in patients with pheochromocytomas. J Chromatogr 344:313, 1985
383. Tasseron SJA, Fiolet JWT, Willebrands AF: Evaluation of a radioenzymatic method for determination of plasma catecholamines. Clin Chem 26:120, 1980
384. Plouin PF, Dudos JM, Menard J et al: Biochemical tests for diagnosis of phaeochromocytoma: urinary versus plasma determinations. Br Med J 282:853, 1981
385. Bravo EL, Tarazi RC, Gifford RW et al: Circulating and urinary catecholamines in pheochromocytoma: diagnostic and pathophysiologic implications. N Engl J Med 301:682, 1979
386. Karlberg BE, Hedman L: Value of the clonidine suppression test in the diagnosis of pheochromocytoma. Acta Med Scand 714:15, 1986
387. Gifford RW, Bravo EL, Manger WM: Diagnosis and management of pheochromocytoma. Cardiology 72:126, 1985
388. Brandstetter K, Krause U, Beyer: Preliminary results with the clonidine suppression test in the diagnosis of pheochromocytoma. Cardiology 72:157, 1985
389. Karlberg BE, Hedman L, Lennquist S et al: The value of the clonidine-suppression test in the diagnosis of pheochromocytoma. World J Surg 10:753, 1986
390. Taylor HC, Mayes D, Anton AH: Clonidine suppression test for pheochromocytoma: examples of misleading results. J Clin Endocrinol Metab 63:238, 1986
391. Bravo EL, Tarazi RC, Fouad FM, et al: Clonidine suppression test: a useful aid in the diagnosis of pheochromocytoma. N Engl J Med 305:623, 1981
392. Welch TJ, Sheedy PF, van Heerden JA et al: Pheochromocytoma: value of computed tomography. Radiology 148:501, 1983
393. Radin DR, Ralls PW, Boswell WD et al: Pheochromocytoma: detection by unenhanced CT. AJR 146:741, 1986
394. Greenberg M, Moawad AH, Wieties BM et al: Extraadrenal pheochromocytoma: detection during pregnancy using MR imaging. Radiology 161:475, 1986
395. Fisher MR, Higgins CB, Andereck W: MR imaging of an intrapericardial pheochromocytoma. J Comput Assist Tomogr 9:1103, 1985
396. Shapiro B, Copp JE, Sisson JC et al: Iodine-131 metaiodobenzylguanidine for the locating of suspected pheochromocytoma: experience in 400 cases. J Nucl Med 26:576, 1985
397. Lynn MD, Shapiro B, Sisson JC, et al: Pheochromocytoma and the normal adrenal medulla: improved visualization with I-123 MIBG scintigraphy. Radiology 156:789, 1985
398. Shulkin BL, Shapiro B, Francis IR et al: Primary extra-adrenal pheochromocytoma positive I-123 MIBG imaging with negative I-131 MIBG imaging. Clin Nucl Med 11:851, 1986
399. Shulkin BL, Shen SW, Sisson JC et al: Iodine 131 MIBG scintigraphy of the extremities in metastatic pheochromocytoma and neuroblastoma. J Nucl Med 28:315, 1987
400. Lynn MD, Braunstein EM, Wohl RL et al: Bone metastases in pheochromocytoma: comparative studies of efficacy of imaging. Radiology 160:701, 1986
401. Swenson SJ, Brown MJ, Sheps SG et al: Use of ^{131}I-MIBG scintigraphy in the evaluation of suspected pheochromocytoma. Mayo Clin Proc 60:299, 1985
402. Koizumi M, Endo K, Sakahara H et al: Computed tomography and ^{131}I-MIBG scintigraphy in the diagnosis of pheochromocytoma. Acta Radiol Diagn 27:305, 1986
403. Fischer M, Galanski M, Winterberg B et al: Localization procedures in pheochromocytoma and neuroblastoma. Cardiology 72:143, 1985
404. Gouch IR, Thompson NW, Shapiro B et al: Limitations of ^{131}I-MIBG scintigraphy in locating pheochromocytomas. Surgery 98:115, 1985
405. Stenstrom G, Kutti J: The blood volume in pheochromocytoma patients before and during treatment with phenoxybenzamine. Acta Med Scand 218:381, 1985
406. Stenstrom G, Haljamae H, Tisell LE: Influence of pre-operative treatment with phenoxybenzamine on the incidence of adverse cardiovascular reactions during anaesthesia and surgery for phaeochromocytoma. Acta Anaesthesiol Scand 29:797, 1985
407. Bornemann M, Hill SC, Kidd GS: Lactic acidosis in pheochromocytoma. Ann Intern Med 105:880, 1986
408. Venkata C, Meese R, Hill SC: Failure of alpha methyltyrosine to prevent hypertensive crisis in pheochromocytoma. Arch Intern Med 145:2114, 1985
409. Imperato-McGinley J, Gautier T, Ehlers K et al: Reversibility of catecholamine-induced dilated cardiomyopathy in a child with a pheochromocytoma. N Engl J Med 316:793, 1987
410. Chimori K, Miyazaki S, Nakajima T et al: Preoperative management of pheochromocytoma with the calcium-antagonist nifedipine. Clin Ther 7:372, 1985

411. Zimmerman ID, Biron RE, MacMahon HE: Pheochromocytoma of the urinary bladder. N Engl J Med 249:25, 1953
412. Carney JA, Sizemore GW, Sheps SG: Adrenal medullary disease in multiple endocrine neoplasia, type 2: Pheochromocytoma and its precursors. Am J Clin Pathol 66:279, 1976
413. Brennan MF, Keiser HR: Persistent and recurrent pheochromocytoma: the role of surgery. World J Surg 6:397, 1982
414. Van Heerden JA, Sheps SG, Hamberger B et al: Pheochromocytoma: current status and changing trends. Surgery 91:367, 1982
415. James RE, Baker HL, Scanlon PW. The roentgenological aspects of metastatic pheochromocytoma. Am J Radiol 115:783, 1972
416. Lewi HJE, Reid R, Mucci B et al: Malignant phaeochromocytoma. Br J Urol 57:394, 1985
417. Scott WH, Reynolds V, Green N et al: Clinical experience with malignant pheochromocytoma. Surg Gynecol Obstet 154:801, 1982
418. Broder LE, Carter SK: Pancreatic islet cell carcinoma: II. Results of therapy with streptozotocin in 52 patients. Ann Intern Med 79:108, 1973
419. Feldman JM: Treatment of metastatic pheochromocytoma with streptozotocin. Arch Intern Med 143:1799, 1983
420. Feldman JM: In reply to a Letter to the Editor by Gross DJ, Schlank E, and Ipp E. Arch Intern Med 145:368, 1985
421. Gross DJ, Schlank E, Ipp E: Letter to the Editor regarding streptozotocin therapy for malignant pheochromocytoma. Arch Intern Med 145:368, 1985
422. McEwan A, Shapiro B, Sisson JC et al: Radio-iodobenzylguanidine for the scintigraphic location and therapy of adrenergic tumors. Semin Nucl Med 15:132, 1985
423. Feldman JM, Frankel N, Coleman RE: Platelet uptake of the pheochromocytoma-scanning agent ^{131}I-meta-iodobenzylguanidine. Metabolism 33:397, 1984
424. Vetter H, Fischer M, Muller-Rensing R et al: [^{131}I]-meta-iodobenzylguanidine in treatment of malignant pheochromocytomas. Lancet 2 (8341):107, 1983
425. Keiser HR, Goldstein DS, Wade JL et al: Treatment of malignant pheochromocytoma with combination chemotherapy. Hypertension 7:1–18, 1985
426. Manger TJ, Tobes MC, Wieland DW et al: Metabolism of Iodine-131 meta-iodobenzylguanidine in patients with metastatic pheochromocytoma. J Nucl Med 27:37, 1986
427. Goldstein DS, Stull R, Eisenhofer G et al: Plasma 3,4-dihydroxyphenylalanine (Dopa) and catecholamines in neuroblastoma or pheochromocytoma. Ann Intern Med 105:887, 1986
428. Averbuch S, Steakley C, Gelmann E et al: Malignant pheochromocytoma: treatment with a combination of cyclophosphamide, vincristine and darcarbazine. Proc ASCO 6:241, 1987
429. Finklestein JZ, Klemperer MR, Evans A et al: Multiagent chemotherapy for children with metastatic neuroblastoma: a report for children's cancer study group. Med Pediatr Oncol 6:179, 1979
430. Taub MA, Osburne RC, Georges LP et al: Malignant pheochromocytoma: severe clinical exacerbation and release of stored catecholamines during lymphoma chemotherapy. Cancer 50:1739, 1982
431. Oberndorfer S: Karzinoide: Tumoren des Dunndarms. Frankf Z Pathol 1:426, 1907
432. Masson P: Carcinoid (argentaffin-cell tumors) and nerve hyperplasia of appendicular mucosa. Am J Pathol 4:181, 1928
433. Kultschitzky N: Zur Frage über den Bau des Darmkanals. Arch Mikrosk Anat 49:7, 1897
434. Maton PN, Hodgson HJF: Carcinoid tumors and the carcinoid syndrome. In Bouchier IAD, Allan RN, Hodgson HJF et al (eds): Textbook of Gastroenterology, p 620. London, Bailliere-Tindall, 1984
435. Bolande RP: The neurocrestopathies: A unifying concept of disease arising from neural crest maldevelopment. Hum Pathol 5:409, 1974
436. Pearse HGE: The APUD concept and hormone production. Clin Endocrinol Metab 9:211, 1980
437. Moertel CG: An odyssey in the land of small tumors. J Clin Oncol 5:1503, 1987
438. Black WC III: Enterochromaffin cell types and corresponding carcinoid tumors. Lab Invest 19:473, 1968
439. Carney JA, Go VLW, Fairbanks VF et al:The syndrome of gastric argyrophil carcinoid tumors and nonantral gastric atrophy. Ann Intern Med 99:761, 1983
440. Feldman JM, O'Dorisio TM: The role of neuropeptides and serotonin in the diagnosis of carcinoid tumors. Am J Med 81:41, 1986
441. Falkmer S, Martensson H, Nobin A et al: Peptide hormones in various types of gastro-entero-pancreatic tumors; immunohistochemical patterns and evolutionary background. In Bresciani F, King RJB, Lippman ME et al (eds): Progress in Cancer Research and Therapy, vol 31, p 597. New York, Raven Press, 1984
442. Pearse AGE, Tabor TT: Embryology of the diffuse neuroendocrine system and its relationship to the common peptides. Fed Proc 38:2288, 1979
443. Williams ED, Sanders M: The classification of carcinoid tumors. Lancet 1:238, 1963
444. Dayal Y: Endocrine cells in the gut and their neoplasms. In Norris HT (ed): Contemporary Issues in Surgical Pathology, vol IV, p 267. New York, Churchill Livingstone, 1983
445. Dayal Y, Wolfe HJ: Regulatory substances in clinically nonfunctioning gastrointestinal carcinoids. In Falkmers S, Hakanson R, Sundler F (eds): Evolution and Tumor Pathology of the Neuroendocrine System, p 497. Amsterdam, Elsevier Science Publishers, 1984
446. Wilander E, Ed-Salhy M, Lundquist M: Argyrophilic reaction in rectal carcinoids. Acta Pathol Microbiol Scand [A] 91:85, 1983
447. Iwafuchi M, Watanabe H, Yanaihara N et al: Immunohistochemical and ultrastructural characteristics of gastric carcinoids. Biomed Res 4:307, 1983
448. Buchanan KD, Johnston CF, O'Hare MMT et al: Neuroendocrine tumors. Am J Med 81(6B):14, 1986
449. Weiss NS, Yang CP: Incidence of histologic types of cancer of the small intestine. JNCI 78:653, 1987
450. Maton PN: The carcinoid tumor and the carcinoid syndrome. In Becker K (ed): Principles and Practice of Endocrinology and Metabolism. Philadelphia, JB Lippincott, 1987
451. Moertel CG, Dockerty MB, Judd ES: Carcinoid tumors of the vermiform appendix. Cancer 21:270, 1968
452. Thompson GB, van Heerden JA, Martin JK et al: Carcinoid tumors of the gastrointestinal tract: presentation, management and prognosis. Surgery 98:1054, 1985
453. Editorial. Bronchial adenomas. Br Med J 282:252, 1981
454. Hasleton PS, Gomm S, Blair V et al: Pulmonary carcinoid tumours: a clinico-pathological study of 35 cases. Br J Cancer 54:963, 1986
455. Soga J, Tazawa K: Pathologic analysis of carcinoids. Histologic reevaluation of 62 cases. Cancer 28:990, 1971
456. Moertel CG, Hanley JA: Combination chemotherapy trials in metastatic carcinoid and malignant carcinoid syndrome. Cancer Clin Trials 2:327, 1979
457. Johnson LA, Lavin PT, Moertel CG et al: Carcinoids: the prognosis effect of primary site histologic type variations. J Surg Oncol 33:81, 1986
458. Wilander E: Achylia and the development of gastric carcinoids. Virch Arch Anat Pathol 394:151, 1981
459. Borch K, Renvall H, Liedberg G: Gastric endocrine cell hyperplasia and carcinoid tumors in pernicious anemia. Gastroenterology 88:638, 1985
460. Hodges JR, Isaacson P, Wright R: Diffuse enterochromaffin-like (ECL) cell hyperplasia and multiple gastric carcinoids: a complication of pernicious anemia. Gut 22:237, 1981
461. Solcia E, Capella L, Baffa R et al: Endocrine cells of the gastrointestinal tract and related tumors. Pathobiol Ann 9:163, 1979
462. Ekman L, Hansson E, Havu N et al: Toxicological studies on omeprazole. Scand J Gastroenterol 20(108):53, 1985
463. Eberle F, Grun R: Multiple endocrine neoplasm Type I (MEN 1). Adv Intern Med Pediatr 46:75, 1981
464. Ballard F, Frame B, Hartsock RJ: Familial multiple endocrine adenoma-peptic ulcer complex. Medicine 43:481, 1964
465. Johnson L, Weaver M: Von Recklinghausen's disease and gastrointestinal carcinoids. JAMA 245:2496, 1981
466. Wheeler MH, Curley IR, Williams ED: The association of neurofibromatosis, pheochromocytoma, and somatostatin-rich duodenal carcinoid tumor. Surgery 100:1163, 1986
467. Davis Z, Moertel CG, McIlrath DC: The malignant carcinoid syndrome. Surg Gynecol Obstet 137:637, 1973
468. Norheim I, Oberg K, Theodorsson-Norheim E et al: Malignant carcinoid tumors. Ann Surg 206:115, 1987
469. Thorson AH: Studies on carcinoid disease. Acta Med Scand 334:81, 1958
470. Feldman JM: Carcinoid tumors and syndrome. Semin Oncol 14:237, 1987
471. Kahler HJ, Heilmeyer L: Klinikund pathophysiologie des Karzinoids und Karzinoid-syndroms unter besonderer beruck sichtigung der Pharmacologie des 5-hydroxyptamins. Ergeb Med Kinderheik 16:291, 1961
472. Leveston SA, McKeel DW Jr, Buckley PG et al: Acromegaly and Cushing's syndrome associated with a foregut carcinoid. J Clin Endocrinol Metab 53:682, 1981
473. Thorson A, Bjork G, Bjorkman G et al: Malignant carcinoid of the small intestine with metastases to the liver, valvular disease of the right heart (pulmonary stenosis and tricuspid regurgitation without septal defect), peripheral vasomotor symptoms, bronchoconstriction and an unusual type of cyanosis. Am Heart J 47:795, 1954
474. Pernow B, Waldenstrom J: Paroxysmal flushing and other symptoms caused by 5-hydroxytryptamine and histamine in patients with malignant tumors. Lancet 2:951, 1954
475. David G, Grahame-Smith OG: The Carcinoid Syndrome. London, William Heinemann Medical Books, 1972
476. Frolich JC, Bloomgarden ZT, Oates JA et al: The carcinoid flush. Provocation by pentagastrin and inhibition by somatostatin. N Engl J Med 19:1055, 1978
477. Roberts LJ, Marney SR, Oates JA: Blockade of the flush associated with metastatic gastric carcinoid by combined H_1 and H_2 receptor antagonists: Evidence for an important role of H_2 receptors in human vasculature. N Engl J Med 300:236, 1979
478. Peart WS, Robertson JS, Andrews TM: Facial flushing produced in patients with carcinoid syndrome by intravenous adrenaline and noradrenaline. Lancet 2:175, 1959
479. Levine RJ, Sjoredson A: Pressor aminos and the carcinoid flush. Ann Intern Med 58:818, 1963
480. Adamson AR, Grahame-Smith DG, Peart WS et al: Pharmacological blockade of carcinoid flushing provoked by catecholamines and alcohol. Lancet 2:293, 1967
481. Oates JS, Sjoerdsma A: A unique syndrome associated with secretion of 5-hydroxytryptophan by metastatic gastric carcinoids. Am J Med 32:333, 1962
482. Knowlessar OD, Law DH, Steisenger MH: Malabsorption syndrome associated with carcinoid tumors. Am J Med 27:673, 1959
483. Roberts WC, Sjoerdsma A: The cardiac disease associated with carcinoid syndrome (carcinoid heart disease) Am J Med 36:5, 1964
484. Schiller VL, Fishbein MC, Siegel RJ: Unusual cardiac involvement in carcinoid syndrome. Am Heart J 112:1322, 1986
485. Wong VW, Melmon KL: Ophthalmic manifestations of the carcinoid flush. N Engl J Med 277:406, 1967
486. Waldenstrom J: Clinical picture of carcinoidosis. Gastroenterology 35:565, 1958

487. Feldman JM, Jones RS: Carcinoid syndrome from gastrointestinal carcinoids without liver metastases. Ann Surg 196:33, 1982
488. Ricci C, Patrassi N, Massa R et al: Carcinoid syndrome in bronchial adenoma. Am J Surg 126:671, 1973
489. Moertel CG, Beahrs O, Woolmer LB et al: Malignant carcinoid syndrome associated with noncarcinoid tumors. N Engl J Med 273:244, 1965
490. McCaughan BC, Martini H, Bains MS: Bronchial carcinoids—review of 124 cases. J Thor Cardiovasc Surg 89:8, 1985
491. Moertel CG, Suer WG, Doherty MG et al: Life history of the carcinoid tumor of the small intestine. Cancer 14:901, 1961
492. Cheek RC, Wilson H: Carcinoid tumors. Curr Probl Surg 11:4, 1970
493. Sjoerdsma A: Serotonin. N Engl J Med 261:181, 231, 1959
494. Campbell ACP, Gowenlock AH, Platt DS et al: A 5-hydroxytryptophan-secreting carcinoid tumor. Gut 4:61, 1963
495. Feldman JM: Serotonin metabolism in carcinoid tumors: Incidence of 5-hydroxytryptophan-secreting tumors. Gastroenterology 75:1109, 1978
496. Warner RRP: Carcinoid tumor. In Berk JE, Haubrich WS, Kalser MH, Roth JLA, Schnaffner F (eds) Gastroenterology, Vol 3, 4th ed, p. 1874. Philadelphia, Saunders, 1985
497. Grahame-Smith DG: Natural history and diagnosis of the carcinoid syndrome. Clin Gastroenterol 3:575, 1974
498. Ahlman H, Dahlstrom A, Gronstad K et al: The pentagastrin test in the diagnosis of the carcinoid syndrome. Ann Surg 201:81, 1985
499. Creutzfeldt W, Stockman F: The carcinoid syndrome. Am J Med 82(suppl 5B):4–16, 1987
500. Oates JA, Melman K, Sjoerdsma M et al: Release of a kinin peptide in the carcinoid syndrome. Lancet 2:514, 1964
501. Oates JA, Pettinger WA, Doctor RB: Evidence for the release of bradykinin in the carcinoid syndrome. J Clin Invest 45:173, 1966
502. Melman K, Lovenberg W, Sjoerdsma A: Identification of lysylbradykinin as the peptide formed in vitro by carcinoid tumor kallikrein. Clin Chim Acta 12:292, 1965
503. Lucas KJ, Feldman JM: Flushing in the carcinoid syndrome and plasma kallikrein. Cancer 58:2290, 1986
504. Robert LJ, Marney SR, Oates JA: Blockade of the flush associated with metastatic gastric carcinoid by combined histamine H_1 and H_2 receptor antagonists. N Engl J Med 300:236, 1979
505. Wilkin JK, Roundtree CB: Blockade of the carcinoid flush with cimetidine and clonidine. Arch Dermatol 118:109, 1982
506. Sandler M, Karim SM, Williams ED: Prostaglandins in amine-peptide-secreting tumors. Lancet 2:1053, 1968
507. Smith AG, Greaves MW: Blood prostaglandin activity associated with noradrenaline-provoked flush in the carcinoid syndrome. Br J Dermatol 90:547, 1974
508. Jaffe BM, Landon C: Prostaglandin E and F in endocrine diarrheagenic syndromes. Ann Surg 84:516, 1976
509. Metz SA, McRae JR, Robertson PR: Prostaglandins as mediators of paraneoplastic syndromes. Metabolism 30:299, 1981
510. Oates JA: The carcinoid syndrome. N Engl J Med 315:702, 1986
511. Hakanson R, Bengmark S, Brondin E et al: Substance P-like immunoreactivity in intestinal carcinoid tumors. In Van Euler US, Pernow B (eds): Substance P, p 55. New York, Raven Press, 1977
512. Theodorsson-Norheim E, Norheim I, Oberg K et al: Neuropeptide K: a major tachykinin in plasma and tumor tissues from carcinoid patients. Biochem Biophys Res Commun 131:77, 1985
513. Conlon JM, Deacon CF, Richter G et al: Measurement and partial characterization of the multiple forms of neurokinin A-like immunoreactivity in carcinoid tumors. Regul Pept 13:183, 1986
514. Emson PC, Gilbert RFT, Martensson H et al: Elevated concentrations of substance P and 5-HT in patients with carcinoid tumors. Cancer 54:715, 1984
515. Norheim I, Theodorsson-Norheim E, Brondin E et al: Tachykinins in carcinoid tumors: their use as a tumor marker and possible role in carcinoid flush. J Clin Endocrinol Metab 63:605, 1986
516. Schaffalitsky de Muckadell OB, Aggestrup S, Stentoft P: Flushing and plasma substance P concentration during infusion of synthetic substance P in normal man. Scand J Gastroenterol 21:498, 1986
517. Feldman JM, Plank JW: Gastrointestinal and metabolic function in patients with the carcinoid syndrome. Am J Med Sci 273:43, 1977
518. Hendrix TR, Atkinson M, Clifton JA, et al: The effect of 5-hydroxytryptamine on intestinal motor function in man. Am J Med 23:886, 1957
519. Donowitz M, Binder JH: Jejunal fluid and electrolyte secretion in carcinoid syndrome. Am J Dig Dis 20:1115, 1975
520. Herxheimer H: Influence of 5-hydroxytryptomine on bronchial function. J Physiol 122:49p, 1953
521. Feldman JM, Lee EM: Serotonin content of foods: effect on urinary excretion of 5-hydroxyindoleacetic acid. Am J Clin Nutr 42:639, 1985
522. Feldman JM, Butler SS, Chapman BA: Interference with measurement of 3-methoxy-4-hydroxymandelic acid and 5-hydroxyindoleacetic acid by reducing metabolites. Clin Chem 20:607, 1974
523. Sjoerdsma A, Weissbach H, Udenfriend H: Simple test for diagnosis of metastatic carcinoid (argentaffinoma). JAMA 159:397, 1955
524. Feldman JM: Urinary serotonin in the diagnosis of carcinoid tumors. Clin Chem 32:840, 1986
525. Hussain MN, Sole MJ: A simple, specific radioenzymatic assay for picogram quantities of serotonin or acetylserotonin in biological fluids of tissues. Anal Biochem 111:105, 1981
526. Feldman JM, Davis JA: Radioenzymatic assay of platelet serotonin, dopamine and norepinephrine in subjects with normal and increased serotonin production. Clin Chem Acta 109:275, 1981
527. Wilkin JK: Flushing reactions: consequences and mechanisms. Ann Intern Med 95:468, 1981
528. Jeffree MA, Barter SJ, Hemingway AP et al: Primary carcinoid tumors of the ileum: the radiological appearances. Clin Radiol 35:451, 1985
529. Banks NH, Goldstein MH, Dodd G: The roentgenologic spectrum of small intestinal carcinoid tumors. Am J Roentgenol 123:274, 1975
530. Picus D, Glazer HS, Levitt RG et al: Computed tomography of abdominal carcinoid tumors. Am J Roentgenol 143:581, 1984
531. Goldstein HM, Miller M: Angiographic evaluation of carcinoid tumors in the small intestine: the value of epinephrine. Radiology 115:23, 1975
532. Gould M, Johnson RJ: Computed tomography of abdominal carcinoid tumour. Br J Radiol 59:881, 1986
533. McCarthy SM, Stark DD, Moss AA et al: Computed tomography of malignant carcinoid disease. J Comput Assist Tomogr 8:846, 1984
534. Lackey BM, Fishman EK, Jones B et al: Computed tomography of abdominal carcinoid tumor. J Comput Assist Tomogr 9:38, 1985
535. Sako M, Lunderquist A, Owman T et al: Angiographic and computed tomographic appearance of secondary carcinoid tumor of the liver. Cardiovasc Intervent Radiol 5:90, 1982
536. Feldman JM, Blinder RA, Lucas KJ et al: Iodine-131 metaiodobenzylguanidine scintigraphy of carcinoid tumors. J Nucl Med 27:1691, 1986
537. Godwin JD: Carcinoid tumors: An analysis of 2837 cases. Cancer 36:560, 1975
538. Brookes VS, Waterhouse JAH, Pawel DJ: Malignant carcinoids of the small intestine — a ten-year survey. Br J Surg 55:405, 1968
539. Orloff, MJ: Carcinoid tumors of the rectum. Cancer 28:175, 1971
540. Van Sickle DG: Carcinoid tumors—Analysis of 61 cases. 11 cases of carcinoid syndrome. Cleve Clin Q 39:79, 1972
541. Caldarola VT, Jackman RJ, Moertel CG et al: Carcinoid tumors of the rectum. Am J Surg 107:844, 1964
542. Peskin GW, Kaplan EL: The surgery of carcinoid tumors. Surg Clin North Am 49:137, 1969
543. Sjoerdsma H, Loyenberg W, Engelman K et al: Serotonin now: clinical implications of inhibiting its synthesis with parachlorophenylalanine. Ann Intern Med 73:607, 1970
544. Moertel CG: Treatment of the carcinoid tumor and the malignant carcinoid syndrome. J Clin Oncol 1:727, 1983
545. Stathopoulous GB, Karvountzis GG, Yiotis J: Tamoxifen in carcinoid syndrome. N Engl J Med 305:52, 1981
546. Myers CF, Ershler WB, Tannenbaum MA et al: Tamoxifen and carcinoid tumor. Ann Intern Med 96:383, 1982
547. Moertel CG, Engstrom PF, Schutt AJ: Tamoxifen therapy for metastatic carcinoid tumor: A negative study. Ann Intern Med 100:531, 1984
548. Thulin L, Samnegard H, Tyden G et al: Efficacy of somatostatin in a patient with carcinoid tumor. Lancet 2:43, 1978
549. Long RG, Peters JR, Bloom SR et al: Somatostatin, gastrointestinal peptides and the carcinoid syndrome. Gut 22:549, 1981
550. Dharmsathaphorn K, Sherwin RS, Calaland S et al: Somatostatin inhibits diarrhea in the carcinoid syndrome. Ann Intern Med 92:68, 1980
551. Davis GR, Camp RG, Raskin P et al: Effect of somatostatin infusion on jejunal water and electrolyte transport in a patient with secretory diarrhea due to malignant carcinoid syndrome. Gastroenterology 78:346, 1980
552. Bauer W, Briner U, Doefner W et al: SMS-201-995, a very potent and selective octapeptide of somatostatin with prolonged actions. Life Sci 31:1183, 1982
553. Pless J, Bauer W, Briner U et al: Chemistry and pharmacology of SMS-201-995, a long-acting octopeptide of somatostatin. Scand J Gastroenterol 21(Suppl 119):54, 1986
554. Kutz K, Nuesch J, Rosenthaler J: Pharmacokinetics of SMS-201-995 in healthy subjects. Scand J Gastroenterol 21(Suppl 119):65, 1986
555. Maton P, O'Dorisio TM, Howe BA et al: Effect of a long-acting somatostatin analogue (SMS-201-995) in a patient with pancreatic cholera. N Engl J Med 312:17, 1985
556. Vinnik AI, Tsai ST, Moattari AR et al: Somatostatin analogue (SMS-201-995) in the management of gastroenteropancreatic tumors and diarrhea syndromes. Am J Med 81:23, 1986
557. Kvols LK: Metastatic carcinoid tumors and the carcinoid syndrome. Am J Med 81:49, 1986
558. Maton PN, Gardner JD, Jensen RT: The use of the long-acting analogue SMS-201-995 in patients with pancreatic islet cell tumors. Dig Dis Sci (in press)
559. Kvols LK, Moertel CG, O'Connell MJ et al: Treatment of the malignant carcinoid syndrome: evaluation of a long-acting somatostatin analogue. N Engl J Med 315:663, 1986
560. Kvols LK, Buck M, Moertel LG et al: Treatment of metastatic islet cell carcinoma with a somatostatin analogue (SMS-201-995). Ann Intern Med 107:162, 1987
561. Marsh HM, Martin JK, Kvols LK et al: Carcinoid crisis during anesthesia: successful treatment with the somatostatin analogue. Anesthesiology 66:89, 1987
562. Martin JK, Moertel CG, Adson MA et al: Surgical treatment of functioning metastatic carcinoid tumors. Arch Surg 118:537, 1983
563. Stockman F, von Tomatowski HJ, Reimold WV et al: Hepatic artery embolization for

treatment of endocrine gastrointestinal tumors with liver metastases. Z Gastroenterol 22:652, 1984
564. Martensson H, Norbin A, Bengmarks S et al: Embolization of the liver in the management of metastatic carcinoid tumors. J Surg Oncol 27:152, 1984
565. Mitty HA, Warner RRP, Newman LH et al: Control of carcinoid syndrome with heaptic artery embolization. Radiology 155:623, 1985
566. Maton PN, Camilleri M, Friggin G et al: The role of hepatic arterial embolization in the carcinoid syndrome. Br Med J 287:932, 1983
567. Moertel CG, May GR, Martin JK et al: Sequential hepatic artery occlusion and chemotherapy for metastatic carcinoid tumor and islet cell carcinoma. Proc Am Soc Clin Oncol 4:80, 1985
568. Oberg IL, Funa K, Alma GV: Effects of leukocyte interferon on clinical symptoms and hormone levels in patients with mid gut carcinoid tumors and carcinoid syndrome. N Engl J Med 309:129, 1983
569. Naunheim KS, Zeitals J, Kaplan EL et al: Rectal carcinoid tumors—Treatment and prognosis. Surgery 94:670, 1983
570. Aranha GV, Greenlee HB: Surgical management of carcinoid tumors of the gastrointestinal tract. Ann Surg 46:429, 1980
571. Gaitan-Gaitan A, Riden WD, Rush RS: Carcinoid tumor—cured by radiation. Int J Radiat Oncol Biol Phys 1:9, 1975
572. Keane TS, Rider WP, Harwood HR et al: Whole-body radiation in the management of the metastatic carcinoid tumor. Int J Radiat Oncol Biol Phys 7:1519, 1981
573. Kvols LK, Buck M: Chemotherapy of the metastatic carcinoid and islet cell tumors: a review. Am J Med 82:77, 1987
574. Van Hazel GA, Rubin J, Moertel CG: Treatment of metastatic carcinoid tumor with dactinomycin or dacarbazine. Cancer Treat Rep 67:583, 1983
575. Moertel CG, Rubin J, O'Connell MJ: Phase II study of cisplatin therapy in patients with metastatic carcinoid tumor and the malignant carcinoid syndrome. Cancer Treat Rep 70:1459, 1986
576. Kelsen D, Fiore J, Heelar R et al: Phase II trial of etoposide in APUD tumors. Cancer Treat Rep 71:305, 1987
577. Oberg K, Norheim I, Lind E et al: Treatment of malignant carcinoid tumors with human leukocyte interferon: long-term results. Cancer Treat Rep 70:1297, 1986
578. Engstrom PF, Lavin PT, Folsch E et al: Streptozotocin plus fluorouracil versus doxorubicin therapy for metastatic carcinoid tumors. J Clin Oncol 2:1255, 1984
579. Bukowski RM, Stephens R, Oishi N et al: Phase II trials of 5-FU, adriamycin, cyclophosphomide and streptozotocin in metastatic carcinoid. Proc Ann Soc Clin Oncol 2:130, 1983
580. Kelsen DG, Cheng E, Kemeny N et al: Streptozotocin and adriamycin in the treatment of APUD tumors (carcinoid, islet cell and medullary thyroid) Proc Am Assoc Can Res 23:433, 1982
581. Kvols LK, Buck M: Chemotherapy of endocrine malignancies. Semin Oncol 14:343, 1987
582. Reubi JC, Maurer R, von Werder K et al: Somatostatin receptors in human endocrine tumors. Cancer Res 47:551, 1987
583. Oberg K, Norheim I, Alm G et al: Long-term treatment of malignant carcinoid tumors with human leukocyte interferon. In Stewart WE (ed): Biology of the Interferon System, p 433. New York, Elsevier, 1985
584. Oberg K, Ericksson B, Norheim I: Interferon treatment of neuroendocrine gut tumors. J Clin Oncol 6:80, 1987
585. Zollinger RM, Ellison EH: Primary peptic ulcerations of the jejunum associated with islet cell tumors of the pancreas. Ann Surg 142:709, 1955
586. Gregory RA, Tracy HJ, French JM et al: Extraction of a gastrin-like substance from a pancreatic tumor in a case of Zollinger-Ellison syndrome. Lancet 1:1045, 1960
587. Gregory RA, Grossman MI, Tracy HJ et al: Nature of the gastric secretagogue in Zollinger-Ellison tumors. Lancet 2:543, 1967
588. Gregory RA, Tracy JH, Agarwal KL: Amino acid constitution of two gastrins isolated from Zollinger-Ellison tumor tissue. Gut 10:603, 1969
589. McGuigan JE, Trudeau WL: Immunochemical measurement of elevated levels of gastrin in the serum of patients with pancreatic tumors of the Zollinger-Ellison variety. N Engl J Med 278:1308, 1968
590. Stremple JF, Meade RC: Production of antibodies to synthetic human gastrin I and radioimmunoassay of gastrin in the serum of patients with the Zollinger-Ellison syndrome. Surgery 64:165, 1968
591. Stadil F, Stage JG: The Zollinger-Ellison syndrome. Clin Endocrinol Metab 9:433, 1979
592. Grossman MI (ed): Peptic Ulcer, pp 141–151. Chicago, Yearbook Medical Publishers, 1981
593. Buchanan KD, Johnston CF, O'Hare MMT et al: Neuroendocrine tumors: A European view. Am J Med 81(Suppl 6B):14, 1986
594. Jensen RT, Gardner JD, Raufman JP et al: Zollinger-Ellison syndrome. NIH combined clinical staff conference. RT Jensen, moderator). Ann Intern Med 98:59, 1983
595. Zollinger RM, Ellison EC, Fabri PJ et al: Primary peptic ulcerations of the jejunum associated with islet cell tumors: Twenty-five-year appraisal. Ann Surg 192:422, 1980
596. Thompson JC, Reeder DD, Villar HV et al: Natural history and experience with diagnosis and treatment of the Zollinger-Ellison syndrome. Surg Gynecol Obstet 140:721, 1975
597. Jensen RT, Doppman JL, Gardner JD: Gastrinoma in the Exocrine Pancreas: Biology, Pathobiology and Diseases, p 727. New York, Raven Press, 1986
598. Ellison EH, Wilson SD: The Zollinger-Ellison syndrome: Re-appraisal and evaluation of 260 registered cases. Ann Surg 160:512, 1964
599. Regan PT, Malagelada JR: A reappraisal of clinical, roentgenographic, and endoscopic features of the Zollinger-Ellison syndrome. Mayo Clin Proc, 53:19, 1978
600. Stage JG, Stadil F: The clinical diagnosis of the Zollinger-Ellison syndrome. Scand J Gastroenterol 14(53):79, 1979
601. Bonfils S, Landor JH, Mignon M et al: Results of surgical management in 92 consecutive patients with Zollinger-Ellison syndrome. Ann Surg 194:692, 1981
602. Johnson LR: Gut hormones on growth of gastrointestinal mucosa. In Chey WY, Brooks FD (eds): Endocrinology of the Gut, p 163. Thorofare, NJ, Charles B Slack, 1974
603. Neurburger PH, Lewin M, Bonfils S: Parietal and chief cell populations in 4 cases of the Zollinger-Ellison syndrome. Gastroenterology 63:937, 1972
604. Sum P, Perey BJ: Parietal cell mass (PCM) in a man with Zollinger-Ellison syndrome. Can J Surg 12:285, 1969
605. Wright HK, Hersh T, Floch MH et al: Impaired intestinal absorption in the Zollinger-Ellison syndrome independent of gastric hypersecretion. Am J Surg 119:150, 1970
606. Creutzfeldt W, Arnold R, Creutzfelt A et al: Pathomorphological, biochemical and diagnostic aspects of gastrinomas (Zollinger-Ellison syndrome). Hum Pathol 6:47, 1975
607. Dockray GJ, Walsh JH, Passaro E Jr: Relative abundance of big and little gastrins in the tumors and blood of patients with Zollinger-Ellison syndrome. Gut 16:353, 1975
608. Yalow RS, Berson SA: Size and charge distinctions between endogenous human plasma gastrins in peripheral blood and heptadecapeptide gastrins. Gastroenterology 58:609, 1970
609. Dockray GJ, Walsh JH: Amino terminal gastrin fragment in serum of Zollinger-Ellison syndrome patients. Gastroenterology 68:222, 1975
610. Rehfeld JF, Stadil F: Gel filtration studies on immunoreactive gastrin in serum from Zollinger-Ellison patients. Gut 14:369, 1973
611. Walsh JH, Grossman MI: Gastrin. N Engl J Med 292:1324, 1975
612. Eysselein VE, Maxwell V, Peedy T et al: Similar and stimulatory palennies of synthetic human big and little gastrins in man. J Clin Invest 73:1284, 1984
613. Thompson JC, Lewis BG, Weiner I et al: The role of surgery in the Zollinger-Ellison syndrome. Ann Surg 197:594, 1983
614. Stabile BE, Morrow DJ, Passaro E Jr: The Gastrinoma triangle: Operative implications. Am J Surg 147:25, 1984
615. Norton JA, Doppman JL, Collen MJ et al: Prospective study of gastrinoma localization and resection in patients with Zollinger-Ellison syndrome. Am J Surg 204:468, 1986
616. Deveney CW, Deveney KS, Stark D et al: Resection of gastrinomas. Ann Surg 198:546, 1983
617. Deveney CW, Deveney KS, Way LW: The Zollinger-Ellison syndrome—23 years later. Ann Surg 188:384, 1978
618. Malagelada JR, Edis AJ, Adson MA et al: Medical and Surgical options in the management of patients with gastrinoma. Gastroenterology 84:1524, 1978
619. Stabile BE, Passaro E Jr: Benign and malignant gastrinoma. Am J Surg 149:144, 1985
620. Fox PS, Hofmann JW, Wilson SD et al: Surgical management of the Zollinger-Ellison syndrome. Surg Clin North Am 54:395, 1974
621. Hofmann JW, Fox PS, Wilson SD: Duodenal wall tumors and the Zollinger-Ellison syndrome. Arch Surg 107:334, 1973
622. Zollinger RM, Martin EW, Carey LC et al: Observations on the postoperative tumor growth behavior of certain islet cell tumors. Ann Surg 184:525, 1976
623. Wolfe MM, Alexander RW, McGuigan JE: Extrapancreatic, extraintestinal gastrinoma. N Engl J Med 306:1533, 1982
624. Friesen SR: Tumors of the endocrine pancreas. N Engl J Med 306:580, 1982
625. Larsson LI, Rehfeld JR, Goltermann N: Gastrin in the human fetus. Distribution and molecular forms of gastrin in the antro-pyloric gland area, duodenum, and pancreas. Scand J Gastroenterol 12:869, 1977
626. Solcia E, Capella C, Buffa R et al: Pathology of the Zollinger-Ellison syndrome. In Fengolio LM, Wolff M (eds): Progress in Surgical Pathology, vol 1, p 119, 1980
627. Creutzfeldt W: Endorine tumors of the pancreas: clinical and morphological patterns In Fitgerald PS, Morrison AB (eds): The Pancreas, p 208, Baltimore, Williams & Wilkins, 1980
628. Fox PS, Hofmann JW, Decosse JJ et al: The influence of total gastrectomy on survival in malignant Zollinger-Ellison tumors. Ann Surg 180:558, 1974
629. Friesen SR: The development of endocrinopathies in the prospective screening of two families with MEN-1. World J Surg 3:753, 1979
630. Larsson LI, Ljungberg O, Sundler F et al: Antropyloric gastrinoma associated with pancreatic nesidioblastosis and proliferation of islets. Virchows Arch 360:305, 1973
631. Harmon JW, Norton JA, Collen MJ et al: Removal of gastrinomas for control of Zollinger-Ellison syndrome. Ann Surg 200:396, 1984
632. Ballard HS, Frame B, Hartsock RJ: Familial multiple adenoma peptic ulcer complex. Medicine 43:481, 1964
633. Zollinger RM, Ellison EC, D'Dorisio TM et al: Thirty years' experience with gastrinoma. World J Surg 8:427, 1984
634. Mukai K, Greider MH, Grotting JC et al: Retrospective study of 77 pancreatic endocrine tumors using the immunoperoxidase method. Am J Surg Pathol 6:387, 1982
635. Larsson LI. Classification of pancreatic endocrine tumors. Scand J Gastroenterol 14(53):15, 1978
636. Larsson LI, Grimelius L, Hakanson R et al: Mixed endocrine pancreatic tumors producing several peptide hormones. Am J Pathol 79:271, 1975
637. Heitz PU, Kasper M, Polak JM et al: Pancreatic endocrine tumors. Hum Pathol 13:263, 1982
638. Larsson LI: PP-producing and mixed endocrine pancreatic tumors. In Bloom SR (ed): Gut Hormones, p 605. London, Churchill Livingston, 1978
639. Blackburn AM, Bryant MG, Adrian TE et al: Pancreatic tumors produce neurotensin. J Clin Endocrinol Metab 52:820, 1981

640. Bloom SR, Adrian TE, Bryant MG et al: Pancreatic polypeptide: A marker for Zollinger-Ellison syndrome. Lancet 1:1155, 1978
641. Lamers CBH, Diemel JM, Roeffen W. Serum levels of pancreatic polypeptide in Zollinger-Ellison syndrome and hyperparathyroidism from families with multiple endocrine adenamotosis Type I. Digestion 18:297, 1978
642. O'Dorisio TM, Howe BH, Howard JM et al: Plasma concentration of human pancreatic polypeptide (HPP), motilin, neurotensin, somatostatin, and prolactin in 30 consecutive cases of Zollinger-Ellison syndrome. Dig Dis Sci 29(1):S60, 1984
643. Taylor IL, Rotter J, Walsh JH et al: Is pancreatic polypeptide a marker for Zollinger-Ellison syndrome. Lancet 1:845, 1978
644. Yamaguchi K, Abe A, Miyakawa S et al: Multiple hormone production in endocrine tumors in the pancreas. In Miyoshi H (ed): Gut Hormones, p 343. Amsterdam, Elsevier North-Holland Biomedical Press, 1979
645. Maton PN, Gardner JD, Jensen RT: The incidence and etiology of Cushing's syndrome in patients with Zollinger-Ellison syndrome. N Engl J Med 315:1, 1986
646. Greider MH, Rosai J, McGuigan JE: The human pancreatic islet cells and their tumors: II. Ulcerogenic and diarrheogenic tumors. Cancer 33:1423, 1974
647. Martin ED, Notet F: Pathology of endocrine tumors of the GI tract. Clin Gastroenterol 3:511, 1974
648. Niewenhuijzen-Knuseman AC, Knijnenburg G, Ribiere GB et al: Morphology and immunohistochemically-defined endocrine function of pancreatic islet cell tumors. Histopathology, 2:389, 1978
649. Wolfe MM, Jain DK, Edgerton JR: Zollinger-Ellison syndrome associated with persistent normal fasting serum gastrin concentrations. Ann Intern Med 103:215, 1985
650. Wolfe MM, Jensen RT: Zollinger-Ellison syndrome. N Engl J Med 317:1200, 1987
651. Aoyagi T, Summerskill SHJ: Gastric secretion with ulcerogenic islet cell tumor. Arch Intern Med 117:667, 1966
652. Deveney CW, Deveney KS, Jaffe BM et al: Use of calcium and secretin in the diagnosis of gastrinoma (Zollinger-Ellison syndrome). Ann Intern Med 87:680, 1979
653. Malagelada JR, Davis CS, O'Fallon WM et al: Laboratory diagnosis of gastrinoma. Mayo Clin Proc 57:211, 1982
654. Isenberg JI, Walsh JH, Grossman MI: Zollinger-Ellison syndrome. Gastroenterology 65:140, 1973
655. Van Heerden JA, Bernatz PE, Rovelstad RA: The retained antrum—clinical considerations. Mayo Clin Proc 46:25, 1971
656. Korman MG, Scott DG, Hansky J et al: Hypergastrinemia due to excluded gastric antrum: A proposed method for differentiation from Zollinger-Ellison syndrome. Aust NZ J Med 3:266, 1972
657. Chaudhuri TK, Shirazi SS, Condon RE: Radioisotope scan—A possible aid in differentiating retained gastric antrum from Zollinger-Ellsion syndrome in patients with recurrent peptic ulcer. Gastroenterology 65:697, 1973
658. Isenberg JI, Walsh JH, Passaro E Jr et al: Unusual effect of secretin on serum gastrin, serum calcium, and gastric acid secretion in a patient with suspected Zollinger-Ellison syndrome. Gastroenterology 62:626, 1972
659. Hansky J, Soveny C, Korman MG: Effect of secretin on serum gastrin as measured by immunoassay. Gastroenterology 61:62, 1971
660. McGuigan JE, Wolfe MM: Secretin injection test in the diagnosis of gastrinoma. Gastroenterology 79:1324, 1980
661. Lamers CBH, Van Tongeren JHM: Comparative study of the value of calcium, secretin, and meal-stimulated increase in serum gastrin in the diagnosis of the Zollinger-Ellison syndrome. Gut 18:128, 1979
662. Slaff JI, Howard JM, Maton PN et al: Prospective assessment of provocative gastrin tests in 81 consecutive patients with Zollinger-Ellison syndrome. Gastroenterology 90:1637, 1986
663. Ganguli PC, Elder JB, Polak MJ et al: Antral gastrin cell hyperplasia in peptic ulcer disease. Lancet 1:1288, 1974
664. Polak JM, Stagg B, Pearse AGE: Two types of Zollinger-Ellison syndrome: Immunofluorescent, cytochemical, and ultrastructural studies of the antral and pancreatic gastrin cells in different clinical states. Gut 13:501, 1972
665. Friesen SR, Schimke RN, Pearse AGE. Genetic aspects of Z-E syndrome: Prospective studies in two kindreds: antral gastrin cell hyperplasia. Ann Surg 176:370, 1972
666. Friesen SR, Tomita T: Pseudo-Zollinger-Ellison syndrome. Hypergastrinemia, hyperchlorohydria without tumor. Ann Surg 194:481, 1981
667. Lamers CBH, Ruland CM, Joosten HJM et al: Hypergastrinemia of antral origin in duodenal ulcer. Dig Dis Sci 23:998, 1978
668. Taylor IL, Calam JK, Roth JI et al: Family studies of hypergastrinemic hyperpepsinogenemic I duodenal ulcer. Ann Intern Med 95:421, 1981
669. Fuerle G, Ketterer H, Becker HD et al: Circadian serum gastrin concentrations in control persons and in patients with ulcer disease. Scand J Gastroenterol 7:177, 1972
670. Fox PS, Hofmann JW, DeCosse JJ et al: The influence of total gastrectomy on survival in malignant Zollinger-Ellison tumors. Ann Surg 180:558, 1974
671. Mignon M, Ruszniewski R, Haffar S et al: Current approach to the management of tumoral process in patients with gastrinoma. World J Surg 10:702, 1986
672. McCarthy DM. The place of surgery in the Zollinger-Ellison syndrome. N Engl J Med 302:1844, 1980
673. Richardson CT, Peters MN, Feldman M et al: Treatment of the Zollinger-Ellison syndrome with exploratory laparotomy, proximal gastric vagotomy, and H_2-receptor antagonists. Gastroenterology 89:357, 1985
674. Norton JA, Sugarbaker PH, Doppman JL et al: Aggressive resection of metastatic disease in selected patients with malignant gastrinoma. Ann Surg 203:352, 1986
675. Hancke S: Localization of hormone-producing gastrointestinal tumors by ultrasonic scanning. Scand J Gastroenterol 53:115, 1979
676. Shawker TH, Doppman JL, Dunnick NR et al: Ultrasound investigation of pancreatic islet cell tumors. J Ultrasound Med 1:193, 1982
677. Damgaard-Petersen K, Stage JG: CT scanning in patients with Zollinger-Ellison syndrome and carcinoid syndrome. Scand J Gastroenterol 53:117, 1979
678. Dunnick NR, Doppman JL, Mills SR et al: Computed tomographic detection of nonbeta pancreatic islet cell tumors. Radiology 135:117, 1980
679. Stark DP, Moss AA, Goldberg HI et al: CT of pancreatic islet cell tumors. Radiology 150:491, 1984
680. Krudy AG, Doppman JL, Jensen RT et al: Localization of islet cell tumors by dynamic CT. Am J Radiol 143:585, 1984
681. Wank SA, Doppman JL, Miller DL et al: Prospective study of the ability of computerized axial tomography to localize gastrinomas in patients with Zollinger-Ellison syndrome. Gastroenterology 92:905, 1987
682. Ruszniewski P, Mignon M, Rene E et al: Localization of tumoral process in Zollinger-Ellison syndrome (ZES): a retrospective study in 76 patients. Gastroenterology 90:1610, 1986
683. Roche A, Raisonnier A, Gillon-Savouret MC: Pancreatic venous sampling and arteriography in localizing insulinomas and gastrinomas: Procedure and results in 55 cases. Radiology 145:621, 1982
684. Maton PN, Miller DL, Doppman JL et al: Role of selective angiography in the management of Zollinger-Ellison syndrome. Gastroenterology 92:913, 1987
685. Burcharth F, Stage JG, Stadil F et al: Localization of gastrinoma by transhepatic portal catheterization and gastrin assay. Gastroenterology 77:440, 1979
686. Glowniak JR, Shapiro B, Vinnik AI et al: Percutaneous transhepatic venous sampling of gastrin. N Engl J Med 307:293, 1982
687. Cherner JA, Doppman JL, Norton JA et al: Prospective assessment of selective venous sampling for gastrin to localize gastrinomas. Ann Intern Med 105:841, 1986
688. Sigel B, Coelho MCU, Nyhus LM et al: Detection of pancreatic tumors by ultrasound during surgery. Arch Radiol 117:1058, 1982
689. Charboneau WJ, James EM, Van Heerden JA et al: Intraoperative realtime ultrasonographic localization of pancreatic insulinomas. J Ultrasound Med 2:251, 1983
690. Cromack DT, Norton JA, Sigel B et al: The use of high-resolution intraoperative ultrasound to localize gastrinomas: an initial report of a prospective study. World J Surg 11:648, 1987
691. Comi R, Norton JA, Doppman JL et al: Insulinoma in The Exocrine Pancreas: Biology, Pathobiology and Diseases, p 745. New York, Raven Press, 1986
692. Friesen SR: Effect of total gastrectomy on the Zollinger-Ellison tumor: Observation by second-look operations. Surgery 62:609, 1967
693. Friesen SR: Treatment of the Zollinger-Ellison syndrome. Am J Surg 143:331, 1982
694. Howard JM, Chremos AN, Collen MJ et al: Famotidine, a new potent long acting histamine H_2-receptor antagonist: comparison with cimetidine and ranitidine in the treatment of Zollinger-Ellison syndrome: Gastroenterology 88:1026, 1985
695. Vinayek R, Howard JM, Maton PN et al: Famotidine in the therapy of gastric hypersecretory states. Am J Med 81:49, 1986
696. McArthur KE, Collen MJ, Cherner JA et al: Omeprazole as a single daily dose is effective therapy in Zollinger-Ellison syndrome. Gastroenterology 88:939, 1985
697. Lamers CBH, Lind T, Moberg S et al: Omeprazole in Zollinger-Ellison syndrome. Effects of a single dose and a long-term treatment in patients resistant to histamine H_2-receptor antagonists. N Engl J Med 310:758, 1984
698. Collen MJ, Howard JM, McArthur KE et al: Comparison of ranitidine and cimetidine in the treatment of gastric hypersecretion. Ann Inter Med 100:52, 1984
699. McCarthy DM, Hyman PE: Effect of isopropamide on response to oral cimetidine in patients with Zollinger-Ellison syndrome. Dig Dis Sci 27:353, 1982
700. Mignon M, Vallot J, Galmiche JP et al: Interest of a combined antisecretory treatment, cimetidine and pirenzepine in the management of severe forms of Zollinger-Ellison syndrome. Digestion 20:56, 1980
701. McCarthy DM, Peiken SR, Lopatin RN: Hyperparathyroidism—A reversible cause of cimetidine-resistant gastric hypersecretion. Br Med J 1:765, 1979
702. Gogel HK, Buckman MT, Cadieux D et al: Gastric secretion and hormonal interactions in multiple endocrine neoplasms Type I. Arch Intern Med 145:855, 1985
703. Norton JA, Cornelius MJ, Doppman JL et al: Effect of parathyroidectomy in patients with hyperparathyroidism and Zollinger-Ellison syndrome and multiple endocrine neoplasia–Type I—A prospective study. Surgery 102:958, 1987
704. Jensen RT: Basis for failure of cimetidine in patients with Zollinger-Ellison syndrome. Dig Dis Sci 29:363, 1984
705. Bonfils S, Mignon M, Gratton J: Cimetidine treatment of acute and chronic Zollinger-Ellison syndrome. World J Surg 3:597, 1979
706. Stadil F, Stage JG: Cimetidine and the Zollinger-Ellison (ZE) syndrome. In Wastell C, Lance P (eds): Cimetidine, pp 91–104. London, Churchill Livingstone, 1978
707. Deveney CW, Stein S, Way LW: Cimetidine in the treatment of Zollinger-Ellison syndrome. Am J Surg 146:116, 1983
708. McCarthy DM: Report on the United States experience with cimetidine in Zollinger-Ellison syndrome and other hypersecretory states. Gastroenterology 74:453, 1978
709. Stabile BE, Ippoliti AF, Walsh JH et al: Failure of histamine H_2-receptor antagonist therapy in Zollinger-Ellison syndrome. Am J Surg 145:17, 1983
710. Mignon M, Vallot T, Hervoir P et al: Ranitidine versus cimetidine in the management of Zollinger-Ellison syndrome. In Riley AJ, Salmon PR (eds): Ranitidine, p 169. Amsterdam, Excerpta Medica, 1982
711. Jensen RT, Collen MJ, McArthur KE et al: Comparison of the effectiveness of ranitidine and cimetidine in inhibiting acid secretion in patients with gastric hypersecretory states. Am J Med 77:90, 1984
712. Delcher JC, Soule JC, Mignon M et al: Effectiveness of omepraxole in seven patients

with Zollinger-Ellison syndrome resistant to histamine H_2-receptor antagonists. Dig Dis Sci 31:693, 1986

713. Lloyd-Davis KA, Rutgerssan K, Solvell L: Omeprazole in Zollinger-Ellison syndrome: Four-year international study. Gastroenterology 90:1523, 1986
714. Raufman JP, Collins SM, Pandol SJ et al: Reliability of symptoms in assessing control of gastric acid secretion in patients with Zollinger-Ellison syndrome. Gastroenterology 84:108, 1983
715. Maton PN, Frucht H, Vinayek R et al: Medical management of patients with Zollinger-Ellison syndrome who have previous gastric surgery. Gastroenterology 94:294–300, 1988
716. McCarthy DM, Olinger EJ, May RJ et al: H_2-Histamine receptor blocking agents in the Zollinger-Ellison syndrome. Ann Intern Med 87:668, 1977
717. McArthur KE, Raufman JP, Seaman JJ et al: Cimetidine pharmacokinetics in patients with Zollinger-Ellison syndrome. Gastroenterology 93:69, 1987
718. Ziemniak JA, Madura M, Adamonis AJ et al: Failure of cimetidine in Zollinger-Ellison syndrome. Dig Dis Sci 28:976, 1983
719. Jensen RT, Collen MJ, Allende HD et al: Cimetidine induced impotence and breast changes in patients with gastric hypersecretory states. N Engl J Med 308:883, 1983
720. Creutzfeldt W, Stockmann F, Conlon JM et al: Effect of short- and long-term feeding of omeprazole on rat gastric endocrine cells. Digestion 35(1):84, 1986
721. Maton PN, McArthur KE, Wank SA et al: Long-term efficacy and safety of omeprazole in patients with Zollinger-Ellison syndrome. Gastroenterology 90:1537, 1986
722. Thompson NW, Lloyd RU, Nishiyama RH et al: MEN-1 pancreas: a histological and immunohistochemical study. World J Surg 8:561, 1984
723. Vogel SB, Wolfe MM, McGuigan JE et al: Localization and resection of gastrinomas in Zollinger-Ellison syndrome. Ann Surg 205:550, 1987
724. Norton JA: Invited Commentary. World J Surg 8:575, 1984
725. Thompson NW: Surgical considerations in the MEN-1 syndrome. In Johnston IDA, Johnston NW (eds): Endocrine Surgery, p 144. London, Butterworths International Medical Reviews, 1983
726. Friesen SR, Tomita T, Kimmel JR: Pancreatic polypeptide update: Its role in detection of the trait for multiple endocrine adenopathy syndrome, type I and pancreatic polypeptide-secreting tumors. Surgery 94:1028, 1983
727. Von Schrenk T, Howard JM, Doppman JL et al: Prospective study of chemotherapy in patients with metastatic gastrinoma. Gastroenterology 94:1326–1334, 1988
728. Moertel CG, Hanley JA, Johnson LA: Streptozotocin alone compared with streptozotocin plus fluorouracil in the treatment of advanced islet-cell carcinoma. N Engl J Med 303:1189, 1980
729. Broder LE, Carter SK: Pancreatic islet cell carcinoma. Ann Intern Med 79:108, 1973
730. Buchanan KD, O'Hare MMT, Russel CJF et al: Factors involved in the responsiveness of gastrointestinal apudomas to streptozotocin. Dig Dis Sci 31:511S, 1986
731. Moertel CG, Lavin PT, Hahn RG: Phase II trial of doxorubicin for advanced islet cell carcinoma. Cancer Treat Rep 66:1567, 1982
732. Bukowski RM, McCracken JD, Balcerzak SP et al: Phase II study of chlorozotocin in islet cell carcinoma. Cancer Chemother Pharmacol 11:48, 1983
733. Bonfils S, Ruszniewski P, Haffar S et al: Chemotherapy of hepatic metastases (HM) in Zollinger-Ellison syndrome (ZES). Report of a multicenteric analysis. Dig Dis Sci 31:51, 1986
734. Carrasco CH, Chuang VP, Wallace S: Apudoma metastatic to the liver: Treatment by hepatic artery embolization. Radiology 149:79, 1983
735. Shepherd JJ, Senator GB: Regression of liver metastases in patients with gastrin secreting tumor treated with SMS 201-995. Lancet 2:274, 1986
736. Bonfils S, Ruszniewski P, Laucouret H et al: Long-term management of Zollinger-Ellison syndrome with SMS-201-995, a long acting somatostatin analog. Program the 6th International Symposium on Gastrointestinal Hormones. Can J Physiol Pharmacol July 6–10:63, 1986
737. Erickson B, Oberg K, Alm G et al: Treatment of malignant endocrine pancreatic tumors with human leukocyte interferon. Lancet 2:1307, 1986
738. Barton JC, Hirschowitz BI, Maton PN et al: Bone metastases in malignant gastrinoma. Gastroenterology 91:1179, 1986
739. Reubi JC: Somatostatin analogue inhibits chondrosarcoma and insulinoma tumor growth. Acta Endocrinol 109:108, 1985
740. Whipple AO: The surgical therapy of hyperinsulinism. J Int Chir 3:237, 1938
741. Galbut DL, Markowitz AM: Insulinoma: diagnosis, surgical management and long-term followup. Am J Surg 139:682, 1980
742. Giercksky KE, Halse J, Mathisen W et al: Endocrine tumors of the pancreas. Scand J Gastroenterol 15:129, 1980
743. Boden G: Insulinoma and glucagoma. Semin Oncol 14:253, 1987
744. Service FJ, Dale AJ, Elveback LR et al: Insulinoma: Clinical and diagnostic features of 60 consecutive cases. Mayo Clin Proc 51:417, 1976
745. Glickman MH, Hart MJ, White TT: Insulinoma in Seattle: 39 cases in 30 years. Am J Surg 140:119, 1980
746. Nelson RL, Rizza RA, Service FJ: Documented hypoglycemia for 23 years in a patient with insulinoma. JAMA 240:1891, 1978
747. Merimee T, Tyson JE: Hypoglycemia in man. Diabetes 26:161, 1977
748. Danforth DN, Gorden P, Brennan MF: Metastatic insulin-secreting carcinoma of the pancreas: clinical course and the role of surgery. Surgery 96:1027, 1984
749. Kahn CR, Rosen SW, Weintraub BD et al: Ectopic production of chorionic gonadotropin and its subunits by islet cell tumors: a specific marker for malignancy. N Engl J Med 297:565, 1977
750. Lloyd RV, Mervak T, Schmidt D et al: Immunohistochemical detection of chromogranin and neuron-specific enolase in pancreatic endocrine neoplasms. Am J Surg Pathol 8:607, 1984
751. Chejfic G, Falkmer S, Grimelius L et al: Synaptophysin, a new marker for pancreatic neuroendocrine tumors. Am J Surg Pathol 11:241, 1987
752. Skrabanek P, Powell D: Ectopic insulin and Occam's razor: reappraisal of the riddle of tumor hypoglyemia. Clin Endocrinol 9:141, 1978
753. Shetty MR, Boghassian HM, Duffell D et al: Tumor induced hypoglycemia. A result of ectopic insulin production. Cancer 49:1920, 1980
754. Norton JA, Sigel B, Baker AR et al: Localization of an occult insulinoma by intraoperative ultrasonography. Surgery 97:381, 1985
755. Dunnick NR, Long JA, Krudy A et al: Localizing insulinomas with combined radiographic methods. AJR 135:747, 1980
756. Rayfield EJ, Goldberg IJ, Gregerich EW et al: Transportal blood sampling for preoperative localization of insulinoma. Mt Sinai J Med 50:258, 1983
757. Cho KJ, Vinnik AI, Thompson NK et al: Localization of the source of hyperinsulinism. AJR 139:237, 1982
758. Doppman JL, Brennan MF, Dunnick NR et al: The role of pancreatic venous sampling in the localization of occult insulinomas. Radiology 138:557, 1981
759. Norton JA, Cromack DT, Shawker TH et al: Intraoperative ultrasonographic localization of islet cell tumors: a prospective comparison to palpation, Ann Surg 207:160, 1988
760. Tutt GO Jr, Edis AJ, Servie FJ et al: Plasma glucose monitoring during operation for insulinoma—A critical reappraisal. Surgery 88:351, 1980
761. Kudlow JE, Albisser AM, Angel A et al: Insulinoma resection facilitated by the artificial endocrine pancreas. Diabetes 27:774, 1978
762. Eckhauser FE, Cheung PS, Vinik AI et al: Nonfunctioning malignant neuroendocrine tumors of the pancreas. Surgery 100:978, 1986
763. Vinik AI, Strodel WE, Eckhauser FE et al: Somatostatinomas, PPomas, Neurotensinomas. Semin Oncol 14:263, 1987
764. Mekhjian HS, O'Dorisio TM: VIPoma syndrome. Semin Oncol 14:282, 1987
765. Kane MG, O'Dorisio TM, Krejs GJ: Production of secretory diarrhea by intravenous infusion of vasoactive intestinal peptide. N Engl J Med 309:1482, 1983
766. Parker CM, Hanke CW, Madura JA et al: Glucagonoma syndrome: case report and literature review. J Derm Surg Oncol 10:884, 1984
767. Clark ES, Carney JA: Pancreatic islet cell tumor associated with Cushing's syndrome. Am J Surg Pathol 8:917, 1984
768. Rasbach DA, Hammond JM: Pancreatic islet cell carcinoma with hypercalcemia. Am J Med 78:337, 1985
769. Guillemin R, Brazeau P, Bohlen P et al: Growth hormone-releasing factor from a human pancreatic tumor that caused acromegaly. Science 27:774, 1978
770. Norton JA, Kahn CK, Schiebinger R et al: Amino acid deficiency and the skin rash associated with glucagonoma. Ann Intern Med 91:213, 1979
771. Abravia C, De Bartolo M, Katzen R et al: Disappearance of glucagonoma rash after surgical resection, but not during dietary normalization of serum amino acids. Am J Clin Nutr 39:351, 1984
772. Peterson LL, Shaw JC, Acott KM et al: Glucagonoma syndrome: in vitro evidence that glucagon increases epidermal arachidonic acid. J Am Acad Dermatol II:468, 1984
773. Santangelo WC, Unger RH, Orci L et al: Somatostatin analog-induced remission of necrolytic migratory erythema without changes in plasma glucagon concentration. Pancreas 1:464, 1986
774. Krejs GJ, Orci L, Conlon M et al: Somatostatinoma syndrome (biochemical, morphological, and clinical features). N Engl J Med 301:285, 1979
775. Ganda PO, Weir GC, Soeldner JS et al: Somatostatinoma: a somatostatin-containing tumor of the endocrine pancreas. N Engl J Med 296:963, 1977
776. Bhathena SJ, Higgins GA, Recant L: Glucagonoma and glucagonoma syndrome. In Unger RH, Orci L (eds): Glucagon, p 413. New York, Elsevier North Holland, 1981
777. Kessinger A, Lemon HM, Foley JF: The glucagonoma syndrome and its management. J Surg Oncol 9:419, 1977
778. Strauss GM, Weitzman SA, Aoki TT: Dimethyltriazenoimidazole carboximide therapy of malignant glucagonomas. Ann Intern Med 90:57, 1979
779. Marynick SP, Fagadau WR, Duncan LA: Malignant glucagonoma syndrome: Response to chemotherapy. Ann Intern Med 93:453, 1980
780. Prinz RA, Budrinath K, Banerji M et al: Operations and chemotherapeutic management of malignant glucagon producing tumors. Surgery 90:713, 1981
781. Awrich AE, Peetz M, Fletcher WS: Dimethyltriazenomidazole carboxamide therapy of islet cell carcinomas of the pancreas. J Surg Oncol 17:321, 1981
782. Kurose T, Seino Y, Ishida LT et al: Successful treatment of metastatic gastrinoma with dacarbazine. Lancet 1:621, 1984
783. Oberg K, Lindstrom H, Alm G, Lundquist G: Successful treatment of therapy-resistant pancreatic cholera with human leukocyte interferon. Lancet 1:725, 1985
784. Anderson JV, Bloom SR: Treatment of malignant endocrine tumors with human leukocyte interferon. Lancet 1:97, 1987
785. Wermer P: Endocrine adenomatosis: peptic ulcer in a large kindred. Am J Med 35:205, 1963
786. Ballard HS, Frame B, Hartsock RT: Familial multiple endocrine adenoma—peptic ulcer complex. Medicine 43:481, 1964
787. Loeb JN: Polyglandular disorders. In Wyngaarden JB, Smith LH (eds): Cecil Textbook of Medicine, p 1304, Philadephia, WB Saunders, 1982
788. Brandi ML, Aurbach GD, Fitzpatrick LA et al: Parathyroid mitogenic activity in plasma from patients with familial multiple endocrine neoplasia type I. N Engl J Med 314:1287, 1986

789. Leight GS, Hensley MI: Management of familial hyperparathyroidism. Prog Surg 18:106, 1987
790. Eberle F, Grun R: Multiple endocrine neoplasia type I. Adv Intern Med Pediatr 5:76, 1981
791. Wells SA Jr, Farndon JR, Dale JK et al: Longterm evaluation of patients with primary parathyroid hyperplasia managed by total parathyroidectomy and heterotopic autotransplantation. Ann Surg 192:451, 1980
792. Prinz RA, Gamvros OI, Seller D et al: Subtotal parathyroidectomy for primary chief cell hyperplasia of the multiple endocrine neoplasia type I syndrome. Ann Surg 193:26, 1981
793. Rizzoli R, Green J, Marx SJ: Primary hyperparathyroidism in familial multiple endocrine neoplasia type I. Long-term follow-up of serum calcium levels after parathyroidectomy. Am J Med 78:467, 1985
794. Thompson NW, Lloyd RV, Nishiyama RH et al: MEN 1 pancreas: a histological and immunohistochemical study. World J Surg 8:561, 1984
795. Schmid JR, Labhart A, Rossier PH: Relationship of multiple endocrine adenomas to the syndrome of ulcerogenic islet cell adenomas (Zollinger-Ellison). Am J Med 31:343, 1961
796. Lamers CB, Stadil F, Tongren JMV: Prevalence of endocrine abnormalities in patients with the Zollinger-Ellison syndrome and their families. Am J Med 64:607, 1981
797. Eisenberg AA, Wallerstein H: Pheochromocytoma of the suprarenal medulla (paraglioma). A clinicopathological study. Arch Pathol 14:818, 1932
798. Hazard JB, Hawk WH, Crile G Jr: Medullary (solid) carcinoma of the thyroid—Clinicopathologic entity. J Clin Endocrinol Metab 19:704, 1979
799. Norton JA, Wells SA Jr: Medullary thyroid carcinoma and multiple endocrine neoplasia type-II syndromes. In Friesen S (ed): Surgical Endocrinology, 2nd ed. Philadelphia, JB Lippincott, 1988
800. Copp DH: Evidence for calcitonin—New Hormone from parathyroid that lowers blood calcium. Endocrinology 70:638, 1962
801. Steiner AL, Goodman AD, Powers SR: Study of a kindred with pheochromocytoma, medullary thyroid carcinoma, hyperparathyroidism and Cushing's disease. Multiple endocrine neoplasia, type 2. Medicine 47:371, 1968
802. Tashjian AH Jr, Howland BG, Melvin KEW et al: Immunoassay of human calcitonin. Clinical measurement, relation to serum calcium and studies in patients with medullary carcinoma. N Engl J Med 283:890, 1970
803. Jackson CE, Block MA, Greenawald KA et al: The two-mutational event theory in medullary thyroid cancer. Am J Hum Genet 31:704, 1979
804. Wolfe HJ, Melvin KEW, Cervi-Skinner SJ et al: C-cell hyperplasia preceding medullary thyroid carcinoma. N Engl J Med 189:437, 1973
805. Sipple JH: The association of pheochromocytoma with carcinoma of the thyroid gland. Am J Med 31:163, 1961
806. Williams ED: A review of 17 cases of carcinoma of the thyroid and pheochromocytoma. J Clin Pathol 18:288, 1965
807. Schimke RN, Hartmann WH: Familial amyloid-producing medullary thyroid carcinoma and pheochromocytoma. A distinct genetic entity. Ann Intern Med 63:1027, 1965
808. Manning PC, Molnar GD, Black BM et al: Pheochromocytoma, hyperparathyroidism and thyroid carcinoma occurring coincidentally. N Engl J Med 268:68, 1963
809. William ED, Pollock DJ: Multiple mucosal neuromata with endocrine tumors: A syndrome alluded to von Recklinghausen's disease. J Pathol Bacteriol 91:71, 1966
810. Gorlin RJ, Sedano HO, Vickers RA et al: Multiple mucosal neuromas, pheochromocytomas and medullary carcinoma of the thyroid—a syndrome. Cancer 22:293, 1986
811. Chong GC, Beahrs DLT, Sizemore GW et al: Medullary carcinoma of the thyroid gland. Cancer 35:695, 1975
812. Grun R, Eberle F: Ergebn Inner Mediz Kind 46:151, 1981
813. Carney JA, Sizemore GW, Sheps SG: Adrenal medullary disease in multiple endocrine neoplasia type 2. Am J Clin Pathol 66:279, 1976
814. Keiser HR, Beaven MA, Doppman J et al: Sipple's syndrome: Medullary thyroid carcinoma, pheochromocytoma and parathyroid disease. Ann Intern Med 78:561, 1973
815. Valk TW, Frager MS, Gross MD et al: Spectrum of pheochromocytoma in multiple endocrine neoplasia: A scintigraphic portrayal using ^{131}I-metaiodobenzylguanidine. Ann Intern Med 94:762, 1981
816. Wells SA Jr, Baylin SG, Leight GS et al: The importance of early diagnosis in patients with hereditary medullary thyroid carcinoma. Ann Surg 195:505, 1982
817. Wells SA Jr, Baylin SB, Gann DW et al: Medullary thyroid carcinoma: Relationship of method of diagnosis to pathological staging. Ann Surg 188:377, 1978
818. Melvin KEW, Miller HH,Tashjian AH Jr: Early diagnosis of medullary carcinoma of the thyroid by means of calcitonin assay. N Engl J Med 285:1115, 1971
819. Wells SA Jr, Baylin SG, Linehan WM et al: Provocative agents and the diagnosis of medullary carcinoma of the thyroid gland. Ann Surg 188:139, 1978
820. Wells SA Jr, Baylin SG, Johnsrude IS et al: Thyroid venous catheterization in the early diagnosis of familial medullary thyroid carcinoma. Ann Surg 196:505, 1982
821. Farndon JR, Fagraeus L, Wells SA Jr: Recent developments in the management of phaechromocytoma. In Johnston IDA, Thompson NW (eds): Endocrine Surgery, pp 189–201. London, Butterworths, 1983
822. Jackson CE, Talpos GB, Kanbouris A et al: The clinical course after definitive operation for medullary thyroid carcinoma. Surgery 94:995, 1983

ALFRED E. CHANG
STEVEN A. ROSENBERG
ELI J. GLATSTEIN
KAREN H. ANTMAN

CHAPTER 40 *Sarcomas of Soft Tissues*

Soft tissues refer to the extraskeletal connective tissues of the body that connect, support, and surround other discrete anatomic structures. This portion of the body mass lying between the epidermis and parenchymal organs includes the organs of locomotion, such as muscles and tendons, and a wide variety of supportive tissue structures, such as fibrous tissue, fat, and synovial tissue. The soft somatic tissues are ubiquitous and comprise over 50% of the body weight. The over 400 muscles in the human body comprise about 40% of adult body weight.

Soft tissue sarcomas refer to a large variety of malignant tumors arising in the soft tissues that are grouped because of similarities in pathologic appearance, clinical presentation, and behavior. A combination of embryologic, functional, and morphologic characterizations of the soft tissue sarcomas are needed to define this tumor group.

Virtually all tumors included in the soft tissue sarcomas (from the Greek *sarkoma*, meaning fleshy growth) arise from a common embryonic ancestry, the primitive mesoderm (Table 40-1). Nine to 13 days after fertilization of the ovum, the human embryo undergoes a transition from a phase of increasing cell number to a phase of morphologic organization into the endoderm, ectoderm, and mesoderm, the three primary germ layers of the embryo.[1] Within these layers are established commitments to developmental potentials that far precede morphologic differentiation of the cells.

The primitive mesoderm gives rise to a variety of organs, such as the kidney, ureter, oviducts, uterus, gonads, and heart, and a wide range of hematopoietic, lymphatic, and reticuloendothelial tissues. The primitive mesenchyme, a loose network of cells and intercellular matrix within the mesoderm, is largely responsible for the development of the common connective tissues of the body listed in Table 40-1. Tumors of these connective tissues are referred to as soft tissue sarcomas. Because of similarities in anatomic sites of origin, clinical presentation, and clinical behavior, tumors arising in Schwann cells, a class of cells surrounding peripheral nerves that arise from the neural tube of the primitive ectoderm, are also included in the category of soft tissue sarcomas.

Malignant tumors are categorized as sarcomas or carcinomas based on whether they arise from connective tissue (sarcomas) or epithelial tissue (carcinomas). This differentiation is imprecise, and many sarcomas arise from tissues that fit the morphologic criteria of epithelium. Epithelium is a morphologic, not embryologic, term that is used to designate cellular structures that cover or line surfaces on or in the body and may arise from ectoderm, endoderm, or mesoderm. The endothelium lining the vascular and lymphatic channels and the mesothelium lining the body cavities and visceral organs are two types of epithelium that arise from the mesoderm. These epithelial structures give rise to malignant tumors that resemble and behave like tumors that develop from connective tissue cells. For this reason, tumors arising from the endothelium and the mesothelium are included in the category of sarcomas.

In summary, sarcomas arise largely, although not exclusively, from mesodermal structures and largely, although not exclusively, from connective tissue cells. Some sarcomas arise from ectodermal structures, and some arise from epithelium.

This chapter describes the natural history and treatment of the soft tissue sarcomas. All visceral organs contain a con-

TABLE 40-1. Embryonic Derivation of the Soft Tissue and Bony Sarcomas

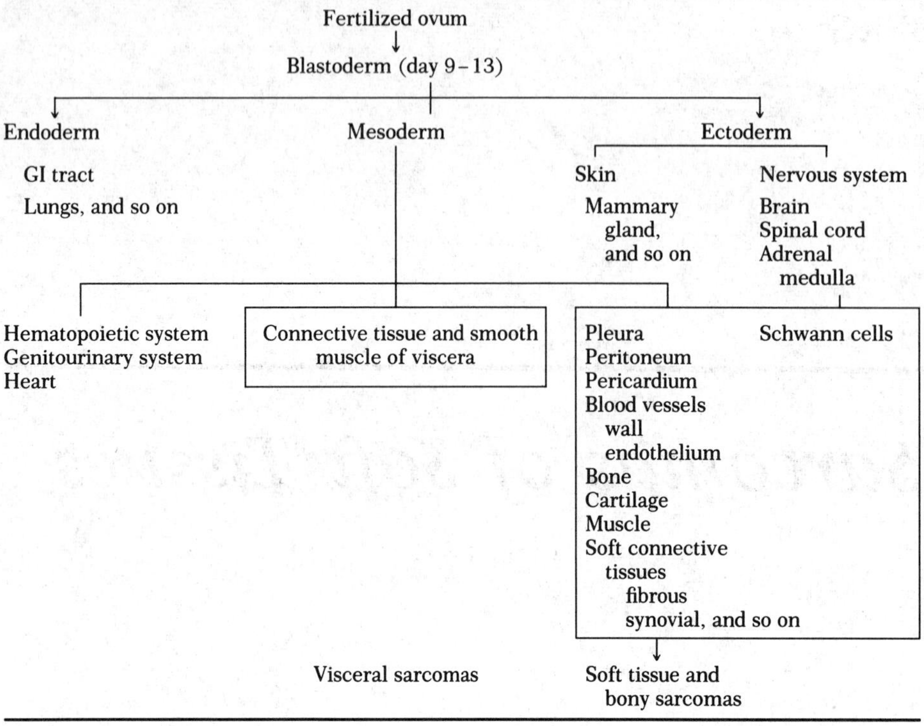

nective tissue stroma that can undergo malignant transformation. These visceral sarcomas are discussed in the chapters dealing with individual organ systems.

INCIDENCE OF SARCOMAS

Approximately 5100 new cases of soft tissue sarcoma and 2800 deaths from this disease were reported in the United States in 1986.[2] The annual age-adjusted incidence was 2 per 100,000. Data from New Zealand suggests that both the incidence and mortality from soft tissue sarcomas has been increasing (from 1.3 per 100,000 men in 1955 to 2.2 per 100,000 men in 1977) in that country, although no change in incidence was seen in Denmark during the same period.[3,4] There appears to be no sex or racial pattern of these cancers in the United States.

Soft tissue sarcomas comprise 0.7% of all cancers, although these tumors comprise 6.5% of all cancers in children under the age of 15.[2] Soft tissue sarcomas rank fifth in cancer incidence in children under the age of 15, behind leukemia, central nervous system cancers, lymphomas, and sympathetic nervous system cancers. Soft tissue sarcomas rank fifth as a cause of cancer death in this age group behind leukemia, nervous system cancers, renal cancer, and bone cancer.

EPIDEMIOLOGY

Little is known about epidemiologic or etiologic factors of importance in patients with soft tissue sarcomas. There is no proven genetic predisposition to the development of soft tissue sarcomas, though Li and Fraumeni have reported four kindreds with pairs of young children (three sets of sibs and one set of cousins) with soft tissue sarcomas.[5] This incidence exceeded that expected on a chance basis ($p = 0.06$). Howard and Casten reported two brothers who developed rhabdomyosarcoma of the orbit.[6] Only 1 in 100 to 400 cases of childhood rhabdomyosarcoma are associated with other relatives developing this cancer.[5,7]

There have been several reports of an association of childhood sarcomas with a small increased incidence of other familial cancers (especially breast cancer) that tended to occur in mothers younger than 30 years of age.[5,7–13] Other, rather unconvincing evidence for a link between breast cancer and sarcomas was the report of breast cancer as a second primary tumor in 2 of 24 women with liposarcoma.[14] The lymphangiosarcoma of the arm in women after mastectomy and axillary lymph node ablation (Steward-Treves syndrome) almost certainly does not represent evidence of an etiologic correlation between mammary cancer and sarcoma of soft tissue, but rather the development of lymphangiosarcoma in lymphedematous arms.[15]

Although Sloane and Hubbel have reported an increased incidence of congenital defects in children with soft tissue sarcomas, this association was not seen by Li and Fraumeni.[7,16]

Soft tissue sarcomas are thought to occur with slightly increased frequency in patients with a variety of genetically transmitted diseases, such as the basal cell nevus syndrome, tuberous sclerosis, Werner's syndrome, intestinal polyposis and Gardner's syndrome.[13,17–21] Patients with multiple neurofibromatosis (Von Recklinghausen's disease) have approximately a 15% chance of developing a neurofibrosarcoma.[18]

Although many patients with soft tissue sarcomas present

with a recent history of trauma, there is no known etiologic relationship, and it is likely that minor trauma merely calls a pre-existing lesion to the patient's attention.

Chemical carcinogens, such as 3-methylcholanthrene, and viruses can cause soft tissue sarcomas in experimental animals, but there is no convincing link between these factors and sarcomas in humans. Studies in Sweden in 1979 and 1981 linked environmental exposure to phenoxyacetic acids (a class of herbicides) and chlorophenols (wood preservatives) to a sixfold increase in the risk of developing soft tissue sarcoma.[22,23] These studies were based on small numbers of patients, however, and a more recent analysis of over 350,000 Swedish agricultural and forestry workers potentially exposed to these chemicals failed to confirm this association.[24] A recent case-control study from New Zealand failed to find an association between exposure to phenoxyherbicides and the incidence of soft tissue sarcomas, and an analysis of data from Denmark also cast doubt on this association.[3,4] Because of the early Swedish reports, there was concern that Vietnam veterans exposed to Agent Orange, a mixture of two commercial phenoxyacetic acid herbicides containing trace amounts of dioxins, might have an increased incidence of soft tissue sarcomas. Two separate studies, however, have failed to show a significant correlation.[25,26]

Sarcomas have a tendency to occur in areas previously exposed to ionizing irradiation, although sarcomas in radiation therapy fields are uncommon. In 1980, Kim and associates could find only 13 cases in the world literature of fibrosarcoma of the chest wall in women undergoing radiation therapy after mastectomy for breast cancer.[27] The latent period of these lesions ranged from 4 to 24 years after radiation exposures from 2000 to 7800 rad. An additional seven cases were described by Kuten and colleagues in 1985.[28] Sixteen cases of radiation-induced sarcomas of the chest wall occurred at the M.D. Anderson Hospital in Houston between 1944 and 1984, representing 5% of the 331 sarcomas of the chest wall that were seen during that period.[29] Similar findings were presented in a report by O'Neil and colleagues, who reviewed 11 patients with soft tissue fibrosarcomas after irradiation of the chest wall for breast cancer.[30]

Halperin and colleagues reported 5 cases of bone or soft tissue sarcomas occurring more than 5 years after treatment of Hodgkin's disease.[31] Two of these patients had received radiation therapy alone, 2 were treated with a combination of radiation and chemotherapy, and 1 received chemotherapy alone. Four cases of soft tissue sarcoma and 1 case of osteosarcoma occurred, with latent periods of 6 to 11 years. These authors calculated the risk of developing a sarcoma in 5-year survivors of Hodgkin's disease to be 0.9%.

Osteosarcomas appear to be the most common sarcomas induced by radiation. Arlen and associates summarized 50 cases of postradiation osteosarcoma, and in a long-term follow-up of 455 persons who painted luminous watch dials with radiomesothelium, 26 developed osteosarcoma.[32,33]

Sarcomas are associated with foreign body implantations in rodents. Sporadic reports of this phenomenon in humans have also appeared.[34] Ott has tabulated all cases published before 1966.[35] The responsible foreign bodies were mainly metal implants, bullets, shrapnel pieces, bone transplants, and so forth, with latent periods of up to 40 years. The true incidence of foreign-body-induced sarcomas is probably minimal, because no sarcomas were seen among 11,000 women who underwent augmentation mammoplasty with a variety of materials or in 281 patients who underwent prosthetic replacement for facial defects.[36,37]

SITES OF SOFT TISSUE SARCOMAS

Because of the ubiquitous nature of the connective tissues, soft tissue sarcomas can arise anywhere in the body. Visceral sarcomas arise from the connective stroma found in all organs and are rarer than sarcomas originating from somatic sites. Visceral sarcomas are not considered here. Sites of somatic soft tissue sarcomas from nine reported series are presented in Table 40-2.[38-46] Approximately 60% of sarcomas occur in the extremities. The ratio of lower-extremity to upper-extremity tumors is 3:1. About 75% of lower-extremity sarcomas originate at or above the knee. Other sites include the head and neck regions, which account for approximately 9% of these tumors, and the trunk (31%). Within the trunks, approximately 40% of tumors are located in the retroperitoneum, and the remaining tumors are located in the abdominal wall, chest wall, mediastinum, and breast. Generally, treatment approaches for patients with

TABLE 40-2. Sites of Soft Tissue Sarcomas

	Sites				
Study	*Head and Neck*	*Trunk/ Retroperitoneum*	*Upper Extremity*	*Lower Extremity*	*Total*
Shieber et al (1961)[38]*	16	39	20	50	125
Hare et al (1963)[39]	42	34/5	32	48	161
Ferrell et al (1972)[40]	8	19	15	36	78
Sears et al (1980)[41]	12	16	6	26	60
Abbas et al (1981)[42]	24	66/38	42	81	251
Lindberg et al (1981)[43]	26	74	63	137	300
Potter et al (1985)[44]	12	48/36	59	152	307
Torosian et al (1987)[45]	21	92/90	81	208	492
ACS Survey (1987)[46]	406	872/568	594	2110	4550
Total	567	1997	912	2848	6324
(%)	(9)	(32)	(14)	(45)	(100)

*Author, year of report, and reference number.

soft tissue sarcomas must consider the site of the origin of the tumor.

PATHOLOGIC CLASSIFICATION

Each of the soft tissues can give rise to benign and malignant groups of tumors. The transformation of a benign soft tissue tumor into a malignant sarcoma is rare. Because of the many different soft tissues, a variety of histologically distinct, but often grossly similar, sarcomas have been identified.[47-50] The pathologic classification presented in Table 40-3, based on the putative cell of origin of each tumor, has been suggested by Enzinger and Weiss.[50] Pathologic classifications based on the appearance of the predominant cell in the lesion (*i.e.*, round cell or spindle cell sarcomas) are less useful and should not be employed. In general, each of the sarcomas tends to reflect the morphologic appearance of the cell of origin, and the tendency of these tumors to dedifferentiate results in a variety of overlapping patterns that can make them very difficult to distinguish from one another. Competent pathologists often disagree on the cell of origin of an individual tumor.[51,52] The great variation in the reported incidence of various subtypes of soft tissue sarcomas probably reflects differences in opinion among pathologists rather than factual differences.

There are tumors arising from the soft tissues that are grossly similar to the sarcomas but rarely metastasize. Many of these tumors (*i.e.*, desmoid tumors or dermatofibrosarcoma protuberans) are capable of aggressively invading local

TABLE 40-3. Histologic Classification of Soft Tissue Tumors

I. Tumors and Tumor-Like Lesions of Fibrous Tissue
- A. Benign
  - 1. Fibroma
  - 2. Nodular fasciitis (including intravascular and cranial types)
  - 3. Proliferative fasciitis
  - 4. Proliferative myositis
  - 5. Fibroma of tendon sheath
  - 6. Elastofibroma
  - 7. Nuchal fibroma
  - 8. Nasopharyngeal fibroma
  - 9. Keloid
- B. Fibrous tumors of infancy and childhood
  - 1. Fibrous hamartoma of infancy
  - 2. Myofibromatosis (solitary, multicentric)
  - 3. Fibromatosis colli
  - 4. Infantile digital fibromatosis
  - 5. Infantile fibromatosis (desmoid type)
  - 6. Giant cell fibroblastoma
  - 7. Gingival fibromatosis
  - 8. Calcifying aponeurotic fibroma
  - 9. Hyalin fibromatosis
- C. Fibromatoses
  - 1. Superficial fibromatoses
    - a. Palmar and plantar fibromatosis
    - b. Penile (Peyronie's) fibromatosis
    - c. Knuckle pads
  - 2. Deep fibromatoses
    - a. Abdominal fibromatosis
    - b. Extra-abdominal fibromatosis
    - c. Intra-abdominal fibromatosis
    - d. Mesenteric fibromatosis (Gardner's syndrome)
    - e. Postradiation fibromatosis
    - f. Cicatricial fibromatosis
- D. Malignant
  - 1. Adult fibrosarcoma
  - 2. Congenital and infantile fibrosarcoma
  - 3. Inflammatory fibrosarcoma
  - 4. Postradiation fibrosarcoma
  - 5. Cicatricial fibrosarcoma

II. Fibrohistiocytic Tumors
- A. Benign
  - 1. Fibrous histiocytoma
    - a. Cutaneous (dermatofibroma)
    - b. Deep
  - 2. Atypical fibroxanthoma
  - 3. Juvenile xanthogranuloma
  - 4. Reticulohistiocytoma
  - 5. Xanthoma
- B. Intermediate
  - 1. Dermatofibrosarcoma protuberans
  - 2. Bednar tumor
- C. Malignant
  - 1. Malignant fibrous histiocytoma
    - a. Storiform–pleomorphic
    - b. Myxoid (myxofibrosarcoma)
    - c. Giant cell (malignant giant cell tumor of soft parts)
    - d. Inflammatory (malignant xanthogranuloma, xanthosarcoma)
    - e. Angiomatoid

III. Tumors and Tumor-Like Lesions of Adipose Tissue
- A. Benign
  - 1. Lipoma (cutaneous, deep, and multiple)
  - 2. Angiolipoma
  - 3. Spindle cell and pleomorphic lipoma
  - 4. Lipoblastoma and lipoblastomatosis
  - 5. Angiomyolipoma
  - 6. Myelolipoma
  - 7. Intramuscular and intermuscular lipoma
  - 8. Lipoma of tendon sheath
  - 9. Lumbosacral lipoma
  - 10. Interneural and perineural fibrolipoma
  - 11. Diffuse lipomatosis
  - 12. Cervical symmetrical lipomatosis (Madelung's disease)
  - 13. Pelvic lipomatosis
  - 14. Hibernoma
- B. Malignant
  - 1. Liposarcoma, predominantly
    - a. Well-differentiated
      - (1) Lipoma-like
      - (2) Sclerosing
      - (3) Inflammatory
    - b. Myxoid
    - c. Round cell (poorly differentiated myxoid)
    - d. Pleomorphic
    - e. Dedifferentiated

IV. Tumors of Muscle Tissue
- A. Smooth muscle
  - 1. Benign
    - a. Leiomyoma (cutaneous and deep)
    - b. Angiomyoma (vascular leiomyoma)
    - c. Epithelioid leiomyoma (benign leiomyoblastoma)
    - d. Intravenous leiomyomatosis
    - e. Leiomyomatosis peritonealis disseminata
  - 2. Malignant
    - a. Leiomyosarcoma
    - b. Epithelioid leiomyosarcoma (malignant leiomyoblastoma)

(*continued*)

TABLE 40-3. Histologic Classification of Soft Tissue Tumors (*continued*)

- B. Striated muscle
  - 1. Benign
    - a. Adult rhabdomyoma
    - b. Genital rhabdomyoma
    - c. Fetal rhabdomyoma
  - 2. Malignant
    - a. Rhabdomyosarcoma, predominantly
      - (1) Embryonal (including botryoid)
      - (2) Alveolar
      - (3) Pleomorphic
      - (4) Mixed
    - b. Ectomesenchymoma (rhabdomyosarcoma with ganglion cell differentiation)

V. *Tumors and Tumor-Like Lesions of Blood Vessels*

- A. Benign
  - 1. Hemangioma
    - a. Capillary (including juvenile)
    - b. Cavernous
    - c. Arteriovenous
    - d. Venous
    - e. Epithelioid (angiolymphoid hyperplasia, Kimura's disease)
    - f. Granulation tissue type (pyogenic granuloma)
  - 2. Deep hemangioma (intramuscular, synovial, perineural)
  - 3. Hemangiomatosis
  - 4. Glomus tumor
  - 5. Hemangiopericytoma
  - 6. Papillary endothelial hyperplasia (intravascular vegetant hemangioendothelioma of Masson)
- B. Intermediate
  - 1. Hemangioendothelioma
    - a. Epithelioid
    - b. Spindle cell
    - c. Malignant endovascular papillary angioendothelioma
- C. Malignant
  - 1. Hemangiosarcoma
  - 2. Kaposi's sarcoma
  - 3. Malignant glomus tumor
  - 4. Malignant hemangiopericytoma

VI. *Tumors of Lymph Vessels*

- A. Benign
  - 1. Lymphangioma
    - a. Cavernous
    - b. Cystic (cystic hygroma)
  - 2. Lymphangiomatosis
  - 3. Lymphangiomyoma and lymphangiomyomatosis
- B. Malignant
  - 1. Angiosarcoma

VII. *Tumors and Tumor-Like Lesions of Synovial Tissue*

- A. Benign
  - 1. Giant cell tumor of tendon sheath
    - a. Localized (nodular tenosynovitis)
    - b. Diffuse (florid synovitis)
- B. Malignant
  - 1. Synovial sarcoma (malignant synovioma), predominantly
    - a. Biphasic (fibrous and epithelial)
    - b. Monophasic (fibrous or epithelial)
  - 2. Malignant giant cell tumor of tendon sheath

VIII. *Tumors of Mesothelial Tissue*

- A. Benign
  - 1. Localized fibrous mesothelioma (subserosal fibroma)
  - 2. Multicystic peritoneal mesothelioma
  - 3. Mesothelioma of the genital tract (adenomatoid tumor)
- B. Malignant
  - 1. Diffuse and localized mesothelioma, predominantly
    - a. Epithelial
    - b. Fibrous
    - c. Biphasic

IX. *Tumors and Tumor-Like Lesions of Peripheral Nerves*

- A. Benign
  - 1. Traumatic neuroma
  - 2. Morton's neuroma
  - 3. Neuromuscular hamartoma
  - 4. Nerve sheath ganglion
  - 5. Neurilemoma (benign schwannoma)
  - 6. Neurofibroma, solitary
    - a. Localized
    - b. Diffuse
    - c. Pacinian
    - d. Pigmented
  - 7. Granular cell tumor
  - 8. Neurofibromatosis (von Recklinghausen's disease)
    - a. Localized
    - b. Plexiform
    - c. Diffuse
  - 9. Pigmented neuroectodermal tumor of infancy (retinal anlage tumor)
  - 10. Ectopic meningioma
  - 11. Nasal glioma
  - 12. Neurothekeoma
- B. Malignant
  - 1. Malignant schwannoma, including malignant schwannoma with rhabdomyoblastic differentiation (malignant Triton tumor), glandular malignant schwannoma, and epithelioid malignant schwannoma
  - 2. Peripheral tumors of primitive neuroectodermal tissues (Neuroepithelioma)
  - 3. Malignant pigmented neuroectodermal tumor of infancy (retinal anlage tumor)
  - 4. Malignant granular cell tumor

X. *Tumors of Autonomic Ganglia*

- A. Benign
  - 1. Ganglioneuroma
  - 2. Melanocytic schwannoma
- B. Malignant
  - 1. Neuroblastoma
  - 2. Ganglioneuroblastoma
  - 3. Malignant melanocytic schwannoma

XI. *Tumors of Paraganglionic Structures*

- A. Benign
  - 1. Paraganglioma (solitary, multiple, familial)
- B. Malignant
  - 1. Malignant paraganglioma

XII. *Tumors and Tumor-Like Lesions of Cartilage and Bone-Forming Tissues*

- A. Benign
  - 1. Panniculitis ossificans
  - 2. Myositis ossificans
  - 3. Fibrodysplasia (myositis) ossificans progressiva
  - 4. Extraskeletal chondroma
  - 5. Extraskeletal osteoma
- B. Malignant
  - 1. Extraskeletal chondrosarcoma
    - a. Well-differentiated
    - b. Myxoid (chordoid sarcoma)
    - c. Mesenchymal
  - 2. Extraskeletal osteosarcoma

XIII. *Tumors and Tumor-Like Lesions of Pluripotential mesenchyme*

- A. Benign
  - 1. Mesenchymoma
- B. Malignant
  - 1. Malignant mesenchymoma

(*continued*)

TABLE 40-3. Histologic Classification of Soft Tissue Tumors (*continued*)

XIV. Tumors and Tumor-Like Lesions of Disputed or Uncertain Histogenesis

A. Benign
1. Congenital granular cell tumor
2. Tumoral calcinosis
3. Myxoma (cutaneous and intramuscular)
4. Aggressive angiomyxoma
5. Amyloid tumor
6. Parachordoma

B. Malignant
1. Alveolar soft part sarcoma
2. Epithelioid sarcoma
3. Clear cell sarcoma of tendons and aponeuroses (malignant melanoma of soft parts)
4. Extraskeletal Ewing's sarcoma

XV. Unclassified Soft Tissue Tumors and Tumor-Like Lesions

Enzinger FM, Weiss SW: Soft Tissue Tumors, 2nd ed. St. Louis, CV Mosby, 1988.

tissues in a fashion characteristic of true sarcomas. It is important to distinguish these locally aggressive, nonmetastasizing lesions from those that are truly benign or malignant because of the therapeutic implications. Injury may provoke proliferative lesions in soft tissues. These can mimic soft tissue tumors, and because of their high mitotic rate, they are often difficult to distinguish from malignant lesions. An example is myositis ossificans.

For each histologically distinct malignant sarcoma, the tendency to metastasize depends on the grade of the tumor. In general, low-grade sarcomas are capable of aggressive, invasive local growth but tend not to disseminate. High-grade tumors are more likely to metastasize. In a survey of 4550 sarcoma patients, Lawrence and colleagues found approximately 33% of the tumors had a low-grade classification and the others were high-grade lesions.[46] Assigning a pathologic grade to an individual tumor as a means of predicting clinical behavior has not been easy. The general criteria for grading —mitotic rate, nuclear morphology, degree of cellularity, cellular anaplasia or pleomorphism, and the presence of necrosis—are not readily quantifiable. However, sarcomas of the various histologic types can be assigned a numerical grade. The range of grades attributed to the more common types of sarcoma is presented in Figure 40-1.[50]

Costa and colleagues at the National Cancer Institute (NCI) correlated histologic features, such as histologic type, number of mitoses, degrees of necrosis, pleomorphism, cellularity, and matrix of the primary lesion, with the overall prognoses of these patients.[53] Stratified analyses revealed that the degree of necrosis was the single best histopathologic parameter that predicted both the time to recurrence and the overall survival of patients ($p = 0.025$ and $p = 0.002$, respectively). These authors proposed a grading system using the degree of necrosis to distinguish aggressive lesions. Grade II lesions were high-grade tumors with either no or minimal necrosis, and Grade III lesions were high-grade lesions with moderate or marked necrosis.[53] When using this criterion alone, a significant difference was seen between the prognoses of patients with Grades II and III lesions. This system was independently confirmed by Lack and co-workers, who reviewed 300 extremity sarcomas and found the degree of necrosis to be the most significant determinant in predicting time to recurrence and overall survival.[54] However, there was only a 64% concordance rate in assigning a grade to 87 extremity soft tissue sarcomas that were previously reviewed by Costa and colleagues.[54]

A somewhat more elaborate grading system has been proposed by Trojani and associates using tumor differentiation, mitosis count, and the degree of tumor necrosis to predict the prognoses of patients with high-grade sarcomas.[55] Using this grading system, Coindre and co-workers reported a 75% concordance in grading 25 soft tissue sarcomas between an experienced panel of pathologists and a study group of 15 pathologists who had not been involved in the development of the grading system.[51] Despite more accurate grading criteria, there are still observer-related variations in grade determination. In time, it is expected that a standard grading system will be developed which will be reproducible.

Routine light microscopy, histochemistry, electron microscopy, and tissue culture studies all play a role in distinguishing one tumor subtype from another. In recent years, much progress has been made in the pathologic classification of the soft tissue sarcomas; a variety of new lesions have been identified and characterized.[50] The classification in

FIG. 40-1. Soft tissue sarcomas. Estimated range of degree of malignancy based on histologic type and grade. Grade within the overall range depends on specific histologic features such as cellularity, cellular pleomorphism, mitotic activity, amount of stroma, infiltrative or expansive growth, and necrosis. (Enzinger FM, Weiss SW: Soft Tissue Tumors, 2nd ed. St Louis, CV Mosby, 1988)

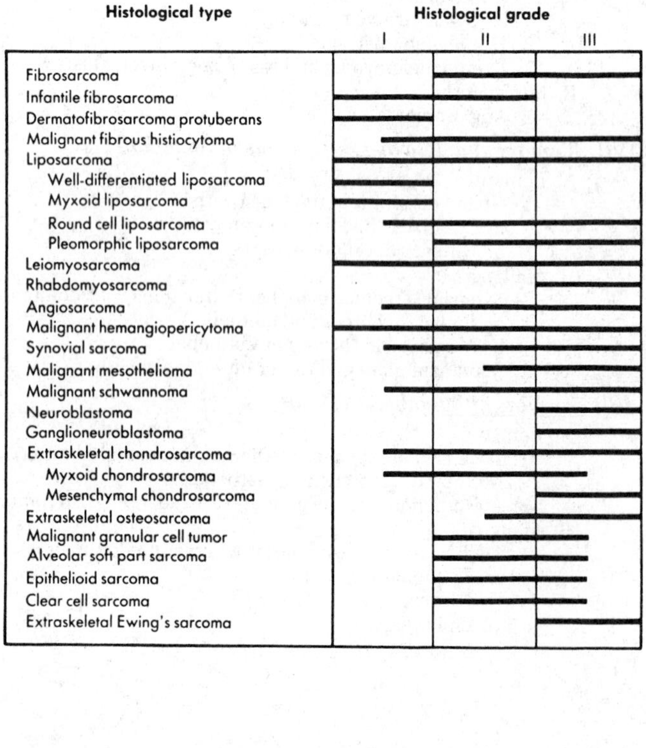

Table 40-3 distinguishes tumors that are benign, tumors that are benign with aggressive local growth requiring vigorous local treatment, and malignant tumors. Frequently, it is difficult to assign definite cells of origin for all benign and malignant tumors. In these instances, the assignment made in the classification in Table 40-3 has been quite arbitrary. Highly undifferentiated tumors may be designated as soft tissue sarcoma, type unspecified. For some tumors, such as epithelioid sarcomas and alveolar soft-part sarcomas, the cells of origin are unknown even though the tumors are not poorly differentiated. This is indicated in Table 40-3.

The pathologist may not feel comfortable with any specific histologic designation and may report the tumor as sarcoma, unclassified type, and this may apply even to a Grade 1 lesion. Knowledge of the histologic grade is critical to developing the proper management strategy, and the clinician should review the slides with the pathologist and obtain a statement about grade, even if the pathologist does not wish to specify cell type.

MALIGNANT LESION CLASSIFICATION

Competent pathologists differ in attaching a histogenic label to types of soft tissue sarcomas. These disagreements confound attempts to compare reports from different institutions about the incidence of histologic subtypes, frequency of tumors at different anatomic sites, stage of disease at presentation, frequency of local failure with different treatment modalities, and frequency of distant metastasis. This is particularly evident in Table 40-4, which collates the relative frequency of the various histopathologic types in several series.[38-40,44,56-63] The large differences in the incidence of different histopathologic types almost certainly reflect the differences in diagnostic criteria used by the pathologists. For example, in the series reported by Shieber and Graham and by Ferrell and Frable, there are no lesions that are considered as unclassifiable sarcomas.[38,40] In contrast, Hare and Cerny had 28.5%, Pack and Ariel had 36.4%, and Potter and co-workers had 9.5% unclassifiable sarcomas.[39,44,56] A further example of these disparities is illustrated by the 5.4% incidence of fibrosarcomas in the series by Pack and Ariel, compared with the 37% to 44% incidence of fibrosarcomas in the series reported by Simon and Enneking, Hare and Cerny, and Shieber and Graham.[38,39,56,59]

Changes in histologic classification of lesions, such as the recognition of a separate category of malignant fibrous histiocytomas, has also lead to wide variations in the reported incidence of soft tissue sarcomas. For example, in the five series listed in Table 40-4 published before 1972, no cases of malignant fibrous histiocytomas were reported. Since 1972, this lesion has gained increasing recognition, and the 20.4% incidence reported in the series by Simon and Enneking in 1976 is comparable to the 17.5% incidence reported by Lindberg and associates, 22.8% reported by Potter and co-workers, 15.6% reported by Suit, 14.6% reported by Collin and colleagues, and 25.9% reported by Lawrence and colleagues.[44,47,59,61-63]

Presant and colleagues reviewed 216 consecutive sarcoma patients in the Southeastern Cancer Study Group experience and found concordance in histopathologic diagnoses in only 66% of cases.[52] The diagnoses of the primary member institution and a pathology review panel were compared. Coindre and co-workers reported only a 61% concordance among pathologists in assigning histologic type in 25 soft tissue sarcomas.[51] The available evidence indicates that the histopathologic grade is the most important indicator of the biologic behavior of soft tissue sarcomas and is of more value to the clinician than is the exact histopathologic type.[50,53-55] When histologic grade is accounted for, most soft tissue sarcomas have a common biologic behavior. In the series of 211 high-grade extremity sarcomas reviewed by Potter and co-workers, histologic subtype was not a significant determinant of disease-free or overall survival (Fig. 40-2).[64] The difficulties in pathologic classification and its negligible importance in arbitrating therapy compel the treatment of soft tissue sarcomas as a group.

TABLE 40-4. Relative Incidence (%) of Histologic Types of Soft Tissue Sarcomas in Various Studies

	Study											
	Shieber and Graham[38] (1962)	*Hare and Cerny[39] (1963)*	*Pack and Ariel[56] (1964)*	*Martin et al[57] (1965)*	*Ferrell and Frable[40] (1972)*	*Shiu et al[58] (1975)*	*Simon and Enneking[59] (1976)*	*Russell et al[60] (1977)*	*Lindberg et al[61] (1977)*	*Suit[62] (1983)*	*Potter et al[44] (1984)*	*Collins et al[63] (1986)*
Sites	All	All	All	All	All	Extremity	Extremity	All	All	All	All	Extremity
Total no. of cases	125	200	717	398	117	297	54	1215	166	315	307	315
Type of Soft-Tissue Sarcomas												
Unclassified	0	28.5	36.4	14.8	0	7.1	5.6	10.0	6.0	16.5	9.5	1.0
Liposarcoma	16.0	11.5	14.6	26.9	17.0	27.6	18.5	18.2	12.7	15.2	18.3	33.9
Rhabdomyosarcoma	16.0	5.0	13.9	20.6	30.0	17.5	5.6	19.3	9.6	4.1	2.9	9.2
Synoviosarcoma	0.8	2.5	8.4	3.0	2.5	14.1	5.6	6.9	10.2	3.8	19.5	12.6
Neurofibrosarcoma	3.2	0	6.4	0	0	5.4	0	4.9	19.3	6.0	6.8	7.6
Fibrosarcoma	44.0	43.0	5.4	24.1	33.0	20.2	37.0	19.0	13.3	16.8	3.6	12.3
Angiosarcoma	4.8	0	2.6	0.3	0	2.0	0	2.7	1.2	3.2	1.6	1.2
Leiomyosarcoma	6.4	6.5	0	6.3	4.0	2.4	0	6.5	4.2	7.6	11.4	3.8
Mesenchymoma	0	0	0	0	0	0.3	0	0.3	0	0.9	0	0
Malignant fibrous histiocytoma	0	0	0	0	0	1.0	20.4	10.5	17.5	15.6	22.8	14.6
Other	8.8	3.0	12.1	4.0	13.5	2.4	7.4	1.7	6.0	10.2	3.6	3.4

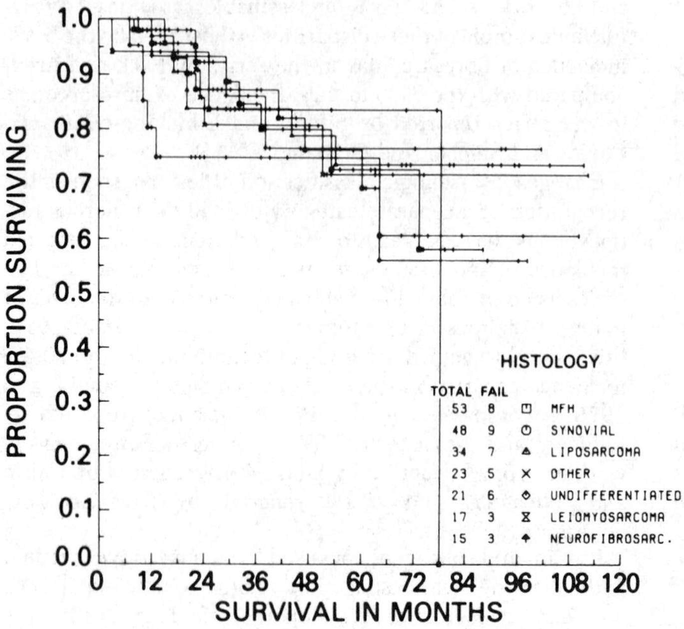

FIG. 40-2. Actuarial analysis of overall survival for 211 patients with high-grade extremity sarcomas categorized by histologic subtype. There are no significant differences between the groups. (Potter DA, Kinsella T, Glatstein E et al: High grade soft tissue sarcomas of the extremities. Cancer 58:190–205, 1986)

BENIGN TUMORS OF SOFT TISSUE

BENIGN TUMORS OF FIBROUS ORIGIN

There are many variants of fibrous tumors that are nonmalignant and do not metastasize. Most are successfully treated by simple excision and do not recur. Some tumors in this category, such as nodular fasciitis, can be mistaken for true fibrosarcomas. Others, such as extra-abdominal desmoid tumors, require special attention because aggressive local therapy is necessary to prevent recurrence.

Fibroma

"Fibroma" has been applied to any benign fibrous growth. Many congenital malformations and reparative tissue growths fall into this category. With increased understanding of the variants of fibrous tissue neoplasms, fewer tumors are called fibromas, and the term is now restricted to benign, encapsulated, fibrous nodules that seldom grow larger than a few centimeters in diameter. A subcutaneous or soft fibroma (fibroma molle) is a pedunculated subcutaneous growth composed of fibrous tissue and fat covered by epidermis. Fibroma durum is a pedunculated lesion, often arising in the oral mucosa, that may result from malocclusion or malfitting dentures. All of these lesions should be treated by simple excision. They rarely recur.

Elastofibroma

Elastofibroma is a rare lesion that usually occurs under the scapular muscles and frequently attaches to the ribcage.[65–68] Many are not noticed, and one series found them present in 10% of 235 autopsy cases.[66] The lesions are totally benign and do not recur after simple enucleation.

Palmar and Plantar Fibromatosis

Tumor-like proliferations of the palmar and plantar aponeuroses can give rise to tumor-like nodules.[69–72] Only the palmar fibromatosis (Dupuytren's contracture) is associated with flexion contractures. Heredity affects incidence, and lesions occur six times as often in men as in women. The lesions grow slowly as localized nodular enlargements that can infiltrate the fascia and involve overlying skin and subcutaneous tissue. The lesions are benign, although they have a tendency to recur after simple excision. Consequently, small nodules should be left untouched. If excision is necessary, attempts should be made to widely excise the palmar or plantar fascia.

Juvenile Aponeurotic Fibroma (Keasby Tumor)

This form of fibromatosis affects the palms or soles of children and young adults.[73–75] The lesion can infiltrate and overgrow subcutaneous fat and muscle, but metastases never occur. The lesions invade locally and have a tendency to recur after limited excision. Thus, attempts to achieve negative microscopic margins should be made.

Congenital Generalized Fibromatosis

This generalized condition, usually present at birth, is characterized by multiple, widely scattered, nodular and infiltrating fibroblastic lesions, diffusely present in the superficial and deep tissues, viscera, and bone.[76–78] The disease is usually fatal because of vital organ involvement.

Fibrous Hamartoma of Infancy

Fibrous hamartoma occurs predominantly in boys and presents in the first year of life with a solitary mass in the axilla, upper extremity, head, or neck.[79] These lesions are situated almost exclusively in the dermis or subcutaneous fat and can become large. Local excision is almost always curative: this lesion does not metastasize.

Fibromatosis Colli

This distinctive form of fibromatosis develops in the sternocleidomastoid muscle of newborn or very young children. In many cases, a small lump in the sternocleidomastoid muscle noticed in the newborn disappears spontaneously.[80,81] If, however, the lesion persists for several months after birth, it will increase in size and often lead to the development of neck contractures. Untreated cases can result in very large growths, with subsequent spread to the trachea and surrounding organs. These lesions should be excised and often require removal of the entire sternocleidomastoid muscle.

Penile Fibromatosis

Also called Peyronie's disease, penile fibromatosis involves a circumscribed fibrous thickening arising in the connective tissue sheath that separates the corpus cavernosum from the tunic albuginea.[82] It causes pain and curvature of the penis on penile erection. Surgical excision of the fibrous tissue is the preferred treatment.

Nodular Fasciitis

This benign lesion, also called pseudosarcomatous or proliferative fasciitis, should be treated by simple excision. Its morphologic appearance causes it to be confused with fibrosarcoma.[83-86] These lesions generally arise in the subcutaneous fascia or the superficial portions of the deep fascia. The growth of these lesions is frequently rapid after they appear. Maximum size is usually achieved within a few weeks and then growth stops. These lesions rarely grow larger than 5 cm and are often asymptomatic. Fewer than 10% recur after simple excision.

Desmoid Tumors

Desmoid tumors, also known as aggressive fibromatosis or musculoaponeurotic fibromatosis, derive primarily from fascial sheaths and musculoaponeurotic structures throughout the body. They differ from most fibrous growths by their tendency to infiltrate extensively into surrounding structures.[87-102]

The term "abdominal desmoid tumor" refers to lesions found in the muscular aponeurotic structures of the abdominal wall, especially in postpartum women.[90] The lesions are thought to be reparative and to have been initiated by the effects of pregnancy on the abdominal wall musculature. If the lesions are resected with good margins, they do not recur. Because of the anatomic location, the lesions are usually seen when they are small, and surgical resection is straightforward.

Extra-abdominal desmoid tumors may present more problems to the physician because they occur in sites where wide-field radical resection is not technically feasible; if attempted, it may be associated with appreciable morbidity. These lesions are not uncommon around the shoulder girdle, inguinal region, and lower extremities. They are unencapsulated, infiltrate locally, and are destructive but do not metastasize. Histopathologically, these lesions are primarily fibroblastic with elongated, thin, delicate nuclei, which appear virtually normal. Mitotic figures are uncommon, usually less than 1 per 50 high-power field.

The preferred treatment for extra-abdominal desmoid is wide-field resection, with care to achieve negative margins in all dimensions.[103] Local recurrence of these lesions, where margins were close or positive, occurs in 50% to 75% of the cases. In situations in which wide resection is not feasible, radiation therapy may be an effective treatment. James Ewing, in 1928, commented that desmoid tumors responded to radiation, but slowly, and that this treatment could be considered for lesions not amenable to surgical resection.[91] Successful treatment by radiation has been reported in an incidental way in describing results of large surgical series.[92]

Benninghoff and Robbins described the treatment of 4 patients with desmoid tumors, 3 of whom were treated after incomplete surgery and 1 for frank recurrent tumor.[93] Radiation doses were modest, but good responses were obtained at least in 3 of 4 patients. Greenberg and co-workers reported long-term control in 8 or 9 patients with desmoid tumors treated by radiation alone or in combination with surgery.[94] Wara and associates reported on a series of 16 patients with desmoid tumors, 12 of whom were treated for gross tumor (*i.e.*, tumor masses greater than 5 cm).[96] Two of these 12 died of disease, but the remaining 10 were alive without tumor 2 to 6 years after treatment. Of the 4 patients treated after incomplete surgical resection (no palpable tumor), there was 1 local recurrence at 2 years; the other 3 patients were free of evident disease at 2 to 4 years.

Suit and Russell described the results of treatment of 4 patients with desmoid tumor, 2 of whom had massive local disease and 2 of whom were treated after incomplete surgery.[97] All 4 remained disease free for 5 years. Seventeen patients treated by radiation therapy for desmoid tumors at the Massachusetts General Hospital and followed for more than 12 months were reported by Kiel and Suit.[98] Ten were treated by radiation alone and 7 by radiation and surgery. There have been 3 local failures; 2 of 10 after radiation and 1 of 7 after radiation and surgery. However, 2 of the failures developed after doses of only 22 and 24 Gy. Of 15 patients who received doses >50 Gy, there has been 1 local failure (follow-up, 12–96 months). For the patient who has uncertain or minimally positive margins at the first resection, and re-resection is not feasible, the patient should be observed and treatment implemented at the first sign of regrowth. In these circumstances local failure is not universal; a worthwhile proportion of patients may be able to avoid high-dose radiation treatment. At the Massachusetts General Hospital eight patients with uncertain or minimally positive margins after resection have been followed, and only one recurred (this patient was reresected and is now free of disease).[98]

There are reports that hormonal or antihormonal medication may achieve long-term remission of desmoid tumors. Kinzbrunner and colleagues described a patient with a 16-kg desmoid tumor of the back that regressed to a 5 × 5 × 2 cm mass in 2 weeks with treatment with tamoxifen, 20 mg four times daily.[99] Further, Lanari described a small series of patients with desmoid tumors treated successfully with progesterone.[100] In yet another approach, Waddell and Gerner reported that administration of indomethacin and ascorbic acid could cause regression of desmoid tumors.[101] Because of these reports and the limited toxicity of these approaches, the use of these agents in the treatment of desmoid tumors deserves further clinical study.

BENIGN TUMORS OF STRIATED MUSCLE

Rhabdomyoma

These are extremely rare benign tumors of skeletal muscle, generally occurring in the tongue, neck muscles, larynx, uvula, nasal cavity, axilla, vulva, and heart.[104,105] These tumors are treated by simple excision.

BENIGN TUMORS OF SMOOTH MUSCLE

Leiomyoma

Leiomyomas rarely occur outside of the uterus and the gastrointestinal tract.[106,107] They can occur in the skin and subcutaneous tissues and probably arise from the smooth muscle of small blood vessels in these tissues. These lesions are treated by simple excision.

Epithelioid Leiomyoma

Epithelioid leiomyoma (leiomyoblastoma) are most frequently found in the wall of the gastrointestinal tract, especially in the stomach. They are similar to other smooth muscle tumors but may become very large and hemorrhagic and exhibit small cystic areas. Simple excision is almost always curative.

BENIGN TUMORS OF ADIPOSE TISSUE

Lipomas

Lipomas are among the most common of all benign neoplasms and arise in any location where fat is normally present. These lesions may occur in deep tissue, although they are usually subcutaneous in origin. They are characteristically multilobulated masses of fatty tissue that vary from small nodules to large masses weighing several kilograms.

Multiple lipomatosis is a condition of diffuse overgrowths that may occur throughout the body. These are not true tumors and are probably a result of fat metabolism disorders.

Spindle cell lipomas are rare benign tumors that occur almost exclusively in the neck and shoulders of males.[108] The major importance of these tumors is their tendency to be confused with liposarcomas.

Angiolipomas are lipomas containing a network of many small capillaries and are usually quite painful.[109] Some angiolipomas are of an infiltrating variety and require a wider margin of resection than most lipomas.

The treatment for lipomas is simple enucleation. Recurrence is extremely unusual after this limited treatment is used.

Lipoblastomatosis

This rare abnormality, also called adipose hamartomatosis, is found in infants. It consists of lobular soft tissue growths separated by partitions of loose fibrous tissue.[91,110,111] About 10% of these lesions recur after simple local excision, but they have no tendency to metastasize.

Atypical Lipoma

Atypical lipomas are a recent designation applied to subcutaneous lipomatous neoplasms that display cytologic atypia not seen in most lipomas.[112–115] These lesions occur in either the subcutaneous or deep muscular layers. Simple excision cures virtually all subcutaneous lesions, although simple excision of deep muscular lesions often results in local recurrence that may require re-excision. These lesions have no tendency to metastasize and can be controlled by re-excision.

Hibernoma

Hibernomas are an unusual type of lipoma that are thought to arise from vestiges of brown fat similar to the glandular, brown adipose tissue occurring in certain hibernating animal species.[116] These are benign tumors and should be treated by simple excision.

BENIGN TUMORS OF SYNOVIAL TISSUE

Giant Cell Tumor of Tendon Sheath

These benign lesions, also called localized nodular tenosynovitis, are usually solitary and arise from either the tendon sheath, joints or bursae of the hand, palm, or wrist.[117,118] These soft tissue lesions can produce atrophy of the bony cortex or actual erosion into adjacent bone. Simple excision is the treatment of choice. Villonodular synovitis is probably related to giant cell tumor of tendon sheath but almost always occurs in joints and presents with pain and swelling. This benign tumor-like growth erodes the bone and appears to be a primary bone tumor. The synovium of the affected joint is generally diffusely involved, and total synovectomy is the treatment of choice.

Ganglion

Ganglions are multilocular, fibrous-walled cysts, usually occurring on the dorsal aspect of the wrist. These lesions form as a result of synovial tissue that has become pinched off and undergoes degeneration. Simple excision is almost always curative.

BENIGN TUMORS OF NEURAL TISSUE

Neurilemoma

These are benign, encapsulated tumors, also called schwannomas, that almost always occur as solitary lesions.[50,119] The most common site of origin is the eight cranial nerve (acoustic neuroma), although cranial peripheral nerves are often affected. This is also the most common benign neoplasm of the spinal canal. These lesions often grow with an easily demonstrable flattened nerve seen along its capsule. These lesions rarely recur when resected locally. Every effort should be made to preserve the nerve involved if this nerve is of clinical significance (*e.g.*, the facial nerve). These lesions arise from Schwann cells, although they are different from neurofibromas.

Neurofibroma

Neurofibromas are thought to arise from Schwann cells, although they differ from neurilemomas in that they tend not to be encapsulated and have a much softer consistency. They may also occur at many different sites. These lesions may be locally infiltrative, although simple excision is almost always curative.

Multiple neurofibromas are a feature of Von Recklinghausen's disease, which is an autosomal dominant disorder that occurs once in 3000 live births.[120–129] In this condition, neurofibromas may occur in virtually all sites of the body and be associated with virtually any peripheral nerve or intraspinal nerves. Plexiform neurofibromas may result in massive enlargement of an extremity. About 10–15% of patients with Von Recklinghausen's disease develop a malignant schwannoma, and these malignant tumors can arise in benign, superficial neurofibromas. Neurofibromas in Von Recklinghausen's disease should be removed either for cosmetic reasons or if they become painful or undergo rapid enlargement. In a recent long-term study of 212 patients with neurofibromatosis, 57 developed malignant tumors; 21 patients developed cancers of the central nervous system, 6 developed cancers of the peripheral nervous system, and the remainder developed cancers at other sites.[129]

BENIGN TUMORS OF VASCULAR TISSUE

Hemangioma

Hemangiomas are vascular neoplasms that can occur anywhere in the body.[130–132] About 75% are present at birth, and about 60% occur in the head and neck area. The majority of hemangiomas of infancy will spontaneously regress. Some lesions grow rapidly during the early months of life and may be a source of some concern, although virtually all disappear by about 5 years of age. These lesions may be primarily composed of capillaries or widely dilated veins (cavernous hemangioma). These lesions do not metastasize, and simple excision will often be curative, although it is not necessary except for cosmetic reasons. In some instances, the hemangioma may exhibit rapid growth and abut on or compromise vital structures. In these instances, low-dose radiation confined to the hemangioma may be used. Efforts should be made to use techniques that limit the dose to the vascular process itself. Radiation treatment for these lesions is rarely indicated, and even large medical centers probably would not see more than three or four cases per decade for which radiation treatment would be warranted.

Lymphangioma

These lesions are similar to hemangiomas, although the vascular spaces do not contain blood cells. These lesions can occur virtually anywhere in the body. Cystic hygromas are lymphangiomas of the neck. Virtually all lesions require surgical excision. The extent of the procedure should be dictated by the location and the desire to achieve a reasonable cosmetic result.

Glomus Tumors

The normal glomus is a 1-mm end organ arteriovenous anastomosis.[133–136] This organ enlarges into a painful and tender mass. About 15% are present in the subungual regions, although any location in the skin and soft tissue is possible. Local excision is usually curative, and metastases do not occur. Glomus tumors may be located along the larger vessels. A common syndrome is that of the glomus tumor near the jugular foramen, designated as a glomus jugulari. These lesions are not resectable and are effectively treated by radiation therapy (5000 cGy delivered over about 5 weeks). Lesions regress slowly, but permanent control of the process is regularly achieved.

Infantile Hemangiopericytomas

Although hemangiopericytomas in the adult are more benign in their behavior than most soft tissue sarcomas, these tumors can definitely metastasize and will therefore be considered under the truly malignant lesions.[136,137] However, hemangiopericytomas that occur in infancy appear to be benign lesions without significant metastatic potential. These tumors occur almost exclusively in the skin and may have evidence of infiltrative growth outside the main tumor mass. These lesions generally do not recur after wide local excision.

BENIGN TUMORS OF HISTIOCYTIC TISSUE

In recent years, significant improvement in our understanding and recognition of tumors of presumed histiocytic origin has taken place largely due to the work of Stout and colleagues.[49,50] Variants of these tumors have received over 30 different names in a variety of nomenclature systems. These tumors are composed wholly or in part of cells with the morphologic characteristics of histiocytes and with various fibroblastic components. It is thought that these tumors are of purely histiocytic origin, but that histiocytes in these lesions can differentiate toward fibroblastic morphology.

Dermatofibroma

These are common soft tissue lesions also called sclerosing hemangioma or fibrous xanthoma of skin, that are usually about 1 cm in diameter and occur in the dermis. Simple excision is always curative.

Fibrous Histiocytoma

Many variants of this lesion, also called fibrous xanthoma, exist.[49,50,138] Superficially located histiocytic lesions behave in a very benign manner, although deep, benign histiocytomas may invade locally into surrounding tissue. These lesions can occur anywhere in the body. Superficial lesions are always cured by simple excision; a wider margin of normal tissue should be obtained for deep, benign fibrous histiocytomas. Local recurrence is uncommon.

Atypical Fibrous Histiocytomas

Although superficial fibrous histiocytomas are always totally benign and cured by simple excision, deep fibrous histiocytomas may have a more atypical morphologic appearance and are more ominous in their tendency to recur locally.[139–141] Although superficial lesions may occasionally fit the criteria for atypical histiocytoma (3 of 18 atypical fibrous histiocytomas reported by Soule and co-workers), almost all are located deep in soft tissue or muscle.[139] Despite the absence of obvious anaplasia, a rapidly growing, deeply occurring fibrous histiocytoma may achieve a diameter of 6 cm or greater; over half of these lesions will recur after simple excision. These lesions usually do not metastasize, although very rare reports of metastases following many local recurrences for lesions with this histology have been reported. Recommended therapy includes wide local excision, with negative microscopic margins in all directions. Recurrent local extension of these tumors, especially in the retroperitoneal area, can lead to death as a result of inadequate local treatment at first resection.

Dermatofibrosarcoma Protuberans

These lesions can occur in any part of the body.[142–147] The exact histogenesis is not known, although a histiocytic origin is likely. These lesions most often begin as indurated nodules in the skin that grow slowly and are therefore often ignored until they are large. They show an extremely aggressive tendency to invade surrounding local tissue; they should be regarded as malignant neoplasms. They do not metastasize, however, even after multiple recurrences. About 50% will recur after simple excision, and a wide excision including a wide margin of surrounding tissue should be achieved in therapy.[147] The first resection is of major importance, because tumor spread at the inadequate first resection may lead to uncontrollable local growth. These benign lesions may ultimately lead to amputation of extremities or even death because of extensive invasion of vital organs. Many of the comments regarding use of radiation therapy discussed under the treatment of desmoid tumors may apply here as well.[94–98] In a review of the NCI experience with locally aggressive but nonmetastasizing soft tissue tumors seen between 1975 and 1982, Glenn and co-workers identified 35 cases that were completely resected. Twenty patients received radiation therapy postoperatively, and 1 tumor recurred. One recurrence was seen in 15 patients treated by surgery alone. Follow-up in this study ranged from 12 to 97 months, with a median of 36 months.

If surgical treatment of dermatofibrosarcoma protuberans is not feasible or requires a very radical procedure, consideration should be given to radiation therapy in combination with conservative surgery, or radiation therapy alone in special circumstances can be used.[148]

BENIGN TUMORS OF MESOTHELIAL TISSUE

Mesothelioma

The cells lining the pleura, peritoneum, and pericardium are mesothelial cells. Although most tumors of mesothelial tissue are malignant, benign tumors can occur, usually in the pleura. These lesions project outwardly from the viscera or parietal pleura into the adjacent cavity but do not infiltrate aggressively into local tissue. These may grow to be quite large, and simple excision is usually curative.

BENIGN TUMORS OF UNCERTAIN TISSUE ORIGIN

Granular Cell Myoblastoma

These small tumors rarely grow larger than 6 cm and can be cured by local excision.[149] When these lesions develop beneath the epidermis or mucous membranes, they can lead to squamous tissue proliferation, possibly mimicking a squamous cell carcinoma.

Mesenchymoma

These benign tumors, also referred to as hamartoma or mixed mesodermal tumor, are composed of at least two different mesenchymal elements.[150] Lesions often contain smooth muscle, skeletal muscle, fat, and angiomatous and osseous tissue in various combinations. Though most lesions are malignant, rare benign forms have been described. Benign tumors are generally small, and none of the individual elements contain cells with atypical or anaplastic appearance. Local excision is adequate therapy.

Myxoma

Myxoma is thought to arise from embryonic rests and is composed of spindle cells imbedded in a mucinous intercellular matrix.[151,152] It can occur in any of the soft tissues, bone, or occasionally in the heart and genitourinary tract. When these lesions develop in the soft tissues, they are generally in close relationship to a large muscle or aponeurosis. They are cured by local excision. Deep tumors can sometimes infiltrate contiguous structures, although even in this situation local resection is almost always curative.

There are many other less common benign tumors of soft tissue.[50]

DIAGNOSIS OF SOFT TISSUE SARCOMAS

Soft tissue sarcomas most often present as asymptomatic soft tissue masses. Because these lesions arise in compressible tissues and are often far from vital organs, symptoms are few until the lesions are quite large, compared with the anatomic part. For example, a sarcoma will often present at 8 to 15 cm in the thigh or buttock, 3 to 4 cm in the wrist, but only 0.5 to 1 cm around the digits. Symptoms generally result from pressure or traction on adjacent nerves or muscles. There are no reliable physical signs to distinguish between benign and malignant soft tissue lesions; consequently, all soft tissue lumps that persist or grow should be biopsied. Even very soft and pliable subcutaneous lumps, thought to be lipomas, can occasionally prove surprising. Leaving soft tissue lumps in place without biopsy is justified only if they have been present and unchanged for many years before being observed by the physician.

The nature of the biopsy of soft tissue sarcomas is an important aspect of the overall management of these patients. Because the biopsy site must be removed in any definitive resection, care should be taken to place the biopsy incision at a location and orientation that will not compromise subsequent surgical excision.

Aspiration or needle biopsy should not play a major role in the diagnosis of primary soft tissue sarcoma. Despite detailed descriptions of the histopathologic characteristics of the various sarcomas of soft tissue by Enzinger and Weiss, Hajdu, and other pathologists, the subtle distinctions necessary to distinguish benign from malignant variants and distinguish among the several types of soft tissue sarcomas are often not possible with the small samples obtained by needle techniques.[47,50] A large sample of tissue is often necessary to assign the accurate diagnosis and grade of soft tissue sarcomas. Special studies (*e.g.*, tissue culture and electron microscopy) that may be necessary for accurate diagnosis rarely are obtained from tissue in a needle biopsy. Because therapy is often determined by the histologic grade of the lesion, a generous sample of tissue is necessary.

Soft tissue sarcomas grow in the path of least resistance and push surrounding tissue before them. This surrounding tissue forms a pseudocapsule and always contains invasive prongs of malignant tissue. For this reason, shelling out soft tissue sarcomas is never curative. In fact, excision through the pseudocapsule often spreads tumor into surrounding tissue and can greatly complicate further surgical treatment. For this reason, excisional biopsy is an appropriate means of establishing a diagnosis only for soft tissue sarcomas smaller than 3 cm in diameter. The appropriate surgical technique for diagnosing any soft tissue sarcoma larger than 3 cm in diameter is an incisional biopsy. This technique allows for the acquisition of a generous wedge of tissue from the lesion and minimally disrupts the surrounding tissue planes. The incisional biopsy should be performed through a carefully placed small incision so as not to compromise subsequent radical excision of the lesion. Care should be taken to obtain excellent hemostasis. Hematomas resulting from biopsies of soft tissue sarcomas can spread tumor along their paths.

Although most experienced surgeons consider an incisional biopsy preferable to a limited excisional biopsy for the diagnosis of soft tissue sarcomas, a survey of surgical practices in the United States conducted by The American College of Surgeons showed that roughly half of the sarcomas were biopsied by excision.[46] This practice did not change during two intervals surveyed, 1977 to 1978 and 1983 to 1984 (Table 40-5). Only 20% of patients had a diagnosis established by incisional biopsy during these same periods.

The importance of the adequate placement of the biopsy incision cannot be overemphasized. Improper placement may preclude proper radical resection of the lesion and may lead to large increases in the radiation fields necessary to encompass all areas of possible spread. Incisions on the extremities should be placed longitudinally, so as not to compromise the muscle group excisions that may subsequently be necessary. At other sites, the incision should be parallel to the long axis of the underlying principal muscle. Biopsies of lesions in the buttocks should be placed as inferiorly as possible to allow for subsequent development of skin flaps if hemipelvectomy is necessary.

Planning surgical resection or radiation therapy requires a careful and detailed determination of the pattern of local spread and assessment of the tissues probably involved by microscopic disease. The physical examination determines the approximate size of the lesion, attachment to deep or superficial structures, relationship of the tumor to prior biopsy sites, functional status of the part, and presence of prior injury or concurrent medical disease that would confound the execution of the desired surgery or radiation. The radiographic evaluation of the patient with soft tissue sarcoma should include these procedures:[153–161]

1. Xerogram or soft tissue radiograph of the affected part
2. CT, MRI, or ultrasound through the affected region
3. CT or full-chest tomogram
4. Arteriogram in certain instances
5. Radionuclide bone scan

The most important diagnostic procedures in assessing the pattern of involvement of the primary lesion are CT (Fig. 40-3) or MRI scans (Fig. 40-4). High quality CT or MRI scans are essential because these techniques permit accurate delineation of the muscle compartment or anatomic structures involved by gross disease.

Chang and colleagues performed a prospective evaluation of preoperative CT and MRI scans in patients with extremity

TABLE 40-5. Biopsy Techniques Used for Sarcoma Diagnosis

Type of Biopsy	*1977–1978*		*1983–1984*	
	No.	*%*	*No.*	*%*
None	319	13.5	380	11.0
Needle	114	4.8	311	9.0
Incisional	466	19.8	753	21.8
Excisional	1210	51.4	1644	47.6
Other	139	5.9	278	8.0
Unknown	107	4.5	91	2.6
Total	2355	100.0	3457	100.0

Lawrence W Jr, Donegan WL, Nachimuth N et al: Adult soft tissue sarcomas. A pattern of care survey of the American College of Surgeons. Ann Surg 205:349–359, 1987

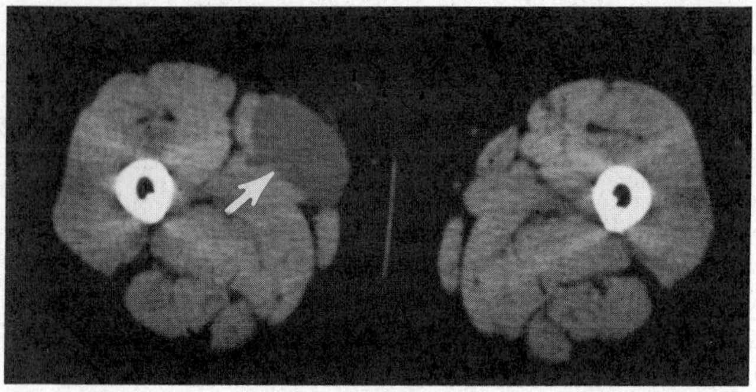

FIG. 40-3. Computed tomography scan of midthigh region in patient with a myxoid liposarcoma (*white arrow*). Transaxial orientation demonstrates relation to underlying muscle groups.

sarcomas.[160] Operative findings were correlated with the scans. Both CT and MRI were found to be comparable in evaluating the tumor's relationship to major neurovascular and skeletal structures. However, MRI demonstrated better visual contrast between tumor and muscle. MRI also has the advantage of displaying anatomy in coronal and sagittal views, whereas CT is restricted to transaxial views. Bland and colleagues reported that MRI was significantly better than CT in predicting resectability of 53 soft tissue sarcomas in various sites.[161] This was a result of the multiplanar imaging and improved visual contrast afforded by MRI.[161]

Arteriography can also delineate the position and status of major vessels and the local extent of disease, and it is particularly useful for estimating the proximity of tumor to major vessels, for determining the pattern of displacement or deviation of vessels, and for determining the encasement of a vessel by tumor, resulting in abrupt, irregular change in the caliber of the vessel, which is characteristic of neoplastic involvement.[157-159] The late venous phase can show the venous drainage, which should be controlled intraoperatively early in the course of surgery to prevent major embolization of tumor cells. An arteriogram is of minimal benefit in planning the treatment of recurrent tumors or the reoperation of incompletely excised lesions.

FIG. 40-4. T1-weighed MRI scan of same patient shown in Figure 40-3. This scan demonstrates excellent tumor to muscle contrast for this myxoid liposarcoma. The coronal image is helpful in defining the longitudinal extent of the tumor in the thigh.

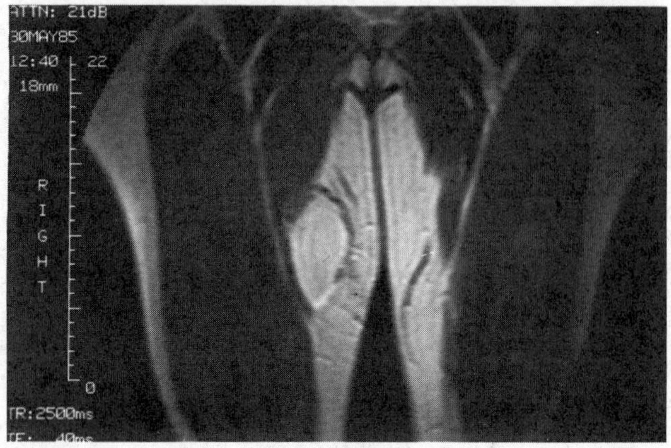

Although sarcomas rarely invade bone, assessment of soft tissue reaction in the periosteum and at the margin of soft tissues may be estimated by bone scan.[46,161a] A positive scan does not mean that the tumor has invaded bone or periosteum. A positive scan may simply be the consequence of periosteal reaction to the increased blood flow of a nearby tumor. This could serve as a guide to wide resection near the bone or to removing periosteum or a portion of the bone in the area that is positive on scan in those patients treated by surgery alone. Patients with positive bone scan and no radiographic periosteal reaction who are being treated by radiation and surgery should not have stripping of periosteum unless operative findings reveal fixation of the lesion to the bone.

Sarcomas of soft tissue infrequently metastasizes to regional lymph nodes, and lymphangiography is rarely indicated.[165]

TABLE 40-6. AJC Staging System for Soft Tissue Sarcomas

T Primary tumor	
T1 Tumor less than 5 cm	
T2 Tumor 5 cm or greater	
G Histologic grade of malignancy	
G1 Low	
G2 Moderate	
G3 High	
N Regional lymph nodes	
N0 No histologically verified metastases to regional lymph nodes	
N1 Histologically verified regional lymph node metastasis	
M Distant metastasis	
M0 No distant metastasis	
M1 Distant metastasis	
Stage I	
Stage IA G1T1N0M0	Grade 1 tumor less than 5 cm in diameter with no regional lymph node or distant metastases
Stage IB G1T2N0M0	Grade 1 tumor 5 cm or greater in diameter with no regional lymph node or distant metastases
Stage II	
Stage IIA G2T1N0M0	Grade 2 tumor less than 5 cm in diameter with no regional lymph node or distant metastases
Stage IIB G2T2N0M0	Grade 2 tumor 5 cm or greater in diameter with no regional lymph node or distant metastases
Stage III	
Stage IIIA G3T1N0M0	Grade 3 tumor less than 5 cm in diameter with no regional lymph node or distant metastases
Stage IIIB G3T2N0M0	Grade 3 tumor 5 cm or greater in diameter with no regional lymph node or distant metastases
Stage IV	
Stage IVA G1–3T1–2N1M0—	Tumor of any grade or size with histologically verified metastasis to regional lymph nodes, but no distant metastases
Stage IVB G1–3T1–2N0–1M1	Clinically diagnosed distant metastases

From the American Joint Committee Staging Manual, 1987.

TABLE 40-7. Local Control and Disease-free Survival in 220 Patients with Soft Tissue Sarcoma Treated at MGH by Radiation and Surgery According to AJC Stage*

AJC Stage	No. of Patients	5-Year Actuarial Results† Local Control	Disease-free Survival
IA	17	1.00	1.00
IB	30	.93	.88
IIA	40	.88	.83
IIB	66	.85	.52
IIIA	33	.93	.87
IIIB	69	.79	.39
IVA	3	1.00	1.00
Total	258	.88	.66

Suit HD, Mankin HJ, Willett G et al: Limited surgery and external irradiation in soft tissue sarcomas. In Recent Concepts in Sarcoma Treatment. Proceedings of the International Symposium on Sarcomas, Tarpon Springs, FL, October 8–10, 1987. The Netherlands, Kluwer Academic Publishers, 1988.

*Excludes patients with distant metastases (Stage IVB) and patients with sarcomas arising from thoracic, abdominal, pelvic, and retroperitoneal sites.

TABLE 40-9. Predicted Survival According to Stages, Based on 397 Extremity Sarcoma Patients

Stage	Probability of Survival: 2 Years	5 Years
IA	0.99	0.97
IB	0.95	0.89
IIA	0.88	0.73
IIB	0.73	0.45
III	0.37	0.08

Enneking WF, Spanier SS, and Goodman MA: The surgical staging of musculoskeletal sarcoma. J Bone Joint Surg [Am] 62:1027–1030, 1980.

STAGING OF SOFT TISSUE SARCOMAS

The single most important prognostic factor in patients with soft tissue sarcomas is the histologic grade of the primary lesion.[50,53–55,60] Grades are assigned from Grade I (well-differentiated) to Grade III (poorly differentiated). The difficulties in assigning grades to sarcomas were considered in Pathologic Classification.

In the staging system for soft tissue sarcomas proposed by the American Joint Committee for Cancer Staging and End Results, the histologic grade is the most important determinant of stage.[60,60a] The system is based on four parameters: G or histopathologic grade, T, N, and M. Details of the staging system, which was revised in 1987, are presented in Table 40-6. G1, G2, and G3 lesions are sarcomas that are well-differentiated, moderately differentiated, or poorly differentiated, respectively. T1 lesions are less than 5 cm; T2 lesions are equal to or greater than 5 cm. N1 lesions have been proved to have metastatic disease in regional lymph nodes, and M1 lesions show clinical evidence of distant metastasis. Accordingly, all lesions that are G1 and T1–2 and are N0M0 are Stage I. Similarly, all lesions that are G2 and T1–2 and are N0M0 are Stage II, and all lesions that are G3 and T1–2 and are N0M0 are Stage III. All lesions that are N1 become Stage IVA, without regard to grade or size. The correlation of this staging system with prognosis in 220 patients with soft tissue sarcomas of all sites, excluding retroperitoneum, treated at the Massachusetts General Hospital is presented in Table 40-7.[60a]

TABLE 40-8. Enneking System for Staging of Sarcomas of Soft Tissues or Bone

Stage	Characteristic
Stage I	Low grade
IA	Intracompartmental
IB	Extracompartmental
Stage II	High grade
IIA	Intracompartmental
IIB	Extracompartmental
Stage III	Any grade
	N1 or M1

Enneking WF, Spanier SS, and Goodman MA: The surgical staging of musculoskeletal sarcoma. J Bone Joint Surg [Am] 62:1027–1030, 1980.

An alternate staging system has been proposed by Enneking and colleagues (Table 40-8).[162] In this system, patients are categorized as Stage I (low-grade, no metastases), Stage II (high-grade, no metastases), or Stage III (either grade with regional or distant metastases). In addition, tumors are designated "A" if they are contained within an anatomic compartment and are designated "B" if they extend across fascial planes. The correlation of survival with stage of disease using this schema in 397 patients with sarcomas of the extremity is shown in Table 40-9.[162] This staging system is practical only for extremity sarcomas.

Factors thought to be of prognostic importance in patients with soft tissue sarcomas are listed in Table 40-10.[44,60,62,163] The site of a soft tissue sarcoma often influences resectability, and thus, local control and cure. Lesions in the trunk, especially those in the retroperitoneum, mediastinum, and head and neck, often involve vital structures before they become clinically apparent. They are usually large, and local control by any approach is less likely for these tumors than for tumors on the extremity or torso. In the extremity, the exact site of the lesion is also of prognostic importance. Proximal lesions are generally less curable than distal lesions. In the series reported by Simon and Enneking, local recurrences after surgery alone in the buttock, groin, thigh, and areas below the knee were 38%, 14%, 15%, and 0, respectively (Table 40-11).[59]

Size is an important parameter, both for freedom from distant metastases and for local control. Among subjects

TABLE 40-10. Prognostic Factors for Patients with Primary Soft Tissue Sarcomas

Histologic grade
Site (proximal versus distal; extremity versus trunk)
Size
Lymph node involvement

TABLE 40-11. Anatomical Site Correlated with Local Recurrence Rate in Soft Tissue Sarcomas of the Extremities

Anatomical Site	*No. of Patients*	*% Total*	*Number with Recurrence*	*Number Without Recurrence*	*% Recurrence*
Lower extremity	(53)				
Intrapelvic	2	3	2	0	100
Buttock	8	11	3	5	38
Groin	7	10	1	6	14
Thigh	26	37	4	22	15
Knee	3	4	0	3	0
Below knee	7	10	0	7	0
Upper extremity	(17)				
Shoulder girdle	4	6	2	2	50
Arm	7	10	0	7	0
Below elbow	6	9	1	5	17

Simon MA, Enneking WF: The management of soft-tissue sarcomas of the extremities. J Bone Joint Surg [Am] 58:317, 1976.

whose treatment controlled the primary lesion, distant control decreased rapidly with tumor size (Table 40-12).[44,60,62,164] Size is a major factor in achieving local control by surgery alone for tumors in some anatomic sites (*e.g.*, head, neck, or retroperitoneum), and it is a dominant factor in the results of radiation alone. For radiation combined with surgery, local control did not depend on size for the lesions up to 150 mm.

Soft tissue sarcomas rarely spread to regional lymph nodes. In a review of 374 patients referred to the NCI during 24 years, only 3 patients (2.6%) had evidence of metastases to draining lymph nodes before gross dissemination of disease.[165] In a review of over 2500 patients in the world literature, Weingrad and Rosenberg analyzed the incidence of lymph node metastases from each of the major histologic types of soft tissue sarcomas (Table 40-13).[165] In general, about 5% of patients with soft tissue sarcomas developed nodal metastases at any point in the course of their disease, although in patients with synovial cell sarcoma and rhabdomyosarcoma the incidence was higher. Patients with involvement of draining lymph nodes had a substantially poorer prognosis than did those whose lymph nodes were not involved. Mazeron and Suit recently reported an incidence of regional lymph node involvement of 5.9% in 323 patients with Stage MO soft tissue sarcoma.[166] There was no regional node involvement in patients with Grade 1 sarcomas compared with 2% and 12% for Grades 2 and 3, respectively. In their series, the 19 patients who had nodal involvement had a 32% 5-year survival rate.

Rosenberg and co-workers reported an inverse correlation between prognosis and the number of perioperative blood transfusions administered to patients who underwent resections of localized high-grade sarcomas of the extremities.[167] The number of transfusions represented a prognostic variable independent of tumor size. This observation requires confirmation by others.

The histologic cell of origin of soft tissue sarcomas is not of major prognostic importance if lesions of equivalent grade are compared. Similarly, there appears to be no prognostic importance attached to the age or sex of patients with soft tissue sarcomas, except that fibrosarcomas occurring in children tend to have a better prognosis than those in adult patients, even when allowances are made for grade and size.[168] Further, liposarcoma may be less aggressive in children.[169]

TABLE 40-12. Actuarial Distant Control Rates at 5 Years Among 141 Patients with G2–3 Sarcoma of Soft Tissue with Control of Primary Lesion After Treatment by Radiation and Surgery

Tumor Size (mm)	*No. of Patients*	*Actuarial Distant Control (5 years)*
<25	16	0.92
26–50	42	0.76
51–100	47	0.67
101–150	17	0.42
>150	19	0.26
Total	141	0.64

TABLE 40-13. Incidence of Lymph Node Metastases in Patients with Soft Tissue Sarcomas

Histology	*No. of Series*	*No. of Patients*	*Incidence of Lymph Node Metastases*	
			No.	*%*
Liposarcoma	7	288	15	5.7
Fibrosarcoma	14	1083	55	5.1
Rhabdomyosarcoma	13	888	108	12.2
Synoviosarcoma	13	535	91	17.0
Unclassifiable	5	125	11	8.8
Neurofibrosarcoma	2	60	0	0

Weingrad DW, Rosenberg SA: Early lymphatic spread of osteogenic and soft-tissue sarcomas. Surgery 84:231–240, 1978.

TABLE 40-14. Clinically Involved Distant Metastatic Sites at Time of Diagnosis of Sarcoma

Metastatic Sites	1977–1978		1983–1984	
	No.	%	No.	%
Bone	126	22.6	191	23.7
Lung	186	33.3	275	34.1
Liver	83	14.9	126	15.7
Brain	19	3.4	22	2.7
Other	144	25.8	193	23.9
Total	558	100.0	807	100.0

Lawrence W, Donegan WL, Natarajan N et al: Adult soft tissue sarcomas. A pattern of care survey of The American College of Surgeons. Ann Surg 205:349–359, 1987.

NATURAL HISTORY OF SOFT TISSUE SARCOMAS

COMMON FEATURES

The poor prognosis of most patients with soft tissue sarcomas is due to the tendency of these lesions to invade aggressively into surrounding tissues and for early hematogenous dissemination, usually to the lungs. Soft tissue sarcomas invade locally along anatomic planes, such as nerve fibers, muscle bundles, fascial planes, and blood vessels. Most patients with soft tissue sarcomas present without obvious clinical metastases. In 565 soft tissue sarcoma patients admitted to Memorial Sloan-Kettering Hospital between 1983 and 1985, 128 (22.7%) had evidence of metastases at presentation.[170] At the Massachusetts General Hospital between 1971 and 1981, 28 (10.3%) of 272 patients who presented with a primary sarcoma were found to have distant metastases.[171] In the American College of Surgeons survey, 1365 (23.5%) of 5812 patients who presented with soft tissue sarcoma had evidence of distant metastases.[46] The lung was the most frequent site of distant metastases, accounting for 33% of the metastatic lesions, followed by bone and liver (Table 40-14).[46]

Because the appropriate diagnosis is often not appreciated or suspected before biopsy, many soft tissue sarcomas are initially treated by shelling out the lesion through the pseudocapsule. In the American College of Surgeons survey, approximately half of sarcomas were biopsied by this procedure or by excision (see Table 40-5). Only 20% of the sarcomas were diagnosed by incisional biopsy. Excisional biopsy is inadequate as sole therapy, and over 90% of these patients will have local recurrences.

The pattern of recurrence in patients with soft tissue sarcomas is a function of the primary site of the lesion. Potter and associates analyzed 307 patients referred to the NCI between 1975 and 1982, who underwent complete surgical resection of high-grade soft tissue sarcomas, often in combination with chemotherapy and radiation therapy.[44] The pattern of recurrence in the 107 patients is shown in Table 40-15. Patients with retroperitoneal sarcomas had a greater tendency to recur with disseminated disease throughout the abdomen, and patients with truncal sarcomas had a higher local recurrence rate than was seen in patients with primary lesions in the extremities. Among the entire group with recurrences, the lung was the predominant site (52%) of the first isolated recurrence; isolated local recurrence was seen in 20% of patients. In the American College of Surgeons survey, treatment failures in patients without metastases at initial diagnoses and with total gross resections of the soft tissue sarcomas occurred in 452 (37%) of 1209 patients.[46] Isolated locoregional recurrence occurred in 236 (52.2%) of these patients. This high rate may reflect inadequate surgical resection or inadequate adjunctive treatments that were administered. In this study, at least 25% of the patients had limited local excisions for the treatment of the primary tumor when no distant disease was documented.

The time until local recurrence is fairly constant in most reported series. Figure 40-5 shows the results of Cantin and co-workers, who demonstrated that approximately 80% of all lesions that recur after surgery do so within 2 years.[172] In 54 patients treated surgically by Simon and Enneking, all local recurrences occurred by 30 months after definitive resection.[59] Lindberg and associates also reported that 80% of local recurrences occurred in the first 2 years and 100% by 3 years.[173] Shiu and associates reported 87% of local recurrences within the first 2 years.[58] Gerner and associates reported that 82% of local recurrences were evident by 2 years at Roswell Park Memorial Institute.[174]

Patients undergoing amputation or radical local excision have local recurrence rates of about 20%.[58,59] In older series from Memorial Sloan-Kettering Hospital, local recurrences were seen in 59% of patients undergoing conservative excision, compared with 25% for those undergoing radical excision.[172] At the M.D. Anderson Hospital, patients undergoing conservative excision had a 77% local recurrence rate, compared with 28% for those undergoing radical excision.[57] These series were not randomized, and these figures are highly influenced by patient selection factors. In general,

TABLE 40-15. Frequency of Initial Recurrence Pattern by Site of Primary Sarcoma

Primary Site	Extremity No. (%)	Retroperitoneal No. (%)	Trunk No. (%)	Breast No. (%)	Head and Neck No. (%)	Total No. (%)
Isolated lung	43 (70)	3 (17)	5 (29)	3 (75)	2 (50)	56 (52)
Isolated local	7 (10)	5 (30)	7 (41)	0	2 (50)	21 (20)
Isolated other	11 (15)	1 (6)	2 (12)	1 (25)	0	15 (14)
Multiple	4 (5)	8 (47)	3 (18)	0	0	15 (14)
Total	65 (100)	17 (100)	17 (100)	4 (100)	4 (100)	107 (100)

Potter DA, Glenn J, Kinsella T et al: Patterns of recurrence in patients with high-grade soft tissue sarcoma. J Clin Oncol 3:353–366, 1985.

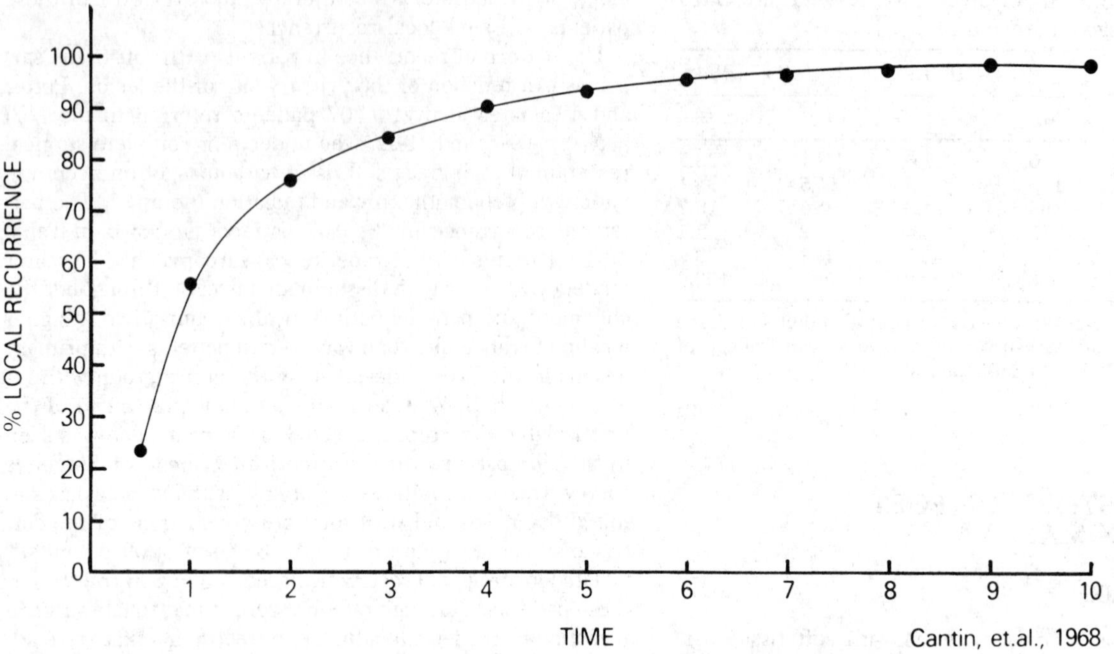

FIG. 40-5. Time course of local recurrence following definitive treatment for soft tissue sarcomas. (Data presented as the percentage of local recurrences of those who will ultimately experience recurrences) (Cantin J, McNeer GP, Chu FC et al: The problem of local recurrence after treatment of soft tissue sarcoma. Ann Surg 168:47–53, 1947)

however, the larger the surgical excisions in all directions from the tumors the lower the local recurrence rates.

Spread to draining lymph nodes is an uncommon finding. In a review by Weingrad and Rosenberg of more than 30 series, 5.8% of almost 3000 patients developed lymph node metastases some time during their course (Table 40-13). These figures reflect the incidence of lymph node metastases at any time during the course of the disease; spread to lymph nodes in the early stages is less frequent. There was a 3.2% incidence of nodal spread in almost 6000 patients analyzed in the American College of Surgeons survey.[46] Mazeron and Suit reported a 5.9% incidence of regional nodal involvement in 323 patients with Stage M0 sarcoma.[166] The incidence of lymph node metastases is somewhat higher for epithelioid sarcomas (20–40%), in synovial cell sarcoma (17%), and in rhabdomyosarcoma (12%) than for most other histologic types.

Before 1977, when surgery was the primary modality of treatment, the overall 5-year survival rate in most reported series of patients with soft tissue sarcoma was approximately 50% (Table 40-16).[38,39,56–60,163,174–176] Widespread disease beyond the lungs was often found at autopsy.

UNIQUE FEATURES OF HISTOLOGIC SUBTYPES

Despite the common biologic behavior of equivalent-grade soft tissue sarcomas, there are some features that are unique to individual histologic types.

TABLE 40-16. Soft Tissue Sarcomas: Results of Surgical Excision Alone

		Survival Before 1977 (%)	
*Study**	*No. of Patients*	*5-Year*	*10-Year*
Task Force, AJC[60]	1215	41	30
Surgery Branch, NCI (before 1975)[175]	66	48	44
Gerner et al[174]	155	50	26
Shieber and Graham[38]	125	27	22
Martin and Ariel[57]	183	40	
Pack and Cerny[56]	717	39	
Hare[39]	200	39	
Shiu et al[58]	297	55	41
Suit et al[163]	100	52	
Simon and Enneking[59]	54	62	
Markhede et al[156]	97	59	

*Groups and reference number.

Fibrosarcoma

Before 1965, fibrosarcoma was the most common diagnosis of soft tissue sarcoma.[177,178] Since that time, the recognition of a larger variety of subtypes of soft tissue sarcoma has significantly decreased this diagnosis. As stated by Stout and Lattes, "One should try to restrict the term 'fibrosarcoma' to growths that are composed of cells and fibers derived from fibrocytes and exclude all the fibrous growths derived from other types of cells acting as facultative fibroblasts."[49] Although some pathologists distinguish fibroblastic fibrosarcoma from pleomorphic fibrosarcoma largely by the uniformity of the herringbone pattern of the tumor and the number of mitotic figures, this is mainly a reflection of grading.[47] Because of the changing definition of fibrosarcoma, earlier series undoubtedly contain sarcomas that would now be identified as other histologic types.[177-180] Infantile fibrosarcomas are extremely rare. There have been 3 cases of inoperable infantile fibrosarcoma that have completely responded to chemotherapy.[181,182]

Rhabdomyosarcoma

Rhabdomyosarcoma accounts for about 15% of all sarcomas.[183-188] Because the skeletal muscle accounts for approximately 40% of adult body weight, this tumor, on a per weight basis, is one of the rarest of all tumors. Striated muscle cells are highly differentiated cells that rarely undergo mitosis in the postnatal period, which probably accounts for the low incidence of these malignancies.

The three categories of rhabdomyosarcoma are pleomorphic, alveolar, and embryonal. Many tumors contain several histologic patterns, and the assignment of a specific subtype is often nebulous. Because the alveolar and embryonal types usually occur in childhood, they are often referred to as juvenile-type rhabdomyosarcomas. "Botryoid" indicates the gross appearance of a subset of embryonal rhabdomyosarcomas that have a polypoid or grapelike appearance. Embryonal rhabdomyosarcomas with botryoid features are commonly found in the urogenital tract of infants and children, although these tumors have also been noticed in the oral and nasal pharynx. Embryonal tumors occasionally are found in adult and elderly patients. Lloyd and associates reported a series of 54 cases of embryonal rhabdomyosarcomas in patients 20 years or older.[188] Embryonal rhabdomyosarcomas are the most common soft tissue sarcomas of children. Discussion of these tumors is presented elsewhere.

Alveolar rhabdomyosarcomas are distinguished by slit-like alveolar spaces in the tumor.

Pleomorphic rhabdomyosarcomas generally present in adulthood, although they can appear in childhood. They are very rare adult sarcomas that arise within skeletal muscles. The most common sites of pleomorphic rhabdomyosarcomas are the extremities. These are often highly anaplastic lesions, having both small and large cells with one or many bizarre nuclei. Their diagnosis has changed dramatically in recent years. A review of Hajdu of 214 sarcomas originally diagnosed as pleomorphic rhabdomyosarcoma led to a reclassification of 93 of these lesions as other histologic subtypes, mainly malignant fibrous histiocytoma.[47]

The distinction between pleomorphic rhabdomyosarcoma and other pleomorphic sarcomas can be aided by immunohistochemical staining using antibodies specific for constituent proteins of sarcomeric muscle.[189-191]

Leiomyosarcoma

Leiomyosarcomas are malignant neoplasms that arise from smooth muscle. Because these tumors can arise from the walls of both small and large blood vessels, they can occur anywhere in the body.[192-195] Leiomyosarcomas also occur in the viscera, arising from either smooth muscle in the viscera (*e.g.*, the uterus) or from vessels in these organs. Leiomyosarcomas commonly arise in the retroperitoneum, where they are highly aggressive neoplasms.

Liposarcoma

Liposarcomas are malignant lesions of adipose tissue.[196-201] The incidence in men exceeds that in women by about 1.5:1. Multicentric liposarcomas have been described. In a series of 97 patients with liposarcomas reported by Kindbloom and co-workers, 11 patients had a second liposarcoma that developed at a site remote from the first tumor.

Four subtypes of liposarcomas are generally recognized: well-differentiated, myxoid, lipoblastic (or round cell), and pleomorphic. Some authors also refer to fibroblastic liposarcomas as a fifth subtype. Well-differentiated liposarcomas can exhibit aggressive local invasion, and can infrequently metastasize late in their course. Round cell or lipoblastic or epithelioid sarcomas are composed of uniform round cells and are highly vascular. These are highly malignant lesions, and like the pleomorphic liposarcomas, they have only a 20% to 30% 5-year survival rate in most reported series.

Synovial Sarcoma

Synovial sarcomas are malignant neoplasms that arise from tendosynovial tissue and occur most commonly in the second through fourth decades.[202-206] The lower extremities are the most common sites of synovial sarcomas. It can occur in any muscle, not usually close to joints. Although extremities are the most common sites, lesions can occur in the abdominal wall and in other skeletal muscles of the trunk. The two synovial sarcomas generally recognized are the monophasic and biphasic types. Monophasic synovial sarcomas are characterized by sheaths of monotonous spindle cells; the biphasic variety has slit-like spaces or clefts present within the tumor. These clefts are lined by cuboidal or tall columnar epithelial cells and sometimes resemble carcinomas. Calcified areas often appear within the synovial sarcomas and lead to a characteristic x-ray appearance of this type of soft tissue sarcoma. Some authors consider epithelioid and clear cell sarcomas to be variants of synovial cell sarcoma, although these are considered separately in this chapter.

Cagle and colleagues reviewed 45 synovial cell sarcoma patients and were able to identify high-risk and low-risk patients based on percent of glandularity and mitotic rates.[207] Low-risk patients, identified as having >50% glandular features and <15 mitoses per 10 high-power fields, had a 100% survival rate. High-risk patients, with <50% glandular features and >15 mitoses per 10 high-power fields, had a 37% survival rate.

Neurofibrosarcomas

Neurofibrosarcomas are malignant tumors of neural sheath origin. They have also been referred to as neurogenic sarcomas, malignant schwannomas, and malignant neurilemmomas.[128,208] These tumors can occur anywhere in the body.

Neurofibrosarcomas are frequently found in association with Von Recklinghausen's disease, a chronic, progressive disease inherited as a Mendelian-dominant trait and associated with multiple neurofibromas and skin pigment changes, which are characterized as cafe-au-lait spots.[120–128] About 10% of patients with neurofibromatosis develop sarcomatous changes during their lifetimes, often in preexisting, benign masses.

Angiosarcomas

Hemangiosarcomas and lymphangiosarcomas arise from blood and lymphatic vessels, respectively.[209–215] These are almost uniformly high-grade lesions. They are uncommon, however, comprising only 2% of all soft tissue sarcomas. In 1948, Stuart and Treves reported six cases of lymphangiosarcoma in lymphedematous arms after radical mastectomy.[15,216–218] In 1972, Woodward and colleagues reported 23 cases of lymphangiosarcoma associated with chronic lymphedema seen at the Mayo Clinic and reviewed the world literature of 163 cases reported up to that time.[216] The cases of postmastectomy lymphangiosarcoma occurred at an average age of 63.9 years and at an average of 10 years and 3 months after mastectomy. Because of the diffuse nature of these tumors, most physicians recommend radical amputation, either shoulder disarticulation or forequarter amputation, for patients who develop lymphangiosarcoma in the upper extremity after mastectomy.[216–218]

Hemangiosarcomas may occur anywhere in the body but often arise in skin and superficial soft tissue, which contrasts sharply with the deep location of most soft tissue sarcomas.[50] Of 366 hemangiosarcomas, 33% arose in the skin and 25% in the soft tissues. Fifty percent of cutaneous hemangiosarcomas are localized in the head and neck region. These are extremely aggressive tumors despite multimodality therapy, one series of 72 patients reported by Holden and co-workers had a 12% 5-year survival rate.[219]

Hemangiopericytoma

Malignant hemangiopericytoma is a malignant sarcoma thought to arise from the pericyte cells of smooth muscle origin that lie around small vessels.[136,137,220–222] Benign and malignant hemangiopericytomas exist, and the rarity of these lesions has led to considerable confusion in distinguishing between benign and malignant variants. Hemangiopericytomas should be treated as other sarcomas. In most series, approximately 50% 5-year survival rates are recorded.

Kaposi's Sarcoma

In 1872, Kaposi described "multiple idiopathic pigmented sarcomas of the skin" that "arise in the skin, without any known local or systemic cause."[223,224] These tumors are thought to arise from endothelial cells and present as raised pigmented lesions of the skin. Four separate clinical types of Kaposi's sarcoma have been recognized (Table 40-17).[225] The classic Kaposi's sarcoma occurs in elderly men of Mediterranean or Jewish extraction living in the United States or Europe.[226–229] This is a rare tumor, and in 1965, Reynolds and colleagues reported a series of only 70 patients collected during 38 years.[226] These lesions usually start as a reddish nodule on the lower extremity. The disease is generally indolent and can be palliated with radiation therapy if necessary. Approximately 20% of these patients die as a direct result of Kaposi's sarcoma, usually because of gastrointestinal or pulmonary involvement.[223] Many of these patients developed second malignancies, often lymphomas, and in one series, death from secondary primaries, often lymphoreticular neoplasms, was as great a threat to life as was mortality from the Kaposi's sarcoma itself.[224,230]

In 1950, interest in Kaposi's sarcoma was renewed when a second form of the disease was described by Kaminer and

TABLE 40-17. Kaposi's Sarcoma: Comparison of Clinical Manifestations

Type	*Population*	*Male to Female Ratio*	*Clinical Characteristics*	*Course*
Classic	Jewish, Italian heritage (age 50–80 yr)	15:1	Lower extremity cutaneous lesions	Indolent; 10–15-year survival
African	Young adult (age 25–40 yr)	13:1	Lower-extremity nodular cutaneous lesions	Indolent, locally aggressive disease
	Children (age 2–13 yr)	3:1	Generalized lymphadenopathy, cutaneous lesions rare	Rapidly progressive; 2–3-year survival
Renal transplant	Iatrogenic immunosuppressed patient	2.3:1	Localized cutaneous or disseminated	Indolent or progressive; fatal in 30%
Epidemic	AIDS patients	20:1	Disseminated mucocutaneous lesion and visceral involvement	Fulminant; <20% 2-year survival

Adapted from Krigel RL, Friedman-Kien AE: Kaposi's Sarcoma in AIDS. In DeVita VT, Hellman S, Rosenberg SA (eds): AIDS. Etiology, Diagnosis, Treatment, and Prevention, pp 185–211. Philadelphia, JB Lippincott, 1985.

Murray, who compiled 43 cases of Kaposi's sarcoma in Bantu men in Africa.[231] In selected areas of Africa, Kaposi's sarcoma is a common neoplasm, representing between 3% and 9% of all reported malignancies.[229,232] This disease can be more aggressive than the American or European Kaposi's sarcoma. These lesions can respond to chemotherapy with dactinomycin, vincristine, and dacarbazine (DTIC).[224]

Another type of Kaposi's sarcoma is associated with renal transplantation; the first case was reported in 1969.[233] Since then, a number of renal allograft recipients have been reported to develop Kaposi's sarcoma after the onset of immunosuppressive therapy. The incidence of Kaposi's sarcoma in patients undergoing renal transplantation appears to be 0.4%, which represents between 150 to 200 times the expected incidence of this tumor in the general population. The average time to development of Kaposi's sarcoma after transplantation is about 16 months. The extent of the tumor correlates with the degree of depression of cellular immunity. In some cases the tumors have regressed because of reduction or changes in immunosuppressive therapy.[235-237]

The Kaposi's sarcoma associated with acquired immune deficiency syndrome (AIDS) has been called epidemic Kaposi's sarcoma. The initial reports of epidemic Kaposi's sarcoma appeared in 1981.[238] The clinical features of these patients are reminiscent of Kaposi's sarcoma of immunosuppressed renal transplant patients, underscoring the opportunistic nature of this tumor. Approximately 48% of all homosexual males with AIDS present with or will eventually develop Kaposi's sarcoma. By comparison, only about 4% of all heterosexual intravenous drug users with AIDS and about 12% of Haitian AIDS patients develop epidemic Kaposi's sarcoma.[225] None of the hemophiliac patients with AIDS have developed Kaposi's sarcoma. This form of the disease can be extremely virulent, and death from the disease or related complications of immune deficiency occurs in most patients. Kaposi's sarcoma in AIDS is reviewed in Chapter 57.

Malignant Fibrous Histiocytoma

Malignant fibrous histiocytoma was characterized by O'Brien and Stout as a group of tumors having a common origin from tissue histiocytes.[138,239-244] This diagnosis has achieved great popularity in recent years, and many cases previously diagnosed as pleomorphic rhabdomyosarcoma or undifferentiated fibrosarcoma are now categorized as malignant fibrous histiocytoma. A wide spectrum of fibrous histiocytomas exists, from those that are benign to those that are highly atypical to those that are frankly malignant. In many recent series, malignant fibrous histiocytoma is the most common diagnosis attached to soft tissue sarcomas.

These tumors are more common in adults, with 40% occurring in the sixth and seventh decades of life and with less than 5% occurring in patients under 20 years of age.[245-247]

Alveolar Soft Part Sarcoma

Alveolar soft part sarcomas were described by Christopherson in 1952.[248-250] These tumors have a unique histologic appearance, but the cell of origin is unknown. These are true malignant sarcomas with no benign counterpart, although they tend to have a more protracted course than most other sarcomas. Although most patients will ultimately die of the disease, 5-year survival rates of 60% are common. Many patients develop metastatic disease that progresses slowly over the course of 5 to 15 years before death.

The tumor commonly arises in the thigh in adults and in the head and neck region in children.[50] In 143 patients reviewed by the Armed Forces Institute of Pathology (AFIP), 44% of the tumors arose in the lower extremities, 27% in the head and neck area, 17% in the upper extremities and 11% in the trunk.[50]

Epithelioid Sarcoma

Epithelioid sarcomas are of unknown origin and occur almost exclusively in the extremities, usually in the hand or foot associated with aponeurotic structures.[251-256] These tumors differ in their natural history from most other sarcomas in that they have a greater tendency to spread to noncontiguous areas of skin, subcutaneous tissue, fat, and bone. In addition, these tumors have a high propensity to spread to draining lymph nodes. Chase and Enzinger reviewed 241 cases of epithelioid sarcoma in which the most common initial sites of metastases were the lymph nodes (48%) and lungs (24%).[256] A more aggressive course was associated with a proximal or axial tumor location, increased tumor size or depth, hemorrhage, mitotic figures, necrosis, or vascular invasion. More favorable behavior was observed when the tumor arose in distal extremities in younger individuals or in female patients between the ages of 10 and 49. Long-term survival is similar to or perhaps slightly better than for most other soft tissue sarcomas. Recommended therapy for these patients is wide excision, often involving amputation of the extremity and regional lymph node dissection.

TREATMENT OF SOFT TISSUE SARCOMAS

Surgery alone, surgery combined with radiation, surgery combined with radiation and intra-arterial chemotherapy, or radiation alone have all been used for the treatment of soft tissue sarcomas. There has been an intense and sustained interest in evaluating treatment strategies that preserve limbs of patients with sarcomas of soft tissue of the extremities and reduce the extent of resection for patients who have lesions on the torso or in the head and neck region by combining less than radical surgery with radiation and chemotherapy.

A National Institues of Health consensus conference in 1984 reviewed a variety of limb-sparing approaches, which included surgery plus adjunctive radiation therapy or chemotherapy, for the treatment of high-grade extremity sarcomas.[257] They concluded that limb-sparing treatment for some of these sarcoma patients was an effective treatment option. The available data indicate that the results of these conservative approaches were equivalent to those obtained by more radical surgical procedures in selected subgroups of patients.

In discussing the rationale for combining these modalities, the results are presented in terms of frequency of local control, survival, and complications. Important technical aspects are delineated for currently employed strategies.

SURGERY

The essential ingredient in any surgical approach designed to maximize local control is to achieve adequate negative surgical margins. Until the late 1940s and the early 1950s, the surgical approach to the patient with sarcoma of a soft tissue was a local excision, which removed the grossly evident tumor mass with little or no margin of adjacent normal tissue. This is a "marginal excision." The local failure rate for this procedure is approximately 86% (range, 50–93%), as indicated in Table 40-18.[58,59,174,176] Improvement to reduce local failure rates emphasized the use of more extensive surgical procedures to obtain wider margins of normal tissue. Wide local excisions, which entail soft tissue resections for the most part, are associated with local recurrences of 49% when surgery alone is performed (Table 40-18). More radical procedures, such as amputation or muscle compartmental excisions, are associated with an even lower local failure rate of 14% (range, 7–18%), as documented in four separate series (Table 40-18).

Resection of a soft tissue sarcoma requires that the tumor be located so that an acceptably wide margin of normal tissue can be obtained between the edge of the tumor and the adjacent critical, nonresectable structures, such as major nerves, vessels, bone, and important tendons. This guideline does not apply to many anatomic sites, such as the groin, knee, popliteal space, most portions of the leg, the ankle, many sites within the head and neck area, supraclavicular area, some axillary sites, the elbow region, and most of the forearm, wrist, and hand. Because of the inability to obtain a clear margin at those sites and still retain acceptable function, approximately half of patients with extremity sarcomas were subjected to amputation at institutions with a large experience in sarcoma surgery. This is shown in Table 40-19, in which the proportion of patients with sarcomas of the extremity treated by radical resection or amputation at the University of Florida in Gainesville or at Memorial Hospital in New York are given.[58,59]

The combined results from four centers of amputation for the treatment of sarcoma of soft tissue showed that local control was obtained in 40 of 40 patients with lesions of the leg or foot.[58,59,176,258] In these patients, the level of amputation was well above the lesion and, in most instances, above the level of the proximal joint. These results can be taken as the benchmark for local control results for sarcomas of the distal extremities. If the level of amputation is closer to the tumor (*e.g.*, thigh lesions), about 10% of patients fail locally. In the University of Florida and Goteborg series, 5% and 89% local failure rates were documented after adequate and inadequate margins were obtained, respectively (Table 40-20).[59,176]

Sites of failure among 464 patients treated by surgery alone at three institutions are shown in Table 40-21.[58,176,259] The total local failure rate was 19%; 35% developed distant metastases. These figures are a fair indication of the best that can be accomplished by surgery alone for sarcoma of soft tissue in extremities, although patient selection factors can influence these results. The proportion of patients amputated in the three centers shown in Table 40-21 were 47%, 16%, and 50%, respectively; which was 41% in the combined study.[58,176,258] Thus, an average local control rate of 81% was achieved but only with a high rate of amputation.

The more conservative procedures have been employed in combined modality treatments to reduce local recurrences and yet perform limb-sparing surgery. These treatments have been adopted by many institutions with extensive experience in sarcoma surgery. For example, the percentage of limb-sparing procedures being performed at Memorial Sloan-Kettering Cancer Center has increased since 1975, when approximately 50% of all extremity sarcoma patients received amputations. Between 1982 and 1984, 83% of patients had limb-sparing operations, and only 17% had amputations.[260] In recommending a limb-sparing procedure, the physician must inform the patient that the risk of local fail-

TABLE 40-19. Local Control of Soft Tissue Sarcomas of the Extremities by Radical Surgery

Series Factors	*Simon and Enneking*[58]	*Shiu* et al[59]
Total number of patients	54	297
Radical local resection	25 (46%)	158 (53%)
Amputation	29 (54%)	139 (47%)
Local control		
Radical local resection	88%	72%
Amputation	79%	93%
Overall	83%	82%

TABLE 40-18. Local Recurrence Rate After Surgery Alone

	Local Failures/Total No. of Patients (%)		
*Study**	*Marginal Excision*	*Wide Excision*	*Radical Excision*
Simon et al[59]	3/6 (50)	7/20 (35)	3/43 (7)
Markehede et al[176]†	16/21 (76)		5/76 (7)
Gerner et al[174]	54/58 (93)	15/25 (60)	3/38 (8)
Shiu et al[58]‡			54/297 (18)
Total	73/85 (86)	22/45 (49)	65/454 (14)

*Group and reference number.
†Two patients received preoperative radiation therapy.
‡Eighteen patients had adjunctive radiation therapy.

TABLE 40-20. Adequacy of Margins of Radical Surgery Related to Local Failure Rate

Study	*Negative Margins*	*Positive Margins*
	Number Local Failures/ Total Failures (%)	
Simon and Enneking[59]	1/46 (2)	8/8 (100)
Markhede et al[176]	5/76 (7)	16/19 (84)
Total	6/122 (5)	24/27 (89)

ure may be higher than for amputation. Further, some of the patients who have local failures may develop distant metastases from the regrowing sarcomas. This will be considered with data on salvage surgery for local and distant failures following initial primary therapy.

Technical Aspects of Surgery

EXTREMITY SARCOMAS. A categorization of surgical procedures by Enneking is useful in carefully defining the nature of the surgical procedure performed (Table 40-22).[261] Surgical procedures for soft tissue sarcomas can be categorized into four types:

1. *Intracapsular excision*: This surgical procedure involves removal of the tumor by directly incising the tumor capsule. This procedure leaves gross tumor behind and is of diagnostic value only.
2. *Marginal excision*: All gross tumor including the pseudocapsule is excised locally. Soft tissue sarcomas tend to grow by radial expansion and compress normal structures around them. This pseudocapsule gives the gross appearance of compartmentalization of the tumor from surrounding structures, but invasion of local tissues occurs through the pseudocapsule. The local recurrence rate following treatment by marginal excision alone is close to 90% (Table 40-18).
3. *Wide excision:* The tumor is removed along with a margin of normal surrounding tissue in continuity with the tumor. This procedure does not, however, imply removal of entire structures within which the tumor may be found. The local recurrence rate following treatment by wide resection alone is approximately 50%.
4. *Radical resection:* Tumor is removed with all tissue in the anatomic compartment occupied by the tumor. The excision takes place by dissecting along planes that are separated from the tumor and its tissues of origin by at least one uninvolved anatomic plane in all directions. The resected specimen includes the origin and insertion of all muscles and any bones or joints that are contained within the anatomic compartment of resection. This procedure may involve amputation, although nonablative procedures can also fulfill the criteria for radical resection (Fig. 40-6). The local recurrence rate after these procedures is approximately 14%.

In the treatment of soft tissue sarcomas of the extremities, a variety of amputative procedures can be employed.

1. *Amputations of the foot:* Although amputations of digits, ray amputations, transmetatarsal amputation, and Syme amputations at the level of the ankle joint are all accepted amputations for ischemic lesions of the foot, they often do not give an adequate margin for soft tissue sarcomas in the foot and should be combined with adjuvant radiation therapy to maximize the changes for obtaining local control.
2. *Below-knee amputation:* This amputation is usually performed about a third the distance between the knee and the ankle and involves division of the tibia and fibula. Muscles to the ankle or foot are transected. This amputation is the treatment of choice for any substantive soft tissue sarcoma of the foot. The weight-bearing portions of the foot tolerate radiation therapy poorly, and therefore, amputation is often the best treatment for these lesions.
3. *Above-knee amputation:* Amputation through the thigh can be performed at any level distal to the lesser trochanter. Major muscle groups of the thigh are transected. This amputation is of little value for tumors occurring above the knee and is often indicated for tumors of the leg.
4. *Hip disarticulation:* This amputation involves disarticulation of the hip joint with complete removal of the femur. Most muscles attached to the lower extremity are removed entirely. It is often suitable for patients with lesions of the middle and distal thigh.
5. *Hemipelvectomy:* This operation involves removal of the entire lower extremity and hemipelvis with disar-

TABLE 40-21. Patterns of Failure in Patients with Extremity Sarcomas Treated by Surgery Alone

Institution	*No. of Patients*	*Follow-up (Years)*	*Amputation (%)*	*Local Failure ± Distant Metastases (%)*	*Distant Metastases (%)*
Memorial Sloan-Kettering Hospital[58]*	297	5–24	139 (47)	54 (18)	88 (30)
University of Goteborg[176]†	97	3–23	17 (16)	20 (21)	46 (27)
University of Florida at Gainesville[259]	70	2–19	35 (50)	14 (20)	27 (39)
Total	464	2–24	191 (41)	88 (19)	161 (35)

*Eighteen patients received adjunctive radiation therapy.
†Series includes four patients with truncal sarcomas; two patients received preoperative radiation therapy.

TABLE 40-22. Surgical Procedures for Soft Tissue Extremity Sarcomas

	How Margin Achieved			
Margin	*Limb-Salvage*	*Amputation*	*Plane of Dissection*	*Microscopic Appearance*
Intracapsular	Intracapsular piecemeal excision	Intracapsular amputation	Within lesion	Tumor at margin
Marginal	Marginal en bloc excision	Marginal amputation	Within reactive zone-extracapsular	Reactive tissue ± microsatellites
Wide	Wide en bloc excision	Wide through-bone amputation	Beyond reactive zone through normal tissue within compartment	Normal tissue ± "skips"
Radical	Radical en bloc resection	Radical disarticulation	Normal tissue extracompartmental	Normal tissue

Adapted from Enneking WF, Staging of musculoskeletal neoplasms. In Current Concepts of Diagnosis and Treatment of Bone and Soft Tissue Tumors. Heidelberg, Springer-Verlag, 1984.

ticulation of the sacroiliac joint and pubic symphysis (Fig. 40-7). All major muscles that attach to the lower extremity, except the iliopsoas, are removed. This operation is often applied to the treatment of proximal thigh and buttock lesions. A conventional hemipelvectomy uses a posterior flap of skin and subcutaneous tissue overlying the buttock. For lesions of the buttock, however, it is possible to construct an anterior flap that includes part of the quadriceps muscles and the femoral vessels. The use of anterior-flap hemipelvectomies has greatly extended the application of this procedure.

6. *Modified hemipelvectomy:* Preservation of the iliac wing, if possible, improves patient rehabilitation. This procedure is similar to the standard hemipelvectomy, except that the sacroiliac joint is preserved and the iliac bone is excised from an area below the level of the sciatic notch (Fig. 40-8). This operation does, however, involve transection of muscles in the buttock and is not suitable for lesions in this area. Internal hemipelvectomy can be performed with removal of the innominate bone and adjacent muscles but with preservation of the ipsilateral lower extremity.[262]
7. *Extended hemipelvectomy:* Lesions of the iliac wing may sometimes be situated too close to the sacroiliac joint to permit its disarticulation. Extension of the standard hemipelvectomy to include excision of the sacral ala at the level of the lateral vertebral bodies adds little in morbidity to this procedure and often adds several centimeters of margin from the tumor.
8. *Amputations of the upper extremities:* These procedures follow the principles enunciated for those of the lower extremities. Below-elbow amputations are often used for the treatment of tumors of the hand and wrist. Above-elbow amputations are used for tumors of the forearm. Disarticulation of the shoulder joint is an operation reserved for distal arm and elbow lesions. Forequarter amputation is applied to the treatment of lesions of the shoulder girdle or the proximal arm. This operation includes removal of the entire upper extremity, including both the scapula and clavicle.

Other nonamputative surgical procedures used in the treatment of patients with soft tissue sarcomas of the extremities should also be known to the surgical oncologist.

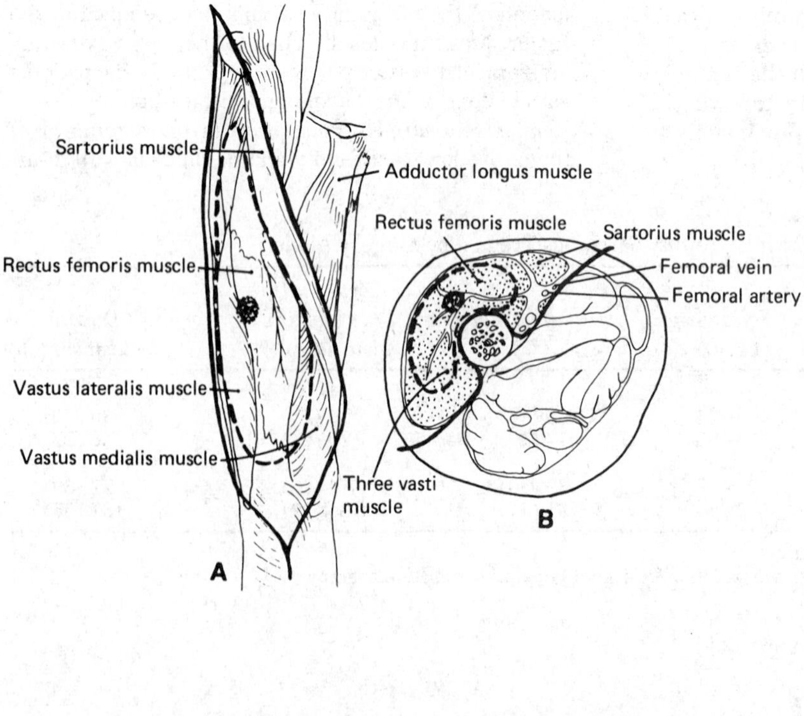

FIG. 40-6. Schematic drawing of the anterior thigh (**A**) and transverse section through the thigh (**B**) illustrating the anatomical extent of a radical resection, without amputation, of a soft tissue sarcoma lying within the rectus femoris muscle. (Courtesy of Dr. Martin Malawer)

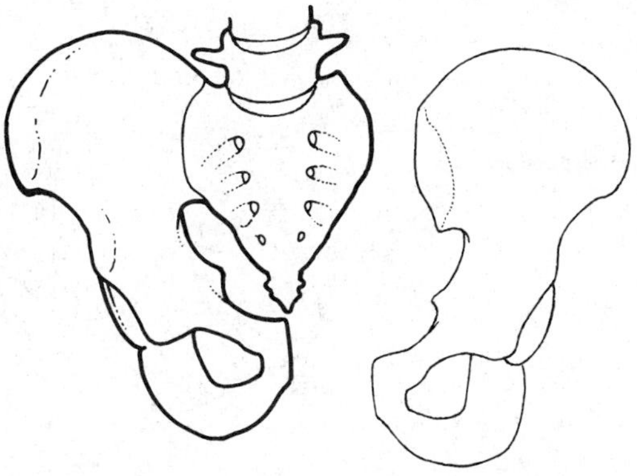

FIG. 40-7. In a hemipelvectomy, removal of the entire lower extremity including the hemipelvis is performed by disarticulation of the sacroiliac joint and symphysis pubis. This approach may be required for large soft tissue tumors of the buttock and anterior or lateral proximal thigh. (Sugarbaker PH, Nicholson TH: Atlas of Extremity Sarcoma Surgery. Philadelphia, JB Lippincott, 1984)

Wide Excision. This is one of the most common surgical procedures performed for extremity sarcomas. In the American College of Surgeons survey, approximately half of all sarcomas were treated with this surgical procedure (Table 40-23).[46] As indicated in Table 40-18, this procedure results in local control only 50% of the time if used alone. Therefore, wide excision is often employed with adjunctive radiation therapy. In performing wide excision of soft tissue sarcomas, sound surgical principles should be adhered to (Fig. 40-9A–D).

Surgery should include wide excision of all normal tissue in the tumor area including, if possible, several centimeters of normal tissue in all directions and excision of all skin and subcutaneous tissue near the tumor. All previous scars, areas of previous biopsy, and any areas that may have contained hematoma from previous biopsies should be resected. Surgical excision of the sarcoma should be completed without spilling of tumor, which can severely compromise the ability to deliver effective radiation therapy.

FIG. 40-8. In a modified hemipelvectomy, there is preservation of the iliac wing. The sacroiliac joint is preserved and the iliac bone divided at the sciatic notch. This operation is appropriate for large soft tissue tumors of the proximal medial thigh. (Sugarbaker PH, Nicholson TH: Atlas of Extremity Sarcoma Surgery. Philadelphia, JB Lippincott, 1984)

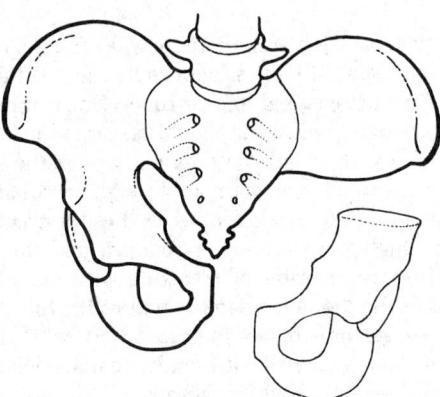

TABLE 40-23. Surgical Procedures Used in Sarcoma Patients Without Metastases at Time of Diagnosis

	1977–1978		*1983–1984*	
Procedures	*No.*	*%*	*No.*	*%*
Wide local resection	879	52.4	1412	56.7
Limited local resection	455	27.1	583	23.4
Anatomic compartmental resection	168	10.0	249	14.8
Amputation	108	6.4	138	8.2
More than one type of surgery	69	4.1	108	6.4
Total	1679	100.0	2490	100.0

Lawrence W, Donegan WL, Natarajan N et al: Adult soft tissue sarcomas. A pattern of care survey of the American College of Surgeons. Ann Surg 205:349–359, 1987.

If desired, place a tourniquet on the extremity above the lesion before ligation of the venous outflow, as a first part of the surgical procedure. There is no convincing evidence that this reduces the distant spread of these tumors. Because these tumors rarely metastasize to draining nodes, lymph node dissection should be confined to those patients with clinically suspicious and biopsy-proven nodal involvement. However, patients with epithelioid sarcoma should have the regional draining lymph nodes resected or treated by appropriate radiation therapy.

Placement of metallic clips as a guide to the limits of the surgical dissection is essential in all nonamputative sarcoma resections. These clips serve as important markers to the radiation therapist, allowing identification of the entire dissected area in the treatment field as the radiation portal is constructed.

Muscle compartmental excision. Some anatomic sites (*e.g.*, the thigh and leg) contain compartments that are bounded by the fascia and its extensions. Because it is unusual for sarcomas to transgress these fascial boundaries, excision of the entire anatomic compartment containing the tumor is often successful in eradicating all local tumor. These procedures are classified as radical nonamputative excisions (see Table 40-22), and according to the American College of Surgeons survey, they were performed in approximately 10% to 15% of patients (see Table 40-23).[46] In the thigh there are three major compartments bounded by the fascia lata and its extensions: the anterior compartment, including the quadriceps muscle (see Fig. 40-7); the medial compartment, including the adductor muscles; the posterior compartment, including the hamstring muscles.

The anterior thigh compartment consists of the quadriceps and sartorius muscles and the femoral artery, vein, and nerve. Excision of the anterior compartment leads to significant loss of motion and stability of the knee. In these situations hamstring transfers can be performed to provide needed muscular movement at the knee. The medial thigh compartment consists of the gracilis, adductor brevis, adductor longus, adductor magnus, and the pectineus muscles. The obturator nerve supplies this compartment. In addition, the profunda femorus artery must be sacrificed when this com-

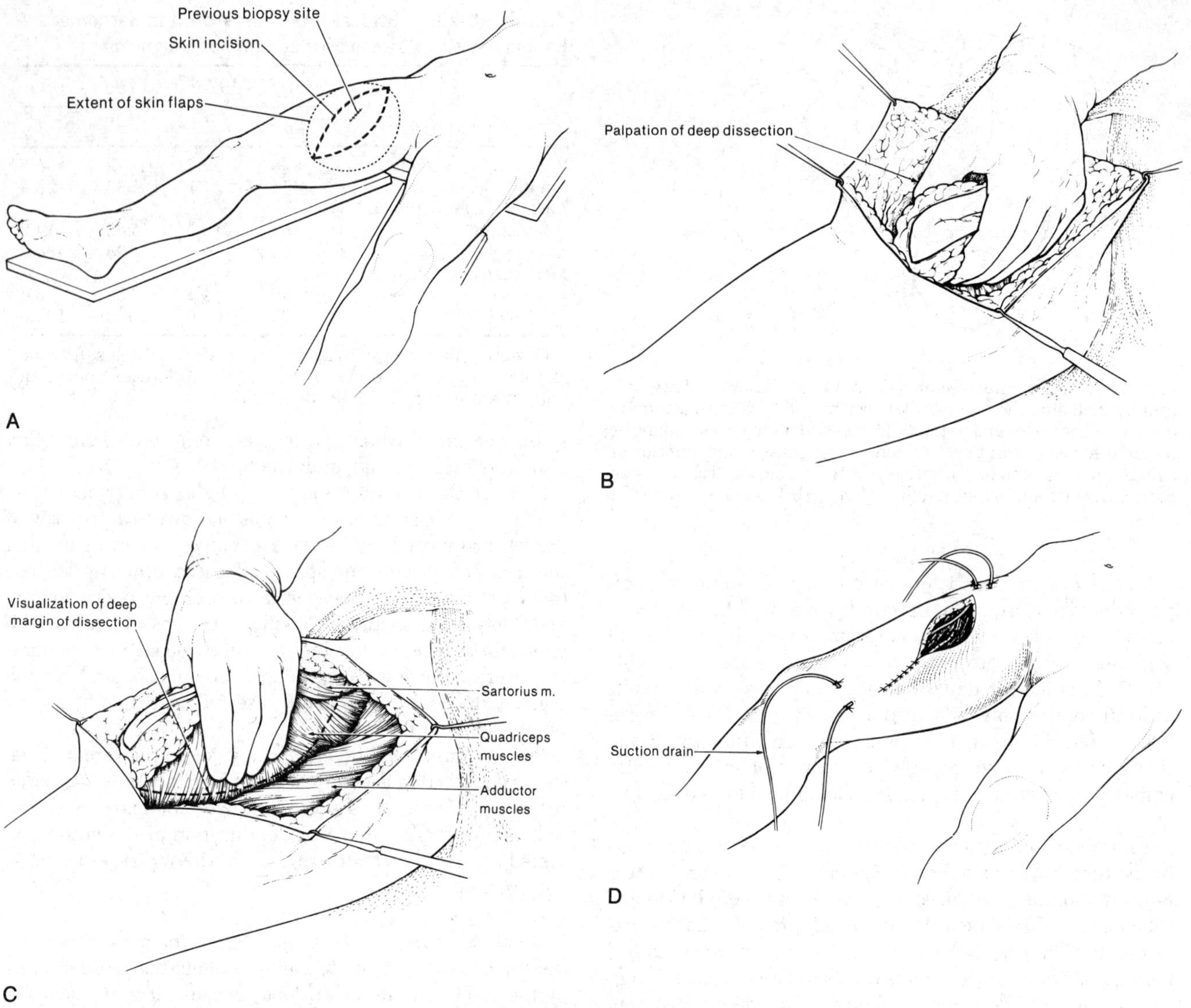

FIG. 40-9. Wide excision of an anterior thigh sarcoma. **A**. Elliptical skin incision encompassing previous biopsy incision(s) or drain site(s) is made. Subcutaneous skin flaps are developed to the lateral extent of the muscle margins. **B**. Palpation of the tumor within the muscle is constantly needed to localize the mass and achieve a margin of at least 2 cm in all directions. Removal of the tumor without visualization of the mass is important. **C**. Visualization of the deep margin is obtained and the muscle divided. **D**. The extent of the dissection is marked with clips for subsequent planning of radiation fields. The skin flaps are closed over suction drains to allow apposition of the flaps to the surgical bed.

partment is resected. The posterior compartment consists of the semimembranosus, semitendinosus, and biceps femorus muscles and the posterior portion of the adductor magnus muscle and the sciatic nerve.

Several atlases of extremity surgery for patients with soft tissue sarcomas detail the performance of these surgical procedures.[156,263]

TRUNCAL SARCOMAS. The same general principles guiding the surgical therapy of extremity lesions also apply to truncal sarcomas.[264–269] There are unique therapeutic features of these lesions, however, that require special consideration. The anatomic location of most truncal sarcomas precludes surgical excision with margins wide enough to ensure local control, especially for sarcomas in the head and neck region and for mediastinal and retroperitoneal tumors. For this reason, surgical excision should be aimed at removing all gross tumor with as much marginal tissue in the expected areas of local spread as is compatible with reasonable morbidity. Radiation therapy should be used in the treatment of virtually all high-grade truncal sarcomas, and the surgeon should outline the margins of resection with metallic clips. For tumors of the thoracic or abdominal walls, full-thickness excisions, except for skin, are indicated.[267,268,270,271] Replacement of the abdominal wall with synthetic materials does not preclude subsequent radiation therapy.

Sarcomas of the retroperitoneum present a unique surgical challenge.[272-277] These tumors tend not to cause symptoms until they are quite large, with extensive local invasion. Delamater reported on a patient with an abdominal liposarcoma that reached 275 lbs., and reports of tumors reaching 60 lbs. are not rare.[278,279] Most retroperitoneal sarcomas weigh several pounds when diagnosed and extensively invade local tissues. The most common diagnoses in the retroperitoneum are liposarcoma and leiomyosarcoma.

Evaluation of patients with retroperitoneal sarcomas should include ultrasound studies, CT, intravenous pyelogram, and when necessary, gastrointestinal contrast studies. Arteriography is often of use to delineate the blood supply of the tumor. Venacavography should be employed if invasion of the vena cava is suspected.

It is rarely possible to achieve negative microscopic margins in the excision of retroperitoneal sarcomas. An attempt should be made to remove all gross tumor, even if this involves resection of a kidney or other intra-abdominal structures. In a 20-year retrospective review of 78 patients with retroperitoneal sarcomas treated between 1951 and 1971 at Memorial, Fortner and colleagues reported the necessity of en bloc excision of adjacent organs in 75% of patients.[280] The colon or kidney were the organs most often resected. This was similar to the experience reported by McGrath and co-workers from the Medical College of Virginia, where complete resection of tumors required en bloc excision of adjacent organs in 68% of the cases; kidney and colon were the organs most often resected.[277] The role of postoperative radiation therapy is unclear.

Reported 5-year survival rates following treatment of retroperitoneal sarcomas vary from 16% to 37% (Table 40-24). The majority of series included patients with all grades of sarcoma. Low-grade tumors have an indolent course. Storm and colleagues reported a 5-year survival rate of 54% for low-grade tumors, compared with a 23% survival rate for high-grade tumors.[274] The major problem is the high frequency of local recurrence. Abbas and co-workers reported a local recurrence rate of 63%.[281] In a series of 36 patients reported by the NCI, 17 had recurrences.[269] Of these 17 patients, 12 had locally recurrent disease, either alone or in conjunction with recurrence in other sites.[269]

The ability to achieve complete resection of all gross disease may improve cure rates. McGrath reported a 70% 5-year survival rate after complete resections, compared with an 8% survival rate for patients undergoing partial excisions or biopsies only.[277] Complete resection of all gross disease was possible in only 49% of these patients in a combined series (Table 40-24).

TABLE 40-24. Treatment Results for Retroperitoneal Sarcomas

*Study**	*No. of Patients*	*No. with Complete Resection (%)*	*5-Year Overall Survival*
Braasch and Mon[272]	37	13 (35)	16%
Cody et al[273]	68	45 (66)	25%
Storm et al[279]	54	28 (52)	33%
Glenn et al[338]	48	37 (77)	43%†
Karakousis et al[275]	68	27 (39)	30%
Bose[276]	29	6 (21)	20%
McGrath et al[277]	47	18 (38)	33%
Total	351	174 (49)	

*Group and reference number.
†Three-year overall survival.

The roles of adjuvant radiation therapy and chemotherapy have not been established, and although widely used, there is no evidence that results are better than from surgical resection alone. A prospective randomized trial at the NCI comparing intraoperative radiotherapy to postoperative external-beam irradiation in 35 patients with resectable retroperitoneal soft tissue sarcomas revealed no difference in therapeutic effectiveness.[282] Innovative combined-modality approaches are needed for retroperitoneal sarcomas.

RADIATION THERAPY

Radiotherapy Alone

Radiation therapy alone in the management of soft tissue sarcomas has been limited to patients who have locally advanced, inoperable, recurrent, or metastatic disease. In general, the radiation doses used have been somewhat low by modern standards, and the intention of radiation therapy was predominantly palliative. Nonetheless, there were reports documenting objective regression and occasional local control of large, inoperable tumors. In 1951, Cade reported that unresectable sarcomas in 6 of 22 patients were locally controlled with radiotherapy alone; they survived from 5 to 26 years after treatment.[283] Windeyer and co-workers similarly reported the results of treating 58 patients with fibrosarcomas.[284] Using doses between 60 and 80 Gy, they treated 11 patients with large, unresectable tumors with radiation therapy alone and an additional 11 with radiation therapy for postsurgical recurrences. Fourteen of these 22 patients had complete regression of their tumors, and 27% of the tumors were locally controlled for many years.

In a series of 35 patients from the M.D. Anderson Hospital, high-dose radiation therapy alone was given for soft tissue sarcomas.[285] Doses ranged from 70 to 75 Gy. The overall local recurrence rate was 66%, and 7 of 10 patients with extremity sarcomas had recurrences. In a series from the Massachusetts General Hospital (MGH) 54 patients were treated with primary radiation therapy for soft tissue sarcomas.[286] Of the 26 patients who were treated with doses greater than 65 Gy, 61% were locally controlled at 4 years. The majority of lesions smaller than 5 cm were controlled. However, of the 28 patients treated with doses less than 65 Gy, only 2 patients were alive and free of disease for more than 2 years. An analysis of the MGH experience with radiotherapy alone ($\geq$65 Gy) reported by Tepper and Suit showed an inverse relationship between tumor size and ability to obtain local control (Table 40-25).[287] For tumors $<$5 cm, 5 to 10 cm, and $>$10 cm, the local control rates with radiotherapy alone were 88%, 53%, and 33%, respectively.

There are data that demonstrate that the dose required to inactivate a tumor increases with the number of viable tumor cells, thus, radiation therapy given to microscopic disease is much more effective than treatment of gross disease.[288]

Local control can be achieved by radiotherapy alone, but it

TABLE 40-25. Relationship of Size of Lesion to Local Control Achieved by Radiotherapy Alone*

Size of Legion	No. of Patients	No. Locally Controlled (%)
<5 cm	8	7 (88)
5–10 cm	17	9 (53)
>10 cm	10	3 (33)
Total	35	19 (54)

*Tumor dose of ≥6500 rad.

Tepper JE, Suit HD: Radiation therapy of soft tissue sarcomas. Cancer 55:2273–2277, 1985.

usually requires very aggressive treatment with very high doses of radiation, which carry significant risks of adverse sequellae. Even so, the local control rates achieved with radiotherapy alone appear to be inferior to those obtained with surgery. Thus, radiation therapy should be used as a primary modality only in patients who have lesions that are not amenable to standard treatments because of tumor size, anatomic location, medical inoperability, or refusal of a patient to agree to conventional treatment. A special situation may occur if desmoid tumors cannot be resected; several series have shown that excellent, local control was achieved with radiation therapy alone.[289–291]

Combining Radiotherapy and Surgery

The rationale for combining surgery with adjuvant radiation therapy is to employ conservative surgery and moderate-dose radiation therapy to preserve the function of the area involved, especially limbs. Radiation therapy is used to treat microscopic tumor extending into the adjacent tissues beyond the primary tumor mass, achieving the same results as a more radical resection. A distinct advantage to this approach is that the treatment volume for radiation therapy is designed to encompass the surrounding tissues at risk for tumor involvement, such as nerves, vessels, tendons, and bone, which would otherwise limit the ability to perform an adequate local resection. Theoretically combined therapy offers both a high degree of local control and improved functional and cosmetic results, especially in the extremities. This expectation has been realized in clinical practice in several different series.[43,44,292,293]

In 1951, Cade reported a survival rate of 61% in a series of 80 patients treated with wide excision followed by radiation therapy, compared with 27% (6 of 22) with amputation.[283] Thus, he championed the use of radiation therapy in combination with wide local excision. Results of combined-modality treatment from recent literature are shown in Tables 40-26 and 40-27.

Although several reports show excellent results from combining limb-sparing surgery with radiotherapy for high-grade sarcomas of the extremities, it is still unclear if radiation therapy should be administered before, during, or after the surgical procedure. It is obvious that combining radiation therapy with conservative surgery has avoided ablative surgical procedures and maintained local control in the majority of patients (85%). Moreover, by eliminating the need for generous surgical margins, the functional results are excellent. Additional research is needed to define the aggressiveness of each modality and to relate results to grade, histologic type, tumor size, and anatomic site.

For most low-grade (Grade I) sarcomas that can be excised with reasonable margins, there is no clear evidence that radiation therapy is beneficial. In recommending treatment for patients with low-grade sarcomas, the pivotal issues are the adequacy of the surgical resection and the closeness with which the patient can be followed. The low-grade sarcomas are frequently very slow in manifesting local recurrences, often requiring many years before recurrences are seen. Only if there are problems with the patient's reliability for follow-up should surgery be combined with radiation therapy.

PREOPERATIVE RADIATION THERAPY. There are several theoretical advantages of preoperative radiation therapy combined with conservative surgery in the management of soft tissue sarcomas. First, inactivation of tumor cells by radiation therapy may decrease the risks of tumor implantation in the surgical wound and subsequently decrease metastatic spread from any tumor cells that enter vascular spaces during surgery. Second, the volume to be treated can be limited to clinically and radiologically evident tumor and the adjacent tissues at risk for microscopic extension, without any necessity for encompassing all the tissues that are manipulated during the surgical procedure itself. Third, in many instances, the mass will be smaller at the time of surgery after responding to radiation therapy, which facilitates conservative resection. Fourth, an inoperable sarcoma

TABLE 40-26. Local Control and Survival After Preoperative Radiation Therapy for Extremity Soft Tissue Sarcomas

Study*	No. of Patients	Follow-up (Years)	Local Failure ± Distant Metastases (%)	5 Year Disease-Free Survival (%)
Massachusetts General Hospital[294]	90	1–18	15 (17)	67 (74)
M.D. Anderson[295]	27	≥5	2 (7)	15 (56)
University of Florida[296]	19	1–5	1 (5)	11 (58)
Pooled Data	136		18 (13)	93 (68)

*Group or institution and reference number.

TABLE 40-27. Local Recurrence Rate with Conservative Surgery and Postoperative Radiation Therapy

*Study**	*No. of Patients*	*Follow-up (Years)*	*Dose (Gy)*	*Patients with Local Recurrence (%)*	*5-Year Disease-Free Survival (%)*
University California, San Francisco[292]	29	>2	50–75	3 (10)	68
M.D. Anderson[43]	300	2–7	60–75	67 (22)	68
National Cancer Institute[44]†	129	1–8	63	10 (8)	60
Massachusetts General Hospital[293]†	123	1–12	60–68	16 (12)	65
Pooled Data	581			96 (17)	

*Group institution and reference numbers.
†Extremity sites only.

may be made resectable by regression with radiation therapy.

The major disadvantages of preoperative radiation therapy are the delay in surgical resection (a psychological disadvantage for some patients), a risk of compromising wound healing, and the necessity for the radiation therapist to have planned and executed radiotherapy before surgical resection. Often, an initial excision is carried out by a surgeon who is removing a piece of tissue for diagnosis. In some instances, the diagnosis of a sarcoma comes as a surprise, and many of the potential benefits of preoperative radiation therapy simply cannot be realized because of a suboptimal biopsy procedure. Nonetheless, there are several series that demonstrate that planned preoperative radiation therapy in patients with high-grade sarcomas can yield excellent results (see Table 40-26).[294–296] In some instances, the radiation-induced shrinkage of an inoperable tumor resulted in these tumors becoming resectable.[285,297,298]

POSTOPERATIVE RADIATION THERAPY. Radiation therapy in combination with surgery is most commonly employed in the postoperative period. For patients for whom postoperative radiation therapy is planned, the amount of surgical resection itself remains a matter of some controversy. Although it is clear that all gross tumor should be removed, some physicians advocate a minimal excision of surrounding normal tissues, and others advocate the widest excision possible that is compatible with reasonable limb function. The crucial issue is that larger surgical excisions not only remove more normal tissue, but also require the use of wider radiation fields; thus, wide excisions may ultimately reduce the functional result that can be achieved. For lesions that are located in the groin, popliteal space, ankle, elbow, forearm, wrist, hand, or foot, the margins are necessarily close at some point in the dissection. For lesions that occur in very fleshy parts of the body, the margins can be more generous. Expansion of local operations to include vascular reconstruction or bone replacement procedures has been advocated in recent years.[299–303]

The advantages of postoperative radiation therapy include immediate surgery, which can be a psychological advantage for some patients; no radiation-induced delay in wound healing; and an entire specimen available for histopathologic investigation. Moreover, the exact size and pattern of extension of the tumor are interpreted definitively.

The conservative surgical procedure itself has a moderate probability of achieving local control if the surgeon is able to get around the tumor with a negative margin. Adjuvant radiation therapy can minimize the necessity of wide margins, thereby optimizing function, and maximize the probability of local control. However, in encompassing all tissues manipulated by the surgeon, the postoperative treatment volume is usually larger than that used for preoperative radiation. Moreover, if there is a delay in starting radiation therapy, as for wound healing, there could ultimately be a larger number of residual tumor cells. A prolonged delay in wound healing may allow residual microscopic tumor to become palpable.

There are several published series demonstrating the results of surgery with postoperative radiation therapy (see Table 40-27).[4,43,292,293] One of the earliest and largest came from the M.D. Anderson Hospital, where over 300 patients with soft tissue sarcomas were treated.[43] The surgery consisted of conservative excision, usually a simple "shelling out," with removal of the gross tumor and a limited amount of normal tissue. Patients received a dose between 60 and 70 Gy during 6 to 7 weeks. In general, no attempt was made to include the entire muscle or anatomic compartment in the treatment field. The local recurrence rate for patients treated with combined conservative surgery and postoperative radiotherapy was 22%; 20% for those with extremity sarcomas. In the patients who had extremity sarcomas, most of the recurrences occurred in the fleshy portions of the extremity, where lesions typically were large and extended for significant distances along fascial planes. The disease-free survival rate at 5 years was 61% for all primary sites; for the extremities, it was 69%. For head and neck sarcomas, it was 63%, but for retroperitoneal disease, only 33%. Local failure rates ranged from 10% for Stage I to 28% for Stage III tumors. Distant metastases developed in 5% of patients with Stage I, in 29% with Stage II, and in 43% with Stage III tumors. The investigators reported significant complications in 7% of the patients, including soft tissue necrosis, traumatic fractures of bone within the radiation field, fibrosis with limitation of motion, nerve and vascular injuries, and moderate edema. Nonetheless, of those with extremity tumors undergoing such treatment, 85% of the patients maintained functional limbs.

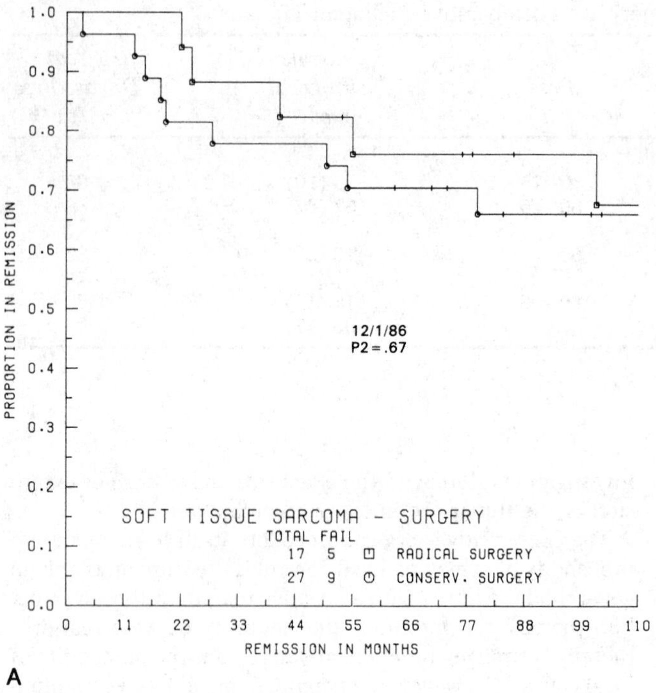

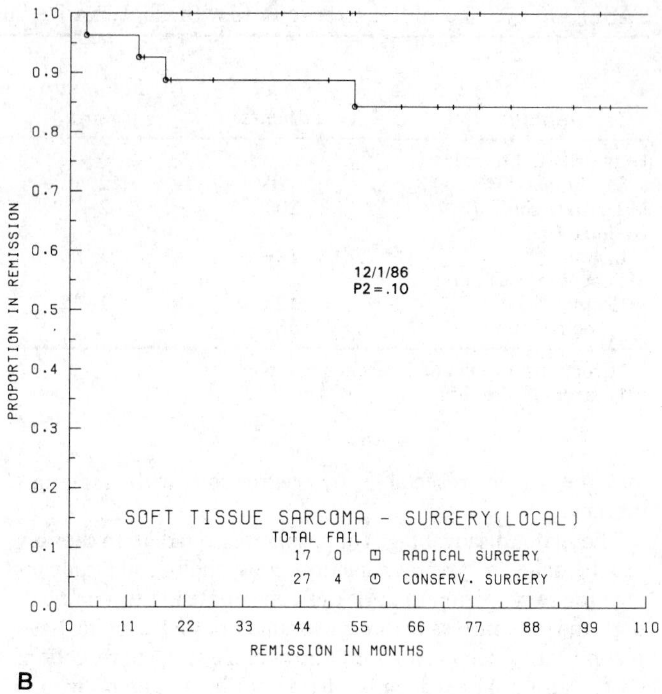

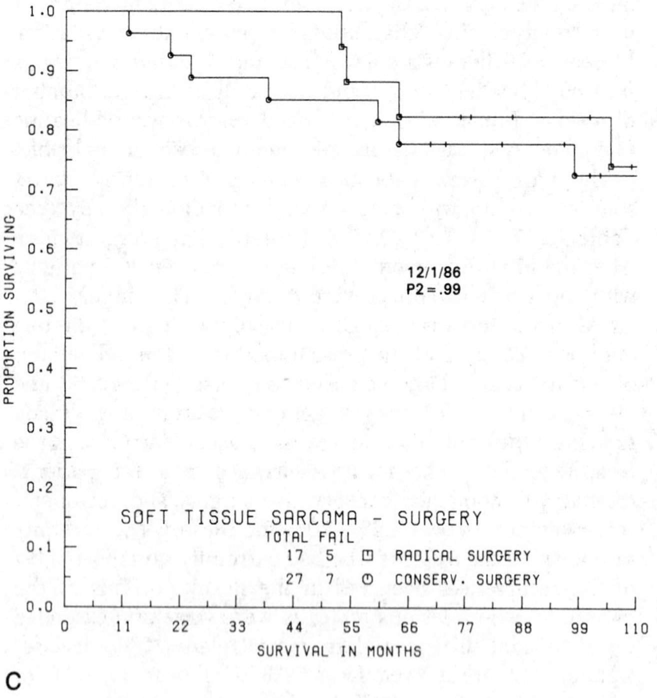

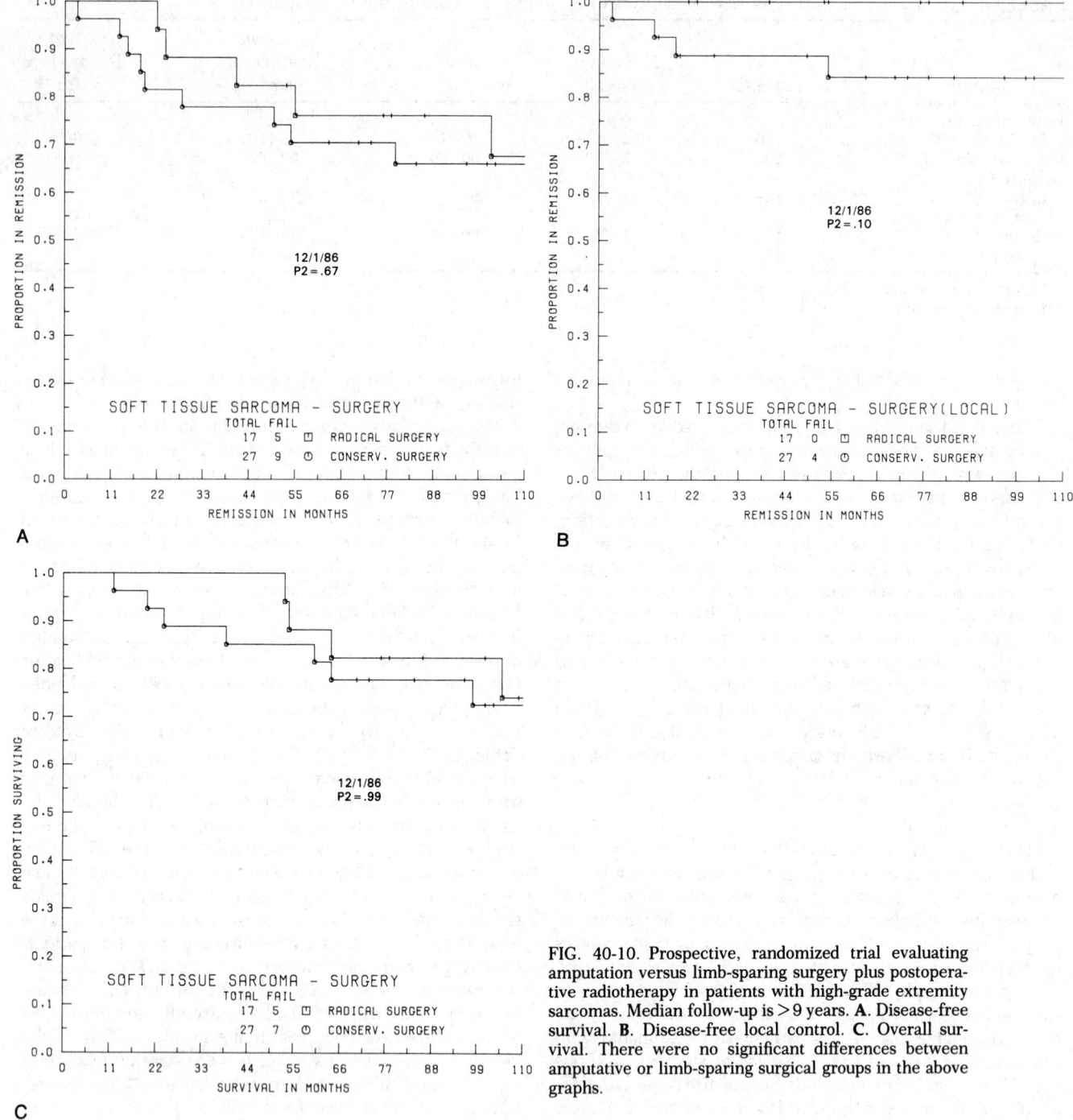

FIG. 40-10. Prospective, randomized trial evaluating amputation versus limb-sparing surgery plus postoperative radiotherapy in patients with high-grade extremity sarcomas. Median follow-up is >9 years. **A.** Disease-free survival. **B.** Disease-free local control. **C.** Overall survival. There were no significant differences between amputative or limb-sparing surgical groups in the above graphs.

In a smaller series from the University of California at San Francisco, 29 patients with extremity sarcomas were treated with surgery and postoperative radiation therapy.[292] The majority had Grade III tumors. The dose usually ranged between 55 and 70 Gy. Radiation fields were designed to cover the surgical bed with a generous margin; no effort was made to treat the entire involved muscle group from origin to insertion. The 5-year determinant survival rate was 81%, and the 5-year relapse-free survival rate was 68%. The local control rate was 90%. No patient required amputation due to radiation sequellae.

In this particular series, it was demonstrated that radiation can sterilize microscopic disease and reduce the local recurrence rate in patients undergoing simple excision of soft tissue sarcomas. Of the patients undergoing conservative excision and postoperative radiation therapy, 22 had microscopically positive margins of resection; yet only 3 of these 22 patients developed a local recurrence after postoperative radiation therapy. In contrast, of 14 nonirradiated patients treated with conservative surgery alone in whom margins were positive, 11 developed local recurrences.

It is difficult to assess the precise influence of size, grade, histology, and anatomic site in comparing patients from different series. To overcome some of these potential biases, Rosenberg and colleagues conducted a randomized prospective clinical trial evaluating limb-sparing surgery plus postoperative radiotherapy compared with amputation in patients with high-grade extremity sarcomas at the NCI.[258] The dose of radiation therapy employed for the patients undergoing limb-sparing surgery was usually 63 Gy. All patients received postoperative adjuvant chemotherapy. Forty-three patients were entered into the trial with a median follow-up of >9 years. There were 17 patients randomized to amputative surgery and 27 to limb-sparing surgery plus postoperative radiotherapy (randomization weighted 2:1 in favor of conservative surgery). There were four local recurrences in the group receiving limb-sparing surgery plus radiation and none in the amputation group (Fig. 40-10). Despite this finding, the 5-year disease-free and overall survival rates for the two groups were comparable, in the range of 70% to 80% (Fig. 40-10).

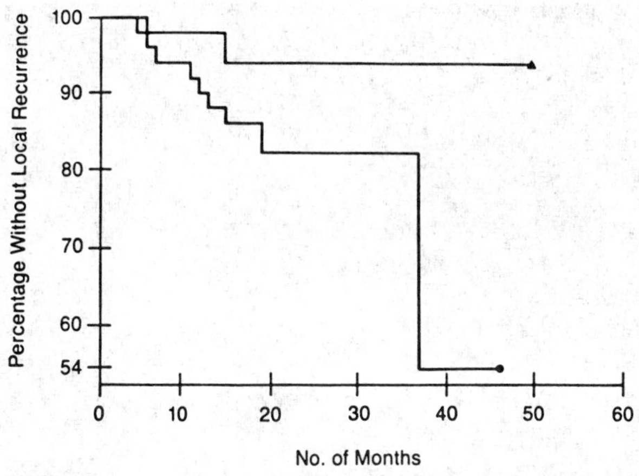

FIG. 40-11. Prospective, randomized evaluation of brachytherapy in 117 patients with extremity and superficial truncal sarcomas. Time to local recurrence is plotted for patients who received brachytherapy (triangle; $n = 52$) and no brachytherapy (circle; $n = 65$) ($p = 0.06$). (Brennan MF, Hilaris B, Shiu MH et al: Local recurrence in adult soft-tissue sarcoma, a randomized trial of brachytherapy. Arch Surg 122:1289–1293, 1987)

INTRAOPERATIVE BRACHYTHERAPY. A less commonly employed approach combining surgery and radiation therapy is the use of intraoperative brachytherapy.[304] This requires a surgery and radiotherapy group with expertise in this technique. Brennan and colleagues reported a trial evaluating the efficacy of intraoperative brachytherapy in adult patients with operable soft tissue sarcomas of the extremities or superficial trunk at Memorial Hospital.[305] Temporary implants of iridium-192 (^{192}Ir) were employed using after-loading techniques. Usually, this consisted of a single-plane implant. A total of 117 patients were prospectively randomized to receive or not receive intraoperative brachytherapy. With median follow-up of only 16 months, 2 of 52 patients receiving brachytherapy developed local recurrences, compared with 9 of 65 in the group not receiving brachytherapy ($p = 0.06$) (Fig. 40-11). It appeared that a significant improvement in local control was demonstrated in those patients receiving brachytherapy. No survival differences were seen between the two groups during the short follow-up period.

The advantages and disadvantages of brachytherapy are somewhat similar to those for preoperative radiation therapy; however, an additional advantage is that the complete treatment is considerably shorter, because the radiation is given during the time of surgery and the immediate week or so thereafter. The treatment necessitates detailed planning and exceptionally close cooperation between the surgeon and the radiation therapist. Nonetheless, the results achieved with brachytherapy in this study are comparable to the best reports of treatment using external-beam radiotherapy.

Technical Aspects of Radiation Therapy

The most commonly employed technique in the treatment of soft tissue sarcomas is the combined use of surgery and postoperative radiation therapy. This approach mandates an adequate resection of all gross disease. A shell-out procedure, which involves the excision of the tumor around its pseudocapsule, is suboptimal. Giuliano and Eilber have documented persistent macroscopic tumor in approximately 50% of the patients at the time of re-excision of previous shell-out operative sites.[306] Therefore, a planned re-excision of the operative sites should always be performed if the initial excision is deemed inadequate.

Radiation portals should be designed to treat muscle groups from origin to insertion in order to encompass the entire fascial plane, which may be potentially contaminated by tumor cells within postoperative hematomas.[307] Whether this is actually better than a 5- to 10-cm margin around the tumor bed is unclear. For the occasional tumor involving a subcutaneous primary location without muscle involvement, an 8- to 10-cm margin around the initial tumor volume should be employed. If preoperative radiation therapy is used, an 8- to 10-cm margin around the tumor mass in all dimensions should be obtained.

For primary tumors of the extremities, the only contraindications to limb-sparing surgery and radiation therapy are lesions that are so extensive that negative margins cannot be obtained; gross invasion of a joint; extensive involvement of several compartments of the extremity; or invasion of major neurovascular or bony structures beyond the scope of grafting or reconstruction.

More commonly, radiation therapy is planned postoperatively after wound healing. It is essential to establish the extent of disease as seen by the surgeons who carried out the surgery and the apparent site of origin, possible residual tumor, tumor spillage, or hemorrhage. Ideally, the radiotherapist should directly observe the surgery.

In planning the radiation therapy, it is essential to simulate the patient in a treatment position. This necessitates immobilizing the extremity in a reproducible position at the time of simulation. In most instances, this means making a cast to immobilize the extremity in the exact same position each

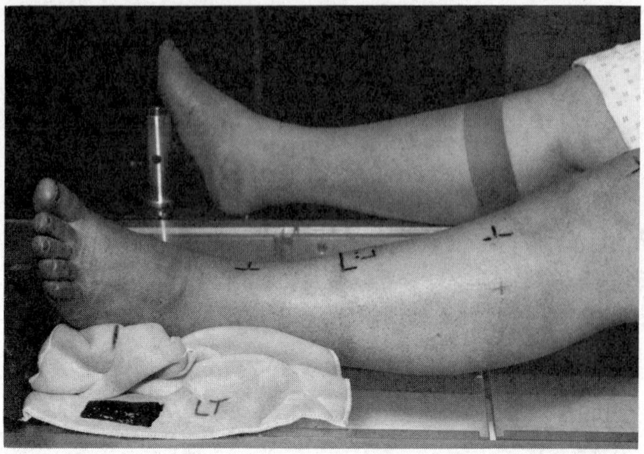

A

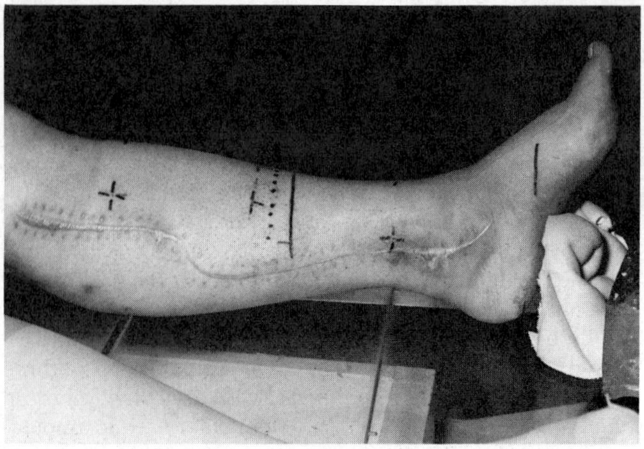

B

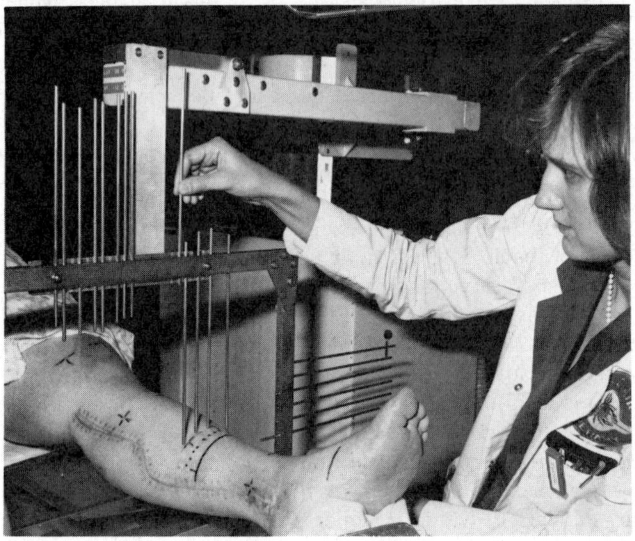

C

FIG. 40-12. **A**. Patient with a sarcoma of the left leg. A cast has been individually molded to surround her foot and ankle such that the foot will always be in exactly the same position for each day's treatment. This is done at the time of simulation, which is a mock-up procedure during which the positioning and measurements required for treatment are determined, although treatment is not actually carried out. Diagnostic x-rays are taken that mimic exactly what will be done with the megavoltage x-ray beam. **B**. Medial view of the left leg. The scar can be seen, and several reference points have been marked on the skin. Again, the cast and its relationship to supporting the foot can be seen. **C**. After positioning, it is important to determine the contour of what is being irradiated. Because the tissues vary in their thickness at any one level and because radiation is continuously attenuating as it transverses tissue, the thickness of the tissue at different levels in the radiation field will result in differing doses. To know what the discrepancies are, contours are taken at various levels. In this view, a mechanical device is being used to outline the contour at various levels in differing directions. Once the contours have been determined, then dose calculations can be made for the various levels that have been determined.

day with respect to the table top (Fig. 40-12A–C). When large fields are needed, the patient should not be turned because rotation of an extremity around a major joint may occur in more than one plane. If very long fields are required, treating isocentrically with pairs of matching fields, either using a shifting match-line technique or the match-line wedge technique.[308] The match-line wedge technique allows shifting the angle of obliquity in such a way that matching may occur in different planes; this can be an advantage in designing radiation fields that correspond to an anatomic compartment. For this reason, the match-line wedge technique has some theoretical advantage over simply shifting the match line 1 cm every 10 Gy, as is commonly done.

Every attempt is made to define the tumor volume in order to optimize the radiation portals (Figs. 40-13 and 40-14). Customized, individually shaped blocks are cut out for each patient to optimize the tumor volume, and the process adds secondary collimation beyond what a linear accelerator itself can offer. Generous use of clips placed at the time of surgery to define the extent of resection allow the therapist to see at simulation where the surgeon has been, and in many instances, allow for planning of oblique fields, which spare unmanipulated tissues but incorporate tissues that were handled at surgery. It is often surprising to see how far beyond the surgical scar some of the clips may appear. At the time of simulation, the scar is marked with wire in order to visualize on simulator films how the scar will be treated within the radiation field. If the radiation port strikes the scar perpendicularly, rather than tangentially, then tissue-equivalent bolus material should be applied superficially to increase the dose to the scar. The reason for this is simply to be certain that the skin-sparing effects of high-energy x-rays, applied perpendicularly to the skin, do not work to the patient's disadvantage by underdosing the scar itself.

An attempt is made to spare at least 33% of the circumference of the extremity from the direct radiation field to optimize function and minimize lymphedema. Every effort is made to exclude joints from the radiation field if the surgery permits. If the scar crosses the joint, at least some of the joint is blocked out, unless the joint was entered surgically. Active involvement of the physical therapist with the patient is essential from the beginning to motivate the patient. This is more than mere "lip service"; it is essential to maximize the function of the extremity, muscles, and joints.

In the postoperative setting, tumor doses of 63 Gy at

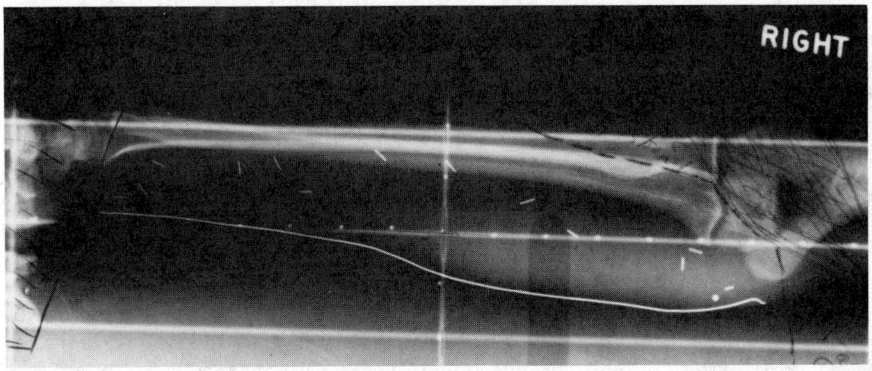

A

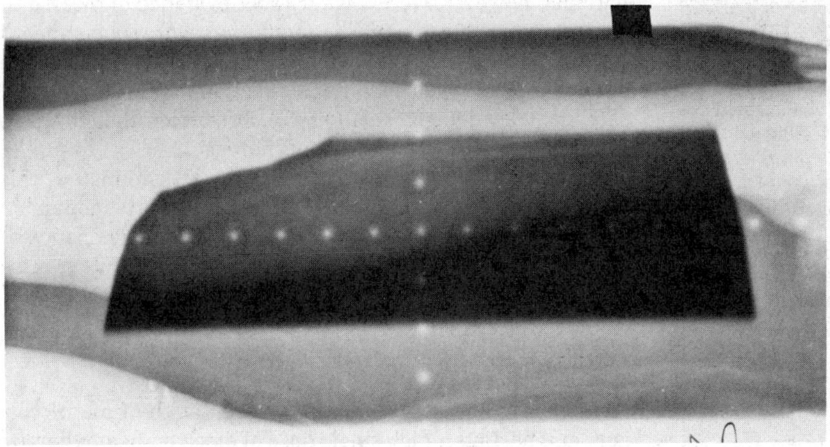

B

FIG. 40-13. **A**. On a different patient, a simulation process is demonstrated. Metallic clips have been placed throughout the course of the surgeon's exploration to show exactly where the surgeon has been. A piece of wire corresponds to the forearm of this particular patient showing where the scar is in relation to the treatment field. It occurs right at the edge of the tissue being treated. The cross-mark represents the center of the radiation field, which is situated in the middle of the soft tissue of the forearm itself. The forearm has been positioned carefully in such a way that the radius and ulna superimpose on the same plane. Thus, one edge of the radiation field corresponds to the bony structures themselves, leaving soft tissue above that line which is outside the radiation field. A dotted line represents a customized block that is cut to protect approximately half of the elbow joint, keeping it outside the high-dose radiation volume. **B**. Port film on the same patient taken with 4 MeV x-rays in the treatment position. This image matches up to the simulator film seen in **A**.

1.8 Gy per day are recommended. If there is gross residual disease, an increase in the total dose to approximately 70 to 75 Gy can be used. In order to do this, shrinking-field techniques should be employed to minimize the volume receiving the highest dose. Generally, the first volume reduction is done at 45 Gy, and if a second volume reduction is needed, it can be made at 63 Gy.

Lesions of the hand and foot are frequently able to be treated with conservative surgery and radiation therapy.[309] The radiation therapy in such instances has to be planned very carefully, and it frequently necessitates high-energy electrons for at least part of the treatment. Nonetheless, lesions of the hand and foot do not always have to be amputated automatically, because conservative surgery and radiation therapy can frequently achieve an excellent functional result. Similar principles apply to sarcomas of the head and neck region.

Lesions of the chest or abdominal wall can frequently be treated with high doses of radiation therapy postoperatively using a combination of x-rays and electrons. Doses frequently range from 60 to 70 Gy or even higher, depending on the volume and exact location. However, for retroperitoneal sarcomas, dose limitations usually reflect the tolerance of the small bowel and kidney. Generally, doses in excess of 55 Gy carry a considerable risk of small bowel injury.

For patients who are to receive preoperative radiation therapy, a dose of 45 to 50 Gy is recommended, at the rate of 1.8 Gy each day. Additional postoperative boosts may be given, either intraoperatively or postoperatively, depending on the surgical findings and pathologic margins. The total dose for such patients can go to 70 Gy.

INTRA-ARTERIAL CHEMOTHERAPY, RADIATION THERAPY, AND SURGERY

Eilber and associates at UCLA have reported their extensive experience with preoperative intra-arterial doxorubicin and radiation for the treatment of sarcomas of the extremity.[310] The rationale for this approach is to regionally deliver an active chemotherapeutic agent that has direct cytotoxic and potentially radiosensitizing effects on the tumor. In their early experience, intra-arterial doxorubicin was given at 30 mg/day during 24 hours for 3 consecutive days. On the following day, radiation therapy was started, and 3.5 Gy fractions were administered daily for 10 days for a total dose of 35 Gy. At 1 to 2 weeks after completion of the radiation, an en bloc resection of all gross disease was performed.

A total of 77 patients with high-grade extremity sarcomas were treated; 74 (96%) were able to have limb-salvage surgery. Local tumor recurrence was noticed in only 3 (4%) patients. However, complications occurred in 25 patients (35%), with 14 (17%) requiring a second operative procedure. These complications consisted mainly of bone fractures and wound slough. Because of this high complication

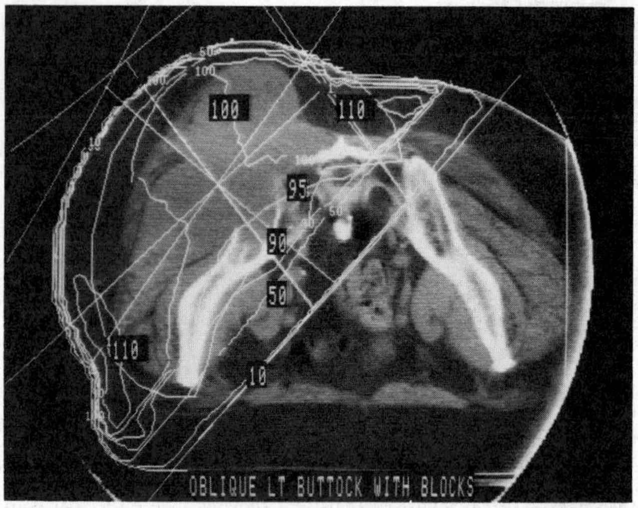

FIG. 40-14. CT cut for a patient with a large buttock sarcoma. The patient is prone, and the extensive soft tissue mass, which could not be resected, is seen. The patient is being treated with obliqued fields designed to treat the entire ilium on the right as well as the soft tissue mass. The fields are wedged, to account for the contour of the buttock itself, and the fields are slightly offset, so that the 50% isodose lines from each field direction coincide within the pelvis. The numbers represent different isodose curves, on this particular slice (one of many sequential cuts), and they can be seen to relate closely to the soft tissue mass itself. The intention is to take this entire volume to a dose of approximately 75 Gy. In this particular instance, treatment was carried out twice a day.

rate, the preoperative radiation therapy regimen was reduced to 1.75 Gy. Subsequently, an additional 105 patients were treated with this regimen, 102 (97%) were able to undergo limb-salvage surgery. Complications were reduced, with reoperation required in 6 (6%) patients. Local recurrences were seen in 9 (8%) patients. With this combined preoperative regimen, more than 96% of the patients with high-grade extremity tumors were able to have nonamputative surgery with acceptable local control.

Denton and colleagues at the University of Alabama reported a local recurrence rate of 3% in 30 patients with soft tissue and bony extremity sarcomas using a similar regimen. The mean follow-up was only 22 months.[311] Results achieved with this approach are comparable to standard multimodality approaches; however, no comparative randomized trials have been performed. Lokich reported the use of preoperative systemic chemotherapy in combination with radiation therapy in 3 patients with bulky soft tissue sarcomas and noticed marked tumor regression in 2 patients.[312]

Other investigators have reported on the use of regional arterial chemotherapy alone or in conjunction with hyperthermic perfusion as a preoperative adjunct or as primary therapy for unresectable tumors.[313–315] The advantages of regional chemotherapy in these approaches have not been definitively demonstrated. Didolkar and colleagues reported that intra-arterial doxorubicin achieved similar regional tissue levels as intravenously administered drug in an animal model.[316] It is difficult to assess the efficacy of preoperative intra-arterial chemotherapy from any of the published studies.

Fast-Neutron Therapy

At least two reports have emerged on the treatment of locally advanced sarcomas treated with fast-neutron therapy. Salinas and co-workers from the M.D. Anderson Hospital reported 20 (69%) of 29 patients with advanced soft tissue sarcomas who achieved local control of their tumor with fast-neutron therapy.[317] Four patients developed complications. Pelton and colleagues from the University of Washington reported that 16 patients with unresectable soft tissue sarcomas were treated with fast neutrons, including 11 who had no evidence of metastatic disease and who were treated with curative intent. These patients received a mixture of neutrons and photons. Local control was achieved in approximately 60%, with no relapses seen after 30 months. Only 4 patients, however, were alive without evidence of disease. A common complication of treatment was severe subcutaneous fibrosis, which in 2 patients necessitated skin grafts. One patient who received abdominal radiation for retroperitoneal sarcomas developed a small bowel obstruction thought to be related to radiation enteritis and fibrosis.

Although neutron therapy is still investigational in this country, fast-neutron therapy for patients with inoperable soft tissue sarcomas appears to offer a reasonable chance of local control and potential long-term survival, but its precise role must still be defined.

Intraoperative Radiation Therapy

Intraoperative radiation therapy is used at the time of surgery and permits a high single dose of electron-beam therapy to be delivered directly to the tumor bed, after moving as many incidental structures out of the radiation field as possible. For soft tissue sarcomas, its use has been predominantly for primaries in the retroperitoneum; it has not shown any significant benefit over conventional surgery and postoperative radiation therapy in terms of survival or freedom from relapse. Large single doses are potentially a source of long-term complications to ureters and especially to nerves. In a randomized study, the NCI was unable to show the benefit of intraoperative radiation therapy over external-beam therapy postoperatively in terms of survival or disease-free survival.[282] Intraoperative radiation therapy was able to reduce the frequency of radiation enteritis in these patients. However, because many of these patients developed sarcomatosis of the peritoneum, the precise role of intraoperative radiation therapy remains investigational at this time.

Radiation Sensitizers, Radiosensitivity, and Radioresistance

For most sarcomas, complete surgical resection is recommended if it can be accomplished without excessive morbidity; however, if a patient has a sarcoma that is not amenable to resection, it is still possible that radiation therapy alone can control the local disease.

Although frequently radiation therapy is said not to be indicated in the management of soft tissue or bony sarcomas because the tumor is "radioresistant," there are data demonstrating that this concept is fallacious. Tepper and Suit reported a series of 35 patients who had soft tissue sarcomas that were treated with doses of 65 Gy or more (see Table 40-25).[287] For lesions smaller than 5 cm, 7 of 8 achieved local control. For those lesions between 5 and 10 cm, 9 of 17 achieved local control. For lesions greater than 10 cm, only 3 of 10 achieved local control.

Kinsella and Glatstein from NCI reported a series using a variety of intravenous radiosensitizers in the management of unresectable sarcomas, both soft tissue and bony in origin.[319] The vast majority of these tumors were large, over 10 cm; the median size was 14 × 14 cm. Kinsella and Glatstein were able to achieve local control (freedom from all symptoms and no further growth) in 22 of 29 patients who had extensive disease for at least 1 year. They demonstrated that many tumors were radiosensitive but radio-unresponsive. Radiosensitive refers to specific parameters (D_o, D_q, or n) that are obtained from in vitro cell survival curves. Whether the tumor is sensitive or resistant depends on the exact quantitative parameters derived from such studies. Often a tumor is called radioresistant, but the tumor is really radio-unresponsive, that is, the tumor does not demonstrate any decrease in size (exactly how much is unspecified) seen relatively quickly (also unspecified) after some modest doses of radiation therapy (also unspecified). The concept of a radioresponsive or radio-unresponsive tumor is 40 years old and was useful for distinguishing tumors that shrank quickly, such as lymphomas or seminomas, from those that did not. In their review of 29 patients with massive sarcomas treated with either hypoxic cell sensitizers or halogenated pyrimidines, the NCI reported patients in whom all the cells were destroyed pathologically, but in whom the mass never regressed. In some instances, the patients survived well over 5 years without any growth of tumor after irradiation.

The precise role of radiation sensitizers in the management of these tumors is still an area of active investigation. The important point is that all the tumor cells can apparently be destroyed, even if the mass does not necessarily regress in size. A significant component of a sarcomatous mass may be represented by the matrix or stroma of the tumor. Depending on the extent of a tumor's composition, the death of tumor cells is not necessarily accompanied by measurable regression. Thus, some sarcomas can be radiosensitive, but not necessarily radioresponsive. Examples of this phenomenon have been seen in a variety of other tumors, such as testis cancer treated with chemotherapy or massive mediastinal Hodgkin's disease. Radiosensitive and radioresistant should be defined very carefully, and the words must be used with precision.

CHEMOTHERAPY

Adjuvant Chemotherapy

Despite adequate local treatment, most patients with high-grade soft tissue sarcomas will ultimately have recurrences with metastatic disease, usually in the lungs. For this reason, effective systemic adjuvant treatments should be given soon after the definitive treatment of local disease.

A variety of factors have made it difficult to accumulate reliable information about the adjuvant treatment of patients with high-grade soft tissue sarcomas. The relatively infrequent incidence of these tumors has made it difficult for any individual institution to accumulate enough patients to perform reliable adjuvant studies. Difficulties in assigning histologic type and grade impede comparison of different series. In addition, soft tissue sarcomas can occur virtually anywhere in the body, and sarcomas at different sites often have a different natural history and prognosis. Thus, accounting for the site of origin is important in evaluating adjuvant treatment trials. Despite these obstacles, a series of historically controlled and prospective, randomized studies of adjuvant chemotherapy have been reported.

NONRANDOMIZED TRIALS. Although difficult to interpret, several historically controlled trials have suggested the efficacy of adjuvant chemotherapy.[320-323] Sordillo and colleagues at Memorial Sloan-Kettering Hospital reported 64 adult patients with soft tissue sarcomas who received adjuvant chemotherapy with a six-drug combination regimen (ALOMAD) after surgery.[320] Their chemotherapy regimen consisted of vincristine, high-dose methotrexate with citrovorum factor rescue, doxorubicin, DTIC, and dactinomycin. The actuarial 3-year survival rate was 85% for patients who received adjuvant chemotherapy, which was interpreted by these authors as an improvement compared with the historical controls.

In another nonrandomized trial, Das Gupta and coworkers reported on the results of 113 adult patients with primary soft tissue sarcomas treated by adjuvant chemotherapy with a two-drug combination of doxorubicin and DTIC.[321,322] Doxorubicin was administered to a maximum cumulative dose of 500 mg/m^2. Dacarbazine was continued for 1 year. The 5-year continuous disease-free survival in patients receiving chemotherapy was 74%, compared with 50% for patients treated with surgery alone ($p = 0.05$).

Weisenberger and associates at UCLA reported on the results of patients with soft tissue sarcomas treated with preoperative intra-arterial infusion of doxorubicin followed by postoperative adjuvant chemotherapy.[323] Postoperative chemotherapy consisted of vincristine, methotrexate with citrovorum rescue, and doxorubicin. A total cumulative doxorubicin dose of 500 mg/m^2 was administered. Thereafter, vincristine and high-dose methotrexate were given monthly for 1 year. Of 62 patients in their series, 28 received postoperative chemotherapy. Six (21%) of the 28 patients who received postoperative chemotherapy relapsed, with a median time to relapse of 12 months, and 16 (47%) of the 34 patients who did not receive postoperative chemotherapy relapsed, with a median time to relapse of 4.5 months. The authors concluded that an improvement in disease-free survival was seen in those patients who received postoperative chemotherapy. There are difficulties in drawing meaningful conclusions from these studies because they were nonrandomized, and therefore patient selection factors that were involved in selecting chemotherapy for the treatment of some patients and not others may have biased the results.

PROSPECTIVE RANDOMIZED TRIALS. Several randomized trials evaluating adjuvant chemotherapy in patients

TABLE 40-28. Randomized Soft Tissue Sarcoma Adjuvant Chemotherapy Trials

Study*	No. of Patients	Site	Grade†	Chemotherapy‡	Median Follow-Up (Years)	5-Year Disease-Free Survival (%)		5-Year Survival (%)	
						Chemo	*No Chemo*	*Chemo*	*No Chemo*
ECOG; DFCI/MGH[333]	75	Extremity, head and neck, truncal, retroperitoneal, other	2.3	Dox	4	74	62	68	66
Mayo Clinic[328]	61	Extremity, head and neck, truncal retroperitoneal, visceral	All	Dox, VCR, DTIC/VCR, CYC, DACT	5.4	70§	50	71	71
EORTC[329]	326	Extremity, head and neck, truncal, retroperitoneal visceral	All	CYVADIC	3	67§,‖	52	79	74
Scandinavian Sarcoma Group[329a]	156		3,4	Dox					
Intergroup Sarcoma Committee[329b]	114	Extremity, head and neck, truncal, retroperitoneal	2,3	Dox					
UCLA[332]	114	Extremity	3	Dox	2.5	78	74		
Picci et al[331]	77	Extremity	2,3	Dox		68§	41	87§	67
NCI[335]	67	Extremity	2,3	Dox,CYC,MTX	7.1	75§	54	82	60
NCI[269]	72	Head and neck, truncal, retroperitoneal	2,3	Dox,CYC,MTX	5.9	57	51	60	58

*Group or institution and reference number. ECOG = Eastern Cooperative Oncology Group, DFCI = Dana Farber Cancer Institute, MGH = Massachusetts General Hospital, EORTC = European Organization for Research on Treatment of Cancer, UCLA = University of California of Los Angeles, NCI = National Cancer Institute.

†Grading performed by each institution. Mayo Clinic and Scandinavian Sarcoma Group used Broder's Grades 1–4; all other institutions had a 1–3 system.

‡Dox = doxorubicin, VCR = vincristine, DTIC = dacarbazine; CYC = cyclophosphamide; CYVADIC = cyclophosphamide, VCR, Dox, DTIC.

§Significantly different from no chemotherapy group.

‖Three-year results.

with soft tissue sarcomas have been reported.[257,269,324–336] Table 40-28 summarizes these trials. There are many factors in the conduct of these trials that make direct comparisons difficult to interpret. These factors influence the patient populations that are involved in each trial and include differences in primary sites of sarcoma, histologic grading, and chemotherapy regimens.

Since 1975, the NCI has studied the role of adjuvant chemotherapy in patients with high-grade soft tissue sarcomas.[257,269,324–326,335,336] Trials were conducted for patients with extremity tumor; head, neck, and trunk lesions; and retroperitoneal sarcomas. All patients in these trials had wide surgical excisions with removal of all gross tumor. All patients with extremity sarcomas received limb-sparing surgery, and all patients with head, neck, trunk and retroperitoneal sarcomas underwent postoperative radiation therapy.

The standard chemotherapy regimen used in the early NCI trials included doxorubicin, cyclophosphamide, and high-dose methotrexate. Doxorubicin and cyclophosphamide were administered monthly. After a maximum cumulative dose of doxorubicin (500–550 mg/m²) was achieved, six cycles of high-dose methotrexate with leucovorin rescue were administered. Chemotherapy was begun as soon as the wound healed, usually within 2 to 3 weeks after surgery. In patients who received the chemotherapy in conjunction with radiation therapy, the first chemotherapy dose was given 3 days before the first dose of radiation. Sixty-seven patients with soft tissue sarcomas of the extremities were randomized into a treatment protocol in which patients received either chemotherapy or no chemotherapy.[324] After a median follow-up of 4.5 years, results were reported that revealed a significantly improved disease-free and overall survival advantage for patients receiving chemotherapy.[325]

Subsequent analysis, with a median follow-up of 7.1 years, is illustrated in Figure 40-15A–C.[335] The 5-year disease-free survival for patients receiving chemotherapy was 75%, compared with 54% for no chemotherapy ($p2 = 0.037$). The 5-year overall survival for patients in this trial was 80% and 60% for the chemotherapy and no chemotherapy groups, respectively, with a trend toward improved survival in the chemotherapy arm ($p2 = 0.124$). In this trial, the adjuvant

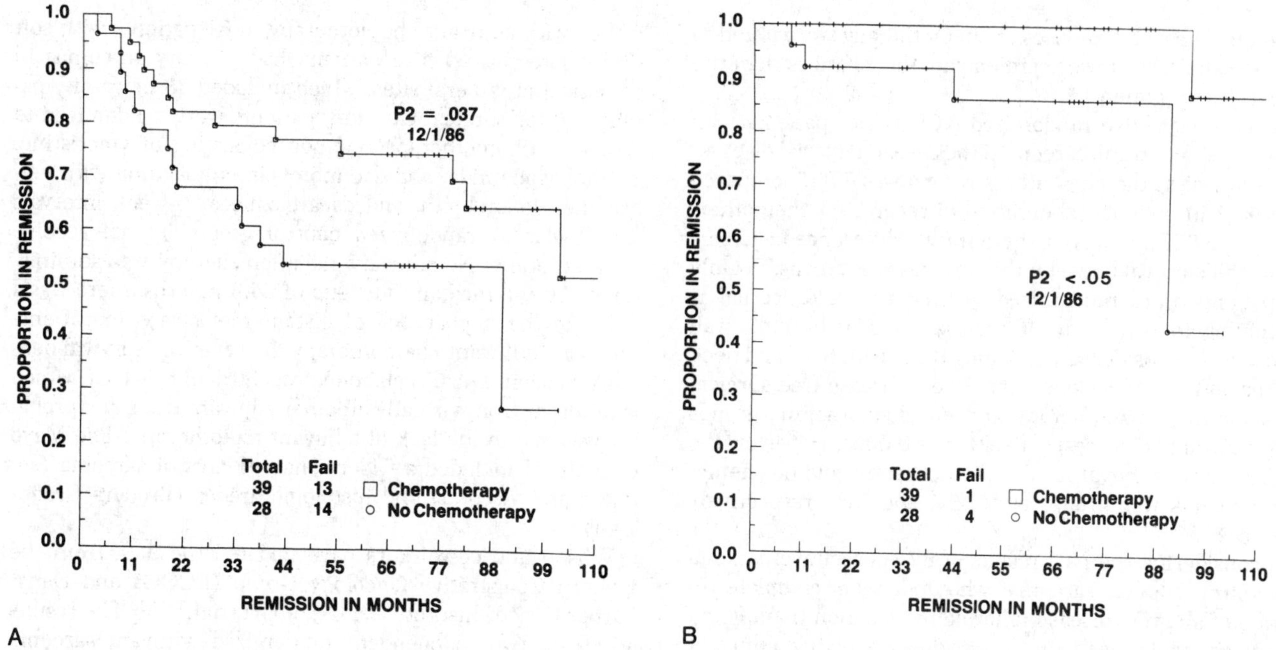

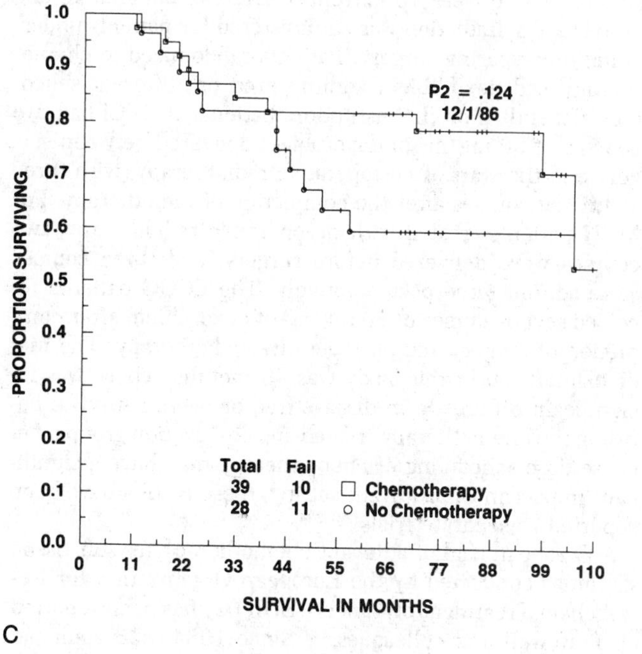

FIG. 40-15. Prospective, randomized trial evaluating adjuvant chemotherapy versus no chemotherapy in patients with high-grade extremity sarcomas at a median follow-up time of 7.1 years. **A.** Disease-free survival was significantly improved in patients who received chemotherapy ($p = 0.037$). **B.** Time to local recurrence. Local recurrences were significantly decreased by chemotherapy ($p < 0.05$). **C.** There was a trend for improved survival in patients who received chemotherapy versus no chemotherapy ($p = 0.124$).

chemotherapy resulted in improved local control rates ($p2 < 0.05$). There were no local recurrences in the patients undergoing amputation. Along the 23 patients who had limb-sparing surgery and chemotherapy, there was only 1 local recurrence, compared with 4 local recurrences in 17 patients who had limb-sparing surgery without chemotherapy.

The impact of chemotherapy on local recurrence may be a direct effect or may be indirectly related to the radiosensitizing properties of doxorubicin. The results of this trial indicated an improved disease-free survival in patients treated with adjuvant chemotherapy, with a trend toward improved overall survival. Toxicity with the chemotherapy regimen used in the early NCI trials consisted of nausea and vomiting and a significant incidence of cardiomyopathy due to doxorubicin.[337] A subsequent trial comparing this chemotherapy regimen to reduced cumulative doses of doxorubicin (350 mg/m^2) and cyclophosphamide (3500 gm/m^2) without high-dose methotrexate was performed at the NCI.[335] Eighty-eight patients with high-grade extremity sarcoma were randomized to receive the reduced-dose regimen or standard regimen. With a median follow-up of 4.4 years, the 5-year disease-free and overall survival for patients treated with reduced doses of chemotherapy was 72% and 75%, respectively, and was not significantly different from the high-dose regimen. The reduced doses of chemotherapy were found to be associated with fewer cardiomyopathic changes than the higher-dose regimen.[338]

In the prospective randomized NCI trial of patients with head, neck, and trunk sarcomas, the 3-year actuarial disease-free survival in the chemotherapy arm was 77%, compared with 49% in patients randomized to receive no chemotherapy ($p = 0.075$); however, there was no difference in actuarial overall survival between the two treatment arms.[269] Only 31 patients were randomized in this trial, and accrual is continuing in this study. If only patients with trunk wall lesions were considered (excluding those with head and neck lesions and breast lesions), the 3-year disease-free survival rates for the chemotherapy and no chemotherapy groups were 90% and 45%, respectively ($p = 0.006$). However, the 3-year overall survival for the chemotherapy and no chemotherapy trunk wall groups were 85% and 73%, respectively ($p = 0.18$).[269]

In considering the NCI results of 37 consecutive patients with retroperitoneal sarcomas who underwent complete resection of all gross disease followed by radiation therapy, no advantage could be seen in patients receiving adjuvant chemotherapy when considering either the entire group of patients or the subset of 15 of these patients who were entered into a prospective randomized trial testing the efficacy of adjuvant chemotherapy.[336] The toxicity of the adjuvant chemotherapy in combination with abdominal radiation therapy was substantial, and this trial was discontinued after 15 patients were randomized.

To summarize the NCI studies, a significant improvement in disease-free survival, with a trend toward improved overall survival, was seen in patients with extremity soft tissue sarcomas randomized to receive adjuvant chemotherapy.[335] Improvement due to adjuvant chemotherapy was also seen in patients with trunk wall lesions, although no improvement could be seen in patients with retroperitoneal sarcomas.[269,336]

Two prospective, randomized studies that examined only high-grade extremity sarcomas were reported by Picci and colleagues and Eilber and colleagues.[331,332] In the report by Picci, 77 patients with high-grade soft tissue sarcomas of the extremities were entered into a protocol evaluating doxorubicin given as an adjuvant to a cumulative dose of 450 mg/m^2. The primary tumor was treated by amputation or limb-sparing surgery in conjunction with adjuvant radiation therapy. All patients were then randomized to receive or not receive adjuvant doxorubicin. Early results of this trial revealed a significant disease-free survival advantage for patients receiving adjuvant chemotherapy.[331a] Subsequent follow-up confirmed a significant disease-free and overall survival advantage for patients treated with adjuvant chemotherapy, compared with no chemotherapy (Table 40-28).[331] In the trial by Eilber and colleagues, high-grade extremity sarcoma patients were given preoperative chemotherapy involving intra-arterial doxorubicin (30 mg/day $\times$ 3) plus radiotherapy and then randomized to receive postoperative doxorubicin (total dose, 450 mg/m^2) or no chemotherapy. There was no demonstrated disease-free or overall survival benefit after a median follow-up of 30 months.[332]

Edmonson and co-workers reported the Mayo Clinic experience with adjuvant chemotherapy in 61 patients with soft tissue sarcomas. These patients had primary sarcomas in somatic and visceral sites, which included 48 extremity patients. After surgical excision, patients were randomized to receive a chemotherapy regimen consisting of vincristine, cyclophosphamide, and dactinomycin, alternating with vincristine, doxorubicin, and dacarbazine at 6-week intervals for 1 year. A randomized control group did not receive chemotherapy. No adjuvant radiation therapy was administered. After a median follow-up of 64.3 months, there was a delay in the appearance of distant metastases in patients receiving adjuvant chemotherapy; however, no survival benefit was seen. Local recurrence was 30% in this trial, which is different from virtually all other adjuvant trials and probably was due to the lack of adjuvant radiotherapy. The Mayo Clinic trial included a wider range of sites of sarcoma (somatic and visceral) and histologic grades (Broders Grades 1–4).

Wilson and co-workers have updated the data from the Eastern Cooperative Oncology Group (ECOG) and Dana-Farber Cancer Institute (DFCI)/MGH trial.[330,333] The results are from two independent randomized adjuvant sarcoma studies. There were 75 extremity sarcoma patients among both studies. Radiation was administered for patients undergoing limb-sparing surgery. Patients randomized to chemotherapy had doxorubicin administered on different schedules, depending on the institution. Patients at DFCI had two courses of 90 mg/m^2 of doxorubicin delivered between surgery and the start of postoperative radiotherapy, with three additional courses after the completion of radiotherapy. For MGH patients treated with preoperative radiotherapy, two courses were delivered before surgery, and three courses were administered postoperatively. The ECOG patients received seven courses of 70 mg/m^2 of doxorubicin after completion of surgery and postoperative radiotherapy. The median follow-up in this study was 49 months. There was no significant difference in disease-free or overall survival between the chemotherapy-treated and observation groups. Because dose scheduling of chemotherapy may have a significant impact in the adjuvant setting, these results have been reported as separate trials.[327,334]

A European trial of adjuvant chemotherapy for soft tissue sarcomas conducted by the European Organization for Research on Treatment of Cancer (EORTC) has been reported by Bramwell and colleagues.[329] Since 1984, 326 adult patients with localized sarcomas of various sites and histological grades (including low-grade tumors) were entered into a prospective, randomized trial of adjuvant chemotherapy. After resection of the primary tumor, in some cases followed by radiotherapy, patients were randomized to receive or not receive eight courses of adjuvant chemotherapy of cyclophosphamide, vincristine, doxorubicin, and dacarbazine (CYVADIC). The median follow-up was 28 months. There was no significant improvement in disease-free or overall survival for the group receiving adjuvant (CYVADIC) chemotherapy. This was also true for the subgroup of patients with extremity sarcomas. However, the authors of this study caution that these conclusions are preliminary and require further follow-up.

Another European trial, conducted by the Scandinavian

Sarcoma Group, randomized patients with high-grade soft tissue sarcomas to receive or not receive adjuvant doxorubicin.[329a] A total of 156 patients have entered this trial with a trend of improved disease-free survival in one of the groups ($p = 0.10$). The results of this study are still preliminary.

In 1983, The Intergroup Sarcoma Committee was formed to pool the resources of various American cooperative groups. A randomized study that allocated patients with high-grade soft tissue sarcomas of all nonvisceral sites to no further treatment or to adjuvant doxorubicin therapy was initiated. As of 1987, 114 patients have been randomized. Preliminary results of the first 81 patients demonstrated no statistical difference in disease-free or overall survival between the groups that received adjuvant chemotherapy, compared with no chemotherapy.[329b] However, there was a trend toward improved disease-free survival in the chemotherapy-treated group ($p = 0.06$). These results are too preliminary to draw any conclusions.

The value of adjuvant chemotherapy for the treatment of patients with high-grade soft tissue sarcomas is unresolved. The NCI and other trials indicated an improved disease-free survival advantage with a trend toward improved survival in patients with extremity sarcomas treated with adjuvant chemotherapy.[328,331,335] However, some trials have not reported significant improvement in disease-free or overall survival with adjuvant chemotherapy.[332,333] There are several prospective, randomized studies which require further follow-up to draw meaningful conclusions.[329,329a,329b] For now, adjuvant chemotherapy in the treatment of high-grade soft tissue sarcomas of the extremities should be administered in the context of prospective clinical trials. There is currently little evidence that adjuvant chemotherapy is of value in patients with head, neck, trunk, and retroperitoneal sarcomas.

Treatment of Recurrent Sarcomas

Potter and associates reviewed the initial sites of tumor recurrence after primary treatment of a soft tissue sarcomas in 307 patients referred to the NCI.[44] These patients underwent complete surgical resection, often in combination with postoperative chemotherapy and radiation therapy. A total of 107 (35%) patients recurred locally or developed distant metastases; the sites of disease are identified in Table 40-14. The lung was the predominant site of first recurrence in 52% of these patients, followed by isolated local recurrences (20%). The pattern of recurrence depended on the primary site of the sarcoma. Patients with sarcomas of the head and neck, retroperitoneum, and chest or abdominal wall had a higher local recurrence rate, compared with extremity sites. In the American College of Surgeons survey, there were 452 (37%) of 1209 treatment failures in patients without metastases at the initial diagnoses who had total gross resection of their soft tissue sarcomas.[46] Among patients with recurrent disease, 236 (52%) had isolated locoregional recurrences; and 83 (18%) had isolated lung recurrences. Approximately 80% of all recurrences became evident within 5 years.

Aggressive surgical management of isolated local recurrences should be attempted. A thorough evaluation for evidence of disseminated disease must be performed before contemplating resection of a local recurrence. In the NCI experience, 20 (96%) of 21 isolated local recurrences were surgically resectable. Figures 40-16A and 40-16B shows the actuarial continuous disease-free and overall survival of patients who were rendered free of disease after resection of a local recurrence. The 3-year survival was 69%. Shiu and associates were able to resect 35 (81%) of 43 isolated locally recurrent extremity sarcomas, with a subsequent 5-year survival rate of 45%.[58] Giuliano and co-workers reported that 35 (92%) of 38 patients surgically rendered free of a local recurrence of an extremity or truncal (excluding retroperitoneal) sarcoma had a 5-year actuarial survival rate of 87%.[339] In the American College of Surgeons survey, the 5-year sur-

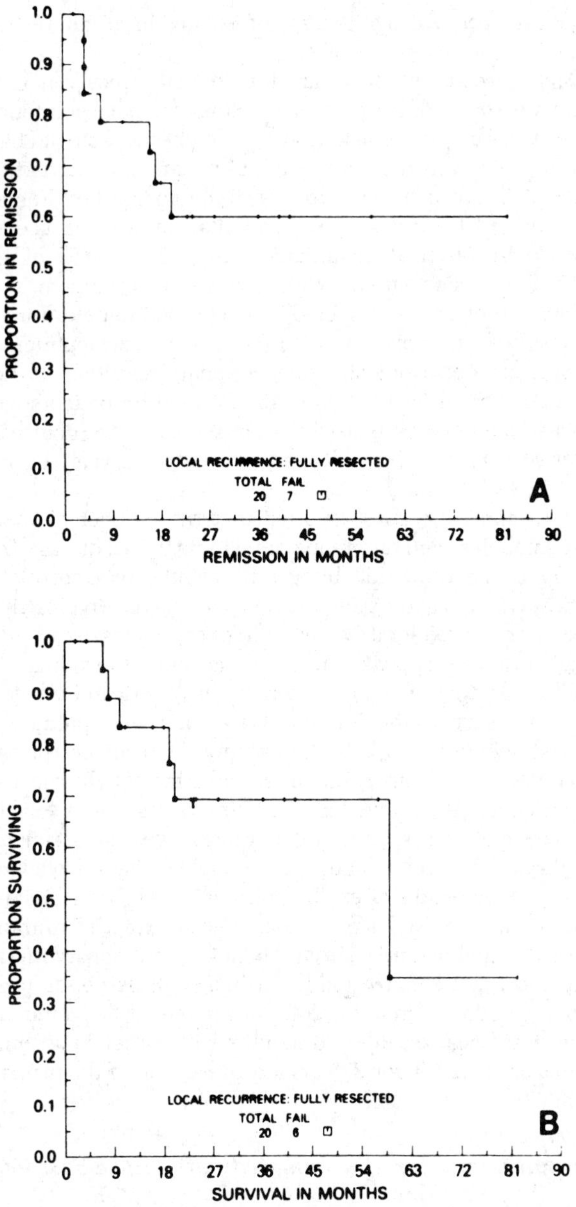

FIG. 40-16. Disease-free survival (**A**) and overall survival (**B**) in patients with high-grade sarcomas who underwent resection of isolated locally recurrent disease. (Potter DA, Glenn J, Kinsella T et al: J Clin Oncol 3:353–366, 1985)

vival rate after salvage therapy of isolated local failures was 61%.[46]

Metastasectomy for isolated pulmonary recurrences is clearly warranted. Patients who are found to have pulmonary metastases by plain chest x-ray film or chest CT should have a thorough evaluation for extrapulmonary tumor, particularly in the primary site, to determine operability. For extremity and truncal sarcoma patients, this can be accomplished by physical examination and CT or MRI of the primary site. For patients with retroperitoneal sarcomas, an evaluation of the liver should be performed to determine if metastases are present. Patients with extrapulmonary tumors are not candidates for pulmonary resection. In Potter's analysis of NCI patients, 40 (72%) of 56 patients with isolated pulmonary metastases were rendered free of disease after surgery, which resulted in an actuarial 3-year survival rate of 38% (Figs. 40-17A,B).

Roth and colleagues reported that the number of metastatic nodules seen on preoperative tomograms, disease-free interval, and tumor doubling time significantly correlated with survival in soft tissue sarcoma patients undergoing their first thoracic exploration for pulmonary metastases.[340] No single criterion appears sufficiently accurate to exclude any individual patient from resection. In the American College of Surgeons survey, the 5-year survival rate after pulmonary metastasectomy was 21%.[46] Resection of recurrent pulmonary metastases can result in survival benefit. In the NCI experience, 29 patients had two or more resections for pulmonary metastases, resulting in a 22% 3-year actuarial survival rate after the second thoracotomy.[341] There have been no operative deaths after 254 pulmonary resections for metastases at the NCI since 1978. Because of the minimal morbidity and potential survival benefit of pulmonary metastasectomy, patients treated for primary soft tissue sarcomas should be closely monitored for development of pulmonary metastases at least every 6 months with either lung tomograms or chest CT for 3 years after resection of the primary tumor.[342]

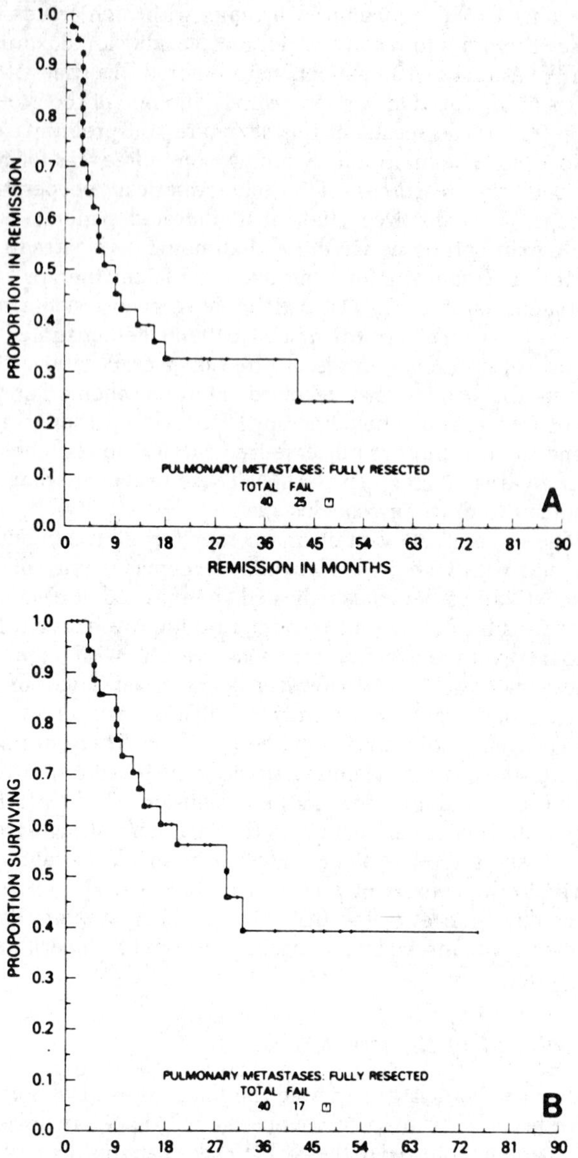

FIG. 40-17. Disease-free survival (**A**) and overall survival (**B**) in patients with high-grade sarcomas who underwent resection of isolated pulmonary metastases. (Potter DA, Glenn J, Kinsella T et al: J Clin Oncol 3:353–366, 1985)

Chemotherapy for Disseminated Soft Tissue Sarcomas

Soft tissue sarcomas constitute a heterogenous class of neoplasms with divergent response rates to available chemotherapy. Regimens including vincristine, dactinomycin, and cyclophosphamide result in response rates of 80% or more in previously untreated embryonal and alveolar rhabdomyosarcoma, and combination chemotherapy is now established in the primary treatment of these lesions. Of the classic adult soft tissue sarcomas, malignant fibrous histiocytoma and synovial sarcomas generally have the highest response rates to doxorubicin based combination chemotherapy. The lowest response rates are observed in angiosarcomas, extra skeletal chondrosarcomas, and in leiomyosarcomas of gastrointestinal origin. Mesotheliomas and Kaposi's sarcoma clearly differ from the classic soft tissue sarcomas and are not discussed in this section.

Widely divergent response rates for a given drug or combination reflect the mix of histologies included on the trial, dose and schedule of administration, prior therapy, and biases introduced by the small numbers of patients in some studies. Publication bias (*i.e.*, negative studies frequently are never reported) probably also plays a role, particularly in nonrandomized studies.

Single-Agent Chemotherapy

COMMERCIALLY AVAILABLE AGENTS. Table 40-29 summarizes the activity of various single agents in soft tissue sarcoma. Single-agent doxorubicin, clearly the most active commercially available single agent has a response rate of 15% to 35% in various studies.[343–349] A dose-response relationship has been observed in nonrandomized (and in combination in randomized trials, with dose rates of 60 to 70

TABLE 40-29. Commercially Available Agents for Soft Tissue Sarcoma by Class in Order of Response Rate

Drug	*Study**	*Cases*	*%RR†*	*mg/m²*
Anthracyclines	Total	356	26	
Doxorubicin	Blum[343]	130	34	60–90 q 3 wk
	O'Bryan[344]	49	31	60–75 q 3 wk
	O'Bryan[345]	82	28	25–70 q 3 wk
	Schoenfeld[346]	66	27	70 q 3 wk
	Borden[347]	93	19	70 q 3 wk
	Borden[347]	92	16	15 q wk
	Cruz[348]	41	15	15/d × 3 q 2 wk
	Creagan[349]	15	13	20–25/d × 3 q 3 wk
Antimetabolites				
Methotrexate, high dose	Total	76	13	
	Rosen[350]	1	1/1	8000/wk
	Vaughan[351]	14	14	5–12,000/2 wk
	Isakoff[352]	6	17	1.5–10,000
	Karakousis[353]	18	5	2–4000/4 wk
	Van Hoff[354]	26	20	Review
	Frei[355]	9	0/9	3–7.5/wk
	Ambinder[356]	2	0/2	2–10,000/1–4 wk
Methotrexate, standard dose	Total	81	21	
	Andrews[357]	19	10	
	Subramanian[358]	41	37	
	Buesa[359]	21	0	
Bleomycin	Amato[360]	32	6	
Actinomycin	Golbey[361]	30	17	
5-Fluorouracil	Gold[362]	8	12	
Vinkas				
Vincristine	Total	22	27	
	Selawry[363]	15	40	
	Korbitz[364]	7	0	
Etoposide	Total	40	8	
	Radice[365]	34	6	
	Bleyer[366]	6	16	
Alkylating Agents				
Dacarbazine (DTIC)	Rosenberg[367]	109	16	
Cisplatin	Total	103	12	
	Bramwell[368]	17	0	
	Karakousis[369]	13	23	
	Samson[370]	42	7	
	Thigpen[371]	19	5	
	Gershenson[372]	12	42‡	
Cyclophosphamide	Total	82	8	
	Bergsagel[373]	12	16	
	Korst[374]	3	0	
	Bramwell[375]	67	8	

*Group and reference numbers.
†% RR = percent response when the denominator includes at least 10 cases.
‡Gynecologic sarcomas only.

mg/m² every 3 weeks superior to dose rates of 50 mg/m² or less every 3 weeks.[344–346,376,377] Doxorubicin administered by continuous infusion over 4 days in combination regimens has been reported to be less cardiotoxic and equally effective as bolus dosing in some, but not in other, studies.[378–381]

Dacarbazine (DTIC) has a single-agent response rate of 16% and seems most active in leiomyosarcomas.[367] Nausea may be decreased by administration as a continuous infusion.

INVESTIGATIONAL AGENTS. Reports of response rates for investigational agents are shown in Tables 40-30 and 40-31. Clearly the most active agent is ifosfamide. Phase II trials of ifosfamide in patients failing a doxorubicin-containing regimen result in a response rate of 20% to 40%.[375,409–416]

EORTC compared 5 g/m² of ifosfamide with cyclophosphamide at 1.5 g/m² in 123 patients (59% with no prior chemotherapy) and observed less myelotoxicity ($p = 0.004$) and an enhanced response rate for IFF in sarcomas (Table 40-32).[375]

Ifosfamide is a cyclophosphamide analogue with one chloroethyl group emanating from each of the nitrogen atoms. Animal studies and human Phase I and II trials for lymphoma and small cell lung cancer have shown an apparent lack of cross resistance with cyclophosphamide.[448–450] Ifosfamide, especially in fractionated doses, has a better therapeutic

TABLE 40-30. Investigational Single Agents for Soft Tissue Sarcoma by Class in Order of Response Rate

Drug	*Reference*	*No. Evaluable*	*% Responding*
Anthracyclines			
Carminomycin	382	48	27
Azotomycin	383, 384	28	18
AMSA	385–388	9	11
Iclarubicin	389	23	4
AZQ	390–391	85	1
Mitoxantrone	392–393	115	1
Antimetabolites			
Cycloleucine	394, 396	118	11
Chlorozotocin	360, 397–402	160	6
Cytembena	403, 404	24	4
PALA/5-fluorouracil	405, 406	23	0
Baker's antifol	407, 408	30	0
Alkylating Agents			
Ifosfamide	375, 409–416	218	30*
Methyl-CCNU	417, 418	85	6
Hexamethylmelamine	419–422	88	5
Dibromodulcitol	423, 424	34	3
Dianhydrogalacitol	425	28	0
Gallium nitrate	426	31	0
Vinca & Related Compounds			
VM-26	365, 366, 427	33	3
Vindesine	428, 429	3	0
Miscellaneous			
DDMP	430	15	7
Piperazinedione	431–433	22	5
ICRF 159	423	29	5
MGBG	360, 434	54	2
Pyazofurin	435–437	47	0
Maytansine	423, 438	44	0
Bruceantin	360	34	0
Homoharingtonin	439	16	0
Biologicals			
Hu interferon	440, 441	36	3
Interleukin-2	442	6	0

*Includes 6% CRs.

index than cyclophosphamide in animal models of sarcoma, and in humans, ifosfamide is less myelosuppressive than cyclophosphamide.[451] Ifosfamide is activated by liver microsomes via hydroxylation of the number 4 ring carbon[452–453] at half the rate of equimolar cyclophosphamide because of a lower affinity for the activating enzymes ($K_m = 19.4$ mM and 40 mM, respectively).[452–453] After a single 5-g/m² dose of ifosfamide, a biexponential plasma decay with a terminal half life of 15.2 hours (twice that of cyclophosphamide) was observed. Because activation by ring hydoxylation proceeds more slowly, a higher proportion of the ifosfamide dose is dechloroethylated, producing nonalkylating metabolites. Thus, an approximately fourfold larger dose is required.

Ifosfamide is usually given at 5 to 10 g/m² per course, compared with 0.6 to 1.5 g/m² for cyclophosphamide. Higher ifosfamide dosages produce more acrolein, resulting in a higher incidence of bladder mucosa irritation and cystitis. Cystitis may be exacerbated by the antidiuretic effect of

TABLE 40-31. Ifosfamide for Failed Soft Tissue Sarcomas in Order of Dose Delivered per Course

*Study**	*g/m²*	*Schedule*	*Dose/Course*	*%CR*	*%RR*	*Evaluated*
Klein[409]	2.5–3.5	/d × 5	12.5–17.5		33	11
Czownicki[410,411]	1.25–2.5	/d × 5	12.5	8	38	13
Scheulen[412]	2.5	/d × 5	12.5	12	31	16
McGrath[413]	1.8	/d × 5	9.0	0	22	18
Antman[414]	2.0–2.5	/d × 4	8–10	0	36	28
Stuart[415]	5 or 8	d1	8.0	15	38	40
Pratt[416]	1.6	/d × 5	8.0	4	33	24
Bramwell[375]	5.0	d1	5.0	3	18	68
Total				6	30	218

*Group and reference number.

TABLE 40-32. Randomized Chemotherapy Trials for Soft-Tissue Sarcoma

	Group	Regimen*	No. of Patients	%CR	%RR	Comments
Studies Comparing the Addition of DTIC						
Omura[443]	GOG	A	80	6	16	Uterine sarcomas only
		AD	66	11	24	
Lerner[444]	ECOG	A	34	3	18	
		AD	32	3	44	Leiomyosarcomas only
Borden[347]	ECOG	A q 3 wk	93	6	19	A 15 mg/m²/wk
		A q wk	92	4	16	A 70 mg/m² q 3 wk
		AD	95	6	30	
Benjamin[445]	SWOG	ACVD	221	14	52	
		ACVAd	224	12	40	
Studies Evaluating the Addition of Cyclophosphamide						
Schoenfeld[346]	ECOG	A	66	6	27	A 70 mg/m²
		ACV	70	4	19	A 50 mg/m²
		CVAd	64	2	11	A 0 mg/m²
Baker[446]	SWOG	AD	79	14	32	
		ADC	95	13	35	
		ADAd	98	9	24	
Muss[447]	GOG	A	50	1	19	
		AC	54	2	20	
Studies Evaluating Dose and Schedule						
Baker[380]	SWOG	AD	135	7	19	Bolus
		AD	143	10	18	Continuous infusion
Bodey[376]	SWOG	ADCV	27	15	67	A 50 mg/m²; C 500 mg/m²
		ADCV	24	33	71	A 80 mg/m²; C 800 mg/m²
Pinedo[377]	EORTC	ADCV	71	20	38	Full dose rate
		AD-CV	74	5	14	Half dose rate
Studies Evaluating Ifosfamide						
Bramwell[375]	EORTC	I	68	3	18	5 g/m²
		C	67	1	8	1.5 g/m²

*A = doxorubicin; Ad = dactinomycin (actinomycin D); C = cyclophosphamide; D = DTIC; I = ifosfamide; V = vincristine.

ifosfamide. Significant cystitis (without diminished cytotoxicity) can be avoided by sodium-2-mercapto-ethanesulfonate (mesna) or N-acetyl cysteine.[410] Both agents protect ureters, renal pelvis, collecting tubules, and the bladder. A third option, intravesical irrigation, protects only the bladder. Mesna is a sulfhydryl compound that is inactive as the dimensa form in the circulation and reactivated in the kidney. Mesna does not appear to interfere with the antitumor effect of ifosfamide. Because mesna's half-life of about 2 hours is considerably smaller than that of ifosfamide (15 hours), mesna must be continued after completion of the ifosfamide.[453]

Lethargy, somnolence, paresthesias, mild depression, and disorientation, persisting 48 to 72 hours after completion of the infusion may result from intoxication by a metabolite of ifosfamide chloroacetaldehyde, structurally similar to chloral hydrate.[454–456] Recovery is generally complete. CNS toxicity may be enhanced by intensive antiemesis and potent narcotics, and it may be less common when ifosfamide is given by continuous infusion.[457] Metabolic acidosis, azotemia, and a proximal Fanconi syndrome usually resolves spontaneously 1 to 5 days after the completion of therapy.

Combination Chemotherapy

RANDOMIZED STUDIES. Table 40-32 summarizes published data evaluating combination chemotherapy in sarcomas. Doxorubicin appears to be the most active commercially available single agent, with a response rate of 20% to 40%. Two randomized studies have compared single-agent doxorubicin with a combination of doxorubicin and DTIC.[354,444,445] Women with measurable gynecologic sarcomas treated with 60 mg/m² of doxorubicin, with or without 250 mg/m/day × 5 of DTIC, had response rates of 24% and 16%, respectively; responses lasted a median of 5.3 months and 4.2 months, respectively. Omura and colleagues concluded that the increased (predominantly gastrointestinal) toxicity of DTIC was not justified by the trend toward an increased response rate.[102] In the ECOG randomized study of doxorubicin compared with doxorubicin and DTIC, the response rate of the combination was significantly higher than that of the single agent given either weekly or every 21 days, although the survival of the two groups was statistically similar.[354,445]

In contrast, there was no advantage for the addition of cyclophosphamide to single-agent doxorubicin in a GOG and an ECOG study nor to doxorubicin and DTIC in a SWOG study.[353] The cyclophosphamide containing arm was found to be significantly inferior in the ECOG study, presumably because of the lower dose of doxorubicin used in the combination, and no better in the GOG and SWOG studies.

Three studies evaluated the role of dose and schedule. In a SWOG study of bolus doxorubicin and DTIC compared with the same combination given as a continuous infusion to avoid cardiotoxicity, the two schedules were equally effective.

TABLE 40-33. Nonrandomized Combination Chemotherapy for Untreated Sarcomas

*Combination**	Study†	*Institute‡*	*No. Evaluable*	*%CR*	*%RR*
Doxorubicin-Based Combinations					
AD	Total		732	9	26
	Gottlieb[458]	SWOG	100	5	41
	Baker[446]	SWOG	79	15	33
	Borden[347]	ECOG	95	6	30
	Omura[443]	GOG	66	11	24
	Saiki[459]	SWOG	114	9	24
	Baker[380]	SWOG	278	9	19
ADC	Total		182	13	49
	Benjamin[379]	MDAH	46	15	59
	Blum[460]	DFCI	23	17	56
	Baker[446]	SWOG	97	11	34
	Ikeda[461]	Japan	16	6	31
ADV	Total		161	7	32
	Gottlieb[462]	SWOG	107	10	42
	Creagan[349]	Mayo Clinic	54	2	11
ADVC	Total		399	15	46
	Yap[463,464]	SWOG	125	17	50
	Benjamin[445]	MDAH	60	13	37
	Bui[465]	France	60	7	48
	Pfeffer[466]	Hadassah	31	13	39
	Pinedo[377]	EORTC	60	13	37
	Choi[467]	Hong Kong	12	17	33§
	Bodey[376]	MDAH	51	23	69
ADVC–Ad	Lopez[468]	Rome	40	10	30
ACV	Schoenfeld[346]	ECOG	70	4	19
ACVAd	Benjamin[445]	MDAH	224	12	40
ADAd	Baker[446]	SWOG	98	10	24
A + methyl-CCNU	Rivkin[469]	SWOG	41	7	49
AV + methyl-CCNU	Shiu[470]	MSKCC	22	0	45
A + streptozotocin	Chang[471]	UMCC	14	0	14
Ifosfamide-Based Combinations					
IVAd	Otten[472]	SIOP	33	92	94
IAD	Elias[473]	DFCI	62	10	52
IA	Schutte[474]	EORTC	125	NA	36
IP	Biernbaum[475]	Essen	12	17	50
IE	Wellens[476,477]	Duisburg	13	15	54
IV	DeKraker[478]	Amsterdam	9	22	78
DDP Combinations					
Total			219	6	38
AP	Klippstein[a479]	Frankfurt	18	21	44
APC	Edmonson[480]	Mayo Clinic	20	0	35
APC	Cormier[481]	Mayo Clinic	20	0	25
APCB	Edmonson[482]	Mayo Clinic	50	0	34
AP Mitc	Edmonson[483]	Mayo Clinic	63	0	43
APV	Biernbaum[475]	Essen	16	19	50
PI	Biernbaum[475]	Essen	12	17	50
P/DTIC	Piver[484]	RPMI	20	20	35‖
Methotrexate Combinations					
Total			463	5	30
AM	Presgrave[485]	Austria	36	0	28
AMV	Kaufman[486]	RPMI	14	7	21
AMVD	Kaufman[486]	RPMI	5	0	40
AMVDad	Shiu[470]	MSKCC	41	0	32
AMVAd	Shiu[470]	MSKCC	32	0	44
AM Mustard	Subramanian[358]	Marsden	22	15	41
AMC	Presant[487]	C. of Hope	105	6	25
AMC/ADV	Presant[487]	C. of Hope	32	16	34
AMCDV	Lynch, Shiu[470,488]	MSKCC	36	11	25
AMC	Lowenbraun[489]		140	3	30

(continued)

TABLE 40-33. Nonrandomized Combination Chemotherapy for Untreated Sarcomas (*continued*)

*Combination**	Study†	*Institute‡*	*No. Evaluable*	*%CR*	*%RR*
Dactinomycin-based combinations					
Total			298	1	11
AdVC	Jacobs[490]	UCSF	17	6	47
AdVC	Schoenfeld[346]	ECOG	64	2	11
AdVC	Creagan[349]	Mayo Clinic	61	2	8
ADL	Cruz[348]	MDAH	25	0	4
AdIV	Cruz[348]	MDAH	26	0	0
AdL + cycloleucine	Golbey[361]	RPMI	25	0	0
AdL + chloroambucil	Golbey[361]	RPMI	40	0	13
AdM + chlorambucil	Golbey[361]	RPMI	40	0	20

*A = doxorubicin; Ad = dactinomycin (actinomycin D); C = cyclophosphamide; D = DTIC; (HD)M = (high-dose) methotrexate; I = ifosfamide; L-PAM) melphalan.

†Group and reference number.

‡UCSF = University of California, San Francisco; ECOG = Eastern Cooperative Oncology Group; COG = Gynecologic Oncology Group; SIOP = International Society of Pediatric Oncology; SWOG = Southwest Oncology Group; MDAH = M.D. Anderson Hospital, Houston; EORTC = European Organization for Research and Treatment of Cancer; MSKCC = Memorial Sloan Kettering Cancer Center, NYC; UMCC = University of Maryland Cancer Center; RPMI = Roswell Park Memorial Institute, Rochester, NY.

§Gastrointestinal sarcomas only.

||Gynecologic sarcomas only.

However, there were nine episodes of clinical congestive heart failure in the bolus arm, compared with four in the continuous-infusion arm. These differences are not statistically significant.

In a study randomizing patients between standard-dose cyclophosphamide, vincristine, doxorubicin, and DTIC (CYVADIC) and higher-dose CYVADIC with treatment in a protected environment, there was a favorable trend in the response rates for the higher-dose therapy, particularly for complete responses.[376] There was no significant difference observed in survival. However, when Pinedo compared full dose CYVADIC with doxorubicin and DTIC, alternating with cyclophosphamide and vincristine, the full-dose schedule had a significantly superior response rate.[377]

A study by the EORTC randomized patients between 1.5 g/m² of cyclophosphamide and 5 g/m² of ifosfamide. Although response rates were surprisingly low in both arms, the response rate for ifosfamide was about twice that for cyclophosphamide and patients had less toxicity.[375]

NONRANDOMIZED STUDIES. Sequential nonrandomized studies from M.D. Anderson Hospital have suggested an improved response rate with combination therapy, including cyclophosphamide, doxorubicin, vincristine, and DTIC (CYVADIC), although the addition of vincristine has never been shown to improve the response rate (Table 40-33).[445,458,462] The observed increased response rate with the addition of cyclophosphamide has not been confirmed in randomized studies.[346,446,447] A response rate of 56% was also observed for an intensive combination of cyclophosphamide, doxorubicin, and DTIC at the DFCI, with a small percentage of long-term disease-free survivors among patients with disseminated disease.[460] A few long-term disease-free survivors (approximately 33% of the complete responders) have also been observed in an English study and the M.D. Anderson series.[358,463,464]

The role of ifosfamide in combination regimens for previously untreated sarcoma is not yet defined. Of 33 newly diagnosed patients with Stages III and IV rhabdomyosarcomas who were given vincristine, dactinomycin, and ifosfamide (3 g/day × 2), 27 responded completely and 4 partially. The response rate of 94%, with 79% responding completely, was superior to their previous standard regimen.[472] A DFCI study of mesna, doxorubicin, ifosfamide, and DTIC (MAID) in 87 evaluable patients resulted in 12% complete responses and an overall response rate of 54% (95% confidence limits, 43–65).[131] Of the inoperable primaries, 77% responded, compared with 42% for metastatic lesions ($p = 0.026$). CNS relapse occurred during continued peripheral response in 3 patients. Five of 8 patients who underwent resection after partial or minimal response remain disease-free after a short follow-up period.

Myelotoxicity was dose limiting. Leukocyte nadirs of <500/μl occurred after completion of 26% of the courses. Platelet nadirs of <50,000, seen in 19% of patients, were significantly associated with the DTIC dose ($p = 0.03$). Moderate to severe nausea and vomiting, with standard antiemetics, occurred in only 3%, and moderate to severe mucositis occurred in 2%. Eight patients had cumulative doxorubicin doses between 420 and 750 mg/m² with no observed congestive heart failure.

A Scandinavian study documented a response rate of 36% for doxorubicin and ifosfamide.[474] An intergroup CALGB/SWOG study of doxorubicin and DTIC with or without ifosfamide and mesna is currently accruing patients.

It is difficult to assess whether there is any advantage of adding cisplatin or methotrexate to a doxorubicin-based combination without a randomized trial. The single-agent response rate of these agents in adult soft tissue sarcomas suggests that without therapeutic synergy, there may be no advantage. Response rates in doxorubicin-containing combinations do not appear superior to those without methotrexate or cisplatin.

Based on these data, patients with newly diagnosed recurrent or metastatic sarcomas who are not candidates for surgical salvage should be placed on protocols to identify more active regimens. Without appropriate clinical trials, the goals of therapy must be carefully considered. Three studies have observed that about 33% of the complete responders may survive disease-free after intensive chemotherapy, and a combination of chemotherapy and surgery can augment the percentage of complete responders.[358,464,465] If this approach is to be successful, a trial of two cycles of intensive chemotherapy begun at the first documentation of recurrence will rapidly distinguish between those destined to have a high-quality response and those who will not. However, if therapy is to be palliative, treatment can be withheld until symptoms develop.

The optimal standard regimen in terms of response rate is a schedule of doxorubicin (70 mg/m^2) and DTIC (1 g/m^2). The dose should be divided over two days. Doxorubicin cardiotoxicity and DTIC-associated nausea may both be diminished by delivery of these doses by a 4 day continuous infusion through a central line to avoid doxorubicin skin ulceration. For palliation of sick or elderly patients, doxorubicin as a single agent is probably preferable. In general, the highest tolerated dose should be given during the first two cycles. If there is disease progression, further cycles can be canceled, thus avoiding the considerable toxicity of inactive therapy. Failed patients should be placed on Phase II studies, because there is currently no comercially available salvage agent or combination with a response rate greater than 20% that would justify the toxicity.

QUALITY OF LIFE ISSUES

Medical decision-making should be predicated on an understanding of the influence of treatments on survival. If different treatments result in equivalent survival outcomes, the effects of these treatments on the quality of life may help in choosing the most appropriate treatment for an individual patient.[491] One example is the treatment of patients with high-grade extremity soft tissue sarcomas in which there is a choice between limb-sparing surgery combined with adjuvant therapy or amputation (Fig. 40-18). In a prospective, randomized study at the NCI, Rosenberg and colleagues demonstrated that the overall survival rates of these two treatment modalities are equivalent.[257] Although intuition predicts that the limb-sparing approach should result in improved quality of life over amputation and should therefore be offered to a patient, there are few data available to determine the functional capacity and quality of life for patients who have had either treatment.

To address this issue, Sugarbaker and co-workers performed a detailed assessment of the quality of life in 26 patients undergoing limb-sparing surgery or amputation for soft tissue sarcomas of the extremity at the NCI.[492] Psychosocial and clinical assessments were used to measure the impact of treatment on psychosocial adjustment, daily activities, economic status, mobility, pain, sexual relationships, and treatment trauma. Analysis of this study revealed no evidence of improved quality of life in patients undergoing limb-sparing surgery plus irradiation compared with amputation.

In a study reported by Weddington and colleagues, the psychological outcome of 33 patients with extremity sarcoma who underwent amputation or limb-sparing surgery were evaluated.[493] A battery of standard psychosocial assessment tests were employed and revealed no psychological advantage of limb-sparing surgery to amputation. These studies appear to indicate that the impact of amputation or limb-sparing surgery are equivalent, an idea that is contrary to intuition. This may be a result of insensitive tools in the assessment of "quality of life," a difficult concept to measure, or these studies may reflect the ability of an amputee to compensate and adjust to a lost limb. It appears that there is no compelling reason to attempt a limb-sparing approach instead of an amputation for every patient with a high-grade sarcoma because the impact of these treatments on survival and quality of life are equivalent. If there is concern about obtaining adequate tumor margins with a limb-sparing procedure, amputation should be performed.

Multimodality treatment of soft tissue sarcomas has resulted in significant improvements in patient survival. The optimal combination of surgery, radiation therapy, and chemotherapy has not been defined. Evaluation of the impact of various combined modality treatments on the quality of life of patients will become an important determinant in optimizing therapy so long as survival results are not affected. In a group of 65 patients with extremity sarcomas undergoing multimodality, limb-sparing therapy at NCI, serial quality of life evaluations performed every 6 months revealed changes in economic status, sexual activity, and functional activity over the course of 1 year after surgery.[494] The combination of chemotherapy plus radiation therapy

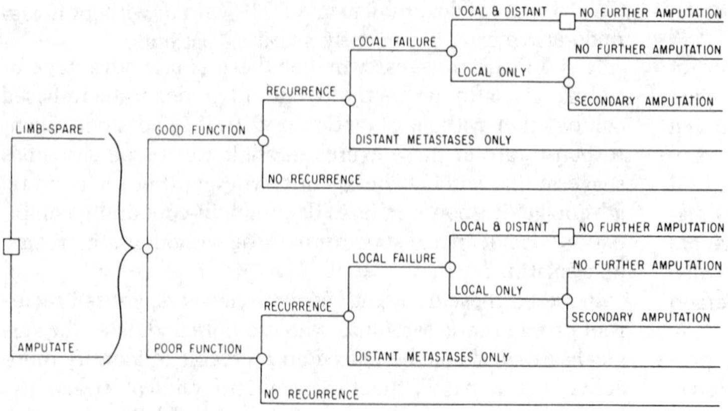

FIG. 40-18. Decision tree for extremity sarcoma. Square node on left is decision node with two strategies, limb-spare and amputate. Complex tree structure applies to each strategy, although probabilities and values would differ. Each circle denotes chance event showing set of mutually exclusive possibilities. (Moskowitz AJ, Pauker SG: A decision analytic approach to limb-sparing treatment of adult soft tissue and osteogenic sarcoma. Cancer Treat Rep 3:11–26, 1985)

given postoperatively resulted in a significantly increased incidence of wound problems, compared with chemotherapy alone.

Prospective, randomized studies have been initiated at Memorial Sloan-Kettering Cancer Center and at NCI, assessing the efficacy of postoperative radiation therapy compared with no radiation therapy in patients with extremity sarcoma undergoing limb-sparing surgery plus postoperative adjuvant chemotherapy. These trials will determine if postoperative radiation therapy can be avoided, potentially improving the quality of life for these patients. Treatment planning based on patients' needs can be more rationally decided on if more information about the impact of treatments on the quality of life is available.

REFERENCES

1. Patten BM: Human Embryology. New York, McGraw-Hill, 1968
2. 1986 Cancer Facts and Figures. American Cancer Society, 1986
3. Smith AH, Pearce NE, Fisher DO et al: Soft tissue sarcoma and exposure to phenoxyherbicides and chlorophenols in New Zealand. JNCI 73:1111–1117, 1984
4. Lynge E, Storm HH, Jensen OM: The evaluation of trends in soft tissue sarcoma according to diagnostic criteria and consumption of phenoxyherbicides. Cancer 60:1896–1901, 1987
5. Li FP, Fraumeni JF Jr: Soft-tissue sarcomas, breast cancer, and other neoplasms. A familial syndrome? Ann Intern Med 71:747–752, 1969
6. Howard GM, Casten VG: Rhabdomyosarcoma of the orbit in brothers. Arch Ophthalmol 70:319, 1963
7. Li FP, Fraumeni JF Jr: Rhabdomyosarcoma in children: Epidemiologic study and identification of a familal cancer syndrome. JNCI 43:1365–1373, 1969
8. Li FP, Tucker MA, Fraumeni JF Jr: Childhood cancer in sibs. J Pediatr 88:419–423, 1976
9. Miller RW: Deaths from childhood leukemia and solid tumors among twins and other sibs in the United States, 1960–1967. JNCI 45:203, 1971
10. Chabalko JJ, Creagon ET, Fraumeni JF Jr: Epidemiology of selected sarcomas in children. JNCI 53:675, 1974
11. Remzi D, Kendi S: Rhabdomyosarcoma of the prostate in childhood. Turk J Pediatr 8:143–149, 1966
12. Bottomley RH, Condit PT: Cancer families. Cancer Bull 20:22–24, 1968
13. Fraumeni JF Jr, Vogel CL, Easton JM: Sarcomas and multiple polyposis in a kindred. A genetic variety of hereditary polyposis? Arch Intern Med 121:57–61, 1968
14. Enterline HT, Culberson JD, Hochlin DB et al: Liposarcoma. A clinical and pathological study of 53 cases. Cancer 13:931–950, 1960
15. Stewart FW, Treves NP: Lymphangiosarcoma in postmastectomy lyphedema: A report of six cases in elephantiasis chirurgica. Cancer 1:64–81
16. Sloane JA, Hubbel MM: Soft tissue sarcomas in children associated with congenital anomalies. Cancer 23:175–182, 1969
17. Schjweisguth O, Gerard-Marchant R, Lemerle J: Naevomatose baso-cellulaire association a un rhabdomyosarcome congenital. Arch Fr Pediatr 25:1083–1093, 1968
18. Heard G: Malignant disease in von Recklinghausen's neurofibromatosis. Proc R Soc Med 56:502–503, 1963
19. Reed WB, Nickel WR, Campion G: Internal manifestations of tuberous sclerosis. Arch Dermatol 87:715–728, 1963
20. Epstein CJ, Martin GM, Schultz AL et al: Werner's syndrome. A review of its symptomatology, natural history, pathologic features, genetics and relationship to the natural aging process. Medicine (Baltimore) 45:177–221, 1966
21. Usui M, Ishii S, Yamawaki S et al: The occurrence of soft tissue sarcomas in three siblings with Werner's syndrome. Cancer 54:2580–2586, 1984
22. Hardell L, Sandstrom A: Case-control study: Soft-tissue sarcomas and exposure to phenoxyacetic acids or chlorophenols. Br J Cancer 39:711–717, 1979
23. Eriksson M, Hardell L, Berg NO, et al: Soft tissue sarcomas and exposure to chemical substances: A case-referent study. Br J Ind Med 38:27–33, 1981
24. Wiklund K, Holm LE: Soft tissue sarcoma risk in Swedish agricultural and forestry workers. JNCI 76:229–234, 1986
25. Greenwald P, Kovasznay B, Collins DN et al: Sarcomas of soft tissue after Vietnam service. JNCI 73:1107–1109, 1984
26. Kang H, Enzinger F, Breslin P et al: Soft tissue sarcomas and military service in Vietnam: A case-control study. JNCI 79:693–699, 1987
27. Kim K, Tidrick RT, Skeel RT et al: Fibrosarcoma of the chest wall following mastectomy and radiation therapy for mammary carcinoma. Breast Dis Breast 6:26–30, 1980
28. Kuten A, Sapir D, Cohen Y et al: Postirradiation soft tissue sarcoma occurring in breast cancer patients: Report of seven cases and results of combination chemotherapy. J Surg Oncol 28:168–171, 1985
29. Souba WW, McKenna RJ, Meis J et al: Radiation-induced sarcomas of the chest wall. Cancer 57:610–615, 1986
30. O'Neil NB, Cocke W, Mason D et al: Radiation-induced soft tissue fibrosarcoma: Surgical therapy and salvage. Ann Thorac Surg 33:625–628, 1982
31. Halperin EC, Greenberg MS, Suit HD: Sarcoma of bone and soft tissue following treatment of Hodgkin's disease. Cancer 53:232–236, 1984
32. Arlen M, Higinbotham NL, Huvos AG et al: Radiation-induced sarcoma of bone. Cancer 28:1087–1099, 1971
33. Martland HS, Humphries RE: Osteogenic sarcoma in dial painters using luminous paint. Arch Pathol 7:406–417, 1929
34. Brand KG: Foreign body induced sarcomas. In Becker FF (ed): Cancer, pp 485–511. New York, Plenum Press, 1975
35. Ott G: Fremd Körpersarkome. Exp Med Pathol Klin 32:1, 1970
36. de Cholnky T: Augmentation mammaplasty: Survey of complications in 10,941 patients by 265 surgeons. Plast Reconstr Surg 45:573, 1970
37. Rubin LR, Bromberg BE, Walden RH: Long-term human reaction to synthetic plastics. Surg Gynecol Obstet 132:603, 1971
38. Shieber W, Graham P: An experience with sarcomas of the soft tissues in adults. Surgery 52:295, 1962
39. Hare HF, Cerny MF: Soft tissue sarcoma: A review of 200 cases. Cancer 16:1332, 1963
40. Ferrell HW, Frable WJ: Soft part sarcomas revisited. Review and comparison of a second series. Cancer 30:475–480, 1972
41. Sears HF, Hopson R, Inouye W et al: Analysis of staging and management of patients with sarcoma. Ann Surg 191:488–493, 1980
42. Abbas JS, Holyoke ED, Moore et al: The surgical treatment and outcome of soft tissue sarcoma. Arch Surg 116:765–769, 1981
43. Lindberg RD, Martin RG, Romsdahl MM et al: Conservative surgery and postoperative radiotherapy in 300 adults with soft-tissue sarcomas. Cancer 47:2391–2397, 1981
44. Potter DA, Glenn J, Kinsella T et al: Patterns of recurrence in patients with high-grade soft tissue sarcomas. J Clin Oncol 3:353–366, 1985
45. Torosian MH, Friedrich C, Godbold J et al: Soft tissue sarcomas: Initial characteristics and prognostic factors in patients with and without metastic disease. Semin Surg Oncol 4:13–19, 1988
46. Lawrence W Jr, Donegan WL, Nachimuth N et al: Adult soft tissue sarcomas. A pattern of care survey of the American College of Surgeons. Ann Surg 205:349–359, 1987
47. Hajdu SI: Pathology of Soft Tissue Tumors. Philadelphia, Lea & Febiger, 1979
48. Mirr JM: The soft tissues. In Coulson WF (ed): Surgical Pathology. Philadelphia, JP Lippincott, 1978
49. Stout AP, Lattes R: Tumors of the soft tissue. In Atlas of Tumor Pathology, 2nd series, Washington, DC, Armed Forces Institute of Pathology, 1967
50. Enzinger FM, Weiss SW: Soft Tissue Tumors. St. Louis, CV Mosby, 1988
51. Coindre JM, Trojani M, Contesso G et al: Reproducibility of a histopathologic grading system for adult soft tissue sarcoma. Cancer 58:306–309, 1986
52. Presant CA, Russell WO, Alexander RW et al: Soft-tissue and bone sarcoma histopathology peer review: The frequency of disagreement in diagnosis and the need for second pathology opinions. The Southeastern Cancer Study Group experience. J Clin Oncol 4:1658–1661, 1986
53. Costa J, Wesley RA, Glatstein E et al: The grading of soft tissue sarcomas. Results of a clinicohistopathologic correlation in a series of 163 cases. Cancer 53:530–541, 1984
54. Lack EE, Steinberg SM, White DE et al: Extremity soft tissue sarcomas: Analysis of prognostic variables with emphasis on reproducibility of tumor typing and grading (submitted)
55. Trojani M, Contesso G, Coindre JM et al: Soft tissue sarcomas of adults, Study of pathological prognostic variables and definition of a histopathological grading system. Int J Cancer 33:37–42, 1984
56. Pack GI, Ariel IM: Treatment of cancer and allied diseases. In Tumors of the Soft Somatic Tissues and Bone, vol VIII. New York, Harper & Row, 1964
57. Martin RG, Butler JJ, Albores-Saavedra J: Soft tissue tumors: Surgical treatment and results. In Tumors of Bone and Soft Tissue. Chicago, Year Book Medical Publishers, 1965
58. Shiu MH, Castro EB, Hajdu SI et al: Surgical treatment of 297 soft tissue sarcomas of the lower extremity. Ann Surg 182:597, 1975
59. Simon MA, Enneking WF: The management of soft tissue sarcomas of the extremities. J Bone Joint Surg [Am] 58:317, 1976
60. American Joint Committee Staging Manual, 1987

60a. Suit HD, Mankin JH, Willett G et al: Limited surgery and external irradiation in soft tissue sarcomas. In Recent Concepts in Sarcoma Treatment. Proceedings of the International Symposium on Sarcoma Treatment. Proceedings of the International Symposium on Sarcomas, Tarpon Springs, FL, October 8–10, 1987. The Netherlands, Kluwer Academic Publishers, 1988

61. Lindberg RD, Martin RG, Romsdahl MM et al: Conservation surgery and radiation therapy for soft tissue sarcomas. In Martin RG, Ayala AG (eds): Management of Primary Bone and Soft Tissue Tumors. Chicago, Year Book Medical Publishers, 1977
62. Suit HD: Patterns of failure after treatment of sarcoma of soft tissue by radical surgery or by conservative surgery and radiation. Cancer Treat Symp 2:241–246, 1983

63. Collins C, Hadju SI, Godbold J et al: Localized, operable soft tissue sarcoma of the lower extremity. Arch Surg 121:1425–1433, 1986
64. Potter DA, Kinsella T, Glatstein E et al: High grade soft tissue sarcomas of the extremities. Cancer 58:190–205, 1986
65. Jarvi OH, Saxen E: Elastofibroma dorsi. Acta Pathol Microbiol Immunol Scand [Suppl] 144:83–84, 1961
66. Jarvi OH, Lansimies PH: Subclinical elastofibromas in the scapular region in an autopsy series. Acta Pathol Microbiol Immunol Scand [A] 83:87–108, 1975
67. Jarvi OH, Saxen AE, Hopsu-Havu VK et al: Elastofibroma: A degenerative pseudotumor. Cancer 23:42–63, 1969
68. Stemmermann GN, Stout AP: Elastofibroma dorsi. Am J Clin Pathol 37:490–506, 1962
69. Conway H: Dupuytren's contracture. Am J Surg 87:10, 1954
70. Luck JV: Dupuytren's contracture. J Bone Joint Surg [Am] 41:635, 1959
71. Skoog T: Dupuytren's contracture: Pathogenesis and surgical treatment. Surg Clin North Am 47:433–444, 1967
72. Allen RA, Woolner LB, Ghormley RK: Soft-tissue tumors of the sole: With special reference to plantar fibromatosis. J Bone Joint Surg [Am] 37:14–26, 1955
73. Allen PM, Enzinger FM: Juvenile aponeurotic fibroma. Cancer 26:857–867, 1970
74. Goldman RL: The cartilage analogue of fibromatosis (aponeurotic fibroma): Further observations based on 7 new cases. Cancer 26:1325–1331, 1970
75. Keasbey LE: Juvenile aponeurotic fibroma (calcifying fibroma). Cancer 6:338–346, 1953
76. Bartlett RC, Otis RD, Haakso AO: Multiple congenital neoplasms of soft tissues. Report of 4 cases in 1 family. Cancer 14:913–920, 1961
77. Beatty EC: Congenital generalized fibromatosis in infancy. Am J Dis Child 103:620, 1962
78. Teng P, Warden MJ, Cohn WL: Congenital generalized fibromatosis (renal and skeletal) with complete spontaneous regression. J Pediatr 62:748–753, 1963
79. Enzinger FM: Fibrous hamartoma of infancy. Cancer 18:241–251, 1965
80. Chandler A: Muscular torticollis. J Bone Joint Surg [Am] 30:566, 1948
81. Brown JB, McDowell F: Wry-neck facial distortion prevented by resection of fibrosed sternomastoid muscle in infancy and childhood. Ann Surg 131:721–733, 1950
82. Smoth BH: Peyronie's disease. Am J Clin Pathol 45:670, 1966
83. Allen PW: Nodular fasciitis. Pathology 4:9–26, 1972
84. MacKenzie DH: The Differential Diagnosis of Fibroblastic Disorders, pp 21, 106, Oxford Blackwell Scientific Publications, 1970
85. Soule EH: Proliferative (nodular) fasciitis. Arch Pathol 73:437, 1962
86. Hutter RVP, Stewart FW, Foote FW Jr: Fasciitis: A report of 70 cases with follow-up proving the benignity of the lesion. Cancer 15:992–1003, 1962
87. MacKenzie DH: The Differential Diagnosis of Fibroblastic Disorders. Oxford, Blackwell Scientific Publications, 1970
88. Das Gupta TK, Brasfield RD, O'Hara J: Extra-abdominal desmoids. Ann Surg 170:109, 1969
89. Enzinger FM, Shiraki M: Musculoaponeurotic fibromatosis of the shoulder girdle. Cancer 20:113, 1967
90. Brasfield RD, Das Gupta TK: Desmoid tumors of the anterior abdominal wall. Surgery 65:241, 1969
91. Ewing J: Neoplastic Disease. Philadelphia, WB Saunders, 1928.
92. Musgrove JE, McDonald JR: Extra-abdominal desmoid tumors: A differential diagnosis and treatment. Arch Pathol 45:513–540, 1948
93. Benninghoff D, Robbins R: The nature and treatment of desmoid tumors. Am J Roentgenol Rad Ther Nucl Med 91:132–137, 1964
94. Greenberg HM, Goebel R, Weichselbaum RR, et al: Radiation therapy in the treatment of aggressive fibromatoses. Int J Radiat Oncol Biol Phys 7:305–310, 1981
95. Kirchmer JT Jr, Woma FJ Jr: Desmoid tumors of the abdominal wall. South Med J 70:1136, 1977
96. Wara WM, Phillips TL, Hill DR et al: Desmoid tumors—treatment and prognosis. Radiology 124:225–226, 1977
97. Suit HD, Russell WO: Radiation therapy of soft tissue sarcomas. Cancer 36:759–764, 1975
98. Kiel KD, Suit HD: Radiation therapy in the treatment of aggressive fibromatoses (desmoid tumors). Cancer 54:2051–2055, 1984
99. Kinsbrunner B, Ritter S, Domingo J et al: Remission of rapidly growing desmoid tumors after tamoxifen therapy. Cancer 52:2201–2204, 1983
100. Lanari A: Effect of progesterone on desmoid tumors (aggressive fibromatosis). N Engl J Med 309:1523, 1983
101. Waddell WR, Gerner RE: Indomethacin and ascorbate inhibit desmoid tumors. J Surg Oncol 15:85–90, 1980
102. Khorsand J, Karakousis CP: Desmoid tumors and their management. Am J Surg 149:215–218, 1985
103. Kofoed H, Kamby C, Anagnostaki L: Aggressive fibromatosis. Surg Gynecol Obstet 160:124–127, 1985
104. Czernobilsky B, Cornog JL, Enterline HT: Rhabdomyoma: Report of case with ultrastructural and histochemical studies. Am J Clin Pathol 49:782–789, 1968
105. Morgan JJ, Enterline HT: Benign rhabdomyoma of the pharynx: A case report, review of the literature, and comparison with cardiac rhabdomyoma. Am J Clin Pathol 42:174–181, 1964
106. Lendrum AC: Painful tumors of the skin. Ann R Coll Surg Engl 1:62–67, 1947
107. Stout AP: Solitary cutaneous and subcutaneous leiomyoma. Am J Cancer 29:435–469, 1937
108. Enzinger FM, Harvey DA: Spindle cell lipoma. Cancer 36:1852–1859, 1975
109. Lin JJ, Lin F: Two entities in angiolipoma. A study of 459 cases of lipoma with review of infiltrating angiolipoma. Cancer 34:720–727, 1974
110. Chung EB, Enzinger FM: Benign lipoblastomatosis. An analysis of 35 cases. Cancer 32:482–491, 1973
111. Alba-Greco M, Garcia RL, Vuletin JC: Benign lipoblastomatosis. Ultrastructure and histogenesis. Cancer 45:511, 1980
112. Evans HL, Soule EH, Winkelmann RK: Atypical lipoma, atypical intramuscular lipoma, and well-differentiated retroperitoneal liposarcoma. A reappraisal of 30 cases formerly classified as well-differentiated liposarcoma. Cancer 43:574–584, 1979
113. Dionne GP, Seemayer TA: Infiltrating lipomas and angiolipomas revisited. Cancer 33:732–738, 1974
114. Enzinger FM: Benign lipomatous tumors simulating a sarcoma. In Martin RG, Ayala AG (eds): Management of Primary Bone and Soft Tissue Tumors, pp 11–24. Chicago. Year Book Medical Publishers, 1977
115. Kindblom LG, Angervall L, Stener B et al: Intermuscular and intramuscular lipomas and hibernomas: A clinical, roentgenologic, histologic, and prognostic study of 46 cases. Cancer 33:754–762, 1974
116. Mesara BW, Batsakis JC: Hibernoma of the neck. Arch Otolaryngol 85:95, 1967
117. Jones FE, Soule EH, Coventry MB: Fibrous xanthoma of synovium (giant cell tumor of tender sheath, pigmented nodular synovitis). J Bone Joint Surg [Am] 51:76, 1969
118. Gehwheiler JA, Wilson VW: Diffuse biarticular pigmented villonodular synovitis. Radiology 93:137, 1969
119. Slooff JL, Kernohan JW, MacCarty CS: Primary Intramedullary Tumors of the Spinal Cord and Filum Terminale. Philadelphia, WB Saunders, 1964
120. D'Agostino A: Sarcomas of the peripheral nerves and somatic soft tissues associated with multiple neurofibromatosis. Cancer 16:1015, 1963
121. Buck BE: Congenital neurogenous sarcoma with rhabdomyosarcomatous differentiation. J Pediatr Surg 12:581–582, 1977
122. Hammond JA: Detection of malignant change in neurofibromatosis by gallium-67 scanning. Can Med Assoc J 119:352–353, 1978
123. Herman J: Sarcomatous transformation in multiple neurofibromatosis. Ann Surg 131:206, 1950
124. Hunt K: Neurofibrosarcoma complicating Von Recklinghausen's disease. J Ky Med Assoc 74:346–349, 1976
125. Lee C: Malignant degeneration of thoracic neurofibromata. NY State J Med 75:347–352, 1972
126. Wander JW, Das Gupta TK: Neurofibromatosis. Curr Probl Surg 14:1–81, 1977
127. Riccardi VM: Medical progress. Von Recklinghausen neurofibromatosis. N Engl J Med 305:1617–1626, 1981
128. Nambisan RN, Rao U, Moore R et al: Malignant soft tissue tumors of nerve sheath origin. J Surg Oncol 25:268–272, 1984
129. Sorensen SA, Mulvihill JJ, Nielsen A: Long-term follow-up of Von Recklinghausen neurofibromatosis survival and malignant neoplasms. N Engl J Med 314:1010–1015, 1986
130. Allen PW, Enzinger FM: Heamangioma of skeletal muscle: An analoysis of 89 cases. Cancer 29:8–22, 1972
131. Lister WA: The natural history of strawberry nevi. Lancet 1:1429–1434, 1938
132. Modlin JJ: Capillary hemangiomas of the skin. Surgery 38:169–180, 1955
133. Riveros M, Pack GT: The glomus tumors—report of 20 cases. Ann Surg 133:394, 1951
134. Carroll RE, Berman AT: Glomus tumors of the hand: Review of the literature and report of 28 cases. J Bone Joint Surg [Am] 54:691–703, 1972
135. Shugart RR, Soule EH, Johnson EW: Glomus tumor. Surg Gynecol Obstet 117:334–340, 1963
136. Stout AP: Tumors featuring pericytes: Glomus tumor and hemangiopericytoma. Lab Invest 5:217–223, 1965
137. Enzinger FM, Smith BH: Hemangiopericytoma. An analysis of 106 cases. Hum Pathol 7:61–82, 1976
138. Soule EH, Enriquez P: Atypical fibrous histiocytoma, malignant fibrous histiocytoma, malignant histiocytoma, and epithelioid sarcoma. A comparative study of 65 tumors. Cancer 30:128, 1972
139. Kempson RL, McGavran MH: Atypical fibroxanthomas of the skin. Cancer 17:1463–1471, 1964
140. Kauffman SL, Stout AP: Histiocytic tumors (fibrous xanthoma and histiocytoma) in children. Cancer 14:469–482, 1961
141. O'Brien JE, Stout AP: Malignant fibrous xanthomas. Cancer 17:1445–1458, 1964
142. Brenner W, Schaefler K, Habrans C et al: Dermatofibrosarcoma protuberans metastatic to a regional lymph node. Report of a case and review. Cancer 36:1897–1902, 1975
143. Burkhardt BR, Soule EH, Winkelman RK et al: Dermatofibrosarcoma protuberans: Study of 56 cases. Am J Surg 111:638–644, 1966
144. Taylor HB, Helwig EB: Dermatofibrosarcoma protuberans: A study of 115 cases. Cancer 15:717–725, 1962
145. McPeak CJ, Druz T, Nicastri AD: Dermatofibrosarcoma protuberans: An analysis of 86 cases—five with metastasis. Ann Surg 166:803, 1967
146. Glenn J, Potter D, Kinsella T et al: Unpublished results, 1985
147. Roses DF, Valensi Q, LaTrenta G et al: Surgical treatment of dermatofibrosarcoma protuberans. Surg Gynecol Obstet 162:449–452, 1986
148. Rinck PA, Habermalz HJ, Loceck H: Effective radiotherapy in one case of dermatofibrosarcoma protuberans. Strahlentherapie [Sonderb] 158:681–685, 1982

149. Strong EW, McDivitt RW, Brasfield RD: Granular cell myoblastoma. Cancer 25:415–422, 1970
150. Le Ber MS, Stout AP: Benign mesenchymomas in children. Cancer 15:598–605, 1962
151. Stout AP: Myxoma, the tumor of primitive mesenchyme. Ann Surg 127:706–719, 1948
152. Enzinger FM: Intramuscular myxoma. Am J Clin Pathol 43:104, 1965
153. Martel W, Abell MR: Radiologic evaluation of soft tissue tumors. A retrospective study. Cancer 32:352–366, 1973
154. Berger PE, Kuhn JP: Computed tomography of tumors of the musculoskeletal system in children. Clinical applications. Radiology 127:171–175, 1978
155. Neifeld JP, Walsh JW, Lawrence W Jr: Computed tomography in the management of soft tissue tumors. Surg Gynecol Obstet 155:535–540, 1982
156. Lawrence W Jr, Neifeld JP, Terz JJ: Manual of Soft Tissue Tumor Surgery. New York, Springer-Verlag, 1983
157. Levin DC, Watson RC, Baltaxe HA: Arteriography in diagnosis and management of acquired peripheral soft-tissue masses. Radiology 103:53–58, 1972
158. Hudson TM, Haas G, Enneking WF et al: Angiography in the management of musculoskeletal tumors. Surg Gynecol Obstet 141:11–21, 1975
159. de Santos LA, Wallace S, Finklestein JB: Angiography and lymphangiography in peripheral soft tissue sarcomas. In Martin RG, Ayala AG (eds): Management of Primary Bone and Soft Tissue Tumors. Chicago, Year Book Medical Publishers, 1977
160. Chang AE, Matory YL, Dwyer AJ et al: Magnetic resonance imaging versus computed tomography in the evaluation of soft tissue tumors of the extremities. Ann Surg 205:340–348, 1987
161. Bland KI, McCoy DM, Kinard RE et al: Application of magnetic resonance imaging and computerized tomography as an adjunct to the surgical management of soft tissue sarcomas. Ann Surg 205:473–481, 1987
161a. Enneking WF: Preoperative staging of sarcomas. Cancer Treat Symp 3:67–70, 1985
162. Enneking WF, Spanier SS, Goodman MA: The surgical staging of musculoskeletal sarcoma. J Bone Joint Surg [Am] 62:1027–1030, 1980
163. Suit HD, Russell WO, Martin RG: Sarcoma of soft tissue: Clinical and histopathologic parameters and response to treatment. Cancer 35:1478–1483, 1975
164. Suit HD, Mankin HJ, Schiller AL et al: Staging systems for sarcoma of soft tissue and sarcoma of bone. Cancer Treat Symp 3:29–36, 1985
165. Weingrad DW, Rosenberg SA: Early lymphatic spread of osteogenic and soft-tissue sarcomas. Surgery 84:231–240, 1978
166. Mazeron JJ, Suit HD: Lymph nodes as sites of metastases from sarcomas of soft tissue. Cancer 60:1800–1808, 1987
167. Rosenberg SA, Seipp CA, White DE et al: Perioperative blood transfusions are associated with increased rates of recurrence and decreased survival in patients with high-grade soft-tissue sarcomas of the extremities. J Clin Oncol 3:698–709, 1985
168. Soule EH, Pritchard DJ: Fibrosarcoma in infants and children: A review of 110 cases. Cancer 40:1711–1721, 1977
169. Shmahler BM, Enzinger FM: Liposarcoma occurring in children. An analysis of 17 cases and review of the literature. Cancer 52:567–574, 1983
170. Brennan MF: Presentation, demographics and prognostic factors of soft tissue sarcoma. In Shiu MH, Brennan MF (eds): Surgical management of soft tissue sarcoma, Lea and Febiger (in press)
171. Suit HD: Patterns of failure after treatment of sarcoma of soft tissue by radical surgery or by conservative surgery and radiation. Cancer Treat Symp 2:241–246, 1983
172. Cantin J, McNeer GP, Chu FC et al: The problem of local recurrence after treatment of soft tissue sarcoma. Ann Surg 168:47–53, 1968
173. Lindberg RD, Martin RG, Romsdahl MM: Surgery and postoperative radiotherapy in the treatment of soft tissue sarcomas in adults. Am J Roentgenol Rad Ther Nucl Med 123:123–129, 1975
174. Gerner RE, Moore GE, Pickren JW: Soft tissue sarcomas. Ann Surg 181:803–808, 1975
175. Rosenberg SA, Kent H, Costa J et al: Prospective randomized evaluation of the role of limb-sparing surgery, radiation therapy, and adjuvant chemoimmunotherapy in the treatment of adult soft-tissue sarcomas. Surgery 84:62–69, 1978
176. Markhede G, Angervall L, Stener B: A multivariate analysis of the prognosis after surgical treatment of malignant soft tissue tumors. Cancer 49:1721–1733, 1982
177. Pritchard DJ, Soule EH, Taylor WF et al: Fibrosarcoma: Clinicopathologic and statistical study of 199 tumors of the soft tissues of the extremities and trunk. Cancer 33:888–897, 1974
178. Stout AP: Fibrosarcoma: The malignant tumor of fibroblasts. Cancer 1:30–63, 1948
179. Pritchard DJ, Soule EH, Taylor WF et al: Fibrosarcoma: Clinicopathological and statistical study of 199 tumors of soft tissues of extremities and trunk. Cancer 33:880, 1974
180. Castro EB, Hajdu SI, Fortner JG: Surgical therapy of fibrosarcoma of extremities. Arch Surg 107:284, 1973
181. Grier HE, Perez-Atayde AR, Weinstein JH: Chemotherapy for inoperable infantile fibrosarcoma. Cancer 56:1507–1510, 1985
182. Delepine N, Cornille H, Desbois JC et al: Complete response of congenital fibrosarcoma to chemotherapy. Lancet 1:1453–1454, 1986
183. Soule EH, Geitz M, Henderson EH: Embryonal rhabdomyosarcoma of the limbs and limb girdles. A clinico-pathologic study of 61 cases. Cancer 23:1338–1346, 1969
184. Maurer HM, Moon T, Donaldson M et al: The intergroup rhabdomyosarcoma study. Cancer 40:2015, 1977
185. Ariel IM, Briceno M: Rhabdomyosarcoma of the extremities and trunk: Analysis of 150 patients treated by surgical resection. J Surg Oncol 7:269–287, 1975
186. Linscheid RL, Soule EH, Henderson ED: Pleomorphic rhabdomyosarcoma of the extremities and limb girdles: A clinico-pathologic study. J Bone Joint Surg [Am] 47:715–725, 1965
187. Albores-Saavedra J, Martin RG, Smith JL: Rhabdomyosarcoma: A study of 35 cases. Ann Surg 157:186–197, 1963
188. Lloyd RV, Hajdu SI, Knapper WH: Embryonal rhabdomyosarcoma in adults. Cancer 51:557–565, 1983
189. Agamanolis DP, Dasu S, Krill CE: Tumors of skeletal muscle. Hum Pathol 17:778–795, 1986
190. Osborn M, Hill C, Altmannsberger M et al: Monoclonal antibodies to titin in conjunction with antibodies to desmin separate rhabdomyosarcomas from other tumor types. Lab Invest 55:101–108, 1986
191. De Jong Ash, Van Kessel-Van Vark M, Alsus-Lutter Che: Hum Pathol 18:298–303, 1987
192. Stout AP, Hill WT: Leiomyosarcoma of the superficial soft tissues. Cancer 11:844–854, 1958
193. Abwasi OE, Dozois RR, Weiland LH, et al: Leiomyosarcoma of the small and large bowel. Cancer 42:1375, 1978
194. Kevorkian J, Cento DP: Leiomyosarcoma of large arteries and veins. Surgery 73:390, 1973
195. Wile AG, Evans HL, Romsdahl MM: Leiomyosarcoma of soft tissue: A clinicopathologic study. Cancer 48:1022–1032, 1981
196. Enterline HT, Culberson JD, Rochlin DB et al: Liposarcoma. A clinicopathologic study of 53 cases. Cancer 11:932–950, 1960
197. Spittle MF, Newton KA, Mackenzie DH: Liposarcoma. A review of 60 cases. Br J Cancer 24: 696, 1971
198. Kindblom L, Angervall L, Svendsen P: Liposarcoma. A clinicopathologic, radiographic and prognostic study. Acta Pathol Microbiol Immunol Scand 253:1, 1975
199. Ackerman LV: Multiple primary liposarcomas. Am J Pathol 20:789–793, 1944
200. Enzinger FM, Winslow DJ: Liposarcoma. A study of 30 cases. Virchows Arch [A] 335:367–388, 1962
201. Reszel PA, Soule EH, Coventry MB: Liposarcoma of the extremities and limb girdles. A study of 222 cases. J Bone Joint Surg [Am] 48:229, 1966
202. Cadman NL, Soule EH, Kelly PJ: Synovial sarcoma: An analysis of 134 cases. Cancer 18:613–627, 1965
203. Gerner RE, Moore GE: Synovial sarcoma. Ann Surg 181:22–25, 1975
204. Hajdu SI, Shiu MH, Fortner JG: Tendosynovial sarcoma. A clinicopathological study of 136 cases. Cancer 39:1201–1217, 1977
205. Crocker DW, Stout AP: Synovial sarcoma in children. Cancer 12:1123–1133, 1959
206. Mobergen G. Nilsonne U, Friberg S: Synovial sarcoma. Acta Orthop Scand [Suppl] 11:3, 1968
207. Cagle LA, Mirra JM, Storm FK et al: Histologic features relating to prognosis in synovial sarcoma. Cancer 59:1810–1814, 1987
208. Storm FK, Eilber FR, Mirra J et al: Neurofibrosarcoma. Cancer 45:126–129, 1980
209. Girard C, Johnson WC, Graham JH: Cutaneous angiosarcoma. Cancer 26:868–883, 1970
210. Gulesserian HP, Lawton RL: Angiosarcoma of the breast. Cancer 24:1021–1026, 1969
211. Dunegan LJ, Tobon H, Watson CG: Angiosarcoma of the breast: A report of two cases and a review of the literature. Surgery 79:57–59, 1976
212. Woodward AH, Ivins JC, Soule EH: Lymphangiosarcoma arising in chronic lymphedematous extremities. Cancer 30:562–572, 1972
213. Rosai J, Sumner HW, Kostianovsky M et al: Angiosarcoma of the skin. A clinicopathologic and fine structural study. Hum Pathol 7:83, 1976
214. Maddox JC, Evans L: Angiosarcoma of skin and soft tissue: A study of forty-four cases. Cancer 48:1907–1921, 1981
215. Morales PH, Lindberg RD, Barkley HT: Soft tissue angiosarcomas. Int J Radiat Oncol Biol Phys 7:1655–1659, 1981
216. Woodward AH, Ivins JC, Soule EH: Lymphangiosarcoma arising in chronic lymphadematous extremities. Cancer 30:562–572, 1972
217. Silverberg SG, Kay S, Koss LG: Postmastectomy lymphangiosarcoma: Ultrastructural observations. Cancer 27:100–108, 1971
218. Nemoto T, Stubbe N, Gaeta J et al: Pathogenesis of lymphangiosarcoma following mastectomy and irradiation. Surg Gynecol Obstet 489–494, 1969
219. Holden CA, Spittle MF, Jones EW: Angiosarcoma of the face and scalp, prognosis and treatment. Cancer 59:1046–1057, 1987
220. Mira JG, Chu FCH, Fortner JG: The role of radiotherapy in the management of malignant hemangiopericytoma. Report of eleven new cases and review of the literature. Cancer 39:1254–1259, 1977
221. Stout AP: Hemangiopericytoma (a study of 25 new cases). Cancer 2:1027–1954, 1949
222. O'Brien PH, Brasfield RD: Hemangiopericytoma. Cancer 14:249–252, 1965
223. Hood AF, Farmer ER, Weiss RA: Kaposi's sarcoma. Johns Hopkins Med J 151:222–239, 1982
224. Steis RG, Broder S: The clinical relationship between immunodeficiency diseases and cancer with special emphasis on acquired immunodeficiency syndrome (AIDS) and Kaposi's sarcoma. In DeVita VT Jr, Hellman S, Rosenberg SA (eds): Important Advances in Oncology 1985. Philadelphia, JB Lippincott, 1985

225. Krigel RL, Friedman-Kien AE: Kaposi's sarcoma in AIDS. In DeVita VT Jr, Hellman S, Rosenberg SA (eds): AIDS. Etiology, Diagnosis, Treatment and Prevention, pp 185–211. Philadelphia, JB Lippincott, 1985
226. Reynolds WA, Winkelmann RK, Soule EH: Kaposi's sarcoma: A clinicopathologic study with particular reference to its relationship to the reticuloendothelial system. Medicine (Baltimore) 44:419–443, 1965
227. Rothman S: Remarks on sex, age and racial distribution of Kaposi's sarcoma and on possible pathogenetic factors. Acta Unio Int Contra Cancrum 18:326–329, 1962
228. Dorffel J: Histogenesis of multiple idiopathic hemorrhagic sarcoma of Kaposi. Arch Dermatol Syph 26:608–634, 1932
229. Oettle AG: Geographical and racial differences in the frequency of Kaposi's sarcoma as evidence of environmental or genetic causes. Acta Unio Int Contra Cancrum 18:330–363, 1962
230. O'Brien PH, Brasfield RD: Kaposi's sarcoma. Cancer 19:1497, 1966
231. Kaminer B, Murray JF: Sarcoma idiopathicum multiples haemorrhagicum of Kaposi, with special reference to its incidence in the South African Negro, and two case reports. Afr J Clin Sci 1:1–25, 1950
232. Loethe F: Kaposi's sarcoma in Uganda Africans. Acta Pathol Microbiol Immunol Scand [Suppl] 161:1–71, 1963
233. Siegel JH Janic R, Alper JC et al: Disseminated visceral Kaposi's sarcoma. JAMA 207:1493, 1969
234. Stribling J, Wertzner S, Smith GV: Kaposi's sarcoma in renal allograft recipients. Cancer 42:442, 1978
235. Zisbrod A, Hairnov M, Schanzer H et al: Kopsi's sarcoma after kidney transplantation. Transplantation 30:383, 1980
236. Penn I: Kaposi's sarcoma in organ transplant recipients. Transplantation 27:8, 1979
237. Myers BD, Kessle E, Levi D et al: Kaposi's sarcoma in kidney transplant recipients. Arch Intern Med 133:387, 1974
238. Hymes K, Cheung T, Greene JB et al: Kaposi's sarcoma in homosexual men: A report of eight cases. Lancet 2:598–600, 1981
239. O'Brien JE, Stout AP: Malignant fibrous xanthomas. Cancer 17:1445–1458, 1964
240. Wasserman TH, Stuart ID: Malignant fibrous histiocytoma with widespread metastases. Autopsy study. Cancer 33:141–146, 1974
241. Kearney MM, Soule EH, Ivins JC: Malignant fibrous histiocytoma. A retrospective study of 167 cases. Cancer 45:167–178, 1980
242. Weiss SW, Enzinger FM: Malignant fibrous histiocytoma. An analysis of 200 cases. Cancer 41:2250–2266, 1978
243. Leite C, Goodwin JW, Sinkovics JG et al: Chemotherapy of malignant fibrous histiocytoma: A Southwest Oncology Group report. Cancer 40:2010–2014, 1977
244. Reagan MT, Clowry LJ, Cox JD et al: Radiation therapy in the treatment of malignant fibrous histiocytoma. Int J Radiat Oncol Biol Phys 7:311–315, 1981
245. Weiss SW: Malignant fibrous histiocytoma. A reaffirmation. Am J Surg Pathol 6:773–784, 1982
246. Bertoni F, Capanna R, Biagini R et al: Malignant fibrous histiocytoma. An analysis of 78 cases located and deeply seated in extremities. Cancer 56:356–367, 1985
247. Raney RB, Allen A, O'Neill J et al: Malignant fibrous histiocytoma of soft tissue in childhood. Cancer 57:2198–2201, 1986
248. Christopherson WM, Foote FW, Stewart FW: Alveolar soft part sarcomas: Structurally characteristic tumors of uncertain histogenesis. Cancer 5:100, 1952
249. Lieberman PH, Foote FW, Stewart FW et al: Alveolar soft-part sarcoma. JAMA 198:1047–1051, 1966
250. Unni KK, Soule EH: Alveolar soft part sarcoma. An electron microscopic study. Mayo Clin Proc 50:592–598, 1975
251. Bryan RS, Soule EH, Dobyns JH et al: Primary epithelioid sarcoma of the hand and forearm. A review of thirteen cases. J Bone Joint Surg [Am] 56:458–465, 1974
252. Peimer AC, Smith RJ, Sirota RL et al: Epithelioid sarcoma of the hand and wrist: Patterns of extension. J Hand Surg [Am] 2:275–282, 1977
253. Prat J, Woodruff JM, Marcove RC: Epithelioid sarcoma. An analysis of 22 cases indicating the prognostic significance of vascular invasion and regional lymph node metastasis. Cancer 41:1472–1487, 1978
254. Enzinger FM: Epithelioid sarcoma. A sarcoma simulating a granuloma or a carcinoma. Cancer 26:1029–1041, 1970
255. Shimm DS, Suit HD: Radiation therapy of epithelioid sarcoma. Cancer 52:1022–1025, 1983
256. Chase DR, Enzinger FM: Epithelioid sarcoma. Am J Surg Pathol 9:241–263, 1985
257. National Institutes of Health Consensus Development Panel on Limb-Sparing Treatment of Adult Soft Tissue Sarcomas and Osteosarcomas: Introduction and Conclusions. Cancer Treat Symp 3:1–5, 1985
258. Rosenberg SA, Tepper J, Glatstein E et al: The treatment of soft tissue sarcomas of the extremities. Prospective randomized evaluations of (1) limb-sparing surgery plus radiation therapy compared with amputation and (2) the role of adjuvant chemotherapy. Ann Surg 196:305–315, 1982
259. Simon MA, Spainer SS, Enneking WF: Management of adult soft-tissue sarcomas of the extremities. Surg Annu 1:363–402, 1979
260. Brennan MF, Shiu MH, Collin C et al: Extremity soft tissue sarcomas. Cancer Treat Symp 3:71–81, 1985
261. Enneking WF: Staging of musculoskeletal neoplasms. In Current Concepts of Diagnosis and Treatment of Bone and Soft Tissue Tumors. Heidelberg, Springer-Verlag, 1984
262. Karakousis CP: Internal Hemipelvectomy. Surg Gynecol Obstet 158:279–282, 1984
263. Sugarbaker P: Atlas of Extremity Surgery. Philadelphia, JB Lippincott, 1985
264. Greager JA, Das Gupta TK: Adult head and neck soft-tissue sarcomas. Otolaryngol Clin North Am 19:565–572, 1986
265. Mc Kenna WG, Barnes MM, Kinsella TJ et al: Combined modality treatment of adult soft tissue sarcomas of the head and neck. Int J Radiat Oncol Biol Phys 13:1127–1133, 1987
266. Weber RS, Benjamin RS, Peters LJ et al: Soft tissue sarcomas of the head and neck in adolescents and adults. Am J Surg 152:386–392, 1986
267. King RM, Pairolero PC, Trastek VF et al: Primary chest wall tumors: Factors affecting survival. Ann Thorac Surg 41:597–601, 1986
268. Greager JA, Patel MK, Briele HA et al: Soft tissue sarcomas of the adult thoracic wall. Cancer 59:370–373, 1987
269. Glenn J, Kinsella T, Glatstein E et al: A randomized prospective trial of adjuvant chemotherapy in adults with soft tissue sarcomas of the head and neck, breast and trunk. Cancer 55:1206–1214, 1985
270. Shiu MH, Flanebaum L, Hajdu SI et al: Malignant soft tissue tumors of the anterior abdominal wall. Arch Surg 115:152–155, 1980
271. Graeber GM, Snyder RJ, Fleming AW et al: Initial and long-term results in the management of primary chest wall neoplasms. Ann Thorac Surg 34:664–673, 1982
272. Braasch JW, Mon AB: Primary retroperitoneal tumors. Surg Clin North Am 47:663, 1967
273. Cody HS, Turnbull AD, Fortner JG et al: The continuing challenge of retroperitoneal sarcomas. Cancer 47:2147–2152, 1981
274. Storm FK, Sondak VK, Economou JS: Sarcomas of the retroperitoneum. In Eilber FR, Morton DL, Sondak VK et al (eds): The Soft Tissue Sarcomas, pp 239–248. New York, Grune & Stratton, 1987
275. Karakousis CP, Velez AF, Emrich LJ: Management of retroperitoneal sarcomas and patient survival. Am J Surg 150:376–380, 1985
276. Bose B: Primary malignant retroperitoneal tumors: Analysis of 30 cases. Can J Surg 22:215–220, 1979
277. McGrath PC, Neifield JP, Lawrence W et al: Improved survival following complete excision of retroperitoneal sarcomas. Ann Surg 200:200–204, 1984
278. Delamater J: Mammoth tumor. Cleve Med Gazette 1:31, 1859
279. Enzinger FM, Winslow DJ: Liposarcoma. A study of 30 cases. Virchows Arch [A] 335:367–388, 1962
280. Fortner JG, Martin S, Hajdu S et al: Primary sarcoma of the retroperitoneum. Semin Oncol 8:180–184, 1981
281. Abbas S, Holyoke ED, Moore R et al: The surgical treatment and outcome of soft-tissue sarcoma. Arch Surg 116:765–769, 1981
282. Kinsella TJ, Sindelar WF, Lack E et al: Preliminary results of a randomized study of adjuvant radiation therapy in resectable adult retroperitoneal soft tissue sarcomas. J Clin Oncol 6:18–25, 1988
283. Cade SS: Soft tissue tumors: Their natural history and treatment. Proc R Soc Med 19:19–36, 1951
284. Windeyer SB, Dische S, Mansfield CM: The place of radio-therapy in the management of fibrosarcoma of the soft tissues. Clin Radiol 17:32–40, 1966
285. Lindberg RD: Soft tissue sarcoma. In Fletcher GH (ed): Textbook of Radiotherapy, pp 922–942. Philadelphia, Lea & Febiger, 1980
286. Suit HD: Sarcomas of soft tissue. In The 3rd Annual Current Approaches to Radiation Oncology, Biology, and Physic, pp 138–141. San Francisco, University of California, 1983
287. Tepper JE, Suite HD: Radiation therapy of soft tissue sarcomas. Cancer 55:2273–2277, 1985
288. Todoroki T, Suit HD: Effect of fractionated irradiation prior to conservation and radical surgery on therapeutic gain in spontaneous fibrosarcoma of the C3H mouse. J Surg Oncol 31:279–286, 1986
289. Leibel SA, Ware WM, Hill DR, et al: Desmoid tumors: Local control and patterns of relapse following radiation therapy. Int J Radiat Oncol Biol Phys 9:1167–1171, 1983
290. Greenberg HM, Goebel R, Weichselbaum RR, et al: Radiation therapy in the treatment of aggressive fibromatoses. Int J Radiat Oncol Biol Phys 7:309–319, 1981
291. Kiel KD, Suit HD: Radiation therapy in the treatment of aggressive fibromatoses (desmoid tumors). Cancer 54:2051–2055, 1984
292. Leibel SA, Transbaugh RF, Wara WM et al: Soft tissue sarcomas of the extremities. Survival patterns of failure with conservative surgery and post-operative irradiation compared to surgery alone. Cancer 50:1076–1083, 1982
293. Suit HD, Mankin HJ, Wood WC et al: Pre-operative, intra-operative, and post-operative radiation in the treatment of primary soft tissue sarcoma. Cancer 55:2659–2667, 1985
294. Suit HD, Mankin HJ, Schiller AL et al: Results of treatment of sarcoma of soft tissue by radiation and surgery at Massachusetts General Hospital. Cancer Treat Symp 3:43–47, 1985
295. Lindberg R: Treatment of localized soft tissue sarcomas in adults at M.D. Anderson Hospital and Tumor Institute (1960–1981). Cancer Treat Symp 3:59–65, 1985
296. Enneking WF, McAuliffe JA: Adjunctive preoperative radiation therapy in treatment of soft tissue sarcomas: A preliminary report. Cancer Treat Symp 3:37–42, 1985
297. Atkinson L, Garvan JM, Newton NC: Behavior and management of soft tissue sarcomas. Cancer 16:1552–1562, 1963
298. Suit HD, Proppe KH, Mankin HJ et al: Pre-operative radiation therapy for sarcoma of soft tissue. Cancer 47:2269–2274, 1981
299. Fortner JG, Kim DK, Shiu MH: Limb-preserving vascular surgery for malignant tumors of the lower extremity. Arch Surg 112:391–394, 1977
300. Imparato AM, Roses DF, Francis KC et al: Major vascular reconstruction for limb

salvage in patients with soft tissue and skeletal sarcomas of the extremity. Surg Gynecol Obstet 147:891–896, 1978
301. Morton DL, Eilber FR, Townsend CM Jr et al: Limb salvage from a multidisciplinary treatment approach for skeletal and soft tissue sarcomas of the extremity. Ann Surg 184:268–278, 1976
302. Steed DL, Peitzman AB, Webster MW et al: Limb sparing operations for sarcomas of the extremities involving critical arterial circulation. Surg Gynecol Obstet 164:493–498, 1987
303. Nambisan RN, Karakousis CP: Vascular reconstruction for limb salvage in soft tissue sarcomas. Surgery 101:668–677, 1987
304. Shiu MH, Turnbull AD, Nori D et al: Control of locally advanced extremity soft tissue sarcomas by function-saving resection and brachytherapy. Cancer 53:1385–1392, 1984
305. Brennan MF, Hilaris B, Shiu MH et al: Local recurrence in adult soft-tissue sarcoma. Arch Surg 122:1289–1293, 1987
306. Giuliano AE, Eilber FR: The rationale for planned reoperation after unplanned total excision of soft-tissue sarcomas. J Clin Oncol 3:1344–1348, 1985
307. Tepper JE, Rosenberg SA, Glatstein E: Radiation therapy technique in soft tissue sarcomas of the extremity—policies at the National Cancer Institute. Int J Radiat Oncol Biol Phys 8:263–273, 1982
308. Fraass BA, Tepper JE, Glatstein E et al: Clinical use of a match-line wedge for adjacent megavoltage radiation field matching. Int J Radiat Oncol Biol Phys 9:209–216, 1983
309. Kinsella TJ, Loefler JS, Fraass BA et al: Extremity preservation by combined modality therapy in sarcomas of the hand and foot: An analysis of local control, disease-free survival and function result. Int J Radiat Oncol Biol Phys 9:1115–1119, 1983
310. Eilber FR, Guiliano AE, Huth J et al: Limb salvage for high grade soft tissue sarcomas of the extremity: Experience at The University of California, Los Angeles. Cancer Treat Symp 3:49–57, 1985
311. Denton JW, Dunham WK, Salter M et al: Preoperative regional chemotherapy and rapid-fraction irradiation for sarcomas of the soft tissue and bone. Surg Gynecol Obstet 158:545–551, 1984
312. Lokich JJ: Preoperative chemotherapy in soft tissue sarcoma. Surg Gynecol Obstet 148:512–516, 1979
313. Stehlin JS, de Ipolyi PD, Giovanella BC et al: Soft tissue sarcomas of the extremity. Multidisciplinary therapy employing hyperthermic perfusion. Am J Surg 130:643–646, 1975
314. Krementz ET, Carter RD, Sutherland CM et al: Chemotherapy of sarcomas of the limbs by regional perfusion. Ann Surg 185:555–564, 1977
315. Karakousis CP, Lopez R, Catane R et al: Intraarterial adriamycin in the treatment of soft tissue sarcomas. J Surg Oncol 13:21–27, 1980
316. Didolkar MS, Kanter PM, Baffi RR et al: Comparison of regional versus systemic chemotherapy with adriamycin. Ann Surg 187:332–336, 1978
317. Salinas R, Hussey DH, Fletcher GH et al: Experience with fast neutron therapy for locally advanced sarcomas. Int J Radiat Oncol Biol Phy 6:267–272, 1980
318. Pelton JG, Del Rowe JD, Bolen JW et al: Fast neutron radiotherapy for soft tissue sarcomas: University of Washington experience and review of the world's literature. Am J Clin Oncol 9:397–400, 1986
319. Kinsella TJ, Glatstein E: Clinical experience with intravenous radiosensitizers in unresectable sarcomas. Cancer 59:908–915, 1987
320. Sordillo PP, Magill GB, Shiu MH et al: Adjuvant chemotherapy of soft part sarcomas with ALOMAD (S4). J Surg Oncol 18:345–353, 1981
321. Das Gupta TK, Patel MK, Chaudhuri PK et al: The role of chemotherapy as an adjuvant to surgery in the initial treatment of primary soft tissue sarcomas in adults. J Surg Oncol 19:139–144, 1982
322. Das Gupta TK: Tumors of the Soft Tissues. East Norwalk, CT, Appelton-Century-Crofts, 1983
323. Weisenburger TH, Eilber FR, Grant TT et al: Multidisciplinary "limb salvage" treatment of soft tissue and skeletal sarcomas. Int J Radiat Oncol Biol Phys 7:1495–1499, 1981
324. Rosenberg SA, Tepper J, Glatstein E et al: Prospective randomized evaluation of adjuvant chemotherapy in adults with soft tissue sarcomas of the extremities. Cancer 52:424–434, 1983
325. Rosenberg SA: Prospective randomized trials demonstrating the efficacy of adjuvant chemotherapy in adult patients with soft tissue sarcomas. Cancer Treat Rep 68:1067–1078, 1984
326. Rosenberg SA, Chang AE, Glatstein E: Adjuvant chemotherapy for treatment of extremity soft tissue sarcomas: Review of National Cancer Institute experience. Cancer Treat Symp 3:83–88, 1985
327. Antman K, Suit H, Amato D et al: Preliminary results of a randomized trial of adjuvant doxorubicin for sarcomas: Lack of apparent difference between treatment groups. J Clin Oncol 2:601–608, 1984
328. Edmonson JH, Felming TR, Ivins JC et al: Randomized study of systemic chemotherapy following complete excision of nonosseous sarcomas. J Clin Oncol 2:1390–1396, 1984
329. Bramwell V, Rousse J, Steward A et al: European experience of adjuvant chemotherapy for soft tissue sarcoma: Interim report of a randomized trial of CYVADIC versus control. In Recent Concepts in Sarcoma Treatment. Proceedings of the International Symposium on Sarcomas, Tarpon Springs, FL October 8–10, 1987. The Netherlands, Kluwer Academic Publishers (in press)
329a. Alvegard TA: Adjuvant chemotherapy with adriamycin in high grade malignant soft tissue sarcoma—Scandanavian randomized study. Proc ASCO 5:125, 1986
329b. Baker LH: Adjuvant therapy for soft tissue sarcomas. In Ryan JR, Baker L (eds): Recent Concepts in Sarcoma Treatment. Proceedings of the International Symposium on Sarcomas, Tarpon Springs, FL, October 8–10, 1987. The Netherlands, Kluwer Academic Publishers (in press)
330. Antman K, Amato D, Lerner H et al: Adjuvant doxorubicin for sarcoma: Data from The Eastern Cooperative Oncology Group and Dana-Farber Cancer Institute/Massachusetts General Hospital Studies. Cancer Treat Symp 3:109–115, 1985
331. Picci P, Bacci G, Gherlinzoni F et al: Results of a randomized trial for the treatment of localized soft tissue tumors of the extremities in adult patients. In Ryan JR, Baker L (eds): Recent Concepts in Sarcoma Treatment. Proceedings of the International Symposium on Sarcomas, Tarpon Springs, FL October 8–10, 1987. The Netherlands, Kluwer Academic Publishers (in press)
331a. Gherlinzoni F, Bacci G, Picci P et al: A randomized trial for the treatment of high-grade soft-tissue sarcomas of the extremities: Preliminary observations. J Clin Oncol 4:552–558, 1986
332. Eilber FR, Giuliano AE, Huth JF et al: Adjuvant adriamycin in high-grade extremity soft-tissue sarcoma—a randomized prospective trial. Proc ASCO 5:125, 1986
333. Wilson RE, Wood WC, Lerner HL et al: Doxorubicin chemotherapy in the treatment of soft-tissue sarcoma. Arch Surg 121:1354–1359, 1986
334. Lerner HJ, Amato DA, Savlov ED et al: Eastern Cooperative Oncology Group: A comparison of adjuvant doxorubicin and observation for patients with localized soft tissue sarcoma. J Clin Oncol 5:613–617, 1987
335. Chang AE, Kinsella T, Glatstein E et al: Adjuvant chemotherapy for patients with high-grade soft-tissue sarcomas of the extremities. J Clin Oncol 6:1491–1500, 1988
336. Glenn J, Sindelar WF, Kinsella T et al: Results of multimodality therapy of resectable soft tissue sarcomas of the retroperitoneum. Surgery 97:316–325, 1985
337. Dresdale A, Bonow RO, Wesley R et al: Prospective evaluation of doxorubicin-induced cardiomyopathy resulting from postsurgical adjuvant treatment of patients with soft tissue sarcomas. Cancer 52:51–60, 1983
338. Ettinghausen SE, Bonow RO, Palmeri ST et al: Prospective study of cardiomyopathy induced by adjuvant doxorubicin therapy in patients with soft-tissue sarcomas. Arch Surg 121:1445–1451, 1986
339. Giuliano AE, Eilber FR, Morton DL: The management of locally recurrent soft-tissue sarcoma. Ann Surg 196:87–91, 1982
340. Roth JA, Putnam JB, Wesley MN et al: Differing determinants of prognosis following resection of pulmonary metastases from osteogenic and soft tissue sarcoma patients. Cancer 55:1361–1366, 1985
341. Rizzoni WE, Pass HI, Wesley MN et al: Resection of recurrent pulmonary metastases in patients with soft-tissue sarcomas. Arch Surg 121:1248–1252, 1986
342. Pass HI, Dwyer A, Makuch R et al: Detection of pulmonary metastases in patients with osteogenic and soft-tissue sarcomas: The superiority of CT scans compared with conventional linear tomograms using dynamic analysis. J Clin Oncol 3:1261–1265, 1985
343. Blum RH: An overview of studies in adriamycin (NSC-123127) in the United States. Cancer Chemother Rep 6:247–251, 1975
344. O'Bryan RM, Luce JK, Talley RW et al: Phase II evaluation of adriamycin in human neoplasia. Cancer 32:1–8, 1973
345. O'Bryan RM, Baker LH, Gottlieb JE et al: Dose response evaluation of adriamycin in human neoplasia. Cancer 39:1940–1948, 1977
346. Schoenfeld D, Rosenbaum C, Horton J et al: A comparison of adriamycin versus vincristine and adriamycin, and cyclophosphamide for advanced sarcoma. Cancer 50:2757–2762, 1982
347. Borden EC, Amato D, Enterline HT et al: Randomized comparison of adriamycin regimens for treatment of metastatic soft tissue sarcomas. J Clin Oncol 5:840–850, 1987
348. Cruz AB Jr, Thames EA Jr, Aust JB et al: Combination chemotherapy for soft tissue sarcomas: A phase III study. J Surg Oncol 11:313–323, 1979
349. Creagan ET, Hahn RG, Ahmann DL et al: A clinical trial adriamycin (NSC 123127) in advanced sarcomas. Oncology 34:90–91, 1977
350. Rosen G, Caparros B, Nirenberg A et al: High-dose methotrexate (HDMTX) with citrovorum factor rescue (CFR) in the treatment of radiation-induced sarcomas. Proc AACR 1983:194, 1981
351. Vaughn C, McKelvey E, Balcerzak S et al: High-dose methotrexate with leucovorin rescue plus vincristine in advanced sarcoma: A Southwest Oncology Group study. Cancer Treat Rep 68:409–410, 1984
352. Isacoff WH, Eilber F, Tabbarah H et al: Phase II clinical trial with high-dose methotrexate therapy and citrovorum factor rescue. Cancer Treat Rep 62:1295–1304, 1978
353. Karakousis CP, Rao U, Carlson M: High-dose methotrexate as secondary chemotherapy in metastatic soft-tissue sarcomas. Cancer 46:1345–1348, 1980
354. Von Hoff DD, Rozencwieg M, Louie AC et al: "Single"-agent activity of high-dose methotrexate therapy with citrovorum factor rescue. Cancer Treat Rep 62:233–235, 1978
355. Frie E, Blum R, Pitman S et al: High-dose methotrexate with leucovorin rescue: Rationale and spectrum of antitumor activity. Am J Med 68:370–375, 1979
356. Ambinder EP, Perloff M, Ohnuma T et al: High-dose methotrexate followed by citrovorum factor reversal in patients with advanced cancer. Cancer 43:1177–1182, 1979
357. Andrews N, Wilson W: Phase II study of methotrexate (NSC 740) in solid tumors. Cancer Chemother Rep 51:471–474, 1967
358. Subramanian S, Wiltshaw E: Chemotherapy of sarcoma—A comparison of three regimes. Lancet 1:683–686, 1978

359. Buesa JM, Mouridsen HT, Santoro A: Treatment of advanced soft tissue sarcomas with low-dose methotrexate: A phase II trial by the European Organization for Research on Treatment of Cancer (EORTC) Soft Tissue and Bone Sarcoma Group. Cancer Treat Rep 68:683–694, 1984
360. Amato DA, Borden EC, Shiraki M et al: Evaluation of bleomycin, chlorozotocin, MGBG, and bruceantin in patients with advanced soft tissue sarcoma, bone sarcoma, or mesothelioma. Invest New Drugs 3:397–401, 1985
361. Golbey R, Li MC, Kaufman RF: Actinomycin in the treatment of soft part sarcomas. (abstr) James Ewing Society Scientific Program, 1968
362. Gold G, Hall T, Shnider B et al: A clinical study of 5-fluorouracil. Cancer 19:935–939, 1959
363. Selawry OS, Holland JF, Wolman IJ: Effect of vincristine (NSC-67574) on malignant solid tumors in children. Cancer Chemother Rep 52:497–499, 1968
364. Korbitzs BC, Davis HL Jr, Ramirez G et al: Low doses of vincristine (NSC-67574) for malignant disease. Cancer Chemother Rep 53:249–254, 1969
365. Radice PA, Bunn PA Jr, Ihde DC: Therapeutic trials with VP-16 and VM26. Cancer Treat Rep 63:1231–1239, 1979
366. Bleyer WA, Chard RL, Krivit W et al: Epipodophyllotoxin therapy of childhood neoplasia. A comparative phase II analysis of VM26 and VP16-213. Proc AACR 19:373, 1978
367. Rosenberg SA, Suit HD, Baker LH: Sarcomas of soft tissue. In Cancer, Principles and Practice of Oncology, 2nd ed, p 1243. DeVita VT Jr, Hellman S, Rosenberg SA (eds): Philadelphia, JB Lippincott, 1985
368. Bramwell VHC, Brugarols A, Mouridsen HT et al: EORTC. Phase II study of cisplatinum in CYVADIC-resistant soft tissue sarcoma. Eur J Cancer 15:1511–1513, 1979
369. Karakousis CP, Holterman OA, Holyoke ED: Cisdichlorodiamineplatinum (II) in metastatic soft tissue sarcomas. Cancer Treat Rep 63:2071–2075, 1979
370. Samson MK, Baker LH, Benjamin RS et al: Cisdichlorodiamineplatinum (II) in advanced soft tissue and bony sarcomas. A Southwest Oncology Group study. Cancer Treat Rep 63:2027–2028, 1979
371. Thigpen JT, Blessing JA, Wilbanks GD: Cisplatin as second-line chemotherapy in the treatment of advanced or recurrent leiomyosarcoma of the uterus. Am J Clin Oncol 9:18–20, 1986
372. Gershenson DM, Kavanagh JJ, Copeland LJ et al: Cisplatin therapy for disseminated mixed mesodermal sarcoma of the uterus. J Clin Oncol 5:618–621, 1987
373. Bergsagel DE, Levin WC: A prelusive clinical trial of cyclophosphamide. Cancer Chemother Rep 8:120–134, 1960
374. Korst DR, Johnson D, Frenkel EP et al: Preliminary evaluation of the effect of cyclophosphamide on the course of human neoplasms. Cancer Chemother Rep 7:1–12, 1960
375. Bramwell V, Mouridsen H, Santoro G et al: Cyclophosphamide vs ifosfamide; Final report of a randomized phase II trial in adult soft tissue sarcoma. Eur J Cancer Clin Oncol 23:311–321, 1987
376. Bodey GP, Rodreguez V, Murphy WK et al: Protected environment—prophylactic antibiotic program for malignant sarcoma: Randomized trial during remission induction chemotherapy. Cancer 47:2422–2429
377. Pinedo HM, Branwell VHC, Mouridson MD et al: CYVADIC in advanced soft tissue sarcoma: a randomized study comparing two schedules. A study of the EORTC Soft Tissue and Bone Sarcoma Group. Cancer 53:1825–1832, 1984
378. Legha S, Benjamin RS, Mackay B et al: Reduction of doxorubicin cardiotoxicity by prolonged continuous intravenous infusion. Ann Intern Med 96:133–139, 1982
379. Benjamin R, Yap B, Frazier O Jr et al: Combination chemotherapy for sarcomas with cyclophosphamide and continuous infusion adriamycin and dacarbazine (CI-CYA-DIC) with surgical intensification (abst). Proc AACR/ASCO 22:526, 1981
380. Baker LK, Green S, Ryan J et al: Combined modality therapy for disseminated soft tissue sarcoma, phase III. Proc ASCO 6:138, 1987
381. Brennan MF, Friedrich C, Almadrones L et al: Prospective randomized trial examining the cardiac toxicity of adjuvant doxorubicin in high grade extremity sarcomas. In Sydney Salmon (ed): Adjuvant Therapy of Cancer V, pp 745–754. Orlando, Grune & Stratton, 1987
382. Perevodchikova NI, Lichinister MR, Gorbunova VA: Phrase II clinical study of carminomycin: Its activity against soft tissue sarcomas. Cancer Treat Rep 61:1705–1707, 1977
383. Chang P, Wiernik PH: Phase II study of azotomycin in sarcomas. Cancer Treat Rep 61:1719, 1979
384. Weiss AJ, Ramirez G, Grage T et al: Phase II study of azotomycin (NSC-56654). Cancer Chemother Rep 52:611–614, 1968
385. Dejager R, Bodey JJ, Dupont D et al: Phase I study of oral 4′-(9-acrindylamino-methanseulfon-m-anididide). Proc ASCO 20:429, 1979
386. Legha SS, Gutterman JU, Hall SW et al: Phase I clinical investigation of 4′-(9-acridinylamino)methanesulfon-m-anisidide (NSC 249992), a new acridine derivative. Cancer Res 38:3712–3716, 1978
387. Von Hoff DD, Howser D, Gormley P et al: Phase I study of methanesulfonamide, N-(4-9-acridinylamino)-3-methoxyphenyl)-(m-AMSA) using a single-dose schedule. Cancer Treat Rep 62:1421–1426, 1978
388. Schneidere R, Sklanoff R, Ochoa M: Phase I trial of AMSA (4′[acrindylamino]-methansulfon-m-anisidide). Proc AACR 20:114, 1979
389. Bertrand M, Multhauf P, Bartolucci A et al: Phase II study of aclarubicin in previously untreated patients with advanced soft tissue sarcoma: Cancer Treat Rep 69:725–726, 1985
390. Zidar B, Baker L, Rivkin S et al: A phase II study of diaziquone in advanced soft tissue and bony sarcoma. A Southwest Oncology Group (SWOG) study. Cancer Treat Rep 69:1035–1036, 1985
391. Chan C, Bartolucci A, Brenner D et al: Phase II trial of diaziquone in anthracycline-resistant adult soft tissue and bone sarcoma patients: A Southeastern Cancer Study Group trial. Cancer Treat Rep 70:427–428, 1986
392. Presant C, Gams R, Bartolucci A et al: Treatment of metastatic sarcomas with mitroxantrone. Cancer Treat Rep 68:813–814, 1984
393. Bull FE, Von Hoff DD, Balcerzak SP et al: Phase II Trial of mitoxantrone in advanced sarcomas: A Southwest Oncology Group study. Cancer Treat Rep 69:231–233, 1985
394. Aust J, Andrews N, Schroeder J et al: Phase II study of 1-aminocyclopentanecarboxylic acid (NSC 1026) in patients with cancer. Cancer Chemother Rep 54:237–241, 1970
395. Savlov ED, MacIntyre JM, Knight E et al: Comparison of doxorubicin with cycloleucine in the treatment of sarcomas, Cancer Treat Rep 65:21–27, 1981
396. Johnson R: Preliminary phase II trials with 1-aminocyclopentance carboxylic acid (NSC-1026). Cancer Chemother Rep 32, 1963
397. Mouridsen HT, Bramwell VH, Lacave J et al: Treatment of advanced soft tissue sarcomas with chlorozotocin: A phase II trial of the EORTC soft tissue and bone sarcoma group. Cancer Treat Rep 65:509–511, 1981
398. Kovach JS, Moertel CG, Schutt AF: A phase I study of chlorozotocin (NSC 178248). Cancer 43:2189–2196, 1979
399. Gralla RJ, Tan CTC, Young CW: Phase I trial of chlorozotocin. Cancer Treat Rep 63:17–20, 1979
400. Presant CA, Bartolucci AA: Phase II evaluation of chlorozotocin in metastatic sarcomas. Med Pediatr Oncol 12:25–27, 1984
401. Sordillo PP, Magill GB, Gralla RJ et al: Chlorozotocin: Phase II evaluation in patients with advanced sarcomas. Canceer Treat Rep 65:513–514, 1981
402. Talley RW, Samson MK, Brownlee RW et al: Phase II evaluation of chlorozotocin in advanced human cancers. Eur J Cancer 17:337–343, 1981
403. Baker LH, Samson MK, Izbicki RM: Phase I and II evaluation of cytembena in disseminated epithelial ovarian cancer and sarcomas. Cancer Treat Rep 60:1389–1391, 1976
404. Matejovsky Z: Effects of cytembena in the treatment of malignant musculoskeletal tumors. Neoplasma 18:473–480, 1971
405. Presant CA, Ardalan B, Multhauf P: Continuous five-day infusion of PALA and 5FU: A pilot phase II trial. Pediatr Oncol 11:162–163, 1983
406. Kurzrock R, Yap BS, Plager C et al: Phase II evaluation of PALA in patients with refractory metastatic sarcomas. Am J Clin Oncol 7:305–307, 1984
407. Rodriquez V, Gottlieb J, Burgess MA et al: Phase I studies with Baker's antifol (BAF) (NSC 139105). Cancer 38:690–694, 1976
408. Thigpen JT, O'Bryan RM, Benjamin RS et al: Phase II trial of Baker's antifol in metastatic sarcoma. Cancer Treat Rep 61:1485–1487, 1977
409. Klein HO, Wickramanayake, Dias P et al: High-dose ifosfamide and mesna as continuous infusion over five days—a phase I/II trial. Cancer Treat Rev (Suppl A) 10:167–173, 1983
410. Czownicki Z, Utracka-Hatka B: Clinical studies with uromitexan—an antidote against urotoxicity of holoxan. Preliminary results. Nowotwory 30:377–383, 1980
411. Czownicki Z, Utracka-Hutka B: Contribution to the treatment of malignant tumors with ifosfamide. In Burkeret H, Voight HC (eds): Proceedings of the International Holoxan Symposium, pp 109–111. Dusseldorf, Asta-Werke, 1977
412. Scheulen M, Niederle N, Seeber S: Results of a clinical phase II study on the use of ifosfamide in refractory malignant diseases. Comparison of the uroprotective effect of uromitexan and forced diuresis with alkalization of the urine. New experience with the oxazaphosphorines with special reference to the uroprotector uromitexan, p 40. In Burkert H, Bielefeld, Nagel GA (eds): 1980
413. Magrath IT, Sandlund JT, Rayner A et al: Treatment of recurrent sarcomas with ifosfamide (IF). Proc ASCO 4:136, 1985
414. Antman K, Montella D et al: Phase II trial of ifosfamide with mesna in previously treated metastatic sarcoma. Cancer Treat Rep 69:499–504, 1985
415. Stuart-Harris R, Harper PG, Kay SB et al: High-dose ifosfamide by infusion with mesna in advanced soft tissue sarcoma. Cancer Treat Rev (Suppl A) 10:163–164, 1983
416. Pratt C, Horowitz M, Meyer W et al: Phase II trial of ifosfamide (IFOS) with mesna in patients with pediatric malignant solid tumors. Proc ASCO 4:234, 1985
417. Creagan ET, Hahn JHRG, Ahmann DL et al: A comparative clinical trial evaluating the combination of actinomycin D, cyclophosphamide, and vincristine, and a single agent, methyl-CCNU, in advanced sarcomas. Cancer Treat Rep 60:1385–1386, 1976
418. Tranum BP, Haut A, Rivkin SE et al: A phase II study of methyl-CCNU in the treatment of solid tumors and lymphomas in the Southwest Oncology Group. Cancer 35:1148–1153, 1974
419. Borden EC, Larson P, Ansfield FJ et al: Hexamethylmelamine. A new drug with activity in solid tumors. Eur J Cancer 9:195–202, 1973
420. Blum RH, Livingston RB, Carter SK: Hexamethylmelamine. A new drug with activity in solid tumors. Eur J Cancer 9:195–202, 1973
421. Bedikian AY, Valdivieso M, Bodey GP et al: Hexamethylmelamine treatment of sarcomas and lymphomas. Med Pediatr Oncol 3:401–406, 1977
422. Sooriyaarachchi GS, Ramirez G, Roley EL et al: Hemangiopericytoma of the uterus. J Surg Oncol 10:399–406, 1978
423. Borden EC, Ash A, Enterline HT et al: Phase II evaluation of dibromodulcitol, ICRF-159, and maytansine for sarcomas. Am J Clin Oncol 5:417–410, 1982

424. Conroy JF, Roda PI, Prasavinichai S: Dibromodulcitol in the treatment of metastic hemangiopericytoma. Am J Clin Oncol 5:453–456, 1982
425. Kimball JC, Cangir A: A phase II trial of dianhydrogalactitol in advanced soft tissue and bony sarcomas. A Southwest Oncology Group study. Cancer Treat Rep 63:553–554, 1979
426. Saiki J, Stephens R, Fabian C et al: Phase II evaluation of Gallium nitrate (NSC-15200) in soft tissue and bone sarcomas. Proc AACR/ASCO 22:525, 1981
427. Bleyer WA, Krivit W, Chard RL et al: Phase II study of VM-26 in acute leukemia, neuroblastoma, and other refractory childhood malignancies: A report from the Children's Cancer Study Group. Cancer Treat Rep 63:977–981, 1979
428. Rossof AH, Chandra G, Walter J et al: Phase II trial of vindesine (desacetyl vinblastine amide sulfate) in advanced metastatic cancer. Proc AACR 20:146, 1979
429. Currie VE, Wong PP, Krakoff IH et al: Phase I trial of vindesine in patients with advanced cancer. Cancer Treat Rep 62:1333–1336, 1978
430. Alberto P, De Jager RL, Brugarolas A et al: Phase II study of diamino-dichlorophenyl-methylpyprimidine with folinic acid protection and rescue. Proc AACR 20:323, 1979
431. Benjamin RS, Keating MJ, Valdivieso M et al: Phase I–II study of piperazinedione in adults with solid tumors and acute leukemia. Cancer Treat Rep 63:939–943, 1979
432. Thigpen T, Blessing JA, Homesley HD et al: Phase II trial of piperazinedione in treatment of advanced or recurrent uterine sarcoma, a GOG study. Am J Clin Oncol 8:350–2, 1985
433. LaGasse L, Thigpen T, Morrison F: Phase II trial of piperazinedione in treatment of advanced endometrial carcinoma, uterine sarcoma, and vulvar carcinoma (abstr). Proc ASCO 20:388, 1979
434. Sordillo PP, Magill GB, Walt S: Phase II trial of methylglyoxal-bix-guanylhydrazone (methyl-GAG) in patients with soft-tissue sarcomas. Am J Clin Oncol 8:316–318, 1985
435. Gralla RJ, Sordillo PP, Magill GB: Phase II evaluation of pyrazofurin in patients with metastatic sarcoma. Cancer Treat Rep 62:1573, 1978
436. Salem PA, Bodey GP, Burgess MA et al: A phase I study of pyrazofurin. Cancer 40:2806–2809, 1977
437. Cormier WJ, Hahn RG, Edmonson JH et al: Phase II study in advanced sarcoma: randomized trial of pyrazofurin versus combination cyclophosphamide, doxorubicin and cis-dichlorodiammineplatinum (II) (CAP). Cancer Treat Rep 64:655, 1980
438. Blum RH, Kahlert T: Maytansine: A phase I study of an ansamacrolide with antitumor activity. Cancer Treat Rep 62:435–438, 1978
439. Ajani JA, Dimery I, Chawla SP et al: Phase II studies of homoharringtonine in patients with advanced malignant melanoma; sarcoma; and head and neck, breast, and colorectal carcinomas. Cancer Treat Rep 70:375–379, 1986
440. Haris JE, Das Gupta TK, Vogelzang N et al: Treatment of soft tissue sarcoma with fibroblast interferon—American Cancer Society/Illinois Cancer Council study. Cancer Treat Rep 70:293–294, 1986
441. Schuff-Werner P, Bartsch H, Schreml W et al: soft tissue sarcoma with recombinant alpha-interferon (abstr). Antiviral Res 1:93, 1984
442. Rosenberg SA, Lotze MT, Muul LM et al: A progress report on the treatment of 157 patients with advanced cancer using lymphokine-activated killer cells and interleukin-2 or high-dose interleukin-2 alone. N Engl J Med 316:890–897, 1987
443. Omura GA, Major FJ, Blessing JA et al: A randomized study of adriamycin with and without dimethyl trazenoimidazole carboxamide in advanced uterine sarcomas. Cancer 52:626–632, 1983
444. Lerner H, Amato D, Stevens C et al: Leiomyosarcoma: The Eastern Cooperative Oncology Group experience with 222 patients. Proc AACR 24:142, 1983
445. Benjamin RS, Gottlieb JA, Baker LH et al: CYVADIC vs CYVADACT—a randomized trial of cyclophosphamide (CY), vincristine (V), and adriamycin (A) plus either dacarbazine (DIC) or actinomycin-D (DACT) in metastatic sarcomas. Proc AACR 17:256, 1976
446. Baker LH, Frank J, Fine G et al: Combination chemotherapy using adriamycin, DTIC, cyclophosphamide, and actinomycin D for advanced soft tissue sarcomas: A randomized comparative trial. J Clin Oncol 5:851–861, 1987
447. Muss HB, Bundy B, DiSaia PJ et al: Treatment of recurrent of advanced uterine sarcoma—a randomized trial of doxorubicin vs doxorubicin and cyclophosphamide. Cancer 55:1648–1653, 1985
448. Brock N: Pharmacological studies with ifosfamide—a new oxazaphosphorine compound. In Semonsky M, Hejzler M, and Masak S (eds)? Advances in Antimicrobial and Antineoplastic Chemotherapy, vol 2, pp 749–756. Baltimore, University Park Press, 1972.
449. Cabanillas F, Hagemeister FB, Bodey GP et al: IMVP-16: An effective regimen for patients with lymphoma who have relapsed after initial combination chemotherapy. Blood 60:693–697, 1982
450. Morgan LR, Posey LE, Rainey J et al: Ifosfamide: A weekly dose-fractionated schedule in bronchogenic carcinoma. Cancer Treat Rep 65:693–695, 1981
451. Goldin A: Ifosfamide in experimental tumor systems. Semin Oncol 9:14–23, 1972
452. Allen LM, Creaven PJ: Effect of microsomal activation on interaction between iphosphamide and DNA. J Pharm Sci 61:2009–2011, 1972
453. Allen LM, Creaven PJ, Nelson RL: Studies on the human pharmacokinetics of isophosphamide (NSC-109724). Cancer Treat Rep 60:451–458, 1976
454. Cohen MH, Creaven PJ, Tejada F et al: Phase I clinical trial of isophosphamide (NSC-109724). Cancer Chemother Rep 59:751–755, 1975
455. Heim ME, Fiene R, Schick E et al: Central nervous side effects following ifosfamide monotherapy of advanced renal carcinoma. J Cancer Res Clin Oncol 100:113–116, 1982
456. Pratt CB, Green AA, Horowitz M et al: Central nervous system toxicity following ifosfamide treatment for children with malignant solid tumors. Proc AACR 26:184, 1985
457. Antman KH, Montella D, Rosenbaum C et al: Phase II trial of ifosfamide with mesna in previously treated metastatic sarcoma. Cancer Treat Rep 69:499–502, 1985
458. Gottlieb JA, Baker LH, Quagliana JM et al: Chemotherapy of sarcomas with a combination of adriamycin and dimethyltrazeno-imidazole-carboxamide. Cancer 30:1632–1638, 1972
459. Saiki J, Baker LH, Rivkin SE et al: A useful high-dose intermittent schedule of adriamycin and DTIC in the treatment of advanced sarcomas. Cancer 58:2196–2197, 1986
460. Blum R, Corson J et al: Successful treatment of metastatic sarcomas with cyclophosphamide, adriamycin, and DTIC (CAD). Cancer 46:1722–1726, 1980
461. Ikeda K, Ogawa M, Inagaki J et al: A combination chemotherapy with adriamycin, cyclophosphamide and DTIC (ACD) for advanced adult soft part sarcoma. Gan To Kagaku Ryoho 11:235–239, 1984
462. Gottlieb JA, Baker LH et al: Adriamycin (NSV-123127) used alone and in combination for soft tissue and bony sarcomas. Cancer Chemother Rep 6:271–282, 1975
463. Yap B, Baker LH, Sinkovics JG et al: Cyclophosphamide, vincristine, adriamycin, and DTIC (CYVADIC) combination chemotherapy for the treatment of advanced sarcomas. Cancer Treat Rep 64:93–98, 1980
464. Yap BS, Sinkovics JG, Benjamin RS et al: Survival and relapse patterns of complete responders in adults with advanced soft tissue sarcomas (ASTS). Proc AACR/ASCO 20:352, 1979
465. Bui NB, Chauvergne J, Hocke C et al: analysis of a series of sixty soft tissue sarcomas in adults treated with a cyclophosphamide-vincristine-adriamycin-dacarbazine (CY-VADIC) combination. Cancer Chemother Pharmacol 15:82–85, 1985
466. Pfeffer MR, Sulkes A, Biran S: Treatment of advanced soft tissue sarcomas with a modified CYVADIC protocol. Oncology 41:308–313, 1984
467. Choi TK, NG A, Wong J: Doxorubicin, dacarbazine, vincristine, and cyclophosphamide in the treatment of advanced gastrointestinal leiomyosarcoma. Cancer Treat Rep 69:443–444, 1985
468. Lopez M, Di Lauro L, Papaldo P et al: Alternating combination chemotherapy of advanced soft tissue sarcomas in adults. Am J Clin Oncol 7:539–542, 1984
469. Rivkin SE, Gottlieb JA, Thigpen T et al: Methyl-CCNU and adriamycin for patients with metastatic sarcomas. A Southwest Oncology Group study. Cancer 46:446–451, 1980
470. Shiu MH, Magill GB, Hopfan S: Recent trends in treatment of soft issue sarcomas—Appendix A. In Hajdu SI (ed): Pathology of Soft Tumors, pp 537–542. Philadelphia, Lea & Febiger, 1979
471. Chang P, Wiernik PH: Combination chemotherapy with adriamycin and streptozotocin. Clin Pharmacol Ther 20:606–610, 1976
472. Otten J, Falmant F, Rodary C et al: Effectiveness of combination of ifosfamide, vincristine and actinomycine D in inducing remission in rhabdomyosarcoma in children. For the RMS group of the International Society of Pediatric Oncology (SIOP). Proc ASCO 4:236, 1985
473. Elias AD, Antman K, Ryan L: Doxorubicin (DOX), ifosfamide (IFF), and DTIC with mesna uroprotection for advanced untreated sarcoma. Proc ASCO 6:134, 1987
474. Schutte J, Dombernowsky P, Santoro A et al: Adriamycin (A) and ifosfamide (I), a new effective combination in advanced soft tissue sarcoma; preliminary report of a phase II study of the EORTC soft tissue and bone sarcoma group. Proc ASCO 5:145, 1986
475. Bierbaum W, Bremer K, Firusian N, et al: Chemotherapeutische Behandlungsmoglichkeiten bei forgeschrittenen Sarkomen. Dtsch Med Wochenschr 106:1181–1185, 1981
476. Wellens W, Mussgnug G, Havets L et al: The combination ifosfamide/VP-16-213 in therapy of small cell bronchogenic carcinoma and other malignant tumors. In Burkert H, Nagel G, (eds): Beitrage zur Onkologie, vol 5, pp 81–87. Basel, S Karger, 1980
477. Wellens W, Donhuijsen-Ant R, Habets L et al: Therapie progredienter Sarkome mit Etososid und Ifosfamide. Etoposide Symposium. Aktuel Onkol Zuckschwerdt (Munchen) 4:159–164, 1981
478. de Kraker J, Voute PA: Ifosfamide and vincristine in pediatric tumors. A phase II study. Eur Paediatr Haematol Oncol 1:47–50, 1984
479. Klippstein TH, Mitrou PS, Kochendorfer KJ et al: High-dose adriamycin (ADM) and cis-platinum (DDP) in advanced soft-tissue sarcomas and invasive thymomas: A pilot study. Cancer Chemoterh Pharmacol 13:78–81, 1984
480. Edmonson JH, Hahn RG, Schutt AJ et al: Cyclophosphamide, doxorubicin, and cisplatin combined in the treatment of advanced sarcomas. Med Pediatr Oncol 11:319–321, 1983
481. Cormier WJ, Hahn RG, Edmonson JH: Phase II study in advanced sarcoma: Randomized trial of pyrazofurin vs combination cyclophosphamide, doxorubicin, and cis-dichlorodiammineplatinum (II) (CAP). Cancer Treat Rep 64:655–658,
482. Edmonson JH, Creagan ET, Kvols LK et al: Failure of bleomycin to improve the therapeutic effects of a combination of cyclophosphamide, doxorubicin, and cisplatin (CAP) in advanced sarcomas. Med Pediatr Oncol 12:264–266, 1984
483. Edmonson JH, Long HJ, Richardson RL et al: Phase II study of a combination of mitomycin, doxorubicin and cisplatin in advanced sarcomas. Cancer Chemother Pharmacol 15:181–182, 1985
484. Piver MS, Shashikant BL, Patsner B: Cis-diamminedichloroplatinum plus dimethyltriazenoimidazole carboxamide as second- and third-line chemotherapy for sarcomas of the female pelvis. Gynecol Oncol 23:371–375, 1986

485. Presgrave P, Woods RL, Tattersall MN et al: Combination chemotherapy of adult soft tissue sarcomas with a combination of doxorubicin and methotrexate. Cancer Treat Rep (in press)
486. Kaufman JH, Catane R, Douglass HO: Combined adriamycin, vincristine, and methotrexate. NY State J Med:742–743, 1977
487. Presant CA, Lowenbraun S, Bartolucci AA et al: Metastatic sarcomas: Chemotherapy with adriamycin, cyclophosphamide, and methotrexate alternating with actinomycin D, DTIC, and vincristine. Cancer 47:457–465, 1981
488. Lynch G, Magill GB, Sordillo PP et al: Combination chemotherapy of advanced sarcomas in adults with Cyomad. Cancer 50:1724–1727, 1982
489. Lowenbraun S, Moffitt JS, Smalley R et al: Combination chemotherapy with adriamycin, cyclophosphamide and methotrexate in metastatic sarcomas (abstr). Proc ASCO 18:289, 1977
490. Jacobs EM: Combination chemotherapy of metastatic testicular germinal cell tumors and soft part sarcomas. Cancer 25:324–332, 1970
491. Moskowitz AJ, Pauker SG: A decision analytic approach to limb-sparing treatment for adult soft tissue and osteogenic sarcoma. Cancer Treat Symp 3:11–26, 1985
492. Sugarbaker PH, Barofsky I, Rosenberg SA et al: Quality of life assessment of patients in extremity sarcoma clinical trials. Surgery 91:17–23, 1982
493. Weddington WW, Segraves KB, Simon MA: Psychological outcome of extremity sarcoma survivors undergoing amputation or limb salvage. J Clin Oncol 3:1393–1399, 1985
494. Chang A, Culnane M, Lampert M et al: Quality of life changes in soft tissue sarcoma patients undergoing multimodality treatment. Proc ASCO 6:254, 1987

KAREN H. ANTMAN
HARVEY I. PASS
ABRAM RECHT

CHAPTER 41 *Benign and Malignant Mesothelioma*

Because malignant mesothelioma is strongly associated with a widely distributed environmental carcinogen, asbestos, it has assumed an importance in the medical and lay literature out of proportion to its annual incidence of approximately 2200 cases in the United States.[1-3] Eight million living Americans have been occupationally exposed between 1940 and 1970, and many public and private buildings contain asbestos.[4] An estimated 10% to 15% of the schools in the United States were insulated with asbestos between 1946 and 1972.[5,6] Of the 70,000 tons of asbestos used in the United States yearly, about half is incorporated into cement for water conduits, which usually contain 10% to 20% asbestos.[7,8] Flooring products, automobile brake linings, roof shingles, insulation, packing plastic, and textiles contain asbestos. Veins of asbestos run through talc deposits, and asbestos has been identified as a contaminant in industrial and body talc. The use of talc has been associated with the development of ovarian cancer.[9] Many urban water reservoirs contain high levels of asbestos-like fibers, presumably a result of erosion of asbestos-cement pipe systems or of dumping mine wastes, as in Lake Superior, which supplies drinking water for Duluth, MN.[7,8]

An increased incidence of mesothelioma is detectable in a population about 15 years after first exposure and rises steadily to 5.5 per 1000 person-years 40 to 45 years after first exposure.[10-13] Despite legislation limiting industrial exposure to asbestos since 1970, an estimated 19,000 to 80,000 new cases of asbestos-associated mesothelioma are expected to occur between 1980 and 2030.[14,15]

EPIDEMIOLOGY

The strength of asbestos and its resistance to combustion were recognized in antiquity.[16] Finnish pottery dating from approximately 2500 BC contains asbestos. There are several references to a tablecloth that Charlemagne allegedly threw into the fireplace after meals, later pulling it clean from the fire. Chinese cloth "purified by fire" is also described by Marco Polo. Recognition of the medical hazards of asbestos may also date from antiquity, because Pliny observed that asbestos mine slaves had poorer health than other mining slaves.[16]

In 1898, pulmonary scarring in asbestos workers from French and English asbestos textile mills, was reported, with death occurring 10 to 15 years after beginning work in the factories.[17] Although the cause of the pulmonary fibrosis remained controversial through the 1920s because of unsanitary conditions and endemic tuberculosis, Cooke began using the term *asbestosis* in 1927.[18] In 1930, the causal association of asbestos and asbestosis was definitively established by Merewether and Price, based on a series of cases from the London Chest Hospital.[19] England promptly introduced limits on allowable industrial levels of asbestos exposure.

Although additional cases of asbestosis were expected over the next 10 to 20 years from asbestos levels allowed before 1930, many experts believed that the asbestos problem had been solved.

Asbestosis did become less common, allowing asbestos workers to survive long enough to develop a more insidious disease, cancer. Case reports of lung cancer in patients with asbestosis appear as early as 1935.[20,21] The disturbing number of lung cancers observed in autopsy series from the London Chest Hospital during the late 1940s and early 1950s was initially dismissed by some as a result of referral patterns of rare diseases to a specialty hospital. A causal association was supported by Merewether's observation of a 14% incidence of lung cancer in an autopsy series of patients with asbestosis, tenfold higher than in patients with silicosis.[22] In 1955, Doll reported a case-control study that established the association between asbestos and lung cancer.[23] The association between lung cancer and smoking was definitively established 3 years later.

The existence of mesothelioma was debated by pathologists before 1960.[24] In 1942, Stout and Murray showed that mesothelial cells differentiate in tissue culture into both the epithelial and sarcomatous variants observed clinically.[25] In the late 1940s, case reports appeared of mesotheliomas arising in patients with asbestosis. In 1960, however, Wagner and colleagues reported 47 cases of mesothelioma in a South African crocidolite mining community.[26] All but two patients had had asbestos contact, thereby establishing the pathologic entity of mesothelioma and its causal association with asbestos exposure. Particularly noteworthy is the fact that of the first 33 patients described, 22 had only an indirect residential exposure.

RISK OF ASBESTOS-RELATED MALIGNANCY

By 1960, the risk of interstitial lung fibrosis, lung cancer, and mesothelioma after asbestos exposure was established. However, the full scope of the problem was not yet recognized. Although *primary* asbestos workers, including miners and textile workers, were known to be at risk, Wagner's original paper in 1960 had also suggested the possibility of a bystander risk.[26] Many of Wagner's patients lived within a half mile of an asbestos mine or mill but had not worked with asbestos directly. In 1964, Selikoff and colleagues, observing that asbestos fibers did not "respect job classifications," predicted that those who worked directly with asbestos products (*i.e., secondary* exposure) and those in the vicinity where asbestos was being used (*i.e., tertiary* exposure) would be at risk.[10] Although the ratio of peritoneal to pleural mesotheliomas in heavily exposed asbestos workers is approximately 3:2, the usual ratio of 2:5 observed in most large series is probably because of the larger number of transiently exposed individuals.

Mesotheliomas developing in wives and children of asbestos workers prompted studies that showed significant asbestos levels in the homes of some asbestos workers.[27] Presumably, asbestos was brought into the home on hair and on clothing, which went into the family laundry. Asbestos workers were required to shower and change clothing before leaving work only after 1972, when industrial standards were legislated. Up to 33% of the household contacts of asbestos workers had findings characteristic of asbestos exposure on chest x-ray films.[11] Asbestos-related neoplasms have arisen in three or more members of some families, suggesting the possibility of a genetic predisposition.[28,29] The risk of mesothelioma in asbestos workers is 8% to 13% and approximately 1% in household contacts of asbestos workers.[11] Because asbestos workers had an average of three to four family members, the total risk for household exposure may be as high as 4% per family. Thus, up to 33% of mesothelioma cases may occur in family members of asbestos workers. The risk of mesothelioma in persons residing within a half mile of asbestos mines and mills has not been quantitated.

Asbestos rarely has been implicated as the cause of mesotheliomas in children younger than 20 years. Many patients between the ages of 20 and 40 report exposure during childhood, frequently to an occupationally exposed parent or by attending an elementary or high school cited for high levels.[30–33] Mesothelioma can develop 20 years or less after the first exposure, but the peak incidence occurs after 35 to 45 years. The cumulative lifetime risk of developing mesothelioma rises as a constant multiplied by the third or fourth power of years since first exposure.[34–35] Although not inherently more susceptible to carcinogenesis, younger persons survive long enough to have a high cumulative lifetime risk. Dose and duration of exposure appear to be linearly related to risk.[35]

ASBESTOS LEGISLATION

When the association of asbestos exposure and pulmonary fibrosis was established in 1930, Great Britain enacted legislation limiting industrial asbestos exposure. By 1970, the scope of the asbestos problem had been broadly defined. That same year in the United States, the Occupational Safety and Health Act (OSHA) and the Clean Air Act limiting the levels of asbestos exposure in the workplace were enacted. The initially acceptable standard, an average of 12 fibers, >5 μm long, per milliliter of air during 8 hours, was decreased to 5 such fibers in 1971, 2 in 1976, and is currently 0.2. However, the current U.S. standard ignores fibers of <5 μm long, which constitute the bulk of asbestos dust in the air. When levels exceed permissible limits, respirators, protective clothing, and shower and changing facilities become mandatory. Cases of mesothelioma have developed after relatively brief or low-level exposures, and many investigators believe that there may be no threshold level below which asbestos exposure is safe on which to base workplace standards.

Because mesothelioma is not currently curable, screening asbestos workers for mesothelioma is not considered cost effective.[36] Clinicians considering the diagnosis of malignant mesothelioma should take a detailed exposure history, emphasizing the interval from 20 to 50 years before diagnosis and including possible household exposure. Brief exposures may be long forgotten. The patient must be promptly informed of the diagnosis and its cause, because the statute of limitations for workman's compensation can be as short as 30 days.[37]

ETIOLOGY

ASBESTOS-RELATED CARCINOGENESIS

Intratracheal or intrapleural asbestos readily induces lung cancer and mesotheliomas in laboratory animals.[38–43] About 67% of the daily dose of inhaled asbestos is expectorated or swallowed. Thus, most inhaled asbestos is excreted in the feces.[7,8] Of the remaining 33%, which initially lodges in the distal airways, only 25% remains after 1 month. Asbestos can be cleared from the tracheal-bronchial tree by ciliary action in the trachea, ingestion by macrophages, or penetration through the endothelial lining into the interstitial tissue.[7,8] Short fibers are cleared more readily than long fibers. Fibers that remain preferentially accumulate in the lower third of the lungs adjacent to the visceral pleura.

Carcinogenesis appears to be dependent on physical rather than chemical properties of asbestos.[44–46] The ratio of length to width of the fiber is critical in the development of tumors in laboratory animals.[47] Thick fibers are deposited in the upper respiratory tract and are cleared efficiently, but thin fibers are carried into the terminal airways.[46] Chrysotile, with a relatively large cross-sectional diameter because of its serpentine configuration, tends to be deposited more proximally than the needle-like amphiboles.[8,46] Similar fibers, such as fiberglass or aluminum oxide, are potent carcinogens in laboratory animals.[45] Because amphibole asbestos is virtually indestructible, once in situ, "exposure" continues for the remainder of the patient's lifetime. In contrast, serpentine asbestos can be degraded gradually. These properties may partially explain the observation that amphibole asbestos (crocidolite and amosite) are considerably more potent carcinogens than the serpentine chrysotile.[48–50]

Asbestos, a poor mutagen, can produce chromosomal abnormalities.[51] Asbestos induces mesothelial proliferation in vitro, but malignant transformation has not been demonstrated. Asbestos, particularly chrysotile, can be cytotoxic, presumably because magnesium ions in fibers interact with the plasmalemma and damage cell lysosomal membranes.[51] (Neoplasms, however, cannot arise from cells which are killed directly). Asbestos activates complement by the alternative pathway, which results in leukocyte accumulation and accelerates collagen and reticulin production in tissue culture.[8] The fibers effectively adsorb and transport carcinogens (*e.g.*, in cigarette smoke) into endothelial cells. The alveolar macrophage, which phagocytizes asbestos, may transform polycyclic hydrocarbons into active carcinogens, or incomplete engulfment of fibers may cause lysosomal liberation of oxygen-free radicals. Although asbestos is believed to promote lung cancer, its action in mesothelioma is unknown.[8] Asbestos-induced epithelial neoplasia in hamster trachea organ cultures can be inhibited in vitro by retinal methyl ethers.[52]

NON-ASBESTOS-ASSOCIATED MESOTHELIOMAS

Asbestos does not appear to cause benign mesotheliomas of any site. In contrast, asbestos contact is documented in perhaps 50% to 67% of patients with malignant pleural mesothelioma. Although one series exists with no reported exposure, up to 90% of patients report prior contact in series from coastal areas with shipping industries in the United States and England or from South African and Canadian mining areas.[26,30,48,53] Some patients with no history of asbestos contact may have had a long-forgotten or cryptic exposure. The findings of 100 to 500 asbestos bodies per 1 g of lung tissue in urban residents at autopsy suggest that incidental asbestos contact is common.[54–58] Asbestos or ferruginous bodies consist of a hemosiderin and glycoprotein-coated fiber core, usually asbestos in human lungs. On the other hand, some mesothelioma patients with no known asbestos contact have no asbestos bodies on careful examination of lung tissue taken at autopsy, supporting a lack of occult exposure. There is no evidence that smoking affects the risk of developing mesothelioma.

Testicular and epididymal mesotheliomas in the laboratory are induced by hydroxyamic acid derivatives, nitrosamines, and fibers with similar length to width ratios, such as fiberglass.[44,45,59,60] About 25 published cases of pleural and peritoneal mesothelioma have developed after radiation exposure, usually from treatment of a prior malignancy.[61,62] In two patients, mesothelioma developed adjacent to deposits of thorium dioxide (thorotrast) still visible on chest x-ray films after extravasation during diagnostic procedures years earlier.[63,64] In reported cases, a median of 16 years (range, 7–36 years) has elapsed between irradiation and detection of mesothelioma. A high incidence of mesothelioma (22 per 10,000 persons of age > 25) observed in the Anatoli region of Turkey has been attributed to zeolite, a silicate ubiquitous in the soil and sometimes sprayed onto homes.[65–68] Other conditions associated anecdotally with the development of mesothelioma have been recurrent diverticulosis, tuberculosis, beryllium exposure, and chemical and lipoid aspiration pneumonia.[69,70]

LOCALIZED MESOTHELIOMA

Localized malignant sarcomatous mesotheliomas have rarely been described. Benign solitary fibrous tumors of the pleura are approximately a third as common as diffuse malignant mesotheliomas.[71,72] Other anatomical locations in which benign epithelial mesotheliomas have risen are the peritoneal cavity, the tunica vaginalis testis, and the atrioventricular node.[73–76] Many pathologists believe that benign mesotheliomas arise from subsurface connective tissue, rather than from the mesothelial lining. Thus they have been called submesothelial fibromas, localized fibrous mesothelioma, or solitary fibrous tumor of the pleura.[72,77,78] Benign mesotheliomas are most common in patients aged 40 to 70 years old. Up to 35% have been associated with hypertrophic pulmonary osteoarthropathy (particularly lesions > 10 cm) and 4% with hypoglycemia. Benign mesotheliomas range from 1 to 36 cm in diameter (Figs. 41-1 and 41-2). Many were pedunculated, and 80% arise from the visceral pleura. Associated effusions can be serosanguineous. (If the pathologic findings are ambiguous, biopsy of a clinically uninvolved area of pleura may document diffuse malignant disease.) Although usually cured if completely resected, there have been recur-

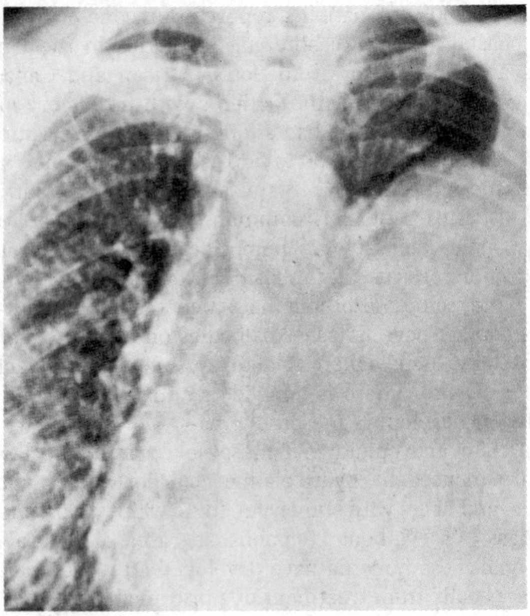

FIG. 41-1. Radiographic appearance of large benign mesothelioma. (Martini N, McCormack PM, Bains MS, et al: Pleural mesothelioma. Ann Thorac Surg 43:113, 1987)

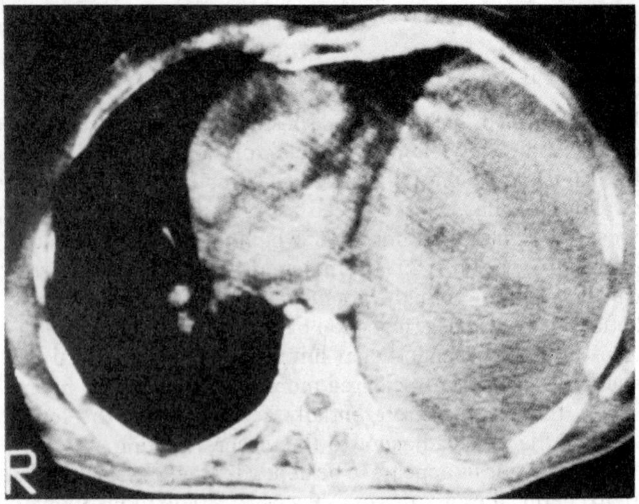

FIG. 41-2. Computed tomographic appearance of the benign mesothelioma depicted in Figure 41-1. (Martini N, McCormack PM, Bains MS, et al: Pleural mesothelioma. Ann Thorac Surg 43:113, 1987)

rences after several decades.[79,80] Although histologically benign, 12% of the patients die of extensive local tumor.[72,77,81] A few patients have recalled an asbestos exposure, probably not exceeding the incidence of exposure in the general population.

DIFFUSE MALIGNANT MESOTHELIOMA

PLEURAL MESOTHELIOMA

Mesothelioma characteristically develops in men 50 to 80 years old (median, 60 years).[81] The ratio of men to women is 2.5:1, presumably reflecting workplace exposure. At the time patients first seek medical attention for dyspnea, nonpleuritic chest wall pain, or both, most will have a large freely movable unilateral pleural effusion on chest x-ray films (Fig. 41-3).[30,82] Approximately 60% arise on the right, and fewer than 5% of patients present with bilateral involvement. Some patients are asymptomatic with an effusion that is found on chest x-ray films taken for another indication.

Pleural plaques or interstitial fibrosis is visible on the chest x-ray films in only about 20% of patients with pleural mesothelioma, despite a history of asbestos contact in 50% to 70%. However, calcifications can be documented on CT scans in almost 50% and at autopsy in up to 87% (Fig. 41-4).[81,83] Lung volume loss can frequently be seen on CT scan, even with early disease.[83,85–88] With more advanced disease, scoliosis with contracture of the ipsilateral hemithorax becomes apparent on x-ray films.

Shortness of breath and chest pain can be controlled initially by repeated thoracenteses and minor narcotics, but pleural fluid eventually becomes loculated or disappears as the tumor obliterates the pleural space.[89] Pleurodesis is usually unsuccessful and renders any subsequent surgical resection technically difficult. With advanced disease, dyspnea increases out of proportion to chest x-ray or pulmonary function values. Because hypoxia results from shunting of blood through a poorly aerated lung, therapeutic oxygen is of little use.

Mesothelioma tends to be locally invasive. Painful chest wall masses, which develop in about 10% of patients with

FIG. 41-3. Nodular left-sided diffuse pleural mesothelioma. (Martini N, McCormack PM, Bains MS, et al: Pleural mesothelioma. Ann Thorac Surg 43:113, 1987)

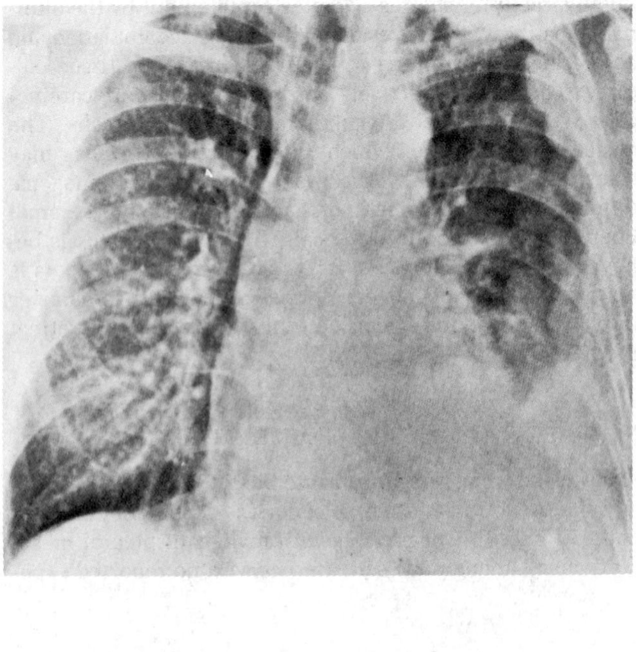

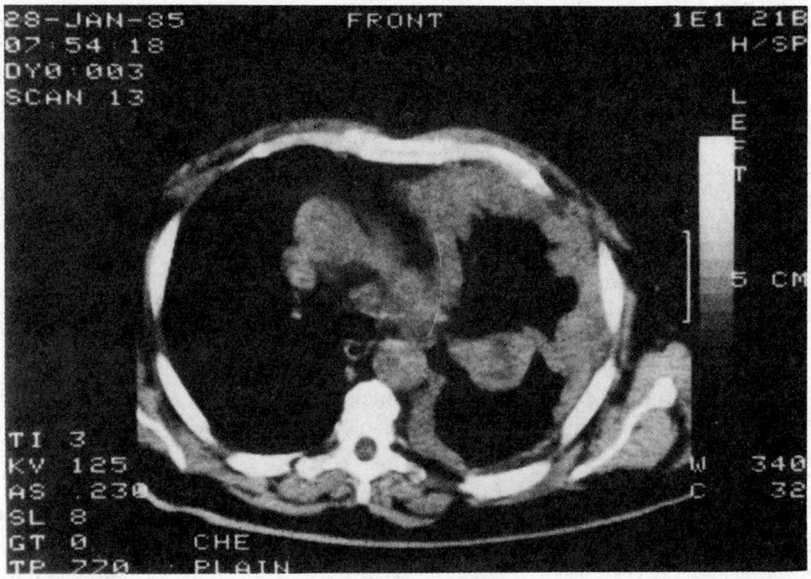

FIG. 41-4. Computed tomographic appearance of diffuse pleural mesothelioma revealing fissural extension, thickened pleura, and encasement of lung. (DaValle MJ, Faber LP, Kittle CF, et al: Extrapleural pneumonectomy for diffuse, malignant mesothelioma. Ann Thorac Surg 42:612, 1986)

thoracentesis, chest tube drainage, or thoracotomy tracts, can sometimes be managed with radiotherapy.[81,89,90] Direct extension to ribs, esophagus, vertebrae, nerves, and the superior vena cava causes pain, dysphagia, cord compression, bracheal plexopathy, Horner's syndrome, or superior vena caval syndromes, respectively.[30] Daily fevers with no documented source of infection are common complications. Fever is usually accompanied by significant weight loss, poor performance status, and early death. Clotting abnormalities are common. Disseminated intravascular coagulation, massive thromboses of extremities, thrombophlebitis with and without pulmonary emboli, and Coombs'-positive hemolytic anemia have all been observed in up to 20% of patients with peritoneal mesothelioma.[62] In the immediate perioperative period in patients with advanced or uncontrolled tumor, these complications have resulted in a significant morbidity and mortality.

After a median of 6 to 18 months in various series (range, weeks to 16 years), patients die, usually of respiratory failure. Small bowel obstruction from direct extension through the diaphragm develops in about 33%. A few patients die of pericardial or myocardial involvement.[30] Prognostic variables associated with significantly prolonged survival include age less than 55 or 65 years; 0–1 performance status, epithelial histology, lack of chest pain at diagnosis, and therapy with pleuropneumonectomy and chemotherapy.[91,92]

PERITONEAL MESOTHELIOMA

Patients with peritoneal mesothelioma present with ascites, pain, or an abdominal mass or some combination of the three.[31,53,62,93] The tumor often remains confined to the abdomen until late in the course and even then is more likely to spread to one or both pleural cavities than to disseminate widely. Chest x-ray films reveal pleural plaques in about 50% of patients with peritoneal primaries.[83] The median survival of untreated patients in most series is short, 4 to 12 months, although a rare, well-differentiated papillary variant found in younger women and a syndrome of recurrent intraperitoneal mesothelial cysts have both been associated with prolonged survival.[94–97]

MESOTHELIOMA OF THE TUNICA VAGINALIS

About half of the more recently reported cases developed after an asbestos exposure. Patients present with a hydrocoel or "hernia," and the diagnosis is established at the time of surgery. There may be diffuse involvement or lymph node involvement in the abdomen at the time of diagnosis. Mesotheliomas arising in the tunica vaginalis testes appear to have a more indolent disease course.[73]

PATHOLOGY

Because mesotheliomas develop in tissues of mesodermal embryologic origin, they are generally classified as soft tissue sarcomas.[98,100] Initial misdiagnosis is common, and pathologic opinion appears particularly diverse if litigation is involved. Asbestos exposure should not be used in the diagnosis of mesothelioma, given the 50% of patients with no known exposure and the common development of other neoplasms in asbestos workers.

Discrete nodules and plaques of firm, grayish tumor visible early in the disease eventually coalesce, obliterating the parietal and visceral surfaces and forming a rind as thick as 5 cm. Although only superficially invading the lung, mesothelioma encases and constricts the lung. Extension into major fissures and invasion of the chest wall, pericardium, and diaphragm occur relatively early.[43,101,102] At autopsy, thoracic regional nodes are involved in up to 70% of cases, with occasional extension to cervical nodes.[101] Often small, clinically unsuspected, hematogeneous metastases are evident in liver, lung, and less commonly, in kidney, adrenal, and bone.[89,101] Without careful postmortem examination, hematogeneous metastases may be missed.

Biopsy, pleurectomy, or pneumonectomy specimens should be extensively sampled. Fixation in neutral buffered formalin should be instituted promptly. A small piece should be fixed in glutaraldehyde for electron microscopy. Histologically, malignant mesothelioma may be epithelial, sarcomatoid, or mixed.[43,101,103,104] Fifty percent to 60% are epithelial, appearing tubular, papillary, solid, or vacuolated. Tumor cells of the sarcomatoid variant are ovoid to spindle shaped, with cellularity and hyperchromatism similar to that of fibrosarcomas. In the mixed type, both epithelial and sarcomatoid patterns are present, although extensive sampling may be required to demonstrate the minor component. A biphasic pattern is virtually pathognomonic of malignant mesothelioma.

DIAGNOSIS

Cytologic evaluation, needle biopsies, and sections from cell blocks on pleural or ascitic fluids provide documentation of malignancy but usually do not distinguish adenocarcinoma from mesothelioma. Electron microscopy of either needle-biopsy or cytocentrifuge specimens from pleural fluid may establish the mesothelial origin of the malignant tumor. Because the risk of lung cancer in smokers with an asbestos exposure exceeds that of mesothelioma by 5 : 2, sputum cytologic and bronchoscopic examinations may document a bronchogenic adenocarcinoma.[11] Thoracoscopy or peritonoscopy-directed biopsies may provide sufficient tissue for diagnosis. Generally, a generous open pleural biopsy obtained at the time of careful surgical inspection and exploration is required to establish the diagnosis. If possible, a sample of uninvaded lung should be obtained for counting of asbestos fibers.[56,105] Because such a thoracotomy may make a subsequent surgical resection technically difficult, the procedure should be done by a surgeon prepared to do definitive surgical resection.

DIFFERENTIAL DIAGNOSIS

Other malignant tumors or benign inflammatory and reactive processes producing mesothelial hyperplasia may mimic mesothelioma.[43,103] Repeated cytologic examination or biopsy may be required for an accurate diagnosis. Benign processes do not invade normal tissues and lack cytologic atypia and hyperchromatism. Although mesothelioma is uncommon, adenocarcinomas from primary breast, ovary, stomach, kidney, or prostate cancers frequently metastasize to the pleura and are often extremely difficult to distinguish cytologically and histologically from the epithelial variant of mesothelioma. Pseudomesothelioma, metastatic adenocarcinoma with extensive pleural involvement, may grossly mimic mesothelioma.[106] The sarcomatoid variant of mesothelioma must be distinguished from other primary sarcomas, such as fibrosarcoma, malignant fibrous histiocytoma, malignant schwannoma, and hemangiopericytoma. Synovial sarcoma and carcinosarcomas may histologically resemble the mixed pattern of a diffuse mesothelioma, but they are usually distinguished grossly because they present as localized masses in the lung.

Autopsy, a valuable diagnostic aid in some cases, requires skilled performance and experienced interpretation to exclude other occult primary carcinomas. Advanced malignant mesothelioma tends to form peripheral visceral masses, mimicking primary carcinomas.[43,101,107] Asbestos fiber counts and postmortem examinations may have legal and epidemiologic value.

Histochemical Methods

Two of the three procedures used to detect mucopolysaccharides are particularly helpful. The periodic acid-Schiff stain (PAS), used before and after diastase (D) digestion, is the single most reliable histochemical method available.[43,101,103,107] Strongly PAS-D-positive *neutral* mucopolysaccharides in intracellular secretory and intra-acinar vacuoles occur in most adenocarcinomas; the reaction effectively excludes a diagnosis of mesothelioma. Appropriate controls for D activity and the distinction of vacuoles from stained stroma and other structures are essential. Alcian blue at pH 2.5 and colloidal-iron stain detect acidic mucopolysaccharides in adenocarcinomas and mesothelioma.[101,103,107] Removal of hyaluronic acid in intracellular and secretory vacuoles by digestion with hyaluronidase is characteristic of mesothelioma, but stromal hyaluronic acid is nonspecifically characteristic of many tumors. Myer's mucicarmine method, which stains weakly acidic mucopolysaccharides pink or red, is not fully reliable because mesotheliomas may stain strongly only in some laboratories. Under most staining conditions, intracellular and intercellular secretory vacuoles stain weakly or not at all in mesotheliomas but strongly in many adenocarcinomas.

Immunohistochemistry

Immunoperoxidase stains may be effectively applied to formalin-fixed, paraffin-embedded tumor tissue. In most mesotheliomas, immunoperoxidase detection, using monoclonal antibodies against keratin proteins, is strongly reactive, with diffuse cytoplasmic staining, perinuclear accentuation with ring formation, and staining of the tumor cell periphery.[108–111] Both epithelial and spindle-shaped tumor cells of mixed and sarcomatoid variants are often stained, reflecting the transitional patterns of differentiation observed on electron microscopy.[112] Staining of adenocarcinoma cells is usually sparse, with the periphery of the tumor cell more prominent than the perinuclear area. However, breast cancer may stain strongly for keratin. Immunoperoxidase staining for carcinoembryonic antigen (CEA) is usually weak or absent in mesotheliomas and in renal, prostate, and some ovarian and endometrial carcinomas, but it is moderate to strong in most other adenocarcinomas.[108,109]

Electron Microscopy

Cells of the epithelial variant are polygonal with many long, slender, branching surface microvilli, desmosomes, abundant tonofilaments, and intracellular lumen formation.[112,113]

TABLE 41-1. Staging

I	Within the "capsule" of the parietal pleura: ipsilateral pleura, lung, pericardium, diaphragm.
II	Invading chest wall or mediastinum: esophagus, heart, opposite pleura. + Lymph nodes within the chest.
III	Through diaphragm to peritoneum. Opposite pleura. + Lymph nodes outside the chest.
IV	Distant blood-borne metastases.

Butchart EG, Ashcroft T, Barnsley WC et al: Pleuropneumonectomy in the management of diffuse malignant mesothelioma of the pleura: Experience with 29 patients. Thorax 31:15, 1976.

Adenocarcinomas of the lung, breast, and upper gastrointestinal tract have short, stubby surface microvilli, fewer tonofilaments, and microvillous rootlets or lamellar bodies.[114,115] Ovary and endometrial carcinomas lack intracytoplasmic lumens, have few tonofilaments, and may have features of intestinal metaplasia (*e.g.*, abundant mucin droplets, numerous cilia, and dense core granules).[114,115]

Sarcomatoid cells, with elongated nuclei and abundant rough endoplasmic reticulum, are separated by matrix containing collagen fibers. Stromal cells appear spindle or ovoid with both sarcomatoid and epithelial features, characteristic of the biphasic nature of mesothelioma.[112,113]

STAGING

Butchart and others have proposed various staging systems for malignant mesothelioma (Table 41-1), but none predict survival with statistical significance.[116] A CT scan of the primary tumor to assess the extent of disease is indicated if treatment is contemplated.[83] Although brain, bone, and liver metastases or extension into other serosal surfaces is present in more than half of patients at autopsy, they are uncommon at presentation, and extensive baseline evaluation is not warranted without symptoms or laboratory abnormalities. Pulmonary function tests may document restrictive lung disease resulting from encasement of the lung and assess the potential tolerance for pneumonectomy. Obstructive spirometric changes are unrelated to mesothelioma or asbestosis.[117] If the histologic results are equivocal, additional diagnostic studies may identify an occult primary adenocarcinoma or a tumor in a location rarely involved by malignant mesothelioma.[101,103,107,118] A markedly elevated serum CEA suggests a diagnosis other than mesothelioma.

SURGICAL MANAGEMENT

DIAGNOSTIC SURGERY

It is sometimes difficult to obtain an accurate histologic confirmation of mesothelioma from pleural fluid cytology or needle biopsy specimens, but the diagnosis of mesothelioma has such a poor prognosis that an unequivocal tissue diagnosis is mandatory. This usually requires surgical intervention, either a thoracoscopy or thoracotomy, despite the risk of seeding the biopsy site or surgical scar with tumor.[119] For patients who are not candidates for radical surgery, thoracoscopy usually obtains sufficient tissue for histochemical analysis. If preoperative studies suggest Stage I mesothelioma in a good-risk patient with asbestos exposure, most surgeons combine the diagnostic and therapeutic surgical interventions in one stage.[120] Generous biopsies can be performed at the inception of the exploration, using frozen sections to differentiate mesothelioma from adenocarcinoma. Bronchoscopy should be performed in all patients suspected of mesothelioma to rule out endobroncheal disease, which is rare in mesothelioma.[121]

The role of mediastinoscopy in patients with suspected mesothelioma is undefined. Some surgeons believe it is unnecessary because nodes can be removed with the lung. Other surgeons believe that, because positive nodes indicate Stage III disease, surgery would be contraindicated. Nevertheless, if radical extrapleural pneumonectomy is contemplated, mediastinoscopy is recommended, because 20% of patients with mesothelioma have mediastinal lymph node involvement.[121]

PHILOSOPHY OF SURGICAL INTERVENTION

Some physicians advocate supportive care alone after definitive biopsy because reported cures with any treatment remain anecdotal. Others feel strongly that these patients should be referred to institutions with research programs.

Radical Surgery

The staging of mesothelioma has been inconsistent. Nevertheless, it is clear that radical surgery should be entertained in patients who have Stage I disease, defined by Butchart as a tumor confined within the capsule of the parietal pleura, involving only the ipsilateral lung, pericardium, and diaphragm (see Table 41-1).[116] As stated by Ginsberg, there are different categories of Stage I disease, which may include a very diffuse process without mediastinal or chest wall invasion or a very early tumor associated with pleural effusion.[122] Only Stage I disease is associated with long-term survival. To clarify which types of Stage I disease are associated with long-term survival and respond to radical surgery, further classification is necessary. Cases in which tumor extends beyond the confines of the parietal pleural capsule, with invasion of neighboring structures, are probably not amenable to radical surgery because of significant amounts of residual tumor.

Palliative Surgery

Diffuse malignant mesothelioma is usually associated with chest wall pain and recurrent effusions.[123] More than half of patients will present with large pleural effusions causing dyspnea. Pleurectomy has been associated with the resolution of recurrent effusions in 88% of patients although the usual management techniques have not been scrutinized in this disease (see Chapter 62). Surgery itself probably has no role in the palliation of the pain associated with chest wall invasion. The pain is better treated with non-narcotic analgesics, anti-inflammatory agents, or opiates.[124]

PREOPERATIVE EVALUATION

Any patient being considered for surgical therapy must be able to withstand pneumonectomy and prolonged anesthesia. Cardiac status should be screened by ECG, and the patient questioned for signs of acquired heart disease that may need further noninvasive investigation. Adequate pulmonary reserve is crucial, and pulmonary function tests should be performed in all cases. An FEV_1 greater than 2 liters per second is desirable; if the FEV_1 is less than 2 liters per second, quantitative ventilation-perfusion scanning should be performed to investigate whether residual FEV_1 following pneumonectomy will be greater than or equal to 1 liter per second. As with primary lung cancer, good-risk patients usually have good nutritional status. Although not agreed upon, some surgeons believe that age greater than 65 years is a contraindication to surgery.[120]

SURGICAL TECHNIQUES

Benign Pleural Mesothelioma

Benign pleural mesotheliomas usually have a sharp separation between tumor and compressed lung, and resection can be performed without pulmonary resection.

Malignant Pleural Mesothelioma

PLEURECTOMY. Pleurectomy has been strongly advocated by the Memorial Sloan-Kettering Cancer Center (MSKCC) group.[121] The procedure is necessarily palliative, because gross tumor is left behind in most instances. DaValle uses pleurectomy in patients with minimal invasion of the visceral pleura (free pleura space without tissue invasion) for attempted cure.[120] Extrapleural dissection of the parietal pleura is begun after a generous posteriorlateral thoracotomy. The pleura is stripped from the apex of the lung to the diaphragm, along with the pericardium, as necessary. Most of the mediastinum and chest wall pleura can be removed, but the diaphragmatic pleura usually cannot be completely resected. Hemostasis is controlled as the procedure is performed, and blood replacement is frequently necessary. Two large intercostal catheters are used to drain blood and to manage peripheral bronchopleural fistulae. Large fistulae are suture-ligated to allow maximum expansion of the underlying lung with underwater seal drainage. Operative mortality is low (1%), but complications include bronchopleural fistulae, hemorrhage, and subcutaneous emphysema.

EXTRAPLEURAL PNEUMONECTOMY. Extrapleural pneumonectomy is a more radical procedure, which includes en bloc removal of the parietal pleura, lung, pericardium, and diaphragm (Fig. 41-5). The approach can be either by posterolateral thoracotomy (in the sixth interspace) or thoracoabdominal incision (in the sixth or seventh interspace), with subdiaphragmatic blunt dissection of the peritoneum. The latter approach allows easier resection of the diaphragm and avoids the lower counter-thoracotomy incision needed if the posterolateral incision is used. Extrapleural dissection to the hilum, early entry into the pericardium retrosternally to accomplish intrapericardial pneumonectomy, and use of double-lumen anesthesia were described by DaValle.[120] Diaphragmatic resection is followed by reconstruction using dacron or gortex material to prevent abdominal content herniation. Right-sided pericardial resections are usually reconstructed to prevent cardiac herniation. Intercostal tube drainage after pneumonectomy is optional.

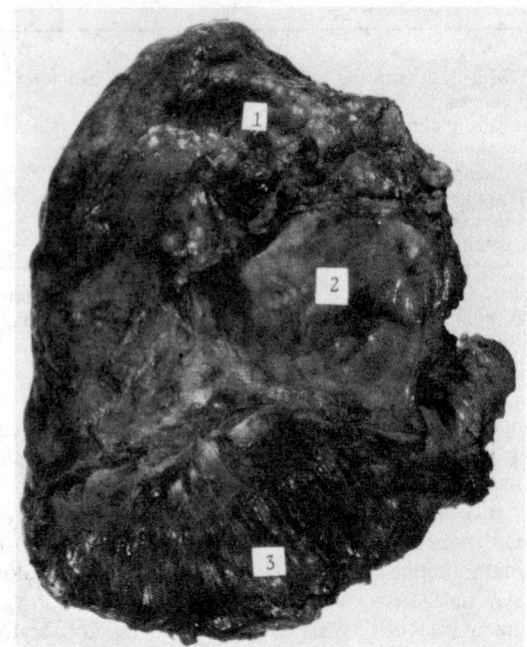

FIG. 41-5. Extrapleural pneumonectomy specimen. 1, lung and tumor; 2, pericardium; 3, diaphragm. (DaValle MJ, Faber LP, Kittle CF, et al: Extrapleural pneumonectomy for diffuse, malignant mesothelioma. Ann Thorac Surg 42:612, 1986)

Operative mortality, earlier reported to be as high as 27% to 31%, is now 5% to 9%.[125–127] Serious complications have been seen in 25% of the patients, including bronchopleural fistulae and empyema, vocal cord paralysis, chylothorax, arrhythmia, and respiratory insufficiency.[120]

Peritoneal Mesothelioma

Surgery is appropriate for treatment of bowel obstruction or for localized or slowly recurrent cystic mesothelial tumors.[125] Multimodality therapy has produced extended survival in selected patients with peritoneal mesothelioma.[31,62] (See below.)

RESULTS OF SURGICAL INTERVENTION

Palliation

There is poor documentation of the results of palliative surgical intervention for mesothelioma. Law controlled 22 of 25 recurrent effusions by pleurectomy and reported objective relief of pain and dyspnea lasting weeks to months.[124] The use of the surgery as a debulking procedure before further

TABLE 41-2. Survival After Extrapleural Pneumonectomy

No. of Patients	*% 2-Year Survival*	*Reference*
62	37	127
29	10	116
17	35	128
33	24	120

therapy must be viewed with skepticism until controlled trials confirm its efficacy.

Survival

Survival figures after pleurectomy or extrapleural pneumonectomy are difficult to interpret due to the different treatment philosophies and ways in which patients are selected for these operations. Thus, they should be considered separately. The MSKCC series, which combines pleurectomy for debulking with brachytherapy, reports a 2-year survival rate of 40%, with a median survival of 21 months.[121,129] Law, in a series of 28 patients, reports a 2-year survival rate of 32% after pleurectomy alone, with a median survival of 20 months.[124] The median survival for 23 patients after pleurectomy performed by DaValle was 11.2 months.[120] Lewis reports an older series of patients with a median survival of 6.7 months after pleurectomy.[126] Because the degree of tumor debulking was variable in the pleurectomy series, the potential impact of radical surgery is probably more accurately assessed by long-term survival after extrapleural pneumonectomy (Table 41-2). However, the 2-year survival data are probably not significantly different between pleurectomy and extrapleural pneumonectomy.

In the future, studies of surgery in mesothelioma will standardize the operative approach and establish a registry of cases. These are the goals of the Lung Cancer Study Group. This group plans to address the questions of morbidity, mortality, and long-term survival after standard extrapleural pneumonectomy, and it will also assess quality of life, rate of local recurrence, and influences of cell type and nodal status, thus establishing a more uniform staging system. With this data base, adjuvant therapies can be evaluated prospectively and results can be meaningfully interpreted.

RADIATION THERAPY

PLEURAL MESOTHELIOMA

Because of the variable presentation and natural history of pleural mesothelioma, the benefits of irradiation in controlling symptoms and extending survival are difficult to evaluate. This is illustrated by one of the earliest reports on the treatment of pleural mesotheliomas by radiotherapy.[130] Three patients were treated at the University of Iowa Hospital in the 1950s with orthovoltage irradiation. One patient treated postoperatively for residual gross disease with 2500 roentgen had a symptom-free interval of over 4 years before disease recurred in the mediastinum. One of two patients treated with 2000 roentgen had a transient symptomatic improvement. The patient who did not respond to external irradiation did, however, have a complete local response to installation of radioactive colloidal gold (^{198}Au) and died 2 years later of distant metastases. In other series one patient treated with radiotherapy for gross residual intrathoracic disease (and later metastases) survived 7.5 years after diagnosis, and another survived 8 years after biopsy and radiotherapy.[131,132]

In a more recent series, 116 patients without evidence of extrathoracic disease were seen at the Brompton and Royal Marsden Hospitals (London) from 1971 through 1980.[124] Sixty-four patients received no active treatment. Twelve patients, all with disease confined to one hemithorax, received 50 to 55 Gy of megavoltage irradiation (after surgery in 8); 28 patients had surgery alone; and 12 patients had chemotherapy (after surgery in 8). There were no significant differences in survival from the onset of symptoms among these groups, with 1-year survival rates of 75% to 100%, 2-year survivals of about 33%, and 4-year survivals of 0 to 11%. One patient had a dramatic response to radiotherapy and was alive without recurrence of effusions or symptoms 4 years after treatment. Two other radiotherapy recipients had control of recurrent pleural effusions until their demise. Thus, doses of radiation that would ordinarily be considered inadequate for the treatment of large malignant tumors occasionally have unexpected effectiveness in this disease. Treatment results must be interpreted keeping in mind the enormous variation in the behavior and growth rate of the disease from patient to patient and the bias in the selection of patients for treatment.

It is difficult to establish a dose-response curve for either palliation of symptoms or long-term local disease control. A series from the Joint Center for Radiation Therapy in Boston reviewed 29 treatment courses from 1968 to 1980.[90] The degree of relief of pain, dyspnea, and other symptoms correlated with radiation dose. Doses of 40 Gy or greater produced significant or complete symptomatic relief in 4 of 6 patients (compared with 1 of 23 for patients treated with a lower dose). In a series from the Institut Gustave-Roussy (Villejuif, France), 12 of 14 patients received doses of 35 to 50 Gy, given in 3.3-Gy fractions three times each week; some patients also underwent surgery or were given chemotherapy.[133] Four patients were alive at 1 to 41 months after radiotherapy; survival for the other 10 patients was 1 to 37 months (median, 15 months), with 4 of 10 with evidence of tumor regression in the treated areas. In a series from Thomas Jefferson Medical School in Philadelphia, 2 of 9 patients had local control 20 and 40 months, respectively, after treatment giving 60 Gy to the entire ipsilateral pleura, mediastinum, and involved areas of lung in three courses of 20 Gy over a total of 10 weeks with a split-course technique.[134] Currently employed radiotherapy techniques and doses can achieve responses in perhaps 67% of all patients with pleural mesothelioma, but most responses are temporary.

The histologic subtype of the tumor appears to have little influence on outcome in patients treated primarily with radiotherapy. In a MSKCC series of patients with disease confined to the hemithorax treated primarily with radiotherapy from 1939 to 1972, 15 patients with the epithelial subtype of mesothelioma had a median survival of 8 months, compared with a median survival of 9 months in 7 patients with the fibrosarcomatous subtype.[135] In comparison, when treated primarily with surgery, median survival appeared longer in the epithelial subtype (21 months) than in the fibrosarcomatous subtype (11 months).

The volume of disease likely substantially determines the effectiveness of radiotherapy. However, this factor is poorly described in most series. Voss and colleagues described 11 "intermediate" and 3 "late-stage" patients treated with doses of 40 to 60 Gy to an entire hemithorax and mediastinum.[136] In the intermediate stage, tumor extended to the mediastinum or pericardium, but the lung and hilar and mediastinal nodes were still uninvolved, and there was only insignificant and superficial involvement of the visceral pleura. No difference in survival was seen between these groups (average, 10 months; range 4–24 months for all patients).

Radiotherapy has also been used to prevent seeding of biopsy tracts and surgical wounds. In one series, a postoperative dose of 21 Gy delivered to the chest wall in 3 fractions over 48 hours with electrons prevented seeding of the thoracoscopy scar in 24 patients treated prophylactically, compared with seeding in 7 of 16 similar, untreated patients.[137]

The incidence of side-effects of radiotherapy depends on the dose given and the proportion of the treated organs in the target volume. Careful treatment planning and the use of mixed photon–electron schemes help reduce pulmonary toxicity. Several series have reported no acute or chronic complications from the use of radiotherapy alone.[90,133] Radiation pneumonitis is seen infrequently, perhaps due to short survival periods.[134] Transient radiation-induced hepatitis and esophagitis have been reported.

Radioactive colloids (^{198}Au or chromic phosphate-^{32}P) have been instilled into the pleural space in selected patients. Pleural effusions have disappeared for up to 3.5 years.[139] However, it is unclear how often these tumors respond. In one series, all six patients treated with ^{32}P were alive at 12 months or longer, but the exact lengths of survival were not described.[140] Neither agent is well suited for the treatment of bulky tumor masses. ^{198}Au, which has a half-life of 2.7 days, emits 90% of its energy as beta particles (electrons) of 0.96 MeV. These have a range in tissue of less than 5 mm. ^{32}P is a pure beta emitter with a half-life of 14.3 days. Maximum tissue penetration is only 8 mm, with most of the energy deposited in the first 1 to 2 mm. Both agents have been used in combination with surgery or other forms of radiotherapy, but their roles appear to be very limited.

RADIATION THERAPY TECHNIQUES

The radiation target volume in patients with disease limited to the hemithorax must be very large. Field borders should clear the first rib superiorly; extend below the diaphragmatic reflection of the pleura inferiorly, which is usually at about the inferior border of the 12th thoracic vertebra; extend laterally to clear the bony rib cage; and cross the midline by at least 2 cm to include the full width of the mediastinum. However, it is common to increase the field size to adequately cover masses extending through the chest wall or diaphragm or to treat the entire heart because of pericardial involvement. The placement of surgical clips in areas of residual gross disease at the time of thoracotomy can be of immeasurable help in designing appropriate treatment portals and also allow the use of boost fields with acceptable morbidity. CT scanning is valuable in delineating areas of gross disease, especially in patients not explored surgically, but it may miss small tumor nodules or be unable to distinguish surgical changes from tumor.[141,142]

Doses of 40 to 50 Gy should be given to the entire pleural surface (except for the reflections within the lung) and the mediastinal nodes. Other structures, such as the pericardium, should be included as clinically indicated. To do this without exceeding the tolerance of the lung, techniques for matching photon and electron beams have been described.[134,141,143] Briefly, blocks are placed in the photon beams to protect most of the lung volume, and then electron beams of adequate energy (usually 10–15 MeV) are used to treat the shielded portions of the pleura and chest wall. CT scans are usually employed to measure chest wall and patient thickness. Tissue compensators are used to achieve a more homogeneous dose. An example of this type of treatment field is shown in Figure 41-6, with a dose distribution for this plan found in Figure 41-7.

Many patients will be treated initially with combined-modality protocols or later with chemotherapy. Chemotherapy, especially doxorubicin, may potentiate the effects of radia-

FIG. 41-6. Anterior port film of photon field for treatment of pleural mesothelioma. A, chest wall–lung interface; B, lung block; C, liver block. (Kutcher GJ et al: Int J Radiat Oncol Biol Phys 13:1747–1752, 1987)

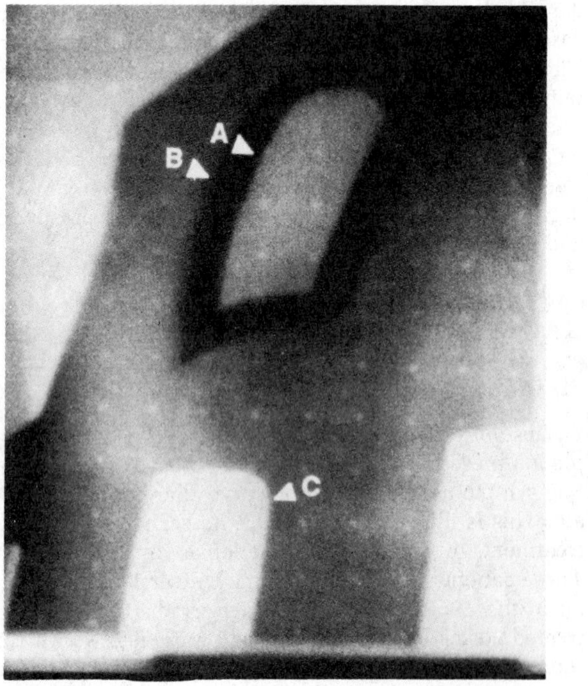

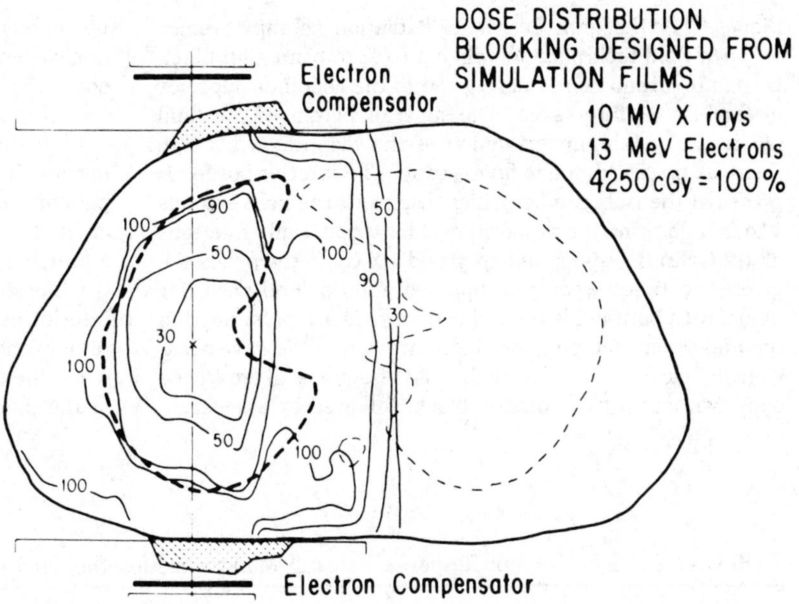

FIG. 41-7. Transverse dose distribution for treatment of pleural mesothelioma with photons and electrons. (Kutcher et al: Technique for external beam treatment for mesothelioma. Int J Radiat Oncol Biol Phys 13:1747–1752, 1987)

tion on normal tissues, even when the two modalities are separated by weeks or months. When fractions of 1.8 to 2 Gy are given five times weekly, reasonable precautions limit the dose to more than 50% of the heart to 40 Gy, the spinal cord to 45 Gy, the esophagus to 45 to 50 Gy, and the underlying lung to 20 Gy. Portions of the liver and other abdominal structures may be blocked, but care must be taken to not block areas of disease.

A single case of complete regression of disease lasting 78 months following fast-neutron therapy has been reported.[144] However, the depth-dose characteristics of current neutron machines is such that only very thin patients could be treated with a pure neutron technique. Neutrons or other particle therapies may therefore play some role in the treatment of pleural mesothelioma in the future, especially for boost doses.

PERITONEAL MESOTHELIOMA

Surgical and autopsy studies have shown that peritoneal mesothelioma involves all peritoneal surfaces, often with masses of 5 cm or more.[102,107] Sites of local invasion include the liver, abdominal wall, diaphragm, retroperitoneum, gastrointestinal tract, and bladder. Seeding of laparotomy scars and biopsy tracts has also been observed. The tumor is most often confined to the peritoneal cavity at the time of initial diagnosis and remains there for much or all of the subsequent clinical course.[62,107,145] Hence, effective local therapy may have a substantial impact on the survival of patients with this disease. Despite its use in the few reported long-term survivors of this disease, the role of radiation therapy remains unclear.

Intraperitoneal instillation of radioactive colloidal gold (^{198}Au) was first reported to improve the symptoms of peritoneal mesothelioma in 1955.[146] Nine other patients treated by the administration of colloidal ^{198}Au have been reported; their outcomes were summarized by Legha and Muggia.[147] Two of the nine were disease-free for 3.5 and 5 years, respectively. Four other patients were reported to have clinical improvement of symptoms, but two patients had no improvement. Rose and colleagues suggested that clinical improvement might be due to several effects, including death of free-floating malignant mesothelioma cells, production of fibrous tissue around tumor nodules and serosal surfaces, elimination of small tumor implants, and obliterative endarteritis of blood vessels of the serosal surface of peritoneum.[146] The concentration of radiocolloid is generally greatest in the pelvis and lateral gutters, but adhesions from prior surgery and tumor can cause adherence of loops of bowel that may result in inhomogeneous spread of the radiocolloid.[148,149] The major complication associated with intraperitoneal instillation of radiocolloids is small bowel obstruction, which occurs in 2% to 10% of patients with ovarian carcinoma treated with surgery and radiocolloid alone.[150,151] When external-beam irradiation is also given to the pelvis, as many as 33% of patients may develop bowel complications.[152,153]

Radiation Therapy Techniques

Neither ^{198}Au nor ^{32}P treatment gives a substantial dose to cells within grossly visible tumor masses. For example, the estimated dose from 20 mCi of ^{32}P is 180 Gy at 0.04 mm, but only 43 Gy at 1 mm and 17 Gy at 2 mm.[157] The distribution of a radiotracer or contrast material should be tested before the therapeutic administration of these agents.

Megavoltage external radiotherapy can deliver a homogeneous dose to the entire abdominal cavity and its contents. Several techniques have been described and used predominantly for the therapy of ovarian carcinoma.[158–161] The first report was the "moving-strip" technique, which has been shown to have higher morbidity than "open-field" techniques.[162] At the Joint Center for Radiation Therapy, we use an open-field technique in which a 67% transmission block is used to attenuate the dose given to the abdomen superior to the L5–S1 interspace. The superior border of the field clears the maximum excursion of the diaphragm by 1 to 2 cm, as observed under fluoroscopy. The inferior border is placed at the ischial tuberosities. Laterally, the field extends 1 to 2 cm beyond the properitoneal fat stripe. Daily fractions of 1.2 Gy in the upper abdomen and 1.8 Gy in the pelvis are given five times weekly to opposed anterior and posterior fields, with both fields treated daily. Doses are prescribed to the mid-separation point on the central axis. (We have occasionally treated patients with 1 Gy fractions given twice daily, without a transmission block, followed by a separate pelvic boost. This has been well-tolerated initially, but it is unclear whether it has any long-term advantages.) Total doses of 30 Gy in the upper abdomen and 45 Gy in the pelvis are given in 5 weeks. Full-thickness kidney blocks are added to both anterior and posterior fields at 18 Gy. Shielding of a portion of the liver after 20 to 27 Gy has been used in some patients in the past, but rarely now. When intraperitoneal chemotherapy is used, the transmission block is omitted and a uniform daily dose of 1.2 Gy is given to a total dose of 30 Gy. Blocks are also placed over a portion of the heart and the inferior pelvis lateral to the abdominal cavity to protect the femoral heads and soft tissue. Treatment breaks are given when the total leukocyte count drops to 1500 to 2000/mm³ or the platelet count drops below 75 to 100,000/mm³.

TABLE 41-3. Single-Agent Response Rates in Malignant Mesothelioma

Agent	*No. Evaluable*	*No. Responding*	*Response Rate (%)*	*References*
Anthracyclines				
Doxorubicin	164	29	18	163–175
Detorubicine	21	9	43	176
Alkylating Agents				
Cyclophosphamide	14	4	28	166,177–180
Mechlorethamine	6	2		147,149,181–184
Thiotepa	7	1		149,165,177,184,185
Melphalan	3	2		180,185
Procarbazine	6	2		163,186
Mitomycin C	12	2	17	187,188
Dacarbazine (DTIC)	4	1		166,189,190
Cisplatin	49	5	10	163,191–196
Dibromodulcitol	5	0		197–198
Nitrosoureas				
BCNU	2	0		199,200
Methyl-CCNU	3	0		201–203
ACNU	2	0		204
Streptozotocin	1	0		163
Vincas & Related Compounds				
Etoposide (VP-16)	8	0		205–207
Vindesine	37	1	3	208,209
Antimetabolites				
5-Fluorouracil	28	4	14	132,166,168,210
Methotrexate				
high-dose	9	4		211
standard	1	0		200
Baker's antifol	3	0		212
Dichloromethotrexate	1	0		213
5-Azacytidine	7	0		163,214,215
Bleomycin	6	1		171,213
Actinomycin D	3	0		69,188
Ara-C, high-dose	1	1		216
Miscellaneous				
Maytansine	5	0		198,213
Methyl-G	2	1		213
Glucosamine	2	0		166,184
Hydroxyurea	2	0		180,188
DDMP	2	0		217
Bruceantin	1	0		218
M-AMSA	19	1	5	219
Cyclolencine	7	2		171
AZQ	20	0	0	220

CHEMOTHERAPY

Defining reliable response rates to standard agents from the published data is difficult. Mesothelioma was rarely reported before 1960, when Wagner established the association of mesothelioma and asbestos exposure.[26] Over the next 2 decades, a few single-institution series of patients treated with various chemotherapy regimens appeared in the literature. Most of these mesotheliomas were not strictly measurable. Pleural thickening on chest x-ray films was frequently obscured by effusions, which are notoriously unreliable in determining responsiveness to therapy.

The wide availability of CT scanning, the increased frequency of the diagnosis of the disease, and the development of multi-institutional cooperative group trials allow a more systematic approach. Nevertheless, the reported response rate of mesothelioma to doxorubicin (Adriamycin) varies from 0 to 40% (Table 41-2).[165-175] Higher response rates are observed in studies from large cancer centers, to which are often referred younger, better performance status patients with less advanced disease. Intensive supportive care facilitates higher-dose treatment. In addition, relatively small, positive studies are reported promptly, but larger series with lower response rates may never be published. The early report of responses to 5-fluorouracil in two of three patients is a particularly good example.[166] Ten years later, a larger, negative study used approximately half of the dose rate of the positive study (400–600 versus 1000 mg/m^2 for 5 days). Thus, the response rate for an optimal dose remains unclear.

SINGLE-AGENT STUDIES

Data from single-agent studies are shown in Table 41-3. Response rates are included in the table when the number of evaluable patients exceeded 10. Doxorubicin and cyclophosphamide appear to have some activity against mesothelioma. Methotrexate with rescue, 5-azacytidine, and 5-flourouracil have also been reported to have single-agent activity. Cisplatin alone does not appear to be significantly active, with only 5 of 49 patients responding in several Phase II studies.

COMBINATION CHEMOTHERAPY

Response rates for doxorubicin- or cisplatin-containing regimens range from of 30% to 40% among 10 to 20 patients in single-institution series to 0 to 14% for cooperative group trials for the same combinations (Tables 41-4 and 41-5).[92,170,171,188,195,228,229] The response rates for doxorubicin-containing regimens shown in Table 41-4 and for non-doxorubicin-containing combinations in Table 41-5 do not differ significantly from the 18% response rate of single-agent doxorubicin (Table 41-3). A large intergroup randomized trial of doxorubicin and cyclophosphamide, with or without dacarbazine (DTIC), observed response rates of 7% in both arms.[229] This study accrued advanced-stage patients simultaneously with a second study of ipsilateral radiotherapy with or without doxorubicin for Stage I and II mesotheliomas. The response rates may be artificially low because patients with good prognoses were treated on a competing study. In another study, early peritoneal mesotheliomas were markedly more responsive to chemotherapy than advanced disease.[31]

Possible synergy between cisplatin and other agents has been seen in the treatment of other human primary cancers, such as testis and small cell lung cancers. A combination of cisplatin and mitomycin C was designed at Mt. Sinai Hospital based on in vitro sensitivity to the two agents when human malignant mesothelioma xenographs were serially transplanted in nude mice and tested against a series of single agents. At doses of 50 and 10 mg/m^2, respectively of cispla-

TABLE 41-4. Doxorubicin-containing Combinations

*Other Agents in Combination**	*No. Evaluable*	*No. Responding*	*Response Rate (%)*	*References*
VCR	6	0		167
DTIC	8	4		172,221
5-AZA	36	8	27	92,213,222
ACT-D	3	0		223
ICRF	1	1		224
DDP	29	7	29	225,226
CPA	6	1		163,188
CPA,VCR	15	5	33	163,167,237
CPA ± DTIC	81	6	7	228,229
CPA,DTIC,VCR	30	8	21	149,203,230
CPA,DTIC,VCR,ACT-D	5	1		180
CPA,MTX,VCR,VP-16	12	2	17	231
DTIC,VCR	4	0		202
High-dose MTX,VCR	5	3		188
Radiotherapy	10	8†		232
Other agents	66	7	11	170,171
Total	337	66	20%	

*CPA = cyclophosphamide; VCR = vincristine; ACT-D = actinomycin D; DTIC = dacarbazine; MTX = methotrexate; DDP = cisplatin; VP-16 = etoposide; 5-AZA = 5-azacytidine.

†Patients with "response or stable disease."

TABLE 41-5. Non-Doxorubicin-containing Combination Chemotherapy in Malignant Mesothelioma

Drug*	No. Responding	No. Evaluable	References
CPA + VCR	0	1	188
CPA + VCR + ACT-D	0	4	202
CPA + VCR + ACT-D + DTIC	1	14	149
CPA + VCR + 5-FU	0	2	184,235
CPA + VBL + 5-FU	2	9	236
CPA + VCR + 5-FU + MTX	4	7	169,174,186,237
DDP + CPA + MTX	1	9	213
DDP + 5-FU	0	12	213,238
DDP + VBL + BLEO	0	1	239
DDP + MIT C	10	32	226,233
DDP + High-dose MTX	4	6	211
VCR + High-dose MTX	6	9	240
5-FU + Methyl-CCNU	0	2	188,213
5-FU + VBL + BCNU + MTX	0	1	241
VBL + BLEO	0	2	163,188
Rubidizone + DTIC	0	23	242
Total	28 (21%)	134	

*CPA = cyclophosphamide; VCR = vincristine; ACT-D = actinomycin D; DTIC = dacarbazine; 5-FU = 5-fluorouracil; MTX = methotrexate; DDP = cisplatine; VBL = vinblastine; BLEO = bleomycin; MIT C = mitomycin C; BCNU = carmustine; CCNU = carmustine.

tin and mitomycin C, 4 of 12 patients responded.[233] Cisplatin analogues, carboplatin and iproplatin, tested in these cell lines, exhibited some activity that did not correlate totally with sensitivity to cisplatin.[234] The Cancer and Leukemia Group B Cooperative Group randomized patients with measurable mesothelioma to cisplatin and mitomycin C or to cisplatin and doxorubicin. The objective response rates (13%) were similar.[226]

INTRACAVITARY DELIVERY

An alternate strategy is intraperitoneal administration of chemotherapy. Delivery of high intra-abdominal concentrations of agents is intended to capitalize on a steep dose-response curve to enhance local control.[31,243–245] The major theoretical obstacle to this approach is the shallow depth of free-surface drug diffusion. Laboratory models document peeling of the tumor surface with repetitive treatment. In addition, substantial intravenous drug concentrations are obtained from peritoneal absorption of some drugs, such as cisplatin. The combination of free-surface diffusion and intracapillary drug flow may be more efficacious than intravenous treatment alone.

COMBINED-MODALITY THERAPY

Because surgery or radiotherapy alone has resulted in only a few anecdotal long-term mesothelioma survivors, intensive combined-modality approaches are being studied at several institutions.[31,246,247]

PLEURAL MESOTHELIOMA

Radiation therapy has been employed as an adjunct to surgery or as the sole treatment for many patients with pleural mesothelioma because of the tendency of this disease to spread beyond the limits of complete surgical resection. In a MSKCC report of 41 patients between 1976 and 1982, after as complete a parietal pleurectomy as possible, residual disease was still found on the diaphragm of patients (49%), the visceral pleura (51%), the mediastinum (49%), the chest wall (27%), and the lung (5%).[129] Seventy-eight percent of all explored patients had residual gross disease after surgery. Radical pleuropneumonectomy can remove further disease in some patients, but many patients have residual microscopic or gross tumor after even the most aggressive surgical resection.

The use of intraoperative brachytherapy to give a boost dose of radiation to residual areas of gross disease after surgical exploration has substantial theoretical appeal, because it can increase tumor kill while avoiding sensitive normal structures. This approach has been pioneered by Hilaris at MSKCC.[121,129] Forty-one patients were treated between 1976 and 1982 with aggressive surgical exploration, permanent ^{125}I implantation if the volume of residual disease was small (4 patients), or temporary ^{192}Ir implantation if disease was more diffuse (11 patients). Because 9 patients underwent complete resection of all gross disease, and thus no implant was attempted, a boost was possible in only 47% of patients who might have benefited from it. Seven patients also had installation of ^{32}P 5 to 7 days postoperatively. All patients then received 45 Gy in 4.5 weeks of external-beam irradiation to the entire hemithorax 4 to 6 weeks postoperatively. A mixed photon–electron technique was used to minimize the dose given to the lung parenchyma. Some patients also received chemotherapy. The median survival for all patients was 21 months (range, 6–32 months), with 1-year and 2-year survivals of 65% and 40%, respectively. Disease-free survival, however, was much lower, 44% at 1 year and 13% at 2 years. Isolated local failure was found in 7 patients (17%). Twenty-two patients had distant failure, accompanied by an unstated number of local recurrences. The local control rate was not analyzed by whether brachytherapy or ^{32}P was used or not. Four patients developed complications probably caused by radiotherapy (pneumonitis, pulmonary fibrosis, pericardial effusion, and esophagitis). In principle, intraoperative electron-beam or brachytherapy boosts may improve local control, but in practice, little advantage has yet been demonstrated.

It is unclear whether combining chemotherapy and radiotherapy in the treatment of pleural mesothelioma is more effective than radiotherapy or chemotherapy alone. One study of 10 patients employed doxorubicin (60 mg/m^2 given every 3 weeks), with a course of radiotherapy given with the first, third, fifth, and seventh doses.[138] Each course was 10 Gy in five fractions over 1 week. Despite the unorthodox fractionation scheme, one patient had an objective partial response for 8 months, and three patients had symptomatic improvements lasting 8 to 25 months. The longest response occurred in a patient with limited disease, as assessed by their radiologic staging system; however, fibrosis developed in the irradiated hemithorax without causing symptoms. One patient developed cardiac failure at 14 months, which may have been related to treatment.

Fourteen patients were treated at Mt. Sinai Medical School with both sequential and concurrent doxorubicin (15 mg/m^2) and low-dose radiotherapy (17–26 Gy).[92] One patient had a complete response lasting 68 months from treatment but then relapsed both locally and with bone metastases. Two patients had partial responses for 12 and 18 months, respectively, and 4 patients had stabilization or improvement of symptoms lasting 3 to 6 months. Survival from treatment was 29% at 1 year and 12% at 2 years. Three to 6 months were needed to assess the extent of the responses. Patients with the biphasic subtype and high performance status appeared to be more likely to respond than patients with other subtypes or those with poorer performance. Toxicity was limited to one patient who developed radiation pneumonitis and pericarditis. There is a randomized intergroup study (ECOG, RTOG, SECSG, and SWOG) that is attempting to examine the benefit of doxorubicin given *after* the completion of radiotherapy in patients with disease limited to the hemithorax.

At M.D. Anderson Hospital in Texas, 20 patients with mesothelioma were initially treated with cyclophosphamide, doxorubicin, and DTIC. Five who achieved a partial response underwent surgical resection. The patients were recently treated, and follow-up was short at the time of publication.[228]

In the Dana-Farber Cancer Institute and Joint Center for Radiation Therapy experience, only one of five patients with pleural mesothelioma treated with curative intent following pleurectomy was a long-term survivor. After surgery, she received 50.75 Gy to a limited thoracic field for treatment of residual disease, estimated to weigh less than 10 g. Two years after treatment, she developed an intrathoracic recurrence superior to this field, and was without disease 3 years later after further radiotherapy of 50 Gy.[90] The remaining four patients had larger tumor burdens after pleurectomy; despite the addition of chemotherapy and other radiotherapy modalities, all four died rapidly after progression or persistence of local disease. At the Dana-Farber Cancer Institute, selected patients have undergone pleuropneumonectomy. Postoperative chemotherapy was followed by external-beam radiotherapy to the mediastinum and chest wall. In a multivariate analysis, survival was significantly prolonged for patients who underwent pleuropneumonectomy and chemotherapy.[91]

PERITONEAL MESOTHELIOMA

The median survival in most series for peritoneal mesothelioma has been 8 to 12 months after diagnosis.[93,101,248] The rare forms of well-differentiated papillary peritoneal mesothelioma and cystic peritoneal mesothelioma are both associated with long survival, even without treatment. However, these patients always have readily apparent tumors by physical examinations or CT scans and may have considerable morbidity from tumor bulk.[94–97] In contrast, some of the patients treated with combined-modality therapy have no disease detectable by CT.

The first long-term survivors reported were among 12 patients treated at Memorial Sloan-Kettering Cancer Center from 1952 to 1970.[154,155] Four patients received whole-abdominal irradiation (1660–3050 cGy to upper abdomen and 3900–4600 cGy to pelvis) and intraperitoneal ^{32}P (10–15 mCi). Three of the four were given chemotherapy in addition. They survived 1, 9, 10, and 18+ years. At the time of the last report, the single survivor, who had originally presented with right supraclavicular adenopathy and diffuse peritoneal disease, had developed recurrent disease 16.5 years after treatment.[155] The other eight patients in this series were treated with various combinations of more limited radiotherapy and chemotherapy, and all rapidly died of their illness.[154]

Several groups have used systemic chemotherapy in addition to radiotherapy. Chahinian and colleagues described two patients treated with intravenous doxorubicin and low-dose limited-field radiotherapy.[92] Neither patient responded to treatment. On the other hand, one of four patients treated with surgery, radiotherapy, and chemotherapy had no tumor by follow-up CT scan six years after treatment.[247] One patient treated with surgery, radiotherapy, and intravenous cyclophosphamide, doxorubicin, and DTIC (both before and after radiotherapy) at the Dana Farber Cancer Institute and Joint Center for Radiation Therapy remains alive and well 9 years from the end of treatment. However, two other patients treated with surgery, whole abdominal irradiation (WAI), and different regimens of intravenous chemotherapy died soon after treatment.[31,62]

A second series of patients treated at the Dana Farber Cancer Institute and Joint Center for Radiation Therapy between 1982 and 1985 were initially evaluated by CT. The protocol surgeon was unwilling to attempt resection in 7 of

13 patients with bulky tumors. The remaining six patients underwent resection of all lesions > 1 cm and placement of either a Tenchkoff catheter or a Port-a-Cath intraperitoneal access device. Two of these six patients had received prior debulking surgery and intravenous chemotherapy. All six received doxorubicin (20–50 mg) and cisplatin (20–100 mg/m^2), separately administered intraperitoneally for a total of 8 to 12 treatments. At the time of the second laparotomies for removal of the access devices, all six patients had at least an objective 50% decrease in the size of the tumor. None of the seven patients who presented with inoperable tumor had more than a minimal response to chemotherapy. Chemotherapy was followed by whole-abdominal irradiation in five of six patients.[31,156] One patient did not receive radiation because of prior limited-field irradiation for Hodgkin's disease. Patients received 30 Gy to the upper abdomen and 30 to 46 Gy to the pelvis. Four of the six patients (including three who received irradiation) remain disease-free at 36, 48, 60, and 61 months after diagnosis.[31,156]

Toxicity from this intensive program was substantial. Nausea and vomiting and myelosuppression occurred transiently in all patients during irradiation. Life-threatening complications from intraperitoneal chemotherapy included *Salmonella* diarrhea, an intraperitoneal hemorrhage, allergic reaction to cisplatin, and *Staphylococcus aureus* peritonitis. One patient requires chronic intravenous hyperalimentation to correct malabsorption. With this single exception, toxicity was limited to the period of active treatment, with the remaining three patients having completely normal performance status. Thus, a substantial percentage of early-stage peritoneal mesotheliomas may respond to intensive combined-modality therapy.[31]

NEW TREATMENT PROTOCOLS

Treatment protocols for pleural mesothelioma should be regarded as investigational until prolonged survival of the treatment group or significant palliation can be documented. Because mesothelioma is now regarded as uniformly fatal, any significant percentage of disease-free survivors would obviate the need for randomized trials. In the interim, randomized trials of chemotherapeutic regimens are needed to define an optimal treatment. Any regimen with a substantial response rate could then be integrated into a multimodality program, introducing the possibility of extended palliation or cure of this lethal tumor.

REFERENCES

1. Hinds MW: Mesothelioma in the United States. Incidence in the 1970s. J Occup Med 20:469-471, 1978
2. Cusano MM, Young JL (eds): 55 years of cancer incidence in Connecticut: 1935–79. Bethesda, National Institutes of Health, 1986
3. Young JL, Percy CL, Asire AJ (eds): Surveillance, epidemiology and end results: Incidence and mortality data, 1973–1977. Bethesda, National Institutes of Health, 1981
4. Hogan MD, Hoel DG: Estimated cancer risk associated with occupational asbestos exposure. Risk Analysis 1:67–76, 1981
5. Irving KF, Alexander RG, Bavley H: Asbestos exposures in Massachusetts public schools. Am Ind Hyg Assoc J 41:270, 1980
6. Spooner, CM: Asbestos in schools—a public health problem. N Engl J Med 301:782, 1979
7. Craighead JE: Asbestos-associated disease. Arch Pathol Lab Med 206:544, 1982
8. Craighead JE, Mossman BT: The pathogenesis of asbestos-associated diseases. N Engl J Med 306:1446, 1982
9. Cramer DW, Welch WR, Scully RE et al: Ovarian cancer and talc: A case-control study. Cancer 50:372, 1982
10. Selikoff IJ, Churg J, Hammond EC: Asbestos exposure and neoplasia. JAMA 188:142, 1964
11. Selikoff IJ: Cancer risk of asbestos exposure. In Origins of Human Cancer, p 1765. Cold Springs Harbor, Cold Springs Harbor Laboratory, 1977
12. Selikoff IJ, Hammonds EC, Seidman H: Mortality experience of insulation workers in the United States and Canada, 1943–76. Ann NY Acad Sci 330:195–203, 1979
13. Selikoff IJ, Hammond EC, Seidman H: Latency of asbestos disease among insulation workers in the United States and Canada. Cancer 46:2736–2740, 1980
14. Walker AM, Loughlin JE, Freidlander ER et al: Projections of asbestos-related disease, 1980–2009. J Occup Med 25:409–425, 1983
15. Nicholson WJ, Perkel G, Selikoff IJ: Occupational exposure to asbestos: Population at risk and projected mortality, 1980–2030. Am J Ind Med 3:259–311, 1982
16. Lee DHK, Selikoff IJ: Historical background to the asbestos problem. Environ Res 18:300, 1979
17. Women Inspectors of Factories, Annual Report for 1898, p 170. London, Her Majesty's Stationery Office, 1899
18. Cooke WE: Pulmonary asbestosis. Br Med J 2:1024, 1927
19. Merewether ERA, Price CV: Report on Effects of Asbestos Dust in the Lungs and Dust Suppression in the Asbestos Industry. London, Her Majesty's Stationery Office, 1930
20. Gloyne SR: Two cases of squamous carcinoma of the lung occurring in asbestosis. Tubercle 17:5, 1935
21. Lynch KM, Smith WA: Pulmonary asbestosis: III. Carcinoma of lung in asbesto-silicosis. Am J Cancer 14:56, 1935
22. Merewether ERA: Annual Report of the Chief Inspector of Factories for the Year 1947. London, Her Majesty's Stationery Office, 1947
23. Doll R: Mortality from lung cancer in asbestos workers. Br J Ind Med 12:81, 1955
24. Robertson HE: Endothelioma of the pleura. Cancer Res 8:317, 1924
25. Stout AP, Murray MR: Localized pleural mesothelioma. Arch Pathol 34:951, 1942
26. Wagner JC, Sleggs EA, Marchand P: Diffuse pleural mesothelioma and asbestos exposure in the North Western Cape Province. Br J Ind Med 17:260, 1960
27. Vianna NJ, Polan AK: Non-occupational exposure to asbestos and malignant mesothelioma in females. Lancet 1:1061–1063, 1978
28. Risberg B, Nickels J, Wagermark J: Familial clustering of malignant mesothelioma. Cancer 45:2422, 1980
29. Li FP, Lokich J, Lapey J et al: Familial mesothelioma after intense asbestos exposure at home. JAMA 240:467, 1978
30. Antman KH, Blum R, Greenberger J et al: Multimodality therapy for mesothelioma based on a study of natural history. Am J Med 68:356, 1980
31. Antman K, Osteen R, Klegar K et al: Early peritoneal mesothelioma: Treatable malignancy. Lancet 1:977, 1985
32. Brenner J, Sordillo PP, Magill GB: Malignant mesothelioma in children: Report of seven cases and review of the literature. Med Pediatr Oncol 8:329, 1981
33. Grundy GW, Miller RW: Malignant mesothelioma in childhood: Report of 13 cases. Cancer 30:1216, 1972
34. Peto J, Henderson BE, Pike MC: Trends in mesothelioma incidence in the United States and the forecast epidemic due to asbestos exposure during World War II. In Peto R, Schniderman M (eds): Quantification of Occupational Cancer. Banbury Report, vol 9, p 51. Cold Springs Harbor, Cold Springs Harbor Laboratory, 1981
35. Peto J, Seidman H, Selikoff IJ: Mesothelioma mortality in asbestos workers: Implications for models of carcinogenesis and risk assessment. Br J Cancer 44:001, 1981
36. McNeil BJ, Eddy DM: The costs and effects of screening for cancer among asbestos-exposed workers. J Chronic Dis 35:351, 1982
37. Carey TS, Hadler NM: The role of the primary physician in disability determination for Social Security insurance and workers' compensation. Ann Intern Med 104:706–710, 1986
38. Churg A, Warnock ML, Bensch KG: Malignant mesothelioma arising after direct application of asbestos and fiber glass to the pericardium. Am Rev Respir Dis 118:419, 1978
39. Croft W: Environmental asbestos and mesotheliomas in dairy calves (abstr 742). Proc AACR 24:188, 1983
40. Donham KJ, Berg JW, Will LA et al: The effects of long-term asbestos ingestion on the colon of F344 rats. Cancer 45:1073, 1980
41. Donham KJ, Will LA, Denman D et al: The combined effects of asbestos ingestion and localized X-irradiation of the colon in rats. J Environ Pathol Toxicol Oncol 45:299, 1984
42. Humphrey E, Ewing S, Wrigley J et al: The production of malignant tumors of the lung and pleura in dogs from intratracheal asbestos instillation and cigarette smoking. Cancer 47L:1994, 1981
43. Kannerstein M, Churg C, MCaughey WTE: Asbestos and mesothelioma: A review. In Sommers SC, Rosen PP (eds): Pathology Annual, vol 13, p 81. New York, Appleton-Century-Crofts, 1978
44. Lee KP, Barras CE, Griffith FD et al: Pulmonary response and transmigration of inorganic fibers by inhalation exposure. Am J Pathol 102:314–323, 1981
45. Stanton MF, Layard M, Tegeris A et al: Carcinogenicity of fibrous glass: Pleural response in relation to fiber dimension. JNCI 58:589–603, 1977
46. Wagner JC, Berry G, Skidmore JW et al: The effects of the inhalation of asbestos in rats. Br J Cancer 29:252–269, 1974

47. Pooley FD: Minerology of asbestos: The physical and chemical properties of the dusts they form. Semin Oncol 8:243, 1981
48. McDonald AD, McDonald JC: Epidemiology of malignant mesothelioma. In Antman K, Aisner J (eds): Asbestos Related Malignancy, pp 31–56. Orlando, Grune & Stratton, 1987
49. McDonald JC, McDonald AD: Epidemiology of mesothelioma from estimated incidence. Prev Med 6:426–446, 1977
50. Wagner JC, Berry G, Polley FD: Mesotheliomas and asbestos type in asbestos textile workers: A study of lung contents. Br Med J 285:603–606, 1982
51. Lechner J, Tokiwa T, Currn R et al: Effects of asbestos on cultured human lung epithelial and mesothelial cells. Proc AACR 24:58, 1983
52. Mossman BT, Craighead JE: Asbestos-induced epithelial changes in organ cultures of hamster trachea: Inhibition by retinyl methyl ether. Science 207:311, 1980
53. Brenner J, Sordillo PP, Magill GB et al: Malignant peritoneal mesothelioma: Review of 25 patients. Am J Gastroenterol 75:311, 1981
54. Langer AM, Selikoff IJ, Sastre A: Chrysotile asbestos in the lungs of persons in New York City. Arch Environ Health 22:1765, 1971
55. Thomson JG, Kaschula ROC, MacDonald RR: Asbestos as a modern urban hazard, S Afr Med J 37:77, 1963
56. Churg A: Fiber counting and analysis in the diagnosis of asbestos-related disease. Hum Pathol 13:381, 1982
57. Churg AM, Warnock ML: Asbestos and other ferruginous bodies. Their formation and clinical significance. Am J Pathol 102:447–456, 1981
58. Mowe G, Gylseth B, Hartveit F et al: Fiber concentration in lung tissue of patients with malignant mesothelioma. A case-control study. Cancer 56:1089–1093, 1985
59. Allaben WT, Burger GT, Weis CT et al: N-Hyroxy-N-2-acylaminofluorene-induced mesothelioma, mammary adenocarcinomas, and zymbal's gland carcinomas in Sprague-Dawley rats. Proc AACR 22:101, 1981
60. Berman JJ, Rice JM: Mesotheliomas and proliferative lesions of the testicular mesothelium produced in Fischer, Sprague-Dawley and Buffalo rats by methyl(acetoxymethyl)nitrosamine (DMN-OAc). Vet Pathol 16:574, 1979
61. Antman KH, Corson JM, Li FP et al: Malignant mesothelioma following radiation exposure. J Clin Oncol 1:695, 1983
62. Antman K, Pomfret E, Aisner J et al: Peritoneal mesothelioma: Natural history and response to chemotherapy. J Clin Oncol 1:386, 1983
63. Dahlgren S: Effects of locally deposited colloidal thorium dioxide. Ann NY Acad Sci 145:786, 1967
64. Maurer R, Egloff B: Malignant peritoneal mesothelioma after cholangiography with thorotrast. Cancer 36:1381, 1975
65. Artvinli M, Baris YI: Malignant mesothelioma in a small village in the Anatolian region of Turkey: An epidemiologic study. JNCI 63:17, 1979
66. Suzuki Y: Malignant mesothelioma induced by asbestos and zeolite in the mouse peritoneum. Proc AACR 24:61, 1983
67. Lilis R: Fibrous zeolites and endemic mesothelioma in Cappadocia, Turkey. J Occup Med 23:548–550, 1981
68. Rohl AN, Langer AM, Moncure G et al: Endemic pleural disease associated with exposure to mixed fibrous dust in Turkey. Science 216:518–520, 1982
69. Oels HC, Harrison EG, Carr DT et al: Diffuse malignant mesothelioma of the pleura: A review of 37 cases. Chest 60:564–570, 1971
70. Meyniard O, Boissonnas A, Laisne MJ et al: Pneumopathie chronique a l'huile de parafine et modifications pleurales. Rev Fr Mal Respir 8:259, 1980
71. Legha SS, Muggia FM: Pleural mesothelioma: Clinical features and therapeutic implications. Ann Intern Med 87:613–621, 1977
72. Briselli M, Mark EJ, Dickersin GR: Solitary fibrous tumors of the pleura: Eight new cases and review of 360 cases in the literature. Cancer 47:2678, 1981
73. Antman K, Cohn S, Green M: Malignant mesothelioma of the tunica vaginalis testic. J Clin Oncol 2:447, 1984
74. DeKlerk DP, Nime F: Adenomatoid tumors (mesothelioma) of testicular and paratesticular tissue. Urology 6:635, 1975
75. Fenoglio JJ, Jacobs DW, McAllister HA: Ultrastructure of the mesothelioma of the atrioventricular node. Cancer 40:721, 1977
76. Scully R, Mark EJ, McNeely BU (eds): Case record of the Massachusetts General Hospital. N Engl J Med 306:32, 1982
77. Dalton WT, Zolliker AS, McCaughey WTE et al: Localized primary tumors of the pleura. An analysis of 40 cases. Cancer 44:1465, 1979
78. Scharifker D, Kaneko M: Localized fibrous "mesothelioma" of pleura (sub-mesothelial fibroma). A clinicopathologic study of 18 cases. Cancer 43:627, 1979
79. DeLaria G, Jensik R, Faber LP et al: Surgical management of malignant mesothelioma. Ann Thorac Surg 26:375, 1978
80. Utley JR, Parker JC, Hahn RS et al: Recurrent benign fibrous mesothelioma of the pleura. J Thorac Cardiovasc Surg 65:830–834, 1951
81. Antman KH: Clinical presentation and natural history of benign and malignant mesothelioma. Semin Oncol 8:313, 1981
82. Antman KH: Malignant mesothelioma. N Engl J Med 303:200, 1980
83. Grant DC, Seltzer SE, Antman KH et al: Computer tomography of malignant pleural mesothelioma. J Comput Assist Tomogr 7:626, 1983
84. Meurman L: Asbestos bodies and pleural plaques in a Finnish series of autopsy cases. Acta Pathol Microbiol Immunol Scand (Suppl) 181:7–107, 1966
85. Alexander E, Clark RA, Colley DP et al: CT of malignant pleural mesothelioma. Am J Roentgenol 137:287, 1981
86. Cohen BA, Efremidis A, Chahinian AP et al: Computer tomography of the chest of diffuse malignant pleural mesothelioma. Am Rev Respir Dis 123:131, 1981
87. Kreel L: Computed tomography in mesothelioma. Semin Oncol 8:302, 1981
88. Mirvis S, Dutcher JP, Haney PJ et al: CT of malignant pleural mesothelioma. Am J Roentgenol 140:665, 1983
89. Elmes PC, Simpson M: The clinical aspects of mesothelioma. Q J Med 45:427, 1976
90. Gordon W, Antman K, Greenberger J et al: Radiation therapy in the management of patients with mesothelioma. Int J Radiat Oncol Biol Phys 8:19, 1982
91. Antman K, Shemin R, Ryan L et al: Malignant mesothelioma: Prognostic variables in a registry of 180 patients, the Dana-Farber Cancer Institute and Brigham and Women's Hospital experience over two decades, 1965–1985. J Clin Oncol 6:147, 1988
92. Chahinian AP, Pajak T, Holland J et al: Diffuse malignant mesothelioma: Prospective evaluation of 69 patients. Ann Intern Med 96:746, 1982
93. Moertel C: Peritoneal mesothelioma. Gastroenterology 63:346, 1972
94. Katsube Y, Mukai K, Silverberg SG: Cystic mesothelioma of the peritoneum: A report of five cases and review of the literature. Cancer 50:1615, 1982
95. Moore JH, Crum CP, Chandler JG et al: Benign cystic mesothelioma. Cancer 45:2395, 1980
96. Fischbein A, Yasunosuke S, Selidoff I et al: Unexpected longevity of a patient with malignant pleural mesothelioma: Report of a case. Cancer 42:1999, 1978
97. Foyle A, Al-Jabi M, McCaughey WTE: Papillary peritoneal tumors in women. Am J Surg Pathol 5:241, 1981
98. Robbins SL, Cotran RS: Pathologic Basis of Disease, 2nd ed, p 144. Philadelphia, WB Saunders, 1979
99. Russell WO, Cohen J, Enzinger F et al: A clinical and pathological staging system for soft tissue sarcomas. Cancer 40:1562, 1977
100. Stout AP, Lattes, R: Tumors of the soft tissues. In Atlas of Tumor Pathology, p 176. Washington, DC, Armed Forces Institute of Pathology, 1967
101. Kannerstein M, McCaughey WTE, Churg J et al: A critique of the criteria for the diagnosis of diffuse malignant mesothelioma. Mt Sinai J Med (NY) 44:485, 1977
102. McCaughey WTE: Criteria for diagnosis of diffuse mesothelial tumors. Ann NY Acad Sci 132:603, 1965
103. Kannerstein M, Churg J, Magner D: Histochemistry in the diagnosis of malignant mesothelioma. Ann Clin Lab Sci 3:207, 1973
104. Winslow DJ, Taylor HB: Malignant peritoneal mesotheliomas. Cancer 13:127, 1960
105. Roggli VL, Greenberg SD, McLarty JL et al: Asbestos body content of the larynx in asbestos workers: A study of five cases. Arch Otolaryngol 106:533, 1980
106. Harwood TR, Grecey DR, Yokoo H: Pseudomesotheliomatous carcinoma of the lung. A variant of peripheral lung carcinoma. Am J Clin Pathol 65:159, 1976
107. Kannerstein M, Churg J: Peritoneal mesothelioma. Hum Pathol 8:83, 1977
108. Corson JM, Pinkus GSS: Mesothelioma: Profile of keratin proteins and caracinoembryonic antigen; an immunoperoxidase study of 20 cases and comparison with pulmonary adenocarcinomas. Am J Pathol 108:80, 1982
109. Said JW, Nash G, Lee M: Immunoperoxidase localization of keratin, proteins, carcinoembryonic antigen, and factor VIII in adenomatoid tumors: Evidence for a mesothelial derivation. Hum Pathol 13:1106, 1982
110. Said JW, Nash G, Lee M: Keratin proteins and carcinoembryonic antigen in lung carcinoma. An immunoperoxidase study of 54 cases with ultrastructural correlations. Hum Pathol 14:17, 1983
111. Schlegel R, Banks-Schlegel S, McLeod JA et al: Immunoperoxidase localization of keratin in human neoplasms. Am J Pathol 101:41, 1980
112. Suzuki Y, Churg C, and Kannerstein M: Ultrastructure of human malignant diffuse mesothelioma. Am J Pathol 85:241, 1976
113. Bolen JW, Thorning D: Mesotheliomas. A light and electron microscopical study concerning the histogenic relationships between the epithelial and the mesenchymal variants. Am J Surg Pathol 4:451, 1980
114. Warhol MJ, Hickey WF, Corson JM: Malignant mesothelioma: Ultrastructural distinction from adenocarcinoma. Am J Surg Pathol 6:307, 1982
115. Warhol MJ, Hunter NJ, Corson JM: An ultrastructural comparison of mesotheliomas and adenocarcinomas of the ovary and endometrium. Int J Gynecol Pathol 1:125, 1982
116. Butchart EG, Ashcroft T, Barnsley WC et al: Pleuropneumonectomy in the management of diffuse malignant mesothelioma of the pleura: Experience with 29 patients. Thorax 31:15, 1976
117. Weill H. Asbestos-associated diseases. Science, public policy and litigation. Chest 84:601–608, 1983
118. McDonald AD, Magner D, Eyssen G: Primary malignant mesothelial tumors in Canada, 1960–1968. Cancer 31:869, 1973
119. Shearin JC Jr, Jackson D: Malignant pleural mesothelioma: Report of 19 cases. J Thorac Cardiovasc Surg 31:53, 1981
120. DaValle MJ, Faber LP, Kittle CF et al: Extrapleural pneumonectomy for diffuse, malignant mesothelioma. Ann Thorac Surg 42:612, 1986
121. Martini N, McCormach PM, Baines MS et al: Pleural mesothelioma. Ann Thorac Surg 43:113, 1987
122. Ginsberg RJ: Diffuse malignant mesothelioma: A therapeutic dilemma. Ann Thorac Surg 42:608, 1986
123. Law MR, Hodson ME, Turner-Warurch M: Malignant mesothelioma of the pleura: Clinical aspects and symptomatic treatment. Eur J Respir Dis 65:162, 1984
124. Law MR, Gregor A, Hodson ME et al: Malignant mesothelioma of the pleura: A study of 52 treated and 64 untreated patients. Thorax 39:255–259, 1984
125. Osteen RT: Surgical treatment of peritoneal mesothelioma. In Antman K, Aisner J (eds): Asbestos-Related Malignancy, pp 339–356. Orlando, Grune & Stratton, 1987

126. Lewis RJ, Sisler GE, Mackenzie JW: Diffuse, mixed malignant pleural mesothelioma. Ann Thorac Surg 31:53–60, 1981
127. Woern H: Mopeglichkeiten und Ergebnisse der chirurgischen Behandlung des malignen Pleuramesothelioms. Thoraxchirurgie 22:391–393, 1974
128. Bamler KJ, Maassen W: Malignen Pleuramesothelioms. Thoraxchirurgie 22:386, 1974
129. Hilaris BS, Dattatreyudu N, Kwong E et al: Pleurectomy and intraoperative brachytherapy and postoperative radiation in the management of malignant pleural mesothelioma. Int J Radiat Oncol Biol Phys 10:325–331, 1984
130. Ehrenhaft JL, Sensenig DM, Lawrence MS: Mesotheliomas of the pleura. J Thorac Cardiovasc Surg 40:393–409, 1960
131. Ratzer ER, Pool JL, Melamed MR: Pleural mesotheliomas: Clinical experience with thirty-seven patients. Am J Roentgenol 99:863–880, 1967
132. Porter JM, Cheek JM: Pleural mesothelioma: Review of tumor histogenesis and report of 12 cases. J Thorac Cardiovasc Surg 55:882–890, 1968
133. Eschwege F, Schlienger M: La radiotherapie des mesotheliomes pleuraux malins: A propos de 14 cas irradies a dose elevees. J Radiol Electrol 54:255–259, 1973
134. Dobelbower RR, Strubler KA, Vaisman I: Clinical applications of high energy electron beams: The pancreas, pleura, and spine. In Zuppinger A, Bataini JP, Irigaray JM et al (eds): High Energy Electrons in Radiation Therapy, pp 91–97. Berlin, Springer-Verlag, 1980
135. Wanebo HJ, Martini N, Melamed MR et al: Pleural mesothelioma. Cancer 38:2481–2488, 1976
136. Voss A-C, Wollgens P, Untucht HJ: Das Pleuramesotheliom aus strahlentherapeutischer Sicht. Strahlentherapie [Sonderb] 148:329–332, 1974
137. Boutin C, Irrisson M, Rathelot P et al: L'extension parietale des mesotheliomas pleuraux malins diffus apres biopsies: Prevention par radiotherapie locale. Press Med 12:1823, 1983
138. Sinoff C, Falkson G, Sandison AG et al: Combined doxorubicin and radiation therapy in malignant pleural mesothelioma. Cancer Treat Rep 66:1605–1607, 1982
139. Richart R, Sherman CD: Prolonged survival in diffuse pleural mesothelioma treated with Au^{198}. Cancer 12:799–805, 1959
140. Brady LW: Mesothelioma—the role for radiation therapy. Semin Oncol 8:329–334, 1981
141. Bricout PB, Engler MJ: Computerized tomography scanning and the planning of high-dose radiotherapy for pleural mesothelioma: A report of five patients. Int J Radiat Oncol Biol Phys 7:821–826, 1981
142. Godwin JD, Rusch VW, Shuman WP: Role of CT in management of mesothelioma (abstr). Radiology 165:197–198, 1987
143. Kutcher GJ, Kestler C, Greenblatt D et al: Technique for external beam treatment for mesothelioma. Int J Radiat Oncol Biol Phys 13:1747–1752, 1987
144. Blake PR, Catterall M, Emerson PA: Pleural mesothelioma treated by fast neutron therapy. Thorax 40:72–73, 1985
145. Jones DEC, Silver D: Peritoneal mesotheliomas. Surgery 86:556–560, 1979
146. Rose RG, Palmer JD, Lougheed MN: Treatment of peritoneal mesothelioma with radioactive colloidal gold. Cancer 8:478–481, 1955
147. Legha SS, Muggia FM: Therapeutic approaches in malignant mesothelioma. Cancer Treat Rev 4:13–23, 1977
148. Leichner PK, Rosenshein N, Leibel SA et al: Distribution and tissue dose of intraperitoneal administered radioactive chromic phosphate (^{32}P) in New Zealand white rabbits. Radiology 134:729–734, 1980
149. Kaplan WD, Zimmerman RE, Bloomer WD et al: Therapeutic intraperitoneal ^{32}P: A clinical assessment of the dynamics of distribution. Radiology 138:683–688, 1981
150. Piver SM: Radioactive colloids in the treatment of stage IA ovarian cancer. Obstet Gynecol 40:42–44, 1972
151. Pezner RD, Stevens KR, Tong D et al: Limited epithelial carcinoma of the ovary treated with curative intent by the intraperitoneal installation of radiocolloids. Cancer 42:2563–2571, 1978
152. Klaassen D, Starreveld A, Shelly W et al: External beam pelvic radiotherapy plus intraperitoneal radioactive chromic phosphate in early stage ovarian cancer: A toxic combination. Int J Radiat Oncol Biol Phys 11:1801–1804, 1985
153. Lederman GS, Rosen EM, Scott P et al: P^{32} for gynecologic cancers: Survival and complications (abstr). Proc ASCO 6:111, 1987
154. Rogoff EE, Hilaris BS, Huvos AG: Long-term survival in patients with malignant peritoneal mesothelioma treated with irradiation. Cancer 32:656–664, 1973
155. Cain J, Nori D, Huvos A et al: The role of radioactive colloids in malignant peritoneal mesothelioma. Gynecol Oncol 16:263–274, 1983
156. Lederman GS, Recht A, Herman T et al: Long-term survival in peritoneal mesothelioma: The role of radiotherapy and combined modality treatment. Cancer 59:1882–1886, 1987
157. Cross WG: Table of Beta Dose Distributions, AECL Report #2793. Chalk River, Ontario, 1967
158. Delclos L, Braun EJ: Whole abdominal irradiation by cobalt-60 moving strip technique. Radiology 81:632–641, 1963
159. Glatstein E, Fuks Z, Bagshaw M: Diaphragmatic treatment in ovarian carcinoma: A new radiotherapeutic technique. Int J Radiat Oncol Biol Phys 2:357–362, 1977
160. Flick H, Lichter A, Order S: Maximal radiation therapy by a new treatment technique for stage III ovarian cancer. Int J Radiat Oncol Biol Phys 4:441–443, 1978
161. Einhorn N, Von Hamos K, Hindmarsh T et al: Radiation therapy of ovarian carcinoma: Presentation of a six-field technique. Radiother Oncol 7:125–131, 1986
162. Fazekas J, Maier JG: Irradiation of ovarian carcinomas: A prospective comparison of the open-field and moving strip techniques. Am J Roentgenol 120:118–123, 1974
163. Aisner J, Van Echo DA, Wiernik PH: Unpublished data
164. Benjamin RS, Wiernik PH, Bachur NR: Adriamycin: A new effective agent in the therapy of disseminated sarcomas. Med Pediatr Oncol 1:63–76, 1975
165. Bonadonna G, Beretta G, Tancini G et al: Adriamycin (NCS 123127) studies at the Instituto Nazionale Tumori, Milan. Cancer Chemother Rep 6:231–245, 1975
166. Gerner RE, Moore GE: Chemotherapy of malignant mesothelioma. Oncology 30:152–155, 1974
167. Gottlieb JA, Baker LH, O'Bryan RM et al: Adriamycin (NSC 123127) used alone and in combination for soft tissue and bony sarcomas. Cancer Chemother Rep 6:271–282, 1975
168. Harvey VJ, Slevin ML, Ponder BA et al: Chemotherapy of diffuse malignant mesothelioma: Phase II trials of single-agent 5-fluorouracil and adriamycin. Cancer 54:961–964, 1984
169. Kucuksu N, Thomas W, Ezdinli E: Chemotherapy of malignant diffuse mesothelioma. Cancer 37:1265–1274, 1976
170. Lerner H, Amato D, Shiraki M et al: A prospective study of adriamycin programs in malignant mesothelioma. Proc ASCO 2:230, 1983
171. Lerner H, Schoenfeld D, Martin A et al: Malignant mesothelioma: The Eastern Cooperative Oncology Group (ECOG) experience. Cancer 52:1981–1985, 1983
172. Mischler NE, Chuprevich T, Johnson RO et al: Malignant mesothelioma presenting in the pleura and peritoneum. J Surg Oncol 11:185–191, 1979
173. O'Bryan RM, Luce JK, Talley RW et al: Phase II evaluation of adriamycin in human neoplasia. Cancer 32:1–8, 1973
174. Stock RJ, Fu YS, Carter JR: Malignant peritoneal mesothelioma following radiotherapy for seminoma of the testis. Cancer 44:914–919, 1979
175. Van Dyk JJ, Van Der Merwe AM et al: Adriamycin in the treatment of cancer. S Afr Med J 50:61–66, 1976
176. Colbert N, Izrael V, Vannetzel JM et al: A prospective study of detorubicin in malignant mesothelioma. Proc Am Soc Clin Oncol 4:127(abstr), 1985
177. Butt WO: Mesothelioma of the pleura. J Can Assoc Radiol 13:40–49, 1962
178. DiPietro S, Gennari L: Successful cyclophosphamide treatment in a case of diffuse pleural mesothelioma. Tumori 49:69–73, 1963
179. Hichock HT: Mesothelioma of the pleura. IR J Med Sci 3:453–456, 1970
180. Yap BS, Benjamin RS, Burgess MA et al: The value of adriamycin in the treatment of diffuse malignant pleural mesothelioma. Cancer 42:1692–1696, 1978
181. Cafrey PF, Lucido JL: The clinical and pathologic aspects of pleural mesotheliomas. Surgery 49:690–695, 1961
182. Champion P: Two cases of malignant mesothelioma after exposure to asbestos. Am Rev Respir Dis 103:821–826, 1971
183. Gray FW, Tom BCK: Diffuse pleural mesothelioma: A survival of one year following nitrogen mustard therapy. J Thorac Cardiovasc Surg 44:73–77, 1962
184. Jara F, Takita H, Rao UN: Malignant mesotheliom: Clinicopathologic observation. NY State J Med 77:1885–1888, 1977
185. McGowan L, Bunnag B, Arias LF: Mesothelioma of the abdomen in women; monitoring of therapy by peritoneal fluid study. Gynecol Oncol 3:10–14, 1975
186. Falkson G, de Villiers PC, Falkson HC: N-isopropyl-L-2-methylhydrazino-p-toluamide hydrochloride (NSC 77213) for the treatment of cancer patients. Cancer Chemother Rep 46:7–16, 1965
187. Kelsen D, Bajorin D, Mintzer D: Phase II trial of mitomycin C in malignant mesothelioma. Proc ASCO 4:146, 1985
188. Antman K, Blum R, Greenberger J et al: Multimodality therapy for mesothelioma based on a study of natural history. Am J Med 68:356–362, 1980
189. Gottlieb JA, Benjamin RS, Baker LH et al: Role of DTIC (NSC 45388) in the chemotherapy of sarcomas. Cancer Treat Rep 60:199–203, 1976
190. Gottlieb JA, Serpick AA: Clinical evaluation of 5-(3,3-dimethyl-1-triazeno) imidazole-4-carboxamide in malignant melanoma and other neoplasms: Comparison of twice-weekly and daily administration schedules. Oncology 25:225–233, 1971
191. Dabouis G, Le Mevel B, Corroller J: Treatment of diffuse pleural malignant mesothelioma by cis-dichloro diammine platinum (CDDP) in nine patients. Cancer Chemother Pharmacol 5:209–210, 1981
192. Daboys G, Delajartre MB, Le Mevel BP: Treatment of diffuse pleural malignant mesothelioma by cis-diamine dichloro platinum (CCDP): Preliminary results in eleven patients. Med Oncol Soc (Nice) 52:98, 1979
193. Hayes DM, Cvitkovic E, Golbey RB et al: High dose cisplatinum diaminedichloride. Cancer 39:1372–1381, 1977
194. Rossoff AH, Slayton RE, Perlia CP: Preliminary clinical experience with cisdiamine dichloroplatinum (II) (NSC 119875 CACO). Cancer 30:1451–1456, 1972
195. Samson MK, Baker LH, Benjamin RS et al: Cis-dichlorodiammineplatinnum (III) in advanced soft tissue and bony sarcomas: A Southwest Oncology Group study. Cancer Treat Rep 63:11–12, 1979
196. Mintzer D, Kelson D, Frimmer D et al: Phase II trial of high dose cisplatin in patients with malignant mesothelioma. Proc ASCO 3:258, 1984
197. Andrews NC, Weiss AJ, Ansfield FT et al: Phase I study of dibromodulcitol (NSC 104800). Cancer Chemother Rep 55:61–65, 1971
198. Borden E, Ash A, Rosenbau C et al: Phase II evaluation of dibromodulcitol (DBD), ICRF 159, and maytansine in sarcomas and mesotheliomas. Proc AACR/ASCO 21:479, 1980
199. Iriarte PV, Hananian J, Cortner JA: Central nervous system leukemia and solid tumors of childhood: Treatment with 1,3-bis(2-chlorethyl)-1-nitrosourea (BCNU). Cancer 19:1187–1194, 1966
200. Kovarik JL: Primary pleural mesothelioma. Cancer 38:1816–1825, 1976
201. Chang P, Levine MA, Wiernik PH et al: A phase II study of intravenously administered methyl CCNU in the treatment of advanced sarcomas. Cancer 37:615–619, 1976
202. Creagen ET, Hahn RG, Ahmann DL et al: A comparative clinical trial evaluating the

combination of adriamycin, DTIC and vincristine, the combination of actinomycin D, cyclophosphamide and vincristine, and a single agent, methylCCNU, in advanced sarcomas. Cancer Treat Rep 60:1385–1387, 1976
203. Spremulli E, Wampler G, Regelson E et al: Chemotherapy of malignant mesothelioma. Cancer 40:2038–2045, 1977
204. Saijo N, Nishiwaki Y, Kawase I et al: Effect of ACNU on primary lung cancer, mesothelioma and metastatic pulmonary tumors. Cancer Treat Rep 62:139–141, 1978
205. Falkson G, Falkson H: Clinical trial of the oral form 4'-dimethylepipodophyllotoxin-p-D-ethylidene glucoside (NSC 141540) VP-16-213. Proc AACR 15:160, 1978
206. Nissen NI, Dombernowsky P, Hansen HH et al: Phase I clinical trial of an oral solution of VP16-213. Cancer Treat Rep 60:943–945, 1976
207. Nissen NI, Larsen V, Pederson H et al: Phase I clinical trial of a new antitumor agent, 4'dimethylepipodophyllotoxin-9-(4,6-O-ethylidene-beta-D-glucopyranoside) (NSC 141540). Cancer Chemother Rep 56:769–777, 1972
208. Boutin C, Irisson M, Guerin J et al: Phase II trial of vindesin on malignant pleural mesothelioma. Cancer Treat Rep (in press)
209. Kelsen D, Gralla R, Cheng E et al: Vindesine in the treatment of malignant mesothelioma: A phase II study. Cancer Treat Rep 67:821–822, 1983
210. Riddell RJ: Three cases of mesothelioma. Med J Aust 2:554–559, 1966
211. Djerassi I, Kim JS, Kassarov L et al: Response of mesothelioma to large doses of methotrexate with rescue (HDMTX-CT) used alone or with cis platinum. Proc Am Soc Clin Oncol 4:191, 1985
212. Thigpen JT, O'Bryan RM, Benjamin RS et al: Phase II trial of Baker's antifol in metastatic sarcoma. Cancer Treat Rep 61:1485–1487, 1977
213. Chahinian AP, Ambinder RM, Mandel EM et al: Evaluation of 63 patients with diffuse malignant mesothelioma. Proc AACR/ASCO 21:360, 1980
214. Vogler WR, Arkun S, Velez-Garcia E: Phase I study of twice-weekly azacytidine (NSC 102816). Cancer Chemother Rep 58:895–899, 1974
215. Vogler WR, Miller DS, Keller JW: 5-Azacytidine (NSC 1082116): A new drug for the treatment of myeloblastic leukemia. Blood 48:331–337, 1976
216. Kirshner J, Delosantos R, Ziegler P et al: Phase I/II study of high dose ara-C (HDA) in solid tumors. Proc ASCO 3:44, 1984
217. Price LA, Hill BT: Clinical use of DDMP (2,4-diamino)-6-(3'5'-dichlorophenyl)-6-methylpyrimidine. Proc AACR 17:15, 1976
218. Garnick MB, Blum RH, Canellos GP et al: Phase I trial of Brucceantin. Cancer Treat Rep 63:1929–1932, 1979
219. Falkson G, Vorobiof DA, Lerner JH: A phase II study of m-AMSA in patients with malignant mesothelioma with cyclophosphamide, adriamycin and vincristin. Cancer Chemother Pharmacol 4:135, 1980
220. Eagan R, Frytak S, Richardson R et al: Phase II trial of aziridinylbenzopuinone (AZQ, NSC 182986) in malignant mesothelioma Cancer Treat Reports 70:429, 1986
221. Gottlieb J, Baker L, Quagliana J et al: Chemotherapy of sarcomas with a combination of adriamycin and dimethyl triazeno imidazole carboxamide. Cancer 30:1632–1638, 1972
222. Chahinian AP, Holland JF, Mandel EM: Chemotherapy for malignant mesothelioma with adriamycin and continuous infusion of 5-azacytidine. Cancer Treat Rep 62:1108–1109, 1978
223. Brenner DE, Chang P, Wiernik PH: Adriamycin and actinomycin-D therapy for advanced sarcomas. Cancer Treat Rep (in press)
224. Chlebowski R, Pugh R, McCracken J et al: A phase I–II trial of combination therapy with adriamycin (ADR) and ICRF. Proc Am Assoc Cancer Research 20, 1979
225. Zidar B, Pugh R, Schiffer L et al: Treatment of six cases of mesothelioma with doxorubicin and cis-platinum. Cancer 52:1788–1791, 1983
226. Chahinian AP, Antman K, Aisner J et al: Cisplatin with adriamycin or mitomycin for malignant mesothelioma: A randomized phase II trial (abstr). Proc ASCO 6:183, 1987
227. Fer M, Beatty P, Richardson R et al: Combination chemotherapy of malignant mesothelioma with cyclophosphamide, adriamycin and vincristine. Cancer Chemother Pharmacol 4:135, 1980
228. Dhingra H, Valdivieso M, Tannir N et al: Combined modality treatment for mesothelioma with cytoxan (CTX), adriamycin (ADR), and DTIC (CYADIC) and adjuvant surgery (abstr). Proc ASCO 2:205, 1983
229. Samson M, Baker L, Wasser L et al: Randomized comparison of cyclophosphamide, DTIC and adriamycin (CIA) vs. cyclophosphamide and adriamycin (CA) in patients with advanced malignant mesothelioma: A sarcoma intergroup study. Proc ASCO 4:128, 1985
230. Gottlieb JA, Bodney GP, Sinkovics JG et al: An effective new four-drug combination regimen (CY-VA-DIC) for metastatic sarcomas. Proc AACR/ASCO 15:162, 1974
231. Jett JR, Eagan RT: Chemotherapy for malignant mesothelioma: CAMEO. Am J Clin Oncol 5:429–431, 1982
232. Sinoff C, Falkson G, Sandison AG et al: Malignant pleural mesothelioma: Combined adriamycin and radiation therapy—a feasibility study. Proc AACR/ASCO 2:524, 1981
233. Chahinian AP, Norton L, Szrajer L et al: Mitomycin C and cisplatin in human malignant mesothelioma xenografts in nude mice: Clinical correlation. Proc AACR 24:151, 1983
234. Chahinian AP, Szrajer L, Malamud S et al: Comparative activity of three platinum analogs against human malignant mesothelioma (HMM) xenografts in nude mice. Proc AACR 26:261, 1985
235. Tucker WG, Talley RW, Brownlee RW et al: Preliminary trials with combination therapy of cyclophosphamide (NSC 26271), vincristine (NSC 67574) and 5-fluorouracil (NSC 19893). Cancer Chemother Rep 52:593–596, 1968
236. Chahinian AP, Holland JF: Treatment of diffuse malignant mesothelioma: A review. Mt Sinai J Med (NY) 45:54–67, 1978
237. Gerner RE, Moore GE: Multiple drug therapy for malignant solid tumors in adults. Cancer Chemother Rep 57:237–239, 1973
238. Ellerby RA, Ansfield FJ, Davis HL: Preliminary report of phase I clinical experience with combined cis-diaminedichloride platinum (II) (PPD) and 5FU. Recent Results Cancer Res 48:153–159, 1974
239. Samson MK, Baker LH, Devos JM et al: Phase I clinical trial of combined therapy with vinblastine (NSC 49842), bleomycin (NSC 125066) and cis-dichloro-diamine-platinum (II) (NSC 119875). Cancer Treat Rep 60:91, 1976
240. Dimitrov NV, Egner J, Balcueva E et al: High-dose methotrexate with citrovorum factor and vincristine in the treatment of malignant mesothelioma. Cancer 50:1245–1247, 1982
241. Omura GA, Roberts GA: Combination therapy of solid tumors using 1,3-bis(2-chlorethyl)-1-nitrosourea (BCNU), vincristine, methotrexate and 5-fluorouracil. Cancer 31:1374–1381, 1973
242. Zidar BL, Benjamin RS, Frank J et al: Combination chemotherapy for advanced sarcomas of bone and mesothelioma utilizing rubidazone and DTID: A Southwest Oncology Group study. Am J Clin Oncol 6:71–74, 1983
243. Tattersall M, Fox R, Newlands E et al: Intracavitary doxorubicin in malignant effusions. Lancet Feb 17:390, 1979
244. Howell SB, Pfeifle CL, Wung WE et al: Intraperitoneal cisplatin with systemic thiosulfate protection. Ann Intern Med 97:845–851, 1982
245. Antman K, Osteen R, Montella D: A Phase I Trial of Intracavitary Doxorubicin (Adriamycin) Alternating with Cisplatin, pp 167–178. In Howell S (ed) Intra-arterial and Intracavitary Chemotherapy. Boston, Martinus Nijhoff, 1984
246. McCormack P, Nagasaki F, Hilaris BS et al: Surgical treatment of pleural mesothelioma. J Thorac Cardiovasc Surg 84:834–842, 1982
247. Taylor RA, Johnson LP: Mesothelioma: Current perspectives. West J Med 134:379–383, 1981
248. Chang PSF, Balfour T, Bourker J et al: Peritoneal mesothelioma. Br J Surg 62:576–580, 1975
249. Elmes PC, McCaughey WTE, Eade OL: Diffuse mesothelioma of the pleura and asbestos. Br Med J 1:350–353, 1965

MARTIN M. MALAWER

MICHAEL P. LINK

SARAH S. DONALDSON

CHAPTER 42 *Sarcomas of Bone*

Malignant tumors arising from the skeletal system are rare, representing only 0.2% of all primary cancers. Approximately 2100 new cases occur in the United States annually.[1] Osteosarcoma and Ewing's sarcoma are the two most common bone tumors; they occur mainly during childhood and adolescence.[2-4] Other mesenchymal (spindle-cell) neoplasms (fibrosarcoma, chondrosarcoma, and malignant fibrous histiocytoma) that characteristically arise after skeletal maturity are less common.[5-18] These are sometimes associated with underlying benign bony tumors, previous radiation, or primary bone disease.[5-16] Most experience in the management of bony neoplasms has been obtained with osteosarcoma. As a result, the surgical, chemotherapeutic, and radiotherapeutic principles developed in the treatment of osteosarcomas form the basis of the management strategy for most of the spindle-cell neoplasms.

During the 1980s, there has been an explosion of clinical knowledge and experience in the management of bony neoplasms.[18-28] The development of centers with specific interest in these tumors has played an important role in the understanding and surgical management of these lesions and in the development of multimodality treatment regimens.[24-27] A surgical staging system that permits standardized preoperative evaluation, analysis, and end-result reporting has been developed.[28]

Although amputation has been the standard treatment of most bony sarcomas, limb-sparing surgery has been developed for both malignant and aggressive benign tumors.[29-39] Advances in orthopedics, bioengineering, radiographic imaging, radiotherapy, and chemotherapy have contributed to safer, more reliable surgical procedures.[40-80] Computed tomography (CT) and magnetic resonance imaging (MRI) permit extremely accurate evaluation of the local anatomy and enhance the possibility of safe resection.[81-88] Limb-sparing surgery is considered safe and routine for a large number of carefully selected patients, and a recently developed evaluation system to determine a patient's functional status is undergoing multi-institutional testing.[28] This system permits evaluation and comparison of the various limb-sparing procedures and types of surgical reconstructions.

Paralleling these advances, adjuvant chemotherapy has dramatically increased overall survival; specifically, the bleak 15% to 20% survival rate with surgery alone during the 1960s rose to 55% to 80% with adjuvant treatment regimens in the 1980s.[49-52,89-91] Multidrug regimens are now essential treatment. The timing, mode of delivery, and different combinations of these agents are being investigated at many centers. Preoperative chemotherapy regimens, administered by the intravenous or intra-arterial route, and postoperative regimens are being evaluated for their effect on the tumor and their impact on the choice of operative procedure and on overall survival.[92-99]

This chapter focuses on malignant spindle-cell tumors. Ewing's sarcoma is presented in detail in Chapter 47. Benign tumors are described briefly.[2,3] Emphasis is placed on natural history and surgical staging of tumors. Patient selection for amputation or limb-sparing surgery and limb-sparing procedures are considered, and the roles of adjuvant chemotherapy and radiotherapy are detailed.

CLASSIFICATION AND TYPES OF BONE TUMORS

Bone consists of cartilaginous, osteoid, fibrous tissue, and bone marrow elements. Each tissue can give rise to benign or malignant spindle-cell tumors.[2-4] The classification of bone tumors is based on cell type and the recognized products of proliferating cells. The classification, described by Lichtenstein and modified by Dahlin, is presented in Table 42-1.[3,55] Jaffe recommends that each tumor be considered a separate clinico-pathologic entity.[4] Radiographic, histologic, and clinical data are necessary to form an accurate diagnosis and to determine the degree of activity and malignancy of each lesion.

Cartilage tumors are lesions in which cartilage is produced. They are the most common bone tumors. *Osteochondroma* is the most common benign cartilage tumor; between 1% and 2% of solitary osteochondromas become malignant.[56,57] *Enchondroma* is a benign cartilage tumor that occurs centrally; malignant transformation may occur in an adult. *Chondrosarcoma,* the most common malignant cartilage tumor, is either intramedullary or peripheral. Ten percent are secondary, arising from an underlying benign lesion.[2] Most chondrosarcomas are low-grade tumors, although 10% will dedifferentiate into high-grade spindle-cell sarcomas, or rare mesenchymal chondrosarcomas.[2,56]

Osteoid tumors are lesions in which the stroma produces osteoid. The benign forms are *osteoid osteoma* and *osteoblastoma.* Osteoid osteomas are never malignant. Osteoblastomas rarely metastasize; when they do, it is only after multiple local recurrences.[58] *Osteosarcomas* are the most common primary malignant tumors of the bone. Histologically they are composed of malignant spindle cells and osteoblasts that produce osteoid or immature bone. Several variants are now recognized.[59] Parosteal, periosteal, and low-grade intraosseous osteosarcoma are histologically and radiographically distinct from the classic central medullary osteosarcomas and have a more favorable prognosis.[60-62]

Fibrous tumors of bone are rare. *Desmoplastic fibroma* is a locally aggressive, nonmetastasizing tumor, analogous to fibromatosis of soft tissue.[5,6] Fibrosarcoma of bone appears histologically as its soft-tissue counterpart. Many sections are necessary to demonstrate the lack of osteoid production. If osteoid is present, the lesion is classified as an osteosarcoma. *Malignant fibrous histiocytoma* (MFH), the bony counterpart of soft-tissue MFH, is rare.[7-9] The pathology of bone and soft-tissue MFH is similar, consisting of a storioform pattern with a histiocytic component. *Giant cell tumors* are of unknown origin; originally called benign, they are now

TABLE 42-1. General Classification of Bone Tumors*

Histologic Type†	Benign	Malignant
Hematopoietic (41.4%)		Myeloma Reticulum cell sarcoma
Chondrogenic (20.9%)	Osteochondroma Chondroma Chondroblastoma Chondromyxoid fibroma	Primary chondrosarcoma Secondary chondrosarcoma Dedifferentiated chondrosarcoma Mesenchymal chondrosarcoma
Osteogenic (19.3%)	Osteoid osteoma Benign osteoblastoma	Osteosarcoma Parosteal osteogenic sarcoma
Unknown origin (9.8%)	Giant cell tumor	Ewing's tumor Malignant giant cell tumor Adamantinoma
	(Fibrous) histiocytoma	(Fibrous) histiocytoma
Fibrogenic (3.8%)	Fibroma Desmoplastic fibroma	Fibrosarcoma
Notochordal (3.1%)		Chordoma
Vascular (1.6%)	Hemangioma	Hemangioendothelioma Hemangiopericytoma
Lipogenic (<0.5%)	Lipoma	
Neurogenic (<0.5%)	Neurilemmoma	

Adapted from Dahlin DC: Bone Tumors: General Aspects and Data on 6,221 Cases, 3rd ed. Springfield, IL, Charles C. Thomas, 1978.

*Classification based on Lichtenstein: Classification of primary tumors of bone. *Cancer* 4:335–351, 1951.

†Distribution based on Mayo Clinic experience.

considered a low-grade sarcoma. They have a high rate of local recurrence and malignant transformation.[63,64]

Tumors presumably arising from bone marrow elements are the *round cell sarcomas*. The two most common are Ewing's sarcoma and, more rarely, a non-Hodgkin's lymphoma. These are discussed in Chapters 47, 48, and 49.

RADIOGRAPHIC EVALUATION AND DIAGNOSIS

Radiographic evaluation, clinical history, and histologic examination are necessary for an accurate diagnosis. Bone scans, angiography, and CT are rarely helpful in determining a diagnosis but are important in delineating the extent of local involvement.

A systematic approach to the radiographic evaluation of skeletal lesions has been described by Madewell and colleagues, who studied and correlated several hundred radiographic and pathologic specimens.[65] They considered the radiograph as the gross specimen from which a detailed histologic interpretation could be made and biologic activity accurately diagnosed. According to their system, a bone tumor is evaluated by five radiographic parameters.

ANATOMICAL SITE

Specific anatomical sites of the bone give rise to specific lesions. Johnson explained this by a field theory, which hypothesizes that the most active cells of a certain area of bone give rise to tumors characteristic of that area.[66] Figure 42-1 summarizes the sites of common bone tumors. In general, spindle-cell sarcomas are metaphyseal, and round cell sarcomas tend to be diaphyseal.

BORDERS

The border reflects the growth rate and the response of the adjacent normal bone to the tumor. Most tumors have a characteristic border. Benign lesions (*e.g.*, nonossifying fibromas and unicameral bone cysts) have well-defined borders and narrow transition areas that are often associated with a reactive sclerosis. Aggressive or benign tumors, (*e.g.*, chondroblastoma and giant cell tumors) tend to have faint borders and wide zones of transition with very little sclerosis, indicating rapid growth. Poorly delineated or absent margins indicate aggressive or malignant lesions.

BONE DESTRUCTION

Bone destruction is the hallmark of a bone tumor. Three patterns of bone destruction have been described; geographic, moth-eaten, and permeative.[67] In general, these patterns are found in the tubular bone rather than in the flat bone, and they represent a combination of cortical and cancellous destruction, which are caused by the increasing growth rate of the underlying tumor.

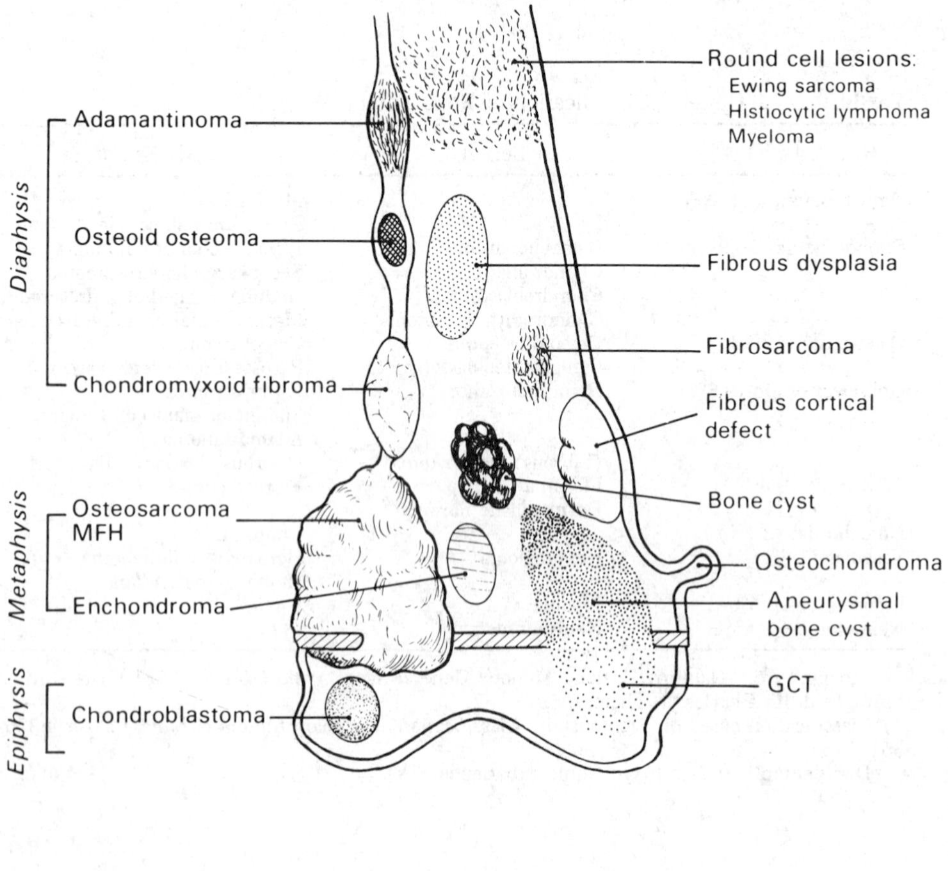

FIG. 42-1. Common anatomical sites of bone tumors. (Modified from Madewell JE, Ragsdale ED, Sweet DE: Radiographic and pathologic analysis of solitary bone lesions. Radiol Clin North Am 19:715–814, 1981)

MATRIX FORMATION

Calcification of the matrix or new bone formation can produce an area of increased density within the lesion. Calcification typically appears as flocculent or stippled rings or clusters. The appearance of new bone varies from dense sclerosis, which obliterates all evidence of normal trabeculae, to small, irregular, circumscribed masses described as "wool" or "clouds." Calcification and ossification may appear in the same lesion. Neither type of matrix formation per se is diagnostic of malignancy.

PERIOSTEAL REACTION

Periosteal reaction is indicative of malignancy, but not pathognomonic of particular tumor. In malignant tumors, periosteal reaction is discontinuous and thin, with multiple laminations; either a parallel or perpendicular pattern may be present.

The radiographic parameters of benign and malignant tumors are quite different. Benign tumors have round, smooth, well-circumscribed borders. There is no cortical destruction and usually no periosteal reaction. Malignant lesions have irregular, poorly defined margins. There is evidence of bone destruction and a wide area of transition with periosteal reaction. Soft-tissue extension is common.

NATURAL HISTORY

Tumors arising in bone have characteristic patterns of behavior and growth that distinguish them from other malignant lesions.[68,88] These patterns form the basis of a staging system and current treatment strategies. These principles and their relationship to management, as formulated by Enneking, are described here.[68,88]

BIOLOGY AND GROWTH

Spindle-cell sarcomas form a solid lesion that grows centrifugally. The cells in the periphery of this lesion are the least mature. In contradistinction to a true capsule that surrounds a benign lesion and is composed of compressed normal cells, the malignant tumor is usually enclosed by a pseudocapsule and consists of compressed tumor cells and a fibrovascular zone of reactive tissue with an inflammatory component that interdigitates with the normal tissue adjacent to and beyond the lesion. The thickness of the reactive zone varies with the degree of malignancy and histogenic type. The histologic hallmark of sarcomas is their potential to break through the pseudocapsule to form satellite lesions of tumor cells. This characteristic distinguishes a nonmalignant from a malignant mesenchymal tumor.

High-grade sarcomas have a poorly defined reactive zone that may be invaded and destroyed by the tumor (Fig. 42-2). In addition, there may be tumor nodules in tissue that appears to be normal and is not contiguous with the main tumor. These nodules are skip metastases. Although low-grade sarcomas regularly demonstrate tumor interdigitation into the reactive zone, they rarely form tumor nodules beyond this area.

The three mechanisms of growth and extension of bone tumors are compression of normal tissue, resorption of bone by reactive osteoclasts, and direct destruction of normal tissue. Benign tumors grow and expand by the first two mechanisms, but direct tissue destruction is characteristic of malignant bone tumors. Local anatomy influences tumor growth by setting the natural barriers to extension. In general, bone sarcomas take the path of least resistance. Most benign bone tumors are unicompartmental; they remain confined and may expand the bone in which they arose. Malignant bone tumors are bicompartmental; they destroy the overlying cortex and go directly into the adjacent soft tissue. The determination of anatomic compartment involvement has become more important with the advent of limb-preservation surgery.

Based on biologic considerations and natural history, Enneking classified bone tumors into five categories, each of which shares clinical characteristics and radiographic patterns and requires similar surgical procedures.[68,118]

Benign, latent: Lesions that grow slowly during normal growth of the individual and then stop, with a tendency to heal spontaneously. They never become malignant and heal rapidly if treated by simple curettage. Surgery is not indicated unless they become symptomatic.

Benign, active: Lesions that grow progressively. Simple curettage leaves a reactive rim with some tumor and has a high recurrence rate. Wide excision through normal bone results in local control in approximately 95% of all cases.

Benign, aggressive: Lesions that are locally aggressive but do not metastasize. The tumor extends through the capsule into the reactive zone. Local control can be obtained only by removing the lesion with a margin of normal bone beyond the reactive zone.

Malignant, low grade: Lesions that have a low potential to metastasize. Histologically, there is a pseudocapsule. Tumor nodules exist within the reactive zone but rarely beyond. Local control can be accomplished only by removal of all tumor and reactive tissue with a margin of normal bone. These lesions can be treated successfully by surgery alone.

Malignant, high grade: Lesions that grow rapidly and metastasize early. Tumor nodules are often found within and beyond the reactive zone and at some distance in the normal tissue. Surgery is necessary for local control, and systemic therapy is warranted to prevent distant metastasis.

METASTASES

Bone tumors, unlike carcinomas, disseminate almost exclusively through the blood; bones lack a lymphatic system. There have been only rare reports of early lymphatic spread to regional nodes.[18,100] Lymphatic involvement, which has been noticed in 10% of cases at autopsy, is a poor prognostic sign.[69] McKenna reported that 6 (3%) of 194 patients with

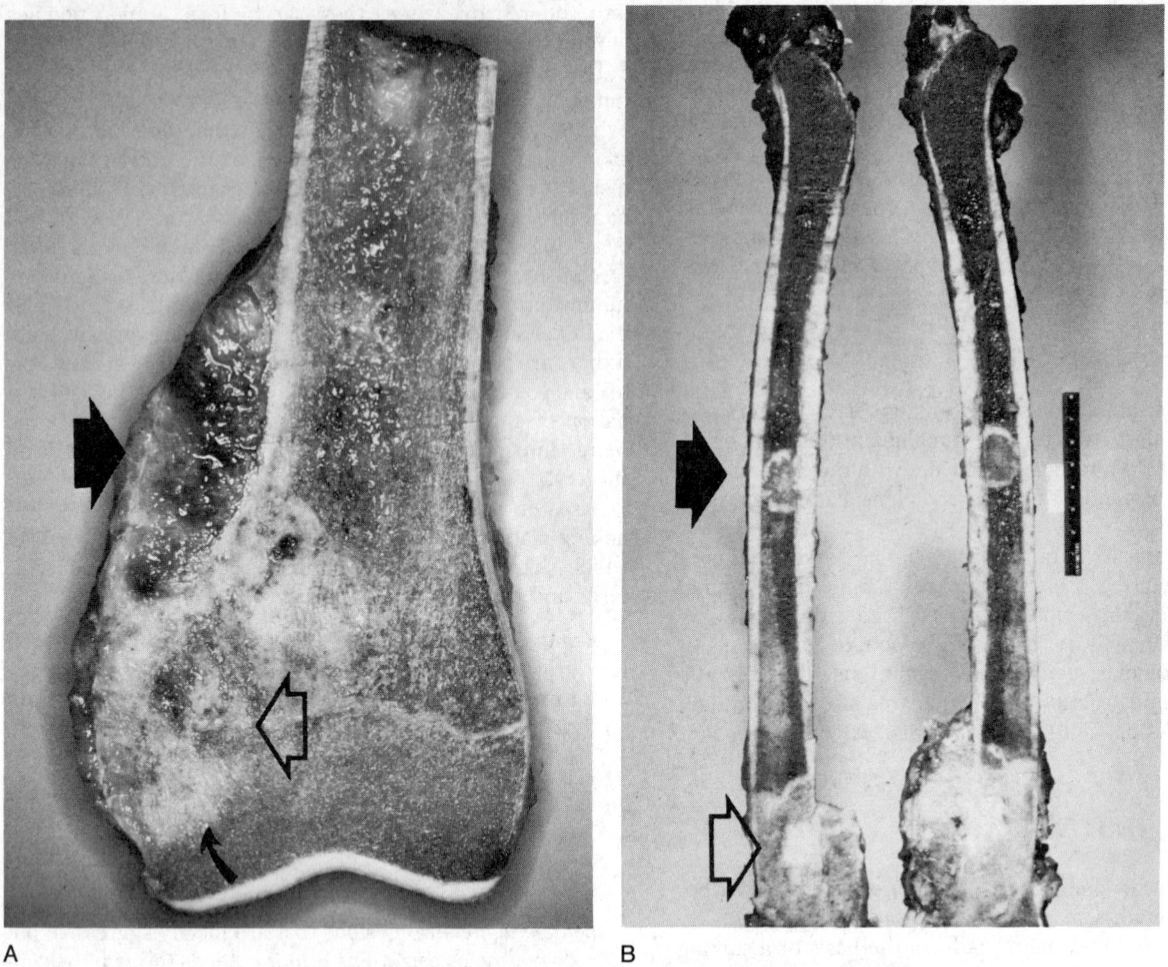

FIG. 42-2. Common patterns of local growth of osteosarcoma. Gross specimens of two femoral osteosarcomas. **A**. Typical osteosarcoma. The majority of osteosarcomas arise within the metaphysis and have a large extraosseous (soft tissue) component (*solid arrow*). This tumor has arisen within the metaphysis and involves the epiphysis by direct destruction (*open arrow*) through the growth plate and also by tracking along the cortex and then back into (*curved solid arrow*) the epiphysis. **B**. Skip metastasis. A separate tumor (*solid arrow*) nodule not in continuity with the main tumor (*open arrow*) mass is termed a 'skip' metastasis. This is a poor prognostic sign for survival.

osteosarcoma who underwent amputation demonstrated lymph node involvement. None of these patients survived 5 years.[70] Hematogeneous spread is manifested by pulmonary involvement in its early stages and secondarily by bony involvement.[70–75] Bone metastases are occasionally the first sign of dissemination. With the use of adjuvant chemotherapy, the skeletal system has become a more common site of initial relapse.[45,101, 102]

SKIP METASTASES

Skip metastases, which are tumor nodules located within the same bone as the main tumor but not continuous with it, are most often seen with high-grade sarcomas. Transarticular skip metastases are located in the joint adjacent to the main tumor.[76] A skip lesion develops by the embolization of tumor cells within the marrow sinusoids; in effect, they are local micrometastases that have not passed through the circulation (Fig. 42-2). Transarticular skips are believed to occur through periarticular venous anastomoses. The clinical incidence of skip metastases is less than 1%.[77] These lesions predict poor survival.[76,77]

LOCAL RECURRENCE

Local recurrence of either a benign or malignant lesion is due to inadequate removal of the primary tumor. The aggressiveness of the tumor determines which surgical procedure is required for local control. Ninety-five percent of all local recurrences, regardless of histology, develop within 24

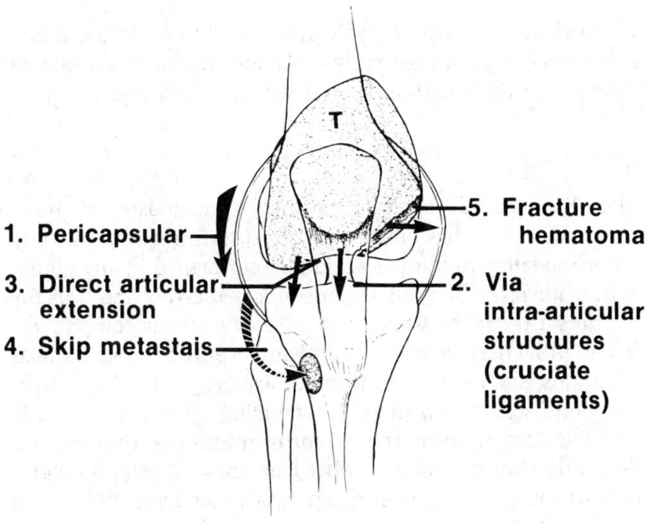

FIG. 42-3. Mechanisms of articular involvement by high grade bone sarcomas.

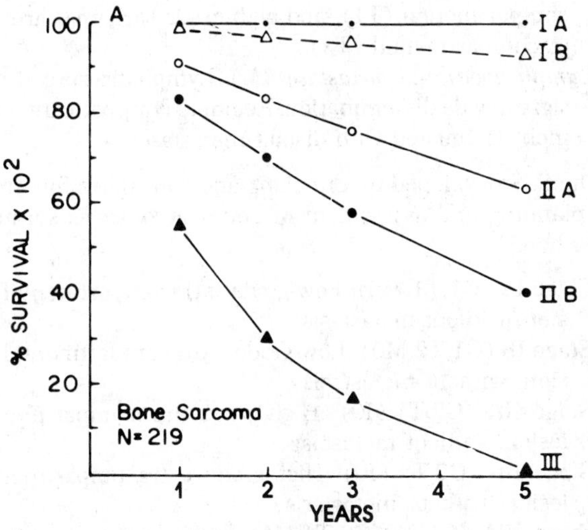

FIG. 42-4. Survival rates of patients over a 5-year period with bone sarcoma according to stage of disease. (Enneking WF, Spanier SS, Goodman MA: A system for the surgical staging of musculoskeletal sarcoma. Clin Orthop 153:106–120, 1980)

months of attempted removal.[68,78,79] Local recurrence of a high-grade sarcoma decreases overall survival prospects substantially. Local recurrence in patients who have undergone therapy may be associated with an even poorer prognosis.[74]

JOINT INVOLVEMENT

The articular cartilage is thought to be a natural barrier to direct articular extension by tumor. In a careful study of 45 macrosections of primary bone sarcomas, Simon reported 17 (38%) with articular extension.[80] He described three mechanisms: pericapsular, direct extension along intra-articular structures, and direct extension through the articular cartilage. Pathologic fracture, which creates direct communication from tumor bone to joint cartilage, is a fourth mechanism (Fig. 42-3).

STAGING BONE TUMORS

In 1980, the Musculoskeletal Tumor Society (MSTS) adopted a Surgical Staging System (SSS) for bone sarcomas (Table 42-2). The system is based upon the fact that all types of mesenchymal sarcomas of bone behave similarly. The SSS described by Enneking and colleagues is based on the GTM classification: grade (G), location (T), and lymph node involvement and metastases (M).

Surgical grade (G): "G" represents the histologic grade of a lesion and other clinical data that are used to make a surgical determination of low grade (G1) or high grade (G2) (Fig. 42-4).

Surgical site (T): "T" represents the site of the lesion, which may be intracompartmental (T1) or extracompartmental (T2). A compartment is an anatomic structure or space bounded by natural barriers to tumor extension. The significance of T1 lesions are easier to define clinically, surgically, and radiographically than that of T2 lesions, and there is a higher chance of adequate removal of T1 tumors by nonamputative procedures. In general, low-grade bone sarcomas are intra-

TABLE 42-2. Surgical Staging* of Bone Sarcomas

Stage	*Grade*	*Site*
IA	Low (*G*1)	Intracompartmental (*T*1)
IB	Low (*G*1)	Extracompartmental (*T*2)
IIA	High (*G*2)	Intracompartmental (*T*1)
IIB	High (*G*2)	Extracompartmental (*T*2)
III	Any G Regional or distant metastasis (M_1)	Any (*T*)

Enneking WF, Spanier SS, Goodman MA: A system for the surgical staging of musculoskeletal sarcoma. Clin Orthop 153:106–120, 1980.

*G = grade
*G*1 is any low-grade tumor;
*G*2 is any high-grade tumor.
T = site
*T*1 intracompartmental location of tumor.
*T*2 extracompartmental location of tumor.
M = regional or distal metastases.
*M*0 represents no metastases.
*M*1 represents any metastases.

compartmental (T1), and high-grade sarcomas are extracompartmental (T2).

Lymph nodes and metastases (M): Lymphatic spread is a sign of wide dissemination. Regional lymphatic involvement is equated with distant metastases.

The SSS developed by Enneking and colleagues for surgical planning and assessment of bone sarcomas is summarized here:

Stage IA (G1,T1,M0): Low-grade intracompartmental lesion, without metastasis
Stage IB (G1,T2,M0): Low-grade extracompartmental lesion, without metastasis
Stage IIA (G2,T1,M0): High-grade intracompartmental lesion, without metastasis
Stage IIB (G2,T2,M0): High-grade extracompartmental lesion, without metastasis
Stage IIIA (G1, or G2,T1,M1): Intracompartmental lesion, any grade, with metastasis
Stage IIIB (G1 or G2,T2,M1): Extracompartmental lesion, any grade, with metastasis

PREOPERATIVE EVALUATION

If the plain radiographs suggest an aggressive or malignant tumor, staging studies should be performed before biopsy. All radiographic studies are influenced by surgical manipulation of the lesion, making interpretation more difficult.[39,68] More important, the biopsy site may be in a location that is not optimal for subsequent en bloc removal or radiotherapy.[24,103,104] Bone scintigraphy, MRI, CT, and angiography are required to delineate local tumor extent, vascular displacement, and compartmental localization.[42–46,68,78,82–88]

BONE SCANS

Bone scintigraphy assists in determining polyostotic involvement, metastatic disease, and intraosseous extension of tumor.[42–45] Malignant bone tumors, although solitary, may in rare cases present with skeletal metastasis.[46] Skip metastases are rarely detected by bone scans because they are small and localized in the fatty marrow and do not excite cortical response.[76,77]

Appreciation of the intraosseous extension of a bone tumor is important in surgical planning. Watts has recommended removal of bone 6 to 7 cm beyond the area of scintigraphic abnormality.[32] This has been accepted as a safe margin for limb-sparing procedures.

CT SCANS

CT allows accurate determination of the intraosseous and extraosseous extensions of skeletal neoplasms.[40–44] It accurately depicts the transverse relationship of a tumor. By varying window settings, cortical bone, intramedullary space, adjacent muscles, and extraosseous soft-tissue extension can be studied. CT scans should include the entire bone and the adjacent joint. Infusion of intravenous contrast material permits identification of the adjacent large vascular structures. CT evaluations must be individualized. To obtain the maximum benefit of image reconstruction, the surgeon should discuss the information desired with the radiologist.

MRI

MRI has several advantages in the diagnoses of bone sarcomas.[81–88] It has better contrast discrimination than any other modality, and imaging can be performed in any plane. MRI is ideal for imaging the medullary marrow and thus for the detection of the tumor and the extraosseous component. It has proven especially helpful in several difficult clinical situations, such as detecting small lesions, evaluating a positive bone scan when the corresponding plain radiograph is negative, determining the extent of infiltrative tumors, and detecting skip metastases. MRI has quickly become invaluable in the planning of limb-sparing procedures.[86,88]

ANGIOGRAPHY

The technique of arteriography for bone lesions differs from that used for arterial disease. A minimum of two views (biplane) is necessary to determine the relationship of the major vessels to the tumor.[105] The late venous phase, which yields information on large veins, is helpful if ligation is planned, and it may occasionally demonstrate tumor thrombi. Because experience with limb-sparing procedures has increased, it has become essential to determine individual vascular patterns before resection. This is especially crucial for tumors of the proximal tibia, where vascular anomalies are common.[106] Angiography is the most reliable means of determining vascular anatomy and displacement; MRI and CT better demonstrate extraosseous extension.

MRI and CT (transverse data), combined with bone scans and angiography, allow the physician to develop a three-dimensional construct of the local tumor area before surgery and to formulate a detailed surgical approach (Fig. 42-5).

BIOPSY TECHNIQUE AND TIMING

The biopsy of a suspected bone tumor must be performed with great care and skill.[103,104] This principle cannot be overemphasized. The consequences of a poorly executed biopsy are often the deciding factor in the choice between a limb-salvage procedure or an amputation. Murray and colleagues, from M.D. Anderson Hospital and Tumor Institute, judged that only 19% of patients referred to that institution for treatment of primary bone sarcomas had properly placed biopsies.[24] All of these patients had open (incisional) biopsies, but 92% of these procedures performed at M.D. Anderson during the same period were needle biopsies. Similarly, Mankin compared the results of biopsies performed at the referring institution with those performed at the treatment center.[104] In this study, which involved 329 patients, a major error in diagnosis occurred in 60% of the patients from referring hospitals, and 18.2% of the referred patients had to have less than optimal treatment because of problems related to the biopsy. In 8.5%, the prognosis and outcome were considered to have been adversely affected by the biopsy.

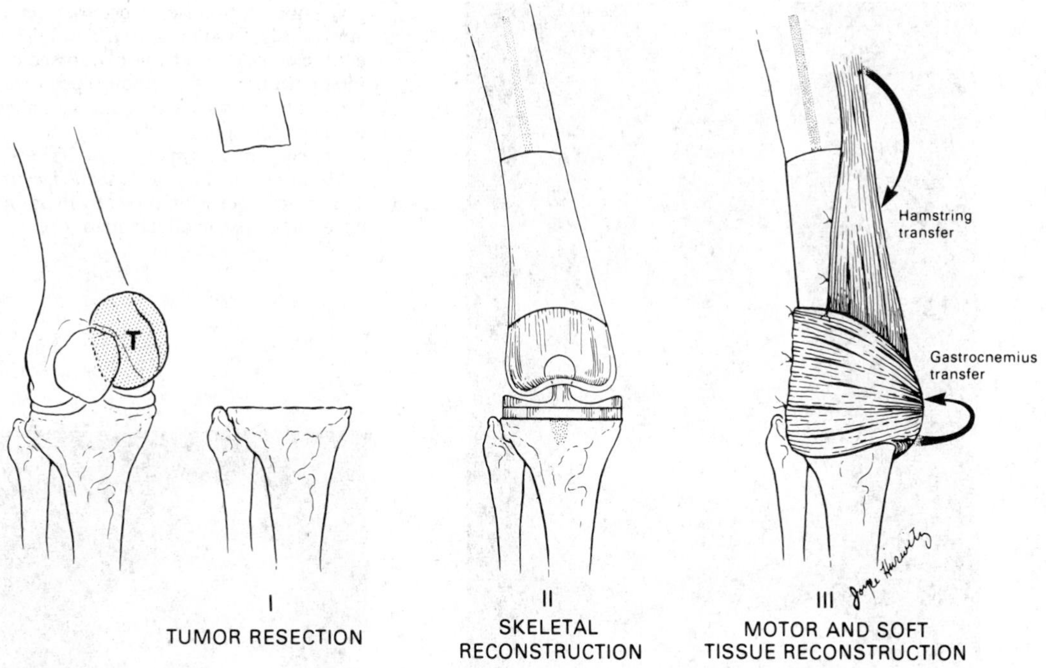

FIG. 42-5. Schematic diagram of the three phases of a limb-sparing procedure.

The biopsy should be performed by the surgeon who will make the ultimate decision about the operative procedure. Patients who probably have primary bony malignancies should be referred to a regional cancer center for biopsy.

Trephine or core biopsy often obtains an adequate specimen for diagnosis.[107-109] Multiple samples can be obtained from the same puncture site by slightly changing the angle of approach. Radiographs should document the position of the trochar. Core biopsy is preferred if a limb-sparing option exists, because it causes less local contamination than does open biopsy. Core biopsy is especially helpful in difficult areas such as the spine, pelvis, and hips. If a core biopsy is inadequate, a small incisional biopsy can be performed.

Every precaution should be taken to avoid contamination when performing an open biopsy. A tourniquet is used if feasible. If a soft-tissue component is present, there is no need to biopsy the underlying bone. To decrease subsequent hemorrhage, polymethylmethacrylate (PMMA) is used to plug a cortical window; Gelfoam is used in the soft tissue. The overlying pseudocapsule is carefully closed to ensure maximum hemostasis. If it is necessary to biopsy the underlying bone, it is essential to use a small, rounded cortical window. This is especially true for a tumor that requires primary radiotherapy. Large segments will not reossify, often leading to fracture and the need for amputation. Regardless of the technique used, tumor cells will contaminate all tissue planes and compartments transversed, and all biopsy sites must be removed en bloc when the tumor is resected or irradiated.

Frozen-section analyses are obtained on all biopsy specimens. Many bone tumors can be adequately sectioned with a microtome. The purpose of the initial frozen-section biopsy is to determine whether enough viable tumor has been obtained to yield satisfactory paraffin sections for interpretation. If there are no tumor cells, additional specimens must be obtained. Frozen-section studies may also suggest that additional material is necessary for electron microscopic studies or for special staining techniques.

Interest has recently been renewed in frozen-section diagnosis and immediate surgery. Though the idea is attractive, there is no evidence that this procedure increases survival. Its major advantage is to decrease the risk of tumor microextension and contamination in a bloodless field, provided that a tourniquet has been used.[68,109]

RESTAGING AFTER PREOPERATIVE CHEMOTHERAPY

With the advent of preoperative chemotherapy for osteosarcoma, a need has developed to evaluate the clinical and radiographic response of the tumor before surgery. The staging and preoperative clinical studies previously described are used for evaluating tumor response[110-114] Because of possible sampling errors, serial needle biopsies are unreliable, but the useful methods of preoperative evaluation are delineated.

CLINICAL EVALUATION

Pain often decreases following the induction of chemotherapy. Alkaline phosphatase levels also decrease. The tumor

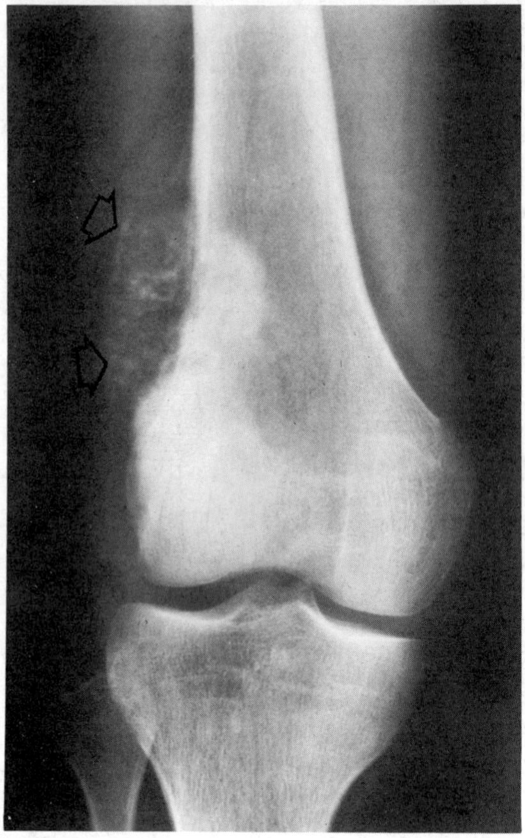

A

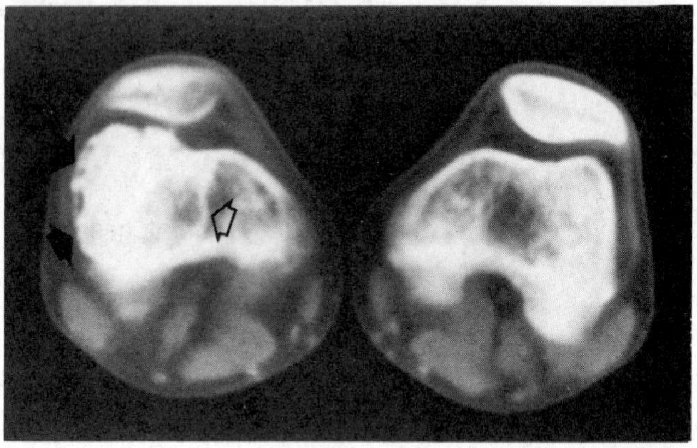

B

FIG. 42-6. Response of osteosarcoma to preoperative chemotherapy. **A**. Plain radiograph of a distal femoral osteosarcoma showing early calcification of the extraosseous component. Note the beginning peripheral ossification (*open arrows*). **B**. CT scan of the distal femur demonstrating increasing ossification and rimming of the soft tissue component (*solid arrows*) and a sclerotic rim within the medullary component (*open arrow*). These changes are considered typical of tumor necrosis with secondary reparative (healing) response. The extraosseous component will often not shrink due to the persistence of the extracellular matrix.

decreases in size, especially if little matrix is present. Conversely, an increase of pain, elevation of alkaline phosphatase, or increasing tumor size are obvious signs of tumor progression.

PLAIN RADIOGRAPHY

There is a good correlation between radiographic response and the amount of necrosis.[112,113] Smith described the radiographic responses seen on serial radiographs: increased ossification of tumor osteoid, marked thickening and new bone formation of the periosteum and tumor border (giving a more benign appearance), and decrease in soft tissue mass.[113] The healing ossification is usually solid, homogeneous, and regular, and it is easily differentiated from tumor osteoid.[112] There are less significant changes within the intramedullary component, including increased sclerosis and lysis caused by necrosis and hemorrhage.

ANGIOGRAPHY

Following chemotherapy, there is a marked decrease in vascularity.[111,112] Chuang examined 53 patients and reported that those with a complete angiographic response had greater than 90% necrosis; among those with a partial response, necrosis ranged from 40% to 78%.[112] He concluded that angiographic evaluation was as reliable as pathologic evaluation and that the angiographic features were the best clinical criteria for the evaluation of tumor response.

CT SCANS

The most consistent finding in patients responding to therapy is a decrease in soft-tissue mass and the development of a rimlike calcification similar to that seen on plain radiographs (Fig. 42-6).[110] Changes in marrow are not helpful in evaluating response. There have been no studies using MRI for the evaluation of neoadjuvant chemotherapy.

BONE SCINTIGRAPHY

Bone scan changes are difficult to evaluate. A decrease in activity generally indicates a favorable response; however, reparative bone formation, signalled by increased activity, may be misleading. Dynamic bone scans, which are based on tumor blood flow and regional plasma clearance by bone and soft tissue, may allow more valid evaluations.[114] Regions that show a greater than 20% decrease in ^{99m}TcMDP plasma clearance are reported to be associated with necrotic tumor.

SURGICAL MANAGEMENT OF SKELETAL TUMORS

Surgical removal, including curettage, resection, and amputation, is the traditional method of managing skeletal neoplasms. Limb-sparing techniques were developed during the early 1970s.[20–22,28–39] Marcove described cryosurgery for some bony tumors.[115–117] Enneking and colleagues formu-

TABLE 42-3. Classification of Surgical Procedures for Bone Tumors*

Margin	*Local*	*Amputation*
Intralesional	Curettage or debulking	Debulking amputation
Marginal	Marginal excision	Marginal amputation
Wide	Wide local excision	Wide throughbone amputation
Radical	Radical local resection	Radical disarticulation

Enneking WF, Spanier SS, Goodman MA: A system for the surgical staging of musculoskeletal sarcoma. Clin Orthop 153:106–120, 1980.
*Classified by the type of margin achieved and whether it is obtained by a local or ablative procedure.

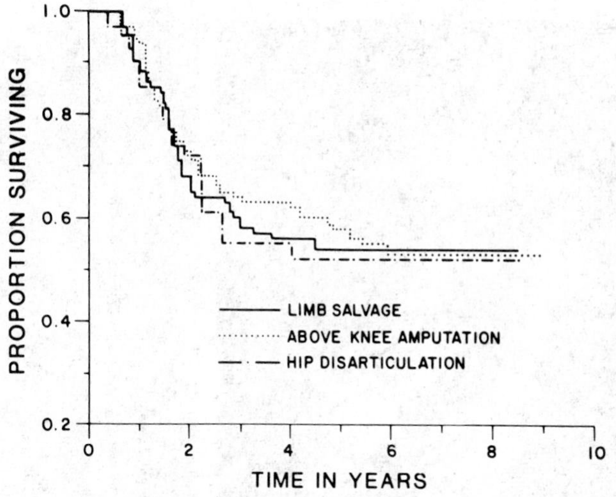

FIG. 42-7. Length of survival versus type of operative procedure for 227 patients (pooled data) with high grade osteosarcoma of the distal femur (Kaplan-Meier analysis). There is no survival difference for patients treated by hip disarticulation, above-knee amputation, or a limb-sparing procedure. (Simon MA, Aschliman MA, Thomas N, et al: Limb-salvage treatment versus amputation for osteosarcoma of the distal end of the femur. J Bone Joint Surg 68 [Am]: 1331–1337, 1986)

lated a classification of surgical procedures based on the surgical plane of dissection in relation to the tumor (Table 42-3) and the method of accomplishing its removal (Table 42-4). The scheme summarized permits meaningful comparisons of surgical procedures, analysis of end results, and gives surgeons a common language.[68,78,118]

Intralesional: An intralesional procedure passes through the pseudocapsule of the neoplasm directly into the lesion. Macroscopic tumor is left, and the entire operative field is potentially contaminated. Curettage is an intralesional procedure.

Marginal: A marginal procedure is one in which the entire lesion is removed in a single piece. The plane of dissection passes through the pseudocapsule or reactive zone around the lesion. When performed for a sarcoma, it leaves macroscopic disease.

Wide (Intracompartmental): A wide excision, commonly called en bloc resection, includes the entire tumor, the reactive zone, and a cuff of normal tissue. The entire tumor origin structure is not removed, and in patients with high-grade sarcomas, this procedure may leave skip nodules.

Radical (Extracompartmental): The entire tumor and the structure of origin of the lesion are removed. The plane of dissection is beyond the limiting fascial or bony borders.

Any of these procedures may be accomplished by a limb-sparing procedure or by amputation. Amputation may entail a marginal, wide, or radical excision, depending upon the plane through which it passes. An amputation does not necessarily remove all cancer, but it can achieve a specific margin. The local anatomy determines how the margin is obtained, and the aim of preoperative staging is to assess local tumor extent and important local anatomy to enable the surgeon to evaluate the feasibility of any surgical procedure. In general, benign bone tumors may be treated adequately by curettage or a marginal excision. Malignant tumors require either wide or radical removal, either an amputation or an en bloc procedure.

LIMB-SPARING SURGERY

Limb-salvage surgery is a safe operation in selected individuals (Fig. 42-7).[23-36,119-121] This technique may be used for all spindle-cell sarcomas, regardless of histogenesis. Between 30% and 80% of individuals with osteosarcoma can be treated successfully with this technique.[24,26,28,32,39,118] The

TABLE 42-4. Relationship of Surgical Procedure, Plane of Dissection, and Residual Disease for Musculoskeletal Tumors

Type	*Plane of Dissection*	*Result*
Intralesional	Piecemeal debulking or curettage	Leaves macroscopic disease
Marginal	Shell out en bloc through pseudocapsule or reactive zone	May leave either "satellite" or "skip" lesions
Wide	Intracompartmental en bloc with cuff of normal tissue	May leave "skip" lesions
Radical	Extracompartmental en bloc, entire compartment	No residual

Enneking WF, Spanier SS, Goodman MA: A system for the surgical staging of musculoskeletal sarcoma. Clin Orthop 153:106–120, 1980.

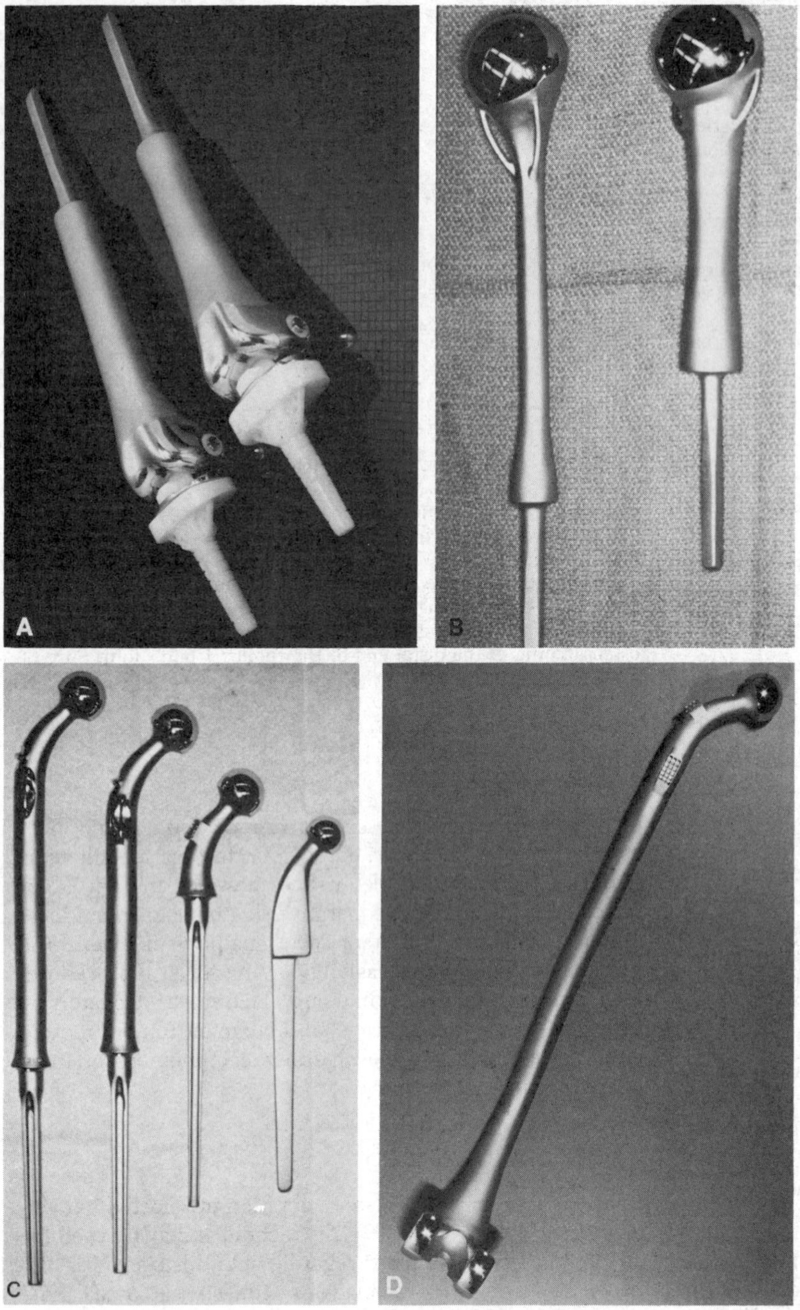

FIG. 42-8. Prostheses used in selective patients for skeletal reconstruction when a limb-sparing procedure has been performed. Different length replacements are necessary to reconstruct the various resection defects. **A**. Segmental distal femoral replacements with a total knee component. **B**. Segmental proximal humeral replacements. **C**. Segmental proximal femoral replacements. **D**. Total femoral replacement.

successful management of localized sarcomas requires careful coordination of staging studies, biopsy, surgery, and preoperative and postoperative chemotherapy or radiation therapy.

Successful limb-sparing procedures consist of three surgical phases (see Fig. 42-5)[120]

1. *Resection of tumor:* This strictly follows the principles of oncologic surgery. Avoiding local recurrence is the criterion of success and the main determinant of the amount of bone and soft tissue to be removed.
2. *Skeletal reconstruction:* The average skeletal defect following adequate bone tumor resection measures 15 to 20 cm. Techniques of reconstruction vary and are independent of the resection, although the degree of resection may favor one technique over the other (Figs. 42-8 and 42-9).
3. *Soft-tissue and muscle transfers:* Muscle transfers are performed to cover and close the resection site and to restore motor power. Adequate skin and muscle coverage is mandatory. Distal tissue transfers are not used because of the possibility of contamination.

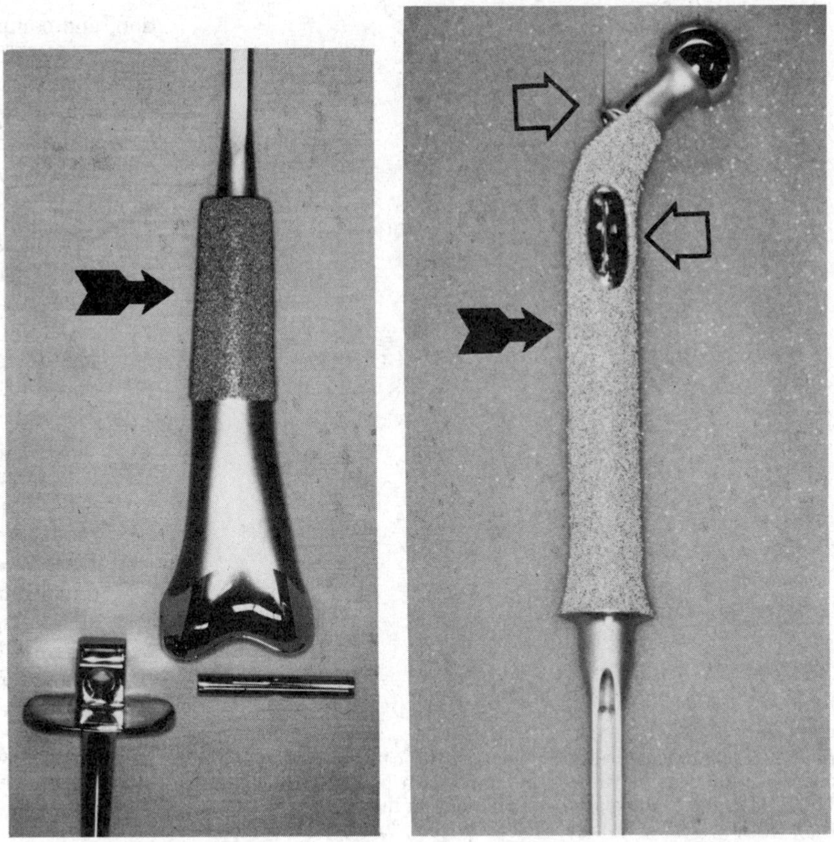

FIG. 42-9. **A**. A distal femoral replacement with a rotating-hinge knee (Kinematic) with porous coating of the segmental component. The purpose of this coating is to allow bony ingrowth into the metal in order to provide additional fixation of the prosthesis to the remaining femur and increase longevity of the prosthesis. **B**. Porous coated (*solid arrow*) segmental prosthesis of the proximal femur. Note the loops (*open arrow*) for the temporary attachment of the hip musculature. The use of biological ingrowth material at this level is for the purpose of soft tissue attachments as well as for bony ingrowth. (Courtesy of Howmedica, Inc. Rutherford, NJ).[123]

Guidelines for Limb-Sparing Resection

The guidelines and techniques of limb-sparing surgery summarized here are based on the preceding surgical maneuvers.

1. No major neurovascular tumor involvement.
2. Wide resection of the affected bone, with a normal muscle cuff in all directions.
3. En bloc removal of all previous biopsy sites and all potentially contaminated tissue.
4. Resection of bone 6 to 7 cm beyond abnormal uptake as determined by CT or MRI.
5. Resection of the adjacent joint and capsule.
6. Placement of the tourniquet proximal to the lesion, if possible.
7. Adequate motor reconstruction, accomplished by regional muscle transfers.
8. Adequate soft-tissue coverage.

Types of Skeletal Reconstruction

Large skeletal defects are reconstructed following tumor resection by several different methods. Osteoarticular defects are most often reconstructed by segmental, custom prostheses that are fixed to the remaining intramedullary bone by PMMA. The newer knee prostheses allow some rotation, as well as flexion and extension. This mobility decreases the forces on the bone–cement interface and thus lessens the risk of loosening (Fig. 42-9). Within the past few years, there has been interest in adding porous coating to the prosthesis in order to obtain biological in-growth, in the hope of obtaining long-term, perhaps even permanent, fixation (Fig. 42-9).[37,122–124] In addition, titanium, a new alloy with superior metallurgical properties, has been introduced. Most of these devices can be custom made within several weeks. In the hope of eliminating even this delay, modular systems that can be assembled in the operating room are now being evaluated.[37,122]

Alternative methods of segmental replacement include large autografts or allografts, used to obtain an arthrodesis, or osteoarticular allografts that may replace the affected joint.[33,122,124,125] Allografts placed over prostheses have been used. In general, allografts have been successful for low-grade sarcomas or giant cell tumors of bone that do not require chemotherapy or radiotherapy.

Contraindications for Limb-Sparing Surgery

1. *Major neurovascular involvement:* Although vascular grafts may be used, the adjacent nerves are usually at risk, making successful resection less likely. In addition, the magnitude of resection in combination with vascular reconstruction is often prohibitive.

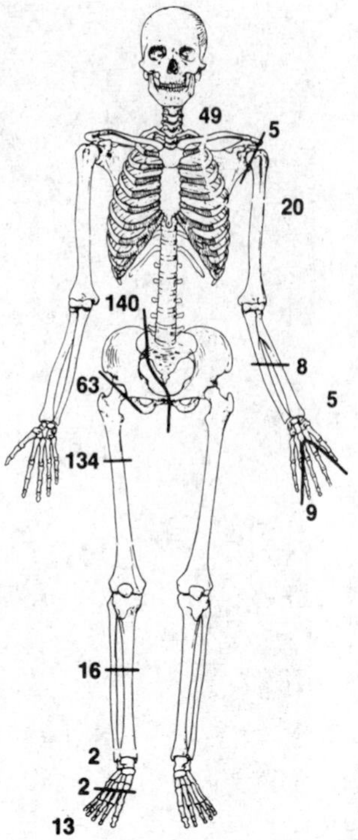

FIG. 42-10. Surgical levels of amputation for cancer (NIH experience) in 466 patients treated by amputation between 1954 and 1986. (Malawer MM, Baker A: Amputations for tumor. In Evarts CM (ed): Surgery of the musculoskeletal system, 2nd ed. New York, Churchill Livingstone [in press])[128]

2. *Pathologic fractures:* A fracture through a bone affected by a tumor spreads tumor cells by the hematoma beyond accurately determined limits. The risk of local recurrence increases under such circumstances (Fig. 42-10).
3. *Inappropriate biopsy sites:* An inappropriate or poorly planned biopsy jeopardizes local tumor control by contaminating normal tissue planes and compartments.
4. *Infection:* The risk of infection following implantation of a metallic device or allograft in an infected area is prohibitive. Sepsis jeopardizes the effectiveness of adjuvant chemotherapy.
5. *Immature skeletal age:* The predicted leg length discrepancy should not be greater than 6 to 8 cm. Upper-extremity reconstruction does not depend on skeletal maturity.
6. *Extensive muscle involvement:* There must be enough muscle remaining to reconstruct a functional extremity.

Evaluation of Limb-Sparing Procedures

A comprehensive and reliable evaluation schema and rating system of limb-sparing procedures has recently been developed.[126,127] The system sets forth six primary factors that depend on the unique considerations of major functional anatomical regions. The primary factors are motion, pain, stability/deformity, strength, emotional acceptance/function, and complications. Extensive analysis using these criteria was performed on all 1323 patients presented at the Third International Symposium on Limb Salvage. The mean follow-up of these patients was 47.8 months. The most common tumors were osteosarcoma, chondrosarcoma, and giant cell tumor, together comprising 70% of all tumors in these patients. The functional results are summarized:

1. *Periacetabular pelvic resections:* "Internal hemipelvectomy" had a higher recurrence rate than resection in other anatomic regions. Arthrodesis of the femur to the ilium produced the best results. Prosthetic and allograft reconstruction had an extremely high incidence of complications, especially infection.
2. *Modular versus customized devices:* There were no significant differences in the functional results of modular or customized prostheses. A significant problem with both systems was the lack of soft-tissue reattachments.
3. *Resections about the knee:* There were no overall functional differences between arthrodesis, osteoarticular allografts, prosthetic arthroplasty, and rotationplasty. All were better than a prosthetic limb after an above-knee amputation. Each, however, had unique limitations that were not reflected in the overall ratings.

Based on this experience, this system has been modified and will continue to be evaluated at international symposia.

AMPUTATIONS

An amputation provides definitive surgical treatment in patients in whom a limb-sparing resection is not a prudent option. A significant number of patients still require amputation, despite the advent of limb-sparing surgery. Amputations for cancer, in contrast to those performed for other causes, tend to be at a higher (more proximal) anatomical level, to occur in younger people (reflecting the incidence of bone sarcomas), and to be technically more difficult.[128] The resultant psychological and cosmetic losses are also more substantial. Figure 42-10 describes the amputation experience of the National Cancer Institute over the past 30 years; 89% of these procedures were done for sarcomas.[128] Fifty-five percent of the lower-extremity amputations were either hip disarticulations or hemipelvectomies. One half of the upper-extremity amputations were interscalpulothoracic (forequarter) resections. Osteosarcoma accounted for 33% of all amputations. Large lesions around the pelvis or proximal femur usually require amputation, but most sarcomas of the shoulder girdle and knee can now be resected. Amputation techniques are well-described elsewhere.

CRYOSURGERY

Cryosurgery is the use of liquid nitrogen at −196°C following curettage of a tumor cavity in order to kill the remaining tumor cells.[115–117,129–132] Necrosis occurs between −20°C and −40°C.[128] In general, a double freeze and thaw cycle is required (Fig. 42-11). The aim of this technique is to enhance local tumor control following a careful curettage and thus avoid resection of the involved bone. Cryosurgery was

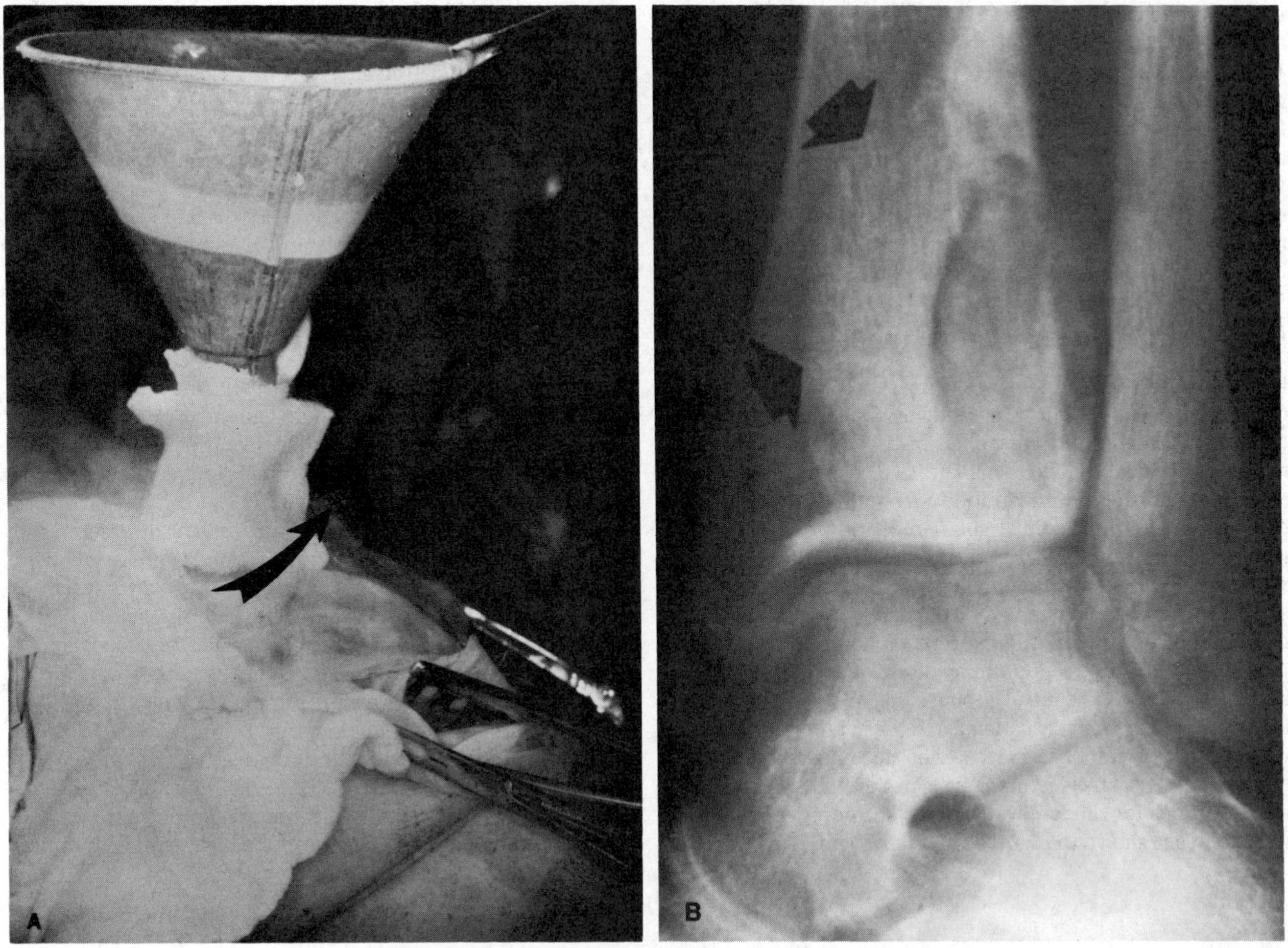

FIG. 42-11. Cryosurgery. **A**. An intraoperative photograph demonstrating the direct-pour method of cryosurgery developed by Marcove at Memorial Sloan-Kettering for aggressive and low grade malignant tumors of bone. After thorough curettage of the lesion, liquid nitrogen is poured directly into the cavity through the funnel. This assures complete contact of the liquid nitrogen with the walls of the cavity in order to kill any remaining tumor cells. The temperature of the freeze is monitored by thermocoules (*arrow*); −20°C to −40°C is necessary for cryonecrosis. **B**. Giant cell tumor of the distal tibia treated by curettage, cryosurgery, and bone graft. Radiograpy at 18 months demonstrates the typical halo effect (*arrows*) of liquid nitrogen. This area of increased sclerosis represents a rim of necrotic bone which indicates the extent of the original freeze. Presumably, any tumor cell remaining within the cavity or in the bony interstices following curettage were killed by the application of liquid nitrogen.

initially developed by Marcove at Memorial Hospital for the treatment of metastatic bone tumors.[115,117] Marcove has applied this technique to the treatment of aggressive benign tumors, specifically giant cell tumors, and more recently to low-grade sarcomas and chordomas.[130-132] The local recurrence rate after cryosurgery for these aggressive benign tumors has decreased from <40% to <10%.[115-117] This technique is not used for high-grade sarcomas.

CHEMOTHERAPY FOR BONE SARCOMAS

Before the advent of effective adjuvant chemotherapy, the outlook for patients with osteosarcoma was dismal. The overwhelming majority of patients who presented without evidence of metastases and were treated only with surgery ultimately developed metastases and died.[133-137] A review of the literature published in 1972 summarized experience with 1337 patients in 11 studies conducted between 1946 and 1971.[137] Approximately half of the patients developed metastatic disease—virtually always in the lung—within 6 months after surgery of the primary tumor, and more than 80% developed recurrent disease. Fewer than 20% of the patients survived 5 years. The inescapable conclusion from these studies is that 80% of patients presenting without overt metastases had microscopic subclinical metastases at the time of diagnosis. Thus, the expectation that fewer than 20% of patients would survive beyond 5 years appeared to be reasonable; this expectation served as the background for trials of adjuvant chemotherapy conducted in the 1970s and 1980s. By the late 1970s, the prognosis for patients with osteosarcoma was improving, and this improvement was largely attributed to the beneficial effects of adjuvant chemotherapy. However, investigators from the Mayo Clinic and elsewhere challenged the apparent contribution of adjuvant chemotherapy, reporting that the prognoses of patients diagnosed and treated with or without adjuvant therapy at that institution had apparently improved over time.[138-144]

MULTI-INSTITUTIONAL OSTEOSARCOMA STUDY

In an effort to resolve the controversy over adjuvant therapy of osteosarcoma, the Multi-Institutional Osteosarcoma Study (MIOS), a randomized controlled trial, was conducted between 1982 and 1984.[89,90] The objective of this study was to determine if the administration of multiagent adjuvant chemotherapy after surgical ablation of the primary tumor would significantly improve the relapse-free survival and survival for patients with nonmetastatic osteosarcoma of the extremity compared with a concurrent, nonadjuvantly treated control group. Patients were randomized to receive intensive multiagent chemotherapy for 1 year or assigned to an observation-only control group (Fig. 42-12). The study included 36 randomized patients and 77 additional patients who declined randomization but who accepted therapy according to one of the treatment arms of the study. Event-free survival times for randomized patients according to assigned treatment are shown in Figure 42-13A. In Figure 42-13B, the event-free survivals according to treatment for nonrandomized patients are superimposed upon those for randomized patients. The event-free survivals of all patients in the control group of this trial, who were treated only with surgery of the primary tumor, recapitulated the historical experience before 1970; more than half of these patients developed metastases within 6 months of diagnosis, and more than 80% of these patients developed recurrent disease within 2 years of diagnosis. The life tables from the observation groups of the MISO are superimposable on the historical control curves generated at many institutions before the 1970s. However, the projected disease-free survivals for patients treated with adjuvant chemotherapy in the MIOS was 64% at 2 years and 60% at 4 years—virtually the same whether randomized or nonrandomized patients are considered. Among the randomized patients, the disease-free survival advantage for patients treated with immediate adjuvant chemotherapy after surgery is highly significant.

Virtually all patients developing recurrent disease on the observation arm of the MIOS were treated aggressively with surgical metastasectomy and chemotherapy after relapse. This resulted in a remarkable prolongation of survival after relapse and the apparent cure of a substantial proportion of these patients. The overall survival for patients on the MIOS is not yet certain, but with a maximum follow-up of close to 5 years, no difference in overall survival according to treatment can yet be demonstrated among the randomized patients. However, if randomized and nonrandomized patients are pooled according to the treatment administered, a trend favoring a survival advantage for patients treated with imme-

FIG. 42-12. Chemotherapy regimen of the Multi-Institutional Osteosarcoma Study. Adjuvant chemotherapy is begun 2 weeks after definitive surgery of the primary tumor. (Link M, et al: The effect of adjuvant chemotherapy on relapse-free survival in patients with osteosarcoma of the extremity. N Engl J Med 314:1600–1606, 1986)

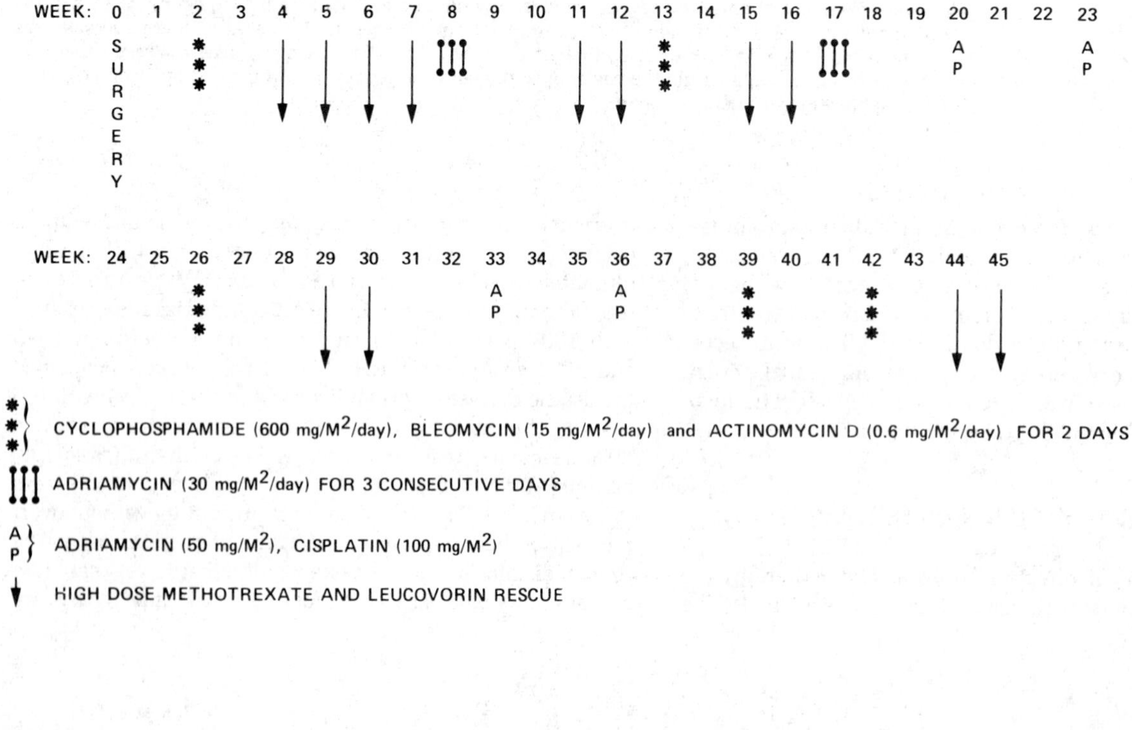

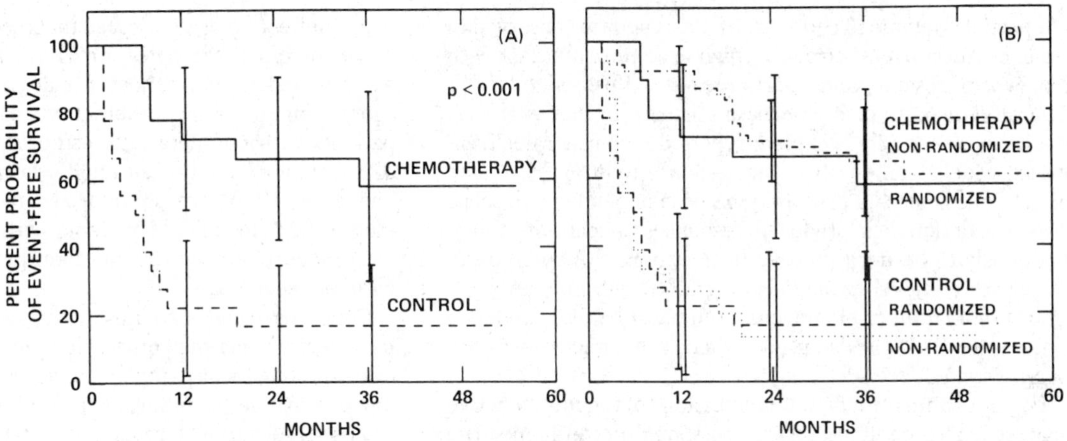

FIG. 42-13. Results from the Multi-Institutional Osteosarcoma Study. **A.** Life table analysis of event-free survival after surgery for patients accepting randomization. The difference in event-free survival is significant ($p < 0.001$). **B.** Life tables of event-free survival for patients declining randomization but electing therapy according to one of the study treatments superimposed on the life tables for patients accepting randomization. Ninety-five percent confidence intervals at 1, 2, and 3 years are shown for all life tables.

diate adjuvant chemotherapy is apparent. Comparable results were obtained in a similar randomized study conducted at UCLA where only 20% of patients treated without postoperative adjuvant chemotherapy survived without recurrence, compared with 55% of patients surviving relapse-free in the group receiving postoperative chemotherapy.[91]

It is apparent that the natural history of osteosarcoma has not changed in the past two decades, because fewer than 20% of patients treated only with surgery of the primary tumor can be expected to survive relapse-free. The bleak historical experience that served as the background for many uncontrolled adjuvant trials in the 1970s appears to be equally valid as a control for studies in the 1980s and beyond. Microscopic, subclinical metastatic disease can be presumed to exist in virtually all patients at the time of diagnosis. Although the more favorable results from the Mayo Clinic for patients treated without adjuvant chemotherapy remain unexplained, it is apparent from the MIOS and UCLA studies that the administration of adjuvant chemotherapy has a significant favorable influence on survival and should be recommended for all osteosarcoma patients.

ADJUVANT CHEMOTHERAPY

The rationale for adjuvant chemotherapy of osteosarcoma is derived from experimental evidence that microscopic metastatic disease can be eradicated if the treatment is initiated when the total body burden of metastatic tumor is sufficiently low.[145-149] The strategy of adjuvant chemotherapy after surgical removal of the primary tumor has been applied successfully in the management of other childhood tumors, but osteosarcoma is a relatively drug-resistant neoplasm, and results of studies of the activity of single agents and drugs in combination against macroscopic osteosarcoma have been disappointing (Table 42-5). Few drugs have produced responses in more than 15% of patients, and most responses

TABLE 42-5. Representative Studies Pooled Data for Single-Agent Chemotherapy Response in Overt, Primary or Metastatic Osteosarcoma

Agent	*Responders/Evaluable Patients*	*% PR + CR**
Cyclophosphamide	4/28	15
Melphalan (L-PAM)	5/32	15
Mitomycin C	3/23	13
Vincristine/vinblastine	0/21	0
Uracil mustard	0/10	0
Hydroxyurea	0/10	0
Procarbazine	0/10	0
DTIC	2/14	14
Adriamycin	28/109	26
5-Fluorouracil (5-FU)	0/11	0
Cisplatin	8/24	33
Dactinomycin	4/26	15
Methotrexate	0/14	0
High-dose methotrexate plus vincristine and leucovorin		
Every 3 weeks	11/26	42
Every week	9/11	82†
Ifosfamide	6/18	33

Adapted with permission from Bode U, Levine AS: The biology and management of osteosarcoma. In Levine AS (ed): Cancer in the Young, pp 575–602. New York, Masson Publishing USA, 1982.

* PR = partial response; CR = complete response. CR is less than 10% of total response rate in all major trials.

† May include some patients who concurrently received surgery or coned-down radiation to metastases.

are partial. Notable exceptions are the responses observed in trials of Adriamycin, cisplatin, high-dose methotrexate with leucovorin rescue, and more recently, ifosfamide.[150–157a] The effectiveness of high-dose methotrexate, however, has not been universally accepted; reported response rates have varied widely, ranging from no response to 80%.[155–158] The effectiveness of this drug may be dose-dependent, because dose escalation has produced responses in patients found previously to be unresponsive to treatment.[93] A steep dose-response relationship may also pertain to Adriamycin.[150,159] The combination of bleomycin, cyclophosphamide, and dactinomycin (BCD) is also used, although its effectiveness has been disputed.[160]

Logic dictates that the application of agents inactive against macroscopic osteosarcoma should not influence the natural history of this disease. Experimental evidence, however, suggests that eradication of microscopic metastases is possible, even with drugs that are marginally effective or even ineffective against gross macroscopic tumors.[145–149,161] Nevertheless, the hopeless prognosis for patients with osteosarcoma led to the enthusiastic application of the available agents, singly or in combination, as adjuvant therapy for patients with nonmetastatic osteosarcoma. Results of some of the important adjuvant chemotherapy trials of the 1970s and early 1980s are summarized in Table 42-6. Approximately 60% to 65% of patients with osteosarcoma treated with modern adjuvant chemotherapy regimens will survive without recurrence.

Concerns have been raised that adjuvant chemotherapy for osteosarcoma may only delay, not prevent relapse. However, the results of many of the adjuvant studies reported in Table 42-6, some followed beyond 10 years, suggest that relapse-free survival rates have stable plateaus beyond 4 years and that relapses after 3 years are infrequent. The majority of patients surviving 3 years without evidence of recurrence are probably cured. The favorable impact of post-

TABLE 42-6. Reported Results of Representative Trials of Adjuvant Chemotherapy for Osteosarcoma

*Adjuvant Regimen**	Investigators	No. of Patients	% Relapse-Free	References
HDMTX, VCR (Study I)	DFCI	12	42	(94,224–226)
HDMTX, VCR + BOG†	NCI	39	38	(227, 228)
ADRIA	CALGB	88	39	(159,229,230)
ADRIA + HDMTX†	CALGB	62	50	(231,235b)
ADRIA + HDMTX (Study II)	DFCI	22	59	(94,225,226)
ADRIA + VCR + (weekly) (Study III)	DFCI	46	60	(94,95,225,226)
ADRIA + VCR + (HDMTX or IDMTX)	CCSG	166	38	(232,235b)
CONPADRI I (CTX, VCR, ADRIA, PAM, HDMTX)	SWOG	43	49	(233–235)
COMPADRI II (CTX, VCR, ADRIA, PAM, HDMTX)	SWOG	53	35	(234,235)
COMPADRI III (CTX, VCR, ADRIA, PAM, HDMTX)	SWOG	84	38	(234,235)
ADRIA + HDMTX + CTX	Stanford	29	47 (2 year) 13 (4 year)	(236)
ADRIA + HDMTX + CTX (OSTEO 72)	St. Jude	26	50	(237,238)
ADRIA + HDMTX + CTX (OSTEO 77)	St. Jude	51	51	(238)
ADRIA + CDDP	Roswell Park	22	64	(96,239)
HDMTX + VCR or no adjuvant therapy‡	Mayo Clinic	38	40 (chemotherapy) 44 (no chemotherapy)	(144)
BCD + HDMTX + ADRIA + CDDP or no adjuvant therapy§	MIOS	36 randomized 77 nonrandomized	64 (chemotherapy) 17 (no chemotherapy)	(89,90)
BCD + HDMTX + VCR + ADRIA (+intra-arterial ADRIA + XRT) or no adjuvant therapy	UCLA	59	55 (chemotherapy) 20 (no chemotherapy)	(91)
Whole-lung irradiation 2000 rad or no adjuvant treatment‖	EORTC	86	43 (with treatment) 28 (without treatment)	(143,240,241)
Whole-lung irradiation (+Dactinomycin) or no adjuvant treatment†	Mayo Clinic	53	40	(14)
HDMTX + VCR + ADRIA + CTX (T4–T5 pooled)	MSKCC	52 (under 21 years)	48	(97,162,163)

Adapted with permission from Link, MP: Adjuvant therapy in the treatment of osteosarcoma. In DeVita VT, Hellman S, Rosenberg SA (eds): Important Advances in Oncology 1986, pp 193–207. Philadelphia, J. B. Lippincott, 1986.

*Abbreviations: HDMTX = high-dose methotrexate (5 g/m² or more) + leucovorin rescue; VCR = vincristine; BCG = bacillus Calmette-Guerin; ADRIA = Adriamycin; IDMTX = intermediate-dose methotrexate (750 mg/m²) + leucovorin rescue; CTX = cyclophosphamide; PAM = phenylalanine mustard; CDDP = cisplatin; DFCI = Dana-Farber Cancer Institute; NCI = National Cancer Institute; CALGB = Cancer and Acute Leukemia Group B; CCSG = Children's Cancer Study Group; SWOG = Southwest Oncology Group; MIOS = Multi-Institutional Osteosarcoma Study; UCLA = University of California, Los Angeles; EORTC = European Organization for Research on Treatment of Cancer; MSKCC = Memorial Sloan-Kettering Cancer Center.

†Randomized study; no significant difference in relapse-free survival for patients on each treatment arm of study.

‡Randomized study; no significant difference in relapse-free survival for patients receiving or not receiving adjuvant HDMTX.

§Randomized study; difference in results of treatments highly significant ($p < 0.01$).

‖Randomized study; difference in results of treatment significant at 6% level.

operative adjuvant chemotherapy on the natural history of osteosarcoma is incontrovertible. Adjuvant therapy should be a component of treatment for all patients with this disease.

PRESURGICAL CHEMOTHERAPY

Presurgical chemotherapy has been used with increasing frequency during the past decade in the management of osteosarcoma. This strategy evolved concurrently with limb-sparing procedures. Initial attempts at limb salvage at the Memorial Sloan-Kettering Cancer Center in 1973 involved the fabrication of customized endoprostheses for select patients undergoing en bloc resection. While the prosthesis was being made, a process requiring up to 3 months, chemotherapy was administered to prevent tumor progression.[162] Retrospectively, patients treated with presurgical chemotherapy fared better than did patients treated during the same period with immediate surgery and postoperative adjuvant therapy.[163] Upon histologic evaluation, the response to preoperative chemotherapy by the tumor was found to be a powerful prognostic factor; unfavorable responders were likely to develop distant metastases, despite continued use of chemotherapy after surgery.[164] The prognostic significance of tumor response to preoperative chemotherapy was confirmed in a study (COSS-80) conducted by the German Society for Pediatric Oncology (GPO).[98,165] Patients at high risk for recurrent disease could be identified early in treatment based on the poor response of the primary tumor to presurgical chemotherapy.

Although the initial impetus for presurgical chemotherapy was limb salvage, several theoretical advantages of presurgical chemotherapy apply to all patients with osteosarcoma (Table 42-7).[163] Because chemotherapy is administered very soon after biopsy and diagnosis, treatment of the micrometastases known to be present in the majority of patients can be instituted early. This offers a substantial advantage over the traditional adjuvant approach, in which the administration of systemic chemotherapy is delayed by a month or more for surgery and wound healing. Earlier administration of systemic treatment may reduce the emergence of drug-resistant cells in the micrometastases.[166,167] For the surgeon, presurgical chemotherapy has some advantages, because it allows time for fabrication of prostheses and may effect a reduction of bulky tumors, thereby increasing the feasibility of limb-salvage surgery in select patients.

TABLE 42-7. Considerations for Presurgical and Postsurgical Chemotherapy Regimens

Timing of Chemotherapy	*Advantages*	*Disadvantages*
Preoperative Chemotherapy	Early institution of systemic therapy against micrometastases	High tumor burden (not optimal for first-order kinetics)
	Reduced chance of spontaneous emergence of drug-resistant clones in micrometastases	Increased probability of the selection of drug-resistant cells in primary tumor, which may metastasize
	Reduction in tumor size, increasing the change of limb salvage	Delay in definitive control of bulk disease; increased chance for systemic dissemination
	Provides time for fabrication of customized endoprosthesis	
	Less chance of viable tumor being spread at the time of surgery	Psychological trauma of retaining tumor
	Individual response to chemotherapy allows selection of different risk groups.	Risk of local tumor progression with loss of a limb-sparing option
Postsurgical Chemotherapy	Radical removal of bulk tumor decreases tumor burden and increases growth rate of residual disease, making S-phase-specific agents more active and optimizing conditions for first-order kinetics.	Delay of systemic therapy for micrometastases No preoperative in vivo assay of cytotoxic response
	Decreased probability of selecting a drug-resistant clone in the primary tumor	Possible spread of viable tumor by surgical manipulation

TABLE 42-8. Histologic Grading of the Effect of Preoperative Chemotherapy on Primary Osteosarcoma

Grade	*Effect*
I	Little or no effect identified
II	Areas of acellular tumor osteoid, necrotic, or fibrotic material attributable to the effect of chemotherapy, with other areas of histologically viable tumor
III	Predominant areas of acellular tumor osteoid, necrotic, or fibrotic material attributable to the effect of chemotherapy with only scattered foci of histologically viable tumor cells identified
IV	No histologic evidence of viable tumor identified within the entire specimen

Reproduced with permission from Rosen G et al: Primary osteogenic sarcoma: Eight-year experience with adjuvant chemotherapy. J Cancer Res Clin Oncol (Suppl) 106:55–67, 1983.

ASSESSMENT OF TUMOR RESPONSE

Assessment of the response of primary tumors has been based on clinical and radiographic data; however, the histologic appearance of the resected tumor specimen after presurgical chemotherapy has emerged as the standard for measuring response.[90,97,164,168–170] Several systems for grading the effect of preoperative chemotherapy have been proposed, all of which are based on the degree of cellularity and necrosis in the resected specimen. The grading system designed at Memorial Hospital by Huvos has been used widely (Table 42-8).[97,164] Grade III and IV responses (>95% and 100% necrosis, respectively), indicating extensive to complete response in the primary tumor, are considered favorable. Grade I and II responses (<50% and 50–95%, respectively), indicating minimal destruction of the tumor, are unfavorable (Fig. 42-14). The grading system used by the GPO identifies six categories of response.[168] In the COSS-80 study, favorable response was defined as greater than 50% tumor destruction after presurgical chemotherapy; however,

FIG. 42-14. Two histologic effects of preoperative chemotherapy. **A.** An H & E section demonstrating a typical high-grade osteosarcoma (×200). Note the typical osteoid (*solid curved arrows*) being made by malignant stroma cells (*open arrow*). **B.** Photomicrograph demonstrating complete tumor cell necrosis. There are no viable cells remaining in this section; the lacunae are empty, and only the extracellular matrix (osteoid and tumor bone) remains. Osteosarcomas may not shrink much despite complete necrosis due to the persistence of their extracellular matrix.

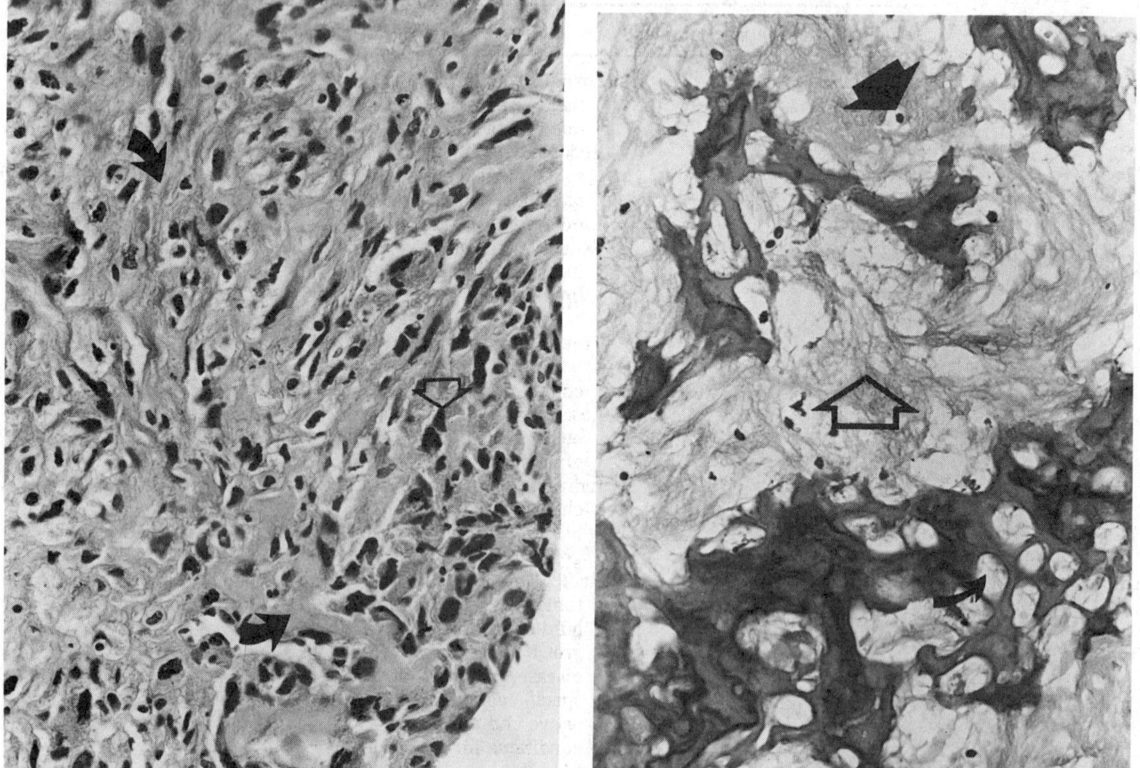

A B

in more recent GPO studies, 90% destruction is required.[90] The grading system used at M.D. Anderson Hospital divides response into three categories: no effect or doubtful effect with less than 40% tumor necrosis; partial effect with 40% to 60% tumor destruction; and definite effect, in which more than 60% of the tumor is destroyed and fibrovascular regeneration is present.[169]

Grading systems are necessarily imprecise and subject to sampling errors. However, with scrupulous attention to adequate sectioning from many sites of the surgical specimen, the degree of response can be reliably assessed.

TAILORING POSTOPERATIVE CHEMOTHERAPY

The use of presurgical chemotherapy to customize the postoperative adjuvant therapy, based on the response of the primary tumor as determined by histologic examination, is called *tailoring.*[170] This strategy was pioneered at the Memorial Hospital in the T-10 protocol (Fig. 42-15).[97,171] Patients were treated preoperatively with high-dose methotrexate, the BCD combination, and Adriamycin. Those with favorable (Grades III and IV) histologic responses continued to receive the same agents postoperatively (T-10B regimen). Patients demonstrating unfavorable (Grades I and II) histologic responses were treated on regimen T-10A, consisting of Adriamycin and cisplatin along with the BCD combination (without high-dose methotrexate) postoperatively (Fig. 42-15). Although only 39% of patients achieved a favorable histologic response to presurgical chemotherapy (51% if only patients younger than 21 were analyzed), virtually all of the favorable responders were projected to survive free of recurrence.[97,171] The patients who initially demonstrated an unfavorable histologic response were switched to the cisplatin-containing regimen, and almost 85% were projected to remain relapse-free at 3 years. Overall, 90% of patients treated on the T-10 regimen with tailored therapy were projected to remain disease-free at 3 years. Moreover, a significant difference in outcome could no longer be detected between favorable and unfavorable responders to presurgical chemotherapy, supporting the contention that poor responders were "salvaged" by the administration of alternative chemotherapy postoperatively. The outcome for patients on the T-10 protocol is the best yet reported for the treatment of osteosarcoma. Several other trials using presurgical chemotherapy have been reported (Table 42-9).

In a recent study, the Children's Cancer Study Group (CCSG) attempted to duplicate the T-10 regimen in a multi-institutional setting. Results were not as favorable as those initially reported from Memorial Hospital; only 30% of the patients demonstrated favorable responses by the primary tumor. These patients fared extremely well; 90% were projected to remain disease-free at 2 years. Twenty-nine percent of the patients demonstrated intermediate response (50–95% necrosis). The largest group of patients (41%) had

FIG. 42-15. The T-10 regimen from the Memorial Hospital. **A**. All patients receive the initial 16-week regimen. The presurgical chemotherapy regimen features four weekly courses of high dose methotrexate and leucovorin rescue followed by resection of amputation. Patients undergoing endoprosthetic replacement receive 16 weeks of presurgical chemotherapy. **B**. Postoperative chemotherapy is determined by the histologic grade of response of the primary tumor to presurgical chemotherapy. Patients achieving an unfavorable response in the primary tumor (Grades I and II) receive T-10A regimen postoperatively, featuring Adriamycin, cisplatin, and the BCD combination. Patients achieving a favorable response (Grades III and IV) receive the T-10B regimen postoperatively and continue to receive high dose methotrexate along with Adriamycin and the BCD combination. (Rosen G, et al: Primary osteogenic sarcoma: Eight year experience with adjuvant chemotherapy. J Cancer Res Clin Oncol 106[Suppl]:55–67, 1983)

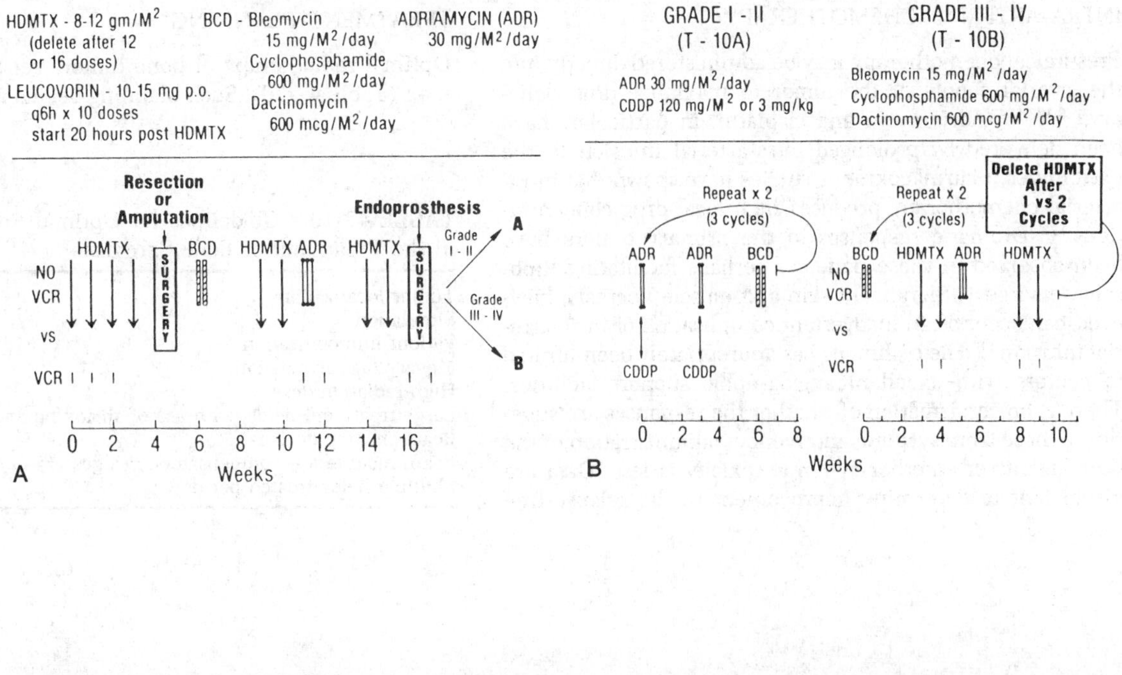

TABLE 42-9. Reported Results of Representative Trials of Presurgical Chemotherapy for Osteosarcoma

*Adjuvant Regimen**	*Investigators*	*No. of Patients*	*% Relapse-Free*	*References*
HDMTX + VCR + ADRIA + BCD (T-7)	MSKCC	55 (under 21 years)	80	97,163
HDMTX + VCR + ADRIA + BCD (depending on response) (T-10)	MSKCC	79 (under 21 years)	92	97,171
ADRIA + HDMTX + (BCD or CDDP) ± Interferon (COSS-80)†	GPO	116	68	98,165
HDMTX + ADRIA + CDDP	Mount Sinai	25	77	242
HDMTX + VCR + ADRIA + BCD + CDDP (depending on response) (CCSG-82)	CCSG	192	61	170
HDMTX + ADRIA + CDDP + IFOS (COSS-82)	GPO	125	58	99,172

* HDMTX = high-dose methotrexate (12 g/m^2 or more) + leucovorin rescue; VCR = vincristine; ADRIA = Adriamycin; CDDP = cisplatin; BCD = bleomycin, cyclophosphamide, actinomycin D combination; MSKCC = Memorial Sloan-Kettering Cancer Center; GPO = German Society of Pediatric Oncology; CCSG = Children's Cancer Study Group.

† Randomized study; no significant difference in relapse-free survival for patients on each treatment arm of study.

unfavorable responses, and only 40% of these patients survived without recurrence, despite the change in their postoperative management. The overall 61% disease-free survival rate at 2 years for patients on the CCSG study is disappointing, compared with the initial results from Memorial Hospital, and suggests that presurgical chemotherapy with tailoring of treatment based on responsiveness of the primary tumor does not lead to improved outcome. The COSS-82 trial by the GPO tested the strategy of custom tailoring therapy, and as in the CCSG trial, the results suggest that patients demonstrating poor response of the primary tumor have poor prognoses and that treatment of poor responders with salvage regimens does not improve their prognoses. Investigators of the GPO concluded that active agents (*e.g.*, cisplatin) should *not* be withheld from the initial therapy of newly diagnosed patients. Thus, the value of presurgical chemotherapy, with or without tailoring, in the treatment of osteosarcoma has not been demonstrated conclusively. A study designed to test this question is being conducted by the Pediatric Oncology Group.

INTRA-ARTERIAL CHEMOTHERAPY

Presurgical chemotherapy may be administered directly into the arterial supply of the tumor to maximize drug delivery.[169,173,174] Adriamycin and cisplatin, in particular, have been delivered by prolonged intra-arterial infusion to the extremities. Pharmacokinetic studies have shown that intra-arterial chemotherapy produces high local drug concentrations.[173] Dramatic responses in the primary tumors have been observed in these patients, perhaps facilitating limb-salvage surgery. Significant skin and muscle necrosis, however, can occur as an inadvertent complication of intra-arterial infusion.[26] The technique has appropriately been limited to centers with excellent angiographic support facilities. There is no confirmation of whether the responses are superior to those from systemic intravenous administration of the same agents or whether systemic toxicity is less. Data are insufficient to determine improvement in the relapse-free survival time and in the number of candidates suitable for limb-salvage surgery.

RADIOTHERAPY FOR BONE TUMORS

In keeping with the multidisciplinary, multimodal approach to the treatment of bone tumors, all patients should be evaluated by a radiation oncologist and by an orthopedic and medical (or pediatric) oncologist before decisions concerning therapy are made. Close communication between members of the care team is crucial. If an ablative approach is not recommended or is refused or if the tumor is judged unresectable because of its location, radiation may become the primary therapy. In addition, tumors of the axial skeleton and facial bones are treated by a combination of limited surgery and radiotherapy. The round cell tumors of bone, primary lymphoma, and Ewing's sarcoma are best managed by definitive radiation treatment; only occasionally is surgery required.

TREATMENT PLANNING

Optimal radiotherapy of bone tumors require careful planning (Table 42-10). Such planning begins with tumor locali-

TABLE 42-10. Guidelines for Optimal Radiotherapy in the Treatment of Bone Sarcomas

Tumor localization
Simulation
Patient immobilization
Megavoltage irradiation
High radiation dose
Large treatment fields, with use of shrinking and cone-down fields
Beam-shaping devices
Beam modifiers—compensators, wedges
Multiple fields treated per day

zation and accurate definition of the clinical and radiographic extent of the tumor and of all tissue at risk for microscopic involvement. Precise, three-dimensional definition is required. This evaluation is identical to that done for surgical evaluation. These composite studies are used to establish the maximal tumor dimensions.

With the clinical physicist, decisions are then made concerning the optimal choice of radiation beam (*e.g.*, photon or electron), technique (*e.g.*, external beam, brachytherapy, or intraoperative therapy), beam modifiers (*e.g.*, compensators or wedge filters), and immobilization system. All patients should undergo simulation and be treated with megavoltage therapy units. There is no role for orthovoltage (low KeV x-ray) in the management of primary tumors of bone.

Patient immobilization is essential to optimal radiotherapy. The patient should be placed in a comfortable position on the treatment table. The precise patient setup should be planned using three points for reproducibility.[174b] Immobilization devices such as casts, shells, vacuum pillows, and sandbags are frequently necessary.[175] Molding techniques that require a cast of the anatomic site to be treated are preferred when treatment fields are complex and the radiation course is lengthy.

DOSE AND VOLUME CONSIDERATIONS

Large treatment volumes that include the entire clinical and radiographic extent of tumor plus a generous margin for microscopic or subclinical extension of disease are needed. For tumors that tend to spread along the medullary canal (lymphoma, Ewing's sarcoma), the standard radiation field involves the entire bone. Investigations are under way to ascertain if it is possible to irradiate only the area of gross tumor in patients who are known to respond to multi-agent chemotherapy given before radiotherapy, on the assumption that chemotherapy can sterilize presumed microscopic disease.[175a] If large fields are needed, it is desirable to use an extended source-to-skin distance (SSD), in order to enable the entire radiation field to fit into one portal. If extended distances are not possible and two radiation fields must be abutted, it should be done through areas of microscopic, rather than gross, disease. Match lines should be routinely moved every 1000 cGy.

The irradiated field should encompass at least the same volume of tissue that would be resected, plus an allowance of approximately 2 cm for patient movement and dose fall-off at the margin of the field. Extremity fields should be planned with a strip of tissue purposely out of the beam to allow for lymphatic and venous return and to decrease morbidity. This nonirradiated strip should overlie the lymphatic drainage, which is located medially in both the lower and upper extremities.

Because high doses are often necessary in the treatment of malignant bone tumors, a shrinking field technique is advised. This allows treatment of large areas of subclinical disease with a moderate radiation dose and coning treatment of the gross tumor with a higher, sterilizing dose.

Additional principles involve using multiple beam-shaping devices so that shaped fields can be designed to conform to the individual tumor volume and patient anatomy. Multiple fields should be used to optimize the radiation dosage, and all fields must be treated every day. Beam modifiers, including compensating filters and wedge filters, should be employed to account for individual variations in patient thickness. Hyperfractionation allows the administration of higher tumor doses while protecting nearby sensitive normal structures, such as the spinal cord, from the late effects of radiotherapy.

COMPLICATIONS OF RADIATION

The complications of radiation are directly related to treatment dose and volume. Reactions occurring during the early stages of treatment are usually reversible and not of major significance. These include erythema, dry desquamation of the skin, and epilation. More serious late reactions include fibrosis, contracture, atrophy, impaired growth, secondary fracture, and radiation-induced sarcoma. Fibrosis and contracture can be minimized and possibly avoided by embarking upon an active physical therapy program during radiation therapy; such a program should be continued after radiation therapy. If possible, avoid treating across a joint space and try to avoid treating an open epiphysis. The risk of secondary fracture increases when there has been such an extensive destruction of bone that remodeling and repair do not reconstitute the affected part. For tumors of weight-bearing bones, partial weight-bearing and protective bracing are important until reossification occurs.

BENIGN BONE TUMORS

Some benign bone tumors are difficult to differentiate from their malignant counterparts. They have a significant rate of local recurrence and may undergo malignant transformation. The oncologist may be called upon to establish the correct diagnosis of a benign bone tumor or to treat local recurrence. Several benign tumors deserve special consideration in this regard.

OSTEOCHONDROMAS

Osteochondromas are the most common benign bone tumor. These tumors are characteristically sessile or pedunculated, arising from the cortex of a long tubular bone adjacent to the epiphyseal plate. Osteochondromas are usually solitary, except in patients with multiple hereditary exostosis. Plain radiographs are usually diagnostic, and no further tests are required. Sessile osteochondromas are difficult to diagnose, especially if they occur in unusual sites such as the distal posterior femur, where they must be differentiated from a parosteal osteosarcoma. Bone scintigraphy and CT are helpful in distinguishing between these two entities.

Osteochondromas "grow" with the individual until skeletal maturity is reached. Growth of an osteochondroma during adolescence therefore does not signify malignancy. Pain is not a sign of malignancy during childhood or adolescence, although in adults it is a significant warning sign. Pain in a child may be due to a local bursitis, mechanical irritation of adjacent muscles, or pathologic fracture.

Between 1% and 2% of solitary osteochondromas undergo

malignant transformation; patients with multiple hereditary exostosis are at higher risk.[2,4,56,57] Malignant tumors arising from a benign osteochondroma are usually low-grade chondrosarcomas. Proximal osteochondromas are at a higher risk to undergo malignant transformation than are distal lesions. Surgical removal is recommended only for symptomatic osteochondromas and for those arising along the axial skeleton and pelvic or shoulder girdles.

ENCHONDROMAS

Enchondromas are composed of mature hyaline cartilage that arises within a bone (Fig. 42-16). They may be solitary or multiple (Ollier's disease) and have been reported in most bones.[3,4] Their biological potential is often overestimated or underestimated. Pathologic interpretation of cartilage tumors is more difficult than for other bone tumors; it is particularly difficult to differentiate a benign enchondroma from a Grade I chondrosarcoma.[10,11,176] Malignant transformations do occur, but the rate is difficult to determine.[177] Lesions of the pelvis, femur, and ribs are generally at higher risk for malignant transformation than are lesions at more distal sites.

FIG. 42-16. Enchondroma. Typical enchondroma occurring in the diaphysis of the femur. There is minimal cortical response to the tumor without evidence of bony destruction. Endosteal scalloping (*arrow*) indicates an active lesion. The differentiation from a low grade intramedullary chondrosarcoma is based on clinical symptoms and histology as well as radiographic changes.

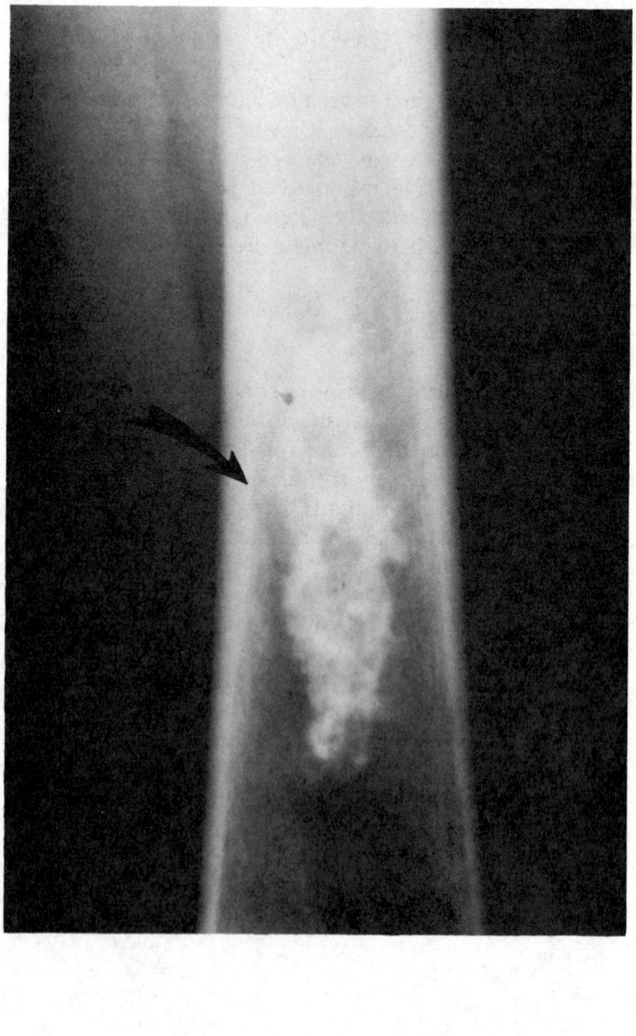

Pain is a sign of local aggressiveness and possible malignancy. Enchondromas of the hands and feet are always benign, but cartilage tumors of the pelvic or shoulder girdles are often malignant, even though the histologic results appear benign.[3] Plain radiographs may help in this differentiation. Radiographic scalloping is a sign of local aggressiveness. Bone scintigraphy is not helpful in differentiating a low-grade chondrosarcoma from an "active" enchondroma. Patient age is an important indicator of possible malignancy; enchondromas rarely undergo malignant transformation before skeletal maturity. Painful, benign-appearing proximal enchondromas in an adult are often malignant. The correlation of symptoms, plain radiographic findings, and histologic examination is crucial.

CHONDROBLASTOMA, OSTEOBLASTOMA, AND OSTEOID OSTEOMA

Chondroblastoma and osteoblastoma are characterized by immature but benign chondroid and osteoid production, respectively. Either may undergo malignant transformation in rare cases.[58,177] Osteoid osteomas are small (<1 cm), painful, bone-forming tumors that are always benign. It is essential that the oncologist is able to differentiate them from their malignant counterparts, chondrosarcoma and osteosarcoma. Chondroblastomas appear radiographically in the epiphysis of a child; conversely, primary chondrosarcomas in adults are rarely epiphyseal. Although osteoblastomas may be found in any bone, lesions in the spine and skull account for 50% of all reported cases. Osteoblastomas must be differentiated from osteosarcomas and osteoid osteoma (Fig. 42-17).

Both chondroblastomas and osteoblastomas are considered aggressive, benign lesions with a high recurrence rate following simple curettage.[2-4,177] Local control can be obtained by primary resection; however, routine resection cannot be recommended for tumors adjacent to a joint. Marcove reported 5% to 10% local recurrence rate when curettage is combined with cryosurgery.[178] This method has avoided the need for resection and extensive reconstruction in select patients. Osteoid osteomas are treated by simple excision.

ANEURYSMAL BONE CYST

Aneurysmal bone cysts (ABC) are benign tumors of children, occurring typically before skeletal maturity.[2-4] They never become malignant. ABC often involve the metaphyseal regions of the long bones or the vertebrae. Radiographically, they are eccentric, lytic, and expansile, characterized by cortical destruction and periosteal elevation (Fig. 42-18). ABC can grow rapidly and appear extremely aggressive, and differentiation from a primary malignancy may be difficult. Differential diagnosis should include giant cell tumor and telangiectatic osteosarcoma. ABC may contain some osteoid; however, careful examination reveals this to be reactive and not neoplastic. Approximately 33% of ABC arise in conjunc-

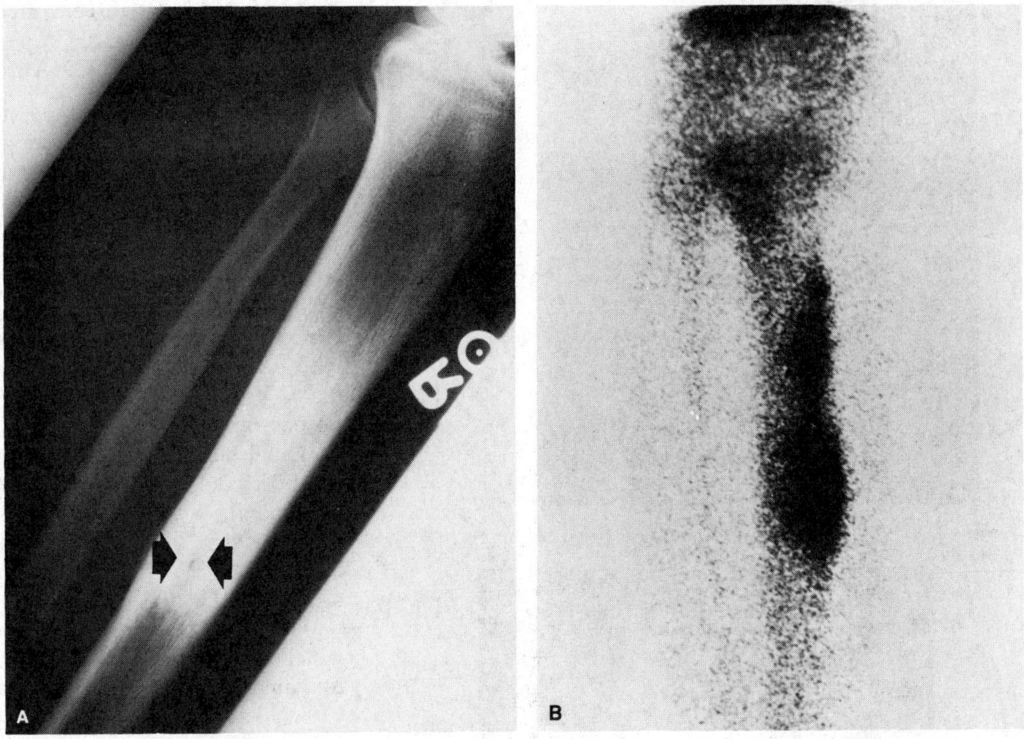

FIG. 42-17. Osteoid osteoma. **A**. Osteoid osteomas are characteristically a small lesion, represented radiographically as a small radiolucent nidus between 1 and 5 mm in diameter (*arrow*) surrounded by a large amount of reactive, that is, non-neoplastic sclerotic bone. Tomograms are often necessary to demonstrate the nidus. **B**. Bone scans will always demonstrate marked uptake that corresponds with the nidus as well as the reactive bone. The main radiologic differential is a sclerosing osteosarcoma.

tion with (*i.e.*, underlying) another bony neoplasm.[177–180] The classical treatment is simple curettage and bone graft, which has a recurrence rate of 20% to 35%.[4] Wide curettage may decrease the recurrence rate to approximately 10%. Marcove recommends curettage and cryosurgery as the primary treatment. Radiation therapy is recommended for difficult lesions of the vertebral bodies in which surgical extirpation may be hazardous for recurrent tumors and for lesions in surgically inaccessible sites.[3,180,181]

DESMOPLASTIC FIBROMA

This is an extremely rare bone tumor; only 50 cases have been reported.[177] It is characterized by abundant collagen formation and a fibrous stroma, without evidence of mitosis or pleomorphism. It presents radiographically as an osteolytic lesion with well-defined margins, and it must be differentiated from primary fibrosarcoma of bone. Treatment is en bloc resection; curettage has a significant rate of local recurrence.

HISTIOCYTOSIS X

Langerhans' cell histiocytosis is a more descriptive and recently accepted term to describe the disease commonly referred to as histiocytosis X. The solitary or multifocal osseous lesions (Greenberger Stage IA and B) were formerly referred to as eosinophilic granuloma.[182a] Histiocytosis X can be difficult to diagnose because it can radiographically mimic a primary bone malignancy.

Almost any bone can be involved. Radiographically, it appears as a lytic, destructive defect, with poorly defined margins. Periosteal elevation occurs in half of all cases. This combination of characteristics strongly resembles that of Ewing's sarcoma or osteomyelitis. If arising in a flat bone, specifically the pelvis, there may be a large soft-tissue component. For a solitary lesion arising in an extremity, curettage is usually curative.

Tumors involving the orbit, skull, or facial bones are best treated by low-dose radiotherapy in the range of 600 to 1000 cGy.[181–184] Local recurrences have been reported following 450 cGy, but they are rare following 600 cGy.[182] Megavoltage equipment should be used. Specific indications for radiation therapy are lesions of the gingiva, mandible and maxilla; diabetes insipidus; local recurrence following surgery; and lesions located in inaccessible sites. Vertebral body lesions do not require treatment unless they are symptomatic. Lesions of the mastoid respond less well to radiotherapy alone and therefore are best treated by curettage and postoperative radiotherapy.

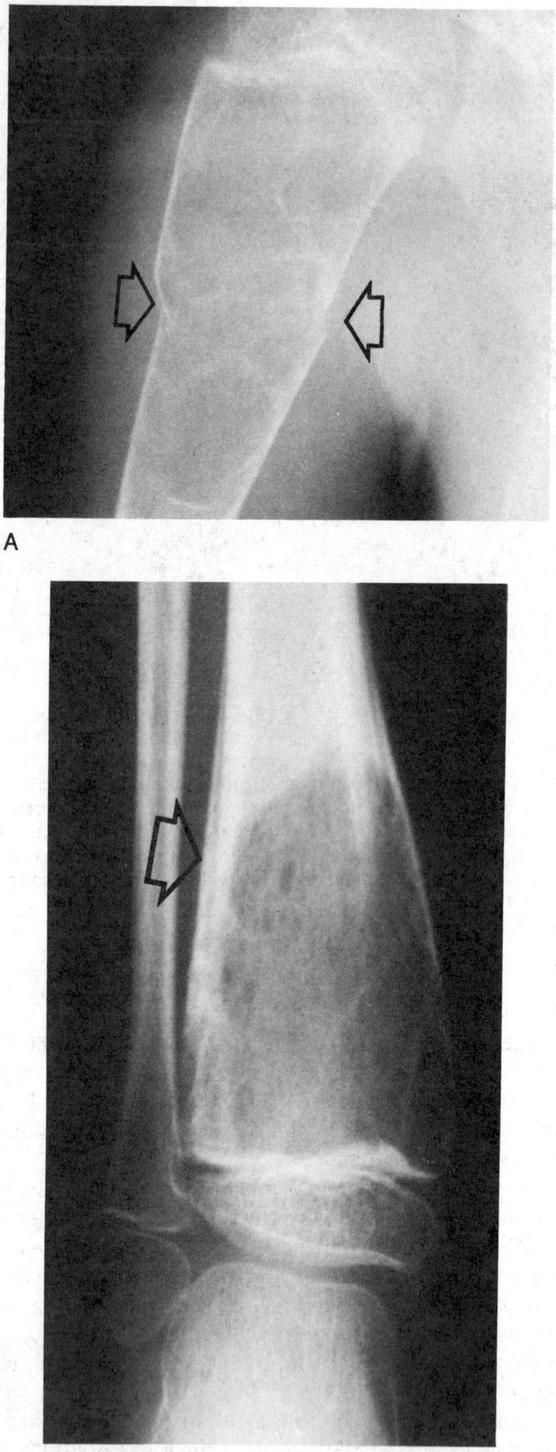

FIG. 42-18. **A.** Unicameral bone cyst of the proximal humerus. Unicameral bone cysts are radiolucent lesions occurring in the metaphysis or diaphysis of long bones. There is no evidence of matrix formation, and unicameral bone cysts are rarely expansile. The majority of unicameral bone cysts present with a small fracture (*arrow*); otherwise they tend to be asymptomatic. The proximal humerus is the most common site. **B.** Aneurysmal bone cyst. Aneurysmal bone cysts are eccentric, expansile lesions occurring in the metaphysis of a long tubular bone and occasionally in a flat bone. Note the sclerotic well-defined border denoting a benign lesion. The main differential diagnosis is a giant cell tumor.

MALIGNANT BONE TUMORS

CLASSIC OSTEOSARCOMA

Osteosarcoma is a high-grade, malignant spindle-cell tumor arising within a bone. Its distinguishing characteristic is the production of tumor osteoid or immature bone directly from a malignant spindle-cell stroma.[2,3,59,183]

Clinical Characteristics

Osteosarcoma typically occurs during childhood and adolescence. In patients older than 40 years, it is usually associated with a preexistent condition, such as Paget's disease, irradiated bones, multiple hereditary exostosis, or polyostotic fibrous dysplasia.[2,183–186] Bones of the knee joint and the proximal humerus are the most common sites, accounting for 50% and 25%, respectively, off all osteosarcoma.[177] In general, 80% to 90% of osteosarcomas occur in the long tubular bones; the axial skeleton is rarely affected.[2,4,56,184,187,188,188a] Less than 1% are found in the hands and feet.[2]

With the exception of serum alkaline phosphatase levels, which are elevated in 45% to 50% of these patients, laboratory findings are usually not helpful.[187] Furthermore, elevated alkaline phosphatase per se is not diagnostic, because it is also found in association with other skeletal diseases. Pain is the most common complaint. Physical examination demonstrates slight tenderness and a firm soft-tissue mass fixed to the underlying bone. There is no effusion in the adjacent joint, and motion is normal. Incidence of pathologic fracture is less than 1%, and systemic symptoms are rare.

Radiographic Characteristics

Typical findings are increased intramedullary radiodensity (tumor bone or calcified cartilage), an area of radiolucency (nonossified tumor), a pattern of permeative destruction with poorly defined borders, cortical destruction, periosteal elevation, and extraosseous extension with soft-tissue ossification.[187,188,188a] This combination of characteristics is not seen in any other lesion. Wilner classified 600 radiographs of osteosarcoma seen at Memorial Sloan-Kettering into three broad categories: sclerotic (32%), osteolytic (22%), and mixed (46%) (Fig. 42-19).[188a] Though there was no statistically significant difference among overall survival rates among these types, the patterns are important to recognize. The sclerotic and mixed type offer few diagnostic problems. Errors of diagnosis most often occur with pure osteolytic tumors. The differential diagnosis of osteolytic osteosarcoma includes giant cell tumor, ABC, and MFH.[189] In a series of 305 patients with osteosarcomas, DeSantos and Edeiken reported that 42 (13.5%) were purely lytic.[189] Most commonly they presented as an ill-defined lesion with a moderate-to-large soft-tissue component. Nine of the lesions had benign radiographic features.

Clinical and Prognostic Considerations

Before the era of adjuvant chemotherapy, treatment consisted of amputation. Metastasis to lungs and other bones

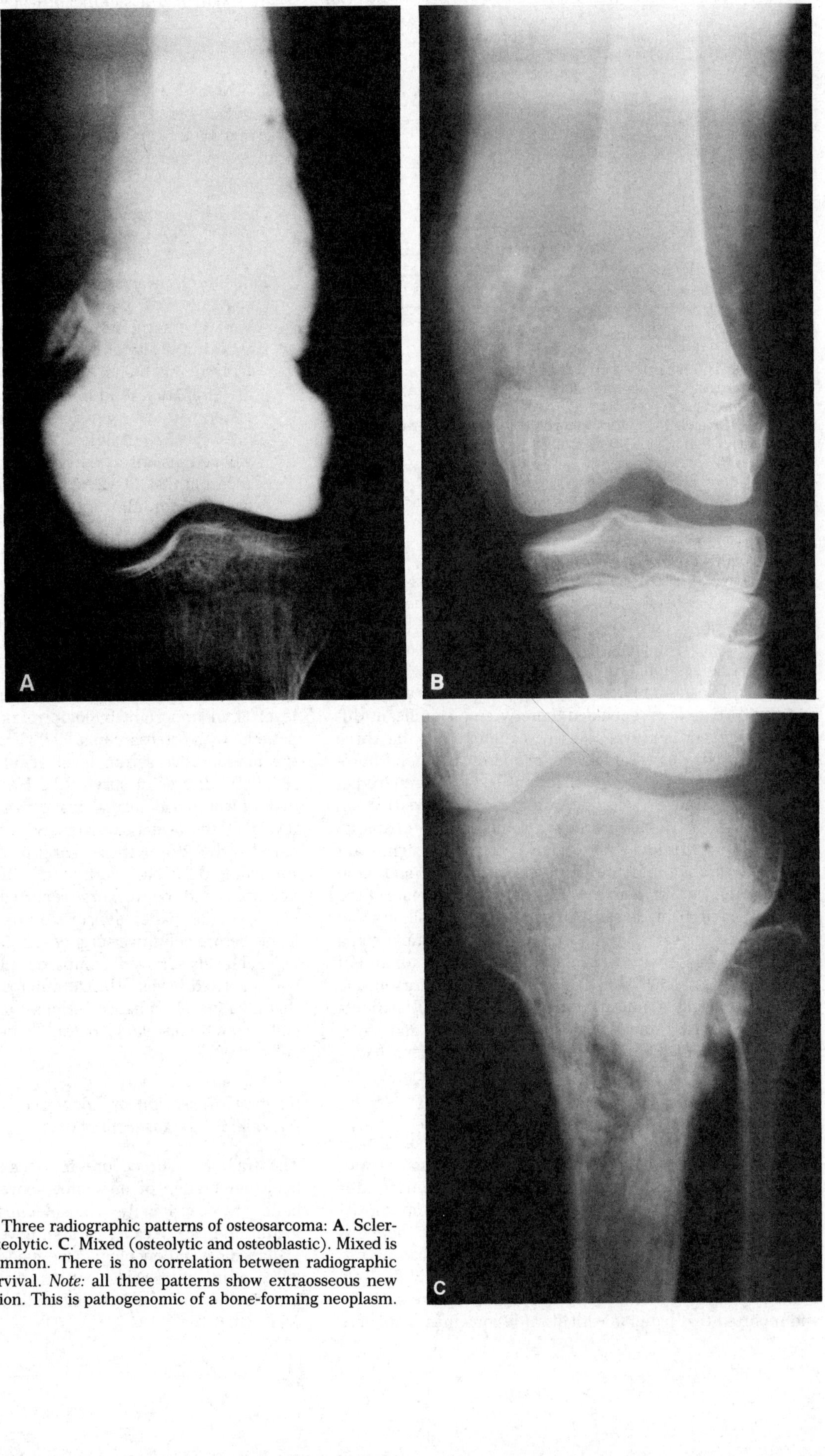

FIG. 42-19. Three radiographic patterns of osteosarcoma: **A**. Sclerosing. **B**. Osteolytic. **C**. Mixed (osteolytic and osteoblastic). Mixed is the most common. There is no correlation between radiographic type and survival. *Note:* all three patterns show extraosseous new bone formation. This is pathogenomic of a bone-forming neoplasm.

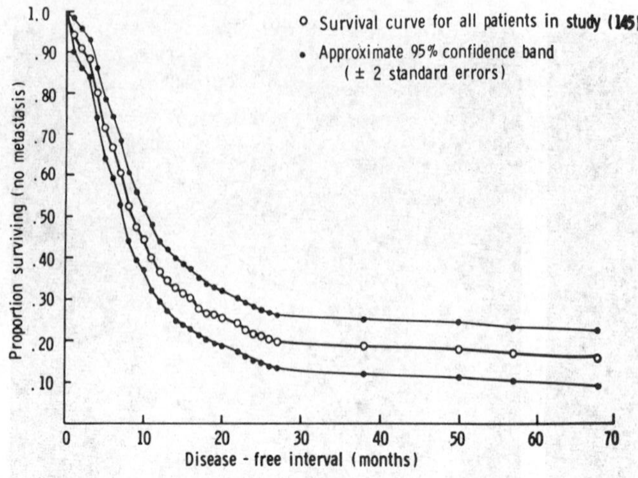

FIG. 42-20. The historical survival curve for 145 patients with osteosarcoma treated by surgery alone at Memorial-Sloan Kettering Cancer Center, as reported by Marcove and associates. (Marcove RC, Mick V, Hajek JV, et al: Osteogenic sarcoma under the age of twenty-one. J Bone Joint Surg [Am] 48:1–26, 1966)[71]

usually occurred within 24 months. Many series show an overall survival of 5% to 20% at 2 years (Fig. 42-20).[71-74] This pattern has been altered by adjuvant chemotherapy and aggressive thoracotomy for pulmonary disease.[45,101,190] Metastases may now appear at less common sites and disease-free intervals are longer.[190]

In 1968, Lockshin reviewed the experience of 100 authors during 50 years and concluded there was no significant difference between survival rates of patients with the three histogenic subtypes (osteoblastic, chondroblastic, and fibroblastic) or between those whose lesions had a different radiographic appearance (sclerotic, osteolytic, or mixed).[191] In addition, size of tumor, patient age, and degree of malignancy did not correlate with survival.[191] The most significant variable was anatomic site. Patients with pelvic and axial lesions had lower survival rates than those with tumors of the extremities, probably because of surgical inaccessibility and incomplete removal. Patients with tumors of the tibia had a significantly higher survival rate than those with tumors of the distal femur (35% and 16%, respectively). Larson and colleagues, using a multifactorial analysis of all patients from the Swedish Cancer Registry between 1958 and 1968, similarly concluded that patients with tibial lesions had a better survival rate than those with femoral lesions (38.1% and 15.1%, respectively), because the former were less advanced at the time of treatment.[192]

Marcove, reviewing 145 patients under the age of 21 who underwent surgery without adjuvant chemotherapy at Memorial Sloan-Kettering, noted no statistically significant differences with regard to race, sex, or duration of symptoms.[71] Younger patients developed metastases sooner, but this made no difference in overall survival. Location had no impact on 5-year survival. Brostrom evaluated 52 patients treated by surgery alone.[193] He studied tumor size and site and reported that patients with distal lesions measuring less than 10 cm had a significantly higher survival ($p < 0.01$) than those with proximal lesions greater than 10 cm (43% and 12%, respectively).

CHANGING PATTERN OF METASTASIS. The classic pattern and time frame of metastatic dissemination of osteosarcoma have been somewhat modified by the use of adjuvant chemotherapy and thoracotomy. These trends are summarized.

Disease-free interval: The first sign of metastatic disease may appear later than the previous median of approximately 6 months, often after 24 months.

Pulmonary metastasis: Guiliano and colleagues reported that only 47% of patients treated with surgery and adjuvant chemotherapy developed pulmonary disease as their initial site of relapse, compared with 95% treated with surgery alone.[101] Pulmonary nodules at the time of dissemination tend to be fewer, and they may be associated with a longer disease-free interval.

Extraskeletal sites: Before chemotherapy, no patients developed lesions at extrapulmonary sites first. Giuliano reported that 11 (27.5%) of 40 patients who had been treated with adjuvant chemotherapy developed extrapulmonary metastasis before pulmonary lesions, and an equal number developed pulmonary and extrapulmonary lesions simultaneously.[101] Bone involvement occurred in 14 (61%) of 23 patients with extrapulmonary lesions. The non-pulmonary sites were epidural (3), brain (2), and other (4).

ALKALINE PHOSPHATASE. Serum alkaline phosphatase level is an important biologic marker of tumor activity in patients with osteosarcoma.[194,195] Francis demonstrated that the preoperative serum level of alkaline phosphatase is a reliable indicator of survival.[187] He reviewed 155 patients, 46% of whom had normal preoperative alkaline phosphatase levels. Of the 2-year survivors, 85% had normal levels, compared with 12% of those dying of disease. Of the 10-year survivors, 93% had normal alkaline phosphatase levels. Scranton and co-workers reported similar findings; 16 (42%) of 38 patients had elevated alkaline phosphatase levels before definitive surgery; 12 (54%) of 22 patients with normal levels survived, compared with only 3 (18.7%) of 16 with elevated levels. Electronmicroscopy has demonstrated that alkaline phosphatase is found predominantly along the cell membrane and outer lamella of osteosarcoma cells.[194-196]

Surgical Resection of Localized Extremity Osteosarcoma

The traditional procedure for localized osteosarcoma has been amputation of one joint above the tumor-containing bone or, occasionally, transmedullary amputation.[2,3,71-73] Within the past decade, parallel developments in radiology, orthopedics, and oncology have made nonamputative procedures an option in select patients.[20-33] The impetus was the introduction of effective chemotherapeutic agents in the early 1970s.[47-52]

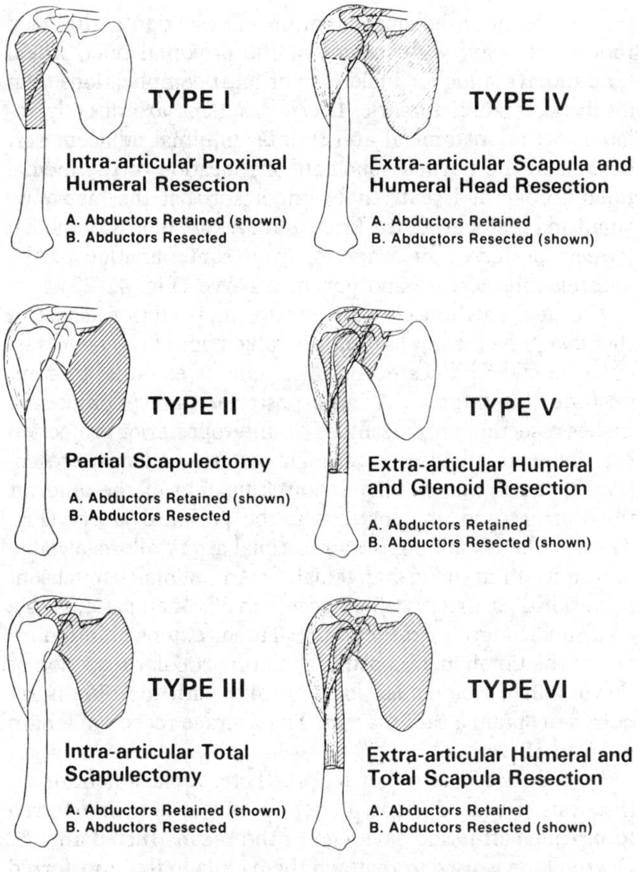

FIG. 42-21. Schematic of proposed surgical classification of shoulder girdle resections. In general, Types I–III are for benign or low grade tumors, whereas Types IV–VI are for high grade tumors. A and B denote the status of the abductor mechanism. A, intact; B, partially or completely excised. Types I–III and Types IV–VI are intra-articular and extra-articular resections, respectively.[197]

Recently, a surgical classification of shoulder girdle resections has been described (Fig. 42-21).[197] This classification is useful for all limb-sparing procedures of the shoulder girdle. Osteosarcomas arising from the proximal humerus should be treated by a Type VB resection (Fig. 42-21).

PROXIMAL HUMERUS. Adequate resection of the proximal humerus requires removal of 15 to 20 cm of the humerus and shoulder joint with the deltoid, rotator cuff, and portions of the biceps and triceps muscles. The procedure involves suspension of the arm, motor reconstruction, and provision of adequate soft-tissue coverage (Fig. 42-22).

Proximal humeral lesions should not be biopsied through the deltopectoral interval, because this contaminates the subscapularis and pectoralis muscles and the area adjacent to the axillary sheath. Biopsy under fluoroscopy through the anterior third of the deltoid by a trochar is preferred. Angiography is the most useful preoperative study. If the neurovascular bundle is clear, resection is feasible. All other structures can be removed. The major contraindications to local resection are tumor involvement of the lymph nodes or chest wall, pathologic fracture, or massive soft-tissue contamination.

Resectability is determined by early exploration of the neurovascular structures by division of the pectoralis major. This approach does not jeopardize formation of an anterior flap in patients who require forequarter amputation. Preservation of the musculocutaneous nerve is important. The short biceps muscle, responsible for elbow flexion, is the most important muscle left after resection. Extra-articular resection of the glenohumeral joint by medial scapulosteotomy is safer than intra-articular resection. A custom prosthesis is used for reconstruction. Soft-tissue reconstruction and suspension are essential to avoid postoperative pain, instability, and fatigue (Fig. 42-22). Suspension by dacron tape and muscle transfers are effective. Hand and wrist function is normal following resection, shoulder motion is minimal, but stable; and scapulothoracic motion provides some internal and external rotation. Cosmetic appearance is acceptable and can be enhanced with the use of a shoulder pad.

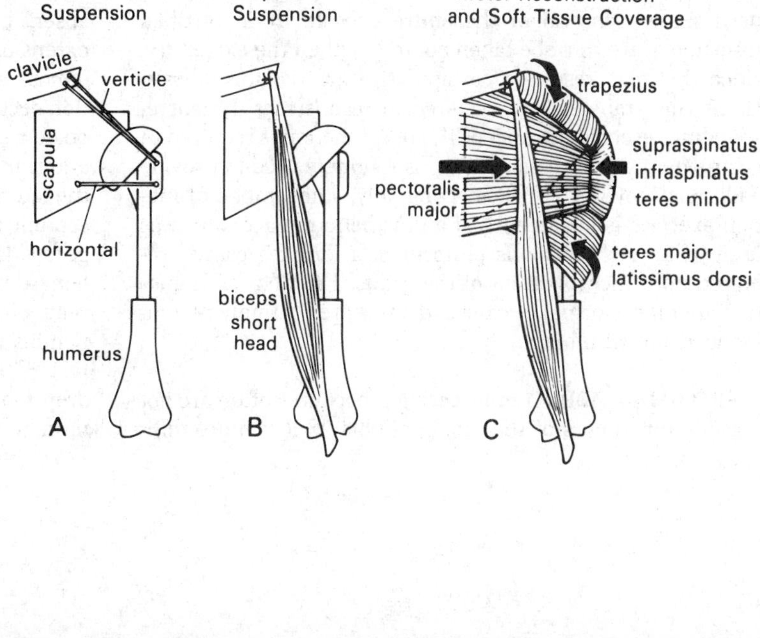

FIG. 42-22. Technique of shoulder girdle reconstruction following resection for high grade sarcomas of the proximal humerus. Dual suspension, that is, both dynamic and static methods, are necessary to recreate shoulder stability. Dacron tape (**A**) and multiple muscle transfers (**B,C**) are used.

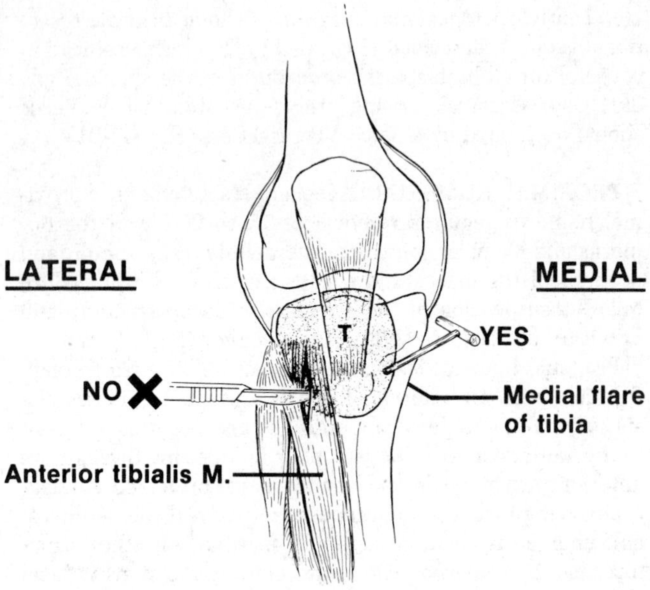

FIG. 42-23. Biopsy technique of proximal tibial sarcomas. The biopsy should always be performed medially so as to avoid contamination of the anterior tibial muscles.

DISTAL FEMUR. Adequate en bloc resection includes 15 to 20 cm of the distal femur and proximal tibia and portions of the adjacent quadriceps (see Fig. 42-5)[120] Biplane angiography is crucial to determine popliteal vessel involvement. Biopsy must avoid the sartorial canal and the knee joint. Contraindications to resection are popliteal vessel involvement, massive soft-tissue contamination from a previous biopsy, or fracture. Large tumors requiring removal of the entire quadriceps or hamstrings can be adequately reconstructed by an arthrodesis.

The operative procedure begins with exploration of the popliteal vessels. Care should be taken to preserve the sural vessels, the neurovascular pedicle to the gastrocnemius muscles. The corresponding vasti muscle is removed en bloc adjacent to the extraosseous tumor component. If an effusion is present, extra-articular resection is performed; this necessitates removal of the entire capsule from its tibial insertion. Care must be taken not to lengthen the extremity, since this may result in postoperative arterial thrombosis. Hamstring transfers are required to reconstruct the corresponding resected quadriceps if motor function is required. A gastrocnemius transposition flap is routinely used to provide additional coverage.[199] Postoperatively, knee range-of-motion exercise is begun early if a prosthetic replacement was used. If an arthrodesis is performed, a long-leg cast is required until incorporation of the grafts. Hip and ankle motion are often normal. A cane and brace are routinely recommended for 12 months.

PROXIMAL TIBIA. Limb-sparing procedures often are not feasible for tumors of the proximal tibia.[200] It is more difficult to obtain an adequate margin of resection and a good functional result with lesions of the proximal tibia, which tend to have a higher incidence of local complications than do distal femoral tumors. These problems are directly related to the anatomical constraints: minimal adjacent soft tissue and the normal subcutaneous location of the medial tibial border. It is extremely important that the biopsy be small and that it avoid the knee joint. A core biopsy of medial flare is preferred in order to avoid contamination of the anterior musculature and peroneal nerve (Fig. 42-23).

The popliteus muscle adjacent to the posterior aspect of the tibia prevents direct tumor involvement of the neurovascular bundle.[200,201] Lateral angiography is essential to demonstrate this interval. A large posterior tumor component makes resection unadvisable. The anteroposterior projection can delineate anomalous vascular patterns. Adequate resection of the proximal tibia requires ligation of the anterior tibial artery and, in most cases, the peroneal artery (Fig. 42-24). The remaining posterior tibial artery allows a viable extremity in a young individual.[200] An anomalously absent posterior tibial artery, which occurs in 5% of all patients, is a contraindication for resection.[202] Tumor extension often involves the tibiofibular capsule.[200] Extra-articular resection of the proximal tibiofibular joint en bloc with the tibia is required to obtain a safe margin. The average resection length is 15 to 18 cm.

Reconstruction is either by prosthetic replacement or arthrodesis. The medial gastrocnemius is routinely transferred to provide soft-tissue coverage of the reconstructed area.[199] Dacron tape is used to reattach the patella to the transferred gastrocnemius and prosthesis.[200]

PROXIMAL FIBULA. Tumors of the proximal fibula require the same evaluation as proximal tibial lesions.[202] Unique considerations are early soft-tissue extension, proximity to the lateral tibial condyle, necessity of ligating the anterior and peroneal arteries, sacrifice of the peroneal nerve, and tumor infiltration of the tibiofibular joint capsule. Large tumors are often unresectable. Biplane angiography is necessary to determine anomalous vascular patterns and vascular displacement. Bone scintigraphy with multiple rotation views of the proximal tibia is essential to determine bony involvement of the adjacent tibial plateau. Contraindications to resection are direct tibial involvement, an anomalously absent posterior tibial artery, and intra-articular knee joint extension of the tumor. Due to the multiple musculotendonous attachments of the proximal fibula, muscle infiltration occurs along muscle planes beyond visible borders. Adequate resection includes the fibula, the tibiofibular joint, the anterior and lateral muscle compartments, and a portion of the lateral gastrocnemius, the soleus, and the intermuscular septum (Fig. 42-25). Wide excision of all adjacent muscle groups is mandatory (Fig. 42-26). No reconstruction of the bony defect is required. The lateral collateral ligament is reattached to the lateral joint capsule, and a lateral gastrocnemius transposition flap is used to close the resultant defect.[199] Following surgery, the only functional deficit is a drop foot, which is treated by an orthosis. Knee function is normal.[202]

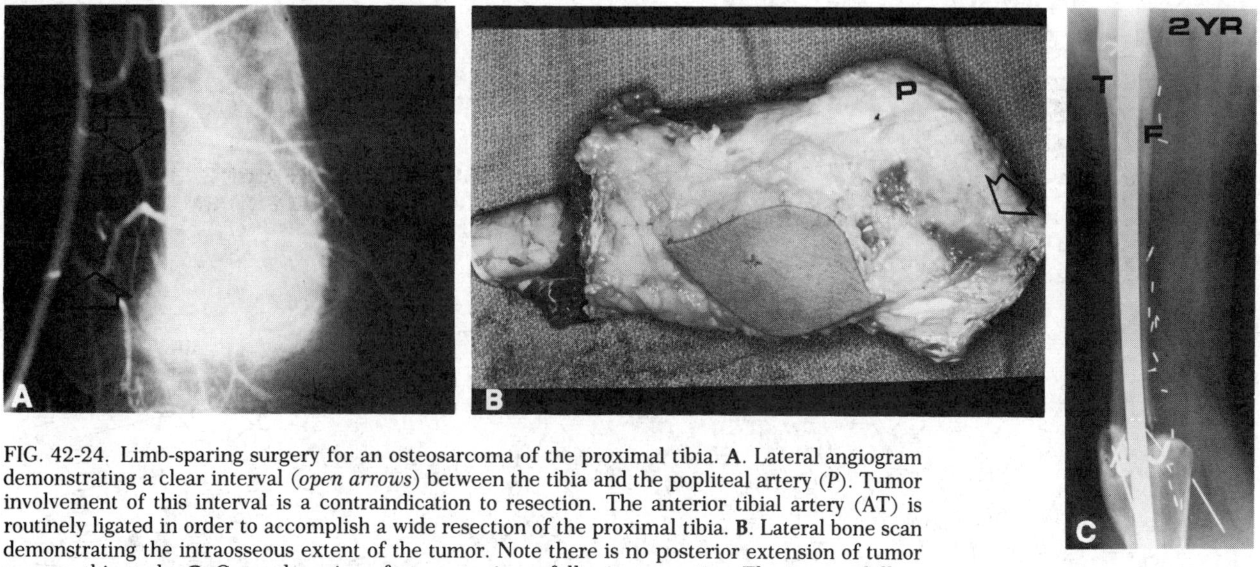

FIG. 42-24. Limb-sparing surgery for an osteosarcoma of the proximal tibia. **A**. Lateral angiogram demonstrating a clear interval (*open arrows*) between the tibia and the popliteal artery (*P*). Tumor involvement of this interval is a contraindication to resection. The anterior tibial artery (AT) is routinely ligated in order to accomplish a wide resection of the proximal tibia. **B**. Lateral bone scan demonstrating the intraosseous extent of the tumor. Note there is no posterior extension of tumor seen on this study. **C**. Coronal section of gross specimen following resection. The intramedullary extent of tumor (*black arrows*) corresponds with the bone scan (**B**). The biopsy site is clearly seen (BX).

PELVIS AND PROXIMAL FEMUR. Osteosarcomas of the pelvis and proximal femur are less common than those occurring at other anatomic areas, accounting for 10% and 5%, respectively, of all osteosarcomas (Fig. 42-27).[177] Tumors arising from these structures are often large, involve important structures, and are difficult to resect. Hemipelvectomy is often required for pelvic tumors, and modified hemipelvectomy is used for tumors of the proximal femur.[128] The limb-sparing options, if feasible, are all functionally superior to amputation at this level.[126,127] A poorly planned biopsy often contaminates the extrapelvic structures, making a hemipelvectomy the only safe option. The technique of pelvic biopsy is shown in Figure 42-28. Detailed anatomic and surgical considerations are discussed in the section of chondrosarcomas, which more commonly arise in these sites.

Limb-Sparing Surgery and Amputation

Limb-sparing surgery is the preferred treatment for many patients with osteosarcomas and other high-grade bone sarcomas.[23,107,119,122,128] Amputations are reserved principally for patients in whom the primary tumor is deemed unresectable.[128] Tremendous experience and data have been obtained in the past 5 years about the crucial factors dictating a limb-sparing procedure or an amputation.[107–109,126,127] Several considerations govern limb-salvage procedures:[23]

Local recurrence: The chance of local recurrence should not be higher than that associated with amputation.

Survival: Overall survival should not be jeopardized, either by treatment delay or by an ineffective adjuvant treatment program.

Function: The result of reconstruction should be functional, with minimal long-term morbidity and need for additional surgery. The psychological impact and duration of rehabilitation must be considered.

Many studies have demonstrated that the risk (<5%) of local recurrence in patients who have undergone limb-sparing surgery is the same or less than the risk in those treated by amputation.[23,26–28,126] These were *carefully* selected patients, however, and the procedures were performed in institutions whose staff was familiar with the techniques. Similarly, the reported continuous disease-free survival rates are the same or better than those in large series of patients undergoing amputation alone.[26,27,30,33,36,38,52,53] If the criteria for patient selection are met, despite the variations among institutions, limb-salvaging is a safe procedure. Eilber and colleagues from UCLA reported 64 (78%) of 83 consecutive patients with malignant skeletal tumors who were treated by a limb-sparing resection, with no difference in overall survival compared with those treated by amputation.[26] The overall local recurrence rate was 2.7%. Eckardt and coworkers, from the same institution, reported their experience specifically with Stage IIB osteosarcoma between 1972 and 1984. Seventy-eight (67%) of 116 patients were treated by a limb-sparing resection; the local recurrence rate was 3.8%.[23]

The functional advantages of limb-sparing surgery merit careful consideration. Preservation of the upper humerus following resection of a proximal humeral sarcoma, for example, leaves a normal hand and elbow that are far superior to any prosthesis. Except for lack of shoulder motion, function is essentially normal. The advantage of such a procedure

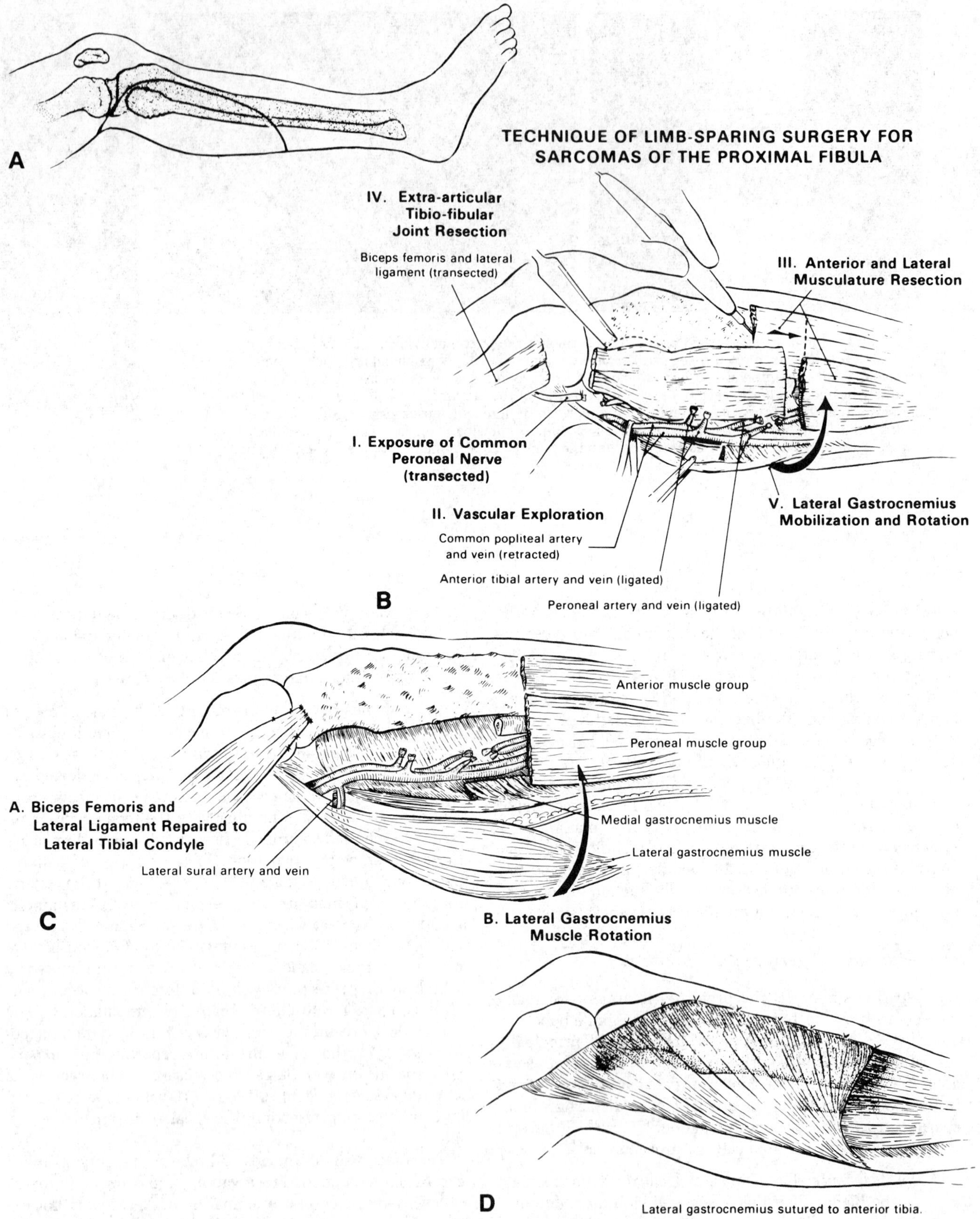

FIG. 42-25. Technique of limb-sparing surgery for sarcomas of the proximal fibula. **A.** Utilitarian incision. **B.** Steps of resection of tumor. **C.** Resection defect. Note that both the anterior tibial and peroneal arteries have been ligated and the anterior and lateral muscle compartments removed. The defect is closed routinely by a lateral gastrocnemius muscle transfer. **D.** Bony reconstruction is not necessary. (Malawer MM: Surgical management of aggressive and malignant tumors of the proximal fibula. Clin Orthop [in press])

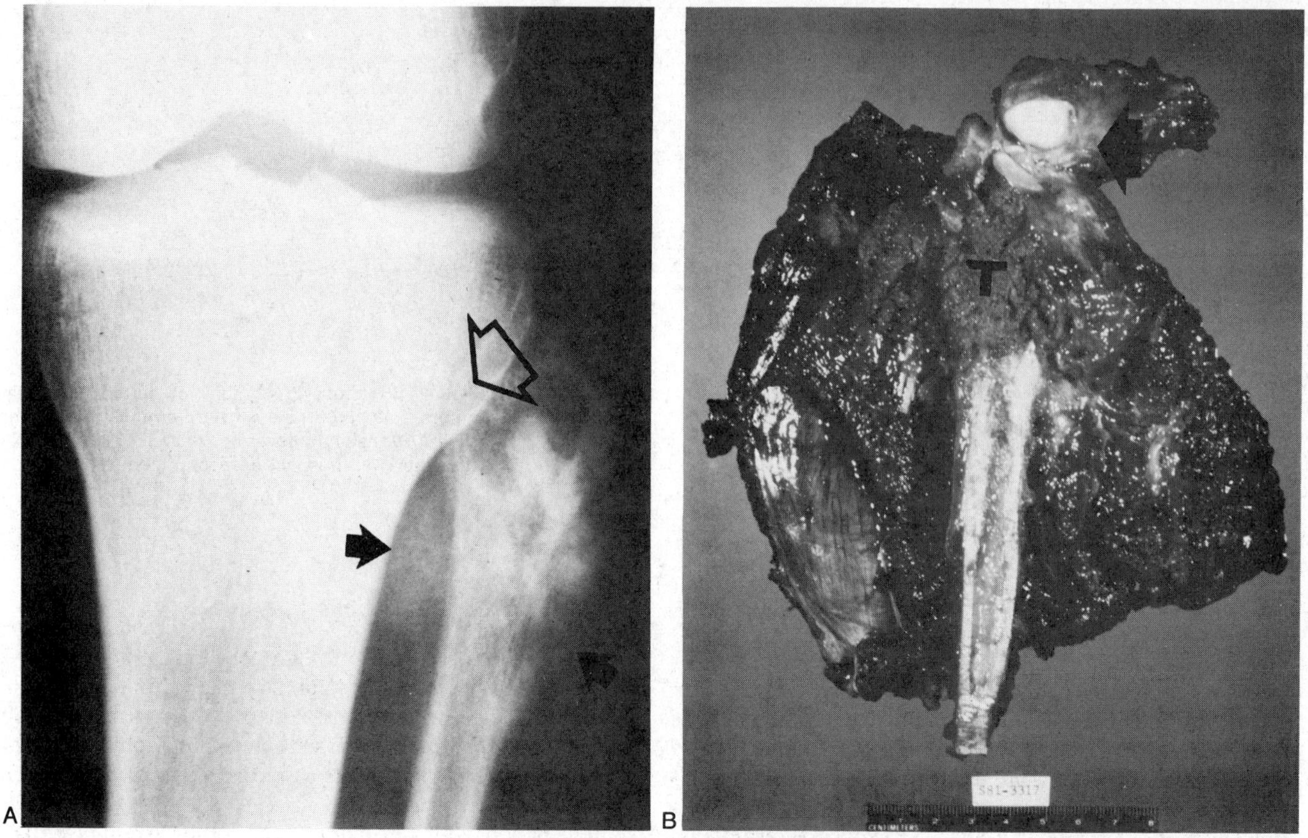

FIG. 42-26. **A**. Osteosarcoma of the proximal fibula. Plain radiograph of the knee demonstrating an osteosarcoma of the proximal fibula. Note the large soft tissue component (*solid arrows*) and the intimate relationship to the proximal tibiofibular joint. Tumors arising from the proximal fibula can often be treated by a limb-sparing procedure. (Malawer MM: Surgical management of aggressive and malignant tumors of the proximal fibula. Clin Orthop 186:172–181, 1984).[202] **B**. Gross specimen of a fibula resection for an osteosarcoma. An extra-articular resection was performed. The libiofibular joint (*solid arrow*) was opened and demonstrated pericapsular tumor extension. This is a common finding and emphasizes the need for routine extra-articular resection for sarcomas of the proximal fibula. T, tumor. (Malawer MM: Surgical management of aggressive and malignant tumors of the proximal fibula. Clin Orthop 186:172–181, 1984)

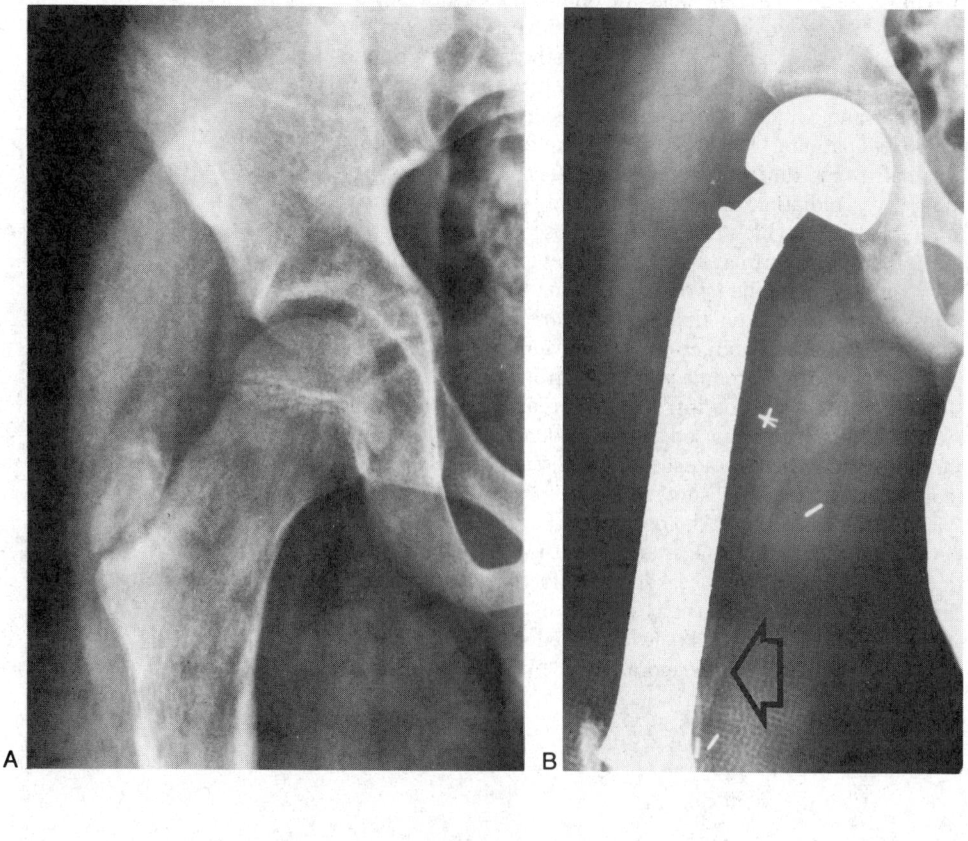

FIG. 42-27. Osteosarcoma of the proximal femur. **A**. Plain radiograph of an osteolytic osteosarcoma of the proximal femur. Note the mottled destruction of the intertrochanteric area with lateral cortical destruction. **B**. Postoperative radiograph demonstrating a custom proximal femoral replacement with porous coating to permit soft tissue as well as bony incorporation. (*Open arrow*, bone graft)

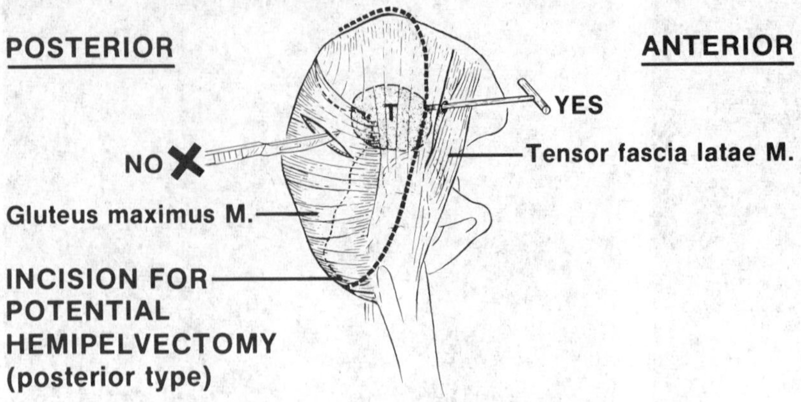

FIG. 42-28. Biopsy technique of buttock and iliac tumors. The potential posterior hemipelvectomy flap (*dotted line*) should never be violated. A small biopsy from the lateral aspect is recommended.

over forequarter amputation is obvious. Similarly, the functional advantages of preservation of the lower extremity following proximal femoral resection or pelvic resection are far superior to a hemipelvectomy. Initially, there was concern regarding the functional outcome of limb-sparing procedures about the knee. Enneking reported that resections followed by reconstruction at this site by several different modalities all had a higher functional ratings than amputation in a multi-institutional study using a standard evaluation scheme.[122]

ADJUVANT THERAPY. The initial impetus to limb-sparing surgery in the mid-1970s was the introduction of Adriamycin and methotrexate.[203] Surgeons decided that adjuvant therapy might allow something less than radical surgery. Today, most surgeons intuitively feel that adjuvant chemotherapy permits limb-sparing surgery to be performed more safely by decreasing the risk of local recurrence rate. Can a narrower surgical margin be a safe one with adjuvant chemotherapy? Although many surgeons believe this is possible, some data suggest that adjuvant chemotherapy has a beneficial effect and other data suggest that it does not.[26,74]

Eilber and colleagues reported an encouragingly low 2.6% (5 of 183 patients) local recurrence rate for high-grade bone and soft-tissue tumors and concluded that it was due to preoperative radiation and intra-arterial and postoperative chemotherapy, which destroyed microscopic disease at the periphery of the primary tumor.[26] Although the exact modality responsible for the favorable outcome was undetermined, these authors doubted that it was more accurate surgery. Conversely, Picci and co-workers evaluated, by detailed mapping, 50 osteosarcoma specimens from patients who had followed two different intravenous preoperative regimens (Fig. 42-29). They reported a high incidence (63%) of viable tumor within the extraosseous soft tissue.[204] The authors concluded that a wide surgical margin is required because viable tumor is often at the periphery. Because all preoperative chemotherapeutic agents entail the risk of increased local morbidity, skin breakdown, infection, and possible tumor progression with the possibility of losing a nonamputative option, additional studies are needed to determine the relationship between preoperative chemotherapy and the choice of surgical margin.

Treatment Considerations

LOCALIZED EXTREMITY DISEASE. Management requires the expertise of a multidisciplinary team familiar with the various management options. Patients with a suspected diagnosis of osteosarcoma (based on radiographic findings) should be referred to centers with treatment programs *before* biopsy.

The patient with a primary tumor of the extremity without evidence of metastases requires surgery to control the pri-

FIG. 42-29. The percentage of viable tumor in each preferential site found in those patients with viable tumor following preoperative treatment for osteosarcoma as reported by Picca and colleagues (n = 50 patients). (Picci P, Bacci G, Companacci M, et al: Histological evaluation of necrosis in osteosarcoma induced by chemotherapy, regional mapping of viable and nonviable tumor. Cancer 56:1515–1521, 1985)

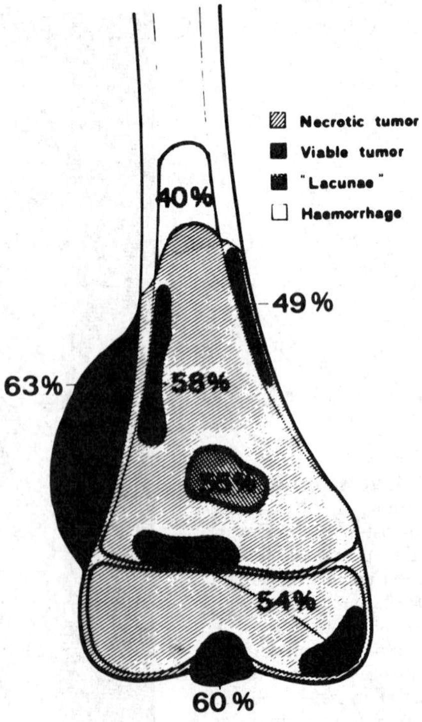

mary tumor and chemotherapy to control micrometastatic disease. The choice between amputation and limb-sparing resection must be made by an experienced orthopedic oncologist. Routine amputations are no longer performed; all patients should be evaluated for limb-sparing options. Studies are being conducted to compare surgery followed by adjuvant chemotherapy and presurgical chemotherapy with delayed surgery of the primary tumor. Intensive, multi-agent chemotherapeutic regimens, as used in the T-10 and Multi-Institutional Osteosarcoma studies, have provided the best results to date (see Figs. 42-12 and 42-15).[90,97,171] Patients who are judged unsuitable for limb-sparing options may be candidates for presurgical chemotherapy; those with a good responses may then become suitable candidates for limb-sparing operations. The management of these patients mandates close cooperation between chemotherapist and surgeon.

PELVIC TUMORS AND UNRESECTABLE DISEASE. In some pelvic and most vertebral primary tumors, complete resection is often not possible. Most pelvic osteosarcomas can be treated by a hemipelvectomy; more centrally located pelvic tumors, especially those involving the sacrum, are unresectable. Only a few pelvic osteosarcomas can be treated by limb-sparing resection (internal hemipelvectomy). Contraindications to resection are unusually large extraosseous extensions with sacral plexus or major vascular involvement. On rare occasions, vertebral and sacral resections have been attempted.[205,206] In general, these tumors cannot be resected with negative margins and are best treated by radiotherapy and chemotherapy.[205-207] Some success has been achieved with systemic or intra-arterial chemotherapy, which is administered to convert apparently inoperable tumors into lesions that can be ablated surgically.[208,209] Patients with primary tumors of the axial skeleton have had poor prognoses because local control was not achieved. The prognoses for these patients may improve with a more aggressive surgical approach and more effective chemotherapy. Patients whose tumors can be completely resected should be approached with curative intent, and radiotherapy provides significant palliation in patients with unresectable primary tumors.

METASTATIC PULMONARY DISEASE AT DIAGNOSIS. Metastatic disease detected during the initial diagnosis does not preclude a curative treatment strategy, although the presence of extrathoracic metastases makes cure extremely unlikely. In general, the surgical principles outlined for the treatment of relapsing patients apply equally to the patient presenting with macroscopic metastases. Newly diagnosed patients have not been exposed to chemotherapy and are thus less likely to have drug-resistant tumors, and several options are therefore available.

For the patient presenting with resectable disease (*i.e.*, usually fewer than 15 pulmonary nodules and a primary tumor of the extremity), the traditional approach has been resection of all evidence of macroscopic disease by median sternotomy and limb amputation or resection, followed by intensive adjuvant chemotherapy. The tumor burden is thereby reduced to a minimum before the application of adjuvant therapy. Some investigators have favored treatment with chemotherapy, followed weeks or months later by definitive surgery for residual macroscopic disease in primary and metastatic sites.[210,211] Arguments advanced to justify this approach are similar to those used to support the strategy of preoperative chemotherapy in general, and the theoretical advantages and disadvantages of this strategy as discussed for patients with nonmetastatic osteosarcoma apply here as well. The risk for the patient with metastases is that growth of tumor nodules in the face of chemotherapy may render small, operable metastases unresectable and prevent cure. Primary treatment with chemotherapy may be appropriate, however, in patients with inoperable metastases, which may respond sufficiently to allow complete resection. Patients with widespread unresectable metastases are also best treated first with chemotherapy, with definitive surgery reserved for those achieving a satisfactory response. Because these patients usually require surgery for the primary tumor as a palliative procedure, early surgery may be recommended despite unresectable pulmonary disease.

RECURRENT DISEASE AFTER CURATIVE ATTEMPT. Historically, patients developing recurrent disease had poor prognoses and were treated palliatively; most patients died within 1 year of the development of metastatic disease. Because more than 85% of metastases occur in the lung, surgical resection of tumor nodules can be readily accomplished. With the advent of CT scans of the chest, metastatic nodules can be detected when quite small and more easily resectable, although in most cases the surgeon will discover more lesions at thoracotomy than anticipated from the CT scan.[212] In many patients, the lungs are likely to be the only site of metastases, especially in cases in which recurrences appear more than 1 year after diagnosis and in which the metastatic lesion is solitary. In such cases, the recurrent tumors are likely to behave more indolently and may not further metastasize. These patients have been cured by thoracotomies alone.

Complete surgical resection of all overt metastatic disease is a prerequisite for long-term salvage after relapse.[213-216] Patients not treated by thoracotomies have little hope for cure, because complete responses of macroscopic metastases to chemotherapy are rare.[213,214] The completeness of surgical resection is an important determinant of outcome, because patients left with measurable or microscopic disease at the resection margins are unlikely to be cured.[213]

CHEMOTHERAPY AND METASTATIC DISEASE. Many investigators have recommended chemotherapy for the management of metastatic osteosarcoma to destroy residual microscopic tumor deposits after surgical treatment of overt metastases.[210,217,218] For patients who develop recurrent disease within 1 year of initial surgery, the possibility of additional microscopic metastatic disease is quite high, and further chemotherapy is indicated. Long-term survival has been reported for some patients with recurrent osteosarcoma who were treated only with surgery without further chemotherapy.[213-215] These survivors were more likely to be patients suffering late relapses with solitary pulmonary nodules.

If overt metastatic disease is discovered, a thorough search for all metastatic lesions is essential. The discovery of unresectable extrathoracic metastases or unresectable pulmonary disease is a contraindication to aggressive thoracotomy, and the patient should be treated palliatively. Radiotherapy may be particularly useful in this context. In some patients with unresectable disease, an aggressive approach with curative intent may still be indicated. Chemotherapy, with or without radiotherapy, rarely eradicates all metastatic disease; nonetheless, some patients with inoperable metastases may respond sufficiently to allow for complete resection of disease at a later date, and occasionally, patients with unresectable pulmonary metastases are cured with chemotherapy or high-dose radiotherapy alone.

Patients found to have resectable lung disease should undergo thoracotomies to remove all evidence of disease. Bilateral disease may be approached by staged bilateral thoracotomies or a median sternotomy. The role of adjuvant chemotherapy after thoracotomy should be studied; it is probably indicated for patients with more than three lesions appearing 6 months to 1 year after initial surgery and for patients whose metastatic disease has not been completely resected or for those with evidence of pleural disruption by tumors. Repeat thoracotomies may be required for subsequent recurrence and should be performed if all disease can be resected.

Radiation Therapy for Osteosarcoma

Experience with primary radiotherapy for osteosarcomas was obtained in the 1950s and early 1960s. Primary radiotherapy with delayed amputation gained acceptance in 1955, when Cade advocated this approach for patients in whom there was no evidence of metastases 4 to 6 months after radiotherapy.[243] This approach was designed to circumvent amputation in the majority of patients who were destined to suffer an early relapse. Radiation doses were 7000 to 8000 cGy in 7 to 9 weeks at 1000 cGy per week. There were a few patients in Cade's series whose disease was initially controlled with irradiation alone, and amputation was eventually performed. The 5-year survival rate was 21.6%. Other investigators followed a similar regime, using various radiation doses and schemas (Table 42-11). Surgical specimens of many of the patients managed in this fashion were found to have no histologic evidence of their tumor.[244–246] The ability of high radiation doses to sterilize some tumors was associated, however, with significant necrosis of normal tissue.

Overall success with preoperative radiation followed by ablative surgery was usually suboptimal; most patients relapsed shortly after treatment. This led Jenkin and colleagues to recommend limiting radiation to patients who had unresectable tumors or to those being treated for palliation only.[247,248] Beck and co-workers observed no survival advantage for preoperative radiation followed by surgery over surgery alone; furthermore, only 43% of their patients obtained any palliative benefit from radiotherapy.[249] No benefit has been derived from radiation delivered under conditions of local tissue hypoxia, split-course radiotherapy, or radiation with hydrogen peroxide or cytotoxic drug therapy.[250–252] However, radiotherapy has been successful in treating facial lesions, for palliation, and possibly as a postoperative adjuvant.

MAXILLA OR MANDIBLE. Osteosarcomas arising from facial bones, specifically the maxilla or mandible, have a different biology and natural history from those located elsewhere in the body. There is a lower risk of dissemination, but tumors arising in these sites have a high rate of local recurrence when treated by surgery alone. Clark and colleagues reported on 66 patients with maxillary or mandibular primary tumors; 43 died, most with primary local recurrence.[253] Chambers and Mahoney have suggested preoperative radiotherapy for such patients.[254] They reported a 73% survival rate at 5 years for 33 patients treated with high-dose radiotherapy (either interstitial technique or external beam) followed immediately by wide surgical excision (hemiman-

TABLE 42-11. Series of Primary Radiation Followed by Delayed Surgery for Osteosarcoma

No. of Patients	*Dose*	*Machine*	*Survival*	*References*
133	7000–8000 cGy/7–9 wk, 1000 cGy/wk	2 MV	21.8%	243
10	10,000 cGy, 180 cGy/fraction	^{60}Co or 2 MV	60%	245
92	6000–8000 rad in 230 rad/fractions	2 MV	21.8%	244a
16	1600–10,500 cGy in 200 cGy/fraction	Orthovoltage and 2 MV	75% (1–16 yr) FU	244b
54	variable	variable	27.5%	244c
23	1800–12,000 cGy/ 2–29 wk	Orthovoltage and 2 MV	26%	244d
27	5000–6000 cGy in 25–30 fractions		0	247
27	5000–6000 cGy/5–6 wk repeated ×1 7000–8000 cGy/8–9 wk	Orthovoltage or 1–4 Mv	23%	249

dibulectomy and resection of surrounding soft tissues). Long-term survival after surgery alone was between 35% and 45%.[255] The high local recurrence rates after surgery are explained by difficulties in achieving adequate surgical margins. The increased survival after combined-modality treatment supports the fact that high radiation doses can eradicate microscopic disease. Both deFries and co-workers and Abbiyik reported similar improved survival rates using a combination of preoperative radiation, resection, and chemotherapy.[256,257] Conversely, Livolsi reported on five patients irradiated in the postoperative period for osteosarcoma of the maxilla, all of whom died.[258] The long delay between the completion of surgery and the start of postoperative radiotherapy may have contributed to the poor results.

PALLIATION. Radiation therapy is extremely beneficial for patients requiring palliation of metastatic bony sarcomas, tumors at axial sites that are unresectable, and advanced, inoperable lesions of the pelvis or extremities. A novel approach using high-dose-per-fraction radiation and intra-arterial 5′-bromodeoxyuridine (BUdR) as a radiosensitizer was undertaken by the Stanford Group.[259] Pulsed 48-hour BUdR infusions were performed before each 600-cGy radiation fraction, with a total radiation dose to the primary site of 4200 to 4800 cGy in 5 weeks (7–8 fractions). Infusions of methotrexate and leucovorin were administered simultaneously. Local control was achieved in seven (78%) of the nine patients treated.[260] However, local tissue toxicity was excessive, including subcutaneous fibrosis, nonhealing traumatic fractures, peroneal neuropathy, and atrophy. Because the patients were treated with an unusual fractionation scheme using large fractions and with intravenous chemotherapy, the specific role of the BUdR in either local control or the excessive toxicity was not established.

Kinsella used the intravenous radiosensitizers of BUdR, iododeoxyuridine (IUDR), or misonidazole with high-dose radiotherapy, in various fractionation schemes, usually with chemotherapy, in patients with large, unresectable primary or metastatic sarcomas.[261] Twenty-one (75%) of 29 patients achieved local control, defined as no symptoms and no tumor growth. These studies demonstrated the efficacy of radiation therapy in obtaining long-term local control and palliation. They lend support to further clinical investigations using radiation sensitizers with high-dose radiotherapy.

ADJUVANT PULMONARY IRRADIATION. Variable results have been achieved from the use of adjuvant pulmonary radiation in patients with primary osteosarcoma.[240,262–269] Breur and colleagues performed a randomized trial comparing amputation plus adjuvant whole-lung irradiation with amputation alone in 86 patients.[240,264–266] The midplane pulmonary lung dose was 1750 cGy, given in 10 fractions in 12 days, which with long correction equalled slightly less than 2000 cGy. They found a significant benefit in the 3-year disease-free survival rate among patients younger than 17 years of age who received adjuvant radiation therapy. Forty-eight percent of these patients survived without disease, compared with 28% in the group receiving surgery alone. This study is now being extended to the European Organization for Research on the Treatment of Cancer (EORTC) in a trial comparing amputation and lung irradiation, surgery and adjuvant chemotherapy, and all three treatments.[264–266] Conversely, Rab and colleagues used a lower midplane radiation dose of 1500 cGy with concomitant dactinomycin in a randomized study and failed to show a survival benefit over amputation alone.[267] No toxicity was seen. Similarly, Jenkin reported no benefit from 1500 cGy given in 14 days of pulmonary irradiation with simultaneous dactinomycin, and Caceres and co-workers found no advantage over adjuvant doxorubicin alone.[268,269]

Variants of Classic Osteosarcoma

Dahlin has identified 11 variants of the classic osteosarcoma.[59] These accounted for 268 (28%) of 1021 cases reviewed at the Mayo Clinic. Osteosarcoma arising in the jaw bones, the most common variant, is characterized by well-differentiated cells with a low metastatic potential.[59] Excluding tumors arising secondary to Paget's disease, irradiation, or dedifferentiation of a chondrosarcoma, parosteal and periosteal osteosarcomas are the most common variants of classic osteosarcoma arising in the extremities. In contrast to classic osteosarcoma, which arises within a bone (intramedullary), both arise on the surface of the bone (juxtacortical).

PAROSTEAL OSTEOSARCOMA. Parosteal osteosarcoma (POS) is a distinct variant of conventional osteosarcoma, accounting for 4% of all osteosarcomas.[60] It arises from the cortex of a bone and usually occurs in older individuals. It has a better prognosis than classical osteosarcoma.

There is a slight predominance of POS in women. The distal posterior femur is involved in 72% of all cases; the proximal humerus and proximal tibia are the next most frequent sites. POS metastasizes slowly and has an overall survival rate of 75% to 85%.[60,270] Unni and colleagues noticed that all patients who died of tumor lived more than 5 years. The natural history of POS is progressive enlargement and late metastasis. POS presents as a mass and occasionally is associated with pain. In contrast with conventional osteosarcoma, the duration of symptoms varies from months to years. Unni reported that 50 of 79 patients had complaints longer than 1 year, and 33% of this group had pain for more than 5 years.[270] Tumor size, location, and duration of symptoms did not correlate with survival.[60]

Radiographic Analysis. Roentgenograms characteristically show a large, dense, lobulated mass broadly attached to the underlying bone, without involvement of the medullary canal. If mature enough, the tumor may encircle the entire bone (Fig. 42-30). The periphery of the lesion is characteristically less mature than the base. Ahuja emphasized that intramedullary extension is difficult to determine from plain radiographs.[60] Unni emphasized that high-grade foci did not usually alter the roentgenographic appearance of these tumors.[270]

Pathology and Grading. POS is characterized by well-formed lamellar or woven bone with a mature spindle-cell stroma with few signs of malignancy. The cellularity of the

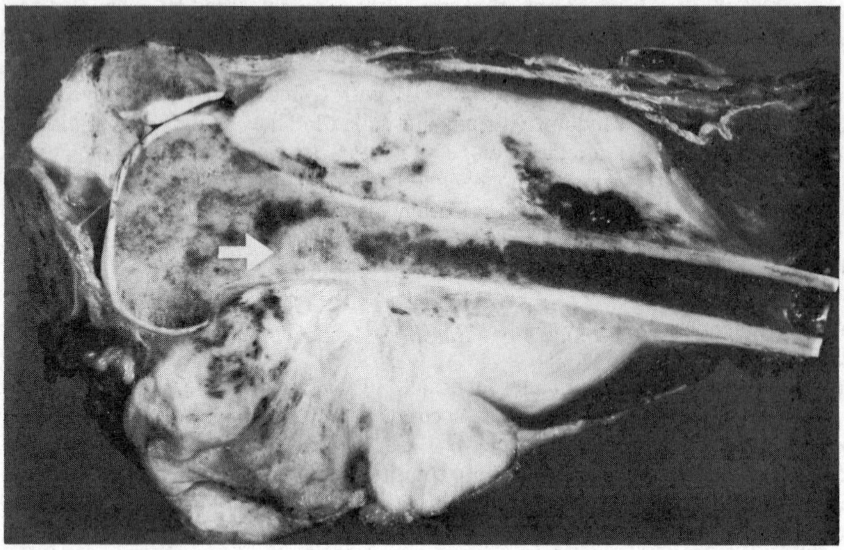

FIG. 42-30. Parosteal osteosarcoma with intramedullary extension (*arrow*). Large parosteal osteosarcoma of the distal femur treated by an above-knee amputation. The patient refused treatment for 4 years before amputation. Intramedullary extension is a sign of advanced disease.

spindle-cell components varies; it is not usually anaplastic, and there are few mitoses.[2-4,59,60] The differential diagnoses include osteochondroma, myositis ossificans, and conventional osteosarcoma. Cortical tumors of the posterior femur should always be suspected of malignancy; this is a rare location for a benign osteochondroma. In contrast to sarcoma, myositis ossificans is rarely attached to the underlying bone. In addition, the periphery is more mature, both radiographically and histologically.

Ahuja reviewed all the POS at Memorial Sloan-Kettering from 1934 to 1975 and described three grades: Grade I (low grade), Grade II (intermediate), and Grade III (high grade).[60] He emphasized the importance of evaluating the fibroblastic, cartilaginous, and osseous components independently. Of 24 patients, 8 were Grade I, 10 were Grade II, and 6 were Grade III. Unni from the Mayo Clinic reviewed 79 patients and reported that 18 (23%) were Grade II and 7 (9%) had high-grade foci.[270] Neither Unni nor Ahuja could distinguish the three grades on plain radiographs. The survival rate of patients with Grade III tumors is similar to that of patients with conventional osteosarcoma.

Intramedullary involvement does not necessarily imply a worse prognosis, although this may be the case in patients with high-grade lesions.[60] Eleven (46%) of 24 patients reviewed by Ahuja had medullary involvement, and the patients with medullary involvement who had a local resection all had a local recurrence.

Treatment. Wide excision of the tumor is the treatment of choice. This may be accomplished either by an amputation or a limb-sparing procedure. There has been no experience reported of preoperative chemotherapy or radiotherapy. Parosteal osteosarcomas are often amenable to limb preservation because of their distal locations, low-grade status, and lack of local invasiveness. If the adjacent neurovascular bundle is free of tumor, resection is feasible. Vascular displacement is not a contraindication for resection. The major surgical decision usually is whether to remove the entire end of the bone and the adjacent joint or to preserve the joint. Small lesions can be resected with joint preservation, but if the medullary canal is involved, the joint usually cannot be preserved. A second factor mitigating against joint preservation is extensive cortical involvement. Techniques of resection and reconstruction are similar to those described for conventional osteosarcoma. The major difference is that only a small amount of soft tissue usually needs to be resected; consequently, good functional results are obtained. Grade III parosteal lesions may warrant systemic therapy because of the risk of metastasis.

PERIOSTEAL OSTEOSARCOMA. Periosteal osteosarcoma is a rare cortical variant of osteosarcoma that arises superficially on the cortex, most often on the tibia shaft.[61] Radiographically, it is a small, radiolucent lesion with some evidence of bone spiculation. The cortex is characteristically intact, with a scooped-out appearance and a Codman's triangle (Fig. 42-31). Histologically, periosteal osteosarcomas are relatively high-grade chondroblastic osteosarcoma, composed of malignant cartilage with areas of anaplastic spindle cells and osteoid production. Unni and colleagues, in a report of 23 cases, found periosteal osteosarcomas to be 33% as frequent as the parosteal variant.[61] The largest tumor measured 2.5 × 3.5 cm. Four of the 23 patients died of metastatic disease. Treatment is similar to that of other high-grade lesions, and en bloc resection should be performed when feasible; otherwise, amputation is indicated. Table 42-12 contrasts the characteristics of periosteal tumors with those of conventional osteosarcoma.

OSTEOSARCOMA AND PAGET'S DISEASE. Approximately 1% of patients with Paget's disease will develop a primary bone sarcoma.[185,186] Greditzer reported 41 sarcomas among 4415 patients with Paget's disease followed at the Mayo Clinic; 35 were osteosarcomas and 6 were fibrosarcomas.[186] The average patient age was 64, and the most common sites were the pelvis, femur, and humerus. Half

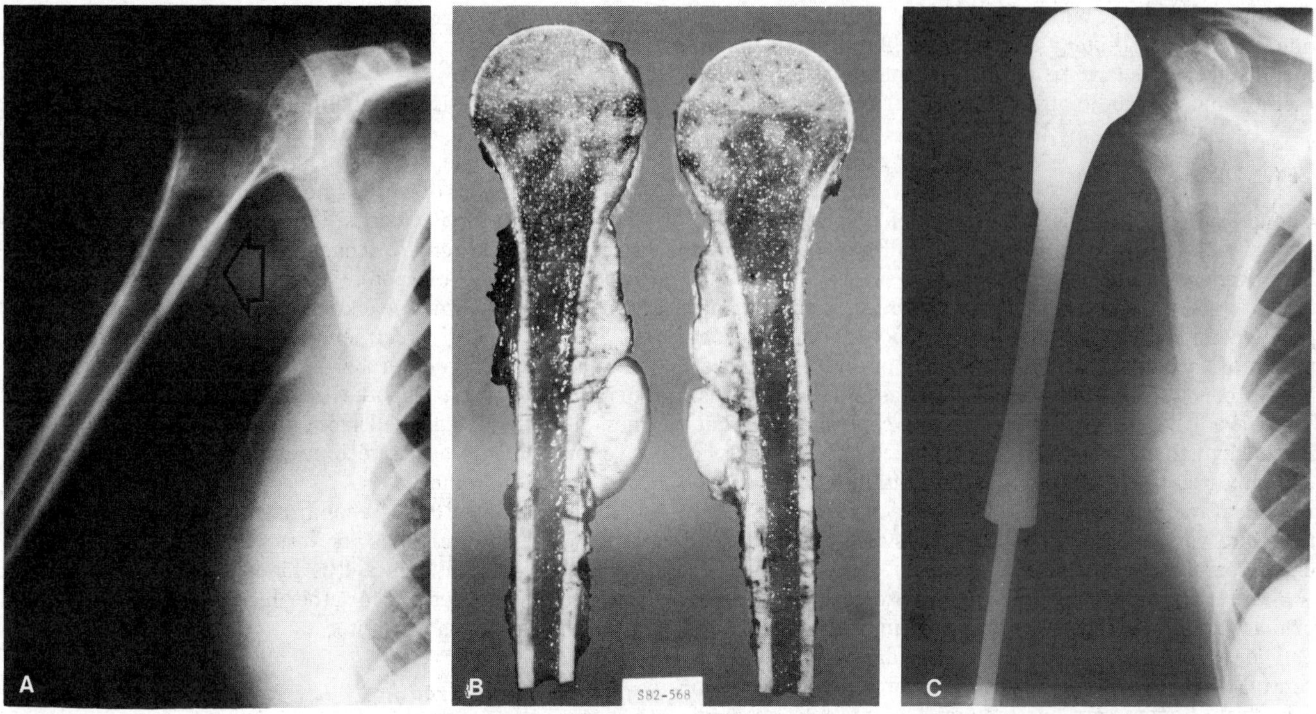

FIG. 42-31. Periosteal osteosarcoma. **A**. Typical radiograph of a periosteal osteosarcoma of the humerus. Note the cortical location with a scooped-out defect of the lateral aspect of the shaft and the diaphyseal location. **B**. Longitudinal section of the gross specimen following a limb-sparing resection. Note that the tumor seems to arise on the outer cortex without any evidence of cortical involvement. **C**. Postoperative radiograph. A custom prosthesis was used to reconstruct the defect. Soft-tissue reconstruction was as described in Figure 42-8. (Dunham WK, et al: Periosteal osteosarcoma. Cancer [in press])

were osteolytic; the remainder had a mixed pattern. Cortical destruction and a soft-tissue component were the most common signs reported; periosteal elevation was rare. Most patients with this condition present with pain; disease in a patient with known Paget's disease who complains of increasing pain, especially when it is localized, should be evaluated radiographically. The diagnosis is usually made by plain radiography and confirmed by biopsy. Traditionally, less than 8% of patients survive, and most deaths occur within 2 years.[186a] Treatment is similar to that recommended for adolescent patients with osteosarcoma without metastatic disease.

SMALL CELL OSTEOSARCOMA. This rare variant of osteosarcoma resembles a Ewing's sarcoma and is often classified as an "atypical" Ewing's sarcoma.[271,272] Characteristically, there are areas of osteoid and upon occasion chondroid formation. Differentiation from either Ewing's sarcoma or the typical osteosarcoma is important, because its response to treatment is poorly defined. Sim and colleagues

TABLE 42-12. Radiographic and Clinical Differential of Classical, Parosteal, and Periosteal Osteosarcoma

Type of Tumor	*Common Anatomical Site*	*Location*	*Radiographic Appearance*	*Histology*	*Metastases*
Classical	Distal femur Proximal tibia	Intramedullary	Destructive, osteoblastic/osteolytic	High-grade (fibroblastic, chondroblastic and osteoblastic)	Early
Parosteal	Posterior distal femur	Cortical	Dense, homogeneous new bone	"Mature" bone and fibroblastic stroma, low grade	Late
Periosteal	Proximal tibia and humerus	Cortical	"Scooped-out" lesion with calcification	Chondroblastic high grade	Intermediate

recommend surgery, but at the Pediatric Branch of the National Cancer Institute, these tumors, like other pediatric round cell tumors, are treated by a combination of radiation therapy and chemotherapy.[271,272]

CHONDROSARCOMA

Chondrosarcoma is the second most common primary malignant spindle-cell tumor of bone.[2] Chondrosarcomas form a heterogeneous group of tumors whose basic neoplastic tissue is cartilaginous, without evidence of direct osteoid formation. Occasionally, bone formation will occur from differentiation of cartilage. If there is evidence of direct osteoid or bone production, the lesion is classified as an osteosarcoma. There are five types of chondrosarcoma: central, peripheral, mesenchymal, differentiated, and clear cell.[2–4,10] The classic chondrosarcomas are central (arising within a bone) or peripheral (arising from the surface of a bone). The other three are variants and have distinct histologic and clinical characteristics.

Both central and peripheral chondrosarcomas can arise as primary tumors or secondary to underlying neoplasms. Seventy-six percent of primary chondrosarcomas arise centrally.[2,10–12,178] Secondary chondrosarcomas most often arise from benign cartilage tumors. The multiple forms of benign osteochondromas or enchondromas have a higher rate of malignant transformation than the corresponding solitary lesions.[11,12,57,176]

Clinical Characteristics

Half of all chondrosarcomas occur in persons older than 40 years.[2,177] Only 3.8% occur in patients younger than 20 years.[2] The most common sites are the pelvis (31%), femur (21%), and shoulder girdle (13%).[11,12,177,178] Chondrosarcomas are the most common malignant tumors of the sternum and scapula. The clinical presentation varies. Peripheral chondrosarcomas may become quite large without causing pain, and local symptoms develop only because of mechanical irritation. Pelvic chondrosarcomas are often large and present with pain referred to the back or thigh, sciatica caused by sacral plexus irritation, urinary symptoms from bladder neck involvement, or unilateral edema due to iliac vein obstruction. They may also present as a painless abdominal mass. Conversely, central chondrosarcomas present with dull pain, and a mass is rare. Pain, which indicates active growth, is an ominous sign of a central cartilage lesion. This cannot be overemphasized. An adult with a plain radiograph suggestive of a benign enchondroma who has pain probably has a chondrosarcoma.

Variants of Chondrosarcoma

CLEAR CELL CHONDROSARCOMA. This is the rarest form of chondrosarcoma. It is a slow-growing, locally recurrent tumor resembling a chondroblastoma but with some malignant potential.[280] It usually occurs in adults. The most difficult clinical problem is early recognition; it is often confused with chondroblastoma. Metastases occur only after several local recurrences. Primary treatment is wide excision, and systemic therapy is not required.

MESENCHYMAL CHONDROSARCOMA. This is a rare, aggressive variant of chondrosarcoma, characterized by a biphasic histologic pattern of small, compact cells intermixed with islands of cartilaginous matrix.[281–283] These have a predilection for flat bones; long, tubular bones are rarely affected.[177] They tend to occur in the younger age group and have high metastatic potential. Harwood reported 8 of 17 patients died within 1 year of diagnosis.[281] The 10-year survival rate is 28%.[281] Treatment is surgical removal combined with adjuvant chemotherapy. This entity responds favorably to radiotherapy. It is hypothesized that the round cell component, like other round cell sarcomas, is relatively radiosensitive, but radiotherapy is recommended if the tumor cannot be completely removed.[281]

Approximately 10% of chondrosarcomas may dedifferentiate into fibrosarcomas or osteosarcomas.[2,10,11,56] This occurs in older patients and is fatal. Surgical treatment is similar to that described for other high-grade sarcomas, and adjuvant therapy is warranted.

Histology and Grading

Chondrosarcomas are graded I, II, and III. The majority of chondrosarcomas are either Grade I or II.[1,10–12,176–178] The metastatic rate of moderate-grade lesions is 15% to 40%; in high-grade lesions it is 75%.[1,10–12,85,176] Grade III lesions have the same metastatic potential as osteosarcomas.[11,178]

Because cartilage tumors are difficult to grade histologically, some investigators have attempted to apply cytologic, histochemical, and biochemical analyses.[10,176,177,273,274] Sanerkin described a combination of cytologic and histologic criteria.[176] He emphasized that cytologic analysis evaluates nuclear abnormalities better than conventional histologic sections, but histologic evaluation of the bone-tumor interface is the best predictor of local aggressiveness. Kricberg performed a retrospective study of DNA content of 45 chondrosarcomas as an indicator of malignancy by evaluating diploid (normal) and hyperploid (abnormal increase) DNA and correlating this to 10-year survival rates.[275] Regardless of tumor grade, size, and location, patients with diploid DNA had better prognoses than those with hyperploid DNA. A preliminary report assessing the malignancy of cartilage tumor by flow cytometry to determine the percentage of diploid, tetraploid, and aneuploid cells indicated that it may be a promising method of grading chondrosarcomas.[276]

Radiographic Analyses

Central chondrosarcomas have two distinct radiologic patterns.[277] One is a small, well-defined lytic lesion with a narrow zone of transition and surrounding sclerosis with faint calcification. This is the most common malignant bone tumor that can appear radiographically benign. The second type has no sclerotic border and is difficult to localize. The key sign of malignancy is endosteal scalloping. It is difficult to diagnose on plain radiographs and may go undetected for a long time. In contrast, peripheral chondrosarcoma is recognized easily as a large, calcified mass protruding from a bone. Its differential diagnosis includes large benign osteochondroma, parosteal osteosarcoma, and juxtacortical myositis ossificans. Correlation of clinical, radiographic, and histologic data is essential for an accurate diagnosis and evaluation of the aggressiveness of cartilage tumor. In general, proximal or axial location, skeletal maturity, and pain indicate malignancy, even though the cartilage may appear to be benign.

Prognosis

Metastatic potential tends to correlate with the histologic grade of the lesion.[10–12,178] Marcove reported on long-term follow-up of 113 chondrosarcomas of the proximal femur and pelvis.[178] The survival rates in patients with Grades I, II, and III lesions were 47%, 38%, and 15%, respectively; the overall survival rate was 52%. There was no significant difference between Grades I and II; however, the mortality rate for Grade III was significantly higher ($p < 0.02$) than for the other two. Eleven of 59 deaths occurred after 5 years. He emphasized that the meaningful survival interval should be considered 10 or 15 years. There were no relationships between grade of tumor and age, size, sex, or location. There was no statistical difference between primary and secondary chondrosarcomas. Adequacy of surgical removal was the main determinant of recurrence. In general, chondrosarcomas occurring during childhood had worse prognoses than those occurring during adulthood.[278]

In a review of 125 chondrosarcomas at the Instituto Ortopedico Rizzoli, Gitellis reported that the adequacy of treatment was the main determinant of local recurrence, length of survival, and length of disease-free interval.[13] Patients adequately treated had a 6% local recurrence rate, but the recurrence rate among those inadequately treated was 69%. The 10-year survival rates were 78% (adequately treated) and 61% (inadequately treated). There was no relationship between local recurrence and grade.

In general, peripheral chondrosarcomas have a lower grade than central lesions. Gitellis and co-workers reported that 43% of the peripheral lesions were Grade I, compared with 13% of the central lesions. The 10-year survival rate among those with peripheral lesions was 77%, but 32% among those with central lesions. Secondary chondrosarcomas arising from osteochondromas also have a low malignant potential; 85% are Grade I. Garrison reported only 3% of 75 patients with secondary chondrosarcoma from an osteochondroma developed metastases, although 12% died of local recurrence.[57]

Treatment

The treatment of chondrosarcoma is surgical removal.[10,12,178,278,279] There have been no reports of effective adjuvant chemotherapy. Resection guidelines for high-grade chondrosarcomas are similar to those for osteosarcoma. The shoulder and pelvic girdle are the most common sites for chondrosarcoma, and these sites, combined with the fact chondrosarcomas tend to be low grade, make them amenable to limb-sparing procedures. Lesions of the ribs and sternum are treated by wide excision. Cryosurgery, a technique using liquid nitrogen after thorough curettage of the lesion, has recently been used for central, low-grade chondrosarcomas.[116,117] There have been few reports of effective radiation therapy for axial chondrosarcomas. High-grade chondrosarcomas may warrant adjuvant chemotherapy.

LIMB-SPARING PROCEDURES. The four most common sites of chondrosarcomas are the pelvis, proximal femur, shoulder girdle, and diaphyseal portions of long bones.

Pelvis. The pelvis consists of three areas: ilium, periacetabulum, and pubic rami (Fig. 42-32). Each site may be resected independently of the others.[29,279] Resections are classified Type I (iliac wing), Type II (acetabulum), and Type III (pubic rami, pelvic floor). Bone scan most accurately determines specific bony involvement, and CT delineates the extraosseous component (Fig. 42-33). Contraindications to resection are vascular (iliac artery and vein), peritoneal, and sacroiliac joint or sarcoplexus involvement.

The retroperitoneal space is explored first to determine resectability. Type I resection is performed by a supra-acetabular osteotomy and disarticulation of the sacroiliac joint. Type II resection may require removal of the femoral head; intra-articular involvement of the hip joint by tumor is evaluated by arthotomy before finalizing the surgical plan. Types II and III resections require mobilization of the iliac vessels and femoral nerve, and care must be taken to protect these structures. The Type III procedure requires mobilization of the bladder and urethra before resection. Bilateral pelvic floor resection may be used for chondrosarcomas arising from the midline of the symphysis pubis, in which case urethral resection and reconstruction may be required. Partial cystectomy may be necessary.

Despite the magnitude of resection, pelvic reconstruction is less complex than that at other anatomical sites. Types I and III resection do not require bony reconstruction. In Type

FIG. 42-32. Segmental resection for pelvic tumors.

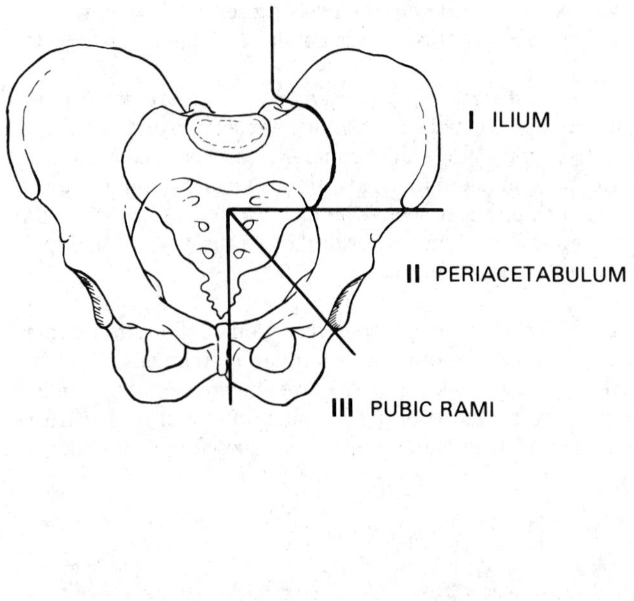

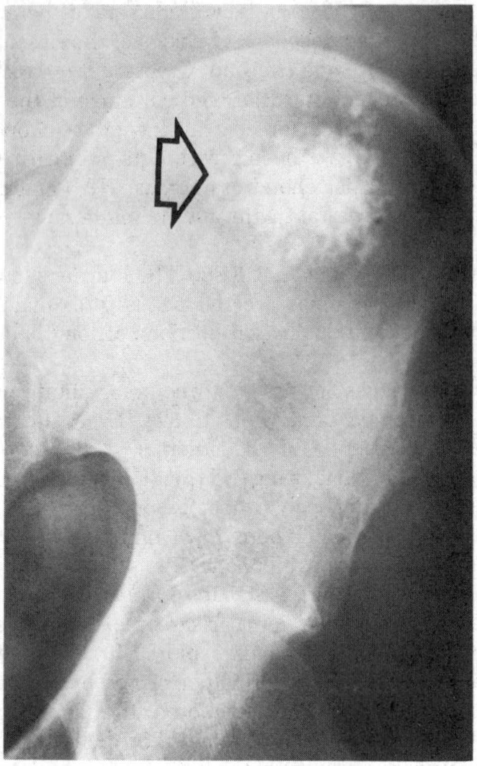
A

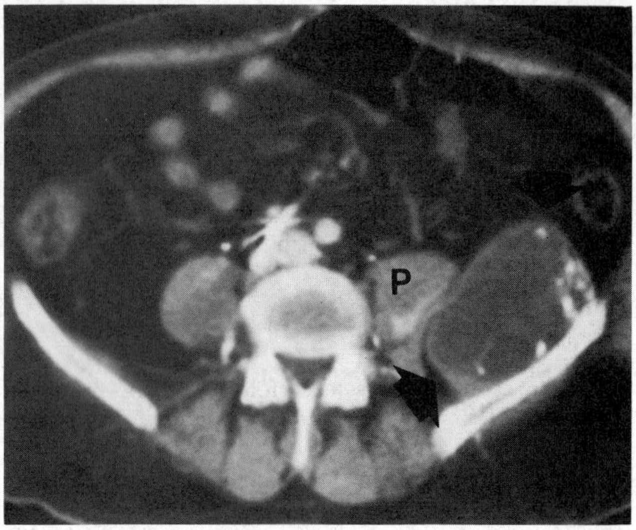

B

FIG. 42-33. Chondrosarcoma of the pelvis. **A**. Plain radiograph demonstrating a small area of calcification within the ilium suggestive of a small intraosseous chondrosarcoma. **B**. CT scan of the same area that surprisingly demonstrated a large chondrosarcoma (*solid arrows*) arising from the ilium, displacing the psoas muscle medially. The small area of calcification (*small solid arrow*) correlated with the plain radiograph (**A**).

I, the adductor musculature is closed to the abdominal wall muscles, and in Type III, the perineal muscles are approximated to the adductor muscles. The periacetabular area is reconstructed either by intentionally creating a nonunion of the femur and the remaining portion of the ilium or pubic rami or by performing a primary arthrodesis. Recently, a unique custom prosthesis, called a saddle prosthesis, has been utilized in replacing the acetabulum. This provides for immediate reconstruction of the pelvis and hip joint.

Long-term results of these procedures have been published by Enneking, who reported that local recurrence was only 4% if adequate margins were obtained.[29] Function was nearly normal if the hip joint was preserved. If the hip joint was removed and fusion was obtained, results were good.

Proximal Femur. Chondrosarcoma of the proximal femur can often be treated successfully by resection and prosthetic replacement. A lateral trephine biopsy is recommended. Care must be taken to avoid intra-articular contamination. A posterior approach should be avoided because of potential contamination of the posterior flap, in the event a hemipelvectomy is required.

Shoulder. The technique of resection of chondrosarcomas of the proximal humerus is similar to that described for osteosarcomas. In low-grade, intracompartmental (Stage IA) tumors, preservation of the deltoid, rotator cuff musculature, and glenoid is possible, and alternatives for reconstruction are more variable. Endoprosthesis, fibula autografts, and allografts all have a high rate of success.[34–39,125–127]

Tibia, Femur, and Humerus. A central diaphyseal chondrosarcoma can be adequately treated by segmental resection without sacrificing the adjacent joint. Because the ends of the bones are not involved, function is excellent. Reconstruction is performed by allografts or autografts combined with internal fixation.

CRYOSURGERY. Marcove pioneered the technique of cryosurgery for bone tumors. This method involves thorough curettage and cryotherapy of the cavity with liquid nitrogen.[115–117] With increasing experience, he has expanded use of the technique for treating low-grade intramedullary cartilage tumors and for some high-grade lesions. He has treated 30 chondrosarcomas with only one local recurrence. Cryosurgery preserves bone stock and avoids resection.

RADIATION THERAPY FOR CHONDROSARCOMA. Unresectable or inoperable chondrosarcomas arising within the axial skeleton and pelvic or shoulder girdle can be controlled, and in some cases cured, by radiation therapy. A combination of radiotherapy and surgery have been shown to be successful for chondrosarcomas of the facial bones and skull.

Although chondrosarcomas have generally been considered radioresistant, there are data to show that some are radiocurable.[284] Among 38 patients undergoing radical irradiation, with or without concurrent chemotherapy, at the Princess Margaret Hospital, 5-year and 10-year actuarial survival rates of 41% and 36%, respectively, were achieved. Median survival was 46 months.[284] A 48% 5-year actuarial survival rate was obtained in the group with well-differentiated and moderately differentiated histologic specimens. Conversely, for those with unfavorable (mesenchymal and poorly differentiated) histology, the 5-year survival rate was only 22%. Radical radiotherapy was defined as a minimum of 40 Gy in 4 weeks or more of megavoltage therapy. Of the 38 patients treated, 17 developed local recurrence. The authors recommend 50 Gy in 4 weeks, with treatment to the whole bone if possible, or at least a 5-cm margin of normal bone. They are now evaluating the effect of concurrent combination chemotherapy in an attempt to improve local control.

McNaney and colleagues, from M.D. Anderson Hospital and Tumor Institute, reported 20 patients with chondrosarcoma treated with photons or neutrons, with or without chemotherapy.[285] The doses of radiation administered ranged from 4000 to 7000 cGy. Thirteen (65%) of 20 are surviving at 30 months. Among the 11 patients treated with radiotherapy alone, 6 (54%) survived. Six patients, all of whom had received photon therapy alone, developed local recurrences. There were no local failures among the four patients treated with a mixed beam of photons and neutrons.

Following radical irradiation, the clinical regression of tumor is slow and may take months to complete. Radiographically, the affected bone never returns to normal. The combination of extremely slow regression of tumor with a persistent radiologic defect makes follow-up and assessment of the response difficult. Unfortunately, there are no rebiopsy data to document long-term sterilization of these tumors. Radiotherapy for chondrosarcoma can provide palliation. In such cases, doses in the range of 5000 cGy over 4 to 5 weeks, or its equivalent, are necessary; low doses for symptomatic relief are ineffective.[286]

Ryall and co-workers used radiation and the radiosensitizer Razoxane (ICRF 159) in eight patients with 12 chondrosarcomas. Seven tumors in five patients achieved complete or partial remission after 4500 to 6000 cGy. Two of the responders were disease-free 2.5 years after treatment.[276a]

Data about the relationship between dose and tumor control are lacking; however, it seems apparent that prolonged local control requires a high radiation dose. Treatment planning requires documentation by CT of the extent of soft-tissue disease.

There is some experience using radioactive ^{35}S for treatment of metastatic chondrosarcoma.[2,287] ^{35}S is selectively taken up by chondrocytes and bone marrow, causing tumor necrosis. Because of reports of associated ^{35}S-induced bone marrow suppression and severe aplastic anemia, this technique is not recommended.[2,287]

The treatment of chondrosarcomas of the maxilla, mandible, and skull entails irradiation and surgery, a combination that has a better potential for improving local control than surgery alone. Local recurrence rates as high as 85% have been reported for head and trunk lesions.[286,288] Among 18 patients with tumors of the head and neck, the Memorial group reported local recurrence in 11 (61%).[288a] The high local recurrence rate reflects the anatomic constraints on the surgical procedure. The use of radiation and surgery should substantially reduce the local recurrence and is currently being studied.

GIANT CELL TUMOR OF BONE

Giant cell tumor (GCT) is an aggressive, locally recurrent tumor with a low metastatic potential.[14–16,63–64,177,287] It consists of spindle-shaped and ovoid cells uniformly interspersed with multinucleated giant cells. Giant cell sarcoma of bone is a term that refers to the de novo, malignant GCT, not the tumor that arises from the transformation of a giant cell tumor previously thought to be benign. These two lesions are separate clinical entities.

Clinical Characteristics

GCT occur slightly more often in females than in males. Pain, mass, local tenderness, and decreased motion in the adjacent joint are the most common clinical symptoms. Eighty percent of these tumors in the long bones occur after skeletal maturity, and 75% develop around the knee joints.[2,3,63] Effusions or pathologic fractures, uncommon with other sarcomas, are common with GCT. GCT occasionally occur in the vertebrae (2–5%) and the sacrum (10%).[2–4]

Grading and Pathology

Jaffe attempted to grade GCT: Grade I (completely benign), Grade II (borderline), and Grade III (frankly sarcomatous).[4] In general, Grades I and II do not correlate well with biologic behavior. There is also a poor correlation between the histologic pattern and the tendency for recurrence or malignant transformation.[14,15,63,177] Nineteen percent to 25% of GCT have some osteoid production.[177] When osteoid formation is noticed, care must be exercised in differentiating a GCT from an osteosarcoma. Conversely, an osteosarcoma with giant cells may be misinterpreted as a benign GCT. There is no correlation between osteoid formation and increased risk of recurrence or metastasis. Necrosis or hemorrhage is often noticed. Neither has a relationship to malignant potential or local recurrence rate.[63]

Natural History

Although GCT are rarely malignant de novo (2–8%), they may undergo transformation and demonstrate malignant potential histologically and clinically after multiple local recurrences.[14–16,177,288] Between 8.6% and 22% of known GCT become malignant following local recurrence.[14–16,177,288] This rate decreases to less than 10% if patients who have undergone radiotherapy are excluded from the series. Hutter reported that 40% of malignant GCT were malignant at the first recurrence.[15] The remainder had become malignant by the second or third recurrence; thus, each recurrence increases the risk of malignant transformation of typical GCT, especially if the transformation occurs after radiation therapy. Local recurrence of a GCT is determined by the adequacy of surgical removal rather than by histologic grade.

Radiographic and Clinical Evaluation

GCT are eccentric lytic lesions without matrix production. They have poorly defined borders with a wide area of transition. They are juxtaepiphyseal with a metaphyseal component. Although the cortex is expanded and appears to be destroyed at surgery, it is usually found to be attenuated but intact. Periosteal elevation is rare; soft-tissue extension is common.

Treatment

Treatment of GCT of bone is surgical removal. Resection is curative in 90% of these tumors, but curettage, with or without bone grafts, has a recurrence rate of 40% to 75%.[14-16,63,283,289] Johnson and Dahlin reported a recurrence rate of 29% within 1 year of curettage and of 54.1% within 5 years.[16] Although en bloc excision offers a reliable cure, routine resection is not recommended.[289] Primary resection of a joint has a significant morbidity, but it is recommended for GCT of the proximal radius and fibula, distal ulna, tubular bones of the hand and foot, coccyx, sacrum, and pelvic bones.

Under certain situations, it is reasonable to perform a curettage. Goldenberg recommends that small tumors with an intact cortex and symptoms of less than 2 to 3 months' duration be treated by curettage.[63] If the lesion heals, resection is avoided. In general, curettage does not rule out a later curative resection. The modern technique of curettage is more extensive than that previously performed. Curettage is accomplished through a large cortical window, equal to the length of the bony defect, using both mechanical curettage and a mechanical burr. This extensive technique has been called *curettage/resection* and has significantly decreased the rate of local recurrence to approximately 25%.

Amputation is reserved for massive recurrence, malignant transformation, or infection. Due to the risk of malignant transformation, lack of effectiveness, and possibility of pathologic fracture, radiation is used only for surgically inaccessible sites.[14,63] Treatment of GCT of the vertebrae and sacrum must be individualized. A combination of surgical excision and cryosurgery or radiotherapy is required to eradicate the tumor and prevent neurological impairment.[105,107]

CRYOSURGERY. Cryosurgery has been used more successfully for GCT than for any other type of bone tumor (Fig. 42-15).[115-117,290] Marcove developed the technique of cryosurgery because of the high recurrence rates after curettage and the significant risk of sarcomatous degeneration in GCT treated by irradiation. He found cryosurgery effective in eradicating the tumor while preserving joint motion and avoiding resection or amputation. He recently reported a 17-year experience of 100 GCT treated by thorough curettage and cryosurgery.[117] He reported a recurrence rate of 16% in the first 50 cases and 2% in the second 50 cases. The major complication of cryosurgery are necrosis of the adjacent bones, which may develop a late pathologic fracture, and delayed union. The rate of secondary pathologic fractures has been decreased by a combination of PMMA augmentation, bone graft, internal fixation of the cavity, and postoperative use of a long-leg brace with a quadrilateral socket.[290] Persson from Sweden reported curettage with PMMA augmentation of the bony defect with bony necrosis due to the heat of polymerization. This technique may provide better local control than curettage alone.[291] Recently, pooled data from several institutions using PMMA and curettage shows a 10% to 15% local recurrence rate.[292]

RADIATION THERAPY. Radiation is recommended for inoperable lesions and local recurrences that develop despite definitive surgery.

There has been a long-term and justified apprehension about patients developing malignant and fatal neoplasms after radiation.[293-297] This concern was supported by Dahlin from the Mayo Clinic, who reported that malignant degeneration ultimately appeared in 37 patients treated with radiation alone or in combination with a surgical procedure.[293] The average time for malignant change was approximately 9 years. McGrath has presented data from the Bristol Tumor Registry that substantiate this concern.[294] Neither of these studies break down the radiation dose to bone in those patients who did and those who did not develop malignant changes. It is known that some of these patients were treated with orthovoltage radiation and that multiple courses were given. The Princess Margaret Hospital group has reported that local tumors have been controlled in 13 of 14 patients with GCT who were treated with one course of megavoltage radiation. Disease in 12 patients was controlled for longer than 5 years.[295] They have observed no instance of malignant transformation. Larsson and colleagues reported three patients with GCT of the spine and sacrum treated by moderate doses of radiotherapy; all have done well.[296]

MALIGNANT FIBROUS HISTIOCYTOMA

Clinical Characteristics

Malignant fibrous histiocytoma (MFH) is a high-grade bone tumor histologically similar to its soft-tissue counterpart.[7-9] It is a disease of adulthood. The most common sites are the metaphyseal ends of long bones, especially around the knee. Serum alkaline phosphatase levels are normal. Pathologic fracture is common. Huvos emphasized that a lytic metaphyseal lesion with a pathologic fracture in an adult with a normal serum alkaline phosphatase level suggests a primary MFH rather than an osteosarcoma or fibrosarcoma.[9] MFH disseminates rapidly. Spanier reported 9 of 11 patients died of the tumor. The average disease-free survival was 6 months.[7] She reported 3 (33%) of 9 patients with pulmonary metastases had lymph node dissemination. She hypothesized that lymphatic spread was due to the histiocytic component of the tumor.

Radiographic Characteristics

MFH is an osteolytic lesion associated with marked cortical disruption, minimal cortical or periosteal reaction, and no evidence of matrix formation.[9] The extent of the tumor routinely exceeds plain radiographic signs. McCarthy and coworkers, reporting on 35 patients with MFH, noticed that four tumors were multicentric and four were associated with bone infarcts.[8]

Treatment

There have been only a few reports regarding the efficacy of chemotherapy for MFH of bone.[298,299] Bacci and colleagues reported 12 patients treated by surgery and chemotherapy, compared with 18 patients treated with surgery alone over the same time at the Istituto Ortopedico Rizzoli.[298] The disease-free survival rates were 59% (7 of 12 patients) and 5% (1 of 18 patients), respectively. Gerado reported three patients with MFH treated by preoperative chemotherapy; a Grade IV response (100% necrosis) was obtained in all three.[299] Due to the extremely poor prognosis of MFH, chemotherapy is justified. Although there are only limited data, there are striking similarities to the results seen with osteosarcoma.

FIBROSARCOMA OF BONE

Clinical Characteristics

Fibrosarcoma is a rare entity characterized by interlacing bundles of collagen fibers (herringbone pattern) without any evidence of tumor bone or osteoid formation.[5] Fibrosarcoma occurs in middle age. The long bones are most affected, but 15% of tumors are found in the bones of the head and neck.[177] Fibrosarcomas occasionally arise in conjunction with an underlying disease such as fibrous dysplasia, Paget's Disease, bone infarcts, osteomyelitis, and postirradiation GCT.[5] Fibrosarcoma may be either central or cortical (periosteal). The histologic grade is a good indicator of metastatic potential. Huvos reported overall survival rates of 27% and 52% for central and peripheral lesions, respectively.[5] Late metastases do occur, and 10-year and 15-year survival rates vary. In general, periosteal tumors have a better prognosis than central lesions.

Radiographic Features

Fibrosarcoma is a radiolucent lesion that shows minimal periosteal and cortical reaction. The radiographic appearance closely correlates with the histologic grade of the tumor.[5] Low-grade tumors are well-defined, but high-grade lesions demonstrate indistinct margins and bone destruction similar to osteolytic osteosarcoma. Plain radiographs usually underestimate the extent of the lesion. Pathologic fracture is common (30%) owing to the lack of matrix formation. Differential diagnosis included GCT, ABC, MFH, and osteolytic osteosarcoma.[5,6]

CHORDOMA

Clinical Characteristics

Chordoma is a rare neoplasm arising from notochordal remnants in the midline of the neural axis and involving the adjacent bone. The ends of the spine are the most common sites. The sacrococcus and the base of the skull near the spheno-occipital area are most commonly involved, accounting for 50% and 35%, respectively, of all chordomas.[177] Histologically, the physaliferous cell is pathognomonic. Large areas of syncytial strands of cells lying in a mass of mucus are typical. Myxoid chondrosarcoma and metastatic carcinoma must be differentiated from chordoma. This tumor is highly fatal because of the high rate of local recurrence and local complications.[300-303] Death is most commonly due to local disease.[300] Gray and colleagues reviewed 222 cases from the literature and noticed that only two patients were disease-free at 10 years.[303] Average survival was 5.7 years. Mindell emphasized the main malignant potential of chordomas resides in their critical locations adjacent to important structures, their locally aggressive nature, and their extremely high rate of recurrence.[300] Chordomas at the base of the skull are often described as chondroid chordomas. Patients with lesions at this site tend to survive longer than those with sacrococcygeal tumors.

The most common complaint of patients with sacrococcygeal tumors is dull pain; constipation is an occasional symptom. Bladder and sensory loss are late complaints. Clinical suspicion is the key to early diagnosis. Rectal examination characteristically reveals a large presacral mass. Spheno-occipital tumors present with signs of cranial nerve or pituitary dysfunction. CT is essential for accurate evaluation. (Fig. 42-34). Myelography is used to determine intraspinal extension. A transrectal biopsy should not be performed because of potential contamination. A small midline posterior incision or trochar biopsy is recommended.

Treatment

The first surgical procedure has the best chance of cure.[302,303] Inadequate surgery results in local recurrence, with little chance of subsequent surgical removal. Sacrococcygeal tumors are best removed by a combined abdominosacral approach, as described by Localio and colleagues.[302,303] They emphasized wide excision of the sacrum one level higher than the lesion. A lateral position is used. The rectum can be mobilized and the iliac vessels controlled anteriorly. The rectum may be removed with the sacrum if necessary. Guterberg and colleagues reported that if only half of the first sacral vertebra remains bilaterally, the pelvic girdle is still stable enough to allow immediate mobilization.[304] Recently DeVries reported two long-term survivors (7 and 10 years) following cryosurgery for sacral chordomas.[305]

RADIATION THERAPY. Because local recurrence is common with chordomas, radiation therapy is an integral treatment modality, particularly for tumors of the base of skull and spheno-occipital region. Results of conventional

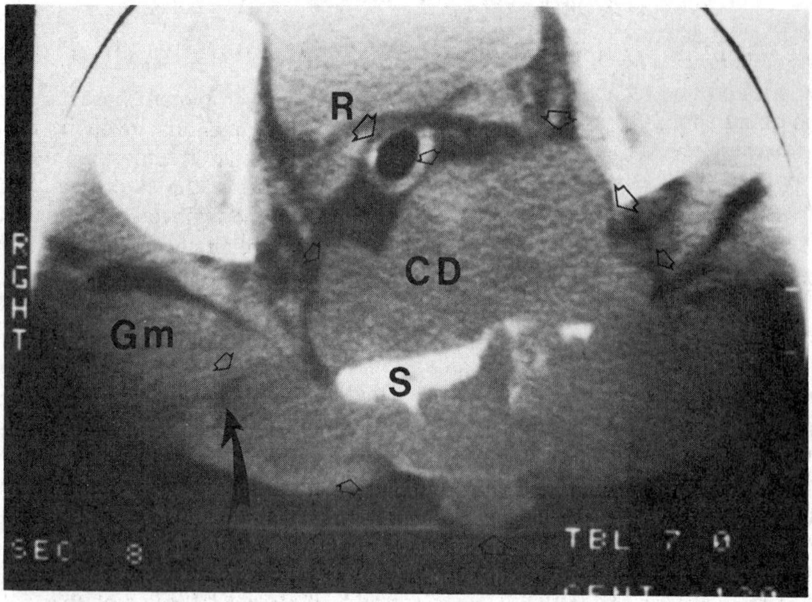

FIG. 42-34. Computed tomography of a chordoma arising within the sacrum (*s*). There is destruction of the body of the sacrum with a huge soft tissue component (outlined by small arrows). The tumor (*CD*) extends to the rectum (*R*) and is infiltrating the gluteus maximus (*Gm*) muscle (*black arrow*). These are typical findings of a sacrococcygeal chordoma, which explains the difference in obtaining local control. Differential diagnosis includes metastatic carcinoma and giant cell tumor of the sacrum.

radiation therapy have been disappointing. Heffelfinger and co-workers reported on 36 patients with nonchondroid varieties of chordomas of the base of skull, none of whom were rendered free of disease by surgery, radiation, or a combination thereof.[306] However, the chondroid variant is more sensitive; of 19 patients with chondroid chordomas, seven were alive and six were disease-free. Other investigators reported on five patients with cervical chordomas; only one was alive and disease-free 5 years after radiation and surgery.[307]

Amendola and colleagues reported on 21 patients with a 5-year survival rate of 50% but a disappointing 10-year survival of only 20%. This is not surprising, because chordomas are relatively slow-growing.[308] Long-term survival without tumor regrowth beyond 10 years is relatively rare.[309] Amendola emphasized the importance of using CT in planning the radiation field, of high radiation doses (*i.e.*, 5500–7000 cGy with megavoltage equipment), and of irradiation immediately after surgery to prolong local control, rather than reserving it until recurrence. The Massachusetts General Hospital (MGH) experience of 48 patients is similar to that reported by others; 50% of the patients survived 5 years or more.[310] Radiation doses varied from 4500 to 8040 cGy, but even with high doses, there was a 45% incidence of local recurrence.

Investigators at MGH and the University of California now advocate using precision heavy-charged-particle irradiation, particularly for chordoma of the basosphenoid region and cervical spine. The MGH experience included 63 patients, 39 with chordomas and 24 with low-grade chondrosarcoma of the basosphenoid region and cervical spine who had been treated with proton-beam radiation therapy at a median tumor dose of 69 CGE.[311] Of the 50 patients with base of skull tumors, six have relapsed. Three of these had chordomas. The increased efficacy using heavy-charged particles is encouraging.[311,312]

SMALL ROUND CELL SARCOMAS OF BONE

Round cell sarcomas of bone behave differently and require different therapeutic management than spindle-cell sarcomas.[313,314] These tumors consist of poorly differentiated small cells without matrix production. They present radiographically as osteolytic lesions. These lesions are best treated with radiation and chemotherapy; surgery is reserved for special situations. Non-Hodgkin's lymphoma and Ewing's sarcoma are the two most common small cell sarcomas. The differential diagnosis of all round cell sarcomas includes metastatic neuroblastoma, metastatic undifferentiated carcinoma, histiocytosis, small cell osteosarcoma, osteomyelitis, and multiple myeloma.

LYMPHOMAS OF BONE

Clinical Characteristics

Lymphoma of bone (previously called reticulum cell sarcoma of bone) accounts for only 5% of the primary bone tumors. In general, lymphoma presenting in bone is a sign of disseminated (Stage IV) disease; occasionally, it may be a solitary lesion defined as "involvement of single extralymphatic organ or site (Stage IE)."[313–314] Reimer at the National Cancer Institute reported that only 1 of 12 patients presenting with bone lymphomas had a solitary lesion.[313] Sweet and colleagues from the University of Chicago reported that 50% of so-called solitary lesions were associated with disease elsewhere.[314] Sweet presented a useful algorithm for the evaluation and treatment of bone lymphomas. He emphasized that all patients with a presumed solitary lymphoma of bone should undergo a thorough evaluation for other involvement.

Treatment is based on the pathologic stage. Stage IE lesions require local radiotherapy and have a reported 90% cure rate.[313] If there is evidence of more advanced disease, chemotherapy is required. The role of surgery is limited to obtaining adequate tissue for diagnosis and treatment of pathologic fracture. The technique of biopsy is important to avoid secondary fracture through potentially irradiated bone. Biopsy of a suspected round cell tumor should always include a frozen section and additional material for electron microscopy, tissue culture, and other special studies. Patients presenting with pathologic fractures usually require a primary resection. To prevent late fractures, all patients treated with radiotherapy should be protected with a brace until reossification occurs.

Radiation Therapy

Local control of the primary tumor with retention of good function of the affected part is commonly achieved following radiation therapy. Radiation therapy is administered to the entire bone and soft-tissue component with a dose of 4000 cGy and a boost to the original tumor area of 5000 cGy. Regional lymph nodes should be included in the radiation port if they are adjacent to the area treated or if clinically involved. Mendenhall and colleagues, from the University of Florida, achieved local and regional control in all irradiated sites in 21 patients with primary bone lymphoma.[315] Two patients relapsed in apparently uninvolved regional lymph node sites that had not been included in the primary treatment portal.

Because most patients with lymphoma of bone have extensive or systemic disease, combination chemotherapy should be part of the treatment. Investigators from Dana-Farber Cancer Center reported on 11 children who had been treated with radiation and chemotherapy consisting of Adriamycin, prednisone, and oncovin, with an 8-year actuarial lymphoma-free survival of 100% and a disease-free survival rate of 79%, for an overall actuarial survival of 90%.[316] There were no relapses. This is consistent with experience from the Bone Tumor Center in Bologna, Italy, where 23 (88%) of 26 patients survived disease-free following radiation and chemotherapy (Adriamycin, vincristine, and cyclophosphamide), with no local relapses at a median follow-up of 7.5 years.[317] In the Dana Farber experience, however, two patients developed second bone tumors, 5 and 7.5 years after beginning therapy. With improvements in survival, the late effects of treatment in these long-term survivors must be considered when therapeutic strategies are planned.

REFERENCES

1. Silverberg E, Lubera, J: Cancer Statistics, 1987. CA 37:2–20, 1987
2. Dahlin DC: Bone tumors: General Aspects and Data on 6,221 Cases, 3rd ed. Springfield, IL Charles C Thomas, 1978
3. Lichtenstein L: Bone Tumors, 5th ed. St Louis, CV Mosby, 1977
4. Jaffe HL: Tumors and Tumorous Conditions of the Bone and Joints. Philadelphia, Lea & Febiger, 1958
5. Huvos AG, Higinbotham NL: Primary fibrosarcoma of bone. A clinicopathologic study of 130 patients. Cancer 35:837–847, 1975
6. Wilner D: Fibrosarcoma. In Wilner D (ed): Radiology of Bone Tumors and Allied Disorders, III, pp 2291–2324. Philadelphia, WB Saunders, 1982
7. Spanier SS, Enneking WF, Enriquez P: Primary malignant fibrous histiocytoma of bone. Cancer 36:2084–2098, 1975
8. McCarthy EF, Matsuno T, Dorfman HD: Malignant fibrous histiocytoma of bone: A study of 35 cases. Hum Pathol 10:57–70, 1979
9. Huvos AG: Primary malignant fibrous histiocytoma of bone. Clinicopathologic study of 18 patients. NY State J Med 76:552–559, 1976
10. Shives TS, Wold LE, Dahlin DC et al: Chondrosarcoma and its variants. In Sim FH (ed): Diagnosis and Treatment of Bone Tumors: A Team Approach (Mayo Clinic Monograph), pp 211–217. Thorofare, NJ, Charles B Slack 1983
11. Marcove RC: Chondrosarcoma: Diagnosis and treatment. Orthop Clin North Am 8:811–819, 1977
12. Pritchard DJ, Lunke RJ, Taylor WF et al: Chondrosarcoma: A clinicopathologic statistical analysis. Cancer 45:149–157, 1980
13. Gitellis S, Bertoni F, Chieti PP et al: Chondrosarcoma of bone. J Bone Joint Surg [Am] 63:1248–1256, 1981
14. Dahlin DC, Cupps RE, Johnson EW Jr: Giant cell tumor: A study of 195 cases. Cancer 25:1061–1070, 1970
15. Hutter VP, Worcester JN Jr, Francis KC et al: Benign and malignant giant cell tumor of bone. A clinicopathological analysis of the natural history of the disease. Cancer 15:653–690, 1962
16. Johnson EW Jr, Dahlin DC: Treatment of giant cell tumor of bone. J Bone Joint Surg [Am] 41:895–904, 1959
17. Nascimento AG, Huvos AC, Marcove RC: Primary malignant giant cell tumor of bone: A study of eight cases and review of the literature. Cancer 44:1393–1402, 1979
18. Weingard DN, Rosenberg SA: Early lymphatic spread of osteogenic and soft-tissue sarcomas. Surgery 84:231–240, 1978
19. Enneking WF, Spanier SS, Goodman MA: A system for the surgical staging of musculoskeletal sarcoma. Clin Orthop 153:106–120, 1980
20. Marcove RC, Rosen G: En bloc resection for osteogenic sarcoma. Cancer 45:3040–3044, 1980
21. Malawer MM: Distal femoral osteogenic sarcoma, principles of soft tissue resection and reconstruction in conjunction with prosthetic replacement (adjuvant surgery). In Chao EYS (ed): Design and Application of Tumor Prosthesis for Bone and Joint Reconstruction, pp 297–309. New York, Thieme-Stratton, 1983
22. Morton DL, Eilber FR, Townsend CM Jr et al: Limb salvage from a multidisciplinary treatment approach for skeletal and soft tissue sarcomas of the extremity. Ann Surg 184:268–278, 1976
23. Enneking WF, Dunham WK: Resection and reconstruction for primary neoplasms involving the innominate bone. J Bone Joint Surg [Am] 60:731–746, 1978
24. Marcove RC, Lewis MM, Rosen G et al: Total femur and total knee replacement: A preliminary report. Clin Orthop 126:147–152, 1977
25. Eilber F, Morton DL, Eckardt J et al: Limb salvage for skeletal and soft tissue sarcomas: Multidisciplinary preoperative therapy. Cancer 53:2579–2584, 1984
26. Eilber FR, Eckhardt J, Morton DL: Advances in the treatment of sarcomas of the extremity. Current status of limb salvage. Cancer 54:2695–2701, 1984
27. Simon MA, Aschliman MA, Thomas N et al: Limb-salvage treatment versus amputation for osteosarcoma of the distal end of the femur. J Bone Joint Surg [Am] 68:1331–1337, 1986
28. Enneking WF: Modification of the system for functional evaluation of surgical management of musculoskeletal tumors. In Enneking WF (ed):Limb-sparing Surgery for Musculoskeletal Tumors, pp 626–639. New York, Churchill Livingstone, 1987
29. Enneking WF, Dunham WK: Resection and reconstruction for primary neoplasms involving the innominate bone. J Bone Joint Surg [Am] 60:731–746, 1978
30. Marcove RC, Lewis MM, Rosen G et al: Total femur and total knee replacement. A preliminary report. Clin Orthop 126:147–152, 1977
31. Mankin HJ, Fogelson FS, Thrasher AZ et al: Massive resection and allograft transplantation in the treatment of malignant bone tumors. N Engl J Med 294:1247–1255, 1976
32. Watts HG: Introduction to resection of musculoskeletal sarcomas. Clin Orthop 153:31–38, 1980
33. Enneking WF, Shirley PD: Resection–arthrodesis for malignant and potentially malignant lesions about the knee using an intramedullary rod and local bone graft. J Bone Joint Surg [Am] 59:223–235, 1977
34. Janeck CJ, Nelson CL: Enbloc resection of shoulder girdle: Technique and indications. Report of a case. J Bone Joint Surg [Am] 54:1754–1758, 1972
35. Francis KC, Worcester JN Jr: Radical resection for tumors of the shoulder with preservation of a functional extremity. J Bone Joint Surg [Am] 44:1423–1429, 1962
36. Marcove RC, Lewis MM, Huvos AG: en bloc upper humeral-interscapular resection: The Tikhoff-Linberg procedure. Clin Orthop 124:219–228,1977
37. Chaos EYS, Ivins JC: Design and Application of Tumor Prosthesis for Bone and Joint Reconstruction: The Design and Application. New York, Thieme-Stratton, 1983
38. Malawer MM, Sugarbaker PH, Lambert M et al: Limb-salvage surgery for tumors of the proximal humerus and shoulder girdle. The Tikhoff-Linberg procedure and its modifications. Surgery 97:518–528, 1985
39. Sim FH, Bowman WE, Chao EYS: Limb-salvage surgery and reconstructive techniques. In Sim FH (ed): Diagnosis and Treatment of Bone Tumors: A Team Approach (A Mayo Clinic Monograph), pp 75–105. Thorofare, NJ, Charles B Slack, 1983
40. de Santos LA, Bernardino ME, Murry JA: Computed tomography in the evaluation of osteosarcoma: Experience with 25 cases. AJR 132:535–540, 1979

41. Destouet JM, Gilula LA, Murphy W: Computed tomography of long bone osteosarcoma. Radiology 131:439–445, 1979
42. Mckillop JH, Etcubanas E, Goris ML: The indications for and limitations of bone scintigraphy in osteogenic sarcoma: A review of 55 patients. Cancer 48:1133–1138, 1981
43. Levine E: Computed tomography of musculoskeletal tumors. CRC Crit Rev Diagn Imaging 16:279–309, 1981
44. Rosenthal DI: Computed tomography in bone and soft tissue neoplasms: Application and pathologic correlation. CRC Crit Rev Diag Imaging 18:243–278, 1982
45. Goldstein H, McNeil BJ, Zufall E et al: Changing indications for bone scintigraphy in patients with osteosarcoma. Radiology 135:177–180, 1980
46. Bacci G, Picci P, Calderoni P et al: Full-lung tomograms and bone scanning in the initial work-up of patients with osteogenic sarcoma. A review of 126 cases. Eur J Cancer Clin Oncol 18:967–971, 1982
47. Jaffe N, Link MP, Cohen D et al: High-dose methotrexate in osteogenic sarcoma. NCI Monogr 56:201–206, 1981
48. Cortes EP, Holland JF, Wang JJ et al: Amputation and Adriamycin in primary osteosarcoma. N Engl J Med 291:998–1000, 1974
49. Rosen G, Marcove RC, Caparros B et al: Primary osteogenic sarcoma. The rationale for preoperative chemotherapy and delayed survey. Cancer 43:2163–2177, 1979
50. Rosen G, Caparros B, Huvos AC et al: Preoperative chemotherapy for osteogenic sarcoma: Selection of postoperative adjuvant chemotherapy based upon the response of the primary tumor to preoperative chemotherapy. Cancer 49:1221–1230, 1982
51. Muggia F, Catani R, Lee YJ et al: Factors responsible for therapeutic success in osteosarcoma. In Jones S, Salmon S (eds): Adjuvant Therapy for Cancer, 2nd ed. New York, Grune & Stratton, 1979
52. Cortes EP, Holland JP: Adjuvant chemotherapy for primary osteogenic sarcoma. Surg Clin North Am 61:1391–1404, 1981
53. Rosen G, Murphy ML, Huvos AG et al: Chemotherapy, en bloc resection and prosthetic replacement in the treatment of osteogenic sarcoma. Cancer 37:1–11, 1976
54. Goorin AM, Frei II E, Abelson HT: Adjuvant chemotherapy for osteosarcoma: A decade of experience. Surg Clin North Am 61:1379–1389, 1981
55. Lichenstein L: Classification of primary tumors of bone. Cancer 4:335–341, 1951
56. Spjut HJ, Dorfman HD, Fechner DE et al: Tumors of bone and cartilage. In Atlas of Tumor Pathology, 2nd series. Washington, DC, Armed Forces Institute of Pathology, 1971
57. Garrison RC, Unni KK, Mcleod RA et al: Chondrosarcoma arising in osteochondroma. Cancer 49:1890–1897, 1982
58. Merryweather R, Middlemiss JH, Sanerkin NG: Malignant transformation of osteoblastoma. J Bone Joint Surg [Br] 62:381–384, 1980
59. Dahlin DC, Unni KK: Osteosarcoma of bone and its important recognizable varieties. Am J Surg Pathol 1:61–72, 1977
60. Ahuja SC, Villacin AB, Smith J et al: Juxtacortical (parosteal) osteogenic sarcoma. J Bone Joint Surg [Am] 59:632–647, 1977
61. Unni KK, Dahlin DC, Beaubout SW: Periosteal osteogenic sarcoma. Cancer 37:2476–2485, 1976
62. Unni KK, Dahlin DC, McLeod RA et al: Intraosseous well-differentiated osteosarcoma. Cancer 40:1337–1347, 1977
63. Goldenberg RR, Campbell CJ, Bongfiglio M: Giant cell tumor of bone. An analysis of two hundred and eighteen cases. J Bone Joint Surg [Am] 52:619–664, 1970
64. Johnson EW, Dahlin DC: Treatment of giant cell tumor of bone: An evaluation of 24 cases treated at the Johns Hopkins hospital between 1925–1955. Orthopedics 62:187–191, 1969
65. Madewell JE, Ragsdale BD, Sweet DE: Radiographic and pathologic analysis of solitary bone lesions. Radiol Clin North Amer 19:715–814, 1981
66. Johnson LC: A general theory of bone tumors. Bull NY Acad Med 19:164–171, 1953
67. Lodwick GS: The bone and joints. In Atlas of Tumor Radiology. Chicago, Year Book Medical Publishers, 1971
68. Enneking WF: Musculoskeletal Tumor Surgery, Vol I, pp 1–60. New York, Churchill Livingstone, 1983
69. Jeffree GM, Price CHG, Sissins HA: The metastatic spread of osteosarcoma: Br J Cancer 32:87–107, 1975
70. McKenna RJ, Schwinn CP, Soong KY et al: Sarcomata of the osteogenic series (osteosarcoma, fibrosarcoma, chondrosarcoma, parosteal osteosarcoma and sarcomata) arising in abnormal bone: An analysis of 552 cases. J Bone Joint Surg [Am] 48:1–26, 1966
71. Marcove RC, Mike V, Hajack JV et al: Ostegenic sarcoma under the age of twenty-one. J Bone Joint Surg [Am] 52:411–423, 1970
72. Sweetnam R: Surgical management of primary osteosarcoma. Clin Orthop 111:57–64, 1975
73. Campanacci M, Bacci G, Bertoni F et al: The treatment of osteosarcoma of the extremities: Twenty years' experience at the Instituto Ortopedico Rizzoli. Cancer 48:1569–1581, 1981
74. Reference deleted.
75. Brostrom L-A: On the natural history of osteosarcoma. Aspects of diagnosis, prognosis and endocrinology. Acta Ortho Scand (Suppl) 183:1–38, 1980
76. Enneking WF, Kagan A: Intramarrow spread of osteosarcoma. In Management of Primary Bone and Soft Tissue Tumors, pp. 171–177. Chicago, Year Book Medical Publishers, 1976
77. Malawer MM, Dunham WF: Skip metastases in osteosarcoma: Recent experience. J Surg Oncol 22:236–245, 1983
78. Enneking WF, Spanier SS, Malawer MM: The effect of the anatomic setting on the results of surgical procedure for soft parts sarcoma of the thigh. Cancer 47:1005–1022, 1981
79. Simon MA, Spanier SS, Enneking WF: The management of soft tissue tumors of the extremities. J Bone Joint Surg [Am] 60:317, 1976
80. Simon MA: Intra-articular extension of adult primary bone sarcomas: Implications for limb-sparing surgical procedures. In Chao EYS, Ivins JS (eds): Tumor Prosthesis for Bone and Joint Reconstruction. The Design and Application. New York, Thieme-Stratton, 1983
81. Bohndorf K, Reiaer M, Lochner B et al: Magnetic resonance imaging of primary tumours and tumour-like lesions of bone. Skeletal Radiol 15:511–517, 1986
82. Cohen MD, Weetman RM, Provisor AG et al: Efficacy of magnetic resonance imaging in 139 children with tumors. Arch Surg 121:522–529, 1986
83. Turner DA: Nuclear magnetic resonance in oncology. Semin Nucl Med 15:210–223, 1985
84. Zimmer WD, Berquist TH, McLeod RA et al: Bone tumors: Magnetic resonance imaging versus computed tomography. Radiology 155:709–718, 1985
85. Powers JA: Magnetic resonance imaging in marrow diseases. Clin Orthop 206: 79–85, 1985
86. Sundaram M, McGuire MH, Herbold DR: Magnetic resonance imaging of osteosarcoma. Skeletal Radiol 16:23–29, 1987
87. Easton EJ, Powers JA: Musculoskeletal Magnetic Resonance Imaging. Thorofare, NJ, Charles B Slack, 1986
88. Patterson H, Springfield DS, Enneking WF: Radiologic Management of Musculoskeletal Tumors. New York, Springer-Verlag, 1986.
89. Link MP: Adjuvant therapy in the treatment of osteosarcoma. In DeVita VT, Hellman S, Rosenberg SA (eds): Important Advances in Oncology, pp 193–207. Philadelphia, JB Lippincott, 1986
90. Link MP, Goorin AM, Miser AW et al: The effect of adjuvant chemotherapy on relapse-free survival in patients with osteosarcoma of the extremity. N Engl J Med 314:1600–1606, 1986
91. Eilber F, Guiliano A, Eckardt J et al: Adjuvant chemotherapy for osteosarcoma: A randomized prospective trial. J Clin Oncol 5:21–26, 1987
92. Edmonson J, Creagan E, Gilchrist G: Phase II study of high dose methotrexate in patients with unresectable metastatic osteosarcoma. Cancer Treat Rep 65:538–539, 1981
93. Rosen G, Nirenberg A: Chemotherapy for osteogenic sarcoma: An investigative method, not a recipe. Cancer Treat Rep 66:1687–1697, 1982
94. Dahlin DC: The problems in assessment of new treatment regimens of osteosarcoma. Clin Orthop 153:81–85, 1980
95. Goorin A, Perez-Atayde A, Gebhardt A et al: Weekly high dose methotrexate and doxorubicin for osteosarcoma: The Dana Farber Cancer Institute/The Children's Hospital–Study III. J Clin Oncol 5:1178–1184, 1987
96. Ettinger LJ, Douglas HO, Mindell ER et al: Adjuvant adriamycin and cisplatin in newly diagnosed, non-metastatic osteosarcoma of the extremity. J Clin Oncol 4:353–362, 1986
97. Rosen G, Marcove RC, Huvos AG et al: Primary osteogenic sarcoma: 8-year experience with adjuvant chemotherapy. J Cancer Res Clin Oncol (Suppl) 106:55–67, 1983
98. Winkler K, Beron G, Kotz R et al: Neoadjuvant chemotherapy for osteogenic sarcoma: Results of a cooperative German/Austrian study. J Clin Oncol 2:617–624, 1984
99. Winkler K, Beron G, Delling G et al: Neoadjuvant chemotherapy of osteosarcoma: Results of a randomized cooperative trial (COSS-82) with salvage chemotherapy based on histological tumor response. J Clin Oncol (in press)
100. Tobias JD, Pratt CB, Parham DM et al: The significance of calcified regional lymph nodes at the time of diagnosis of osteosarcoma. Orthopedics 8:49–52, 1985
101. Giuliano AE, Feig S, Eilber F: Changing metastatic patterns of osteosarcoma. Cancer 54:2160–2164, 1984
102. Jaffe N, Smith E, Abelson H et al: Osteogenic sarcoma. Alterations in the pattern of pulmonary metastases with adjuvant chemotherapy. J Clin Oncol 1:251–254, 1983
103. Enneking WF: Editorial: The issue of the biopsy. J Bone Joint Surg [Am] 64:1119–1120, 1982
104. Mankin HJ, Lange TA, Spanier S: The hazards of biopsy in patients with malignant primary bone and soft-tissue tumors. J Bone Joint Surg [Am] 64:1121–1127, 1982
105. Hudson TM, Hass G, Enneking WF et al: Angiography in the management of musculoskeletal tumors. Surg Gynecol Obstet 141:11–21, 1975
106. Malawer MM, McHale KA: Limb-sparing surgery for high grade malignant tumors of the proximal tibia: Surgical technique and a new method of extensor mechanism reconstruction. Abstracts of 4th International Symposium on Limb-salvage Surgery in Musculoskeletal Oncology. Presented in Kyoto, Japan, 1987
107. Moore TM, Meyers MH, Patzakis MJ et al: Closed biopsy of musculoskeletal lesions. J Bone Joint Surg [Am] 61:374–380, 1979
108. Schajowicz F, Derqui JC: Puncture biopsy in lesions of the locomotor system. Review and results in 4050 cases, including 941 vertebral punctures. Cancer 21:5331–5487, 1968
109. Springfield DS, Goodman MA: Biopsy of musculoskeletal lesions. Orthopedics 3:868–870, 1980
110. Mail JT, Cohen MD, Mirkin LD et al: Response of osteosarcoma to preoperative intravenous high-dose methotrexate chemotherapy: CT evaluation. AJR 144:89–93, 1985
111. Jaffe N, Knapp J, Chuang VP et al: Osteosarcoma: Intra-arterial treatment of the

primary tumor with cis-diamminedichlorplatinum II (CDP): Angiographic, pathologic, and pharmacologic studies. Cancer 51:402–407, 1983
112. Chuang VP, Benjamin R, Jaffe N et al: Radiographic and angiographic changes in osteosarcoma after intra-arterial chemotherapy. AJR 139:1065–1069, 1982
113. Smith J, Heelan RT, Huvos AG et al: Radiographic changes in primary osteogenic sarcoma following intensive chemotherapy. Radiology 143:355–360, 1982
114. Sommer H-J, Knop J, Heise U et al: Histomorphometric changes of osteosarcoma after chemotherapy: Correlation with ^{99}Tc Methylene diphorphonate functional imaging. Cancer 59:252–258, 1987
115. Marcove RC, Lyden JP, Huvos AC et al: Giant cell tumor treated by cryosurgery. Report of 25 cases. J Bone Joint Surg [Am] 55:1633–1644, 1973
116. Marcove RC, Stovell P, Huvos AC et al: The use of cryosurgery in the treatment of low and medium grade chondrosarcoma: A preliminary report. Clin Orthop 122:147–156, 1977
117. Marcove RC: A 17-year review of cryosurgery in the treatment of bone tumors. Clin Orthop 163:231–233
118. Enneking WF, Spanier SS, Goodman MA: A system for the surgical staging of musculoskeletal sarcoma. Clin Orthop 153:106–120, 1980
119. Marcove RC, Rosen G: En bloc resection for osteogenic sarcoma. Cancer 45:3040–3044, 1980
120. Malawer MM: Distal femoral osteogenic sarcoma, principles of soft tissue resection and reconstruction in conjunction with prosthetic replacement (adjuvant surgery). In Chao EYS (ed): Design and Application of Tumor Prothesis for Bone and Joint Reconstruction, pp. 297–309. New York, Thieme-Stratton, 1983
121. Morton DL, Eilber FR, Townsend CM Jr et al: Limb salvage from a multidisciplinary treatment approach for skeletal and soft tissue sarcomas of the extremity. Ann Surg 184:268–278, 1976
122. Enneking WF: Concluding material. In Enneking WF (ed): Limb-sparing Surgery for Musculoskeletal Tumors, pp 624–639. Churchill Livingstone, New York, 1987
123. Malawer MM, Meller I: Porous-coated segmental prosthesis for large tumor defects—a prosthesis based upon immediate fixation (PMA) and extracortical bone fixation: Analysis of 20 consecutive patients. Presented at Annual Meeting of the Musculoskeletal Tumor Society, Toronto, 1987
124. Heck DA, Chao EY, Sim FH et al: Titanium fibermetal segmental replacement prostheses and radiographic analysis and review of current status. Clin Orthop 204:266–285, 1987
125. Mankin HJ, Fogelson FS, Thrasher AZ et al: Massive resection and allograft transplantation in the treatment of malignant bone tumors. N Engl J Med 294:1247–1255, 1976
126. Enneking WF: A system for the functional evaluation of the surgical management of musculoskeletal tumors. In Enneking WF (ed): Limb-sparing Surgery for Musculoskeletal Tumors, pp 5–19. New York, Churchill Livingstone, 1987
127. Miller G: Opening remarks. In Enneking WF (ed): Limb-sparing Surgery for Musculoskeletal Tumors, pp 5–19. New York, Churchill Livingstone, 1987
128. Malawer MM, Baker A: Amputations for tumor. In Evarts CM (ed): Surgery of the Musculoskeletal System, 2nd ed. New York, Churchill Livingstone (in press)
129. Marcove RC, Mirra JM: Principles and techniques of treatment. In Mirra JM (ed): Bone Tumors, Diagnosis and Treatment, pp. 578–614. Philadelphia, JB Lippincott, 1980.
130. Marcove RC, Miller TR: Treatment of primary and metastatic bone tumors by cryosurgery. JAMA 207:189, 1969
131. Marcove RC, Searfoss, Whitmore WF et al: Cryosurgery in the treatment of bone metastases from renal cell carcinoma. Clin Orthop 127:220, 1977
132. deVries J, Oldhoff J, Hadders HN: Cryosurgical treatment of sacrococcygeal chordoma; report of four cases. Cancer 58:2348–2354, 1986
133. Marcove RC, Mike V, Hajek JV et al: Osteogenic sarcoma under the age of 21. A review of 145 operative cases. J Bone Joint Surg [Am] 25:411–423, 1970
134. Mike V, Marcove RC: Osteogenic sarcoma under the age of 21: Experience at Memorial Sloan-Kettering Cancer Center. In Terry WD, Windhorst D (eds): Immonotherapy of Cancer: Present Status of Trials in Man. New York, Raven Press, 1978
135. Gehan EA, Sutow WW, Uribe-Botero G et al: Osteosarcoma: The MD Anderson experience, 1950–1974. In Terry WD, Windhorst D (eds): Immunotherapy of Cancer: Present Status of Trials in Man, pp 271–282. New York, Raven Press, 1978
136. Uribe-Botero G, Russell W, Sutow W et al: Primary osteosarcoma of bone: A clinicopathological investigation of 243 cases, with necropsy studies in 54. Am J Clin Pathol 67:427–435, 1977
137. Frieman MA, Carter SK: The therapy of osteogenic sarcoma: Current status and thoughts for the future. J Surg Oncol 4:482–510, 1972
138. Taylor WF, Ivins JC, Dahlin DC et al: Osteogenic sarcoma experience at the Mayo Clinic, 1963–1974. In Terry WD, Windhorst D (eds): Immunotherapy of Cancer: Present Status of Trials in Man. New York, Raven Press, 1978
139. Taylor WF, Ivins JC, Dahlin DC et al: Trends and variability in survival from osteosarcoma. Mayo Clinic Proc 53:697–700, 1978
140. Taylor WF, Ivins J, Pritchard D et al: Trends and variability in survival among patients with osteosarcoma: A 7-year update. Mayo Clin Proc 60:91–104, 1985
141. Strander H, Adamson U, Aparisi T et al: Adjuvant interferon treatment of human osteosarcoma. Recent Results Cancer Res 68:40–44, 1979
142. Rab GT, Ivins JC, Childs DS et al: Elective whole lung irradiation in the treatment of osteogenic sarcoma. Cancer 38:939–942, 1976
143. Breuer K, Cohen P, Schweisguth O et al: Irradiation of the lungs as an adjuvant therapy in the treatment of osteosarcoma of the limbs: An EORTC randomized study. Eur J Cancer 14:461–471, 1978
144. Edmonson J, Green S, Ivins J et al: A controlled pilot study of high-dose methotrexate as post-surgical adjuvant treatment for primary osteosarcoma. J Clin Oncol 2:152–156, 1984
145. Schabel FM: Rationale for adjuvant chemotherapy. Cancer 39:2875–2882, 1977
146. Schabel FM: Experimental basis for adjuvant chemotherapy. In Salmon SE, Jones SE (eds): Adjuvant Therapy of Cancer, pp 3–14. Amsterdam, Elsevier, 1977
147. Schabel FM Jr: *In vivo* leukemic cell kill kinetics and "curability" in experimental systems. In The proliferation and Spread of Neoplastic Cells, pp 379–408. Baltimore, Williams & Wilkins, 1968
148. Schabel FM Jr: The use of tumor growth kinetics in planning "curative" chemotherapy of advanced solid tumors. Cancer Res 29:2385–2388, 1969
149. Laster WR Jr, Mayo JG, Simpson-Herren L, et al: Success and failure in the treatment of solid tumors: II. Kinetic parameters and "cell cure" of moderately advanced carcinoma 755. Cancer Chemother Rep 54:169–188, 1969
150. Cortes EP, Holland JF, Wang JJ et al: Doxorubicin in disseminated osteosarcoma. JAMA 211:1132–1138, 1972
151. Nitschke R, Starling KA, Vats T et al: Cis-diamminedichloroplatinum (NSC-119875) in childhood malignancies: A Southwest Oncology Group study. Med Pediatr Oncol 4:127–132, 1978
152. Ochs JJ, Freeman AI, Douglas HO et al: Cis-dichlorodiammineplatinum (II) in advanced osteogenic sarcoma. Cancer Treat Rep 62:239–245, 1978
153. Baum ES, Gaynon P, Greenberg L et al: Phase II study of cis-dichlorodiammineplatinum (II) in childhood osteosarcoma: Children's Cancer Study Group report. Cancer Treat Rep 63:1621–1627, 1979
154. Gasparini M, Rouesse J, van Oosterom A et al: Phase II study of cisplatin in advanced osteogenic sarcoma. Cancer Treat Rep 69:211–213, 1985
155. Jaffe N, Farber S, Traggis D et al: Favorable response of metastatic osteogenic sarcoma to pulse high dose methotrexate with citrovorum rescue and radiation therapy. Cancer 31:1367–1373, 1973
156. Pratt C, Howarth C, Ransom J et al: High dose methotrexate used alone and in combination for measurable primary and metastatic osteosarcoma. Cancer Treat Rep 64:11–20, 1980
157. Jaffe N, Frei E, Traggis D et al: Weekly high-dose methotrexate—citrovorum factor in osteogenic sarcoma. Cancer 39:45–50, 1977
157a. Marti C, Kroner T, Remagen W et al: High-dose ifosfamide in advanced osteosarcoma. Cancer Treat Rep 69:115–117, 1985
158. Edmonson J, Creagan E, Gilchrist G: Phase II study of high dose methotrexate in patients with unresectable metastatic osteosarcoma. Cancer Treat Rep 65:538–539, 1985
159. Cortes EP, Holland JF, Wang JJ et al: Amputation and Adriamycin in primary osteosarcoma. N Engl J Med 291:998–1000, 1974
160. Mosende C, Gutierrez M, Caparros B et al: Combination chemotherapy with bleomycin, cyclophosphamide and dactinomycin for the treatment of osteogenic sarcoma. Cancer 40:2779–2786, 1977
161. Frei E, Jaffe N, Skpper H et al: Adjuvant chemotherapy of osteogenic sarcoma: Progress and perspectives. In Salmon SE, Jones SE (eds): Adjuvant Therapy of Cancer, pp 49–64. Amsterdam, Elsevier, 1977
162. Rosen G, Murphy ML, Huvos AG et al: Chemotherapy, en bloc resection, and prosthetic bone replacement in the treatment of osteogenic sarcoma. Cancer 37:1–11, 1976
163. Rosen G, Marcove RC, Caparros B et al: Primary osteogenic sarcoma. The rationale for preoperative chemotherapy and delayed surgery. Cancer 43:2163–2177, 1979
164. Huvos A, Rosen G, Marcove RC: Primary osteogenic sarcoma. Pathologic aspects in 20 patients after treatment with chemotherapy, en bloc resection and prosthetic bone replacement. Arch Pathol Lab Med 101:14–18, 1977
165. Winkler K, Beron G, Kotz R et al: Adjuvant chemotherapy in osteosarcoma—effects of cisplatinum, BCD, and fibroblast interferon in sequential combination with HD-MTX and Adriamycin. Preliminary results of the COSS 80 study. J Cancer Res Clin Oncol (Suppl) 106:1–7, 1983
166. Goldie JH, Coldman AJ: A mathematical model for relating the drug sensitivity of tumors to their spontaneous mutation rate. Cancer Treat Rep 63:1727–1733, 1979
167. DeVita VT: The relationship between tumor mass and resistance to chemotherapy. Cancer 51:1209–1220, 1983
168. Salzer-Kuntschik M, Delling G, Beron G et al: Morphological grades of regression in osteosarcoma after polychemotherapy—Study COSS 80. J Cancer Res Clin Oncol (Suppl) 106:21–24, 1983
169. Jaffe N, Prudich J, Knapp J, et al: Treatment of primary osteosarcoma with intra-arterial and intravenous high-dose methotrexate. J Clin Oncol 1:428–431, 1983
170. Provisor A, Nachman J, Krailo M et al: Treatment of non-metastatic osteogenic sarcoma of the extremities with pre- and post-operative chemotherapy. Proc Am Soc Clin Oncol 6:217, 1987
171. Rosen G, Caparros B, Huvos AG et al: Preoperative chemotherapy for osteogenic sarcoma: Selection of post-operative based on the response of the primary tumor to preoperative chemotherapy. Cancer 49:1221–1230, 1982
172. Winkler K, Beron G, Delling G et al: Selective postoperative (pOp) adjuvant chemotherapy (CT) after agressive vs. mild preoperative (prOp) CT in osteosarcoma. Proc Am Soc Clin Oncol 5:128, 1986
173. Jaffe N, Knapp J, Chuang VP et al: Osteosarcoma: Intra-arterial treatment of the primary tumor with cis-diammine-dichloroplatinum II (CDP): Angiographic, pathologic and pharmocologic studies. Cancer 51:402–407, 1983

174. Jaffe N, Robertson R, Ayala A et al: Comparison of intra-arterial cis-diamminedicholoroplatinum II with high dose methotrexate and citrovorum factor rescue in the treatment of primary osteosarcoma. J Clin Oncol 3:1101-1104, 1985
174a. Martinez A, Donaldson SS, Bagshaw MA: Special set-up and treatment techniques for the radiotherapy of pediatric malignancies. Int J Radiat Oncol Biol Phys 2:1007-1016, 1977
175. Watkins DMB: Radiation Therapy Mold Technology. Toronto, Pergamon Press, 1981
176. Sanerkin NG: The diagnosis and grading of chondrosarcoma of bone. A combined cytologic and histologic approach. Cancer 45:582-594, 1980
177. Huvos AG: Bone Tumors. Diagnosis, Treatment and Prognosis. Philadelphia, WB Saunders, 1979
178. Marcove RC, Mike V, Hutter RVP et al: Chondrosarcoma of the pelvis and upper end of femur. J Bone Joint Surg [Am] 54:561-572, 1972
179. Bacci G, Springfield D, Picci P et al: Adjuvant chemotherapy for malignant fibrous histiocytoma in the femur and tibia. J Bone Joint Surg [Am] 67:620-625, 1985
180. Nobler MP, Higginbotham NL, Phillips RF: The cure of aneurysmal bone cyst: Irradiation superior to surgery in an analysis of 33 cases. Radiology 90:1185-1192, 1968
181. Cassady JR: Radiation therapy in less common primary bone tumors. In Jaffe N (ed): Solid Tumors in Childhood, pp 205-214. Littleton, MA, PSG Publishing, 1979
182. Anonsen CK, Donaldson SS: Langerhans' cell histiocytosis of the head and neck. Laryngoscope 97:537-542, 1987
182a. Greenberger JS, Crocker AC, Vawter G et al: Results of treatment of 127 patients with systemic histiocytosis (Letterer-Siwe syndrome, Schuller-Christian syndrome and multifocal eosinophilic granuloma). Medicine [Baltimore] 60:311-338, 1981
183. Dahlin DC, Coventry MB: Osteosarcoma, a study of 600 cases. J Bone Joint Surg [Am] 49:101-110, 1967
184. Richter MP, D'Angio GJ: The role of radiation therapy in the management of children with histiocytosis X. Am J Pediatr Hematol Oncol 3:161-163, 1981
185. Wick MR, Siegal GP, Unni KK et al: Sarcomas of bone complicating osteitis deformas (Paget's disease), 50 years' experience. Am J Surg Pathol 5:47-59, 1981
186. Greditzer HG, McLeod RA, Unni KK et al: Bone sarcomas in Paget's disease. Radiology 146:327-333, 1983
186a. Huvos AG, Wooard HQ, Cahan WG et al: Postradiation osteogenic sarcoma of bone and soft tissues, a clinicopathologic study of 66 patients. Cancer 55:1244-1255, 1982
187. Francis KC, Kohn H, Malawer MM: Osteogenic sarcoma. J Bone Joint Surg [Am] 55:754, 1976
188. Enneking WF: Musculoskeletal Tumor Surgery, vol VII, pp 1021-1125. New York, Churchill Livingstone, 1983
188a. Wilner D: Osteogenic sarcoma (osteosarcoma). In Wilner D (ed): Radiology of Bone Tumors and Allied Disorders, pp 1897-2095. Philadelphia, WB Saunder, 1982
189. de Santos LA, Edeiken B: Purely lytic osteosarcoma. Skeletal Radiol 9:1-7, 1982
190. Jaffe N, Smith E, Abelson HT et al: Osteogenic sarcoma: Alterations in the pattern of pulmonary metastases with adjuvant chemotherapy. J Clin Oncol 1:251-254, 1983
191. Lockshin MD, Higgins TT: Prognosis in osteogenic sarcoma. Clin Orthop 58:85-103, 1968
192. Larsson SE, Lorentzon R, Wedron H et al: The prognosis in osteosarcoma. Int Orthop 5:305-310, 1981
193. Brostrom L, Strander H, Nisonne U: Survival in osteosarcoma in relation to tumor size and location. Clin Orthop 167:250-254, 1982
194. Levine AM, Rosenberg SA: Alkaline phosphatase levels in osteosarcoma tissue are related to prognosis. Cancer 44:2291-2293, 1979
195. Levin AM, Trich T, Rosenberg SA: Osteosarcoma cells in tissue culture: II. Characterization and location of alkaline phosphatase activity. Clin Orthop 3:33-41, 1975
196. Scranton PE Jr, DeCicco FA, Totten RS et al: Prognostic factors in osteosarcoma. A review of 20 years' experience at the University of Pittsburgh Health Center Hospitals. Cancer 36:2179-2191, 1975
197. Malawar MM, Meller I, Dunham WK: Proposed surgical classification of shoulder girdle resections for bone and soft tissue tumors: Description for a new system and analysis of 38 patients. Presented at American Society of Shoulder and Elbow Surgery, New Orleans, 1987
198. Malawer MM, Sugarbaker, PH et al: The Tikhoff-Linberg procedure and its modifications. In Sugarbaker PH (ed): Atlas of Sarcoma Surgery, Chap 14. Philadelphia, JB Lippincott, 1984
199. Malawer MM, Price WM: Gastrocnemius transposition flaps in conjunction with limb-sparing surgery for primary sarcomas around the knee. Plast Reconstr Surg 73:741-750, 1984
200. Malawer MM, McHale KA: Limb-sparing surgery for high grade tumors of the proximal tibia and a new method of extensor mechanism reconstruction. 4th International symposium on limb-salvage in musculoskeletal oncology. Kyoto, Japan, 1987
201. Hudson TM, Springfield DS, Schiebler M: Popiteus muscle as a barrier to tumor spread: Computer tomography and angiography. J Computer Assist Tomogr 8:498-501, 1984
202. Malawer MM: Surgical management of aggressive and malignant tumors of the proximal fibula. Clin Orthop 186:172-181, 1984
203. Rosen G: Preoperative chemotherapy in osteogenic sarcoma. In Enneking, WF (ed): Limb-sparing Surgery for Musculoskeletal Tumors, pp 260-267. New York, Churchill Livingstone, 1987
204. Picci P, Bacci G, Companacci M et al: Histological evaluation of necrosis in osteosarcoma induced by chemotherapy, regional mapping of viable and nonviable tumor. Cancer 56:1515-1521, 1985
205. Martin NS, Williamson J: The role of surgery in the treatment of malignant tumors of the spine. J Bone Joint Surg [Br] 52:227-237, 1970
206. Sterner B: Total spondylectomy in chondrosarcoma arising in the seventh thoracic vertebra. J Bone Joint Surg [Br] 53B:288-295, 1971
207. Sterner BL, Johnson OE: Complete removal of three vertebra for giant-cell tumor. J Bone Joint Surg [Br] 53:278-287, 1971
208. Maobiglet GM, Benjamin R, Patt YZ et al: Intra-arterial cis-platinum for patients with inoperable skeletal tumors. Cancer 48:1-4, 1981
209. Sundaresan N, Rosen G, Fortner JG et al: Preoperative chemotherapy. and surgical resection in the management of posterior paraspinal tumors. J Neurosurg 58:446-450, 1983
210. Rosen G, Huvos A, Mosende C et al: Chemotherapy and thoracotomy for metastatic osteogenic sarcoma. Cancer 41:841-849, 1978
211. Pratt C, Champion J, Senzern et al: Treatment of unresectable or metastatic osteosarcoma with cisplatin or cisplatin-doxorubicin. Cancer 56:1930-1933, 1985
212. Creagan E, Frytak S, Pairolero P et al: Surgically proven pulmonary metastases not demonstrated by computed chest tomography. Cancer Treat Rep 62:1404-1405, 1978
213. Putnam JB, Roth J, Wesley M et al: Survival following aggressive resection of pulmonary metastases from osteogenic sarcoma: Analysis of prognostic factors. Ann Thorac Surg 36:516-523, 1983
214. Goorin A, Delorey M, Lack E et al: Prognostic significance of complete surgical resection of pulmonary metastases in patients with osteogenic sarcoma: Analysis of 32 patients. J Clin Oncol 2:425-431, 1984
215. Meyer WH, Schell MJ, Kumar APM et al: Thoracotomy for pulmonary metastatic osteosarcoma. An analysis of prognostic indicators of survival. Cancer 59:374-379, 1987
216. Telander R, Pairolero P, Pritchard D et al: Resection of pulmonary metastatic osteogenic sarcoma in children. Surgery 84:335-341, 1978
217. Weichselbaum R, Cassady J, Jaffe N et al: Preliminary results of aggressive multimodality therapy for metastatic osteosarcoma. Cancer 40:78-83, 1977
218. Beattie E, Martini N, Rosen G: The management of pulmonary metastases in children with osteogenic sarcoma with surgical resection combined with chemotherapy. Cancer 35:618-621, 1975
219. Martini N, Huvos A, Mike V et al: Multiple pulmonary resections in the treatment of osteogenic sarcoma. Ann Thorac Surg 12:271-280, 1971
220. Spanos P, Payne W, Ivins J et al: Pulmonary resection for metastatic osteogenic sarcoma. J Bone Joint Surg [Am] 58:624-628, 1976
221. Giritsky A, Etcubanas E, Mark J: Pulmonary resection in children with metastatic osteogenic sarcoma. J Thorac Cardiovasc Surg 73:354-362, 1978
222. Rosenberg S, Flye M, Conkle D et al: Treatment of osteogenic sarcoma. II. Aggressive resection of pulmonary metastases. Cancer Treat Rep 63:753-756, 1979
223. Han M-T, Telander R, Pairolero P et al: Aggressive thoracotomy for pulmonary metastatic osteogenic sarcoma in children and young adolescents. J Pediatr Surg 16:928-933, 1981
224. Jaffe N, Frei E, Traggis D et al: Adjuvant methotrexate and citrovorum-factor treatment of osteogenic sarcoma. N Engl J Med 291:994-997, 1984
225. Jaffe N, Frei E, Watts H et al: High dose methotrexate in osteogenic sarcoma: A 5-year experience. Cancer Treat Rep 62:259-264, 1978
226. Frei E, Jaffe N, Link M et al: Adjuvant chemotherapy of osteogenic sarcoma: Progress, problems and prospects. In Jones S, Salmon S (eds): Adjuvant Therapy of Cancer II, pp 355-363. New York, Grune & Stratton, 1979
227. Rosenberg SA, Chabner BA, Young RC et al: Treatment of osteogenic sarcoma. I. Effect of adjuvant high-dose methotrexate after amputation. Cancer Treat Rep 63:739-751, 1979
228. Bode U, Levine AS: The biology and management of osteosarcoma. In Levine AS (ed): Cancer in the Young, pp 575-602. New York, Masson Publishing USA, 1982
229. Cortes EP, Holland JF, Glidewell O: Amputation and adriamycin in primary osteosarcoma: A 5-year report. Cancer Treat Rep 62:271-277, 1978
230. Cortes EP, Holland JF, Glidewell O: Adjuvant therapy of operable primary osteosarcoma — Cancer and Leukemia Group B experience. Recent Results Cancer Res 68:16-24, 1979
231. Cortes E, Necheles TF, Holland JF et al: Adjuvant chemotherapy for primary osteosarcoma: A Center and Leukemia Group B experience. In Salmon S, Jones S (eds): Adjuvant Therapy of Cancer III, pp 201-210. New York, Grune & Stratton, 1981
232. Krailo M, Ertel I, Makley J et al: A randomized study comparing high dose methotrexate with moderate dose methotrexate as components of adjuvant chemotherapy in childhood nonmetastatic osteosarcoma: A report from the Children's Cancer Study Group. Med Pediatr Oncol 15:69-77, 1987
233. Sutow WW, Sullivan MP, Fernbach DJ et al: Adjuvant chemotherapy in primary treatment of osteogenic sarcoma. A Southwest Oncology Group study. Cancer 36:1598-1602, 1975
234. Sutow WW, Gehan EA, Dyment PG et al: Multidrug adjuvant chemotherapy for osteosarcoma: Interim report of the Southwest Oncology Group studies. Cancer Treat Rep 62:265-269, 1978

235. Herson J, Sutow WW, Elder K et al: Adjuvant chemotherapy in nonmetastatic osteosarcoma: A Southwest Oncology Group study. Med Pediatr Oncol 8:343–352, 1980
235a. Goorin A, Delorey M, Geiber R et al: The Dana-Farber Cancer Institute/The Children's Hospital adjuvant chemotherapy trials for Osteosarcoma: Three sequential studies. Cancer Treat Rep 3:155–159, 1986
236. Etcobanas E, Wilbur JR: Adjuvant chemotherapy for osteogenic sarcoma. Cancer Treat Rep 62:283–287, 1978
237. Pratt CB, Rivera G, Shanks E, et al: Combination chemotherapy for osteosarcoma. Cancer Treat Rep 62:251–257, 1978
238. Pratt CB: Personal Communication
239. Ettinger LJ, Douglass HO, Higby DJ et al: Adjuvant Adriamycin and cis-diamminedichloroplatinum (cis-platinum) in primary osteosarcoma. Cancer 47:248–254, 1981
240. Breur K, van der Schueren E: Adjuvant therapy in the management of osteosarcoma: Need for critical reassessment. Recent Results Cancer Res 68:5–15, 1979
241. van der Schueren E, Breur K: Role of lung irradiation in the adjuvant treatment of osteosarcoma. Recent Results Cancer Res 80:98–102, 1982
242. Weiner M, Harris M, Lewis M et al: Neoadjuvant high-dose methotrexate, cisplatin, and doxorubicin for the management of patients with nonmetastatic osteosarcoma. Cancer Treat Rep 70:1431–1432, 1986
242a. Sutow WW, Herson J, Perez C: Survival after metastasis in osteosarcoma. NCI Monogr 56:227–231, 1981
242b. Marcove R, Martini N, Rosen G: The treatment of pulmonary metastasis in osteogenic sarcoma. Clin Orthop 111:65–70, 1975
242c. Levine AS, Appelbaum FR, Echelberger C et al: Metastatectomy followed by multiagent intensive chemotherapy in osteosarcoma. Proc ASCO 1:47, 1982 Pratt CB: Outcome of patients failing adjuvant chemotherapy for osteosarcoma. Cancer Bull 34:101–103, 1982
243. Cade S: Osteogenic Sarcoma: A study based on 133 patients. JR Coll Surg Edinb 1:79–111, 1955
244. Lee ES, MacKenzie DH: Osteosarcoma: A study of the value of preoperative megavoltage radiotherapy. Br J Surg 51:252–274, 1964
244a. Farrell C, Reventos A: Experience in treating osteosarcoma at the Hospital of the University of Pennsylvania. Radiology 83:1080–1083, 1964
244b. Sweetnan R, Knowelden J, Seedon H: Bone sarcoma: Treatment by irradiation, amputation, or a combination of the two. Br Med J 2:363–367, 1971
244c. Phillips TL, Sheline GE: Radiation therapy of malignant bone tumors. Radiology -92:1537–1545, 1969
245. Allen CV, Stevens KR: Preoperative irradiation for osteogenic sarcoma. Cancer 31:1365–1366, 1973
246. Gaitan-Yanguas M: A study of the response of osteogenic sarcoma and adjacent normal tissues to radiation. Int J Radiat Oncol Biol Phys 7:593–595, 1981
247. Jenkin RD: Radiation treatment of Ewing's sarcoma and osteogenic sarcoma. Can J Surg 20:530–536, 1977
248. Jenkin RDT, Allt WEC, Fitzpatrick PJ: Osteosarcoma. An assessment of management with particular reference to primary irradiation and selective delayed amputation. Cancer 30:393–400, 1972
249. Beck JC, Wara WM, Bovill EG et al: The role of radiation therapy in the treatment of osteosarcoma. Radiology 120:163–165, 1976
250. Suit HD: Radiation therapy given under conditions of local tissue hypoxia for bone and soft tissue sarcoma. In MD Anderson Hospital: Tumors of Bone and Soft Tissue, pp 143–163. Chicago, Year Book Medical Publishers, 1965
251. Scanlon PW: Split-dose radiotherapy for radioresistant bone and soft tissue sarcoma: Ten years' experience AJR 114:544–552, 1972
252. Lee ES: Treatment of bone sarcoma. Proc R Soc Med 64:1179–11180, 1971
253. Clark JL, Unni KK, Dahlin DC et al: Osteosarcoma of the jaw. Cancer 51:2311–2316, 1983
254. Chambers RG, Mahoney WD: Osteogenic sarcoma of the mandible: Current management. Am Surg 36:463–471, 1970
255. Suit HD: Role of Therapeutic radiology in cancer of bone. Cancer 35:930–935, 1975
256. deFries HO, Perlin E, Leibel SA: Treatment of osteogenic sarcoma of the mandible. Arch Otolaryngol 105:358–359, 1970
257. Akbiyik N, Alexander LL: Osteosarcoma of the maxilla treated with radiation therapy and surgery. J Natl Med Assoc 73:355–356, 1981
258. Livolsi VA: Osteogenic sarcoma of the maxilla. Arch Otolaryngol 103:485–488, 1977
259. Goffinet DR, Kaplan HS, Donaldson SS et al: Combined radiosensitizer infusion and irradiation of osteogenic sarcoma. Radiology 117:211–214, 1975
260. Martinez A, Goffinet DR, Donaldson SS et al: Intra-arterial infusion of radiosensitizer (BUdR) combined with hypofractionated irradiation and chemotherapy for primary treatment of osteogenic sarcoma. Int J Radiat Oncol Biol Phys 11:123–128, 1985
261. Kinsella TJ, Glatstein E: Clinical experience with intravenous radiosensitizers in unresectable sarcomas. Cancer 59:908–915, 1987
262. Weichselbaum RR, Cassady JR: Radiation therapy in osteosarcoma. In Jaffe N (ed): Solid Tumors in Childhood, pp 183–190. Boca Raton, FL, CRC Press, 1983
263. Newton KA, Barrett A: Prophylactic lung irradiation in the treatment of osteogenic sarcoma. Clin Radiol 29:493–496, 1978
264. Breur K, Cohen P, Schweisguth O et al: Irradiation of the lungs as an adjuvant therapy in the treatment of osteosarcoma of the limbs. An EORTC randomized study. Eur J Cancer 14:461–471, 1978
265. Breur K, Schweisguth O, Cohen P et al: Prophylactic irradiation of the lungs to prevent development of pulmonary metastases in patients with osteosarcoma of the limbs NCI Monogr 56:233–236, 1981
266. Breur K, van der Schueren E: Adjuvant therapy in the management of osteosarcoma: Need for critical reassessment. Recent Results Cancer Res 68:5–15, 1978
267. Rab GT, Luins JC, Child DS et al: Elective whole lung irradiation in the treatment of osteogenic sarcoma. Cancer 38:949–942, 1976
268. Jenkins RDT: The treatment of osteosarcoma with radiation: Current indications. In Management of Primary Bone and Soft Tissue Tumors, pp 151–162. Chicago, Year Book Medical Publishers, 1976
269. Caceres E, Zaharia M, Moran M et al: Adjuvant whole lung radiation with or without adriamycin treatment in osteogenic sarcoma. Cancer Treat Rep 62:297–299, 1978
270. Unni KK, Dahlin DC, Beaubout SW et al: Parosteal osteogenic sarcoma. Cancer 37: 2466–2475, 1976
271. Martin SE, Dwyer A, Kissane JM et al: Small-cell osteosarcoma. Cancer 50:990–996, 1982
272. Sim FH, Unni Ku, Beaubout JW et al: Osteosarcoma with small cells simulating Ewing's tumor. J Bone Joint Surg [Am] 61:207–215, 1979
273. Mankin HJ, Cantley KD, Lipielo L et al: The biology of human chondrosarcoma. I. Description of the cases, grading, and biochemical analyses. J Bone Joint Surg [Am] 62:160–176, 1980
274. Mankin HJ, Cantley KD, Schiller AL et al: The biology of human chondrosarcoma: II. Variations in chemical composite among types and subtypes of benign and malignant cartilage tumors. J Bone Joint Surg [Am] 62:176–188, 1980
275. Krocberg A, Zelterberg A, Soderberg G: A comparative study of cellular DNA content and clinicopathologic features. Cancer 50:577–583, 1982
276. Alho A, Connor JF, Mankin HJ et al: Assessment of malignancy of cartilage tumors using flow cytometry. A preliminary report. J Bone Joint Surg [Am] 65:779–785, 1983
277. Edeiken J: Bone tumors and tumor-like conditions. In Edeiken J (ed): Roentgen Diagnosis of Diseases of Bone, 3rd ed, pp 30–414. Baltimore, Williams & Wilkins, 1981
278. Aprin H, Riserborough EJ, Hall JE: Chondrosarcoma in children and adolescents. Clin Orthop 166:226–232, 1982
279. Steel HH: Partial or complete resection of the hemipelvis: An alternative to hindquarter amputation for periacetabular chondrosarcoma of the pelvis. J Bone Joint Surg [Am] 60:719–730, 1978
280. Unni KK, Dahlin DC, Beaubout JW et al: Chondrosarcoma: Clear-cell variant. A report of 16 cases. J Bone Joint Surg [Am] 57:676–683, 1976
281. Harwood AR, Krajbich JI, Fornasier VL: Mesenchymal chondrosarcoma: A report of 17 cases. Clin Orthop 158:144–148, 1981
282. Huvos AG, Rosen G, Dabska M et al: Mesenchymal chondrosarcoma: A clinicopathologic analysis of 35 patients with emphasis on treatment. Cancer 51:1230–1237, 1983
283. Mankin HJ, Doppelt SH, Sullivan TR et al: Osteoarticular and intercalary allograft transplantation in the management of malignant tumors of bone. Cancer 50:613–630, 1982
284. Krochak R, Harwood AR, Cummings BJ et al: Results of radical radiation for chondrosarcoma of bone. Radiother Oncol 1:109–115, 1983
285. McNaney D, Lindberg RD, Ayala AG et al: Fifteen-year radiotherapy experience with chondrosarcoma of bone. Int J Radiat Oncol Biol Phys 8:187–190, 1982
286. Harwood AR, Krajbich JI, Fornasier VL: Radiotherapy of chondrosarcoma of bone. Cancer 45:2769–2777, 1980
286a. Ryall RDH, Bates T, Newton KA et al: Combination of radiotherapy and RA 20X and (ICRF 159) for chondrosarcoma. Cancer 44:891–895, 1979
287. Marcove RC: The Surgery of Tumors of Bone and Cartilage, 2nd ed. New York Grune & Stratton, 1984
288. Nascimento AG, Huvos AC, Marcove RC: Primary malignant giant cell tumor of bone study of eight cases and review of the literature. Cancer 44:1393–1402, 1979
288a. Arlen M, Tollefsen HR, Huvos AS et al: Chondrosarcoma of the head and neck. Am J Surg 120:456–460, 1970
289. Campanacci M, Giunti A, Olmi R: Giant-cell tumors of bone: A study of 209 cases with long-term follow-up in 130. Ital J Orthop Traumatol 1:249–277, 1977
290. Marcove RC, Weiss L, Vaghaiwall M et al: Cryosurgery in the treatment of giant cell tumor of bone: A report of 52 consecutive cases. Clin Orthop 134:275–289, 1978
290a. Malawer MM, Dunham WK, Zaleski T et al: The management of aggressive and low grade malignant bone tumors by cryosurgery: Analysis of 40 consecutive cases. In Enneking WF (ed): Limb-sparing Surgery for Musculoskeletal Tumors, pp 498–510. New York, Churchill Livingstone, 1987
291. Persson BM, Wouters HW: Curettage and acrylic cementation in surgery of giant cell tumor of bone. J Bone Joint Surg [Am] 120:125–133, 1976
293. Dahlin DC, Cupps RE, Johnson EW: Giant cell tumor: A study of 195 cases. Cancer 25:1061–1070, 1970
294. McGrath PH: Giant cell tumor of the bone: An analysis of fifty-two cases. J Bone Joint Surg [Br] 54:216–229, 1972
295. Bell RS, Harwood AR, Goodman SB et al: Supervoltage radiotherapy in the treatment of difficult giant cell tumors of bone. Clin Orthop 174:208–216, 1983
296. Larsson SE, Lorenzton R, Boquist L: Giant cell tumors of the spine and sacrum causing neurological problems. Clin Orthop 111:201–211, 1975

297. Tountas AA, Fornasier VL, Harwood AR et al: Post-irradiation sarcoma of bone. Cancer 43:182–187, 1979
298. Bacci G, Springfield D, Picci P et al: Adjuvant chemotherapy for malignant fibrous histiocytoma in the femur and tibia. J Bone Joint Surg [Am] 67:620–625, 1985
299. Heeten GJ, Koops HS, Kamps WA et al: Treatment of malignant fibrous histiocytoma of bone. A plea for primary chemotherapy. Cancer 56:37–40, 1985
300. Mindell ER: Current concept review. Chordoma. J Bone Joint Surg [Am] 63:501–505, 1981
301. Localio AS, Eng K, Ranson JHC: Abdominosacral approach for retrorectal tumors. Am Surg 179:555–560, 1980
302. Localio AS, Francis KC, Rossano PC: Abdominosacral resection of sacrococcygeal chordoma. Ann Surg 166:394–400, 1967
303. Gray SW, Singhabhandhu B, Smith RA et al: Sacrococcygeal chordoma: Report on a case and review of the literature. Surgery 78:573, 1975
304. Guterberg B, Romanus B, Sterner BL: Pelvic strength after major amputation of the sacrum. An experimental study. Acta Orthop Scand 47:635–642, 1976
305. DeVries J, Oldhoff J and Hadders, HN: Cryosurgery treatment of sacrococcyceal chordoma. Report of four cases. Cancer 58:2348–2354, 1986
306. Heffelfinger MJ, Dahlin DC, MacCarthy CS et al: Chordomas and cartilaginous tumors of the skull base. Cancer 32:410–420, 1973
307. Sundaresian N, Galicich JH, Chu FCH et al: Spinal chordoma. J Neurosurg 50:312–319, 1979
308. Amendola BE, Amendola MA, Oliver E et al: Chordoma: Role of radiation therapy. Radiology 158:839–843, 1986
309. Cummings BJ, Hodson ID, Bush RS: Chordoma: The results of megavoltage radiation therapy. Int J Radiat Oncol Biol Phys 9:633–642, 1983
310. Rich TA, Schiller A, Suit HD et al: Clinical and pathologic review of 48 cases of chordoma. Cancer 56:182–187, 1985
311. Austin-Seymour M, Munzenrider J, Goitein M et al: Proton radiation therapy of chordoma and low grade chondrosarcoma of the base of the skull and cervical spine. Int J Radiat Oncol Biol Phys (Suppl 1) 12:98, 1986
312. Raffel C, Wright DC, Gutin PH et al: Cranial chordomas: Clinical presentation and results of operative and radiation therapy in twenty-six patients. Neurosurgery 17:703–710, 1985
313. Reimer RR, Chabner BAC, Young RC et al: Lymphoma presenting in bone. Results of histopathology, staging and therapy. Ann Intern Med 87:50–55, 1977
314. Sweet DL, Moss DP, Simon MA et al: Histiocytic lymphoma (reticulum-cell sarcoma) of bone. Current strategy for orthopedic surgeons. J Bone Joint Surg [Am] 63:79–84, 1981
315. Mendenhall NP, Jones JJ, Kramer BS et al: The management of primary lymphoma of bone. Radiother Oncol 9:137–1137, 1987
316. Loeffler JS, Tarbell NJ, Kozakewich H et al: Primary lymphoma of bone in children: Analysis of treatment results with Adriamycin, prednisone, Oncovin (APO), and local radiation therapy. J Clin Oncol 4:496–501, 1986
317. Bacci G, Jaffe N, Emiliani E et al: Therapy for Primary non-Hodgkin's lymphoma of bone and a comparison of results with Ewing's sarcoma. Ten years' experience at the Instituto Orthopedico Rizzoli. Cancer 57:1468–1472, 1986

JENNIFER A. K. PATTERSON
ROY G. GERONEMUS

CHAPTER 43 *Cancers of the Skin*

Basal cell carcinoma and squamous cell carcinoma are the most common forms of skin cancer. They usually occur on the sun-exposed skin of the head, neck, and hands. Diagnosis is facilitated by the appropriate biopsy method, and treatment is essentially curative in the early stages of the disease. However, any skin cancer may be fatal because of local invasion or because of local and distant metastases. It is therefore essential that malignant cutaneous neoplasms be diagnosed early. A comprehensive annual cutaneous examination should be performed on all patients, regardless of the reason for which they sought medical attention, and any potentially malignant lesions should be biopsied.

EPIDEMIOLOGY AND PATHOGENESIS

Nonmelanoma skin cancer is the most common malignant neoplasm in the United States. According to statistics published by the American Cancer Society, more than 500,000 newly diagnosed skin cancers were reported in the United States in 1987.[1] This figure, however, grossly underrepresents the true prevalence of the disease since the majority of malignant cutaneous neoplasms are diagnosed and treated in an outpatient setting and do not require hospitalization. Such cases are not recorded in any tumor registry. It is also estimated that there were 2000 deaths from nonmelanoma skin cancer in 1987.[1]

Basal cell carcinoma is the most frequent type of skin cancer in whites, outnumbering the second most common type, squamous cell carcinoma, by a ratio of more than 3:1. The majority of basal cell carcinomas are found on sun-exposed skin areas of individuals with fair skin who sunburn easily. The lesions usually appear in later life, and most series report a higher rate in men than in women. Basal cell carcinomas are uncommon in deeply pigmented individuals, in whom squamous cell carcinoma is the most common skin cancer.

The two main etiological factors, the amount of sunlight exposure and the susceptibility of the skin to ultraviolet light (UVL), are responsible for the low incidence of skin cancers in England as compared with Australia (similar skin type but difference in sun exposure),[2] and the higher incidence of skin cancer in African albinos than in normally pigmented individuals living in the same country (different skin type but same sun exposure).[3,4]

The known etiological factors in the generation of nonmelanoma skin cancer include exposure to UVL, chemical carcinogens, viral carcinogens, and ionizing radiation; chronic irritation or inflammation; and an immunosuppressed state. Each of these is discussed below.

EXPOSURE TO ULTRAVIOLET (SOLAR) LIGHT

Abundant evidence supports the combined effect of UVL, immune system function, and the protection afforded by melanin in the development of malignant cutaneous neoplasms. Sun-exposed areas of the body *(the head, neck, and hands)* are most prone to skin cancer. Squamous cell carcinoma of the head and neck occurs almost exclusively in areas that receive maximal ultraviolet radiation. Laboratory

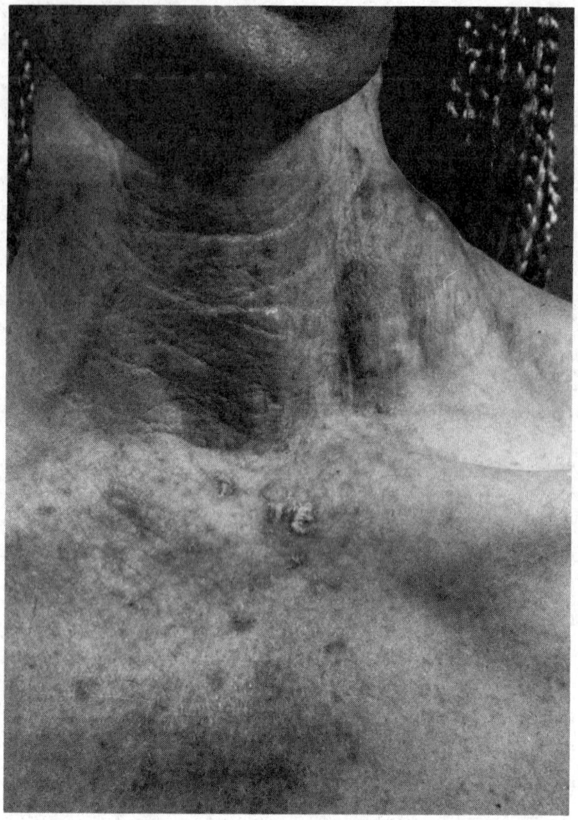

FIG. 43-1. Severe sun damage, solar keratoses, and squamous cell carcinomas on sun-exposed skin of a black albino man.

evidence for this common clinical observation was adduced by Urbach, who placed in sunlight a mannequin head covered with a chemical dosimeter for UVL.[5] Individuals with outdoor occupations, such as sailors, ranchers, farmers, and gardeners, have a higher incidence of skin cancer than persons with indoor occupations; those with indoor occupations who spend considerable time outdoors in recreational pursuits have a higher incidence than those who do not. Neoplasms develop on the trunk in men who go shirtless in the sun, while women are more likely to have neoplasms on the legs below the dress line. The incidence of solar keratoses and sun damage on the hand and forearm of automobile drivers correlates with local driving practices; in Australia the right arm is more often affected than the left arm.[6]

Persons with certain skin types and bodily complexions are more susceptible to the effects of UVL than others. White persons of Irish, Scottish, or English descent who have red or light blond hair, blue or green eyes, and white skin that freckles but does not tan are particularly susceptible.[7] Dark-skinned persons are protected from solar damage by the substantial amount of melanin in the skin, but albinos of the same race develop multiple aggressive cutaneous neoplasms (Fig. 43-1).[3,4] The proclivity to sun damage within groups of the same complexion is affected by degree of exposure to sunlight. Whites of Irish, Scottish, or English descent living in areas of the world that receive large amounts of sunlight are more affected than those living in areas of less sunlight.[2] A 1-year study comparing the incidence of solar keratoses in residents of Melbourne, Australia, and a town one degree north of Melbourne, hence closer to the equator, found a 14.2% greater incidence in residents of the town closer to the equator.[8] The ozone layer in the stratosphere absorbs ultraviolet radiation of 320 nm and less. The protective effect of the ozone layer increases with distance from the equator because the rays penetrate at a more oblique angle and are filtered more effectively.[5]

In addition to the protective effects of melanin and the ozone layer, the immune system likely plays a substantial role in susceptibility or nonsusceptibility to solar radiation damage. Kripke observed that skin cancers induced in mice by ultraviolet radiation are highly antigenic. Most are therefore rejected by the host's immune system when transplanted into a normal, genetically identical animal, but are tolerated in the primary host.[9] Mice exposed to ultraviolet radiation that did not develop skin cancers tolerated the transplanted tumor—that is, they were unable to reject the highly antigenic transplant.[9] Thus, UVL produced a systemic alteration that interfered with the immunologic rejection of UVL-induced skin cancers implanted at nonirradiated sites.[10] The alteration consisted of an increase in number of suppressor lymphocytes and perturbation of Langerhans cells, the immunocompetent cells of the epidermis. These changes in cell populations led to an altered response to antigens applied topically at irradiated sites, and to other antigens applied to nonirradiated skin.[11,12] Such local and systemic immunologic alterations, produced on a daily basis by UVL exposure, are thought to be of importance in the induction of cutaneous neoplasms because the immune surveillance against tumor antigens is greatly perturbed.

EXPOSURE TO CHEMICAL CARCINOGENS

Sir Percivall Pott, in 1775, observed the carcinogenic effect of soot in causing scrotal cancer in chimney sweeps.[13] Among the many topical agents now recognized as chemical carcinogens are tar, pitch, crude paraffin oil, lubricating oil, anthracene, creosote, and fuel oil.[14] Application of these various hydrocarbons will induce skin cancers in rodents.[15] The use of topical nitrogen mustard as therapy for cutaneous T-cell lymphoma[16] and of systemic 8-methoxypsoralen for the treatment of psoriasis,[17] may also predispose to the formation of skin cancers.

Arsenic is a well-known chemical carcinogen. The incidence of cancers is increased in areas with an abnormally high amount of arsenic in the drinking water.[18] Occupational exposure (as in the manufacture or agricultural use of insecticides and the smelting of several kinds of metal ores) or medicinal exposure to arsenic (*e.g.*, in Fowler's solution, Donovan's solution, Asiatic pills for the treatment of asthma or syphilis)[19] predispose to the development of arsenical keratoses, skin cancers, and systemic malignancies. In fact, the arsenic content is increased in the lesions of Bowen's disease (squamous cell carcinoma in situ).[20]

Chemical carcinogenesis in the skin can be divided into two distinct stages, initiation and promotion. Initiation results from limited exposure to a specific agent or carcinogen; the process is irreversible, and the cellular changes are heritable. Promotion requires repeated exposure to promoting agents at frequent intervals. If the interval between exposures is quite long, the effects are reversible. Promoters induce tumor development only after initiation, even if a long interval separates the two episodes. Exposure to promoting agents in the absence of or prior to initiation will not result in tumor formation.[21]

EXPOSURE TO VIRAL CARCINOGENS

Many viruses can induce tumors in animal hosts. For example, the Shope papillomavirus acts with a cofactor, probably an environmental agent, to produce papillomas and carcinomas in cottontail rabbits in the Mississippi Valley. Similar neoplasms have been induced in domestic rabbits experimentally exposed to the Shope papillomavirus and methylcholanthrene.[22] In man, many subtypes of human papillomavirus have been found in verrucae,[23] lesions of bowenoid papulosis,[24] and genital neoplasms.[25]

Human papillomavirus type 5 is the virus most commonly found in benign lesions of patients with epidermodysplasia verruciformis. The HPV-5 genome has also been found in cancers developed from these lesions, and the papillomaviruses therefore appear potentially oncogenic in humans.[26] A specific combination, order, and "dosage" of oncogenic factors besides the virus, such as exposure to UVL and a decrease in cell-mediated immunity, is probably required to induce the carcinomas.

EXPOSURE TO IONIZING RADIATION

In the past, inappropriate radiation therapy (γ, Grenz, and x-rays) led to chronic radiodermatitis, often associated with the appearance of radiation-induced cancers.[27] In many cases the therapy was given for benign or cosmetic conditions, such as acne or to remove hair. This often resulted in alopecic, dry atrophic skin with telangiectasias and patchy areas of hypopigmentation and hyperpigmentation. In 1952, Sulzberger et al reported that superficial x-ray treatment (60–100 kV; half-value layer of 0.5–1.0 mm aluminum) for benign lesions, if given in small fractionated doses to a total dose of 1000 R or less, caused no untoward effects.[28] Severe radiodermatitis is rare today because radiation therapy units are calibrated accurately, personnel are more knowledgeable about dosages, fractionation, and adverse effects, and benign conditions are no longer treated with superficial irradiation.

In 1957 Totten et al reported on 105 consecutive patients admitted for treatment of skin cancers.[29] Six of 21 patients with squamous cell carcinoma and 14 of 84 with basal cell carcinomas had coexisting chronic radiodermatitis. Three of the six squamous cell carcinomas were caused by occupational exposure to irradiation from therapy units. It is known that such skin cancers can be experimentally induced in animals by ionizing radiation.

CHRONIC IRRITATION OR INFLAMMATION

Malignant cutaneous neoplasms often develop in areas of chronic scarring, ulceration, or sinus formation,[30–34] such as burn scar (Marjolin's ulcer),[35] chronic osteomyelitic sinus,[36,37] decubitus ulcers,[38] and in skin areas affected by lupus erythematosus.[39] The site of the malignant lesion therefore corresponds to the distribution of the previous assault. For example, an entity called Kangri ulcer develops on the chest, abdomen, and thighs of the Kashmiri as a result of infrared burns received from hot earthenware pots held against the skin for warmth.[40] Another habit that predisposes to chronic irritation and neoplasia is the chewing of tobacco or betel nuts in some Asian groups, which causes squamous cell carcinoma of the lips and oral cavity.[40]

IMMUNE SYSTEM FUNCTION

Patients with a defective immune system are prone to develop malignant cutaneous neoplasms de novo.[41] Individuals who have undergone organ transplantation and are on immunosuppressive therapy (*e.g.*, cytotoxics, corticosteroids) commonly develop skin cancers,[42–44] as do those on other immunosuppressive therapy (*e.g.*, chemotherapeutic agents to treat systemic malignancies).[45] There is also an increased incidence of cutaneous malignancies—basal cell carcinoma, squamous cell carcinoma, and malignant melanoma—in patients with lymphoma, leukemia, or myeloma.[46] The behavior of these neoplasms is often aggressive,[47,48] and there may be multiple lesions. The increased incidence of cutaneous malignancies in such patients is thought to be due to immunosuppression, as evidenced by anergy and a decreased percentage of T-lymphocytes, and hence to the inability of the host to reject the cutaneous neoplasm.[49] UVL incident on the skin causes perturbation of the Langerhans cells and induces suppressor T-cells. These factors contribute to the increased frequency of skin cancers in immunosuppressed patients. Individuals with the acquired immunodeficiency syndrome also have an increase in suppressor T-cells relative to the helper subset. The occasional development of a malignant cutaneous neoplasm in AIDS patients has been reported recently;[50] these neoplasms may be more aggressive in their biologic behavior.[51]

CLINICAL PRESENTATION, PATHOLOGY, AND NATURAL HISTORY

BASAL CELL CARCINOMA

Basal cell carcinoma is a malignant cutaneous neoplasm that arises from the basal cell layers of the epidermis and adnexal structures. More than 95% of these neoplasms occur in patients over the age of 40,[52] although cases have been reported in children.[53] Basal cell carcinomas develop on hair-bearing skin, most commonly on sun-exposed areas; approximately 85% are found on the head and neck area and the remaining 15% on the trunk and limbs.[52,54] Pruritus and bleeding are common symptoms, and patients frequently complain of a bleeding sore that heals partially and then ulcerates again. More than one basal cell carcinoma may be present synchronously. A 5-year prospective study of 1000 patients treated for one basal cell carcinoma found that 36% of the individuals developed a second basal cell carcinoma.[55] It therefore behooves the physician to perform a complete

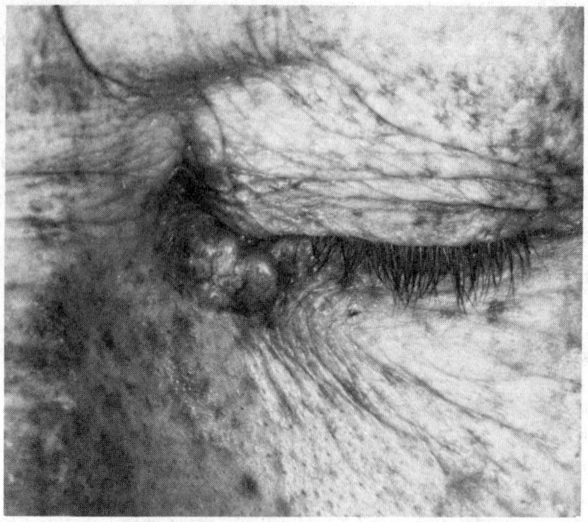

FIG. 43-2. Nodular basal cell carcinoma at medial canthus of eye. Note telangiectasias and sun-damaged skin.

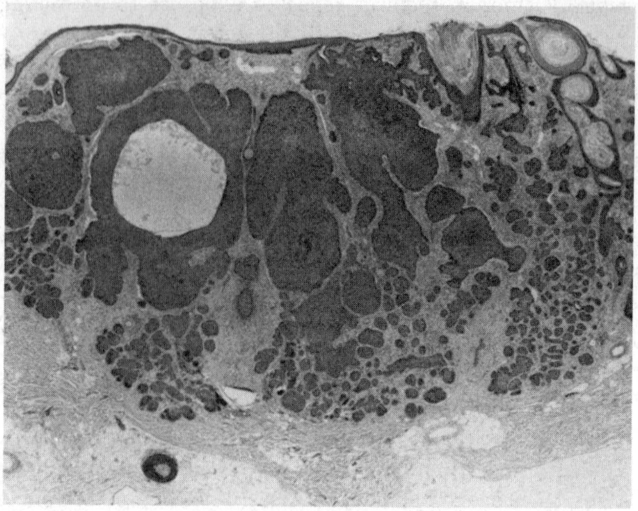

FIG. 43-4. Basal cell carcinoma, 3 mm depth. Hematoxylin and eosin stained section of nodular type.

cutaneous examination annually on each patient and to biopsy any suspicious lesions, since the etiological factor of solar damage, for example, affects many areas of the body and thus predisposes to neoplasms elsewhere.

Tumor Subtypes

There are various subtypes of basal cell carcinoma with differing clinical presentation, histologic appearance, differentiation, and biologic behavior. The most common type of basal cell carcinoma is the *nodulo-ulcerative* basal cell carcinoma, which emerges as a flesh-colored, cream to pink, waxy papule with prominent surface telangiectasias (Fig. 43-2). As the lesion grows, central erosion or ulceration and crusting occur, surrounded by a pearly, rolled, translucent border (Color Fig. 43-1). This clinical presentation has also been called a "rodent ulcer" (Fig. 43-3). Histologic examination of a nodulo-ulcerative basal cell carcinoma reveals large islands of monomorphous basaloid cells in the dermis (Fig. 43-4). These cellular aggregates vary in size and shape. The basaloid cells resemble keratinocytes of the basal layer but have large oval hyperchromatic nuclei, scant cytoplasm, and no intercellular bridges. There are no abnormal mitoses.[56] The peripheral cell layer of the tumor aggregate often shows palisading, but the inner cells are arranged haphazardly. The aggregates of neoplastic cells are embedded in a characteristic fibroblastic stroma, often in association with amyloid[57,58] and mucin-amyloid deposits and mucin deposits. It is thought that the mucin deposits are extracted during fixation and dehydration of the biopsy specimen, producing an artifactual retraction of the neoplasm from its stroma.[56] This finding is often used as an aid in the histologic diagnosis of basal cell carcinoma. This solid type of basal cell carcinoma is undifferentiated. However, since the neoplasm arises from the pluripotential basal cell, many will demonstrate differentiation toward hair structures (keratotic type), sebaceous glands (cystic type), or apocrine or eccrine glands (adenoid type). Since there is no difference in the biologic behavior of differentiated and undifferentiated basal cell carcinomas, such terminology seems unnecessary. The term *basal cell carcinoma with sebaceous differentiation,* for example, expresses the diagnosis quite clearly when more information on the histologic type is sought.

FIG. 43-3. Large ulcerated basal cell carcinoma (rodent ulcer) on neck. Note rolled borders.

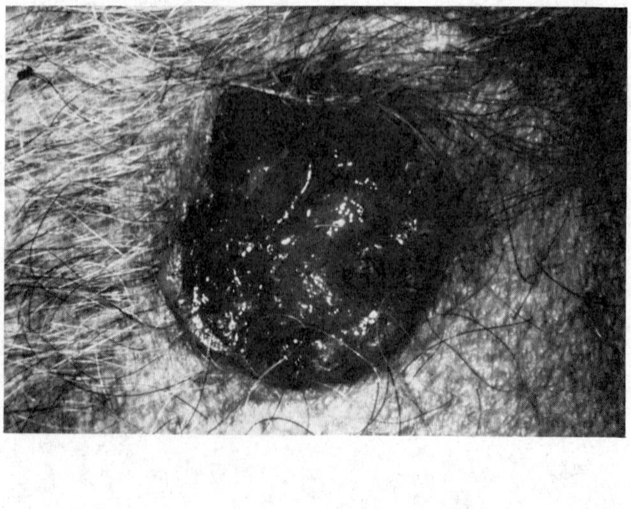

The exception to this rule is the nodulo-ulcerative basal cell carcinoma with basosquamous differentiation. This lesion exhibits squamous metaplasia, including large polygonal eosinophilic cells and foci of keratinization. It is associated with aggressive biologic behavior and a tendency to metastasize.[59]

Pigmented basal cell carcinomas are similar to nodulo-ulcerative lesions but may vary in color from blue through tan, brown, or black, depending on the number of melanocytes and thus the amount of melanin present in the neoplasm (Fig. 43-5). It is often difficult to differentiate these lesions clinically from malignant melanoma (Color Fig. 43-2). An excisional biopsy should be performed to ensure an adequate pathologic specimen.

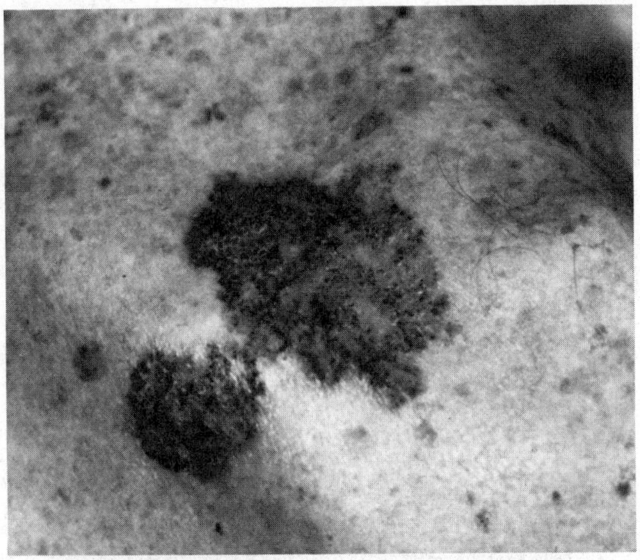

FIG. 43-5. Pigmented basal cell carcinoma on posterior shoulder. Note concomitant solar damage.

Superficial basal cell carcinomas occur commonly on the trunk and manifest clinically as ill-defined red scaly macules; occasionally they are pigmented (Color Fig. 43-3). Superficial basal cell carcinomas increase in size to form crusted, occasionally ulcerated, scaly erythematous patches, but are never indurated. The differential diagnosis includes psoriasis, nummular dermatitis, squamous cell carcinoma in situ (Bowen's disease), extramammary Paget's disease, and solar keratosis. Histologic examination reveals multiple foci of buds of neoplastic cells emanating from the undersurface of the epidermis. As in the nodulo-ulcerative basal cell carcinoma, there is peripheral palisading of the neoplastic cells and separation of tumor aggregates from the stroma.

Morphea-form and *sclerosing* types of basal cell carcinoma appear as single, flat, indurated, off-white, ill-defined macules (Color Fig. 43-4). As the lesion enlarges into a plaque, the smooth, shiny surface may become depressed (Color Fig. 43-5). Examination of a punch biopsy specimen discloses a dense fibrous connective tissue stroma in which small groups and narrow strands of basaloid cells are embedded. There is little or no stromal retraction or peripheral palisading. These lesions must be differentiated histologically from metastatic breast carcinoma[60] and desmoplastic trichoepithelioma.[61] A shave biopsy is inappropriate for this type of basal cell carcinoma.

An *infiltrative* type of basal cell carcinoma has been described.[62] The lesion has an opaque yellowish white color and blends subtly with the surrounding normal skin. Histologically, the neoplasm is poorly circumscribed with angular, spiky neoplastic aggregates in the superficial portion and strands four to eight cell layers thick forming the bulk of the neoplasm in the reticular dermis and subcutis. There is no differentiation or peripheral palisading, and the stroma is similar to that of the surrounding normal skin.

Fibroepithelial tumor of Pinkus, another type of basal cell carcinoma,[63] manifests as a flesh-colored papule without epidermal change. It is often located on the trunk. Microscopic examination of a typical lesion reveals long thin strands of basal cell carcinoma emanating from the basal layer of the epidermis and anastomosing within a dense fibrous dermal connective tissue stroma.

Natural History

The natural history and biologic behavior of basal cell carcinoma depend on the histologic type. The fibroepithelial tumor of Pinkus and the superficial basal cell carcinoma may remain stable or grow slowly over a number of years to eventually result in a nodulo-ulcerative basal cell carcinoma. The nodulo-ulcerative type also grows slowly over several years, invading locally by peripheral and deep extension, especially along nerve sheaths and the embryonal fusion planes. Ulceration may be extensive, with secondary bacterial infection, and vital organs may be destroyed, leading to death, if the neoplasm is not treated in time (Fig. 43-6). Morphea-form, sclerosing, basosquamous, and infiltrative types of basal cell carcinoma are biologically more aggressive[64,59,62] and more difficult to treat because of indistinct lateral margins and deep infiltration.

Basal cell carcinoma rarely metastasizes; the incidence is only 0.0028% of all basal cell carcinomas in Australia and New Zealand.[65] Primary tumors that metastasize typically are located on the head and neck, are large, are locally invasive, and are not cured with repeated surgery and radiation therapy.[66] Once metastasis is recognized, the mean survival time is approximately 1 year. Dissemination of the neoplasm (both epithelial and stromal elements) occurs via lymphatics and veins. Most metastases are found in regional lymph nodes (68%), but bone, lung and liver are all involved in up to 20% of cases.[67]

FIG. 43-6. Basal cell carcinoma invasive into the frontal lobe.

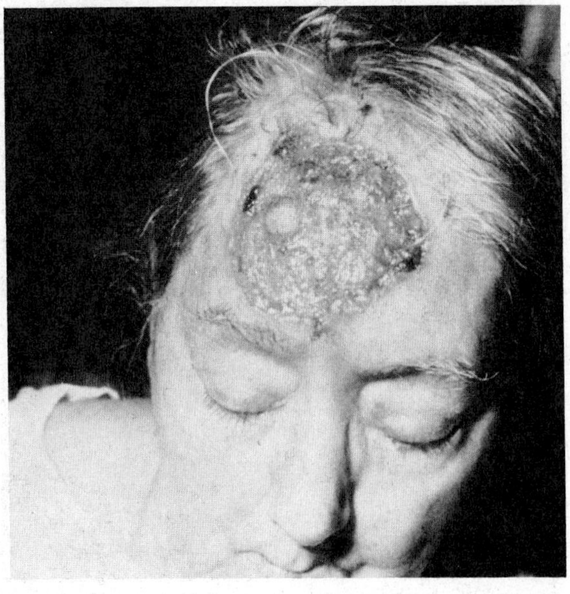

SQUAMOUS CELL CARCINOMA

Squamous cell carcinoma of the skin is a malignant neoplasm that arises from keratinocytes of the epidermis. Rarely, it arises de novo from normal-appearing skin; more commonly it develops from sun-damaged skin or, occasionally, from a preexisting cutaneous lesion, such as an area of chronic radiodermatitis,[29] solar keratosis, arsenical keratosis, a thermal burn scar (*e.g.*, Kangri ulcer),[40] hydrocarbon (tar) keratosis, a chronic cicatrix (scar), a lesion of discoid lupus erythematosus,[39] a smallpox vaccination scar, a chronic ulcer (*e.g.*, venous stasis ulcer, decubitus ulcer),[38] a pilonidal sinus,[34] a site of chronic osteomyelitis,[37] a burn scar (Marjolin's ulcer)[35] (Fig. 43-7), porokeratosis of Mibelli,[68] or a site of epidermodysplasia verruciformis.[69] Squamous cell carcinoma occurs on any part of the skin and mucous membranes but is seen most commonly on sun-exposed areas (Fig. 43-8).

Squamous cell carcinoma in situ, Tis (Table 43-1), represents intraepidermal carcinoma in which the neoplasm is confined to the epidermis. Atypical keratinocytes with large hyperchromatic and pleomorphic nuclei extend from the basal to the cornified layers. Clinically, squamous cell carcinoma in situ manifests as an erythematous, scaly, well-defined patch without induration (Fig. 43-9). Erythroplasia of Queyrat, described in 1911, is now considered to be carcinoma in situ of the penis. Another form of carcinoma in situ is Bowen's disease, first described in 1912.[70] Bowen's disease may be associated with prior arsenic ingestion when the

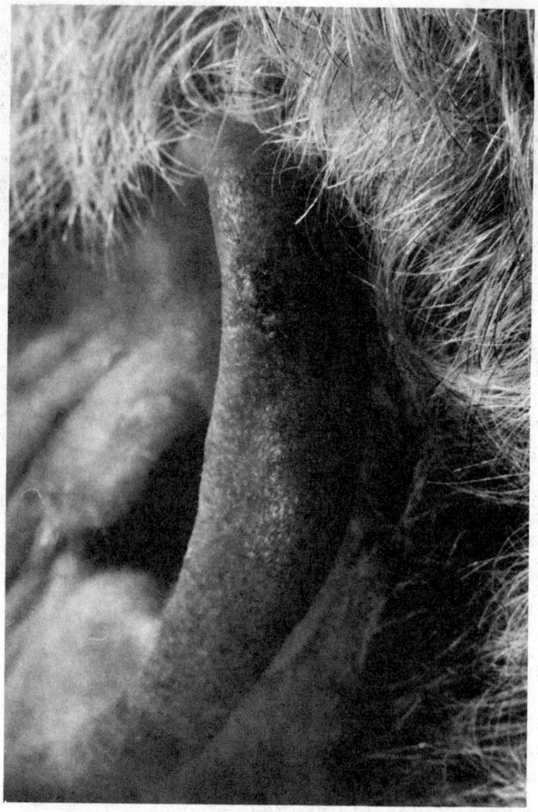

FIG. 43-8. Squamous cell carcinoma on the sun-exposed helix of the ear in a man.

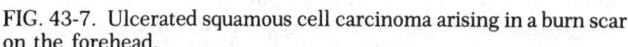

FIG. 43-7. Ulcerated squamous cell carcinoma arising in a burn scar on the forehead.

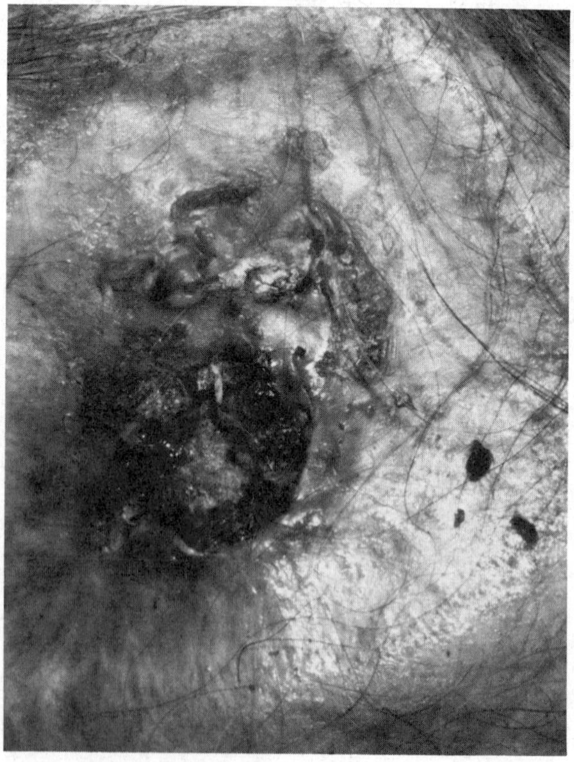

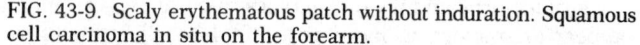

FIG. 43-9. Scaly erythematous patch without induration. Squamous cell carcinoma in situ on the forearm.

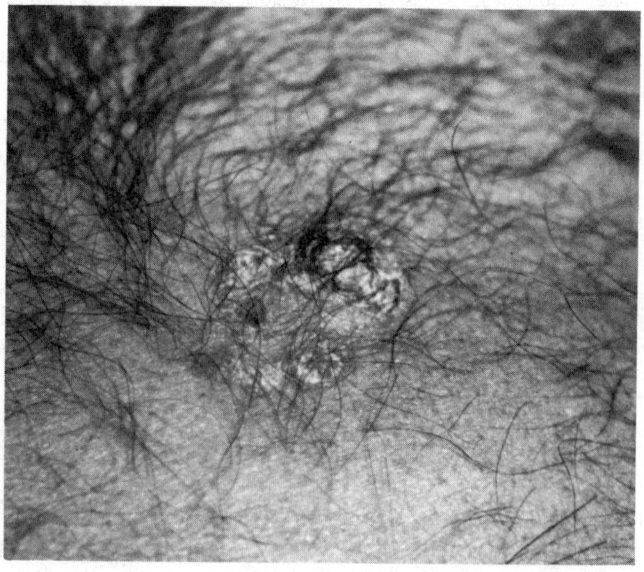

TABLE 43-1. TNM Classification for Squamous Cell Carcinoma and Basal Cell Carcinoma

Primary Tumor (T)	
Tx	Minimum requirements to assess the primary tumor cannot be met
Tis	Carcinoma in situ
T0	No primary tumor present
T1	Tumor 2 cm or less in its largest dimension, strictly superficial or exophytic
T2	Tumor more than 2 cm but not more than 5 cm in its largest dimension or with minimal infiltration of the dermis, irrespective of size
T3	Tumor more than 5 cm in its largest dimension or with deep infiltration of the dermis, irrespective of size
T4	Tumor involving other structures such as cartilage, muscle, or bone
Nodal Involvement (N)	
	The nodal involvement for cervical nodes is identical to that of the head and neck cancers; this can also be applied to other nodal regions.
Nx	Minimum requirements to assess the regional nodes cannot be met
N0	No evidence of regional lymph node involvement
N1	Evidence of involvement of movable homolateral regional lymph nodes
N2	Evidence of involvement of movable contralateral or bilateral regional lymph nodes
N3	Evidence of involvement of fixed regional lymph nodes
Distant Metastasis (M)	
Mx	Minimum requirements to assess distant metastasis cannot be met
M0	No (known) distant metastasis
M1	Distant metastasis present (specify site: pulmonary, osseus, hepatic, brain, lymph nodes, bone marrow, pleura, skin, eye, other)
Staging	
I	Localized T1
II	Regional nodal involvement (first chain of drainage)
III	Distant metastases
Tumor Grade	
G1	Well differentiated
G2	Moderately well differentiated
G3–G4	Poorly to very poorly differentiated

lesion is located on non-sun-exposed skin.[20] In the past Bowen's disease was sometimes thought to be associated with an internal malignancy.[71–73] However, such an association is not supported by reports in the literature to date.[74]

Carcinoma in situ may remain quiescent for years or may gradually evolve into the plaque stage (superficial squamous cell carcinoma) with the development of ulceration, a scaly crust, and a verrucous or papillated surface (Fig. 43-10). Eventually, an infiltrating squamous cell carcinoma is manifest as a firm endophytic erythematous ulcerated neoplasm with an elevated nodular border. This grows locally into the subcutis, muscle, periosteum, and along nerves, and invades blood vessels and lymphatic channels. The biologic behavior and depth and rate of invasion correlate with the degree of cellular differentiation. The differential diagnosis includes keratoacanthoma, other cutaneous neoplasms, granulomas, and an ulcer of atypical mycobacterial or deep fungal etiology.

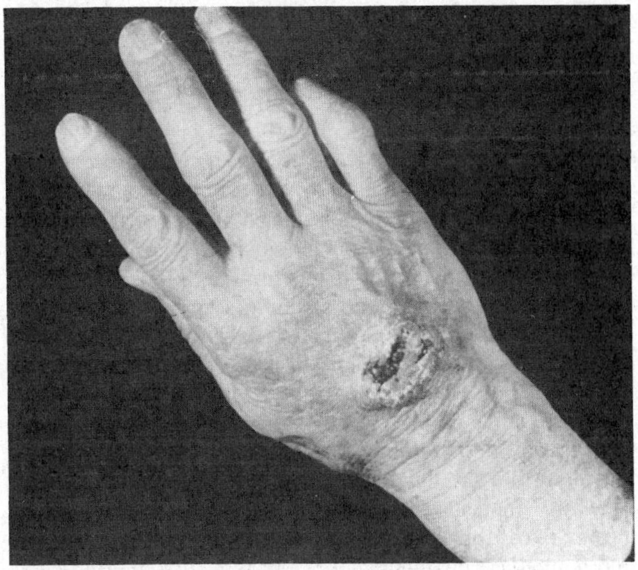

FIG. 43-10. Squamous cell carcinoma on the dorsum of the hand.

Histologically squamous cell carcinoma is composed of tongues, strands, and broad sheets of atypical keratinocytes emanating from the epidermis. The term *superficial squamous cell carcinoma* describes a neoplasm confined to the upper reticular dermis; *infiltrating squamous cell carcinoma* denotes involvement of the lower reticular dermis and eventually the subcutaneous tissue.[75] The neoplasm is graded as well, moderately, or poorly differentiated or as a spindle cell neoplasm. A well-differentiated neoplasm has sheets of large, polygonal cells with abundant eosinophilic cytoplasm and pleomorphic, hyperchromatic nuclei with few mitoses or prominent nucleoli. There is evidence of keratinization (dyskeratosis, horn pearls) and preservation of the intercellular bridges. Poorly differentiated (anaplastic) neoplasms exhibit marked cellular atypism with many abnormal mitoses. Spindle cell neoplasms may be difficult to diagnose as squamous cell carcinomas. In this case, immunoperoxidase studies with antikeratin antibodies will demonstrate reactivity in squamous cell carcinoma but not in malignant melanoma, Kaposi's sarcoma, atypical fibroxanthoma (malignant fibrous histiocytoma), or leiomyosarcoma.[76,77]

Squamous cell carcinoma metastasizes to regional lymph nodes and eventually to distant sites, including bone, brain, and lungs. The likelihood of metastasis depends on the anatomical site, previous inflammation or injury at that site, duration and size of the lesion, depth of dermal invasion, and degree of differentiation of the squamous cell carcinoma. In a review of 63 patients with squamous cell carcinoma of the trunk and extremities,[75] 14% had either local recurrence or metastases that proved fatal (five patients). The biologic behavior of the neoplasms correlated best with the level of dermal invasion and the vertical tumor thickness: in all cases of recurrence, the primary tumors were 4 mm or more thick and involved the lower reticular dermis or deeper structures.[75] Lesions that caused death of the host were at least 10 mm in maximum thickness. Large, less differentiated lesions also have a greater probability of recurrence.[78] The noninvasive squamous cell carcinomas (Clark levels I, II, III) did not recur.[78]

Squamous cell carcinomas arising from normal skin may be rapidly invasive and metastasize frequently, but those developing in sun-damaged skin may have a lower incidence of metastasis, although there are reports in the literature of metastasizing squamous cell carcinomas arising in solar keratoses.[79] Squamous cell carcinomas arising in modified skin, such as the vulva, glans penis, oral mucosa, or anus, have a higher rate of metastasis, as do lesions arising in sites of chronic cutaneous injury such as thermal burns and decubitus ulcers. The literature to date is somewhat confusing on this point, but Moller et al,[80] summarize the probable frequency of metastasis as follows: for primary squamous cell carcinoma of the skin, 3%; for primary mucocutaneous (lips and genitalia) squamous cell carcinoma, 11%; and for secondary squamous cell carcinoma developing in burn scars, osteomyelitic foci and the like, 10% to 30%.

Epstein et al studied approximately 6900 cases of squamous cell carcinoma recorded and followed up by the California Tumor Registry.[81] Of 142 patients with metastatic disease at the time of diagnosis, the metastatic involvement was noted in 2.5% within 1 month of the appearance of the primary lesion, in 40% by 6 months, and in 70% by 1 year. Survival figures reflect the biologically aggressive behavior of these neoplasms—only 25% of patients with metastases were alive at 5 years, 13% at 10 years, and 8% at 15 years.[81] Epstein has stressed the potentially malignant behavior of all cutaneous squamous cell carcinomas, whatever their etiology, including those arising in sun-damaged and PUVA-treated skin.[82]

Tumor Subtypes

Verrucous carcinoma is a low-grade squamous cell carcinoma.[83] It grows slowly as an exophytic, verrucous, fungating lesion that may eventuate in a locally invasive neoplasm. This type of squamous cell carcinoma arises in the oral cavity (oral florid papillomatosis); in the anogenital region (giant condyloma acuminatum of Buschke and Lowenstein), especially on the glans penis and foreskin of uncircumcised males; and on the plantar surface of the foot (epithelioma cuniculatum).

Solar (actinic) keratoses are very common lesions found on the sun-exposed skin of elderly white people.[84] There are usually several to multiple lesions appearing as red to tan, scaly, ill-defined macules on the face, dorsa of the hands, extensor aspect of the forearms, and on the scalp of bald men (Fig. 43-11). The differential diagnosis includes seborrheic keratosis and lesions of discoid lupus erythematosus. Lesions of solar keratoses arise in sun-damaged skin in which there may be cutaneous furrows and yellow discoloration because of the severe solar elastosis (dermatoheliosis). Solar keratoses are often asymptomatic but may produce local irritation. Any change—induration, erythema, erosion, or increased size—may denote eventual progression of the solar keratosis to a squamous cell carcinoma. The analogous lesion appearing on the vermilion border of the lip (usually the lower lip, which has the greater sun exposure) is termed *actinic cheilitis.*

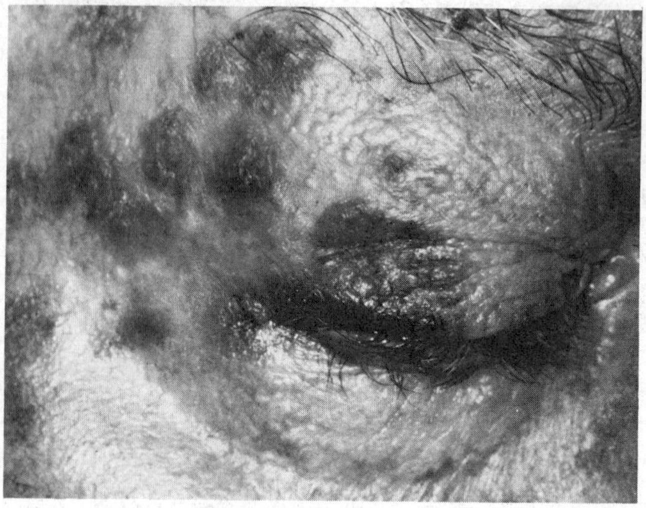

FIG. 43-11. Several solar keratoses on the right temple and upper eyelid.

A variable number of atypical keratinocytes are seen in the atrophic or hyperplastic epidermis on biopsy of a solar keratosis. There may be alternating areas of orthokeratosis and parakeratosis since the adnexal structures often are not involved in the neoplastic process and therefore keratinize normally. Often there is irregular downward proliferation with budding of the epidermal keratinocytes into the papillary dermis. Most of the keratinocytes are pleomorphic with large, irregular, hyperchromatic nuclei and are arranged in a totally disorganized fashion. There may also be evidence of premature keratinization. Thus, the microscopic changes of squamous cell carcinoma can be found in the full thickness of the epidermis, but are confined to it.

Keratoses caused by factors other than solar radiation include chronic cicatricial (scar) keratosis, chronic radiation keratosis, thermal keratosis, hydrocarbon (tar) keratosis, and arsenical keratosis. *Arsenical keratoses* develop at sites of trauma and friction, especially on the palms and soles. The multiple, hard, yellowish, hyperkeratotic papules range in diameter from 2 to 10 mm. All the keratoses are considered possible precursor lesions of squamous cell carcinoma and should be followed closely with expeditious biopsies of changing (*e.g.*, indurated) areas. Histologic examination reveals changes similar to those of a solar keratosis, but there may also be features associated with the predisposing condition, such as sequelae of late radiation damage in the dermis and subcutaneous tissue underlying a chronic radiation keratosis.

A *cutaneous horn* (cornu cutaneum) is a descriptive term for any exophytic keratinous nodule projecting from the skin (Fig. 43-12). The lesions are usually hard and conical (resembling an animal's horn) with a papular erythematous base. These lesions represent a cutaneous neoplasm, usually

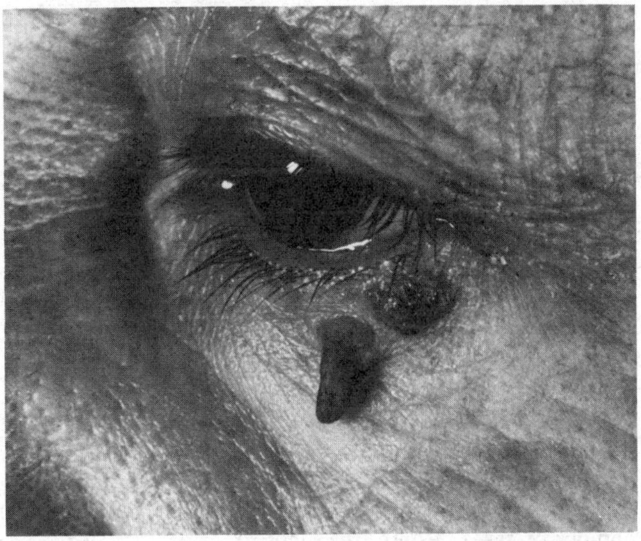

FIG. 43-12. Cutaneous horn on left lower eyelid. Differential diagnosis includes verruca, solar keratosis, and basal cell carcinoma.

a verruca vulgaris, a hyperplastic (digitate) solar keratosis, a keratoacanthoma, or a squamous cell carcinoma with an overlying hyperkeratosis. All such lesions should be biopsied (by excision or deep shave) because an accurate diagnosis can only be made on histologic examination.

Leukoplakia is a morphological term which describes a white patch or plaque on the oral, genital, or anal mucosa that cannot be rubbed off.[85] The white appearance is attributed to the hydration of the hyperkeratotic lesion. *Candida albicans* is often a secondary invader in these lesions. Leukoplakia may be idiopathic, may represent a benign inflammatory process such as lichen planus, or may be secondary to mechanical or chemical irritation from, for example, ill-fitting dentures, pipe smoking, or tobacco chewing. All cases of leukoplakia should be biopsied if there is no improvement with treatment or removal of the inciting agent. In one study 20% of lesions biopsied revealed squamous cell carcinoma in situ or invasive squamous cell carcinoma.[86] The vermilion border of the lip is the most common site of leukoplakia. In the United States, the overall prevalence of leukoplakia is 43:1000 white men over age 35 years.[87] It therefore behooves the physician to biopsy or follow very carefully lesions of leukoplakia in this population since an accurate diagnosis of a malignant neoplasm or benign hyperkeratosis can only be made on histologic examination. This is especially important when one considers the poor prognosis of squamous cell carcinoma of lip. Boddie et al reported a 32% metastasis rate and a 20% mortality in patients less than 40 years old followed for 5 years or more with squamous cell carcinoma of the lower lip.[88]

Erythroplakia is a red, sharply delineated patch in the oral mucosa that invariably represents either carcinoma in situ or invasive squamous cell carcinoma.[89] Areas of erythroplakia may be intermingled with leukoplakia and must always be biopsied. Application of 1% toluidine blue to the suspicious area will aid in recognition and delineation of the erythroplakic area.[90]

Keratoacanthoma is considered a benign self-limiting cutaneous keratinocytic neoplasm. Some, however, consider it to be a very well-differentiated squamous cell carcinoma that regresses spontaneously because of host immune factors. The clinical and histologic differential diagnosis includes squamous cell carcinoma.[91]

A keratoacanthoma usually develops as a single lesion on the sun-exposed skin of an elderly person.[92] A history of preceding trauma is common.[93] The lesion develops as an exophytic-endophytic, firm, dome-shaped nodule up to 2.5 cm in diameter with a central keratin-filled crater and surrounding heaped-up epithelial borders overhanging the crater (Fig. 43-13). The nodules grow rapidly to full-sized lesions within 6 to 8 weeks, followed by gradual involution over 2 to 6 months. It is thought that a keratoacanthoma arises from the hair follicles[94] and that the pattern of growth and regression follows the cyclic history of the hair follicle.[95]

There are six types of keratoacanthoma, as follows[96]:

1. Solitary keratoacanthoma: found in 95% of patients.
2. Ferguson-Smith type: numerous, frequently ulcerated, self-healing lesions that appear over a period of time.
3. Grzybowski type: numerous small lesions.
4. Witten and Zak type: both Grzybowski and Ferguson-Smith types occur.
5. Giant, massive, or confluent keratoacanthoma: large lesions, possibly derived by coalescence of adjacent lesions.
6. Keratoacanthoma centrifugum marginatum: lesions characterized by marked peripheral growth and extension with central healing.

FIG. 43-13. Keratoacanthoma on left temple of an elderly woman.

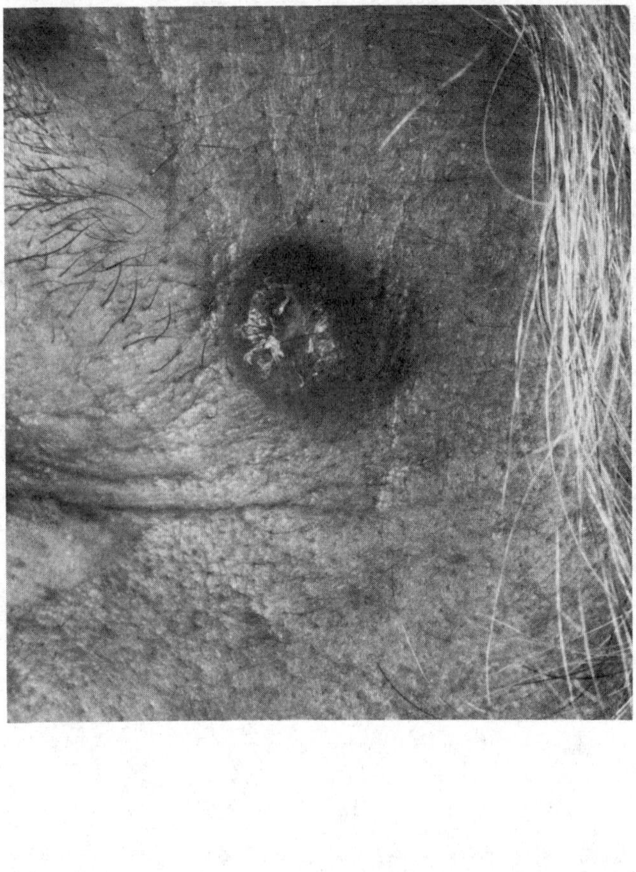

The major histologic feature that distinguishes keratoacanthoma from squamous cell carcinoma is the different and distinctive architectural patterns seen on examination of an appropriate biopsy specimen.[91]

OTHER NONMELANOMA SKIN CANCERS

APOCRINE CARCINOMA. Carcinoma of the apocrine glands is rare; only 28 cases were reported in the literature up to 1978.[97,98] It occurs most commonly in the axilla but can also arise from apocrine glands of the vulva and from modified apocrine glands such as Moll's glands on the eyelids and the ceruminal glands of the external auditory meatus.[99] Clinically, apocrine carcinoma appears as a red or purple, single or multinodular, firm, rubbery or cystic dermal mass ranging from 1.5 to 8.0 cm in diameter. These neoplasms are most common in the sixth decade and produce discomfort rather than pain.[98] Biopsy reveals an adenocarcinoma of varying differentiation. In a well-differentiated neoplasm, there are well-developed glandular structures lined by cells showing evidence of decaptitation secretion, periodic acid—Schiff (PAS)-positive, diastase-resistant granules,[100] and iron-positive granules.[101] Apocrine carcinoma can invade locally, metastasize to regional lymph nodes, and sometimes cause death from widespread disease.[98]

ECCRINE CARCINOMA. Carcinoma of the eccrine glands is also rare; over a period of 20 years 35 cases of primary eccrine adenocarcinoma were diagnosed from 450,000 consecutive skin biopsy specimens.[102] There is no characteristic clinical appearance or location. The average patient age at presentation is 60 years. Five distinct histologic variants have been identified: eccrine porocarcinoma,[103] syringoid eccrine carcinoma,[104] mucinous eccrine carcinoma,[105] clear cell carcinoma,[106] and microcystic adnexal carcinoma.[107,108] The histologic differential diagnosis includes metastatic adenocarcinoma. Microscopic examination reveals well-differentiated tubular structures with single or double cell layers, anaplastic epithelial cells, and mucinous stroma. The lumina in some of the tubules may be lined with an eosinophilic, PAS-positive, diastase-resistant cuticle.[109] Eccrine gland carcinomas are locally destructive, recur after treatment, and can metastasize to regional and distant lymph nodes.[102]

SEBACEOUS CARCINOMA. Sebaceous gland carcinoma is uncommon, possibly representing 0.2% to 4.6% of all cutaneous neoplasms.[110] It manifests clinically as a slow-growing, hard yellow nodule often arising from the meibomian glands or glands of Zeis of the eyelid. However, it may occur elsewhere on the face, scalp, or the rest of the body. Histologically, irregular lobules of well-differentiated sebaceous cells are admixed with atypical undifferentiated and sebaceous cells containing hyperchromatic, pleomorphic nuclei. The differential diagnosis includes basal cell carcinoma with sebaceous differentiation, and sebaceous adenoma.[109] Sebaceous carcinoma of the eyelid often invades locally and can metastasize.[111] Occasionally malignant sebaceous neoplasms arising elsewhere will metastasize or even cause death.[112]

MERKEL CELL TUMOR. The Merkel cell tumor was originally described as a trabecular carcinoma[113] but proved to be derived from Merkel cells after electron microscopic study demonstrated membrane-bound, dense-core neurosecretory granules in the cytoplasm.[114] This primary cutaneous neuroendocrine carcinoma occurs most frequently as a dermal nodule or plaque on the head, neck, or lower extremities of an elderly person. Anastomosing cords and strands of neoplastic cells are seen in the dermis and subcutis. The individual cells are monomorphous with round vesicular nuclei and scanty, ill-defined cytoplasm. The granules in the neoplastic cells are argyrophilic. The histologic differential diagnosis includes basal cell carcinoma, eccrine carcinoma, metastatic oat cell carcinoma, and lymphoma.

Merkel cell tumors can recur locally, may metastasize to regional lymph nodes even in the absence of local recurrence, and may metastasize to distant sites, including the central nervous system.[115] Death occurs in a significant number of cases despite treatment.[116]

EXTRAMAMMARY PAGET'S DISEASE. Extramammary Paget's disease is a rare cutaneous neoplasm that occurs in the elderly. It develops more frequently in women and predominantly involves aprocrine gland–bearing areas, especially the vulva, scrotum, and perianal areas. The lesions develop as erythematous scaly patches that progress to crusted, pruritic, erythematous plaques. The clinical differential diagnosis includes squamous cell carcinoma in situ, and superficial fungal infection.[117]

Extramammary Paget's disease is generally thought to be an adenocarcinoma of the epidermis, from which it extends into the contiguous epithelium of hair follicles and eccrine sweat ducts.[118] The individual Paget cells are large with round or oval nuclei and abundant pale cytoplasm. Occasionally the nucleus is found at the cell periphery and is indented (signet-ring cells). The cells are distributed in a pagetoid pattern (singly) and in groups of various sizes and shapes throughout the epidermis and epithelia of the adnexa.[118] The histologic differential diagnosis includes squamous cell carcinoma in situ (pagetoid Bowen's disease) and superficial spreading malignant melanoma.[118]

Rarely, extramammary Paget's disease may result from direct extension into the skin of an adenocarcinoma from a contiguous organ such as the genitourinary or gastrointestinal tract.[118] In a retrospective analysis of 197 cases of extramammary Paget's disease, 12% of patients had a concurrent internal malignancy,[119] and 26% of patients died of the disease or an associated internal malignancy.[119]

SYNDROMES ASSOCIATED WITH MALIGNANT CUTANEOUS NEOPLASMS

Xeroderma pigmentosum is a rare disease of autosomal recessive inheritance that occurs in approximately 1 in 250,000 of the general population. It is characterized by severe sun sensitivity, photophobia, cutaneous pigmentary changes, advanced solar damage, and malignant cutaneous neoplasms, especially basal cell carcinoma, squamous cell carcinoma, and malignant melanoma (Fig. 43-14). There may be asso-

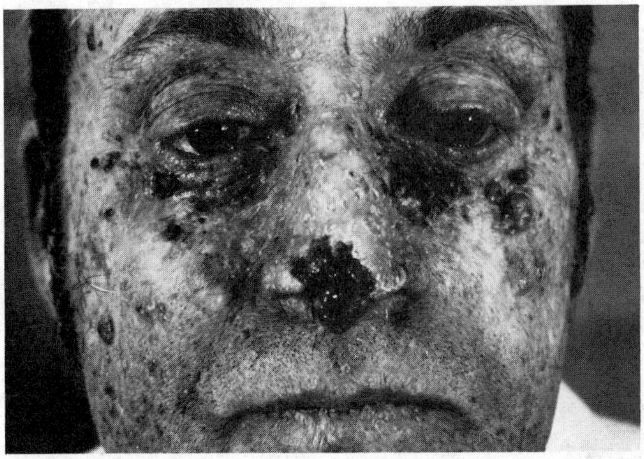

FIG. 43-14. Severe solar damage and multiple basal cell and squamous cell carcinomas in man with xeroderma pigmentosum.

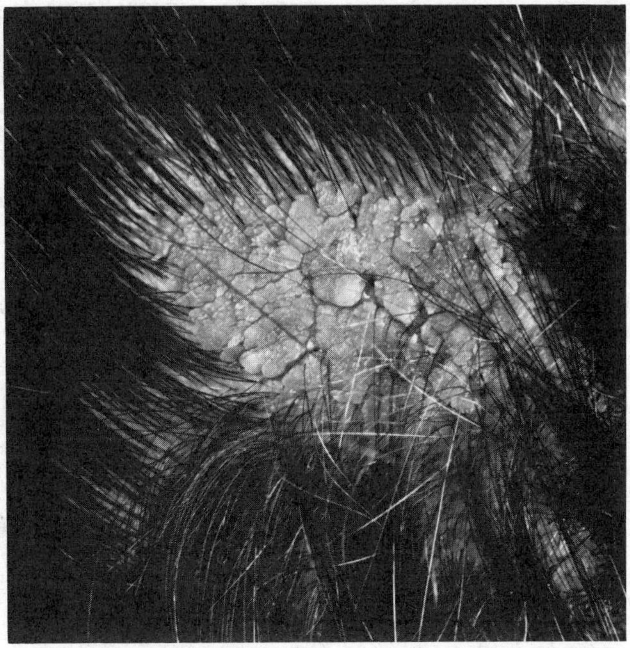

FIG. 43-15. Nevus sebaceus of Jadassohn on scalp. Note alopecia and verrucous surface.

ciated ocular and neurologic abnormalities.[120] Most cell strains from patients with xeroderma pigmentosum are unable to excise ultraviolet-induced pyrimidine dimers adequately,[121] which results in cutaneous malignancies from the unrepaired UVL-damaged DNA. The residual repair capacity of these patients is expressed as unscheduled DNA synthesis and confirmed by complementary methods (post-UVL exposure colony-forming ability and DNA-incising capacity).[122] There is a clear correlation between the onset and severity of symptoms and the residual repair capacity.[123] Miniscule amounts of UVL exposure appear sufficient to cause a malignancy, since squamous cell carcinoma of the tongue has been reported in two black patients with xeroderma pigmentosum.[124]

Nevus sebaceus of Jadassohn usually manifests as a single oval alopecic orange-yellow plaque on the scalp of a child.[125] At puberty the lesion becomes verrucous (Fig. 43-15), and in adult life both malignant cutaneous neoplasms and benign neoplasms such as syringocystadenoma papilliferum may develop.[126] Malignant neoplasms include basal cell carcinoma, apocrine carcinoma, squamous cell carcinoma, and adnexal carcinoma with possible pilar differentiation.[127] Basal cell carcinomas appear to behave in a biologically benign manner in this context, but the other neoplasms metastasize or recur locally and can lead to death.

Torre's syndrome was first described in 1967 in a patient with more than 100 cutaneous lesions of sebaceous adenoma, sebaceous carcinoma, and basal cell carcinoma in association with carcinoma of the ampulla of Vater and primary carcinoma of the colon.[128] Multiple keratoacanthomas may also be seen in these patients,[129] and there may be a strong family history of carcinoma.[130] Sebaceous carcinomas associated with Torre's syndrome do not metastasize.[131]

Epidermodysplasia verruciformis is a rare familial disease that starts in childhood with disseminated multiple scaly red, brown or achromic macules resembling tinea versicolor and flat wart-like lesions. The lesions are especially prominent on the face, neck, dorsa of the hands and feet, wrists, and knees. In about 10% of epidermodysplasia verruciformis families, more than one sibling will be affected, and about 10% of the patients have consanguineous parents. It has been suggested that epidermodysplasia verruciformis is linked to a rare, recessive, abnormal allele of an autosomal gene.[132] At least 15 types of papillomavirus particles, most commonly HPV types 5, 8, 20, and 17, have been detected in the benign lesions.[132]

In about 30% of patients with epidermodysplasia verruciformis, the benign lesions progress to large verrucous plaques and nodules of squamous cell carcinoma in the third and fourth decades of life (Fig. 43-16).[69] Since most patients have impaired cell-mediated immunity and the carcinomas arise in sun-exposed areas of the skin, the etiology of malignant neoplasms may be multifactorial and include viral, genetic, immunologic, and environmental causes. Of great interest is the detection of the HPV-5 genomes as free DNA molecules (not integrated into the cellular genome) in the lesions of epidermodysplasia verruciformis, indicating the oncogenic potential and possible role of HPV-5 in malignant transformation.[132] The resulting squamous cell carcinomas are locally invasive but do not appear to metastasize.

The *basal cell nevus syndrome* is a genetic form of basal cell carcinoma under the control of a single autosomal dominant gene that has complete penetrance and variable expressivity.[133] About 60% of patients do not have an affected parent. It has been suggested that this syndrome fits the Knudson two-hit hypothesis,[134] in which expression of the autosomal dominant gene requires solar radiation damage.[135]

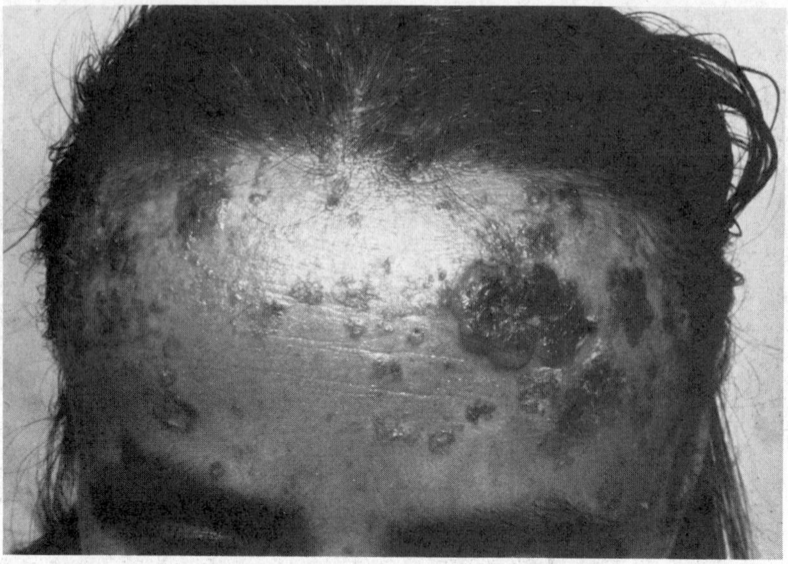

FIG. 43-16. Multiple lesions of in situ and superficial squamous cell carcinoma on the face of a woman with epidermodysplasia verruciformis.

In the basal cell nevus syndrome several to hundreds of basal cell carcinomas appear on the skin between puberty and age 35 years. The lesions may be superficial, nodular, or nodulo-ulcerative and often occur on the trunk. Most lesions remain quiescent, but some may become locally aggressive.[136] In 65% of patients an associated finding is asymmetric palmar or plantar pits measuring 1 to 3 mm in diameter (Fig. 43-17). The pits develop in the young adult patient and result from premature desquamation of the corneal layer overlying foci of basaloid cells thought to be a forme fruste of basal cell carcinoma.[137,138] Other associated clinical findings include odontogenic keratocysts of the jaw, mild ocular hypertelorism, calcified falx cerebri, rib anomalies, and an enlarged occipitofrontal head circumference. Less common findings have recently been reviewed.[139]

CLINICAL AND LABORATORY INVESTIGATIONS

In all patients presenting with a malignant cutaneous neoplasm, the following information should be elicited: duration of the lesion(s); the presence of associated symptoms (*e.g.*, pruritus, pain); changes occurring in the lesion; skin type, hair color, and eye color; history of sun exposure (blistering sunburn, ability or inability to tan); occupational and recreational history; past medical history (including arsenic ingestion, radiation therapy, osteomyelitis, thermal burn, chronic venous ulcer); ethnic background (*e.g.*, Celtic, Scandinavian); the presence of other coexisting disease or carcinoma; organ transplantation; state of the immune system; and the family history of cutaneous or other malignancies.

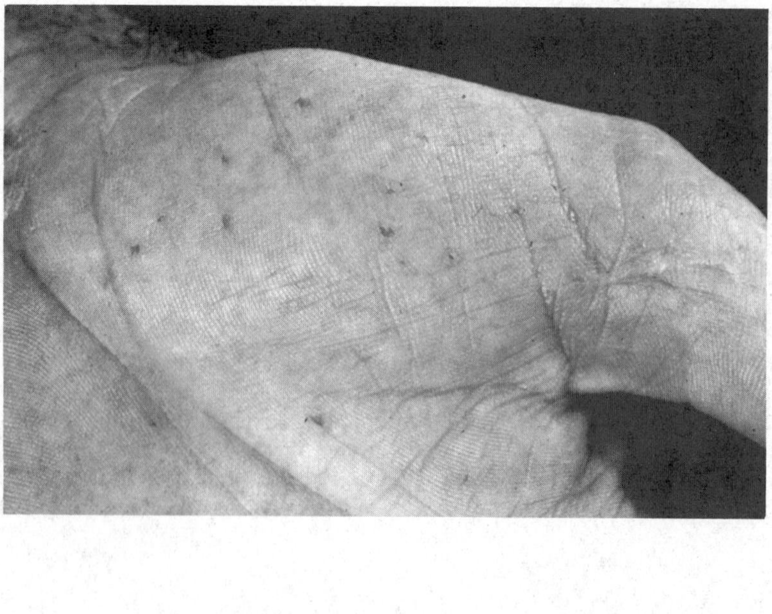

FIG. 43-17. Pits on the palm of a patient with basal cell nevus syndrome.

A thorough cutaneous examination should be undertaken that includes a scalp examination with the aid of a blow-dryer to expose the scalp, and examination of the mucous membranes (oral cavity, penis, perianal area, and vulva), ears, palms, soles, and interdigital clefts. This comprehensive examination may disclose other suspicious lesions, including malignant melanoma, unrecognized by the patient. Other signs of disease should be sought, such as palmar pits of the basal cell nevus syndrome and the flat warts of epidermodysplasia verruciformis. Manifestations of solar damage to date should be assessed, including cutaneous atrophy, telangiectasias, scaling erythema, wrinkles, solar elastosis, cutis rhomboidalis nuchae, solar lentigines, freckles, and so forth.

The site and extent of the neoplasm should be recorded on an anatomical diagram to include full morphologic description and accurate measurements made with calipers. Regional and distant lymph node groups should be evaluated by palpation. An adequate and expeditious biopsy of the neoplasm and involved nodes is essential; aspiration cytology may be of help in assessing the cutaneous lesion and lymph nodes. Biopsy specimens are processed for routine histologic studies and for immunoperoxidase staining. The latter is especially useful in the histologic diagnosis of spindle cell carcinoma, the differential of which includes squamous cell carcinoma, malignant melanoma, and malignant fibrous histiocytoma.[76,77]

Screening blood tests should be performed to assess possible immunosuppression, anemia, hepatic metastases, coagulation disorders, and markers of malignancy, such as lactate dehydrogenase levels. In some cases, an anergy panel and tests for cell-mediated immunity, including T-lymphocyte subset values, may be useful.

Imaging studies such as chest radiography, lymphangiography, liver-spleen scan, computed tomography, and magnetic resonance imaging should be performed as indicated in the individual case to assess local and distant spread of the neoplasm and to detect any associated disease.

Once these investigations are complete, the neoplasm can be appropriately diagnosed and staged with the TNM classification (see Table 43-1). Appropriate therapy can then be planned.

BIOPSY AND TREATMENT PLANNING

Biopsy of a lesion suspected of being malignant provides essential information for the appropriate treatment of a skin cancer. The microscopic interpretation of the tissue specimen allows the physician to choose the correct therapeutic approach from among the several available.

BIOPSY TECHNIQUES

The four principal biopsy techniques used for cutaneous malignancies are the shave biopsy, in which a superficial portion of the tumor is sliced with a scalpel; the punch biopsy, in which a cylindrical instrument is placed into the reticular dermis or subcutaneous tissue to obtain a deeper specimen; the incisional biopsy, in which a portion of the tumor is removed with a scalpel; and the excisional biopsy, in which the entire lesion is excised for histologic analysis. The technique selected in an individual case should yield the optimal pathologic specimen to facilitate accurate diagnosis. In some instances the correct diagnosis cannot be made from a superficial biopsy specimen. For example, the diagnosis of squamous cell carcinoma might be missed in a superficial shave biopsy since the pathologist can assess only the atypical keratinocytes that extend to the base of the specimen. Because squamous cell carcinomas extend into the papillary dermis and often the reticular dermis, a deep punch biopsy or incisional biopsy is indicated in such cases. In other instances, such as pigmented basal cell carcinoma, where the differential diagnosis includes malignant melanoma, an incisional or excisional biopsy is required to rule out the more serious malignancy. For the evaluation of nodulo-ulcerative basal cell carcinomas, a shave biopsy is usually adequate. If morphea-form or infiltrating basal cell carcinoma is considered clinically, a deep biopsy should be performed to obtain sufficient tissue for histologic evaluation of tumor cells in the dermis. A shave biopsy of a morphea-form basal cell carcinoma would not readily permit differentiation of this entity from a benign process such as a scar or a desmoplastic trichoepithelioma, which may have a similar histologic appearance.[61]

Although keratoacanthomas are considered benign neoplasms, it is of value to discuss the biopsy of these lesions. A keratoacanthoma is often difficult to diagnose histologically since it can be confused with a squamous cell carcinoma. The histopathologist relies on the gross architectural pattern of a keratoacanthoma to distinguish it from a squamous cell carcinoma. Thus, the surgeon must begin the biopsy at the edge of the keratoacanthoma and extend it to the center of the lesion. This "paramedian biopsy" is equivalent to taking a wedge-shaped portion of the lesion, which is often concentric.

The recommended approaches for biopsy of possible malignant cutaneous neoplasms are outlined in Table 43-2.

Biopsies of cutaneous lesions are performed in an outpatient setting using local anesthesia such as 1% or 2% Xylocaine without epinephrine or Xylocaine with epinephrine in

TABLE 43-2. Biopsy Techniques for Cutaneous Malignancies

Tumor	*Biopsy Technique*
Basal cell carcinoma	
Nodulo-ulcerative	Shave biopsy
Superficial	Shave biopsy
Cystic	Shave biopsy
Pigmented	Punch or excisional biopsy
Morphea-form (sclerosing) or infiltrating	Punch, incisional, or excisional biopsy
Squamous cell carcinoma	Punch, incisional, or excisional biopsy
Keratoacanthoma	Paramedian, incisional, or excisional biopsy
Adnexal neoplasms	Punch, incisional, or excisional biopsy

a concentration of 1:100,000. These biopsies are usually uncomplicated, and the postoperative morbidity is limited to mild oozing or superficial infection.

TREATMENT PLANNING

Once the histologic diagnosis has been made, numerous factors must be considered in determining the appropriate therapeutic approach. As outlined in Table 43-3, there are many choices in the treatment of cutaneous carcinomas. The therapeutic choice is often based not only on the histologic type of tumor, but also on its anatomical location and the general health and age of the patient. The anatomical considerations include certain areas that have a higher predilection for recurrences and certain areas that are more amenable to healing by secondary intention. Carcinomas in the embryonic fusion planes, such as the periorbital, perinasal, and periauricular areas, are notorious for their high rate of recurrence after treatment.[141] Therefore, the physician must choose the technique with the highest cure rate. Other anatomical considerations include the final cosmetic appearance of the wound and the anatomical function of the area after removal of the carcinoma. Zitelli has outlined those areas which are likely to heal well by secondary intention and those where cosmetically unacceptable results may occur.[142] Secondary intention healing of convex surfaces such as the nose, lips, cheeks, chin, and helix of the ear often leads to unacceptable scars, whereas concave areas involving the nose, eye, ear, and temple often heal well by secondary intention, with very acceptable cosmetic results. In convex areas and in areas where functional impairment from healing is of concern, such as the eyes and lip, excisional surgery or skin flaps or grafts may be required.

The general medical status of the patient must be carefully considered. In patients with a coagulopathy or who are receiving medical anticoagulation therapy, the tumor should be removed by a bloodless method such as cryosurgery, radiation therapy, or carbon dioxide laser excision or vaporization. For very debilitated patients, fractionation of radiation therapy in 10 to 15 office visits may not be possible. In such cases techniques requiring one or two office visits, such as curettage and electrodesiccation or surgical excision, would be preferable.

TABLE 43-3. Treatment Approaches to Nonmelanoma Skin Cancer

Carcinoma	*Treatment*
Basal Cell Carcinoma	
Nodular	Curettage and electrodesiccation
	Cryotherapy
	Excision
	Mohs' micrographic surgery (in anatomical sites of high recurrence)
	Radiation therapy
Superficial	Curettage and electrodesiccation
	Cryotherapy
	Excision
	Topical chemotherapy
	Radiation therapy
	Laser vaporization
Morphea-form, infiltrating	Excision
	Mohs' micrographic surgery
Recurrent	Mohs' micrographic surgery
Basosquamous differentiation	Excision
Squamous Cell Carcinoma	
In situ (Bowen's disease)	Curettage and electrodesiccation
	Cryotherapy
	Excision
	Radiation therapy
	Laser vaporization
	Mohs' micrographic surgery
Invasive	Excision
	Radiation therapy
	Mohs' micrographic surgery
Verrucous carcinoma	Excision
	Mohs' micrographic surgery
Adnexal Carcinoma	
Eccrine carcinoma, apocrine carcinoma, sebaceous carcinoma, Merkel cell tumor, extramammary Paget's disease	Excision
	Mohs' micrographic surgery

TREATMENT MODALITIES

CURETTAGE, ELECTRODESICCATION, AND LASER VAPORIZATION

Dermatologists commonly use curettage and electrodesiccation to treat basal cell carcinomas and superficial squamous cell carcinomas. The technique is based on the difference in consistency between the tumor and the surrounding normal tissue. A curette is used to debulk and delineate the tumor from the surrounding normal skin. As the curette, a moderately sharp, oval- or round-tipped instrument with a handle, is stroked firmly across the visible tumor, the periphery and depth of the tumor can be determined from the difference in consistency between tumor and normal tissue as indicated by sound and texture: normal dermis is firm and has a gritty sound on curettage, whereas tumor is very soft and produces no sound on curettage. After curettage, the lesion is electrodesiccated. Accepted standards of care indicate that the procedure of curettage followed by electrodesiccation should be repeated two or three times.[143] However, some physicians have achieved good results with curettage alone for many basal cell carcinomas.[144]

Cure rates with this technique range from 77% to 97%.[145] The best results have been achieved with superficial and nodular basal cell carcinomas in areas of low recurrence. Curettage and electrodesiccation is more likely to fail in recurrent tumors and in primary basal and squamous cell carcinomas in embryonic fusion planes. Use of electrodesiccation and curettage is also limited in certain anatomical areas because of cosmetic considerations. Postoperative wound contracture around the eyelids and mouth may lead to distortion of these anatomical structures as the electrodesiccated wound heals by secondary intention (Fig. 43-18). In these anatomical areas, surgical excision, Mohs' micrographic surgery followed by reconstructive surgery, cryotherapy, or radiation therapy should be considered.

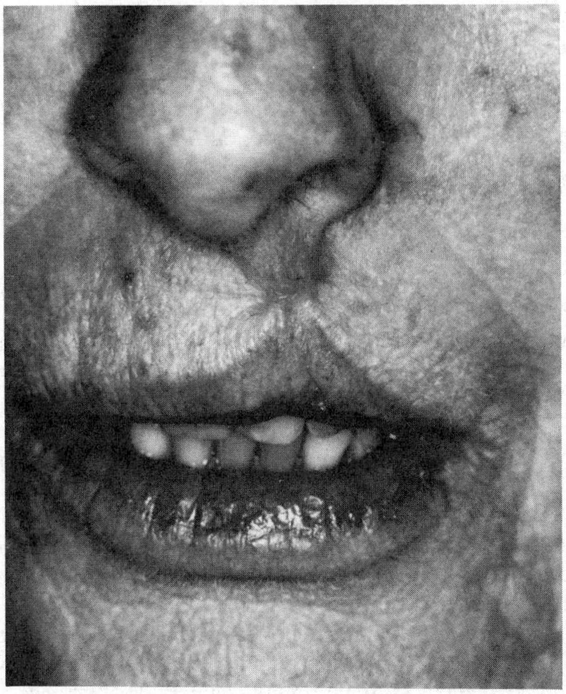

FIG. 43-18. Electrodesiccation and curettage of basal cell carcinoma of upper lip 6 months previously has resulted in upward contracture and distortion of lip.

Curettage may be helpful in determining which lesions are too deep to respond to electrodesiccation and curettage. During the course of a treatment, the physician may find the curettage extending deeply into the subcutaneous tissue. In this circumstance it is best to consider an alternative therapy to define the peripheral and deep margins of the tumor.

Immediately after curettage and electrodesiccation, tumor has been found to persist in 12% to 30% of midfacial basal cell carcinomas.[146] The persistent tumor was seen on microscopic examination. By contrast, 5-year cure rates in the range of 85% to 97% have been reported with this technique. This discrepancy suggests that other factors, perhaps an immunologic response or an inflammatory reaction secondary to surgery, may be responsible for the high success rate of this technique.

A multivariate analysis by Dubin and Kopf identified certain factors associated with an increased risk of recurrence after curettage and electrodesiccation.[147] These factors included location of a lesion on the forehead, ears, eyes, nose, or face, and increasing lesion diameter. Previous treatment of any type and advanced patient age also correlated with a higher recurrence rate.[147]

Curettage and electrodesiccation remains the simplest method of treating superficial cutaneous carcinomas. With appropriate patient selection, a high cure rate should be achieved with curettage and electrodesiccation of uncomplicated carcinomas.

A similar technique entails using a carbon dioxide (CO_2) laser in place of electrodesiccation.[148] The CO_2 laser is an infrared laser beam emitted at 10,600 nm. When the beam is defocused, it can be used to vaporize cutaneous lesions such as basal cell carcinomas, superficial squamous cell carcinomas, and premalignant lesions such as solar keratoses.[148,149] Laser vaporization may be used in conjunction with curettage.

Some physicians prefer CO_2 laser vaporization to electrodesiccation because of the bloodless field, diminished postoperative pain, and less scarring. However, this modality has not been fully assessed or compared with electrodesiccation, since the data on long-term cure rates for superficial malignant cutaneous neoplasms treated by laser vaporization are not yet available.

SURGICAL EXCISION

Surgical excision with primary closure of the wound is an effective treatment for all types of skin cancer in almost all anatomical locations. Complete excision of a tumor has the advantage of allowing microscopic evaluation of the tumor margins. Most surgical excisions are performed in an elliptical fashion along Langer's cleavage lines, which allows for a good cosmetic result. Usually the cancer is excised under local anesthesia with a scalpel or curved scissor.

Elliptical excisions can be performed with minimal complications and discomfort to the patient. If the relaxed skin tension lines or Langer's lines are followed, the final scar is barely perceptible on facial surfaces. It is more prominent on the chest or back, where greater tension on the wound can result in a wider scar. The decision to perform elliptical excisions must be made with consideration of the other therapeutic modalities available, the biologic nature of the lesion to be excised, and the anatomical location of the lesion. Elliptical excisions are easily performed on the trunk, extremities, cheeks, forehead, chin, and scalp. Special consideration must be given to excision of lesions from the lip, eyelids, alar rim of the nose, and the ears. A wedge-shaped excision may be preferable so that these important anatomical areas are not distorted with healing.

Most skin cancers can be excised relatively easily. However, specialized training may be required. Most primary cutaneous neoplasms involving cosmetically important areas, such as the nose, eyes, lip, and ears, can be excised. Recurrent basal and squamous cell carcinomas, morpheaform and infiltrating basal cell carcinomas, and certain adnexal tumors are preferably removed by Mohs' micrographic surgery instead of simple excision.

The surgical margins for excision of cutaneous malignancies vary from a few millimeters for basal cell carcinomas to several centimeters for a Merkel cell carcinoma. Since the basal cell carcinoma is unlikely to metastasize, narrow margins of 3 to 5 mm are usually acceptable. Morphea-form, infiltrating, or recurrent basal cell carcinomas should be excised with margins wider than 1 cm if Mohs micrographic surgery is not utilized. Squamous cell carcinomas, eccrine carcinomas, and Merkel cell carcinomas all can metastasize and therefore require wider margins of excision. Unlike malignant melanoma, the clinical margins for these tumors with the potential to metastasize have not been well defined. It is clear, however, that greater margins should be taken with tumors that involve broad areas or extend deep into the underlying subcutaneous tissue. In a neoplasm with potential

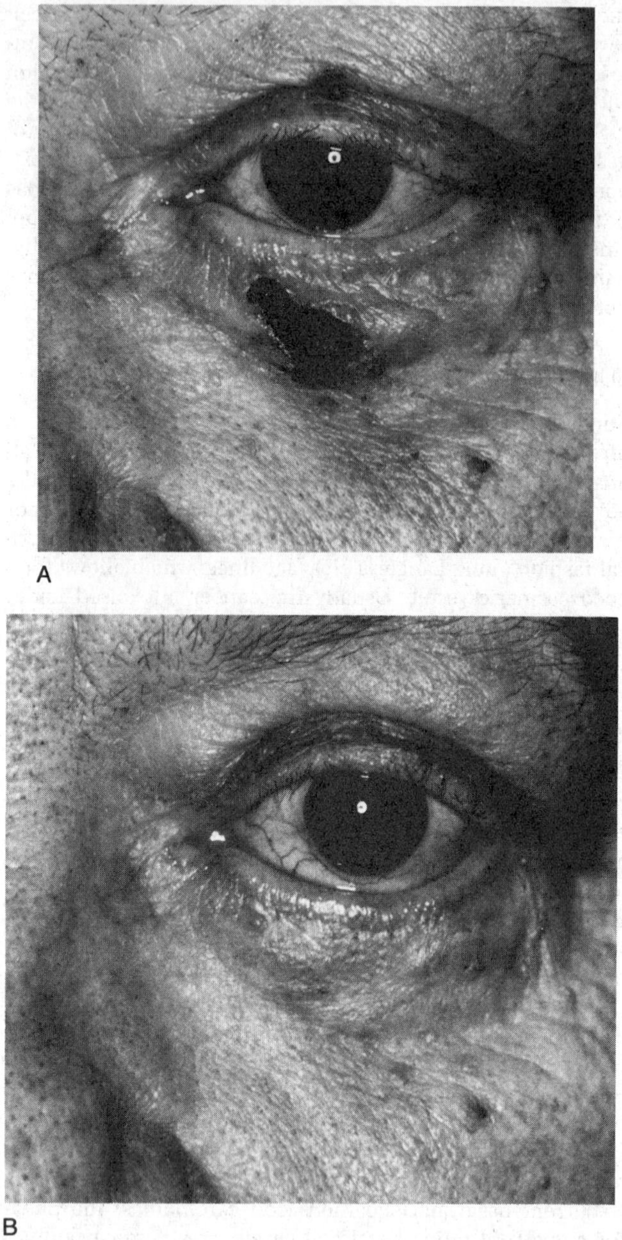

FIG. 43-19. **A.** Basal cell carcinoma of the left lower eyelid that was subsequently treated by Mohs' surgery. **B.** Appearance of the left lower eyelid after full-thickness skin grafting. Very good cosmetic result achieved with graft from left upper eyelid.

for metastatic spread, clinical evaluation of the regional lymph nodes is mandatory. However, lymph node dissection is required only when there is clinically palpable lymphadenopathy.

Occasional skin tumors that are very large or are in critical anatomical areas may not be suitable for excision with primary wound closure. For example, when an elliptical or wedge-shaped excision might result in an ectropion of an eyelid (Fig. 43-19) or distortion of the lip or nose, a skin graft or flap should be considered. Skin grafts are either split-thickness or full-thickness. Split-thickness grafts, usually taken with a mechanical dermatome, are used to cover very large surgical defects and areas where there is minimal vascularity, such as the perichondrium or periosteum.[150] The disadvantages of split-thickness grafting are (1) the color match is usually poor and (2) a donor site results that heals by secondary intention over a 2- to 4-week period. Conversely, split-thickness grafts are easy to create and are usually well accepted by noninfected recipient sites.

Full-thickness grafts require primary closure of the donor site (often the posterior auricular area, eyelid, or neck for defects on the face) (Fig. 43-20). Full-thickness grafts are necessary when a good color match is important. These grafts contract less than split-thickness grafts.[150] Both split-thickness and full-thickness grafts are immobilized after surgery to prevent bleeding and movement of the graft over the recipient site. Skin grafts are usually accepted by the recipient site within 5 to 7 days and mature over a 2- to 3-month period, at which time they become cosmetically acceptable.

Another alternative to elliptical or wedge-shaped excisions and skin grafting is the placement of a skin flap. In contrast to a skin graft, which receives its blood supply from the recipient surgical site, a skin flap carries its own vascular supply. A pedicle of tissue remains attached at the base and the tissue is rotated or advanced to cover the surgical wound. The simplest and most common skin flap is the rotation flap, in which adjacent skin is rotated across the defect. Rotation flaps can be designed in various shapes to adapt to the anatomical location and the size of the wound being treated. Other flap techniques include transposition, advancement, and island flaps.[151] Also of use is the microvascular free flap, in which tissue is transferred from one part of the body to another, with the donor artery and vein anastomosed to the corresponding artery and vein in the area being reconstructed.[152]

MOHS' MICROGRAPHIC SURGERY

Mohs' micrographic surgery is a specialized technique in which serial horizontal sections of excised tissue are systematically mapped and microscopically evaluated by frozen section examination. Because margins are checked thoroughly at the time of surgery, this technique is a major improvement in the treatment of difficult and recurrent skin cancers. The technique was first described by Dr. Frederick Mohs in the late 1930s, when it was known as *Mohs' chemosurgery*.[153] Originally, a chemical fixative (zinc chloride paste) was used to fix the tumor in situ. The tumor was then serially removed and carefully mapped and color coded. Horizontal sections of the excised neoplasm were then prepared by the frozen tissue technique and examined by light microscopy. The margins (deep and peripheral) of the neoplasm were evaluated, and areas of tumorous involvement were noted on the color-coded maps of the removed tissue. These steps were then repeated in areas identified as still containing tumor until the entire neoplasm was removed and all margins were free of tumor (Fig. 43-21).

The fixed-tissue technique, although effective, was time-consuming and eventually was modified to eliminate the step of chemical fixation.[154] The current procedure, known as

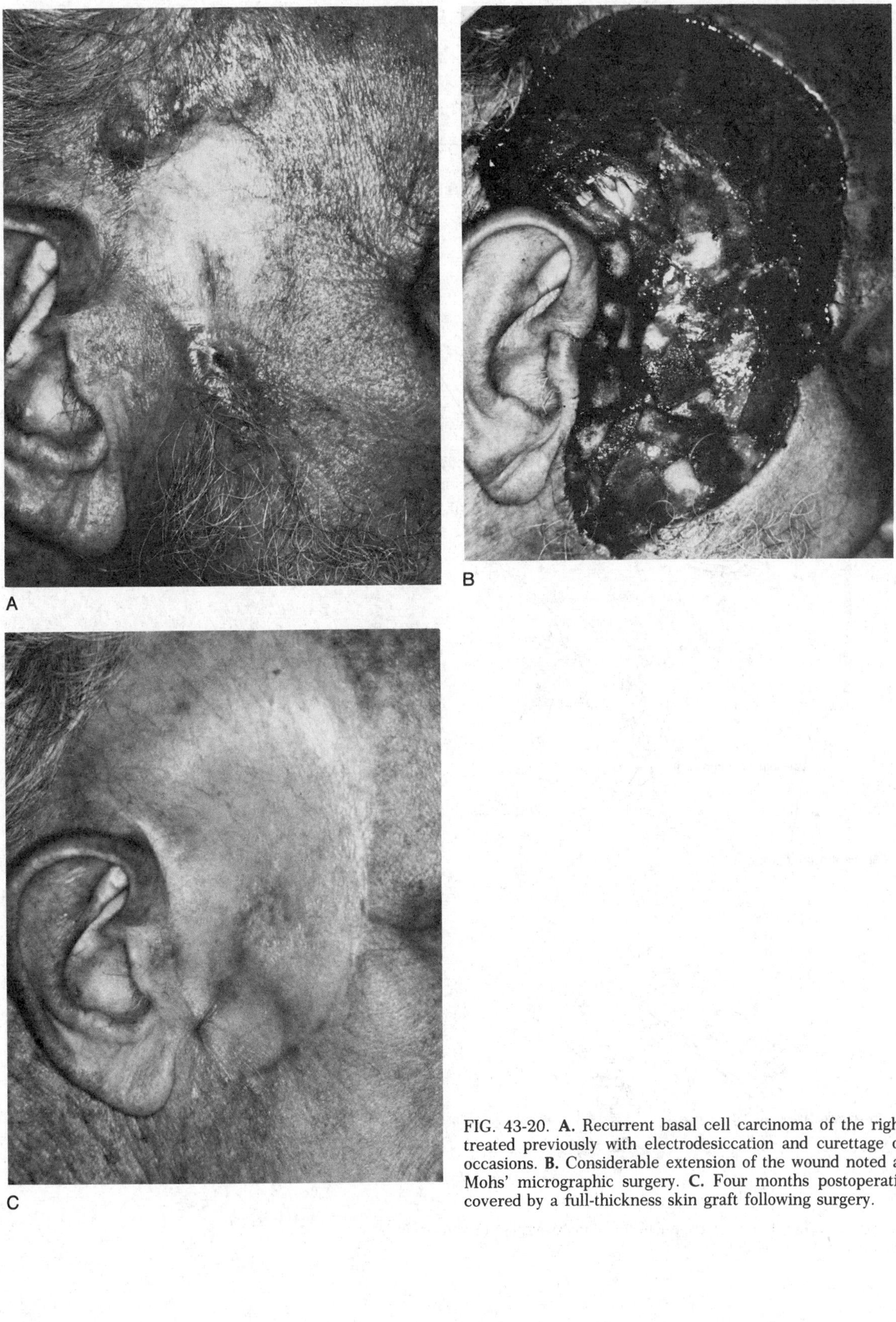

FIG. 43-20. **A.** Recurrent basal cell carcinoma of the right cheek that was treated previously with electrodesiccation and curettage on three separate occasions. **B.** Considerable extension of the wound noted after six stages of Mohs' micrographic surgery. **C.** Four months postoperatively. Defect was covered by a full-thickness skin graft following surgery.

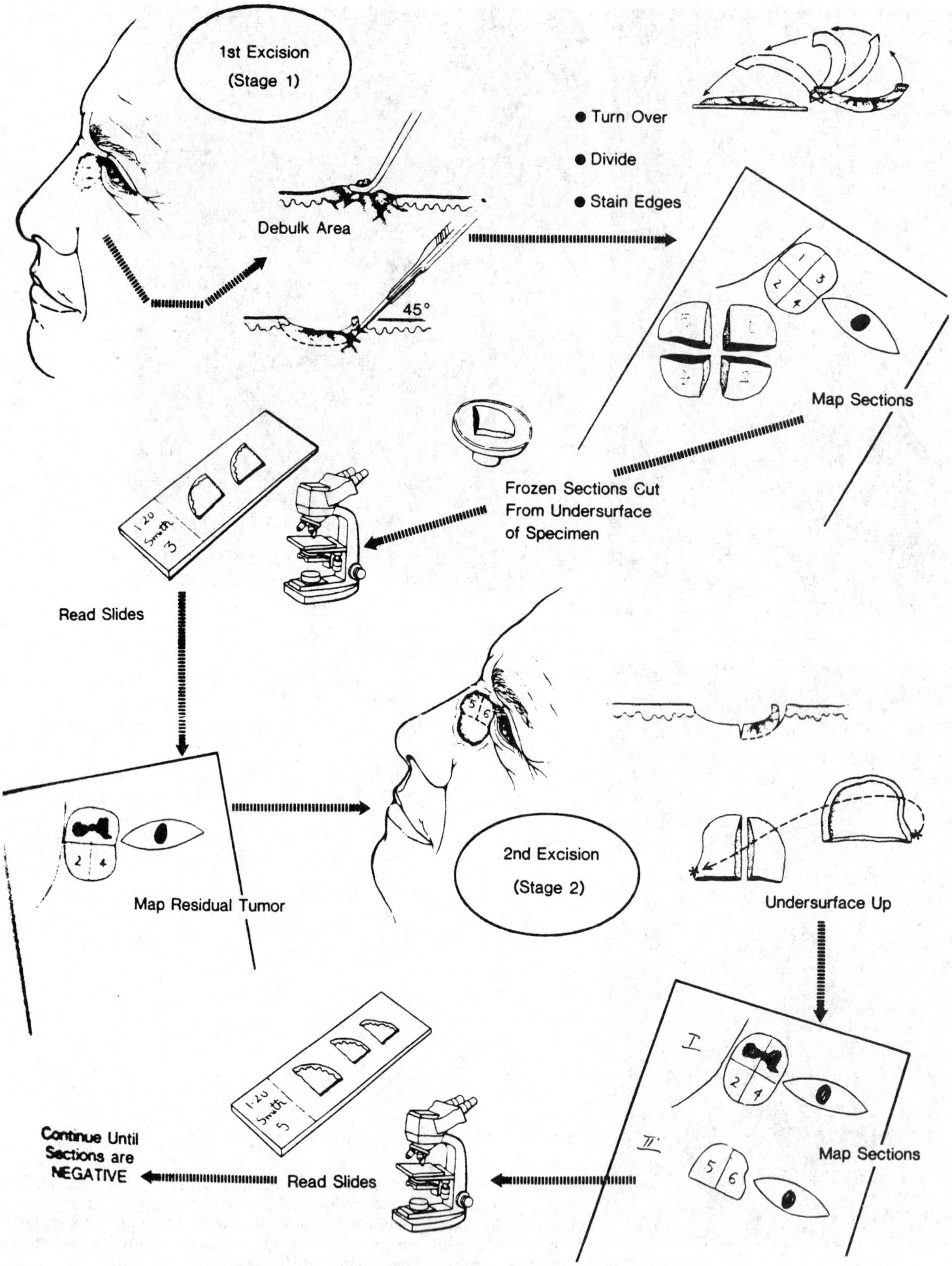

FIG. 43-21. Schematic representation of technique of Mohs' surgery. (Swanson N: Mohs surgery. Arch Dermatol 119:761, 1983)

Mohs' micrographic surgery, is therefore performed on fresh tissue. Mohs' surgery has the highest cure rate of all the therapeutic modalities available for treatment of nonmelanoma skin cancer. The cure rate is approximately 99% for primary basal cell carcinomas and 96% to 98% for recurrent basal cell carcinomas.[155]

There are many advantages to the Mohs' technique:

1. The horizontal sectioning and examination of 100% of the true peripheral and deep margins ensures complete removal of the tumor. Such margin control therefore obviates removal of normal tissue.
2. The complete circumspection of the tissue margins is superior to that achieved with standard processing and step-sectioning by pathologists, or routine frozen section examination, in which only 1/1000th of the margin may be evaluated.[156]
3. Removal of a layer of tissue can take 15 minutes to 1 hour. The duration of the procedure depends on the size of the neoplasm and the number of stages required. Most patients are therefore treated in an outpatient setting, with tumor-free margins achieved within several hours.
4. Many defects can heal by secondary intention. However, if necessary, wound reconstruction can be performed immediately after Mohs' surgery. Thus, a good cosmetic result is obtained with primary closure, skin flap, or skin graft, with the benefit of an assured tumor-free wound. Complex repairs may require hospitalization so that the surgeon can work with a specialized plastic surgeon, oculoplastic surgeon, or head and neck surgeon.
5. The cure rate with Mohs' surgery for recurrent cutaneous neoplasms is dramatically higher than the cure rate achieved with other treatment modalities.[157] This technique traces the spread of tumor cells within the scar tissue of recurrences and ensures complete removal of the infiltrating neoplasm. This is especially important, since recurrent tumors often spread microscopically far beyond the clinical margins. Margin control is very difficult to achieve with routine histologic sections or vertically cut frozen sections.
6. Mohs' surgery is very effective in the treatment of morphea-form and infiltrating basal cell carcinomas (Fig. 43-22) as well as primary tumors in areas of high recurrence. These areas include embryonic fusion planes such as the medial canthi, periauricular skin, and paranasal skin.
7. The Mohs' technique spares normal tissue when primary lesions are removed in cosmetically important areas such as the nasal tip, and in areas where there is significant concern about postoperative reconstruction, such as the eyelids and lips.[158]
8. Patients with deeply or widely invasive tumors benefit

FIG. 43-22. **A.** Extensive infiltrating destructive morpheaform basal cell carcinoma of the left cheek. **B.** Extension of the tumor noted far beyond the clinical margins as defined by Mohs' micrographic surgery.

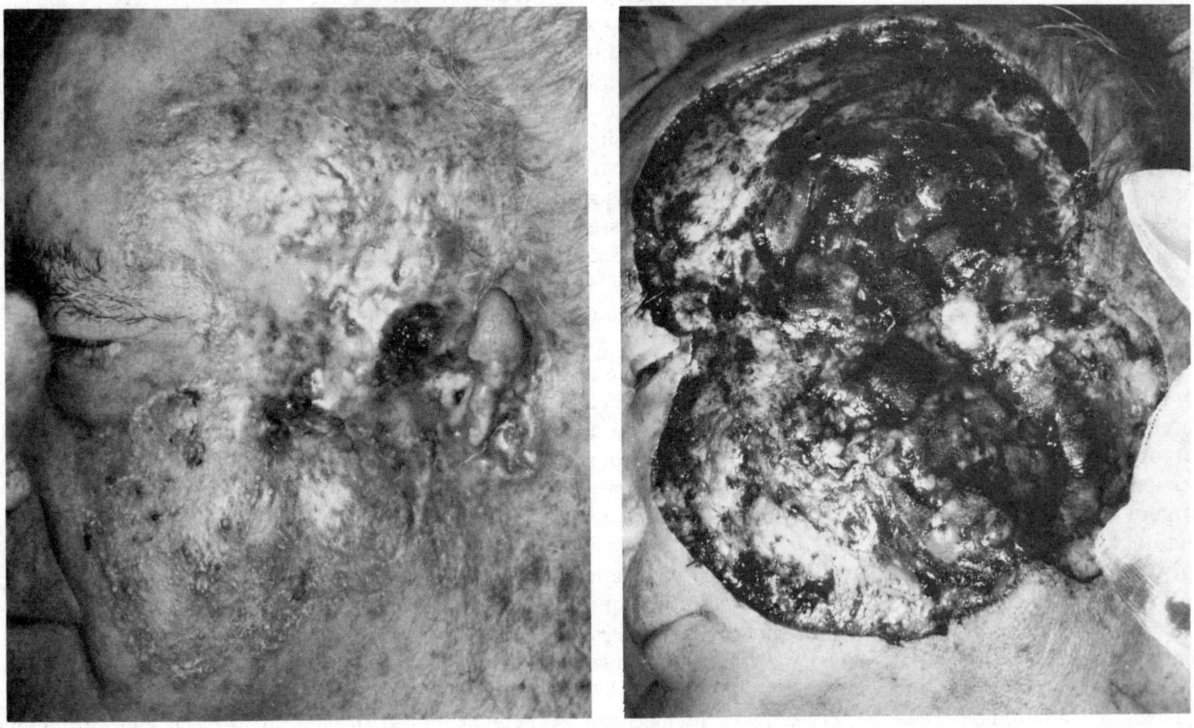

A B

from Mohs' surgery because the technique maps out and ensures total removal of tumor involving subcutaneous tissue, cartilage, muscle, nerves, and bone.

9. Squamous cell carcinoma of the digits and male genitalia was treated in the past by amputation. Such mutilating surgery can be avoided (if the neoplasm is limited in its depth) by careful but thorough Mohs' surgery, with sparing of the normal tissue.[159,160]

The defect produced by the thorough examination and removal of all neoplastic tissue can often be extremely large and potentially devastating to the patient. In-depth discussion of the procedures involved and photographic illustrations of other patients' appearances after Mohs' surgery, repair possibilities, and the like will help the patient tolerate the morbidity inherent in these procedures.

Other tumors that can be treated with Mohs' surgery include verrucous carcinoma, extramammary Paget's disease, Bowen's disease of the genitalia, dermatofibrosarcoma protuberans, keratoacanthomas, and various other adnexal carcinomas.[107, 160–164]

CRYOSURGERY

Cryosurgery with liquid nitrogen has been used for 25 years as an effective treatment for various cutaneous carcinomas in selected patients. This nonsurgical technique requires liquid nitrogen at −196.5°C, a pyrometer, and thermocouple needles.[165] The tumor is anesthetized with local anesthesia and liquid nitrogen is sprayed on the center of the tumor for several seconds until the complete surface area of the tumor, with an additional 3 to 5-mm border, is frozen. The temperature of the pyrometer, measured by the thermocouples in the neoplasm, should reach −50°C.[166] The liquid nitrogen is applied to the tumor with a cotton applicator stick, by open aerosol, or by directed aerosol via a plastic cone attached to the cryosurgical unit. The cone directs the spray to the midpoint of the tumor and allows the tumor to be frozen in a shorter period of time. With the open spray, the freezing time is approximately 1 minute for a medium-size tumor and the thawing time (the amount of time required for the tissue to retain its normal turgor) is about 2 minutes. If the plastic cone is used to direct the spray, the freezing time can be as short as 15 seconds, with a thawing time of 60 seconds. A double freeze–thaw cycle is recommended for cutaneous malignancies.

Effectively administered cryosurgery is a good treatment for many basal cell carcinomas and superficial squamous cell carcinomas. It is particularly valuable for patients in whom surgery is contraindicated. The cure rate for cryosurgery of a primary basal cell carcinoma is in excess of 90%.[167] Cryosurgery is most effective for primary basal and superficial and in situ squamous cell carcinomas of the skin. Cryosurgery is not the optimal treatment for morphea-form and infiltrating basal cell carcinomas, recurrent basal cell and squamous cell carcinomas, tumors with ill-defined borders, tumors more than 2 cm in diameter, and infiltrating squamous cell carcinomas.

Favorable anatomical sites for cryosurgery include the eyelids, ears, face, neck, and trunk.[168] Particular care must be taken when treating tumors involving the embryonic fusion planes such as the nasolabial fold, inner canthi of the eyes, and the periauricular areas. These anatomical sites usually require a wider margin of freezing to help prevent recurrence since there is often deep cryptic infiltration. Some clinicians consider cryosurgery of the legs to be contraindicated because of the prolonged healing time. Cryosurgery should, of course, be avoided in patients with cold sensitivity (*e.g.*, cryoglobulinemia).

The morbidity following cryosurgery is moderate and includes edema, oozing, erosions, hemorrhage, and secondary infection.[167] The latter two complications are quite rare. The treated area heals by secondary intention with a favorable cosmetic result apart from hypopigmentation (Fig. 43-23). Scar formation has been reported, but it is usually not of cosmetic concern.

CHEMOTHERAPY

Topical chemotherapy with 5-fluorouracil (5-FU) has been established as effective treatment for precancerous skin conditions as well as for certain cutaneous carcinomas.[169] 5-FU is a fluoronated pyrimidine that inhibits the methylation of deoxyuradilic acid to thymidylic acid, thus interfering with the synthesis of DNA and RNA. There is a subsequent deficiency in DNA synthesis, which results in cell death. Inhibition of DNA and RNA synthesis is most notable in rapidly proliferating (*e.g.*, neoplastic) cells as compared to cells with a normal rate of metabolism.

5-FU is applied topically as a cream or lotion twice a day for a period of several weeks, producing a dramatic inflammatory response in the precancerous and malignant areas. The inflammation is allowed to persist for 2 to 3 weeks of treatment for the face and scalp; longer periods of time are required on other parts of the body. The physician should evaluate the patient at this time to ensure that the desired response has been achieved. Concentrations of the 5-FU cream can be increased to achieve an inflammatory response if lower concentrations have been unsuccessful. Concentrations of 5-FU usually begin at 1% or 2% and may be increased to 5% if the desired inflammatory response has not been achieved. The lower concentrations are usually appropriate for the face and scalp, whereas the 5% concentration is often necessary for the extremities or trunk. The use of 5-FU on the extremities or trunk can also be enhanced with the concomitant use of topical 13-*all-trans*-retinoic acid (tretinoin cream). Sun avoidance is required during this treatment because of an induced photosensitivity. Once the desired inflammatory response has been achieved, the area is treated with topical corticosteroids to alleviate any discomfort or discoloration of the skin.

Complications from this treatment are rare, although occasionally posttreatment erythema and pigmentary changes of the skin may occur. Contact sensitivity to the vehicle used in the cream or lotion may develop. The patient should be carefully examined following 5-FU treatment and any persistent or newly noted lesions should be biopsied to rule out underlying carcinoma.[169] The best results with 5-FU have been achieved in superficial basal cell carcinomas on the trunk and extremities. The use of 5-FU in all other types of

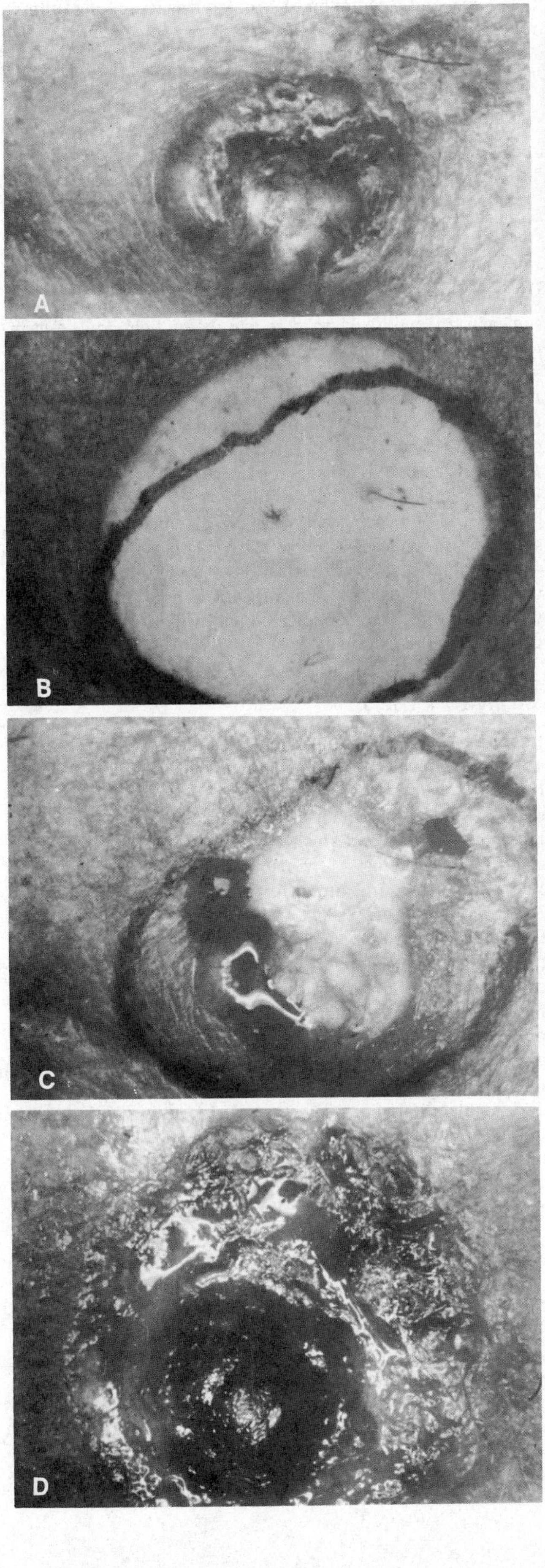

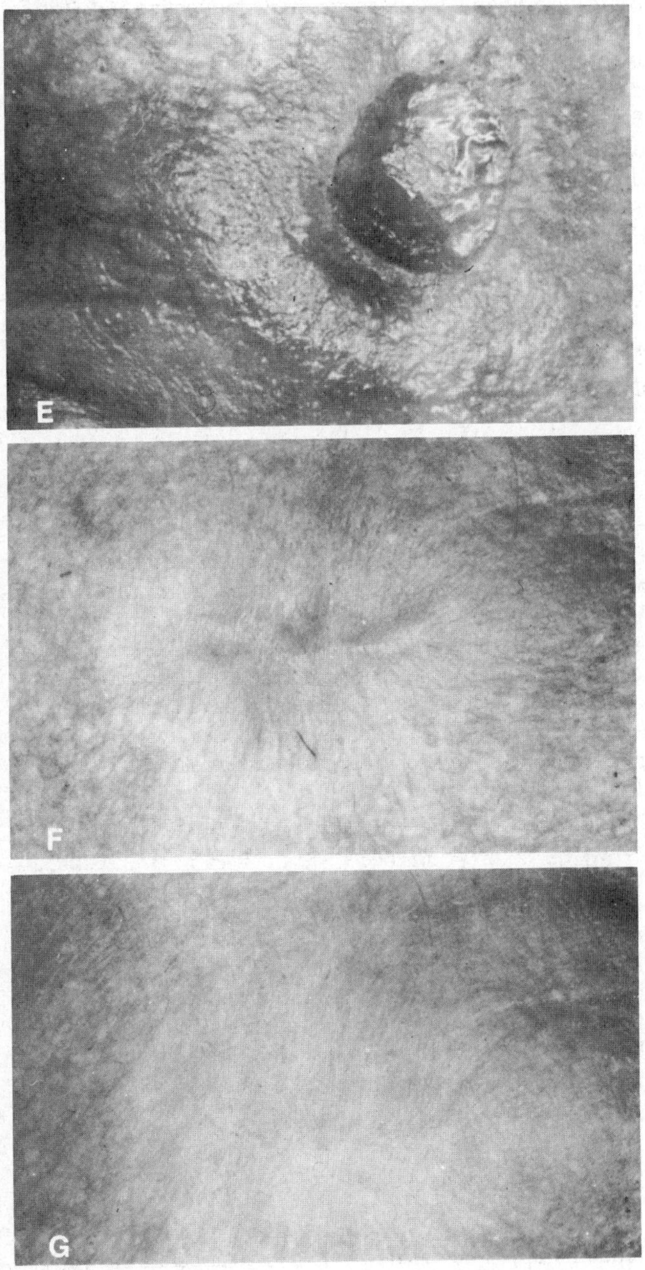

FIG. 43-23. **A.** Basal cell carcinoma over zygoma before therapy. **B.** Lesion frozen by liquid nitrogen. Marking pen outlines treatment fields. **C.** Lesion thawing 1½ minutes after nitrogen spray stopped. **D.** Necrosis 1 week after cryosurgery. **E.** Early healing 3 weeks after cryosurgery. **F.** Scar with linear hypertrophic element 3 months after cryosurgery. **G.** One year after cryosurgery; hypopigmented scar with no hypertrophy.

basal cell carcinoma has been generally ineffective and, if it is used, one must be aware of the possibility of recurrence. The use of 5-FU in other types of cutaneous malignancies is not indicated.[170]

5-FU has also been used in combination with topical immunotherapeutic agents such as 2-4-dinitrochlorobenzene (DNCB). This combination has been used in a limited number of studies to treat squamous cell carcinoma in situ (Bowen's disease). The results were moderately successful, but recurrences did occur.[171]

Systemic chemotherapy has not proved to be very effective so far in the treatment of nonmelanoma skin cancer. Treatment of metastatic basal cell carcinoma, an uncommon sequela of this tumor, has included systemic 5-FU, cisplatin, and several other agents.[172,173] These studies cannot be effectively evaluated because only small numbers of patients have been treated. Systemic chemotherapy will probably never play a role in the treatment of any primary or recurrent basal cell carcinoma.

Chemotherapy for squamous cell carcinoma and adnexal tumors of the skin has generally been unsuccessful and without significant support for its use. It may, however, be useful as adjunctive therapy when metastases occur. For example, a recent preliminary study suggested the use of isotretinoin, a vitamin A derivative, as treatment for advanced primary squamous cell carcinomas.[174] However, not enough data are currently available to support the use of isotretinoin for this indication.

In 1988 Weiss et al reported that tretinoin cream may be of value in reducing damage to the skin induced by sunlight.[175] The photodamage was diminished with daily use of the retinoic acid for periods of time ranging from several weeks to several months. Histologic examination of the skin following use of this topical agent for more than 1 year revealed a thickened epidermis and new collagen formation in the papillary dermis.[176] Topical retinoic acid may also be of help in diminishing the existing solar keratoses and other signs of solar-induced damage of the skin such as lentigines and fine wrinkling.[175]

IMMUNOTHERAPY AND OTHER EXPERIMENTAL MODALITIES

Immunotherapy is not currently used to treat cutaneous carcinomas. Recent studies on the use of interferon to treat cutaneous neoplasms have, however, suggested that immunotherapy may become a standard therapy in the future.[175] A preliminary study demonstrated that local injection of α_2-interferon into basal cell carcinomas can provide at least a short-term remission of the tumor. Long-term follow-up is not yet available, nor has α_2-interferon been tried in more difficult basal cell carcinomas, such as the morphea-form or recurrent tumors. The minimal morbidity noted with these injections did suggest that its use may be of value in the future if long-term effectiveness can be demonstrated.

Another immunotherapeutic approach is the use of 2-4-dinitrochlorobenzene (DNCB) in the treatment of basal cell carcinoma.[178] Again, insufficient data are available to support its use at present. Similarly, recall agents including purified protein derivative (PPD), *Trichophyton, Candida,* pertussin, and streptokinase-streptodornase, among others, may also show efficacy in the treatment of uncomplicated cutaneous carcinomas when more data are available on their use.[179]

Limited but exciting data suggest that photodynamic therapy may be effective in the treatment of cutaneous malignancies. This technique entails tumor-specific or systemic injection of a photosensitizing substance that is relatively selectively retained by the malignant tumor as compared to the surrounding skin.[180,181] When exposed to a penetrating visible light source, the photosensitizing substance undergoes a photodynamic reaction that destroys the tumor cells and spares the surrounding normal skin. The photosensitizing substance utilized to date has been hematoporphyrin derivative or dihematoporphyrin ether. The bulk of the early work on this technique used the hematoporphyrin derivative in combination with a red laser light at a wavelength of approximately 600 to 700 nm. Limited studies have demonstrated effectiveness in both basal and squamous cell carcinomas and in Bowen's disease; however, long-term follow-up is not yet available. The technique has been limited by a generalized photosensitivity that the patients experience on systemic injection of the porphyrins. This therapeutic regimen, which has not yet received Food and Drug Administration approval, may be of significant benefit in patients in whom surgery is contraindicated and in patients whose disease encompasses a wide area.

RADIATION THERAPY

Radiation therapy is an excellent modality for the treatment of selected basal cell and squamous cell carcinomas. Both types of carcinomas are radiosensitive. However, the decision to treat with radiation, as with desiccation and curettage, cryosurgery, and any other modality, is based on anatomical site, histology of the neoplasm, patient age, cure and recurrence rates, and anticipated final cosmetic appearance. Many patients prefer radiation therapy because (1) there is no pain with treatment, (2) there is less psychological trauma since the patient continues to function well in his own environment without experiencing the temporary disfigurement or defect of other modalities, (3) no surgery is necessary (many patients are fearful of any invasive procedures), and (4) no hospitalization is required. The physician may opt for this modality in cases where the patient is elderly or debilitated, a poor surgical risk, or on anticoagulation therapy, or for very large lesions. In such cases, surgery may result in a poor cosmetic result because of the large area or depth of the defect, which may require excision of involved bone.[182] Radiation therapy has a distinct advantage over other modalities because uninvolved tissue is preserved and a lesser defect is produced (Fig. 43-24). Disadvantages of the treatment include alopecia (always permanent when cancericidal doses are used) in hair-bearing areas, possible dysfunction of sweat glands in the treated area, no tissue available for pathologic examination and margin control, and multiple patient visits.

Lesions on the trunk and extremities may be treated by radiation therapy. Most, however, are cured with a better cosmetic result using cryosurgery, excision, or curettage and

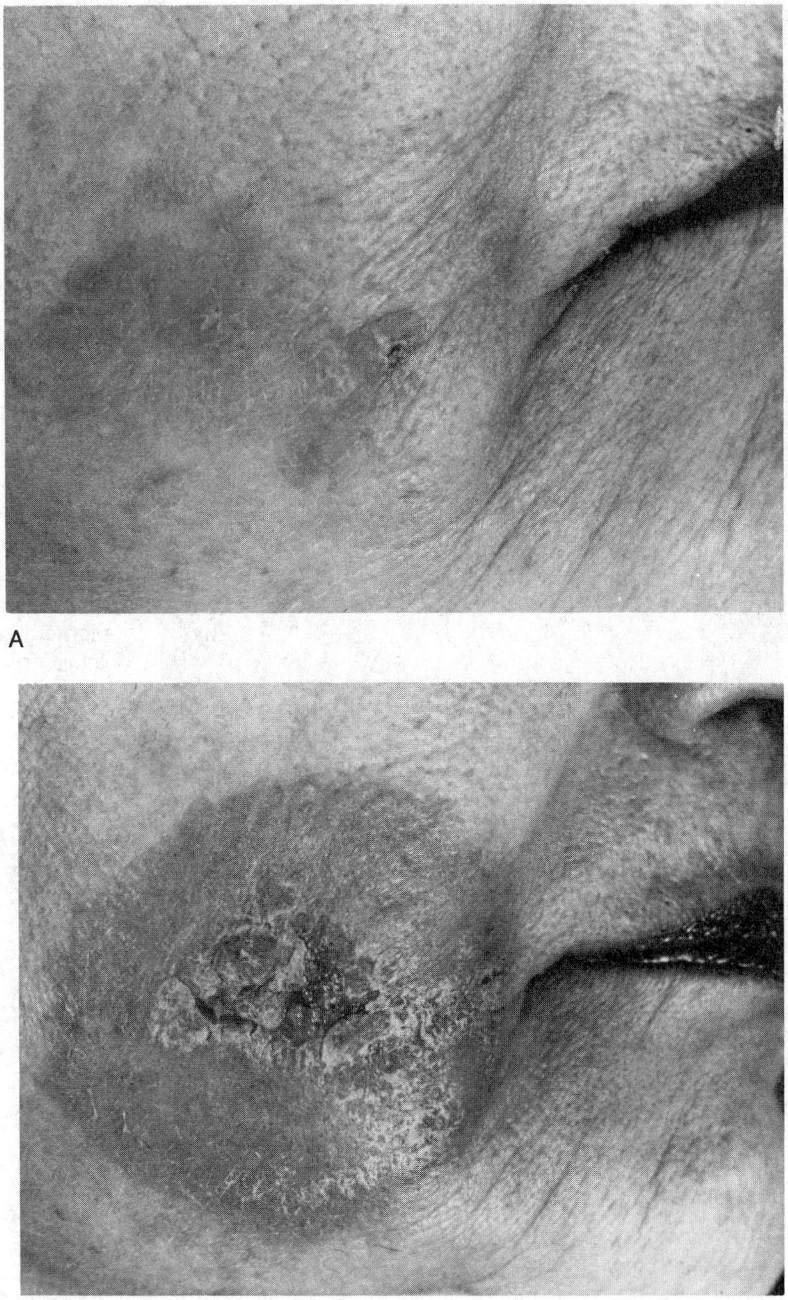

A

B

FIG. 43-24. **A.** Squamous cell carcinoma in situ of right cheek. **B.** Erythema, erosion, and exudate following 10 treatments of 400 R each, fractionated over 3 weeks, 50 kV, D1/2 of 10 mm and half value layer of 0.9 mm aluminum.

electrodesiccation. Indeed, the scarring resulting from radiation therapy in these areas is often of poor quality. Radiation therapy is often the best modality for the treatment of malignant cutaneous neoplasms on the nose (especially the tip), ear, lip, and eyelid, including the medial and lateral canthi (Figs. 43-25 to 43-27). Radiation usually does not produce the contour changes, hypertrophic scars, keloids, defects (with resultant need for flaps and grafts), contractures, ectropion, or epiphora that may occur following treatment with other modalities. Again, lesions along the embryonal fusion planes—the nasolabial fold, retroauricular sulcus, and periorbital areas—infiltrate deeply but can be cured by radiation therapy with relatively good results.

A biopsy should always be performed before radiation therapy is initiated to confirm the diagnosis and document the type of neoplasm. Radiation therapy is most appropriate for primary squamous cell carcinomas and basal cell carcinomas, although recurrences (of neoplasms treated by other modalities previously) can also be treated.[183] Usually morphea-form basal cell carcinomas are too ill-defined, both in depth and in peripheral borders, to be treated by radiation therapy. However, cases have been reported to respond well

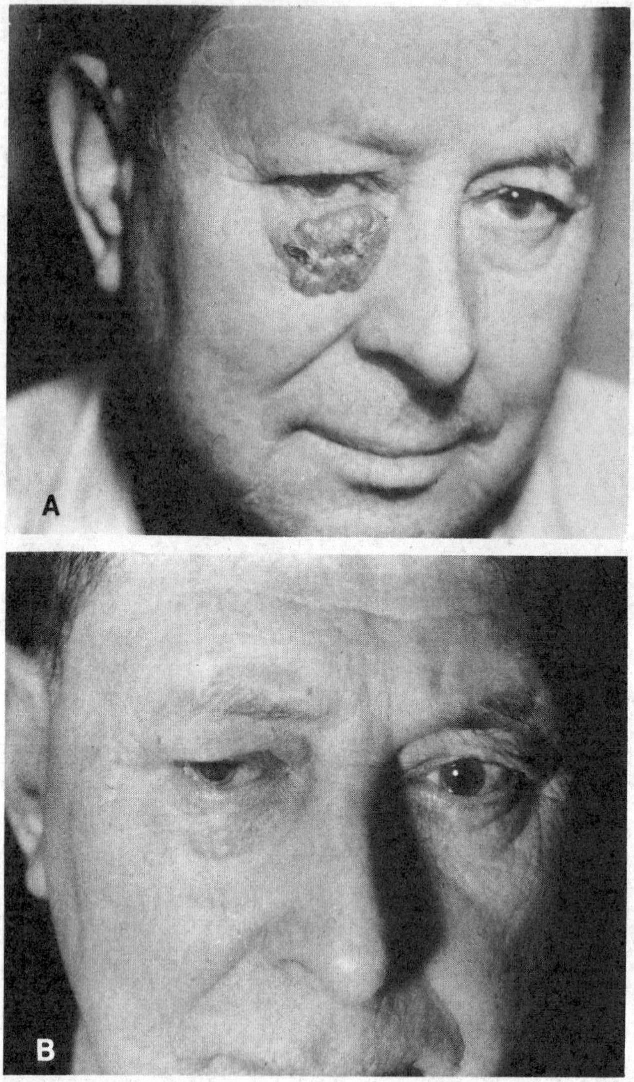

FIG. 43-25. **A.** A nodular basal cell carcinoma involving lower eyelid. **B.** Same patient 15 months after radiation therapy.

without recurrences.[184] It is inappropriate to treat a recurrence with radiation therapy if the lesion was previously treated with this modality because (1) the lesion may be radioresistant and (2) the area will already have received a large dose of radiation, making healing and final cosmetic appearance less than optimal.[28] The depth of the biopsied neoplasm should be measured with a micrometer and reported by a pathologist. This is important information which is required to plan the radiation therapy. Often this is not possible since only a shave biopsy is available for assessment. Studies have shown, however, that most basal cell carcinomas measure 5 mm or less in depth.[185]

Published reports of cure and recurrence rates show that most modalities are successful in the treatment of cutaneous neoplasms. Knox et al followed patients (with 894 tumors) for 5 years.[186] Cure rates were 96.4%, 95.7%, and 97.5% for basal cell carcinomas less than 2 cm diameter and 91.9%, 93.3%, and 99.5% for squamous cell carcinomas of a similar size treated by irradiation, excisional surgery, and curettage and electrodesiccation. Knox et al remarked that the higher cure rate following curettage and electrodesiccation might have reflected case selection; the larger and more infiltrative lesions were treated with surgery or irradiation.[186] Kopf reported the 5-year recurrence rates for 1818 patients treated by various modalities as follows: 19.8% for curettage and electrodesiccation, 9.3% for radiation therapy, and 8.9% for surgical excision.[52] The high recurrence rate for curettage and electrodesiccation was attributed to performance of this treatment by residents in training, whereas the other two types of treatments were carried out under exceedingly close faculty supervision.[52] These observations reinforce the fact that no treatment can be successful unless performed by an experienced, knowledgeable physician.

The cosmetic appearance of an irradiated site can look worse with time, as judged by physicians,[187] although many patients find the cosmetic appearance acceptable (Fig. 43-28). For this reason, radiation therapy is offered only to patients over the age of 45 unless there are extenuating circumstances. There may be hypopigmentation and hyperpigmentation with telangiectases and atrophy of the skin (chronic radiodermatitis).[188] In addition, a pseudorecidive

FIG. 43-26. **A.** Ulcerated basal cell carcinoma of eyelid. **B.** Results after radiation therapy.

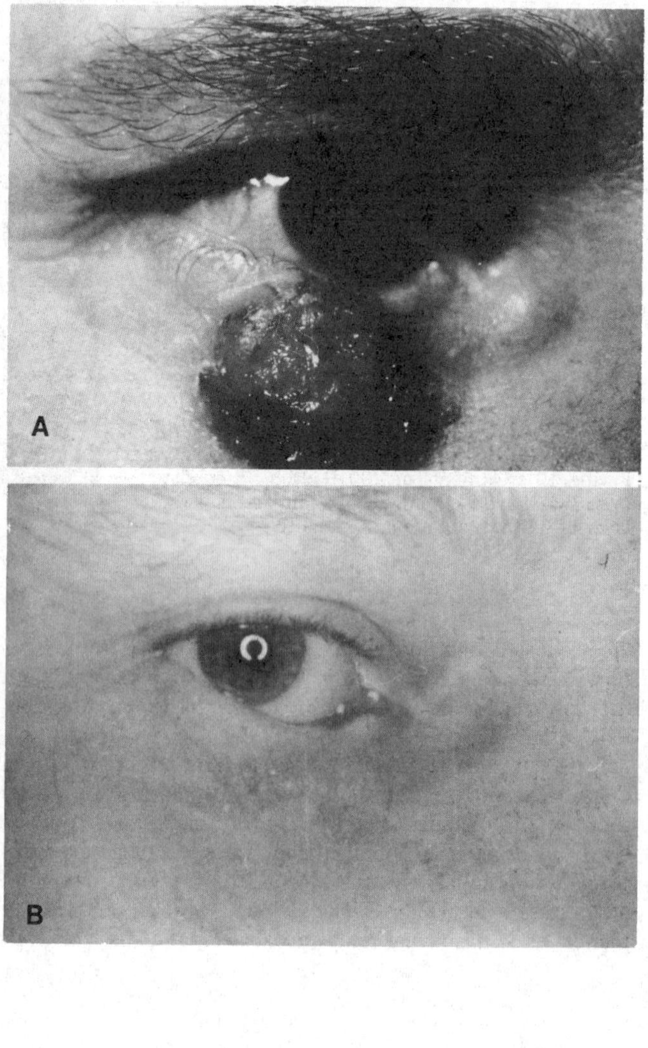

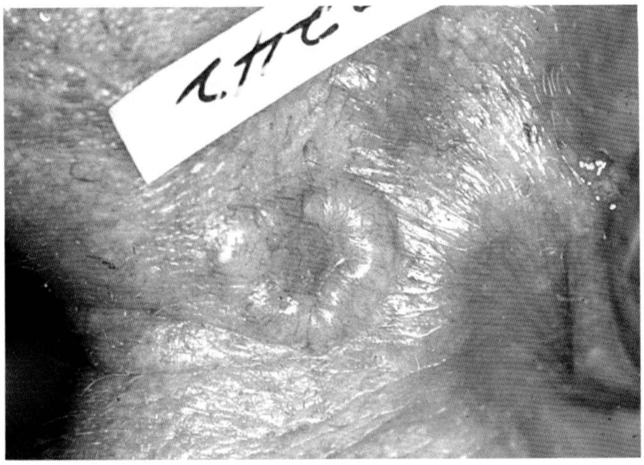

Color FIG. 43-1. Nodulo-ulcerative basal cell carcinoma.

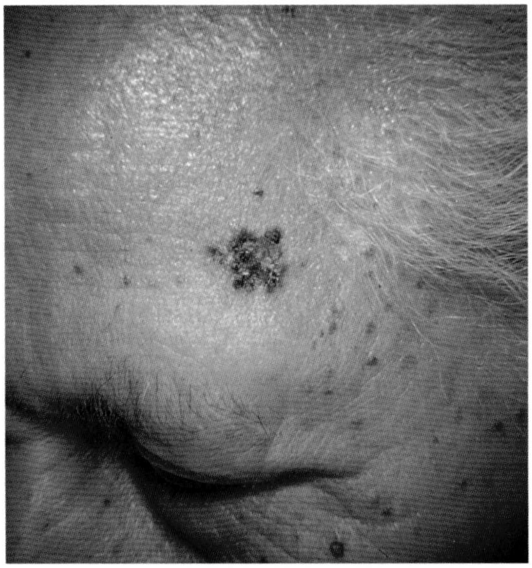

Color FIG. 43-2. Pigmented basal cell carcinoma.

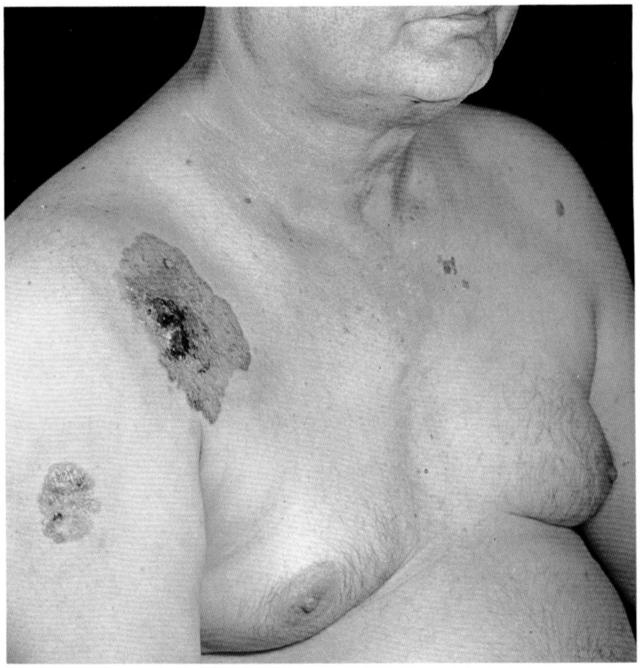

Color FIG. 43-3. Superficial basal cell carcinomas.

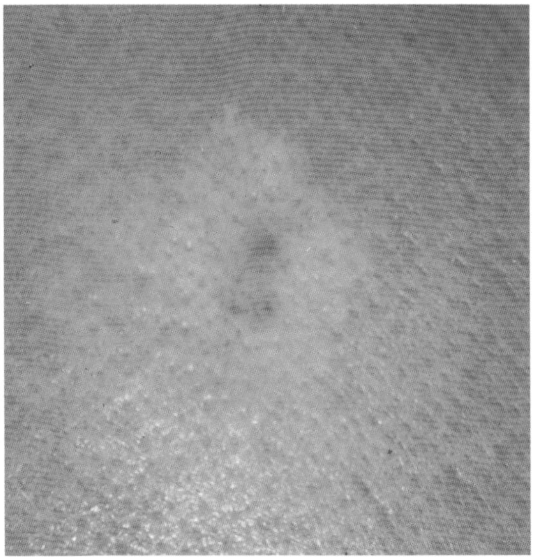

Color FIG. 43-4. Morpheaform basal cell carcinoma. The entire pale area has been infiltrated by carcinoma; the margins are indistinct.

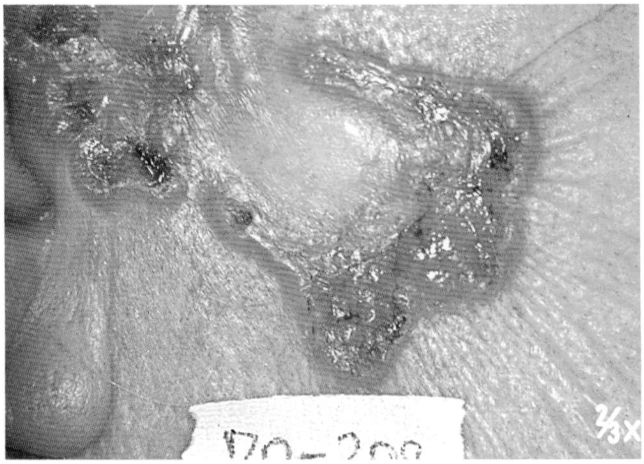

Color FIG. 43-5. Sclerosing basal cell carcinoma that damaged the facial nerve.

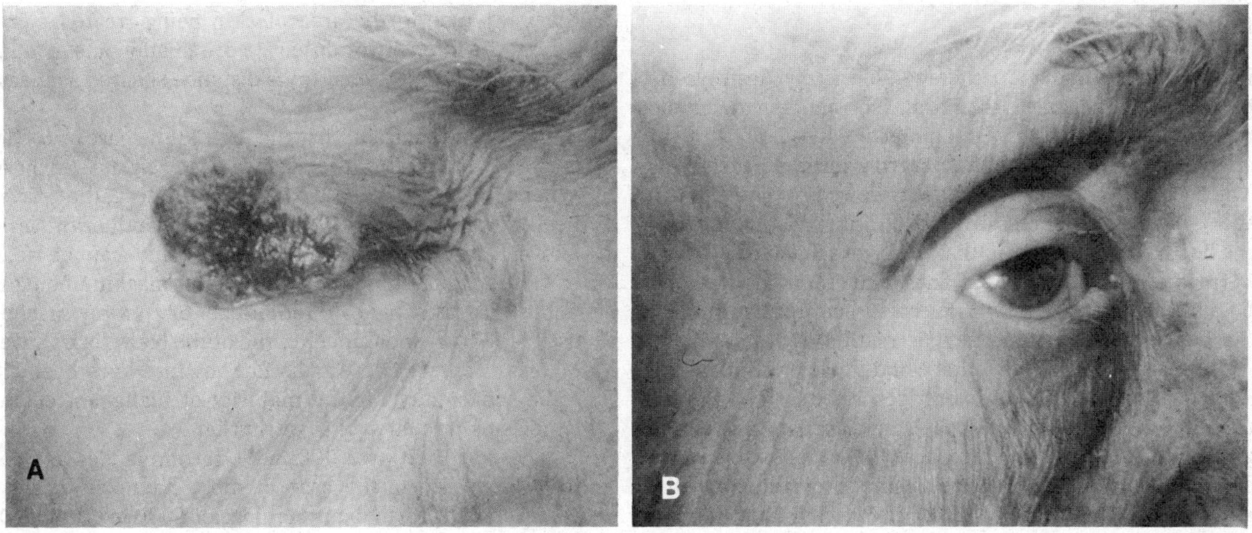

FIG. 43-27. **A.** Squamous cell carcinoma of the eyelid in an 86-year-old woman. **B.** Results 7 months after radiation therapy.

may occur when benign epidermal keratoses develop in and then spontaneously disappear from irradiated areas.[188,189] Of course, these must be differentiated from recurrence of the neoplasm.

It is important to ask each patient about previous radiation therapy to the area, either for a previous neoplasm or for benign conditions such as acne, hair removal, or tinea capitis. Other treatments to the site should also be documented. The neoplasm is then palpated and a portal is cut in a lead shield to expose the neoplasm plus at least a 0.5-cm-diameter border of normal tissue on all sides of the lesion. This should allow adequate treatment of neoplasm not clinically obvious. If the neoplasm is recurrent or occurs in an embryonal fusion plane, a wider margin is necessary. The portal is cut with serrated edges to blur the otherwise well-defined border between treated and normal skin. If there is any doubt about the clinical margins, several biopsy specimens can be taken to map out the neoplasm before treatment. The x-rays are directed onto the skin via a cone of lead glass placed on the lead surrounding the portal, thus minimizing scatter radiation. The skin overlying the eyes, thyroid gland, and gonads is covered with lead shields for each treatment, thus preventing exposure of these sites to radiation; "stray" radiation has been reported to be insignificant.[187] Additional shielding is required to protect areas from the exit dose of radiation: internal nasal shields are used when treating the skin of the nose, a gum shield of lead is used when treating the lip, and an internal brass-, gold-, or silver-plated lead shield over the globe (with local anesthesia for the eye) is used when treating eyelid lesions.

FIG. 43-28. Appearance of right nose after radiation therapy for basal cell carcinoma 11 years before.

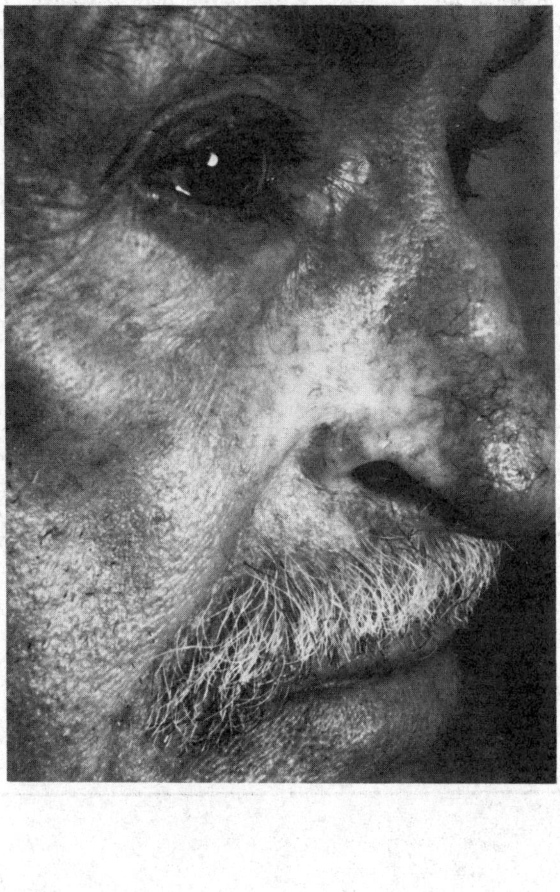

Patients are warned of potential problems of therapy, which include loss of eyelashes when treating an eyelid, mucositis when treating the nose, and erythema and an exudative reaction at any treatment site. The treated area should be bathed gently with plain water washes, and no cosmetics or moisturizers should be applied. Friction from clothing or other sources should be avoided in the irradiated area, and the treated skin should be protected from cold, sun, and wind.

At follow-up visits after radiation therapy the patient is examined for other neoplasms and again urged to stay out of the sun and to use effective sun blocks.

Radiation Technology

Ideally applied radiation therapy selectively destroys neoplastic tissue and spares the normal surrounding area. Selection of the appropriate radiation quality, dose, and fractionation is now possible with modern radiologic technology. The theory of this has been well reviewed.[190] The *quality* of the x-ray beam denotes the penetrating characteristics of the beam. It is selected so that the entire depth of the lesion is treated but with as rapid an attenuation of the beam as possible in the underlying normal tissue, thus minimizing the possibility of chronic radiodermatitis.

The two factors of kilovoltage and filtration influence the x-ray quality, which is commonly described by the term *half-value layer* (HVL). The HVL is defined as that thickness of a given filter material which reduces the intensity of a narrow beam of photons to 50% of the original exposure. Superficial x-ray therapy has an HVL of 0.7 to 2.0 mm aluminum and contact therapy has an HVL of 2 to 4 mm aluminum. More penetrating x-ray qualities are rarely needed for cutaneous lesions.

The selection of the appropriate combination of kilovoltage, filter, and HVL is the most important decision in treatment planning. This has been simplified by the use of the half-value depth (D½), which is defined as the tissue depth (expressed in mm) at which 50% of the surface dose is absorbed. The radiation quality is selected so that the D½ corresponds to the depth of the neoplasm. Most of the radiation will then be absorbed by the neoplasm, with rapid attenuation in the underlying normal tissue. Here, the softer radiation will cause fewer late radiation sequelae such as telangiectases, hypopigmentation and hyperpigmentation, and so forth. Superficial x-ray therapy with a D½ of 7 to 10 mm is appropriate for the majority of cutaneous neoplasms since 50% of all basal cell carcinomas and selected squamous cell carcinomas infiltrate to a depth of 2 mm or less, and 75% to 5 mm or less.[185]

The D½ rule does not apply to skin directly over bone or cartilage since these structures exhibit increased absorption in the soft x-ray range. In these areas, a softer radiation quality should be selected. D½ is influenced by size of field, target-to-skin distance (TSD), and HVL. The TSD is the distance measured in centimeters from the anode (target) of the x-ray tube to the area of skin being treated. For hard x-rays, the intensity or dose rate of radiation at a given point is inversely proportional to its distance squared as measured from the target.

It can be seen, then, that the dose to the base of the lesion is exactly one-half of the surface dose (air dose, exposure). When 5000 R is delivered as the surface dose, the base of the neoplasm receives 2500 rad. Once the depth of the lesion is known, the appropriate radiation quality can be selected from the calibration data of the x-ray machine being used. Table 43-4 presents calibration data of an x-ray machine in use at the Skin and Cancer clinic of the New York University Medical Center. These radiation qualities have been shown to be satisfactory for the majority of malignant cutaneous neoplasms treated at this institution.

A dose of 2,000 to 3,000 rad is recommended as the dose to be delivered to the base of most cutaneous neoplasms, corresponding to an exposure dose of 4000 to 6000 R. Delivery of this amount of radiation in one treatment would result in severe radiation sequelae and possible recurrence. The total dose is therefore fractionated as a course of smaller doses delivered over a period of time. This ensures that the rapidly dividing neoplastic cells are destroyed while allowing the normal cells time to repair the damage incurred. Based on the studies of Strandquist[191] and von Essen,[193] protocols have been developed to deliver cancericidal doses of superficial x-ray therapy fractionated over a period of time resulting in optimal cosmetic appearance (fewer manifestations of chronic radiodermatitis) and the lowest recurrence rates. For example, a basal cell carcinoma of 7 mm depth and 2 cm diameter was once treated at the Skin and Cancer Clinic at New York University Medical Center with a course of 5 × 680 R for a total of 3400 R delivered over 2 weeks. The long-term cosmetic appearance was considered suboptimal, and now a higher (4000 R) dose is given as 10 × 400 R over 3½ weeks. The cosmetic appearance is better, and the recurrence rate (very low) is comparable. At other institutions 5000 R is given over 2 weeks fractionated as 10 × 500 R—*i.e.*, the patient receives therapy on each weekday.[190] All of these protocols are associated with a high cure rate and low recurrence rate.

Most malignant cutaneous neoplasms are treated with superficial or standard x-ray therapy (*e.g.*, 50 kV, HVL=0.96

TABLE 43-4. Calibration Data for Soft X-ray Machine with Beryllium Window

TSD (cm)	*D½ (mm)*	*mA*	*kV*	*Filter (mm Al)*	*HVL (mm Al)*	*Dose per Treatment (R)*	*Time to Deliver Treatment (2-cm-diameter area) (sec)*
15	1.9	25	29	0.3	0.15	100	13
30	2.5	25	29	0.3	0.17	100	50
15	5.8	25	43	0.6	0.44	100	12
30	6.1	25	43	0.6	0.47	100	46
15	10.2	25	50	1.0	0.93	100	12
30	10.5	25	50	1.0	0.96	100	50
15	15	25	50	2.0	1.7	100	24
30	16	25	50	2.0	1.8	100	120

mm aluminum, D½=10.2 mm tissue) because the photons produced exhibit minimal penetration and rapid attenuation in tissue.[194] However, certain selected cutaneous neoplasms, such as smaller lesions on the eyelids and elsewhere, may be treated by contact x-ray (ultrashort distance) with 50 to 60 kV and an HVL of 2 to 4 mm aluminum.[195] This regimen was proposed in 1931 by Chaoul. There is a very short target-to-skin distance (1.5–3.0 cm), and the incident x-rays are absorbed mostly by the lesion because of rapid attenuation of the incident radiation. Excellent results have been achieved with this type of x-ray therapy. Contact therapy has now largely been superseded by soft x-ray units with beryllium windows. These versatile machines are now used most frequently in dermatologic therapy. They have a range of 10 to 50 or 100 kV, and lower inherent filtration with resultant higher dose rates. Modern machines are fitted with fixed kV–filter combinations and interlock mechanisms to avoid errors in delivery of treatment from x-ray machines with potentially extremely high output.

Some cutaneous neoplasms may be treated with electron beam therapy (4–15 MeV) since the electrons produced will treat the superficial cutaneous neoplasm but spare the deep tissues.[196,197] The rapid fall-off in dose at depth results in protection of normal tissues, giving excellent cosmetic and functional results. This type of radiation therapy may be more precise than x-ray therapy but is not widely available, is more expensive, and the machine must undergo a lengthy recalibration for each case. However, it has proved to be of great use in treating certain difficult cutaneous neoplasms, such as a large lesion overlying the skull or cartilage of an elderly patient, where there is a risk of bone or cartilage necrosis if low-energy photons are used.[196] Radium molds and implants have been used in the past to deliver radiation to such lesions, but these devices may be hazardous to both patient and staff. The use of molds and implants has now been discontinued in most centers.

PREVENTION

The majority of malignant cutaneous neoplasms and resultant deaths could be prevented if the main etiological factor, sunlight, were avoided. People of all ages must protect their skin from damaging solar radiation by staying out of the sun, wearing loose cotton clothing, and applying sunscreens with a sun protection factor of 15 or more to all exposed areas. The sunscreen should be renewed every 2 hours or more often if it is washed off by excessive sweating or swimming. Sunscreens protect the skin by absorbing and scattering incident radiation. The most widely used chemical sunscreens contain para-aminobenzoic acid (PABA), PABA esters, benzophenones, cinnamates, salicylates, and anthranilates. Most sunscreens (*e.g.*, PABA and PABA esters) absorb and filter out the sunburn-producing UVB radiation (290–320 nm). Only benzophenones and, less so, anthranilates absorb in the UVA range (320–400 nm).[198] The principles of photoprotection and available products are reviewed elsewhere.[199]

The sun protection factor, or SPF, in sunscreens is defined as the ratio of the UVL dose required to produce the minimal erythema reaction through the sunscreen to the UVL dose required to produce the same minimal erythema reaction without the sunscreen. The SPF number therefore indicates the factor by which the sunscreen decreases the amount of UVL reaching the skin. An individual using a sunscreen with an SPF of 15 can stay in the sun 15 times longer than without the sunscreen before achieving the same degree of erythema.

TABLE 43-5. Skin Type Assessment

Skin Type	*Sunburn and Tanning History*
I	Always burns, never tans
II	Always burns, minimal tan
III	Burns often, tans gradually (light brown)
IV	Burns minimally, tans well (moderate brown)
V	Burns rarely, tans profusely (dark brown)
VI	Never burns, deeply pigmented (black)

Skin type is an important factor in predisposition to solar damage and the development of cutaneous malignancies. Persons with a light complexion, blond hair, and blue eyes are much more prone to problems than darker-skinned individuals since the former have little cutaneous melanin to protect against the harmful ultraviolet radiation. Skin type can be assessed from sunburn and tanning history (Table 43-5).

It has been estimated that regular use of a sunscreen with an SPF of 15 during the first 18 years of life would reduce the lifetime incidence of basal cell carcinomas and squamous cell carcinomas by 78%.[200] This would, of course, also decrease the risk of sunburn, photo-aging, and malignant melanoma. It is therefore essential that all the public, including young children, be educated and made aware of the risks of overexposure to sunlight. Mass educational programs in the workplace, schools, colleges, clubs, parent-teacher associations, and the like are needed to disseminate this information to children and adolescents and their caretakers. Light-skinned children should be encouraged to use sunscreen lotion and to reapply it frequently.

Blistering sunburns in childhood lead to a greatly increased incidence of malignant melanoma in later life.[201] Such burns are common in white children, adolescents, and college students who live in the temperate northern states of the United States and vacation in the south or in snow states. The sudden intense exposure of their skin to strong sun does not allow time for the development of adaptive UVB pigmentation (tanning) or of thickened stratum corneum to decrease UVB transmission.[202] Sitting on a beach under an umbrella does not protect the skin from rays reflected from the sand. Because ultraviolet rays penetrate through cloud and through three feet of water, and are reflected off concrete, snow, and bright sand, protection from hazy diffuse or reflected UVL as well as from obvious strong direct sunlight is needed.

Monthly at-home examinations with full-length and hand-held mirrors to inspect all areas of the body are useful for detecting skin changes. Any change in preexisting lesions or the appearance of new lesions should be brought to the attention of a physician as soon as possible. Comprehensive annual cutaneous examinations by a dermatologist to check for cutaneous malignant neoplasms that have been ignored or not noticed are advisable.

TANNING SALONS. A misguided school of thought believes that "you can never be too rich or too tan," equating a tan with health, leisure, and affluence. In truth, of course, a tan denotes potential skin damage and cancer but these individuals not only will roast on the beach, but also will take expensive, poorly supervised "treatments" at a tanning parlor. The lamps used in artificial tanning units emit UVA (320–400 nm), which has been shown in animal studies to cause immunologic, degenerative, and neoplastic alterations of the skin[11,12] and cataracts and retinal damage of the eye. Clients of tanning parlors subject themselves to an increased risk of UVA damage, cumulative with that of everyday exposure to sunlight. Clients who are not given goggles or who remove them (to prevent raccoon eyes) are at risk for cataract formation and retinal damage.

Most tanning sessions are scheduled by time regardless of output of the sun-lamps. This practice is especially dangerous because 15 minutes in the unit on Monday may be inconsequential if the bulbs are near the end of their lifetime and their energy output is low, but once the bulbs have been changed, the same 15 minutes in the same unit on Tuesday may cause a severe blistering burn.

Artificial tanning can increase the risk of adverse cutaneous drug photosensitivity reactions in individuals taking drugs such as antibiotics, antihypertensives, oral hypoglycemic agents, and diuretics. Individuals with photosensitive diseases such as lupus erythematosus and porphyria may experience a severe exacerbation after the tanning session. Artificial light treatments, including the use of home sunlamps, should be avoided unless prescribed for therapeutic reasons (*e.g.*, for the treatment of psoriasis) and closely supervised by a physician.

REFERENCES

1. Silverberg E, Lubera J: Cancer statistics, 1987. CA 37:2, 1987
2. Eastcott DF: Epidemiology of skin cancer in New Zealand. Natl Cancer Inst Monogr 10:141, 1963
3. Luande J, Henschke CI, Mohammed N: The Tanzanian human albino skin: Natural history. Cancer 55:1823, 1985
4. Okoro AN: Albinism in Nigeria. Br J Dermatol 92:485, 1975
5. Urbach F: Geographic distribution of skin cancer. J Surg Oncol 3:219, 1971
6. Foley P, Lanzer D, Marks R: Are solar keratoses more common on the driver's side? Br Med J 295:18, 1986
7. Hall AF: Relationship of sunlight, complexion and heredity to skin carcinogenesis. Arch Dermatol Syphilol 61:589, 1950
8. Marks R, Selwood TS: Solar keratoses: The association with erythemal ultraviolet radiation in Australia. Cancer 56:2332, 1985
9. Kripke ML: Antigenicity of murine skin tumors induced by ultraviolet light. J Natl Cancer Inst 53:133, 1974
10. Kripke ML, Fisher MS: Immunologic parameters of ultraviolet carcinogenesis. J Natl Cancer Inst 57:211, 1976
11. Kripke ML: Photoimmunology: The first decade. Curr Probl Dermatol 15:164, 1986
12. Kripke ML: Immunology and photocarcinogenesis. J Am Acad Dermatol 14:149, 1986
13. Potter M: Percivall Pott's contribution to cancer research. Natl Cancer Inst Monogr 10:1, 1963
14. Hueper WC: Chemically induced skin cancers in man. Natl Cancer Inst Monogr 10:377, 1963
15. Yuspa SH: Chemical carcinogenesis related to the skin. Prog Dermatol 15:1, 16:1, 1981
16. Lee LA, Fritz KA, Golitz L et al: Second cutaneous malignancies in patients with mycosis fungoides treated with topical nitrogen mustard. J Am Acad Dermatol 7:590, 1982
17. Stern RS, Thibodeau LA, Leinerman RA et al: Risk of cutaneous carcinoma in patients treated with oral methoxsalen photochemotherapy for psoriasis. N Engl J Med 300:809, 1979
18. Yeh S: Relative incidence of skin cancer in Chinese in Taiwan: With special reference to arsenical cancer. Natl Cancer Inst Monogr 10:81, 1963
19. Arhelger SW, Kremen AJ: Arsenical epitheliomas of medicinal origin. Surgery 30:977, 1951
20. Graham JH, Mazzanti GR, Helwig EB: Chemistry of Bowen's disease: Relationship to arsenic. J Invest Dermatol 37:317, 1961
21. Marks F, Furstenberger G: Experimental evidence that skin carcinogenesis is a multistep phenomenon. Br J Dermatol 115 (suppl 31):1, 1986
22. Rous P, Kidd JG, Smith WE: Experiments on the cause of rabbit carcinomas derived from virus-induced papillomas. J Exp Med 96:159, 1953
23. Lutzner MA: The human papillomaviruses. Arch Dermatol 119:631, 1983
24. Ikenberg H, Gissmann L, Gross G et al: Human papillomavirus type 16–related DNA in genital Bowen's disease and in bowenoid papulosis. Int J Cancer 32:563, 1983
25. Obalek S, Jablonska S, Orth G: HPV-associated intraepithelial neoplasia of external genitalia. Clin Dermatol 3:104, 1985
26. Ostrow RS, Bender M, Niimura M et al: Human papillomavirus DNA in cutaneous primary and metastasized squamous cell carcinomas from patients with epidermodysplasia verruciformis. Proc Natl Acad Sci USA 79:1634, 1982
27. Pack GT, Davis J: Radiation cancer of the skin. Radiology 84:436, 1965
28. Sulzberger M, Baer RL, Borota A: Do roentgen-ray treatments as given by skin specialists produce cancers or other sequelae? Arch Dermatol Syph 65:639, 1952
29. Totten RS, Antypas PG, Dupertuis SM et al: Pre-existing roentgen-ray dermatitis in patients with skin cancer. Cancer 10:1024, 1957
30. Glass RL, Spratt JS Jr, Perez-Mesa C: Epidermoid carcinomas of lower extremities. Arch Surg 89:955, 1964
31. Bowers RF, Young JM: Carcinoma arising in scars, osteomyelitis and fistulae. Arch Surg 80:564, 1960
32. Treves N, Pack GT: The development of cancer in burn scars. Surg Gynecol Obstet 51:749, 1930
33. McAnally AK, Dockerty MB: Carcinoma developing in chronic draining cutaneous sinuses and fistulas. Surg Gynecol Obstet 88:87, 1949
34. Cruickshank AH, McConnell EM, Miller DG: Malignancy in scars, chronic ulcers and sinuses. J Clin Pathol 16:573, 1963
35. Giblin T, Pickrell K, Pitts W et al: Malignant degeneration in burn scars: Marjolin's ulcer. Ann Surg 162:291, 1965
36. Sedlin ED, Fleming JL: Epidermoid carcinoma arising in chronic osteomyelitic foci. J Bone Joint Surg [Am] 45:827, 1963
37. Hejna WF: Squamous cell carcinoma developing in the chronic draining sinuses of osteomyelitis. Cancer 18:128, 1965
38. Mustoe T, Upton J, Marcellino V et al: Carcinoma in chronic pressure sores: A fulminant disease process. Plast Reconstr Surg 77:116, 1986
39. Rattner H, Bluefarb SM, Johnson HJ: Squamous cell epithelioma superimposed on a patch of chronic discoid lupus erythematosus. Arch Dermatol 73:601, 1956
40. Mulay DM: Skin cancer in India. Natl Cancer Inst Monogr 10:215, 1963
41. Walder BK, Robertson MR, Jeremy D: Skin cancer and immunosuppression. Lancet 2:1282, 1971
42. Hoxtell EO, Mandel JS, Murray SS et al: Incidence of skin carcinoma after renal transplantation. Arch Dermatol 113:436, 1977
43. Koranda FC, Dehmel EM, Kahn G et al: Cutaneous complications in immunosuppressed renal homograft recipients. JAMA 229:419, 1974
44. Penn I, Halgrimson CG, Starzl TE: *De novo* malignant tumors in organ transplant recipients. Transplant Proc 3:773, 1971
45. Westburg SP, Stone OJ: Multiple cutaneous squamous cell carcinomas during immunosuppressive therapy. Arch Dermatol 107:893, 1973
46. Berg JW: The incidence of multiple primary cancers: 1. Development of further cancers in patients with lymphoma, leukemias and myeloma. J Natl Cancer Inst 38:741, 1967
47. Turner JE, Callen JP: Aggressive behavior of squamous cell carcinoma in a patient with preceding lymphocytic lymphoma. J Am Acad Dermatol 4:446, 1981
48. Weimar VM, Ceilley RI, Goeken JA: Aggressive behavior of basal and squamous cell cancers in patients with chronic lymphocytic lymphoma or chronic lymphocytic leukemia. J Dermatol Surg Oncol 5:609, 1979
49. Penn I: Immunosuppression and skin cancer. Clin Plast Surg 7:361, 1980
50. Slazinski L, Stall JR, Matthews CR: Basal cell carcinoma in a man with acquired immunodeficiency syndrome. J Am Acad Dermatol 11:140, 1984
51. Sitz KV, Keppen M, Johnson DF: Metastatic basal cell carcinoma in acquired immunodeficiency syndrome–related complex. JAMA 257:340, 1987
52. Kopf AW: Computer analysis of 3531 basal cell carcinomas of the skin. J Dermatol 6:267, 1979
53. Milstone EB, Helwig EB: Basal cell carcinoma in children. Arch Dermatol 108:523, 1973
54. Rahbari H, Mehregan AH: Basal cell epitheliomas in usual and unusual sites. J Cutan Pathol 6:425, 1979
55. Robinson JK: Risk of developing another basal cell carcinoma: A 5-year prospective study. Cancer 60:118, 1987
56. Lever WF, Schaumberg-Lever G: Tumors of the epidermal appendages. In: Histopathology of the Skin, 6th ed, p 564. Philadelphia, JB Lippincott, 1983

57. Weedon D, Shand E: Amyloid in basal cell carcinomas. Br J Dermatol 101:141, 1979
58. Hashimoto K, Brownstein MH: Localized amyloidosis in basal cell epithelioma. Acta Derm Venereol (Stockh) 53:331, 1973
59. Farmer ER, Helwig EB: Metastatic basal cell carcinoma: A clinicopathologic study of 17 cases. Cancer 46:748, 1980
60. Ackerman AB, Niven J, Grant-Kels JM: Metastatic carcinoma from the breast vs. morphea-like basal cell carcinoma. In: Differential Diagnosis in Dermatopathology, p 134. Philadelphia, Lea & Febiger, 1982
61. Brownstein MH, Shapiro L: Desmoplastic trichoepithelioma. Cancer 40:2979, 1977
62. Siegle RJ, MacMillan J, Pollack S: Infiltrative basal cell carcinoma: A nonsclerosing subtype. J Dermatol Surg Oncol 12:830, 1986
63. Pinkus H: Premalignant fibroepithelial tumors of the skin. Arch Dermatol Syph 67:598, 1953
64. Caro MR, Howell JB: Morphea-like epithelioma. Arch Dermatol Syph 63:471, 1952
65. Paver K, Poyzer K, Burry N: The incidence of basal cell carcinomas and their metastases in Australia and New Zealand. Aust J Dermatol 14:53, 1973
66. Soffer D, Kaplan H, Weshler Z: Meningeal carcinomatosis due to basal cell carcinoma. Hum Pathol 16:530, 1985
67. Cannon JR, Schneidman DW: Recent developments in adnexal pathology. In Moschella SL (ed): Dermatology Update, p 217. New York, Elsevier, 1982
68. Shrum JR, Cooper PH, Greer KE et al: Squamous cell carcinoma in disseminated superficial actinic porokeratosis. J Am Acad Dermatol 6:58, 1982
69. Lutzner MA: Epidermodysplasia verruciformis: An autosomal recessive disease characterized by viral warts and skin cancer. A model for viral oncogenesis. Bull Cancer (Paris) 65:169, 1978
70. Bowen JT: Precancerous dermatosis. J Cutan Dis 30:241, 1912
71. Callen JP, Headington J: Bowen's and non-Bowen's squamous intraepidermal neoplasia of the skin: Relationship to internal malignancy. Arch Dermatol 116:422, 1980
72. Graham JH, Helwig EB: Bowen's disease and its relationship to systemic cancer. Arch Dermatol 80:133, 1959
73. Peterka ES, Lynch FW, Goltz RW: An association between Bowen's disease and internal cancer. Arch Dermatol 84:623, 1961
74. Arbesman H, Ransohoff DF: Is Bowen's disease a predictor for the development of internal malignancy? A methodological critique of the literature. JAMA 257:516, 1987
75. Friedman HI, Cooper PH, Wanebo HJ: Prognostic and therapeutic use of microstaging of cutaneous squamous cell carcinoma of the trunk and extremities. Cancer 56:109, 1985
76. Penneys NS, Nadji M, Ziegels-Weissman J et al: Prekeratin in spindle cell tumors of the skin. Arch Dermatol 119:476, 1983
77. Kahn H, Baumal R, From L: Role of immunohistochemistry in the diagnosis of undifferentiated tumors involving the skin. J Am Acad Dermatol 14:1063, 1986
78. Immerman SC, Scanlon EF, Christ M et al: Recurrent squamous cell carcinoma of the skin. Cancer 51:1537, 1983
79. Fukamizu H, Inoue K, Matsumoto K et al: Metastatic squamous-cell carcinomas derived from solar keratosis. J Dermatol Surg Oncol 11:518, 1985
80. Moller R, Reymann F, Hou-Jensen K: Metastases in dermatological patients with squamous cell carcinoma. Arch Dermatol 115:703, 1979
81. Epstein E, Epstein NE, Bragg K et al: Metastases from squamous cell carcinomas of the skin. Arch Dermatol 97:245, 1968
82. Epstein E: Malignant sun-induced squamous cell carcinoma of the skin. J Dermatol Surg Oncol 9:505, 1983
83. Ackerman LV: Verrucous carcinoma of the oral cavity. Surgery 23:670, 1948
84. Tindall JP: Skin changes and lesions in our senior citizens: Incidences. Cutis 18:359, 1976
85. Pindborg JJ: Pathology of oral leukoplakia. Am J Dermatopathol 2:277, 1980
86. Waldron CA, Shafer WG: Leukoplakia revisited: A clinicopathologic study of 3256 leukoplakias. Cancer 36:1386, 1975
87. Bouquot JE, Gorlin RJ: Leukoplakia, lichen planus and other oral keratoses in 23,616 white Americans over the age of 35 years. Oral Surg Oral Med Oral Pathol 61:373, 1986
88. Boddie AW Jr, Fischer EP, Byers RM: Squamous carcinoma of the lower lip in patients under 40 years of age. South Med J 70:711, 1977
89. Shafer WG, Waldron CA: Erythroplakia of the oral cavity. Cancer 36:1021, 1975
90. Mashberg A: Reevaluation of toluidine blue application as a diagnostic adjunct in the detection of asymptomatic oral squamous carcinoma: A continuing prospective study of oral cancer: III. Cancer 46:758, 1980
91. Ackerman AB, Niven J, Grant-Kels JM: Keratoacanthoma vs. squamous cell carcinoma. In: Differential Diagnosis in Dermatopathology, p 122. Philadelphia, Lea & Febiger, 1982
92. Rook A, Whimster I: Keratoacanthoma—a thirty year retrospect. Br J Dermatol 100:41, 1979
93. Ghadially FN, Barton BW, Kerridge DF: Etiology of keratoacanthoma. Cancer 16:603, 1963
94. Ghadially FN: The role of hair follicle in origin and evolution of some cutaneous neoplasms in man and experimental animals. Cancer 14:801, 1986
95. Whiteley HJ: Effect of hair growth cycle on experimental skin carcinogenesis in rabbit. Br J Cancer 11:196, 1957
96. Ghadially FN: Keratoacanthoma. In Fitzpatrick TB, Eisen AZ, Wolff K et al (eds): Dermatology in General Medicine, 3rd ed, p 766. New York, McGraw-Hill, 1987
97. Baes H, Suurmond D: Apocrine sweat gland carcinoma: Report of a case. Br J Dermatol 83:483, 1970
98. Warkel RL, Helwig EB: Apocrine gland adenoma and adenocarcinoma of the axilla. Arch Dermatol 114:198, 1978
99. Neldner KH: Ceruminoma. Arch Dermatol 98:344, 1968
100. Elliott GB, Ramsey DW: Sweat gland carcinoma. Ann Surg 144:99, 1956
101. Kipkie GF, Haust MD: Carcinoma of apocrine glands. Arch Dermatol 78:440, 1958
102. Mehregan AH, Hashimoto K, Rahbari H: Eccrine adenocarcinoma: A clinicopathologic study of 35 cases. Arch Dermatol 119:104, 1983
103. Mishima Y, Morioka S: Oncogenic differentiation of the intraepidermal eccrine sweat duct: Eccrine poroma, poroepithelioma and porocarcinoma. Dermatologica 138:238, 1969
104. Lipper S, Peiper SC: Sweat gland carcinoma with syringomatous features: A light microscopic and ultrastructural study. Cancer 44:157, 1979
105. Mendoza S, Helwig EB: Mucinous (adenocystic) carcinoma of the skin. Arch Dermatol 103:68, 1971
106. Liu Y: The histogenesis of clear cell papillary carcinoma of the skin. Am J Pathol 25:93, 1949
107. Lupton GP, McMarlin SL: Microcystic adnexal carcinoma: Report of a case with 30 year old follow-up. Arch Dermatol 122:286, 1986
108. Nickoloff BJ, Fleischmann HE, Carmel J et al: Microcystic adnexal carcinoma: Immunohistologic observations suggesting dual (pilar and eccrine) differentiation. Arch Dermatol 122:290, 1986
109. Lever WF, Schaumberg-Lever G: Tumors of the epidermal appendages. In: Histopathology of the skin, 6th ed, p 575. Philadelphia, JB Lippincott, 1983
110. Urban FH, Winkelmann RK: Sebaceous malignancy. Arch Dermatol 84:63, 1961
111. Boniuk M, Zimmerman LE: Sebaceous carcinoma of the eyelid, eyebrow, caruncle and orbit. Trans Am Acad Ophthalmol Otolaryngol 72:619, 1968
112. King, DT, Hirose FM, Gurevitch AW: Sebaceous carcinoma of the skin with visceral metastases. Arch Dermatol 115:862, 1979
113. Toker C: Trabecular carcinoma of the skin. Arch Dermatol 105:107, 1972
114. Tang C-K, Toker C: Trabecular carcinoma of the skin: An ultrastructural study. Cancer 42:2311, 1978
115. Meland NB, Jackson IT: Merkel cell tumor: Diagnosis, prognosis and management. Plast Reconstr Surg 77:632, 1986
116. Sidhu GS, Feiner H, Flotte TJ et al: Merkel cell neoplasms: Histology, electron microscopy, biology and histogenesis. Am J Dermatopathol 2:101, 1980
117. Bart RS, Kopf AW. Tumor conference #57: Extramammary Paget's disease. J Dermatol Surg Oncol 11:870, 1985
118. Jones RE Jr, Austin C, Ackerman AB: Extramammary Paget's disease: A critical re-examination. Am J Dermatopathol 1:101, 1979
119. Chanda JJ: Extramammary Paget's disease: Prognosis and relationship to internal malignancy. J Am Acad Dermatol 13:1009, 1985
120. Robbins JH, Kraemer KH, Lutzner MA et al: Xeroderma pigmentosum: An inherited disease with sun sensitivity, multiple cutaneous neoplasms, and abnormal DNA repair. Ann Intern Med 80:221, 1974
121. Cleaver JE: Defective repair replication of DNA in xeroderma pigmentosum. Nature 218:652, 1968
122. Thielmann HW, Edler L, Popanda O et al: Xeroderma pigmentosum patients from the Federal Republic of Germany: Decrease in post-UV colony-forming ability in 30 xeroderma pigmentosum fibroblast strains is quantitatively correlated with a decrease in DNA-incising capacity. J Cancer Res Clin Oncol 109:227, 1985
123. Jung EG: Xeroderma pigmentosum. Int J Dermatol 25:629, 1986
124. Wade MH, Plotnick H: Xeroderma pigmentosum and squamous cell carcinoma of the tongue: Identification of two black patients as members of complementation group C. J Am Acad Dermatol 12:515, 1985
125. Mehregan AH, Pinkus H: Life history of organoid nevi: Special reference to nevus sebaceus of Jadassohn. Arch Dermatol 91:574, 1965
126. Wilson-Jones E, Heyl T: Naevus sebaceus: A report of 140 cases with special regard to the development of secondary malignant tumors. Br J Dermatol 82:99, 1970
127. Domingo J, Helwig EB: Malignant neoplasm associated with nevus sebaceus of Jadassohn. J Am Acad Dermatol 1:545, 1979
128. Torre D: Multiple sebaceous tumors. Arch Dermatol 98:549, 1968
129. Reiffers J, Laugier P, Hunziker N: Sebaceous hyperplasia keratoacanthomas, epitheliomas of the face and cancer of the colon: A new entity? Dermatologica 153:23, 1976
130. Finan MC, Connolly SM: Sebaceous gland tumors and systemic disease: A clinicopathologic analysis. Medicine 63:232, 1984
131. Leonard DD, Deaton WR Jr: Multiple sebaceous gland tumors and visceral carcinomas. Arch Dermatol 110:917, 1974
132. Orth G: Epidermodysplasia verruciformis: A model for understanding the oncogenicity of human papillomaviruses. In: Papillomaviruses. CIBA Found Symp 120:157, 1986
133. Anderson DE, Taylor WB, Falls HF et al: The nevoid basal cell carcinoma syndrome. Am J Hum Genet 19:12, 1967
134. Knudson AG Jr: Mutation and cancer: Statistical study of retinoblastoma. Proc Natl Acad Sci USA 68:820, 1971
135. Howell JB: Nevoid basal cell carcinoma syndrome: Profile of genetic and environmental factors in oncogenesis. J Am Acad Dermatol 11:98, 1984
136. Southwick GJ, Schwartz RA: The basal cell nevus syndrome: Disasters occurring among a series of 36 patients. Cancer 44:2294, 1979
137. Howell JB, Mehregan JB: Pursuit of the pits in the nevoid basal cell carcinoma syndrome. Arch Dermatol 102:586, 1970
138. Howell JB, Freeman RG: Structure and significance of the pits with their tumors in the nevoid basal cell carcinoma syndrome. J Am Acad Dermatol 2:224, 1980
139. Gorlin RJ: Nevoid basal-cell carcinoma syndrome. Medicine 66:98, 1987

140. Goldberg LH, Altman A: Benign skin changes associated with chronic sunlight exposure. Cutis 34:33, 1984
141. Mohs F, Lathrop T: Modes of spread of cancer. Arch Dermatol 66:427, 1952
142. Zitelli J: Wound healing by secondary intention: A cosmetic appraisal. J Am Acad Dermatol 9:407, 1983
143. Popkin GL: Electrosurgery. In Epstein E, Epstein E Jr (eds): Skin Surgery, 6th ed, p 164. Philadelphia, WB Saunders, 1987
144. McDaniel W: Therapy for basal cell epitheliomas by curettage only: Further study. Arch Dermatol 119:901, 1983
145. Spiller WF, Spiller RF: Treatment of basal cell carcinoma by curettage and electrodesiccation. J Am Acad Dermatol 11:808, 1984
146. Salasche S: Curettage and electrodesiccation in the treatment of midfacial basal cell epithelioma. J Am Acad Dermatol 8:496, 1983
147. Dubin N, Kopf A: Multivariate risk score for recurrence of cutaneous basal cell carcinoma. Arch Dermatol 119:373, 1983
148. Wheeland RG, Bailin PL: Dermatologic applications of the argon and carbon dioxide laser. Curr Concepts Skin Dis 5:5, 1984
149. Wheeland RG, Bailin PL, Ratz JL et al: Carbon dioxide laser vaporization and curettage in the treatment of large or multiple superficial basal cell carcinomas. J Dermatol Surg Oncol 13:119, 1987
150. Stegman S, Tromovitch T, Glugau R: Chapter 12 Grafts. In: Basics of Dermatologic Surgery, p 96. Chicago, Year Book Medical Publishers, 1982
151. Jackson I: Chapter 1, General Considerations. In: Local flaps in Head and Neck Reconstructive Surgery. St Louis, CV Mosby, 1985
152. Harii K: Chapter 3, Free Skin Flap Transfer. In: Microvascular tissue transfer: Fundamental techniques and clinical applications. New York, Igaku-Shoin, 1983
153. Mohs FE: Chemosurgery for skin cancer: Fixed and fresh tissue techniques. Arch Dermatol 11:211, 1976
154. Tromovitch TA, Stegman S: Microscopically controlled excision of skin tumors. Chemosurgery (Mohs) fresh tissue technique. Arch Dermatol 110:231, 1974
155. Robins P: Chemosurgery: A surer method to treat basal cell epithelioma. Consultant 14:137, 1974
156. Davidson TM, Nahum AM, Haghihi P et al: The biology of head and neck cancer. Arch Otolaryngol 110:193, 1984
157. Menn H, Robins P, Kopf A et al: The recurrent basal cell epithelioma. Arch Dermatol 103:628, 1971
158. Mohs FE, Swanson N, Tromovitch T, Stegman S: Reconstruction post-microscopically controlled excision. Aesthet Reconstr Fac Plastic Surg 6:3, 1981
159. Mohs FE, Snow SN, Messing EM et al: Microscopically controlled surgery in the treatment of carcinoma of the penis. J Urol 133:961, 1985
160. Mikhail GR: Bowen's disease and squamous cell carcinoma of the nail bed. Arch Dermatol 110:267, 1970
161. Mohs FE, Sahl W: Chemosurgery for verrucous carcinoma. J Dermatol Surg Oncol 5:302, 1979
162. Mohs FE, Blanchard L: Microscopically controlled surgery for extramammary Paget's disease. Arch Dermatol 115:706, 1979
163. Harvey JT, Anderson RS: The management of Meibomian gland carcinoma. Ophthalmic Surg 13:56, 1982
164. Peters CW, Hanke CW, Pasarell HA et al: Chemosurgical reports: Dermatofibrosarcoma protruberans of the face. J Dermatol Surg Oncol 8:823, 1982
165. Lubritz RR: Cryosurgery of benign and premalignant lesions. In Zacarian SA (ed): Cryosurgical Advances in Dermatology and Tumors of the Head and Neck. Springfield, IL, Charles C Thomas, 1977
166. Lubritz R: Superficial Cryosurgery. In Epstein E, Epstein E Jr (eds): Skin Surgery, 6th ed. Philadelphia, WB Saunders, 1987
167. Zacarian SA: Chapter 7, Cryosurgery for cancer of the skin. In: Cryosurgery for Skin cancer and Cutaneous disorders, p 157. St Louis, CV Mosby, 1985
168. Zacarian SA: Cryosurgery for head and neck tumors. Compr Ther 5:48, 1979
169. Odom R: Fluorouracil. In Epstein E, Epstein E Jr (eds): Skin Surgery, 6th ed, p 396. Philadelphia, WB Saunders, 1987
170. Goette DK: Topical chemotherapy with 5-fluorouracil. J Am Acad Dermatol 4:633, 1981
171. Raat JH, Krown SE, Pinske CM et al: Treatment of Bowen's disease with topical dinitrochlorobenzene and 5-fluorouracil. Cancer 37:1633, 1976
172. Coker DD, Elias EG, Virvathana T et al: Chemotherapy for metastatic basal cell carcinoma. Arch Dermatol 119:44, 1983
173. Woods RL, Stewart JF: Metastatic basal cell carcinoma: Report of a case responding to chemotherapy. Cancer 52:1583, 1983
174. Lippman S, Meyskens F: Treatment of advanced squamous cell carcinoma of the skin with isotretinoin. Ann Intern Med 107:499, 1987
175. Weiss JS, Ellis CN, Headington JT et al: Topical Tretinoin improves photoaged skin: A double-blind vehicle-controlled study. JAMA 259:527–532, 1988
176. Kligman AM, Grove GL, Hirose R et al: Topical tretinoin for photoaged skin. J Am Acad Dermatol 15:836–859, 1986
177. Greenway H, Cornell RG, Tanner AJ et al: Treatment of basal cell carcinoma with intralesional interferon. J Am Acad Dermatol 15:437, 1986
178. Klein E, Holterman OA, Helm F et al: Immunologic approaches to the management of primary and secondary tumors involving the skin and soft tissues: Reviews of a ten year program. Transplant Proc 7:297, 1975
179. Holterman OA, Papermaster BW, Walker MJ et al: Regression of cutaneous neoplasms following delayed-type hypersensitivity challenge reactions to microbial antigens or lymphokines. J Med 6:157, 1975
180. Dougherty TJ, Weishaupt KR, Boyle DG: Photoradiation therapy of human tumors. In Regan JD, Parrish JA (eds): The Science of Photomedicine, p 625. New York, Plenum Press, 1982
181. Dougherty TJ: Photodynamic therapy (PDT) of malignant tumors. CRC Crit Rev Oncol Hematol 2:83, 1984
182. Farina A, Leider M: Treatment of complicated cutaneous malignant neoplasms by modern radiotherapy: Principles, practice and results. J Dermatol Surg Oncol 4:759, 1978
183. Goldschmidt H, Sherwin WK: Office radiotherapy of cutaneous carcinomas: II. Indications in specific anatomic regions. J Dermatol Surg Oncol 9:47, 1983
184. Bart RS, Kopf AW, Gladstein AH: Treatment of morphea-type basal cell carcinomas with radiation therapy. Arch Dermatol 113:783, 1977
185. Atkinson HR: Skin carcinoma depth and dose homogeneity in dermatological x-ray therapy. Aust J Dermatol 6:208, 1962
186. Knox JM, Freeman RG, Duncan WC et al: Treatment of skin cancer. South Med J 60:241, 1967
187. Bart RS, Kopf AW, Petratos MA: X-ray therapy of skin cancer: Evaluation of a "standardized" method for treating basal cell epitheliomas. In: Sixth National Cancer Conference Proceedings, p 559. Philadelphia, JB Lippincott, 1968
188. Baer RL, Kopf AW: Complications of therapy of Basal cell epitheliomas, p 7. In: Year Book of Dermatology 1964–65. Chicago, Year Book Medical Publishers, 1965
189. Traenkle HL: Management of skin cancer: Basal cell epithelioma. NY State J Med 69:863, 1968
190. Goldschmidt H, Sherwin WK: Office radiotherapy of cutaneous carcinomas: I. Radiation techniques, dose schedules and radiation protection. J Dermatol Surg Oncol 9:31, 1983
191. Strandquist M: Studien über die kumulative Wirkung der Röntgenstrahlen bei Fraktionierung. Acta Radiol [Suppl] (Stockh) 55, 1944
193. von Essen CF: A spatial model of time–dose–area relationships in radiation therapy. Radiology 81:881–883, 1963
194. Cipollaro AC, Crossland PM: Chapter 11, Practical X-ray Therapy Techniques. In: X-rays and Radium in the Treatment of Diseases of the Skin, 5th ed., p 161. Philadelphia, Lea & Febiger, 1967
195. Domonkos AN: Treatment of eyelid carcinoma. Arch Dermatol 91:364, 1965
196. Grosch E, Lambert HE: The treatment of difficult cutaneous basal and squamous cell carcinomata with electrons. Br J Radiol 52:472, 1979
197. Viravathana T, Prempree T, Sewchand W et al: Technique and dosimetry in the management of extensive basal-cell carcinomas of the head and neck region by irradiation with electron beams. J Dermatol Surg Oncol 6:290, 1980
198. Pathak MA, Fitzpatrick TB, Greiter FJ et al: Principles of photoprotection in sunburn and suntanning, and topical and systemic photoprotection in health and diseases. J Dermatol Surg Oncol 11:575, 1985
199. Pathak MA: Sunscreens. J Dermatol Surg Oncol 13:739, 1987
200. Stern RS, Weinstein MC, Baker SG: Risk reduction for nonmelanoma skin cancer with childhood sunscreen use. Arch Dermatol 122:537, 1986
201. Lew RA, Sober AJ, Cook N et al: Sun exposure habits in patients with cutaneous melanoma: A case control study. J Dermatol Surg Oncol 9:981, 1983
202. Kaidbey KH, Kligman AM: Sunburn protection by long-wave ultraviolet radiation–induced pigmentation. Arch Dermatol 114:46, 1978

CHARLES M. BALCH

ALAN HOUGHTON

LESTER PETERS

CHAPTER 44 *Cutaneous Melanoma*

Cutaneous melanoma is becoming a more common disease. In 1987 an estimated 26,000 individuals developed melanoma, and almost 6,000 died. In the past decade the incidence of melanoma increased faster than that of any other cancer except lung cancer in women. The reasons for the increased incidence are unclear but may relate to a combination of increased recreational exposure to sunlight, an increased amount of ultraviolet B irradiation from sunlight that reaches the earth's surface, and early detection of melanoma. This is a disease that is largely confined to whites, in whom the U.S. age-adjusted incidence rate is about 10 per 100,000, but threefold higher (30 per 100,000) in some geographic areas.[1-3] In 1935, only 1 in 1500 individuals developed melanoma. By 1980 this ratio has dramatically dropped to 1:250, and by 1987 to 1:135. Assuming that present trends continue, the figure will be 1:90 by the year 2000 (Fig. 44-1).[4]

Fortunately, most new cases of melanoma are diagnosed early in the clinical course of the disease, when it can be cured with simple surgical treatment. Over 90% of melanomas can be recognized as malignant by experienced observers; therefore, it behooves each physician to know the clinical characteristics of melanoma so that biopsies can be performed on suspicious moles or skin lesions as early as possible. Histologic verification and microstaging are essential before embarking on treatment. The options for therapy range from very conservative surgical treatment for early lesions to more radical approaches for biologically aggressive melanomas. Judgment, experience, and knowledge of the prognostic factors are essential for choosing the most appropriate treatment for individual patients.

CLINICAL CHARACTERISTICS

HIGH-RISK POPULATIONS

The typical melanoma patient has a fair complexion and a tendency to sunburn rather than tan, even after a relatively brief exposure to sunlight.[5,6] The importance of these features was delineated in a case–control study in which 287 women with melanoma were compared with 574 age-matched controls.[5] Red hair was associated with a tripling of relative risk, blond hair with a 60% increase in risk, and fair skin with a doubling of risk. There was a greater than threefold increase in risk for patients with more than 20 nevi.

A patient with a melanoma has a higher risk of developing a second primary melanoma than an individual in the general population has of developing a melanoma.[7] This risk varies from 3% to 5% in different series,[8-10] a 900 times higher risk than that of the general population.[11] A patient with multiple dysplastic nevi or a familial form of melanoma is at even greater risk of developing multiple primary melanomas than are other patients.[8,12,13]

Familial melanomas are uncommon but have been well documented, and individuals in such families constitute an identifiable high-risk group.[9,13-18] Between 4% and 10% of patients described a history of melanoma among their first-

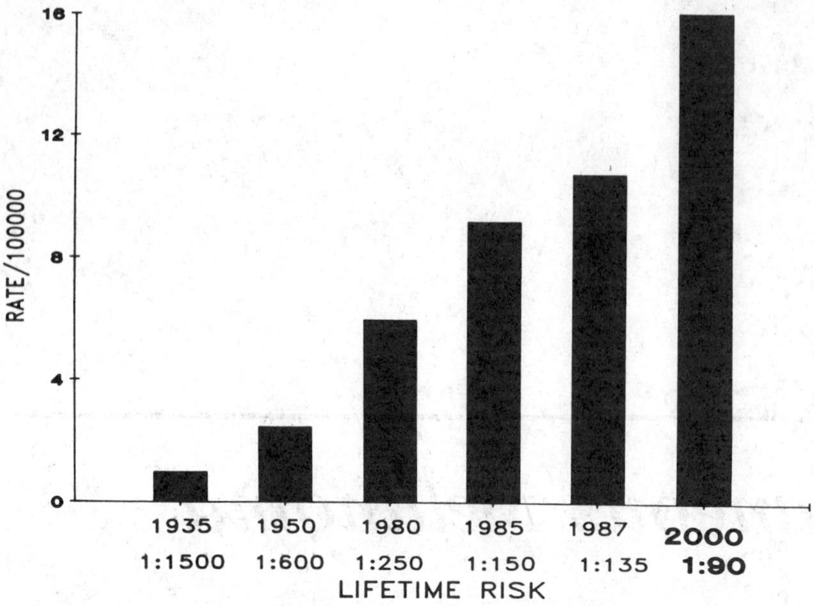

FIG. 44-1. Past, current, and projected lifetime risk of an individual in the United States developing malignant melanoma. (Rige DS et al: The rate of malignant melanoma in the US: Are we making an impact? J Am Acad Dermatol [in press])

degree relatives.[14] Clark et al[19] described an autosomal dominant hereditary occurrence of melanoma, originally termed the B-K mole syndrome and now referred to as the dysplastic nevus syndrome, familial type.[20] Patients with this syndrome typically have between 10 and 100 pigmented lesions, located predominantly on the trunk, buttocks, or lower extremities. Genetic factors may play an important role in the predisposition to melanoma, perhaps through genes controlling some aspect of immune response to melanoma antigens.[14,21,22] Melanoma-prone patients appear to have increased frequencies of certain blood, complement, and HLA phenotypes.[14,21,23–26]

SIGNS AND SYMPTOMS

Melanomas can be located anywhere on the body, but they most commonly occur on the lower extremities in women and on the trunk in men. Several journal articles have described and illustrated some of the clinical characteristics of melanoma,[27–30] examples of which are shown in Color Figure 44-1. Typical features of cutaneous melanomas include (1) variation in color, (2) an irregular, raised surface, (3) an irregular perimeter with indentations, and (4) ulceration of the surface epithelium. Although melanomas may have a variety of clinical appearances, the common denominator is their changing nature. Therefore, any pigmented lesion that undergoes a change in size, configuration, or color should be considered a melanoma, and an excisional biopsy should be performed.

GROWTH PATTERNS

A convenient way to categorize melanomas is by their growth patterns.[27,31,32] Different growth patterns represent distinct pathologic entities and have unique clinical features that should be distinguishable by the experienced clinician. The different categories of melanoma are all distinct from benign lesions, and each portends a different prognosis. Obviously, histologic confirmation is essential before any definitive treatment plans are made. The four major growth patterns are superficial spreading melanomas, nodular melanomas, lentigo maligna melanomas, and acral lentiginous melanomas.

SUPERFICIAL SPREADING MELANOMA. Superficial spreading melanoma constitutes the majority of melanomas (about 70% in most series).[27,31–33] The lesions generally arise in a preexisting nevus. A history of slowly evolving change of the precursor lesion over 1 to 5 years is not uncommon, with more rapid growth developing in the months before diagnosis. Superficial spreading melanomas can occur at any age after puberty. A typical superficial spreading melanoma first appears as a deeply pigmented area in a brown junctional nevus. The lesion may take on a "lacy" appearance. Often there are patches of regression recognizable by an amelanotic area. Early in its evolution, a superficial spreading melanoma is generally a flat lesion. It may develop an irregular surface, usually asymmetrically, depending on the vertical growth phase that develops as it enlarges. As the lesion grows, the surface may become glossy. Notching or indentation of the perimeter is characteristic especially as the lesion enlarges.

NODULAR MELANOMA. Nodular melanoma is the second most common growth pattern in most series (15% to 30% of patients).[27,31–33] Nodular melanomas are more aggressive than superficial spreading melanomas and usually develop more rapidly. They can occur at any age but usually appear in middle age, and are most common on the trunk or head and neck. Men are more likely to have nodular melanomas than women, whereas the opposite is true for superficial spreading melanomas. Nodular melanomas are usually 1 cm to 2 cm in diameter, but can be much larger. They commonly begin in uninvolved skin, rather than arising from preexisting nevi.

Nodular melanomas are generally darker than superficial spreading melanomas, more uniform in coloration, and more raised or dome-shaped. The typical nodular melanoma is a blue-black lesion that often resembles a blood blister or hemangioma. It may have other shadings of red, gray, or purple. About 5% of nodular melanomas lack pigment altogether (*i.e.*, are amelanotic) and have a fleshy appearance. Nodular melanomas are often symmetric, but sometimes they appear as irregularly shaped plaques. They lack the radial (horizontal) growth phase typical of the other melanotic growth patterns and therefore have discrete, sharply demarcated borders, often with irregular perimeters. Nodular melanomas that are polypoid, with a stalk or cauliflower appearance, are particularly aggressive lesions.[34]

LENTIGO MALIGNA MELANOMA. Lentigo maligna melanoma does not have the same propensity to metastasize as other melanomas and therefore appears to be a separate entity.[32,35,36] Lentigo maligna melanomas constitute a small percentage of melanomas (usually 4%–10%) and are typically located on the face in older caucasian women.[37] Usually lentigo maligna melanomas have been present for long periods of time (5–15 years). They are generally large (>3 cm), flat lesions that occur in an older age group, being uncommon before the age of 50 years. Almost all are located on the face or neck; a few occur on the back of the hands or the lower legs. They are typically tan-colored lesions with different shades of brown. Irregular mottling or flecking may appear as the lesions enlarge, with areas of dark brown or black in some parts and areas of regression in others. Lentigo maligna melanomas can have extremely convoluted borders with prominent notching and indentation, which generally represent areas of regression. The diagnosis of lentigo maligna melanoma requires the presence of sun-related changes in both the epidermis and dermis.[32,36,37]

ACRAL LENTIGINOUS MELANOMA. Acral lentiginous melanoma characteristically occurs on the palms or soles or beneath the nail beds.[28,38–42] However, not all plantar or volar melanomas are acral lentiginous melanomas: a minority are superficial spreading melanomas or nodular melanomas.[43–46] Acral lentiginous melanomas occur in only 2% to 8% of whites with melanomas[47] but in a substantially higher proportion (35%–60%) of dark-skinned patients, such as blacks, Asians, and Hispanics.[41,48–51]

The majority of acral lentiginous melanomas are located on the sole of the foot.[40] They are generally large, with an average diameter of about 3 cm.[39] Acral lentiginous melanomas generally occur in older people, with the average patient's age in the 60s. The lesions evolve over a short time, from a few months to several years, with an average of 2.5 years. Initially they appear as tan or brown flat stains on the palm or sole, often resembling lentigo maligna melanomas. The haphazard array of color is characteristic. A minority of acral lentiginous melanomas have a flesh-colored appearance and can be misdiagnosed as granulomas. Ulceration is not uncommon, and fungating masses can result from neglected lesions. Like lentigo maligna melanomas, these lesions often have very irregular, convoluted borders. However, acral lentiginous melanomas are much more aggressive than lentigo maligna melanomas and are more likely to metastasize.

Acral lentiginous melanomas also include subungual melanomas, an infrequent presentation of cutaneous melanoma.[43–45,52,53] Subungual melanoma develops in only 2% to 3% of white patients but in a higher proportion of dark-skinned patients. It occurs equally in men and women and is most often diagnosed in older patients (median age, 55–65 years). Over three fourths of subungual melanomas involve the great toe or the thumb. The most common sign of an early subungual melanoma is a brown to black discoloration under the nail bed.

BIOLOGIC AND PATHOLOGIC FEATURES

BIOLOGY OF MELANOCYTES

A number of biologic features of melanocytes are relevant to the biology of melanoma. Melanocytes arise from the neural crest early in fetal development, and by 4 to 6 weeks they have migrated to their final destinations in the skin, uveal tract, meninges, and ectodermal mucosa.[54,55] It is not clear whether the ability of melanocyte precursors to migrate readily through tissues during development is related to traits that determine the capacity of melanoma to metastasize rapidly and widely.[55]

In adults, most melanocytes are found at the epidermal–dermal junction of the skin and in the eye, but melanocytes can be found in the meninges, along the alimentary and respiratory tracts, and even in lymph nodes.[56,57] More than 90% of melanomas arise in the skin, although a small percentage arise in the eye. However, melanoma can arise from the meninges, respiratory tract, gallbladder, and other odd sites,[56] although such instances are rare. Approximately 4% of melanomas have no known primary site, and although the majority of these presumably come from primary lesions in the skin that have completely regressed, some unknown primary melanoma may arise from undiagnosed internal sites.

Melanocytes synthesize the pigment melanin in distinct, specialized organelles called melanosomes. The presence of melanosomes, detected by electron microscopy, or of pigment in an undifferentiated tumor can help in the diagnosis of melanoma. Melanin is synthesized using the enzyme tyrosinase, and some intermediates in the melanin synthetic pathway can be cytotoxic.[58,59] This phenomenon has led to research into new strategies for treatment with compounds that augment the production of toxic metabolites in the melanin pathway.[60]

The regulation of growth and differentiation of melanocytes and melanoma cells is an area of active research that may eventually lead to novel pharmacologic or biologic approaches to therapy. Melanocytes and melanoma cells express a range of receptors for known growth factors and produce ligands for these receptors. Growth factors and receptors that have been found to be expressed in melanocytes include nerve growth factor and its receptor,[61] epidermal growth factor and transforming growth factor-alpha,[62,63] platelet-derived growth factor, transferrin receptor, and insulin receptor.[64] Basic fibroblast growth factor has been found to stimulate the growth of mature normal melanocytes in tissue culture,[65] and melanoma cells produce a melanocyte growth factor that is similar to basic fibroblast growth factor.[66,67] The role, if any, of growth factors such as basic fibroblast growth factor or of growth factor receptors in the pathogenesis of melanoma remains to be determined.

The ability of melanocytes to produce melanin and the identification of well-defined characteristics such as tyrosinase activity, melanosomes, and melanocyte differentiation antigens have provided markers for the differentiation of melanoma cells.[68] Differentiation of melanoma cells and melanocytes can be induced by a number of agents,[68–71] and melanoma is one of the best-defined cell systems outside of the hematopoietic lineages in which to study tumor differentiation.

GENETIC ALTERATIONS IN MELANOMA

As a general rule, metastatic melanoma cells are highly aneuploid, whereas normal melanocytes are diploid. Melanoma cells from both primary and metastatic lesions have been found to contain nonrandom chromosomal alterations involving the short arm of chromosome 1 (1p), both arms of chromosome 6, and chromosome 7.[72–83] The occurrence of these alterations suggests that there are genes in these chromosomal locations that are necessary for malignant transformation of melanocytes. Specific genetic loci that are implicated in growth or malignant transformation of melanocytes have not yet been identified. Genes that code for potential oncogenes are of particular interest because they code proteins that can result in malignant transformation.[84] No oncogene has been clearly implicated in the pathogenesis of melanoma, although activated oncogenes of the *ras* family have been detected in melanoma cells.[85–87] When activated *ras* genes are expressed in normal cultured melanocytes, the melanocytes acquire a number of traits that are characteristic of melanoma cells.[88] Preliminary evidence had implicated rare alleles of *ras* in several types of cancer, including melanoma, but follow-up studies have not confirmed the association in melanoma.[89,90]

Preliminary evidence has also suggested that a trait of melanoma is closely linked to the Rh blood group locus on the short arm of chromosome 1 in certain familial melanoma clusters.[91] The linkage was not statistically significant and needs to be confirmed in more detailed and extensive genetic studies of familial melanoma patients.

In addition to these nonrandom chromosomal abnormalities in melanoma patients, analysis of polymorphic genetic loci has shown the widespread loss of alleles throughout the genome in cultured metastatic melanoma cells.[92] Approximately one fourth of genetic loci examined had lost one allele or the other. Since there is evidence that melanoma can arise from a single cell, this segregation of genetic material appears to start in the primary lesion, but random losses appear to continue during metastasis.[93]

EPIDEMIOLOGY, STAGING, AND PROGNOSIS

EPIDEMIOLOGY

Exposure to ultraviolet (UV) rays emitted by the sun is considered to be the major cause of cutaneous melanoma.[94] A causal association is supported by the demographic pattern of occurrence in humans, by the observation that DNA is sensitive to damage by solar radiation,[95] by sporadic induction of melanomas in animals through the use of dual exposure to chemical carcinogens and UV light,[96,97] and by evidence that the immune system may be depressed by UV rays.[98]

In humans, the patterns of melanoma occurrence that suggest sunlight as a cause include (1) an inverse relation between the incidence of melanoma and the degree of skin pigmentation, (2) higher incidence rates in persons residing closer to the equator,[99,100] (3) increases in the incidence of certain types of melanomas in anatomical sites exposed to sunlight,[101] and (4) migration studies suggesting that risk increases with immigration to an area of more intense sun exposure.[102] Inability to tan, higher frequency of sunburns, and younger age at first sunburn have also been associated with a predisposition to melanoma.[5] Finally, lentigo maligna melanomas occur almost exclusively on sun-exposed parts of the body and in elderly persons, suggesting cumulative sunlight exposure as a contributing etiological factor.

However, several observations are not consistent with UV irradiation being the sole cause of melanoma.[103] First, the incidence of melanoma does not consistently increase across geographic areas with increasing sunlight exposure, although the relationship may be skewed by the variable mix of people of different ethnic backgrounds and skin color. Second, melanoma more commonly affects the white-collar, educated, urban individual than the outdoor or blue-collar worker. Third, most melanomas occur in relatively young persons who have not had years of constant exposure to sunlight. Finally, some melanomas occur in relatively unexposed anatomical sites such as the palms, soles, and trunk areas normally covered by bathing suits. These observations are inconsistent with assigning cumulative sunlight exposure as the only etiological factor, although it is possible that brief, intense exposure may contribute to or initiate carcinogenic events.

For both superficial spreading melanomas and nodular melanomas, the pattern of risk suggests that susceptibility to sunburn determines the risk to the same or greater degree than the actual incidence of sunburn events does. Cumulative sunlight exposure has not been a consistent finding in many epidemiologic studies to date. However, no major environmental factors other than UV irradiation have yet been identified as contributing substantially to the increasing incidence of cutaneous melanoma. The inheritable combination of light skin color and freckling also suggests that genetically determined host susceptibility may play a more important role in the etiology of cutaneous melanoma than was previously appreciated. The above characteristics are consistent with the two-step model of UV-ray carcinogenesis in which the initiation and promotion events result in melanoma in a genetically susceptible subpopulation of individuals.

Both the incidence of and mortality from cutaneous melanoma are rising steadily among white populations throughout the world.[48,94,104] In most studies, the incidence is doubling every 6 to 10 years. It is estimated that by the year 2000, one in 90 caucasians in the United States will develop a melanoma during their lifetime (see Fig. 44-1).[5] In Queensland, Australia, the incidence has increased from 15 per 100,000 persons (the highest incidence in the world) in the 1963 to 1968 period to 28.4 per 100,000 persons in the 1979 to 1980 period[105,106]; In Sweden, it has increased from 2.5 per 100,000 in 1958 to 11.6 per 100,000 in 1980.[107] In contrast to this high incidence in fair-skinned populations, the incidence in Chinese persons is only 0.8 per 100,000.[48,108,109]

CHANGES IN THE NATURAL HISTORY OF MELANOMA

The incidence of melanoma has been increasing rapidly, especially during the past two decades. A detailed analysis involving 1648 Stage I melanoma patients treated over a period of 27 years revealed major changes in the clinical and pathologic features of the disease.[110] There was a steady increase in the proportion of patients initially diagnosed as having localized disease (73% before 1960, compared with 81% by 1980). Melanomas have thus become thinner, less invasive, less ulcerative, and more curable. In fact, the majority of melanomas now seen at many institutions measure less than 1 mm thick,[110,111] and more melanomas exhibit a radial growth phase with a superficial spreading growth pattern. The median thickness of melanomas decreased from about 3.0 mm before 1960 to less than 1.0 mm during the period 1981 to 1982 (Fig. 44-2).[110] There was a significant increase during this period of melanomas located on the trunk in men (from 40% to 56%, p = 0.004) and a corresponding decrease in head and neck melanomas in men (from 36% to 17%, p = 0.001). No significant change in site distribution was observed for any major anatomical area in women. The changes in distribution patterns in men probably resulted both from earlier diagnosis and from changes in the biologic nature of the disease.

STAGING SYSTEMS

MICROSTAGING. Microstaging is now an integral part of the staging and clinical management of melanoma. Two methods have been used. In the Breslow microstaging method, the thickness of the lesion is measured with an ocular micrometer to determine the total vertical height (not just the depth) of the melanoma, from the granular layer to the area of deepest penetration.[112] If the lesion is ulcerated, measurements should be made from the surface of the ulcer to the deepest part of the lesion. The Clark microstaging method categorizes different levels of invasion that reflect increasing depth of penetration into the dermal layers of the subcutaneous fat (*i.e.*, levels II, III, IV, or V).[27]

Although both tumor thickness and level of invasion can predict the risk of metastases, data from several institutions have clearly demonstrated that tumor thickness is a relatively more accurate and reproducible prognostic parameter than level of invasion. Significant regression of the tumor invalidates the prognostic value of these microstaging methods.

ORIGINAL THREE-STAGE SYSTEM. The original and most widely used classification system involves three stages: Stage I for localized melanoma, Stage II for regional metastases, and Stage III for distant metastases.[113,114] The system is simple and easy to recall, but does not incorporate such important disease criteria as tumor thickness that allow for more accurate staging. A major limitation of this system is that 85% or more of melanoma patients diagnosed now have clinically localized disease (Stage I). This disproportionate number of patients in one stage defeats the purpose of a classification system designed to categorize metastatic risk.

NEW STAGING SYSTEM ADOPTED BY AJC. The American Joint Committee on Cancer (AJC) has worked for more than a decade to develop uniform staging systems for all

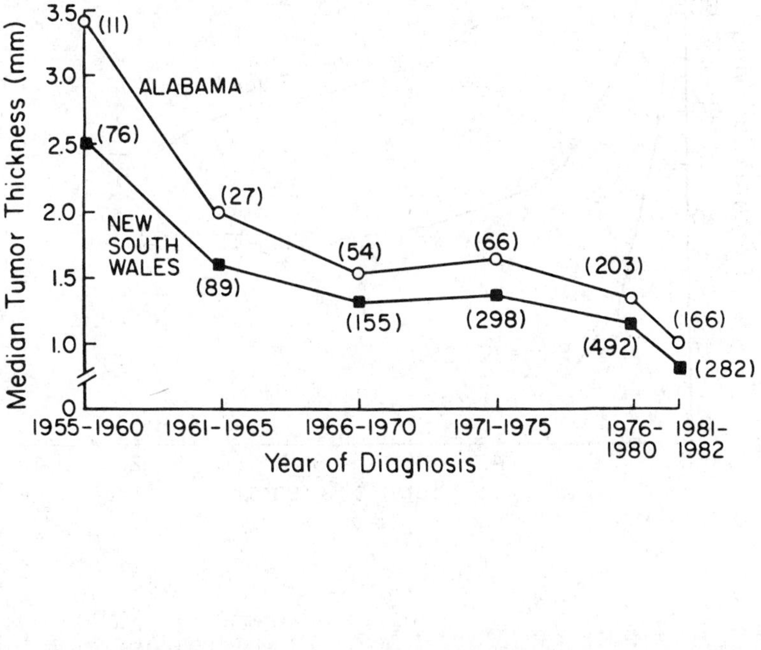

FIG. 44-2. Changes in the median tumor thickness of melanomas treated from 1955 to 1982 (number of patients in parentheses). (Balch CM, Shaw HM, Soong S-J, et al: Changing trends in the clinical and pathological features of melanoma. In Balch CM, Milton GW [eds]: Cutaneous Melanoma: Clinical Management and Treatment Results Worldwide, p 313. Philadelphia, JB Lippincott, 1985)

TABLE 44-1. New Staging System for Melanoma Adopted by the American Joint Committee on Cancer*

Stage	*Criteria*
IA:	Localized melanoma ≤ 0.75 mm or level II† (T1N0M0)
IB:	Localized melanoma 0.76 mm to 1.5 mm or level III† (T2N0M0)
IIA:	Localized melanoma 1.5 mm to 4 mm or level IV† (T3N0M0)
IIB:	Localized melanoma >4 mm or level V† (T4N0M0)
III:	Limited nodal metastases involving only one regional lymph node basin, or less than 5 in-transit metastases but without nodal metastases (any T, N1M0)
IV:	Advanced regional metastases (any T, N2M0) or any patient with distant metastases (any T, any N, M1 or M2)

*Ketcham AS, Balch CM: Classification and staging systems. In Balch CM, Milton GW (eds): Cutaneous Melanoma: Clinical Management and Treatment Results Worldwide, p 55. Philadelphia, JB Lippincott, 1985.

†When the thickness and level of invasion criteria do not coincide within a T classification, thickness should take precedence.

cancer types. In its extensive retrospective studies of melanoma, many factors influencing treatment results were identified, and based on these, a four-stage system was adopted (Table 44-1.)[115,116] Basically, this system divides clinically localized melanomas into two groups according to microstaging criteria, with the result that the metastatic risk categories are more evenly grouped among four stages (Fig. 44-3). Thus the AJC staging system provides a more useful and practical classification for clinicians treating melanoma.

PROGNOSTIC FEATURES OF MELANOMA

Many aspects of melanoma are known to predict the risk of metastatic disease. A prognostic factors analysis of melanoma is therefore essential to identify the dominant variables that can be used for evaluating results of clinical research trials involving adjunctive systemic therapy, and for making certain surgical decisions. Also, when evaluating treatments, it is important to account for those prognostic variables that can accurately categorize patients into different risk groups for metastatic disease. Otherwise, differences (or lack of differences) between treatment regimens may not be due to the treatments themselves, but may merely reflect imbalances of prognostic factors.

This section reviews a prognostic factors analysis involving more than 4,000 patients with cutaneous melanoma treated at the University of Alabama in Birmingham (UAB) and the University of Sydney Melanoma Unit (SMU) over a 25-year period (1955–1980).[117] The median follow-up of all patients was 8 years.

Clinically Localized Melanoma (AJC Stages I and II)

Characteristics of 3505 patients with localized melanoma were submitted to both single and multifactorial statistical analysis to determine which clinical and pathologic features of melanoma would predict the risk of metastases.[117]

ANATOMICAL LOCATION OF PRIMARY LESION. Melanomas were divided evenly among the four major anatomical locations: 46% were on the upper and lower extremities and 52% occurred on the trunk or head and neck. Patients with melanomas on the extremities had a better survival rate than those with melanomas on the trunk or head and neck ($p < 0.00001$), and those with melanomas on the upper extremities had a slightly better survival rate than those with melanomas on the lower extremities ($p = 0.08$). Analysis of anatomical subsites revealed additional differences in prognosis. Among patients with melanomas in the head and neck region, those with melanomas on the scalp had worse prog-

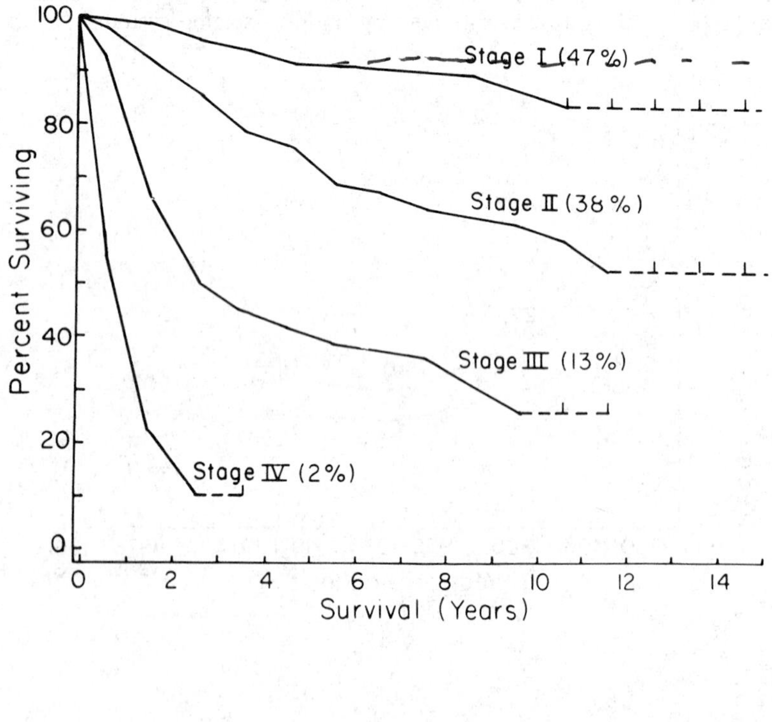

FIG. 44-3. Fifteen-year survival results for more than 4000 melanoma patients treated at the University of Alabama in Birmingham and the Sydney Melanoma Group who are subgrouped according to the new four-stage system proposed by the American Joint Commission on Cancer. The distribution of patients is shown in parentheses. Note that the patients with clinically localized melanoma (Stage I by the original three-stage system) have now been divided into two stages according to tumor thickness and level of invasion (newly designated Stages I and II). (Ketcham AS, Balch CM: Classification and staging systems. In Balch CM, Milton GW [eds]: Cutaneous Melanoma: Clinical Management and Treatment Results Worldwide, p 55. Philadelphia, JB Lippincott, 1985)

noses than those with lesions on the face or neck. These differences remained, even after accounting for sex and tumor thickness.[35,117] There was no sex difference in prognosis for patients with lesions on these head and neck subsites. There was no survival difference between patients with back lesions and those with chest lesions, even when subgrouped by sex. Patients with melanomas on the hands and feet had significantly worse prognoses than those with lesions on the arms or legs.[117-119] Women with extremity melanomas had better prognoses than men ($p < 0.00001$). Part of this sex difference in prognosis could be accounted for by the higher proportion of men with ulcerated melanomas (29% vs. 19%).

SEX. Numerous studies have shown that women with melanoma have a better survival rate than men.[48,117-125] In this analysis, women with melanoma had a statistically significant ($p < 0.00001$) survival advantage over men. However, a primary reason for better survival rates in women was that their melanomas occurred more commonly on the extremities (a more favorable prognostic site) and were less frequently ulcerated.

TUMOR THICKNESS. The total vertical height of a melanoma is the single most important prognostic factor in Stage I and II melanoma.[120,126-128] Total vertical lesion height is a quantitative parameter that can define subsets of patients with different survival rates ($p < 0.00001$). Numerous lesion thickness subsets were analyzed for their prognostic value (*e.g.*, <1 mm, 1 to 4 mm, >4 mm); only one subset was found to be more discriminating than those originally advocated by Breslow.[128] As demonstrated by actuarial survival curves, a more significant survival difference was found when 4 mm was used as a cutoff point, rather than 3 mm.[117,120] However, there are apparently no "natural breakpoints,"[129] but rather statistically defined subgroups that vary from one data set to another, depending on the number of patients, the duration of follow-up, and the distribution of other factors (*e.g.*, ulceration, anatomical site of primary lesion, and sex). The large number of patients in the UAB–SMU series has permitted the derivation of a simple nonlinear mathematical model that describes the relationships between tumor thickness and 10-year mortality as a continuous event (Fig. 44-4).[130]

LEVEL OF INVASION. There is an inverse correlation between increasing level of melanoma invasion and survival. The level of invasion is a significant prognostic factor by single-factor analysis ($p < 0.00001$), and it will differentiate patients at various risks for metastases.

COMPARISON OF LEVEL VERSUS THICKNESS AS PROGNOSTIC INDICATORS. A direct comparison of the level of invasion and thickness microstaging methods was made by subdividing each level of invasion into thickness categories. Within levels III, IV, and V, gradations of thickness influenced survival (Fig. 44-5). Converse relationships were not observed when subsets of melanoma thickness were analyzed by levels of invasion. For example, the 5-year survival rates for patients with level III, IV, or V lesions that measured 1.5 to 4.0 mm were not significantly different. These observations demonstrate that tumor thickness is a more accurate prognostic factor than level of invasion.[48,118,119,120-123,126,127,131-135]

ULCERATION. Ulcerated melanomas appear to be more aggressive lesions biologically, since they invade through the epidermis rather than pushing it upward. Thus, the presence of ulceration in microscopic sections of melanoma was a significant adverse determinant of survival ($p < 0.00001$) in the UAB–SMU study.[117] Patients with ulcerated Stage I and II melanomas had a 10-year survival rate of 50%, whereas those with nonulcerated Stage I and II lesions had a 78% 10-year survival rate ($p < 0.0001$). Men had a higher proportion of ulcerated lesions than women (29% versus 19%). There was a positive correlation between ulceration and thickness ($p < 0.0001$). The median tumor thickness of ulcerated lesions was 3 mm, whereas for nonulcerated lesions it was 1.3 mm. Lesions more than 1.5 mm thick were associated with a 44% incidence of ulceration.

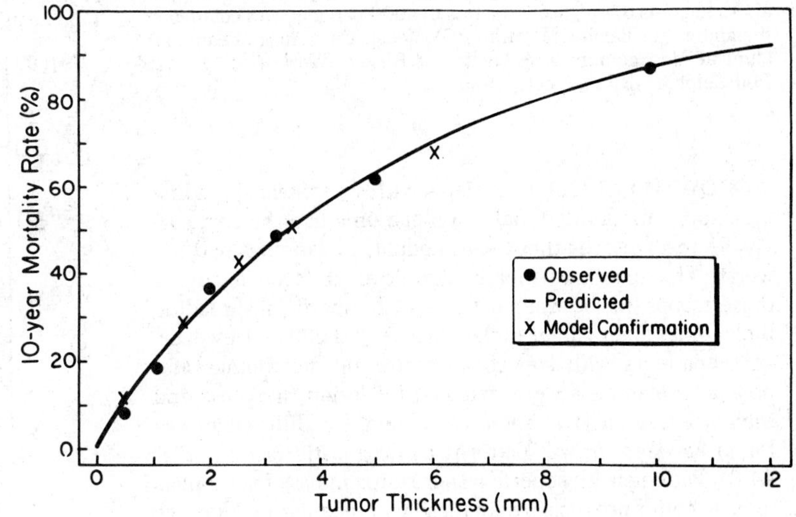

FIG. 44-4. Observed and predicted 10-year mortality rate based on a mathematical model derived from tumor thickness.[117] The mathematical model is $9(T) = 1 - 0.966.e^{-0.2016T}$ and is described elsewhere in more detail.[130] The solid line represents that predicted by the model, and the closed circles demonstrate the actual observed survival for 2627 patients. The accuracy of the model was confirmed by applying it to 747 Stage I melanoma patients from the World Health Organization Melanoma Group (data that were not used in the derivation of the model). The linear nature of the curve demonstrates that there are no natural breakpoints but rather a continuous correlation survival with tumor thickness. (Balch CM, Soong S-J, Shaw HM, et al: An analysis of prognostic factors in 4000 patients with cutaneous melanoma. In Balch CM, Milton GW [eds]: Cutaneous Melanoma: Clinical Management and Treatment Results Worldwide, p 321. Philadelphia, JB Lippincott, 1985)

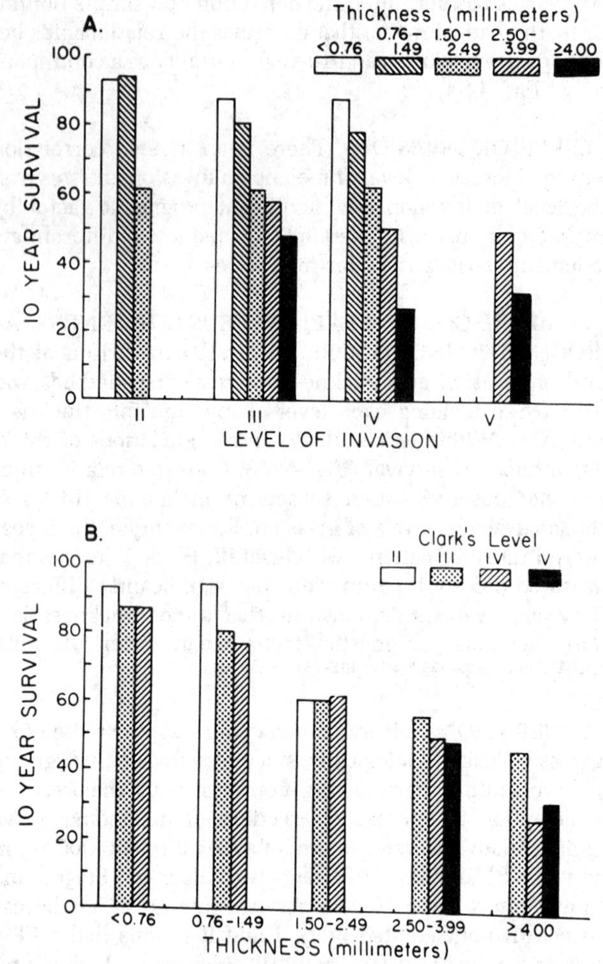

FIG. 44-5. Comparison of two microstaging methods (tumor thickness versus level of invasion. **Top.** Ten-year survival rates for Stage I melanoma patients according to levels of invasion subgrouped by tumor thickness. There were statistically significant differences in survival rates for patients with lesions of various thicknesses within levels III, IV, and V. **Bottom.** Ten-year survival rates for Stage I melanoma patients according to tumor thickness subgrouped by levels of invasion. There were no statistically significant differences in survival rates for patients with lesions of various levels of invasion within each thickness subgroup. (Balch CM, Soong S-J, Shaw HM, et al: An analysis of prognostic factors in 4000 patients with cutaneous melanoma. In Balch CM, Milton GW [eds]: Cutaneous Melanoma: Clinical Management and Treatment Results Worldwide, p 332. Philadelphia, JB Lippincott, 1985)

GROWTH PATTERN. Patients with superficial spreading melanoma and lentigo maligna melanoma had the best survival rates, whereas those with nodular melanomas had the worst. The most statistically significant difference among these groups was between patients with superficial spreading melanomas and nodular melanomas ($p < 0.0001$). However, when patients with superficial spreading melanomas and nodular melanomas were matched for lesion thickness and their 10-year survival rates calculated, no difference was found between growth patterns as prognostic factors (Fig. 44-6). Patients with superficial spreading melanomas appear to have better prognoses than those with nodular melanomas only because the former lesions are thinner. Those with lentigo maligna melanomas constituted only a small number of patients (4%). These lesions were all located on the face or neck and were generally thinner lesions. When lesions were matched by thickness, patients with lentigo maligna melanoma lesions had better prognoses than those with melanomas of other growth patterns.[35,36] Even patients with lentigo maligna melanoma lesions 3 mm thick or greater had an 80% 10-year survival rate. It should be emphasized that other characteristics of lentigo maligna melanomas (*e.g.*, face and neck locations, chronic skin damage, older patient age) may in fact contribute to the distinctiveness of this growth pattern as much as its histologic appearance.

AGE. The median age of patients with Stage I and II melanomas was 45 years. Advanced age at the time of diagnosis correlated significantly with a shortened length of survival ($p < 0.00001$). Patient age also correlated with melanoma thickness ($p < 0.00001$): older patients had thicker lesions. The median lesion thickness for melanoma patients in the third decade of life was 1.1 mm, whereas it was 1.5 mm for those in the fifth decade and 2.8 mm for those in the seventh decade.

MULTIFACTORIAL ANALYSIS. The above clinical and pathologic parameters were simultaneously compared for their prognostic strength by multifactorial analysis. The influence of these factors on survival was examined in a cohort of 2151 patients with AJC Stage I and II disease for whom information was available for all prognostic factors being analyzed. Five major factors influenced survival: (1) *thickness* of melanoma, (2) the type of *initial surgical manage-*

FIG. 44-6. Ten-year survival rates for Stage I melanoma patients according to growth pattern and tumor thickness. In patients with melanomas of equivalent tumor thickness, those with nodular and superficial spreading melanomas had similar survival rates and those with lentigo maligna melanomas had a much more favorable prognosis. (Balch CM, Soong S-J, Shaw HM, et al: An analysis of prognostic factors in 4000 patients with cutaneous melanoma. In Balch CM, Milton GW [eds]: Cutaneous Melanoma: Clinical Management and Treatment Results Worldwide, p 336. Philadelphia, JB Lippincott, 1985)

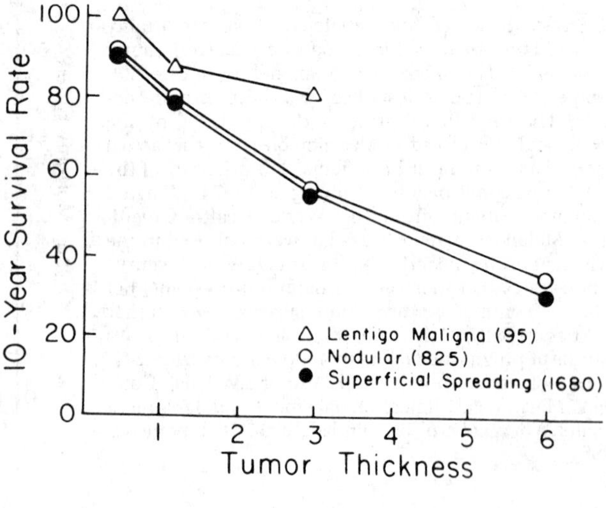

ment (primary excision alone versus excision plus elective lymph node dissection), (3) pathologic *stage,* (4) melanoma *ulceration* (presence or absence), and (5) anatomical *location* (upper extremity, lower extremity, trunk, or head and neck). Three other variables also correlated to a lesser extent with survival or nonsurvival in certain subgroups of patients: (1) level of *invasion,* (2) *sex,* and (3) tumor *regression* (presence or absence).

Most other major studies utilizing multifactorial analysis have established tumor thickness to be the most important prognostic factor in Stage I and II melanoma patients.[48,118,119,121,123,131–137] Ulceration was found to be another strong prognostic factor in seven other patient series.[119,122,123,132,133,135,136,138] Three series confirmed that anatomical location of the primary lesion was a major prognostic factor.[118,119,132]

Other factors analyzed by multifactorial analysis that emerged as important variables overall or within selected subgroups in other series included sex[121,122,137] and age of the patient,[132] as well as tumor features such as lymphocytic infiltration,[122,131] tumor diameter,[122,123,134] cell type,[122,135] the presence of microscopic satellites,[138] mitotic activity,[118,123,131–137] and level of invasion.[132] The timing of the biopsy prior to first definitive treatment was found to have a significant influence on survival in one series.[122]

Metastatic Melanoma in Regional Lymph Nodes (AJC Stage III)

Twelve prognostic factors of melanoma were examined in a series of 551 patients with nodal metastases who were treated at UAB and SMU in the past 20 years.[117]

SEX. The majority (69%) of patients with AJC Stage III melanomas were men, whereas men constituted a minority of Stage I and II patients (44%). There were no differences in survival rates between male and female patients with Stage III melanoma, even when the data were cross-analyzed by other categories.

ANATOMICAL LOCATION OF PRIMARY LESION. Primary melanomas accompanied by nodal metastases occurred in anatomical locations distributed throughout the body, with 56% arising in axial locations (trunk or head and neck). Patients with melanomas on the trunk constituted the largest group (35% of the entire series). There was no statistically significant difference in survival rates for patients with Stage III melanoma when subgrouped by anatomical sites.

NUMBER OF METASTATIC NODES. There was a direct correlation between number of metastatic nodes and survival. Patients with one metastatic node had a better survival rate than patients with two or more metastatic nodes.[139] Data from patients with different numbers of nodal metastases were analyzed for survival differences. The greatest differences in this series were between patients with one metastatic node (37% of patients), patients with two to four nodes (41%), and patients with five or more nodes (22%) (Fig. 44-7). The 3-year survival rates of these patient subgroups were 65%, 43%, and 22%, respectively ($p < 0.001$). Ten-year survival rates demonstrated that only patients with one positive node had a reasonable prospect of cure: 40% were alive at 10 years, whereas only about 13% of patients with two or more metastatic nodes were alive at 10 years.

ULCERATION. Ulceration was the most important characteristic that predicted the risk of subsequent nodal metastases in AJC Stage I and II patients and continued to be an important predictive factor once nodal metastases had occurred.[139,140] The 3-year survival rate for patients with Stage III ulcerative melanomas was only 29%, compared with 61% for those with nonulcerative melanomas ($p = 0.0002$). For each category of nodal metastasis, ulceration in the primary lesion implied a worse prognosis than if the melanoma had an intact overlying epithelium. Patients with one positive node and no ulceration of the primary melanoma had a 50% 10-year survival rate, the most favorable prognosis of any Stage III patient subgroup.

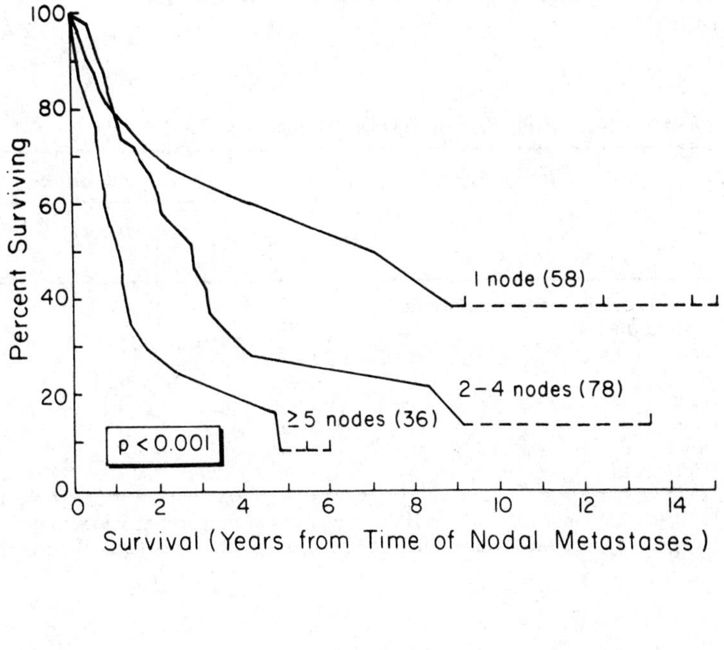

FIG. 44-7. Survival for all Stage III (AJC) melanoma patients according to the number of metastatic nodes. (Balch CM, et al: A multifactorial analysis of melanoma patients with lymph node metastases [stage II]. Ann Surg 193:377, 1981)

TUMOR THICKNESS. The median thickness for Stage III melanomas was 3.6 mm, compared with 1.5 mm for Stage I and II lesions ($p < 0.001$). Forty-nine percent of patients with Stage III disease had thick melanomas (>4 mm thick). A significant relationship was identified between thickness and ulceration. Patients with nonulcerative melanomas 4 mm thick or less had a relatively more favorable 5-year survival rate than patients whose lesions were greater than 4 mm thick (57% versus 44%, respectively); patients with ulcerated melanomas greater than 4 mm thick had only an 8% 5-year survival rate.

MULTIFACTORIAL ANALYSIS. Each of the above prognostic factors was examined for its predictive value for metastatic risk and survival in Stage III melanoma patients.[117,139] By single-factor analysis, the most significant prognostic variables were (1) the *number of nodes,*(2) the presence or absence of *ulceration* of the primary melanoma, (3) *thickness* of the primary melanoma (≤ or >4 mm), and (4) the patient's *age.* The multifactorial analysis confirmed that the number of nodes ($p = 0.0005$), ulceration ($p < 0.00001$), and age ($p = 0.05$) were the dominant prognostic variables; tumor thickness had a borderline correlation ($p = 0.0686$) in the combined data but a stronger correlation in the SMU data ($p = 0.01$). All other factors had a p value greater than 0.10.

The number of metastatic nodes was first shown to be of prognostic significance in a multifactorial analysis by Cohen and associates.[141] Later, both Day and associates[142] and Callery and associates[143] demonstrated that tumor thickness and the number of metastatic nodes were dominant independent variables in Stage III patients. Cascinelli and colleagues[121] identified the extent of nodal metastases (*i.e.,* confined to or invading through the lymph node capsule) and the number of metastatic nodes as the most significant factors in a multifactorial analysis of 530 Stage III patients.[144]

Metastatic Melanoma at Distant Sites (AJC Stage IV)

The data on 200 patients with distant metastases treated at UAB were analyzed for predictive factors affecting survival rates.[145]

SITE OF DISTANT METASTASES. The locations of distant metastases were an important prognostic factor when examined by single-factor analysis ($p = 0.0001$). The skin, subcutaneous tissues, and distant lymph nodes were the most common first sites of relapse, which occurred in 59% of patients. In 23% of patients, nonvisceral metastases at these sites were the sole manifestation of disease (14% for skin sites, 5% for subcutaneous sites, and 4% for distant lymph nodes). The median duration of survival for the entire patient group was 7 months, with 25% alive at 1 year. There was no difference in survival among patients with metastases at any combination of these three sites. The next most common site of first relapse was the lungs (36% of patients). Patients with isolated lung metastases had the longest median survival duration (11 months) of patients with metastases at distant sites. The brain, liver, and bone were the next most common sites of first relapse. The median duration of survival for these patients was very poor, ranging from 2 to 6 months, with a 1-year survival rate of only 8% to 10%. The presence of visceral metastases had an overriding influence on survival, since patients with combined visceral and nonvisceral metastases had the same poor prognoses as those with visceral metastases alone.

NUMBER OF METASTATIC SITES. Patients with a single distant metastasis had a longer survival than patients with metastases at two sites or three or more (see Fig. 44-7). The number of metastatic sites was the most significant factor influencing survival in patients with distant metastases by single-factor analysis ($p < 0.00005$). The median survival time was 7 months for patients with one metastatic site, 4 months for those with two sites, and 2 months for those with three or more metastatic sites. Similarly, the 1-year survival rate was 36% for patients with one metastatic site, 13% for patients with two sites, 0 for patients with three or more sites. Within the single-site group, patients with metastases to the lungs, skin, subcutaneous tissues, or distant lymph nodes had a better survival rate than patients with metastases to any other single site (Table 44-2).

SEX. Once melanoma progressed to distant metastases, there was no correlation whatsoever between patient sex and

TABLE 44-2. First Site of Distant Metastases*

Site		*Site Alone*		*Plus Other Sites*	
	Overall (%)	*Incidence (%)*	*Median Survival (mo)*	*Incidence (%)*	*Median Survival (mo)*
Skin, subcutaneous tissues, distant lymph nodes	59	23	7.2	36	5.0
Lung	36	11	11.4	25	4.0
Brain	20	8	5.0	12	1.4
Liver	20	3	2.4	17	2.0
Bone	17	3	6.0	14	4.0
Other	12	2	2.2	10	2.0
Widespread	4		2.4		2.4

*Balch CM, Soong S–j, Shaw HM: An analysis of prognostic factors in 4000 patients with cutaneous melanoma. In Balch CM, Milton GW (eds): Cutaneous Melanoma: Clinical Management and Treatment Results Worldwide, p 321. Philadelphia, JB Lippincott, 1985.

the clinical courses ($p = 0.98$). Survival curves for male and female patients with AJC Stage IV melanoma were superimposable.

REMISSION DURATION. The length of remission was not a statistically significant factor, by single-factor analysis, in predicting the clinical course of disease when the survival rates were calculated from the onset of distant metastases ($p = 0.25$).

MULTIFACTORIAL ANALYSIS. Each of the prognostic factors was examined for its predictive value for metastatic risk and survival rate.[145] Only the number of metastatic sites and the location of the sites (visceral, nonvisceral, or both) correlated with survival rates in a single-factor analysis. When all factors were analyzed in a Cox regression analysis, the dominant factors for Stage IV melanoma patients were (1) the *number of metastatic sites* (one, two, or three or more; $p = 0.00001$), (2) the *remission duration* (<12 months versus ≥12 months; $p = 0.019$) and (3) the *site of metastases* (visceral versus nonvisceral, $p = 0.019$). These results were the same even after administration of palliative chemotherapy was accounted for. There were no histologic criteria of the primary melanomas that predicted the patients' clinical courses once distant metastases had developed.

Another multifactorial analysis of Stage IV patients was performed by Presant et al.[146] They found that the following were all significant determinants of survival: high performance (activity) status, no liver involvement, female sex, and bone involvement only.

MANAGEMENT OF THE PRIMARY MELANOMA

INDICATIONS FOR AND TECHNIQUES OF BIOPSY

Biopsies for melanomas can be either excisional or incisional.[147] Whichever technique is utilized, full-thickness biopsy into the subcutaneous tissue must be performed to permit microstaging of the lesion (for thickness and level of invasion). Shave or curette biopsies are absolutely contraindicated for lesions suspected of being melanomas.

EXCISIONAL BIOPSIES. An excisional biopsy is indicated for a suspicious lesion that is not large (*i.e.,* <1.5 cm in diameter) and is situated so that the amount of skin excised is not critical (*e.g.,* on the trunk). The lesion should be excised with an elliptical incision that includes a narrow margin (2 mm) of normal-appearing skin. Taking slightly larger margins (*e.g.,* 1 cm) of skin may be insufficient for a malignant lesion and excessive for a benign one.

The direction of the biopsy incision is important, since a biopsy that is not oriented properly may necessitate a skin graft when an elliptical incision and primary closure might have been possible. The biopsy incision should be oriented so that it can be reexcised with optimal skin margins and minimal skin loss if the lesion proves to be malignant. The excisional biopsy technique is illustrated in Figure 44-8.

INCISIONAL BIOPSIES. Incisional biopsies should be performed when the amount of skin removed is critical (*e.g.,* for lesions on the face, hands, or feet). They may also be

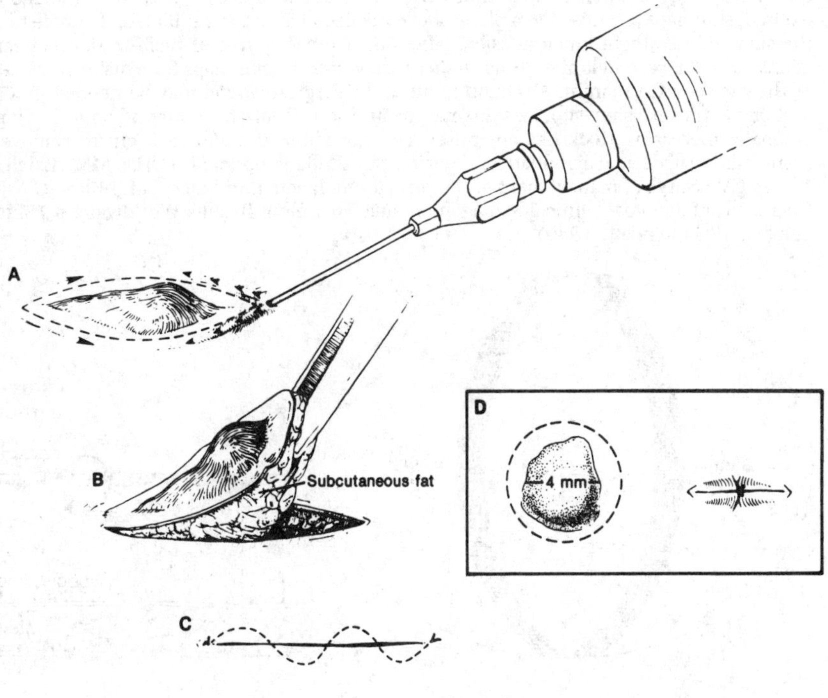

FIG. 44-8. Technique of excisional biopsy for melanoma. **A.** The suspicious lesion is infiltrated with local anesthetic elliptically around but not into the lesion itself (**B**). The entire lesion is excised with a narrow rim (1–2 mm) of normal-appearing skin around it, including the underlying subcutaneous fat. Care is taken to avoid crushing the specimen with forceps. **C.** The incision is closed after hemostasis has been completed. This can be performed with a subcuticular closure using synthetic absorbable sutures or with simple interrupted nylon sutures. **D.** An alternative approach for small lesions. An excision with a 6-mm punch is an inexpensive and expedient office procedure. The lesion is completely excised with the punch biopsy instrument, and the skin edges are closed with a single 4-0 nylon suture. (Urist MM, Balch CM, Milton GW: Surgical management of the primary melanoma. In Balch CM, Milton GW [eds]: Cutaneous Melanoma: Clinical Management and Treatment Results Worldwide, p 74. Philadelphia, JB Lippincott, 1985)

indicated for large lesions, for which an excisional biopsy would be a formidable procedure. An incisional biopsy can be made with a scalpel, but usually a 6-mm punch biopsy is preferred to take a full-thickness core of skin and subcutaneous tissues from the most raised or irregular area of the lesion. The biopsy specimen should not be taken at the periphery of the lesion unless there are areas of raised nodularity at this location. No decrease in survival rates or increase in local recurrence rates have been observed in our experience with the incisional approach.[147] Moreover, an incisional biopsy is a simple, expedient office procedure and yields representative tissue if done properly. And, just as important, such an approach is more cost-effective than inpatient biopsies, especially those performed under general anesthesia. Others have similarly found no increased risk with such an approach.[148,149]

SURGICAL MARGINS OF EXCISION

Local control of a primary melanoma requires wide excision of the tumor or biopsy site with a margin of normal-appearing skin. Until recently, the routine surgical approach was to excise all primary melanomas with a 3- to 5-cm margin and apply a split-thickness skin graft to the defect. However, it has become increasingly clear that the risk of local recurrence correlates more with tumor thickness than with the margins of surgical excision.[127,150–153] It therefore seems more rational to excise melanomas using surgical margins that vary according to tumor thickness and ulceration, since these factors correlate best with the risk for local recurrence.

The earliest lesion is a melanoma in situ.[154] This is a noninvasive tumor that does not metastasize but can recur locally.[155] Although the natural history of these noninvasive lesions is not completely understood, there is a risk of local recurrence (either as an in situ melanoma or as an invasive melanoma) if they are not reexcised after biopsy.[155,156] It is therefore recommended that the biopsy site of an in situ melanoma be excised, usually with a 0.5- to 1-cm margin of skin.

For thin melanomas (<0.76 mm thick), there has been only minimum risk of local recurrence in all reported patient series,[127,147,148,150,152,156–158] despite wide variations in margins of excision. In other words, survival is not influenced by the size of the resection margins. This does not mean that reexcision is unnecessary, but that the minimum "safe" margin has not been established in any scientific study. At present, a wide excision consisting of a 1- to 2-cm minimum margin of skin is recommended by many melanoma surgeons.[127,147,152,156,157,159–161] This can be performed as a generous elliptical excision with primary skin closure (Fig. 44-9). In a recent study of 936 patients with melanomas less than 1 mm thick, there was not a single local recurrence, even though conservative margins (≤2 cm) of excision were used in 61% of patients.[147] For intermediate and thick melanomas (*i.e.*, >1.0 mm thick), a 3-cm margin is usually employed. The risk of local recurrence may exceed 10% to 20% for melanomas more than 4 mm thick.[127,152,158,161] Since lentigo maligna melanomas have a low risk for recurrence and generally occur on the face, they can be safely excised with a 1-cm margin of excision.

Results of the first randomized surgical study involving

FIG. 44-9. Technique of excising a primary melanoma with an elliptical excision and primary skin closure. **A.** The surgical margin consists of a 3-cm radius of normal-appearing skin surrounding the biopsy site or the lateral margin of the intact melanoma. The long axis of the incision should be three to four times the width of the incision. After the melanoma is excised, skin flaps are raised in a plane above the deep fascia for a sufficient distance to close the skin edges without undue tension. The most extensive area of mobilization is near the center of the flaps, and it often is necessary to mobilize the skin flaps for a distance twice that of the excised skin margin. A suction drain in the surgical wound may be needed. **B.** Cross-section of the excision site. A skin margin of 3 cm from the tumor is shown. Flaps of gradually increasing thickness are raised for an additional 1 cm to 2 cm to remove any surrounding subdermal lymphatics. Excising the fascia is optional. (Urist MM, Balch CM, Milton GW: Surgical management of the primary melanoma. In Balch CM, Milton GW [eds]: Cutaneous Melanoma: Clinical Management and Treatment Results Worldwide, p 78. Philadelphia, JB Lippincott, 1985)

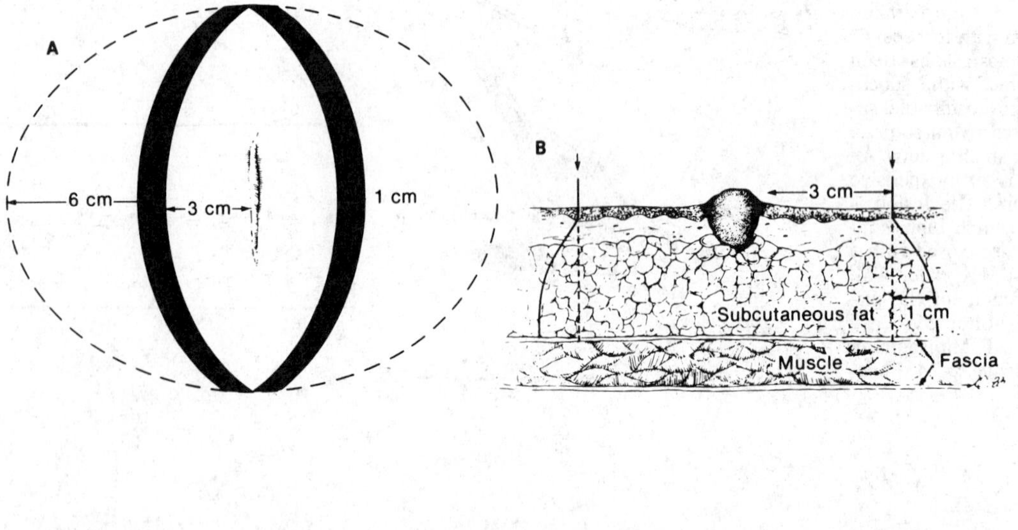

surgical margins for melanomas less than 2 mm thick have recently been reported from the World Health Organization (WHO) Melanoma Group.[162] In a study of 612 evaluable patients who were randomly assigned to either a 1- or a 3-cm surgical margin of excision, there were no local recurrences in the group with melanomas less than 1 mm thick. There were three local recurrences in the group of patients with melanomas 1.0 to 2.0 mm thick; in all three cases narrow surgical excision margins had been used. These results demonstrate conclusively that a narrow excision for thin melanomas is safe.

Special Sites

FINGER AND TOES. A melanoma on the skin of a digit or beneath the fingernail must be removed by digital amputation. When such a biopsy-confirmed lesion is located on the fingers (especially the thumb), it is important to save as much of the digit as possible to maximize function. The amount that can be saved depends on the extent of the lesion (some have significant nail bed or paronychial involvement) and the location of its proximal border. In general, amputations of digits are performed proximal to the distal interphalangeal joint of the thumb and at the middle interphalangeal joint of the fingers, as long as the lesions are small and confined to the nail bed. For a melanoma located on a toe, amputation of the entire digit at the metatarsal-phalangeal joint is indicated; this generally does not cause any significant morbidity.

SOLE OF THE FOOT. A melanoma on the plantar surface of the foot often involves a sizable defect in a weight-bearing area. If possible, a portion of the heel or ball of the plantar surface should be retained to bear the greatest burden of pressure. Where possible, the deep fascia over the extensor tendons should be preserved as a base for the skin coverage.

EAR. For a small suspicious lesion of the helix, the preferred initial procedure for diagnosis is excisional biopsy, followed by a wedge reexcision if the diagnosis of melanoma is confirmed. A partial amputation may be necessary for larger lesions. Total amputation of the ear should be restricted to cases of widespread local disease or disease that recurs after partial amputation.

FACE. Facial lesions usually cannot be excised with more than a 1-cm margin because of adjacent vital structures. In these cases, the surgeon should use his best judgment based on the width and thickness of the melanoma and its exact location on the face. The expected local recurrence rate after surgery is 4%. Radiation therapy has been used with some success for lentigo maligna melanomas located on the face.[163]

ROLE OF RADIATION THERAPY

Superficial contact x-ray therapy has been used in Europe for over 60 years in the treatment of cutaneous melanoma. This technique results in extremely high incident doses of radiation, often in excess of 100 Gy, with very rapid fall-off (approximately 50% at 1 mm), and is therefore suitable only for superficial lesions. Conventional radiation therapy has little role in the initial treatment of primary melanoma, except perhaps for the lentigo maligna melanomas. Harwood in 1983 reported results in a series of 28 patients with lentigo maligna melanomas who had been treated definitively with conventionally fractionated radiation therapy at Princess Margaret Hospital from 1958 to 1982.[163] Only two had recurrences, although some lesions took up to 24 months to regress completely after irradiation.

LOCAL RECURRENCES

A local recurrence is defined as any tumor that occurs within 5 cm of the scar of a previously excised melanoma. This definition is important in analyzing the risk factors involved and the influence of the surgical margins of excision of the primary melanoma. Local recurrences should be considered as retained extensions of the primary tumor. They are distinct from satellites and in-transit metastases that are intralymphatic in origin and occur between the primary tumor site and the regional lymph nodes.

Risk Factors in Local Recurrences

In general, patients at highest risk for local recurrence have melanomas that have metastasized or melanomas with poor prognostic features. One analysis of local recurrence demonstrated that AJC Stage I and II patients at highest risk had melanomas with any of the following features: (1) 4 mm or more thick (13% prevalence), (2) ulceration (11.5%), or (3) location on the foot, hand, scalp, or face (5%–12%).[147] The overall risk for local recurrence is extremely low, only 3.2% in collected series involving 3520 patients.[147] Local recurrences usually develop within 5 years after excision of the primary melanoma but sometimes occur as late as 10 years afterward.[153,164]

Management of Local Recurrences

Comparative studies of treatment alternatives have not been performed for local recurrences. There are three options: (1) surgical excision, (2) isolated limb perfusion with regional chemotherapy and hyperthermia, or (3) radiation therapy. A single local recurrence, especially in a patient with a previously excised melanoma having favorable prognostic features, can probably be excised with a generous surgical margin and no further treatment. On the other hand, a patient who has multiple recurrences (either simultaneous or sequential) or whose primary tumor had poor prognostic features (*e.g.*, >4 mm thick, especially with ulceration) might be considered for isolated limb perfusion, because the risk of additional recurrences and in-transit metastases are substantially increased.[165] In patients for whom surgical excision is not feasible, such as those whose lesions have recurred on multiple occasions, electron beam radiation therapy delivered with a rapid-fraction technique might be considered. Few data on treatment results are available.

Local recurrences imply a poor prognosis and are usually

the first sign that metastases will develop, since most patients with local recurrences subsequently develop metastatic disease.[147,158,166] In one series of 95 patients with local recurrences, the median survival was 3 years, and the 10-year survival rate was only 20%.[147]

REGIONAL METASTATIC MELANOMA

DIAGNOSIS AND CLINICAL EVALUATION

Regional metastases are the most common indication of metastatic melanoma. The physician managing melanoma must be vigilant in making the diagnosis and instituting prompt treatment, because some patients can be cured. Moreover, effective palliation can be provided even to those with incurable disease. Any adenopathy suspected of harboring metastatic disease should be investigated. If the index of suspicion for metastatic disease is low, the node may be monitored by frequent examination until a diagnosis can be made. In some instances, either fine-needle or open biopsy is warranted if the examination results are equivocal or close follow-up is not possible.

Surgical excision of metastatic nodes is the only effective treatment for cure or control of local disease. Some surgeons prefer to excise only clinically demonstrable metastatic nodes. This type of excision has been termed a therapeutic or delayed lymph node dissection. Other surgeons choose to excise even normal-appearing nodes because of the risk of occult or microscopic metastases. This excision has been termed an elective lymph node dissection (also called an immediate or prophylactic lymph node dissection). Surgical treatment for established nodal metastases is best described by discussing each of the major lymph node basins where metastatic melanoma can occur. Later sections described the management of in-transit metastases and the rationale for elective lymph node dissection for micrometastases in the lymph nodes.

SITE-SPECIFIC NODAL DISEASE

Ilioinguinal Nodal Metastases

RATIONALE FOR DISSECTION. The surgical technique for ilioinguinal lymph node dissection has been described and illustrated.[167-170] There are two contiguous node-bearing basins in the ilioinguinal area that might contain metastatic melanoma. The first is composed of the femoral nodes located within the femoral triangle. The second nodal basin is composed of the iliac and obturator lymph nodes.

In patients with demonstrable nodal metastases, a combined dissection of the iliac and femoral lymph nodes is recommended because at least 25% of patients with femoral nodal metastases will have iliac nodal involvement as well.[171,172] There is some controversy concerning the benefit of iliac lymph node dissection. Some surgeons have stated that patients with melanoma of the lower extremities cannot be cured if their nodal metastases extend above the inguinal ligament, and that a combined ilioinguinal lymph node dissection is associated with a higher risk of leg edema and wound complications, compared with excision of the inguinal nodes alone.[173] Others have demonstrated that some patients with iliac nodal metastases either can be cured or experience prolonged survival (9%–30% 5-year survival rate) with ilioinguinal lymph node dissection, particularly patients with microscopic metastases in the inguinal nodes.[171,172,174,175] Excision of the obturator lymph nodes is important, because they can also be metastatically involved.[170,176]

COMPLICATIONS AND THEIR MANAGEMENT. In an analysis of 58 patients who underwent inguinal groin dissections, the short-term complications were relatively infrequent and of short duration.[177] Leg edema was a frequent long-term complication (26%) of patients but was largely confined to the thigh; only 8% of patients had edema of the lower leg. Seroma occurred in 23% of patients despite the use of suction catheters, but treatment with simple incision and drainage was generally straightforward. Pain (5%) and functional deficit (3%) were uncommon. Only one patient (2%) had persistent severe edema. The occurrence of a wound complication extended hospitalization by an average of 2.1 days. Increasing age was the only risk factor for the development of one or more wound complications.

Residual edema can be a debilitating sequel of inguinal node dissection. Three series have now shown a decreased rate of leg edema after groin dissection as a result of using preventive measures that included perioperative antibiotics, elastic stockings, leg elevation exercises, and diuretics.[169,177,178] Vigorous prophylactic measures are important because it is difficult to reverse the progression of edema. The patients in one series in whom this prophylactic regimen was followed had a strikingly lower rate of leg edema than those who did not (7% versus 46%, $p < 0.004$).[178]

Axillary Nodal Metastases

RATIONALE FOR DISSECTION. The surgical technique for axillary node dissection has been described and illustrated.[167,179-181] The most important feature of this operation is the completeness of the dissection, which should include the level III lymph nodes medial to the pectoralis minor muscle. A partial axillary node dissection is simply not in the patient's best interest; moreover, little additional morbidity or operative time is incurred with a complete axillary node dissection.

COMPLICATIONS AND THEIR MANAGEMENT. The complication rate for axillary node dissection is quite low. The most frequent complication is wound seroma.[177,179,180] In a series of 98 radical axillary node dissections in melanoma patients treated at UAB,[177] wound-related complications included infections (7%), seroma (27%), nerve dysfunction or pain (22%), and hemorrhage (1%). Wound-related complications extended the average hospitalization by less than 1 day. Long-term complications included arm edema (1%), pain at the operative site (6%), and functional deficit (9%). Analysis of risk factors showed that increasing age was significantly associated with wound complications, whereas female sex or obesity only approximated statistical significance as predictive factors.

Cervical Nodal Metastases

RATIONALE FOR DISSECTION. Metastases to lymph nodes from primary melanomas in the head and neck area via lymphatics are fairly predictable.[167] Melanomas anterior to the pinna of the ear generally metastasize to the parotid, submandibular, submental, upper jugular, and posterior triangle (spinal accessory and transverse cervical) lymph nodes. Lesions inferior to the lateral commissure of the lip will spread to cervical lymph nodes rather than to parotid nodes. Melanomas occurring on the scalp posterior to the pinna of the ear usually spread to occipital, postauricular, posterior triangle, or jugular chain nodes.

Radical neck dissection is recommended when nodal metastases are clinically evident. The surgical technique for this operation has been described elsewhere.[167,182-184]

MODIFIED NECK DISSECTION. Although no comparative study has evaluated modified versus radical neck dissection for melanoma, many surgeons have adopted the modified approach because of favorable results in patients with squamous cell carcinoma.[185,186] Modified neck dissection is generally reserved for patients undergoing elective neck dissection, but patients with limited metastatic disease are also considered, except when the disease occurs in the posterior triangle near the spinal accessory nerve. Several variations of a basic technique have been described.[186-191] Modified neck dissection differs from the radical neck dissection discussed above only in that the spinal accessory nerve and the sternomastoid muscle are spared.

There are two advantages to modified neck dissection. First, there is better shoulder function and no shoulder drop. Second, the cosmetic result is better. Studies evaluating the functional results of modified neck dissection have shown a good cosmetic result; however, 30% of patients do not retain full spinal accessory nerve function.[192]

COMPLICATIONS AND THEIR MANAGEMENT. A review of complications after radical neck dissection for melanoma revealed that short-term complications (seroma, pain, and skin slough) were relatively common, occurring in 10% to 19% of patients. Long-term problems (neck pain and functional deficit) occurred in only 6% to 7% of patients.[177]

A chylous leak can occur even when great care is used to detect leaks prior to closing the neck wound. Once the leakage rate is less than 50 ml/day, it will usually stop within 7 to 10 days.

Parotid Lymph Node Dissection

RATIONALE FOR DISSECTION. Parotid lymph node metastases may be extraglandular or intraglandular. The most common extraglandular nodal metastases are in the preauricular nodes and the nodes located about the tail of the parotid gland. Metastatic intraglandular nodes are generally found within the substance of the parotid gland and are usually located superficial to the seventh cranial nerve.

Melanomas arising on the scalp or face, anterior to the pinna of the ear, and superior to the commissure of the lip are at risk of metastasizing to parotid lymph nodes.[193] This parotid chain of nodes is contiguous to the cervical nodes; for this reason, it is generally advisable to combine neck dissection with parotid lymph node dissection when parotid nodes are involved by metastatic disease. The exception to this rule might be a tumor arising immediately over the parotid gland and requiring wide local excision, thus necessitating parotid dissection to avoid injury to the seventh cranial nerve. Details of the surgical technique have been previously published.[167,194,195]

COMPLICATIONS AND THEIR MANAGEMENT. Complications after parotidectomy are uncommon when the principles outlined in the preceding paragraphs are followed. The incidence of facial nerve injury is proportional to the extent of dissection and the type and amount of tumor.[196-198] For elective dissection of parotid tumors in general, temporary paralysis of the facial nerve is reported to occur in 10% to 20% of patients and permanent paralysis in 1% to 3%. When recognized during surgery, facial nerve injury should be repaired by primary anastomosis or nerve grafting from the contralateral greater auricular nerve. Seromas and salivary fistulas are uncommon and usually self-limited. Gustatory sweating (Frey's syndrome) occurs more often than is generally reported but poses problems only in about 5% of patients.[197]

MANAGEMENT OF IN-TRANSIT METASTASES

Diagnosis

In-transit metastases are located between the primary melanoma and the first major regional nodal basin. They probably originate from melanoma cells trapped in lymphatics. Although in-transit metastases may occur in deeper lymphatics, they are usually observed as either subcutaneous or intracutaneous metastases (*i.e.,* satellitosis).

The number and location of in-transit metastases and the presence or absence of regional nodal metastases have various implications for survival. Patients with few in-transit metastases have better prognoses than those with multiple lesions. In the Tulane Medical Center series, patients with four or fewer lesions had better outcomes than those with five or more lesions.[199] Regional nodal metastases occur in about two thirds of patients with in-transit metastases and, if present, are associated with a lower survival rate.[200,201]

The reported incidence of in-transit metastases varies. This variation is partly due to the different definitions of in-transit metastases, the referral patterns of the reporting institution, and the proportion of patients with high-risk melanomas. Centers that practice isolated limb perfusion report a substantially higher incidence of in-transit metastases than those that do not. The actual incidence is probably 2% in most current surgical practices. The 10% to 20% incidence reported in some series in the 1960s and early 1970s[173,174,202,203] probably resulted from the fact that the majority of melanomas diagnosed at that time were thicker, more likely to be ulcerated, and associated with a higher risk for nodal metastases than the average melanomas diagnosed in the 1980s.

Treatment Options

The treatment for in-transit metastases is not standardized. The treatment chosen depends primarily on the number and location of lesions in the integument, the presence of metastases elsewhere, the risk of the treatment, and whether previous metastases have been treated successfully. Aggressive local treatment is more effective than presently available systemic treatment. The treatment options are described below.

SURGERY. Surgery may be considered for one or a few lesions. Even when multiple lesions are present, excision of larger metastases (*i.e.*, >2 cm) may prevent or relieve symptoms. Usually, a regional lymph node dissection is performed in patients with in-transit metastases, if it has not been done earlier, since there is a substantial risk of nodal metastases. Amputation of an extremity is rarely indicated, and only when other treatments have failed and the patient is quite symptomatic with pain, bleeding, or odor.

ISOLATED LIMB PERFUSION. Isolated limb perfusion is probably the treatment of choice for most patients with in-transit metastases involving an extremity. Sometimes dramatic results can occur, in terms of both local disease control and prolongation of life.[165] There was some evidence that prophylactic perfusion increased survival rates in one prospective controlled clinical trial.[204]

REGIONAL CHEMOTHERAPY INFUSION. Intra-arterial infusion of decarbazine (DTIC) or cisplatin can reduce tumor burden in some patients.[205-207] It may be considered for lesions of the extremities if isolated limb perfusion has previously failed or is unavailable. Partial response rates of 40% to 50% have been reported, but the response durations were short.

RADIATION THERAPY. In-transit metastases too extensive for surgical excision can often be effectively controlled by radiation therapy. Wide fields and the use of an electron beam of 6 to 9 MeV with an appropriate bolus to eliminate skin sparing are recommended. Postoperative irradiation is also indicated after excision of in-transit metastases that recurred after previous excision. The choice of dose fractionation schedules and the role of adjuvant hyperthermia in the treatment of metastatic melanoma are discussed later in this chapter.

INTRALESIONAL IMMUNOTHERAPY. Some of the first successful treatments using nonspecific immunotherapy were for in-transit metastases. Immunotherapy has been administered as intralesional injections of a variety of agents, including bacillus Calmette-Guérin (BCG), vaccinia virus, DNCB, or other agents.[208-210]

SYSTEMIC CHEMOTHERAPY. In most instances, systemic DTIC chemotherapy (alone or in combination) offers little chance of success for controlling in-transit metastases. Tumor growth can be temporarily arrested in a few patients, but rarely for more than a few months. Systemic chemotherapy may be considered for multiple lesions, especially if the lesions are symptomatic and if other treatment alternatives described above cannot be used or have previously failed.

ELECTIVE LYMPH NODE DISSECTION

Rationale

The issue of elective lymphadenectomy is one of the most important controversies in the management of patients with melanoma. Two randomized prospective studies involving patients with only extremity melanomas did not demonstrate any survival advantage for elective lymphadenectomy, while three nonrandomized studies on patients with melanomas at all anatomical sites showed a statistically significant improvement in survival for a subgroup of patients with intermediate thickness melanomas.[211] Although it is unanimously agreed that not all melanoma patients need ELND, a continuing debate centers on two issues: (1) Is it possible to identify accurately a subgroup of melanoma patients at high risk for microscopic regional nodal metastases? (2) What is the optimal timing of dissection (immediate versus delayed) if such a high-risk group can be identified? Prospective randomized studies are in progress to resolve these issues. In the meantime, consideration of elective lymphadenectomy is justified in selected patients with intermediate thickness melanomas in whom the benefit is sufficiently high and the morbidity sufficiently low that such treatment might be warranted in individual cases.

Elective lymphadenectomy has the theoretical major advantage of treating nodal metastases at a relatively early stage in the natural history of the disease, when the tumor burden is generally less than several million cells. The disadvantage is that some patients may be subjected to surgery when they do not have nodal metastases. Conversely, the advantage of delayed, therapeutic lymphadenectomy is that only patients with demonstrable metastases undergo major operations. The great disadvantage, however, is that treatment is delayed until the metastases are clinically palpable, corresponding to a much greater tumor burden (*i.e.*, many billions of metastatic cells). As a consequence, the chances for cure are diminished. Thus, by the time regional nodal metastases can be detected clinically, 70% to 85% of patients will have distant micrometastases of which they will eventually die.[139]

Patient Selection

Before defining risk factors for occult metastatic disease in melanoma patients with clinically normal lymph nodes, it is important to categorize patients biologically into three groups: (1) those patients with melanoma localized to the primary lesion site, (2) those with local disease plus possible regional nodal micrometastases, and (3) those with local disease plus distant micrometastases, irrespective of whether they also have nodal micrometastases. The intuitive surgical strategies are wide excision of the primary lesion site as the sole procedure for patients in the first group, and removal of regional nodes containing microscopic or occult metastases for patients in the second group. However, regardless of the surgical treatment of the primary and regional sites, the survival of patients in the third category is dictated by the presence of micrometastases at distant sites.

Tumor thickness provides a quantitative estimate of the risk for occult metastatic melanoma at regional and distant sites (Fig. 44-10). In fact, melanoma thickness is the most important but not the sole guide for selecting patients who might benefit from elective lymphadenectomy.[127] The major advantage of basing surgical decisions on tumor thickness is that tumor thickness provides a quantitative estimate of the risk for occult metastatic melanoma in both regional and distant sites.[112,117,120,126–128] Thin melanomas (<0.76 mm) are associated with localized disease and a 95% or greater cure rate. Elective lymphadenectomy would provide no therapeutic benefit in such patients. Patients with intermediate thickness melanomas (0.76 mm to 4 mm) have an increased risk (up to 60%) of harboring occult regional metastases but a relatively low risk (<20%) of distant metastases (see Fig. 44-10). Patients with these lesions might therefore benefit from elective lymphadenectomy.[112,126,127,211–216] Patients with thick melanomas (≥4 mm) not only are at high risk for regional nodal micrometastases (>60%), they are also at high risk (>70%) for occult distant disease at the time of initial presentation.[112,120,127,140,211,214] These patients do poorly as a group, since the distant metastases in most instances negate the benefit of surgical excision of the regional lymph nodes. The treatment goal of removing these nodes is

FIG. 44-10. Estimated biologic risk that microscopic metastases will become clinically evident in regional nodes (within 3 years) and at distant sites (within 5 years) for melanomas subgrouped by thickness categories. (Balch CM: Surgical management of regional lymph nodes in cutaneous melanoma. J Am Acad Dermatol 3:511, 1980)

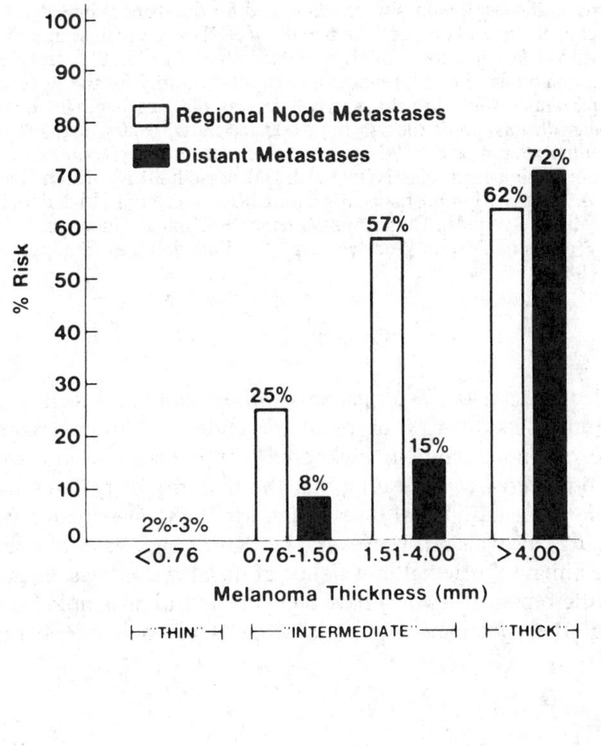

palliative, and the operation might be deferred until nodal metastases become clinically evident. Some surgeons prefer to perform elective lymphadenectomy as expectant palliation in patients with thick melanomas to avoid the probability (about 30%) of a second operation for lymph node metastases.[214] Elective lymphadenectomy might also be justified as a staging procedure to document the pathologic status of the lymph nodes in patients with thick melanomas prior to entry into clinical trials involving systemic adjuvant chemotherapy or immunotherapy.

The anatomical site of the melanoma is also an important criterion in predicting the risk for regional nodal micrometastases. Patients with melanomas on the extremities have more favorable prognoses, whereas those with melanomas on the trunk or head and neck area are at higher risk of microscopic metastatic disease, even with equivalent tumor thicknesses. Extremity melanomas in women have less biologic potential for metastasis than extremity lesions of equivalent thickness in men. Patients with melanomas on the trunk or head and neck area fare worse regardless of sex.[124,125,211,217] Finally, ulcerative melanomas have a higher risk for micrometastases than their nonulcerated counterparts, even when matched for other prognostic parameters such as tumor thickness.[126,213,218,219] The growth pattern is also important to consider in the surgical decision-making process. Lentigo maligna melanomas have a low biologic risk for metastases, so elective lymphadenectomy is not recommended in these patients.[217,220]

The decision to perform elective lymphadenectomy is made selectively, based on the estimated risk of nodal metastases in regional lymph nodes and at distant sites. Elective lymphadenectomy for extremity melanomas in women is usually not recommended unless the tumor thickness is at least 1.5 mm or more.[211] The procedure is recommended more liberally for patients at higher risk, such as men with extremity melanomas and men or women with melanomas located on the trunk or head and neck area. A recommendation for elective lymphadenectomy might be considered in these latter patients whose tumor thickness is as low as 1.0 mm. In patients with melanomas more than 4 mm thick, the likelihood of distant microscopic metastases is so high that it negates any potentially curative benefit of a regional operation.

Tumor thickness should not be the sole criterion for making surgical treatment decisions. Other factors, such as the presence or absence of tumor ulceration, the patient's sex and age, the anatomical location of the melanoma, and the operative risk, should be considered when making the decision to perform elective lymphadenectomy in an individual patient.

Identifying Regional Lymph Nodes at Risk

Since melanomas located on the trunk and on the head and neck area have unpredictable lymphatic drainage, it is difficult to decide which nodal basin is at risk for metastatic disease. In many patients, this problem has been surmounted by performing a radionuclide cutaneous scan that can accurately define the location of nodes that are the primary drainage site for a melanoma located anywhere on the trunk.[221-224] Either all of the regional nodes should be removed, or a policy of monitoring multiple nodal sites at risk should be followed. An elective lymphadenectomy of two nodal basins (*e.g.*, bilateral axillary dissection) for trunk melanomas may be warranted in highly selected cases, but removing more than two nodal basins or performing a bilateral cervical dissection as an elective procedure is never indicated. Bilateral inguinal dissection is usually not performed electively because of its attendant side-effects, especially edema of the extremities and genitalia.

Results of Treatment

Results of a prospective but nonrandomized trial of elective lymphadenectomy performed on 1319 surgically treated patients at SMU demonstrated an improved survival rate for those with intermediate thickness melanomas ranging from 0.76 to 4.0 mm (Fig. 44-11).[126,211,212,215] For patients with extremity melanomas, the benefit was greater in men than in women.[211,217] A similar analysis of 676 patients treated at UAB during the past 25 years also demonstrated a benefit of elective lymphadenectomy in patients who had intermediate thickness melanomas ranging from 1.5 to 4.0 mm (see Fig. 44-11).[35,112,126,140,211,217] Men with melanomas 0.76 to 1.5 mm thick had the same trend toward an improved survival rate, but this was not statistically significant, largely because the sample size was smaller (Table 44-3). A retrospective data analysis from the Duke Medical Center and the Memorial Sloan-Kettering Cancer Center also demonstrated an improved survival rate for patients with intermediate thickness melanomas who underwent elective lymphadenectomy,[213,216] although a similar analysis from the University of Pennsylvania did not.[220]

Patients with melanomas located on axial sites (trunk, head and neck) are at higher risk for metastases than patients with extremity melanomas.[211,212] There have been no randomized prospective trials of the benefits of elective lymphadenectomy for axial melanomas. In our view, it is incorrect to extrapolate the data from patients with extremity melanomas and apply them to the treatment of patients with axial melanomas. The UAB and SMU data indicate an improved survival rate for patients with axial melanomas of intermediate thickness (0.76 to 4 mm) who underwent elective lymphadenectomy. The risk of regional nodal metastases is greater and the benefit of elective lymphadenectomy is even more apparent in this patient group than in patients with extremity melanomas (see Table 44-3).[35,211,212,217] Hansen and McCarten, in a retrospective analysis of 50 patients with head and neck melanomas, also demonstrated an apparent improved survival rate after elective lymphadenectomy in patients with melanomas more than 1.5 mm thick.[225]

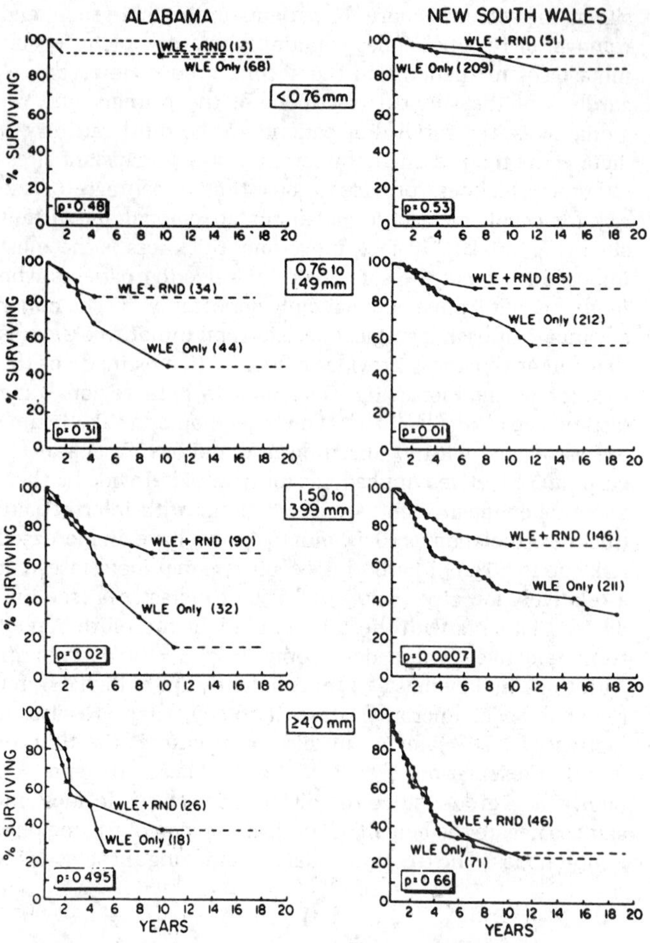

FIG. 44-11. Actuarial survival curves calculated over 20 years for clinical AJC Stage I and Stage II melanoma patients at the University of Alabama in Birmingham and the University of Sydney Melanoma Unit. Patients are subgrouped by tumor thickness and initial surgical management (wide local excision [WLE] ± elective lymph node dissection [RND]). The number of patients in each group is shown in parentheses. P values were calculated for differences between each pair of survival curves. The benefit of RND was greatest in patients with 1.50 to 3.99 mm thick melanomas. For 0.76 to 1.49 mm melanomas, the differences were significant only for the Australian patients. Note that the survival curves did not begin to diverge significantly until the 5th to 8th postoperative years. Patients with thin melanomas (<0.76 mm) and thick melanomas (≥4.00 mm) did not benefit from an RND. (Balch CM, Cascinelli N, Milton GW, et al: Elective lymph node dissection: Pros and cons. In Balch CM, Milton GW [eds]: Cutaneous Melanoma: Clinical Management and Treatment Results Worldwide, p 135. Philadelphia, JB Lippincott, 1985)

Other Considerations

Some investigators have argued that the number of metastatic lymph nodes identified by the pathologist is quite small after elective lymph node dissection. The proportion of patients with demonstrable metastatic disease in surgically excised nodes has ranged from 10% to 25% in different series.[226-228] Within thickness categories, this figure ranged from less than 5% for patients with melanomas less than 1.5 mm thick to 40% or more for patients with melanomas exceeding 3.0 mm in thickness.[127,214,216] These results can be interpreted as indicating that the majority of patients have no metastatic nodal disease and are being overtreated with surgical excision. However, the figures significantly underestimate the actual prevalence of nodal metastases, because micrometastases may have been present in unsampled areas of the specimens. Multiple sections of each lymph node

TABLE 44-3. Ten-Year Survival Rates of Clinical Stage I Melanoma Patients Treated at the Sydney Melanoma Unit, Australia, and the University of Alabama, Birmingham*

Tumor Thickness (mm)	*Extremity Melanomas*			*Trunk and Head and Neck Melanomas*		
	WLE Only	*WLE and RND*	*p=*	*WLE Only*	*WLE and RND*	*p=*
<0.76	94% ± 5% (n = 142)	100% ± 0% (n = 26)	0.230	86% ± 6% (n = 135)	83% ± 8% (n = 38)	0.343
0.76–1.49	74% ± 8% (n = 125)	92% ± 4% (n = 66)	0.042	56% ± 10% (n = 131)	80% ± 7% (n = 51)	0.049
1.50–3.99	54% ± 7% (n = 114)	80% ± 6% (n = 107)	0.005	33% ± 6% (n = 129)	64% ± 7% (n = 129)	0.0008
≥ 4.0	30% ± 10% (n = 33)	44% ± 13% (n = 34)	0.400	22% ± 9% (n = 56)	26% ± 13% (n = 38)	0.806

WLE = wide local excision, RND = elective (prophylactic) regional node dissection.
*Balch CM, Cascinelli N, Milton GW: Node dissection: Pros and cons. In Balch CM, Milton GW (eds): Cutaneous Melanoma: Clinical Management and Treatment Worldwide, p 131. Philadelphia, JB Lippincott, 1985.

would be needed to be sure that micrometastases were not present.

A more accurate approach is to analyze the incidence of regional nodal metastases in a follow-up evaluation of patients treated initially by wide excision alone. In a retrospective analysis of patients treated at UAB, those with melanomas more than 1.5 mm thick and who underwent wide excision of the melanoma as the only initial surgical management had a 57% risk of developing clinically detectable nodal micrometastases within 3 years of diagnosis (see Fig. 44-10).[127] This percentage is more than double the percentage of patients with occult nodal metastases found on examination of randomly sectioned lymph nodes after elective lymph node dissection and is substantiated in part by the studies of Lane and colleagues[229] and Das Gupta,[230] who examined serial sections of nodes removed electively and found occult metastases in 42%.

Results of Randomized Clinical Trials Involving Elective Lymphadenectomy

Two prospective trials to evaluate elective lymphadenectomy in the treatment of Stage I and II melanoma have been performed: an international cooperative study conducted by the WHO Melanoma Group[231–233] and a study by surgeons at the Mayo Clinic.[234] Both studies included patients with melanomas of all thicknesses and did not specifically address the potential benefit of elective lymphadenectomy in the subgroup of patients with intermediate thickness melanomas, as described above.

The WHO Melanoma Group study involved 553 patients with Stage I or II primary melanoma in the distal two thirds of the limbs. Of these patients, 286 (52%) were randomly assigned to undergo wide excision of the primary melanoma as initial treatment and node dissection only if regional nodal metastases became clinically detectable; 267 (48%) underwent wide excision plus elective lymphadenectomy. The two groups were matched according to the major prognostic criteria. No differences in survival were noted between the two groups (Fig. 44-12). Because subgroups of patients may have benefited from elective lymphadenectomy, survival was evaluated according to prognostic criteria: sex, invasion levels III and IV, tumor thickness, and ulceration. No significant survival differences were noted in any of these subgroups. However, a separate analysis of the data demonstrated a 22% increase in the 10-year survival rate in a small subgroup with intermediate-risk lesions.[211]

Surgeons at the Mayo Clinic conducted a clinical study from 1972 to 1976 in which 171 patients with Stage I melanoma were randomly assigned to one of three treatment groups: (1) 62 patients underwent no nodal dissection, (2) 55 underwent elective lymphadenectomy delayed 30 to 60 days after the primary melanoma excision, and (3) 54 underwent elective lymphadenectomy concomitantly with excision of the primary melanoma.[234] Patients with lesions of the head and neck and midline trunk were excluded.

In this study, the subgroup of patients who did not undergo elective lymphadenectomy was older, consisted of more males, and had worse tumor prognostic features (deeper invasion, thicker lesions, and more nodular lesions) than did the two subgroups that underwent elective nodal dissection. The subgroup treated with immediate nodal dissection had more sites involving the trunk than did the other subgroups. None of these differences was statistically significant, although the subgroup with intact nodes was biased toward an unfavorable prognosis. Six characteristics were analyzed: initial surgical treatment, age, sex, anatomical site, tumor thickness, and growth pattern. The only factors that were significantly related to survival were tumor thickness ($p < 0.0001$) and growth pattern ($p = 0.02$).

When overall survival and disease-free survival of the three surgical treatment groups were compared, there were no significant differences.[234] The 5-year survival rate was 85% in patients in whom the nodes were left intact, 85% in patients from whom the nodes were removed immediately, and 91% in patients who underwent delayed nodal dissection. Survival and disease-free survival rates were significantly related to the thickness of the lesion.

Thus, both the Mayo Clinic and the WHO Melanoma Group studies indicated no benefit from routine elective

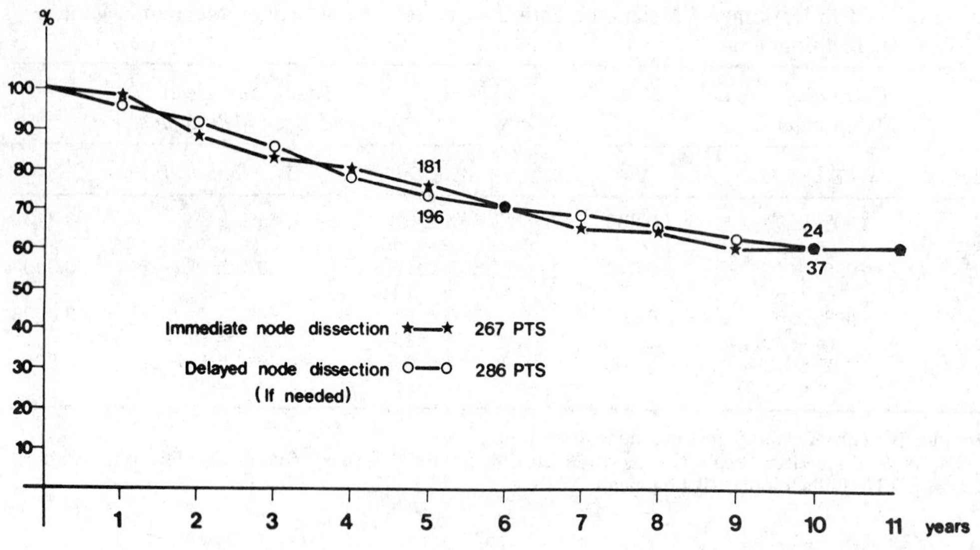

FIG. 44-12. Survival of 553 patients with Stage I and Stage II melanoma of the extremies (World Health Organization Who Melanoma Group Study Trial #1), analyzed according to initial surgical treatment. There was no survival advantage for elective (immediate) node dissection in this group of patients overall. (Veronesi U et al: Delayed regional lymph node dissection in stage I melanoma of the lower extremities. Cancer 49:2420, 1982)

lymphadenectomy for patients with Stage I or II melanoma involving the extremities. However, different conclusions can be legitimately derived from the results of the two trials,[211,217] and these can only be resolved by continuing to perform randomized clinical trials using current stratification criteria and extending these studies to all anatomical sites, but confining participation to patients with intermediate thickness melanomas. Multi-institutional surgical trials are now being conducted in North America and Europe to assess the optimal timing of lymphadenectomy (immediate versus delayed if necessary) in a randomized prospective manner for intermediate thickness melanomas.

ROLE OF ADJUVANT RADIATION THERAPY FOR REGIONAL METASTATIC MELANOMA

The role of radiation therapy as a surgical adjuvant after therapeutic node dissection or as an alternative to elective lymphadenectomy in the treatment of regional metastatic disease in patients with intermediate to thick melanomas has not been clearly defined. The rationale for considering radiation therapy in this context is as follows. Elective lymphadenectomy, while effectively reducing regional recurrence rates, is associated with varying degrees of morbidity and does not offer any survival advantage in patients with thick primary tumors.[211,215] On the other hand, therapeutic dissection of pathologically involved nodes is associated with a local recurrence rate of up to 50% in patients with head and neck melanomas.[185,235]

In view of the management problems associated with uncontrolled local-regional disease and the extent of elective dissections required for scalp and facial primary sites, a study was initiated at the University of Texas M. D. Anderson Cancer Center to evaluate the role of radiation therapy in the treatment of clinically uninvolved lymph drainage areas in patients at high risk of nodal metastases, or as an adjunct to surgery in patients undergoing therapeutic nodal dissections. From January 1983 through July 1987, 67 patients with cutaneous malignant melanoma of the head and neck region were entered into the study. The patients were divided into three groups. Group I consisted of 27 patients with intermediate to thick primary melanomas (≥1.5 mm; median, 4 mm) who had no clinically palpable lymphadenopathy. After wide local excision, these patients received elective irradiation to the tumor bed and draining lymphatics of 30 Gy D_{max} delivered in five fractions over 2½ weeks with electron beams of appropriate energy. Group 2 consisted of 15 patients with previously untreated disease who presented with clinically positive lymphadenopathy. These patients received either preoperative (24 Gy D_{max} delivered in four fractions over 2 weeks) or postoperative (30 Gy D_{max} delivered in five fractions over 2½ weeks) radiation therapy. Group 3 consisted of 25 patients who presented with recurrent regional and/or local disease but without evidence of distant metastases. These patients were treated in the same manner as group 2 patients.

Results of the study as of March 1988 are as follows: The actuarial 2-year local and regional control rates for groups 1, 2, and 3 are 95%, 83%, and 85%, respectively. Corresponding disease-free survival rates are 75%, 55%, and 52%. The great majority of failures have been due to distant metastases. Local-regional control rates are significantly better than those reported previously after surgery alone in comparable patients, and treatment morbidity has been minimal.

However, further experience with adjuvant radiation therapy and longer follow-up are required before radiation therapy can be recommended beyond the confines of a clinical trial. Any influence of adjuvant radiation therapy on survival is likely to be limited to the same subset of patients as might benefit from elective lymphadenectomy—that is, those with no clinically positive nodes and with primary tumors of intermediate thickness. Although a borderline significant survival advantage was observed in a small randomized trial comparing therapeutic lymph node dissection with and without radiation therapy,[236] the difference could be accounted for by an imbalance in prognostic factors between the groups.

METASTATIC MELANOMA AT DISTANT SITES

SITES AND PATTERNS OF METASTASES

Melanoma can metastasize to almost every major organ and tissue. The average survival time is very short when metastases are detected in multiple visceral sites. Autopsy series have revealed that the lung is involved in 70% to 87% of cases, the liver in 54% to 77%, bowel in 26% to 58%, the brain in 36% to 54%, the heart in 40% to 45%, the adrenal glands in 36% to 54%, the kidney in 35% to 48%, and bone in 23% to 49% (Table 44-4).[236,237] The large majority of patients die with disseminated disease involving multiple organ sites; the actual cause of death is often respiratory failure or brain complications.[238,239] In clinical series, metastases to the lung, liver, brain, and bone have been recognized with frequencies ranging from 11% to 36%, well below the frequencies reported in autopsy series.[145,238–246] Metastases to the heart, adrenals, pancreas, and kidney have been detected only infrequently in clinical series (<1% of cases), although abdominal visceral metastases are now identified at higher frequencies with the use of computed tomography (CT) and magnetic resonance (MR) imaging. These studies suggest that the clinical evaluation of patients often underestimates the extent of metastastic disease and actual tumor burden.

The site of the first distant metastasis is an important prognostic variable (see Table 44-4). Following treatment for primary or regional disease, the most frequent distant sites for first recurrence are skin, subcutaneous tissues, and distant lymph nodes (up to 59% of patients).[117,247] This pattern of recurrence confirms the importance of a careful physical examination in monitoring patients with AJC Stage I, II, or III melanoma who are free of disease. The median survival of patients with skin, subcutaneous tissue, and distant lymph node metastases is 7 months, but there is wide variability in survival in this group of patients. The second most frequent site for first relapse is the lung (up to 36% of patients); patients with lung involvement have a median survival of 11 months. The liver, brain, and bone comprise the next most frequent sites of recurrence, and the median survival time for these patients ranges from only 2 to 6 months. In general, patients with visceral metastases (with or without skin, subcutaneous tissue, or lymph node involvement) do very poorly. In the UAB series, more than 80% of patients with visceral metastases were dead within 1 year, and almost all died within 2 years.[117] Patients with lung metastases as the only visceral metastatic site generally fared better (median survival, 11.4 months) than patients with tumors at other visceral sites.

In the UAB series,[117,145] the median survival time of patients with a single distant metastatic site was 7 months. For those with two sites it was 4 months, and for those with three sites it was 2 months. Disease-free intervals of 1 year[145] and 2 years[248] have been associated with longer survival.

TABLE 44-4. Common Distant Sites of Metastatic Melanoma*

Site	*Clinical Series*† (%)	*Autopsy Series*† (%)
Skin, subcutaneous, lymph nodes	42–59	50–75
Lungs	18–36	70–87
Liver	14–20	54–77
Brain	12–20	36–54
Bone	11–17	23–49
GI tract	1–7	26–58
Heart	<1	40–45
Pancreas	<1	38–53
Adrenals	<1	36–54
Kidneys	<1	35–48
Thyroid	<1	25–39

*Adapted from Balch CM, Milton GW: Diagnosis of metastatic melanoma at distant sites. In Balch CM, Milton GW (eds): Cutaneous Melanoma: Clinical Management and Treatment Results Worldwide, p 221. Philadelphia, JB Lippincott, 1985.

†References: 145, 238, 240, 241, 242, 243, 244, 245, 246, and 250.

DIAGNOSTIC EVALUATION FOR METASTATIC DISEASE

The evaluation for metastatic disease in patients who are clinically free of tumors should include a careful physical examination, chest x-ray, and liver function tests. The serum lactate dehydrogenase (LDH) level is a useful marker for widespread metastases, especially for the detection of liver disease.[243,249,250] Blood in the stool and abdominal and gastrointestinal (GI) symptoms should be investigated as possible indications of metastases. Particular attention should be paid to signs or symptoms of central nervous system involvement. In all patients with systemic melanoma metastases, there should be a high index of suspicion for associated brain, spinal cord, or meningeal metastases.

Extensive radiographic evaluation of patients with AJC Stage I, II, or III melanomas who are free of disease rarely reveals metastases. Thus, chest tomography, upper GI series and barium enema, abdominal ultrasound, intravenous pyelography, brain CT, and radionuclide scans of brain, bone, and liver rarely reveal metastases in the absence of symptoms, signs, or abnormal standard test results (*e.g.*, chest x-ray hemogram, and liver function tests including LDH).[244,251–260] The rate of false-positive tests makes extensive evaluations costly. Likewise, conventional scanning with ^{67}Ga is not a sufficiently sensitive or specific screening test, although it can detect metastatic melanoma.[261–265]

Although metastases can remain stable for months, even without treatment, progression of existing tumors or appearance of new tumors can occur rapidly, sometimes accompanied by precipitous clinical deterioration. Patients need to be evaluated at frequent intervals by medical personnel who are familiar with the patient's diagnosis and condition. Despite the poor prognoses and the availability of a number of prognostic indicators for patients with systemic metastases, it is often difficult to predict the course of an individual patient's disease. Periods of stability without evident tumor growth can be interrupted by a medical emergency, such as seizure due to intracranial hemorrhage from a brain metastasis or acute GI bleeding from a small bowel lesion.

TABLE 44-5. Treatment Options for Systemic Metastatic Melanoma*

Treatment Option	*Site of Metastases*	*Comments*
Surgery	Superficial lesions Brain Symptomatic visceral Occasional lung	Best for solitary lesions, especially symptomatic; low-risk patients
Radiation therapy	Superficial lesions Brain Bone	Treatment of symptomatic lesions
Chemotherapy	Systemic metastases	Skin, subcutaneous tissue, lymph node, and lung lesions most responsive
Limb perfusion	Local recurrences	Restricted to extremity lesions; requires major surgery
Hyperthermia	Liver lesions Large superficial lesions	Experimental treatment
Intralesional therapy	Skin lesions	Experimental treatment; can be locally effective for dermal metastases
Systemic immunotherapy	Systemic metastases	Experimental treatment

*Adapted from Balch CM, Milton GW: Treatment for advanced metastatic melanoma. In Balch CM, Milton GW (eds): Cutaneous Melanoma: Clinical Management and Treatment Results Worldwide, p 251. Philadelphia, JB Lippincott, 1985.

TREATMENT MODALITIES

Patients with systemic metastases (AJC Stage IV) have poor prognoses. The mean survival time is about 6 months,[117,145,248] and cure is not a realistic aim. Treatment of this group of patients should include careful evaluation for the potential role of surgery, radiation therapy, and systemic therapy.[266] General guidelines for choosing treatment modalities are presented in Table 44-5. Selection of treatment options should take into account the general medical condition of the patient, the potential for prevention or relief of symptoms, and improvement in the quality of life. The median age of patients with melanoma, approximately 45 years, is young relative to the age of the majority of adult cancer patients. Careful consideration must be given to the impact of prognosis and treatment for these patients, who are frequently primary providers for their families and who have full-time occupations.

No Treatment

No treatment is an important option, especially in asymptomatic patients, those who are terminally ill, and the elderly. There are two situations for which no treatment is a major consideration. First, in asymptomatic patients with tumors in favorable sites, such as the lung or bone (but not brain), the physician may elect to observe these lesions if they are growing slowly and not causing symptoms. Quality of life is maintained in this instance, and treatment can be deferred until the lesions begin to progress, either in size or multiplicity, or the patient develops symptoms. Second, for patients who are terminally ill or extremely old, the benefit to risk ratio is small. The decision to forgo treatment can be difficult; it is often best made by the patients themselves, assisted by close relatives or medical or nursing advisors. Naturally, a patient should not be denied treatment in an individual circumstance when there is a reasonable expectation that the treatment will be successful and the risk or toxicity is low.

Surgery

Surgery is a very effective palliative treatment for isolated metastases, especially since melanoma often metastasizes sequentially and effective chemotherapy is not presently available. Surgical excision of metastatic melanoma probably gives the patient the best, quickest, and longest lasting palliation. On some occasions, the palliative effect can last for 5 to 10 years.[242,267–269] The favorable experience with surgical resection of distant metastases in selected patients treated at four institutions is shown in Table 44-6.

The obvious limitation of surgery is that it is a local form of treatment, and the patient will eventually die from metastatic disease elsewhere. Careful patient selection is therefore important. Observation for several weeks may provide relevant information about the rate of tumor growth and the presence of other metastases, which could emerge during the observation period. Surgery should be confined to patients with accessible lesions limited in sizes and number, and in whom the operation can be safely performed. Some examples of accessible lesions include isolated visceral metastases (especially brain) and occasional lung metastases. Gastrointestinal metastases that are causing obstructions and most superficially located lesions in the skin, subcutaneous tissues, or distant lymph nodes are also amenable to this approach. Liver metastases are associated with such a short survival (2–4 months) that surgical excision is generally not indicated.

The choice of surgical excision as a means of palliation depends on the site of the disease and the duration of antici-

TABLE 44-6. Median Survival (months) of Melanoma Patients After Complete Surgical Resection of Distant Metastases

Site[267]	*M. D. Anderson Hospital*[242]	*Memorial Hospital*[268]	*Univ. of Alabama Hospitals*[269]	*Roswell Park Institute*[267]
Skin, subcutaneous	23 (64)	25 (12)	17 (13)	31 (25)
Lung	16 (26)	19 (17)	9 (17)	9 (13)
Brain	15 (16)	7.5 (5)	8 (17)	5 (4)
GI (excluding liver)	18 (9)	15 (12)	8 (5)	8 (3)
Overall 2-year survival	15%	21%	16%	31%

Number of patients in parentheses.

pated survival. If the patient's life is likely to be measured in weeks, surgical ablation of a large growth is not justified, whereas longer anticipated survival makes excision of gross disease worth considering. Each case has to be considered on its own merit.

Radiation Therapy

Over the past decade, a large number of retrospective clinical studies on the role of radiation therapy for metastatic and recurrent melanoma have been published.[270–283] The majority of these reports have documented higher complete response rates (approximately 50%) for cutaneous and/or lymph node metastases with the use of larger doses per fraction than the norm of 2 Gy given five times per week in conventional radiation therapy. In an extensive analysis of 204 cutaneous or lymph node lesions in 114 patients with recurrent metastatic melanomas treated with a variety of different dose fractionation schedules, Overgaard et al[283] concluded that, within the ranges of time and dose studied, the probability of a complete response depended most significantly on size of dose per fraction and volume of disease. In contrast to an earlier analysis by Trott et al,[284] Overgaard and associates found that overall duration of treatment had little influence on tumor response. Overgaard et al[283] also analyzed their fractionation data according to the method described by Douglas and Fowler[285] and employed an empirically optimized tumor volume correction factor to derive a dose–response function for percent–complete response versus the volume-corrected extrapolated total dose (ETD_{vol}), where $ETD_{vol} = \frac{D \times (d + 2.5)}{2.5} \times M^{-0.33}$ (D = total dose given in fractions each of d size; M = mean tumor diameter in cm) (Fig. 44-13). According to this formula, treatment of 4-cm-diameter nodes with 6 × 6 Gy would be expected to produce a complete response rate of approximately 40%.

The addition of hyperthermia has been shown in several series to increase the complete response rate to an average of 70% to 80% without an apparent increase in treatment-related toxicity.[286–288] However, effective, controlled hyperthermia is difficult to achieve even in superficial tumors and essentially impossible to achieve in deep lesions, and its use should be restricted to defined clinical protocols. Excellent results have also been reported with fast-neutron therapy. In a series of 87 lesions in 68 patients, Blake et al[289] reported a 71% complete response rate with a subsequent recurrence rate of only 9%. A 22% complication rate was observed, however. Another approach using concomitant cisplatin and radiation therapy offered no advantage over radiation therapy alone in a small pilot study.[290]

Chemotherapy

Very few chemotherapeutic agents have demonstrated antitumor activity against metastatic melanoma. In a review of Phase II trials supported by the National Cancer Institute, only 2 of 30 tested drugs resulted in a response rate greater than 10% (with 80% confidence limits) in melanoma patients.[291] The best single agents for treatment of melanoma, DTIC and nitrosoureas, produce objective response rates between 10% and 20%. Complete responses are uncommon. Patients who respond to treatment have a longer survival than nonresponders.[292–294]

FIG. 44-13. Dose–response relation showing the probability of achieving complete response as a function of volume-corrected extrapolated total dose (ETD_{vol}). The horizontal bar indicates the 95% confidence limits of the 50% complete response probability. (Overgaard J et al: Some factors of importance in the radiation treatment of malignant melanoma. Radiotherapy Oncology 5:187, 1986)

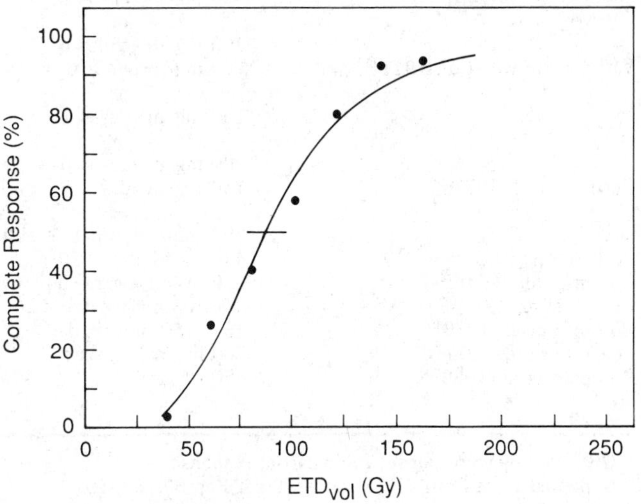

Responses are observed most frequently in patients with skin, subcutaneous tissue, lymph node, and lung metastases, which are associated with longer median survival time than metastases at other sites.[117] It is therefore difficult to distinguish a potential survival advantage due to treatment from that related to other prognostic indicators, and no survival advantage associated with treatment has been shown to be independent from other prognostic factors.

The evaluation of experimental systemic treatments for melanoma should take into account the following prognostic factors for metastatic disease: (1) site of tumor (skin, subcutaneous tissues, lymph nodes, and lung versus nonlung visceral sites) and (2) the number of organs or tissues involved with disease (one, two, three or more). Occasionally, individual skin or subcutaneous lesions that are small (several millimeters in diameter) can wax and wane without treatment. It is therefore important to choose sizable indicator lesions that can be confidently measured. Spontaneous regression that would fit the criterion for objective response to treatment (*i.e.*, more than 50% decrease in the product of the greatest perpendicular diameters of measurable lesions, lasting at least 1 month) occurs very infrequently when measurable indicator lesions are used.

SINGLE AGENT CHEMOTHERAPY. Dacarbazine (DTIC) remains the most active agent for the treatment of systemic melanoma. The response rate is in the range of 15% to 25% (Table 44-7), and patients with skin, subcutaneous tissue, and lymph node involvement respond most frequently.[293–305] Lung metastases are also relatively responsive to DTIC, but liver and brain metastases rarely respond. The median duration of response is 5 to 6 months. Complete responses have been observed in only about 5% of 580 patients entered into Phase III trials, and the majority of these responses occurred in patients with subcutaneous and lymph node metastases.[306] A minority (31%) of patients who achieved complete response survived and remained disease free at 6 years. Overall, only 1% to 2% of patients treated with DTIC sustain long-term complete responses.

The major side-effects of DTIC are nausea and vomiting. The development of effective antiemetic regimens has had a major impact on the rate of occurrence side-effects of DTIC. In one study, metoclopramide alone (2.0 mg/kg given intravenously [IV] over 15 minutes, beginning 30 minutes before DTIC infusion) markedly reduced the number of emetic episodes in 60% to 90% of patients.[307] The combination of lorazepam (1.5 mg/m^2 given 45 minutes before chemotherapy), dexamethasone (20 mg given IV 40 minutes before chemotherapy), and metoclopramide (3 mg/kg given IV 30 minutes before and 90 minutes after therapy) appears to be an even more effective antiemetic regimen.[308] The major side-effects are diarrhea, restlessness, sedation, and enuresis.

Other side-effects of DTIC include local pain at the injection site; neutropenia and thrombocytopenia, which are usually mild and occur between day 10 and 14; flu-like symptoms; and diarrhea. Photosensitivity reactions occur infrequently, and life-threatening liver failure due to hepatic necrosis and veno-occlusive disease has been seen rarely. DTIC may be given as a 10-day, 5-day, or 1-day regimen. Recommended doses are (1) 850 mg/m^2 given IV for 1 day every 3 weeks, (2) 250 mg/m^2/day given IV for 5 days every

TABLE 44-7. Evaluation of DTIC in Patients with Metastatic Melanoma*

Study, Year	*Dose/Schedule*	*No. of Evaluable Patients*	*No. of CR and PR*	*Response Rate (%)*
Wagner et al, 1971[295]	4.5 mg/kg/day × 10	393	100	28
Luce, 1972[293]	250 mg/m^2/day × 5	125	20	16
Nathanson et al, 1971[296]	2 or 4.5 mg/kg/day × 10	115	32	28
Costanza et al, 1972[297]	150 mg/m^2/day × 5	51	9	18
Moon et al, 1975[298]	300 mg/m^2/day × 6			
	or			
	100 mg/m^2 q8h × 6	46	12	26
Van der Merwe et al, 1971[299]	100 mg/m^{2}q8h × 6			
	or			
	150 mg/m^2/day × 10			
	or			
	300 mg/m^2/day × 6	29	8	28
Gottlieb et al, 1971[300]	150 mg/m^2/day × 5			
	or			
	350–450 mg/m^2 biweekly	25	3	12
Burke et al, 1971[301]	4.5 mg/kg/day × 10	20	4	20
Cowan et al, 1971[302]	650–1450 mg/m^2 q4–6wk	20	4	20
Gerner et al, 1973[303]	3.5–5.3 mg/kg/day × 10	15	3	20
Costanza et al, 1976[304]	150–250 mg/m^2/day × 5	110	21	19
Costanza et al, 1977[294]	200 mg/m^2/day × 5	127	9	15
Pritchard et al, 1980[305]	850 mg/m^2	57	14	25
Total		1133	239	21

CR = complete response, PR = partial response.
*Adapted from Comis RL: Cancer Treat Rep 60:165, 1976.

3 weeks, or (3) 4.5 mg/kg/day given IV for 10 days, repeated every 4 weeks. There is no evidence that response rates or duration are affected by schedule or daily dose. With the advent of effective antiemetic regimens, the 1-day schedule repeated every 3 weeks is generally well tolerated and can be administered in an appropriate outpatient setting. Dose can be escalated as tolerated, depending on neutropenia and thrombocytopenia, since hematologic toxic reactions are not usually cumulative.

The nitrosoureas are a second group of agents with defined activity against melanoma. Response rates are between 10% and 18%. Carmustine (BCNU),[309,310] lomustine (CCNU)[311-314] and semustine (methyl-CCNU)[315,316] are the most studied of this class. Sites of responses are similar to those responding to DTIC (skin, subcutaneous tissues, lymph nodes, and lungs). There is no indication that brain metastases have a measurable response to nitrosoureas, despite the lipid solubility and ability of nitrosoureas to cross the blood–brain barrier.

Cisplatin[317-319] and the related compound carboplatin[320] have recently been shown to have activity against melanoma. Taxol, a plant product that promotes microtubule assembly, has produced partial responses in 4 of 12 patients with metastatic melanoma in a Phase I trial.[321] Numerous other chemotherapeutic agents have been evaluated in patients with metastatic melanoma; most have not demonstrated activity.[291]

COMBINATION CHEMOTHERAPY FOR SYSTEMIC METASTATIC MELANOMA. There is no compelling evidence that combination therapy is better than DTIC alone. Because the toxicity of DTIC alone is mild when the drug is accompanied by effective antiemetic therapy, it is important to demonstrate some therapeutic gain for potentially more toxic combination regimens. DTIC in combination with a variety of other single agents has yielded response rates in the range of those for DTIC alone (15%–25%).[322] Despite an initial encouraging report of high response rates for a combination of cisplatin, vinblastine, and bleomycin (PVB),[323] confirmatory trials and randomized studies comparing PVB with DTIC showed no advantage for the combination.[324,325] Responses of short duration were observed in patients with metastases in nonlung visceral sites (including the liver), sites that only rarely respond to DTIC. Randomized studies of combination chemotherapy plus or minus the immunomodulators BCG or levamisole have shown no advantages of immunomodulators.[326,327] A number of other nonrandomized Phase II studies have recently reported high response rates for combination chemotherapy, and responses have been observed in patients with liver metastases, particularly with regimens that include cisplatin.[328,329]

HIGH-DOSE CHEMOTHERAPY WITH OR WITHOUT AUTOLOGOUS BONE MARROW TRANSPLANTATION. Chemotherapy dose may be a crucial factor in establishing responses, particularly for alkylating agents, and high-dose chemotherapy is being actively investigated in the treatment of advanced melanoma. Most studies to date have been Phase I trials. High-dose chemotherapy with or without autologous bone marrow rescue has been reported in small numbers of patients. Responses have been observed in 22% to 27% of patients treated with high-dose BCNU and in over 60% of patients treated with high-dose melphalan or combinations of alkylating agents.[330-336] The toxicity of these regimens is severe and associated with fatality in up to 35% of patients treated with very high doses; life-threatening toxic reactions occur primarily at extramedullary sites (*e.g.*, liver and lung) when autologous bone marrow rescue is used and even in some studies where autologous marrow rescue has not been necessary. In trials with adequate follow-up, median durations of responses have been short, and long-term remissions in tumors of nonlung viscera have been infrequent.

High-dose cisplatin (60–150 mg/m^2) in combination with WR 2721 (ethiofos), a thiol derivative that protects normal host tissues but has no known antitumor activity itself, has been reported to give an objective response rate of 53% (19 of 36 patients, including patients with metastatic sites in the liver), considerably better than the response rate observed with cisplatin alone.[318,337] No complete responses were observed, and the median duration of response was 4 months. Intrahepatic infusion of cisplatin combined with chemoembolization with polyvinyl sponge for liver metastases has been reported to produce responses in 25% to 50% of patients, with response durations of between 2 and 19 months.[338] The preliminary results of these trials suggest that systemic or regional high-dose chemotherapy with certain agents may lead to higher response rates and induce responses in sites that are usually resistant to treatment. However, these studies are at an early stage, and toxicity is high, unacceptably so in some circumstances. Median response durations so far remain short. Phase II studies need to be performed to evaluate more critically the potential efficacy, including duration and sites of response, and toxicity of these regimens.

Immunologic Agents

Systemic therapy for melanoma, both as adjuvant therapy and for treatment of disseminated disease, still remains unsatisfactory. Nevertheless, patients with metastatic or high-risk disease should be considered for enrollment in investigational studies because of a lack of effective standard therapy and because of evidence that the immune system can influence the pathogenesis of melanoma.

A number of immunologic and biologic agents have been tested in patients with metastatic melanoma, and some immunologic agents have demonstrated antitumor activity (Table 44-8). The rapid evolution of recombinant DNA technology to produce cytokines such as interferons and interleukins and hybridoma methodology to develop monoclonal antibodies is allowing purified reagents to be produced in large quantities for clinical trials. The availability of these agents and the development of assays to measure them are allowing better studies about their pharmacology, their mechanisms of action and their effects on various components of the immune system. Among this class of agents, the type I interferons (specifically recombinant α-interferon) have been most extensively studied, but Phase II clinical studies are in progress to evaluate interleukin-2 (IL-2), with or without

TABLE 44-8. Immunologic Modalities with Antitumor Activity in Phase I/II Trials

Study, Year	*Therapy*	*No. of Evaluable Patients*	*Objective Responses*	
			CR	*PR*
Kirkwood and Ernstoff, 1986[339]	rIFN-α2b	23	0	8
Creagan et al, 1986[340]	rIFN-αA	96	4	18
Robinson et al, 1984[341]	rIFN-α2	63	6	6
Robinson et al, 1986[342]	rIFN-α2	45	4	6
Coates et al, 1986[343]	rIFN-α2	15	0	0
Dorval et al, 1987[344]	rIFN-α2b	24	2	5
Rosenberg et al, 1987[345]	IL-2	16	0	5
West et al, 1987[346]	IL-2	10	0	5
Rosenberg et al, 1987[345]	IL-2 plus LAK cells	26	2	4
Schroff et al, 1987[388]	Anti-mCSP (mAb 9.2.27)	32	0	6
Houghton et al, 1985[347]	Anti-GD3 (mAb R24)	21	0	4
Goodman et al, 1985[348]	Anti-*p*97 and anti-mCSP (mAb 96.5 and mAb 48.7)	5	0	0
Cheung et al, 1987[349]	Anti-GD2 (mAb 3F8)	9	0	2

CR = complete response, PR = partial response, rIFN = recombinant interferon, IL-2 = interleukin-2, LAK = lymphokine-activated killer cell, mCSP = melanoma chondroitin sulfate photeoglycan, mAB = monoclonal antibody.

adoptive immunotherapy, and monoclonal antibodies. Another area of intensive investigation is active immunotherapy by vaccination with modified melanoma cells or purified components of melanoma cells. Evidence is mounting that vaccination can induce an immune response to melanoma, and trials are under way to evaluate potential efficacy of vaccines as adjuvant therapy.

α-INTERFERONS. Initial clinical investigations of α-interferons in patients with cancer used a purified preparation obtained from virus-stimulated buffy coat leukocytes. The purification of small quantities of α-interferons required huge amounts of blood products and resulted in a final product that was less than 2% pure. Production was complicated by the fact that α-interferons are a family of at least 20 proteins with a high degree of identity (>80%) in amino acid sequences. The isolation of genes coding for leukocyte α-interferons allowed clinical studies of the pure (>95%) recombinant materials to begin in 1983. Although responses were infrequently observed in trials using purified natural α-interferon, trials using recombinant α-interferons have confirmed that these agents have antitumor activity against melanoma (see Table 44-8).[339] Toxicity is manifested mainly by flu-like symptoms, myalgia, chills, and fever, with an accompanying drop in performance status during treatment with high doses. Continued treatment is generally associated with a decrease in side-effects. Objective response rates average between 10% and 20% (Table 44-8). Responses have been generally partial and short-lived and have occurred mainly in skin, subcutaneous tissue, lymph node, and lung sites. Occasional long-term complete responses have been observed.[340,350] α-Interferon is currently being evaluated in combination with cytotoxic agents, other immunologic agents such as IL-2 and monoclonal antibodies, and in adjuvant trials.

INTERLEUKIN-2 AND ADOPTIVE IMMUNOTHERAPY. A large body of evidence has demonstrated that rejection of established tumors can be mediated by cellular immune responses.[351] Initial observations in experimental animal models, using both immunogenic and nonimmunogenic tumors, showed that high doses of IL-2 can induce tumor regressions of established micrometastases in liver and lung.[352] When lymphocytes are activated by IL-2, they acquired enhanced lytic activity for tumor cells and are called lymphokine-activated killer (LAK) cells.[353] The addition of LAK cells to treatment with high doses of IL-2 has produced higher therapeutic efficacy in animal models than is achieved with either treatment alone.[352,354–356] These experimental studies in animal models led Rosenberg and coworkers to design Phase I trials to evaluate IL-2 and activated lymphocytes individually and then in combination.[345]

Initial studies of the combination of high-dose bolus injections of IL-2 plus LAK cells from the National Cancer Institute demonstrated antitumor effects in patients with advanced cancer, including patients with disseminated melanoma.[357] Follow-up studies reported objective responses in 6 (26%) of 23 melanoma patients treated with

THE CLINICAL SPECTRUM OF CUTANEOUS MELANOMA

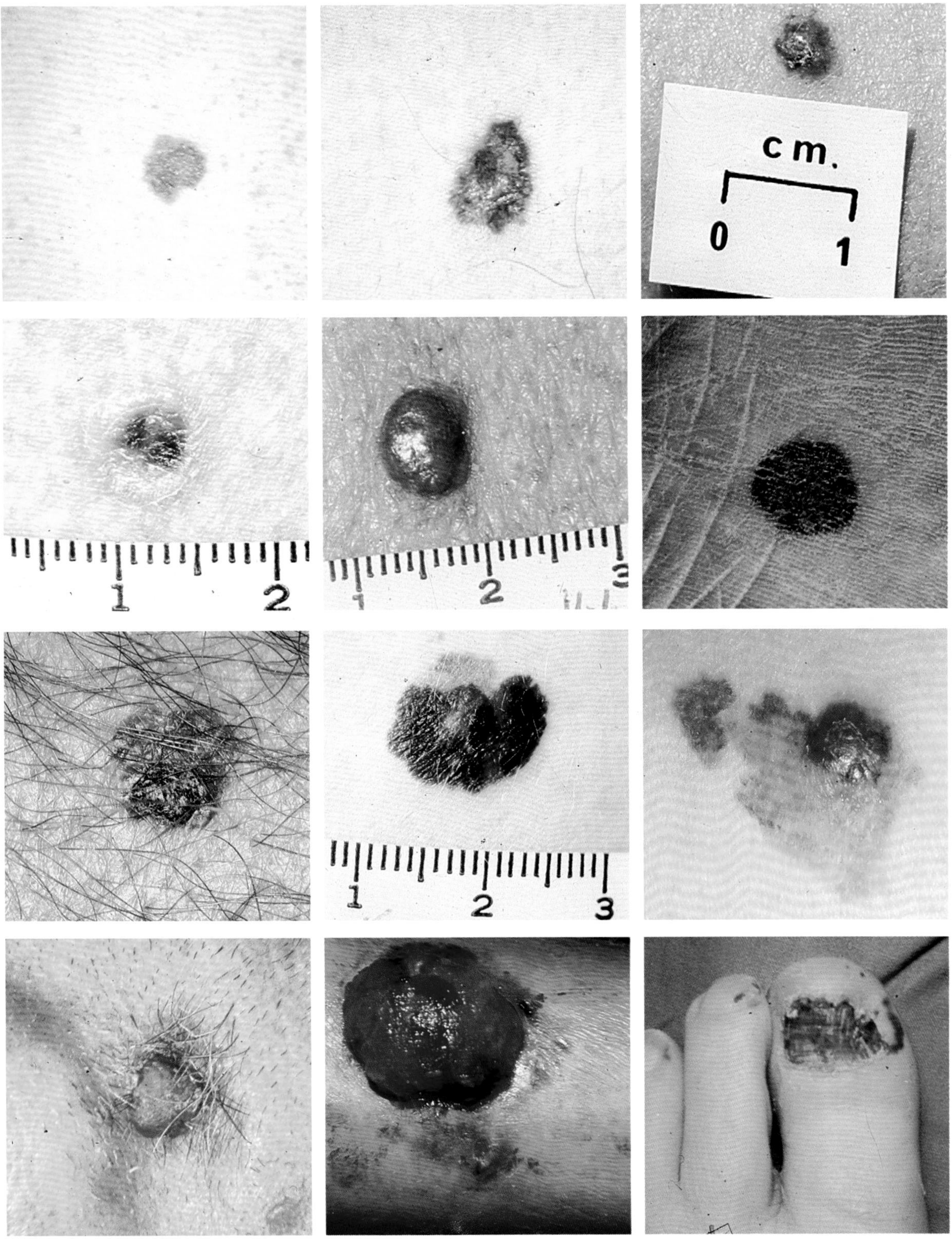

Color FIG. 44-1.

bolus injections of IL-2 plus LAK cells, including two complete responses, and in 5 (31%) of 16 patients treated with high-dose IL-2 alone.[345] A more recent update of results is presented in Tables 17-18 and 17-19 in this book. It is important to note that complete and durable responses have been observed. In confirmatory studies using an identical treatment regimen of IL-2 plus LAK cells, 6 (19%) of 32 patients responded.[358] In addition, 5 of 10 patients had objective responses when treated with continuous-infusion high-dose IL-2 alone in a Phase I trial.[346] In each of these trials objective responses have occurred in liver and other metastatic sites that are relatively resistant to systemic therapy. The toxic effects of high-dose IL-2 can be severe, and include oliguria, confusion, arrhythmia, hypotension, and, infrequently, myocardial infarction.[345,358] Continuous infusion of IL-2 may be associated with more manageable toxic reactions, but efficacies of different dose schedules need to be compared.[346] Ongoing studies will determine the response rates and durations achieved with alternative doses and schedules, with particular reference to the rate and duration of complete responses; will compare the efficacy of IL-2 plus LAK versus IL-2 alone; and will evaluate the effectiveness of combination therapy with monoclonal antibodies or other cytokines utilized together with IL-2.

A number of strategies are being pursued to evaluate the potential role of specific cytotoxic and helper T-lymphocytes in tumor regression in animal models.[359,360] Cytotoxic T-lymphocytes that specifically kill or proliferate in response to autologous melanoma cells can be isolated from patients with advanced melanoma.[361–370] Animal models have shown substantial antitumor activity for adoptive immunotherapy using lymphocytes isolated from tumor sites (tumor-infiltrating lymphocytes, or TIL). Animals were primed with either cyclophosphamide or total body irradiation and injected with IL-2–expanded TIL and IL-2.[371] Much lower doses of IL-2 were needed to attain the equivalent antitumor effects seen in animals treated with high-dose IL-2 plus LAK cells. Based on these preclinical studies, clinical evaluation of adoptive immunotherapy with TIL and IL-2 is under way (see Chap. 17).[372]

MONOCLONAL ANTIBODIES. Several different approaches to cancer therapy with monoclonal antibodies (mAb) are being explored.[373] Two strategies are being pursued in the treatment of melanoma: treatment with mAb alone to activate the host immune system against the tumor, and treatment with mAb conjugated to a cytotoxic agent, either a radioisotope or the toxin ricin A chain, to deliver the agent to the tumor. Although a much larger number of antigen systems have been defined,[374,375] four antigens expressed on the surface of melanoma cells have been most thoroughly investigated as targets for therapy: (1) the p97 antigen, a 97,000-dalton glycoprotein that has sequence identity with transferrin[376]; (2) the melanoma chondroitin-sulfated proteoglycan, a high molecular weight glycoprotein, composed of a core protein of 250,000 daltons, whose size is greater than 500,000 daltons after the addition of carbohydrates; (3) the glycolipid GD3, a ganglioside that contains sialic acid and other carbohydrate residues attached to a lipid core structure; and (4) the ganglioside GD2, which differs from the GD3 ganglioside only in the addition of an *N*-acetylgalactosamine sugar residue.

Phase I studies of mouse mAb alone have shown that mAb can reach tumor sites after systemic administration,[346,348–350,377,378] and in some cases there is evidence that inflammatory responses can be induced.[348,350] Toxicity has generally been mild to moderate, and maximum tolerated doses have not yet been defined for most unconjugated mAb. Objective responses have been observed in preliminary trials of IgG3 subclass mAb against GD3 gangliosides (partial responses in 4 of 21 patients)[348,379] and GD2 gangliosides (objective responses in 2 of 9 patients).[350] These two mAb are notable because they mediate activation of human complement, kill target melanoma cells in the presence of human peripheral blood mononuclear cells (antibody-dependent cellular cytotoxicity), and induce inflammatory responses at tumor sites.[348,350] More studies are needed to establish response rates, response durations, and responsive sites for both anti-GD3 and anti-GD2 mAb.

A pilot trial of mAb Fab fragments against the p97 antigen conjugated to ^{131}I has been reported.[380] Up to 500 mCi of radioisotope was administered, and the primary dose-limiting toxic effects (thrombocytopenia and neutropenia) were due to marrow irradiation.[380] Ricin, a natural product of beans from the plant *Ricinus communis*, is an extremely potent inhibitor of protein synthesis. Ricin is composed of two chains, designated A and B, that are disulfide linked. The A chain is able to inhibit protein synthesis; the B chain mediates binding to the cell surface. The ricin A chain has been conjugated to mAb,[381] and Phase I trials have demonstrated generally mild toxicity (flu-like symptoms and hepatic enzyme elevations).[382] A Phase II study in 46 patients with melanoma has been completed; one complete response and three partial responses were observed.[383]

Because most antimelanoma mAb are of mouse origin, they have generally induced a human IgG response to the mouse immunoglobulin.[346,348–350,384] Two methods are being explored to bypass the human antimouse immunoglobulin response. First, genes coding for mouse mAb can be genetically manipulated to construct chimeric mAb composed of mouse antigen-binding regions ligated to human immunoglobulin sequences.[385] A second approach is to derive human mAb to melanoma antigens. Human mAb to the gangliosides GD2 and GD3 have been isolated,[386–388] and a pilot trial of intralesional injection of the human anti-GD2 mAb has reportedly shown regression of skin lesions.[386]

Mouse mAb conjugated to radioisotopes are being evaluated for the diagnosis of regional and distant metastases in patients with melanoma.[389] Although the primary focus in most of these studies has been to determine whether tumor sites can be identified, useful information about isotope dosimetry at tumor sites and in critical normal tissues (*e.g.*, marrow) has been elicited in some cases.[380] In addition to evaluating systemic disease, radiolabeled mAb are being evaluated as agents to detect regional metastases by lymphoscintigraphy.[390,391]

Three different isotopes have been evaluated for diagnostic imaging: ^{131}I,[391–393] ^{111}In,[390,394–402] and ^{99m}Tc.[397,402,403] Each isotope offers advantages and disadvantages for imaging, nonspecific uptake by organs such as the liver, isotope half-life, and stability of mAb–isotope conjugates in the patient. In the majority of studies whole IgG has been injected. Fragments of IgG, either Fab[380,390,392] or $F(ab')_2$,[397,402,403] generally have shorter half-lives in the circulation and may allow better tumor to normal tissue ratios of isotope in a shorter period of time. Side-effects of imaging with radiolabeled mAb have been rare. Overall, between 40% and 87% of tumors have been imaged with mAb labeled with radioisotopes; sensitivity is generally better at higher mAb doses.[390,392,394,395,397–403] It is not yet possible to determine the potential diagnostic role of radiolabeled mAb in the evaluation of patients for metastatic melanoma. In nude mouse models bearing human melanoma xenografts, imaging with ^{111}In-labeled mAb against the p97 or melanoma proteoglycan antigens has no advantage over imaging with ^{67}Ga, a standard radioisotope occasionally used in the evaluation of melanoma metastases.[404] However, there are limitations to extrapolating data from mouse models to human studies. Further clinical trials to compare radiolabeled-mAb imaging with physical examination and standard diagnostic procedures will be necessary to assess the role of diagnostic imaging with radiolabeled mAb.

ACTIVE IMMUNIZATION—TUMOR VACCINES. Tumor vaccines have a long history, but the search for effective methods to induce active immunity against tumors has been difficult. Repeated attempts have been made to inhibit the outgrowth of tumors and influence the natural history of melanoma using tumor cells themselves or extracts of tumor cells.[405] Most clinical studies have been performed in patients with regional lymph node metastases or high-risk primary lesions. The rationale for using melanoma vaccines comes from the identification of cell surface antigens on melanoma cells that can be recognized by antibodies in sera or lymphocytes from patients with melanoma.[406]

A number of problems exist in the construction of tumor vaccines, including weak immunogenicity of tumor antigens, heterogeneity of antigen expression in tumors, and the ability of tumors to escape an immune response.[407–411] Immunization with irradiated allogeneic melanoma cells, either alone or in combination with BCG, has mainly elicited antibodies against major histocompatibility alloantigens and not against more restricted tumor antigens.[411–413] Although most studies have not reported an improvement in survival,[414–416] the largest study of this kind (in 719 patients) has suggested improved survival rates in patients injected with neuraminidase-treated allogeneic melanoma cells and BCG compared to survival in untreated historical controls.[417,418] Prospective randomized studies are needed to determine whether this protocol can confer disease-free survival and survival advantage.

Strategies have been developed to augment the immune response to tumor antigens by infecting tumor cells with nonpathogenic viruses. Viral proteins presented on the cell membrane of tumors have been shown to augment the immunogenicity of tumor antigens.[419] Several centers have investigated the immunogenicity of lysates derived from tumor cells infected with Newcastle disease virus, vaccinia virus, and vesicular stomatitis virus.[420–430] Vaccines have been safe, and preliminary studies have suggested in some cases that vaccinated patients have improved survival over historical controls.[421,422,428,429] However, prospective randomized clinical trials are necessary to evaluate the effects of vaccines on the clinical course of melanoma.

Studies in mice bearing transplantable tumors have demonstrated that a population of T-lymphocytes can actively suppress an immune response to tumors, and this population of suppressor T-lymphocytes can be abrogated by low doses of cyclophosphamide.[431] Studies in humans also suggest that low-dose cyclophosphamide can enhance humoral and cell-mediated response to challenge with tumor antigens, and some vaccine trials are beginning to incorporate pretreatment with cyclophosphamide.[432–434]

A major effort is underway to immunize with purified preparations of potentially immunogenic molecules from melanoma cells. Gangliosides, the major acidic glycolipid of melanoma cells, have been shown to induce antibody responses after immunization.[435,436] Of particular interest, the ganglioside GM2 can induce IgM antibody responses in the majority of immunized patients, and prospective randomized studies are underway to evaluate GM2 vaccines.[436] Genes that code for melanoma antigens can be used to construct recombinant vaccines using vaccinia virus as vector. The p97 glycoprotein antigen is immunogenic in primates immunized with a recombinant vaccine constructed by transfecting the p97 gene into a vaccinia virus vector.[437]

INTERLESIONAL THERAPY. A high proportion of skin lesions have been shown to regress after injection with nonspecific inflammatory agents such as BCG. The first study of this sort was reported by Morton in 1971,[438] and subsequent investigations confirmed that injection of BCG into superficial cutaneous lesions leads to responses both at the injected sites (in approximately two thirds of lesions) and occasionally at uninjected sites (in 21% of lesions, in proximity to injected lesions).[439–442] Other agents, including purified protein derivative,[443] methanol-extracted residue,[444] and dinitrochlorobenzene,[445] have produced similar results. Intralesional therapy is most likely to lead to regression of small dermal lesions; the response of subcutaneous or large tumors is substantially lower.

Endocrine Therapy

At present, there appears to be little role for endocrine therapy in the treatment of melanoma. Although melanoma tissues and cell lines can demonstrate binding of estrogen and other steroids, it is unclear whether melanoma cells can express estrogen receptor–binding proteins or whether tyrosinase, the enzyme that controls melanin synthesis, binds estrogen. If tyrosinase accounts for estrogen binding,[446] the role of endocrine therapy lacks biologic support at this time. Clinical reports of responses to tamoxifen are mainly anecdotal, and larger trials have demonstrated minimal or no activity for tamoxifen, the antiandrogen cyproterone acetate, and medroxyprogesterone acetate.[447–451]

CURRENT STATUS OF ADJUVANT THERAPY

Advances in melanoma treatment over the past decade have evolved primarily from more detailed knowledge about prognostic factors of primary and metastatic lesions. Within the larger group of melanoma patients who undergo potentially curative surgical resection, subgroups can be identified who are at high risk for recurrence and for the development of systemic metastases. Patients with thick primary melanomas (≥4.0 mm thick), in-transit lesions, and regional lymph node involvement are at particular risk. Once distant metastases develop, most patients will die of the disease. The investigation of adjuvant systemic treatment that can prevent melanoma recurrence remains a critical area of research.[405,452] The rationale and general principles for adjuvant treatment of cancer are based on the premise that treatment, whether chemotherapy or immunotherapy, is more effective when the tumor cell population is small.[453-455]

Chemotherapeutic agents with demonstrated activity against advanced melanoma have been evaluated in patients with local and regional melanoma who are surgically rendered free of disease. The agents with the best established activity against advanced melanoma, DTIC and the nitrosoureas, have been studied as adjuvant therapies in a number of randomized trials (Table 44-9).[405,456-476] No statistical advantage in survival or disease-free survival has been identified in treated patients. In the realm of immunotherapy, the nonspecific immunomodulators BCG and *Corynebacterium parvum* have been studied most intensively. Although initial reports suggested that patients treated with BCG and *C. parvum* did better than historical or nonrandomized controls, randomized studies have shown no measurable benefit from adjuvant treatment with either agent (see Table 44-9). Combinations of DTIC and BCG have also demonstrated no efficacy, nor have randomized trials of transfer factor, a dialyzed extract from leukocytes, or of the nonspecific immunomodulator levamisole. However, nonrandomized adjuvant trials with melanoma-specific tumor cell vaccines have shown encouraging results, and these vaccines are now being tested in a series of Phase III studies.[413-421,429,430]

Adjuvant treatment for melanoma should be considered only in clinical research protocols. It is recommended that the option of experimental adjuvant treatment be considered for patients with AJC Stage I, II, or III melanoma who are free of disease but who are at high risk for recurrence. Current investigations of adjuvant treatment include (1) treatment with cytokines (α-interferon and IL-2); (2) active immunization by modified melanoma cells, lysates of virus-infected melanoma cells, melanoma cell extracts, or purified melanoma antigens; (3) high-dose chemotherapy with autologous bone marrow transplantation; (4) therapy with a single cytotoxic drug or with combinations that have activity against advanced metastatic melanoma; and (5) regional perfusion with or without hyperthermia.

SITE-SPECIFIC MANAGEMENT OF DISTANT METASTASES

Skin, Subcutaneous Tissues, and Distant Lymph Nodes

The most common sites of distant metastases are the skin and subcutaneous tissues.[145,242,243] Lesions are usually 0.5 to 2.0 cm in diameter and are readily detectable on physical examination. Occasionally it may be clinically difficult to distinguish a cutaneous metastasis from a second primary melanoma. Many patients retain remarkably good health despite large numbers of subcutaneous metastases.

Distant metastases can occur in any lymph node chain. Superficial nodal metastases are easily diagnosed on physical examination. Those within the thorax can usually be detected on chest radiographs, with CT or tomography used as confirmatory studies, whereas abdominal metastatic nodes are usually detected with CT or ultrasonography.[255,477,478] When nodal metastases occur in the retroperitoneum, the pelvis, or the mediastinum, they can become quite large and cause symptoms by invading or displacing adjacent tissues.[255,479,480]

Once distant nodal metastases (one or a few) have been isolated, surgical excision is the treatment of choice, providing a safe, quick, and effective treatment (see Table 44-6). Distant nodal metastases should usually be excised before they become bulky and symptomatic, when they would require even more extensive surgery. They should be excised with a rim of normal-appearing tissue (usually 0.5–1.0 cm) to minimize the risk of recurrence. Sequential metastases can be excised surgically unless they are multiple or appear in rapid succession. For multiple or recurrent lesions, radiation therapy may be considered as a second option.[270-283] Radiation therapy might also be considered for symptomatic nodal or soft tissue metastases in surgically inaccessible sites (*e.g.*, mediastinum, retroperitoneum, pelvis). Systemic therapy, either experimental or standard chemotherapy, might be considered for widespread multiple lesions or symptomatic deep lymph nodes not accessible to radiation therapy. Approximately 40% of patients with metastases localized to the skin, subcutaneous tissues, or lymph nodes without visceral involvement will survive more than 1 year, and a finite but small proportion (5%–10%) of these patients will be alive at 5 years. Overall, patients with metastases confined to the skin, subcutaneous tissues, lymph nodes, or lungs survive longer and response better to surgery, radiation therapy, or systemic therapy than patients with involvement of other visceral sites, but most patients in both groups do not survive beyond 3 years.

Lung, Pleura, and Mediastinum

The second most common initial sites of metastasis are the lungs and pleura (see Table 44-2). Nearly all patients with disseminated melanoma will develop metastases in the chest before death. These lesions are evaluated with chest radiography preoperatively and during follow-up, while suspicious intrathoracic metastases are further evaluated with tomography, CT, or bronchoscopy.

For screening purposes, standard chest radiography (upright posteroanterior and lateral views) is sufficiently sensitive and cost-effective to be used for all melanoma patients. The yield of the more expensive pulmonary tomography or CT is too low and the cost too high to justify their use when the chest radiographs are normal.[244,478,481] Evaluation of suspicious metastases begins when one or more lesions are seen on chest radiographs, the usual presentation of pulmonary metastases from melanoma.[145,243,482-485] Most patients have multiple pulmonary nodules; only 22% have solitary nodules.[485] Hilar and mediastinal adenopathy frequently accompanies pulmonary metastases.[486] Patients with hilar

TABLE 44-9. Randomized Clinical Trials Evaluating Adjuvant Therapy for Melanoma

Study Group or Institution	*No. of Patients*	*Treatments Evaluated*	*Results*
Central Oncology Group[456]	174	1. DTIC 2. Control	No benefit of DTIC
WHO/Melanoma Group[457]	761	1. DTIC 2. BCG 3. DTIC + BCG 4. Control	No difference
National Cancer Institute[458]	181	1. Methyl-CCNU 2. BCG 3. BCG + TCV 4. Control	No difference
Southeastern Cancer Study Group (SEG)[405]	136	1. *C. parvum* 2. DTIC + *C. parvum*	No difference
GIF, France[459]	248	1. BCG 2. BCG + CCNU, DTIC, VM26	No difference
Southwestern Cancer Study Group[460]	217	1. BCNU, hydroxyurea, TIC (BHD) 2. BHD + BCG	BHD alone better than combined with BCG
Massachusetts General Hosp.[461]	70	1. DTIC 2. BCG 3. DTIC + BCG	DTIC + BCG better than DTIC alone ($p < 0.05$)
UCLA[462]	66	1. DTIC 2. DTIC + BCG	No difference
Roswell Park Memorial Institute[463]	84	1. DTIC + estrogen 2. BCG 3. Control	No difference
St. Louis Hosp.[464]	77	1. BCNU, actinomycin + vinblastine (BAV) 2. BAV + BCG + *C. parvum*	No difference
Eastern Cooperative Oncology Group[465]	60	1. DTIC 2. DTIC + BCG	No difference
Vanderbilt[466]	60	1. BCG + DTIC 2. BCG + CCNU	No difference
Canadian Cooperative Group[467]	57	1. BCG + DTIC 2. Control	No difference
EORTC[468]	200	1. DTIC 2. Levamisole 3. Control	No difference
SEG[469]	260	1. *C. parvum* 2. Control	Survival benefit for melanomas > 3 mm ($p = 0.01$)
Alberta[470]	152	1. Oral BCG 2. ID BCG	No difference overall
Christie Hosp.[471]	115	1. IV *C. parvum*	No difference overall
UCLA[462]	137	1. BCG 2. Control	No difference
UCSF[472]	203	1. Levamisole 2. Control	No difference
UCLA[473]	139	1. BCG 2. Tumor cell vaccine + BCG 3. Control	No difference
Memorial Hosp., N.Y.[405]	48	1. BCG 2. *C. parvum*	No difference
Cleveland Clinic[474]	36	1. Transfer factor	No difference
SEG[405]	237	1. BCG 2. *C. parvum*	No difference
Eastern Oncology Group[475]	98	1. BCG 2. Control	No difference
Pennsylvania State [476]	116	1. BCG 2. *C. parvum*	Significant improvement with *C. parvum* in relapse rate and survival for Stage II only

*Balch CM, Hersey P: Current status of adjuvant therapy. In Balch CM, Milton GW (eds): Cutaneous Melanoma: Clinical Management and Treatment Results Worldwide, p 197. Philadelphia, JB Lippincott, 1985.

nodules or lymphangitic spread have a particularly rapid disease course, with an average survival of about 1 month.

Whole-lung tomograms or CT scans of the chest are of value in evaluating suspicious chest lesions or in determining whether the metastatic disease seen on chest radiographs is also present elsewhere in the chest.[478,487–490] Bronchoscopy with biopsy may be considered in a few patients when the diagnosis of pulmonary lesions is in doubt (*i.e.*, when pulmonary lesions could be due to metastatic disease, fungal disease, benign tumors, or bronchogenic carcinoma), especially when symptoms suggest bronchial involvement (*e.g.*, a productive cough, or a centrally located or cavitary lesion).

The treatment of choice is influenced by the site and number of thoracic metastases. For solitary pulmonary metastases in asymptomatic patients, surgical excision may be indicated if no new lesions appear during an observation period of 3 to 4 weeks and if the tumor has a relatively slow growth rate. Morton et al have recommended excision of solitary metastases when the tumors have a doubling time exceeding 40 days.[491] Whole-lung tomograms or CT scans are essential, for often a patient with a solitary lesion appearing on chest radiographs actually has other pulmonary or intrathoracic lesions as well.[485,489,492] The operation is safe (<1% mortality), but careful patient selection is important, as only a minority of patients will benefit. Surgical excision of solitary pulmonary metastases is justified in selected patients, however, because truly long-term survival can be achieved.[242,267–269,492–497] The median postoperative survival ranges from 16 to 24 months, with 5-year survival rates of 12% to 21% in some large series. Not all institutions have had such favorable results (see Table 44-6).[498,499]

Another justification for excising solitary pulmonary lesions is to confirm that they do not represent a second primary malignancy or a benign process. This situation can occur in up to one third of patients whose workups culminate in thoracotomies.[492,494]

Patients who are not candidates for surgery, such as those with multiple, slow-growing tumors, might be followed with no treatment at all while the tumors are asymptomatic. If the pulmonary metastases grow rapidly, especially if multiple visceral sites are also involved or if the patient is symptomatic, an initial course of chemotherapy might be given. However, the response rate for DTIC chemotherapy is particularly poor for pulmonary metastases, and there is no evidence that the drug prolongs life.[250,500]

Brain and Spinal Cord

Melanoma ranks behind lung and breast carcinoma as the third most common tumor that metastasizes to the brain.[501] The brain is the initial site of metastases in 12% to 20% of patients and is usually associated with widespread visceral disease (Fig. 44-14).[145,240,246,250,502–505] At autopsy, cerebral metastases are present in 36% to 54% of patients.[230–240,241,250] The hemispheres are generally involved equally, with the cerebrum, usually the frontal lobe, involved most frequently, followed by the cerebellum, base of the brain, and spinal cord. Hydrocephalus is associated with about 33% of posterior fossa lesions. Cerebral metastases are solitary in only about 25% of patients.[246,504–507] An unusual feature of cerebral metastases is their propensity for hemorrhage, which occurs much more frequently than with other histologic types of metastases. Hemorrhage occurs in 33% to 50% of patients with melanoma metastases involving the brain.[504,508–510]

Headaches, alterations of mental status, and focal neurologic deficits are the most common symptoms of brain metastases.[245,502,505,507,508,511,512] A headache resulting from brain metastases characteristically begins as a mild ache, often in the morning. Seizures are more common in patients with melanoma metastases in the brain than in patients with other types of brain tumors but occur in only about 25% to

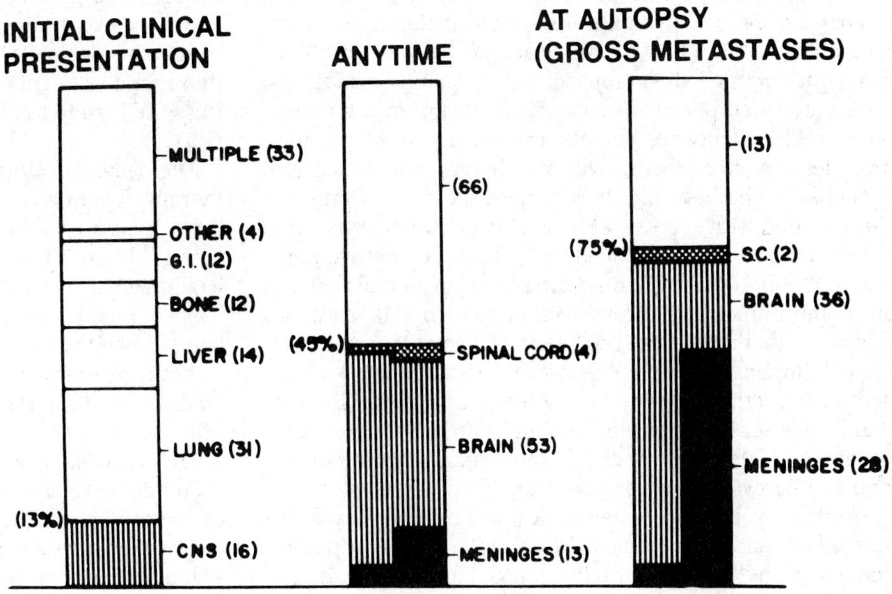

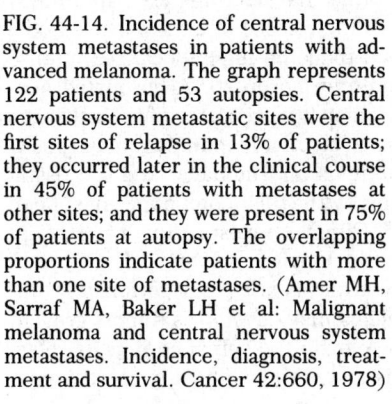

FIG. 44-14. Incidence of central nervous system metastases in patients with advanced melanoma. The graph represents 122 patients and 53 autopsies. Central nervous system metastatic sites were the first sites of relapse in 13% of patients; they occurred later in the clinical course in 45% of patients with metastases at other sites; and they were present in 75% of patients at autopsy. The overlapping proportions indicate patients with more than one site of metastases. (Amer MH, Sarraf MA, Baker LH et al: Malignant melanoma and central nervous system metastases. Incidence, diagnosis, treatment and survival. Cancer 42:660, 1978)

37% of melanoma patients with brain involvement.[508,511-513] It is also common for these melanoma patients to present with either subarachnoid or intracerebral hemorrhages.[504,508,509,514-519]

Routine brain scans are not useful for detecting occult metastases in asymptomatic patients in any disease stage. This was demonstrated in five separate series involving 504 patients with local or regional disease: not a single true-positive brain scan was obtained, whereas there were 11 (2%) false-positive brain scans.[245,252,254,520,521] In patients with Stage IV melanomas, cerebral metastases were detected by brain scan in 11% to 16% of patients studied, but all patients with positive scans had antecedent symptoms.[245,258,504,522]

The radiologic diagnosis of symptomatic melanoma metastases of the central nervous system (CNS) has been reviewed in several published series.[504,509] The best single test for the diagnosis of intracerebral metastases is CT with contrast agent enhancement.[504,509,512,523-525] The accuracy and sensitivity of the study makes it unnecessary in most cases to obtain either a radionuclide brain scan or electroencephalogram, unless equivocal findings warrant these complementary studies. Unlike CT, MR imaging does not produce artifacts from bone images, and it offers an advantage over CT for tumors at the superior vertex, posterior fossa, middle fossa, base of the skull, and orbits.

Leptomeningeal metastases can occur, usually in association with other distant metastases. Most melanoma patients with leptomeningeal involvement have signs or symptoms involving multiple areas, suggesting disseminated CNS disease. Signs and symptoms can result from involvement of the brain, cranial nerves, or spinal nerves.[526] Diagnosis depends on cytologic examination of spinal fluid. Single spinal fluid examinations have been shown to be positive in approximately one half of affected patients, but repeated spinal fluid assays have been positive in most patients.[526] Spinal fluid LDH levels, especially isoenzyme LDH-5, can be useful for diagnosis when infectious etiology is absent.[527]

Corticosteroids are the mainstay of initial treatment for brain metastases, the most effective being dexamethasone (up to 100 mg/day). This can reduce the edema around the tumor and relieve symptoms in most patients, at least temporarily.[528-530] The steroid dose can be tapered off in some patients and then stopped, but frequently symptoms are exacerbated during withdrawal, requiring maintenance on steroids. Eighty-six percent of patients with multiple brain lesions treated with radiation therapy remain steroid dependent, whereas only 33% of patients with solitary lesions treated with surgery with or without radiation therapy have remained steroid dependent.[513] Lack of improvement or exacerbation of symptoms during a trial of steroids can be due to intratumor hemorrhage with intracerebral hematoma. Radiation therapy is the treatment of choice for multiple tumors. Surgical excision with cranial irradiation is the most definitive treatment option for a solitary metastasis. Chemotherapy generally is not effective for brain metastases from melanoma,[250,502,511,529] although intrathecal chemotherapy needs to be evaluated more carefully.[526]

Surgical excision is preferred for solitary and surgically accessible lesions. A craniotomy is a relatively safe procedure (with an operative mortality of less than 5%) that alleviates symptoms in most patients and prevents further neurologic damage in patients with demonstrable metastases. It should be considered for some patients with symptomatic brain metastases, even when there is limited disease at other sites, since their estimated life span can exceed 2 to 3 months and their neurologic status usually improves. Whole brain irradiation is generally given postoperatively.[242,269,502,503] Although this combined approach appears to improve survival rates compared with surgery alone, there is a paucity of data concerning the use of adjunctive irradiation.

Survival in different series averages about 7 months for surgically treated patients (see Table 44-6) and ranges from 2 to 20 months.[242,258,267-269,501-503,505-508,531-534] Satisfactory improvement in neurologic condition occurs in the majority of patients. Survival results are influenced by remission duration, neurologic status at time of surgery, and the presence of metastases at other sites.[535] Although long-term survival is uncommon, a few patients will live 3 years or more after surgery.[246,506,508,533,536-538]

Radiation therapy should be considered if the lesions are multiple or located in an area that would preclude a safe operation. Brain metastases present a challenging radiotherapeutic management problem. Approximately half of all patients achieve objective improvement in functional status, but overall survival is of only 3 to 6 months from initiation of therapy. Changes in fractionation schedule either to high dose per fraction[275,539,540] or to accelerated twice daily treatment with dose escalation[541] have not yielded consistently improved results over those obtained with the regimen most commonly prescribed for brain metastases, 30 Gy delivered in 10 fractions over 2 weeks. In the subset of patients who have brain metastases only, without visceral disease, long-term survival is possible, and high-dose, large dose per fraction treatment schedules carrying a high risk of late brain injury should be avoided in these patients.

Two new strategies aimed at selective radiosensitization of melanoma metastases in the brain exploit kinetic and metabolic differences between the tumor and normal brain tissue. Halogenated pyrimides such as bromodeoxyuridine (BUdR) and iododeoxyuridine (IUdR) are incorporated into the DNA of proliferating cells, sensitizing them to conventional radiation therapy.[542] This approach is currently being tested in a Phase I/II study by the Radiation Therapy Oncology Group (RTOG).

The second strategy is based on boron neutron capture therapy. Thermal and epithermal neutrons are captured by the isotope boron-10 with the release of an α particle and a recoil lithium-7 nucleus, producing highly localized intense irradiation of cells containing boron-10. A boronated analogue of phenylalanine (which is a precursor of melanin) has been shown to concentrate selectively in melanoma deposits in both experimental animals and humans, and successful neutron capture therapy with this compound has been achieved in animals.[543] Clinical investigation of this approach is most advanced in Japan.

Spinal metastases are a devastating but fortunately unusual occurrence. Paraplegia may develop as tumors grow in one or more areas close to or in the spinal cord or its roots. The most common site is extradural. Clinically, the development of paraplegia may be preceded by back pain or radicular nerve pain with weakness or numbness of the leg or urinary incontinence.[512] It may progress to complete and irreversible paralysis within 24 hours.

Surgical decompression of obstructing spinal cord lesions is indicated in selected patients, although there is evidence that radiation therapy might be an effective alternative in some patients.[512,544] High doses of corticosteroids should be given as well. Early treatment intervention is essential, since the best results for both surgical and irradiation treatments have been achieved in patients with mild neurologic symptoms; there have been very few treatment responses in totally paraplegic patients. Patients with symptomatic but nonobstructive disease might be considered for radiation treatment of the local area.[277] Usually, this type of disease is caused by the extension of bone metastases into the surrounding spinal cord.

Gastrointestinal Tract

Melanoma is one of the types of tumors that most frequently metastasize to the GI tract. Metastases to the GI tract usually occur simultaneously in multiple sites. The individual lesions are exophytic or polypoid submucosal nodules that can be umbilicated or undergo central cavitation.[545–549] Metastases in the GI tract are difficult to detect with radiologic studies, so the routine use of these studies is not indicated for screening purposes.

Early involvement of the GI tract usually causes vague and subtle symptoms. Only occasionally do some acute and potentially catastrophic symptoms occur. The most common clinical manifestations are due to (1) chronic bleeding, resulting in anemia, anorexia, and weight loss, (2) obstruction of the small bowel, resulting in abdominal pain, nausea, and vomiting, or (3) acute bleeding, causing hematemesis or melena.[244,250,547,550–556]

Intussusception is a frequent cause of obstructive symptoms and other abdominal complaints. Numerous cases have been reported in the literature.[547,554,555,557] Intussusception usually follows a chronic or subacute course, characterized by an insidious onset. The triad of abdominal cramps, nausea without vomiting, and abdominal distention was the most consistent symptom complex in one series.[557] Frequently, the typical signs of palpable abdominal mass, bloody stools, and abdominal tenderness are lacking in these patients.

The diagnosis of GI metastases is usually made with barium contrast radiography or, more recently, with endoscopy. Several reviews have addressed the radiologic detection of metastatic melanoma involving the GI tract.[547–549,558] All patients undergoing an upper GI series for abdominal complaints should have a small bowel follow-through examination, since metastases are most likely to be present in this area. If the small bowel series is normal but there is strong clinical suspicion of metastases, a small bowel enteroclysis can be performed.

One of the most common symptoms of GI metastases is chronic bleeding. In anemic patients, this can be treated with repeated blood transfusions. Systemic therapy can be considered for patients with multiple GI lesions. Surgical excision is the treatment of choice for solitary metastases, if the patient's condition permits and there are no other visceral metastases.

Surgery is recommended for most patients with the acute complications of obstruction, massive bleeding, or perforation. These complications cannot be treated by other modalities, and the only alternative is to allow the patient to die. The final decision depends on the patient's overall condition, but symptoms can be successfully alleviated in most cases, and survival after surgical excision of the metastases averages 4 to 8 months.[240,242,244,267–269,550–555,557] In patients with multiple GI metastases, only lesions causing immediate symptoms should be removed unless those remaining are relatively few and can be safely excised. Survival of 2 to 5 years after excision of GI metastases has been reported in a few patients, most of whom underwent palliative excision of symptomatic solitary gastric or intestinal metastases.[240,242,267–269,550–555]

Obstruction is usually due to large polypoid lesions that mechanically obstruct the bowel or act as leading points for intussusception.[552,555,557] These submucosal lesions are generally removed with bowel resections or, occasionally, enterotomies, depending on the sites and numbers of lesions.

Massive or repeated episodes of bleeding requiring transfusions are uncommon and are likely to result from gastric metastases. Surgical treatment in most instances consists of segmental bowel resection or partial gastrectomy, although sometimes more extended surgery is required.[242,246,267–269,550–552,554]

Liver, Biliary Tract, and Spleen

Hepatic metastases occur in 5% to 20% of patients with metastatic melanoma in different clinical series but are found in the majority of cases at autopsy.[145,240,246,250,559] It is unusual for isolated liver metastases to occur in patients with cutaneous melanoma. Patients with liver metastases generally have widespread melanoma with liver involvement. The prognosis for these patients is poor (median survival of 2 to 4 months), and treatment options are few.

Screening tests for liver metastases should consist only of the history, physical examination, and measurement of serum liver chemistries. These are sufficiently accurate and the most cost-effective of all available tests. Numerous studies now clearly document the futility of using liver scintigraphy, ultrasound, or CT to screen for occult liver metastases in melanoma patients.[244,245,252,254,520,521,560] They are therefore neither warranted nor cost-effective as screening tests in patients with local or regional melanoma.

The patterns of abnormal liver chemistries that suggest liver metastases are elevated LDH and/or alkaline phosphatase levels in the presence of normal or only slightly elevated serum glutamic-oxaloacetic transaminase or bilirubin levels.[243,250,522,561] Measuring LDH levels is a clinically useful and specific test for detecting metastatic melanoma.[243] When liver metastases are suspected, the confirmatory radiologic tests to be considered are (1) radionuclide liver scintigraphy, (2) ultrasound, (3) CT, or (4) hepatic arteriography.[562] The studies actually used depend on availability and cost at individual hospitals, the interpretive skills of the radiologists, and the generation of equipment available, which is especially important for CT scanners and ultrasound units. Most comparative studies have found that abdominal CT scans are somewhat more accurate and reliable than ultrasound and radionuclide liver scans for evaluation of liver masses.[255,563–565]

Metastatic melanoma involving the gallbladder or bile ducts is found in 4% to 20% of patients at autopsy.[246,250,251] It can involve the serosal surfaces or appear as polypoid masses arising from the mucosa within the gallbladder. Rarely, these metastases can cause symptoms of cholecystitis manifested as fixed filling defects on a cholecystogram.[547,566–569] Patients with symptoms of gallbladder metastases should be considered for cholecystectomy if metastasis is confined to the gallbladder and if they are medically fit and have life expectancies exceeding several months. Short-term relief of symptoms is usually successful, but all reported patients have died within a year.[567–569]

Melanoma is one of the few tumors that metastasizes to the spleen.[240,244,246] It may rarely cause splenomegaly but is more often diagnosed as an incidental finding on liver-spleen scintigraphy or abdominal CT, or at laparotomy. Most patients with splenic metastases (up to 88%) have concomitant liver or pancreatic metastases.

Bone

Bone metastases occur infrequently (11% to 17%) in most clinical series but are more commonly observed in autopsy series (see Table 44-4).[240,246,570,571] Skeletal metastases generally occur in patients with widespread metastatic disease but occasionally represent the first evidence of recurrence.[570,571] The life span of these patients is short, but effective palliative treatment can be achieved in many cases, so it is worthwhile to pursue the diagnosis. In the asymptomatic melanoma patient, particularly with AJC Stage I or II disease, the yield of occult bone metastases on bone scan is too low to justify it as a screening procedure.[245,252,520–522,572]

Bone metastases from melanoma are medullary in location and destructive in nature. They generally appear osteolytic on radiographs and provoke little if any bone formation. Patterns of bone metastases have been described elsewhere.[570,571,573] Axial metastases account for up to 80% of bone lesions and are most common in the spine.[246,570,571] When they involve the vertebral body, there are often compression fractures that may lead to neurologic symptoms such as radicular back pain, paresthesia or paresis of the legs, or urinary retention. About 10% of lytic lesions occur in weight-bearing bones, which could result in pathologic fractures.[246,571]

Skeletal radionuclide scintigraphy has clearly established itself over radiographic surveys as the initial study for evaluating suspected bone metastases. However, abnormalities detected on bone scans are nonspecific and must be correlated with radiographic studies and patient histories (for fractures, trauma, arthritis, etc.) to distinguish between benign and malignant causes. It may be necessary to perform a bone biopsy to establish the diagnosis before instituting treatment.

The average life span of melanoma patients with bone metastases is 4 to 6 months, and even shorter when other sites are involved as well.[145,570,571] The treatment chosen depends on (1) the degree of symptoms, (2) the location and magnitude of bone lesions, and (3) the expected life span. Symptomatic metastases generally involve non-weight-bearing bones, particularly the spine or ribs. In these cases, radiation therapy to the lesions will usually give relief for up to 6 months; however, the fields should generally be restricted to the area of symptomatic involvement. A high-dose, short-course schedule will minimize patient travel time and hospitalization.[277,574] Currently available chemotherapy is not generally effective for palliation of skeletal metastases.[575]

Irradiation is effective in palliating the pain of bone metastases in the great majority of patients. A fractionation schedule of 30 Gy in 10 fractions is usually recommended, although it has not been established to be the optimum in any comparative study. More abbreviated schedules, such as 20 Gy in five fractions, are effective but are not recommended for spinal or pelvic bone metastases requiring large fields because of acute GI toxicity. Pathologic fractures in long bones should be stabilized before radiation therapy is initiated. In weight-bearing long bones judged radiographically to be at risk for pathologic fracture, prophylactic internal fixation is advisable. Radiation therapy should be initiated immediately after surgery in these patients to minimize the period of hospitalization. Wound healing is not compromised by the recommended dose of 30 Gy in 10 fractions delivered with megavoltage beams.

Patients with compression fractures of the vertebrae that result in cord compression require prompt diagnosis and treatment to avoid paralysis. Treatment may entail decompressive laminectomy with postoperative radiation therapy or irradiation alone, depending on the extent of the disease and the patient's overall medical condition.

Kidneys and Urinary Tract

Although metastatic melanoma frequently appears in the kidneys and urinary tract at autopsy, metastases in these sites rarely cause clinically recognizable symptoms, and usually these symptoms are terminal manifestations of the disease. Solitary or symptomatic metastases that are amenable to treatment do, however, occur occasionally.

Renal metastases generally occur as multiple, small (3–10 mm) cortical nodules that are usually asymptomatic but can cause hematuria or melanuria. Some may be large enough to cause obstructive lesions with hydronephrosis or bleeding.[576] Although patients with bladder metastases commonly have multiple subepithelial pedunculated or sessile lesions, solitary lesions can occur.[577–581]

Kidney and urinary tract metastases generally are asymptomatic until the terminal stages of disease, and death usually occurs within 1 to 4 months after the clinical diagnosis is made. Metastatic melanoma can occasionally mimic primary renal or bladder carcinomas, both endoscopically and radiographically.[579] The most common symptom prompting a urinary tract investigation is gross or microscopic hematuria.[240,246] In the majority of patients, the diagnosis of metastases can be made by intravenous pyelography, cystography, cystoscopy, or radiologic imaging techniques (CT or ultrasound). Occasionally, cytologic examination of the urine will reveal melanoma cells.[582]

Bladder metastases can be treated by transurethral resection or partial cystectomy, depending on their number, size, and location.[577] Symptoms usually can be relieved, but survival after treatment averages only 3 to 6 months. Rarely do patients survive more than 1 year. Kidney and ureteral metastases causing bleeding or obstruction can be treated by ureteronephrectomy in selected patients,[576,583] or by a ureteral stent if the patient is not a candidate for surgery. In most cases, survival averages only 4 months.

Prostate and urethral metastases can also cause hematuria, dysuria, or hesitancy.[584] Symptomatic prostatic metastases occur rarely but can be treated by transurethral resection or open prostatectomy.[576,584] Obstructive urethral disease can also be decompressed by a suprapubic cystostomy in poor-risk patients.

Metastases from Unknown Primary Sites

A small proportion of melanoma patients present with metastatic disease in the lymph nodes or at distant sites, but no detectable primary site. Patients presenting with occult primary melanoma comprise between 1% and 12% of patients with metastatic disease.[139,585-591] About two thirds of these patients present with tumors in lymph nodes (most frequently in the axilla) and one third with distant metastases (most frequently in the skin, subcutaneous tissues, lungs, and brain).

All patients with occult primary melanoma should be examined carefully for potential sequestered primary lesions, especially in the eye and scalp. In this group of patients, it is important to get a careful history of prior treatment for nevi. About 10% to 20% of patients will describe previous nevi within the lymphatic drainage areas of metastatic lymph nodes. Approximately one third of patients have undergone treatment for pigmented lesions, often by nondiagnostic procedures such as curettage or diathermy.[236,592] Any available biopsy specimens from previously excised pigmented lesions should be reevaluated by an experienced pathologist, because occasionally these will turn out to be well-differentiated primary melanomas on review. However, two thirds of patients give no history of suspicious pigmented lesions. There is a high likelihood that a high proportion, if not most, of these patients have had primary cutaneous melanoma lesions that have completely regressed. Careful skin examinations can reveal areas of depigmentation or leukoderma in up to one third of patients, and biopsies of these sites can show the same triad—fibrosis, mononuclear cell infiltrates, and melanophages.[593] Patients with occult primary melanoma should be examined for areas of regressed primary lesions characterized by patches of depigmentation; examination can be facilitated by a Wood's ultraviolet lamp. A second explanation for the phenomenon of unknown primary melanoma is that some melanomas can arise de novo in lymph nodes and viscera. Melanocytes can occasionally be found around lymph nodes, in meninges, and in a variety of viscera.[56,57]

The survival rate of patients with unknown primary lesions is no different from that of patients with metastatic cutaneous melanoma when matched for prognostic factors. When appropriate, surgical management should be considered first. Lymphadenectomy for nodal disease can be associated with long-term survival similar to the results seen in patients with cutaneous metastases to lymph nodes; survival is generally better if only one node is involved than if multiple nodes contain tumors. Two-year survival rates of 30% to 40% can be observed in patients with skin and subcutaneous metastases from both cutaneous and unknown primary sites.[236,588]

A small proportion of melanoma patients present with metastatic disease either in lymph nodes or at distant sites, and no primary site can be detected. Patients presenting with occult primary melanoma comprise between 1% and 12% of patients with distant metastatic disease.[139,585-591] Overall, about two thirds of patients with unknown primary melanomas present with tumor in lymph nodes (most frequently in the axilla) and one third with distant metastases (most frequently skin, subcutaneous tissue, lung, and brain).

REFERENCES

1. McLeod GR, David NC, Little JH et al: Melanoma in Queensland, Australia: Experience in the Queensland Melanoma Project. In Balch CM, Milton GW (eds): Cutaneous Melanoma: Clinical Management and Treatment Results Worldwide, p 379. Philadelphia, JB Lippincott, 1985
2. Roush GC, Schymurs M, Holford TR: Risk for cutaneous melanoma in recent Connecticut birth cohorts. Am J Public Health 75:679, 1985
3. Redman JC, Mora DB: Malignant melanomas of the skin diagnosed and treated in Albuquerque, New Mexico in 1980. J Dermatol Surg Oncol 8:41, 1982
4. Rigel DS, Kopf AW, Friedman RJ: The rate of malignant melanoma in the US: Are we making an impact? J Am Acad Dermatol 17:1050, 1987
5. Beral V, Evans S, Shaw H et al: Cutaneous factors related to the risk of malignant melanoma. Br J Dermatol 109:165, 1983
6. Gellin GA, Kopf AW, Garfinkel L: Malignant melanoma: A controlled study of possibly associated factors. Arch Dermatol 99:43, 1969
7. Scheibner A, Milton GW, McCarthy WH et al: Multiple primary melanoma: A review of 90 cases. Aust J Dermatol 23:1, 1982
8. Bellet RE, Vaisman I, Mastrangelo MJ et al: Multiple primary malignancies in patients with cutaneous melanoma. Cancer 40:1974, 1977
9. Lynch HT, Frichot BC III, Lynch J et al: Family studies of malignant melanoma and associated cancer. Surg Gynecol Obstet 141:517, 1975
10. Moseley HS, Giuliano AE, Storm FK et al: Multiple primary melanoma. Cancer 43:939, 1979
11. Veronesi U, Cascinelli N, Bufalino R: Evaluation of the risk of multiple primaries in malignant cutaneous melanoma. Tumori 62:127, 1976
12. Elder DE, Goldman LI, Goldman SC et al: Dysplastic nevus syndrome: A phenotypic association of sporadic cutaneous melanoma. Cancer 46:1787, 1980
13. Wallace DC, Exton LA, McLeod GRC: Genetic factor in malignant melanoma. Cancer 27:1262, 1971
14. Acton RT, Balch CM, Budowle B et al: Immunogenetics of melanoma. In Reisfeld RA, Ferrone S (eds): Melanoma Antigens and Antibodies, p 1. New York, Plenum Press, 1982
15. Greene MH, Reimer RR, Clark WH Jr et al: Precursor lesions in familial melanoma. Semin Oncol 5:85, 1978
16. Lynch HT, Frichot BC III, Lynch JF: Familial atypical multiple mole–melanoma syndrome. J Med Genet 15:352, 1978
17. Reimer RR, Clark WH Jr, Greene MH et al: Precursor lesions in familial melanoma: A new genetic preneoplastic syndrome. JAMA 239:744, 1978
18. Wallace DC, Beardmore GL, Exton LA: Familial malignant melanoma. Ann Surg 177:15, 1973
19. Clark WH Jr, Reimer RR, Greene M et al: Origin of familial malignant melanomas from heritable melanocytic lesions: "The B-K mole syndrome." Arch Dermatol 114:732, 1978
20. Elder DE, Green MH, Guerry D et al: The dysplastic nevus syndrome: Our definition. Am J Dermatopathol 4:455, 1982
21. Acton RT, Balch CM, Barger BO et al: The occurrence of melanoma and its relation-

ship with host, lifestyle and environmental factors. In Costanzi JJ (ed): Malignant Melanoma 1, p 151. The Hague, Martinus Nijhoff, 1983
22. Clark DA, Necheles T, Nathanson L et al: Apparent HL-A5 deficiency in malignant melanoma. Transplantation 15:326, 1973
23. Barger BO, Acton RT, Soong S-j et al: Increase of HLA-DR4 in melanoma patients from Alabama. Cancer Res 42:4276, 1982
24. Budowle B, Barger BO, Balch CM et al: Associations of properdin factor B with melanoma. Cancer Genet Cytogenet 5:247, 1982
25. Pandey JP, Johnson AH, Funderberg HH et al: HLA antigens and immunoglobulin allotypes in patients with malignant melanoma. Hum Immunol 2:185, 1981
26. Walter G, Brachtel R, Hilling M: On the incidence of blood group O and Gm phenotypes in patients with malignant melanoma. Hum Genet 49:71, 1979
27. Clark WH Jr, Ainsworth AM, Bernardino EA et al: The developmental biology of primary human malignant melanomas. Semin Oncol 2:83, 1975
28. Milton GW, Balch CM, Shaw HM: Clinical characteristics. In Balch CM, Milton GW (eds): Clinical Melanoma: Clinical Management and Treatment Results Worldwide, p 13. Philadelphia, JB Lippincott, 1985
29. Mihm MC Jr, Fitzpatrick TB, Lane-Brown MM et al: Early detection of primary cutaneous malignant melanoma: A color atlas. N Engl J Med 289:989, 1973
30. Sober AJ, Fitzpatrick TB, Mihm MC Jr et al: Early recognition of cutaneous melanoma. JAMA 242:2795, 1979
31. Clark WH Jr, From L, Bernardino EA et al: The histogenesis and biologic behavior of primary human malignant melanomas of the skin. Cancer Res 29:705, 1969
32. McGovern VJ, Murad TM: Pathology of melanoma: An overview. In Balch CM, Milton GW (eds): Cutaneous Melanoma: Clinical Management and Treatment Results Worldwide, p 29. Philadelphia, JB Lippincott, 1985
33. Mihm MC Jr, Clark WH Jr, From L: The clinical diagnosis, classification and histogenetic concepts of the early stages of cutaneous malignant melanomas. N Engl J Med 284:1078, 1971
34. Manci EA, Balch CM, Murad TM et al: Polypoid melanoma, a virulent variant of the nodular growth pattern. Am J Clin Pathol 75:810, 1981
35. Urist MM, Balch CM, Soong S-j, et al: Head and neck melanoma in 536 clnical stage I patients: A prognostic factors analysis and results of surgical treatment. Ann Surg 200:769, 1984
36. McGovern VJ, Shaw HM, Milton GW et al: Is malignant melanoma arising in a Hutchinson's melanotic freckle a separate entity? Histopathology 4:235, 1980
37. Clark WH Jr, Mihm MC Jr: Lentigo maligna and lentigo-maligna melanoma. Am J Pathol 55:39, 1969
38. Arrington JH III, Reed RJ, Ichinose H: Plantar lentiginous melanoma: A distinctive variant of human cutaneous malignant melanoma. Am J Surg Pathol 1:131, 1977
39. Coleman WP III, Loria PR, Reed RJ et al: Acral lentiginous melanoma. Arch Dermatol 116:773, 1980
40. Krementz ET, Reed RJ, Coleman WP et al: Acral lentiginous melanoma: A clinicopathologic entity. Ann Surg 195:632, 1982
41. Seiji M, Takahashi M: Acral melanoma in Japan. Hum Pathol 13:607, 1982
42. Sondergaard K, Olsen G: Malignant melanoma of the foot: A clinicopathological study of 125 primary cutaneous malignant melanomas. Acta Pathol Microbiol Immunol Scand [A] 88:275, 1980
43. Feibleman CE, Stoll H, Maize JC: Melanomas of the palm, sole and nailbed: A clinicopathologic study. Cancer 46:2492, 1980
44. Paladugu RR, Winberg CD, Yonemoto RH: Acral lentiginous melanoma: A clinicopathologic study of 36 patients. Cancer 52:161, 1983
45. Patterson RH, Helwig EB: Subungual malignant melanoma: A clinical-pathologic study. Cancer 46:2074, 1980
46. Hughes LE, Horgan I, Taylor BA et al: Malignant melanoma of the hand and foot: Diagnosis and management. Br J Surg 72:813, 1985
47. Lopansri S, Mihm MC Jr: Clinical and pathological correlation of malignant melanoma. J Cutan Pathol 6:180, 1979
48. Balch CM, Soong S-j, Shaw HM: A comparison of worldwide melanoma data. In Balch CM, Milton GW (eds): Cutaneous Melanoma: Clinical Management and Treatment Results Worldwide, p 507. Philadelphia, JB Lippincott, 1985
49. Balch CM, Urist MM, Maddox WA et al: Melanoma in the Southern United States: Experience at the University of Alabama in Birmingham. In Balch CM, Milton GW (eds): Cutaneous Melanoma: Clinical Management and Treatment Results Worldwide, p 397. Philadelphia, JB Lippincott, 1985
50. Reintgen DS, McCarty KM Jr, Cox E et al: Malignant melanoma in black American and white American populations: A comparative review. JAMA 248:1856, 1982
51. McCarthy WH, Shaw HM, Milton GW et al: Melanoma in New South Wales, Australia: Experience at the Sydney Melanoma Unit. In Balch CM, Milton GW (eds): Cutaneous Melanoma: Clinical Management and Treatment Results Worldwide, p 371. Philadelphia, JB Lippincott, 1985
52. Pack GT, Oropeza R: Subungual melanoma. Surg Gynecol Obstet 124:571, 1967
53. Papachristou DN, Fortner JG: Melanoma arising under the nail. J Surg Oncol 21:219, 1982
54. Weston JA: The migration and differentiation of neural crest cells. Adv Morphol 8:41, 1970
55. Le Douarin N: Migration and differentiation of neural crest cells. Curr Top Dev Biol 61:31, 1980
56. Woodruff JM: Pathology of malignant melanoma: Part I. Clin Bull 6:15, 1976
57. Ridolfi RL, Rosen PP, Thaler H: Nevus cell aggregates associated with lymph nodes: Estimated frequency and clinical significance. Cancer 39:164, 1977
58. Wick MM, Byers L, Frei E III: L-dopa: Selective toxicity for melanoma cells in vitro. Science 197:468, 1977
59. Pawelek JM, Lerner AB: 5,6-dihydroxyindole is a melanin precursor showing potent cytotoxicity. Nature 276:627, 1978
60. Morrison ME, Yagi MJ, Cohen G: In vitro studies of 2,4-dihydroxyphenylalanine, a prodrug targeted against malignant melanoma cells. Proc Natl Acad Sci USA 82:2960, 1985
61. Sherwin SA, Sliski AH, Todaro GJ: Human melanoma cells have both nerve growth factor and nerve growth factor-specific receptors on their cell surfaces. Proc Natl Acad Sci USA 76:1288, 1979
62. Marquardt H, Todaro G: Human transforming growth factor: Production by a melanoma cell line, purification, and initial characterization. J Biol Chem 257:5220, 1982
63. Houghton AN, Real FX, Davis LJ et al: Phenotypic heterogeneity of melanoma: Relation to the differentiation program of melanoma cells. J Exp Med 164:812, 1987
64. Herlyn M, Clark WH, Rodeck V et al: Biology of tumor progression in human melanocytes. Invest Pathol 56:461, 1987
65. Halaban R, Ghosh S, Baird A: bFGF is the putative growth factor for human melanocytes. In Vitro Cell Dev Biol 23:47, 1987
66. Eisinger M, Marko O, Ogata S-I et al: Growth regulation of human melanocytes: Mitogenic factors in extracts of melanoma, astrocytoma and fibroblast cell lines. Science 229:984, 1985
67. Ogata S-I, Furuhashi Y, Eisinger M: Growth stimulation of human melanocytes: Identification and characterization of melanoma-derived melanocyte growth factor (M-McGF). Biochem Biophys Res Commun 146:1204, 1987
68. Houghton AN, Eisinger M, Albino AP et al: Surface antigens of melanocytes and melanomas: Markers of melanoma differentiation and melanoma subsets. J Exp Med 156:1755, 1982
69. Wong G, Pawelek J: MSH promotes the activation of pre-existing tyrosinase molecules in Cloudman S91 melanoma cells. Nature 255:644, 1975
70. Mufson RA, Fisher PB, Weinstein IB: Effect of phorbol ester tumor promoters on the expression of melanogenesis in B-16 melanoma cells. Cancer Res 39:3915, 1979
71. Houghton AN, Real FX, Davis LJ et al: Phenotypic heterogeneity of melanoma: Relation to the differentiation program of melanoma cells. J Exp Med 154:812, 1987
72. Becher R, Gibas Z, Karakousis C et al: Nonrandom chromosome changes in malignant melanoma. Cancer Res 43:5010, 1983
73. Becher R, Gibas Z, Sandberg AA: Chromosome 6 in malignant melanoma. Cancer Genet Cytogenet 9:173, 1983
74. Trent JM, Rosenfeld SB, Meyskens FL: Chromosome 6q involvement in human malignant melanoma. Cancer Genet Cytogenet 9:177, 1983
75. Pathak S, Drwinga HL, Hsu TC: Involvement of chromosome 6 in rearrangements in human malignant melanoma cell lines. Cytogenet Cell Genet 36:573, 1983
76. Balaban G, Herlyn M, Guerry D et al: Cytogenetics of human malignant melanoma and premalignant lesions. Cancer Genet Cytogenet 11:429, 1984
77. Reichmann A, Martin P, Levin B: Chromosome $6q^{-}$ in metastatic melanoma involving the large bowel. Cancer Genet Cytogenet 13:275, 1984
78. Rey JA, Bello MJ, de Campos JM: Cytogenetic findings in a human malignant melanoma metastatic to the brain. Cancer Genet Cytogenet 16:179, 1985
79. Herlyn M, Thurbin J, Balaban G et al: Characteristics of cultured human melanocytes isolated from different stages of tumor progression. Cancer Res 45:5670, 1985
80. Balaban GB, Herlyn M, Clark WH Jr et al: Karyotypic evolution in human malignant melanoma. Cancer Genet Cytogenet 19:113, 1986
81. Pedersen MI, Bennett JW, Wang N: Nonrandom chromosome structural aberrations and oncogene loci in human malignant melanoma. Cancer Genet Cytogenet 20:11, 1986
82. Cowan JM, Halaban R, Lane AT et al: The involvement of 6p in melanoma. Cancer Genet Cytogenet 20:255, 1986
83. Ohyashiki JH, Ohyashiki K, Gibas Z et al: Cytogenetic findings in a malignant melanoma and its derived cell line. Cancer Genet Cytogenet 23:77, 1986
84. Bishop JM: The molecular genetics of cancers. Science 235:305, 1987
85. Albino AP, LeStrange R, Oliff AI et al: Transforming *ras* genes from human melanoma: A manifestation of tumor heterogeneity? Nature 308:69, 1984
86. Padua RA, Barrass N, Currie GA: A novel transforming gene in a human malignant melanoma cell line. Nature 311:671, 1984
87. Albino AP: The role of oncogenes in the pathogenesis of malignant melanoma. In Nathanson L (ed): Basic and Clinical Aspects of Malignant Melanoma, p 3. Boston, Martinus Nijhoff, 1987
88. Albino AP, Houghton AN, Eisinger M et al: Class II histocompatibility antigen expression in human melanocytes transformed by Ha-MSV and Ki-MSV retroviruses. J Exp Med 164:1710, 1986
89. Krontiris TG, DiMartino NA, Colb M et al: Unique allelic restriction fragments of the human Ha-*ras* locus in leukocyte and tumor DNA of cancer patients. Nature 313:369, 1985
90. Gerhard DS, Dracopoli NC, Bale SJ et al: Evidence against Ha-*ras*-1 involvement in sporadic and familial melanoma. Nature 325:73–75, 1987
91. Greene MH, Goldin LR, Clark WH Jr et al: Familial cutaneous malignant melanoma: Autosomal dominant trait possibly linked to the Rh locus. Proc Natl Acad Sci USA 80:6071, 1983
92. Dracopoli NC, Houghton AN, Old LJ: Loss of polymorphic restriction fragments in malignant melanoma: Implications for tumor heterogeneity. Proc Natl Acad Sci USA 82:1470, 1985
93. Dracopoli NC, Alhadeff B, Houghton AN: Loss of heterozygosity at autosomal and

X-linked loci during tumor progression in a patient with melanoma. Cancer Res 47:3995, 1987
94. Lee JAH: The causation of melanoma. In Balch CM, Milton GW (eds): Cutaneous Melanoma: Clinical Management and Treatment Results Worldwide, p 303. Philadelphia, JB Lippincott, 1985
95. Lee JAH: Melanoma and exposure to sunlight. Epidemiol Rev 4:110, 1982
96. Berkelhammer J, Oxenhandler RW: Evaluation of premalignant and malignant lesions during the induction of mouse melanomas. Cancer Res 46:2923, 1987
97. Pawlowski A, Haberman HF, Menon IA: Junctional and compound pigmented nevi induced by 9,10-demethyl-1, benzanthracene in skin of albino guinea pigs. Cancer Res 36:2813, 1976
98. Kripke ML, Fisher MS: Immunologic parameters of ultraviolet carcinogenesis. JNCI 57:211, 1976
99. Crombie IK: Variation of melanoma incidence with latitude in North America and Europe. Br J Cancer 40:774, 1979
100. Lee JAH: Melanoma in cancer epidemiology and prevention. In Schottenfeld D, Fraumeni JF Jr (eds): Cancer: Epidemiology and Prevention, p 984. Philadelphia, WB Saunders, 1982
101. Elwood JM, Gallagher RP: Site distribution of malignant melanoma. Can Med Assoc J 128:1400, 1983
102. Katz L, Ben-Tuvla S, Steinitz R: Malignant melanoma of the skin in Israel: Effect of migration. In Magnus K (ed): Trends in Cancer Incidence, p 419. Washington, DC, Hemisphere, 1982
103. Newell GR: Is ultraviolet irradiation the sole cause of melanoma? Melanoma Lett 5:4, 1987
104. Jensen OM, Bolander AM: Trends in malignant melanoma of the skin. World Health Stat Q 33:2, 1980
105. Greene A: Incidence and reporting of cutaneous melanoma in Queensland. Aust J Dermatol 23:105, 1982
106. McLeod GR, Davis NC, Little JH et al: Melanoma in Queensland, Australia: Experience in the Queensland Melanoma Project. In Balch CM, Milton GW (eds): Cutaneous Melanoma: Clinical Management and Treatment Results Worldwide, p 379. Philadelphia, JB Lippincott, 1985
107. Eldh J, Boeryd B, Suurkula M et al: Melanoma in Sweden: Experience at the University of Goteborg. In Balch CM, Milton GW (eds): Cutaneous Melanoma: Clinical Management and Treatment Results Worldwide, p 469. Philadelphia, JB Lippincott, 1985
108. Crombie IK: Radical differences in melanoma incidence. Br J Cancer 40:185, 1979
109. Lam K-H, Wong J: Melanoma in Hong Kong: Experience at the Queen Mary Hospital. In Balch CM, Milton GW (eds): Cutaneous Melanoma: Clinical Management and Treatment Results Worldwide, p 495. Philadelphia, JB Lippincott, 1985
110. Balch CM, Shaw HM, Soong S-j et al: Changing trends in the clinical pathological features of melanoma. In Balch CM, Milton GW (eds): Cutaneous Melanoma: Clinical Management and Treatment Results Worldwide, p 313. Philadelphia, JB Lippincott, 1985
111. Balch CM, Soong S-j, Milton GW et al: A comparison of prognostic factors and surgical results in 1,786 patients with localized (stage I) melanoma treated in Alabama, USA, and New South Wales, Australia. Ann Surg 196:677, 1982
112. Breslow A: Thickness, cross-sectional areas and depth of invasion in the prognosis of cutaneous melanoma. Ann Surg 172:902, 1970
113. Goldsmith HS: Melanoma: An overview. CA 29:194, 1979
114. McNeer G, Das Gupta TK: Prognosis in malignant melanoma. Surgery 56:512, 1964
115. Beahrs OH, Myers MH: Manual for Staging of Cancer, American Joint Committee on Cancer, p 117. Philadelphia, JB Lippincott, 1983
116. Ketcham AS, Balch CM: Classification and staging systems. In Balch CM, Milton GW (eds): Cutaneous Melanoma: Clinical Management and Treatment Results Worldwide, p 55. Philadelphia, JB Lippincott, 1985
117. Balch CM, Soong S-j, Shaw HM, et al: An analysis of prognostic factors in 4000 patients with cutaneous melanoma. In Balch CM, Milton GW (eds): Cutaneous Melanoma: Clinical Management and Treatment Results Worldwide, p 321. Philadelphia, JB Lippincott, 1985
118. Day CL Jr, Sober AJ, Kopf AW: A prognostic model for clinical stage I melanoma of the lower extremity: Location on foot as independent risk factor for recurrent disease. Surgery 89:599, 1981
119. Day CL Jr, Sober AJ, Kopf AW: A prognostic model for clinical stage I melanoma of the upper extremity: The importance of anatomic subsites in predicting recurrent disease. Ann Surg 193:436, 1981
120. Balch CM, Murad TM, Soong S-j et al: A multifactorial analysis of melanoma: Prognostic histopathological features comparing Clark's and Breslow's staging methods. Ann Surg 188:732, 1978
121. Cascinelli N, Morabito A, Bufalino R, et al: Prognosis of stage I melanoma of the skin. Int J Cancer 26:733, 1980
122. Drzewiecki KT, Andersen PK: Survival with malignant melanoma: A regression analysis of prognostic factors. Cancer 49:2414, 1982
123. Schmoeckel C, Bockelbrink A, Bockelbrink H et al: Low- and high-risk malignant melanoma: I. Evaluation of clinical and histological prognosticators in 585 cases. Eur J Cancer Clin Oncol 19:227, 1983
124. Shaw HM, McGovern VJ, Milton GW et al: Histologic features of tumors and the female superiority in survival from malignant melanoma. Cancer 45:1604, 1980
125. Shaw HM, McGovern VJ, Milton GW et al: Malignant melanoma: Influence of site of lesion and age of patient in the female superiority in survival. Cancer 46:2731, 1980
126. Balch CM, Soong S-j, Milton GW et al: A comparison of prognostic factors and surgical results in 1,786 patients with localized (stage I) melanoma treated in Alabama, USA, and New South Wales, Australia. Ann Surg 196:677, 1982
127. Balch CM, Murad TM, Soong S-j et al: Tumor thickness as a guide to surgical management of clinical stage I melanoma patients. Cancer 43:883, 1979
128. Breslow A: Thickness, cross-sectional areas and depth of invasion in the prognosis of cutaneous melanoma. Ann Surg 172:902, 1970
129. Day CL Jr, Lew RA, Mihm MC Jr et al: The natural break points for primary-tumor thickness in clinical stage I melanoma. N Engl J Med 305:1155, 1981
130. Soong S-j: A computerized mathematical model and scoring system for predicting outcome in melanoma patients. In Balch CM, Milton GW (eds): Cutaneous Melanoma: Clinical Management and Treatment Results Worldwide, p 353. Philadelphia, JB Lippincott, 1985
131. Day CL Jr, Sober AJ, Kopf AW et al: A prognostic model for clinical stage I melanoma of the trunk: Location near the midline is not an independent risk factor for recurrent disease. Am J Surg 142:247, 1981
132. Eldh J, Boeryd B, Peterson LE: Prognostic factors in cutaneous malignant melanoma in stage I: A clinical, morphological and multivariate analysis. Scand J Plast Reconstr Surg 12:243, 1978
133. Prade M, Bognel C, Charpentier P et al: Malignant melanoma of the skin: Prognostic factors derived from a multifactorial analysis of 239 cases. Am J Dermatopathol 4:411, 1982
134. Schmoeckel C, Bockelbrink A, Bockelbrink H et al: Low- and high-risk malignant melanoma: II. Multivariate analyses for a prognostic classification. Eur J Cancer Clin Oncol 19:237, 1983
135. van der Esch EP, Cascinelli N, Preda F et al: Stage I melanoma of the skin: Evaluation of prognosis according to histologic characteristics. Cancer 48:1668, 1981
136. Cox EB: Prognostic factors in malignant melanoma. In Seigler HF (ed): Clinical Management of Melanoma, p 279. The Hague, Martinus Nijhoff, 1982
137. Hacene K, Le Doussal V, Brunet M et al: Prognostic index for clinical stage I cutaneous malignant melanoma. Cancer Res 43:2991, 1983
138. Day CL Jr, Sober AJ, Kopf AW et al: A prognostic model for clinical stage I melanoma of the upper extremity: The importance of anatomic subsites in predicting recurrent disease. Ann Surg 193:436, 1981
139. Balch CM, Soong S-j, Murad TM et al.: A multifactorial analysis of melanoma: III. Prognostic factors in melanoma patients with lymph node metastases (stage II). Ann Surg 193:377, 1981
140. Balch CM, Soong S-j, Murad TM et al: A multifactorial analysis of melanoma: II. Prognostic factors in patients with stage I (localized) melanoma. Surgery 86:343, 1979
141. Cohen MH, Ketcham AS, Feix EL et al: Prognostic factors in patients undergoing lymphadenectomy for malignant melanoma. Ann Surg 186:635, 1977
142. Day CL Jr, Sober AJ, Lew RA et al: Malignant melanoma patients with positive nodes and relatively good prognoses: Microstaging retains prognostic significance in clinical stage I melanoma patients with metastases to regional nodes. Cancer 47:955, 1981
143. Callery C, Cochran AJ, Roe DJ: Factors prognostic for survival in patients with malignant melanoma spread to the regional lymph nodes. Ann Surg 196:69, 1982
144. Cascinelli N, Nava M, Vaglini M et al: Melanoma in Italy: Experience at the National Cancer Institute of Milan. In Balch CM, Milton GW (eds): Cutaneous Melanoma: Clinical Management and Treatment Results Worldwide, p 447, Philadelphia, JB Lippincott, 1985
145. Balch CM, Soong S-j, Murad TM et al: A multifactorial analysis of melanoma: IV. Prognostic factors in 200 melanoma patients with distant metastases (stage III). J Clin Oncol 1:126, 1983
146. Presant CA, Bartolucci AA, Southeastern Cancer Study Group: Prognostic factors in metastatic malignant melanoma: The Southeastern Cancer Study Group experience. Cancer 49:2192, 1982
147. Urist MM, Balch CM, Milton GW: Surgical management of the primary melanoma. In Balch CM, Milton GW (eds): Cutaneous Melanoma: Clinical Management and Treatment Results Worldwide, p 71. Philadelphia, JB Lippincott, 1985
148. Bagley FH, Cady B, Lee A et al: Changes in clinical presentation and management of malignant melanoma. Cancer 47:2126, 1981
149. Jones WM, Williams WJ, Roberts MM et al: Malignant melanoma of the skin: Prognostic value of clinical features and the role of treatment in 111 cases. Br J Cancer 22:437, 1968
150. Cascinelli N, van der Esch EP, Breslow A et al: Stage I melanoma of the skin: The problem of resection margins. Eur J Cancer 16:1079, 1980
151. Day CL Jr, Mihm MC Jr, Sober AJ et al: Narrower margins for clinical stage I malignant melanoma. N Engl J Med 306:479, 1982
152. Elder DE, Guerry D IV, Heiberger RM et al: Optimal resection margin for cutaneous malignant melanoma. Plast Reconstr Surg 71:66, 1983
153. Milton GW, Shaw HM, Farago GA et al: Tumour thickness and the site and time of first recurrence in cutaneous malignant melanoma (stage I). Br J Surg 67:543, 1980
154. Ackerman AB: Malignant melanoma in situ: The fat, curable stage of malignant melanoma. Pathology 17:298, 1985
155. Jones RE Jr, Cash ME, Ackerman AB: Malignant melanomas mistaken histologically for junctional nevi. In Ackerman AB (ed): Pathology of Malignant Melanoma, p 93. New York, Masson, 1981
156. Kelly JW, Sagebiel RW, Calderon W et al: The frequency of local recurrence and microsatellites as a guide to re-excision margins for cutaneous malignant melanoma. Ann Surg 6:759, 1984

157. Breslow A, Macht SD: Optimal size of resection margin for thin cutaneous melanoma. Surg Gynecol Obstet 145:691, 1977
158. Roses DF, Harris MN, Rigel D et al: Local and in-transit metastases following definitive excision for primary cutaneous malignant melanoma. Ann Surg 198:65, 1983
159. Schmoeckel C, Bockelbrink A, Bockelbrink H et al: Low- and high-risk malignant melanoma: Prognostic significance of the resection margin. Eur J Cancer Clin Oncol 19:237, 1983
160. Cosimi AB, Sober AJ, Mihm MC: Conservative surgical management of superficially invasive cutaneous melanoma. Cancer 53:1256, 1984
161. Milton GW, Shaw HM, McCarthy WH: Resection margins of melanoma. Aust NZ J Surg 55:225, 1985
162. Veronesi U, Cascinelli N, Adamus J et al: Primary cutaneous melanoma 2 mm less in thickness: Results of a randomized study comparing wide with narrow surgical excision. A preliminary report. N Engl Med 318:1159, 1988
163. Harwood AR: Conventional fractionated radiotherapy for 51 patients with lentigo maligna and lentigo maligna melanoma. Int J Radiat Oncol Biol Phys 9:1019, 1983
164. Briele HA, Beattie CW, Ronan SG et al: Late recurrence of cutaneous melanoma. Arch Surg 118:800, 1983
165. Krementz ET, Ryan RF, Carter RD et al: Hyperthermic regional perfusion for melanoma of the limbs. In Balch CM, Milton GW (eds): Cutaneous Melanoma: Clinical Management and Treatment Results Worldwide, p 171. Philadelphia, JB Lippincott, 1985
166. Elias EG, Didolkar MS, Goel IP et al: A clinicopathologic study of prognostic factors in cutaneous malignant melanoma. Surg Gynecol Obstet 144:327, 1977
167. Balch CM, Urist MM, Maddox WA: Management of metastatic melanoma. In Balch CM, Milton GW (eds): Cutaneous Melanoma: Clinical Management and Treatment Results Worldwide, p 93. Philadelphia, JB Lippincott, 1985
168. Das Gupta TK: Radical groin dissection. Surg Gynecol Obstet 129:1275, 1969
169. Holmes EC, Moseley HS, Morton DL et al. A rational approach to the surgical management of melanoma. Ann Surg 186:481, 1977
170. Karakousis CP: Ilioinguinal lymph node dissection. Am J Surg 141:299, 1981
171. Dasmahapatra KS, Karakousis CP: Therapeutic groin dissection in malignant melanoma. Surg Gynecol Obstet 156:21, 1983
172. Finck SJ, Giuliano AE, Mann BD et al: Results of ilioinguinal dissection for stage II melanoma. Ann Surg 196:180, 1982
173. McCarthy JG, Haagensen CD, Herter FP: The role of groin dissection in the management of melanoma of the lower extremity. Ann Surg 179:156, 1974
174. Fortner JG, Booher RJ, Pack GT: Results of groin dissection for malignant melanoma in 220 patients. Surgery 55:485, 1964
175. Karakousis CP, Lawrence JE, Rao UR: Groin dissection in malignant melanoma. Am J Surg 152:491, 1986
176. Harris MN, Gumport SL, Berman IR et al: Ilioinguinal lymph node dissection for melanoma. Surg Gynecol Obstet 136:33, 1973
177. Urist MM, Maddox WA, Kennedy JE et al: Patient risk factors and surgical morbidity after regional lymphadenectomy in 204 melanoma patients. Cancer 51:2152, 1983
178. Karakousis CP, Heiser MA, Moore RH: Lymphedema after groin dissection. Am J Surg 145:205, 1983
179. Chretien PB, Ketcham AS, Hoye RC et al: Axillary dissection with preservation of the pectoralis major muscle. Ann Surg 173:554, 1971
180. Harris MN, Gumport SL, Maiwandi H: Axillary lymph node dissection for melanoma. Surg Gynecol Obstet 135:936, 1972
181. Yonemoto RH, Thompson WC, Byron RL et al: Complete axillary node dissection with preservation of the pectoralis major muscle. Arch Surg 102:578, 1971
182. Bakamjian VY, Miller SH, Poole AG: A technique for radical dissection of the neck. Surg Gynecol Obstet 144:419, 1977
183. Beahrs OH: Surgical anatomy and technique of radical neck dissection. Surg Clin North Am 57:663, 1977
184. Martin HE, Del Balle B, Ehrlich H et al: Neck dissection. Cancer 4:441, 1951
185. Byers RM: The role of modified neck dissection in the treatment of cutaneous melanoma of the head and neck. Arch Surg 121:138, 1986
186. Turkula LD, Woods JE: Limited or selective nodal dissection for malignant melanoma of the head and neck. Am J Surg 148:446, 1984
187. Becker GD, Parell GJ: Technique of preserving the spinal accessory nerve during radical neck dissection. Laryngoscope 89:827, 1979
188. Bocca E, Pagnataro O: A conservative technique in radical neck dissection. Ann Otol Rhinol Laryngol 76:975, 1967
189. Calearo CV, Teatini G: Functional neck dissection: Anatomical grounds, surgical technique, clinical observations. Ann Otol Rhinol Laryngol 92:215, 1983
190. Jesse RH, Ballantyne AJ, Larson D: Radical or modified neck dissection: A therapeutic dilemma. Am J Surg 136:516, 1978
191. Lingeman RE, Helmus C, Stephens R et al: Neck dissection: Radical or conservative. Ann Otol Rhinol Laryngol 86:737, 1977
192. Schuller DE, Reiches NA, Hamaker RC et al: Analysis of disability resulting from treatment including radical neck dissection or modified neck dissection. Head Neck Surg 6:551, 1983
193. Storm FK, Eilber FR, Sparks FC et al: A prospective study of parotid metastases from head and neck cancer. Am J Surg 134:115, 1977
194. Beahrs OH, Adson MA: The surgical anatomy and techniques of parotidectomy. Am J Surg 95:885, 1958
195. Woods JE: Parotidectomy: Points of technique for brief and safe operation. Am J Surg 145:678, 1983
196. Dunn EJ, Kent T, Hines J, et al: Parotid neoplasms: A report of 250 cases and review of the literature. Ann Surg 184:500, 1976
197. Powell ME, Clairmont AA: Complications of parotidectomy. South Med J 76:1109, 1983
198. Woods JE: The facial nerve in parotid malignancy. Am J Surg 146:493, 1983
199. Sutherland CM, Mather FJ, Krementz ET: Factors influencing survival among patients with regional melanoma treated by regional perfusion. AISMO 3rd Rome International Symposium, p 130, 1985
200. Stehlin JS Jr, Smith JL Jr, Jing B et al: Melanomas of the extremities complicated by in-transit metastases. Surg Gynecol Obstet 122:3, 1966
201. Treidman L, McNeer G: Prognosis with local metastasis and recurrence in malignant melanoma. Ann NY Acad Sci 100:123, 1963
202. Moore GE, Gerner RE: Malignant melanoma. Surg Gynecol Obstet 132:427, 1971
203. Stehlin JS Jr, Clark RL: Melanoma of the extremities: Experiences with conventional treatment and perfusion in 339 cases. Am J Surg 110:366, 1965
204. Ghussen F, Nagel K, Groth W et al: A prospective randomized study of regional extremity perfusion in patients with malignant melanoma. Ann Surg 200:764, 1984
205. Calvo DB III, Patt YZ, Wallace S et al: Phase I–II trial of percutaneous intra-arterial *cis*-diamminedichloroplatinum (II) for regionally confined malignancy. Cancer 45:1278, 1980
206. Einhorn LH, McBride CM, Luce JK et al: Intra-arterial infusion therapy with 5-(3,3-dimethyl-1-triazeno)imidazone-4-carboxamide (NSC-45388) for malignant melanoma. Cancer 32:749, 1973
207. Savlov ED, Hall TC, Oberfield RA: Intra-arterial therapy of melanoma with dimethyl triazeno imidazole carboxamide (NSC-45388). Cancer 28:1161, 1971
208. Karakousis CP, Choe KJ, Holyoke ED: Biologic behavior and treatment of in-transit metastasis of melanoma. Surg Gynecol Obstet 150:29, 1980
209. Morton DL, Eilber FR, Holmes EC et al: BCG immunotherapy of malignant melanoma: Summary of a seven-year experience. Ann Surg 180:634, 1974
210. Shingleton WW, Seigler HF, Stocks LH et al: Management of recurrent melanoma of the extremity. Cancer 35:574, 1975
211. Balch CM, Cascinelli N, Milton GW et al: Elective node dissection: Pros and cons. In Balch CM, Milton GW (eds): Cutaneous Melanoma: Clinical Management and Treatment Results Worldwide, p 131. Philadelphia, JB Lippincott, 1985
212. Milton GW, Shaw HM, McCarthy WH et al: Prophylactic lymph node dissection in clinical stage I cutaneous malignant melanoma: Results of surgical treatment in 1319 patients. Br J Surg 69:108, 1982
213. Reintgen DS, Cox EB, McCarty KM Jr et al: Efficacy of elective lymph node dissection in patients with intermediate thickness primary melanoma. Ann Surg 198:379, 1983
214. Schneebaum S, Briele HA, Walker MJ et al: Cutaneous thick melanoma: Prognosis and treatment. Arch Surg 122:707–711, 1987
215. McCarthy WH, Shaw HM, Milton GW: Efficacy of elective lymph node dissection in 2,347 patients with clinical stage I malignant melanoma. Surg Gynecol Obstet 161:575, 1985
216. Wanebo HJ, Woodruff J, Fortner JG: Malignant melanoma of the extremities: A clinicopathologic study using levels of invasion (microstage). Cancer 35:666, 1975
217. Balch CM: The role of elective lymph node dissection in melanoma: Rationale, results and controversies. J Clin Oncol 6:163, 392, 1988
218. Balch CM, Wilkerson JA, Murad TM et al: The prognostic significance of ulceration of cutaneous melanoma. Cancer 45:3012, 1980
219. McGovern VJ, Shaw HM, Milton GW et al: Ulceration and prognosis in cutaneous malignant melanoma. Histopathology 6:399, 1982
220. Elder DE, DuPont G, Van Horn M et al: The role of lymph node dissection for clinical stage I malignant melanoma of intermediate thickness (1.51–3.99 mm). Cancer 56:413–418, 1985
221. Fee HJ, Robinson DS, Sample WF et al: The determination of lymph shed by colloid fold scanning in patients with malignant melanoma: Preliminary study. Surgery 84:626, 1978
222. Sullivan DC, Croker BP, Harris CC et al: Lymphoscintigraphy in malignant melanoma: Tc-antimony sulfur colloid. AJR 137:847, 1981
223. Meyer CM, Lecklitner ML, Logic JR et al: Technetium-99m sulfur colloid cutaneous lymphoscintigraphy in the management of truncal melanoma. Radiology 131:205, 1979
224. Logic JR, Balch CM: Defining lymphatic drainage patterns with cutaneous lymphoscintigraphy. In Balch CM, Milton GW (eds): Cutaneous Melanoma: Clinical Management and Treatment Results Worldwide, p 159. Philadelphia, JB Lippincott, 1985
225. Hansen MG, McCarten AB: Tumor thickness and lymphocytic infiltration in malignant melanoma of the head and neck. Am J Surg 128:557, 1974
226. Goldsmith HS, Shah JP, Kim DH: Prognostic significance of lymph node dissection in the treatment of malignant melanoma. Cancer 26:606, 1970
227. Gumport SL, Harris MN: Results of regional lymph node dissection for melanoma. Ann Surg 179:105, 1974
228. Sugarbaker EV, McBride CM: Melanoma of the trunk: The results of surgical excision and anatomic guidelines for predicting nodal metastasis. Surgery 80:22, 1976
229. Lane N, Lattes R, Malm J: Clinicopathological correlations in a series of 117 malignant melanomas of the skin of adults. Cancer 11:1025, 1958
230. Das Gupta TK: Results of treatment of 269 patients with primary cutaneous melanoma: A five-year prospective study. Ann Surg 186:201, 1977
231. Veronesi U, Adamus J, Bandiera DC et al: Inefficacy of immediate node dissection in stage I melanoma of the limbs. N Engl J Med 297:627, 1977

232. Veronesi U, Adamus J, Bandiera DC et al: Stage I melanoma of the limbs: Immediate versus delayed node dissection. Tumori 66:373, 1980
233. Veronesi U, Adams J, Bandiera DC et al: Delayed regional lymph node dissection in stage I melanoma of the skin of the lower extremities. Cancer 49:2420, 1982
234. Sim FH, Taylor WF, Pritchard DJ et al: Lymphadenectomy in the management of stage I malignant melanoma: A prospective randomized study. Mayo Clin Proc 61:697, 1986
235. Bowsher WG, Taylor BA, Hughes LE: Morbidity, mortality and local recurrence following regional node dissection for melanoma. Br J Surg 73:906, 1986
236. Creagan ET, Cupps RE, Ivins JC et al: Adjuvant radiation therapy for regional nodal metastases from malignant melanoma: A randomized prospective study. Cancer 42:2206, 1978
237. Lee YT: Malignant melanoma: Patterns of metastasis. CA 30:137, 1980
238. Budman DR, Camacho E, Wittes RE: The current causes of death in patients with malignant melanoma. Eur J Cancer 14:327, 1978
239. Patel JK, Didolkar MS, Pickren JW et al: Metastatic pattern of malignant melanoma: A study of 216 autopsy cases. Am J Surg 135:807, 1978
240. Amer MH, Al-Sarraf M, Vaitkevicius VK: Clinical presentation, natural history and prognostic factors in advanced melanoma. Surg Gynecol Obstet 149:687, 1979
241. De la Monte SM, Moore GW, Hutchins GM: Patterned distribution of metastases from malignant melanoma in humans. Cancer Res 43:3427, 1983
242. Feun LG, Gutterman J, Burgess MA et al: The natural history of resectable metastatic melanoma (stage IVA melanoma). Cancer 50:1656, 1982
243. Finck SJ, Giuliano AE, Morton DL: LDH and melanoma. Cancer 51:840, 1983
244. Meyer JE, Stolbach L: Pretreatment radiographic evaluation of patients with malignant melanoma. Cancer 42:125, 1978
245. Roth JA, Eilber FR, Bennett LR et al: Radionuclide photoscanning: Usefulness in preoperative evaluation of melanoma patients. Arch Surg 110:1211, 1975
246. Das Gupta T, Brasfield R: Metastatic melanoma: A clinicopathological study. Cancer 17:1323, 1964
247. Sacre R, Lejeune FJ: Patterns of metastases distribution in 173 stage I and II melanoma patients. Anticancer Res 2:47, 1982
248. Nambisan RN, Alexiou G, Reese PA et al: Early metastatic patterns and survival in malignant melanoma. J Surg Oncol 34:248, 1987
249. Garg R, McPherson TA, Lentle B et al: Usefulness of an elevated serum lactate dehydrogenase value as a marker for hepatic metastases in malignant melanoma. Can Med Assoc J 120:1114, 1979
250. Einhorn LH, Burgess MA, Vallejos C et al: Prognostic correlations and response to treatment in advanced metastatic malignant melanoma. Cancer Res 34:1995, 1974
251. Muss HB, Richards F II, Barnes PL et al: Radionuclide scanning in patients with advanced malignant melanoma. Clin Nucl Med 4:516, 1979
252. Aranha GV, Simmons RL, Gunnarsson A et al: The value of preoperative screening procedures in stage I and II malignant melanoma. J Surg Oncol 11:1, 1979
253. Thomas JH, Panoussopoulous D, Liesmann GE, et al: Scintiscans in the evaluation of patients with malignant melanoma. Surg Gynecol Obstet 149:574, 1979
254. Evans RA, Bland KI, McMurtrey MJ et al: Radionuclide scans not indicated for stage I melanoma. Surg Gynecol Obstet 150:532, 1980
255. Doiron MJ, Bernardino ME: A comparison of non-invasive imaging modalities in the melanoma patient. Cancer 47:2581, 1981
256. Au FC, Maier WP, Malmud LS et al: Preoperative nuclear scans in patients with melanoma. Cancer 53:2095, 1984
257. Iscoe N, Kersey P, Gapski J et al: Predictive value of staging investigations in patients with clinical stage I malignant melanoma. Plast Reconstr Surg 80:233, 1987
258. Lewi HJ, Roberts MM, Donaldson AA et al: The use of cerebral computer assisted tomography as a staging investigation of patients with carcinoma of the breast and malignant melanoma. Surg Gynecol Obstet 151:385, 1980
259. Ardizzoni A, Grimaldi A, Repetto L et al: Stage I–II melanoma: The value of metastatic workup. Oncology 44:87, 1987
260. Zartman GM, Thomas MR, Robinson WA: Metastatic disease in patients with newly diagnosed malignant melanoma. J Surg Oncol 35:163, 1987
261. Milder MS, Frankel RS, Bulkley BG et al: Gallium-67 scintigraphy in malignant melanoma. Cancer 32:1350, 1973
262. Romolo JL, Fischer SG: Gallium-67 scanning compared with physical examination in the preoperative staging of melanoma. Cancer 44:468, 1979
263. Berkerman C, Hoffer PB, Bitran JD: The role of gallium-67 in the evaluation of cancer. Semin Nucl Med 14:296, 1984
264. Rossleigh MA, McCarthy WH, Milton GW et al: The role of gallium-67 studies in the management of malignant melanoma. Med J Aust 140:401, 1984
265. Kirkwood JM, Meyers JE, Vlock DR et al: Tomographic gallium-67 citrate scanning: Useful new surveillance for metastatic melanoma. Ann Surg 198:102, 1983
266. Balch CM, Milton GW: Treatment for advanced metastatic melanoma. In Balch CM, Milton GW (eds): Cutaneous Melanoma: Clinical Management and Treatment Results Worldwide, p 251. Philadelphia, JB Lippincott, 1985
267. Hena MA, Emrich LJ, Nambisan RN, et al: Effect of surgical treatment of stage IV melanoma. Am J Surg 153:270, 1987
268. Overett TK, Shiu MH: Surgical treatment of distant metastatic melanoma: Indications and results. Cancer 56:1222, 1985
269. Wornom IL, Smith JW, Soong S-j, et al: Surgery as palliative treatment for distance metastases of melanoma. Ann Surg 204:181, 1986
270. Habermalz HJ, Fischer JJ: Radiation therapy of malignant melanoma: Experience with high individual treatment doses. Cancer 38:2258, 1976
271. Hornsey S: The relationship between total dose, number of fractions and fraction size in the response of malignant melanoma in patients. Br J Radiol 51:905, 1978
272. Overgaard J: Radiation treatment of malignant melanoma. Int J Radiat Oncol Biol Phys 6:41, 1980
273. Harwood AR, Cummings BJ: Radiotherapy for malignant melanoma: A re-appraisal. Cancer Treat Rev 8:271, 1981
274. Harwood AR, Dancuart F, Fitzpatrick PJ et al: Radiotherapy in nonlentiginous melanoma of the head and neck cancer. Cancer 48:2599, 1981
275. Katz HR: The results of different fractionation schemes in the palliative irradiation of metastatic melanoma. Int J Radiat Oncol Biol Phys 7:907, 1981
276. Lobo PA, Liebner EJ, Chao JJ et al: Radiotherapy in the management of malignant melanoma. Int J Radiat Oncol Biol Phys 7:21, 1981
277. Strauss A, Dritschilo A, Nathanson L et al: Radiation therapy of malignant melanomas: An evaluation of clinically used fractionation schemes. Cancer 47:1262, 1981
278. Trott KR, von Lieven H, Kummermehr J et al: The radiosensitivity of malignant melanomas: II. Clinical studies. Int J Radiat Oncol Biol Phys 7:15, 1981
279. Adam JS, Habeshaw T, Kirk J: Response rate of malignant melanoma to large fraction irradiation. Br J Radiol 55:605, 1982
280. Doss LL, Memula N: The radioresponsiveness of melanoma. Int J Radiat Oncol Biol Phys 8:1131, 1982
281. Johanson CR, Harwood AR, Cummings BJ et al.: 0-7-21 radiotherapy in nodular melanoma. Cancer 51:226, 1983
282. Overgaard J, von der Masse H, Overgaard MA: A randomized study comparing two high-dose per fraction radiation schedules in recurrent or metastatic melanoma. Int J Radiat Oncol Biol Phys 11:1837, 1985
283. Overgaard J, Overgaard M, Hansen V et al: Some factors of importance in the radiation treatment of malignant melanoma. Radiother Oncol 5:183, 1986
284. Trott KR, von Lieven H, Kummermehr J et al: The radiosensitivity of malignant melanomas: I. Experimental studies. Int J Radiat Oncol Biol Phys 7:9, 1981
285. Douglas BG, Fowler JF: The effect of multiple small doses of x-rays on skin reactions in the mouse and a basic interpretation. Radiat Res 66:401, 1976
286. Kim JH, Hahn EW, Ahmed SA: Combination hyperthermia and radiation therapy for malignant melanomas. Cancer 50:478, 1982
287. Perez CA, Emami B: Review of human clinical data on treatment of superficial tumors with irradiation and hyperthermia. In: Physical Aspects of Hyperthermia. Med Phys Monogr (in press)
288. Overgaard J, Overgaard MA: Clinical trial evaluating the effect of simultaneous or sequential radiation and hyperthermia in the treatment of malignant melanoma. In Overgaard J (ed): Hyperthermia Oncology, vol 1. London, Taylor & Francis, 1984
289. Blake PR, Catterall M, Errington RD: Treatment of malignant melanoma by fast neutrons. Br J Surg 72:517, 1985
290. Dewit L, Bartelink H, Rumke P: Concurrent *cis*-diamminedichloroplatinum (II) and radiation treatment for melanoma metastases: A pilot study. Radiother Oncol 3:303, 1985
291. Marsoni S, Hoth D, Simon R: Clinical drug development. An analysis of phase II trials, 1970–1985. Cancer Treat Rep 71:71, 1987
292. Comis RL: DTIC (NSC-45388) in malignant melanoma: A perspective. Cancer Treat Rep 64:1123, 1976
293. Luce JK: Chemotherapy of malignant melanoma. Cancer 30:1604, 1972
294. Costanza ME, Nathanson L, Schoenfeld D et al: Results with methyl-CCNU and DTIC in metastatic melanoma. Cancer 40:1010, 1977
295. Wagner DE, Ramirez G, Weiss AJ: Combination phase I–II study of imidazole carboxamide (NSC-45388). Oncology 26:310, 1971
296. Nathanson L, Wolter K, Horton J: Characteristics of prognosis and response to an imidazole carboxamide in malignant melanoma. Clin Pharmacol Ther 12:955, 1971
297. Costanza ME, Nathanson L, Lenhard R et al: Therapy of malignant melanoma with an imidazole carboxamide and bischloroethyl nitrosourea. Cancer 30:1457, 1972
298. Moon JH, Gailanai S, Cooper MR et al: Comparison of the combination of 1,3-bis(2-chloroethyl)-1-nitrosourea (BCNU) and vincristine with two dose schedules of 5-(3,3-dimethyl-1-triazeno) imidazole 4-carboxamide (DTIC) in the treatment of disseminated malignant melanoma. Cancer 35:368, 1975
299. Van der Merwe AM, Falkson G, Van Eden EB: Metastatic malignant melanoma: Imidazole carboxamide in its treatment. Med Proc 17:399, 1971
300. Gottlieb JA, Serpick AA: Clinical evaluation of 5-(3,3-dimethyl-1-triazeno) imidazole 4-carboxamide in malignant melanoma and other neoplasms: Comparison of twice weekly and daily administration schedules. Oncology 25:255, 1971
301. Burke PJ, McCarthy NWH, Milton GW: Imidazole carboxamide therapy in advanced malignant melanoma. Cancer 27:744, 1971
302. Cowan DH, Bersagel DE: Intermittent treatment of metastatic malignant melanoma with high-dose 5-(3,3-dimethyl-1-triazeno) imadazole-4-carboxamide (NSC-45388). Cancer Chemother Rep 55:175, 1971
303. Gerner RE, Moore GE: Study of 5-(3,3-dimethyl-1-triazeno) imadazole-4-carboxamide (NSC-45388) given intravenously in the treatment of malignant melanoma in Uganda. Cancer Chemother Rep 55:143, 1973
304. Costanza J: DTIC (NSC-45388) studies in the Southwest Oncology Group. Cancer Treat Rep 60:189, 1976
305. Pritchard KI, Quirt IC, Cowan DH et al: DTIC therapy in metastatic malignant melanoma: A simplified dose schedule. Cancer Treat Rep 64:1123, 1980
306. Hill GJ Jr, Krementz ET, Hill HZ: Dimethyl triazeno imidazole carboxamide and combination therapy for melanoma: IV. Late results after complete response to chemotherapy. Cancer 53:1299, 1984

307. Tyson LB, Clark RA, Gralla RJ: High-dose metoclopramide: Control of dacarbazine-induced emesis in a preliminary trial. Cancer Treat Rep 66:2108, 1982
308. Kris MG, Gralla RJ, Clark RA et al: Antiemetic control and prevention of side-effects of anti-cancer therapy with lorazepam or diphenhydramine when used in combination with metoclopramide plus dexamethasone: A double-blind, randomized trial. Cancer 60:2816, 1987
309. Ramirez G, Wilson W, Grage T et al: Phase II evaluation of 1,3-bis(2-chloroethyl-nitrosourea) (BCNU; NSC-409962) in patients with solid tumors. Cancer Chemother Rep 56:787, 1972
310. DeVita VT, Carbone PP, Owens AH Jr et al: Clinical trials with 1,3,-bis(2-chloroethyl)-1-nitrosourea, NSC-409962. Cancer Res 25:1875, 1965
311. Ahmann DL, Hahn RG, Bisel HF: A comparative study of 1-(2-chloroethyl)-3-cyclohexyl-1-nitrosourea (NSC-79037) and imidazole carboxamide (NSC-45388) with vincristine (NSC-67574) in the palliation of disseminated malignant melanoma. Cancer Res 32:2432, 1972
312. Hoogstraten B, Gottlieb JA, Caoili E et al: CCNU (1-(2,chloroethyl)-3-cyclohexyl-1-nitrosourea, NSC-79037) in the treatment of cancer. Cancer 32:38, 1973
313. Ahmann DL, Hahn RG, Bisel HF: Evaluation of 1-(2-chloroethyl-3-4-methyl-cyclohexyl)-1-nitrosourea (methyl-CCNU, NSC-95441) versus combined imidazole carboxamide (NSC-45388) and vincristine (NSC-67574) in palliation of disseminated melanoma. Cancer 33:615, 1974
314. Wasserman TH, Slavik M, Carter SK: Review of CCNU in clinical cancer therapy. Cancer Treat Rev 1:131, 1974
315. Young RC, Canellos GP, Chabner BA, et al: Treatment of malignant melanoma with methyl-CCNU. Cancer Pharmacol Ther 15:617, 1974
316. Wasserman TH, Slavik M, Carter SK: Methyl-CCNU in clinical cancer therapy. Cancer Treat Rev 1:251, 1974
317. Chang P, Knapper WH: Metastatic melanoma of unknown primary. Cancer 49:1106, 1982
318. Al-Sarraf M, Fletcher W, Oishi N et al: Cisplatin hydration with and without mannitol diuresis in refractory disseminated malignant melanoma: A Southwest Oncology Group study. Cancer Treat Rep 66:31, 1982
319. Goodnight JE Jr, Moseley HS, Eilber FR et al: *cis*-Dichlorodiammineplatinum (II) alone and combined with DTIC for treatment of disseminated malignant melanoma. Cancer Treat Rep 63:2005, 1979
320. Evans L, Casper ES, Rosenbluth R: Phase II trial of carboplatin in advanced malignant melanoma. Cancer Treat Rep 71:171, 1987
321. Wiernik PH, Schwartz EL, Einzig A et al: Phase I trial of taxol given as a 24-hour infusion every 2 days: Responses observed in metastatic melanoma. J Clin Oncol 5:1232, 1987
322. Wittes RE, Wittes JT, Golbey RB: Combination chemotherapy in metastatic malignant melanoma: A randomized study of three DTIC-containing combinations. Cancer 41:415, 1978
323. Nathanson L, Kaufman SD, Carey RW: Vinblastine infusion, bleomycin, and *cis*-dichlorodiammine-platinum chemotherapy in metastatic melanoma. Cancer 48:1290, 1981
324. National Cancer Institute of Canada Melanoma Group: Vinblastine, bleomycin, and *cis*-platinum for the treatment of metastatic malignant melanoma. J Clin Oncol 2:131, 1984
325. Luikart SD, Kennealey GT, Kirkwood JM: Randomized phase III trial of vinblastine, bleomycin, and *cis*-dichlorodiammine-platinum versus dacarbazine in malignant melanoma. J Clin Oncol 2:164, 1984
326. Costanzi JJ, Al-Sarraf M, Groppe C et al: Combination chemotherapy plus BCG in the treatment of disseminated malignant melanoma: A Southwest Oncology Group study. Med Pediatr Oncol 10:251, 1982
327. Costanzi JJ, Fletcher WS, Balcerzak SP et al: Combination chemotherapy plus levamisole in the treatment of disseminated malignant melanoma: A Southwest Oncology Group study. Cancer 53:833, 1984
328. Del Prete SA, Maurer LH, O'Donnell J: Combination chemotherapy with cisplatin, carmustine, dacarbazine, and tamoxifen in metastatic melanoma. Cancer Treat Rep 68:1403, 1984
329. McClay EF, Mastrangelo MJ, Bellet RE: Combination chemotherapy and hormonal therapy in the treatment of malignant melanoma. Cancer Treat Rep 71:465, 1987
330. Phillips GL, Fay JW, Herzig GP et al: Intensive 1,3-bis(2-chloroethyl)-1-nitrosourea (BCNU) with autologous bone marrow transplantation therapy of refractory cancer: A preliminary report. Exp Hematol 7:372, 1979
331. Thomas MR, Robinson WA, Glode LM et al: Treatment of advanced malignant melanoma with high-dose chemotherapy and autologous bone marrow transplantation: Preliminary results. Phase I study. Am J Clin Oncol 5:611, 1982
332. Lazarus HM, Herzig RH, Graham-Pole J et al: Intensive melphalan chemotherapy and cryopreserved autologous bone marrow transplantation for the treatment of refractory cancer. J Clin Oncol 1:359, 1983
333. Spitzer G, Dicke K, Zander AR et al: High-dose chemotherapy with autologous bone marrow transplantation. Cancer 54:216, 1984
334. Tchekmedyian NS, Tait N, van Echo D et al: High-dose chemotherapy without autologous bone marrow transplantation in melanoma. J Clin Oncol 4:1811, 1986
335. Phillips GL, Fay JW, Herzig GP et al: Intensive 1,3-bis(2-chloroethyl)-1-nitrosourea (BCNU), NSC-409962 and cryopreserved autologous marrow transplantation for refractory cancer: A phase I–II study. Cancer 52:1792, 1983
336. Antman K, Eder JP, Elias A et al: High dose combination alkylating agent preparative regimen with autologous bone marrow support: The Dana-Farber Cancer Institute/Beth Israel Hospital experience. Cancer Treat Rep 71:119, 1987
337. Glover D, Glick JH, Weiler C et al: WR2721 and high-dose cis-platin: An active combination in the treatment of metastatic melanoma. J Clin Oncol 5:574, 1987
338. Mavligit G, Carrasco C, Papadopoulos N et al: Regression of ocular melanoma metastatic to the liver after chemoembolization with *cis*-platinum and polyvinyl sponge. Proc Am Soc Clin Oncol 6:830, 1987
339. Kirkwood JM, Ernstoff M: Therapeutic option with recombinant interferons: Lessons drawn from studies of human melanoma. Semin Oncol 13:48, 1986
340. Creagan ET, Ahman DL, Frytak S et al: Recombinant leukocyte A interferon (rIFN-alpha A) in the treatment of disseminated malignant melanoma: Analysis of complete and long-term responding patients. Cancer 58:2576, 1986
341. Robinson WA, Kirkwood J, Harvey H et al: Effective use of recombinant α_2 interferon in metastatic malignant melanoma. Proc Am Soc Clin Oncol 3:60, 1984
342. Robinson WA, Mughal TI, Thomas MR et al: Treatment of metastatic melanoma with recombinant interferon alpha 2. Immunobiology 172:275, 1986
343. Coates A, Rallings M, Hersey P et al: Phase II study of recombinant alpha-2 interferon in advanced malignant melanoma. J Interferon Res 6:1, 1986
344. Dorval T, Palangie T, Jouve M et al: Treatment of metastatic malignant melanoma with recombinant interferon alpha-2b. Invest New Drugs 5:561, 1987
345. Rosenberg SA, Lotze MT, Muul LM et al: A progress report on the treatment of 157 patients with advanced cancer using lymphokine-activated killer cells and interleukin-2 or high-dose interleukin-2 alone. N Engl J Med 316:889, 1987
346. West WH, Tauer KW, Yanelli JR et al: Constant infusion recombinant interleukin 2 adoptive immunotherapy of advanced cancer. N Engl J Med 316:898, 1987
347. Houghton AN, Mintzer D, Cordon-Cardo C et al: Mouse monoclonal IgG3 antibody detecting GD3 ganglioside: A phase I trial in patients with malignant melanoma. Proc Natl Acad Sci USA 82:1242, 1985
348. Goodman GE, Beaumier P, Hellstrom I et al: Pilot trial of murine monoclonal antibodies in patients with advanced melanoma. J Clin Oncol 3:340, 1985
349. Cheung N-K, Lazarus H, Miraldi FD et al: Ganglioside GD2 specific monoclonal antibody 3F8: A phase I study in patients with neuroblastoma and malignant melanoma. J Clin Oncol 5:1430, 1987
350. Kirkwood JM, Ernstoff M: Potential application of the interferons on oncology: Lesions drawn from studies of human melanoma. Semin Oncol 13:48, 1986
351. Truitt RL, Gale RP, Bortin MM: Cellular immunotherapy of cancer. Prog Clin Biol Res 244:1, 1987
352. Rosenberg SA, Mule JJ, Spiess PJ et al: Regression of established pulmonary metastases and subcutaneous tumor mediated by the systemic administration of high-dose recombinant interleukin 2. J Exp Med 161:1169, 1985
353. Grimm EA, Mazumder A, Zhang HZ et al: Lymphokine-activated killer phenomenon: Lysis of natural killer resistant fresh solid tumor cells by interleukin-2-activated autologous human peripheral blood lymphocytes. J Exp Med 155:1823, 1982
354. Mule JJ, Shu S, Schwarz SL: Successful adoptive immunotherapy of established pulmonary metastases with LAK cells and recombinant interleukin 2. Science 255:1487, 1984
355. Mule JJ, Shu S, Rosenberg SA: The antitumor efficacy of lymphokine-activated killer cells and recombinant interleukin 2 in vivo. J Immunol 135:646, 1985
356. Lafreniere R, Rosenberg SA: Successful immunotherapy of experimental hepatic metastases with lymphokine-activated killer cells and recombinant interleukin 2. Cancer Res 45:3755, 1985
357. Rosenberg SA, Lotze MT, Muul LM et al: Special report: Observations on the systemic administration of autologous lymphokine-activated killer cells and recombinant interleukin-2 to patients with metastatic cancer. N Engl J Med 313:1485, 1985
358. Dutcher JP, Creekmore S, Weiss GR et al: Phase II study of high dose interleukin-2 and lymphokine activated killer cells in patients with melanoma. Proc Am Soc Clin Oncol 6:970, 1987
359. Greenberg PD: Therapy of murine leukemia with cyclophosphamide and immune Lyt 2+ cells: Cytolytic T cells can mediate eradication of disseminated leukemia. J Immunol 136:1917, 1986
360. Greenberg PD, Kern DE, Cheever MA: Therapy of disseminated murine leukemia with cyclophosphamide and immune Lyt 1 + 2 − T cells: Tumor eradication does not require participation of cytotoxic T cells. J Exp Med 161:4303, 1985
361. Anichini A, Fossati G, Parmiani G: Clonal analysis of cytotoxic T lymphocyte response to autologous human metastatic melanoma. Int J Cancer 35:683, 1985
362. De Vries JE, Spits H: Cloned cytolytic T lymphocyte (CTL) lines reactive with autologous melanoma cells: I. In vitro generation, isolation, and analysis of phenotype and specificity. J Immunol 132:510, 1984
363. Herin M, Lemoine C, Weynant P et al: Production of stable cytolytic T lymphocyte (CTL) against autologous human melanoma. Int J Cancer 39:390, 1987
364. Hersey P, MacDonald M, Schibeci S et al: Clonal analysis of cytotoxic T lymphocytes (CTL) against autologous melanoma: Classification based on phenotype, specificity, and inhibition of monoclonal antibodies to T cell structures. Cancer Immunol Immunother 22:15, 1986
365. Fossati G, Anichini A, Parmiani G: Melanoma cell lysis by human CTL clones: Differential involvement of T3, T8 and HLA antigens. Int J Cancer 39:689, 1987
366. Anichini A, Fossati G, Parmiani G: Heterogeneity of clones from a human metastatic melanoma detected by autologous cytotoxic T lymphocyte clones. J Exp Med 163:215, 1986
367. Itoh K, Tilden AB, Balch CM: Interleukin 2 activation of cytotoxic T lymphocytes infiltrating into human metastatic melanoma. Cancer Res 46:3011, 1986

368. Muul LM, Spiess PJ, Director EP et al: Identification of specific cytolytic immune responses against autologous tumors in humans bearing malignant melanoma. J Immunol 138:989, 1987
369. Mukherji B, MacAlister TJ: Clonal analysis of cytotoxic T cell response against human melanoma. J Exp Med 158:240, 1983
370. Knuth A, Danowski B, Oettgen HF et al: T cell mediated cytotoxicity against autologous malignant melanoma: Analysis with interleukin 2 dependent T cell cultures. Proc Natl Acad Sci USA 81:3511, 1984
371. Rosenberg SA, Spiess PJ, Lafreniere R: A new approach to adoptive immunotherapy of cancer with tumor-infiltrating lymphocytes. Science 233:1318, 1986
372. Topalian S, Solomon D, Avis FP et al: Immunotherapy of patients with advanced cancer using tumor infiltrating lymphocytes in recombinant interleukin-2: A pilot study. J Clin Oncol 6:839, 1988
373. Houghton AN, Scheinberg DA: Monoclonal antibodies: Potential applications to the treatment of cancer. Semin Oncol 13:165, 1986
374. Melanoma Workshop: Workshop on monoclonal antibodies to melanoma-associated antigens. Hybridoma 1:266–402, 1982
375. Houghton AN, Cordon-Cardo C, Eisinger M: Differentiation antigens of melanoma and melanocytes. Int Rev Exp Pathol 28:217, 1986
376. Rose TM, Plowman GD, Teplow DB et al: Primary structure of the human melanoma-associated antigen p97 (melanotransferrin) deduced from the mRNA sequence. Proc Natl Acad Sci USA 83:1261, 1986
377. Oldham RK, Foon KA, Morgan AC et al: Monoclonal antibody therapy of malignant melanoma: In vivo localization in cutaneous metastasis after intravenous administration. J Clin Oncol 2:1235, 1984
378. Schroff RW, Woodhouse CS, Foon KA et al: Intratumor localization of monoclonal antibody in patients with melanoma treated with antibody to a 250,000 dalton melanoma-associated antigen. JNCI 74:299, 1985
379. Houghton AN, Vadhan S, Wong G et al: Clinical study of a mouse monoclonal antibody directed against GD3 ganglioside in patients with melanoma. Proc Am Soc Clin Oncol 5:231, 1986
380. Larson SM, Carrasquillo JA, Krohn KA et al: Localization of 131-I labeled p97-specific Fab fragments in human melanoma as a basis for radiotherapy. J Clin Invest 72:2101, 1983
381. Vitteta ES, Fulton RJ, May RD et al: Redesigning nature's poisons to create antitumor reagents. Science 238:1098, 1987
382. Spitler LE, Del Rio M, Khentigan A et al: Therapy of patients with malignant melanoma using a monoclonal antimelanoma antibody-ricin A chain immunotoxin. Cancer Res 47:1717, 1987
383. Spitler LE: Clinical trials of immunotoxin. In: Proceedings of the Second International Congress on Monoclonal Antibody, vol 1, p 26, 1987
384. Schroff RW, Foon KA, Beatty SM et al: Human anti-mouse immunoglobulin response in patients receiving monoclonal antibody therapy. Cancer Res 45:879, 1985
385. Morrison SL, Oi V: Transfer and expression of immunoglobulin genes. Annu Rev Immunol 2:239, 1984
386. Irie RF, Morton DL: Progression of cutaneous metastatic melanoma by intralesional injection with human monoclonal antibody to ganglioside GD2. Proc Natl Acad Sci USA 83:8694, 1986
387. Yamaguchi H, Furukawa K, Fortunato S et al: Cell surface antigens of human melanoma recognized by human monoclonal antibodies. Proc Natl Acad Sci USA 84:2416, 1987
388. Schroff RW, Morgan AC Jr, Woodhouse CS et al: Monoclonal antibody therapy in malignant melanoma: Factors effecting in vivo localization. J Biol Response Mod 6:457, 1987
389. Carrasquillo JA, Krohn KA, Beaumier P et al: Diagnosis of and therapy for solid tumors with radiolabeled antibodies and immune fragments. Cancer Treat Rep 68:317, 1984
390. Lotze MT, Carrasquillo JA, Weinstein JN et al: Monoclonal antibody imaging of human melanoma: Radioimmunodetection by subcutaneous or systemic injection. Ann Surg 204:223, 1986
391. Nelp WB, Eary JF, Jones RF et al: Preliminary studies of monoclonal antibody lymphoscintigraphy in malignant melanoma. J Nucl Med 28:34, 1987
392. Larson SM, Carrasquillo JA, McGuffin RW et al: Use of I-131 labeled, murine Fab against a high molecular weight antigen of human melanoma: A preliminary experience. Radiology 155:487, 1985
393. Bajorin D, Yeh S, Wong G et al: Pharmacokinetics, distribution and radiolocalization of ^{131}I-labeled mouse monoclonal antibody R24. Proc Am Assoc Cancer Res 28:385a, 1987
394. Murray JL, Rosenblum MG, Sobol RE et al: Radioimmuno-imaging in malignant melanoma with indium-111 labeled monoclonal antibody 96.5. Cancer Res 45:2376, 1985
395. Halpern SE, Dillman RO, Witztum KF et al. Radioimmunodetection of melanoma utilizing indium-111 96.5 monoclonal antibody: A preliminary report. Radiology 155:493, 1985
396. Rosenblum MG, Murray JL, Haynie TP et al: Pharmacokinetics of indium-111 labeled anti-p97 monoclonal antibody in patients with metastatic malignant melanoma. Cancer Res 45:2382, 1985
397. Siccardi AG, Buraggi GL, Callegaro L et al: Multicenter study of immunoscintigraphy with radiolabeled monoclonal antibodies in patients with melanoma. Cancer Res 46:4817, 1986
398. Murray JL, Rosenblum MG, Lamki L et al: Clinical parameters related to optimal tumor localization of indium-111 labeled mouse antimelanoma monoclonal antibody ZME-018. J Nucl Med 28:25, 1987
399. Rosenblum MG, Murray JL, Lamki L et al: Comparative clinical pharmacology of indium-111 labeled murine monoclonal antibodies. Cancer Chemother Pharmacol 20:41, 1987
400. Kirkwood JM, Neumann RD, Zoghbi SS et al: Scintigraphic detection of metastatic melanoma using indium-111/DTPA conjugated anti-gp240 antibody (ZME-018). J Clin Oncol 5:1247, 1987
401. Taylor, A Jr, Milton W, Eyre H, et al: Radioimmunodetection of human melanoma with indium-111 labeled monoclonal antibody. Natl Cancer Inst Mongr 3:25, 1987
402. Paganelli G, Riva P, Moscatelli G et al: Improved immunoscintigraphy by subcutaneous injection of ^{99m}Tc or indium-111 labeled F(ab')2 fragments of an anti-melanoma monoclonal antibody. Int J Radiat Appl Instrum [B] 13:423, 1986
403. Cerny T, Owens SE, Mackenzie SA et al: Immunoscintigraphy with ^{99m}Tc labelled $F(ab)_2$ fragments of anti-melanoma monoclonal antibody (225.28S) in patients with metastatic malignant melanoma. Eur J Nucl Med 13:130, 1987
404. Chan SM, Hoffer PB, Maric N et al: Comparison of gallium-67 indium-111 monoclonal antibody (96.5, ZME-018) in detection of human melanoma in athymic mice. J Nucl Med 28:1441, 1987
405. Balch CM, Hersey P: Current status of adjuvant therapy. In Balch CM, Milton GW (eds): Cutaneous Melanoma: Clinical Management and Treatment Results Worldwide, p 197. Philadelphia, JB Lippincott, 1985
406. Old LJ: Cancer immunology: The search for specificity. G.H.A. Clowes Memorial Lecture. Cancer Res 41:361, 1981
407. Morton DL, Nizze RJ, Gupta RK et al: Active specific immunotherapy of malignant melanoma. In Kim JP, Jim BS, Park J-G (eds): Current Status of Cancer Control and Immunobiology, p 152. Seoul, Korea, 1987
408. Resifeld RA, Ferrone S: Melanoma Antigens and Antibodies. New York, Plenum Press, 1982
409. Natali PG, Cavaliere R, Bigotti A et al: Antigenic heterogeneity of surgically removed primary and autologous metastatic human melanoma lesions. J Immunol 130:1462, 1983
410. Houghton AN, Real FX, Davis LJ et al: Phenotypic heterogeneity of melanoma: Relation to the differentiation program of melanoma cells. J Exp Med 164:812, 1987
411. Livingston PO, Oettgen HF, Old LJ: Specific active immunotherapy in cancer treatment. In Mihich E (ed): Immunological Approaches to Cancer Therapeutics, p 363. New York, John Wiley & Sons, 1982
412. Livingston PO, Takeyama H, Pollack MS et al: Serological responses of melanoma patients to vaccines derived from allogeneic cultured melanoma cells. Int J Cancer 31:567, 1983
413. Livingston PO, Kaelin K, Pinsky CM: The serologic response of patients with stage II melanoma to allogeneic melanoma cell vaccines. Cancer 56:2194, 1985
414. Fisher RI, Terry WD, Hodes RJ et al: Adjuvant immunotherapy or chemotherapy for malignant melanoma. Surg Clin North Am 61:1267, 1981
415. Eilber FR, Morton DL, Holmes EC et al: Adjuvant immunotherapy with BCG in treatment of regional lymph node metastases from malignant melanoma. N Engl J Med 294:237, 1976
416. Golub SH, Forsythe AB, Morton DL: Sequential examination of lymphocyte proliferative capacity in patients with malignant melanoma receiving BCG immunotherapy. Int J Cancer 19:19, 1977
417. Seigler HF, Cox E, Mutzner F et al: Specific active immunotherapy for melanoma. Ann Surg 190:366, 1979
418. Cox EB, Vollmer RT, Seigler HF: Melanoma in the Southeastern United States: Experience at The Duke Medical Center. In Balch CM, Milton GW (eds): Cutaneous Melanoma: Clinical Management and Treatment Results Worldwide, p 407. Philadelphia, JB Lippincott, 1985
419. Austin FC, Boone CW: Virus augmentation of the antigenicity of tumor cell extracts. Adv Cancer Res 301, 1979
420. Lindemann J: Viruses as immunological adjuvants in cancer. Biochem Biophys Acta 355:49, 1974
421. Cassel WA, Murray DR, Phillips HS: A phase II study on the postsurgical management of state II malignant melanoma with a Newcastle disease virus oncolysate. Cancer 52:856, 1983
422. Murray DR, Cassel WA, Torbin AH, et al: Viral oncolysate in the management of malignant melanoma: II. Clinical studies. Cancer 40:680, 1977
423. Wallack MK: Specific immunotherapy with vaccinia oncolysates. Cancer Immunol Immunother 12:1, 1981
424. Wallack MK: Specific tumor immunity produced by the injection of vaccinia viral oncolysates. J Surg Res 33:11, 1982
425. Wallack MJ, Meyer M, Baurgoin A et al: A preliminary trial of vaccinia oncolysate in the treatment of recurrent melanoma with serologic response to the treatment. J Biol Response Mod 2:586, 1983
426. Wallack MK, McNally KR, Leftheriotis E: A Southeastern Cancer Study Group phase I/II trial with vaccinia melanoma oncolysates. Cancer 57:649, 1986
427. Wallack MK, Bash JA, Leftheriotis E et al: The positive relationship of clinical and serologic responses to vaccinia melanoma oncolysate. Arch Surg 122:1460, 1987
428. Hersey P, Edwards A, D'Alessandro G et al: Phase II study of vaccinia melanoma cell lysates (VMCL) as adjuvant to surgical treatment of state II melanoma: II. Effects on cell mediated cytotoxicity and leukocyte dependent antibody activity. Cancer Immunol Immunother 22:221, 1986
429. Hersey P, Edwards A, Coates A et al: Evidence that treatment with vaccinia mela-

noma cell lysates (VMCL) may improve survival of patients with state II melanoma. Cancer Immunol Immunother 25:257, 1987
430. Livingston PO, Albino AP, Chung TJC et al: Serological response of melanoma patients to vaccines prepared from VSV lysates of autologous and allogeneic cultured melanoma cells. Cancer 55:713, 1985
431. North RJ: Cyclophosphamide-facilitated adoptive immunotherapy of an established tumor depends on elimination of tumor-induced suppressor T-cells. J Exp Med 35:1063, 1982
432. Livingston PO, Hoffman MK, Enker WE: Inhibition of suppressor cell activity in melanoma patients by cyclophosphamide. Proc Am Assoc Clin Oncol 3:58, 1984
433. Berd D, Mastrangelo MJ, Engstrom PF et al: Augmentation of the human immune response by cyclophosphamide. Cancer Res 42:4862, 1982
434. Berd D, Danna V, Maguire HC, et al: Induction of cell mediated immunity to autologous melanoma cells and regression of metastases after treatment with a melanoma cell vaccine preceded by cyclophosphamide. Cancer Res 46:2572, 1986
435. Jones PC, Sze LL, Liu PY et al: Prolonged survival for melanoma patients with elevated IgM antibody to oncofetal antigen. JNCI 66:249, 1981
436. Livingston PO, Natoli EJ, Calves MJ et al: Vaccines containing purified GM2 ganglioside elicit GM2 antibodies in melanoma patients. Proc Natl Acad Sci USA 84:2911, 1987
437. Estin CD, Stevenson US, Plowman GD et al: Recombinant vaccinia virus vaccine against the human melanoma antigen p97 for use in immunotherapy. Proc Natl Acad Sci USA 85:1052, 1988
438. Morton DL: Immunological studies with human neoplasms. J Reticuloendothel Soc 10:137, 1971
439. Mastrangelo MJ, Bellet RE, Berd D: Immunology and immunotherapy of human cutaneous malignant melanoma. In Clark WH Jr, Goldman LI, Mastrangelo MJ (eds): Human Malignant Melanoma, p 355. New York, Grune & Stratton, 1979
440. Pinsky CM, Hirshaut Y, Oettgen HF: Treatment of malignant melanoma by intra-tumoral injection of BCG. Natl Cancer Inst Monogr 39:255, 1973
441. Mastrangelo MJ, Sulit HL, Prehn LM: Intralesional BCG in the treatment of metastatic malignant melanoma. Cancer 37:684, 1976
442. Klein E, Holterman OA: Immunotherapeutic approaches to the management of neoplasms. Natl Cancer Inst Monogr 35:379, 1972
443. Klein E, Holterman OA, Helm F et al: Immunologic approaches to the management of primary and secondary tumors involving the skin and soft tissues: Review of a ten year program. Transplant Proc 7:297, 1975
444. Krown SE, Hilal EY, Pinsky CM: Intralesional injection of the methanol extraction residue of Bacillus Calmette-Guérin (MER) into cutaneous metastases of malignant melanoma. Cancer 42:2648, 1978
445. Cohen MH, Felix E, Jessup J et al: Treatment of metastatic melanoma by intralesional injection of BCG: Treatment of metastatic melanoma by intralesional injection of BCG, organic chemicals of *C. parvum*. In Crispen RG (ed): Neoplasm Immunity Mechanisms, p 121. Philadelphia, Franklin Institute Press, 1975
446. Hakim AA: Correlation between tyrosine hydoxylase activity, melanogenesis, and estradiol binding in human melanoma cells. Res Exp Med (Berl) 180:99, 1982
447. Rose C, Pedersen L, Mouridsen HT: Endocrine treatment with antiestrogen, anti-androgen or progestagen of advanced malignant melanoma: Three consecutive phase II trials. Eur J Cancer Clin Oncol 21:1171, 1985
448. Wagstaff J, Thatcher N, Rankin E et al: Tamoxifen in the treatment of metastatic melanoma. Cancer Treat Rep 66:1171, 1982
449. Leichman CG, Samson MK, Baker LH: Phase II trial of tamoxifen in malignant melanoma. Cancer Treat Rep 66:1447, 1982
450. Telhaug R, Klepp O, Bremer O: Phase II study of tamoxifen in patients with metastatic malignant melanoma. Cancer Treat Rep 66:1437, 1982
451. Creagan ET, Ingle JN, Ahmann DL et al: Phase II study of high-dose tamoxifen (NSC-180973) in patients with disseminated melanoma. Cancer 49:1353, 1982
452. Pinsky CM, Oettgen HF: Surgical adjuvant therapy for malignant melanoma. Surg Clin North Am 61:1259, 1981
453. Skipper HE, Schabel FM Jr, Wilcox WS: Experimental evaluation of potential anti-cancer agents: XII. On the criteria and kinetics associated with "curability" of experimental leukemia. Cancer Chemother Rep 35:1, 1964
454. Schabel FM: Concepts from systemic treatment of micrometastases. Cancer 35:15, 1975
455. Schabel FM: Rationale for adjuvant chemotherapy. Cancer 39:2875, 1977
456. Hill GJ III, Moss SE, Golomb FM et al: DTIC and combination therapy for melanoma: III. DTIC (NSC 45388) surgical adjuvant study COG protocol 7040. Cancer 47:2556, 1981
457. Veronesi U, Adamus J, Aubert C et al: A randomized trial of adjuvant chemotherapy and immunotherapy in cutaneous melanoma. N Engl J Med 307:913, 1982
458. Fisher RI, Terry WD, Hodes RJ et al: Adjuvant immunotherapy or chemotherapy for malignant melanoma. Surg Clin North Am 61:1267, 1981
459. Misset JL, Delgado M, DeVassal F et al: Immunotherapy or chemotherapy as adjuvant treatment for malignant melanoma: A.G.I.F. trial. In Salmon SS, Jones SE (eds): Adjuvant Therapy of Cancer III, p 225. New York, Grune & Stratton, 1981
460. Quagliana J, Tranum B, Neidhardt J et al: Adjuvant chemotherapy with BCNU, Hydrea and DTIC (BHD) with or without immunotherapy (BCG) in high-risk melanoma patients. Proc Am Assoc Cancer Res 21:399, 1980
461. Wood WC, Cosimi AB, Carey RW et al: Randomized trial of adjuvant therapy for "high risk" primary malignant melanoma. Surgery 83:677, 1978
462. Kaiser LR, Burk MW, Morton DL: Adjuvant therapy for malignant melanoma. Surg Clin North Am 61:1249, 1981
463. Holtermann OA, Karakousis CP, Berger J et al: Adjuvant therapy with DTIC and Estracyt or BCG in malignant melanoma. Soc Clin Oncol 21:400, 1980
464. Banzet P, Jacquillat C, Civatte J et al: Adjuvant chemotherapy in the management of primary malignant melanoma. Cancer 41:1240, 1978
465. Cunningham TJ, Schoenfeld D, Nathanson L et al: A controlled ECOG study of adjuvant therapy in patients with stage I and II malignant melanoma. In Salmon SS, Jones SE (eds): Adjuvant Therapy of Cancer II, p 507. New York, Grune & Stratton, 1979
466. Knost JA, Reynolds V, Greco FA et al: Adjuvant chemoimmunotherapy: Stage I/II malignant melanoma. J Surg Oncol 19:165, 1982
467. Quirt IC and National Cancer Institute of Canada Melanoma Study Group: Randomized controlled trial of adjuvant chemoimmunotherapy with DTIC and BCG after complete excision of primary melanoma with a poor prognosis of melanoma metastases. Can Med Assoc J 128:929, 1983
468. Czarnetski BM, Macher E, Berendt H et al: Current status of melanoma chemotherapy and immunotherapy. Recent Results Cancer Res 80:264, 1982
469. Balch CM, Smalley RV, Bartolucci AA et al: A randomized prospective clinical trial of adjuvant *C. parvum* immunotherapy in 260 patients with clinically localized melanoma (stage I): Prognostic factors analysis and preliminary results. Cancer 49:1079, 1982
470. Paterson AHG, Williams D, Jerry LM et al: Reduced incidence of loco-regional recurrences in melanoma using BCG immunotherapy after surgery. Proc Am Soc Clin Oncol 1:170, 1982
471. Thatcher N, Mene A, Banerjee SS et al: Randomized study of *Corynebacterium parvum* adjuvant therapy following surgery for (phase III) malignant melanoma. Br J Surg 73:111, 1986
472. Spitler LE, Sagebiel R: A randomized trial of levamisole versus placebo as adjuvant therapy in malignant melanoma. N Engl J Med 303:1143, 1980
473. Silberman AW, Morton DL: Adjuvant therapy following surgery for primary malignant melanoma. In Costanzi JJ (ed): Malignant Melanoma, p 207. The Hague, Martinus Nijhoff, 1983
474. Bukowski RM, Deodhar S, Hewlett JS et al: Randomized controlled trial of transfer factor in stage II malignant melanoma. Cancer 51:269, 1983
475. Cunningham TJ, Schoenfeld D, Nathanson L et al: A controlled ECOG study of adjuvant therapy in patients with stage I and II malignant melanoma. In Salamon SS, Jones SE (eds): Adjuvant Therapy of Cancer II, p 507. New York, Grune & Stratton, 1979
476. Lipton A, Harvey HA, Lawrence B et al: *Corynebacterium parvum* vs. BCG adjuvant immunotherapy in human malignant melanoma. Cancer 51:57, 1983
477. Bernardino ME, Goldstein HM: Gray scale ultrasonography in the evaluation of metastatic melanoma. Cancer 42:2529, 1978
478. Heaston DK, Putman CE: Radiographic manifestations of thoracic malignant melanoma. In Seigler HF (ed): Clinical Management of Melanoma, p 62. The Hague, Martinus Nijhoff, 1982
479. Braman SS, Whitcomb ME: Endobronchial metastasis. Arch Intern Med 135:543, 1975
480. Feldman L, Kricun ME: Malignant melanoma presenting as a mediastinal mass. JAMA 241:396, 1979
481. Curtis A McB, Ravin CE, Deering TF et al: The efficacy of full-lung tomography in the detection of early metastatic disease from melanoma. Diagn Radiol 144:27, 1982
482. Chen JTT, Dahmash NS, Ravin CE et al: Metastatic melanoma to the thorax: Report of 130 patients. AJR 137:293, 1981
483. Gromet MA, Ominsky SH, Epstein WL et al: The thorax as the initial site for systemic relapse in malignant melanoma: A prospective survey of 324 patients. Cancer 44:776, 1979
484. Simeone JF, Putman CE, Greenspan RH: Detection of metastatic malignant melanoma by chest roentgenography. Cancer 39:1993, 1977
485. Webb WR, Gamsu G: Thoracic metastasis in malignant melanoma: A radiographic survey of 65 patients. Chest 71:176, 1977
486. Webb WR: Hilar and mediastinal lymph node metastases in malignant melanoma. AJR 133:805, 1979
487. Chang AE, Schaner EG, Conkle DM et al: Evaluation of computed tomography in the detection of pulmonary metastases: A prospective study. Cancer 43:913, 1979
488. Mintzer RA, Malave SR, Neiman HL et al: Computed vs. conventional tomography in evaluation of primary and secondary pulmonary neoplasms. Radiology 132:653, 1979
489. Neifeld JP, Michaelis LL, Doppman JL: Suspected pulmonary metastases: Correlation of chest x-ray, whole lung tomograms, and operative findings. Cancer 39:383, 1977
490. Schaner EG, Chang AE, Doppman JL et al: Comparison of computed and conventional whole lung tomography in detecting pulmonary nodules: A prospective radiologic–pathologic study. AJR 131:51, 1978
491. Morton DL, Joseph WL, Ketcham AS et al: Surgical resection and adjunctive immunotherapy for selected patients with multiple pulmonary metastases. Ann Surg 178:360, 1973
492. Cahan WG: Excision of melanoma metastases to lung: Problems in diagnosis and management. Ann Surg 178:703, 1973
493. Cline RE, Young WG Jr: Long term results following surgical treatment of metastatic pulmonary tumors. Am Surg 36:61, 1970
494. McCormack, Martini N: The changing role of surgery for pulmonary metastases. Ann Thorac Surg 28:139, 1979
495. Thayer JO Jr, Overholt RH: Metastatic melanoma to the lung: Long-term results of surgical excision. Am J Surg 149:558, 1985

496. Vidne BA, Richter S, Levy MJ: Surgical treatment of solitary pulmonary metastasis. Cancer 38:2561, 1976
497. Morrow CE, Vassilopoulos PP, Grage TB: Surgical resection for metastatic neoplasms of the lung: Experience at the University of Minnesota Hospitals. Cancer 45:2981, 1980
498. Mathisen DJ, Flye MW, Peabody J: The role of thoracotomy in the management of pulmonary metastases from malignant melanoma. Ann Thorac Surg 27:295, 1979
499. Wilkins EW Jr, Head JM, Burke JF: Pulmonary resection for metastatic neoplasms in the lung: Experience at the Massachusetts General Hospital. Am J Surg 135:480, 1978
500. Presant CA, Bartolucci AA, Smalley RV et al: Cyclophosphamide plus 5-(3,3-dimethyl-1-triazeno)-imidazole-4-carboxamide (DTIC) with or without *Corynebacterium parvum* in metastatic malignant melanoma. Cancer 44:899, 1979
501. Vieth RG, Odom GL: Intracranial metastases and their neurosurgical treatment. J Neurosurg 23:375, 1965
502. Amer MH, Al-Sarraf M, Baker LH et al: Malignant melanoma and central nervous system metastases: Incidence, diagnosis, treatment and survival. Cancer 42:660, 1978
503. Fell DA, Leavens ME, McBride CM: Surgical versus nonsurgical management of metastatic melanoma of the brain. Neurosurgery 7:238, 1980
504. Ginaldi S, Wallace S, Shalen P et al: Cranial computed tomography of malignant melanoma. AJR 136:145, 1981
505. Pennington DG, Milton GW: Cerebral metastasis from melanoma. Aust NZ J Surg 45:405, 1975
506. Bullard DE, Cox EB, Seigler HF: Central nervous system metastases in malignant melanoma. Neurosurgery 8:26, 1981
507. Posner JB, Chernik NL: Intracranial metastases from systemic cancer. Adv Neurol 19:579, 1978
508. Bremer AM, West CR, Didolkar MS: An evaluation of the surgical management of melanoma of the brain. J Surg Oncol 10:211, 1978
509. Enzmann DR, Kramer R, Norman D et al: Malignant melanoma metastatic to the central nervous system. Radiology 127:177, 1978
510. Gildersleeve N Jr, Koo AH, McDonald CJ: Metastatic tumor presenting as intracerebral hemorrhage: Report of 6 cases examined by computed tomography. Radiology 124:109, 1977
511. Carella RJ, Gelber R, Hendrickson F et al: Value of radiation therapy in the management of patients with cerebral metastases from malignant melanoma: Radiation Therapy Oncology Group brain metastases study I and II. Cancer 45:679, 1980
512. Posner JB: Management of central nervous system metastases. Semin Oncol 4:81, 1977
513. Byrne TN, Cascino TL, Posner JB: Brain metastases from melanoma. J Neuroncol 1:313, 1983
514. Hayward RD: Malignant melanoma and the central nervous system: A guide for classification based on the clinical findings. J Neurol Neurosurg Psychiatry 39:526, 1976
515. Hayward RD: Secondary malignant melanoma of the brain. Clin Oncol 2:227, 1976
516. McCann WP, Weir BKA, Elvidge AR: Long-term survival after removal of metastatic malignant melanoma of the brain: Report of two cases. J Neurosurg 28:483, 1968
517. McNeel DP, Leavens ME: Long-term survival with recurrent metastatic intracranial melanoma: Case report. J Neurosurg 29:91, 1968
518. Scott M: Spontaneous intracerebral hematoma caused by cerebral neoplasms: Report of eight verified cases. J Neurosurg 42:338, 1975
519. Wolpert SM, Zimmer A, Schechter MM et al: The neuroradiology of melanomas of the central nervous system. AJR 101:178, 1967
520. Felix EL, Sindelar WF, Bagley DH et al: The use of bone and brain scans as screening procedures in patients with malignant lesions. Surg Gynecol Obstet 141:867, 1975
521. Thomas JH, Panoussopoulous D, Liesmann GE et al: Scintiscans in the evaluation of patients with malignant melanomas. Surg Gynecol Obstet 149:574, 1979
522. Muss HB, Richards F II, Barnes PL et al: Radionuclide scanning in patients with advanced malignant melanoma. Clin Nucl Med 4:516, 1979
523. Bardfeld PA, Passalaqua AM, Braunstein P et al: A comparison of radionuclide scanning and computed tomography in metastatic lesions of the brain. J Comput Assist Tomogr 1:315, 1977
524. Holtas S, Cronqvist S: Cranial computed tomography of patients with malignant melanoma. Neuroradiology 22:123, 1981
525. Solis OJ, Davis KR, Adair LB, et al: Intracerebral metastatic melanoma: CT evaluation. Comput Tomogr 1:135, 1977
526. Wasserstrom WR, Glass JP, Posner JP: Diagnosis and treatment of leptomeningeal metastases from solid tumors: Experience with 90 patients. Cancer 49:759, 1982
527. Fleisher M, Wasserstrom WR, Schold SC et al: Lactic dehydrogenase isoenzymes in the cerebrospinal fluid of patients with systemic cancer. Cancer 47:2654, 1981
528. Fletcher JW, George EA, Henry RE, et al: Brain scans, dexamethasone therapy, and brain tumors. JAMA 232:1261, 1975
529. Gottlieb JA, Frei E III, Luce JK: An evaluation of the management of patients with cerebral metastases from malignant melanoma. Cancer 29:701, 1972
530. Ruderman NB, Hall TC: Use of glucocorticoids in the palliative treatment of metastatic brain tumors. Cancer 18:298, 1965
531. Atkinson L: Melanoma of the central nervous system. Aust NZ J Surg 48:14, 1978
532. Cooper JS, Carella R: Radiotherapy of intracerebral metastatic malignant melanoma. Radiology 134:735, 1980
533. Hafstrom L, Jonsson P-E, Stromblad L-G: Intra-cranial metastases of malignant melanoma treated by surgery. Cancer 46:2088, 1980
534. Winston KR, Walsh JW, Fischer EG: Results of operative treatment of intracranial metastatic tumors. Cancer 45:2639, 1980
535. Galicich JH, Sundearesan N, Arbit E et al: Surgical treatment of single brain metastasis: Factors associated with survival. Cancer 45:381, 1980
536. Bauman ML, Price TR: Intracranial metastatic malignant melanoma: Long-term survival following subtotal resection. South Med J 65:344, 1972
537. Mandybur TI: Intracranial hemorrhage caused by metastatic tumors. Neurology 27:650, 1977
538. Reyes V, Horrax G: Metastatic melanoma of the brain: report of a case with unusually long survival period following surgical removal. Ann Surg 131:237, 1950
539. Ziegler JC, Cooper JS: Brain metastases from malignant melanoma: Conventional vs. high-dose-per-fraction radiotherapy. Int J Radiat Oncol Biol Phys 12:1839, 1986
540. Vlock DR, Kirkwood JM, Leutzinger C et al: High dose fraction radiation therapy for intracranial metastases of malignant melanoma. Cancer 49:2289, 1982
541. Choi KN, Withers R, Rotman M: Metastatic melanoma in brain: Rapid treatment or large dose fractions. Cancer 56:10, 1985
542. Szybalski W: X-ray sensitization by haloprimidines. Cancer Chemother Rep 58:539-557, 1974
543. Hatanaka H, (ed): Neutron capture therapy, in: Proceedings of the Second International Symposium on Neutron Capture Therapy, Teikyo University, Tokyo, October 1985. Niigata, Japan, Nishimura Co, 1986
544. Young RF, Post EM, King GA: Treatment of spinal epidural metastases: Randomized prospective comparison of laminectomy and radiotherapy. J Neurosurg 53:741, 1980
545. Booth JB: Malignant melanoma of the stomach: Report of a case presenting as an acute perforation and review of the literature. Br J Surg 52:262, 1965
546. Das Gupta TK, Brasfield RD: Metastatic melanoma of the gastrointestinal tract. Arch Surg 88:969, 1964
547. Goldstein HM, Beydoun MT, Dodd GD: Radiologic spectrum of melanoma metastatic to the gastrointestinal tract. AJR 129:605, 1977
548. Oddson TA, Rice RP, Seigler HF et al: The spectrum of small bowel melanoma. Gastrointest Radiol 3:419, 1978
549. Thompson WH: Radiographic manifestations of metastatic melanoma to the gastrointestinal tract, hepatobiliary system, pancreas, spleen and mesentery. In Seigler HF (ed): Clinical Management of Melanoma, p 133. The Hague, Martinus Nijhoff, 1982
550. Fraser-Moodie A, Hughes RG, Jones SM et al: Malignant melanoma metastases to the alimentary tract. Gut 17:206, 1976
551. Giler S, Kott I, Urca I: Malignant melanoma metastatic to the gastrointestinal tract. World J Surg 3:375, 1979
552. Goodman PL, Karakousis CP: Symptomatic gastrointestinal metastases from malignant melanoma. Cancer 48:1058, 1981
553. Harris MN: Massive gastrointestinal hemorrhage due to metastatic malignant melanoma of small intestine. Arch Surg 88:1049, 1964
554. Klausner JM, Skornick Y, Lelcuk S et al: Acute complications of metastatic melanoma to the gastrointestinal tract. Br J Surg 69:195, 1982
555. Macbeth WAAG, Gwynne JF, Jamieson MG: Metastatic melanoma in the small bowel. Aust NZ J Surg 38:309, 1969
556. Shah SM, Smart DF, Texter EC Jr et al: Metastatic melanoma of the stomach: The endoscopic and roentgenographic findings and review of the literature. South Med J 70:379, 1977
557. Karakousis C, Holyoke ED, Douglass HO Jr: Intussusception as a complication of malignant neoplasm. Arch Surg 109:515, 1974
558. Beckly DE: Alimentary tract metastases from malignant melanoma. Clin Radiol 25:385, 1974
559. Felix EL, Bagley DH, Sindelar WF et al: The value of the liver scan in preoperative screening of patients with malignancies. Cancer 38:1137, 1976
560. Seigler HF, Fetter BF: Current management of melanoma. Ann Surg 186:1, 1977
561. Garg R, McPherson TA, Lentle B et al: Usefulness of an elevated serum lactate dehydrogenase value as a marker of hepatic metastases in malignant melanoma. Can Med Assoc J 120:1114, 1979
562. Bernardino ME, Thomas JL, Barnes PA et al: Diagnostic approaches to liver and spleen metastases. Radiol Clin North Am 20:469, 1982
563. MacCarty RL, Stephens DH, Hattery RR et al: Hepatic imaging by computed tomography: A comparison with ^{99m}Tc-sulfur colloid, ultrasonography, and angiography. Radiol Clin North Am 17:137, 1979
564. Smith TJ, Kemeny MM, Sugarbaker PH et al: A prospective study of hepatic imaging in the detection of metastatic disease. Ann Surg 195:486, 1982
565. Snow JH Jr, Goldstein HM, Wallace S: Comparison of scintigraphy, sonography, and computed tomography in the evaluation of hepatic neoplasms. AJR 132:915, 1979
566. Balthazar EJ, Javors B: Malignant melanoma of the gallbladder. Am J Gastroenterol 64:332, 1975
567. Bowdler DA, Leach RD: Metastatic intrabiliary melanoma. Clin Oncol 8:251, 1982
568. McFadden PM, Krementz ET, McKinnon WMP et al: Metastatic melanoma of the gallbladder. Cancer 44:1802, 1979
569. Shimkin PM, Soloway MS, Jaffe E: Metastatic melanoma of the gallbladder. AJR 116:393, 1972
570. Fon GT, Wong WS, Gold RH et al: Skeletal metastases of melanoma: Radiographic, scintigraphic, and clinical review. AJR 137:103, 1981
571. Stewart WR, Gelberman RH, Harrelson JM et al: Skeletal metastases of melanoma. J Bone Joint Surg [Am] 60:645, 1978
572. Devereux D, Johnston G, Blei L et al: The role of bone scans in assessing malignant melanoma in patients with stage III disease. Surg Gynecol Obstet 151:45, 1980

573. Steiner GM, MacDonald JS: Metastases to bone from malignant melanoma. Clin Radiol 23:52, 1972
574. Tong D, Gillick L, Hendrickson FR: The palliation of symptomatic osseous metastases: Final results of the study by the Radiation Therapy Oncology Group. Cancer 50:893, 1982
575. Harrelson JM: Orthopaedic considerations in the treatment of malignant melanoma. In Seigler HF (ed): Clinical Management of Melanoma, p 435. The Hague, Martinus Nijhoff, 1982
576. McKenzie DJ, Bell R: Melanoma with solitary metastasis to ureter. J Urol 99:399, 1968
577. Das Gupta T, Grabstald H: Melanoma of the genitourinary tract. J Urol 93:607, 1965
578. deKernion JB, Golub SH, Gupta RK et al: Successful trans-urethral intralesional BCG therapy of a bladder melanoma. Cancer 36:1662, 1975
579. Goldstein HM, Kaminsky S, Wallace S et al: Urographic manifestations of metastatic melanoma. Radiology 121:801, 1974
580. Sheehan EE, Greenberg SD, Scott R Jr: Metastatic neoplasms of the bladder. J Urol 90:281, 1963
581. Weston PAM, Smith BJ: Metastatic melanoma in the bladder and urethra. Br J Surg 51:78, 1964
582. Woodard BH, Ideker RE, Johnston WW: Cytologic detection of malignant melanoma in urine. Acta Cytol 22:350, 1978
583. Nakazono M, Iwata S, Kuribayashi N: Disseminated metastatic ureteral melanoma: A case report. J Urol 114:624, 1975
584. Lowsley OS: Melanoma of the urinary tract and prostate gland. South Med J 44:487, 1951
585. Baab GH, McBride CM: Malignant melanoma: The patient with an unknown site of primary origin. Arch Surg 110:896, 1975
586. Chang P, Knapper WH: Metastatic melanoma of unknown primary. Cancer 49:1106, 1982
587. Das Gupta T, Bowden L, Berg JW: Malignant melanoma of unknown primary origin. Surg Gynecol Obstet 117:341, 1963
588. Giuliano AE, Moseley HS, Morton DL: Clinical aspects of unknown primary melanoma. Ann Surg 191:98, 1980
589. Milton GW, Shaw HM, McCarthy WH: Occult primary malignant melanoma: Factors influencing survival. Br J Surg 64:805, 1977
590. Reintgen DS, McCarty KS, Woodard B et al: Metastatic malignant melanoma with an unknown primary site. Surg Gynecol Obstet 156:335, 1983
591. Mundth ED, Guralnick EA, Raker JW: Malignant melanoma: A clinical study of 427 cases. Ann Surg 162:15-28, 1965
592. Elder DE: Metastatic melanoma. Pigment Cell 8:182, 1987
593. Elder DE, Ainsworth AM, Clark WH Jr: The surgical pathology of primary cutaneous malignant melanoma. In Clark WH Jr, Goldman LI, Mastrangelo MJ (eds): Human Malignant Melanoma, p 55. New York, Grune & Stratton, 1979

DANIEL M. ALBERT
JOHN D. EARLE
JOSE A. SAHEL

CHAPTER 45 *Intraocular Melanomas*

Intraocular melanomas are the most common primary ocular malignancy in whites. They arise from uveal melanocytes (*i.e.*, mature melanin-producing and melanin-containing cells) residing in the uveal stroma. These cells originate from the neural crest and possess long, dendrite-like processes. Other proliferations of pigmented cells can occur in the eye: the pigmented epithelia of the iris, ciliary body, and retina can undergo a reactive or neoplastic proliferation, forming adenomas or adenocarcinomas.[1-2] This chapter deals exclusively with uveal melanomas.

EPIDEMIOLOGY

The annual age-adjusted incidence of nonskin melanomas as reported in the Surveillance, Epidemiology and End Results (SEER) Program during 1973 to 1977 was 0.7/100,000 population in the United States.[3] Similar figures were reported from epidemiologic studies conducted in New England (0.69/100,000 residents in 1984),[4] the Swedish west coast (0.72/100,000 over the period 1956 to 1975),[5] and Iceland (0.7/100,000 in males and 0.5/100,000 in females over the period 1955 to 1979).[6] Ocular tumors make up 30% to 79% of noncutaneous melanomas.[7,8] In the Third National Cancer Survey, conducted in 1969 to 1971, the precise anatomical origin of ocular melanomas was unspecified in about 25% of cases, 73% of the tumors arose within the globe (mainly from the choroid), and 2% developed from the conjunctiva. Melanoma accounted for 70% of all eye malignancies, followed in frequency by the childhood tumor retinoblastoma (13%). In persons over the age of 20, melanoma was the reported diagnosis for 80% of all primary ocular cancers.[8] Data from the Connecticut Tumor Registry,[9] the Missouri Department of Health,[7] China,[10] the SEER Program,[3] New England,[4] Ireland,[6] Finland,[11] and the ocular melanoma task force[12] are similar to those reported by the Third National Cancer Survey.[8]

The annual age-adjusted incidence of ocular melanomas is about one-eighth that of skin melanomas in the United States.[13] The recently observed increase in the incidence of cutaneous melanomas has not been observed for uveal melanomas.[5,6,10] Although the incidence increases steadily by decade, with a peak in the seventh decade, uveal melanomas can occur before the age of 20, as illustrated by 101 of the 6359 cases on file at the Registry of Ophthalmic Pathology at the Armed Forces Institute of Pathology (AFIP).[4,10,14,15] Whites have an eightfold greater risk for ocular melanomas than blacks (compared to a sixfold greater risk for skin melanomas),[12] and a threefold greater risk than certain Asian populations.[13,16] Although Scotto et al found that the overall risk of ocular melanomas did not vary by sex, Jensen[15] and Gislason et al[6] noted a predominance of males.[6] Ocular and skin melanoma show similar age patterns, with more women affected at younger ages and more men later in life.[13] The Third National Cancer Survey indicated a left-sided excess of 18% for ocular melanomas in males and a right-sided excess in females.[8]

ETIOLOGY AND HISTOGENESIS OF OCULAR MELANOMAS

As for most human cancers, the specific causes of ocular melanomas are unknown. However, epidemiologic, electron microscopic, and experimental data allow characterization of risk factors, predisposing conditions, and hypothetical genetic or oncogenic causes.

PREDISPOSING CONDITIONS

Ocular and oculodermal melanocytosis (*i.e.*, nevus of Ota) predispose to the development of uveal melanomas. In 4.6% of reported cases of nevus of Ota, malignant transformation was recorded,[17-21] and except for a single anecdotal case,[18] the melanoma occurred in the pigmented eye. Rare cases of uveal melanomas have been reported in patients with neurofibromatosis.[21,22] Evidence that nevi are the origin of most choroidal melanomas has been provided by Yanoff and Zimmerman[23] and others.[24,25] Yet a nevus-like configuration associated with choroidal melanoma may in some cases be explained by other mechanisms, such as (1) flattening of normal uveal melanocytes or of tumor cells, (2) a secondary proliferative effect of the malignancy, or (3) common oncogenic stimuli.[25-27] The last two mechanisms have been postulated in a few cases of bilateral diffuse melanocytic tumors of the uvea in patients with systemic carcinoma.[25,28]

In rare instances, a familial increased occurrence of uveal melanoma has been recorded.[29] Data on the occurrence of uveal melanocytic tumors in patients with the dysplastic nevus syndrome are controversial,[29-33] but in general support periodic ophthalmoscopic examination of these patients.[25,26] Cytogenetic studies of uveal melanoma tissues from 19 patients suggest that recessive alleles at some chromosome 2 loci may be important in the oncogenesis of these tumors.[34]

ONCOGENIC STIMULI

Certain electron microscopic and biomolecular studies of ocular melanomas suggest an etiologic role of viruses.[35] Viruses such as the feline sarcoma virus have been used successfully in the induction of animal ocular melanoma models.[35-38] In a study of a single population of chemical workers, a statistically significant and higher than expected incidence of ocular melanomas was found.[9] Nicotine has been incriminated in the unusual incidence of uveal melanomas in males.[39] Various chemicals, including nickel bisulfide, platinum, methylcholanthrene, ethionine, *N*-2-fluorenylacetamide, radium, and *N*-methyl-*N*-nitrosourea, have been reported to induce ocular melanomas in animals.[36-45] A possible connection among Parkinson's disease, levodopa therapy, and malignant melanoma has been mentioned.[46] The role of hormonal factors and pregnancy has been suggested in anecdotal reports, but no epidemiologic or biologic support exists for these factors.[25,47]

A recent case–control study lends support to the etiological role of sunlight exposure.[48] These data, contradicting previous studies,[8,49] could account for the high association between light iris color and the presence of iris melanocytic lesions.[50]

HISTOPATHOLOGY, PROGNOSTIC PARAMETERS, AND NATURAL HISTORY

CHOROIDAL AND CILIARY BODY MELANOMAS

Cytologic and Histologic Classification

The accurate diagnosis of uveal melanoma is generally easily made by the experienced histopathologist. In rare cases, differentiation from metastatic carcinoma may be facilitated by immunohistochemical labeling of S100 protein. This technique is not helpful in differentiating other neural crest–derived tumors (schwannomas, neurofibromas, and leiomyomas).[25] In 1931 Callender recognized major cell types in the spectrum of cells composing uveal melanomas and thus provided a cytologic classification clearly correlated with prognosis after enucleation.[51] The different cell types are as follows.[25,51,52]

Spindle A cells are uniform, cohesive cells with a small, slender, spindle-shaped nucleus often showing a longitudinal fold in the nuclear membrane. The nucleoli are not distinct, and mitotic figures are rare. The cell borders are difficult to identify.

Spindle B cells are plumper, cohesive spindle cells with larger ovoid nuclei containing a coarse chromatin network and a conspicuous nucleolus. Mitotic figures are seen more frequently. The cell borders are difficult to discern.

Spindle A and B cells may be arranged in rows or palisades, constituting the classic fascicular pattern, which is now regarded as having no prognostic significance per se.[25,53] A careful reappraisal of 90 pure spindle A melanomas by McLean et al[54] found that 15 had cytologic features of benignity whereas the other 75 had larger, hyperchromatic nuclei with frequent mitotic activity associated with histologic features of malignancy (*e.g.*, invasiveness) and greater size. In the revised AFIP classification of uveal melanomas, the spindle A and B subtypes are no longer separated.[53]

Epithelioid cells were described by Callender as larger, more pleomorphic, poorly cohesive, polygonal cells with abundant acidophilic cytoplasm. The nuclei are round and contain large single or multiple nucleoli. Mitotic figures are abundant. A type consisting of small cells with less cytoplasm and a smaller nucleus is now included in this category because it has other typical features of epithelioid cells such as large eosinophilic nucleoli and lack of cohesiveness.[55]

According to this cytologic characterization, uveal melanomas are divided into three categories:

1. Spindle cell melanomas type A, B, or both, accounting for 30% of intraocular tumors.
2. Mixed cell melanomas containing both spindle and epithelioid cells.
3. Epithelioid cell melanomas, accounting for 5% of intraocular tumors.

The major cell types described by Callender are part of a continuous spectrum, and the pathologist's identification of a particular cell type involves subjective judgment.[56,57] This issue was addressed by Gamel et al, who described a more objective method of assessing uveal melanomas histopathologically.[58] This method, which uses computerized cytomorphometry, mainly entails evaluating the inverse of the standard deviation of the nucleolar area (ISDNA). This appears to be the best objective cytologic measure of a tumor's malignant potential ($p > 0.001$).[59] Work by Gamel et al has corroborated the well-documented prognostic value of Callender's classification.[51,53,55,59–64]

Paul and co-workers reviewed 2652 cases accessioned at the AFIP by 1959 and found that 95% of patients with spindle A tumors, 85% of those with spindle B tumors, 60% of those with mixed tumors, and 83% of those with epithelioid tumors were alive 5 years after enucleation.[61] At 15 years after enucleation the survival rates were respectively 85%, 80%, 46%, and 34%.[61] McLean et al, in a review of 3432 cases from the AFIP, found that the overall mortality from metastasis 15 years after enucleation was 46%. The mortality of patients with mixed cell melanomas was three times that of patients with pure spindle cell lesions.

In Jensen's series of 302 cases reported from Denmark that had been observed for 25 years, 150 (50%) of the patients died of metastatic melanoma.[15,65,66] Less than 1% of patients with spindle A tumors died of metastatic disease; 63% with mixed tumors died; and in 71% with epithelioid tumors the cause of death was metastatic melanoma.

Natural History

GROWTH RATE. Little is known about the natural history of uveal melanomas; until recently, all patients underwent enucleation immediately after the diagnosis.[25,67,68] Data on the growth pattern of small melanomas from series of patients observed by Gass and others have contributed to our knowledge of the rate of intraocular tumor growth prior to treatment.[69,70] These findings and other selected reports[71,72] suggest a Gompertzian (exponential) growth curve, as postulated by Manschot et al.[73] The doubling time of uveal tumors may vary from 2 months or less[70–72,74] to several years.[68–70] In rapidly growing tumors, a high mitotic activity and the presence of epithelioid cells have been documented.[70,72,74]

Rarely, spontaneous regression of a choroidal melanoma has been described.[75]

INTRAOCULAR SPREAD. Small melanomas grow from a discoid to a hemispherical shape. They progressively obliterate the choriocapillaris and displace Bruch's membrane and the retina inward. When Bruch's membrane is disrupted, the tumor grows in the subretinal space in a mushroom configuration. The retinal pigment epithelium overlying the tumors undergoes early changes, including drusen formation and orange pigment (lipofuscin) accumulation.[76,77] The neurosensory retina is frequently detached and in some instances infiltrated by tumor cells, which can eventually seed into the vitreous.

Anterior tumors are more likely to affect the lens and to seed the posterior chamber. The zonule, lens, iris, anterior chamber, and angle may be involved. A secondary glaucoma may result from obstruction of the outflow pathways by tumor cells, cell debris, and phagocytic cells swollen with ingested cell debris (melanomalytic glaucoma).[77,78] The tumor may infiltrate, through the scleral spur, into the anterior chamber.

Although the sclera is thought to be an effective barrier against extraocular extension, scleral infiltration by tumor cells along ciliary vessels and nerves and along the vortex veins is frequent (32.3% of large melanomas in a series reported by Shammas and Blodi[79]). Approximately 5% of melanomas grow diffusely in the plane of the uvea or circumferentially along the root of the iris. They induce a slight thickening of the uvea (approximately 3–5 mm) and are often unsuspected or diagnosed late when secondary glaucoma or extraocular spread occur. The latter may be adjacent to or within the optic nerve or can occur anteriorly about the limbus.[80]

EXTRAOCULAR EXTENSION. Although extrascleral extension may be observed with small tumors,[81,82] it is more likely to occur when the tumor has reached a larger size. In a study by Shammas and Blodi, extrascleral extension was observed in 18% of tumors exceeding 10 mm in diameter.[82] The overall incidence of transscleral extension was determined to be about 13% among 1842 malignant melanomas studied by Starr and Zimmerman.[83] These authors noted a tenfold increase in the incidence of postoperative recurrence if the tumor extended to the surgical margin. Other rare paths of extraocular spread include the optic nerve[84] and the lumen of the vortex veins.[85]

As would be expected from the absence of lymphatics in the eye, lymphatic spread has not been demonstrated. Hematogenous dissemination to the liver is a frequent form of metastatic spread.[16,25,86,87] Patients with preexisting liver damage are more likely to be affected.[88,89] Some clones of melanoma cells with a preferential propensity for liver metastasis mediated by cell surface properties have been characterized.[90,91] Metastases to other sites (lung, heart, gastrointestinal tract, lymph nodes, pancreas, skin, central nervous system, bones, spleen, adrenal, kidneys, ovaries, thyroid) generally occur in association with liver metastases.

In a series of studies, Zimmerman and McLean found that most deaths from metastatic disease occurred in the first 5 years after enucleation, with a peak mortality in the second and third years (about 8% per year).[25,55,67,92–94] In a conclusion that remains controversial, they incriminated enucleation as a risk factor, and suggested two principal mechanisms: (1) dissemination of tumor cells during traumatic operations, as demonstrated experimentally by Fraunfelder et al[95]; and (2) decreased host resistance to disseminated tumor cells. This latter mechanism has been called by Niederkorn et al the "loss of intraocular induced concomitant immunity" mediated by cytotoxic T-lymphocytes.[96,97]

Zimmerman and McLean's assumptions have been challenged by several investigators. Seigel et al concluded that the statistical data can be interpreted differently, and that no evidence presently suggests that the existing pattern of treatment be altered.[98] Manschot and Van Peperzeel,[73] Kersten and Blodi,[99] and Davidorf[100] pointed out that most melanomas are diagnosed only when they have reached a relatively large size and concomitantly given rise to metastases, and only then are enucleated. The clinical consequences of these controversies are the use of less traumatic techniques for enucleation and new impetus to the search for alternative treatments.[77,101]

Prognostic Assessment of Choroidal and Ciliary Body Melanomas

In most studies the second most important prognostic parameter after the number of epithelioid cells is the largest tumor diameter.[25,55,62,63,79,102] This is followed, according to Seddon et al, by the location of the anterior margin of the tumor, invasion of the line of transsection, and the degree of pigmentation.[62,63] Shammas and Blodi,[79] in a study of 253 choroidal and ciliary body melanomas for which a follow-up of 5 years or more was available, identified nine factors that significantly influenced prognosis:

Age of the patient at enucleation
Location of the tumor
Location of its anterior border
Largest tumor diameter in contact with the sclera
Height of the tumor
Integrity of Bruch's membrane
Cell type
Pigmentation
Scleral infiltration by tumor cells

McLean et al,[64] using a multivariate analysis, reached similar conclusions for small melanomas. Parameters that significantly influenced prognosis were cell type, largest dimension, scleral extension, and mitotic activity. A single factor analysis identified three additional factors of significance: degree of scleral invasion, optic nerve invasion, and pigmentation. In most studies increased pigmentation has been associated with increased mortality.[16,61,64,79] However, in a multivariate analysis these last three parameters appear statistically related to cell type and tumor size.[59,62,63,75]

In summary, all studies show that the prognosis of a patient with a choroidal or ciliary body melanoma is adversely affected if

the tumor contains epithelioid cells.
the tumor involves the ciliary body.
the largest tumor dimension exceeds 10 mm.
the tumor extends to the sclera.
numerous mitotic figures are present.

DISTINGUISHING FEATURES OF IRIS MELANOMAS

Malignant melanoma of the iris is rare in comparison to melanomas of the rest of the uvea; the estimated ratios range from 1:6 to 1:30.[16,103–106] Many patients (17%–33%) give a long history of a noticeable pigmented iris lesion prior to clinical diagnosis, interpreted by many physicians as suggesting that the tumor arose from a preexisting nevus.[107–112] Zimmerman believes that the difference in size between tumors of the iris and other uveal tumors is the most critical feature affecting tumor behavior. Iris melanomas are invariably small lesions, usually much smaller than the posterior uveal tract tumors that come to clinical attention.[107,113] Iris melanomas grow more slowly than posterior uveal melanomas. Kasten et al,[114] applying the scheme proposed by Apple and Blodi for choroidal melanomas,[115] suggested that the slow growth rate is related to the small size of iris melanomas. This slow growth probably accounts for occasional cases of recurrences, metastases, or death from disease several years or decades after the onset of symptoms.[114]

Both the older literature and more recent reports stress the relatively benign behavior and good prognosis of iris melanomas compared with melanomas of the choroid and ciliary body. The latter are associated with a mortality tenfold higher than the mortality from iris melanomas.[55] Green, reviewing 783 cases from the literature, noted 18 (2.29%) reported deaths from metastatic disease.[14] In two recent clinicopathologic studies, 138 and 107 patients with a previous diagnosis of iris melanomas had no tumor-related deaths.[106,107] These series emphasize that many lesions previously called melanomas are actually nevi. Jakobiec and Silbert reclassified 138 lesions with a former diagnosis of melanomas, into a nine-part classification including only three malignant categories corresponding to only 13% of lesions.[106] In a similar series of 107 such tumors, a ten-part classification derived from Jakobiec and Silbert was applied. Only 10% of the lesions were considered melanomas.[107] Nevertheless, in the prognostic assessment of iris melanomas, one should remember that local spread of some melanocytic tumors, even with "benign" cytology, may lead to sight-threatening complications such as refractory secondary glaucoma.[106,107,111]

DIAGNOSIS OF UVEAL MELANOMAS

CHOROIDAL AND CILIARY BODY MELANOMAS

The diagnosis of choroidal and ciliary body melanomas has reached a high degree of accuracy at eye centers where experienced clinicians and modern ancillary testing facilities are available. This is well illustrated by a comparison of the misdiagnosis rates among the eyes on file at the AFIP: 19% (of 529 eyes) until 1962, 20% (of 208 eyes) between 1963 and 1970, 6.4% (of 744 eyes) between 1970 and 1980.[116–119] During the 11-year period of the last study, the rate of misdiagnosis declined from 12.5% to 1.4%.[119] Between 1954 and 1977 the misdiagnosis rate was 2.6% (of 224 eyes) at the Mayo Clinic.[120] In this series, in addition, six clinically unsuspected melanomas were found.[119] This high rate of correct clinical diagnosis is particularly impressive because only outpatient procedures (including clinical examination, ultrasound, and fluorescein angiography) were used. No biopsies were performed, as is done for many other tumors. A review of 395 eyes enucleated during a 50-year period, drawn from the pathology files of Ohio State University, revealed a misdiagnosis rate of 10.9% in the period 1931 to 1959 that decreased to 1.7% in the period 1960 to 1981. Nine percent of choroidal melanomas were unsuspected preoperatively; all were in eyes with opaque media.[121] In a series of 400 consecutive patients referred to the oncology unit of the Wills Eye Hospital with an incorrect diagnosis of melanoma (*i.e.*, patients proved to have a pseudomelanoma), the correct diagnosis was reached through clinical evaluation in 397 cases (99%).[122] In that series, the most commonly encountered conditions mimicking a melanoma included suspicious choroidal nevi (26.5%), peripheral disciform degeneration (11%), congenital hypertrophy of the retinal pigment epithelium (9.5%), and choroidal hemangioma (8%). Most metastatic carcinomas had been correctly diagnosed by the referring ophthalmologists.[123]

The cornerstone of diagnosis of posterior uveal melanoma remains clinical examination and, in particular, indirect ophthalmoscopy through a dilated pupil. Fundus contact lens examination and the use of a three-mirror lens can be extremely helpful.[77] Scleral transillumination as advocated by Reese is also a useful aid.[76] Pigmented conjunctival lesions such as conjunctival melanoma, staphylomas, scleral ectasia, hematoma, cellular blue nevi, and ocular melanocytosis may mimic extraocular extension of uveal melanomas.[124] Visual field studies are of little help, especially in distinguishing melanomas from choroidal nevi.[56,77,124] Although clinical examination by an experienced observer remains the most important test in establishing the presence of an ocular melanoma, ancillary diagnostic testing can be extremely valuable.[28,77,124]

Fluorescein angiography and monochromatic photography have proved useful in differentiating among subretinal or choroidal hemorrhage, hemangioma, and melanoma. Although no angiographic pattern is pathognomonic, features of value include early mottling fluorescence, orange pigment over the margin of the tumor, progressive fluorescence of the lesion with late staining, and multiple pinpoint leaks that increase in size.[28,77] Breaks in Bruch's membrane and retinal invasion can be detected from abnormalities such as a "double circulation" pattern.[28,77,125]

The combined use of A- and B-mode ultrasound (US) techniques is of great value in confirming the clinical diagnosis of choroidal melanoma, especially in the presence of opaque media.[77,122,126,127] The B-mode US characteristics useful in differentiating melanomas from metastases or hemangiomas are acoustic hollowness, choroidal excavation, and orbital shadowing.[77] Small tumors elevated less than 2 mm to 3 mm cannot be evaluated accurately. In large tumors, US provides valuable size data for serial measurements.[128] Extrascleral extension can be detected by contact B-mode US.[129] The usefulness of radioactive phosphorus (^{32}P) in determining malignancy is more controversial. In addition, it probably has limited indications for use in routine cases in which adequate support for a diagnosis of ocular melanoma can be obtained with less complicated procedures.[77,130-135]

Radiologic examination, including computed tomography (CT), is useful in evaluating the presence and size of extraocular extension of tumor.[136,137] Images of uveal melanoma have been obtained by magnetic resonance imaging. This promising imaging modality will probably become more useful with the increase in availability and use of thin-section imaging and surface coils.[138-140]

Electrophysiologic testing usually is not indicated, although some authors report that the electrooculogram is reduced in eyes of patients with choroidal melanoma.[141-143]

Immunologic testing does not yet offer reliable results.[144-146] Using the indirect immunoperoxidase method, Felberg et al found that 78% of patients with uveal malignancy had tumor-associated antibodies (TAA), whereas 24% of controls tested positive for TAA.[147] Unfortunately, TAA assays could not be used to separate primary from secondary uveal tumors. However, surveillance of melanoma-associated antigens and carcinoembryonic antigens may be useful for monitoring recurrences or metastatic disease.[148,149]

In a review of 51 consecutive patients who had undergone enucleation for a choroidal melanoma and 50 patients with simulating lesions, Char and colleagues found that the ophthalmoscopic examination was the most accurate diagnostic modality, allowing correct diagnosis of choroidal melanomas in all patients with clear media.[150] Subretinal fluid, orange pigmentation, and collar-button configuration occurred more often with melanomas than with other lesions. In 63% of melanoma patients, fluorescein angiography was diagnostic, and in 82%, A- and B-mode US was diagnostic.

In some dubious cases, fine needle aspiration biopsy has been proposed.[151] However, the interpretation of aspirates may be difficult, and subsequent tumor cell seeding in the needle track has been reported.[152]

Despite ancillary examinations, the differential diagnosis of small tumors may be difficult. Careful follow-up of such patients at short intervals with photography, fluorescein angiography, and US is advocated in order to demonstrate tumor growth.[28]

Patients with suspected intraocular melanoma should undergo a physical examination and metastatic workup. Clinical laboratory studies should include routine blood work, chest radiography, and liver enzyme measurements. CT should be performed if other tests suggest liver involvement.[86,87,127,153-155] Liver US and liver-spleen scans may be useful.

IRIS MELANOMAS

Iris tumors are visible not only to the ophthalmologist but also to the patient, family, and friends.[113] Patients frequently are aware of a spot on the iris that has been present for many years but has only recently shown growth. The ophthalmologist can examine the lesion carefully with a slit-lamp biomicroscope and gonioscopy, and with the aid of serial iris fluorescein photography can determine the size and vasculature of the tumor.[156] Iris tumors are usually small, discrete lesions, but they may be diffuse and infiltrative or even multiple.[103,106,107] Only a few clinical findings—vascularity, involvement of the ciliary body, and secondary glaucoma—are helpful in distinguishing benign from malignant iris melanocytic tumors.[106,107] The differential diagnosis includes entities characterized by diffuse increased pigmentation (*e.g.*, melanosis, siderosis bulbi, heterochromia iridis, foreign bodies encapsulated by fibrous tissue, iris cysts, essential iris atrophy, peripheral anterior synechia, tumors of the retinal pigment epithelium, leiomyomas, granulomas—as seen in tuberculosis, herpes, or sarcoidosis—metastatic neoplasms, syphilitic gummas, and nevoxanthoendothelioma.[157-159]

TREATMENT OF UVEAL MELANOMAS

PRETREATMENT CLINICAL STAGING

In light of current knowledge it is useful to discuss the treatment of choroidal and ciliary body melanomas in terms of tumor size—small tumors, <10 mm in diameter *and* <2

TABLE 45-1. Histopathologic Classification of Choroidal and Ciliary Body Melanocytic Tumors

IRIS

Pretreatment Clinical Classification (cTNM)

Primary Tumor (T)

TX	Minimum requirements to assess the primary tumor cannot be met
T0	No evidence of primary tumor
T2	Tumor involving not more than one quadrant, with extension into the anterior chamber angle
T3	Tumor involving more than one quadrant, with extension into the anterior chamber angle
T4	Tumor with extraocular extension

Regional Lymph Nodes (N)

NX	Minimum requirements to assess the regional lymph nodes cannot be met
N0	No evidence of regional lymph node involvement
N1	Evidence of involvement of the regional lymph nodes

Distant Metastases (M)

MX	Minimum requirements to assess the presence of distant metastases cannot be met
M0	No evidence of distant metastases
M1	Evidence of distant metastases

CILIARY BODY

Pretreatment Clinical Classification (cTNM)

Primary Tumor (T)

TX	Minimum requirements to assess the primary tumor cannot be met
T0	No evidence of primary tumor
T1	Tumor limited to the ciliary body
T2	Tumor with extension into the anterior chamber and/or iris
T3	Tumor with extension into the choroid
T4	Tumor with extraocular extension

Regional Lymph Nodes (N)

NX	Minimum requirements to assess the regional lymph nodes cannot be met
N0	No evidence of regional lymph node involvement
N1	Evidence of involvement of the regional lymph nodes

Distant Metastases (M)

MX	Minimum requirements to assess the presence of distant metastases cannot be met
M0	No evidence of distant metastases
M1	Evidence of distant metastases

CHOROID

Pretreatment Clinical Classification (cTNM)

Primary Tumor (T)

TX	Minimum requirements to assess the primary tumor cannot be met
T0	No evidence of primary tumor
T1	Tumor not more than 10 mm in its greatest dimension, and/or with an elevation of not more than 3 mm
T1a	Tumor not more than 7 mm in its greatest dimension and with an elevation of not more than 2 mm
T1b	Tumor more than 7 mm but not more than 10 mm in its greatest dimension and with an elevation of more than 2 mm but not more than 3 mm
T2	Tumor more than 10 mm but not more than 15 mm in its greatest dimension and with an elevation of more than 3 mm but not more than 5 mm
T3	Tumor more than 15 mm in its greatest dimension or with an elevation of 5 mm or more
T4	Tumor with extraocular extension
	Note: When dimension and elevation show a difference in classification, the highest category should be used for classification.

Regional Lymph Nodes (N)

NX	Minimum requirements to assess the regional lymph nodes cannot be met
N0	No evidence of regional lymph node involvement
N1	Evidence of involvement of regional lymph nodes

Distant Metastases (M)

MX	Minimum requirements to assess the presence of distant metastases cannot be met
M0	No evidence of distant metastases
M1	Evidence of distant metastases

mm in elevation; medium-sized tumors, 10 to 15 mm in diameter *and* 2 to 5 mm in elevation; and large melanomas, >15 mm in diameter *and* >5 mm in elevation.[25,77] This division by size is followed for the remainder of this chapter.

Comparisons of results from various series would benefit from uniform staging of uveal tumors. The American Joint Committee on Cancer has developed a staging classification of uveal melanomas based on the TNM system (Table 45-1).[26,160]

TREATMENT OF CHOROIDAL AND CILIARY BODY MELANOMAS

In the late 19th century, enucleation became the standard and almost universally accepted treatment for all choroidal or ciliary body melanomas.[161] Even today, early enucleation continues to have its ardent advocates.[72,162] However, in the last 10 years enucleation has been reassessed as a conventional means of treating malignant melanomas of the choroid and ciliary body. This reassessment has resulted from (1) the development of newer and more precise diagnostic tests for recognizing malignant melanomas and the serial documentation of their size; (2) more information about clinical and pathologic features that determine survival; (3) additional observations about the natural course of untreated ciliary body and choroidal melanomas; (4) therapeutic developments other than enucleation to treat these tumors without destroying the eye; and (5) disagreements to the value and risks of enucleation.[25,38,55,62,63,68,69,72,77,92–101,115,127]

Most authors today agree that the goals of an ophthalmologist treating a uveal melanoma should be to destroy or inactivate the neoplasm, to maintain useful vision in the involved eye, to use a treatment with few side effects, and most important, to provide the patient with the best prognosis for life among the treatment alternatives that are available.[77,127,163] Beyond these rather basic statements, many controversies will continue until results from prospective randomized treatment trials are collected.[77,101,127,164,165] Therefore, the treatment ultimately selected is determined by the specific findings in the individual case with regard to tumor size, location, and growth rate, the preferences of the ophthalmologist, and the desires of the patient.

Small Melanomas

The choices open to the physician treating a small choroidal or ciliary body melanoma include (1) observation; (2) some method of local treatment, such as radiation therapy, photoradiation, cryotherapy, ultrasonic hyperthermia, local resection, and so forth; and (3) enucleation.

OBSERVATION. An accumulating body of evidence indicates that the risks in observing these tumors are low (Table 45-2).[56,68,69,75,77,165–168] Serial examination every 3 months without intervention seems appropriate if the melanoma is asymptomatic, the diagnosis is equivocal, no growth is seen on serial ophthalmoscopic, photographic and US examinations, and, in elderly or seriously ill patients, the tumor is growing slowly.[77,125,165,168]

If the tumor shows progression, particularly rapid growth or an increase in size beyond 10 mm in diameter and 2 mm in elevation, or if the lesion results in significant impairment of vision, treatment is indicated.

PHOTOCOAGULATION. In this method, the xenon arc, the argon laser, or photoradiation with red light after photosensitization with hematoporphyrin derivatives can be used.[77,165,169–175] Some success with photocoagulation has been documented histologically in small series.[77,169–176] The following criteria for selecting patients with melanoma for photocoagulation treatment were suggested by Meyer-Schmickerath[169] and Vogel[170] and adapted by Shields.[77]

TABLE 45-2. Observation Versus Enucleation of Small Tumors of the Choroid and Ciliary Body

Aspect Evaluated	*Char et al*[69]	*Gass*[70]*	*Shields*[70]	*Davidorf et al*[168]	*McLean et al*[164]	*Shammas et al*[79]	*Barr et al*[166]	*Thomas et al*[167]	*Seddon et al*[62]
No. of eyes	20	100	150	38	37	129	16	27	267
Management	Observation; enucleation if growth	Observation; enucleation or further follow-up if growth	Observation; enucleation if growth	Enucleation	Enucleation	Enucleation	Enucleation	Enucleation	Enucleation
Follow-up	1–19 yr prior to enucleation; average 4.5 yr after enucleation	>8 yr	2–5 yr	>5 yr	6 yr	5 yr	6 yr	10 yr	8 yr
Evidence of growth	45%	36%	10%–15%						
Deaths from metastases	. . .	3%	. . .	5% 5 yr 19% 10 yr	25%	8% 5 yr 10% 10 yr	11%	10%	12% 5 yr 18% 10 yr

*Gass assumed that tumors exhibiting no growth over 5 years were actually nevi.

1. The diagnosis of melanoma and evidence of growth should be documented thoroughly.
2. The tumor should not be greater than 5 diopters in elevation and 6 disc diameters at its greatest diameter.
3. The tumor must be surrounded completely, without damaging the fovea or the optic disc.
4. The patient must have clear ocular media and a sufficient mydriasis to enable photocoagulation to be performed.
5. The tumor surface should not have large retinal vessels.

Photocoagulation requires several outpatient treatment sessions and is carried out after mydriasis and (for xenon photocoagulation) induction of retrobulbar anesthesia. A double confluent row of heavy coagulation is repeated three times at monthly intervals to encircle the tumor and to obliterate the choroidal vasculature supplying the lesion. The tumor subsequently becomes necrotic with gray discoloration and a surrounding chorioatrophic scar.

Long-term complications of photocoagulation include retinal vascular obstruction, visual field defect, macular pucker, cystoid macular edema, choroid neovascularization, vitreous hemorrhage, and retinal detachment.[77,170] Recurrences may appear, usually within 2 years of treatment. In a 20-year follow-up of 54 patients with uveal melanoma, Vogel reported that 63% were alive, although only 46% were considered cured by photocoagulation. Twenty percent of patients subsequently underwent enucleation. Of the 20 patients (37%) who died, eight did so as a result of metastatic disease, three died of other causes, and in nine patients the cause of death was undetermined.[170] Shields reports that among 35 patients treated between 1976 and 1979, 25 retained useful vision, five had poor vision, and five subsequently underwent enucleation. There were no tumor-related deaths.[77]

Photocoagulation seems best suited for small posterior melanomas located within 3 mm of the optic disc or fovea. In such lesions radiation-induced retinopathy may cause visual loss.[77] The patient's wish to avoid radiation therapy or enucleation may be the deciding factor.

Reports on hematoporphyrin phototherapy are too preliminary to provide conclusive data.[172-176]

RADIATION THERAPY. For lesions meeting the clinical criteria for choroidal melanomas that are no larger than about 10 mm in height or 15 mm in diameter, brachytherapy is an acceptable therapeutic option. Before 1930, Moore used radon-222 seeds to treat choroidal melanomas.[177] In the 1960s Stallard popularized cobalt-60 as a brachytherapy source.[178] Although dosimetry was still relatively crude, the use of standardized plaques became common because of the long half-life of ^{60}Co. Results in large series of patients managed in similar fashion thus became available, demonstrating the equivalence with enucleation within the limits of balancing the prognostic factors in these retrospective analyses. Markoe et al used the Cox proportional hazards model to compare results in 100 patients treated with ^{60}Co plaques with results in enucleated patients. Survival was better for the plaque-treated patients, although not statistically significant. Vision deteriorated in a roughly linear fashion: approximately 40% had vision better than 20/200 visual acuity at 5 years.[179]

In 1976 Sealy and co-workers first reported using iodine-125 for choroidal melanomas.[180] In 1979, Packer and Rotman suggested ^{125}I as the isotope of choice for brachytherapy of choroidal melanomas, based on the ease of shielding the adjacent structures and the safety of medical personnel.[181] Garretson et al reported results in 26 patients treated with ^{125}I plaques who were followed up for a minimum of 2 years (mean, 45 months).[181a] One patient died at 21 months. Visual acuity remained within two Snellen lines of preoperative levels in 54%. Of the 12 who lost more than two lines of acuity, retinal changes developed in 8 and cataracts in 3. Enucleation accounted for the loss of vision in the last patient. Enucleation was necessary in a single patient because of tumor growth.

Lommatsch, utilizing beta particles from ruthenium-106/rhubidium-106, has published results comparable to those achieved with ^{125}I or ^{60}Co plaque.[182] He notes "successful" treatment in 131 of 205 cases.

The Collaborative Ocular Melanoma Study (COMS), involving some 30 clinical centers and six central units carefully monitoring quality, is conducting two randomized clinical trials. The first trial compares enucleation with ^{125}I brachytherapy for melanomas 3 to 8 mm in height and up to 16 mm in diameter. Eligible patients randomized to irradiation receive treatment with ^{125}I sources in a gold-backed plaque shielding the posterior tissues. A dose of 100 Gy is delivered at 50 to 125 cGy per hour at the apex of the tumor (for tumors 5–8 mm high and to 5 mm for tumors 3–5 mm high). The second trial tests the value of preoperative external beam irradiation (2000 cGy delivered in five fractions) versus enucleation alone for patients with larger tumors.[127]

Heavy charged particle beams are being investigated, utilizing cyclotron-produced protons at Massachusetts General Hospital and synchrocyclotron-generated helium ions at the Lawrence Laboratory at Berkeley. These beams were selected because of their sharp penumbra and the Bragg peak, describing the greater deposition of energy at a depth. Both facilities use careful patient evaluation prior to treatment and sophisticated immobilization procedures that allow precise positioning of ports, guided by x-ray confirmation of the tumors, the bases of which are marked by tantalum rings sutured to the sclera around the margin demonstrated by transillumination and indirect ophthalmoscopy. For treatment, generally 4000 to 10,000 cGy (^{60}Co equivalent dose corrected for relative biological effect [RBE] with a factor of 1.1) is delivered in five fractions over 8 to 10 days at Harvard. At Berkeley, 7000 or 8000 cGy (^{60}Co equivalent dose corrected for RBE 1.3) is delivered in five fractions. With a relatively short follow-up period, Saunders et al have reported that irradiation failed locally in 5 of 75 patients, and 18% had neovascular glaucoma. Twenty patients received 70 Gy equivalent. Because of the high local failure rate, the dose was increased to 80 Gy equivalent for the remaining 55 patients. The mean follow-up at the time of reporting was only 18 months. Local recurrence was detected in 4 of 20 patients treated with 70 Gy equivalent and in 1 of 55 treated to 80 Gy equivalent (mean follow-up in the latter group was 14 months). Of the 42 patients followed up for more than a year, 10 had vision worse than 20/200.

Between 1975 and 1981, 128 patients were treated at Lawrence Laboratory. The results were reported after a median follow-up of 5.4 years. Vision appeared to be declining linearly, with 69% of patients having at least 20/200 visual acuity at 5 years. Eight eyes were enucleated because of complications (6%), and metastases had developed in 20.5% of patients.[184] Poorer outcome was seen for thicker tumors and tumors located nearer the optic disk and fovea.[185]

OTHER LOCAL NONSURGICAL TECHNIQUES. Preliminary reports on the experimental use of ultrasonically induced hyperthermia noted tumor regression in most cases.[186,187] This technique has been used in association with radiation in exceptional instances, with good results.[188–190]

Lincoff and co-workers obtained discouraging results with cryotherapy of ocular melanomas in four patients.[191] Anecdotal reports of successful treatments for small peripheral melanomas exist.[77,165,192,193]

LOCAL RESECTION. Peyman and co-workers have developed a technique of local sclerochorioretinal resection for choroidal melanomas.[194–197] After a series of photocoagulation treatments around the tumor to create a firm chorioretinal adhesion or an area of bare sclera, the tumor is removed surgically, along with the adjacent sclera and retina. The defect is replaced by a scleral graft. Peyman has suggested that surgical candidates should have

1. no evidence of metastatic disease;
2. the ability to tolerate general anesthesia;
3. a tumor base no larger than 12 mm and tumor location at least three disc diameters from the optic disc;
4. exudative retinal detachment no larger than one third of the fundus;
5. clear media.

After local resection, one third of the eyes (11 of 35) needed enucleation because of complications, including vitreous hemorrhage and retinal detachment. Most authors note that patients treated by local resection are also amenable to radiation therapy.[77,165] Local resection has not been adopted widely.

Iridocyclectomy has proved useful in the treatment of ciliary body melanomas in several series.[77,198,199] In the series of Forrest and associates, of 107 iridocyclectomies for ciliary body melanoma, 6% of the patients had subsequent enucleation. The majority of problems related to surgical management or to the tumor area occurred within 4 years of surgery.[198] In contrast to resection of choroidal melanomas, iridocyclectomy is widely accepted for the treatment of ciliary body melanomas.

ENUCLEATION. In the case of patients with a healthy second eye, enucleation is advised if the tumor shows evidence of rapid progression, and invasion of the optic nerve or extraocular extension is suspected.[77] Other considerations, including loss of central vision, failure of previous conservative treatment, and the patient's wishes, may make enucleation a reasonable choice.[165]

Large Melanomas of the Choroid and Ciliary Body

There is at present general agreement that it would be inadvisable to treat cases of large melanoma by methods other than enucleation.[200] Possible exceptions include patients with only one sighted eye, rare patients in whom vision can be salvaged, and patients who refuse enucleation.[201] Abramsom and Ellsworth recommend local irradiation in these latter difficult cases.[201] Some authors recommend external irradiation prior to enucleation in related cases.[202–204] This method is currently being evaluated in the COMS study.[125]

Zimmerman and associates have suggested that when enucleation is carried out, the "no-touch" technique of Fraunfelder should be considered.[77,205] This method was designed to minimize the possibility of seeding of tumor cells into the blood vessels during enucleation. The authors claim that this technique avoids intraocular pressure elevations above 15 mm before complete freezing occurs around the tumor. Subsequently, cryotherapy prevents flow of fluid and blood to or from the tumor prior to the manipulation necessary for enucleation. Although most surgeons do not use the "no-touch" technique, it is increasingly recognized that enucleation should be carried out by a person skilled and experienced in the procedure, and that surgery should be done with a minimum of manipulation.

Medium-sized Melanomas of the Choroid and Ciliary Body

Treatment of medium-sized tumors is the subject of current controversy. Although general agreement exists that observation of small melanomas carries little risk and that large melanomas should be treated by enucleation, there is less consensus regarding medium-sized melanomas. To date, good results with radiation therapy (versus enucleation, see Table 45-2) using various modalities have been reported. This method is unequivocally advocated in patients with only one sighted eye, in patients whose eyes retain useful vision, and in patients who refuse enucleation. However, in most cases, both options remain possible, and personal choice is often the deciding factor. For these reasons, a nationwide, prospective, randomized comparison of radiation versus enucleation has been undertaken under the auspices of the National Eye Institute "in order to demonstrate that either radiation or enucleation offers a better chance for survival, or that there is no difference in survival." In this 15-year multiple-center study, tumors 3 to 8 mm in height *and* no more than 16 mm in basal diameter will be randomized.[125]

Immunotherapy and chemotherapy have not yet been established as significantly useful modalities for primary or adjuvant treatment of medium-sized melanomas of the choroid or ciliary body.[206–209]

Tumors with Extrascleral Extension

Patients with extrascleral extension of an intraocular tumor have a poor prognosis.[83] Affeldt and co-workers reported that two thirds of 60 patients followed up after enucleation for uveal melanoma with extrascleral extension eventually died of metastatic disease.[208] Attempts should be made to detect extraocular extension preoperatively with CT and US. At the time of surgery the episcleral surface should be carefully inspected. These visual and imaging findings can be eventually confirmed by frozen section study.[25] Excision of adjacent Tenon's capsule and orbital tissue is then performed.

The indications for primary or secondary exenteration remain controversial since no clear evidence exists for an increase of life expectancy after exenteration as compared to enucleation. Of 15 patients who underwent exenteration in the series reported by Starr and Zimmerman, only one survived longer than 13 months.[83] Affeldt et al did not conclude that exenteration within 2 months after enucleation is beneficial.[127,208] Shammas and Blodi in 1977 reported good results of exenteration, particularly if the operation was performed promptly after recognition of residual tumor in the orbit.[82] However, a subsequent study of long-term results at the same institution showed little improvement in survival. Adjuvant therapy will likely find increasing use in these cases in the future.[77,209–212]

Metastatic Disease

Metastatic disease is observed in about 2% of patients at the time of diagnosis.[12,86,87] Fournier and co-workers and Gronemeyet et al have suggested that local resection of solitary hepatic metastases in patients with uveal melanoma may be an effective palliative treatment and possibly lead to longer survival.[211,212] Others have recently reported prolonged periods of remission after hepatic artery embolization.[213] These tentative treatments are yet anecdotal. Metastatic melanoma is incurable at present and usually is treated palliatively with chemotherapy and radiation therapy, similar to metastatic cutaneous melanomas.

TREATMENT OF IRIS MELANOMAS

In the past 30 years, gradual recognition of the better prognosis of iris melanomas has led to a conservative approach. Every effort is made to avoid enucleation in most cases.[77,104–109] According to the clinical situation different options are possible.

OBSERVATION. If the following factors are present, surgical intervention is not necessary:

1. There is no clinical evidence that the lesion is progressing.
2. There is a lack of pronounced neovascularization.
3. The lesion is not producing any visual disturbances.
4. No significant complications, such as hemorrhage into the anterior chamber, trabecular involvement, secondary glaucoma, or an obvious extension outside the eye, are evident.
5. The lesion arises in the patient's better eye.
6. The lesion is situated near the pupil.

CONSERVATIVE EXCISION. The anecdotal nature of reports on photocoagulation of iris melanomas does not allow definitive conclusions to be drawn.[214–217] If there is evidence of tumor growth, surgery should be considered.

In 1958 Reese pointed out that iris melanoma, with or without ciliary body involvement, seldom metastasized or spread by seeding. Iris melanomas are capable of local extension and infiltration. Subsequently, interest developed in the use of iridectomy, iridocyclectomy, and corneoscleroiridosclerectomy, with grafting, as an alternative to enucleation.[76,77] Although some authors advocate diagnostic needle biopsy of the iris lesion, this is usually not performed because of the risk of tumor dissemination.[106,154,155,218]

The object of excisional iridectomy is to remove the tumor entirely without allowing tumor cells to disseminate in the eye or the incision. In general, the procedure is similar to that described by Reese, in which a limbal incision is made that is large enough to allow removal of the lesion by basal iridectomy under direct observation.[76] Iridectomy of peripheral tumors should be performed before the lesion extends to the trabecular meshwork.[107] If the trabecular meshwork is involved in the quadrant of the tumor, inducing secondary glaucoma, iridotrabeculectomy is indicated. When the iris tumor extends to the ciliary body, iridocyclectomy must be considered, as advocated by Raubitscheck[217] and Verhoeff[218] many years ago and introduced into clinical practice through the efforts of Muller and Stallard.[219–221] A basic technique for resecting the iris tumor together with involved ciliary body has been described by Jones.[222] Many cases requiring more than iridectomy for iris tumor removal also require an operation more extensive than iridocyclectomy. Examples are patients in whom the tumor not only invades the ciliary body, but also fills the chamber angle and is adjacent to the tissue in the angle or to the cornea itself. In such cases the surgeon should consider corneoscleroiridocyclectomy with or without a corneoscleral graft.[77] An alternative method not requiring a transplant has been described by Sears.[223]

Surgical complications include intraocular hemorrhage, hypotony, subluxation of the lens, cataract, late detachment of the retina, corneal edema, macular edema, and vitreous loss. If the excision is incomplete, tumor may recur. When metastases occur after iridocyclectomy, it is difficult to assess the role of surgery in their causation.[113]

ENUCLEATION. Enucleation for an iris melanoma is now exceptional but must be considered in individual cases if the following conditions exist:

1. The melanoma is clearly growing and involves more than half the iris and anterior chamber angle.
2. The tumor, growing in a blind eye, is too bulky to be removed by excision.
3. There is a secondary glaucoma refractory to medical treatment in an eye with a melanoma involving more than half the iris.
4. Extraocular extension is present.
5. The tumor has recurred after previous iridectomy or

iridocyclectomy and is judged unsuitable for further treatment.

In the case of extraocular spread or metastatic disease, the treatment is the same as for advanced choroidal or ciliary body melanoma.

REFERENCES

1. Rawles ME: Origin of pigment cells from neural crest in mouse embryo. Physiol Zool 20:248–266, 1947
2. Zimmerman LE: Melanocytes, melanocytic nevi and melanocytomas. Invest Ophthalmol 4:11–41, 1965
3. Young JL, Percy CL, Asire AJ et al: Cancer Incidence and Mortality in the United States, 1973–1977. Cancer Inst Monogr 57:1–187, 1981
4. Egan EM, Seddon JM, Gragoudas ES et al: Uveal melanoma in New England: Profile of cases diagnosed in 1984. Presented at the Massachusetts Eye and Ear Infirmary Alumni Association Award Meeting, Cambridge, Mass, April 9, 1987
5. Abrahamson M: Malignant melanoma of the choroid and the ciliary body 1956–1975. Acta Ophthalmol (Copenh) 61:600–610, 1982
6. Gislason I, Magnusson B, Tulinius H: Malignant melanoma of the uvea in Iceland 1955–1979. Acta Ophthalmol (Copenh) 63:385–394, 1985
7. Chang JC: Personal communication, October 4, 1983, Missouri Department of Social Services, Division of Health
8. Cutler SJ, Young JL (eds): Third National Cancer Survey: Incidence Data. Natl Cancer Inst Monogr 41:1–454, 1975
9. Albert DM, Puliafito CA, Fulton AB et al: Increased incidence of choroidal malignant melanoma occurring in a single population of chemical workers. Am J Ophthalmol 89:323–337, 1980
10. Kuo PK, Puliafito CA, Wang KM et al: Uveal melanoma in China. In Ni C, Albert DM (eds): Ocular Tumors and Other Ocular Pathology. Int Ophthalmol Clin 22(3):57–71, 1982
11. Teikari JM, Rairio I: Incidence of choroidal melanoma in Finland in the years 1973–1980. Acta Ophthalmol (Copenh) 63:661–665, 1985
12. Graham BJ, Daune TD: Meetings, conferences, symposia: Report of ocular melanoma task force. Am J Ophthalmol 90:728–733, 1981
13. Scotto J, Fraumeni JF, Lee JAH: Melanomas of the eye and other noncutaneous sites. JNCI 56:489–491, 1976
14. Barr CC, McLean IW, Zimmerman LE: Uveal melanomas in children and adolescents. Arch Ophthalmol 95:2133–2134, 1981
15. Jensen OA: Malignant melanoma of the uvea in Denmark 1943–1952: A clinical, histopathological and prognostic study. Acta Ophthalmol [Suppl] 75:1–220, 1963
16. Haukulin T, Teppo L, Saxen F: Cancer of the eye: A review of trends and differentials. World Health Stat Q 31:143–158, 1978
17. Albert DM, Scheie HG: Nevus of Ota with malignant melanoma of the choroid. Arch Ophthalmol 69:774, 1963
18. Blodi FC: Ocular melanocytosis and melanoma. Am J Ophthalmol 80:389, 1975
19. Dutton JJ, Anderson RL, Schelper RL et al: Orbital malignant melanoma and oculodermal melanocytosis: Report of two cases and review of the literature. Ophthalmology 91:497–507, 1984
20. Gonder JR, Shileds JA, Albert DM et al: Uveal malignant melanoma associated with ocular and oculodermal melanocytosis. Ophthalmology 89:953–960, 1982
21. Yanoff M, Zimmerman LE: Histogenesis of malignant melanomas of the uvea: III. The relationship of congenital ocular melanocytosis and neurofibromatosis to uveal melanomas. Arch Ophthalmol 77:331–336, 1967
22. Gartner S: Malignant melanoma of the choroid in von Recklinghausen's disease. Am J Ophthalmol 23:73–78, 1940
23. Yanoff M, Zimmerman LE: Histogenesis of malignant melanomas of the uvea: II. Relationship of uveal nevi to malignant melanomas. Cancer 20:497–507, 1967
24. Volcker HE, Naumann GO: Multicentric primary malignant melanomas of the choroid: Two separate malignant melanomas of the choroid and two uveal nevi in one eye. Br J Ophthalmol 62:408–413, 1978
25. Zimmerman LE: Malignant melanoma of the uveal tract, in Spencer WH (ed): Ophthalmic Pathology, Vol 3, pp 2072–2139. Philadelphia, WB Saunders.
26. Sahel JA, Albert DM: Choroidal nevi. In Ryan SJ (ed): Retinal Disease. St Louis, CV Mosby (in press)
27. Albert DM, Lahav M, Packer S et al: Histogenesis of malignant melanomas of the uvea: Occurrence of nevus-like structures in experimental choroidal tumors. Arch Ophthalmol 92:318–323, 1974
28. Gass JDM: Stereoscopic Atlas of Macular Diseases, pp 182–195. St Louis, CV Mosby, 1987
29. Walker JP, Wecker JJ, Albert DM et al: Uveal malignant melanoma in three generations of the same family. Am J Ophthalmol 88:723–726, 1979
30. Albert DM, Chang MA, Lamping K et al: The dysplastic nevus syndrome: A pedigree with primary malignant melanomas of the choroid and skin. Ophthalmology 92:1728–1734, 1985
31. Albert DM, Searl SS, Forget B et al: Uveal findings in patients with cutaneous melanoma. Am J Ophthalmol 95:474–479, 1987
32. Rodriguez-Sains RS: Ocular findings in patients with dysplastic nevus syndrome. Ophthalmology 93:661–665, 1986
33. Taylor MR, Guerry D IV, Dondl EE et al: Lack of association between intra-ocular melanoma and cutaneous dysplastic nevi. Am J Ophthalmol 98:478–482, 1984
34. Mukai S, Dryja TP: Loss of alleles at polymorphic loci on chromosome 2 in uveal melanoma. Cancer Genet Cytogenet 22:45–53, 1986
35. Albert DM: The association of viruses with uveal melanoma. Trans Am Ophthalmol Soc 77:367–421, 1980
36. Albert DM, Shadduck JA, Lin HS et al: Animal models for the study of uveal melanomas. Int Ophthalmol Clin 20(2):143–160, 1980
37. Albert DM: Need for animal models of human diseases of the eye. Am J Pathol 101:177–185, 1980
38. Albert DM: Ocular melanoma: A challenge to visual science. Friedenwald Lecture. Invest Ophthalmol Vis Sci 23:550–580, 1982
39. Keeney AH, Waddell WJ, Perraut TC: Carcinogenesis and nicotine in malignant melanoma of the choroid. Trans Am Ophthalmol Soc 80:131–142, 1987
40. Albert DM, Gonder JR, Papale J et al: Induction of ocular neoplasms in Fisher rats by intraocular injection of nickel subsulfide. Invest Ophthalmol Vis Sci 22(6):768–782, 1982
41. Evgenyeva TP: Pigmented tumors in rats induced by introduction of platinum and cellophane films into the chamber of the eye. Biull Eksp Biol Med (Moscow) 74:75–77, 1972
42. Patz A, Wulff LB, Rogers SW: Experimental production of ocular tumors. Am J Ophthalmol 48:98–111, 1959
43. Benson WR: Intraocular tumor after ethionine and *N*-2-fluorenyl-acetamide. Arch Pathol 73:404–406, 1962
44. Taylor GH, Dougherty TF, Mays CW et al: Radium-induced eye melanomas in dogs. Radiat Res 51:361–373, 1972
45. Albert DM, Puliafito CA, Haluska FG et al: Induction of ocular neoplasms in Wistar rat by *N*-methyl-*N*-nitrosourea. Exp Eye Res 42:83–86, 1986
46. Van Rens GH, De John P, Demols E et al: Uveal malignant melanoma and levodopa therapy in Parkinson's disease. Ophthalmology 89:1464–1466, 1982
47. Seddon JM, MacLaughlin DT, Albert DM et al: Uveal melanomas presenting during pregnancy and the investigation of estrogen receptors in melanomas. Br J Ophthalmol 66:695–704, 1982
48. Tucker MA, Shields JA, Hartge P et al: Sunlight exposure as risk factor for malignant melanoma. N Engl J Med 313:789–792, 1985
49. Edwood JM, Lee JA, Walter SD et al: Relationship of melanoma and other skin cancer mortality to latitude and ultraviolet radiation in the United States and Canada. Int J Epidemiol 3:325–332, 1972
50. Kliman GH, Augsburger JJ, Shields JA: Association between iris color and iris melanocytic lesions. Am J Ophthalmol 100:547–548, 1985
51. Callender GR: Malignant melanotic tumors of the eye: A study of histologic types in 111 cases. Trans Am Acad Ophthalmol Otolaryngol 36:131–142, 1931
52. Zimmerman LE, Sobin LH: International Histological Classification of Tumours, No. 24. Histological Typing of Tumors of the Eye and its Adnexa. Geneva, World Health Organization, 1980
53. McLean IW, Foster WD, Zimmerman LE, Gamel JW: Modifications of Callender's classification of uveal melanoma at the Armed Forces Institute of Pathology. Am J Ophthalmol 96:502–509, 1983
54. McLean IW, Zimmermann LE, Evans RM: Reappraisal of Callender's spindle A type of malignant melanoma of choroid and ciliary body. Am J Ophthalmol 86:557–564, 1978
55. McLean IW, Foster WD, Zimmerman LE: Uveal melanoma: Location, size, cell type and enucleation as risk factors in metastasis. Hum Pathol 13:123–132, 1981
56. Gass JDM: Problems in the differential diagnosis of choroidal nevi and malignant melanomas. The XXXIII Edward Jackson Memorial Lecture. Am J Ophthalmol 83:299–323, 1977
57. Gamel JW, McLean IW: Quantitative analysis of the Callender classification of uveal melanoma cells. Arch Ophthalmol 95:686–691, 1977
58. Gamel JW, McLean IW: Modern developments in histopathologic assessment of uveal melanomas. Ophthalmology 91:679–684, 1984
59. Gamel JW, McLean IW, Greckey RA et al: Objective assessment of the malignant potential of intraocular melanomas with standard microslides stained with hematoxylin-eosin. Hum Pathol 16:689–692, 1985
60. Wilder HC, Callender GR: Malignant melanoma of the choroid: Further studies on prognosis by histologic type and fiber content. Am J Ophthalmol 22:851–855, 1939
61. Paul EV, Parnel BL, Fraker M: Prognosis of malignant melanomas of the choroid and ciliary body. Int Ophthalmol Clin 5(2):387–402, 1968
62. Seddon JM, Albert DM, Lavin PT et al: A prognostic factor study of disease-free interval and survival following enucleation for uveal melanoma. Arch Ophthalmol 101:1894–1899, 1983
63. Lavin PT, Albert DM, Seddon JM: A deficit survival analysis to assess the natural history of uveal melanoma. J Clin Dis 37:481–487, 1984
64. McLean IW, Foster WD, Zimmerman LE: Prognostic factors in small malignant melanomas of choroid and ciliary body. Arch Ophthalmol 95:48–58, 1977
65. Jensen OA: Malignant melanomas of the human uvea: Recent follow-up of cases in Denmark, 1943–1952. Acta Ophtholmol 48:1113–1128, 1970
66. Jensen OA: Malignant melanomas of the human uvea: 25-year follow-up of cases in Denmark, 1943–1952. Acta Ophthalmol 60:161–182, 1982
67. Curtin VT, Cavender JC: Natural course of selected malignant melanomas of the choroid and ciliary body. Mod Probl Ophthalmol 12:523–527, 1974

68. McLean IW, Foster WD, Zimmerman LE et al: Inferred natural history of uveal melanoma. Invest Ophthalmol Vis Sci 19:760–770, 1980
69. Char DH, Heilbron DL, Juster RR et al: Choroidal melanoma growth patterns. Br J Ophthalmol 67:575–578, 1983
70. Gass JDM: Comparison of uveal melanoma growth rates with mitotic index mortality. Arch Ophthalmol 103:924–931, 1985
71. Fribert TR, Finchberg E, McQuaig S: Extremely rapid growth of a primary choroidal melanoma. Arch Ophthalmol 101:1375–1377, 1983
72. Sahel JA, Pesavento R, Frederick A Jr et al: Uveal melanoma arising de novo over a 16-month period. Arch Ophthalmol 106(3):381–385, 1988
73. Manschot WA, Van Peperzeel HA: Choroidal melanoma: Enucleation or observation? A new approach. Arch Ophthalmol 98:71–77, 1980
74. Augsburger JJ, Gonder JR, Amsel J et l: Growth rates and doubling time of posterior uveal melanomas. Ophthalmology 91:1709–1715, 1984
75. Lambert JR, Char DM, Howes E Jr et al: Spontaneous regression of a choroidal melanoma. Arch Ophthalmol 104:732–734, 1986
76. Reese AB: Tumors of the Eye, 3rd ed, pp 174–262. Hagerstown, Md, Harper & Row, 1976
77. Shields JA: Diagnosis and Management of Intraocular Tumors, pp 75–254. St Louis, CV Mosby, 1983
78. Yanoff M: Glaucoma mechanisms in ocular malignant melanomas. Am J Ophthalmol 70:898–904, 1970
79. Shammas HF, Blodi FC: Prognostic factors in choroidal and ciliary body melanomas. Arch Ophthalmol 95:63–69, 1977
80. Font RL, Spauding AG, Zimmerman LE: Diffuse malignant melanoma of the uveal tract: A clinicopathologic report of 56 cases. Trans Am Acad Ophthalmol Otolaryngol 72:877–894, 1968
81. Duffin RM, Straatsma BR, Foos RY et al: Small malignant melanoma of the choroid with extraocular extension. Arch Ophthalmol 99:1027–1030, 1981
82. Shammas HF, Blodi FC: Orbital extension of choroidal and ciliary body melanomas. Arch Ophthalmol 93:2002–2005, 1977
83. Starr HJ, Zimmerman LE: Extrascleral extension and orbital reoccurrence of malignant melanomas of the choroid and ciliary body. Int Ophthalmol Cent V(2):369–385, 1962
84. Chess J, Albert DM, Bellows AR et al: Uveal melanoma: Case report of extension through the optic nerve to the surgical margin in the orbital apex. Br J Ophthalmol 68:272–275, 1984
85. Ruiz RS: Early treatment in malignant melanomas of the choroid. In Brockhurst RJ, Boruchuff SA, Hutchinson BT et al (eds): Controversy in Ophthalmology, pp 604–610. Philadelphia, WB Saunders, 1977
86. Pack JM, Robertson DM: Metastases from untreated uveal melanomas. Arch Ophthalmol 104:1624–1625, 1986
87. Wagoner MD, Albert DM: The incidence of metastases from untreated ciliary body and choroidal melanoma. Arch Ophthalmol 100:939–940, 1982
88. Zimmerman LE: Letter: Gamma-glutamyl transpeptidase in the prognosis of patients with uveal malignant melanomas. Am J Ophthalmol 96:409–411, 1983
89. Pascal SG, Saulenas AM, Fournier GA et al: An investigation into the association between liver damage and metastatic uveal melanoma. Am J Ophthalmol 100:448–453, 1985
90. Fidler IJ, Nicolson CL: Organ selectivity for implantation survival and growth of B16 melanoma. JNCI 57:1199–1201, 1976
91. Donoso LA, Nagy RM, McFall RC et al: Metastatic choroidal melanoma: Hepatic binding protein reactivity toward a liver-metastasizing clone. Arch Ophthalmol 101:787–790, 1983
92. Zimmerman LE, McLean IW, Foster WD: Does enucleation of the eye containing a malignant melanoma prevent or accelerate the dissemination of tumour cells? Br J Ophthalmol 62:420–425, 1978
95. Fraunfelder FT, Boozman FW, Wilson RS et al: No-touch technique for intraocular malignant melanomas. Arch Ophthalmol 95:1616–1620, 1977
96. Niederkorn JY, Streilen JW: Intracamerally induced concomitant immunity: Mice harboring progressively growing intraocular tumors are immune to spontaneous metastases and secondary tumor challenge. J Immunol 131:2587–2594, 1983
97. Niederkorn JY: Enucleation-induced metastasis of intraocular melanoma in mice. Ophthalmology 91:692–700, 1984
98. Seigel D, Myers M, Ferris F III et al: Survival rates after enucleation of eyes with malignant melanomas. Am J Ophthalmol 87:761–765, 1979
99. Kersten RC, Blodi FC: Prognosis of choroidal melanomas. Ophthalmic Forum 1:21–27, 1983
100. Davidorf FH: The melanoma controversy: A comparison of choroidal, cutaneous and iris melanomas. Surv Ophthalmol 25:373–377, 1981
101. Albert DM: Editorial: Toward resolving the ocular melanoma controversy. Arch Ophthalmol 97:431–432, 1979
102. Kidd MN, Cyness RW, Patterson CC et al: Prognostic factors in malignant melanomas of the choroid: A retrospective survey of cases occurring in Northern Ireland between 1965 and 1980. Trans Ophthalmol Soc UK 105:114–121, 1986
103. Holland G: Zur Klinik und Pathologie der Pigmenttumoren der Iris. Klin Monatsbl Augenheilkd 150:359–370, 1967
104. Rones B, Zimmerman LE: The prognosis of primary tumors of the iris treated by iridectomy. Arch Ophthalmol 60:193–205, 1958
105. Sunba MN, Rahi AHS, Morgan G: Tumors of the anterior uveal tract: I. Metastasizing malignant melanoma of the iris. Arch Ophthalmol 98:82–85, 1980
106. Jakobiec FA, Silbert G: Are most iris 'melanomas' really nevi? Arch Ophthalmol 99:2117–2132, 1981
107. Colt CA, Sahel JA, Seddon J et al: Reappraisal of clinicopathologic evaluation of iris melanomas (in press)
108. Reese AB: Tumors of the Eye, 3rd ed, pp 229–262. Hagerstown, Md, Harper & Row, 1977
109. Cleasby GW: Malignant melanoma of the iris. Arch Ophthalmol 60:403–417, 1958
110. Arentsen JJ, Green WR: Melanoma of the iris: Report of 72 cases treated surgically. Ophthalmic Surg 6:23–32, 1975
111. Green WR: The uveal tract. In Spencer WH (ed): Ophthalmic Pathology, Vol 3, pp 1322–1342. Philadelphia, WB Saunders, 1986
112. Ashton N: Primary tumors of the iris. Br J Ophthalmol 48:65–68, 1964
113. Zimmerman LE: Histologic considerations in the management of the iris and ciliary body. Ann Ist Barraquer 10:27–56, 1972
114. Kasten RC, Tse DT, Anderson R: Iris melanoma: Nevus or malignancy? Surv Ophthalmol 29:423–433, 1985
115. Apple D, Blodi FC: Pathologic observations and clinical approach to uveal melanomas. In Nicholson D (ed): Ocular Pathology Update, pp 213–226. New York, Masson Publishing USA, 1980
116. Ferry AP: Lesions mistaken for malignant melanoma of the posterior uvea: A clinicopathologic analysis of 100 cases with ophthalmoscopically visible lesions. Arch Ophthalmol 72:463–469, 1964
117. Shields JA, Zimmerman LE: Lesions simulating malignant melanoma of the posterior uvea. Arch Ophthalmol 89:466–471, 1973
118. Zimmerman LE: The 1972 Bedell Lecture. Problems in the diagnosis of malignant melanomas of the choroid and ciliary body. Am J Ophthalmol 75:917–929, 1973
119. Chang M, Zimmerman LE, McLean IW: The persisting pseudomelanoma problem. Arch Ophthalmol 102:726–727, 1984
120. Robertson DM, Campbell RJ: Errors in the diagnosis of malignant melanoma of the choroid. Am J Ophthalmol 87:269–275, 1979
121. Davidorf FH, Letson AD, Weiss ET et al: Incidence of misdiagnosed and unsuspected choroidal melanomas. Arch Ophthalmol 101:410–412, 1983
122. Shields JA, Augsburger JJ, Brown GC et al: The differential diagnosis of posterior uveal melanoma. Ophthalmology 87:518–522, 1980
123. Flindall RJ, Drance SM: Visual field studies of benign choroidal melanoma. Arch Ophthalmol 81:41–44, 1969
124. Donoso LA, Shields JA, Nagy RM: Epibulbar lesions simulating extraocular extension of uveal melanoma. Ann Ophthalmol 14:1120–1123, 1982
125. Augsburger JJ, Golden MI, Shields JA: Fluorescein angiography of choroidal malignant melanomas with retinal invasion. Retina 4:232–241, 1986
126. Coleman DJ, Abramson DH, Jack RL et al: Ultrasonic diagnosis of tumors of the choroid. Am J Ophthalmol 91:344–354, 1974
127. Collaborative Ocular Melanoma Study: Manual of Procedures. Baltimore, July 15, 1986
128. Nicholson DH, Frazier-Byrne S, Chin MT: Echographic and histologic tumor height measurements in uveal melanoma. Am J Ophthalmol 100:456–457, 1985
129. Martin JA, Robertson DM: Extrascleral extension of choroidal melanoma diagnosed by ultrasound. Ophthalmology 90:1334–1339, 1983
130. Shields JA: Current approaches to the diagnosis and management of choroidal melanomas. Surv Ophthalmol 21:443–463, 1977
131. Shields JA, McDonald PR, Leonard BC et al: The diagnosis of uveal malignant melanoma in eyes with opaque media. Am J Ophthalmol 83:95–105, 1977
132. Wollensak J, Heinrich M: In vivo and in vitro measurement of P32 uptake in the ocular tissue in cases of malignant melanoma. Graefes Arch Clin Exp Ophthalmol 217:35–44, 1981
133. McLean IW, Shields JA: Prognostic value of ^{32}P uptake in posterior uveal melanomas. Ophthalmology 87:543–548, 1980
134. Boniuk M, Ruiz RS: Viewpoints: The ^{32}P test in the diagnosis of ocular melanoma. Surv Ophthalmol 24:671–678, 1980
135. Goldberg B, Kara GB, Previtte LR: The use of radioactive phosphorus (^{32}P) in the diagnosis of ocular tumors. Am J Ophthalmol 90:817–828, 1980
136. Mafee MF, Peyman GA, McKusick MA: Malignant uveal melanoma and similar lesions studied by computed tomography. Radiology 156:403–408, 1985
137. Peyster RG, Augsburger JJ, Shields JA et al: Choroidal melanoma: comparison of CT, fundoscopy and ultrasound. Radiology 136:675–680, 1985
138. Sobel DF, Kelly W, Kjos BO et al: MR imaging of orbital and ocular disease. AJNR 6:259–264, 1983
139. Mafee MF, Peyman GA, Grisdano JF et al: Malignant melanoma and simulating lesions: MR imaging evaluation. Radiology 160:773–780, 1986
140. de Keiser RJ, Vielvoye GJ, de Wolff-Rouendahl D: Nuclear magnetic resonance imaging of intraocular tumors. Am J Ophthalmol 102:438–441, 1986
141. Markoff JI, Shakin E, Shields JA et al: The electrooculogram in eyes with choroidal melanoma. Ophthalmology 88:1112–1125, 1981
142. Staman JA, Fitzgerald CR, Dawson WW et al: The EOG and choroidal malignant melanoma. Doc Ophthalmol 49:1–10, 1980
143. Ponte F, Lauicella M: On the lack of correlation between the ERG and EOG alterations in malignant melanoma of choroid. Doc Ophthalmol Proc Ser 13:87–92, 1977
144. Char DH: Inhibition of leukocyte migration with melanoma-associated antigen in choroidal tumors. Invest Ophthalmol Vis Sci 16:176–179, 1977
145. Brownstein S, Phillips TM, Lewis MG: Specificity of tumor-associated antibodies in serum of patients with uveal melanoma. Can J Ophthalmol 13:190–193, 1978

146. Felberg NT, Donoso LA, Federman JL: Tumor-associated antibodies in the serum of patients with ocular melanoma. Ophthalmology 87:529–533, 1980
147. Felberg NT, Pro-Landazuri JM, Shields JA et al: Tumor-associated antibodies in the serum of patients with ocular melanoma. Arch Ophthalmol 97:256–259, 1979
148. Donoso LA, Felberg NT, Edelberg K et al: Metastatic uveal melanoma: An ocular melanoma-associated antigen in the serum of patients with metastatic disease. J Immunol 7:273–283, 1986
149. Meyer F, Naron D, Zonix S: The role of carcinoembryonic antigen in surveillance of patients with choroidal malignant melanoma: A prospective study. Ann Ophthalmol 19:24–25, 1987
150. Char DH, Stone RD, Irvine AR et al: Diagnostic modalities in choroidal melanoma. Am J Ophthalmol 89:223–230, 1980
151. Augsburger JJ, Shields JA, Folberg R et al: Fine needle aspiration biopsy in the diagnosis of intraocular cancer: Cytologic-histologic correlations. Ophthalmology 92:39–49, 1985
152. Karcioglu ZA, Gordon RA, Karcioglu GC: Tumor seeding in ocular fine needle aspiration biopsy. Ophthalmology 92:1763–1767, 1985
153. Felberg NT, Shields JA, Maguire J et al: Gamma-glutamyl transpeptidase in the prognosis of patients with uveal malignant melanoma. Am J Ophthalmol 95: 467–473, 1983
154. Donon CA, Nagy RG, Brochman RJ et al: Metastatic uveal melanoma: Hepatic cell-surface enzymes, isoenzymes, and serum sialic acid levels in early metastatic disease. Arch Ophthalmol 101:791–794, 1983
155. Donoso LA, Bend D, Augsburger JF: Metastatic uveal melanoma: Pretherapy serum liver enzyme and liver scan abnormalities. Arch Ophthalmol 103:796–798, 1985
156. Jakobiec FA, Depot MJ, Henkind P et al: Fluorescein angiographic patterns of iris melanocytic tumors. Arch Ophthalmol 100:1288–1299, 1982
157. Ferry AP: Lesions mistaken for malignant melanoma of the iris. Arch Ophthalmol 74:9–18, 1965
158. Shields JA, Sanborn GE, Augsburger JJ: The differential diagnosis of malignant melanoma of the iris: A clinical study of 300 patients. Ophthalmology 90:716–720, 1983
159. Gupta K, Hoepher JA, Streeten BW: Pseudomelanoma of the iris in herpes simplex keratitis. Ophthalmology 93:1524–1527, 1986
160. Beras OH, Myers MH: Manual for Staging of Cancer, 2nd ed, pp 197–208. Philadelphia, JB Lippincott, 1983
161. Fuchs E: Das Sarcom des Uvealtractus. Wein, Wilhelm Braumueller, 1882
162. Kersten RC: Management of choroidal malignant melanoma at Iowa. Ophthalmologica 189:24–35, 1984
163. Shields JA, Augsburger JJ, Brady CW et al: Cobalt plaque therapy of posterior uveal melanomas. Ophthalmology 89:1201–1212, 1982
164. Char DH: Therapeutic options in uveal melanomas. Am J Ophthalmol 98:796–799, 1984
165. Char DH: Management of choroidal melanoma and retinoblastoma. In Kanski JJ, Morse PM (eds): Disorders of the Vitreous, Retina and Choroid, pp 122–146. Butterworth International Medical Review—Ophthalmology. London, Butterworth, 1983
166. Barr CC, Sipperley JO, Nicholson DH: Small melanomas of the choroid. Arch Ophthalmol 96:1580–1582, 1978
167. Thomas JV, Green WR, Maumenee AE: Small choroidal melanomas: A long-term follow-up study. Arch Ophthalmol 97:861–864, 1979
168. Davidorf FH, Lang JR: The natural history of malignant melanoma of the choroid and ciliary body: Small versus large tumors. Trans Am Acad Ophthalmol Otolaryngol 79:310–320, 1975
169. Meyer-Schwickerath G: The preservation of vision by treatment of intraocular tumors with light coagulation. Arch Ophthalmol 66:458–466, 1961
170. Vogel MH: The application of photocoagulation in the treatment of malignant melanomas of the choroid. Ophthalmic Forum 1(4):46–47, 1983
171. Foulds WS, Danato BF: Low-energy long-exposure laser therapy in the management of choroidal melanoma. Graefes Arch Clin Exp Ophthalmol 224:26–31, 1986
172. Lin LH, Ni C: Hematoporphyrin phototherapy for experimental intraocular malignant melanoma. Arch Ophthalmol 101:301–303, 1983
173. Gomer CJ, Doinon DR, White L et al: Hematoporphyrin derivative photoradiation induced damage to normal and tumor tissue of the pigmented rabbit eye. Curr Eye Res 3:229–237, 1984
174. Tse DT, Dutton JJ, Weingeist TA et al: Hematoporphyrin photoradiation therapy for intraocular and orbital malignant melanoma. Arch Ophthalmol 102:833–838, 1984
175. Bruce RA Jr: Evaluation of hematoporphyrin photoradiation therapy to treat choroidal melanomas. Lasers Surg Med 4:59–64, 1984
176. Vogel MH: Histopathologic observations of photocoagulated malignant melanomas of the choroid. Am J Ophthalmol 74:466–474, 1972
177. Moore RF: Choroidal sarcoma treated by the intraocular insertion of radon seeds. Br J Ophthalmol 14:14–152, 1930
178. Stallard HB: Radiotherapy for malignant melanoma of the choroid. Br J Ophthalmol 50:147–155, 1966
179. Markoe AM, Brady LW, Shields JA et al: Malignant melanoma of the eye: Treatment of posterior uveal lesions by Co-60 plaque radiotherapy versus enucleation. Radiology 156:801–803, 1985
180. Sealy R, Le Roux PLM, Rapley F et al: The treatment of ophthalmic tumors with low energy sources. Br J Urol 49:551–554, 1976
181. Packer S, Rotman M: Radiotherapy of choroidal melanoma with iodine-125. Ophthalmology 87:582–590, 1980
181a. Garretson BR, Robertson DM, Earle JD: Choroidal melanoma treatment with iodine-125 brachytherapy. Arch Ophthalmol 105(10):1394–1397, 1987
182. Loammatsch PK: B-irradiation of choroidal melanoma within $^{106}R/^{106}Rh$ applicators: 16 years' experience. Arch Ophthalmol 101:713–717, 1983
183. Saunder WH, Char DH, Quivey JM: Precision high dose radiotherapy: Helium ion treatment of uveal melanoma. Int J Radiat Oncol Biol Phys 11:227–233, 1985
184. Gragoudas ES, Seddon JW, Egan KM et al: Long-term results of proton beam radiated uveal melanomas. Ophthalmology 94:395–453, 1987
185. Seddon JM, Gragoudas ES, Polivogianis L et al: Visual outcome after proton beam irradiation of uveal melanoma. J Ophthalmol 93:666–674, 1986
186. Finger PT, Packer S, Svitra P et al: Hyperthermic treatment of intraocular tumors. Arch Ophthalmol 102:1477–1481, 1986
187. Burgess JE, Chang S, Svitra PP et al: Effects of hyperthermia on experimental choroidal melanoma. Br J Ophthalmol 69:854–860, 1985
188. Finger PT, Packer S, Svitra PP et al: Thermoradiotherapy for intraocular tumors. Arch Ophthalmol 103:1574–1578, 1985
189. Riedel KG, Svitra PP, Seddon JM et al: Proton beam irradiation and hyperthermia: Effects on experimental choroidal melanoma. Arch Ophthalmol 103:1862–1869, 1985
190. Coleman DJ, Lizzi FL, Burgess SE et al: Ultrasonic hyperthermia and radiation in the management of intraocular malignant melanoma. Am J Ophthalmol 101:635–642, 1986
191. Lincoff H, McLean T, Long R: The cryosurgical treatment of intraocular tumors. Am J Ophthalmol 63:389–390, 1977
192. Abramson DH, Lisman RD: Cryopexy of a choroidal melanoma. Ann Opthalmol 11:1418–1421, 1979
193. Hidayat AA, LaPiana FG, Kramer KK et al: The effect of rapid freezing on uveal melanomas. Am J Ophthalmol 103:66–80, 1987
194. Peyman GA, Ericson ES, Axelrod AJ et al: Full-thickness eyewall resection in primates: An experimental approach to the treatment of choroidal melanoma. Arch Ophthalmol 89:410–412, 1973
195. Peyman GA, Apple DJ: Local excision of a choroidal malignant melanoma: Full-thickness eyewall resection. Arch Ophthalmol 92:216–218, 1974
196. Peyman GA: Eye wall resection. Ophthalmic Forum 1(4):38–41, 1983
197. Peyman GA, Juarez CI, Diamond FG et al: Ten year experience with eye wall resection for unveal malignant melanomas. Ophthalmology 91:1720–1723, 1984
198. Forrest AW, Keyser RB, Spencer WH: Iridocyclectomy for melanomas of the ciliary body: A follow up study of pathology and surgical mortality. Trans Am Acad Ophthalmol 85:1237–1249, 1978
199. Damato BE, Foulds WS: Ciliary body tumors and their management. Trans Ophthalmol Soc UK 103:256–264, 1986
200. Blodi FC: Ophthalmology. JAMA 243:2202–2203, 1980
201. Abramson DH, Ellsworth RM: Treatment of choroidal melanomas. Bull NY Acad Med 54:849–854, 1978
202. Char DH, Phillips TL: Pre-enucleation irradiation of uveal melanoma. Br J Ophthalmol 69:177–179, 1985
203. Wilson RS: Ocular melanoma: Surgical experience with "no touch" enucleation. South Med J 76:202–204, 1983
204. Smith GM: Ocular melanoma and immunotherapy. Ophthalmologica (Basel) 178:111–113, 1979
205. The TH, deGast GC, Huiges HA et al: Immunologic aspects of melanoma. Ophthalmologica (Basel) 175:25–27, 1977
206. Stark WJ, Rosenthal AR, Mullins GM et al: Simultaneous bilateral uveal melanomas responding to BCNU therapy. Trans Am Acad Ophthalmol Otolaryngol 75:70–83, 1971
207. Liu HS, Refojo MF, Albert DM: Experimental combined systemic and local chemotherapy for intraocular malignancy. Arch Ophthalmol 98:905–908, 1980
208. Affeldt JC, Minckler DS, Azen SP et al: Prognosis of malignant melanoma of the choroid and ciliary body. Int Ophthalmol Clin 5(2):389–402, 1962
209. Kersten RC, Tse D, Anderson RL et al: Role of orbital exenteration in malignant melanoma with extrascleral extension. Ophthalmology 92:436–443, 1985
210. Haye Ch: Traitement chirurgical des melanomes malins. In Haye Ch (ed): Conduite a tenir devant une tumeur maligne de la choroide. Bull Soc Ophthalmol Fr 197–211, 1986
211. Fournier GA, Albert DM, Arrigg CA et al: Resection of solitary metastasis: Approach to palliative treatment of hepatic involvement with choroidal melanoma. Arch Ophthalmol 102:80–82, 1984
212. Gronemeyer U, Enger Mann R, Thiede A: Erfolgreiche Entfernung einer Lebersmetastase 15 Jahre nach Enukleation wegen Aderhaut melanom. Fortschr Ophthalmol 81:363–364, 1984
213. Carrasco CH, Wallace S, Charnsangavny C et al: Treatment of hepatic metastases in ocular melanoma: Embolization of the hepatic artery with polyvinyl sponge and asplatin. JAMA 255:3152–3154, 1986
214. Wilson RS, Fraunfelder FT, Hanna C: Recurrent tapioca melanoma of the iris and ciliary body treated with Argon laser. Am J Ophthalmol 82:213–217, 1976
215. Cleasby GW, van Wertenbrugge JA: Treatment of iris melanoma by photocoagulation: A case report. Ophthalmic Surg 18:42–44, 1987
216. Krzystolik Z, Czerniak B, Stanislaw W: Proby rozpoznawania czerniakow wewnqtrzgalkowych za pomocq biopsji aspiracyjnej cienkoiglowej. Klin Oczna 84:279–282, 1982
217. Raubitschek E: Über Iristumoren. Klin Monatsbl Augenheilkd 52:683–694, 1914

218. Verhoeff FH: Sarcoma of the iris. Trans Am Ophthalmol Soc 31:270–271, 1933
219. Muller HK, Sollner F, Lund OE: Erfahrungen bei der operativen von Tumoren der Iriswurzel und des Ciliarkorpers. Ber Dtsch Ophthalmol Ges Heidelberg 63:194–199, 1961
220. Stallard HB: Partial cyclectomy. Br J Ophthalmol 45:797–802, 1961
221. Stallard HB: Partial iridocyclectomy and sclerectomy. Br J Ophthalmol 50:656–659, 1966
222. Jones IS: Iridocyclectomy and corneoscleroiridocyclectomy. In Reese AB (ed): Tumors of the Eye, 3rd ed, pp 238–239. Hagerstown, Md, Harper & Row, 1976
223. Sears ML: Technique for iridocyclectomy. Am J Ophthalmol 66:42–44, 1968

VICTOR A. LEVIN

GLENN E. SHELINE

PHILIP H. GUTIN

CHAPTER 46 *Neoplasms of the Central Nervous System*

INCIDENCE AND CLASSIFICATION

The true incidence and frequency of primary intracranial and spinal axis tumors are not precisely known because some tumors considered rare or uncommon or "benign" by tumor registries have not been recorded until recently. Extrapolating from available Surveillance, Epidemiology and End Results (SEER) registry data for the period 1978 to 1984,[1] the combined incidence of primary intracranial and spinal axis tumors is between 2 and 19/100,000 per year, depending on age. There is an early peak (3.1/100,000) between ages 0 to 4 years, a trough (1.8/100,100) between ages 15 to 24 years, and then a steady rise in incidence that plateaus (17.9 to 18.7/100,000) at 65 to 79 years of age.

The tremendous diversity in primary intracranial and spinal axis tumors is a function of the diversity of phenotypically distinct cells capable of transformation into tumors. Table 46-1 lists the hypothetical 15 cell types that can give rise to primary intracranial and spinal tumors. This list must not be accepted unquestioningly, since adherents to monoclonal causation for cancer would argue that it does not reflect the occurrence of mixed tumors such as astrocytoma–oligodroglioma and astrocytoma–ependymoma tumors. The existence of these histologically mixed phenotypic tumors would imply that these tumors arise from a common stem cell prior to its divergence into astrocytes, oligondendrocytes, and ependymocytes. Further complicating diagnostic and subsequent therapeutic efforts is the fact that these tumors arise in different locales within the cranium and spinal axis, and various types predominate at different ages. The relative frequency of the seven most common families of intracranial tumors is given in Table 46-2, and for spinal tumors, in Table 46-3.[2]

Although central nervous system (CNS) tumors are the primary solid neoplasms of childhood, the second leading cause of cancer-related death in children less than 15 years old, and the third leading cause of cancer-related death in adolescents and adults between the ages of 15 and 34, the majority of intracranial tumors occur in persons over the age of 45. Table 46-4 lists the frequency of intracranial tumors by tumor type and age at first presentation. Glioblastoma, rare in persons less than 15 years old, increases in incidence to 8.8% of all malignant intracranial tumors after the age of 45. The incidence of most glial tumors other than glioblastoma multiforme actually decreases with increasing age.

Differentiated or "benign" meningiomas increase from 0.2% of all primary intracranial tumors in patients less than 24 years old to 39% of tumors in patients more than 65 years old.[3] Table 46-4 shows a different pattern for malignant meningiomas, the prevalence of which increases from 0.2% in children to 2.4% in persons over age 60.

Overall, spinal cord tumors account for less than 15% of brain tumors. The same tumor types that occur in the brain affect the spinal cord, although the frequency of specific tumors is strikingly different. Schwannomas and meningiomas account for approximately one half of spinal tumors, with schwannomas being slightly more frequent; both types occur almost exclusively in adults. Gliomas constitute 20% of spinal tumors, and the majority are ependymomas with a predilection for the cauda equina. Other less common spinal tumors are the lipomas, dermoids, and hemangioblastomas.

TABLE 46-1. Classification of Primary Intracranial Tumors by Cell of Origin

Normal Cell	*Tumor*
Astrocyte	Astrocytoma, astroblastoma, glioblastoma, spongioblastoma
Ependymocyte	Ependymoma, ependymoblastoma
Oligodendrocyte	Oligodendroglioma
Microgliocyte	Reticulum cell sarcoma or microglioma
Arachnoidal fibroblasts	Meningioma
Nerve cell or neuroblast	Ganglioneuroma, neuroblastoma, retinoblastoma
External granular cell or neuroblast	Medulloblastoma
Schwann cell	Schwannoma (neurinoma)
Melanocyte	Melanotic carcinoma
Choroid epithelial cell	Choroid plexus papilloma or carcinoma
Pituitary	Adenoma
Endothelial cell or "stromal" cell	Hemangioblastoma
Primitive germ cells	Germinoma, pinealoma, teratomas, cholesteatoma
Pineal parenchymal cells	Pinealcytoma
Notochordal remnants	Chordoma

At UCSF, which has a large primary CNS tumor program, almost 10% of spinal tumors originate as metastases from an intracranial primary CNS tumor. The majority represent spinal subarachnoid seeding from medulloblastoma and ependymoma, less commonly from anaplastic astrocytoma, glioblastoma multiforme, and germinoma.

EPIDEMIOLOGY OF CNS TUMORS

GENETICS

For the majority of brain tumors, a genetic predisposition is lacking. Some exceptions are neurofibromatosis (von Recklinghausen's disease), tuberous sclerosis, familial polyposis (Turcot's syndrome), and the Osler-Weber-Rendu syndrome; the last two entities are quite rare.

Neurofibromatosis is inherited as an autosomal dominant disorder with incomplete penetrance. Patients with neurofibromatosis develop cutaneous lesions (café au lait), subcutaneous neurofibromas, bony and mesenchymal abnormalities, and a variety of brain tumors. Acoustic neurinomas, especially bilateral acoustic neurilemmomas, anterior optic nerve gliomas, and a spectrum of gliomas from well-differentiated astrocytoma to glioblastoma multiforme have been observed in families with neurofibromatosis. Recent studies have shown that a gene near the centromere of chromosome 17 is responsible for a kindred of 15 in Utah.[4] Some cases of bilateral acoustic neurinoma also are associated with meningioma and loss of chromosome 22.[5]

TABLE 46-2. Frequency of Primary Intracranial Brain Tumors*

Type	*Frequency (%)*
Glioblastoma multiforme	30
"Astrocytoma"	20
Other "gliomas" (ependymoma, oligodendroglioma, medulloblastoma)	7
Meningioma	18
Nerve sheath (*e.g.*, neurinoma)	9
Pituitary	5
Other (unspecified)	11

* Data from Tables 3-1C, 3-5, and 3-6A of Office of Biometry and Epidemiology (1977).

TABLE 46-3. Distribution of Primary Spinal Tumors

Tumor	*Percentage*
Neurilemmoma	29
Meningioma	25.5
Ependymoma	12.8
Sarcomas	11.9
Astrocytoma	6.5
Vascular tumors	6.2
Chordomas	4
Epidermoids	1.4
Other*	2.7

Slooff et al.[2]

* Lipoma and subarachnoid seeding from primary intracranial tumor.

Another phakomatosis associated with brain tumors is tuberous sclerosis. Tuberous sclerosis is a hereditary disease with cutaneous, neurologic, cardiac, and renal abnormalities. Tuberous sclerosis is normally obvious in youngsters. It is characterized by acneiform skin lesions, angiofibromas, periungual fibromas, epilepsy, periventricular hamartomas composed of abnormal glia, and in some cases mental retardation. Gliomas may be associated with tuberous sclerosis; the most common type is an uncommon ganglioglioma.

With greater sophistication in genetic investigations it is likely that specific abnormalities of the genome will be found for many types of brain tumor. Already a significant number of nonrandom chromosomal changes have been observed in a number of tumors. One of the earliest chromosomal abnormalities was seen in meningiomas at chromosome 22.[6,7] Studies with gliomas have shown double minutes, gains at No. 7, losses at No. 10 and No. 22, and gonosomes, and abnormalities at No. 9[8]; others have found increased copy numbers of chromosome 7 (the genomic locus for *erb*-B[9]) and duplication of the long arm of No. 9 and translocation of the short arm of No. 9 associated with secretion of a specific protease.[10] Medulloblastomas have shown extra copies of chromosome 11 and marker chromosomes 8q+, 17p+, and 20q+.[11] Ependymomas are associated with a duplication of the long arm of chromosome 12.[12]

As we learn more about oncogene function and the specific association of chromosomal loci with structural proteins and enzymes, it is likely that we will understand not only the genetics of tumor development, but also the entire panoply of tumor growth control.

CHEMICAL CAUSES

Although brain tumors can be experimentally induced in rodents, the association of chemical exposure and brain

TABLE 46-4. Frequency of Intracranial Tumors as a Function of Age Range

	Age Ranges						
Histology	*0–9*	*10–19*	*20–29*	*30–39*	*40–49*	*50–59*	*60–74*
Astrocytoma	60	59	76	81	86	87	91
"Low-grade"	9.8	7.1	7.1	4.9	2.5	1.5	1.8
"Astrocytoma"	28.0	31.7	40.4	41.9	38.2	31.1	28.8
Anaplastic	18.5	10.9	11.0	12.8	9.6	8.3	11.0
Mixed	2.5	2.7	2.8	3.4	2.2	2.1	0.7
Glioblastoma	1.3	7.4	14.4	18.2	32.9	44.2	51.0
Medulloblastoma	21	10	5.5	2.3	1.0	0.1	0
Ependymoma*	8.7	2.7	4.3	1.8	0.8	1.3	0.5
Oligodendroglioma	1.1	4.0	5.0	6.4	6.2	3.6	1.6
Embryonal/teratoid†	1.0	1.3	0.3	0.3	0	0	0
Meningioma‡	0.2	0.4	1.2	1.7	1.2	2.0	2.4

Data based on unpublished SEER program search 1978–1984.
* Includes differentiated and anaplastic ependymoma.
† Includes germinoma, mixed embryonal pinealomas, and malignant teratomas.
‡ Underestimate, since SEER does not include many "benign" tumors in its registry; these are probably malignant meningiomas.

tumors in humans is limited to a small number of occupations. An increased incidence of brain tumors over that expected has been observed among anatomists[13]; in farm workers in Italy after 1960, suggesting that exposure to pesticides, herbicides, and fertilizers may somehow be related to the development of brain tumors[14]; and in workers in various petrochemical industries.[15,16] In 1987 McLaughlin et al, using data from a Swedish Cancer Registry, found that the standardized incidence ratio for intracranial gliomas was increased among male dentists, agricultural research workers, public prosecuters, female physicians, other health care employees, welders, metal cutters, glass, porcelain, and ceramic workers, and women employed in wool mills.

Although many of the observed associations are interesting, it is difficult to know how much credibility to assign these statistical observations. Aside from a known association between vinyl chloride and gliomas, there is no common chemical or environmental thread among the above observations.[15]

VIRAL CAUSES

Viruses have been implicated directly only in the development of gliomas in rats, dogs, and monkeys. In all cases direct CNS injection of the virus is required. In rats, the avian sarcoma virus produces glial tumors[18]; in dogs, the Rous sarcoma virus leads to gliosarcomas[19]; and in owl monkeys, a human polyoma virus (JC virus) produces glial neoplasms. Although a direct association between virus exposure and the subsequent development of CNS tumors has not been established in humans, patients with primary CNS lymphoma have been observed to have a high rate of infection with Epstein-Barr (EB) virus and evidence of EB virus in their tumor tissue.[20]

TRAUMA

CNS neoplasia, like most cancers, appears to be unassociated with prior trauma. It has been suggested that the incidence of meningiomas is higher in patients with a prior history of head trauma, but this was not supported by a recent prospective study.[21]

IRRADIATION, CHEMOTHERAPY, AND IMMUNOSUPPRESSION

The incidence of CNS tumors following irradiation or chemotherapy for a prior malignancy is small. The literature records several examples of astrocytomas occurring 3 to 7 years after cranial–spinal irradiation and chemotherapy for acute lymphocytic leukemia (ALL) and craniopharyngioma[22–24]; unfortunately, none of the reports contain sufficient information to allow determination of risk assessment. In non-Hodgkin's lymphoma, 1 of 44 second malignancies was an astrocytoma.[25] Again, no measure of risk assessment is possible, although the infrequent reporting suggests that these events are uncommon to rare. Meningiomas have been reported in association with scalp irradiation for tinea capitis.[26,27] The risk of meningiomas was as high as 21% in one study.[26]

Transplant recipients are at substantially increased risk for developing primary CNS histiocytic lymphoma; the reason is unknown.

ANATOMICAL AND CLINICAL CONSIDERATIONS

The clinical presentation of the various tumors is best appreciated by considering the relationship of signs and symptoms to anatomy. Although this chapter cannot include all manners of presentation, an attempt is made to provide a basis for appreciating and understanding the more common presentations. For a more detailed presentation of neurologic signs and symptoms of intracranial tumor the reader is referred to *Principles of Neurology* by Adams and Victor.[29]

For the convenience of the reader, basic anatomical drawings of the cerebral lobes (Fig. 46-1), sagittal brain (Fig.

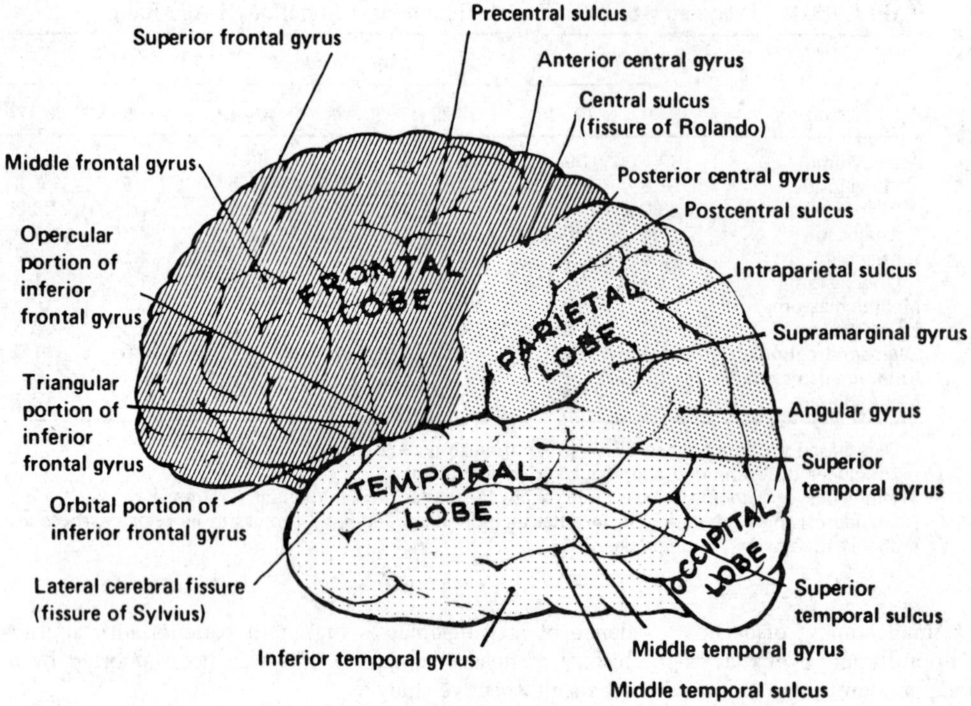

FIG. 46-1. Lobes and major gyri and sulci of the cerebrum. (Chusid JG: Correlative Neuroanatomy and Functional Neurology. Los Altos, CA, Lange, 1973)

46-2), ventral brain stem (Fig. 46-3), and a cross-section of the spinal cord (Fig. 46-4) are included.[30]

INTRACRANIAL TUMORS

The spectrum of tumors originating in the brain, cranial nerves, and leptomeninges is quite diverse. All tumor types listed in Table 46-1 may produce intracranial tumors. The most common primary tumors are the gliomas, which include glioblastoma multiforme, anaplastic astrocytoma, astrocytoma, oligodendroglioma, ependymoma, and mixed astrocytoma–oligodendroglioma and astrocytoma–ependymoma tumors. Table 46-5 shows the breakdown of tumors by location in children and adults.

Patients with intracranial tumors, unlike patients with vascular thromboembolic disease of the brain, rarely present with "classic" anatomically distinct neurologic syndromes. Brain tumors are far less stereotypic with respect to location and size. Intracranial tumors produce symptoms primarily by two mechanisms: (1) mass effect (and increased intracranial pressure), due either entirely to the tumor or to the tumor and surrounding edema, and (2) infiltration and destruction of normal tissue.

General Signs and Symptoms

Intracranial tumors can produce general signs and symptoms due to an increase in intracranial pressure and focal signs

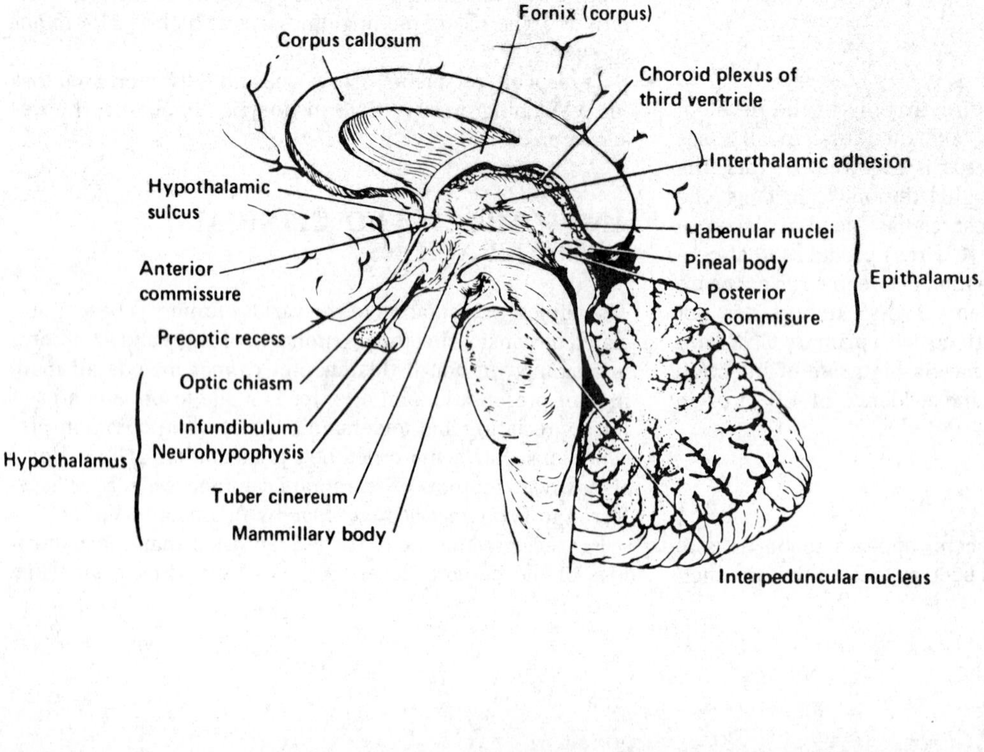

FIG. 46-2. Sagittal section taken through splenium of corpus callosum through the brain stem and cerebellum. (Chusid JG: Correlative Neuroanatomy and Functional Neurology. Los Altos, CA, Lange, 1973

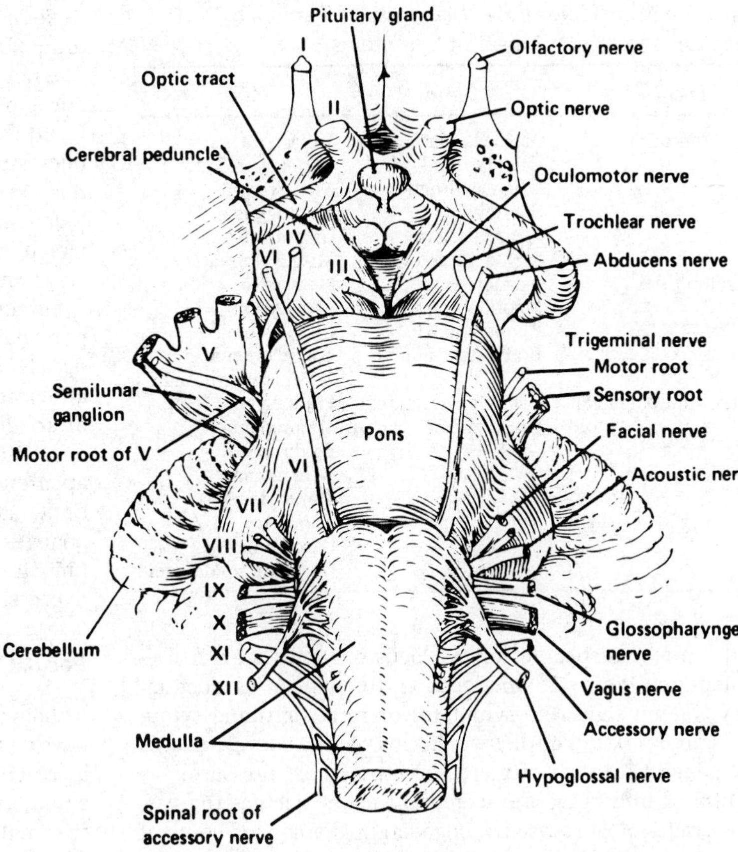

FIG. 46-3. Ventral brain stem showing relationships to cranial nerves. (Chusid JG: Correlative Neuroanatomy and Functional Neurology. Los Altos, CA, Lange, 1973

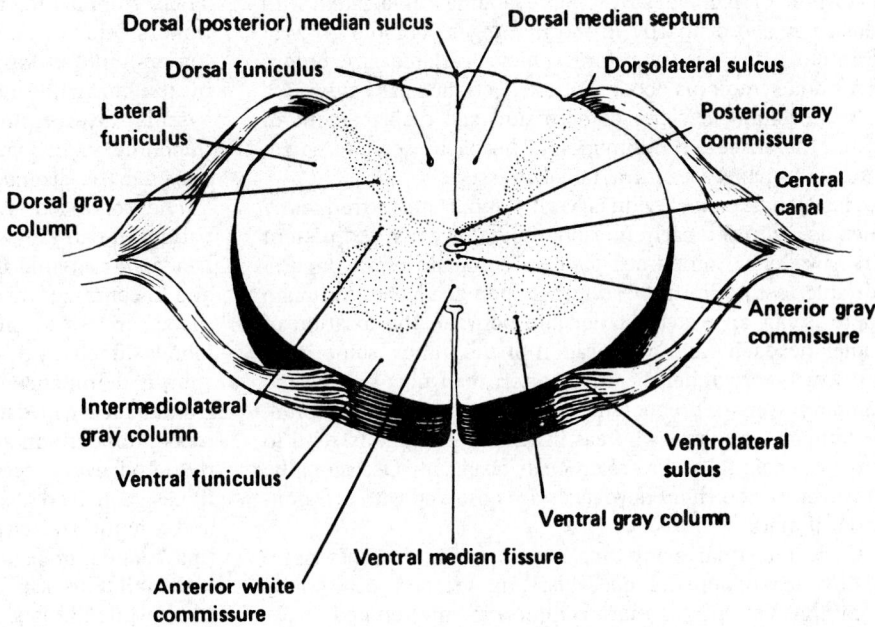

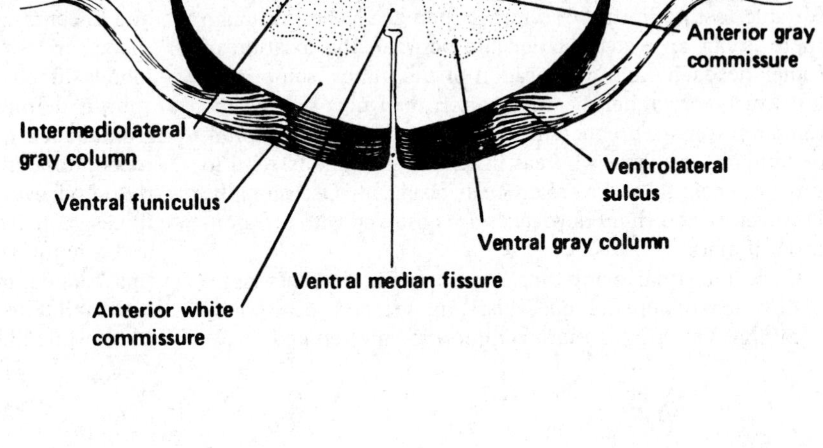

FIG. 46-4. Cross-section of thoracic spinal cord showing relationships of spinal nerves to intraspinal tracts.

TABLE 46-5. Differential Diagnosis of Tumors by Location and Age at Onset of Symptoms

Location	*Child*	*Adult*
Supratentorial	Astrocytoma Glioblastoma Oligodendroglioma Sarcoma Neuroblastoma Mixed glioma	Metastatic Glioblastoma Astrocytoma Meningioma Oligodendroglioma Mixed glioma
Infratentorial	Astrocytoma Medulloblastoma Ependymoma Brain stem glioma	Metastatic Astrocytoma Glioblastoma Ependymoma Brain stem glioma
Sellar and parasellar	Craniopharyngioma Optic glioma	Pituitary Meningioma Epidermoid
Base of skull		Neurinoma Meningioma Chordoma Carcinoma Dermoid, epidermoid

and symptoms specific for the locus of tumor growth. Depending on their size and location, tumors can produce either general signs and symptoms or focal signs and symptoms, or a mixture of the two. In this section we will discuss the general features of increased intracranial pressure.

Typical infiltrative intracerebral tumors, such as the various grades of astrocytoma, oligodendroglioma, and some of the more primitive neuroectodermal tumors, can produce headache, gastrointestinal upset such as nausea and vomiting, personality changes, and slowing of psychomotor function. These may be the only clinical indications of tumor.

Because headache is a common presenting symptom in patients with intracranial tumor, it is important to appreciate clinical patterns and their localizing value. Brain parenchyma does not have pain-sensitive structures, and tumor pain (headache) has been attributed to local swelling and distortion of pain-sensitive nerve endings associated with blood vessels, primarily in the meninges. Tumors grow at different rates and therefore achieve variable size before signs and symptoms occur. But once a tumor has achieved a critical volume causing compression and displacement of brain, the onset and diminution of headache seem to correlate with changes in intracranial pressure.

Headaches can vary in severity and quality; frequently they occur in the early morning hours or when the patient first awakens. Sometimes patients complain of an uncomfortable feeling in the head rather than headache. Although there is not an exact relationship between the location of tumor headache and the location of the tumor, some rules are worth remembering. More often than not, frontal and temporal tumors produce headache in frontal, retro-orbital, or temporal regions, whereas infratentorial tumors tend to produce occipital and retroauricular headache. Occasionally, however, retro-orbital headaches are observed with infratentorial tumors.

Gastrointestinal symptoms are common. Patients complain of loss of appetite, queasiness, nausea, and occasionally vomiting. Vomiting is more common in children and in patients harboring infratentorial tumors rather than supratentorial tumors. Although textbooks discuss projectile vomiting as a not infrequent generalized symptom of brain tumors, in our experience it is common in children but rare in adults. From the literature and from discussions with experienced neurosurgeons, it seems that vomiting is less frequent today than in past years; this may reflect the fact that patients today are diagnosed earlier and receive glucocorticoids, which can dramatically modify many of the generalized signs and symptoms of brain tumors.

Sometimes the only presenting symptoms are changes in personality, mood, mental capacity, and concentration. On occasion merely a slowing of psychomotor activity is the antecedent symptom of intracranial tumor. Patients with brain tumors tend to sleep longer at night and nap during the day. Often these changes in function and activity will be apparent to the family and the examiner but not to the patient; at other times, only the patient will recognize the changes in mental function. None of these symptoms are unique to brain tumors; they could easily be confused with depression, neurasthenia, or other psychological problems.

Focal Cerebral Syndromes

Although less than 10% of patients presenting with seizures have a brain tumor as the etiology of the seizure, seizures are a presenting symptom in approximately 20% of patients with supratentorial brain tumors. With rapidly growing infiltrative malignant gliomas, they are likely to take the form of focal motor or sensory seizures, although generalized seizures are also common. In patients with slowly growing astrocytomas, oligodendrogliomas, or meningiomas, generalized seizures may antedate the clinical diagnosis by months to years. The value of the focal seizure as a means of tumor localization is quite high, sufficiently so that one should consider tumor as causative until proven otherwise.

The distribution of infiltrative parenchymal tumors in the brain is directly related to the mass of the lobe or region. Thus, frontal tumors occur more commonly than parietal tumors, which in turn occur more often than temporal lobe tumors, and so forth. Anatomical or regional involvement by tumors, while not completely stereotypic as with CNS vascular disease, nonetheless has certain features that help the clinician distinguish and localize such tumors, or at least consider the diagnosis.

The frontal lobe syndrome varies markedly from patient to patient. It can range from personality change to a picture of headache and mild slowing of contralateral hand movements and to contralateral spastic hemiplegia, marked elevation in mood, or loss of initiative and dysphasia (if the dominant lobe is affected). Assuming the normal pattern of left hemisphere dominance, unilateral tumors affecting the right frontal lobe can cause left hemiplegia, slight elevation in mood, difficulty in adapting to new situations, loss of initiative, and even occasional primitive grasp and sucking reflexes. Left frontal lobe tumors can cause right hemiplegia and a nonfluent dysphasia with or without some apraxia of lips, tongue, or hand movements.

Bifrontal disease, a condition usually associated with infiltrative gliomas and primary CNS lymphomas, can cause variable degrees of bilateral hemiplegia, spastic bulbar palsy, severe impairment of intellect, lability of mood, dementia, and prominent primitive grasping, sucking, and snout reflexes.

Symptoms of temporal lobe syndromes, like those of frontal lobe syndromes, can range from subliminal symptoms detectable only with careful testing of perception and spatial judgment to severe impairment of recent memory. Homonymous quadrantanopsia, auditory hallucinations, and even aggressive behavior can occur as a result of tumors of either temporal lobe. Involvement of the nondominant temporal lobe can, in addition, result in minor perceptual problems and spatial disorientation. Dominant temporal lobe involvement can lead to dysnomia, impaired perception of verbal commands, and even a full-blown fluent Wernicke-like aphasia. Bilateral disease, involving both temporal lobes, is rare in comparison to the bilaterality of frontal lobe tumors, which readily cross through the corpus callosum. This is fortunate, as bitemporal tumor involvement is devasting, producing impairment of memory (especially recent memory) and sometimes leading to dementia.

Parietal lobe syndromes affect sensory and perceptual functions more than motor modalities, although mild hemiparesis is sometimes seen with extensive parietal lobe tumors. Tumors impinging on either parietal lobe can produce a decrease in the perception of cortical sensory stimuli that may vary from mild sensory extinction, observable only with testing, to a more severe sensory loss (with deep tumors) that leads to hemianesthesia or other hemisensory abnormalities. There also may be a homonymous hemianopsia or visual inattention. In addition, involvement of the nondominant parietal lobe can lead to perceptual abnormalities and, in severe cases, to anosognosia and a dressing apraxia. Unilateral dominant parietal lobe tumors lead to alexia, dysgraphia, and certain types of apraxia.

Occipital lobe tumors can produce contralateral homonymous hemianopsia or visual aberrations that take the form of imperception of color, object size, or object location. Bilateral occipital disease can produce cortical blindness.

The classic disconnection syndromes associated with corpus callosum lesions are rarely seen in patients with brain tumors. The main reason for this is that even though infiltrative gliomas frequently cross the corpus callosum in the region of the genu or the splenium, the involvement of additional structures complicates neurologic interpretation, obscuring classic disconnection syndromes. With respect to partial lesions, in general, interruption of association fibers in the anterior part of the corpus callosum causes a failure of the left hand to carry out spoken commands. Lesions in the splenium of the corpus callosum interrupt visual fibers connecting the right occipital lobe and left angular gyrus, resulting in inability to read or name colors.

Symptoms related to thalamic tumors vary as a function of tumor size and whether the tumor produces secondary blockage of cerebrospinal fluid (CSF) flow and hydrocephalus. Tumors in the thalamus and, less commonly, in the basal ganglia can reach 3 to 4 cm in diameter before the patient has symptoms severe enough to seek medical attention. Typically patients present with headaches resulting from hydrocephalus and increased intracranial pressure secondary to trapping of the lateral horn of one of the ventricles. In addition or independently, patients may have a mild sensory abnormality on the contralateral side that is detected only by testing of sensory extinction; rarely, they may have a severe neuropathic pain syndrome. Patients may complain of intermittent paresthesias on the contralateral side; because the paresthesias are episodic and seizure-like, anticonvulsant drugs are sometimes used and actually may be beneficial. With more involvement of the basal ganglia, contralateral intention tremor and hemiballistic-like movement disorders can be observed. It is uncommon for thalamic tumors to manifest in a manner typical of thalamic strokes unless bleeding into the tumor has occurred.

FOCAL INFRATENTORIAL SYNDROMES

The brain stem, composed of the medulla oblongata and the pons, has both nuclear groups and traversing axons. Tumors invading or compressing the brain stem can produce dire consequences; even a small increase in size — 1 to 2 mm — may lead to death or devastating signs and symptoms. Tumors can be primarily intrinsic or intrinsic with exophytic components in the fourth ventricle, peripontine cisterns, or both locations. Cranial nerve involvement, therefore, can be at the nuclear level or at the level of the cranial nerve as it leaves the brain stem.

The most common tumor of the brain stem is an astrocytoma (glioma). In 90% of patients the initial clinical manifestations are cranial nerve palsies involving the sixth and seventh cranial nerves on one side. These nerve palsies usually are followed by involvement of long tracts, resulting in hemiplegia, unilateral limb ataxia, ataxia of gait, paraplegia, hemisensory syndromes, gaze disorders, and occasionally hiccups. Less commonly, long tract signs precede the cranial nerve abnormalities; this presentation is more likely with confined intrinsic brain stem lesions.

The midbrain, juxtaposed between the pons and cerebral hemispheres, encompasses the tectum, cerebral peduncles, and cerebral aqueduct. If the midbrain is involved, obstructive hydrocephalus can occur, producing vomiting, drowsiness, and cerebellar signs. Patients with medullary tumors have a more rapidly progressive course and are more likely to have seventh, ninth, tenth, and sixth (usually late) cranial nerve deficits, along with dysarthria, personality change, and head tilt. Unlike what is seen with the expansive posterior fossa tumors, headache, vomiting, and papilledema occur late.

Fourth ventricular tumors, because of their location, tend to produce obstructive hydrocephalus early in their development. This produces profound headache and vomiting and associated disturbances of gait and balance. With rapidly progressing lesions, cerebellar herniation may develop.

Tumors of the cerebellum have valuable localizing signs and symptoms. In slowly growing tumors, the initial symptoms may be headache and nausea, due to increased intracranial pressure, and mild imbalance in gait or ataxia of a limb. In more rapidly growing cerebellar tumors, there may be quite prominent morning headache, vomiting, a stumbling gait with frequent falling, nystagmus and dizziness, and visual symptoms caused by papilledema. Abnormal posturing of the head is often seen in children but not in adults. In children, the head is tilted back and away from the side of the tumor. Posturing of the head indicates unilateral cerebellar–foramen magnum herniation. Bilateral sixth nerve palsies are uncommon. Midline lesions in and around the cerebellar vermis lead to truncal and gait ataxia, whereas lesions in a cerebellar hemisphere lead to unilateral appendicular ataxia, most readily observed in upper extremity movements.

Tumors of the base of the skull, although not particularly common, are important since many are curable by surgery. Table 46-6 summarizes the salient clinical features of seven of the more common clinical syndromes.[30]

A classic base of skull tumor presentation is that associated with acoustic neurilemmomas (schwannoma), the most frequent cause of the cerebellopontine (CP) angle syndrome. Almost all such patients have involvement of the auditory or vestibular portions of the eighth nerve; more than 50% have facial weakness, disturbance of taste, and sensory loss of the face; approximately 40% have ataxia of gait; and fewer than 25% have unilateral appendicular ataxia. Deafness and vestibular dysfunction due to damage to the auditory and vestibular nerve branches is characteristic of these tumors, which can attain a very large size before they are discovered.

Another group of tumors manifested by rather distinct signs and symptoms are those that occur in or near the sella turcica. Table 46-7 summarizes the location, frequency, and selected salient features of sellar and parasellar tumors.[31] Many patients with tumors of the sellar region present with defects of the visual field(s), less commonly with blindness and optic atrophy. The visual field abnormality is usually a partial or complete bitemporal hemianopsia in the case of intrasellar tumors such as pituitary adenomas. With lesions that expand from below the optic chiasm, the upper temporal quadrants are affected first. Patients can also present with scotomas in either eye. With long-standing, slowly progressive disease, unilateral or bilateral optic atrophy can be observed. Expansion of tumor may involve the hypothalamus and compress the third ventricle, leading to obstructive hydrocephalus and signs of increased intracranial pressure such as headache and nausea and vomiting.

Some of the pituitary tumors produce secondary signs and symptoms because they elaborate hormones that create various syndromes of endocrine hyperactivity (Table 46-8). A small number of pituitary tumors produce no detectable hormones or hormones in quantities that assume no clinical significance. It is uncommon today for patients with endocrine-active tumors to present with large tumors; it is more common for patients with endocrine-inactive tumors to seek medical attention because of optic chiasmal compression–hypopituitarism as a consequence of a large mass. Compression leads to detectable hyposecretion of specific cells; production of growth hormone is most sensitive, followed closely by gonadotropins. Cells producing thyroid-stimulating hormone (TSH) and adrenocorticotropic hormone (ACTH) are much more resistant, and their function is impaired only at a later stage of growth.

To conclude this section, the reader should review Table 46-5, which summarizes the differential diagnosis of tumors by location in children and adults. It is intended to serve as a guide and is not by any means an exhaustive enumeration of all possible tumors that can occur in those locations. For a more extensive description of CNS tumor pathology, the reader is referred to Rubinstein and Russell's textbook on neuropathology,[32] or the AFIP's *Brain Tumors of the Central Nervous System*, by Rubinstein.[33] For a more extensive de-

TABLE 46-6. Differential Diagnosis of Tumors at the Base of the Skull

Site of Lesion	*Associated Tumors*	*Clinical Findings*
Anterior parts	Carcinomas invasive from frontal and ethmoid sinuses, meningiomas	Unilateral anosmia, frontal lobe syndrome, seizures
Superior orbital	Meningiomas, carcinoma of nasopharnyx	3rd, 4th, 5th, 6th nerve lesions with ophthalmoplegia and pain and hypesthesia in 5_1 distribution
Cavernous sinus	Chondromas, meningiomas, sellar and parasellar tumors	3rd, 4th, 6th, sometimes 5th nerve involvement with ophthalmoplegia
Apex of petrous temporal bone	Cholesteatoma, chondroma, meningioma, neurinoma, sarcoma	5th and 6th nerve involvement with sensory and motor findings and diplopia
Sphenoid and petrous bones	Meningioma, chondroma, nasopharyngeal carcinoma, metastasis	3rd, 4th, 6th nerve lesions resulting in ophthalmoplegia; 5th may be associated with trigeminal neuralgia syndrome
Jugular foramen	Glomus jugular tumors, neurinomas, chondromas cholesteatoma, meningioma, nasopharyngeal carcinoma	9th, 10th, 11th nerves producing difficulty with swallowing, speaking, and weakness of strap muscles of neck
Cerebellopontine angle	Neurinoma, meningioma, cholesteatoma, metastatic cerebellar tumors	7th nerve lesions causing loss of hearing, vertigo, and nystagmus; cerebellar lesions producing ataxia of limbs and gait; 5th, 7th and occasionally 9th and 12th nerve lesions; brain stem symptoms and signs of increased intracranial pressure

Adapted from Bingas.[30]

TABLE 46-7. Clinical Syndromes Associated with Tumors of Sellar Region

Tumor	Disorders of: Anterior Pituitary Gland	Disorders of: Hypothalamus	Incidence and Degree	Syndromes
In the sella				
Adenoma				Cushing's disease, acromegaly, gigantism
Active	+			
Inactive	+	±		Forbes-Albright syndrome, hypopituitarism
Chondroma	+			
Metastasis	+			
Craniopharyngioma			Regular, clinical	
Intrasellar	+			
Intrasellar and suprasellar	+	+		
Close to sella				
Suprasellar craniopharyngioma		+	Regular, clinical	Adiposogenital dystrophy (Frohlich)
Suprasellar meningioma		±		
Suprasellar epidermoid				
Optic pathway glioma		±	Rare	Russell's syndrome
Hypothalamic glioma		+	Frequent	Precocious puberty
Hypothalamic hamartoma		+	Clinical	
Pineal tumors		+	Frequent, clinical	
Tumors with aqueductal obstruction and hydrocephalus		+		Cushingoid
Remote from sella				
Cerebral hemispheres	±	±	Rare	
Meningioma glioma			Latent	

Fahlbusch R, Marguth F: Endocrine disorders associated with intracranial tumors. In Vinken PJ, Bruyn GW (eds): Handbook of Clinical Neurology; Tumors of the Brain and Skull, part I, vol 16, p 345. Amsterdam, North Holland, 1974.

scription of the neurology of CNS tumors, a standard textbook of neurology, such as *Principles of Neurology*, by Adams and Victor,[29] should be read.

Acute and Life-Threatening Syndromes Caused by Intracranial Tumors

Since the brain and the spinal cord are surrounded by a rigid skull and dural membranes, expanding lesions within or abutting the brain or spinal cord can cause displacement of vital structures, leading, in the brain, to respiratory arrest and death, and in the spinal cord to paraplegia or quadriplegia.

In order to understand the sequence of events leading to temporal lobe–tentorial (uncal) herniation and cerebellar–foramen magnum herniation, one must have a visual image of intracranial anatomy. The tentorium cerebelli forms a rigid tissue partition between the cerebral hemispheres above and the cerebellum and brain stem below. Through this opening passes the midbrain centrally and the third nerve anterolaterally. Immediately lateral to the third nerve lies the medial portion of the temporal lobe called the uncus. An expanding mass lesion situated above the tentorium may displace the uncus medially and inferiorly beneath the tentorium. Table 46-9 summarizes the neurologic findings and pathologic causes of the events that make up the temporal lobe–tentorial herniation syndrome.[29]

TABLE 46-8. Clinical Syndromes Produced by Endocrine-Active Pituitary Adenomas

Hormone Produced	*Clinical Syndrome*
Prolactin	Amenorrhea and galactorrhea, impotence
Growth hormone	Giantism and acromegaly
ACTH	Cushing's disease, Nelson's syndrome (following adrenalectomy)
TSH (rare)	Hyperthyroidism

A rapid increase in the volume of the supratentorial compartment leading to herniation can be caused by a number of different factors. A very rapidly growing glioblastoma can produce this picture, although it is more usual for it to occur as a terminal or near-terminal event following ineffective therapy for the tumor. It can also occur when there is a dramatic increase in the amount of edema associated with metastasis to the brain or with hyponatremia and hypo-osmolar syndromes. Sometimes the injudicious use of parenteral hypo-osmolar 5% dextrose in water will be sufficient to produce an abrupt increase in brain edema, and temporal lobe herniation. We have also seen temporal lobe herniation follow a group of shortly spaced seizures. Presumably the seizures, which are associated with hypoventilation, produce a local hypoxia around the tumor, with a resulting increase in brain edema.

Mass lesions in the infratentorial compartment can displace brain tissue upward through the tentorium, but more commonly they force brain tissue downward through the foramen magnum. In this situation, the cerebellar tonsils move caudally through the foramen magnum and in so doing wedge against the medulla, causing the findings summarized in Table 46-10.

TABLE 46-9. Temporal Lobe-Tentorial (Uncal) Herniation

Neurologic Findings	*Pathologic Cause*
Pupillary dilation and ptosis	Compression of ipsilateral oculomotor nerve between herniating tissue and petroclinoid ligament
Ipsilateral hemiplegia	Compression of contralateral cerebral peduncle against tentorium (Kernohan's notch)
Contralateral hemiplegia	Compression of ipsilateral cerebral peduncle; when associated with compression of contralateral peduncle, bilateral corticospinal tract signs will be present
Homonymous hemianopia	Compression of posterior cerebral artery against the tentorium can lead to occipital ischemia or infarction and contralateral homonymous hemianopia; occasionally bilateral field cuts will occur
Midbrain syndrome: Cheyne-Stokes respirations, stupor-coma, bipyramidal signs, decerebrate rigidity, dilated fixed pupils, gaze paresis, altered oculocephalic reflexes	Crushing of midbrain between herniating temporal lobe and leaf of tentorium associated with vascular occlusion and perivascular hemorrhages
Coma, rising blood pressure, bradycardia	Rising intracranial pressure and hydrocephalus as the aqueduct is compressed and the subarachnoid space becomes compromised

Adapted from Adams and Victor.[29]

Cerebellar–foramen magnum herniation frequently results from, or is contributed to by, obstructive hydrocephalus. Emergency removal of fluid from the more cephalad ventricular system may relieve symptoms and be lifesaving. Surgical intervention is indicated only if the cause of the herniation is treatable. In the case of cerebellar–foramen magnum herniation aggravated by acute obstructive hydrocephalus, ventricular–peritoneal shunting is frequently necessary. The procedure must be done carefully, however, since too rapid a change in the CSF dynamics can lead to a rapid and damaging movement of the brain that can lead to occlusion of posterior cerebral arteries and brain stem injury.

These two herniation syndromes can and will lead to death unless there is prompt intervention. The immediate intravenous administration of hyperosmotic agents such as mannitol or urea and large doses of synthetic glucocorticoids such as dexamethasone or methylprednisolone should be instituted promptly to reduce intracranial pressure and avert impending death.

TABLE 46-10. Cerebellar-Foramen Magnum Herniation

Neurologic Findings	*Pathologic Cause*
Head tilt, stiff neck, posturing of neck, or paresthesias over the neck	Downward displacement of inferior hemispheres through the foramen magnum; may be unilateral or bilateral
Tonic extensor spasms of limbs and body (cerebellar "fits") and later coma	Compressive effects of cerebellum or hydrocephalus on the upper brain stem
Respiratory arrest	Medullary compression

Adapted from Adams and Victor.[29]

Hemorrhage into a tumor is not as common as might be expected, although the incidence of intratumor hemorrhage may increase because of iatrogenic thrombocytopenia associated with the current use of chemotherapy in the treatment of brain tumors. Primary tumors that most commonly bleed de novo are glioblastoma and oligodendrogliomas; of the metastatic tumors, those from the lung, melanoma, hypernephroma, and choriocarcinoma are most likely to be associated with intratumoral hemorrhage. Temporizing treatment of signs and symptoms of intratumoral hemorrhage entails the use of osmotic agents and glucocorticoids, but if the hemorrhage is extensive and life-threatening, operation and decompression are indicated. Under no circumstances should a lumbar puncture be performed in any patient with an acute herniation syndrome. In fact, lumbar puncture should never be done indiscriminately. The indications for lumbar puncture are covered in another section.

SPINAL AXIS

In order to understand the clinical presentation of tumors of the spinal axis, one must appreciate the local anatomy (see Fig. 46-4) and how tumors might manifest with respect to anatomy. The cranial dura is firmly adherent to the skull (with the exception of dural duplications of the falx and tentorium), and normally no extradural space exists between dura and skull. An entirely different anatomical relationship in the spinal canal accounts for a well-defined extradural space containing epidural fat and blood vessels. Through the intervertebral foramina this extradural space communicates with adjacent extraspinal compartments, such as the mediastinum and retroperitoneal space. With rare exceptions, extradural tumors are metastatic, reaching the extradural space through intervertebral foramina.

Tumors arising inside of the dural tube (intradural tumors)

may originate within the spinal cord (intramedullary) or outside the spinal cord (extramedullary). The two common extramedullary intradural tumors, neurilemmoma (schwannoma) and meningioma, are attached respectively to sensory nerve roots and dura, and involve the spinal cord by compression.

Neurology of Spinal Cord Tumors

A spinal tumor produces two kinds of effects, local (focal) and distal (remote). Local effects indicate the tumor's location along the spinal axis; distal effects reflect involvement of motor and sensory long tracts within the spinal cord. Table 46-11 summarizes the clinical findings useful in localizing a spinal cord tumor.

Distal effects are common to all spinal tumors sooner or later, and symptoms and signs are confined to structures innervated below the spinal cord level of involvement. Although neurologic manifestations commonly begin unilaterally, a full-blown Brown–Séquard syndrome of cord hemisection can rarely occur. More characteristic are motor changes: weakness and spasticity, if the tumor lies above the conus medullarus, or weakness and flaccidity if the tumor is at or below the conus. Typically, sensory impairment begins distally in the feet. Impairment of bladder function occurs later in tumors above the conus but may be an early manifestation of tumors in or below the conus. As a rule, the upper level of impaired long tract function is several segments below the actual site of tumor involvement.

Local manifestations may reflect bone involvement, pain constituting the cardinal symptom of metastatic tumors. Involvement of spinal roots produces pain, sensory impairment, and weakness with atrophy in the appropriate radicular distribution. Less often, involvement of spinal gray matter produced either by extensive pressure from extramedullary tumors or by direct damage from intramedullary tumors causes segmental sensory and motor changes.

TABLE 46-11. Clinical Manifestations of Spinal Cord Tumors

Location	*Findings*
Foramen magnum	11th and 12th cranial nerve palsies, ipsilateral arm weakness early, cerebellar ataxia, neck pain
Cervical	Ipsilateral arm weakness with leg and opposite arm in time; wasting and fibrillation of ipsilateral neck, shoulder girdle, and arm; decreased pain and temperature sensation in upper cervical regions early; pain in cervical distribution
Thoracic	Weakness of abdominal muscles, sparing of arms, unilateral root pains, sensory level with ipsilateral changes early and bilateral with time
Lumbosacral	Root pain in groin region and/or sciatic distribution, weakened proximal pelvic muscles, impotence, bladder paralysis, decreased knee jerk and brisk ankle jerk
Cauda equina	Unilateral pain in back and leg, becoming bilateral when the tumor is quite large; bladder and bowel paralysis

Historically, tumors at or near the foramen magnum have been diagnosed incorrectly more often than spinal tumors at any other site. This is due to the fact that foramen magnum tumors can mimic such diverse conditions as multiple sclerosis, amyotrophic lateral sclerosis, and cervical disk disease. The frequency of delayed diagnoses of these tumors justifies the dictum that myelography or, more recently, magnetic resonance (MR) imaging is indicated as a diagnostic measure in any neurologic disease that can be accounted for by a lesion at or below the foramen magnum.

Occasionally a cervical intramedullary tumor will mimic syringomyelia, producing dissociated sensory loss, weakness and wasting in the arms and hands, and variable long tract involvement. In most cases the clinical signs of a spinal tumor do not indicate whether it is extradural or intradural.

As a rule, the rate at which symptoms develop can be helpful in distinguishing extradural from intradural tumor. A history of days to a few weeks characterizes metastatic extradural tumors, and a longer course, often many months, reflects the slower growth of intradural tumors. A history of previously diagnosed cancer or other system involvement can also be helpful.

NEURODIAGNOSTIC TESTS

NEUROIMAGING

The diagnosis of intracranial tumor requires radiographic confirmation. Recent technological advances in radiology are well suited for imaging the brain and spinal cord. Fifteen years ago, the imaging modalities commonly used to confirm the diagnosis of tumor were (1) skull radiography, to evaluate shift in the calcified midline pineal, hyperostosis or bone erosion, or, in children, bone mottling indicating long-standing increased intracranial pressure; (2) radionuclide brain scintigraphy, which demonstrated tumors on the basis of increased permeability of capillaries within a tumor to tracer compared to normal brain capillaries, which excluded the tracer; (3) arteriography, by which tumors could be specifically identified on the basis of abnormal tumor vessels, or less specifically by displacement of normal vessels; and (4) pneumoencephalography, which, by the distribution of air injected into the ventricular system and cisterns, could be used to demonstrate tumors within or impinging on the ventricular system or cisterns.

Today, the much more sensitive and descriptive techniques of MR imaging and computed tomography (CT) are widely available. Both techniques can demonstrate intracranial and spinal lesions, and both produce cross-sectional digital images. The depicted anatomy and pathology is based on numerical computerized representations of certain physical properties of the tissue.[34] The CT image is composed of pixels based on the attenuation of x-rays, which in turn are dependent on the electron density of the tissue being studied. MR imaging also produces an image based on pixels, but, unlike CT, the pixel intensity of MR imaging is based on proton density, T1 and T2 relaxation times, and flow (blood flow). Thus, the MR image represents a complex interrelationship of four parameters; furthermore, data acquisition can be manipulated by the operator to a greater degree than with CT. CT and MR imaging also differ in that MR imaging data can be acquired in any plane desired, including oblique planes, in a primary fashion so that there is no compromise of spatial or contrast detail. CT scans for all practical purposes can be acquired only in the axial or half-axial planes. Computer-generated reformations are required to generate alternative views such as orthogonal or off-axis images, all of which will exhibit degradation of both spatial and contrast detail.

MR imaging is in general more sensitive than CT. As clinical experience and laboratory benchwork expands, the pathologic correlates of the MR image are rapidly becoming better understood. Non-contrast-enhanced MR imaging is in general more sensitive than even contrast-enhanced CT. One limitation to MR imaging, however, is the not infrequent inability of this modality to differentiate between tumor and surrounding edema. An MR study performed without contrast material also fails to indicate the degree of blood–brain barrier defect (vessel leakiness) associated with the tumor. By the time this chapter is published, at least one paramagnetic agent will be in clinical use. This agent is a gadolinium molecule chelated to a diethelyne triaminopenta-acetic acid (DTPA). Gd-DTPA will cross leaky tumor capillaries and provide a T1-weighted MR image with high signal intensity in any situation in which there are leaky vessels. If the study is performed immediately after injection of Gd-DTPA, there will also be enhancement of normal vascular structures that dissipates rapidly as the contrast material equilibrates with the extravascular pool.

In addition to the inability to distinguish between tumor and surrounding edema, the non-contrast-enhanced MR image is also relatively limited in comparison to CT in depicting small meningiomas, which can be isointense with normal brain tissue, and in demonstrating seeding of tumor along the subependymal and subarachnoid spaces. These limitations make MR imaging particularly unattractive for interval evaluation of patients who have undergone tumor therapy. These are the patients in whom the degree of vessel leakiness is of importance in evaluating response to therapy and in whom the possibility of tumor seeding is much greater. With the availability of Gd-DTPA, MR imaging will be the most effective means of evaluating patients with tumors, both before and after therapy. This is due to both the increased contrast and spatial sensitivity associated with this modality and the ability to image the tumor in a plane that optimizes the relationship of abnormal tissues to normal adjacent structures. For example, a subfrontal lesion is best viewed in the coronal plane rather than in the axial plane.

The availability of modern imaging equipment varies with the economies of various communities and states. If MR imaging is unavailable, CT performed after the administration of iodinated contrast material is the imaging method of choice. If neither CT nor MR imaging is available, radionuclide scintigraphy with ^{99m}Tc-DTPA and even occasionally plain skull radiography are useful.

Approximately 50% of patients with low-grade gliomas may present with tumors that do not enhance on CT. Some in fact may not be detectable with CT because they are isodense with brain. In these cases the differential sensitivity of MR imaging, even without the use of a paramagnetic contrast agent, is clearly evident. Figure 46-5, a CT scan of a patient with a seizure disorder, was interpreted as normal both prospectively and retrospectively and before and after contrast agent administration. The MR image is clearly abnormal. Stereotactic biopsy demonstrated a well-differentiated astrocytoma.

The possibility of obtaining high-quality coronal images without the artifact associated with beam hardening through bone makes MR imaging particularly attractive for evaluating lesions of the base of the skull and the posterior fossa. Figure 46-6 is a high-quality MR image of a patient with a pituitary adenoma. Although this lesion would be readily identified on CT, the relationships to the optic chiasm and infundibulum would not be as clear.

In the posterior fossa, the lack of artifact and the availability of sagittal and coronal planes make MR imaging uniquely suited for demonstrating and characterizing neoplasms. Both intra-axial and extra-axial masses are easily distinguished and their relationship to the ventricular cisternal systems is easily assessed.

In the evaluation of intracranial tumors, cerebral angiography is used much less frequently than in the past. Angiography may be used to confirm an impression gained from MR imaging or CT that the lesion in question is a vascular malformation or aneurysm rather than a neoplasm. Angiography may be used before surgery to determine and obliterate the vascular supply to lesions such as meningiomas. Angiography is almost never performed as a roadmapping procedure before surgery.

In the evaluation of both inframedullary and extramedullary spinal cord lesions, high-quality MR imaging is the diagnostic study of choice. Except for drop metastases, it is much more sensitive than myelography. Once Gd-DTPA is incorporated into the MR examination, the indications for myelography will be extremely limited. Preliminary studies have already indicated that the sensitivity of MR imaging in the evaluation of drop metastases to the spinal axis following gadolinium is nothing short of spectacular. Current experience with MR imaging has indicated that it can demonstrate tumors not visible with myelography, so we can anticipate earlier detection of intramedullary or extramedullary spinal cord tumors. Spinal cord tumors can be much more reliably distinguished from syrinxes than in the past (Fig. 46-7). Also, the frequent association of cysts with intramedullary cord tumors can be identified so that if appropriate, a shunting procedure can be performed on the cyst even if the tumor cannot be removed.

Myelography is in general more reliable than plain MR or CT in demonstrating drop metastases. In the detection of extramedullary lesions such as meningiomas, neurinomas, and chordomas, MR imaging, even without the use of contrast agents, is the most sensitive technique available. With agents such as Gd-DTPA, it is the definitive examination.

A unique and particularly important application of sagittal MR imaging is in therapy planning. The sagittal MR image can be superimposed on the port film for accurate localization of the tumor for appropriate port design. The use of MR imaging should be requisite in planning the treatment of any base of skull or posterior fossa lesion.

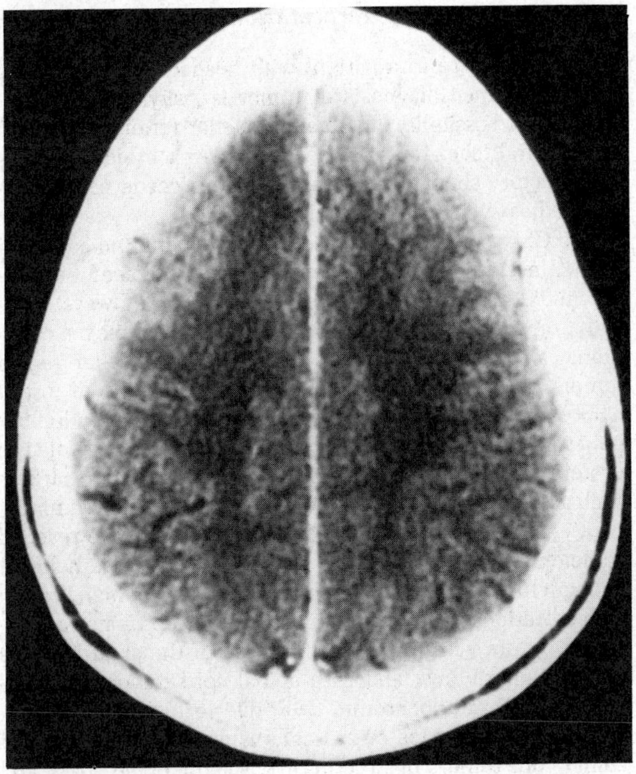

A

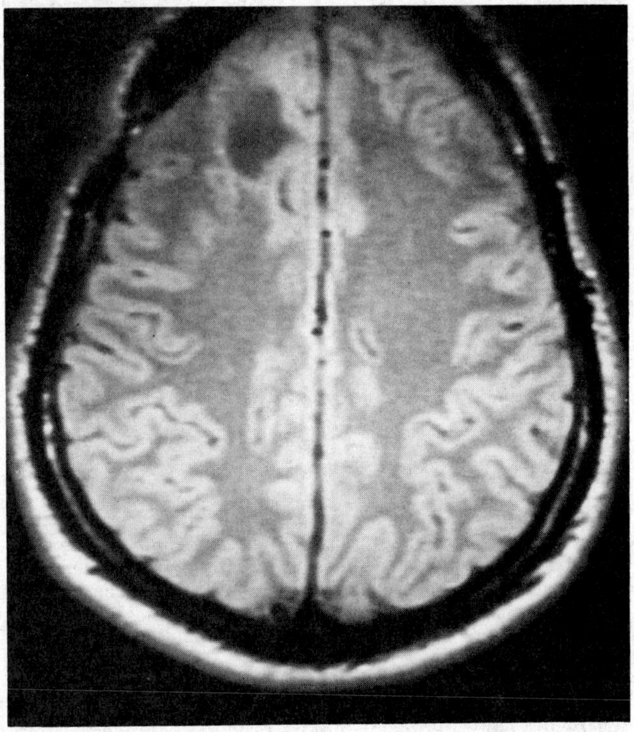

B

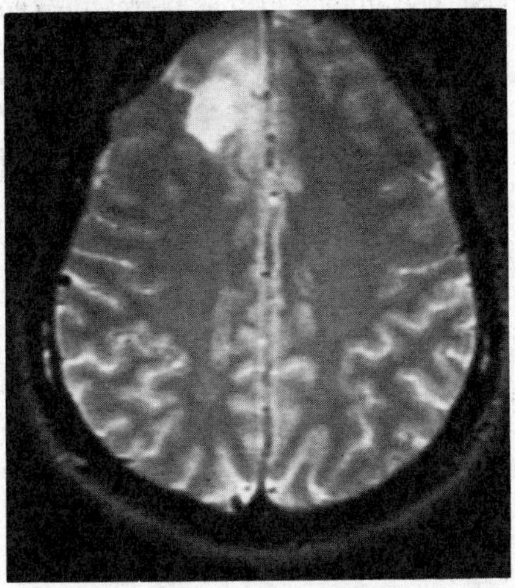

C

FIG. 46-5. A young man presented with a single focal seizure that generalized into a major motor seizure. **A.** A postcontrast axial CT demonstrates a poorly defined area of low density involving the most anterior portion of the corona radiata extending anteriorly to the gray matter on the right. No contrast enhancement, sulcal effacement, or mass effect is present. **B.** Following this CT scan, a T2-weighted (TR 2000, TE 20) axial MR scan was performed that shows an area of decreased signal intensity at the gray–white junction at the most anterior medial aspect of the right frontal lobe. On the second echo (TR 2000, TE 60) **C**, the lesion exhibits high signal intensity. On biopsy the tumor was found to be a well-differentiated astrocytoma.

TANGENT SCREEN, PERIMETRY, AUDIOMETRY, AND ELECTROENCEPHALOGRAPHY

Few of the ancillary tests used in the past are needed today because of the sophisticated neuroimaging techniques that allow precise tumor localization. However, there still remain instances in which other and less expensive testing can be of help to the practitioner.

Testing for abnormalities of the visual system is part of the neurologic examination. At times, however, the results of confrontation visual field testing need quantification for greater accuracy and to observe the effects of treatment. Formal visual field testing is done using tangent screens; scotomas and field defects are tested with perimetry. Figure 46-8 schematically presents the common visual field abnormalities and their anatomical localization.

Deafness is quantified with formal audiometric testing. This can be helpful in the diagnosis of acoustic neurinomas. The electrical equivalent of auditory signals can be observed by recording over the brain stem. These signals, called auditory evoked responses, correlate well with lesions in the brain stem and can be used to follow patients with brain stem tumors. Similar evoked potentials measured over the visual cortex following visual stimuli are of much less value in the evaluation or follow-up of patients with brain tumors.

The electroencephalogram (EEG) once had a place in the

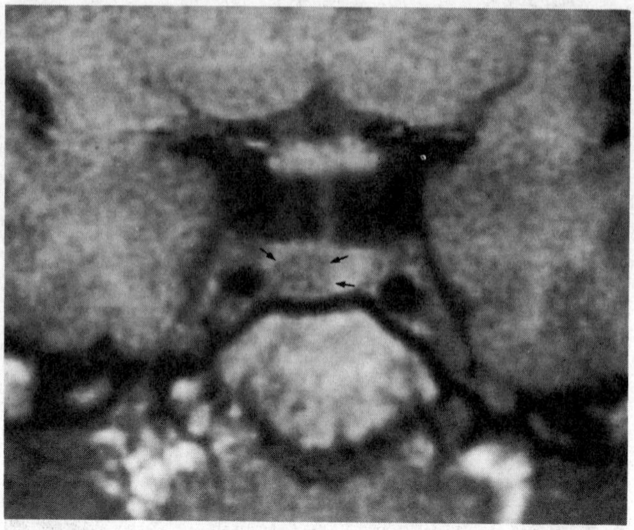

FIG. 46-6. A 30-year-old woman presented with hyperprolactinemia. Coronal T1-weighted (TR 600, TE 20) 3-mm thick section scan of the pituitary gland demonstrates a low intensity lesion 9 mm in diameter (*arrows*) involving the right-hand side of the pituitary fossa. It displaced the gland and the stalk to the left. Findings are typical of a pituitary microadenoma.

diagnosis and follow-up of intracranial neoplasms.[36] Characteristically, supratentorial tumors produce polyphasic slow-wave (theta and delta waves) activity, which had some localizing value. Infratentorial lesions are sometimes associated with high-voltage slow waves, seen particularly in anterior EEG leads. Today the EEG has no value in the diagnosis of brain tumors. Its major value is in the diagnosis of seizure disorders and in following the rare patient whose neurologic deterioration may be related to subclinical seizures rather than tumor growth.

TUMOR AND CSF MARKERS

The measurement of body fluids for products or body responses to tumor has been attempted for diagnostic reasons and to quantify responses to therapy. For patients with intracranial and spinal tumors, examination of peripheral blood and cerebrospinal fluid (CSF) has proved helpful in many instances.

Specific Markers

Pituitary tumors often produce endocrinologic abnormalities measurable by very sensitive radioimmunoassays. Polycythemia associated with a tumor of the posterior fossa (cerebellum) may be useful as presumptive evidence of hemangioblastoma. Some parasellar and pineal region embryonal tumors secrete unique hormones and proteins. β-Human chorionic gonadotropic hormone (β-hCG) and α-fetoprotein (AFP) are examples of hormones associated with trophoblastic tissue and yolk sac, respectively.[37,38] Measurement of polyamines such as putrescine in the CSF has proved helpful in following the cause of tumors located near the ventricle or spinal subarachnoid space.

Indications for and Interpretation of CSF Examination

Lumbar puncture in a patient with headache, papilledema, and a presumed diagnosis of tumor is risky because it increases the possibility of a fatal cerebellar-foramen magnum or temporal lobe–tentorial herniation. As a basic rule, lumbar puncture should follow rather than precede neuroimaging studies such as MR imaging and CT.

The CSF examination is useful in following the course of intracranial tumors that have a propensity to seed the subarachnoid space and spread through the CSF pathways. Typically, medulloblastoma, ependymoma, choroid plexus carcinoma, and some embryonal pineal and suprasellar region tumors have a high enough likelihood of spread to justify CSF examinations. In these cases, CSF obtained by lumbar puncture should be examined for malignant cells (cytology), protein and glucose concentrations, and specific markers such as β-hCG and AFP. These tests will determine if malignant cells are in the CSF or if tumor deposits have reached sufficient size (high protein concentrations can be helpful) to begin to block CSF subarachnoid pathways. A high protein concentration with normal glucose values and a normal cytology occurs with tumors of the base of the skull, such as acoustic neurinoma, and with spinal cord tumors. The appearance of xanthochromic CSF, due to high protein content, with an absence of red cells is quite characteristic of spinal cord tumors obstructing the subarachnoid space and producing stasis of the CSF in the caudal lumbar sac.

Measurement of CSF polyamines such as putrescine can be valuable since elevated polyamine levels frequently precede clinical and neuroimaging evidence of tumor progression.[39] The major use of these measurements is to monitor therapy and possible recurrence rather than for initial diagnosis.

EVALUATION OF PATIENTS WITH INTRACRANIAL TUMORS DURING THERAPY

Critical to the evaluation of the efficacy of any therapy for brain tumors is the reliability of the measurement of tumor growth (deterioration) or tumor regression (response). Before MR imaging became available, sequential neurologic examinations, CT, and radionuclide scintigraphy were used to evaluate tumor response and regrowth.[36] Later, with improvements in CT scanners, and to reduce the cost of therapy evaluations, contrast-enhanced CT became the major method of evaluating tumor response and regrowth. For patients that do not have contrast-enhanced CT scans, MR imaging is a logical alternative. However, the extreme sensitivity of MR imaging to changes in brain water content can work to a disadvantage in the evaluation of regrowth. If a tumor appears smaller on MR imaging it can correctly be assumed that the tumor is responding to treatment, but if a lesion appears larger post irradiation, the increase in size may only reflect demyelination from irradiation and the replacement of myelin by water. The use of Gd-DPTA or other technological advances will be necessary before MR imaging can be used reliably to assess tumor regrowth in the post irradiation period.

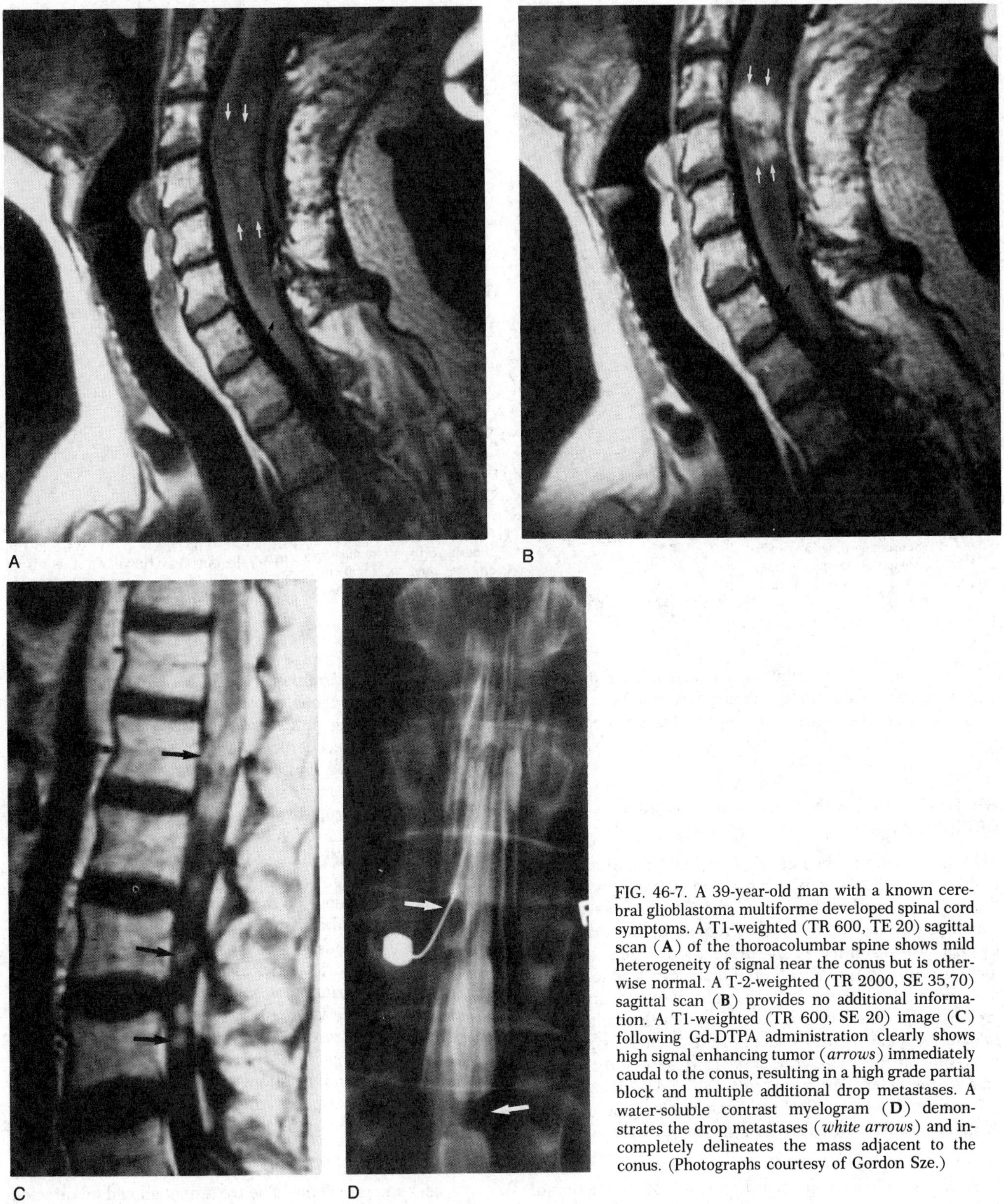

FIG. 46-7. A 39-year-old man with a known cerebral glioblastoma multiforme developed spinal cord symptoms. A T1-weighted (TR 600, TE 20) sagittal scan (**A**) of the thoroacolumbar spine shows mild heterogeneity of signal near the conus but is otherwise normal. A T-2-weighted (TR 2000, SE 35,70) sagittal scan (**B**) provides no additional information. A T1-weighted (TR 600, SE 20) image (**C**) following Gd-DTPA administration clearly shows high signal enhancing tumor (*arrows*) immediately caudal to the conus, resulting in a high grade partial block and multiple additional drop metastases. A water-soluble contrast myelogram (**D**) demonstrates the drop metastases (*white arrows*) and incompletely delineates the mass adjacent to the conus. (Photographs courtesy of Gordon Sze.)

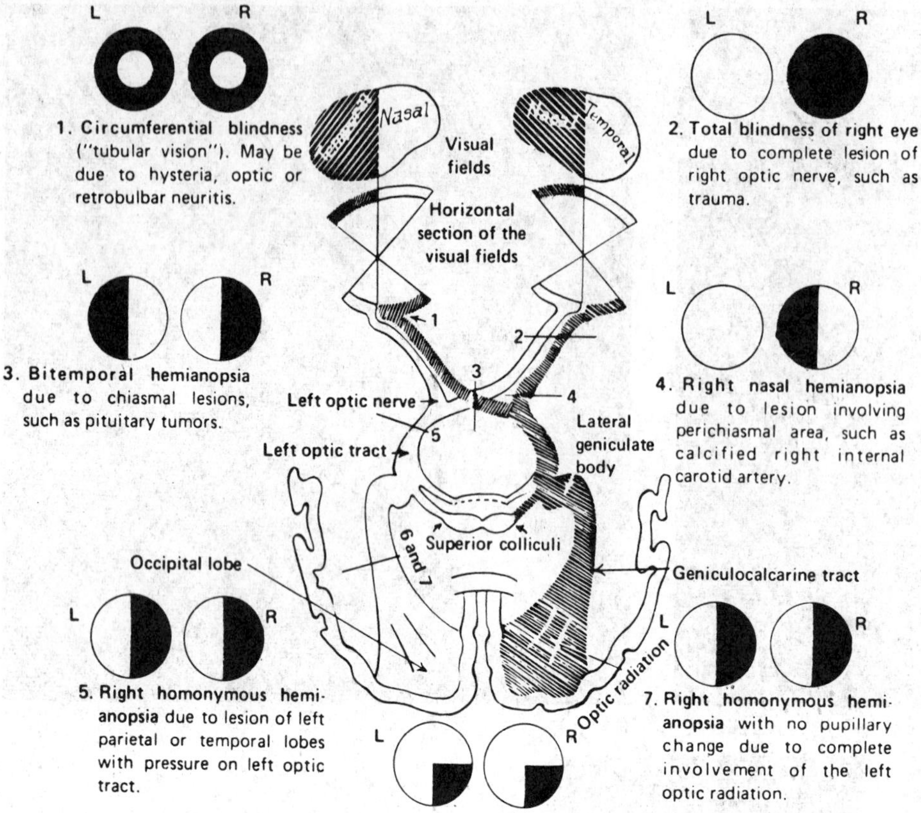
L
R
1. Circumferential blindness ("tubular vision"). May be due to hysteria, optic or retrobulbar neuritis.
Nasal
Temporal
Visual fields
Horizontal section of the visual fields
L
R
2. Total blindness of right eye due to complete lesion of right optic nerve, such as trauma.
L
R
3. Bitemporal hemianopsia due to chiasmal lesions, such as pituitary tumors.
Left optic nerve
Left optic tract
1
2
3
4
5
Lateral geniculate body
L
R
4. Right nasal hemianopsia due to lesion involving perichiasmal area, such as calcified right internal carotid artery.
Superior colliculi
6 and 7
Occipital lobe
Geniculocalcarine tract
Optic radiation
L
R
5. Right homonymous hemianopsia due to lesion of left parietal or temporal lobes with pressure on left optic tract.
L
R
L
R
7. Right homonymous hemianopsia with no pupillary change due to complete involvement of the left optic radiation.

FIG. 46-8. The visual pathways and the effects lesions can have on the visual fields. (Chusid JG: Correlative Neuroanatomy and Functional Neurology. Los Altos, CA, Lange, 1973)

For the correct interpretation of results of therapy and to improve patient care, understanding factors other than cell division is important; these factors are discussed below.

FACTORS THAT MAY PRODUCE CLINICAL DETERIORATION

The most common causes of neurologic deterioration in brain tumor patients undergoing radiation therapy or chemotherapy are growth of the tumor and increased peritumoral edema. Both cause an increased pressure in the cranial cavity that is transmitted primarily to the adjacent brain; in turn, hydrostatic pressure on the brain can lead to impairment of cerebral blood flow. The clinical result can be progressive impairment of functioning brain with resultant neurologic deficits. Manifestations may include signs and symptoms of increased intracranial pressure and temporal lobe or cerebellar herniation (see Tables 46-6 and 46-7).

Neurologic deterioration without neuroimaging evidence of tumor growth can occur for a number of reasons.

1. Hydrocephalus can occur as a result of obstruction of the ventricular system at the aqueduct of Sylvius, the fourth ventricle, or the foramen of Monro; except for obstruction of the foramen of Monro, obstructive hydrocephalus most often results from infratentorial tumors. Occasionally, hydrocephalus is caused by a cerebral subarachnoid convexity block due to infiltrative tumor (carcinomatosis, CNS leukemia, arachnoiditis). Hydrocephalus is usually treated with a ventricular shunting procedure, although administration of high-dose glucocorticoids may temporarily ameliorate the associated signs and symptoms.
2. Hemorrhage into a tumor, although rare, can occur as either an abrupt event or stepwise deterioration over hours. It is more likely to occur in a hypertensive patient. The incidence of intratumoral bleeding may increase as more patients undergo myelotoxic chemotherapy and develop thrombocytopenia. The treatment for intratumoral hemorrhage is high-dose glucocorticoids initially, followed by surgery if necessary.
3. Fluid imbalance, particularly hyponatremia, can accentuate peritumoral edema. A common cause of hyponatremia is the use of excessive amounts of parenteral dextrose–water solutions. Salt-wasting syndromes, except in the immediate postoperative period, are uncommon in patients with brain tumors. In either case, the treatment is fluid restriction and, if herniation appears imminent, parenteral hyperosmotic therapy.
4. Hypertension can also accentuate intratumoral and peritumoral edema. The treatment should be directed to control of the hypertension. Occasionally high-dose glucocorticoids and hyperosmotic agents are needed. However, these agents may aggravate the hypertension or put undue stress on the cardiovascular system and hence should be used with caution.
5. Radiation therapy can cause deterioration in several

ways (see section Radiation Therapy, under Treatment Modalities). Early in the course of radiation therapy, peritumoral edema (or demyelination) may cause progression of neurologic deficit, requiring an increase in glucocorticoid dosage. From 1 to 12 weeks (usually 6 to 12 weeks) after the completion of radiation therapy, a transient encephalopathy, with signs and symptoms of increased intracranial pressure, drowsiness, nausea, and exacerbation of preexisting neurologic deficit, can occur.[40] This self-limited encephalopathy responds to steroids and resolves within several weeks without specific deficit. Steroids can then be discontinued. This delayed syndrome, observed in about 14% to 20% of patients completing a course of cranial irradiation, sometimes can be distinguished from tumor regrowth only by temporizing and finding that the patient's condition improves. This characteristic syndrome is not unique to brain tumors; it is also observed in leukemic children following prophylactic cranial irradiation. From a few months to 10 years or more after radiation therapy (commonly 1 to 2 years), radiation necrosis can occur. Necrosis is generally associated with an increased neurologic deficit that may or may not mimic tumor recurrence. Either atrophy or increased mass effect is seen on CT. (See section on Radiation Therapy, under Treatment Modalities, for further discussion of adverse effects of irradiation.)

6. Seizures can complicate the evaluation of brain tumor response and progression. The occurrence of seizures may suggest (rightly or wrongly) that the tumor is growing, and may result in an increase of the neurologic deficit apart from any direct effect of the tumor. Recovery from any increase in weakness and mental dullness may take several hours to a week in postictal patients who are already brain injured. Even subclinical seizures can cause deterioration, persisting for hours to days, which will resolve with control of the seizures. The EEG is usually diagnostic in these cases, and the treatment consists of better control of seizures. In this regard, we believe that patients receiving long-term chemotherapy frequently require higher doses of anticonvulsants because of deleterious drug interactions and increased degradation of the anticonvulsant drugs caused by drug-induced hepatic changes.
7. Infection can produce neurologic deterioration independent of tumor growth. Examples, although uncommon in brain tumor patients, are meningitis and cerebral abscess. The former is usually diagnosed from the presence of fever and meningismus; the latter, if in the same area as the tumor, is difficult to distinguish from a tumor undergoing changes. CT, MR imaging, and cerebral angiography can be helpful in establishing the correct diagnosis. The more common causes of meningitis include pneumonia and urinary tract infections.
8. Metabolic disorders, anemia, fatigue, and emotional depression can cause clinical deterioration, including an increase in focal deficit on testing, that is difficult to distinguish from tumor progression. Such conditions generally produce no alteration on brain scans (CT, MR imaging, or radionuclide scintigraphy), which, therefore, are useful in establishing the diagnosis, or at least in ruling out tumor progression as the cause of the deterioration.

It should be kept in mind that patients harboring responsive tumors also show clinical evidence of deterioration after a course of chemotherapy. In our experience, at least 10% of patients who eventually respond to therapy become significantly worse at the end of a first course of chemotherapy, and transient deterioration is occasionally observed even during the second year of continuous chemotherapy. Paradoxically, this clinical worsening early in therapy may result from an increase in tumor bulk due to "effective" therapy. Several factors contribute:

a. The brain is surrounded by a rigid skull.
b. The cell mass may increase when doomed cells either form giant cells or undergo one or more successful cell divisions before dying.
c. The CNS has an inefficient mechanism for disposing of dead cells produced by either chemotherapy or irradiation.
d. Edema, probably caused by irritative products of cell lysis, may be present within the tumor mass and in adjacent brain.

Glucocorticoids May Produce Clinical Improvement

Theoretically, tumor regression should result in clinical improvement because of a reduction in the size of the tumor mass. However, if the neurologic deficit is caused by infiltration with destruction of neural tissue, rather than by compression and displacement of brain, clinical improvement may be negligible or nonexistent, despite oncolytic effectiveness.

Aside from the benefits of radiation therapy and chemotherapeutic agents, clinical improvement is most likely to occur as a result of glucocorticoid administration. Thus, in order to assess accurately the effects of radiation therapy and chemotherapy in patients with intracranial tumors, glucocorticoid administration must be closely controlled.

GLUCOCORTICOID USE. Administration of glucocorticoids is usually begun before surgery for brain tumor. If adequate surgical decompression is achieved, the steroid dosage can be tapered rapidly and discontinued within the first week or two after the operation. Some patients require steroid maintenance because a large volume of tumor remains, because tumor occupies the brain stem or spinal cord, or because of steroid dependence resulting from long-term prior use.

Patients who no longer require glucocorticoids after surgery may need them during or after radiation therapy. Reactive edema may occur during radiation therapy, and occasionally there is a transient period of drowsiness and increased deficit at 6 to 12 weeks after completion of a course of irradiation. The delayed radiation reaction usually resolves within a few weeks; observation of the patient's subsequent clinical course is the only way to distinguish it with certainty from tumor progression.

Except for the situations cited above, a patient's glucocorticoid requirement is most likely related to tumor growth or regression. The lowest dosage of glucocorticoid that will maintain a patient at his or her maximum level of comfort and function should be sought. Ordinarily this is determined by decreasing the dosage until symptoms increase or become apparent, then increasing the dosage until they subside. If the patient continues to do well, periodic attempts should be made to decrease the dosage. Keeping the dosage as low as tolerable minimizes the side-effects of steroids and allows earlier recognition of tumor growth. If the patient becomes worse from physiologic stress, such as a severe infection, glucocorticoid requirements generally increase, but should be returned to the original level when the stress resolves.

If deterioration is secondary to tumor growth or treatment-induced effects, glucocorticoids may have to be increased to keep the patient comfortable. For example, 3 mg/day of dexamethasone may have the desired effect for a patient with stabilized disease; however, a patient whose condition is deteriorating may require dexamethasone dosages of 64 mg/day or more.

Changes in glucocorticoid dosage affect the evaluation of the clinical state and response to cytotoxic treatment. A decrease in steriod requirement suggests improvement, assuming that the previous dosage was actually required. An increase in dosage suggests deterioration. Because an increased steroid dosage may (1) improve the neurologic status, (2) reduce the size of the lesion seen on neuroimaging, and (3) reduce the size of the tumor and the degree of contrast enhancement on CT, an attempt should be made to document tumor recurrence before increasing the glucocorticoid dosage; this would rule out transient causes of deterioration, such as seizures or infection, so that a rational decision for change in treatment can be made.

TREATMENT MODALITIES

SURGERY

No other modality can reduce tumor bulk as quickly as surgery. Advances in imaging, pharamacologics for brain edema, neuroanesthesia, and surgical magnification, illumination, and instrumentation have made operative approaches to tumors in even the most remote corners of the CNS possible and reasonably safe. The goal of brain tumor surgery is to completely resect and thereby cure the tumor. In the sections of this chapter which follow, such cures will be seen to be not uncommon. If surgical cure is not possible (as, for example, in most gliomas), tumor bulk reduction and consequent decompression of the brain is the next goal and when possible should be the first therapeutic modality for the tumor.

An extremely important byproduct of cytoreductive surgery is the acquisition of adequate tissue for histopathologic examination. In our opinion, only very rarely should brain tumors be treated with radiation or chemotherapy in the absence of a definitive tissue diagnosis. In patients with tumors thought to be inaccessible by open craniotomy or in patients in whom open craniotomy is deemed unhelpful, a needle biopsy should be performed under CT or ultrasound (US) guidance. We have found CT-guided stereotaxy to be the most facile method for obtaining tissue with a needle.

Surgical Planning

The first step in surgical planning is adequate imaging. CT is the premier imaging modality for CNS tumors. MR imaging is rapidly becoming imperative for optimal imaging of tumors of the skull base and posterior fossa, and for the lower grade gliomas. The intrinsic characteristics of a tumor's appearance and its relative position in the brain as shown on a technically adequate CT or MR imaging study can often narrow the diagnostic possibilities to one or two choices.

Cerebral angiography is important in surgical planning for tumors that may encircle critical cerebral blood vessels, like basal meningiomas, or for tumors that can be extremely vascular, like hemangioblastomas, meningiomas, and glomus tumors. For such lesions, angiography done in temporal proximity (24–48 hours) to the planned surgical procedure can be combined with embolization of the tumor's blood supply, in many instances making the surgical procedure technically easier.

The final selection of a surgical approach is made after adequate imaging studies have been performed, a differential diagnosis has been developed, and the patient's general condition has been assessed. In the era of modern neuroanesthesia, it is rare that a craniotomy is prohibited because of poor general medical status. The design of an appropriate scalp incision and bone flap is the final preoperative decision.

Preoperative and Anesthetic Management

Patients should be placed on anticonvulsants (diphenylhydantoin is preferred), and corticosteroids (commonly dexamethasone) should be administered for a few days preoperatively to reduce cerebral edema and thereby facilitate cerebral retraction for perfect exposure. Blood levels of anticonvulsants should be monitored to ensure that the therapeutic range has been achieved; such monitoring should be continued for at least 1 year. Corticosteroids should be continued into the postoperative period and then tapered when possible.

Patients undergoing craniotomy are operated on under general anesthesia, with the anesthetic agents selected for their lack of effect on intracranial pressure. In general, the head is rigidly held with pin fixation to minimize movement as the surgeon is looking through the operating microscope, where the slightest movement is dramatically amplified. Once the patient has been intubated and the pin fixation device applied to the head, positioning is attended to with care, as poor positioning can blight the remainder of the procedure. Patients are operated on in the supine, lateral decubitus, prone, or sitting position, depending to some extent on the tumor location and to a greater extent on the surgeon's preferences and habits. No matter what the patient's position, all pressure points are carefully padded. Just before the procedure is begun, mannitol (1 g/kg body weight) is administered and hyperventilation to a P_{CO_2} of 25 to 30 torr is accomplished for definitive reduction of intracranial pressure in preparation for brain retraction.

Craniotomy for Supratentorial Tumors

The bony opening is designed such that it is generous enough to facilitate surgery. The bone flap is centered over the tumor when a transcortical approach is planned (*e.g.*, in glioma resections) or positioned to provide access to the route of approach—for example, over the interhemispheric fissure for falx meningiomas or the floor of the middle fossa for certain tumors in the tentorial incisura. For tumors in the region of the third ventricle, the choice of surgical approach varies according to the specific purpose of the surgery and the experience of the operator. In all cases, the scalp flap is designed to fully accommodate the bone flap and the vascular supply to the scalp is given careful consideration in the design.

After the scalp incision is made and the scalp flap reflected, bur holes are drilled and connected with a hand saw or power saw. The bone flap can be turned back, attached to the temporalis muscle (osteoplastic flap) and its blood supply, or removed completely (free flap). The dura is opened only after the brain has been completely softened by mannitol diuresis and intraoperative hyperventilation. Sometimes a few minutes' wait is necessary to secure maximum decompression, and this (typically) short wait can be critical to the success of the subsequent surgical approach.

The dura is reflected back and the tumor is approached. The surgeon can be confused by a field of normal-appearing cortex when seeking to expose a small subcortical lesion. In this situation intraoperative US is invaluable in delineating the position of a small tumor, and a cortical incision can be made directly over the lesion, thereby minimizing cortical injury. After the cortical incision is made in one of the overlying gyri or at the point where an approach around the brain to a deep tumor is to begin, self-retaining brain retractors are placed, and the operating microscope is brought to the field to provide essential magnification and illumination. Tumor is usually removed with grasping instruments, sponges, and suction. Removal of firm, adherent, or calcified tumor tissue is facilitated by use of the Cavitron ultrasonic aspirator (CUSA), which ultrasonically disrupts the tumor at its tip and sucks it away. Tumor in locations where access is limited (*e.g.*, the third ventricle) and space to use graspers and other instruments is not available are sometimes best treated with the carbon dioxide laser, which vaporizes tumor tissue with a "hands off" technique. Laser removal of tumor is slow, however, and is reserved for special circumstances.

When maximal tumor removal has been achieved, all bleeding points are carefully coagulated, the retractors are removed, and closure is begun. The dural incision is sutured, the bone flap is wired back into position, and the muscle and scalp are reapproximated in several layers. In the rare situation in which brain swelling is worrisome at the time of closure, a catheter is left in the subdural space to measure the intracranial pressure. All patients are monitored in the intensive care unit for at least one night after surgery, and CT is performed within 48 hours to evaluate the success of the tumor resection. Serum electrolytes and osmolality are measured frequently in the postoperative period to ensure that the patient is relatively dehydrated through the first several days, and to detect the possible onset of inappropriate secretion of antidiuretic hormone or of diabetes insipidus.

Craniotomy for Posterior Fossa Tumors

Through a midline or paramedian vertical incision, the occiput and, commonly, the dorsal aspects of the first and second cervical vertebrae are exposed. A generous craniotomy is done unilaterally or bilaterally to accommodate an approach through the vermis or through, over, or around the cerebellar hemisphere. A laminectomy of C1 and sometimes C2 is done in certain midline approaches to improve tumor exposure or extend the decompression.

Instrumentation for posterior fossa tumor surgery is the same as that discussed in the previous section on supratentorial tumor resection techniques. The carbon dioxide laser is sometimes more helpful than the CUSA instrument in posterior fossa tumor resections because of the tight working space. Closure entails suturing multiple layers of muscle and muscle fascia. The bone is not replaced. Principles of postoperative care are similar as for supratentorial tumor resection.

Stereotaxic Tumors Biopsy

For intrinsic tumors of the deep midline (*e.g.*, pontine or corpus callosum gliomas), for deep tumors of the dominant hemisphere, or for very diffuse, nonfocal tumors, surgical resection is not practical. In these situations needle biopsy for diagnosis is essential. There is no longer any reason to perform a full craniotomy solely to obtain a biopsy specimen. Tissue can be obtained through a needle directed by hand through a bur hole under CT guidance or a needle directed by a number of devices which incorporate US technology. However, in our opinion, nothing is as simple or as accurate as CT-directed stereotaxic biopsy.

A number of CT-guided stereotaxic systems are in common use, and several have also been adapted for guidance by MR imaging.[41,42] Figure 46-9 shows the general sequence of events using the Brown–Roberts–Wells guidance technique. Typically, the patient undergoes CT with a rigid array of bars affixed tightly to the skull to minimize movement. Local anesthesia is generally used in adults, and general anesthesia in children. The CT scan shows the lesion to be biopsied and shows the localizing rods, thereby relating the target to a volume encompassed by the rods. This relationship is formalized by digitizing the position of the target and the position of the rods, and the coordinates for a trajectory to the target are created in a way specific to the individual stereotaxic system used.

The target is approached through a bur hole or a (smaller) twist drill hole. The biopsy instrument is guided to the target by means of an adjustable stereotaxic arc placed on the patient's head in a defined relationship to the former position of the localizing rods used for the CT scan. A fragment of tissue is aspirated or grasped for removal, and a frozen section confirms the acquisition of diagnostic material and frequently suggests a working diagnosis. Experienced sur-

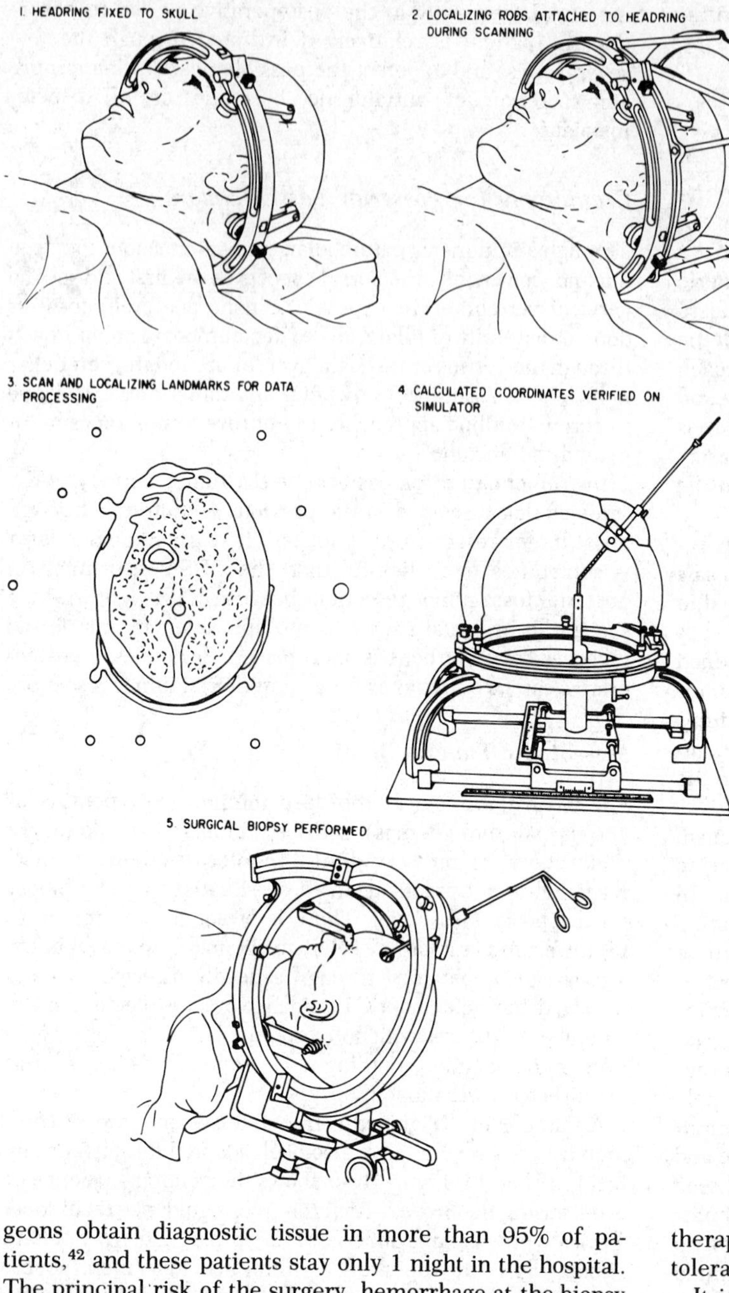
1. HEADRING FIXED TO SKULL
2. LOCALIZING RODS ATTACHED TO HEADRING DURING SCANNING
3. SCAN AND LOCALIZING LANDMARKS FOR DATA PROCESSING
4. CALCULATED COORDINATES VERIFIED ON SIMULATOR
5. SURGICAL BIOPSY PERFORMED

FIG. 46-9. Steps and typical equipment used for CT-guided stereotactic biopsy. The equipment depicted here is part of the Brown-Roberts-Wells guidance technique. (Weiss MH: Clinical Neurosurgery. Proceedings of the Congress of Neurological Surgeons. Baltimore, Williams & Wilkins, 1983)

geons obtain diagnostic tissue in more than 95% of patients,[42] and these patients stay only 1 night in the hospital. The principal risk of the surgery, hemorrhage at the biopsy site, occurs in only a small number of patients.[42] Occasionally, cerebral edema is exacerbated by the procedure.

RADIATION THERAPY

The large majority of primary CNS neoplasms are unifocal, and hence an effective local therapy might be expected to be curative. However, the majority of primary CNS lesions infiltrate a considerable distance, often poorly demarcated even by CT or MR imaging, into normal CNA tissue. Thus, curative therapy means including a substantial amount of normal tissue within the target volume, and CNS tolerance to irradiation becomes a limiting factor. Unfortunately, many of these tumors require relatively high doses, often exceeding CNS tolerance. Before proceeding to the radiation therapy of specific tumor types, we will examine CNS tolerance.

It is clinically and prognostically useful to consider CNS reactions to irradiation according to time of appearance: (1) acute reactions, occurring during or very shortly after radiation therapy; (2) early delayed reactions, appearing a few weeks to 2 or 3 months after radiation therapy; and (3) late delayed reactions, typically appearing several months to many years later.[43]

With conventional fractionation (*i.e.*, 1.8–2.0 Gy/day, five times per week), total doses up to 60 Gy to the whole brain usually are tolerated without clinically significant acute reactions. With reduction of total dose to 30 Gy, fractions as high as 6 Gy given twice weekly also are well tolerated. However, two increments of 7.5 Gy on successive days or single doses of 10 Gy have been reported to cause severe complications. Acute reactions usually are manifested by increased intracranial pressure or exacerbation of the focal signs and symptoms of the lesion treated. These reactions probably are due to edema. With conventional therapy they are usually self-limited, but patients may need and benefit from corticosteroid therapy. However, there is no evidence of long-term benefit from such therapy.

Early delayed reactions, like acute reactions, usually are transient and disappear without definitive therapy. There is some evidence that these reactions are the result of transient demyelination. Here also corticosteroid therapy may be useful in ameliorating symptoms. A worsening of signs and symptoms during this period of time must not be interpreted as necessarily indicating treatment failure[40] and the need for a change of therapy. Early delayed reactions in the brain are probably analogous to the transient radiation myelopathy that may occur after irradiation of the spinal cord.

Late delayed reactions range from asymptomatic narrowing of large vessels to loss of function, frank necrosis, and secondary neoplasia. These reactions tend to be irreversible and often progressive. Clinical findings, of course, depend on the area and volume of brain irradiated. The lesions may present with loss of volume due to atrophy, as a glial reaction masquerading as a space-occupying tumor, or as a low-density, enhancing or mineralized area on CT. As a rule, white matter is more sensitive than gray matter. The child's brain, especially before 2 or 3 years of age, when development and myelination are incomplete, is thought to be more radiosensitive than the adult brain. Postirradiation narrowing of large intracranial arteries has been reported but fortunately is rare. It may be asymptomatic. For example, we have seen asymptomatic narrowing of both internal carotid arteries as they pass through the cavernous sinus, 10 years after a dose of 45 Gy (1.2 Gy/day) was administered to a 17-year-old patient with Cushing's disease. On the other hand, if the arterial compromise is sufficient, a stroke may ensue. Other rare but reported late reactions are secondary neoplasms such as fibrosarcoma, meningioma, and gliomas.

Necrotizing leukoencephalopathy and mineralizing microangiopathy are two late delayed syndromes that occur in children with acute lymphocytic leukemia (ALL) treated with cranial irradiation and aggressive chemotherapy. Necrotizing leukoencephalopathy, the more ominous after the two syndromes, appears 4 to 12 months after CNS prophylactic therapy for ALL. Dementia, drooling, dysarthria, and dysphasia may occur. The majority of patients survive, but often with permanent neurologic impairment. Some patients show complete clinical recovery, others die. This type of injury has been seen with doses as low as 24 Gy delivered in 1.5- to 2.0-Gy fractions in conjunction with chemotherapy. Although necrotizing leukocephalopathy has not been reported with radiation doses less than 24 Gy, and occurs in less than 1% or 2% of patients receiving intrathecal methotrexate or high-dose intravenous methotrexate, the combination of all three therapies may lead to an incidence as high as 40% to 50%.[44] Methotrexate appears to be most neurotoxic when given during or after radiation therapy. CT scans show paraventricular hypodensity, ventricular dilatation, widening of sulci, and calcification within cerebral white matter; such CT findings also may be evident in asymptomatic patients who have received intensive CNS prophylaxis for ALL.

In children with ALL treated with CNS prophylaxis, mineralizing microangiopathy generally is associated with mild, often subclinical and transient neurologic dysfunction. It primarily affects gray matter and is characterized by dystrophic calcification of basal ganglia and subcortical zones. Calcium deposition may appear within the walls of small blood vessels, which may become occluded and surrounded by mineralized and necrotic brain tissue.

There have been numerous reports of impaired intellectual function in children who have received radiation therapy for tumors of the brain or for ALL. It seems clear that some patients will exhibit a decreased level of intellectual function, but it is often difficult to determine the specific role of factors such as the tumor and its location, elevated intracranial pressure, surgery, radiation therapy, chemotherapy, psychological stress, reduced school attendance, and the adequacy of efforts to rehabilitate. Some studies have suggested that mental retardation is more common in patients with tumors of the hypothalamic region, thalamic regions, or brain stem, and less than 5 years old. Meadows et al reported a study of children with ALL who had received cranial prophalyxis consisting of 24 Gy whole brain irradiation and intrathecal methotrexate.[45] These children were compared with a group treated at an earlier date without cranial irradiation and with a group that had received chemotherapy for Wilms' tumor but without cranial irradiation. After 3 years, approximately 60% of those with ALL who had received cranial irradiation had a decrement in IQ of 10 or more points. Children less than 5 years old and those with initial IQ scores of 110 or more showed a greater decrement in IQ score than did older children or those whose IQ scores were initially lower. Ochs et al compared ALL patients who had received intrathecal methotrexate plus 18 Gy whole brain irradiation with another group that had received intrathecal methotrexate plus intravenous methotrexate without irradiation and found a decrease in verbal and performance IQ scores in approximately 40% of each group. Other studies have indicated that 18 to 24 Gy cranial irradiation plus intrathecal methotrexate results in performance scores around 8 to 9 points lower than in patients who received intrathecal methotrexate alone. It appears that relatively low-dose whole brain irradiation in young children, especially in conjunction with chemotherapy, can cause a modest but measurable decrease in intellectual function. It is important that such deficit be recognized early and remedial action, such as special schooling, be undertaken early.

Although we are convinced that high-dose irradiation (*e.g.*, 60 Gy conventionally fractionated) may cause some degree of intellectual impairment in adults, data on adults are sparse. Such impairment appears to be accentuated by concurrent or subsequent multiple-agent chemotherapy. Also, it seems more prominent in those who have undergone whole brain as compared with partial brain irradiation, which is one reason for avoiding whole brain irradiation when possible. A recent report by Maire et al on adult patients with primary intracranial tumors showed that during the first 4 months after partial or whole brain irradiation (about three fourths of these patients also received chemotherapy), full-scale IQ coefficients were normal.[47] Between 5 and 30 months after irradiation there was intellectual deterioration which subsequently disappeared. Full-scale IQ scores fell after 30 months, but recovery was seen in four of five patients less than 30 years old and in two patients between 30 and 50 years old, who returned to work early after treatment. Maire et al recommended early neuropsychological testing with psychological assistance when indicated, and an early return to work.

Further studies in children and adults are needed to determine the incidence and precise cause or causes of intellectual deterioration following irradiation of the CNS. Such studies should aid in preventing or reducing intellectual impairment and should provide aid in dealing with it when it does occur.

Frank radiation necrosis may occur a few months to many years after irradiation of the CNS. The frequency of radiation necrosis as a function of dose and fractionation, however, is not well documented. A review by Sheline et al suggested that threshold doses with conventional fractionation (1.8–2.0 Gy per fraction per day) are approximately 45 Gy for 10 fractions, 60 Gy for 35 fractions, and 70 Gy for 60 fractions.[48] That review also suggested that the isoeffective dose is equal to the total dose times $N^{-0.4} \times T^{-0.03}$, where N is the number of fractions and T is the total time in days. It was cautioned that it might be unwise to use such a formula to extrapolate to very small or very large numbers of fractions, or to very short or long overall treatment times. Marks et al reported on 139 patients who received irradiation for primary brain tumors with at least 45 Gy (1.8–2.0 Gy/day).[49] Reinterpretation and recalculation of their data indicates that (1) for total doses ≤57.6 Gy, there was no necrosis in 51 patients; (2) for total doses between 57.6 and 64.8 Gy, there were two instances of necrosis in 60 patients; and (3) for total doses between 64.8 and 75.6 Gy, there were five instances in 28 patients, for an incidence of about 20%.

Delayed Radiation Myelopathy of the Spinal Cord

Various studies have indicated that a total dose of 50 Gy delivered in 25 fractions over 5 weeks generally is safe. It is widely believed that the cervical spinal cord is more tolerant than the thoracic cord, and that the incidence of injury is related to the length of the cord irradiated. Good experimental evidence to support these two concepts, however, is lacking. Certainly, overlapping of radiation portals that included only short segments of the spinal cord has led to catastrophe. Various isoeffect formulas have been derived for the spinal cord. Wara et al used an Ellis type formula, in which the exponent for N was −0.377 and that for T was −0.058.[50] Van der Kogel concluded that the isoeffect formula should have an N exponent of −0.4, and that for treatment times up to about 6 weeks, the time factor was essentially negligible. These isoeffect formulas predict that spinal cord tolerance will continue to increase with decreasing fraction size. However, Ang et al found that for the rat spinal cord, reduction of dose per fraction from 2.0 to 1.3 Gy did not result in a further increase in spinal cord tolerance.[52] Until more data are available on fraction sizes of less than 1.8 or 2.0 Gy, hyperfractionated or accelerated radiation therapy with doses in the 1.0 to 1.2 Gy range, and in which the total dose is calculated on the basis of an isoeffect formula, should be approached with caution. Furthermore, Ang et al reported that repair of radiation-induced sublethal damage in the rat spinal cord requires more than 4 hours for completion.[52]

Tumor Target Volume

The appropriate target volume varies widely according to the specific pathology, and for certain histologic types it is the subject of considerable debate. In defining the target volume, radiographic information, especially from CT and MR imaging, is used in conjunction with consultation among the neurosurgeon, radiation oncologist, neuroradiologist, and neuropathologist. Some tumors, such as certain meningiomas, pituitary adenomas, and chordomas, may be treated with tight fields—that is, with minimal margins for uncertainty. On the other hand, tumors such as astrocytomas, anaplastic astrocytomas, and glioblastomas multiforme may require large margins for uncertainty of the distance of tumor infiltration beyond that identified by available diagnostic techniques. For these lesions, we usually include a margin of 2 to 3 cm beyond the enhancing volume on CT and at least 1 cm beyond the T2-weighted MR image, using whichever volume is larger. Others have advocated whole brain irradiation for lesions such as glioblastoma multiforme. Our approach is based on several considerations: (1) The vast majority of these lesions, when they recur, do so at the primary tumor site. (2) Injury to normal brain should be kept to a minimum. (3) Various randomized trials and historical data have failed to show that whole brain irradiation improves the survival rate. (4) CT studies have shown that recurrences are within a 2-cm margin of the primary site in 90% of patients.[53] (5) CT performed shortly before death has shown that the microscopic tumor extent was within a 2-cm margin in 80% of patients. (6) Serial biopsies have shown that isolated tumor cell infiltration may extend at least as far as T2 prolongation abnormalities.[54] (7) Choucair et al found that only 1.1% of patients presented with multiple lesions (405 glioblastomas multiforme, 630 anaplastic gliomas).

Certain neoplasms, such as medulloblastoma and malignant ependymoma, require treatment of the entire craniospinal axis. In our technique for irradiation of the cranial-spinal axis the intracranial contents, including the upper one or two segments of the cervical cord, are treated through opposed lateral fields. The spine is treated through one or two posterior fields, depending on the size of the individual. The lateral cranial fields are angled so that the lower border parallels the upper border of the adjacent spinal field, and the inferior border abuts the superior edge of the spinal field in midplane. Suitable individualized blocks are used to protect the face, nasal passages, and nasopharynx from needless irradiation. When two posterior spinal fields are used, as is usually the case, a simple gap is calculated so that the 50% isodose lines meet at the level of the spinal cord. After every 10 Gy to the spinal cord, the junction lines are moved 0.5 to 1 cm. This is accomplished by expanding the lateral skull fields and moving the posterior spinal fields caudally without changing their dimensions. A fixed block at the inferior margin of the caudal spinal field serves to keep the lower edge of the irradiated volume at the same location.

CHEMOTHERAPY

The use of anticancer agents in the treatment of intracranial and spinal tumors is established for many primary tumors. For parenchymal CNS tumors, however, controversy surrounds the concept of limited antitumor efficacy for agents with restricted blood–brain barrier permeability.[56] Supporting the concept is the fact that many infiltrative primary CNS tumors (*e.g.,* gliomas) have cellular regions within brain with apparently intact, normal-appearing brain capillaries. In addition, the actual extent of capillary breakdown accounting for the leakage responsible for positive contrast CT and radionuclide brain scans is quite small.[57] While drug delivery to portions of any primary tumor would be expected to occur to the same extent as with non-CNS tumors, delivery (via diffusion) to infiltrative regions distant from leaky tumor capillaries would be expected to be compromised. Diffusion, a slow process, cannot produce significant drug concentrations unless plasma drug levels are sustainable for prolonged periods of time and the diffusing drug is relatively stable in the tumor tissue as it diffuses.

A secondary supporting argument is that most agents with antitumor activity against CNS tumors readily cross the blood–brain barrier.[58] For example, all of the non-sugar-containing chloroethylnitrosoureas (CENU) such as BCNU, CCNU, PCNU, and ACNU have shown efficacy as single agents, whereas sugar-containing CENU are less effective.[28] Procarbazine, another commonly used agent, also crosses the blood–brain barrier and is active.[59] Agents such as bleomycin, Adriamycin, cisplatin, vincristine, and mithramycin have either shown no activity or have activity limited to primitive childhood and embryonal tumors.

Whether ease of passage through the blood–brain barrier is an absolute or relative advantage is somewhat academic, given the paucity of chemotypes with demonstrable antitumor activity. Even a small pharmacokinetic disadvantage takes on disproportionate importance when the selective cytotoxicity of a drug is small. This may well be the case with many of the drugs used since they share narrow therapeutic indices because of dose-limiting systemic toxicity.

With respect to drugs for CNS tumors, many of the available anticancer drugs can be toxic to the CNS if given at very high doses or in a manner that circumvents the blood–brain barrier.[60] The blood–brain barrier protects the brain from many potentially toxic compounds. If it did not exist, CNS toxicity rather than myelotoxicity or gastrointestinal toxicity would be dose-limiting for most drugs.

Pharmacokinetic considerations for intracranial nonparenchymal tumors and extramedullary spinal tumors are less dependent on the ability of chemotherapeutic agents to cross the blood–brain barrier, since many of these tumors take their blood supply from meningeal blood vessels, which are significantly more permeable than brain blood vessels.

Regional Drug Delivery Considerations

Under most circumstances, regional drug delivery produces greater drug exposure than systemic intravenous (IV) or oral administration. With respect to intracranial and spinal tumors, the regional delivery takes the form of intra-CSF therapy, intra-arterial infusion, and intratumoral therapy.

Therapy by the CSF route (usually by ventricular reservoir) is a form of regional drug delivery that is used to treat meningeal neoplasia resulting from primary or secondary tumor invasion of the subarachnoid space and, less commonly, one of the ventricular cavities. It is frequently but not always associated with malignant cells floating in the CSF.

The advantages of intra-CSF therapy are high local drug levels, low systemic toxicity, and the ability to increase the frequency of treatments. However, delivery of drugs through the CSF can be dangerous and is associated with a high morbidity. The drugs commonly used are methotrexate, cytosine arabinoside, and thiotepa. All three drugs have been reported to produce CNS damage ranging from fever and chills to leukoencephalopathy and myelitis. Efficacy is limited when lesions are large (≥5 mm in diameter) or when CSF pathways are blocked and CSF flow is diverted.

Of concern in the use of CSF therapy is that slow clearance of drug can lead to increased neurotoxicity. Normally we find, after injection into a ventricular reservoir and pumping the reservoir 5 times, the CSF distribution and flow of radionuclide-labeled albumin in the ventricle is well-distributed and the half-time from ventricle to cisterna magnum is approximately 60 minutes. In many cases, obvious hydrocephalus is not apparent on neuroimaging, but a physiologic slowing of CSF flow (and presumably CSF absorption) is present. This slowing of CSF flow can lead to (1) poor distribution in the subarachnoid CSF for drugs with high capillary clearance, such as cytosine arabinoside, and (2) a greater likelihood of serious CNS toxicity for a drug such as methotrexate.

Another form of regional therapy is the intra-arterial administration of anticancer drugs through either carotid or vertebral arteries. The advantage of this approach is an increased uptake during the first passage of drug through tumor capillaries. Increased efficacy would be expected for patients whose tumors lie within the perfusion territory of the infused artery. Contrary to what might be thought, systemic toxicity will not be reduced unless the total administered dose is reduced, since the actual amount of drug taken up by the tumor is a small fraction of the injected dose. On the other hand, focal brain and retinal morbidity is increased, as was demonstrated by the clinical trials with BCNU[61] and cisplatin.[62] Because of the controversial results of clinical trials, this form of treatment is not recommended except under controlled experimental conditions.

Intratumoral therapy is regional therapy that, at best, is applicable for cystic tumors with a narrow rim of surrounding tumor. Pharmacokinetic considerations implicate problems with (1) maintenance of tumor cavity drug levels, (2) diffusion distances from the cavity to the outer margin of tumor, (3) nonspecific biodegradation and binding of drug or drug products, and (4) the need for repeated treatments. Modern clinical trials evaluating this form of regional therapy have not been published.

CLASSIFICATION AND TREATMENT OF CNS TUMORS BY ANATOMICAL LOCATION

CEREBRAL ASTROCYTOMAS

Pathologic Classification

This section will deal primarily with classification of astrocytomas of varying degrees of aggressiveness, ranging from juvenile pilocytic astrocytoma to glioblastoma multiforme. The slower growing or lesser aggressive lesions are often referred to as "low grade" or "benign," while the more rapidly progressive neoplasms are referred to as "high grade" or "malignant." However, with the exception of juvenile pilocytic astrocytomas and the limited number of astrocytomas that can be completely resected, even the "benign" astrocytomas are highly lethal. For low-grade astrocytomas, Bloom reported 10-year survival rates of 6% to 10%.[63] Laws et al reported 10-year and 20-year survival rates of about 21% and 16% for patients with subtotally resected low-grade cerebral astrocytomas[64]; expected survival for a comparable group of age- and sex-matched normal individuals would have been around 95% at 10 years. Liebel et al reported 10-year survival rates of 35% and 11%, depending on whether or not radiation therapy had been used.[65]

Many classification systems for astrocytomas have been advanced. In general, these have followed one of two different approaches. The first approach, and one we highly advocate, is based on the presumed cell of origin. The other is based on grading the degree of malignancy. The most widely used grading system is the Kernohan–Sayre system,[66] in which astrocytomas are graded from I to IV, with Grade IV representing the most malignant tumors. Although patients with Kernohan–Sayre Grade I or II disease have significantly longer median survival times than patients with Grade III or IV disease, the system is not prognostically useful for separating Grades I and II and Grades III and IV. The difference in 5-year survival for Grades I and II in the large Mayo Clinic series reported in 1984 by Laws et al was not statistically significant.[64] Fazekas actually reported a higher survival rate for patients with Grade II disease than for patients with Grade I disease.[67] Furthermore, the large randomized trials reported during the last decade for malignant gliomas have failed to find a difference in survival for Grade III versus Grade IV. In the RTOG/ECOG prospective randomized trial of 626 patients, the median survival time for patients with Grade III astrocytomas was 10 months, versus 9 months for those with Grade IV astrocytoma.[68] On the other hand, when these same cases were histologically grouped as astrocytoma with anaplastic foci versus glioblastoma multiforme, there were marked differences in both median survival time and 18-month survival rates; these were 28 months and 62%, respectively, for anaplastic astrocytoma, versus 8 months and 15% for glioblastoma multiforme. Similar differences between anaplastic astrocytoma (or malignant astrocytoma) and glioblastoma multiforme has been reported in older retrospective studies from UCSF,[69] Stanford,[70] and Jefferson.[71]

Thus, while the Kernohan–Sayre grading system is of limited usefulness, histologic features are of considerable prognostic significance. The UCSF experience shows a clear separation of survival curves for patients with incompletely resected astrocytomas, with survival decreasing in the following order: juvenile pilocytic astrocytoma, astrocytoma, anaplastic astrocytoma, and glioblastoma multiforme. Preliminary data (R. D. Davis et al, unpublished observations, 1987) suggest that anaplastic astrocytomas can be histologically separated into two different prognostic groups, which Davis et al have termed moderately anaplastic and highly anaplastic astrocytoma. The survival curves for patients with highly anaplastic astrocytoma and those with gemistocytic astrocytoma are virtually superimposable and lie between those for the moderately anaplastic astrocytoma and glioblastoma multiforme.

Surgery

RATIONALE. Data from animal experiments suggest, and a large clinical experience with tumors at many sites would confirm,[42,72] that maximal surgical resection improves the results of subsequent radiation therapy and chemotherapy. This principle would seem to apply to the treatment of astrocytomas. Gross total surgical resection was among the dominant factors favoring longer survival in a large series of patients with Grade 1 or Grade 2 astrocytomas treated at the Mayo Clinic.[73] The second Brain Tumor Study Group trial of radiation and chemotherapy regimens showed a correlation between the extent of surgical resection and subsequent survival rates in patients with the more malignant astrocytomas.[74] Salcman's review of older reports on the results of treatment in more than 600 patients with such malignant gliomas who received only surgical treatment confirms this correlation.[80] Andreou et al approached the problem from a different perspective, looking at the impact of amount of tumor present on postoperative CT on the subsequent "useful survival" (Karnofsky Performance Score >30), and found a significant inverse correlation.[75]

A number of factors might be responsible for the improved clinical outcome when astrocytomas are aggressively resected. An assiduous resection can remove 90% of a typical astrocytoma, thereby decompressing the brain and substantially reducing the tumor cell burden, which when killed by subsequent therapies serves as a nidus for cerebral edema because of the indolent dead cell removal in the brain.[76,77] In addition, aggressive surgical resection reduces the number of separate cell populations in these very heterogeneous tumors, thereby eliminating some already radioresistant and chemoresistant populations; reduces the probability of further mutation toward resistance by lowering the overall number of tumor cells; and reduces the number of cells in regions remote from blood vessels, regions where chemotherapeutic agents cannot penetrate and where hypoxia can (theoretically) confer radioresistance.[78]

SURGICAL PRINCIPLES. The surgery for cerebral astrocytomas is complicated by the intra-axial location of these tumors. Therefore, careful preoperative planning of the surgical exposure is critical. The goal of every craniotomy for a cerebral astrocytoma is gross total resection, and adequate exposure should be achieved for this purpose, although sometimes aggressive resection proves impossible at the time of the operation. Tumors are approached through an incision in the crest of an overlying gyrus, the selection of which is aided by intraoperative US images. Self-retaining retractors are placed to gently retract both sides of the cortical incision (generally about 3 cm long), then the operating microscope is brought in for the approach through the subcortical white matter to the tumor. The tumor is resected with suction, with two-point coagulation forceps, with grasping instruments, with the CO_2 laser, or with the CUSA; the resection proceeds from the inside out, so that surrounding normal white matter is minimally disturbed. The glistening peritumoral white matter is easily spotted through the microscope as each of the tumor's margins is reached, and it is at this interface that the resection is stopped. Hemostasis is sometimes difficult to achieve, but must be perfect. Hemispheric tumor cysts can be drained and, when possible, fenestrated into an adjacent ventricle to prevent reaccumulation. Tumors not amenable to resection because of their location or their diffuseness should be biopsied stereotaxically. Again, there is no indication for a craniotomy when the purpose is merely to biopsy (and not resect) a tumor.

REOPERATION. Accumulating evidence indicates that reoperation for resection of cerebral astrocytomas at the time of recurrence can be efficacious.[79–81] The rationale cited above for the aggressive initial resection of cerebral astrocytomas seems to fit equally well the prospect for reresection at recurrence. This is only true, however, if there is some treatment modality (*e.g.*, chemotherapy, brachytherapy) that the patient can receive after the reoperation, and most often there is.

Salcman et al, based on their experience with reoperation on all patients who were to receive further therapy for recurrence of malignant glioma, propose that a relatively nonselective approach might be rational, given that reoperation is safe and, in their experience, of potential benefit despite the patient's age, performance status, tumor grade, or interval between initial surgery and recurrence.[80] Salcman et al emphasized that reoperation is technically more demanding than the initial surgery because tissues are compromised by previous therapy, and consequently the postoperative infection rate is high.[80]

Young and co-workers argue for more rigid selection criteria when choosing candidates for reoperation on recurrent malignant gliomas.[79] They found that patients with Karnofsky Performance Scores (KPS) above 60 and an interval between the initial surgery and recurrence of at least 6 months had the longest survival rates after reoperation. Harsh et al considered the effect of reoperation on subsequent high-quality survival (KPS at least 70) in patients with recurrent malignant gliomas.[81] Age and preoperative KPS affected the duration of high-quality survival in this study: a relatively young age and high performance scores were advantageous. Because their data also suggest that reoperation can significantly enhance the effects of chemotherapy on recurrent brain tumors, Harsh et al do not suggest confining reoperation to young patients in excellent condition, but suggest instead simply using these factors as guidelines in the broader therapeutic picture.

Radiation Therapy

When administering radiation therapy for the astrocytomas, it is our policy to use local rather than whole brain irradiation, for reasons outlined earlier. Nevertheless, the target volumes may be relatively large, as in the treatment of infiltrating astrocytoma, anaplastic astrocytoma, and glioblastoma multiforme. The target volume is shaped to the location and dimensions of the volume thought to be at risk. Depending on size and location, the portals may be co-axial opposed or more complex, using multiple fields and wedge fibers. All fields are treated daily with megavoltage radiation. The daily dose increment is 1.8 to 2.0 Gy. The more differentiated astrocytomas receive a total dose of approximately 55 Gy, whereas lesions such as anaplastic astrocytoma and glioblastoma multiforme receive a total dose of 60 Gy.

For the cystic cerebellar astrocytomas, where tumor is confined to a resectable mural nodule, the control rate for surgical resection alone approaches 100% and irradiation is not recommended. Similarly, in a UCSF series[82] of 12 patients with completely resected juvenile pilocytic astrocytoma, the 10-year survival rate was 100%. For incompletely resected and irradiated juvenile pilocytic astrocytoma, the UCSF 5- and 10-year progression-free survival rates were about 90% and 80%, respectively. We have no data on incompletely resected and nonirradiated juvenile pilocytic astrocytoma; hence, evaluation of the efficacy of radiation therapy for this tumor is uncertain.

Although there has not been a prospective randomized trial, retrospective reviews of other types of low-grade astrocytoma suggest that postoperative radiation therapy is of value for incompletely resected lesions. For incompletely resected tumors at UCSF,[65] the 5- and 10-year recurrence-free survival rates following incomplete resection alone were 19% and 11%, respectively. With the addition of postoperative radiation therapy, these rates increased to 46% and 35%. Fazekas reported 5-year survival rates of 41% with irradiation and 13% without irradiation.[67] Laws et al reported a 5-year survival rate of 49% for patients who received at least 40 Gy versus a 34% survival rate ($p = 0.05$) for those who received lesser doses or no irradiation.[64] They concluded that "radiation therapy was of clear benefit, primarily in older patients with incompletely removed tumors (based on a step down regression analysis)."

Retrospective studies also have indicated that the survival from anaplastic astrocytoma is superior to survival from glioblastoma multiforme and that irradiation is a benefit. Marsa et al reported a mean survival time of 20 months for patients with malignant astrocytoma versus 9 months for patients with glioblastoma multiforme; the 5-year actuarial survival rates were 19% and 0%, respectively.[70] The UCSF investigators reported a 5-year recurrence-free survival of 18% for patients with irradiated anaplastic astrocytomas versus 0% for patients with nonirradiated disease.[69] At UCSF the survival time was longer for irradiated than for nonirradiated glioblastoma multiforme; however, none of the patients survived 5 years.

In 1978 Walker et al reported the only prospective randomized clinical trial in which patients with malignant gliomas were randomized to receive or not to receive postoperative radiation therapy.[83] This study was carried out by the United States Brain Tumor Study Group (BTSG) and included 222 patients, of whom 90% had glioblastoma multiforme and 9% had anaplastic astrocytoma. The median survival times were 14 weeks without radiation therapy versus 36 weeks with radiation therapy ($p = 0.001$). The 12-month survival rates were 24% with radiation therapy and 3% without. Thus, even in patients with glioblastoma multiforme a survival advantage accrues from radiation therapy. When data from several BTSG clinical trials were combined, a

TABLE 46-12. Survival Time for Studies That Combined Radiation and Chemotherapy for Patients with Anaplastic Astrocytoma or Glioblastoma Multiforme Whose Karnofsky Performance Scores ≥60

		Survival Percentile	
Treatment	*%GM*	*50%*	*25%*
BCNU(85)	81	51 wk	78 wk
BCNU(86)	89	50 wk	75 wk
BCNU(68)	66	43 wk	
BCNU(87)	45	55 wk	
CCNU(88)	100	55 wk	
CCNU(88)	0	106 wk	
CCNU(89)	68	55 wk	
CCNU(90)	100	51 wk	
CCNU(91)	41	43 wk	
MeCCNU(85)	82	42 wk	73 wk
STZ(93)	79	43 wk	78 wk
PCB(86)	89	47 wk	83 wk
CDDP(93)	77	53 wk	
CCNU-PCB(89)	63	50 wk	
BCNU-PCB(93)	79	50 wk	
HU-BCNU-PCB-VM26(93)	78	50 wk	
MeCCNU-DTIC(68)	68	42 wk	

MeCCNU = methyl CCNU; STZ = streptozotocin; DTIC = dimethyl imidazole carboxamide; VM26 = etoposide; CDDP = cis-diaminedichloroplatinum.

regimen of 60 Gy delivered in 6 to 7 weeks was found to yield a better survival rate than 50 Gy in 5 to 6 weeks.[84] The combined RTOG/ECOG study referred to earlier failed to find further improvement in survival when the total dose was increased from 60 to 70 Gy. These data, together with the desire to limit the adverse effects of irradiation, have led us to limit the total dose to 60 Gy for anaplastic astrocytoma and glioblastoma multiforme when the radiation is conventionally fractionated.

Chemotherapy

Few patients with astrocytoma receive chemotherapy; most are never offered the option. Nonetheless, astrocytomas have been the most extensively treated of primary intracranial tumors.

Controlled (randomized) clinical trials have demonstrated the efficacy of a number of drugs when combined with irradiation as adjuvant therapy. Table 46-12 summarizes the results of controlled (randomized) clinical trials of adjuvant chemotherapy.[68,85–91,93] Efficacy has been shown for BCNU,[94] CCNU,[95] PCNU,[96] procarbazine,[59] streptozocin,[93] and the combination of CCNU, procarbazine, and vincristine.[97,98] Lesser activity has been shown for some of the newer agents such as AZQ[99] and spiromustine.[100]

The era of controlled clinical trials for malignant astrocytomas began with the inception of the BTSG in 1967. Shortly afterward, the EORTC established a comparable group. In addition, other national and regional cooperative groups have conducted controlled chemotherapy trials. Tables 46-12 to 46-14 summarize selected data from these groups.[58,60,101–103] Some groups report survival from initiation of therapy, others report time to tumor progression (TTP). Whereas some groups defined histologic groups and separated glioblastoma multiforme from anaplastic astrocytoma, others combined the two groups in the same study. Thus, it is somewhat difficult to compare studies.

In addition to histology, other factors influence the likelihood and duration of response. Major known factors are age, performance status, and extent of surgical resection at onset of therapy. For instance, younger patients are more likely to respond and for a longer period of time; better performance status patients do best; and patients who have more extensive surgical resection do better than those who do not have surgery or have had a biopsy only.[104]

With consideration for the above covariates, it is still clear that adjuvant chemotherapy following surgery and radiation therapy for glioblastoma and anaplastic astrocytomas increases both TTP and survival time. Less precise information is available with respect to response because of differing criteria used by the various groups. However, most investigators agree on the definition of deterioration or tumor progression. Thus, TTP and survival are more universal measures for controlled clinical trials. In many ways TTP is a more pure measure of efficacy since, at the time of initial progression, many patients receive other forms of therapy. Survival, however, is a better measure of the social usefulness of the additional life conferred by the therapy.

For comparison to the clinical trials presented in Table 41-12, we generated Kaplan-Meier representations of a group of 251 consecutive patients at UCSF for survival as a function of histology. Patients with glioblastoma had a median survival of 15 months, those with highly anaplastic astrocytomas and gemistocytic astrocytomas had a median survival of more than 55 months, and those with well-differentiated (also referred to as moderately anaplastic) astrocytomas had a median survival of 4.3 years.

In trying to understand gains in chemotherapy, it is important to appreciate that chemotherapy appears to benefit mostly the lower 50th percentile of patients, and especially those below the 25th percentile. This is reasonable, since in vitro tumor drug sensitivity assays suggest that approximately 60% of tumors are resistant to a given agent.[105,106]

With respect to specific recomendations, it is best to be tentative. Nitrosourea-based drug combinations appear superior to monotherapy, although even this conclusion is based on only one controlled study by the Northern California Oncology Group. In that study, postirradiation BCNU was compared with the PCV combination.[98] The last analysis (conducted by NCOG headquarters in April 1988) showed that the greatest benefit for chemotherapy, based on TTP and survival, was in patients with PCV-treated anaplastic astrocytomas. For patients with glioblastoma multiforme, TTP and survival at the 50th percentile were respectively 37 and 50 weeks for PCV and 34 and 59 weeks for BCNV; for the 25th percentile the figures were 72 and 94 weeks for PCV and 43 and 71 weeks for BCNU. This was more significant ($p = 0.02$), however, for anaplastic tumors. TTP and survival at the 50th percentile were 126 and 157 weeks for PCV and 63 and 82 weeks for BCNU; for the 25th percentile they were 317 weeks and not attained (>320 weeks) for PCV and 142 and 214 weeks for BCNU.

It is clear that more approaches need to be consid-

TABLE 46-13. Time to Tumor Progression for Glioblastoma Multiforme in Patients with Karnofsky Performance Scores ≥60

	TTP, Percentile		
Treatment	50%	25%	*p Value*
BCNU–RT + HU–BCNU[101]	41 wk	74 wk	0.04
BCNU–RT–BCNU[101]	31 wk	52 wk	
RT + HU–BCNU[58,102] *	34 wk	43 wk	0.106 NS
RT + HU–PCV[58,102] *	37 wk	72 wk	
FU–CCNU–RT + HU + MISO–PCB–VCR–BCNU–FU[102]	41 wk	59 wk	

HU = hydroxyurea; PCV = CCNU, procarbazine (PCB), vincristine (VCR); FU = fluorouracil; P = p value; NS = not significant.
* This analysis was performed 4/6/88 on the previously reported data set.

ered to improve on the results cited in Tables 46-12 to 46-14. As a rule, new protocols for controlled trials usually come from Phase II studies of chemotherapy efficacy against recurrent or progressive astrocytomas. Table 46-15[36,58,76,94,96–98,100,107–115] summarizes many of the published studies and several recently completed at UCSF. It is apparent that responses and stable tumors are more common in patients with nonglioblastoma anaplastic astrocytoma who are available for treatment at recurrence. Some selection process is undoubtedly taking place among patients with recurrences and progression; precisely what is not currently known.

In many ways the results in Table 46-15 are disappointing. As was the case with adjuvant therapy of previously untreated astrocytomas, the nitrosoureas, alone and in combination, are the most active for recurrent and progressive tumors. It is quite disappointing that drugs designed specifically for gliomas, such as AZQ and spiromustine, are only mediocre agents in the clinic. Furthermore, from the studies reported in Table 46-15 it is evident that, even though the number of patients benefiting from chemotherapy is quite high in some studies, among patients with responsive or stable tumors the duration of benefit has shown only modest gains over the past decade. This failure of chemotherapy is likely a function of de novo and emergent resistance tumor cell subclones.

One bright spot that recently emerged is the use of the combination of two polyamine inhibitors, DFMO and MGBG, for anaplastic astrocytomas.[113] In a study by Levin et al, patients with recurrent or progressive disease who had been heavily pretreated with nitrosoureas responded and stabilized on the combination for a median time to progression of 52 weeks; the median time to progression for the stable group was similar at 50 weeks. Since that study, additional patients have been treated; as of September 1, 1987, 21 of 29 patients with anaplastic astrocytomas have stabilized or responded with a median duration of 49 weeks. These studies are exciting in that they open new therapeutic opportunities, since these polyamine inhibitors can interact with other agents that act on DNA to improve their efficacy.

TABLE 46-14. Time to Tumor Progression for Anaplastic Astrocytoma Other Than Glioblastoma Multiforme in Patients with Karnofsky Performance Scores ≥60

	TTP, Percentile		
Treatment	50%	25%	*p Value*
BCNU–RT + HU–BCNU[101]	50 wk	74 wk	NS
BCNU–RT–BCNU[101]	72 wk	94 wk	
RT + HU–BCNU[58,102] *	63 wk	142 wk	0.023
RT + HU–PCV[58,102] *	126 wk	317 wk	

HU = hydroxyurea; PCV = CCNU, procarbazine (PCB), vincristine (VCR); FU = fluorouracil; P = p value; NS = not significant.
* This analysis was performed 4/6/88 on the previously reported data set.

BRAIN STEM GLIOMAS

Clinical and Pathologic Considerations

Tumor involvement of the brain stem is due, in order of decreasing frequency, to astrocytoma, glioblastoma, and ependymoma. These tumors can be primarily central and intrinsic (type I) or central with exophytic components in the fourth ventricle (type II), peripontine cisterns (type III), or in both locations (type IV). Furthermore, central lesions can be diffuse and infiltrative or focal; the latter carry a better prognosis. Cranial nerve involvement, therefore, can be at the nuclear level or at the level of the cranial nerve as it leaves the brain stem. The initial manifestations of a brain stem glioma are unilateral palsies of the sixth and seventh cranial nerves in approximately 90% of patients. Cranial nerve involvement is usually followed by long tract signs such as hemiplegia, unilateral limb ataxia, ataxia of gait, paraplegia, hemisensory syndromes, gaze disorders, and occasionally hiccups. Less commonly, long tract signs precede the cranial nerve abnormalities; this is more likely with confined central intrinsic lesions (type I).

If the tumor is a well-differentiated or anaplastic astrocytoma it is likely to involve the midbrain and produce hydrocephalus, vomiting, drowsiness, and cerebellar signs; if the tumor is a glioblastoma it more frequently involves the medulla. Children with glioblastoma characteristically have a rapidly progressive course and are likely to have seventh, ninth, tenth, and sixth cranial nerve deficits along with dysarthria, personality change, and head tilt. Unlike what occurs with expansive posterior fossa tumors, headache, vomiting, and papilledema occur late.

TABLE 46-15. Chemotherapy of Recurrent and Progressive Supratentorial Astrocytomas

Treatment	Percent, R + S		
	GM	*AA*	*GM + AA**
		% (MTP, wk)	
BCNU[58,94]	29(22)	64(22)	
CCNU[107]			42(23)
PCNU[96]	33(8)	69(28)	
PCB[76]			50(26)
BIC[108]	20(NA)	23(22)	
AZQ (24-h inf)†	50(18)	47(16)	
AZQ[109]			24(24)
BCNU–VCR[110]			41(17)
BCNU–PCB[36]	46(17)	56(23)	
CCNU,PCB,VCR[97,98]	45(15)	65(27)	
BCNU,FU[113]		89(32)	
BCNU,FU,HU,MP[114]	55(23)	71(46)	
PCB,FU,HU,MP‡	33(16)	50(20)	
CYCLE (BCNU–FU, PCB, CCNU–PCB)‡		95(41)	
DFMO–MGBG[113]	—	74(50)	
Melphalan (oral)	0(NA)	7(NA)	
Melphalan (IV)§	0(NA)	0(NA)	
Spiromustine[100]			27(5)
AZQ–BCNU[115]	28(9)	80(37)	
AZQ–PCB[115]	31(25)	53(42)	

* GM and AA were not analyzed separately because histologies were not separated, or too few patients were found in each group to separate activity by histology. PCB = procarbazine.
† Chamberlain et al, unpublished observations, 1987.
‡ Levin et al, unpublished observations, 1987.
§ Prados et al, unpublished observations, 1987.

The prognosis for patients with brain stem gliomas as a group is poor, with 5-year survival rates varying between 0% and 38% and a median survival time of less than 1 year in most series.[116,117] Certain patients do better than others. For instance, patients with type II tumors do better than those with infiltrative type I tumors. Patients with moderately anaplastic exophytic tumors do better than those with higher grade anaplastic tumors.

Surgery

Modern imaging of the CNS with CT and particularly MR imaging has improved the capability for definitive diagnosis of brain stem tumors. Lesions previously difficult to distinguish from brain stem glioma, such as clivus tumors, foramen magnum meningiomas, multiple sclerosis, occult arteriovenous malformations, and brain stem abscesses, usually can now be excluded; thus, the place for surgery in the management of these tumors is increasingly indefinite. It appears that brain stem gliomas accessible through the floor of the fourth ventricle or presenting on the lateral surface of the pons can be safely biopsied for prognostic information; furthermore, associated symptomatic cysts can be drained. Any attempt at complete resection of these tumors is foolish. There is some enthusiasm for stereotaxic needle biopsy of brain stem gliomas using CT and MR imaging guidance, since early reports indicate a low complication rate.[118] Although we have considerable expertise at our center in both microsurgical and stereotaxic techniques, many brain stem gliomas are still treated without tissue diagnosis.

Radiation Therapy

Irradiation is the conventional treatment for brain stem gliomas. In addition to improving survival, radiation therapy can improve the symptoms and signs due to tumor in 75% to 80% of patients. Modern diagnostic imaging (*e.g.*, MR imaging) has reduced the likelihood of misdiagnosis and allows the radiation oncologist to tailor his field to encompass the tumor with a relatively small margin.

Irradiation is started shortly (2–3 weeks) after the diagnosis has been established. The standard fractionation is 8 to 9 Gy/week to a total dose of 50–60 Gy given in five daily fractions per week. Treatment is usually via parallel opposed portals, with the tumor dose calculated at the midline on the central axis of the beam. The irradiated volume is based on the CT or, preferably, MR imaging appearance and includes a margin of normal tissue not less than 1 to 2 cm around the tumor. As a rule, the lower border of the field is at the inferior border of the second cervical vertebral body and the upper border is around the superior aspect of the third ventricle. The anterior border is near the anterior clinoid process and the posterior border is about 1 to 2 cm beyond the apparent extent of the tumor. Radiation blocks are used to protect the nasopharnyx.

Because of the relatively poor results obtained with conventional radiation dose schedules, with or without chemotherapy, new hyperfractionation protocols designed to deliver higher doses to these patients are being evaluated. A recently closed protocol at UCSF utilized 1 Gy twice a day, with a minimum 4-hour interval between fractions, to a total dose of 72 Gy. Preliminary results in approximately 50 patients indicate that, with this treatment, a 2-year survival rate of 50% may be expected. Because the results in children appear significantly better than those previously achieved and no obvious radiation-induced toxicity has been observed, a new protocol (BTRC 8725) has been initiated using the same hyperfraction schedule with an increase in the total dose to 78 Gy.

Chemotherapy

Chemotherapy for brain stem gliomas, like chemotherapy for cerebral astrocytomas, is primarily nitrosourea-based.[103] Chemotherapy has infrequently been used as an adjuvant to irradiation. A randomized Childrens Cancer Group Study (CSG) compared radiation therapy with radiation therapy followed by CCNU, VCR, and prednisone.[119] The median survival time was 11 months, and there was no difference between the two groups. In another trial, 5-FU and CCNU given before radiation therapy and HU and misonidazole given during radiation therapy were evaluated.[120] In that study TTP (32 weeks) and survival time (44 weeks) were not better than in the initial CSG study.

Certain therapies have been evaluated for recurrent or progressive brain stem gliomas.[103] Some benefit has been demonstrated, but the extent of benefit was not well established. In a recent study, 5-FU, CCNU, HU, and 6-MP were used to treat children and adults with recurrent or progressive brain stem gliomas.[121] Approximately 69% of 13 patients responded or had stabilized disease with a relapse-free survival time of 25 weeks; the overall survival time was 27 weeks. This is somewhat worse than would be expected for supratentorial gliomas. Currently, we are evaluating a combination of BCNU and DFMO. Unfortunately, new chemotherapeutic leads are not obvious.

CEREBELLAR ASTROCYTOMAS

Clinical and Pathologic Considerations

Astrocytomas arising in the cerebellum are considered separately since their prognosis is consistently better than that for astrocytomas arising in the cerebrum or brain stem. These tumors, which occur most frequently during the first two decades of life, arise in the vermis or more laterally in a cerebellar hemisphere. Usually cerebellar astrocytomas are well circumscribed. They can be cystic, solid, or an admixture of polycystic and solid.

Histologically, the majority are low grade and lack features commonly associated with anaplasia; many are pilocytic in appearance, and, histologically, some are juvenile pilocytic astrocytomas. In a series of 451 pediatric cases reported from the Hospital for Sick Children of Toronto,[122] cerebellar astrocytomas accounted for 25% of all posterior fossa tumors; 99 (89%) of the 111 cerebellar astrocytomas were low grade and nearly all were vermian in origin.

Since most of these tumors arise in the vermis, the clinical presentation is similar to that of medulloblastoma, with truncal ataxia, headache, nausea and vomiting, and, in the very young, split cranial sutures and head enlargement from increased intracranial pressure.

Surgery

Cystic cerebellar astrocytomas are exposed through a posterior fossa craniectomy. The cyst is located with a cannula and then exposed via an incision through the cerebellar folia. Self-retaining retractors are placed into the cyst. With the aid of the operating microscope, the cyst is examined and the vascular, firm mural module is identified, dissected, and removed. The nonneoplastic cyst wall is not excised.

Solid cerebellar astrocytomas are carefully separated from surrounding cerebellar white matter, again using the improved visualization offered by the operating microscope. The texture and appearance of the tumor are usually distinct and distinction from white matter is usually not difficult, so the only barrier to complete resection is deep penetration of the tumor into the dentate nucleus, cerebellar peduncles, or brain stem.

Radiation Therapy

The same radiation principles as apply to cerebral astrocytomas also apply for cerebellar astrocytomas. Completely resected cerebellar astrocytomas do not require radiation therapy. The remainder are treated with total doses of 50 to 60 Gy, depending on histology and the patient's age.

Chemotherapy

Since surgery alone or surgery and irradiation are frequently curative, chemotherapy has not been needed except for cases of recurrence after surgery and irradiation, or if the tumor is histologically highly anaplastic. When chemotherapy is used, our approach has been to use nitrosourea-based therapies as outlined in the section on Cerebral Gliomas.

In the past decade we have used irradiation and adjuvant polydrug chemotherapy to treat five patients who had cerebellar glioblastoma multiforme (three) or highly anaplastic astrocytomas (two). All patients received a nitrosourea, but the chemotherapy combinations varied, depending on which program was being used at the time for supratentorial gliomas. A specific chemotherapy program for the cerebellar gliomas has not been developed for evaluation. Table 46-16 summarizes the patient age, treatment, and outcome in these five cases.

For recurrent or progressive tumors, we have had experience with ten patients. Table 46-16 also summarizes the characteristics of these patients and the outcome of treatment. Again, the patients were treated with protocols being used at the time for supratentorial gliomas. The median survival of this group of patients from first treatment with chemotherapy was 18 months; the 25th percentile survival was 32 months.

OPTIC GLIOMAS

Clinical and Pathologic Considerations

Nearly all gliomas of the optic nerve and chiasm are discovered before the age of 20 years, and most before the age of 10 years.[123] In some cases there is a family kindred of neurofibromatosis. Lewis et al found that of 217 patients with

TABLE 46-16. Chemotherapy for Recurrent Cerebellar Astrocytomas at UCSF Between 1977 and 1987

Patient	*Age*	*Diagnosis*	*Treatment(s)*	*Survival (mo)*
Ajuvant Chemotherapy				
J.C.	13	HAA	RT–CYCLE	+ 51.9
T.S.	25	GM	RT–BUDR–PCV	+ 45.2
J.L.	8	GM	RT–8422	+ 22.2
C.H.	15	GM	RT–8422	+ 19.2
M.J.	13	HAA	RT–PCV	21.9
Chemotherapy at Progression				
R.C.	31	MG	CYCLE	9.9
G.T.	29	HAA	BCNU,PCV,8422	17.5
S.M.	38	AA	BFHM	10.2
W.C.	19	GM	8522,ACNU,PCB	+ 19.9
J.R.	25	HAA	CYCLE,AraC,TEPA	32.2
H.M.	4	MG	CCNU	+151.6
M.P.	11	AA	BCNU,CYCLE	+111.9
C.L.	33	AA	BCNU	6
M.S.	38	LG	PCV	5.3
J.G.	42	JPA	CYCLE,HME	30.5

PCV = CCNU, procarbazine (PCB), vincristine; CYCLE = BCNU, 5-fluorouracil, CCNU, PCB; BTRC 8422 = 6-thioguanine, PCB, dibromodulcitol, CCNU, vincristine; 8522 = 6-thioguanine, PCB, dibromodulcitol, CCNU, 5-fluorouracil, hydroxyurea; HME = ellipitinium; BUDR = bromodeoxyuridine; ACNU = intraventricular ACNU; AraC = intraventricular cytosine arabinoside; TEPA = intraventricular thio-TEPA; BFHM = BCNU, 5-fluorouracil, hydroxyurea, 6-mercaptopurine.

neurofibromatosis evaluated prospectively by ophthalmologic examination and neurodiagnostic studies, gliomas along the anterior visual pathway occurred in 15% and were occasionally bilateral.[124] Of interest was the fact that 67% of these tumors were neither suspected clinically nor obvious on ophthalmologic examination.

With respect to the location of optic gliomas, Housepian et al reported that 25% involved one optic nerve, 73% the chiasm, and 3% the optic tracts.[125] In another series, 25% involved the chiasm alone, 33% the chiasm and hypothalamus, and 42% the chiasm and optic nerves or tracts.[126] Clinically, these tumors produce loss of visual acuity (70%), strabismus and nystagmus (33%), visual field impairment (bitemporal hemianopsia, 8%), developmental delay, macrocephaly, ataxia, hemiparesis, proptosis, and precocious puberty. Funduscopic evaluation demonstrates a range of findings from normal optic disks through venous engorgement to disk pallor due to atrophy. Tumors involving the chiasm frequently grow to involve the hypothalamus, causing a diencephalic syndrome that is characterized by emaciation (especially in children between 3 months and 2 years of age), motor overactivity, and euphoria.

Pathologically, these tumors range from primarily piloid and stellate astrocytes, with or without oligodendroglia, through the gamut of malignant astrocytomas to glioblastoma multiforme; pilocytic tumors are most common and glioblastomas quite rare. Optic gliomas typically appear as fusiform expansions of any part of the nerve; they tend to bridge through the optic foramen and expand as dumbbell-shaped tumors within the skull. The nerve can be infiltrated by tumor originating in the chiasm, the walls of the third ventricle, or the hypothalamus. Often the tumors found in patients with neurofibromatosis affect a single optic nerve and are grossly normal appearing although infiltrated by tumor and surrounded by a fibrous stroma. In most other cases of optic glioma, the nerve is infiltrated by tumor cells and irregularly thickened in appearance.

Diagnosis is best made from MR imaging, which should utilize images in the sagittal plane. CT is satisfactory for diagnosis but is not as sensitive or descriptive as MR imaging, which also shows hypothalamic involvement more clearly.

Surgery

Unilateral tumors of the optic nerve (as opposed to the chiasm) should be resected, particularly when there is profound visual loss or when proptosis is disfiguring.[127] A transcranial approach to the orbit is preferred, permitting complete resection of the tumor-infiltrated nerve from the chiasm to the globe and sparing the globe for an optimum cosmetic effect.[127] The involved nerve is inspected through a unilateral craniotomy and the nerve sectioned at the chiasm. The orbit is then unroofed and the optic nerve's attachment to the globe exposed and divided, allowing the tumor to be removed.

Smaller tumors of the optic nerve, chiasm, or the nerve and chiasm must sometimes be biopsied when radiographic studies cannot definitively exclude meningioma or other diagnoses. Subtotal resection of larger tumors of these structures is occasionally necessary for decompression, but resection of the chiasm with resultant blindness is never indicated.

Radiation Therapy

There is some controversy regarding the treatment of optic nerve gliomas since some patients with incomplete surgical resections have shown no disease progression with 10 to 20 years of follow-up.[123] That same report noted cases of chiasmal tumors that, after biopsy confirmation, showed no progression for more than a decade.

The UCSF experience with optic gliomas treated in the megavoltage era was reviewed recently.[128] Of the 38 cases, 9 were confined to a single optic nerve; the remainder involved the chiasm with or without extension to the hypothalamic area, optic nerves, or optic tracts. Most of the tumors were slow-growing but progressive. Eight patients eventually died of chiasmal tumor. The deaths occurred as late as 18 years after diagnosis and were all in patients with chiasmal lesions. Three of the deaths were in adults with rapidly progressive disease, proven to be glioblastoma multiforme in the two cases in which biopsy or autopsy was performed. Of the five patients initially untreated, three demonstrated tumor progression in 2 to 7 years, and in the other two who underwent biopsies, proof of the nature of the lesion was lacking. Four of the nine with lesions limited to one optic nerve received radiation therapy, with no demonstrable benefit. One patient who received radiation therapy and one who did not ultimately failed.

Excluding two postoperative deaths, there were 27 patients with tumors of the chiasm. Six of the seven who did not receive radiation showed disease progression, and the nature of the lesion in the seventh patient was unknown, since biopsy was not performed. There were nine treatment failures among the 20 patients who received radiation therapy; however, three of the treatment failures occurred in the adults with very aggressive, nonresponsive tumors. Furthermore, disease was controlled in seven of the eight patients who received a dose of 50 to 55 Gy, whereas treatment failed in five of nine patients who received 46 Gy or less. Within the limits of the visual examination conducted, there were 22 evaluable patients with chiasmal lesions. Improvement occurred in six of 17 irradiated patients but in none of the five nonirradiated patients. The mean follow-up period for the UCSF patients was 9.4 years.

It was concluded that optic gliomas confined to a single nerve are sometimes a surgical problem and are not likely to benefit from radiation therapy. On the other hand, the histologically similar tumors that involve the chiasm do benefit from radiation therapy. They should be treated with limited portals to a dose of at least 50 Gy. These data and conclusions are consistent with others reported in the literature.[129–131]

OLIGODENDROGLIOMAS

Clinical and Pathologic Considerations

The peak occurrence of oligodendrogliomas is in persons aged 30 to 49 years. Although oligodendrogliomas are most common (80%) in the cerebral hemispheres, approximately 15% occur in the third or lateral ventricles or protrude into a ventricle from the thalamus.[131] Grossly these tumors are frequently well demarcated and in 20% of cases they are cystic.

Oligodendrogliomas have a 10% likelihood of spreading through the CSF pathways. Like astrocytomas, they vary in malignancy. Attempts have been made to grade oligodendrogliomas on an A through D scale[132]; however, Grades A through C vary so little in survival that this division seems unnecessary. A designation of differentiated or highly anaplastic may be sufficient. These tumors frequently have both astrocytic and/or ependymal elements seen at biopsy; such tumors are called mixed gliomas.

Clinically, oligodendrogliomas manifest in the fashion typical of hemispheral astrocytomas. However, two features distinguish them from astrocytomas: the antecedent history, averaging 7 to 8 years, tends to be longer; and seizures are more common, occurring in 70% to 90% of patients by the time of diagnosis. Provisional diagnosis may be made by CT or MR neuroimaging, but histologic confirmation is necessary and almost always possible. Somewhat helpful is the fact that approximately 50% of oligodendrogliomas have scattered calcification, usually related to intrinisic blood vessels, that is evident on CT scans.

Surgery

The surgical resection of hemispheric oligodendrogliomas follows the same principles as for cerebral astrocytomas; gross total removal is the goal when this is consistent with good neurologic outcome. The margins of oligodendrogliomas can appear to be more distinct than those of astrocytomas, but generally they are infiltrative, and surgical cure remains unlikely. Frequently oligodendrogliomas recur in the previous operative site. Under these circumstances, reoperation may be advisable, particularly if followed by chemotherapy.

Radiation Therapy

Although there has been no randomized clinical trial evaluating the efficacy of radiation therapy for oligodendroglioma, retrospective reviews have indicated a benefit. An earlier review[133] disclosed 5- and 10-year survival rates of 85% (11/13) and 55% (6/11) for patients who received radiation therapy versus 31% (4/13) and 25% (2/8) for those who did not. At 5 years the difference was statistically significant ($p = 0.02$). Although this was not a randomized trial, selection factors were sought. There was no correlation between the use of irradiation and tumor location, extent of resection, histologic diagnosis, patient's age, duration of symptoms, or presence of tumor calcification. A more recent review (KE Wallner et al, unpublished observations, 1987) yielded 5- and 10-year actuarial survival rates of 78% and 56% for patients with pure oligodendroglioma who had received at least 45 Gy, versus 54% and 18% for those not irradiated. The survival curve for patients with irradiated mixed tumors (*i.e.*, oligodendroglioma-astrocytoma) was virtually identical to that for the irradiated pure tumors. Only two patients with mixed tumors did not receive irradiation. All patients who died of disease had evidence of recurrence at the primary tumor site; one of these also had intraventricular seeding. One patient, not initially irradiated, had evidence of spinal seeding. Six of ten patients with pure oligodendrogliomas in whom histologic studies were repeated at the time of recurrence or at autopsy showed progression to either an anaplastic astrocytoma or glioblastoma multiforme. The experience with cerebral oligodendrogliomas at McGill University Hospitals[134] also supports the use of postoperative radiation therapy.

The current policy at UCSF is to give postoperative radiation therapy whenever resection is thought incomplete, which is usually the case. Generous but less than whole brain target volumes are utilized. The daily increment is approximately 1.8 Gy and the total dose is about 55 Gy.

Chemotherapy

As with radiation trials, prospective clinical chemotherapy trials of patients with oligodendroglioma have not been published. There are, however, individual patients reported within trials for malignant astrocytomas. In those reports chemotherapy was limited to the treatment of recurrent well-differentiated and moderately anaplastic oligodendrogliomas and primary treatment of the highly anaplastic oligodendrogliomas with surgery, radiation therapy and chemotherapy.

Since many of these isolated patients came from our own published reports, we reviewed our experience over the past decade. Table 46-17 summarized TTP and survival results of treatment of oligodendrogliomas that had been treated at recurrence. In our series, the median time to first recurrence was 2.4 years; patients treated with chemotherapy at recurrence had a median survival of an additional 1.4 years. These results are similar to those reported for well-differentiated (moderately anaplastic) astrocytomas. Table 46-18 summarizes results of mixed tumor treatments, which are very similar. The median time to first recurrence was 1.8 years and the median time from recurrence to death was an additional 1.6 years for those treated with chemotherapy at recurrence.

EPENDYMOMA

Clinical and Pathologic Considerations

Ependymomas arise from ependymal cells and tend to occur along ventricular surfaces. Ependymal rests are also seen in the obliterated central canal of the spinal cord, the filum terminale, and white matter adjacent to a ventricular surface (usually a highly angled surface).[32] Some 60% of intracranial ependymomas are infratentorial and 40% are supratentorial.[135] Of the infratentorial sites, the fourth ventricle is most commonly involved. Extension into the subarachnoid space occurs in 50% of these cases, and encasement of the medulla and upper cervical cord can occur. The lumbosacral spinal axis is also a common site.

TABLE 46-17. UCSF Series of 21 Patients with Oligodendoglioma Tumors Treated for Recurrence with Chemotherapy* Between 1977 and 1987†

	50%	25%
Time to first tumor recurrence (n = 21)	2.4 yr	3.8 yr
Time from recurrence to death (n = 12)	1.4 yr	2.8 yr

* Chemotherapy included nitrosourea-based therapies, the combination of DFMO-MGBG, procarbazine, and thio-TEPA. In addition, 4/12 underwent reoperation before starting chemotherapy.

† Median age was 37 years (range 19–62 years).

TABLE 46-18. UCSF Series of 53 Patients with Mixed Oligodendoglioma-Astrocytoma Tumors Treated for Recurrence with Chemotherapy* Between 1977 and 1987†

	50%	25%
Time to first tumor recurrence (n = 53)	1.8 yr	4.9 yr
Time from recurrence to death (n = 20)	1.6 yr	>2.0‡ yr

* Chemotherapy included nitrosourea-based therapies, the combination of DFMO–MGBG, procarbazine, AZQ, and thio-TEPA. In addition, 4/20 had a reoperation before starting chemotherapy.

† Median age was 35 years (range 1–63 years).

‡ The 25% has not been reached, as 10/20 have not failed yet.

Of the supratentorial ependymomas, 50% are primarily intraventricular and the remainder are parenchymal, arising from rests. Most of the intraventricular tumors arise in the lateral ventricles; a few arise in the third ventricle (25%).

Ependymomas can be classified in various ways. From a practical viewpoint, ependymomas are either differentiated and therefore low grade, or they are anaplastic, higher grade, and more likely to disseminate through the CSF pathways. Fortunately, the former are far more common.

The clinical presentation of patients with ependymomas depends on the location of the tumor. Intraventricular tumors frequently cause increased intracranial pressure and hydrocephalus. As a result, headache, nausea and vomiting, papilledema, ataxia, and vertigo are found in most patients at presentation. Focal neurologic signs and symptoms are more often seen with extraventricular supratentorial ependymomas.

Either MR imaging or CT is sufficient to establish the anatomical diagnosis before surgery. The presence of calcium in a fourth ventricular tumor is highly suggestive but not diagnostic of an ependymoma. Surgical exploration and biopsy are essential for the selection of appropriate treatment. For anaplastic ependymomas, staging myelography and examination of the CSF for cytologic evidence of malignancy are essential.

Surgery

Approximately half of hemispheric ependymomas arise from the wall of the lateral ventricle and half appear to be intraparenchymal, arising perhaps from remote fetal ependymal cell rests.[136] Hemispheric ependymomas tend to be cystic and, even when not, are frequently well circumscribed from surrounding brain, allowing gross total resection. A wide craniotomy permits a transcortical exposure of the tumor through a cortical incision placed to avoid injury to vital brain. The tumor is removed using the operating microscope, and every effort is made to minimize bleeding into the ventricular cavity. At the end of the resection the ventricular system is gently irrigated free of blood and blood clots to prevent mechanical obstruction to CSF flow, to prevent blockage of the CSF absorptive bed (arachnoid granulations), and to reduce the irritation of bloody CSF to the brain.

Ependymomas arising from the floor of the fourth ventricle are approached through a wide bilateral suboccipital craniectomy and laminectomy of C1. The tumor is exposed by retracting the cerebellar tonsils laterally and splitting the inferior aspect of the vermis, although frequently a tongue of tumor is visible over the dorsal aspect of the medulla and upper cervical spinal cord before the tonsils are retracted. The dorsal convexity of the tumor comes into view as the cerebellar vermis is divided, and its attachment to the floor of the fourth ventricle can then progressively be exposed and evaluated. Firm attachment precludes a gross total resection, as does infiltration of the tumor into the cranial nerves of the cerebellopontine angle via the foramen of Luschka. Tumor is removed to the extent possible using illumination and magnification afforded by the operating microscope.

Radiation Therapy

Postoperative radiation therapy improves the survival rate in patients with ependymoma and anaplastic (high-grade) ependymoma. There is, however, considerable debate in the literature as to how extensive the radiation volume should be: Should it include only the primary tumor site, the entire ventricular system, the entire intracranial space, or the entire cerebrospinal axis? Most authors agree that for anaplastic ependymomas, the entire axis should be treated. The current policy at UCSF is to give a dose of about 54 Gy to the primary tumor site and 35 to 40 Gy to the remainder of the axis. If spread within the brain is demonstrated, the entire brain receives the 54 Gy dose. Myelography is routinely performed and any area of gross involvement is boosted to 50 Gy. Various authors have reported 5-year survival rates for anaplastic or high-grade ependymoma that range from 10% to 50%. Even with such radiation doses, at least 50% of patients develop a local recurrence.

For low-grade ependymoma the recommendations of various authors range from irradiation only of the primary tumor site to whole-axis radiation therapy.[43] Much of the debate has arisen because of the varied patient populations included in individual reviews. In some reviews, the incidence of meningeal seeding has been based on clinical evidence, whereas others have reported on autopsy data. Of the last 41 low-grade ependymomas treated at UCSF with local tumor site irradiation after surgery, there have been two instances of dissemination to the spine, but in both cases treatment also failed at the primary site.[137] The 5- and 10-year survival rates for those who received more than 45 Gy (approximately 50 Gy in most cases) were 75% (21/28) and 58% (15/26), respectively. The main source of failure was recurrence at the primary tumor site. Based on such evidence and the greater precision in determining tumor extent now available through high quality CT and MR imaging, it is our policy to use a generous target volume for low-grade supratentorial ependymomas and to administer a dose of at least 54 Gy. If the tumor has arisen in the posterior fossa (*i.e.*, infratentorially), the remainder of the cerebrospinal axis is irradiated if CSF cytology studies reveal malignant cells, or the preliminary myelogram shows evidence of seeding. Pretreatment myelograms are not obtained routinely in patients with low-grade supratentorial tumors.

Chemotherapy

For primary treatment of anaplastic ependymomas, we have been utilizing cranial-spinal axis irradiation with oral hydroxyurea followed by six courses of polydrug chemotherapy (BTRC 8422) with 6-thioguanine, procarbazine, DBD, CCNU, and vincristine. Since 1983, when we first started using this approach, we have treated seven patients (four fourth ventricle tumors, two spinal cord tumors, one frontal tumor), with only one failure to date.

There have been few published reports of chemotherapy for recurrent differentiated or anaplastic ependymomas. For many years we have treated recurrent ependymomas with BCNU as monotherapy. Results were comparable to those achieved with astrocytomas. Subsequent to those trials, we used dibromodulcitol (DBD) as monotherapy, primarily for BCNU failures.[138] A summary of both series is given in Table 46-19.

MENINGIOMAS

Clinical and Pathologic Considerations

Meningiomas arise from arachnoidal cells in the meninges, especially in areas of the arachnoid villi. In some series meningiomas make up 39% of primary CNS tumors.[27] These tumors are most frequently located along the sagittal sinus and over the cerebral convexity. Table 46-20[139] summarizes the frequency of these tumors according to location.

Meningiomas are extra-axial, intracranial (and sometimes spinal) tumors that produce symptoms and signs through compression of adjacent brain tissue and cranial nerves. They frequently also produce hyperostosis. Table 46-21 summarizes the symptoms and signs associated with these tumors.

Histologically, the large majority of meningiomas are differentiated, with low proliferative capacity and limited invasiveness. Less commonly, meningiomas are more anaplastic, with a higher proliferative capacity and greater invasiveness. Even though the difference in the 30-minute bromodeoxyuridine labeling index in situ for the differentiated meningiomas may be less than 1%, versus 3% to 4% for anaplastic meningiomas,[140] biologically the anaplastic meningiomas behave considerably differently from the more differentiated meningiomas.

Surgery

The general perception that meningiomas are surgically resectable gives these tumors an undeserved reputation of be-

TABLE 46-19. Chemotherapy for Recurrent Ependymoma: UCSF Experience

	TTP Percentile	
Treatment	*50%*	*25%*
BCNU (11/14)	56 wk	102 wk
Dibromodulcitol (9/12)[138]	67 wk	85 wk

[(Responder + stable)/all patients].

TABLE 46-20. Sites of Predilections of Meningiomas Within Intracranial Regions

Site	*Number*
Parasagittal	65
Convexity	54
Sphenoidal ridge	53
Olfactory groove	29
Suprasellar	28
Posterior fossa	23
Spinal	18
Periauricular	12
Temporal fossa	8
Falx	7
Chorioidal	6
Gasserian	5
Multiple	2
Combined with neurinomas	2
Intraorbital	1

Cushing, et al.[139] H, Eisenhardt L: Meningiomas, Vol I. Their Classification, Regional Behavior, Life History and Surgical End Results, p 73. Springfield, IL, Charles C Thomas, 1938.

nignity. Although meningiomas generally are well circumscribed and do not invade adjacent brain, they can occur virtually anywhere in the CNS, and access sometimes is achievable only by deep retraction. In addition, these tumors may be extremely vascular and can surround important structures like cranial nerves and major arteries at the skull base. Such characteristics can preclude a smooth operation, and total removal is commonly not possible. Simpson in 1957 reported on a large series of surgically resected meningiomas and noted that even when there was a perceived total resection, the recurrence rate was 9%.[141] In 1985 a series from Massachusetts General Hospital indicated that "total resection" was followed by a 7% recurrence rate at 5 years, 20% at 10 years, and 32% at 15 years.[142]

Nevertheless, in dramatic contrast to the much more common cerebral gliomas, certain meningiomas are surgically resectable, and the neurosurgeon is generally more favorably disposed toward tackling a meningioma than operating on yet another glioma. The neurosurgeon's zeal must be tempered with an understanding of the risks of removing a particular meningioma in a particular location and an understanding of the impact of this meningioma on the well-being of the particular patient, since these tumors are commonly exceedingly slow-growing and the patients are often elderly. In other words, the presence of a meningioma is not an absolute indication for surgery; and when surgery is undertaken in an elderly patient, partial removal is sometimes adequate.

TABLE 46-21. Neurologic Findings Associated with Meningiomas as a Function of Their Location

Site	*Presentation*
Sphenoidal ridge	Nonpulsating, painless unilateral exophthalmos; unilateral visual loss; ophthalmoplegia; ICP
Cerebral convexity	Altered mentation, ICP, seizures
Intraventricular	Hydrocephalus, headache, mental changes, visual field abnormalities
Olfactory groove	Central scotoma, ipsilateral optic atrophy, contralateral papilledema, ipsilateral loss of smell, altered mentation, focal motor abnormalities
Tuberculum sellae	Loss of vision, bitemporal hemianopsia, papilledema or optic atrophy
Other basilar sites	See Table 46-5
Cerebellar convexity	ICP, cerebellar findings
Cerebellar-pontine angle	Cerebellar findings, hearing loss
Foramen magnum	No findings, spastic paresis and sensory findings in upper extremities

ICP = increased intracranial pressure.

PREOPERATIVE PLANNING. The preoperative preparation of the patient is as described in the section on Surgery, under Treatment Modalities, as are the surgical planning and the intraoperative anesthetic management. However, the planning of surgery for meningiomas must be extremely assiduous, as a detailed knowledge of surgical anatomy is of the utmost importance in these tumors. A preoperative angiogram to assess overall tumor vascularity and to identify arterial feeders is important. In many instances, angiography is combined with embolization of the tumor's blood supply. The angiogram is obtained within 24 to 48 hours of the operative procedure, so that alternate vascular routes to the tumor do not have time to develop.

SURGICAL PRINCIPLES. Feeding arteries that could not be occluded by embolization are addressed first at the operation if they are accessible. These arteries are both meningeal and cerebral in origin. The tumor is retracted away from surrounding normal brain progressively as the tumor bulk is reduced by the use of the CUSA or, for very vascular tumors, the cutting loop of the electrocoagulation unit or the CO_2 laser. Since meningiomas at individual sites pose special surgical problems, brief descriptions of techniques used for resection of meningiomas at the more common sites follow.

Cerebral Convexity. A large bone flap is made around the tumor. A dural incision circumscribes the tumor several centimeters from its edge, and the dura attached to the tumor is used to retract the tumor from the brain as microdissection frees the adhesions between the tumor and surrounding brain. Removal of the interior of the tumor facilitates separating the tumor margin from the adjacent brain. When the mass is lifted free, its bed must be inspected for minute bleeding points before closure is begun.

Parasagittal and Falx. Parasagittal meningiomas are those abutting the midline, and the difficulties in their removal are related to the risk to critical draining veins to the sagittal sinus, possible involvement of the sagittal sinus with tumor, and the often massive overlying bony erosion or hyperostosis. The patent sagittal sinus cannot be transected for a complete tumor removal except in its anterior one third, so a careful study of the preoperative arteriogram, looking for the patency of the sinus and for the position of the draining veins in the region, is absolutely critical.

The parasagittal meningioma is removed like the convexity tumors through a bone flap that abuts the midline and with gradual separation of the tumor from the surrounding brain, progressively reflecting the mass toward the sagittal sinus. Some advocate opening the sagittal sinus for removal of tumor that has grown through its wall; others advocate resecting and grafting the involved sagittal sinus wall. In our opinion these dangerous maneuvers are not usually indicated since recurrence-free survivals after subtotal resection of these lesions are long,[142] and since the tumor may grow to completely occlude the sinus, allowing complete resection later with a lesser risk to life.

Falx meningiomas do not involve the sagittal sinus but simply occupy the falx below the sinus, often becoming bilateral. The bone flap is made to overlie the midline to an extent depending on the tumor's laterality, and deep retraction between major draining veins into the interhemispheric fissue exposes the tumor, the attachment of which on the falx is circumscribed. The tumor is progressively dissected free and removed. Major complications of resection of falx meningiomas relate to interruption of draining veins and consequent cerebral edema and venous infarction.

Figure 46-10 shows CT scans from a patient with a convexity meningioma before and after surgical resection.

Olfactory Groove and Tuberculum Sellae. Olfactory groove meningiomas grow very large before their neurologic sequelae are anything but vague. Surgery therefore is carried out through a large bifrontal bone flap based low on the forehead. The broad, sessile base of the tumor is attacked first so that the tumor's blood supply, penetrating through the frontal base, is interrupted. Then the tumor's bulk is reduced by internal coring and the tumor is freed from surrounding normal brain and pulled forward for removal, with attention to protection of the optic nerves, carotid artery, and anterior cerebral arteries on the tumor's posterior aspect.

Tuberculum sellae meningiomas are smaller at presentation because of their proximity to the optic apparatus, but they are also sessile and receive their blood supply through their base. For this reason, the initial attack on these tumors also entails undercutting of their base. Internal coring and teasing the tumor forward are performed in a similar fashion as for the olfactory groove meningiomas, and attention to the safety of the optic apparatus and the anterior cerebral and carotid arteries is equally critical.

Sphenoid Ridge, Outer Third. These tumors can be a problem purely of tumor mass, purely of massive temporal hypertosis from en plaque tumor invading bone, or a combination of both. When it is present, the tumor mass insinuates itself into the sylvian tissue; its removal through a frontotemporal craniotomy is complicated only by the tumor's adherence (on its medial aspect) to sylvian veins. Tumor hyperostosis without bulky tumor is addressed only for severe cosmetic deformity or for visual impairment from exophthalmos (exposure keratitis and malignant chemosis) or compression of the optic nerve in the optic canal. Thickened bone is removed through a frontotemporal craniotomy; the lateral sphenoid wing, the lateral wall and roof of the orbit, and involved temporal bone are removed. Surgical cure is not possible.

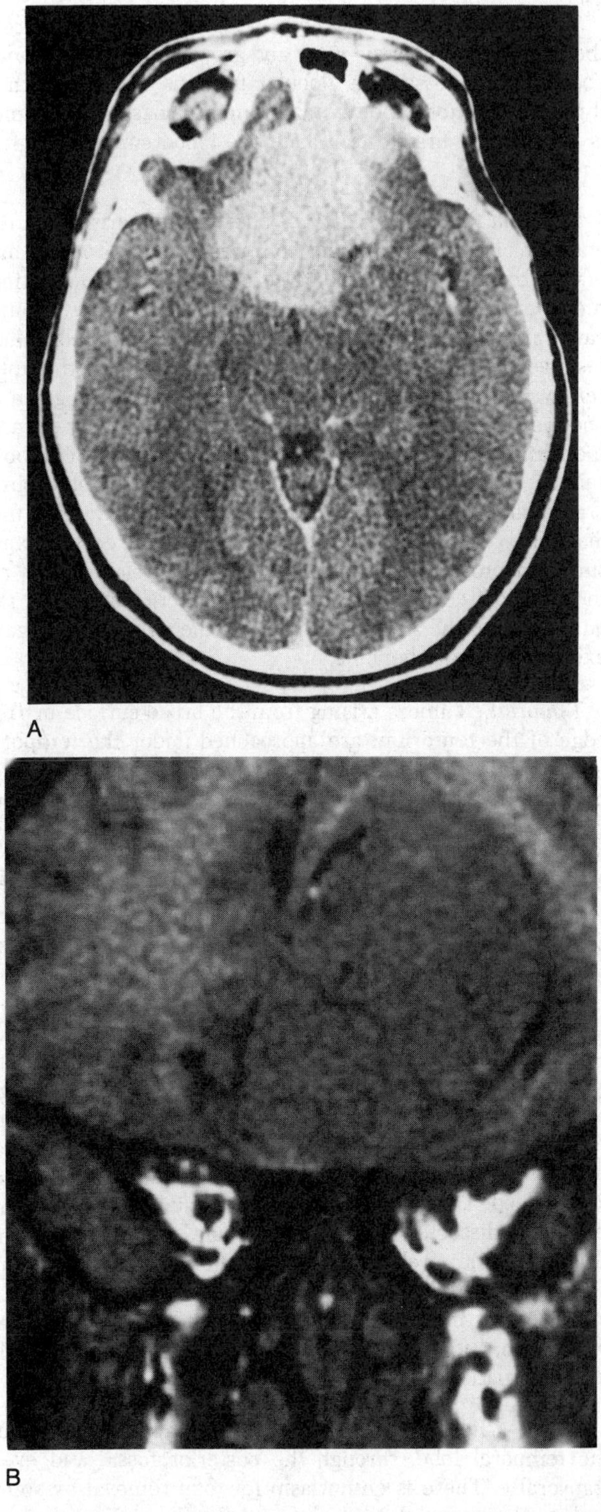

FIG. 46-10. A 32-year-old woman presented with decreased sense of smell and taste, headache, and decreasing vision on the left. Axial **A**. contrast-enhanced CT scan demonstrates a large olfactory grove meningioma. **B**. A T1-weighted sagittal MRI scan (TR 600, TE 20) demonstrates a large low intensity subfrontal mass.

Sphenoid Ridge, Middle Third. These tumors arise from the edge of the sphenoid ridge and grow into both the frontal and temporal fossa in a globular fashion. The approach is through a frontotemporal craniotomy; the base of the tumor is approached first to eliminate the blood supply. Surgical cure is likely.

Sphenoid Ridge, Inner Third. These tumors arise from the anterior clinoid process and compress the optic nerve and encase the carotid and middle cerebral arteries. In addition, medial sphenoidal meningiomas can grow diffusely into the cavernous sinus and optic canal. Only when the tumor manifests very early because of optic nerve compression is total removal even feasible. After a preoperative angiogram is obtained to assess carotid and middle cerebral artery encasement and tumor blood supply (with the possibility of embolization), the tumor is approached through a frontotemporal craniotomy and its lateral aspect is resected. Careful medially directed microdissection is done with the goal of exposure and protection of vital structures and slow tumor removal. Most commonly a complete resection is out of the question, and the surgeon stops when the risk of the surgery exceeds potential benefits.

Tentorial. Tumors arising from the broad surface or free edge of the tentorium are approached under the temporal lobe or under the occipital lobe, depending on their placement. In the more posterior lesions a posterior fossa craniectomy is sometimes done along with the occipital craniectomy, so that the approach can be both above and below the tumor. In all cases the principle of removal is incision of the tentorium around the tumor and gradual bulk reduction and separation of the tumor from surrounding brain. Venous sinuses and critical draining veins, particularly the vein of Labbe, must be protected.

Cerebellopontine Angle. Lateral posterior fossa meningiomas arise from the petrous bone and are exposed through a posterior fossa craniectomy by retracting the cerebellum medially. The tumor's base is addressed after the lower cranial nerves are identified and internal decompression is accomplished. The seventh and eighth cranial nerves are identified and dissected free of the capsule, which is removed from adjacent cerebellum. Finally, the tumor's attachment on the petrous bone is coagulated. Ventrally situated CP angle lesions may be marked by extreme adherence to the brain stem, and no attempt at complete removal is justifiable in this situation.

Clivus. Clival meningiomas have been approached under the temporal lobe, through the posterior fossa, and even transorally. There is enthusiasm for total removal by some authors; but since these tumors involve cranial nerves and important arterial perforators to the brain stem, a more conservative approach, internal decompression of the tumors, seems prudent.

Radiation Therapy

Two separate, partially overlapping reviews of the USCF experience have been reported. Included in the initial report were 84 patients thought to have undergone complete resection and 92 in whom the resection was thought incomplete.[50] Nearly 60% of patients with complete removal had been followed up at least 5 years, and no recurrence had developed. In contrast, with subtotal removal alone, 74% of 58 patients showed progressive growth of the meningioma. However, among the 34 patients with subtotal removal followed by radiation therapy, only 29% had shown progression, even though a greater percentage of these had been followed up for 5 years or longer: 53% of patients who had undergone subtotal resection followed by radiation therapy had been followed up for at least 5 years, versus 38% of those who underwent subtotal resection alone.

The second UCSF report considered patients treated from 1968 to 1978. Fifty-one were thought to have had total resection, with a 4% recurrence rate.[143] Eighty-four patients were known to have had an incomplete resection, and of these, 54 received postoperative radiation therapy. The recurrence rate in the irradiation group was 32%, versus 60% in those not irradiated ($p < 0.05$). The median time to recurrence was 125 months with irradiation and 66 months without ($p = < 0.05$). The two subtotal resection groups appeared to be comparable with respect to factors such as age, sex ratio, and tumor location. Solan and Kramer have suggested that patients with meningiomas of benign histology do equally as well whether they are treated with radiation therapy initially or at the time of progression.[144] This observation was based on only nine patients, two of whom died of intercurrent disease, and only three others had been observed for more than 5 years. The UCSF data, however, suggest that radiation therapy as part of initial treatment is preferable; of 16 irradiated for progression, two died of intercurrent disease, six died as a direct result of the recurrent meningioma, and one was alive with progressive disease. Although we have not recently reviewed results for patients with malignant meningioma, it is our impression that these patients do poorly. In this respect our results are in agreement with those of Solan and Kramer, who reported that of seven patients with malignant meningioma, five died, four within 9 months of diagnosis.

It is our current policy to recommend radiation therapy for patients with incompletely resected meningioma. The target volume is limited to a fairly narrow margin beyond the volume defined by CT as modified by a discussion with the neurosurgeon regarding the site(s) where tumor was left behind. With malignant meningioma the margin is more generous. Various field arrangements are utilized, depending on the volume and its location. These range from simple opposed fields to complex fields using wedge filters; with small tumors, even arc rotation with wedges may be used. The daily tumor dose is 1.8 Gy. With meningioma, the total dose is usually about 55 Gy, with an increase to 60 Gy for malignant meningioma.

Chemotherapy

There is currently no place for chemotherapy for newly diagnosed and nonirradiated meningiomas. This is due to (1) the lack of chemotherapy trials, and (2) the fact that there is little real need for chemotherapy except in the most intransigent recurrences. For patients who present with histologically malignant meningiomas, the situation is only slightly different. Because of the potentially lethal consequences of malignant meningioma, we have been treating these patients with aggressive surgery, focal irradiation, and eight courses of combination chemotherapy with cyclophosphamide, Adriamycin, and vincristine.

In the past 5 years we have treated five patients at the time of recurrence of meningioma and four patients with malignant meningioma in an adjuvant setting. Disease has progressed in four patients but none of the latter.

We expect that chemotherapy will be of value in both patients with recurrences and those with malignant meningiomas. However, the precise chemotherapy regimen is yet to be determined.

PRIMARY CNS LYMPHOMA

Clinical and Pathologic Considerations

Primary CNS lymphoma has variously been called microglioma, reticulum cell sarcoma, and histocytic lymphoma.[145] Histologically, the last designation is most correct, as most of these tumors are currently considered to be B-cell lymphomas of the histiocytic (large cell or large cell immunoblastic) type. In some cases the Epstein–Barr virus has been found in biopsy material.[17]

In the past, the majority of patients with primary CNS lymphomas had no predisposing immunosuppressive disorder. However, primary CNS non-Hodgkin's lymphoma has been seen in patients with inherited immunosuppressive disorders (ataxia–telangiectasia, Wiskott–Aldrich syndrome, and SCID), acquired immunosuppression (SLE, tuberculosis, and vasculitis), patients on immunosuppressive drug regimens (transplant patients), and those with Epstein–Barr virus infection.[17,146–148] Unfortunately, these tumors are assuming greater importance because of their association with immunodeficiency states. Before the AIDS era, CNS lymphomas represented only 1% of all lymphomas. In transplant recipients, CNS lymphomas accounted for 50% of lymphomas. As a result of the AIDS epidemic, primary CNS lymphoma has become more prevalent and, by some estimates, will become the most common primary CNS tumor by 1991.[149] (For additional information concerning lymphomas and the CNS, see chapter 44.)

Clinically, primary CNS lymphomas are more prevalent in males than in females. Prior to the AIDS epidemic the peak occurrence of these tumors was in the fourth to sixth decades of life. Because of AIDS-associated CNS lymphomas, the age for the peak incidence is decreasing, and these tumors are becoming more common in the third and fourth decades. The average time from onset of disease to diagnosis is approximately 1 to 2 months. In a recent literature review, Murray et al found that 52% of cases were supratentorial, 34% were multiple, 12% were cerebellar, 2% were in the brain stem, and less than 0.5% were spinal.[150]

Since the level of clinical concern will determine how quickly the diagnosis is made and how long symptoms are allowed to progress, patterns of presentation vary from series to series. The following categories of symptoms have been observed: (1) those due to increased intracranial pressure, such as headache, nausea, and vomiting; (2) those associated with deficits in higher cortical function, including personality change, psychiatric manifestations, and dementia; (3) focal neurologic deficits; and (4) seizures. Most prevalent are symptoms and signs of confusion, lethargy, and memory loss, followed by focal findings of hemiparesis or dysphasia.

The appearance of these lesions on contrast-enhanced CT and MR imaging is sometimes distinctive. Multiple lesions and homogeneous enhancement or signal in the paraventricular regions, basal ganglia, thalamus, or corpus callosum is suggestive of CNS lymphoma. Sometimes the extent of disease appears disproportionate to the neurologic deficit. Many tumors have minimal if any mass effect. The differential diagnosis of AIDS-associated CNS lymphoma must include the many opportunistic fungal and parasitic infections also common to AIDS. But, as with gliomas, the diagnosis is made by biopsy.[151]

CSF examination is sometimes helpful to identify specific cytoplasmic immunoglobulins. Although specific CSF abnormalities are seen in less than 30% of patients with primary CNS lymphomas, pleocytosis, increased protein concentration, low glucose, positive cytology, and specific monoclonal antibody staining of surface markers may be helpful.

Surgery

Because a tissue diagnosis is essential and surgery is not curative for patients with multiple lesions or small or poorly accessible lesions (in, for example, the thalamus, corpus callosum, or deep dominant hemisphere), these patients may undergo only a CT-guided stereotaxic biopsy. Large single hemispheric lesions should be surgically reduced, as should the largest of multiple lesions, if intracranial pressure cannot otherwise be controlled. CSF shunting procedures are sometimes necessary when there is diffuse meningeal tumor invasion and consequent communicating hydrocephalus.

Radiation Therapy

Radiation therapy of primary CNS lymphoma generally results in prompt clinical and radiographic improvement. The duration of improvement, however, may be surprisingly short, lasting only 12 to 24 months on average. Usually this is followed by local recurrence. Based on experience with extraneural lymphoma, tumor doses of around 40 to 45 Gy have frequently been used; however, it is obvious from the high local recurrence rate that such doses are inadequate. Most patients have received whole brain irradiation, whereas others have received irradiation only to the primary tumor site, and a smaller group has received CNS cranial–spinal axis therapy. Mean survival rates[43] pooled from a number of reports were 40 months, 25 months, and 18 months for irradiation of primary tumor only, whole brain, and the entire axis, respectively. The inverse relationship between the extent of CNS irradiated and mean survival time probably reflects patient selection, with those having the more favorable lesions receiving the more limited irradiation. Although some investigators have advocated treatment of the entire cranial–spinal axis, the incidence of spinal cord seeding is small, and most patients, including those who develop spinal seeding, experience failure at the primary site. Therefore, it is unlikely that prophylactic irradiation of the entire cranial–spinal axis would have a significant impact on survival.

When data from various reports in the literature are combined, the 1-, 2-, 3-, and 5-year survival rates are 66%, 43%, 28%, and 7%. The recurrence-free 5-year survival rate is around 3% (8 of 245 reported patients). AIDS-related CNS lymphomas appear to respond to irradiation much as do other CNS lymphomas; however, AIDS patients are much more likely to die relatively soon of causes other than the CNS lymphoma.

The current policy, admittedly somewhat arbitrary, at UCSF is to irradiate the entire brain to a dose of about 40 Gy, then boost the primary tumor site(s) plus a margin to an additional 20 Gy. Although the clinical significance of tumor cells in the CSF has not been established, if they are present the spine is irradiated to a total of about 40 Gy. If myelography shows spinal cord involvement, an additional boost of 10 Gy is given to the involved area.

Chemotherapy

Chemotherapy is of proven efficacy in the treatment of systemic lymphoma. A variety of agents and approaches have been used to treat primary CNS lymphoma, with variable results.[150,151]

Glucocorticoids in some cases cause the temporary disappearance of contrast-enhancing lesions on CT. This effect may be due to the direct cytolytic effect of glucocorticoids or to stabilization of the blood–brain barrier.

Unfortunately, chemotherapy trials to date have been sporadic and have enrolled small numbers of patients. Although in some studies chemotherapy has been given as an adjuvant to radiation therapy, most trials have been conducted in patients with disease recurrence or progression. No defined clinical chemotherapy trials have provided sufficient information to permit judgment of relative merit.

Regimens used include nitrosoureas, procarbazine, mustard compounds, high-dose methotrexate, high-dose cytosine arabinoside, CHOP (cytoxan, Adriamycin, vincristine, prednisone), VENP or VEMP (vincristine, cytocan, procarbazine or 6-mercaptopurine), PCV (CCNU, procarbazine, vincristine), and osmotic blood–brain barrier opening with cytoxan, methotrexate, procarbazine, and dexamethasone. From the reports it appears that all regimens are capable of inducing remissions, although the resilience of remission in terms of duration is variable. Randomized cooperative trials are necessary to consolidate these observations and provide a more rational basis for future treatments.

PRIMITIVE NEUROEPITHELIAL TUMORS

Clinical and Pathologic Considerations

The treatment of primitive neuroepithelial tumors is controversial and complex. Much of the controversy is based on the failure to understand that multiple entities are included in this pathologic diagnosis. Furthermore, controversy surrounds the classification of these tumors.[152] Primitive cells that remain undifferentiated or exhibit varying degrees of neuronal or glial differentiation are the hallmark of these tumors. Conceptually, these tumors can be viewed as developmentally aberrant brain cells. Thus, primitive neuroepithelial tumors can be divided according to the following classification schema: medulloepithelioma, neuroblastoma, spongioblastoma, ependymoblastoma, pineoblastoma, and medulloblastoma. With the exception of the medulloblastoma, primitive neuroepithelial tumors are rare.

Recently it has been proposed that all neoplasms showing primitive poorly differentiated neuroepithelial cells be called primitive neuroectodermal tumors, regardless of location or cell type. Because of the infrequency of these tumors and the present controversy surrounding an all-inclusive classification schema, it is best to refer to each histiotype separately.

Clinically, however, these tumors do share some common and disquieting features. As a rule they are highly proliferative, malignant tumors that tend to spread throughout the neuraxis like medulloblastoma. As a result, a complete CNS evaluation, including contrast-enhanced CT of the entire brain, CSF cytology, and metrizimide myelography, must be performed prior to the initiation of treatment.

Surgery

The initial therapy for primitive neuroectodermal tumors is surgical bulk reduction whenever feasible. Surgical principles are the same as those for astrocytoma, described earlier.

Radiation Therapy

Primitive neuroepithelial tumors do metastasize and should be treated as medulloblastomas, with cranial-spinal axis irradiation. The doses are similar to those used for medulloblastomas, except that the primary tumor should receive 54 Gy at 1.8 Gy/day, with the remainder of the axis receiving 30 to 40 Gy, depending on the age and size of the patient.

Within this category is a distinct pathologic and clinical entity that differs from the primary neuroectodermal tumors, namely the primary cerebral neuroblastoma. Berger et al reviewed the results of treatment for 11 patients with this diagnosis and found that after local irradiation to total doses of 50 Gy, given at 1.8 Gy/day, 7 of the 11 patients were alive with no evidence of tumor progression.[153] Of the 6 patients with cystic tumors, none had recurrent disease, while 4 of the 5 patients with solid tumors had recurrences. Currently we recommend that patients with primary cerebral neuroblastoma should receive only craniospinal axis irradiation only if postoperative assessment shows spread of tumor beyond the site of origin. If the tumor is localized, local focal irradiation is the treatment of choice.

Chemotherapy

Because primitive neuroepithelial tumors are uncommon, there are no controlled chemotherapy trials. Literature reports of isolated cases and small series indicate that drugs active against medulloblastoma are active against these tumors as well.

MEDULLOBLASTOMA

Clinical and Pathologic Considerations

Medulloblastoma appears more similar to the primitive neuroectodermal tumors of childhood than to the gliomas. The cell of origin of these tumors is a matter of controversy, but medulloblastoma probably originates from germinative neuroepithelial cells in the roof of the fourth ventricle.[32] Consistent with its embryonal nature is the observation that 50% to 60% of medulloblastomas occur in the first decade of life, with a peak at ages 5 to 9 years (see Table 46-4). A second, but lesser, peak occurs between 20 and 30 years.

The typical location for childhood medulloblastoma is in the cerebellum, mostly in the midline and posterior vermis (Fig. 46-11); many encroach on the cisterna magnum and the fourth ventricle. In adolescents and adults there is an increasing tendency for tumors to be laterally placed in the cerebellar hemispheres. Regardless of where in the cerebellum they occur, the tendency for metastatic spread of medulloblastoma is relatively high. At presentation up to 30% of patients will have positive cytology or myelographic evidence of spinal metastasis.[154,155] Extra-CNS metastasis is less common, occurring in less than 5% of cases; most metastases are to long bones.[154]

Based on bromodeoxyuridine 30-minute labeling indices, medulloblastoma would be considered a highly proliferative tumor, since its labeling index is approximately 14%, as compared to gliomas, which have a labeling index ranging from less than 1% to 10%.[140]

The overall disease-free 5-year survival rate for patients with medulloblastoma is approximately 50%.[116,154,156–159] However, the extent of disease at initial diagnosis defines risk. When risk factors are considered, survival is dramatically altered. Poor risk factors are defined as (1) a less than 75% resection, (2) metastasis to spinal cord, cerebrum, leptomeninges, or seeding of the cerebellum, (3) positive CSF cytology 2 weeks after surgery, and (4) age under 4 years.[116,156] Sometimes included as a poor risk factor is invasion of the brain stem by tumor.[157] Of the poor risk factors, two need explanation. Resection of less than 75% is an imprecise measure of remaining tumor; CT or MR imaging measurement of residual tumor volume would be better. However, in most cases, if the surgeon can remove more than 75% of tumor, the resection is usually a gross total resection. Poor risk associated with age 4 years and younger relates to the toxicity of irradiation to the developing CNS. Most radiation therapists will not treat young children with full doses of craniospinal irradiation.

The disease-free survival of poor-risk patients after craniospinal irradiation, with or without chemotherapy, is approximately 25% to 30%.[158] Good-risk patients, on the other hand, have 5-year disease-free survival rates of 66% to 70%.[159]

At relapse, the major site of first recurrence is the posterior fossa in more than 50% of cases, the frontal lobe in nearly 20%, bone in 10% to 15%, and other cerebral and suprasellar regions in 10% to 15%.[160]

Surgery

Although hydrocephalus associated with medulloblastoma obstructing the fourth ventricle can be relieved with a preresection CSF diversion, it is more usual to defer shunting and control increased intracranial pressure with corticosteroids. In up to 60% of cases, aggressive resection of the tumor will relieve hydrocephalus. An occipital bur hole is commonly

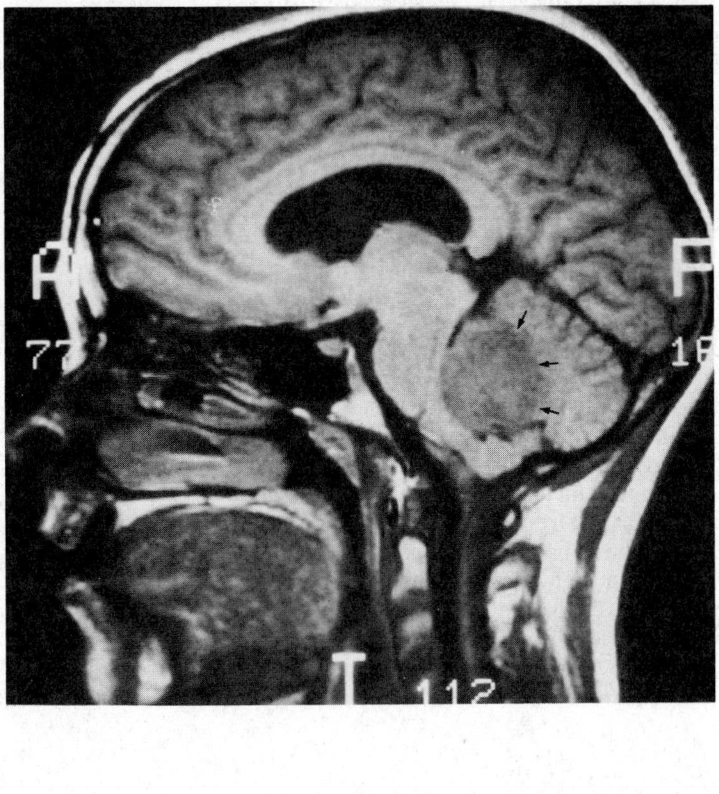

FIG. 46-11. A young girl presented with headache and gait ataxia. A T1-weighted sagittal MRI scan (TR 600, TE 20) demonstrates a large low intensity mass involving the inferior aspect of the cerebellum in the midline and extending to and filling the fourth ventricle. There is arcuate stretching and displacement of the medulla and secondary hydrocephalus. Well-circumscribed nature and location of the tumor are fairly characteristic for medulloblastoma.

placed at surgery, before the posterior fossa is exposed, to allow cannulation of the ventricles for drainage of CSF to lower the increased intracranial pressure to allow the dura to be safely opened.

Surgery for medulloblastoma is carried out with the patient prone or in a sitting position. The prone position is preferred, especially in children. The incision and bony exposure are usually made in the midline, but a paramedian incision and unilateral bony removal are used when the tumor is limited to one hemisphere, particularly in adults. The more commonly used midline craniectomy extends down through the foramen magnum, and a laminectomy of C1 (and, rarely, C2) is performed to decompress herniated cerebellar tonsils or to remove a caudally extending tongue of tumor over the dorsum of the spinal cord.

After the dura is opened the cerebellar tonsils are retracted laterally. The purplish gray tumor usually is first seen in the foramen of Magendie. The floor of the fourth ventricle is separated from the tumor with a cottonoid pledget. The pledget is advanced to protect the floor of the fourth ventricle as the tumor is resected.

The thinned cerebellar vermis is progressively incised in the midline until the dorsum of the tumor is exposed. The tumor is generally soft and moderately vascular, and is readily removed with suction irrigation, the Cavitron ultrasonic aspirator (CUSA), or laser, with the operating microscope used for magnification and illumination. Cooperative clinical studies have yielded relatively convincing evidence that an aggressive (gross total) removal is associated with an improved prognosis for the patient.[157] Dissection is continued laterally to remove tumor from the cerebellar hemispheres and ventrally to remove tumor from the fourth ventricle. When the obstructive hydrocephalus has been relieved, the CSF will be seen flowing from the aqueduct of Sylvius superiorly. Medulloblastoma rarely invades the floor of the fourth ventricle; when it does, careful laser surgery can be attempted to remove it. Closure is carried out in multiple layers with particular attention to a tight dural closure to decrease the risk of pseudomeningocele (bulging wound) formation and the risk of aseptic meningitis, and consequent communicating hydrocephalus from spilled blood products. Postoperative CSF shunting for hydrocephalus is necessary in about 30% to 40% of patients.

Radiation Therapy

At present, entire cranial–spinal axis irradiation is the treatment of choice for medulloblastoma. Although medulloblastoma generally is considered one of the most radiosensitive tumors of the CNS, radiation doses of 50 to 55 Gy, in daily fractions of about 1.8 Gy, to the primary tumor site in the posterior fossa results in disease control in only 60% to 80% of patients. In fact, local recurrence is the chief cause of treatment failure for medulloblastomas. It appears that the dose to the remainder of the axis for subclinical disease need not be that high. Most authors have reported using doses of 30 to 40 Gy for the spinal cord and 35 to 45 Gy for the remainder of the brain. These doses are usually reduced by around 10 Gy for children less than 2 or 3 years old. In the past 4 years we have been using prophylactic doses, distant from the primary tumor site, as low as 24 Gy. To date, nearly 50 patients have been so treated, and of the 17 patients in whom recurrence developed, only one had evidence of seeding to the spinal axis at *initial* recurrence.

In the past decade, reported 5-year survival rates have ranged from around 30% to 40% up to 85%. The higher survival rates, 75% to 85%, have been reported for patients who underwent gross total resection of tumor, in whom the brain stem was not involved, myelography was negative, and who received posterior fossa doses greater than 50 Gy. Preliminary results are available for the large, multi-institutional randomized trials conducted by the U.S. Children's Cancer Study Group (CCSG) and the European International Society of Pediatric Oncology (SIOP).[116,159] Both of these studies compared postoperative radiation therapy alone with postoperative radiation therapy plus chemotherapy. The chemotherapy consisted of vincristine, given weekly during radiation therapy, plus eight courses of vincristine and CCNU cycled every 6 weeks after completion of radiation therapy. In addition, patients in the CCSG study received prednisone. The 54-month disease-free survival rates for the CCSG study were 59% with and 49% without the chemotherapy. The SIOP studies had survival rates of 55% with and 43% without radiation therapy at 54 months. These trials demonstrated that extent of disease, extent of resection, and age were prognostic factors. Chemotherapy benefited primarily high-risk patients, i.e., those less than 2 years of age, those who underwent subtotal excision, M stages M1 to M5, and those with larger lesions. It may be that the improved prognosis with chemotherapy is due to a need for higher doses with larger tumors and a tendency to reduce the radiation dose for children less than 2 years of age.

The necessity of keeping the posterior fossa radiation dose as high as possible has been discussed. As the survival of children with medulloblastoma has improved there has been a greater appreciation of late complications such as neuropsychological dysfunction, impaired growth of the spine, and pituitary–hypothalamic dysfunction. Although it is difficult to sort out the precise role played by radiation in the late complications, it seems prudent to reduce the prophylactic radiation therapy dose in good risk patients as low as possible, consistent with prevention of subsequent seeding. At UCSF the current policy is to treat the entire cranial-spinal axis concurrently. The posterior fossa receives a total of 54 Gy at 1.8 Gy/day. Admittedly still experimental, we are carrying the remainder of the brain and spinal cord to 25 Gy at 1.8 and 1.6 Gy per day, respectively.

The incidence and degree of endocrine dysfunction appear dose-related, with a threshold of around 25 to 30 Gy. Growth hormone deficiency is the most frequent endocrine dysfunction post irradiation. All children who undergo irradiation to the hypothalamic–pituitary axis should be evaluated for pituitary function before, and periodically after, irradiation; early detection of a deficiency permits appropriate hormonal replacement therapy before irreversible damage has occurred.

Chemotherapy

Medulloblastomas are responsive to wide variety of antineoplastic agents including vincristine, nitrosoureas, pro-

TABLE 46-22. Efficacy of Single-Agent Chemotherapy for Recurrent and Progressive CNS Medulloblastoma

Treatment	*Response*
Adriamycin[160]	0/6
AZQ[99,116]	6/21
BCNU[110,162]	2/6
CCNU[94,95,163-165]	12/15
PCNU[166]	0/4
Procarbazine[76]	3/4
Cisplatinum[167-169]	11/27
Carboplatin[170]	6/14
Cyclophosphamide[171]	7/7
Dibromodulcitol[138]	15/29
Methotrexate (IV)[172-174]	5/13
Vincristine[175-182]	11/15
Tenoposide (VP16)[183]	1/1

Response = CR, PR, or SD.

carbazine, dibromodulcitol, cyclophosphamide, methotrexate, cisplatin, and various drug combinations. Table 46-22[76,94,95,99,110,138,160,183] summarizes some of the single agents and their observed response rates for CNS medulloblastoma when treated at recurrence or for progressive disease. For extra-CNS disease, these same agents have activity, although drugs such as cyclophosphamide, methotrexate, Adriamycin, and vincristine may be more active than the nitrosoureas and procarbazine (personal observations).

Table 46-23[184-190] summarizes some of the drug combinations that have been used for recurrent or progressive CNS medulloblastoma. Since some reports do not provide the length of response, one cannot be sure whether combinations provide a more lasting response than single agents. What is clear, however, is that better treatments are needed for recurrent and progressive disease.

As adjuvant therapy to surgery and irradiation, chemotherapy has not shown dramatic benefit. In part this reflects the fact that patients who receive craniospinal irradiation do not tolerate high-dose aggressive chemotherapy protocols well because of reduced bone marrow reserves. If the poor-risk patients from the CCSG and SIOP trials are examined for benefit from chemotherapy, it is apparent that those who received adjuvant chemotherapy did better. In an attempt to improve the tolerance to cytotoxic agents, we conducted a nonrandomized trial of preradiation procarbazine and hydroxyurea during reduced craniospinal irradiation.[156] In that study we found that reducing the craniospinal radiation dose to 25 Gy to the spinal axis and 25 to 35 Gy to the whole brain was not detrimental with respect to disease-free survival or recurrence patterns in good-risk and poor-risk patients. Continued efforts to reduce spinal axis irradiation and improved chemotherapy are clearly requisites for improving survival, especially in poor-risk medulloblastoma patients.

TABLE 46-23. Efficacy of Combination Chemotherapy for Recurrent and Progressive CNS Medulloblastoma

Treatment	*Response*
CCNU–PCB–VCR(PCV)[184]	10/16
VCR–MTX–BCNU[185]	4/4
VM26–CCNU–Pred[186]	2/3
MUS–VCR–Pred–PCB(MOPP)[187]	8/10
VCR–Pred–PCB(OPP)[188]	3/12
VCR–CYT[189]	4/8
VCR–BCNU–Dex–MTX(iv)[190]	8/8
6TG–PCB–DBD–CCNU–VCR*	3/8

* VA Levin et al, unpublished observations, 1987.

The incidence of systemic metastasis varies between 10% and 30%,[157,158] although the figure of 10% is closest to our experience. Most extra-CNS metastases are to long bones and ribs with lymph nodes being a distant second site. In the Park[157] and Lowery[158] series the median time to the development of extra-CNS metastasis was 10 to 12 months; in our more recent study it was 18 months (M. C. Chamberlain et al, unpublished observations, 1987). In the Park study, 17% of ventriculoperitoneal shunted patients developed systemic metastases, compared to only 4% of unshunted patients. In Lowery's series 30% of patients developed systemic metastases, and none had been shunted previously. Except in patients with rampant disease, we did not find an association between ventriculoatrial or ventriculoperitoneal shunting, with or without an inline filter, and systemic metastases. It is important to remember that bone metastases can be the only evidence of recurrence in nonshunted patients years after their initial presentation with CNS disease.

Many will benefit from aggressive polydrug chemotherapy. Our preference has been the combination of cyclophosphamide, Adriamycin, and vincristine; in all, 7 patients treated responded for a median duration of 17 months and 2 continue at 34, and 62 months without evidence of disease (M. C. Chamberlain et al, unpublished observation 1987). Other combinations with good activity are cyclophosphamide and vincristine[191] or vincristine, actinomycin, and cyclophosphamide.[192]

PINEAL REGION TUMORS

Clinical and Pathologic Considerations

The pineal gland is located in the posterior portion of the third ventricle. Tumors in this region are rare, accounting for less than 1% of intracranial tumors, although in children they constitute 3% to 8% of intracranial tumors.[193] The peak incidence of germ cell tumors is in the second decade, and few present after the third decade.[194] Table 46-24 summarizes the types of tumors found in the pineal region.[195] In all series, germinomas are the most common, accounting for 33% to 50% of pineal tumors (the higher frequencies are

TABLE 46-24. Classification of Pineal Region Tumors

I. Tumors of germ cell origin
- A. Germinoma (atypical teratoma, dysgerminoma, seminoma)
- B. Embryonal carcinoma
  1. Extraembryonic structures
     a. Endodermal sinus tumors (yolk sac tumor)
     b. Choriocarcinoma
  2. Embryonic endoderm, mesoderm, ectoderm
     a. Immature teratoma
     b. Mature teratoma

II. Tumors of pineal parenchymal cells
- A. Pineoblastoma
- B. Pineocytoma

III. Tumors of glial and other cell origin

IV. Nonneoplastic cysts and masses

Adapted from Herrick.[195]

seen in Japan). Gliomas are second, accounting for about 25% of pineal tumors; astrocytomas are the most common of the glial neoplasms arising at this site.

Neurologic signs and symptoms are due to obstructive hydrocephalus and involvement of ocular pathways. Major symptoms are headache, nausea and vomiting, lethargy, and diplopia. Signs are primarily ocular but can include ataxia and hemiparesis. The major ocular manifestation is paralysis of conjugate upward gaze (Parinaud's syndrome), although pupillary and convergence abnormalities, deviation, and papilledema are also seen.

We believe that determination of tumor histology and extent of disease are critical for optimal management of pineal region tumors. Figure 46-12 is a schema that we use to evaluate and stage patients with pineal region tumors.

The prognosis for these tumors varies, depending on the histology and size of tumor and extent of disease at presentation. Typically, patients with mature teratomas do quite well with surgery alone, germinomas do best with radiation, and the remaining tumors have variable courses ranging from months to years before recurrence.

Surgery

Because pineal tumors are near the very center of the brain, they are among the most difficult brain tumors to remove; and it is this factor that has given rise to some controversy in their management. There are those who promulgate decompressing the nearly invariable obstructive hydrocephalus with a shunt and then irradiating the tumor without a tissue diagnosis. However, because of an increasingly favorable experience with microsurgical approaches to the pineal region, the current recommendation is to obtain a tissue diagnosis and, when possible, to carry out a gross total resection of the tumor.[196] Resection is particularly important for pineal masses that may be relatively radioresistant or do not require radiation therapy, such as teratomas, arachnoid cysts, and meningiomas.

A variety of surgical approaches to the pineal region have been described: (1) through the dilated lateral ventricle, (2) through the posterior corpus callosum, (3) under the occipital lobe, and (4) through the posterior fossa over the cerebellum.[197] The most commonly used microsurgical approaches today are the infratentorial, supracerebellar approach described first by Horsley, later by Krause, and recently resurrected and modernized by Stein,[197] and the supratentorial approach under the occipital lobe described by Poppen and popularized recently by Clark.[197] Both have been associated with low morbidity and mortality in experienced hands.

The place of CT-guided (stereotaxic) biopsy in the diagnosis of pineal region tumors is unclear. While such biopsies have been described as relatively safe,[198] there is a risk that tissue sampling of these heterogeneous tumors may not accurately depict the correct histologic nature of the tumor. Without an accurate histologic diagnosis treatment planning may be erroneous or inadequate. In its favor is the advantage of rapid tissue diagnosis and shortened hospital stay.

Radiation Therapy

With certain notable exceptions (*e.g.*, benign teratomas), radiation therapy has an established role in the treatment of

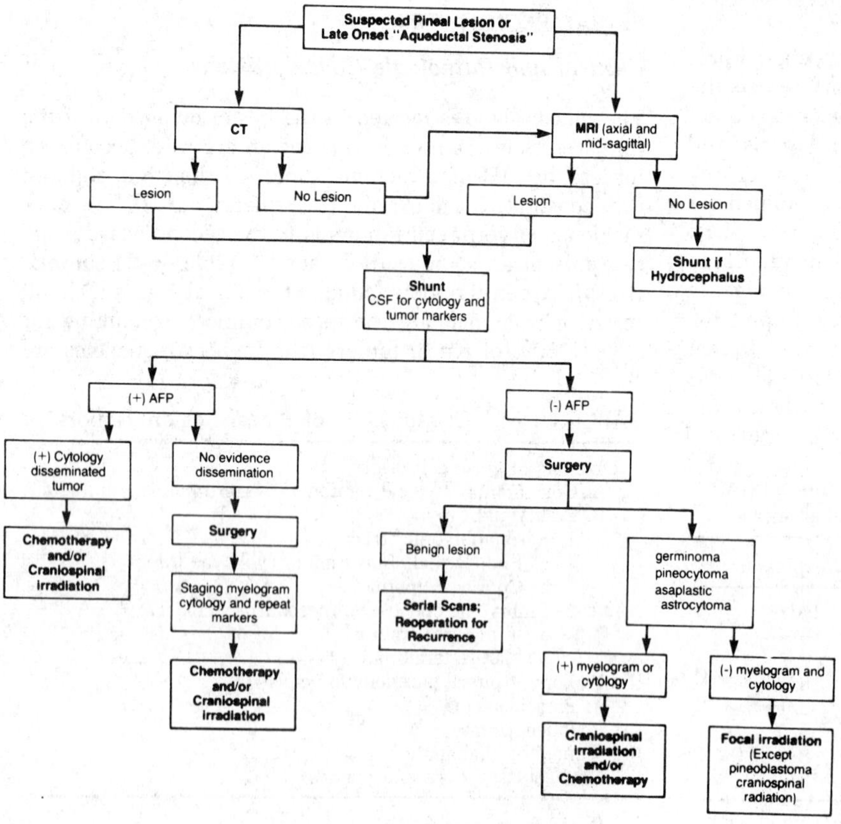

FIG. 46-12. Treatment and evaluation schema for pineal region tumors. (Edwards MSB, Hudgins RJ, Wilson CB et al: Pineal region tumors in children. J Neurosurg 68:689–697, 1988)

pineal and suprasellar tumors of pineal parenchymal cell origin or germ cell origin. Because of location, infiltrative nature, and tendency to seed throughout the leptomeningis, complete surgical extirpation is often not possible. In the past, high mortality and morbidity rates associated with biopsy or attempted resection, especially with older surgical techniques, often led to the use of radiation therapy without histologic confirmation. In such cases, response to low-dose radiation therapy, measurement of AFP and β-hCG, and CSF cytology were used to provide diagnostic information. In recent years there has been a growing tendency to increase the use of biopsy and of attempted resection. While theoretically surgery might be expected to increase the incidence of CSF seeding, there is no proof that this will occur. A review[43] of older literature suggests that the incidence of spinal seeding increases from around 3% for unbiopsied tumors to about 23% when tumors of these regions have undergone biopsy.

Survival rates vary with histology and extent of disease, age, radiation volume, and dose to the primary tumor site. According to a multi-institutional survey by Wara et al, the survival of patients with pineal parenchymal cell tumors was 21% (3/14) compared with 72% (26/36) for those with germinoma (199). This survey, as well as that of Jenkin et al, indicated that patients less than 25 to 30 years of age have survival rates of 65% to 80% versus 35% to 40% for older patients.[119] This finding may reflect the increased incidence of true germinomas in younger patients. In a literature review, Salazar et al found a recurrence-free survival rate for patients with whole brain irradiation of 76%, compared with 61% for irradiation to the ventricular system and 51% for smaller volumes.[200] Analysis of those data[43] showed a 90% survival rate for patients with whole brain irradiation and a tumor dose of at least 50 Gy; if smaller fields were used or the dose to the primary tumor site was less than 50 Gy, the survival was 33%.

At some institutions, if the histological diagnosis is unknown and CSF cytology and myelography are negative, the primary tumor site, with a generous margin that includes at least the third ventricle, receives a dose of about 25 Gy at 1.8 Gy per fraction. The CT or MR imaging study is then repeated. If substantial regression has occurred, it is assumed that the lesion is a germinoma and the whole brain is given an additional dose of approximately 25 Gy. If there is little or no response by CT or MR imaging, either an additional 30 Gy is given to the primary field or surgical resection is, if possible, carried out.

The current UCSF paradigm for management of pineal region tumors differs somewhat from the above and is outlined in Figure 46-17. If hydrocephalus is present, patients are placed on corticosteroids. A shunt is placed only if corticosteroids fail to relieve the symptoms of raised intracranial pressure. An open operation with the goal to resect the tumor is preferred to a CT-guided stereotaxic biopsy. Occasionally, in a patient with widely disseminated disease, a stereotaxic biopsy may be indicated. The approach (supratentorial vs intratentorial) is planned on the basis of the MR imaging study. At the time of craniotomy an external ventricular drain with ICP monitor is placed in the lateral ventricle and CSF removed to lower intracranial pressure and measure CSF tumor markers (β-hCG and AFP). A tumor biopsy is obtained, and, based on the findings at operation and the histologic diagnosis, a decision is reached regarding the aggressiveness of tumor resection.

Additional therapy is planned based on the histology, CSF markers, and staging CT/MR imaging study and myelogram: localized germinomas (2-cell pattern) are treated with 25 Gy to the ventricular system and an additional 25 Gy to the tumor with a 1–2-cm margin. If the germinoma is disseminated, systemic chemotherapy or craniospinal irradiation therapy is administered. Nongerminoma malignant germ cell tumors, whether localized or disseminated, are treated with systemic chemotherapy (× 6 courses), followed by restaging studies. At restaging, localized tumors receive focal radiation therapy, and disseminated tumors receive craniospinal radiation (54 Gy to the tumor and 45 Gy to the ventricular system; 35 Gy to the spinal cord and 45 Gy to any localized spinal cord tumors).

Biopsy-verified tumors with little or no tendency to metastasize to the spinal cord, such as teratomas, parietal cell carcinomas, pineocytoma, and low-grade glioma, are treated by resection or with local radiation fields only. Cranial–spinal axis irradiation is reserved for tumors that have a high tendency to cord involvement (such as pineal blastoma), for those with positive CSF cytology, or those with myelographic demonstration of spinal cord involvement.

Chemotherapy

The chemotherapy for glial neoplasms is similar to that covered in earlier sections. Chemotherapy for germ cell tumors is in flux but is encouraging. The most effective regimens use cisplatin and bleomycin,[201] although good results have been reported with actinomycin D, methotrexate, vinblastine, and cisplatin.[194,196] At times the results appear paradoxical, since patients with systemic seminoma treated with cisplatin, bleomycin, and vinblastine have developed brain metastases while receiving chemotherapy.

For nongerminoma malignant germ cell tumors (*e.g.*, endodermal sinus tumors), the combination of cisplatin, bleomycin, and VP-16 has been found to be quite effective in Phase II studies at UCSF (M. S. B. Edwards and A. Ablin, unpublished observations, 1987).

Occasional patients with recurrent germ cell tumors that have failed cisplatin-bleomycin-vinblastine therapies have responded to our BTRC 8422 protocol (6-thioguanine, procarbazine, dibromodulcitol, CCNU, and vincristine).

Much work needs to be done to elucidate the best drug combinations and use of chemotherapy in these patients.

PITUITARY ADENOMAS

Clinical and Pathologic Considerations

Pituitary tumors tend to produce neuroendocrine or neurological symptoms and signs. Anatomically, tumors arising from the pituitary can compress the pituitary; grow out of the sella to compress and invade the optic chiasm; and, if growth is unabated, can extend into the temporal lobe, third ventricle, and/or the posterior fossa. The chief finding in most patients is visual loss initially characterized by a bitemporal hemianopia. Headache occurs in about 20%. Less frequent are ocular palsies due to compression or invasion of the cavernous sinus.

Neuroendocrine abnormalities can be associated with tumor compression of the pituitary and/or hypersecretion of hormones. Table 46-7 summarizes some of the more common syndromes and their endocrine abnormalities. Sexual impotence in the male and amenorrhea and galatorrhea in the female are commonly associated with hyperprolactinemia. Growth hormone hypersecretion is associated with acromegaly or giantism, depending on the age of the patient. ACTH hypersecretion results in Cushing's disease. Elements of hypothyroidism, adrenal insufficiency, and growth hormone deficiency may follow compression of the pituitary gland by growth of an adenoma.

The diagnosis of a pituitary tumor is based on (1) sensitive radioimmunoassays, (2) CT scans, and, most recently, (3) MR imaging studies. Figure 46-6 is an MR image of a pituitary adenoma before surgery. Pituitary adenomas are classified as endocrine inactive or endocrine active. The majority secrete one or, occasionally, two hormones. The reported incidence of the various types of pituitary adenomas depends on the institutions referral patterns. Of 800 cases operated on at UCSF between 1970 and 1981, 79% (630/800) were endocrine-active; of these, 52% were prolactin-secreting (331/630), 27% growth hormone-secreting, 20% ACTH-secreting, and only 0.3% were TSH-secreting (202). Undifferentiated cell adenomas are considered to be either nononcocytic (null) or oncocytic (oncocytoma) tumors.

Of prognostic importance are the functional status of the tumor and how large or invasive it is. Table 46-14 is the grade and staging system used at UCSF.[202]

Surgery

The goal of surgery for the larger (usually, but not always endocrine inactive) pituitary tumors is to decompress the visual pathways and reduce tumor bulk, whereas the goal for hypersecreting adenomas is normalization of the hypersecretion with preservation of remaining normal pituitary function. For larger, nonsecreting pituitary adenomas, surgical cure is not possible; nor is it necessary since radiation therapy adjuvant to surgery is usually curative. In contradistinction, whenever possible, the hypersecreting adenoma should be resected in its entirety, since the effects of hypersecretion can be devastating and response to radiotherapy is slow and less predictable (see below).

The operative approach of choice for most pituitary tumors is transsphenoidal because it is safer and better tolerated than the alternative transcranial (frontal craniotomy) approach.[203] The transsphenoidal approach is possible for tumors occupying the sella turcica and even in those with fairly large medial suprasellar extension as long as the tumor is soft (the usual case) and can drop into the sella with progressive resection. Tough, woody suprasellar tumors and those with extension laterally into the middle fossa or arteriorly beneath the frontal lobes must be resected by craniotomy.

Radiation Therapy

Microadenomas of the pituitary, usually diagnosed because of endocrine hypersecretion, may be totally resected. Complete resection is confirmed through serial endocrine evaluations. When the adenoma is completely resected, there is no indication for radiotherapy. Many adenomas, particularly the endocrine-inactive lesions, may be relatively large and have invaded adjacent structures such as the cavernous sinus, optic chiasm, or the third ventricle, and not be completely resectable. Occasionally a patient may be medically inoperable or may refuse surgery. Unless the adenoma is completely resectable, radiation therapy should be considered to control mass effect and growth or to control endocrine hypersecretion.

Radiation therapy controls tumor growth in at least 95% of patients with nonfunctioning adenomas or with prolactenomas. This is also true for the larger growth hormone secreting adenomas. At UCSF, patients with large nonfunctioning adenomas or prolactinomas associated with visual field deficits had a 60% recurrence rate, as demonstrated by visual field changes within 5 years after incomplete resection alone.[204] This was reduced to about 4% by the addition of radiation therapy. In patients with modest visual field defects involving not more than one quadrant, surgery or radiation therapy alone were approximately equally effective in restoring vision; approximately two thirds of patients treated by either method had return of normal vision in the involved eye(s). With larger visual field defects, restoration of vision was better in those who received preradiotherapy surgical decompression than in those treated by radiotherapy alone. In patients with acromegaly and visual field defects, normal vision was achieved by irradiation alone in about two thirds (10/15).

Conventional radiotherapy is less effective in controlling endocrine hypersecretion than in controlling growth of pituitary adenomas. Eastman et al treated 47 acromegalic patients with radiotherapy alone.[205] The response, as measured by fasting growth hormone concentrations, was slow but progressive. Seventy-three percent achieved FGH levels <10 ng/ml by 5 years, and 81% by 10 years. If 5 ng/ml was used as the indicator of normal function, the 5- and 10-year rates decreased to 42% and 69%, respectively. Orth et al[206] reported on 44 patients with Cushing's disease treated by conventional radiation therapy (40 to 50 Gy/5 weeks), of whom 23 were cured and required no further treatment. They subsequently reported on 15 children treated with radiation therapy alone, of whom 12 were cured by radiation therapy.[207]

The data on control of prolactin secretion by conventional radiotherapy is more difficult to interpret. It appears that irradiation will decrease prolactin levels of about 80% on average but that only about 30% of patients will achieve normal levels, even after several years. It may be that hypothalamic injury with resultant loss of prolactin-inhibiting hormone results in a continued stimulus of normal pituitary cells to secrete prolactin.

With occasional exceptions, in cases of massive tumors, at UCSF pituitary adenomas are treated by coronal arc rotation using megavoltage radiation and moving wedge filters. The

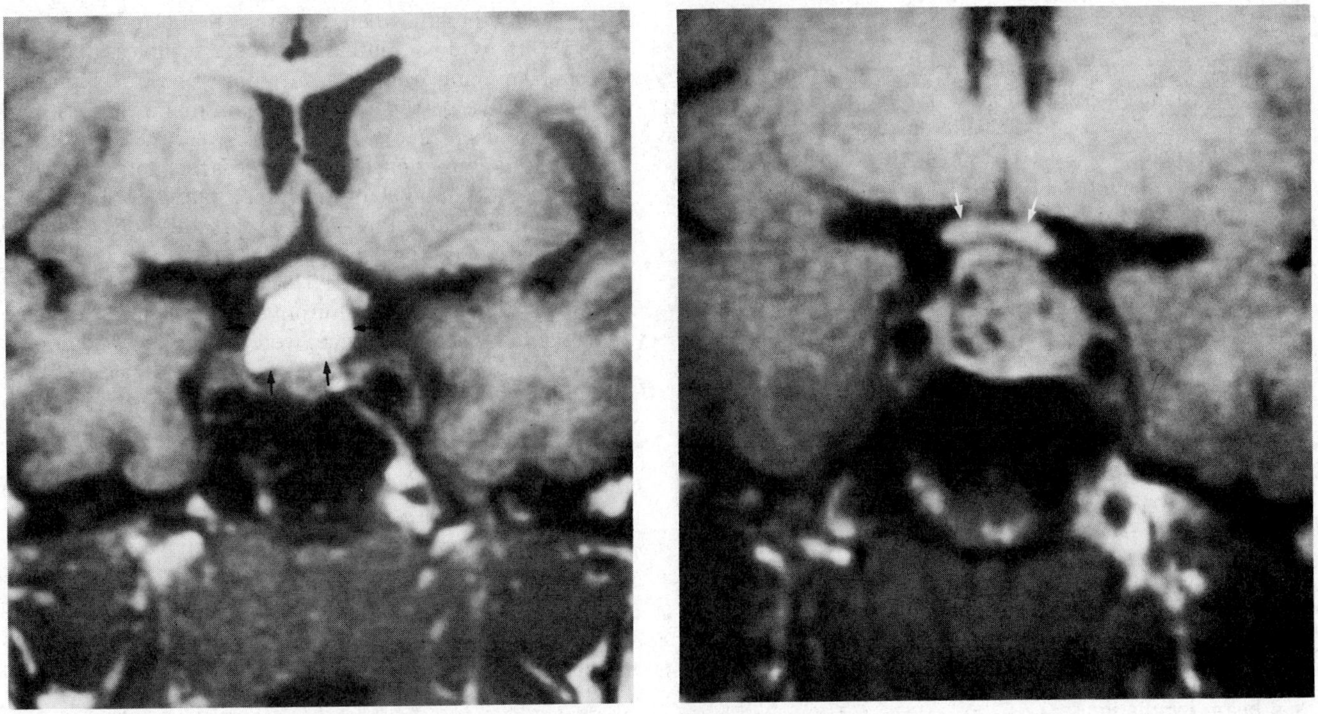

A B

FIG. 46-13. Craniopharyngiomas are solid (**A**) or cystic (**B**). **A.** T1-weighted (TR 600, TE 20) coronal scan demonstrates a 0.5 cm supracellar lesion abutting the chiasm (*black arrows*). Lesion is isointense with brain tissue except for multiple punctate areas of low signal intensity, which represent calcifications. Calcium appears as low signal intensity on magnetic resonance because of the lack of mobile hydrogen protons. **B.** T1-weighted (TR 600, TE 20) coronal scan of a cystic supracellar craniopharyngioma that deforms the chiasm. The high signal intensity represents hemorrhagic and cholesterol material. No calcifications are demonstrable.

usual setup includes two 110° arcs with 30° wedge filters. The field sizes are such as to include the target volume in the 95% isodose line. Careful attention is given to reproducibility of setup and avoidance of inclusion of the eyes. The neck is flexed so that the plane of rotation is behind the eyes. During simulation, markers are placed on the eyelids. The eye is approximately 25 mm long. Three tattoo marks are placed and used for alignment with laser beams. Both arcs are treated daily, with a daily dose of 1.8 Gy, calculated at the 95% isodose line. In almost all cases the total dose is carried to 45 Gy in 25 fractions over 5 weeks. The limited available dose response data indicate that lower doses yield higher recurrence rates. This combination of fraction size and total dose controls tumor growth in over 95% of cases; hence, a larger dose is not indicated. Larger fractions or greater total doses lead to a higher incidence of optic nerve or optic chiasm injury. The optic chiasm appears especially sensitive to radiation injury in patients with acromegaly; Bloom and Kramer reported 5 instances of visual complication in 40 acromegalic patients, largely in those with daily increments of 2.0 Gy and total doses of 50 Gy.[208] With a daily increment of 1.8 Gy and a total of 45 Gy at the 95% isodose line, injury to optic apparatus or adjacent brain is rare. Hypopituitarism, however, may develop as a late complication, years after completion of radiotherapy. Hypopituitarism is more likely to occur in patients who have had surgery and postoperative radiation therapy than in those who have been treated by radiation therapy or surgery alone. Since hypopituitarism is largely correctible by hormone replacement therapy, patients treated for pituitary adenomas should be observed by an endocrinologist for the remainder of their lives.

CRANIOPHARYNGIOMAS

Clinical and Pathologic Considerations

Craniopharyngiomas occur primarily in children. These tumors arise from cell rests that are remnants of Rathke's pouch at the juncture of the infundibular stalk and the pituitary. Most of these tumors become symptomatic only after they have attained a diameter of about 3 cm. Usually they are cystic at the time of presentation. They may compress the optic chiasm or pituitary and extend up into the third ventricle. The cyst is high in proteinaceous material and calcium and is easily seen by either CT scan or MR imaging study. Figure 46-13 shows MR images of typical solid and cystic craniopharyngiomas.

Clinically, craniopharyngiomas increase intracranial pressure and hypopituitary-hypothalamic-chiasmal dysfunction. Symptoms vary and may include, in children, obesity, delayed development, decreased vision and optic atrophy, field defects, and papilledema.

Surgery

Craniopharyngiomas are usually treated by a microsurgical procedure done via a right frontal craniotomy. Large craniopharyngiomal cysts that enter and enlarge the sella turcica can be drained and resected through a transsphenoidal procedure. The goal of most surgeons is total removal, but some do a more conservative operation and depend on the excellent results of radiation therapy discussed below. Aggressive removal nearly guarantees some injury to the pituitary gland and stalk, with subsequent temporary or permanent diabetes insipidus and elements of hypopituitarism. Patients thus injured face a lifetime of taking replacement hormones and using inhaled desmopressin acetate (DDAVP) spray for the control of diabetes insipidus. However, patients whose vision was affected by the craniopharyngioma can expect improvement following surgery. The mortality of craniopharyngioma resection is very low.

In Europe, a few centers are treating craniopharyngioma cysts with stereotaxic puncture and the instillation of colloidal therapeutic radioisotopes, particularly yttrium-90.[209] Such treatments are also being tried in this country with colloidal ^{32}P. Intracystic therapy may be a good treatment for craniopharyngioma cysts recurring after conventional external beam irradiation.

Radiation Therapy

Although debate exists regarding the extent to which total excision should be attempted, numerous reports attest to the efficacy of postoperative radiation therapy in the decompressed or incompletely resected craniopharyngioma. Data from the Columbia Presbyterian Hospital series[210,211] and from UCSF will be presented. At Columbia-Presbyterian, 43 children were treated by total resection, subtotal resection, or minimal resection. Those treated by total resection did not receive postoperative radiation therapy, whereas some of the other 2 groups (6 of 20 subtotal and 8 of 9 minimal resection) were irradiated. In the total resection group, the actuarial survival rate was 100% at 10 years; however, the actuarial relapse-free survival was 77% at 5 years and 47% at 10 years. For children with less than total resection, the relapse-free survival rates at 5 and 10 years were 14% and 7% without irradiation, and 78% and 78% when radiation therapy was given. In that series, the actuarial survival rates for adults at 5 and 10 years were: total resection alone, 59% and 24%; subtotal resection without irradiation, 37% and 31%; subtotal resection with radiation, 91% and 76%; there were only 2 patients with minimal resection without radiation therapy, and both of these failed to survive 5 years; minimal resection plus radiotherapy, 81% and 73%. The local recurrence rates after irradiation were 47% for a total dose of 50 Gy or less versus 26% for doses of 55 to 56 Gy. It was recommended that, for patients thought to have had a total resection but in whom a postoperative CT scan showed residual tumor, the total dose for children be 50 Gy in 6 weeks, and for adults 55 Gy in 6½ weeks. For gross residual disease, the recommended dose was 55 Gy in 6½ weeks for children and 60 to 65 Gy in 7 to 7½ weeks for adults.

At UCSF,[212] the treatment policy has been total resection without radiotherapy when such resection could be accomplished with minimal morbidity. Patients with less than total resection, ranging from cyst decompression to subtotal resection, receive postoperative radiation therapy. In 74 consecutive patients, reported in 1986, 7 were thought were to have had total resection, and 67 had less than total resection. One of the former and 6 of the latter groups have had recurrence. With a mean follow-up of 4 years, this policy resulted in a remission (clinically improved, neurologically stable, and decreased tumor size) in 91% of patients. There were 2 operative deaths and 1 death from uncontrolled disease. The remainder of the 7 recurrences were controlled by additional surgical procedures. Of the 52 patients with preoperative visual field deficits, 93% showed improvement, which in 33% represented a return to normal visual fields. Hypoadrenalism increased from 24% to 45% after treatment, but the rates of hypothyroidism and of diabetes insipidus were the same as before treatment. The radiation therapy target volume is based largely on CT scanning and uses relatively small margins around demonstrated tumor. The technique varies according to size and location of residual tumor, but most patients are treated by bicoronal arcs with moving wedge filters, similar to the method used for pituitary adenomas. All fields are treated daily, with a daily increment of 1.8 Gy. Generally, the total dose is 55 Gy. In children less than 3 years of age, it is recommended that, if possible, irradiation be delayed until they are older.

CEREBELLOPONTINE ANGLE NEURILEMMOMAS

Clinical and Pathologic Considerations

The major tumors occurring in this region are the acoustic nerve tumors and meningiomas. Meningiomas have been covered previously; therefore, the discussion that follows will be limited to acoustic neurilemmomas (schwannoma, neurofibroma). These tumors originate on the eighth cranial nerve, nearly always on the vestibular division, at the point where the nerve acquires its reticulin and schwann cell investment. Within the skull, this transition zone occurs in the internal auditory foramen and causes local erosion of the internal auditory meatus. Slow growth characterizes these tumors; therefore, they can grow to substantial size before clinical symptoms lead to diagnosis. Frequently they occupy the posterior fossa at the angle between the cerebellum and pons. By compression, they can affect the seventh, fifth, and, less often, the ninth and tenth cranial nerves alone or in various combinations. When large enough they can compress the medulla and obstruct the CSF, leading to hydrocephalus.

Acoustic neurilemmomas are the most common in the fifth decade and can be associated with familial neurofibromatosis. In the latter instance they occur earlier, in late childhood and adolescence, and may be bilateral.

In a series from the Massachusetts General Hospital[29] it was found that auditory and vestibular branch involvement occurred in 98%, facial weakness with disturbances of taste in 56%, sensory loss over the face in 56%, gait abnormality in 41%, and appendicular ataxia in 20%.

Diagnosis by skull radiography is suggestive, but definitive diagnosis is best made with MR imaging or CT scan done in conjunction with the CSF administration of metrizamide contrast.

Surgery

The aim of surgery for acoustic neurilemmomas is complete resection, and presently there are two commonly used approaches—the translabyrinthine and the transoccipital (posterior fossa).[213] Since the translabyrinthine approach assumes complete deafness on the side of the operation because it transgresses the middle ear, and since larger tumors are difficult to remove through this approach, the translabyrinthine route is usually reserved for smaller tumors that have already caused complete or nearly complete deafness.

The translabyrinthine route requires only a small incision behind the ear, through which the petrous bone is gradually removed with a high-speed drill until the facial nerve is exposed to the point where it can be separated from the tumor and protected. The dura of the posterior fossa is easily seen and can be opened to gain access to larger tumors. Surgical experts in this approach can remove very large tumors this way, but most neurosurgeons defer to a posterior fossa approach for larger tumors. Many avoid the translabyrinthine approach and use the transoccipital posterior fossa route for all tumors, but certainly the larger tumors or very small tumors with some useful preserved hearing are generally approached through the posterior fossa. In patients with smaller tumors and preserved hearing, there is a small chance that hearing can be preserved or even improved after posterior fossa surgery.

The transoccipital approach requires a unilateral posterior fossa craniectomy, after which the dura is opened and the cerebellum retracted medially to expose the cerebellopontine angle. The lower cranial nerves are protected while tumor is removed and the porus acusticus unroofed in an effort to identify the facial nerve and, in smaller tumors, the acoustic nerve as well. Once the facial nerve is identified, the remainder of the tumor is removed in a usually long and tedious operation that fully tests the surgeon's microsurgical skill.

Acoustic neurilemmomas can be completely removed through the posterior fossa in nearly every instance, and life-threatening complications are rare except in patients with very large tumors. As mentioned above, preservation of the acoustic nerve is rare in even small tumors, but the facial nerve is in continuity at the end of most acoustic tumor resections; therefore, any postoperative paresis or paralysis tends to be temporary. When the facial nerve is divided during surgery, it is sutured together when possible, or a nerve graft is placed between the stumps. Facial paralysis with no evidence of recovery within a few months is treated by surgical reinnervation, wherein another cranial nerve, usually a branch of the accessory nerve, is joined to the facial nerve peripherally. Bilateral acoustic tumors are seen with central neurofibromatosis and present difficult problems in surgical decision-making.[214] In general, a conservative approach is taken, treating the largest tumor when symptoms absolutely require it. Bilateral aggressive tumor resections lead to complete deafness and carry the possibility of bilateral facial nerve paralysis, a horrifying cosmetic and functional problem.

Radiation Therapy

There have been few reports on the role of radiation therapy for treatment of acoustic neurilemmomas. A recent review of the UCSF experience disclosed 124 patients of whom 62 were thought to have had a total resection and did not receive irradiation.[82] There was only one recurrence among these 62 patients. The 15-year actuarial survival rate was 98%, and 15-year relapse-free survival was 94%. In patients who had a subtotal resection, the 15-year relapse-free survival rates were 94% with irradiation ($\geq$45 Gy) versus 41% without; the corresponding 15-year survival rates were 100% and 67%, respectively ($p = 0.01$ for relapse-free and 0.016 for overall survival differences). There was no recurrence in three patients with biopsy plus >45 Gy irradiation. On the other hand, 4 of 7 patients who were irradiated for disease progression after having had resection alone subsequently developed a second recurrence. It was concluded that irradiation should follow subtotal resection. The target volume includes a narrow margin around residual tumor. Usually, treatment is given via two beams at right angles to each other and with wedge filters. Both fields are treated daily with an increment of 1.8 Gy, and the total dose is carried to approximately 55 Gy.

GLOMUS JUGULARE TUMORS

Clinical and Pathologic Considerations

These tumors arise from glomus tissue in the adventitia of the jugular bulb (glomus jugulare) or along Jacobson's nerve in the temporal bone, sometimes multifocally. The tumor invades temporal bone diffusely, but growth is characteristically slow. Sometimes they are endocrine active, with a carcinoid or pheochromocytoma-like syndrome.[215]

Glomus jugulare tumors, because they occur in the jugular foramen, commonly cause lower cranial nerve palsies and early symptoms of hoarseness and difficulty in swallowing. Later, facial weakness, hearing loss, and atrophy of the tongue become prominent. Pulsating tinnitus may also be a presenting symptom, and a pulsating mass can sometimes be seen behind the eardrum.

A presumptive radiologic diagnosis of glomus tumor can be made with CT or MR imaging, with jugular neurilemmoma being the main differential diagnosis. Since glomus tumors require a tremendous blood supply, particularly via the ascending pharyngeal artery, cerebral angiography provides the definitive diagnosis. Since preoperative tumor embolization is essential to surgical removal of glomus tumors, the diagnostic angiogram should be performed just before surgery whenever possible.

Histopathologically, numerous vascular channels are distinctive. The background is composed of clear cells clumped in a fibrous matrix. A small percentage of glomus tumors are malignant.

Surgery

The treatment of glomus jugulare tumors is a matter of some controversy, with advocates for radiation,[216] surgery, and the combination.[217] Most agree that resection should be attempted and that in most cases gross surgical resection, if not cure, is a realistic goal.

Surgery on glomus tumors is most frequently done by a neurosurgeon and a head and neck surgeon together after preoperative embolization. The base of the skull in the region of the jugular foramen is first exposed and neurovascular structures identified and mobilized through a high transverse cervical incision. When the incision is extended behind the pinna and a mastoidectomy completed, the facial nerve can be protected, and the entire tumor bulb as well as the jugular bulb and internal jugular vein can be seen passing through the base of the skull. Finally, after a suboccipital craniectomy, the sigmoid sinus above and the jugular vein below can be ligated, and the segment between them excised with the attached tumor.[205] Complications of this procedure include CSF leak and cranial nerve (particularly facial) palsy.

Radiation Therapy

Even though glomus tumors are histologically benign, irradiation is effective and certainly is indicated for symptomatic lesions that cannot be totally resected. These tumors tend to regress very slowly and success of radiotherapy is generally measured by amelioration of symptoms and absence of disease progression. The dose required for control is relatively modest. Kim et al reported a series of 40 patients with such lesions and added a literature survey.[218] They reported a control rate with subtotal resection and postoperative radiation therapy of 85%. When radiation therapy only was used for inoperable or recurrent tumors, control was obtained in 88%. Their composite data, including cases from the literature, showed a 22% recurrence rate for doses less than 40 Gy, compared with a 2% rate for doses equal to or greater than 40 Gy in 4 weeks.

At UCSF, incompletely resected lesions are usually treated with 1.8 Gy/day, to a total of about 45 Gy in 5 weeks. Depending on the precise location of the lesion, therapy usually makes use of a pair of wedged portals.

CHORDOMAS

Clinical and Pathologic Considerations

Chordomas occur along the pathway of the primitive notochord, which extends, in human embryos, from the tip of the dorsum sellae to the coccyx. Chordomas are extradural, multilobulated tumors, varying in consistency from very soft to woody and cartilaginous. They are pseudoencapsulated and may invade through the basal dura.

The typical chordoma is composed of cord-like rows of distended, vacuolated (physaliferous) cells. A variant, the chondroid chordoma, has distinctly chondroid elements and may be less aggressive.[219] None of the histopathologic characteristics of tumor aggressiveness (cellularity, pleomorphism, mitoses) seems to be predictive in chordoma.

The diagnosis of clivus chordomas cannot be made without radiological tests and is often delayed because symptoms are nonspecific and vague. At onset, there is usually headache and intermittent diplopia; and these vague symptoms are often not reported, allowing the tumor to grow to an enormous size before the diagnosis is made. Gradually, headache (upper clivus tumors) and neck pain (lower clivus tumors) worsen. Superiorly placed tumors go on to cause diplopia and facial numbness as the cavernous sinus and Meckel's cave are invaded. Lower clivus tumors compress the lower cranial nerves and later the brain stem.

The differential diagnosis of cranial chordoma includes basal meningioma, neurilemmoma (schwannoma), nasopharyngeal carcinoma, pituitary adenoma, and craniopharyngioma. MR imaging usually results in a working diagnosis of chordoma, but surgical biopsy (and resection) is mandatory.

Surgery

Surgery for cranial chordomas is obligatory to obtain diagnostic tissue, to enhance the effectiveness of subsequent radiation therapy, and to improve the patient's clinical condition. With an aggressive surgical resection, a favorable effect on the severe headaches and neurologic deficits associated with chordomas can be anticipated.

Intracranial chordomas occur at the base of the skull, a region relatively remote from surgical access. Consequently, a variety of innovative approaches have been developed by neurosurgeons and head and neck surgeons, and these procedures are commonly done with both types of specialist in attendance.

For midline lesions of the upper clivus that extend into the sella and/or sphenoid sinus a transseptal, transsphenoidal approach (as for pituitary tumors) is best. Large, compressive, transdural extensions of these upper clivus tumors into the interpeduncular cistern must be removed through a transcranial, subtemporal, intradural approach. For the more lateralized upper clival tumor and some lateralized midclival tumors, an approach through the appropriate maxillary sinus (midfacial degloving) is useful. For midline tumors of the midclivus and lower clivus, transoral resection is commonly used. Sometimes a combination of exposures is necessary for very large tumors.

A potentially serious complication of the transsphenoidal, transmaxillary, and transoral approaches is CSF leak and consequent meningitis. Therefore, every attempt must be made to keep the dura intact during these procedures. The incidence of dural invasion by cranial chordomas may be as high as 50%, however, so an inadvertent entry into the dura during resection is sometimes unavoidable. Careful intraoperative patching of the leak with fat and muscle grafts, followed by postoperative spinal CSF drainage, is essential.

Cranial chordomas frequently recur after surgery and radiation therapy. In this situation, reoperation directed toward symptomatic improvement is the only treatment option. Reoperations are complicated by surgical scarring and tissue compromise from radiation.

Radiation Therapy

Chordoma and low-grade chondrosarcoma of the base of skull, clivus, or axial skeleton are not amenable to complete surgical resection. Because of the proximity of dose-limiting critical CNS structures such as optic nerves or chiasm, other cranial nerves, brain stem, temporal lobe or spinal cord, charged particles such as protons or helium ions are often used to deliver higher tumor doses than are possible with low-LET radiation therapy while keeping the dose to neighboring critical structures at a safe level.

Tumor doses of 60 to 75 Gy-equivalent (GyE) can be achieved depending on site and extent of disease with a resultant local control rate in the range of 65% to 75% and actuarial survival of 70% at 5 years (J. Castro et al, unpublished observations, 1987). Precise beam delivery techniques, highly reproducible patient positioning, and very accurate compensation for tissue in homogeneities in the beam path are required. Computerized treatment planning is based on CT and MR data, collimator and compensator design, and known isodose distributions in bone and soft tissues. To maximize tumor dose relative to dose to adjacent critical structures, the physical parameters of charged particles must be considered. These include relatively sharp lateral beam edges with dose decreased from 90% to 10% in about 10 to 12 mm (depending on beam size and depth of penetration) and an abrupt distal decrease from 90% to 10% over about 7 mm. The depth of penetration can be altered to suit the clinical situation by varying the energy of the beam or interposition of bolus material in the beam path. Charged particle beams can be made to halt in front of a critical structure such as the spinal cord by appropriate compensation techniques; and, in combination with other lateral or oblique beams, a target volume may be "wrapped" around a critical structure.

At University of California Lawrence Berkeley Laboratory (UCLBL), 67 patients have been treated with helium beams between 1976 and 1986. Thirty-seven had chordoma or chondrosarcoma of the base of skull or clivus; 68% (25/37) have local control with follow-up ranging from 4 to 115 months (median = 28 months). In this group, the mean tumor dose was 65 GyE. An additional 20 patients had similar tumors of the cervical (10/20), thoracic (8/20), or lumbar (2/20) spine. Of these patients, 70% (14/20) have local control of their tumors with follow-up ranging from 2 to 70 months (median = 15 months). In this group, the mean tumor dose was 68 GyE. Ten patients had sacral tumors, of whom 7 have local tumor control from 22 to 117 months (median = 42 months). The mean tumor dose was 75 GyE. Thus, of the 67 patients, 69% (46/67) have local control. There have been 9 major complications, including brain and cranial nerve (6 patients), spinal cord (1 patient), and other major nerve injury (2 patients) for a 13% incidence. For the total group, the actuarial (Kaplan-Meier) survival is 67% at 3 years; the projected 3-year actuarial local control rate is 65%.

HEMANGIOBLASTOMAS AND HEMANGIOMAS

Clinical and Pathologic Considerations

The hemangioblastoma accounts for approximately 2% of intracranial tumors, arising most frequently in the cerebellar hemispheres and vermis. Usually solitary, these tumors can be multiple and may also occur in the brain stem, spinal cord, and supratentorial compartment. Cerebellar hemangioblastoma can be sporadic or occur as a familial disorder as part of the Von Hippel–Lindau complex that is transmitted as an autosomal dominant disorder with varying degrees of penetrance. Other entities associated with familial hemangioblastoma are hypernephroma, polycystic kidneys, pancreatic cysts, pheochromocytoma, and erythrocytosis.

Cerebellar hemangioblastomas usually are recognized in the third decade, causing symptoms of increased intracranial pressure and symptoms and signs of cerebellar dysfunction. Gait disturbance and imbalance are particularly common. Clinical progression is slow, as these tumors enlarge very slowly.

The hemangioblastoma probably arises during embryonic life from primitive endothelial cells around the fourth ventricle. The tumor is composed of numerous capillary and sinusoidal channels lined with endothelial cells. Interspersed are nests of lipid-laden pseudoxanthoma cells. The tumor is generally cystic and contains proteinaceous, xanthochromic fluid. The cyst contains a red (vascular), firm mural nodule, the apparent source of the fluid. The cyst wall is a glial, nonneoplastic reaction to the secreted fluid. Occasional hemangioblastomas (brain stem and spinal cord particularly) are without cysts.

Surgery

The diagnosis can be made, in most cases, with CT or MR imaging. Angiography, to confirm the diagnosis, is normally done before surgery. Cerebellar hemangiomablastoma tumors are readily approached and excised with the cyst drained and the entire solid portion carefully dissected and removed. Solid hemangioblastomas of the brain stem are exceedingly vascular, and their removal is associated with high mortality; even biopsy can be associated with percipitous bleeding and significant morbidity. Such tumors are sometimes irradiated with or without a confirmatory biopsy.

Radiation Therapy

Sung et al reported the experience at Columbia-Presbyterian Hospital on the radiotherapy for cerebellar hemangioblastoma.[220] Twenty-three patients received radiation therapy using coaxial bilateral ports. About half received doses of 36 Gy or less, and the other half (12/23) received doses of 40 to 55 Gy in 4 to 6½ weeks. The 5-, 10-, and 15-year survival rates for the lower dose group were 54.5%, 27.3%, and 8.1%, respectively. With the higher dose the survival rates were 90.5%, 56.5%, and 56.5%, respectively. They recommended postoperative radiotherapy for incompletely excised tumors and for tumors recurring after "total" excision. The recommended dose was 45 to 50 Gy in 4½ to 5 weeks. Our experience, although more limited, is consistent with that of Sung et al, and we concur with their recommendations.

CHOROID PLEXUS PAPILLOMA AND CARCINOMA

Clinical and Pathologic Considerations

These rare tumors occur most often in children under 12 years, although they can occur at any age. Nearly half of these tumors are found in patients under the age of 20 years.

The tumor is an irregularly lobulated reddish mass, which on histopathologic examination is apparently normal choroid plexus. Very rarely, these tumors show malignant features and are then classified as choroid plexus carcinoma.

In children, choroid plexus papillomas most frequently occur in the lateral ventricles. In adults, the fourth ventricular papilloma is the most common site. Third ventricle tumors are very rare. Since papillomas tend to grow slowly within ventricles, they expand to fill the ventricle and block CSF flow. In addition, papillomas are thought to secrete CSF. Thus, choroid plexus papillomas (and carcinomas) can produce hydrocephalus (1) secondary to obstruction of the CSF, (2) by CSF overproduction by the tumor, or (3) by damage to the CSF resorptive bed from recurrent hemorrhages. As a result, increased intracranial pressure without focal findings is the most common presentation; fourth ventricular tumors can also be associated with focal findings of ataxia and nystagmus.

Although choroid plexus papillomas and carcinomas extensively seed throughout the ventricular and subarachnoid spaces, seeding from papillomas is usually subclinical while that from carcinomas is frequent and dramatically symptomatic. These tumors are easily seen by both CT scan and MR image study. In patients with anaplastic changes, we advocate staging by myelography and examination of the CSF.

Therapy for anaplastic tumors should be approached in a manner similar to that for medulloblastoma and malignant ependymomas. Because of the aggressive nature of the more anaplastic tumors, therapy must be equally aggressive requiring radiation and, in some cases, intraventricular chemotherapy.

Surgery

The treatment of choroid plexus papillomas is total surgical excision. This is accomplished for fourth ventricular tumors through a standard suboccipital craniectomy. For lateral ventricular tumors the approach is through an ipsilateral high posterior parietal craniotomy and transcortical approach to the ventricular trigone, the usual tumor site. In either instance the surgeon attempts first to reduce the tumor's abundant blood supply to facilitate resection. Nearly half the cases of hydrocephalus are ameliorated by the surgery, and the others require shunting.

Choroid plexus papillomas of the third ventricle are exceedingly rare but can be approached through a variety of surgical exposures of the third ventricle. The problems of removal of fourth ventricular choroid plexus tumors are similar to those associated with suboccipital removal of medulloblastomas or ependymomas as discussed above.

Choroid plexus tumors of the lateral ventricle are approached through a high parietal cortical incision and transcortical approach to the ventricular trigone. The predilection of these tumors for the left side makes this more worrisome. Hydrocephalus is the rule and simplifies the exposure when retraction into the ventricle is established. Tumor arteries and veins are identified via the operating microscope and then coagulated, after which smaller tumors are removed intact and larger tumors removed piecemeal. Persistent hydrocephalus in the postoperative period requires shunting.

Radiation Therapy

These lesions are generally considered "radioresistant," and there is little information regarding their response to irradiation; the use of irradiation is anecdotal. Naguib et al reported a case of chorid plexus papilloma with extensive involvement of the mastoid bone, hence, inoperable.[221] This patient received 49.5 Gy in 32 treatments over a period of 33 days. Serial CT scans showed that 16 months after completion of the radiotherapy the mass was markedly reduced in size. Such anecdotes suggest that radiation therapy to the primary tumor site may be tried for an inoperable choroid plexus papilloma. With choroid plexus carcinoma, consideration must be given to treating the entire cerebrospinal axis. With a normal myelogram and negative CSF cytology studies, we have recommended radiation therapy to the primary tumor site with intrathecal and systemic chemotherapy but have no data to support this approach.

Chemotherapy

Normally, chemotherapy is not used for choroid plexus papillomas. However, for the more anaplastic tumors, we have increasingly utilized chemotherapy adjuvant to surgery and irradiation to prevent the inevitable recurrence and CSF dissemination common with choroid plexus carcinomas. As with many of the less common tumors discussed, there are no chemotherapeutic guidelines and few reports to guide the therapist.

Initially, we used chemotherapy only for recurrent disease. We have used combinations of cyclophosphamide, Adriamycin, and vincristine, as well as nitrosourea-based combinations. We have seen transient responses and disease control with both. We have also utilized intraventricular chemotherapy with low-dose methotrexate (2 mg/day × 5 days) and/or cytosine arabinoside (20–30 mg/day × 3 days) to stave subarachnoid spread. As a result of this experience, we currently advocate the use of adjuvant chemotherapy with a nitrosourea-based combination after irradiation and the use of concomitant intraventricular chemotherapy. During irradiation we have used intraventricular cytosine arabinoside, and methotrexate after irradiation. Further study and additional approaches are worthy of consideration as well.

SPINAL AXIS TUMORS

Clinical and Pathologic Considerations

Some of the clinical features of spinal axis tumor localization and diagnosis have been covered previously. Most primary spinal axis tumors produce symptoms and signs as a result of spinal cord and nerve root compression rather than because of parenchymal invasion.

The reported frequency of primary spinal cord tumors is between 10% and 19% of all primary CNS tumors.[222] While the largest number of spinal axis tumors are extradural, the majority of **primary** spinal axis tumors are intradural. Of intradural tumors, the intradural-extramedullary neurilemmomas and meningiomas are the commonest (see Table 46-3). Neurilemmomas and meningiomas are normally intradural, but occasionally they may present as extradural tumors. Other intradural-extramedullary tumors are vascular tumors, chordomas, and epidermoids.

Intramedullary tumors have the same cellular origins as the other CNS tumors covered previously. In terms of frequency, ependymomas occur in about 40% of patients with intramedullary tumors; next most common are the astrocytomas of low- and mid-anaplasia. These are followed in frequency by less common histologies such as oligodendroglioma, ganglioglioma, medulloblastoma, and various hemangiomas and hemangioblastomas.

Table 46-25 classifies spinal axis tumors by location. Different tumor types exhibit a predilection for certain spinal regions, but, taken altogether, spinal tumors are distributed fairly evenly along the spinal axis. Approximately half of spinal tumors involve the thoracic spinal canal, 30% the lumbosacral spine, and the remainder the cervical spine, including the foramen magnum. Some tumors, like the neurilemmomas, occur with greatest frequency in the thoracic region, although they can be found throughout the spine and often extend through an intervertebral foramen to acquire a dumbbell configuration.

Meningiomas are dura-based and arise preferentially at the foramen magnum and in the thoracic spine. Astrocytomas are distributed throughout the spinal cord, whereas most ependymomas involve the conus medullarus and cauda equina. Spinal chordomas are characteristically sacral.

Clinically, patients with spinal axis tumors present with a sensorimotor spinal tract syndrome, a painful radicular spinal cord syndrome, or a central syringomyelic syndrome.[29] In the **sensorimotor presentation,** symptoms and signs result from compression of the spinal cord. The onset is gradual over weeks to months, initial presentation is asymmetric, and motor weakness predominates. The level of impairment determines the muscle groups involved. Because of external compression, dorsal column involvement occurs with paresthesia and abnormalities of pain and temperature on the side contralateral to the motor weakness.

Radicular spinal cord syndromes occur also because of external compression and infiltration of spinal cord roots. The main symptom is sharp, "knifelike" pain in the distribution of a sensory nerve root. The intense pain is frequently of short duration, with pain that is more aching in nature persisting for longer periods of time. The pain typically is exacerbated by coughing and sneezing or other maneuvers that increase intracranial pressure. Local paresthesia and impairment of sensations of pain and touch are common, as are weakness and muscle wasting. Not uncommonly, these findings antedate cord compression by months.

Spinal tumors, particularly intramedullary tumors, can produce **syringomyelic dysfunction** by destruction and cavitation within the central gray matter of the cord. This produces lower motor neuron destruction and attendant segmental muscle weakness, wasting, and loss of reflexes. There is also a dissociated sensory loss of pain and temperature sensation with preservation of touch. With extension of the lesion, however, touch, vibration, and position sense are affected.

TABLE 46-25. Classification of Spinal Tumors by Their Location in Relation to the Spinal Cord and Dura Mater

Location	*Usual Tumor Types*
Extradural	Metastatic (carcinoma, lymphoma, melanoma, sarcoma), chordoma
Intradural	
Extramedullary	Schwannoma*, meningioma
Intramedullary	Astrocytoma, ependymoma†

* May extend along nerve root into extradural and extraspinal spaces.

† Ependymomas originating from the filum terminale and involving the cauda equina, not intramedullary in the strictest sense, are included here by custom.

Surgery

The use of the operating microscope is as essential for spinal cord tumor surgery as it is for brain tumor surgery. In addition, other surgical adjuncts like intraoperative ultrasound, the CO_2 laser, and the CUSA, the uses of which were emphasized above when discussing brain tumor surgery, are equally valuable for the resection of spinal cord tumors. US is particularly useful for examining the spinal cord through an intact or open dura to assess the level of maximum tumor involvement or to differentiate tumor cysts from solid tumor masses.

SURGICAL PLANNING. MR imaging is rapidly replacing myelography and CT scanning for the diagnosis, localization, and characterization of spinal tumors (see Fig. 46-7). In all but vascular tumors (e.g., hemangioblastoma) where angiography is needed or tumors that cause extensive bony destruction (e.g., metastasis) where CT scanning might be helpful, a technically excellent MR study is most often sufficient for preoperative planning for spinal tumors. Important in localization is not only determination of the spinal level of the tumor but also its exact relationship to the spinal cord. Corticosteroids are given before, during, and after spinal cord tumor surgery to help control spinal cord edema.

REMOVAL OF INTRADURAL EXTRAMEDULLARY TUMORS. Meningiomas and neurilemmomas (schwannomas) occur in the intradural extramedullary spinal compartment. Most of these tumors can be completely resected (cured), since through a laminectomy exposure they can be easily separated and rotated away from the spinal cord, already displaced, but not invaded, by tumor.

Neurilemmomas arise from spinal rootlets (most often dorsal rootlets), and their removal includes sections of those rootlets involved. Neurilemmomas can grow along the nerve root in a "dumbbell" fashion through a neural foramen; and, while some of these extraspinal tumor extensions can be removed by extending the initial laminectomy exposure laterally, some must be resected at a separate operation through a thoracotomy, costotransversectomy or retroperitoneal approach.

Meningiomas in most cases can be removed through a posterior (laminectomy) approach, since they are commonly lateral or anterolateral; even the more anteriorly placed tumors cause enough lateral displacement of the spinal cord to allow access for resection without traction on the spinal cord. The uncommon tumor directly anterior to the spinal cord must sometimes be approached anteriorly or anterolaterally. Anteriorly situated meningiomas at the foramen magnum are sometimes unresectable because of their encasement of the vertebral artery.

REMOVAL OF INTRAMEDULLARY TUMORS. The most common intramedullary tumors are ependymoma and astrocytoma. Hemangioblastoma is another (infrequent) tumor occurring in the spinal intramedullary compartment. Surgery is the principal treatment for all these tumors, with the exception of astrocytomas that are anaplastic.

Intramedullary tumors are approached via laminectomy; and, after the dura is opened, a longitudinal myelotomy is made over the widened region of spinal cord and the incision deepened several millimeters to the tumor surface. Dissection planes around the tumor are sought microsurgically and, in the case of ependymomas, usually found and extended gradually around the tumor's surface as removal of the central tumor bulk (by CO_2 laser or CUSA) causes the tumor to collapse. Generally, such tumors are completely removed. Tumors with indefinite dissection planes (usually low-grade astrocytomas) cannot be completely removed, but bulk reduction can cause long-term palliation. If frozen section shows a tumor to be malignant, surgery is aborted, and radiation therapy is the treatment.

Hemangioblastomas are extremely vascular tumors, so the tumor margins are addressed first. Feeding arteries are coagulated and the tumor dissected and removed en bloc. The dorsal location of most of these tumors and the commonly associated cyst simplifies the removal to some extent.

Radiation Therapy

Radiation therapy is generally recommended for incompletely resected neoplasms of the spinal axis; see above for considerations relative to specific histologic types. As a rule, radiation doses are kept low enough so that the risk of injury to the spinal cord is less than that from the neoplasm itself. Generally, this means doses of 50 to 55 Gy; however, for lesions involving only the cauda equina and for situations where irreversible and complete transverse myelopathy has occurred, higher doses are permissible.

Chemotherapy

There have been no reports of controlled clinical trials of chemotherapy for primary spinal axis tumors. It would be logical to assume that drugs active against intracranial astrocytomas, oligodendrogliomas, and ependymomas would be equally efficacious against these same lesions in the spinal cord. Along with reports of chemotherapy activity against intracranial tumors, anecdotal cases have been included.

Our own experience suggests that palliation is possible for astrocytomas with nitrosourea-based chemotherapy regimens. No therapy, however, is clearly superior. For drop metastases from ependymomas, we have used BCNU and DBD as single agents with some benefit[138] (Levin et al, unpublished observations; see Table 46-19).

For drop metastases from medulloblastoma, a variety of drugs have been found to be beneficial—specifically, cyclo-phosphamide, carboplatin, methotrexate, procarbazine alone and in combination, and vincristine. For the most part, these drugs have produced palliation for variable times, from weeks to many months.

In general, the use of intraventricular and intrathecal chemotherapy is limited to microscopic deposits. Biodistribution in the subarachnoid CSF can be limited in the face of intradural-extramedullary tumors. In addition, deposits of 5 mm in diameter or greater are not likely to benefit because of limitations in diffusion coupled with transcapillary loss of drug in the tumor.

Portions of the section on Anatomical and Clinical Considerations were adapted with permission from Levin VA, Wilson CB: Clinical characteristics of cancer in the brain and spinal cord. In Crook ST, Prestayko A (eds): Cancer and Chemotherapy, Vol II: Introduction to Neoplasia and Antineoplastic Chemotherapy, p 167; New York, Academic Press, 1981. We thank Michael Edwards, Steven Leibel, David Norman, and Joseph Castro for writing or editing portions of this chapter; Irene Asturias for typing much of the chapter; and Pamela Silver Johnson for providing unpublished data from UCSF studies.

REFERENCES

1. SEER search performed for this chapter between 1978-1984
2. Sloof JL, Kernohan JW, MacCary CS: Primary Intramedullary Tumors of the Spinal Cord and Filum Terminale. Philadelphia, WB Saunders, 1964
3. Percy AK, Elveback LR, Okazaki H et al: Neoplasms of the central nervous system: Epidemiologic considerations. Neurology 22:40, 1972
4. Barker D, Wright E, Nguyen K et al: Gene for von Recklinghausen neurofibromatosis is in the pericentromeric region of chromosome 17. Science 236:1100, 1987
5. Seizinger BR, Rouleau G, Ozelius LJ et al: Common pathogenetic mechanism for three tumor types in bilateral acoustic neurofibromatosis. Science 236:317, 1987
6. Mark J: Chromosomal patterns in human meningiomas. Eur J Cancer 6:489, 1970
7. Zankl H, Zang KD: Cytology and cytogenetical studies on brain tumors: III. Ph¹-like chromosomes in human meningiomas. Humangenetik 12:42, 1971
8. Bigner SH, Bjerkvig R, Laerum OD: DNA content and chromosomal composition of malignant human gliomas. Neurol Clin 3:769, 1985
9. Henn W, Blin N, Zang KD: Polysomy of chromosome 7 is correlated with over-expression of the erbB oncogene in human glioblastoma cell lines. Hum Genet 74:104, 1986
10. Liepkalns VA, Icard-Liepkalns C, Sommer AM et al: Properties of cloned human glioblastoma cells: Release of a specific protease. J Neurol Sci 57:257, 1982
11. Freidman HS, Schold C Jr: Rational approaches to the chemotherapy of medulloblastoma. In Vick NA, Bigner DD (eds): Neurologic Clinics, p 843. Philadelphia, W.B. Saunders, 1985
12. Neville BG, Berry AC, Stoddart Y: A case of malignant spinal cord ependymoma in association with a duplication of part of the long arm of chromosome 12. J Med Genet 22:154, 1985
13. Stroup NE, Blair A, Erikson GE: Brain cancer and other causes of death in anatomist. JNCI 77:1217, 1986
14. Musicco M, Filippini G, Bordo BM et al: Gliomas and (occupational) exposure to carcinogens: Case–control study. Am J Epidemiol 116:782, 1982
15. Moss AR: Occupational exposure and brain tumors. J Toxicol Environ Health 16:703, 1985
16. Bovet P, Lob M: Cancer mortality among the workers of a Swiss rubber goods factory: Epidemiological study, 1955–1975. Schweiz Med Wochenschr 110:1277, 1980
17. McLaughlin JK, Malker HS, Blot WJ et al: Occupational risks for intracranial gliomas in Sweden. JNCI 78:253, 1987
18. Copeland DD, Bigner DD: Glial-mesenchymal tropism of in vivo avian sarcoma virus neuro-oncogenis in rats. Acta Neuropathol (Berl) 41:23, 1978
19. Wodinski I, Kensler CJ, Rall DP: The induction and transplantation of brain tumors in neonate beagles. Proc AACR, p 99, 1969
20. Hochberg RH, Miller G, Schooley RT et al: Central nervous system lymphoma related to Epstein-Barr virus. N Engl J Med 309:745, 1983
21. Annegers JF, Laws ER Jr, Kurland LT et al: Head trauma and subsequent brain tumors. Neurosurg 4:203–205, 1979
22. Raffel C, Edwards MS, Davis RL et al: Post irradiation cerebellar glioma: Case report. J Neurosurg 62:300

23. Malone M, Lumley H, Erdohazi M: Astrocytoma as a second malignancy in patients with acute lymphoblastic leukemia. Cancer 57:979, 1986
24. Sogg RL, Donaldson SS, Yorke CH: Malignant astrocytoma following radiotherapy of a craniopharyngioma. J Neurosurg 48:622, 1978
25. Poster DS, Bruno S: The occurrence of second primary neoplasms in patients with non-Hodgkin's lymphomas. IRCS Med Sci: Cancer 8:554, 1980
26. Rubinstein AB, Shalit MN, Cohen M et al: Radiation-induced cerebral meningioma: A recognizable entity. J Neurosurg 61:966, 1984
27. Spallone A, Gagliardi FM, Vagnozzi R: Intracranial meningiomas related to external cranial irradiation. Surg Neurol 12:153, 1979
28. Levin VA, Wilson CB: Clinical characteristics of cancer in the brain and spinal cord. In Crook ST, Prestayko A (eds): Cancer and Chemotherapy: Introduction to Neoplasia and Antineoplastic Chemotherapy, Vol II, p 167. New York, Academic Press, 1981
29. Adams RD, Victor M: Principles of Neurology, p 586. New York, McGraw-Hill, 1977
30. Bingas B: Tumours of the base of the skull. In Vinken PJ, Bruyn GW (eds): Handbook of Clinical Neurology. Vol. 17: Tumors of the Brain and Skull, p 136. Amsterdam, North Holland, 1974
31. Fahlbusch R, Marguth F: Endocrine disorders associated with intracranial tumors. In Vinken PJ, Bruyn GW (eds): Handbook of Clinical Neurology; Tumors of the Brain and Skull, part I, vol 16, p 345. Amsterdam, North Holland, 1974
32. Russell DJ, Rubinstein LJ: Pathology of Tumors of the Nervous System, 4th ed. Baltimore, Williams & Wilkins, 1977
33. Rubinstein LJ: The Armed Forces Institute of Pathology Fascicle on Brain Tumors of the Central Nervous System, US Government Printing Office, 1972
34. Brant-Zawadzki M, Norman D (eds): Magnetic Resonance Imaging of the Central Nervous System. New York, Raven Press, 1987
35. Norman D, Enzmann D, Levin VA et al: Computerized tomographic scanning in the evaluation of malignant gliomas under therapy. Radiology 121:85, 1976
36. Levin VA, Crafts D, Wilson CB et al: BCNU and procarbazine treatment for malignant brain tumors. Cancer Treat Rep 60:243, 1976
37. Edwards MSB, Davis RL, Laurent JP: Tumor markers and cytologic features of cerebrospinal fluid. Cancer 56:1773, 1985
38. Inoue HK, Naganuma H, Ono N: Pathobiology of intracranial germ-cell tumors: Immunochemical, immunohistochemical, and electron microscopic investigations. J Neuro-Oncol 5:105, 1987
39. Marton LJ, Edwards MS, Levin VA et al: CSF polyamines: A new and important means of monitoring medulloblastoma. Cancer 47:757, 1981
40. Hoffman WF, Levin VA, Wilson CB: Evaluation of malignant glioma patients during the postirradiation period. J Neurosurg 50:624, 1979
41. Heilbrun MP: Computed tomography–guided stereotactic systems. Clin Neurosurg 31:564–581, 1984
42. Apuzzo MLJ, Chandrasoma PT, Cohen D et al: Computed imaging stereotaxy: Experience and perspective related to 500 procedures applied to brain masses. Neurosurgery 20:930–937, 1987
43. Leibel SA, Sheline GE: Radiation therapy for neoplasms of the brain. J Neurosurg 66:1, 1987
44. Bleyer WA, Griffin TW: White Matter Necrosis, Mineralizing Microangiopathy, and Intellectual Abilities in Survivors of Childhood Leukemia. In Gilbert HA, Kagan AR (eds): Radiation Damage to the Nervous System, p 155. New York, Raven Press, 1980
45. Meadows AT, Gordon J, Massari DJ et al: Declines in IQ scores and cognitive dysfunction in children with acute lymphocytic leukemia treated with cranial irradiation. Lancet 1:1015, 1981
46. Ochs J, Ch'ien L, Parvey L et al: Comparison of central nervous system (CNS) toxicity between two methods of CNS prophylaxis—1800 R cranial radiation and moderate dose methotrexate infusion (MDMTX)/gm/m²—in childhood acute lymphocytic leukemia. Proc Am Soc Clin Oncol 2:75, 1983
47. Maire JPh, Coudin B, Guerin J et al: Neuropsychologic impairment in adults with brain tumors. Am J Clin Oncol 10:156, 1987
48. Sheline GE, Wara WM, Smith V: Therapeutic irradiation and brain injury. Int J Radiat Oncol Biol Phys 6:1215, 1980
49. Marks JE, Baglan RJ, Prassad SC et al: Cerebral radionecrosis: Incidence and risk in relation to dose, time, fractionation and volume. Int J Radiat Oncol Biol Phys 7:243, 1981
50. Wara WM, Sheline GE, Newman H et al: Radiation therapy of meningiomas. Am J Roentgenol Radium Ther Nucl Med 123:453, 1975
51. Van der Kogel AJ, Barendsen GW: Late effects of spinal cord irradiation with 300 kV x-rays and 15 MeV neutrons. Br J Radiol 47:393, 1974
52. Ang KK, Van der Kogel AJ, van der Scheuren E: Lack of evidence for increased tolerance of rat spinal cord with decreasing fraction doses below 2 Gy. Int J Radiat Oncol Biol Phys 11:105, 1985
53. Hochberg FH, Pruitt A: Assumptions in the radiotherapy of glioblastoma. Neurology 30:907, 1980
54. Kelly PJ, Dauman-Duport C, Kispert DB et al: Imaging-based stereotaxic serial biopsies in untreated intracranial glial neoplasms. J Neurosurg 66:865, 1987
55. Choucair AK, Levin VA, Gutin PH et al: Development of multiple lesions during radiation therapy and chemotherapy in patients with gliomas. J Neurosurg 65:654, 1986
56. Levin VA: Pharmacokinetics and CNS Chemotherapy. In Hellmann K, Carter SK (eds): Fundamentals of Cancer Chemotherapy, p 28. New York, McGraw-Hill, 1986
57. Levin VA, Patlak CS, Landahl HD: Heuristic modeling of drug delivery to malignant brain tumors. J Pharmacokinet Biopharm 8:257, 1980
58. Levin VA: Chemotherapy of primary brain tumors. In Vick NA, Bigner DD (eds): Neuro-Oncology, Neurologic Clinics of North America, Third edition, p 855. Philadelphia, W.B. Saunders, 1985
59. Kumar ARV, Renaudin J, Wilson CB et al: Procarbazine hydrochloride in the treatment of brain tumors. J Neurosurg 40:365, 1974
60. Weiss HD, Walker MD, Wiernik PH: Neurotoxicity of commonly used antineoplastic agents. N Engl J Med 291:75, 1974
61. Feun LG, Wallace S, Yung WK et al: Phase I trial of intracarotid BCNU and cisplatin in patients with malignant intracerebral tumors. Cancer Drug Deliv 1:239–245, 1984
62. Stewart DJ, Grahovac Z, Benoit B et al: Intracarotid chemotherapy with a combination of 1,3-*bis*(2-chloroethyl)-1-nitrosourea (BCNU), *cis*-diaminedichloroplatinum (cisplatin), and 4′-O-demethyl-1-O-(4,6-O-2-thenylidene-beta-D-glucopyranosyl) epipodophyllotoxin (VM-26) in the treatment of primary and metastatic brain tumors. Neurosurgery 15:828–833, 1984
63. Bloom HJG: Intracranial tumors: Response and resistance to therapeutic endeavors 1970–1980. Int J Radiat Oncol Biol Phys 8:1083, 1982
64. Laws ER Jr, Taylor WF, Clifton MB et al: Neurosurgical management of low-grade astrocytoma of the cerebral hemispheres. J Neurosurg 61:665, 1984
65. Leibel SA, Sheline GE, Wara WM et al: The role of radiation therapy in the treatment of astrocytomas. Cancer 35:1551, 1975
66. Kernohan JW, Sayre GP: Tumors of the central nervous system. Atlas of Tumor Pathology, Section 10, Fascicle 35. Washington, DC: Armed Forces Institute of Pathology, 1952
67. Fazekas JT: Treatment of grade I and II brain astrocytomas: The role of radiotherapy. Int J Radiat Oncol Biol Phys 2:661, 1977
68. Chang CH, Horton J, Schoenfeld D et al: Comparison of postoperative radiotherapy and combined postoperative radiotherapy and chemotherapy in the multidisciplinary management of malignant gliomas. Cancer 52:997, 1983
69. Sheline GE: Radiation therapy of primary tumors. Semin Oncol 2:29, 1975
70. Marsa GW, Goffinet DR, Rubinstein LJ et al: Megavoltage irradiation in the treatment of gliomas of the brain and spinal cord. Cancer 36:1681, 1975
71. Kramer S: Radiation therapy in the management of malignant gliomas. In: Cancer of the Central Nervous System. Proceedings of the Seventh National Cancer Conference, p 823. Philadelphia, JB Lippincott, 1983
72. Gastrointestinal Tumor Study Group: Adjuvant therapy of colon cancer: Results of a prospectively randomized trial. N Engl J Med 310:737–743, 1984
73. Laws ER, Taylor WF, Clifton MB et al: Neurosurgical management of low-grade astrocytoma of the cerebral hemispheres. J Neurosurg 61:665–673, 1984
74. Waller MD, Alexander E Jr, Hunt WE et al: Evaluation of BCNU and/or radiotherapy in the treatment of anaplastic gliomas: A cooperative clinical trial. J Neurosurg 49:333–343, 1978
75. Andreou J, George AE, Wise A et al: CT prognostic criteria of survival after malignant glioma surgery. Am J Neuroradiol 4:488, 1983
76. Kumar ARV, Hoshino T, Wheeler KT et al: Comparative rates of dead tumor cell removal from brain, muscle, subcutaneous tissue, and peritoneal cavity. JNCI 52:1751, 1974
77. Gutin PH, Leibel SA, Wara WM et al: Recurrent malignant gliomas: Survival following interstitial brachytherapy with high activity iodine-125 sources. J Neurosurg 67:864–873, 1987
78. DeVita VT Jr: The relationship between tumor mass and resistance to chemotherapy: Implication for surgical adjuvant treatment of cancer. Cancer 51:1209, 1983
79. Young B, Oldfield EH, Markesbery WR et al: Reoperation for glioblastoma. J Neurosurg 55:917, 1981
80. Salcman M, Kaplan RS, Ducher TB et al: Effect of age and reoperation on survival on the combined modality treatment of malignant astrocytoma. Neurosurg 10:454, 1982
81. Harsh GR, Levin VA, Gutin PH et al: Reoperation for recurrent glioblastomas and anaplastic astrocytomas. Neurosurg 21:615–621, 1987
82. Wallner KE, Wara WM, Sheline GE et al: Efficacy of postoperative irradiation for incompletely excised acoustic neuromas. J Neurosurg 67:858–863, 1987
83. Walker MD, Alexander E Jr, Hunt WE et al: Evaluation of BCNU and/or radiotherapy in the treatment of anaplastic gliomas: A cooperative clinical trial. J Neurosurg 49:333, 1978
84. Walker MD, Strike TA, Sheline GE: An analysis of dose-effect relationship in the radiotherapy of malignant gliomas. Int J Radiat Oncol Biol Phys 5:1725, 1979
85. Walker MD, Green SB, Byar DP et al: Randomized comparison of radiotherapy and nitrosoureas for the treatment of malignant glioma after surgery. N Engl J Med 303:1323, 1980
86. Green SB, Byar DP, Walker MD et al: Comparison of carmustine, procarbazine, and high-dose methylprednisolone as additions to surgery and radiotherapy for the treatment of malignant glioma. Cancer Treat Rep 67:1, 1983
87. Nelson DF, Schoenfeld D, Weinstein AS et al: A randomized comparison of misonidazole sensitized radiotherapy plus BCNU and radiotherapy plus BCNU for treatment of malignant glioma after surgery: Preliminary results of an RTOG study. Int J Radiat Oncol Biol Phys 9:1143, 1983
88. Paoletti P, Cuna GRD, Knerich R et al: Multidisciplinary treatment for central nervous system tumors with nitrosourea compounds. Acta Neurochir 41:287, 1978
89. Eyre HJ, Quagliana JM, Eltringham JR et al: Randomized comparisons of radiotherapy and CCNU versus radiotherapy, CCNU plus procarbazine for the treatment of malignant gliomas following surgery. J Neuro-Oncol 1:171, 1983

90. Adinolfi D, Buoncristiani P, Casotto A et al: Multidisciplinary treatment for brain tumors. J Neurosurg Sci 22:111, 1978
91. E.O.R.T.C. Brain Tumor Group: Effect of CCNU on survival rate of objective remission and duration of free interval in patients with malignant brain glioma: Final evaluation. Eur J Cancer 14:851, 1978
92. Feun LG, Steward DJ, Maor M et al: A pilot study of *cis*-diamminedichloroplatinum and radiation therapy in patients with high grade astrocytomas. J Neuro-oncol 1:109, 1983
93. Shapiro WR: Therapy of adult malignant brain tumors: What have the clinical trials taught us? Semin Oncol 13:38, 1986
94. Wilson CB, Gutin PH, Boldrey EB et al: Single-agent chemotherapy of brain tumors. Arch Neurol 33:739, 1976
95. Fewer D, Wilson CB, Boldrey EB et al: Phase II study of 1-(2-chloroethyl)-3-cyclohexyl-1-nitrosourea (CCNU) in the treatment of brain tumors. Cancer Chemother Rep 56:421, 1972
96. Levin VA, Resser K, McGrath L et al: PCNU treatment for recurrent malignant gliomas. Cancer Treat Rep 68:969, 1984
97. Gutin PH, Wilson CB, Kumar ARV et al: Phase II study of procarbazine, CCNU, vincristine combination chemotherapy in the treatment of malignant brain tumors. Cancer 35:1398, 1975
98. Levin VA, Wara WM, Davis RL et al: Phase III comparison of chemotherapy with BCNU and the combination of procarbazine, CCNU, and vincristine administered after radiation therapy with hydroxyurea to patients with malignant gliomas. J Neurosurg 63:218, 1985
99. Schold SC, Friedman HS, Bjornsson TD et al: Treatment of patients with recurrent primary brain tumors with AZQ. Neurology 34:615, 1984
100. Prados MD, Rodriguez L, Seager M et al: Phase II study of spirohydantoin mustard for the treatment of recurrent malignant gliomas. Cancer Treat Rep 71:1105–1106, 1987
101. Levin VA, Wilson CB, Davis R et al: Phase III comparison study of BCNU, hydroxyurea and irradiation for the treatment of primary malignant gliomas. J Neurosurg 51:526, 1979
102. Levin VS, Wara WM, Davis RL et al: NCOG protocol 6G91: Seven drug chemotherapy and irradiation for patients with glioblastoma multiforme. Cancer Treat Rep 70:739, 1986
103. Fulton DS, Levin VA, Wara WM et al: Chemotherapy of pediatric brain stem tumors. J Neurosurg 54:721, 1981
104. Byar DP, Green SB, Strike TA: Prognostic factors for malignant glioma. In Walker MD (ed): Oncology of the Nervous System, p 379. Boston, Martinus Nijhoff, 1983
105. Rosenblum ML, Gerosa MA, Wilson CB et al: Stem cell studies of human brain tumors. J Neurosurg 58:170, 1983
106. Thomas DGT, Darling JL, Paul EA et al: Assay of anti-cancer drugs in tissue culture: Relationship of relapse free interval (RFI) and in vitro chemosensitivity in patients with malignant cerebral glioma. Br J Cancer 51:525, 1985
107. Rosenblum ML, Reynolds AF, Smith KA et al: Chloroethyl-cyclohexyl-nitrosourea (CCNU) in the treatment of malignant brain tumors. J Neurosurg 39:306, 1973
108. Levin VA, Crafts D, Wilson CB et al: Imidazole carboxamides: Relationship of lipophilicity to activity against intracerebral murine glioma 26 and preliminary phase II clinical trial of 5-(3,3-bis chloroethyl)-1-triazeno)-imidazole-4-carboxamide (NSC-82196) in primary and secondary brain tumors. Cancer Chemother Rep 59:107, 1975
109. Decker DA, Al-Sarraf M, Kresge C et al: Phase II study of aziridinylbenzoquinone (AZQ:NSC-182986) in the treatment of malignant gliomas recurrent after radiation. Preliminary report. J Neuro-oncol 3:19, 1985
110. Fewer D, Wilson CB, Boldrey EB et al: Chemotherapy of brain tumors: Clinical experience with carmustine and vincristine. JAMA 222:549, 1972
111. Levin VA, Hoffman WF, Pischer TL et al: BCNU-5-fluorouracil combination in the treatment of recurrent malignant brain tumors. Cancer Treat Rep 62:2071, 1978
112. Levin VA, Phuphanich S, Liu H-C et al: Phase II study of combined BCNU, 5-fluorouracil, hydroxyurea, and 6-mercaptopurine (BFHM) for the treatment of malignant gliomas. Cancer Treat Rep 70:1271, 1986
113. Levin VA, Chamberlain MC, Prados MD et al: Phase I-II study of eflornithine and mitoguazone combined in the treatment of recurrent primary brain tumors. Cancer Treat Rep 71:459, 1987
114. Chamberlain MC, Prados MD, Silver P et al: A phase II trial of oral melphalan in recurrent primary brain tumors. Am J Clin Oncol 11:52–54, 1988
115. Schold SC Jr, Mahaley MS Jr, Vick NA et al: Phase II diaziquone-based chemotherapy trials in patients with anaplastic supratentorial astrocytic neoplasms. J Clin Oncol 5:464, 1987
116. Allen JC, Bloom J, Ertel I et al: Brain tumors in children: Current cooperative and institutional chemotherapy trials in newly diagnosed and recurrent disease. Semin Oncol 13:110, 1986
117. Eifel PJ, Cassady JR, Belli JA: Radiation therapy of tumors of the brainstem and midbrain in children: Experience of the Joint Center For Radiation Therapy and Children's Hospital Medical Center (1971–1981). In J Rad Oncol Biol Phys 13:847, 1987
118. Coffey RJ, Lunsford LD: Stereotactic surgery for mass lesions of the midbrain and pons. Neurosurgery 17:12, 1985
119. Jenkin D: Posterior fossa tumors in childhood: Radiation treatment. Clin Neurosurg 30:203, 1983
120. Levin VA, Edwards MS, Wara WM et al: 5-fluorouracil and CCNU followed by hydroxyurea, misonidazole and irradiation for brain stem gliomas: A pilot study of the Brain Tumor Research Center and Children's Cancer Group. Neurosurgery 14:679, 1984
121. Rodriguez L, Prados M, Fulton D et al: Treatment of recurrent brain stem glioma and other CNS tumors with 5-fluorouracil, CCNU, hydroxyurea, and 6-mercaptopurine. Neurosurgery 22:691–693, 1988
122. Humphreys RP: Posterior cranial fossa brain tumors in children. In Youmans JR (ed): Youmans Neurological Surgery, p 2747. Philadelphia, W.B. Saunders, 1982
123. Walsh FB, Hoyt WF: Clinical Neuro-ophthalmology, p 2076. Baltimore, Williams & Wilkins, 1969
124. Lewis RA, Gerson LP, Axelson KA et al: von Recklinghausen neurofibromatosis. II. Incidence of optic gliomata. Ophthalmology 91:929–935, 1984
125. Housepian EM, Trokel SL, Jakobiec FO et al: Tumors of the orbit. In Youmans JR (ed): Youmans Neurological Surgery, p 3024. Philadelphia, W.B. Saunders, 1982
126. Packer RJ, Sutton LN, Bilaniuk LT et al: Treatment of chiasmatic/hypothalamic gliomas of childhood with chemotherapy: an update. Ann Neurol 23:79–85, 1988
127. Housepian EM: Surgical treatment of unilateral optic nerve gliomas. J Neurosurg 31:604, 1969
128. Wong JYC, Uhl V, Wara WM et al: Optic gliomas: A re-analysis of the UCSF experience. Cancer 60:1847–1855, 1987
129. Montgomery AB, Griffin T, Parker RG et al: Optic nerve glioma: the role of radiation therapy. Cancer 40:2079, 1977
130. Danoff BF, Kramer S, Thompson N: The radiotherapeutic management of optic nerve gliomas in children. Int J Radiat Oncol Biol Phys 6:45, 1980
131. Horowich A, Bloom HJG: Optic gliomas: Radiation therapy and prognosis. Int J Radiat Oncol Biol Phys 11:1067, 1985
132. Ludwig CL, Smith MT, Godfrey AD et al: A clinicopathologic study of 323 patients with oligodendrogliomas. Ann Neurol 19:15–21, 1986
133. Sheline GE, Boldrey E, Karlsberg P et al: Therapeutic considerations in tumors affecting the central nervous system: oligodendrogliomas. Radiology 82:84, 1964
134. Chin HW, Hazel JJ, Kim TH et al: Oligodendrogliomas. I. A clinical study of cerebral oligodendrogliomas. Cancer 45:1458, 1980
135. Kernohan JW, Sayre GP: Tumors of the central nervous system. Atlas of Tumor Pathology, Section 10, Fascicle 35. Washington, DC: Armed Forces Institute of Pathology, 1952
136. Svien HJ, Mabon RF, Kernohan JW et al: Ependymoma of the brain: Pathologic aspects. Neurology 3:1, 1953
137. Wallner KE, Wara WM, Sheline GE et al: Intracranial ependymomas: Results of treatment with partial or whole brain irradiation without spinal irradiation. Int J Radiat Oncol Biol Phys 12:1937, 1986
138. Levin VA, Edwards MSB, Gutin PH et al: Phase II evaluation of dibromodulcitol in the treatment of recurrent medulloblastoma, ependymoma, and malignant astrocytoma. J Neurosurg 61:1063, 1984
139. Cushing H, Eisenhardt L: Meningiomas, Vol I. Their Classification, Regional Behavior, Life History and Surgical End Results, p 73. Springfield, IL, Charles C Thomas, 1938
140. Hoshino T, Nagashima T, Murovic J et al: Cell kinetic studies of in situ human brain tumors with bromodeoxyuridine. Cytometry 6:627, 1985
141. Simpson D: The recurrence of intracranial meningiomas after surgical treatment. J Neurol Neurosurg Psychiat 20:22, 1957
142. Mirimanoff RO, Dosoretz DE, Linggood RM et al: Meningioma: Analysis of recurrence and progression following neurosurgical resection. J Neurosurg 62:18, 1985
143. Barbaro NM, Gutin PH, Wilson CB et al: Radiation therapy in the treatment of partially resected meningiomas. Neurosurgery 20:525, 1987
144. Solan MJ, Kramer S: The role of radiation therapy in the management of intracranial meningiomas. Int J Radiat Oncol Biol Phys 11:675, 1985
145. Schaumberg HH, Plank CR, Adams RD: The reticulum cell sarcoma-microglioma group of brain tumors. A consideration of their clinical features and therapy. Brain 95:199, 1972
146. Schneck SA, Penn I: De novo brain tumors in renal transplant recipients. Lancet 1:983, 1971
147. Pitchenik AE, Fischl MA, Walls KW: Evaluation of cerebral-mass lesions in acquired immunodeficiency syndrome. N Engl J Med 308:1099, 1983
148. Payan MJ, Gambarelli D, Routy JP et al: Primary lymphoma of the brain associated with AIDS. Acta Neuropathol 64:78, 1984
149. Rosenblum ML, Levy RM, Bredesen DE et al: Primary central nervous system lymphomas in patients with AIDS. Ann Neurol 23 Suppl 513–16, 1988
150. Murray K, Kun L, Cox J: Primary malignant lymphoma of the central nervous system. J Neurosurg 65:600, 1986
151. Neuwelt EA, Frenkel EP, Gumerlock MK et al: Developments in the diagnosis and treatment of primary CNS lymphoma. Cancer 58:1609, 1986
152. McComb RD, Burger PC: Pathologic Analysis of Primary Brain Tumors. In Vick NA, Bigner DD (eds): Neurologic Clinics, p 711. Philadelphia, W.B. Saunders, 1985
153. Berger MS, Edwards MD, Wara WM et al: Primary cerebral neuroblastoma: Long-term follow-up review and therapeutic guidelines. J Neurosurg 59:418, 1983
154. Bloom HJG: Medulloblastoma in children: Increasing survival rates and further prospects. Int J Radiat Oncol Biol Phys 8:2023, 1982
155. Deutsch M: The impact of myelography on the treatment results for medulloblastoma. Int J Radiat Oncol Biol Phys 10:999, 1984
156. Levin VA, Rodriguez LA, Edwards MSB et al: Treatment of medulloblastoma with procarbazine, hydroxyurea, and reduced radiation doses to whole brain and spine. J Neurosurg 68:383–387, 1988
157. Park TS, Hoffman HJ, Hendrick EB et al: Medulloblastoma: Clinical presentation and

management. Experience at the Hospital for Sick Children, Toronto, 1950–1980. J Neurosurg 58:543, 1983
158. Lowery GS, Kimball JC, Patterson RB et al: Extraneural metastases from cerebellar medulloblastoma. Am J Ped Hem/Oncol 4:259, 1982
159. Bloom HJG, Thornton H, Schweisguth O: SIOP medulloblastoma and high grade ependymoma therapeutic clinical trails: Preliminary results (1975–1981). In: Pediatric Oncology, C Raybaud, R Clement, G Lebreuli, JL Bernard (eds). Amsterdam, Excerpta Medica, 1982, p 309
160. Benjamin RS, Wiernik PH, Bachur NR: Adriamycin chemotherapy: Efficacy, safety, and pharmacologic basis of an intermittent single high-dose schedule. Cancer 33:19–27, 1974
161. Kun LE, D'Souza B, Tefft M: The value of surveillance testing in childhood brain tumors. Cancer 56(7 suppl):1818, 1985
162. Shapiro WR: Chemotherapy of primary malignant brain tumors. Cancer in Children 35:965, 1975
163. Ward HWC: Central nervous system tumors of childhood treated with CCNU, vincristine and radiation. Med Ped Oncol 4:315, 1978
164. Garrett MJ, Hughs HJ, Ryall RDH: CCNU in brain tumors. Clin Radiol 25:183, 1974
165. Ward HWC: CCNU in the treatment of recurrent medulloblastoma. Br Med J 1:642, 1974
166. Hancock C, Allen J, Tan CTC: Phase II trial of PCNU in children with recurrent brain tumors and Hodgkin's disease. Cancer Treat Rep 68:441, 1984
167. Walker RW, Allen JC: Treatment of recurrent primary intracranial childhood tumors with cis-diamminedi-chloroplatinum. Ann Neurol 14:371, 1983
168. Bertolone SJ, Baum E, Krivit W et al: Phase II trial of cisplatinum diamino dichloride (CPDD) in recurrent childhood brain tumors: A CCSG trial. Proc Am Assoc Cancer Res 2:72, 1983
169. Sexauer CL, Kahn A, Burger PC et al: Cis-platinum in recurrent pediatric brain tumors: A POG Phase II study. Cancer 56:1497, 1985
170. Allen JC, Walker R, Luks E et al: Carboplatin and recurrent childhood brain tumors. J Clin Oncol 5:459, 1987
171. Allen JC, Helson L: High-dose cyclophosphamide chemotherapy for recurrent CNS tumors in children. J Neurosurg 55:749, 1981
172. Rosen G, Ghavimi F, Nirenberg A et al: High-dose methotrexate with citrovorum factor rescue for the treatment of central nervous system tumors in children. Cancer Treat Rep 61:681, 1977
173. Djerassi I, Kim JS, Shulman K: High-dose methotrexate-citrovorum factor rescue in the management of brain tumors. Cancer Treat Rep 61:691, 1977
174. Mooney C, Souhami R, Pritchard J: Recurrent medulloblastoma: Lack of response to high-dose methotrexate. Cancer Chemother Pharmacol 10:135, 1983
175. Haddy TB, Ferbach DJ, Watkins WL et al: Vincristine in uncommon malignant disease in children. Cancer Chemother Rep 41:41, 1964
176. Lassman LP, Pearce GW, Gang J: Effect of vincristine sulfate on the intracranial gliomata of childhood. Br J Surg 53:774, 1966
177. Lampkin BC, Maurer AM, McBride BH: Response of medulloblastoma to vincristine sulfate: A case report. Pediatrics 39:761, 1967
178. Smart CR, Ottoman RE, Rochlin DB et al: Clinical experience with vincristine in tumors of the central nervous system and other malignant diseases. Cancer Chemother Rep 52:733, 1968
179. Afra D: Vincristine therapy in malignant glioma recurrencies. Neurochirurgia 16:189, 1973
180. Van Eys J, Cangir A, Coody D et al: MOPP regimen as primary chemotherapy for brain tumors in infants. J Neurol Oncol 3:237, 1985
181. Rosenstock JG, Evans AE, Schut L: Response to vincristine of recurrent brain tumors in children. J Neurosurg 45:135, 1976
182. Christ WM, Ragab AH, Vietti TJ et al: Chemotherapy of childhood medulloblastoma. Am J Dis Child 13:639, 1976
183. Skylansky BD, Mann-Kaplan RS, Reynolds BF et al: 4'-Demethyl-epipodophyllotoxin--D-thenylidene-glucoside (PTG) in the treatment of malignant intracranial neoplasms. Cancer 33:460, 1974
184. Crafts DC, Levin VA, Edwards MS et al: Chemotherapy of recurrent medulloblastoma with combined procarbazine, CCNU, vincristine. J Neurosurg 49:589, 1978
185. Duffner PK, Cohen ME, Thomas PRM et al: Combination chemotherapy in recurrent medulloblastoma. Cancer 43:41, 1979
186. Seiler RW: Combination chemotherapy with VM26 and CCNU in primary malignant brain tumors of children. Helv Paediat Acta 35:51–56, 1980
187. Cangir A, Van Eyes J, Berry DH et al: Combination chemotherapy with MOPP in children with recurrent brain tumors. Med Ped Oncol 4:253, 1978
188. Cangir A, Ragab AH, Steubner P et al: Combination chemotherapy with vincristine, procarbazine, prednisone with or without nitrogen mustard (MOOP vs OPP) in children with recurrent brain tumors. Med Ped Oncol 12:1, 1984
189. Freidman HS, Mahaley MS, Schold SC Jr et al: The efficacy of vincristine and cyclophosphamide in the therapy of recurrent medulloblastoma. Neurosurgery 18:335, 1986
190. Thomas PR, Duffner PK, Cohen ME et al: Multimodality therapy for medulloblastoma. Cancer 45:666, 1980
191. Christ WM, Ragab AH, Vietti TJ et al: Chemotherapy of childhood medulloblastoma. Am J Dis Child 13:639, 1976
192. Nathanson L, Kovacs SG: Chemotherapeutic response in metastatic medulloblastoma: Report of two cases and a review of the literature. Med Pediat Oncol 4:105, 1978
193. Hoffman HJ: Pineal region tumors. Prog Exp Tumor Res 30:281, 1987
194. Matsutani M, Takakura K, Sano K: Primary intracranial germ cell tumors: Pathology and treatment. Prog Exp Tumor Res 30:307, 1987
195. Herrick MK: Pathology of Pineal Tumors. In Neuwelt EA (ed): Diagnosis and Treatment of Pineal Region Tumors, p 31. Baltimore, Williams & Wilkins, 1984
196. Edwards MSB, Levin VA: Chemotherapy of Third Ventricle tumors. In Appuzzo M (ed): Third Ventricular Tumors, p 838. Baltimore, Williams & Wilkins, 1987
197. Schmidek HH, Waters A: Pineal masses: Clinical features and management. In Wilkins RH, Rengachary SS (eds): Neurosurgy, p 688. New York, McGraw-Hill, 1985
198. Pecker J, Scarabin J-M, Vallee B et al: Treatment in tumours of the pineal region: Value of stereotaxic biopsy. Surg Neurol 12:341, 1979
199. Wara WM, Fellows CF, Sheline GE et al: Radiation therapy for pineal tumors and suprasellar germinomas. Radiology 124:221, 1977
200. Salazar OM, Castro-Vita H, Bakos RS et al: Radiation therapy for tumors of the pineal region. Int J Radiat Oncol Biol Phys 5:491, 1979
201. Matsukado Y, Abe H, Tanaka R et al: [Cisplatin, vinblastine and bleomycin (PVB) combination chemotherapy in the treatment of intracranial malignant germ cell tumors — a preliminary report of a phase II study — The Japanese Intracranial Germ Cell Tumor Study Group]. Gan No Rinsho 32:1387, 1986
202. Wilson CB: Surgical Management of Endocrine-Active Pituitary Adenomas. In Walker MD (ed): Oncology of the Nervous System, p 117. Boston, Martinus-Nijhoff, 1983
203. Ross DA, Wilson CB: Results of transsphenoidal microsurgery for growth hormone-secreting pituitary adenoma in a series of 214 patients. J Neurosurg 68:854–867, 1988
204. Sheline GE, Tyrrell JB: Pituitary Tumors. In Perez CA, Brady LW (eds): Principles and Practice of Radiation Oncology, p 1108. Philadelphia, J.B. Lippincott, 1987
205. Eastman RC, Gorden P, Roth J: Conventional supervoltage irradiation is an effective treatment for acromegaly. J Clin Endocrin Metab 48:931, 1979
206. Orth DN, Liddle GW: Results of treatment in 108 patients with Cushing's syndrome. N Engl J Med 285:243, 1971
207. Jennings AS, Liddle GW, Orth DN: Results of treating childhood Cushing's disease with pituitary irradiation. N Engl J Med 297:957, 1977
208. Bloom B, Kramer S: Conventional Radiation Therapy in the Management of Acromegaly. In Black P, et al (eds): Secretory Tumors of the Pituitary Gland, Vol 1, p 179. New York, Raven Press, 1984
209. Strauss L, Sturm V, Georgi P et al: Radioisotope therapy of cystic craniopharyngiomas. Int J Radiat Oncol Biol Phys 8:1581, 1982
210. Sung DI, Chang CH, Harisiadis L et al: Treatment results of craniopharyngiomas. Cancer 47:847, 1981
211. Carmel PW, Antunes J, Chang CH: Craniopharyngiomas in children. Neurosurgery 11:382, 1982
212. Baskin DS, Wilson CB: Surgical management of craniopharyngiomas. J Neurosurg 65:22, 1986
213. Buchheit WA, Delgado TE: Tumors of the Cerebellopontine Angle: Clinical Features and Surgical Management. In Wilkins RH, Rengachary SS (eds): Neurosurgery, p 720. New York, McGraw-Hill, 1985
214. Martuza RL, Ojemann RG: Bilateral acoustic neuromas: Clinical aspects, pathogenesis, and treatment. Neurosurgery 10:1, 1982
215. Farriro JB III, Hyams VL, Benke RH et al: Carcinoid apudoma arising in glomus jugulare tumors. Laryngoscope 90:110, 1980
216. Simko TG, Griffin TW, Gerdes AJ et al: The role of radiation therapy in the treatment of glomus jugulare tumors. Cancer 42:104, 1978
217. Gardner G, Cocke EW Jr, Robertson JT et al: Glomus jugulare tumors: Combined treatment. Part I. J Laryngol Otol 95:437, 1981
218. Kim J-A, Elkon D, Lim M-L et al: Optimum dose of radiotherapy for chemodectomas of the middle ear. Int J Radiat Oncol Biol Phys 6:815, 1980
219. Heffelfinger MJ, Dahlin DC, MacCarty CS et al: Chordomas and cartilaginous tumors at the skull base. Cancer 32:410, 1973
220. Sung DI, Chang CH, Harisiadis L: Cerebellar hemangioblastomas. Cancer 49:553, 1982
221. Naguib MG, Chou SH, Mastri A: Radiation therapy of a choroid plexus papilloma of the cerebellopontine angle with bone involvement. J Neurosurg 54:245, 1981
222. Connolly ES: Spinal cord tumors in adults. In Youmans JR (ed): Youmans Neurological Surgery, p 3196. Philadelphia, W.B. Saunders, 1982

PHILIP A. PIZZO
MARC E. HOROWITZ
DAVID G. POPLACK
DANIEL M. HAYS
LARRY E. KUN

CHAPTER 47 *Solid Tumors of Childhood*

Despite their rarity, childhood cancers have enlightened the epidemiology, genetics, etiology, and treatment of both pediatric and adult malignancies. There are, however, striking and important differences in the types of malignancies that occur in children compared with adults.

CHILDHOOD CANCER

EPIDEMIOLOGY

Approximately 6500 new cases of childhood cancer are diagnosed each year in the United States. Cancer is second only to accidents as the leading cause of death in children younger than 15 years of age. Table 47-1 lists the relative incidence of the most common childhood cancers. Leukemias and lymphomas comprise almost 48% of pediatric cancers, followed by tumors of the central nervous system (20%), the sympathetic nervous system, soft tissues, kidney, bone, liver, eye, and germ cells. These malignancies often have a high growth fraction and a propensity for rapid growth. In contrast to adults, carcinomas are rare during childhood. Pediatric tumors are characterized by unique age peaks, and some have sex, genetic, race, and geographic predilections.

Age is important in pediatric cancer in at least three ways. First, as shown in Table 47-2, the predominant type of childhood cancer varies according to the age of the child. The incidence of several cancers peaks soon after birth (*e.g.*, neuroblastoma, retinoblastoma), suggesting the role of prenatal events, but other tumors (*e.g.*, lymphomas, bone tumors) increase in frequency with age, suggesting that postnatal events are important. Second, histologically identical malignancies can behave very differently at different ages. For example, neuroblastoma, the most common tumor of infancy, has an excellent prognosis when it occurs in infants younger than 1 year of age, but it has a dismal prognosis in older children. Whether these differences reflect biologic properties of the host or the tumor is an unresolved but important issue. Third, the age of the child at diagnosis may predict the tumor's malignant potential. For example, sacrococcygeal tumors rarely have malignant elements when they are diagnosed at birth. However, if diagnosis is delayed until after the child is 2 months old or older (because the mass is intrapelvic and not directly visible), 50% to 70% of these tumors will be malignant.

Sex influences the incidence and outcome of certain pediatric cancers. Most pediatric neoplasms have a male predominance (Table 47-1), although for some tumors, such as Ewing's sarcoma and rhabdomyosarcoma, this does not become apparent until after the age of 13 years. Teratomas are an exception because almost 75% occur in girls, but their potential for malignancy is higher in boys.

Race also influences the distribution and outcome of several pediatric cancers. The cancer rate for black children is approximately 20% less than that for white children. For example, Ewing's sarcoma rarely occurs in American and African blacks. Testicular cancer is also distinctly unusual in black children, and the early age peak observed in white children with acute lymphocytic leukemia (ALL) is not observed in blacks. On the other hand, the prognosis for black children who do develop ALL appears to be worse than for white children, probably because of the predominance of T-cell leukemia in black patients.

During recent years, the geographical diversity of cancer has become better appreciated. For example, although Burkitt's lymphoma accounts for nearly half of the childhood

TABLE 47-1. Incidence of Childhood Cancers

Malignancy	*Rate* *Rate* *(per million/yr)*	*Ratio* *Sex (M:F)*	*Race (W:B)*	*Peak Age* *Peak Age (yr)*
Leukemia				
Acute lymphocytic	24.7	1.3	2.4	2–5
Acute nonlymphocytic	5.0	1.2	1.0	<2
Lymphomas				
Non-Hodgkin's	9.3	2.9		6–16
Hodgkin's	7.5	3.0	1.6	>10
Central Nervous System Tumors				
Gliomas	13.4	>1.0	1.1	Constant
Medulloblastoma	4.9	1.6	0.8	5–10
Ependymoma	2.1	>1.0	2.6	<5
Solid Tumors				
Neuroblastoma	8.0	1.4	1.6	<3
Wilms' tumor	6.9	0.9	0.9	<5
Retinoblastoma	3.0	<1.0	0.8	<3
Rhabdomyosarcoma	3.7	>1.2	0.9	Bimodal: 2–6 and 14–18
Ewing's sarcoma	2.1	>1.0	>1.0	10–18
Osteosarcoma	3.1	>1.0	1.2	10–18
Primary hepatic	1.6	>1.3		Bimodal: <2 and >14
Germ cell teratoma	0.4	0.3	0.8	Bimodal <2 and >14

cancers in Uganda, it is rare outside of the "Burkitt's belt." Conversely, neuroblastoma appears to be exceedingly rare in the Burkitt's belt. Retinoblastoma accounts for only 1% of the childhood cancers in the United States but is far more common in India. Hepatic tumors, which are very rare in the United States, are considerably more frequent in the Far East. The distribution of Hodgkin's disease by subtype also appears to vary geographically, with the more aggressive varieties predominating in developing countries. Some of these differences reflect racial and genetic factors, whereas others are due to variations in the environment and various oncogenic cofactors, like Epstein-Barr virus (EBV), hepatitis B virus, and human T-lymphotropic virus (HTLV).

Geographic clusters of childhood cancers have also been reported, the most famous of which was the putative concentration of childhood leukemia in a single parish in Niles, Illinois, in 1963. A number of such clusters have been described over the years to suggest an association of the malignancy with environmental factors (*e.g.*, viruses, chemical pollution). Most have not held up to detailed investigation, but the recent cluster of leukemia in Woburn, Massachusetts, implicating chemical water pollution is noteworthy and suggests the need for continuing vigilance and research.

Ecogenetics is the study of the interaction between environmental and genetic factors in carcinogenesis, particularly of genetic variations in response to environmental agents. Table 47-3 details environmental agents that interact with specific genetic traits or defects and result in a malignant phenotype. Environmental factors include chemicals, radiation, and viruses, and the genetic predisposition may be created by a sporadic mutation or familial transmission.

GENETICS AND BIOLOGY

The importance of genes and inheritance is exemplified in many childhood cancers. In some families, several members are affected by either the same tumor or by various types of cancers. Certain human tumors are clearly inheritable. For example, approximately 40% of retinoblastomas appear to be inherited as an autosomal dominant trait with high penetrance. Wilms' tumor and neuroblastoma may also be bilateral and inheritable. In spite of this dominant pattern of transmission, it is gene loss that leads to malignancy. The genetic information in the "retinoblastoma locus" on chromosome 13q14 acts to suppress the development of retinoblastoma, and if both alleles are lost (*i.e.*, a recessive mutant), the normal suppression of this tumor is lost and retinoblastoma occurs. In familial retinoblastoma, a loss of both retinoblastoma alleles is transmitted, leading to the expression of disease. In patients who have one copy of the allele, which can effectively suppress the development of retinoblastoma, a mutation, loss, or inactivation of this allele results in retinoblastoma. Similar modes of genetic oncogenesis appear to occur in patients with Wilms' tumor, osteosarcoma, hepatoblastoma, and rhabdomyosarcoma (Table 47-4).[1]

Some genetic disorders are associated with an increased incidence of cancer. For example, children with trisomy 21 (Down's syndrome) have a tenfold increase in the incidence of acute lymphocytic leukemia; those with Klinefelter's syndrome (XXY) have a greater than 60-fold increase in their incidence of breast cancer. Patients with chromosome fragility and defective DNA repair (xeroderma pigmentosa,

TABLE 47-2. Predominant Pediatric Cancers by Age and Site

Tumors	*Newborn (<1 yr)*	*Infancy (1–3 yr)*	*Children (3–11 yr)*	*Adolescents and Young Adults (12–21 yr)*
Leukemias	Congenital leukemia AML AMMoL CML, juvenile	ALL AML CML, juvenile	ALL AML	AML ALL
Lymphomas	Very rare	Lymphoblastic	Lymphoblastic Undifferentiated	Lymphoblastic Undifferentiated—Burkitt's Hodgkin's
Solid Tumors				
CNS	Medulloblastoma Ependymoma Astrocytoma Choroid plexus papilloma	Medulloblastoma Ependymoma Astrocytoma Choroid plexus papilloma	Cerebellar astrocytoma Medulloblastoma Astrocytoma Ependymoma Craniopharyngioma	Cerebellar astrocytoma Astrocytoma Craniopharyngioma Medulloblastoma
Head and neck	Retinoblastoma Rhabdomyosarcoma Neuroblastoma MNET	Retinoblastoma Rhabdomyosarcoma Neuroblastoma	Rhabdomyosarcoma Lymphoma	Lymphoma Rhabdomyosarcoma
Thoracic	Neuroblastoma Teratoma	Neuroblastoma Teratoma	Lymphoma Neuroblastoma Rhabdomyosarcoma	Lymphoma Ewing's Rhabdomyosarcoma
Abdominal	Neuroblastoma Mesoblastic nephroma Hepatoblastoma Wilms' (>6 mos)	Neuroblastoma Wilms' Hepatoblastoma Leukemia	Neuroblastoma Wilms' Lymphoma Hepatoma	Lymphoma Hepatocellular carcinoma Rhabdomyosarcoma
Gonadal	Yolk sac tumor of testis (endodermal sinus tumor) Teratoma Sarcoma Botryoides Neuroblastoma	Rhabdomyosarcoma YST of testis Clear cell sarcoma kidney	Rhabdomyosarcoma	Rhabdomyosarcoma Dysgerminoma Teratocarcinoma, teratoma Embryonal carcinoma of testis Embryonal cell and endodermal sinus tumors of ovary
Extremity	Fibrosarcoma	Fibrosarcoma Rhabdomyosarcoma	Rhabdomyosarcoma Ewing's	Osteosarcoma Rhabdomyosarcoma Ewing's sarcoma

Bloom's syndrome, Franconi's anemia) have an increased risk of cancer.

Many translocations specific for malignancies have been identified (Table 47-5). Some translocations are associated with oncogenes (*myc* and the 8 : 14 translocation of Burkitt's lymphoma), and some oncogenes are uniquely associated with certain tumors (N-*myc* in neuroblastoma). The genome of every normal cell contains at least 30 proto-oncogenes.[2] Although the gene product of every oncogene is not known, it is apparent that some of their products play a role in the regulation of cell growth. Thus, the activation or mutation of oncogenes or their translocation next to sites important in growth regulation contribute to malignancy. Although many of the examples in which alteration of growth factors and differentiation contribute to the expression of neoplasia have been in pediatric tumors, the genetic mechanism being elucidated clearly has relevance to adult tumors (Table 47-6).

Certain pediatric tumors have an increased association with congenital disorders, malformations, or syndromes (Table 47-7). Patients with these disorders should be followed with the awareness that they may be at risk for developing a cancer. Because congenital findings may be associated with an inheritable malignancy, such as retinoblastoma and MEN syndromes, genetic counseling of the patient and family is important.

Genetic disorders that alter the immune system (ataxia telangiectasia, Wiskott-Aldrich syndrome) are associated with an increased risk of cancer. The increased occurrence of lymphoma in patients with acquired immune deficiency syndrome (AIDS) emphasizes the integral association between immunoregulation and cancer.

In addition to genetically mediated or transmitted factors, prenatal exposure to certain drugs or substances have been associated with a heightened risk for developing cancer. For example, the fetal alcohol or hydantoin syndromes have been associated with neuroblastoma, and prenatal exposure to diethylstilbestrol increases the risk for adolescent girls to develop a clear cell adenocarcinoma of the vagina.

Some pediatric tumors have the interesting biological property of undergoing spontaneous regression. This is most

TABLE 47-3. Genetic-Environmental Interactions (Ecogenetics) in Tumors of the Young

Environmental Agent	*Genetic Trait*	*Tumor or Outcome*
Ionizing radiation	Ataxia-telangiectasia with lymphoma	Radiation toxicity
	Retinoblastoma	Sarcoma
	Nevoid basal-cell carcinoma syndrome	Basal cell carcinoma
Ultraviolet radiation	Xeroderma pigmentosum	Skin cancer, melanoma
	Cutaneous albinism	Skin caner
	Hereditary dysplastic nevus syndrome	Melanoma
Stilbestrol	XO Turner's syndrome	Adenosquamous endometrial carcinoma
Androgen	Fanconi's pancytopenia	Hepatoma
Iron	Hemochromatosis	Hepatocellular carcinoma
Tyrosine	Tyrosinemia	Hepatocellular carcinoma
Monosaccharides	Glycogen storage disease type I	Hepatic adenoma
Epstein-Barr virus?	Purtilo X-linked lymphoproliferative syndrome	Burkitt's and other lymphomas
Papillomavirus type 5	Epidermodysplasia verruciformis	Skin cancer

Mulvihill JJ: Clinical genetics of pediatric cancer. In Pizzo PA, Poplack DG (eds): Principles and Practice of Pediatric Oncology, p 21. Philadelphia, JB Lippincott, 1989.

common in neuroblastoma, but it has also been noted in retinoblastoma, histiocytosis, sacrococcygeal teratoma, and hepatoblastoma. Study of the genetic controls that affect this differentiation process are central to developing new treatment modalities for these neoplasms. For example, N-*myc* amplification correlates with the stage of neuroblastoma, and lowering N-*myc* expression in vitro with cis-retinoic acid causes differentiation of these cells into more mature neural cells. This suggests that future therapeutic strategies should focus on the differentiation of tumor cells rather than their destruction.

UNUSUAL CLINICAL MANIFESTATIONS

Although most children with cancer come to medical attention because of growing masses, the signs and symptoms of cancer can sometimes be subtle, nonspecific, or confusing and can result in delays in diagnosis and treatment (Table 47-8).

TABLE 47-4. Pediatric Malignancies with Recognized Recessive Genetic Alterations

Tumor	*Chromosomal Alterations*
Retinoblastoma	13q14
Osteosarcoma	13q14
Wilm's tumor	11p13
Embryonal tumors of Beckwith-Wiedermann syndrome	11p
Acoustic neuroma and meningioma	22
Meningioma	22

Israel MA: Molecular and cellular biology of pediatric malignancies. In Pizzo PA, Poplack DG (eds): Principles and Practice of Pediatric Oncology, p 50. Philadelphia, JB Lippincott, 1989.

Several pediatric tumors are biologically active and produce a variety of oncofetal proteins and other substances that may have diagnostic or prognostic value. These indicators, listed in Table 47-9, are measured in serum or in urine. Only rarely do these substances directly affect the patient.

Some pediatric cancers may present with bilateral involvement (Wilms' tumor, retinoblastoma), making thorough examination important before any surgical procedures are performed. Some nonmalignant processes can also be confused with a cancer (*e.g.*, histoplasmosis with lymphoma, osteomyelitis with bone tumors), and some cancers can mimic other malignancies (*e.g.*, neuroblastoma mimics acute lymphoblastic leukemia in the bone marrow or peripheral blood).

PROGNOSTIC FACTORS

Most pediatric cancers can be divided into good and poor prognostic categories. Although the stage, site, and extent of disease have provided the traditional means for classifying patients, additional refinements have been achieved using tumor histology, immunologic typing, and molecular analysis. The identification of risk groups permits therapy to be tailored so that patients likely to do well can receive less intensive and less toxic regimens, and more intensive therapies can be restricted to patients with a poorer prognosis. However, prognostic factors are dynamic and, in some cases, artificial, because improvements in therapy may modify or even nullify previously important risk factors.

Histologic variants of specific pediatric neoplasms have been recognized and correlated with prognosis. For example, Wilms' tumors can now be divided into favorable and unfavorable histologic variants, which correlate with prognosis (*e.g.*, 57% of patients with unfavorable histology die of their tumors compared with 7% of patients with favorable histol-

TABLE 47-5. Cytogenetic Rearrangements in Selected Pediatric Hematopoietic Tumors

Tumor Type	*Chromosomal Rearrangement*
Hematopoietic Tumors	
Acute lymphoblastic leukemia	
Pre-B-cell leukemia	t(1:19)(q23;p13.3)
B-cell leukemia	t(2:8), t(8;14), t(8;22)
	t(11:14)(q13;q23)
Not defined	t(4:11)(q21:q32)
Acute T-cell lymphocytic leukemia	t(11;14)(p13;q13)
Acute nonlymphocytic leukemia	
Acute myelogenous leukemia (M2)	t(8;21)(q22;q22)
Acute promyelocytic leukemia (M3)	t(15;17)(q25;q22)
Acute monoblastic leukemia (M5)	11q, t(9;11)(p21;q23)
Acute nonlymphocytic leukemia with basophils	t(6;9)
Acute nonlymphocytic leukemia with eosinophils	inv(16)(p13q22)
Chronic myelogeneous leukemia	t(9;22)(q3:i;q11)
Non-Hodgkin's lymphoma	
B-cell lymphoma	
Burkitt's lymphoma	t(8:14)(q24;q23)
	t(2:8)(p13;q24)
	t(8:22)(q24;q11)
Large cell lymphoma	del(6) (q21) + 7
T-cell lymphoma	inv(14) (q11.2:q32.2)
	t(8:14)(q2:i;q11.2)
	t(14:14)(q11.2;q32)
Solid Tumors	
Germ cell tumors	i(12p)
Retinoblastoma	del(13) (q14)
Osteogenetic sarcoma	del(13) (q14)
Wilms' tumor	del(11) (p13); t(3;17)
Neuroblastoma	del(1) (p32) (p36), DM, HSR
Rhabdomyosarcoma	3p,t(2:13)(q37;q14), t(2,11)
Ewing's sarcoma	t(11;22)(q24;q12)
Peripheral neuroepithelioma	t(11;22)(q24;q12)
Synovial sarcoma	t(X;18)(q22.1;q11.2)

Israel MA: Molecular and cellular biology of pediatric malignancies. In Pizzo PA, Poplack DG (eds): Principles and Practice of Pediatric Oncology, p 41. Philadelphia, JB Lippincott, 1989.

TABLE 47-6. Oncogenes Located near Structural Genetic Rearrangements in Selected Pediatric Malignancies

Oncogene	*Genetic Rearrangement*	*Tumor*
myc	t(8;14)(q24;q32)	Burkitt's lymphoma
abl	t(9;22)(q34;q11)	Chronic myelogenous leukemia
N-*myc*	DM, HSR	Neuroblastoma
rel	t(2;11)(q37;q14)	Rhabdomyosarcoma
ets	t(11;22)(q24;q12)	Neuroepithelioma

Israel MA: Molecular and cellular biology of pediatric malignancies. In Pizzo PA, Poplack DG (eds): Principles and Practice of Pediatric Oncology, p 49. Philadelphia, JB Lippincott, 1989.

ogy). Similar prognostic correlations can be achieved with immunologic classification (*e.g.*, children with the common acute leukemia antigen, CALLA, on their lymphoblasts fare better than those lacking this antigen). Molecular analysis has permitted the determination of gene rearrangements in children with null cell leukemias, further clarifying the cell lineage and guiding treatment. Pathologic diagnosis and molecular analysis have become particularly important in defining the small, round cell tumors of childhood (*i.e.*, neuroblastoma, rhabdomyosarcoma, Ewing's sarcoma, lymphoma, peripheral neuroectodermal tumors), not only in clarifying important prognostic features, but also in directing new therapeutic approaches. For example, recognition that peripheral neuroepithelial tumors share a t(11;22) abnormality and an oncogene profile with Ewing's sarcoma, rather than with the histologically similar neuroblastoma, has helped to define more appropriate treatment regimens.

MANAGEMENT

The successful management of pediatric cancer requires a carefully orchestrated team comprising a pediatric oncologist; a surgeon; a radiotherapist; diagnostic specialists in radiology, nuclear medicine, pathology, and clinical laboratory data; pediatric, medical, and surgical subspecialty consultants; nurses; pharmacists; and the supportive care services of specialists in physical, respiratory, recreation, and occupational therapy. Because the child with cancer is under enormous physical and emotional stress, appropriate psychosocial resources for the patient and family are important for optimal therapy.

Therapy for certain pediatric tumors has become more specialized, raising the question of whether all children with cancer should be treated at pediatric cancer centers. The complexity of most treatment protocols and the support services necessary to deliver and monitor them has, however, consistently demonstrated a significant survival advantage for children treated in a specialty center compared with a community hospital.[3] An alternative is a shared management plan in which the daily primary care is coordinated by community physicians who work under the guidance of a specialty treatment center.

Although the major modalities of therapy—surgery, radiation, and chemotherapy—are the same for pediatric and adult neoplasms, several features distinguish their application in children.

Surgery

Two principles guide management. First, with rare exception, no child should be considered to have disease that is so far advanced that cure can be ruled out. Second, although there should be no hesitation to perform a radical procedure for cure, every attempt should be made to minimize disability and deformity. With the use of preoperative or neoadjuvant chemotherapy or radiotherapy, tumors resectable with difficulty or loss of function (*i.e.*, hepatoma, rhabdomyosarcoma) have been converted into more readily resectable lesions. Limb-sparing procedures also provide important alter-

TABLE 47-7. Childhood Cancers Associated with Congenital Syndromes or Malformations

Syndrome or Anomaly	*Tumor*
Aniridia	Wilms' tumor
Hemihypertrophy	Wilms' tumor, hepatoblastoma, adrenocortical carcinoma
Genitourinary abnormalities (including testicle maldescent)	Wilms' tumor, Ewing's sarcoma, nephroblastoma, testicular carcinoma
Beckwith-Wiedmann syndrome	Wilms' tumor, neuroblastoma, adrenocortical carcinoma
Dysplastic nevus syndrome	Melanoma
Nevoid basal cell carcinoma syndrome	Basal cell carcinoma, medulloblastoma, rhabdomyosarcoma
Poland's syndrome	Leukemia
Trisomy-21 (Down's syndrome)	Leukemia, retinoblastoma
Bloom's syndrome	Leukemia, gastrointestinal carcinoma
Severe combined immune deficiency disease	EBV-associated B-lymphocyte lymphoma/leukemia
Wiscott-Aldridge syndrome	EBV-associated B-lymphocyte lymphoma
Ataxia telangiectasia	EBV-associated B-lymphocyte lymphoma, gastric carcinoma
Retinoblastoma	Wilms' tumor, osteosarcoma, Ewing's sarcoma
Fanconi's anemia	Leukemia, squamous cell carcinoma
Multiple endocrine neoplasia syndromes (MEN I,II,III)	Anenomas of islet cells, pituitary, parathyroid, and adrenal glands Submucosal neuromas of the tongue, lips, eyelids Pheochromocytomas, medullary carcinoma of the thyroid Malignant schwannoma, nonappendiceal carcinoid
Neurofibromatosis (von Recklinghausen's syndrome)	Rhabdomyosarcoma, fibrosarcoma, pheochromocytomas, optic glioma, meningioma

natives for children with extremity lesions and have become increasingly important with improvements in survival.

Attention should be given to the general principles of pediatric and cancer surgery. In particular, care must be exercised to avoid excessive blood loss because the common tumors of childhood are both large and vascular, either originating in vascular organs (hepatoma) or surrounding major blood vessels, such as the vena cava and aorta (neuroblastoma, Wilms' tumor). Surgical technique must be meticulous and presurgical planning must anticipate a vascular catastrophe. Blood replacement must be readily accomplished. If rapid transfusion is necessary, however, the blood should be warmed to 37°C and its pH buffered to 7.4 to avoid the potential for a cardiac arrest that can occur when large volumes of cold, relatively acid, bank blood [10°C, pH 7.0] are administered to the small child. The surgeon and anesthesiologist must be aware that what is considered insignificant blood loss in an adult may be life-threatening in a small child whose circulating blood volume is small. For example, the loss of 400 ml of blood in a 1-year-old child represents half of the child's blood volume.

Another important difference between children and adults is the greater heat loss that occurs when a child is anesthetized, primarily because of the proportionally large body surface area of children. Hypothermia, cardiac irritability, metabolic acidosis, and clotting abnormalities can result from excessive heat loss. To avoid this, both the operating room and the child should be kept warm and monitored carefully.

Radiation Therapy

As with adults, the primary goal of radiation therapy in children is to deliver an effective tumoricidal dose while sparing as much normal tissue as possible. This goal is more difficult to achieve in young children because of potential growth retardation and second malignancies.

In order to deliver technically acceptable irradiation, careful treatment planning and simulation are essential, as is immobilization and sedation, particularly for the young or uncooperative child. Ketamine anesthesia is particularly useful in young children, especially for those who require multiple treatments.

Although children often tolerate the acute radiation reactions better than adults, late changes in skeletal and soft tissue development are important and unique consequences. Treatment planning should attempt to create symmetry wherever possible, particularly in visible areas, such as the head and neck, or in the spine. Inadequate attention to symmetrical irradiation of growing bone results in abnormal development that may not become apparent until the child enters the pubertal growth phase (*e.g.*, vertebral asymmetry resulting in scoliosis). In addition, soft tissues, teeth, and visual structures may fail to develop normally after irradiation. For example, decreased muscle mass can lead to imbalance and relative asymmetry. Blood vessels and other structures with the radiation field, such as the thyroid and pituitary glands, may develop imperfectly. Brain tissue may be particularly susceptible to late effects, especially when

TABLE 47-8. Nonspecific Clinical Findings Associated with or the Sole Manifestation of a Childhood Cancer

Clinical Findings	*Tumor*
Eye or orbit	
Strabismus	Retinoblastoma
Leukokoria ("cat's eye")	Retinoblastoma
Heterochromia—anisocoria and Horner's syndrome	Neuroblastoma
Opsoclonus—myoclonus ("dancing eyes") or acute cerebellar encephalopathy	Neuroblastoma
Proptosis	Neuroblastoma, lymphoma, retinoblastoma, rhabdomyosarcoma
Chronic sinusitis or otitis media	Rhabdomyosarcoma, nasopharyngeal carcinoma
Chronic diarrhea (Verner-Morrison syndrome)	Neuroblastoma, MEN II
Skin	
"Blueberry muffin" nodules	Neuroblastoma
Seborrheic dermatitis	Histiocytosis
Nodular "blueberry" lips	MEN II
Hypertension	Neuroblastoma, carcinoid, APUD tumors, pheochromocytoma, Wilms'
Virilization	Hepatoblastoma, arrhenoblastoma, adrenal rest tumors, gonadoblastoma
Feminization	Chorioepithelioma, teratoma, hepatoblastoma, adrenal tumor, nongestational choriocarcinoma, embryonal cell carcinoma, granulosa thecal cell tumors

radiation is combined with neurotoxic drugs like methotrexate. Similarly, radiation therapy may exacerbate chemotherapy-induced toxicities, such as doxorubicin-induced cardiomyopathy or cyclophosphamide-related hemorrhagic cystitis. The most sobering consideration is that therapeutic irradiation increases the risk of second tumors.

Chemotherapy

One of the most important features distinguishing pediatric from adult neoplasms is their general chemosensitivity and the possibility that a cure can be attained with combination chemotherapy. Analyses confirm continued improvements during the last decade in the numbers of children with cancer who are being cured.[4] The drugs used in children are usually the same as those used in adults. Combination chemotherapy is the rule and, for the most part, higher dosages of chemotherapeutic agents are employed in children, because, except for newborns, their tolerance of the acute side-effects of chemotherapy is greater than that of adults. Many chemotherapeutic regimens in children consist of more intensive and frequent drug administrations, with less dose modifications for myelosuppression or infection, than in adults. However, appropriate dose adjustment and modification is necessary on a regular basis to account for the normal growth of children. Brain growth relative to body surface area is completed by the age of 3 years, and dosages of intrathecal drugs should have an upper limit based on age rather than body surface area.

Many chemotherapy regimens in children are given over prolonged periods, frequently from 1 to 3 years. Efforts are being directed at defining good risk patients for whom shorter durations of therapy may suffice. Nonetheless, for many children extended courses of treatment are necessary. In attempting to adjust schedules so that school attendance and daily activities can be normal, many treatment protocols use oral therapy patients who are receiving maintenance therapy. Two problems should be considered with oral therapy. First, absorption of oral chemotherapy may result in decreased bioavailability of the chemotherapeutic agent, which can contribute to treatment failure. Second, children, particularly adolescents, may not take medications, necessitating careful monitoring of pediatric cancer patients.

Because long-term survival is achievable in children, and because growing organs may be more susceptible to long-term damage, careful consideration must be given to the chemotherapeutic agents used in children. The magnitude of long-term complications from regimens administered a decade ago are only now being appreciated. The pediatric-oncologist should anticipate the future impact of current strategies.

Supportive Care

The treatment program for the child with cancer cannot focus only on tumor reduction and the physical side-effects of therapy. Every attempt must be made to assure that the child will survive as a functional member of the family and society, and a comprehensive support matrix must offer the child every opportunity to grow and mature as normally as

TABLE 47-9. Biological Markers and Pediatric Tumors

Tumors	*AFP**	*hCG*	*Ferritin*	*Catecholamines*	*NSE*	*LDH*	*Alkaline Phosphatase*	*Polyamine*	*Cystathionine*	*CEA*
Germ cell tumor	+	+				+				+
Liver tumor	+	+	+						+	+
Neuroblastoma			+	+	+	+			+	+
Ewing's sarcoma						+				
Osteosarcoma						+	+			
Medulloblastoma					+			+		
Lymphoma						+				

* AFP = alpha-1-fetoprotein; hCG = human chorionic gonadotropin; NSE = neuron-specific enolase; LDH = lactate dehydrogenase; CEA = Carcinoembryonic antigen; + = reported to be elevated in some or all patients with active disease.

possible. This requires a coordinated school program with educational monitoring and psychological counseling; psychosocial support for the patient, siblings, and family; and occupational, recreational, and physical therapy.

WILMS' TUMOR

EPIDEMIOLOGY AND GENETICS

The annual incidence of Wilms' tumor is 7 per million children younger than 16 years of age, a statistic that varies little from one part of the world to another.[5] One child in ten thousand will develop Wilms' tumor; 350 new cases are diagnosed yearly in the United States, comprising approximately 5% of childhood cancers. The sex ratio is 1 : 1 worldwide; however, a slight preponderance of girls was seen in the National Wilms' Tumor Study (NWTS).[5] The median age at diagnosis in the NWTS experience was 39 months for patients with unilateral tumors and 26 months for those with bilateral tumor.

Congenital anomalies associated with Wilms' tumor include aniridia, hemihypertrophy, malformation of the genitalia (*e.g.*, cryptorchidism, hypospadias, pseudohermaphroditism, gonadal dysgenesis), the Beckwith-Wiedemann, Drash, and Perlman malformation syndromes, and neurofibromatosis.

Case reports and the records of the NWTS-1 document the occurrence of familial Wilms' tumor in about 1% of cases.[5] The mode of inheritance is thought to be autosomal dominant with variable penetrance. According to the "two-hit" mutation model, the pathogenesis of Wilms' tumor lies in the loss of a functioning gene by mutations at homologous loci. Cytogenetic characterization of both somatic and tumor cells from patients with Wilms' tumor has identified the location of this gene at band p13 of chromosome 11. Although the somatic cells of most patients are karyotypically normal, those with aniridia often have a deletion at 11p13 or half-normal levels of catalase, an enzyme mapped to that region of chromosome 11. This constitutional chromosomal abnormality, the "first-hit," may involve enough of the chromosome to be cytogenetically detectable, as is the case with associated aniridia, or may involve only a point mutation at the Wilms' tumor locus. Efforts to map band p13 on chromosome 11 and determine the structure and function of the Wilms' tumor "recessive oncogene" will probably yield a detailed understanding of the molecular basis of this tumor.

PATHOLOGY

Wilms' tumor usually presents as a large mass, the surface of which is smoother than the more irregular and nodular neuroblastoma. The tumor mass is often surrounded by a fibrous pseudocapsule composed of compressed, atrophic renal tissues and may contain cystic areas and necrosis and hemorrhage. Calcification is uncommon. The tumors are most often unicentric, but in the NWTS experience, 7% are multifocal in one kidney and 5.4% involved both kidneys either at the time of presentation or subsequently. Rarely, the tumor is extrarenal, occurring in the retroperitoneum, pelvis, or inguinal region. The local extension of tumor through the capsule and into the perinephric fat is common. Tumor invades the renal vein in 10% of patients, and tumor thrombus may extend to the right atrium. Spread to the lymph nodes of the renal hilum or the perinephric lymph nodes occurs in approximately 20% of patients and is prognostically unfavorable.

As a consequence of its derivation from the metanephric blastema, the histologic spectrum of Wilms' tumor is broad. The typical histologic pattern is triphasic, which includes blastemal, epithelial and stromal cells, with undifferentiated spindle cells surrounding epithelial cell tubules of various sizes and shapes, sometimes forming abortive glomeruli. Biphasic patterns composed of stromal and blastemal cells and monophasic tumors consisting of one cell type are also encountered.[7] A monophasic epithelial Wilms' tumor with papillary or tubular differentiation may be difficult to distinguish from an undifferentiated renal cell carcinoma. Because Wilms' tumor rarely poses a problem in recognition, ultrastructural and immunohistochemical studies, often essential for other childhood tumors, have little utility. Ultrastructurally, the tumor is characterized by numerous desmosomes, cilia, and distinctive flocculent densities surrounding the tumor cells.

There is a subgroup of patients with Wilms' tumor who have *anaplastic tumors*. The tumor cells are characterized by extreme nuclear atypia (anaplasia), which correlates with a poor prognosis. Two sarcomatous variants, clear cell sarcoma and rhabdoid tumor also confer poor prognoses. Anaplasia is recognized by hyperdiploid miotic features, threefold or greater nuclear enlargement, and hyperchromasia of enlarged nuclei. Even a single focus of anaplasia correlates with an adverse prognosis. These histologic markers of hyperploidy have been supported by flow cytofluorometric studies of DNA content in Wilms' tumor.[8] Anaplasia is present in approximately 5% of tumors overall, is rare (2%) in children younger than 2 years, and increasingly frequent in older children, until the incidence reaches 13% in those older than 5 years. Relapses were seen in 27 (55%) of 49 NWTS 1 and NWTS 2 Stage I–III children with anaplastic tumors compared with 101 (14%) of 720 patients with nonanaplastic or "favorable histology" tumors. Stage I patients with anaplastic tumors do as well as those with histologically favorable tumors.

Clear cell sarcoma of the kidney, a distinct entity, occurs in the same age group as Wilms' tumor, but it has a poorer prognosis, with relapse common even in the Stage I patients. The tumor consists of nests of polygonal to stellate cells with small nuclei, inconspicuous nucleoli, and pale vesicular cytoplasm, which forms cords separated by a fine vascular network. This variant of Wilms' tumor has been associated with a high rate of skeletal metastasis and was originally called the "bone-metastasizing renal tumor of childhood."

Rhabdoid tumor of the kidney is a monomorphous tumor with cells containing prominent acidophilic cytoplasm, similar to rhabdomyoblasts, but does not contain ultrastructural features of muscle and immunohistochemical markers. This tumor has no relationship to rhabdomyosarcoma. The cell of origin is unknown, and it may occur outside the kidney. The median age at diagnosis of the cases seen in the NWTS was

13 months, with a range of 2 months to 5 years. Simultaneous primitive neuroectodermal tumors of the brain have developed in children with this variant. The outlook for children with rhabdoid tumor of the kidney is poor. Fewer than 20% of the patients survive, and aggressive chemotherapy has not altered this.

Nephroblastomatosis, a small cluster of blastemal cells, tubules, or stromal cells that is usually situated at the periphery of the renal lobe is thought to be the precursor lesion of Wilms' tumor. Its presence in a kidney biopsy specimen should indicate close clinical follow-up to detect possible evolution of bilateral Wilms' tumor.

Congenital mesoblastic nephroma is a tumor of the newborn or young infant. It is composed of bundles of spindle cells with an interdigitating margin that extends into the renal parenchyma. Although these tumors are usually curable by surgery alone, there are subtypes that contain more cystic components and have a higher mitotic index, indicating a metastatic potential. The tumor has been diagnosed in utero by ultrasound and may be associated with polyhydramnios. This tumor is curable by a standard surgical approach that results in a histologically proven complete resection. Rarely, the tumor may infiltrate the perirenal structures, including the liver. Care must be taken in the resection of tumor infringing upon the capsule of the liver because hemostasis may be difficult to achieve and uncontrollable bleeding may result.

CLINICAL PRESENTATION AND NATURAL HISTORY

Wilms' tumor most frequently presents as an asymptomatic flank or abdominal mass, usually detected on a routine physical exam or discovered by parents when bathing the child. The differential diagnosis includes hydronephrosis, neuroblastoma, and other tumors that present with an abdominal component or organomegaly, such as leukemia, lymphoma, and hepatoma. Wilms' tumor is rare after the age of 7 years. A characteristic presentation of rapid abdominal enlargement, anemia, hypertension, and occasionally, fever with egg-shell calcification visible on plain x-ray films has been attributed to sudden subcapsular hemorrhage. Of 164 patients, 68% presented with abdominal mass, 29% with abdominal pain, 26% with hematuria, 18% with fever, and 14% with anorexia. Elevated blood pressure is present in approximately 25% of patients and is caused by elevated renin.

On physical examination, the abdominal mass of Wilms' tumor is smoother in outline and usually more confined to one side of the abdomen than the irregular and nodular mass of neuroblastoma (Table 47-10). Nonetheless, Wilms' tumor may be bilateral or may grow large enough that it can be felt on both sides of the abdomen. Tumor involvement can be extensive, with infiltration through the renal capsule or invasion into the renal vein (8–40%) through the vena cava to the heart.

Metastatic disease is evident at diagnosis in approximately 15% of patients with Wilms' tumor. The most common sites of hematogenous metastasis are the lung (85%) and liver (15%). Brain metastasis has been diagnosed as a site of recurrence, but this is very rare. With the exception of those with clear cell sarcoma, bone metastasis is uncommon. The regional lymph nodes are involved in 15% to 25% of patients. Positive nodes are associated with unfavorable histology (*i.e.*, anaplasia) and a relatively poor prognosis. In node-positive Wilms' tumor of a favorable histologic pattern, mortality is 17% compared with 97% survival for patients with negative nodes.[9]

EVALUATION

The child with an abdominal mass should be examined thoroughly to arrive at the most likely preoperative diagnosis, assess the local and distant extent of the tumor, and prepare the patient for surgery.

Physical evaluation for evidence of concomitant congenital anomalies should be sought (Table 47-10). Distended abdominal veins may indicate occlusion of the inferior vena cava by tumor thrombus. Routine laboratory studies should also include tests for urine catecholamines. The diagnostic imaging workup of the child with a Wilms' tumor is controversial. The most sensitive tests are not necessarily the best because the very successful treatment of Wilms' tumor is founded on the chest x-ray films and intravenous pyelograms (IVP). The abdominal ultrasound can provide a very accurate assessment of the mass and detect tumor thrombi in renal veins. Ultrasound can delineate tumor extension to the inferior vena cava or right atrium. Abdominal computed tomography (CT) provides the most precise means to assess the tumor lesion. Magnetic resonance imaging (MRI) is useful for diagnosing and staging Wilms' tumor and may replace other techniques because it is noninvasive and does not employ ionizing radiation.

Metastatic workup should include four-view chest x-ray films. The use of lung CT is controversial and not advocated by the NWTS for low-risk children. Should a patient with low-stage disease whose only site of metastasis is a lung nodule, visible on CT scan but not chest x-ray films, be upstaged and treated more aggressively? There are no data to support such an approach, and the majority of Stage I and II patients assessed by chest x-ray films alone are cured. In addition, focal atelectasis or granulomas are indistinguishable from metastatic tumor. Treatment for Stage IV patients with lung disease includes irradiation of the entire thorax; whether patients with lung metastases demonstrated only by CT scan require this therapy is unknown. Postoperatively, patients with a histologic diagnosis of clear cell sarcoma should be staged with bone scan and CT of the brain. This is unnecessary for other variants of Wilms' tumor. The diagnosis of rhabdoid tumor of the kidney warrants brain CT because of its association with brain metastases and primary brain tumors.

STAGING AND PROGNOSTIC FACTORS

A clinicopathologic grouping that determined the extent of tumor at diagnosis and surgery was used in NWTS 1 and 2. Analysis of these clinical trials has resulted in the staging system shown in Table 47-11. Unfavorable histologic types, distant metastasis and lymph node involvement continue to affect prognosis adversely.[10]

TABLE 47-10. Characteristic Features of Wilms' Tumor and Neuroblastoma

Characteristic Features	*Wilms' Tumor*	*Neuroblastoma*
Age of presentation	3.6 years (rare before 6 months)	<2 years (most common tumor of infancy)
Associated congenital anomalies	Aniridia, hemihypertrophy, genitourinary abnormalities	Rare: Beckwith-Wiedmann syndrome, nisidioblastosis, von Recklinghausen's syndrome
Clinical presentation	Smooth, bulging flank mass; may enlarge rapidly; usually confined to one side	Firm and irregular flank mass frequently crossing the midline of abdomen, often fixed
Radiological findings	Intrarenal mass with calyceal distortion and displacement but little change in axis of the kidney	Outward and downward displacement of kidney, "drooping lily," with microcalcifications
Tumor markers	None	VMA, HVA, catechols, ferritin, NSE
Metastases	Lungs, lymph nodes, liver, brain, bone (rare)	Liver, bone, bone marrow, lymph nodes

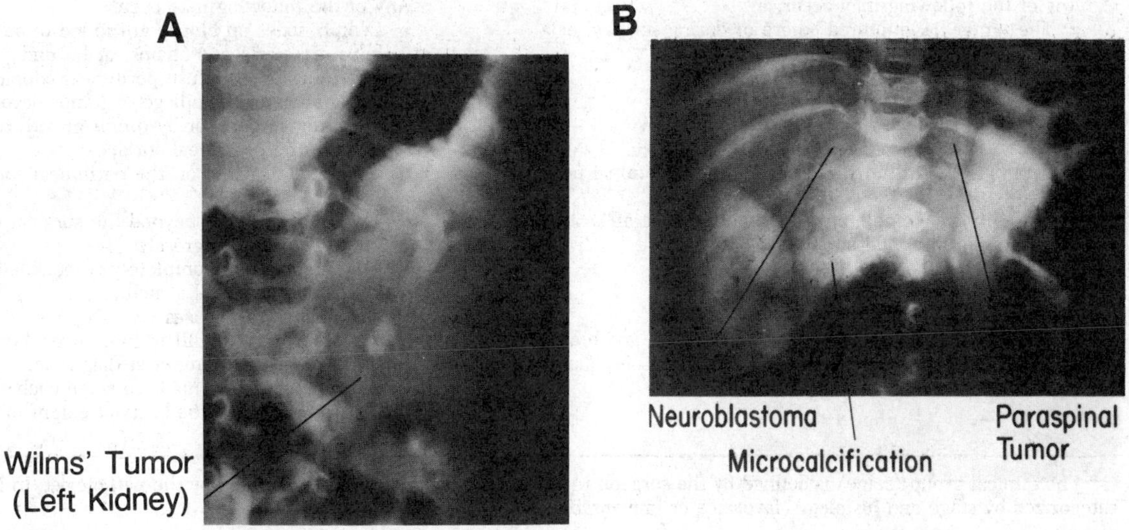

TREATMENT

The advances in treating Wilms' tumor reflect integration of improved methods of surgery, radiation therapy, and chemotherapy. Optimal treatment of the patient requires that the pediatric, radiation, and surgical oncologists begin to coordinate their efforts during the initial diagnostic and staging workup.

Surgery

The goal of surgery is to remove the primary tumor, even if there are distant metastases. Two questions require consideration preoperatively. First, is the mass too large for safe resection without tumor rupture? Second, is there any evidence for bilateral involvement?

Approximately 5% to 15% of patients have tumors that are too large for safe primary surgical resection. These tumors cross the midline, appear to be fixed to adjacent structures, or were not visualized on IVP. In the past, radiation therapy was used to achieve preoperative tumor shrinkage, and although it was effective, it frequently delayed surgery. More recently, preoperative chemotherapy (1.0 mg/m² of vincristine for infants or 1.5 mg/m² for children, administered every 5–7 days) has been shown to substantially shrink the tumor mass in 80% of patients within 2 to 3 weeks, making subsequent surgery safe and effective.

If preoperative chemotherapy or radiation therapy is being considered, a definitive diagnosis should first be established by either a needle biopsy or an open biopsy through a small retroperitoneal incision. Biopsy by one of these methods minimizes the possibility of tumor contaminating the entire abdominal cavity and eliminates the possibility of a false diagnosis and unnecessary therapy.

The possibility of bilateral Wilms' tumors (5% of cases) should be determined preoperatively. The prognosis for patients with bilateral disease is good (approximately an 87% survival rate), even if the tumors are not entirely resectable. Surgery should remove all tumor only if adequate renal parenchyma can be left on one or both sides. Treatment for bilateral Wilms' tumor should be individualized, and many different approaches have been successful. For example, in patients with a large tumor on one side and a small tumor on the other, nephrectomy is indicated for the larger lesion and

TABLE 47-11. Staging Systems for Wilms' Tumor

*Clinical Grouping (NWTS 1 and 2)**	*Clinical Staging (NWTS 3)*
I. Tumor limited to the kidney and completely resected. The surface of the renal capsule is intact. The tumor was not ruptured before or during removal. There is no residual tumor apparent beyond the margins of resection.	I. Tumor limited to the kidney and completely resected. The surface of the renal capsule is intact. The tumor was not ruptured before or during removal. There is no residual tumor apparent beyond the margins of excision.
II. Tumor extends beyond the kidney but is completely resected. There is local extension of the tumor: penetration beyond the pseudocapsule into the perirenal soft tissues or periaortic lymph node involvement. The renal vessel outside the kidney substance is infiltrated or contains tumor thrombus. There is no residual tumor apparent beyond the margins of resection.	II. Tumor extends beyond the kidney but is completely excised. There is regional extension of the tumor: penetration through the outer surface of the renal capsule into the perirenal soft tissues. Vessels outside the kidney substance are infiltrated or contain tumor thrombus. The tumor may have been biopsied or there has been local spillage of tumor confined to the flank. There is no residual tumor apparent at or beyond the margins of excision.
III. Residual nonhematogenous tumor confined to the abdomen. Any of the following may occur:	III. Residual nonhematogenous tumor confined to the abdomen. Any of the following may occur:
a. The tumor has ruptured before or during surgery, or a biopsy has been performed.	a. Lymph nodes on biopsy are found to be involved in the hilus, the periaortic chains, or beyond.
b. Implants are found on peritoneal surfaces.	b. There has been diffuse peritoneal contamination by the tumor such as by spillage of tumor beyond the flank before or during surgery, or by tumor growth that has penetrated through the peritoneal surface.
c. Lymph nodes are involved beyond the abdominal periaortic chains.	c. Implants are found on the peritoneal surfaces.
d. The tumor is completely resectable because of local infiltration into vital structures.	d. The tumor extends beyond the surgical margins either microscopically or grossly.
	e. The tumor is not completely resectable because of local infiltration into vital structures.
IV. Hematogenous metastases. Deposits beyond group III in lung, liver, bone, and brain.	IV. Hematogenous metastases. Deposits beyond stage III in lung, liver, bone, and brain.
V. Bilateral renal involvement either initially or subsequently.	V. Bilateral renal involvement at diagnosis. An attempt should be made to stage each side according to the above criteria on the basis of extent of disease before biopsy.

* The clinical group (stage) is defined by the surgeon in the operating room and is confirmed by the pathologist. In NWTS, patients are categorized by stage and histology (favorable or unfavorable).

partial nephrectomy for the smaller one. In patients with two large primary tumors, biopsy followed by chemotherapy and radiation therapy with subsequent resection of the residual tumors should be considered. Bilateral nephrectomy and renal transplant has not been especially successful, and this approach is indicated only if all other measures have failed.

In patients deemed surgically resectable, good exposure should be obtained with a generous transabdominal incision that, if necessary, should extend into the thorax. The renal vein should be ligated before beginning extensive dissection, although this does not appear to affect prognosis. Avoid rupture of the tumor during surgery because operative spill, which occurs in 16% of cases, appears to increase the risk of abdominal recurrence. This liability may be overcome if the peritoneal surfaces are irradiated after the spill. Perhaps the greatest hazard in the resection of Wilms' tumor is hemorrhage due to injury to the vena cava. The cava should be isolated above and below the tumor so that damage to it can be quickly controlled. Tumors that invade the liver capsule usually are totally resectable because they rarely penetrate deeply into the liver parenchyma.

After the tumor is removed with a long segment of ureter, the hilar and local para-aortic lymph nodes should be biopsied, and any enlarged or suspicious nodes should be removed. Although lymph node biopsy is important in staging, retroperitoneal lymph node dissection is not of proven value and has potential morbidity.

Tumor extending into the vena cava can usually be removed with venotomy and traction. If the tumor segment in the inferior vena cava is completely obstructed, it is best left in situ. If the tumor embolus extends into the heart, removal can be accomplished by inserting a finger into an opening in the right atrial appendage while the embolus is withdrawn from below. Rarely, cardiac bypass is necessary to remove the tumor embolus.

For very large or hemorrhagic tumors, surgical resection may be accomplished more effectively after embolization of the renal artery with gelfoam particles, which reduce renal vascularity and shrink tumor bulk. This procedure should be considered if the patient presents with gross hematuria but has a resectable primary tumor.

During surgery, the contralateral kidney should be carefully examined after it has been mobilized and its capsule has been opened. If, after resection of the primary tumor, an easily removable contralateral lesion is found, it should be excised if sufficient renal tissue can be left behind to maintain renal function. If this cannot be safely guaranteed, the contralateral nodule should be biopsied.

The liver and the remainder of the abdomen should be inspected for metastases, and the tumor bed or areas of extension or residual disease should be outlined with metallic chips. Although tumor resection is important, a small volume of residual tumor does not appear to adversely affect prognosis. Thus, heroic efforts to remove the last vestiges of tumor are not indicated.

Surgical extirpation of pulmonary nodules is of benefit if the resection can be accomplished without compromising pulmonary function. Similarly, surgical resection also has been successful in eradicating liver and brain metastases.

Radiation Therapy

The role of radiation therapy has become more sharply defined in recent years. Improved chemotherapy has eliminated postoperative irradiation of early staged patients. Radiation therapy is used conservatively because of the toxic effects of large irradiation fields in very young children. There is a potential for growth disturbances, and hepatic, pulmonary, or cardiac damage can result from irradiation used in conjunction with chemotherapy. Because of the anticipated long survival of patients with Wilms' tumor, there is appropriate concern about the risk of developing second malignancies.[11]

Radiation therapy has been effective in virtually eliminating abdominal failure because of microscopic or gross residual disease. In conjunction with chemotherapy, irradiation has achieved a high proportion of disease control in cases with pulmonary metastases. Preoperative radiation therapy had proven the value of diminishing large tumors before resection, diminishing operative spill and improving disease-free survival. The efficacy and reduced toxicity of preoperative chemotherapy has supplanted preoperative radiation.

The use of postoperative radiation therapy is dictated by operative stage and histology. The NWTS 1 and 2 trials have shown that postoperative radiation therapy is not necessary for Stage I patients, regardless of age, who have favorable histologic patterns if they are treated with adjuvant vincristine and dactinomycin. Whether or not children with Stage II Wilms' tumors with favorable histologic patterns should receive postoperative radiation therapy is being addressed by the NWTS 3, which randomizes patients to either no radiation or 2000 cGy to the renal fossa. The goal of diminishing radiation-related sequelae must be balanced against the ability to control abdominal disease with postoperative irradiation. Unlike pulmonary metastases, abdominal failure is rarely treated successfully.

FIG. 47-1. Dosimetry for hemiabdominal irradiation. Note inclusion of the para-aortic lymph nodes and full width of the vertebral body within the 90% volume. Dosimetry depicts dose configuration for a field identical but contralateral to that shown.

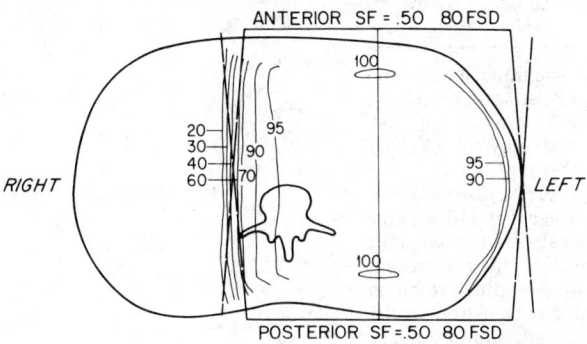

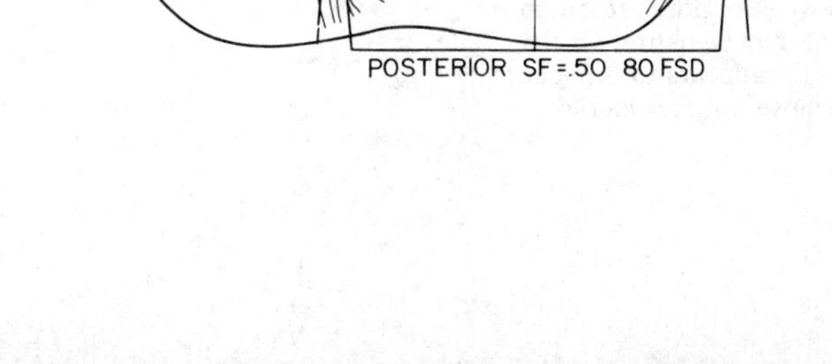

Patients with favorable Stage III tumors (and some would include Stage II patients with intraoperative spillage) require postoperative radiation therapy. In an attempt to reduce toxicity, the NWTS 3 has compared low-dose (1000 cGy) with higher-dose (2000 cGy) treatment for Stage III (favorable) patients; the option of additional boost therapy to gross residual disease may observe interpretation of this trial.

Postoperative radiation therapy is recommended for all patients with unfavorable histologic patterns, regardless of stage, and for patients with Stage IV tumors. Abdominal treatment in Stage IV presentations should be defined by the extent of abdominal disease. Radiation treatment of pulmonary metastases is independent of "abdominal stage."

Radiation therapy ports should be tailored to the extent of disease found at surgery. Whole abdominal irradiation is used only in patients with abdominal spill (Fig. 47-1). Residual disease or documented lymph node involvement requires tumor bed irradiation, generally as hemiabdominal therapy to encompass the initial tumor and para-aortic volume. It is important to include the full width of the vertebrae to encompass the retroperitoneal nodes and to avoid asymmetric closure of the vertebral epiphyses.

The dosage for postoperative irradiation has been defined in part by NWTS and major institutional trials. Patients with gross residual disease (Stage III or IV) require 2000 cGy to overt disease sites, preferably fractionated at approximately 150 cGy per day. It is possible that tumors with favorable histologic patterns may require only 1000 cGy; data is yet unavailable to confirm this reduction. In tumors with unfavorable histologic patterns, dose levels of 2000 to 2700 cGy are appropriate; the occurrence of abdominal failures despite 2000 cGy suggests that the higher dose may be necessary.

Radiation to extrarenal and extra-abdominal sites has been integrated into treatment planning for patients with Stage IV Wilms' tumor. Patients with pulmonary metastases should receive 1200 to 1500 cGy whole-lung irradiation, with only the growth centers of the humeri blocked. If this treatment follows abdominal or renal fossa irradiation, care must be taken to avoid normal tissues such as the remaining kidney or liver. Patients with hepatic, brain, or bone involvement are treated with irradiation.

Chemotherapy

Wilms' tumor was found to be responsive to dactinomycin in the 1960s. Other active agents include vincristine, doxorubicin (Adriamycin), cyclophosphamide, and cisplatin with response rates of 63%, 60%, 27%, and 16%, respectively. Successive studies by single institutions, collaborative groups, and the NWTS have identified the following principles of treatment:

1. *Stage I FH or Anaplastic and II FH:* Chemotherapy with dactinomycin and vincristine is superior to either alone. Radiotherapy is not needed.[12]
2. *Stage III FH and IV FH:* Chemotherapy with dactinomycin, vincristine, and doxorubicin and postoperative irradiation.[12]

3. *Stage II, III, and IV anaplastic tumors:* Chemotherapy with dactinomycin, vincristine, doxorubicin, and possibly cyclophosphamide (pending results from NWTS IV) and postoperative irradiation.
4. *Clear cell sarcoma, Stage I–IV:* Chemotherapy with vincristine and dactinomycin and irradiation.
5. *Stage V (bilateral) Wilms' tumor:* The surgical goal should be to preserve enough functioning renal parenchyma generally by removing the kidney with the major involvement and only a portion of the less affected kidney. Bilateral nephrectomy and kidney transplantation should be a last resort. Postoperative radiation therapy should be considered for both renal fossae, although lack of residual disease may make this unnecessary. The adjuvant schedules and radiation treatment should be dictated by the histology and extent of residual disease.

The results of NWTS 3 are summarized in Table 47-12. Because relapse after 2 years from diagnosis is very rare, the majority of disease-free children at this point are cured. NWTS 4, now underway, will determine if there is an advantage to single-dose or divided-dose dactinomycin and doxorubicin. It will also evaluate a 6-month treatment for patients with Stage II, III, or IV tumors. The International Society of Pediatric Oncology (SIOP) focused on the preoperative treatment of Wilms' tumor with radiation therapy or with chemotherapy. Results have been excellent. The group found that residual tumor at the time of surgery is a negative prognostic indicator.

The toxicity of therapy, both acute and long-term, has influenced treatment. Seventeen toxic deaths in NWTS 2 resulted primarily from leukopenia (7) and liver failure (4). Because 4 of 47 infants (<1 year old) died of leukopenia, chemotherapy doses have been decreased by 50% for this age group. Long-term side-effects of the disease and its treatment include cardiomyopathy caused by the interaction between doxorubicin and radiation, skeletal growth disturbances after irradiation, and radiation-induced nephritis in the remaining kidney.

Most children in the United States with Wilms' tumor are treated on the NWTS. Although almost 90% of Wilms' tumor patients are curable and tolerate therapy well, the child with this disease deserves to be managed by a team experienced in pediatric cancer.

NEUROBLASTOMA

Neuroblastoma represents frustration and hope to those who treat cancer in children. Cure is elusive for the majority of children (>1 year old) with this disease who present with disseminated tumor. In spite of improved chemotherapeutic regimens that can result in complete responses, recurrence is common in older patients. However, because the molecular genetics of this tumor are better understood than for any other human cancer, there is an implicit promise of more effective and less toxic treatments.

EPIDEMIOLOGY AND GENETICS

Neuroblastoma is the fourth most common pediatric malignancy, with an annual incidence of 10 cases per million

TABLE 47-12. Results in Randomized NWTS 3 Patients

			2-Year Survival (%)	
Stage/Histology	*Regimen*	*No.*	*Relapse Free*	*Overall*
I/FH*	AMD + VCR, 10 wk vs. 6 mo.	469	90 vs 93	98
II/FH	15 mo. AMD + VCR vs. AMD + VCR + ADR† (±RT)	262	91 vs. 90	99 vs. 93
II/FH	AMD + VCR ± ADR No RT vs. 200 cGy†	262	90 vs. 91	95 vs. 96
III/FH	AMD + VCR vs. AMD + VCR + ADR† (15 mo; +RT)	264	77 vs. 88	88 vs. 95
III/FH	AMD + VCR ± ADR 1000 vs. 2000 cGy†	264	82 vs. 83	92 vs. 91
Any IV, any UH	AMD + VCR + ADR vs. AMD + VCR + ADR + CTX (15 mo; +RT)	291	63 vs. 69	78 vs. 80

Adapted from D'Angio GJ, Beckwith JB, Breslow N et al: Wilms' tumor (nephroblastoma and renal embryoma). In Pizzo PA, Poplack DG (eds): Principles and Practice of Pediatric Oncology. Philadelphia, JB Lippincott, 1989.

* FH = favorable histology; UH = unfavorable histology; ADM = dactinomycin; VCR = vincristine; ADR = doxorubicin; CTX = cyclophosphamide; RT = radiation therapy.

† Comparisons denoted are collapsed regimens from the factorial design; persistent disease at last follow-up Stage IV was scored as relapse. Data indicate that, in general, FH Stages II and III patients can be treated successfully with the less intensive regimens and that better treatment is needed for patients with UH or metastases, especially those with rhabdoid tumors. Stage I/FH children present particular problems for analysis. These results show the less intensive 10-week regimen to be no worse than 6 months, but other analyses suggest that 6 months of treatment may be better. Of the four possible treatment combinations for Stage III/FH, AMD+VCR+1000 cGy appears to produce inferior results when both relapse-free survival and infradiaphragmatic relapse are considered.

children. In the United States it comprises 8% of cancers diagnosed in children under 15 years of age. The incidence is significantly less in African than in American black children, raising the possibility that environmental factors are important and may be responsible for the increased incidence of neuroblastoma between 1943 and 1980. Alcohol, hair coloring products, and certain medicines used during pregnancy may be prenatal risk factors for neuroblastoma.

The median age at diagnosis of neuroblastoma is 2 years. Half of all malignancies diagnosed in the first month of life and a third during the first year are neuroblastoma. The mortality of neuroblastoma occurring in the first year of life is far lower than that in the older child, suggesting the unique biology of this tumor. Microscopic nodules of primitive neuroblasts, usually larger than 3 mm and occasionally invading blood vessels, referred to as "neuroblastoma in situ," have been observed at autopsy in infants dying before 3 months old of other causes at 40 to 200 times the expected incidence. Autopsy examination of the adrenal glands of 92 18-week to 20-week fetuses demonstrated "neuroblastoma in situ" in all. It is clear that a normal phase in the embryogenesis of the adrenal gland, which is histologically similar to neuroblastoma, may persist into the first year of life. It is not understood how this relates to the observed spontaneous regression of neuroblastoma, especially Stage IV-S, or to the high rate of cure of the less than 1-year-old infant with a tumor indistinguishable from the usually fatal lesion seen in older children.

Molecular geneticists are studying neuroblastoma as a paradigm for elucidating the biology of differentiation and its relationship to oncogenesis.[13] The "two-hit" hypothesis, which postulates that malignancy is a function of prezygotic and postzygotic mutations, may be relevant to neuroblastomas. Neuroblastoma has been associated with the genetic diseases neurofibromatosis, Beckwith-Wiedemann syndrome (omphalocele, macroglossia, visceromegaly, neonatal hypoglycemia), nisidioblastosis, and trisomy 18 and with teratogenic syndromes caused by in-utero exposure to alcohol and hydantoins. These associations are very rare, indicating that they may be coincidental. Although familial neuroblastoma, characterized by multiple primaries, very young age at presentation, and autosomal dominant inheritance, is uncommon, its existence establishes that a germ-line mutation may promote tumorigenesis. Siblings and offspring of nonfamilial neuroblastoma patients are at low risk for developing the disease. A specific constitutional karyotypic abnormality has not been identified in familial neuroblastoma.

Progress has been made in the understanding of the chromosomal abnormalities of the neuroblastoma cell. Human neuroblastomas are characterized cytogenetically by partial monosomy for the short arm of chromosome 1 (1p−) and abnormality of chromosome 17. In addition, double-minutes (DM) and homogeneously staining regions (HSR), cytogenetic evidence of gene amplification, and variability in modal chromosome number, ranging from hypodiploidy (<46 chromosomes) to hypertetraploidy (>92 chromosomes), are evident. Chromosome 1 abnormalities, specifically deletions at 1p22, are a common feature of a diverse group of pediatric solid tumors. The amplified genes identified within neuroblastoma cells as HSR and DM are homologous to the v-*myc* and c-*myc* oncogenes and designated as N-*myc*. This gene is normally present in a single copy on chromosome 2. The number of copies of the N-*myc* oncogene is related to the clinical aggressiveness of the tumor and is a prognostic indicator independent of stage and age, the number of copies does correlate with the stage of the tumor and progression-free survival at 18 months from diagnosis. Amplification of N-*myc* has been detected in 30% of untreated neuroblastomas. The N-*myc* copy number is an intrinsic biologic property of each patient's tumor, remaining consistent within the tumor, in tumors at different sites, and over time, uninfluenced by treatment.[14] The product of N-*myc* gene is yet to be identified, but it is probably related to the growth of the neuroblastoma cell.

Other oncogenes implicated in pathogenesis include N-*ras*, identified initially in human neuroblastoma cell line SK-N-SH, and c-*src*, which expresses the enzyme tyrosyl kinase. The understanding of the molecular pathogenesis of neuroblastoma is increasing faster than that for most other human cancers, leading to predictions that this will lead to molecular biologically based therapy.[13] Even today the relationship of the chromosomal content of neuroblastoma to prognosis has clinical utility. The DNA content of neuroblastoma cells, analyzed by flow cytometry, was shown by Look and colleagues to reliably predict response to chemotherapy in patients younger than 1 year old at diagnosis.[15] Favorable prognosis has been correlated with aneuploidy.

The status of the immune system in patients with neuroblastoma has been studied. Although mild lymphopenia and leukopenia have been demonstrated at diagnosis, no general humoral or cellular immune defects have been detected. Natural killer (NK) cell activity is depressed in neuroblastoma patients. Clinical trials using the methanol-extracted residue of bacillus Calmette-Guerin (BCG), with BCG-treated and neuraminidase-treated tumor cells, to provoke an antitumor immune response in patients have not demonstrated the benefit for this immunotherapy.

Monoclonal antibodies have been raised to antigens on the surface of human neuroblastoma cells in order to develop reagents that will have immunodiagnostic and immunotherapeutic utility. The cell-surface glycosphingolipid disganglioside GD_2 is an abundant antigen on neuroblastoma cells. Monoclonal antibodies to GD_2 recognize neuroblastoma cells relatively specifically without cross-reacting with normal marrow or lymphoid cells.[16] With this monoclonal antibody, Cheung and co-workers were able to detect as few as 0.01% neuroblastoma cells in the marrow. They were able to identify neuroblastoma cells in the bone marrow in 74% of 35 neuroblastoma patients, while conventional histologic techniques and clonogenic assays detected 27% and 55%, respectively. Shedding of GD_2 into the plasma of patients with neuroblastoma may be useful for monitoring responses to therapy. ^{131}I-tagged monoclonal antibodies to GD_2 can ablate human neuroblastoma xenograft tumors in nude mice. Monoclonal antibodies to other neuroblastoma antigens include 5A7 to a cytoplasmic antigen and CE7, KP-NAC8, 5G3, 6-19, and UJ13A to cell-surface antigens. ^{131}I-coupled monoclonal antibodies have been administered as treatment for neuroblastoma. Responses were seen in patients with disseminated disease, but those with large tumor masses were resistant to this therapy. Substantial bone marrow toxicity was incurred, and issues of delivery and dosimetry must be addressed before the potential of this approach can be realized. Monoclonal antibodies may be useful in purging tumor cells from bone marrow for use in autologous bone marrow transplant regimens.

Neuroblastoma has a biological characteristic unique among human cancers, the capacity to spontaneously differentiate and regress. Residual microscopic tumor left in the bed of a resected, localized neuroblastoma rarely results in recurrence of the disease. Disseminated neuroblastoma has spontaneously regressed in a subset of very young children with disease metastatic to the liver, skin, or bone marrow, but not involving bone, designated as Stage IV-S neuroblastoma by D'Angio, Evans, and Koop.[17] Histologic evidence of neuroblastoma having differentiated into mature ganglion cells is found in tumors removed from patients during second-look surgical procedures after induction chemotherapy and in older children with isolated mediastinal or abdominal masses, detected incidentally and found to be pure ganglioneuroma.

This phenomenon has stimulated laboratory investigation into the mechanisms of differentiation of neuroblastoma cells. In cultured neuroblastoma cells, agents such as prostaglandin E1, 3′, 5′-cyclic nucleotide phosphodiesterase inhibitors, thyroid hormone, and Bu_2cAMP that increase the intracellular cAMP levels, decrease the mitotic rate and increase the degree of differentiation. Differentiating agents, including cyclophosphamide, vincristine, the phosphodiesterase inhibitor papaverine, and the thymidylate synthetase inhibitor trifluromethyl-2-deoxyuridine, used in the treatment of neuroblastoma have resulted in good antitumor responses, but the role of the differentiating agents could not be ascertained because the patients got simultaneous high-dose chemotherapy. Retinoic acid also differentiates neuroblastoma cells in vitro. It probably interacts through a cytoplasmic retinoic-acid-binding protein or by the glycosylation of cell surface constituents. No clinical studies with this agent have been performed.

PATHOLOGY AND BIOLOGICAL MARKERS

Neuroblastoma is thought to be derived from the embryonic neural crest. The presumptive stem cell of the neural crest, the sympathogon, differentiates into sympathoblasts, the cells of origin of neuroblastoma, and into its more mature forms, ganglioneuroblastoma and ganglioneuroma, and the chromaffin or nonchromaffin paraganglionic cells, the progenitors of pheochromocytomas and paragangliomas. As a "small, round, blue cell" tumor, neuroblastoma consists of dense nests of cells separated by fibrovascular bundles. Hemorrhage, necrosis, and calcification are frequent. Other microscopic features include Homer-Wright neural rosettes with a central fibrillar core and a fibrillary intercellular matrix that can be shown ultrastructurally to be neural cell processes. In the more-differentiated tumor, ganglion cells are present. They are large cells with prominent nucleoli and generous cytoplasm that are scattered throughout a fibrillar matrix. Ganglioneuroblastoma contains areas of neuroblastoma and ganglion cells; ganglioneuroma has ganglion cells, Schwann cells, and nerve bundles. It is important for the pathologist to take multiple sections of a ganglioneuroma to exclude neuroblastoma.

The characteristic electron microscopic finding of neuroblastoma is the dense core granule (catecholamine or neurosecretory granule), which is a 50-mm to 200-mm membrane-bound unit found in the periphery of the cytoplasm. The ultramicroscopic appearance of the neural rosettes is that of peripherally clustered tumor nuclei surrounding a mass of neuritic processes or neuropil.

Neuroblastoma can be difficult to distinguish from other small round cell tumors of childhood, including Ewing's sarcoma, lymphoma, rhabdomyosarcoma, and other peripheral neurally derived neoplasms such as the peripheral neuroepithelioma or Askin's tumor. Table 47-13 lists some of the features that will help distinguish these tumors. Neuroblastoma also exhibits formaldehyde-induced florescence as the catecholamine metabolites form isoquinolone compounds when exposed to formaldehyde, and glyoxylic acid provides a rapid and sensitive assay. Identification of specific cellular constituents, such as enzymes (*i.e.*, neuron-specific enolase) or surface antigens, by sensitive immunoperoxidase techniques, in which paraffin-embedded, formaldehyde-fixed tissues may be used with specific antisera, have become an integral part of the pathologist's workup of the small, round, blue cell tumor.

An often useful adjunct to tissue examination in the diagnosis of neuroblastoma is detection of tumor markers in the blood or urine. The most commonly used is the urinary excretion of tumor-produced catecholamines. Urinary vanilmandelic acid (VMA) and homovanillic acid (HVA) are elevated in at least 65% of neuroblastoma patients. When both

TABLE 47-13. Special Diagnostic Techniques for Small, Round, Blue Tumors of Childhood

		Immunocytochemistry						
Tumors	*Electron Microscopy*	*NSE**	*LEU 7*	*HSAN 1.2*	*Desmin*	*Myoglobin*	*Vimentin*	*CCA*
Neuroblastoma	Dense core neurosecretory granules, neural tubules or filament	+	+	+	−	−	+	−
Lymphoma	Lack of cell attachments, glycogen and dense core granules	−	−/+	−	−	−	+/−	+
Ewing's sarcoma	Cytoplasmic glycogen	−	−	−	−	−	+	−
Peripheral neuroepithelioma	Neurites and dense core granules	+	−	+	−	−	+	−
Rhabdomyosarcoma	Intermediate filaments, fibrillar collagen stroma	+/−	−	−	+	+	+	−

* NSE = neuron-specific enolase;

TABLE 47-14. Primary Site of Neuroblastoma According to Age

Primary Site of Tumor	Age at Diagnosis	
	≤12 Months	>13 Months
Head and neck	5%	2–3%
Thoracic	20%	10–15%
Abdominal	55%	70–75%
Pelvic	5%	5%
Other (or unknown)	15%	2–13%

metabolites are sought, more than 90% of patients will be identified. Pretreatment measurements correlate with prognosis. Higher levels of catecholamine metabolites are found in patients with more extensive disease. For Stage IV patients, a ratio of VMA to HVA of >1.5 is associated with a better prognosis. Patients whose neuroblastomas arise from the dorsal root ganglions are nonsecretors of catecholamines. The most reliable method for detection of catecholamine metabolites is a 24-hour urine test. The LaBrosse spot test, which screens for VMA in the urine, is associated with a relatively high false-negative rate because it requires a high concentration of VMA in the samples. Dietary restrictions are not necessary for a reliable 24-hour urine catecholamine quantitation, but catecholamine medications should be avoided. In Japan, mass screening of infants 6 to 7 months old using VMA spot tests has been successful in the early detection of neuroblastoma.[18]

Neuron-specific enolase is elevated in the majority of neuroblastoma patients. Higher levels in those with more advanced disease are prognostic of a poorer outcome. Serum ferritin elevation also correlates with a poorer prognosis. Cystathionine is elevated in the urine of at least 50% of neuroblastoma patients. As with the other biomarkers, lower levels were associated with a better prognosis.

CLINICAL PRESENTATION AND DIAGNOSIS

Neuroblastoma can occur anywhere along the sympathetic nervous system. The most common site of primary tumor is within the abdomen, either in an adrenal gland (40%) or in a paraspinal ganglion (25%); thoracic (15%) and pelvic (5%) primaries account for the rest. Thoracic primaries are more common in children younger than 1 year old (Table 47-14). Metastatic disease is identified in half the infants and 75% of the older children at diagnosis. The most common sites of metastases are lymph nodes, bone marrow, bone, liver, and subcutaneous tissue. Lung metastases are rare.

The signs and symptoms at presentation depend on the primary and metastatic sites. The most common presentation, that of a large abdominal or flank mass that is firm, irregular, and crosses the midline must be distinguished from Wilms' tumor. Thoracic neuroblastoma presents as a posterior mediastinal mass and is usually found coincidentally when a chest radiograph is obtained for other reasons, although it occasionally causes respiratory symptoms or signs of thoracic spinal cord compression from local extension (Fig. 47-2). Neuroblastoma arising from the cervicothoracic ganglion is often confused with benign lymphadenopathy, but the presence of Horner's syndrome or heterochromia irides from sympathetic dysfunction suggests the true diagnosis. Pelvic neuroblastoma arising from the organ of Zuckerkandl may present as a palpable mass alone or with symptoms related to bladder or vascular compression.

Several unusual presentations of neuroblastoma are noteworthy. First the firm, subcutaneous, blue-tinged nodules, reminiscent of the blueberry muffin sign associated with congenital rubella, are most often encountered in the neonate with neuroblastoma. Second is the opsoclonus-polymyoclonus syndrome of acute cerebellar and truncal ataxia and dancing eyes, which is associated with persistent neurological sequelae but limited tumor; it indicates a favorable prognosis. A third unusual symptom is that of intractable, watery diarrhea and hypokalemia caused by vasoactive intestinal peptide (VIP) produced by ganglioneuroblastoma and measured in the plasma of these patients. Olfactory neuroblastoma (esthesioneuroblastoma) arises in the nasal cavity and presents with obstruction. It is most commonly seen in adults.

Neuroblastoma has an unusual predisposition to periorbital metastasis, which presents with proptosis and ecchymosis. This is secondary to sphenoid bone involvement or invasion of the retrobulbar tissues. Intracranial metastasis other than direct extension from bony lesions of the skull are rare. The so-called cerebral neuroblastoma is a supratentorial tumor of primitive neuroectoderm that is more closely related to a family of primary central nervous system tumors.

Bone marrow involvement with neuroblastoma is common

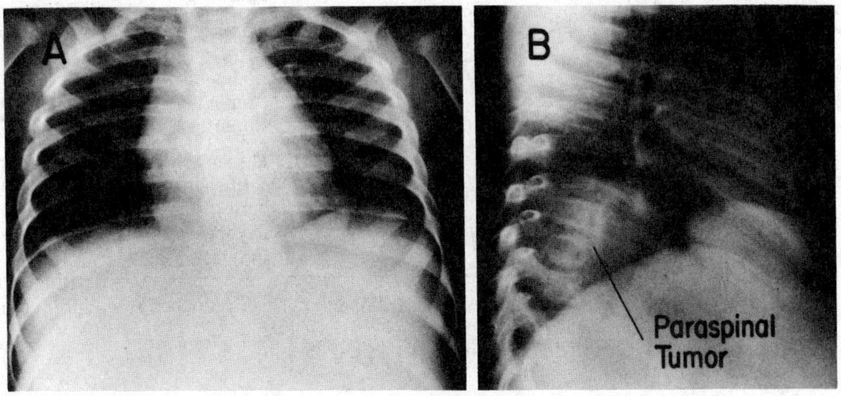

FIG. 47-2. Chest roentgenograph in frontal (**A**) and lateral (**B**) projections demonstrating paravertebral pleural displacement. Size of the thoracic component can be appreciated on the lateral projection.

and may be difficult to distinguish from acute leukemia or other solid tumors, like rhabdomyosarcoma, metastatic to marrow. Neuroblastoma cells are more likely to be PAS-negative and form rosettes, but the clinical tests and tissue histopathology usually confirm the diagnosis.

In some neuroblastoma patients, no primary tumor site can be found. This is most common in the unique syndrome (Stage IV-S) that occurs in infants younger than 1 year old. It is characterized by small or undetectable tumors, usually of the adrenal, with skin, hepatic, or bone marrow (but not bone) metastases that may undergo spontaneous regression. Hepatic enlargement may be very significant, causing symptoms that necessitate therapeutic intervention.[19]

A bone marrow aspirate and, if necessary, a biopsy may provide tumor for diagnostic pathologic studies and adjunctive laboratory analysis such as flow cytometry for establishing the DNA index, which may be clinically useful.[15]

Although other small, round, blue cell tumors metastatic to the bone marrow may have similar histologic features, a diagnosis of neuroblastoma may be confirmed if abnormal urine catecholamine excretion is found in conjunction with the marrow findings, this often obviates a major surgical procedure. A careful search of many slides must be undertaken before the marrow can be declared uninvolved. Examination of slides of the buffy coat made from 1 to 2 ml of heparinized marrow may increase the yield.

CT is the best imaging modality for neuroblastoma and should be performed for every patient to determine the location and extent of the primary and metastatic lesions. CT detects abdominal neuroblastoma with an extremely high sensitivity, and calcifications are seen in approximately 85% of patients. The IVP is less sensitive than a CT scan in the evaluation of an abdominal mass and should not be done routinely. Bilateral adrenal calcifications detected in an otherwise asymptomatic child with an abnormal birth history are probably due to neonatal adrenal hemorrhage. Experience with MRI of neuroblastoma visualizes the tumor in many planes, demonstrates the vascular anatomy, improves the definition of the intraspinal extension, aiding the determination of resectability.

Nuclear medicine scans of use in evaluating neuroblastoma include the technetium-99m methylene diphosphonate bone scan, which should be performed on every child with neuroblastoma because it is more sensitive than the conventional skeletal survey. Bone scanning agents are frequently taken up by extraosseus tumor, further aiding in the metastatic workup. ^{131}I-meta-iodobenzylguanidine (MIBG), which has been used in the diagnosis and treatment of pheochromocytoma because of its preferential uptake by cells with adrenergic secretory vesicles, allows the imaging of most neuroblastomas and is being investigated for the treatment of this disease.

The laboratory evaluation of neuroblastoma should include a complete blood count and coagulation studies. Coagulopathy is not uncommon in patients with disseminated disease and may be caused by intravascular coagulation. Both hypocoagulability and hypercoagulability have been described.

STAGING

There have been several staging systems for neuroblastoma (Table 47-15). Because of the prognostic influence of regional lymph node involvement and the importance of the initial surgical procedure in determining further treatment,

TABLE 47-15. Staging Systems for Neuroblastoma

*Evans Staging System**		*Pediatric Oncology Group Staging System*	
Stage I:	Tumor confined to the organ structure of origin.	Stage A:	Complete gross excision of primary tumor, margins histologically negative or positive. Intracavitary lymph nodes not intimately adhered to and removed with resected tumor must be histologically free of tumor. If primary is in abdomen (including pelvis), liver must be histologically free of tumor.
Stage II:	Tumors extending in continuity beyond the organ or structure of origin but not crossing the midline. Regional lymph nodes on the homolateral side may be involved.	Stage B:	Incomplete gross resection of primary. Lymph nodes and liver must be histologically free of tumor as Stage A.
Stage III:	Tumors extending in continuity beyond the midline. Regional lymph nodes may be involved bilaterally.	Stage C:	Complete or incomplete gross resection of primary. Intracavitary nodes histologically positive for tumor.† Liver histologically free of tumor.
Stage IV:	Remote disease involving skeleton, soft tissues, distant lymph node groups, etc.	Stage D:	Disseminated disease beyond intracavitary nodes, in bone marrow, bone, liner, skin, or lymph nodes beyond cavity containing primary tumor.
Stage IV-S:	Patients with local Stage I or II disease but who have remote disease confined to one or more of the following: liver, skin, and bone marrow (without radiographic evidence of bone metastases on complete skeletal survey).		

* Staging systems from Evans A, D'Angio GJ, Randolph JA: A proposed staging for children with neuroblastoma. Cancer 27:347, 1971.

† Intracavitary nodes = nodes in same cavity as primary.

TABLE 47-16. POG Stage Distribution by Age of Patient

POG Stage	<365 Days Old No. (%)	>365 Days Old No. (%)	Total
A	16 (18.4)	13 (8.7)	29 (12.2)
B	10 (11.5)	10 (6.6)	20 (8.4)
C	19 (21.8)	20 (13.4)	39 (16.5)
D	42 (48.3)	107 (71.3)	149 (62.9)
Total	87 (36.7)	150 (63.3)	237 (100)

the Pediatric Oncology Group (POG) has recently adopted a modification of the staging system advocated by Hayes and co-workers at St. Jude Children's Research Hospital based on the surgical-pathologic staging of patients with clinically localized disease, a concept originally advocated by Pinkel in 1958.[20] It is important that investigators working in this field be able to compare results of treatment protocols, and a working group has been established to develop a common system. Discussion of the treatment of neuroblastoma is based on the POG system and the age of the patient at diagnosis, a strong independent prognostic factor (Tables 47-16 and 47-17).

THERAPY

Successful treatment of the child with neuroblastoma requires a carefully considered multidisciplinary approach. The initial diagnostic workup will establish whether the disease is disseminated or localized. In the patient with localized disease, the operation is key to defining the local extent of tumor and to completely resecting the tumor. Radiation therapy plays a role in the treatment of the patient with localized disease and the palliative management of the patient with disseminated disease unresponsive to chemotherapy. Chemotherapy is central in the management of those with unresectable local tumor or metastatic disease.

Surgery

The surgical approach depends on site, stage, and age of the patient. Among those with cervical, mediastinal, and to a lesser extent, pelvic tumors, complete excision is usually feasible and should be aggressively pursued. The same approach is occasionally possible for a primary abdominal tumor, particularly if it is small or laterally placed. In contrast, most localized abdominal neuroblastomas extend centrally and surround the major branches of the aorta, making the tumors unresectable by conventional surgical procedures. Every large series contains some long-surviving patients in whom these tumors were literally "carved" away from the central vessels, but there are more patients for whom this did not result in cure. In general, abdominal tumors are biopsied, and a second or third attempt is made to remove them after intensive chemotherapy or radiotherapy. If complete gross resection can be carried out during a second or third procedure, the patient will probably survive. These procedures may be instrumental in creating a favorable-prognosis group.

TABLE 47-17. Three-Year Disease-free Survival of Patients with Neuroblastoma by Age and Stage

POG Stage	3-Year Disease-free Survival (%) <12 Months	3-Year Disease-free Survival (%) >12 Months
A	>90	>90
B	85	80
C	90	<20
D	90	<20

Among patients with metastatic disease, an early aggressive attempt to resect the primary tumor does not increase survival. In patients in whom metastatic disease can be controlled, successful secondary excisions of the primary tumors produce relatively extensive survival times.

In patients with functional neuroblastomas, early excision of the major tumor mass is essential to ameliorate symptoms. Surgery for patients with Stage IV-S disease should be conservative. After all disseminated disease is eliminated by chemotherapy or spontaneously, the remaining primary tumor mass is usually excised, although this has never been demonstrated to be necessary. Surgical procedures have been devised to relieve intra-abdominal pressure in patients with Stage IV-S disease by employing plastic sheets to create an artificial ventral "hernia."

Radiation Therapy

The value of radiation therapy for neuroblastoma has been inadequately defined. In Stage II (partially comparable to POG Stage B) neuroblastoma, the indications for radiation therapy are controversial. There have been reports of 60% to 100% survival rates for children after incomplete resection and irradiation for Stage II or III neuroblastoma. Rosen reported 26 of 28 disease-free survivors (17 of 19 older than 1 year old) after postoperative irradiation and chemotherapy.[21] Other studies have found no benefit from the addition of radiation therapy. Current treatments have avoided irradiation for Stage B patients known to have no obvious regional node involvement.

For Stage III disease, radiation seems to improve survival rates. Impressive survival rates have been reported by Jacobsen (71% of 14 patients) and Rosen (81% of 16 patients).[21] Both groups of patients received systematic regional irradiation and intensive chemotherapy. Rosen recorded 5 of 7 disease-free survivors who were Stage II patients older than 1 year of age.[21]

Radiation therapy in Stage III cases requires attention to

lymph node status. Hayes has reported survival in 16 (62%) of 26 Evans' Stage III patients with negative lymph node status, compared with[11] (33%) of 33 patients with lymph node metastases.[20] In children older than 1 year, only 4 of 23 survived. In contrast, Rosen's series documented survival in 21 (84%) of 25 cases with lymph node metastases, including 12 of 15 with Stages II or III who were older than 1 year of age.[21] The difference in the two series raises questions. Irradiation was used in Rosen's institution; surgery and chemotherapy alone were used by Hayes.

Chemotherapy

Neuroblastoma is usually chemoresponsive and in some instances curable. The complete and partial response rates vary for the most common single agents: cyclophosphamide (59%), cisplatin (46%), epipodophyllotoxins (30%), vincristine (24%), dacarbazine (14%), melphalan (24%) and ifosfamide (20%). Green, Hayes, and Hustu at the St. Jude Children's Research Hospital gave children with disseminated neuroblastoma cyclophosphamide (150 mg/m^2) for 7 days followed by doxorubicin (35 mg/m^2) on day 8, based on the hypothesis that cyclophosphamide, active in all phases of the cell cycle, would increase the proportion of cells in the DNA synthetic phase of the cell cycle, making them more vulnerable to the cytotoxic effects of doxorubicin, an S-phase-specific agent.[22] Fifty-two percent of the 68 patients had complete responses, and 18% had partial responses, a better result than achieved when these two agents are used in other schedules. These investigators also demonstrated that cisplatin (90 mg/m^2) on day 1 and VM-26 (100 mg/m^2) 48 hours later was a very active combination, with complete and partial responses in 15 of 22 children with tumors resistant to cyclophosphamide and doxorubicin. The excellent response rates observed in the St. Jude studies may have been influenced by the interval of only 1 to 2 weeks between courses of chemotherapy. The interval was based on recovery from myelosuppression, the criteria to begin the next course was an absolute granulocyte count of 500 cells/mm^3. This dose frequency may be very important in the treatment of tumors like neuroblastoma that have a rapid doubling time.

Treatment by Age and Stage

Careful clinical studies have resulted in guidelines for the treatment of the child with neuroblastoma. These guidelines are determined by the stage, and for Stage C or D patients, by age greater or less than 1 year at diagnosis.

POG STAGE A. Surgical excision of the tumor, with no chemotherapy or radiotherapy, will cure more than 90% of Stage A patients, whether the resection margins are positive or not. In a prospective POG study of Stage A patients who received surgery alone 84 of 92 children are recurrence free (Fig. 47-7).

POG STAGE B. If the tumor is localized, without histologic evidence of nodal or hepatic involvement, but it is unresectable because of its relationship to vital structures, treatment with chemotherapy followed by a second surgical procedure is often successful and avoids more radical surgery. Forty-six of 58 patients treated with cyclophosphamide and doxorubicin every 21 days for 4 months, followed by a second-look surgical excision of residual tumor, were rendered disease-free.[20] Cisplatin and VM-26 were given to 7 patients who had residual disease; 4 of them achieved disease-free status. Of 50 patients rendered disease free by chemotherapy and a later surgical procedure, 46 remain in remission. Thus, 79% of Stage B patients are disease free, with a median follow-up of more than 36 months. Equivalent results have been documented with postoperative irradiation from Stage II patients (including Stage B and an undefined proportion of Stage C), with disease-free survival of 75% to 80%.

STAGE C AND D, <1 YEAR. Infants with gross residual tumor, which is local, metastatic to nodes or liver, or disseminated, may be treated very successfully with chemotherapy, with or without radiotherapy. Approximately half of those with Stage D disease treated with cyclophosphamide, dacarbazine, vincristine, and doxorubicin survived for more than 36 months from diagnosis in two Children's Cancer Study Group, (CCSG) protocols. In a series reported by Kretschmar and colleagues, 10 of 11 infants with Stage D disease treated with various chemotherapy regimens survived 2.5 to 13 years from diagnosis.[23] At St. Jude Children's Research Hospital, 49 Stage C or D infants were treated with 4-month courses of cyclophosphamide and doxorubicin as described above. Sixty-five percent responded completely. Ten of 12 who had residual disease with that combination had complete responses to cisplatin and VM-26. Of 31 infants diagnosed since 1979, when cisplatin and VM-26 became available, all achieved complete remission, and 28 survived 16 to 93 months (median, 59 months). The strategy of using the less toxic drugs first and reserving cisplatin, VM-26 and, on occasion, radiotherapy for the minority of patients who do not respond completely, cures 90% of patients with the least toxicity possible.

EVANS STAGE IV-S. The treatment of Stage IV-S patients remains controversial. Some of these patients have spontaneous regressions of their tumors without treatment, but about 40% will die of progressive disease. Frequently these babies will have huge livers, causing mechanical problems with respiration and making an open surgical approach difficult. The diagnosis can be determined by percutaneous biopsy, and radiotherapy or chemotherapy may shrink the mass. Surgical resection of the primary tumor followed by short-term chemotherapy or low-dose irradiation are potentially useful strategies, but no data exists on which to base guidelines. However, if the primary tumor and metastatic lesions regress, there is no evidence that resection of the residual primary disease increases survival rates. If a no-treatment approach is adopted, the patient should be watched very closely for progression of disease. The infant younger than 2 months old may be a greater risk for failure.

STAGE C, >1 YEAR. Most of these children have Evans Stage III disease, although the converse is not true, with only half of all Evans Stage III patients having POG Stage C tumors. For this reason, it is not easy to apply the results of treatment of patients treated as Evans Stage III without lymph node staging. Results of the treatment of Evans Stage III patients are varied, with Rosen reporting 1.5 years or more survival in 8 patients treated with a 4-drug or 6-drug regimen, compared with 2 of 7 other patients who survived with a 4-drug or 5-drug treatment and radiation therapy.[21] Hayes and colleagues reported the survival of only 1 of 15 Stage C patients treated with cyclophosphamide, doxorubicin or cyclophosphamide, and vincristine, largely without irradiation.[20] The same investigators incorporated cisplatin and VM-26 into the regimen, and 7 of 11 patients attained complete remission, with 5 having no evidence of disease 6, 6, 22, 82, and 87 months from diagnosis.

The POG is currently evaluating the role of radiation therapy in Stage C patients. The early data suggest a role for regional nodal irradiation. The previously documented poor prognosis compelled new trials with more aggressive chemotherapy in conjunction with radiation therapy.

STAGE D, >1 YEAR. Unfortunately, the majority of children with neuroblastoma fall into this category and the results of treatment have been poor. Because they have disseminated disease, chemotherapy is the primary treatment. Single institutions and collaborative groups have explored protocols with increasingly intensive multidrug chemotherapy regimens, which include cyclophosphamide, doxorubicin, cisplatin, VM-26, vincristine, and DTIC. Complete or partial responses are achieved in the majority of patients, and a gradual increase in duration of disease-free survival has been demonstrated over the past 10 years. In spite of this, less than 25% of patients survive free of disease at 2 years from diagnosis.[24] This has encouraged treatment with supralethal doses of chemotherapy and total-body irradiation, with autologous or allogeneic bone marrow transplant rescue. Preliminary results with this approach suggest that it provides modest improvement at best. In one study, 15 of 45 patients were disease-free, with some patients surviving as long as 4 years, but with a median follow-up of less than 12 months from diagnosis.[25] In another report 7 of 29 patients were disease-free for 23 to 48 months from treatment. Both the POG and CCSG have protocols underway to compare the efficacy of the bone marrow transplant and a nontransplant, intensive-chemotherapy approach.

Because improved outcomes depend on more effective chemotherapy, both collaborative groups are evaluating experimental drugs in newly diagnosed patients. Traditionally, Phase II studies have been performed in patients who have failed chemotherapy. The likelihood of finding agents active in these drug-resistant tumors is low. By testing new drugs in a "Phase II window" before initiating other therapy, new agents may be identified.[26]

Most children with Stage D neuroblastoma respond initially to treatment, and a minority may enjoy long-term survival. Therefore, treatment should proceed with curative intent.

RETINOBLASTOMA

Retinoblastoma, the most common primary tumor of the eye in children, has many important distinguishing features. Arising from the nuclear layer of the retina, tumors may be multifocal, bilateral, congenital, inherited, or acquired. Patients may have unique chromosomal abnormalities, and tumors can undergo spontaneous regression. Patients with the inherited form of retinoblastoma also appear to be at increased risk for second, nonocular malignancies.

The estimated annual incidence of retinoblastoma is between 1 in 15,000 to 1 in 34,000 live births. According to the Third National Cancer Survey and SEER, there are approximately 11 new cases of retinoblastoma per million children under 5 years of age. There are approximately 200 new cases each year in the United States, 90% of which are diagnosed in children (see Table 47-1). The disease is bilateral in 40 to 60 cases. Although retinoblastoma accounts for only 1% of pediatric tumors, it serves as an important model for understanding the genetics of oncogenesis.

EPIDEMIOLOGY AND GENETICS

The mean age of presentation for retinoblastoma is 17 months, with 80% diagnosed before the age of 4 years. Although the tumor has been described in adults, it is quite rare in children older than 5 years. Retinoblastoma occurs in hereditary, nonhereditary, and chromosomal deletion forms. The retinoblastoma gene may be transmitted from parent to child or acquired as a new mutation. No family history of retinoblastoma is found in 90% of patients.

The hereditary form of retinoblastoma accounts for approximately 40% of cases, and it is inherited as a highly penetrant, autosomal dominant trait. A two-mutation hypothesis explains the genetics of inherited retinoblastoma. The first mutation occurs in the germinal cells, and the second occurs in the somatic cells. In the sporadic form of the disease, both mutations occur in the somatic cells. It is presumed that the timing of the mutational event in embryonic development determines whether the entire retinal anlage or only that of one eye is affected. Accordingly, the majority of patients with the hereditary form of retinoblastoma have bilateral disease, although unilateral disease may occur in almost 25% of these patients. Overall, approximately 30% of patients with retinoblastoma have bilateral disease, and 70% have unilateral involvement. Eleven patients with bilateral retinoblastoma subsequently developed pineoblastoma, suggesting that genetic susceptibility to transformation can be conferred to ectopic neuroblastic photoreceptors in the pineal gland (trilateral retinoblastoma).

The majority of patients with retinoblastoma lack appreciable chromosomal abnormalities in most autosomal cells. A deletion on the long arm of chromosome 13 within band 13q14 has been observed in a small number of patients with retinoblastoma, some of whom have a syndrome that includes mental retardation, microcephaly, skeletal abnormalities, and dysmorphic features. Using recombinant DNA probes, which are homologous to unique loci on human chromosome 13, a specific retinoblastoma locus (Rb-1) has been defined, confirming that chromosome loss, or loss and reduplication, can lead to the expression of a recessive mutation. Dryja and co-workers examined tumor tissue obtained from 8 patients with retinoblastoma, none of whom had a family history of this disease.[27] Four of these eight tumors demonstrated chromosome 13 homozygosity, which had no correlation with the degree of tumor differentiation or whether the tumors were multifocal or unifocal.

The tight linkage of the retinoblastoma (Rb) gene locus to the genetic locus of esterase D, assigned to 13q14, has demonstrated that the two independent genetic events consist of the loss or inactivation of wild-type alleles. Within the 13q14 band locus of the retinoblastoma gene, the loss of one Rb allele is insufficient for tumorogenesis, but the loss of both alleles by nondisjunction or point mutation is associated with tumor production.

The genetic susceptibility for oncogenesis in patients with the inheritable form of retinoblastoma is further underscored by the fact that these patients have an increased risk for developing second malignancies that are unrelated to radiation or chemotherapy exposure. The predominant second cancers include osteosarcoma, fibrosarcoma, Ewing's sarcoma, and Wilms' tumor.[28] Patients with bilateral retinoblastoma have a 15% to 20% chance of developing a second, nonocular neoplasm 1 to 40 years after their treatment for retinoblastoma. Fibroblasts from patients with the genetic form of retinoblastoma have increased radiation sensitivity and defective DNA repair. Fibroblasts from siblings of patients with retinoblastoma also have this radiation sensitivity pattern. The complementary sequences to the retinoblastoma gene have been cloned and demonstrate deletion at the 13q14 Rb locus in some patients with osteosarcoma, offering an explanation for the close association of these two malignancies.[29]

The incidence of second malignancies increases over time. For irradiated patients, the incidence of second tumor was 20% at 10 years, 50% at 20 years, and approximately 90% at 30 years. For nonirradiated patients, the incidence of second malignancies was 10% at 10 years, 30% at 20 years, and 68% at 30 years. Based on a series of 882 patients, the cumulative index of second malignancies was 2% at 12 years after diagnosis and 4.2% at 18 years after diagnosis. This incidence was doubled in patients with the genetic form of retinoblastoma.

Genetic counseling is important for patients with the genetic form of retinoblastoma. Assuming that the mutation is a germinal event, the risk for bearing an affected child may be as high as 50%. This is straightforward if there is a family history of the disease but more difficult for sporadic cases, because these may be either hereditable or nonhereditable. Bilateral cases, even without a family history, are always the hereditary type, and the offspring of affected patients have a 50% risk of having retinoblastoma. Of the unilateral cases, 10% to 12% have the hereditary form, and the first child of a survivor has a 5.6% chance of having the disease (Fig. 47-3).

Parents of an affected child should always have a fundoscopic examination. If a child with retinoblastoma is born to physically sound parents, the risk of a second child having retinoblastoma is 1% if the first child had unilateral retinoblastoma and 6% if the child had bilateral disease. The use of restriction fragment length polymorphism may facilitate diagnosis and permit prenatal and postnatal prediction of susceptibility to the hereditable form of retinoblastoma.

Nonprogressive retinal lesions (retinomas) have been described in patients presumed to carry the retinoblastoma gene. These retinomas consist of translucent, gray, elevated masses that extend from the retina into the vitreous cavity and are frequently associated with calcified foci and pigment-epithelium hyperplasia. In a recent survey of 34 individuals with retinomas and 5 with phthisis bulbi, which is also associated with retinoblastoma, 67% had a family history of retinoblastoma, and 23 (68%) of their offspring developed retinoblastomas. Although retinoma may represent a mutation of a more mature retinoblast, making it nonmalignant, its detection should prompt genetic counseling and follow-up of the affected individual.

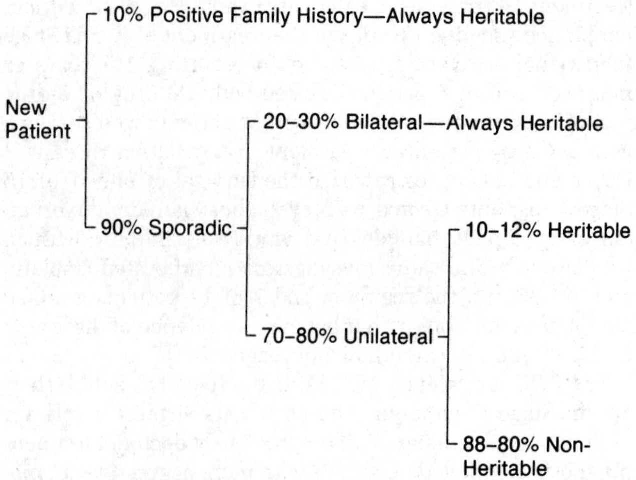

FIG. 47-3. Flow diagram of statistical probabilities for a newly diagnosed patient with retinoblastoma. (Donaldson SS, Egbert PR: Retinoblastoma. In Pizzo PA, Poplock DG [eds]: Principles and Practice of Pediatric Oncology, p 557. Philadelphia, JB Lippincott, 1989)

PATHOLOGIC AND ANATOMICAL CONSIDERATIONS

Retinoblastoma, putatively arising from the outer layer of the retina, consists of small, round cells with scanty cytoplasm and chromatin-rich nuclei. Histologic examination shows similarity with neuroblastoma and medulloblastoma, including aggregation around blood vessels, necrosis, calcification, and Flexner-Winterstainer rosettes. Tumors are often multifocal, averaging four to five lesions in as many as 84% of the patients. This multifocality, as well as the predilection of retinoblastoma to invade the optic nerve, influences treatment planning.

Endophytic and exophytic local extension of retinoblastoma are recognized. Endophytic growth is characterized by extension into the vitreous cavity, and exophytic growth invades the subretinal space, with consequent retinal detachment. With endophytic extension, tumor fragments can break away from the main tumor mass to form vitreous seeds, a poor prognostic finding.

The vast majority of patients with retinoblastoma have disease restricted to the eye and orbit. Local tumor growth usually involves the choroid or the sclera if subretinal seeds cross Brach's membrane. The highly vascular choroid is involved in more than 25% of patients and, although this serves as a potential site for dissemination, it is not as serious as scleral involvement. Scleral involvement usually occurs by direct extension from the choroid or by spread along emissary veins.

Glaucoma can result from tumor growth in a retinal detachment that pushes the iris forward to occlude the trabecu-

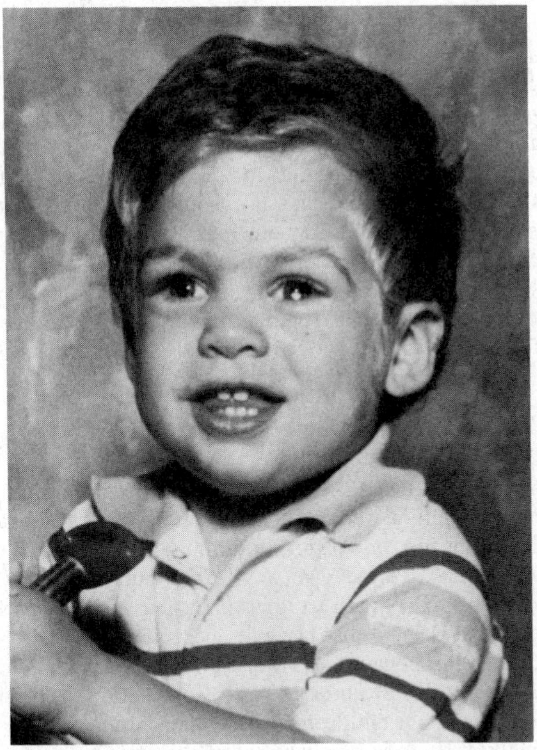

FIG. 47-4. Child exhibiting leukokoria in the left eye, the most common presenting sign of retinoblastoma. (Donaldson SS, Egbert PR: Retinoblastoma. In Pizzo PA, Poplock DG [eds]: Principles and Practice of Pediatric Oncology, p 560. Philadelphia, JB Lippincott, 1989)

lar network. It can also result if a neovascular membrane grows on the iris and over the trabecular network, blocking the egress of aqueous fluid. Iris neovascularization may be exacerbated by radiation therapy.

Of particular concern is extension of retinoblastoma cells through the lamina cribrosa and into or along the optic nerve. If the tumor extends just 10 to 22 mm along the optic nerve, invasion into the meninges is almost always a consequence, a particularly poor prognostic feature.

Slightly more than half of the deaths with retinoblastoma are due to distant tumor metastases, although 47% of deaths are a consequence of direct intracranial extension. As with neuroblastoma, hematogenous metastases most often involve bones, bone marrow, and lymph nodes; pulmonary metastases are uncommon.

CLINICAL PRESENTATION

In children without a known family history, 75% present with either leukocoria or "cat's eye" reflex (Fig. 47-4), strabismus, or poor vision due to vascular involvement, vitreous seeds, or retinal detachment (see Table 47-8). In patients with unilateral retinoblastoma, strabismus is the most frequent early sign. Less commonly, children may present with proptosis, a painful inflamed eye, cervical adenopathy, or symptoms referable to sites of metastatic disease. It is imperative that infants and children with these symptoms undergo a careful ophthalmologic evaluation. Young children do not complain of loss of vision, and intraocular tumors are not painful unless there is also glaucoma or inflammation. Any child with a known family history of retinoblastoma or retinomas should be examined at birth and at regular intervals thereafter. Of 158 infants with retinoblastoma diagnosed during the first 6 months of life (mean age, 3.6 years), 60% had leukocoria, and 68% had bilateral disease. Many of these patients had advanced disease despite their early evaluation.

In young children suspected of having retinoblastoma, examination of the retina may need to be performed under general anesthesia. This is particularly important if tumor involvement includes the ora serrata or if the tumor cannot be visualized because of retinal detachment or vitreous hemorrhage obscuring the tumor mass. The differential diagnosis includes visceral larva migrants (toxocara granuloma), Coats' disease, retrolental fibroplasia, and persistent hyperplastic primary vitreous. However, findings of calcification, which occurs in 50% to 75% of patients, or vitreous seedings are most compatible with retinoblastoma. Orbital CT scan can detect calcification in more than 80% of patients, and in children younger than 3 years of age in whom the diagnosis is suspected, CT-detected calcification is virtually diagnostic. Two dimensional B-scan ultrasonography is of particular value in demonstrating mass lesions in the posterior segment of the fundus because retinoblastoma has a high internal acoustic reactivity due to the pressure of calcium and the interface between necrotic and viable areas.

EVALUATION

Examination of the child with retinoblastoma should determine the extent of local disease and metastatic disease. Careful examination of both retinas by direct and indirect ophthalmoscopy is essential, and the extent of orbital disease and intracranial extension should be assessed by CT scan. Ultrasound and orbital polytomography may also be used to assess orbital disease. MRI can determine the extent of orbital and CNS involvement. Patients should have a lumbar puncture for cytocentrifuge CSF examination, a bone marrow aspirate, and a biopsy. Patients with extensive orbital involvement should have bone scans. Lactic acid dehydrogenase may be elevated in the aqueous humor of patients with retinoblastoma.

Because of the predominance of intraocular disease and because of improved survival, treatment planning and staging has been focused on the management of local disease and on preserving the eye and vision. The most widely used grouping (staging) system for retinoblastoma assesses the likelihood of local tumor control and preservation of vision but does not predict survival. As outlined in Table 47-18, this grouping system divides patients according to the likelihood of preserving vision after radiation therapy based on tumor size, the number and location of lesions, and vitreous seeding. In this system, tumor size is expressed by comparison with the optic disk (1.5 mm diameter). Each eye should be evaluated separately to assess the most effective therapy and to determine if there is any potential for preserving or restoring useful vision. Although this system is useful in guiding management of intraocular disease, it does not predict survival for patients with advanced (Group V) disease at presentation.

A histologically based staging system, which considers intraocular and extraocular tumor extension and which corre-

TABLE 47-18. Reese-Ellsworth Clinical Grouping System for Retinoblastoma

Group I: Very Favorable
1. Solitary tumor, less than 4 disc diameters* in size, at or beyond equator.
2. Multiple tumors, none over 4 disc diameters in size, all at or behind equator.

Group II: Favorable
1. Solitary tumor, 4 to 10 disc diameters in size, at or behind equator.
2. Multiple tumors, 4 to 10 disc diameters in size, at or behind equator.

Group III: Doubtful
1. Any lesion anterior to equator.
2. Solitary tumors larger than 10 disc diameters behind equator.

Group IV: Unfavorable
1. Multiple tumors, some larger than 10 disc diameters.
2. Any lesion extending anteriorly to ora serrata.

Group V: Very Unfavorable
1. Massive tumors involving over half the retina.
2. Vitreous seeding.

Reese AB, Ellsworth RM: The evaluation and current concepts of retinoblastoma therapy. Trans Am Acad Ophthalmol Otolaryngol 67:164–172, 1963.
* 1 disc diameter = 1.6 mm.

lates with patient survival, has been adopted by St. Jude Children's Research Hospital (Table 47-19). This staging system permits the integration of multimodal treatment planning for patients with advanced local disease, but is based on results of enucleation.

TREATMENT PLANNING

Treatment planning must consider unilateral or bilateral involvement; the size, number, and location of local tumors; tumor extension into the choroid, sclera, or optic nerve; and evidence of extraocular disease. The goal of therapy for patients with localized disease (Ellsworth–Reese Stages I and II or St. Jude Stages I, IIA, and IIB) is local control with surgery or radiation therapy. Unfortunately, most children with unilateral involvement present with far advanced disease and with little potential for preserving vision. Patients with advanced local disease may require postoperative treatment to the orbit or contiguous extension sites of the CNS. The management of patients with bilateral disease depends on the extent and group of disease in each eye. It is no longer appropriate to enucleate the most severe eye in patients with bilateral involvement. With modern radiotherapy, vision may be spared.

TABLE 47-19. St. Jude Children's Research Hospital Staging System

I. Tumor (unifocal or multifocal) confined to retina
  A. occupying 1 quadrant or less
  B. occupying 2 quadrants or less
  C. occupying more than 50% of retinal surface
II. Tumor (unifocal or multifocal) confined to globe
  A. with vitreous seeding
  B. extending to optic nerve head
  C. extending to choroid
  D. extending to choroid and optic nerve head
  E. extending to emissaries
III. Extraocular extension of tumor (regional)
  A. extending beyond cut end of optic nerve (including subarachnoid extension)
  B. extending through sclera into orbital contents
  C. extending to choroid and beyond cut end of optic nerve (including subarachnoid extension)
  D. extending through sclera into orbital contents and beyond cut end of optic nerve (including subarachnoid extension)
IV. Distant metastases
  A. extending through optic nerve to brain
  B. blood-borne metastases to soft tissue and bone
  C. bone marrow metastases

Pratt CB: Management of malignant solid tumors in children. Pediatr Clin North Am 19:1141–1155, 1972.

Surgery

ADVANCED UNILATERAL DISEASE. Most children with sporadic unilateral retinoblastoma have advanced intraocular disease at the time of presentation, often with little or no vision in the affected eye. While the potential for visual preservation exists with irradiation, at least 50% of patients with advanced local disease will subsequently require enucleation, either because of irradiation-induced complications or inadequate local tumor control. Enucleation is the treatment of choice for children with advanced unilateral disease, especially if there is involvement of the optic nerve head or if the child has glaucoma. If enucleation is performed, at least 10 mm of the optic nerve should be resected to remove any disease that may have extended along the nerve. If microscopic examination detects evidence of tumor along the nerve tract, local irradiation should be administered. An artificial eye can be fitted in 6 weeks. In children younger than 3 years of age, the orbit ceases to grow normally after enucleation and, as the face grows, the orbit becomes more sunken in appearance.

LESS ADVANCED DISEASE. Patients with limited unilateral or bilateral tumors (usually less than 4 disc diameters) may be candidates for photocoagulation or cryotherapy instead of enucleation combined with radiation. Photocoagulation by the technique of Meyer-Schwicherath obliterates small tumors and destroys their blood supply. This procedure requires direct visualization of the tumor and is best restricted to posterior tumor masses. The tumor mass must be easily distinguished from the optic nerve head or macula, must not involve the choroid, and must not have a large nutrient vessel. The technique is used in cases with residual or recurrent disease after irradiation. Although successful, photocoagulation can be complicated by retinal detachment and hemorrhage.

Cryotherapy has been occasionally successfully used for primary treatment; it is more often employed for excision of residual or recurrent disease after irradiation. It is applied by a probe placed directly on the conjunctiva or sclera through a small incision in the conjunctiva. The position of the probe is guided by ophthalmoscopy, and the tumor can be observed to whiten as it freezes. Of 138 retinoblastomas treated in one study, the overall success with cryotherapy was 70%, with a 93% survival. Cryotherapy was useful as a primary modality in small (less than 4 disk diameters) tumors (20 of 21

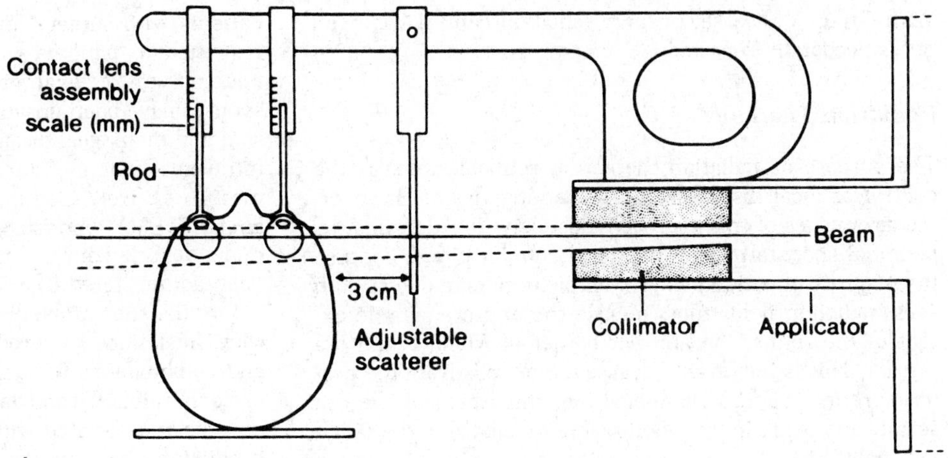

A

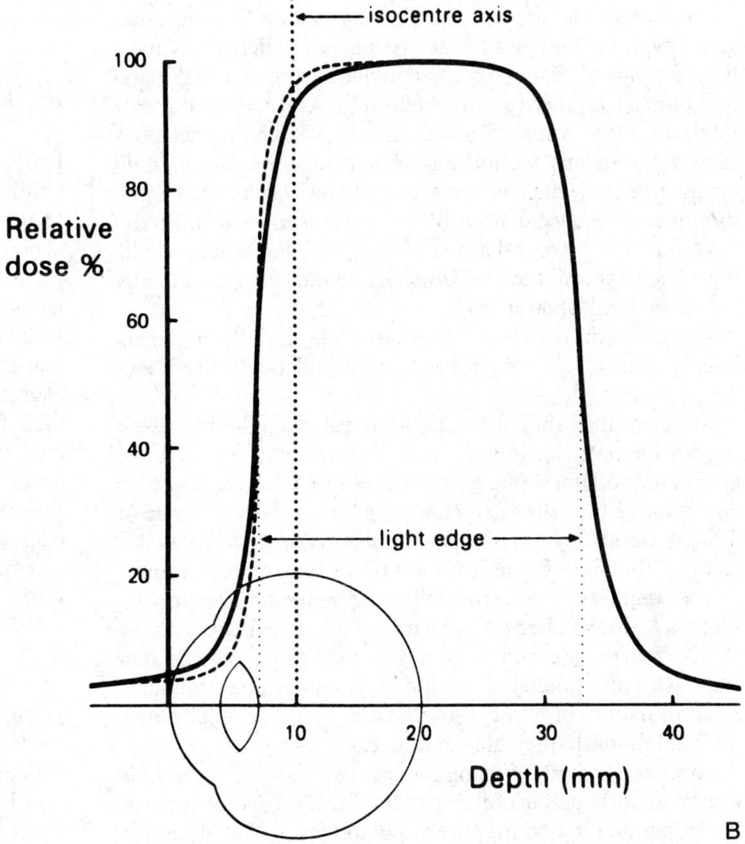

B

FIG. 47-5. Diagram of a modified Utrecht method for achieving full retinal irradiation in bilateral retinoblastoma. A stabilizing arm attached directly to the linear accelerator (at the collimator). **A**. The device assumes accurate placement of the eyes related to the incident beam, idealizing homogeneous irradiation of the retina (to the level of the ora serrata anteriorly) while avoiding direct irradiation of the lens. **B**. Dosimetry within the eye.

cured) and for radiation failures (58 of 66). Successful cryotherapy is limited, however, by the size, location, and elevation of the tumor. It is ineffective in the treatment of vitreous seeds. Peripheral lesions may not be effectively treated by cryotherapy.

BILATERAL DISEASE. The treatment plan for patients with bilateral disease depends on the extent of tumor involvement in each eye. If one eye has lost vision or has clearly established optic nerve head involvement, it should be enucleated, and the less involved eye should be irradiated. If vision is present and imaging studies show no obvious optic nerve involvement, both eyes may be treated by irradiation. For Group I, II, and III patients with bilateral retinoblastoma treated with irradiation, tumors were controlled in 73% to 80% of the cases. If both eyes are severely affected at the time of presentation, it is preferable to administer a trial of bilateral irradiation, because the possibility for some preservation or restoration of vision exists.

Although the 5-year survival of patients presenting with Group IV or V disease is 88%, the chance for satisfactory tumor control and preservation of vision is low (29%). Recent experience with improved radiation therapy techniques and liberal use of phototherapy or cryotherapy have resulted in disease control in almost 80%, including Group IV cases.

With Group V disease, primary radiation control has been only anecdotally reported.

Radiation Therapy

The purpose of radiation therapy in retinoblastoma is the control of local disease while preserving vision. However, the advantages of this approach must be weighed against its potential short-term and long-term complications. Because the majority of patients have multiple tumors in one or both eyes, radiation fields must include the entire anatomic extent of the retina, the anterior border of which is the ora serrata. This is important because tumor cells from the posterior retina may be channeled into the region of the ora serrata and result in local failure if not included in the radiation field.

Radiation treatment planning requires the joint efforts of the radiation therapist, ophthalmologist, and anesthesiologist. Several techniques for external-beam radiotherapy have been employed. Concerns about including the lacrimal gland and direct conjunctival effects limit general use of anterior fields to cases with advanced disease (including vitreous seeding). Modern techniques permit accurate lateral field arrangements, which assure adequate coverage of the retina, diminish direct irradiation of the optic lens, and limit the degree of late xerophthalmia (Fig. 47-5). Excellent results have been reported by the Utrecht group using a technically precise lateral photon field.

Young children should be anesthetized, usually requiring ketamine to assure immobilization and relatively fixed ocular positioning.

No firm radiation dose-response relationship has been proved for retinoblastoma. Most clinical series report doses between 3500 and 5000 cGy delivered in 17 to 25 fractions and given 4 to 5 times weekly over 4 to 5 weeks. Doses of 5000 to 5600 cGy have been administered in 5 to 5.5 weeks using 200-cGy fractions with a 4.6 mV linear accelerator.

The regression patterns following radiation therapy include a "cottage cheese" appearance due to calcium deposition or shrinkage and a homogeneous, gray, nonvascular mass with an annulus of atrophic pigment around the bone. Determination of tumor sterilization requires experience and serial ophthamologic examinations.

Localized radiation, using radioactive plaques or particle radiation, although useful in patients with recurrent tumors, is comparable to cryotherapy or phototherapy. Local modifications, such as addressing less than the full retinal surface, should be used for primary control only in the unusual unilateral, limited-size, unifocal tumors. Patients who have residual orbital or optic nerve tumor after surgery should receive wide-field (orbit and optic nerve) irradiation after enucleation. In general, a dosage of 5000 to 5500 cGy is delivered in 200-cGy fractions over 5 to 6 weeks. At higher doses, optic atrophy may occur. Full cranial or craniospinal irradiation is indicated for patients with brain or dural extension.

Chemotherapy

Although chemotherapy was first used in patients with retinoblastoma in 1953, its role remains undefined. Because effective local control and survival is achieved in 90% of patients with surgery and radiation, chemotherapy is best restricted to patients with locally extensive (choroidal or optic nerve), regional, or distant disease. Unfortunately, responses have been unsatisfactory. Patients with CNS extension and meningeal disease may benefit from intrathecal or intraventricular methotrexate. The agents that have been most extensively used in retinoblastoma include triethanolamine (TEM), vincristine, nitrogen mustard, cyclophosphamide, doxorubicin, and methotrexate. TEM has most often been administered by way of an intracarotid route, usually before the start of irradiation, although without proven efficacy. Ifosfamide has produced short-term partial responses, and combinations of cyclophosphamide and dactinomycin, cyclophosphamide and doxorubicin, and cisplatin and VM-26 have been associated with mixed or partial responses. Preirradiation chemotherapy has also been used for children with extensive intraocular tumors.

PRIMARY HEPATIC TUMORS

Primary malignancies of the liver, although infrequent in childhood, pose a considerable therapeutic and diagnostic challenge. One to two hepatic tumors per million children occur annually in the United States, with hepatoblastoma predominating in children younger than 5 years of age and hepatocellular carcinoma (HCC) in older children. As with Wilms' tumor, hepatoma most often presents as an asymptomatic abdominal mass that is found in a routine physical examination or discovered coincidentally by parents. Fewer than 25% of patients experience symptoms of abdominal pain, weight loss, or malaise, but when these symptoms occur they are usually associated with advanced disease.[30] The primary objective is to distinguish a hepatic malignancy from benign hepatic tumors, non-neoplastic hepatomegaly, and other causes of abdominal enlargement, particularly Wilms' tumor and neuroblastoma.

From a survey of 656 hepatic tumors in children, 423 (64%) were malignant, 54% were hepatoblastomas, 35% were hepatocellular sarcomas, and 11% were sarcomas (Table 47-19). Hemangiomas and hamartomas account for approximately 75% of the benign liver tumors, and almost 90% of these lesions occur in infants younger than 6 months old (Table 47-20). Benign vascular tumors can reach considerable size in infancy and may have an alarming clinical presentation, including high-output congestive heart failure due to arteriovenous shunting, hemorrhage, and bleeding with evidence of platelet consumption (the Kasabach-Merritt syndrome), and shock may occur after the rupture of a vascular tumor mass. Cavernous hemangioma, characterized by vascular spaces lined by a single layer of flat endothelial cells, often with evidence of old and new thrombus formation, and hemangioendotheliomas, composed of many small vascular channels lined by one or more layers of endothelial cells, are the two most important benign lesions that should be distinguished from malignant hepatic tumors. Although hemangioendotheliomas can occasionally be found at multiple sites within the liver, the metastatic potential of these tumors is exceedingly low. Benign hemangiomas can be treated with steroids and, if they fail to respond, low doses of

TABLE 47-20. Frequency of Benign and Malignant Hepatic Tumors in Children: Selected North American Series

Tumor Type	*Number*	*Percentage of Total*
Malignant		
Hepatoblastoma	227	34.6
Hepatocellular carcinoma	148	22.5
Sarcoma*	45	6.8
Benign		
Adenoma	13	2
Focal nodular hyperplasia	12	2
Vascular tumors	118	18
Mesenchymal hamartoma	53	8
Other	40	6

Greenberg M, Filler RM: Hepatic tumors. In Pizzo PA, Poplack DG (eds): Principles and Practice of Pediatric Oncology, p 570. Philadelphia, JB Lippincott, 1989.

* Sarcomas often arose from extrahepatic biliary tree.

radiation are generally successful in causing shrinkage; surgical resection is rarely necessary.

Hepatic sarcoma is a rare malignancy that constitutes approximately 10% of the primary hepatic tumors of childhood. The most common presenting symptom is abdominal pain. Evaluation should include a thorough determination of the extent of abdominal disease to guide resection and a search for metastases, especially in lung and bone. Tumors are classified as undifferentiated (embryonal) sarcomas if there is no evidence of specific differentiation and the malignant elements are mysenchymal, having a myxoid background and stellate cells. If there is evidence of differentiation, a more specific diagnosis may be assigned, such as rhabdomyosarcoma if striated muscle cells are present.

Treatment should begin with an aggressive attempt at complete resection. These tumors are relatively responsive to chemotherapy, and patients given therapy similar to that developed for rhabdomyosarcoma may experience long-term survival.

EPIDEMIOLOGY AND GENETICS

Hepatic tumors occur more often in boys and occur in two age peaks. Virtually all hepatoblastomas occur before 5 years of age, with 65% occurring in children younger than 2 years old. Anecdotal reports have associated hepatoblastoma with the fetal alcohol syndrome or the maternal use of oral contraceptives. One familial case of hepatoblastoma has been reported. Hepatoblastoma has been described in association with the Beckwith-Wiedemann syndrome and its incomplete variants. In addition, both hepatoblastoma and Wilms' tumor can occur synchronously. Homozygosity for a mutant allele at the 11p locus, corresponding to the so-called WAGR locus (Wilms', anidridia, genital malformation, and mental retardation) has been shown in biopsy tissue and in explants from two cases of hepatoblastoma.

HCC rarely occurs in infants and has its peak childhood incidence during adolescence. HCC is associated with preexisting cirrhosis and chronic hepatitis caused by the hepatitis B virus (HBV), an association that is particularly prominent in countries where there is a high prevalence of HBV infection, such as Japan. HBV sequences are integrated into the DNA of these HCC. Perinatal transmission of HBV has been associated with the onset of HCC 6 to 7 years later, suggesting that the latency period may be shorter in children than in adults. Epidemiologic studies suggest that control of HBV transmission and infection may eventually decrease the incidence of HCC in both adults and children.

A variety of syndromes and congenital malformations have been associated with primary hepatic tumors, including hemihypertrophy, osteopetrosis, DeToni-Fanconi syndrome, neurofibromatosis, ataxia telangiectasia, lipid storage disease, glycogen storage disease, hereditary tyrosinemia, biliary atremia secondary to extrahepatic biliary atresia, and the homozygous ZZ and heterozygous phenotypes of alpha-1-antitrypsin deficiency states. Hepatoblastoma has presented with virilization in fewer than 25 boys. Prolonged use of anabolic steroids, especially the C17 alkylated forms (*e.g.*, oxymetholone, methyltestosterone, testosterone enanthate, methandieone) have been associated with HCC. Although alpha-fetoprotein (AFP) is commonly detected in the serum of patients with hepatoblastoma, it is unusual to find evidence of elevated levels of choriogonadotropin (hCG). However, hCG can be detected in children with evidence of virilization, and immunoperoxidase staining has confirmed that hepatoma cells produce the hCG, although these cells may not be the same ones producing AFP. Estrogen and progesterone receptors have also been found in hepatoblastoma.

PATHOLOGY

Hepatoblastoma and HCC are both epithelial neoplasms. Hepatoblastomas are generally divided into tumors that consist of fetal or immature hepatic epithelial cells and tumors that consist of mixtures of epithelial and mesenchymal elements. The tumor cells have a high nuclear to cytoplasmic ratio, compact amphophilic or basophilic cytoplasm, and evidence of miotic activity. Most commonly, the tumor cells are arranged in cords two to three cells thick and have a sheet-like configuration. Acinar or pseudoglandular components can sometimes be defined, although a mixed epithelial-mesenchymal variant of hepatoblastoma, accounting for nearly 30% of hepatoblastomas, can have a spindle cell component. Osteoid and extramedullary hematopoiesis are frequently observed in these mixed tumors. Although the epithelial component appears to be a prognostic determinant for patients with mixed hepatoblastomas, embryonal cells influence the malignant potential of these tumors. Less commonly, the tumor may appear more anaplastic, consisting of sheets of loosely connected cells with scant cytoplasm and a high mitotic rate.

HCC in children may be histologically identical to that seen in adults, although an important variant has been recently defined. This rare tumor, called fibrolamellar carcinoma, occurs primarily in younger patients (mean age, 25; range, 5–35 years) and is characterized by deeply eosinophilic neoplastic hepatocytes, many of which contain intracellular hyaline globules and distinct pale bodies surrounded by fibrous bands, often with a lamellar configuration. Fibrolamellar carcinoma presents as a single tumor nodule and has a much more favorable prognosis (median survival, 32 months) than other forms of HCC. Nonetheless, it is important to distinguish fibrolamellar carcinomas from benign hepatic adenomas, because survival depends on surgical resection.

HCC has a distinctive ultrastructural appearance characterized by large, round, centrally placed nuclei, prominent nucleoli, abundant large mitochondria, and microvilli on the plasma membrane.

By the time of presentation, tumor masses are usually quite large, regardless of histologic type, and frequently involve the right lobe of the liver. Spread to other parts of the liver usually occurs by direct extension, but may also take place through intrahepatic vascular or lymphatic channels. Extrahepatic tumor spread usually occurs by way of the regional lymph nodes in the porta hepatis, and the lungs are the primary sites of metastatic disease.

CLINICAL PRESENTATION

A palpable abdominal mass in the right upper quadrant is the predominant finding in more than 90% of patients with primary hepatic tumors. Usually, there are no other physical signs or symptoms.[30] Severe osteopenia with back pain and pathologic features of weight bearing bones can occur. Isosexual precocity, although uncommon, can be seen in approximately 3% of the hepatoblastomas that secrete beta-hCG.

In contrast, abdominal pain is more frequent in patients with HCC and the mean duration of symptoms before presentation is only 1 to 2 months. Hemoperitoneum with an acute abdominal crisis may be the primary presentation.

In patients with localized hepatic tumors, most routine laboratory tests are normal. Anemia or thrombocytopenia are important findings because they may indicate that the mass is a benign vascular tumor with associated bleeding or platelet consumption. Thrombocytosis can be seen in both hepatoblastoma and HCC. Polycythemia, with hemoglobin levels higher than 16 g/100 ml may occur in patients with HCC due to the extrarenal production of erythropoietin. In patients with hepatic tumors, the SGOT and alkaline phosphatase may be slightly elevated, but the serum bilirubin is elevated in only 5% of patients with hepatoblastoma, compared with almost 25% of those with HCC.

An alpha-globulin, AFP is produced normally by embryonic hepatocytes and is present in the serum for the first few days after birth. Elevated alpha-fetoprotein has been described in 40% of children with HCC and in 67% of children with hepatoblastomas. The protein is not specific for hepatic tumors and can be elevated in the serum of children with embryonal testicular carcinoma and teratomas. Cystanthioninuria has also been described in children with primary hepatic neoplasms, but it can also be found in patients with neuroblastoma. Serum ferritin levels are elevated in 97% of patients with HCC, but they are also elevated in 87% of patients with uncomplicated cirrhosis. Although not useful diagnostically, serum ferritin levels have been observed to fall with tumor response, and to rise with tumor progression. Rarely, the serum hCG levels may be elevated in patients with virilization and hepatomas. The level of unsaturated vitamin-B_{12}-binding protein is elevated in the fibrolamellar variant of HCC and increases with disease progression.

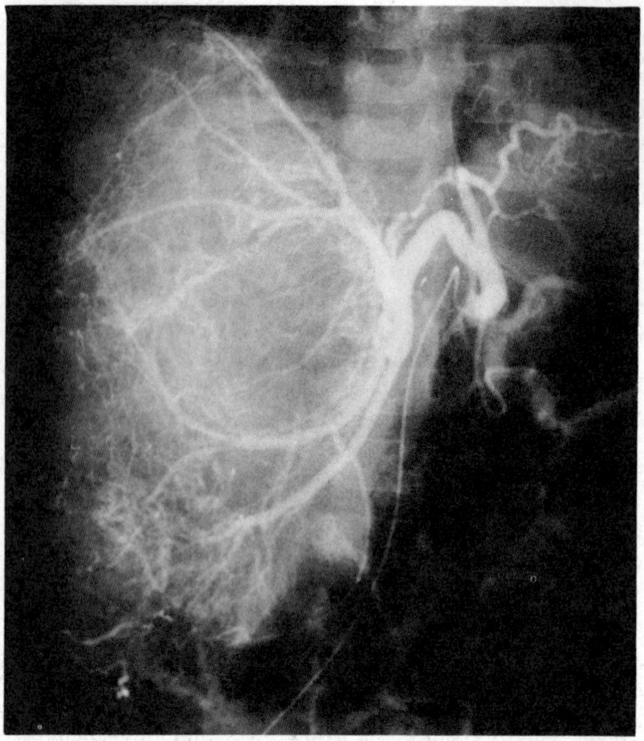

FIG. 47-6. Celiac arteriogram in 1½-year-old boy with abdominal distention for 3 months. Celiac axis is displaced to the left by a large vascular mass containing many tumor vessels and involving the inferior portion of the right lobe of the liver. A second mass can be seen in the left lobe. At surgery both lobes were involved by hepatoblastoma, and resection was not possible.

Because the primary goal of the initial evaluation is to define the extent of disease and to differentiate a primary hepatic tumor from the other abdominal masses that may occur in children, a chest x-ray film, abdominal radiograph, and IVP should be obtained. Ultrasound radionuclide liver scan, CT, and to a lesser extent, arteriography are important in delineating the contour and extent of the tumor (Fig. 47-6). Both hepatoblastoma and HCC have diffused hyperechoic patterns, in contrast to benign lesions, which are usually less ectogenic. CT scanning is important in defining the extent of tumor and potential operability. Characteristically, tumor masses have lower attenuation than surrounding tissue, although tumors may be isodense. CT scanning is of particular value in assessing the left lobe of the liver, a site hard to define by arteriography. Experience with MRI of the liver is limited but appears very promising.

Once a diagnostic mainstay, arteriography is now best used to define the vascular anatomy of a centrally located tumor or to determine the tumor margins not defined by CT scanning. Except in the case of a typical hepatic hemangioma, angiography rarely obviates the need for surgery. Surgical exploration is always necessary to provide a definitive diagnosis and to determine malignancy and resectability.

TREATMENT PLANNING

A staging system, based on surgical resectability, correlates with outcome (Table 47-21, Fig. 47-7). This approach is

TABLE 47-21. Clinical Grouping of Malignant Hepatic Tumors

Designation	*Criteria*
Group I	Complete resection of tumor by wedge resection lobectomy, or by extended lobectomy as initial treatment
Group IIA	Tumors rendered completely resectable by initial irradiation and/or chemotherapy
Group IIB	Residual disease confined to one lobe
Group III	Disease involving both lobes of the liver
Group IIIB	Regional node involvement
Group IV	Distant metastases, irrespective of the extent of liver involvement

Greenberg M, Filler R: Hepatic tumors. In Pizzo PA, Poplack DG (eds): Principles and Practice of Pediatric Oncology, p 576. Philadelphia, JB Lippincott, 1989.

verified by the fact that cure of primary hepatic neoplasms requires complete resection. From a surgical viewpoint, the liver can be divided into lobes and segments according to its vascular supply. The right lobe of the liver contains about 70% of the total liver mass, and each segment of the left lobe represents an additional 15%. Because of the liver's remarkable ability to regenerate, it is possible to remove as much as 85% of the total liver at one time and still expect complete regeneration of liver cell mass within 3 weeks in infants and within 3 months in children after surgery. Thus, tumors contained in one lobe of the liver and those arising in the right lobe that do not extend beyond the medial segment of the left lobe are amenable to surgical resection. Improvements in anesthesia and surgical techniques and in vigilant management before, during, and after surgery have minimized the hazards of hepatic resection.

Surgery

BIOPSY. Although excision is preferred, some tumors may be unresectable, because many liver segments are involved or because the hepatic arterial and venous inflow and outflow tracts are involved with tumors. In such cases, preoperative chemotherapy, with or without radiation, may render the tumor resectable. Before beginning such therapy, however, histologic diagnosis is essential. Although an open liver biopsy has been employed, a needle biopsy is quite satisfactory and avoids the need for general anesthesia, although hemorrhage may occur. Some recommend preoperative chemotherapy in patients with an elevated AFP who have CT scans and anteriograms suggesting hepatoma.

OPERATIVE TECHNIQUE. The recommended procedure for hepatic resection in children is similar to that used in adults. A thoracoabdominal approach is preferred because it offers excellent exposure and precludes the development of negative intrathoracic pressure, which may cause the aspiration of air into an open venous system. This approach also provides excellent visualization of the entire supradiaphragmatic inferior vena cava, into which an internal venous shunt can be placed so that liver blood flow can be isolated in the event of catastrophic hemorrhage.

Once the porta hepatis is dissected, the vessels and ducts to the lobe to be excised are ligated and divided. The liver is mobilized by dividing the diaphragmatic attachments, and the diaphragm may be divided radially to the vena cava. Tapes are passed around the vena cava above and below the liver to ensure control of excessive bleeding. Before the hepatic veins are isolated, the liver capsule is incised along a lobar or segmental division, and the liver substance is divided bluntly. Bridging vessels and bile ducts are ligated as they are encountered. Because of the very short extrahepatic length

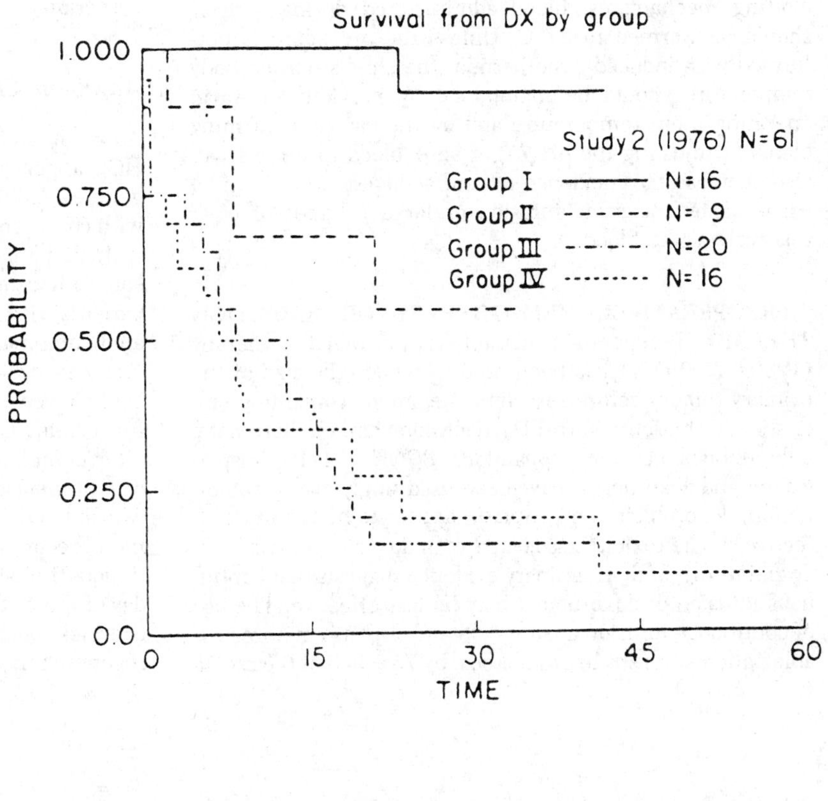

FIG. 47-7. Life table analysis of survival in a mixed population of children with hepatoblastoma and hepatocellular carcinoma. Shown is correlation between survival probability and clinical grouping 0 to 60 months after diagnosis and treatment. (Greenberg M, Filler RM: Hepatic tumors. In Pizzo PA, Poplock DG [eds]: Principles and Practice of Pediatric Oncology, p 576. Philadelphia, JB Lippincott, 1989)

of the hepatic veins in children, they should be approached by dissection through the liver substance rather than at their exit from the liver. By this technique, inadvertent venous injury, which can result in difficult to control bleeding, can be minimized. Large vessels and ducts are individually ligated on the raw surface of the remnant lobe. Sump and Penrose drains are placed in the liver bed, and the incision is closed. If the gallbladder remains, it should be drained with a cholecystostomy.

Profound hypothermia with circulatory arrest has been used as an adjunct to surgery in a difficult hepatectomy. Before division of the liver, cardiopulmonary bypass is instituted and hypothermia is induced. With the child's body temperature at 20°C, the circulation can be stopped for as long as 60 minutes, and resection and repair of vascular structures can be performed in a bloodless operative field. Alternatively, a normothermic, isolated hepatic circulatory arrest in which the lower thoracic aorta, porta hepatis, and the vena cava above or below the liver are clamped to effectively stop liver circulation has also been used as an adjunct to hepatic resection. Hemodilution is another procedure that produces an essentially bloodless exposure and permits the return of the patient's own red blood cells after surgery. These techniques should be considered for children with very large tumors or with tumors adjacent to the hepatic veins.

INTRAOPERATIVE MANAGEMENT. The most frequent and serious intraoperative problem is hemorrhage. Even without uncontrolled bleeding, the loss of one blood volume (up to 800 ml in a 10-kg child) is not unusual. Accurate measurement of blood lost in surgical sponges and by suction and measurement of intra-arterial blood pressure, central venous pressure, and urine output is necessary to estimate replacement volumes. Because hypothermia tends to cause cardiac irritability, metabolic acidosis, and abnormal blood clotting mechanisms, blood administered during surgery should be warmed to 37°C. Unless the procedure is performed with induced hypothermia, the child's normal body temperature should be maintained by providing a warm operating room temperature and by the use of a warming blanket. Adjusting the pH 7.0 of bank blood to pH 7.4 will also decrease the incidence of cardiac arrest, which can be triggered by the rapid infusion of large volumes of cold, relatively acidic blood.

PREOPERATIVE CHEMOTHERAPY OR RADIATION THERAPY. Preoperative chemotherapy or radiation therapy (1200–2000 cGy) has been used to reduce the size of the primary tumors before resection. Regimens containing vincristine, 5-fluorouracil (5-FU), dactinomycin, methotrexate, chlorambucil, cyclophosphamide, BCNU, VP-16, cisplatinum, and doxorubicin have been used singly and in combination, doxorubicin, and cisplatin appear to be the most effective.[31] The toxicity associated with doxorubicin has been dose limiting, and preliminary evidence suggests that continuous infusion of doxorubicin may be less effective. The use of continuous-infusion doxorubicin and cisplatin in unresectable patients has shrunk tumor size by 75% in 5 of 6 patients treated preoperatively, rendering each surgically resectable. Even with metastatic disease, the combination of chemotherapy, surgery, and radiation therapy can result in complete responses and long-term survival.

The preoperative chemotherapy and survival rates are not as promising for HCC. Only a third of patients with HCC are surgically resectable, and only a third of these are long-term survivors. Doxorubicin, VP-16, and 5-FU can induce partial remissions, but they are generally short-lived.

POSTOPERATIVE MANAGEMENT. Despite advances in surgical techniques, surgical morbidity and mortality are still high. Between 11% and 25% of the patients die during or after hepatic resections.[30] Blood loss was the most common intraoperative and postoperative complication. A single blood-stained dressing may represent significant blood loss in an infant, but too vigorous volume replacement may result in pulmonary edema. Other postoperative complications include subphrenic abscess, wound infection, biliary fistula, and small bowel obstruction.

Hepatic resection may result in a variety of metabolic derangements, particularly hypoglycemia and coagulopathies. These problems can usually be avoided by the continuous intravenous infusion of 10% dextrose postoperatively, with daily infusion of albumen for the first postoperative week and the administration of vitamin K.

Radiation Therapy

The role of preoperative and postoperative radiation therapy is less defined than that for surgery and chemotherapy. When employed, doses range between 1200 and 2000 cCy. Although used for preoperative therapy in patients failing to respond to chemotherapy, radiation therapy may be better used for the treatment of microscopic residual disease after resection.

Adjuvant Chemotherapy

Approximately 50% of children with hepatoblastomas or HCC appear to be cured after complete tumor resection. In general, children with hepatoblastoma do better than those with HCC. The use of preoperative chemotherapy in patients with inoperative tumors should further improve these results. Metastatic disease is an important cause of death in patients with residual tumor. The CCSG and the POG evaluated combination chemotherapy consisting of pulses of vincristine, cyclophosphamide, and doxorubicin, alternating every 3 weeks with vincristine, cyclophosphamide, and 5-FU for 1 year. Of 16 patients who received adjuvant therapy after complete surgical resection, only 1 patient developed distant metastases, compared with 7 of 11 historical controls who did not receive adjuvant chemotherapy. Among the regimens recommended are cisplatin (20 mg/m^2/day) by continuous infusion for 5 days with doxorubicin (25 mg/m^2/day) for 3 days. Treatments are given every 3 to 4 weeks for 6 cycles, beginning 3 to 4 weeks after surgery, permitting regeneration of hepatic tissue.

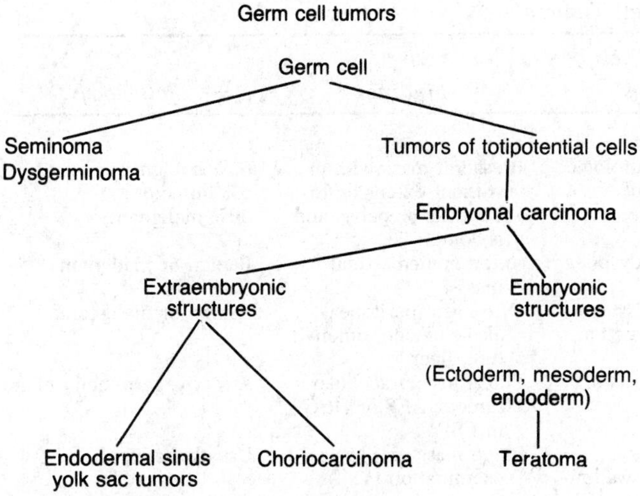

FIG. 47-8. Histogenesis of germ cell tumors.

GERM CELL TUMORS

The germ cell tumors of infants and children reflect the transformation of primordial cells that have failed to migrate to their predestined location. The totipotent germ cells normally arise from the yolk sac of the 4-week-old human embryo and migrate along the gonadal ridge to the gonadal anlage before their final descent into the pelvis. During embryogenesis, some of these germ cells fail to complete this migration and come to rest along the dorsal midline of the embryo. The primordial germ cells give rise to both an undifferentiated cell line and a primitive, committed germ cell line. The undifferentiated germ cell undergoes differentiation into either embryonic (*i.e.,* somatic cells) or the extraembryonic cells of yolk sac, chorion, and alantoin cells. Malignant transformation of these cells gives rise to tumors that reflect their embryonic features. Tumors of the embryonic germ cells are the teratomas and consist of each of the embryonic cell layers of ectoderm, mesoderm, and endoderm. On the other hand, tumors of extraembryonic cells have trophoblastic features, as in choriocarcinoma, or characteristics of the yolk sac endoderm and extraembryonic mesoderm, as in embryonal adenocarcinoma of the infantile testis (Fig. 47-8).

EPIDEMIOLOGY AND GENETICS

Germ cell tumors comprise approximately 3% of childhood neoplasms and have a bimodal age distribution. Almost 67% arise in extragonadal sites. Extragonadal teratomas and yolk sac tumors of the testis occur in infants and young children. Ovarian teratomas and dysgerminomas have their peak incidence during adolescence.

Karyotypic analysis has demonstrated duplication or loss of the short arm of chromosome 1. The malignant potential of histologically benign-appearing teratomas may be suggested by the DNA index, aneuploidy, and presence of C-*myc* oncogene. Germ cell tumors can occur with hematologic malignancies in children.

TABLE 47-22. Comparative Characteristics by Pathologic Types

Tumor Type	*Characteristic Histology*	*Frequency*	*Most Common Locations*	*Markers* AFP*	*Markers* HCG
Germinoma	Large round cells, vesicular nuclei, clear eosinophilic cytoplasm; monotonous pattern	+	Ovary, anterior mediastinum, pineal, undescended testes	−	−
Embryonal carcinoma	Poorly differentiated, epithelial appearance; solid or glandular, anaplasia, necrosis	++	Testes, young adult	+	+
Yolk-sac tumor (endodermal sinus tumor)	Papillary, reticular or solid pattern; papillary projections with perivascular sheaths (Schiller-Duval bodies)	+++	Testes, infant: sacrococcygeal, ovary	+	−
Choriocarcinoma	Cytotrophoblasts (large round cells, clear cytoplasm, vesicular nuclei) and syncytiotrophoblasts (syncytia with abundant cytoplasm); hemorrhage, necrosis	+	Mediastinal, ovary, pineal	−	+
Teratoma	Immature to well-differentiated tissues foreign to anatomic site with lack of organization; benign or immature may contain other malignant components	++++	Sacrococcygeal midline structures	−	−
Polyembryoma	Embryoid bodies, resembling embryos with amniotic cavity, yolk sac, and embryonic disc	+	Ovary, anterior mediastinum	+	+
Gonadoblastoma	Large germ cells surrounded by smaller Sertoli cells containing hyaline bodies and calcium	+	Dysgenic gonads	−	−

Ablin A, Isaacs H Jr: Germ cell tumors. In Pizzo PA, Poplack DG (eds): Principles and Practice of Pediatric Oncology, p 716. Philadelphia, JB Lippincott, 1989.
* AFT = alpha-fetoprotein; HCG = human chorionic gonadotropin.

TABLE 47-23. Comparative Clinical Presentations of Germ Cell Tumors

Tumor	*Age*	*Relative Frequency (%)*	*Symptoms*	*Findings*	*Pathology*
Extragonadal					
Sacrococcygeal	Infants	41	Constipation, neurologic abnormalities of bladder or lower extremities	Presacral mass with or without extension to buttocks or pelvis and abdomen	65% benign 5% immature 30% malignant
Mediastinal		6	Cough, wheeze, dyspnea	Anterior mediastinal mass	Benign or malignant
Abdominal	<2 yr	5	Secondary to pressure pain, GU obstruction, constipation*	Often retroperitoneal; also stomach, omentum, liver	Benign or malignant
Intracranial	Children	6	Headache, paralysis of upward gaze, incoordination	Pineal or supracellular tumors; AFP or HCG in CSF*	Any type germ cell tumor
Head and neck	Infants	4	Pressure-related; respiratory or swallowing difficulty	Large mass on physical examination	Usually benign
Vagina	<3 yr	1	Blood-tinged vaginal discharge	Polyoid mass from vagina	Usually malignant
Gonadal					
Ovarian	10–14 yr	29	Abdominal pain, nausea, vomiting, constipation, GU symptoms	Abdominal pelvic mass; calcifications in 50%; often + AFD or HCG	Any type germ cell tumor
Testicular	Infants, postpubertal	7	Painless swelling of testis	Testicular mass; metastases to lung in infants	Any type germ cell tumor 82% malignant 18% benign infants mostly yolk sac tumors

Ablin A, Isaacs H Jr: Germ cell tumors. In Pizzo PA, Poplack DG (eds): Principles and Practice of Pediatric Oncology, p 719. Philadelphia, JB Lippincott, 1989.
* GU = genitourinary; AFP = alpha-fetoprotein; HCG = human chorionic gonadotropin.

ANATOMICAL AND PATHOLOGIC CONSIDERATIONS

The classification and comparative pathology of germ cell tumors are shown in Tables 47-22 and 47-23.

Teratomas

Teratomas are composed of tissues that are derived from three germinal layers, the endoderm, mesoderm, and ectoderm. They may be solid or cystic and are classified histologically as mature, immature, and malignant.[32] Mature teratomas consist of well-differentiated tissues (*e.g.*, brain, skin, gastrointestinal, bone) and are benign. Immature teratomas contain embryonic tissue, usually neuroglia or neural tube-like structures, in addition to mature tumors. Teratomas with malignant potential may contain elements of germinoma, choriocarcinoma, endodermal sinus tumor, or embryonal carcinoma. There may be a mixture of mature, embryonic and unequivocally malignant elements, making examination of multiple histological sections mandatory.

Teratomas in infants and young children are primarily extragonadal. Of 245 patients with 254 teratomas admitted to the Boston Children's Hospital Medical Center from 1928 to 1982, 49% were detected in the newborn period. Sacrococcygeal teratomas were most common (40%), followed by ovary (37%), head and neck (6%), retroperitoneum (5%), mediastinum (4%), CNS (4%), testes (3%), and liver or trunk (1%) teratomas.

The vast majority (50–75%) of sacrococcygeal teratomas are diagnosed at birth, and nearly 75% occur in girls. Although every teratoma has the potential to become malignant, 75% to 82% are benign at presentation. Most tumors are diagnosed within the first 2 months after birth (90% at birth) and are almost invariably benign. Approximately 11% to 19% of teratomas contain immature but not frank malignant elements; these tumors have an increased likelihood of malignant degeneration.

Sacrococcygeal tumors can be external or internal (*i.e.*, presacral) and 44% of them have an external component and an intrapelvic or intra-abdominal extension. In 10% of patients, they can be entirely presacral.[33] Tumors that are entirely or predominantly external have a lower malignant potential than presacral tumors, 8% of which are malignant, or intrapelvic or intra-abdominal tumors, approximately 20% of which are malignant.

Sacrococcygeal teratomas vary in size from small localized lesions to massive tumors. Rarely, the tumor is so large in utero that a cesarean section is necessary for delivery, and death of the child due to uncontrolled hemorrhage has been reported during vaginal delivery if the tumor ruptures.

Germinoma

Germinomas are uniform in appearance, consisting of large, round cells with vesicular nuclei and clear or finely granular eosinophilic-staining cytoplasm separated by vascular fibrous septal-containing lymphocytes and focal granulomas.

The most common sites in children are the ovary, anterior

mediastinum, and pineal gland, and the tumor is the predominant histologic type found in dysgenetic gonads and undescended testes. Germinomas account for 10% of ovarian tumors in children and 15% of all germ cell tumors.

Embryonal Carcinoma and the Endodermal Sinus Tumor

Endodermal sinus tumor, or yolk-sac tumor, is the most common malignant germ cell tumor found in children. It is characterized by a labyrinthine glandular pattern consisting of flat epithelial cells and rounded papillary processes with a central capillary (Schiller-Duval body). The tumor represents a proliferation of both yolk-sac endoderm and extraembryonic mesenchyme. It was first recognized as a distinct entity by Teilum, because of its similarity to the endodermal sinus found in rat placenta. Although the vast majority of yolk-sac tumors present as infant testicular tumors, yolk-cell tumors occurring as pure or component portions of mixed germ cell tumors are rather common in the ovaries of young girls and in a number of extragonadal sites, including the sacrococcygeal area, pelvis, mediastinum, liver, retroperitoneum, vagina, and CNS.

Choriocarcinoma, Gonadoblastoma, Polyembryoma

Choriocarcinoma is an uncommon, highly malignant tumor consisting of gestational forms, arising from placenta, and nongestational forms, arising from extraplacental tissues in a non-gravid individual. In an infant, choriocarcinoma may present as a congenital tumor arising from a maternal placental primary tumor and transmitted to the fetal bloodstream; it presents as a mediastinal or ovarian tumor in young children or as a placental tumor in the pregnant adolescent. Choriocarcinomas consist of cytotrophoblasts, which are large round cells with clear cytoplasms and variable venicular nuclei, and syncytitrophoblasts, which are larger cells with vacuolated cytoplasm and irregular nuclei which form syncytia.

Gonadoblastoma is a rare germ cell tumor that occurs almost exclusively during the first two decades of life in dysgenetic gonads, usually in association with a Y chromosome. Almost 33% of these tumors are associated with germinomas. Gonadoblastomas consist of large germ cells surrounded by smaller round, darkly staining Sertoli cells, forming microfollicles consisting of hylanine bodies and calcium deposits.

Polyembryoma is a rare tumor that consists of embryoid bodies comparable to presomatic embryos. They stain positive for both AFP and hCG, suggesting both embryonic and extraembryonic differentiation.

CLINICAL EVALUATION AND TREATMENT PLANNING

Depending on the anatomic site, histologic type, and stage, surgery is combined with radiation or chemotherapy in the management of children with germ cell tumors. The surgical considerations are appropriate for each tumor.

Radiation Therapy

Radiation therapy can be highly curative, even in limited doses, for a number of germ cell tumors. However, in the more common yolk-sac tumors and embryonal carcinomas, or the malignant teratomas of extra-gonadal origin, the role of radiation therapy is less certain. Few patients with malignant sacrococcygeal teratomas have been long-term survivors. Similar data supports use of regional radiation therapy for other extragonadal tumors poorly controlled with surgery or chemotherapy.

Doses of radiation for germinomas may be limited to 25 Gy for patients with microscopic disease or to 35 Gy for large tumors. With endodermal sinus tumors (YST), effective local control has only been achieved at doses of 40 to 45 Gy or higher.

Chemotherapy

Methotrexate was the first chemotherapeutic agent to demonstrate efficacy against germ cell tumors, producing a 47% complete response rate in gestational choriocarcinoma. A number of agents have since been evaluated, both singly and in combination, with remarkable results in some germ cell tumors. Among the agents that have been used are vincristine, dactinomycin, cyclophosphamide, vinblastine, bleomycin, cisplatin, doxorubicin, and more recently, ifosfamide and VP-16. The most commonly employed combinations are VAC (vincristine, dactinomycin, cyclosphamide), VAB (vinblastine, dactinomycin, bleomycin), or PVB (cisplatin, vinblastine, bleomycin). For testicular tumors in adults, PVB combinations have been the standard, with complete response rates of 70% and overall response rates of 100%. Combinations of PVB plus doxorubicin have also been employed. For ovarian germ cell tumors in adults, PVB combinations have proven superior to VAC regimens for patients with endodermal sinus tumor and those with Stage III or IV disease of any cell type.

Similar regimens have been employed for germ cell tumors occurring in children. Adjuvant VAC chemotherapy has been most extensively used, particularly for children with ovarian tumors and endodermal sinus tumors. Other combinations have also demonstrated efficacy, particularly those with cisplatin, bleomycin, and doxorubicin in addition to vincristine, dactinomycin, and cyclophosphamide.

Vinblastine, bleomycin, cisplatin, dactinomycin, cyclophosphamide, and doxorubicin were evaluated in treating 79 children with poor-risk germ cell tumors; 39% had evidence of metastatic disease at diagnosis. Approximately 69% of these patients had complete responses and 27% attained partial responses. After 4 years, 45% of the patients are free of disease.

Epipodophyllotoxin and ifosphamide have been evaluated as salvage agents for both adults and children with germ cell tumors, particularly in conjunction with high-dose cisplatin. More intensive regimens using high doses of melphalan, VP-16, and cyclophosphamide have also been administered in conjunction with autologous bone marrow reconstitution. Regimens using ifosphamide and VP-16 in conjunction with cisplatin, bleomycin, cyclophosphamide, dactinomycin, doxorubicin, and vinblastine are being explored.[34]

Specific Management Strategies

SACROCOCCYGEAL TUMORS. For infants with external masses in the sacrococcygeal area, the differential diagnosis includes meningomyelocele, chordoma, duplication of the rectum, neurogenic tumors, lipoma, vestigial tail, and hemangioma. In infants without external masses, asymmetrical intergluteal folds warrant a careful rectal examination to search for a presacral lesion. The incidence of malignancy when the diagnosis is established before the infant is 2 months of age is 10% in boys and 7% in girls. If diagnosis is delayed until the infant is older than 2 months, 67% of boys and 47% of girls develop malignant tumors. A careful rectal exam is essential in the evaluation of these infants. With more advanced presacral or intrapelvic involvement, particularly when the diagnosis is delayed, infants may develop bowel or bladder dystonia as a consequence of the tumor mass. Albeit rarely, invasion of the lumbosacral plexus or spinal cord may result in lower extremity weakness and pain. Approximately 20% of infants with advanced local involvement have pulmonary metastases at the time of diagnosis.

Radiographic examination of the pelvis may demonstrate calcification in the tumor mass or the destruction of the sacrum. A barium enema, a CT scan, and an IVP should also be performed to evaluate the intrapelvic extent of tumor. A chest x-ray film should always be obtained to assess the presence of metastatic disease.

The serum AFP level is elevated in malignant sacrococcygeal tumors. Of 61 infants with teratoma, the AFP level was normal in 96% with mature lesions but was elevated in 97% of those with malignant elements. It is important to monitor AFP levels, even in patients whose sacrococcygeal tumor was initially benign, because late recurrences may develop. Serum ferritin may also be elevated in patients with germ cell tumors and, although not tumor-specific, may serve as another biologic marker.

The operative approach depends on whether the tumor is primarily extrapelvic or there is intrapelvic or intra-abdominal extension. For lesions that are predominantly external, a one-stage posterior sacral approach, in which the coccyx and possibly the lower sacrum are removed, is the treatment of choice. However, for lesions that extend into the pelvis, a two-stage procedure is generally necessary. An anterior approach through the abdomen is taken so that the superior extent of the tumor can be defined and removed. For the second stage, the child is positioned face downward and a V-shaped incision is made over the upper buttocks. The lower sacrum is divided, and with the coccyx attached to the specimen, the previously mobilized intrapelvic mass is delivered. Then, the lower part of the mass is separated from the rectum, and finally, the skin is incised posteriorly behind the mass so that the tumor can be removed intact. The major surgical complication is massive bleeding. In most children, anal and urinary sphincter functions are not impaired.

The success of therapy correlates most closely with the histologic type and the surgical resectability of the primary tumor. With few exceptions, patients with benign, resectable tumors survive with surgery alone. If local, benign recurrence takes place, re-excision can be curative. In contrast, fewer than 10% of children whose tumors have malignant components or who have surgically unresectable tumors survive.

MEDIASTINAL GERM CELL TUMORS. Mediastinal tumors are usually located in the anterior superior mediastinum, but they rarely can be located posteriorly. Occurrence in the mediastinum is related to the fact that the urogenital ridge in the embryo extends past C6 to L4. These tumors are often asymptomatic but may result in tracheobronchial compression hemoptysis or hormone production.

In boys, most lesions are endodermal sinus tumors, but (pure and malignant-element) teratomas have been described. Chest CT scanning is the imaging procedure of choice, and the differential diagnosis must include thymomas, thymic cysts, lymphomas, lymphangiomas, lipomas, bronchial and enteric cysts, and neurogenic tumors.

Most mediastinal germ cell tumors can be approached by a unilateral thoracotomy or a median sternotomy. Complete excision is necessary except for immature teratomas with neuroglial elements in young children; in older children, this can be highly malignant.

ABDOMINAL GERM CELL TUMORS. The primary sites are in the retroperitoneum, but can involve the stomach, omentum, and liver. Patients may present with vague abdominal complaints or bleeding, and abdominal germ cell tumors must be distinguished from Wilms' tumor, neuroblastoma, lymphoma, or rhabdomyosarcoma.

HEAD AND NECK. The oral cavity is the site of almost 6% of germ cell neoplasms. They are usually found at birth, and most are benign. Intracranial germ cell tumors account for 0.5.%–2% of brain tumors in children. They arise in the pineal area but also involve the suprasellar and infrasellar regions.

TESTICULAR TUMORS. Approximately 7% of germ cell tumors and 1% of all childhood cancers arise in the testes. About 77% of testicular tumors originate from germ cells; 25% of these are benign. Three types of testicular cancer are found in children: endodermal sinus tumors (or yolk-sac carcinoma), Teilum's tumor, and adenocarcinoma with clear cells. Less frequent are embryonal carcinoma, which is histologically similar to the tumor in adults, and teratocarcinoma; both are more likely to occur during puberty. Choriocarcinomas and seminomas are unusual in children; the youngest patient described being 8 years old. Although testicular tumors account for less than 1% of childhood tumors, they are much less common in American and African blacks and in Asians. An increased incidence of congenital anomalies, particularly of the genitourinary tract, is associated with patients with testicular germ cell tumors.

Most infants and young boys with cancer of the testes present with a painless mass that usually has been growing slowly for months. Almost all of these children, particularly those with endodermal sinus tumors, are younger than 2 years of age. Testicular tumors rarely occur in adolescents.

Nearly 25% of infants with a malignant tumor will also have a hydrocele, making transillumination potentially misleading. Physical examination usually reveals a hard, painless testicular mass, 2 cm or greater in diameter, not involving the scrotal wall or spermatic cord. The possibility of distant spread, particularly to lymph nodes in the inguinal and supraclavicular regions and retroperitoneum, should be carefully assessed. The scrotum should be carefully examined for evidence of direct extension to the scrotal skin and to determine if the mass is in the testis or in a paratesticular site.

Although endodermal sinus tumors tend to remain confined to the testes for a relatively long period, unlike embryonal carcinoma and teratocarcinoma, early diagnosis is critically important. However, the relative rarity of these tumors and a lack of awareness that testicular cancer can occur in young infants makes delays in diagnosis of up to 3 months common.

Once a testicular mass is suspected, a biopsy should be done as soon as possible. An inguinal incision should be made, and the spermatic cord should be exposed and occluded at the internal abdominal ring with a noncrushing vascular clamp before manipulation of the testis. If a gross diagnosis of neoplasm can be made when the testis is delivered into the wound, radical orchiectomy is performed by ligating and dividing the spermatic cord at the internal ring and removing the mass with the entire cord. If the testicular mass is obviously benign (hydrocele), appropriate treatment is provided and the testis is returned to the scrotum. In cases in which the diagnosis is uncertain, the testis is walled off with sponges and an incisional biopsy is performed. Frozen section diagnosis is used to determine further treatment. It is unnecessary to excise a portion of the scrotum unless the tumor has been previously biopsied in situ or if the extragonadal tissues are grossly involved. If retroperitoneal lymph node dissection is contemplated, placement of a nonabsorbable suture on the ligated spermatic cord will aid in defining the distal end of the inguinal dissection during lymphadenectomy.

The physician must determine whether the tumor is restricted to the scrotum and, if not, whether the retroperitoneal lymph nodes or distant sites are involved. This will dictate retroperitoneal node dissection, radiation, or chemotherapy. The major sites of metastases for testicular germ cell cancers are the lungs, liver, lymph nodes, and CNS.

A variety of staging systems are used, and in evaluating reports from different centers, the distinction between clinical staging and pathologic staging should be recognized, although they are usually the same for boys with this neoplasm.

Virtually all patients with embryonal adenocarcinoma of the testis and 90% of patients with nonseminomatous testicular tumors have elevated serum levels of hCG and AFP. Measurement of AFP and hCG before and after surgery, and then at least monthly, can assess tumor burden or recurrence.

Retroperitoneal node dissection has been recommended for accurate pathologic staging of testicular tumors. For example, of adults with Stage I embryonal carcinoma, 53% actually had Stage II disease after retroperitoneal lymphadenectomy. However, for endodermal sinus tumor, the results of node dissection have been quite different. Positive nodes were found in only 4 of 53 node dissections in clinical Stage I patients. Therefore, node dissection for staging purposes is useful only for those children in whom retroperitoneal node involvement is suspected by ultrasound or CT scan or for patients without lung metastases in whom AFP of hCG remains elevated.

After radical orchiectomy and clinical staging are completed, further therapy, possibly including retroperitoneal node dissection, chemotherapy, and irradiation, is considered. Approximately 80% of children will have Stage I disease and 20% will have Stage II or Stage III disease.

The value of node dissection in the treatment of endodermal sinus tumor is not clear cut. Current data suggest that radical orchiectomy alone is comparable to orchiectomy plus retroperitoneal node dissection for children younger than 36 months of age with Stage I embryonal carcinoma or endodermal sinus tumor. However, other data describe a cure rate (84%) after orchiectomy plus node dissection that is nearly twice the cure rate after orchiectomy alone (48%). These discrepancies may be due to inclusion of older patients in the early studies, histologic differences in the study populations, and the fact that less radical orchiectomies are performed than in the past. On the basis of current data, retroperitoneal lymphadenectomy is not recommended for patients with Stage I disease, particularly for children younger than 2 years of age.

However, when retroperitoneal lymph nodes are the site of metastatic disease (Stage II), lymphadenectomy appears to increase survival. Considerable controversy surrounds the value of bilateral or unilateral lymphadenectomy. The cross-communications between the lymphatic channels of the testes support the need for bilateral retroperitoneal node dissection, but very few patients have had negative ipsilateral nodes and positive contralateral nodes. Survival figures for patients with germ cell neoplasms receiving unilateral or bilateral adenectomies were comparable. Thus, unilateral dissection is recommended if no gross tumor is discovered. When ipsilateral nodes are grossly positive, bilateral adenectomy is advised, or a modified (superior aspect only) node dissection on the contralateral side can be performed, minimizing the possibility of retrograde ejaculation, a disturbing complication of bilateral adenectomy if both second lumbar sympathetic ganglia are excised. Although some reports raise doubts about the safety of this procedure in small children, experience indicates that retroperitoneal node dissection is tolerated well. A simple midline, paremedian, or transverse abdominal incision generally gives adequate exposure in children.

Approach to the Child with an Undescended Testicle. Although the incidence of an undescended testis is 0.23%, the risk for developing testicular cancer in these cases is 20 to 40 times that in a normal testis. Almost 20% of the tumors that occur in cryptorchid patients do so in the descended testis. This suggests that there may be a genetic predisposition to develop testicular cancer in patients with an undescended testis or that a basic defect in gonadogenesis accounts for both failure of the testis to descend and for subsequent oncogenesis.

Tumors of all germ cell types can arise in cryptorchid testis and can occur in adulthood (median age, 38 years). However, seminomas appear to be more common in the undescended testis than in the scrotal testis.

There is debate about orchiopexy in the child with an undescended testis. Although it is clear that orchiopexy will not prevent the development of testicular cancer, especially because it can arise in the contralateral descended testis, it does make the testis more accessible for palpation and monitoring. Because these patients have a higher risk for developing cancer, periodic evaluation is important. If the diagnosis of a crytorchid testis is not made until after puberty, when dysgenesis and atrophy are probable, orchiectomy is recommended.

OVARIAN TUMORS. Gynecologic malignancies are extremely rare in children and adolescents and differ in their clinical presentation and histology from those occurring in adults. Ovarian tumors are the most common, yet only account for 1% of cancers in girls younger than 17 years of age; non-ovarian malignant tumors are even less common. The peak incidence is between 10 and 14 years of age.[35] Unlike the pattern in adults, approximately 90% of pediatric gynecologic tumors are immature, and only 10% are differentiated carcinomas.

The ovary descends from the abdomen into the bony pelvis during puberty, and in younger children and in most adolescents, an ovarian tumor presents as an abdominal mass. The longer infundibular pedicle in the child also facilitates torsion of an enlarged ovary, resulting in abdominal pain. In the adolescent, abdominal pain can also be due to endometriosis, a diagnosis that is frequently overlooked. Symptoms can include constipation or genitourinary complaints. Rarely, tumors may produce hCG and can mimic signs of pregnancy. Non-neoplastic cysts comprise 25% to 35% of the ovarian masses, of which half are follicular and half are simple, parovarian, or luteal. In an infant, an adnexal mass is likely to be a non-neoplastic cyst. Mesonephric duct cysts (Gartner's duct cysts) and paramesonephric duct cysts can present as abdominal or pelvic masses. When associated with symptoms, or if the cystic mass is larger than 4 cm, laparoscopy or laparotomy is indicated.

The remaining 65% to 75% of ovarian tumors are true neoplasms, of which 33% are malignant. Germ cell tumors account for 60% to 89% of the ovarian tumors in children and adolescents (compared with 20% in adults) and are more likely to be malignant in younger children and infants. With increasing age, tumors of the sex cord stroma (granulosa-theca cell tumor, Sertoli-Leydig cell tumors) and tumors of common epithelial origin increase in frequency; in adolescents 15 to 17 years old, nearly 33% of ovarian neoplasms will be epithelial tumors. Most benign tumors occur in prepubertal patients, although malignant tumors occur after 13 years of age.

A calcified ovarian mass is found in nearly half of the patients, particularly those with benign teratomas. These can be demonstrated with pelvic ultrasound, and abdominal and chest CTs should be performed to rule out evidence of metastatic disease. Levels of hCG can be elevated with embryonal carcinoma and choriocarcinoma, and AFP increases in patients with endodermal sinus tumor.

The staging for ovarian tumors in children is modified from the International Federation of Gynecology and Obstetrics as follows:

Stage I: Disease limited to one or both ovaries. Capsule intact. Peritoneal fluid negative for malignant cell.
Stage II: Disease including or beyond the ovarian capsule with local pelvic extension. Retroperitoneal nodes and peritoneal fluid negative for malignant cells.
Stage III: Positive retroperitoneal nodes or malignant cells in the peritoneal fluid or abdominal extension.
Stage IV: Extra-abdominal dissemination.

In children, the ovaries are in the abdomen, and if there are malignant ascites, they are classified as Stage III disease. Approaches to management are based on the patient's tumor type and extent.

Mature Cystic (Dermoid) or Solid Teratoma. The benign neoplasm accounts for approximately 40% of ovarian tumors and is the most common tumor in older adolescents. These tumors are frequently unilateral in children, but in adults, nearly 25% are bilateral. Approximately 40% to 50% of mature teratomas are calcified, and diagnosis is usually suggested by a plain abdominal radiograph and ultrasonography. Malignant degeneration is rare in children. Therapy consists of oophorocystectomy with the preservation of as much ovarian tissue as possible. Oophorectomy is indicated only when there is torsion, rupture, or if the mass is so large that normal ovarian tissue cannot be reconstructed.

Immature Teratomas. These teratomas account for 7.4% of childhood ovarian neoplasms and most commonly occur around the age of 11 years. The tumors are composed of variable amounts of incompletely differentiated germ cell elements, most commonly of neural origin. Immature teratomas may not be clinically or grossly distinguishable from benign cysts or solid teratomas, and scrupulous histologic examination is important. Teratomas containing immature elements can become malignant, and survival is closely correlated with stage. Approximately 50% of patients with immature teratomas have measurable levels of AFP. These tumors tend to be radioresistant, and treatment has included surgery (salpingo-oophorectomy for unilateral lesions) and chemotherapy with VAC.

Dysgerminomas. These tumors comprise 16% of germ cell tumors. They are rare before the age of 10 and occur most frequently in prepubertal and young adolescent girls; nearly 50% of these tumors occur before the age of 20. These tumors are usually surrounded by a dense capsule and may be bilateral in 5% to 10% of patients. Dysgerminomas are endocrinologically inactive; hormonal symptoms signal an undetected teratocarcinoma with chorioepitheliomatous elements. Dysgerminomas are generally considered low-grade malignancies, although spread may occur if the tumor extends through the capsule and involves lymph nodes or blood vessels.

Treatment planning should take into account that dysgerminomas are highly radiosensitive tumors. If the tumor is well encapsulated, a salpingo-oophorectomy is recommended and has been associated with a 96% survival. More advanced disease may require hysterectomy and bilateral oophorectomy. Wide-field, low-dose irradiation or chemotherapy (VAC or PVB) are indicated if the tumor has penetrated through the ovarian capsule. Disease has recurred 5 to 34 years after treatment.

Embryonal Cell Carcinoma. This carcinoma accounts for 6% of ovarian neoplasms, is highly malignant, and occurs primarily in girls 13 to 14 years of age. Almost 60% of these tumors are associated with endocrinologic manifestations, including precocious puberty, abnormal vaginal bleeding, and hirsutism.[36] Both hCG and AFP are detectable in patients with this tumor. Because the survival for patients whose tumor has been completely resected, usually with salpingo-oophorectomy, is only 50%, adjuvant chemotherapy (VAC) is indicated.

Endodermal Sinus or Yolk-Sac Tumors. Like embryonal cell carcinomas, YST are highly malignant germ cell tumors, primarily occurring in older adolescents. AFP is detectable in virtually all cases. The fact that less than 20% of patients with localized and completely resected tumors are curable with surgery alone is testimony to the high malignant potential of these tumors. All patients, even with completely resectable tumors, should receive VAC or PVB chemotherapy. Mixed germ cell tumors are infrequent and are treated according to the most malignant element present.

Mesenchymal Sex Cord Stromal Tumors. Stromal tumors account for approximately 13% of ovarian tumors in children. The granulosa-theca cell tumor is the most common type and most often presents with precocious pseudopuberty and an abdominal mass, particularly in premenarcheal girls. Postmenarcheal girls may present with menstrual abnormalities or with virilization. In contrast to the typical thecal tumor in adults, the histologic picture in children consists of a diffuse or solid pattern with larger cells and prominent luteinization of cellular components; Call-Exner bodies and "coffee bean"nuclei are inconspicuous. This tumor follows a benign course in children and is usually effectively treated with a unilateral salpingo-oophorectomy. Sertoli cell tumor (androblastoma) is extremely rare and is benign and effectively treated with a salpingo-oophorectomy.

Epithelial ovarian neoplasms are rarely found in premenarcheal girls, and even when they occur in adolescents, their malignant potential is less than in adults. Because of their rarity, specific therapeutic guidelines distinct from those used in adults are not defined.

CERVICAL AND VAGINAL TUMORS. Vaginal or cervical neoplasms are rare in children. In infants and young children, vaginal tumors are more likely to be rhabdomyosarcoma (the botryoides variant) than carcinomas. However, with increasing age, evidence of cervical intraepithelial neoplasias (CIN) has been observed with frequencies of up to 31 of 1000 female adolescents. The current recommendation is for sexually active adolescents to have PAP smears annually.

In the early 1970s, an increased frequency of clear cell adenocarcinoma was observed in young women whose mothers had received diethylstilbestrol (DES) in an attempt to prevent fetal wastage. Although the survival rate for women with clear cell adenocarcinomas is 80% to 90%, this is closely correlated with the extent and stage of disease at diagnosis, and in-utero exposure to DES should be recognized as a significant risk factor. It is also important to recognize that the incidence of vaginal adenosis and adenocarcinoma depends on the age of the fetus at the time of in-utero exposure to DES and the dose and duration of DES treatment. As many as 20% to 90% of exposed girls can have vaginal adenosis, defined as mucinous columnar cells or metaplastic squamous cells, with or without mucinous droplets in the vaginal scrapings. Present recommendations call for all exposed girls to have pelvic examinations by an experienced gynecologist by the age of 14 or after menarche. This should include careful examination, cytologic samplings of the cervix and vagina, iodine staining of the vagina, and colposcopy and biopsy of suspicious lesions. Follow-up examinations should be performed annually. The treatment of clear cell sarcoma requires radical surgery, including vaginectomy, hysterectomy, and lymphatic resection.

RHABDOMYOSARCOMA

Rhabdomyosarcoma, putatively derived from the unsegmented, undifferentiated mesoderm, accounts for approximately 5% to 10% of all solid tumors in children. It is the most common soft tissue sarcoma in children younger than 15 years, with an annual incidence of 4.5 per million white children and 1.3 per million black children. Survival for children with rhabdomyosarcoma, like that for children with Wilms' tumor, has greatly improved since the incorporation of chemotherapy into treatment programs. With current multidisciplinary regimens, the overall 2-year survival rate for children with rhabdomyosarcoma is approximately 70%.

Rhabdomyosarcoma can occur in infants, children, or adolescents, and because its presentations are varied, is best not considered as a single entity. The extent of the tumor at diagnosis, its histology, and the primary site are each important factors for treatment planning and prognosis. During the last decade, many hundreds of patients have been entered into multi-institutional trials organized by the Intergroup Rhabdomyosarcoma Study (IRS), and much of our present understanding of the natural history, pathology, and treatment of rhabdomyosarcoma is derived from these studies.

EPIDEMIOLOGY AND GENETICS

Rhabdomyosarcoma appears to have two age peaks of occurrence, the first in children between 2 and 6 years of age and the second during adolescence, between 14 and 18 years. The early peak is primarily due to the occurrence of tumors in the head and neck region and the genitourinary tract. The late peak is predominately accounted for by primary tumors of the male genitourinary tract; tumors of the head and neck region, trunk, and extremity are also common in this group. Orbital tumors occur at any age.

As with other pediatric malignancies, rhabdomyosarcoma has been associated with several congenital disorders, including neurofibromatosis, Gorlin's basal cell nevus syndrome, and the fetal alcohol syndrome. A small number of families have also been described with an increased frequency of breast cancer in the relatives of children with rhabdomyosarcoma. Other familial associations have been reported, including an excess incidence of rhabdomyosarcoma in the siblings of children with brain tumors and adrenal cortical carcinoma.

There has been work on the characterization of the molecular and cytogenetic lesions of rhabdomyosarcoma, although this lags behind the progress made in neuroblastoma. Alterations in chromosome 3p24–21 were identified by banding techniques. In addition, there is a translocation t(2;13)(q37;q14) in alveolar rhabdomyosarcoma. Work with human rhabdomyosarcoma cell lines led to the identification of intracellular peptides that modulate cell growth, the transforming growth factors (TGF), tumor cell inhibitory factors (TIF), and of the transforming oncogene N-*ras*.

Human rhabdomyosarcoma xenograft lines were grown in the flanks of immunosuppressed mice to investigate the mechanisms of resistance of rhabdomyosarcoma to cytotoxic chemotherapy. Vincristine resistance may be related to the production of an altered tubuli subunit. In addition, the level of activity of a DNA repair enzyme correlates with the sensitivity of the rhabdomyosarcoma xenograft lines to the nitrosourea, methyl-CCNU. Human xenograft tumors have been invaluable for the rational development of new approaches to the treatment of rhabdomyosarcoma. The identification of melphalan as an active agent in the xenograft model has had its activity confirmed in Phase II clinical studies.

PATHOLOGY

The head and neck are sites for approximately 38% of rhabdomyosarcomas, with the orbit being the most common single location. The next most common sites include the genitourinary tract (21%), extremities (18%), trunk (7%), and retroperitoneum (7%). The sites of primary involvement are related to the age of the child. Histologic subtype of rhabdomyosarcomas vary according to both age and site.

Since the description in 1946 of rhabdomyosarcoma as a tumor of skeletal muscle, significant advances have been made in the histopathologic classification of this tumor and in correlating subtypes with clinical behavior and prognosis. Three major subtypes of rhabdomyosarcoma exist: embryonal, alveolar, and pleomorphic. The embryonal histologic subtype accounts for approximately 50% to 60% of childhood rhabdomyosarcoma and is characterized by variable numbers of large acidophilic myoblast cells and a large number of primitive round cells and spindle-shaped cells showing little myoblastic differentiation. The tumor stroma is usually loose and edematous. Compared with fetal tissue, the embryonal variant most closely resembles the developing muscle of a 7- to 1-week-old fetus. Although cross-striations can facilitate the diagnosis, they often are not visible by light microscopy. Sarcoma botryoides, although grossly distinguished by polypoid, edematous, and myxoid appearance, is histologically similar to embryonal rhabdomyosarcoma. The characteristic feature of the botryoides variant is the cambium layer of Nicholoson, a multilayered band of spindle cells with relatively little cytoplasm that lies parallel to and just below the mucosal surface of the tumor.

Alveolar rhabdomyosarcoma, the second most common subtype, is distinguished by a unique tissue pattern reminiscent of pulmonary alveoli. Tumor cells and giant multinucleated cells line septae and protrude into an open alveolar space. The alveolar subtype typically occurs in older children and young adults, is much more likely to occur in the extremities or perineal sites, is more likely to spread to the lymph nodes, and has a worse prognosis than the more common embryonal rhabdomyosarcoma.

Pleomorphic rhabdomyosarcoma is rarely seen in children, occurring primarily in adults aged 30 to 50 years. It is a more differentiated tumor composed of haphazardly and compactly arranged spindle cells and multinucleated giant cells.

A pathologic classification was developed by the IRS. This classification divides tumors into favorable and unfavorable histologies by cytologic features rather than the tissue pattern. There are two unfavorable histologic categories. The first, called anaplastic, is similar to that described for Wilms' tumor and is characterized by the presence of enlarged, bizarre mitotic figures and diffuse nuclear hyperchromatism with pleomorphism. It can be found focally or diffusely throughout the tumor. The second, called monomorphous, is characterized by round cells of uniform size with constant cytologic features. Tumors that contain neither anaplastic nor monomorphic features are histologically favorable. Of 405 cases evaluated from the first IRS trial, 330 (81.5%) were categorized as favorable, and 75 (18.5%) were categorized as unfavorable. This histologic grading was used to evaluate the prognosis of 261 patients with localized rhabdomyosarcoma on the second IRS trial, and 89% of the 211 patients with favorable histologic subtypes survived, compared with 72% of those with unfavorable cytologic features. If both the cytologic and tissue patterns are evaluated by light microscopy, a group of patients with a less favorable prognosis can be defined. Of 171 patients with completely resected rhabdomyosarcoma, 40 (23%) had either unfavorable cytology features or the alveolar subtype. The recurrence rate for these patients was 43%, compared with 15% for patients whose tumors did not have these unfavorable features. Analyses may permit the selection of patients who are at increased risk for tumor recurrence and who may profit from additional or more intensive therapy. However, the IRS criteria have not yet been fully validated.

An independent study at the National Cancer Institute and St. Jude Children's Research Hospital evaluated the IRS cytologic criteria in conjunction with the classical histologic classification (embryonal or alveolar) and other criteria (*e.g.*, solid variant of alveolar rhabdomyosarcoma) and demonstrated that the monomorphous or solid variant of alveolar rhabdomyosarcoma is associated with an aggressive clinical course, as is alveolar rhabdomyosarcoma of any cytologic type. Although various percentages of alveolar histologic features have been used by pathologists to diagnose "alveolar" rhabdomyosarcoma, it now is apparent that any amount confers a poor prognosis. Therefore, the "0% standard" is being used in IRS III to diagnose alveolar rhabdomyosarcoma for the assignment of treatment.

CLINICAL PRESENTATION

Rhabdomyosarcoma may occur at any body site containing striated muscle or its mesenchymal anlage. In infants, a frequent presentation is a grape-like, clustered polypoid vaginal mass, the botryoides variant of embryonal rhabdomyosarcoma. In young patients, the most common presentation is a mass in the head and neck region or genitourinary tract. In adolescence, rhabdomyosarcoma often presents as a painless extremity or truncal mass or as a nontender scrotal swelling that may be separate from the testis. Intra-abdominal lymph node metastases, which occur in as many as 26% of patients with paratesticular rhabdomyosarcoma, may sometimes present as an abdominal mass. The only sites not recognized by the IRS as probable primary tumors are brain, bone, and lung.

Rhabdomyosarcoma may present as a tumor mass or it may be discovered coincidentally during the evaluation of more nonspecific clinical symptoms. For example, a retroperitoneal rhabdomyosarcoma may present as an abdominal mass, with or without ascites, or it may present as an acute abdomen mimicking acute appendicitis. Rhabdomyosarcoma of the biliary tract, which is usually the botryoides type, most frequently presents with asymptomatic, direct hyperbilirubinemia due to biliary obstruction, but it may also present with symptoms of acute cholecystitis or "relapsing hepatitis."

Rhabdomyosarcoma is the most common malignancy involving the bladder, prostate, or vagina in children. The clinical presentation may be as an asymptomatic abdominal or perineal mass, with tumor encroachment or obstruction. Symptoms include increased frequency of urination, urinary retention, or hematuria.

Rhabdomyosarcoma is also the most common nonocular orbital tumors in children, usually presenting with proptosis, but rarely with evidence of direct extension into the central nervous system, perhaps because of its early diagnosis or containment by the bony orbit. In contrast, tumors of the middle ear may present as either a polypoid or botryoid mass associated with ear pain and chronic otitis media, as a hemorrhagic discharge from the ear canal, or with evidence of a cranial nerve palsy. Contiguous extension into the central nervous system by primary parameningeal rhabdomyosarcoma may result in cranial nerve palsies, increased intracranial pressure, and meningeal symptoms. Tumors of the nasopharynx can be subtle in their presentation, including airway obstruction, sinusitis, epistaxis, local pain, and dysphagia. The rich lymphatics of the nasopharynx contribute to contiguous and distant spread. The CNS is the most common site of invasion by nasopharyngeal rhabdomyosarcoma.

Rhabdomyosarcoma spreads by either direct extension to contiguous structures, such as parameningeal extension to the CNS, or by lymphatic and hematogenous metastasis. The margins of the primary tumor are often indistinct because of its pseudocapsule and are difficult to define on physical examination and at surgery. The incidence of lymph node metastases varies according to primary site in most series. However, there appears to be a particularly high incidence of lymph node involvement associated with primary lesions of the genitourinary tract (20%), paratesticular region (26%), extremity and perineum (10–17%), but the incidence of lymph node metastasis from other sites appears to be lower (*e.g.*, 4% in the orbit).

The most common sites of hematogenous spread are lungs, bone, bone marrow, and liver. Because this occurs at initial diagnosis in 10% to 20% of patients, pretreatment examination should include a careful evaluation of the extent of the primary tumor and a detailed investigation of potential metastatic sites. In addition to special radiographic studies of the primary site, patients should have a bone scan, chest CT scan, bilateral bone marrow biopsies, and aspirates. Patients with head and neck primaries should also have a head CT scan and spinal fluid examination. MRI scan may assist in defining the extent of the primary and its resectability.

STAGING

The staging system for rhabdomyosarcoma used most commonly is the IRS clinical-pathologic grouping system, which is based on the extent of the extirpative surgery, except in cases of distant dissemination (Table 47-24). Although this has been a useful approach to directing treatment, it obviates analysis of the local characteristics of the tumor, such as size and invasiveness, and incorporates results of therapy (*i.e.*, extent of operative resection) in outcome analysis. The IRS Committee analyzed IRS II patients retrospectively restaged using a presurgical system. They confirmed the validity of staging by the degree of involvement of contiguous organs or structures, tumor size of >5 cm, and the presence of metastatic disease. Furture IRS studies seek to prospectively evaluate a prospective TNM staging system. A clinically relevant staging system is necessary to assess results from different treatment centers.

TREATMENT PLANNING

The therapeutic plan for patients with rhabdomyosarcoma is determined by the primary site of involvement, histologic classification, and the clinical group or stage. Certain primary sites, such as the orbit, parameningeal, vagina, and prostate, are usually best managed by an initial biopsy followed by primary irradiation and adjuvant chemotherapy. Conversely, the management of limited trunk, extremity, and paratesticular lesions usually includes the removal of all gross disease followed by adjuvant chemotherapy with irradiation as needed.

Among patients with bladder or prostate lesions, the overall bladder salvage rate on the same IRS regimens has been approximately 35%, and the mortality has been 20% to 30%, which is higher than the mortality associated with standard primary surgical approaches. Primary uterine tumors are a distinct group (older patients) and apparently not very responsive to chemotherapy. Primary chemotherapy has

TABLE 47-24. Most Commonly Used Staging Systems for Rhabdomyosarcoma

Intergroup Rhabdomyosarcoma Study

Clinical Grouping System

GROUP I	Localized disease, completely resected Regional nodes not involved a. Confined to muscle or organ of origin b. Contiguous involvement-infiltration outside the muscle or organ of origin, as through fascial planes
GROUP II	Regional disease a. Grossly resected tumor with microscopic residual disease. No evidence of gross residual tumor. No clinical or microscopic evidence of regional node involvement b. Regional disease, completely resected (regional nodes involved completely resected with no microscopic residual) c. Regional disease with involved nodes, grossly resected, but with evidence of microscopic residual
GROUP III	Incomplete resection or biopsy with gross residual disease
GROUP IV	Metastatic disease present at onset

TGNM System

Summary of pretreatment clinical staging based on clinical, radiographic and laboratory examination (plus histologic biopsy):

A. Localized tumor with favorable histology and clinical negative nodes
B. Locally extensive tumor with favorable histology and clinically negative lymph nodes
C. Any size tumor with clinically involved regional lymph nodes and/or unfavorable histology
D. Distant metastasis

TUMOR - T(site)1 - confined to anatomic site of origin
(a) <5 cm in size
(b) >5 cm in size
T(site)2 - extension and/or fixation to surrounding tissues
(a) <5 cm in size
(b) >5 cm in size

HISTOLOGY - G1 - favorable histology (mixed, undifferentiated, embryonal, botyroid, other)
G2 - unfavorable histology (alveolar)
GX - insufficient tumor for histologic classification

Regional Lymph Nodes -
N0 - regional nodes not clinically involved
N1 - regional nodes *clinically* involved by neoplasm
NX - clinical status of regional nodes unknown (especially sites that preclude regional lymph node evaluation)

METASTASES - M0 - no distant metastasis
M1 - (sites) metastases present; subscript indicates site(s)

Subscript for T(site)	Subscript for M(site)
hn - head and neck	dn - distant nodes
or - orbit	lu - lung or positive pleural effusion
ex - extremities	li - liver
ex-lg - limb girdle	b - bone
gu - pelvic GU	m - marrow
te - paratesticular	n - CNS or positive CSF
ot - other (includes trunk, retroperitoneal and perineum)	s - soft tissue other than nodes
	p - peritoneum or positive ascitic fluid

clearly achieved its goal in eliminating anterior pelvic exeneration for patients with vaginal tumors.

Because the prognosis and approach to management vary according to the primary tumor sites, the general principles of management will first be considered and then applied to specific sites of disease.

SURGERY

The efficacy of radiation therapy and chemotherapy has had a major impact on the surgical procedures now recommended for rhabdomyosarcoma. Before the development of these modalities, radical operations were the only means to achieve tumor control; however, even with extensive and often disabling surgery, local recurrence rates were high and cure rates were low. Not only are some limited surgical procedures now adequate, but the timing and extent of these procedures are important for retaining high rates of survival and improving functional results.

The exact role of surgery varies with the location, size, and extent of the tumor at presentation. Surgical extirpation is indicated if removal of the primary tumor imposes no major functional disability or if excision of the primary tumor permits the elimination of postoperative irradiation by completely excising the tumor or permits a reduction in the dose without increasing functional deficit by eliminating all but microscopic disease. This approach is especially appropriate in the treatment of rhabdomyosarcoma of the extremity, for which Group I and II tumors without lymph node metastases have a much better prognosis then Group III tumors. However, patients with large, invasive extremity tumors (without evidence of metastatic disease) do poorly even after amputation.

If only partial tumor removal is possible, particularly if

removal would result in significant long-term disability, initial surgery should be limited to biopsy, preferably with sampling of regional lymph nodes. This is especially true in the treatment of orbital tumors, for which biopsy followed by radiation and chemotherapy has resulted in excellent long-term survival. Sampling of clinically uninvolved regional nodes is recommended for tumors of the genitourinary tract, paratesticular region, extremities, and perineum. Node groups with apparent involvement are biopsied regardless of the primary site, except for patients with Stage IV disease.

Preoperative chemotherapy or radiation therapy to reduce the size of the tumor, followed by removal of the residual tumor at a second operation, is currently under evaluation in the treatment of genitourinary rhabdomyosarcomas. The goals of this approach are the preservation of bladder function and achievement of long-term survival.

Radiation Therapy

Reports in the 1960s established the efficacy of high-dose, wide-field irradiation to achieve local control of rhabdomyosarcomas in children. With megavoltage equipment, orbital rhabdomyosarcoma could be controlled in 90% of patients with appropriate doses and volumes of radiation therapy.

Local control was achieved in 96% of the 27 patients treated with conservative, function-preserving surgery plus combination chemotherapy and high-dose, large-volume radiation therapy, with doses of 5500 to 6500 cGy to the primary tumor site. This approach has been confirmed in many studies. Concern about the relative toxicity of radiation therapy with chemotherapy and surgery has curtailed the use of more aggressive irradiation in growing children.

The IRS analyzed the role of radiation therapy in the local tumor control of 524 children with rhabdomyosarcoma and showed that radiation therapy was not required for patients whose primary tumor was totally excised and who had no microscopic residual disease (Group I).

For more advanced disease, radiation therapy is important for local and regional disease control. Overall local tumor control in patients with local residual disease (Stages II and III) is well documented in 75% to 90% of those treated with adequate irradiation and chemotherapy.

Both principles of treatment include wide volumes, using prechemotherapy or preoperative tumor extent to determine irradiation fields. Wide margins are important; 60% local or regional failure in paramengineal tumors are due primarily to inadequate irradiation volumes. Inclusion of regional lymph nodes with documented involvement is important; irradiation of clinically uninvolved nodes is controversial.

Greater than 95% local control can be achieved for microscopic disease (Stage II) with 4000 cGy. For patients with "gross" or "bulky" disease (Stage III), doses in excess of 5000 to 5500 cGy are required. Daily fractions of 150 to 180 cGy are effective and well tolerated.

In selected patients, brachytherapy may be of value. Particularly for pelvic tumors, the use of intracavitary irradiation may facilitate disease control with less damage to surrounding normal tissues.

Chemotherapy

After the routine use of systemic chemotherapy, the long-term survival for children with rhabdomyosarcoma was poor, and cure was largely restricted to a few favorable anatomic sites, such as the orbit. The utility of adjuvant chemotherapy in patients who had been rendered disease-free with surgery or radiation therapy has been convincingly demonstrated. The survival for patients receiving vincristine plus dactinomycin was 82%, compared with 47% for patients not receiving chemotherapy.

Many chemotherapeutic agents have single-agent activity in rhabdomyosarcoma (Table 47-25), although the most commonly used regimens include combinations of vincristine, dactinomycin, and cyclophosphamide. Refinements of the chemotherapy regimens for rhabdomyosarcoma have been generated by the IRS studies. Data accrued from the first of these cooperative trials (IRS I) supported the following conclusions.

1. Adjuvant chemotherapy with vincristine, dactinomycin, and oral cyclophosphamide (VAC) (Table 47-26) eliminates the need for postoperative radiation therapy in patients whose tumors were totally excised and who had no evidence of residual microscopic disease (Group I).
2. A two-drug regimen (vincristine + dactinomycin) was

TABLE 47-25. Response of Rhabdomyosarcoma to Single Agents

Drug	*No. of Evaluable Patients*	*CR*	*PR*	*% CR + PR/ Total*
Dactinomycin	14		6	43
Cyclophosphamide	26	2	11	42
Vincristine	42	3	10	31
Doxorubicin	40	2	11	33
Cisplatin	19	1	3	21
VP-16 (Etoposide)	5		1	20
DTIC	9		2	22
Methotrexate	6	1	2	50
Melphalan (newly diagnosed)	13		10	77
Melphalan (recurrent)	13		2	8
Ifosfamide	8		2	25

* CR = complete response (100% disappearance); PR = partial response (50–99% disappearance).

TABLE 47-26. Drug Doses and Schedules in Clinical Use

Intergroup Rhabdomyosarcoma Study
Vincristine, 2.0 mg/m² (maximum, 2.0 mg) IV weekly for 6 to 10 weeks
Doxorubicin (Adriamycin), 30 mg/m² IV daily × 2
Cyclophosphamide, 10 mg/kg IV daily × 3
Dactinomycin, 0.015 mg/kg (maximum, 5.0 mg) IV daily × 5
Pediatric Branch, NCI
Vincristine, 2.0 mg/m² (maximum, 2.0 mg) IV weekly for 6 weeks
Doxorubicin, 35–45 mg/m² IV daily × 2
Cyclophosphamide, 900 mg/m² IV daily × 2
St. Jude Children's Research Hospital
Doxorubicin, 60 mg/m² IV
Dacarbazine (DTIC), 250 mg/m² IV daily × 5
Vincristine, 2.0 mg/m² (maximum, 2.0 mg) IV weekly for 6 weeks
Dactinomycin, 1.5 mg/m² IV × 1
Cyclophosphamide, 200 mg/m² IV or PO daily × 5

as effective as three drugs (VAC) for patients with grossly resected but microscopic residual disease (Group II) treated with radiation.

3. Doxorubicin did not improve the outcome when added to pulse VAC (vincristine, dactinomycin, and intravenous cyclophosphamide) for patients with gross residual (Group III) or disseminated (Group IV) disease. However, doxorubicin was not given in an optimal schedule.

The relapse-free survival rates at 3 years were 82% to 84% for Group I, 63% to 72% for Group II, 54% to 61% for Group III, and only 17% to 23% for Group IV patients (Table 47-27). Preliminary conclusions drawn from the data generated from 511 patients in IRS I reported in 1983 include the following:

1. The chemotherapy regimen for Group I patients could be simplified, because a two-drug regimen (vincristine + dactinomycin) appeared as effective (83% 2-year relapse-free survival) as the three-drug VAC regimen (87% 2-year relapse-free survival).
2. A moderately more intensive regimen of vincristine and dactinomycin was as good as or better (81% 2-year relapse-free survival) than a pulse VAC regimen of vincristine, dactinomycin, and intravenous cyclophosphamide (70% 2-year relapse-free survival) for Group II patients, all of whom had postoperative irradiation.
3. Treatment of Groups III and IV patients remains a problem. In this trial, the addition of doxorubicin to the VAC regimen did not result in a major improvement in survival. The preliminary results for Group IV patients showed the 3-year survival in IRS II to be 32%, compared with 17% to 23% in IRS I.[37]

TABLE 47-27. Actuarial Survival at Three Years: Results of The Intergroup Rhabdomyosarcoma Studies I and II

Prognostic Factors	*IRS I*	*IRS II*
Clinical Group		
I	79	88
II	68	77
III	42	68
IV	18	32
Histologic Type		
Embryonal		69
Alveolar		56
Other		66
Primary Site		
Orbit	91	93
Genitourinary (GU)	74	
GU (mainly Group III)		64
Cranial parameningeal	53	71
Other head/neck	59	69
Trunk	53	57
Extremity	53	56
Retroperitoneum–pelvis	39	46
Total	686	956

For patients with advanced disease, new approaches to treatment are being explored. The most prominent are new drugs, such as cisplatin, VP-16, and DTIC, added to the current chemotherapy regimen of vincristine, dactinomycin, cyclophosphamide, and doxorubicin, and the intensification of chemotherapy, particularly doxorubicin and cyclophosphamide, with or without total-body irradiation and autologous bone marrow rescue. General conclusions from the St. Jude Children's Research Hospital study of preirradiation chemotherapy in the treatment of rhabdomyosarcoma are that the approach does not jeopardize overall survival and does allow the assessment of chemotherapy response independently. Those patients with chemotherapy-resistant tumors were unlikely to be locally controlled with irradiation. This identifies subsets of patients who may be approached with experimental techniques such as hyperfractionation or brachytherapy.

Analysis of many studies suggests that many of the patients who are disease-free at 2 years will remain in remission. However, if relapse occurs, the long-term survival rate is poor (2%), emphasizing the need to maximize primary treatment regimens and to develop better salvage protocols.

Management of Specific Tumors

HEAD AND NECK PRIMARIES. Embryonal tumors (78%) predominate in the head and neck region, including the botryoid variant in the pharynx, larynx, maxillary sinus, and middle ear. Alveolar tumors are found in 9.5% of cases; extraosseous Ewing's sarcoma is found in 2.5%; and 10% are undifferentiated.

Before the routine use of chemotherapy and adequate irradiation, the long-term survival of patients with head and neck primaries was poor (9–15%), with metastases occurring by both the hematogenous and lymphatic routes. After combined modality therapy, the 3-year disease-free survival for patients with rhabdomyosarcoma of the head and neck region (Groups I–III) rose to 66%.

In spite of these improvements, the potential long-term complications of therapy are of concern because the mean age of children with head or neck rhabdomyosarcoma is less than 10 years. In particular, the use of high-dose local radiotherapy and prophylactic whole-brain radiation can cause major complications for these children, and the facial, dental, mucosal, and endocrine complications of high-dose radiotherapy, especially if administered with chemotherapy, are well known.

EYE AND ORBIT. The orbit is the most common site for rhabdomyosarcomas of the head and neck region, accounting for approximately 25% of these tumors. Since the institution of multimodality therapy for orbital rhabdomyosarcomas 91% of patients are disease-free at 3 years. Orbital tumors are usually confined to the orbit and surrounding structures and rarely metastasize to distant sites, local nodes, or the CNS if properly irradiated. Although most orbital tumors are only biopsied and are thus classified as Group III tumors, orbital exenteration is unnecessary because of the efficacy of radiotherapy and chemotherapy, except for local recurrence after conventional therapy.

Whether radiation should be administered before or in conjunction with systemic chemotherapy is controversial. The IRS protocols used simultaneous therapy. The total radiation dose is comparable to that prescribed for other sites, and the minimal volume usually includes the entire bony limits of the orbit. For treatment of limited disease, this field usually extends from the supraorbital ridge superiorly, to the infraoptic foramen interiorly, and across the midline to the inner canthus of the opposite eye. To avoid chronic keratoconjunctivitis, radiation therapy should be delivered with the eyelids open. Because the preauricular and upper cervical nodes appear to be negative in most cases, their inclusion in the irradiated field is unnecessary.

Adjuvant chemotherapy is necessary for all patients with orbital rhabdomyosarcoma. Treatment with radiation alone results in hematogenous metastases in approximately 33% of the patients. The most common therapy uses vincristine plus dactinomycin.

Ninety percent of the children whose orbits have been irradiated for rhabdomyosarcoma developed evidence of a cataract 1 to 4 years after completion of therapy. Enophthalmus, stenosis of the lacrimal duct, keratoconjunctivitis, photophobia, or conjunctivitis were seen in 20% of these patients. Secondary surgery was necessary in approximately 33% of these patients to improve functional results after radiotherapy; enucleation has been required in 8% of cases.

PARAMENINGEAL RHABDOMYOSARCOMA. The parameningeal sites include the middle ear, auditory canal, mastoid, nasal cavity, paranasal sinuses, pharynx, pterygopalatine fossa, and the infratemporal fossa. Patients with parameningeal tumors who were enrolled in the IRS I protocol had a significantly lower 3-year relapse-free survival (46%) than those with other head and neck primaries. The reason for treatment failure in 35% of these patients was tumor invasion into the CNS. This was a particularly ominous event, because none of the patients who developed this pattern of relapse survived. Detailed analysis of these patients suggested that these local treatment failures were probably a reflection of inadequate radiation dose (13 of 19 patients received less than 5000 cGy) and volume (11 of 19 patients had less than adequate volume). After using adequate treatment fields and doses > 5000 cGy, parameningeal tumor extension occurred in less than 5% of the patients. Rhabdomyosarcoma arising in a parameningeal site has a propensity for contiguous extension into the CNS, but radiation ports that include potential extension sites control the tumor in many patients. Current treatment planning includes higher radiation doses and more carefully planned radiation ports based on extensive imaging studies before chemotherapy. Intrathecal chemotherapy for patients with parameningeal disease may be unnecessary if the radiation ports are adequate. These modifications have resulted in a significant reduction in local failures and CNS extension in patients with primary parameningeal rhabdomyosarcoma.

OTHER HEAD AND NECK TUMORS. Rhabdomyosarcoma can arise in the scalp, neck, parotid, oropharynx, larynx, or cheek. Surgical resection with margins that are sufficient to eliminate the need for radiation therapy are rarely possible without unacceptable functional or cosmetic consequences. Thus, primary radiation and chemotherapy form the cornerstone of management for these patients. Of 36 patients with primaries in these areas (Groups I–III), 27 (75%) have remained disease-free for 3 or more years after therapy. Four of 5 failures had received no irradiation or <1500 cGy. Only 2 of 37 patients with nonorbital, nonparameningeal primaries of the head (excluding the neck) on IRS I have relapsed.

PRIMARY TUMORS OF THE TRUNK. The trunk is the primary site in 7% to 9% of patients. The prognosis for this group, influenced by the type, extent, and location of the tumor at diagnosis, is not as favorable as that for patients with head and neck primaries. Of 30 patients, 14 tumors occurred on the chest wall, 10 were paraspinal, and 6 were on the abdominal wall; 15 of the 30 patients remained disease-free at 5+ years. The prognosis appeared to be best for patients with paraspinal tumors (7 of 10 surviving disease-free) and poorest for those with chest wall tumors (5 of 15 survived disease-free). Only 3 of 12 patients with alveolar tumors have remained disease-free, in contrast to 12 of 18 patients with nonalveolar tumors. Of 18 patients with retroperitoneal tumors treated with multimodality therapy, 14 had a greater than 50% tumor response; however, only 4 remained alive and free of active tumor.

As expected, patients with localized tumors of the trunk (Groups I and II) fare better (9 of 14 surviving disease-free) than those with extensive local or disseminated tumor at diagnosis (6 of 16 disease-free survivors). Because of the poorer prognosis for patients with gross residual disease, complete surgical removal of the tumor is recommended and should be possible in many of these patients without unacceptable consequences. Such procedures are frequently recognized as incomplete, because microscopic residual disease is found in the detailed examination of the specimen. If the tumor is completely excised with adequate margins and there is no microscopic disease, postoperative irradiation is not necessary. Use of electron-beam irradiation and interstitial techniques and the judicious use of photon irradiation to minimize normal tissue damage are particularly important. Because the major reason for failure in this group is distant dissemination, adjuvant chemotherapy is essential.

PRIMARY TUMORS OF THE EXTREMITY. Approximately 16% of rhabdomyosarcomas occur in the extremities. In contrast to tumors of the head and neck region, rhabdomyosarcoma of the extremity is more common in adolescents, is associated with a high incidence of relapse, and has a low survival rate. Early studies suggested that upper extremity and distal lesions had a better prognosis than lower extremity and proximal lesions, an observation which is supported in the IRS I study, in which 44% of patients with lower extremity lesions relapsed, compared with 30% of those with upper extremity disease.

Rhabdomyosarcoma of the extremity is distinct in two important ways: the high incidence of alveolar cells (44% compared with 16% for all other sites); and the high incidence of lymph node metastasis (17% compared with none for orbit lesions and 3% for head and neck primaries). The importance of histologic types is reflected in the higher relapse rate (65%) for patients with Stage I or II disease whose extremity tumors were alveolar, compared with 33% for patients with nonalveolar tumors, although their initial response rates were similar.

Although wide surgical resection should be performed if it can be accomplished without causing a major functional defect, amputation, especially of the upper extremity, is rarely required. Delayed amputation may be necessary if significant uncorrectable growth discrepancy occurs in the lower extremity after cure of the lesion. Because of the high incidence of regional lymphatic spread, a lymph node biopsy is recommended. The radiation guidelines are similar to those for other sites, although care must be taken to avoid circumferential irradiation with its attendant risk of long-term vascular and lymphatic complications.

The major problem in the treatment of patients with alveolar rhabdomyosarcoma continues to be the failure to control systemic disease. Current regimens for patients with extremity lesions use more intensive chemotherapy schedules.

PRIMARY TUMORS OF THE GENITOURINARY SYSTEM. The genitourinary tract is the primary site of approximately 20% of rhabdomyosarcomas. The principal genitourinary sites are the prostate, bladder, vagina, and paratesticular tissues. The overall survival was 70% to 75% for patients with genitourinary primaries. As with other sites, the overall survival of patients with genitourinary tumors is related to stage; relapse rate is 19% for patients with localized, grossly resected bladder and prostate tumors, compared with 39% for patients with Group III or IV disease at diagnosis. The most common histologic type is embryonal, although the botryoid variant occurs frequently in these sites. Lymph node metastases are common but site-specific. For example, 26% of patients with paratesticular primaries have para-aortic node involvement, compared with a lower incidence for vaginal primaries. The role of retroperitoneal node dissection is an area of controversy, particularly in view of its long-term complications. It is generally recommended that regional nodes be sampled, especially in patients with paratesticular primaries, and if they are positive, patients should receive radiation therapy.

Although the survival of patients with tumors at these sites has improved markedly with the addition of combination chemotherapy to pelvic surgery and radiation therapy, the long-term sequelae of these therapies in young children are significant. The use of primary chemotherapy (pharmacologic debulking) followed by limited surgery and irradiation has been evaluated for treatment of the primary tumors of the genitourinary tract. This sequencing has eliminated anterior pelvic exenteration for many children with vaginal tumors. Among patients with localized bladder or prostate lesions, the overall bladder salvage rate on the IRS regimens has been approximately 35%; the mortality of 20% to 30% with attempted bladder salvage seems higher than that associated with standard primary exenteration approaches. Primary uterine tumors are a distinct group (older age) and apparently not very responsive.[38]

Radiation therapy seeks to include the pelvic disease with maximal sparing of the femoral heads, acetabulum, and bowel. Coordination of radiation with cyclophosphamide is important to minimize short-term and long-term bladder complications. Rotational and multiple-field techniques should be used. Brachytherapy may be possible in selected cases. Dose and volume considerations are comparable to other sites. If para-aortic node biopsies and lymphangiogram are negative, radiation to these regional nodes may be omitted. If positive, however, these lymph nodes should be included in the radiation fields.

EWING'S SARCOMA

In 1921, James Ewing described a vascular, hemorrhagic bone tumor composed of small, round cells without associated osteoid formation that usually occurred in the midshaft of the long bones or in the flat bones of the trunk. Although Ewing's sarcoma, the second most common primary bone tumor of childhood, was originally thought to arise from the endothelial cell, recent evidence suggests that it is probably derived from primitive neural tissue. Molecular and cytogenetic studies of this tumor produced important clues regarding the molecular pathogenesis of this disease. Multimodality therapy has increased the proportion of long-term disease-free survivors from less than 15% to more than 50% over the past two to three decades.

EPIDEMIOLOGY AND BIOLOGY

Ewing's sarcoma occurs most frequently in the second decade of life and is rare before 5 or after 30 years of age (Fig. 47-9). The incidence in males is equal to that in females until age 13 years, when, as with osteosarcoma, males predominate. As with osteosarcoma, epidemiologic studies demonstrate that taller individuals are more likely to develop Ewing's sarcoma, suggesting that its development is in some way linked to growth.

The incidence of Ewing's sarcoma in the United States for white children younger than 15 years of age is 1.7 cases per million per year. A striking epidemiologic finding is the exceedingly low incidence of Ewing's sarcoma in African and American blacks and Chinese. Ewing's sarcoma has not been associated with congenital syndromes, but an association with skeletal anomalies (*i.e.*, enchondroma, aneurysmal bone cyst) and genitourinary anomalies (*i.e.*, hypospadias,

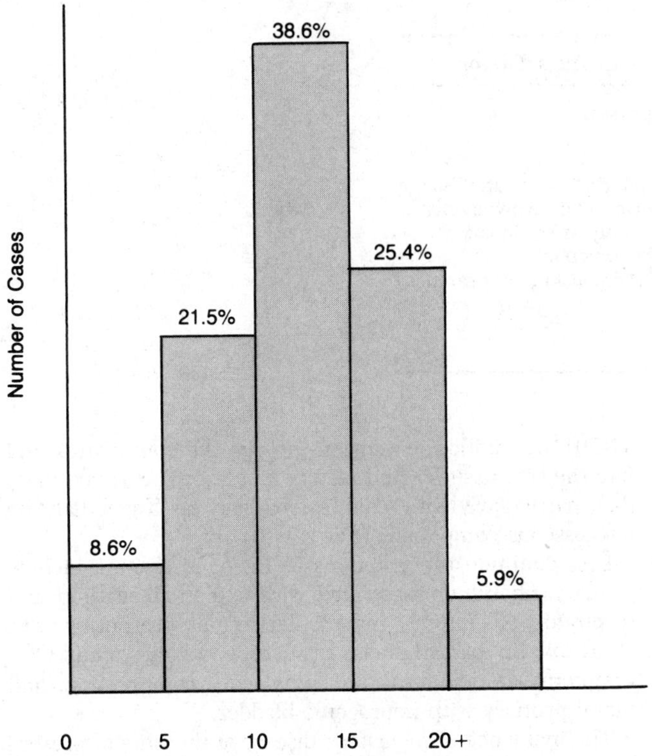

FIG. 47-9. Age distribution of 303 cases of Ewing's sarcoma of bone in the Intergroup Ewing's Sarcoma Study (IESS).

duplication of the renal collecting system) has been reported. Ewing's sarcoma has also been associated with retinoblastoma.

A chromosomal translocation, t(11:22), is a characteristic abnormality of Ewing's sarcoma. In a series of 13 karyotyped tumors, 9 demonstrated this translocation and 2 others contained a deletion on chromosome 22. The translocation is indistinguishable from that reported in peripheral neuroepithelioma by Whang-Peng and colleagues.[39] This has given rise to the hypothesis that these entities have a common histogenesis. This is further supported by the demonstration of neuroectoderm-associated antigens on Ewing's cell lines in culture and identical patterns of proto-oncogene expression as seen in peripheral neuroepithelioma.

PATHOLOGY

Ewing's sarcoma is an undifferentiated round cell tumor possessing no unique morphologic markers. It is diagnosed only after the exclusion of the other small, round, blue cell tumors of childhood, which include primary sarcoma of bone (including small cell osteosarcoma and mesenchymal and myxoid chondrosarcoma), primitive sarcoma of bone, rhabdomyosarcoma, lymphoma, neuroblastoma, and peripheral neuroepithelioma. Refinements in electron microscopic, immunocytochemical, cytogenetic, and molecular genetic techniques have increased the sensitivity with which these tumors can be identified, consequently shrinking the numbers of cases left in the Ewing's "waste basket." Biopsy should ensure that adequate tissue is obtained for these special studies. Tissue for electron microscopy is best fixed in glutaraldehyde and in alcohol for immunocytochemistry. The thin-needle biopsy may compromise an accurate diagnosis.

By light microscopy, Ewing's sarcoma is a diffuse mass of homogenous tumor cells. There is often a biphasic population, with larger, clear cells and smaller, darker cells. Marked vascularity and widespread coagulative necrosis are typical features. The tumor infiltrates bone with surprisingly little destruction. Tumor margins are usually infiltrative or "pushing." A filigree pattern in which finger-like processes of compact, basophilic cells intertwine correlates with poorer survival.[40]

The cells of Ewing's sarcoma are approximately the size of histiocytes, two to three times the size of a small lymphocyte, and have a centrally placed ellipsoid or spherical nucleus with a delicate nuclear membrane. The nuclear chromatin is usually faintly stippled, and the nucleoli are inconspicuous. The cytoplasm of Ewing's sarcoma is devoid of organelles, but cytoplasmic glycogen is usually demonstrable by electron microscopy or the periodic acid-Schiff (PAS) stain with light microscopy. A large cell variant consisting of larger, more pleomorphic cells with conspicuous nucleoli demonstrates the same clinical behavior as typical Ewing's sarcoma. An unusual pattern of intramyofiber skeletal muscle invasion by tumor cells seen in a few patients is a negative prognostic factor.

Ewing's sarcoma is a diagnosis of exclusion that will be made with decreasing frequency by pathologists who, using electron microscopy and immunocytochemistry, diligently search for clues to a tumor's histogenesis. This can be a source of frustration for the oncologist who must determine treatment for patients with tumors that have limited "history," such as primitive sarcomas of bone and peripheral neuroepithelioma. A rational approach is to treat the Ewing's family of tumors in a uniform manner until there is data to indicate that specific subsets have biological differences that warrant a unique approach.

TABLE 47-28. Distribution of Primary Sites in Ewing's Sarcoma

Primary Site	*Frequency (%)*	
Pelvis/sacrum	20.5	
Pelvis		17.2
Sacrum		3.3
Proximal extremity	31.4	
Humerus		10.6
Femur		20.8
Distal extremity	27.1	
Tibia		10.6
Fibula		12.2
Radius + ulna		2.0
Hands + feet		2.3
Other	14.1	
Rib		6.9
Vertebrae		4.9
Skull/face		2.8
Scapula		4.0
Clavicle		1.7
Other		0.7

TABLE 47-29. Typical Radiographic Characteristics

Feature	*Osteosarcoma*	*Ewing's Tumor*
Location in bone	Metaphyseal	Diaphyseal
Involvement of long bones	Yes	Yes
Involvement of flat bones	Rare	Yes
Diffuse medullary cavity involvement	Rare	Common ("moth-eaten" or permeative involvement)
New bone formation	Yes	No—only as secondary phenomenon
Periosteal reaction	Yes ("Codman triangle") or spiculation	Yes ("onionskin" appearance)
	Not prominent but may be present	Yes

NATURAL HISTORY AND EVALUATION

Although Ewing's sarcoma most commonly presents in the femur and bones of the pelvis, it can affect any bone. Unlike osteosarcoma, it often originates in the axial skeleton. Table 47-28 lists the distribution and frequency of primary sites of patients enrolled in the first Intergroup Ewing's Sarcoma Study.[40]

Most patients with Ewing's sarcoma seek medical attention because of pain and swelling of the affected bone or region. Systemic symptoms, such as fatigue, weight loss, and intermittent fever, may be present, especially in patients with metastatic disease. The duration of symptoms before presentation may be measured in weeks or months and is often prolonged in patients who have primary sites in the axial skeleton. When intratumor hemorrhage and necrosis occur, the tumor can become fluctuant, erythematous, and warm, mimicking infection. Frequently the entire medullary cavity of the affected bone is involved with the tumor (Table 47-29). In addition, extension through the bony cortex and into the soft tissues often results in a large soft tissue mass that, particularly with axial lesions, may be larger than the intraosseous component (Fig. 47-10).

FIG. 47-10. Radiographs of typical osteosarcoma and Ewing's tumor. **A**. Ewing's tumor of ulna. Note diaphyseal involvement with no tumor-related new bone and extensive permeative appearance. **B**. Classic osteosarcoma of femur in frontal and lateral projections. Typical metaphyseal location with new bone formation, lack of permeation, Codman's triangle, and spiculation are evident.

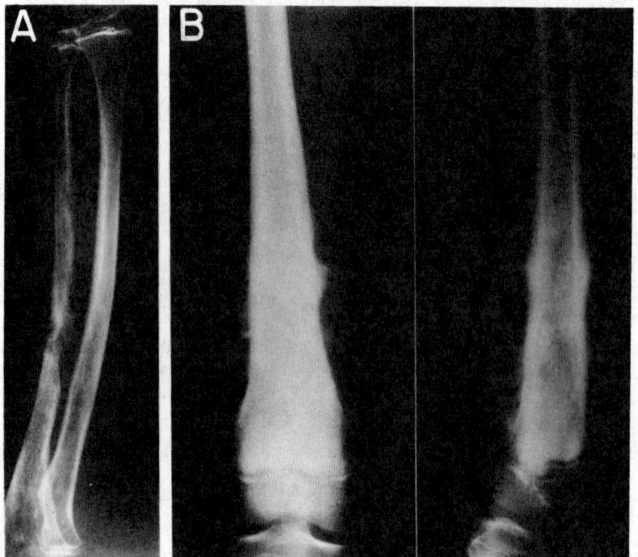

Less common presentations of Ewing's sarcoma include primary rib tumor associated with a pleural effusion and respiratory symptoms, mandibular lesions presenting with chin and lip parasthenias, primary vertebral tumor with symptoms of nerve root or spinal cord compression, and sacral primary with neurogenic bladder.

The incidence of metastatic disease at the time of presentation in patients with Ewing's sarcoma ranges from 14% to 50%, depending on the thoroughness of the metastatic workup and the referral base of the reporting institutions. Metastasis is predominantly hematogenous, although lymph node involvement may occur. The lung is the most common site of metastatic disease at presentation and the most frequent site of initial relapse. CNS involvement is detected in fewer than 1% of patients and is the site of first relapse in fewer than 5% of patients. More commonly, the CNS is involved as a result of direct intracranial or intraspinal extension of bony metastatic disease.

The importance of the initial diagnostic biopsy in a patient with a suspected Ewing's sarcoma should be emphasized. The soft tissue component of the tumor is often viable and will yield a better specimen than the frequently necrotic intramedullary component of the tumor. Electron microscopy and immunocytochemistry must be employed for an accurate diagnosis. The surgical or pediatric oncologist should tell the pathologist the suspected diagnosis before surgery.

The diagnostic evaluation should include a CT scan of the primary tumor and lungs. The use of MRI may complement the CT scan in defining the primary tumor. Experience with this technology suggests that it may be overly sensitive, exaggerating the size of the lesion, resulting in overly generous radiation ports. Until experience with MRI accumulates, it should not replace the CT. A radionuclide bone scan is essential to find bony metastases. The bone marrow should be assessed with a bone aspirate and biopsy. In the event of a pelvic lesion, bone marrow distant from the primary site must be sampled to determine if there has been dissemination. Although there is no specific serum marker for Ewing's sarcoma, lactic dehydrogenase (LDH) is frequently elevated in those with more advanced disease, which has negative prognostic implications.

STAGING AND PROGNOSTIC FACTORS

There is no uniformly accepted staging system for Ewing's sarcoma. A system based on a TNM concept is more appropriate for this disease than a system based on the extent of disease after a surgical procedure, because the approach to the local control of this tumor is rarely surgical. Experience suggests that the size of the lesion has prognostic importance. Eighty-seven percent of patients with tumor (T) confined to bone were alive at 5 years compared with 20% of patients with an extraosseous component. Node involvement (N) is very rare. The presence of metastatic disease (M) dramatically reduces the likelihood of survival; bone or marrow involvement is more ominous than lung metastasis alone.

The most favorable prognostic factors are a distal primary tumor, normal serum LDH, and absence of metastatic disease at presentation. Pelvic and sacral sites for primary tumors and metastatic disease are the least favorable factors. A partial or complete response to initial chemotherapy is a strong predictor of long-term disease control.

Treatment

Every patient with Ewing's sarcoma should be treated with curative intent. Even patients with widely metastatic disease can, if not cured, have excellent responses to therapy, which may translate into years of disease control. Successful treatment requires close coordination among the surgeon, chemotherapist, and radiotherapist to ensure the most effective approach to controlling the primary lesion and the inevitable dissemination of the tumor.

Surgery

With surgical therapy alone, the long-term survival rates of patients in most early series was less than 10%, with failure usually caused by distant metastatic disease. The success of adjuvant chemotherapy in preventing distant failure in patients with Ewing's sarcoma and the effectiveness of radiation therapy in controlling the primary site of disease has resulted in abandoning surgery as the sole primary modality of therapy. Before improved radiation equipment, patients whose initial treatment included surgery lived longer than patients who did not have surgery. A retrospective analysis revealed that 57 of the 334 patients had either partial or complete resection of the tumor, and patients whose tumors had been resected lived longer than those who did not have surgery. Although these data must be cautiously evaluated for their potential selection bias, they do suggest that the role of surgery in the primary management of Ewing's sarcoma deserves evaluation. Balanced against this is the excellent local control attained with megavoltage irradiation and the low frequency of therapy-induced functional deficits if careful treatment planning was used.[41] There are, however, no controlled data that compare the advantages and disadvantages of surgery and radiation for the primary treatment of Ewing's sarcoma.

The generally accepted indications for primary surgical resection of Ewing's sarcoma used at some institutions are a lesion in an expendable bone, such as the rib, clavicle, fibula, or individual bones of the feet, or a lesion in the pelvic region, although surgery will usually follow initial chemotherapy. Amputation may be indicated if there is an unmanageable pathologic fracture or if the tumor arises at or below the knee in a young child (>6 years old) and a major uncorrectable functional deformity is expected from radiation therapy. Although most patients with metastatic disease die, an aggressive surgical or radiotherapeutic approach to the patient with a solitary pulmonary metastasis may be indicated.

The two goals of therapy, tumor control and preservation of function, guide the management of an individual lesion. If a major functional loss, such as sacrifice of the peroneal nerve in resection of a fibular lesion, is likely to result from surgery, then irradiation is usually preferred.

Radiation Therapy

James Ewing initially described the tumor's susceptibility to radium. It has since been recognized that this tumor is highly responsive to radiation therapy. Before the availability of chemotherapy, local control of Ewing's sarcoma was attained in 44% to 86% of patients with radiation doses greater than 4000 to 5000 cGy, even though long-term survival was low (16% to 25%).

With the addition of effective chemotherapy and local irradiation, local recurrence of Ewing's sarcoma is less than 10% for distal extremity lesions and 20–40% for patients with proximal extremity or pelvis primaries. Coordinated therapy has increased the control of microscopic systemic disease and markedly increased survival.[41] In a report of 193 patients treated on the first Intergroup Ewing's Sarcoma Study, the overall local control rate was 90%, and the survival had increased to 56% at 3 + years. These results have been corroborated in other studies.

Local control with primary irradiation and chemotherapy appears to depend upon tumor size. Failure occurred in 2 of 20 patients with lesions <8 cm in diameter, compared with 9 of 30 patients with larger primary tumors. Disease-free survival differed even more: 72% of patients with <8 cm lesions at 5 years compared with 22% of patients with larger lesions. Local failures with pelvic primary tumors were only 8% for <5 cm tumors, compared with 17% for larger lesions. There are significant differences in local control and survival with lesions greater or smaller than 100 mL in volume.

Radiation therapy is the primary mode of therapy for most local lesions. In conjunction with chemotherapy, doses of >50 to 55 Gy achieve tumor control in 80% to 85% of instances. Overall survival and local control have been improved by adding chemotherapy to radiation.

In order to maintain function, a meticulous radiation technique is required. Necessary technical aspects include megavoltage apparatus, immobilization techniques for daily reproducition, and the use of beam-modifying devices, including compensators, wedge filters, and individually constructed blocks. In addition, appropriate treatment of an extremity lesion includes the preservation of an unirradiated strip of skin and soft tissue in order to prevent late lymphedema and contractures (Fig. 47-11). With the use of moderate-dose radiation therapy and systemic chemotherapy, the functional

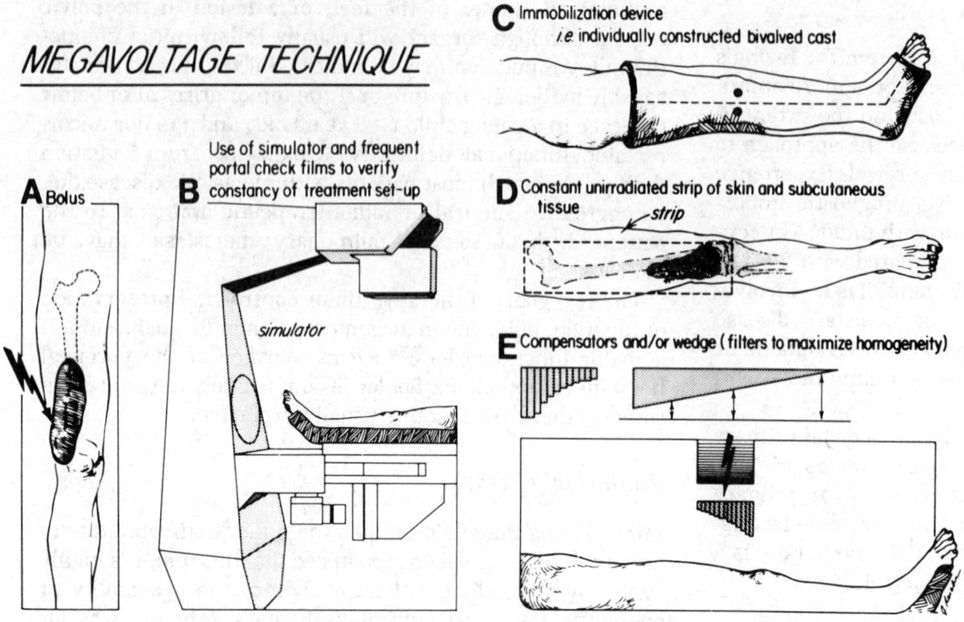

FIG. 47-11. Composite figure demonstrating some of the technically essential features for optimum results. Included are sparing of an adequate strip of skin and subcutaneous tissue to avoid late constrictive fibrosis and edema, use of appropriate treatment simulation and portal verification, appropriate immobilization during treatment, and use of wedges and compensators for homogeneity of treatment.

results achieved in 29 patients who survived 2 years showed that only 18% of the patients had a severe functional deficit when doses of 5000 cGy were combined with chemotherapy. Higher doses of radiotherapy or less conventional radiation techniques in combination with chemotherapy, however, have resulted in a higher incidence (62.5%) of severe functional disability.

Second cancers occur in the radiation field in 3% to 18% of patients. The incidence appears to be related to total radiation dose, to radiation energy (orthovoltage), and to the use of chemotherapy.

Integration of Radiation Therapy and Chemotherapy

Current treatment protocols for Ewing's sarcoma often begin with three to five cycles of chemotherapy before irradiation. This allows for the assessment of the response to chemotherapy. Early institution of radiotherapy should be considered in a patient with progressive spinal cord compression or airway obstruction caused by the tumor. Doxorubicin (Adriamycin) and dactinomycin, commonly used chemotherapeutic agents in Ewing's sarcoma, interact with radiation, potentially exacerbating local toxicity and necessitating treatment interruptions, with negative consequences for local control. These problems may be decreased by delaying irradiation for a few days after the drugs are given and carefully planning radiation treatment.

Chemotherapy

Before the use of adjuvant chemotherapy, long-term survival of patients with Ewing's sarcoma was rare. In the largest prechemotherapy series, only 36 (9.6%) of 374 patients treated with surgery or radiation therapy survived for 5 years. As with Wilms' tumor and rhabdomyosarcoma, single-agent chemotherapy trials were initiated in the 1960s with highly encouraging results. As shown in Table 47-30, many agents appear to be active against Ewing's sarcoma, with

TABLE 47-30. Phase II Studies in Ewing's Sarcoma

Agent	*Response (no. responding/total)*	*Response Rate (%)*
Cyclophosphamide	19/37	51
Doxorubicin	24/58	41
Ifosfamide	10/31	32
Vincristine	3/10	30
Dactinomycin	3/9	33
BCNU	6/18	33
5-Fluorouracil	5/16	31
Etoposide	3/10	30
Cisplatin	2/27	7
Melphalan (high-dose)	9/11	82
Ifosfamide/etoposide	16/17	94

TABLE 47-31. Correlation of Local Control and Disease-free Survival with Site of Primary Disease

Site	*No. of Patients*	*Local Control (%)*	*NED Survival (%)*
Pelvis	37	31 (84)	14 (38)
Humerus	24	19 (79)	12 (50)
Femur	43	40 (93)	22 (51)
Tibia	22	20 (91)	15 (68)
Fibula	25	24 (96)	17 (68)
Ribs	10	9 (90)	6 (60)
Skull and spine	12	12 (100)	12 (100)
Others	20	18 (90)	14 (70)

cyclophosphamide and doxorubicin consistently the most active. Few new agents have been developed for the treatment of this and other pediatric cancers, possibly because drugs are tested against tumors resistant to multiple drugs and radiation. This makes the report of complete and partial responses in 16 of 17 patients with recurrent Ewing's sarcoma to ifosfamide and etoposide by Miser and co-workers at the NCI particularly striking.[42]

In 1973, a multi-institutional randomized trial, the first Intergroup Ewing's Sarcoma Study (IESS-I), was initiated. Patients without evidence of metastatic disease were treated on one of three treatment regimens. Local tumor control was planned with radiation therapy to the entire involved bone in doses ranging from 4500 to 4400 cGy, depending on the patient's age, followed by a boost of 1000 cGy to gross radiographically demonstrable tumor. Daily dose fractionation was 200 cGy, delivered 5 days each week. In addition to local therapy, patients were randomly assigned to receive adjuvant chemotherapy with vincristine, dactinomycin, cyclophosphamide (VAC), and doxorubicin (regimen 1); VAC without doxorubicin (regimen 2); or VAC plus bilateral pulmonary irradiation, which consisted of midplane dose of 1500 to 1800 cGy (regimen 3). The duration of chemotherapy was 1.5 to 2 years. The survival of patients on this study are listed in Table 47-31. Important results included the following:

1. The survival rate after 3 years was 56% for the entire group.
2. The addition of doxorubicin to VAC significantly improved the disease-free survival at 2 years (72% compared with 36%).
3. The addition of pulmonary irradiation to VAC decreased pulmonary recurrence if compared with VAC alone, but it was less effective than the combination of VAC plus doxorubicin.
4. The local control and disease-free survival was related to treatment and to primary site. Pelvic, humeral, and femur lesions had the poorest outcome; rib lesions were intermediate; and the best results were seen in patients with primary lesions below the knee and in the skull or spine.
5. A filigree histologic pattern was associated with the poorer prognosis.

Of 44 patients with metastatic disease or advanced regional disease treated with VAC plus doxorubicin and irradiation to both primary and metastatic sites, 31 (70%) responded completely. Of these, 18 (41%) remained disease-free at a median of 34 months.

The second Intergroup Ewing's Sarcoma Study (IESS II) evaluated the role of a more intensive regimen, which relied heavily on the two most active agents, cyclophosphamide and doxorubicin. Preliminary communications suggest improvement over the IESS I for patients with pelvic primaries but not for those with metastatic disease.

Single-institution studies have played a major role in the development of therapy for Ewing's sarcoma. These studies furthered the concepts of dose intensity and preirradiation chemotherapy. Seventy-nine percent of patients with localized disease treated with aggressive chemotherapy and local irradiation or surgery were free of disease at a median of 41 months from beginning therapy.

Investigators at the NCI tested a strategy that maximized the use of cyclophosphamide and doxorubicin to achieve complete remission followed by irradiation to the primary and metastatic sites of disease, which was followed by total-body irradiation and autologous bone marrow reconstitution to prevent systemic recurrence. Twenty (83%) of 24 patients achieved a complete response, and 6 remain free of disease more than 5 years later. In another study with higher doses of drugs, 30 to 31 of these high-risk patients completely responded. Seventeen remain disease-free, with a median time on the study of 24 months; 9 failed in metastatic sites and 4 failed locally.[42] A study in progress is testing the efficacy of the intensive vincristine, doxorubicin, and cyclophosphamide regimen in combination with the non-cross-resistant pair, ifosfamide and etoposide, and irradiation to the primary site and, if feasible, metastatic lesions.

Hayes and co-investigators at the St. Jude Children's Research Hospital, using a cytokinetically based, sequential, moderate-dose cyclophosphamide and doxorubicin regimen based on their experience with neuroblastoma, report complete responses in patients with metastatic disease and a disease-free survival rate comparable to that achieved with more intense regimens.[43] This approach is being tested by the POG in a larger group of patients.

Although several groups have been very successful in achieving complete responses, the actuarial disease-free survival curves have continued to drop in a relatively steady fashion for years after diagnosis. The disheartening experience of diagnosing a relapse in a Ewing's sarcoma patient as much as 10 to 15 years after their initial treatment is all too familiar to those who treat this disease. This phenomenon is not commonly seen with the other childhood sarcomas. It is reasonable to speculate that the molecular abnormality that gives rise to this tumor is predisposed by a somatic defect that favors oncogenesis and that the late recurrence is, in fact, a new tumor. Recent epidemiologic evidence that demonstrates a high rate of development of second malignancies, most often osteosarcoma, in survivors of Ewing's sarcoma further suggests a somatic cell defect that predisposes to tumor formation. The solution to this disease probably depends on elucidating the molecular defects that give rise to it.

PERIPHERAL NEUROECTODERMAL TUMORS

Peripheral neuroectodermal tumors (PNET) constitute a heterogeneous group of neoplasms arising in either supportive structures or neuronal tissue. A number of entities are represented in this nosology, including neuroepithelioma, adult neuroblastoma, primitive neuroectodermal tumors of bone, or malignant small cell tumors of the thorasopulmonary region ("Askin's tumor").

EPIDEMIOLOGY AND GENETICS

PNET are malignancies of adolescents and young adults. The tumor shares a number of characteristics with Ewing's sarcoma, including the presence of a unique chromosomal translocation [t(11;22)(q24;q12)] and the fact that it is rare in black children.[44,45] PNET usually arise on the extremities, pelvis, or chest wall and tend to metastasize widely. Although they have the chromosomal translocation found in Ewing's sarcoma, PNET bear histopathologic similarity to neuroblastoma and high levels of enzymes that are important for the synthesis of catecholamine, including choline acetyltransferase, suggests that PNET may arise in the parasympathetic nervous system. Moreover, unlike neuroblastoma and CNS tissue, cell lines from PNET express a high level of class I histocompatibility antigens. PNET are distinguished by a variety of biological and molecular features that suggest that these tumors are closely associated with Ewing's sarcoma (Table 47-32).

PATHOLOGY

Like neuroblastoma and Ewing's sarcoma, PNET are highly cellular and consist of a monotonous pattern of primitive-appearing round cells, the vast majority of which lack any evidence of neural differentiation. On occasion, electron microscopy will reveal evidence of dense core granules, neurites, neurotubules, and neurofilaments in prominent Golgi's apparatus. Immunocytochemical staining is positive for neuron-specific enolase (NSE). PNET can be confused with Ewing's sarcoma if light microscopic evidence of neuronal differentiation is lacking.

CLINICAL PRESENTATION AND EVALUATION

The chest wall is the most common site for PNET. The trunk, abdomen, and pelvis are the other primary sites. PNET usually present in a mass, sometimes painful, and when invading the chest wall, are often associated with a malignant pleural effusion. If the tumor involves the paraspinal region, extension into the spinal cord must be considered. PNET arising in the extremities or pelvis are similar to Ewing's sarcoma, with bony involvement of a soft tissue mass and pain. The most common sites of metastases are bone, bone marrow, lung, and lymph nodes.

As with other solid tumors of childhood, the initial goal of evaluation is to determine the extent of local tumor involve-

TABLE 47-32. Comparison of Neuroepithelioma with Neuroblastoma and Ewing's Sarcoma

Variable	*Neuroblastoma*	*Neuroepithelioma*	*Ewing's Sarcoma*
Clinical Presentation			
Age	<4	Adolescence	Adolescence
Site	Abdominal	Thoracic, extremity, pelvis	Thoracic, extremity, pelvis
Biological Markers			
Cytologic features of neural differentiation	+	±	−
EM features of neural differentiation	+	±	−
Neurotransmitters	Adrenergic	Cholinergic	Cholinergic
Surface HLA expression	−	+	+
Cytogenetic Characteristics			
Chromosomal translocation	−	t(11;22) (q24;q11-12)	t(11;22) (q24;q11-12)
Gene amplification	+	−	−
Oncogene Expression			
N-*myc*	+	−	−
c-*myc*	−	+	+

Israel MA, Miser JS, Triche TJ et al: Neuroepithelial tumors. In Pizzo PA, Poplack DG (eds): Principles and Practice of Pediatric Oncology, p 624. Philadelphia, JB Lippincott, 1989.

ment and whether there is evidence of metastatic spread. Because of the site of origin and pattern of spread, the differential diagnosis includes rhabdomyosarcoma, Ewing's sarcoma, neuroblastoma, and the less common tumors of bone in children, including small cell osteosarcoma, mesenchymal chondrosarcoma, spindle cell bone tumor, osteogenic sarcoma, lymphoma of bone, and malignant fibrous histiocytoma of bone.

Evaluation includes a bone scan, chest CT scan, MRI of the primary lesion, bone marrow aspirate and biopsy, and careful pathologic evaluation of tumor tissue.

TREATMENT PLANNING

Because PNET is emerging as a distinct clinical entity, clearly defined guidelines for management are evolving. However, an approach similar to that used for Ewing's sarcoma seems appropriate at this time.

Surgery

Data to support debilitating surgery do not exist. If the primary tumor is amenable to complete resection without functional impairment of the patient, surgery may be a viable option. However, no effect of surgery on patient outcome has been identified.

Radiation Therapy

Local control has been achieved with high-dose, large-volume irradiation in conjunction with chemotherapy. Because large fields, often including segments of the lung(s) or heart, are necessary, careful treatment planning is essential to avoid morbidity. Guidelines are similar to those used for Ewing's sarcoma and rhabdomyosarcoma.

Chemotherapy

Recent clinical trials suggest that PNET respond to combination chemotherapy in a manner analogous to Ewing's sarcoma. Using vincristine, doxorubicin, and cyclophosphamide induction and consolidation, an objective response (>50% reduction of tumor volume) was observed in 14 of 15 patients.[44] However, even when combined with local irradiation and subsequent intensification with chemotherapy and total-body irradiation, relapses still occurred in patients with more extensive tumor involvement.

Because responses have been observed with the combination of ifosfamide and VP-16 in patients who had recurrences after treatment with vincristine, doxorubicin, cyclophosphamide, and high-dose total-body irradiation, current studies are exploring the integration of ifosfamide and VP-16 into the primary treatment regimen of patients with PNET.

LESS COMMON SARCOMAS OF CHILDHOOD AND ADOLESCENCE

Approximately 25% of all soft tissue sarcomas in children have a histologic pattern other than rhabdomyosarcoma, comprising nearly 3% of all tumors in children. Although these types of sarcomas are more commonly seen in adults, the prognosis may be better for children. The difference in prognosis is most pronounced for infants and younger children whose tumors often have a benign behavior and excellent prognosis with surgery alone. Soft tissue sarcomas that occur in adolescents, on the other hand, often have a behavior similar to those in adults.

The most common sites for soft tissue sarcomas are the extremities and trunk, especially the retroperitoneum. The usual approach to the treatment of these tumors in adults is wide surgical excision. Radiation therapy is usually added postoperatively. Although debated, the role of adjuvant chemotherapy appears to be useful for patients with resectable, high-grade soft tissue sarcomas of the extremities.

The approach to children with similar tumors is less clearly defined. Indeed similar histologic patterns may have a very different biologic behavior in children, and the morbidity of radiation in a small and rapidly growing child is likely to be greater than in an adult. Moreover, it is more difficult to perform functionally successful limb-sparing procedures in young growing children.

Most of the data about the treatment of children with nonrhabdomyosarcomatous soft tissue sarcomas comes from retrospective analyses of the experiences of a single institutions. Although valuable, careful prospective multi-institutional studies are needed to determine the roles of radiation therapy and chemotherapy in the treatment of these diseases. The POG is addressing these issues in a prospective multi-institutional trial. The ability to surgically extirpate the tumor is the most important prognostic factor. In a retrospective review of 62 cases of childhood soft-tissue sarcomas other than rhabdomyosarcoma treated at St. Jude, 84% survived with no evidence of disease if the tumor could be completely removed, but only 1 of 26 patients survived if gross tumor remained after resection.[47]

FIBROSARCOMA

Although rare, fibrosarcoma is one of the most common nonrhabdomyosarcomatous soft tissue sarcomas in children and adolescents. It occurs most frequently in the extremity, often in the distal segments. Incidence of fibrosarcoma has two age peaks, one in infants and children younger than 5 years of age, and the second in patients 10 to 15 years of age. It appears that fibrosarcoma in infants has a more benign course.

Fibrosarcoma is a spindle cell tumor with a characteristic herringbone pattern, or regularly interweaving fascicles of parallel arrays of tumor cells. Important features are evidence of mitoses, nuclear pleomorphism, and increased basophilia of individual, sometimes anaplastic, tumor cells. Cells are densely packed, but reticulin stain reveals a regular pattern of stromal collagen fibers not easily appreciated by light microscopy. The differential diagnosis includes fibromatosis (which can be exceedingly aggressive locally, but which does not metastasize), nodular fasciitis, myositis ossificans, and inflammatory pseudotumor among the nonmalignant conditions and neurofibrosarcoma and poorly differentiated embryonal rhabdomyosarcoma among malignant tumors.

Of 52 cases of congenital fibrosarcoma, 37 occurred on an extremity and 15 on the trunk. Of the patients with extremity tumors, 92% were free of metastatic disease, and 95% were alive, in spite of a 27% local recurrence rate. Congenital fibrosarcomas of the trunk appear to be more aggressive, with 20% of patients developing metastases, and 26% dying of their disease. The standard therapy for fibrosarcoma is surgical extirpation by wide local excision, usually without additional therapy. The use of radiation and chemotherapy in the local management of congenital fibrosarcoma is restricted to situations in which surgical removal is not possible.

There is no evidence that adjuvant chemotherapy is indicated in the treatment of congenital fibrosarcoma and nonmetastatic fibrosarcoma of young children. Several recent reports document that at least some of these tumors are sensitive to chemotherapy, and for patients who have unresectable metastatic or primary disease, chemotherapy may be useful. Several combinations of chemotherapy have been used: vincristine, doxorubicin, and cyclophosphamide; vincristine, dactinomycin, and cyclophosphamide; the combination of ifosfamide and etoposide is notable since it has resulted in complete regressions of metastatic fibrosarcoma.[44]

NEUROFIBROSARCOMA

Neurofibrosarcomas, malignant tumors of nerve sheath origin, account for approximately 5% to 10% of all nonrhabdomyosarcomatous soft tissue sarcomas in children. Neurofibrosarcoma occurs in association with a dominantly inherited syndrome, neurofibromatosis (von Recklinghausen's disease). Approximately 5% to 16% of patients with von Recklinghausen's disease develop neurofibrosarcoma.

Although superficially similar in appearance to fibrosarcoma, neurofibrosarcoma is a more aggressive tumor. The cells are usually more variable in size and shape, a herringbone pattern is absent, and typical features of adult neurofibrosarcomas often can be found in some areas of the tumor (*i.e.*, a myxoid stroma, palisading of nuclei, and occasionally well-defined organoid arrays of nuclei). These features, common in benign schwannomas, are far less conspicuous in the malignant counterpart, but can be diagnostic when present. Diagnosis is best established by electron microscopy. The most common primary sites of neurofibrosarcoma appear to be the extremities (42%), retroperitoneum (25%), and trunk (21%).[46]

As with fibrosarcoma, surgery plays a key role in the management of children with neurofibrosarcoma. Postoperative irradiation may be indicated if surgery does not attain negative margins. The role of chemotherapy in the treatment of patients with neurofibrosarcoma is unclear.[47] Experience with extremity tumors in a small number of adults at the NCI suggests that a regimen of doxorubicin and cyclophosphamide may be effective in the adjuvant treatment of localized, grossly removed neurofibrosarcoma. Although chemotherapy can produce tumor regressions in patients with gross local and metastatic disease, no regimen appears to enhance disease-free survival in patients with advanced disease. The combination of ifosfamide and etoposide, a regimen highly active in the treatment of recurrent small, round cell tumors of neural origin, has produced partial tumor regressions in two of the four patients with recurrent neurofibrosarcoma thus far evaluated.[44]

MALIGNANT FIBROUS HISTIOCYTOMA

Although malignant fibrous histiocytoma (MFH) was the most common histologic diagnosis in the NCI series of adults with extremity sarcomas, accounting for 53 (25%) of 211 patients, it is much less common in children. At St. Jude, only 5 (8%) of the 62 cases of nonrhabdomyosarcomatous soft tissue sarcoma were diagnosed as MFH.[47] The typical microscopic appearance of MFH resembles fibrosarcoma, but it is distinguished by marked cellular pleomorphism, multiple cell types (especially lipid-laden tumor cells), and a more malignant appearance. A storiform pattern of tumor cells, described as radiating fascicles of tumor cells at right angles from one another, is virtually diagnostic of this tumor.

Because of the rarity of this tumor in childhood, the approach to treatment of this malignancy is based on the adult experience. The accepted initial management is wide local excision of the tumor. Limb-sparing operations with radiation to the tumor bed have been as successful as amputations for tumors in the extremities. The role of adjuvant chemotherapy is not yet established in children with MFH. Of 7 patients with MFH, 2 had their tumor completely removed and were then treated with adjuvant chemotherapy; both were alive 1.4 and 9 years later. In contrast, comparable survival without adjuvant chemotherapy have also been described.

Vincristine, dactinomycin, and cyclophosphamide, with or without doxorubicin, has produced objective tumor regressions in patients with advanced disease. Four of the 5 patients with Group III or IV disease had complete or partial tumor regressions, and 2 remained disease-free at 4.6 and 5.4 years. Responses to ifosfamide plus etoposide have also been seen.

SYNOVIAL SARCOMA

Synovial sarcoma accounted for 29% of the nonrhabdomyosarcomatous soft tissue sarcomas at St. Jude. The most common anatomical location is the lower extremity, often in the thigh and the knee; the next most common site is the upper extremity. Approximately 15% to 20% occur on the head, neck, or trunk.

Synovial cell sarcomas can have two components, a spindle cell fibrous stroma virtually indistinguishable from fibrosarcoma and a distinct glandular component with absolute epithelial differentiation.

Significant prognostic features are small tumor size (<5-cm diameter); a primary site in the hand, foot, or knee; a younger age; and a predominant epithelioid pattern. The disease-free survival rate for adult patients with localized tumors of the extremities is approximately 70%. Eight of the 18 patients treated at St. Jude were alive in follow-up.

Because this tumor is relatively rare in children, the optimal treatment guidelines have not yet been established. Wide local excision is the treatment of choice to control the primary tumor. Radiation therapy may improve control with microscopically inadequate margins; treatment planning should seek to assure normal function and normal growth by maximal sparing of bone and normal soft tissue. The effectiveness of radiation in the control of bulky disease has not yet been established.

The benefit of adjuvant chemotherapy in the treatment of synovial sarcoma in children and young adults is not clear; however, adjuvant cyclophosphamide and doxorubicin administered postoperatively to adult patients was beneficial. Tumor regressions in patients with advanced disease have been documented with several chemotherapy regimens. Although these treatment plans have usually included cyclophosphamide and doxorubicin, a regimen of vincristine, dactinomycin, and cyclophosphamide has also been advocated. Objective tumor regressions have been seen with the combination regimen of ifosfamide and etoposide.[44]

HEMANGIOPERICYTOMA

Hemangiopericytoma, a tumor that presumably arises from the pericyte cells that surround vascular channels, accounts for approximately 3% of all soft tissue sarcomas in children. It can be either benign or malignant. The most common primary sites are the extremities, especially the lower extremities; the retroperitoneum is the second most common site of disease, followed by the head and neck region and the trunk. The most common sites of secondary disease are the lungs and bone.

The behavior of this tumor in older children is similar to that of hemangiopericytoma in adult patients. The overall 5-year survival rate for adults varies from 30% to 70%. The therapeutic approach is wide local excision. Adjuvant chemotherapy has been of value in adults with this disease. As with other soft tissue sarcomas, radiotherapy is used if complete surgical removal of the tumor cannot be accomplished.

Responses to chemotherapy have been reported with the use of vincristine, cyclophosphamide, doxorubicin, dactinomycin, methotrexate, mitoxantrone, and other alkylating agents. Although there is no randomized study confirming the role of adjuvant chemotherapy in this disease, the high incidence of metastatic disease and relative chemoresponsiveness of the tumor had led many investigators to treat these patients with chemotherapy after extirpation of the primary tumor.

Hemangiopericytoma may rarely occur in infants, and although similar in histologic appearance to the adult form, infantile hemangiopericytoma usually follows a more benign course. These tumors usually arise in the subcutis; however, occasionally they may have extensive local infiltration or metastasize. The treatment of choice for infantile hemangiopericytoma is surgery alone if the tumor is localized; however, complete regression of metastatic disease in patients with this entity has been seen with chemotherapy.

ALVEOLAR SOFT PART SARCOMA

Alveolar soft part sarcoma (ASPS) is a rare sarcoma that usually occurs in individuals between the ages of 15 and 35 years. Although 6 of the 62 patients in the St. Jude series had ASPS, the actual incidence in children and adolescents is probably lower.[47] The tumor usually occurs in the skeletal muscle of the extremities in adults; however, the head and neck region is a common site in children.

The most distinctive feature of ASPS is the presence of PAS-positive, diastase-resistant inclusions in the cytoplasm, which show a regular crystalline structure. That some inclusions closely resemble neurosecretory granules provokes suspicion that the tumor may be neuroepithelial, but immunocytochemistry is inconclusive in this regard.

Alveolar soft part sarcoma usually presents as a slow-growing, painless mass. The clinical course of patients with ASPS is indolent but usually progressive. The most common sites of metastatic disease are lung, brain, bone, and lymph nodes.

The initial therapeutic approach is complete local excision alone, with radiation and chemotherapy reserved for the treatment of recurrent disease. Many patients eventually relapse and subsequently die of disease. This ominous fact strongly suggests that new approaches to the prevention of relapses are needed in the treatment of this disorder.

LEIOMYOSARCOMA

Leiomyosarcoma is rare in childhood, accounting for less than 2% of soft tissue sarcomas in children. The most common primary sites of disease are the retroperitoneum, vascular tissue, peripheral soft tissue, and the gastrointestinal tract.

The tumor cells are elongate, with cigar-shaped nuclei and brightly eosinophilic cytoplasm (due to the content of myofilaments), and they are closely packed in parallel arrays. The appearance is superficially similar to fibrosarcoma, but the eosinophilic nuclei, resembling smooth muscle in normal tissues, and usual monotonous regularity of tumor cells are distinct.

The most common approach to the treatment is local excision. The role of chemotherapy and radiation therapy in children is undefined. If complete extirpation of the tumor can be achieved, the prognosis is usually good for tumors arising outside of the gastrointestinal tract; however, tumors arising in this site generally have a poor prognosis. Leiomyosarcomas of the colorectal region in children, although extremely rare, appear to have a relatively good prognosis if the tumor can be successfully excised.

LIPOSARCOMA

Although it is primarily a disease of adults, with a peak age of incidence between 40 and 60 years, liposarcomas may occur in children, most often in the early part of the second decade of life. The tumor rarely affects infants and young children, in whom its behavior is almost always benign. The two most common primary sites are the extremities and the retroperitoneum. The tumor may be well-differentiated, myxoid, round cell, or pleomorphic (in increasing degree of malignancy and decreasing survival). Most tumor cells are fibroblastic; only rare cells show conspicuous lipoblastic differentiation. The distinction from MFH can be difficult, but the presence of a myxoid stroma, conspicuous small blood vessels, and scant mitotic activity are all typical of liposarcoma.

The treatment of choice for localized liposarcoma is wide local excision. Local recurrences may ultimately result in the death of the patient because of extension of the tumor into vital structures. The role of adjuvant chemotherapy in the treatment of liposarcomas of childhood is undefined. Radiation appears to be effective in the control of microscopic disease in adults.

THE HISTIOCYTOSES

The histiocytoses are an uncommon group of clinically diverse syndromes that share a histopathology characterized by granuloma formation with the infiltration and proliferation of histocytes. The classic clinical triad of the histiocytosis X syndromes includes a solitary lytic lesion of bone (eosinophilic granuloma); a chronic disorder characterized by exophthalmos, diabetes insipidus, and skeletal lesions (Hand-Schuller-Christian syndrome); and an acute fulminant disseminated disorder of young children manifested by skin lesions, hepatosplenomegaly, lymphadenopathy, mastoiditis, osteolytic lesions, pneumonitis, anemia, thrombocytopenia, and fever (Letterer-Siwe disease).[48] The clinical and biologic diversity has made it difficult to characterize and classify histiocytosis as a neoplastic or non-neoplastic disorder and has contributed to the controversy about its appropriate management.

BIOLOGIC CONSIDERATIONS

The infiltration and accumulation of cells in the monocyte or macrophage series into a target tissue can be a primary or secondary event, and not all diseases associated with histiocytic infiltration are classified as histiocytoses.

Histiocytes arise from the uncommitted bone marrow stem cell and differentiate along the granulocyte macrophage axis. One of the primary functions of normal histiocytes is phagocytoses of aged red blood cells, microbes, or tumor cells, and erythrophagocytosis is a common finding in many of the histiocytoses of childhood. The characteristic findings of histiocytoses may be the result of diverse pathogenic mechanisms. For example, in "histiocytosis-X," now known as Langerhans' cell histiocytosis, the proliferation and accumulation of histiocytes is the result of immunologic stimulation of the Langerhans' cell. It does not appear that these histiocytes are truly malignant, and improvement has been noticed with the administration of thymic extracts. In the cases of infection-associated hemophagocytic syndrome, the macrophage appears to be reacting to a foreign antigen, and this histiocytosis reverses when the infection and its antigenic stimulation abates. In contrast, other histiocytoses may represent a genetic abnormality (*e.g.*, familial erythrophagocytic lymphohistiocytosis) or a clonal neoplastic proliferation (*e.g.*, malignant histiocytosis).

PATHOLOGY

To clarify this diverse group of histiocytoses, the Histiocytosis Society has recently developed a classification system based on pathologic examination that divides the histiocytoses into three classes (Table 47-33).

In Class I histiocytoses, the central cell has the histopathologic feature of the Langerhans' cell and this designation replaces those syndromes previously referred to as histiocytosis X (*i.e.*, eosinophilic granuloma, Hand-Schuller-Christian syndrome, and Letterer-Siwe disease). The lesions associated with Langerhans' cell histiocytosis are granulomatous and are highlighted by the presence of Langerhans' cells with Birbeck granules, which can be seen by electron microscopy.

Class II histiocytoses include all the other nonmalignant histiocytoses in which the mononuclear phagocyte is not a Langerhans' cell. These are reactive histiocytoses that are usually associated with a mixed lymphohistiocytic infiltrate, generally in the sinusoids, cortex, and paracortex, but without effacement of nodal architecture. The infiltrating histiocytes appear normal, and they have low nuclear to cytoplasmic ratios, mature nuclear chromatin, inconspicuous nucleoli, and abundant cytoplasm. The two disorders categorized in Class II histiocytoses, the infection-associated hemophagocytic syndrome (IAHS) and familial erythrophagocytic lymphohistiocytosis (FEL), are hallmarked by erythrophagocytosis and the secondary accumulation of histocytes.

Class III histiocytosis is a true neoplasm, of which malignant histiocytosis is the best known disease. Lymph nodes in Class III histiocytosis are characterized by nodal effacement and infiltration with cells containing reticular chromatic patterns, prominent nucleoli, and basophilic cytoplasm. Erythrophagocytosis may be observed in Class III histiocytosis, but it is not as prominent as in Class II.

CLINICAL PRESENTATION, DIAGNOSIS, AND TREATMENT

Class I Histiocytoses

As seen in Table 47-34, the Langerhans' cell histiocytosis has a variable presentation and clinical course and can undergo regression and exacerbation within the same patient. In acute disseminated histiocytosis, the skin is involved in 70% to 100% of patients and is characterized by a scaling, eczematoid rash over the trunk, neck, groin, and scalp.[48,49] Scalp lesions are not infrequently misdiagnosed as a seborrheic dermatitis. There is often a petechial component, and in rare cases, skin lesions can also antedate more widespread disease. A syndrome referred to as regressing atypical histiocytosis has been described and is characterized by nodulo-ulcerative skin lesions composed of atypical histiocytes, monocytes, and multinucleated giant cells with erythrophagocytosis. However, these patients have cutaneous disease only, and the skin lesions are both indolent and characterized by spontaneous regressions and recurrences. Recognition of this disorder is important in order to avoid unnecessary treatment.

Lytic bone lesions serve as the clinical hallmark of Langerhans' histiocytoses and occur with a frequency comparable to skin disease, most commonly involving the flat bones and vertebrae, frequently with pain and functional impairment. In approximately 33% of patients, there is evidence of bilateral osteomastoiditis with bilateral suppurative discharge. Skeletal survey is a more reliable diagnostic and follow-up tool in these patients than radionuclide bone scans.

Histiocytic infiltration into the reticuloendothelial system results in generalized lymphadenopathy. Enlargement of the liver and spleen, particularly if associated with functional abnormalities, carries an ominous prognosis. Although hepatosplenomegaly is infrequent in initial presentation, it develops in nearly half of patients with disseminated histiocytosis, sometimes with jaundice and occasionally with the onset of cirrhosis.[50] Similarly, pulmonary findings are infre-

TABLE 47-33. Classification of the Childhood Histiocytoses

Class	*I*	*II*	*III*
Pathological findings	Granulomatous lesions, yellow-brown, in involved tissues, including skin	Infiltration of lymph nodes, without effacement of nodal architecture	Invasive infiltration of lymph nodes
Cellular characteristics of the lesions	Langerhans cells with cleaved nuclei and Birbeck granules seen by electron microscopy, cell surface antigens (not found on normal macrophages) include S-100 protein and OKT-6; mixed with varying proportions of eosinophils; multinucleated giant cells sometimes seen	Morphologically normal, reactive macrophages with prominent erythrophagocytosis; varying proportions of lymphocytes also seen in lesions	Neoplastic macrophages or neoplastic macrophage precursors
Diseases included	Langerhans cell histiocytosis*	Infection-associated hemophagocytic syndrome (IAHS); familial erythrophagocytic lymphistiocytosis (FEL)	Malignant acute monocytic leukemia
Diagnostic finding	Birbeck granules in cells of the lesions, defining the cells as Langerhans cells	Histopathologically benign, activated macrophages	Histopathologically neoplastic macrophages stain positively for acid phosphatase and nonspecific esterase.
Proposed pathophysiologic mechanisms of the histiocytosis	Immunologic stimulation of a normal antigen-processing cell—the Langerhans cell—in a somehow uncontrolled manner	Secondary histiocytic reaction to an unknown antigenic stimulation (FEL) or an infectious agent (IAHS), with erythrophagocytosis possibility reflecting foreign antigens absorbed on erythrocytes	Neoplasm; clonal autonomous uncontrolled proliferative process

Ladisch S, Jaffe ES: The histiocytoses. In Pizzo PA, Poplack DG (eds): Principles and Practice of Pediatric Oncology, p 494. Philadelphia, JB Lippincott, 1989.

* Previously known as histiocytosis X and its related syndromes of eosinophilic granuloma, Hand-Schuller-Christian syndrome, and Letterer-Siwe disease.

quent at initial diagnosis, but some pulmonary manifestations, particularly a diffuse interstitial infiltrate, develop during the disease course in nearly 67% of patients. Buccal and gingival infiltration occurs in about 40% of patients and is manifested as loose or floating teeth. More ominous are hematologic abnormalities, including anemia and thrombocytopenia.

Of patients with generalized disease, 25% to 50% develop diabetes insipidus during their disease course. Nonetheless, the classic Hand-Schuller-Christian syndrome, which includes diabetes insipidus, exophthalmos, and geographic skull lesions, is found in fewer than 10% of patients with disseminated histiocytosis. The presence of diabetes insipidus is rarely associated with radiographic abnormalities of the sella turcica.

Diagnosis requires biopsy and electron microscopy to determine the presence of Birbeck granules and to eliminate other disorders that may cause lytic bone lesions, especially metastatic neuroblastoma.

Two prognostic features stand out. First, mortality is higher for children younger than 2 years of age at the time of diagnosis. Second, organ dysfunction, especially if multiple organ systems are involved, decreases survival. These factors influence approaches to therapy.

The treatment of patients with monostotic bone lesions is the most straightforward and includes surgical biopsy or curettage. Low-dose megavoltage irradiation (500–1000 cGy) is recommended only for lesions that are surgically inaccessible, including vertebral bodies or sites adjacent to major growth plates.

The treatment of patients with generalized involvement is more controversial. Which patients should be treated? If treatment is undertaken, should it be with chemotherapy or immunotherapy? What should be the intensity and duration of therapy? These questions are complicated by the clinical diversity of Langerhans' cell histiocytosis and the chance that the disease may undergo a spontaneous regression. While treating the underlying process, care should be taken to avoid iatrogenic morbidity. Symptomatic or palliative therapy should not be overlooked, because disabling prob-

TABLE 47-34. Clinical, Prognostic, and Therapeutic Aspects of the Major Childhood Histiocytoses

Class	*LCH* *I*	*IAHS* *II*	*FEL* *II*	*MH* *III*
Clinical presentation	Wide spectrum, from mild discomfort related to lesions (lytic bone lesions, chronic otitis, diabetes insipidus) to generalized symptoms including fever and weight loss	Irritability, fever, wasting	Irritability, fever, wasting sometimes with a coagulopathy	Irritability, fever wasting
Diagnostic findings	Birbeck granules in lesional cells	Morphologically normal macrophages, documented infection, and negative family history	Morphologically normal macrophages and negative search for infection, sometimes positive family history	Malignant macrophages
Prognosis	Variable, but a self-resolving disease process in most cases	Excellent, providing underlying infection is controlled	Extremely poor; uniformly rapidly fatal	Up to 75% survival at 40 months reported with appropriate therapy
Recommended treatment	None to mild radiation or chemotherapy (vinblastine and steroids) for certain lesions	Avoidance of all immunosuppressive therapy	Experimental	Doxorubicin in a combination chemotherapy regimen

Ladisch S, Jaffe ES: The histiocytoses. In Pizzo PA, Poplack DG (eds): Principles and Practice of Pediatric Oncology, p 499. Philadelphia, JB Lippincott, 1989.

lems, such as diabetes insipidus, progressive destruction of a weight-bearing bone, extensive and progressive mandibular involvement, mastoid disease, and proptosis, can often be resolved with a short course of local irradiation.

Present systemic treatment options include chemotherapy, immunotherapy, and low-dose, total-body irradiation. A variety of drugs (chlorambucil, vincristine, and methotrexate, with or without prednisone) yield complete and partial response rates of 40% to 60%. The overall response rates to combination chemotherapy do not appear to be clearly superior to single-drug schedules in most series, although one study did suggest that combination therapy was preferable for children younger than 2 years of age who had extensive disease. Conversely, combination regimens are likely to be associated with more toxicity. Some investigators recommend withholding chemotherapy from patients who have multifocal disease limited to the skeleton or skin. Patients with more extensive disease, particularly those with evidence of hepatic dysfunction, require chemotherapy with agents such as vinblastine (for infants <1 year of age) or vinblastine plus prednisone and 6-mercaptopurine for older children. The provocative observation that some children with Langerhans' cell histiocytosis improved with thymus extract raises the possibility that immunotherapy or reconstitution may play a role in future treatment programs.

Class II Histiocytoses

FEL is an autosomal-recessive disorder characterized by fever, irritability, leptomeningeal involvement, hepatosplenomegaly, and abnormal liver dysfunction, with bone marrow findings of histiocytic and lymphocytic infiltration, and prominent erythrophagocytosis. FEL occurs primarily in young infants, and families with several affected members have been described. Unlike histiocytosis X, FEL is distinguished by a variety of immunologic abnormalities, including depressed antibody levels, anergy, and defective lymphocyte proliferation. In one family, plasma-mediated inhibition of cellular immunity was described, which was correlated with the plasma triglyceride level, raising the question of whether the immune abnormalities were primary or secondary phenomena. Furthermore, clinical and immunologic improvement was observed with plasma-exchange transfusion in a patient with FEL. An increase of acidic glycosphingolipids and a decrease of alpha-galactosidase activity suggest that FEL may be associated with unique quantitative and qualitative abnormalities of the hepatic gangliosides. FEL is generally a rapidly progressive disorder and is frequently complicated by thrombocytopenia and a disseminated intravascular coagulopathy. Progressive neurologic deterioration and brain atrophy with perivascular infiltration of the brain and meninges by lymphocytes and histiocytes can occur. An X-linked histiocytosis has also been described in which there is nodal infiltration by macrophages and plasma cells with hypergammaglobulinemia.

Because of its rapidly fulminant course and lymphohistiocytic infiltration suggesting a malignant neoplasm, cytotoxic therapy has been employed for FEL. Although transient improvements have been observed with combination regimens similar to those used for acute leukemia, remissions are rarely sustained, and the patients die. Two approaches have been explored as alternatives to chemotherapy: plasma exchange and bone marrow transplantation. Plasma exchange is based on the presence of circulating immunosuppressive activity in patients with FEL. After exchange transfusion, a reduction in plasma-inhibiting activity and some reversal of the depressed cellular immunity was observed, but these responses were not sustained. Bone marrow transplantation is based on the hypothesis that FEL represents an uncontrolled proliferation of lymphocytes and histiocytes. Bone marrow transplantation has been successful in one patient, but additional experience is necessary.

IAHS is also considered a Class II histiocytosis. The clinical appearance of IAHS is similar to FEL, and the diagnosis rests on presence of an infection and a negative family history for this disease. Like FEL, there is striking erythrophagocytosis in the bone marrow of children with IAHS, and with the absence of Birbeck granules on electron microscopy, this distinguishes IAHS from Langerhans' cell histiocytosis.

The keys to the successful therapy of children with IAHS are the discovery of the infectious agent and the avoidance of immunosuppressive therapy.

Class III Histiocytosis

Acute monocytic leukemia and malignant histiocytosis fall into this category. Malignant histiocytosis is a nonfamilial, rapidly fatal disorder characterized by fever, generalized tender lymphadenopathy, hepatosplenomegaly, subcutaneous inflammatory infiltration, pancytopenia, and a Coombs'-positive hemolytic anemia. A characteristic finding is erythrophagocytosis in the bone marrow, liver, and spleen, along with histiocytic infiltration of the subcapsular and medullary regions of lymph nodes. Immunochemical analysis has demonstrated that malignant histiocytosis cells stain positively for the S-100 protein (a CNS-specific protein), that many contain evidence of kappa or lambda chains, and that many are lysosome negative, suggesting that they are derived from T-zone histiocytes rather than from the monocyte-macrophage axis. Cytogenetic analysis of malignant histiocytes from the bone marrow of an infant with malignant histiocytosis revealed a translocation [t(8:16)(p11;p13)], which disappeared after clinical remission.

For patients with malignant histiocytosis and FEL, intervention is clearly necessary. However, a continuing issue is whether this should be with prednisone alone or with regimens including vincristine and cyclophosphamide. Prolonged responses have been observed in some patients with malignant histiocytosis treated with combination chemotherapy, including vincristine, prednisone, cyclophosphamide, doxorubicin, vinblastine, bleomycin, methyl-CCNU, and cytosine arabinoside, although the overall mortality of these patients remains quite high (68%).

Additional insights into the immunology and classification of the histiocytoses are necessary, and continued exploration of immune replacement or its mediation are important objectives.

CARCINOMAS AND OTHER LESS COMMON TUMORS OF CHILDHOOD

Many of the tumors that are common in adults occur only rarely in children. Principles for evaluation and management are generally similar to those for adults. Some insights about the pediatric aspects of those tumors are offered here.

HEAD AND NECK TUMORS

Nasopharyngeal Carcinoma

This carcinoma is a rare neoplasm in North America. It is more common in black than white teenagers. In children, rhabdomyosarcoma and non-Hodgkin's lymphomas are much more common nasopharyngeal tumors. Nasopharyngeal carcinoma appear to be closely associated with Epstein-Barr virus. Management includes radiation (6000–7000 cGy) and chemotherapy (*e.g.*, 5-FU, methotrexate, bleomycin, cisplatin). In patients with localized involvement, a disease-free survival of 78% has been reported.

Oropharyngeal Tumors

Squamous cell carcinoma of the tongue and oral cavity are extremely rare in children, but the incidence is increasing because of the use of smokeless tobacco products. It has been estimated that as many as 8% to 30% of male high-school and college students regularly use smokeless tobacco, often beginning at 12 years old. The use of these products should be discouraged by physicians caring for teenagers and young adults.

Ameloblastoma

Ameloblastoma or adamtanoma is a rare tumor that arises in the mandible, maxilla, or rarely, long bones. The primary therapeutic modality is surgery and radiation. The role of chemotherapy is not established.

Larynx

The most common childhood tumor involving the larynx is rhabdomyosarcoma, and squamous cell tumors of the larynx occur only rarely.

TUMORS OF THE LUNG AND THORAX

Lung Cancer

Although rare, more that 100 cases of primary lung cancers in children have been reported. These include bronchogenic carcinoma, usually of the undifferentiated or adenocarcinomatous type, primarily in adolescents. Bronchial adenomas have also been described, the primary treatment for which is surgical resection.

Pulmonary blastoma, a rare subpleural neoplasm has been described in children. It can metastasize and may respond to combination chemotherapy.

Thymoma

To be considered a tumor of the thymus gland, neoplastic epithelial cells must be demonstrable, because many malignant and nonmalignant processes are associated with thymomas. Included are both Hodgkin's and non-Hodgkin's lymphomas, germ cell tumors, carcinoids, thymolipomas, myasthenia gravis, autoimmune diseases (*e.g.*, polymyositis, SLE, rheumatoid arthritis), and endocrine disorders (*e.g.*, hyperparathyroidism, Addison's syndromes, panhypotuitarism).

Thymomas are usually slowly growing tumors found in the anterior mediastinum. Diagnosis may be heralded by nonspecific symptoms, including cough, dyspnea, and in advanced cases, evidence of a superior vena cava syndrome. Thymomas are locally invasive, but metastases can occur in lymph nodes, bone, liver, kidney, or brain.

Thymomas are generally radiosensitive and treatment includes 3500 to 4500 cGy given over 3 to 6 weeks. Thymomas have responded to doxorubicin, cisplatin, and alkylating agents. Most authorities reserve chemotherapy for patients not responding to local therapy. Survival appears to be 65% to 83% for patients with locally confined tumors and 30% to 54% for invasive tumor.

Breast Cancer

The majority of breast tumors in pediatric patients are benign, the most common being the fibroadenomas that occur in adolescents. Although these tumors can become quite large (cystosarcoma phylloides), they are almost always benign.

Although uncommon, carcinomas of the breast have been described in both boys and girls. They do not appear to be different from adult tumors, and the recommendations for therapy are the same.

ENDOCRINE TUMORS

Endocrine tumors comprise 4% to 5% of childhood neoplasms, the majority of which are benign or low-grade malignancies. Most of these tumors do not secrete hormones, 40% to 45% arising from gonadal origins, 30% from the thyroid, and 20% from the pituitary gland. Less commonly, tumors involve the parathyroids, adrenal gland, and the gastroenteropancreatic unit. Although most of these tumors are sporadic and of embryonic origin, a smaller percentage may be familial (*e.g.*, medullary carcinomas of the thyroid, pheochromocytoma), among which are the genetically transmitted syndromes of multiple endocrine neoplasia (MEN).

The majority of thyroid cancers in children are papillary or follicular, usually presenting as an asymptomatic solitary nodule or cervical adenopathy. Although a trial of thyroid suppression is recommended by some, the 14% to 40% incidence of carcinoma in children with thyroid nodules should prompt surgical resection. The 10-year survival is better for younger patients with thyroid carcinoma (83%) than for adults (60%).

Adrenal carcinomas are also rare in childhood (<0.5% of pediatric tumors) and occur primarily in children younger than 8 years old. These tumors are endocrinologically active, causing either Cushing's syndrome, virilization, or feminization; aldosterenomas are rare in children. One of the primary objectives is to distinguish carcinoma from a benign adenoma. Carcinomas are usually larger and more inhomogeneous by CT and ultrasound at the time of diagnosis. Tumors weighing less than 100 g have an excellent prognosis, but those weighing more than 500 g have a very poor prognosis. Surgery is the treatment of choice, and awareness that tumors may be bilateral in up to 10% of cases is important. For patients with extensive local or metastatic disease in kidney, lymph nodes, liver, lung, mesentery, brain, or bone, chemotherapy with 5-FU, dactinomycin, cyclophosphamide, and op′DDD should be administered. Inhibitors of steroid synthesis (*e.g.*, aminoglutethimate, metapyrone, ketoconazole) or glucocorincoid antiagonists (*i.e.*, RU 486) may be useful. If hypoaldosteronism or hypocortisolism develops, after treatment with mitolane, fludrocortisone or hydrocortisone replacement may be necessary. Studies are in progress using suramin, an antiparasitic agent that, as a side-effect, can cause the necrosis of the adrenal cortex. Preliminary results are encouraging.

MEN syndromes are exceedingly rare in pediatrics but have been described in families. MEN type I consists of tumors of the pituitary, parathyroid, and pancreas (in particular, the ZE syndrome); MEN II consists of medullary carcinoma of the thyroid and pheochromocytoma (MEN IIa) and a familial syndrome that also includes mucosal neuromas and a Marfan-like body habitus (MEN IIb) (Table 47-35).

RENAL CELL CARCINOMA

Renal cell carcinoma (clear cell carcinoma, renal cell adenocarcinoma, hypernephroma) is the most common primary kidney tumor in adults, but it is rare in children, occurring with an annual incidence of 4 per million. Renal cell carcinoma has been seen in patients with the von Hippel-Lindau syndrome, tuberous sclerosis, and a constitutional chromosome translocation. There is a high frequency of abnormalities, t(3:8)(p14; p24), of chromosome 3.

The four patterns of pathology are papillary, solid, cystic, and sarcomatous, although these have little prognostic impact. The cellular morphology includes clear cell, granular cell, and sarcomatoid types.

Unlike Wilms' tumor, in which the presenting mass is often asymptomatic, renal cell carcinoma usually presents with abdominal or flank pain and hematuria. The average age of patients with renal cell carcinoma is 11 years, but it has been described in children as young as 14 months.

Among the most important prognostic factor is stage. Children with Stage I disease had a 100% survival; Stage II had a 66% survival; Stage III had 43% survival; and Stage IV had a

TABLE 47-35. Comparison of Clusters of Involved Tumors in MEN Syndromes

Site of Origin	*MEN I*	*MEN IIa*	*MEN IIb**
Pituitary gland	Prolactinoma Somatotropinoma Corticotropinoma		
Thyroid gland		C-cell hyperplasia Medullary carcinoma	Medullary carcinoma
Parathyroid glands	Parathyroid hyperplasia–adenoma	Parathyroid hyperplasia–adenoma	
Adrenal cortex	Adrenal adenoma–hyperplasia		
Adrenal medulla		Pheochromocytoma	Pheochromocytoma
Gastroenteropancreatic unit	Gastrinoma Insulinoma VIPoma Glucagonoma		Mucosal neuromas, ganglioneuromas
Other	PPoma Lipomas Carcinoids		

Chrousos GP: Endocrine tumors. In Pizzo PA, Poplack DG (eds): Principles and Practice of Pediatric Oncology, p 750. Philadelphia, JB Lippincott, 1989.
* Characterized also by marfanoid habitus.

12% survival rate. This is related to the therapeutic approaches. Radical nephrectomy with resection of the kidney, adrenal gland, surrounding perinephric fat, Gerota's fascia, and regional lymph nodes, is the treatment for localized renal cell carcinoma. The role of radiotherapy is unclear for children, although some physicians have advocated 4000 to 4500 cGy postoperatively for children with Stage II disease. Chemotherapy has not been particularly successful, but interferon and the use of interleukin-2 (IL-2) with lymphokine-activated killer (LAK) cells have been successful in adults; data for children, however, are lacking.

GASTROINTESTINAL TRACT

Carcinomas of the stomach, colon, gallbladder, and pancreas have been described in children, although their incidence is strikingly low.[51] These tumors are usually not suspected in children. Because the tumors are so rare in children, the treatments are similar to those used in adults.

CANCERS OF THE SKIN

Melanoma is the most common skin cancer in children, followed by basal and squamous cell carcinoma. Ionizing irradiation is an important risk factor and contributes to the regional distribution of these cancers.

The familial occurrence of melanoma in individuals with the dysplastic nevus syndrome is recognized. These nevi are usually located on the trunk but can occur in the scalp or extremities. Approximately 10% of patients with these lesions will develop melanomas.

The clinical appearance of melanomas and their local and metastatic spread is similar in children to that of adults. Biopsy is necessary for diagnosis, but whether it is incisional or excisional depends on the location and size of the lesion. If the lesion is a melanoma, a wide excision is necessary. Curettage or cryotherapy can be used for basal cell or squamous cell carcinomas. As in adults, chemotherapy has been used for patients with melanoma who have evidence of regional lymph node involvement.[52] The use of IL-2 and LAK cells in adults with melanoma suggests therapeutic utility for children or adolescents with evidence of extensive disease.

Pediatricians should recommend decreased sun exposure, the use of sunscreens for children and teenagers, and the removal of congenital nevi.

REFERENCES

1. Koufos A, Hansen MF, Copeland NG et al: Loss of heterozygosity in three embryonal tumours suggests a common pathogenetic mechanism. Nature 316:330–334, 1985
2. Bishop JM: The molecular genetics of cancer. Science 253:305–311, 1987
3. Meadows AT, Kramer S, Hopson R et al: Survival in childhood acute lymphocytic leukemia: Effect of protocol and place of treatment. Cancer Invest 1:49–55, 1983
4. Miller RW, McKay FW: Decline in US childhood cancer mortality, 1950 through 1980. JAMA 251:1567–1570, 1984
5. Breslow NE, Beckwith JB: Epidemiological features of Wilms' tumor: Results of the National Wilms' Tumor Study. JNCI 68:429–436, 1982
6. Mannens M, Slater RM, Heyting C: Regional localization of DNA probes on the short arm of chromosome 11 using aniridia-Wilms' tumor-associated deletion. Hum Genet 75:180–187, 1987
7. Beckwith JB: Wilms' tumor and other renal tumors of childhood: An update. J Urol 136:320–324, 1986
8. Douglass EC, Look AT, Webber B et al: Hyperdiploidy and chromosomal rearrangements define the anaplastic variant of Wilms' tumor. J Clin Oncol 4:975–981, 1986
9. Sutow WW, Breslow NE, Palmer NR et al: Prognosis in children with Wilms' tumor metastasis prior to or following primary treatment. Am J Clin Oncol 5:339–347, 1982
10. Breslow NE, Churchill G, Nesmith B et al: Clinicopathologic features and prognosis for Wilms' tumor patients with metastases at diagnosis. Cancer 58:2501–1511, 1986
11. D'Angio GJ, Evans A, Breslow N et al: The treatment of Wilms' tumor: Results of the Second National Wilms' Tumor Study. Cancer 47:2302–2311, 1981
12. D'Angio GJ, Evans AE, Breslow N et al: The treatment of Wilms' tumor. Results of the National Wilms' Tumor Study. Cancer 38:633–646, 1976
13. Israel MA: The evolution of clinical molecular genetics. Neuroblastoma as a model. Am J Pediatr Hematol Oncol 8:163–172, 1986
14. Brodeur GM, Hayes FA, Green AA et al: Consistent N-*myc* copy number in simultaneous or consecutive neuroblastoma samples from sixty individual patients. Cancer Res 47:4248–4253, 1987
15. Look AT, Hayes FA, Nitschke R et al: Cellular DNA content as a predictor of response to chemotherapy in infants with unresectable neuroblastoma. N Engl J Med 311:231–235, 1984
16. Cheung NK, Von Hoff DD, Strandjord SE et al: Detection of neuroblastoma cells in bone marrow using GD_2 specific monoclonal antibodies. J Clin Oncol 4:363–369, 1986
17. D'Angio GJ, Evans AE, Koop CE: Special pattern of widespread neuroblastoma with a favourable prognosis. Lancet 1:1046–1049, 1971

18. Sawada T, Kidowaki T, Sakamoto I et al: Neuroblastoma. Mass screening for early detection and its prognosis. Cancer 53:2631–2735, 1984
19. Evans AE, Chatten J, D'Angio GJ et al: Review of 17 IV-S neuroblastoma patients at the Children's Hospital of Philadelphia. Cancer 45:833–839, 1980
20. Hayes FA, Green A, Hustu HO et al: Surgicopathologic staging of neuroblastoma: Prognostic significance of regional lymph node metastases. J Pediatr 102:59–62, 1983
21. Rosen E, Cassady JR, Frantz C et al: Neuroblastoma: The Joint Center for Radiation Therapy/Dana-Farber Cancer Institute/Children's Hospital Experience. J Clin Oncol 2:719–732, 1984
22. Green AA, Hayes FA, Hustu HO: Sequential cyclophosphamide and doxorubicin for induction of complete remission in children with disseminated neuroblastoma. Cancer 48:2310–2317, 1981
23. Kretschmar CS, Frantz CN, Rosen EM et al: Improved prognosis for infants with stage IV neuroblastoma. J Clin Oncol 2:799–803, 1984
24. Kushner BH, Helson LH: Coordinated use of sequentially escalated cyclophosphamide and cell-cycle-specific chemotherapy (N4SE protocol) for advanced neuroblastoma: Experience with 100 patients. J Clin Oncol 5:1746–1751, 1987
25. Philip T, Bernard J, Zucker J et al: High-dose chemoradiotherapy with bone marrow transplantation as consolidation treatment in neuroblastoma. An unselected group of stage IV patients over 1 year of age. J Clin Oncol 5:266–271, 1987
26. Horowitz ME, Etcubanas E, Christensen M et al: Phase II testing of melphalan in children with newly diagnosed rhabdomyosarcoma: A model for anticancer drug development. J Clin Oncol 6:308–314, 1988
27. Dryja TP, Cavenee W, White R et al: Homozygosity of chromosome 13 in retinoblastoma. N Engl J Med 310:550–553, 1984
28. Benedict WF, Murphree AL, Banerjee A et al: Patient with 13 chromosome deletion: Evidence that the retinoblastoma gene is a recessive cancer gene. Science 219:973–975, 1983
29. Friend SH, Bernards R, Rogelj S et al: A human DNA segment with properties of the gene that predisposes to retinoblastoma and osteosarcoma. Nature 232:643–646, 1986
30. Exelby PR, Filler RM, Grosfeld JL: Liver tumors in children in the particular reference to hepatoblastoma in hepatocellular carcinoma. American Academy of Pediatric Surgical Section Survey, 1974. J Pediatr Surg 10:329–337, 1975
31. Douglass EC, Green AA, Wrenn E et al: Effective cisplatin (DDP) based chemotherapy in the treatment of hepatoblastoma. Med Pediatr Oncol 13:187–190, 1985
32. Isaacs H: Perinatal (congenital and neonatal) neoplasms: A report of 110 cases. Pediatr Pathol 3:165–216, 1985
33. Noseworthy J, Lack EE, Kozakewich HP et al: Sacrococcygeal germ cell tumors in childhood: An updated experience with 118 patients. J Pediatr Surg 16:358–364, 1981
34. Hawkins EP, Finegold MJ, Hawkins HK et al: Nongerminomatous malignant germ cell tumors in children: A review of 89 cases from the Pediatric Oncology Group, 1971–1984. Cancer 58:2579–2584, 1986
35. Raney BB, Jr, Sinclair L, Uri A et al: Malignant ovarian tumors in children and adolescents. Cancer 59:1214–1220, 1987
36. Kurman RJ, Norris HJ: Germ cell tumors of the ovary. Pathol Annu 13:291–325, 1978
37. Maurer HM, Beltangady M, Gehan EA et al: The Intergroup Rhabdomyosarcoma Study-I. A final report. Cancer 61:209–220, 1988
38. Hays DM, Shimada H, Raney RB et al: Sarcomas of the vagina and uterus: The Intergroup Rhabdomyosarcoma Study. J Pediatr Surg 20:718–724, 1985
39. Whang-Peng T, Triche TJ, Knutsen T et al: Chromosomal translocation in peripheral neuroepithelioma. N Engl J Med 311:584–585, 1984
40. Kissane JM, Askin FB, Foulkes M et al: Ewing's sarcoma of bone: Clinicopathological aspects of 303 cases from the Intergroup Ewing's Sarcoma Study. Hum Pathol 14:773–779, 1983
41. Razek A, Perez CA, Tefft M et al: Intergroup Ewing's Sarcoma Study. Local control related to radiation dose, volume, and site of primary lesion in Ewing's sarcoma. Cancer 46:516–521, 1980
42. Miser JS, Kinsella TJ, Triche TJ et al: Ifosfamide with MESNA uroprotection and etopside: An effective regimen in the treatment of recurrent sarcomas and other tumors of children and young adults. J Clin Oncol 8:1171–1198, 1987
43. Hayes FA, Thompson EI, Parvey L: Metastatic Ewing's sarcoma: Remission, induction and survival. J Clin Oncol 5:1199–1204, 1987
44. Miser JS, Kinsella TJ, Triche TJ et al: Treatment of peripheral neuroepithelioma in children and young adults. J Clin Oncol 5:1752–1758, 1987
45. Whang-Peng J, Triche TJ, Knutsen T et al: Cytogenetic characterization of selected small round cell tumors of childhood. Cancer Genet Cytogenet 21:185–208, 1986
46. Raney RB, Schnaufer L, Zeigler M et al: Treatment of children with neurogenic sarcoma. Cancer 59:1–5, 1987
47. Horowitz ME, Pratt CB, Webber BL et al: Therapy of childhood soft tissue sarcomas other than rhabdomyosarcoma: A review of 62 cases treated at a single institution. J Clin Oncol 4:559–564, 1986
48. Writing Group of the Histiocyte Society: Histiocytosis syndromes in children. Lancet 1:208–209, 1987
49. Greenberger JS, Crocker AC, Vawter G et al: Results of treatment in 127 patients with systemic histiocytosis (Letterer-Siwe syndrome, Schuller-Christian syndrome and multifocal eosinophilic granuloma). Medicine 60:311–338, 1981
50. Lahey ME: Histiocytosis X. An analysis of prospective factors. J Pediatr 87:184–189, 1975
51. Rao BN, Pratt CB, Fleming ID et al: Colon carcinoma in children and adolescents: A review of thirty cases. Cancer 55:1322–1326, 1985
52. Hayes FA, Green AA: Malignant melanoma in childhood: Clinical course and response to chemotherapy. J Clin Oncol 2:1229–1234, 1984

DAVID G. POPLACK

LARRY E. KUN

J. ROBERT CASSADY

PHILIP A. PIZZO

CHAPTER 48 *Leukemias and Lymphomas of Childhood*

There have been major advances in the treatment of children with leukemia and lymphoma. The record of therapeutic achievements in these diseases constitutes one of the true success stories of modern clinical oncology. The improvement in the outlook for children with acute lymphoblastic leukemia (ALL) is perhaps the most dramatic example. More than half of the children with this disease, a disorder that was uniformly fatal only 40 years ago, now are alive and free of disease more than 5 years after their initial diagnosis, and most of these patients are considered cured. Thirty years ago the major concern was developing better methods of inducing complete remission, today the focus has shifted to issues facing long-term survivors. In acute nonlymphocytic leukemia (ANLL) of childhood, considerable improvement has occurred, but curative therapy for the majority of these children remains elusive. However, progress in treating the childhood non-Hodgkin's lymphomas (NHL) has been striking. Before the 1970s, fewer than 30% of children obtained long-term, disease-free survival. Currently, about 60% of children with NHL are considered curable.[1] Improvement has resulted from innovative application of the principles of combination chemotherapy and the combined modality approach.

These diseases have served as a paradigm for the treatment of many adult malignancies in that many commonly accepted treatment principles and practices, including combination chemotherapy, central nervous system (CNS) preventive therapy, and hematologic and nonhematologic supportive care, were developed from the experience with pediatric malignancies, particularly ALL. Many new therapies, including bone marrow transplantation and in vitro immunotherapy, were initially introduced as treatments for these childhood cancers.

Intensive biologic, immunologic, and cytogenetic characterization has contributed significantly to our understanding of these disorders. For example, information about the differentiation status of malignant lymphoid cells, derived in part from technical advances such as immunophenotyping with monoclonal antibodies and determination of immunoglobulin and T-cell-receptor gene rearrangement, has provided a more rational means of classifying these disorders. Similarly, application of the type of molecular biologic methods that led to the demonstration of oncogene expression in Burkitt's lymphoma cells is likely to help elucidate the cause of lymphoid and nonlymphoid malignancies.

EPIDEMIOLOGY AND ETIOLOGY

Acute leukemia is the most common malignancy in children. Each year in the United States, approximately 2000 cases are diagnosed. ALL makes up 75% of these cases; ANLL accounts for most of the remaining cases. Chronic myelogenous leukemia (CML) is rare and makes up less than 5% of all childhood leukemias.[2]

ALL has a peak incidence between 2 and 6 years of age. Historically, this age peak has developed at different times in different countries. Because these times appear to correspond to major periods of industrialization in these countries, it has been suggested that they represent exposure to new environmental leukemogens. This peak-age phenomenon was first noted in Great Britain in the 1920s, in the United States in 1940s, and in Japan in the 1960s, but it has not yet been seen in relatively unindustralized countries. The increased peak incidence of ALL in whites in the United States is not observed in blacks. This difference, which may reflect a difference in susceptibility to environmental leukemogens, is largely responsible for the observation that acute leukemia is almost twice as common in white than in nonwhite children.

In ANLL there is no peak-age incidence in childhood. The two forms of CML in childhood tend to occur at somewhat different ages. The median age of onset for the juvenile form is approximately 2 years of age, whereas the Philadelphia chromosome-positive (Ph^1-positive) type more commonly appears in older children.[3] Both ANLL and CML occur with similar frequency in whites and nonwhites.

ALL occurs more commonly in boys, a disparity greatest in pubertal children. In children younger than 5 years of age, ANLL occurs more commonly in girls; between ages 5 to 15 years, the incidence in each sex is equal; thereafter males are affected more frequently.

There has been considerable interest in reports of "leukemic clusters," the occurrence of a greater than expected number of leukemia cases within a given geographical area or time period. Although the demonstration of bona fide clustering would have profound epidemiologic implications, most studies have been unable to confirm this phenomenon.

A variety of possible causative factors for leukemia have been examined, including environmental and genetic factors, viruses, and immunodeficiency states. Irradiation and exposure to toxic chemicals are the most studied environmental factors that predispose to leukemia. The increased incidence of leukemia observed in survivors of atomic bomb explosions in Hiroshima and Nagasaki in 1945 is well known. Persons closest to the hypocenters of these explosions had the highest incidence of leukemia, and for exposure to doses of more than 100 R, the dose-response relationship was linear. The type of leukemia that developed corresponded to the age at exposure. ALL was more common in children. Although atomic bomb survivors had no increase in the incidence of leukemia in children exposed to radiation in utero, more recent data have demonstrated an increased risk to children exposed to diagnostic radiation, particularly in the first trimester. A higher incidence of leukemia was noted in several early studies to have resulted from radiation used to treat thymic enlargement in neonates, tinea capitis infection, and ankylosing spondylitis. The association of alkylating agents used for treating childhood malignancy with the development of adult leukemia is well documented. The incidence of therapy-induced leukemia is higher in those persons who also have received concomitant radiotherapy. Chronic exposure to toxic chemicals (*e.g.* benzene) has been associated with the development of leukemia, usually ANLL. There is considerable controversy about the potential risks associated with exposure to ionizing radiation from routine nuclear power plant emissions.

There is evidence for the role of genetic factors in leukemogenesis. The incidence of leukemia is increased in children with certain constitutional chromosomal abnormalities. Children with trisomy 21 (Down's syndrome) have approximately 15 times more risk of developing leukemia than individuals in the general population. ALL is most commonly observed, although ANNL may occur, particularly in neonatal cases. The development of leukemia in children with Down's syndrome is believed to reflect the presence of an unstable genome that is more susceptible to other leukemogenic factors (*e.g.*, viruses). The observation that fibroblasts from Down's syndrome children are transformed more readily in vitro by SV40 virus supports this thesis. The same observation has been made in fibroblasts of children with Fanconi's syndrome, a rare, recessively transmitted disorder characterized by a variety of congenital abnormalities and frequently associated with the development of acute myelomonocytic leukemia. Patients with Bloom's syndrome, another recessively transmitted chromosomal fragility disorder, characterized by short stature and photosensitive telangiectatic erythema, have a higher incidence of leukemia, usually ANLL. The development of leukemia in these patients may be a consequence of genetic recombination of somatic cell chromosomes.

Patients with ataxia-telangiectasia, an immunodeficiency disease in which abnormalities of chromosomes 14 and 7 have been observed, are at an increased risk of lymphoid malignancy, including ALL. The loci of three rearranging T-cell-receptor genes, alpha (chromosome 14), beta, and gamma (chromosome 7), are at chromosomal positions susceptible to breakage and rearrangement in patients with ataxia-telangectasia. The extent to which immune deficiency contributes to the genetic predisposition of patients to develop malignancy is not known.

The risk of leukemia is increased in children with Klinefelter's syndrome and the trisomy G syndrome. Leukemia has been associated with a variety of less-well-characterized chromosomal abnormalities. The increased risk of leukemia in children born to relatively older women may be related to the existence of subtle karyotypic abnormalities in aging mothers. An increased risk of leukemia has also been observed in several genetically determined congenital syndromes that are not associated with known karyotypic abnormalities, including the Rubinstein-Taybi syndrome, Schwachman's syndrome, Poland's syndrome, and neurofibromatosis.

The development of leukemia in more than one family member has been documented. The risk of leukemia is four times greater among siblings of leukemic children than in the general population. Those at highest risk for the development of leukemia are identical twins of children with the disease. Their risk may be as high as 25%, but it diminishes with age, and after the age of 7 years, the risk of leukemia for the unaffected twin returns to that of the general population. Although these observations strongly imply a genetic basis for the increased risk of leukemia, other factors, such as common exposure to a leukemogenic prenatal or postnatal event, cannot be excluded.

There has been intense interest in the possible role of viruses in the development of human leukemia. Certain RNA viruses can cause leukemia in avian, murine, bovine, feline, and nonhuman primate species. Study of vertically transmitted leukemogenic viruses in the murine system led to the viral-oncogene hypothesis, which has been proposed as a model for the viral initiation of human leukemia. Evidence linking viruses to the development of human leukemia was somewhat circumstantial and consisted of the rare finding of C-type viral particles in human leukemic tissue, identification of virus-like particles from marrow, plasma, and urine of leukemia patients, and demonstration of reverse transcriptase and 70S high-molecular-weight RNA in human leukemia cells. Recently, a human T-cell lymphoma–leukemia virus (HTLV-1) has been consistently isolated from and linked specifically to a rare, clinically distinctive, and aggressive form of adult T-cell lymphoma–leukemia prevalent in the Southeastern United States, the Caribbean basin, and parts of Japan. HTLV-1 has not been identified in childhood leukemias; however, its discovery has confirmed the potential role of retroviruses in human leukemogenesis. The role of DNA viruses, particularly the Epstein-Barr virus (EBV), in lymphoid malignancy has been studied. The relationship of EBV to Burkitt's lymphoma is discussed later in this chapter.

A relationship between immunodeficiency and the development of leukemia has been established. Children with the Wiskott-Aldrich syndrome, congenital hypogammaglobulinemia, and severe combined immunodeficiency disease all have an increased incidence of lymphoid malignancy, including leukemia. Presumably impaired immune surveillance eventually permits the development of malignancy. The increased risk of leukemia in ataxia-telangiectasia patients probably is related both to impaired immunity and genetic factors. Chronic use of immunosuppressive agents has also been associated with the development of leukemia. The role that immune dysfunction plays in the development of leukemia in patients without a recognized immunodeficiency syndrome is not known. Abnormalities in the immune system of newly diagnosed patients with ALL have been observed, but whether they precede or are a consequence of the leukemia is unclear.

ACUTE LYMPHOBLASTIC LEUKEMIA

CLINICAL PRESENTATION AND DIAGNOSIS

The presenting signs and symptoms of the child with ALL (Table 48-1) reflect the degree to which the bone marrow has been infiltrated with leukemic lymphoblasts and the extent of extramedullary spread. The most common symptoms and physical findings, resulting from anemia, thrombocytopenia, and neutropenia, include pallor and fatigue, anorexia, petechiae, purpura, bleeding, and infection. Localized or generalized lymphadenopathy, hepatomegaly, and splenomegaly are the consequence of extramedullary leukemic spread. Overt symptoms of CNS leukemia are relatively rare at the time of initial diagnosis. Leukemic infiltration of the periosteum and bone frequently occurs, and bone pain, often manifesting as a limp or refusal to walk, is quite common in young children. The duration of symptoms in children presenting with ALL varies from days to months. Because children most frequently present with relatively nonspecific symptoms, ALL clinically may mimic a number of childhood conditions, including infectious mononucleosis, idiopathic thrombocytopenic purpura, pertussis and parapertussis, chronic viral infections (*e.g.*, cytomegalovirus, acute infectious lymphocytosis), and rheumatoid arthritis. ALL may be confused with aplastic anemia. Very rarely it may present as the hypereosinophilic syndrome. ALL also must be differentiated from other pediatric malignancies that may involve bone marrow, including non-Hodgkin's lymphoma, rhabdomyosarcoma, retinoblastoma, and neuroblastoma.

Replacement of normal bone marrow elements by leukemic cells produces an abnormal hemogram in most newly diagnosed patients (Table 48-1). Anemia and thrombocytopenia occur in more than two thirds of patients. The peripheral leukocyte count may be normal or even low, but approximately one third of patients have an initial leukocyte count >20,000/mm³. An increased leukocyte count at diagnosis connotes a poor prognosis. Leukemic cells may be seen in the peripheral blood; however, morphologic assessment of these cells is often misleading. Careful examination of a bone marrow aspirate is mandatory to make a diagnosis. On rare occasions, a bone marrow biopsy may be necessary. Although the presence of greater than 5% lymphoblasts indicates leukemia, most laboratories require a minimum of 25% leukemic blast cells in the bone marrow aspirate to confirm the diagnosis.[3] A definitive diagnosis requires careful morphologic examination of marrow aspirate smears stained with Romanovsky stain and detailed cytochemistry studies using myeloperoxidase or Sudan black, periodic acid-Schiff (PAS), and nonspecific esterase stains. Although use of these special stains will help to distinguish ALL from

TABLE 48-1. Symptoms, Physical Findings, and Laboratory Features in Children with ALL

Clinical or Laboratory Feature	*% of Patients*
Symptoms and Physical Findings	
Fever	61
Bleeding (*e.g.*, petechiae or purpura)	48
Bone pain	23
Lymphadenopathy	50
Splenomegaly	63
Hepatosplenomegaly	68
Laboratory Features	
Leukocyte count (/mm³)	
<10,000	53
10,000–49,000	30
>50,000	17
Hemoglobin (g/dl)	
<7.0	43
7.0–11.0	45
>11.0	12
Platelet count (/mm³)	
<20,000	28
20,000 to 99,000	47
>100,000	25
Lymphoblast morphology	
L1	84
L2	15
L3	1
Immunologic markers	
Non-T, non-B	80
T	18
B	1

Miller DR: Acute lymphoblastic leukemia. Pediatr Clin North Am 27:269–291, 1980.

TABLE 48-2. Morphologic and Cytochemical Characteristics of ALL and ANLL

Characteristics	*ALL*	*ANLL*
Nuclear/cytoplasmic ratio	High	Low
Nuclear chromatin	Finely dispersed	Spongy
Nucleoli	0–2	2–5
Granules	Absent	Present
Auer rods	Absent	May be present
Cytoplasm	Blue	Blue gray
Cytochemical reaction		
Peroxidase test	–	–
Sudan black B test	–	–
Periodic acid-Schiff test	–	–
Naphthol ASD chloracetate esterase test	–	–
Alpha-naphthylacetate esterase test	–	–

ANLL in most cases (Table 48-2), immunophenotyping, biochemical analysis (*e.g.*, TdT determination), and cytogenetic analyses should be performed.

In addition to a detailed history, physical examination, and hematologic evaluation, newly diagnosed leukemia patients require other laboratory studies, including uric acid level and electrolyte level determinations, kidney and liver function studies, and appropriate radiologic studies. Hyperuricemia, a consequence of increased purine metabolism in leukemic cells, is often present at diagnosis or provoked by initiation of treatment. Adequate hydration, alkalinization, and treatment with the xanthine oxidase inhibitor allopurinol are required to prevent uric acid nephropathy. Leukemic-cell lysis frequently produces elevated serum lactate dehydrogenase (LDH) levels, LDH levels are prognostically important. Abnormal liver function tests may be present at diagnosis, presumably the result of leukemic infiltration of the liver. A variety of metabolic abnormalities also may be seen on initial presentation including hyperkalemia, hypomagnesemia, and hypocalcemia or hypercalcemia. Low serum immunoglobulins have been reported in as many as 30% of newly diagnosed patients with ALL. Whether this represents a preexisting condition or is a consequence of the disease is not clear. Leukemic cells are capable of suppressing immunoglobulin synthesis in vitro, suggesting that in some patients this mechanism may play a role.

Chest x-ray films may reveal the presence of a mediastinal mass, particularly in high-risk patients. Leukemic infiltrates of the periosteum and bone may produce typical changes that are usually seen in the long bones. Bone lesions may be present radiographically even if there is no pain. Although it has been suggested that bone lesions at diagnosis are a poor prognostic sign, this has not been confirmed. Rarely, the bone lesions of ALL will mimic osteomyelitis.

EXTRAMEDULLARY LEUKEMIA

Extramedullary leukemic spread may be clinically overt or detectable only by invasive diagnostic procedures. Extramedullary disease is important because it may cause local morbidity and because an extramedullary relapse frequently heralds bone marrow relapse, presumably as a result of spread to the bone marrow from the involved site. The themes of current treatment strategies are to prevent extramedullary relapse and to treat it aggressively if it occurs.

The two most important sites of extramedullary spread are the CNS and the testes. Ovarian leukemia, perhaps because of inaccessibility to detailed physical examination, is rarely detected. Extramedullary disease can also occur in the liver, spleen, kidneys, gastrointestinal tract, and lung.

Central Nervous System Leukemia

The significance of CNS leukemia became apparent in the late 1950s and 1960s when, with better systemic treatment and longer survival, the CNS became the most frequent site of initial relapse. The incidence of CNS disease was as high as 75% to 80%. CNS disease was difficult to eradicate, CNS relapse was frequent, and almost invariably, CNS disease was rapidly followed by bone marrow relapse. The recognition of this latter phenomenon led to the development of effective CNS preventive therapy that improved the prognoses of children with this disease.

CNS leukemia is believed to develop either by hematogenous "seeding" of circulating leukemic cells or by direct spread of leukemic cells from involved cranial bone marrow. CNS leukemia initially involves the meninges; deeper invasion of the brain parenchyma occurs in more advanced disease. Overt CNS leukemia occurs in fewer than 5% of children at diagnosis and rarely is symptomatic.[4] Symptomatic patients manifest a variety of signs and symptoms of increased intracranial pressure, including headache, nausea, vomiting, lethargy, irritability, nuchal rigidity, and papilledema. Cranial nerve palsies also may occur (most commonly of the sixth or seventh cranial nerves), often as an isolated event. More unusual presentations include the hypothalamic-obesity syndrome, diabetes insipidus, ataxia due to cerebellar involvement, and symptoms related to subdural or even epidural leukemic infiltration. Any unexplained neurologic sign or symptom in a patient with ALL requires evaluation to exclude CNS leukemia.

The diagnosis of CNS disease is made by cytologic examination of cerebrospinal fluid (CSF) obtained by lumbar puncture. CSF should be examined after cytocentrifugation, a technique that concentrates the leukemic cells and increases diagnostic sensitivity tenfold. Relying solely on the demonstration of a pleocytosis in CSF is insufficient and potentially misleading. In symptomatic patients, CSF pressure is usually elevated, and hypoglycorrhachia and increased CSF protein levels are common. The heightened awareness of the possibility of CNS relapse has made surveillance lumbar punctures routine, and CNS leukemia is more commonly diagnosed in the asymptomatic patient, in whom CSF pressure and chemistries may be normal and CSF leukemic-cell counts relatively low. Although skull x-ray films, the computed tomography (CT) brain scan, head magnetic resonance imaging (MRI), and the electroencephalogram (EEG) may occasionally be abnormal in the patient with overt CNS leukemia, none of these tests are reliable for diagnosis.

Testicular Leukemia

The incidence of testicular leukemia increased in the 1970s with improved survival of ALL patients. The testes constitute an important site of relapse, and although clinically demonstrable testicular disease is rarely evident at the initial diagnosis, occult testicular involvement has been reported to occur in up to 25% of newly diagnosed boys. Overt testicular recurrence, presenting as painless testicular enlargement, may occur in up to 15% of boys undergoing chemotherapy and in one earlier study was reported in approximately 40% of boys who have successfully completed a 2.5-year to 3-year course of treatment.[5,6] Although the overall incidence of testicular disease may be significantly lower on current therapeutic protocols, biopsy-proven, occult testicular leukemia has been found in as many as 15% of asymptomatic boys upon completion of chemotherapy, an observation consistent with relatively high incidence of late, overt relapses in such patients.

Testicular disease is more likely to occur in boys with a high initial leukocyte count (>20,000/mm³), prominent lymphadenopathy and splenomegaly, T-cell disease, or significant thrombocytopenia (<30,000/mm³).[7] The diagnosis of clinically suspected testicular leukemia is made by wedge biopsy. Testicular recurrence frequently is followed by systemic relapse, particularly when the testicular relapse has occurred during or immediately after maintenance chemotherapy. Isolated testicular relapse occurring 6 months or longer after cessation of therapy is usually unilateral and is associated with a relatively good prognosis when treated appropriately.

MORPHOLOGIC CLASSIFICATION

The considerable variation in the morphologic appearance of ALL cells has led to numerous attempts to subclassify the disease. The system proposed by the French-American-British (FAB) cooperative working group, which divides lymphoblasts into three categories, has been most useful (Table 48-3).[8] L1 lymphoblasts are smaller, with little cytoplasm and inconspicuous nucleoli or none at all. L2 lymphoblasts are larger, with abundant cytoplasm and prominent nucleoli. Leukemic cells of the L3 type are cytomorphologically identical to Burkitt's lymphoma cells. Approximately 85% of childhood ALL cases have L1 lymphoblasts, 14% are L2, and 1% are L3. The L2 lymphoblast is the most common type in adults. Concordance among observers using this system is high, and the FAB classification has prognostic value.[8,9] L1 lymphoblasts are associated with a higher remission induction rate and prolonged remission and survival. L2 cells convey a poor prognosis independently of other prognostic variables. Patients with the L3 variety have the least favorable prognosis. With the possible exception of L3 cells, which ordinarily possess surface immunoglobulin and other B-cell markers, there is no apparent correlation between FAB classification and immunologic cell-surface markers.[8]

IMMUNOPHENOTYPES

Immunologic techniques have permitted the identification of distinct immunologic subtypes of ALL and have confirmed that ALL is a heterogeneous disease in which leukemic transformation and clonal expansion may occur at different stages in lymphoid differentiation. Initially, using standard immunologic methods for surface membrane characterization, three forms of ALL were identified. Approximately 20% of patients had T-cell lymphoblasts, 1% to 2% had lymphoblasts with B-cell characteristics, and the vast majority of patients were found to have lymphoblasts that lacked definable T-cell or B-cell markers. Further classification using heterologous antisera and monoclonal antibodies detected a common leukemia-associated antigen (CALLA) on the leukemic cells of approximately 80% of the children with "non-T, non-B-cell" leukemia, and designated these as having "common ALL" to differentiate them from the antigen-negative, non-T, non-B-cell group with "null cell" ALL.

Clinical differences were apparent among the immunologic subtypes of ALL. Children with common ALL had a relatively good prognosis, faring better than those with null cell ALL. T-cell ALL was found to have distinctive clinical features, frequently occurring in older boys presenting with a high initial leukocyte count and a mediastinal mass. T-cell ALL is associated with a poor prognosis; however, it is unclear whether any immunologic subtype is a significant independent prognostic variable.

More sophisticated immunologic methods have revealed that the majority of non-T, non-B lymphoblasts are actually early B cells. In addition to possessing intracytoplasmic immunoglobulin, these cells are capable of differentiating in vitro into cells with B-cell markers, and they demonstrate immunoglobulin gene rearrangement indicative of precursor cells committed to the B-cell lineage.[10] Approximately 20% to 30% of B-cell-precursor ALL cases have lymphoblasts that are cytoplasmic μ heavy-chain positive. These "pre-B-cell"

TABLE 48-3. FAB Classification of Lymphoblastic Leukemia

Cytologic Features	*L1*	*L2*	*L3*
Cell size	Small cells predominate	Large, heterogeneous in size	Large and homogeneous
Nuclear chromatin	Homogeneous in any one case	Variable—heterogeneous in any one case	Finely stippled and homogeneous
Nuclear shape	Regular, occasional clefting or indentation	Irregular, clefting and indentation common	Regular—oval to round
Nucleoli	Not visible, or small and inconspicuous	One or more present, often large	Prominent, one or more vesicular
Amount of cytoplasm	Scanty	Variable, often moderately abundant	Moderately abundant
Basophilia of cytoplasm	Slight or moderate, rarely intense	Variable, deep in some	Very deep
Cytoplasmic vacuolation	Variable	Variable	Often prominent

Bennett JM, Catovsky D, Daniel MT et al: French-American-British (FAB) Cooperative Group proposals for the classification of acute leukemia. Br J Haematol 33:351-358, 1976.

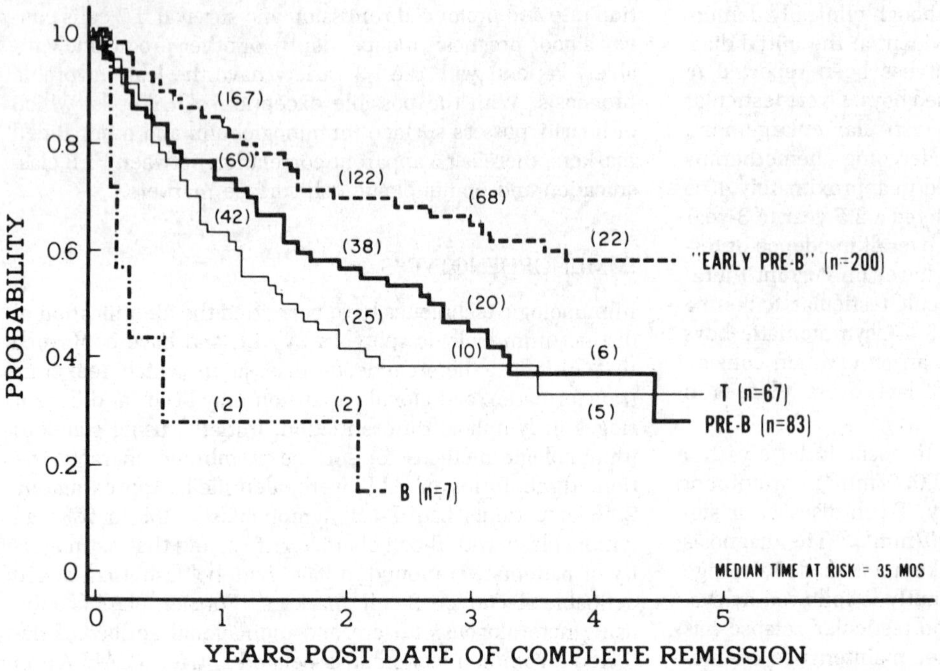

FIG. 48-1. Duration of continuous complete remission in childhood ALL for patient groups with early pre-B, pre-B, and B-cell leukemia. Data from Pediatric Oncology Group study (ALinC 13). (Crist WM, Grosse CE, Pullen J et al: Immunologic markers in childhood acute lymphocytic leukemia. Semin Oncol 12: 105–121, 1985)

ALL cases represent a relatively mature stage of development and are distinguished from $c\mu^-$ early pre-B-cell cases of ALL.[11] Pre-B-cell ALL has a worse prognosis than the early pre-B-cell type (Fig. 48-1).[11]

Using recombinant DNA technology for analysis of immunoglobulin gene rearrangement in B-cell-precursor ALL and monoclonal antibodies for immunophenotyping different B-cell antigens, investigators have defined distinct stages of differentiation for B-cell-precursor ALL (Fig. 48-2).[11] In addition, heteroantisera and monoclonal antibodies have defined different subsets of normal thymocytes that correspond to different stages of intrathymic differentiation, "early," "common," and "late."[12] Typing with these antibodies demonstrated that T-cell leukemias were derived from each of these different "stages" of differentiation.

Molecular biologic analysis of the genes encoding the T-cell receptor provided a useful marker of T-cell differentiation like the immunoglobulin gene rearrangement in B-cell-precursor ALL. Rearrangement of the gamma and beta T-cell-receptor loci are seen in T-cell lymphoblasts derived from the earlier stage of T-cell development, alpha mRNA expression appearing in more mature T lymphoblasts.[13] Although most ALL cells can be readily classified as B-cell or T-cell lineage, some leukemic cells coexpress cell surface marker antigens or molecular markers, suggesting that traditional views of lineage classification may be overly restrictive.[13,14] Although changes in blast-cell immunophenotype have been reported at relapse, this appears to be the exception.

CYTOGENETICS

Abnormal karyotypes have been reported in as many as 90% of children with ALL.[15] The abnormalities are ordinarily restricted to the leukemia cells, a finding consistent with the clonal nature of the disease. Abnormalities in both chromosome number and structure have been observed. Approximately 67% of patients have diploid or pseudodiploid karyotypes. The remaining 33% of patients manifest hyperdiploidy, which is associated with a relatively good prognosis.[16] Translocations, the most common structural abnormality observed, occur in approximately 40% of patients. They are associated with a poor prognosis. More commonly observed translocations include the t(8;14) (specific for B-cell ALL), t(9;22), t(4;11), and t(1;19) abnormalities. The typical translocation, t(9;22)(q34;q11), observed in the 5% of children with Ph[1]-positive ALL is similar to that seen in CML. In Ph[1]-positive ALL, a disorder with a poor prognosis, the Ph[1] chromosome is not found in remission and occurs only in the leukemic lymphoid line. There are also differences at the molecular level (see Chap. 53).[16] Chromosomal abnormalities appear to have considerable prognostic importance. Chromosomal studies are usually normal during remission; the presence of aneuploid cells is believed to herald relapse.

BIOCHEMISTRY

Study of a number of enzymes indicate that they may be useful in the diagnosis and classification of ALL. Terminal deoxynucleotidyl transferase (TdT), a DNA polymerizing enzyme, is not found in normal lymphocytes but is present in lymphoblasts of both T-cell and non-T, non-B-cell types. TdT expression is variable in B-cell ALL. TdT determination may help to discriminate ALL from ANLL, in which it is rarely present; however, TdT activity has no prognostic significance in ALL.

Several purine pathway enzymes, whose activity is abnormal in certain childhood immunodeficiency states, have specific patterns of expression that correlate with immunologic subtypes of ALL.[17] For example, T-cell lymphoblasts have elevated adenosine deaminase (ADA), but lower 5′-nucleotidase and purine nucleoside phosphorylase activity than non-T, non-B lymphoblasts.[17] These findings raised the possibility that selective therapy, aimed at taking advantage of

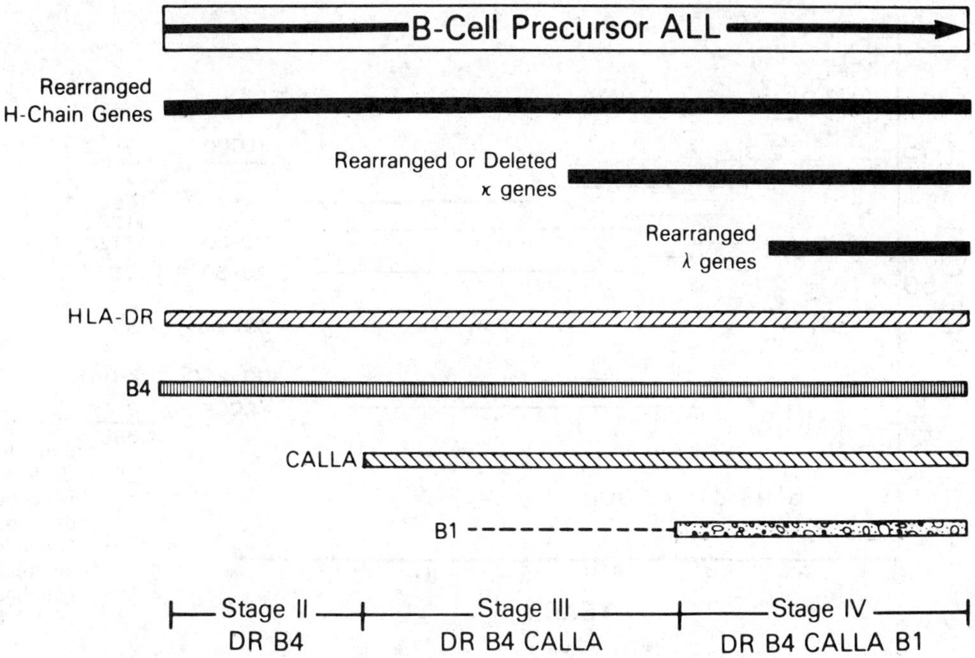

FIG. 48-2. Phenotypic subgroupings of B-cell-precursor ALL based on immunoglobulin gene rearrangement and monoclonal antibody reactivity. The monoclonal antibodies shown, DR, B4, CALLA, and B1, react with antigens that appear at various stages in the process of normal B-cell differentiation. The majority of cases of non-T-cell ALL can be classified into the three stages shown. The Stage II phenotype is seen more commonly in very young children (< 2 years old); Stage IV disease is more common in adults. Stage I (the theoretical, earliest stage of B-cell-precursor ALL) is not shown.[110] (Nadler LM, Korsmeyer SJ, Anderson KC, et al: B cell origin of non-T cell acute lymphoblastic leukemia. A model for discrete stages of neoplastic and normal pre-B cell differentiation. J Clin Invest 74:332, 1984)

these enzyme abnormalities, might be of value. Deoxycoformycin, an ADA inhibitor, has undergone clinical trials and has been used for in vitro marrow purging.

Abnormalities in various lysozomal enzymes have been observed in ALL. Elevated LDH activity has been observed in ALL at diagnosis; low serum LDH levels correlate with longer remissions and better prognoses.

Glucocorticoid receptor numbers correlated with in vitro sensitivity. Greater numbers of glucocorticoid receptors have been found on non-T, non-B-cell lymphoblasts. Low glucocorticoid receptor numbers are associated with a poor response to induction therapy and a shorter remission duration.

PROGNOSTIC FACTORS

The initial leukocyte count and age at diagnosis of ALL are universally accepted as the two most reliable indicators of prognosis for remission duration and survival.[18] There is a linear relationship between initial leukocyte count and outcome; children with higher leukocyte counts have poorer prognoses (Fig. 48-3). Very young children (<2 years of age) and older patients (>10 years of age) have relatively poor prognoses; children in the intermediate age group have the best prognoses. The worst prognosis is for infants younger than 1 year of age.[19,20] These children present with a higher incidence of poor prognostic features (*e.g.*, increased initial leukocyte count, massive organomegaly, thrombocytopenia, CNS leukemia at diagnosis) and appear to be biologically unique.[19]

Other factors correlate with prognosis, including sex, race, organomegaly, lymphadenopathy, mediastinal mass, initial hemoglobin, initial platelet count, FAB morphologic classification, immunophenotype, serum immunoglobulin levels at diagnosis, CNS leukemia at diagnosis, the rapidity of attaining complete remission, chromosomal status, serum LDH, and human leukocyte antigen (HLA) type.[16,18,21] When subjected to multivariate analysis, however, many of these features are found to be dependent variables.[18,21] A recent retrospective study of the relative order of significance and interrelationship of factors predictive for disease-free survival in a group of 1419 children treated for ALL between 1978 and 1983 revealed, after multivariate analysis, that the factors of greatest importance were initial leukocyte count, sex (girls fare better than boys), mediastinal mass, the marrow response on day 14 of induction treatment, age, initial platelet count, hematomegaly, and FAB morphologic classification.[18] Cytogenetics and immunophenotypic subgroup were found to be important in other studies.[11,16] The prognostic importance of some factors may vary somewhat from study to study. A number of factors may be responsible for this, including differences in treatment and in the patient populations.

Most current protocols use prognostic criteria (*e.g.*, initial leukocyte count, age at diagnosis) to stratify patients at diagnosis into different risk groups. Staging of this type permits

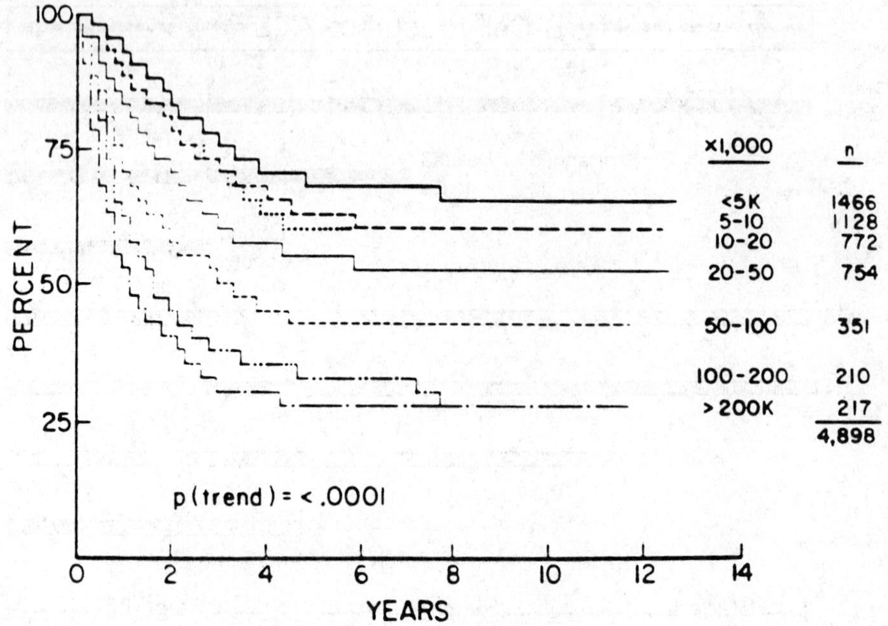

FIG. 48-3. Continuous complete remission duration of children with acute lymphoblastic leukemia, stratified according to initial white blood cell count. Data from 4898 children treated by the Children's Cancer Study Group. (Hammond D, Sather H, Nesbit M et al: Analysis of prognostic factors in acute lymphoblastic leukemia. Med Pediatr Oncol 14:1224–1234, 1965)

selective application of treatment to different risk groups. High-risk patients are treated with more aggressive chemotherapy regimens, but low-risk patients receive less-intensive therapy, designed to be equally effective and yet avoid the toxicities and complications of aggressive therapy.

No single system of ALL staging has been universally accepted. An example is shown in Figure 48-4, which illustrates the event-free survival curves for patients treated on a current Children's Cancer Study Group series of protocols that stratify patients into five risk groups: good, average, poor (primarily on the basis of initial leukocyte count, age at diagnosis and FAB classification), infants, and patients presenting with lymphomatous features, a group at high risk of treatment failure, particularly CNS relapse.[18]

TREATMENT

As our understanding of ALL has increased, evaluation and treatment of children with this disease has become more complex. An appropriate patient workup requires more sophisticated techniques (*e.g.*, immunophenotyping, cytogenetic analysis, biochemical assays) and stratification of patients

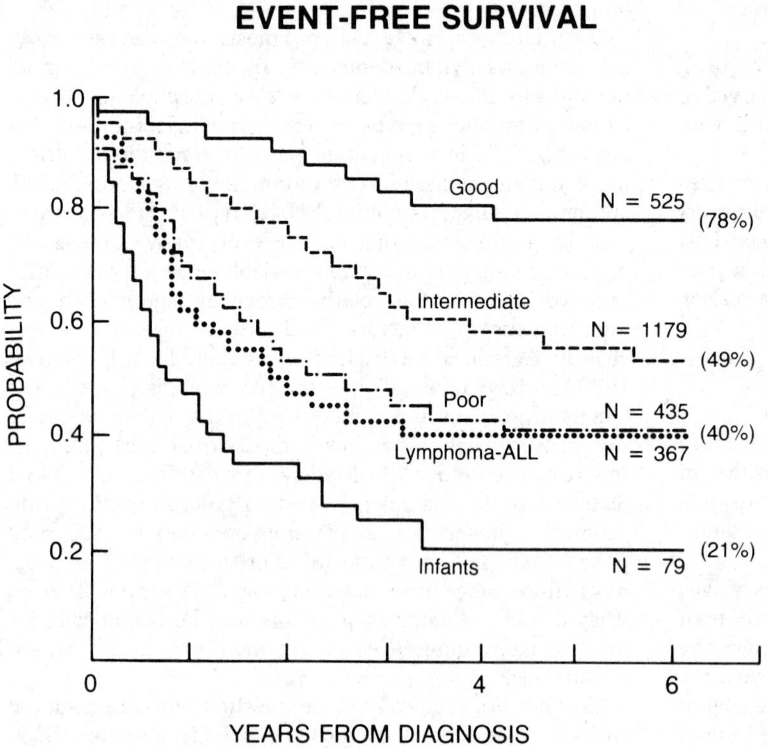

FIG. 48-4. Event-free survival for children with ALL stratified into five prognostic groups. Children's Cancer Study Group. (With permission of Dr. W. A. Bleyer)

into various risk groups for appropriate therapy. Recognition of the biological heterogeneity of ALL makes it inappropriate to define a standard ALL treatment regimen. Combination chemotherapy remains the primary therapeutic modality, with evolving indications for limited radiation therapy. The principles used to manage all patients with ALL are somewhat similar. Current treatment is divided into four phases: remission induction, CNS preventive therapy, consolidation, and maintenance.

Remission Induction

The first goal of ALL treatment is induction of complete remission, defined as the lack of any evidence of leukemia on physical examination and hematologic evaluation. The bone marrow must be normocellular, with <5% lymphoblasts, and peripheral blood counts should be within the range of normal values. There must be no detectable CNS or other extramedullary disease. It has been estimated that patients with clinically overt ALL have approximately 10^{12} leukemic cells, whereas patients in remission have less than 10^{10} blast cells. In these terms, remission induction requires a reduction in the number of leukemic cells by at least 99%. Although prednisone and vincristine traditionally have been the most widely used two-drug combination, capable of inducing remission in approximately 80% to 90% of patients, it is now clear that it is inadequate. The addition of a third agent, either L-asparaginase or daunorubicin, raises the induction rate to 90% to 100% and significantly prolongs remission. The addition of a fourth induction agent, usually the anthracycline daunorubicin, together with intensive consolidation therapy, improves remission duration, even in patients with poor risk features.[22] Most induction regimens are approximately 4 weeks. There is evidence that the rapidity of cytoreduction correlates with remission duration.

Central Nervous System Prophylaxis

The concept of CNS preventive therapy is based on the assumption that undetectable CNS leukemia is present in most patients at the time of diagnosis, residing in that "sanctuary site" protected by the blood–brain barrier from cytotoxic concentrations of most systemically administered antileukemic agents. Studies in the 1960s aimed at prevention of CNS leukemia demonstrated that administration of 2400 cGy of cranial irradiation and intrathecal methotrexate after remission induction reduced the incidence of overt CNS leukemia to 10% or less. Although this approach was universally adopted in the 1970s, the adverse effects of CNS irradiation on neurologic and intellectual functions prompted a reappraisal of this strategy. There is now a large body of data documenting long-term side effects, including CT-detected brain abnormalities, impaired intellectual and psychomotor function, and neuroendocrine dysfunction, in a proportion of patients treated with 2400 cGy of cranial irradiation and intrathecal chemotherapy, which stimulated a search for an alternative, safer method of CNS prophylaxis. A number of approaches have been studied, including using lower doses of cranial radiation (1800 cGy) with intrathecal methotrexate; periodic intrathecal methotrexate during maintenance with intensive systemic chemotherapy; triple intrathecal chemotherapy with methotrexate, cytosine arabinoside, and hydrocortisone; intermediate-dose methotrexate alone or with concomitant intrathecal methotrexate; or high-dose methotrexate alone.

It is now apparent that the risk of developing CNS leukemia depends on certain predictive factors at presentation. Characteristics associated with an increased risk of CNS leukemia include a high initial leukocyte count, T-cell disease, thrombocytopenia, profound lymphadenopathy or hepatosplenomegaly, and patients who are either very young or black.[4,19] The recognition of different risk groups led to the concept of tailoring CNS preventive therapy, using equally effective, less-intensive CNS treatment if possible. For example, it is now clear that 1800 cGy is as effective as 2400 cGy in providing CNS protection in regimens that use cranial radiation plus intrathecal chemotherapy, although it is not clear if reduction in radiation dose will be associated with a lower incidence of adverse CNS sequellae. It now appears that cranial irradiation is not necessary for patients with a good prognosis; intrathecal methotrexate alone offers adequate protection for this group of children with a low risk of CNS relapse.[23]

The combination of intrathecal and moderate-dose intravenous methotrexate, maintenance intrathecal triple chemotherapy (methotrexate, cytarabine, and hydrocortisone), and high-dose methotrexate alone appear to provide equivalent protection to that offered by cranial irradiation and intrathecal methotrexate for patients at an intermediate risk of CNS relapse. Triple intrathecal chemotherapy given frequently and continuing throughout maintenance is as effective as 2400 cGy of cranial irradiation plus intrathecal methotrexate in patients with ALL without lymphomatous presentations or T-cell disease. In high-risk patients the majority of published data indicates the necessity of cranial irradiation and intrathecal methotrexate to prevent CNS relapse.[4] The preliminary results of a randomized study comparing very high-dose methotrexate infusions with cranial irradiation and intrathecal methotrexate indicate that equivalent CNS protection can be obtained in both average and high-risk patients, raising the possibility that cranial irradiation in high-risk patients may eventually be obviated by aggressive chemotherapy.[193]

Maintenance and Consolidation Therapy

After remission induction, additional treatment is necessary. Without maintenance treatment the overwhelming majority of patients relapse within 1 to 2 months. Methotrexate and 6-mercaptopurine are the two drugs most frequently administered during maintenance. Usually, 6-mercaptopurine is given on a daily basis; methotrexate is given intermittently (*e.g.*, once or twice weekly). The value of adding agents to standard 6-mercaptopurine and methotrexate maintenance therapy has been controversial, and the data have been somewhat contradictory. The addition of intermittent pulses of vincristine and prednisone appears to prolong remission, although the value of this approach after intensive induction therapy is not totally clear. The intensive, weekly use of L-asparaginase may add to the effectiveness of maintenance treatment. Other approaches include the repeated use of pulses of intensive combinations of agents periodically during maintenance and sequential intensive multiagent therapy.[24]

The choice of an appropriate maintenance regimen may differ for different risk groups. While 6-mercaptopurine and methotrexate may be adequate for certain good-risk patients, more intensive maintenance therapy appears to be optimal in treating poor-risk patients. To improve cytoreduction early in maintenance, many regimens now include a period of intensified therapy, shortly after remission induction, with drugs that will minimize the development of cross resistance. Intensive remission "consolidation" therapy of this type has improved treatment success even in patients with poor prognoses.[24,25] A West German study that used both intensive induction and consolidation and "reinduction" and "reconsolidation" phases of therapy early in maintenance obtained prolonged disease-free survival in approximately 70% of children, with significantly improved results in poor-prognosis patients.[25]

Drug dosage is an important consideration in maintenance therapy. Longer remissions occurred in patients randomized to receive full-dose maintenance therapy with 6-mercaptopurine, methotrexate, and cyclophosphamide than in those treated with the same agents administered at half dose. Orally administered 6-mercaptopurine and methotrexate have profound variations in bioavailability, suggesting that this may be a mechanism of treatment failure for some patients.

The optimal duration of maintenance treatment is not identified. The majority of centers treat patients for 2.5 to 3 years. A randomized study demonstrated that 5 years of maintenance treatment has no advantage over 3 years.[26] The optimal duration of treatment appears to be different for girls and boys; in one study 1.5 years of therapy was sufficient for girls but inadequate for boys. It is likely that the intensity of therapy has bearing on the optimal duration of treatment. Because much of the information on which the current policy of 2.5 to 3 years of maintenance therapy is based was derived from less-intensive therapeutic regimens than many currently in use, additional study of this important question is needed.

The outlook for patients who successfully complete a full 2.5-year to 3-year course of treatment is good. Approximately 80% of these patients can expect to remain disease free. The greatest number of relapses occur in the first year after discontinuing chemotherapy. After 4 years "off" treatment, relapse is unusual.

TREATMENT OF RELAPSE

Bone Marrow Relapse

Bone marrow relapse is the most frequent source of treatment failure in patients with ALL. Reinduction of remission is possible in the majority of patients who suffer an initial marrow relapse; however, most patients experience subsequent relapse and eventually die of the disease. Nevertheless, many patients can achieve prolonged second remissions, justifying an aggressive treatment approach to the child in relapse. Multiple-drug induction regimens are the most effective. The best results have been obtained with a four-drug combination, which includes vincristine, prednisone, L-asparaginase, and daunorubicin and produces remissions in 90% of patients.

In addition to the intensity of the reinduction regimen, a variety of other factors influence the remission induction rate for relapsed patients. Children whose relapses occur more than 6 months after completion of chemotherapy regimens have a better chance of achieving and maintaining prolonged second remissions than do children who relapse while receiving maintenance therapy. Second remissions are also more easily induced in patients who received suboptimal induction or maintenance therapy as initial treatment for their disease or who had longer first remissions.

A second course of CNS preventive therapy is necessary for patients in second remission. Without additional CNS prophylaxis in these patients, almost 50% will suffer CNS relapse. In previously irradiated patients, intrathecal chemotherapy has been found to be an effective form of second CNS prophylaxis.

Unfortunately, second or subsequent remissions, particularly in children relapsing on treatment, are usually short. However, it has been reported that prolonged second remissions (>2 years) can be obtained with aggressive chemotherapy in 10% to 25% of patients who relapse on therapy and in almost 33% of patients who relapse after elective cessation of therapy.[27]

Bone marrow transplantation is another approach used to treat relapsed patients (Fig. 48-5; see Chap. 66, sect 6). A report from the Seattle transplant group on the long-term follow-up of a group of patients with ALL who received allogeneic bone marrow transplantation indicated that, with a minimum follow-up of more than 5 years, 27% of the patients transplanted in second or subsequent remissions and

FIG. 48-5. Disease-free survival of children receiving transplants for ALL. Patients were stratified according to their disease status at the time of transplantation. (Brochstein JA, Kernan NA, Groshen S et al: Allogeneic bone marrow transplantation after hyperfractionated total-body irradiation and cyclophosphamide in children with acute leukemia. N Engl J Med 317:1618–1624, 1987)

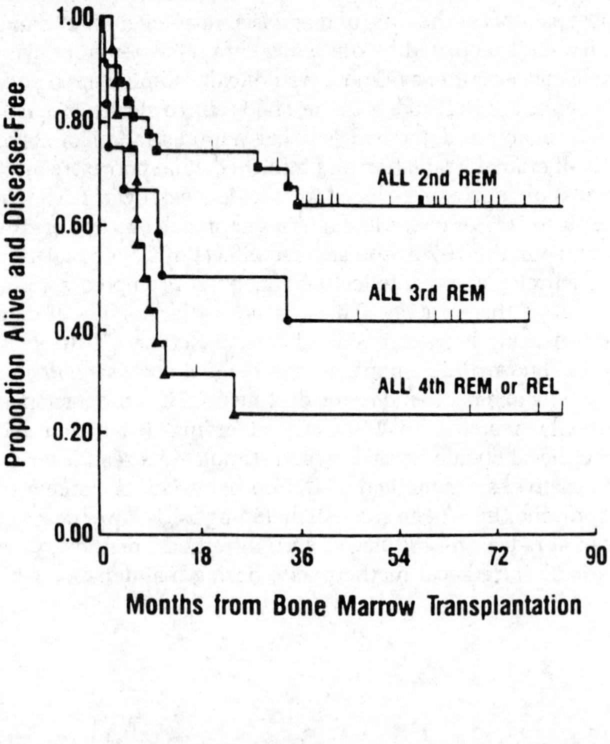

15% of patients transplanted in relapse were alive and free of disease.[28] Other studies, with shorter follow-up, have reported long-term disease-free survival in 40% or more of patients transplanted during second remission.[29] Allogeneic bone marrow transplantation is feasible for approximately one third of relapsed patients, those fortunate enough to have an HLA-identical sibling. The encouraging results suggest that in relapsed patients with tissue-compatible siblings, bone marrow transplantation must be given strong consideration as the treatment of choice.[27]

Methods of crossing the histocompatibility barrier are being studied in a number of centers and, if successful, ultimately may increase the applicability of bone marrow transplantation. Autologous transplantation with remission marrow treated in vitro with leukemia-specific monoclonal antibodies is also being investigated. Relapse-free survival can be achieved in approximately 20% of relapsed patients using this approach.

Central Nervous System Relapse

Although CNS preventive therapy has dramatically reduced its incidence, CNS relapse remains a significant cause of treatment failure in ALL, occurring as an isolated relapse, concomitantly with bone marrow relapse, or with recurrence in another extramedullary site (*e.g.*, testes). Intrathecal methotrexate, alone or together with cytosine arabinoside and hydrocortisone, produces CNS remission (*i.e.*, clearance of CSF lymphoblasts) in more than 90% of patients. Unless followed by craniospinal irradiation or by maintenance intrathecal chemotherapy, relapse ensues within 3 to 4 months. Continued periodic administration of intrathecal chemotherapy on a maintenance schedule may prolong CSF remission, but relapse usually occurs.[4] Craniospinal irradiation, at doses of 2400 to 2500 cGy (150 cGy daily) to the cranial vault and approximately 1200 to 1800 cGy to the spinal axis, administered shortly after induction of a CSF remission, is effective in achieving durable control of established meningeal leukemia.[4] Treatment of CNS disease may be less effective in patients who received CNS irradiation previously; re-irradiation, in particular, poses a greater risk for delayed neurotoxicity.[30]

Other therapeutic approaches include intraventricular chemotherapy and intraventricular chemotherapy with low-dose craniospinal irradiation.[4] Administration of methotrexate by means of an indwelling subcutaneous Ommaya reservoir has a number of technical and pharmacologic advantages and produces longer remissions than intralumbar therapy alone. High-dose methotrexate and high-dose cytarabine have been effective in inducing CSF remission in patients with overt meningeal leukemia. New intrathecal agents are also being developed. Because isolated CNS relaps, often heralds a bone marrow relapse intensification of systemic therapy at the time of isolated CNS relapse is considered essential.

Testicular Relapse

Testicular relapse requires treatment with radiotherapy. Unilateral disease frequently has been followed by relapse in the contralateral testes, particularly in patients with early testicular relapse during therapy.[6] Bilateral testicular radiotherapy is indicated for all patients. A dosage of 2400 cGy is considered adequate, although rare cases of local recurrence have been reported. In the past, testicular recurrence frequently was followed by systemic relapse and was associated with a poor prognosis. The more recent practice of intensifying systemic therapy or reinducing patients at the time of isolated testicular relapse has produced a dramatic improvement, and prolonged disease-free survival is now possible.

SUPPORTIVE CARE

The provision of optimal supportive care is a vital element in the treatment of the child with ALL. Appropriate use of blood component therapy, an aggressive approach to detection, prevention, and management of infectious complications, maintenance of the metabolic and nutritional needs of the patient, and comprehensive, continuous psychosocial support for both patient and family are mandatory (see Chaps. 59 and 61).

LATE EFFECTS OF TREATMENT

The increased survival of children with ALL has focused attention on the late effects of antileukemia therapy. Recognition of adverse sequelae is particularly important now that it is possible to define good-risk patients for whom less intensive but equally effective therapy may be designed.

Of particular concern are the effects of CNS preventive therapy on neurologic and intellectual function. There is ample evidence of adverse CNS sequelae, including CT-demonstrated brain abnormalities, impairment of intellectual function, and abnormal neuroendocrine function, in patients treated with cranial irradiation and intrathecal chemotherapy.[30] The incidence of these abnormalities is related to the intensity and duration of CNS preventive therapy. For example, the highest reported incidence of brain abnormalities occurred in patients receiving cranial irradiation and maintenance intrathecal therapy. In contrast, for patients who received intermediate-dose intravenous methotrexate and intrathecal methotrexate, changes detected by CT scan are not apparent or are very infrequent. It is unclear whether the lower dose of cranial radiation used in many current treatment regimens (*i.e.*, 1800 cGy) will avoid or diminish some of the sequelae seen after the conventional 2400 cGy dose. There are some indications, however, that the use of 1800 cGy with intrathecal methotrexate may also have adverse CNS sequelae.

Studies have confirmed significant decrements in the IQs of children receiving CNS preventive therapy with cranial irradiation and intrathecal methotrexate, with greater impairment in those patients who were youngest during CNS treatment.[30] In one prospective study patients randomized to CNS preventive therapy with 2400 cGy and intrathecal methotrexate showed a progressive decline in verbal IQ and significantly impaired academic achievement, findings not observed in patients randomized to receive high-dose systemic methotrexate infusions alone. Memory dysfunction and impaired attentional processing and frontal lobe function have also been documented.[30]

The relative contributions of radiation and chemotherapy to adverse CNS sequelae is unclear. The interaction of methotrexate and cranial irradiation in producing CNS toxicity was best illustrated in an early study of patients given 2400 cGy of cranial irradiation and maintenance chemotherapy that included different doses of systemic methotrexate, the higher doses of intravenous methotrexate were associated with a considerably higher incidence of necrotizing leukoencephalopathy than observed with conventional doses of methotrexate for maintenance. Children treated for overt CNS disease are at a higher risk for neurologic and neuropsychologic sequelae.[30] Neuroendocrine abnormalities, particularly decreased growth hormone responses to provocative stimuli and blunted basal pulsatile growth hormone output, are the presumed result of radiation-induced damage of the hypothalamic-pituitary axis and may cause the short stature of some children receiving treatment. Careful monitoring of patients at risk for possible adverse CNS sequelae, with periodic neurologic examination, CT brain scans, and psychometric testing is advocated.[30] Recognition of the potential of CNS preventive therapy to produce adverse neurotoxic sequelae has provided the stimulus for a variety of ongoing studies seeking equally effective but less toxic alternative methods of CNS preventive therapy (see CNS Preventive Therapy).

The reproductive capacity of children exposed to prolonged antileukemic therapy has been evaluated, and the majority of boys and girls treated with conventional chemotherapy (not including cyclophosphamide) appear to maintain gonadal function and undergo normal pubertal progression. However, boys who have received testicular irradiation have a high rate of testicular endocrine failure and may require androgen replacement therapy. As survival times increase, more patients face the prospect of parenthood. Although scarce, the available evidence suggests no increase in birth defects in the offspring of mothers or fathers previously treated for ALL.

Damage to other systems may occur during therapy, but fortunately, long-term post-treatment toxicity is unusual. For example, liver function tests frequently are elevated during the chronic methotrexate therapy of maintenance treatment. However, abnormal liver function persisting after therapy rarely occurs, and if it does, frequently it is associated with chronic hepatitis B viral disease. Although treatment with anthracyclines carries the possibility of cardiac toxicity, most protocols use limited cumulative doses of this agent. Thus, the overall incidence of this complication in leukemic children is believed to be extremely low.

Second malignancies have been reported in ALL, but their incidence is exceedingly low. There are, however, an increasing number of brain tumors, mostly secondary malignant gliomas that are rarely documented in other disease settings, diagnosed in children after CNS preventive therapy including cranial irradiation.

For most children with ALL, the majority of therapy can be administered on an outpatient basis, and despite its length, treatment is usually compatible with a reasonably normal life-style. Most patients do not experience significant late sequelae and tolerate treatment well. In those areas in which particular therapeutic modalities have been found to be associated with significant problems, studies of alternative, less toxic strategies are underway.

TREATMENT OBSTACLES

Despite the dramatic improvements in therapy, many treatment obstacles must be overcome before cure becomes a reality for all patients.

Continued efforts must be made to define more precisely those clinical and biologic features of greatest prognostic value. This will permit more accurate delineation of patient subgroups requiring more or less intensive therapy. The most important problem is the need for improved treatment of patients in the poor-risk category. Although efforts to intensify therapy for these patients appear promising, greater understanding of the disease that affects them is needed. The group of patients failing current therapy is known to be biologically heterogeneous, manifesting differences in clinical presentation and in the cytogenetic, immunologic, and molecular features of their disease. The application of molecular biologic methods to the study of drug resistance may ultimately provide valuable information about the mechanisms of treatment failure.

Major emphasis also must be placed on identifying the causes of treatment failure. Almost half of the children with ALL relapse, most during maintenance therapy. Recent studies, suggesting that variation and limitations in drug bioavailability may be partially responsible for treatment failure during maintenance, require confirmation.

Molecular biological techniques, such as assessment of immunoglobulin and T-cell-receptor gene rearrangement, are being used to study ALL. These techniques, possibly with methodology incorporating "in situ hybridization," may permit identification of residual leukemia in otherwise morphologically normal marrows, but further technical refinements are required.[31]

Because attention also must focus on the development of more effective treatment for the relapsed patient, the role of bone marrow transplantation in the treatment of ALL is likely to increase. Recent successes in the use of partially mismatched donors offers the possibility of totally crossing the HLA barrier. The role of autologous marrow transplantation may expand as newer methods of in vitro purging (*e.g.*, radiolabeled monoclonal antibodies or biologics) become available.

The recognition that some forms of adult leukemia (*e.g.*, hairy cell, CML) respond to certain types of interferons stimulated investigation of biologics for treating lymphoid leukemia. Clinical studies of interleukin-2-(IL-2) have only recently been initiated. Another exciting potential use for biologics is in the area of molecularly cloned hematopoietic growth factors. Preclinical and early clinical studies with granulocyte-macrophage colony-stimulating factor (GM-CSF) and granulocyte colony-stimulating factor (G-CSF) confirm the potential of these agents to shorten the duration and severity of chemotherapy-induced myelosuppression. These agents may allow intensified chemotherapy for patients with ALL at high risk of treatment failure.

ACUTE NONLYMPHOCYTIC LEUKEMIA

ANLL represents approximately 25% of all cases of acute leukemia in children. Although considerable progress has been made in the treatment of childhood ANLL in the past decade, the prognosis for children with this disease, although appreciably greater than that for adults, is significantly worse than for children with ALL. ANLL shares many features with the adult form of the disease (see Chap. 52). With some minor differences, the biology of ANLL is similar in children and adults, with the possible exception of neonatal leukemia.

Approximately 50% to 70% of children are classified as having acute myelogenous leukemia, and 20% to 40% have acute myelomonocytic leukemia.[32] The FAB system of morphologic classification is equally applicable to childhood ANLL (see Chap. 52). There is some evidence that patients in the FAB M5a (acute monoblastic leukemia) and M5b (acute monocytic leukemia) subcategories have a less favorable prognosis.[33] The responses to treatment of the other FAB subtypes are similar.

Mixed-lineage leukemia has been reported in cases presenting as childhood ANLL; its clinical significance is not clear.[14] Acute megakaryocytic leukemia (M7), recently added to the FAB classification system, occurs more commonly in children with Down's syndrome. There are some cytogenetic differences between childhood and adult ANLL. The −5, 5q−, and −7 abnormalities often seen in adults are rare in children. In contrast, t(11q) and a t19 are common in children but unusual in adults. An extra chromosome 8 is the most common abnormality in both age groups. Chromosomal patterns appear to have prognostic implications. Trisomy 8 and the t(8:21) abnormality are associated with a high rate of complete remission; abnormalities of chromosome 7 are associated with a low rate of remission induction. There is some preliminary evidence that indicates that the patterns of in vitro marrow growth are different in children.

Information about the influence on prognosis of factors such as age, sex, and leukocyte count has been somewhat conflicting. Very young age (<1 year) and high leukocyte count (>20,000/mm^3) are unfavorable prognostic factors for attaining complete remission.[32,34] Age at diagnosis, initial leukocyte count, and FAB classification affect remission duration.[32] Children older than 2 years of age have a better prognosis than younger children, with those between 3 and 10 years of age having the best prognosis. The very poor prognosis for children younger than 2 years may be related to the observation that the M4 and M5 FAB categories occur more often in these children.[33]

Because ANLL and ALL have similar clinical presentations but quite different therapies and prognosis, it is important for the clinician to distinguish between them. In addition to use of special stains (*e.g.*, myeloperoxidase or Sudan black, PAS, specific esterase), determining TdT activity (usually lacking in ANLL) and immunophenotyping with myeloid-specific monoclonal antibodies may be of help.[35] Once the diagnosis of ANLL is established, the FAB subtype should be determined, because this classification system has some prognostic value and because certain FAB subcategories present unique clinical problems. For example, patients with the M3 (promyelocytic leukemia) subtype frequently develop a disseminated intravascular coagulation-like syndrome.

As in adults, the most effective regimens for remission induction include cytosine arabinoside plus an anthracycline (usually daunorubicin), either in a two-drug combination or with additional drugs such as 6-thioguanine, prednisone, vincristine, or 5-azacytidine. To induce a complete remission, it is usually necessary to produce profound marrow aplasia. As a consequence, the potential for morbidity and mortality from infection is great, necessitating aggressive supportive care measures. Induction morbidity may be higher with doxorubicin (Adriamycin) than with daunomycin. In most centers, complete remission can be induced in approximately 75% of children.

CNS leukemia appears to be more common at diagnosis in ANLL than in ALL, occurring in <5% to 20% of patients.[36] Perhaps the overall incidence of CNS relapse has been lower than for ALL because of the shorter survival of children with ANLL.[36] It has also been suggested that CNS leukemia is seen more frequently in children than in adults; this also may be because of the shorter survival time of adults with this disease. CNS disease appears to be more common in patients with very high initial leukocyte counts and with the monoblastic subtype.[36] Several studies have indicated benefit of CNS preventive therapy, using intrathecal chemotherapy with methotrexate or with cytosine arabinoside or cranial irradiation with intrathecal methotrexate.[33,37]

As in ALL maintenance, chemotherapy has been employed in childhood ANLL in an attempt to prolong the duration of the initial remission. Although a variety of strategies have been used, most regimens produced median remissions of less than 2 years. More recent studies, using intensive treatment, have shown improvement, with approximately 40% of children achieving prolonged event-free survival (Table 48-4).[33,37] Although these studies used extensive postremission therapy, data conclusively demonstrating the value of maintenance therapy in childhood ANLL do not exist, and definition of the optimal duration of treatment in this disease requires a comprehensive prospective study. A trial designed to answer this question is being conducted by the Children's Cancer Study Group.

Many centers perform bone marrow transplantation for patients who achieve an initial remission and have a histocompatible sibling donor (see Chap. 66). This approach is very promising. The Children's Cancer Study Group has compared bone marrow transplantation to conventional ANLL maintenance chemotherapy in a nationwide comparative study. The results demonstrated a statistically significant better disease-free survival rate at 3 years for transplantation (46%) than for chemotherapy (36%). Because some intensive chemotherapy programs have achieved results similar to those obtained for transplantation, there is controversy about the optimal postremission strategy. Most centers suggest marrow transplantation for those patients who have an appropriately matched HLA-compatible allogeneic sibling donor.

TABLE 48-4. VAPA Intensive Sequential Maintenance Therapy*

Sequence 1 *Drugs*	*Sequence 2* *Drugs*	*Sequence 3* *Drugs*	*Sequence 4* *Drugs*
Adriamycin, 45 mg/m^2 Day 1, IV	Adriamycin, 30 mg/m^2 Day 1, IV	Vincristine, 1.5 mg/m^2 (maximum single dose 2 mg) Day 1, IV	Cytosine arabinoside, 200 mg/m^2 Days 1–5, continuous IV infusion
Cytosine arabinoside, 200 mg/m^2 Days 1–5, continuous infusion	Azacytidine, 150 mg/m^2 Days 1–5, continuous IV infusion	Methylprednisolone, 800 mg/m^2 Days 1–5, IV	
		6-Mercaptopurine, 500 mg/m^2 Days 1–5 IV	
		Methotrexate, 7.5 mg/m^2 Days 1–5, IV	

*Duration of maintenance therapy is approximately 14 months; all sequences are given four times at 3- to 4-week intervals.

NEONATAL LEUKEMIA

Neonatal leukemia occurs in the first month of life. It is a rare disorder in which the majority of cases are considered ANLL. Neonatal or so-called congenital leukemia may be associated with Down's syndrome or other chromosomal abnormalities. Congenital leukemia frequently presents with infiltration of the skin, usually nodular in appearance, which may be ecchymotic as a result of concomitant thrombocytopenia. Leukemia infiltration of the lungs, liver, and spleen are common. The initial leukocyte count is frequently greater than 100,000/mm^3. The prognosis for neonatal leukemia has been poor. Although complete remissions have been obtained, they are usually short, and long-term survivors have not been reported. There is, however, little experience treating these children with the type of intensive combination chemotherapy regimens used to treat older children with ANLL.

Patients with neonatal leukemia and Down's syndrome pose a particularly unique problem. A number of these children have been documented in whom the disease has resolved spontaneously over a matter of weeks or months. Some researchers have suggested that this disorder represents a defect in the regulation of granulopoiesis and should be considered a myeloproliferative syndrome. However, some patients with this transient disorder have experienced recurrences that have proven fatal. The relationship between these processes is unclear.

CHRONIC MYELOGENOUS LEUKEMIA

CML is relatively rare in childhood, accounting for from 1% to 5% of childhood leukemias.[2] The two major forms are the adult form, which typically is seen in adolescents, and the juvenile form, which occurs mainly in infants. Adult CML is discussed in depth in Chapter 52. The juvenile form of the disease occurs less frequently and differs biologically and clinically from adult CML (Table 48-5).

Juvenile CML is a disease of infancy, rarely occurring after 5 years of age. Typically it presents with symptoms of fatigue, pallor, and recurrent infection. An eczematoid facial rash, prominent and frequently suppurative lymphadenopathy, thrombocytopenia, and hemorrhagic manifestations at diagnosis also differentiate juvenile CML from the adult form. The Ph^1 chromosome, a hallmark of adult CML, is lacking in juvenile CML. The leukocyte is usually <100,000/mm^3. These features, the presence of thrombocytopenia and a relatively low myeloid to erythroid ratio, which reflects the hyperplasia of both lines in the bone marrow, are useful in distinguishing juvenile from adult CML.[2]

In juvenile CML, in-vitro bone marrow culture yields a predominance of monocytic colonies, suggesting that it is a form of myelomonocytic leukemia. Juvenile CML is also associated with a number of erythroid abnormalities, including a persistently high fetal hemoglobin and other findings similar to those seen in fetal erythrocytes, suggesting that there is disordered regulation of erythropoiesis. Immunologic abnormalities have also been noticed. Unlike adult CML, which has its characteristic chronic phase, the juvenile form of the disease follows a course of progressive deterioration that does not have a terminal blastic phase. In its later stages, profound erythroid hyperplasia is seen.

Treatment for juvenile CML is totally unsatisfactory; most patients survive less than 1 year from diagnosis. Neither radiotherapeutic nor chemotherapeutic intervention have altered the natural history of this disease, although bone marrow transplantation has been attempted successfully.

NON-HODGKIN'S LYMPHOMA

All malignant lymphomas not considered to represent Hodgkin's disease have been designated as non-Hodgkin's lymphoma (NHL). The use of this negative terminology has not helped to clarify what we now appreciate is not a single entity, but a heterogenous group of diseases with differing clinical presentations, behaviors, pathologies, and prognoses.

The childhood non-Hodgkin's lymphomas differ in many respects from their adult counterparts. For example, pediatric lymphomas are virtually always diffuse, rather than nodular; extranodal, rather than nodal; and have the propensity for early, widespread and noncontiguous dissemination. "Conversion" to a leukemic presentation and the development of primary CNS relapse are also more frequently seen in children. Immunologic studies indicate that B-cell lymphomas predominate in adult NHL, but both B-cell and T-

TABLE 48-5. Features of the Adult and Juvenile Forms of Chronic Myelogenous Leukemia

Feature	Adult Form	Juvenile Form
Age at onset (median)	14.2 years	22.5 months
Sex (M:F)	6:1	2:1
Philadelphia chromosome	Present	Absent
Physical findings		
Facial rash	Absent	Present
Lymphadenopathy	Occasional	Frequent, with tendency to suppuration
Splenomegaly	Marked	Mild to moderate
Hemorrhagic manifestations	Absent	Frequent
Hematologic findings		
Initial leukocyte count	Usually >100,000/mm³	Usually <100,000/mm³
Thrombocytopenia at diagnosis	Uncommon	Frequent
Monocytosis	Absent	Usually present
Fetal hemoglobin levels	Normal	30%–70%
Erythrocyte I antigen	Normal	Reduced
Erythrocyte enzymes	?	Increased fetal enzyme systems Decreased carbonic anhydrase
Ineffective erythropoiesis	Absent	Present
Marrow M:E ratio	10:1–50:1	2:1–5:1
Leukocyte alkaline phosphatase	Decreased	Decreased or lower limit of normal
Serum vitamin B_{12} level	Increased	Increased
Colony-forming characterizations	Predominantly granulocytic	Almost exclusively monocytic
Urine and serum muramidase	Slightly elevated	Markedly elevated
Immunologic abnormalities	None	Increased immunoglobulin levels High incidence of antinuclear and anti-IgG antibodies
Response to busulfan	Good	Poor
Median survival	2.5–3 years	<9 months
Terminal phase	Blast crisis	Erythroid hyperplasia; intense normoblastemia

Poplack DG: Acute lymphoblastic leukemia. In Pizzo PA, Poplack DG (eds): Principles and Practice of Pediatric Oncology. Philadelphia, JB Lippincott, 1989.

cell lymphomas are common in childhood. There is considerable evidence that childhood NHL arises from less-differentiated lymphoid stem cells, and as a consequence, tumors in both age categories with identical cell surface markers may behave very differently. For example, B-cell tumors in children have a rapidly fatal outcome unless treated aggressively, whereas in adults, these tumors often have a more indolent course. Two-2 year disease-free survival in children usually constitutes cure, but continuing relapse is seen even after 10 years in adults, especially those with certain nodular lymphomas.

EPIDEMIOLOGY AND ETIOLOGY

NHL is approximately 1.5 times as common as Hodgkin's disease in childhood and represents the third most common childhood malignancy. It has an annual incidence in the Unites States of approximately 9 cases per million white children younger than 15 years old and approximately 5 per million black children. There is a striking male to female ratio of 2.5:1 to 3:1. The peak incidence occurs between the ages of 7 to 11 years. Involvement before 3 years of age is uncommon.

Although the precise cause of NHL is unknown, there is evidence that genetics and immunologic, viral, and environmental factors play important roles. A number of inherited and acquired conditions predispose the child to development of lymphoma. The association between inherited immunodeficiency disease and lymphoma is well documented. NHL made up more than half of all malignancies that occurred in a large group of children with a variety of genetic immunodeficiency conditions. The genetically determined immunodeficiency syndromes with the greatest risk of lymphoma are ataxia-telangiectasia, Wiscott-Aldrich Syndrome common variable immunodeficiency disease, severe combined immunodeficiency disease (SCID), and the X-linked lymphoproliferative syndrome. In some of these immunodeficiency states, chromosomal abnormalities contribute to the increased risk of lymphoid malignancy. For example, translocation of the long arm of chromosome 14 (14q+) is frequently seen in ataxia-telangiectasia. Involvement of chromosome 14 is common in neoplasms of B-cell origin. The X-linked recessive syndrome described by Purtilo is associated with a variety of sequelae, including fatal infection with infectious mononucleosis of lymphoid malignancy, particularly Burkitt's lymphoma. EBV appears to be important in the pathogenesis of the lymphomas that develop in these immunodeficiency states; most contain EBV genomes.

Acquired immunodeficiency also is associated with the development of lymphoma. Patients undergoing chronic immunosuppressive therapy with kidney transplantation have an increased risk of a form of NHL that arises most often in the CNS. Patients with acquired immune deficiency syndrome (AIDS) also have an apparent increased risk of lymphomas, some of which have the typical histologic pattern and chromosomal abnormalities of Burkitt's lymphoma.

Both EBV and malaria have been associated with the development of Burkitt's lymphoma in African children. The retrovirus HTLV-1 has been implicated in the pathogenesis of adult T-cell leukemia. However, retroviruses have not been definitively linked to the pathogenesis of childhood lymphomas.

Chronic treatment with hydantoin drugs, including phenytoin (Dilantin), has been associated with development of both pseudolymphomas and true malignant lymphomas, including both Hodgkin's disease and NHL. NHL also has occurred as a second malignancy in patients treated with chemotherapy or radiotherapy for Hodgkin's disease.

PATHOLOGIC AND IMMUNOLOGIC CLASSIFICATION

As noted previously, virtually all pediatric NHL are diffuse. Using the Rappaport classification with suitable modification, most pediatric NHL can be grouped histologically in one of three major categories (Table 48-6). Lymphoblastic lymphomas, the most common, comprise over one third of all cases. These tumors characteristically present with supradiaphragmatic disease and anterior mediastinal involvement. Undifferentiated lymphomas, the next most common form of NHL in children, include both the undifferentiated Burkitt's and non-Burkitt's types. These tumors frequently present with intra-abdominal disease. The third and least common histologic type includes the so-called histiocytic or large lymphoid cell tumors. These tumors are morphologically and immunologically heterogeneous. Large cell lymphomas may occur at a variety of nodal and extranodal sites, including Waldeyer's ring and bone.

Immunologic classification is extremely important in childhood NHL. Lymphoblastic lymphomas are neoplasms of the precursors of functional T cells. Cells from these tumors invariably contain TdT and express T-cell markers. Studies using monoclonal antibodies capable of delineating the various stages of intrathymic differentiation indicate that the malignant T cells in lymphoblastic lymphoma have characteristics of the intermediate to late stages of intrathymic development. In contrast, T-cell ALL lymphoblasts more frequently display characteristics of early thymocyte precursors.

TABLE 48-6. Distribution of Histopathologic Types of Diffuse Lymphomas in Childhood

Histologic Classification	*Approximate Frequency (%)*
Lymphoblastic	30–50
Convoluted	
Nonconvoluted	
Undifferentiated	20–40
Burkitt's	
Non-Burkitt's, pleomorphic	
Histiocytic (large lymphoid cell)	15–20
Unclassifiable	5–10
Total	100

Murphy SB: Classification, staging and end results of treatment of childhood non-Hodgkin's lymphoma: Dissimilarities from lymphomas in adults. Semin Oncol 7:332–339, 1980.

The majority of undifferentiated childhood lymphomas are derived from B cells and can be shown to have surface immunoglobulin. This includes Burkitt's and the non-Burkitt's lymphomas. Many of the histiocytic or large lymphoid cell tumors also express B-cell characteristics.

For practical purposes, then, childhood NHL can be divided into two major immunologic groups:

1. Lymphoblastic lymphomas, which usually present with supradiaphragmatic disease with or without extrathoracic involvement, are of T-cell origin.
2. Nonlymphoblastic lymphomas, which generally arise within the abdominal cavity, GI tract, or Waldeyer's ring, include several morphologic subtypes (*e.g.*, undifferentiated Burkitt's and non-Burkitt's, histiocytic or large cell) and are most often B-cell tumors.

Lymphoma or Leukemia?

Childhood NHL and ALL are closely related disorders. Distinguishing between them is difficult. A significant number of patients who present with characteristic lymphomatous features, such as an anterior mediastinal mass or massive lymphadenopathy, also have bone marrow involvement. In addition, the malignant T cells from patients with lymphoblastic lymphoma cytomorphologically are indistinguishable from those of ALL; those of Burkitt's lymphoma are similar to those of B-cell ALL. The basis for separating NHL from ALL has been arbitrary, using criteria such as the presence or absence of circulating malignant cells or the extent of bone marrow involvement (*i.e.*, >5% or >25% malignant cells in the marrow), rather than more relevant biologic differences.[38,39] Different definitions have been used by different centers, creating obvious heterogeneity within groups of patients presumed to have the same disease and complicating intrainstitutional comparison of treatment results.

Although these arbitrary methods of separating NHL from ALL have been appropriately criticized, they continue to be used. The distinction between T-cell ALL and T-cell lymphoblastic lymphoma is particularly difficult. Immunophenotyping with monoclonal antibodies that detect T-cell antigens expressed at different stages of T-cell maturation demonstrated that these disorders arise from different stages of T-cell differentiation. Because this distinction does not apply in every case, however, it does not provide a reliable method upon which to delineate between these two disorders. Indeed, it is unclear whether NHL and ALL of the same immunologic type actually require different therapy.

CLINICAL PRESENTATION

Childhood NHL can arise in any of the variety of sites containing lymphoid tissue, including lymph nodes, Peyer's patches, Waldeyer's ring, the thymus, and bone marrow, and in certain extralymphatic sites, including bone, skin, and the orbit. Extranodal disease is much more common in children, nodal presentation occurring in only approximately 15% of patients.

Intra-abdominal disease is most common. More than one

third of affected children present either with gastrointestinal involvement alone or with widespread intra-abdominal disease.[38,40] Symptoms for this group range from right lower-quadrant pain, nausea, vomiting, and other symptoms typical of the intussusception seen in children with ileocecal and appendiceal tumors to the rapid onset of diffuse abdominal pain, rapidly enlarging abdominal mass, development of malignant ascites, and progressive weight loss, all frequently observed in children with widespread intra-abdominal disease.

Approximately 25% of children with NHL present with mediastinal involvement. These tumors are typically T-cell lymphoblastic lymphomas.[38,39] These children are characteristically adolescent boys with cervical or supraclavicular lymphadenopathy, or with symptoms resulting from local tumor compression. Lymphoblastic lymphomas have a propensity for rapid spread to bone marrow, the CNS, and the gonads. Pleural effusions may be evident at presentation.

Less frequently, children present with regionally limited disease involving the tonsil, nasopharynx, or other portions of Waldeyer's ring, with or without involvement of cervical lymph nodes. Other regional sites include the bones, skin, gonads, or CNS. Systemic symptoms, including unexplained, widely fluctuating fevers, drenching night sweats, and significant weight loss are relatively common, particularly in children with more advanced disease.[40]

Childhood NHL are rapidly growing, and clinical symptoms and signs are usually short-lived, rarely extending more than 6 to 8 weeks before presentation. The histologic subtype, immunologic surface characteristics, and natural history can often be predicted by the mode of clinical presentation.

BURKITT'S LYMPHOMA

Burkitt's lymphoma is a malignant proliferation of lymphoid cells that have B-cell phenotypes. Originally described in East Africa, Burkitt's lymphoma makes up a significant portion of the undifferentiated B-cell lymphomas in childhood. The malignant B cells express surface immunoglobulins, almost always IgM, in association with either the kappa or lambda light chain, and react with monoclonal antibodies specific for B cells.[41] They possess HLA-DR antigens and frequently express the CALLA antigen, but do not contain TdT.

Burkitt's cells manifest a characteristic cytogenetic abnormality in which genetic material from the distal segment of the long arm of chromosome 8 is translocated to chromosome 14, t(8;14). More rarely, "variant" translocations can be demonstrated, t(8;22) or t(2;8). It is now known that the proto-oncogene C-*myc*, found on chromosome 8, is translocated to the immunoglobulin heavy-chain locus on chromosome 14 [in t(8;14)] or, in the case of variant translocation, to either the kappa or lambda immunoglobulin light-chain loci on chromosomes 2 and 22, respectively. As a consequence of these translocations, C-*myc* becomes abnormally expressed, an event believed to result in the maintenance of the malignant cells in their proliferative state.[38] The molecular genetic findings in Burkitt's lymphoma have provided perhaps the best clues to date about the molecular mechanisms involved in the pathogenesis of human malignancy.

There are some major differences between American (sporadic) and African (endemic) Burkitt's tumor (Table 48-7). Perhaps the most readily apparent differences are in the clinical presentation. The typical presentation of African Burkitt's lymphoma, a large tumor of the maxilla or mandible, with or without orbital involvement, is rarely seen in the United States, even in patients with Burkitt's histologic pattern. The majority of children with American Burkitt's tumors present with massive abdominal disease, occasionally combined with CNS or bone marrow involvement at presentation. The latter form is uncommon in African children with this disease. Involvement of the peripheral lymph nodes, pleura, and kidneys is also noticed quite frequently in American patients.

These tumors also differ biologically. EBV DNA and nuclear antigen are usually noticed in tumor cells of African children but are rare in American patients. Cell lines from American Burkitt's tumors appear to lack EBV receptors. The t(8;14) translocation is found in both forms of the disease; however, there appears to be a difference in the location of the breakpoint on chromosome 8. In African tumors, the breakpoint occurs at some distance "upstream" of the gene, but in North American tumors, it is usually within the gene or its flanking sequences. The reasons for the differences between African and non-African Burkitt's

TABLE 48-7. Comparison of Burkitt's Lymphoma in Africa and the United States

Africa (Equatorial)	*United States*
Very common (100 per 1 million children)	Very rare (1–2 per 1 million children)
Distribution relates to climate and geography	Distribution apparently unrelated to climate and geography
Nearly always associated with EBV*	Uncommonly associated with EBV
t(8:14) very common	t(8:14) very common
Jaw tumors common, marrow involvement rare	Jaw tumors rare, marrow involvement common
50% prolonged survival with CTX* alone	50% prolonged survival with combination therapy (COM)*
Isolated CNS relapse common with CTX therapy	Isolated CNS relapse uncommon with CTX or COM therapy
Multiple relapses not incompatible with eventual prolonged disease-free survival	Survival uncommon after relapse

Magrath IT: Malignant non-Hodgkin's lymphomas. In Pizzo PA, Poplack DG (eds): Principles and Practice of Pediatric Oncology. Philadelphia, JB Lippincott, 1989.

*EBV = Epstein-Barr virus; CTX = cyclophosphamide; COM = cyclophosphamide, vincristine, methotrexate.

tumors are unclear. Differences in racial or epidemiologic factors have been suggested, as has the possibility that they represent etiologically separate entities.[38] The incidence of Burkitt's tumor in childhood NHL varies among different series.

In view of its relatively different natural history, a separate staging system has been proposed for Burkitt's lymphoma, one that is based on the extent of disease. This system appears to separate prognostic groups in both African and American tumors; however, because of their different clinical presentations, the number of patients in the various stages differs considerably. For example, the large number of jaw tumors in African children help to account for relatively higher numbers of patients in Stages A and B. In contrast, Stages A and B are relatively uncommon in American children, the majority of whom have Stage C and D disease.[38]

PRETREATMENT EVALUATION AND STAGING

A rapid and expeditious assessment of disease extent is mandatory to permit treatment to begin with as little delay as possible. In addition to needing a detailed history and physical examination, the child who presents with a possible lymphoma requires a complete blood and platelet count with careful examination of the peripheral smear for circulating blasts. Posteroanterior and lateral chest x-ray films should be obtained to assess mediastinal, hilar, pericardial, or pleural involvement. The trachea and bronchi should be evaluated for patency and displacement. CT scan of the mediastinum is helpful.

Bone marrow aspiration and biopsy will frequently establish the diagnosis and obviate the need for more invasive surgical intervention. Bilateral bone marrow biopsies and aspirates are advocated to maximize detection of marrow involvement.[38] Lumbar puncture should be performed and a cytocentrifuged CSF specimen should be examined for malignant cells. Baseline liver and renal function studies and serum chemistries, including uric acid determination, are indicated. Measurement of serum LDH is useful, because it correlates with tumor burden. The level of soluble IL-2 receptor in serum also appears to be a reliable prognostic factor, particularly for B-cell lymphomas.

The role of surgery is limited to lymph node biopsy or, perhaps, incisional or excisional biopsy of a mass. Staging laparatomy is not indicated because chemotherapy is the major treatment modality. However, laparotomy may be necessary for biopsy or therapy in many children. For example, in those children with regionally limited disease affecting the terminal ileum and caecum, with or without mesenteric nodes, an ileotransverse colorectomy and anastamosis can be both diagnostic and therapeutic. In the more frequently seen child with massive abdominal involvement, surgery usually will be limited to biopsy. At the time of biopsy, tissue should be obtained for histopathologic study, including imprints, immunophenotyping, and cytogenetics.

Mandatory and optional staging procedures for the child in whom a diagnosis of NHL has been confirmed are shown in Table 48-8. Traditional staging systems are of limited value in childhood NHL. Although used in the past and shown to have some prognostic significance if treatment was limited

TABLE 48-8. Staging Procedures for Non-Hodgkin's Lymphoma

Mandatory
CBC, platelet count, differential
Chest x-ray (posteroanterior and lateral)
Bone marrow aspirates and biopsy
Lumbar puncture with cytocentrifuge examination of CSF
Liver function tests
Serum electrolytes, BUN, creatinine, and uric acid levels
Optional (depending on clinical circumstances)
Bone scan and skeletal survey
Intravenous urogram
Barium studies of the GI tract
Myelography
CT scan
Lymphangiography*
Ultrasonography

*Rarely indicated.

to the local modalities or surgery and irradiation, the Ann Arbor classification, devised for Hodgkin's disease, has many deficiencies when applied to childhood NHL. Most pediatric lymphomas are extranodal, rather than nodal. In addition, unlike Hodgkin's disease, NHL in the child is not orderly or predictable in its pattern of spread or relapse, and prognosis is not readily determined by the number of sites affected. As an example, solitary mediastinal involvement carries a relatively poor prognosis. The frequency of leukemic involvement also suggests that a system that relies primarily on anatomic extent of lymph node disease has limited value in childhood NHL.

Murphy and others have proposed alternative systems that answer many of these problems and are clearly superior to the Ann Arbor system (Table 48-9).[39] These systems share some common features. They do not distinguish between primary nodal and extranodal presentations for staging purposes, and they all recognize that bone marrow involvement and CNS disease carry a poor prognosis. A system, originally designed for Burkitt's lymphoma, includes a Stage AR that recognizes the good prognosis of patients with more than 90% resection of intra-abdominal disease. Certain problems remain, however, even with these improved systems. For example, the systems fail to make distinctions between patients within a given stage who may differ prognostically. Thus, a patient with Stage I axillary nodal disease may have a far better prognosis than another Stage I patient whose primary disease is in the orbit, a site with a high propensity for subsequent meningeal spread.[39] No system has incorporated current knowledge regarding the histopathologic or immunologic characteristics of these tumors.

Many institutions no longer use a recognized system. For example, the Children's Cancer Study Group classifies children with NHL on the basis of whether they have localized or nonlocalized disease. In this definition, patients with localized disease have tumor limited either to a single extranodal site, with or without positive regional nodes, or to lymph nodes in one or two adjacent lymphatic regions. All other tumors, including mediastinal disease, are classified as nonlocalized disease. Localized disease in this system corresponds to Stage I and Stage II disease in the Murphy and Wollner systems and encompasses those children with a particularly favorable prognoses. This system, although less

TABLE 48-9. Clinical Staging Systems for Childhood Lymphomas

Stage	*Memorial Sloan-Kettering (Wollner)*	*St. Jude Children's Research Hospital (Murphy)*	*Stage*	*National Cancer Institute (Ziegler, Magrath)*
	One single site	A single tumor (extranodal) or single anatomic area (nodal), with the exclusion of mediastinum or abdomen	A	Single solitary extra-abdominal site
I	Two or more sites on the same side of the diaphragm	A single tumor (extranodal) with regional node involvement Two or more nodal areas on the same side of the diaphragm Two single (extranodal) tumors with or without regional node involvement on the same side of the diaphragm A primary G1 tract tumor, usually in the ileocecal area, with or without involvement of associated mesenteric nodes only	B	Multiple extra-abdominal sites
II	Disseminated disease without marrow or CNS involvement	Two single tumors (extranodal) on opposite sides of the diaphragm Two or more nodal areas above and below the diaphragm All the primary intrathoracic tumors (mediastinal, pleural, thymic) All extensive primary intra-abdominal disease All paraspinal or epidural tumors, regardless of other tumor site(s)	C	Intra-abdominal tumor
V	Any of the above with bone marrow and/or CNS involvement	Any of the above with initial CNS or bone marrow involvement	D	Intra-abdominal tumor with involvement of ≥1 extra-abdominal site
			AR	Intra-abdominal tumor with >90% of tumor surgically resected

elaborate, effectively separates patients with limited disease from those with extensive tumor involvement.

TREATMENT

Chemotherapy

Before the 1970s, the overall survival of children with NHL was very poor; fewer than 30% of patients survived 5 years after diagnosis. Most of these children had limited, localized disease that was controllable with surgery, radiotherapy, or both. The introduction of aggressive, multiagent chemotherapy dramatically improved treatment results so that approximately two thirds of children with this disease are now considered curable. Combination chemotherapy is the most important treatment modality. Although the use of surgery or radiotherapy was modestly effective in patients with limited disease (*e.g.*, a simple extra-abdominal, extrathoracic tumor site, or those with totally resected abdominal tumor), many of these patients experienced relapse. The pattern of relapse, with frequent recurrences at sites significantly distant from the radiation field, including bone marrow, suggested that failure occurred because of widespread occult disease. The addition of combination chemotherapy to patients with limited disease raised the overall survival figures for this group to approximately 90%. Systemic chemotherapy is indicated for all patients with childhood NHL, even when the disease is limited.

Chemotherapy is capable of inducing remissions in 85% to 95% of all patients.[39] Children with this disease are at greatest risk of relapse within the first year from diagnosis. Relapse after 2 years of disease-free survival is unusual.

For purposes of treatment, childhood NHL is usually divided into the lymphoblastic, T-cell lymphomas and the nonlymphoblastic, usually B-cell, tumors. The therapeutic approaches to the lymphoblastic lymphomas usually involve intensive treatment similar to that initially designed for the treatment of high-risk leukemias. Many of the treatment protocols used are based on the LSA_2-L_2 protocol. This intensive ten-drug regimen combined chemotherapy with moderate doses of radiation to treat sites of bulk disease. Using this and similar protocols, long-term disease-free survival can be obtained in approximately 60% to 80% of patients with extensive disease and approximately 90% or more of patients with limited-stage disease.

Evidence that the therapy of children with lymphoblastic lymphomas should be different than that for the other nonlymphoblastic (usually B-cell) lymphomas of childhood was obtained in a randomized trial performed by the Children's Cancer Study Group. It compared the effectiveness of the LSA_2-L_2 protocol to the COMP regimen, which includes cyclophosphamide, vincristine, methotrexate, and prednisone and was originally developed for patients with Burkitt's lymphoma. Most patients in both treatment groups also received radiation therapy to sites of bulk disease. Patients with nonlocalized lymphoblastic lymphoma obtained a 76% 2-year disease-free survival rate when treated with LSA_2-L_2, compared with a 26% rate in patients treated with COMP. In contrast, in nonlocalized nonlymphoblastic lymphoma, 57% of patients treated with COMP achieved 2-year disease-free survival, compared with 28% of those children who received LSA_2-L_2 therapy. For patients with localized disease, however, histologic subtype did not appear to have prognostic significance. In this group, the less toxic four-drug COMP regimen was as effective as the more intensive ten-drug LSA_2-L_2 treatment (89% versus 84%, respectively).

The APO regimen (Table 48-10) achieved an excellent 2-year survival rate of 82%. Patients with Burkitt's lymphoma, however, fared poorly with this therapy. Anthracyclines in particular appear to be an important component in successful treatments of lymphoblastic lymphoma. However, the results of one recent small study using an approach similar to that used to treat ALL, without anthracyclines but including cytarabine and VM-26, predicted a disease-free survival at 4 years of 73%.

Treatment for the nonlymphoblastic lymphomas, the majority of which are B-cell tumors, usually involves regimens incorporating cyclophosphamide, vincristine, prednisone, intermediate-dose or high-dose methotrexate, and doxorubicin. Other drugs (*i.e.*, VM-26, cytarabine, BCNU) are sometimes employed. CNS preventive therapy is also used. An NCI regimen using cyclophosphamide, vincristine, prednisone, and doxorubicin alternating with prolonged methotrexate infusions is effective both for lymphoblastic and nonlymphoblastic lymphomas, producing a disease-free survival at 3 years of approximately 60%. Another regimen studied at St. Jude Children's Cancer Research Hospital used the same agents, also incorporating sequenced high-dose methotrexate and cytosine arabinoside infusions, to treat children with advanced stages of Burkitt's lymphoma. Therapy lasted only 6 months. The protocol was effective, but patients with bone marrow involvement and CNS disease at diagnosis fared significantly worse.

CENTRAL NERVOUS SYSTEM PREVENTIVE THERAPY

The CNS has been an initial site of relapse in almost one third of children with NHL. It is therefore evident that some form of CNS preventive therapy is warranted for most patients. CNS spread is less common in patients with limited disease (*e.g.*, Stage I or II disease) and more frequent with widespread disease. It may be possible to avoid CNS preventive therapy in certain patients with limited disease without the risk of subsequent CNS relapse. This has been suggested for patients with totally resected abdominal disease and non-Burkitt's, nonmediastinal, limited (Stage I) nodal disease that is not close to the meninges.[38] However, without a definitive study, the ability to predict patients at risk for CNS relapse in the limited-disease category is not ideal, and for this reason most centers treat all patients with some form of CNS preventive therapy. Intrathecal therapy or cranial irradiation has been used. Although the relative efficacy of each form has not been carefully studied in a randomized fashion, there is evidence that intrathecal chemotherapy alone is highly effective and that cranial irradiation is not necessary. In the Children's Cancer Study Group comparative LSA_2-L_2 versus COMP study, the use of intrathecal chemotherapy alone was associated with an incidence of isolated CNS disease of only 6%. In the NCI study (see above) the inclusion of intrathecal chemotherapy with both methotrexate and cytosine arabinoside reduced the incidence of primary CNS relapse from approximately 20% to 2%.

Radiotherapy

Although radiation therapy plays an important role in the treatment of adult non-Hodgkin's lymphomas, its role in pediatric NHL is limited. Various emergency situations, including acute respiratory distress, superior vena cava syndrome, spinal cord compression, orbital proptosis, and cranial nerve palsy are effectively treated with radiation therapy.

Because childhood NHL is appropriately viewed as a systemic disease, chemotherapy is the major form of treatment. Although involved-field, high-dose irradiation administered to patients with limited disease (excluding the mediastinum) in combination with one of several multiagent systemic regimens has been associated with a high level of local control and substantial overall success (see Table 48-9), recent data indicates that good treatment results can be obtained in early-stage and advanced-stage patients without additional irradiation. "Bulk site" irradiation to all known disease sites in patients with widespread lymphoma usually produces unacceptable additive toxicity if combined with systemic chemotherapy. The use of irradiation to treat localized childhood NHL is no longer warranted. A recent study by the Pediatric Oncology Group (POG) randomized patients with localized disease to receive either a 6-month course of reduced intensity chemotherapy alone or that treatment with involved-field radiotherapy. The projected disease-free survival for all patients is 95% at 2 years. Patients who received radiotherapy fared no better and incurred significantly greater toxicity.

Duration of Therapy

The optimal duration of therapy for children with NHL is not known. The majority of centers treat patients for approximately 18 months to 2 years. Late relapses are relatively rare, and it is unlikely that longer periods of treatment will be advantageous. A review of current treatment results indicates no obvious difference from shorter durations of treatment. The West German BFM Study 83/86 treats all patients for 12 weeks with excellent overall results. The St. Jude study for patients with advanced disease and the POG study for limited disease used approximately 6 months of treatment. In the NCI study (see above) patients with total abdominal disease resection and those with limited non-lymphoblastic disease also received only 6 monthly cycles of maintentance treatment.

Complications of Therapy

Treatment of children with NHL may be associated with both acute and chronic complications. In addition to the usual acute risks of multiagent systemic chemotherapy, such as infection from myelosuppression and hemorrhage from thrombocytopenia, patients with large tumor burdens are at risk for developing severe and potentially life-threatening metabolic complications. Impairment of renal function is a

TABLE 48-10. Several Chemotherapy Regimens in Use for Childhood Non-Hodgkin's Lymphoma

LSA_2/L_2 (Modified)	*COMP*	*APO*	*NCI 77-04*
Induction Cyclophosphamide, 1.2 g/m^2 IV, Day 1 Vincristine, 2.0 mg/m^2 IV (maximum dose, 2.0 mg) Days 3, 10, 17, and 24 Methotrexate, 6.25 mg/m^2 IV Days 5, 31, and 34 Daunomycin, 60 mg/m^2 IV Days 12 and 13 Prednisone, 60 mg/m^2 PO (maximum dose, 60 mg) Days 3–30 *Consolidation* Cytosine arabinoside, 100 mg/m^2 IV daily for 5 days (Mon–Fri) for 2 wk Thioguanine, 50 mg/m^2 PO 8–12 h after each cytosine arabinoside injection Asparaginase, 6000 IU/m^2 IM Daily for 14 days after completion of cytosine arabinoside and thioguanine Methotrexate, 6.25 mg/m^2 IT Twice, 3 days apart, beginning 2 to 3 days after last dose of asparaginase Carmustine, 60 mg/m^2 IV Single dose given 2 to 3 days after completion of methotrexate *Maintenance* 1. Thioguanine, 300 mg/m^2 PO, Days 1–4 Cyclophosphamide, 600 mg/m^2 IV, Day 5 2. Hydroxyurea, 2.4 g/m^2 PO, Days 1–4 Daunomycin, 45 mg/m^2 IV, Day 5 3. Methotrexate, 10 mg/m^2 IV, Days 1–4 Carmustine, 60 mg/m^2 IV, Day 5 4. Cytosine arabinoside, 150 mg/m^2 IV, Days 1–4 Vincristine, 2.0 mg/m^2 IV (maximum dose, 2.0 mg), Day 5 5. Methotrexate, 6.25 mg/m^2 IT, 2 doses given at 3 days apart Repeat maintenance cycles 1–5	*Induction* Cyclophosphamide, 1.2 g/m^2 IV, Day 1 Vincristine 2.0 mg/m^2 IV, (maximum dose, 2.0 mg) Days 3, 10, 17, and 24 Methotrexate, 6.25 mg/m^2 IT Days 5, 31, and 34 Methotrexate, 300 mg/m^2 IV (60% of dose as IV push, 40% as 4-h infusion) on day 12 Prednisone, 60 mg/m^2 PO (maximum dose, 60 mg) Days 3–30 *Maintenance* Cyclophosphamide, 1.0 g/m^2 IV Day 1 Vincristine, 1.5 mg/m^2 IV (maximum dose, 2 mg) Days 1 and 4 Methotrexate, 6.25 mg/m^2 IT Day 1 (excluded from first maintenance cycle) Methotrexate, 300 mg/m^2 IV (60% of dose as IV push, 40% as 4-h infusion) Day 15 Prednisone, 60 mg/m^2 PO (maximum dose, 60 mg) Days 1–5 (excluded from first maintenance cycle) Repeat maintenance cycle every 28 days	*Induction* Vincristine, 1.5 mg/m^2 IV (maximum dose, 2.0 mg) Days 1, 8, 15, 22, and 29 Adriamycin, 75 mg/m^2 IV Days 1 and 22 Prednisone, 40 mg/m^2 PO Days 1–29 (taper over last 7 days) *Consolidation* Vincristine, 2.0 mg/m^2 (maximum dose, 2.0 mg) Day 1 of weeks 6 and 9 Adriamycin, 30 mg/m^2, IV Day 1 of weeks 6 and 9 Asparaginase, 56,000 IU/m^2 IV (pts <6 yr); 28,000 IU/m^2 IV (pts >6 yr) Days 1, 3, 5, 7 and 9 during weeks 7 and 8 Prednisone, 120 mg/m^2 PO Days 1–5 of weeks 6 and 9 6-Mercaptopurine, 225 mg/m^2 PO Days 1–5 of weeks 6 and 9 *CNS Preventive Therapy* (follows Consolidation) Cranial radiation (2400 rad in 13 fractions) over 17 days Methotrexate IT, 12 mg/m^2 (maximum 12 mg) 5 doses given at intervals during periods of cranial radiation, then given every 18 wk during maintenance *Maintenance* Vincristine, 2.0 mg/m^2 IV (maximum dose, 2.0 mg), Day 1 Adriamycin, 30 mg/m^2 IV, Day 1 Prednisone, 120 mg/m^2 PO, Days 1–5 } Repeat every 3 weeks 6-Mercaptopurine, 225 mg/m^2 PO, Days 1–5 When total Adriamycin dose of 450 mg/m^2 has been reached replace with methotrexate 7.5 mg/m^2 PO Days 1–5. Continue 3-wk cycles until 2 yr of complete remission	CYCLE 1 *Systemic Therapy* Cyclophosphamide, 1,2 g/m^2 IV, Day 1 Methotrexate (begins on Day 10), 300 mg/m^2 IV (over first hour), then 60 mg/m^2 IV hourly for next 41 h, followed by calcium leukovorin 48 mg/m^2 IV, then 12 mg/m^2 IV every 6 h until plasma methotrexate levels $<5 \times 10^{-8}$ M. *Intrathecal Therapy* Cytosine arabinoside, 30 mg/m^2 IT Days 1, 2, 3, and 7 Methotrexate, 12.5 mg/m^2 IT (maximum dose, 12.5 mg) Day 10, 6–8 hours after commencement of systemic methotrexate infusion CYCLES 2 TO 6 *Systematic Therapy* (Begins when granulocyte count $\geq$1500/mm^3) Cyclophosphamide, 1.2 g/m^2 IV, Day 1 Adriamycin, 40 mg/m^2 IV, Day 1 Vincristine, 1.4 mg/m^2 IV, Day 1 (maximum dose 2.0 mg) Prednisone, 40 mg/m^2 IV or PO, Days 1–5 Methotrexate and calcium leucovorin Day 10, as in cycle 1 *Intrathecal Therapy* CYCLES 2 AND 3 Cytosine arabinoside, 30 mg/m^2 IT Days 1 and 2 Methotrexate, 12.5 mg/m^2 IT (maximum dose 12.5 mg), Day 3 and on Day 10 6–8 h after commencement of systemic methotrexate infusion CYCLES 4, 5, AND 6 Cytosine arabinoside, 45 mg/m^2 IT, Day 1 Methotrexate 12.5 mg/m^2 IT (maximum dose 12.5 mg), Day 10 Patients with Burkitt's lymphoma/undifferentiated lymphoma, stages A,B,AR, stop therapy after 6 cycles. All other patients are treated for a total of 15 cycles. CYCLES 7 TO 15 Cyclophosphamide, 1.2 mg/m^2 IV, Day 1 Adriamycin, 40 mg/m^2 IV, Day 1 Vincristine, 1.4 mg/m^2 IV (maximum dose 2.0 mg), Day 1 Prednisone, 40 mg/m^2 IV or PO, Days 1–5 Methotrexate and calcium leucovorin on Day 14 as in cycle 1 Cycles are repeated on Day 28 or when granulocyte count is $\geq$1500/mm^3 and platelet count $\geq$75,000/mm^3

significant threat. Compromised renal function, frequently as a result of infiltration of the kidneys with tumor, may be present initially. Many patients also present with uric acid nephropathy. Initial treatment of these patients requires expert medical care. Optimal hydration, alkalinization, and treatment with allopurinol is mandatory. Even when the uric acid level is normalized, there is the possibility of developing the acute tumor lysis syndrome in the immediate postchemotherapy period. This syndrome is characterized by azotemia, hyperphosphatemia, and hypocalcemia, presumably occurring as a result of the liberation of tumor breakdown products into the bloodstream. Patients may develop florid renal failure for which hemodialysis is required. Without proper management, hyperkalemia, hyperphosphatemia, and hypocalcemia may be life-threatening.

In addition to these unique disease-related complications, there is the possibility of toxicities associated with the various chemotherapeutic agents used to treat NHL. Anthracycline-induced cardiomyopathy is a well-recognized complication related to cumulative drug dose. Cyclophosphamide administration carries the risk of bladder toxicity, gonadal failure, and sterility. Damage to other organs, such as the liver and CNS, is also possible. However, with refinements in therapy, such as elimination of radiation therapy and the shorter duration of treatment, the risks for adverse long-term sequelae have decreased.

Therapeutic Challenges

Despite the impressive advances made in the treatment of children with NHL in the past decade, a number of unresolved issues and therapeutic challenges remain. Perhaps the major task is to improve the treatment for patients with widely disseminated disease, a group with a very poor prognosis. Attempts to intensify therapy for this group of patients have failed. Whether more intensive chemotherapy schedules can be designed with currently available drugs or whether future improvements await the development of effective new drugs is unclear.

One possible approach is bone marrow transplantation, which may be of value in poor-prognosis patients with widespread disease. A current POG study is evaluating the role of bone marrow transplantation in Stage IV patients who achieve a complete remission and who have a matched donor.

The eventual impact of agents recently introduced into childhood NHL treatment, such as high-dose cytarabine, ifosfamide, and epipodopholotoxins remains to be determined. Whether biological agents such as interleukin-2 will have an impact is also unknown. There is a considerable interest in using molecularly cloned hematopoietic growth factors, which may lessen the severity of chemotherapy-induced myelosuppression, in combination with more intensive chemotherapy.

Continuing studies at the molecular level investigating the role of oncogenes in the cause of these diseases is vital. Molecular phenotyping may provide a more rational approach to therapy in the future.

HODGKIN'S DISEASE

Hodgkin's disease is uncommon in childhood. Approximately 10% to 15% of all cases occur in patients younger than 16 years. The consequences of stage-specific therapeutic plans devised for adults may be more problematic in the child. This section covers only features of particular relevance to Hodgkin's disease in children.

EPIDEMIOLOGY AND ETIOLOGY

The incidence of Hodgkin's disease increases throughout the pediatric age range. The majority of pediatric cases occur in children 11 years of age or older.[42] Hodgkin's disease is rarely seen in children younger than the age of 4. A striking predominance of boys is seen in prepubertal children. Beginning in early adolescence, however, an increasing number of girls are affected.

The cause of Hodgkin's disease remains obscure. Although an increased incidence of this disease has been noticed in children with a number of hereditary conditions, including ataxia-telangiectasia, Chediak-Higashi syndrome, Wiskott-Aldrich syndrome, and congenital agammaglobulinemia, Hodgkin's disease is not seen as frequently in these conditions as non-Hodgkin's lymphoma.

Suspicion of an infectious cause for Hodgkin's disease has been fostered by a number of reported associations, including reports of case clustering, a higher incidence in patients with infectious mononucleosis, and the bimodal incidence curve of the disease. There is no conclusive evidence to confirm case clusters in children; the other associations are believed to represent the interplay of several factors other than common infections.

There is an increased incidence of Hodgkin's disease among siblings of affected patients, especially if they are of the same sex. An association between certain HLA antigens and the disease has also been reported. These two observations suggest that genetic factors play a role. A difference in the age peaks of Hodgkin's disease in industrialized and underdeveloped countries suggest that environmental factors may also be important. Although a significant relationship between the number of tonsillectomies performed in children with Hodgkin's disease has been noticed by some, this relationship has not been confirmed.

Children and young adults receiving phenytoin for control of seizures are at risk for both a lymphoma-like syndrome that usually reverses with cessation of the drug and the development of true malignant lymphomas and Hodgkin's disease.

A link between socioeconomic status and Hodgkin's disease has been suggested. The incidence of Hodgkin's disease is correlated with higher family income and educational status and with smaller family size.

PATHOLOGY AND CLINICAL PRESENTATION

The proportion of histologic subtypes of Hodgkin's disease is different in children. The incidence of both lymphocyte-predominant and nodular-sclerosis patterns is greater in American children than in adults; the lymphocyte-depleted histologic pattern is extremely uncommon in childhood.

Children usually present with disease above the diaphragm, principally in the cervical or mediastinal nodes. Isolated axillary lymph node involvements are infrequent.[42] Subdiaphragmatic presentations are usually Stage I lymphocyte-predominant cases originating in inguinal lymph nodes.

PRETREATMENT EVALUATION

The principles of the diagnostic workup for the child with Hodgkin's disease are similar to those for adults (see Chap. 49). Lymphangiography is a feasible procedure in the majority of children, and its diagnostic accuracy in the pediatric population has been substantiated, with a 98% correlation between lymphangiographic and histopathologic results. The yield is approximately 15% above that of CT alone. In the very young child, however, lymphangiography is understandably a more difficult procedure. Lymphangiography is critical in cases potentially treated by primary irradiation. Although desirable in all instances, its impact upon treatment is limited to institutions using combined therapy for pediatric Hodgkin's disease.

Indications for staging laparotomy are controversial, and arguments for and against its use are considered in Chapter 49. Reviews of staging laparotomies with splenectomy in the pediatric population have demonstrated changes in the clinical stage in from approximately 15% to almost 50% of cases.[43] In lymphocyte-predominant disease limited to the neck, the yield of laparotomy is sufficiently low to obviate its use. Approximately 20% of all clinical Stage I cases have occult infradiaphragmatic disease at laparotomy; with NS disease, 16% of laparotomies have been positive. In Stage II, apparently supradiaphragmatic disease, the incidence of histologically positive disease is higher (30%).

Although it is evident that staging laparotomy frequently provides information unobtainable by other means, there has been considerable concern about the morbidity of the procedure in the pediatric population. Overwhelming postsplenectomy infection has been reported to occur in as many as 10% of children with Hodgkin's disease. The use of polyvalent pneumococcal vaccine has been recommended, and routine prophylactic antibiotic therapy with penicillin or erythromycin appears to have markedly reduced the incidence of postsplenectomy infection in children at risk (see Chap. 59, sect. 5).[42]

The impact of laparotomy and splenectomy has been greatest in radiation therapy series, with suggested improvement of disease-free survival and relapse-free survival.[44] In centers selectively using combined modality therapy, the advantage of laparotomy is largely to identify site(s) of abdominal disease for inclusion in "local" irradiation fields. Systemic use of chemotherapy and extended-field, low-dose irradiation has achieved 85% survival in all childhood presentations without laparotomy; relapse-free survival in clinical Stages I, II, and III approaches 90%.[45] With selected use of primary radiotherapy or combined modality therapy, appropriate emphasis on diminishing long-term complications of treatment requires the additional information that laparotomy and splenectomy provide.

THERAPY

Optimal therapy for children with Hodgkin's disease is controversial. The major goal in the treatment of Hodgkin's disease in children is to achieve cure with the least morbidity possible. Available data indicate that the use of combined modality therapy for patients in all stages of disease, except perhaps those with Stage I or certain presentations of Stage IV disease, results in the highest survival rate with the lowest risk of relapse.[45,46] Universal application of this approach, however, may inappropriately expose patients to added complications from both modalities.[47]

Complications of irradiation in childhood include structural alterations such as limitation in growth and development of bones, muscles, and soft tissues, thyroid dysfunction, and an increase in the risk of second malignancies, particularly solid tumors.[42] Radiation to the spleen may cause functional asplenia. Although serious cardiac, pulmonary, and gastrointestinal complications have been reported, if radiation treatment is carefully administered and appropriately fractionated, the incidence of clinically overt visceral sequelae is low.

Complications of MOPP chemotherapy include a high incidence of sterility, particularly in postpubertal men. Although data are scanty, fertility problems will eventually occur in prepubertal boys. Ovarian function may also be compromised, although younger prepubertal and pubertal girls appear to be less susceptible to these effects than older, postpubertal women. Chemotherapy-induced myelosuppression also carries the risk of infection. Finally, there is a significant incidence of acute myelogenous leukemia after MOPP treatment, which may be exacerbated by previous or concurrent extensive irradiation. Other treatment regimens, such as ABVD (Adriamycin, bleomycin, vincristine, and DTIC), may achieve similar disease control with potentially less risk of secondary tumors. However, the use of ABVD carries the potential risk of anthracycline-induced cardiac damage. The combined use of MOPP and ABVD may be more effective and has been well-tolerated in children.

Concern about treatment sequelae has, to a considerable degree, shaped current treatment philosophy for children with Hodgkin's disease. A variety of treatment policies have been recommended, including high-dose, involved-field irradiation, with a greater likelihood of relapse, requiring secondary treatment, but less somatic dysfunction than more extended irradiation volumes; extended-field or total nodal high-dose irradiation, with excellent disease control but considerable morbidity in young or prepubertal children; routine use of intermediate-dose, involved-field irradiation and chemotherapy with MOPP, ABVD, or MOPP plus ABVD, with perhaps the highest relapse-free survival rates, but with the risk of secondary leukemias; and chemotherapy alone.[42,43,45] The specifics of these strategies and the controversies surrounding them are discussed in detail in Chapter 49.

It is clear, however, that to achieve an optimal balance

between maximizing disease-free survival and minimizing treatment complications for the child with Hodgkin's disease, therapy must be tailored according to the patient's age and stage of disease. Children beyond puberty represent the majority of pediatric Hodgkin's patients. For this group, growth changes are of relatively less concern. Therefore, extended field irradiation has been advocated for patients with pathologic Stage I or IIA disease, with chemotherapy reserved for children who might relapse after initial irradiation.[42] Traditionally, older children with Stage III disease have received initial combined-modality therapy, although controversy exists about treatment of patients, especially boys, with minimal Stage IIIA disease (see Chap. 53).[42,46] In cases with large mediastinal disease, B symptoms, or disease beyond Stage IIIA, there is relative agreement on the use of primary chemotherapy, usually with added involved-field irradiation.[42,45,46]

Defining optimal treatment for the younger child has been more difficult. Younger children with pathologic Stage I LP disease limited to the neck have an excellent disease-free survival rate after involved-field or limited extended-field ("mini-mantle") treatment. Treatment of this favorable-prognosis group in this fashion reduces the likelihood of significant cardiac, pulmonary, and structural effects from irradiation, and by eliminating chemotherapy, prevents those adverse sequelae associated with combined-modality treatment. In Stages I and IIA disease, managed with local fields only, relapse rates of >30% are common even with surgical staging. Although patients in these categories appear to respond well to chemotherapy if they relapse, the excellent overall survival must be balanced against the frequency of necessary combined therapy in a group selected for minimal irradiation.

In young children with extensive disease, most centers favor chemotherapy to diminish the pronounced growth changes associated with large-volume, full-dose radiation therapy. Involved-field or extended-field irradiation using limited doses (1500–2500 cGy) appear to add to efficacy with far less likelihood of major structural consequences.[45–47] A group of children treated with 1500 cGy to 2500 cGy of total nodal irradiation followed by six cycles of MOPP chemotherapy had a 93% relapse-free survival rate (Fig. 48-6).[47]

Treatment with chemotherapy alone may achieve equivalent results, with less concern about toxicities of combined treatment and potentially lower rates of secondary malignancies. In children data to support this approach are not plentiful. In adults, DeVita and co-workers noted that 22 of 23 patients with Stages IIA and IIIA disease were disease-free survivors following MOPP therapy alone.[48] Other series have also yielded encouraging early results using chemotherapy alone. The possibility of eliminating irradiation in selected patients (*i.e.*, those with stages II and III disease of mixed-cell type) is appealing if it can be demonstrated that chemotherapy alone offers equivalent efficacy with less morbidity.

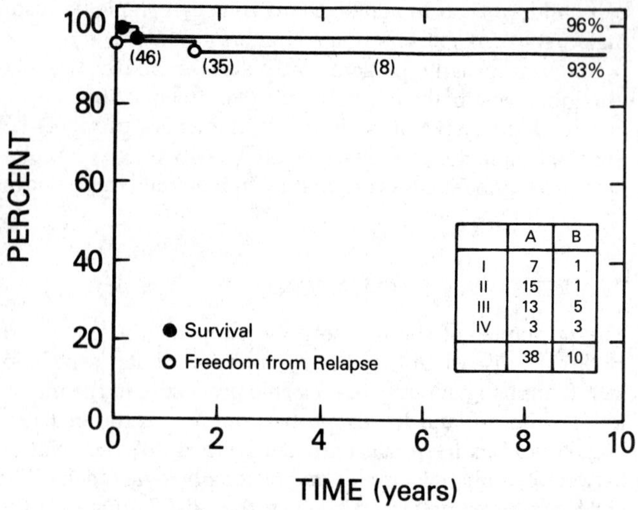

FIG. 48-6. Kaplan-Meier plot of overall survival and disease-free survival among 48 children treated with low-dose irradiation and MOPP. (Donaldson SS: Hodgkin's disease: Treatment with low-dose radiation and chemotherapy. In Frontiers in Radiation Therapy and Oncology, pp 122–133. Basel, S Karger, 1982)

THERAPEUTIC IMPROVEMENTS

The advances made in treating adult Hodgkin's disease have also been translated into dramatically improved survival in children. Overall 5-year survival has progressively improved, so that most centers are achieving rates of approximately 90%. Accurate staging, selective use of single-modality therapy with extended-field irradiation or chemotherapy in clinical trial settings, and improved combined-modality programs have been responsible for this success. However, considerable controversy exists about what constitutes optimal treatment, primarily because of the morbidity associated with combined-modality treatment.

REFERENCES

1. Anderson JR, Wilson JF, Jenkin DJ et al: Childhood non-Hodgkin's lymphoma: The results of a randomized therapeutic trial comparing a 4-drug regimen (COMP) with a 10-drug regimen LSA_2-L_2. N Engl J Med 308:559–565, 1983
2. Smith KL, Johnson W: Classification of chronic myelocytic leukemia in children. Cancer 34:670–679, 1974
3. Altman A, Altman AJ: Chronic leukemias of childhood. Pediatr Clin North Am 35: 1988
4. Bleyer WA, Poplack DG: Prophylaxis and treatment of leukemia in the central nervous system and other sanctuaries. Semin Oncol 12:131–148, 1985
5. Russo A, Schiliro G: The enigma of testicular leukemia: A critical review. Med Pediatr Oncol 14:300–306, 1986
6. Bowman WP, Aur RJA, Hustu HO et al: Isolated testicular relapse in acute lymphocytic leukemia of childhood: Categories and influence on survival. J Clin Oncol 2:924–929, 1984
7. Miller LP, Miller DR: Acute lymphoblastic leukemia in children: Current status, controversies, and future perspective. CRC Crit Rev Oncol Hematol 1:129–197, 1986
8. Bennett JM, Catovsky D, Daniel MT et al: French-American-British (FAB) Cooperative Group: The morphological classification of acute leukemias—concordance among observers and clinical correlation. Br J Haematol 47:553–561, 1981
9. Miller DR, Krailo M, Bleyer WA et al: Prognostic implications of blast cell morphology in childhood acute lymphoblastic leukemia: A report from the Children's Cancer Study Group. Cancer Treat Rep 69:1211–21, 1985
10. Korsmeyer SJ, Arnold A, Bakshi A et al: Immunoglobulin gene rearrangement and cell surface antigen expression in acute lymphocytic leukemia of T-cell and B-cell precursor origins. J Clin Invest 71:301–313, 1983
11. Crist WM, Grosse CE, Pullen J, Cooper MD: Immunologic markers in childhood acute lymphocytic leukemia. Semin Oncol 2:105–121, 1985
12. Foon KA, Todd RF III: Immunologic classification of leukemia and lymphoma. Blood 68:1–31, 1986
13. Felix CA, Wright JJ, Poplack DG et al: T-cell receptor α-, β-, and γ-genes in T-cell and pre-B cell acute lymphoblastic leukemia. J Clin Invest 80:545–556, 1987

14. Mirro J, Zipf TF, Pui C et al: Acute mixed lineage leukemia: Clinicopathologic correlations and prognostic significance. Blood 65:1115–1123, 1985
15. Williams DL, Raimondi S, Rivera G et al: Presence of clonal chromosome abnormalities in virtually all cases of acute lymphoblastic leukemia. N Engl J Med 10:640–641, 1985
16. Look AT: The emerging genetics of acute lymphoblastic leukemia: Clinical and biologic implications. Semin Oncol 12:92–104, 1985
17. Poplack DG, Blatt J, Reaman G: Purine pathway enzyme abnormalities in acute lymphoblastic leukemia. Cancer Res 41:4821–4823, 1981
18. Hammond GD, Sather H, Bleyer WA et al: Stratification by prognostic factors in the design and analysis of clinical trials for acute lymphoblastic leukemia. Haematology and blood transfusion. In Buchner, Schellong, Hiddemann (eds): Acute Leukemias. Berlin, Springer-Verlag, 1987
19. Reaman G, Zeltzer P, Bleyer WA et al: Acute lymphoblastic leukemia in infants less than one year of age: A cumulative experience of the Children's Cancer Study Group. J Clin Oncol 3:1513–1521, 1985
20. Crist W, Pullin J, Boyett J et al: Clinical and biologic features predict a poor prognosis in acute lymphoid leukemias in infants: A Pediatric Oncology Group Study. Blood 67:135–140, 1986
21. Sather HN: Statistical evaluation of prognostic factors in ALL and treatment results. Med Pediatr Oncol 14:158–165, 1986
22. Steinherz PG, Gaynon P, Miller DR et al: Improved disease-free survival of children with acute lymphoblastic leukemia at high risk for early relapse with the New York regimen—a new intensive therapy protocol: A report from the Children's Cancer Study Group. J Clin Oncol 4:744–752, 1986
23. Bleyer WA, Coccia PF, Sather HN et al: Reduction in central nervous system leukemia with a pharmacokinetically derived intrathecal methotrexate dosage regimen. J Clin Oncol 1:317–325, 1983
24. Riehm H, Gadner H, Henze G et al: Acute lymphoblastic leukemia: Treatment results in three BFM studies (1970–1981). In Murphy SB, Gilbert JR (eds): Leukemia Research: Advances in Cell Biology and Treatment, pp. 251–263. New York, Elsevier, 1983
25. Henze G, Langermann HJ, Fengler R et al: Acute lymphoblastic therapy study BFM 70/81 in children and adolescents: Intensified reinduction therapy for patients with different risk for relapse. Klin Padiatr 194:195–203, 1982
26. Nesbit ME, Sather HN, Robison LL et al: Randomized study of 3-years versus 5-years of chemotherapy in childhood acute lymphoblastic leukemia J Clin Oncol 1:308–316, 1983
27. Butturine A, Rivera GK, Bortin MM et al: Which treatment for childhood acute lymphoblastic leukaemia in second remission? Lancet 1:429, 1987
28. Thomas ED, Sanders JE, Flowinoy N et al: Marrow transplantation for patients with acute lymphoblastic leukemia: A long-term follow-up. Blood 62:1139–1141, 1983
29. Sanders JE, Thomas ED, Buckner CD et al: Marrow transplantation for children with acute lymphoblastic leukemia in second remission. Blood 70:324–326, 1987
30. Poplack DG, Brouwers, P: Adverse Sequelae of central nervous system therapy. Clin Oncol 4:263–285, 1985
31. Wright JJ, Poplack DG, Bakhski A et al: Gene rearrangements as markers of clonal variation and minimal residual disease in acute lymphoblastic leukemia. J Clin Oncol 5:735–741, 1987
32. Lampkin BC, Woods W, Strauss R et al: Current status of the biology and treatment of acute non-lymphocytic leukemia in children (Report from the ANLL Strategy Group of Children's Cancer Study Group) Blood 61:215–228, 1983
33. Weinstein HJ, Mayer RJ, Rosenthal DS et al: Chemotherapy for acute myelogenous leukemia in children and adults: VAPA update. Blood 62:315–319, 1983
34. Creutzig U, Ritter J, Riehm H et al: Improved treatment results in childhood acute myelogenous leukemia: A report of the German cooperative study AML-BFM-78. Blood 65:298, 1985
35. Griffin JD, Mayer RJ, Weinstein HJ et al: Surface marker analysis of acute myeloblastic leukemia: Identification of differentiation-associated phenotypes. Blood 62:557–563, 1983
36. Pui CH, Dahl GV, Kalwinsky DK et al: Central nervous system leukemia in children with acute nonlymphoblastic leukemia. Blood 66:1062–1067, 1985
37. Grier HE, Gelber RD, Camitta BM et al: Prognostic factors in childhood acute myelogenous leukemia. J Clin Oncol 5:1026, 1987
38. Magrath I: Malignant non-Hodgkin's lymphomas in children. In Pizzo PA, Poplack DG (eds): Principles and Practice of Pediatric Oncology. Philadelphia, JB Lippincott, 1988
39. Murphy SB: Classification, staging and end results of treatment of childhood non-Hodgkin's lymphoma: Dissimilarities from lymphomas in adults. Semin Oncol 7:332–339, 1980
40. Link MP: Non-Hodgkin's lymphoma in children. Pediatr Clin North Am 32:699–720, 1985
41. Magrath IT: Biological features of pediatric non-Hodgkin's lymphomas. In Ford RJ, Fuller L, and Hagermeister (eds): Hodgkin's Disease and Non-Hodgkin's Lymphoma. New Perspectives in Immunotherapy, Diagnosis and Treatment, pp 201–212. New York, Raven Press, 1984
42. Mauch PM, Weinstein H, Botnick L et al: An evaluation of long-term survival and treatment complications in children with Hodgkin's disease. Cancer 51:925–932, 1983
43. Donaldson SS, Kaplan HS: A survey of pediatric Hodgkin's disease at Stanford University: Results of therapy and quality of survival. In Rosenberg SA, Kaplan HS (eds): Malignant Lymphomas: Etiology, Immunology, Pathology, Treatment, pp 571–590. New York, Academic Press, 1982
44. Russell KJ, Donaldson SS, Cox RS et al: Childhood Hodgkin's disease: Patterns of relapse. J Clin Oncol 2:80–87, 1984
45. Jenkin D, Doyle J: Paediatric Hodgkin's disease—late results and toxicity. Int J Radiat Oncol Biol Phys 13:92, 1987
46. Lange B, Littman P: Management of Hodgkin's disease in children and adolescents. Cancer 51:1371–1377, 1983
47. Donaldson SS, Kaplan HS: Complications of treatment of Hodgkin's disease in children. Cancer Treat Rep 66:977–989, 1982
48. DeVita VT, Simon RT, Hubbrd SM et al: Curability of advanced Hodgkin's disease with chemotherapy: Long-term follow-up of MOPP-treated patients at NCI. Ann Intern Med 92:587–595, 1980

SAMUEL HELLMAN

ELAINE S. JAFFE

VINCENT T. DeVITA, Jr.

CHAPTER 49 *Hodgkin's Disease*

ETIOLOGY AND EPIDEMIOLOGY

In the United States a minority of patients with lymphomas have Hodgkin's disease. Between 7000 and 7500 patients are diagnosed with this disease annually. There appears to be a bimodal incidence curve for Hodgkin's disease in economically developed countries.[1] Correa and colleagues[2] recognized that, in economically underdeveloped countries, the overall incidence of Hodgkin's disease is lower than in developed countries, but incidence before the age of 15 is higher, with only a modest increase throughout adolescence and young adulthood. Associated with this disparity is a difference in the distribution of histologic subgroups, with nodular sclerosing Hodgkin's disease underrepresented in these countries. In Japan, the first peak of Hodgkin's disease that is usually seen in developed countries is absent.

Cole and colleagues[3] have postulated that the dual-peak incidence of Hodgkin's disease supports the hypothesis that this disease is the result of two etiologic processes: a biologic agent of low infectivity that causes the disease in young adults, and a mechanism similar to that of other lymphomas in the older age group. An alternative explanation is that these data reflect a variation in host response to a single etiologic mechanism. There is an increased risk of Hodgkin's disease with increasing educational level of the patient. The relative risk varied from 0.7 to 1.8, depending on the educational level.

The potential infectious nature of Hodgkin's disease has been a topic of discussion since its earliest description. *Mycobacterium tuberculosis* was early suspected to be the etiologic organism because of the high incidence of tuberculosis in patients with this disease. The idea was first advanced seriously by Sternberg in 1898,[4] and others have added to the discussion.[5-8] Since that time, considerable epidemiologic evidence that suggests an infectious etiology, particularly a virus, has been found. A number of studies have addressed the possibility of an increased risk of Hodgkin's disease in infectious mononucleosis.[9-12] A small but consistent increase in the incidence of Hodgkin's disease has been noted after this disease (Table 49-1). This relationship is supported by the identification of cells resembling the Reed–Sternberg cell (described in the section on pathology) in infectious mononucleosis. While the latter disease is known to be caused by the Epstein–Barr virus, no convincing evidence has yet been produced for the role of that virus in Hodgkin's disease.[13]

A variety of hypotheses have been set forth to explain the unusual presentation of Hodgkin's disease. Because of the similarity of the disease to the then newly described graft-versus-host disease (GVHD) seen in bone marrow transplantation, Kaplan and Smithers[14] speculated that the process might include an interaction between normal lymphocytes and antigenically different neoplastic cells. Expanding on this notion, it has been suggested that T lymphocytes may be infected by either a single or a number of viruses that alter their antigenicity.[15] Uninvolved T cells would then react against these altered cells, resulting in an autoimmune response similar to GVHD. Schwartz and Beldotti[16] have shown that chronic GVHD often resulted in lymphoma in mice, and this hypothesis suggests a similar consequence in humans. Others have suggested an altered B-cell response secondary to a virus infection.[17] Whatever the pathogenesis, Hodgkin's disease has a number of unusual characteristics that require explanation, including the axial distribution of

TABLE 49-1. Risk of Developing Hodgkin's Disease After Infectious Mononucleosis

Source	*Size of Population at Risk*	*Observed*	*Expected*	*Years of Follow-up*	*Reference*
US soldiers	2,437	2	1	22	9
Connecticut	4,529	5	1	16	10
Denmark	17,000	17	6	—	11

lymph node disease as opposed to the more centrifugal distribution seen in non-Hodgkin's lymphomas, the large number of nonmalignant lymphocytes and eosinophils intermixed with the malignant cells, frequent lymphoid hyperplasia either preceding or adjacent to the disease, and the early and persistent derangement of cell-mediated immunity.

Clustering of Hodgkin's disease has been reported by Vianna and associates.[18,19] Whether such clusters are significant or a matter of chance has been discussed by a number of investigators. Population-based studies, using cancer registries in Connecticut and California, have made a rather convincing argument that the reported clusters of Hodgkin's disease have occurred by chance alone.[20,21] A study that repeated the methodology of Vianna and co-workers in a different location failed to confirm the findings.[22] Although these studies do not confirm an infectious etiology, there nevertheless have been some suggestions that this might be the case.[23] Studies investigating the association of Hodgkin's disease with childhood factors that decrease the exposure to infectious agents at an early age have shown that the risk of Hodgkin's disease is higher under certain circumstances. Risk-reducing factors known to decrease or delay early exposure to infections include fewer siblings, single-family houses, early birth order, and fewer playmates. For example, the incidence of clinical mononucleosis is associated with these factors because this disease becomes clinically relevant with infections after early childhood, rather than the inapparent infections seen with early exposure. This finding suggests that there may be an infectious origin having different consequences depending on the age of infection.[23]

Other unexplained factors are associated with the increased risk of acquiring Hodgkin's disease, including increased risk in woodworkers; the relationship between Hodgkin's disease, tonsillectomy, and appendectomy; and the association of Hodgkin's disease with certain HLA antigens.[24–29] Because viruses of both the DNA and RNA type have been associated with lymphomas and leukemias in animals and in humans, they have been the prime suspects for the etiology of Hodgkin's disease, and cell cultures taken from patients with Hodgkin's disease have been found on occasion to contain viral information in their genomes. However, while suggestive, none of these findings have provided definitive proof. Recently, the similarity of the immune defect so characteristically found in Hodgkin's disease patients (see below) to infections associated with human retroviruses has raised the possibility of an association with such an agent.[30] Gallo and colleagues have recently noted a strong association between antibodies in Hodgkin's disease patients and a herpes-like DNA virus (HBLV), which was first observed in conjunction with B-cell lymphomas in patients with acquired immune deficiency syndrome (AIDS) (personal communication).

HISTORY

Hodgkin's disease has a special place in the history of the understanding of cancer because so many principles important to modern diagnosis, staging, and treatment were first used in the management of this disease.[31] Thomas Hodgkin's historic paper, "On Some Morbid Appearances of the Absorbent Glands and Spleen,"[32] was read before the Medical and Chiruorgical Society on January 10 and 24, 1832. Hodgkin described six cases of his own and added a discussion of a case described by Thomas Carswell in 1828. A watercolor painting of the morbid anatomy of this case by Carswell was on display during Hodgkin's presentations. Like many later discoverers of new diseases, Hodgkin was certain that other anatomists must have noticed the same disorder; he commented to fellow anatomists that such cases "can scarcely have failed to have fallen under their observation in the course of cadaveric inspection," and, indeed, such observations had been made.

Hodgkin's unique contribution was in the recognition that he was dealing with a primary disease of the lymphatic glands and not a secondary response to inflammation. His certainty about this was remarkable enough in its day but especially so because he was aware that two of his patients had other illnesses (tuberculosis in case 1 and syphilis in case 3) that might have accounted for the pathology. Also remarkable is the fact that Hodgkin described the entity based on the now well-known natural history of this disease but without the aid of a microscope. Subsequent analysis of material from Hodgkin's patients (preserved in the Gordon Museum at Guy's Hospital Medical School, London) confirmed that four of the seven cases were indeed Hodgkin's disease; Carswell's case could not be confirmed in the absence of tissue, and, in the remaining two cases, syphilis and lymphosarcoma were thought to be the causes of the adenopathy.[31]

However, Hodgkin's contribution would have fallen into oblivion if not for the unselfish behavior of Sir Samuel Wilks. In the course of his description of primary and secondary amyloidosis, also a first, he noted a variant associated with "a peculiar enlargement of lymphatic glands frequently associated with diseases of the spleen." He was clearly under the impression that his observation was original; however, by the time he completed writing his paper, he became aware of Hodgkin's work through mention of it in another paper by

Bright[33] and diligently tracked it down, noting, "It is only to be lamented that Dr. Hodgkin did not affix a distinct name to this disease, for by so doing, I should not have experienced so long an ignorance (which I believe I share with many others) of a very remarkable class of cases." Wilks' paper in 1865 was entitled, "Enlargement of the Lymphatic Glands and Spleen (or, Hodgkin's Disease)," thereby immortalizing Thomas Hodgkin.[34]

Hodgkin's description was the first of a distinct malignancy of the lymphatic system and preceded the description of leukemia by Craigie,[35] Bennett,[36] and Virchow[37] by 61 years; and of reticulum cell sarcoma by Roulet[38] by 98 years. These important descriptions were also largely microscopic delineations of causes of adenopathy other than Hodgkin's disease. Another feat similar to that of Dr. Thomas Hodgkin was not to follow for 126 years, when Burkitt[39] was to describe the lymphoma that bears his name, based on its unique clinical presentation in patients in central Africa.

The history of the discovery of the pathognomonic giant cells of Hodgkin's disease has been reviewed in detail by Kaplan.[31] Wilks[34] had the benefit of a microscope and had examined the histology of some of his cases, but noted only that "the microscope showed masses of cells and fibres as of new tissue." Greenfield[40] contributed the first low-power drawings of the appearance of those cells in 1878; Goldmann,[41] using Ehrlich's staining procedures, recognized the acidophilic nature of the nucleolus of the cells in 1892; and Sternberg[4] also described the cells in 1898. However, it was Reed[42] who most clearly illustrated the appearance of the multinuclear giant cells with excellent drawings from her eight cases in 1902, and, appropriately, the cells have since been known as Reed–Sternberg cells. The malignant nature of the disease was generally agreed upon when the clonal origin of the malignant cell was confirmed by cytogenetic analysis of cell lines by Sief and Spriggs in 1967.[44]

PATHOLOGY

CLASSIFICATION

Hodgkin's disease is unique among cancers because the tumor palpated by the physician contains primarily normal lymphocytes, plasma cells, and fibrous stroma of the lymph node, with only a scattering of the characteristic malignant cells of Hodgkin's disease, the Reed–Sternberg cells, and their mononuclear variants. The diagnosis of Hodgkin's disease should rarely be made in the absence of Reed–Sternberg cells, although the presence of such cells, by itself, is not pathognomonic of the disease. Cells resembling Reed-Sternberg cells have been found in reactive lymphoid hyperplasias such as infectious mononucleosis, non-Hodgkin's lymphomas, and nonlymphoid malignancies, including carcinomas and sarcomas.[45,46]

The historic evolution of the diagnosis and classification of Hodgkin's disease is shown in Table 49-2. Since the detailed descriptions by Sternberg and Reed, Hodgkin's disease has been recognized as a form of lymphoreticular malignancy with distinctive clinical and pathologic features.[4,42] Histologically, one sees a polymorphous admixture of cytologically abnormal cells (Reed–Sternberg cells and their mononuclear variants) and a variety of apparently normal reactive elements. The Reed–Sternberg cell is large, with two or more mirror-image nuclei, each containing a single prominent nucleolus (Fig. 49-1). In the first clinically useful subclassification of Hodgkin's disease, developed by Jackson and Parker,[47] cases were divided into three groups: paragranuloma, granuloma, and sarcoma. This classification identified the 10% of cases with the most favorable and least favorable prognoses (paragranuloma and sarcoma, respectively), but approximately 80% of cases remained in the category of granuloma. A major advance occurred in 1966 when Lukes and colleagues[48] proposed a new histologic classification that appeared to correlate well with clinical stage and aggressiveness of disease. This scheme was later simplified into the Rye classification, which is now widely accepted and used by both pathologists and clinicians. These two classifications are compared in Table 49-3. In the Rye classification, Hodgkin's disease is divided into four categories: lymphocyte-predominant, mixed cellularity, lymphocyte-depleted, and nodular sclerosis. The first three categories differ primarily in the relative proportion of neoplastic mononuclear and Reed–Sternberg cells to reactive elements, especially lymphocytes. An indolent natural history and prolonged survival appear to be directly related to the ratio of lymphocytes to abnormal cells in diagnostic biopsies. The fourth category, nodular sclerosis (shown in Fig. 49-2), has distinctive clinical and morphologic features that were

TABLE 49-2. Landmarks in the Description of Hodgkin's Disease

Author	*Year*	*Observation*
Hodgkin[32]	1832	"On some morbid appearance of the absorbent glands and spleen"
Wilks[34]	1865	"Cases of the enlargement of the lymph glands and spleen (or Hodgkin's disease)"
Langhans[414]	1872	First description of histologic features of Hodgkin's disease,
Greenfield[40]	1878	including a description of giant cells and intense fibrous bands
Pell[415]	1887	Described cyclical fever in Hodgkin's disease
Sternberg,[4] Reed[42]	1898	First definitive description of Hodgkin's disease and clear illustrations of the cells bearing their names
Parker et al[416]	1932	Described the absence of response to tuberculin in the presence of tuberculosis in Hodgkin's disease
Jackson[417]	1937	First histopathologic classification of Hodgkin's disease
Lukes et al[48]	1963	Described the current histopathologic classification of Hodgkin's disease

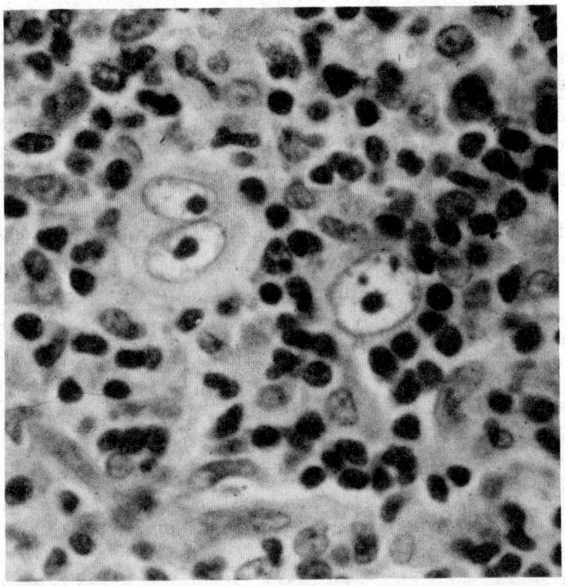

FIG. 49-1. Characteristic Reed–Sternberg cell and mononuclear variant of Hodgkin's disease. (Hematoxylin and eosin; magnification ×400)

first hinted at by Greenfield in 1878[40] but more clearly described by Lukes in 1963.[49] Although the histologic subtype of Hodgkin's disease does correlate with stage and natural history, with modern advances in treatment, histology has become less important as a guide to clinical management and therapy.

In lymphocyte-predominant Hodgkin's disease, the lymph node architecture is usually effaced, although a remnant of normal lymph node may remain. The cellular proliferation is composed of benign-appearing lymphocytes with or without benign histiocytes. The growth pattern may be diffuse or nodular, the nodules being considerably larger than those of follicular lymphomas. It is often necessary to examine multiple sections to identify diagnostic Reed–Sternberg cells. However, variant cells, termed *L* and *H* variants, may be more frequent and may lead one to suspect the diagnosis. These cells often have multilobated nuclei and have been called *popcorn* cells because of their resemblance to a popped kernel of corn. Fibrosis is usually not seen. The lymphocyte-predominant subtype is more common in men than in women and often occurs in the younger age groups (less than 35 years of age). Most patients have clinically localized disease and are asymptomatic, and the prognosis is usually favorable.

TABLE 49-3. Histologic Classification of Hodgkin's Disease Comparing the Jackson and Parker[47] Classification to that of Lukes, Butler, and Hicks[48]

Jackson and Parker (1944)	*Lukes and Butler (1966)*
Paragranuloma (10%)*	Lymphocytic predominant (15%)
Granuloma (80%)	Nodular sclerosis (70%)
	Mixed cellularity (10%)
	Lymphocyte depleted (5%)
	1. Diffuse fibrosis
	2. Reticular type
Sarcoma (10%)	

*The figures in parentheses indicate percentage of patients in various subcategories in the National Cancer Institute population.

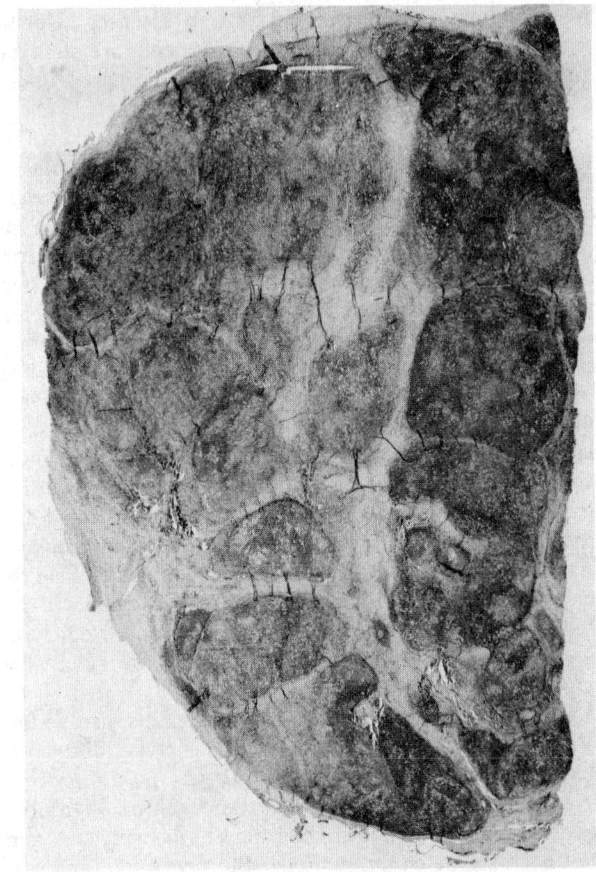

FIG. 49-2. Lymph node, nodular sclerosing Hodgkin's disease. Cellular nodules are surrounded by dense fibrous bands. (Hematoxylin and eosin; magnification ×8)

The original Lukes and Butler scheme subdivided lymphocyte-predominant Hodgkin's disease into nodular and diffuse subtypes. This distinction was obliterated by the Rye modification but appears to be important in the light of new information that links the nodular subtype to the B-cell arm of the immune system. Moreover, progressive transformation of germinal centers is a relatively recently described[50,51] entity that is often associated with lymphocyte-predominant Hodgkin's disease of the nodular subtype. In patients with this subtype of the disease, the architecture of the lymph nodes is altered by large nodules that contain dispersed follicular center cells in clusters and ill-defined islands; Reed–Sternberg cells and *L* and *H* variants, however, are absent. Progressive transformation of germinal centers can be seen before or concurrently with lymphocyte-predominant Hodgkin's disease or may follow it in other sites.[50–52] The association of this lesion with nodular lymphocyte-predominant Hodgkin's disease supports the concept that the latter may be closely linked with the B-cell system. The diagnosis of progressive transformation of germinal centers should alert the clinician to the possible development of lymphocyte-predominant Hodgkin's disease.

In lymphocyte-depleted Hodgkin's disease, Reed–Sternberg cells and "pleomorphic" variant cells are plentiful in proportion to normal lymphocytes. The original Lukes and Butler scheme included two subtypes of lymphocyte-depleted Hodgkin's disease: diffuse fibrosis and reticular. The reticular subtype contained sheets of pleomorphic neoplastic cells, making it difficult to distinguish from a high-grade non-Hodgkin's lymphoma.[53] Indeed, recent studies have indicated a lower incidence of lymphocyte-depleted Hodgkin's disease than previously reported and have suggested that some cases previously diagnosed as lymphocyte-depleted Hodgkin's disease may have represented large cell immunoblastic lymphomas.[54] Lymphocyte-depleted Hodgkin's had been considered a distinct clinicopathologic entity occurring in older patients with minimal peripheral adenopathy and widespread abdominal disease.[55] However, this syndrome is now in question because of the finding that high-grade diffuse lymphomas were commonly misclassified as Hodgkin's disease in older series. This same difficulty may be responsible for the finding, in these same studies, that a significantly worse prognosis was associated with the lymphocyte-depleted type.[54] When stringent criteria are employed, lymphocyte-depleted Hodgkin's disease accounts for only 5% of all cases in current series.

Most cases of lymphocyte-depleted Hodgkin's disease fall into the diffuse fibrosis subtype. In this subtype, diffuse fibroblastic proliferation may be prominent, and the process may even have a sarcomatous appearance. Normal lymphocytes are sparse, but neutrophils may be conspicuous and foci of necrosis are common. Reed–Sternberg cells and variants are present but may be difficult to detect because of the marked fibroblastic reaction. Lymphocyte-depleted Hodgkin's disease is the most common category seen in association with the acquired immunodeficiency syndrome. Such patients usually have widespread disease with involvement of liver and bone marrow.[56–58] The absence of an effective lymphocytic response may contribute to aggressive clinical and pathologic behavior.

The nodular sclerosis category is distinctive both morphologically and clinically. From the histologic standpoint, two features distinguish this form of Hodgkin's disease from all others. The first is the presence of a particular variant of the Reed–Sternberg cell, the so-called lacunar cell.[59,60] In formalin-fixed tissue, the abundant pale cytoplasm often retracts and gives the appearance of a cell in space. The second feature seen in most, but not all, cases is a thickened capsule with a proliferation of orderly collagenous bands that divide the lymphoid tissue into circumscribed nodules (Fig. 49-2). In some cases, the sclerosis is absent or minimal, but the presence of numerous lacunar cells, often in focal nodular aggregates, has led some investigators to refer to this as the *cellular phase* of nodular sclerosis. Strum and Rappaport have observed progression from the cellular phase to classic nodular sclerosis with fibrous bands in sequential biopsies. Nodular sclerosis is the only form of Hodgkin's disease that is more common in women than in men. It occurs most frequently in adolescents and young adults and is unusual in patients over 50 years old. The process has a striking propensity to involve lower cervical, supraclavicular, and mediastinal lymph nodes. Patients with nodular sclerosis, particularly those with localized tumors, usually have good prognoses.

This category can be further subclassified according to the frequency of the malignant cells relative to normal lymphocytes. In the lymphocyte-depleted subtype, malignant cells are extremely numerous. Marked necrosis accompanied by acute inflammatory cells is seen in the center of cellular nodules. The neoplastic "histiocytes" palisading this necrosis may, to the unwary, mimic necrotizing granulomas. Fibrous bands may be inconspicuous, although capsular fibrosis is evident. Because of the frequent sheets of malignant cells, this subtype also has been referred to as the *syncytial variant.* The lymphocyte-depleted subtype, although not clearly an independent prognostic indicator,[54,62] correlates with advanced stage at presentation and the presence of B symptoms.[63] Bulky mediastinal disease is often associated with this subtype.

Mixed cellularity Hodgkin's disease is characterized by an inflammatory background rich in lymphocytes, plasma cells, eosinophils, and histiocytes.[64,65] The Reed–Sternberg cells and their mononuclear counterparts are of the classical variety, with prominent inclusion-like nucleoli, and represent 5 to 15 cells per high-power field. Because of the inflammatory background, the differential diagnosis often includes peripheral T-cell lymphoma, and immune markers may be necessary to resolve this point. A relatively high percentage of patients will have Stage III or IV disease. To some extent, mixed cellularity Hodgkin's disease has been used to include all cases of Hodgkin's disease that do not readily fall into another category.[48] This "wastebasket" approach should be avoided, and such cases should be considered unclassifiable or not further subclassified.

CRITERIA REQUIRED FOR HISTOLOGIC DIAGNOSIS

Needle core biopsies of the liver and bone marrow are frequently obtained for staging Hodgkin's disease. To diagnose involvement, one should see atypical mononuclear cells or Reed–Sternberg cells in the appropriate inflammatory environment.[64] In a patient with an established primary diagnosis, Reed–Sternberg cells are not required. However, a polymorphous cellular infiltrate in the absence of atypical cells with prominent nucleoli is a nonspecific finding and should not be considered evidence of disease.

In the bone marrow, the atypical cells are frequently distributed in a markedly fibrotic background. Indeed, the marrow may be replaced by diffuse fibrosis, and atypical cells may be difficult to observe.[66] For this reason, bone marrow aspirates are usually not useful in the diagnosis of Hodgkin's disease in the bone marrow.

Most subtypes of Hodgkin's disease preferentially involve the T-cell–dependent zones of the lymphoid system.[63] In partially involved lymph nodes, the paracortex, and in the splenic white pulp, the periarteriolar lymphoid sheath and marginal zone are preferentially involved. The thymus gland itself is frequently involved by nodular sclerosing Hodgkin's disease and may undergo cystic degeneration secondary to involvement.[67] Therefore, a thymic cyst should be carefully examined microscopically for evidence of occult Hodgkin's disease. Hodgkin's disease tends to involve axial or central lymph node groups. Mesenteric lymph nodes, Waldeyer's ring, and epitrochlear lymph nodes are rarely involved.

A non-necrotizing epithelioid granulomatous reaction frequently accompanies Hodgkin's disease.[60,68] It may be found in involved lymph nodes and can be so extensive that it obscures the presence of Hodgkin's disease. Sarcoid-like granulomas can be seen throughout the lymphoreticular system (that is, in the spleen, liver, and bone marrow). This granulomatous response by itself does not indicate evidence of occult involvement. In fact, patients with granulomas, stage for stage have an improved prognosis over patients without such a reaction.[65] Thus, the granulomas may represent a positive response to the disease.

CELLULAR ORIGIN OF HODGKIN'S DISEASE

The precise cellular origin of Hodgkin's disease has not yet been firmly established, but theories have included derivation from a B-lymphocyte, T-lymphocyte, or macrophage/reticulum cell line.[69–72] Hodgkin's disease is characterized by functional deficits in T-cell–mediated immune responses, often early in the course of disease and prior to therapy.[73,74] The lymphocytes within Hodgkin's lesions are usually identifiable as T cells, predominantly CD4-positive cells.[75] In the past, a B-cell origin had been proposed based on the presence of either surface or cytoplasmic immunoglobulins.[76] However, there is a lack of evidence of monoclonality and/or synthesis or immunoglobulin associated with Reed–Sternberg cells. The immunoglobulin is probably passively absorbed via IgG Fc receptors present on the neoplastic cells and later internalized into the cytoplasm. Internalization of cytophilic antibody has been shown in vitro, and similar binding in vivo might result in the presence of immunoglobulin on the surface of and within the neoplastic cells.[71]

Later observations suggested that the Reed–Sternberg cell might be related to the "histiocytic" system, in particular, to an antigen-presenting cell rather than a phagocytic cell.[77] Although Reed–Sternberg cells have Ia antigens and Fc receptors, they have never been observed to be phagocytic. They also lack the lysosomal enzymes characteristic of phagocytic cells. Rather, the cytochemical profile of Reed–Sternberg cells resembles that of interdigitating reticulum cells, which are involved in antigen presentation to T cells and are usually identified in the lymph node paracortex. An interesting feature is that normal lymphocytes, particularly T cells, tend to form rosettes with Reed–Sternberg cells. This tendency resembles a phenomenon normally demonstrated by T cells and histiocytes.

A useful diagnostic feature, which does not necessarily shed light on the cell of origin of Hodgkin's disease, is the reactivity of Reed–Sternberg cells and their mononuclear counterparts with Leu M1, a monoclonal antibody that reacts with normal granulocytes.[79] This reagent works in paraffin-embedded sections and thus has considerable clinical utility. Reactivity is positive in most cases, with the exception of the lymphocyte-predominant variant, which is usually negative. Leu M1 detects a sugar sequence containing lacto-*N*-fucopenatose.

Recently, investigators have established Hodgkin's disease–derived cell lines that share many of the phenotypic characteristics of freshly isolated Reed–Sternberg cells.[80] The cells express Ia antigens and form rosettes with T lymphocytes but usually lack demonstrable Fc and C3 receptors. Moreover, they fail to secrete lysozyme or perform phagocytosis. However, they do appear to fit the hypothesis of Reed–Sternberg cells as antigen-presenting cells, as they form rosettes with and can present antigen to normal T lymphocytes.[81] A monoclonal antibody, Ki-1 (CD30), which was prepared against these Hodgkin's-derived cell lines, also reacts with Hodgkin's cells in frozen sections of involved nodes.[82] In normal lymphoid tissues, this monoclonal antibody stains rare small mononuclear cells. The antibody is not entirely specific for Hodgkin's cells, also staining certain high-grade T-cell immunoblastic lymphomas.[83,84] The CD30 antigen is also expressed on activated T cells, B cells, and Epstein–Barr virus–transformed cell lines. Thus, the CD30 antigen is unlikely to shed light on the cell of origin of Hodgkin's disease.

More recent hypotheses have come full circle to present evidence for a lymphoid origin for Hodgkin's disease. Although Reed–Sternberg cells do not express lineage-specific markers, they do express antigens characteristic of activated T or B lymphocytes. The cells express interleukin-2 receptors, transferrin receptors, HLA–DR antigens, and Ki-1, all features of activated lymphocytes.[85] The application of molecular probes has yielded further support for a lymphoid origin. Clonal rearrangements of T-cell receptor β-chain genes and immunoglobulin genes have been shown in several instances, in particular, in those cases containing numerous malignant cells or enriched for malignant cells.[86–89] Clonal rearrangements have not been seen in the background lymphocytes. Rearrangements of the T-cell γ-chain gene should not be misconstrued as evidence for a clonal T-cell origin. The T-γ gene has a limited number of V genes —only seven or eight. Thus, a polyclonal population of T cells, when probed with T-γ, will show a discrete number of bands. These bands should not be misinterpreted as evidence of monoclonality.[90]

In contrast to most subtypes of Hodgkin's disease, the nodular subtype of lymphocyte predominant appears more closely related to the B-cell system than to the T-cell system. Affected lymph nodes contain large numbers of polyclonal B lymphocytes, and this subtype of Hodgkin's disease often coexists with or is preceded by a process known as *progressive transformation of germinal centers*.[52] It has been suggested that the atypical cells express B1 (CD20) and contain J chain, further supporting a B-cell derivation.[91–93] Rare cases of nodular lymphocyte-predominant Hodgkin's disease have progressed to a diffuse large cell lymphoma–like picture, and in those cases studied, a B-cell origin has been shown.[94]

NATURAL HISTORY OF HODGKIN'S DISEASE

Most patients with Hodgkin's disease present to their physicians with superficial adenopathy and are asymptomatic. The lymph node enlargement is usually painless, rubbery, matted, or discrete, and is most commonly located in the

TABLE 49-4. Clinical Features of the Lymphoma

Hodgkin's Disease	*Non-Hodgkin's Lymphoma*
Lymph node disease "centripetal," tends to be in axial lymph nodes	Lymph node disease "centrifugal," noncontinuous
Epitrochlear nodes. Waldeyer's ring, testicular and gastrointestinal sites uncommon	More common involvement of epitrochlear nodes, Waldeyer's ring, testes, and gastrointestinal tract
Mediastinal presentation in over 50% of patients	Mediastinal presentation less common (~20%)
	Distinct syndrome of T-cell lymphoblastic lymphoma with mediastinal presentation most commonly in 2nd or 3rd decades
Abdominal nodal involvement uncommon in asymptomatic but common in older patients or when fever or night sweats present	Abdominal lymph node involvement common
Commonly localized; contiguous nodal disease	Rarely localized nodal disease (<10%)
Bone marrow involvement uncommon	Bone marrow involvement common
Liver involvement uncommon; when present, spleen almost always involved; is rare without fever or night sweats	Liver commonly involved in follicular lymphoma, rare in diffuse lymphoma

neck and supraclavicular areas. It is sometimes detected during a physical examination for another reason.

A second common presentation is during routine chest roentgenogram taken for another purpose, as mediastinal Hodgkin's disease is quite common. Table 49-4 contrasts the clinical features of Hodgkin's disease with those of the non-Hodgkin's lymphomas. Emphasized here is the centripetal and axial nature of the lymph nodes; the neck, supraclavicular and mediastinal presentations being common, while subdiaphragmatic presentations are less common. There may be associated symptoms in as many as 40% of Hodgkin's disease patients. These systemic symptoms are fever, night sweats, weight loss, or pruritus, with fever being the most common.[95,96] Frequently, the patient will give a history of the adenopathy waxing and waning before clinical presentation.

DIFFERENTIAL DIAGNOSIS OF LYMPH NODES

Peripheral lymphadenopathy can be the cause of confusion to the physician, and it is often not easy to separate the great variety of causes. In general, Hodgkin's disease lymph nodes are firm, especially those associated with nodular sclerosis. They may be matted, rubbery, or hard. The location of the lymph nodes is important. A display of the lymph node areas is shown in Figure 49-3. Soft, flat, elliptical, 0.5- to 1.0-cm submandibular lymph nodes may normally be palpable in the submandibular and submental regions, as are soft elliptical 0.5-cm nodes in the superficial jugular and posterior cervical chain.[97] These are seen commonly, especially in young patients, in whom they are associated with infectious disease in the mouth or pharynx. Specific infections can be confused with Hodgkin's disease, most commonly, mononucleosis and occasionally toxoplasmosis. Adenopathy resulting from infection usually causes firm and often tender spherical enlargement of lymph nodes. The presence of tenderness favors an infectious origin, although infectious lymph nodes are not always tender. Biopsy should be performed on persistent nodes larger than 1 cm that are spherical and firm and present for longer than 4 to 8 weeks, as well as on discrete, hard, nontender, matted nodes, especially in older patients. Lymph nodes in the neck may be due to other tumors. Nasopharyngeal cancers often drain to the posterior cervical lymph nodes and make their first presentation as enlargements of these nodes. Thyroid cancer often presents primarily with lymph node involvement. The supraclavicular lymph nodes drain both the thorax and abdomen. The left side is more commonly associated with lesions of the abdomen while the right side is more commonly associated with intrathoracic disease, either malignant or infectious. Isolated axillary lymph node involvement may be related to local infection or other tumors such as non-Hodgkin's lymphoma or breast cancer.

THORACIC PRESENTATIONS

Mediastinal lymphadenopathy is quite common in Hodgkin's disease, occurring in approximately 50% of patients. Its highest frequency occurs in young women.[95] The differential diagnosis of mediastinal or hilar adenopathy is complex. Mediastinal adenopathy alone may be due to benign or malignant masses arising from mediastinal structures. In young people, malignant tumors to be considered include other lymphomas and testicular tumors. When hilar lymphadenopathy is also present, a pulmonary source of the problem should be sought. This category includes both infections and sarcoid and malignant tumors. Formerly, Hodgkin's disease of the thymus was considered a separate entity called *granulomatous thymoma*. As a result of careful studies, this now appears to be Hodgkin's disease involvement of the thymus gland and should be considered no different than other mediastinal Hodgkin's disease.

ABDOMINAL PRESENTATIONS

While Hodgkin's disease often involves the spleen, liver, and retroperitoneal lymph nodes, primary presentation in these sites is less common and more often associated with the non-Hodgkin's lymphomas. When Hodgkin's disease does present primarily within the abdomen, it is usually asso-

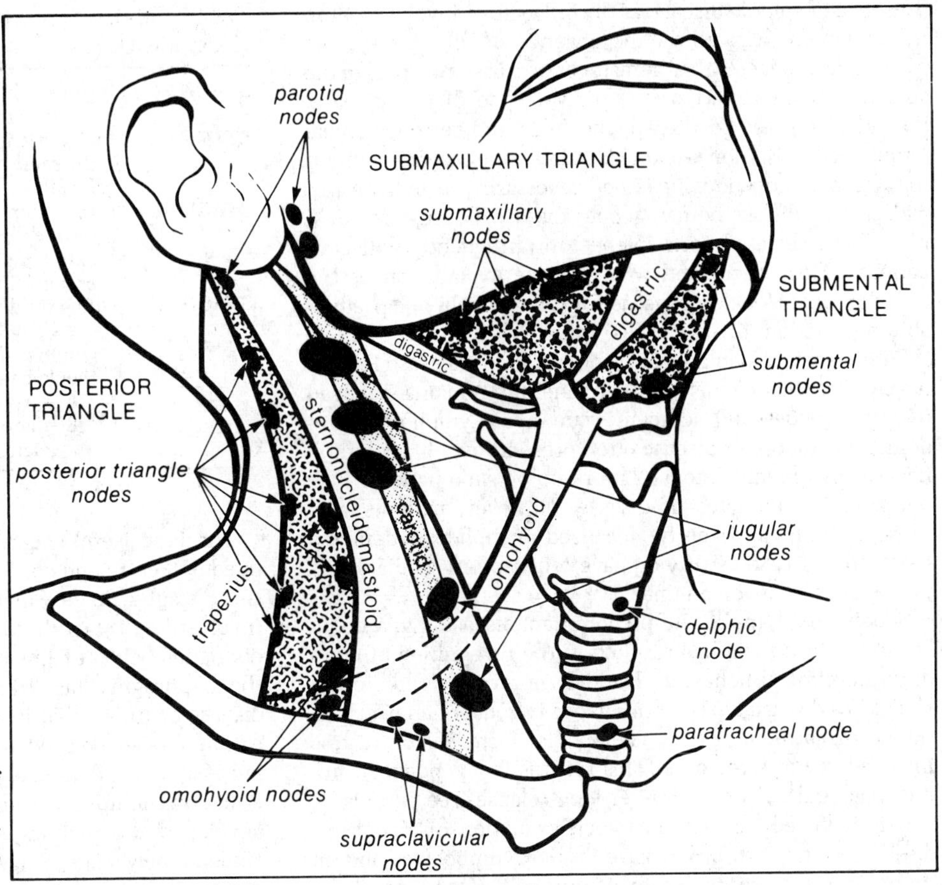

FIG. 49-3. Anatomical subdivisions of the neck depicting lymph node areas. (Adapted from Sade HH: Palpable cervical lymph nodes. JAMA 168:496, 1958)

ciated with systemic symptoms—in patients over the age of 40 years—and with mixed cellularity or lymphocyte-depleted histology. The diagnosis of abdominal Hodgkin's disease is usually made at laparotomy as a part of the staging workup or in the diagnostic evaluation for fever of undetermined origin, and occasionally for unexplained splenomegaly. Hodgkin's disease can involve the retroperitoneal lymph nodes but rarely the mesenteric nodes or Peyer's patches. These presentations are much more common in the non-Hodgkin's lymphomas.

OTHER CLINICAL PRESENTATIONS

Hodgkin's disease should be considered in the differential diagnosis of superior vena cava syndrome and acute spinal cord compression. These conditions seldom are manifested on initial presentation, but they are much more commonly associated with advancing disease. Hodgkin's disease rarely presents as solitary central nervous system disease, Waldeyer's ring, or as testicular masses. These presentations, like intestinal involvement, are far more common in the non-Hodgkin's lymphomas.[98,99]

DISEASE EVOLUTION

Initially, Hodgkin's disease was thought to be capricious in its presentation, natural history, and lymph node involvement. It was first suspected by the Swiss radiotherapist Gilbert[100,101] to spread by contiguity. His work was expanded by Peters, Kaplan, and others,[102–105] who tested the value of prophylactic radiotherapy to lymph nodes adjacent to those involved with disease. With the advent of bipedal lymphangiography in the early 1960s and routine use of staging laparotomy, a better understanding of the evolution of this disease was reached.[106–108]

Hodgkin's disease appears to be contiguous, involving the adjacent lymph nodes first. It may extend to the adjacent viscera and, if unchecked, disseminate to the spleen, bone marrow, liver, bone, and other organs in a fashion somewhat resembling metastases from epithelial cancers.[109] Left cervical lymph node involvement is more common than right-sided and is more often associated with involvement of the retroperitoneal lymph nodes. However, in 15% of patients with involvement of the left cervical nodes and retroperitoneum, the mediastinal lymph nodes are not involved. This skipping of the mediastinum led to the suggestion that Hodgkin's disease sometimes does not spread by contiguity. Kaplan suggested that spread to the left cervical region was due to retroperitoneal nodes' being involved through retrograde spread from the supraclavicular fossa to the thoracic duct.[109] While this hypothesis has been questioned because of the physiologic pressure required to develop retrograde flow, a close association clearly exists between these two sites of involvement.[110–114] The spleen may be involved with tumor when the remainder of the abdomen is normal; this will be discussed further in the section on staging laparotomy. The presence of splenic disease as the only site of involvement in the abdomen, as well as the absence of afferent splenic lymphatics, suggests that hematogenous dissemination to the spleen may be a part of the early course of this disease. Spread of disease to the splenic hilar and retroperitoneal lymph nodes is then assumed. While splenic involvement may be hematogenous, it is not necessarily an indicator of widespread, diffuse hematogenous disease, because regional radiation associated with splenectomy frequently will cure patients. Most important, whatever the explanation, is the orderliness of Hodgkin's disease. It is contiguous and predictable not random or capricious, in its spread.

Patients with nodular sclerosing Hodgkin's disease tend to have upper thoracic disease that generally remains localized in lymph nodes and adjacent structures. Lymphocyte-predominant Hodgkin's disease often presents as solitary lymph node involvement. Extensive work-up on such patients may not reveal other sites of disease. However, patients who present with apparently localized lymphocyte-depleted Hodgkin's disease usually do have other, often subdiaphragmatic, sites of involvement.[115,116]

Subdividing lymphocyte-predominant disease into a nodular and diffuse form has resulted in the recognition of quite different clinical behavior. The diffuse form acts like other Hodgkin's disease types, with relapse infrequent and early in the post-treatment period. The nodular form, in contrast, is involved in more relapses. This form is independent of initial stage and occurs even after long relapse-free periods.[117]

It is believed that the histologic evolution of Hodgkin's disease occurs with progressive loss of lymphocytes and an increase in the number of malignant cells. One type of the disease probably begins as lymphocyte-predominant disease and evolves into mixed cellularity and eventually lymphocyte-depleted Hodgkin's disease. In patients who present initially with nodular sclerosing disease, a progressive depletion of lymphocytes and an increase in the number of malignant cells will develop.[118] The reasons for this development, however, are unknown.

Histologic characteristics and stage are correlated. Lymphocyte-predominant and nodular sclerosing Hodgkin's disease are more commonly seen in Stages I and II disease, whereas mixed cellularity and lymphocyte-depleted disease are more common in advanced stages. Untreated Hodgkin's disease is rare today because both chemotherapy and radiation therapy are effective curative treatments. As Craft[119] described, if the disease is left untreated, the course is brief, measuring 1 to 2 years with fewer than 5% of patients alive at 5 years.

DIAGNOSIS AND STAGING

Hodgkin's disease can be diagnosed securely only with a biopsy. Occasionally, multiple biopsies are necessary for proper diagnosis because reactive hyperplasia of lymph nodes adjacent to those involved by tumor may lead to biopsy of a node that is easily accessible but uninvolved.[120] Needle aspiration of lymph nodes is never adequate for initial diagnosis because it is impossible to subclassify the disease with the limited amounts of biopsy material provided.

TABLE 49-5. Ann Arbor Staging Classification for Hodgkin's Disease

STAGE I	Involvement of a single lymph node region (I) or a single extralymphatic organ or site (I_E)
STAGE II	Involvement of two or more lymph node regions on the same side of the diaphragm (II) or localized involvement of an extralymphatic organ or site (II_e)
STAGE III	Involvement of lymph node regions on both sides of the diaphragm (III) or localized involvement of an extralymphatic organ or site (III_E) or spleen (III_S) or both (III_{Se})
STAGE IV	Diffuse or disseminated involvement of one or more extralymphatic organs with or without associated lymph node involvement. The organ(s) involved should be identified by a symbol: A = Asymptomatic B = Fever, sweats, weight loss >10% of body weight

The first useful staging for Hodgkin's disease was developed by Peters and colleagues.[121] It divided the patients into three stages. Stage I included patients with a single site of involvement. Stage II comprised patients with two or more contiguous sites of involvement, but limited to one side of the diaphragm. Stage III included those with extensive nodal disease or tumor that involved visceral organs. This classification was elaborated on and modified because its initial purpose was to delineate patients who were most suitable for radiation therapy treatment.[95] In 1965, a staging system was developed at a meeting in Rye, New York. This system included a new stage, Stage IV, for patients with disseminated disease outside the lymph node system.[122] This was modified at the Ann Arbor Staging Conference in 1970, as shown in Table 49-5.[123]

The Ann Arbor version modifies the previous classification in two major ways. First, based on therapeutic data provided by Musshoff, patients whose disease has spread contiguously from lymph nodes to adjacent organs are not considered to be in Stage IV; they are classified by the extent of lymph node involvement (Stage I–III) followed by the subscript *E*, which denotes direct extension.[124] Second, involvement of the spleen is indicated by the subscript *S*. In all systems, patients are classified further as either *A* or *B* on the basis of the absence or presence of constitutional symptoms such as fever higher than 38°C for three consecutive days, night sweats, or unexplained loss of more than 10% of body weight. At the Ann Arbor meeting, it was decided that pruritus, previously considered an important systemic symptom, did not by itself have prognostic value and was not sufficient to include a patient in the B category.

Table 49-6 outlines the proper staging procedures.[125] Staging starts with a detailed history and physical examination. The history must be careful to determine the presence or absence of systemic symptoms and to note whether symptoms suggest extranodal involvement. Physical examination should record the extent of lymph node involvement. Basic laboratory tests include evaluation of renal and hepatic function as well as the more important complete blood count, erythrocyte sedimentation rate, and serum alkaline phosphatase. Roentgenographic studies include the chest roentgenogram and thoracic computed tomography (CT) to evalu-

TABLE 49-6. Required Evaluation Procedures in Staging Hodgkin's Disease

1. Adequate surgical biopsy, reviewed by an experienced hematologist
2. A detailed history recording duration and the presence or absence of fever, unexplained sweating and its severity, unexplained pruritus, and unexplained weight loss
3. A careful and detailed physical examination; special attention to all node-bearing areas, including Waldeyer's ring, and determination of size of liver and spleen
4. Necessary laboratory procedures
   a. Complete blood count, including an erythrocytic sedimentation rate
   b. Serum alkaline phosphatase
   c. Evaluation of renal function
   d. Evaluation of liver function
5. Radiologic studies including
   a. Chest roentgenogram (posterior–anterior and lateral)
   b. Chest and abdominal computed tomography scan
   c. Bilateral lower extremity lymphogram
   d. Views of skeletal system to include thoracic and lumbar vertebrae, the pelvis, proximal extremities, and any areas of bone tenderness

ate mediastinal lymphadenopathy and any extension of such adenopathy into the surrounding viscera. Abdominal involvement is evaluated using the lower extremity lymphogram and abdominal CT. With the advent of CT, the routine use of the bipedal lymphogram has been questioned. The Stanford group[126] has shown that the sensitivity appears similar for both tests. However, specificity appears better for lymphangiography. The lymphogram, while more labor intensive, can be used during laparotomy to ensure the removal of nodes in question and can identify abnormal nodes when they are not enlarged. The CT scan is easier to administer and more valuable in the assessment of hepatic portal and celiac lymph nodes.

Bone marrow biopsy, not aspiration, is required. Bone marrow biopsy is particularly important in symptomatic patients and in those with bone lesions, bone pain, hypercalcemia, or an elevated serum alkaline phosphatase.[127–131] Isotope scanning of the liver, spleen, and bone may be helpful in defining sites of additional disease.[131] Gallium scanning may be useful, especially with the recently developed higher-dose (7–10 mCi) imaging on a triple-peak Anger camera. Single-photon emission CT (SPECT) has resulted in the occasional finding of unexpected disease but is more useful in determining suspected recurrence in previously treated patients.[132] Magnetic resonance imaging (MRI) may prove useful. Recent evidence suggests that lymphomatous involvement of lymph nodes may have a different MRI pattern than fibrosis. This finding, like gallium scanning, may be more important in evaluating patients for recurrence following treatment.

STAGING LAPAROTOMY

Staging laparotomy was originally developed by the Stanford group to provide information about the patterns of involvement in subdiaphragmatic Hodgkin's disease.[108] Its justification is that it may alter therapy.[133] If the procedure is done, it must be carried out by physicians skilled in the technique who will perform it in a consistent fashion.[134,135] It should include detailed inspection of the abdomen. The removed spleen should be sectioned in 0.3-cm slices. If disease is identified in the spleen, the total number of nodules should be enumerated. In all cases, the weight of the spleen should be determined. Examination of the liver should include a wedge biopsy of the right lobe as well as three needle biopsies of both the right and left lobes, and a biopsy of any grossly abnormal hepatic lesions. After inspection and palpation of the nodal groups, a biopsy should be taken of the right and left para-aortic and iliac nodes regardless of their character on palpation and even if they appear normal on lymphangiography. Of course, suspicious nodes identified on lymphangiography should be removed. In addition, lymph nodes should be removed from the splenic hilar, portal hepatic, mesenteric, and iliac regions. At one time, oophoropexy, the placement of the ovaries out of their normal position to shield them from pelvic irradiation, was recommended in young female patients. This method is no longer recommended, because the use of pelvic irradiation has been nearly eliminated. Iliac bone marrow biopsy should be performed at the time of operation.

It is not possible to review the information gained from routine use of staging laparotomy. The early studies noted that alterations in treatment were made as frequently as 35% of the time as a result of the findings obtained at surgical staging.[136] Currently, CT, MRI, and modern gallium scanning are all useful in lymph node evaluation and may reduce this number somewhat. While laparotomy may change the stage, it should be only part of routine staging when the change in stage is likely to result in a change of therapy, as indicated in the section on treatment by stage. Thus, the treatment approaches in use at any institution should influence the judgment as to whether laparotomy should be performed.

It is important to note that the major site of occult disease in the abdomen is in the spleen, and none of these studies evaluates splenic involvement. Even splenic enlargement is poorly predictive of involvement.[137] A recent review of 692 patients staged by laparotomy seen at the Joint Center for

TABLE 49-7. Upstaging of 552 Clinical Stage I and II Patients by Clinical Parameter

Subgroup	*% Pathologic Stage III–IV*	*Level (Cox Multi)*
Gender		
M	29	0.004
F	18	
Symptomatic stage		
A	21	0.02
B	34	
Sites		
1	17	0.0006
≥2	27	
Age		
≤39	23	0.09
≥40	30	
Histology		
LP/NS	23	NS
MC/LD	27	

Adapted from Mauch P et al.[418]

TABLE 49-8. Downstaging of 140 Clinical Stage III–IV Patients by Clinical Parameters

Subgroup	*Pathologic Stage I–II*	*Level (Cox Multi)*
Symptomatic stage		
A	55	0.001
B	22	
Age		
≤39	48	0.01
≥40	21	
Gender		
M	43	NS
F	40	
Sites		
1	52	NS
≥2	40	
Histology		
NS/LP	55	0.004
MC/LD	28	

Adapted from Mauch P et al.[418]

Radiation Therapy (JCRT) between April 1969 and December 1986 by Mauch and colleagues indicates that there is still considerable change of stage as a result of staging laparotomy (Mauch et al, in preparation). Table 49-7 shows the extent of upstaging of clinical Stages I and II patients and indicates the importance of a variety of prognostic features. In general, men are more likely to have Stage III disease, as are patients who are symptomatic or have more than one site of involvement. The group with the most favorable prognosis, asymptomatic female patients with only a single site of supradiaphragmatic involvement, were found to have Stage III disease only 6% of the time. No other subgroup had less than an 18% likelihood of occult subdiaphragmatic disease. The use of staging laparotomy was equally important for patients of clinical Stage III or IV (Table 49-8). Reduction of stage occurred in more than half of those without systemic symptoms. A similar frequency in downstaging was found for patients with favorable histology or who were less than 40 years of age.

A further subclassification of the Ann Arbor staging system has been proposed by Desser and associates.[138,139] They analyzed patients with Stage III disease to determine whether the location of involved abdominal sites influenced survival. They found that patients with disease limited to the spleen or splenic, celiac, or portal nodes (anatomic substage III_1) had a more favorable survival rate than did those patients with involvement of para-aortic, iliac, or mesenteric nodes (anatomic substage III_2).

COMPLICATIONS OF STAGING LAPAROTOMY

Staging laparotomy is a major surgical procedure with established morbidity and mortality.[140–142] Institutions with the most extensive experience report mortality statistics as low as 0.5%.[143] Nevertheless, one study of a cooperative hospital experience reported a 27% morbidity and a 6.6% mortality.[144] Morbidity may include wound infection, subphrenic abscess, pulmonary embolus, stress ulcer, gastrointestinal bleeding, pulmonary infection, and wound dehiscence. The recent JCRT review of 692 patients revealed 0.3% mortality, small-bowel obstruction in 1.3%, wound or subdiaphragmatic abscess in 1.3%, and bleeding in 0.4% (Mauch et al, in preparation).

Staging laparotomy and splenectomy need special consideration in children. Although the complication rate is similar to that observed in adults,[145] of great concern is the increased incidence of severe, sudden, overwhelming infection seen in children after staging laparotomy and splenectomy.[140–142,146–148] The risk of this complication increases as age decreases below 10 years. Therefore, it seems prudent to be selective in the use of such procedures in the very young.[149,150]

It has been suggested that splenectomy allows the patient to tolerate chemotherapy or radiation more easily. While it is true that the blood counts may be higher, this does not appear to affect response or survival rates.[151–154] At present, no evidence suggests that splenectomy improves the ability to administer chemotherapy, increases the response rate, or alters the survival rate.[125] Laparotomy does, however, treat the involved spleen. The reduction of the irradiated field required may permit the physician to avoid irradiating a significant portion of the stomach, intestine, left kidney, and left lower lobe of the lung. Post-treatment laparotomy as a guide to further management has had mixed results and should not be considered a useful routine procedure.[155,156]

Patterns of Anatomical Distribution

Figure 49-4 shows the frequency of sites of involvement of Hodgkin's disease in 285 consecutive patients evaluated using full pathologic staging by the Stanford University

FIG. 49-4. Hodgkin's disease showing the anatomical distribution of sites of involvement in 285 consecutive, unselected, previously untreated cases. (Adapted from Kaplan HS, Dorfman RF, Nelson TS et al: Staging laparotomy and splenectomy in Hodgkin's disease: Analysis of indications and patterns of involvement in 285 consecutive, unselected patients. Natl Cancer Inst Monogr 36:291, 1973)

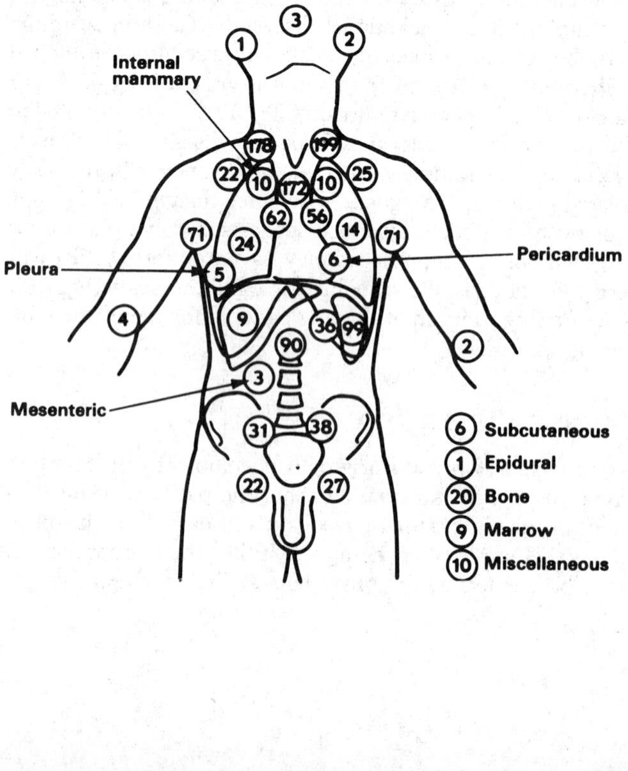

group.[137] These data emphasize the rarity of nonaxial locations such as epitrochlear, popliteal, and mesenteric nodes. The prominence of the supraclavicular and mediastinal sites as well as the spleen is shown. Pleural effusions with low specific gravity and low protein content are usually simple transudates. Neither these nor exudative pleural effusions can be regarded as indicative of pleural invasion of Hodgkin's disease. Such a diagnosis requires histologic confirmation by either pleural biopsy or open thoracotomy. Often, these effusions are the consequence of hilar or pulmonary involvement. Pericardial involvement may occur as a result of direct invasion from mediastinal lymphadenopathy.

Liver involvement without splenic involvement is rare in Hodgkin's disease. The risk of liver involvement increases as the size of the involved spleen increases. Liver involvement is unusual in patients who have normal-sized spleens even if the spleens are involved in Hodgkin's disease,[95,125] Bone marrow involvement with Hodgkin's disease is associated with extensive tumor and usually with systemic symptoms.[157,158] Usually, leukopenia, anemia, or thrombocytopenia are not seen, although an elevated alkaline phosphatase may give some hint of bone marrow involvement. It is necessary to take a bone marrow biopsy, using either an open surgical technique or a cutting needle. The bones themselves may be involved, especially in patients with advanced disease. Rarely, one can see local invasion of the bone by adjacent lymphadenopathy. The bone lesions are usually osteolytic but may be osteoblastic and quite characteristic. Radioisotopic bone scans may reveal focal areas of increased uptake when conventional roentgenograms are normal.[159] Such findings are not definite evidence of involvement and must be confirmed histologically. Involvement of the bone should not be equated with involvement of the marrow unless there is other evidence of widely disseminated disease. Musshoff and Boutis[160] have demonstrated long-term disease-free survival in patients with isolated bone lesions when treated appropriately with radiotherapy.

Involvement of the skin, subcutaneous tissue, and breast can occur with Hodgkin's disease.[161] The disease rarely involves the central nervous system,[99,162,163] although invasion of the epidural space can occur by extension through the intervertebral foramina from para-aortic lymph nodes, with neurologic symptoms and pain being the predominant clinical features. In contrast to the other malignant lymphomas, Hodgkin's disease rarely arises in the gastrointestinal tract. Compression of the ureters from lymphadenopathy may occur. Unusual urologic complications of Hodgkin's disease are lipoid nephrosis and amyloid nephrosis, which may occur at a time when no other clinical manifestations of persistence or recurrence may be detected.[164,165] They have been reported to regress with effective antitumor treatment.[166]

IMMUNOLOGIC ABNORMALITIES

The first systematic study of the capacity of patients with Hodgkin's disease to react to a battery of antigens was reported in 1956 by Schier and associates.[167] They reported that the delayed reactivity to purified tuberculin, *Trichophyton gypseum, Candida albicans*, and mumps skin test antigens was severely depressed. Lamb and colleagues[168] first suggested that the absence of a skin test response might indicate that anergy was related to the primary disease process itself. The first definitive study of the question of the relationship of anergy to the stage of Hodgkin's disease awaited the modern era of staging in 1967.[169] Response to two or more antigens in patients with Stage I disease was similar to controls, and responsiveness decreased with increasing stage. It was concluded that anergy was the consequence of progressive Hodgkin's disease.

In 1965, studies of in vitro lymphocyte response to various antigens also showed a striking impairment in the lymphoblastic transformation capacity of peripheral blood lymphocytes from patients with Hodgkin's disease.[170] Lymphocyte transformation once again diminished with increasing stage. Refinement of techniques for measuring in vitro lymphocyte response showed that defects were present even in patients with the earliest stages of disease,[171,172] and, in the 1970s, techniques for phenotyping lymphocytes localized the defect to T lymphocytes. The capacity to form spontaneous E-rosettes with uncoated sheep erythrocytes, a characteristic of T cells, for example, is impaired in Hodgkin's disease. That the defect might be due to the effect of suppressor cells was highlighted by Bobrove and co-workers[173] and Twomey and colleagues,[174] who reported that in vitro response of lymphocytes to antigens was increased when mononuclear cells were removed by passage through glass wool. Goodwin and associates[175] also found that the inhibitory activity of glass-adherent cells in culture could be reduced by adding indomethacin, leading to the suggestion that production of prostaglandin E_2 by suppressor cells could be responsible for lymphocyte hyporesponsiveness. Increased sensitivity to suppressor responses has been reported by other investigators as well.[176–179] The ratio of CD4- to CD8-positive T-cell subsets has recently been shown to be somewhat depressed at diagnosis; in those patients with long-lasting remissions, there is a redistribution of the T-cell subsets with a significant increase in the CD8 population, particularly those expressing the natural killer phenotype—that is, coexpressing both Leu-7 and CD8.[180,181]

Increasing numbers of long survivors provided the opportunity to restudy anergy and in vitro lymphocyte responsiveness in patients who have been successfully treated. Studies at the National Cancer Institute (NCI) in a well-defined and substantial population of uniformly staged and treated patients showed that anergy did not influence prognosis within a given stage; after successful treatment, anergy to recall antigens was reversible, although response to neoantigens remained suppressed.[137,182,183] Fisher and co-workers[185] have shown that, although the total number of circulating lymphocytes in patients who have been in remission for anywhere from 1.3 to 12.8 years (mean, 6.5 years) was not different from normals, the percentage of E-rosetting cells and the response to concanavalin-A and phytohemagglutinin were significantly depressed when compared to normal controls. Patients with normal numbers of T cells also had depressed in vitro response to antigens and were abnormally sensitive to the suppressor effects of concanavalin-A–activated lymphocytes and suppressor monocytes when compared to normal controls. This defect also persisted for long disease-free periods.[184,185] That this defect seems to be related to the disease itself is reinforced by the fact that patients with other types of lymphomas treated with a similar chemotherapy regimen did not have evidence of such a defect.[186,187]

Lymphopenia is common in advanced stages of Hodgkin's disease and is also induced by treatment, particularly by radiotherapy. Its most profound effect is in depressing the CD4:CD8 ratio. Radiotherapy-induced lymphopenia returns to normal within 12 to 111 months after cessation of treatment.[188-190] Because the CD8-positive population appears relatively unaffected by radiotherapy, and the CD4-positive lymphocyte population regenerates very slowly after treatment is discontinued, the profound deficiency in T-helper cells induced by radiotherapy may explain the clinical features of immunodeficiency, with an excess of herpes zoster infection during the first and second years after cessation of radiotherapy.[191-194] The immunologic profiles of patients with Hodgkin's disease before and after treatment are summarized in Table 49-9.[187]

A number of other immunologic abnormalities have been noted. Although the response of peripheral blood monocytes to interleukin-2 appears to be normal, decreased production of interleukin-2 by peripheral blood mononuclear cells has been reported.[195] Natural killer cell activity is also diminished at the time of diagnosis but improves with successful therapy.[196-198] Studies of polymorphonuclear leukocyte function in Hodgkin's disease reveal a persistent abnormality in neutrophil killing attributable to an intrinsic, although unexplained, defect in the leukocyte.[199,200]

With better definition of the immunologic defect in Hodgkin's disease, and in contrast to older reports, some workers have reported that immunologic abnormalities may serve as prognostic indicators.[201-203] A study by Van Rijswijk and associates[203] showed that, while crude estimates of immune capacity such as skin test reactivity, total lymphocyte counts, and total number of T cells and B cells did not relate to prognosis, lymphocyte response in mixed lymphocyte cultures did have prognostic importance, especially when coupled with age, and it may be useful as an initial prognostic indicator.[204,205] However, these studies suffer from the fact that they consistently include fewer than 50 patients, the patients have a variety of disease stages, and the patients are treated in a variety of ways. These studies, therefore, do not lend themselves to consistent conclusions about the value of immunologic testing as part of the staging work-up.

In contrast to the defects in delayed hypersensitivity, most studies of humoral response have shown that the antibody response of B cells and that B-cell numbers are normal in all but patients with the most advanced Hodgkin's disease, although (as discussed below) B-cell function is affected by therapy. In the early study by Schier and associates,[167] it was reported that 12 patients had normal antibody response to mumps vaccine. In the study by Brown and colleagues,[169] a normal antibody response to tularemia antigen was noted, even though there was no evidence of hypersensitivity to the tularemia skin test. Also, antibody responses to pneumococcal polysaccharides in patients with Hodgkin's disease who were known to be unresponsive to dinitrochlorobenzene (DNCB) were normal.[167,206,207]

B-cell function, however, is affected by treatment. While splenectomy alone does not alter B-cell function, the combination of splenectomy and chemotherapy, or splenectomy, chemotherapy, and radiotherapy, diminished B-cell function, as measured by antibody response to several bacterial antigens. Weitzman and colleagues measured antibody response to *Haemophilus influenza* type B in patients who had received radiation therapy, chemotherapy, or both after splenectomy.[208] Antibody titers were reduced significantly in patients receiving multimodality therapy or combination chemotherapy alone, but they were not significantly reduced in those who received radiotherapy alone. Patients who underwent splenectomy but had not yet begun treatment had normal antibody responses. Immunoglobulin levels, likewise, were normal in untreated patients, but chemotherapy significantly reduced levels of IgM, an effect that was potentiated in the group undergoing splenectomy. Minor and coworkers[209] examined the response of 41 successfully treated patients to pneumococcal vaccine, all of whom had undergone splenectomy. The postimmunization antibody level was significantly lower for 10 of 12 serotypes measured. Antibody recovery was time dependent from the end of treatment, with several patients in remission more than three years having normal responses. Pneumococcal sepsis was seen in one case and meningitis in another despite vaccination.

A recent study by Siber and colleagues[44] examined more

TABLE 49-9. Immunologic Profiles of Patients with Hogdkin's Disease Before and After Successful Treatment

	Untreated Active Disease	*Disease-Free Survivors*
Delayed hypersensitivity skin tests		
Recall antigens	Anergic	Reactive
Neoantigens	Anergic	Anergic
E-rosette formation	Decreased	Decreased
Mitogen-induced T-cell proliferation	Decreased	Decreased
Prostaglandin-mediated suppression	Present	Absent
Sensitivity to suppressor monocytes	Increased	Increased
Sensitivity to suppressor T cells	Increased	Increased
CD4 : CD8 T-cell ratio	Decreased	Decreased

Data from Fisher RI.[187]

closely the issue of pretreatment vaccination of patients with Hodgkin's disease. Fifty-one patients were vaccinated with the 14-valent Pneumococcus vaccine, combined with *Haemophilus influenza* type B and meningococcus type C. Their response was compared to normal control samples and to control patients rendered asplenic for reasons other than the staging of Hodgkin's disease. They found that the geometric mean of natural antibodies to these bacterial polysaccharides was not significantly different among the three groups. Peak response to vaccination also did not vary, with the exception of the response to meningococcal group C, which was significantly lower in patients with Hodgkin's disease. Persistence of antibody levels in Hodgkin's disease patients was also similar to that of healthy controls, asplenic controls, and patients treated with radiation therapy only. However, patients who received either chemotherapy or chemotherapy plus radiotherapy had more significant and rapid declines in antibody levels, to 10% to 20% of peak levels, as well as declines in the levels of natural antibodies. Timing of splenectomy was not important to the development of antibody response, but the timing of initiation of treatment was significant. Patients receiving chemotherapy or combined modality therapy less than 10 days after vaccination had significantly lower antibody responses. The authors concluded that antibody response in patients with untreated Hodgkin's disease is normal, and is not affected by either the stage or the procedures used for staging the disease. Vaccination of all patients 10 to 14 days before the initiation of chemotherapy is therefore appropriate.[210,211] Because there is no response to booster vaccinations within the first year, boosters are not recommended, although no data are available to evaluate the effect of booster vaccination at a later time.[33] It should be reemphasized, however, that neither immunization nor antibiotic prophylaxis can be guaranteed to prevent the development of sepsis due to encapsulated microorganisms in patients with Hodgkin's disease whose staging included splenectomy and who have been heavily treated with chemotherapy and/or radiotherapy. Vaccinated patients and antibiotic-treated patients should remain alert to the risk.

Taken in full, the data indicate that the functional defect in the immune system in Hodgkin's disease appears simultaneously with the appearance of the disease itself. The defect is aggravated by treatment, particularly radiotherapy, and persists in a variable, time-dependent way, with some recovery occurring after treatment is discontinued. With the exception of rare cases of autoimmune hemolytic anemia and autoimmune thrombocytopenia, a mildly increased incidence of herpes zoster, and the rare occurrence of overwhelming sepsis related to splenectomy and therapy, the immune system of patients with Hodgkin's disease appears to function quite well, given the large number of immune defects that have been described. Opportunistic infections are relatively rare, and second malignancies appear to be more a function of the use of a combined chemotherapy and radiotherapy regimen than the underlying immune defect itself. Placed, now, in the context of the defect found in patients with AIDS, these immunologic abnormalities have more importance with reference to the etiology of the disease itself than as a complicating factor. It is ironic that in Hodgkin's disease, a disease with a defect in T-cell immunity, the major functional immunologic residuum after successful treatment is converted to a defect in humoral immunity.

CLINICAL IMMUNOLOGIC DISORDERS IN HODGKIN'S DISEASE

In comparison to lymphocytic lymphomas, monoclonal protein spikes are less common in Hodgkin's disease. In a study by Ko and Pruzanski[212] of 1246 patients identified in a screening process to have M components in their serum, 62 (0.05%) were found to have lymphomas. In a study of 71 patients with Hodgkin's disease, unexplained positive Coombs' test results were noted in 7 male patients;[213] all had extensive disease (Stages III and IV), and 6 had constitutional symptoms. The Coombs' test results were positive at initial diagnosis in 3 patients and at the time of relapse in 4. Only 3 patients in this group had overt hemolysis. The authors re-emphasized that, when autoimmune hemolytic anemia occurs in lymphoma patients, it is associated with advanced stages. In their series, the antibody was characterized in 3 patients, all of whom fulfilled the criteria for IgG with anti-I^t specificity, as described by Booth and colleagues in 1966.[214] This antibody may be unique for Coombs' test–positive hemolytic anemia associated with Hodgkin's disease.

Waddell and Cimo[215] and Jones[216] were able to locate a total of only 36 cases of idiopathic thrombocytopenic purpura (ITP) in the English literature. An additional case with platelet-associated IgG has been reported by Berkman and co-workers.[217] For 7 patients, no further analysis was done because the data reported were not sufficient to characterize the syndrome. In 3 of the cases, the diagnosis of ITP antedated the diagnosis of lymphoma. In the remaining 24 patients, ITP occurred either at the time of the diagnosis or subsequent to it. The authors pointed out several characteristic features of ITP associated with Hodgkin's disease: (1) Although ITP occurs predominantly in women, ITP associated with Hodgkin's disease is more common in men. (2) ITP associated with Hodgkin's disease appears to be more severe and resistant to treatment than ITP alone or in association with other illnesses. Only 6 of 23 patients, for example, responded to steroids, although 6 of 10 patients who underwent splenectomy specifically for ITP appeared to have a good and durable response. (3) Autoimmune hemolytic anemia, a frequent accompaniment of ITP occurring in other disorders, was present in only 3 of 24 patients in the series. (4) ITP occurred after splenectomy had been performed for staging purposes in 11 reviewed patients. This finding indicates that the antibody responsible for thrombocytopenia can be produced in sites other than the spleen. (5) All the patients with a recorded histology had either nodular sclerosing or mixed cellularity Hodgkin's disease. (6) Most patients develop ITP while in remission after successful radiotherapy or chemotherapy, and the occurrence of ITP did not necessarily indicate relapse. Because most reported cases occurred after splenectomy, the combination of corticosteroids and immunosuppressive drugs is required for treatment. Six patients were treated this way and 4 had excellent response; the other 2 patients had useful responses.

Autoimmune neutropenia has rarely been reported to be associated with Hodgkin's disease. In a recent report by Heyman and Walsh,[218] isolated neutropenia developed in a patient who was asplenic and had been treated 4 years previously for Stage IIA Hodgkin's disease. Bone marrow examination revealed myeloid hyperplasia, and the serum was positive for antigranulocyte antibodies. No evidence existed of recurrent Hodgkin's disease. The two prior reported cases also occurred after splenectomy, suggesting that the spleen plays no role in this disorder and that splenectomy should not be considered as a form of treatment.

RADIATION THERAPY OF HODGKIN'S DISEASE

The extreme radiation responsiveness of the lymphomas was noted shortly after the discovery of x-rays. Pusey,[219] in 1902, reported a series of patients with Hodgkin's disease treated with radiation. In the early part of the century, therapy was limited by the equipment available. The machines had poor depth-dose characteristics and caused extensive skin reactions, thus limiting their usefulness. Despite this drawback, there was a great deal of interest in using radiation on this tumor. Teschendorf,[220] Voorhoeve,[221] and Kruchen[222] described therapy for such patients. It was Gilbert[100,101] who laid the foundation for the principles of modern radiation therapy. Despite the availability of only orthovoltage radiation. Gilbert recognized the importance of treating all involved disease with the maximum dose possible if cure was the goal of treatment. He suggested that, to the extent possible, one should treat adjacent sites because of the frequency of adjacent recurrence. These are the principles of radiotherapy today. Gilbert's technique was followed in Toronto and reported by Peters in 1950.[102] Subsequently, she has reported on patients who were alive as long as 20 years after treatment, indicating that patients could be cured with radiation because there were no recurrences in those patients who were disease-free 10 years after treatment.[103] Peters also first described the staging system for the disease detailed earlier in this chapter. The dose to the involved areas in these reports depended on the site and extent of the disease; the higher doses were given when the disease was relatively localized. The concept of irradiation of adjacent nodal groups with lower doses of radiation was used by Peters. In 1963 Easson and Russell published an article entitled, "The Cure of Hodgkin's Disease."[223] This work reported the long-term results of local treatment of both Hodgkin's disease and localized non-Hodgkin's lymphomas. As indicated in the title, the emphasis of the paper was that Hodgkin's disease could be cured. Other authors in the early 1950s and 1960s also reported the results of localized radiation; however, it was Kaplan and his group at Stanford who systematically studied the role of radiation therapy in the treatment of Hodgkin's disease and devised new techniques using supervoltage radiation to treat the disease.[208,224-229] These pioneering studies form the basis of much of what we know today of the curability of Hodgkin's disease.

Figure 49-5 is redrawn from Kaplan[228] to indicate that,

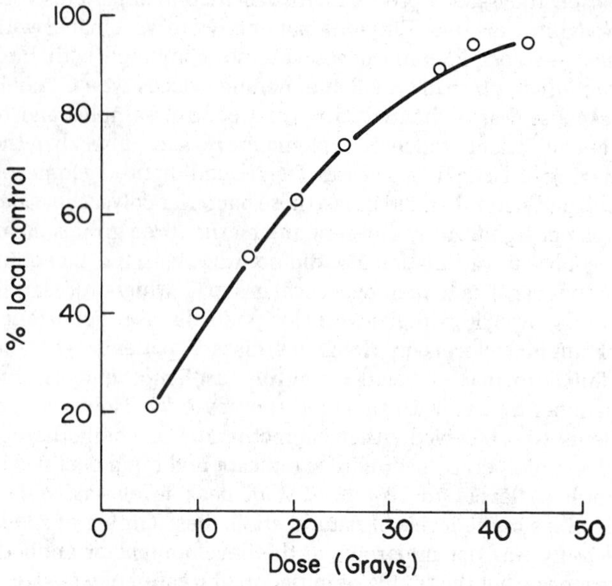

FIG. 49-5. Risk of recurrence in the treatment field after radiotherapy related to dose.

although low doses of radiation cause tumors to disappear, high doses are required to ablate them permanently. Hodgkin's disease, like all other tumors, has a dose–response curve. This was a very important concept, because the prevailing attitude at the time was that, since the disease was so responsive to radiation but, of course, incurable, one should give low doses and make local nodal masses regress while "saving" the radiation tolerance for the required subsequent therapies when the disease reappeared. Such a philosophy of treatment confirmed the self-fulfilling prophecy of the incurability of Hodgkin's disease. As can be seen from the figure, when high doses were given, local recurrence was very uncommon.

The Stanford group provided evidence, suspected by Gilbert and Peters, of the orderliness and continuity of the initial presentation of Hodgkin's disease, as well as of its subsequent extension.[227,229] The adaptation of modern supervoltage techniques for the treatment of Hodgkin's disease for the first time allowed high doses of radiation to be given in extensive volumes, and careful beam direction and shielding allowed such treatment to be tolerated by normal tissues.

Generally, it is recommended that local tumor masses receive "boost therapy" to a minimum dose of 4000 to 4400 rad, whereas apparently uninvolved areas treated for subclinical disease appear to be controlled adequately with doses of 3000 to 3500 rad. Other data suggest that 3000 rad may be sufficient.[230] The dose–time relationship for Hodgkin's disease is less well known. Because of normal tissue tolerance, patient acceptance, and tumor control, tumor doses of between 150 and 220 rad/day given five times a week appear to be most appropriate. When a significant interruption in treatment occurs, it appears that larger doses should be given.[231] Supervoltage radiation must be used to deliver the wide-field radiation required. This method has the advantages of spared skin, increased depth-dose, and sharp beam edges with reduced lateral scatter. A basic tool for the treatment of patients with Hodgkin's disease is the modern linear

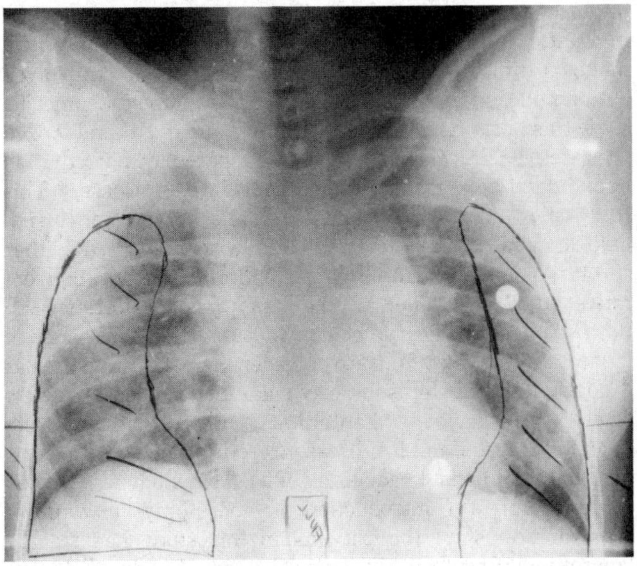

FIG. 49-6. Simulated film for radiation treatment fields in a patient with mediastinal Hodgkin's disease. Dark lines indicate shielding blocks.

accelerator, which provides x-ray beams in the 4-MeV to 8-MeV range. Although cobalt units can be used, conventionally available cobalt units have significant limitations. When used at distances of less than 80 cm, they tend to have poor depth-dose characteristics. They often have far less well defined beam edges, because of the large source and short treatment distances. This latter factor causes significantly greater irradiation of adjacent and apparently shielded tissues.

Hodgkin's disease treatment may be divided into three volumes to be irradiated: the mantle, the para-aortic area, and the pelvis.[232] The mantle technique has been well described by the Stanford group. It is an attempt to treat in continuity the lymph nodes of the neck, axilla, and mediastinum—including the occipital and preauricular lymph nodes—in one contiguous treatment volume. To do this, a wide field is placed on the patient and individually made blocks are fashioned to shield the normal tissues that are not to be treated. For this technique to be done accurately, not only is the supervoltage linear accelerator required, but a treatment-planning simulator or localizer must be available as well. This must allow the duplication of therapy fields using diagnostic-quality radiation so that detailed radiographs can be made for the fabrication of the blocks. Such a simulator film is shown in Figure 49-6 with the appropriate block outlines. The check films are made on the supervoltage machine. However, because of the radiation energy, this film, while useful for check purposes, is much less satisfactory than the simulator films. These blocks can be made to conform to the divergent x-ray beam so that the edge of the field can be as sharp as possible. The mantle treatment irradiates a large volume of normal tissues; therefore, care must be taken to limit the unnecessary normal tissue irradiation while at the same time ensuring adequate irradiation of the tumor volume. This procedure requires careful evaluation and planning, using diagnostic x-rays, CT scans, simulation, and dosimetric calculations and measurements. The normal tissue tolerance of the lung and heart has been evaluated in the course of treatment of Hodgkin's disease.[233-235] Whole-lung irradiation, to a maximum dose of 1650 rad in 150-rad fractions, is used frequently when the ipsilateral hilum is involved with tumor. The whole heart should not be treated unless evidence of pericardial involvement exists. Under normal circumstances, a significant portion of the cardiac silhouette can be shielded. It is very important that the "matchline" between the mantle and the para-aortic area does not allow overlap of a portion of the spinal cord. If this overlap occurs, the dose that is received can cause significant neurologic damage. The geometry involved in proper field arrangement for the matchline can be more complicated than is immediately apparent. Techniques to match these particular fields properly have now been described.[236] Treatments of the para-aortic nodes and pelvis are frequently done together as described by the Stanford group.[237,238] It is the experience of others that this treatment is better tolerated when divided into a para-aortic field and a separate pelvic field. In either circumstance, the para-aortic field must be wide enough to include the para-aortic lymph nodes as demonstrated on the lymphogram.

Most modern radiotherapeutic technique has been influenced by the results of laparotomy. As discussed earlier, laparotomy is only of value if the results may alter therapy. It allows removal of the spleen and the placement of radiopaque clips on the splenic pedicle, so that the radiotherapy field may be tailored accurately to this volume. The normal right side of the para-aortic field, as shown in Figure 49-7, does not treat the porta hepatitis; if it is to be treated, the field must be extended laterally. The same considerations for field overlap apply between the para-aortic and pelvic fields; however, these fields are less critical, because this overlap is placed below the level of the spinal cord. Considerations for the pelvic field include the treatment of the lymph nodes with as little radiation as possible to important sacral and pelvic bone marrow. The place for pelvic treatment has been markedly reduced because, as will be discussed, Stages I and II supradiaphragmatic Hodgkin's disease can be treated without pelvic irradiation, and, for Stage III disease, total nodal irradiation has only a limited role. If the pelvic field is to be treated, the amount of marrow irradiated may be greatly reduced by careful blocking and by the use of linear accelerators rather than cobalt units. Adequate covering of the inguinal and femoral lymph nodes must be ensured, and the testes should be shielded. For women, a central block can be placed and the ovaries moved to the midline by tacking them either in front or in back of the uterus, a technique first described by Trueblood and colleagues.[239] However, this procedure is rarely used because pelvic irradiation is no longer applied in the primary treatment of supradiaphragmatic Hodgkin's disease.

While individual preference in technique may have a role, most important are the general principles of careful beam definition, detailed patient positioning, use of simulators, individually constructed shielding techniques, and, finally, verification of dose, usually using thermoluminescent dosimetry. Small technical considerations, such as the position of the arm, can greatly influence the amount of normal tissue treated and must be considered carefully. With Hodgkin's disease as with other malignancies, maximum cure with

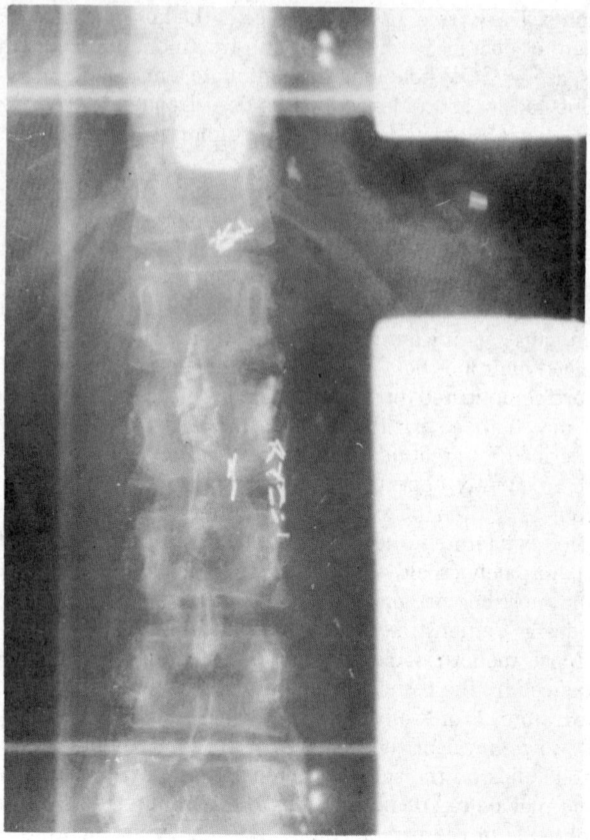

FIG. 49-7. Normal para-aortic field in treating a patient with Hodgkin's disease below the diaphragm. Field for porta hepatic nodes not involved.

minimal complications can occur only when all the technical aspects of radiotherapy are considered carefully. This fact has been substantiated in a review of the pattern of radiation treatment relating recurrence to technical inadequacies. This study found that the facility at which treatment was given significantly affected recurrence rate. Even among university medical centers, technical differences were noted that had a significant effect on relapse-free survival. The rates of in-field or marginal recurrence varied from 0% to 11% at different centers among patients with identical-stage disease, and the relapse rate varied from 10% to 39% ($p=0.0006$). These differences did not relate to variation in staging procedures. However, when portal films were reviewed in a random sample of patients treated for curative intent, in more than one third of the cases, the treatment portal films did not adequately cover the disease, and more than half of these patients had experienced relapse. For patients with adequate portals, relapse rate was only 14% over a 4-year period.[230,240] Thus, it seems prudent for every oncologist to know the success rate of the radiotherapist with whom he or she works.

RESULTS OF RADIATION THERAPY

With the results of radiation therapy reported by Peters and associates[102,103] and Easson and Russell,[223] the question of whether uninvolved areas ought to be irradiated becomes an important one. In 1966, Peters[104] carefully analyzed her data in an attempt to answer this question. Review of these data makes it difficult to prove that irradiation of the uninvolved lymph nodes in Stage I or IIA disease affects the outcome. To study this point further, the Stanford group did a randomized prospective clinical trial (L1) that compared local irradiation to extended field irradiation in Stages I and II disease.[95] This study showed no significant difference between involved-field and extended-field irradiation with respect to either survival or freedom from relapse. A similar national collaborative study also failed to show significant differences.[241] Both of these studies preceded, in part, the use of staging laparotomy and also failed to consider the para-aortic area as a contiguous site for supraclavicular node disease. A new trial was introduced at Stanford (H1) in which the alternatives for Stages I and IIA disease were involved-field irradiation and total nodal irradiation (TNI). This study was started 1 year before the introduction of laparotomy at Stanford; therefore, most of the patients in this study had staging laparotomy. Results of this study showed a highly significant difference in relapse-free survival in favor of TNI, although overall survival was not affected.[95]

Total nodal irradiation is far more extensive than the intended irradiation of subclinical contiguous disease in Stages I and IIA patients. Surely, for supradiaphragmatic disease, pelvic irradiation might be eliminated. This deletion would be important, as it would greatly reduce the amount of bone marrow irradiated and would limit the dose to the gonads. Such a technique for supradiaphragmatic Stages I and IIA patients has been recommended at the JCRT.[127] The results of such treatment are shown in Figure 49-8. Relapse-free and overall survivals for Stages IA and IIA patients are 82% and 93%, respectively. Review of the 315 patients treated in this manner with a median follow-up of 9 years reveals only 3% pelvic nodal recurrences. This result would seem to indicate that the pelvis can be spared irradiation, while the patient still derives the value of extended field irradiation. The importance of pelvic sparing, even in patients who eventually fail and require chemotherapy, is important because it allows shielding of significant bone marrow. This method permits adequate chemotherapy dosage and a decreased likelihood for tumor induction or fatal infection.[242] These studies were done in laparotomy-staged patients in whom the spleen had been removed.

As long-term follow-up increases, it appears that survival of patients with early-stage Hodgkin's disease is independent of initial treatment. Freedom from relapse is, of course, quite dependent on initial therapy, but salvage therapy is so good that overall survival is unaffected. As an example, Figure 49-9 describes the results of patients treated at Stanford with involved fields as compared to those treated by extended-field irradiation. Chemotherapy with a regimen of nitrogen mustard, vincristine, procarbazine, and prednisone (MOPP) for such radiation failures is quite successful (Table 49-10).[243–245]

The goal of treatment is to cure the most patients with the least therapy in order to avoid complications to the greatest extent possible. Because, as shown in Figure 49-9, only 32% of those patients treated by involved fields avoid relapse, 68% will require chemotherapy. Chemotherapy, especially

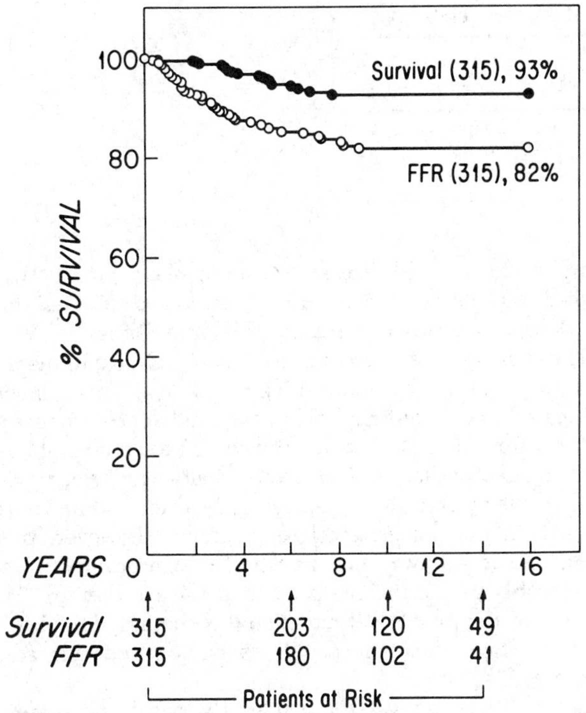

FIG. 49-8. Survival and freedom from first relapse (*FFR*) for pathologic Stage IA–IIA patients treated with mantle and para-aortic–splenic pedicle irradiation. Median follow-up time was 9 years. (Mauch PM et al: Stage IA–IIA supradiaphragmatic Hodgkin's disease: Prognostic factors in surgically staged patients treated with mantle and para-aortic irradiation [in preparation])

when combined with extensive irradiation, may be accompanied by untoward late complications.[246] We believed that most patients with Stages I and II supradiaphragmatic disease treated by radiation should receive extended-field irradiation. Accumulating data suggest that this irradiation need not include the para-aortic field.

Data from the M.D. Anderson Hospital,[247] the European Organization for the Research and Treatment of Cancer (EORTC),[248] and Memorial Hospital pediatric studies[249] have indicated that relapse-free survival was similar in laparotomy-staged patients treated with a mantle field only as compared to those treated more extensively. It is important to note that in all of these studies, the patients were usually selected for having no or only minimal mediastinal involvement. The EORTC included only patients under 40 years old with nodular sclerosis or lymphocyte-predominant histology, an erythrocyte sedimentation rate (ESR) of less than 70, and only one or two sites of involvement. Thus, these data must be used with caution for patients with more extensive disease. While the para-aortic field is not associated with significant long-term toxicity, it does cause acute symptoms; increases the amount of bone marrow involved; and, in the pediatric patient, results in a significant amount of damage to growth in the axial spine. Avoid its use if possible.

A separate subgroup of Stages I and II patients has a higher likelihood for relapse. These patients have large mediastinal masses.[250] Review of such patients at the JCRT revealed that, of 315 Stage IA and IIA patients treated with mantle or para-aortic fields, 35 had mediastinal masses greater than one third of the total chest diameter (Table 49-11). Patients relapsed both within the initial treatment volume as well as in adjacent untreated lymph nodes, and extranodal relapse occurs primarily in the lung. These patients are more likely to experience recurrence even at involved sites separate from the mediastinum (Table 49-12).

Authors disagree as to the best treatment for patients with large mediastinal masses. Significant numbers of patients with large mediastinal masses who fail to respond to radiation only may be salvaged with chemotherapy, and their ultimate results are similar to those patients treated by combined modalities initially. However, treatment with initial irradiation often requires extensive irradiation of the heart and lung to include the large mediastinal mass, which in

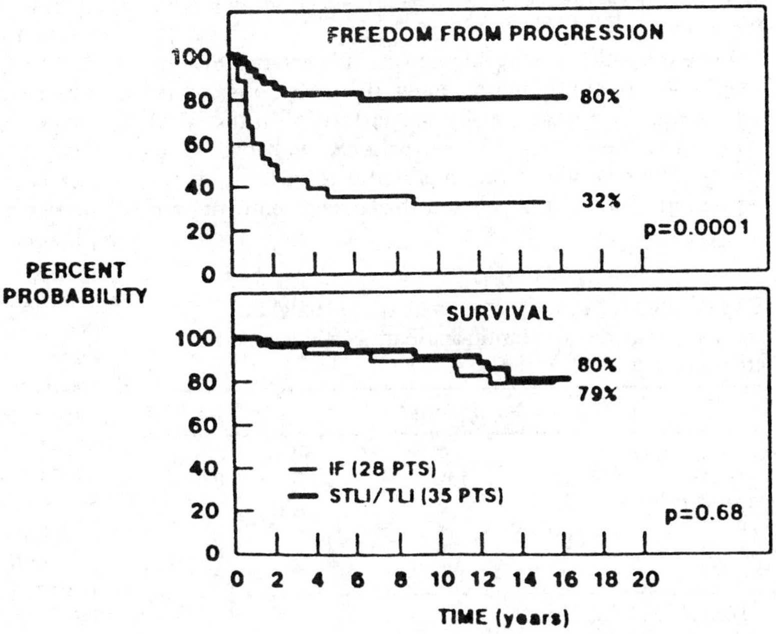

FIG. 49-9. Involved-field (*IF*) versus extended-field irradiation. (Rosenberg SA, Kaplan HS: The evolution and summary results of the Stanford randomized clinical trials of the management of Hodgkin's disease. Int J Radiat Oncol Biol Phys 11:5–22, 1985)

TABLE 49-10. MOPP for Hodgkin's Disease Relapse After Initial Radiation Therapy

Author (Reference)	*Initial Stage*	*No. of Patients*	*% 5-Year FFR*	*% 5-Year Survival*
Timothy et al[243]	IA–IIIA	33	85	92
Portlock[244]	IA–IIIA	46	50	58
Mauch et al[245]	IA–IIIA	28	70	70

FFR = freedom from relapse.

itself can be the source of significant morbidity. Despite this drawback, with the careful use of thoracic CT scanning, patients may be selected for radiation therapy only.[251] Thus, it appears that the treatment of patients with large mediastinal masses needs to be individualized to maximize cure while avoiding unnecessary complications of either radiation of combined-modality treatment. The prognostic importance of large mediastinal masses has been confirmed by others.[252–255] Fortunately, most patients with Stages I and IIA disease have no, or little, mediastinal involvement. For this group, the relapse-free survival is 86% and the overall survival is 93%, using a technique that spares the pelvis from irradiation.[264] There appears to be a subgroup of patients with disease limited only to the mediastinum. These patients rarely (2 of 22) have large masses and enjoy excellent prognoses, with an 85% relapse-free and 100% overall actuarial survival at 8 years.[255,256]

Extensive mediastinal involvement causes a number of additional problems for patients. Such patients appear to be anesthesia risks, with difficulty occurring during extubation,[257] and, thus, the risk–benefit ratio of laparotomy increases. Although this risk can be greatly reduced by irradiating the mass before exploratory laparotomy, such irradiation by its nature involves a significant amount of heart and lung. This provides another reason for treating such patients with primary chemotherapy, restricting radiation to a limited role as a boost technique at the end of the chemotherapy. If such a program is accepted, there appears to be no need for a laparotomy. Appropriate management for these patients is described when treatment for each stage is described.

While the data for subdiaphragmatic-presentation Stages I and IIA disease are far more limited, the results of extended field treatment appear equally satisfactory.[258] In the JCRT experience, there were 15 such patients, with two recurrences. The question of the importance of histology is not certain. In general, it is believed that mixed cellularity and

TABLE 49-11. Influence of Mediastinal Hodgkin's Disease Treated with Mantle and Para-aortic Irradiation on Relapse

	No. of Patients	*% 14-yr FFR*
No mediastinal disease	142	87
Mediastinal disease		
≤1/3	138	85
>1/3	35	53

Data from Mauch et al.[419]

lymphocyte-depleted disease are more likely present with higher-stage disease when carefully evaluated. JCRT results for Stages I and IIA patients are shown in Table 49-13.

The first curative attempt at treatment of Stage III disease was presented in the Stanford (L2) protocol. This protocol compared the convention of low dose irradiation—palliative therapy for a disease that was considered to be incurable—with radical irradiation to all lymph node-bearing areas, including the spleen. Relapses occurred earlier and more frequently in the palliatively treated groups; however, their ultimate survival was not statistically significantly lower, presumably because of the success of salvage therapy. The success of the total nodal radiation was the first demonstration that Stage III patients could, in fact, be cured with radiation only.[224]

Figure 49-10 reveals the actuarial survival and relapse-free survival for laparotomy-staged IIIA patients from the JCRT. Despite the increased accuracy of staging, more than 50% of the patients so treated will experience relapse.[259] While many of these patients can be salvaged by subsequent combination chemotherapy, initial treatment with combined-modality therapy is associated with an overall improvement in survival (Fig. 49-10). Attempts to subdivide these patients into Stages III_1A and III_2A demonstrate the important prognostic significance of this substaging. But even Stage III_1 patients have a significant likelihood of failure when treated with radiation only (Fig. 49-11). Perhaps the only group associated with an excellent relapse-free survival are those Stage III_1A patients with fewer than five splenic nodules, because in the JCRT experience, those patients, treated with radiation only, had a 70% freedom from first relapse and an overall survival of 100%. Total lymphoid irradiation in the hands of the Stanford group has been associated with a better relapse-free survival in Stage III patients. These data are better than those from both Yale and the JCRT. Possible reasons for this difference include a larger proportion of nodular sclerosis patients seen at Stanford and the routine irradiation of the liver employed there for treating patients with splenic involvement.

Treatment of Stages IIB and IIIB Hodgkin's disease with radiation alone can result in some long-term, relapse-free survival (approximately 30% in the Stanford L1 and L2 protocols using total nodal irradiation). While there is general agreement that radiation therapy alone is unsatisfactory treatment for Stage IIIB disease, the data suggest that, in surgical Stage IIB disease, irradiation alone may have the same results as combined-modality treatment.[95,260,261]

A recent report combines the Stanford and JCRT results for such patients. In this series, 103 patients were treated with radiation therapy only with a 7-year freedom from relapse of 74% and overall survival of 87%. While the freedom

TABLE 49-12. Relapse Frequency With and Without Mediastinal Disease

	Initial Sites	*Relapses*	*% Relapse*
No mediastinal disease	85	1	1.1
Mediastinal disease <⅓ all sites	124	4	3.2
Mediastinal sites alone	50	1	2.0
Nonmediastinal sites	74	3	4.1
Mediastinal disease >⅓ all sites	92	16	17.4
Mediastinal sites alone	25	10	40.0
Nonmediastinal sites	67	6	9.0

from relapse with combined-modality treatment was better (84%), the overall survival was the same.[262]

COMPLICATIONS OF RADIATION TREATMENT

Complications of treatment are related to the technique used, dose administered, and irradiated volume. Most of the complications associated with irradiation are seen in the mantle field.[263] Following such irradiation, usually no immediate changes are apparent on the chest roentgenogram or in clinical function. With time, a paramediastinal pulmonary density that outlines the irradiated field may be seen on roentgen film. These signs are usually without symptoms, although the patients occasionally may develop dry cough or dyspnea on exertion. A more important potential complication is acute radiation pneumonitis. This side-effect depends very much on the volume of the lung irradiated and the total dose given. Some changes in pulmonary function after irradiation can be seen if looked for carefully; however, symptomatic radiation pneumonitis is much less common if one is careful to restrict the pulmonary volume irradiated. When whole-lung irradiation is required, the dose should be restricted to less than 1650 rad. For example, of 315 Stages IA and IIA patients treated with mantle (and para-aortic) irradiation at the JCRT, only 16 (5.1%) developed symptomatic radiation pneumonitis.[264] Symptoms associated with this condition include shortness of breath, cough, and occasional fever. If a large volume of lung has been irradiated to high doses, these changes may become progressive and sometimes fatal. In an attempt to reduce pulmonary complications, a variety of techniques has been used. Radiation therapy has been given to large pulmonary masses and interrupted at approximately 1500 rad to allow time for the mass to shrink; the radiation then was continued after a 2- or 3-week hiatus using smaller fields. Similarly, whole-lung irradiation has been given to patients with hilar lymph node involvement, using either transmission blocks that allow only a portion of the dose to reach the lungs, or fields that include the whole lungs but only to tolerable doses.[95] Both of these techniques have allowed pulmonary irradiation without complications, although long-term follow-up reveals some persistent effects.[265]

Cardiac complications of radiation therapy in Hodgkin's disease were first reported by the Stanford group.[235] By limiting the volume of pericardium irradiated, keeping the radiation fraction less than 250 rad, and limiting the total dose, such complications have become uncommon, with only 9 cases of pericarditis in 315 patients treated in the JCRT series.[264] When the whole heart is irradiated to doses of greater than 3000 rad, as many as 50% of the patients will develop pericardial complications.[233] It is very important to avoid treating the whole pericardium, but if whole-pericardium irradiation is required, the dose must be limited. Technique is also important. If patients are treated primarily through anterior portals, a much larger dose is received to the anterior-placed heart. Such techniques have resulted in significant cardiac complications and should be avoided.[266] New methods of cardiac evaluation have revealed abnormal ventricular ejection fractions in some patients long after mediastinal irradiation.[267,268] The symptom complex seen is largely that of pericarditis and, in some patients, continued pericardial fluid causing tamponade or eventual pericardial fibrosis. Both of these conditions can be treated surgically. Some evidence suggests that early coronary artery disease may be a consequence of mediastinal irradiation.[269] This

TABLE 49-13. Influence of Histology on Prognosis for Stage I and IIA Hodgkin's Disease

Histology	*Patients*	*Relapses*	*Dead*
Lymphocyte predominant	34	2 (6%)	0
Nodular sclerosis	150	25 (17%)	7
Mixed cellularity	79	17 (22%)	8
Lymphocyte depleted	3	0	0

FIG. 49-10. Actuarial and relapse-free (*FFR*) survival for laparotomy Stage IIIA patients treated with combined-modality therapy (*CMT*) versus total nodal irradiation (*TNI*). (Mauch PM et al: Unpublished data)

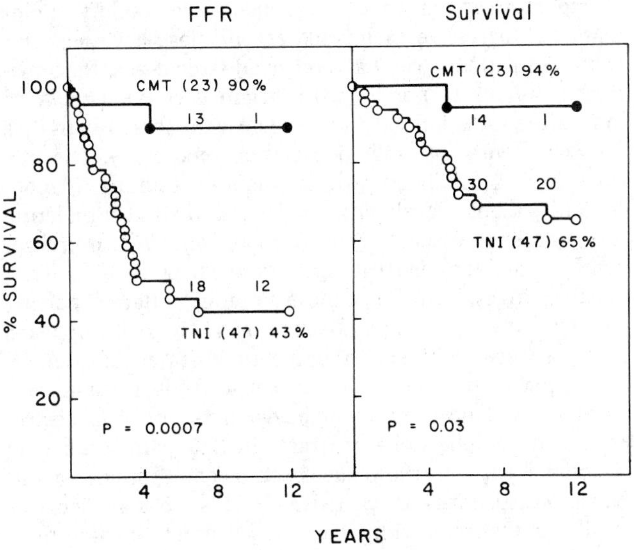

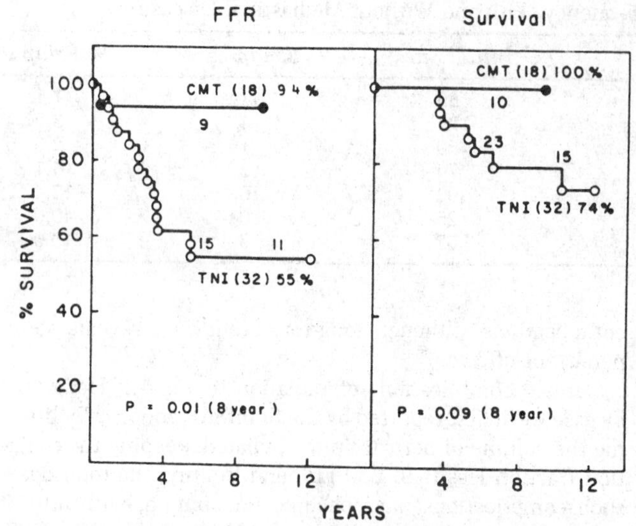

FIG. 49-11. Results of total nodal irradiation (*TNI*) versus combined-modality therapy (*CMT*) for pathologic Stage III_1A Hodgkin's disease patients. FFR = freedom from relapse. (Mauch PM et al, unpublished data)

possibility is currently being reviewed. Thus far, in a large epidemiologic study, no significant increase in cardiac-related deaths in Hodgkin's disease patients is evident.[270]

The most common neurologic complication seen with irradiation is Lhermitte's sign. This transient complication of radiation therapy consists of numbness, tingling, or "electric" sensations, which are produced or exacerbated by head flexion. Carmel and Kaplan[233] reported an incidence of 15% in their patients treated with mantle fields. These symptoms are transitory and are not associated with permanent sequelae. The pathogenesis is unknown. Spinal cord transection can occur when a portion of the spinal cord is included in both the mantle and para-aortic fields. If overlap is avoided, this complication does not occur at the doses of 3600 to 4000 rad used. Radiation fibrosis in the brachial plexus rarely has been seen. This complication usually arises when high doses of radiation are given to large neck and axillary tumor masses. Progressive motor and sensory loss have been recorded in patients who have received large doses. Rare malignant tumors of nerve sheath origin have been reported long after radiation therapy.[271] These tumors usually are associated with both radiation and chemotherapy. The thyroid gland is irradiated with the mantle, resulting in about 30% of patients developing an elevated thyroid-stimulating hormone level without T_3 or T_4 reduction.[272] With prompt supplemental thyroid treatment, clinical hypothyroidism has occurred in less than 5% of these patients.[264] Rare hyperthyroidism and exophthalmos also are seen. Thyroid neoplasms rarely are seen with such therapeutic doses of radiation.[273]

Complications related to para-aortic fields are quite uncommon, and, if the doses and fields are as described, gastrointestinal complications are rare. In 315 para-aortic field irradiation patients, there have been 8 complications (small-bowel obstructions) at the JCRT.[264] This 2.5% incidence is similar to that seen with laparotomy without radiation therapy. Pelvis treatment alone may cause persistent thrombocytopenia or leukopenia. This complication is quite rare with current techniques that use well-collimated linear accelerators and judicious blocks. Infectious complications of treatment are seen when total nodal irradiation and splenectomy are used.

CHEMOTHERAPY OF HODGKIN'S DISEASE

Hodgkin's disease is curable by combination chemotherapy. Single drugs play no role in the treatment of newly diagnosed patients with this disease because, under almost any medical circumstance, experienced oncologists can select a combination drug treatment program from the large number of options displayed in the tables in this chapter[274-325] that can fit the condition of the patient; the use of drugs in combination is a requirement to effect substantial remission rates and durable remissions.

The story of the cure of Hodgkin's disease by chemotherapy goes back to the beginnings of chemotherapy itself. The perplexing influence of disease variables on the interpretation of the efficacy of drugs was noted by Osler in his text in 1892.[326] Fowler's solution, containing arsenic, was thought to be effective against Hodgkin's disease at that time, but Osler skillfully sorted out the variable natural history of Hodgkin's disease from a true therapeutic effect. Nitrogen mustard was the first useful chemical and was used as treatment for lymphomas in 1943 by Goodman and associates.[327] The results, published after the World War II, were exciting; they showed marked dissolution of lymph nodes in patients with Hodgkin's disease treated with this alkylating agent. Subsequent studies rapidly confirmed the results.[328,329] There was palpable excitement over the possibilities these results augured for potential cure of widespread cancers with drugs. However, as it became apparent that relapse and death were universal, excitement was overtaken by a gloom and pessimism that handicapped clinical trials of new approaches to cure lymphomas and other cancers for almost two decades.

The period between 1942 and 1963 saw the introduction of a number of new drugs—the alkylating agents, corticosteroids, the antifols, the vinca alkaloids, and a drug almost entirely specific for Hodgkin's disease, procarbazine[330-334]—all of which were to be the tools of the first attempts to cure advanced Hodgkin's disease by combination chemotherapy. By 1963, clinical studies had also shown that continued treatment (maintenance treatment) after a response was attained by one or another drug could prolong remissions but did not prolong survival.[335] Patients who experienced relapse without maintenance drug treatment could be retreated with the primary drug with some success. In the seminal study, reported by Carbone and co-workers,[336] patients were also grouped for the first time according to the quality of their initial response; complete remissions were separated from partial responses, and the striking advantage of complete remission was noted. These early observations provided the ethical basis for future studies that allowed patients who achieved complete remission after combination chemotherapy to be followed with no further therapy, and to

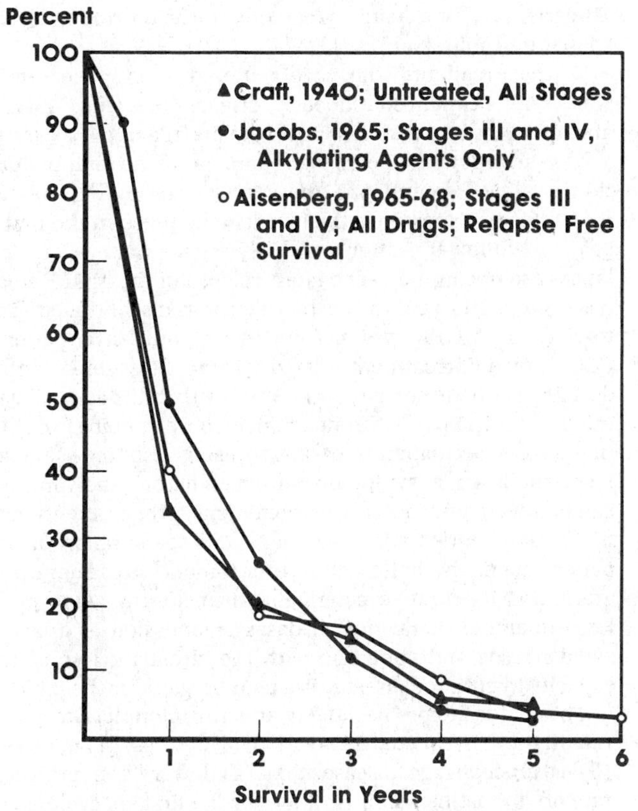

FIG. 49-12. Three survival curves of patients with advanced Hodgkin's disease treated with single-agent chemotherapy compared to a group left untreated. (DeVita VT Jr: Consequences of the chemotherapy of Hodgkin's disease. Cancer 47:1, 1981)

test the quality of the remission and, ultimately, the capacity of drug combinations to cure the disease.

These early studies, however, did not provide any evidence of or confidence in the capacity of chemotherapy to cure Hodgkin's disease as shown in Figure 49-12. This figure compares the only available series of untreated patients of all stages[337] to results using alkylating agents alone[338] and to a more modern series using all the drugs applied in later combination programs in sequence.[339] The shapes of the curves are similar. Median survival was approximately 1 year, and less than 5% of patients were alive at 5 years.

The first intensive drug combination program for Hodgkin's disease used vincristine, methotrexate, cyclophosphamide, and prednisone (MOMP) given for 2.5 months.[339] The goal of this pilot protocol was to test the safety of such an approach. Only 14 patients were studied, but the data showed the approach to be safe and a high complete remission rate was achieved. In 1965, Lacher and Durant[340] published the results of the administration of a two-drug combination, vinblastine and chlorambucil. A complete remission rate of approximately 40% was reported. However, this difference was not a significant improvement over the response achieved with vinblastine alone, and no further reports of this study or treatment program have been published.

In 1964, as experience with procarbazine accrued, the MOMP program was modified in several ways. The duration of treatment was lengthened to 6 months, and procarbazine was substituted for methotrexate.[340] This program was named MOPP.[341] The use of MOPP in the first 43 patients with advanced Hodgkin's disease produced an 80% complete-remission rate (a four-fold increase over results achieve with the best single agents), and the remissions were durable. In this and later reports, it was noted that asymptomatic patients responded better than those with constitutional symptoms; patients previously treated with single-agent chemotherapy responded less well to MOPP than did previously untreated patients[342-346] and, curiously enough, previous exposure to radiotherapy did not seem to compromise the patients' ability to respond to chemotherapy. In fact, a consistently better response rate has been noted in most series for patients who experience relapse from radiotherapy compared to those with equivalent stages of disease who were previously untreated.[347,348]

Each of the agents in the MOPP regimen was selected based on its antitumor activity when used as a single agent, and the drugs were given in full dose and according to their optimal schedule with the exception that rest intervals were spaced between cycles to allow marrow recovery. Drugs were also selected to minimize overlapping toxicity to any single organ. Therefore, vincristine was selected over its analog vinblastine, even though vinblastine was the favored drug, because vincristine has less marrow toxicity (however, vincristine produced more neurotoxicity). The four drugs were given over a 2-week period. The intervals between cycles were constructed around intervals known from experimental studies to be required for recovery of bone marrow.[349] Thus, a complete cycle of MOPP consisted of a 2-week treatment period and a 2-week recovery period. A minimum of six cycles were given every 29 days until the patients achieved a complete remission or tumor grew despite treatment.

Three features of MOPP were unique at the time: (1) the goal of the program was to cure rather than to palliate, as had been the practice in the preceding 2 decades; (2) the cyclic use of combination chemotherapy for 6 months exceeded the duration of any prior treatment in adult tumors; and (3) it was the first regimen to make use of the sliding scale to adjust drug doses for marrow suppression. The sliding scale was designed to permit the administration of each cycle on time, with maximum allowable doses of each agent, and to preserve both the dose rate and the integrity of the drug combination.[342] Provisions for delaying subsequent cycles were made only if toxicity was severe enough to require omission of drugs from that cycle. The sliding scale had an interesting effect on dosing in the MOPP and other combination chemotherapy studies and is now used in all clinical protocols. Usually, after two cycles at full or near-full doses, patients have significant myelosuppression, and doses in the third cycle must be reduced according to the sliding scale to administer the third cycle on schedule. The impact of reducing doses in the third cycle was to allow the use of full or near-full doses in the fourth or later cycles. The net effect is preservation of dose rate by not prolonging intervals between cycles. The standard practice has been to administer a minimum of six cycles of treatment or enough cycles to attain a complete remission plus two additional cycles. The average duration of administration for six cycles in the NCI program was 5.8 months, and the omission of any drugs from

TABLE 49-14. MOPP Regimen*

Drug	Dose	Schedule
Nitrogen mustard	6.0 mg/m²IV	Days 1 and 8
Vincristine (Oncovin)	1.4 mg/m² IV	Days 1 and 8
Procarbazine	100.0 mg/m² PO	Days 1 through 14
Prednisone†	40.0 mg/m² PO	Days 1 through 14

*Repeat cycle every 28 days for a minimum of six cycles. Complete remission must be documented before discontinuing therapy.
†Used only in cycles 1 and 4. However, in the National Cancer Institute's current MOPP trials, prednisone is administered in every cycle.

the program was rare at NCI. The MOPP regimen is shown in Table 49-14 and its sliding scale for dose modification is shown in Table 49-15.

The MOPP regimen was considered high-dose, long-duration chemotherapy in 1964. However, subsequent calculations of its dose intensity, using the methods of Hryniuk and Bush[350,351] and DeVita and colleagues[352] to calculate doses on the basis of mg/m²/wk—which takes into account the impact of treatment-free intervals on total dose delivered over time—show that the MOPP program used at NCI had a dose intensity of 70% relative to a hypothetical version of MOPP that would use the same four drugs, in their full doses, continuously, without rest intervals, over 6 months.[352] This finding is true of all cyclically administered drug combination programs. In practice, because of the tendency to delay intervals between cycles of therapy to allow recovery of blood counts to pretreatment levels, all cytotoxic drug combinations in the clinic today are given at a reduced dose vis-à-vis their optimal single drug schedules.

The early results of the use of MOPP have been confirmed by others, and the durable remissions have been maintained in the NCI study over the past 20 years.[353] Table 49-16 shows the results of the original series after 20 years of follow-up: 198 patients with diagnoses of Hodgkin's disease were treated with MOPP; all are at risk for a minimum of 10 years and 140 patients are at risk for more than 15 years. This study population has more patients with poor prognostic features than more recent studies—an important point in comparing results. For example, 88% of patients were classified as having B symptoms, a variable that carries a poor prognosis independent of all other prognostic factors. Most recent studies have about one third asymptomatic patients. Since this 1980 report, pathologists at NCI have reviewed the histologic material of these patients and have found that ten patients in the original study who had been diagnosed as having lymphocyte-depleted Hodgkin's disease would now be classified as having diffuse large cell lymphomas.[354] These 10 patients are evaluated separately in the current analysis, shown in Table 49-15.

Of those patients who have achieved a complete remission, 64% remain continuously disease-free (Fig. 49-13), and, of all treated patients, 54% remain free of disease after a 20-year follow-up. Forty-eight percent of the total population is alive. The relapse-free survival curve (Fig. 49-13) illustrates that most negative events take place in the first 4 years of follow-up, after which the curve flattens and relapses are uncommon. The latest relapse in the MOPP study has occurred 11 years after treatment was discontinued. The toxicity of MOPP was not excessive; only five patients (2.5%) died of treatment-related toxicity. Most importantly, despite the neurotoxicity associated with full doses of vincristine (1.4 mg/m² with no artificial dose capping), no patients were permanently paralyzed using a sliding-scale adjustment based on symptoms. Although nausea and vomiting can be severe with all drug combinations, proper attention to motivation, antiemetics, sedation, and reassurance of the patient about the finite nature of a 6-month treatment program, and its curative potential, can make the acute problems tolerable. Reduction of doses or omission of drugs to avoid nausea and vomiting, with the attendant loss of the capacity to cure the disease, is a poor bargain for the patient.

The major factors negatively affecting complete response rate in the 20-year study were (1) B symptoms, (2) male sex, (3) advanced-stage disease, and (4) lower than projected rate of vincristine administration for the first six cycles. The most important variables for predicting complete remission duration were (1) B symptoms, (2) age, (3) rapidity with which complete response was achieved (patients requiring five cycles or less had significantly longer remissions), (4) number of external sites of disease, and (5) liver or pleural involvement. The impact of being symptom-free is dramatic in the NCI study. All of the asymptomatic patients with Stages IIIA (10 patients) and IVA (13 patients) disease attained a complete remission in the NCI study, and only 2 have experienced relapse in over 15 years of follow-up.

In the 1960s, it was fashionable to give additional chemotherapy after a maximum response was attained to maintain this response (maintenance chemotherapy), especially since there was no expectation of cure. In all studies of maintenance chemotherapy, doses of drugs are invariably reduced and given at intervals more widely spaced than in the induction program, raising the question of their capacity to do anything but suppress residual disease for brief periods. A study at NCI in which patients who achieved complete remission were randomized to further treatment with MOPP, no further treatment, or treatment with nitrosourea (BCNU)

TABLE 49-15. Sliding Scale for Dose Adjustment in the MOPP Regimen

Leukocyte Count	*Platelet Count*	*Dose Adjustment**
>4000/mm³	100,000/mm³	100% all drugs
3000–4000/mm³	100,000/mm³	100% vincristine, 50% nitrogen mustard and procarbazine
2000–3000/mm³	50,000–100,000/mm³	100% vincristine, 25% nitrogen mustard and procarbazine
1000–2000/mm³	50,000/mm³	50% vincristine, 25% nitrogen mustard and procarbazine
<1000/mm³	50,000/mm³	No therapy

*No prednisone dose adjustment is required for bone marrow suppression.

TABLE 49-16. Twenty-Year MOPP Follow-Up Study by the National Cancer Institute

	1980 Analysis[346]	*1986 Analysis 198 Original Patients*[353]	*Patients with Hodgkin's Disease in 1986 Analysis*
No. of evaluable patients	198	198	188
No. of complete responders	159 (80%)	160 (81%)	157 (84%)
No. of induction failures	39 (20%)	38 (19%)	31 (16%)
No. of relapses	52 (33%)	57 (36%)	56 (34%)
No. continuously free of disease	107 (54%)	103(52%)	101 (54%)
No. dead	98 (49%)	106 (54%)	98 (52%)
With Hodgkin's disease	75	76	68
Free of disease	23	30	30
No. alive	100 (51%)	92 (46%)	90 (48%)
With Hodgkin's disease		2	2
Free of disease		90	88

showed maintenance treatment to be ineffective. A recent update of this study 20 years later reconfirmed the results. A total of nine studies of maintenance treatment after remission with MOPP show that it adds nothing to overall relapse-free survival, and maintenance chemotherapy is not recommended if patients have achieved a complete remission after a minimum of six cycles of treatment or two additional cycles of treatment have been given after complete remission was documented.[344,345] With the introduction of effective systemic therapy, all stages of Hodgkin's disease were potentially curable, and, indeed, data from NCI's Surveillance, Epidemiology and End Results Program (SEER) confirm the impact of treatment on survival rates since 1973 (Fig. 49-14), and on mortality rates (Fig. 49-15).

In the 25 years since the inception and confirmation of the efficacy of the MOPP program, therapeutic research in clinical trials in advanced Hodgkin's disease has taken three major directions: (1) the development of modifications of MOPP, aimed at retaining efficacy while reducing toxicity; (2) the development of new combinations constructed of drugs with different mechanisms of action and known to be non–cross-resistant to the drugs in the MOPP program; and (3) the use of these non–cross-resistant drug combinations in alternating cycles with MOPP, or MOPP modifications, to avoid early treatment failures and circumvent the development of drug resistance. Although this approach preceded the publication of the Goldie–Coldman somatic mutation hypothesis[355] (see Chap. 16), the authors' articulation of the potential problem presented by the spontaneous development of drug resistance in cancer cells has had a significant impact on the design of the most recent drug combination programs.

The complete literature on combination chemotherapy is summarized in Tables 49-17 and 49-18, which list published results with all major programs that are modifications of the MOPP program (Table 49-17) and all published randomized trials of MOPP versus modifications of MOPP or non–cross-resistant combinations (Table 49-18). Abbreviations and acronyms for all drug programs in this chapter are shown in Table 49-19, and details for doses and schedules are in Tables 49-20, 49-21, and 49-22. Acute toxicity for most of these programs is similar but varies in intensity depending on the mix of drugs. Readers are advised to refer to the original publications for details of administration of the program they select to become familiar with the side-effects.

Interpretation of these trials is complicated by different

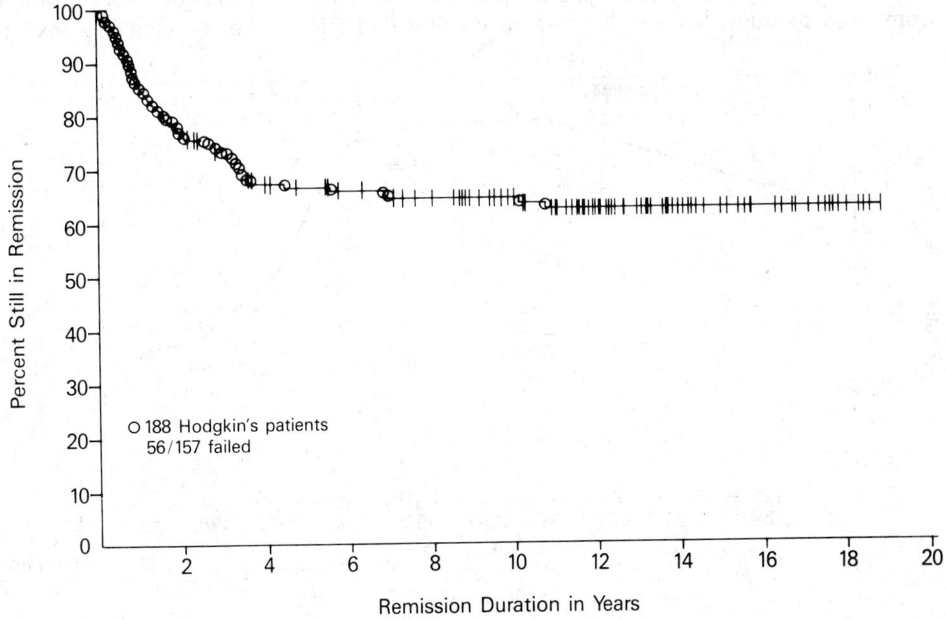

FIG. 49-13. Remission duration in 188 patients with Hodgkin's disease.

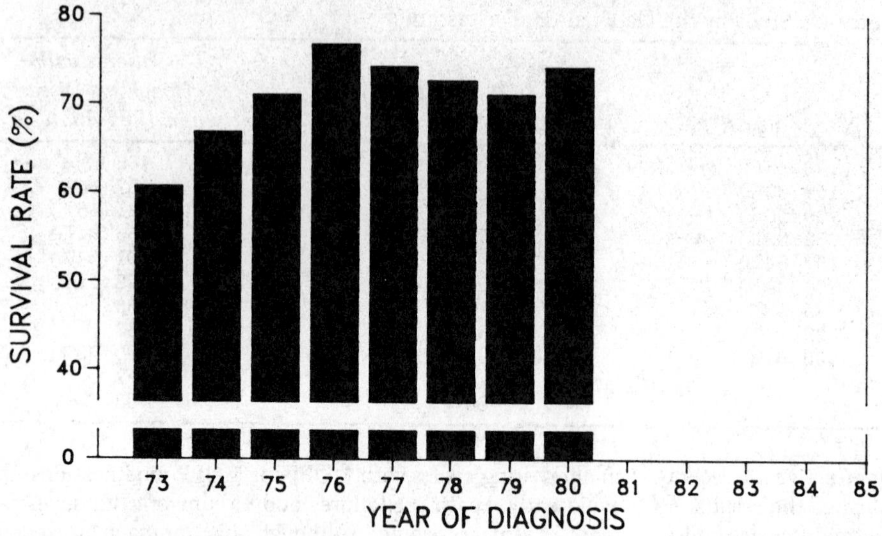

FIG. 49-14. Five-year relative survival rates of white men and women with Hodgkin's disease.

mixes of disease variables, different approaches to staging, and inclusion of varying fractions of previously treated patients. Fairly uniform agreement now exists on the impact of these variables, and the practitioner needs to temper the evaluation and selection of a treatment program by the mix of the variables in reported studies. The strongest disease variable known is the absence of symptoms. Other variables, such as stage and number of sites of involvement within a stage, tend to reflect tumor volume, with greater volume imparting a worse prognosis. While prior chemotherapy affects the capacity to achieve a complete response to combination chemotherapy, patients who experience relapse after treatment with radiotherapy almost always have better prognoses than newly diagnosed patients of the same stage. Varying approaches to staging, particularly whether patients have been surgically staged, alters the stage designation and changes the interpretation of the results. For example, yesterday's clinical Stage II patients, are often today's surgical Stage III patients. A study reporting superior results in Stage III patients needs to have a careful analysis of its staging practices. Comparison of results from different time periods are difficult not only because staging methods have changed from study to study, but also because an investigation encompassing a decade will have used a varying mix of approaches to staging within the study population. The most pernicious variable of all, however, has been dose modification.[352] Dose modification is nearly ubiquitous in clinical studies and in practice, and the method and extent are often not recorded or reported. Only recently has it been possible to estimate the true impact of dose modification on outcome in lymphomas and other tumors. This aspect will be discussed further later in the chapter.

The first series of studies that followed the NCI report showed MOPP to be superior to nitrogen mustard used continuously for 6 months in a controlled trial.[276] MOPP also proved superior to a new five-drug combination and to the same five drugs used one by one in sequence,[274,275] even though the complete remission rates with the latter two regimens was similar to that with MOPP. This study provided important early evidence that complete remission rates alone did not necessarily reflect the true quality of the remissions, and duration of remission after all therapy is discontinued is the most important end prognostic factor. Investigators from Stanford University[356] also replicated the results of MOPP, using it as reported from NCI. However, they thought that toxicity from vincristine at doses used at

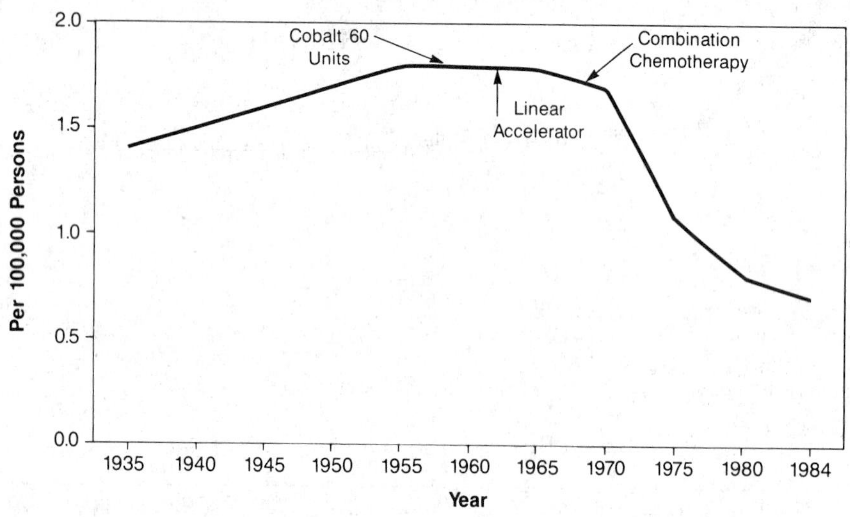

FIG. 49-15. National mortality from Hodgkin's disease related to introduction of radiotherapy and chemotherapy, 1935–1984.

TABLE 49-17. Modifications in MOPP as Primary Treatment

Author	Regimen*	Prior Therapy	No. of Patients	CR (%)	DFS (%/yr)	NED (%/yr)	OS (%/yr)
Sutcliffe et al[301]	MVPP	RT; No CT	133	82	60/5	49/5	76/5
Wagstaff et al[302]	MVPP	None	114	74	86/5†	64/5†	70/5
Pavlovsky et al[303,304]	CVPP vs CCVPP	Yes	160‡	78	66/6§		69/7
			143‡	82	52/6§		57/7
Gams et al[305,306]	BVCPP	RT; No CT	188	68	55/4§	48/4§	NS
Dady et al[307–309]	ChlVPP	None	59	73	63/5†	46/5†	66/5
		RT	32	91	76/5	69/5	76/5
		CT and/or RT	20	55	9/5	<1/5	15/5
Lister et al[310]	MVPP vs TNI	No	32	88	96/10	84/10	91/10
			21	95	70/10	67/10	86/10
Crowther et al[311]	MVPP vs MVPP + RT	No	26	88	87/5	77/5	84/5
			30	100	90/5	90/5	80/5
Gams et al[312]	BVCPP vs BVCPP–ADB	RT	93	69	77/5	63/5	68/NS
			90	64	78/5	69/5	67/NS
Propert et al[313–315]	COPP vs CVPP vs MOPP vs MVPP	None	260	64‖	56/10‖		44/10‖
	As above	RT	132	77‖	56/10‖		44/10‖
Vinciguerra et al[316]	CVPP vs ABOS vs CVPP–ABOS	RT only	44	72	51/5¶	55/5¶	
			29	70	64/5¶	61/5¶	
			40	82	64/5¶	68/5¶	
Druker et al[317]	ChlVPP	None or RT	19	89	74/5		
Armitage et al[318]	ChlVPP	None or RT	44	76	97/3	82/3	
Prosnitz et al[319–321]	MVVPP or MOPP	None or RT	151	82**	85/15†,**	67/15†,**	54/15†,**
Wegener et al[322]	MOPP–CAVmP	None	47	68	80/2†	70/3†	86/3
Klimo and Connors[323–325]	MOPP–ABV	No	76	98	91/4		

CR = complete response; CT = chemotherapy; DFS = disease-free survival; FOD = free of disease; NS = not specified; OS = overall survival; RT = radiotherapy; TNI = total nodal irradiation.

*See Table 49-19 for explanation of acronyms.

†Radiation administered to sites of bulky disease after CR induction in some or all patients.

‡Forty-seven of 303 patients had Stage I–IIA disease.

§Maintenance CT after CR induction given in some or all patients.

‖No significant difference in CR rate was seen in untreated patients among the four regimens. In patients previously treated with RT, nitrogen mustard–containing regimens produced a significantly higher CR rate [86% versus 66%]. DFS and OS were not significantly different among patients in any group with any of the regimens.

¶No significant difference in DFS or OS among patients given chlorambucil maintenance when compared to no further therapy.

**Data not provided on CR rate, DFS, or percentage of patients FOD by treatment group [MOPP versus MVVPP].

NCI was too severe, and they recommended the now widely adopted practice of limiting the dose of vincristine to no more than 2 mg/dose regardless of body weight or surface area. Omitting prednisone from MOPP reduced the effectiveness, as was shown in one controlled trial comparing MOPP to MOP.[279] Although one uncontrolled study from Stanford did not show this effect,[357] the population of patients at Stanford was composed largely of patients who had relapsed following radiation therapy and is not comparable to most other studies.

In the decade of additional studies designed to reduce the side-effects of MOPP by substituting or adding additional drugs, many combinations have been tested and none has improved the results. Three combinations have emerged with effects equivalent to MOPP but with different side-effects, making them useful under certain circumstances: MVPP,[301,302] ChlVPP[307–309] and BCVPP.[305,306] ChlVPP is an attractive variant of the MOPP program. It substitutes chlorambucil for nitrogen mustard and vinblastine for vincristine. It produces somewhat less nausea and vomiting and much less neurotoxicity, although the degree of myelosuppression is similar. At last report, 191 patients have been treated with CHlVPP since 1975. The complete remission rate was 73% for 59 previously untreated patients with advanced-stage disease, and 91% for patients who experienced relapse after previous treatment with radiotherapy. The 59 patients with advanced disease who received no other treatment besides ChlVPP had a disease-free survival of 64%, which is comparable to the NCI MOPP. However, 40% of this population was asymptomatic compared to only 12% in the NCI study. Another variant (LOPP) substitutes chlorambucil for nitrogen mustard. In a controlled trial comparing LOPP to MOPP, the programs were found to be equivalent,[290,291] but the results with both arms were quite inferior to those reported elsewhere, a difference apparently, related to inadequate dosing. Some concern has arisen about the carcinogenic effects of oral chlorambucil compared to nitrogen mustard. The results with MVPP, which substitutes vinblastine for vincristine, also appear equivalent to MOPP results but with less neurotoxicity and more myelotoxicity. Interpretation of long-term results of MVPP are complicated by the use of two- and four-drug maintenance treatment in all responders. Both ChlVPP and MVPP are reasonable alternatives to MOPP for older patients who are less able to tolerate the neurologic side-effects of vincristine or for those patients with intractable nausea and vomiting.

The BCVPP regimen substitutes vinblastine and cyclophosphamide for vincristine and nitrogen mustard and also adds the nitrosourea BCNU. The Eastern Cooperative Oncology Group (ECOG)[284] conducted a randomized comparison

TABLE 49-18. Randomized Studies Evaluating MOPP, MOPP Modifications, or MOPP and ABVD Drugs as Primary Treatment

Author	*Regimen**	*Prior Therapy*	*No. of Patients*	*CR (%)*	*DFS (%/yr)*	*FOD (%/yr)*	*Survival (%/yr)*
Stutzman et al[274,275]	MOPP vs	Yes	81	63	M = 11 mo		50/2
	VPBCP† vs		89	62	M = 7 mo		50/2
	VPBCP‡		77	53	M = 7 mo		50/2
Huguley et al[276]	MOPP vs	Yes	61	48	38/4	34/4	52/4
	HN2		47	13	16/4	50/4	30/4
Coltman et al[277,278]	MOPP vs	Yes	42	71	62/4.6 yr	NS	M = 6.0 yr
	MOPP LDB vs		111	85	M = 3.8 yr	NS	M = 8.3 yr
	MOPP HDB		35	82	M = 3.2 yr	NS	M = 5.3 yr
Goldman[279,280]	MOPP vs	Yes	49	73	69/5	51/5	51/5
	MOP		42	36	33/5	12/5	24/5
Bonadonna et al[281,282]	MOPP vs	RT only	41	63	79/5§	56/5§	67/5
	ABVD		35	72	80/5	63/5§	73/5
Jones et al[283]	MOPP LDB vs	RT only	121	66	61/5	48/5	59/5
	MOP-BAP#1		160	77	68/5	60/5	70/5
Bakemeier et al[284]	MOPP vs	RT 8%	146	73‖	61/5	37/5	57/5
	BCVPP		147	76‖	51/5	46/5	51/5
Straus et al[285]	MOPP–ABVD	None	37	78¶	90/3‖	70/3‖	87/4
	CAD MOPP–ABV		34	82¶	93/3‖	76/3‖	92/4
BNLI[286,287]	British MOPP	None	40	72	30/5	NS	80/5
	vs TNI		47	90	45/5		90/5
Bonadonna et al[288,289]	MOPP vs	RT only	43	74	45/8	36/8	64/8
	MOPP–ABVD		45	89	73/8	65/8	84/8
Hancock[290]	MOPP vs	None	157	60	33/5		
	LOPP		142	69	32/5		66/5
							68/5
Hancock et al[291]	LOPP vs	None	**	58			
	MOPP–British		**	70			
	EVAP						
Bonadonna[292]	MOPP/ABVD	None		91‡‡			
	MA/MA			90			
Longo et al[293]	MOPP vs	None	44	100	91/3	91/3	91/3
	subtotal nodal RT		41	95	67/3	63/3	78/3
Somers et al[294]	MOPP vs	None	95	60	65/4§	39/4	62/4
	2MOPP/2ABVD (8 cycles)		95	61	72/4§	44/4	75/4
Canellos et al[295]	MOPP vs	None	49	69	48/3		
	ABVD vs		49	81	64/3		
	MOPP–ABVD		50	82	64/3		
Brusamolino et al[296]	MOPP–ABVD	None	50	80	77/4	62/4	86/4
Young et al[297]	MOPP vs	None	59	92	74/7	67/7	80/8
	MOPP–CABS		59	90	79/7	71/7	76/8
Glick et al[298]	MOPP–ABVD vs	None	NS††	85	64/4	NS	81/4
	BCVPP vs		NS††	75	66/4	NS	74/4
	BCVPP–XRT		NS††	68	63/4	NS	74/4
Canadian NCI[299]	MOPP & ABVD vs MOPP/ABV						

BNLI = British National Lymphoma Investigation; CR = complete response; DFS = disease-free survival; FOD = free of disease; OD = overall survival; M = median; NS = not specified; RT = radiotherapy; TNI = total nodal irradiation; XRT = x-ray irradiation.

*See Table 49-19 for explanation of acronyms.

†Simultaneous administration.

‡Sequential administration.

§Radiation administered to sites of bulky disease after CR induction in some or all patients.

‖Maintenance chemotherapy after CR induction given in some or all patients.

¶All patients received 200 to 300 rad of radiotherapy to bulky disease as part of the induction regimen.

**Data on 167 randomized patients were evaluated in this report.

††Data on 305 randomized patients were evaluated in this report.

‡‡Relapse has occurred in 20% of 209 patients.

TABLE 49-19. Acronyms

ABOS: Doxorubicin, bleomycin, vincristine, streptozocin
ABV: Doxorubicin, bleomycin, vinblastine
ABVD: Adriamycin, bleomycin, vinblastine, DTIC
ADB: Doxorubicin, dacarbazine, bleomycin
ADBC: Adriamycin, DTIC, bleomycin, CCNU
B-CAVe: Bleomycin, CCNU, Adriamycin, velban
BCNU: 1,3-bis(2-chlorethyl)-1-nitrosourea
BCVPP: BCNU, cyclophosphamide, velban procarbazine, prednisone
BVCPP: BCNU, velban cyclophosphamide, procarbazine, prednisone
BVCPP-B: BCNU, velban, cyclophosphamide, procarbazine, prednisone, bleomycin
BVDS: Bleomycin, velban, Adriamycin, streptozocin
BVPP: BCNU, vincristine, procarbazine, prednisone
CABS: CCNU, Adriamycin, bleomycin, streptozocin
CAD: CCNU, doxorubicin, vindesine
CAVmP: Cyclophosphamide, doxorubicin, teniposide, prednisone
CBVD: CCNU, bleomycin, vinblastine, doxorubicin
CCNU:: (1-(2-chloroethyl)-3-cyclohexyl-1-nitrosourea)
CCVPP: CCNU, cyclophosphamide, velban, procarbazine, prednisone
CEM: CCNU, etoposide, methotrexate
CEP: CCNU, etoposide, prednimustine
CEVD: CCNU, etoposide, vindesine, doxorubicin
Ch1VPP: Chlorambucil, vinblastine, procarbazine, prednisone
CVB: CCNU, velban, bleomycin
CVPP: Cyclophosphamide, velban, procarbazine, prednisone
DTIC: 5-(3,3-dimethyl-1-triazine) imidazole-4-carboxamide
EVA: etoposide, vincristine, doxorubicin
EVAP*: Etoposide, vinblastine, Adriamycin, prednisone
EVAP†: Etoposide, vinblastine, arabinosyl cytosine, cisplatin
HN2: Nitrogen mustard
LOPP: Chlorambucil, vincristine, procarbazine, prednisone
MABOP: Nitrogen mustard, Adriamycin, bleomycin, vincristine, prednisone
Methyl GAG: methylglyoxal bis(guanylhydrazone)dihidro-chloride
MIME: Mitogauzone, ifosphamide, methotrexate, etoposide
MOP: Nitrogen mustard, vincristine, prednisone
MOP–ABV: Nitrogen mustard, vincristine, procarbazine, doxorubicin, bleomycin, vinblastine
MOP-BAP: Nitrogen mustard, vincristine, procarbazine, bleomycin, doxorubicin, prednisone
MOPLACE: Methotrexate, vincristine, prednisone, leucovorin, cytosine arabinoside, cyclophosphamide, etoposide
MOPP: Nitrogen mustard, vincristine, procarbazine, prednisone
MOPPHDB: Nitrogen mustard, vincristine, procarbazine, prednisone, high-dose bleomycin
MOPPLDB: Nitrogen mustard, vincristine, procarbazine, prednisone, low-dose bleomycin
MTX-CHOP: Methotrexate, cyclophosphamide, doxorubicin, vincristine, prednisone
MVPP: Nitrogen mustard, vinblastine, procarbazine, prednisone
MVVPP: Nitrogen mustard, vincristine, vinblastine, procarbazine, prednisone
PAVe: Procarbazine, phenylalanine mustard, velban
PCVP: Procarbazine, cyclophosphamide, vinblastine, prednisone
SCAB: Streptozocin, CCNU, doxorubisine, bleomycin
VABCD: Vinblastine, doxorubicin, bleomycin, CCNU, dacarbazine
VPBCP: Vincristine, procarbazine, vinblastine, chlorambucil, prednisone

* British EVAP regimen.
† National Cancer Institute's EVAP salvage regimen.

of BCVPP and MOPP in a population of patients with advanced disease, of whom 35% were asymptomatic, and MOPP was used in reduced doses and at wider intervals. A maximum vincristine dose of 2 mg was also employed in the MOPP arm of the study. The complete response rates for the two regimens were identical, but the duration of complete remission with BCVPP was significantly longer than with the reduced version of MOPP in previously untreated patients. Life-threatening hematologic toxicity was slightly more severe with BCVPP, probably because of the addition of BCNU, but BCVPP treatment resulted in less gastrointestinal and neurologic toxicity. Recent follow-up of this population indicates a higher incidence of acute leukemia in the BCVPP than the MOPP arm — again, most likely due to the addition of the nitrosourea. The addition of BCNU with greater acute toxicity and long-term side-effects makes this combination too toxic for routine use.

TABLE 49-20. Alternatives to MOPP*: Minor Variations

MVPP
Nitrogen mustard 6 mg/m² IV days 1, 8
Vinblastine 10 mg days 1, 8, 15
Procarbazine 100 mg/m² days 1–15 (not to exceed [NTE] mg/day)
Prednisone 40 mg days 1–15
Repeat every 28 days

British MOPP (BNLI)
Nitrogen mustard 6 mg/m² IV days 1, 8 (NTE 15 mg/dose)
Vincristine (Oncovin) 1.4 mg/m² IV days 1, 8 (NTE 2 mg/dose)
Procarbazine 100 mg/m² PO days 1–10 (NTE 200 mg/day)
Prednisone 25 mg/m² PO days 1–14 (NTE 60 mg/day)

LOPP (BNLI)
Chlorambucil 10 mg/day PO days 1–10
Vincristine (Oncovin) 1.4 mg/m² IV days 1, 8 (NTE 2 mg/dose)
Procarbazine 100 mg/m² PO days 1–10 (NTE 200 mg/day)
Prednisone 25 mg/m² PO days 1–14

MVVPP
Nitrogen mustard 0.4 mg/kg IV day 1
Vincristine 1.4 mg/m² IV days 1, 8, 15
Vinblastine 6 mg/m² IV days 22, 29, 36
Procarbazine 100 mg (total) PO days 22–43
Prednisone 40 mg days 1–22; then taper 14 days
Repeat every 57 days

CVPP
Cyclophosphamide 300 mg/m² IV days 1,8
Vinblastine 10 mg IV days 1, 8, 15
Procarbazine 100 mg/m² PO days 1–15
Prednisone 40 mg/m² PO days 1–15†
Repeat every 28 days

BVCPP
BCNU 100 mg/m² IV day 1
Vinblastine 5 mg/m² IV day 1
Cyclophosphamide 600 mg/m² IV day 1
Procarbazine 50 mg PO day 1; 100 mg/m² PO days 2–10
Prednisone 60 mg/m² PO days 1–10
Repeat every 28 days

Ch1VPP
Chlorambucil 6 mg/m² PO days 1–14 (NTE 10 mg/day)
Vinblastine 6 mg/m² IV days 1–8 (NTE 10 mg/dose)
Procarbazine 100 mg/m² PO days 1–14 (NTE 150 mg/day)
Prednisone 40 mg/m² PO days 1–14 (25 mg/m² for children)

B-MOPP (low-dose bleomycin)
Bleomycin 2 U/m² IV days 1, 8
Nitrogen mustard 6 mg/m² IV days 1, 8
Vincristine (Oncovin) 1.4 mg/m² IV days 1, 8 (NTE 2 mg/dose)
Procarbazine 100 mg/m² PO days 1–10 (round to nearest 50 mg)
Prednisone 40 mg/m² PO days 1–10‡

* See Table 49-19 for explanation of acronyms.
† Cycles1 and 4 only.
‡ Cycles 1, 4, 7, and 10 only.

In other commonly tested MOPP variants, known by the

TABLE 49-21. Non–cross-resistant Alternatives to MOPP*

ABVD Doxorubicin (Adriamycin) 25 mg/m^2 IV days 1, 15 Bleomycin 10 U/m^2 IV days 1, 15 Vinblastine 6 mg/m^2 IV days 1, 15 Dacarbazine 375 mg/m^2 IV days 1, 15 Repeat every 28–35 days	B-CAVe Bleomycin 5 U/m^2 IV days 1, 28, 35 CCNU 100 mg/m^2 PO day 1 Doxorubicin (Adriamycin) 60 mg/m^2 IV day 1 Vinblastine 5 mg/m^2 IV day 1 Repeat every 42 days
BVDS Bleomycin 5 U/m^2 days 1, 15 Vinblastine 6 mg/m^2 IV days 1, 15 Doxorubicin 30 mg/m^2 IV day 1 Prednisone 40 mg/m^2 PO days 1–6 Repeat every 28 days	CEP CCNU 80 mg/m^2 PO day 1 Etoposide (VP-16) 100 mg/m^2 days 1–5 Prednimustine 60 mg/m^2 days 1–5 Repeat every 28 days
CABS (also known as SCAB) CCNU 100 mg/m^2 PO day 1 Doxorubicin (Adriamycin) 45 mg/m^2 IV day 1 Bleomycin 15 U/m^2 IV days 1, 8 Streptozocin 500 mg/m^2 IV days 1–5 Repeat every 28 days	CVB CCNU 100 mg/m^2 PO day 1 Vinblastine mg/m^2 IV days 1, 8 Bleomycin 15 U/m^2 IM days 1, 8 Repeat every 28 days
CEM CCNU 100 mg/m^2 PO day 1 Etoposide (VP-16) 100 mg/m^2 days 1–3, 21–23 MTX 30 mg/m^2 days 1, 8, 21, 28	
EVAP (British regimen) Etoposide (VO-16) Vinblastine Doxorubicin (Adriamycin) Prednisone	EVAP (NCI salvage regimen) Etoposide (VO-16) 120 mg/m^2 days 1, 8, 15 Vinblastine 4 mg/m^2 days 1, 8, 15 Arabinosyl cytosine 30 mg/m^2 days 1, 8, 15 Platinol (cisplatin) 40 mg/m^2 days 1, 8, 15 Repeat every 28 days
MOP-BAP Nitrogen mustard 6 mg/m^2 IV days 1, 8 Vincristine (Oncovin) 1.4 mg/m^2 IV days 1, 8 (NTE 2 mg/dose) Bleomycin 2 U/m^2 IV days 1, 8 Adriamycin (doxorubicin) 30 mg/m^2 IV days 1, 15 Prednisone 100 mg/m^2 PO days 2–7, 9–12 (round to nearest 50 mg)† Repeat every 28 days	
VABCD Vinblastine 6 mg/m^2 IV q 3 wk Doxorubicin (Adriamycin) 40 mg/m^2 q 3 wk Bleomycin 15 U q wk (NTE 300 U total dose) CCNU 80 mg/m^2 q 6 wk Dacarbazine 800 mg/m^2 q 3 wk	

*See Table 49-19 for explanation of acronyms.
†Cycles 1, 4, 7, and 10 only.

acronym CVPP, various doses of parenteral cyclophosphamide and vinblastine were combined with various doses of oral procarbazine and prednisone in a variety of schedules. The overall complete remission rate in collected studies is approximately 70% (range 62%–74%), and the actuarial 4-year relapse-free survival rates range from 50% to 60%.[314,358] These results do not represent an improvement over MOPP, MVPP, or ChlVPP, since toxicities are similar to that of MOPP with the exception of peripheral neuropathy and extravasation sequelae.

The Cancer and Leukemia Group B (CALGB) studied four-drug regimens differing from BCVPP in that BCNU or CCNU was substituted for nitrogen mustard, or CCNU was substituted for nitrogen mustard, in the CVPP regimen. These studies have resulted in an average of 68% complete response rate and four-year relapse-free survivals of 50% to 70%.[354,359,360]

The Southwest Oncology Group (SWOG) conducted a study comparing MOPP to MOPP plus bleomycin.[277,278] The complete response rate with MOPP, in this first SWOG study, was 70% compared to that with MOPP–bleomycin of 87%, and MOPP–bleomycin was thought to be the superior treatment. The latter program was selected for the next study as the control and it was compared to a new version of MOPP referred to as MOPP–BAP,[283] in which half of the dose of nitrogen mustard is replaced with half of the dose of adriamycin. The complete response rate with MOPP–bleomycin in the second study was not comparable to the first SWOG study, decreasing to 67%, which was inferior to the complete response rate for MOPP–BAP of 77%. Based

TABLE 49-22. MOPP Hybrid Combinations*

MA/MA
Nitrogen mustard 6 mg/m² IV day 1
Vincristine (Oncovin) 1.4 mg/m² IV day 1 (NTE 2 mg/dose)
Procarbazine 100 mg/m² PO days 1–7
Prednisone 40 mg/m² days 1–7
Doxorubicin (Adriamycin) 25 mg/m² IV day 15
Bleomycin 10 U/m² IV day 15
Vinblastine 6 mg/m² IV day 15
Dacarbazine 375 mg/m² IV day 15
Repeat every 28–35 days
MOPP/ABV
Nitrogen mustard 6 mg/m² day 1
Vincristine (Oncovin) 1.4 mg/m² day 1 (NITE 2 mg/dose)
Procarbazine 100 mg/m² days 1–7
Prednisone 40 mg/m² days 1–14
Doxorubicin (Adriamycin) 35 mg/m² day 8
Vinblastine 6 mg/m² day 8
Bleomycin 10 U/m² day 8
Repeat every 28 days

*See Table 49-19 for explanation of acronyms.

on these results, MOPP–BAP was said to be superior; however, superiority once again came at the expense of a sharp decline in the complete response rate for the control arm in each study, with the complete response rate of MOPP–BAP not being significantly better than that of the MOPP-only arm in the original SWOG study. While these trends could be accounted for if the later studies shifted to treating patients with poorer prognostic factors, the data indicate the opposite. Once again, alterations in doses and schedules seem the more likely explanation, with physicians reducing doses of more familiar programs as they learn to anticipate the toxicity.

Thus, by and large, the addition of drugs to MOPP has not made it more useful than adequate doses of MOPP or MOPP equivalents, like ChlVPP or MVPP. Adding drugs adds significant risks, and the risk of using a BCNU as part of treatment in newly diagnosed patients does not appear justified by the results.

The first new regimen of importance was the ABVD regimen (doxorubicin, bleomycin, vinblastine and dacarbazine) developed by Bonadonna and others.[292,361–363] In the first comparison of ABVD with MOPP as initial therapy for advanced disease, a 71.5% complete remission rate was obtained with the former, which was not significantly different from the 63% remission rate obtained with the latter.[282,292] No significant difference in the disease-free or overall survival was noted. Bonadonna and associates[281,288,289] then compared alternating cycles of MOPP and ABVD to treatment with MOPP alone for patients with Stage IV Hodgkin's disease. They randomized 88 Stage IV patients to receive either 12 monthly cycles of MOPP or 6 cycles of MOPP alternating monthly with 6 cycles of ABVD. This population had a predominance of two favorable prognostic factors. Twenty percent of the patients had experienced relapse after radiotherapy alone; 30% were in the asymptomatic category. A complete remission was obtained in 74.4% of patients with MOPP alone and 88.9% of patients with MOPP/ABVD; the difference was not significant. Although greater differences in complete response rate in favor of MOPP/ABVD were noted in patients over age 40 who had no prior radiotherapy, lymphocyte-depleted histology, B symptoms, more than three nodal sites involved, or bulky tumor, none of the differences were significant. The median number of cycles required to achieve a complete remission was five for both treatment arms, which was greater than the median number of cycles (three) required to achieve remission in the MOPP-treated patients at NCI. Disease-free and overall survival was significantly different between the two groups and favored MOPP–ABVD. The 8-year freedom from progression was 35.9% and 64.6% for the MOPP and MOPP–ABVD groups, respectively. Of the total of 72 complete responders, 45.1% in the MOPP group and 72.6% in the MOPP–ABVD group were continuously disease-free at 8 years. The total survival of the complete responders was significantly different in favor of MOPP–ABVD when only death from Hodgkin's disease was considered. When all deaths were considered, the differences were not significant (61.9% for MOPP; 76.2% for MOPP–ABVD) after 8 years of observation. The toxicity of MOPP–ABVD was more unacceptable to patients than that of MOPP alone. Only 7% of MOPP patients refused to complete treatment, compared with 22% of MOPP–ABVD patients. The doses in the MOPP arm were once again markedly reduced, and the result with MOPP in this study was inferior to those at NCI and in prior (8C) MOPP studies from the Milan group (see discussion of dose intensity below).

The CALGB recently reported the early results of a comparison of MOPP with ABVD and MOPP–ABVD in a group of patients with previously untreated advanced Hodgkin's disease with Stages $IIIA_2$–IVB.[364] MOPP–ABVD patients received 6 cycles of each regimen for a total of 12 cycles, whereas the other patients received less prolonged therapy but a minimum of 6 cycles. Once again, an extraordinary rate of dose reduction in the MOPP arm was allowed. In addition to capping the vincristine dose, projected doses of vincristine were reduced by 30% by the third cycle, and the doses of nitrogen mustard and procarbazine were reduced by 56% and 61% respectively, by the third cycle. Calculations of dose intensity have not been reported, so the impact of prolonging the intervals between cycles was not assessed. The complete response rate for MOPP–ABVD was 82%, compared with 69% for the reduced version of MOPP. However, the complete response rate for ABVD, 81%, was identical to that with MOPP–ABVD. Failure-free survival of 36 months was significantly better with MOPP–ABVD (64%) compared with MOPP (48%), but it was identical to that obtained with ABVD alone (64%). No significant difference in disease-free or overall survival among the regimens has yet emerged with a median follow-up of only 2 years. The data suggest an early failure-free survival advantage for MOPP–ABVD compared to the reduced version of MOPP, but no advantage of MOPP–ABVD over ABVD alone.

The ECOG also compared MOPP–ABVD to their BCVPP regimen alone or with low-dose radiation therapy added to initially involved sites in patients with advanced Hodgkin's disease. In an interim evaluation of 294 patients, complete response rates among the therapeutic options were found to be similar (68%–76%), and no differences in projected 3-year disease-free survival of complete responders (66%) was observed. These data support the contention that ABVD is superior to MOPP when dose intensity of MOPP is suboptimal, but they do not support the concept that alternating cycles of non–cross-resistant combinations improved the results of an adequately used four-drug combination. The data also strongly support the view that investigator bias in regard to anticipated toxicity can radically alter dosing practices and outcome.

Others have studied alternating non–cross-resistant regimens that include combinations other than ABVD. The most prominent study is that of Connors and Klimo,[323–325] which features a MOPP–ABVD variant in which dacarbazine is omitted and all drugs other than prednisone are given within 8 days (MOPP–ABV hybrid). Six courses of treatment are given after which response is assessed. Patients in complete remission at that time receive two more treatment courses. Partial responders receive radiotherapy to a single nodal area or to residual disease, or further MOPP–ABV for more extensive residual disease. In the Connors and Klimo study, complete response was attained in 96% of 74 evaluable patients, and the actuarial relapse-free survival for complete responders, after more than 5 years off treatment, was 90%. However, the complete response rate includes the 15% of the patients who had radiotherapy to residual disease, and almost 40% of the patients in this study population were asymptomatic. This regimen is currently part of a prospective randomized trial in Canada comparing it to MOPP–ABVD as used in Milan. Bonadonna[292] is also testing alternating half cycles of MOPP and ABVD (MA–MA) compared to their original MOPP–ABVD program. Early results show comparable complete remission rates for MA–MA but greater ease of administration.

A study testing the utility of alternating cycles of two non–cross-resistant drug combinations has also been conducted at the NCI and recently reported.[297] MOPP was compared, in a randomized trial, with MOPP–CABS (CCNU, Adriamycin, bleomycin, and streptozotocin). In this study, cycles of CABS were alternated with MOPP, but, in both arms of the study, the projected numbers of cycles for remission induction was 6 instead of 12 as in the Milan trial. One hundred twenty-seven patients were randomized, 64 to MOPP and 63 to MOPP–CABS, of whom 59 and 56, respectively, were evaluable. The complete response rate is 92% for MOPP and 88% for MOPP–CABS, an insignificant difference. At 5 years of follow-up, the results of both arms were equal and equivalent to or slightly better than the original MOPP study. Dose intensity of the MOPP program in this study exceeded that of the original NCI MOPP study because dose escalation was allowed.

Three other studies have routinely added radiotherapy to the chemotherapy of advanced Hodgkin's disease to sites known to be previously involved with tumor. Wagener and associates[322] studied 50 advanced-stage patients in a nonrandomized trial in which MOPP was alternated with CAVmP (cyclophosphamide, doxorubicin, Vm 26, and prednisone). Three cycles of each regimen were given on an alternating schedule, after which consolidation radiotherapy was given to initially involved sites. The complete response after chemotherapy was only 68%; 87% were in complete remission after radiotherapy. Actuarial 3-year survival of the total group of complete responders was 94%, and relapse-free survival was 73%. The authors concluded that the treatment was no more effective than MOPP in achieving complete remission but that it may be superior in terms of survival. No direct comparison has been made to MOPP. Farber, Prosnitz and colleagues[319–321] recently updated results of 102 previously untreated Stages IIIB and IV patients and 82 patients who experienced relapse after radiotherapy. Initially, patients were treated with nitrogen mustard, vincristine, vinblastine, procarbazine, and prednisone (MVVPP) for three cycles over 6 months; this regimen was followed by low-dose radiation to the initial sites of disease. Later in the study, the chemotherapy was changed to MOPP–ABVD and, ultimately, to a randomization between MOPP and MVVPP before radiotherapy. The three regimens were found to be equivalent. The overall complete response rate was 82% and the 15-year actuarial survival of all treated patients was 54% (71%, if only deaths from Hodgkin's disease are considered). Strauss and associates[285] reported no differences in outcome between patients treated with low-dose radiotherapy to involved sites combined with MOPP–ABVD or CAD (CCNU, phenylalanine mustard, and vindesine) alternated with MOPP–ABVD; they concluded that disease-free and overall survival in the study were similar to those reported for MOPP alone, although early results were more encouraging.

IMPACT OF DOSE INTENSITY ON OUTCOME IN HODGKIN'S DISEASE

From the foregoing review, it should be apparent that dosing practices in clinical studies have been inconsistent. While drugs were added and substituted at will, and schedules manipulated frequently, the total dose and dose rate themselves were never examined prospectively as independent variables in any of the studies reported.[352] A retrospective report by Carde and colleagues[365] from Stanford University noted that lower doses were related to poorer outcome. The dose and dose rate of nitrogen mustard, vincristine, and procarbazine in MOP as used at Stanford (Stanford physicians omit prednisone out of fear of radiation pneumonitis) were important variables both in the ability to attain complete remission and in survival. A regression analysis showed that the mean of the total dose, and the dose rate of three cytotoxic agents combined, had a significant impact on complete remission rate, particularly in patients with B symptoms, strongly supporting the contention that preservation of the integrity of the combination is important. Also, patients who received less than 65% of the projected dose of nitrogen mustard had significantly poorer survival than those who received more than 65% of the projected dose. Another report from Stanford indicated that, in their hands, MOPP failures often achieved good palliation with the use of single–alkylating-agent chemotherapy as salvage treatment, which also suggested that significant underdosing with alkylating agents was occurring during their initial use of MOPP.[366]

To compare results across studies in Hodgkin's disease, the NCI group followed the practice of Hryniuk and Bush[350,351] in converting doses in the MOPP program to mg/m^2/wk for each drug and averaging the doses of the three cytotoxic drugs to obtain an average dose intensity over

TABLE 49-23. MOPP Regimen Alterations in Relative Dose Intensity

Versions	*Cycle Intervals (Weeks)* 4	5	6	8
I MOPP, standard	1	0.80	0.67	0.50
II VCR total, 2 mg PCZ scaled up; 14 days	0.92	0.74	0.61	0.46
III VCR total, 2 mg PCZ scaled up; 10 days	0.82	0.66	0.55	0.41

the 6-month MOPP treatment duration.[351] In comparing one study to another, the program with the highest average dose intensity is used as the standard, and the dose intensity of other studies is reported as the decimal fraction of the dose intensity of the standard, or the relative dose intensity (RDI). Calculating RDI has several advantages over comparing percentages of projected dose delivered in each study, the most prevalent practice. The percentages of projected dose delivered may be similar, but the projected dose within each study may vary, as is true for vincristine in most trials. It is also possible to compare the impact of dose intensity of individual cytotoxic drugs or the average RDI of all the drugs in the combination. However useful the method is in ranking dosing practices, it is imprecise as applied to clinical studies for two important reasons: (1) Data on actual doses delivered are rarely given in sufficient detail to make the necessary calculations, a practice that could be corrected by making such data a requirement of publication; and (2) the end points used to determine the effects of dose reduction on outcome are often imprecise. Studies are reported at different time intervals and normally give data only on relapse-free survival and overall survival of those patients who attained a complete remission. The most sought-after data on outcome is the fraction of all treated patients who survive free of recurrence more than 5 years from the end of treatment. These data must often be extrapolated using the complete remission rate and published relapse-free survival curves.

Examples of the impact of ad hoc alterations in the MOPP program are shown in Table 49-23. Version I is used at NCI. It has the highest dose intensity of any reported program and is used as the reference standard. Giving version I with an extra week between cycles results in a 20% reduction in the average dose intensity per cycle. Version II, used in many clinical studies, limits the dose of vincristine to a total of 2 mg, in effect a full dose for a person of 1.43 m^2 body surface area; procarbazine is scaled up in dose slowly, a practice used in the clinic to reduce nausea and vomiting. If given on schedule, version II has an 8% decrease in average dose intensity. Version III is used in some clinical trials and by many practicing oncologists. The schedule of administration of procarbazine is shortened to 10 days along with the other dose modifications already mentioned. This practice results in an average decrease in RDI of 18% if it is given on schedule. In practice, however, MOPP is rarely given on schedule. MOPP in practice, and in most clinical trials cited, is more often given at 5-week intervals, with a resulting decrease in dose intensity of up to 34%, a reduction in the range that causes a loss of over half of the cure rate in almost all animal models. It should be noted that, in some studies, additional significant changes are made, such as omission of a drug entirely, usually vincristine or procarbazine, from the combination.

Table 49-24 shows data on intended and actual dose intensity in studies using MOPP. It was possible to estimate actual dose intensity in only five of the eight studies shown. No consistent effect of intended or actual dose intensity is noted on the complete response rate. However, the relationship between dose intensity and the fraction of patients who remain free of disease is more revealing. Reductions in actual dose intensity of 29% and 38% in the ECOG and Milan studies, respectively, resulted in 33% and 35% decreases in overall disease-free survival. A regression analysis yields a correlation coefficient of 0.88 ($p<0.02$) (Fig. 49-16). The difference in outcome between MOPP and the next three programs shown in Figure 49-16 is significant at the $p<0.001$ level.

As an example of the impact of ad hoc alteration of doses in a clinical trial, we can return to the Milan trial comparing MOPP to MOPP–ABVD.[289] The complete remission and overall survival rates are not significantly different between the two programs, but the relapse-free survival was superior for MOPP–ABVD. The results with MOPP, however, were among the worst ever reported. Fifty percent of all patients in the MOPP arm of the Milan study experienced relapse in the first 24 months compared to only 34% of patients at NCI over a 14-year follow-up. Asymptomatic patients made up a

TABLE 49-24. MOPP Regimens for Hodgkin's Disease: Dose Intensity and Outcome

Study/Author	*Relative Dose Intensity vs NCI MOPP*	*Actual Relative Dose Intensity*	*Complete Remission (%)*	*% Patients Free of Disease (yr)*	
NCI/DeVita	1.0	0.85	84	55	(15)
Stanford/Carde	0.95	0.64*	72	30†	(5)
BNLI/Goldman	0.82	—	52	30	(5)
SEG/Huguley	0.82	0.64	46	16	(2)
CALGB/Nissen	0.81	—	74	37	(5)
ECOG/Bakemeier	0.77	0.60	73	37	(5)
Milan/Bonadonna	0.76	0.53–0.66	74	36	(8)
SWOG/Frel	0.70	—	78	31	(5)

*Actual relative dose intensity from a prior paper.
†Estimate made from patients with marrow Stage IV.

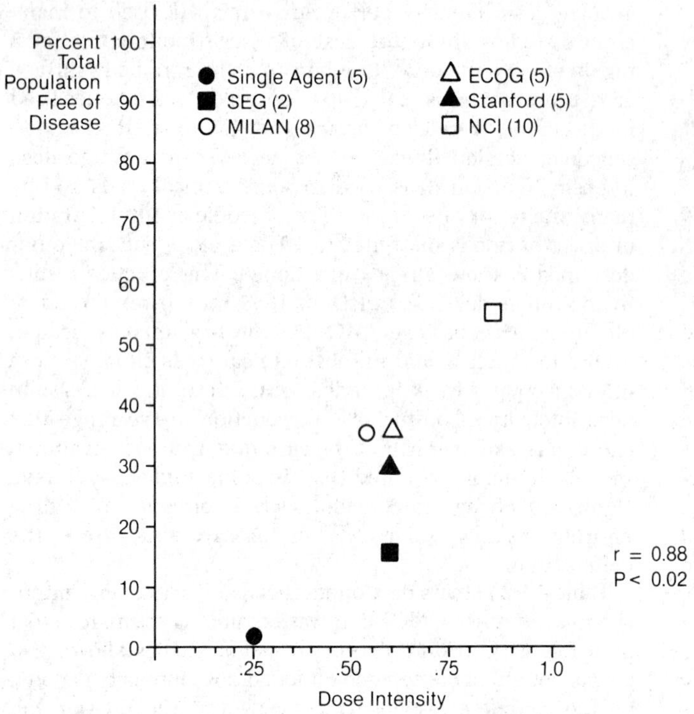

FIG. 49-16. Relative dose intensity compared to disease-free survival of patients with Hodgkin's disease in MOPP programs.

substantially larger portion of the study population in Milan than at NCI, but, rather than the 96% relapse-free survival rate reported by others, only 35% of asymptomatic Stage IIIA patients treated with MOPP in the Milan trial remain free of disease. The dose and dose rate of vincristine were significant variables with an impact on survival in the NCI study. In the Milan study, 35% of patients experienced a 50% reduction of the dose of vincristine, and, in 9% of patients, the integrity of the combination was entirely disrupted as vincristine was permanently discontinued. The problem with dose rate in the study is also emphasized by the median time to attain a complete remission with MOPP, 5 months in the Milan trial, compared to 3 months in the NCI study; time to attain a complete remission was also a significant variable predicting durability of remission in the NCI study. A reason for these dose reductions can be found in the study design. The newer program, MOPP–ABVD, was designed as a 12-month treatment program. MOPP is normally given for 6 months, but, in the Milan trial, it was extended to 12 months to make it comparable in length to MOPP–ABVD without pretesting the capability of patients to tolerate MOPP for 12 months. Most patients cannot tolerate vincristine and the other MOPP drugs for a 12-month period, and sharp dose reduction appeared to have occurred in anticipation of the side-effects attendant to 12 months of MOPP. The other study comparing MOPP to ABVD and MOPP–ABVD, the CALGB trial, suffers from similar ad hoc dose reductions. While the data from the CALGB trial comparing MOPP to MOPP–ABVD and ABVD are not yet available in sufficient detail to calculate relative dose intensity, considering the reported reductions in percent of projected doses discussed earlier, the skewed results are probably dose related as well.

The data on the impact of reduction of doses are derived from published reports of clinical trials conducted primarily at major medical centers. Reduction in doses should not, therefore, be interpreted as a practice limited to physicians in private practice. Nonetheless, the example having been set by the nation's clinical investigators, it is my experience that dose alterations are commonly made in practice as well. The information in Table 49-25 is representative of office practices and chart instruction.

TABLE 49-25. Investigator/Practitioner-initiated Modifications of MOPP Regimen

1. Use of "ideal" body weight in calculation of body surface area (BSA).
2. Rounding of BSA (example: 1.98 m^2 becomes 1.9).
3. Multiplication errors of $m^2 \times$ BSA.
4. Rounding of dose to fit a certain size vial of IV drug (example: 11.8 mg of HN2 becomes 10 mg to fit vial size).
5. Rounding of procarbazine dose to fit 50-mg size capsules, almost always lower (example: 1.78 m^2 BSA gets 150 mg/day).
6. Limit maximum dose regardless of height and weight; vincristine dose maximum is 2 mg in all but NCI studies.
7. Procarbazine dose is given on first 3 days in escalating dose (example: 50 mg, 100 mg, 150 mg, then full dose).
8. Omit a drug from a combination.
9. Drug administration intervals are lengthened to fit holidays or vacations (*e.g.*, 2-week rest period is lengthened to 4 to circumvent Christmas/New Year's) or to await complete return of blood count to normal.

SELECTION OF TREATMENT FOR ADVANCED HODGKIN'S DISEASE

Hodgkin's disease is indeed curable by chemotherapy, but at least four active drugs in combination are required for cure. When the available data are adjusted for differences in staging, the mix of asymptomatic and symptomatic patients, the use of concomitant radiotherapy, and dose adjustments, there are no significant differences in long-term outcome between MOPP, MVPP, ChlVPP, and ABVD, and one of these programs should be used alone as the initial treatment for most previously untreated patients with advanced Hodgkin's disease. To date, data are insufficient to support the contention that adding more drugs to the MOPP program or alternating MOPP with ABVD or other combinations produces superior long-term results compared to four drugs used in adequate doses. The impressive results with MOPP/ABVD by Klimo and Connors and Prosnitz require confirmation in a study testing the value of adding radiation therapy to sites of prior involvement or residual disease, a process that carries a greater risk of developing serious malignancies, especially tumors in the treatment field.

The choice of which of the suggested programs to use is based on toxicity. The acute toxicities of MOPP and ABVD are roughly equivalent, although the unwarranted fear most physicians have of vincristine-induced neuropathy and the slightly greater nausea and vomiting associated with MOPP often lead to greater dose reductions of MOPP with less therapeutic effect, as mentioned earlier. The most useful MOPP substitute is the ChlVPP regimen, which appears to preserve dose intensity because of fewer acute side-effects and produces equivalent long-term results to MOPP. The worldwide experience with ChlVPP is, however, minimal. The long-term leukemogenic effect of substituting chlorambucil for nitrogen mustard while retaining procarbazine is not yet known. Both MOPP and ChlVPP are reported to be more leukemogenic than ABVD, although the shorter follow-up of most ABVD studies does not allow a final conclusion. The limiting and irreversible cardiopulmonary toxicity associated with the use of adriamycin and bleomycin in ABVD is significant, especially in a young population, and may be a serious concern when ABVD is planned to be coupled with radiation therapy to the mediastinum. It should be noted that the highest risk of leukemia occurs in patients who receive extensive x-irradiation coupled with combination chemotherapy, a practice that should be discouraged in patients with early-stage disease, except for those with massive mediastinal involvement. This practice remains unproven when added to the site of residual disease in patients with advanced Hodgkin's disease successfully treated with drugs alone.

SALVAGE CHEMOTHERAPY FOR ADVANCED HODGKIN'S DISEASE

One of the most difficult problems faced by oncologists is the proper approach to managing patients with Hodgkin's disease who experience relapse after their primary treatment. Relapse occurs under three general circumstances: (1) Relapse as a Stage III or IV disease after primary treatment with radiotherapy for localized disease; (2) relapse after a chemotherapy-induced complete remission; and (3) failure to attain a complete remission with primary combination chemotherapy. Some general guidelines prove useful in the management of these patients. As pointed out in the discussion of the initial treatment of advanced Hodgkin's disease, it is apparent that patients who fail to respond to radiotherapy respond well to one of the primary treatment programs—MOPP, ChlVPP, MVPP, or ABVD—with a frequency and durability superior to patients who present de novo with the same stage of disease. One of these programs should be used in full doses and according to appropriate schedules. Marrow toxicity may be more severe if prior radiotherapy has been extensive. While the risk of secondary leukemia is high in this group and will approach 10% at 10 years, the benefits far outweigh the risks.

The choice of treatment for patients who experience relapse after combination chemotherapy-induced complete remission is based on the length of the initial remission. Patients with remissions in excess of 1 year have a high complete response rate to retreatment with the same regimen (93% in the NCI study),[367] and this phenomenon is generalizable to any initial treatment program.[336,368] About 35% of such patients have long disease-free survivals with retreatment. That this subgroup of patients is still so responsive to the same drug program indicates that drug resistance was not the likely reason for failure; inadequate dosing is the most plausible explanation. It is important, therefore, that the second round of treatment be administered at full doses or as near as safety will allow, using the sliding scale.

It has been argued that it would be more sensible to cross the patient over to a non–cross-resistant primary treatment program at this point to reduce any problems with residual drug-resistant cell lines, however minimal; indeed, this can be done. Among MOPP-treated patients who experience relapse after a long remission, treatment with ABVD yields results similar to those at NCI using MOPP again. The issue has two facets to consider. First, the results of the use of a cross-over regimen do not seem to be superior compared to the reuse of the primary regimen. Second, treatment with a second non–cross-resistant regimen is fine if it works. If, however, the patient experiences relapse once more, the second regimen is then not available for retreatment, although, in truth, scant data are available on the capacity to cure patients by crossing over to a non–cross-resistant regimen after their second relapse.

Of greater importance is the patient's tolerance to the primary regimen. Because dosing is the most important issue in administering the second set of induction chemotherapy, the choice of which regimen to use should be guided by the physician's knowledge of the capacity of that particular patient to tolerate the primary treatment. If the patient was treated with MOPP, for example, and marrow suppression was so severe that full doses were not possible, a second six cycles of MOPP is not likely to be any easier to administer, and the selection of ABVD might be a better choice, although marrow sensitivity to drugs is often a generic problem and is usually also severe with any second program. If a patient experienced severe neurotoxicity from the initial treatment with MOPP, then MVPP or ChlVPP could be used for retreatment instead of MOPP because vinblastine is substituted for vincristine in these regimens, and the general results are roughly equivalent. If nausea and vomiting were the obstacle to administering full doses, as they are occasionally, ChlVPP could be the superior choice for retreatment. It now also appears likely that the issue of adequate dosing in patients with marrow compromise by prior therapy may be solved by the use of colony-stimulating factors (CSFs) concomitant with induction or reinduction chemotherapy. The studies to determine their utility in lymphoma therapy are in progress,

Retreatment with ABVD after initial long remission is complicated by the inability to proceed with another set of full doses of adriamycin and bleomycin without the risk of severe cardiac and pulmonary compromise, and cross over to another primary regimen is preferable.

Patients who experience relapse after complete remissions lasting less than 1 year are only relatively resistant to chemotherapy, with 29% of such patients achieving a second complete remission with MOPP in the NCI series. However, these remissions are not as durable as those in patients with long first remissions, and patients who experience relapse in less than 1 year should be crossed over to a secondary regimen like ABVD. Once again, experience with ABVD in Milan indicates that some 20% of such patients can be salvaged using ABVD in MOPP failures.[369] Recent data from centers using autologous bone marrow transplantation (ABMT) as support to high-dose chemotherapy are encouraging. Although data are meager (see Chap. 65), these programs are yielding high complete remission rates, and disease-free survival is occurring at twice the frequency reported with cross over to a non–cross-resistant regimen alone without ABMT support. In young patients who have short first remissions, especially those with poor prognostic factors and for whom cure is unlikely, high-dose drug treatment with or without total body irradiation and with ABMT support should be considered an option equal to the use of a non–cross-resistant regimen alone.

While complete remissions are reported with cross-over treatment in patients for whom initial treatment fails to produce a remission, or whose tumors grow during primary treatment, the remissions are infrequent and rarely durable. Such patients should be considered candidates for high-dose chemotherapy with ABMT even if retreatment with a standard regimen induces a remission. Reduction of disease to a minimum puts the patient in a favorable circumstance to respond to high-dose chemotherapy with ABMT support. Patients experiencing relapse with extensive bone marrow involvement require chemotherapy to eradicate the marrow disease before consideration is given to ABMT, since the various purging techniques are being assessed only as a tool to reduce microscopic residual marrow disease.

Physicians should be aware that the salvage treatment of Hodgkin's disease is changing rapidly because of the improvements in the use of ABMT as supportive care and the availability of CSFs. More facile, less toxic use of high-dose chemotherapy with ABMT should soon make it possible to consider its use in all patients experiencing relapse from, or failing to respond to, the primary combination chemotherapy program. The widespread availability of CSFs may also make ABMT unnecessary by making it possible to administer full doses of chemotherapy for initial treatment programs, thereby improving results with primary treatment, or by making salvage treatment more effective.

The selection of a particular salvage treatment program for a patient no longer responsive to standard regimens is complicated by the heterogeneity of the available data. The

TABLE 49-26. Salvage Treatments for Patients Failing to Respond to MOPP Regimen

Author	*Regimen**	*No. of Patients*	*CR (%)*	*Median Duration (mo)*	*% FOD/mo*	*Comments*
Vinciguerra et al[370]	BVDS	10	30	NS	—	1 pt/DFS NS
Goldman & Dawson[369,371]	CVB	39	26	NS	—	10 of 10 patients relapse by 5 yr
Santoro et al[361,362]	ABVD	54	59	17	22/60	
Papa et al[363]	ABVD	18	55	>36	50	9 of 10 patients FOD @ 9–60 mo
Weiss et al[372]	CBVD	20	45	10	15/12	3 patients FOD @ 8, 12, & 16 mo
Tannir et al[373]	ABDIC	34	35	47	19/36	
Einhorn et al[374]	VABCD	18	44	>30	28/30	
Piga et al[375]	ABVD	39	30	>25	30/>52	
Harket et al[376]	B-CAVe	48	44	24.3	21/46	
	ABVD	55	38	>25	21/35	
Santoro et al[377,378]	CEP	58	40	15	NS	
	CEP–ABVD	21	67	>24	NS	
Cervantes et al[379]	CEP	15	27	5.5	—	2 patients FOD @ 7, 18 mo
Mandelli et al[380]	PCVP	11	72	>8	54/9	
Richards et al[381]	EVA	19	31	15	26/7	3 of 5 patients in CR given RT
Garbes et al[382]	MTX-CHOP	11	36	18	—	1 patient FOD @ 8 yr
Hagemeister et al[383]	MIME	47	23	NS	NS	
Pfreundschuh et al[383a]	CEVD	32	44	>10	22/36	
Tseng et al[384]	CEM	32	13	>33	—	3 patients FOD @ 6, 24, 44 mo after consolidation
Schulman[385]	MOPLACE	30	17	NS	NS	
Levi[386]	SCAB	17	35	>8	29/>8	
Longo[387]	$EVAP^2$	27	33	12	—	9 of 9 patients in relapse by 24 mo

CR = complete remission; DFS = disease-free survival; FOD = free of disease; NS = not specified; RT = radiation therapy.
*See Table 49-19 for explanation of acronyms.

literature is summarized in Table 49-26,[361,363,369–388] where the results of 19 studies are portrayed. Few of the reports encompass a population of patients greater than 30. Further, the problem of small numbers is compounded in all studies by the extensive mixture of important disease variables and prior response duration. However, the same general theme runs through these data. The best results are attained in patients who experience relapse asymptomatically, who have recurrent nodal disease, and who had attained a prior complete remission of long duration. But long-term complete remissions are unusual in the programs illustrated in Table 49-25 among patients with B symptoms and extensive visceral or marrow disease, especially if they have failed to respond to one of the prior treatment programs.

The use of ABVD as a MOPP salvage treatment has already been mentioned. The CEP (lomustine, etoposide, and prednimustine) salvage program, also developed by the Milan group, is the most interesting among those in Table 49-26. It works as well or better than any other regimen, and all the drugs are administered by the oral route.[377–379] CEP has also been used effectively with MOPP or ABVD in alternating cycles in patients who fail to respond to either ABVD or MOPP, respectively. Most of the other programs in Table 49-26 do not have follow-up periods adequate to determine long-term results or have had no follow-up report, suggesting that long-term results did not prove the program useful. The results with the ABDIC,[373] VABCD,[374] and B-CAVe[376] regimens are interesting enough to warrant consideration (see Table 49-21 for doses and schedules). ABDIC and VABCD contain adriamycin, bleomycin, dacarbazine, CCNU, and prednisone and, therefore, resemble ABVD except for the inclusion of a nitrosourea. They are most useful in patients not responding to MOPP but may not be superior to ABVD alone; no data are available for comparison. The patient population in the VABCD study was more uniform and the results easier to interpret. Fifteen patients, for example, had Stage IV disease, 11 with systemic symptoms. Eight complete remissions occurred in this group and five remained disease-free at the time of the report. B-CAVe also has three of the ABVD drugs plus the nitrosourea, CCNU, but not dacarbazine. Forty-four percent of patients who did not respond to the MOPP regimen had a complete remission, and a quarter of these patients had not progressed at 4 years, although not all were disease-free. No other program has emerged as a major improvement over these regimens. Thus, for those who fail to respond to MOPP, the choices are ABVD, ABVD-like combinations, or CEP. For patients who do not respond to ABVD, CEP appears to be the treatment of choice, although the PCVP program (procarbazine, cyclophosphamide, vinblastine, and prednisone), which resembles the MOPP program,[380] may be a useful alternative cross-over regimen after ABVD failure. Physicians are once again urged to use these programs in their recommended doses and schedules.

THE TREATMENT OF STAGE IIIA DISEASE

Several studies now support the use of combination chemotherapy alone for treatment of Stage IIIA disease not associated with bulky mediastinal disease. A 94% 10-year disease-free survival was reported for patients with asymptomatic disease in the original NCI study, which is essentially identical to the 96% 10-year disease-free survival for patients with Stage IIIA disease reported by Lister and associates[310] and the 91% reported by Crowther and associates[311] using MVPP as the drug treatment. Results in the Lister study were significantly better than the 60% 10-year disease-free survival obtained with total nodal irradiation alone, and the results of the chemotherapy alone were identical to that obtained with combined-modality therapy in the Crowther study. It would appear, therefore, that combination chemotherapy alone is optimal for patients with Stage IIIA disease. However, for asymptomatic patients with bulky mediastinal masses or other evidence of massive tumor involvement, combined-modality treatment may be superior to either modality alone.

USE OF CHEMOTHERAPY IN EARLY-STAGE DISEASE

The success of chemotherapy alone in patients with Stage IIIA disease, and the demonstration of significant activity of chemotherapy in early-stage disease in NCI-sponsored studies in Uganda, East Africa,[389] led to the initiation of a pilot study at the NCI Baltimore Cancer Research program in 1976. In this trial, patients with surgical Stage IB to IIIA disease were randomized to treatment with extended-field radiotherapy followed by six cycles of MOPP, or MOPP alone.[390] A complete remission occurred in 94% of patients with combined-modality therapy and in 80% of those treated with MOPP alone. Two of three MOPP failures subsequently achieved complete remission with radiotherapy. Of the 15 patients treated with MOPP alone, one nonresponder died of progressive Hodgkin's disease at 57 months, and one partial responder, given radiation as salvage therapy; died of acute leukemia at 78 months. The remaining 13 patients continue in their first remission at 10.5+ years, although 1 of those patients developed squamous cell carcinoma of the lung that has apparently been cured by surgery. To date, there is no significant difference in outcome between the two groups with respect to disease-free or overall survival. The NCI is now conducting a study randomizing patients with early-stage disease (without massive mediastinal involvement) to MOPP chemotherapy alone or radiotherapy. Eighty-six patients with Stages IA and IIB involvement have been randomly allocated to treatment with six cycles of MOPP, or subtotal radiation therapy after staging laparotomy. In an interim evaluation with a median observational period of 40 months,[391] all MOPP-treated patients had achieved complete remission and only four had experienced relapse. The complete response rate was 95% for the radiotherapy group, but one third have suffered relapse. Death had occurred in 9% of the MOPP group and 22% of the radiation-treated group. There was a significant difference in relapse-free survival in favor of the MOPP group, but overall survival was not significantly different.

HODGKIN'S DISEASE IN AIDS AND AIDS-RELATED COMPLEX

Controversy exists concerning whether Hodgkin's disease is part of the spectrum of AIDS, although most authorities believe there is no evidence to suggest that this is true. However, HIV-positive patients with Hodgkin's disease usually present with advanced stage, advanced histology, and B symptoms. In contrast to HIV-negative patients, Hodgkin's disease tissues from HIV-positive patients are depleted of helpet T lymphocytes and infiltrated with suppressor T cells. Response to chemotherapy has been poor.[392-394]

COMPLICATIONS OF THERAPY OF HODGKIN'S DISEASE

The major consequence of the treatment of Hodgkin's disease is its cure. The availability of populations of long-term survivors has allowed investigators to describe numerous side-effects that warrant attention on the part of the physician. A detailed list of reported complications in long-term survivors is found in Table 49-27 and reviewed in detail in reference 394. More extensive discussions of the complications of treatment can be found in Chapters 58 and 59. Despite the extensive nature of the list of side-effects, the lives of long-term survivors are quite normal, because many side-effects represent minor annoyances that may be easily corrected, occur in few patients, or represent only the potential for future problems. The most serious problem is the risk of developing secondary leukemia and solid tumors in the treatment field. This complication is discussed in Chapter 59. Table 49-28 summarizes the relative risk of the development of leukemia under different treatment circumstances.

Risk increases dramatically whenever combination chemotherapy and extensive radiation therapy are used together. This practice can be avoided in most cases by using each modality in its optimal way (see the section on treatment by stage). The patient is done a disservice if radiotherapy doses or fields are compromised because salvage treatment with chemotherapy is effective or if chemotherapy will be given concomitantly, except in children (see Chap. 47). Using chemotherapy in full doses minimizes the number of drugs and programs that patients need to be exposed to as well. The problem of fertility and treatment is discussed in Chapter 59.

TABLE 49-27. Long-term Complications in Patients Cured of Hodgkin's Disease

Complication	*Etiology and Risk Factors*	*Management and Prevention*
Immunologic dysfunction	Underlying disease, therapy	Appropriate vaccinations
Herpes zoster-varicella	Underlying disease, therapy	Systemic antiviral therapy, zoster immune globulin
Pneumococcal sepsis	Splenectomy Functional asplenia post radiation therapy (RT)	Pretherapy pneumonococcal vaccine, selected antibiotic prophylaxis, avoid unnecessary staging splenectomy
Nonlymphocytic leukemia	Therapy, age above 40	Avoid combined modality therapy for HD, supportive care, low-dose chemotherapy, aggressive therapy +/− bone marrow transplant
Myelodysplastic syndromes	Therapy, age above 40	Same as above
Non-Hodgkin's lymphoma	Therapy	Aggressive combination CT (i.e., MACOP-B)
Solid tumors	Direct or indirect RT exposure	Conventional management
Thymic hyperplasia	Underlying disease, therapy	Resection
Hypothyroidism	Direct or indirect RT exposure	Hormone replacement, thyroid suppression during therapy (?)
Thyroid cancer	Direct or indirect RT exposure, chronic thyroid stimulation	Thyroid suppression
Male infertility	Therapy, underlying disease	Attempt sperm storage, testicular shielding during RT, suppression of spermatogenesis during CT (?), alternative chemotherapy regimens
Male impotence	Therapy, underlying disease	Counseling, trial of testosterone
Female infertility	Therapy	Oophoropexy, ovarian suppression during therapy (?), cyclic estrogen replacement
Female impotence	Therapy, underlying disease	Counseling, cyclic estrogen replacement
Pericarditis, acute	Mediastinal RT, recall with chemotherapy (CT) post-RT	Appropriate RT shielding and technique, avoid doxorubicin post-RT, anti-inflammatory medication, pericardiocentesis
Pericarditis, chronic	Mediastinal RT	Appropriate RT shielding and technique, pericardiectomy
Cardiomyopathy	Mediastinal RT, doxorubicin, recall with CT post-RT	Appropriate RT shielding and technique, avoid doxorubicin post-RT, monitor for early signs of toxicity, limit cumulative doxorubicin dose, supportive medical management
Pneumonitis, acute	Direct or indirect RT, bleomycin, nitrosoureas, recall with CT post-RT	Appropriate RT shielding and technique, monitor for early signs of toxicity, avoid known toxic drugs, avoid excessive pO_2
Pneumonitis, chronic	Same as above	Supportive management
Avascular necrosis	Steroid therapy, underlying disease (?)	Anti-inflammatory medications, joint surgery
Growth retardation	Pediatric RT	Minimize RT, use symmetric RT fields
Dental caries	Salivary change post-RT	Maintaiin good oral hygiene, daily fluoride treatments

TABLE 49-28. Relative Importance of Various Risk Factors for Secondary Acute Myelocytic Leukemia Following Therapy for Hodgkin's Disease

*Therapy Category**	*Relative Risk*	*% Cumulative Risk at 10 Years*
Radiation therapy (RT) alone	Very low	0
Induction chemotherapy alone		
MOPP	Low	2–3
BCNU regimens	Intermediate	3–6
ABVD	Low	?
Combined-modality therapy		
Limited field RT plus MOPP	Low	2–3
Extensive RT plus MOPP	High	4–8
Salvage therapy	High	5–15
Age greater than 40	Very high	25–40
Maintenance therapy		
All therapy	High	5–10
Prolonged alkylating agents	Very high	10–30

*See Table 49-19 for explanation of acronyms.

NEW DRUGS AND BIOLOGICS IN HODGKIN'S DISEASE

From the foregoing discussion on salvage treatment, it should be apparent that testing of new agents for Hodgkin's disease presents a challenging problem.[395] Because treatment of newly diagnosed patients has been so successful and some patients are curable with second-line therapy or with high doses of chemotherapy with ABMT as support, the patient who fails to respond to all available treatment is a poor subject for new drug testing. Bone marrow reserve is usually minimal, and the advanced nature of the disease makes long-term observation difficult. This is a problem faced by oncologists in all tumors that respond well to chemotherapy such as childhood leukemia and testicular cancer. Nonetheless, there is some experience with agents in early clinical trials in Hodgkin's disease and these are summarized in Table 49-29.[396–403a] Details of the dose, side-effects and mechanism of action of these drugs are discussed in Chapter 18. Patients with advanced Hodgkin's disease should be referred to institutes conducting these trials for therapy.

Treatment with biologics should be considered as an alternative to chemotherapy because the side-effects of the two modalities are often different. The experience with biologics in Hodgkin's disease is, however, not extensive. Some useful responses and one complete remission have been reported with the use of isotopic immunoglobulins directed against ferritin.[403b] Recent improvement in labeling with isotopes other than ^{131}iodine may improve the effectiveness of this approach. The use of interleukin-2 plus lymphokine-activated killer cells in Hodgkin's disease is in its early stages. Some investigators have begun to combine less toxic analogues of active drugs with standard agents in standard combinations to test retention of efficacy, with reduced overall toxicity, as a way of introducing new agents. Given the heterogeneity of previously treated patients few useful data have yet to emerge from this approach.

TABLE 49-29. New Agents for the Treatment of Hodgkin's Disease

Gallium nitrate[396]
Amsacrine[399]
Diaziquone (aziridinylbenzoquonone, AZQ)[400]
Mitoxantrone[401]
Spirogermanium[398]
Carboplatin[395]
Methyl-bis-quanyl hydrazene (mitoquazone, methyl-GAG)[397]
Anthracycline analogues (aclacinomycin, 4′-demethoxy-daunorubicin, 4′-deoxydoxorubicin)[402–403a]

COMBINED RADIATION AND CHEMOTHERAPY IN HODGKIN'S DISEASE: STAGES I, II, AND III

Chemotherapy has been used in combination with radiation in the treatment of Stages I and II Hodgkin's disease. While some of these data show a tendency to reduce the rate of relapse as compared to radiation alone, overall survival is not affected[403c,404] because salvage chemotherapy used for radiation relapse saves a significant number of these patients. Combined chemotherapy and extensive radiation is associated with significant long-term complications[405–407] and mortality of approximately 10% in groups of patients receiving extensive radiation and chemotherapy. Figure 49-17[407] shows the recent JCRT experience, which will be discussed in greater detail in Chapter 60, Section 7. Combined radiation and chemotherapy is increasing in use in Stage IIIA Hodgkin's disease.[411–413] Because total nodal irradiation fails in more than 50% of patients, chemotherapy alone is the desired treatment for patients without bulky disease.[408–409] For those patients with initial bulky disease, if irradiation is to be used to supplement chemotherapy, it should be restricted in volume to those sites. A special group of patients comprises those with mediastinal involvement greater than one third the diameter of the chest. Here, combined-modality treatment is clearly indicated because patients with large mediastinal masses account for most relapses in supra-

FIG. 49-17. Actuarial risk of fatal complications after initiation of the last course of treatment. Treatments with total nodal irradiation (TN1) and MOPP, extended-field irradiation and MOPP, and radiation therapy (RT) alone are compared. (Mauch PM, Canellos GP, Rosenthal DS: Reduction of fatal complications from combined modality therapy in Hodgkin's disease. J Clin Oncol 3:501–505, 1985)

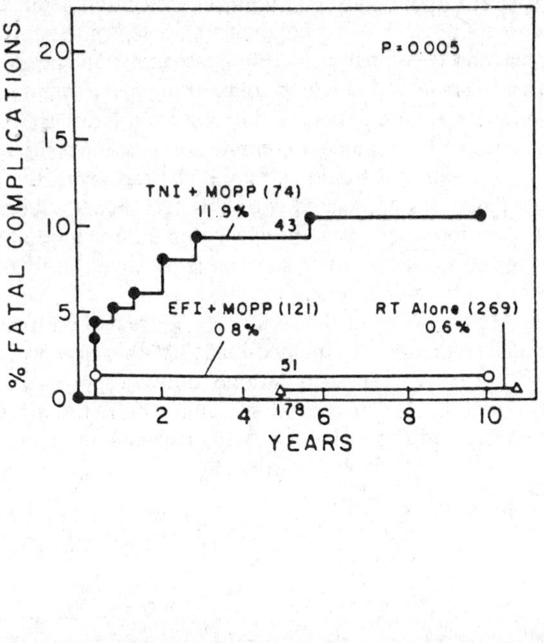

diaphragmatic Stages I and IIA, and the major sites of chemotherapy failure are those with large-bulk disease.[252-255, 410] Combined-modality therapy seems appropriate in this group.

The techniques of combining radiation and chemotherapy vary. While some studies administer all the radiation and then all the chemotherapy, others divide the chemotherapy, giving the radiation after two or three cycles, and then finally completing the chemotherapy. An important principle of treatment is to be sure that at least one treatment modality is administered with appropriate time–dose considerations and the other serves as an adjuvant. Thus, for patients with Stage II disease with a large mediastinal mass, the full course of chemotherapy should be administered and the radiation reserved as an adjuvant to the initial site of bulky disease. Extensive radiation given before chemotherapy may limit the amount of chemotherapy given. This pitfall should be avoided if possible.

CURRENT RECOMMENDATIONS FOR TREATMENT OF HODGKIN'S DISEASE BY STAGE

Based on the previous data, the following recommendations for treatment appear appropriate.

Laparotomy-staged patients with pathologic Stages I and IIA supradiaphragmatic disease and without large mediastinal masses should be treated with mantle radiation. For most patients, para-aortic fields should also be included. Exceptions to this rule may be those patients without evidence of mediastinal disease and having nodular sclerosis of lymphocyte-predominant histology. Continued use of the para-aortic field in these patients is uncertain and must be left to individual judgment.

Clinical Stages I and IIA patients with large mediastinal masses should be spared laparotomy and splenectomy and treated with combination chemotherapy initially, then with radiation to areas of previous bulky disease (mediastinum). Such a treatment technique means that, in patients presenting initially with large mediastinal masses, laparotomy is not indicated because it will not significantly alter therapy and does have an anesthesia risk. Full-dose chemotherapy should be given with the radiation volume restricted. The total dose of radiation under these circumstances may be reduced to 3500 to 4000 rad. Subdiaphragmatic disease is almost invariably diagnosed by laparotomy. Such disease should be treated with para-aortic and pelvic irradiation for pelvic or inguinal presentation. Those patients who present with disease in the periaortic nodes produce a complicated problem, since appropriate treatment would be total nodal radiation. Because of complications associated with this technique, especially when chemotherapy must be given for failure, one should consider seriously whether such patients should be treated with primary chemotherapy.

Patients with Stage IIB disease may be treated with subtotal nodal radiation. Combined-modality therapy probably should not be used in such patients unless they have large mediastinal disease or their B symptoms do not abate with the mantle radiation therapy field. Patients with clinical Stage IIB disease who have not been evaluated by laparotomy should be treated primarily with chemotherapy, with radiation reserved for sites of previous bulk disease.

Radiation therapy alone is not indicated in most Stage III patients. The possible exception is Stage IIIA patients having only splenic involvement; the radiation would be administered following laparotomy and splenectomy. If such patients have only a few splenic nodules, radiation alone may be used as an alternative to chemotherapy. For the remainder of Stage III patients, chemotherapy is the treatment of choice. Radiation should not be added in these groups: it should be limited, and used only to augment treatment to initial sites of bulk disease.

Radiation therapy should be limited in children. The data (from Memorial Sloan-Kettering Cancer Center)[249] indicate that the para-aortic fields can be omitted in pathologic Stages I and IIA pediatric Hodgkin's disease patients. A volume reduction even further than the mantle is desirable if possible, because the radiation produces significant retardation of bone growth. This drawback must be balanced against the risks of recurrence, especially in the very young. When radiation is given, not only must the volume be limited, but care should be taken to attempt symmetrical irradiation in order to limit the deformities produced by unilateral asymmetric bone growth. In general, for the very young, we recommend chemotherapy with avoidance of radiation as much as possible. For the young adolescent with supradiaphragmatic presentation following pathologic staging, mantle fields offer the best treatment success with the fewest complications.

REFERENCES

1. MacMahon B: Epidemiological evidence of the nature of Hodgkin's disease. Cancer 10:1045–1054, 1957
2. Correa P, O'Conor GT, Berard CW et al: International comparability and reproducibility in histologic subclassification of Hodgkin's disease. JNCI 50:1429–1435, 1973
3. Cole P, MacMahon B, Aisenberg A: Mortality from Hodgkin's disease in the United States. Evidence for the multiple etiology hypothesis. Lancet 2:1371–1376, 1968
4. Sternberg C: Uber eine eigenartige unter dem Bilde der Pseudoleukamie verlaufende Tuberculose des lymphatichon Apparates. Ztschr Heilk 19:21–90, 1898
5. Steiner PE: Hodgkin's disease: search for infective agent and attempts at experimental reproduction. Arch Pathol 17:749–763, 1934
6. L Esperance ES: Experimental innoculation of chickens with Hodgkin's nodes. J Immunol 16:37–60, 1929
7. Van Rooyan CE: Etiology of Hodgkin's disease with special reference to B. Tuberculosis avis. Br Med J 1:50–51, 1933
8. Van Rooyan CE: Recent experimental work on the etiology of Hodgkin's disease. Br Med J 2:519–524, 1934
9. Miller RW, Beebe: Infectious mononucleosis and the empirical risk of cancer. JNCI 50:315–321, 1973
10. Connolly RR, Chistene BW: A cohort study of cancer following infectious mononucleosis. Cancer Res 34:1172–1178, 1974
11. Rosdahl N, Larsen SO, Clemmensen J: Hodgkin's disease in patients with previous mononucleosis, 30 years' experience. Br Med J 2:253–256, 1974
12. Munoz N, Davidson RJ, Witthoff B et al: Infectious mononucleosis and Hodgkin's disease. Int J Cancer 22:10–13, 1978
13. Nonoyama M, Kawai Y, Huang CH et al: Epstein–Barr virus DNA in Hodgkin's disease, American Burkitt's lymphoma and other human tumors. Cancer Res 34:1228–1231, 1974
14. Kaplan HS, Smithers DW: Auto-immunity and homologous disease in mice in relation to the malignant lymphomas. Lancet 2:1–4, 1959
15. Order SE, Hellman S: Pathologenesis of Hodgkin's disease. Lancet 1:571–573, 1972
16. Schwartz RS, Beldotti L: Malignant lymphomas following allogenic disease: Transition from an immunological to a neoplastic disorder. Science 149:1511–1514, 1965
17. DeVita VT: Lymphocyte reactivity in Hodgkin's disease: A lymphocyte civil war. N Engl J Med 289:801–802, 1973

18. Vianna NJ, Greenwald P, Davies JNP: Extended epidemic of Hodgkin's disease in high school students. Lancet 1:1209–1210, 1971
19. Vianna JH, Polan AK: Epidemiological evidence for transmission of Hodgkin's disease. N Engl J Med 289:499–502, 1973
20. Smith PG, Pike MC, Kinlam LJ et al: Contacts between young patients with Hodgkin's disease: A case control study. Lancet 2:59–62, 1977
21. Zack MM, Heath CW Jr, Andrews MD et al: High school contact among persons with leukemia and lymphoma. JNCI 59:1343–1349, 1977
22. Gutterman S, Cole P, Levitan TR: Evidence against transmission of Hodgkin's disease in high schools. N Engl J Med 300:1000–1011, 1979
23. Gutensohn N, Cole P: Childhood social environment and Hodgkin's disease. N Engl J Med 304:135–140, 1981
24. Milham S Jr, Hesser J: Hodgkin's disease in woodworkers. Lancet 2:136–137, 1967
25. Vianna NJ, Greenwald P, Davies JNP: Tonsillectomy and Hodgkin's disease: The lymphoid tissue barrier. Lancet 1:431–432, 1971
26. Bierman HR: Human appendix and neoplasia. Cancer 21:109–118, 1968
27. Hyams L, Wynder EL: Appendectomy and cancer risk: An epidemiological evaluation. J Chronic Dis 21:319–415, 1968
28. Lilly F, Pincus T: Genetic control of murine viral leukemogenesis. In Klein G, Weinhouse S (eds): Advances in Cancer Research. Vol 17, pp 231–277. New York, Academic Press, 1977
29. Graff KS, Simons RM, Yankee RA et al: HLA antigens in Hodgkin's disease: Histopathologic and clinical correlations. JNCI 52:1087–1090, 1974
30. Longo DL, DeVita VT Jr: Lymphomas. In Pinedo HM (ed): Cancer Chemotherapy 1982, the EORTC Cancer Chemotherapy Annual 4. Amsterdam, Elsevier, 1982
31. Kaplan HS: Hodgkin's Disease, 2nd ed. Cambridge, Harvard University Press, 1980
32. Hodgkin T: On some morbid appearances of the absorbent glands and spleen. Med-Chir Trans 17:68–114, 1832
33. Bright R: Observations on abdominal tumours and intumescence. Guy's Hosp Rep 3:401–460, 1838
34. Wilks S: Cases of enlargement of lymphatic glands and spleen (or Hodgkin's disease), with remarks. Guy's Hosp Rep 11:56–67, 1865
35. Craigie D: Case of disease of the spleen, in which death took place in consequence in the presence of purulent matter in the blood. Edinburgh Med Surg J 64:400–413, 1845
36. Bennett JH: Case of hypertrophy of the spleen and liver in which death took place from suppuration of the blood. Edinburgh Med Surg J 64:413–423, 1845
37. Virchow R: Weisses blut, Neue Notizen aus den Geb der Naturund Heikunde. (Froriep's neue Notizen) 36:151–156, 1845
38. Roulet F: Dasprinare Retothelsarkom der Lymphkonten. Virchows Arch Pathol Anat 277:15–47, 1930
39. Burkitt D: A sarcoma involving the jaws in African children. Br J Surg 46:218–223, 1958
40. Greenfield WS: Specimens illustrative of the pathology of lymphadenoma and leucocythemia. Trans Pathol Soc London 29:272–304, 1878
41. Goldmann EE: Beitrug zu der Lehre von dem malignen Lymphom. Centr Allg Pathol Anat 3:665–690, 1892
42. Reed DM: On the pathological changes in Hodgkin's disease, with especial reference to its relation to tuberculosis. Johns Hopkins Hosp Rev 10:133–196, 1902
43. Ewing J: Neoplastic Diseases. Philadelphia, WB Saunders, 1928
44. Seif GSF and, Spriggs AI: Chromosome changes in Hodgkin's disease. J Nat Cancer Inst 39:557–470, 1967
45. Lukes RJ, Tindle BH, Parker JW: Reed–Sternberg-like cells in infectious mononucleosis. Lancet 2:1000–1004, 1969
46. Strum SB, Dark JK, Rappaport H: Observations of cells resembling Sternberg–Reed cells in conditions other than Hodgkin's disease. Cancer 26:176–190, 1970
47. Jackson H Jr, Parker F Jr: Hodgkin's disease. II. Pathology. N Engl J Med 231:35–44, 1944
48. Lukes RJ, Butler JJ, Hicks ED: Natural history of Hodgkin's disease as related to its pathologic picture. Cancer 19:317–344, 1966
49. Lukes RJ: Relationship of histiologic features to clinical stages in Hodgkin's disease. Am J Roentgenol 90:944–955, 1963
50. Poppema S, Kaiserling E, Lennert K: Hodgkin's disease with lymphocyte predominance, nodular type (nodular paragranuloma) and progressively transformed germinal centers—A cytohistological study. Histopathology 3:295, 1979
51. Poppema S, Kaiserling E, Lennert K: Nodular paragranuloma and progressively transformed germinal centers. Ultrastructural and immunohistologic findings. Virchows Arch [B] 31:211–225, 1979
52. Burns BF, Colby TV, Dorfman RF: Differential diagnostic features of nodular L&H Hodgkin's disease, including progressive transformation of germinal centers. Am J Surg Pathol 8:253–261, 1984
53. Miller TP, Byrne GE, Jones SE: Mistaken clinical and pathologic diagnoses of Hodgkin's disease: A Southwest Oncology Study Group. Cancer Treat Rep 66:645, 1982
54. Kant JA, Hubbard SM, Longo DL et al: The pathologic and clinical heterogeneity of lymphocyte-depleted Hodgkin's disease. J Clin Oncol 4:284, 1986
55. Neiman RS, Rosen PJ, Lukes RJ: Lymphocyte-depleted Hodgkin's disease. A clinopathological entity. N Engl J Med 288:751–755, 1973
56. Schoeppel SL, Hoppe RT, Dorfman RF et al: Hodgkin's disease in homosexual men with generalized lymphadenopathy. Ann Intern Med 102:68–70, 1985
57. Ioachim HL, Cooper MC, Hellman GC: Lymphomas in men at high risk for acquired immune deficiency syndrome (AIDS). Cancer 56:2831–2842, 1985
58. Jaffe ES, Clark J, Steis R et al: Lymph node pathology of HTLV and HTLV-associated neoplasms. Cancer Res (Suppl) 45:4662s–4664s, 1985
59. Anagnostou D, Parker JW, Taylor CR et al: Lacunar cells of nodular sclerosing Hodgkin's disease. An ultrastructural and immunohistologic study. Cancer 39:1032–1043, 1977
60. Kadin ME, Glatstein E, Dorfman RF: Clinicopathologic study of 117 untreated patients subject to laparotomy for the staging of Hodgkin's disease. Cancer 27:1277–1294, 1971
61. Strum SB, Rappaport H: Interrelations of the histologic types of Hodgkin's disease. Arch Pathol 91:127–134, 1971
62. DeVita VT Jr, Simon RM, Hubbard SM et al: Curability of advanced Hodgkin's disease with chemotherapy. Ann Intern Med 92:587–595, 1980
63. Mann RB, Jaffe ES, Berard CW: Malignant lymphomas—A conceptual understanding of morphologic diversity. A review. Am J Pathol 94:105–191, 1979
64. Lukes RJ: Criteria for involvement of lymph node, bone marrow, spleen, and liver in Hodgkin's disease. Cancer Res 31:1755–1764, 1971
65. Colby TV, Hoppe RT, Warnke RA: Hodgkin's disease: A clinicopathologic study of 659 cases. Cancer 49:1848–1858, 1981
66. Grogan TM: Hodgkin's disease. In Jaffe ES (ed): Surgical Pathology of Lymph Nodes and Related Organs, pp 86–134. Philadelphia, WB Saunders, 1985
67. Rosai J, Levine GD: Tumors of the thymus. Atlas of Tumor Pathology. Second Series, Fascicle 13. Washington DC, Armed Forces Institute of Pathology, 1976
68. Kadin ME, Donaldson SS, Dorfman RF: Isolated granulomas in Hodgkin's disease. N Engl J Med 283:859–861, 1970
69. Order SE, Hellman S: Pathogenesis of Hodgkin's disease. Lancet 1:571–573, 1972
70. DeVita VT: Lymphocyte reactivity in Hodgkin's disease: A lymphocyte civil war. N Engl J Med 289:801–802, 1973
71. Kadin ME, Stites DP, Levy R et al: Exogenous immunoglobulin and the macrophage origin of Reed–Sternberg cells in Hodgkin's disease. N Engl J Med 299:1208–1214, 1978
72. Kaplan HS, Gartner S: "Sternberg–Reed" giant cells of Hodgkin's disease: Cultivation in vitro, heterotransplantation, and characterization as neoplastic macrophages. Int J Cancer 19:511–525, 1977
73. Corder MP, Young RC, DeVita VT: Delayed hypersensitivity in patients with cancer. N Engl J Med 285:522–524, 1971
74. Corder MP, Young RC, Brown RS et al: Phytohemagglutinin-induced lymphocyte transformation: The relationship to prognosis of Hodgkin's disease. Blood 39:595–602, 1972
75. Poppema S, Bhan AK, Reinherz EL et al: In situ immunologic characterization of cellular constituents in lymph nodes and spleens involved by Hodgkin's disease. Blood 59:226–232, 1982
76. Garvin AJ, Spicer SS, Parmley RT et al: Immunohistochemical demonstration of IgG in Reed–Sternberg and other cells in Hodgkin's disease. J Exp Med 139:1077–1083, 1974
77. Kadin ME: Possible origin of the Reed–Sternberg cell from an interdigitating reticulum cell. Cancer Treat Rep 66:601–608, 1982
78. Braylan RC, Jaffe ES, Berard CW: Surface characteristics of Hodgkin's lymphoma cells. Lancet II 7891:1328–1329, 1974
79. Hsu S, Jaffe ES: Leu M1 and peanut agglutinin stain the neoplastic cells of Hodgkin's disease. Am J Clin Pathol 82:29–32, 1984
80. Diehl V, Kirschner HH, Burrighter H et al: Characteristics of Hodgkin's disease-derived cell lines. Cancer Treat Rep 66:615–632, 1982
81. Fisher RI, Bates SE, Bostick-Bruton F et al: Neoplastic cells obtained from Hodgkin's disease are potent stimulators of human primary mixed lymphocyte cultures. J Immunol 130:2666, 1983
82. Stein H, Gerdes J, Schwab U et al: Identification of Hodgkin and Sternberg–Reed cells as a unique cell type derived from a newly detected small-cell population. Int J Cancer 30:445–459, 1982
83. Hecht TT, Longo DL, Cossman J et al: Production and characterization of a monoclonal antibody that finds Reed–Sternberg cells. J Immunol 134:4231, 1984
84. Stein H, Mason DY, Gerdes J et al: The expression of the Hodgkin's disease associated antigen Ki-1 in reactive and neoplastic lymphoid tissue: Evidence that Reed–Sternberg cells and histiocytic malignancies are derived from activated lymphoid cells. Blood 66:848–858, 1985
85. Hsu S, Yang K, Jaffe ES: Phenotypic expression of Hodgkin's and Reed–Sternberg cells in Hodgkin's disease. Am J Pathol 118:209–217, 1985
86. Weiss L, Strickler JG, Hu E et al: Immunoglobulin gene rearrangements in Hodgkin's disease. Hum Pathol 17:1009–1014, 1986
87. Sundeen JT, Lipford E, Uppencamp M et al: Rearranged antigen receptor genes in Hodgkin's disease. Blood 70:96–103, 1987
88. Greisser H, Feller A, Lennert K: Rearrangement of the B chain of the T-cell receptor and immunoglobulin genes in lymphoproliferative disorders. J Clin Invest 78:1179–1184, 1986
89. Brinker MG, Poppema S, Buys C et al: Clonal immunoglobulin gene rearrangements in tissues involved by Hodgkin's disease. Blood 70:186–189, 1987
90. Uppenkamp M, Pittaluga S, Lipford EH et al: Limited diversity and selection of rearranged gama genes in polyclonal T cells. J Immunol 138:1618, 1987
91. Pinkus GS, Said JW: Hodgkin's disease, lymphocyte predominance type, nodular—A distinct entity? Unique staining profile for L&H variants of Reed–Sternberg cells defined by monoclonal antibodies to leukocyte common antigen, granulocyte-specific antigen, and B-cell–specific antigen. Am J Pathol 118:1–6, 1985
92. Stein H, Hansmann L, Lennert K et al: Reed–Sternberg and Hodgkin cells in

lymphocyte-predominant Hodgkin's disease of nodular subtype contain J chain. Am J Clin Pathol 86:292–297, 1986
93. Timens W, Visser L, Poppema S: Nodular lymphocyte predominance type of Hodgkin's disease is a germinal center lymphoma. Lab Invest 54:457–461, 1986
94. Sundeen JT, Cossman J, Klein M: Lymphocyte predominant Hodgkin's disease nodular subtype with coexistent "large cell lymphoma": Histological progression or composite malignancy? Am J Surg Pathol (in press)
95. Kaplan HS: Hodgkin's Disease, 2nd ed. Cambridge, Harvard University Press, 1980
96. Rosenberg SA, Diamond HD, Jaslowitz B et al: Lymphosarcoma: A review of 1269 cases. Medicine 40:31, 1961
97. Sage HH: Palpable cervical lymph nodes. JAMA 168:496–498, 1958
98. Buskirk SJ, Evans RG, Banks PM et al: Primary lymphoma of the testis. Int J Radiat Oncol Biol Phys 8:1699–1703, 1982
99. Sapozink MD, Kaplan HS: Intracranial Hodgkin's disease. Report of 12 cases and review of the literature. Cancer 52:1301–1307, 1982
100. Gilbert R: La roentgentherapie de la granulomatose maligne. J Radiol Electrol 9:509–513, 1925
101. Gilbert R: Radiotherapy in Hodgkin's disease (malignant granulomatosis): Anatomic and clinical foundations: Governing principles: Results. Am J Roentgenol 41:198–241, 1939
102. Peters MV: A study of survival in Hodgkin's disease treated radiologically. Am J Roentgenol 63:299–311, 1950
103. Peters MV, Middlemiss KCH: A study of Hodgkin's disease treated by irradiation. Am J Roentgenol 79:114–121, 1958
104. Peters MV: Prophylactic treatment of adjacent areas in Hodgkin's disease. Cancer Res 26:1232–1243, 1966
105. Kaplan HS: The radical radiotherapy of regionally localized Hodgkin's disease. Radiology 78:553–561, 1962
106. Kinmouth JB, Taylor GW, Harper RK: Lymphography: A technique for its clinical use in the lower limbs. Br Med J I:930–942, 1955
107. Lee BJ, Nelson JH, Schwarz G: Evaluation of lymphangiography, inferior venocavography and intravenous pyelography in the clinical staging and management of Hodgkin's disease and lymphosarcoma. N Engl J Med 271:327–337, 1964
108. Glatstein E, Guernsey JM, Rosenberg SA et al: The value of laparotomy and splenectomy in the staging of Hodgkin's disease. Cancer 24:709–718, 1969
109. Kaplan HS: On the natural history, treatment and prognosis of Hodgkin's disease. Harvey Lectures, 1968–1969, pp 215–259. New York, Academic Press, 1970
110. Glatstein E, Trueblood HW, Enright LP et al: Surgical staging of abdominal involvement in unselected patients with Hodgkin's disease. Radiology 97:425, 1970
111. Desser RK, Moran EM, Ultmann JE: Staging of Hodgkin's disease and lymphoma. Med Clin North Am 57:479, 1973
112. Rosenberg SA: A critique of the value of laparotomy and splenectomy in the evaluation of patients with Hodgkin's disease. Cancer Res 31:1737, 1971
113. Prio AJ, Hellman S, Moloney WC: The influence of laparotomy on management decisions in Hodgkin's disease. Arch Intern Med 130:844, 1972
114. DeVita VT: The role of staging laparotomy in combined modality therapy of Hodgkin's disease. World J Surg 2:105–107, 1978
115. Peters MV, Alison RE, Buch RS: Natural history of Hodgkin's disease as related to staging. Cancer 19:308–346, 1966
116. Johnson RE, Thomas LB, Chretien P: Correlation between clinico-histologic staging and extranodal relapse in Hodgkin's disease. Cancer 25:1071–1075, 1970
117. Regula DP, Hoppe RT, Weiss LM: Nodular and diffuse types of lymphocyte predominant Hodgkin's disease. N Engl J Med 318:214–219, 1988
118. Strum SB, Rappaport H: Interrelationships of the histologic types of Hodgkin's disease. Arch Pathol 91:127–134, 1971
119. Craft CB: Results with roentgen ray therapy in Hodgkin's disease. Bull Staff Meet Univ Miami Hosp 11:391–409, 1940
120. Slaughter DP, Economou SG, Southwick HW: The surgical management of Hodgkin's disease. Ann Surg 148:705–710, 1958
121. Peters MV, Hasselbach R, Brown TC: The natural history of the lymphomas related to the clinical classification. In Zarafonetis CJD (ed): Proceedings of the International Conference on Leukemia–Lymphoma, pp 357–370. Philadelphia, Lea and Febiger, 1968
122. Lukes RJ, Craver LF, Hall TC et al: Report of the nomenclature committee. Cancer Res 26:311, 1966
123. Carbone PP, Kaplan HS, Musshoff K et al: Report of the committee on Hodgkin's disease staging. Cancer Res 31:1860–1861, 1971
124. Musshoff K, Ronemann H, Bourlis L et al: Die extranodulare Lymphogranulomatose. Diagnose, Therapie und Prognose bei zwei unterschiedlichen Formen de Organ Befalls. Ein Beitrag zur Stadienein teilung des morbus Hodgkin Forschr. Geb Roentgenstr 109:776–786, 1968
125. Young RC, Anderson T, DeVita VT: The treatment of Hodgkin's disease: Emphasizing programs at the Clinical Center, National Institutes of Health. Curr Probl Cancer 1:1–29, 1977
126. Castellino RA: Imaging techniques for staging abdominal Hodgkin's disease. Cancer Treat Rep 66:697–700, 1982
127. Redman HC, Glatstein E, Castellino RA et al: Computed tomography as an adjunct in the staging of Hodgkin's disease and non-Hodgkin's lymphomas. Radiology 124:381–385, 1977
128. Breeman RS, Castellino RA, Harell GS et al: CT-pathologic correlations in Hodgkin's disease and non-Hodgkin's lymphoma. Radiology 126:159–166, 1978
129. Jones SE, Tobias DA, Waldman RS: Complete tomographic scanning in patients with lymphoma. Cancer 41:480–486, 1978
130. Aisenberg AC: The staging of Hodgkin's disease. J Exp Clin Cancer Res 2:209–212, 1983
131. Mellor JA, Simmons AV, Barnard DL et al: A retrospective evaluation of mediastinal tomograms, isotope liver scans and isotope bone scans in the staging and management of patients with lymphoma. Cancer 52:2227–2229, 1983
132. Tumeh SS, Rosenthal DS, Kaplan WD et al: Lymphoma: Evaluation with Ga-67 SPECT. Radiology 164:111–114, 1987
133. John RE: Is staging laparotomy routinely indicated in Hodgkin's disease? Ann Intern Med 75:459, 1971
134. Kinsella TJ, Glatstein E: Staging laparotomy and splenectomy for Hodgkin's disease: current status. Cancer Invest 1:87–91, 1983
135. Lacher MJ: Routine staging laparotomy for patients with Hodgkin's disease is no longer necessary. Cancer Invest 1:93–99, 1983
136. Piro AJ, Hellman S: Laparotomy alters treatment in Hodgkin's disease. Natl Cancer Inst Monogr 36:307–311, 1973
137. Kaplan HS, Dorfman RF, Nelson TS et al: Staging laparotomy and splenectomy in Hodgkin's disease: Analysis of indications and patterns of involvement in 285 consecutive, unselected patients. Natl Cancer Inst Monogr 36:291–301, 1973
138. Desser RK, Golomb HM, Ultmann JE et al: Prognostic classification of Hodgkin's disease in pathologic Stage III, based on anatomic considerations. Blood 49:883–893, 1977
139. Stein RS, Golomb HM, Diggs CH et al: Anatomic substages of Stage III-A Hodgkin's disease. Ann Intern Med 92:159–165, 1980
140. Rosner F, Zarrabi MH: Late infections following splenectomy in Hodgkin's disease. Cancer Invest 1:57–65, 1983
141. Coker DD, Morris DM, Coleman JJ et al: Infection among 210 patients with surgically staged Hodgkin's disease. Am J Med 75:97–109, 1983
142. Notter DT, Grossman PL, Rosenberg SA et al: Infections in patients with Hodgkin's disease: A clinical study of 300 consecutive adult patients. Rev Infect Dis 2:761–800, 1980
143. Desser RL, Ultmann JE: Risk of severe infection in patients with Hodgkin's disease or lymphoma after diagnostic laparotomy and splenectomy. Ann Intern Med 77:143–147, 1972
144. Meeker WR, Richardson JD, West W et al: Critical evaluation of laparotomy and splenectomy in Hodgkin's disease. Arch Surg 105:222, 1972
145. Jenkin RRT, Berry MP: Hodgkin's disease in children. Semin Oncol 7:202–211, 1980
146. Chilcote RR, Baehner RH, Hammond D: Septicemia and meningitis in children splenectomized for Hodgkin's disease. N Engl J Med 295:798–800, 1976
147. Slaven R, Nelson TS: Complications of staging laparotomy for Hodgkin's disease. Natl Cancer Inst Monogr 36:457, 1973
148. Donaldson SS, Kaplan HS: Complications of treatment of Hodgkin's disease in children. Cancer Treat Rep 66:977–989, 1982
149. Mauch PM, Weinstein H, Botnick L et al: An evaluation of long-term survival and treatment complications in children in Hodgkin's disease. Cancer 51:925–932, 1983
150. Lange B, Littman P: Management of Hodgkin's disease in children and adolescents. Cancer 51:1371–1377, 1983
151. Salzman JR, Kaplan HS: Effect of splenectomy on hematologic tolerance during total lymphoid radiotherapy of patients with Hodgkin's disease. Cancer 27:471–478, 1971
152. Panattiere RJ, Coltman CA: Splenectomy effects on chemotherapy in Hodgkin's disease. Arch Intern Med 131:363–366, 1973
153. Panattiere RJ, Coltman CA, Delaney FC: Splenectomy, chemotherapy and survival in Hodgkin's disease. Arch Intern Med 137:341–343, 1977
154. Ihde DC, DeVita VT, Canellos GP et al: Effect of splenectomy on tolerance to combination chemotherapy in patients with lymphoma. Blood 47:211–222, 1976
155. Sutcliffe SB, Wrigley PFM, Timothy AR et al: Posttreatment laparotomy as a guide to management in patients with Hodgkin's disease. Cancer Treat Rep 6:759–765, 1982
156. Kostraba NC, Peterson BA, Kennedy BJ et al: Laparotomy in the reevaluation of patients with advanced Hodgkin's disease. Cancer Treat Rep 65:685–687, 1981
157. Myers CE, Chabner BA, DeVita VT et al: Bone marrow involvement in Hodgkin's disease: Pathology and response to MOPP chemotherapy. Blood 44:197–204, 1974
158. Rosenberg SA: Hodgkin's disease of the bone marrow. Cancer Res 31:1733–1736, 1971
159. Ferrant A, Rodhain J, Michaux L et al: Detection of skeletal involvement in Hodgkin's disease: a comparison of radiography bone scanning and bone marrow biopsy in 38 patients. Cancer 35:1346–1353, 1975
160. Musshoff K, Boutis L: Therapy results in Hodgkin's disease. Freiburg I Br 1948–1966. Cancer 21:1100–1113, 1968
161. Rubins J: Cutaneous Hodgkin's disease: Indolent causes and control with chemotherapy. Cancer 42:1219–1221, 1978
162. Valtysson G, Fisher-Beckfield P, Carbone PP: Cerebellar degeneration with Hodgkin's disease. Cancer 29:246–249, 1979
163. Young RC, Howser DM, Anderson T et al: Central nervous system complications of non-Hodgkin's lymphoma. The potential role for prophylactic therapy. Am J Med 66:246–249, 1979
164. Moorthy AV, Zimmerman SW, Burkholder PM: Nephrotic syndrome in Hodgkin's disease. Evidence for pathogenesis alternative to immune complex deposition. Am J Med 61:471–477, 1976
165. Yum MN, Edwards JL, Kleit S: Glomerular lesions in Hodgkin's disease. Arch Pathol 99:645–649, 1975

166. Longo DL, DeVita VT Jr: Lymphomas. In Pinedo HM, Chabner BA (eds): Cancer Chemotherapy 1984, The EORTC Cancer Chemotherapy Annual 6. New York, Elsevier-Dutton, 1984
167. Schier WW, Roth A, Ostroff J: Hodgkin's disease and immunity. Am J Med 20:94–99, 1956
168. Lamb D, Pilney F, Kelly WD et al: A comparative study of the incidence of anergy in patients with carcinoma, leukemia, Hodgkin's disease and other lymphomas. J Immunol 89:555–558, 1962
169. Brown RS, Haynes HA, Foley HJ et al: Hodgkin's disease. Immunological, clinical and histologic features of 50 untreated patients. Ann Intern Med 67:291–302, 1967
170. Hersh EM, Oppenheim JJ: Impaired lymphocyte transformation in Hodgkin's disease. N Engl J Med 273:1006–1012, 1965
171. Matchett KM, Huang AT, Kremer WB: Impaired lymphocyte transformation in Hodgkin's disease. Evidence for depletion or circulating T-lymphocytes. J Clin Invest 52:1908–1917, 1973
172. Levy RA, Kaplan HS: Impaired lymphocyte function in untreated Hodgkin's disease. N Engl J Med 290:181–186, 1974
173. Bobrove AM, Fuks Z, Strober S et al: Quantitation of T and B lymphocytes and cellular immune function in Hodgkin's disease. Cancer 36:169–179, 1975
174. Twomey JJ, Laughter AH et al: Hodgkin's disease. An immunodepleting and immunosuppressive disorder. J Clin Invest 56:467–475, 1975
175. Goodwin JS, Messner RP, Barkhurst AD et al: Prostaglandin-producing suppressor cells in Hodgkin's disease. N Engl J Med 297:963–968, 1977
176. Engleman EG, Hoppe R, Kaplan HS et al: Suppressor cells of a mixed lymphocyte reaction in healthy subjects and patients with Hodgkin's disease and sarcoidosis. Clin Res 20:513A, 1978
177. Hillinger SM, Herzig GP: Impaired cell-mediated immunity in Hodgkin's disease mediated by suppressor lymphocytes and monocytes. J Clin Invest 61:1620–1627, 1978
178. Fuks Z, Strober W, King DP et al: Reversal of cell surface abnormalities of T lymphocytes in Hodgkin's disease after *in vitro* incubation in fetal sera. J Immunol 117:1331–1335, 1976
179. Fuks Z, Strober S, Kaplan HS: Interaction between serum factors and T-lymphocytes in Hodgkin's disease. N Engl J Med 295:1273–1278, 1976
180. Lauria F, Foa R, Gobbi M et al: Increased proportion of suppressor/cytotoxic (OKT8+) cells in patients with Hodgkin's disease in long-lasting remission. Cancer 52:1385–1388, 1983
181. Bjorkholm M, Holm H, Mellstedt H: Immunologic profile in patients with cured Hodgkin's disease. Scand J Haematol 18:361–368, 1977
182. Young RC, Corder MP, Haynes HA et al: Delayed hypersensitivity in Hodgkin's disease. A study of 103 patients. Am J Med 52:63–71, 1972
183. King GW, Yanes B, Hurtubise PE et al: Immune function of successfully treated lymphoma patients. J Clin Invest 57:1451–1460, 1976
184. VanHaelen CP, Fisher RR: Increased sensitivity of T-cells to regulation by normal suppressor cells persist in long-term survivors with Hodgkin's disease. Am J Med 72:385–390, 1982
185. Fisher RI, DeVita VT, Bostick F et al: Persistent immunologic abnormalities in long-term survivors of advanced Hodgkin's disease. Ann Intern Med 92:595–599, 1980
186. VanHaelen CPJ, Fisher RI: Increased sensitivity of T-cells to regulation by normal suppressor cells persists in long-term survivors in Hodgkin's disease. Am J Med 72:385–390, 1982
187. Fisher RI: Implications of persistent T-cell abnormalities for the etiology of Hodgkin's disease. Cancer Treat Rep 66:4, 681–687, 1982
188. Fuks Z, Strober S, Bobrove AM et al: Longterm effects of radiation on T and B lymphocytes in peripheral blood of patients with Hodgkin's disease. J Clin Invest 58:803–814, 1976
189. Van Rijswijk RE, Sybesma JP, Kater L: A prospective study of the changes in the immune status before, during and after multiple agent chemotherapy for Hodgkin's disease. Cancer 53:637–644, 1983
190. Van Rijswijk RE, Sybesma JP, Kater L: A prospective study of the changes in immune status following radiotherapy for Hodgkin's disease. Cancer 53:62–69, 1984
191. Lauria F, Raspadori D, Foa R et al: Normal T-lymphocyte function in patients with Hodgkin's disease in long-lasting remission. Tumori 72:75–80, 1986
192. Liberati AM, Ballatori E, Fizzotti M et al: Immunologic profile in patients with Hodgkin's disease in complete remission. Cancer 59:1906–1913, 1987
193. Schulof RS, Bockman RS, Garofalo JA et al: Multivariant analysis of T-cell functional defects in circulating serum factors in Hodgkin's disease. Cancer 48:964–973, 1981
194. Posner MR, Reinherz EL, Breard J et al: Lymphoid subpopulations of peripheral blood and spleen in untreated Hodgkin's disease. Cancer 48:1170–1176, 1981
195. Ford RJ, Tsao J, Kouttab NM et al: Association of an interleukin abnormality with the T-cell defect in Hodgkin's disease. Blood 64:386–392, 1984
196. Frydecka I: Natural killer cell activity during the course of disease in patients with Hodgkin's disease. Cancer 56:2799–2803, 1985
197. Ruco LP, Procopio A, Uccini S et al: Natural killer activity in spleens and lymph nodes in patients with Hodgkin's disease. Cancer Res 42:2063–2068, 1982
198. Levy S, Tempe JL, Aleksijevic A et al: Depressed NK cell activity of peripheral blood mononuclear cells in untreated Hodgkin's disease: Enhancing effect of interferon in vitro. Scand J Haematol 33:386–390, 1984
199. Al-Hadithy H, Cawley JC, Addison IE et al: Neutrophil function in advanced Hodgkin's disease: Effective therapy. Leukemia Res 6:261–267, 1982
200. Corberand J, Benchekroun S, Nguyen F et al: Polymorphonuclear functions in Hodgkin's disease patients at diagnosis, in remission, and in relapse. Cancer Res 42: 1595–1559, 1982
201. Van Rijswijk REN, Sybesma B, Kater L: Prospective study of the changes in the immune status before, during, and after multi-agent chemotherapy for Hodgkin's disease. Cancer 51:637–644, 1983
202. Van Rijswijk REN, Sybesma B, Kater L: Prospective study of the changes in the immune status following radiotherapy for Hodgkin's disease. Cancer 53:62–69, 1984
203. Van Rijswijk REN, DeMeijer AJ, Sybesma B et al: Five year survival in Hodgkin's disease: The prospective value of immune status at diagnosis. Cancer 57:1489–1496, 1986
204. Faquet GB, Davis HC: Survival in Hodgkin's disease: The role of immunocompetence in other major risk factors. Blood 59:938–945, 1982
205. Haybittle JL, Hayhoe FGJ, Easterling MJ et al: Review of British national lymphoma investigation studies of Hodgkin's disease and development of prognostic index. Lancet 1:967–972, 1985
206. Kelly WD, Good RA, Varco RI et al: The altered response to skin homographs and to delayed allergens in Hodgkin's disease. Surg Forum 9:785–789, 1958
207. Aisenberg AC, Leskowitz S: Antibody formation in Hodgkin's disease. N Engl J Med 26:1269–1272, 1963
208. Weitzman SA, Aisenberg AC, Siber GR, Smith DH: Impaired humoral immunity in treated Hodgkin's disease. New England J Med 297:245–248, 1977b
209. Minor DR, Schiffman G, McIntosh LS: Response of patients with Hodgkin's disease to pneumococcal vaccine. Ann Intern Med 90:887–892, 1979
210. Hays DM, Ternberg JL, Chen TT et al: Complications related to 234 staging laparotomies performed in the intergroup Hodgkin's disease in childhood study. Surgery 96:471–478, 1984
211. Donaldson SS, Vosti KL, Berberich FR et al: Response to pneumococcal vaccine among children with Hodgkin's disease. Rev Infect Dis 3:S133–S143, 1981
212. Ko HS, Pruzanski W: M components associated with lymphoma: A review of 62 cases. Am J Med Sci 272:175–183, 1976
213. Levine AM, Thorton P, Forman SJ et al: Positive Coombs test in Hodgkin's disease. Significance and implications. Blood 55:607–611, 1980
214. Booth PB, Jenkins WJ, Marsh WL: Anti-It: A new antibody of the I blood group system occurring in certain Melanesian sera. Br J Haematol 12:341–344, 1966
215. Waddell CC, Cimo PL: Idiopathic thrombocytopenia purpura occurring in Hodgkin's disease after splenectomy. A report of two cases and review of the literature. Am J Haematol 7:381–387, 1979
216. Jones SE: Autoimmune disorders and malignant lymphoma. Cancer 31:1092–1098, 1973
217. Berkman AW, Woog JJ, Kickler TS et al: Serial determinations of anti-platelet antibodies in a patient with Hodgkin's disease and autoimmune thrombocytopenia. Cancer 51:2057–2060, 1983
218. Heyman MR, Walsh TJ: Autoimmune neutropenia in Hodgkin's disease. Cancer 59:1903–1905, 1987
219. Pusey WA: Cases of sarcoma and of Hodgkin's disease treated by exposures to x-rays: A preliminary report. JAMA 38:166–170, 1902
220. Teschendorf W: Veber Bestrahlung der ganzen menschluchen Korpers bel Blutkrankheiten. Strahlenther Onkol 26:720–729, 1927
221. Voorhoeve N: La lymphogranulomatose maligne. Acta Radiol 4:567–589, 1925
222. Kruchen C: Beltrag zur Rontgentheraple der Lymphogranulomatose mit besonder Berucksichtigung der neuren klinischen Ergelnisse. Strahlenther Onkol 31:623–670, 1929
223. Easson EC, Russell MH: The cure of Hodgkin's disease. Br Med J 1:1704, 1963
224. Kaplan HS: Long-term results of palliative and radical radiotherapy of Hodgkin's disease. Cancer Res 26:1250–1252, 1966
225. Kaplan HS: Role of intensive radiotherapy in the management of Hodgkin's disease. Cancer 19:356–367, 1966
226. Kaplan HS: Clinical evaluation and radiotherapeutic management of Hodgkin's disease and the malignant lymphomas. N Engl J Med 278:892–899, 1968
227. Kaplan HS: On the natural history, treatment and prognosis of Hodgkin's disease. Harvey Lectures 1968–1969, pp 215–259. New York, Academic Press, 1970
228. Kaplan HS: Evidence for a tumorocidal dose level in the radiotherapy of Hodgkin's disease. Cancer Res 26:1221–1224, 1966
229. Rosenberg SA, Kaplan HS: Evidence for an orderly progression in the spread of Hodgkin's disease. Cancer Res 26:1225–1231, 1966
230. Hanks GE, Kinzie JJ, Herring DR et al: Patterns of care outcome studies in Hodgkin's disease: Results of the national practice and implications for management. Cancer Treat Rep 66:805–808, 1982
231. Landberg T, Liden K, Forslo H: Split-course radiation therapy of mediastinal Hodgkin's disease. TSD and CRE concepts. Acta Radiol 12:33–39, 1973
232. Page V, Gardner A, Karsmark CJ: Physical and dosimetric aspects of the radiotherapy of the malignant lymphomas. I. The mantle technique. Radiology 96:609–618, 1970
233. Carmel RJ, Kaplan HS: Mantle irradiation in Hodgkin's disease. An analysis of technique, tumor irradiation and complications. Cancer 37:2812–2825, 1976
234. Kaplan HS, Stewart HR: Complications of intensive megavoltage radiotherapy for Hodgkin's disease. Natl Cancer Inst Monogr 36:439–444, 1973
235. Stewart HR, Cohn KE, Fajardo LF et al: Radiation-induced heart disease: A study of twenty-five patients. Radiology 89:302–310, 1967
236. Lutz WP, Larsen RD: Technique for match mantle and paraaortic fields. Int J Radiat Oncol Biol Phys 9:1753–1756, 1983

237. Page V, Gardner A, Karsmark CJ: Physical and dosimetric aspects of the radiotherapy of malignant lymphoma. II. The inverted Y technique. Radiology 96:619–626, 1970
238. Lutz WR, Larsen RD: Technique to match mantle and paraaortic fields. Int J Radiat Oncol Biol Phys 5 (Suppl 2):159, 1979
239. Trueblood HW, Enright LP, Roy GR et al: Preservation of ovarian function in pelvic irradiation for Hodgkin's disease. Arch Surg 100:236–237, 1970
240. Kinzle JJ, Hanks GE, Maclean CJ et al: Patterns of care study: Hodgkin's disease relapse rates and adequacy of portals. Cancer 52:2223–2226, 1983
241. Collaborative Study. Survival and complications of radiotherapy following involved and extended field therapy of Hodgkin's disease. Stage I and II–a collaborative study. Cancer 38:288–305, 1976
242. Mauch PM, Canellos GP, Rosenthal DS et al: Reduction of fatal complications from combined modality therapy in Hodgkin's disease. J Clin Oncol 3:501–505, 1985
243. Timothy AR et al: Hodgkin's disease: Combination chemotherapy for relapse following radical radiotherapy. Int J Radiat Oncol Biol Phys 5:165–169, 1979
244. Portlock CS: Impact of salvage treatment on initial relapses in patients with Hodgkin's disease Stages I–III. Blood 51:825–833, 1978
245. Mauch P et al: The influence of initial pathologic stage on the survival of patients who relapse from Hodgkin's disease. Blood 56:892–897, 1980
246. Mauch PM, Canellos GP, Rosenthal DS et al: Reduction of fatal complications from combined modality therapy in Hodgkin's disease. J Clin Oncol 3:501–505, 1985
247. Hagemeister FB, Fuller LM, Sullivan JA, et al: Treatment of patients with Stages I and II non-mediastinal Hodgkin's disease. Cancer 50:2307–2313, 1982
248. Carde P, Burgers JM, Henry-Amar M et al: Clinical Stages I and II Hodgkin's disease: A specifically tailored therapy according to prognostic factors. J Clin Oncol 6: 239–252, 1988
249. Mandell LR, Tan C, Groshen S et al: Can paraaortic radiation be omitted in pathologically staged IA and IIA pediatric Hodgkin's disease? (in press)
250. Mauch P, Goodman R, Hellman S: The significance of mediastinal involvement in early stage Hodgkin's disease. Cancer 42:1039–1045, 1978
251. Hoppe RT: The management of Stage II Hodgkin's disease with a large mediastinal mass: A prospective program emphasizing irradiation. Int J Radiat Oncol Biol Phys 11:349–355, 1985
252. Thar TL, Million RR, Hausner RJ et al: Hodgkin's disease Stage I and II: Relationship of recurrence to size of disease, radiation dose and number of sites involved. Cancer 43:1101–1105, 1979
253. Hoppe RT, Coleman CN, Kaplan HS et al: Hodgkin's disease, pathologic Stage I and II, the prognostic importance of initial sites of disease and extent of mediastinal involvement. Proc Am Soc Clin Oncol 21:471, 1980
254. Velentjas E, Barrett A, McElwain TJ et al: Mediastinal involvement in early-stage Hodgkin's disease. Eur J Cancer 16:1065–1068, 1980
255. Mauch P, Gorshein D, Cunningham J et al: Influence of mediastinal adenopathy on site and frequency of relapse in patients with Hodgkin's disease. Cancer Treat Rep 66:809–817, 1982
256. Leslie NT, Mauch P, Hellman S: Radiation therapy in the treatment of early Hodgkin's disease. Cancer (in press)
257. Piro AJ, Weiss DR, Hellman S: Mediastinal Hodgkin's disease: A possible danger for intubation anesthesia. Int J Radiat Oncol Biol Phys 1:415–419, 1976
258. Krikorian JG, Portlock CS, Mauch PM: Hodgkin's disease presenting below the diaphragm: A review. J Clin Oncol 4:1551–1562, 1986
259. Mauch P, Goffman T, Rosenthal DS et al: Stage III Hodgkin's disease: Improved survival with combined modality therapy as compared with radiation therapy alone. J Clin Oncol 3:1166–1173, 1985
260. Rosenberg SA, Kaplan HS, Gladstein EJ et al: Combined modality therapy of Hodgkin's disease. A report of the Stanford trials. Cancer 42:991–1000, 1978
261. Goodman R, Mauch P, Piro A et al: Stages IIB and IIB Hodgkin's disease: Results of combined modality treatment. Cancer 40:8489, 1977
262. Crnkovich MJ, Leopold K, Hoppe RT et al: Stage I to IIB Hodgkin's disease: the combined experience at Stanford University and the Joint Center for Radiation Therapy. J Clin Oncol 5:1041–1049, 1987
263. Hellman S, Mauch P, Goodman RL et al: The place of radiation therapy in the treatment of Hodgkin's disease. Cancer 42:971–978, 1978
264. Mauch PM et al: Stage IA–IIA supradiaphragmatic Hodgkin's disease: Prognostic factors in surgically staged patients treated with mantle and para-aortic irradiation (in preparation)
265. Zucali R, Pagnoni AN, Zanini M et al: Radiological and spirometric evaluation of mediastinal and pulmonary late effects after radiotherapy and chemotherapy for Hodgkin's disease. J Eur Radiother 2:169, 1981
266. Appelfield MM, Slawson RG, Spicer KM et al: Long-term cardiovascular evaluation of patients with Hodgkin's disease treated by thoracic mantle radiation therapy. Cancer Treat Rep 66:1003–1013, 1982
267. Mauch P, Hellman S, Belli JA: Cardiac effects of mediastinal irradiation. N Engl J Med 309:378, 1983
268. Burns RJ, Bar-Schlomo BZ, Druck MN et al: Detection of radionuclide cardiomyopathy by gated radionuclide angiography. Am J Med 74:297–303, 1983
269. Annest LS, Anderson RP, Li W et al: Coronary artery disease following mediastinal radiation therapy. J Thorac Cardiovasc Surg 85:257–263, 1983
270. Bowin JF, Hutchinson GB: Coronary heart disease after irradiation for Hodgkin's disease. Cancer 49:2470–2475, 1982
271. Foley KM, Woodruff J, Ellis F et al: Radiation induced malignant and atypical schwannomas. Ann Neurol 7:311–318, 1979
272. Kinsella TJ, Fraass BE, Glatstein E: Late effects of radiation therapy in the treatment of Hodgkin's disease. Cancer Treat Rep 66:991–1001, 1982
273. McDougall IR, Coleman CN, Burke JS et al: Thyroid carcinoma after high-dose external radiotherapy for Hodgkin's disease. Cancer 45:2056–2060, 1980
274. Stutzman L, Glidewell O: Multiple chemotherapeutic agents for Hodgkin's disease. JAMA 225:1202–1211, 1973
275. Luce JK, Frei E, Gehan EA et al: Chemotherapy of Hodgkin's disease. Arch Intern Med 131:391–395, 1973
276. Huguley CM, Durant JR, Moores RR et al: A comparison of nitrogen mustard, vincristine, procarbazine and prednisone (MOPP) vs nitrogen mustard in advanced Hodgkin's disease. Cancer. 36:1227–1240, 1975
277. Coltman CA Jr, Jones SE, Grozea PN et al: Bleomycin in combination with MOPP for management of Hodgkin's disease: Southwest Oncology Group experience. In Carter SK, Crooke ST (eds): Bleomycin: Current Status and New Developments, pp 227–242. Orlando, FL, Academic Press, 1978
278. Coltman CA Jr, Jones SE, Grozea PN et al: Bleomycin in combination with MOPP in the management of advanced Hodgkin's disease: A Southwest Oncology Group experience. In Sikic BI, Rosenscweig M, Carter SK (eds): Bleomycin Chemotherapy, pp 137–153. Orlando, FL, Academic Press, 1985
279. British National Lymphoma Investigation: Value of prednisone in combination chemotherapy of stage IV Hodgkin's disease. Br Med J 3:413–414, 1975
280. Goldman JM: Combination chemotherapy for Stage IV Hodgkin's disease (report #14). Clin Radiol 32:531–535, 1981
281. Bonadonna G, Santoro A, Bonfante V et al: Cyclic delivery of MOPP and ABVD combinations in stage IV Hodgkin's disease: Rationale, background studies and recent. Cancer Treat Rep 66:881–887, 1982
282. Bonadonna G: Chemotherapy strategies to improve the control of Hodgkin's disease (Rosenthal Award Lecture). Cancer Res 42:4309–4320, 1982
283. Jones SE, Haut A, Weick JK et al: Comparison or adriamycin containing chemotherapy (MOP-BAP) with MOPP–bleomycin in the management of advanced Hodgkin's disease. Cancer. 51:339–347, 1983
284. Bakemeier RF, Anderson JR, Costello W et al: BCVPP chemotherapy for advanced Hodgkin's disease: Evidence for greater duration of complete remission, greater survival and less toxicity than with a MOPP regimen. Ann Intern Med 101:447–456, 1984
285. Straus DJ, Myers J, Lee BJ et al: Treatment of advanced Hodgkin's disease with chemotherapy and irradiation. Am J Med 76:270–278, 1984
286. British National Lymphoma Investigation: Initial treatment of Stage IIIA Hodgkin's disease: Comparison of radiotherapy with combined chemotherapy. Lancet 1: 991–996, 1976
287. Haybittle JL, Eastering MJ, Hudson BV et al: Review of British National Lymphoma Investigation studies of Hodgkin's disease: Development of a prognostic index. Lancet 1:967–972, 1985
288. Santoro A, Bonadonna G, Bonfante V et al: Alternating drug combinations in the treatment of advanced Hodgkin's disease. N Engl J Med 306:770–775, 1982
289. Bonadonna G, Valagussa P, Santoro A: Alternating non–cross-resistant combination chemotherapy with ABVD or MOPP in Stage IV Hodgkin's disease: A report of eight year results. Ann Intern Med 104:739–746, 1986
290. Hancock BW: Randomized study of MOPP (mustine, oncovin, procarbazine, prednisone) against LOPP (leukeran substituted for mustine) in advanced Hodgkin's disease. Radiother Oncol 7:215–221, 1986
291. Hancock BW, Vaughan-Hudson B, Vaughan-Hudson G: Randomized study of LOPP (leukeran, oncovin, procarbazine, prednisone) and LOPP alternating with EVAP (etoposide, velbe, adriamycin, prednisone) in advanced Hodgkin's disease: Preliminary results. (Meeting abstract) Third International Conference on Malignant Lymphoma, June 10–13, 1987
292. Bonadonna G: Hodgkin's disease: The Milan Cancer Institute experience with MOPP and ABVD. (Meeting abstract) Third International Conference on Malignant Lymphoma. June 10–13, 1987
293. Longo D, Glatstein E, Young R et al: Randomized trial of MOPP chemotherapy vs subtotal nodal radiation therapy in patients with laparotomy documented early stage Hodgkin's disease. Proc Am Soc Clin Oncol 6:206, 1987
294. Somers R, Henry-Amar M, Carde P et al: MOPP vs alternating MOPP/ABVD in advanced Hodgkin's disease (HD). Proc Am Soc Clin Oncol 7:236, 1988
295. Canellos GP, Propert K, Cooper R et al: MOPP vs ABVD vs MOPP alternating with ABVD in advanced Hodgkin's disease: A prospective CALGB trial. Proc Am Soc Clin Oncol 7:230, 1988
296. Brusamolino E, Lazzarino M, Canevari A, et al: Alternating non–cross resistant chemotherapy (MOPP–ABVD) in advanced Hodgkin's disease. Proc Am Soc Clin Oncol 7:239, 1988
297. Young RC, Longo DL, Glatstein E et al: Hodgkin's disease: NCI trials addressing the remaining challenges. Third International Conference on Malignant Lymphoma. June 10–13, 1987, p 29. Lugano, Switzerland, 1987
298. Glick J, Tsaitis A, Chen A et al: A randomized ECOG trial of alternating MOPP–ABVD vs BCVPP vs BCVPP plus radiotherapy (RT) for advanced Hodgkin's disease. Proc Am Soc Clin Oncol 7:223, 1988
299. Bergsagel D: Personal communication, 1988
300. Nicholson WM, Beard MEJ, Crowther D et al: Combination chemotherapy in generalized Hodgkin's disease. Br Med J 3:7–10, 1970
301. Sutcliffe SB, Wrigley PFM, Peto J et al: MVPP chemotherapy regimen for advanced Hodgkin's disease. Br Med J 1:679–683, 1978

302. Wagstaff J,. Steward W, Jones M et al: Factors affecting remission and survival in patients with advanced Hodgkin's disease treated with MVPP. Hematol Oncol 4: 135–147, 1986
303. Morgenfeld M, Somoza N, Magnasco J et al: Combined chemotherapy cyclophosphamide, vinblastine, procarbazine and prednisone (CVPP) versus CVPP plus CCNU (CCVPP) in Hodgkin's disease. Cancer 43:1579–1586, 1979
304. Pavlovsky S, Morgenfeld M, Somoza N et al: Long-term follow-up of two chemotherapy protocols in Hodgkin's disease. Medicina 41:15–21, 1981
305. Durant JR, Gams RA, Velez-Garcia E et al: BCNU, velban, cyclophosphamide, procarbazine, and prednisone (BVCPP) in advanced Hodgkin's disease. Cancer 42:2101–2110, 1978
306. Gams RA, Durant JR, Bartolucci AA: Chemotherapy for advanced Hodgkin's disease: Conclusions from the Southeastern Cancer Study Group. Cancer Treat Rep 66: 899–905, 1982
307. McElwain TJ, Toy J, Smith E et al: A combination of chlorambucil, vinblastine, procarbazine and prednisolone for treatment of Hodgkin's disease. Br J Cancer 36:276–280, 1977
308. Kaye SB, Juttner CA, Smith IE et al: Three years' experience with ChlVPP (a combination of drugs for low toxicity) for the treatment of Hodgkin's disease. Br J Cancer 39:168–174, 1979
309. Dady PJ, McElwain TJ, Auston DE et al: Five years' experience with ChlVPP effective low-toxicity combination chemotherapy for Hodgkin's disease. Br J Cancer 45:851–859, 1982
310. Lister TA, Dorreen MS, Faux M et al: The treatment of stage IIIA Hodgkin's disease. J Clin Oncol 1:745–749, 1983
311. Crowther D, Wagstaff J, Deakin D et al. A randomized study comparing chemotherapy alone with chemotherapy followed by radiotherapy in patients with pathologically staged IIIA Hodgkin's disease. J Clin Oncol 2:892–897, 1984
312. Gams RA, Omura GA, Velez-Garcia E et al: Alternating sequential combination chemotherapy in the management of advanced Hodgkin's disease. A Southeastern Cancer Study Group trial. Cancer 58:1963–1968, 1986
313. Cooper MR, Pajak TF, Nissen N et al: A new effective four-drug combination of CCNU (1-[2-Chloroethyl]-3-Cyclohexyl-1-Nitrosourea) (NSC-79038), vinblastine, prednisone, and procarbazine for the treatment of advanced Hodgkin's disease. Cancer 46:654–662, 1980
314. Cooper MR, Pajak TF, Gottlieb AJ et al: The effects of prior radiation therapy and age on the frequency and duration of complete remission among various four-drug treatment for advanced Hodgkin's disease. J Clin Oncol 2:748–755, 1984
315. Propert KJ, Cooper MR, Spurr C et al: Combination chemotherapy with vinca alkaloids and alkylating agents for Stage III and IV Hodgkin's disease (HD): Ten years of follow-up (CALGB 7251). Proc Am Soc Clin Oncol 5:192, 1986
316. Vinciguerra V, Propert KJ, Coleman M et al: Alternating cycles of combination chemotherapy for patients with recurrent Hodgkin's disease following radiotherapy a prospectively randomized study by the Cancer and Leukemia Group B. J Clin Oncol 4:838–846, 1986
317. Druker BJ, Canellos GP: Chlorambucil, vinblastine, procarbazine and prednisone (ChlVPP): An effective but less toxic regimen than MOPP for advanced stage Hodgkin's disease (HD). Proc Am Assoc Cancer Res 27:198, 1986
318. Armitage J, Vose J, Weisenburger D et al: ChlVPP: An effective and well tolerated alternative to MOPP. Proc Am Soc Clin Oncol 6:A771, 1987
319. Farber LR, Prosnitz LR, Cadman EC et al: Curative potential of combined modality therapy for advanced Hodgkin's disease. Cancer 46:1509–1517, 1980
320. Prosnitz LR, Farber LR, Kapp DS et al: Combined modality therapy for advanced Hodgkin's disease: Long-term follow-up data. Cancer Treat Rep 66:871–879, 1982
321. Prosnitz LR, Farber LR, Scott J et al: Combined modality therapy for advanced Hodgkin's disease: A 15-year follow-up data. J Clin Oncol 6:603–612, 1988
322. Wagener DJT, Marion J, Burgers V et al: Sequential non–cross-resistant chemotherapy regimens (MOPP and CAVmP in Hodgkin's disease Stage IIIB and IV. Cancer. 52:1558–1562, 1983
323. Klimo P, Connors JM: MOPP/ABV hybrid program: Combination chemotherapy based on early introduction of seven effective drugs for advanced Hodgkin's disease. J Clin Oncol 3:1174–1182, 1985
324. Connors JM, Klimo P: MOPP/ABV hybrid chemotherapy for advanced Hodgkin's disease. Semin Hematol 24:35–40, 1987
325. Klimo P, Connors JM: An update on the Vancouver experience in the management of advanced Hodgkin's disease treated with the MOPP/ABV-hybrid program. Semin Hematol (in press)
326. Osler W: The Principles and Practice of Medicine. New York, D Appleton and Company, 1892
327. Goodman LS, Wintrobe MM, Dameshek W et al: Nitrogen mustard therapy. Use of methyl bis (B-chloroethyl) amine hydrochloride and tris (B-chloroethy) amine hydrochloride for Hodgkin's disease lymphosarcoma, leukemia, certain allied and miscellaneous disorders. JAMA 132:126–132, 1946
328. Alpert LP, Petersen SK: The use of nitrogen mustard in the treatment of lymphomata. Bull US Army Med Dept 7:187–194, 1947
329. Damesheck W, Weisfuse L, Stein T: Nitrogen mustard therapy in Hodgkin's disease. Analysis of 50 consecutive cases. Blood 4:338–379, 1949
330. Bollag, Grunberg E: Tumor inhibitory effects of a new class of cytotoxic agents: Methyl hydrazine derivatives. Experientia 19:751, 1963
331. Mathe G, Schweisguth O, Schneider M et al: Methylhydrazine in the treatment of Hodgkin's disease. Lancet 2:1077, 1963
332. Martz G, D'Alessandri A, Keel HJ et al: Preliminary clinical results with a new anti-tumor agents RO 4-6467 (NSC 77213). Cancer Chemother Rep 33:5–14, 1963
333. Falkson G, deVillieb PC, Falkson HC: N-Isopropyl-(2-methyl-hydrazine)-p-toluamide (MIH). Proc Soc Exp Biol Med 120:561–565, 1965
334. DeVita VT, Serpick A, Carbone PP: Preliminary clinical studies with ibenzmethyzin. Clin Pharmacol Tera 7:542–546, 1966
335. Scott JL: The effect of nitrogen mustard and maintenance chlorambucil in the treatment of advanced Hodgkin's disease. Cancer Chemother Rep 27:27–32, 1963
336. Carbone PP, Spurr C, Schneiderman M et al: Management of patients with malignant lymphoma, a comparative study with cyclophosphamide and vinca alkaloids. Cancer Res 28:811–822, 1968
337. Craft CB: Results with roentgen ray therapy in Hodgkin's disease. Bull Staff Meet Univ Miami Hosp 11:391–409, 1940
338. Jacobs EM, Peters FC, Luce JK et al: Mechlorethamine HCL and cyclophosphamide in the treatment of Hodgkin's disease. Cancer Chemother Rep 27:27–32, 1963
339. Aisenberg AC, Qazi R: Improved survival in Hodgkin's disease. Cancer 37: 2323–2329, 1976
340. Lacher MJ, Durant JR: Combined vinblastine and chlorambucil therapy of Hodgkin's disease. Ann Intern Med 62:468–476, 1965
341. DeVita VT, Serpick A: Combination chemotherapy in the treatment of advanced Hodgkin's disease. Proc Am Assoc Cancer Res 8:13, 1967
342. DeVita VT, Serpick AA, Carbone PP: Combination chemotherapy in the treatment of advanced Hodgkin's disease. Ann Intern Med 73:891–895, 1970
343. Lowenbraun S, DeVita VT, Serpick AA: Combination chemotherapy with nitrogen mustard, vincristine, procarbazine, and prednisone in previously treated patients with Hodgkin's disease. Blood 36:704–717, 1970
344. DeVita VT: Consequences of the chemotherapy of Hodgkin's disease. Cancer 47: 1–13, 1981
345. Frei E III, Luce JK, Gamble JF et al: Combination chemotherapy in advanced Hodgkin's disease: Induction and maintenance of remission. Ann Intern Med 79:376–382, 1973
346. DeVita VT, Simon RM, Hubbard SM et al: Curability of advanced Hodgkin's disease with chemotherapy. Long-term follow up of MOPP treated patients at NCI. Ann Intern Med 92:587–595, 1980
347. Canellos GP, Young RC, DeVita VT et al: Combination chemotherapy of advanced Hodgkin's disease in relapse following extensive radiotherapy. Clin Pharmcol Ther 13:750–754, 1972
348. Cadman E, Bloom AF, Prosnitz A et al: The effective use of combined modality therapy for the treatment of patients with Hodgkin's disease who relapsed following radiotherapy. Am J Clin Oncol 6:313–318, 1983
349. DeVita VT: Cell kinetics and the chemotherapy of cancer. Cancer Chemother Rep 3:23–33, 1971
350. Hryniuk W, Bush H. The importance of dose intensity in chemotherapy of metastatic breast cancer. J Clin Oncol 2:1281–1288, 1984
351. Hryniuk WM: Average relative dose intensity and the impact on design of clinical trials. Semin Oncol (in press)
352. DeVita VT, Hubbard SM, Longo DL: The chemotherapy of lymphomas: Looking back, moving forward—the Richard and Hinda Rosenthal Foundation Award Lecture. Cancer Research 47:5810–5824, 1987
353. Longo DL, Young RC, Wesley M et al: Twenty years of MOPP chemotherapy for Hodgkin's disease. J Clin Oncol 4:1295–1306, 1986
354. Morgenfeld M, Somoza N, Magnasco J et al: Combined chemotherapy cyclophosphamide, vinblastine, procarbazine and prednisone (CVPP) vs CVPP plus CCNU (CCVPP) in Hodgkin's disease. Cancer 43:1579, 1979
355. Goldie JH, Coldman AJ, Gudauskas GA: Rationale for the use of alternating non–cross-resistant chemotherapy. Cancer Chemother Pharmacol 2:101–105, 1979
356. Moore ME, Jones SE, Bull JM et al: MOPP chemotherapy for advanced Hodgkin's disease: Prognostic factors in 81 patients. Cancer 32:52–60, 1973
357. Jacobs C, Portlock CS, Rosenberg SA: Prednisone in MOPP chemotherapy for Hodgkin's disease. Br Med J 2:1469, 1976
358. Diggs Ch, Wiernik PH, Levi JA et al: Cyclophosphamide, vinblastine, procarbazine and prednisone with CCNU and vinblastine maintenance for advanced Hodgkin's disease. Cancer 39:1949, 1977
359. Gibbs GE, Peterson BA, Kennedy BJ et al: Long term survival of patients with Hodgkin's disease. Arch Intern Med 141:897, 1981
360. Nissen IN, Pajak FT, Glidewell O et al: A comparative study of a BCNU containing 4-drug program versus MOPP versus 3-drug combinations in advanced Hodgkin's disease. Cancer 43:31–40, 1979
361. Santoro A, Bonadonna G: Prolonged disease-free survival in MOPP-resistant Hodgkin's disease after treatment with adriamycin, bleomycin, vinblastine and dacarbazine (ABVD). Cancer Chemother Pharmacol 2:101–105, 1979
362. Santoro A, Bonfante V, Bonadonna G: Salvage chemotherapy with ABVD in MOPP-resistant Hodgkin's disease. Ann Intern Med 96:139–143, 1982
363. Papa G, Mandelli F, Anselmo AP et al: Treatment of MOPP-resistant Hodgkin's disease with adriamycin, bleomycin, vinblastine and dacarbazine (ABVD). Eur J Cancer 9:803–806, 1982
364. Canellos GP, Propert K, Cooper R et al: MOPP vs ABVD vs MOPP alternating with ABVD in advanced Hodgkin's disease: A prospective randomized CALGB trial. Proc Am Soc Clin Oncol 1988
365. Carde P, MacKintosh R, Rosenberg SA: A dose and time response analysis of the treatment of Hodgkin's disease with MOPP therapy. J Clin Oncol 1:146–153, 1983
366. Mead GM, Harker WG, Kushlan P et al: Single agent palliative chemotherapy for end-stage Hodgkin's disease. Cancer 50:829–835, 1982

367. Fisher RI, DeVita VT, Hubbard SM et al: Prolonged disease-free survival in Hodgkin's disease with MOPP reinduction after first relapse. Ann Intern Med 90: 761–763, 1979
368. Portlock CS, Rosenberg SA, Galtstein E et al: Impact of salvage treatment on initial relapses in patients with Hodgkin's disease Stages I to II. Blood 51:825–833, 1978
369. Goldman JM, Dawson AA: Chemotherapy for advanced resistant Hodgkin's disease (letter). Lancet 2:252, 1981
370. Vinciguerra V, Coleman M, Jarowski CI et al: A new combination chemotherapy for resistant Hodgkin's disease. JAMA 237:33–35, 1977
371. Goldman JM, Dawson AA: Combination chemotherapy for advanced resistant Hodgkin's disease. Lancet 2:1224–1227, 1975
372. Weiss J, von Roemling H, Peters HJ et al: Chemotherapie bei Vorbehandeltem morbus Hodkin mit Lomustin, Bleomycin, Vinblastin und Dexamethason. Dtsch Med Wschr 108:1428–1432, 1983
373. Tannir N, Hagemeister F, Valasquez W et al: Long-term follow-up with ABDIC salvage chemotherapy of MOPP-resistant Hodgkin's disease. J Clin Oncol 1: 432–439, 1983
374. Einhorn LH, Williams SD, Stevens EE et al: Treatment of MOPP-refractory Hodgkin's disease with vinblastine, doxorubicin, bleomycin, CCNU, and dacarbazine. Cancer 51:1348–1352, 1983
375. Piga A, Ambrosetti A, Todeschini et al: Doxorubicin, bleomycin, vinblastine and dacarbazine (ABVD) salvage of mechlorethamine vincristine, prednisone, and procarbazine (MOPP)-resistant advanced Hodgkin's disease Cancer Treat Rep 58: 947–951, 1984
376. Harker GW, Kushlan P, Rosenberg SA: Combination chemotherapy for advanced Hodgkin's disease after failure of MOPP: ABVD and B-CAV-e. Ann Intern Med 10:440–446, 1984
377. Bonadonna G, Viviani S, Valagussa P et al: Third-line salvage chemotherapy in Hodgkin's disease. Semin Oncol 12:23–25, 1985
378. Santoro A, Viviani SS, Valagussa P et al: CCNU, etoposide, & predni- mustine (CEP) in refractory Hodgkin's disease. Semin Oncol 13:23–26, 1986
379. Cervantes F, Reverter JC, Montserrat E et al: Treatment of advanced resistant Hodgkin's disease with lomustine, etoposide and prednimustine. Cancer Treat Rep 70:665–667, 1986
380. Mandelli F, Cimino G, Mauro FR et al: Prognosis and management of patients affected by multi-pre-treated Hodgkin's disease. Haematology 71:205–208, 1986
381. Richards MA, Waxman JH, Ganesan TS et al: EVA treatment for recurrent or unresponsive Hodgkin's disease. Cancer Chemother Pharmacol 18:51–53, 1986
382. Garbes ID, Gomez GA, Tan T et al: Salvage chemotherapy for advanced Hodgkin's disease. Med Pediatr Oncol 15:45–48, 1987
383. Hagemeister FBN, Tannir N, McLaughlin P et al: MIME chemotherapy (Methyl-GAG, ifosfamide, methotrexate, etoposide) as treatment for recurrent Hodgkin's disease. J Clin Oncol 5:556–561, 1987
383a. Pfrendschuh MG, Schoppe WD, Fuchs R et al: Lomustine, etoposide, vindesine, and dexamethasone (CEVD) in Hodgkin's lymphoma refractory to cyclophosphamide, vincristine, procarbazine, and prednisone (COPP) and doxorubicin, bleomycin, vinblastine, and dacarbazine (ABVD): A multi-center trial of the German Hodgkin Study Group. Cancer Treat Rep 71:1203–1207, 1987
384. Tseng A, Jacobs C, Coleman CN et al: Third-line chemotherapy for resistant Hodgkin's disease with lomustine, etoposide, and methotrexate. Cancer Treat Rep 71:475–478, 1987
385. Schulman P, Propert K, Cooper MR et al: Phase II study of MOPLACE in previously treated Hodgkin's disease. Proc Soc Clin Oncol 6:A742, 1987
386. Levi JA, Wiernik PH, Diggs CH: Combination chemotherapy of advanced previously treated Hodgkin's disease with streptozoticin, CCNU, adriamycin and bleomycin. Med Pediatr Oncol 3:33–40, 1977
387. Longo D: Personal communication, 1988
388. Olweny CLM, Katongole-Nvidda E, Kirre C et al: Childhood Hodgkin's disease in Uganda. A 10-year experience. Cancer 42:787, 1978
389. O'Dwyer PJ, Wiernik PH, Stewart MB et al: Treatment of early stage Hodgkin's disease: A randomized trial of radiotherapy plus chemotherapy versus chemotherapy alone. In Cavalli F, Bonadonna G, Rozensweig N (eds): Malignant Lymphomas in Hodgkin's Disease: Experimental and Therapeutic Advances, pp 329–336. Boston, Martinus Nijhoff, 1985
390. Longo D, Gladstein E, Young R et al: Randomized trial of MOPP chemotherapy versus subtotal nodal radiation therapy in patients with laparotomy-documented early stage Hodgkin's disease. Proc Am Soc Clin Oncol 6:206, 1987
391. Gill PS, Levine AM, Kiarlo M et al: AIDS-related malignant lymphomas: Results of prospective drug trials. J Clin Oncol 5:1322, 1987
392. Prior E, Goldberg AF, Conjalka MS et al: Hodgkin's disease in homosexual men. An AIDS-related phenomenon? Am J Med 81:1085, 1986
393. Unger PD, Strauchen JA: Hodgkin's disease in AIDS complex patients. Cancer 58:821, 1986
394. Bookman MA, Longo DL: Complications in patients treated for Hodgkin's disease. Cancer Treat Rev 13:77–111, 1986
395. Louie AC, Cavalli F, Rozensweig M: New agents for Hodgkin's and non-Hodgkin's lymphoma in malignant lymphomas and Hodgkin's disease: Experimental and therapeutic advances. In Cavalli F, Bonadonna G, Rozensweig M (eds): Malignant Lymphomas in Hodgkin's Disease: Experimental and Therapeutic Advances, pp 493–511. Boston, Martinus Nijhoff, 1985
396. Warrell RP, Coonley CJ, Straus DJ et al: Treatment of patients with advanced malignant lymphoma using gallium nitrate administered as a seven-day continuous infusion. Cancer 51:1982–1987, 1983
397. Knight WAT, Fabian C, Costanzi J et al: Methylglyoxal-bis guanylhydrazone (methyl GAG, MGBG) in lymphoma and Hodgkin's disease. Invest New Drugs 1:235–237, 1983
398. Espana P, Kaplan R, Robichaud K et al: Phase II study of spiroglimanium (Spiro G) in lymphoma patients. Proc Am Soc Clin Oncol 1:166, 1982
399. Weick JK, Jones SE, Ryan DH: Phase II study of amsacrine (m-AMSA) in advanced lymphomas: A Southwest Oncology Group study. Cancer Treat Rep 67:489–492, 1983
400. Case ED, Hayes DM: Phase II study of arizidinybenzo-quinone in refractory lymphoma. Cancer Treat Rep 67:993–996, 1983
401. Coltman CA, McDaniel TM, Balcerzak SP et al: Mitoxantone hydrochloride (NSC-310739) in lymphoma. A Southwest Oncology Group study. Invest New Drug 1:65–70, 1983
402. Warrell RP, Kempen SJ: Clinical evaluation of a new anthracyline antibiotic aclacinomycin-A in patients with advanced malignant lymphoma. Am J Clin Oncol 6:81–84, 1983
403. Coonley CJ, Warrell RP, Straus DJ et al: Clinical evaluation of 4-demethoxydaunorubicin in patients with advanced malignant lymphoma. Cancer Treat Rep 67: 949–950, 1983
403a. Rosensweig M, Crespeigne N, Kenis Y: Phase I trial with 4′deoxydoxorubin (esonibicen). Invest New Drug 1:309–313, 1983
403b. Lenhard RE, Order SE, Spunberg JJ: Isotopic immunoglobulin: A new systemic therapy for advanced Hodgkin's disease. J Clin Oncol 3:1296–1300, 1985
403c. Hoppe RT, Coleman CN, Cox RS et al: The management of Stages I–II Hodgkin's disease with irradiation alone or combined modality therapy: The Stanford experience. Blood 59:455–465, 1982
404. Mauch P, Rosenthal DS, Canellos GP et al: Improved survival for Stage IIA and IIB Hodgkin's disease patients treated with combined radiation therapy and chemotherapy. Ann Intern Med (in press)
405. Canellos GP, Arseneau JC, DeVita VT et al: Second malignancies complicating Hodgkin's disease in remission. Lancet 1:947–949, 1975
406. Coleman CN, Williams CJ, Flint A et al: Hematological neoplasia in patients treated for Hodgkin's disease. N Engl J Med 300:452–458, 1979
407. Mauch PM, Canellos GP, Rosenthal DS et al: Reduction of fatal complications from combined modality therapy in Hodgkin's disease. J Clin Oncol 3:501–505, 1985
408. DeVita VT Jr, Lewis BJ, Rozencweig M et al: The chemotherapy of Hodgkin's disease: Past experiences and future directions. Cancer 42:979–990, 1978
409. Lister TA, Dorreen NS, Faux M et al: The treatment of stage IIIA Hodgkin's disease. J Clin Oncol 1:745–749, 1983
410. Mauch P, Goodman R, Hellman S: The significance of mediastinal involvement in early stage Hodgkin's disease. Cancer 42:1039–1045, 1978
411. Glick JH: The treatment of Stage IIIA Hodgkin's disease: What is the role of combined modality therapy? Int J Radiat Oncol Biol Phys 4:781–787, 1978
412. Prosnitz LR, Montalvo RL, Fischer DB: Treatment of Stage IIIA Hodgkin's disease is radiotherapy alone adequate? Int J Radiat Oncol Biol Phys 4:781–787, 1978
413. Russell KJ, Donaldson SS, Cox RS et al: Childhood Hodgkin's disease: Patterns of relapse. J Clin Oncol 2:80–87, 1984
414. Langhans T: Das Maligne Lymphosarkom (Pseuddukamie). Virchows Arch [A] 54:509–537, 1872
415. Pell PK: Zur Symptomatologie der sogenannten Pseudoleukamie II. Pseudoleukamie oder chronisches Ruckfallsfieber? Berlin Klin Wchnschr 24:644–646, 1887
416. Parker F Jr, Jackson H Jr, Fitzhugh G et al: Studies of diseases of the lymphoid and myeloid tissues, IV. Skin reactions to human and avian tuberculin. J Immunol 22:277–282, 1932
417. Jackson H Jr: Classification and prognosis of Hodgkin's disease and allied disorders. Surg Gynecol Obstet 64:465–467, 1937
418. Mauch P et al: Hodgkin's disease: Current controversies in staging and treatment. ASTRO Refresher Course, October 1987
419. Mauch PM et al: Unpublished data
420. JAMA 168:496, 1958
421. Kaplan HS, Dorfman RF, Nelson TS et al: Staging laparotomy and splenectomy in Hodgkin's disease: Analysis of indications and patterns of involvement in 285 consecutive, unselected patients. Natl Cancer Inst Monogr 36:291, 1973
422. Rosenberg SA, Kaplan HS: The evolution and summary results of the Stanford randomized clinical trials of the management of Hodgkin's disease: 1962–1984. Int J Radiat Oncol Biol Phys 11:5–22, 1985
423. Mauch PM et al: Unpublished data

VINCENT T. DEVITA, JR.
ELAINE S. JAFFE
PETER MAUCH
DAN L. LONGO

CHAPTER 50 *Lymphocytic Lymphomas*

ETIOLOGY AND EPIDEMIOLOGY

The lymphomas are the seventh most common causes of death from cancer in the United States.[1] About 30,000 new cases of lymphocytic lymphoma occur each year. Because of a young average age of the lymphoma population (42 years), the total in person-years of life lost each year ranks the lymphomas fourth in terms of economic impact among cancers in the United States. The incidence of lymphomas appears to be increasing each year.[2,3] The reasons for the increase are not entirely clear; however, there is some contribution from patients infected with human immunodeficiency virus (HIV). This number may greatly increase over the next few years if projections about the acquired immunodeficiency syndrome (AIDS) epidemic are accurate. Studies of the epidemiology of lymphomas have been hampered in the past by the lack of worldwide, standard, histopathologic classifications of the disease.

In the United States there is a steady increase in the incidence of the lymphocytic lymphomas from childhood through age 80 years, and in the United States lymphocytic lymphoma is more common in males (8.1:100,000) than in females (5.7:100,000).[4-6] The incidence rates for lymphocytic lymphomas also show marked variations from country to country, ranging from 1:100,000 in rural Poland to 9.1:100,000 in the non-Jewish population of Israel.[7] Lymphocytic lymphomas appear more frequently in younger age groups in Egypt than in American or European countries. In Africa and New Guinea Burkitt's lymphoma is very common, whereas in the United States, Great Britain, and tropical Latin America this lymphoma is very rare.

The cause of the lymphomas is unknown. There is convincing evidence that viruses cause certain types of lymphomas in rodents, birds, cats, and cows.[8-11] Marek's disease, a lymphoma of chickens, is caused by a herpes-like deoxyribonucleic acid (DNA) virus and can now be prevented by vaccines.[12] A horizontally transmitted type C retrovirus of cows is a highly infectious cause of bovine lymphosarcoma.[13] Inbreeding appears to play an important role in the viral etiology of these animal cancers. In humans there is a strong association between the Epstein–Barr virus (EBV) and the lymphoma described by Burkitt in East Africa (anti-EBV antibodies have been identified in the serum of patients and complementary viral DNA in the DNA of Burkitt cells), but the association is not as strong for Burkitt's lymphoma diagnosed in the United States.[14] Cells cultured from patients with Hodgkin's disease and some patients with diffuse lymphocytic lymphoma have been shown to express type C ribonucleic acid (RNA) virus particles and appear to contain viral information such as protein coat antigens and viral reverse transcriptase.[15,16] All of these observations have supported a viral etiology of lymphomas in humans but have not provided definitive proof. Several alternatives could be considered based on these earlier studies: a true causative relation, contamination of tissue cultures by ubiquitous viruses, or infection by virus in vivo or expression of viral genes after the cell has been altered by malignant transformation.

The most convincing evidence for viral etiology of human malignant lymphoma has come from the recent studies of a distinct clinicopathologic entity, adult T-cell leukemia/lymphoma (ATL), which is endemic in southwestern Japan and now identified in other parts of the world as well.[17-19] The striking geographic distribution and clustering of these patients might have suggested a viral cause. However, convincing proof has come from the work of Gallo and his co-workers, who, in 1978, identified a unique type C RNA tumor virus in certain patients with mature T-cell malignancies.[20-22] This virus was termed human T-cell leukemia/lymphoma virus (HTLV). HTLV was shown to be a unique, exogenously acquired retrovirus that is not closely related to any known animal retroviruses in terms of antigenicity, amino acid sequence, and nucleic acid sequence homology. Although HTLV first was isolated from the neoplastic cells of patients thought to have an aggressive variant of mycosis fungoides (MF), it subsequently was recognized that the disease in these patients was identical to ATL as described in Japan.[23] Subsequent studies demonstrated an association between ATL and HTLV in Japan as well as in other endemic areas such as the Caribbean and southeastern United States.[24-27]

Subsequent to the identification of HTLV and its association with ATL, four other members of this family of human retroviruses have been described. The original member is called HTLV-I. HTLV-II was identified in a patient with atypical T-cell hairy cell leukemia (HCL).[28] It has been isolated from very few patients and is not clearly associated with a distinct clinicopathologic disease entity. HTLV-III (or human immunodeficiency virus [HIV-1]) is the causative agent of AIDS.[29,30] HTLV-IV (or HIV-2) has been isolated from West African patients with AIDS, but its role in disease pathogenesis is not yet clear.[31,32] Recently HTLV-V, a putative causative virus for certain cutaneous T-cell lymphomas (CTCL), was described.[33] Data on its epidemiology are not available.

The precise mechanism by which HTLV-I infection leads to malignant transformation in vivo is unknown. In vitro transformation appears to be linked to viral replication[34]; however, fresh tumor cells from patients with HTLV-I–associated ATL rarely express viral messenger RNA (mRNA). It is clear that the HTLV-I genome can interact with certain host genes,[35] for example, interleukin-2 (IL-2) and the IL-2 receptor,[36] and it appears possible that transformation in vivo may be related to the activation by the virus of a cellular oncogene called *rel* that is not normally expressed in mature post-thymic T cells (Ruscetti, Longo DL, unpublished observations).

Because many patients in endemic areas are infected with HTLV-I but few go on to develop ATL, there appear to be host factors that affect transformation of lymphocytes by HTLV-I. In fact, strong evidence supporting such host-related genetic factors is emerging. HTLV-I has recently been isolated from the neurons of patients suffering from tropical spastic paraparesis, a disease with epidemiology similar to that of ATL.[37] A preliminary study in Japan of patients infected with HTLV-I appears to demonstrate that patients who develop ATL have a high incidence of expressing certain HLA antigens (A26, DQw3) and those who develop myelopathy express a distinct HLA haplotype (A11 or A26, Bw52 or Bw54, Cw1, DQw3).[38] Such strong linkage disequilibrium suggests that the major histocompatibility complex (MHC) is involved in the pathogenesis of HTLV-I–related disease.

In addition to the B-cell tropic EBV and the T-cell tropic HTLV retrovirus family, a third virus type associated with lymphoma has recently been isolated from a patient with AIDS and lymphoma by Gallo and his colleagues.[39] HBLV appears to be a B-cell tropic virus related to the herpesvirus family and is capable of transforming human B cells in vitro. Its role in human lymphomagenesis has not yet been defined.

The search for a viral etiology of lymphoma and other cancers also has led to the identification of retroviral *onc* genes, which appear to be similar to human cellular genes involved in the regulation of cellular differentiation and growth. Recent work has suggested that such oncogenes may be implicated in the pathophysiology and development of lymphomas. For example, the quinacrine and Giemsa banding techniques[40] had demonstrated that in patients with both endemic and nonendemic Burkitt's lymphomas, there is a translocation of a portion of chromosome 8 onto chromosome 14,8q − :14q+.[41,42] More important, this translocation results in the translocation of the c-*myc* oncogene into the immunoglobulin heavy-chain locus.[42] Moreover, the less common 8:2 and 8:22 translocations are associated with the juxtaposition of the same oncogene, c-*myc*, with the light-chain loci, kappa and lambda, respectively.[43] Such translocations might result in the oncogene coming under the influence of a promoter region in the activated immunoglobulin genes in this Ig-synthesizing B-cell lymphoma, culminating in the transformation of the cell. Similar translocations also have been identified in murine plasmacytomas, and changes in chromosome 14 also have been reported in other B-cell lymphomas.[44-46] There have now been five recurring chromosome translocations involving the immunoglobulin genes associated with lymphoproliferative diseases: t(8;14) [and less commonly, t(2;8) and t(8;22)] involving *myc* associated mainly with Burkitt's and diffuse small noncleaved cell (non-Burkitt's) lymphomas; the inverted 14 involving the locus for the alpha chain of the T-cell antigen receptor[47]; t(14;18) involving *bcl2* on chromosome 18 (whose capacity to transform cells has not yet been demonstrated) associated with follicular lymphomas; t(11;14) involving *bcl1* on chromosome 11 (which has not yet been identified) associated with chronic lymphocytic leukemia (CLL); and t(14;19) (the gene involved on chromosome 19 is not known) associated with CLL.[48] Only in the t(14;19) cases of CLL does the translocation appear to make an important impact on prognosis; patients with t(14;19) have more aggressive disease than those without.

A hereditary influence on the incidence of lymphomas is suggested by their higher incidences in patients with inherited immunologic deficiency diseases, and by a small increase in the incidence in families of patients with immunologic disorders.[49] In one study a significant increase in the incidence of Hodgkin's disease was noted in siblings of the index case, particularly in siblings of the same sex.[50] A slight increase in the incidence of lymphomas has been noted in large series of patients with collagen vascular diseases as compared with the general population adjusted for age.[51] This increased incidence approached 10% in patients with long-standing Sjögren's syndrome, who tend to develop diffuse aggressive lymphomas or immunoblastic sarcomas.[52-54]

Lymphoma-like syndromes associated with lymphadenopathy have been found in patients who take phenytoin in order to control seizures.[55] Although in most cases the disease regresses when the patient stops taking phenytoin, a small fraction proceeds to develop malignant lymphomas of several varieties, including Hodgkin's disease. Such observations suggest that the drug is acting on patients with an inherited tendency to develop the disease. Patients who are chronically immunosuppressed by drugs, particularly those who have received renal transplants, have a higher incidence of diffuse aggressive lymphomas and immunoblastic sarcomas, often in the brain.[56,57] Except for the higher incidence of Hodgkin's disease in siblings and the influence of phenytoin on the development of lymphomas, it is difficult to separate the influence of inheritance per se from immunosuppression, which may be of etiologic importance without an inherited background. For example, lymphomas occur with an increased frequency in many congenital and acquired immunodeficiency diseases. The incidence of lymphoma in graft-versus-host disease, iatrogenic immune suppression, AIDS, and autoimmune disease argues strongly for immune dysregulation in lymphoma etiology. Chronic antigenic stimulation has been thought to play a role in the development of lymphomas in certain animal models, but there are no convincing data in humans. Some patients with nontropical sprue may develop primary T-cell lymphomas in the gastrointestinal (GI) tract, perhaps related to the gluten stimulation. It was recently shown that the immunoglobulin gene rearrangements in about 25% of patients with CLL (by inference, diffuse, small lymphocytic lymphomas) result in the production of immunoglobulins that share kappa chain idiotypes, the structures unique to the antigen recognition site.[58] Thus these tumors rearrange V-kappa genes nonstochastically. This could represent evidence that tumors in different people result from the transformation of a B cell that recognizes a common or similar antigen.

It is now clear that many, if not all, lymphomas that occur in the setting of acquired or congenital immunodeficiency are associated with EBV as a causative agent.[59] Most individuals infected with EBV harbor the virus in B lymphocytes, which are infected by way of their cell surface receptor for the C3d component of complement. The polyclonal B-cell infection is normally controlled by T lymphocytes that eliminate the infected B cells.[60] When T-cell deficiency exists, EBV-infected B cells can proliferate, and usually one clone escapes immune surveillance to become autonomously proliferating, perhaps owing in some cases to genetic translocations that juxtapose oncogenes with expressed cellular genes like immunoglobulin, as discussed earlier.

The increased incidence of lymphoma among Midwestern farmers born after 1900 and dying before age 65 years has raised the possibility that relatively recent changes in agricultural techniques and practices, such as the increased use of pesticides and fertilizers, may play a role in the cause of lymphoid neoplasia.[61]

Although it appears that ionizing radiation can cause malignant lymphoma in humans, the mechanism of neoplastic transformation and the condition under which it occurs have not been clearly delineated. An increased prevalence of lymphocytic lymphoma has been demonstrated in survivors of the atomic bomb in Hiroshima who were exposed to 100 or more rad.[62,63] An increased incidence of lymphoma has been demonstrated in patients irradiated for ankylosing spondylitis.[64] In both groups the ratio of observed to expected cases of lymphoma was 2:1. Patients with Hodgkin's disease treated with radiation therapy and chemotherapy have an increased risk of developing secondary large-cell lymphoma, often involving the GI tract.

TABLE 50-1. Disease with a Predisposition to Develop Lymphomas

Klinefelter's syndrome
Chediak–Higashi syndrome
Ataxia telangiectasia syndrome
Wiscott–Aldrich syndrome
Swiss-type agammaglobulinemia
Common variable immunodeficiency disease
Acquired hypogammaglobulinemia
Iatrogenic immunosuppression
Sjögren's syndrome
Rheumatoid arthritis and systemic lupus erythematosus
Acquired immunodeficiency syndrome
X-linked lymphoproliferative syndrome

Investigations of the association of histocompatibility antigens with lymphoma report an association with HLA-B12 antigen.[65,66] Klinefelter's syndrome has been associated with large-cell lymphoma, and Chediak–Higashi syndrome has been associated with an increased risk of lymphoreticular malignancy.[67,68] The disease that have been shown to predispose to the development of lymphomas are listed in Table 50-1.

MICROSCOPIC AND FUNCTIONAL ANATOMY OF NORMAL LYMPHOID TISSUES

The principal cellular component of lymphoid tissue is the lymphocyte.[69] Lymphoid cells are widely distributed throughout the body, both singly and in centers of aggregation.[70] Primary lymphoid organs in which these cells are generated include the bone marrow and thymus. The secondary lymphoid organs populated by differentiated lymphoid cells include lymph nodes, spleen, Waldeyer's ring (the oropharyngeal lymphoid tissues), and lymphoid aggregates in the lamina propria and submucosa of the respiratory and GI tracts; in the latter location they are referred to as Peyer's patches. Sometimes lymphoid elements associated with epithelium in the respiratory and GI tracts are referred to as the mucosa-associated lymphoid tissues and gut-associated lymphoid tissues.[71] Lymphoid cells also populate bone marrow, as cohabitants of the numerous hematopoietic elements. In addition to these major sites of aggregation and proliferation, lymphoid cells are distributed as normally inconspicuous interstitial elements in essentially all tissues except the central nervous system (CNS).

Other cells of the lymphoreticular system include reticular supporting cells, dendritic and interdigitating reticulum cells, and cells of the monocyte–macrophage series. The reticular cells provide the basic three-dimensional matrix of lymph nodes by virtue of their long cytoplasmic processes joined by tight junctions or desmosomes. Within this matrix the functional cells of the lymphoid and monocyte–macrophage series migrate, proliferate, and serve as the primary arm of the host immunologic defense apparatus. The lymphoreticular system is thus the anatomical basis of cell-mediated and humoral immunity.

Normally both the lymphoid and monocytic cells of the lymphoreticular system originate in the bone marrow and from there migrate by way of the blood and lymphatic vessels to populate other lymphoreticular tissues.[69] T cells are processed through the thymus gland, whereas B cells are processed through the mammalian equivalent of the avian bursa of Fabricius, probably the fetal liver. Although T cells and B cells constitute the two major components of lymphocytic series, there are minor populations of other lymphocytes, such as natural killer (NK) cells that may develop independently. Monocytes also originate in the bone marrow and, like lymphocytes, circulate and eventually populate extramedullary tissues as cells of the monocyte–histiocyte series.[72] These three populations of lymphoreticular cells (T cells, B cells, and monocyte–macrophages) serve different functions in the system and are, to some degree, compartmentalized anatomically (Fig. 50-1). The malignant lymphomas frequently mirror these normal anatomical distributions in their spread throughout the lymphoreticular system.[73] The pattern of spread of the lymphomas is thus not random but mimics patterns of normal lymphocyte circulation and distribution.

Functionally, T cells are regarded as the basis of the cell-mediated immune system.[74] Cytotoxic T cells may directly lyse specific target cells, such as tumor cells or virally infected cells. Other subpopulations of T cells subserve an immunoregulatory function and act as helpers or suppressors for B cells, macrophages, and other T cells. T lymphocytes recognize antigen when it is associated with the membrane-bound products of the MHC. Some T cells (CD4-positive cells) predominantly recognize antigen in association with class II MHC antigens, whereas other cells (CD8-positive cells) recognize antigen in association with class I MHC antigens.

B cells form the basis of the humoral immune system.[75] These cells express membrane-bound immunoglobulin and, as differentiated B cells or plasma cells, secrete immunoglobulin. The ability to phagocytize particulate material is the hallmark of macrophages and monocytes.[76] These cells play a major role in the processing of antigens and the presentation of antigens to lymphocytes. Dendritic reticulum cells and interdigitating reticulum cells are thought to be related to monocyte–macrophages. However, these cells are involved in antigen presentation and do not subserve a phagocytic function.[77,78] The dendritic reticulum cells are localized in lymphoid follicles, whereas interdigitating reticulum cells are the antigen-presenting cells of the T-cell system and are found in the paracortex. Langerhans' cells, most conspicuous in the skin but also found in other sites such as lymph nodes, are closely related to interdigitating reticulum cells[79] and present antigen to T lymphocytes.

IDENTIFICATION OF LYMPHOID CELLS

Normal and neoplastic cells of the immune system can be distinguished by characteristic surface markers. The neoplastic cells frequently retain the phenotypic markers of their normal counterparts. Thus these features can be used to aid in the characterization and subclassification of lymphoid malignancies (Table 50-2). Surface markers may be antigens acquired during differentiation without recognized specific functions. However, in many instances these markers have been functionally characterized and can be recognized as specific membrane receptors or other structures of functional significance.

In 1975 Kohler and Milstein[80] showed that normal murine B lymphocytes could be fused with murine myeloma cells, producing a hybridoma cell line that would secrete an antibody of predefined specificity indefinitely. The hybridoma cell line used the machinery of the myeloma cell, but the specificity of the antibody produced was derived from the normal B cell with which it was fused. The resulting monoclonal antibody is of extraordinary specificity because it is

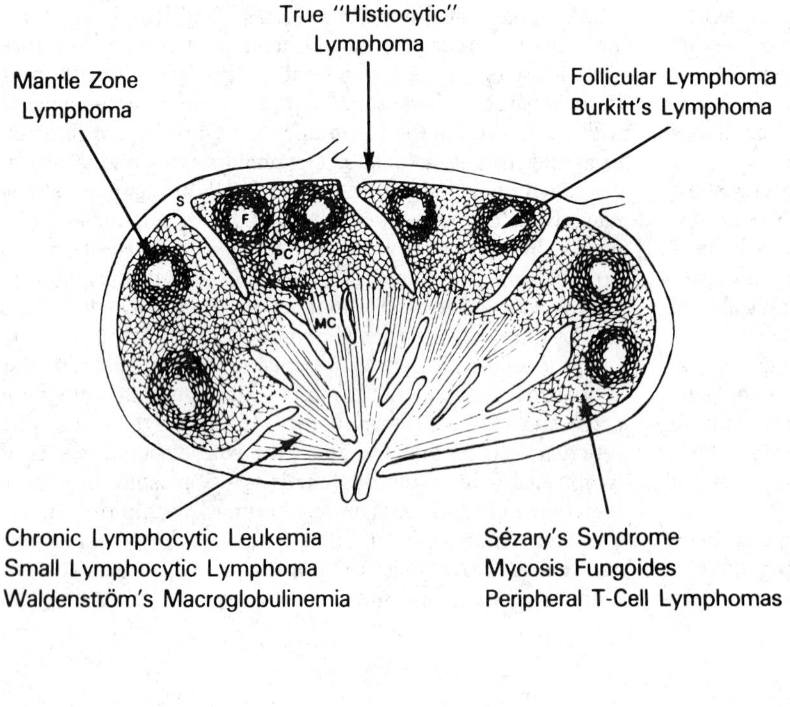

FIG. 50-1. Schematic diagram of normal lymph node illustrating anatomical and functional compartments of the immune system. Malignant lymphomas can be related to compartments as shown. S, sinuses; F, follicles; PC, paracortex; MC, medullary cords. (Modified from Mann RB et al: Malignant lymphomas: A conceptual understanding of morphologic diversity. Am J Pathol 94:1–3, 1979)

TABLE 50-2. Cellular Origin of Malignant Lymphomas

Neoplasms of B-Cell Origin	*Neoplasms of T-Cell Origin*	*Neoplasms of Histiocytic Reticulum Cell Origin*
Chronic lymphocytic leukemia (98%)	Chronic lymphocytic leukemia (2%) Large granular lymphocyte leukemia (T gamma lymphoproliferative disease)	Monocytic leukemia
Small lymphocytic (well-differentiated) lymphoma	Mycosis fungoides/Sézary syndrome	Malignant histiocytosis
Lymphocytic lymphoma, intermediate and/or small cleaved cell types (mantle zone lymphoma)	Diffuse aggressive lymphomas of adults (15%) Peripheral T-cell lymphomas Mixed-cell type Large cell, immunoblastic	True histiocytic lymphomas
Follicular lymphomas	Adult T-cell leukemia/lymphoma	
Diffuse aggressive lymphomas of adults (85%) Mixed-cell type Large-cell type* Large-cell immunoblastic Small noncleaved cell* Burkitt's (small noncleaved cell) lymphoma	Angiocentric lymphomas (lymphomatoid granulomatosis) (polymorphic reticulosis)	Dendritic reticulum cell sarcomas Interdigitating reticulum cell sarcomas
Acute lymphocytic leukemias† (75%) Lymphoblastic lymphomas (10%)†	Acute lymphocytic leukemias† (25%) Lymphoblastic leukemias (85%)†	

* Majority of cases, 95%.
† These malignancies are of stem cell origin; they have an immature phenotype but are committed to B- or T-cell differentiation, respectively.

directed against a single antigenic determinant. Additionally, the hybridoma cell line allows for a nearly unlimited supply of the antibody. This technology has produced an ever-increasing battery of reagents that can identify the antigenic determinants of lymphoreticular cells.

Previously a complex variety of assays was used to detect lymphocyte surface markers or receptors.[81] For example, the E rosette assay was used to detect T lymphocytes that have receptors for sheep erythrocytes. The EAC (erythrocyte, antibody, and complement) rosette assay was used to detect cells (B cells and monocytes) that bear receptors for the C3d complement receptor. However, the advent of the monoclonal antibody technology has rendered many of these cumbersome assays obsolete. Now monoclonal antibodies have been developed that recognize these specific structures. Thus antibodies to CD2 (T11, Leu5) recognize the sheep erythrocyte receptor, and antibodies to CD21 (B2, HB5) recognize the C3d receptor.[82,83]

A somewhat bewildering aspect of this technology is the enormous number of monoclonal antibodies published and available through commercial and private sources. In many cases monoclonal antibodies bear different names but immunoprecipitate identical antigens and are of identical specificity. An international nomenclature has been developed that follows the pattern used for the naming of HLA-related antigens, and the use of such commonly agreed-on terminology is invaluable in comparing reagents and results. Monoclonal antibodies of comparable specificity belong to the same group or "cluster of differentiation" and bear the same "CD" name. Thus antibodies to the T3 complex on T cells linked to T-cell antigen receptor are termed CD3 (T3, OKT3, anti-Leu4).[82,83]

Monoclonal antibodies can be used in immunofluorescence or immunohistochemical assays to identify both normal and neoplastic lymphoid cells. As currently performed, the cell preparation is incubated with an antibody to the molecule of interest, the nonadherent antibody is washed off, and adherent antibody is detected by either fluorescence or a linked enzymatic reaction that gives a colored product. The advantage of immunohistochemical or immunocytochemical techniques (*i.e.*, those on which tissue sections or cytologic preparations from cell suspensions, respectively, are used) is that the in situ organization and cell morphology can be seen, as well as immunologic phenotype. This is useful when one considers that neoplasms rarely are pure populations of neoplastic cells—a variety of normal cell types are invariably present. Thus if one were trying to decide whether a lymphoma was of B- or T-cell origin, a positive result with an antibody to CD3 would be suggestive of T-cell origin only if the tumor cells were positive; many B-cell lymphomas contain large numbers of infiltrating T cells. Although not a substitute for hematoxylin and eosin (H&E) morphologic examination, the use of immunohistochemistry is a valuable adjunct to accurate diagnosis.[84]

Complementary information can be gained by using a flow cytometer or fluorescent-activated cell analyzer to quantitate the expression of surface antigens on cells.[85] Labeling of cells is conceptually the same as in immunohistochemistry, except that the second antibody is conjugated to a fluorescent molecule, such as fluorescein or rhodamine, instead of to an enzyme. Cells in suspension are passed single file through a glass chamber through which laser light of an appropriate wavelength is passed. The amount of fluorescence on a given cell in sensed quantitatively, which is directly proportional to the number of antibody molecules bound, and hence to the expression of surface antigen. Measurement of cell size is made at the same time. Current models allow the quantitation of two antigens on a single cell through the concurrent use of two antibodies tagged with molecules that fluoresce at different wavelengths. The flow cytometer provides enumerations of cell size, number, and fluorescent intensity that can be plotted together in various ways. Using a flow cytometer, one can look at a statistically significant, reproducible sample of tens of thousands of cells in seconds, which allows one to characterize a given preparation with numerous antibodies. The optical system is unbiased and sensitive (it can detect on the order of a few thousand molecules on the cell surface with a high-affinity antibody), and the output can be stored in computers as raw data, allowing for sophisticated manipulation and analysis. Analyzers capable of looking at three or four parameters at once are in development.

Most antibodies currently available work only in suspension or in frozen preparations, as the processing for paraffin sections can significantly alter the antigenic determinants. However, some antigens are preserved in paraffin, such as the leukocyte common antigen (T200 or CD45), which is useful in differential diagnosis of lymphoma and undifferentiated carcinoma.[86,87]

T cells have been especially well characterized with monoclonal antibodies, which can be used to identify not only the stage of differentiation of the cell, but also its functional capabilities (Fig. 50-2).[88] Functional studies have suggested that there were distinct T-cell populations, the so-called helper and suppressor cells.[89,90] Helper T cells are required for the terminal differentiation of a B cell into a plasma cell and provide help for immunoglobulin secretion. In contrast, suppressor cells can reverse this process and inhibit antibody production. Helper cells also promote the differentiation of cytotoxic T cells. Most CD4-positive cells are helper cells and recognize antigen in the context of class II MHC.[74] Conversely, CD8-positive cells constitute the cytotoxic/suppressor subset and recognize antigen in the context of class I. In normal peripheral blood CD4-CD8 ratio is approximately 2:1, whereas in normal lymph nodes it is approximately 3.5 or 4:1. Most malignancies of T-cell origin usually express, preferentially, either a CD4- or a CD8-positive phenotype. However, these antigens are not clonal markers and should not be interpreted as such. For reasons as yet undetermined, the vast majority of mature T-cell malignancies have a CD4-positive phenotype.[91,92]

Monoclonal antibodies can also be used to delineate developmental stages of T-cell differentiation.[93,94] Early T cells lack CD4 and CD8 antigens and then coexpress them. Immature T cells express transferrin receptors identified by T9.[95] This marker has no lineage specificity, since most proliferating cells have such receptors. Two of the earliest markers with some lineage specificity include the E rosette receptor (CD2) and CD7.[96] Both of these markers can be expressed before rearrangement of the T-cell antigen receptor. This feature also raises a question as to marker specificity, and some have reported expression of CD2 and CD7 in acute myelogenous leukemia blasts.[97] The CD1 (T6) antigen is found on cortical thymocytes but is absent on mature T cells.[93] Interestingly, this antigen is expressed on Langerhans' cells of the skin.[79] The CD5 antigen found on all normal T cells is also expressed on a subpopulation of normal B cells.[98] It is useful in the characterization of B-cell malignancies because it is expressed in some tumors (such as B-cell CLL) but not others.[99]

The hallmark of a B lymphocyte is the expression of surface immunoglobulin, which is a product of cell synthesis and consists of one or more heavy chains and only one type of light chain per lymphocyte. Surface immunoglobulin, like other surface markers, can be detected by a variety of immunochemical techniques. Reactive B-cell proliferations are polyclonal, with a ratio of kappa to lambda expression of approximately 2:1. B-cell lymphomas are monoclonal and express only a single light chain type. When all the cells express a given light chain, the correlation with malignancy is excellent. However, when using very sensitive techniques, such as immunoglobulin gene rearrangement studies, one must be cautious in equating monoclonality with malignancy. Under some conditions, particularly in association with immunodeficiency, a monoclonal population may be detected and may undergo spontaneous regression.[100]

Fewer monoclonal antibodies have been developed against B cells and B-cell subsets (Fig. 50-3).[83] Monoclonal antibod-

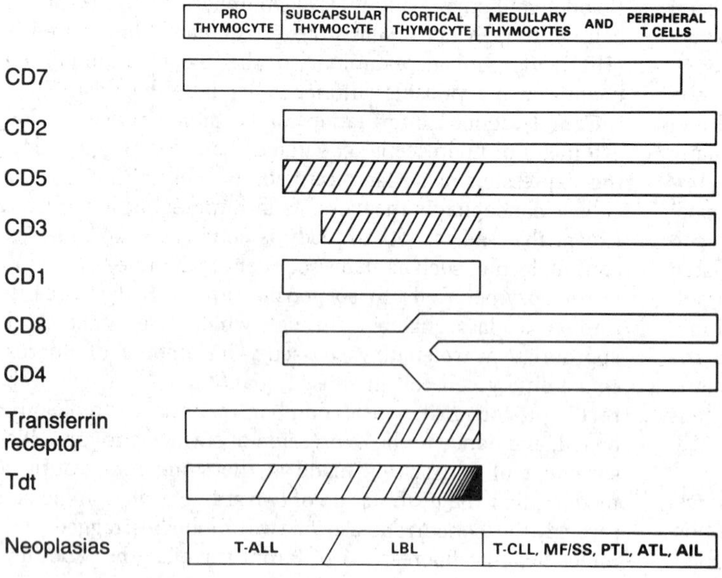

FIG. 50-2. Monoclonal antibodies can be used to identify different developmental and functional T-cell subpopulations. Monoclonal antibodies are identified according to CD groups established by international nomenclature panel. Neoplasias of T-cell origin can be related to sequential stages of T-cell differentiation. (Modified from Cossman J et al: Diversity of immunologic phenotypes of lymphoblastic lymphoma. Cancer Res 43:4486, 1983)

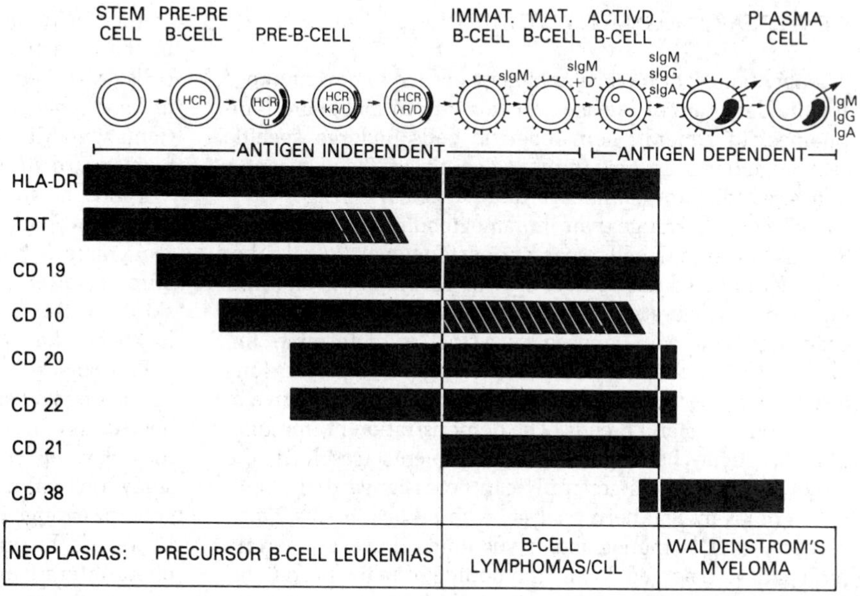

FIG. 50-3. Schematic diagram demonstrating molecular genetic and immunophenotypic correlates of normal B-cell differentiation. Monoclonal antibodies are identified according to CD groups established by international nomenclature panel. Steps of heavy and light chain immunoglobulin gene rearrangement are shown. B-cell malignancies can be related to sequential stages of B-cell differentiation. HCR, heavy chain rearrangement; kappa R/D, kappa light chain rearrangement or deletion; lambda R/D, lambda light chain rearrangement or deletion; u, mu heavy chain synthesis.

ies with broad reactivity against normal B cells include CD20 (b1), CD19 (B4), and CD22 (Leu14).These antigens are usually absent at the plasma cell stage. However, they are expressed in immature B cells before the acquisition of immunoglobulin on the cell membrane.[101,102] The so-called common acute lymphoblastic leukemia antigen (cALLa) (CD10) was initially described on tumor cells from approximately 70% of patients with acute lymphoblastic leukemia (ALL).[103] Such leukemias lacked markers of mature T or B lymphocytes and were termed non-T, non-B, or common acute lymphoblastic leukemias (cALL). Subsequent studies capable of identifying immunoglobulin gene rearrangement have shown that these cells are, in fact, committed to B-cell differentiation, although they lack surface or cytoplasmic immunoglobulin.[104] Although it was initially postulated that this antigen might be tumor specific, subsequent studies showed that cALLa was present on normal B-cell precursor cells in the bone marrow. Further studies have shown that this antigen is expressed on many B-cell malignancies, including Burkitt's lymphoma and most follicular lymphomas.[99,105] Although normal peripheral blood B cells do not stain with J5, this antibody will stain follicular center cells when sensitive techniques are used.[106] Further studies have shown that not only is CD10 not tumor specific, but it is also not lineage specific. It stains neoplastic cells from a small percentage (10%–20%) of cases of T-cell lymphoblastic lymphoma and leukemia.[94,105] It is present at a low density on normal peripheral blood polymorphonuclear leukocytes as well.[107]

Most monoclonal antibodies reactive with monocytes and macrophages also react with cells of the granulocytic series. Included in this category are the monoclonal antibodies to CD11 and CD15.[108–110] Antibodies with greater specificity for the monocyte–macrophage fraction include the CD14 group, but these stain many B cells as well.[111]

Several monoclonal antibodies are available that detect the so-called common leukocyte antigen (CD45).[86,87] This antigen is expressed on all normal lymphoreticular cells. Although these antibodies are not useful in the subclassification of lymphoreticular malignancies, they are useful in the differentiation of malignant lymphomas from nonlymphoid neoplasms such as carcinomas and sarcomas. All of these antibodies react with an antigen of approximately 200,000 daltons. However, they vary in their ability to stain paraffin-embedded or cryostat sections.

Terminal deoxynucleotidyl transferase (TdT) is a DNA polymerase that catalyzes the addition of deoxyribonucleotide triphosphate to the 3′ hydroxy end of single-stranded polydeoxyribonucleotide or oligodeoxyribonucleotide primers.[112] This enzyme is present in immature or primitive lymphoid cells of both T- and B-cell origin. The enzyme is found in low levels in normal bone marrow. Mature peripheral blood B and T lymphocytes and phytohemagglutinin-stimulated lymphocytes do not contain detectable TdT. This enzyme has been identified in the cells of nearly all patients with ALL and lymphoblastic lymphoma and in the cells of some cases of blastic crisis of chronic myelogenous leukemia, so-called lymphoblastic crisis.[113] TdT determinations may be performed on fresh or frozen tissues in cell suspension and can be identified biochemically or with antisera reactive with TdT antigenically.[114]

The demonstration of various hydrolytic enzymes by cytochemical and histochemical techniques has been useful in the identification of certain cells of the lymphoreticular system.[115] The most helpful assays are those for nonspecific esterase (NSE), acid phosphatase (AP), and tartrate-resistant phosphatase (TRAP). Diffuse activity for NSE and AP is characteristic of monocytes–macrophages, whereas antigen-presenting cells have a more punctate and localized reaction pattern. Normal T lymphocytes also display punctate reactivity for NSE (at an acid *p*H) and AP. However, some reactivity may be seen in both normal and neoplastic B lymphocytes. Thus these cytochemical markers are not reliable for the determination of immunologic phenotype of lymphoid cells. TRAP is a characteristic feature of the cells of leukemic reticuloendotheliosis (HCL).[116]

GENE REARRANGEMENT STUDIES

The technology of molecular biology has led to new methods for the detection of lineage and clonality in malignant lymphomas. In general, hematopoietic cells undergo specific rearrangements of their immunoglobulin or T-cell receptor genes, as they are committed to a particular lineage.[117-120] Thus B cells rearrange their immunoglobulin genes, whereas T cells undergo T-cell receptor rearrangement. Cells that have not initiated this process are in a germline or "undifferentiated" configuration. As a consequence, the detection of a rearrangement can be used as a tool to determine lineage.[121,122] For example, the cellular origin of HCL was long a subject of speculation because it had features suggestive of both monocytes and B cells. The demonstration of immunoglobulin light-chain gene rearrangements resolved the issue.[122] Lymphomas generally can be assigned to T- or B-cells groups by Southern analysis with probes for the T-cell receptor and immunoglobulin subunits. However, certain pitfalls have emerged. While the finding of rearranged light-chain genes appears to be diagnostic of B lineage, occasionally heavy-chain genes are rearranged in T or myeloid neoplasms[123,124] for unknown reasons. Also, the presence of rearranged T-cell receptor genes is not entirely specific for T lineage. For example, rearranged beta-chain genes have been seen in otherwise clear-cut B-cell lymphomas.[125] Also, the T gamma gene is problematic as a clonal marker, since its limited number of V regions gives rise to distinct bands on Southern analysis even in polyclonal populations.[126] Nevertheless, only hematopoietic cells rearrange these genes, and so this kind of analysis can be helpful in the differential between poorly differentiated carcinoma and lymphoma.

The sequences of DNA involved in these rearrangements are detected by the Southern blot technique. Because of the sensitivity of the method, it is a powerful tool in the detection of clonality within a lymphoid proliferation. Intact cellular DNA is isolated and cut into many small fragments by restriction enzymes that are highly specific for certain nucleotide sequences. The restriction fragments can be size-separated with agarose gel electrophoresis, and a fragment containing a particular sequence can be detected by using a radioactively labeled, cloned DNA probe that is complementary to the sequence of interest. Because of the innumerable possible rearrangements, in a population of normal, polyclonal lymphocytes no one rearrangement pattern would predominate, and a probe would label a smear of fragments of all sizes. However, the nature of the Southern method is such that if greater than 1% to 5% of the cells are of monoclonal origin, a single restriction fragment will be labeled above the background. In this way a change in a restriction fragment size from the germline can be used as a marker for a clone of cells derived from a particular lymphocyte.[100] Moreover, because each clone has a unique rearrangement pattern, Southern blot analysis is particularly useful in examining sequential specimens. If one establishes the rearrangement pattern of the primary lesion, in looking at the subsequent biopsies one can determine not only that they contain a clonal population of lymphoid cells, but whether or not the clone is identical to the original one.

Another important potential clinical use is in staging and in the detection of even small numbers of lymphomatous cells. It has been shown, for example, that clonal populations of T lymphocytes can be detected in lymph nodes from patients with MF that had been called negative for involvement by standard surgical pathology techniques.[127]

It must be borne in mind, however, that the demonstration of a clonal population of lymphocytes is not always proof of malignancy. For example, lymphomatoid papulosis is a chronic, often self-remitting illness that is limited to the skin, usually without clinical progression to malignancy, and has been shown to contain clonally rearranged T cells.[128]

Particularly in the setting of immunodeficiency, clonal populations must be viewed with caution. For example, it has been noted that patients with the Wiskott–Aldrich syndrome may develop transient serum monoclonal spikes. In one study a clonal proliferation of B cells was also identified by gene rearrangement in a lymph node from one patient.[100] However, this individual never developed a malignant lymphoproliferative disorder. EBV can immortalize B cells both in vitro and in vivo, and in the setting of immunodeficiency these clones may be expanded and identifiable by Southern blot analysis.[129] However, if immunocompetence can be restored, these clones may regress, as has been demonstrated in renal transplant recipients.[130] A second mutational event is probably required for the true malignant transformation of such expanded B-cell clones. In fact, such a sequence may indeed be involved in the pathogenesis of high-grade B-cell tumors (Burkitt's high-grade B-cell and Burkitt's-like) that occur in patients with AIDS.[131]

For these reasons one must be careful to use the information these techniques provide only with the benefit of relevant clinical information. The finding of a faint T beta gene rearrangement in a pleural effusion from a patient with a known T-cell lymphoma, in which the rearranging band matches the size of that in the previous biopsy, can be interpreted as diagnostic of the presence of lymphoma in the pleural fluid. The same finding in a patient with AIDS is of unknown significance. Moreover, as these techniques become more widely available, clinical correlation studies will need to be done. For example, it is currently unknown whether the demonstration of occult disease in lymph nodes of MF patients has any effect on prognosis, or whether it is simply a reflection of the ability of the neoplastic cells to circulate throughout the lymphoid system.

Molecular biology techniques have recently been made dramatically more sensitive at detecting very few residual tumor cells, particularly those that express chromosomal translocations for which there are probes available (*e.g.*, t(14;18) in follicular lymphoma). Using the polymerase chain reaction to amplify the sequences detected by the probe, it is now possible to reliably identify residual tumor representing only 1 cell in 100,000 in mixed-cell populations.[132] This technique is currently being used to monitor the completeness of purging of tumor cells from bone marrow in extracorporeal depletion experiments, and if carefully applied to bone marrow and lymph node aspirates, it could alter the criterion for determining complete remission (CR) in lymphoma.

Normal T- and B-Cell Development and Their Relation to Malignancy

With a combination of cell surface phenotyping, enzyme histochemistry, and Southern and Northern molecular biology techniques it is possible to roughly map the stages of differentiation of lymphoid cells and relate those stages to the phenotypes of particular lymphocytic lymphomas[133] (see Figs. 50-2 and 50-3).

T cells arise from a pluripotent stem cell by way of a lymphoid stem cell and undergo maturation in the thymus. The earliest committed T cells express surface receptors for T9 (transferrin receptor) and T10 antibodies and contain terminal transferase. These cells are located in the thymic cortex and constitute about 5% of all thymocytes. With further maturation these cells lose T9, acquire CD1, and concurrently express T10, CD4, and CD8 antigens. Such cells contain no terminal transferase but message for rearranged beta chains of the T-cell antigen receptor and CD3, the nonpolymorphic seven-chain receptor–associated molecule is detectable in the cytoplasm, but protein is not yet expressed on the cell surface. A fraction of these cells also express low-affinity IL-2 receptors. In all, such CD4- and CD8-positive cells (also called double-positive thymocytes) constitute around 80% to 85% of thymocytes and are located in the cortex. In the medulla, which makes up about 10% of the thymocyte population, the phenotype of the thymocytes is indistinguishable from peripheral mature T cells. These cells lose CD1, express CD3 and antigen receptors (mainly alpha chain–beta chain heterodimers), and lose either CD8 to become class II MHC-restricted helper T cells, or CD4 to become class I MHC-restricted cytotoxic or suppressor T cells. Throughout their maturation in the thymus, T cells express CD2 and CD7 (see Fig. 50-2).

Malignancies that arise in early or subcapsular cortical thymocytes are usually T-cell ALL. Lymphoblastic lymphomas may have the phenotype of early or common cortical thymocytes. All the other T-cell lymphomas arise from cells with mature or post-thymic phenotype. The majority of tumors that arise from mature cells bear CD4, and include ATL, MF, Sézary's syndrome (SS), angiocentric immunoproliferative lesions, most so-called peripheral T-cell lymphomas (which include diffuse large-cell, immunoblastic, and mixed lymphomas by Working Formulation terminology), and about half of the cases of T-cell CLL. A few peripheral T-cell lymphomas, about half of the cases of T-cell CLL, and some cases of T-gamma lymphoproliferative disease (also known as large granular lymphocytic leukemia and occasionally called T-cell CLL) express CD8. T-gamma lymphoproliferative disease is heterogeneous, including some CD3-positive and some CD3-negative cases. Its rarity interferes with thorough subclassification. However, even those that express CD3 have more similarity to a subset of NK cells than T cells in that they may also express OKM1, LeuM1, T10, Fc receptors, asialo-GM1, Leu7, and NKH-1. In general, those that express CD3 are associated with neutropenia and often rheumatoid arthritis and autoantibody formation, and those that do not express CD3 less frequently have neutropenia and autoimmune phenomena.[134] More complete discussion of T-CLL, T-prolymphocytic leukemia, and T-gamma lymphoproliferative disease is in Chapter 53.

Somewhat less is known about B-cell development and the role of the host in shaping it. Fewer B-cell–specific antibodies are available, so most of what is known about B-cell maturation relates to the steps of immunoglobulin gene rearrangement and expression of surface immunoglobulin. The earliest B cell expresses Ia, cALLa, and B4 on the surface and terminal transferase intracellularly, and has rearranged its heavy-chain genes. Subsequently it acquires B1 surface expression and then sequentially expresses cytoplasmic mu heavy chains, rearranges kappa light chains, rearranges lambda light chains, and loses terminal transferase. This represents the pre–B-cell stage of development. The cell becomes recognizable as an immature B cell when it loses cALLa expression and expresses surface IgM. The cell then acquires surface B2 expression and places surface IgD on the membrane as well as IgM. All subsequent steps in B-cell development are driven by exposure to antigen. After contacting antigen the immunoglobulin genes undergo a class switch and express the isotype they ultimately secrete. Then they lose B2 and then B1 and surface immunoglobulin, they acquire PC-1 and PCA-1, which are plasma cell markers, and they secrete immunoglobulin. This is the life history of follicular center B cells, those cells that most commonly give rise to lymphocytic lymphomas (see Fig. 50-3). There is another subpopulation of B cells whose relation with follicular center B cells is unclear. Many of the events in the maturation of follicular center B cells after exposure to antigen are assisted by factors produced by helper T cells. Immunoglobulin class switch is T cell mediated. However, mantle zone B cells appear to be more independent of the influence of T cells. They express CD5, a pan T-cell marker, and do not appear capable of switching to immunoglobulin isotypes other than IgM after exposure to antigen.

Most ALL originate from pre–B cells. Burkitt's lymphoma and leukemia arise from the surface IgM-positive immature B cell. Most follicular and diffuse B-cell lymphomas arise from mature or activated B cells. Waldenström's macroglobulinemia and multiple myeloma originate from cells near terminal differentiation. CLL cells express CD5, as do cells of diffuse intermediately differentiated lymphocytic lymphoma (which are also cALLa positive). This may mean that these tumors derive from mantle zone rather than follicular center B cells.

Although it is possible to phenotype malignancies of lymphocytes, the correlation of the phenotype with a histology is not complete. Diffuse large-cell lymphoma may be the most heterogeneous, including some tumors of B-cell, T-cell, and histiocytic origin. Furthermore, the clinical course of disease is not accurately predicted by the stage of developmental arrest of a particular tumor. For example, ATL is a tumor of mature, post-thymic T cells but is every bit as aggressive clinically (or perhaps more so) than lymphoblastic lymphoma, which is derived from a more immature cell. Similarly for B cells, Burkitt's leukemia is the B-cell leukemia with the poorest prognosis, yet it is derived from a maturer cell than cALL. Therefore, although phenotyping can be useful in certain ways, it does not provide information that is more valuable to the clinician than the interpretation of H&E-stained tissue examined under a light microscope by an experienced hematopathologist.

PATHOLOGY OF LYMPHOCYTIC LYMPHOMAS

The classification of neoplastic lymphoid disorders has undergone significant evolution over the past 150 years (Table 50-3).[135-147] Since the 1960s the Rappaport classification (Table 50-4) of lymphocytic lymphoma has been widely used and has probably been the most popular classification for clinicians.[145,148] The approach used by this classification first divided lymphomas by pattern, whether nodular or diffuse, and then by cytologic subtypes. Tumors were termed well differentiated lymphocytic based on the degree to which the neoplastic cells resembled normal lymphocytes.

Lymphomas composed of large cells with abundant cytoplasm were termed "histiocytic" and were thought to be derived from histiocytes or phagocytic cells. The term "undifferentiated" was used for lymphomas of intermediate cell size that failed to demonstrate evidence of either "lymphoid" or "histiocytic" origin.

Although the Rappaport classification was quite popular among clinicians, it became the subject of considerable controversy, for it was proposed at a time when relatively little was known about the normal immune system. As scientists discovered the functional and ontogenetic heterogeneity of the normal immune system, people questioned the scientific validity of the Rappaport approach. The concepts of well differentiated and poorly differentiated were inaccurate as applied in the Rappaport scheme, as was the use of the term "histiocytic" for a tumor of transformed lymphoid cells.

New classifications were proposed that attempted to address the scientific inaccuracies of the Rappaport scheme and to relate these tumors more closely to the normal immune system (Table 50-5).[149-154] For example, the classification of Lukes and Collins proposed that immunologic subtypes could be recognized by morphologic features alone.[151] Although certain features, such as follicle formation by the neoplastic cells, were found to be reliable indicators of follicular B-lymphocyte origin,[155] cytologic features were shown to be unreliable for predicting T- or B-cell phenotype in the diffuse lymphomas.[156]

The use of six different pathologic classifications for lymphocytic lymphomas throughout the world obviously makes the international analysis and comparison of clinical trials extremely difficult. A new classification system was proposed, based on an international study comparing the six major systems, as shown in Tables 50-4 and 50-5.[157] The basic approach is similar to that of the Rappaport scheme in that lymphomas are classified on the basis of pattern—follicular or diffuse—and cytologic composition. Although immunologic terminology is not used, correlations with immunologic phenotype, when established, can be drawn. It has been proposed that this formulation not be viewed as an alternative classification, but rather as a common language that might be used by all clinical investigators to translate from one classification scheme to another. This classification will be used throughout the rest of this chapter. However, an attempt will also be made to relate these tumors to the normal immune system, when this information is available.

A diagnosis of lymphocytic lymphomas in the Working Formulation is based on morphologic features only but has predictive value for survival.[158,159] Low-grade lymphomas are usually characterized by an indolent clinical course and relatively long survival with or without aggressive therapy. In contrast, the intermediate- and high-grade lymphomas have an aggressive natural history with short survival unless treated vigorously.[160] In low-grade lymphocytic lymphoma, involvement is usually found at sites where the normal counterparts of these lymphocytic lymphoma cells are located.[161]

TABLE 50-3. Landmarks in the Description of the Lymphocytic Lymphomas

Author	*Year*	*Observation*
Craigie[135] Bennett[136] Virchow[137]	1845	Described the first cases of leukemia
Virchow[137]	1845	Distinguished lymphosarcoma from leukemia. Included cases described by Hodgkin in the lymphosarcoma group
Bilroth[138]	1871	Coined phrase "malignant lymphomas"
Dreschfeld[139] Kundradt[140]	1892	Developed histologic criteria for diagnosing lymphosarcoma
Brill, Baehr, Rosenthal et al[141] Symmers[142]	1925	Described giant follicular lymphoma and considered it a benign disease ("Brill–Symmers disease")
Roulet[143]	1930	Developed histologic criteria for diagnosing reticulum cell sarcoma. Considered it a malignancy of the supporting cells of the lymph node
Gall, Mallory[144]	1942	Developed criteria for distinguishing benign hyperplasia from malignant follicular lymphoma
Rappaport et al[145]	1956	Described different cell types within follicular lymphomas and termed them "nodular lymphomas"
Burkitt[146]	1958	Described lymphoma of the jaw in Africa, which bears his name
Uchiyama et al[147]	1977	Described adult T-cell leukemia/lymphoma, later shown to be associated with HTLV-I

TABLE 50-4. A Working Formulation of Lymphocytic Lymphoma for Clinical Use: Recommendations of an Expert International Panel and Comparisons to the Rappaport Scheme

Working Formulation	*Rappaport Terminology*
Low Grade	
A. Malignant lymphoma Small lymphocytic Consistent with chronic lymphocytic leukemia Plasmacytoid	Diffuse well-differentiated lymphocytic
B. Malignant lymphoma, follicular, predominantly small cleaved cell Diffuse areas Sclerosis	Nodular poorly differentiated lymphocytic
C. Malignant lymphoma, follicular mixed, small cleaved and large cell Diffuse areas Sclerosis	Nodular mixed lymphocytic histiocytic
Intermediate Grade	
D. Malignant lymphoma, follicular Predominantly large cell Diffuse areas Sclerosis	Nodular histiocytic
E. Malignant lymphoma, diffuse small cleaved cell	Diffuse poorly differentiated lymphocytic
F. Malignant lymphoma, diffuse mixed, small- and large-cell sclerosis Epithelioid cell component	Diffuse mixed lymphocytic–histiocytic
G. Malignant lymphoma, diffuse Large-cell Cleaved cell Noncleaved cell Sclerosis	Diffuse histiocytic
High Grade	
H. Malignant lymphoma large cell, immunoblastic Plasmacytoid Clear cell Polymorphous Epithelioid cell component	Diffuse histiocytic
I. Malignant lymphoma lymphoblastic Convoluted cell Nonconvoluted cell	Diffuse lymphoblastic
J. Malignant lymphoma small noncleaved cell Burkitt's Follicular areas	Diffuse undifferentiated

For example, follicular lymphomas are derived from follicular B lymphocytes and demonstrate a striking capacity to home to B-cell–dependent portions of the lymphoid system and have a nondestructive growth pattern.[73] The cells readily circulate or disseminate, and patients with this type of lymphocytic lymphoma usually have Stage III or IV disease. However, privileged sites such as testis or CNS are rarely involved by these tumors. Cytologic atypia or anaplasia also is not typical of low-grade lymphocytic lymphoma. Follicular lymphomas may respond to normal immunoregulation, in contrast to the high-grade lymphomas, which are consistently autonomous.[162,163] Patients with follicular lymphoma may have a history of lymph nodes that wax and wane in size, often for many years before diagnosis.[164] Host immunity has been invoked to explain this phenomenon, and in some cases the clinical regression has been preceded by bacterial or viral infection. In contrast, the intermediate- or high-grade lymphomas usually have an aggressive and unrelenting natural history. Extranodal sites and privileged sites are more frequently involved, and B symptoms are more common.

A further complication in the classification of lymphocytic lymphoma is that a significant fraction of patients with lymphocytic lymphoma have divergent histologies in the same or different biopsy sites, up to 33% in some series.[165,166] Commonly one observes a follicular pattern in one site and diffuse pattern in another; in such cases survival is reported to be intermediate between the two.[166] Histologic progression from a low grade to a higher grade during the clinical course is also common in B-cell lymphomas. At the National Institutes of Health (NIH) 37% of patients with a follicular pattern of lymphocytic lymphoma had progression to a diffuse pattern when rebiopsied (greater than 3 months) after initial staging.[167] With modern therapy, eradication of the

TABLE 50-5. Comparison of Commonly Used Classifications for the Lymphocytic Lymphomas

Modified Rappaport Classification (1966)[149,150]		*Lukes and Collins Classification (1974)*[151]		*Kiel Classification (1974)*[152,153]	
Nodular		Undefined cell type		Low-grade malignancy	
Lymphocytic, well differentiated	A*	T-cell type, small lymphocytic	A	Lymphocytic, chronic lymphocytic/leukemia	A
Lymphocytic, poorly differentiated	B	T-cell type, Sézary–mycosis fungoides (cerebriform)		Lymphocytic, other	A
Mixed, lymphocytic and histiocytic	C	T-cell type, convoluted lymphocytic	I	Lymphoplasmacytoid	A
Histiocytic	D	T-cell type, immunoblastic sarcoma (T-cell)	H	Centrocytic	E
Diffuse		B-cell type, small lymphocytic	A	Centroblastic-centrocytic, follicular without sclerosis	B,C,D
Lymphocytic, well differentiated with plasmacytoid features	A	B-cell type, plasmacytoid lymphocytic	A	Centroblastic-centrocytic, follicular with sclerosis	
Lymphocytic, well differentiated with plasmacytoid features	A	Follicular center cell, small cleaved	B-E	Centroblastic-centrocytic, follicular and diffuse, without sclerosis	
Lymphocytic, poorly differentiated	E	Follicular center cell, large cleaved	D-G	Centroblastic-centrocytic, follicular and diffuse, with sclerosis	
Lymphoblastic, convoluted	I	Follicular center cell, small noncleaved	J	Centroblastic-centrocytic, diffuse	F
Lymphoblastic, nonconvoluted	I	Follicular center cell, large noncleaved	D-G	Low-grade malignant lymphoma, unclassified	
Mixed, lymphocytic and histiocytic	F	Immunoblastic sarcoma (B-cell)		High-grade malignancy	
Histiocytic without sclerosis	G	Subtypes of follicular center cell lymphomas	H	Centroblastic	G
Histiocytic with sclerosis	G	1. Follicular		Lymphoblastic, Burkitt's type	J
Burkitt's tumor	J	2. Follicular and diffuse		Lymphoblastic, convoluted cell type	I
Undifferentiated	J	3. Diffuse		Lymphoblastic, other (unclassified) immunoblastic	H
Malignant lymphoma, unclassified		4. Sclerotic with follicles		High-grade malignant lymphoma, unclassified	
Composite lymphoma		5. Sclerotic without follicles		Malignant lymphoma, unclassified (unable to specify "high grade" or "low grade")	
		Histiocytic		Composite lymphoma	
		Malignant lymphoma, unclassified			

*Letters indicate equivalent or related category in the Working Formulation as shown in Table 50-3.

diffuse aggressive component with only the residual low-grade follicular component remaining is now seen. The term "composite lymphoma" has been used to describe various cases with more than one histologic type; a strict definition of composite lymphoma is a lymphoma consisting of the two distinctly different and well-delineated varieties of lymphoma occurring in a single anatomical site or mass.[168] However, most so-called composite lymphomas represent not two distinct tumors but different manifestations of the same clonal proliferation. However, rarely are true composite lymphomas identified, such as the coexistence of Hodgkin's disease and lymphocytic lymphomas in a single site.

MALIGNANT LYMPHOMA, SMALL LYMPHOCYTIC (DIFFUSE WELL DIFFERENTIATED LYMPHOCYTIC)

Diffuse small lymphocytic lymphoma composed of well-differentiated small lymphocytes is the solid tumor counterpart of CLL.[169] If patients with usual peripheral blood manifestations of CLL are excluded, these neoplasms constitute approximately 5% of all lymphocytic lymphomas. The patients, even when aleukemic or subleukemic, often have focal involvement of the bone marrow, liver, and other visceral sites at presentation and usually generalized asymptomatic lymphadenopathy.[73,170] With time, the natural history of this disease seems to be progression to CLL. In the vast majority of patients the malignant cells are monoclonal B lymphocytes and, as in CLL, the neoplastic cells express the p65 membrane protein CD5.[99,171] These neoplastic cells, like normal medullary cord B lymphocytes, may exhibit some functional differentiation toward plasma cells and can be readily induced to secrete monoclonal immunoglobulin after exposure to the phorbol ester 12-*0*-tetradecanoylphorbol-13-acetate.[172] The monoclonal protein expressed on the cell surface and synthesized in the vast majority of cases is IgM, with the light-chain type being kappa more often than lambda.

The disorder known as *Waldenström's macroglobulinemia* can be most readily viewed as a form of small lymphocytic neoplasia with immunoglobulin secretion as its sine qua non (see Chap. 54).[173,174] The cells spontaneously secrete immunoglobulin, resulting in a monoclonal IgM serum spike. Such cases represent approximately 15% of all small lymphocytic lymphomas. Morphologically, the cells usually demonstrate plasmacytoid features, often exhibiting a spectrum, even within a single patient. In contrast to CLL and small lymphocytic lymphomas without plasmacytoid differentiation, the cells are CD5 negative. Clinically, the disease also presents a spectrum from CLL-like features to a form characterized predominantly by lymphadenopathy and hepatosplenomegaly. Heavy-chain diseases corresponding to the three most plentiful classes of immunoglobulins are discussed in the chapter on plasma cell neoplasms.

Small lymphocytic lymphomas may contain moderate numbers of larger cells or prolymphocytes, which may accumulate in growth centers, sometimes imparting a pseudofollicular appearance at low power.[169] If the mitotic rate is not greater than 30 mitoses/20 high-powered field, the prognosis is not adversely affected.[175] However, emergence of a monomorphic proliferation of the larger lymphoid cells indicates progression to a diffuse large-cell lymphoma, so-called Richter's syndrome.[176] This transformation occurs in approximately 1% of patients, but a larger proportion of patients undergo a gradual acceleration in the clinical course of their disease over time. Immunologic studies have now shown that these large cells bear the same surface determinants as the small lymphoid cells of the original disease.[177]

FOLLICULAR (NODULAR) LYMPHOMAS

Follicular lymphomas are those in which the neoplastic cells form circumscribed aggregates that morphologically resemble germinal centers (Fig. 50-4).[178] The nodular pattern may be present throughout the tumor, or it may be manifested only in a portion of the lymphoma that elsewhere is composed of diffuse cellular proliferation.[165,179] Follicular lymphoma can be distinguished from reactive follicular hyperplasia by the total effacement of lymph node architecture by nodular proliferation. The nodules vary little in size and shape and are crowded together with little intervening normal lymphoid parenchyma. They also lack well-defined lymphoid cuffs. In areas of the nodules the neoplastic cells may be either confined to the nodules with normal-appearing cells in the internodular tissue, or present between the nodules as well. In the former situation these neoplasms may be mistaken for benign follicular hyperplasia unless careful scrutiny is given to the cells composing the nodules. Whereas normal germinal centers are composed of cytologically heterogeneous populations representing the entire spectrum of proliferating B cells, neoplastic nodules appear more homogeneous and "clonal." Other useful differential features include polarization and the presence of a "starry sky" in reactive germinal centers but not in follicular lymphomas. It has now been proved that nodular lymphomas are neoplasms of follicular B cells.[155,180]

FIG. 50-4. Effacement of architecture by monotonous nodularity in follicular lymphoma. Compare to predominantly cortical location of follicles in normal lymph node shown in Figure 50-1. (H&E; magnification ×10).

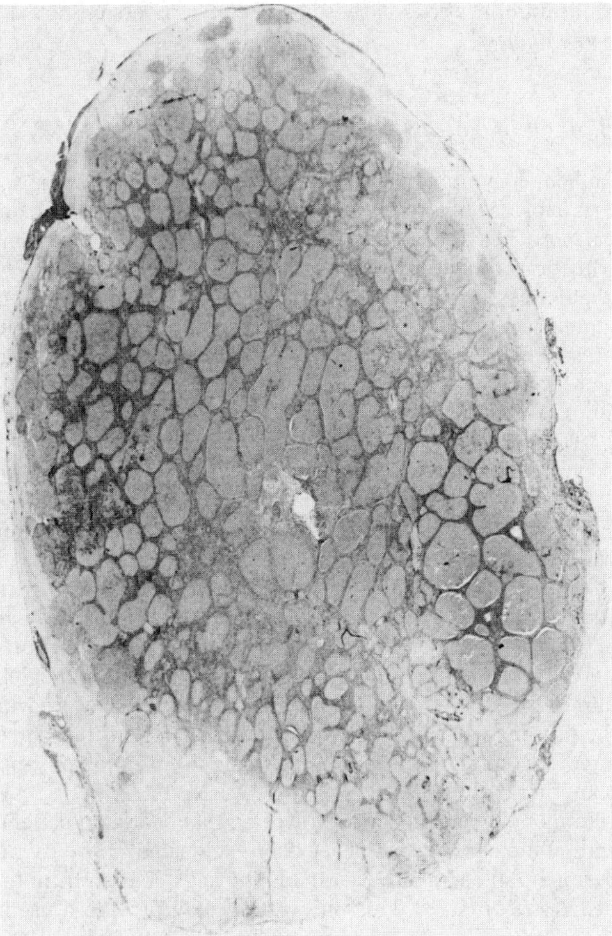

Using the Working Formulation, the cells of follicular lymphomas can be either predominantly small cleaved cells (poorly differentiated lymphocytic), large noncleaved or large cleaved cells (histiocytic), or a mixture of cell types, mixed small cleaved and large cell (mixed lymphocytic–histiocytic). The larger cells appear to be the replicative component of the process wherein the smaller lymphoid cells are relatively indolent but perhaps more motile. These observations also shed light on the clinical behavior of these lymphomas.

Malignant Lymphoma, Follicular, Predominantly Small Cleaved Cell Lymphoma

In this most common type of follicular lymphoma, accounting for approximately 60% of cases, the vast majority of neoplastic cells are small cleaved, indented lymphocytes with only occasional large cells (Fig. 50-5). Mitotic figures are few. Recent studies have demonstrated that monoclonal populations of lymphocytes, identical to those found in lymph nodes involved with tumor, are present in the peripheral blood of many patients with follicular lymphomas who do not otherwise have morphologic evidence of leukemia.[181] When leukemia does appear the lymphoid cells in the peripheral blood exhibit notches in the nucleus ("buttock cells" to some hematologists). The process has been referred to as lymphosarcoma cell leukemia.[182] This term, however, should be avoided because it has been used with biologically and clinically diverse malignant lymphomas that happen to have a leukemic phase.

Malignant Lymphoma, Follicular, Mixed Small Cleaved and Large Cell (Nodular Mixed Lymphoma)

In this form of follicular lymphoma, representing approximately 30% of cases, the large nucleolated cells are more abundant, numbering more than five per high-powered field

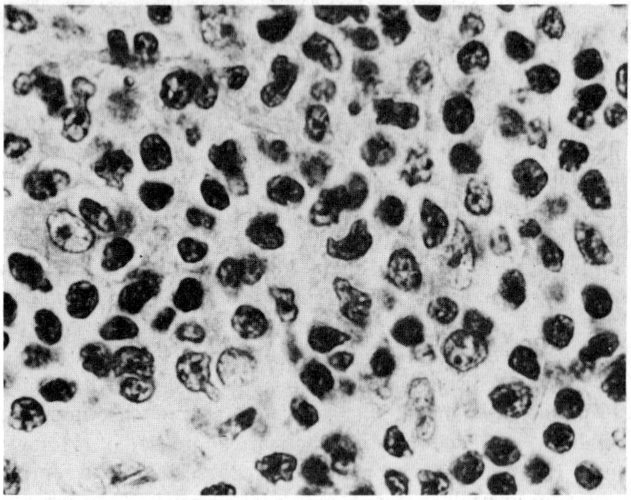

FIG. 50-5. Follicular lymphoma, predominantly small cleaved cell. Atypical lymphocytes are indented and angular. (H&E; magnification ×1000)

and, in some cases, appearing to be admixed in almost equal numbers with smaller lymphoid cells.[183] As with most follicular lymphomas, patients usually have easily detectable disseminated disease at presentation, but it is not uncommon to find only the smaller cleaved lymphoid cells in sites distant from the nodes of origin such as liver or bone marrow. In bone marrow the characteristic paratrabecular location of the lymphoid infiltrates is useful in distinguishing involvement by follicular lymphoma from normal lymphoid nodules that are usually within the marrow space and perivascular in location. This observation underscores the belief that the smaller cells are the migratory component of the normal and malignant lymphoid system and the large cells are the replicative forms.

Malignant Lymphoma, Follicular, Predominantly Large Cell (Nodular Histiocytic Lymphoma)

This is the least common form of nodular lymphomas and accounts for only 10% of cases.[184] The motile small lymphoid cells, seen in appreciable numbers in the other nodular lymphomas, are few in these tumors, and the patients often appear to have localized tumors. Despite their earlier clinical stage at diagnosis, they nevertheless have had, until recently, the least favorable prognosis of all nodular lymphomas because their localized appearance is deceptive and frequent recurrences and progression to diffuse large-cell tumors occur.

Variations in Pattern and Cytology of Follicular Lymphomas

In many cases of follicular lymphoma the nodular growth pattern will be seen in only part of the lesion, and the clinical consequences of a diffuse component vary considerably, depending on the cytologic composition of the tumor.[185] In lymphomas composed predominantly of small cleaved cells, the presence of even a major diffuse component does not adversely affect prognosis.[179] However, in follicular lymphomas of the mixed small cleaved and large-cell type, if the diffuse phase exceeds 50% of the lesion, the tumor appears to behave in a more aggressive manner. In follicular lymphomas composed predominantly of large cells, even if the diffuse component is only focal, the prognosis deteriorates and approximates that of the diffuse aggressive lymphomas.[184]

Variations in histologic composition can be seen not only in a single lymph node, but, as might be expected, in different anatomical sites at the same point in time. Up to one-third of patients with lymphocytic lymphoma who undergo staging laparotomy will exhibit some histologic discordance in different sites.[186,187] Usually these differences are minor, such as follicular, small cleaved and follicular, and mixed small cleaved and large cell, and do not imply a differing prognosis. However, in some cases major histologic discrepancies can be seen, such as follicular, mixed small cleaved and large cell, and diffuse large cell. In such cases treatment should be based on the most aggressive histologic subtype encountered.

The natural history of follicular lymphomas results in progression in time from a follicular to a diffuse growth pattern, as well as a cytologic shift from small, relatively slowly proliferating cells to large, more rapidly proliferating cells. The clinical implications of these histologic progressions are discussed below.

Biology of Follicular Lymphomas

Follicular lymphomas are monoclonal B-cell lymphomas that express only a single light chain, usually kappa, with one or more heavy-chain determinants, most commonly IgM, with or without IgD.[180,188] IgG is the predominant heavy-chain class in less than half the cases. The cells are intimately associated with dendritic reticulum cells, and the presence of dendritic reticulum cells correlates with a follicular growth pattern.[189] The cells express the B-cell antigens CD19, CD20, and CD22. They also usually express cALLa or CD10. In contrast with the small lymphocytic malignancies, they are consistently CD5 negative.[99]

Suspensions prepared from follicular lymphomas may contain 50% or more T lymphocytes, and these cells are within as well as between the neoplastic nodules.[190] The T cells are phenotypically normal with a normal lymph node CD4–CD8 ratio, and there is no evidence that they are part of the neoplastic proliferation. However, they are not functionally inert and retain a capacity to modulate immunoglobulin synthesis by the neoplastic B lymphocytes.[191] Moreover, the presence of numerous T cells in these lesions has correlated with the likelihood of responding to anti-idiotypic antibody therapy.[192]

Immunologic studies have revealed that nearly all patients with follicular lymphomas exhibit "clonal excess" in the peripheral blood and have circulating cells derived from the neoplastic clone.[181] This observation may provide a useful parameter to follow to determine response to treatment as well as for early detection of recurrence. It also implies that truly localized disease in follicular lymphomas is extremely unlikely because of the propensity of the malignant cells to circulate and home.

Cytogenetically, most follicular lymphomas carry the t14;18 chromosomal translocation.[193] The translocation involves the Ig heavy-chains locus on chromosome 14 and a putative new oncogene, *bc1*-2, on chromosome 19.[194] Using molecular probes to *bc1*-2, the translocation can be identified in nearly 100% of cases. The translocation is also found in approximately one-third of diffuse large-cell lymphomas, suggesting that many of these tumors that present with a diffuse growth pattern may be pathogenetically related to follicular lymphomas.[195] The translocation is not found in other low-grade B-cell neoplasms.

Malignant Lymphoma, Diffuse, Small Cleaved Cell Type (Malignant Lymphoma, Poorly Differentiated Lymphocytic, Diffuse)

Diffuse small cleaved cell lymphomas are composed of lymphoid cells that are cytologically similar to the small cleaved lymphocytes of follicular lymphomas. However, in most cases this neoplasm is not simply a consequence of progression to a diffuse growth pattern in a follicular lymphoma. Most cases represent a B-cell lymphoma, initially termed lymphocytic lymphoma of intermediate differentiation[196,197] or mantle zone lymphoma.[198] This tumor is equivalent to diffuse centrocytic lymphoma in the Kiel classification.[199] This lesion seems somewhat more common in southern Europe than in the United States. The clinical behavior is heterogeneous, and clinical aggressiveness correlates with the mitotic rate.[197] Like the low-grade lymphomas, patients usually present with disseminated disease and are in the middle-aged or older-aged groups. A male predominance is usually seen. Despite some heterogeneity in the clinical behavior, unlike most aggressive lymphomas, sustained CR is not seen.[200]

The term "intermediate" had been used to reflect that cytologically, these tumors seemed intermediate between the small lymphocytic and small cleaved lymphomas. In some cases there was an admixture of small round and small cleaved lymphocytes. The growth pattern is diffuse or vaguely nodular. The term "mantle zone lymphoma" stems from the observation that residual naked, normal-appearing germinal centers are often seen, and it has been postulated that the tumor is derived from the cells of the follicular lymphoid cuff or mantle zone.[201]

Immunologically, these are monoclonal B-cell tumors that more often express lambda than kappa, in contrast to most other B-cell neoplasms.[200] Like small lymphocytic neoplasms, the cells are usually CD5 positive but often share with follicular lymphoma the expression of CD10.[99] Phenotypically, mantle zone lymphomas and diffuse centrocytic lymphomas are identical. Correlating with the vaguely nodular growth pattern, a residual meshwork of dendritic reticulum cells may be seen.[189]

TABLE 50-6. Diffuse Aggressive Lymphocytic Lymphomas

Working Formulation	*Rappaport Classification*
Mixed small and large cell	Mixed lymphocytic "histiocytic"
Large cell	"Histiocytic"
Large cell, immunoblastic	"Histiocytic"
Small, noncleaved, non-Burkitt's	Undifferentiated, non-Burkitt's

DIFFUSE AGGRESSIVE LYMPHOMAS

For clinical purposes these lymphomas can be thought of as a group in that they share a common clinical presentation and natural history. They include several subtypes in both the Working Formulation and the Rappaport classification, all of which are diffuse (Table 50-6). They are most common in adults but occur in all age groups and present in both nodal (65%) and extranodal (35%) sites. These tumors tend to disseminate rapidly and, in contrast to the low-grade lymphomas, will involve privileged sites such as the CNS. They also have a destructive growth pattern, and regardless of the immunologic phenotype, one less often sees the selective involvement of T-cell–dependent or B-cell–dependent zones.[161] Their prognosis is distinctly unfavorable unless modern intensive chemotherapeutic regimens can induce a sustained CR.[160] If a CR is attained and maintained beyond 2 years, the likelihood of being cured is high, in contrast to the low-grade lymphomas, which have a continuous relapse rate over time.

Immunologically, these lymphomas are heterogeneous and are composed of morphologically transformed B (85%) and T (15%) lymphocytes. In less than 5% of cases can true histiocytic markers be demonstrated. Immunophenotypic studies of these high-grade lymphomas are often rendered difficult in that only a minority of cells may express markers of cellular differentiation, the cells may exhibit an abnormal phenotype, or, owing to a high metabolic rate, tumor cell viability and recovery may be low. Therefore, using only limited studies, a large proportion of these tumors may appear to be "null," lacking markers of T or B lymphocytes. However, using a large battery of techniques, including Southern blotting for immunoglobulin gene rearrangement and T-cell receptor rearrangement, the cellular origin can be identified in more than 95% of cases.[202]

Both morphologic and immunologic studies have attempted to derive clinically and prognostically useful subclassifications of these high-grade lymphomas. Morphologically, most studies have shown that most diffuse lymphomas composed of follicular center cells (*i.e.*, mixed small cleaved and large-cell, large cleaved, and large noncleaved) have a somewhat better prognosis than other diffuse aggressive lymphomas.[157] However, these differences have not always achieved statistical significance and should not be interpreted to imply that less than intensive chemotherapy is required for these clinically aggressive lymphomas.[203] Reproducibility of these fine morphologic distinctions among different observers or even by the same observer is another problem in developing useful subclassification schemes. Likewise, although immunologic studies have been useful in illustrating the heterogeneity of this group of tumors, immunologic phenotype has not yet proved useful in delineating distinctive clinical and prognostic subtypes.[202]

Malignant Lymphoma, Diffuse, Mixed Small- and Large-Cell (Malignant Lymphoma, Diffuse, Mixed Lymphocytic–"Histiocytic")

In approximately 65% of cases the neoplastic cells of diffuse mixed lymphomas are cytologically identical to those of follicular mixed lymphomas, and it is likely that the tumors are diffuse outgrowths of formerly follicular proliferations. B-cell markers, similar to those found on the cells of follicular lymphomas, may be demonstrable on the cells of these diffuse tumors, and the term "histiocytic" is again a misnomer for the large nucleolated transformed B cell. Adequate biopsy sampling may even reveal focal residual nodularity. Using immunohistochemical studies of frozen sections, many of these tumors are seen to be composed of large monoclonal B cells and admixed phenotypically normal T cells.[204] The T-cell component is believed to represent a host response comparable to that seen in many follicular lymphomas. In extranodal sites, particularly in the retroperitoneum and mesentery, these follicular center cell lymphomas may be associated with extensive sclerosis. These patients have an age distribution similar to those with nodular lymphomas, and the disease is often of advanced clinical stage at the time of diagnosis, with occult disease in the liver, bone marrow, and extranodal sites. However, the natural history of these diffuse lymphomas is more aggressive, and potential for cure exists with appropriate therapy.

In some diffuse lymphomas of mixed cell type (approximately 35%) the cells do not resemble those of nodular lymphomas but appear instead to be a pleomorphic mixture of large and small atypical lymphoid cells. The small cells are atypical but distinctively lymphoid, whereas the larger cells have prominent central nuclei and abundant cytoplasm. An inflammatory background composed of epithelioid histiocytes, plasma cells, and eosinophils may be present. Binucleated forms of large atypical cells may simulate Reed–Sternberg cells, and these cases may be misdiagnosed as Hodgkin's disease, if the fact that the small lymphoid cells also have neoplastic appearance, in contrast to Hodgkin's disease, is not recognized. In the majority of such cases studied the malignant cells have been shown to bear markers of mature or "peripheral" T lymphocytes.[205,206] Cases in which the epithelioid component is very conspicuous have been termed "lymphoepithelioid cell lymphomas" or "Lennert's lymphoma" because Lennert first described these tumors and postulated that they might be related to Hodgkin's disease.[207–209] With time, the epithelioid cell component, which is non-neoplastic, is lost and the tumor may progress to one predominantly composed of the large nucleolated cells, so-called large-cell immunoblastic lymphoma. In contrast to Hodgkin's disease, these peripheral T-cell lymphomas occur in middle-aged or elderly individuals and often present with disseminated disease.[91,210] Clinically, they should be approached as other diffuse aggressive lymphocytic lymphomas.

Malignant Lymphoma, Diffuse, Large-Cell (Diffuse Histiocytic Lymphoma)

This category represents one of the two subtypes in the Working Formulation derived from diffuse "histiocytic" lymphoma of Rappaport. These lymphomas are composed of large lymphoid cells with nuclear diameters greater than those of admixed "starry sky" histiocytes. The cells may have cytologic features of either *large noncleaved* or *large cleaved* follicular center cells. In the noncleaved variant (Fig. 50-6) the nuclei are vesicular with reticulated chromatin and two to three distinct nucleoli, often apposed to the nuclear membrane. The cytoplasm is abundant and slightly amphophilic. The cells of the large cleaved variant have finely dispersed nuclear chromatin, inconspicuous and basophilic nucleoli, and sparse eosinophilic cytoplasm. Sclerosis is frequent in the large cleaved cell variant. Mitoses are usually readily identified in both subtypes. As one might expect, given the follicular center cell characteristics, the vast majority of cases are of B-cell origin.[202] In some cases a lymphoma with a follicular pattern can be identified in another anatomical site, and biopsies obtained for staging may indicate other evidence of an underlying follicular lymphoma, such as paratrabecular small cleaved or mixed lymphoid infiltrates in the bone marrow. Cases with this morphology may carry the t14;18 translocation, further supporting a relation to follicular lymphoma.[211]

Malignant Lymphoma, Diffuse, Large-Cell, Immunoblastic (Diffuse Histiocytic Lymphoma)

This category is composed of all diffuse histiocytic lymphomas in the Rappaport scheme that do not have the cytologic features of large follicular center cells. Various subtypes are described in the Working Formulation.[157] These are all high-grade neoplasms and commonly exhibit a high mitotic rate. The *plasmacytoid* subtype is composed of large pleomorphic cells with abundant, deeply amphophilic and pyroninophilic cytoplasm. The cells appear morphologically plasmacytoid and exhibit eccentric nuclei and prominent central nucleoli. The *clear cell* subtype is composed of cells with abundant, optically clear cytoplasm and distinct nuclear membranes. The *polymorphous* category was proposed to include those lymphomas composed of a pleomorphic population of large lymphoid cells, reflecting the morphologic diversity of T-cell lymphomas described in Japan and elsewhere. The term "epithelioid" is used to refer to those large-cell lymphomas with a high content of epithelioid histiocytes and represents part of the spectrum of Lennert's lymphomas or lymphoepithelioid cell lymphomas. Similar tumors with a more mixed lymphoid composition are also included in the diffuse, mixed small- and large-cell category.

The correlation between morphologic appearance and immunologic subtype is less predictable in these high-grade

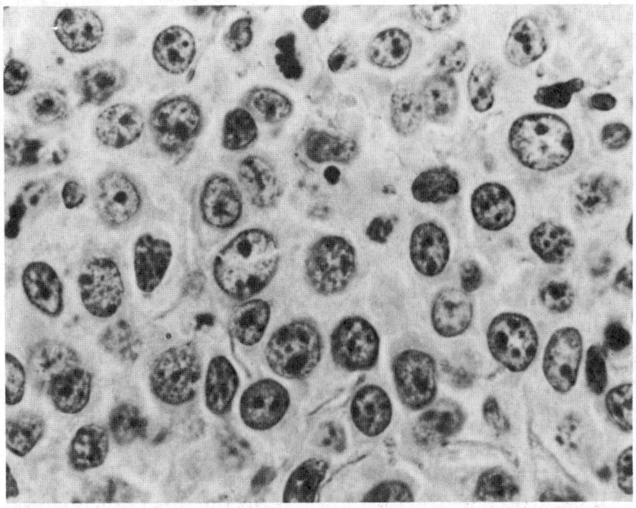

FIG. 50-6. Malignant lymphoma, diffuse, large cell type. Cells resemble large noncleaved follicular center cells and have multiple, prominent, often membrane-bound nucleoli. (H&E; magnification ×1000)

neoplasms. Although one might assume that plasmacytoid features would be indicative of a B-cell phenotype, T-cell lymphomas with plasmacytoid features have been described.[156,212] Similarly, the features of the clear cell, polymorphous, and epithelioid subtypes of immunoblastic lymphomas have been most often associated with lymphomas of T-cell origin but can also be encountered in B-cell neoplasms. Moreover, no clinical significance could be demonstrated for these subtypes of large-cell immunoblastic lymphoma. Thus the use of these additional descriptive terms is optional.

A variant of immunoblastic lymphoma has recently been described that is characterized by the propensity of the malignant cells to invade lymphoid sinuses.[213] Because of the sinusoidal location of the tumor cells, misdiagnosis as malignant histiocytosis or metastatic carcinoma is common. In most cases studied the malignant cells express some T-cell antigens, although the cells have a markedly aberrant phenotype. T-cell gene rearrangement has also been shown in some instances. A consistent feature is the expression of the Hodgkin's disease–associated antigen CD30 detected by Ki-1 and Hefi-1 (see Chap. 49).[213,214] This antigen, although present on the malignant cells of Hodgkin's disease, is also found in activated T and B lymphocytes. This tumor commonly can present in all age groups but appears relatively common in children and young adults.[214] A high incidence of cutaneous disease has been reported.

Malignant Lymphoma, Lymphoblastic (Diffuse Lymphoblastic Lymphoma)

This form of lymphocytic lymphoma is most common in adolescents and young adults and demonstrates a marked male preponderance.[215,216] The neoplastic cells appear blastic with finely distributed nuclear chromatin, small nucleoli, scant cytoplasm, and numerous mitotic figures. The nuclei in some cases are round to oval, whereas in others a variable percentage have nuclei with marked lobulations and convolutions. Many of these patients have mediastinal masses, and a relation to the thymus gland was suggested on clinical grounds long before the discovery of T- and B-cell systems.[217] Progression to ALL is a frequent phenomenon in these patients. The enzyme TdT is a ubiquitous feature of all lymphoblastic malignancies and has been demonstrable in virtually all cases studied.[114] The cells from 85% of cases have T-cell surface markers and share many characteristics with the cells of the 20% to 30% of ALL cases considered the T-cell type (T-ALL).[94] However, most lymphoblastic lymphoma cases have a slightly more differentiated phenotype than seen in T-ALL (see Fig. 50-2) (see Chap. 48). Clinically and cytologically, these neoplasms are closely related as well. Even in those patients who present with solid tissue involvement, a careful workup will often reveal occult marrow involvement. There is also a high risk of infiltration of the leptomeninges, with neoplastic cells demonstrable in the cerebrospinal fluid (CSF). The CSF is a common site of relapse, as in T-ALL, and should be treated prophylactically. Although the disease may appear circumscribed at the time of diagnosis, progression to systemic disease is such a common feature that these patients are now treated in most centers with regimens similar to those used for T-ALL. This approach has significantly improved the prognosis for this high-grade tumor.

In up to 10% of cases the neoplastic cells demonstrate a phenotype similar to that of common ALL or pre–B-cell ALL and are immature lymphoid cells committed to the B-cell lineage.[94] Morphologically, such cases are indistinguishable from the more frequent T-cell lymphoblastic lymphomas. Clinical differences, however, have been observed in that these patients usually do not present with mediastinal disease, and isolated lytic bone lesions have been reported in a number of instances.[94]

Malignant Lymphoma, Small Noncleaved Cell (Diffuse, Undifferentiated, Burkitt's and Non-Burkitt's)

Small noncleaved cell lymphomas are high-grade neoplasms with a high growth fraction and include both *Burkitt's* and *non-Burkitt's* subtypes. Cytologically, these tumors are composed of cells that resemble small noncleaved follicular center cells. Burkitt's lymphoma is characterized by uniform cells of moderate size (15–25 mu) with round to oval nuclei, coarsely reticulated chromatin, and two to five prominent basophilic nucleoli.[218] Each cell possesses a distinct rim of amphophilic and intensely pyroninophilic cytoplasm with the methyl green pyronine stain. Mitoses are numerous, and a "starry sky" pattern is characteristic but not pathognomonic, as it can be encountered in any rapidly proliferating lymphoma. The growth pattern is usually diffuse, but selective involvement of germinal centers can be seen, further supporting a relationship to the B-cell system.[219]

All cases of Burkitt's lymphoma have demonstrated B-cell markers. The cells usually express a mu heavy chain with a single light-chain type. The CD10 antigen is almost invariably present.[105] The presence of C3d receptors varies and correlates with the presence or absence of EBV genome.[220] Endemic Burkitt's lymphomas, which are usually genome positive, express C3d receptors, whereas 85% of nonendemic cases are EBV- and C3d-receptor negative. Burkitt's lymphoma exhibits chromosomal abnormalities involving chromosome 8 and chromosomes 14, 2, and 22 that result in the juxtaposition of the c-*myc* oncogene with the immunoglobulin genes, translocations that may be crucial for the malignant transformation observed.[221,222] The c-*myc* gene is constitutively expressed in Burkitt's lymphoma. The morphologic features of endemic and nonendemic Burkitt's lymphoma are identical. The endemic cases present at a lower median age (7 years) than nonendemic cases (11 years) and more often present in face and jaw bones. An intra-abdominal mass involving the ileocecal region or ovaries is the most common clinical presentation for nonendemic cases. Other extranodal sites frequently involved include kidney, testis, thyroid, and distal long bones. The staging scheme used for Burkitt's lymphoma differs from that used for the other lymphocytic lymphomas. It relates prognosis, in general, to overall tumor burden as well as bone marrow involvement (see Chap. 48). As a high-grade lymphoma with a high growth fraction, Burkitt's lymphoma is potentially curable with appropriate combination chemotherapy.[223]

Small, noncleaved cell (undifferentiated) lymphomas of the *non-Burkitt's* type show a greater degree of nuclear pleomorphism than that considered acceptable for Burkitt's lymphoma but are also high-grade lymphoid neoplasms.[224,225] The mean nuclear diameter is similar to that of Burkitt's lymphoma, 15 to 35 mu, but with greater variation within the tumor cell population; occasional giant cell forms and bizarre cells may be present. The cytologic characteristics are similar to those of Burkitt's as well, but with greater variation in nuclear shape, chromatin condensation, and nucleolar prominence and number. Most frequently there is a single distinct eosinophilic nucleolus. Small noncleaved cell non-Burkitt's lymphomas present most often in adults, median 34 years, and the site of presentation is usually nodal with peripheral lymphadenopathy not uncommon. However, small noncleaved cell lymphomas with nuclear pleomorphism also occur in children, and in this age group are virtually indistinguishable clinically and biologically from classic Burkitt's lymphoma.

Neoplastic cells from approximately 95% of cases express B-cell surface markers. As in classic Burkitt's lymphomas, translocations involving the c-*myc* oncogene are often seen. Both variants of small noncleaved cell lymphomas are the most frequent form of lymphoma seen in association with HIV infection. It has been postulated that the pathogenesis of high-grade B lymphoma in the setting of HIV infection is similar to that of classic Burkitt's lymphoma in Africa.[226] In both settings polyclonal B-cell proliferation occurs in the absence of effective T-cell regulation, possibly leading to the emergence of a malignant clone.

A mature T-cell phenotype is identified in rare cases of small noncleaved non-Burkitt's. This immunologic heterogeneity in concert with some clinicopathologic diversity suggests that, in contrast to Burkitt's lymphoma, this morphologic subtype is not a homogeneous clinicopathologic entity.

MISCELLANEOUS RARE LYMPHOPROLIFERATIVE DISEASES

Adult T-Cell Leukemia/Lymphoma

ATL is a characteristic clinicopathologic entity associated with HTLV-I, a unique type C retrovirus.[23,144] The syndrome was originally described in southwestern Japan, where it was endemic, but has been identified in other parts of the world as well, including the Caribbean and southeastern United States. In the United States it is most common in blacks. The median age at presentation is approximately 45 years, with no sex predilection. The pathologic spectrum of the associated lymphomas is broad and includes several diffuse subtypes in the Rappaport classification and the Working Formulation.[227] However, differences in survival have not been correlated with differences in histologic subtype, and thus ATL is favored as the diagnostic term for this clinicopathologic entity.[227] The most characteristic morphologic feature is the presence of highly pleomorphic and polylobated cells in the peripheral blood. Polylobated and multinucleated cells can also be seen in the lymph nodes, and by this criterion many cases have been classified as large-cell immunoblastic in the Working Formulation. Approximately 65% of patients present with peripheral blood involvement, and a leukemic phase develops in almost 100% at some time during the clinical course. Other common clinical features include generalized lymphadenopathy, hepatosplenomegaly, cutaneous involvement, hypercalcemia, and lytic bone lesions. Biopsies of lytic lesions do not necessarily show involvement by tumor, and marked osteoclastic activity is seen, both in lytic lesions and in routine bone marrow biopsies. These observations support the concept that a lymphokine secreted by neoplastic cells, osteoclast activating factor or an osteoclast activating factor–like substance, is responsible for these manifestations. The skin lesions are papulonodular with or without ulceration. In two-thirds of patients with cutaneous involvement epidermal infiltration resembling Pautrier's microabscesses is observed. However, most cases can readily be distinguished from MF/SS on clinical and epidemiologic grounds.

ATL is a post-thymic T-cell neoplasm that usually expresses a helper antigenic phenotype. However, in vitro the cells actually function as suppressor cells and suppress immunoglobulin synthesis by B cells.[228] They are strongly positive for acid phosphatase, and the activity is not always entirely inhibited by tartrate.[227] Thus TRAP activity is not pathognomonic of HCL.

Mycosis Fungoides/Sézary Syndrome

MF/SS are sometimes referred to collectively as the CTCL.[229] This spectrum of rare T-cell disorders is discussed more fully in Chapter 51.

Angioimmunoblastic Lymphadenopathy

A new clinicopathologic entity was described in 1975 by Lukes and Tindle and Frizzera, Moran, and Rappaport and termed angioimmunoblastic lymphadenopathy (AILD).[230,231]

It was initially construed as a hyperimmune disorder, but more recently questions have been raised as to its potentially neoplastic nature. In 24 patients described by Frizzera and colleagues, the mean age was 68 years. The disease had an acute onset with generalized lymphadenopathy. Hepatosplenomegaly and constitutional symptoms occurred in almost all cases (20 of 24). Rashes and a positive Coombs' test were commonly found. A polyclonal hypergammaglobulinemia was found in 17 of 22 patients. Similar results were reported in the series of Lukes and Tindle. Essential diagnostic features include (a) complete architectural effacement; (b) proliferation of arborizing small blood vessels; (c) polymorphous cellular proliferation of lymphocytes, immunoblasts, plasma cells, and +/− histiocytes and eosinophils; and (d) absence of germinal centers or a few residual "burned out" or hyalinized germinal centers. Other frequent but not essential histologic features are an overall hypocellular appearance with amorphous acidophilic interstitial material. Usually all lymph nodes are involved, and it is important to make the diagnosis only in the appropriate clinical context. Although the disease is progressive and often fatal (median survival, 15 months), the cells are not morphologically malignant. However, up to 50% of patients are found to have overt lymphomas, either during the clinical course or at autopsy.[232] The lymphomas are classified as large-cell immunoblastic in the Working Formulation. To date, cytotoxic treatment has not proved effective in controlling the disease or in preventing progression to lymphoma. Corticosteroid therapy, with or without cyclophosphamide, does provide temporary control in some cases.

Initial observations based on the polyclonal hypergammaglobulinemia and plasmacytosis in these lesions had suggested that AILD might be a hyperimmune disorder of the B-cell system. However, the immunoblastic cells in both AILD and the malignant lymphomas that supervene are Ig negative, and Japanese investigators have described a variant of peripheral T-cell lymphoma that bears a marked resemblance to this lesion.[233] Thus more recently it has been suggested that AILD is a peripheral T-cell lymphoma of helper T-cell origin. Cytogenetic investigations that have shown clonal abnormalities in several patients have also supported a malignant nature for this disease, even early in its course.[234] Clonal rearrangements of the T-cell receptor beta chain gene have provided additional evidence for T-cell origin in some cases and further suggest a neoplastic nature.[235,236] However, immunoglobulin gene rearrangements have been found in some cases, and sequential analysis has shown spontaneous regression of both T-cell and B-cell clones. Thus others have argued that AILD may be an immunoregulatory disorder.[236]

Angiocentric Immunoproliferative Lesions, Lymphomatoid Granulomatosis, Polymorphic Reticulosis, Midline Malignant Reticulosis

These lesions all represent the same histologic process, although initially described as different entities in different anatomical sites. Midline malignant reticulosis (MMR) and polymorphic reticulosis (PMR) are associated with the clinical entity lethal midline granuloma and involve the nose, paranasal sinuses, nasopharynx, and palate.[237,238] Lymphomatoid granulomatosis (LYG) was first described in the lung but involves the sites above in a high percentage of cases.[239] Other frequent sites of involvement include skin, kidneys, central and peripheral nervous system, and GI tract. The lesion common to all is an angiocentric and angiodestructive atypical lymphoreticular infiltrate. The vascular involvement often leads to necrosis, which may be extensive. Atypical lymphoid cells are admixed with plasma cells, eosinophils, and histiocytes. Because of these common histologic features, it has been proposed that these lesions represent the same nosologic entity, and the term "angiocentric immunoproliferative lesions" (AIL) has been proposed.[91,240]

LYG was initially described as a benign disorder with a limited risk of progressing to a malignant lymphoma. Similarly, MMR and PMR were believed to be locally invasive and destructive lesions with a low risk of peripheral dissemination. However, in some series, up to 50% of patients progress to lymphomas of the large-cell immunoblastic type.[241] Moreover, the median survival of LYG patients in one series was only 14 months, and survival was noted to be inversely proportional to the number of large, atypical lymphoreticular cells.[242] These observations have prompted the suggestion that these disorders, at least in some cases, may be neoplastic at onset. In the few cases studied the lymphoid cells have had a mature T-cell phenotype, and thus these processes may represent variants of peripheral T-cell lymphoma.[91,240,243]

Clinically, most cases present in adult life (median age, 50 years); the male-female ratio is 2 : 1. Presenting complaints are usually related to the involved organs: cough, shortness of breath, and nasal discharge; systemic symptoms, including fever, weight loss, and malaise, are common. Patients with localized upper airway disease have been reported to respond to radiation therapy in about 75% of cases without local recurrence or peripheral dissemination. Cyclophosphamide and prednisone have been used in LYG, with up to 50% sustained CR.[241] Patients who have recurrences or undergo histologic progression require more aggressive multiagent systemic chemotherapy, but in such patients, who have usually received prior therapy, survival has been poor.

A grading scheme has recently been proposed for AIL.[240] Grade I lesions have a polymorphic cellular composition and no cellular atypia. Grade II lesions demonstrate some cytologic atypia. Grade III lesions represent clear-cut angiocentric lymphoma. Most patients with grade I disease achieved control of their disease with cyclophosphamide and prednisone, in contrast to patients with grade II disease, the majority of whom progressed to overt lymphoma within 2 years. Patients with grade III disease treated aggressively at onset had a high CR rate.[240]

True Histiocytic Lymphoma/Malignant Histiocytosis

Malignancies of mononuclear phagocytes include acute monocytic leukemia, malignant histiocytosis, and true histiocytic sarcoma. These three malignancies represent a spectrum in terms of their degree of dissemination and can be conceptually related to different stages of maturation and differentiation in the mononuclear phagocytic series.[244]

Acute monocytic leukemia relates to a bone marrow-derived monoblast. This malignancy arises in the bone marrow compartment with secondary involvement of the peripheral blood and usually a markedly elevated white blood cell count. In contrast to acute myeloid leukemia, there is a somewhat higher incidence of involvement of nonhematopoietic sites, with frequent involvement of skin and gingiva. Hepatosplenomegaly and lymphadenopathy are relatively common (25% and 50%, respectively).[245]

Malignant histiocytosis represents a malignancy of mononuclear phagocytes that are intermediate in differentiation between monocytes and monoblasts and fixed tissue histiocytes. In many instances the syndromes of acute monocytic leukemia and malignant histiocytosis may merge, and the distinction may be arbitrary and somewhat semantic. Malignant histiocytosis is a systemic malignancy that involves the entire reticuloendothelial system. Within the lymphoreticular system there is preferential involvement of sites normally populated by histiocytes, such as lymph node sinuses, splenic red pulp, and hepatic sinusoids. Bone marrow involvement is common, and although abnormal cells can be seen in the peripheral blood, if peripheral blood involvement is extensive, a diagnosis of acute monocytic leukemia should be considered. Other frequent sites of involvement include skin and bone.

The end point of the spectrum is histiocytic sarcoma or "true histiocytic lymphoma," which represents a malignancy of the mononuclear phagocytic series at the stage of the fixed tissue histiocyte. As such, the lesions in histiocytic sarcoma represent localized, relatively discrete tumefactions.[246] In addition to the reticuloendothelial system, common sites of involvement include skin and bone.[247]

Histiocytic sarcomas initially confined to the skin have been reported to pursue an indolent clinical course, with spontaneous regression of lesions in some cases.[247] The entity initially described as regressing atypical histiocytosis may represent histiocytic sarcoma with this characteristic presentation.[248] Alternatively, the clinical and pathologic features of these cutaneous lesions are remarkably similar to lymphomatoid papulosis, a chronic self-remitting T-cell lesion of the skin. Poppema had suggested a histiocytic derivation for lymphomatoid papulosis,[249] and, given the high content of lysosomal enzymes in activated T cells, it is not surprising that the distinction between a histiocytic and T-cell derivation has been a difficult one. The current molecular and phenotypic evidence supporting a T-cell derivation for lymphomatoid papulosis is strong, and the natures of "regressing atypical histiocytosis" and isolated histiocytic sarcomas of the skin need to be reassessed in light of this new information.[128]

In the absence of special studies, morphologic evidence of phagocytosis by the neoplastic cells, most commonly erythrophagocytosis, has been proposed as a criterion for determining derivation from mononuclear phagocytes. However, phagocytosis is not reliably seen in most mononuclear phagocytic malignancies. Moreover, it is not a specific finding and has been described in lymphoid, plasmacytic, and even epithelial tumors (reviewed in ref. 244). Even if phagocytosis is observed, it is virtually always clinically insignificant. The clinical syndrome of histiocytic medullary reticulosis, characterized by hepatosplenomegaly, pancytopenia, and jaundice, has been proposed as a manifestation of malignant histiocytosis.[148,250] However, most observers now believe that it is nearly always a manifestation of a hemophagocytic syndrome, usually seen in association with immunodeficiency or another hematopoietic malignancy.[251,252] This syndrome appears pathogenetically related to excessive production of lymphokines capable of stimulating mononuclear phagocytes.[253]

Because of the misinterpretation of hemophagocytic syndromes in the past as "malignant histiocytosis," many literature reports of "malignant histiocytosis" actually represent hemophagocytic syndromes. This appears to be true for many cases of malignant histiocytosis reported in association with acute lymphocytic leukemia. AIL, including LYG, PMR, and MMR, also is often associated with a hemophagocytic syndrome as a terminal event that has been misdiagnosed as malignant histiocytosis.[252] These lesions are now recognized as a variant of peripheral T-cell lymphoma. Because of the underlying T-cell malignancy, there may be an associated immunodeficiency and the subsequent development of a hemophagocytic syndrome. Alternatively, the hemophagocytic syndrome could be due to lymphokine production by neoplastic cells. Familial erythrophagocytic lymphohistiocytosis is another disorder in which the terminal phase of the disease appears to be a hemophagocytic syndrome. The underlying condition appears to be a poorly characterized immunodeficiency.

True histiocytic lymphomas preferentially involve lymph nodes sinuses. However, this feature, too, is not specific and can be seen in certain T-cell immunoblast lymphomas (see above). Indeed, many instances of so-called malignant histiocytosis appear to represent this variant of Ki-1-positive immunoblastic lymphoma.[213]

Enzyme cytochemistry and histochemistry remain a reliable adjunct to morphology in the diagnosis of malignancies of the mononuclear phagocytic system. The cells have diffuse activity for nonspecific esterase, which is usually at least partially fluoride sensitive. Preferable methods for detection of esterase activity include the alpha-naphthyl butyrate esterase reaction because activity will not be observed in myeloid cells. Myeloid cells also contain minimal, if any, activity for alpha-naphthyl acetate esterase. The use of the naphthyl ASD acetate requires the use of fluoride to distinguish myeloid and mononuclear phagocytic cells. Activity for acid phosphatase and beta-glucuronidase is usually present as well. In all cases the activity should be relatively diffuse throughout the cytoplasm and not punctate. Punctate reactivity localized to the Golgi region is more characteristic of lymphoid rather than mononuclear phagocytic cells. Caution should be exercised in the use of enzyme cytochemistry because these enzymes are not specific for mononuclear phagocytes and can be seen in certain carcinomas and sarcomas.

Proliferative lesions of antigen-presenting cells are relatively rare. The principal proliferative lesion of the dendritic cell system is histiocytosis X. Most individuals do not consider histiocytosis X to be a malignancy, but rather consider it to be a proliferative lesion, possibly secondary to immunodeficiency.[254-256] The cells of histiocytosis X have the characteristics of Langerhans' cells, including CD1 expression and Birbeck granules. In contrast to normal Langerhans' cells, the cells also express antigens associated with phagocytic histiocytes such as MY4 (CD14) and LeuM5 (CD11C).

Although the cells of histiocytosis X may sometimes appear cytologically atypical, even with abnormal mitotic figures, histologic features are said not to be an important prognostic indicator in this disease. Prognosis is best correlated with age at presentation and extent of organ system involvement.[255,256] Patients under 2 years of age tend to have a poor prognosis, whereas those older than 6 years have an excellent prognosis. Clinical staging schemes useful in prognosis relate to the extent of organ system involvement. The greater the number of organ systems involved, the poorer is the prognosis.

Recently rare tumors have been described that have a proposed derivation from dendritic reticulum cells[257] and interdigitating reticulum cells,[258,259] respectively. These lesions have been based in lymph nodes and are often associated with an inflammatory background or necrosis, or both. Clinically, they tend to present as local disease, and, although they may be characterized by local recurrence, systemic spread has not been a feature. Because of the rarity of these lesions, it is difficult to make definitive statements about their clinical course.

NATURAL HISTORY OF THE LYMPHOMAS

SUPERFICIAL LYMPH NODE PRESENTATIONS

Eighty percent or more of adult patients with lymphomas present to their physicians with superficial adenopathy. Contrasting clinical features of Hodgkin's disease and the lymphocytic lymphomas are shown in Table 50-7. Lymph node enlargement is usually painless, rubbery, discrete, and located in the neck region. It may have been detected by the patient or found as a result of a physical examination for another reason.

Most patients are asymptomatic, although 20% of patients with the lymphocytic lymphomas and as many as 40% of patients with Hodgkin's disease may have some combination of fever, night sweats, weight loss, or pruritus, with fever being the most common associated symptom.[260,261] Often patients will give a history of waxing and waning adenopathy over periods extending from months to years before diagnosis, with an average duration of 5 months. Isolated axillary or inguinal lymph node presentations occur but are less common than cervical node presentations. It is not possible to make accurate distinctions between the various lymphomas by the size, shape, or feel of the lymph nodes. The distribution of peripheral adenopathy, however, can yield diagnostic information. Involvement of Waldeyer's ring occurs in less than 1% of patients with Hodgkin's disease but is identified in 15% to 33% of patients with the lymphocytic lymphomas and often is associated with lymphomas of the GI tract.[260-262] The higher figure has been found in a series in which lymphatic tissue of Waldeyer's ring is routinely biopsied. Epitrochlear node involvement is unusual in Hodgkin's disease but relatively common in patients with follicular lymphomas. When the patient's medical history is obtained, care should be taken to document the presence or absence of night sweats before the diagnosis is made because anxious patients can have night sweats from anxiety alone. The duration of signs and symptoms, unexplained weight loss, particularly that in excess of 10% of body weight, and a family history of similar or related illnesses such as mononucleosis and immunologic disorders should be noted. During the physical examination the status of lymph nodes in all peripheral sites, including the spleen, should be determined and each site recorded separately.

DIFFERENTIAL DIAGNOSIS OF SUPERFICIAL LYMPHADENOPATHY

The differential diagnosis of adenopathy depends on the age of the patient; the size, shape, and feel of the lymph nodes; and the location of the adenopathy. Palpable lymph nodes usually are found in normal people on careful examination, particularly in the neck region. A display of the lymph node areas of the head and neck region is shown in Figure 50-7.[263] Soft, flat, elliptical submandibular nodes of 0.5 to 1.0 cm are

TABLE 50-7. Clinical Features of the Lymphomas

Hodgkin's Disease	*Lymphocytic Lymphoma*
Lymph node disease "centripetal," tends to be in axial lymph nodes	Lymph node disease "centrifugal" noncontiguous
Epitrochlear nodes, Waldeyer's ring, testicular and gastrointestinal sites uncommon	More common involvement of epitrochlear nodes, Waldeyer's ring, testes, and gastrointestinal tract
Mediastinal presentation in 50% of patients	Mediastinal presentation less common (~20%)
	Distinct syndrome of T-cell lymphoblastic lymphoma with mediastinal presentation most commonly in 2nd or 3rd decades
Abdominal nodal involvement uncommon in asymptomatic but common in older patients or when fever or night sweats present	Abdominal lymph node involvement common
Commonly localized; contiguous nodal disease	Rarely localized nodal disease (<10%)
Bone marrow involvement uncommon	Bone marrow involvement common
Liver involvement uncommon; when present, spleen usually involved; is rare without fever or night sweats	Liver commonly involved in follicular lymphoma, rare in diffuse lymphoma

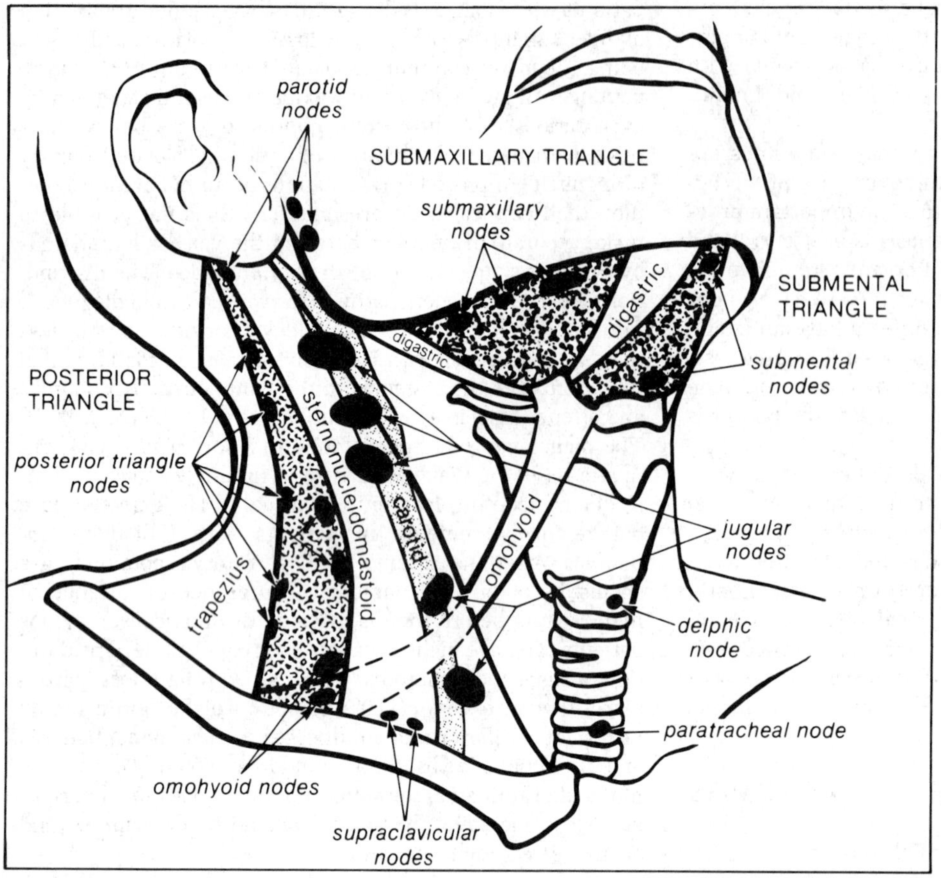

FIG. 50-7. Anatomical subdivisions of the neck depicting lymph node areas. (Adapted from Sade HH: Palpable cervical lymph nodes. JAMA 168:496, 1958)

commonly palpable in the submandibular and submental regions, and soft elliptical nodes of about 0.5 cm are found by careful examination in as many as 50% of normal people in the superficial jugular posterior cervical chain.[263] In young patients superficial adenopathy in the head and neck region is most often related to acute infectious illnesses of the mouth or pharynx. Mononucleosis is a common cause of cervical adenopathy, and, although often associated with pharyngitis, adenopathy can occur without pharyngeal symptoms. Toxoplasmosis can mimic mononucleosis as well; these disorders can be easily diagnosed by standard methods if suspected. Adenopathy resulting from infection usually causes firm, sometimes tender spherical enlargement of nodes that can be easily confused with lymphomas if they are nontender. Generally, a spherical lymph node greater than 1 cm in diameter, thought to be due to an infectious process, that does not diminish in size over a 4- to 8-week period of observation after resolution of the acute process should be biopsied. Discrete hard lymph nodes, particularly if fixed or matted, are more worrisome and should be promptly biopsied for diagnosis, particularly in older people. Hard lymph nodes in the submandibular or submental region in older people are more likely related to tumors of the floor of the mouth or larynx. Nasopharyngeal cancers often drain to and present as posterior cervical lymph node enlargements. Thyroid carcinoma can mimic lymphoma, although the lymph nodes involved with thyroid cancer generally are firmer and often found in the submental and superficial jugular region, an area less commonly involved in isolation by lymphomas.

Because supraclavicular lymph nodes drain regions of the lung and retroperitoneal space, they can reflect either lymphomas or tumors and infectious processes originating in these areas. Isolated axillary lymph node enlargement can be related to local phenomena in the hands or arms, such as infections, trauma, or insect bites. A young male adult with a tumor in an axillary lymph node is most likely to have a lymphoma or a malignant melanoma. In women the same two tumors plus breast cancer are the most likely diagnoses. Isolated inguinal adenopathy is often difficult to separate from the normal 0.5- to 1.0-cm elliptical lymph nodes found in the region of the inguinal ligament, which also are influenced by disorders that occur on the legs and feet. Concomitant enlargement of nodes in the femoral triangle or adenopathy along the external iliac chain should make inguinal adenopathy more suspicious and decrease the threshold for biopsy.

THORACIC PRESENTATIONS

Thoracic adenopathy is relatively common in patients with lymphomas. It may be detected by routine roentgenogram or films taken for another purpose, such as the workup after the discovery of peripheral adenopathy, or because the patient has had a chronic dry, nonproductive cough with or without fever. The overall frequency of mediastinal adenopathy in Hodgkin's disease is 50%. The highest frequency (70%) of mediastinal adenopathy occurs in young women with Hodgkin's disease.[260] The mediastinum is involved in less than 20% of patients with the other lymphomas.[264] Mediastinal adenopathy is a common presenting problem in patients with T-cell lymphocytic lymphomas.[265,266] Involvement of hilar nodes in patients with lymphomas is usually unilateral.

The differential diagnosis of mediastinal and hilar adenopathy includes primary lung disorders and some systemic illnesses that characteristically involve hilar or mediastinal nodes. In the young, mediastinal adenopathy commonly occurs in patients with infectious mononucleosis and sarcoidosis, which in both cases is usually panhilar. In endemic regions histoplasmosis can cause unilateral paratracheal node enlargement that mimics lymphoma but that usually is associated with the node calcification and esophageal symptoms. Unilateral tuberculous adenopathy is not often confused with lymphoma because of the associated Ghon complex. Primary lung cancer is an important part of the differential diagnosis in older people, especially smokers, and usually can be distinguished from lymphomas by the presence of a parenchymal lesion.

ABDOMINAL PRESENTATIONS

Hodgkin's disease and the common lymphomas frequently involve either retroperitoneal lymph nodes or the primary lymphatic tissue of the gut and its mesenteric drainage sites. Patients who present with abdominal lymphoma usually have either a painless mass discovered on physical examination or pain associated with a palpable mass. Some patients present only with splenomegaly and most often have one of the lymphomas, not uncommonly leukemic reticuloendotheliosis (HCL).[267] Rarely, previously untreated patients may present with perforation of a viscus through tumor, or hemorrhage from the upper or lower GI tract. Previously unsuspected abdominal lymphomas are found more often after the staging workup is completed in patients who have superficial lymph node presentations. Patients whose abdominal disease alone prompts their visit to their physicians most often have one of the lymphomas. It is distinctly unusual to be able to palpate significant abdominal adenopathy in patients with Hodgkin's disease because mesenteric lymph node involvement is uncommon. This is not the case for lymphoma. Hodgkin's disease may rarely make its appearance associated with idiopathic thrombocytopenic purpura and splenomegaly, but only a few of the patients with such a presentation have been described.[268]

The most common clinical symptoms and signs in patients with Hodgkin's disease who ultimately have abdominal tumor are fever and weight loss. The diagnosis of Hodgkin's disease is made at laparotomy performed as part of a diagnostic evaluation for fever of undetermined origin. Such patients usually have involvement of the retroperitoneal lymph nodes, and the histologic subtype is likely to be lymphocyte-depleted Hodgkin's disease. The so-called Mediterranean lymphoma often presents with disease in the abdomen. Pathologically, these tumors resemble diffuse plasma cell tumors (see Chap. 54) and often are associated with aberrant production of immunoglobulin heavy chains and malabsorption.[269] Abdominal presentations of lymphoma also may mimic any type of intra-abdominal disease. About two-thirds of the lymphomas that involve the GI tract originate in the stomach, 25% from the small intestine, and the remainder from the colon and rectum.[270]

CUTANEOUS PRESENTATIONS

Lymphocytic lymphomas may involve the skin primarily or secondarily. Although lymphomas of either B-cell or T-cell origin may involve the skin, it is more common for skin lymphoma lesions to be of T-cell origin. Involvement of skin by lymphomas other than CTCL (MF/SS) makes the lymphoma Stage IV; however, the prognosis of the underlying lymphoma is not dramatically affected by cutaneous spread. Skin disease may be indolent (regardless of histologic grade) or may be a component of rapidly progressing systemic disease.

An important subset of patients with cutaneous presentations have a lymphocytic lymphoma that represents a distinct clinicopathologic entity called variously CTCL, MF, and SS. Clinical features of this disease are discussed in Chapter 51.

OTHER CLINICAL PRESENTATIONS

Lymphomas should be included in the differential diagnosis of superior vena cava syndrome (most often Hodgkin's disease or diffuse histiocytic lymphoma), acute spinal cord compression, isolated tumor nodules of the skin, bone tumors, and unexplained anemias. Although these manifestations occur with considerable frequency in patients with widespread advancing tumor, they are uncommon as initial presentations of the disease. Seven percent of testicular masses in older men are lymphomas, usually of the diffuse aggressive variety. They often are associated with CNS and Waldeyer's ring involvement.[271] Because they are highly treatable, but with therapy different from that for testicular cancer, the distinction is important. Lymphomas also present as solitary thyroid nodules, usually in women and in association with Hashimoto's thyroiditis. Solitary brain lymphomas are being reported with increasing frequency, more commonly lymphocytic lymphomas, and associated with AIDS or iatrogenic immunosuppression. More commonly, CNS lymphoma is leptomeningeal disease and occurs in association with bone or bone marrow involvement with a diffuse aggressive lymphoma histology.[272] Such disease commonly presents with symptoms of headache or cranial nerve abnormalities.

DISEASE EVOLUTION

With the advent of modern treatment, patients with lymphoma rarely are left untreated, and the natural history is interrupted, often successfully, by treatment.

CLINICAL EVOLUTION OF LYMPHOCYTIC LYMPHOMAS

The natural history of the lymphocytic lymphomas is quite different from that of Hodgkin's disease. The clinical features of Hodgkin's disease and the lymphocytic lymphomas are compared in Table 50-7. Predictability of spread is less certain in lymphocytic lymphomas, although some tendency toward contiguity of spread has been demonstrated in a series from Stanford.[273] The disease may be unifocal in origin, but, if so, it remains localized so briefly that widespread disease is the rule at the time of diagnosis rather than the exception. A reasonable estimate of the percentage of patients with truly localized lymphomas is 10%, compared with approximately 50% of patients who present with localized Hodgkin's disease. Now that it is apparent that most of the common types of the lymphomas in adults originate from a monoclonal population of B cells, and the anatomic compartmentalization of these cells in lymph nodes is understood more clearly, certain generalizations can be made relating the type of disease to the clinical course of patients with lymphomas.

The most common histologic subgroup of patients with the lymphoma includes those with nodular (follicular) patterns in the lymph node. Patients in this group make up almost half of all cases in most series. When patients with nodular lymphomas present with apparently localized adenopathy, it usually is easy to demonstrate generalized adenopathy with few additional examinations. This propensity to have widespread disease matches the normal tendency of the small, untransformed follicular center B cell to migrate in the circulation. Nonetheless, despite wide dissemination, the follicular small cleaved cell variety of lymphoma is often clinically indolent. An as-yet-undetermined fraction of such patients can be left untreated and around 25% will evidence waxing and waning adenopathy for months to years before unsightly or painful lymph node enlargement or compression of a vital organ requires treatment.[274] In a very small number of low-grade lymphomas spontaneous regression can occur and last for many years.[164] Involvement of the bone marrow and liver, frequently easily demonstrated at initial diagnostic evaluation, does not impart the same adverse prognosis as involvement of these organs by Hodgkin's disease. Several studies have now clearly indicated that there is no difference in survival between patients with widespread disease confined to lymph nodes (Stage III) and those with involvement of lymph nodes, bone marrow, and liver.[275,276]

Patients with diffuse, aggressive lymphomas, although these are also most often of B-cell origin, have a vastly different natural history than patients with nodular lymphomas.[277] In keeping with the lack of motility of transformed follicular B cells, the diffuse large-cell lymphomas (pleomorphic undifferentiated or histiocytic of Rappaport), the second most common type, more often appear to be clinically localized, although the recurrence rate after local treatment indicates otherwise. In contrast to patients with follicular small cleaved cell lymphoma, when tumor is identified in organs such as the bone marrow, liver, and bone, patients with diffuse large-cell lymphomas have aggressive, rapidly fatal illnesses unless treated successfully.

There is now also evidence for a link between follicular small cleaved cell lymphomas and the diffuse large-cell lymphomas of B-cell origin. At the National Cancer Institute (NCI) a series of 515 patients with lymphomas has been analyzed for frequency of histologic evolution.[167,278] The clinical course of 114 of these patients had led to a repeat biopsy more than 3 months after the initial diagnostic biopsy. Among patients with nodular types of lymphoma at diagnosis, repeat biopsies revealed histologic progression in 41%. These results have been confirmed.[279] At Stanford the actuarial risk of histologic conversion is about 60% at 8 years. An autopsy study of patients at the NCI who initially were diagnosed as having follicular lymphomas revealed that fewer than 10% had evidence of exclusively follicular disease at autopsy. Survival after conversion is short unless CR is achieved with chemotherapy. These data indicate that a substantial number of patients with nodular lymphomas will evolve to a diffuse variety as part of the natural history of their disease.

A likely evolution of the lymphoma can be constructed as follows. The follicle-associated cells of B-cell lymphomas (see Fig. 50-1) that initially retain the characteristic of forming follicles are close to normal tissue in their growth characteristics and migrate easily while minimally dedifferentiated. This accounts for the ease of detectability of these cells in other organs (and, indeed, in the peripheral blood) and yet the indolent natural history. Their growth rate and invasive potential, for unknown reasons, remain low, and in time those that are not clonogenic probably die. In time the malignant clonogenic B cells take on the morphologic characteristics of transformed lymphocytes. This transformation may occur slowly over several years, or so rapidly that the evolution antedates diagnosis. These transformed cells are less motile, which accounts for the difficulty in detecting them outside the site of origin with normal staging procedures, but they are more invasive and produce a rapidly fatal disease if growth is unchecked. In the past these histologic types were called reticulum cell sarcomas, and in the more recent Rappaport classification, diffuse histiocytic lymphoma. It also seems likely that follicular small cleaved cell lymphoma subtype evolves to nodular mixed and nodular histiocytic lymphomas of Rappaport as the percentage of large cells increases until, finally, effacement of the lymph node occurs and a pathologic picture of diffuse large-cell lymphoma is observed under the microscope. As with the evolution of the histologic effacement of a lymph node in Hodgkin's disease, the reasons for the varying rate of transformation from nodule-forming indolent lymphocytes to large transformed cells are unknown. However, increased cytogenetic abnormalities have been noted with histologic progression.[280] Lymphomas of diffuse small lymphocytic cells disseminate widely at an early stage but have an indolent course, in keeping with their benign histologic appearance. They evolve to large-cell B neoplasms much less frequency and usually kill patients by causing bone marrow failure, with hypogammaglobulinemia leading to fatal infections.

STAGING OF LYMPHOCYTIC LYMPHOMAS

Patients with lymphocytic lymphoma most frequently present with advanced disease, commonly with liver, bone marrow, or pulmonary parenchymal involvement. Past studies reveal that as few as 10% of all lymphocytic lymphoma

TABLE 50-8. Ann Arbor Staging Classification for Hodgkin's Disease

Stage I
Involvement of a single lymph node region (I) or a single extralymphatic organ or site (IE)

Stage II
Involvement of two or more lymph node regions on the same side of the diaphragm (II) or localized involvement of an extralymphatic organ or site (IIE)

Stage III
Involvement of lymph node regions on both sides of the diaphragm (III) or localized involvement of an extralymphatic organ or site (IIIE) or spleen (IIIS) or both (IIISE)

Stage IV
Diffuse or disseminated involvement of one or more extralymphatic organs with or without associated lymph node involvement. The organ(s) involved should be identified by a symbol: A = asymptomatic; B = fever, sweats, weight loss >10% of body weight.

TABLE 50-9. Staging Lymphocytic Lymphomas: Required Evaluation Procedures

1. Adequate surgical biopsy, reviewed by an experienced hematologist
2. A detailed history recording duration and the presence or absence of fever, unexplained sweating and its severity, unexplained pruritus, and unexplained weight loss
3. A careful and detailed physical examination; special attention to all node-bearing areas, including Waldeyer's ring (indirect laryngoscopy is the procedure of choice) and determination of size of liver and spleen
4. Necessary laboratory procedures
   a. Complete blood count, including an erythrocytic sedimentation rate
   b. Serum alkaline phosphatase
   c. Evaluation of renal function
   d. Evaluation of liver function
5. Radiologic studies include
   a. Chest roentgenogram (posteroanterior and lateral)
   b. Bilateral lower extremity lymphogram
   c. Abdominal-pelvic computed axial tomographic scan
6. Bilateral bone marrow needle biopsies (not just aspirates; biopsy should be performed before aspirate, if both are done together)

patients appear to have true Stage I disease.[281-283] An analysis of stage distribution from the tumor registry at the Harvard Joint Center for Radiation Therapy demonstrated that approximately 15% of patients with lymphocytic lymphoma have Stage I-II disease in contrast to 50% to 60% of patients presenting with Hodgkin's disease. Localized extralymphatic involvement is more common in lymphocytic lymphomas than in Hodgkin's disease and can often occur as an isolated site of involvement (Stage IE) or with adjacent nodes (Stage IIE). There appears to be no difference in prognosis for Stage I or II lymphocytic lymphoma patients with localized extralymphatic involvement.[284,285] Systemic symptoms are less frequently seen in lymphocytic lymphomas than in Hodgkin's disease, and in many studies the presence of systemic symptoms has not been separately analyzed.

The standard staging system used for lymphocytic lymphomas is the same as that proposed for Hodgkin's disease at the Ann Arbor Conference in 1971.[286] This system is summarized in Table 50-8 and reflects both the number of sites of involvement and the presence of disease above or below the diaphragm. Patients can be assigned both a clinical stage and a pathologic stage. The clinical stage is based on initial tissue biopsy studies, physical examination, bone marrow biopsy, and radiographic evaluation. The pathologic stage uses, in addition, invasive surgical procedures such as additional extranodal tissue biopsies, laparoscopy-directed biopsies or staging laparotomy, and splenectomy. Recommendations for proper staging procedures made at the Ann Arbor symposium (and currently modified) are shown in Tables 50-9 and 50-10.[287]

Although the Ann Arbor staging scheme is extremely useful in defining the patient composition in clinical trials (Table 50-8), there is currently considerable uncertainty whether the distinction between the various stages in patients with lymphocytic lymphoma is as prognostically important as it is for Hodgkin's disease. Certain factors not explicitly recognized by the Ann Arbor classification, such as the bulk of the tumor and the specific sites of organ involvement in certain histologic subtypes, may have a more profound influence on the prognosis than does the distinction between Stage III and Stage IV disease.

The value of the Ann Arbor scheme in follicular or low-grade lymphomas is marginal. Patients either have disseminated disease (85%) or localized disease (15%), and the Ann Arbor stages do not identify distinctive groups of patients with different prognoses. It would appear preferable to advocate a system with only two stages for the follicular lymphomas. Those with localized disease (Ann Arbor Stages I and II) may be cured with localized therapy. Those with disseminated disease are responsive to a variety of systemic treatment approaches, and attempts are under way to develop curative therapy (Table 50-11).

The Ann Arbor staging classification is also inadequate in diffuse large-cell or aggressive lymphomas. To say that a patient has Stage II diffuse large-cell lymphoma is to convey

TABLE 50-10. Staging Lymphocytic Lymphomas: Procedures Required Under Certain Circumstances

1. Whole-chest tomography if any abnormality is noted or suspected on the routine chest roentgenogram
2. Abdominal ultrasonogram, inferior cavography, intravenous pyelogram or upper and lower GI contrast studies to supplement lymphographic findings or investigate sites of unexplained symptoms
3. Plain bone radiographs of symptomatic or tender areas
4. Head or spinal CT for neurologic signs or symptoms
5. Exploratory laparotomy and splenectomy, if management decision will depend on the identification of abdominal involvement. Note: Decision to proceed with laparotomy requires knowledge of treatment plan used at institution of record

Useful Ancillary Procedures Not Required for Staging

1. Magnetic resonance imaging (under investigation)
2. Gallium whole-body scans
3. Skeletal scintigrams
4. Hepatic and spleen scintigrams
5. Serum chemistries to include serum calcium and uric acid for overall management of patient
6. Estimates of the patient's delayed hypersensitivity of the tuberculin type

TABLE 50-11. National Cancer Institute Modified Staging Schema for Indolent and Aggressive Lymphomas

Indolent Lymphomas	
Stage I	Localized disease (Ann Arbor Stages I and II)
Stage II	Disseminated disease (Ann Arbor Stages III and IV)
Aggressive Lymphomas	
Stage I	Localized nodal or extranodal disease (Ann Arbor Stage I or IE)
Stage II	Two or more nodal sites of disease or a localized extranodal site plus draining nodes with none of the following: performance status ≤70, B symptoms, any mass >10 cm in diameter (particularly GI), serum LDH > 500, three or more extranodal sites of disease
Stage III	Stage II plus any poor prognostic feature

no useful prognostic information. Such a patient might have small cervical and axillary lymph nodes and an excellent probability of successful treatment outcome, or might have a bulky abdominal mass that may be refractory to treatment. Most workers find that the presence or absence of certain clinical prognostic factors that are basically surrogate measures of tumor bulk are more useful in predicting the course of disease and outcome of treatment. For example, poor performance status, the presence of any mass (particularly involving the GI tract) larger than 10 cm, a serum lactic dehydrogenase (LDH) level over 500 IU/dl, bone marrow involvement, and B symptoms are poor prognostic factors. A more reasonable staging classification for the diffuse aggressive lymphomas would be a three-stage scheme: Stage I is the same as the Ann Arbor Stage I, involvement of a single lymph node group or a single extranodal site; Stage II is disease in more than one lymph node group or extranodal site with none of the poor prognostic factors; and Stage III is disease in more than one lymph node group or extranodal site with one or more of the poor prognostic factors (Table 50-11).

CLINICAL STAGING

Patients should be questioned about the date the lymph node enlargement was first noted and the rate of subsequent tumor growth, as this information may influence the choice of therapy and, indeed, even the decision to institute treatment in patients with low-grade lymphomas. In contrast to Hodgkin's disease, certain clinical correlations must be made during the physical examination. Preauricular nodal enlargement often is associated with disease in the Waldeyer's ring area, which is uncommon in Hodgkin's disease. Indirect laryngoscopy is an absolute requirement of the staging workup. Waldeyer ring involvement often is associated with involvement of the intestine, and GI contrast studies are indicated if the patient appears to have localized disease. Primary lesions in extranodal sites such as bone or skin frequently are associated with involvement of regional nodes. Many patients with skin lesions that occur as primary or secondary lesions have multiple cutaneous lesions that may be remote from one another. Thus a careful inspection of the skin and biopsy of suspicious lesions are necessary, especially in patients with diffuse lymphomas. Primary lymphoma of the testes can often be associated with extension to regional pelvic or para-aortic nodes that may be detected by lymphogram or computed tomography (CT) scan.

The correlation between peripheral blood counts and marrow involvement by lymphoma is poor. Some abnormality in blood counts is found in only 37% of patients with bone marrow infiltration by lymphoma. Approximately one-half of patients with abnormal blood counts will not even have bone marrow involvement on biopsy. Examination of the peripheral smear in patients with lymphoma may yield evidence of malignant cells in approximately 10% of patients, primarily those with low-grade, follicular center cell lymphomas. Chest roentgenograms yield positive information in 26% of patients. The most frequent abnormality is hilar or mediastinal adenopathy, which occurs in only 18% of patients (pleural effusions 8% and parenchymal lesions 4%). Parenchymal lesions and pleural effusions require pathologic verification. A chylous or transudative effusion that lacks malignant cells does not change the pathologic stage of the patient. As in Hodgkin's disease, pulmonary parenchymal lesions usually are associated with concurrent hilar lymph node involvement, and if they involve only one hemithorax, they are considered to be an extension from the lymph nodes and do not necessarily change the patient's stage. Full lung tomograms and CT scans usually are not needed in the search for parenchymal nodes if chest roentgen films are completely normal, in view of the infrequency of parenchymal disease in these patients. They should be done, however, on any patient with extensive mediastinal or hilar adenopathy if the disease is localized to the mediastinum and radiotherapy is to be given alone—both unusual circumstances in patients with lymphocytic lymphoma.

Bone lesions are more common in patients with diffuse aggressive lymphomas than in patients with small-cell lymphomas. Routine roentgenographic studies of bone have largely been replaced by bone scanning, a technique with greater sensitivity. Bone lesions are particularly common in patients with diffuse aggressive lymphoma. In a series from the NCI, 10 (25%) of 40 patients with this diagnosis had bone lesions detected radiologically.[281,288,289] All ten of these lesions were seen on bone scan, whereas bone films showed the lesions in only eight patients. Thus, as an initial procedure, it is unnecessary to do both bone roentgen films and scans. A positive bone scan should be confirmed by plain films and biopsied if possible.

Bipedal lymphography is a particularly valuable procedure in the staging of lymphoma. Filling defects, or absence of filling, with collateral lymphatic drainage are signs of malignant disease, although less specific for lymphoma. An accurate assessment of abdominal lymph nodes has been reported in 83% to 90% of patients studied in a number of large series in which the roentgenographic interpretations were verified by laparotomy.[266,290–294] In patients with a negative study, 20% to 30% had involvement with tumor at laparotomy. A striking feature of the lymphocytic lymphomas is that the frequency of retroperitoneal nodal involvement as demonstrated by lymphography varies sharply with histologic type, and ranges from about 90% for patients with follicular lymphomas to 57% of those with diffuse lymphoma.[281] Most patients with positive lymphograms also have generalized palpable adenopathy, so that an advance in stage occurs in only 10% of the patients as a result of a positive lymphogram. However, the lymphogram provides easy follow-up evaluation of abnormal opacified nodes with plain abdominal films.

The lymphogram is also an accurate predictor of the chances of finding intra-abdominal lymphoma in extranodal sites, or in splenic, portal, or mesenteric lymph nodes. In the NCI series 81% of patients with a positive lymphogram had disease in liver or in lymph nodes outside the para-aortic chain or in ascites fluid.[281] Only 18% of patients with negative lymphograms had similar findings at laparotomy. The group at Stanford has shown a similar positive correlation between lymphogram and mesenteric lymph node involvement. CT scans are virtually the only reliable noninvasive test for diagnosing mesenteric node, porta hepatica, and splenic hilar node involvement, with an overall accuracy of 60%. This is particularly useful in the follicular lymphomas, in which mesenteric node involvement is common. However, the information is required only if radiotherapy is the sole treatment to be given.[290]

Lymphograms are more sensitive than CT scans in detecting para-aortic nodal disease, but neither are completely sensitive in detecting other intra-abdominal sites of nodal disease. In a series comparing CT scans with lymphograms in laparotomy-staged patients, Best and colleagues found that 9 of 45 patients with a negative CT scan and a negative lymphogram had positive abdominal nodes at laparotomy.[295,296] Two patients with a positive CT scan but with negative lymphography had positive lymph nodes at surgery. This reflects the capacity of the CT scan to detect some mesenteric nodes. CT scans appear to provide a true estimate of the size of the involved nodes that are often underestimated by lymphography.[290]

Gallium-67 (^{67}Ga) scanning is of some value in patients with diffuse aggressive lymphomas in whom 60% to 80% of involved nodal sites can be visualized.[297-300] In the small-cell and small cleaved cell lymphocytic lymphomas this test is quite unreliable, with less than 50% of nodal sites known to be involved by tumor detected by the scan. Because ^{67}Ga is taken up by cell by way of the transferrin receptor and the transferrin receptor may be a surrogate measure of proliferative cells, a patient with low-grade disease may demonstrate sites of ^{67}Ga uptake that auger histologic progression to more aggressive histology. Lesions in or near the liver may be obscured by the normal accumulation of ^{67}Ga in the bowel and liver. Iliac lymph nodes are difficult to interpret because of the usual accumulation of ^{67}Ga in the cecum and sigmoid colon. Some have argued that the use of higher doses of ^{67}Ga improves the sensitivity; however, the bowel retention of biliary-excreted isotope makes accurate interpretation of intra-abdominal tracer difficult.

Thus ^{67}Ga scans are a poor substitute for lymphography or other tests such as the CT scan and sonography. However, with technical improvements such as the use of spot films, use of double or triple peak angle camera, and single photon emission CT, ^{67}Ga scanning may add supportive staging information to that obtained with other tests.

One of the major findings of exhaustive staging studies, and indeed an important reason for the decline of interest in staging laparotomy in lymphocytic lymphoma, is the approximately 50% incidence of bone marrow and hepatic involvement.[281] The incidence of bone marrow metastasis in lymphoma is highest in patients with the small-cell lymphocytic lymphomas, follicular or diffuse (40%–100%, depending on the specific type), and lowest in those with diffuse large-cell lymphoma (5%–15%). Each subtype of disease tends to have an identifiable pattern of bone marrow involvement.[301] The follicular lymphomas are characterized by a paratrabecular location of involvement, whereas the T-cell lymphoma infiltrates within the marrow space. Bone marrow involvement in patients with diffuse, aggressive lymphomas is usually widespread and may be associated with focal or diffuse myelofibrosis. Although bone marrow involvement is less frequent in diffuse large-cell lymphoma, its detection is important because of its strong correlation with later spread of disease to the CNS. Up to 35% of patients with large-cell lymphomas and positive bone marrow biopsies may develop CNS spread.[302] Cytologic examination of the spinal fluid should be performed in all patients with diffuse types of lymphoma with bone marrow involvement, since prophylactic therapy of the CNS is indicated in such patients.[303] As with Hodgkin's disease, aspiration of the bone marrow is inadequate for staging purposes. In view of the clinical importance of bone marrow evaluation and the focal nature of metastases, more than one biopsy should be obtained for evaluation. For patients having two biopsies, up to 30% will have positive findings in only one biopsy.[266] Assuming an even chance of obtaining the positive biopsy on the first attempt, a second biopsy should increase the number of positives by up to 15%. Overall, bone marrow biopsy can be expected to advance the stage in approximately 25% of patients to Stage IV because some of those with marrow disease will have been previously classified as Stage IV on the basis of other extranodal sites. The shift to Stage IV predominantly occurs in patients with Stage III disease and in those with follicular and small-cell lymphocytic lymphomas. In these patients it is then unnecessary to proceed with further staging unless documentation of liver involvement will influence the choice of therapy. In most clinical situations this is not the case.

Intensive efforts to identify hepatic metastases in lymphocytic lymphoma have led to the recognition of a surprisingly high incidence of involvement in some categories of disease. The incidence of lymphomatous involvement of the liver in patients who present with lymphocytic lymphoma ranges from 11% to 42%.[281,304,305] The yield increases as the size and number of biopsy specimens increase. Percutaneous biopsy reveals disease in approximately 30% of patients with follicular or diffuse small cleaved cell lymphomas but in only 6% of patients with diffuse large-cell lymphoma. Peritoneoscopy-directed biopsies add an additional 30% after a negative percutaneous biopsy. Laparotomy in patients who have a negative biopsy by a nonsurgical technique (percutaneous biopsy or biopsy at time of peritoneoscopy) reveals an additional 20% with positive liver biopsy, primarily in patients with follicular lymphoma who have a positive lymphogram before biopsy. By all biopsy techniques, patients with diffuse large-cell lymphoma have a much lower incidence of liver metastases then do patients with lymphoma in the other major categories of disease. Percutaneous biopsy is usually the most invasive procedure performed in patients with lymphocytic lymphoma. Laparoscopy with multiple liver biopsies should be done only when there is a strong suspicion of liver involvement in a patient who would otherwise have Stage I or II disease.

In view of the results above, the discussion of staging laparotomy in the lymphocytic lymphomas takes on an entirely different meaning. Most patients with lymphocytic lymphomas will be found to have Stage III or IV disease without a staging laparotomy after the careful use of the sequential staging procedures outlined above.[266,281] The results of a study of 170 consecutively staged and previously untreated patients with lymphocytic lymphoma at the NCI are shown in Table 50-12. A total of 34% of patients were Stage I or II at the time of referral to the NCI. Lymphangiography decreased this number to 23%, bone marrow biopsy further decreased it to 20%, and liver biopsy and laparotomy decreased it to 14%. Only 6% of nodular lymphoma patients remained Stage I or II, as compared with 30% of patients with diffuse lymphomas.

Staging laparotomy and splenectomy were routinely performed in the late 1960s and early 1970s in a number of centers in patients with lymphocytic lymphoma, and considerable staging information is available.[266,281,304–308] One of the larger studies reports on laparotomy findings of 197 patients evaluated at Stanford University Medical Center.[306] Of 51 clinical Stage I or II patients with diffuse histology only 3 (6%) were upstaged to Stage III or IV. In contrast, 16 of 41 (40%) of clinical Stage I or II patients with nodular histology were upstaged. Downstaging was rare in the nodular lymphomas but occurred in 10 of 38 (25%) of patients with clinical Stage III or IV diffuse lymphomas. Another study has reported 61% of clinical Stage I or II nodular lymphocytic lymphomas and 22% of diffuse lymphocytic lymphoma patients being upstaged by surgical staging.[308] Although, as in Hodgkin's disease, it has enhanced our understanding of the behavior of the lymphocytic lymphomas, it should never be performed in general practice as a routine staging procedure. Because patients with lymphocytic lymphoma generally are older than those with Hodgkin's disease, postoperative complications are more common. Although surgical mortality is approximately 0.5%, significant morbidity, primarily pneumonia, pulmonary embolism, pancreatitis, subdiaphragmatic abscesses, or GI bleeding, has been reported in 11% to 40% of patients in three larger series.[266,291–293]

Thus the primary factor that accounts for the limited need for laparotomy in lymphocytic lymphoma is the high yield of less morbid procedures and the recognition that precise definition of involvement probably has limited importance in treatment planning for most patients. Because most patients have easily demonstrated Stage III or IV disease, and because these patients are treated with chemotherapy in most centers, routine staging laparotomy obviously is not indicated. Laparotomy may not even be indicated for the 20% of patients who remain in clinical Stage I or II after sequential staging tests, since increasingly systemic therapy is being used in such patients with excellent results. Laparotomy is used as a diagnostic tool in patients with undiagnosed abdominal masses. One study that evaluated laparotomy as a restaging tool showed that CT scans, lymphograms, and gallium scans overpredict for residual disease, and more patients are actually in CR than appears to be the case after routine restaging.[294] An NCI study of reexploration of residual abdominal masses that had been stable for at least two cycles of chemotherapy demonstrated that the procedure was not necessary.[309]

IMMUNOLOGIC ABNORMALITIES IN PATIENTS WITH LYMPHOMA

Clinically apparent immunologic abnormalities, especially of T cells, may precede the development of malignant lymphomas (see above); however, for most lymphoma patients the usual measures of immunity are normal. Because the early studies of delayed hypersensitivity in lymphoma patients did not reveal distinct abnormalities in patients with lymphocytic lymphomas, there have been fewer studies in these patients and data are surprisingly scarce. Interpretation of results of available studies needs to be qualified as well because, in general, investigators have not allowed for differences among the various histologic subtypes and stages of lymphocytic lymphoma.

The most common immunologic abnormality found in patients with lymphoma is a monoclonal immunoglobulin peak in the serum. With increasingly sophisticated detection methods, it appears that the vast majority of patients with B-cell lymphoma have microgram to milligram quantities of monoclonal immunoglobulin in the serum that is identical in isotype and idiotype to that borne by the malignant cells.[310] In general, the malignant B cells of lymphoma patients do not subserve any normal or abnormal immunologic functions, and the paraprotein is not present in sufficient quantity to affect antibody responses to neoantigens. Rare lymphomas may produce factors with biologic activity; for example, there have been reports of patients with lymphoma

TABLE 50-12. Change in Stage During Sequential Workup of 170 Consecutively Staged, Previously Untreated Patients with Lymphocytic Lymphoma: Percentage of Patients Each Stage After Indicated Procedure[362]

	Stage I	*Stage II*	*Stage III*	*Stage IV*
Clinical stage on referral	13	21	42	24
After lymphogram	8	15	54	24
After bone marrow	7	13	33	48
After closed liver biopsies	6	11	25	58
After laparotomy	6	8	21	65

and leukopenia whose tumor cells produced an inhibitor of myelopoiesis.[311]

Although patients with systemic symptoms or malnutrition may have generalized immunosuppression,[312] there is no consensus that a particular abnormality can be said to be related to the lymphoma. A number of studies have been carried out. Jones and colleagues[313] measured peripheral lymphocyte number, serum immunoglobulins, and delayed hypersensitivity to six recall antigens. In 38 patients with diffuse large-cell lymphoma there were pretreatment abnormalities, including low IgA levels, poor skin test reactivity, and low lymphocyte counts. The abnormalities were more common in patients with advanced-stage disease and B symptoms. Their patients with follicular lymphoma had only skin test abnormalities, and their defects were more selective (only 2 of 6 antigens failed to elicit a response). Similar findings were reported by Advani and associates.[314] Because skin tests are an in vivo measure of CD4+ or helper T-cell function, one might conclude from these studies that lymphoma is associated with some compromise of helper T-cell function and that advanced symptomatic large-cell lymphomas are associated with severe immune dysfunction than asymptomatic follicular lymphomas.

Gajl–Peczalska and co-workers[315] described increased helper-cell function of peripheral blood T cells from lymphoma patients in an assay system measuring immunoglobulin secretion by allogeneic normal B cells. Silver and colleagues[316] concluded that the helper T-cell function of lymphoma patients was mildly defective when they used patient T cells to drive pokeweed mitogen stimulation of normal allogeneic B cells. Whisler and co-workers[317] found that T cells from lymphoma patients responded poorly to the mitogen concanavalin A but that some of them developed enhanced responsiveness after 3 days of preculture, a technique designed to eliminate suppressor-cell function. All of this work is highly phenomenological. Variations in outcome between assay systems do not allow definitive conclusions; however, for most patients with lymphoma, immune defects do not seem to be an important cause or effect of the disease.

Nevertheless, rare patients do manifest significant immune abnormalities that appear to be a consequence of the disease rather than a cause of it. Certain T cell malignancies, most notably some patients with CTCL, continue to subserve immune functions such as helper activity[318] or suppressor activity.[319] Patients with HTLV-I–related ATL have functional helper T-cell deficits that are comparable to those seen in HIV infection and are associated with a significant risk of opportunistic infections from a variety of pathogens, including *Pneumocystis carinii*.[320]

CLINICAL IMMUNOLOGIC DISORDERS IN PATIENTS WITH LYMPHOMA

A clinically significant monoclonal gammopathy has been shown by Moore and colleagues to occur in 6% to 8% of patients with diffuse lymphomas but in only 1% or less of patients with the nodular lymphomas.[321] These incidence figures reflect the origin of the former cells from the immunoglobulin-producing cells of the medullary cords (see Fig. 50-1). This region is thought to be the site of origin of the cells of Waldenström's macroglobulinemia as well as the chronic variety of lymphocytic leukemia and diffuse small lymphocytic lymphomas.

In a study by Ko and Pruzansky of 1246 patients identified in a screening process to have M components in their serum, 62 (0.05%) were found to have lymphomas.[322] Thirty-three of these patients had an elevated level of IgM, 20 had elevated IgG levels, 5 had elevated IgA levels, and 1 had a Bence Jones protein spike. Fifty-four of 67 patients had diffuse lymphomas and only 13 had evidence of nodularity. Nine patients had Hodgkin's disease. An associated decrease in the normal serum globulin levels was noted in 20 patients (IgM, 16; IgG, 4). Seven patients had cryoglobulinemia, five with IgM and two with IgG. Six patients had cold agglutinins identified of IgM type with anti-I specificity.

In a report by Jones in 1973 that focused on immune disorders in lymphoma patients, nine (an incidence of 1.7%) patients with Coombs'-positive autoimmune hemolytic anemia (AIHA) and four (0.4%) cases of idiopathic thrombocytopenia purpura (ITP) were identified.[323] He analyzed four additional cases of Hodgkin's disease with immune disorders previously known to him, two each with AIHA and ITP. In only two patients did the autoimmune disorder precede the diagnosis. AIHA was associated with splenomegaly, systemic symptoms, and, in eight of nine patients with diffuse lymphomas, widely disseminated disease. No patient in their series died of the autoimmune disorder, which could usually be controlled with the drugs used to treat the underlying lymphoma.

TREATMENT OF LYMPHOCYTIC LYMPHOMAS

The treatment approach to a particular patient with a lymphocytic lymphoma is determined by several factors: the tumor histology, the stage of disease, and the physiologic status of the patient.

The influence of tumor histology on the natural history of disease became evident with the introduction by Henry Rappaport in 1956 of a reproducible histopathologic classification for the lymphocytic lymphomas. Subsequent clinical studies confirmed the capacity of the Rappaport diagnosis to convey prognostic information about the disease course and prognosis.[273] The histologic diagnosis is perhaps the best single predictor of the outcome of the disease. A remarkable aspect of Rappaport's achievement is its prescience. The Rappaport scheme was formulated in the absence of systematic clinical data. Only after the use of the Rappaport schema became widespread was it able to be demonstrated that the natural history of the disease was predicted by the Rappaport diagnosis. Minor additions and alterations in the Rappaport system have been necessary throughout the 32 years since its original description, and these have been formalized in a Working Formulation. However, the fundamental insights that created order out of the chaos that had typified lymphoma pathology and the insights that formed the basis for our current clinical approach to lymphoma treatment were Henry Rappaport's insights.

As detailed above, the Working Formulation divides the

lymphocytic lymphomas into histologic grades: low-grade, intermediate-grade, and high-grade. By and large, the clinical course corresponds to histologic grades; however, there are some exceptions and there are some disease entities that have been omitted from the Working Formulation. These imperfections have led us to develop a clinical schema based on the untreated or palliatively treated natural history of the histologic entities that divides the lymphomas into three groups: indolent lymphomas, which on average have a natural history measured in years; aggressive lymphomas, which on average have a natural history measured in months; and highly aggressive lymphomas, which on average have a natural history measured in weeks (Table 50-13). Thus the primary determinant of the treatment approach to an individual patient is the natural history of the particular histologic subtype of lymphocytic lymphoma.

The second major determinant of the treatment approach is the extent of disease. As previously discussed, the Ann Arbor staging scheme for Hodgkin's disease suits the lymphocytic lymphomas poorly, since stepwise progression to contiguous lymph node groups is unusual in the lymphomas. Staging issues vary with the natural history of the lymphoma. For the indolent lymphomas nearly 90% of all patients have widely disseminated disease at presentation, and there are no significant differences in survival between Stage III and Stage IV patients. However, for those with Ann Arbor Stage I or II disease radiation therapy may be curative for the majority. Thus a two-stage system is more appropriate for these patients: Stage I would include Ann Arbor Stages I and II and would imply potential curability with radiation therapy; Stage II would include Ann Arbor Stages III and IV and would imply that localized therapies have no curative potential (see Table 50-11).

For the aggressive lymphomas it is also clear that localized disease is rare (probably less than 20% of all patients), but there are a series of consistent clinical prognostic factors that can affect the prognosis of patients without localized disease. The factors associated with a poor prognosis include the presence of a poor performance status, the presence of B symptoms, the presence of an abdominal mass more than 10 cm in diameter, the presence of three or more extranodal sites of disease, bone marrow involvement, and a serum LDH level over 500 IU/ml. Some series have suggested that age over 55 years is a poor prognostic factor and others include the speed of response to therapy as a prognostic factor, but these are not universal. These clinical prognostic factors are much more important in determining treatment outcome than Ann Arbor stage. Thus, for aggressive lymphomas, a three-stage system seems most appropriate: Stage I is the same as Ann Arbor Stage I; Stage II is the involvement of two or more lymph node regions or localized extralymphatic organ or site (IIE) with none of the poor prognostic factors (poor performance status, B symptoms, mass more than 10 cm, three or more extranodal sites, marrow involvement, LDH over 500); and Stage III is Stage II with one or more of the poor prognostic factors (see Table 50-11).

For the highly aggressive lymphomas the natural history is so short that nearly all patients have disseminated disease at diagnosis, and there is no evidence that clinical staging should make an impact on the treatment approach, which in all cases is high-dose combination chemotherapy.

The final determinant of the treatment approach to individual patients with lymphocytic lymphoma is the physiologic status of the patient. There is no question that the treatments for lymphoma are toxic, but the toxicities are nearly always *dose-related* and predictable. The age range for patients with lymphoma is quite large, and many patients are over the age of 65 years at diagnosis. Lymphomas that occur in older patients are disproportionately those that may be curable with aggressive combination chemotherapy programs. It is important to remember that advanced age per se is not a contraindication to using an effective combination chemotherapy program. Clinical experience suggests that older patients may experience somewhat more myelotoxicity than younger patients when drug doses are administered on the basis of body surface area. Older patients are also more sensitive to the marrow-suppressive effects of radiation therapy. However, myelotoxicity from chemotherapeutic agents is related to dose, and there is nearly always a particular dose of drugs that can be safely administered even to a patient whose marrow is extremely sensitive. It has been our practice to administer the first cycle of drugs to older patients in full doses (or rarely at 80%–90% doses) and to modify subsequent cycles by a sliding scale based on the nadir counts, similar to what is done in younger patients. There is some evidence that the speed of response is an important factor in long-term disease-free survival,[324] and the poorer treatment outcome that has been seen in some series of older patients may be related more to the delivery of inadequate doses of drugs in the first few cycles of treatment than to any feature of the tumor in an older patient. Patients with aggressive lymphomas who do not achieve CR will have a short and unpleasant life because of the lymphoma. Patients with potentially curable disease should therefore not be treated gently out of fear of causing toxici-

TABLE 50-13. National Cancer Institute Clinical Schema for Lymphocytic Lymphomas Based on Natural History of Untreated or Palliatively Treated Patients

Indolent (Median Survival Measured in Years)
Small lymphocytic
Follicular, small cleaved cell
Follicular, mixed
Diffuse, small cleaved cells*
Diffuse, intermediately differentiated (or mantle zone)†
Cutaneous T-cell†
Aggressive (Median Survival Measured in Months)
Follicular, large cell
Diffuse mixed
Diffuse large cell
Diffuse immunoblastic‡
Highly Aggressive (Median Survival Measured in Weeks)
Diffuse small noncleaved cell (Burkitt's)
Diffuse small noncleaved cell (non-Burkitt's)
Lymphoblastic
Adult T-cell leukemia/lymphoma†

*Working Formulation intermediate-grade tumor with an indolent natural history.
†Omitted from the Working Formulation.
‡Working Formulation high-grade tumor with an aggressive natural history.

ties, which in the overwhelming majority of patients are completely reversible. The alternative to effective therapy —gentle palliation—has a uniformly fatal outcome and offers the patient treatment- and disease-related toxicity with no prospect for prolonged survival. Certainly treatment priorities must be adjusted to the seriousness of the disease. Most older patients are willing to cope with acute toxicity for the prospect of disease-free survival, and with the most recent treatment programs treatment-related death is far less common than treatment-induced long-term CR.

The existence of serious underlying medical problems may complicate the choice of therapy for patients with lymphoma. Patients with severe chronic obstructive pulmonary disease should probably not receive a regimen containing bleomycin. Patients with underlying serious renal failure should probably not receive a regimen containing high-dose methotrexate. Patients with a severe cardiomyopathy or severe hepatic dysfunction should probably not receive doxorubicin. For older patients and patients with severe underlying cardiorespiratory disease, tolerance to therapy may be markedly improved by maintaining the hemoglobulin level above 11 g/dl by transfusion, if necessary.

Another increasingly common clinical dilemma is the treatment of an aggressive or highly aggressive lymphoma that occurs in the setting of an underlying immunodeficiency. Lymphomas are the most common malignancy seen in immunodeficient patients. They may evolve in the natural history of Wegener's granulomatosis, Wiscott–Aldrich syndrome, Chediak–Higashi syndrome, Sjögren's syndrome, and just about any other disease of the immune system. Aggressive or highly aggressive lymphocytic lymphomas occur in up to 10% of AIDS patients, and the increasing incidence of AIDS makes the secondary lymphoma an important medical problem. In general, the lymphomas that occur under these conditions are immunoblastic (aggressive) or small noncleaved cell (non-Burkitt's or Burkitt's) in histology. Intensive treatment may be associated with responses, but the probability of long-term survival often depends more on the natural history of the underlying immune system defect than on the lymphoma.

If an underlying medical problem alters the choice of therapy, it is probably best to choose an alternate regimen that does not contain the threatening drug rather than to modify a program on an ad hoc basis by simply omitting the dangerous drug. No one knows the contribution to the overall success of a program that is related to the effects of an individual agent in that program or whether the modified regimen would have the potential to induce long-term disease-free survival. Without such information it would seem more prudent to use an alternative regimen with a known (although perhaps lower) success rate than to create a new program with no record of success.

TREATMENT OF INDOLENT LYMPHOCYTIC LYMPHOMAS

Although the treatment of lymphoma itself is the subject of debate and controversy because of the diverse approaches that show some degree of efficacy, there is no area of lymphoma treatment more controversial than the approach to the indolent lymphocytic lymphomas. There are no subsets of patients with low-grade histologies for which there is unanimity on the best treatment. The major controversy is whether any treatment can induce long-term disease-free survival and alter the natural history of the disease. Rosenberg[325] maintains that there are no treatments for patients with any stage of indolent lymphoma that are likely to cure. However, for early-stage disease there is ample evidence that radiation therapy is a potentially curative modality, and a growing body of evidence supports the use of intensive treatment approaches for various subsets of patients with advanced-stage disease.

Treatment of Early-Stage Indolent Lymphoma (Ann Arbor Stages I, II; NCI Stage I)

Most series of patients with early-stage indolent lymphomas are mainly composed of patients with follicular small cleaved cell and follicular mixed lymphomas, since the other low-grade histologic varieties are rarely localized at presentation. A number of studies have demonstrated the efficacy of radiation therapy in the treatment of clinically staged patients with localized disease. In the Stanford series patients with Stage I or II follicular lymphoma (including some patients with the aggressive follicular large-cell lymphoma) staged with procedures that stopped short of laparotomy in 60% were treated with involved field, extended field, or total nodal radiation therapy. Overall, 54% of the patients were free of disease after 10 years of follow-up.[326] The freedom from relapse was significantly higher in the patients who received total lymphoid radiation than in those who received involved or extended field radiation. Only 10% of the patients who were treated with total lymphoid radiation relapsed. Patients with follicular large-cell lymphoma had significantly poorer survival when treated with radiation therapy alone than did patients with follicular small cleaved cell or follicular mixed lymphoma. Patients under age 40 years had a significantly higher likelihood of being cured of their disease regardless of the field of therapy. If only patients with follicular small cleaved cell or follicular mixed lymphoma undergoing clinical staging are considered, total lymphoid radiation should be able to cure more than three fourths. Patients who are found to have early-stage disease after a negative exploratory laparotomy can achieve comparable long-term disease-free survival with either involved field or total nodal radiation therapy[327]; however, exploratory laparotomy is not indicated solely to allow a reduction in the field of radiation.

A retrospective analysis of results at Yale University with radiation therapy in Stage I or II follicular lymphoma demonstrated an 88% 5-year disease-free survival for Stage I patients and a 61% 5-year disease-free survival for Stage II patients.[285] At St. Bartholomew's Hospital in London, extended field radiation therapy obtained an 83% relapse-free survival at 10 years in Stage I or II follicular lymphoma patients.[328] Using involved field radiation therapy for Stage I patients and total lymphoid radiation therapy for Stage II patients, Gomez and co-workers[329] found an 83% disease-free survival at 10 years. Thus radiation therapy is effective therapy in early-stage disease. The contiguous and noncontiguous nodal relapses seen in patients who receive limited-field radiation in all studies suggests that clinically staged patients should receive total nodal radiation.

The role of combination chemotherapy in the management of early-stage follicular lymphoma is unclear. At least three randomized studies fail to demonstrate that the use of chemotherapy plus radiation therapy is superior to radiation therapy alone,[330-332] but the chemotherapy regimen used in the studies was cyclophosphamide, vincristine, and prednisone (CVP) or one of similar efficacy. In a recent report from the M. D. Anderson Hospital the relapse-free survival was significantly better for patients with Stage I and II follicular lymphoma who received cyclophosphamide, doxorubicin, vincristine, and prednisone (CHOP) chemotherapy with or without radiation (64% at 5 years) than for those treated with radiation alone (37% at 5 years).[333] Thus it is possible that the use of more effective chemotherapy programs might improve on the results obtained with involved-field radiation therapy, or might in fact be useful without added radiation therapy; however, at the moment, the data suggest that total nodal radiation therapy is the treatment of choice in Ann Arbor clinical Stage I or II (or NCI Stage I) follicular small cleaved cell and follicular mixed lymphoma.

Treatment of Advanced-Stage Indolent Lymphoma (Ann Arbor Stages III, IV; NCI Stage II)

The treatment experiences in patients with diffuse small lymphocytic lymphoma, diffuse small cleaved cell lymphoma, and diffuse intermediately differentiated lymphocytic lymphoma (or mantle zone lymphoma) are not extensive, and most of the information about these entities is hidden in larger studies of the more common indolent lymphoma types—follicular small cleaved cell and follicular lymphocytic lymphomas. There is no evidence that the rarer forms of indolent lymphomas (except for CTCL; see Chap. 51) require a distinct treatment approach from the more common follicular small cleaved cell and follicular mixed varieties. Thus the treatment issues are considered to be similar.

The optimal treatment approach to patients with advanced-stage indolent lymphoma is one of the most controversial areas in medical oncology. More than 20 years of painstaking clinical investigation have documented that advanced-stage follicular small cleaved cell lymphoma responds to single- and multiple-agent chemotherapy, radiation therapy, and combined modality treatment approaches; however, the responses are not durable, lasting for a median of around 2 years, with 10% or fewer patients with follicular small cleaved cell lymphoma remaining in remission for 5 years (reviewed in ref. 334). This is an unusual advanced malignancy, in that despite the absence of durable CR, median survival is more than 8 years in some series.[335] The capacity of patients to live so long with such short remissions implies that patients are living with disease. However, the paradox of this indolent lymphoma is that all patients ultimately die of their disease and do so on average more quickly and often than patients with more aggressive lymphomas.[336] There is no convincing evidence that combinations of drugs, with or without radiation therapy, can cure patients with advanced follicular small cleaved cell lymphoma.

In a randomized clinical trial conducted at Stanford, patients were assigned to receive either a single oral alkylating agent (chlorambucil) or CVP or CVP combined with total lymphoid irradiation.[337] Although the CR rate after the first 6 months of treatment was higher in the CVP group, by 4 years the single-agent CR rate was equivalent, and survival was not significantly different in any group at 5 years. Total body irradiation was not more effective than single-agent or combination chemotherapy,[338,339] nor was it superior when given together with CVP.[340] A number of other studies comparing CVP with single agents have also failed to demonstrate a significant advantage to the combination chemotherapy program.[341-343] One promising report by Cadman and colleagues[344] using high-dose pulses of chlorambucil (16 mg/m^2 orally each day for 5 days each month for 12 months) achieved a CR in 78% of 18 patients so treated, and with a median follow-up of nearly 3 years no relapses were reported. However, a recent follow-up report of this series of patients was less encouraging.[345] With a thorough application of careful restaging criteria, the CR rate was only 46% (11 of 24), and with longer follow-up (median 4.2 years) the median duration of remission is 28 months. Studies of maintenance therapies with drugs or immune stimulants have occasionally shown some prolongation of remissions, but never has this been shown to influence survival.[346]

In the midst of all the activity designed to compare various aggressive treatments, Rosenberg at Stanford quietly began managing a selected group of patients with no initial therapy.[325] His patients presented essentially without symptoms and often with a history of many months of gradually enlarging nontender adenopathy. Routinely the patients selected for no initial therapy remained asymptomatic for at least 2 months after their initial evaluation and some had advanced age, concurrent medical problems that made aggressive treatment somewhat riskier, or an extended prior history of spontaneously waxing and waning adenopathy. His criteria for initiating therapy were rapid progression of disease, development of B symptoms or cytopenias related to marrow replacement by disease, and the development of a site of disease that threatened the function of an organ.

The median time to requiring treatment among patients with advanced-stage follicular small cleaved cell lymphoma was 4 years, and the median actuarial survival for the conservatively managed group was 11 years. The actuarial overall survival curves did not differ significantly from those of two prospective randomized studies being carried out at Stanford at the same time, one comparing single-agent chemotherapy, combination chemotherapy, and total body irradiation,[338] and the other comparing the first two arms to combined modality therapy with chemotherapy plus total lymphoid irradiation.[337] Thus the data from conservatively treated patients make it difficult to discern an effect from aggressive treatment. As a result it has become routine to defer initial therapy in patients with advanced-stage follicular small cleaved cell lymphoma, and, when therapy is required by the appearance of progressive or troublesome symptoms, usually that therapy is single-alkylating agent therapy with chlorambucil, alkeran, or cyclophosphamide, with or without pulses of prednisone.

A number of findings color the catholicity of the Stanford

experience. First, many centers have found that their patients with follicular small cleaved cell lymphoma do not fare as well as the selected group of Stanford patients. Data collected in 1919 by Yates suggested that most patients require some form of therapy within the first 2 years of diagnosis.[347] In fact, there may be subsets of patients who, based on histology or clinical features, should be treated aggressively at diagnosis because of a more accelerated natural history. Frizzera and associates[348] found a median survival of only 40 months in patients with neoplastic plasma cells as a component of their follicular lymphoma. Straus and colleagues[349] found that patients with advanced-stage disease at Memorial Sloan-Kettering had a median survival of less than 5 years with conservative treatment. At St. Bart's, poor prognosis patients could be identified on the basis of the presence of B symptoms, anemia, abnormal liver function tests, and hepatosplenomegaly.[328] Thus there may be features associated with a more aggressive clinical course that would identify patients poorly served by conservative management.

In addition, there are certain disadvantages associated with the conservative approach.[336,350] Many patients are adversely affected by the constant and visible enlargement of lymph nodes, which serves as an ever-present reminder of their illness and the uncertainties associated with no therapy. When therapy is finally given, often it is in the form of chronic administration of daily oral alkylating agents with or without radiation therapy, treatment that seriously depletes the nonrenewable marrow stem cell pool[351,352] and can lead to subsequent intolerance to combination chemotherapy or, more seriously, to secondary acute leukemia or myelodysplastic syndromes.[353-356] Thus so-called conservative therapy may be associated with even greater iatrogenic problems than aggressive cyclic combination chemotherapy.

Also to be considered in the management of patients with advanced-stage follicular small cleaved cell lymphoma is the propensity of the disease to evolve to more aggressive lymphomas, especially diffuse large-cell lymphoma.[167,279] Such a transition occurs at a rate of about 8% per year, probably by evolving through follicular mixed and follicular large-cell stages first. When the histology changes, the natural history accelerates. However, by and large, the histologic subtypes to which follicular small cleaved cell lymphomas evolve usually have a higher likelihood of responding to combination chemotherapy with durable CR,[167,184,357] although this is not a universal finding.[358] This tendency to evolve is so pervasive that one autopsy series demonstrated that 95% of the patients with follicular lymphoma who died with lymphoma had undergone evolution to a diffuse histology.[359]

Furthermore, a number of recent studies suggest that improvements in therapy could well result in long-term disease-free survival in patients with advanced-stage follicular small cleaved cell lymphoma. The Stanford experience with total nodal irradiation in patients with laparotomy-documented Stage III disease is instructive.[360,361] The 10-year relapse-free survival of Stage III patients treated with radiation therapy was 40%. For those with so-called limited Stage III disease (no B symptoms, less than five sites of involvement, maximum size of disease <10 cm), the 15-year freedom from relapse was 88%.[361] Most patients relapsed in previously unirradiated lymph node groups, suggesting that the addition of epitrochlear, mesenteric, and Waldeyer's ring fields might have further improved the outcome. Studies by Cox and co-workers[362] and Flippen and associates[363] also suggest that 45% to 50% of patients with Stage III follicular small cleaved cell lymphoma can achieve CR lasting in excess of 5 years with radiation treatment.

The use of combination chemotherapy in patients with advanced-stage follicular small cleaved cell lymphoma has rarely gotten more aggressive than CVP. A feature of the response to CVP is that more than 70% of patients get a complete response, but patients relapse more or less continuously over time until by 5 years fewer than 10% are in remission. The sites of relapse from chemotherapy-induced CR are nearly always previously involved nodal sites of disease,[364] unlike radiation relapses, which occur in previously uninvolved and unirradiated sites. This observation forms the basis for the rationale for combined modality therapy. Radiation therapy appears extremely effective at eradicating disease within the beam field, and relapses occur because disease is disseminated. Combination chemotherapy is effective at eliminating sites of disease affected by subclinical levels of tumor load, but the bulk associated with involved nodes results in the persistence of disease even when the patient appears to be in CR.

The application of the more recent advances in lymphoma treatment (chiefly the new active regimens in diffuse large-cell lymphoma treatment) to patients with advanced-stage follicular small cleaved cell lymphoma has been slow; however, as a result of these treatment advances, the probability of long-term survival appears to be appreciably higher in patients with more virulent tumor. Isolated attempts at improving the chemotherapy treatment of the indolent lymphomas have now begun. The group at the Dana–Farber Cancer Institute used M-BACOD (methotrexate, bleomycin, doxorubicin, cyclophosphamide, vincristine, dexamethasone) in patients with advanced-stage follicular small cleaved cell lymphoma and obtained 5-year disease-free survival around 40%.[365] Case used a program called M-2, consisting of BCNU, cyclophosphamide, vincristine, melphalan, and prednisone, and obtained data projecting an 83% 5-year disease-free survival for complete responders.[366] The short duration of follow-up makes it difficult to be certain of the accuracy of that projection. The Eastern Cooperative Oncology Group demonstrated that the COPP regimen (cyclophosphamide, vincristine, procarbazine, prednisone) achieved CR in 56% of patients with advanced follicular small cleaved cell lymphoma, and 57% of the CR lasted more than 5 years.[367] Thus the results of treatment in advanced-stage follicular small cleaved cell lymphoma appear to be improving with the use of more active combination chemotherapy programs. However, the critics of the curative approach to indolent lymphoma treatment would point out that none of these improvements in CR rate or duration have as yet translated into survival advantages for treated patients. Because the median survival of even palliated patients is up to more than 8 years, such a stringent criterion for efficacy is time-consuming to meet. Nevertheless, it should be clear that survival without disease off all treatment is also an important goal, and the availability of a treatment approach that can achieve durable CR in most patients would probably change the clinical approach to these patients even before the demonstration of a survival advantage.

In an effort to examine the alternative approaches to indolent lymphoma treatment prospectively, the NCI is engaged in a prospective randomized study comparing conservative treatment (no initial therapy) with aggressive combined modality therapy with ProMACE/MOPP flexitherapy followed by low-dose total lymphoid radiation therapy. The patients randomized to receive initial treatment will test the hypothesis that the reason for the inability of drug combination programs to produce a significant fraction of long-term disease-free survivors is due to the failure in dose escalation. The group receiving no initial therapy is closely followed to determine the overall survival; the fraction of patients with indolent follicular lymphomas that can be followed without drug treatment; the number of patients that evolve to follicular mixed, or follicular or diffuse large-cell lymphoma over time; and the success of delayed aggressive treatment in achieving long-term disease-free survival. Clinically aggressive tumor masses are biopsied at intervals to determine the histology. If therapy is required and the histology remains follicular small cleaved cell lymphoma, small-field palliative radiation therapy is used as long as possible. If chemotherapy is required for control of systemic symptoms or for histologic evolution, patients are crossed over to the same treatment as those randomized to initial treatment—ProMACE/MOPP flexitherapy.

More than 100 patients have been entered on this study since 1978.[368] Eighty-six percent of all patients presenting with low-grade histologic subtypes were able to be randomized to aggressive therapy versus conservative therapy. The other 14% had serious enough symptoms at presentation that local treatment was not thought to be appropriate. Among the patients randomized to aggressive combination chemotherapy with ProMACE/MOPP flexitherapy (followed by 24 Gy total lymphoid irradiation for those achieving CR with chemotherapy), 78% achieved CR and 86% of those achieving CR remain in their initial remission with a median follow-up of more than 4 years. Keep in mind that the median remission duration in previous treatment programs was about 2 years. Thus, with median follow-up over twice as long as the average remission duration from previous treatments, only 14% of the complete responders have relapsed.

Of the patients randomized to conservative treatment, 56% have not required systemic treatment, although 39% have received some local radiation to control symptomatic local disease. The 44% of patients who have crossed over to receive aggressive therapy did so a median of 34 months after randomization. About 40% of those crossing over did so because of progressive systemic symptoms, 33% because of histologic conversion to diffuse large-cell or other aggressive lymphoma, and 27% because they had exhausted the limits of local irradiation for symptom control. When these patients were treated with ProMACE/MOPP flexitherapy, their CR rate was only 43%, appreciably less than those who received the therapy at diagnosis. Only two of the complete responders have relapsed, but there is not enough information as yet to predict whether the responses will be as durable with delayed treatment as with immediate treatment. Because the median survival of patients with low-grade lymphoma is about 7 to 9 years in previous NCI studies and the median follow-up on the current study is only about 4.5 years, there is no significant impact of immediate aggressive treatment on overall survival as yet. However, there is considerable difference between the two approaches in terms of patients alive and free of disease. Furthermore, it appears that improvements in therapy can result in prolonged disease-free survival in some patients with follicular and low-grade lymphomas.

The notion that emerges from this study is that aggressive therapy at diagnosis may be curative. Furthermore, it appears that delaying therapy until symptoms demand systemic intervention substantially reduces the chances for a successful treatment outcome. More data on the negative impact of delaying treatment were generated by a retrospective analysis of patients treated at the University of Chicago.[369] Initial aggressive therapy achieved a CR rate of 71%, but aggressive therapy delivered after initial conservative management achieved a CR rate of only 25%. Thus it would appear that delaying aggressive therapy results in some patients becoming less responsive to therapy. It may be that the decision about whether the treatment approach will be palliative or curative must be made at diagnosis. Failing to decide between these options initially is to decide, since palliation is all that can be done if the decision is delayed.

In conclusion, no initial therapy is an acceptable management approach to patients with advanced-stage follicular small cleaved cell lymphoma. However, there is mounting evidence that aggressive treatment at diagnosis may permit a large fraction of patients to enjoy prolonged *disease-free* survival. Patients under the age of 50 years for whom a median survival of 10 years or less represents a significant foreshortening of life expectancy; patients without intercurrent illness; patients with B symptoms, abnormal liver function tests, effusions, or other suggestions of more aggressive disease; and patients initially treated conservatively who undergo histologic conversion to a more aggressive lymphoma should probably receive treatment with a combination chemotherapy program like ProMACE/MOPP with or without total nodal irradiation for those who achieve CR (not necessary in patients with converted histology). The decision about whether to treat aggressively should not be indefinitely delayed after diagnosis. Postponing the decision until symptoms demand treatment appears to substantially reduce the efficacy of the treatment program. Those who believe that they must manage patients conservatively should consider the use of cyclical combination chemotherapy such as CVP to control the disease, since the use of chronic oral alkylating agents such as chlorambucil, although it is well tolerated, is associated with irreversible damage to the marrow stem cells, the possible development of a myelodysplasia or secondary leukemia, and a reduction in the capacity to deliver curative therapy if histologic progression should occur. CVP is not associated with such chronic marrow damage.

Although in the past advanced-stage follicular mixed lymphoma was subject to the same debate about management approach that currently affects follicular small cleaved cell lymphoma patients, it is no longer controversial that patients with Stage III or IV (NCI Stage II) follicular mixed lymphoma should be treated aggressively with curative intent from diagnosis. In the first place, it is clear that the conservative approach is not associated with prolonged survival of follicular mixed patients.[325] In addition, the benefits of the conservative approach in terms of the interval of freedom from therapy for patients with follicular mixed lymphoma are marginal (median time to treatment is only 16 months). Furthermore, the durability of chemotherapy-induced CR in patients with advanced-stage follicular mixed lymphoma initially reported from the NCI[346,370] has been confirmed in several other studies.[341,371,372] We obtained CR in 72% of Stage III or IV follicular mixed lymphoma patients using the C-MOPP regimen (cyclophosphamide, vincristine, procarbazine, prednisone), with the median duration of remissions lasting for about 7 years. At the M. D. Anderson Hospital CHOP-bleomycin followed by involved-field radiation therapy obtained CR in 74% of Stage III and 57% of Stage IV patients.[372] At 4 years 64% of the Stage III complete responders and 48% of the Stage IV complete responders remained free of disease. No patient with an initial LDH under 250 IU/ml relapsed more than 2 years after therapy. The NCI patients also demonstrated that high LDH, B symptoms, and marrow involvement were poor prognostic factors. Even the application of the more sophisticated measures of CR, such as the presence of circulating clonal excess, confirms that CR in follicular mixed lymphoma is durable and complete.[373] The circulating abnormal clone that is readily detectable in nearly 70% of patients with advanced-stage follicular lymphoma disappears with the achievement of clinical CR. In follicular small cleaved cell lymphoma clinical CR is often not accompanied by clearing the malignant clone, and it now appears that this is the harbinger of relapse.[374]

There has been little experience with the more recently developed lymphoma treatment programs in advanced-stage follicular mixed lymphoma, but, extrapolating from the effects of C-MOPP in diffuse large-cell lymphoma and the general correlation between the presence of a large-cell component and curability with combination chemotherapy, it seems likely that the second- and third-generation combination chemotherapy programs would be excellent therapy of advanced-stage follicular mixed lymphoma patients (see below).

The cell cycle kinetics of the individual histologic subtypes is rather distinct.[375] Follicular small cleaved cell lymphomas have the lowest growth fraction and the lowest percentage of cells expressing the transferrin receptor, a rough immunologic correlate of growth fraction. Follicular mixed lymphomas may have a higher growth fraction and more transferrin receptor–positive cells than do follicular small cleaved cell lymphomas, and the follicular and diffuse large-cell lymphomas have the highest growth fraction of tumors of follicular center cell origin. It has been observed in the study of the follicular lymphomas that as the fraction of large cells in the tumor rises, the growth fraction of the tumor increases, the clinical pace of disease becomes more rapid, and the tumor becomes more susceptible to eradication by combination chemotherapy. The behavior of the follicular lymphomas is analogous to bone marrow, another stem cell compartment with two stem cells. In this analogy the tumor has two stem cell populations, the small cleaved lymphocytic stem cell that is not in cycle, but is renewable and sensitive to inhibition but not eradication by combination chemotherapy, and a second stem cell that becomes more prominent as the fraction of large cells increases is nonrenewable, in cell cycle, and sensitive to combination chemotherapy.[357] Thus the explanation for both the more indolent growth and the more remote curability of the follicular small cleaved cell lymphomas relates to cell kinetics and the resistance of the stem cell. The analogy to bone marrow seems apt. Although most chemotherapeutic agents at conventionally tolerable doses can produce transient cytopenias, the marrow stem cell population nearly always fully recovers and repopulates the marrow to the normal level. Similarly, the stem cell for follicular small cleaved cell lymphoma nearly always responds to chemotherapy but continues to regrow and repopulate. A larger fraction of follicular mixed lymphoma patients are curable with combination chemotherapy, which correlates with the larger fraction of large cells and the kinetic advantage to treating a nonrenewable stem cell population. This model is speculative but has the advantage of accurately describing the clinical spectrum and response to treatment of the follicular lymphomas. In addition, if the stem cell compartment of follicular small cleaved cell lymphomas is analogous to that of the bone marrow, it is possible that treatment capable of ablating bone marrow might also ablate follicular lymphoma. This model thus provides conceptual support for treating follicular small cleaved cell lymphoma with a high-dose therapy perhaps with total body irradiation and autologous bone marrow support.

TREATMENT OF AGGRESSIVE LYMPHOCYTIC LYMPHOMAS

The aggressive lymphocytic lymphomas include follicular large-cell, diffuse large-cell (all varieties, including immunoblastic), and diffuse mixed lymphomas. They constitute about 60% of all lymphocytic lymphomas. The majority are of B-cell origin, but about 20% (including nearly 80% of the diffuse mixed lymphomas and some diffuse large-cell and immunoblastic tumors) are of T-cell origin and are sometimes called peripheral T-cell lymphomas. This term is not useful however, in that it does not describe a discrete clinicopathologic entity and conveys no useful prognostic information. In large series of patients treated homogeneously no prognostic significance is associated with lymphomas that express the markers of peripheral T cells.[202] Markers do influence the prognosis of the acute lymphocytic leukemias, which are more immature lymphoid neoplasms.[376]

Although the cell surface phenotype of aggressive lymphomas appears to have little to do with the clinical course of disease, a variety of clinical factors aside from Ann Arbor stage do. Most of the important prognostic factors for the aggressive lymphomas are surrogate measures of tumor burden and bulk.[203,377,378] Although different series vary somewhat in their criteria, nearly all investigators have found that patients with poor prognosis have the following features: poor performance status, one or more tumor masses more than 10 cm in diameter (especially involving the GI tract), multiple (usually more than two or three) extranodal sites of tumor, B symptoms, and serum LDH over 500 IU/ml. In series of patients in which the treatment for older patients is compromised because of age or age-related physiologic intolerance, age can be a prognostic factor. It is not clear whether older patients treated comparably to younger patients have a poorer prognosis. In the early chemotherapy studies male sex was an unexplained poor prognosis factor; however, more recent studies with more effective regimens and larger numbers of patients have not found male sex to be significantly associated with poorer treatment outcome. In general, as treatment has improved, certain factors previously found to negatively influence the prognosis (*e.g.*, bone marrow involvement, anemia) have been found to no longer exert a significant effect.

Treatment of Localized Aggressive Lymphomas

Historically, radiation therapy has been used as the primary modality of treatment for patients with localized aggressive lymphomas. Modern radiotherapeutic techniques for the treatment of lymphomas include the use of opposed- or multiple-field arrangements, treatment simulation, and contoured divergent blocks to protect normal tissue. Considerable local control data per radiation dose exist to aid in formulating a treatment plan for patients receiving radiation therapy alone.[379,380] The data are retrospective and not controlled for tumor bulk or disease response; however, usually 3500 to 4000 cGy delivered in fractionated doses over 4 to 5 weeks is sufficient to achieve local control in patients with follicular lymphoma. However larger doses may be required for patients with bulky tumors and those with a large-cell component to the histology. In the Stanford experience a substantial number of patients developed in-field relapses even with total doses of 5000 cGy.[379] At the Princess Margaret Hospital 80% of patients with medium or large bulky nodal involvement had local control of nodal disease after total doses of 4500 to 5000 cGy.[381]

The efficacy of involved-field radiation therapy in the treatment of patients with Ann Arbor Stage I, IE, II, or IIE aggressive lymphoma varies with the staging techniques used to define eligible patients. Studies in which patients underwent "clinical staging" (*e.g.*, no laparotomy to search for occult disease, occasional studies eschewed liver biopsy) report 5-year survival rates of 65% for Stage I or IE patients, but only 25% for Stage II or IIE patients.[382] On the other hand, Stage I patients whose staging includes laparotomy may have long-term survival approaching 100%.[383] The use of more sensitive noninvasive staging techniques such as CT scanning has improved the reliability of clinical staging to some degree. A more recent series of patients treated with radiation therapy alone had a 10-year relapse-free survival of 75%.[384] The Stanford group made an effort to improve on the outcome of radiation therapy by delivering treatment to nodal fields on both sides of the diaphragm.[377] Five-year disease-free survival rates were 67% for those receiving total or subtotal nodal radiation, but only 25% for those receiving involved-field radiation. For patients with three or more sites of involvement or bulky disease, the more extensive irradiation achieved 5-year survival rates of only 55%. Thus it would appear from these and other large studies from experienced treatment centers like the Joint Center for Radiation Therapy and the Princess Margaret Hospital that radiation therapy alone is most effective in patients whose staging has included exploratory laparotomy and who have small-volume disease in limited stages.

However, in the vast majority of clinical early-stage patients an exploratory laparotomy is not justified simply to decide whether they are treatable with radiation therapy alone. Other investigators have attempted to improve on the results obtained with radiation therapy alone and to save patients from the morbidity associated with exploratory laparotomy by adding combination chemotherapy to radiation therapy in clinically staged patients. Most of the clinically staged patients relapsing from a radiation-induced CR relapsed in sites not previously irradiated or known to be involved with lymphoma. Patients relapsing from large-field irradiation usually relapsed in extranodal sites, making it unlikely that more extensive irradiation would improve disease control.[377] It was presumed that failure to control the disease was due to undetected early systemic spread of disease that may have been controlled with combination chemotherapy.

Nearly all investigators who have used combined modality approaches to the treatment of early-stage aggressive lymphoma have confirmed that the addition of combination chemotherapy is associated with significantly improved results over radiation therapy alone, even when the chemotherapy regimen is not one of those successfully used in the treatment of advanced-stage aggressive lymphoma.[384a] The NCI of Milan randomized patients who had achieved CR with radiation therapy to receive chemotherapy consisting of six cycles of CVP or no further therapy. There was a significant advantage for clinical Stage I, IE, II, or IIE patients receiving the adjuvant chemotherapy (76% versus 45% 5-year disease-free survival).[330] Landberg and colleagues[331] demonstrated similar findings with the use of nine cycles of CVP. Nissen and colleagues[385] administered 6 weeks of induction chemotherapy with streptonigrin, vincristine, and prednisone given concurrently with radiation therapy followed by 3 years of maintenance chemotherapy. They achieved a 5-year disease-free survival of 88% with combined modality therapy, compared with only 32% 5-year disease-free survival from extended-field radiation therapy alone. However, the superiority of combined modality has not been universally supported by prospective randomized trials. The British National Lymphoma Investigation[386] and Stanford[387] have reported studies showing no difference between the outcome of treatment with radiation therapy alone and combined modality therapy. These studies, however, were most likely negative primarily because inadequate chemotherapy programs were used. In their recent retrospective analysis the Stanford investigators demonstrated that combined modality therapy using mainly cyclophosphamide, doxorubicin, vincristine, and prednisone (CHOP) as the chemotherapy component achieved better results than involved-field radiation therapy alone and was comparable to the results achieved with total nodal irradiation.[377] It is also important to avoid the use of chemotherapeutic agents known to synergize with radiation therapy in leukemogenesis, such as the nitrosoureas. Gomez and associates[388] detected some secondary acute leukemias in patients with early-stage aggressive lymphoma treated with total nodal radiation therapy plus chemotherapy with BCNU, nitrogen mustard, and CVP. The tragedy of such second tumors is that the nitrosoureas are not active and have no role in the treatment of aggressive lymphomas, and thus patients were subjected to toxicity without potential for benefit. Despite the second malignancies, the group receiving the combined modality treatment had a 66% disease-free survival rate at 6 years, significantly better than the 45% seen in patients treated with total nodal radiation therapy alone.

In any setting where radiation therapy alone is not adequate therapy, it is appropriate to evaluate chemotherapy alone. Only when neither modality alone is successful should the potential synergistic toxicities of combined modality therapy be considered acceptable. There is little information on the use of combination chemotherapy alone in patients with early-stage diffuse aggressive lymphoma. Cabanillas and co-workers[389] used CHOP combination chemotherapy in patients with Stage I or II disease. The Stage I patients had 100% 5-year relapse-free survival, and the Stage II patients had an 80% 5-year relapse-free survival. Miller and Jones[390] began therapy with CHOP alone and added radiation therapy to more than a third of the patients who were either responding slowly to chemotherapy or required significant dose reductions of chemotherapy because of bone marrow toxicity. Disease-free survival was 84% at 41 months.

The NCI group has been evaluating the efficacy of four cycles of combination chemotherapy with cyclophosphamide, doxorubicin, etoposide, nitrogen mustard, vincristine, procarbazine, and prednisone (ProMACE-MOPP, in which the doses of the myelotoxic drugs are lowered 20%–25% to reduce toxicity) followed by involved-field radiation therapy.[391] Thirty-nine of 41 patients (95%) achieved CR, and all have remained free of disease for a median follow-up period of more than 3 years. This is the first study to use a chemotherapy treatment program that is highly effective in patients with advanced-stage disease. In view of the nearly invariant principle that tumor response is inversely related to tumor burden, it is reasonable to explore in early-stage patients the use of the newer and more active combination chemotherapy programs developed for use in patients with advanced-stage disease. From the available data it appears that chemotherapy is at least as good as radiation therapy in the management of patients with Stage I or IE disease and is superior to radiation therapy in the management of patients with Stage II or IIE disease.

We recommend that patients with localized aggressive lymphoma *not* undergo staging laparotomy. Although the best treatment program has not been defined conclusively by prospective randomized trial, we would suggest that clinically staged early-stage patients with fewer than three sites of disease and no bulky masses receive either CHOP or modified ProMACE-MOPP combination chemotherapy for four to six cycles followed by involved-field radiation therapy if the response to therapy is sluggish (*i.e.*, residual disease is present after cycle 3). Patients with three or more sites of disease, any bulky mass (>10 cm), or other poor prognostic factor (see Table 50-11) should be managed similarly to patients with advanced-stage disease (see below).

Treatment of Advanced-Stage Aggressive Lymphomas

We define advanced-stage aggressive lymphoma as all Ann Arbor Stage III or IV patients plus those patients with Ann Arbor Stage II with one or more of the poor prognostic factors, such as three or more sites of disease, bulky disease, B symptoms, poor performance status, or high serum LDH levels. The treatment of choice for advanced-stage aggressive lymphoma is combination chemotherapy. The treatment for advanced-stage diffuse aggressive lymphomas has improved since the mid-1970s. Before the introduction of MOPP (nitrogen mustard, vincristine, procarbazine, prednisone) and C-MOPP (MOPP with cyclophosphamide replacing nitrogen mustard) by the NCI group, treatment for aggressive lymphomas was primarily single-agent chemotherapy and the 5-year survival was essentially zero. The first significant improvement in treatment outcome came with the use of MOPP and C-MOPP, which induced CR in about 45% of advanced-stage patients, and, amazingly, most patients who achieved CR have remained disease-free for periods up to 24 years.[160] After a median follow-up of nearly 15 years 37% of all treated patients remain free of disease. The durability of the CR was surprising in light of the previous experience with indolent lymphomas (*i.e.*, short remission durations) and the resistance of the aggressive lymphomas to single-agent chemotherapy. However, it has now been widely reproduced in a number of treatment centers and cooperative groups that patients with aggressive lymphomas are much more readily cured of disease than patients with indolent lymphomas. In fact, a patient with aggressive lymphoma has a much higher likelihood of surviving 10 years than a patient with an indolent lymphoma. Research on the development of curative programs for indolent lymphoma has proceeded much more slowly at least in part because of the widespread use of a palliative approach to its management.

On the other hand, treatment programs for aggressive lymphoma have progressed to the point that more than 60% of patients with advanced-stage disease are being cured (Tables 50-14 and 50-15). The treatments have become more intensive, but the minor increase in toxicity has been accompanied by substantial increases in the fraction of patients achieving CR. Unlike in the indolent lymphomas, achieving CR is the only path to prolonged survival with the aggressive lymphomas. Survival with disease in aggressive lymphoma is short.

Initial attempts to improve the treatment programs focused on adding active agents to cyclophosphamide, vincristine, and prednisone. Two regimens named BACOP were developed by adding bleomycin and doxorubicin in slightly different doses and schedules.[392–394] Neither regimen achieved results that were significantly better than those seen with C-MOPP, both were more toxic, and the similarity of results with C-MOPP and BACOP was even documented in a prospective randomized trial.[395]

At about the same time that C-MOPP was reported, Bertino and his colleagues at Yale were developing a program called COMLA,[396] which was devised on the basis of somewhat different assumptions than those underlying C-MOPP. In COMLA a very high dose of cyclophosphamide (1.5 g/m^2)

TABLE 50-14. The Most Active Chemotherapy Programs in Intermediate-Grade Lymphoma

ProMACE-MOPP Flexitherapy	*Day 1*	*Day 8*	*Day 15*	*Days 16–28*
				No therapy
Cyclophosphamide 650 mg/m² IV	x	x		
Doxorubicin 25 mg/m² IV	x	x		
Etoposide 120 mg/m² IV	x	x		
Methotrexate 1.5 mg/m² IV			x with leucovorin rescue	
Prednisone 60 mg/m² PO	x-	---	-x	

Flexible number of cycles until complete response or decreased rate of response, then switch to:

	Day 1	*Day 8*	*Day 14*	*Days 15–28*
				No therapy
Nitrogen mustard 6 mg/m² IV	x	x		
Vincristine 1.4 mg/m² IV	x	x		
Procarbazine 100 mg/m PO	x-	---	-x	
Prednisone 60 mg/m² PO	x-	---	-x	

Same number of cycles as ProMACE, then restart ProMACE.

m-BACOD	*Day 1*	*Day 8*	*Day 15*	*Days 16–21*
				No therapy
Cyclophosphamide 600 mg/m² IV	x			
Doxorubicin 45 mg/m² IV	x			
Vincristine 1 mg/m² IV	x			
Bleomycin 4 mg/m² IV	x			
Methotrexate 200 mg/m² IV		x rescue	x with leucovorin rescue	
Dexamethasone 6 mg/m² PO	xxxxx			

COP-BLAM	*Day 1*	*Day 10*	*Day 14*	*Days 15–21*
				No therapy
Cyclophosphamide 400 mg/m² IV	x			
Doxorubicin 40 mg/m² IV	x			
Vincristine 1 mg/m² IV	x			
Procarbazine 100 mg/m² PO	x-	-x		
Prednisone 40 mg/m²	x-	-x		
Bleomycin 15 mg IV			x	

COP-BLAM III	*Day 1*	*Day 2*	*Day 3*	*Day 4*	*Day 5*
		Cycle A			
Vincristine 1 mg/m²/day IV infusion	x-	-x			
Bleomycin 7.5 mg/m² IV bolus, then 7.5 mg/m²/day IV infusion	x-	---	---	---	-x
Cyclophosphamide 350 mg/m² IV	x				
Doxorubicin 35 mg/m² IV	x				
Prednisone 40 mg/m² PO	x	x	x	x	x
Procarbazine 100 mg/m² PO	x	x	x	x	x

Cycle B

Like Cycle A without bleomycin and without day 2 of vincristine infusion

Week	1	3	7	10	13	16	19	22	25	28	31	34
Cycle	A	B	A	B	A	B	A	B	A	B	A	B

CAP-BOP	*Day 1*	*Day 7*	*Day 15*	*Day 21*
Cyclophosphamide 650 mg/m² IV	x			
Doxorubicin 50 mg/m² IV	x			
Procarbazine 100 mg/m² PO	x-	-x		
Vincristine 1.4 mg/m²			x	
Bleomycin 10 U/m² SC			x	
Prednisone 100 mg PO			x-	-x

Cycles repeated every 3–4 weeks

(continued)

TABLE 50-14. The Most Active Chemotherapy Programs in Intermediate-Grade Lymphoma (*continued*)

ProMACE-CytaBOM	*Day 1*	*Day 8*	*Day 14*	*Days 15–21*
Cyclophosphamide 650 mg/m² IV	x			No therapy
Doxorubicin 25 mg/m² IV	x			
Etoposide 120 mg/m² IV	x			
Cytarabine 300 mg/m² IV		x		
Bleomycin 5 mg/m² IV		x		
Vincristine 1.4 mg/m² IV		x		
Methotrexate 120 mg/m² IV		x with leucovorin rescue		
Prednisone 60 mg/m² PO	x- - - - - - - - - -	- - - - - - - - - - - - -	- - - - - -x	
Cotrimoxazole 2 PO b.i.d. throughout 6 cycles of therapy				

MACOP-B Week	1	2	3	4	5	6	7	8	9	10	11	12
Cyclophosphamide 350	x		x		x		x		x		x	
Doxorubicin 50 mg/m² IV	x		x		x		x		x		x	
Vincristine 1.4 mg/m² IV		x		x		x		x		x		x
*Methotrexate 400 mg/m² IV		x				x				x		
Bleomycin 10 mg/m² IV				x				x				x
Prednisone 75 mg/m² PO o.d.	x- - -	- - -	- - -	- - -	- - -	- - -	- - -	- - -	- - -	- - -	- - -	taper
Cotrimoxazole 2 PO b.i.d.	x- - -	- - -	- - -	- - -	- - -	- - -	- - -	- - -	- - -	- - -	- - -	x

*With leucovorin rescue

was given on day 1 of a 12-week cycle, vincristine was given on days 8 and 15, and weekly doses of the antimetabolites cytosine arabinoside and methotrexate were given for the next 8 weeks. The basic principle was to achieve rapid antitumor effects with the cyclophosphamide and to suppress the outgrowth of dividing cells with the antimetabolites while the marrow was recovering from the cyclophosphamide. This "hit-and-hold" strategy was able to produce long-term disease-free survival and initially had CR rates around 58%.[397] With more prolonged follow-up, however, the treatment outcome was no better than that obtained with C-MOPP.[398] Efforts to improve on COMLA by adding doxorubicin (ACOMLA) have only modestly augmented response rates and survival.[399]

A third line of development in the first generation or first quantum of effective treatment programs also came to light in the mid-1970s. Based on Phase II studies with single-agent doxorubicin, McKelvey and his colleagues[400] developed the CHOP regimen. CHOP gained immediate acceptance in the medical community because it had the highest CR rate (58%) of any regimen reported at that time, it was easy to give (a cycle required only a single office visit each month to deliver intravenous cyclophosphamide, vincristine, and doxorubicin on day 1, and oral prednisone was given for 5 days), and it was easy to take (minimal nausea, only moderate bone marrow toxicity). The initial reports seemed to show, however, that 50% or more of the complete responders had relapsed within the first 2 years, and this was much higher than the relapse rate reported for C-MOPP- and BACOP-induced complete responders. There was concern that the durability of the responses would be limited. Coltman and his colleagues[401] have recently reviewed the experience of the Southwest Oncology Group in which more than 400 patients were treated with CHOP-based programs. The CR rate is 53%, and 30% of all treated patients achieved durable CR with no relapses after 7 years. Armitage and his colleagues[402] have obtained similar results. Efforts to improve on the results with CHOP by adding bleomycin, levamisole, and bacille Calmette-Guérin have had no significant impact on treatment outcome.[403] A large number of CHOP

TABLE 50-15. Prospect for Long-term Survival from More Recent Treatment Programs for Diffuse Aggressive Lymphoma

Regimen	*Complete Responses (CR)*	*Relapse Rate (RR)*	*Potential for Long-term Survival (CR) × (1-RR)*
ProMACE/MOPP flexitherapy	60/75 (80%)	21/60 (35%)	52%
m-BACOD	59/86 (70%)	15/59 (25%)	52%
COP-BLAM	24/33 (73%)	4/24 (17%)	61%
CAP-BOP	37/51 (73%)	11/37 (30%)	51%
COP-BLAM III	43/51 (84%)	4/43 (9%)	76%
MACOP-B	104/125 (84%)	23/104 (21%)	66%
ProMACE-CytaBOM	80/95 (84%)	20/80 (25%)	63%

These studies were conducted and reported at different times. Thus the relapse rates cannot be considered to have reached the maximal level, since the denominators probably still include at least some patients who remain at risk of relapse. Therefore, the calculated potential for long-term disease-free survival for these treatment programs is likely to overestimate the actual potential for cure in some studies, particularly those with the shortest actual patient follow-up.

variants have been developed (*e.g.*, CHOP-bleomycin, CHOP-methotrexate), but none is superior to CHOP alone.[404]

Several other programs less effective than C-MOPP, CHOP, and COMLA have been developed, but they need not be discussed. It would seem valid to lump together MOPP, C-MOPP, BACOP, COMLA, and CHOP and its variants into the first generation of treatment programs. Each regimen appears to be capable of inducing CR in around 50% of patients, and about a third of all patients with advanced-stage aggressive lymphoma appear to be cured by each of them. The vast majority of patients relapsing from CR did so within the first 2 years after completion of treatment, and relapse was nearly always accompanied by death within a few months.

The second step resulting in treatment progress in advanced-stage aggressive lymphoma began with the second generation of treatment programs in the late 1970s. Different research groups set out in quite different directions, yet, like the first-generation programs, the second-generation programs achieved similar rates of success despite their disparate hypotheses. The Dana–Farber Cancer Institute was influenced by the observation that 40% of the patients relapsing from BACOP as they devised it developed CNS disease. Because of the efficacy of systemic high-dose methotrexate in the treatment of CNS lymphoma and the use of dexamethasone (rather than prednisone) to reduce CNS edema in brain tumors (there is little rationale for the choice of one corticosteroid over another), Skarin and his colleagues[405] added high-dose methotrexate (3 g/m^2) and substituted dexamethasone for prednisone in BACOP to get the M-BACOD regimen. M-BACOD induced CR in about 75% of patients, and around 55% appear to be cured. CNS relapse was not a problem with this regimen. Because of the difficulty of administering high-dose methotrexate at 3 g/m^2 in the practice of oncology, Skarin and co-workers lowered the dose of methotrexate to 200 mg/m^2 and administered the drug on days 8 and 15 of the monthly cycle instead of only on day 15 (see Table 50-14). The new regimen was called m-BACOD (to distinguish it from M-BACOD), and, although the follow-up is shorter, it appears that m-BACOD and M-BACOD achieve comparable results but that m-BACOD produces more mucositis and pulmonary infiltrates.[406]

Laurence and colleagues[407] at the New York Hospital also chose to build on BACOP, but took a different tack. They shortened the treatment cycle to 3 weeks and added 10 days of oral procarbazine, which was a component of the first-generation programs MOPP and C-MOPP. Thus they created a six-drug program called COP-BLAM with cyclophosphamide, doxorubicin, and vincristine given intravenously on day 1, prednisone and procarbazine orally for 10 days, and bleomycin given intravenously on day 14. Of their 33 patients, 73% achieved CR, and the plateau of the survival curve appeared to be around 55%.

The NCI group took a different approach. The Norton–Simon hypothesis on the development of drug resistance influenced them to consider individualizing treatment on the basis of the rate of response. The Norton–Simon hypothesis proposed that as a tumor shrinks, there is an increase in the fraction of the remaining tumor cells that might be drug-resistant.[408] Thus smaller tumors may be more resistant to therapy than the tumor at presentation. One should be able to gauge the development of resistance by looking at the rate of tumor response. As the response rate slows and resistance is apparently emerging, one could switch therapy to a combination regimen to which the tumor had not been exposed and to which it was not resistant. Keep in mind that this idea predates the discovery of pleiotropic drug resistance, a phenomenon in which the induction of a single gene conveys resistance to a number of chemically unrelated drugs and the existence of which calls into question the assumption of non-cross-resistance.

Nevertheless, the ProMACE/MOPP flexitherapy scheme was devised based on the idea that a new five-drug program called ProMACE (cyclophosphamide, doxorubicin, and etoposide intravenously on days 1 and 8, prednisone orally on days 1 through 14, high-dose methotrexate intravenously on day 15 with leucovorin rescue) would be delivered for a flexible number of cycles based on the rate of tumor response.[409] Patients whose *rate* of response slowed in response to ProMACE were switched on their next cycle to MOPP chemotherapy, which contained three drugs to which their tumors had not been exposed and, it was hoped, to which the tumors were not resistant. After achieving CR or after the rate of response to MOPP slowed, patients were switched back to ProMACE in an effort to consolidate CR. Although it sounds difficult to gauge the rate of response for individual patients, operationally it was not difficult, and most patients received either two cycles of ProMACE, two of MOPP, and two more of ProMACE, or three cycles of each phase of treatment.

CR was obtained in 77% of patients with Stage III or IV disease. With a median follow-up of more than 6 years, one-third of the patients have relapsed and about half appear to be cured of disease. About 25% of the relapses occurred more than 2 years after therapy, and these patients by and large recurred with indolent lymphoma by histology and clinical course. These results are certainly superior to those obtained with first-generation treatment programs (Fig. 50-8A), but what do the results teach us about the hypothesis on which the program is based? First, about half the patients who achieved CR did so in the first (ProMACE) phase of treatment, about 25% of the complete responders went into remission in the second (MOPP) phase, and 15% went in with the final ProMACE consolidation phase. In 10% of the complete responders we could not tell precisely when the remission was achieved. If patients who respond more slowly to treatment have more resistant disease, as has been suggested in one carefully done study[324] and as predicted by the Norton–Simon hypothesis, one might expect that the relapse rate would be higher for patients who achieve remission later in treatment than for those who achieve remission in the initial phase of treatment. In fact, there appear to be no significant differences in the relapse rate when one examines the phase of treatment in which those who relapsed entered remission. Thus the results do not confirm one of the predictions of the Norton–Simon hypothesis. The ProMACE/MOPP flexitherapy program is better than C-MOPP, but probably because of the incorporation of etoposide, methotrexate, nitrogen mustard, and doxorubicin

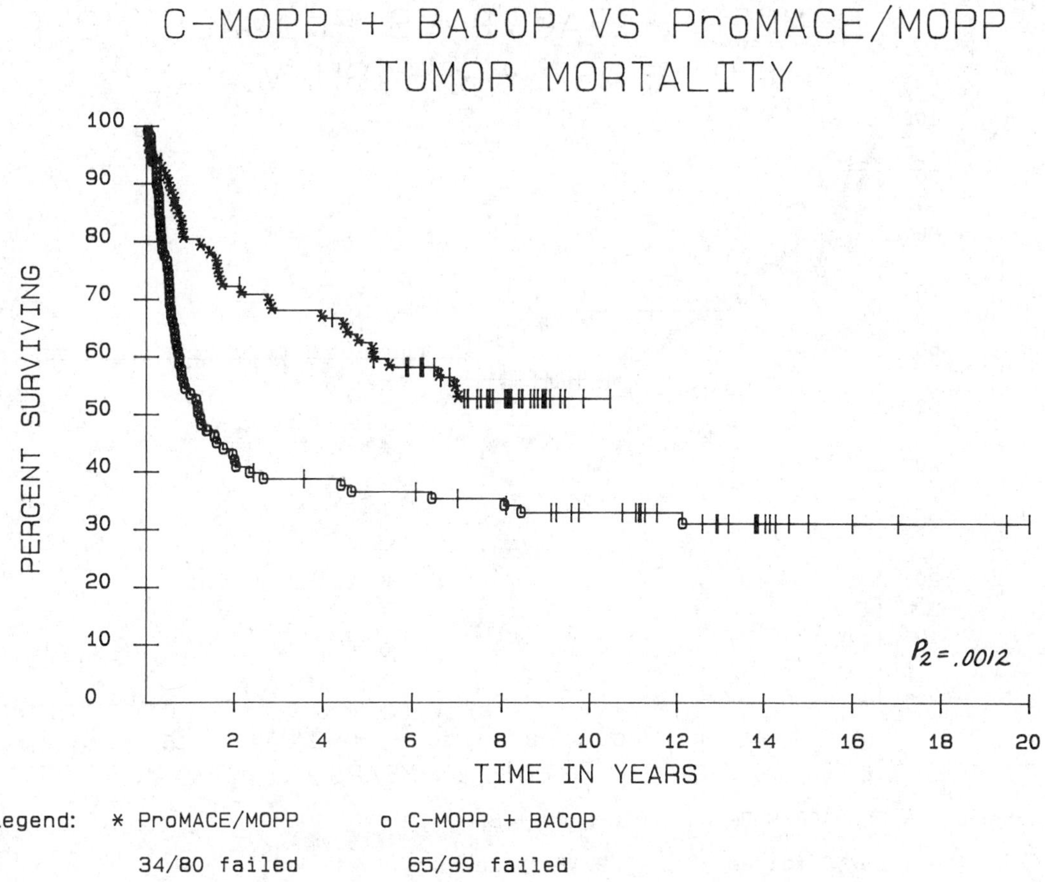

A

FIG. 50-8. Tumor mortality of all patients (**A**) and disease-free survival of diffuse lymphoma patients achieving complete remission with ProMACE/MOPP flexitherapy versus C-MOPP or BACOP. Tumor mortality is significantly lower with the use of ProMACE/MOPP flexitherapy. *(continued)*

rather than because of the unique manner in which it was administered.

Cabanillas and colleagues[410] also attempted to alter the timing of administration of agents to minimize the emergence of drug resistance. Patients were given three cycles of CHOP chemotherapy, and those who did not attain CR were switched to HOAP-bleo, in which cytosine arabinoside and bleomycin substitute for cyclophosphamide. Patients who achieve CR with initial CHOP get OAP-bleo (HOAP-bleo without doxorubicin). Those who complete CHOP and HOAP-bleo then receive IMVP-16 (ifosphamide, methotrexate, etoposide) either as consolidation of CR or as salvage. The CR rate for advanced-stage patients was over 70%. About 80% of CR occurred with initial CHOP therapy, and only 4 of 11 patients receiving HOAP-bleo in the setting of persistent disease achieved CR. There are no data on the durability of the responses based on the phase of treatment in which remission was obtained; however, it is projected that about 50% of advanced-stage patients may be cured by this program.

Thus, with the addition of a larger number of active drugs to the treatment programs, it appears that the second generation of treatment programs for diffuse aggressive lymphoma (M-BACOD, m-BACOD, COP-BLAM, ProMACE/MOPP flexitherapy, CHOP-HOAP-bleo-IMVP-16) are capable of obtaining CR in about 75% of all patients and about half of them are rendered permanently disease-free. These apparent improvements must be carefully examined because these regimens have not been compared in prospective randomized trials and are, therefore, subject to the problems associated with the use of historical controls. Median follow-up varies among studies, and all have included patients less than 2 years from remission induction who must be considered at risk for relapse. Some studies have included Stage I or Stage II patients, or both, who may have a more favorable prognosis, and some have added radiation therapy to sites of bulk disease, a practice that has not been prospectively evaluated and should be discouraged until data support its use. The studies vary in their criteria for patient selection and stratification for known prognostic factors. Despite these potential drawbacks, we believe that the improved remission rates and the consistent durability of remission represent real progress over the first-generation regimens. At the NCI the major difference between the first- and second-generation programs is in the fraction of patients achieving CR. As shown in Figure 50-8B, once remission is achieved, there

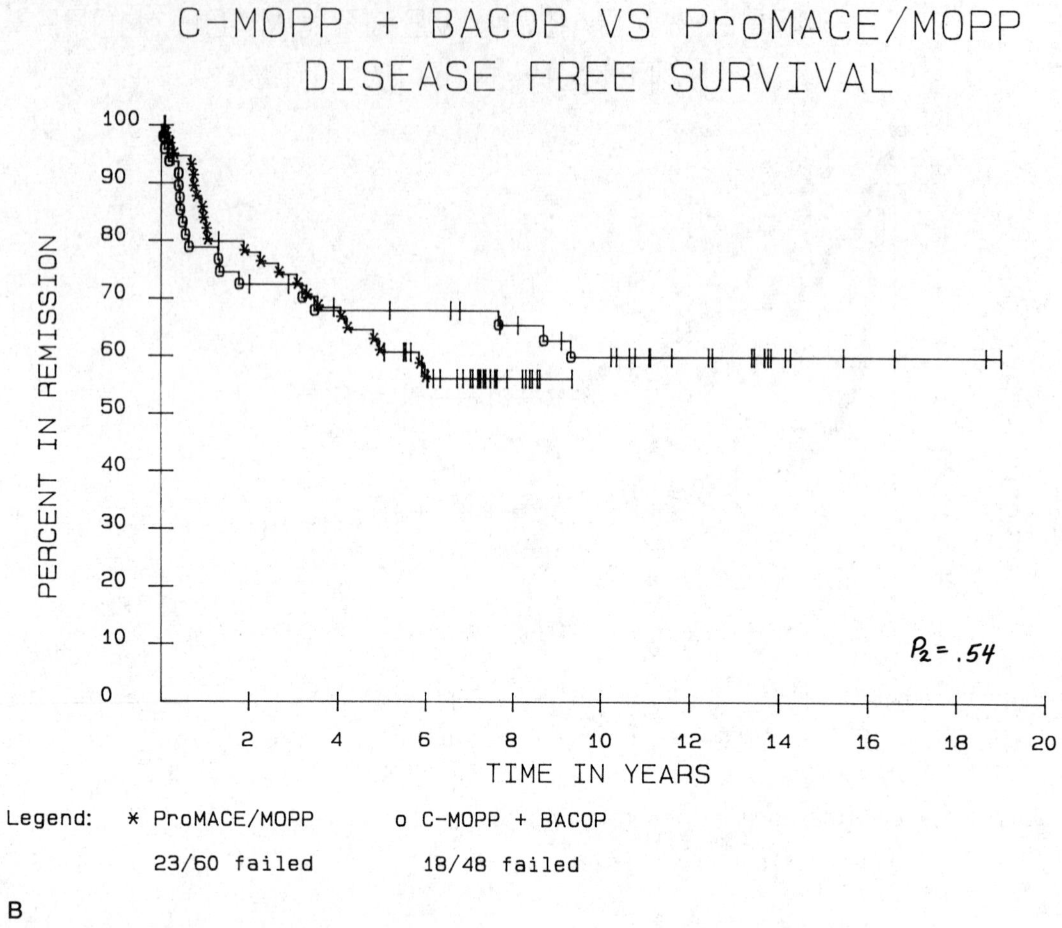

FIG. 50-8 (*continued*). In (**B**), the percentage of patients remaining in their initial chemotherapy-induced complete remission is plotted against time in years from the end of therapy for patients treated with ProMACE/MOPP flexitherapy versus C-MOPP or BACOP. The data suggest that the major difference in outcome between the first and second generation treatment programs is in the fraction of patients achieving complete remission. Once complete remission has been achieved, the probability of remaining free of disease is similar between the regimens. *, ProMACE-MOPP (23 of 60 failed); O, C-MOPP-BACOP (18 of 48 failed).

appears to be no difference in the likelihood of relapse and cure. The improvement in the overall survival between the two programs appears to be solely related to the ability of patients who previously fell in a poor prognostic category to attain CR with the newer programs.

The dominant ideas that have guided the design of the newer third-generation chemotherapy regimens for diffuse aggressive lymphoma are the Goldie-Coldman hypothesis[411] and the Hryniuk dose-intensity hypothesis.[412] Like the Norton-Simon hypothesis, the Goldie-Coldman hypothesis seeks to explain the emergence of drug resistance and to use the explanation in the design of combination chemotherapy treatment programs. Goldie and Coldman drew an analogy between the emergence of drug resistance in tumors and bacteriophage resistance. Delbruck and Luria demonstrated in 1943 that bacteriophage resistance did not occur as a *consequence* of exposure to bacteriophage, but mutation to bacteriophage resistance occurred spontaneously in the bacteria population at a defined frequency and became detectable only under the selective influence of bacteriophage exposure. As applied to tumor biology, the notion would be that drug resistance in tumors does not occur as a consequence of treatment but that each tumor has an intrinsic rate of spontaneous mutation to drug resistance. Those tumors curable with chemotherapy have a low rate of mutation to resistance, and those that are not have a high rate. A major assumption of the Goldie-Coldman hypothesis is that distinct genetic events (mutations) are needed to acquire resistance to separate agents. Here again, the phenomenon of pleiotropic drug resistance presents a difficulty for this theory, since it appears that the activation of one or a small number of genes can convey resistance to a number of structurally unrelated agents. Nevertheless, if one can assume that mutations conveying resistance to some drugs will not convey cross-resistance to others, the Goldie-Coldman hypothesis would predict that a larger fraction of patients with diffuse aggressive lymphomas could be cured if the patients were exposed to the largest possible number of active agents at full dose as early as possible in the treatment course.

The Hryniuk dose-intensity hypothesis is based on a review of treatment outcome in patients with metastatic breast cancer, adjuvant breast cancer, and ovarian cancer. Hryniuk found that treatment outcome was related to the dose-intensity of the treatment programs as measured by the number of milligrams of a particular agent given per week. The introduction of a time frame for agent administration is an important feature of the idea. It has long been appreciated in animal models of cancer treatment that there is a dose–response relation in the successful treatment of responsive tumors. The predictions from the analysis of results obtained in breast cancer and ovarian cancer were that the best chance for obtaining CR will occur when a maximum *rate* of drug delivery is maintained. An oversimplified amalgamation of both ideas is that the use of more drugs at higher doses administered as soon as possible and as frequently as possible will achieve the best results.

The NCI group has tested the Goldie–Coldman hypothesis for advanced-stage diffuse aggressive lymphomas. Because we had treatment experience with ProMACE/MOPP flexitherapy in which ProMACE and MOPP were given in distinct months of the treatment cycle, we believed that the Goldie–Coldman hypothesis would predict the achievement of superior results when the agents of ProMACE/MOPP flexitherapy were used in the same month. Therefore, we tested ProMACE/MOPP days 1 through 8, a program in which cyclophosphamide, doxorubicin, and etoposide are given intravenously on day 1, nitrogen mustard and vincristine are given intravenously on day 8, prednisone is given orally on days 1 through 14, procarbazine is given orally on days 8 through 14, and high-dose methotrexate is given on day 15 of a 28-day treatment cycle.[413] The early results of this treatment program are quite similar to the results obtained with ProMACE/MOPP flexitherapy. About 78% of patients have achieved CR. Certainly giving the drugs in the same month is not superior to giving the drugs in separate monthly cycles. Thus this particular application of the predictions of the Goldie–Coldman hypothesis does not appear to result in an improved treatment outcome. This does not imply that the Goldie-Coldman hypothesis is not correct. The hypothesis is based on a fundamental principle of biology that is irrefutable. However, it may be that we do not have the appropriate agents to exploit the biology, or that by the time patients come to clinical attention, the genetic patterns of resistance are unalterably established. Certainly the Goldie–Coldman hypothesis provides important guidelines for study design that permit much more to be learned from both positive and negative results than protocols empirically designed.

There have been a number of recent attempts to improve treatment outcome through manipulations that augment dose intensity. Baer and co-workers[414] doubled the dose intensity of the cyclophosphamide in COMLA by shortening the cycle to 6 weeks instead of 12. In a small number of patients the CR rate was increased to 80%, and 25% of the complete responders had relapsed with a median follow-up of 26 months. Conclusions are difficult to draw because of the liberal use of radiation therapy, the small number of patients, and the sporadic use of CHOP chemotherapy as consolidation. Nevertheless, the results appear to be superior to those obtained with conventional COMLA and provide support for the idea that maximizing dose intensity may be effective in improving treatments.

Improving the dose intensity of CHOP-bleo did not appear to improve the treatment outcome in a series of patients treated at the M. D. Anderson Hospital.[415] Nonconcurrent series of patients were treated with either conventional doses or maximally tolerated doses of CHOP-bleo. The conventional-dose regimen had a dose intensity of about 80% of the high-dose regimen. Yet the CR rates (75% conventional, 81% high-dose) and overall survival (53% conventional, 48% high-dose) were not significantly different. Because the study was not randomized it is possible that the imbalance in prognostic factors (*e.g.*, there were more Stage I patients on the conventional-dose scheme) contributed to the apparent lack of differences. On the other hand, for CHOP-bleo, 20% differences in dose intensity may not be adequate to augment the treatment outcome. Certainly there are plateaus on some dose–response curves.

There are now four third-generation treatment protocols that appear to have further advanced the standard of expected results. CR rates in excess of 80% with cure of about two-thirds of all patients have been achieved in the most recent protocols. Their major focus was not the addition of new agents, the change apparently most responsible for the second major treatment advance, but the alteration of doses and schedules to augment dose intensity. Coleman and co-workers[416,417] at the New York Hospital formulated COP-BLAM III, a regimen that alters the delivery of vincristine and bleomycin by administering continuous infusions of these agents for 2 and 5 days, respectively, while alternating during every other cycle with bolus vincristine and delivering the other four agents similarly to the original COP-BLAM. CR was obtained in 84% of patients, and the plateau in the survival curve is projected at 70%.

Preliminary results with three other regimens, MACOP-B, ProMACE-CytaBOM, and F-MACHOP, suggest that the use of high doses of many drugs early in intensive short-course treatments will indeed improve results. MACOP-B consists of six drugs.[418,419] Treatment is given weekly for only 12 weeks in which cyclophosphamide and doxorubicin are alternated with vincristine and methotrexate or bleomycin. Prednisone and cotrimoxazole are given orally throughout the 12 weeks of therapy. ProMACE-CytaBOM consists of eight drugs: cyclophosphamide, doxorubicin, and etoposide are given on day 1; cytosine arabinoside, bleomycin, vincristine, and methotrexate are given on day 8; prednisone is given on days 1 through 14, and cycles last for 3 weeks.[413] Cotrimoxazole is given throughout the 17 weeks of therapy. Treatment is given 2 weeks out of 3 for six cycles. F-MACHOP consists of seven drugs (5-fluorouracil, methotrexate, cytosine arabinoside, cyclophosphamide, doxorubicin, vincristine, and prednisone) administered sequentially within the first 3 days of a 3- or 4-week cycle.[420] Thus MACOP-B emphasizes dose intensity; F-MACHOP, early exposure to around twice as many drugs as the usual regimen; and ProMACE-CytaBOM, both dose intensity and more drugs. All three programs achieve CR in 80% or more of patients and only about 20% of complete responders have relapsed within the first 2 years. If these results hold true with longer follow-up, two-thirds of patients may be cured.

Where do we go from here? Perhaps the best approach to charting our path is to carefully analyze what we have learned up to now. In order to compare the dose intensity of each of the three generations of combinations for diffuse aggressive lymphomas in some relevant way, we have used

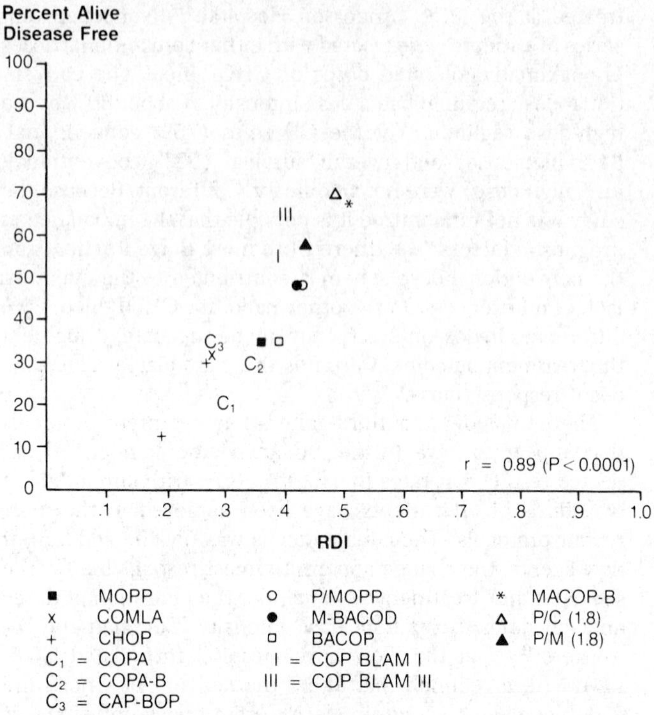

FIG. 50-9. Relation between normalized 9-drug relative dose intensity and disease-free survival in diffuse large cell lymphomas. The 14 most extensively studied treatment programs for diffuse large cell lymphomas use 9 different drugs in some permutation. Each of the 14 regimens was evaluated for its relative dose intensity based on delivery of full doses of all 9 drugs. Of course, none of the programs achieved such an ideal because they used from 4 to 8 drugs. The regimen that had the highest relative dose intensity was MACOP-B. Its dose intensity was arbitrarily rated as 1, and the other regimens were normalized to MACOP-B, thus giving a normalized 9-drug relative dose intensity. The long-term survival of each regimen was plotted against the normalized 9-drug relative dose intensity. A statistically significant correlation was found between dose intensity and disease-free survival.

the method of Hryniuk and Bush to calculate dose intensity of each drug and the average dose intensity of the combinations of drugs. However, because there are nine drugs in use in various ways in the combinations, we have constructed as a standard of comparison a hypothetical nine-drug combination regimen that would use all of the drugs in full doses continuously.[421] The dose intensity of drugs in the various treatment programs is calculated as the decimal fraction of the dose in the hypothetical combination over the same time frame. A zero is assigned to a drug that is omitted from a combination. A value of one has been assigned to methotrexate in all studies analyzed, since although it is used at varying doses in the different programs, all use it at doses that require leucovorin rescue. In addition, steroids are assigned a value of one. When comparisons among programs are made excluding methotrexate and prednisone from the combinations, the average dose intensity changes but the ranking of the programs is not altered. To examine the effect of the three major drugs used in the first-generation programs, compared with second- and third-generation programs, we also calculated two- and three-drug average dose intensities for doxorubicin and cyclophosphamide with and without vincristine separately from the nine-drug dose intensity. It must be kept in mind that these are the *projected* values for dose intensity, not *actual* dose intensity, since the actual amount of drug delivered and the time frame in which it was delivered are never given when results of treatment outcome are reported. The data are depicted in Figure 50-9 and Table 50-16.

Newer regimens have the highest relative dose intensity, and there appears to be a strong correlation between the nine-drug relative dose intensity and outcome (r-0.82, $p < 0.0008$). There was no significant correlation between outcome and two- or three-drug relative dose intensity. The success of the third-generation programs appears to be related to the use of more drugs, early exposure to non-cross-resistant agents, and the high dose intensity. The effects of dosing can be ascertained within some programs. For example, Figure 50-10 shows the impact of dosing on outcome in the CHOP program. This first-generation program may cure a significantly greater fraction of patients treated with full

TABLE 50-16. Two-, Three-, and Nine-Drug Relative Dose Intensities of 11 Primary Programs for Diffuse Aggressive Lymphomas

Regimen	*Duration of Treatment (mo)*	*Percentage of Long-term Survival*	*Percentage of Standard*	*RDI* 9 Drugs	*RDI* 3 Drugs	*RDI* 2 Drugs	*Drug Exposure During First 2 Weeks*
MACOP-B	3	69	1.0	0.51	0.78	0.74	5/6
ProMACE/CytaBOM (1.8)	4.5	70	0.94	0.48	0.50	0.46	8/8
ProMACE/MOPP (1.8)	6	58	0.86	0.44	0.52	0.56	6/7
ProMACE/MOPP	8	48	0.84	0.43	0.50	0.60	5/7
M-BACOD	7	48	0.82	0.42	0.51	0.56	5/6
COP BLAM III	9	65	0.78	0.40	0.58	0.56	6/6
BACOP	6	35	0.76	0.39	0.75	0.69	3/5
COP BLAM I	6	55	0.76	0.39	0.43	0.44	6/6
MOPP	6	35	0.71	0.36	0.58	0.44	4/4
COMLA	9	<33	0.55	0.28	0.25	0.17	2/4
CHOP	6	<30	0.51	0.26	0.46	0.50	4/4

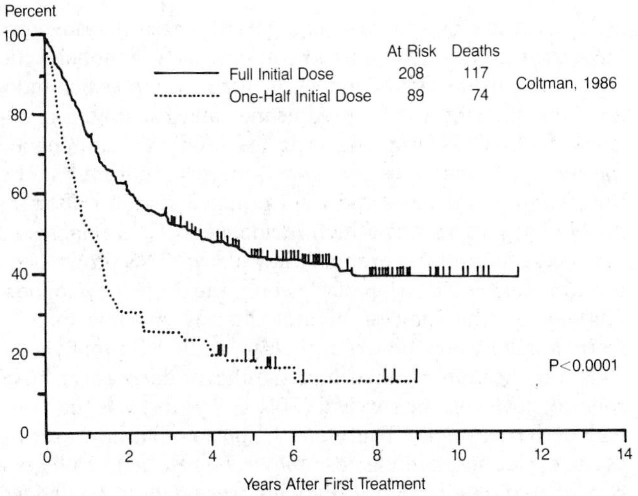

FIG. 50-10. Effect of dose of CHOP on treatment outcome in Southwest Oncology Group studies in advanced stage diffuse large cell lymphoma. The Southwest Oncology Group has conducted a number of studies of the treatment of diffuse large cell lymphoma using CHOP combination chemotherapy and variations on CHOP. A provision in the protocols allows physicians at their discretion to deliver CHOP at one-half the protocol dose if the patient is over age 65 or has other clinical problems that the physician thinks might affect tolerance to chemotherapy. This curve depicts the percentage of all patients surviving as a function of time for those patients receiving initial full dose CHOP versus those receiving initial half-dose CHOP. There is a statistically significant survival advantage to those receiving full-dose CHOP.

doses (41%) than those given low doses of CHOP (12%).[421] Furthermore, it is apparent from Figure 50-9 that so far the curve relating dose intensity to treatment outcome is linear. This implies that further augmentation of dose intensity may well increase the fraction of patients cured. Thus it would appear that we ought to make alterations in our treatment programs to augment dose intensity.

There are two components of dose intensity: amount of drug delivered and interval between administration. Thus one can imagine taking two approaches to augmenting dose intensity: administer the drugs at conventional doses more frequently, or at higher doses at conventional frequency. Because the regimens are primarily limited by marrow suppression, the question really relates to augmenting marrow tolerance. The results with MACOP-B imply that alternating myelotoxic drugs with nonmyelotoxic drugs on alternating weeks may be one fruitful approach to shorten the interval between drug treatment. The NCI has generated some preliminary data with a regimen called short-course ProMACE-CytaBOM, a delta-drug combination with a pattern of alternating weekly drug combinations similar to MACOP-B but with an even higher dose intensity. Myelotoxicity has been milder than anticipated. The augmentation of doses also may be facilitated by a number of biologic agents (*e.g.*, colony-stimulating factors, transforming growth factor-beta) that appear capable of protecting the marrow or enhancing its recovery from chemotherapy-induced suppression.[422,423] The explosion in cancer biology lends special excitement to the prospect of melding of chemotherapeutic and biologic approaches to lymphoma treatment.

TREATMENT OF HIGHLY AGGRESSIVE LYMPHOMAS

The highly aggressive lymphomas are the diffuse small noncleaved cell lymphomas (non-Burkitt's, formerly called diffuse undifferentiated), Burkitt's lymphoma, lymphoblastic lymphoma, and HTLV-I–related ATL. These are very rare tumors in adults. The first three forms of highly aggressive lymphoma are much more common in childhood, and the approaches to their treatment in adults are largely derived from the treatment experiences in children. HTLV-I–related ATL is common in regions where the virus is endemic (*i.e.*, southern Japan and the Caribbean basin). Isolated cases from southeastern United States and émigrés from endemic regions are diagnosed in the United States.[23] The highly aggressive lymphomas are nearly always disseminated at diagnosis; thus the application of a rigid staging schema is not very informative.

The diffuse small noncleaved cell lymphomas (non-Burkitt's) have often been lumped together with diffuse large-cell lymphomas in series reporting treatment results. In general, these lymphomas account for less than 10% of the cases of diffuse lymphomas. The small number prohibits making definitive conclusions about their response to treatment. However, we favor separating them from the diffuse large-cell lymphomas for a variety of reasons. First, their morphology is often difficult to discern from Burkitt's lymphoma. The major difference involves the degree of homogeneity in the nuclei; in Burkitt's lymphoma there is homogeneity and in non-Burkitt's lymphoma there is substantial heterogeneity. Both tumors have a high growth fraction and rapid clinical progression. Second, the distinction from Burkitt's lymphoma is also blurred by the presence of similar cytogenetic abnormalities, particularly t(8;14) involving *c-myc* and the immunoglobulin heavy-chain genes, in non-Burkitt's lymphoma. Third, in our own treatment experience the probability of long-term disease-free survival in diffuse small noncleaved cell, non-Burkitt's lymphoma is slightly less than half that of the other diffuse aggressive lymphomas similarly treated. Therefore, we believe that diffuse small noncleaved cell non-Burkitt's lymphoma in the adult should be treated in a manner similar to that used in Burkitt's lymphoma. Most series of pediatric patients do not make a distinction between non-Burkitt's and Burkitt's varieties of diffuse small noncleaved cell lymphomas, and there is no evidence that the outcome from identical treatment differs.

Lymphoblastic lymphoma is overwhelmingly a tumor of thymocyte origin. It is difficult to distinguish from acute lymphoblastic leukemia on morphologic grounds. Many workers use the degree of bone marrow involvement as the criterion to separate lymphoblastic lymphoma from lymphoblastic leukemia; leukemia is present if neoplastic cells account for 25% or more of the marrow cells. There are certain monoclonal antibodies that have been said to distinguish lymphoblastic leukemia from lymphoma.[424] Lymphoblastic lymphoma has a high propensity to involve the mediastinum (presumably related to thymus origin or tropism), the bone marrow, and CNS, and has a high male preponderance.[425] Abundant experience treating such patients with lymphoma regimens has demonstrated excellent response rates, but nearly all patients relapse and die of progressive disease.[426]

There is no evidence that the natural histories or responses to therapy of lymphoblastic leukemia and lymphoblastic lymphoma are distinct.

There is no serious controversy over the general structure of treatment programs for lymphoblastic and nonlymphoblastic highly aggressive lymphomas. Treatment needs to include a high-dose induction, consolidation, and maintenance phases together with CNS prophylaxis. The major controversy is whether the same therapy is appropriate for both lymphoblastic and nonlymphoblastic histologies. Weinstein and his colleagues[427,428] using the APO regimen and Magrath and his colleagues[429] using the CHOMP regimen would suggest that response to aggressive therapy is similar regardless of histology. Using the APO regimen, 95% of patients with lymphoblastic lymphoma and 98% of patients with nonlymphoblastic lymphoma achieved CR and 60% to 75% of patients enjoy long-term disease-free survival. Weinstein and his colleagues often use radiation therapy to local masses in an effort to improve disease control; however, Camitta and his colleagues[430] have achieved similar long-term survival without radiation. Magrath and co-workers[429] used cycles of cyclophosphamide, doxorubicin, vincristine, prednisone, and high-dose methotrexate for all the histologic groups. The CR rate for all stages and histologies was 89% and the 3-year survival was 60%. Patients with lymphoblastic lymphomas and those with completely resected small non-cleaved cell lymphomas (Burkitt's or non-Burkitt's) had the best prognosis (81%–94% 3-year survival) and those with bulky unresected abdominal disease and bone marrow involvement had the worst.[431]

On the other hand, the LSA2-L2 protocol developed by Wollner and colleagues[432] has been compared with COMP in a prospective randomized trial by the Children's Cancer Study Group, and significant differences in outcome were found between the regimens based on the histology of the lymphoma.[433] The study involved the treatment of 234 children randomized to COMP versus LSA2-L2. For lymphoblastic lymphoma LSA2-L2 was significantly more effective therapy (76% 2-year disease-free survival versus 26% for COMP), but for nonlymphoblastic histologies COMP was more effective (57% versus 28% for LSA2-L2). The Pediatric Oncology Group also found that LSA2-L2 was significantly poorer treatment for nonlymphoblastic lymphomas than for lymphoblastic lymphomas.[434] LSA2-L2 was modified somewhat by Levine and colleagues[435] and used to treat adults with lymphoblastic lymphoma. The CR rate was 73%, but 36% of the complete responders had relapsed at the time of the report and the median remission duration was only 3½ years.

Although there has been a modicum of effort to study adult patients with highly aggressive lymphomas, the information on treatment is substantially less complete. Stanford investigators have taken distinct approaches to lymphoblastic and small noncleaved cell neoplasms. Eighteen adult patients with small noncleaved cell lymphoma were treated with six to ten 3-week cycles of cyclophosphamide, doxorubicin, vincristine, prednisone, and methotrexate with involved-field irradiation to large masses.[436] Patients without extensive disease fared well (100% relapse-free survival at 2 years), but only 41% of patients with disease both within and outside the abdomen were disease free at 2 years. These investigators have used a more leukemia-like approach to lymphoblastic lymphoma in the adult. Induction with cyclophosphamide, doxorubicin, vincristine, prednisone, and asparaginase together with CNS prophylaxis is followed by maintenance therapy with methotrexate and 6-mercaptopurine.[437] The initial regimen delayed the CNS prophylaxis until after induction, and there was a high incidence of CNS relapse. In the second part of the protocol they placed CNS prophylaxis up front during induction but lowered the dose of cyclophosphamide in the interest of ameliorating marrow toxicity from simultaneous induction therapy and CNS prophylaxis. This modification resulted in a significant decrease in CNS relapse; however, the survival (56% at 3 years) was the same with both treatments. Therefore, it appears that the lowering of the cyclophosphamide dose may have resulted in a higher rate of peripheral relapse. Patients were able to be divided into good and poor prognostic groups based on the presence of marrow or CNS disease and a serum LDH level of over 300 IU/ml. Good-prognosis patients had a 5-year freedom-from-relapse rate of 94%. Poor-prognosis patients had a 5-year freedom-from-relapse rate of 19%. Clearly improvement in the therapy for the poor-prognosis group is essential.

Clarkson and his colleagues[438] treated 51 patients with lymphoblastic lymphoma with one of five intensive induction programs between 1971 and 1987. The 5-year survival was 45% and was independent of marrow involvement. The results with lymphoblastic lymphoma were comparable to the results with acute lymphoblastic leukemia treated with the same regimens. When patients with lymphoblastic lymphoma relapse, they are usually refractory to further therapy. However, there is some evidence that salvage leukemia regimens may produce responses. For example, in one small series five of eight relapsed patients achieved a second CR lasting for a median of 9 months when treated with high-dose cytosine arabinoside and m-AMSA.[439]

There are no clear differences in the results of a variety of treatment regimens for lymphoblastic and nonlymphoblastic lymphomas in the adult. The Weinstein APO regimen and the Magrath CHOMP regimen appear to be highly effective in either lymphoblastic or nonlymphoblastic (*i.e.*, small noncleaved cell) histologies and may be expected to be curative in two-thirds or more of patients. LAS2-L2 and the Coleman regimen are effective in lymphoblastic lymphomas. Early CNS prophylaxis is essential in any treatment approach and can be accomplished either by intrathecal drug alone administered by way of an Ommaya reservoir, by cranial irradiation plus intrathecal drug given by way of lumbar puncture, or by way of systemic high-dose methotrexate. Some experimental therapies are under way that use high-dose therapy with bone marrow transplantation.

The data on the treatment of HTLV-I–related ATL are even scantier than the data on the other highly aggressive histologies.[440] Adenopathy, skin involvement, CNS involvement, pulmonary infiltrates, and hypercalcemia (mediated by a T-cell lymphokine) dominate the clinical picture.[23] The disease is rapidly progressive. Most patients respond to treatment programs like ProMACE/MOPP, but CR is durable in a minority of patients. We have seen two patients relapse from a CR lasting for more than 2 years; thus it is uncertain that any treatment has curative potential. The underlying severe immunodeficiency increases the incidence of treatment-related morbidity. We have seen two patients with refractory disease who have responded dramatically to 2′-deoxycoformycin as a single agent.[441] However, both patients died of opportunistic infections while maintaining CR. From all clinical indications ATL is two life-threatening diseases in one. If one can control the neoplasm, one is left with a severe cellular immune defect every bit as severe as those seen in patients with AIDS. A small number of patients will have a more smoldering clinical course characterized by high titers to the HTLV-I viral envelope, fungal infections of the skin, chronic adenopathy, interstitial pneumonitis, chronic renal failure, and strongyloidiasis.[442] Experimental immunotherapies with antibody to the IL-2 receptor alone and conjugated with toxins and isotopes are being tested in humans.[443] Therapeutic progress in this rare tumor will only come as a consequence of further clinical trials in large treatment centers.

TREATMENT OF LYMPHOMAS IN SPECIAL SITES AND SPECIAL CIRCUMSTANCES

The vast majority of lymphomas that occur in the setting of AIDS are highly aggressive tumors, usually of the small noncleaved cell non-Burkitt's variety. Aggressive treatment is usually associated with serious treatment-related toxicity; however, unlike Kaposi's sarcoma, which is a contributor to death in a minority of AIDS patients in whom it occurs, lymphomas in the AIDS patient are nearly always life-threatening. Lymphoma-related symptoms can be effectively controlled with systemic combination chemotherapy, but long-term survival is not a possible outcome, given the underlying disease process.[444]

Lymphomas that involve the CNS are increasing in frequency because of the propensity of this entity to occur in the setting of immunodeficiencies like AIDS. CNS lymphoma usually occurs in one of two forms: primary CNS lymphoma, which causes mass lesions and usually is not associated with systemic lymphoma until late in its course, and secondary (usually meningeal) lymphoma, which usually is not associated with mass lesions and nearly always occurs in the setting of relapsed or growing systemic lymphoma, particularly involving bone or bone marrow or testes.

Primary CNS lymphoma accounts for about 2% of brain tumors and 2% of all lymphomas. It appears on CT scan radiographically as a lesion of increased density (63% or more of cases) and uniformly enhances with contrast, usually homogeneously.[445] The lymphoma often occurs in the frontal lobes or involves deep central brain structures and may produce multiple lesions, leading to confusion with metastatic carcinoma. The most common symptoms are headache, mental changes (memory loss, dementia, personality changes), nausea, vomiting, and seizures. The major neurologic findings are hemipareses, papilledema, visual field defects, and cranial nerve palsies. The CSF usually has a high protein level but no cytologically malignant cells. CNS lymphoma is responsive to radiation therapy,[446] but the median survival is 12 to 18 months, not terribly different from the survival of primary brain neoplasms. After surgical removal of as much tumor as possible, patients are usually treated with whole-brain irradiation to about 4000 cGy with a boost to the primary lesion of about 1500 cGy. Some have advocated radiating the spinal axis, but with a clinical failure rate in the spinal cord of only 4% this practice seems unwarranted. About 90% of relapses are in the CNS and less than 10% relapse solely outside the CNS. Investigators have recently been exploring the use of systemic combination chemotherapy with or without radiation therapy. The regimens usually include methotrexate, which can penetrate the CNS and achieve therapeutic levels in the CSF when given systemically, steroids, nitrosoureas, procarbazine, or high-dose cytosine arabinoside, or a combination of these, with or without osmotic disruption of the blood–brain barrier.[447] To date, most of the treatment experiences are elaborate anecdotes, and while there is appropriate optimism about the use of drugs, it is not clear whether systemic chemotherapy with or without radiation therapy is superior to radiation therapy alone.

Secondary CNS lymphoma (*i.e.*, involvement of the CNS secondary to peripheral disease) most often involves the meninges and is decreasing in incidence dramatically with the appropriate institution of CNS prophylaxis in the high-risk setting. Nearly all cases occur in patients with diffuse lymphoma. If a patient with indolent lymphoma develops CNS signs and symptoms, it nearly always represents histologic evolution to aggressive lymphoma. Although systemic therapy may on occasion be successful at treating meningeal disease, the usual treatment approach is to administer methotrexate, cytosine arabinoside, or thiotepa individually or in combination into the spinal canal either by repeated spinal taps (which requires concurrent cranial irradiation to treat the meninges over the convexities) or by way of an indwelling Ommaya reservoir.[448] The CNS disease is usually treated at the same time that therapy is administered for peripheral disease. It is generally true that meningeal lymphoma can be eradicated, but foreshortened survival is a function of the inability to control the systemic disease. CNS symptoms can also be produced by expanding nodal or extranodal masses that cause cord compression. This complication occurs in about 2% of cases of lymphoma and is best managed by local radiation treatment together with systemic treatment, if the symptoms have an acute onset, but combination chemotherapy alone may be used if the symptoms developed gradually and have not progressed to complete cord block. The decision about whether to use radiation therapy is usually aided by obtaining a magnetic resonance imaging scan to better define the anatomy of the involvement.

Orbital lymphomas are rare and can be a site of spread to or from the CNS. They can usually be managed with excellent local control by radiation therapy,[449] but cataracts are a frequent late complication. High-dose cytosine arabinoside administered by peripheral vein has recently been found to produce CR in a patient with intraocular lymphoma.[450]

The most common extranodal site involved with lymphoma among patients in the United States is the GI tract.[451] By and large, lymphomas that involve the GI tract should be staged and treated like any other lymphomas, and the treatment results appear to be comparable to those obtained in other stage- and bulk-matched patients. The major unanswered question is whether surgical debulking improves the response to chemotherapy and results in improved survival in histologies other than Burkitt's lymphoma. Although data have not been obtained in prospective randomized studies, most investigators find that patients whose disease is resected fare better than those who do not undergo debulking surgery.[452]

SALVAGE TREATMENT OF LYMPHOMAS

Patients with indolent lymphoma who relapse from CR with an indolent lymphoma histology usually receive symptomatic treatment. If indolent lymphoma patients relapse with an aggressive lymphoma, an attempt at curative therapy with a third-generation treatment program appears warranted, since at least a third of such patients achieve long-term remissions from the first-generation programs.[167,279]

Until the mid-1980s patients with aggressive lymphoma relapsing from or failing to achieve CR had a life expectancy of around 4 months. More recently, however, several groups have treated relapsed patients with high-dose chemotherapy with or without total body irradiation followed by autologous bone marrow transplantation, and the results provide perhaps the strongest data in favor of the importance of dose intensity in treatment outcome. For the first time durable second remissions are being obtained in up to 40% of patients.[453-464] With the clinical experience rapidly growing, several issues are clear. First, patients do better if they enter the high-dose phase of therapy with no or minimal residual disease. Second, high-dose cyclophosphamide plus total body irradiation is a well-tolerated and effective marrow ablative regimen in lymphoma, and it appears that certain other agents, such as cytosine arabinoside, can be added to it without significant increase in toxicity. Third, allogenic transplantation is associated with a high rate of treatment-related fatality. Fourth, patients with disease progression in the days leading up to high-dose therapy are unlikely to benefit from the therapy.

One potential limitation of applying autologous bone marrow transplantation to the treatment of aggressive lymphoma is that some patients have marrow involvement at relapse, and even more (perhaps as many as 75%) have occult marrow disease. Several approaches have been taken to purge the marrow of residual tumor cells before reinfusion. Nadler and colleagues[453] have used the monoclonal antibody anti-B1-plus complement to purge marrow of normal and neoplastic B cells before reinfusion in patients prepared with high-dose cyclophosphamide and total body irradiation. With a median follow-up of nearly a year, only 13 of 49 patients have relapsed.[453] Other investigators are using drugs such as hydroperoxycyclophosphamide and ASTA-Z, another cyclophosphamide congener that does not require metabolic activation to exert its cytotoxic effects. A few patients have survived more than a year free of disease after receiving such purged marrow with high-dose cyclophosphamide and total body irradiation, but there is too little experience to say whether this approach will be superior to others that omit marrow purging.

Thus many questions remain. All the series use highly selected patients to study. What fraction of an unselected group of relapsing patients would be eligible for such an approach? Can the efficacy of high-dose cyclophosphamide plus total body irradiation be improved on by adding other drugs or biologic agents? What is the role of purging of bone marrow with in vitro immunotoxins, drugs, or antibody purging techniques? Is the presence of gross marrow disease or prior CNS involvement an absolute contraindication to high-dose treatment? What are the best approaches and regimens to accomplish the debulking before high-dose therapy? These questions need to be addressed before one can place this treatment modality into the proper perspective. Regardless of the answers to the questions, however, it is clear that the introduction of high-dose cyclophosphamide plus total body irradiation with autologous bone marrow rescue has accomplished an unprecedented achievement; some fraction (which we estimate to be between 10% and 40%) of refractory and relapsed patients with aggressive lymphoma have been shown to be curable with this salvage approach and the fraction of patients selected to go through the treatment who benefit from it appears to be high. These are findings on which to build.

An important component of any salvage program will be the conventional-dose regimen that achieves a clinical response before the high-dose therapy. Several new combinations have been tested in small numbers of patients and may hold promise as debulking regimens. They include vindesine, etoposide, and prednisolone[465]; etoposide, BCNU, bleomycin, and methotrexate[466]; cisplatin and etoposide[467]; cisplatin, m-AMSA, and mitoguazone[468]; and ifosphamide, methotrexate, etoposide, and mitoguazone,[469] among others.[470]

TREATMENT OF RARE PROLIFERATIVE DISORDERS OF THE LYMPHATIC SYSTEM

AILD is a rare disease with histologic features that resemble Hodgkin's disease without Reed–Sternberg cells. In some series life expectancy is less than a year.[471] The disease is idiopathic but is associated with diffuse adenopathy, polyclonal serum immunoglobulin elevations, and often a history of allergic or autoimmune disease. Transient responses have been obtained after plasmapheresis, but more typically the disease evolves into an aggressive lymphoma. There is evidence that the cells express elevated levels of N-*ras* mRNA,[472] the significance of which is unknown. The disease appears responsive to prednisone and certain combination chemotherapy programs (*e.g.*, C-MOPP), and there is theoretical support for a therapeutic role for cyclosporin A.

Castleman's disease, angiofollicular lymph node hyperplasia, is most often an asymptomatic condition diagnosed incidentally in young men on chest x-ray as enlarged mediastinal nodes. Sometimes the adenopathy is accompanied by systemic symptoms of fever and weight loss. Frizzera and associates[473] have reported a systemic form of the illness associated with malaise, fever, adenopathy, hepatosplenomegaly, rashes, hypergammaglobulinemia, and, occasionally, CNS symptoms. Although symptomatic therapy was occasionally helpful, the median survival was only 30 months. A case report of a patient with Castleman's disease obtaining CR with high-dose melphalan with autologous bone marrow rescue suggests that aggressive therapy may be lifesaving in this rare disease.[474]

Angiocentric immunoproliferative lesions are on the spectrum of peripheral T-cell disorders that includes lymphomatoid granulomatosis and midline lethal reticulosis. Examination of 23 cases revealed that patients fell into three histologic grades, as noted earlier in the section on the morphology of the immunoproliferative diseases.[240] Treatment of Grade 1 disease with cyclophosphamide and prednisone resulted in long-term survival in 45% of patients and in Grade 2 patients, only 33% long-term survival. Most of the deaths in Grade 1 or 2 patients were from treatment-refractory malignant lymphoma. Grade 3 lesions were thought to be overt angiocentric lymphoma, and seven of the eight patients treated for lymphoma are alive and free of disease.[240] It appears that even the low-grade angiocentric lesions could benefit from aggressive therapy with a lymphoma regimen, since they evolve to lymphoma with a high frequency and their previous treatment appears to result in the emergence of drug-resistant neoplasms.

TREATMENT APPROACHES WITH IMMUNOLOGIC AND BIOLOGIC AGENTS

Biologic approaches to cancer treatment can be said to fall into one of three categories: agents acting indirectly against the tumor (active immunotherapy), agents acting directly on the tumor cell (passive immunotherapy), and agents acting on tumor biology (*e.g.*, antimetastatic agents, differentiation agents). All three classes of biologic therapy have been tried, at least to a limited degree, in patients with lymphoma, and each has had enough preliminary success to warrant further exploration.

The most widely studied cytokine in the treatment of lymphoma is interferon. Studies with crude preparations, purified natural products, and recombinant DNA-derived molecules of interferons of all three classes, alpha, beta, and gamma, have been found to have activity in patients with low-grade lymphoma or CTCL, but not in patients with intermediate- or high-grade lymphoma.[475] Alpha interferon at the maximum tolerated dose (around 30×10^6 U/m^2 daily or three times a week) produces transient partial responses in about 45% of patients. Responses are seen at lower doses but not as frequently, and the duration of response is short at any dose whether or not interferon therapy is continued. The side-effects from interferon therapy are not usually life-threatening but seriously affect the quality of life. They include fevers, chills, headache, nausea, malaise, depression, myelosuppression, and hepatic enzyme elevations. A number of studies are under way that incorporate interferon into a combination chemotherapy induction regimen to assess its impact on CR rate, and at least one study is analyzing the capacity of interferon administered to complete responders to prolong remission duration. A disturbing case report documented the occurrence of a secondary acute leukemia in a lymphoma patient whose only cytotoxic therapy was alpha interferon[476]; thus it is not completely clear that biologic therapies will not also have serious late complications, similar to some chemotherapeutic and radiation therapy programs.

Trials of other cytokines are just beginning. It appears, however, that patients with lymphoma who have been treated with recombinant tumor necrosis factor at or near its maximum tolerated dose have been poorly responsive.[477] Anecdotal responses to high doses of IL-2 have been described, but the number of patients who have received such therapy is too small to make valid conclusions.

Passive immunotherapy has been given in both specific (monoclonal antibodies) and nonspecific (adoptive transfer of lymphokine-activated or alloantigen-activated killer cells) forms. Monoclonal antibodies have been used quite extensively but primarily in pilot studies. The first murine monoclonal antibody ever administered to a human being was given by Nadler and his colleagues[478] to a patient with a B-cell lymphoma. Using an antibody he made to a B-cell tumor, Nadler discovered several features that limit the efficacy of monoclonal antibodies in that first human subject. First, the patient experienced a dramatic clearing of malignant cells from the peripheral blood, but this response was transient. The response fulfilled magnitude criteria but not duration criteria to be considered a partial response. The target antigen was modulated off the surface of the malignant cells, thus rendering useless further therapy directed at that target. The patient developed an antibody response to the murine antibody being used for therapy. This single patient was entirely predictive for the types of response and problems that would be encountered using monoclonal antibodies directed against Leu1 and cALLa in a number of studies in different tumor types, CTCL, CLL, and ALL.[479–481] Press and colleagues[482] addressed one of these problems by using an antibody called 1F5 directed against the CD20 determinant on B cells and B-cell tumors that does not modulate. Among four patients with refractory B-cell lymphoma a brief partial response was seen in one patient who received more than 2 g of antibody.

One of the most interesting uses of monoclonal antibody therapy has been the use of anti-idiotypic antibodies directed against the unique determinants on the antibody molecule expressed by the malignant cell. Levy and his colleagues[192] obtained one complete and two partial responses in the first 11 patients they treated, and the complete responder has remained in complete remission over 5 years. Response did not correlate with antibody isotype or avidity, but antibodies recognizing a combinatorial determinant between the heavy and light chains appeared to be somewhat more effective. In one patient with prolymphocytic leukemia the anti-idiotype had a direct antiproliferative effect on the tumor cells. In other patients responses correlated with the number of host nontumor T cells (particularly CD4+ cells) infiltrating tumor-bearing nodes. In addition to the problem of developing an antimurine antibody response that can limit the efficacy of treatment, anti-idiotype therapy has other barriers to overcome. For example, virtually all patients with B-cell tumors secrete or shed their surface immunoglobulin into the serum at microgram to milligram per deciliter levels. Such circulating targets significantly impair the ability of the antibody to reach tumor cells. In addition, spontaneous mutation in the immunoglobulin genes of B-cell tumors frequently alters the idiotype such that some of the specially developed reagents no longer interact with the malignant cells.[483] Other workers using anti-idiotype antibodies have not been successful in producing meaningful antitumor responses even at very high doses of anti-idiotype antibody aimed at eliminating host antimurine antibody responses.[484] Stevenson and colleagues[485] have taken a particularly clever approach to anti-idiotype therapy. They have used a chimeric univalent anti-idiotype antibody in a patient with follicular lymphoma. The univalency was intended to discourage target modulation, and the human immunoglobulin to which the mouse anti-idiotype was linked was designed to recruit human effector mechanisms. Four injections were given over 11 weeks with only a minor antitumor response. However, there did not appear to be modulation of the target idiotype and no human antimurine antibodies were detected. A recent animal study suggests that certain drugs (*e.g.*, daunomycin) can synergize with the anti-idiotype antibodies by recruiting host cells into the antitumor response.[486] Thus there may be strategies that can overcome the difficulties associated with the generation and delivery of anti-idiotype therapy; however, the expense in time and money to generate unique reagents for each patient and the tendency of the tumors to spontaneously alter the target are serious problems with this approach.

Another clever use of a monoclonal antibody has been the treatment of patients with HTLV-I–related ATL with antibody directed against the alpha IL-2 receptor (Tac) by Waldmann and colleagues.[443] This is the first clinical trial to use an antibody to antagonize the effects of a possible tumor growth factor. Three of nine patients had responses, one of which was complete and lasted for 5 months. Further studies of this approach are indicated in this and other tumors expressing IL-2 receptors and using antibodies against other growth factors in other tumor types.

Efforts to improve the efficacy of antibodies include conjugating them to radioisotopes,[487] toxins,[488] and chemotherapeutic agents.[489] All three types of conjugates have been used in animal tumor models of lymphoma with evidence of in vivo activity. A ^{131}I radioisotope conjugate of T101 has produced some transient partial responses in cutaneous T-cell lymphoma,[490] and an ^{131}I conjugate of an anti-idiotype antibody used at high dose with bone marrow transplantation (because of isotope-related marrow damage) has produced a dramatic anecdotal response at the University of Washington.[491] To date, toxin conjugates have been used only to purge tumor cells from bone marrow ex vivo.[492] Drug conjugates have not been used in patients with lymphoma.

Another idea to improve on the efficacy of antibodies is to use human antibodies or chimeric antibodies with human Fc fragments, as noted earlier. Some have proposed that antibody cocktails might be more efficacious, but there are no data to support this notion. Finally, there is recent experimental evidence that antibodies directed at tumor targets that transduce activation signals on normal lymphocytes (*e.g.*, T-cell antigen receptors; Ia molecules, Ig molecules, and CD20 on B cells) are capable of killing murine tumors in vivo[493] and human tumors in vitro.[494] Human clinical trials of such an approach are just beginning.

In addition to in vivo use, antibodies have also been used in vitro in an effort to eliminate residual tumor cells from the bone marrow in clinical trials of high-dose chemotherapy and radiation therapy followed by marrow transplantation with purged autologous marrow.[495] Patients with relapsed diffuse aggressive lymphoma have uniformly followed a fatal course. With antibody-purged bone marrow transplantation and high-dose therapy, up to 40% of highly selected patients survive 2 years free of disease. Studies are under way to test the generalizability of these findings. No studies have documented that antibody purging contributes to the therapeutic effect. When Burkitt's lymphoma cells that are capable of being detected in a clonogenic assay are used to measure the magnitude of the effects of purging experimentally, there are serious limitations on the magnitude of the killing that is possible.[496] Some tumor cells that survive antibody-plus-complement killing express less target antigen than the original tumor and others do not. Bone marrow cells can exert anticomplement effects that limit lysis of tumor. Some antibodies result in more tumor variants than others. The issue of purging is complicated and has not been systematically addressed in clinical studies. Current studies have focused on alternative methods of using antibodies for purging besides complement-mediated tumor lysis, including magnetically attracting a metal-attached antibody, toxin and drug conjugates, alpha-emitting radioisotope conjugates, and antibody cocktails.

A promising avenue for immunologic treatment of the lymphomas is adoptive cellular therapy. Rosenberg and colleagues[497] have reported responses in two of four patients with lymphoma treated with lymphokine-activated killer (LAK) cells plus IL-2, and Kohler and colleagues[498] obtained CR in a patient treated with cyclophosphamide followed by adoptive transfer of allogeneic MHC-matched alloantigen- and IL-2–activated lymphocytes.[498] A number of types of host cells may be effective in killing lymphoma cells, and some types may enhance antibody killing. There is excellent rationale for the use of lymphokines, cells, and antibodies together, and many models demonstrate synergy when such an approach is combined with chemotherapy. For example, Wiltrout and colleagues[499] have been able to cure 80% of mice bearing advanced-stage renal cell carcinoma with a combination of IL-2 with or without LAK cells plus the chemotherapeutic agent flavone-8-acetic acid. The unprecedented level of antitumor effects in animal models using chemoimmunotherapy in a variety of combinations has produced enormous excitement in clinical research on cancer treatment. There is little doubt that these treatment modalities will be found to have synergistic tumor effects in humans.

A number of recent studies suggest that some maneuvers to elicit specific tumor immunity may have therapeutic benefit in patients with lymphoma. Intralymphatic administration of an autochthonous tumor cell vaccine in dogs was associated with a therapeutic effect.[500] In humans Edelson and colleagues[501] treated 37 patients with CTCL with oral psoralen and then exposed their sensitized peripheral blood cells to ultraviolet light extracorporeally and returned the damaged cells to the patients. Twenty-seven of their patients responded to this vaccination approach, presumably because the damaged cells elicited a host–antitumor immune response. The ultraviolet light is an example of physical xenogenation, but there are also viral and chemical approaches to altering the immunogenicity of tumor cells. Such studies are likely to be conducted in solid tumors in the near future.

Differentiating agents (particularly retinoids) have been tested in some patients with CTCL with a low response rate.[502] However, an interesting small study examined the effects of 3-alpha-hydroxy vitamin D in seven patients with follicular lymphoma.[503] At a dose of 1 μg daily, one clinical complete and three partial remissions were obtained. Dihydroxy D3 has been shown to interact with cytosolic receptors in some leukemia cell lines and to promote differentiation and alter expression of cellular oncogenes. The high frequency of the 14;18 translocation in follicular lymphoma may represent a target for regulation by D3 and its receptor.

A variety of immunologic and biologic approaches have been used in patients with lymphoma, and a burgeoning number of possibilities are ahead of us. The explosion in information about the biology of lymphomas is providing many interesting hypotheses to put to therapeutic trial. Those that have already come to clinical trial have either been modestly disappointing (anti-idiotype antibodies in B-cell lymphoma) or have made an unclear contribution to the ultimate treatment outcome (bone marrow purging with anti-B1 plus complement in salvage lymphoma protocols). This situation is likely to change.

REFERENCES

1. Cancer Facts and Figures 1984, p 8. New York, American Cancer Society, 1983
2. Forty-five years of cancer in Connecticut. In Cusano MM, Young JL Jr (eds): Natl Cancer Inst Monograph 70, p 1935, 1986
3. Devesa SS, Silverman DT, Young JL Jr et al: Cancer incidence and mortality trends among whites in the United States, 1947–84. J Natl Cancer Inst 79:701, 1987
4. Cantor KP, Fraumeni JF: Distribution of non-Hodgkin's lymphoma in the United States between 1950 and 1975. Cancer Res 40:2645, 1980
5. Third National Cancer Survey, 1969 Incidence. Preliminary Report. Department of Health, Education and Welfare, Publ No (NIH) p 71, 1971
6. Higginson J, Muir CS: Epidemiology. In Holland JF, Frei E (eds): Cancer Medicine, p 241. Philadelphia, Lea & Febiger, 1973
7. Anderson RE, Ishida K, Li Y et al: Geographic aspects of malignant lymphoma and multiple myeloma. Am J Pathol 61:85, 1970
8. Kaplan HS: Etiology of lymphomas and leukemia: Role of C-type RNA viruses. Leukemia Res 2:253, 1978
9. Dmochowski L: Viral studies in human leukemia and lymphoma. In Zarafonetis CJD (ed): Proceedings of the International Conference on Leukemia-Lymphoma, p 97. Philadelphia, Lea & Febiger, 1968
10. Kawakami TG, Theilan GH, Dungworth DL et al: "C" type viral particles in plasma of cats with feline leukemia. Science 158:1049, 1967
11. Kawakami TG, Hull SD, Buckley DM et al: C-type virus associated with Gibbon lymphosarcoma. Nature New Biol 235:170, 1972
12. Rapp F: Viruses an etiologic factor in cancer. Semin Oncol 3:49, 1976
13. Van der Maaten MJ, Miller JM, Booth AD: Replicating type-C virus particles in monolayer cell cultures from cattle with lymphosarcoma. J Natl Cancer Inst 52:491, 1974
14. Reedman BM, Klein G: Cellular localization of an Epstein-Barr virus (EBV)-associated complement fixing antigen in producer and non producer lymphoblastoid cell lines. Int J Cancer 11:499, 1973
15. Kaplan HS, Goodenow RS, Gartner BA et al: Biology and virology of the human malignant lymphomas. Cancer 43:1, 1979
16. Epstein AL, Kaplan HS: Biology of the human malignant lymphomas. I. Establishment in continuous culture and heterotransplantation of diffuse histiocytic lymphomas. Cancer 34:1851, 1974
17. Uchiyama T, Yodoi J, Sagawa K et al: Adult T-cell leukemia: Clinical and hematologic features of 16 cases. Blood 50:481, 1977
18. Catovsky D, Greaves MF, Rose M et al: Adult T-cell lymphoma-leukaemia in blacks from the West Indies. Lancet 1:639, 1982
19. Blattner WA, Gibbs WN, Saxinger C et al: Human T-cell leukaemia/lymphoma virus-lymphomareticular neoplasia in Jamaica. Lancet 2:61, 1983
20. Poiesz BJ, Ruscetti FW, Gazdar AF et al: Detection and isolation of type C retrovirus particles from fresh and cultured lymphocytes of a patient with cutaneous T-cell lymphoma. Proc Natl Acad Sci USA 77:7415, 1980
21. Posner LE, Robert-Guroff M, Kalyanaraman VS et al: Natural antibodies to the human T-cell lymphoma virus in patients with T-cell lymphomas. J Exp Med 154:333, 1981
22. Kalyanaraman VS, Sarngadharan MG, Bunn PA et al: Antibodies in human sera reactive against an internal structural protein of human T-cell lymphoma virus. Nature 294:271, 1981
23. Blayney DW, Jaffe ES, Blattner WA et al: The human T-cell leukemia/lymphoma virus associated with American adult T-cell leukemia/lymphoma. Blood 62:401, 1983
24. Robert-Guroff M, Nakao Y, Notake K et al: Natural antibodies to human retrovirus HTLV in a cluster of Japanese patients with adult T-cell leukemia. Science 215:975, 1982
25. Kalyanaraman VS, Sarngadharan MG, Nakao Y et al: Natural antibodies to the structural core protein (p24) of the human T-cell leukemia (lymphoma) retrovirus found in sera of leukemia patients in Japan. Proc Natl Acad Sci USA 79:1653, 1982
26. Blattner WA, Kalyanaraman VS, Robert-Guroff M et al: The human type-C retrovirus, HTLV, in blacks from the Caribbean region, and relationship to adult T-cell leukemia/lymphoma. Int J Cancer 30:257, 1982
27. Blayney DW, Blattner WA, Robert-Guroff M et al: The human T-cell leukemia/lymphoma viruses (HTLV) in the Southeastern United States. JAMA 250:1048, 1983
28. Kalyanaraman VS, Sarngadharan MG, Robert-Guroff M et al: A new subtype of human T-cell leukemia virus (HTLV-II) associated with a T-cell variant of hairy cell leukemia. Science 218:571, 1982
29. Barre-Sinoussi F, Chermann JC, Rey F et al: Isolation of a T-lymphotropic retrovirus from a patient at risk for acquired immune deficiency syndrome (AIDS). Science 220:868, 1983
30. Gallo RC, Salahuddin SZ, Popovic M et al: Frequent detection and isolation of cytopathic retroviruses (HTLV-III) from patients with AIDS and at risk for AIDS. Science 224:500, 1984
31. Kanki PJ, Barin F, M'Boup S et al: New human T-lymphotropic retroviruses related to simian T-lymphotropic virus type III (STLV-III-HGM). Science 232:238, 1986
32. Clavel F, Guetard D, Brun-Vezinet F et al: Isolation of a new human retrovirus from West African patients with AIDS. Science 233:343, 1986
33. Manzari V, Gismondi A, Barillari G et al: HTLV-V: A new human retrovirus in Tac-negative T-cell lymphoma/leukemia. Science 238:1581, 1987
34. Sodroski JG, Rosen CA, Haseltine WA: Trans-acting transcriptional activation of the long terminal repeat of human T-lymphotrophic viruses in infected cells. Science 225:381, 1984
35. Ruscetti FW, Seigel L, Mikovits JA et al: Variable levels of HTLV-I replication and transactivation among cell lines infected with the same virus: Evidence for cellular regulation of HTLV-I transcription. Blood 70:285a, 1987
36. Siekevitz M, Feinberg MB, Holbrook N et al: Activation of interleukin 2 and interleukin 2 receptor (Tac) promoter expression by the transactivator (*tat*) gene product of human T-cell leukemia virus, type I. Proc Natl Acad Sci USA 84:5389, 1987
37. Jacobson S, Raine CS, Mingioli ES et al: Isolation of an HTLV-I-like retrovirus from patients with tropical spastic paraparesis. Nature 331:540, 1988
38. Sonoda S: Relationship of HTLV-I-related adult T-cell leukemia and HTLV-I-associated myelopathy to distinct HLA haplotypes. Jikken Igaku 5:769, 1987
39. Salahuddin SZ, Ablashi DV, Markham PD et al: Isolation of a new virus, HBLV, in patients with lymphoproliferative. Science 234:596, 1986
40. Caspersson T, Zech L, Johansson C et al: Identification of human chromosomes by DNA-binding fluorescent agents. Chromosoma 30:215, 1970
41. Manolov G, Manolova Y: Marker band in one chromosome 14 from Burkitt lymphomas. Nature 237:33, 1972
42. Taub R, Kirsch I, Morton C et al: Translocation of the c-myc gene into the immunoglobulin heavy chain locus in human Burkitt's lymphoma and murine plasmacytoma cells. Proc Natl Acad Sci USA 79:7837, 1982
43. Klein G: Specific chromosomal translocations and the genesis of B cell derived tumors in mice and men. Cell 32:311, 1983
44. Fukuhara S, Rowley JD, Variakojiis D et al: Banding studies on chromosomes in diffuse histiocytic lymphoma: Correlation of 14Q + marker chromosome with cytology. Blood 52:989, 1978
45. Yunis JJ, Oken MM, Kaplan ME et al: Distinctive chromosomal abnormalities in histologic subtypes of non-Hodgkin's lymphoma. N Engl J Med 307:1231, 1982
46. Yunis JJ: The chromosomal basis of human neoplasia. Science 221:227, 1983
47. Denny CH, Hollis GF, Hecht F et al: Common mechanism of chromosome inversion in B- and T-cell tumors: Relevance to lymphoid development. Science 234:197, 1986
48. McKeithan TW, Rowley JD, Shows TB et al: Cloning of the chromosome translocation breakpoint junction of the t(14;19) in chronic lymphocytic leukemia. Proc Natl Acad Sci USA 84:9257, 1987
49. Vianna NJ, Davies JNP, Polan AK et al: Familial Hodgkin's disease: An environmental and genetic disorder. Lancet 7885:854, 1974
50. Grufferman S, Cole P, Smith PG et al: Hodgkin's disease in siblings. N Engl J Med 296:248, 1977
51. Miller DG: The association of immune disease and malignant lymphoma. Ann Intern Med 66:507, 1967
52. Zulman J, Jaffe R, Talal N: Evidence that the malignant lymphoma of Sjogren's syndrome is a monoclonal B-cell neoplasm. N Engl J Med 299:1215, 1978

53. Talal N, Sokoloff L, Barth W: Extra salivary lymphoid abnormalities in Sjogren's syndrome (reticulum cell sarcoma, "pseudolymphoma," macroglobulinemia). Am J Med 43:50, 1967
54. Kassan JS, Thomas TL, Moutsopoulos HM et al: Increased risk, of lymphoma in Sicca syndrome. Ann Intern Med 89:888, 1978
55. Hyman G, Sommers S: The development of Hodgkin's disease and other lymphomas during anticonvulsant therapy. Blood 28:416, 1966
56. Penn I: The incidence of malignancies in transplant recipients. Transplant Proc 7:323, 1975
57. Matas AJ, Hertel BF, Rosai J et al: Post-transplant malignant lymphoma. Distinctive morphologic features related to its pathogenesis. Am J Med 61:716, 1976
58. Kipps TJ, Fong S, Tomhave E et al: High-frequency expression of a conserved kappa light-chain variable-region gene in chronic lymphocytic leukemia. Proc Natl Acad Sci USA 84:2916, 1987
59. List AF, Greco FA, Vogler LB: Lymphoproliferative diseases in immunocompromised hosts: The role of Epstein-Barr virus. J Clin Oncol 5:1673, 1987
60. Tosato G, Blaese RM: Epstein-Barr virus infection and immunoregulation in man. Adv Immunol 37:99, 1985
61. Weisenburger DD: Lymphoid malignancies in Nebraska: A hypothesis. Neb Med J 70:300, 1985
62. Anderson RE, Nishiyama H, Yohei I et al: Pathogenesis of radiation related leukemia and lymphoma. Speculations based primarily on experience of Hiroshima and Nagasaki. Lancet 1:1060, 1972
63. Miller RW: Delayed radiation effects in atomic bomb survivors. Science 166:569, 1969
64. Court Brown WM, Doll R: Leukemia and aplastic anemia in patients irradiated for ankylosing spondylitis. Med Res Council Spec Rep Ser (Lond), No 295, Her Majesty's Stationery Office, 1957
65. Kissmeyer-Nielsen F, Bjorn-Jensen K, Femara RB et al: HLA phenotypes in Hodgkin's disease: Preliminary report. Transplant Proc 3:1287, 1971
66. Dick FR, Fortuny I, Theologides A et al: HL-A and lymphoid tumors. Cancer Res 32:2608, 1972
67. MacSween RNM: Reticulum cell sarcoma and rheumatoid arthritis in a patient with XY/XXY/XXX/Y Klinefelter's syndrome and normal intelligence. Lancet 1:460, 1965
68. Tan C, Etcubanas E, Lieberman P et al: Chediak-Higashi syndrome in a child with Hodgkin's disease. Am J Dis Child 121:135, 1971
69. Greaves MF, Owen JJT, Raff MC: T and B lymphocytes: Origins, Properties, and Roles in Immune Responses. New York, American Elsevier, 1974
70. Weiss L: The Cells and Tissues of the Immune System. Structure, Functions, Interactions. Englewood Cliffs, NJ, Prentice-Hall, 1972
71. Bienenstock J, Befus D: Gut- and bronchus-associated tissue. Am J Anat 170:437, 1984
72. Golde D, Cline MJ: A review and reevaluation of the histiocytic disorders. Am J Med 55:49, 1973
73. Mann RB, Jaffe ES, Berard CW: Malignant lymphomas—a conceptual understanding of morphologic diversity. A review. Am J Pathol 94:103, 1979
74. Royer HD, Reinherz EL: T lymphocytes: Ontogeny, function, and relevance to clinical disorders. N Engl J Med 317:1136, 1987
75. Cooper MD: B lymphocytes: Normal development and function. N Engl J Med 317:1452, 1987
76. VanFurth R, Taeburn JA, van Zwet TL: Characteristics of human mononuclear phagocytes. Blood 54:485, 1979
77. Steinman RM, Nussenzweig MC: Dendritic cells: Features and functions. Immunol Rev 53:125, 1980
78. Tew JG, Thorbecke GJ, Steinman RM: Dendritic cells in the immune response: Characteristics and recommended nomenclature. J Reticuloendothel Soc 31:371, 1982
79. Wood GS, Turner RR, Shiruba RA et al: Human dendritic cells and macrophages: In situ immunophenotypic definition of subsets that exhibit specific morphologic and microenvironmental characteristics. Am J Pathol 119:73, 1985
80. Kohler G, Milstein C: Continuous cultures of fused cells secreting antibody of pre-defined specificity. Nature 256:495, 1975
81. Aiuti F, Cerrottini JC, Coombs RRA et al: Identification, enumeration and isolation of B and T lymphocytes from human peripheral blood. Special Technical Report. Scand J Immunol 3:521, 1974
82. Bernard A, Boumsell L, Dausset J et al: Leucocyte Typing. Human Leucocyte Differentiation Antigens Detected by Monoclonal Antibodies: Specification—Classification—Nomenclature. New York, Springer-Verlag, 1984
83. Reinherz EL, Haynes BF, Nadler LM et al: Leukocyte Typing II: Human B Lymphocytes, Vol 2. New York, Springer-Verlag, 1987
84. Jaffe ES, Cossman J: Immunodiagnosis of lymphoid and mononuclear phagocytic neoplasms. In Rose NR, Friedman H, Fahey JL (eds): Manual of Clinical Laboratory Immunology, 3rd ed, p 779. Washington, American Society of Microbiology, 1986
85. Lovett EJ, Schnitzer B, Keren DF et al: Application of flow cytometry to diagnostic pathology. Lab Invest 540:115, 1984
86. Battifora H, Trowbridge IS: A monoclonal antibody useful for the differential diagnosis between malignant lymphoma and nonhematopoietic neoplasms. Cancer 51:816, 1983
87. Warnke RA, Gatter KC, Phil D et al: Diagnosis of human lymphoma with monoclonal antileukocyte antibodies. N Engl J Med 309:1275, 1983
88. Reinherz EL, Haynes BF, Nadler LM et al: Leukocyte Typing II: Human T Lymphocytes, Vol 1. New York, Springer-Verlag, 1987
89. Broder S, Waldemann TA: Helper activity by lymphocytes derived from patients with the Sezary syndrome. J Clin Invest 58:1297, 1976
90. Broder S, Waldmann TA: The suppressor cell network in cancer. N Engl J Med 299:1281, 1978
91. Jaffe ES: Pathologic and clinical spectrum of post-thymic T-cell malignancies. Cancer Invest 2:413, 1984
92. Weiss LM, Crabtree GS, Rouse RV et al: Morphologic and immunologic characterization of 50 peripheral T cell lymphomas. Am J Pathol 118:316, 1985
93. Reinherz EL, Kung PC, Goldstein G et al: Discrete stages of human intrathymic differentiation: Analysis of normal thymocytes and leukemic lymphoblasts of T-cell lineage. Proc Natl Acad Sci USA 77:1588, 1980
94. Cossman J, Chused T, Fisher R et al: Diversity of immunologic phenotypes of lymphoblastic lymphoma. Cancer Res 43:4486, 1983
95. Goding JW, Burns GF: Monoclonal antibody OKT-9 recognizes the receptor for transferrin on human acute lymphocytic leukemic cells. J Immunol 127:1256, 1982
96. Pittaluga S, Uppenkamp M, Cossman J: Development of T3/T cell receptor gene expression in human pre-T neoplasms. Blood 69:1062, 1987
97. Greaves MF, Chan LC, Furley AJW et al: Lineage promiscuity in hematopoietic differentiation and leukemia. Blood 67:1, 1986
98. Caligaris-Cappio F, Gobbi M, Bofill M et al: Infrequent normal B lymphocytes express features of B-chronic lymphocytic leukemia. J Exp Med 155:623, 1982
99. Cossman J, Neckers LM, Hsu SM et al: Low grade lymphomas: Expression of developmentally regulated B-cell antigens. Am J Pathol 114:117, 1984
100. Arnold A, Cossman J, Bakhshi A et al: Immunoglobulin gene rearrangements as unique clonal markers in human lymphoid neoplasms. N Engl J Med 309:1593, 1983
101. Nadler LM, Korsmeyer SJ, Anderson KC et al: B cell origin of non-T cell acute lymphoblastic leukemia. J Clin Invest 74:332, 1984
102. Loken MR, Shah VO, Dattilio KL et al: Flow cytometric analysis of human bone marrow: II. Normal B lymphocyte development. Blood 70:1316, 1987
103. Greaves MF, Brown G, Rapson NT et al: Antisera to acute lymphoblastic leukemia cells. Clin Immunol Immunopathol 4:67, 1975
104. Korsmeyer SJ, Arnold A, Beach A et al: Immunoglobulin gene rearrangement and cell surface antigen expression in acute lymphocytic leukemias of T-cell and B-cell precursor origins. J Clin Invest 71:301, 1983
105. Ritz J, Nadler LM, Bhan AK et al: Expression of common acute lymphoblastic leukemia antigen (cALLa) by lymphomas of B cell and T cell lineage. Blood 58:648, 1981
106. Hsu SM, Jaffe ES: Phenotypic expression of B lymphocytes. Identification with monoclonal antibodies in normal lymphoid tissues. Am J Pathol 114:387, 1984
107. Cossman J, Neckers LM, Leonard WJ et al: Polymorphonuclear neutrophils express the common acute lymphoblastic leukemia antigen. J Exp Med 157:1064, 1983
108. Breard J, Reinherz EL, Kung PC et al: A monoclonal antibody reactive with peripheral blood monocytes. J Immunol 124:1943, 1980
109. Todd RF, Nadler LM, Schlossman SF: Antigens on human monocytes by monoclonal antibodies. J Immunol 126:1435, 1981
110. Hanjan SN, Kearney JF, Cooper MD: A monoclonal (MMA) that identifies a differentiation antigen on human myelomonocytic cells. Clin Immunol Immunopathol 23:172, 1982
111. Reinherz EL, Haynes BF, Nadler LM et al: Leukocyte Typing II. Human Myeloid and Hematopoietic Cells. New York, Springer-Verlag, Vol 3, 1988
112. Bollum FJ: Terminal deoxynucleotidyl transferase as a hematopoietic cell marker. A review. Blood 54:1203, 1979
113. Kung PC, Long JC, McCaffrey RP et al: Terminal deoxynucleotidyl transferase in the diagnosis of leukemia and malignant lymphoma. Am J Med 64:788, 1978
114. Braziel RM, Keneklis T, Donlon JA et al: Terminal deoxynucleotidyl transferase in non-Hodgkin's lymphoma. Am J Clin Pathol 80:655, 1983
115. Braziel RM, Hsu SM, Jaffe ES: Lymph nodes, spleen, and thymus. In Spicer SS (ed): Histochemistry in Pathologic Diagnosis, p 203. New York, Dekker, 1986
116. Yam LT, Li CY, Lam KW: Tartrate-resistant acid phosphatase isoenzyme in the reticulum cells of leukemic reticuloendotheliosis. N Engl J Med 284:357, 1971
117. Tonegawa S: Somatic generation of antibody diversity. Nature 301:575, 1983
118. Yanagi Y, Yoshikai Y, Leggett K et al: A human T-specific cDNA clone encodes a protein having extensive homology to immunoglobulin chains. Nature 308:145, 1984
119. Hedrick SM, Cohen DI, Nielsen EA et al: Isolation of cDNA clones encoding T-cell specific membrane-associated proteins. Nature 308:149, 1984
120. Hood L, Kronenberg M, Hunkapiller T: T cell antigen receptors and the immunoglobulin gene superfamily. Cell 40:255, 1985
121. Flug F, Pier-Giuseppe P, Bonetti F et al: T-cell receptor gene rearrangements as markers of lineage and clonality in T-cell neoplasms. Proc Natl Acad Sci USA 82:3460, 1985
122. Korsmeyer SJ, Greene WC, Cossman J et al: Rearrangement and expression of immunoglobulin genes and expression of Tac antigen in hairy cell leukemia. Proc Natl Acad Sci USA 80:4522, 1983
123. Cheng GY, Minden M, Toyonaga B et al: T cell receptor and immunoglobulin gene rearrangements in acute myeloblastic leukemia. J Exp Med 163:414, 1986
124. Ha K, Minden M, Hozumi N et al: Immunoglobulin chain gene rearrangement in a patient with T cell acute lymphoblastic leukemia. J Clin Invest 73:1232, 1984
125. Pelicci PG, Knowles DM, Dalla-Favera R: Lymphoid tumors displaying rearrangements of both immunoglobulin and T cell receptor genes. J Exp Med 162:1015, 1985

126. Uppenkamp M, Pittaluga S, Lipford EH et al: Limited diversity and selection of rearranged gamma genes in polyclonal T cells. J Immunol 138:1618, 1987
127. Weiss LM, Hu E, Wood GS et al: Clonal rearrangements of T cell receptor genes in mycosis fungoides and dermatopathic lymphadenopathy. N Engl J Med 313:537, 1985
128. Weiss LM, Wood GS, Trela M et al: Clonal T cell populations in lymphomatoid papulosis: Evidence of a lymphoproliferative origin for a clinically benign disease. N Engl J Med 315:475, 1986
129. Shearer WT, Ritz J, Finegold MK et al: Epstein–Barr virus associated B cell proliferations of diverse clonal origins after bone marrow transplantation in a 12 year old boy with severe combined immunodeficiency. N Engl J Med 312:1151, 1985
130. Starzl TE, Porter KA, Iwatsuki S et al: Reversibility of lymphomas and lymphoproliferative lesions developing under cyclosporin-steroid therapy. Lancet 1:583, 1984
131. Pelicci PG, Knowles DM, Arlin ZA et al: Multiple monoclonal B cell expansions and c-myc oncogene rearrangements in acquired immune deficiency syndrome related lymphoproliferative disorders. J Exp Med 164:2049, 1986
132. Lee M-S, Chang K-S, Cabanillas F et al: Detection of minimal residual cells carrying B t(14;19) by DNA sequence amplification. Science 237:175, 1987
133. Urba WJ, Longo DL: Cytologic, immunologic, and clinical diversity in non-Hodgkin's lymphoma: Therapeutic implications. Semin Oncol 12:250, 1985
134. Chan WC, Link S, Mawle A et al: Heterogeneity of large granular lymphocyte proliferations: Delineation of two major subtypes. Blood 68:1142, 1986
135. Craigie D: Case of disease of the spleen, in which death took place in consequence in the presence of purulent matter in the blood. Edinburgh Med Surg J 64:400, 1845
136. Bennett JH: Case of hypertrophy of the spleen and liver in which death took place from suppuration of the blood. Edinburgh Med Surg J 64:413, 1845
137. Virchow R: Weisses blut, Neue Notizen aus den Geb der Naturund Heikunde. Froriep's neue Notizen 36:151, 1845
138. Bilroth T: Multiple lymphome. Erfolgreiche Behandling mit arsenik. Wien Med Wochengchie 21:1066, 1871
139. Dreschfeld J: Clinical lecture on acute Hodgkin's (or pseudoleucocythemia). Br Med J 1:893, 1892
140. Kundrat H: Uber. Lympho-sarkomatosis. Wien Klin Wchnschr 6:211, 1893
141. Brill NE, Baehr G, Rosenthal N et al: Generalized giant lymphfollicle hyperplasia of lymph nodes and spleen, a hitherto undescribed type. JAMA 84:668, 1925
142. Symmers D: Follicular lymphadenopathy with splenomegaly. A newly recognized disease of lymphatic system. Arch Pathol Lab Med 3:816, 1927
143. Roulet F: Dasprinare Retothelsarkom der Lymphkonten. Virchows Arch Pathol Anat 277:15, 1930
144. Gall EA, Mallory TB: Malignant lymphoma. A clinical pathologic survey of 618 cases. Am J Pathol 18:381, 1942
145. Rappaport H, Winter WJ, Hicks EB: Follicular lymphoma. A reevaluation of its position in the scheme of malignant lymphomas, based on a survey of 253 cases. Cancer 9:792, 1956
146. Burkitt D: A sarcoma involving the jaws in African children. Br J Surg 46:218, 1958
147. Uchiyama T, Yodoi J, Sagawa K et al: Adult T-cell leukemia: Clinical and hematologic features of 16 cases. Blood 50:481, 1977
148. Rappaport H: Tumors of the hematopoietic system. In Atlas of Tumor Pathology, sect III, fasc 8. Washington, DC, Armed Forces Institute of Pathology, 1966
149. Dorfman RF: Classification of non-Hodgkin's lymphomas. Lancet 1:1295, 1974
150. Bennett MH, Farrer–Brown G, Henry K et al: Classification of non-Hodgkin's lymphomas. Lancet 2:405, 1974
151. Lukes RJ, Collin RD: Immunologic characterization of human malignant lymphomas. Cancer 34:1488, 1974
152. Lennert K, Mohri N, Stein H et al: Malignant Lymphomas Other Than Hodgkin's Disease. Berlin, Springer-Verlag, 1978
153. Lennert K, Mohri N, Stein H et al: The histopathology of malignant lymphoma. Br J Haematol 31 (suppl 1):193, 1975
154. Mathe G, Rappaport H, O'Conor GT et al: Histological and cytological typing of neoplastic diseases of hematopoietic and lymphoid tissues. In WHO International Histological Classification of Tumors, No. 14, Geneva, World Health Organization, 1976
155. Jaffe ES, Shevach EM, Frank MM et al: Nodular lymphoma: Evidence for origin from follicular B lymphocytes. N Engl J Med 290:813, 1974
156. Jaffe ES, Strauchen JA, Berard CW: Predictability of immunologic phenotype by morphologic criteria in diffuse aggressive non-Hodgkin's lymphomas. Am J Clin Pathol 77:46, 1982
157. National Cancer Institute Sponsored Study of Classifications of non-Hodgkin's Lymphomas. Summary and description of a working formulation for clinical usage. Cancer 49:2112, 1982
158. Rosenberg SA: Current concepts in cancer. Non-Hodgkin's lymphoma: Selection of treatment on the base of histologic type. N Engl J Med 301:924, 1979
159. Jaffe ES: Relationship of classification to biologic behavior of non-Hodgkin's lymphoma. Semin Oncol 13:3, 1986
160. DeVita VT Jr, Canellos GP, Chabner BA et al: Advanced diffuse histiocytic lymphoma, a potentially curable disease. Lancet 1:248, 1975
161. Jaffe ES: Follicular lymphomas: Possibility that they are benign tumors of the lymphoid system. J Natl Cancer Inst 70:401, 1983
162. Foon KA, Sherwin SA, Abrams PG et al: Treatment of advanced non-Hodgkin's lymphoma with recombinant leukocyte A interferon. N Engl J Med 311:1148, 1984
163. Cohen PJ, Lotze MT, Roberts JR et al: The immunopathology of sequential tumor biopsies in patients treated with interleukin-2. Correlation of response with T-cell infiltration and HLA-DR expression. Am J Pathol 129:208, 1987
164. Krikorian JG, Portlock CS, Cooney DP et al: Spontaneous regression of non-Hodgkin's lymphomas. A report of nine cases. Cancer Res 46:2093, 1980
165. Warnke RA, Kim H, Fuks Z et al: The coexistence of nodular and diffuse patterns in nodular non-Hodgkin's lymphomas: Significance and clinicopathologic correlation. Cancer 40:1229, 1977
166. Fisher RI, Jones RB, DeVita VT Jr et al: Natural history of malignant lymphomas with divergent histologies at staging evaluation. Cancer 47:2022, 1981
167. Hubbard SM, Chabner BA, DeVita VT Jr et al: Histologic progression in non-Hodgkin's lymphoma. Blood 59:258, 1982
168. Kim H, Hendrickson MR, Dorfman RF: Composite lymphoma. Cancer 40:959, 1977
169. Dick FR, Maca RD: The lymph node in chronic lymphocytic leukemia. Cancer 41:282, 1978
170. Pangalis GA, Nathwani BN, Rappaport H: Malignant lymphoma, well differentiated lymphocytic. Its relationship with chronic lymphocytic leukemia and macroglobulinemia in Waldenstrom. Cancer 39:999, 1977
171. Royston I, Majda JA, Baird SM et al: Human T-cell antigens defined by monoclonal antibodies: The 65,000-dalton antigen of T-cells (T65) is also found on chronic lymphocytic leukemia cells bearing surface immunoglobulin. J Immunol 125:725, 1980
172. Cossman J, Necker LM, Braziel RM et al: In vitro enhancement of immunoglobulin gene expression in chronic lymphocytic leukemia. J Clin Invest 73:587, 1984
173. Harrison CV: The morphology of the lymph node in the macroglobulinemia of Waldenstrom. J Clin Pathol 25:12, 1972
174. Dutcher TF, Fahey JL: The histopathology of the macroglobulinemia of Waldenstrom. J Natl Cancer Inst 22:887, 1959
175. Evans HL, Butler JJ, Youness EL: Malignant lymphoma, small lymphocytic type. A clinicopathologic study of 84 cases with suggested criteria for intermediate lymphocytic lymphoma. Cancer 41:1440, 1978
176. Richter MN: Generalized reticular cell sarcoma of lymph nodes associated with lymphatic leukemia. Am J Pathol 4:285, 1928
177. Trump DL, Mann RB, Phelps R et al: Richter's syndrome: Diffuse histiocytic lymphoma in patients with chronic lymphocytic lymphoma. A report of 5 cases and review of the literature. Am J Med 68:539, 1980
178. Nathwani BN, Winberg CD, Diamond LW et al: Morphologic criteria for the differentiation of follicular lymphoma from florid reactive follicular hyperplasia. A study of 80 cases. Cancer 48:1794, 1981
179. Garvin AJ, Simon R, Young RC et al: The Rappaport classification on non-Hodgkin's lymphomas: A closer look using other proposed classifications. Semin Oncol 7:234, 1980
180. Leech JH, Glick AD, Waldron JA et al: Malignant lymphomas of follicular center cell origin in man. I. Immunologic studies. J Natl Cancer Inst 54:11, 1975
181. Ault KA: Detection of small numbers of monoclonal B lymphocytes in the blood of patients with lymphoma. N Engl J Med 300:1401, 1979
182. Come SE, Jaffe ES, Anderson JC et al: Leukemic progression of non-Hodgkin's lymphoma: Clinicopathologic features and therapeutic implications. Am J Med 69:667, 1980
183. Nathwani BN, Metter GE, Miller TP et al: What should be the morphologic criteria for the subdivision of follicular lymphomas? Blood 68:837, 1986
184. Osborne CK, Norton L, Young RC et al: Nodular histiocytic lymphoma: An aggressive nodular lymphoma with potential for prolonged disease-free survival. Blood 56:98, 1980
185. Hoppe RT: Histologic variation in non-Hodgkin's lymphomas: Commentary. Cancer Treat Rep 65:935, 1981
186. Kim H, Dorfman RF: Morphological studies of 84 untreated patients subject to laparotomy for the staging of non-Hodgkin's lymphomas. Cancer 33:657, 1974
187. Lotz HJ, Chabner B, DeVita VT et al: Pathological staging of 100 consecutive untreated patients with non-Hodgkin's lymphomas. Extramedullary sites of disease. Cancer 37:266, 1976
188. Levy R, Warnke R, Dorfman RF et al: The monoclonality of human B-cell lymphomas. J Exp Med 145:1014, 1977
189. Harris NL, Nadler LM, Bhan AK: Immunohistologic characterization of two malignant lymphomas of germinal center type (centroblastic/centrocytic and centrocytic) with monoclonal antibodies: Follicular and diffuse lymphomas of small-cleaved-cell type are related but distinct entities. Am J Pathol 117:262, 1984
190. Jaffe ES, Braylan RC, Nanba K et al: Functional markers: A new perspective on malignant lymphomas. Cancer Treat Rep 61:953, 1977
191. Braziel RM, Sussman E, Neckers LM et al: Induction of immunoglobulin secretion in follicular non-Hodgkin's lymphomas: Role of immunoregulatory T cells. Blood 66:128, 1985
192. Lowder JN, Meeker TC, Campbell M et al: Studies on B lymphoid tumors treated with monoclonal anti-idiotype antibodies: Correlations with clinical responses. Blood 69:199, 1987
193. Yunis JJ, Oken MM, Kaplan ME et al: Distinctive chromosomal abnormalities in histologic subtypes of non-Hodgkin's lymphoma. N Engl J Med 307:1231, 1982
194. Tsujimoto Y, Cossman J, Jaffe ES et al: Involvement of the bcl-2 gene in human follicular lymphoma. Science 228:1440, 1985
195. Weiss LM, Warnke RA, Sklar J et al: Molecular analysis of the t(14;18) chromosomal translocation in malignant lymphomas. N Engl J Med 317:1185, 1987
196. Berard CW, Dorfman RF: Histopathology of malignant lymphomas. In Roschberg SA (ed): Clinics in Hematology, Vol 3, p 39. Philadelphia, WB Saunders, 1974
197. Weisenburger DD, Nathwani BN, Diamond LW et al: Malignant lymphoma, intermediate lymphocytic type: A clinico-pathologic study of 42 cases. Cancer 48:1415, 1981

198. Weisenburger DD, Kim H, Rappaport H: Mantle-zone lymphoma: A follicular variant of intermediate lymphocytic lymphoma. Cancer 49:1429, 1982
199. Swerdlow SH, Habeshaw JA, Murray LJ et al: Centrocytic lymphoma: A distinct clinicopathologic and immunologic entity. Am J Pathol 113:181, 1983
200. Jaffe ES, Bookman MA, Longo DL: Lymphocytic lymphoma of intermediate differentiation—mantle zone lymphoma: A distinct subtype of B-cell lymphoma. Hum Pathol 18:877, 1987
201. Nanba K, Jaffe ES, Braylan RC et al: Alkaline phosphatase-positive malignant lymphomas. Am J Clin Pathol 68:535, 1977
202. Cossman J, Jaffe ES, Fisher RI: Immunologic phenotypes of diffuse, aggressive, non-Hodgkin's lymphomas. Correlation with clinical features. Cancer 54:1310, 1984
203. Fisher RI, Hubbard SM, DeVita VT Jr et al: Factors determining our ability to cure aggressive forms of diffuse lymphomas. Blood 58:45, 1981
204. Jaffe ES, Longo DL, Cossman J et al: Diffuse B cell lymphomas with T cell predominance in patients with follicular lymphoma or "pseudo T cell lymphoma." Lab Invest 50:27A, 1984
205. Jaffe ES, Shevach EM, Sussman EH et al: Membrane receptor sites for the identification of lymphoreticular cells in benign and malignant conditions. Br J Cancer 31:107, 1975
206. Waldron JA, Leech JH, Glick AD et al: Malignant lymphoma of peripheral T lymphocyte origin. Cancer 40:1604, 1977
207. Lennert K, Mestdagh J: Lymphogranulomatosen mit konstant hohem Epitheloidzellgehalt. Virchows Arch [Pathol Anat] 344:1, 1968
208. Burke JS, Butler JJ: Malignant lymphoma with a high content of epithelioid histiocytes (Lennert's lymphoma). Am J Clin Pathol 66:1, 1976
209. Kim H, Jacobs C, Warnke RA et al: Malignant lymphoma with a high content of epithelioid histiocytes. A distinct clinicopathologic entity and a form of so-called "Lennert's lymphoma." Cancer 41:620, 1978
210. Levine AM, Taylor CR, Schneider DR et al: Immunoblastic sarcoma of T-cell versus B-cell origin: I. Clinical features. Blood 58:52, 1981
211. Lipford E, Wright JJ, Urba W et al: Refinement of lymphoma cytogenetics by the chromosome 18q21 major breakpoint region. Blood 70:1816, 1987
212. Muller-Hermelink HK, Steinmann G, Stein H et al: Malignant lymphoma of plasmacytoid T-cells. Morphologic and immunologic studies characterizing a special type of T-cell. Am J Surg Pathol 7:849, 1983
213. Stein H, Mason DY, Gerdes J et al: The expression of Hodgkin's disease associated antigen Ki-1 in reactive and neoplastic lymphoid tissue: Evidence that the Reed-Sternberg cells and histiocytic malignancies are derived from activated lymphoid cells. Blood 66:848, 1985
214. Kadin ME, Sako D, Berliner N et al: Childhood Ki-1 lymphoma presenting with skin lesions and peripheral lymphadenopathy. Blood 68:1042, 1986
215. Barcos MP, Lukes RJ: Malignant lymphoma of convoluted lymphocytes: A new entity of possible T cell type. In Sinks LF, Godden JO (eds): Conflicts in Childhood Cancer: An Evaluation of Current Management, Proceedings, p 147. New York, Alan R Liss, 1975
216. Nathwani BN, Kim H, Rappaport H: Malignant lymphoma, lymphoblastic. Cancer 38:964, 1976
217. Smith JL, Barker CR, Clein GP et al: Characterization of malignant mediastinal lymphoid neoplasm (Sternberg sarcoma) as thymic in origin. Lancet 1:74, 1973
218. Banks PM, Arseneau JC, Gralnick HR et al: American Burkitt's lymphoma: A clinicopathologic study of 30 cases: II. Pathologic correlations. Am J Med 58:322, 1975
219. Mann RB, Jaffe ES, Braylan RC et al: Nonendemic Burkitt's lymphoma: A B-cell tumor related to germinal centers. N Engl J Med 295:685, 1976
220. Magrath IT, Freeman CB, Pizzo P et al: Characterization of lymphoma-derived cell lines: Comparison of cell lines positive and negative for Epstein-Barr virus nuclear antigen: II. Surface markers. J Natl Cancer Inst 64:477, 1980
221. Taub R, Kirsch I, Morton C et al: Translocation of the c-myc gene into the immunoglobulin heavy chain locus in human Burkitt's lymphoma and murine plasmacytoma cells. Proc Natl Acad Sci USA 79:7837, 1982
222. Klein G: Specific chromosomal translocations and the genesis of B cell derived tumors in mice and men. Cell 32:311, 1983
223. Ziegler JL: Treatment results of 54 American patients with Burkitt's lymphomas are similar to the African experience. N Engl J Med 297:75, 1977
224. Grogan TM, Warnke RA, Kaplan HS: A comparative study of Burkitt's and non-Burkitt's "undifferentiated" malignant lymphomas: Immunologic, cytochemical, ultrastructural, cytologic, histopathologic, clinical and cell culture features. Cancer 49:1817, 1982
225. Miliauskas JR, Berard CW, Young RC et al: Undifferentiated non-Hodgkin's lymphomas (Burkitt's and non-Burkitt's types). The relevance of making this histologic distinction. Cancer 50:2115, 1982
226. Croce CM, Tsujimoto Y, Erikson I et al: Biology of disease: Chromosome translocations and B cell neoplasia. Lab Invest 51:258, 1984
227. Jaffe ES, Blattner WA, Blayney DW et al: The pathologic spectrum of HTLV-associated leukemia/lymphoma in the United States. Am J Surg Pathol 8:263, 1984
228. Broder S, Bunn PA Jr, Jaffe ES et al: T-cell lymphoproliferative syndrome associated with human T-cell leukemia/lymphoma virus. Ann Intern Med 100:543, 1984
229. Broder S, Bunn PA Jr: Cutaneous T-cell lymphomas. Semin Oncol 7:310, 1980
230. Lukes RJ, Tindle BH: Immunoblastic lymphadenopathy. A hyper-immune entity resembling Hodgkin's disease. N Engl J Med 292:1, 1975
231. Frizzera G, Moran EM, Rappaport H: Angioblastic lymphadenopathy: Diagnosis and clinical course. Am J Med 59:803, 1975
232. Nathwani BN, Rappaport H, Moran EM et al: Malignant lymphomas arising in angioimmunoblastic lymphadenopathy. Cancer 41:578, 1978
233. Watanabe S, Shimosato Y, Shimoyama M: Adult T-cell lymphoma with hypergammaglobulinemia. Cancer 41:2472, 1980
234. Kaneko Y, Larson RA, Variakojis D et al: Nonrandom chromosome abnormalities in angioimmunoblastic lymphadenopathy. Blood 60:877, 1982
235. Weiss LM, Strickler JG, Dorfman RF et al: Clonal T cell populations in angioimmunoblastic lymphadenopathy and angioimmunoblastic lymphadenopathy-like lymphoma. Am J Pathol 122:392, 1986
236. Lipford EH, Smith HR, Pittaluga S et al: Clonality of angioimmunoblastic lymphadenopathy and implications for its evolution to malignant lymphoma. J Clin Invest 79:637, 1987
237. Kassel SH, Echevarria RA, Guzzo FP: Midline malignant retriculosis (so-called lethal midline granuloma). Cancer 23:920, 1969
238. DeRemee RA, Weiland LH, McDonald TJ: Polymorphic reticulosis, lymphomatoid granulomatosis: Two diseases or one? Mayo Clin Proc 53:634, 1978
239. Liebow AA, Carrington CB, Friedman RJ: Lymphomatoid granulomatosis. Hum Pathol 3:457, 1972
240. Jaffe ES, Lipford EH Jr, Margolick JB et al: Lymphomatoid granulomatosis and angiocentric lymphoma. A spectrum of post-thymic T-cell proliferations. Semin Respir Med (in press)
241. Fauci AS, Haynes BF, Costa J et al: Lymphomatoid granulomatosis, prospective clinical and therapeutic experience over ten years. N Engl J Med 306:68, 1982
242. Katzenstein A, Carrington CB, Liebow AA: Lymphomatoid granulomatosis: A clinico-pathologic study of 152 cases. Cancer 43:360, 1979
243. Nichols PW, Koss M, Levine AM et al: Lymphomatoid granulomatosis: A T-cell disorder. Am J Med 72:467, 1982
244. Jaffe ES: Malignant histiocytosis and true histiocytic lymphomas. In Jaffe ES (ed): Surgical Pathology of Lymph Nodes and Related Organs, p 381. Philadelphia, WB Saunders, 1985
245. Sultan C, Imbert M, Richard MF et al: Pure acute monocytic leukemia. A study of 12 cases. Am J Clin Pathol 68:752, 1977
246. Van der Valk P, Meijer CJLM, Willemze R et al: Histiocytic sarcoma (true histiocytic lymphoma): A clinicopathologic study of 20 cases. Histopathology 8:105, 1984
247. Willemze R, Rinter DJ, Willem A et al: Reticulum cell sarcomas (large cell lymphomas) presenting in the skin. High frequency of true histiocytic lymphoma. Cancer 50:1367, 1982
248. Flynn KJ, Dehner LP, Gajl-Peczalska KJ et al: Regressing atypical histiocytosis: A cutaneous proliferation of atypical neoplastic histiocytes with unexpectedly indolent biologic behavior. Cancer 49:959, 1982
249. Poppema S, Van Voorst Vader PC, Rozenboom-Uiterwijk T et al: Lymphomatoid papulosis. Case report providing evidence for a monocyte-macrophage origin of the atypical cells. Cancer 52:1178, 1983
250. Scott RB, Robb-Smith AHT: Histiocytic medullary reticulosis. Lancet 2:194, 1939
251. Risdall RJ, McKenna RW, Nesbit ME et al: Virus-associated hemophagocytic syndrome—a benign histiocytic proliferation distinct from malignant histiocytosis. Cancer 44:993, 1979
252. Jaffe ES, Costa J, Fauci AS et al: Malignant lymphoma and erythrophagocytosis simulating malignant histiocytosis. Am J Med 75:1741, 1983
253. Simrell CR, Margolick JB, Crabtree GR et al: Lymphokine-induced phagocytosis in angiocentric immunoproliferative lesions (AIL) and malignant lymphoma arising in AIL. Blood 65:1469, 1985
254. Favara BE, McCarthy RC, Mierau GW: Histiocytosis X. In Finefold M (ed): Pathology of Neoplasia in Children and Adolescents, p 126. Philadelphia, WB Saunders, 1986
255. Nezelof C, Frileux-Herbet F, Cronier-Sachot J: Disseminated histiocytosis X, analysis of prognostic factors based on a retrospective study of 50 cases. Cancer 44:1824, 1979
256. Lahey ME: Prognostic factors in histiocytosis X. Am J Pediatr Hematol Oncol 3:57, 1981
257. Monda L, Warnke R, Rosai J: A primary lymph node malignancy with features suggestive of dendritic reticulum cell differentiation. A report of 4 cases. Am J Pathol 122:562, 1986
258. Feltkamp CA, van Heerde P, Feltkamp-Vroom TM et al: A malignant tumor arising from interdigitating cells; light microscopical, ultrastructural, immuno- and enzmehistochemical characteristics. Virchows Arch [Pathol Anat] 393:183, 1981
259. Chan W, Zaatari G: Lymph node interdigitating reticulum cell sarcoma. Am J Clin Pathol 85:739, 1986
260. Kaplan HS: Hodgkin's Disease, 2nd ed. Cambridge, Harvard University Press, 1980
261. Rosenberg SA, Diamond HD, Jaslowitz B et al: Lymphosarcoma: A review of 1269 cases. Medicine 40:31, 1961
262. Banfi A, Bonadonna G, Riece SB et al: Malignant lymphomas of Waldeyer's ring—natural history and survival after radiotherapy. Br Med J 2:140, 1972
263. Sage HH: Palpable cervical lymph nodes: JAMA 168:496, 1958
264. Filly R, Blank N, Castellino RA: Radiographic distribution of intrathoracic disease in previously untreated patients with Hodgkin's disease and non-Hodgkin's lymphoma. Radiology 120:277, 1976
265. Simone JV, Verzosa MS, Rudy JA: Initial features and prognosis in 363 children with acute lymphoblastic leukemia. Cancer 36:2099, 1975
266. Bitran JD, Golomb HM, Ultmann JE et al: Non-Hodgkin's lymphoma, poorly differentiated lymphocytic and mixed cell types: Results of sequential staging procedures, response to therapy, and survival of 100 patients. Cancer 42:88, 1978

267. Golomb H: "Hairy" cell leukemia: An unusual lymphoproliferative disease. Cancer 42:946, 1958
268. Rudders RA, Aisenberg AC, Schiller AL: Hodgkin's disease presenting as "idiopathic" thrombocytopenia purpura. Cancer 30:220, 1972
269. Rappaport H, Ramot B, Hulu N et al: The pathology of so-called Mediterranean abdominal lymphoma with malabsorption. Cancer 29:1502, 1972
270. Dragosics B, Bauer P, Radaszkiweicz T: Primary gastrointestinal lymphomas. A retrospective clinicopathologic study of 150 cases. Cancer 55:1060, 1985
271. Buskirk SJ, Evans RG, Banks PM et al: Primary lymphoma of the testis. Int J Radiat Biol Phys 8:1699, 1982
272. Young RC, Howser DM, Anderson T et al: Central nervous system complications of non-Hodgkin's lymphoma. The potential role for prophylactic therapy. Am J Med 66:435, 1979
273. Jones SE, Fuks Z, Bull M et al: Non-Hodgkin's lymphomas: IV. Clinicopathologic correlation in 405 cases. Cancer 31:806, 1973
274. Portlock CS, Rosenberg SA: No initial therapy for stage III and IV non-Hodgkin's lymphomas of favorable histologic types. Ann Intern Med 90:10, 1979
275. Rosenberg SA, Kaplan HS: Clinical trials in the non-Hodgkin's lymphoma at Stanford University: Experimental design and preliminary results. Br J Cancer 31:456, 1975
276. Roeser HP, Hocker GK, Kynaston B et al: Advanced non-Hodgkin's lymphomas: Response to treatment with combination chemotherapy and factors influencing prognosis. Br J Haematol 30:323, 1975
277. Paryani S, Hoppe RT, Burke JS et al: Extralymphatic involvement in diffuse non-Hodgkin's lymphomas. J Clin Oncol 1:682, 1983
278. DeVita VT: Human models of human disease: Breast cancer and the lymphomas. Int J Radiat Oncol Biol Phys 5:1855, 1979
279. Acker B, Hoppe RT, Colby TV et al: Histologic conversion in the non-Hodgkin's lymphomas. J Clin Oncol 1:11, 1983
280. Rowley JD: Consistent chromosome abnormalities in human leukemia and lymphoma. Cancer Invest 3:267, 1983
281. Chabner BA, Johnson RE, Young RC et al: Sequential non-surgical and surgical staging of non-Hodgkin's lymphoma. Ann Intern Med 85:149, 1976
282. Anderson T, Chabner BA, Young RC et al: Malignant lymphoma: I. The histology and staging of 473 patients at the National Cancer Institute. Cancer 50:2699, 1982
283. DeVita VT, Canellos GP: Treatment of the lymphomas. Semin Hematol 9:193, 1972
284. Reddy S, Saxena VS, Pellettiere EV et al: Early nodal and extra nodal non-Hodgkin's lymphomas. Cancer 40:98, 1977
285. Chen MG, Prosnitz LR, Gonzalez–Serva A et al: Results of radiotherapy in control of stage I and II non-Hodgkin's lymphoma. Cancer 43:1245, 1979
286. Carbone PP, Kaplan HS, Musshoff K et al: Report of the Committee on Hodgkin's disease staging. Cancer Res 31:1860, 1971
287. Young RC, Anderson T, DeVita VT: The treatment of Hodgkin's disease: Emphasizing programs at the Clinical Center, National Institutes of Health. Curr Probl Cancer 1:1, 1977
288. Reimer RR, Chabner BA, Young RC et al: Lymphoma presenting in bone: Results of histopathology, staging and therapy. Ann Intern Med 87:50, 1977
289. Shoji H, Miller T: Primary reticulum cell sarcoma of bone. Significance of clinical features upon prognosis. Cancer 28:1234, 1971
290. Castellino RA, Marglin SI: Imaging of abdominal and pelvic lymph nodes: Lymphography or computed tomography. Invest Radiol 17:433, 1983
291. Castellino RA, Goffinet DR, Blank N et al: The role of radiography in the staging of non-Hodgkin's lymphoma with laparotomy correlation. Radiology 110:329, 1974
292. Dunnick NR, Fuks Z, Castellino RA: Repeat lymphography in non-Hodgkin's lymphoma. Radiology 115:349, 1975
293. Herman TS, Jones SE: Systemic re-staging in the management of non-Hodgkin's lymphoma. Cancer Treat Rep 61:1009, 1977
294. Fuks JZ, Aisner J, Wiernik PH: Restaging laparotomy in the management of non-Hodgkin's lymphomas. Med Pediatr Oncol 10:429, 1982
295. Best JJK, Blackledge G, Forbes WS et al: Computed tomography of abdomen in staging and clinical management of lymphoma. Br Med J 2:1675, 1978
296. Schaner EG, Head GL, Doppman JL et al: Computed tomography in the diagnosis, staging and management of abdominal lymphoma. J Comput Assist Tomogr 1:176, 1977
297. Anderson KC, Leonard RC, Canellos GP et al: High dose gallium imaging in lymphoma. Am J Med 75:327, 1981
298. Longo DL, Schilsky RL, Blei L et al: Gallium-67 scanning has limited usefulness in staging patients with non-Hodgkin's lymphoma. Am J Med 68:695, 1980
299. Moran EJ, Ultmann JE, Ferguson DJ: Staging laparotomy on non-Hodgkin's lymphoma. Br J Cancer 31:228, 1975
300. Turner DA, Fordham EW, Amjad A et al: Gallium-67 imaging in the management of Hodgkin's disease and other malignant lymphomas. Semin Nucl Med 8:205, 1978
301. Chabner BA, Fisher RI, Young RC et al: Staging of non-Hodgkin's lymphoma. Semin Oncol 7:285, 1980
302. Levitt LJ, Dawson DM, Rosenthal DS et al: CNS involvement in the non-Hodgkin's lymphomas. Cancer 45:545, 1980
303. Bunn PA Jr, Schein PS, Banks PM et al: Central nervous system complications in patients with diffuse histiocytic and undifferentiated lymphoma: Leukemia revisited. Blood 47:3, 1976
304. Veronesi U, Musumeci R, Pizzetti F et al: The value of staging laparotomy in non-Hodgkin's lymphomas (with emphasis on the histiocytic type). Cancer 33:446, 1974
305. Castellino R, Bonadonna G, Spinelli P et al: Sequential pathologic staging of untreated non-Hodgkin's lymphomas by laparoscopy and laparotomy combined with marrow biopsy. Cancer 40:2322, 1977
306. Goffinet DR, Warnke R, Dunnick NR et al: Clinical and surgical (laparotomy) evaluation of patients with non-Hodgkin's lymphomas. Cancer Treat Rep 61:981, 1977
307. Chabner BA, Johnson RE, DeVita VT et al: Sequential staging in non-Hodgkin's lymphoma. Cancer Treat Rep 61:993, 1977
308. Heifetz LJ, Fuller LM, Rogers RW et al: Laparotomy findings in lymphangiogram-staged I and II non-Hodgkin's lymphomas. Cancer 45:2778, 1980
309. Surbone A, Longo DL, DeVita VT Jr et al: Residual abdominal masses in aggressive non-Hodgkin's lymphoma after combination chemotherapy: Significance and management. J Clin Oncol (in press)
310. Levy RL, Miller RA: Biological and clinical implications of lymphocyte hybridomas: Tumor therapy with monoclonal antibodies. Annu Rev Med 34:107, 1983
311. Balantine L, Skikne BS, Park CH et al: Malignant lymphocytic lymphoma: Demonstration of a serum inhibitor of myelopoiesis and response to combination chemotherapy. Cancer 52:35, 1983
312. Anderson TC, Jones SE, Soehnlen BJ et al: Immunocompetence and malignant lymphoma: Immunologic status before therapy. Cancer 48:2702, 1981
313. Jones SE, Griffith K, Dombrowski P et al: Immunodeficiency in patients with non-Hodgkin's lymphomas. Blood 49:335, 1977
314. Advani SH, Dinshaw KA, Nair CN et al: Immune dsyfunction in non-Hodgkin's lymphomas. Cancer 45:2843, 1980
315. Gajl–Peczalska KJ, Chartrand SL, Bloomfield CD: Abnormal immunoregulation in patients with non-Hodgkin's malignant lymphomas. Clin Immunol Immunopathol 23:366, 1982
316. Silver BA, Bostick–Bruton FW, Neckers L et al: Deficient helper cell function as a cause of diminished pokeweed mitogen blastogenic responses in patients with non-Hodgkin's lymphomas. Cancer 54:2936, 1984
317. Whisler RL, Balcerzak SP, Murray JL: Heterogeneous mechanisms of impaired lymphocyte responses in non-Hodgkin's lymphomas. Blood 57:1081, 1981
318. Broder S, Edelson RL, Lutzner MA et al: Sezary syndrome: A malignant proliferation of helper T cells. J Clin Invest 58:1297, 1976
319. Broder S, Uchiyama T, Muul L et al: Activation of leukemic prosuppressor cells to become suppressor effector cells. Influence of cooperating normal T cells. N Engl J Med 302:1382, 1981
320. Longo DL, Broder S: Human T-cell leukemia/lymphoma virus (HTLV)-associated adult T-cell leukemia. Med Grand Rounds 3:239, 1984
321. Moore DF, Migliore PH, Shullenberg CC et al: Monoclonal macroglobulinemia in malignant lymphoma. Ann Intern Med 72:43, 1970
322. Ko HS, Pruzanski W: M components associated with lymphoma: A review of 62 cases. Am J Med Sci 272:175, 1976
323. Jones SE: Autoimmune disorders and malignant lymphoma. Cancer 31:1092, 1973
324. Armitage JO, Weisenburger DD, Hutchins M et al: Chemotherapy for diffuse large-cell lymphoma: Rapidly responding patients have more durable remissions. J Clin Oncol 4:160, 1986
325. Rosenberg SA: The low-grade non-Hodgkin's lymphomas: Challenges and opportunities. J Clin Oncol 3:299, 1985
326. Paryani SB, Hoppe RT, Cox RS et al: Analysis of non-Hodgkin's lymphomas with nodular and favorable histologies, stages I and II. Cancer 52:2300, 1983
327. Fuks Z, Glatstein E, Kaplan HS: Patterns of presentation and relapse in the non-Hodgkin's lymphomata. Br J Cancer 31:286, 1975
328. Gallagher CJ, Gregory WM, Jones AE et al: Follicular lymphoma: Prognostic factors for response and survival. J Clin Oncol 4:1470, 1986
329. Gomez GA, Barcos M, Krishnamsetty RM et al: Treatment of early—stages I and II—nodular, poorly differentiated lymphocytic lymphoma. Am J Clin Oncol 9:40, 1986
330. Monfardini S, Banfi A, Bonadonna G et al: Improved five-year survival after combined radiotherapy-chemotherapy for stage I-II non-Hodgkin's lymphoma. Int J Radiat Oncol Biol Phys 6:125, 1980
331. Landberg TG, Hakansson LG, Moller TR et al: CVP remission maintenance in stage I or II non-Hodgkin's lymphomas: Preliminary results of a randomized study. Cancer 44:831, 1979
332. Toonkel LM, Fuller LM, Gamble JF et al: Laparotomy staged I and II non-Hodgkin's lymphomas: Preliminary results of radiotherapy and adjunctive chemotherapy. Cancer 45:249, 1980
333. McLaughlin P, Fuller LM, Velasquez WS et al: Stage I-II follicular lymphoma. Treatment results for 76 patients. Cancer 58:1596, 1986
334. Matis LA, Young RC, Longo DL: Nodular lymphomas: Current concepts. CRC Crit Rev Oncol Hematol 5:171, 1986
335. Anderson T, DeVita VT Jr, Simon RM et al: Malignant lymphoma II. Prognostic factors and response to treatment of 473 patients at the National Cancer Institute. Cancer 50:2708, 1982
336. Longo DL, Young RC, DeVita VT Jr: What is so good about the good prognosis lymphomas? In Williams CJ, Whitehouse JMA (eds): Recent Advances in Medical Oncology, p 223. Edinburgh, Churchill Livingstone, 1982
337. Portlock CS, Rosenberg SA, Glatstein E et al: Treatment of advanced non-Hodgkin's lymphomas with favorable histologies. Preliminary results of a prospective trial. Blood 47:747, 1976
338. Hoppe RT, Kushlan P, Kaplan HS et al: The treatment of advanced stage favorable non-Hodgkin's lymphoma: A preliminary report of a randomized trial comparing

single agent chemotherapy, combination chemotherapy, and whole body radiation. Blood 58:592, 1981

339. Young RC, Johnson RE, Canellos GP et al: Advanced lymphocytic lymphoma. Randomized comparisons of chemotherapy and radiotherapy alone or in combination. Cancer Treat Rep 61:1153, 1977
340. Brereton HD, Young RC, Longo DL et al: A comparison between combination chemotherapy and total body radiation plus combination chemotherapy in non-Hodgkin's lymphoma. Cancer 43:2227, 1979
341. Lister TA, Cullen MH, Beard MEJ et al: Comparison of combined and single-agent chemotherapy in non-Hodgkin's lymphoma of favorable histological type. Br Med J 1 (6112):533 1978
342. Kennedy BJ, Bloomfield CD, Kiang DT et al: Combinations versus successive single agent chemotherapy in lymphocytic lymphoma. Cancer 41:23, 1978
343. Monfardini S, Tancini G, DeLena M et al: Cyclophosphamide, vincristine and prednisone (CVP) versus Adriamycin, bleomycin, and prednisone (ABP) in stage IV non-Hodgkin's lymphomas. Med Pediatr Oncol 3:67, 1977
344. Cadman E, Drislane F, Waldron JA et al: High-dose pulse chlorambucil. Effective therapy for rapid remission induction in nodular lymphocytic poorly differentiated lymphoma. Cancer 50:1037, 1982
345. Portlock CS, Fischer DS, Cadman E et al: High-dose pulse chlorambucil in advanced, low-grade non-Hodgkin's lymphoma. Cancer Treat Rep 71:1029, 1987
346. Longo DL, Hubbard SM, DeVita VT Jr: The non-Hodgkin's lymphomas. In Slevin M, Staquet M (eds): Randomized Trials in Cancer. A Critical Review by Site, p 91. New York, Raven Press, 1985
347. Yates JL: The proper treatment of chronic malignant diseases of the superficial lymph glands. Arch Surg 5:65, 1922
348. Frizzera G, Anaya JS, Banks PM: Neoplastic plasma cells in follicular lymphomas. Clinical and pathologic findings in six cases. Virchows Arch A 409:149, 1986
349. Straus DJ, Gaynor JJ, Leiberman PH et al: Non-Hodgkin's lymphomas: Characteristics of long-term survivors following conservative treatment. Am J Med 82:247, 1986
350. Chabner BA: Nodular non-Hodgkin's lymphoma: The case for watchful waiting. Ann Intern Med 90:115, 1979
351. Botnick LE, Hannon EC, Hellman S: Limited proliferation of stem cells surviving alkylating agents. Nature 262:68, 1976
352. Hellman S, Reincke V, Botnick S et al: Functional organization of the hematopoietic stem cell compartment: Implications for cancer and its therapy. J Clin Oncol 1:227, 1983
353. Dumont J, Thiery JP, Mazabrand A et al: Acute myeloid leukemia following non-Hodgkin's lymphoma: Danger of prolonged use of chlorambucil as maintenance therapy. Nouv Rev Fr Hematol 22:391, 1980
354. Cameron S: Chlorambucil and leukemia. N Engl J Med 296:1065, 1977
355. Casciata DA, Scott DA: Acute leukemia following prolonged cytotoxic agent therapy. Medicine 58:32, 1979
356. Lerner HJ: Acute myelogenous leukemia in patients receiving chlorambucil as long-term adjuvant chemotherapy for stage II breast cancer. Cancer Treat Rep 62:1136, 1978
357. Longo DL, Young RC, Hubbard SM et al: Prolonged initial remission in patients with nodular mixed lymphoma. Ann Intern Med 100:651, 1984
358. Armitage JO, Dick FR, Corder MP: Diffuse histiocytic lymphoma after histologic conversion: A poor prognostic variant. Cancer Treat Rep 65:413, 1981
359. Garvin AJ, Simon RM, Osborne CK et al: An autopsy study of histologic progression in non-Hodgkin's lymphoma: 192 cases from the National Cancer Institute. Cancer 52:393, 1983
360. Glatstein E, Fuks Z, Goffinet DR et al: Non-Hodgkin's lymphoma of stage III extent. Is total lymphoid irradiation appropriate treatment? Cancer 37:2806, 1976
361. Paryani SB, Hoppe RT, Cox RS et al: The role of radiation therapy in the management of stage III follicular lymphomas. J Clin Oncol 2:841, 1984
362. Cox JD, Komaki R, Kun LE et al: Stage III nodular lymphoreticular tumors (non-Hodgkin's lymphomas): Results of central lymphatic irradiation. Cancer 47:2247, 1981
363. Flippen T, McLaughlin P, Conrad FG et al: Stage III nodular lymphomas. Preliminary results of a combined chemotherapy/radiotherapy program. Cancer 51:987, 1983
364. Schein PS, Chabner BA, Canellos GP et al: Non-Hodgkin's lymphoma: Patterns of relapse from complete remission after combination chemotherapy. Cancer 35:354, 1975
365. Anderson KC, Skarin AT, Rosenthal DS et al: Combination chemotherapy for advanced non-Hodgkin's lymphomas other than diffuse histiocytic or undifferentiated histologies. Cancer Treat Rep 68:1343, 1984
366. Case DC Jr: Comparison of M-2 protocol with COP in patients with nodular lymphoma. Oncology 41:159, 1984
367. Ezdinli EZ, Anderson JR, Melvin F et al: Moderate versus aggressive chemotherapy of nodular lymphocytic poorly differentiated lymphoma. J Clin Oncol 3:769, 1985
368. Young RC, Longo DL, Glatstein E et al: Watchful waiting vs aggressive combined modality therapy in the treatment of stage III-IV indolent non-Hodgkin's lymphoma. Proc Am Soc Clin Oncol 6:200, 1987
369. Samuels B, Ultmann J, Pearson M et al: Favorable non-Hodgkin's lymphoma: A fifteen year experience. Proc Am Soc Clin Oncol 6:206, 1987
370. Anderson T, Bender RA, Fisher RI et al: Combination chemotherapy in non-Hodgkin's lymphomas: Results of long-term follow-up. Cancer Treat Rep 61:1057, 1977
371. Ezdinli EZ, Costello WG, Icli F et al: Nodular mixed lymphocytic–histiocytic lymphoma (NM): Response and survival: Eastern Cooperative Oncology Group. Cancer 45:261, 1980
372. Merchant N, McLaughlin P, Fuller L et al: Follicular (nodular) mixed lymphoma: A review of 65 cases. Proc Am Soc Clin Oncol 3:249, 1984
373. Sobel RE, Dillman RO, Collins H et al: Applications and limitations of peripheral blood lymphocyte immunoglobulin light chain analysis in the evaluation of non-Hodgkin's lymphoma. Cancer 56:2005, 1985
374. Lindemalm C, Mellstedt H, Biberfeld P et al: Clonal blood B-cell excess in relation to prognosis in untreated non-leukemic patients with non-Hodgkin's lymphoma. In Cavalli F, Bonadonna G, Rozencweig M (eds): Malignant lymphomas and Hodgkin's disease: Experimental and therapeutic advances, p 225. Boston, Martinus-Nijhoff, 1985
375. Hansen H, Koziner B, Clarkson B: Marker and kinetic studies in the non-Hodgkin's lymphomas. Am J Med 71:107, 1981
376. Sobol RE, Royston I, LeBien T et al: Adult acute lymphoblastic leukemia phenotypes defined by monoclonal antibodies. Blood 65:730, 1985
377. Kaminski MS, Coleman CN, Colby TV et al: Factors predicting survival in adults with stage I and II large-cell lymphoma-treated with primary radiation therapy. Ann Intern Med 104:747, 1986
378. Shipp MA, Harrington DP, Klatt MM et al: Identification of major prognostic subgroups of patients with large-cell lymphoma treated with m-BACOD or M-BACOD. Ann Intern Med 104:757, 1986
379. Fuks Z, Kaplan HS: Recurrence rates following radiation therapy of nodular and diffuse malignant lymphomas. Radiology 108:675, 1973
380. Bush RS, Gospodarowicz M, Sturgeon J et al: Radiation therapy of localized non-Hodgkin's lymphoma. Cancer Treat Rep 61:1129, 1977
381. Bush RS, Gospodarowicz M: The place of radiation therapy in the management of patients with localized non-Hodgkin's lymphoma. In Rosenberg SA, Kaplan HS (eds): Malignant Lymphomas, p. 485. Orlando, Academic Press, 1982
382. Jones SE, Fuks Z, Kaplan HS et al: Non-Hodgkin's lymphomas. V. Results of radiotherapy. Cancer 32:682, 1973
383. Vokes EE, Ultmann JE, Golomb HM et al: Long-term survival of patients with localized diffuse histiocytic lymphoma. J Clin Oncol 3:1309, 1985
384. Levitt SH, Lee CK, Bloomfield CD et al: The role of radiation therapy in the treatment of early stage large cell lymphoma. Hematol Oncol 3:33, 1985
384a. Mauch P, Leonard R, Skarin A et al: Improved survival following combined radiation therapy and chemotherapy for unfavorable prognosis stage I–II non-Hodgkin's lymphomas. J Clin Oncol 3:1301, 1985
385. Nissen NI, Ersboll J, Hansen HS et al: A randomized study of radiotherapy vs radiotherapy plus chemotherapy in stage I-II non-Hodgkin's lymphomas. Cancer 52:1, 1983
386. Phillips DL: Radiotherapy in the treatment of localized non-Hodgkin's lymphoma (BNLI report 16). Clin Radiol 32:543, 1981
387. Glatstein E, Donaldson SS, Rosenberg SA et al: Combined modality therapy in malignant lymphomas. Cancer Treat Rep 61:1199, 1977
388. Gomez GA, Aggarwal KK, Han T: Post-therapeutic acute malignant myeloproliferative syndrome and acute nonlymphocytic leukemia in non-Hodgkin's lymphoma. Cancer 50:2285, 1982
389. Cabanillas F, Bodey GP, Freireich EJ: Management with chemotherapy only of stage I and II malignant lymphoma of aggressive histologic types. Cancer 46:2356, 1980
390. Miller TP, Jones SE: Initial chemotherapy for clinically localized lymphomas of unfavorable histology. Blood 62:413, 1984
391. Longo DL, Glatstein E, DeVita VT Jr et al: Combined modality treatment of patients with stage I diffuse aggressive lymphoma. Proc Am Assoc Cancer Res 28:205, 1987
392. Schein PS, DeVita VT Jr, Hubbard SM et al: Bleomycin, Adriamycin, cyclophosphamide, vincristine, and prednisone (BACOP) combination chemotherapy in the treatment of advanced diffuse histiocytic lymphoma. Ann Intern Med 85:417, 1976
393. Skarin AT, Rosenthal DS, Moloney WC et al: Combination chemotherapy of advanced non-Hodgkin's lymphoma with bleomycin, Adriamycin, cyclophosphamide, vincristine, and prednisone (BACOP). Blood 49:759, 1977
394. Levine AM, Goldstein M, Meyer PR et al: Heterogeneity of response and survival in diffuse histiocytic lymphoma after BACOP therapy (bleomycin, doxorubicin, cyclophosphamide, vincristine, prednisone). Hematol Oncol 3:87, 1985
395. Dupont J, Caray G, Scaglione C et al: A randomized comparison of two chemotherapy regimens: BACOP vs COPP in the treatment of diffuse histiocytic and mixed lymphoma. In Cavalli F, Bonadonna G, Rozensweig M (eds): Malignant Lymphomas and Hodgkin's Disease: Experimental and Therapeutic Advances, p 475. Boston, Martinus Nijhoff, 1985
396. Berd D, Cornog J, DeConti RC et al: Long-term remission in diffuse histiocytic lymphoma treated with combination sequential chemotherapy. Cancer 35:1050, 1975
397. Sweet DL, Golomb HM, Ultmann JE et al: Cyclophosphamide, vincristine, methotrexate and leucovorin rescue, and cytarabine (COMLA) combination sequential chemotherapy for advanced diffuse histiocytic lymphoma. Ann Intern Med 92:785, 1980
398. Gaynor ER, Ultmann JE, Golomb HM et al: Treatment of diffuse histiocytic lymphoma (DHL) with COMLA (cyclophosphamide, oncovin, methotrexate, leucovorin, cytosine arabinoside): A 10-year experience in a single institution. J Clin Oncol 3:1596, 1985
399. Todd M, Cadman E, Spiro P et al: A follow-up of a randomized study comparing two chemotherapy treatments for advanced diffuse histiocytic lymphoma. J Clin Oncol 2:986, 1984

400. McKelvey EM, Gottlieb JA, Wilson HE et al: Hydroxydaunomycin (Adriamycin) combination chemotherapy in malignant lymphoma. Cancer 38:1484, 1976
401. Coltman CA Jr, Dahlberg S, Jones SE et al: CHOP is curative in 30 percent of patients with large cell lymphoma: A 12-year Southwest Oncology Group follow-up. In Skarin AT (ed): Advances in Cancer Chemotherapy: Update on Treatment for Diffuse Large Cell Lymphoma, p 71. New York, Park Row, 1986
402. Armitage JO, Fyfe MA, Lewis J: Long-term remission durability and functional status of patients treated for diffuse histiocytic lymphoma with the CHOP regimen. J Clin Oncol 2:898, 1984
403. Jones SE, Grozea PN, Miller TP et al: Chemotherapy with cyclophosphamide, doxorubicin, vincristine, and prednisone alone or with levamisole or with levamisole plus BCG for malignant lymphoma: A Southwest Oncology Group study. J Clin Oncol 3:1318, 1985
404. Longo DL, DeVita VT Jr: Lymphomas. In Pinedo HM, Chabner BA (eds): Cancer Chemotherapy Annual 6, p 232. Amsterdam, Elsevier, 1984
405. Skarin AT, Canellos GP, Rosenthal DS et al: Improved prognosis of diffuse histiocytic and undifferentiated lymphoma by use of high-dose methotrexate alternating with standard agents (M-BACOD). J Clin Oncol 1:91, 1983
406. Skarin AT, Canellos GP, Rosenthal DS et al: Moderate dose m-BACOD in advanced diffuse large cell lymphoma: An interim report. In Skarin AT (ed): Advances in Cancer Chemotherapy: Update on Treatment for Diffuse Large Cell Lymphoma, p 23. New York, Park Row, 1986
407. Laurence J, Coleman M, Allen SL et al: Combination chemotherapy of advanced diffuse histiocytic lymphoma with the six-drug COP-BLAM regimen. Ann Intern Med 97:190, 1982
408. Norton L, Simon RM: Tumor size, sensitivity to therapy, and the design of treatment schedules. Cancer Treat Rep 61:1307, 1977
409. Fisher RI, DeVita VT Jr, Hubbard SM et al: Diffuse aggressive lymphomas: Increased survival after alternating flexible sequences of ProMACE and MOPP chemotherapy. Ann Intern Med 98:304, 1983
410. Cabanillas F, Burgess MA, Bodey GP et al: Sequential chemotherapy and late intensification for malignant lymphomas of aggressive histological type. Am J Med 74:382, 1983
411. Goldie JH, Coldman AJ: The genetic origin of drug resistance in neoplasms: Implications for systemic therapy. Cancer Res 44:3643, 1984
412. Hryniuk W, Bush H: The importance of dose intensity in chemotherapy of metastatic breast cancer. J Clin Oncol 2:1281, 1984
413. Longo DL, DeVita V Jr, Duffey P et al: Randomized trial of ProMACE-MOPP (day 1, day 8) vs ProMACE-CytaBOM in stage II-IV aggressive non-Hodgkin's lymphoma. Proc Am Soc Clin Oncol 6:206, 1987
414. Baer MR, Stein RS, Greer JP et al: Modified cyclophosphamide, vincristine, methotrexate, leucovorin, and cytarabine (COMLA) in intermediate- and high-grade lymphoma: An effective short course regimen. Cancer Treat Rep 70:785, 1986
415. Lee R, Cabanillas F, Bodey GP et al: A 10-year update of CHOP-Bleo in the treatment of diffuse large-cell lymphoma. J Clin Oncol 4:1455, 1986
416. Coleman M, Boyd DB, Beshevkin M et al: COP-BLAM treatment of large cell lymphoma: A status report. In Skarin AT (ed): Advances in Cancer Chemotherapy: Update on Treatment for Diffuse Large Cell Lymphoma, p 63. New York, Park Row, 1986
417. Coleman M, Gerstein G, Topilow A et al: Advances in chemotherapy for large cell lymphoma. Semin Hematol 24:8, 1987
418. Klimo P, Connors JM: MACOP-B chemotherapy for the treatment of diffuse large-cell lymphoma. Ann Intern Med 102:596, 1985
419. Klimo P, Connors JM: Updated clinical experience with MACOP-B. Semin Hematol 24:26, 1987
420. Amadori S, Guglielmi C, Anselmo AP et al: Treatment of diffuse aggressive non-Hodgkin's lymphomas with an intensive multi-drug regimen including high-dose cytosine arabinoside (F-MACHOP). Semin Oncol 12:218, 1985
421. DeVita VT Jr, Hubbard SM, Longo DL: The chemotherapy of lymphomas: Looking back, moving forward—The Richard and Hinda Rosenthal Foundation Award lecture. Cancer Res 47:5810, 1987
422. Gabrilove J, Jakubowski A, Fain K et al: A phase I/II study of rhG-CSF in cancer patients at risk for chemotherapy-induced neutropenia. Blood 70:135a, 1987
423. Bronchud MH, Scarffe JH, Thatcher N et al: Phase I/II study of recombinant human granulocyte colony-stimulating factor in patients receiving intensive chemotherapy for small cell lung cancer. Br J Cancer 56:809, 1987
424. Bernard A, Boumsell L, Reinherz EL et al: Cell surface characterization of malignant T cells from lymphoblastic lymphoma using monoclonal antibodies: Evidence for phenotypic differences between malignant T cells from patients with acute lymphoblastic leukemia and lymphoblastic lymphoma. Blood 57:1105, 1981
425. Nathwani BN, Diamond LW, Winberg CD et al: Lymphoblastic lymphoma: A clinicopathologic study of 95 patients. Cancer 48:2347, 1981
426. Voakes JB, Jones SE, McKelvey EM: The chemotherapy of lymphoblastic lymphoma. Blood 57:186, 1981
427. Weinstein HJ, Cassady JR, Levey R: Long-term results of the APO protocol (vincristine, doxorubicin [Adriamycin], and prednisone) for the treatment of mediastinal lymphoblastic lymphoma. J Clin Oncol 1:537, 1983
428. Weinstein HJ, Lack EE, Cassady JR: APO therapy for malignant lymphoma of large cell "histiocytic" type of childhood: Analysis of treatment results for 29 patients. Blood 64:422, 1984
429. Magrath IT, Janus C, Edwards BK et al: An effective therapy for both undifferentiated (including Burkitt's) lymphomas and lymphoblastic lymphomas in children and young adults. Blood 63:1102, 1984
430. Camitta BM, Lauer SJ, Casper JT et al: Effectiveness of a six-drug regimen (APO) without local irradiation for treatment of mediastinal lymphoblastic lymphoma in children. Cancer 56:738, 1985
431. Janus C, Edwards BK, Sariban E et al: Surgical resection and limited chemotherapy for abdominal undifferentiated lymphomas. Cancer Treat Rep 68:599, 1984
432. Wollner N, Wachtel AE, Exelby PR et al: Improved prognosis in children with intra-abdominal non-Hodgkin's lymphoma following LSA2-L2 protocol chemotherapy. Cancer 45:3034, 1980
433. Anderson JR, Wilson JF, Jenkin DT et al: Childhood non-Hodgkin's lymphoma. The results of a randomized therapeutic trial comparing a 4-drug regimen (COMP) with a 10-drug regimen (LSA2-L2). N Engl J Med 308:559, 1983
434. Sullivan MP, Boyett J, Pullen J et al: Pediatric Oncology Group experience with modified LSA2-L2 therapy in 107 children with non-Hodgkin's lymphoma (Burkitt's lymphoma excluded). Cancer 55:323, 1984
435. Levine AM, Forman SJ, Meyer PR et al: Successful therapy of convoluted T-lymphoblastic lymphoma in the adult. Blood 61:92, 1983
436. Bernstein JI, Coleman CN, Strickler JG et al: Combined modality therapy for adults with small noncleaved cell lymphoma (Burkitt's and non-Burkitt's types). J Clin Oncol 4:847, 1986
437. Coleman CN, Picozzi VJ Jr, Cox RS et al: Treatment of lymphoblastic lymphoma in adults. J Clin Oncol 4:1628, 1986
438. Slater DE, Mertelsmann R, Koziner B et al: Lymphoblastic lymphoma in adults. J Clin Oncol 4:57, 1986
439. Willemze R, Peters WG, VanHennik MB et al: Intermediate and high-dose ara-c and m-AMSA (or daunarubicin) as remission and consolidation treatment for patients with relapsed acute leukaemia and lymphoblastic non-Hodgkin's lymphoma. Scand J Haematol 34:83, 1985
440. Urba WJ, Longo DL: Clinical spectrum of human retroviral-induced disease. Cancer Res 45:4509, 1985
441. Daenen S, Rojer A, Smit JW et al: Successful chemotherapy with deoxycoformycin in adult T-cell lymphoma/leukaemia. Br J Haematol 58:723, 1984
442. Takatsuki K, Yamaguchi K, Kawano F et al: Clinical diversity in adult T-cell leukemia-lymphoma. Cancer Res 45:4544, 1985
443. Waldmann TA, Goldman CK, Bongiovanni KF et al: Therapy of patients with human T-cell leukemia virus I-induced adult T-cell leukemia with anti-Tac, a monoclonal antibody to the receptor for interleukin-2 (in press)
444. Gill PS, Levine AM, Krailo M et al: AIDS-related malignant lymphoma: Results of prospective treatment trials. J Clin Oncol 5:1322, 1987
445. Jack CR Jr, Reese DF, Scheithauer BW: Radiographic findings in 32 cases of primary CNS lymphoma. Am J Roentgenol 146:271, 1986
446. Amendola BE, McClatchey KD, Amedola MA et al: Primary large-cell lymphoma of the central nervous system. Am J Clin Oncol 9:203, 1986
447. Cohen IJ, Vogel R, Matz S et al: Successful non-neurotoxic therapy (without radiation) of a multifocal primary brain lymphoma with a methotrexate vincristine and BCNU protocol (DEMOB). Cancer 57:6, 1986
448. Giannone K, Greco FA, Hainsworth JD: Combination intraventricular chemotherapy for meningeal neoplasia. J Clin Oncol 4:68, 1986
449. Gordon PS, Juillard GJ, Selch MT et al: Orbital lymphomas and pseudolymphomas: Treatment with radiation therapy. Radiology 159:797, 1986
450. Baumann MA, Ritch PS, Hande KR et al: Treatment of intraocular lymphoma with high-dose ara-C. Cancer 57:1273, 1986
451. ReMine SG, Braasch JW: Gastric and small bowel lymphoma. Surg Clin North Am 66:713, 1986
452. Sheridan WP, Medley G, Brodie GN: Non-Hodgkin's lymphoma of the stomach: A prospective pilot study of surgery plus chemotherapy in early and advanced disease. J Clin Oncol 3:495, 1985
453. Takvorian T, Canellos GP, Ritz J et al: Prolonged disease-free survival after autologous bone marrow transplantation in patients with non-Hodgkin's lymphoma with a poor prognosis. N Engl J Med 316:1499, 1987
454. Armitage JO, Gringrich RD, Klassen LW et al: Trial of high-dose cytarabine, cyclophosphamide, total-body irradiation and autologous marrow transplantation for refractory lymphoma. Cancer Treat Rep 70:871, 1986
455. Philip T, Biron P, Herve P et al: Massive BACT chemotherapy with autologous bone marrow transplantation in 17 cases of non-Hodgkin's lymphoma with a very bad prognosis. Eur J Cancer Clin Oncol 19:1871, 1983
456. Philip T, Biron P, Maraninchi D et al: Role of massive chemotherapy and autologous bone marrow transplantation in non-Hodgkin's malignant lymphoma. Lancet 1:391, 1984
457. Philip T, Biron P, Maraninchi D et al: Massive chemotherapy with autologous bone marrow transplantation in 50 cases of bad prognosis non-Hodgkin's lymphoma. Br J Haematol 60:599, 1985
458. Armitage JO, Jagannath S, Spitzer G et al: High-dose therapy and autologous marrow transplantation as salvage treatment for patients with diffuse large cell lymphoma. Eur J Cancer Clin Oncol 22:871, 1986
459. Phillips GL, Herzig RH, Lazarus HM et al: Treatment of resistant malignant lymphoma with cyclophosphamide, total body irradiation, and transplantation of cryopreserved autologous marrow. N Engl J Med 310:1557, 1984
460. Phillips GL, Herzig RH, Lazarus HM et al: High-dose chemotherapy, fractionated total-body irradiation, and allogeneic marrow transplantation for malignant lymphoma. J Clin Oncol 4:480, 1986
461. Verdonck LF, Dekker AW, van Kempen ML et al: Intensive cytotoxic therapy followed by autologous bone marrow transplantation for non-Hodgkin's lymphoma of high grade malignancy. Blood 65:984, 1985

462. Gorin NC, Jajman A, Douay L et al: Autologous bone marrow transplantation in the treatment of poor prognosis non-Hodgkin's lymphomas. Eur J Cancer Clin Oncol 20:217, 1985
463. Bone marrow auto-transplantation in man: Report of an international cooperative study. Lancet 2:960, 1986
464. Singer CRJ, Goldstone AH: Clinical studies of ABMT in non-Hodgkin's lymphoma. Clin Haematol 15:105, 1986
465. Hancock BW: Vindesine, etoposide (VP-16), and prednisolone (VEP) in relapsed patients with grade II non-Hodgkin's lymphoma. Semin Oncol 2:26, 1985
466. Helms SR, Oblon DJ, Braylon RC et al: Etoposide, carmustine, bleomycin, and methotrexate with leucovorin rescue as retreatment for unfavorable non-Hodgkin's lymphoma. Cancer Treat Rep 69:783, 1985
467. Judson IR, Wiltshaw EA: Cis-dichorodiammineplatinum (cis-platinum) and etoposide (VP-16) in malignant lymphoma—an effective salvage regimen. Cancer Chemother Pharmacol 14:258, 1985
468. Dana BW, Jones SE, Coltman C et al: Salvage treatment of unfavorable non-Hodgkin's lymphoma with cisplatin, amsacrine, and mitoguazone: A Southwest Oncology Group pilot study. Cancer Treat Rep 70:291, 1985
469. Cabanillas F, Hagemeister FB, McLaughlin P et al: Experience with ifosphamide-based regimens for the treatment of malignant lymphomas. In Skarin AT (ed): Advances in Cancer Chemotherapy: Update on Treatment for Diffuse Large Cell Lymphoma, p 85. New York, Park Row, 1986
470. Longo DL, DeVita VT Jr: Lymphomas. In Pinedo HM, Longo DL, Chabner BA (eds): Cancer Chemotherapy and Biological Response Modifiers Annual 9, p 165. Amsterdam, Elsevier, 1987
471. Schauer PK, Straus DJ, Bagley DM Jr et al: Angioimmunoblastic lymphadenopathy: Clinical spectrum of disease. Cancer 48:2493, 1981
472. Klinman DM, Steinberg AD, Mushinski JF: Effect of cyclophosphamide therapy on oncogene expression in angioimmunoblastic lymphadenopathy. Lancet 2:1055, 1986
473. Frizzera G, Peterson BA, Bayrd ED et al: A systemic lymphoproliferative disorder with morphologic features of Castleman's disease: Clinical findings and clinicopathologic correlations in 15 patients. J Clin Oncol 3:1202, 1985
474. Repetto L, Jaiprakash MP, Selby PJ et al: Aggressive angiofollicular lymph node hyperplasia (Castleman's disease) treated with high dose melphalan and autologous bone marrow transplantation. Hematol Oncol 4:213, 1986
475. Urba WJ, Longo DL: Alpha-interferon in the treatment of nodular lymphomas. Semin Oncol 13:40, 1986
476. Warrell RP Jr, Krown SE, Koziner B et al: Acute nonlymphoblastic leukemia after treatment of nodular lymphoma with human leukocyte interferon. Ann Intern Med 98:482, 1983
477. Jakubowski AA, Casper ES, Gabrilove JL et al: Phase I trial of intramuscularly administered tumor necrosis factor in adults with advanced cancer. Proc Am Soc Clin Oncol 6:243, 1987
478. Nadler LM, Stashenko P, Hardy R et al: Serotherapy of a patient with a monoclonal antibody directed against a human lymphoma-associated antigen. Cancer Res 40:3147, 1980
479. Miller RA, Oseroff AR, Stratte PT et al: Monoclonal antibody therapeutic trials in seven patients with T-cell lymphoma. Blood 62:988, 1983
480. Ritz J, Pesando JM, Sallan SE et al: Serotherapy of acute lymphoblastic leukemia with monoclonal antibody. Blood 58:141, 1981
481. Foon KA, Schroff RW, Bunn PA et al: Effects of monoclonal antibody therapy in patients with chronic lymphocytic leukemia. Blood 64:1085, 1984
482. Press OW, Applebaum F, Ledbetter JA et al: Monoclonal antibody 1F5 (anti-CD20) serotherapy in malignant B-cell lymphomas. Blood 69:584, 1987
483. Raffeld M, Neckers L, Longo DL et al: Spontaneous alteration of idiotype in a monoclonal B-cell lymphoma: Escape from detection by anti-idiotype. N Engl J Med 312:1653, 1985
484. Rankin EM, Hekman A, Somers R et al: Treatment of two patients with B cell lymphoma with monoclonal anti-idiotype antibodies. Blood 65:1373, 1985
485. Hamblin TJ, Cattan AR, Glennie MN et al: Initial experience in treating human lymphoma with a chimeric univalent derivative of monoclonal anti-idiotype antibody. Blood 69:790, 1987
486. Hurwitz E, Burowski D, Kashi R et al: A synergistic effect between anti-idiotype antibodies and anti-neoplastic drugs in the therapy of a murine B-cell tumor. Int J Cancer 37:739, 1986
487. Badger CC, Krohn KA, Peterson AV et al: Experimental radiotherapy of murine lymphoma with 131I-labeled anti-Thy 1.1 monoclonal antibody. Cancer Res 45:1536, 1985
488. Gregg EO, Bridges SH, Youle RJ et al: Whole ricin and recombinant ricin A chain idiotype-specific immunotoxins for therapy of the guinea pig L2C B cell leukemia. J Immunol 138:4502, 1987
489. Kulkarni PN, Blair AH, Ghose T et al: Conjugation of methotrexate to IgG antibodies and their $F(ab')_2$ fragments and the effect of conjugated methotrexate on tumor growth in vivo. Cancer Immunol Immunother 19:211, 1985
490. Rosen ST et al: Personal communication, 1989
491. Applebaum F et al: Personal communication, 1989
492. Gorin NC, Douay L, Laporte JP et al: Autologous bone marrow transplantation with marrow decontaminated by immunotoxin T101 in the treatment of leukemia and lymphoma: First clinical observations. Cancer Treat Rep 69:953, 1985
493. Ashwell JD, Longo DL, Bridges SH: T-cell tumor elimination as a result of T-cell receptor-mediated activation. Science 237:61, 1987
494. Beckwith M, Urba WJ, Longo DL: Activation signals produce irreversible growth inhibition in human B-cell lymphoma cell lines (in preparation)
495. Nadler LM, Takvorian T, Botnick L et al: Anti-B1 monoclonal antibody and complement treatment in autologous bone marrow transplantation for relapsed B-cell non-Hodgkin's lymphoma. Lancet 2:421, 1984
496. DeFabritiis P, Bregni M, Lipton J et al: Antigenic heterogeneity among Burkitt's lymphoma cells surviving treatment with monoclonal antibody and complement. Leuk Res 10:35, 1986
497. Rosenberg SA, Lotze MT, Muul LM et al: A progress report on the treatment of 157 patients with advanced cancer using lymphokine-activated killer cells and interleukin 2 or high-dose interleukin 2 alone. N Engl J Med 316:889, 1987
498. Kohler PC, Hank JA, Exten R et al: Clinical response of a patient with diffuse histiocytic lymphoma to adoptive chemoimmunotherapy using cyclophosphamide and alloactivated haploidentical lymphocytes. A case report and phase I trial. Cancer 55:552, 1985
499. Wiltrout RW, Boyd MR, Back TT et al: Flavone-8-acetic acid augments systemic natural killer cell activity and synergizes with interleukin 2 for treatment of murine renal cell cancer. J Immunol (in press)
500. Jeglum KA, Young KM, Barnsley K et al: Intralymphatic autochthonous tumor cell vaccine in canine lymphoma. J Biol Resp Mod 5:168, 1986
501. Edelson R, Berger C, Gasparro F et al: Treatment of cutaneous T-cell lymphoma by extracorporeal photochemotherapy. Preliminary results. N Engl J Med 316:297, 1987
502. Thomsen K, Molin L, Volden G et al: 13-cis-retinoic acid effective in mycosis fungoides. A report from the Scandinavian Mycosis Fungoides Group. Acta Derm Venereol (Stockh) 64:563, 1984
503. Cunningham D, Gilchrist NL, Cowan RA et al: Alfacalcidol as a modulator of growth of low grade non-Hodgkin's lymphomas. Br Med J 291:1153, 1985

PAUL A. BUNN, JR

ZVI FUKS

CHAPTER 51 *Cutaneous Lymphomas*

INTRODUCTION AND T-CELL BIOLOGY

The understanding of the functional, phenotypic, and genotypic properties of normal T lymphocytes and their malignant counterparts led to a better understanding of the biology and classification of T-cell lymphomas.[1-6] Advances in molecular biology and virology led to the discovery of a new T-cell lymphoma termed acute T-cell leukemia/lymphoma (ATL), caused by a type C retrovirus, human T-cell lymphotrophic virus-I (HTLV-I).[7,8] Other T-cell malignancies, including mycosis fungoides (MF) and the Sézary syndrome, may be caused by related viruses. HTLV-V, a putative etiologic virus for the cutaneous T-cell lymphomas (CTCL), was recently described.[9]

T-cell lymphomas in the United States are much less common than B-cell lymphomas. Peripheral T-cell lymphomas, T-cell chronic lymphocytic leukemia (CLL), and T-gamma lymphoproliferative disorders are discussed in other chapters. CTCL is uncommon. The age-adjusted incidence of CTCL in the United States is two to three cases per million persons per year, and there are about 600 total new cases per year.[10,11] The peak incidence is in the sixth decade of life; onset before age 30 is rare. The disease is slightly more common in males, and there is no racial predilection. ATL is rare in the United States, with fewer than 100 cases being reported in the literature. It is uncertain whether the incidence is rising because of an increased prevalence of HTLV-I infection.

Stem cells destined to become T-lymphocytes originate in the bone marrow and migrate to the thymus, where they undergo differentiation under the influence of several thymic hormones.[12] During this differentiation they undergo rearrangement of the T-cell receptor gene loci.[13,14] The exquisite specificity of T cells is a result of this cell surface receptor. The diversity with the ability to recognize millions of antigens is a result of the rearrangement of the gene. The human T-cell receptor has two major subunits, Ti alpha and Ti beta, which are held together by disulfide bonds. These subunits are closely associated with the T3 molecule, which consists of a 25-kd gamma chain and two 20-kd delta and epsilon chains (Fig. 51-1). The Ti subunits form a binding site for antigen and major histocompatibility complex (MHC) through interaction of their variable domains, and the T3 subunits serve a signal transduction function. The Ti receptor subunit proteins are translated from genes that contain variable, diverse, joining, and constant regions (Fig. 51-1). Thus Southern analysis of deoxyribonucleic acid (DNA) from patients' T cells can be used to determine whether malignant cells are T cells and whether there is monoclonal rearrangement of the T-cell receptor gene loci.[6]

Early T-cell cells may express the 3A1 and T11 (CD2) antigens as well as intracellular terminal deoxyribonucleotide transferase (TdT) before rearrangement of the T-cell receptor gene.[13] The T11 antigen is the sheep erythrocyte receptor. This 50-kd surface glycoprotein facilitates T lymphocyte/target cell interactions and activates resting T cells.[15] The ability of the T11 antigen to trigger T-cell activation independent of antigen and MHC is important for amplification of the immune response. The T11 antigen is present on T cells throughout their differentiation. The function of the 3A1 antigen is unknown, and it is lost as the cells mature. The transcription of Ti beta precedes Ti alpha; T3 transcription first occurs at about the same stage, whereas surface T3–Ti appears in the late thymocyte stage.[13]

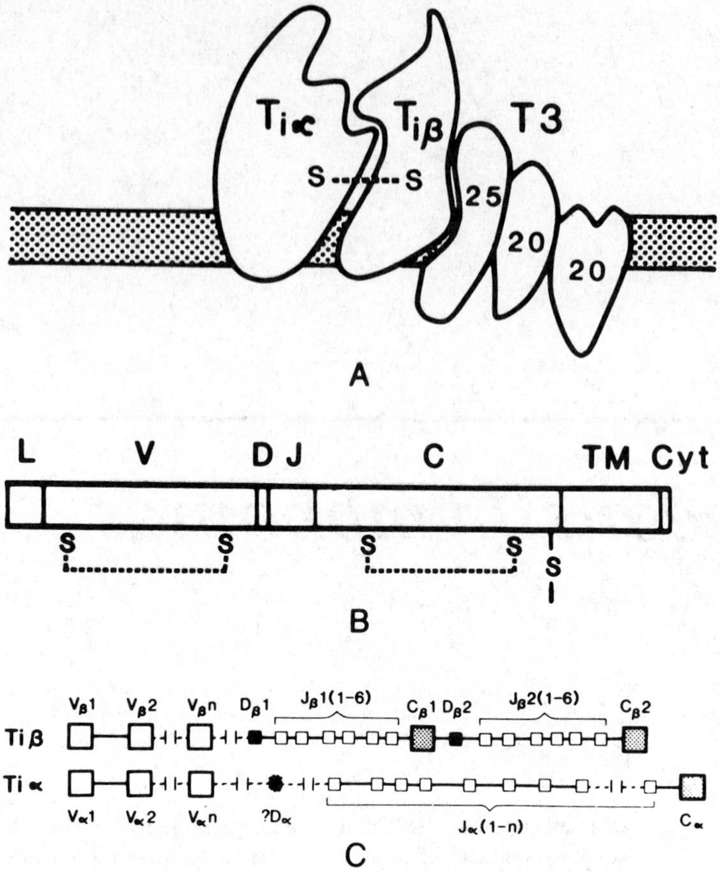

FIG. 51-1. Structure of the human T-cell receptor and its subunits. **A**. Subunit composition of the human T-cell receptor. The Ti α and Ti β subunits are held together by S-S bonds and are most closely associated with the 25-kd γ chain of the T3 molecule. The α and β subunits are anchored in the cell membrane with their transmembrane segments. The T3 complex consists of two additional subunits (δ and ϵ), with molecular weights of 20,000. Although not shown, a recently described 16-kd homodimer (32-kd nonreduced), termed zeta, is also noncovalently associated with the T3-Ti complex. **B**. Structure of the Ti subunits. The predicted primary structure of the β-chain subunit after translation from the cDNA sequence is depicted, as are the variable region leader (*L*), V, D, and J segments, a hydrophobic transmembrane segment (*TM*), and cytoplasmic part (*Cyt*) in the C region, potential intrachain sulfhydryl bonds (*S-S*), and the single SH group (*S*) that can form a sulfhydryl bond with the α subunit. **C**. Scheme of the genomic organization of the human β- and α-chain genes. In the β locus, V indicates the V gene pool located at the 5′ end, at an unknown distance from the $D_{\beta 1}$ element, the $J_{\beta 1}$ cluster, and the $C_{\beta 1}$ constant-region gene. Further downstream, a second $D_{\beta 2}$ element, $J_{\beta 2}$ cluster, and $C_{\beta 2}$ constant-region gene are indicated. A similar nomenclature is used for the Ti α locus in which only a single constant region is found. ?D indicates the uncertainty about the existence of a putative Ti α diversity element. (Reproduced with permission from Royer HD, Reinherz EL: T lymphocytes: Ontogeny, function, and relevance to clinical disorders. N Engl J Med 317:1136–1142, 1987)

The T4 (CD4) and T8 (CD8) surface glycoproteins appear during mid- to late thymocyte development, and eventually cells retain or lose one of these antigens.[12] The $CD4^+$ cells, termed helper/inducer T cells, constitute two-thirds of peripheral blood T cells and bind to invariant regions of Class II MHC antigens. These cells facilitate the differentiation of B cells into antibody-producing plasma cells and facilitate the function of $T8^+$ cytotoxic/suppressor cells. The T4 molecule is also the receptor for the human immunodeficiency virus (HIV, HTLV-III).[16] $T8^+$ cytotoxic/suppressor cells constitute one-third of peripheral blood T cells and have specificity for antigen and Class I MHC antigens. They are responsible for MHC-directed cytotoxicity of virus infected and malignant cells, for graft rejection, for delayed hypersensitivity reactions, and for inhibiting the differentiation of B cells into plasma cells.

T-cell proliferation results from events involving the T3–Ti complex and the binding of interleukin-2 (IL-2) (T-cell growth factor, TCGF) to the IL-2 receptor.[13,17,18] Resting T cells have no IL-2 receptors. After antigen or MHC exposure the number of surface antigen (Ti) receptors decreases while IL-2 receptors increase. In contrast to resting lymphocytes and the low-grade T-cell lymphomas, the HTLV-I–infected malignant cells in ATL constitutively express IL-2 receptors. This may account for the rapid proliferation of these cells.

A small fraction of peripheral blood T cells lack T4 and T8 antigens and express the T3–Ti gamma–delta receptor.[19] These cells have broad natural killer (NK)–like activity. Reports of target granular lymphocytic malignancies derived from this population of cells are now appearing.[20]

CLASSIFICATION OF T-CELL MALIGNANCIES

The Rappaport and Working Formulations[21,22] were not developed for classifying T-cell malignancies. Thus some T-cell malignancies appear in these classifications and others are omitted. The T-cell malignancies can be separated into low, intermediate, and high grades, as in the Working Formulation, and can be distinguished by their phenotypic properties.

The most immature T-cell malignancies are the lymphoblastic lymphomas and T-cell acute lymphoblastic leukemias.[23,24] The malignant cells in these disorders have prethymic or thymic markers and can be considered to be the leukemic or tissue phases of the same disease process, in analogy with CLL and diffuse well-differentiated lymphocytic lymphoma. The malignant cells in these disorders usually have intracellular Tdt and express the 3A1 antigen. Clinically, these disorders are often associated with mediastinal masses and a predilection for CNS involvement. More detailed descriptions may be found elsewhere (see Chaps. 48 and 50). T-cell prolymphocytic leukemia is a rare leukemia derived from intermediate or mature thymocytes and thus may be T4+ T8+ or T4+ T8−.[25]

Malignancies of mature T cells may be of low, intermediate, or high grade. ATL is a high-grade T-cell leukemia/lymphoma with some distinct clinical features described below, caused by the HTLV-I retrovirus.[1,7,8,26] The cells in ATL have the helper/inducer phenotype and constitutively express the IL-2 receptor (IL-2R). All other T-cell lymphomas do not express IL-2R. The peripheral T-cell lymphomas (including T immunoblastic, diffuse T large noncleaved, diffuse T large noncleaved) are intermediate or high grade. These lymphomas do not express immature T-cell markers, almost always express T1, T3, T11, and T4 antigens, and always have monoclonally rearranged T-cell receptor genes.[27]

Low-grade T-cell lymphomas always have a mature T-cell phenotype. CTLL, including MF and the Sézary syndrome, is derived from mature helper/inducer T cells (T1, T3, T11, T4+, T8−).[3-5] The true T-cell CLL cells may be derived from either the helper/inducer or the cytotoxic/suppressor subsets.[28,29] Finally, the cells in the syndrome of T gamma lymphocytosis may be derived from the T8+ cytotoxic/suppressor subset, from NK cells, or perhaps from the T3–Ti gamma subset of T cells.[30-32]

CLINICAL FEATURES OF ADULT T-CELL LEUKEMIA/LYMPHOMA

In the United States the majority of malignant lymphomas are of B-cell origin, whereas in other parts of the world, such as Japan, T-cell lymphomas predominate.[1] In the late 1970s several Japanese investigators recognized a distinct group of T-cell lymphoma patients.[33] These patients were geographically clustered in the southwestern provinces and had an acute fulminant lymphoma characterized by leukemic cells, tissue invasion (including skin), and a rapidly fatal course. The clustering suggested an infectious cause. Several years later Catovsky and associates described a series of black patients from the Caribbean basin who had similar features, often with hypercalcemia.[34]

At the same time a malignant cell line, Hut102, was initiated from a patient with an atypical cutaneous T-cell lymphoma at the National Cancer Institute (NCI).[35] This cell line, which grew without exogenous growth factors, was shown to produce IL-2, to have high expression of IL-2 receptors, and to be infected with HTLV-I.[1,7] Shortly thereafter antibodies to this virus were detected in 100% of the patients with ATL in Japan, the Caribbean, and the United States.[1,36] An identical virus was detected in Japanese patients and cell lines.

The HTLV-I retrovirus from Hut102 and other cell lines has been isolated and completely sequenced.[1] It contains 1096 nucleotides. Long terminal repeats (LTRs) are positioned at the 5′ and 3′ ends, which regulate transcription by providing sites for ribonucleic acid (RNA) polymerase attachment. The proviral RNA next contains gag, pol, and env genes, which encode for the structural proteins, the reverse transcriptase, and the envelope proteins, respectively. The most 3′ region, termed pX, contains a long open reading (LOR) frame which encodes for a protein that acts as a transcriptional activator of the LTR regions and perhaps as an activator for other genes.

There is overwhelming evidence that HTLV-I is the causative agent of ATL.[1] This evidence includes the following: (1) ATL occurs in areas endemic for HTLV-I; (2) ATL patients have anti–HTLV-I antibodies in their serum; (3) HTLV-I proviral genome is monoclonally integrated in malignant ATL cells; (4) infection of normal T4 cells with HTLV-I causes alternations in morphology and independent growth properties characteristic of ATL cells; and (5) proviral integration into these cells and their descendants is monoclonal. However, the actual site of integration varies from patient to patient and from cell line to cell line.

The clinical features of ATL in the United States and the Caribbean are well described.[8,37] Most patients are from the southeastern United States or Hawaii or have emigrated from other endemic regions such as Japan or the Caribbean basin. The disease has not been reported in children; the median age is 35 to 55 with a slight male predominance. The disease tends to have a sudden onset, usually with hypercalcemia or rapidly developing skin lesions. The median interval between the onset of symptoms and a diagnosis of lymphoma is short (median, 2 months). Systemic B symptoms are common, and all patients are Stage IV with involvement of at least one organ (usually skin, gastrointestinal tract, pulmonary system, or central nervous system). Lymphadenopathy is invariably present; massive mediastinal node enlargement is uncommon. Opportunistic infections are extremely common because the patients are immunosuppressed.

Hypercalcemia or evidence of bone resorption, or both, are extremely common ATL. The presence of hypercalcemia imparts a poor prognosis, and the hypercalcemia is extremely difficult to manage without an excellent antitumor response. Osteolytic bone lesions, abnormal bone scans, and elevated alkaline phosphatase levels are other manifestations of the bone-resorbing features of ATL. It appears that the malignant cells secrete an osteoclast-activating, bone-resorbing protein as yet uncharacterized. Vitamin D and parathormone levels are normal.

Many patients with ATL have a T-cell leukemia in which the malignant circulating cells have a characteristic cloverleaf appearance.[26] The peripheral white blood cell count varies from normal to extremely high (>200,000/μl) in these patients. When these cells are present, a morphologic diagnosis is more easily established. The histologic picture in tissue sites is quite variable. The lymphoma may be described as one of several in the Rappaport classification (*e.g.*, diffuse poorly differentiated lymphocytic, diffuse mixed, diffuse histiocytic), and the cell morphology may be quite pleomorphic.[26]

CLINICAL FEATURES OF LOW-GRADE T-CELL LYMPHOMAS

CUTANEOUS T-CELL LYMPHOMA

Patients with low-grade T-cell lymphomas typically have a natural history extending over years to decades, but most patients eventually die of lymphoma or secondary infections unless successfully treated.[3] Aggressive and fulminate variants leading to death shortly after diagnosis have also been described. Mycosis fungoides was first described by Alibert in 1806[38], and derives its name from the mushroom-like appearance of tumors found in the advanced stages of the diseases. The cause is unknown, but recently a putative etiologic retrovirus termed HTLV-V was isolated from a patient-derived cell line.[9] Various environmental factors, chemicals, physical agents, and drugs have also been implicated as causative factors.[10,39]

Cutaneous Manifestations of Disease

Most patients experience periods of months to years (average, 5–10 years)[1,11] of transitory and nonspecific cutaneous manifestations before establishment of a diagnosis of CTCL. This premycotic phase is often misdiagnosed as eczema, neurodermitis, erythema, poikiloderma, parapsoriasis enplaques, or other dermatoses. The most common symptom at this stage is itching, and typically the initial lesions are eczematous, frequently appearing in a bathing trunk distribution. As the disease progresses, the eczematous patches gradually develop into indurated erythematous or hyperpigmented plaques, which have serpiginous and sharply demarcated margins. At this stage a definitive histologic diagnosis is usually attainable. During the plaque phase the disease frequently begins to progress more rapidly as the cutaneous involvement becomes more generalized, with scattered or confluent plaques progressively covering increasing portions of the body surface. Prognostically, it has been shown useful to distinguish between the limited plaque stage (plaques covering less than 10% of the body surface) and the generalized plaque stage (more than 10% of the body surface).[1,40,41] The plaques can grow not only in their surface dimensions, but also in thickness, gradually producing tumors, which can be elevated a few centimeters above the skin surface and are prone to ulceration and secondary infections. Occasionally, however, patients may present with skin tumors, without a history of preexisting plaques (mycosis fungoides d'emblée).[1]

Another common cutaneous variant of CTCL is the generalized erythroderma (l'homme rogue) variant. The erythroderma usually involves most of the skin surface and is accompanied by either skin thickening (lichenification) or, more frequently, skin atrophy. It may appear simultaneously with plaques or tumors, although most often it precedes their appearance. Occasionally it has an explosive onset, frequently confused with allergic reactions or toxic exposures. Extreme itching is most common at this stage, leading to excoriation, skin ulceration, and infection. Patients with erythroderma who have evidence of more than 5% circulating malignant convoluted atypical mononuclear MF (Sézary) cells have the so-called Sézary syndrome.[1,42] Recent studies showed that, when carefully examined, nearly all patients with generalized erythroderma and 13% to 65% of patients with plaque–tumor will have some circulating MF cells.[43–45] Patients with high percentages of circulating Sézary cells have a shorter survival than do those with lower percentages.[44,45] Very rarely patients may present with generalized lichenification without erythroderma (the lichenoid variant).

As to the relative distribution of the various cutaneous types, cumulative data from several large series[41,43,46,47] show that approximately 40% of the patients have limited plaque disease at initial diagnosis, 30% have generalized plaques, 15% tumors, and 15% generalized erythroderma.

Extracutaneous Manifestations of Disease

Staging and autopsy series both confirm that extracutaneous spread is found most often in peripheral blood and lymph nodes. Approximately 45% of CTCL patients present with peripheral lymphadenopathy at the time of initial diagnosis.[41,43,46–48] Enlarged lymph nodes are palpable in 20% of limited plaque, 54% of generalized plaque, 81% of erythematous, and 84% of tumor-stage patients.[46] Histologic evaluation of lymph node biopsies has been somewhat controversial. Previous studies confirmed that patients with effaced lymph node architecture had a worse prognosis than those with dermatopathic lymphadenopathy, who in turn had a worse prognosis than those with normal or reactive nodes.[11,46,47] Subsequent studies, which used cytogenetic analysis, electron microscopy, DNA content analysis, molecular probes for T-cell receptor gene rearrangements, and immunohistopathology, demonstrated at least some malignant "Sézary cells" in the majority of lymph nodes.[5,6,43,48–51] An LN classification recently described by Gazdar and Mathews has provided useful prognostic information.[48] Patients with dermatopathic changes and small numbers of malignant cells (LN1 or LN2) had 5-year survivals of 80%; those with dermatopathic changes and large clusters of paracortical malignant cells (LN3) had 5-year survivals of 30%; and those with effaced nodes (LN4) had 5-year survivals of only 15%. The spread of MF from one lymph node region to another is centripetal, as lymphographic studies showed that most prominent abnormalities are found in distal nodes with less prominent changes centrally.[52] Node biopsy is more important than lymphangiography for routine staging information.[48]

Peripheral blood evaluation should be performed in all patients because it provides prognostic information. Circulating MF cells are present in 90% with erythroderma, 27% with cutaneous tumors, 10% with generalized plaques, and rarely with limited plaques. The presence of high numbers of circulating cells and large cells provides additional prognostic information.[44,45,50]

Visceral involvement, easily identifiable by light microscopy, is found frequently (72%) in the terminal stages of the disease.[1,11] Whereas virtually every organ may become involved, the most common sites of involvement are bone marrow, lung, spleen, and liver. Careful staging at the time of initial presentation revealed[43,48] that 18% had pathologically proven visceral involvement. This observation suggests that the dissemination of the disease is frequently hematogeneous and may occur early in the course of CTCL. Routine evaluations should include only chest x-rays unless signs and symptoms suggest organ involvement. Bone marrow and liver biopsies should be considered for those with peripheral blood involvement or generalized lymphadenopathy.

Staging of CTCL

The most commonly used staging classification system was proposed by the Mycosis Fungoides Cooperative Group (MFCG),[40,41] using a modified TNM system (Table 51-1). This system considers the extent of disease in the skin (T), lymph nodes (N), visceral organs (M), and peripheral blood (B). Patients are then regrouped into stages, with Stage I representing disease limited to the skin as plaques in the absence of palpable lymph nodes; Stage II consists of plaques associated with adenopathy or tumors with or without adenopathy; Stage III represents generalized erythroderma patients; and Stage IV includes patients with biopsy-proven lymph node or visceral involvement, or both. Recent studies from the NCI and the MFCG showed a significant correlation between survival and the MFCG TNM staging classification.[41,43,44,48,49] Prognostically, patients can be divided into three groups. Patients with Stage I or IIa (about 50% of all patients) have a 90% 5-year survival (Fig. 50-1). Stage IIb, III, or IVa patients (approximately 40%) have a median survival of about 5 years. Median survival for Stage IVB patients (about 10% of patients) is only about 2 years.

Natural History

Most CTCL patients have an indolent course, and infection is the most common cause of death primarily because of the breakdown of the normal skin barrier.[3,11] Progressive disseminated lymphoma is the second most common cause of death. Often this occurs after cytologic or histologic transformation into a high-grade lymphoma.[53] This was initially believed to represent the development of a second neoplasm; more recent studies showed that this was evolution of the original malignant clone. CTCL patients are more likely to develop other neoplasms, however. These include second skin cancers (see below), Hodgkin's disease, and myeloid leukemias.[1,3]

LYMPHOMATOID PAPULOSIS AND LYMPHOMATOID GRANULOMATOSIS

Lymphomatoid papulosis and lymphomatoid granulomatosis are other T-cell lymphoproliferative disorders whose nature is poorly understood. Lymphomatoid papulosis is characterized by nodular lymphocytic proliferation in the skin and subcutaneous tissues.[54–56] Histologically, the picture is typical of cutaneous T-cell lymphoma; the cells have similar morphologic, ultrastructural, and phenotypic properties. Clinically, the nodules may appear and disappear spontaneously. The natural history is long; evolution into more typical MF is common. It is not clear whether this is a premalignant or malignant condition since appropriate cytogenetic and molecular studies have not been performed.

Lymphomatoid granulomatosis is characterized by a T-cell lymphocytic proliferation in association with giant cell granuloma formation.[57,58] The skin, lungs, and kidneys are most frequently involved. Cutaneous lesions are usually tumors with a propensity to ulcerate. The disease is often aggressive, and conversion to high-grade T-cell lymphomas is often described. It is unclear whether lymphomatoid granulomatosis is a premalignant or frankly malignant process because there are insufficient cytogenetic and molecular data to draw firm conclusions.

THERAPY OF ATL

Therapy of this disorder is currently unsatisfactory, and patients have a very poor prognosis. Complete remission (CR) has been observed in about 50% of patients given intensive combination chemotherapy regimens such as ProMACE/CytaBOM or M-BACOD.[8] These regimens generally alleviate symptoms such as hypercalcemia and skin lesions; however, long-term remissions are not observed. Opportunistic infections spreading to the central nervous system and relapse are

TABLE 51-1. National Cutaneous T-Cell Lymphoma Workshop Staging Classification*

T	*Skin*	*N*	*Lymph Nodes*	*M*	*Visceral Organs*
T_1	Limited plaques (<10% BSA)†	N_0	No adenopathy; histology negative	M_0	No involvement
T_2	Generalized plaques	N_1	Adenopathy; histology negative	M_1	Visceral involvement
T_3	Cutaneous tumors	N_2	No adenopathy; histology positive		
T_4	Generalized erythroderma	N_3	Adenopathy; histology positive		

Stage I	Limited (IA) or generalized plaques (IB) without adenopathy or histologic involvement of lymph nodes or viscera ($T_1N_0M_0$ or $T_2N_0M_0$)
Stage II	Limited or generalized plaques with adenopathy (IIA) or cutaneous tumors with or without adenopathy (IIB); without histologic involvement of lymph nodes or viscera ($T_{1-2}N_1M_0T_2N_{0-1}M_0$)
Stage III	Generalized erythroderma with or without adenopathy; without histologic involvement of lymph nodes or viscera ($T_4N_{0-1}M_0$)
Stage IV	Histologic involvement of lymph nodes (IVA) or viscera (IVB) with any skin lesion and with or without adenopathy ($T_{1-4}N_{2-3}M_0$ for IVA; $T_{1-4}N_{0-3}M_1$ for IVB).

*Blood involvement should be recorded as absent (B_0) or present (B_1) but is not currently used to determine final stage.

†BSA, body surface area.

major problems. Numerous biologic agents have been evaluated. Unlabeled monoclonal antibodies (T101, anti-Tac), deoxycoformycin, and interferons have not been useful. Antibody conjugates are being evaluated, as are antiviral agents.[59] For the rare patient with an indolent asymptomatic course, observation is reasonable.

THERAPY OF CTCL

Because the cutaneous manifestations represent the major clinical manifestations and the most common source of symptoms in CTCL, topical treatments have been the mainstay of CTCL management. Topical treatments with nitrogen mustard, PUVA (psoralen with ultraviolet light A, or photochemotherapy), and electron beam irradiation have been established as effective, although their impact on survival is still debated. With the increasing realization that CTCL disseminates early, systemic chemotherapy has been increasingly used, but its effectiveness and impact on survival have not yet been established. Interferon has also been established as an effective systemic agent, with an unknown effect on survival. Other biologic and experimental therapies are under investigation.

Radiation Therapy

The first effective topical treatment for CTCL was with small-field soft x-ray radiation introduced by Scholtz in 1902.[60] Early experience demonstrated the outstanding sensitivity of CTCL lesions to radiation, and in fact the MF/Sézary cells are considered among the most radiation sensitive of all cells. Small-field ("spot") orthovoltage radiotherapy is still being used for eradication of symptomatic tumors or plaques in patients with relapsing disease who do not respond to other forms of treatment. The effective local dose is relatively low (800–1550 cGy) given in fractions of 300 to 500 cGy two to four times per week. Although such treatment frequently results in relatively long-term local control, its use is not recommended for patients who have not received previous radiation, since other techniques of radiotherapy and other topical treatments produce better long-lasting therapeutic effects.

Because of the generalized nature of the cutaneous manifestations in most patients, total skin application of topical treatments has been used for many years. Trump and coworkers[61] were the first to suggest the use of total skin irradiation with 2.5 MeV electrons. Electron beam irradiation, produced by linear accelerators, has the same radiobiologic effects as x-rays, but electrons have a limited penetration into the skin. The radiation dose distribution and maximal range of penetration of electrons depend on the electron beam energy. With the 4 to 7 MeV beams generally used for CTCL, the maximal radiation dose is deposited within the first 4 to 5 mm of the surface, whereas only 50% of the dose reaches 11 to 15 mm and little, if any, radiation reaches the tissues at a depth of 20 mm. This method, therefore, represents a highly effective mode of treatment for superficial cutaneous lesions over the entire body surface, with a complete sparing of deeper tissues, thus avoiding the systemic effects of radiation.

To cover the entire body surface, special techniques have been used, such as the four-field, six-field, or rotational treatments.[46,62] Most techniques use a fractionation schedule that delivers 400 cGy total skin dose per week in four treatment sessions,[46] whereas others use 400 cGy in single fraction given once a week.[62] The recommended total dose is 3000 to 3600 cGy in 8 to 9 weeks, and doses in this range should be used for any extent of disease. The high radiation doses are required for induction of CR. The Stanford studies[46] showed that the rate of initial CR in patients with T_1 or T_2 lesions treated with less than 2000 cGy was 55% compared to 92% observed with 3000 to 3600 cGy. Although the initial CR rates in T_3 and T_4 patients was somewhat lower, the dose response effect was still demonstrated (32% versus 80%). The tolerance of treatment is usually good, although nearly all patients who receive 3000 cGy or more develop various degrees of cutaneous erythema and desquamation, and some patients develop lower-extremity or generalized skin edema. These symptoms subside after completion of treatment.

The largest experience with long-term results has been published by the Stanford group.[46,63] A recent update of their experience showed that the continuous unmaintained freedom from relapse at 15 years in 192 patients with T_1 or T_3 lesions was 22%, with 10- and 15-year survival rates of 41% and 32%, respectively.[63] The results differed according to the T stage (Fig. 51-2), with 50% of T_1 patients surviving 15 to 18 years without evidence of relapse, suggesting that some of these patients may have been cured. The Stanford study also demonstrated the effect of radiation dose on survival.[46] Patients with plaques who were treated with doses exceeding 3000 cGy had significantly improved survival compared to patients who were treated with less than 3000 cGy. Essentially similar therapeutic benefits, although with shorter durations of follow-up, have been reported by other groups using total skin irradiation with electrons.

Topical Chemotherapy

Another highly useful treatment for T_1 or T_2 patients is the topical application of aqueous solutions of nitrogen mustard (HN_2). Haserick and colleagues[64] first reported in 1959 regressions of cutaneous lesions after topical application of HN_2. The mechanism of action of this modality is still unknown, since the alkylating properties of HN_2 dissipate shortly after it is dissolved in water, whereas the anti-CTCL effects of aqueous HN_2 are maintained long after its alkylating properties deteriorate.

The technique of topical application of HN_2 requires the dilution of a 10-mg vial in 50 to 100 ml of water. The solution is then applied with cloth or brush to the entire skin surface, sparing only the eyelids, lips, and the rectal and vaginal orifices. More diluted solution can be applied, if necessary, to spared areas and other sensitive regions. Treatment is applied daily for 6 to 12 months, and then the frequency is reduced to three times per week for another year or more. Although the treatment is well tolerated by most patients, about 40% develop delayed hypersensitivity reac-

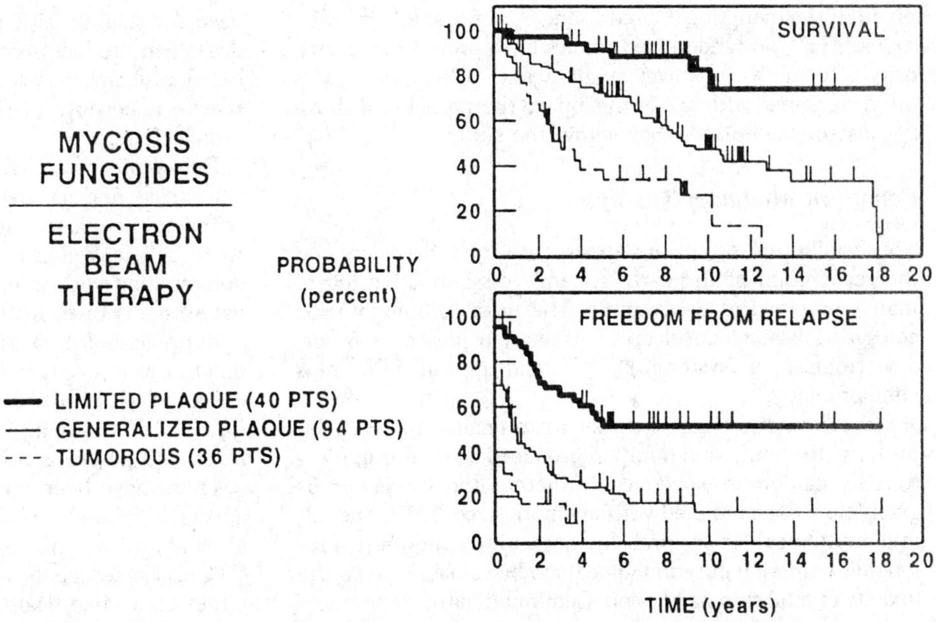

FIG. 51-2. Actuarial survival and relapse-free survival in 192 CTCL patients treated at Stanford University with total skin irradiation with electrons. (Courtesy of Dr. R. T. Hoppe[67])

tions marked by erythematous eruptions and severe pruritus.[47,65] Although the hypersensitivity reaction itself may enhance the beneficial local antineoplastic response, the hypersensitivity reaction is considered to be a limitation to the use of topical HN_2 in CTCL. Several methods of desensitization have been reported,[65] also showing the continued beneficial effects of HN_2 even after desensitization has been achieved. Investigators at Stanford University have recently shown that ointment-based HN_2 in aquaphor or polyethylene glycol (PEG) produces fewer allergic reactions and equivalent response rates.[69] It is also more convenient for the patient because it does not require daily drug mixing.

The largest therapeutic experience with this method has been reported by Vonderheid and co-workers.[47] The overall CR in 243 treated patients was 64%, with 75% to 80% of T_1 or T_2 patients and 54% of T_3 patients responding with CR. However, the continuation of CR required maintenance applications of HN_2, and only 13% of the patients were without relapses after 3 years. In a more recent report Hoppe and associates[65] showed that only 37% of 37 T_1 or T_2 patients responded with CR. Treatment was continued for 1 to 2 years after complete skin clearing, after which it was terminated. The 14-year disease-free survival for all treated T_1 and T_2 patients was 30% and 10%, respectively. Several groups have used topical HN_2 given as adjuvant therapy after total skin electron beam therapy. Preliminary data suggest an advantage for this combined modality over the use of electron beam irradiation alone.[46,66]

PUVA

Topical photochemotherapy (PUVA) has also been used extensively for the management of CTCL. In this method, 8-methoxypsoralen (Methoxalen) is given orally followed by exposure to long-wave ultraviolet A light (UVA).[67,68] Methoxypsoralen is a phototoxic compound that is activated by UVA. Once activated, it binds covalently to DNA and causes cell death. Because UVA does not penetrate beyond the epidermis and papillary dermis, the effects of this photochemotherapy remain confined to the skin.

The 8-methoxypsoralen (0.4–0.6 mg/kg) is taken orally 2 hours before UVA exposure. The UVA exposure (1.5–15 J/cm^2) is adjusted to achieve minimal erythema within 2 days after initial exposure. Treatment is given three times weekly, and, after resolution of skin lesions, maintenance therapy is given once every 2 to 4 weeks. The acute side-effects of PUVA are minimal and include mild nausea, generalized pruritus, and sunburn-like changes. The main long-term complication of PUVA therapy, especially when given in association with other topical therapies, is the development of secondary cutaneous malignancies.[69] This complication raises questions about the advisability of the use of PUVA in early-stage disease.

PUVA therapy is highly effective in clearing skin lesions, and approximately 60% of treated patients in all T stages will achieve CR.[67–70] However, maintenance therapy is required in all CR patients, since its discontinuation results in a prompt relapse. With maintenance therapy durable remissions are observed, with a mean duration after skin clearing of 6 to 16 months.

Systemic Chemotherapy

Chemotherapeutic principles in treating CTCL are similar to those used for the low-grade B-cell lymphoma.[1,3] Objective responses that produce palliation of symptoms (produced by refractory cutaneous lesions, or extracutaneous disease) are frequent (70% response rates), but chemotherapy is not curative. The most active agents include methotrexate, alkylating agents (cyclophosphamide, chlorambucil), etoposide (VP-16), and cisplatin.[1,3,71] Combination chemotherapy produces higher CR rates but is not curative. Regimens commonly used are similar to those used for B-cell lymphomas, including chlorambucil + prednisone, CVP (cyclophosphamide + vincristine + prednisone), or similar regimens.[2,3,72,73] No randomized studies have proved the superiority of combinations over single agents. Chemotherapy is often combined with one of the topical therapies listed above because of the bulk disease within the skin.[73]

Combined Modality Therapy

The inability of topical therapy to cure these disorders and the recognition of the early systemic dissemination led to many combined modality trials. The most commonly used combinations include electron irradiation plus chemotherapy (topical or systemic)[66,74-77] and topical HN_2 plus chemotherapy.[73]

Several studies suggested that maintenance topical HN_2 prolongs the remission duration produced by total skin electron irradiation irrespective of whether the irradiation is given alone or combined with chemotherapy.[66,74,76] The addition of topical HN_2 is probably not curative; however, prolonging remission duration appears to be valuable, given the toxicity of total skin irradiation. Combinations of chemotherapy with total skin irradiation were evaluated in four studies.[74-77] The first three studies demonstrated the feasibility of this approach and provided provocative disease-free and overall survival rates.[74-76] An NCI prospective randomized trial comparing topical HN_2 to combined total skin irradiation plus chemotherapy has completed patient accrual.[77] Preliminary results show a small survival benefit only in patients with Stage I or II.

A nonrandomized trial combining topical HN_2 with systemic chemotherapy (bleomycin + doxorubicin + methotrexate) demonstrated a 70% CR rate (in ten patients), with the longest responses in excess of 5 years.[73]

The combined use of total skin irradiation and chemotherapy currently remains experimental. When using either chemotherapy or irradiation the addition of topical HN_2 is a reasonable approach.

Biologic and Experimental Therapies

Recombinant interferons were shown to be active agents in CTCL, with response rates of about 50% for patients with advanced disease refractory to other treatments and 90% for early-stage untreated patients.[78,79] Whether interferons should be combined with other effective therapies and whether they should be used initially will be determined only by future trials.

Antithymocyte globulin (ATG) was evaluated because of the T-cell nature of the malignant process. It produced transient partial remissions in most treated patients, but ATG is extremely toxic and expensive, considering the short duration of remission.[80] Monoclonal antibodies that react with T-cell antigens were thus logical to evaluate. Clinical studies at Stanford demonstrated transient remissions in several patients without appreciable toxicity.[81] Subsequent studies demonstrated little therapeutic effect primarily because the antigen is rapidly modulated after antibody binding.[82,83] This modulation primarily results from internalization of the antigen–antibody complex. Thus radiolabeled anti–T-cell antibodies are capable of localizing in tumor sites and can be used for staging patients.[84] Radiolabeled antibodies in high doses can produce substantial remissions compared to unlabeled antibody.[85] This approach is still highly experimental, however, because of the myelosuppression caused by free radioisotope.

Deoxycoformycin (DCF) is a potent inhibitor of adenosine deaminase and has been evaluated in a number of chronic lymphoid neoplasms. It has been shown to be active in both hairy cell leukemia and CTCL[86] and is being evaluated in combination with interferon in both of these disorders. Its use remains investigational.

Retinoic and derivatives such as 13-cis-retinoic acid (Accutane) were evaluated in a single trial, and responses were observed in about 50% of patients with advanced disease.[87] Like DCF, it is being evaluated in combination with interferon and its use is investigational.

There have been anecdotal reports of responses to both acyclovir[88,89] and cyclosporine A.[90,91] The response observed after acyclovir have been used to support a viral cause for CTCL. These agents will also remain investigational until larger controlled trials document their value.

Patients with the Sézary syndrome often have large numbers of circulating cells that migrate between the skin, peripheral blood, and lymph nodes.[92] Leukapheresis with removal of large numbers of circulating cells causes transient remissions in some cases.[93] After the development of PUVA therapy, Edelson et al evaluated extracorporeal photophoresis by administering oral methoxsalen 2 hours before leukapheresis.[94] The peripheral blood cells were exposed to UVA light during the leukapheresis. Objective responses were noted in 64% of 37 evaluable patients. As with the agents listed above, the exact mechanism of action is unknown, and further trials are necessary to define the ultimate role of this modality.

The combined use of total skin electron irradiation and wide-field "systemic" irradiation was evaluated in several investigational studies. The Philadelphia group used TNI with skin electron irradiation.[95] Complete responses were observed in most cases. Remission duration was longest in patients with disease confined to the skin. A group in France used 125 cGy of TBI (12.5 cGy twice daily three times weekly) before and after 2400 cGy of total skin electron irradiation.[96] There was considerable myelosuppression, but 8 of 18 patients survived a median of 30+ months without evidence of disease.

REFERENCES

1. Broder S, Bunn PA Jr: Neoplasms of T cell origin: Immunological aspects and therapy. Semin Oncol 7:310, 1980
2. Broder S, Bunn PA Jr, Jaffe ES et al: T cell lymphoproliferative syndrome associated with human T cell leukemia-lymphoma virus. Ann Intern Med 100:543, 1984
3. Sausville EA, Bunn PA Jr: Biologic and clinical spectrum of T-cell neoplasms. In Harrison's Principles of Internal Medicine, Update VII, Oncology, pp 159–189, 1986
4. Broder S, Edelson RL, Lutzner M et al: The Sezary syndrome. A malignant proliferation of helper T cells. J Clin Invest 58:1297, 1976
5. Haynes BR, Metzger RS, Minna JD et al: Phenotypic characterization of cutaneous T-cell lymphoma. N Engl J Med 304:1319, 1981
6. Bertness V, Kirsch I, Hollis G et al: T-cell receptor gene rearrangements as clinical markers of human T-cell lymphomas. N Engl J Med 313:534, 1985
7. Poiesz NJ, Ruscetti FM, Gazdar AF et al: Detection and isolation of type-c retrovirus particles from fresh and cultured lymphocytes of a patients with cutaneous T-cell lymphoma. Proc Natl Acad Sci USA 77:7415, 1980

8. Bunn PA Jr, Schechter GP, Blayney D et al: Clinical course of retrovirus-associated adult T-cell lymphoma in the United States. N Engl J Med 309:257, 1983
9. Manzari V, Gismondi A, Barillari G et al: HTLV-V: A new human retrovirus in Tac-negative T cell lymphoma/leukemia. Science 238:1581, 1987
10. Greene MH, Dalager NA, Lamberg SI et al: Mycosis fungoides: Epidemiologic observations. Cancer Treat Rep 63:596, 1979
11. Epstein EH, Levine DL, Croft JD et al: Mycosis fungoides: Survival prognostic features, response to therapy, and autopsy findings. Medicine (Baltimore) 51:61, 1972
12. Reinherz EL, Schlossman SF: Regulation of the immune response: Inducer and suppressor T lymphocyte subsets in human beings. N Engl J Med 303:370, 1980
13. Royer HD, Reinherz EL: T lymphocytes: Ontogeny, function, and relevance to clinical disorders. N Engl J Med 317:1136, 1987
14. Davis MM, Chin Y-H, Gascoigne NRJ et al: A murine T cell receptor gene complex: Isolation, structure, and rearrangement. Immunol Rev 81:235, 1984
15. Yang SY, Chowaif S, Dupont B: A common pathway for T lymphocyte activation involving both CD3–Ti complex and CD2 sheep erythrocyte receptor determinants. J Immunol 137:1097, 1986
16. McDougal JS, Kennedy MS, Sligh JM et al: Binding of HTLVIII/LAV to T4 and T cells by a complex of the 11K viral protein and the T4 molecule. Science 231:382, 1986
17. Smith KA, Baker PE, Gillis et al: Functional and molecular characteristics of T cell growth factor. Mol Immunol 17:579, 1980
18. Waldmann TA: The structure, function, and expression of interleukin 2 receptors on normal and malignant lymphocytes. Science 232:727, 1986
19. Moingeon P, Ythier A, Goubin G et al: A unique T cell receptor complex expressed on human fetal lymphocytes displaying natural-killer-like activity. Nature 323:638, 1986
20. Oshimi K, Hoshino S, Takahashi M et al: Ti(WT31)-negative, CD3-positive, large granular lymphocyte leukemia with nonspecific cytotoxicity. Blood 71:923, 1988
21. Rappaport H: Tumors of the hematopoietic system. In Atlas of Tumor Pathology, sect III, fasc 8. Washington, DC, Armed Forces Institute of Pathology, 1966
22. Rosenberg S, members of the Non-Hodgkin's Lymphoma Pathologic Classification Project: National Cancer Institute–sponsored study of non-Hodgkin's lymphoma. Cancer 49:2112, 1982
23. Nathwani BN, Kim H, Rappaport H: Malignant lymphoma, lymphoblastic. Cancer 38:964, 1976
24. Weiss LM, Bindl J, Picozzi VJ et al: Lymphoblastic lymphoma, an immunophenotyping study of 26 cases with comparison to T cell acute lymphoblastic leukemia. Blood 67:474, 1986
25. Catovsky D, Okos, Willt–Shaw E et al: Prolymphocytic leukemia of B and T cell type. Lancet 2:232, 1973
26. Jaffe ES, Blattner WA, Blayney DW et al: The pathologic spectrum of HTLV associated leukemia/lymphoma in the United States. Am J Surg Pathol 8:263, 1984
27. Greer JP, York JC, Cousar JB et al: Peripheral T-cell lymphoma: A clinicopathologic study of 42 cases. J Clin Oncol 2:788, 1984
28. Pandolfi F, De Rossi G, Semenzato G et al: Immunologic evaluation of T chronic lymphocyte leukemia cells: Correlations among phenotype, functional activities, and morphology. Blood 59:688, 1982
29. Reinherz EL, Nadler LM, Rosenthal DS et al: T-cell-subset characterization of human T-CLL. Blood 53:1066, 1979
30. Aisenberg AC, Wilkes BM, Harris N et al: Chronic T-cell lymphocytosis with neutropenia: Report of a case studied with monoclonal antibody. Blood 58:818, 1981
31. Kruskall MS, Weitzman SA, Stossel TP et al: Lymphoma with autoimmune neutropenia and hepatic sinusoidal infiltration: A syndrome. Ann Intern Med 97:202, 1982
32. Rumke HC, Miedema F, Ten Berge, IJM et al: Functional properties of T cells in patients with chronic TG lymphocytosis and chronic T-cell neoplasia. J Immunol 129:419, 1982
33. Uchiyama T, Yodoi J, Sagawa K et al: Adult T cell leukemia: Clinical and hematological features of 16 cases. Blood 50:481, 1977
34. Catovsky D, Rose M, Goolden AWG et al: Adult T cell lymphoma-leukemia in blacks from the West Indies. Lancet 1:639, 1982
35. Gazdar AF, Carney DN, Bunn PA et al: Mitogen requirements for the in vitro propagation of cutaneous T cell lymphomas. Blood 55:409, 1980
36. Gallo RC, Kalyanaraman VS, Sarngadharan MG et al: Association of the human type C retrovirus with a subset of adult T-cell cancers. Cancer Res 43:3892, 1983
37. Gibbs WN, Lofters WS, Campbell M et al: Non-Hodgkin's lymphoma in Jamaica and its relation to adult T cell leukemia–lymphoma. Ann Intern Med 106:361, 1987
38. Alibert JLM: Description des maladies de la peau observees a l' Hopital St. Louis. Paris, Barrois, 1806
39. Fischman AB, Bunn PA Jr, Guccion JC et al: Exposure to chemicals, physical and biologic agents in cutaneous T cell lymphomas. Cancer Treat Rep 63:591, 1979
40. Bunn PA Jr, Lamberg SI: Report of the Committee on Staging and Classification of Cutaneous T Cell Lymphomas. Cancer Treat Rep 63:725, 1979
41. Lambert SI, Green SB, Byar DP et al: Clinical staging for cutaneous T cell lymphoma. Ann Intern Med 100:187, 1984
42. Sezary A, Bouvrain Y: Erythrodermine avec presence de cellules monstrueses dans le derme et dans le sang circulant. Bull Soc Fr Dermatol Symp 45:254, 1938
43. Bunn PA Jr, Huberman MS, Whang-Peng J et al: Prospective staging evaluation of patients with T cell lymphoma: Demonstration of high frequency of extracutaneous dissemination. Ann Intern Med 93:223, 1986
44. Schechter GP, Sausville EA, Fischmann AB et al: Evaluation of circulating malignant cells provides prognostic information in cutaneous T cell lymphoma. Blood 69:841, 1987
45. Vonderheid EC, Sobel EL, Nowell PC et al: Diagnostic and prognostic significance of Sezary cells in peripheral blood smears from patients with cutaneous T cell lymphoma. Blood 66:358, 1985
46. Hoppe RT, Cox RS, Fuks ZY et al: Electron beam therapy in the treatment of mycosis fungoides: The Stanford experience. Cancer Treat Rep 63:691, 1979
47. Vonderheid EC, Van Scott EJ, Wallner PE et al: A 10-year experience with topical mechlorethamine for mycosis fungoides: Comparison with patients treated by total-skin electron-beam radiation therapy. Cancer Treat Rep 63:681, 1979
48. Sausville EA, Worsham GF, Matthews MJ et al: Histologic assessment of lymph nodes in mycosis fungoides/Sezary syndrome (cutaneous T cell lymphoma): Clinical correlations and prognostic import of a new classification system. Hum Pathol 16:1098, 1985
49. Sausville EA, Eddy JL, Makuck RW et al: Histopathologic staging at initial diagnosis of mycosis fungoides and the Sezary syndrome: Definition of three distinctive prognostic groups (In press)
50. Van der Loo EM, Meijjer C, Scheffer E et al: Prognostic value of membrane markers and morphometric characteristics of lymphoid cells in blood and lymph nodes from patients with mycosis fungoides. Cancer 48:738, 1981
51. Whang-Peng J, Bunn PA Jr, Knutsen T et al: Clinical implications of cytogenetic studies in cutaneous T cell lymphoma. Cancer 50:1539, 1982
52. Castellino RA, Hoppe RT, Blank N et al: Experience with lymphography in patients with mycosis fungoides. Cancer Treat Rep 63:581, 1979
53. Dmitrovsky E, Bunn PA Jr, Matthews MJ et al: Cytologic transformation in cutaneous T cell lymphoma: A clinicopathologic entity associated with poor prognosis. J Clin Oncol 5:208, 1987
54. Macaulay WL: Lymphomatoid papulosis: A continuing self-healing eruption, clinically benign, histologically malignant. Arch Dermatol 97:23, 1968
55. Lutzner M, Edelsen R, Schein PH et al: Cutaneous T cell lymphomas: The Sezary syndrome, mycosis fungoides, and related disorders. Ann Intern Med 83:534, 1975
56. Weiss LM, Wood GS, Trela et al: Clonal T cell populations in lymphomatoid papulosis. N Engl J Med 315:475, 1986
57. Katzenstein A, Carrington C, Liebow A: Lymphomatoid granulomatosis a clinicopathologic study of 152 cases. Cancer 43:360, 1979
58. Nichols PW, Koss M, Levine AM et al: Lymphomatoid granulomatosis. Prospective clinical and therapeutic experience over 10 years. N Engl J Med 306:68, 1982
59. Kronke M, Pepper JM, Leonard WJ et al: Adult T cell leukemia: A potential target for ricin A chain immunotoxins. Blood 65:1416, 1985
60. Scholtz W: Uber den einfluss der roentgenstrohlen auf die haut in gesundem und krankem zustande. Arch Dermatol 59:421, 1902
61. Trump JG, Wright KA, Evans WW et al: High energy electrons for the treatment of extensive superficial malignant lesions. Am J Roentgenol Radium Ther Nucl Med 69:623, 1953
62. Nisce LA, Safai B, Kim JH: Effectiveness of once weekly total skin electron-beam therapy in mycosis fungoides and Sezary syndrome. Cancer 47:870, 1981
63. Hoppe RT: Long term results of total skin irradiation with electrons for mycosis fungoides (unpublished data)
64. Haserick JR, Richard JH, Grant DJ: Remission of lesions in mycosis fungoides following topical application of nitrogen mustard. Cleve Clin Q 26:144, 1959
65. Hoppe RT, Abel EA, Deneau DG et al: Mycosis fungoides: Management with topical nitrogen mustard. J Clin Oncol 5:1796, 1987
66. Price NM, Hoppe RT, Constantine FS et al: The treatment of mycosis fungoides: Adjuvant topical mechlorethamine after electron-beam therapy. Cancer 40:2851, 1977
67. Gilchrest BA: Methoxsalen photochemotherapy for mycosis fungoides. Cancer Treat Rep 63:663, 1979
68. Roenigk HH: Photochemotherapy for mycosis fungoides: Long-term follow-up study. Cancer Treat Rep 63:669, 1979
69. Abel EA, Sendagorta E, Hoppe RT: Cutaneous malignancies and metastatic squamous cell carcinoma following therapies for mycosis fungoides. J Am Acad Dermatol 14:1029, 1986
70. Abel EA, Sendagorta E, Hoppe RT et al: PUVA treatment of erythrodermic and plaque type mycosis fungoides. Ten year follow-up. Arch Dermatol 123:897, 1987
71. McDonald CJ, Bertino JR: Treatment of mycosis fungoids lymphoma: Effectiveness of infusions of methotrexate followed by oral citrovorum factor. Cancer Treat Rep 62:1009, 1978
72. Grozea PN, Jones SE, McKelvey EM et al: Combination chemotherapy for mycosis fungoides: A Southwest Oncology Group Study. Cancer Treat Rep 63:647, 1979
73. Zakem MH, Davis BR, Adelstein DJ et al: Treatment of advanced stage mycosis fungoides with bleomycin, doxorubicin and methotrexate with topical nitrogen mustard (BAM-M). Cancer 58:2611, 1987
74. Winkler CF, Sausville EA, Ihde DC et al: Combined modality treatment of cutaneous T cell lymphomas: Results of 6 year follow-up. J Clin Oncol 4:1094, 1986
75. Griem ML, Tokars RP, Petras V et al: Combined therapy for patients with mycosis fungoides. Cancer Treat Rep 63:655, 1979
76. Braverman IM, Yager NB, Chen M et al: Combined total body electron beam irradiation and chemotherapy for mycosis fungoides. J Am Acad Dermatol 16:45, 1987
77. Kaye F, Ihde D, Fischmann A et al: A randomized trial comparing conservative and aggressive therapy in mycosis fungoides. Proc ASCO 5:195, 1987
78. Bunn PA Jr, Foon KA, Ihde DC et al: Recombinant leukocyte A interferon: An active agent in advanced refactory cutaneous T-cell lymphomas (mycosis fungoides and Sezary syndrome). Ann Intern Med 101:484, 1984
79. Covielli A, Cavalieri R, Coppola G et al: Recombinant leucocyte A interferon as initial therapy in mycosis fungoides and Sezary syndrome. Proc ASCO 6:189, 1987

80. Edelson RL, Raafat J, Berger CL et al: Antithymocyte globulin in the management of cutaneous T-cell lymphoma. Cancer Treat Rep 63:675, 1979
81. Miller RA, Levy R: Response of cutaneous T-cell lymphoma to therapy with hybridoma monoclonal antibody. Lancet 1:226, 1981
82. Foon KA, Schroff RW, Bunn PA Jr: Monoclonal antibody therapy for patients with leukemia and lymphoma, pp 85–101. In Foon KA, Morgan AC Jr (eds): Monoclonal Antibody Therapy for Human Cancer. Hingham, Mass, Martinus Nijhoff, 1985
83. Dillman RO, Shawler DL, Dillman JB et al: Therapy of chronic lymphocytic leukemia and cutaneous T-cell lymphoma with T101 monoclonal antibody. J Clin Oncol 2:881, 1984
84. Carrasquillo JA, Bunn PA Jr, Keenan AM et al: Radioimmunodetection of cutaneous T-cell lymphoma with 111-In-T101 monoclonal antibody. N Engl J Med 315:673, 1986
85. Rosen ST, Zimmer M, Goldman–Leiken R et al: Radioimmunodetection and radioimmunotherapy of cutaneous T cell lymphomas using an 131I-labeled monoclonal antibody: An Illinois Cancer Council Study. J Clin Oncol 5:562, 1987
86. Grever MR, Leiby JM, Kraut EH et al: Low-dose deoxycoformycin in lymphoid malignancy. J Clin Oncol 3:1196, 1985
87. Kessler JF, Meyskens FL, Levine N et al: Treatment of cutaneous T-cell lymphoma (mycosis fungoides) with 13-cis-retinoic acid. Lancet 1:1345, 1983
88. Scheman AJ, Steinberg I, Taddeini L: Abatement of Sezary syndrome lesions following treatment with acyclovir. Am J Med 80:1199, 1986
89. Resnick L, Schleider–Kushner N, Horwitz SN et al: Remission of tumor stage mycosis fungoides following intravenously administered acyclovir. JAMA 251:1571, 1984
90. (Jensen JR, Thestrup–Pederson K, Zachariae H et al: Cyclosporin A therapy for mycosis fungoides. Arch Dermatol 123:160, 1987
91. Puttick L, Pollock A, Fairburn E: Treatment of Sezary syndrome with cyclosporin A. J R Soc Med 76:1063, 1983
92. Bunn PA Jr, Edelson RL, Ford SS et al: Patterns of cell proliferation and migration in patients with Sezary syndrome. Blood 57:452, 1981
93. Edelson RL, Facktor M, Andrews A et al: Successful management of the Sezary syndrome: Mobilization and removal of extravascular neoplastic T-cell by leukapheresis. N Engl J Med 291:293, 1974
94. Edelson R, Berger C, Gasparro F et al: Treatment of cutaneous T-cell lymphoma by extracorporeal photochemotherapy. N Engl J Med 316:297, 1987
95. Micaily B, Vonderheid EC, Brady L et al: Total electron beam and total nodal irradiation for treatment of patients with cutaneous T-cell lymphoma. Int J Radiat Oncol Biol Phys 11:111, 1985
96. Hariot JC: Personal communication

PETER H. WIERNIK

CHAPTER 52 *Acute Leukemias*

The incidence of acute leukemia in the United States is approximately 4.9 cases: 100,000 population. About 75% of new acute leukemia cases are in adults, and the ratio of new acute nonlymphocytic (ANLL) to acute lymphocytic leukemia (ALL) cases is roughly 6:1. Both ALL and ANLL are slightly more common in males, and the incidence of both is greatest over the age of 65 years. ANLL incidence steadily increases with age, whereas the incidence of ALL in adults remains relatively constant until the age of 65 years, after which it rises sharply. The incidence of ANLL in the elderly appears to be steadily increasing over time. Approximately 900 new cases of ALL and 6300 new cases of ANLL are diagnosed annually in adults in the United States. Mortality rates for the acute leukemias are approximately 80% of the incidence rates.

Acute leukemia, untreated, is a rapidly fatal disease that is characterized by a proliferation and accumulation of abnormal immature blood cell progenitors in the bone marrow and other tissues. The progressive disappearance of normal erythrocytes, granulocytes, and platelets from the blood leads to progressive fatigue, infection, and hemorrhage during the course of the disease. Disease control requires more intensive treatment in adults than in children. Intensive chemotherapy and substantial supportive care, which includes infection prevention and treatment measures, and granulocyte, platelet, and red cell transfusions, are required to affect favorably the course of the disease. This treatment must be administered by a team of trained health care professionals thoroughly knowledgeable in the disease, its treatment, and the complications of both if optimal results are to be obtained. Because of the difficulty and expense of administering proper care to the leukemia patient, the patient's interests are usually best served by referral immediately upon diagnosis to a facility that specializes in leukemia treatment.

Patients with signs and symptoms of anemia, granulocytopenia, and thrombocytopenia, associated with splenomegaly or lymphadenopathy, have been reported since the time of Hippocrates. It was not until the mid-19th century, however, that leukemia was recognized as a distinct disease entity, after Donne made meticulous microscopic studies of the blood of patients and Virchow recorded clinical and autopsy data.[1] The disease was called leukemia by Virchow, who observed that the blood of some patients had a whitish color. The development of cellular stains by Ehrlich in 1877, when he was a medical student, allowed him to recognize lymphocytic, myelocytic, and blastic forms of the disease. Naegeli in 1900 described the myeloblast and divided the blastic leukemias into myelocytic and lymphocytic varieties. Reschad and Schilling-Torgau a decade later described the monocytic variety of blastic leukemia.

Radiation therapy was shown to offer palliation to many patients with chronic leukemia in the second decade of this century. The startling observation that drugs could favorably affect the course of a malignant disease was made in the immediate post-World War II period, when nitrogen mustard was shown to have antilymphoma activity. Soon thereafter, Farber and others[2] demonstrated the antileukemic activity of glucocorticoids and folic acid antagonists in children with ALL. These landmark observations represent the seeds from which modern medical oncology has grown.

Treatments have been developed from which most patients with acute leukemia substantially benefit. Current treatment research has been directed primarily at reducing the toxicity of and prolonging the response to treatment. It is clear that a fraction of treated adults with acute leukemia, perhaps 30% to 35%, is actually cured with drug treatment.

ETIOLOGY

Although the cause of acute leukemia in most patients has not been identified, some predisposing factors, as well as some potential leukemogens, have been defined.

GENETIC FACTORS

The observations that children with Down's syndrome have a 20-fold increased incidence of acute leukemia and that the risk of Down's syndrome is increased among siblings of children with acute leukemia suggest that alterations or reorganization of the information on chromosome 21 can lead to the development of ALL or ANLL.[3] This suspicion is strengthened by the fact that the Philadelphia chromosome (Ph^1), the hallmark of chronic myelocytic leukemia (CML) that terminates as an acute leukemia, results from a translocation of some information from chromosome 21 to some other chromosome, usually chromosome 9.[4] It has been recognized that some patients with acute leukemia who have no history or evidence of CML also have the Ph^1 chromosome. In most cases, the survival of such patients and their response to therapy is somewhat poorer than expected for the type of acute leukemia with which they present (ALL or myelocytic leukemia) but better than expected for blast crisis of CML.[5] In some series, however, outcome of patients with acute leukemia and the Ph^1 chromosome was similar whether or not the acute leukemia was preceded by CML.[6] Thus, de novo acute leukemia with the Ph^1 chromosome may have a common origin with blast crisis of CML.

A number of specific chromosomal aberrations have been identified in patients with acute leukemia. For instance, C-group trisomy has been reported in patients with ANLL,[7] and a patient who, after treatment for ALL, developed ANLL coincident with the emergence of a monosomy-7 marrow clone also has been reported.[8] ANLL patients with monosomy-7 have been described with increasing frequency.[9] The fact that the T-antigen gene of simian virus 40 (SV40) has been demonstrated on human chromosome 7 after transformation of human cell lines in vitro by that virus makes that observation especially intriguing.[10]

Many congenital disorders that have an inherited tendency for chromosomal fragility or an association with unstable chromosome patterns (*e.g.*, aneuploidy) are associated with an increased incidence of ANLL. The list of such diseases is rather long and includes congenital agranulocytosis, Ellis–van Creveld syndrome, celiac disease, Bloom's syndrome, Fanconi's anemia, Wiskott-Aldrich syndrome, Kleinfelter's syndrome, D^1-trisomy syndrome, and von Recklinghausen's neurofibromatosis.[11–19]

Environmental factors known to cause acquired chromosomal breaks (*e.g.*, ionizing radiation), as well as some chemicals (*e.g.*, benzene) and drugs (*e.g.*, some used for cancer treatment or more benign conditions), are associated with an increased incidence of acute leukemia, especially ANLL.[20–24]

VIRUSES

Certain viruses are known to cause acute leukemia in many species of subhuman vertebrates. They may be leukemogenic to their host or may be carried by germ cell or milk to a future generation in which the disease becomes manifest.[25] Whether the inoculated virus leads to the development of acute leukemia apparently depends on many modulating factors, such as age, sex, and strain of the host; quantity of the inoculum; immunologic factors; and the presence or absence of certain environmental cocarcinogens such as chemicals or ionizing irradiation.[26,27]

No conclusive evidence confirms that common varieties of human leukemia are viral diseases. However, molecular biological evidence in support of that theory is mounting. RNA-dependent DNA polymerase (reverse transcriptase) has been detected in human leukemic blood cells but not in normal blood cells. This enzyme is known to be present primarily in oncogenic viruses such as C-type viruses, a group of RNA viruses that can cause leukemia in animals, including primates other than humans.[28] This enzyme allows the virus to synthesize genetic material that can be incorporated into the genome of the infected cell. Viral genetic information then can be passed on through replication of the infected host cell.[29]

Electron microscope and other classic virologic studies have failed to yield evidence of intact C-type viral particles in human leukemia cells. However, the study of two pairs of identical twins, each with one member afflicted with leukemia, revealed that DNA from the patient contained specific polynucleotide sequences not found in the DNA of the healthy twin.[30] These data suggest that alteration of host genetic information may be related to the development of leukemia in humans.

These data, taken with the suspicion that under certain circumstances human-to-human transmission of leukemia may occur, have served to intensify research in the area of viral oncogenesis.[31]

CHEMICALS AND DRUGS

Exposure to a variety of substances has been associated with an increased incidence of acute leukemia, especially ANLL. Turkish cobblers who are chronically exposed to benzene during their work are an example. Drugs that can cause aplastic anemia such as chloramphenicol and phenylbutazone, and anticancer alkylating agents such as melphalan and chlorambucil, have resulted in a 1% to 17% incidence of ANLL within 5 years after initiation of the treatment. The incidence of leukemia varies with the primary disease and the intensity and duration of treatment with these drugs.[23,24] In a recent preliminary report,[32] cigarette smoking has been associated with an increased risk of ANLL.

RADIATION EXPOSURE

Ionizing radiation is the external factor most clearly leukemogenic in both animals and humans. Both ANLL and CML occur with increased frequency after exposure to such radiation; dose–response curves have been established for humans and animals.[33,34] The increased incidence of ALL in humans after exposure to radiation is minimal and is not detected in all studies. Radiologists experienced a tenfold increase in incidence of leukemia prior to the recognition of the need for protection from exposure.[35] Japanese atomic bomb survivors sustained up to a greater than 20-fold increased incidence of ANLL and CML, depending on their distance from the hypocenter of the explosion. The peak incidence of leukemia occurred 5 to 7 years after the explosion, and the incidence of new cases continued above the expected rate for 20 years.[36] Similarly, a 14-fold increased incidence of ANLL has been observed in patients with ankylosing spondylitis who were treated with at least 2000-rad irradiation compared with patients who were not irradiated.[37] Similar data are available for patients therapeutically irradiated for malignant disease.[38] Recent data suggest that as many as 5% to 10% of patients who receive radiation and chemotherapy for Hodgkin's disease develop acute leukemia within 2 to 12 years after their first treatment, with the peak incidence at 6 years.[39] This finding is especially true if many months or years separate the two modalities of treatment. It must be remembered, however, that the number of patients who develop acute leukemia after therapy for another malignant disease is small compared to the number of patients who benefit from the treatment.

SPONTANEOUS REGRESSION

Rarely, babies born with widespread marrow, blood, and organ infiltration with myeloblasts experience a spontaneous complete regression of this phenomenon that is transient or permanent.[40,41] Transient spontaneous regression of ANLL in older patients has rarely been observed and is usually associated with a pyogenic bacterial infection.[42] The mechanism of these phenomena is not known. Careful study of such patients may provide insight into control mechanisms that regulate myeloblast differentiation and the aberrations of these control mechanisms that result in ANLL.

MORPHOLOGIC AND ANATOMIC CONSIDERATIONS

Acute leukemia is subclassified as lymphocytic (ALL) or nonlymphocytic (ANLL) according to the morphology of the marrow and blood leukemic cells. ANLL is subclassified further as acute myelocytic (granulocytic), promyelocytic (progranulocytic), monocytic, myelomonocytic, erythroleukemic, or megakaryocytic by a variety of methods. The major morphologic distinction to be made is between ALL and ANLL, however. This distinction is important for two reasons. First, the response to therapy and prognosis is often better in ALL, and, second, different treatments usually are prescribed for the two diseases. Distinction among the various subtypes of ANLL is more difficult but it is currently possible with greater precision because of new histochemical stains (Table 52-1) and immunologic techniques. Identification of the many varieties of ANLL is becoming more important because several new drugs appear to have more activity against some varieties than against others. In addition, prognosis and clinical features may differ considerably among the various subtypes.

The French-American-British (FAB) morphologic classification scheme is used universally with excellent reproducibility[43] and is described in the following sections and summarized in Table 52-1.

ACUTE LYMPHOCYTIC LEUKEMIA

The blast cells that always infiltrate the bone marrow and often the blood of patients with ALL have several important cytologic features. They are round cells usually with amphophilic cytoplasm. Granules are almost never present in the cytoplasm, although an occasional azurophilic tiny granule may be seen. The nucleus is usually round and contains finely reticulated, homogeneous, open chromatin. It may contain one or two small nucleoli, which are often inconspicuous and difficult to resolve. These cells appear to be essentially undifferentiated. The morphologic variation from cell to cell in a given patient is greater in adults than in children. FAB type L1, with scant cytoplasm, is preponderant in childhood ALL, whereas FAB type L2, with more abundant cytoplasm and more variation in size and shape from cell to cell, is more common in adults. FAB type L3 is characterized by intensely basophilic and vacuolated abundant cytoplasm and is common in leukemia associated with Burkitt's lymphoma, or B-ALL. Certain histochemical stain reactions are characteristic of the blast cells in ALL. Stains for lysosomal granules, such as the myeloperoxidase and Sudan black stains, must give negative reactions to support the diagnosis of ALL. The periodic acid–Schiff (PAS) reagent will reveal clumpy reddish positivity in the cytoplasm of most cells in more than 80% of patients. Various esterase stains yield negative results. The blast cells of more than 95% of patients with ALL contain the enzyme terminal deoxynucleotidyl transferase (TdT). This enzyme may be demonstrated by a biochemical assay of the marrow aspirate, or by an immunofluorescent stain of a marrow or blood smear.[44] With the latter technique, most leukemic lymphoblasts will demonstrate nuclear positivity. Although low levels of TdT activity rarely can be detected biochemically in the marrow aspirate of a patient with ANLL, the fluorescent stain technique will identify only a few positive cells in such a patient. Some patients with the blast crisis of CML will demonstrate significant TdT activity with either technique.[44] Thus, the demonstration of TdT activity in the leukemic cells of a patient with newly diagnosed acute leukemia is convincing evidence that the leukemia is ALL.

Acute lymphocytic leukemia is primarily a disease of the marrow and blood; however, at least 80% of patients have lymphadenopathy, splenomegaly, or both at the time of diagnosis because of infiltration of those organs with leukemic

TABLE 52-1. FAB Classification of the Acute Leukemia

FAB Type	Morphology	Histochemistry
Acute Lymphocytic Leukemia (ALL)		
L 1	Small blasts with scant cytoplasm and little variation in size and shape from cell to cell. The nucleus is round and usually has a single small nucleolus. This is the most common morphology in childhood ALL.	PAS$^+$. Peroxidase$^-$. Acid phosphatase and naphthyl esterase$^+$ in T-ALL.
L 2	Larger cells with more abundant cytoplasm than L1. Significant variation in size and shape among cells. The nucleus may have an irregular shape and often contains multiple nucleoli. This is the most common morphology in adult ALL.	Same as L1.
L 3	Large cells with strongly basophilic cytoplasm that may be vacuolated. Fine chromatin is seen within a round nucleus. Nucleoli are often basophilic and multiple. This morphology is common in leukemia associated with Burkitt's lymphoma.	PAS$^-$. Peroxidase$^-$. Vacuoles are usually oil red 0$^+$.
Acute Nonlymphocytic Leukemia (ANLL)		
M 1	Cells are very undifferentiated, with only occasional cytoplasmic granules. Some promyelocytes are seen. Acute myelocytic leukemia.	Occasional peroxidase$^+$ granules. PAS$^-$.
M 2	Granulated blasts predominate. Small number of monocytoid cells may be present. Differentiation beyond the promyelocyte stage is clearly evident. Auer's bodies may be seen. Acute myelocytic leukemia.	Strongly peroxidase$^+$. PAS$^-$.
M 3	Hypergranular promyelocytes predominate. The cells have large basophilic and eosinophilic granules. Acute promyelocytic leukemia.	Strongly peroxidase$^+$. PAS$^-$.
M 4	Both monocytic and granulocytic precursors are seen. Serum lysozyme is elevated. Acute myelomonocytic leukemia.	Strongly peroxidase$^+$. Some cells may be PAS$^+$.
M 4E	Same as M4, but young eosinophils with small eosinophilic granules and large, basophilic primary granules constitute up to 30% or more of marrow cells. Acute myelomonocytic leukemia.	Same as M4.
M 5A	Large monoblasts with abundant, relatively agranular cytoplasm that may be vacuolated and basophilic are characteristic. More common in children. Acute monoblastic leukemia.	May be peroxidase$^+$ and PAS$^+$. Nonspecific esterase stains are strongly + and inhibited by NaF.
M 5B	The predominant cell has a characteristic twisted, indented, or folded nucleus. More common in adults. Acute monocytic leukemia.	Same as M5A.
M 6	Megaloblastoid red cell precursors predominate, but myeloid blasts are seen also. Multinucleated red cell precursors are common. Erythroleukemia.	Red cell precursors are PAS$^+$. Ringed sideroblasts are seen with iron stains.
M 7	Variable morphology. Megakaryocytic features may not be seen with light microscopy. This rare entity is usually identified with monoclonal antibodies to platelet antigens. Megakaryocytic leukemia.	Variable. Platelet peroxidase can be demonstrated by electron microscopy.

cells. In addition, the liver is palpable in half of adults with ALL.

ACUTE NONLYMPHOCYTIC LEUKEMIA

The blast cells in the marrow and blood of patients with ANLL are usually larger than lymphoblasts, and their variation in size and shape is much greater. Leukemic cells in ANLL have more abundant cytoplasm, and cytoplasmic granulation is usually, but not always, evident. Auer's bodies, reddish-staining abnormal lysosomal granules visible with Wright's stain, are present in the cytoplasm of at least some cells in about 10% of patients (Fig. 52-1). The cell nucleus is relatively large and usually irregular in shape. Usually, some evidence of nuclear or cytoplasmic differentiation is evident. The nuclear chromatin pattern is more heavily reticulated than in the blast cells of ALL, and multiple nucleoli frequently are easily seen within each nucleus. The nucleoli may vary greatly in size within the same nucleus and from cell to cell and are often relatively large. Nucleolar staining characteristics are also variable. The nucleoli may be amphophilic or basophilic but more often are lightly eosinophilic.

ACUTE MYELOCYTIC LEUKEMIA

The leukemic cells in this variant of ANLL are the most uniform of all ANLL variants, although variation in size and shape is still evident. The cytoplasm usually contains fine azurophilic granules, especially in the perinuclear region.

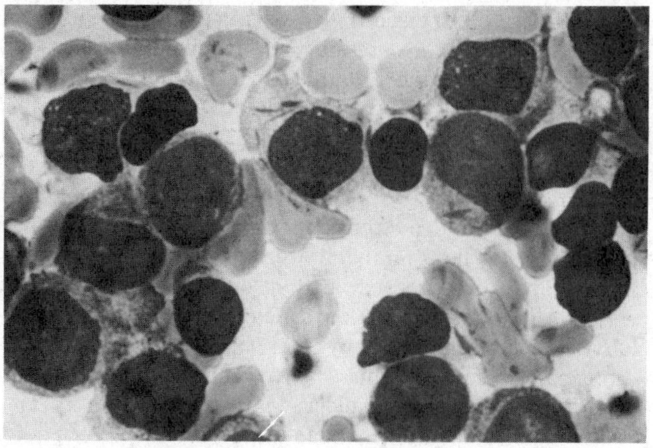

FIG. 52-1. Wright's stained bone marrow aspirate from a patient with FAB type M2 ANLL and the t(8;21) cytogenetic translocation. Many leukemic cells have cytoplasmic Auer rods.

The nucleus is generally round. Lysosomal granule stains such as myeloperoxidase and Sudan black are almost always positive in most cells. Sometimes, however, the granules are so small that they are evident only with electron microscopy. The PAS stain is negative.

Cells of this subtype are designated FAB type M1 when cytoplasmic granules are rarely seen, or FAB type M2 when granulated blasts are preponderant. In addition, differentiation beyond the promyelocyte stage is clearly evident in the latter type.

ACUTE PROMYELOCYTIC LEUKEMIA

The leukemic cells almost always appear heavily granulated with light microscopy and are usually very basophilic with Wright's stain. Electron microscopy is sometimes necessary to demonstrate granules in the microgranular variant.[45] Curiously, the nucleus of the leukemic cell is often lobulated, folded, or highly irregular and suggests a monocytoid morphology. Sometimes, although heavy and bizarre granulation is evident with Wright's stain, the usual lysosomal granule stains give negative reactions. Rarely, ANLL with basophilic differentiation may be mistaken for acute promyelocytic leukemia. The granules in the former stain with toluidine blue.[46] Acute promyelocytic leukemia is classified as M3 in the FAB scheme.

ACUTE MYELOMONOCYTIC LEUKEMIA

In this variant, cells characteristic of acute myelocytic and acute monocytic leukemia are seen in various ratios. In both acute monocytic and myelomonocytic leukemia, muramidase (lysozyme) activity is evident in the leukemic cells.[47] Intramedullary destruction of leukemic cells in these two variants often leads to greatly elevated levels of that enzyme in the blood and urine, which can be detected and quantified with a simple turbidimetric technique.[48] Patients with acute monocytic or myelomonocytic leukemia often have evidence of significant extramedullary leukemic infiltration. Thus, gingival hypertrophy, leukemia cutis, and meningeal leukemia are more common in these variants of ANLL than in others. This characteristic may be related to the greater ability of leukemic cells in these variants to migrate to skin windows.[49]

This disorder is classified as FAB type M4. When abnormal eosinophils are also found in the marrow, the designation M4E is applied.

ACUTE MONOCYTIC LEUKEMIA

The leukemic cells are large with abundant, sparsely granulated or ungranulated cytoplasm, and cytoplasmic buds that mimic pseudopodia may be evident. The nucleus is large and convoluted or folded. Great morphologic variation from cell to cell is evident. The peroxidase and Sudan black stains may show light, punctate positivity in some or most cells. Some cells also show punctate PAS positivity but rarely the "clumpy" positivity of lymphoblasts. Certain esterase stains are usually positive, and sodium fluoride inhibition of cytoplasmic esterase activity is characteristic.[47] Acute monocytic leukemia is FAB type M5.

ERYTHROLEUKEMIA

This variant was first described by Di Guglielmo and is often referred to as the *acute Di Guglielmo syndrome.* A more chronic variant (termed the *chronic* Di Guglielmo syndrome by some) is characterized by less morphologic immaturity initially and may at first glance appear to be a refractory anemia with ineffective erythropoiesis. The chronic Di Guglielmo syndrome becomes indistinguishable from the acute syndrome with time. It therefore seems appropriate to refer to this ANLL variant as *erythroleukemia*, a term suggested by Di Guglielmo himself.

The preponderant proliferating cell in the bone marrow is an abnormal erythroblast. Usually, the morphology of most of the marrow cells is such that the erythrocytic derivation is obvious. Frequently many bizarre abnormal erythrocyte forms are present, and occasionally they may be dominant. In such cases, multinucleated red cells are usually found, and cells often as young as proerythroblasts with three or more nuclei are seen in clumps. The red cell precursors are usually megaloblastic and demonstrate obvious nuclear–cytoplasmic maturation dissociation, represented by relatively mature red cell precursors with little or no hemoglobinization of the cytoplasm, which in such cases stains intensely basophilic with Wright's stain. An iron stain will usually reveal rare or abundant ringed sideroblasts, and the PAS stain frequently demonstrates blocks of cytoplasmic positivity in many abnormal erythrocytes. Erythrocyte PAS positivity does not occur in any other disease, except perhaps extremely rarely in thalassemia major. Ringed sideroblasts may be found on occasion in other variants of ANLL, especially when the leukemia can be related to previous alkylating agent therapy for another malignancy, such as multiple myeloma.[50] In many patients, the abnormal erythroblasts have esterase activity,[51] which is not present in normal erythroblasts. Erythroleukemia is designated M6 in the FAB classification. As erythroleukemia progresses, the erythroid element becomes less obvious, and a morphologic picture more characteristic of acute myelocytic or myelomonocytic leukemia emerges.

Some erythroleukemia patients have a peculiar rheumatic disorder that responds to aspirin but not to antileukemic treatment. In addition, about one quarter of patients have a positive Coombs' test and one third have demonstrable rheumatoid factor.[52] The significance of these findings is unclear.

MEGAKARYOCYTIC LEUKEMIA

This rare variant, designated M7 in the FAB system, has extremely variable morphology and a poor prognosis. Megakaryocytic features may not be seen with light microscopy, and reaction with monoclonal antibodies to platelet antigens may be necessary for diagnosis.

PATHOLOGY

Acute leukemia may result in dysfunction of various organs by direct invasion of leukemic cells or compression of a vital conduit by enlarged lymph nodes or other tissues, or as a consequence of the release of a variety of bioactive substances from leukemic cells.

BONE MARROW

An increased number of blast cells in the bone marrow is necessary to diagnose acute leukemia. The blast count in a normal marrow may be as high as 5%, although blasts are usually very difficult to find in a normal specimen. Therefore, a patient whose marrow contains even a low percentage of blasts should have another examination in a month or so. The marrow may be completely replaced by leukemic cells, or such cells may account for a large minority of marrow-nucleated cells at the time of diagnosis of acute leukemia. Very early in the disease, especially in patients with ALL, leukemic infiltration may vary in degree from site to site. Thus, it may be possible for a marrow aspirate from one iliac crest to be nondiagnostic, while the aspirate from the other is frankly leukemic.

The leukemic infiltration usually results in a hypercellular marrow. The number of nucleated cells usually is increased, and the amount of fat is decreased. However, in many patients whose leukemia is considered secondary to prior radiotherapy or chemotherapy administered for another disease, the marrow aspirate may be hypocellular, or essentially aplastic. Some patients with de novo ANLL, especially elderly ones, who are leukopenic when diagnosed have hypocellular bone marrows. It should be remembered that marrow cellularity cannot be assessed properly by reviewing an aspirate. A marrow biopsy must be studied to determine the true cellularity.

The number of normal elements in a leukemic marrow is almost always reduced. A fairly good inverse relation exists between the number of normal elements and the number of leukemic cells. In ALL, the normal marrow elements have essentially normal morphologic characteristics. In ANLL, however, distinct morphologic abnormalities of the normal elements are often discernible. As an example, cytoplasmic granulation of granulocytes beyond the myelocyte stage may be reduced or absent.[53] Rarely, an acquired Pelger–Hüet nuclear anomaly, principally characterized by a reduction of nuclear segments to two or fewer in mature neutrophils, may be evident. Abnormalities may be evident in the red cell series also. There may be erythroid hyperplasia with or without megaloblastoid maturation, and immaturity of the red cell series may be prominent. Megakaryocyte abnormalities in the form of decreased budding or nuclear morphologic abnormalities may be observed. These erythroid and megakaryocytic abnormalities are quite common in acute myelomonocytic leukemia. Thus, marrow morphology in ANLL often represents a panmyelosis.

A radioisotope marrow scan usually discloses peripheral extension of the active marrow into areas that are largely replaced by fat in the normal adult, such as distal long bones. Isotope uptake in the distal tibia may be as great as in the pelvic bones.

BONES AND JOINTS

The most commonly appreciated radiologic finding in bone in adult acute leukemia is thinning of the cortex of long bones as a result of expansion of the marrow cavity. Osteolytic lesions rarely occur, and the metaphyseal lines commonly seen in children with ALL are not observed in adults. These lines represent functional impairment of the metaphyseal growth centers in the child, and, because these centers are inactive in adults, they are not affected by the expanding marrow cavity. Arthritis secondary to infiltration of synovium by leukemic cells occasionally occurs in children but is rare in adults. However, patients with acute leukemia of all ages may experience a migratory polyarthritis secondary to hyperuricemia. This tendency is especially likely when an unusually large leukemic cell mass exists, as evidenced by an extremely high leukocyte count and hypercellular marrow, or by bulky lymphadenopathy or splenomegaly. In addition, migratory polyarthritis may occur after the administration of a xanthine oxidase inhibitor such as allopurinol, given to reduce uric acid production.

SKIN AND SOFT TISSUE

The most common skin manifestations of acute leukemia are petechiae that result from capillary hemorrhage. They tend to occur on dependent or traumatized areas of the body. Leukemic infiltration of skin (leukemia cutis) may be found in patients who present with high leukocyte counts, or in patients with far advanced disease no longer responsive to therapy. Such infiltration usually results in small (2–5 mm) raised, pinkish nodules that are painless, nontender, and not pruritic. These lesions are most common on the extremities or trunk, but they occasionally involve the face and other areas. They may rarely be massive in size (Fig. 52-2). Leukemia cutis usually occurs when the marrow is frankly infiltrated with leukemic cells, but it rarely may be the only evidence of leukemia.[54] On occasion, the appearance or reappearance of leukemia cutis during hematologic remission may be the first harbinger of relapse. These lesions, like

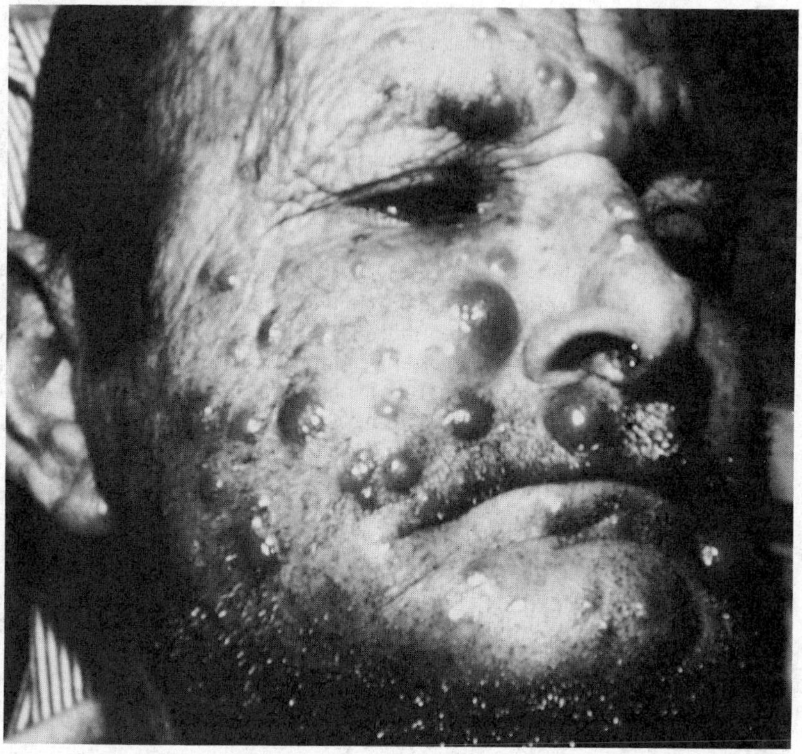

FIG. 52-2. Gross leukemia cutis in a patient with FAB type M4 ANLL.

all extramedullary leukemic lesions, impair prognosis[55] and are more common in patients with acute monocytic or myelomonocytic leukemia. The leukemic cells in these variants of ANLL have been shown to have the greatest potential for migration to soft tissue.[49]

Ecchymoses, characteristic of bleeding secondary to clotting factor deficiencies, may be found on the skin of any acute leukemia patient after local trauma, but they occur most frequently in patients with acute promyelocytic leukemia even in the absence of trauma. Patients with this variant of ANLL often have a disseminated intravascular coagulopathy that can lead to clotting factor depletion. Procoagulant released from the abnormal granules of the leukemic cells in this variant triggers the intravascular clotting.[56]

Chloromas, or granulocytic sarcomas, are focal soft-tissue masses of leukemic cells.[57] They rarely, if ever, occur in ALL and arise in only a few ANLL patients. The term *chloroma* derives from the fact that some of these lesions have a greenish color from the high myeloperoxidase content of the leukemic cells in them. However, most such lesions are not green, and the term *granulocytic sarcoma* seems more appropriate. The lesions often arise from the subperiosteal region of bone—especially ribs, sternum, or orbit—and expand into soft tissue. Lesions unassociated with bone have been observed on the face and in the ovary, breast, and other organs and tissues, including the dura. Most patients with granulocytic sarcomas have only one or two such lesions.

Although patients with granulocytic sarcomas usually have other evidence of ANLL, the lesions may precede bone marrow involvement[58] or occur in patients who never develop evidence of disseminated disease.[59]

The lesions usually are composed primarily of immature leukemic cells. The true character of the lesion may not be appreciated from routine surgical pathology sections stained with hematoxylin and eosin. Such a preparation may be misinterpreted as anaplastic carcinoma, diffuse lymphoma, plasmacytoma, or other lesions, particularly when a granulocytic sarcoma is the first evidence of malignant disease. Whenever biopsy is performed on a suspected granulocytic sarcoma, touch preparations stained with Wright's stain should be made, and the pathologist should be alerted to the possible diagnosis.

Rarely, a nonspecific exfoliative dermatitis[60] may occur at any time during the course of ANLL, and a febrile neutrophilic dermatosis of unknown etiology that responds to steroids also has been reported.[61]

LESIONS OF THE HEAD AND NECK

The most common manifestation of acute leukemia in this area is cervical lymphadenopathy in the patient with ALL. Oropharyngeal infections are common in acute leukemia patients before or during therapy. Periodontal infections are particularly common and, if possible, should be treated before the institution of antileukemic therapy to prevent subsequent septicemia. Every acute leukemia patient should be examined by a dentist shortly after diagnosis and before therapy.[62]

Antileukemic drugs frequently cause oral mucosal ulcerations that are usually minimal but can be extensive. Such lesions tend to become infected, particularly with *Candida albicans*, when the patient is granulocytopenic. Most such infections can be prevented with prophylactic oral antifungal drug administration.

Ocular involvement with ANLL may produce protean complications. Retinal hemorrhages owing to leukemic infiltration or thrombocytopenia may occur. Fundic leukemic infiltrates usually appear as Roth-like spots, whereas thrombocytopenia usually results in hemorrhage alone. Fundic leukemic infiltration, often associated with other evidence of central nervous system (CNS) leukemia, is important to recognize because low-dose irradiation may save the vision in the involved eye.

Gingival hypertrophy, sometimes marked, is common in patients with acute myelomonocytic or monocytic leukemia. The hypertrophy is due to massive infiltration of the gingivae with leukemic cells. The gingivae often become necrotic and superinfected. The degree of gingival hypertrophy usually parallels the activity of the disease in marrow and blood.

CARDIOPULMONARY MANIFESTATIONS

The most common pulmonary lesion secondary to acute leukemia is pneumonia, which can occur whenever the patient is granulocytopenic from disease or its treatment. Pneumonia is most often due to gram-negative bacteria; however, after prolonged granulocytopenia, fungal pneumonia is common. The incidence of pneumonia, especially fungal, may be sharply reduced by conducting therapy in a laminar air-flow room or another ultraclean environment (see below).

The usual signs and symptoms of pneumonia in a granulocytopenic leukemia patient may be lacking because of the lack of granulocytes. Thus, sputum production, cough, and roentgenographic changes may be minimal.[63] Therefore, fever may be the only clue to life-threatening infection.

Some patients with newly diagnosed or relapsed acute leukemia may have impaired respiration secondary to pulmonary capillary plugging with leukemic cells. This tendency is especially true of acute monocytic and myelomonocytic leukemia patients with hyperleukocytosis.[64] Such a patient may present with a sudden asthma-like attack before or after chemotherapy, and histologic examination of the lung often will show capillaries and alveoli engorged with leukemic cells. The prognosis for such patients is poor if the possibility of this complication is not entertained. If it is suspected, low-dose whole-lung irradiation may be lifesaving.

Cardiovascular abnormalities due to leukemic infiltration are rarely clinically important. However, conduction defects, murmurs, pericarditis, and congestive heart failure have been observed rarely as a result of leukemic infiltration of the bundle of His, cardiac valves, pericardium, or myocardium[65]; rare disasters such as rupture of an aortic aneurysm secondary to leukemic infiltration also have been reported.[66]

GASTROINTESTINAL MANIFESTATIONS

Dysphagia, which is common in patients with acute leukemia, may be due to hypopharyngeal infection, especially candidiasis, or to mucosal ulceration secondary to chemotherapy, or both. Rarely, leukemic infiltration of the tonsils or uvula is the cause of dysphagia (Fig. 52-3).[67] Substernal burning and dysphagia are clues to esophagitis caused by *Candida* sp or gram-negative organisms, and the classic radiographic findings of *Candida* esophagitis are seen with both. Occasionally, these lesions are caused by instrumentation of the granulocytopenic patient with unsterile equipment prepared for routine use.[68]

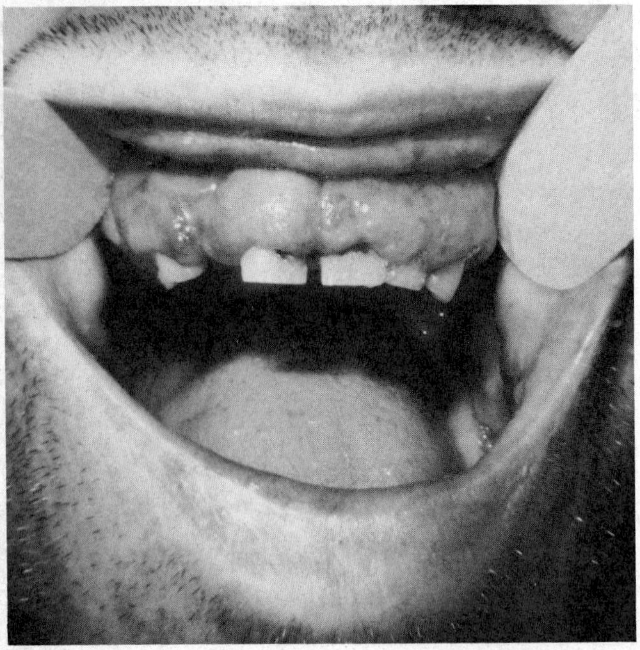

FIG. 52-3. Marked gingival hypertrophy due to leukemic infiltration in a patient with acute monocytic leukemia.

Thrombocytopenic leukemia patients may have significant gastrointestinal bleeding, but this problem is rare since the general acceptance of prophylactic platelet transfusions. Occasionally, hematemesis in a far advanced, relapsed patient is due to leukemic infiltration of the stomach. Irradiation of the stomach may be useful in stopping the bleeding. Usually a 1000-rad dose given in daily fractions is successful.

Small-bowel granulocytic sarcoma may rarely cause obstruction.[69] Although such lesions are often complications of advanced disease, they may be the first manifestation of leukemia.

Perirectal abscess is relatively common in patients with acute monocytic or myelomonocytic leukemia who have not undergone bowel decontamination procedures. The only signs of the lesion may be a small mucosal tear and fever, and the only symptom may be pain on defecation if the patient is severely granulocytopenic.[70] It is important to recognize these lesions, which usually are due to gram-negative bacterial infection, because they may progress rapidly to septicemia if not treated. Typhlitis, or fulminant necrotizing colitis, occurs rarely in acute leukemia patients and may be related to granulocytopenia, cytotoxic therapy, or both. Most reported cases have been recognized only at autopsy. When recognized clinically, surgical intervention can be lifesaving.[71]

GENITOURINARY MANIFESTATIONS

The kidneys may be diffusely enlarged secondary to leukemic infiltration in a small fraction of patients, especially those with ALL. In such cases, the renal cortex is usually more heavily infiltrated than the medulla, and both kidneys are usually involved. Renal failure may result, in which case radiotherapy to the kidneys may rapidly improve renal function.

Occasionally, a patient with acute leukemia presents with renal failure. Uric acid nephropathy is responsible for most such cases and usually occurs in patients with high leukocyte counts (>1,000,000/μl) who have been untreated for a time. The high turnover of leukemic cells leads to more uric acid production than can be solubilized in the normally acid urine. Consequently, urate crystals precipitate in the renal tubules and mechanically impede urine flow.

Urine flow rarely may be obstructed in a male patient by acute prostatism secondary to massive leukemic infiltration of the prostate.[72]

Patients with acute myelomonocytic or monocytic leukemia may have evidence of proximal renal tubular dysfunction secondary to the toxic effects of muramidase (lysozyme) on renal tubular epithelium. The major clinically important manifestation of this problem is potassium wasting, which may lead to severe hypokalemia.[48]

NERVOUS SYSTEM MANIFESTATIONS

Meningeal leukemia is much more common in ALL than in ANLL, and in children than in adults. Prophylactic meningeal leukemia treatment of children and adults with ALL is standard therapy and reduces the incidence to one-quarter or less than that of patients who do not receive prophylaxis. Prevention of meningeal leukemia results in a decrease in systemic relapse as well. Prophylaxis has not been shown to be of value in ANLL.

About 15% of adults with ALL and 5% of those with ANLL will either present with or develop meningeal leukemia sometime during the course of the disease, even if prophylactic therapy was administered.[73] The incidence is higher in acute myelomonocytic leukemia associated with an abnormality of chromosome 16 (usually inversion) than in other variants of ANLL.[74] Headache due to increased intracranial pressure is the most frequent complaint. Because the elevated pressure is distributed evenly within the cranium, a lumbar puncture may be safely performed. Examination of the cerebrospinal fluid (CSF) will reveal, in addition to an elevated opening pressure, increased protein concentration with a normal concentration of glucose. A routine cell count of the CSF may reveal an increased number of cells. The cytocentrifuge (Fig. 52-4) or Millipore filter techniques for examining the CSF will allow stained preparations of concentrated specimens to be examined.[75] This strategy is important for accurate and early diagnosis because these methods may reveal leukemic cells despite a normal routine cell count.

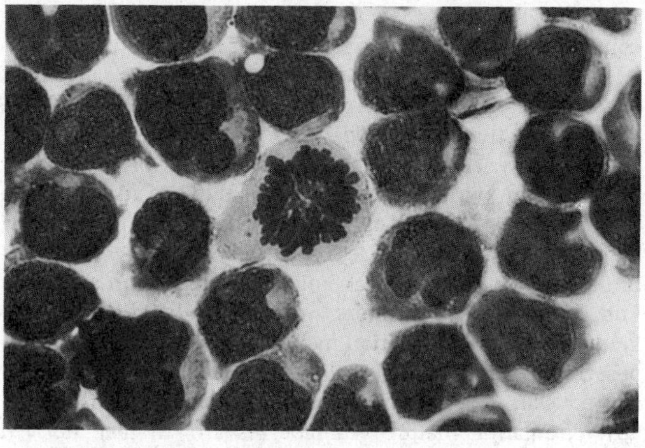

FIG. 52-4. Wright's stained cytocentrifuge preparation of cerebrospinal fluid from a patient with FAB type L2 ALL. The diagnosis of meningeal leukemia was easily made, although routine cell count of the fluid revealed only 2 cells/μl.

Cranial nerve palsies may appear suddenly in an acute leukemia patient secondary to leukemic infiltration of the nerve sheath. The long cranial nerves, VI and VII, are affected most often. The palsy may occur without other clinical evidence of CNS leukemia, and examination of the CSF may be unrevealing. The course of the affected nerve must be irradiated within 24 hours of onset of the palsy if as much function as possible is to be restored.

METABOLIC PATHOLOGY

A number of important metabolic derangements can occur in the acute leukemia patient as a consequence of the disease, its treatment, or both. Two important biochemical causes of renal functional impairment, urate nephropathy and muramidasuria (lysozymuria), have been discussed earlier in this chapter.

Rarely, lactic acidosis complicates acute leukemia.[76] In such cases, the morphologic characteristics of the leukemic cells are often unusual, including prominent cytoplasmic vacuolization. Most patients with lactic acidosis have had poorly controlled leukemia with only brief remissions. Many have had evidence of an unusually large body burden of tumor as evidenced by hyperleukocytosis, massive extramedullary disease, or an extremely hypercellular bone marrow. Some reported patients have, however, been leukopenic. The etiology of lactic acidosis in acute leukemia is unclear, but it may be profound, with arterial blood lactate concentrations as high as 36 mEq/liter. The acidosis has been at least partially corrected by bringing the leukemia under control in all cases in which chemotherapy resulted in a remission, and the degree of acidosis roughly paralleled disease activity in such instances.

Most untreated patients with ANLL have significantly reduced plasma total, low-density lipoprotein concentrations, and high-density lipoprotein cholesterol concentrations. Increased use of cholesterol for membrane synthesis by the expanding leukemic clone has been postulated as a mechanism.[77] The plasma concentrations normalize with remission.

Hypercalcemia secondary to ectopic production of parathyroid hormone or parathyroid hormone fragments by leukemic cells, or other causes, has been observed on occasion in both ANLL and ALL.[78-80] The blood calcium level usually parallels disease activity. Hypocalcemia may also occur and may be more common than hypercalcemia. Hypocalcemia is most common in patients with greatly elevated blood leukemic cell counts and some degree of renal failure. It is usually associated with hyperphosphatemia and hyperphosphaturia. Hypocalcemia in such patients is probably secondary to the increased endogenous phosphorus load that results from the destruction of leukemic cells either as a result of ineffective leukopoiesis, chemotherapy, or both. On the other hand, accelerated bone formation stimulated by leukemic cells may have been the mechanism of hypocalcemia in one ANLL patient.[81]

Hyperkalemia may result from the rapid destruction of a large number of leukemic cells. The sudden elevation of blood potassium levels has caused cardiac arrest in at least one patient.[82] On occasion, hyperkalemia is spurious[83] and results from potassium release by leukemic cells during in vitro clotting. Therefore, serum electrolyte studies should be repeated with anticoagulated blood immediately after venipuncture when elevated blood potassium levels are reported and hyperkalemic effects are not seen on the electrocardiogram.

PATHOLOGY OF THE IMMUNE SYSTEM

Impaired cell-mediated immunity measured by reaction to a variety of intradermal antigens has been observed in 10% to 45% of acute leukemia patients in various studies, but this finding is of little clinical significance. Some investigators believe that the immunoincompetence is a direct effect of the leukemia on the immune system, whereas others consider it a nonspecific manifestation of cachexia that may accompany advanced leukemia. In some, but not all, studies, anergy prior to treatment had a poor prognosis, while intact cell-mediated immunity (or controversion to it during therapy) had a very favorable prognosis.[84,85] Results of current management are unaffected by skin test reactivity.

Abnormalities of the humoral immune system in acute leukemia patients were observed in some studies. In some patients, decreased IgG and increased IgM and IgA levels are present before therapy. These abnormalities usually normalized during the initial phase of chemotherapy, and their significance is unclear. Rarely, an abnormal paraprotein is present in the serum prior to therapy and disappears with successful treatment. Such paraproteins have been reported more frequently with acute monocytic or myelomonocytic leukemia than with other varieties of acute leukemia.[86]

At least two thirds of ANLL patients have a relatively normal ability to develop a primary or secondary antibody response as measured by the development of lymphocytotoxic or anti-red blood cell (ABO) antibodies, or both, after multiple ABO-incompatible platelet transfusions. The ability to develop such antibodies correlates neither with pretreatment blood immunoglobulin levels or skin test reactivity nor with subsequent response to therapy or ultimate prognosis.[87]

Significant elevations of whole complement and C5, C8, and C9 were observed in acute leukemia patients in one study, but the significance of these observations is not known.[88] One mouse model of spontaneously arising acute leukemia, the AKR mouse, is deficient in C5.[89]

NATURAL HISTORY

PATHOGENESIS

Acute leukemia patients, in general, suffer from the lack of normal numbers of normal blood cells more so than from the presence of leukemic cells. Thus, infection and hemorrhage due to insufficient numbers of circulating granulocytes and platelets are the most serious threats to the well-being and life of the patient. Decreased production of granulocytes, platelets, and red cells by the leukemic marrow has classically been attributed to a "crowding" phenomenon, in which the normal marrow stem cell clone is physically crowded out by the unchecked proliferation of the leukemic clone. The mechanism by which proliferation and maturation of normal blood cell precursors is reduced may be more complicated than that explanation implies, however. Some data suggest that leukemic cells may produce certain chalones that inhibit proliferation and differentiation of normal marrow stem cells.[90]

When a patient with acute leukemia achieves complete remission after therapy, the bone marrow and peripheral blood cells become relatively normal morphologically, and the proportions of the various cells within each compartment normalize. The explanation for this observation has been that therapy successfully reduces the body burden of leukemic cells to a point at which it cannot be observed by available techniques, and derivatives of the normal stem cell clone, now relatively unopposed, have repopulated marrow and blood. This explanation is consistent with the widely accepted theory that acute leukemia is a disease that begins with the development of a single malignant clone of cells. Some evidence against this theory has been collected, however. Rare patients who achieve complete remission after chemotherapy for ANLL have been observed to have Auer's bodies in their otherwise morphologically normal mature polymorphonuclear leukocytes.[91] In addition, some patients have been noted to lose the normal granulation of mature polymorphonuclear leukocytes as the first evidence of impending relapse with ANLL,[53,92] and the granulation becomes normal again if another remission is subsequently achieved. The buffy coats from the blood of some patients in complete remission after treatment for ANLL contain significant reverse transcriptase activity, although the peripheral leukocytes appear to be morphologically normal.[93] These data suggest that, in some patients with ANLL, the morphologically normal leukocytes in marrow and blood may be derived from abnormal leukemic cells. Thus it is possible that, in some ANLL patients at least, no normal marrow stem cell exists and that remission results from differentiation and maturation of leukemic cells induced in some unknown manner by treatment. Some naturally occurring leukemic cell differentiation-inducing proteins have been described,[94] and recombinant DNA techniques have demonstrated that, in some ANLL patients in remission after therapy, circulating mature granulocytes are, in fact, derived from the leukemic clone.[95]

Exceptions exist to the general statement that, in most patients, the presence of leukemic cells is less dangerous than the absence of normal cells, and many examples have already been noted.

The presence of leukemic cells in the central nervous system can be life threatening. ANLL patients with a very high peripheral blood blast count (>200,000 blasts/μl) have at least a 25% risk of fatal intracerebral hemorrhage within 24 to 48 hours if not treated.[96] Blood viscosity with such a high concentration of large, sticky cells is increased, and sludging tends to occur at the venous end of the capillary bed. Plugging of the low-pressure side of the capillary network may be caused by these blast cells, and the capillary may rupture. The resultant bleeding will go undetected if it occurs in a tissue such as muscle, but it may be fatal if it occurs in brain. Therefore, the presentation of an ANLL patient with a greatly elevated blood blast count is a medical emergency requiring immediate treatment as discussed below. Patients with ALL who have extreme leukocytosis do not appear to have the same risk because the more rigid lymphoblast has less intrinsic viscosity and does not alter blood viscosity as greatly. Patients with chronic leukemia, except patients with blast crisis of CML, are also not at as great a risk for this complication.

Another manifestation of CNS leukemia is meningeal leukemia. Acute leukemia patients rarely present with this complication but can develop it months or years after treatment, even while in hematologic complete remission, especially if prophylactic treatment for this complication was not part of the initial treatment program (see below).

The pathogenesis of meningeal leukemia has been explained by some as follows. At the time of presentation, the patient has a marrow cavity packed with leukemic cells, including areas of marrow that are usually inactive in the adult (*e.g.*, the marrow of the skull bones). Leukemic cells from skull marrow may rupture through the periosteum and infiltrate the dura. The cells then may migrate down the adventitia of vessels that transverse the space between the dura and pia-arachnoid and infiltrate that membrane. Systemic chemotherapy usually will not cross the so-called blood–brain barrier. Capillary endothelial cells of the brain, unlike other such cells elsewhere in the body, restrict passage of drugs bound to plasma protein and also limit diffusion of drugs in general and lipid-insoluble drugs in particular (such as most antineoplastic agents). Entry of drugs into the brain from CSF is similarly limited by choroid plexus cells. Therefore, systemic chemotherapy may eradicate leukemic cells on the blood side of that barrier (dura) but will not kill cells on the brain side (pia-arachnoid). Leukemic cells in the pia-arachnoid will multiply and, with time, block the flow of CSF. Hydrocephalus will result, and the patient will present with signs and symptoms of increased intracranial pressure.[97] Examination of the CSF will reveal leukemic cells and establish the diagnosis.[98]

A simpler, alternative explanation for this phenomenon has been offered.[99] Leukemic meningitis occurs more frequently in ALL patients who present with high blast counts (>20,000/μl) and low platelet counts (<20,000/μl). It has been suggested that, in such a patient, petechial hemorrhage in the pia-arachnoid may deposit leukemic cells in a pharmacologic sanctuary. Whatever the true pathogenesis of this lesion, prophylactic treatment greatly reduces its clinical incidence, and effective palliative therapy exists for most patients who develop it (see below).

PATTERNS OF SPREAD

Leukemia, at the time of diagnosis, is a disseminated systemic disease. It is therefore difficult to discuss patterns of spread in the way that we do with more common tumors such as those of lung, colon, or breast. Certain useful general statements can be made, however. Parenchymal organ dysfunction secondary to leukemic cell infiltration is not common in acute leukemia. When present, it usually occurs late in the clinical course of a patient who has had relapsed, poorly controlled disease. In addition, extramedullary relapses are more common than extramedullary presentations. A notable exception to this statement is gingival infiltration in a patient with acute monocytic or myelomonocytic leukemia, which is commonly present at the time of diagnosis.

CLINICAL PRESENTATION

ACUTE LYMPHOCYTIC LEUKEMIA

Most adults with ALL are young, in the third or fourth decade of life, and the disease is observed less frequently in succeeding decades. The patient usually gives a history of lassitude for several weeks or more. Moderate signs and symptoms of anemia are present at the time of diagnosis, and some evidence of minor bleeding is elicited from the history or detected by physical examination in one third of patients. The patient is usually not infected, and perhaps 10% of patients feel entirely well. Physical examination reveals generalized minimal or moderate lymphadenopathy in most patients, especially of the cervical region, and minimal or moderate splenomegaly in more than half. The leukocyte count is normal or elevated in at least 85% of patients, but 15% are leukopenic. Approximately 25% of adults with ALL present with a leukocyte count greater than 50,000/μl. The differential leukocyte count reveals at least some lymphoblasts in virtually every patient, and at least 50% of the leukocytes are lymphoblasts in approximately two thirds of patients. The platelet count is reduced in most patients, but it is below 50,000/μl in only one third. Moderate anemia is noted initially in approximately three-fourths of patients. The bone marrow biopsy is hypercellular in virtually all patients, and a smear of the marrow aspirate reveals megakaryocytes and decreased numbers of erythrocyte and granulocyte precursors. The normal cells present generally have normal morphologic characteristics. At least half of the marrow nucleated elements are lymphoblasts in three fourths of patients.

Serum uric acid is elevated in almost all patients, and the degree of elevation roughly parallels the degree of marrow infiltration with lymphoblasts. Serum and urinary muramidase are normal or reduced. The serum lactic dehydrogenase (LDH) activity is usually increased, and is greatly increased in about one third of patients.

In an untreated patient, the blood and marrow blast count will rise almost daily, and the granulocyte and platelet count will fall correspondingly. The rise is usually gradual but at times can be alarming. Patients with ALL rarely have a spontaneous stabilization of disease. Therefore, *preleukemia* and *smoldering leukemia* are terms that rarely, if ever, apply to ALL. It is important to initiate therapy as soon after diagnosis as possible to prevent infection and hemorrhage from complicating management.

ACUTE NONYLMPHOCYTIC LEUKEMIA

ANLL is much more common in adults than is ALL and occurs at any age. In most series, the majority of patients are 35 to 65 years old. Patients with ANLL give a history similar to those with ALL, but the history may be very brief, with only a week or two of symptoms prior to diagnosis. Significant evidence of hemorrhage is more likely to be found in ANLL than in ALL. About one third of ANLL patients have had serious orificial bleeding or have noted petechial rashes that may be confluent in some areas. Patients with acute promyelocytic leukemia commonly present with moderately severe hemorrhage and large areas of cutaneous ecchymoses. Approximately one third of ANLL patients present with a serious or even life-threatening infection, such as a pyogenic abscess or septicemia. Rarely, the patient will be entirely asymptomatic and will be diagnosed after a routine examination. The physical examination is often otherwise entirely normal. Lymphadenopathy is unusual, and splenomegaly is found in less than one quarter of patients. Gingival hypertrophy may be prominent in patients with a monocytic component of the disease and may be the problem for which the patient initially seeks attention. The leukocyte count is low in one third, normal in one third, and elevated in one third of patients at diagnosis; it is less than 50,000/μl in approximately one half of newly diagnosed patients. It is much less common today for a patient to present with extreme hyperleukocytosis ($>$300,000/μl) than it was a decade ago. This difference may result from earlier diagnosis now than previously for a variety of reasons. The differential leukocyte count reveals some blast forms in most patients, but in approximately 10%, no peripheral blasts are noted. The platelet count is usually reduced significantly, and counts of less than 20,000/μl are common. Almost all patients have a moderate reduction of hematocrit to at least 30% to 35%. The peripheral blood granulocyte count is reduced in most patients and is below 1000/μl in at least half when diagnosed.

The bone marrow biopsy is usually hypercellular but may be hypocellular in patients who have developed ANLL after another hematologic disorder such as aplastic anemia or paroxysmal nocturnal hemoglobinuria,[100] or after treatment with radiotherapy, chemotherapy, or both for another malignant disease. Leukemic cells constitute at least 50% of the marrow nucleated elements in most patients at diagnosis. Striking changes may be evident in other marrow elements. Erythroid hyperplasia or bizarre granulation of more mature granulocytes may exist.

The serum uric acid is elevated in approximately half of patients but is usually only 1 to 2 mg/dl above normal. Serum LDH activity is increased in many patients but much less so than in patients with ALL. Serum and urine muramidase may be greatly elevated in acute monocytic leukemia and moderately so in acute myelomonocytic leukemia.[48]

Acute nonlymphocytic leukemia progresses rapidly in most patients if not treated. It is imperative to begin treatment before the blood granulocyte count falls below 1500/μl to 1000/μl if at all possible, because infected ANLL patients have much less of a chance of obtaining a complete remission after treatment than do uninfected patients.[101]

About 10% of patients who eventually are diagnosed as having ANLL present with a hematologic disorder that cannot be completely characterized. Such patients are often elderly and present with complaints referable to anemia or thrombocytopenia. Anemia, leukopenia, and thrombocytopenia may be present in any combination and degree. An occasional blast cell may be seen on the blood smear, and there may be a monocytosis. The bone marrow may be normocellular, hypercellular, or hypocellular. An increased number of sideroblasts (often ringed) may be present, and a maturation arrest at the myelocyte level of leukocyte maturation may be observed together with an excess number of blasts (perhaps 10%–15% of marrow-nucleated elements).[102] The terms *refractory sideroblastic anemia with excess blasts* and *preleukemia* have been applied to these patients. Many patients presenting in this manner, progress over time (months to years) to unequivocal ANLL, especially acute myelomonocytic leukemia. One third to one half of patients with this syndrome will have a clonal karyotypic abnormality usually due to deletion of part of a chromosome 5 or 20 long arm, monosomy 5 or 7, or trisomy 8. Progression to frank leukemia occurs in most patients with abnormal cytogenetics but in only a few patients with a normal karyotype.[103]

A variation of the preleukemic syndrome termed *smoldering leukemia* includes patients with frank ANLL, usually acute myelomonocytic leukemia, whose disease may remain stable for many weeks or months without treatment.[104] The patient demonstrates stable peripheral blood counts above dangerous levels ($>$1500 granulocytes/μl and $>$20,000 platelets/μl) and a marrow blast count of less than 30% to 50% of marrow nucleated elements. It is not clear why the disease does not progress, but treatment may be withheld until progression is evident from serial blood and marrow examinations.

METHODS OF DIAGNOSIS

The work-up for patients with acute leukemia is summarized in Table 52-2. Acute leukemia may be diagnosed from a peripheral blood smear in most cases. In some patients, only a few immature cells will appear on the blood smear, and examination of a marrow aspirate will be necessary to make the diagnosis. However, the marrow should always be examined in a newly diagnosed acute leukemia patient because, in many cases, proper subclassification of the diagnosis will be facilitated, and cellularity can be assessed on biopsy.

TABLE 52-2. Work-up for Patient with Acute Leukemia

- Complete history, including:
  - Family, work, and medical history
  - Radiation and chemical exposure history
- Complete physical examination, with special attention to:
  - Temperature
  - Lymph node–bearing areas and splenic area
  - Optic fundi and cranial nerves
  - Potential sites of infection
  - Skin, including axillae
  - Oropharynx, including gingivae
  - Lungs
  - Perianal area
- Peripheral blood studies
  - Hematocrit, leukocyte count, platelet count
  - Leukocyte differential count
- Bone marrow examination
  - Perform biopsy to determine cellularity
  - Aspirate smears stained with Wright's, Sudan black, and esterase stains; period acid–Schiff reagent; iron stain; and immunofluorescent stain for terminal transferase.
  - Aspirate for karyotyping
- Blood chemistries and other studies
  - Serum electrolytes, uric acid, blood urea nitrogen, and muramidase (lysozyme)
  - Coagulation profile, including fibrinogen level, prothrombin time, and partial thromboplastin time
- Cerebrospinal fluid
  - Routine studies
  - Examine Wright's-stained concentrated specimen
- Radiographs
  - Chest posteroanterior and lateral radiographic films
- Transfusion work-up
  - Determine blood type and human leukocyte antigen type if patient has circulating lymphocytes
  - Do same for family members who are willing to serve as platelet, granulocyte, or marrow donors for patient

Special Work-up of Patient with Acute Lymphocytic Leukemia

- Peripheral blood
  - Determination of B-cell and T-cell surface markers. If not possible, do acid phosphatase stain of blood smear.

The usual site chosen for marrow aspiration and biopsy is the posterior iliac crest. In a grossly obese patient, it may be difficult to perform the procedure at that site. An alternative site for aspiration in such patients is the sternum. Great care must be taken in performing a sternal marrow aspiration because retrosternal bleeding may be serious, even life threatening. Of course, biopsy is never performed on the sternal marrow (Figs. 52-5 and 52-6).

The most important subclassification of acute leukemia to be made is to distinguish between ALL and ANLL because their treatments differ. The distinction is facilitated by interpretation of morphologic characteristics and histochemical stain reactions as discussed in the preceding sections. Determination of TdT activity is extremely helpful because the presence of nuclear TdT activity in most of the leukemic cells strongly supports a diagnosis of ALL.

A careful lumbar puncture with a small bore needle should be performed on newly diagnosed ALL patients and on ANLL patients of the FAB M4E subtype because an occasional patient will present with meningeal leukemia. The CSF should be studied routinely and studied after concentration by cytocentrifugation or Millipore filtration and staining with Wright's stain. The platelet count should be at least 50,000/μl at the time of the procedure. The procedure should be performed, therefore, only after a successful platelet transfusion if the patient presents with a lower count.

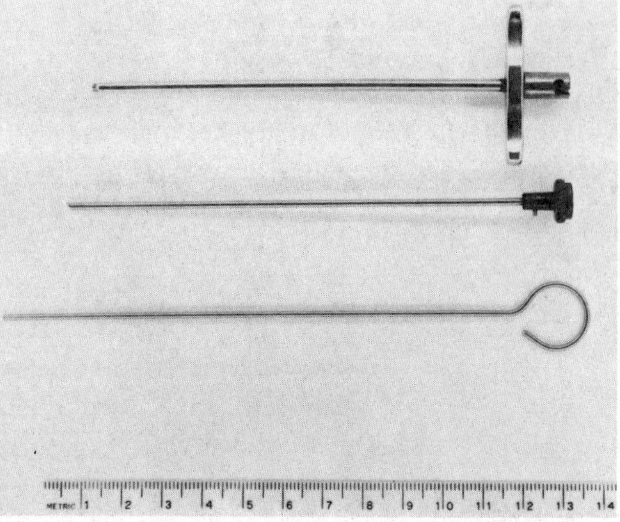

FIG. 52-5. The Jamshidi adult needle for posterior iliac crest marrow aspiration and biopsy. The patient is placed on his or her abdomen, and the posterior iliac spine is located and marked with an indelible pen. The sterile gloved operator swabs the operative site with antiseptic and covers surrounding areas with surgical drapes. Local anesthetic is infiltrated into the operative site down to and including the periosteum. A skin incision a few millimeters in length is made over the marked area with a scalpel. The needle (*top*) with the stylet (*middle*) locked in place is introduced through the incision and advanced through soft tissue to the periosteal surface with a gentle, rotating motion. The instrument should contact the posterior iliac spine at such an angle that it is aimed at the ipsilateral anterior superior iliac spine. The instrument is then advanced with firmer pressure and a rotating counterclockwise-clockwise motion until entrance into the marrow cavity is perceived by sudden decreased resistance, or "give." The stylet is then removed, and a 10-ml syringe is attached to the hub of the needle. Negative pressure is briskly applied to the syringe, and several milliliters of marrow are aspirated. The syringe is quickly removed from the needle and the stylet replaced. A small drop of marrow is quickly placed on each of five specially cleaned cover slips. Each cover slip is covered with a dry cover slip placed so that the corners of each pair form a six-pointed star. The weight of the dry cover slip, without additional pressure, is allowed to spread the drop of marrow aspirate over the surfaces of both cover slips. The pair of cover slips are briskly pulled apart and allowed to air dry. Ten aspirate preparations are now available for staining, after which they may be mounted on glass microscope slides. If a biopsy is also to be done, the needle with stylet in place is withdrawn from the marrow cavity and repositioned through the same skin incision into a slightly different location in the marrow cavity. The stylet is then removed and the needle advanced approximately 5 mm into the marrow cavity. A core of marrow will enter the needle. The needle is then pulled back a few millimeters and its tip advanced at a slightly different angle for a few millimeters. This maneuver severs the specimen from the marrow. The needle is then briskly rotated several times along its long axis in one direction and then in the other. The needle is then removed. The probe (*bottom*) is introduced into the distal end of the needle and the biopsy specimen pushed out through the hub of the needle into a specimen bottle containing formalin and sent to the laboratory. A small gauze dressing is taped to the operative site unless the patient is thrombocytopenic, in which case a pressure dressing is applied. The site must be kept dry for 24 hours.

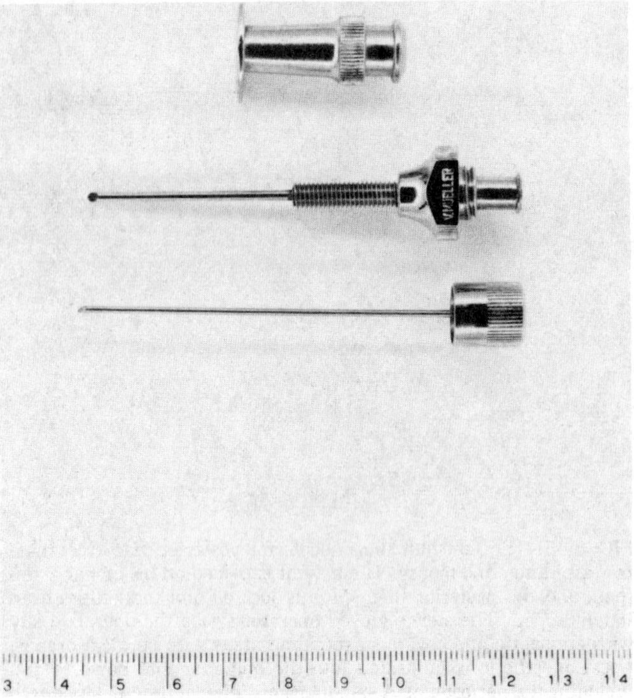

FIG. 52-6. The Illinois needle for sternal marrow aspiration. The sternal angle is identified in the supine patient. The operative site is prepared and anesthetized as described in Figure 52-5. The guard (*top*) is screwed onto the needle and adjusted so that no more than 1 cm of the needle will enter the marrow cavity. The stylet (*bottom*) is inserted into the needle and locked in place. A small skin incision is made with a scalpel just under the ridge of the sternal angle, midpoint from each side of the sternum. The marrow aspiration needle is inserted through the incision at a 45° angle under the sternal angle, in a cephalad direction. When the periosteum is reached, gentle pressure is applied as the needle is rotated clockwise-counterclockwise until a sudden "give" indicates entrance into the marrow cavity. The stylet is then withdrawn, a syringe is attached to the needle, marrow is aspirated, and slides are prepared. The site is then dressed as described in Figure 52-5.

CELL SURFACE ANTIGENS IN ALL

It is important to perform cell surface marker studies on the blast cells of a patient with ALL to identify leukemia-associated antigens.[105] Originally, three ALL groups were described by such methods: (1) B-ALL (surface-associated immunoglobulin SIg$^+$, usually μ heavy chain with κ or λ light chains); (2)T-ALL (receptors for unsensitized sheep erythrocytes allowing rosette formation E$^+$); and (3) non-B, non-T-ALL (SIg$^-$ and E$^-$). Roughly 75% of patients with adult ALL fall into the non-B, non-T category, 20% are T-ALL, and 5% are B-ALL. New monoclonal antibodies developed against a host of leukemia-associated antigens have allowed for the subdivision of non-B, non-T-ALL into at least four important phenotypes, based on the predominance of cells that are either B-cell or T-cell precursors.

1. Common ALL. The common ALL antigen can be demonstrated on the leukemic cell surface (CALLA$^+$). The Ia antigen is also present. Only 50% to 60% of adult ALL patients are CALLA$^+$, whereas at least 80% of children carry this antigen.
2. Pre-B-ALL. The leukemic cells have no surface immunoglobulin, but intracytoplasmic μ chains without light chains can be demonstrated. In addition, the Ia antigen is usually present.
3. Pre-T-ALL. The leukemic cells do not form rosettes with sheep erythrocytes but have some surface antigens characteristic of early T cells. Ia antigen is usually not present.
4. Null cell ALL. The leukemic cells do not form rosettes with sheep red cells, have no surface or cytoplasmic immunoglobulin, and lack CALLA and T-cell antigens. However, they usually possess an antigen characteristic of early B cells (BA-2) and express the Ia antigen. Thus, null cells are probably very early committed B cells. Further evidence for this conclusion derives from experiments in which the culture of some null cells in vitro may result in the expression of CALLA, and some CALLA$^+$ cells express early B-cell markers such as BA-1 or can be induced to express that antigen in vitro.[106,107] In addition, some CALLA$^+$ cells can be induced to produce intracytoplasmic or surface immunoglobulin.[108] For these and other reasons, CALLA$^+$ cells are considered to be "pre-pre-B cells."

Some useful correlations between immunologic phenotype and FAB classification have been made. For instance, most adult ALL patients with FAB type L3 morphology have B-ALL, and virtually no B-ALL patients have L1 morphology.[109] TdT activity is expressed by all ALL cells, except mature T and B cells.

Children and adults with T-ALL or B-ALL have similar survival, which is significantly worse than that of children or adults with non-B, non-T-ALL. However, children with non-B, non-T-ALL usually have better survival rates than do adults with that type of leukemia.[109] It has been reported that children and adults with CALLA$^+$ ALL have the same excellent prognosis, a finding that suggests that the poorer prognosis for adults with non-B, non-T-ALL compared with prognosis of children may be related to the lower incidence of CALLA$^+$ ALL in adults.[110] Controversy exists over this point because some studies have suggested a poorer prognosis for CALLA$^+$ adult ALL than for CALLA$^-$ patients. Another possible explanation for the poor prognosis for adults with ALL compared with children is the fact that as many as one third of adults with ALL express myeloid antigens on the leukemic cell surface,[111,112] a phenomenon that is much less common in childhood ALL. Such hybrid leukemias are associated with a significantly lower complete response rate than typical ALL[112] and constitute a high-risk group.

It should be remembered that no leukemia-specific antigen has yet been discovered. Thus, CALLA is expressed on certain normal tissues, including 2% to 6% of nonmyeloid-nucleated elements of the normal adult bone marrow.[106,113–116] The percentage is often higher in regenerating marrow, a characteristic that can lead to confusion in differentiating between remission and persistent leukemia in some treated patients.

The lack of specificity of CALLA and other leukemia-associated antigens suggests that immunotherapy targeted at them will be associated with toxicity to various normal tissues. Such treatment is likely to be less than completely effective for other reasons. Antibody-induced modulation of the leukemic cell due to internalization of the antigen with loss of its expression has been the most significant problem with the therapeutic use of the anti-CALLA monoclonal antibody J-5 in patients with CALLA$^+$ ALL. In addition, antigens shed from the leukemic cell may block infused antibody, and the clearance of circulating immune complexes may in turn result in significant nephrotoxicity.[117] Also, these antibodies are of murine origin and may cause anaphylactoid reactions when reinfused into patients after the initial exposure. Finally, binding of monoclonal antibodies to antigens expressed on the leukemic cell usually does not result in cytotoxicity unless the antibodies are employed as carriers of nonspecific cytotoxic agents, such as metabolic enzyme inhibitors.[117]

The most promising therapeutic use of monoclonal antibodies is in selective killing of leukemic lymphocytes during in vitro purging of bone marrow for autologous marrow transplantation. Anti–T-cell monoclonal antibodies have also been used in an attempt to eradicate graft-versus-host disease (GVHD) associated with allogeneic bone marrow transplantation either by in vitro treatment of donor marrow or by in vivo treatment of the recipient with steroid-resistant acute GVHD.[117,118]

CELL SURFACE ANTIGENS IN ANLL

The value of cell-surface marker studies in ANLL is being established.[119] It is clear that ANLL is both a morphologic and an antigenically heterogeneous disease, and immunologic subsets with different prognoses are beginning to emerge.[119] Monocytoid cells in acute monocytic or myelomonocytic leukemia usually have Fc-receptors and membrane-bound IgG. Myeloblasts are characteristically Fc-receptor negative.[105] Furthermore, monoclonal antibodies specifically recognizing antigens expressed by monocytoid but not myeloid cells have been developed. Thus, cell surface marker studies in ANLL facilitate subclassification and, in the future, may define functional differences among leukemic cell populations.

ASSESSING PROGNOSIS BEFORE THERAPY

A number of characteristics of the acute leukemia patient at the time of diagnosis have prognostic import. Age is the most consistent factor in de novo patients. Patients over the age of 70 years are less likely to survive the rigors of treatment and achieve a complete response, and all possible supportive care must be given to the elderly patient if treatment is to be successful. It should be remembered that once the elderly patient achieves complete remission, subsequent survival and remission duration can be expected to be as long as in younger patients.[120]

As discussed earlier, several poor prognostic factors for ALL patients have been identified. These include high leukocyte count, the presence of meningeal leukemia or infection at diagnosis, the presence of the Ph[1] chromosome in lymphoblasts, and B-cell markers on lymphoblasts. Except for infection, none of these characteristics impairs the patient's chance of obtaining a complete response to chemotherapy, but they are associated with a propensity for early relapse and impaired overall survival. Those ALL patients with myeloid cell surface markers on leukemic cells have a poor prognosis for complete remission, as well as for overall survival.

Most factors of prognostic import in ANLL affect the likelihood of a complete response to chemotherapy, rather than response duration. An exception is hyperleukocytosis ($>$100,000 leukocytes/μl), which is usually associated with impaired remission duration and survival.[121] Perhaps the single most important negative prognostic factor is prior treatment with radiation or chemotherapy. For unclear reasons, patients with therapy-related "secondary leukemia" have notoriously poor response to chemotherapy; usually, fewer than 15% of such patients achieve complete remission.[122] However, some studies suggest that response to therapy in such patients may be improving with new treatments.[123]

As discussed earlier, the presence of a serious infection at the time of diagnosis significantly reduces the likelihood of achieving complete remission. Although the leukemic cell is as sensitive to chemotherapy as in an uninfected patient, death from uncontrolled infection during chemotherapy is, unfortunately, common. However, if an infected patient achieves complete remission, subsequent prognosis is similar to that of other patients.[120]

The percent labeling index of bone marrow leukemic cells correlated with the probability of complete remission in one study[124] in which young ANLL patients with high labeling indices had the highest complete response rate. Interestingly, in the same study, marrow percent labeling index had no prognostic significance in ALL.

The presence of aneuploidy or other gross karyotypic abnormalities in a patient with ANLL may impair response to chemotherapy. In one study, none of 43 patients with initially abnormal karyotypes achieved a complete response with chemotherapy, in contrast to 37 patients with normal karyotypes, who had a complete response rate of 69%.[125] Cytogenetic abnormalities can be demonstrated in the leukemic cells from most patients with ANLL with newer techniques that involve methotrexate synchronization and prophase banding.[126] Many subtle chromosomal translocations, partial deletions, and inversions disclosed in this manner have important diagnostic and therapeutic implications. Analysis of response, remission duration, and survival data indicates that patients with normal karyotypes, with inversion of chromosome 16 (found in most patients with FAB type M4E)[127] or with translocations involving chromosomes 8 and 21 (found in some patients with FAB type M2) had favorable prognoses. Patients with translocations involving chromosomes 15 and 17, diagnostic of FAB-type M3, had an intermediate prognosis, and patients with most other abnormalities composed an unfavorable prognostic group.[128] In addition, patients with therapy-related myelodysplastic syndromes or ANLL frequently have leukemic cells with specific abnormalities of chromosomes 5 and 7, usually partial or complete deletions.[129]

The prognostic values of colony-forming and colony-stimulating capacities of bone marrow cells from patients with ANLL have been studied[130] and the number of colonies and clusters in both in vitro soft agar marrow and blood cultures

TABLE 52-3. Selected Acute Nonlymphocytic Leukemia (ANLL) Syndromes

Syndrome	FAB Type	Molecular Biology	Karyotype	Incidence	Prognosis	Other
ANLL with abnormal eosinophils	M4E	Disruption of metallothionin gene	Inversion, translocation, or deletion of chr#16	5% of ANLL	Excellent	Increased incidence of CNS leukemia
Biphenotypic leukemia with t(4;11)	L2	Translocation of c-*ets*-1 oncogene to 4q21	t(4;11)(q21;q23)	5% of ANLL	Very poor	Monocytic differentiation inducible in vitro
ANLL with t(9;11)	M5	Translocation of c-*ets*-1 oncogene to 9p22 into alpha interferon gene	t(9;11)(p22;q23)	10% of M5	Better than M5 in general	Young adults
ANLL with t(8;21)	M2	Translocation of c-*ets*-2 to 8q, and of c-*myc* to 21q	t(8;21)(q22;q22)	5%–10% of ANLL	Excellent for CR, average for survival	Auer's bodies common
Acute promyelocytic leukemia	M3	—	t(15;17)(q22;q21.1)	5%–10% of ANLL	Poorer than average	Coagulopathy common
ANLL with abnormal megakaryocytes	M4	Apposition of genes for transferrin and its receptor	Various inversions and rearrangements of chr #3	Rare	Poorer than average	High platelet count or abnormal megakaryocytes
Therapy-related ANLL	Variable	c-*fms*, GM-CSF, or CSF-1 gene may be deleted in -5 or 5q-	Deletion of chr #5 or #7 in whole or in part is common	5% of ANLL	Very poor	Preleukemic phase common

Modified from Koeffler.

was significantly lower at presentation in patients who entered remission than in those who did not. Thus, growth patterns of bone marrow and circulating colony-forming units may be of value in predicting response to chemotherapy.

Most attempts to correlate therapeutic response to morphologic subclass of ANLL fail,[131] and, as suggested above, karyotypic analysis is much more useful in classifying patients with ANLL than are morphologic characteristics (Table 52-3).[132]

As the therapy for a given disease improves, the importance of previously recognized prognostic factors often diminishes. Such may be the case for patients with ANLL.[133] For example, advanced age alone is no longer an absolute deterrent to a successful therapeutic outcome.

TREATMENT

It is very important to remember that some patients with ANLL do not require specific immediate treatment. A small number of patients, as discussed earlier, present with a "smoldering" disease that is not immediately progressive. Such patients are usually elderly and are either entirely clinically well or have only signs and symptoms of anemia that can be corrected with blood transfusion. Although variable degrees of thrombocytopenia and granulocytopenia may be present, platelet and granulocyte counts are above dangerous levels. Bone marrow examination is diagnostic of ANLL, but adequate granulocyte and platelet production is evident. This quiescent status may persist for only a few weeks or for months or years. Weekly blood counts should be performed to determine when the disease becomes progressive so that treatment may be instituted while the patient is still well. Initiation of treatment is indicated when serial studies reveal (1) progressive thrombocytopenia with platelet counts falling to the 30,000/μl to 50,000/μl range, (2) progressive granulocytopenia with the granulocyte count falling below 1,500/μl, or (3) progressive marrow infiltration with leukemic cells to the point that they account for more than 50% of marrow hematopoietic cells.

An ALL patient should begin treatment as soon as the diagnosis is firmly established because the disease almost always progresses steadily. Moreover, compelling evidence suggests that prognosis is directly related to the body burden of tumor in the patient with ALL.

Adult acute leukemia patients should almost always undergo treatment in a facility that has essentially unlimited supportive care capabilities, including access to sufficient quantities of platelets and granulocytes for transfusion and, above all, a multidisciplinary team of physicians, nurses, and pharmacists thoroughly experienced in the management of such patients. Obvious exceptions to this recommendation include patients who refuse the intensive chemotherapy necessary for optimal results, and patients who refuse transfusion of blood products. In addition, patients over the age of 70 years are much less likely to respond favorably to treatment than are younger patients[134] and therefore are often candidates for largely symptomatic care that can be delivered elsewhere. All other patients should be strongly advised to accept treatment at the nearest facility specializing in the management of acute leukemia patients.

MANAGEMENT OF EMERGENCIES

Some readily treatable emergencies may exist at the time acute leukemia is diagnosed. Their recognition and proper management will preclude early death in many patients and allow them to survive long enough to receive an adequate trial of chemotherapy, to which most adult acute leukemia patients will respond.

Hemorrhage

Bleeding in a setting of thrombocytopenia and normal concentrations of clotting factors is most likely the result of the thrombocytopenia. In such cases, the platelet count is usually well below 20,000/μl, but if the platelet count has been falling rapidly, serious hemorrhage may occur with higher platelet counts. Platelet concentrate transfusion will almost always stop the bleeding, although the platelets from 10 or more units of fresh whole blood may be required to do so (see Chap. 59). Such hemorrhage can almost always be prevented by the prophylactic transfusion of fewer platelets (6–8 units) every 2 to 3 days when the platelet count is below 20,000/μl.

Disseminated intravascular coagulation may result in life-threatening bleeding, as discussed earlier. The use of heparin in the treatment and prevention of this problem in acute leukemia patients has generally been accepted,[135,136] although recently it has been challenged.[137] Usually bleeding in acute leukemia patients that is secondary to disseminated intravascular coagulation can be prevented or stopped with low doses of heparin (50 units/kg) given intravenously every 6 hours.[136] Heparin should be administered prophylactically in this dose and schedule before bleeding starts in an acute leukemia patient with laboratory evidence of this syndrome. Such evidence includes a falling plasma fibrinogen concentration below 100 mg/dl and elevated and rising titers of fibrin degradation products. If the blood fibrinogen concentration does not rise within 24 hours or the concentration of fibrin degradation products does not fall in that time, the dose of heparin should be doubled. It may also be necessary to administer fresh frozen plasma in this circumstance. If the platelet count is below 20,000/μl, as is often the case, platelet concentrate transfusions should also be given but only after heparin therapy is well underway. Otherwise, the coagulopathy may be exacerbated. Heparin may be successful in active bleeding secondary to disseminated intravascular coagulation, but prevention is much easier than treatment. The coagulopathy should be controlled before the leukemia is treated, because destruction of leukemic cells will augment the problem.

On occasion surgery is necessary in an acute leukemia patient not in remission. Surgery can usually be performed with minimal blood loss provided that coagulation factor abnormalities can be corrected beforehand, and abundant platelet transfusions to which the patient responds can be provided before and after surgery.[138] The platelet count must be maintained above 50,000/μl if adequate hemostasis is to be maintained.

Infection

A febrile granulocytopenic leukemia patient must be considered to be infected until proved otherwise. Treatment with empiric broad-spectrum parenteral antibiotics should be instituted immediately after the patient is examined and cultures are made.[139] A commonly used empiric antibiotic regimen for this situation is cefaperazone and gentamicin, both given at maximum dose. Appropriate antibiotic changes are made when pretherapy culture results identify a specific organism. When those cultures yield no growth, the patient's clinical response to empiric therapy must serve as a guide to continue, discontinue, or change it. Some authorities recommend adding amphotericin B empirically if the patient has not improved in 4 or 5 days and granulocytopenia persists. Resolution of fever may be the only clue that an infection was treated successfully by the empiric therapy. Because the infected patient is less likely than the uninfected patient to have a favorable outcome after antileukemia treatment, it is necessary to bring the infection under control as much as possible before beginning chemotherapy. It is essential to withhold chemotherapy in an infected ANLL patient who has circulating granulocytes, because the marrow-suppressive drugs used in leukemia treatment may reduce the circulating granulocyte count to zero and impair the patient's chances of surviving the infection (see Chap. 59).

Intracerebral Leukostasis

The likelihood of fatal intracerebral hemorrhage associated with a greatly elevated blood blast count in a patient with ANLL can virtually be eliminated by (1) immediately delivering cranial irradiation, 600 rad in one dose; and (2) placing the patient on hydroxyurea, 3 g/m^2 of body surface area daily, orally for 2 days.[140] The radiation will destroy intracerebral foci of leukemic cells that already may be established, and the drug will cause a rapid fall in the blood blast count over 24 to 48 hours and prevent the reaccumulation of potentially lethal intracerebral lesions. In some cases, leukapheresis with the removal of substantial numbers of blasts from the blood may be as effective.[141]

Urate Nephropathy

Patients with acute leukemia, especially ALL, who have a high leukocyte count will occasionally present with anuria and uremia associated with a greatly elevated serum uric acid concentration. Urine alkalinization, reduction of uric acid production, and even renal dialysis may be necessary to reverse urate nephropathy. The xanthine oxidase inhibitor, allopurinol, should be given three times daily in a dose of 300 mg or 400 mg in such cases. Pyrazinamide, a potent inhibitor of tubular secretion of urate, may be very helpful for patients with serum uric acid levels greater than 20 mg/dl if given at a dose of 1 g every 8 hours for several days. Acetazolamide, 500 mg at bedtime, will keep the urine alkaline overnight and should be given until the serum uric acid is within the normal range. Dialysis should be strongly considered when the blood urea nitrogen (BUN) is greater than 100 mg/dl and rising. To be successful, these potentially lifesaving emergency measures must be undertaken when indicated by the referring physician prior to transfer of the patient to another facility.

ADDITIONAL PREPARATION FOR DEFINITIVE TREATMENT

Chemotherapy designed to induce complete remission will have the greatest chance of success if the patient is brought into stable condition before its initiation. Hemorrhage and infection must be brought under control (discussed earlier) before chemotherapy is begun, if possible. Even if urate nephropathy were not present at the time of diagnosis, it may be precipitated by the rapid destruction of leukemic cells by chemotherapy. Therefore, allopurinol, 100 mg to 200 mg orally three times daily, should be administered for at least 24 hours before beginning chemotherapy. The higher dose is usually only necessary for patients with ALL or those with significant extramedullary leukemic infiltration, such as a mediastinal mass. Allopurinol should be continued until chemotherapy results in leukopenia and marrow hypocellularity, at which time it may be safely discontinued.

All patients with ANLL and some with ALL are likely to undergo a prolonged period of severe granulocytopenia after chemotherapy; therefore, infection prevention methods are of paramount importance. After several showers with topical disinfectants, the patient is placed in strict reverse isolation in a specially cleaned private room. Some physicians prefer to use a laminar air-flow room equipped with a high-efficiency particulate air filter for reverse isolation of acute leukemia patients.[142] These rooms are expensive to build and to operate, but data indicate that ANLL patients treated in them sustain fewer infections and fewer fatal infections during chemotherapy. Patients so treated experience one third to one half the incidence of bacterial pneumonias and virtually no fungal pneumonias, compared with patients undergoing leukemia treatment without mechanical and chemical protection from organisms in their internal and external environments. This finding is especially true if the patient is also placed on a regimen of oral prophylactic antibiotics. A useful regimen consists of trimethoprim–sulfamethoxazole tablets (160 mg of trimethoprim and 900 mg of sulfamethoxazole) given every 8 hours. In addition, nystatin tablets, 4 million units, and nystatin liquid, 1 million units, are given every 4 hours around the clock, beginning 24 hours prior to the first chemotherapy dose and continued through the chemotherapy treatment until the patient is no longer granulocytopenic. This regimen is highly successful in preventing such serious infections as esophageal candidiasis and perirectal abscess and septicemia. The regimen is inexpensive and well tolerated.[143] It may not be wise to use this regimen routinely without a laminar air-flow unit because there may be an increase in the incidence of *Aspergillus* pneumonia in patients receiving the regimen in a standard hospital setting.[144]

SPECIFIC THERAPY FOR ACUTE LYMPHOCYTIC LEUKEMIA

Treatment of ALL in children and adults is usually delivered in four phases: (1) initial or remission induction therapy, (2) consolidation therapy, (3) meningeal leukemia prophylactic therapy, and (4) maintenance therapy. Remission induction therapy is designed to result in complete remission, a state in which it is impossible to make the diagnosis of leukemia. All signs and symptoms of the disease are absent once complete remission has been achieved, and all blood counts are normal. The bone marrow biopsy and aspirate are nondiagnostic and essentially normal also.

Remission induction therapy for adult ALL, usually begun in the hospital, may result in dramatic improvement in hematologic parameters and physical examination in days or in a week or two. Complete remission will not be achieved until 3 weeks or more of treatment have been given, however. Clinical improvement in many patients may be sufficient enough in several days to allow the treatment to be completed in the clinic.

The cornerstone of remission induction treatment for adult ALL is the combination of vincristine and prednisone. Although more than 60% of adults will achieve complete remission with those drugs alone,[145] the complete response rate can be increased by adding an anthracycline such as daunorubicin with or without other agents to that basic regimen.[145–148] A recent example of such success is a study by Linker and associates[149] in which a complete response rate of 94% was achieved in stringently selected group of adults with vincristine, prednisone, daunorubicin, and L-asparaginase. Although encouraging, the study excluded patients with poor prognostic factors such as age greater than 50 years, the presence of the Philadelphia chromosome, and B-cell disease.

Once complete remission is achieved, several additional courses of the initially successful drugs usually are given in an attempt to reduce the now clinically undetectable leukemic cell mass as much as possible (consolidation therapy). In some studies, drugs other than those employed in induction therapy are used for this purpose. The drugs are delivered in doses designed to result in toxicity similar to that experienced with induction therapy, and the schedule of drug administration is such that courses of treatment are delivered as quickly as hematologic recovery from the preceding course will allow. In the Linker study,[148] several combination regimens given in rotation for approximately 9 months were given, using drugs employed for remission induction and others, such as teniposide, cytosine arabinoside, and high-dose methotrexate with leucovorin rescue.

Prophylactic meningeal leukemia therapy usually is delivered immediately before or after consolidation therapy. In one study, patients who received CNS prophylaxis subsequently had an 11% incidence of meningeal leukemia, compared with a 32% incidence in the control group.[146] Thus, meningeal leukemia prophylaxis, which has been eminently successful in children, is also of significant value in adults with ALL. The combination of cranial irradiation and intrathecal methotrexate are commonly used for meningeal leukemia prophylaxis, but, in some studies, intrathecal methotrexate alone has been equally as effective.[146,150,151] In addition, high-dose parenteral methotrexate given with folinic acid rescue may be an effective prophylactic treatment for meningeal leukemia.[152]

Any of these methods may be used to treat meningeal leukemia that develops in an adult with ALL after initial therapy. Some evidence suggests that combination chemotherapy with or without cranial irradiation is superior to single-agent therapy.[153] In refractory patients, systemic high-dose cytosine arabinoside may be helpful.[154] Intrathecal drug may be administered by lumbar puncture or through a reservoir implanted under the scalp that cannulates the third ventricle. The latter approach may be more tolerable for the patient than repeated lumbar punctures, but there is no evidence that therapeutic results are better.

Maintenance treatment begins after consolidation therapy has been completed and the patient has fully recovered. Usually it is carried out in the clinic with doses and schedules of drugs that are not associated with significant acute toxicity. Often, drugs not previously used in the patient's treatment constitute all or at least part of the maintenance regimen. It is not known whether maintenance therapy can be safely discontinued in an adult with ALL who has been in long-term, continuous complete remission. Oral 6-mercaptopurine and methotrexate were employed in the Linker study[149] in which the total duration of postremission therapy was approximately 30 months. Life table analysis of that study predicts that 53% of complete responders will remain in continuous complete remission for at least 3 years. At present it is recommended that postremission therapy be continued for at least 2 to 3 years. A treatment program for adult ALL is given in Table 52-4.

Although the rate of complete response in adult ALL now approaches that of childhood ALL in many studies, the long-term results in adults are poorer. Current therapeutic programs are associated with median remission durations of only 15 to 36 months and median survivals for complete responders of approximately 2 to 4 years.[146,149–152] However, in most recent studies, approximately one third of patients appear to be long-term disease-free survivors, judging from 4 to 5 years of follow-up (Fig. 52-7).[146,150–152]

Multiple therapeutic regimens can induce a second complete response in relapsed adults with ALL almost as frequently as first remissions are obtained.[155] Newer drugs such as amsacrine may be useful in this regard, although this agent seems more useful in ANLL thus far (see below).[156] The duration of second remission is directly related to the duration of first remission,[155] and cure is exceedingly rare. Recently, mitoxantrone has emerged as an active agent in relapsed ALL, and encouraging reports of combinations of that agent with cytosine arabinoside in conventional or high-dose amounts[157] have appeared.

Many investigations of allogeneic bone marrow transplantation for treatment of ALL patients have been reported (see Chap. 66). Thomas and colleagues[158] treated 22 ALL pa-

TABLE 52-4. A Plan for the Treatment of Adult Acute Lymphocytic Leukemia (ALL)

Drug or Irradiation	*Route**	*Dose*	*Schedule*
Induction Therapy			
Vincristine	IV	2 mg/m²	Days 1, 8, 15, 22
Prednisone	PO	60 mg/m²	Days 1 through 28
Daunorubicin	IV	45 mg/m²	Days 1 through 3
L-asparaginase	IM	4000 U/m²	Days 17 through 28
Central Nervous System Prophylaxis			
Whole-brain irradiation		1800-rad total, in 10 fractions	
Intrathecal methotrexate	IT	12 mg/m²	Days 1, 8, 15, 22, 29, 36
Postremission Systemic Therapy†			
RegimenA			
Vincristine	IV	2 mg/m²	Days 1 and 8
Prednisone	PO	60 mg/m²	Days 1 through 14
Daunorubicin	IV	50 mg/m²	Days 1 and 2
L-asparaginase	IM	10,000 U/m²	Days 2, 4, 7, 9, 11, 14
Regimen B			
Etoposide	IV	75 mg/m²	Days 1, 4, 8, 11
Cytarabine	IV	300 mg/m²	Days 1, 4, 8, 11
Regimen C			
Methotrexate	IV	700 mg/m²	42-hour continuous infusion
Calcium leucovorin	IV	15 mg/m²	Every 6 hours × 12 doses, starting at end of methotrexate infusion
Regimen D			
Methotrexate	PO	20 mg/m²	Weekly
6-mercaptopurine	PO	75 mg/m²	Daily

Adapted from Linker et al.[149]

*All intravenous drugs are given by rapid injection except in Regimen C. IM = intramuscularly; IT = intrathecally; IV = intravenously; PO = orally.

†Regimens A and B are given on alternate months for a total of 8 months. Regimen C is given in the 9th month. Regimen D is given for 20 months, beginning after complete hematologic recovery from Regimen C. All doses must be modified according to tolerance.

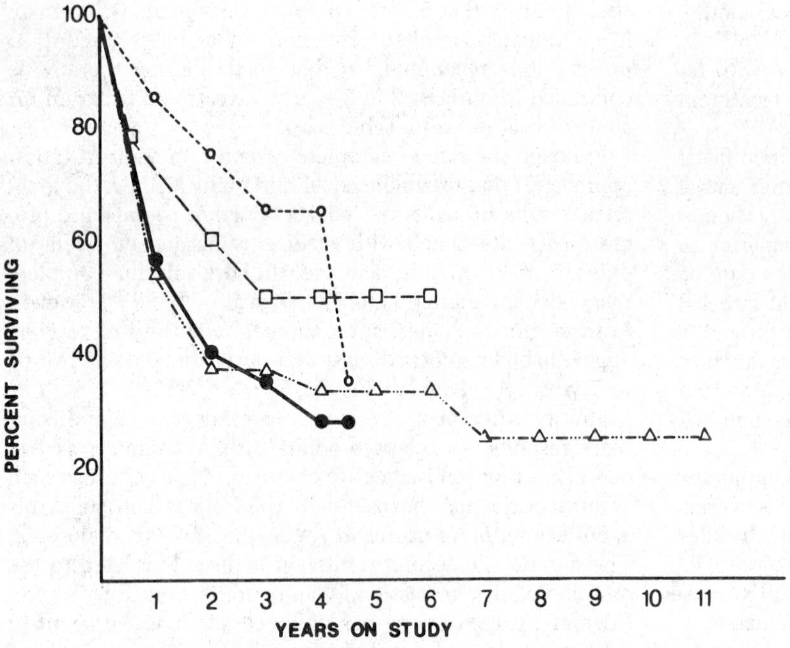

FIG. 52-7. Selected recent results in previously untreated adults with ALL. In some of the studies, subsets had a significantly better outcome than did the entire group. The curves show overall survival of all treated patients as determined by life-table analysis (○- -○). A study by Linker et al.[149] that featured intensive postremission chemotherapy included 81 patients with a median age of 24 years (range, 16–48 years) entered between 1980 and 1986. Patients with the Ph[1] chromosome, B-cell disease, or age greater than 50 years were excluded (□- -□). Another study (by Gingrich et al[148]) of intensive postremission chemotherapy entered 48 patients into the study (no exclusions) who had a median age of 33 years (range, 15–72 years) from 1977 to 1983 (△· · ·△). An update of the MOAD study by Esterhay et al[152] in which no anthracyclines were given and high-dose parenteral methotrexate was the only CNS prophylaxis enrolled 24 patients (no exclusions) with a median age of 31 years (range, 15–60 years) from 1975 to 1980 (●—●). In a study by Weisdorf et al[160] in which 40 patients in complete remission but at high risk for relapse underwent allogeneic marrow transplantation after preparation with cyclophosphamide and fractionated total body irradiation, patients with a median age of 14.2 years (range, 3.6–47.7 years) were entered into this study from 1982 to 1985.

tients in second or subsequent remission and 46 ALL patients with end-stage disease with marrow obtained from a sibling with identical human leukocyte antigen (HLA).[158] Transplantation during remission was generally more successful than transplantation during relapse. Of the 22 patients receiving transplants during remission, 60% have relapsed, but 25% appear cured after follow-up of at least 5 years. The results in these patients (mostly children) who experienced at least one relapse prior to transplantation are superior to those usually reported for chemotherapy alone, but results are poorer in young adults.[159] Results reported for 46 end-stage patients are more provocative. Twelve are alive, disease-free and off all therapy 8 to 11 years after transplantation.[158]

In a recent study of 40 high-risk patients with ALL who received an allogeneic bone marrow transplant during complete remission, the development of acute GVHD was the only factor identified that favorably affected outcome. Eleven of the 40 patients continued disease-free for 2 to 4.5 years after transplantation. The 17 patients who developed GVHD are projected by actuarial analysis to have a 40% overall survival rate at 5 years, which compares favorably with a rate half that for the 23 patients who did not experience acute GVHD.[160] A beneficial effect of GVHD on outcome has been reported by others for ANLL patients who undergo that treatment also.

No comparative studies of marrow transplantation and chemotherapy alone for adults for ALL have been published. Therefore, the relative merits of the two treatment methods cannot be precisely determined at this time.

SPECIFIC THERAPY FOR ANLL

The phases of ANLL treatment are patterned after those of ALL, but many variations on the theme are commonly employed. This is testimony to the fact that, except for remission induction therapy, no single philosophy of management has emerged as clearly superior to another. Thus, controversy exists concerning the value of consolidation and maintenance therapy of patients with ANLL.

Remission induction therapy for ANLL differs from that of ALL in several important ways. The treatment for ANLL is much more toxic, primarily because of the toxicity associated with the most useful drugs, but also because of the greater impairment of normal marrow reserve in the ANLL patient. Thus, although few ALL patients will be required to receive most of their induction therapy in the hospital, most ANLL patients will need to be hospitalized for induction therapy and will recover from it. This is because of the moderate to severe nausea and vomiting usually experienced during the first week of continuous intravenous drug administration, the great susceptibility to infection and bleeding that exists during the subsequent 2 or 3 weeks of drug-induced marrow hypoplasia and resultant pancytopenia, and the frequent laboratory testing necessary to evaluate the results of therapy properly.

The most successful remission induction therapy for ANLL consists of the anthracycline daunorubicin given in conjunction with cytosine arabinoside.[161,162] Daunorubicin treatment alone will result in a 40% to 50% complete response rate, and cytosine arabinoside as a single agent yields a complete response in approximately 25% of patients. Treatment with both drugs given simultaneously yields better results, with complete responses occurring in 65% or more of adult ANLL patients.[163] The drugs have been combined in a variety of ways with equal success. A popular daunorubicin–cytosine arabinoside remission induction regimen for ANLL is outlined in Table 52-5. Some studies suggest that the addition of thioguanine to such a regimen further enhances its efficacy, but this assertion has not been proved.[120,164,165]

Profound marrow hypoplasia and pancytopenia will result

TABLE 52-5. A Plan for the Treatment of Adult Acute Nonlymphocytic Leukemia (ANLL)

Drug	*Route*	*Dose*	*Schedule*
Induction Therapy			
Daunorubicin	IV	45 mg/m²*	Days 1 through 3
Cytarabine	IV	100 mg/m²†	Days 1 through 7
Postremission Systemic Therapy‡			
Option 1§			
Cytarabine, SC, and 6-thioguanine, PO, each at a dose of 100 mg/m², given every 12 hours until severe marrow hypoplasia is achieved. Treatment is repeated every 3 months for a total of 3 years.			
Option 2‖			
Cytarabine, 3 g/m² IV over 1 hour, given every 12 hours for a total of 12 doses. Give a second course as soon as hematologic recovery from the first permits.			
Option 3¶			
Allogeneic bone marrow transplantation.			

*Rapid intravenous (IV) injection.

†Continuous 7-day intravenous infusion.

‡Begin when complete hematologic recovery from induction therapy is evident. PO = orally; SC = subcutaneously.

§Adapted from Dutcher et al.[174] Option 1 is applicable to virtually all patients.

‖Adapted from Cassileth et al,[167] Wolff et al,[171] and Tallman et al.[172] Option 2 is applicable to patients younger than 60 years of age.

¶Option 3 is applicable to patients younger than 40 years of age who have donors that are identical for human leukocyte antigen and negative for mixed leukocyte reaction.

from remission induction therapy. Evidence of marrow recovery usually will be first noted 2 to 3 weeks after the completion of therapy, and 80% of patients who ultimately achieve a complete remission will do so within 1 month after completing the first induction therapy course. Most of the remainder of patients destined to respond completely will do so after the second course. When the marrow becomes repopulated after the first course of treatment, a decision about further induction therapy will have to be made. If the marrow shows evidence of normal megakaryocytic and myeloid regeneration, the marrow should be reassessed in several days. If, at that time, more evidence of normal marrow regeneration is obtained and leukemic blast cells are difficult to find, the blood counts should be followed until they have become normal. At that time, the marrow should be re-examined to confirm complete remission or recurrent leukemia. If the first marrow examined after initial induction therapy appears to be leukemic, retreatment should be withheld until the need for it is confirmed by another marrow examination several days later. This procedure is recommended because a regenerating normal marrow after anthracycline drug administration may appear frankly leukemic because of the large number of megaloblastoid normal myeloblasts present that are destined to mature normally.

Several clues from peripheral blood studies after induction treatment of ANLL may serve as early signals of response or lack of it. The earliest clue of success is a gradual and steady daily rise in the platelet count. A transient rise in platelet count is usually a sign of incomplete response to induction therapy, a suspicion that must be confirmed by marrow examination. A rise in the granulocyte count typically follows a rise in platelet count by several days or more.

Differences of opinion exist as to whether postremission therapy should be administered to the ANLL patient after complete response.[166,167] There is no evidence that both consolidation and maintenance therapy are necessary, so most treatment programs incorporate one or the other. Different drugs than those initially employed are usually recommended for consolidation or maintenance therapy (see Tables 52-4 and 52-5). At least one study suggested that the intensity of remission induction therapy is a more powerful determinant of remission duration than is maintenance therapy.[168] Conversely, some studies employing intensive maintenance therapy have yielded very impressive remission duration results.[169,170]

Currently, much attention centers on intensive short-term consolidation therapy in ANLL, after which no treatment is administered. High-dose cytosine arabinoside in conjunction with other agents is usually the cornerstone of such an approach,[167,171,172] while others have used more complicated schemes.[173] The long-term disease-free survival rate obtained in such studies is on the order of 30% or more of patients who achieved complete remission. Death rates during complete remission have varied from 10% to 20% or more, primarily from the toxicity of treatment. A less aggressive approach that has led to a comparable outcome (25% continuous complete remission rate at 8 years) has employed conventional doses of cytosine arabinoside and 6-thioguanine given every 3 months for 3 years until severe marrow hypoplasia is achieved.[174] The advantage of the latter approach is the lower death rate during remission (6%). All of these studies appear to have yielded results superior to those obtained previously, although most comparisons have been made with historical controls.

Meningeal prophylaxis usually is not employed in the management of adults with ANLL.[175] However, meningeal leukemia is more common in children than adults with ANLL, and prophylaxis is sometimes applied to childhood ANLL. Meningeal leukemia incidence in ANLL appears to have decreased since the general acceptance of treatments employing continuous intravenous infusions of cytosine arabinoside. The reduced incidence may be related to the fact that parenteral infusions of the drug in standard dosage result in therapeutic drug levels in CSF.[176] Thus, standard induction treatment may also be effective meningeal leukemia prophylaxis.

It may be more important from a therapeutic standpoint to subclassify ANLL precisely in the future. Some recent data suggest that induction drug specificity for the various subgroups is emerging. Acute progranulocytic leukemia appears to be highly sensitive to daunorubicin, and acute monocytic leukemia appears to be the only ANLL variant sensitive to etoposide.[177,178]

Data suggesting drug specificity for postremission therapy of the various ANLL subtypes have also begun to appear. Remission duration in acute promyelocytic leukemia may be greater when intensive treatment with 6-mercaptopurine and methotrexate is given during remission than when other equally intensive regimens are administered.[179]

Although results of current treatment of ANLL leave much to be desired, results are infinitely better now than only a few years ago. With treatments such as those outlined in Tables 52-4 and 52-5, approximately 65% of all treated patients and 70% or more of patients less than 50 years of age will achieve a complete response. The median duration of remission for complete responders of all ages is approximately 1 to 1.5 years. More importantly, in some recent studies, approximately one fourth of complete responders appear to be long-term disease-free survivors who are well 8 or more years after initial treatment (Fig. 52-8).

The feasibility of treating ANLL patients in complete remission with bone marrow transplantation has been studied by many investigators,[158,159,180–183] and results with a total of 203 patients from eight centers were reported.[158] Approximately 30% of patients achieve prolonged survival if transplantation is performed during initial relapse or second complete remission. In some studies, results are better if the procedure is performed during first complete remission,[183] and actuarial relapse rates of 0 to 40% have been reported from those investigations. In all studies, the same prognostic factors that affect outcome after chemotherapy alone are operative.

Three prospective controlled comparisons of chemotherapy alone with allogeneic bone marrow transplantation for postremission therapy of adults with ANLL have been reported.[184–186] In each, there was a significantly lower leukemia relapse rate and greater survival rate with transplantation, but the survival difference was significant in only one study.[184]

Only a minority of ANLL patients are presently candidates for the procedure: those under age 40 years who have donors with identical HLA and nonreactive mixed-lymphocyte cultures. Although the prospects for marrow transplantation are encouraging, the comparative studies addressed above and other recent studies of chemotherapy alone[187] have cast doubt on the advisability of performing transplantation on all candidates during first remission because of the initial mortality associated with the procedure. At present, many authorities recommend withholding transplantation until early relapse or second complete remission, since essentially identical results can be obtained at those times or during first

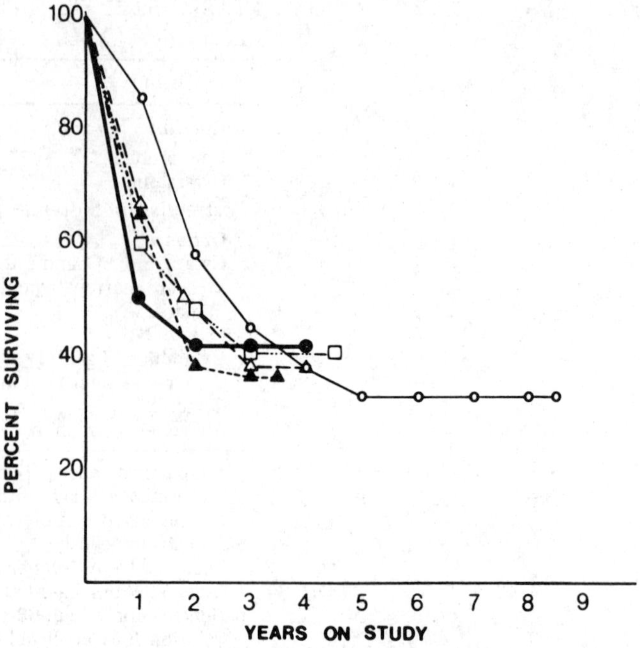

FIG. 52-8. Selected recent results of post-complete-remission therapy of adults with ANLL in first complete remission. The curves show overall survival of all treated patients as determined by life-table analysis (○——○). In a study by Dutcher et al[174] in which severe marrow hypoplasia was induced every 3 months for 3 years with conventional doses of ara-C plus thioguanine, 86 patients were entered into the study from 1978 to 1982 with a median age of 47 years (range, 15–74 years). The death rate during complete remission was 6% (□- · · -□). A study of intensive consolidation therapy for 6 months by Tallman et al[172] included 74 patients with a median age of 48 years (range, 19–75 years) entered into the study from 1982 to 1985. The death rate during complete remission was 22% (△- -△). In a study by Cassileth et al,[167] 35 patients received a single consolidation course of high-dose ara-C plus amsacrine. Patients were entered into the study from 1982 to 1984 and had a median age of 46 years (range, 18–69 years). There was a 17% death rate during remission (●——●). In a study by Santos et al,[182] 18 patients received an allogeneic marrow transplant during the period 1975 to 1979 after preparation with high doses of busulfan and cyclophosphamide. The median age was 25 years (range, 13–41 years). Ten patients (56%) died of transplant-related complications 1.5 to 12.5 months after the transplant (▲- -▲). In a study by Champlin et al,[186] 22 patients who were entered into the study from 1979 to 1983 with a median age of 25 years (range, 15 to 41 years) received an allogeneic transplant after preparation with high-dose cyclophosphamide and total body irradiation. There were nine deaths from transplant-related complications (41%).

remission (see Chap. 66, sect. 6, for a more detailed discussion of bone marrow transplantation).

Immunotherapy with a variety of agents has been studied extensively in ANLL patients. They were based initially on successful studies in mice with leukemia L1210, in which treatment with bacillus Calmette-Guerin (BCG) and irradiated leukemic cells yielded some cures in animals with a minimum body burden of tumor cells.[188] The human experiments presume the existence of a human leukemia–specific antigen or antigens, which have not been identified to date.[189] Most human trials were conducted with patients in chemotherapy-induced remission. Results with BCG were initially encouraging, but enthusiasm for this treatment has waned because larger, controlled trials have now shown no statistically significant effect on remission rate or duration, or on survival for patients treated with various BCG preparations.[189] The same results have been obtained with other similar agents such as *Corynebacterium parvum*.[190] In some small studies, however, modest improvement of postrelapse survival seems to have resulted from immunotherapy for unclear reasons.[189,191] In one study in which neuraminidase-treated allogeneic cells were used as immunotherapy, enhanced remission duration and survival resulted from treatment,[192] but this has not been observed in other studies.[174,193]

TREATMENT OF RELAPSED PATIENTS WITH ACUTE NONLYMPHOCYTIC LEUKEMIA

The treatment of relapsed ANLL patients is unrewarding for the most part. In general, irrespective of treatment, complete responses are obtained in a small minority of patients, are more frequent in patients who previously obtained a long complete remission, and are usually of brief duration.[194,195] Amsacrine has significant activity in relapsed ANLL patients. In one study in which the drug was given in a dose of 75 mg/m^2 to 90 mg/m^2 daily for 7 days, 9 of 30 patients responded with a complete remission.[196] Results are substantially better when the agent is combined with high-dose cytosine arabinoside,[197] but it is not clear that the combination is superior to high-dose cytosine arabinoside alone. Results with amsacrine and etoposide appear to be better than those obtained with amsacrine and high-dose cytosine arabinoside.[198] Therefore, amsacrine deserves further study in ANLL, especially in combination with other agents.

High-dose cytosine arabinoside alone has been studied in relapsed ANLL patients, and complete responses of approximately 50% have been obtained, even in patients judged to be refractory to standard doses of the drug,[199] but the median duration of remission has, again, been only approximately 4 months in most studies. At a dose of 3 g/m^2 every 12 hours for 6 days, toxicity is acceptable in young patients; however, severe conjunctivitis, liver toxicity, and mucosal ulceration have been observed primarily in patients over age 60 years, especially with longer courses or larger doses. Mitoxantrone recently has been shown to have impressive activity in relapsed ANLL when given alone[200] or combined with conventional[201] or high-dose[202] cytosine arabinoside. It is most encouraging that some second complete remissions obtained with mitoxantrone and cytosine arabinoside have been of greater duration than the patient's first remission induced with daunorubicin and the same dose and schedule of cytosine arabinoside. In studies of cytosine arabinoside and mitoxantrone as initial therapy for ANLL, which are still in progress, less alopecia and gastrointestinal toxicity have been noted than usually observed with standard regimens.

The daunorubicin analogue, 4-demethoxydaunorubicin (idarubicin), has activity in ANLL and may lack complete cross resistance with other anthracyclines.[203] The drug is particularly attractive in that it may be given orally.[204] Clinical trials of its efficacy by both oral and intravenous routes, given alone or in combination with cytosine arabinoside, for relapsed or previously untreated ANLL are in progress.

TREATMENT OF MYELODYSPLASTIC SYNDROMES

The FAB classification includes refractory anemia, refractory sideroblastic anemia, refractory anemia with excess blasts (RAEB), chronic myelomonocytic leukemia (CMML), and refractory anemia with progressive transformation (RAEBT) to ANLL in the myelodysplastic syndromes.[205]

Although subclassification of this syndrome by FAB criteria as outlined here is useful, prognosis is more accurately assessed by other methods. In one study,[206] the presence or absence of abnormal localized immature myeloid precursors in the bone marrow biopsy had significantly greater prognostic value than did FAB type.

The pathogenesis of this syndrome is unclear, but two events appear to be involved: proliferation of a clone of genetically unstable pluripotent stem cells and of another inducing chromosomal abnormalities in its descendants.[207]

Immunoregulatory abnormalities have been reported in myelodysplasia. Mitogen-stimulated T-lymphocyte blastogenesis is significantly depressed,[208] and T-cell and B-cell interactions are impaired.[209] The significance of these observations remains to be determined.

Most patients with myelodysplasia need only careful observation and periodic blood transfusion initially. However, with time, blood transfusion requirements increase and platelet transfusions may also be necessary. Treatment for ANLL ultimately will be required by at least one third of patients (especially those with RAEB, CMML, and RAEBT); however, in some, the requirement for intensive treatment may be deferred for variable periods of time by the administration of corticosteroids alone.[210] This possibility is especially likely if cortisol enhances in vitro colony formation from the patient's bone marrow cells. Myelodysplastic patients whose in vitro marrow colony-forming activity is not enhanced by cortisol are unlikely to respond to it and should be treated by other means.

Some patients with this syndrome will respond favorably to small subcutaneous doses of cytosine arabinoside given every 12 hours for 2 to 4 weeks or as a continuous infusion for several days. In some cases, complete remission may be obtained.[211] However, it is not clear that this therapy is as successful as originally reported.[212] Although low-dose cytosine arabinoside has been popularized as a relatively nontoxic treatment for preleukemia, myelodysplastic syndromes, and elderly patients with ANLL, it is clearly myelosuppressive and may not be as productive of complete remission as standard induction therapy with conventional doses of cytosine arabinoside and daunorubicin.[212]

Recently 1,25-dihydroxyvitamin D_3 and 13-cis-retenoic acid have been shown to differentiate marrow cells from patients with the myelodysplastic syndrome in vitro,[213] and 13-cis-retenoic acid improved the circulating granulocyte count in half of treated patients in one small study.[214] Recombinant human granulocyte colony–stimulating factor was reported to increase leukocyte alkaline phosphatase activity significantly in cultured granulocytes from patients with myelodysplastic syndromes.[215] These exciting observations suggest a role for these and other differentiation-inducing agents in the myelodysplastic syndromes.

TREATMENT OF ACUTE LEUKEMIA DURING PREGNANCY

The delivery of normal children by mothers receiving antileukemic therapy has been amply documented.[216,217] Treatment of women in the second or third trimester of pregnancy appears to be safe for the fetus and mother, but outcome for both is compromised when treatment is given during the first trimester.[218] Most children born of mothers who received chemotherapy while pregnant enjoy normal growth and development, and do not appear to be at increased risk for cancer or leukemia for at least the first 17 years of life.[219]

MONITORING RESPONSE TO TREATMENT OF ACUTE LEUKEMIA

The bone marrow must be examined serially to assess the results of chemotherapy properly. However, a wealth of laboratory evidence strongly suggests that a significant number of leukemic cells may still exist when the marrow examination gives normal results. Thus, marrow examination is a relatively crude method of monitoring disease activity. For that reason, much effort has gone into the search for a tumor-specific biomarker of disease activity, the blood level of which might be a more sensitive indicator of residual disease. Plasma levels of a fucosyltransferase specified by the human blood group H gene have been shown to correlate with disease activity in acute leukemia patients[220] but are not clinically helpful. Nor has flow cytometry been routinely useful in monitoring leukemia patients. Perhaps in the future, serial determinations of blood biomarkers will prove to be a more accurate and less painful means of following response to therapy than serial bone marrow aspiration.

Other methods of predicting relapse are under investigation. Principal among these possibilities is a method using premature chromosome condensation, which allows for the determination of the relative number of bone marrow cells in early versus late G_1 phase of the cell cycle.[221] Because normal cells appear to come to rest in early G_1 phase and malignant cells seem to do so in late G_1, determining the fraction of G_1 phase cells of a population that are in late G_1 may indicate repopulation of the marrow with leukemic cells before standard morphologic studies will do so. This potentially useful test is difficult to perform and has been done only in one laboratory on a small number of patients.[221]

FUTURE TREATMENT CONSIDERATIONS

Current treatment of adult acute leukemia is difficult to deliver properly and is quite toxic. There are reasons to believe that therapy will become more specific and less toxic in the near future as second-generation treatments, such as differentiation-inducing agents, and less toxic cytotoxic drugs, such as mitoxantrone, are developed.[222-225] Important potential developments in supportive care, such as improvement in bone marrow transplantation technology, the development of platelets for transfusion devoid of HLA, or other methods to prevent alloimmunization from random-donor platelet transfusions may improve treatment results in acute leukemia dramatically.

Investigation of the bone marrow microenvironment is in its infancy, but important findings of potential clinical relevance have already been reported. Type IV nuclear bodies, which are often found in virally infected tissues, have been identified in marrow fibroblasts obtained from patients with ANLL.[226] It has been postulated that disturbances of the marrow microenvironment may be responsible for leukemic relapse in donor cells or selective failure of engraftment of specific normal cell lines after transplantation, and may also explain t-lymphocyte–depleted, histoincompatible marrow rejection by the allograft recipient's stromal cells that persist despite radiotherapy and chemotherapy. Further knowledge of the marrow microenvironment may be necessary before the next major advance in leukemia treatment can be made.[227]

REFERENCES

1. Gunz FW: The dread leukemias and the lymphomas: Their nature and their prospects. In Wintrobe MM (ed): Blood, Pure and Eloquent, pp 511–517. New York, McGraw-Hill, 1980
2. Farber S, Diamond LK, Mercer RD et al: Temporary remissions in acute leukemia in children produced by folic acid antagonist, 4-aminopteroylglutamic acid (aminopterin). N Engl J Med 238:787, 1948
3. Rosner F, Lee SL: Down's syndrome and acute leukemia: Myeloblastic or lymphoblastic? Am J Med 53:203, 1972
4. Nowell PC, Hungerford DA: Chromosome studies in human leukemia. II. Chronic granulocytic leukemia. JN CI 27:1013, 1961
5. Catovsky D: Ph¹- positive acute leukaemia and chronic granulocytic leukaemia: One or two diseases? Br J Haematol 42:493, 1979
6. Jain K, Arlin Z, Mertelsmann R et al: Philadelphia chromosome and terminal transferase positive acute leukemia. Similarity of terminal phase of chronic myelogenous leukemia and de novo acute presentation. J Clin Oncol 1:669, 1983
7. Hilton HB, Lewis IC, Trowell HF: C-group trisomy in identical twins with acute leukemia. Blood 35:222, 1970
8. Walker LMS, Sandler RM: Acute myeloid leukemia with monosomy-7 follows acute lymphoblastic leukaemia. Br J Haematol 38:359, 1978
9. Kaufmann U, Loffler H, Foerster W et al: Fehlendes Chromosom nr. 7 in der praleukamischen Phase einer Myeloblastenleukose bei einem Kind. Blut 29:50, 1974
10. Croce CM, Girardi AJ, Kaprowski H: Assignment of the T-antigen gene of simian virus to human chromosome C-7. Proc Natl Acad Sci USA 70:3617, 1973
11. Gilman PA, Jackson DP, Guild HG: Congenital agranulocytosis: Prolonged survival and terminal acute leukemia. Blood 36:576, 1970
12. Miller DR, Newstead GJ, Young LW: Perinatal leukemia with a possible variant of the Ellis-van Creveld syndrome. J Pediatr 74:300, 1969
13. Gupte SP, Perkash A, Mahajan CM et al: Acute myeloid leukemia in a girl with celiac disease. Am J Dig Dis 16:939, 1971
14. Sawitsky A, Bloom D, German J; Chromosomal breakage and acute leukemia in congenital telangiectasia, erythema and stunted growth. Ann Intern Med 65:487, 1966
15. Bloom GE, Warner S, Gerald PS et al: Chromosomal abnormalities in constitutional aplastic anemia. N Engl J Med 274:8, 1966
16. Zuelzer WW, Cox DE: Genetic aspects of leukemia. Semin Hematol 6:228, 1969
17. Jackson LG: Chromosomes and cancer: Current aspects. Semin Oncol 5:3, 1978
18. Schade H, Schoeller L, Schultze KWD: D-Trisomie (Patau) mit kongenitaler meyloischer Leukaemie. Med Welt 50:2690, 1966
19. Reich SC, Wiernik PH: Von Recklinghausen neurofibromatosis and acute leukemia. Am J Dis Child 130:888, 1976
20. Conrad RA: Acute myelogenous leukemia following fallout radiation exposure. JAMA 232:1356, 1975
21. Karchmer RK, Caldwell GG, Chin TDY: Acute leukemia following localized irradiation for carcinoma of the larynx. Blood 43:721, 1974
22. Rinsky RA, Smith AB, Hornung R et al: Benzene and leukemia. N Engl J Med 316:1044, 1987
23. Boice JD, Green MH, Killan JY et al: Leukemia and preleukemia after adjuvant treatment of gastrointestinal cancer with semustine (methyl-CCNU). N Engl J Med 309:1079, 1983
24. Greene MH, Harris EL, Gershenson DM et al: Melphalan may be a more potent leukemogen than cyclophosphamide. Ann Intern Med 105:360, 1986
25. Jarrett WFH: Viruses and leukaemia. Br J Haematol 25:287, 1973
26. Rowe WP, Hartley JW, Landes MR et al: Noninfectious AKR mouse embryo cell lines in which each cell has the capacity to produce infectious murine leukemia virus. Virology 46:866, 1971
27. Weiss RA, Fris RR, Katz E et al: Induction of avian tumor viruses in normal cells by physical and chemical carcinogens. Virology 46:920, 1971
28. Gallo RC, Miller N, Saxinger W et al: Primate RNA tumor virus-like DNA synthesized endogenously by RNA-dependent DNA polymerase in virus-like particles from fresh human acute leukemic blood cells. Proc Natl Acad Sci USA 70:3219, 1973
29. Baltimore D: Viral-dependent DNA polymerase in virions of RNA tumor viruses. Nature 226:1209, 1970

30. Baxt W, Yates JW, Wallace HJ Jr: Leukemia-specific DNA sequences in leukocytes of the leukemic members of identical twins. Proc Natl Acad Sci USA 70:2629, 1973
31. Schimpff SC, Brager DM, Schimpff CR et al: Leukemia and lymphoma patients linked by prior social contact. Evaluation using a case-control approach. Ann Intern Med 84:547, 1976
32. Severson RK: Cigarette smoking and leukemia. Cancer 60:141, 1987
33. Brill AB, Tomonaga M, Heyssell RM: Leukemia in man following exposure to ionizing radiation: Summary of findings in Hiroshima and Nagasaki and comparison with other human experience. Ann Intern Med 56:590, 1962
34. Kaplan HS: The role of irradiation in experimental leukemogenesis. NCI Monogr 14:207, 1964
35. March HC: Leukemia in radiologists, ten years later: With review of pertinent evidence for radiation leukemia. Am J Med Sci 242:137, 1961
36. Bizzozero OJ, Johnson KG, Ciocco A: Leukemia in Hiroshima and Nagasaki. N Engl J Med 274:1095, 1966
37. Court-Brown WM, Doll R: Leukemia and aplastic anemia in patients irradiated for ankylosing spondylitis. Med Res Council Spec Rep Ser No. 295, London, Her Majesty's Stationery Office, 1957
38. O'Donnell JF, Brereton HD, Greco FA et al: Acute nonlymphocytic leukemia and acute myeloproliferative syndrome following radiation therapy for non-Hodgkin's lymphoma and chronic lymphocytic leukemia: Clinical Studies. Cancer 44:1930, 1979
39. Blayney DW, Longo DL, Young RC et al: Decreasing risk of leukemia with prolonged follow-up after chemotherapy and radiotherapy for Hodgkin's disease. N Engl J Med 316:710, 1987
40. van Eys J, Flexner JM: Transient spontaneous remission in a case of untreated congenital leukemia. Am J Dis Child 118:507, 1979
41. Zussman WV, Khan A, Shayesteh P: Congenital leukemia. Cancer 20:1227, 1967
42. Wiernik PH: Spontaneous regression of hematologic cancers. NCI Monogr 44:35, 1976
43. Head DR, Cerezo L, Savage RA et al: Institutional performance in application of the FAB classification of acute leukemia. Cancer 55:1979, 1985
44. Bollum FJ: Terminal deoxynucleotidyl transferase as a hematopoietic cell marker. Blood 54:1203, 1979
45. Golomb HM, Rowley JD, Vardiman JW et al: "Microgranular" acute promyelocytic leukemia. A distinct clinical, ultrastructural, and cytogenetic entity. Blood 55:253, 1980
46. Wick MR, Li C-Y, Pierre RV: Acute nonlymphocytic leukemia with basophilic differentiation. Blood 60:38, 1982
47. Bennett JM, Catovsky D, Daniel MT et al: Proposals for the classification of the acute leukaemias. Br J Haematol 33:451, 1976
48. Wiernik PH, Serpick AA: Clinical significance of serum and urinary muramidase activity in leukemia and other hematologic malignancies. Am J Med 46:330, 1979
49. Schiffer CA, Sanel FT, Stechmiller BK et al: Functional and morphologic characteristics of the leukemia cells of a patient with acute monocytic leukemia: Correlation with clinical features. Blood 46:17, 1975
50. Foucar K, McKenna RW, Bloomfield CD et al: Therapy related leukemia. A panmyelosis. Cancer 43:1285, 1979
51. Kass L: Esterase activity in erythroleukemia. Am J Clin Pathol 67:368, 1977
52. Hetzkel P, Gee TS: A new observation in the clinical spectrums of erythroleukemia. A report of 46 cases. Am J Med 64:765, 1978
53. Davis AT, Brunning RD, Quie PG: Polymorphonuclear leukocyte myeloperoxidase deficiency in a patient with myelomonocytic leukemia. N Engl J Med 285:789, 1971
54. Haubenstock A, Zalusky R, Ghali VS et al: Isolated leukemia cutis—A case report. Am J Hematol 24:437, 1987
55. Shaikh BS, Frantz E, Lookingbill DP: Histologically proven leukemia cutis carries a poor prognosis in acute nonlymphocytic leukemia. Cutis 39:57, 1987
56. Andoh K, Kubota T, Takada M et al: Tissue factor activity in leukemic cells. Cancer 59:748, 1987
57. Wiernik P, Serpick AA: Granulocytic sarcoma (chloroma). Blood 35:361, 1970
58. King DJ, Ewen SWB, Sewell HF et al: Obstructive jaundice. An unusual presentation of granulocytic sarcoma. Cancer 60:114, 1987
59. Meis JM, Butler JJ, Osborne BM et al: Granulocytic sarcoma in nonleukemic patients. Cancer 58:2697, 1986
60. Nicolis GD, Helwig EB: Exfoliative dermatitis. Arch Dermatol 108:788, 1973
61. Klock JC, Oken RL: Febrile neutrophilic dermatosis in acute myelogenous leukemia. Cancer 37:922, 1976
62. Peterson DE, Overholser CD Jr: Dental management of leukemia patients. Oral Surg 47:40, 1979
63. Sickles EA, Young VM, Greene WH et al: Pneumonia in acute leukemia. Ann Intern Med 79:528, 1973
64. Lester TJ, Johnson JW, Cuttner J: Pulmonary leukostasis as the single worst prognostic factor in patients with acute myelocytic leukemia and hyperleukocytosis. Ann Intern Med 79:43, 1985
65. Wiernik PH, Sutherland JC, Stechmiller BK et al: Clinically significant cardiac infiltration in acute leukemia, lymphocytic lymphoma, and plasma cell myeloma. Med Pediatr Oncol 2:75, 1976
66. Shifrin EG, Drenger B, Matzner Y et al: Ruptured inflammatory abdominal aortic aneurysm due to acute myelomonoblastic leukemia. J Cardiovasc Surg 28:32, 1987
67. Sklansky BD, Jafek BW, Wiernik PH: Otolaryngologic manifestations of acute leukemia. Laryngoscope 84:210, 1974
68. Greene WH, Moody M, Hartley R et al: Esophagoscopy as a source of Pseudonomas aeruginosa sepsis in patients with acute leukemia: The need for sterilization of endoscopes. Gastroenterology 67:912, 1974
69. Brugo EA, Marshall RB, Riberi AM et al: Preleukekmic granulocytic sarcomas of the gastrointestinal tract. Am J Clin Pathol 68:616, 1977
70. Schimpff SC, Wiernik PH, Block JB: Rectal abscesses in cancer patients. Lancet 2:844, 1972
71. Varki AP, Armitage JO, Feagler JR: Typhilitis in acute leukemia. Successful treatment by early surgical intervention. Cancer 43:695, 1979
72. Frame R, Head D, Lee R et al: Granulocytic sarcoma of the prostate. Two cases causing urinary obstruction. Cancer 59:142, 1987
73. Lister TA, Whitehouse JMA, Beard MEJ et al: Early central nervous system involvement in adults with acute non-myelogenous leukaemia. Br J Cancer 35:479, 1977
74. Holmes R, Keating MJ, Cork A et al: A unique pattern of central nervous system leukemia in acute myelomonocytic leukemia associated with inv(16)(p13q22). Blood 65:1071, 1985
75. Woodruff KH: Cerebrospinal fluid cytomorphology using cytocentrifugation. Am J Clin Pathol 60:621, 1973
76. Wainer RA, Wiernik PH, Thompson WL: Metabolic and therapeutic studies of a patient with acute leukemia and severe lactic acidosis of prolonged duration. Am J Med 55:255, 1973
77. Budd D, Ginsberg H: Hypocholesterolemia and acute myelogenous leukemia. Cancer 58:1361, 1986
78. Cohn SL, Morgan ER, Mallette LE: The spectrum of metabolic bone disease in lymphoblastic leukemia. Cancer 59:346, 1987
79. Gewirtz AM, Stewart AF, Vignery A et al: Hypercalcemia complicating acute myelogenous leukaemia: A syndrome of multiple aetiologies. Br J Haematol 54:133, 1983
80. Zussman J, Brown DJ, Nesbit ME: Hyperphosphatemia, hyperphosphaturia and hypocalcemia in acute lymphoblastic leukemia. N Engl J Med 289:1335, 1973
81. Schenkein DP, O'Neill W, Shapiro J et al: Accelerated bone formation causing profound hypocalcemia in acute leukemia. Ann Intern Med 105:375, 1986
82. Wilson D, Stewart A, Szwed J et al: Cardiac arrest due to hyperkalemia following therapy for acute lymphoblastic leukemia. Cancer 39:2290, 1977
83. Salomon J: Spurious hypoglycemia and hyperkalemia in myelomonocytic leukemia. Am J Med Sci 267:359, 1974
84. Hersh EM, Whitecar JP, McCredie KB et al: Chemotherapy, immunocompetence, immunosuppression and prognosis in acute leukemia. N Engl J Med 285:1211, 1971
85. Greene WH, Schimpff SC, Wiernik PH: Cell-mediated immunity in acute nonlymphocytic leukemia: Relationship to host factors, therapy and prognosis. Blood 43:1, 1974.
86. Van Camp B, Reynaerts PH, Naets JP et al: Transient IgA_1 paraproteinemia during treatment of acute myelomonocytic leukemia. Blood 55:21, 1980
87. Dutcher JP, Schiffer CA, Aisner J, Wiernik PH: Long-term follow-up of patients with leukemia receiving platelet transfusions: Identification of a large group of patients who do not become alloimmunized. Blood 58:1007, 1981
88. Lichtenfeld JL, Wiernik PH, Mardiney MR Jr et al: Abnormalities of complement and its components in patients with acute leukemia, Hodgkin's disease, and sarcoma. Cancer Res 36:3678, 1976
89. Hartveit F: The complement content of the serum of normal as opposed to tumour bearing mice. Br J Cancer 18:714, 1964
90. Boll ITM, Sterry K, Maurer HR: Evidence of a rat granulocyte chalone effect on the proliferation on normal human bone marrow and of myeloid leukemias. Acta Haematol 61:130, 1979
91. Davies AR: Auer bodies in mature neutrophils. J Am Med Assoc 202:895, 1968
92. Cech P, Markert M, Perrin LH: Partial myeloperoxidase deficiency in preleukemia. Blut 47:21, 1983
93. Viola MV, Frazier M, Wiernik PH et al: Reverse transcriptase in leukocytes of leukemic patients in remission. N Engl J Med 294:75, 1976
94. Sachs L: The differentiation of myeloid leukaemia cells: New possibilities for therapy. Br J Haematol 40:509, 1978
95. Fearon ER, Burke PJ, Schiffer CA et al: Differentiation of leukemia cells to polymorphonuclear leukocytes in patients with acute nonlymphocytic leukemia. N Engl J Med 315:15, 1986
96. Fritz RD, Forkner CD Jr, Freireich EJ: The association of fatal intracranial hemorrhage and "blastic crisis" in patients with acute leukemia. N Engl J Med 261:59, 1959
97. Law IP, Blom J: Adult central nervous system leukemia. South Med J 69:1054, 1976
98. Dawson DM, Rosenthal DS, Moloney WC: Neurological complications of acute leukemia in adults. Ann Intern Med 79:541, 1973
99. West RJ, Graham-Pole J, Hardisty RM et al: Factors in the pathogenesis of central nervous system leukaemia. Br Med J 2:311, 1972
100. Jenkins DE Jr, Hartmann RC: Paroxysmal nocturnal hemoglobinuria terminating in acute myeloblastic leukemia. Blood 33:274, 1969
101. Kansal V, Omura GA, Soong S-J: Prognosis in adult acute myelogenous leukemia related to performance status and other factors. Cancer 38:329, 1976
102. Koeffler HP, Golde DW: Human preleukemia. Ann Intern Med 93:347, 1980
103. Clark R, Peters S, Hoy T et al: Prognostic importance of hypodiploid hemopoietic precursors in myelodysplastic syndromes. N Engl J Med 314:1472, 1986
104. Rheingold JJ: Acute leukemia: Its smouldering phase, or leukemia never starts on Thursday. JAMA 230:985, 1974
105. Gordon DS, Hubbard M: Surface membrane characteristics and cytochemistry of the abnormal cells in adult acute leukemia. Blood 51:681, 1978
106. Pachmann K, Penning R, Lau B et al: Detection of CALLA positive cells in the human

normal peripheral blood by microimmunofluorometry and their fate during cultivation in diffusion chambers. Scand J Haematol 30:257, 1983

107. Nadler LM, Ritz J, Bates MP, et al: Induction of human B-cell antigens in non-T cell acute lymphoblastic leukemia. J Clin Invest 70:433, 1982
108. Cossman J, Neckers LM, Arnold A et al: Induction of differentiation in a case of common acute lymphoblastic leukemia. N Engl J Med 307:1251, 1982
109. Bloomfield CD: The clinical relevance of lymphocyte surface markers in adult acute lymphoblastic leukemia. In Bloomfield CD (ed): Adult Leukemia 1, pp 265–308. Boston, Martinus-Nijhoff, 1982
110. Greaves MF: Analysis of the clinical and biological significance of lymphoid phenotypes in acute leukemia. Cancer Res 41:4752, 1981
111. Bettelheim P, Paietta E, Majdic O et al: Expression of a myeloid marker on TdT-positive acute lymphocytic leukemic cells: Evidence by double-fluorescence staining. Blood 60:1392, 1982
112. Sobol RE, Mick R, Royston I et al: Clinical importance of myeloid antigen expression in adult acute lymphoblastic leukemia. N Engl J Med 316:1111, 1987
113. Braun MP, Martin PJ, Ledbetter JA et al: Granulocytes and cultured human fibroblasts express common acute lymphoblastic leukemia-associated antigens. Blood 61:718, 1983
114. Keating A, Whalen CK, Singer JW: Cultured marrow stromal cells express common acute lymphoblastic leukaemia antigen (CALLA): Implications for marrow transplantation. Br J Haematol 55:623, 1983
115. Metzgar RS, Borowitz MJ, Jones NH et al: Distribution of common acute lymphoblastic leukemia antigen in nonhematopoietic tissues. J Exp Med 154:1249, 1981
116. Greaves MF, Hariri G, Newman RA et al: Selective expression of the common acute lymphoblastic leukemia (gp 100) antigen on immature lymphoid cells and their malignant counterparts. Blood 61:628, 1983
117. Ritz J, Schlossman SF: Utilization of monoclonal antibodies in the treatment of leukemia and lymphoma. Blood 59:1, 1982
118. Remlinger K, Martin PJ, Hansen JA et al: Murine monoclonal anti-T cell antibodies for treatment of steroid-resistant acute graft-versus-host disease. Hum Immunol 9:21, 1984
119. Griffin JD, Davis R, Nelson DA et al: Use of surface marker analysis to predict outcome of adult acute myeloblastic leukemia. Blood 68:1232, 1986
120. Wiernik PH, Glidewell OJ, Hoagland HC et al: A comparative trial of daunorubicin, cytosine arabinoside and thioguanine, and a combination of the three agents for the treatment of acute myelocytic leukemia. Med Pediatr Oncol 6:261, 1979
121. Dutcher JP, Schiffer CA, Wiernik PH: Hyperleukocytosis in adult acute nonlymphocytic leukemia; Impact on remission rate and duration, and survival. J Clin Oncol 5:1364, 1987
122. Reiner RR, Hoover R, Fraumeni JF Jr et al: Acute leukemia after alkylating-agent therapy of ovarian cancer. N Engl J Med 297:17, 1977
123. Vaughan WP, Karp JE, Burke PJ: Effective chemotherapy of acute myelocytic leukemia occurring after alkylating agent or radiation therapy for prior malignancy. J Clin Oncol 1:204, 1983
124. Hart JS, George SL, Frei III E et al: Prognostic significance of pretreatment proliferative activity in adult acute leukemia. Cancer 39:1603, 1977
125. Golomb HM, Vardiman JW, Rowley JD et al: Correlation of clinical findings with quinacrine-banded chromosomes in 90 adults with acute nonlymphocytic leukemia. N Engl J Med 299:613, 1978
126. Misawa S, Hogge DE, Oguman N et al: Detection of clonal karyotypic abnormalities in most patients with acute nonlymphocytic leukemia examined using short-term culture techniques. Cancer Genet Cytogenet 22:239, 1986
127. Larson RA, Williams SF, Le Beau M et al: Acute myelomonocytic leukemia with abnormal eosinophils and inv(16) or t(16;16) has a favorable prognosis. Blood 68:1242, 1986
128. Keating MJ, Cork A, Broach Y et al: Toward a clinically relevant cytogenetic classification of acute myelogenous leukemia. Leuk Res 11:119, 1987
129. Le Beau MM, Albain KS, Larson RA et al: Clinical and cytogenetic correlation in 63 patients with therapy-related myelodysplastic syndromes and acute nonlymphocytic leukemia: Further evidence for characteristic abnormalities of chromosomes no. 5 and 7. J Clin Oncol 4:325, 1986
130. Beran M, Reizenstein P, Uden AM: Response to treatment in acute nonlymphatic leukaemia: Prognostic value of colony forming and colony stimulating capacities of bone marrow and blood cells compared to other parameters. Br J Haematol 44:39,1980
131. Foon KA, Naiem F, Yale C et al: Acute myelogenous leukemia: morphologic classification and response to therapy. Leuk Res 3:171, 1979
132. Bitter MA, Le Beau MM, Rowley JD et al: Association between morphology, karyotype, and clinical features in myeloid leukemias. Hum Pathol 18:211, 1987
133. Brandman J, Bukowski RM, Greenstreet R et al: Prognostic factors affecting remission, remission duration, and survival in adult acute nonlymphocytic leukemia. Cancer 44:1062, 1979
134. Walters RS, Kantarjian HM, Keating MJ et al: Intensive treatment of acute leukemia in adults 70 years of age and older. Cancer 60:149, 1987
135. Kantarjian HM, Keating MJ, Walters RS et al: Acute promyelocytic leukemia. Am J Med 80:789, 1986
136. Gralnick HK, Bagley J, Abrel E: Heparin treatment for the hemorrhagic diathesis of acute promyelocytic leukemia. Am J Med 52:167, 1972
137. Goldberg MA, Ginsburg D, Mayer RJ et al: Is heparin administration necessary during induction chemotherapy for patients with acute promyelocytic leukemia? Blood 69:187, 1987
138. Bishop JF, Schiffer CA, Aisner J et al: Surgery in acute leukemia: A review of 167 operations in thrombocytopenic patients. Am J Hematol 26:147, 1987
139. DeJongh CA, Wade JC, Schimpff SC et al: Empiric antibiotic therapy for suspected infection in granulocytopenic cancer patients. A comparison between the combination of moxalactam plus amikacin and ticarcillin plus amikacin. Am J Med 73:89, 1982
140. Grund FM, Armitage JO, Burns CP: Hydroxyurea in the prevention of the effects of leukostasis in acute leukemia. Arch Intern Med 137:1246, 1977
141. Cuttner J, Holland JF, Norton L et al: Therapeutic leukapheresis for hyperleukocytosis in acute myelocytic leukemia. Med Pediatr Oncol 11:76, 1983
142. Schimpff SC, Greene WH, Young VM et al: Infection prevention in acute nonlymphocytic leukemia. Ann Intern Med 82:351, 1975
143. Gurwith MJ, Brunton JL, Lank BA et al: A prospective controlled investigation of prophylactic trimethoprim/sulfamethoxazole in hospitalized granulocytopenic patients. Am J Med 66:248, 1979
144. Wade JC, de Jongh CA, Newman KA et al: Selective antimicrobial modulation as prophylaxis against infection during granulocytopenia. Trimethoprim–sulfamethoxazole vs. nalidixic acid. J Infect Dis 147:624, 1983
145. Barnett MJ, Greaves MJ, Amess JA et al: Treatment of acute lymphoblastic leukaemia in adults. Br J Haematol 64:455, 1986
146. Omura GA, Moffitt S, Vogler WF et al: Combination chemotherapy of adult acute lymphoblastic leukemia with randomized central nervous system prophylaxis. Blood 55:199, 1980
147. Gottlieb AJ, Weinberg V, Ellison RR et al: Efficacy of daunorubicin in the therapy of adult acute lymphocytic leukemia: A prospective randomized trial by Cancer and Leukemia Group B (CALGB). Blood 64:267, 1984
148. Gingrich RD, Burns CP, Armitage JO et al: Long-term relapse-free survival in adult acute lymphoblastic leukemia. Cancer Treat Rep 69:153, 1985
149. Linker CA, Levitt LJ, O'Donnell M et al: Improved results of treatment of adult acute lymphoblastic leukemia. Blood 69:1242, 1987
150. Polli EE: A cooperative study on the therapy of acute lymphoblastic leukemia. Haematologica 64:119, 1979
151. Willemze R, Hillen H, den Ottolander GJ et al: Acute lymfatische Leukemie bij adolelescenten Envolwassenen: Behandelings-Resullaten bij 75 Patienten in de Periode 1970–1977. Ned T Geneesk 123:1782, 1979
152. Esterhay RJ, Wiernik PH, Grove WR et al: Moderate-dose methotrexate, vincristine, asparaginase and dexamethasone for treatment of adult acute lymphocytic leukemia. Blood 59:334, 1982
153. Stewart DJ, Smith TL, Keating MJ et al: Remission from central nervous system involvement in adults with acute leukemia. Cancer 56:632, 1985
154. Morra E, Lazzarino M, Inverardi D et al: Systemic high-dose Ara-C for treatment of meningeal leukemia in adult acute lymphoblastic leukemia and non-Hodgkin's lymphoma. J Clin Oncol 4:1207, 1986
155. Woodruff RK, Lister TA, Paxton AM et al: Combination chemotherapy for haematological relapse in adult acute lymphoblastic leukaemia (ALL). Am J Hematol 4:173, 1978
156. Arlin ZA: Current status of amsacrine (AMSA) combination chemotherapy programs in acute leukemia. Cancer Treat Rep 67:967, 1983
157. Hiddemann W, Kreutzmann H, Donnhuijsen-Ant R et al: High-dose cytosine arabinoside and mitoxantrone (HAM) for the treatment of refractory acute lymphoblastic leukemia. Onkologie 10:11, 1987
158. Thomas ED: Marrow transplantation for malignant disease. J Clin Oncol 1:517, 1983
159. O'Reilly RJ: Allogeneic bone marrow transplantation: Current status and future directions. Blood 62:941, 1983
160. Weisdorf DJ, Nesbit ME, Ramsay NKC et al: Allogeneic bone marrow transplantation for acute lymphoblastic leukemia in remission: Prolonged survival associated with acute graft-versus-host disease. J Clin Oncol 5:1348, 1987
161. Wiernik PH, Serpick AA: A randomized trial of daunorubicin and a combination of prednisone, vincristine, 6-mercaptopurine, and methotrexate in adult acute nonlymphocytic leukemia. Cancer Res 32:2023, 1972
162. Ellison RR, Holland JF, Weil M et al: Arabinosyl cytosine: a useful agent in the treatment of acute leukemia in adults. Blood 32:507, 1978
163. Van Sloten K, Wiernik PH, Schiffer CA et al: Evaluation of levamisole as an adjuvant to chemotherapy for treatment of ANLL. Cancer 51:1576, 1983
164. Gale RP, Cline MJ: High remission-induction rate in acute myeloid leukaemia. Lancet 1:497, 1977
165. Rees JKH, Sandler RM, Challener J et al: Treatment of acute myeloid leukaemia with a triple cytotoxic regime: DAT. Br J Cancer 36:770, 1977
166. Kantarjian HM, Keating MJ, Walters RS et al: Early intensification and short-term maintenance chemotherapy does not prolong survival in acute myelogenous leukemia. Cancer 58:1603, 1986
167. Cassileth PA, Begg CB, Silber R et al: Prolonged unmaintained remission after intensive consolidation therapy in adult acute nonlymphocytic leukemia. Cancer Treat Rep 71:137, 1987
168. Burke PJ, Karp JE, Braine HG et al: Timed sequential therapy of human leukemia based upon the response of leukemic cells to humoral growth factors. Cancer Res 37:2138, 1977
169. Bodey GP, Freireich EJ, McCredie KB et al: Prolonged remissions in adults with acute leukemia following late intensification chemotherapy and immunotherapy. Cancer 47:1937, 1981
170. Weinstein HJ, Mayer RJ, Rosenthal DS et al: Chemotherapy for acute myelogenous leukemia in children and adults: VAPA update. Blood 62:315, 1983

171. Wolff SN, Herzig RH, Phillips GL et al: High-dose cytosine arabinoside and daunorubicin as consolidation therapy for acute nonlymphocytic leukemia in first remission: An update. Semin Oncol 14(suppl 1):12, 1987
172. Tallman MS, Appelbaum FR, Amos D et al: Evaluation of intensive postremission chemotherapy for adults with acute nonlymphocytic leukemia using high-dose cytosine arabinoside with L-asparaginase and amsacrine with etoposide. J Clin Oncol 5:918, 1987
173. Buchner T, Urbanitz D, Hiddemann W et al: Intensified induction and consolidation with or without maintenance chemotherapy for acute myeloid leukemia (AML): Two multicenter studies of the German AML cooperative group. J Clin Oncol 3:1583, 1985
174. Dutcher JP, Wiernik PH, Markus S et al: Intensive maintenance therapy improves survival in adult acute non-lymphocytic leukemia: An eight year follow-up. Leukemia 2:413, 1988
175. Wiernik PH, Schimpff SC, Schiffer CA et al: A randomized comparison of daunorubicin alone with a combination of daunorubicin, cytosine arabinoside, thioguanine, and pyrimethamine for the treatment of acute nonlymphocytic leukemia. Cancer Treat Rep 60:41, 1976
176. van Prooijen R, van der Kleijn E, Haanen C: Pharmacokinetics of cytosine arabinoside in acute myeloid leukemia. Clin Pharmacol Ther 21:744, 1977
177. Bernard J, Weil M, Boiron M et al: Acute promyelocytic leukemia: Results of treatment by daunorubicin. Blood 41:489, 1973
178. Chard RL Jr, Hammond D: 4'-Demethyl-epipodophyllotoxin-D-ethylidene glucoside (VP16-213). Phase II study for refractory acute leukemias of childhood. Proc Am Soc Clin Oncol 18:354, 1977
179. Kantarjian HM, Keating MJ, Walters RS et al: Role of maintenance chemotherapy in acute promyelocytic leukemia. Cancer 59:1258, 1987
180. Durie BGM; Marrow transplantation for acute nonlympho-Jblastic leukemia. N Engl J Med 302:408, 1980
181. Begg CG, Bennett JM, Cassileth PA: Marrow transplantation for acute nonlymphoblastic leukemia. N Engl J Med 302:408, 1980
182. Santos GW, Tutschka PJ, Brookmeyer R et al: Marrow transplantation for acute nonlymphocytic leukemia after treatment with busulfan and cyclophosphamide. N Engl J Med 309:1347, 1983
183. Champlin R, Gale RP: Acute myelogenous leukemia: Recent advances in therapy. Blood 69:1551, 1987
184. Appelbaum FR, Dahlberg S, Thomas ED et al: Bone marrow transplantation or chemotherapy after remission induction for adults with acute nonlymphoblastic leukemia. Ann Intern Med 101:581, 1984
185. Powles RL, Morgenstern G, Clink HM et al: The place of bone marrow transplantation in acute myelogenous leukaemia. Lancet 1:1047, 1980
186. Champlin R, Ho W, Gale RP et al: Treatment of acute myelogenous leukemia: A prospective controlled trial of bone marrow transplantation versus consolidation chemotherapy. Ann Intern Med 102:285, 1985
187. Glucksberg H, Cheever MA, Farewell VT et al: Intensification therapy for acute nonlymphoblastic leukemia in adults. Cancer 52:198, 1982
188. Mathe G, Pouillart P, Lapeyraque F: Active immunotherapy of L1210 leukaemia applied after the graft of tumour cells. Br J Cancer 23:814, 1969
189. Whittaker JA: Immunotherapy in the treatment of acute leukaemia. Br J Haematol 45:187, 1980
190. Eppinger-Helft M, Pavlovsky S, Hidalgo G et al: Chemoimmunotherapy with Corynebacterium parvum in acute myelocytic leukemia. Cancer 45:280, 1980
191. Powles RL, Russell J, Lister TA et al: Immunotherapy for acute myelogenous leukemia: A controlled clinical study 2½ years after entry of the last patient. Br J Cancer 35:265, 1977
192. Holland JF, Bekesi JG, Cuttner J et al: Chemoimmunotherapy in acute myelocytic leukemia. Israel J Med Sci 13:694, 1977
193. Hayat M, Jehn U, Willemze R et al: A randomized comparison of maintenance treatment with androgens, immunotherapy, and chemotherapy in adult acute myelogenous leukemia. Cancer 58:617, 1986
194. Omura GA, Vogler WR, Bartolucci A et al: Treatment of refractory adult acute leukemia with 5-azacytidine plus 2 deoxythioguanosine. Cancer Treat Rep 63:209, 1979
195. Elias L, Shaw MT, Raab SO: Reinduction therapy for adult acute leukemia with adriamycin, vincristine, and prednisone. Cancer Treat Rep 63:1413, 1979
196. Legha SS, Keating MJ, Zander AR et al: 4'-(9-acridinylamino) Methanesulfon-m-Ansidide (AMSA): A new drug effective in the treatment of adult acute leukemia. Ann Intern Med 93:17, 1980
197. Arlin ZA, Ahmed T, Mittelman A et al: A new regimen of amsacrine with high-dose cytarabine is safe and effective therapy for acute leukemia. J Clin Oncol 5:371, 1987
198. Tschopp L, von Fliedner VE, Sauter C et al: Efficacy and clinical cross-resistance of a new combination therapy (AMSA/VP16) in previously treated patients with acute nonlymphocytic leukemia. J Clin Oncol 4:318, 1986
199. Herzig RH, Wolff SM, Lazarus HM et al: High-dose cytosine arabinoside therapy for refractory leukemia. Blood 62:361, 1983
200. Larson RA, Daly KM, Choi KE et al: A clinical and pharmacokinetic study of mitoxantrone in acute nonlymphocytic leukemia. J Clin Oncol 5:391, 1987
201. Paciucci PA, Dutcher JP, Cuttner J et al: Mitoxantrone and Ara-C in previously treated patients with acute myelogenous leukemia. Leukemia 1:565, 1987
202. Hiddemann W, Kreutzmann H, Straif K et al: High-dose cytosine arabinoside and mitoxantrone: A highly effective regimen in refractory acute myeloid leukemia. Blood 69:744, 1987
203. Carella AM, Santini G, Martinengo M et al: 4-demethoxydaunorubicin (idarubicin) in refractory or relapsed acute leukemias. Cancer 55:1452, 1985
204. Smith DB, Margison JM, Lucas SB et al: Clinical pharmacology of oral and intravenous 4-demethoxydaunorubicin. Cancer Chemother Pharmacol 19:138, 1987
205. Economopoulos T, Stathakis N, Foudoulakis A et al: Myelodysplastic syndromes: Analysis of 131 cases according to the FAB classification. Eur J Haematol 38:338, 1987
206. Tricot G, Vlietinck R, Boogaerts A et al: Prognostic factors in the myelodysplastic syndromes: Importance of initial data on peripheral blood counts, bone marrow cytology, trephine biopsy and chromosomal analysis. Br J Haematol 60:19, 1985
207. Raskind WH, Tirumali N, Jacobson R et al: Evidence for a multistep pathogenesis of a myelodysplastic syndrome. Blood 63:1318, 1984
208. Baumann MA, Milson TJ, Patrick CW et al: Immunoregulatory abnormalities in myelodysplastic disorders. Am J Hematol 22:17, 1986
209. Ayanlar-Batuman O, Shevitz J, Traub UC et al: Lymphocyte interleukin 2 production and responsiveness are altered in patients with primary myelodysplastic syndrome. Blood 70:494, 1987
210. Bagby CG Jr, Gabourel JD, Linman JW: Glucocorticoid therapy in the preleukemic syndrome (hemopoietic dysplasia). Ann Intern Med 92:55, 1980
211. Baccarani M, Zaccaria A, Bandini G et al: Low-dose arabinosyl cytosine for treatment of myelodysplastic syndromes and subacute myeloid leukemia. Leuk Res 7:539, 1983
212. Cheson BD, Jasperese DM, Simon R et al: A critical appraisal of low-dose cytosine arabinoside in patients with acute non-lymphocytic leukemia and myelodysplastic syndromes. J Clin Oncol 4:1857, 1986
213. Nagler A, Rikilis I, Tatarsky I et al: Effect of 1,25-dihydroxyvitamin D_3 and 13-cis-retenoic acid on in vitro hematopoiesis in the myelodysplastic syndromes. J Lab Clin Med 110:237, 1987
214. Picozzi VJ, Swanson GF, Morgan R et al: 13-cis retenoic acid treatment for myelodysplastic syndromes. J Clin Oncol 4:589, 1986
215. Yuo A, Kitaggawa S, Okabe T et al: Recombinant human granulocyte colony-stimulating factor repairs the abnormalities of neutrophils in patients with myelodysplastic syndromes and chronic myelogenous leukemia. Blood 70:404, 1987
216. Pizzuto J, Aviles A, Noriega L et al: Treatment of acute leukemia during pregnancy: Presentation of nine cases. Cancer Treat Rep 64:679, 1980
217. Dara P, Slater LM, Armentrout SA: Successful pregnancy during chemotherapy of acute leukemia. Cancer 47:845, 1981
218. Catanzarite VA, Ferguson II JE: Acute leukemia and pregnancy: A review of management and outcome, 1972–1982. Obstet Gynecol Surv 39:663, 1984
219. Reynoso EE, Shepherd FA, Messner HA et al: Acute leukemia during pregnancy: The Toronto leukemia study group experience with long-term follow-up of children exposed in utero to chemotherapeutic agents. J Clin Oncol 5:1098, 1987
220. Khilanani P, Chou TH, Lomen PL et al: Variation of levels of plasma guanosine diphosphate 1-fucose: beta-D galactosyl alpha-2-L frucosyltransferase in acute adult leukemia. Cancer Res 37:2557, 1977
221. Hittelman WN, Vellkoop L, Zander AR et al: Premature chromosome condensation studies in human leukemia: 4. Characterization of albumin density fractionations of bone marrow at presentation, remission, and relapse. Blood 60:1203, 1982
222. Koeffler HP: Review: Induction of differentiation of human acute myelogenous leukemia cells: Therapeutic implications. Blood 62:709, 1983
223. Novogrodsky A, Dvir A, Ravid A et al: Effect of polar organic compounds on leukemic cells. Cancer 51:9, 1983
224. Brennan J, DePersio JF, Abboud CN et al: The exceptional responsiveness of certain myeloid leukemia cells to colony-stimulating activity. Blood 54:1230, 1979
225. Suzuki H: Aclacinomycin A in acute leukemias and lymphomas. Lancet 2:310, 1975
226. Payne CM, Greenberg B, Cromey D et al: Morphological evidence of an altered bone marrow microenvironment in patients with acute nonlymphocytic leukemia and myelodysplastic disorders. Exp Hematol 15:143, 1987
227. Greenberger JS: Future directions in clinical bone marrow transplantation: Interests converge on the bone marrow microenvironment. Br J Haematol 62:603, 1986
228. Koeffler HP: Syndromes of acute nonlymphocytic leukemia. Ann Intern Med 107:748, 1987

PHILIP J. FIALKOW
JACK W. SINGER

CHAPTER 53 *Chronic Leukemias*

CHRONIC MYELOGENOUS LEUKEMIA

Chronic myelogenous leukemia (CML), also called chronic granulocytic leukemia (CGL), is a clonal neoplastic disorder that originates in a pluripotent stem cell. Although the predominant manifestation of the disease is an overproduction of cells in the granulocytic series, abnormalities in all myeloid lineages are often present. For this reason we prefer the term CML to the earlier term, CGL.

ETIOLOGY AND INCIDENCE

The incidence of CML is approximately 1 per 100,000 per year.[1] Although the incidence was higher than expected in a large group of patients treated with irradiation for ankylosing spondylitis[2,3] and in atomic bomb survivors in Hiroshima,[4] most occurrences of this leukemia cannot be ascribed to known physical or chemical leukemogens. CML is not a hereditary disease, and a history of leukemia in a relative of a patient with CML is unusual. In a series of 40 pairs of identical twins in which one twin had CML, there was no instance in which the other twin had CML or any other hematologic disease.[5-8] Adult-type CML occurs rarely during the first decade of life. Thereafter, the disease incidence increases slightly and peaks during the fourth to fifth decade. There may be a slight preponderance of males.[1]

CELLULAR AND MOLECULAR BIOLOGY

The Philadelphia Chromosome

CML is the first human malignancy to be associated with a specific chromosomal abnormality. In 1960 Nowell and Hungerford described the presence in marrow cells of a G group chromosome from which a large portion of the long arm was missing.[9] This truncated chromosome was termed the Philadelphia chromosome, first abbreviated Ph[1] and now Ph. Later Ph was identified as a derivative of chromosome 22 (22q−), and Rowley demonstrated that the missing piece of chromosome 22 was not lost to the cell, but was translocated to the long arm of chromosome 9 (to form 9q+).[10] Subsequently it was shown that a portion of the long arm of chromosome 9 was reciprocally translocated to chromosome 22. Occasional CML patients have complex translocations involving chromosomes in addition to numbers 9 and 22.[11] However, the molecular consequences of these chromosomal changes appear similar to those resulting from the typical Ph translocation.

Clonal Development and Stem Cell Origin of CML

The clonality of a disorder and the differentiative expression of the cell of origin can be assessed by analyzing neoplastic tissues in patients with naturally occurring cellular mosaicism, such as that present in females as a result of X chromosome inactivation. Early in embryogenesis one of the two X chromosomes in XX somatic cells is randomly but stably inactivated. Thus females have two cell populations: one with an active maternally derived X chromosome and one with an active paternally derived X chromosome. Because the locus for the enzyme glucose-6-phosphate dehydrogenase (G6PD) is on a portion of the X chromosome that undergoes inactivation, women who are heterozygous for the usual B gene (Gd^B) and a variant gene such as Gd^A have two cell populations: one with an active Gd^A and synthesis of type A G6PD and the other with an active Gd^B and production of type B enzyme. The two forms of G6PD can be distinguished by electrophoresis. Normal tissues are composed of mixtures of cells and, therefore, manifest both A *and* B G6PDs. In contrast, a neoplasm that develops clonally (*i.e.*, from a single cell) will show only one G6PD, A *or* B.

We and our colleagues have studied 35 patients with Ph-positive CML who were heterozygous for G6PD (refs. 12–14 and unpublished observations, 1985–1988). In each case, granulocytes expressed a single G6PD while normal tissues manifested both A- and B-type G6PD. The conclusion from these data that CML is a clonal disorder has been supported by studies in which other enzymes or chromosomal abnormalities have been used to determine clonality.

The same single G6PD found in CML granulocytes is also present in red cells, platelets, and monocyte–macrophages.[12–14] These observations and the finding of Ph in multiple myeloid lineages demonstrate that CML involves a multipotential stem cell. Additional studies have shown that minority populations of lymphoid cells are also derived from the stem cell involved by CML.[15–17] In contrast, marrow fibroblasts do not arise from the CML stem cell even in the presence of myelofibrosis.[12] Thus marrow fibrosis in CML presumably is the result of an overgrowth of normal fibroblasts, and myelofibrosis is a secondary or reactive process, possibly in response to growth factors released by leukemic cells.

Multistep Pathogenesis

In patients treated with single-agent oral chemotherapy the prevalence of Ph-positive marrow cells is not altered, but in patients given intensive combination chemotherapy there often is a decrease in the frequency of such cells.[18–22] Study of a patient with CML who was heterozygous for G6PD and who was given intensive chemotherapy showed a strong correlation between the frequency of myeloid cells judged to be nonclonal by G6PD assays and the frequency of Ph-negative marrow cells.[23] This and other studies unequivocally demonstrate the presence of substantial numbers of normal nonclonal, Ph-negative cells in patients with CML. However, more recent data suggest that not all Ph-negative cells are nonclonal. Specifically, evidence has been adduced that at least some patients with CML have lymphoid cells derived from the abnormal clone that are nonetheless Ph-negative.[24]

The probable occurrence of clonal yet Ph-negative cells provides strong support for the suggestion that CML has a multistep pathogenesis. According to this hypothesis, an early genetic event(s) results in clonal proliferation of Ph-negative hematopoietic pluripotent stem cells. Presumably these stem cells are genetically unstable, and a later event(s) leads to development of the Ph translocation in one or more descendants of this progenitor clone. A subclone of Ph-positive cells then evolves, and ultimately overt CML is present. Because generally more than 95% of metaphase cells have Ph in patients with Ph-positive CML, it must be assumed that Ph-positive stem cells have a proliferative advantage when compared with their normal counterparts and with clonal, Ph-negative stem cells. Recent molecular studies suggest that this putative selective advantage is related to activation of an oncogene.

Molecular Consequences of the Ph Translocation

As discussed earlier, the formation of Ph involves a reciprocal translocation between the long arms of chromosomes 9 and 22. In order for this translocation to occur, there must first be breaks on both of these chromosomes. As shown in Figure 53-1, the breakpoint on chromosome 22 occurs in a restricted region termed the breakpoint cluster region (*bcr*). The *bcr* is approximately 5.8 kilobases (kb) in length and is within the region of a gene of unknown function.[25–29] In contrast, the breaks in chromosome 9 occur in a relatively

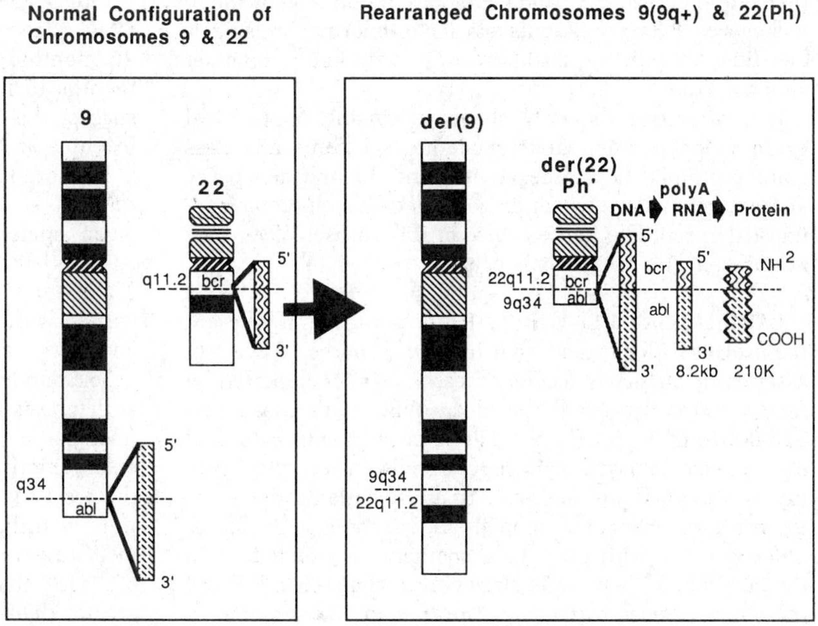

FIG. 53-1. Schematic representation of the translocation between chromosomes 9 and 22. Also shown are the molecular consequences of the Ph translocation—a hybrid DNA joining most of the C-*abl* gene to the 5′ region of the *bcr* gene on chromosome 22, a hybrid mRNA of 8.2 kb and a hybrid protein of 210 kd.

large region 5′ to a cellular oncogene (c-*abl*) that has homology with the v-*abl* oncogene. V-*abl* is associated with the Abelson strain of murine leukemia virus. During formation of Ph the c-*abl* oncogene is translocated to the *bcr* region of chromosome 22, creating a novel fusion gene that encodes an 8.2-kb transcript involving the 5′ segment of *bcr* and the 3′ segment of c-*abl*.[30–34] This "new" deoxyribonucleic acid (DNA) sequence codes for a c-*abl*–related protein (P210) unique to CML that has elevated levels of tyrosine kinase activity.[35,36] The normal c-*abl* protein has low levels of kinase activity. Tyrosine kinase activity is associated with the transforming functions of several oncogenic retroviruses. However, the CML-specific P210 *bcr/abl* protein, unlike the viral (v-*abl*) oncogene product, does not transform NIH/3T3 fibroblasts.[37] Although it is very likely that the *bcr/abl* fusion gene is involved in the pathogenesis of CML, its exact role has not been elucidated.

Clinical Features and Therapy

CML as a clinical disorder is a continuum, but it is generally divided into three stages: chronic phase, accelerated phase, and blast crisis. Although patients may present themselves with advanced disease, the great majority of patients come to medical attention while in chronic phase.

Chronic Phase

CLINICAL FEATURES. The clinical onset of chronic phase CML is generally insidious. Increasing numbers of patients with CML are discovered while still asymptomatic because of the use of automated blood cell counts as health screening tests. The common symptoms of CML at presentation are those of increased metabolism, including fatigue, malaise, weight loss, night sweats, and low-grade fevers. Some patients have symptoms resulting from splenic enlargement, such as early satiety or left upper quadrant pain. More unusual presentations include priapism,[38] gout owing to overproduction of uric acid, and end-organ dysfunction owing to leukostasis.[39] Rarely patients may have abnormal bruising or bleeding caused by qualitative or quantitative platelet abnormalities.[40]

In most cases the only abnormal finding on physical examination is minimal to moderate splenomegaly. Less commonly mild hepatomegaly is found. Lymphadenopathy and extramedullary leukemic nodules called chloromas are unusual except late in the course of the disease. When they are present the prognosis is poor.

LABORATORY FEATURES. Patients with CML present themselves with elevated white blood cell counts (WBCs). In a series of 50 newly diagnosed cases of CML reported by Spiers and colleagues,[41] the mean WBC at diagnosis was 225,000/mm^3 with 61% postmitotic cells (granulocytes and metamyelocytes) and 26% mitotic cells (myelocytes, promyelocytes, and myeloblasts). In most patients there are increased numbers of eosinophils and basophils in the blood. Some patients with CML have spontaneous oscillations in the numbers of their while blood cells and platelets,[42,43] and these occurrences may complicate therapy. Large numbers of hematopoietic progenitor cells capable of granulocytic and erythrocytic colony formation in vitro (CFU-GM and BFU-E, respectively) are also present in the circulation.[44,45] Moreover, sufficient numbers of functional stem cells are present in the blood of CML patients to enable their leukapheresed peripheral blood cells to be used to rescue patients after marrow ablative chemoradiotherapy.[46,47] At diagnosis most patients have a normocytic, normochromic anemia that tends to be severer in patients with higher WBCs. Platelet counts are generally moderately increased, but the platelets may be functionally abnormal when tested by aggregation or by bleeding time measurement. These aberrations usually are not significant clinically, since bleeding disorders rarely occur in patients with CML. Some patients may have prolonged prothrombin times owing to depressed levels of factor V.[48]

Increased bone marrow cellularity with a greatly elevated myeloid-erythroid ratio is found in almost all patients with CML. Fibrosis, although rare at diagnosis, may appear later in the course of the disease and is common in the accelerated phase of CML. Leukocyte alkaline phosphatase (LAP) activity is characteristically low in CML cells, and this finding may be useful in distinguishing CML from leukemoid reactions or other myeloproliferative disorders in which LAP activity is generally elevated.[49] LAP activity may normalize after therapy and increase with infection.[50] Levels in the blood of vitamin B_{12} and B_{12}-binding proteins are greatly elevated.[51] However, the current definitive test for CML is cytogenetic analysis of marrow cells. Ph is found in more than 90% of patients who have classic features of CML at presentation. The great majority of these patients have the usual Ph translocation [t(9;22)]. In about 10% of cases of Ph-positive CML the leukemic cells have a variant translocation, and in a few of these cases the Ph is "masked" and cannot be recognized morphologically.[11,52,53] It is likely that tests with the *bcr* probe will replace chromosome assay as the definitive diagnostic technique for CML.

PROGNOSTIC FEATURES IN CHRONIC PHASE CML. The median duration of chronic phase CML is about 45 months, but the range is wide and varies from a few months to more than 20 years. Retrospective evaluations suggest that chemotherapy does not prolong survival. For example, in an analysis of the survival of CML patients seen at Memorial Sloan-Kettering Institute from 1948 through the mid-1960s, the more recently treated patients who were given single-agent chemotherapy had a median survival of 31 months with or without the addition of splenic irradiation. The median survival of patients in the late 1940s who were treated with splenic irradiation alone or splenic irradiation and ^{32}P was 37 months.[54]

Sokal and co-workers analyzed clinical and laboratory data at diagnosis in 813 patients with CML to determine which findings have prognostic significance (Fig. 53-2).[55] Splenic enlargement of more than 6 cm below the costal margin and the presence of more than 1% blasts in the peripheral blood were identified as the most important independent variables indicating a poor prognosis. Increasing age, a platelet count of more than 700,000/mm^3, basophils plus eosinophils greater than 15%, and karyotypic abnormalities in addition

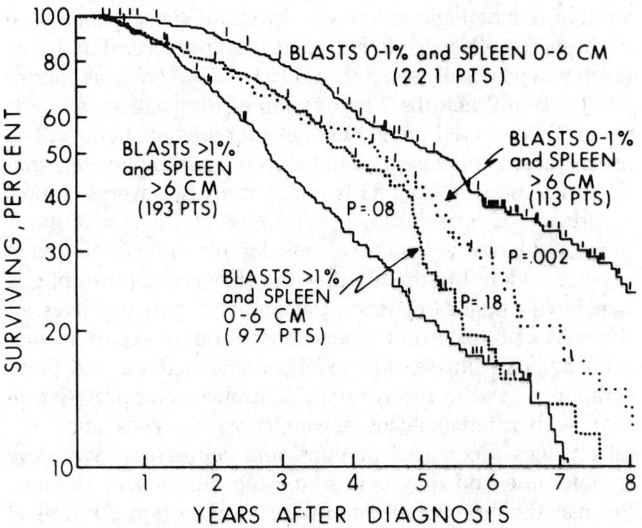

FIG. 53-2. Survival in 624 patients with chronic phase chronic myelogenous leukemia according to spleen size and percentage of circulating blasts at diagnosis. (Sokal JE, Cox EB, Baccarani M, et al: Prognostic discrimination in "good-risk" chronic granulocytic leukemia. Blood 63:789, 1984)

to Ph also were associated with an unfavorable prognosis. From analysis of the findings in these 813 patients and 625 others who were under age 45, Sokal and co-workers defined low- and high-risk groups.[56] Low-risk patients constituted more than one-third of the total, and had a 2-year survival of 90%, an average death rate after 2 years of 17% to 19% per year, and a median survival of 5.5 years. Another third of the patients were in a high-risk group with a 2-year survival of 65% to 70% and an average death rate of 30% to 35% per year. It is important to identify features that are associated with a poor prognosis in chronic phase CML so that subgroups can be defined in which early use of high-risk therapy such as marrow transplantation is justifiable. Unfortunately there are no published data relating assignment of the risk groups defined by Sokal and colleagues to the success of marrow transplantation. However, in the Seattle series the actuarial probability of survival for 3 years after transplantation in the chronic phase was 74% for patients transplanted within 1 year of diagnosis, 56% for patients transplanted 1 to 3 years after diagnosis, and only 38% for patients transplanted 3 or more years after diagnosis.[7] Therefore, although it may be possible to prognosticate accurately on the basis of risk factors present at diagnosis, delay of marrow transplantation could in itself be a major risk factor for decreased subsequent survival. However, the survival advantage for early transplantation found in the Seattle study could not be confirmed by analysis of data from the International Bone Marrow Transplant Registry.

THERAPY FOR CHRONIC PHASE CML. If the WBC is greater than 300,000/mm^3 and symptoms of leukostasis are present,[39] leukapheresis can be used to rapidly reduce blood viscosity.[57–59] Because there is no evidence that maintenance of the WBC in the normal range during the chronic phase of CML prolongs survival, the goal of conventional therapy is to alleviate symptoms.

Treatment regimens for chronic phase CML are outlined in Table 53-1. In most patients symptoms and the WBC can be easily controlled with hydroxyurea at a dose of 1 to 3 g/day.[61,62,66] This drug is usually well tolerated. Most patients will need to take it continuously at a dose adjusted to maintain the WBC between 10,000 and 20,000/mm^3. Side-effects of hydroxyurea are mild and relatively infrequent. They include mild gastrointestinal symptoms, rashes, and headaches.

Busulphan can also be used and has the virtue that, in contrast to hydroxyurea, it can be taken intermittently.[67–70] Treatment is usually initiated at doses of 6 to 8 mg/day and is discontinued when the WBC falls to 20,000 to 30,000/mm^3. Thereafter, the WBC continues to fall for up to several weeks, but it usually stabilizes in a near-normal range. The drug can be reinstituted at low doses when the WBC begins to climb or at 6 to 8 mg/day when the WBC exceeds 50,000/

TABLE 53-1. Treatment of Chronic Phase Chronic Myelogenous Leukemia

Therapy Regimen	*No. of Patients Treated*	*Reference*	*Median Survival (mo)*
None	52	60	36
Hydroxyurea (20 mg/kg/day)	20	61	50+
Hydroxyurea (40–50 mg/kg/day until WBC <50,000, then 20 mg/kg/day or 50 mg/kg biweekly or triweekly)	41	62	51
Busulphan (4 mg/day)	48	63	40
(2–12 mg/day)	26	62	45
(various regimens)	30	64	48
Splenic irradiation	78	60	42
	54	63	30
Combination chemotherapy (various regimens)	139	18–22	48+
Recombinant human interferon 2 alpha (5×10^6 U/m^2/day IM)*	17	65	Not yet known

*Interferon therapy is still considered experimental.

mm^3. Busulphan causes profound marrow hypoplasia in rare patients who have aberrant responses to it and in patients for whom treatment is maintained after normal WBCs are achieved. Occasionally these patients revert to a long-term Ph-negative state after recovery from hypoplasia,[71,72] but others never recover, and die with marrow aplasia. Important but unusual side-effects of busulphan include pulmonary fibrosis, a wasting illness resembling Addison's disease,[73] and, more rarely, cataract formation. The drug also produces irreversible gonadal failure in both sexes, resulting in amenorrhea with menopausal symptoms in women and long-lasting azospermia in men. The amount of busulphan required during the first year after diagnosis has prognostic significance: patients who require higher doses have a shorter survival.[74] Busulphan may increase the complications associated with marrow transplantation; currently most transplantation centers recommend that patients likely to be transplanted receive only hydroxyrurea.

The influence of splenectomy on survival in CML has been evaluated in numerous trials, including randomized, prospective studies.[75–79] The data show that this procedure does not result in an increase in survival or improvement in the quality of life. Similarly, analyses of the outcomes for patients with and without splenectomy who underwent marrow transplantation indicate no survival benefit for splenic removal.[7,80]

When CML is diagnosed in pregnancy and the patient requires symptomatic relief, repeated leukaphereses may be used to control the WBC and to control symptoms in order to spare the fetus from exposure to teratogenic drugs.[57–59] Alternatively, it has been reported that splenic irradiation with pelvic shielding can be used to control disease symptoms without adversely affecting the fetus.[81] Symptomatic relief can usually be obtained with 1200 to 1500 rad given over 2 to 3 weeks. Although splenic irradiation is as effective as busulphan in controlling clinical symptoms, a controlled trial demonstrated shorter survival with splenic irradiation than with chemotherapy.[63]

Death from CML occurs with progression of the disease to accelerated phase or blast crisis (see below). Intensive combination chemotherapy[18–22] and, recently, interferon therapy[65,82] have been used to selectively suppress Ph-positive cells in order to test the hypothesis that this will prevent or delay the onset of disease progression. There have been several studies cumulatively involving more than 100 chronic phase patients in which regimens of intensive combination chemotherapy similar to those used in the treatment of acute myelogenous leukemia were used.[18–22] Although with treatment the frequency of Ph-positive cells decreased in approximately 50% of patients, the frequency of Ph-positive marrow cells began to increase within weeks to months, and the incidence and time to occurrence of blast crisis were not changed.

Several groups have recently reported encouraging results with interferon therapy. In an initial report favorable hematologic responses were noted in 24 of 27 patients treated with human leukocyte (alpha) interferon.[82] The frequency of Ph-positive marrow metaphase cells decreased to below 70% in seven patients. In a subsequent study[65] 14 of 17 patients treated with recombinant alpha$_A$ interferon had favorable hematologic responses. In six of these patients no Ph-positive cells were found on at least one occasion. Interferon was used daily starting at 5×10^6U/m^2 and was continued for 6 to 9 months. Suppression of Ph-positive cells was generally observed after 3 or more months of therapy. The use of recombinant gamma interferon alone and in combination with interferon alpha is under study by several groups.

Although these reports are encouraging, the cost of interferon and its side-effects are considerable. Interferon toxicities are seldom life-threatening, but they are unpleasant and may have a major impact on the quality of patients' lives. At the start of interferon therapy most patients experience an influenza-like illness with myalgias and malaise, but these symptoms tend to resolve with continued therapy.[65] Symptoms such as fatigue, nausea, weight loss, diarrhea, and mental changes (decreased memory and depression) are more troublesome and may persist for the duration of therapy. Because the ultimate effect of interferon therapy on survival is unknown, noninvestigational use of the drug is not currently recommended. Large numbers of patients must be studied in controlled trials to assess the effect of interferon on disease progression and mortality.

Accelerated Phase

Between chronic phase and terminal phase of CML (blast transformation), an intermediate stage of the disease called accelerated phase can be identified in some patients (reviewed in ref. 83). The transition to accelerated phase is rarely abrupt; symptoms in many patients gradually increase over a period of 1 or more months. The presence of at least one of the features listed in Table 53-2 is generally associated with disease acceleration and short survival. Patients who develop new chromosomal abnormalities, the most common of which are duplication of the Ph and a number 17 chromosome composed of two long arms and no short arms (isochromosome 17), are, by definition, considered to be in an accelerated phase of the disease.[85,86] Mean survival time from diagnosis of accelerated phase is approximately 3 months.

TABLE 53-2 Signs and Symptoms of Disease Progression in CML

Difficulty maintaining control of WBC (ref. 83)
Increasing numbers of blood basophils and eosinophils (ref. 83)
Increasing percentage of marrow promyelocytes and blast cells (ref 83)
Increasing anemia (ref. 83)
Falling platelet count (ref. 83)
Persistent thrombocytosis (>10^6/mm^3) (ref. 84)
Karyotypic abnormalities in addition to Ph (refs. 85–87)
Increasing spleen size (ref. 83)
Extramedullary disease ("chloromas") (ref. 88)
Increasing myelofibrosis (ref. 83)
Lymphadenopathy (ref. 88)
Bone pain (ref. 89)
Unexplained fever (ref. 83)
Significant unexplained weight loss (ref. 83)
Night sweats (ref. 83)
Hypercalcemia (refs. 90, 91)

Except for marrow transplantation, which can cure some patients in accelerated phase,[7,92–95] therapy has been generally ineffective. Splenectomy may occasionally be required to control pain and may produce hematologic improvement. Single-agent chemotherapy with hydroxyurea should be used to control the WBC. Not infrequently, doses of hydroxyurea necessary to control very high WBCs in patients in accelerated phase may cause severe marrow hypoplasia.

Blast Crisis

Unless they die with intercurrent diseases or in accelerated phase, almost all patients with CML will enter the terminal stage of the disease, blast crisis (also termed blast transformation). The metamorphosis of CML to this acute leukemia-like phase is manifested by the presence of large numbers of blast cells and a decline of other marrow cellular elements. Cytogenetic and molecular studies indicate that progression to blast crisis occurs by subclonal evolution of chronic phase cells.

The blast cells have myeloid features in about two-thirds of patients.[96,97] In one-third of patients they have lymphoid characteristics such as terminal deoxynucleotidyl transferase (TdT) activity,[98] common acute lymphoblastic leukemia antigen expression,[99,100] and immunoglobulin gene rearrangements,[101] indicating that they are at a differentiative level similar to pre-B cells. Rarely T-cell surface markers are found on lymphoid blast crisis cells.[102,103] Myeloid blast crisis cells may have morphologic and phenotypic features of cells in any myeloid lineage. They are most commonly classified by the French-American-British classification as M2 or M4, but promyelocytic (M3),[104,105] erythroblastic (M6), or megakaryocytic (M7)[106] variants have been seen. Ph is almost always found in blast cells, and commonly there are additional nonrandom abnormalities, such as an extra Ph, an extra chromosome number 8 (trisomy 8), or an isochromosome 17.[85]

In some patients with CML the development of blast crisis is accompanied or preceded by the development of extramedullary tumors, previously called chloromas and now known as granulocytic sarcomas or myeloblastomas.[83,88,89] Common sites of involvement are bone and lymph nodes, but the tumors can occur in the skin, meninges, and gastrointestinal tract.

Rarely patients with CML present themselves with acute lymphoblastic leukemia (ALL), have Ph in the malignant cells, and after treatment lose the characteristics of blast phase. These patients, however, remain Ph-positive. Some of them manifest the classic characteristics of chronic phase CML and others appear to be in accelerated phase. This presentation of CML should not be confused with Ph-positive ALL. Although both leukemias have Ph by cytogenetic analysis, on a molecular level the breakpoints on chromosome 22 in the true ALL cases are different from the breakpoints in CML.[107,108] Thus, on a molecular level, the two disorders are different. Moreover, in patients with Ph-positive ALL, Ph is present only in the malignant blast cells, and these patients become Ph-negative if a remission can be induced. A patient in Ph-positive CML blast crisis with a T-cell phenotype was recently reported in whom the rearranged *bcr*/c-*abl* fusion transcript that had been present in chronic phase was not detected in blast crisis cells.[109] This finding suggests that the *bcr/abl* protein product may not be required for maintenance of the leukemic state in blast crisis.

Therapy of Lymphoid Blast Crisis

The majority of patients with lymphoid blast crisis are TdT positive, and after treatment with regimens similar to those used in ALL, they reenter chronic phase (termed second chronic phase).[98,110] Marrow cells remain Ph-positive in nearly all instances. A typical therapeutic regimen includes vincristine and prednisone followed by L-asparaginase. Maintenance with methotrexate and 6-mercaptopurine may be used with reinduction at 3- to 4-month intervals. Therapy with intrathecal methotrexate should be used, since patients with lymphoid blast crisis have a significant risk of leukemic central nervous system disease.[111] Although remissions can be induced, relapse occurs early and there are few long-term survivors. The best survival prolongations reported to date are in a series of 15 patients with lymphoid blast crisis who were treated with the L10 or L10M protocols at Memorial Sloan-Kettering Institute.[112] Sixty-seven percent of patients achieved a complete remission with a median duration of 7.5 months. The median survival for all patients was 11 months, with responders surviving 15.7 months and nonresponders surviving 4 months. These figures compare favorably with the median survival of 30 weeks in responders to a less aggressive treatment program reported by the Cancer and Leukemia Group B.[113]

Therapy for Myeloid Blast Crisis

Treatment of myeloid blast crisis with regimens similar to those used in acute myeloid leukemia has yielded dismal results.[114–120] Although the blast cell count can be brought under control and marrow aplasia can be produced, in most patients there is a rapid return of blast cells rather than reversion to chronic phase. Results of clinical trials suggest a remission rate of less than 20%. Survival rates for nonresponders and for those who respond by entering second chronic phase are approximately 2 and 6 months, respectively. It was recently reported that a regimen consisting of plicamycin and hydroxyurea may induce a second chronic phase in a substantial proportion of patients with myeloid blast crisis.[121] Unlike traditional combination chemotherapy, this regimen may exert its effect by inducing differentiation in blast cells. Responses are generally seen within 3 weeks of the start of therapy and are best described as a return toward chronic phase. Five of six patients with myeloid blast crisis who were treated with this regimen had responses lasting between 9 and 83 weeks. Toxicity was mild, since remissions occurred without the development of marrow aplasia. More patients must be studied in multicenter trials to confirm these intriguing preliminary results. It is possible that use of this regimen before marrow transplantation for blast crisis will be efficacious, since transplantation is more successful when performed in second chronic phase rather than in frank blast crisis.[7]

Marrow Transplantation

Treatment by marrow transplantation is curative for a proportion of patients with CML, but it is attended by a high early mortality owing to the transplant procedure.[7,93,94,122,123] In this setting the timing of intervention by transplantation is critical, difficult, and heavily influenced by philosophic considerations. Computer programs have been advocated to assist in decision making.[124]

Results of marrow transplantation treatment of patients with CML are summarized in Table 53-3 and also discussed in greater detail in Chapter 66. Initially, marrow transplantation was offered to patients with chronic phase CML who had identical twin (syngeneic) donors. Of the 20 such patients transplanted thus far, 2 died of transplant-related toxicity and 1 died in blast crisis after relapsing at 8 months. The other 17 patients are alive between 5 and 137 months after transplantation.[5–8] Four of the latter patients have relapsed at 13, 22, 25, and 53 months and are alive in chronic phase at 66 to 128 months after transplantation.[7,8]

The factor most strongly associated with success in HLA-matched allogeneic transplantation is the phase of the disease at the time of transplant. Results of hundreds of transplants from several groups suggest that the probability of long-term, disease-free survival is better than 60% for patients transplanted in the chronic phase, less than 30% for patients transplanted in accelerated phase, and about 15% for patients transplanted in the blast phase of the disease. Other factors that influence the success of transplantation include age (procedure-related mortality increases with advancing age and most groups will not transplant patients over the age of 50 during chronic phase) and the interval from diagnosis to transplant (see above).

The published incidence of post-transplant relapse varies between 7% and 30%. The Seattle experience is that 20% of patients transplanted in chronic phase have clinical relapse by 3 years, with a very small relapse probability thereafter. An additional 10% of these patients experienced cytogenetic relapse without hematologic or clinical manifestations of recurrent disease, and in approximately half of these cases the Ph had spontaneously disappeared. The relapse probability for patients transplanted in blast phase is very high (greater than 75% in the Seattle experience), and the probability for patients transplanted in the accelerated phase is intermediate between these two extremes. It is clear that patients who receive T-cell–depleted marrow when transplanted in any phase of CML have a prohibitively high rate of relapse.[126] The reasons for this are not known, but may be associated with a reduced probability of developing a graft-versus-host reaction. The frequencies of relapse in patients with syngeneic donors transplanted in accelerated phase or blast crisis were three of seven and four of eight, respectively.[7] Surprisingly, of 15 patients transplanted before 1985 in a chemotherapy-induced second chronic phase, none has relapsed and the probability of survival is 35% at 5 years. However, one of these patients developed Ph-negative ALL in cells of donor origin nearly 3 years after transplantation.[7,127]

There is a single report of the acquisition of Ph in donor-derived blast cells at relapse after marrow transplantation for CML in blast crisis.[128] Because the *bcr* probe was not available, it was not determined if the donor Ph had a breakpoint identical to the one in original host CML cells. All other evaluable relapses have been in host cells.

The *bcr* rearrangement can be used as a clonal marker for CML, and restriction enzyme analysis of blood DNA with a *bcr* probe may prove the most sensitive test for relapse after marrow transplantation. Moreover, it can be used to determine if a relapse is due to failure to eradicate the original clone, or to emergence of a new clone. Restriction enzyme analyses of cellular DNA with the *bcr* probe of small numbers of patients who relapsed after transplantation suggest that relapses are due to persistence of the original leukemic clone rather than to development of a new Ph.[129]

Because somewhat less than one-third of patients have an HLA-matched family donor, other treatment options have been explored. Using marrow from donors who are mismatched for a single HLA antigen increases the frequency of graft-versus-host disease, but it does not affect long-term survival and enlarges the pool of patients with CML who are candidates for allogeneic marrow transplantation from related donors.[7] Another method of expanding the pool of candidates for transplantation relies on the use of data banks to identify unrelated, HLA-matched donors. Transplants have been performed on 24 patients with chronic phase CML using fully matched or 1-antigen mismatched unrelated donors identified by searches of HLA data banks.[130] Although the data are very preliminary, it appears that survival may be similar to that in patients who receive transplants from sibling donors. A major difficulty is the lack of a sufficiently large donor pool to allow identification of unrelated donors for more than a small percentage of patients.

Another investigational approach to therapy for CML is cryopreservation of chronic phase blood or marrow cells for

TABLE 53-3. Results of Marrow Transplantation Treatment in CML

Disease Stage	*Type of Transplant*	*Reference*	*Relapse Rate (%)*	*Survival >3 Years (% of Patients)*
Chronic	Syngeneic	5–7	25	>90
	Allogeneic	7,93,95	10–30	55–70
Accelerated	Syngeneic	7	43	25
	Allogeneic	7,92,93	30–70	30
Blast crisis	Syngeneic	7	50	16
	Autologous	46,47,119,125	100	0
	Allogeneic	7,94	50–70	0–20
Second chronic phase	Allogeneic	7	15	35

use after ablative therapy in subsequent blast crisis.[46,47,119,125] Use of this procedure resulted in only brief remissions in most patients, often with inadequate hematologic reconstitution. However, occasional patients survived in chronic phase for more than 1 year. Other experimental treatment modalities include the use of chemically purged marrow stored during chronic phase to rescue patients after ablative therapy late in the course of their illnesses. The rationale for chemical purging resides in animal and human studies that suggest that leukemic cells and their progenitors may be preferentially killed by drugs such as 4-hydroperoxy-cyclophosphamide.[131] It may also be possible to accomplish purging by culturing marrow cells in vitro. Recent observations suggest that growth of CML marrow cells in suspension culture (Dexter culture) for several weeks is associated with a selective loss of Ph-positive colony-forming stem cells and with the appearance of Ph-negative colony-forming cells presumably derived from normal stem cells.[132,133] A major problem with all of these approaches is the lack of an ablative therapeutic regimen that can cure advanced stages of CML even when a normal marrow, such as one from a syngeneic or allogeneic donor, is used. Better marrow ablative regimens must be developed for use with allogeneic as well as autologous transplantation.

Ph-NEGATIVE CML

Ph is not detected in about 10% of patients who otherwise present themselves with typical CML. Studies with G6PD of two patients with Ph-negative CML demonstrated that, like the Ph-positive type of CML, the disease developed clonally and involved a stem cell multipotent for granulocytic, erythrocytic, and megakaryocytic differentiation.[134,135] DNA studies of one of the two patients[135] failed to show a *bcr* rearrangement.[136] However, in an important fraction of patients with Ph-negative CML, DNA studies do demonstrate the presence of a *bcr* rearrangement on chromosome 22, the molecular counterpart to Ph.[137–139] The course of the disease in these patients is similar to the course in patients in whom Ph is found. The other Ph-negative patients may have a different disease that is characterized by later onset and shorter survival than are present in Ph-positive CML.[140–142] However, *bcr* probe studies of additional patients with apparent Ph-negative CML are required to better define this disease entity.

JUVENILE CHRONIC MYELOGENOUS LEUKEMIA

Two distinct types of CML occur in children. Patients over the age of 5 years generally have Ph, and their disease is similar to Ph-positive CML in adults. Patients with CML younger than age 4 years usually do not have Ph, and their disease is notably different from CML in older patients. This disorder accounts for approximately 2% to 5% of childhood leukemia. Although generally known as juvenile CML, the disease is actually a subacute myelomonocytic leukemia, and unlike adult CML, it may be inherited.[143,144] The disease has been seen in identical twins, and dominant inheritance was suggested in a family with nine affected children.[145,146]

Splenomegaly is frequent and may be massive. In one series of patients generalized lymphadenopathy was found in 21% of cases, and skin infiltrates with leukemic cells were present in 42% of patients.[145] Infections are frequent in children with juvenile CML. Thrombocytopenia with hemorrhagic manifestations is common early in the disease. The WBC in juvenile CML rarely exceeds 100,000/mm^3. Monocytes generally constitute more than 50% of white blood cells; the other cells are immature granulocytic elements and normoblasts. At presentation most patients have moderate to severe thrombocytopenia, over two-thirds have more than 1% blasts in the blood, and over half have more than 10% blasts in marrow. Unlike adult CML, leukocyte alkaline phosphatase activity is elevated or normal in about 50% of cases. A similar percentage of patients have elevated levels of fetal hemoglobin.[145,147] Ph is not present in these patients, and in a series reported from St. Jude Children's Research Hospital no cytogenetic abnormalities were detected in marrow cells from 14 of 17 patients with juvenile CML.[148] Three patients had an increased number of aneuploid cells, and one of these had a consistent aneuploid abnormality. It has been suggested that some of the patients without cytogenetic abnormalities who survive long-term with no cytotoxic therapy may have a non-neoplastic disorder.[148] These patients with favorable prognoses include two sets of affected siblings who responded to splenectomy alone. In another series 6 of 11 patients had a missing number 7 chromosome (monosomy 7) and a shorter median survival than the patients without cytogenetic abnormalities.[149]

The course of juvenile CML is highly variable, and the survival curve is bimodal.[145] More than 60% of patients in a large series died within 2 years, but 14% survived more than 10 years.[145] Although not tested in a controlled manner, splenectomy is often performed for relief of thrombocytopenia and symptoms caused by splenic enlargement. The value of cytotoxic therapy remains unproved, but some patients may benefit from it.[150] Because some patients can become long-term survivors in the absence of any treatment other than splenectomy, observation after splenectomy may be indicated for those patients who present with platelet counts higher than 100,000/mm^3 and with fewer than 2% blasts in the peripheral blood. In six patients with progressive juvenile CML who received marrow transplants from HLA-matched donors, three are disease-free at 6 to 11 years after transplantation, two others relapsed, and one died of cytomegalovirus pneumonia.[151,152] Marrow transplantation should be considered for any patient who manifests progressive disease.

CHRONIC LYMPHOCYTIC LEUKEMIA—B-CELL TYPE

The great majority of chronic lymphocytic leukemias (CLL) are clonal neoplasms of B-lymphoid cells. Unlike in multiple myeloma, in which plasma cells differentiate from the lymphoid clone, the leukemic cells in CLL do not differentiate beyond the stage of the small B lymphocyte. The latter cells accumulate in blood, marrow, lymph nodes, and spleen. The predominant clinical features of CLL result from enlargement of lymphoid organs owing to accumulation of neoplastic small lymphocytes and decreased function of both the lymphoid and myeloid systems owing to replacement of normal cells by neoplastic lymphocytes. There is a mild to moderate depression in humoral and cell-mediated immunity and a slowly progressive hypofunctioning of marrow.

INCIDENCE AND ETIOLOGY

CLL, the most common leukemia, has an incidence of between 1.8 and 3.0 per 100,000 population.[1] The median age of onset is in the seventh decade, and thereafter, the incidence continues to increase through the ninth decade. The overall age-adjusted incidence rate is 5.2 per 100,000 in the 55-to-59-year range and 30.4 per 100,000 in the 80-to-84-year range.[1] The incidence of CLL in men is about twice that in women and rises from 10.6 per 100,000 in the 55-to-59-year range to 43.7 per 100,000 in the 80-to-84-year range.[1]

Familial CLL has been reported,[153–158] but most cases occur sporadically in individuals without exposure to known leukemogens. The incidence of CLL is not increased after exposure to radiation. CLL, like Waldenström's macroglobulinemia,[159] is more common in families with one of a variety of immunologic disorders (reviewed in ref. 160), although the frequency of antecedent rheumatologic disorders is not higher in CLL patients than in the general population.

CELLULAR BIOLOGY

Immunologic Characterization

CLL is a clonal proliferation of B cells that express surface immunoglobulins (Ig).[161–163] As expected in a clonal neoplasm of B lymphocytes, only a single Ig light-chain type and a single antibody specificity (idiotype) are expressed by the leukemic cells. The number of surface membrane IgM molecules per cell is only about 10% of that expressed on normal circulating B lymphocytes.[163] Cells from most patients have surface IgM molecules, but when tested with conventional protein electrophoresis techniques, serum IgM paraproteins are found in only a small fraction of cases. However, with more sensitive methods, paraproteins in the serum or urine or both are found in nearly all patients with CLL, including some whose tumor cells do not have detectable cell surface Ig.[164] CLL cells have C′3 and Fc receptors and express the B-cell antigens B1 (CD20), B2 (CD21), and T1 (CD5), but not the C3b (CD35) receptor.[161,165,166] The neoplastic cells also express Ia (HLA-DR) determinants.[166] In about 10% of patients with otherwise typical CLL, neoplastic cell surface Ig is not detected; nonetheless, the tumor cells have B-cell type Fc receptors and express B1 antigen.[162] The neoplastic clone of lymphoid cells in these patients is presumably slightly less differentiated than are the clones in the usual type of CLL. In most patients with CLL pre-B cells express the same Ig as the neoplastic B lymphocytes. In many patients the neoplastic cells express T1 (CD5), an antigen found on subsets of normal adult and fetal B cells but not on mature B lymphocytes.[161,166] Most patients with CLL have hypogammaglobulinemia and impaired responses to neoantigens.[167,168]

Studies with G6PD confirm the conclusion reached from investigations with Ig markers that CLL develops clonally.[169] These studies also indicate that myeloid cells and at least the great majority of circulating T lymphocytes are not part of the neoplastic clone in CLL. Nonetheless, numerous studies have demonstrated characteristic T-cell abnormalities in patients with CLL, and these alterations may affect the disease process.[170–173] The proportion of blood T lymphocytes is generally low, but the absolute number of T cells may actually be elevated and reportedly increases with advancing stage of the disease.[174] The ratio of T4+ to T8+ T cells is significantly lower than normal, possibly because of an absolute increase in T8+ cells. Suppressor T cells that infiltrate the marrow in patients with CLL may directly suppress erythropoiesis.[175] In vitro studies suggest that there may be functional abnormalities of circulating T cells such as reduced mitogen responsiveness, decreased responsiveness to interleukin-2 (IL-2) (possibly because of a decrease in the number of IL-2 receptors), and a decrease in IL-2 production after appropriate T-cell activation.[176] T cells in most patients with B-cell CLL also have defective recognition of self and foreign histocompatibility antigens. The absolute number of natural killer cells is depressed in patients with CLL, but it increases with interferon therapy.[177,178] The basis for these T-cell abnormalities in patients with B-cell CLL is not known.

Cytogenetic Abnormalities

Consistent cytogenetic abnormalities are found in about 40% of patients with CLL.[179–184] An extra number 12 chromosome (trisomy 12) is the most common abnormality and is found in familial and sporadic cases. A recent study demonstrated that trisomy 12 was found only in the neoplastic B cells in CLL; B cells with the nonclonal light chain and T cells were cytogenetically normal.[184] Trisomy 12 has also been observed in patients with Waldenström's macroglobulinemia, and this chromosomal aberration may be associated with IgM production by CLL cells.[185]

Although a strong association between advanced stage of disease and presence of cytogenetic abnormalities has been reported in one series,[182] this correlation was not found in a series of patients seen at Roswell Park Memorial Institute.[183] In the former series patients with trisomy 12 required earlier therapeutic intervention and had a shorter survival time than patients with normal karyotypes. In both series the presence of abnormalities in addition to trisomy 12 was strongly correlated with a very short survival time.

Clinical Features and Staging

In the early stages of CLL, when the only abnormality is an absolute lymphocytosis in blood and marrow, patients are asymptomatic and may remain so for many years. As the disease slowly progresses, lymphadenopathy and splenomegaly occur and patients generally complain of fatigue. In late stages of the illness patients may experience symptoms that result from infiltration of neoplastic lymphocytes into non-

TABLE 53-4. Staging of Chronic Lymphocytic Leukemia*

Stage 0:	Blood lymphocytosis, 15,000 mm^3; marrow, 40% lymphocytes
Stage I:	Lymphocytosis with lymphadenopathy
Stage II:	Lymphocytosis with enlarged spleen or liver. Lymphadenopathy is not necessarily present.
Stage III:	Lymphocytosis with anemia. Lymph nodes, liver, and spleen may or may not be enlarged. Anemia may be hemolytic or due to decreased red cell production.
Stage IV:	Lymphocytosis with thrombocytopenia (<100,000/mm^3); anemia and lymphadenopathy. Hepatic and splenic enlargement may be present.

*After Rai et al.[189]

lymphoid organs, such as pleura, orbit, conjunctiva, gonad, liver, pulmonary parenchyma, and Waldeyer's ring. Patients with CLL progressively lose humoral immune function and become increasingly susceptible to systemic infection with encapsulated organisms.[186,187]

Staging and Prognosis

In an analysis of 130 patients with CLL, Boggs and associates[188] found a correlation between tumor burden at the time of diagnosis and survival. In 1975 Rai and colleagues[189] proposed a staging system for CLL that has since been verified and widely adopted (Table 53-4; Fig. 53-3). Patients

FIG. 53-3. Survival by Rai stage in 125 patients with chronic lymphocytic leukemia. (Rai KR, Sawitsky A, Cronkite EP, et al: Clinical staging of chronic lymphocytic leukemia. Blood 46:219, 1975)

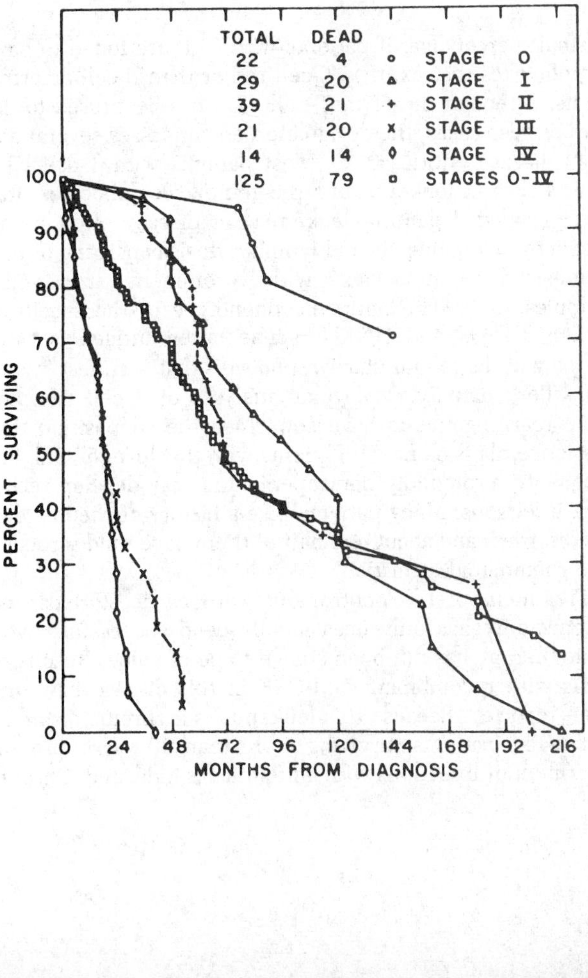

with Stage 0 CLL do not have symptoms attributable to their leukemia; the lymphocytosis is usually discovered when WBC counts are done for other reasons. Patients with Stages 0 through II have similar survival times of generally more than 6 years, whereas patients with Stage III or IV disease survive less than 2 years.

Multiple modifications of this schema have been suggested in efforts to identify subgroups with differing prognoses within Rai stages.[190–195] For example, a lymphocyte count of greater than 50,000/mm^3 suggests a poor prognosis in patients with Rai Stages 0 through II. Binet and co-workers[192] suggest that patients with Stage II disease who have splenomegaly without lymphadenopathy have a better long-term survival. It has also been suggested that patients with immune-mediated platelet destruction who respond to splenectomy may have a better prognosis than other Stage IV patients. Marrow histology may be an independent prognostic parameter: patients who have diffuse marrow infiltration have a significantly poorer prognosis than those who have nodular infiltration.[191,195] Although staging systems are derived from analyses of patients' findings at diagnosis, they can also be used to indicate prognosis later in the course of the illness.[196]

Treatment and Clinical Course

CLL is generally an indolent disease. If deaths from intercurrent illnesses are censored, the median survival of CLL patients is reported to be 9 years.[188] In Rai and co-workers' series the mean interval from diagnosis of Stage 0 CLL to the time at which therapy was needed was 5.3 years.[189] By the time treatment was needed, patients had progressed to Stage II or beyond. Indications for therapy in CLL are symptoms of fatigue, bulky lymphadenopathy, or evidence of progressive marrow infiltration. In the absence of these manifestations, lymphocytosis, even of 100,000/mm^3, is not an indication for therapy. Autoimmune hemolytic anemia or thrombocytopenia is generally considered an indication for cytotoxic therapy after control of the immune destruction is achieved with corticosteroids and, if necessary, with splenectomy.[197]

Treatment regimens for CLL are outlined in Table 53-5. Therapy is usually initiated with daily or pulsed administration of alkylating agents with or without prednisone (reviewed in ref. 199). Chlorambucil or cyclophosphamide may be used either daily or pulsed every 2 weeks.[200,203] Prednisone pulsed for 5 days each month may improve the rapidity of clinical response and the overall response rate.[198,201,204] More intensive therapy has not proved beneficial except late in the course of CLL, when patients are refractory to low doses of alkylating agents. Some of these patients may respond to vincristine, Adriamycin, BCNU, or other antilymphoma drugs. The morbidity of treatment is often substantial owing to poor marrow reserve and general debility.

Splenectomy may be necessary to control autoimmune hemolytic anemia or thrombocytopenia.[197] Although removing an enlarged spleen may reduce red cell transfusion requirements and increase the platelet count, it does not prolong survival.[205–207] Repeated leukaphereses reduce the tumor cell burden and produce symptomatic benefit, but such treatments have no apparent advantage over low-

TABLE 53-5. Treatment of Chronic Lymphocytic Leukemia

Regimen	*Reference*	*Response Rate* (% of Patients)*
Single Agent		
Prednisone (0.8 mg/kg/day with taper over 6 wk)	198	11†
Chlorambucil (0.1–0.2 mg/kg/day)	199	70
Chlorambucil (0.4 mg/kg every other week)	200	64
Chlorambucil (6 mg daily)	201	75
Combination		
Chlorambucil (6 mg/day) + prednisone (30 mg/day)	201	87
Chlorambucil (0.4–0.8 mg/kg/mo) + prednisone (0.8 mg/kg/day for 6 wk)	198	47†
Chlorambucil (0.08 mg/kg/day) + prednisone (0.8 mg/kg/day for 6 wk)	198	38†
Cyclophosphamide (200 mg/m²/day PO × 5 days); vincristine (2 mg, one dose only); prednisone (2 mg/kg/day × 5 days). Repeat every 21 days.	202	72

*Includes all major responses as defined by investigators.
†Rai Stages III and IV only.

dose alkylating agent therapy.[208–210] Low-dose total body irradiation and localized splenic irradiation have also been used in the treatment of CLL. The efficacy of these treatment modalities appears similar to that of alkylating agents, but the hematopoietic toxicity includes sustained pancytopenia.[211–214]

Patients with CLL who have recurrent infections may benefit from prophylactic administration of antibiotics and monthly intravenous immunoglobulin. Because these patients form antibodies poorly, they are less likely to be protected by pneumococcal vaccine.

Although most patients with CLL die of infection or of illnesses unrelated to the leukemia, patients occasionally develop an aggressive, large-cell lymphoreticular neoplasm (Richter's syndrome).[215–219] It is likely, but not definitively proven, that Richter's syndrome results from evolution of the CLL clone rather than from development of a new neoplasm. Typically, the onset of the syndrome is explosive, with fever and enlargement of the liver, spleen, and paraaortic lymph nodes, although any lymph node group can be affected. Most patients die within 2 months despite attempts at therapy. CLL in other patients may slowly or rapidly transform into prolymphocytic leukemia, a more aggressive disease characterized by large cells with nuclear immaturity (see below).[220–225]

Susceptibility to Additional Neoplasms

Patients with CLL have an incidence of nonlymphoid neoplasms that is more than twofold higher than expected.[226–228] Pulmonary neoplasms account for approximately one-third of this excess of cancers. Other malignancies found with increased frequency in patients with CLL include melanoma and other skin cancers and soft tissue sarcomas such as fibrous histiocytomas. Basal cell carcinomas may be more aggressive in patients with CLL than they are in normal hosts.

Experimental Therapies

Recombinant alpha interferon stimulates CLL cells to develop plasmacytoid features and express cytoplasmic Ig.[229] However, results of clinical trials with interferon in CLL have been disappointing, although some patients have had partial responses manifested by decreases in circulating lymphocytes and regression of lymphadenopathy.[230–232] Currently interferon should be used only investigationally for the treatment of CLL, since there are no data suggesting efficacy equivalent to that of oral alkylating agents. Furthermore, toxicity and expense of interferon therapy are substantial.

Administration to patients with CLL of a monoclonal antibody (T101) to the T65 antigen present on T lymphocytes and CLL cells[233,234] or anti-idiotypic antibody to cell surface Ig[235] produced transitory drops in circulating tumor cells. However, most patients had a return to pretreatment levels of peripheral blood CLL cells within 24 to 48 hours. The T65 antigen is rapidly modulated, and this may account for the rapid loss of effectiveness of the unconjugated antibody. Nonetheless, these studies do suggest the use of monoclonal antibodies conjugated to toxins as an experimental treatment modality in CLL.

T-CELL CLL

A small percentage of patients with CLL are found to have lymphocytes that express T-cell rather than B-cell determinants. Although the term T-cell CLL has been used to describe these cases, the designation encompasses several distinct disease entities.[236,237] Most patients with T-cell CLL have a chronic leukemia of large granular lymphocytes (formerly called T-gamma leukemia), a disease often manifested by splenomegaly and lymphocytosis consisting of medium-sized lymphocytes with prominent azurophilic granules.[238–243] The antigenic phenotype of these cells is CD3+, CD8+, and HNK-1+. The latter antigen is associated with large granular lymphocytes that manifest "natural killer" activity. Molecular analyses of T-cell receptor gene rearrangements have confirmed the supposition that the leukemia is clonal.[244] Patients with this form of CLL are frequently profoundly neutropenic and may develop recurrent infections. Many patients give a history of rheumatologic disorders and about one-half of them have mild seropositive rheumatoid arthritis.

Treatment of the neutropenia with corticosteroids and splenectomy has only occasionally been successful. Cytotoxic therapy has not been shown to be of value. Results of trials with recombinant GM-CSF in this disease have not been reported. Because this leukemia is a chronic disorder, with some patients surviving more than 20 years, prompt treatment of infections with antibiotics is indicated. Chronic prophylactic administration of antibiotics may be of benefit in some patients with recurrent infections.

A second disorder often placed in the T-cell CLL category is leukemia of CD4+ (helper) dermatotropic lymphocytes.[236,237] This disease is readily distinguishable from the Sézary syndrome, which is more indolent, related to early mycosis fungoides, and characterized by distinctive circulating atypical lymphocytes in association with erythroderma. T-cell CLL with CD4+ dermatotropic lymphocytes is an aggressive disease. Patients affected with it present themselves with a high WBC and hepatosplenomegaly without lymphadenopathy. They usually develop infiltration of the skin with leukemic lymphocytes. The patients respond poorly to cytotoxic drug therapy but may benefit from intensive leukapheresis if the WBC exceeds 50,000/mm^3. Treatment is ineffective, and most patients succumb within 1 year of diagnosis. Therapeutic modalities now under investigation for this disorder include monoclonal antibodies, interferon, and deoxycoformycin.

PROLYMPHOCYTIC LEUKEMIA

Prolymphocytic leukemia is a rare neoplasm of either T or B cells characterized by a high number of circulating large lymphoid cells with prominent nucleoli but relatively mature chromatin, massive splenomegaly, minimal lymphadenopathy, and a uniformly poor prognosis.[245,246] The disease may evolve from B-cell CLL[220–225] or present de novo. Characteristic features of B-cell prolymphocytic leukemia cells are the presence of cytoplasmic Ig and relatively high levels of expression of surface Ig when compared with CLL cells.

The T-cell type of prolymphocytic leukemia accounts for about 20% of cases. The cells in this form of leukemia can be distinguished by assays of surface antigens (the cells are CD4+ and CD8−).[247,248] Affected patients often develop skin involvement, and like the B-cell prolymphocytic leukemia patients, they respond poorly to therapy.

HAIRY CELL LEUKEMIA

Hairy cell leukemia (HCL), also called leukemic reticuloendotheliosis, is an uncommon B-cell neoplasm characterized by pancytopenia, splenomegaly without lymphadenopathy, and circulating leukemic cells with cytoplasmic projections. A distinguishing feature of the leukemic cells is expression of acid phosphatase that is resistant to tartrate inhibition.[249,250] Typically, it is difficult or impossible to aspirate marrow from patients with HCL because of reticulin fibrosis and infiltration by neoplastic cells. Diagnosis of HCL rests on the demonstration of tartrate-resistant acid phosphatase in blood and marrow cells.

Cellular Biology

Studies of chromosomes,[251] cell surface Ig expression,[252,253] and Ig gene rearrangements[254] in circulating cells from patients with HCL suggest that the leukemic cells are clonally proliferating B-lymphoid cells. "Clonal" rearrangements of genes for Ig heavy and light chains are found in almost all patients with HCL.[254] The neoplastic cells in most cases also express "monoclonal" surface Ig and the B-cell determinants B1 and B4 as well as the PCA-1 antigen, which is found on early plasma cells.[255] Hairy cells do not express the PC-1 antigen found on myeloma cells, but in about 50% of patients the hairy cells express MO-1, an antigen associated with elements in the monocytic and granulocytic series but not associated with normal cells in the B-lymphocyte lineage.[252,255] Leukemic cells from more than one-half of patients with HCL express the antigenic determinant associated with the IL-2 receptor.[255] It has been suggested on the basis of these findings that HCL is a neoplasm of B cells predominantly at the pre–plasma cell level of differentiation.

A few cases have been described in which the characteristic hairy cell is in the T-cell lineage.[256,257] In two patients with T-cell HCL the disease was associated with a retrovirus known as HTLV-II that can infect and transform normal T lymphocytes. In one of the two patients integration of provirus into the neoplastic cells was demonstrated, supporting the hypothesis that the HTLV-II virus is the proximate cause of this disorder.[257] No virus has been associated with B-lymphoid cell HCL.

Clinical Course

The most common complication in patients with HCL is infection.[258–260] Because HCL causes neutropenia and is associated with defects in humoral and cell-mediated immune function, patients are prone to develop pyogenic and opportunistic infections. Common offending bacterial organisms are *Escherichia coli, Pseudomonas aeruginosa,* and *Staphylococcus aureus.* Opportunistic infections with atypical acid-fast bacteria, toxoplasma, legionella, or fungi are often seen. Patients with HCL are also prone to develop "autoimmune" and connective tissue disorders, especially vasculitis (erythema nodosum, cutaneous vasculitis, and polyarteritis nodosa),[261] which may occur in as many as 30% of patients.[262]

Before discovery of effective therapy for HCL, the clinical course of the disease was variable. Some patients had prolonged survival after splenectomy, but if they had only partial responses to splenectomy, the median survival was about 5 years.[263,264] Death was generally caused by infection.

Therapy

The primary indication for therapy in HCL is progressive pancytopenia with infection. Treatment regimens for HCL are outlined in Table 53-6. Splenectomy is the established first therapeutic maneuver for most patients. Removing the spleen, an organ that traps blood cells, results in a return of normal blood cell counts in about 50% of patients with HCL.[264] In most patients there is some improvement in blood cell counts in at least one hemopoietic lineage.[265] The response to splenectomy can be prolonged, especially in patients who have patchy marrow involvement and splenomegaly. However, almost half of Golomb's series of 166 patients needed additional therapy at a median time of 8.3

TABLE 53-6. Treatment of Hairy Cell Leukemia

Regimen	*Reference*	*Patients (No. Treated/No. Evaluable)*	*Response Rate* (% of Patients)*
Splenectomy	264, 265	166/166	CR 42 PR 58
Human recombinant interferon 2 alpha (IFa) (3–12 × 10^6 U/day for 4–6 mo, then 3 × weekly for 12 mo)	266	30/30	CR 30 PR 57
IFa (2 × 10^6 U/m^2 3 × weekly)	267	22/21	CR 0 PR 43†
IFa (2 × 10^6 U 3 × weekly for 18 mo or less)	268	135/128	CR 4 PR 77
Deoxycoformycin (5 mg/m^2 for 2 days every other week)	269	37/27	CR 59 PR 37
Deoxycoformycin (4 mg/m^2 every other week)	270	31/18	CR 83 PR 6

*CR, complete response; PR, partial response.
†PR rate low owing to early reporting of data.

months after splenectomy.[265] Spleen size alone is not an accurate predictor of blood cell count response to splenectomy, since patients with pancytopenia and minimal splenic enlargement may respond to splenectomy with increases in blood counts. However, owing to the availability of other effective therapies, it has been recommended that patients with pancytopenia, a nonpalpable spleen, and a diffusely involved marrow initially receive systemic therapy.[265]

HCL is the only neoplastic disease in which a biologic response modifier, alpha-interferon (produced by recombinant DNA technology), has become the therapeutic agent of first choice. Studies initially reported by Quesada and others[266,271] and later confirmed by other investigators[267,272] indicate that recombinant alpha-interferon given either daily or three times weekly in doses of 2 to 3 × 10^6 U/m^2 produces partial remission in 80% to 90% of patients and complete remission in about 5% of patients. Responses include decrease in spleen size, normalization of blood cell counts, and decrease in the frequency of serious infections. Interferon therapy is generally continued for 12 months. When it is discontinued, about 20% of patients will relapse within the first year, but retreatment is likely to be successful. The role of maintenance therapy is under study. The toxicity of recombinant interferon at doses effective in the treatment of HCL is modest. Most patients initially develop an influenza-like syndrome, but this regresses with continued therapy. Chronic side-effects include mild skin disorders, diarrhea or constipation, nausea, and inflammation at the injection site. About 20% of patients develop reversible but disturbing central nervous system effects such as memory loss, depression, and severe fatigue.

Recent studies suggest that the experimental agent 2′-deoxycoformycin (pentostatin) is a highly effective alternative therapy to interferon in untreated patients with HCL.[269,270,273] Moreover, it appears to be effective in patients who either do not respond or who become refractory to interferon.[274] Unlike interferon, which produces complete remissions in fewer than 10% of cases, 2′-deoxycoformycin, an adenosine deaminase inhibitor, reportedly induces complete remissions in more than 70% of untreated patients.[275] Prospective trials directly comparing therapy with alpha-interferon and 2′-deoxycoformycin are in progress.

REFERENCES

1. Surveillance Epidemiology End Results Incidence and Mortality Data: 1973–1977, NCI Monograph 57, p. 10. Bethesda, Md, National Cancer Institute, 1981
2. Silberber DH, Frohman LA, Duff IF: The incidence of leukemia and related diseases in patients with rheumatoid (ankylosing) spondylitis with x-ray therapy. Arthritis Rheum 3:64, 1960
3. Graham DC: Leukemia following x-ray therapy for ankylosing spondylitis. Arch Intern Med 105:51, 1960
4. Lange RD, Moloney WC, Yamawaki R: Leukemia in atomic bomb survivors. Blood 9:574, 1954
5. Fefer A, Cheever MA, Thomas ED, et al: Disappearance of Ph¹-positive cells in four patients with chronic granulocytic leukemia after chemotherapy, irradiation and marrow transplantation from an identical twin. N Engl J Med 300:333, 1979
6. Fefer A, Cheever MA, Greenberg PD, et al: Treatment of chronic granulocytic leukemia with chemoradiotherapy and transplantation of marrow from identical twins. N Engl J Med 306:63, 1982
7. Thomas ED, Clift RA, Fefer A, et al: Marrow transplantation for the treatment of chronic myelogenous leukemia. Ann Intern Med 104:155, 1986
8. Fefer A: Personal communication. 1988
9. Nowell RC, Hungerford DA: A minute chromosome in human chronic granulocytic leukemia. Science 132:1497, 1960
10. Rowley JD: A new consistent chromosomal abnormality in chronic myelogenous leukemia identified by quinacrine fluorescence and Giemsa staining. Nature 243:290, 1973
11. Sandberg AA: Chromosomes and causation of human cancer and leukemia. XL. The Ph¹ and other translocations in CML. Cancer 46:2221, 1980
12. Fialkow PJ, Jacobson RJ, Papayannopoulou T: Chronic myelocytic leukemia: Clonal origin in a stem cell common to the granulocyte, erythrocyte, platelet and monocyte/macrophage. Am J Med 63:125, 1977
13. Fialkow PJ: Clonal and stem cell origin of blood cell neoplasms. In Lobue J, Gordon AS, Silber R, Muggia FM (eds): Contemporary Hematology/Oncology, p 11. New York, Plenum Press, 1980
14. Fialkow PJ, Singer JW: Tracing development and cell lineages in human hemopoietic

neoplasia. In Weissman IL (ed): Leukemia, Proceedings of Dahlem Konferenzen, p 203. Berlin, Springer-Verlag, 1985
15. Fialkow PJ, Denman AM, Jacobson RJ, Lowenthal MN: Chronic myelocytic leukemia: Origin of some lymphocytes from leukemic stem cells. J Clin Invest 62:815, 1979
16. Martin PJ, Najfeld V, Hansen JA, et al: Involvement of the B-lymphoid system in chronic myelogenous leukemia. Nature 287:49, 1980
17. Bernheim A, Berger R, Preud'Homme JL, et al: Philadelphia chromosome positive blood B lymphocytes in chronic myelocytic leukemia. Leuk Res 5:331, 1981
18. Sharp JC, Joyner MV, Wayne AW, et al: Karyotype conversion in Ph[1]-positive chronic myeloid leukaemia with combination chemotherapy. Lancet 1:1370, 1979
19. Smalley RV, Vogel J, Huguley CM, Miller D: Chronic granulocytic leukemia: Cytogenetic conversion of the bone marrow with cycle-specific chemotherapy. Blood 50:107, 1977
20. Cunningham I, Gee T, Dowling M, et al: Results of treatment with Ph[1]+ chronic myelogenous leukemia with an intensive treatment regimen (L-5 protocol). Blood 53:375, 1979
21. Kantarjian HM, Villekoop L, McCredie B, Keating M, et al: Intensive combination chemotherapy (ROAP 10) and splenectomy in the management of chronic myelogenous leukemia. J Clin Oncol 3:192, 1985
22. Clarkson BD: Chronic myelogenous leukemia: Is aggressive treatment indicated? J Clin Oncol 3:135, 1985
23. Singer JW, Arlin ZA, Najfeld V, et al: Restoration of nonclonal hematopoiesis in chronic myelogenous leukemia following a chemotherapy-induced loss of the Ph[1] chromosome. Blood 56:356, 1980
24. Fialkow PJ, Martin PL, Najfeld V, et al: Evidence for a multistep pathogenesis of chronic myelogenous leukemia. Blood 58:158, 1981
25. Heisterkamp NJ, Stephenson R, Groffen J, et al: Localization of the c-abl oncogene adjacent to a translocation breakpoint in chronic myelocytic leukemia. Nature 306:239, 1983
26. Groffen J, Stephenson JR, Heisterkamp N, et al: Philadelphia chromosomal breakpoints are clustered within a limited region, bcr, on chromosome 22. Cell 36:93, 1984
27. Heisterkamp N, Stam K, Groffen J, et al: Structural organization of the bcr gene and its role in the Ph[1] translocation. Nature 315:758, 1985
28. Leibowitz D, Schaefer-Rego K, Popenoe DW, et al: Variable breakpoints on the Philadelphia chromosome in chronic myelogenous leukemia. Blood 66:243, 1985
29. Popenoe DW, Schaefer-Rego K, Mears JG, et al: Frequent and extensive deletion during the 9,22 translocation in CML. Blood 68:1123, 1986
30. deKlein A, van Kessel A, Grosveld G, et al: A cellular oncogene is translocated to the Philadelphia chromosome in chronic myelocytic leukemia. Nature 300:765, 1982
31. Shtivelman E, Lifshitz B, Gale RP, Canaani E: Fused transcripts of abl and bcr genes in chronic myelogenous leukemia. Nature 315:550, 1985
32. Canaani E, Gale RP, Steiner-Saltz D, et al: Altered transcription of the c-abl oncogene in chronic myelocytic leukemia. Lancet 1:593, 1984
33. Heisterkamp NJ, Stephenson R, Groffen J, et al: Localization of the c-abl oncogene adjacent to a translocation breakpoint in chronic myelocytic leukemia. Nature 306:239, 1983
34. Collins SJ, Kubonishi I, Miyoshi I, Groudine MT: Altered transcription of the c-abl oncogene in K-562 and other chronic myelogenous leukemia cells. Science 225:72, 1984
35. Konopka JB, Watanabe SM, Singer JW, et al: Cell lines and clinical isolates derived from Ph-positive chronic myelogenous leukemia patients express c-abl proteins with a common structural alteration. Proc Natl Acad Sci USA 82:1810, 1985
36. Konupka JB, Watanabe S, Witte ON: An alteration of the human c-abl protein in K562 leukemia cells unmasking associated tyrosine kinase activity. Cell 37:1035, 1984
37. Daley GQ, McLaughlin J, Witte ON, Baltimore D: The CML-specific P210 bcr/abl protein, unlike v-abl, does not transform NIH/3T3 fibroblasts. Science 237:532, 1987
38. Suri R, Goldman JM, Catovsky D: Priapism complicating chronic granulocytic leukemia. Am J Hematol 9:295, 1980
39. Hild DH, Meyers TJ: Hyperviscosity in chronic granulocytic leukemia. Cancer 46:1418, 1980
40. Schafer AI: Bleeding and thrombosis in the myeloproliferative disorders. Blood 64:1, 1984
41. Spiers ASD, Bain BB, Turner JE: The peripheral blood in chronic granulocytic leukaemia. Scand J Haematol 18:25, 1977
42. Vodopick H, Rupp EM, Edwards CL, et al: Spontaneous cyclic leukocytosis and thrombocytosis in chronic granulocytic leukemia. N Engl J Med 286:284, 1972
43. Wheldon TE, Kirk J, Finlay HM: Cyclic granulopoiesis in chronic granulocytic leukemia: A simulation study. Blood 43:379, 974
44. Moore MAS, Williams N, Metcalf D: In vitro colony formation by normal and leukemic human hematopoietic cells. J Natl Cancer Inst 50:603, 1973
45. Goldman JM, Shiota F, Th'ng KH, Orchard KH: Circulating granulocytic and erythroid progenitor cells in chronic granulocytic leukaemia. Br J Haematol 47:7, 1980
46. Goldman JM, Catovsky D, Goolden AWG, et al: Buffy coat autografts for patients with chronic granulocytic leukemia in transformation. Blut 42:149, 1981
47. Haines ME, Goldman JM, Worsley AM, et al: Chemotherapy and autografting for chronic granulocytic leukaemia in transformation: Probable prolongation of survival for some patients. Br J Haematol 58:711, 1984
48. Hasegawa DK, Bennett AJ, Coccia PF, et al: Factor V deficiency in Philadelphia-positive chronic myelogenous leukemia. Blood 56:585, 1980
49. Bennett JM, Rutonberg AM: Diagnostic value of leukocyte alkaline phosphatase: A 3 year experience. Ann Histochem 11:173, 1966
50. Rosner F, Schreiber ZR, Parise F: Leukocyte alkaline phosphatase: Fluctuations with disease status in chronic granulocytic leukemia. Arch Intern Med 130:892, 1972
51. Gilbert HS, Krauss S, Pasternack B, et al: Serum vitamin B_{12} content and unsaturated vitamin B_{12} binding capacity in myeloproliferative disease. Ann Intern Med 71:719, 1969
52. First International Workshop on Chromosomes and Leukemia: Chromosomes in Ph[1] positive chronic granulocytic leukemia. Br J Haematol 39:305, 1978
53. Oshimura M, Sandberg A: Chromosomes and causation of human cancer and leukemia. XXIV. Unusual and complex Ph[1] translocations and their clinical significance. Blood 50:691, 1977
54. Monfardini S, Gee T, Fried J, Clarkson B: Survival in chronic myelogenous leukemia: Influence of treatment and extent of disease at diagnosis. Cancer 31:492, 1973
55. Sokal JE, Cox EB, Baccarani M, et al: Prognostic discrimination in "good-risk" chronic granulocytic leukemia. Blood 63:789, 1984
56. Sokal JE, Baccarani M, Tura S, et al: Prognostic discrimination among younger patients with chronic granulocytic leukemia: Relevance to bone marrow transplantation. Blood 66:1352, 1985
57. Mehta AB, Goldman JM, Kohner E: Hyperleucocytic retinopathy in chronic granulocytic leukaemia: The role of intensive leucapheresis. Br J Haematol 56:661, 1984
58. Vallejos CS, McCredie KB, Britiin GM, Freireich EJ: Biological effects of repeated leukapheresis of patients with chronic myelogenous leukemia. Blood 42:925, 1973
59. Lowenthal RM, Buskard NA, Goldman JM, et al: Intensive leukapheresis as initial therapy for chronic granulocytic leukemia. Blood 46:835, 1975
60. Minot GR, Buckman TE, Isaacs R: Chronic myelogenous leukemia: Age, incidence, duration and benefit derived from irradiation. JAMA 82:1489, 1924
61. Kennedy BJ: Hydroxyurea therapy in chronic myelogenous leukemia. Cancer 29:1052, 1972
62. Rushing D, Goldman A, Gibbs G, et al: Hydroxyurea versus busulphan in the treatment of chronic myelogenous leukemia. Am J Clin Oncol 5:307, 1982
63. Medical Research Council: Chronic granulocytic leukaemia: Comparison of radiotherapy and busulphan therapy. Br Med J 1:201, 1968
64. Bolin RW, Robinson WA, Sutherland J, Hamman RF: Busulphan versus hydroxyurea in long-term therapy of chronic myelogenous leukemia. Cancer 50:1683, 1982
65. Talpaz M, Kantarjian HM, McCredie K, et al: Hematologic remission and cytogenetic improvement induced by recombinant human interferon alpha-A in chronic myelogenous leukemia. N Engl J Med 314:1065, 1986
66. Schwartz JH, Canellos GP: Hydroxyurea in the management of the hematologic complications of chronic granulocytic leukemia. Blood 46:11, 1975
67. Galton DAG: Myeleran in chronic myeloid leukaemia. Lancet 1:208, 1953
68. Koeffler HP, Golde DW: Chronic myelogenous leukemia: New concepts. N Engl J Med 304:1269, 1981
69. Council of Medical Research for Working Party in Therapeutic Trials and Leukaemia. Chronic granulocytic leukaemia: Comparison of radiotherapy and busulphan therapy. Br Med J 1:201, 1969
70. Goldman JM: Management of chronic myeloid leukaemia. Scand J Haematol 37:269, 1986
71. Singer CJR, McDonald GA, Douglas AS: Twenty-five year survival of chronic granulocytic leukaemia with spontaneous karyotype conversion. Br J Haematol 57:309, 1984
72. Appelbaum FR, Najfeld V, Singer JW: Prolonged survival with spontaneous decline in the frequency of Ph[1]-positive cells and subsequent development of mixed Ph[1]-positive and Ph[1]-negative blast crisis. Cancer 51:149, 1983
73. Kyle RA, Schwartz RA, Olner HB, Dameshek W: Syndrome resembling adrenal cortical insufficiency associated with long term busulfan (Myleran) therapy. Blood 18:497, 1981
74. Wareham NJ, Johnson SA, Goldman JM: Relationship of the duration of chronic phase in chronic granulocytic leukaemia to the need for treatment during the first year after diagnosis. Cancer Chemother Pharmacol 8:205, 1982
75. Council of Medical Research for Working Party in Therapeutic Trials and Leukaemia: Randomized trial of splenectomy in Ph[1]-positive chronic granulocytic leukaemia including an analysis of prognostic features. Br J Haematol 54:415, 1983
76. Gomez GA, Sokal JE, Mittelman A, Aungst CW: Splenectomy for palliation of chronic myelocytic leukemia. Am J Med 61:14, 1976
77. Wolf DJ, Silver RT: Splenectomy in chronic myeloid leukemia. Ann Intern Med 89:684, 1978
78. The Italian Cooperative Study Group on Chronic Myeloid Leukemia. Results of a prospective randomized trial of early splenectomy in chronic myeloid leukemia. Cancer 56:445, 1984
79. Ihde DC, Canellos GC, Schwartz JH, DeVita VT: Splenectomy in the chronic phase of chronic granulocytic leukemia. Effects in 32 patients. Ann Intern Med 84:17, 1976
80. Gratwohl A, Goldman J, Gluckman E, Zwaan F: Effect of splenectomy before bone marrow transplantation on survival in chronic granulocytic leukaemia. Lancet 2:1290, 1985
81. Richards HGH, Spiers ASD: Chronic granulocytic leukaemia in pregnancy. Br J Radiol 48:261, 1975
82. Talpaz M, McCredie K, Kantarjian H, et al: Chronic myelogenous leukaemia: Haematological remissions with alpha interferon. Br J Haematol 64:87, 1986
83. Spiers ASD: Metamorphosis of chronic granulocytic leukemia: Diagnosis, classification and management. Br J Haematol 41:1, 1979
84. Mason JE, DeVita VT, Canellos GP: Thrombocytosis in chronic granulocytic leukemia: Incidence and clinical significance. Blood 44:483, 1974
85. Sonta S, Sandberg AA: Chromosomes and causation of human cancer and leukemia. XXIX. Further studies on karyotypic progression in CML. Cancer 41:153, 1978

86. Kohno S, Sandberg AA: Chromosomes and causation of human cancer and leukemia. XXXIX. Usual and unusual findings in Ph[1]-positive CML. Cancer 46:2227, 1980
87. Whang–Peng J, Canellos GP, Carbone PP, Tijo JH: Clinical implications of cytogenetic variants in chronic myelocytic leukemia. Blood 32:755, 1968
88. Terjanian T, Kantarjian H, Keating M, et al: Clinical and prognostic features of patients with Philadelphia chromosome-positive chronic myelogenous leukemia and extramedullary disease. Cancer 59:297, 1987
89. Chabner BA, Haskell CM, Canellos GP: Destructive bone lesions in chronic granulocytic leukemia. Medicine 48:401, 1969
90. Ballard HS, Marcus AJ: Hypercalcemia in chronic myelogenous leukemia. N Engl J Med 282:663, 1970
91. Walter RM, Jr, Greenberg BR: Hypercalcemia in the accelerated phase of chronic myelogenous leukemia. Cancer 46:1174, 1980
92. McGlave PB, Arthur DC, Weisdorf D: Allogeneic bone marrow transplantation as treatment for accelerating chronic myelogenous leukemia. Blood 63:219, 1984
93. Goldman JM, Apperly JF, Jones L, et al: Bone marrow transplantation for patients with chronic myelogenous leukemia. N Engl J Med 314:202, 1986
94. Speck B, Bortin MM, Champlin R, et al: Allogeneic bone marrow transplantation for chronic myelogenous leukemia. Lancet 1:665, 1984
95. McGlave P, Arthur D, Haake R, et al: Therapy of chronic myelogenous leukemia with allogeneic bone marrow transplantation. J Clin Oncol 5:1033, 1987
96. Rosenthal S, Canellos GP, DeVita VT, Gralnick HR: Characteristics of blast crisis in chronic granulocytic leukemia. Blood 49:705, 1977
97. Polli N, O'Brien M, Tavares De Castro J, et al: Characterization of blast cells in chronic granulocytic leukaemia in transformation, acute myelofibrosis and undifferentiated leukaemia. I. Ultrastructural morphology and cytochemistry. Br J Haematol 59:277, 1985
98. Marks SM, Baltimore D, McCaffrey R: Terminal transferase as a predictor of initial responsiveness to vincristine and prednisone in blastic chronic myelogenous leukemia. N Engl J Med 298:812, 1978
99. San Miguel JF, Tavares De Castro J, Matutes E, et al: Characterization of blast cells in chronic granulocytic leukaemia in transformation, acute myelofibrosis and undifferentiated leukaemia. II. Studies with monoclonal antibodies and terminal transferase. Br J Haematol 59:297, 1985
100. Griffin JDG, Todd RF, Ritz J, et al: Differentiation patterns in the blast phase of chronic myeloid leukemia. Blood 61:85, 1983
101. Bakshi A, Minowada J, Arnold A, et al: Lymphoid blast crisis of chronic myelogenous leukemia represents stages in the development of B-cell precursors. N Engl J Med 309:826, 1983
102. Bourinbaiar AA, Georgoulias V, Consolini R, et al: T cell lineage involvement in lymphoid blast crisis of chronic myeloid leukemia. Blood 66:1155, 1985
103. Chan LC, Furley AJ, Ford AM, et al: Clonal rearrangement and expression of the T cell receptor B gene and involvement of the breakpoint cluster region in blast crisis of CGL. Blood 67:533, 1986
104. van der Merwe T, Bernstein R, Derman D, et al: Acute promyelocytic transformation of chronic myeloid leukaemia. Br J Haematol 64:751, 1986
105. Misawa S, Lee E, Schiffer CA, et al: Association of the translocation (15;17) with the malignant proliferation of promyelocytes in acute leukemia and chronic myelogenous leukemia at blastic crisis. Blood 67:270, 1986
106. Williams WC, Weiss GB: Megakaryoblastic transformation of chronic myelogenous leukemia. Cancer 49:921, 1982
107. Rodenhuis S, Smets L, Slater R, et al: Distinguishing the Philadelphia chromosome of acute lymphoblastic leukemia from its counterpart in chronic myelogenous leukemia. N Engl J Med 313:51, 1985
108. Clark SS, MacLaughlin J, Crist WM, et al: Unique forms of the abl tyrosinase kinase distinguish Ph-positive CML from Ph-positive ALL. Science 235:85, 1987
109. Bartram CR, Janseen JWG, Becher R, et al: Persistence of chronic myelocytic leukemia despite deletion of rearranged bcr/c-abl sequences in blast crisis. J Exp Med 144:1389, 1986
110. Janossy G, Woodruff RK, Pippard MJ, et al: Relation of "lymphoid" phenotype and response to chemotherapy incorporating vincristine-prednisone in the acute phase of Ph[1]-positive leukemia. Cancer 43:426, 1979
111. Schwartz JH, Canellos GP, Young RC, DeVita VT: Meningeal leukemia in the blastic phase of chronic granulocytic leukemia. Am J Med 59:819, 1974
112. Jain K, Arlin Z, Mertelsmann R, et al: Philadelphia chromosome and terminal transferase positive acute leukemia: Similarity of terminal phase of chronic myelogenous leukemia and de novo acute presentation. J Clin Oncol 1:669, 1983
113. Coleman M, Silver RT, Pajak TF, et al: Combination chemotherapy for terminal phase chronic granulocytic leukemia: Cancer and Leukemia Group B studies. Blood 55:29, 1980
114. Spiers ADS, Costello C, Catovsky D, et al: Chronic granulocytic leukaemia: Multiple drug chemotherapy for acute transformation. Br Med J 2:77, 1974
115. Vallejos CS, Trujillo JM, Cork A, et al: Blastic crisis in chronic granulocytic leukemia: Experience in 39 patients. Cancer 34:1806, 1974
116. Duhamel G, Najman A, Gorin N, et al: Etude de la transformation aigue dans 45 cas de leucemie myeloide chronique. Nouv Rev Fran de'Hematol 15:301, 1975
117. Pedersen–Bjergaard J, Worm AM, Hainau B: Blastic transformation of chronic myelocytic leukaemia: Clinical manifestations, prognostic factors and results of therapy. Scand J Haematol 18:292, 1977
118. Schiffer CA, DeBelis R, Kasdorf H, Wiernik PH: Treatment of blast crisis of chronic myelogenous leukemia with 5-azacytidine and VP16-213. Cancer Treat Rep 66:267, 1982
119. Preisler HD, Raza A, Hibby D, et al: Treatment of myeloid blast crisis of chronic myelogenous leukemia. Cancer Treat Rep 68:1351, 1984
120. Canellos GP, DeVita VT, Whang–Peng J, Carbone PP: Hematologic and cytogenetic remission of blastic transformation in chronic granulocytic leukemia. Blood 38:671, 1971
121. Koller CA, Miller DM: Preliminary data on the therapy of the myeloid blast phase of chronic granulocytic leukemia with plicamycin and hydroxyurea. N Engl J Med 315:1433, 1986
122. McGlave PB, Arthur DC, Weisdorf D, et al: Allogeneic bone marrow transplantation as treatment for accelerating chronic myelogenous leukemia. Blood 63:219, 1984
123. McGlave P, Arthur D, Haake R, et al: Therapy of chronic myelogenous leukemia with allogeneic bone marrow transplantation. J Clin Oncol 5:1033, 1987
124. Segel GB, Simon W, Lichtman MA: Variables influencing the timing of marrow transplantation in patients with chronic myelogenous leukemia. Blood 68:1055, 1986
125. Buckner CD, Clift RA, Fefer A, et al: Treatment of blastic transformation of chronic granulocytic leukemia by high dose cyclophosphamide, total body irradiation and infusion and cryopreserved autologous marrow. Exp Hematol 2:138, 1974
126. Apperly JF, Jones L, Hale G: Bone marrow transplantation for patients with chronic myelogenous leukemia: T-cell depletion with Campath 1 reduces the incidence of graft-vs-host disease but may increase the risk of leukemic relapse. Bone Marrow Transplant 1:341, 1986
127. Smith JL, Hereema NA, Provisor AJ: Leukemic transformation of engrafted bone marrow cells. Br J Haematol 60:415, 1985
128. Marmont A, Frassoni F, Bacigalupo A, et al: Recurrence of Ph[1]-positive leukemia in donor cells after marrow transplantation for chronic granulocytic leukemia. N Engl J Med 310:903, 1984
129. Ganesan TS, Min GL, Goldman JM, Young BD: Molecular analysis of relapse in chronic myeloid leukemia after allogeneic bone marrow transplantation. Blood 70:873, 1987
130. McGlave P, Scott E, Ramsay N, et al: Unrelated donor bone marrow transplantation for chronic myelogenous leukemia. Blood 70:877, 1987
131. Degliantoni G, Mangoni L, Rizzoli V: In vitro restoration of polyclonal hematopoiesis in chronic myelogenous leukemia after in vitro treatment with 4-hydroperoxycyclophosphamide. Blood 65:753, 1985
132. Dube ID, Kalousek DK, Coulombel L, et al: Cytogenetic studies of early myeloid progenitor compartments in Ph[1]-positive chronic myeloid leukemia. II. Long-term culture reveals the persistence of Ph[1]-negative progenitors in treated as well as newly diagnosed patients. Blood 63:1172, 1984
133. Dube ID, Arlin ZA, Kalousek DK, et al: Nonclonal hemopoietic progenitor cells detected in long-term marrow cultures from a Turner syndrome mosaic with chronic myeloid leukemia. Blood 64:1284, 1984
134. Fialkow PJ, Jacobson RJ, Singer JW, et al: Philadelphia chromosome (Ph[1])-negative chronic myelogenous leukemia (CML): A clonal disease with origin in a multipotent stem cell. Blood 56:70, 1980
135. Kaye FJ, Najfeld V, Singer J, et al: Confirming evidence for the clonal development and stem cell origin of Philadelphia chromosome-negative chronic myelogenous leukemia. Am J Hematol 17:93, 1984
136. Najfeld V, Gordon J, Clark S, et al: Personal communication. 1988
137. Morris CM, Reeve AE, Fitzgerald PH, et al: Genomic diversity correlates with clinical variation in Ph-negative chronic myeloid leukaemia. Nature 320:281, 1986
138. Ganesan TS, Rasool F, Gu AP, et al: Rearrangement of the bcr gene in Philadelphia chromosome-negative chronic myeloid leukemia. Blood 68:959, 1986
139. Kurzock R, Blick MB, Talpaz M, et al: Rearrangement in the breakpoint cluster region and the clinical course of Philadelphia-negative chronic myelogeous leukemia. Ann Intern Med 105:673, 1986
140. Krauss S, Sokal J, Sandberg AA: Comparison of Philadelphia chromosome-positive and -negative patients with chronic myelocytic leukemia. Ann Intern Med 61:625, 1984
141. Ezdinli EZ, Sokal JE, Crosswhite BS, Sandberg AA: Philadelphia chromosome-positive and -negative chronic myelocytic leukemia. Ann Intern Med 72:175, 1970
142. Canellos GP, Whang–Peng J, DeVita VT: Chronic granulocytic leukemia without the Philadelphia chromosome. Am J Clin Pathol 65:467, 1976
143. Altman AJ, Palmer CG, Baehner RL: Juvenile "chronic granulocytic" leukemia: A panmyelopathy with prominent monocytic involvement and circulating monocyte colony-forming cells. Blood 43:341, 1974
144. Holton CP, Johnson WW: Chronic myelocytic leukemia in infant siblings. J Pediatr 72:377, 1968
145. Castro–Malaspina H, Schaison G, Passe H, et al: Subacute and chronic myelomonocytic leukemia in children (juvenile CML). Cancer 54:675, 1984
146. Randall DL, Reiquam CW, Githens JH, Robinson A: Familial myeloproliferative disease: A new syndrome closely resembling myelogenous leukemia in children. Am J Dis Child 110:479, 1965
147. Travis SF: Fetal erythropoiesis in juvenile chronic myelocytic leukemia. Blood 62:602, 1983
148. Brodeur GM, Dow LW, Williams DL: Cytogenetic features of juvenile chronic myelogenous leukemia. Blood 53:812, 1979
149. Ghione F, Mecucci C, Symann M: Cytogenetic investigation in childhood chronic myelocytic leukemia. Cancer Genet Cytogenet 15:317, 1986
150. Lilleyman JS, Harrison JF, Black JA: Treatment of juvenile chronic myeloid leukemia with sequential subcutaneous cytarabine and oral mercaptopurine. Blood 49:559, 1977

151. Sanders JE, Buckner CD, Stewart P, Thomas ED: Successful treatment of juvenile chronic granulocytic leukemia with marrow transplantation. Pediatrics 63:44, 1979
152. Sanders JE: Personal communication
153. Reilly EB, Rapaport SI, Karr NW, et al: Familial chronic lymphocytic leukemia. Arch Intern Med 90:87, 1952
154. Gunz F, Dameshek W: Familial chronic lymphocytic leukemia in a family including twin brothers and a son. JAMA 164:1323, 1957
155. Balttner WA, Strober W, Muchmore AV, et al: Familial chronic lymphocytic leukemia: Immunologic and cellular characterization. Ann Intern Med 84:554, 1976
156. Fraumeni JF, Vogel CL, DeVita VT: Familial chronic lymphocytic leukemia. Ann Intern Med 71:279, 1969
157. Branda RF, Ackerman SK, Handwerger BS et al: Lymphocyte studies in familial chronic lymphatic leukemia. Am J Med 64:508, 1978
158. Neuland CY, Blattner WA, Mann DL, et al: Familial chronic lymphocytic leukemia. J Natl Cancer Inst 71:1143, 1983
159. Seligmann M, Danon F, Mihaesco C, Fudenberg H: Immunoglobulin abnormalities in families of patients with Waldenstrom's macroglobulinemia. Am J Med 43:66, 1967
160. Conley CL, Misiti J, Laster AJ: Genetic factors predisposing to chronic lymphocytic leukemia and to autoimmune disease. Medicine 59:323, 1980
161. Freedman AS, Boyd AW, Bierber FR, et al: Normal cellular counterparts of B cell chronic lymphocytic leukemia. Blood 70:418, 1987
162. Rudders RA: B lymphocyte subpopulations in chronic lymphocytic leukemia. Blood 47:229, 1976
163. Ternynck T, Dighiero G, Follezou J, Binet JL: Comparison of normal and CLL lymphocyte surface Ig determinants using peroxidase-labeled antibodies. I. Detection and quantitation of light chain determinants. Blood 43:789, 1974
164. Deegan MJ, Abraham JP, Sawdyk M, Van Slyck EJ: High incidence of monoclonal proteins in the serum and urine of chronic lymphocytic leukemia patients. Blood 64:1207, 1984
165. Martin PJ, Hansen JA, Siadak AW, Nowinski RC: Monoclonal antibody recognizing normal human T lymphocytes and malignant human B lymphocytes: A comparative study. J Immunol 127:1920, 1981
166. Perri RT, Royston I, LeBien T, Kay NE: Chronic lymphocytic leukemia progenitor cells carry the antigens T65, BA-1 and Ia. Blood 61:871, 1983
167. Cone L, Uhr JW: Immunological deficiency disorders associated with chronic lymphocytic leukemia and multiple myeloma. J Clin Invest 43:221, 1964
168. Foa R, Catovsky D, Brozovic M, et al: Clinical staging and immunological findings in chronic lymphocytic leukemia. Cancer 44:483, 1979
169. Fialkow PJ, Reddy AL, Najfeld V, et al: Chronic lymphocytic leukemia: Clonal origin in a committed B-lymphocyte progenitor. Lancet 2:443, 1978
170. Han T: Studies of correlation of lymphocyte response to PHA with the clinical and immunologic status in chronic lymphocytic leukemia. Cancer 31:280, 1973
171. Schultz EF, Davis S, Rubin AD: Further characterization of the circulating cell in chronic lymphocytic leukemia. Blood 48:223, 1976
172. Kay NE, Oken MM, Perri RT: The influential T cell in B-cell neoplasms. J Clin Oncol 1:810, 1983
173. Kay NE, Kaplan ME: Defective T cell responsiveness in chronic lymphocytic leukemia: Analysis of activation events. Blood 67:578, 1986
174. Davis S: The variable pattern of circulating lymphocyte subpopulations in chronic lymphocytic leukemia. N Engl J Med 294:1150, 1976
175. Mangan KF, D'Alessandro L: Hypoplastic anemia in B cell chronic lymphocytic leukemia: Evolution of T cell-mediated suppression of erythropoiesis in early-stage and late-stage disease. Blood 66:533, 1985
176. Ayanlar-Bateman O, Ebert E, Hauptman SP: Defective IL-2 production and responsiveness by T cells in patients with chronic lymphocytic leukemia of B cell variety. Blood 67:279, 1986
177. Kay NE, Zarling JM: Impaired natural killer activity in patients with chronic lymphocytic leukemia is associated with a deficiency of azurophilic cytoplasmic granules in putative NK cells. Blood 63:305, 1984
178. Foa R, Fierro MT, Lusso P, et al: Reduced NK T-cells in B-cell chronic lymphocytic leukemia identified by three monoclonal antibodies: Leu 11, A10, AB8.28. Br J Haematol 62:151, 1986
179. Najfeld V, Fialkow PJ, Karande A, et al: Chromosome analysis of lymphoid cell lines derived from patients with chronic lymphocytic leukemia. Int J Cancer 26:543, 1980
180. Ross FM, Stockdill G: Clonal chromosome abnormalities in chronic lymphocytic leukemia patients revealed by TPA stimulation of whole blood cultures. Cancer Genet Cytogenet 25:109, 1987
181. Han T, Emrich LJ, Ozwer H, Sandberg AA: Prognostic implications of trisomy 12 and non-trisomy 12 karyotypes in B-cell chronic lymphocytic leukemia. Blood 66:470, 1985
182. Juliusson G, Ost RA, Friberg K, et al: Prognostic information from cytogenetic analysis in chronic B-lympocytic leukemia and leukemic immunocytoma. Blood 65:134, 1985
183. Han T, Ozser H, Sadamori N, et al: Prognostic importance of cytogenetic abnormalities in patients with chronic lymphocytic leukemia. N Engl J Med 310:288, 1984
184. Knuutila S, Elonen E, Teerenhavi L, et al: Trisomy 12 in B cells of patients with B-cell chronic lymphocytic leukemia. N Engl J Med 314:865, 1986
185. Han T, Sandamori N, Takeuchi J, et al: Clonal chromosome abnormalities in patients with Waldenstrom's and CLL-associated macroglobulinemia: Significance of trisomy 12. Blood 62:525, 1983
186. Miller DG, Karnofsky DA: Immunologic factors and resistance to infection in chronic lymphocytic leukemia. Am J Med 31:748, 1961
187. Shaw RK, Szwed D, Boggs D, et al: Infection and immunity in chronic lymphocytic leukemia. Arch Intern Med 106:467, 1960
188. Boggs DR, Sofferman SA, Wintrobe MM, Cartwright GE: Factors influencing the duration of survival of patients with chronic lymphocytic leukemia. Am J Med 40:243, 1965
189. Rai KR, Sawitsky A, Cronkite EP, et al: Clinical staging of chronic lymphocytic leukemia. Blood 46:219, 1975
190. Rozman C, Montserrat E, Feliu E, et al: Prognosis of chronic lymphocytic leukemia: A multivariate survival analysis of 150 cases. Blood 59:1001, 1982
191. Rozman C, Montserrat E, Rodriguez-Fernandez JM, et al: Bone marrow histologic pattern—the best single prognostic parameter in chronic lymphocytic leukemia: A multivariate survival analysis of 329 cases. Blood 64:642, 1984
192. Binet JL, LePorrier M, Dighiero G, et al: A clinical staging system for chronic lymphocytic leukemia. Cancer 40:855, 1977
193. Baccarani M, Cavo M, Gobbi M, et al: Staging of chronic lymphocytic leukemia. Blood 59:1191, 1982
194. Dighiero G, Charron D, Debre P, et al: Identification of a pure splenic form of chronic lymphocytic leukemia. Br J Haematol 41:169, 1979
195. Gray JL, Jacobs A, Block M: Bone marrow and peripheral blood lymphocytosis in the prognosis of chronic lymphocytic leukemia. Cancer 33:1169, 1974
196. Michallet M, Sotto JJ, Moulin J, et al: Management of CLL patients after chlorambucil. Special value of a second RAI staging. Eur J Cancer 16:511, 1980
197. Rubenstein DB, Longo DL: Peripheral destruction of platelets in chronic lymphocytic leukemia: Recognition, prognosis and therapeutic implications. Am J Med 71:729, 1981
198. Sawitsky A, Rai KR, Glidewell O, et al: Comparison of daily versus intermittent chlorambucil and prednisone therapy in the treatment of patients with chronic lymphocytic leukemia. Blood 50:1049, 1977
199. Silver RT: The treatment of chronic lymphocytic leukemia. Semin Hematol 6:344, 1969
200. Knospe WH, Loeb V Jr, Huguley CM Jr: Bi-weekly chlorambucil treatment of chronic lymphocytic leukemia. Cancer 33:555, 1974
201. Han T, Ezdinli EZ, Shimaoka K, Desai DJ: Chlorambucil vs combined chlorambucil-corticosteroid therapy in chronic lymphocytic leukemia. Cancer 31:502, 1973
202. Lipeman M, Votaw ML: The treatment of chronic lymphocytic leukemia with COP chemotherapy. Cancer 41:1664, 1978
203. Ezdinli EZ, Stutzman L: Chlorambucil therapy for lymphomas and chronic lymphocytic leukemia. JAMA 191:100, 1965
204. Galton DAG, Wiltshaw E, Szur L, Dacie JV: The use of chlorambucil and steroids in the treatment of chronic lymphocytic leukaemia. Br J Haematol 7:73, 1961
205. Mentzer S, Osteen RT, Starnes HF, et al: Splenic enlargement and hyperfunction as indications of splenectomy in chronic leukemia. Am J Surg 205:13, 1987
206. Mower WR, Hawkins JA, Nelson EW: Postsplenectomy infection in patients with chronic leukemia. Am J Surg 152:583, 1986
207. Ferrant A, Michaux JL, Sokal G: Splenectomy in advanced chronic lymphocytic leukemia. Cancer 58:2130, 1986
208. Cooper IA, Ding JC, Adams PB, et al: Intensive leukapheresis in the management of cytopenias in patients with chronic lymphocytic leukemia and lymphocytic lymphoma. Am J Hematol 6:387, 1979
209. Curtis JE, Hersh EM, Freireich EJ: Leukapheresis therapy of chronic lymphocytic leukemia. Blood 39:163, 1972
210. Fortuny IER, Hadlock DC, Kennedy BJ, et al: The role of continuous flow centrifuge leucapheresis in the management of chronic lymphocytic leukemia. Br J Haematol 32:609, 1976
211. del Regato JA: Total body irradiation of chronic lymphocytic leukemia. Am J Roentgenol 120:504, 1974
212. Johnson RE: Total body irradiation of chronic lymphocytic leukemia. Cancer 25:523, 1970
213. Parmentier C, Chauvel P, Hayat M, et al: La radiotherapie dans la leucemie lymphoide chronique: I. L irradiation and splenique. Nouv Rev Fr Hematol 14:737, 1974
214. Byhardt RW, Brace KC, Wiernik PH: The role of splenic irradiation in chronic lymphocytic leukemia. Cancer 35:1621, 1975
215. Richter MN: Generalized reticular cell sarcoma of lymph nodes associated with lymphocytic leukemia. Am J Pathol 4:285, 1928
216. Foucar K, Rydell RE: Richter's syndrome in chronic lymphocytic leukemia. Cancer 46:118, 1980
217. Trump DL, Mann RB, Phelps R, et al: Richter's syndrome: Diffuse histiocytic lymphoma in patients with chronic lymphocytic leukemia: A report of 5 cases and review of the literature. Am J Med 68:539, 1980
218. Harousseau JL, Flandrin G, Tricot G, et al: Malignant lymphoma supervening in chronic lymphocytic leukemia and related disorders. Richter's syndrome: A study of 25 cases. Cancer 48:1302, 1981
219. Armitage JO, Dick FR, Corder MP: Diffuse histiocytic lymphoma complicating chronic lymphocytic leukemia. Cancer 41:422, 1978
220. Enno A, Catovsky D, O'Brien M, et al: Prolymphocytoid transformation of chronic lymphocytic leukemia. Br J Haematol 41:9, 1979
221. Stark AN, Limbert HJ, Roberts BE, et al: Prolymphocytoid transformation of CLL: A clinical and immunological study of 22 cases. Leuk Res 10:1225, 1986
222. Kjeldsberg C, Marty J: Prolymphocytic transformation of chronic lymphocytic leukemia. Cancer 48:2447, 1981
223. Melo JV, Catovsky D, Gregory W, Galton DG: The relationship between chronic

lymphocytic leukemia and prolymphocytic leukemia. IV. Analysis of survival and prognostic features. Br J Haematol 65:23, 1987
224. Melo JV, Catovsky D, Galton DA: The relationship between chronic lymphocytic leukemia and prolymphocytic leukemia. I. Clinical and laboratory features of 300 patients and characterization of an intermediate group. Br J Haematol 63:377, 1986
225. Melo JV, Catovsky D, Galton DA: The relationship between chronic lymphocytic leukemia and prolymphocytic leukemia. II. Patterns of evolution of prolymphocytoid transformation. Br J Haematol 64:77, 1986
226. Davis JW, Weiss NS, Armstrong BK: Second cancers in patients with chronic lymphocytic leukemia. J Natl Cancer Inst 78:91, 1987
227. Moayeri H, Han T, Stutzman L, Sokal JE: Second neoplasms with chronic lymphocytic leukemia. NY State J Med 76:278, 1976
228. Knospe WH, Gregory SA, Trobaugh FE Jr, et al: Chronic lymphocytic leukemia: Correlation of clinical course and therapeutic response with in vitro testing and morphology of lymphocytes. Am J Hematol 2:73, 1977
229. Ostlund L, Einhorn S, Robert KH, et al: Chronic B-lymphocytic leukemia cells proliferate and differentiate following exposure to interferon in vitro. Blood 67:152, 1986
230. Faltnek CR, Princier GL, Rossio JL: Relationship of the clinical response and binding of recombinant interferon alpha in patients with lymphoproliferative diseases. Blood 67:1077, 1986
231. O'Connell MJ, Colgan JP, Oken MM, et al: Clinical trial of recombinant leukocyte A interferon as initial therapy for favorable histology non-Hodgkin's lymphomas and chronic lymphocytic leukemia: An Eastern Cooperative Oncology Group study. J Clin Oncol 4:128, 1986
232. Talpaz M, Rosenblum M, Kurzock R, et al: Clinical and laboratory changes induced by alpha interferon in chronic lymphocytic leukemia—a pilot study. Am J Hematol 24:341, 1987
233. Dillman RO, Shawler DL, Dillman JB, Royston I: Therapy of chronic lymphocytic leukemia and cutaneous T-cell lymphoma with T101 monoclonal antibody. J Clin Oncol 2:881, 1984
234. Foon KA, Schroff RW, Bunn PA: Effects of monoclonal antibody therapy in patients with chronic lymphocytic leukemia. Blood 64:1085, 1984
235. Gordon J, Abdul-Ahad AK, Hamblin TJ, et al: Mechanisms of tumor cell escape encountered in treating lymphocytic leukaemia with anti-idiotypic antibody. Br J Cancer 49:547, 1984
236. Huhn D, Thiel E, Rodt H, et al: Subtypes of T-cell chronic lymphatic leukemia. Cancer 5:1434, 1983
237. Knowles DM II: The human T-cell leukemias: Clinical, cytomorphologic, immunophenotypic and genotypic characteristics. Hum Pathol 17:14, 1986
238. Noorloos BV, Pegels HG, van Oers RJ, et al: Proliferation of T gamma cells with killer-cell activity in two patients with neutropenia and recurrent infections. N Engl J Med 302:933, 1980
239. Palutke M, Eisenberg L, Kaplan J, et al: Natural killer and suppressor T-cell chronic lymphocytic leukemia. Blood 62:627, 1983
240. Miedema F, Melief JM: Immunobiology of the expanded T cells in T-cell leukemia and T-gamma lymphocytosis. Leuk Res 10:469, 1986
241. Loughran TP Jr, Kadin ME, Starkebaum G, et al: Leukemia of large granular lymphocytes: Association with clonal chromosomal abnormalities and autoimmune neutropenia, thrombocytopenia and hemolytic anemia. Ann Intern Med 102:169, 1985
242. Semenzanto G, Pizzolo G, Ranucci A, et al: Abnormal expansions of polyclonal large to small size granular lymphocytes: Reactive or neoplastic process? Blood 63:1271, 1984
243. Starkebaum G, Martin P, Singer JW, et al: Chronic lymphocytosis with neutropenia: Evidence for a novel, abnormal T-cell population associated with antibody-mediated neutrophil destruction. Clin Immunol Immunopathol 27:110, 1983
244. Foa R, Pelicci PG, Migone N, et al: Analysis of T-cell receptor beta chain gene rearrangements demonstrates the monoclonal nature of T-cell chronic lymphoproliferative disorders. Blood 67:247, 1986
245. Galton DAG, Goldman JM, Wiltshaw E, et al: Prolymphocytic leukaemia. Br J Haematol 27:7, 1974
246. Bearman RM, Pangalis GA, Rappaport H: Prolymphocytic leukemia: Clinical, histological and cytochemical observations. Cancer 42:2360, 1978
247. Catovsky D, Wechsler A, Matutes E, et al: The membrane phenotype of T-prolymphocytic leukemia. Scand J Haematol 29:398, 1982
248. Matutes E, Talavera G, O'Brien M, Catovsky D: The morphologic spectrum of T-prolymphocytic leukaemia. Br J Haematol 64:111, 1986
249. Bouroncle BA, Wiseman BK, Doan CA: Leukemic reticuloendotheliosis. Blood 13:609, 1958
250. Golomb HM, Catovsky D, Golde DW: Hairy cell leukemia: A clinical review based on 71 cases. Ann Intern Med 89:677, 1978
251. Brito-Babapulle V, Pittman S, Melo JV, et al: The 14q+ marker in hairy cell leukaemia. A cytogenetic study of 15 cases. Leuk Res 10:131, 1986
252. Jansen J, LeBien TW, Kersey JH: The phenotype of the neoplastic cells of hairy cell leukemia studied with monoclonal antibodies. Blood 59:609, 1982
253. Golomb H, Strehl S, Oleske D, Vardiman J: Prognostic significance of immunologic phenotype in hairy cell leukemia: Does it exist? Blood 66:1358, 1985
254. Cleary ML, Good GS, Warnke R, et al: Immunoglobulin gene rearrangements in hairy cell leukemia. Blood 64:99, 1984
255. Anderson KC, Boyd AW, Fisher DC, et al: Hairy cell leukemia: A tumor of pre-plasma cells. Blood 65:620, 1985
256. Saxon A, Stevens RH, Golde DW: T-lymphocyte variant of hairy cell leukemia. Ann Intern Med 88:323, 1978
257. Rosenblatt JD, Golde DW, Wachsman W, et al: A second isolate of HTLV-II associated with atypical hairy cell leukemia. N Engl J Med 315:272, 1986
258. Bouza E, Burgaleta C, Golde DW: Infections in hairy cell leukemia. Blood 51:851, 1978
259. Mackowiak PA, Denman SE, Sutker WL, et al: Infections in hairy cell leukemia: Clinical evidence of a pronounced defect in cell-mediated immunity. Am J Med 78:718, 1980
260. Golomb HM, Hanauer SB: Infectious complications associated with hairy cell leukemia. J Infect Dis 143:639, 1981
261. Westbrook CA, Golde DW: Autoimmune disease in hairy cell leukaemia: Clinical syndromes and treatment. Br J Haematol 61:249, 1985
262. Elkon KB, Hughes GRV, Catovsky D, et al: Hairy cell leukemia with polyarteritis nodosa. Lancet 2:280, 1979
263. Jansen J, Hermans J: Splenectomy in hairy cell leukemia: A retrospective multicenter analysis. Cancer 47:2066, 1981
264. Golomb HM, Vardiman JW: Response to splenectomy in 65 patients with hairy cell leukemia: An evaluation of spleen weight and bone marrow involvement. Blood 61:349, 1983
265. Golomb HM: The treatment of hairy cell leukemia. Blood 69:979, 1987
266. Quesada JR, Hersh EM, Manning J, et al: Treatment of hairy cell leukemia with recombinant a-interferon. Blood 68:493, 1986
267. Jacobs AD, Champlin RE, Golde DW: Recombinant alpha-2 interferon for hairy cell leukemia. Blood 65:1017, 1985
268. Golomb HM, Fefer A, Colde IW, et al: Sequential evaluation of alpha-2b interferon treatment in 128 patients with hairy cell leukemia. Sem Oncol 14(suppl 2):13, 1987
269. Spiers ASD, Moore D, Cassileth PA, et al: Hairy cell leukemia: Complete remissions with pentostatin (2′deoxycoformycin). N Engl J Med 316:825, 1987
270. Kraut EH, Bournocle BA, Grever MR: Low-dose deoxycoformycin in the treatment of hairy cell leukemia. Blood 68:1119, 1986
271. Quesada JR, Reuben J, Manning JT, et al: Alpha interferon for induction of remission in hairy cell leukemia. N Engl J Med 310:15, 1984
272. Golomb HM, Jacobs A, Fefer A: Alpha-2 interferon therapy of hairy cell leukemia: a multicenter study of 64 patients. J Clin Oncol 4:900, 1986
273. Spiers ASD, Parekh SJ, Bishop MB: Hairy cell leukemia: induction of complete remission with pentostatin (2′deoxycoformycin). J Clin Oncol 2:1336, 1984
274. Foon KA, Nakano GM, Koller CA et al: Response to 2′-deoxycoformycin after failure of interferon-alpha in nonsplenectomized patients with hairy cell leukemia. Blood 68:297, 1986
275. Cheson BD, Martin A: Clinical trials in hairy cell leukemia: Current status and future directions. Ann Intern Med 106:871, 1987

SYDNEY E. SALMON
J. ROBERT CASSADY

CHAPTER 54 *Plasma Cell Neoplasms*

DEFINITION

Plasma cell neoplasms are a group of related disorders, each of which is associated with proliferation and accumulation of immunoglobulin-secreting cells that are derived from the B-cell series of immunocytes. Tumor cells in these neoplasms retain the cytoplasmic differentiation of normal plasma cells and are particularly well adapted to high rates of synthesis and secretion of immunoglobulin (Ig). They contain substantial quantities of rough-surfaced endoplasmic reticulum in their cytoplasm and are specialized for rapid rates of antibody production and secretion into the plasma. In the normal immune response, individual plasma cells can synthesize and secrete antibody immunoglobulin at rates up to 100,000 molecules each minute. On the basis of their synthesis and secretion of an electrophoretically homogeneous immunoglobulin (M-component or M-protein) these neoplasms have been hypothesized to be monoclonal—and derived originally from a single transformed B lymphocyte or plasma cell. A large amount of additional laboratory data is now available in support of the concept of monoclonality of origin of B-cell neoplasms. A number of synonyms have also been applied to plasma cell neoplasms (*e.g.*, dysproteinemias, gammopathies, immunoglobulinopathies, monoclonal gammopathies, paraproteinemias, plasma cell dysgrasias). In terms of incidence and severity, the most important malignant plasma cell neoplasm is multiple myeloma.

The plasma cell neoplasms have been best characterized by their monoclonal immunoglobulin products. M-components are seen in both the malignant plasma cell disorders (*e.g.*, multiple myeloma and Waldenström's macroglobulinemia) and in clinically unclear or idiopathic circumstances, and these may be associated with either benign, premalignant, or early malignant disorders. The idiopathic M-proteins are, therefore, best described clinically as monoclonal gammopathies of unknown significance (MGUS).[1] Transient M-components have been observed in patients recovering from pneumonia, hepatitis, and other infections; after drug reactions; after other illnesses; or after bone marrow transplantation. The monoclonal immunoglobulins secreted in malignant plasma cell disorders are the equivalent of homogeneous normal antibody molecules; however, in most instances the antigen to which the monoclonal antibody binds is not known. For those few instances in which the antibody specificity of M-components has been identified, the specificity appears to be random and not focused toward any specific or tumor-associated antigenic stimulus. An M-component can be detected and discriminated from normal immunoglobulins, by serum electrophoresis, when its concentration is about 0.5 g/dl or higher. Detection of a serum M-component is of major diagnostic value in plasma cell disorders. Quantities of Ig in the range of 0.5 g/dl are the product of approximately 10^9 to 10^{10} monoclonal immunoglobulin-secreting cells in the body.[2] A classification of diseases associated with M-component secretion appears in Table 54-1.

There are five major classes of immunoglobulins synthesized by B lymphocytes and plasma cells: IgG, IgA, IgM, IgD, and IgE. Antibody protein molecules in each of these classes have common monomeric structures. Any one antibody molecule has a monomeric structure comprised of two identical heavy (H) chains and two identical light (L) chains, each of which has constant (c) and variable (v) regions of amino acid sequence. The constant regions of the heavy chains for

TABLE 54-1. Classification of Disorders Associated with Monoclonal Immunoglobulin (M-Component) Secretion

Disorder	*M-Component*	
Plasma cell neoplasms		
Multiple myeloma	IgG > IgA > IgD > IgE; ±free L chain or L chain alone (κ > λ); rarely biclonal or without detectable Ig abnormality	
"Solitary" myeloma of bone		
Extramedullary plasmacytoma		
Macroglobulinemia	IgM ± free L chain (κ > λ)	
Heavy-chain disease	γ, α, or μ chain or fragment; δ, or ε	
Primary amyloidosis	Free L chain (λ > κ) or L chain fragment alone or plus IgG, IgA, IgM, or IgD	
Monoclonal gammopathy of unknown significance	IgG, IgM, IgA, or IgD usually without urinary L chain secretion	
Other B-cell neoplasms		
Chronic lymphocytic leukemia	M-component (occasionally secreted) IgM > IgG	
B-cell non-Hodgkin's lymphomas (any morphologic pattern or lymphoid cell types)		
Nonlymphoid neoplasms		
Chronic myelogenous leukemia	No consistent patterns	
Carcinoma of colon, breast, prostate, or other sites		
"Autoimmune" or autoreactive disorders		
Cold agglutinin disease (some	M-component	Antibody activity of M-component
characteristics of	IgMκ most common	Anti-I antigen of RBC membrane
Waldenström's)	IgM	Anti-IgG
Mixed cryoglobulinemia	IgG	Anti-IgG
Hypergammaglobulinemia	IgM	?
Sjögren's syndrome		
Miscellaneous inflammatory storage, or infectious disorders		
Lichen myxedematosus	IgGλ	
Gaucher's disease	IgG	
Cirrhosis, sarcoid, parasitic diseases, renal acidosis	No consistent pattern	

Modified from Ref. 3.

the various classes are γ, α, μ, δ, or ε, respectively. The L chains on the molecule are of either the κ or λ constant region type. The constant regions of the molecule define its class specificity as well as a number of other biologic characteristics (*e.g.*, the ability to fix complement). Separate *c* genes code for the constant regions of the H and L chains for each H chain class and L chain type. The *variable regions* of H and L chains are considered to be structurally related to the region of the specific antigen-binding site of the molecule and are, therefore, unique to each specific antibody. A very large set of *v* genes code for the variable portions of the Ig molecule in relation to the wide variety of antibody specificities present in the normal immune response. The variable region of an M-component can be identified immunologically as having a specific *idiotype*, or unique structural region, that distinguishes it from virtually all other immunoglobulin antibody molecules. Table 54-2 summarizes structural and functional properties of normal immunoglobulins. These properties are generally shared by M-proteins.

Although not clinically practical, radioimmunoassay for the idiotype on a serum M-component could permit detection of the presence of as few as 10^3 to 10^4 neoplastic cells in the body.[2] For all Ig classes other than IgM, the monomeric form of the Ig is secreted and has a molecular mass (M_r) of about 150,000 to 190,000. Immunoglobulin is secreted as a pentameric unit with a M_r of 900,000. As with a number of

TABLE 54-2. Properties of Normal Immunoglobulins

	IgG	*IgA*	*IgM*	*IgD*	*IgE*
Molecular mass	150,000	160,000	900,000	180,000	200,000
Subclasses	4	2	1	2(?)	1
Serum concentration (mg/dl; mean)	1140	180	100	3	0.03
Fixes complement	+	+	+	—	+
Carbohydrate (%)	2.6	5–10	10	10–12	11
T½ (days)	23.6*	5.8	5.1	2.8	2.3

*Half-lite varies proportionally to total serum IgG concentration.

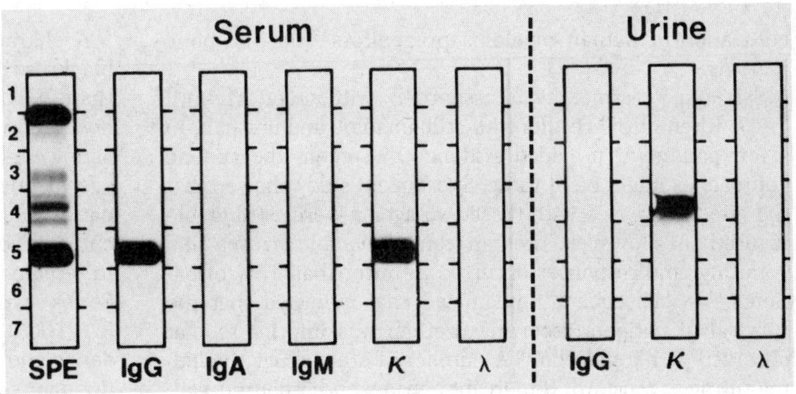

FIG. 54-1. Identification of serum and urine M-components by the immunofixation technique. The legends indicate the specificity of the antiserum used in developing the immunofixation pattern. In this case, the patient can be seen to have an IgGκ serum M-component. Additionally, κ Bence Jones proteinuria is present.

other proteins, immunogloblins are secreted with varying amounts of attached carbohydrate; this also applies to M-components. Whereas myeloma can be diagnosed in patients with any of the Ig types just summarized, IgM M-components are usually associated with other malignant or benign plasma cell disorders. The synthesis of H and L chain is generally well balanced in normal antibody-producing clones. However, in neoplastic clones, biosynthesis of intracellular H and L chain is sometimes "unbalanced," with an excess synthesis of free L chains that are secreted by the cell as L chain dimers of M_r 60,000. Because of their relatively low M_r, L chain dimers are normally filtered by the renal glomerulus, partially reabsorbed and catabolized in the renal tubules, and partially excreted in the urine. Detection of substantial quantities of free light chains in the urine serves as a useful diagnostic test in myeloma and related disorders.

Serum M-components are usually observed as a sharp peak or "spike" in the beta or gamma globulin regions on electrophoresis. Urinary M-components are usually detected in concentrates of 24-hr urine collections, and they migrate similarly on electrophoresis. Definition of an M-component as being monoclonal requires H and L chain typing. This is done with immunoelectrophoresis or immunofixation techniques. Examples of a serum and urine protein electrophoresis and H and L chain typing by immunofixation in a specific myeloma case are depicted in Figure 54-1.

HISTORY

Although skeletal evidence for the existence of myeloma in earlier millennia has been obtained from Egyptian mummies and other anthropological remains, the first published descriptions of major clinical features in a patient with multiple myeloma were made about 1850 in England. A well-respected tradesman, Thomas Alexander McBean, was seen in consultation by Dr. William Macintyre of London in 1845. The patient's symptoms included episodes of fatigue, diffuse bone pain, and urinary frequency. Mcintyre treated McBean during the course of that year and from urinalysis tests, Macintyre detected the presence of a urinary protein with the heat properties often observed for urinary L chains. He diagnosed "mollities and fragilitas ossium" based on the patient's bony symptoms and consulted with Dr. Thomas Watson concerning therapy for his patient.[4] Later that year Dr. Henry Bence Jones also tested urine specimens provided by Macintyre and Watson and corroborated the heat properties of urinary L chains (which we now call *Bence Jones proteins*). Bence Jones thought that the protein was the "hydrated deuteroxide of albumin" and published his findings several years before Macintyre published his case report.[5] Bence Jones also emphasized the potential importance of looking for this urinary protein in other cases with mollities ossium. When the patient died in 1846, a surgeon, Dr. John Dalrymple, examined several vertebrae and a rib from the patient and made both gross and microscopic observations. Woodcuts made from Dr. Dalrymple's drawings were included in his report and have the appearance of myeloma cells.[6]

In 1873, Rustizky independently described a similar patient and employed the term *multiple myeloma* for the first time to focus on the multiple bone tumors that were present.[7] In 1889, Kahler published a major view on multiple myeloma, and the disease became known, particularly in Europe, as Kahler's disease.[8] Ellinger, in 1899, identified the increased serum proteins and sedimentation rate in myeloma.[9] In 1900, Wright published a case report in which he indicated that myeloma did not arise from the red marrow but, rather, was a neoplasm comprising specifically plasma cells.[10] Wright's case was probably also the first one in which x-ray films were used to show diagnostic abnormalities in the patient's ribs.

Other developments that enhanced the diagnosis or understanding of myeloma included the development of bone marrow aspiration in 1929[11] and of electrophoresis to separate serum proteins in 1937.[12] Within several years of the development of electrophoresis, the tall narrow-based spike in the gamma globulin zone was identified in myeloma.[13] In 1938, Magnus-Levy described amyloidosis as a complication of multiple myeloma,[14] and in 1953, Grabar and Williams developed immunoelectrophoresis, which enabled the precise immunologic identification of the H and L chains present in a monoclonal immunoglobulin and, thereby, enhanced the diagnosis of monoclonality of an Ig.[15] In the 1970s, structural evidence for the relationship of amyloid in myeloma to the variable component of L chains was subsequently achieved by Glenner and his colleagues by studying the amino acid sequence of solubilized amyloid fibrils.[16] Additionally, methods for immunoquantitation of the total body burden of tumor cells in myeloma, for definition of its relationship to clinical manifestations of disease, and for provision of a useful staging system were developed,[17] as were methods of cultivation of human myeloma progenitors from the bone marrow.

Systemic treatment was essentially without effect until 1947, when initial results with stilbamadine and urethan, in a few patients,[18] provided evidence that chemotherapeutic approaches might be of value. Subsequent study showed that the effects reported with these two agents were attributable to urethan. However, urethan caused notable nausea and vomiting, and responses occurred in fewer than 15% of patients.[19] A subsequent randomized trial indicated that the survival of patients receiving urethan was inferior to that observed with a placebo.[19] A number of other drugs, including nitrogen mustard, 6-mercaptopurine, and 5-flourouracil, were tried and appeared to be of no value.[20] In 1958, the use of a racemic mixture of D-, and L-phenylalanine mustards (Sarcolysin) was reported to be of use in cases of myeloma by Blokhin and colleagues,[21] and this was subsequently confirmed by others. Subsequently, both the D- and L-isomers of phenylalanine mustard were tested separately, and the antimyeloma activity was found to reside in the L-isomer, melphalan. Bergsagel and colleagues, in the Southwest Oncology Group (SWOG), reported in 1962 that melphalan could induce remissions in about one-third of myeloma patients.[19] Several years thereafter, similar activity was observed with another alkylating agent, cyclophosphamide.[22] Administration of high doses of the glucocorticoid, prednisone, alone on alternate days, was first reported to induce remissions in relapsing or refractory myeloma cases in 1967.[23] The use of melphalan in combination with prednisone was then studied extensively.[24,25] A few other single agents with definite activity in myeloma have subsequently been reported including carmustine (BCNU),[26] doxorubicin,[27] and interferon-α.[28]

INCIDENCE AND MORTALITY

Incidence data in the United States as reported by the Surveillance, Epidemiology, and End Result (SEER) program of the National Cancer Institute for the period 1973 to 1977 indicate that multiple myeloma accounts for 1.1% of all malignancies in whites and 2.1% in blacks.[29] The average annual incidence for myeloma (age-adjusted) in whites is 4.3 : 100,000 and 3.0 : 100,000 in males and females, respectively.[29] In blacks, the incidence is higher, 9.6 : 100,000 and 6.7 : 100,000 in males and females, respectively.[29] Myeloma is the most common lymphoid malignancy in blacks and the second most common in whites, for whom non-Hodgkin's lymphoma ranks first. Incidence and mortality data for myeloma in whites have recently been updated by SEER and have risen considerably in both males and females from the late 1940s to the late 1970s, with net increases of 145% or more.[30] Among women, the increase in myeloma morbidity was exceeded only by that of lung cancer. In 1983–1984 the morbidity for whites with myeloma in the United States was 2.8 : 100,000 in males and 2.1 : 100,000 in females. Incidence figures for multiple myeloma in Western European countries are similar to those for the American white population and have been estimated at 2.6 : 100,000 in England[31] and 3.3 : 100,000 for Sweden.[32]

A characteristic feature of myeloma in both whites and blacks is the increasing incidence with increasing age. Fewer than 2% of the patients are under 40 years of age at diagnosis; however, the disease has been reported to occur in young adults and children.[33] In the United States, the median age of onset is 68 in males and 70 in females.[28] The age patterns for death for myeloma closely parallel the incidence curves; the median age at death is 70 years in males and 71 in females.[34] For 1983–1984, the morbidity for the United States white population with multiple myeloma was 8.7 : 100,000 in males and 5.1 : 100,000 for females.[30] Incidence and mortality appear to have been rising recently, but the data supporting this trend suggest that the apparent increases in myeloma reflect prior underdiagnosis, rather than a true increase in incidence.[30,35]

A similar age distribution is also observed in the related plasma cell disorders of MGUS and Waldenström's macroglobulinemia.[36] The disorder MGUS occurs much more frequently than multiple myeloma, but it can be detected only with specific screening examinations for monoclonal immunoglobulins. Axelsson and colleagues[37] screened for serum M-components in 6995 asymptomatic adults over the age of 25 who composed most of the adult population in four parishes in Sweden.[37] Sera from 1% of these subjects contained M-components, and the prevalence of MGUS in this population increased with age, from 2% of those in the eighth decade to almost 6% of those in the ninth decade. Use of more sensitive screening tests for M-components appears to increase the frequency with which MGUS can be observed.[38] Because MGUS has a long natural history and cases tend to accumulate over time, the annual age incidence is not known.

PATHOGENESIS

In addition to humans, myeloma has been reported to occur in a variety of mammalian species including mice, rats, hamsters, cats, and dogs.[39–45] In rodents, increased susceptibility to plasma cell tumors has been selected fortuitously in some strains compared with others as a result of nonrandom breeding patterns used to create genetic uniformity. An additional factor in various domesticated species, which is probably important, is the prevalence of endogenous retroviruses. General mechanisms by which retroviruses are associated with the development of B-lymphoid neoplasms are through mutagenicity resulting from insertion of viral genomes into cellular DNA[46] and as a result of the transforming ability of certain recombinant retroviruses. In some animal models, retroviruses carry specific oncogenes that play a direct role in malignant transformation.[47] A human B-cell lymphocytotropic virus with oncogenic potential has recently been reported.[48]

MURINE MODELS OF DISORDERS ASSOCIATED WITH M-COMPONENTS

Study of inbred mouse strains has yielded substantial information on both the occurrence of asymptomatic monoclonal gammopathies without obvious tumor formation (perhaps the equivalent of MGUS) and on mechanisms of induction of plasma cell neoplasms.[49] Monoclonal gammopathies (usually IgG) without tumor formation occur spontaneously in approximately 60% of mice of the inbred C57BL/Ka strain within 24 months, whereas BALB/c and CBA/Rij mice have a very low spontaneous incidence of monoclonal gammopathies.[50] Spontaneous plasmacytomas are infrequent findings in old mice, and they are usually encountered as an incidental finding.[50] In contrast with the low spontaneous susceptibility of BALB/c mice to monoclonal gammopathy or spontaneous plasma cell tumors, peritoneal plasmacytomas can be very readily induced in inbred strains.[51–53] However, the C57BL/Ka strain, which expresses spontaneous monoclonal gammopathies, is relatively resistant to plasmacytoma induction.[54] Plasmacytomas can be readily induced in BALB/c mice with the intraperitoneal injection of mineral oils[55,56] or by implantation of solid plastic materials such as lucite.[57] The plasmacytomas develop within oil or foreign-body granulomas in the peritoneum or mesentery, and each plasmacytoma produces a unique M-component. Chemically defined mineral oil alkane components, such as pristane, also induce plasmacytomas,[58] and this process can be facilitated by subsequent infection of the mice with the Abelson virus. Such induced plasmacytomas in mice lead to the production of a growth factor in the peritoneal fluid that sustains the growth of the neoplasm.[59,60] Plasmacytoma growth factors that support the growth of human myeloma cells in culture have been isolated from the splenic macrophages of oil-treated BALB/c mice[61] as well as from a number of other sources.[62–64] Most recently, a human B-cell growth factor interleukin-6 (IL-6; BFS2, IFNβ_2) has been isolated from Epstein-Barr virus (EBV)-infected B cells or monocytes.[65] This IL-6 has been purified and produced by recombinant DNA methods and has been identified as the plasmacytoma growth factor. Interleukin-6 is a 184-amino acid glycoprotein that stimulates the growth of EBV-infected human B cells as well as mouse and rat plasmacytomas. The stimulatory effects of IL-6 on human myeloma cells are currently being studied. A factor that is probably also produced by BALB/c splenic macrophages in plasmacytoma-bearing mice and that inhibits the normal humoral antibody response has also been identified.[66]

The presence of antigenic stimulation by normal bacterial flora has either a direct or an indirect effect on plasmacytoma formation, as there is a marked reduction in the incidence of myeloma in pristane-treated BALB/c mice that have been raised in a germ-free environment,[67] although other lymphoid neoplasms may arise. Germ-free mice have a less-stimulated or less-developed immune apparatus and may lack the B-cell populations most susceptible to myeloma induction. BALB/c mice are also known to harbor oncogenic retroviruses, which may also play a role in myeloma induction. Mouse plasmacytomas contain large numbers of intracisternal A particles[68] that are not seen in normal plasma cells. These particles are considered to represent a distinct group of retroviruses.[69]

Nonrandom chromosomal translocations, as well as the expression or alteration of specific oncogenes, have been observed in murine plasmacytomas. The distal part of chromosome 15 is translocated to chromosome 12 (where the heavy chain genes reside) in several long-term transplanted plasmacytomas.[70,71] A similar phenomenon has been reported in human Burkitt's lymphoma, wherein translocations between the long arm of chromosome 8 (band 24) and the bands on chromosomes 14, 2, and 22 that contain the genetic loci for heavy chain, κ, and λ light chains, respectively.[72] The finding that the translocated component of chromosome 15 in the mouse and of chromosome 8 in man transfers the c-*myc* oncogene to the locus of an immunoglobulin gene suggests that the control of c-*myc* expression is enhanced by this translocation and leads to increased cell proliferation and tumor formation. Abnormal expression and alterations in c-*myc* have recently been reported in human myeloma.[73,74] However, this gene was detected in about one-fourth of the patients studied.[73] These data suggest that the c-*myc* oncogene may have some pathologic role in the evolution of myeloma in humans.[73]

ETIOLOGIC CONSIDERATIONS IN HUMANS

The availability of the aforementioned mouse model of myeloma provides opportunity for comparison of various etiologic factors that also may be relevant in the human disease. Although the cause of multiple myeloma and related plasma cell disorders remains unknown, a series of factors may play a role in pathogenesis. Several lines of evidence suggest that genetic factors may play a role in predisposing individuals to developing myeloma or related disorders. One factor that may implicate genetics is race because of the increased prevalence of the disease in blacks in the United States;[75,76] however, this could also relate to environmental differences. Genetic marker studies carried out to date have yielded only minimal information on the gammopathies. The frequency of HLA antigens of the 4C group appears to be slightly increased in myeloma.[77–80] The incidence of myeloma appears to be increased in first-degree relatives, and familial myeloma has been the subject of a number of case reports. At the Mayo Clinic, during one 6-year period, myeloma was diagnosed in eight siblings of 440 patients with myeloma, an incidence that far exceeds that generally reported.[81] In a review of etiologic factors, the median age and sex ratio of 75 reported familial cases was found to resemble those of nonfamilial cases.[82] In 70% of these cases, siblings were affected, suggesting that inherited susceptibility is recessive. Inasmuch as cases usually have been observed in siblings, and only rarely in spouses,[83,84] it appears that transmission is vertical rather than horizontal. Within a given family, the heavy chain types of M-components differ; however, there is concordance in light chain type in 80% of the cases.[82] Idiopathic monoclonal peaks (MGUS) have been reported sporadically in relatives of patients with myeloma.[81,85–87] Genetic factors in MGUS are also suggested by its relation to selected HLA types and the predominance of the IgG1 subclass as well as by reports of the familial occurrence of myeloma and macroglobulemia.[88–94] At the Mayo Clinic, where 241 patients with MGUS were followed for at least 10 years, MGUS has been evaluated as a precursor to myeloma.[1] During this period 38% of patients had no change in the concentration of the M-component and remained asymptomatic. An additional 35% of the patients died without developing myeloma or any other B-cell neoplasm. In 9%, the M-component increased significantly, but myeloma or a related disorder was not diagnosed. Most importantly, 17% of the patients (44 cases) had a diagnosis established of myeloma, macroglobulinemia, amyloidosis, or lymphoma. Multiple myeloma was the diagnosis in 30 of these 44 cases (68%). This report, as well as anecdotal observations in the literature, implicate MGUS as a premalignant condition. In one fascinating case, a patient received passive serotherapy with horse antiserum to tetanus in the 1930s and subsequently developed a serum M-component that persisted for more than 3 decades before overt myeloma developed. Once the diagnosis was made, it was determined that the serum IgG M-component exhibited antibody activity with specificity directed towards horse α_2-macroglobulin.[95] Such findings and others discussed later under pathogenesis have given rise to a "two-hit hypothesis," wherein antigenic stimulation in a susceptible host is the first hit, giving rise to a benign monoclone. The second hit is postulated to be a mutagenic or transforming event that then gives rise to myeloma from the expanded monoclonal B-cell population.[96]

Environmental or occupational factors in myeloma have been examined in large occupational studies, but these data must be interpreted cautiously because multiple comparisons have been made and some associations may have occurred by chance alone. A case-control study has been reported recently on 100 white myeloma patients and 100 matched controls in seven hospitals in the Baltimore area.[97] Statistically significant positive associations were documented with a history of occupational exposure to petroleum products, with an observed rate of myeloma that was 3.7 times the expected rate (range 1.3–10.3), and to asbestos with an observed rate of 3.5 (range 1.0–12.0). Additionally, among a large number of medications assessed, use of laxatives also appeared to elevate risk of myeloma to 3.5 times the expected rate (range 1.1–11.1). A variety of other industrial exposures, as well as chronic antigenic stimulation, or a history of autoimmune disease or allergy, or of taking various other medications did not appear to increase risk of myeloma in this study. The finding of increased risk with exposure to petroleum products in this study confirms earlier reports of an excessive number of cases of myeloma in workers exposed to petroleum.[1,98] The increased risk of myeloma in petroleum workers is of particular interest in the light of the mineral oil-induced model for plasma cell neoplasms in BALB/c mice. Also relevant to that model is the report of a patient who developed a plasmacytoma in the cutaneous pocket wherein a silastic-covered cardiac pacemaker was installed.[99] Prior reports on 61 patients with asbestosis have documented the occurrence of four cases of myeloma, one of macroglobulinemia, and one of chronic lymphocytic leukemia, suggesting that this known carcinogen for mesothelioma and other pulmonary tumors may also be involved in the induction B-cell neoplasms.[100] Although chronic antigenic stimulation (in disorders such as cholecystitis, osteomyelitis, and after allergen hyposensitization injections) has also been suggested as a predisposing factor for human plasma cell neoplasms;[101] data from various studies are quite inconclusive.[102–118]

As in other hematologic malignancies, a significant association has been observed between high-dose radiation exposure and the subsequent development of myeloma. This has been documented in the studies of survivors of the atomic bombs in Hiroshima and Nagasaki.[119,120] Among 109,000 survivors, 29 myeloma deaths were identified between 1950 and 1976. For persons exposed to 100 cGy, the observed rate of myeloma was about 4.7 times greater than controls, with the excess risk in this high-dose exposure group becoming apparent after a latent period of about 20 years. Associations between myeloma and low-dose irradiation exposure are more controversial than the atomic bomb casualty reports.[119] However, studies of radiologists have also shown excessive mortality resulting from myeloma,[121–123] as have workers in nuclear plants,[122,124] supporting the conclusion that even low-level radiation may be a risk factor for myeloma.

PATHOLOGY

In most instances the morphologic appearance of plasma cells in both malignant and benign disorders is quite similar. Plasma cells are at least two to three times the size of peripheral lymphocytes and are round or egg shaped, with one or more eccentrically placed nuclei containing either diffuse or clumped chromatin (Fig. 54-2). The light microscopic appearance was first drawn by Dalrymple and published from a wood-cut in 1846.[6] Plasma cells contain a highly differentiated cytoplasm that is very rich in rough-surfaced endoplasmic reticulum specialized for Ig synthesis. The cytoplasm normally stains a blue or bluish-purple on Romanovsky-type stains, but occasional myeloma cells stain a reddish-orange and have been called *thesaurocytes* or *flame*

FIG. 54-2. Bone marrow plasma cell in a patient with IgG myeloma. With the exception of a single cell in the neutrophilic series, the remaining cells are all neoplastic plasma cells at varying stages of differentiation.

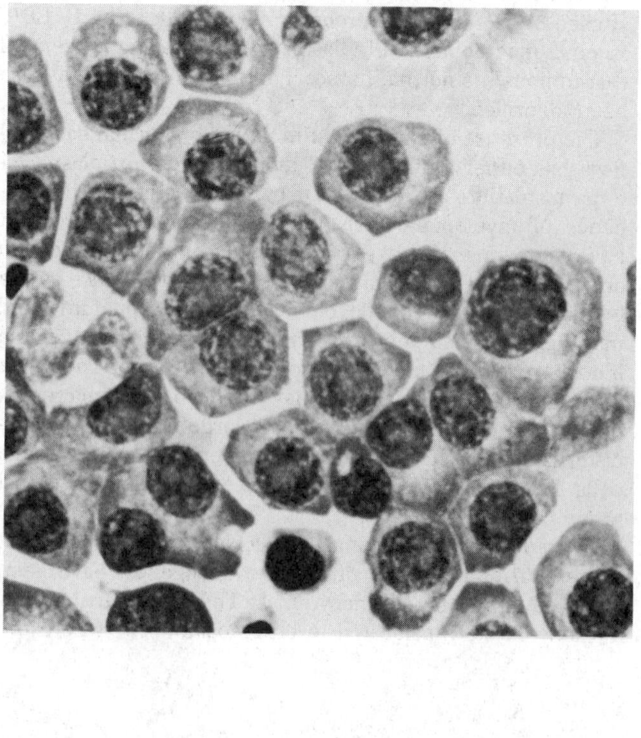

cells.[125,126] Once thought to be diagnostic of IgA myeloma,[126,127] such flame cells are now recognized in any plasma cell proliferation wherein the M-component has a very high carbohydrate content. A perinuclear clear zone (hof) is usually present in plasma cells and is the site of the Golgi apparatus, wherein Ig is packaged and glycosylated for secretion.[128] Occasional other cytoplasmic findings are numerous vacuoles (Mott cells, cells with Russell bodies,[129] grape cells, and morula cells). Electron microscopy has shown this appearance to be caused by protein-filled secretion vacuoles or dilated cisternae in the endoplasmic reticulum. Although the cytoplasm is well differentiated, in malignant plasma cell disorders the nucleus can be relatively less differentiated and, in addition to often having diffuse chromatin, may have several nucleoli and intranuclear inclusions. None of these features absolutely distinguish benign from malignant plasma cell proliferations. Myeloma patients with large numbers of plasmablasts in their marrow may have a poorer prognosis than those with predominantly mature plasma cells. In macroglobulinemia, cells may have a "lymphoplasmacytic" appearance, with morphologic variation in size and characteristics from those of small lymphocytes to large plasma cells. This pattern is occasionally also observed in myeloma. When such lymphoplasmacytic cells are examined with immunofluorescence, they almost all contain large amounts of cytoplasmic M-component. Cell surface Ig usually cannot be demonstrated on plasma cells.

In addition to these conventional morphologic assessments of plasma cells, use of monoclonal antibody reagents, histochemical analyses, and other morphologic approaches have been useful in analyzing plasma cells. Several plasma cell-associated antigens have been identified with specific monoclonal antibodies. Some patients' cells react strongly with antibodies to the common acute lymphocytic leukemia antigen (CALLA); such patients also may have a poorer prognosis.[130] Immunologic and cytogenetic markers have been used to identify a series of characteristics that may be associated with myeloma stem cells.[131] Histochemical stains, including β-glucuronidase and plasma cell acid phosphatase, have been used to assist in identifying plasma cells and in an effort to obtain additional prognostic information.[132] Such stains are usually not required for distinguishing plasma cells from red cell progenitors; however, the plasma cell acid phosphatase may be of some use in distinguishing active myeloma from MGUS.[133,134] Morphologic assessment of the tritiated thymidine-labeling index has been of greater value in distinguishing active myeloma from MGUS and other entities.[135,136] Monoclonal antibody reagents capable of evaluating cells undergoing DNA synthesis[137] and flow cytometry have also been applied to evaluation of plasma cell disorders.[138] The plasma cell β-glucoronidase has been correlated with the extent of disease. With some exceptions, increasing tumor burden is associated with higher plasma cell glucuronidase levels.[139]

Core bone marrow biopsies demonstrate that myeloma cells are present in cords in a reticular network. Involvement of the marrow can be either diffuse or nodular, although diffuse involvement with sheets of plasma cells is somewhat more common.

Amyloid deposits can occasionally be found either in the bone marrow in the vicinity of myeloma cells or in biopsies of soft-tissue plasmacytomas. Other biopsy sites (*e.g.*, the abdominal fat and rectal mucosa) have a higher likelihood of demonstrating the presence of amyloid.[140]

PATHOPHYSIOLOGY AND GROWTH KINETICS OF MYELOMA

The symptoms and signs of multiple myeloma and its effects on the patient result from the effects of secreted products from the myeloma cells (which have a variety of hormonal, immunologic, and physicochemical effects), as well as from the growth kinetics and total-body tumor burden of malignant plasma cells.

HYPERCALCEMIA

In the clinical phase of myeloma, hematogenous dissemination to various skeletal sites is usually extensive and leads to both bone pain and hypercalcemia. Radiographic findings of skeletal destruction are depicted in Figure 54-3. In areas of bone resorption, it appears that the cells adjacent to the bony matrix in the resorption lacunae are osteoclasts, which are separated from the myeloma cells by a membrane. This morphologic finding, plus functional studies using myeloma cell secretion products, provided the basis for the concept that myeloma cells liberated an osteoclast-activating factor responsible for bone destruction.[141,142] Clinical correlations indicate that the production of osteoclast-activating factor by a patient's myeloma cells correlates with the extent of skeletal involvement present.[143] Several bone-resorbing cytokines have been identified including lymphotoxin, tumor necrosis factor (TNF), and interleukin-1 (IL-1). Lymphotoxin has recently been documented as being produced by cultured human myeloma cells. Additionally, antibody neutralization of the myeloma cell-secreted lymphotoxin blocked at least part of the bone-resorbing activity secreted by myeloma cells. Neither TNF nor IL-1 was detected in the myeloma supernatants, nor did antibody to lymphotoxin block the bone-resorbing activity of these latter two peptides.[144]

ANEMIA

Marrow involvement results in the development of a normochromic, normocytic anemia, heralding the symptoms of fatigue and weakness. Reduced red cell production and an increase in the red cell destruction rate have both been observed. High concentrations of serum M-component in the blood lead to rouleux formation and may lead to blood sludging, which further increases hemolysis.

RENAL FAILURE

Renal failure is a common complication of myeloma that can be significant at the time of clinical presentation. When present, it is an adverse prognostic factor that has a negative impact on overall survival. The renal failure appears to be multifactorial and is most frequently correlated with the

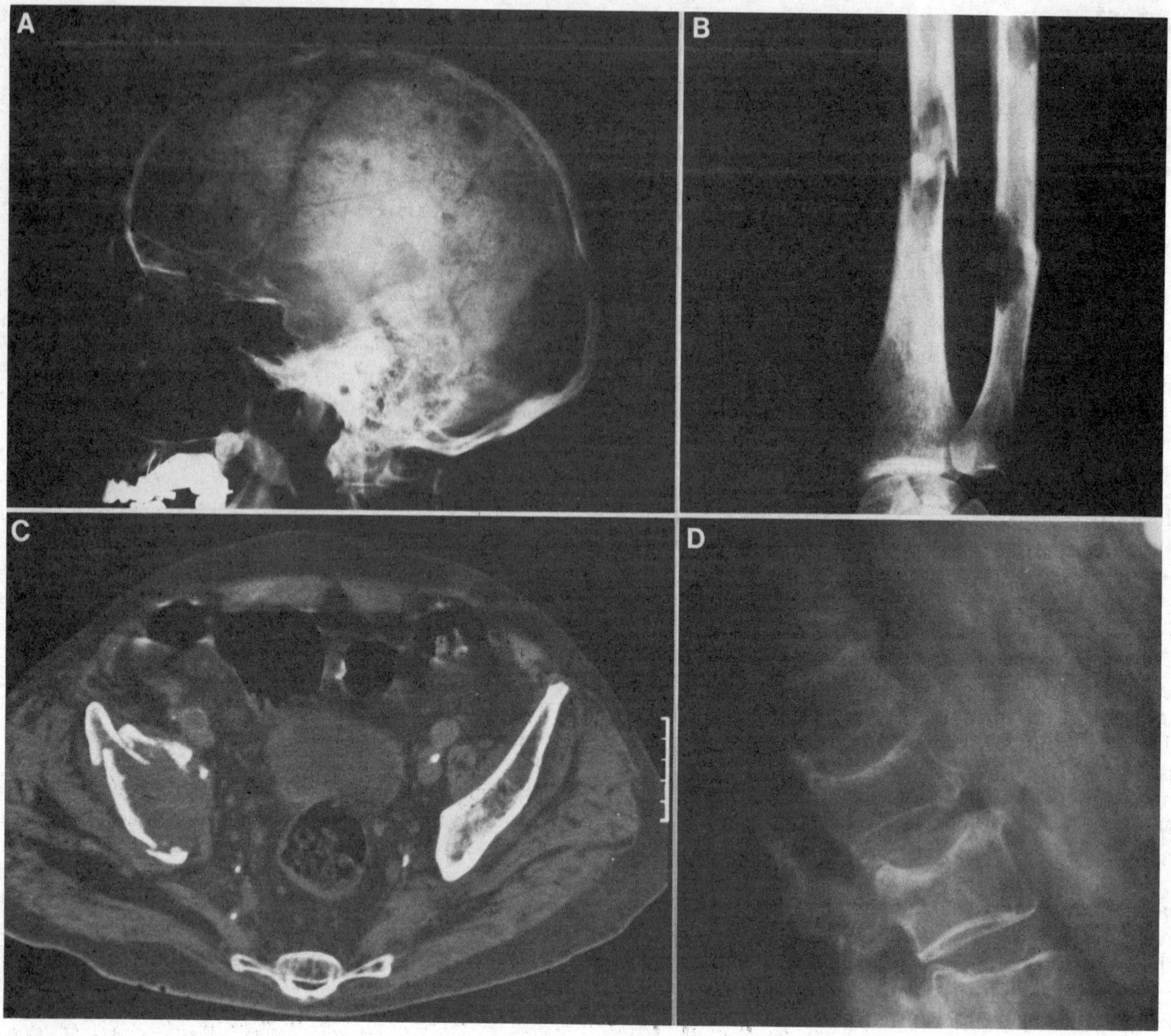

FIG. 54-3. Typical radiographic evidence of bone involvement in myeloma. **A**. Punched out lesions in the skull. **B**. Intramedullary expansile lesions in forearm with fracture. **C**. Pelvic plasmacytoma with fracture and associated soft tissue mass seen on computed tomography. **D**. Vertebral compression fractures in the spine.

presence of Bence Jones proteinuria, hypercalcemia, or both. The presence of λ light chains in the urine is more strongly correlated with renal failure than is the excretion of κ chains, suggesting that they may be more nephrotoxic. Light chains normally pass the glomerulus and are reabsorbed and catabolized in the proximal tubules.[145–147] They appear in large quantities in the urine only when the catabolic rate is exceeded, resulting in an increased fractional proteinuric rate. The excretion of dense (often laminated) tubular casts is a characteristic finding in patients with myeloma kidney.[148] Such casts contain albumin, intact Ig molecules, or Bence Jones proteins.[148–158] The proteinuria present in patients with myeloma kidney comprises monoclonal light chains plus some albumin. Additional factors that sometimes contribute to renal failure are infection, hyperuricemia, or amyloidosis. Amyloid deposition in the kidney usually appears in the blood vessels, basement membranes of the tubules and interstitium, and occasionally in glomeruli. Proteinuria in patients with renal amyloid is often generalized, and this can provide a clue to distinguish the syndrome from that of myeloma kidney.

IMMUNODEFICIENCY

Increased susceptibility to bacterial infections, particularly before treatment, is principally due to an acquired hyporesponsiveness to antigenic stimulation. Reduced serum levels of normal serum antibody immunoglobulins are observed in almost all patients with multiple myeloma, as well as in many MGUS patients.[159] Studies with the mouse model indicate that myeloma cells produce a humoral *PC-factor* that stimulates monocytes and macrophages to produce a second factor, *PIMS*, which inhibits normal antigen-stimulated B-cell proliferation subsequently to antibody production.[160]

Mixing experiments using peripheral blood mononuclear cells from patients with myeloma and those from normal subjects indicates that monocytic cells in the myeloma patient's blood can inhibit normal B-cell Ig synthesis induced with pokeweed mitogen.[161] The precise molecular nature of these immunosuppressive cytokines has yet to be established.

PHYSICOCHEMICAL OR IMMUNOLOGIC EFFECTS OF M-COMPONENTS

M-components in myeloma and related disorders can cause clinically significant abnormalities in blood flow and function.[162] The most common of these phenomena is the hyperviscosity syndrome. Although more common in macroglobulinemia than in myeloma, it results from the presence of a sufficient concentration of an M-protein with a high molecular mass or with a tendency to self-aggregation, and a resultant increase in its intrinisic viscosity. The hyperviscosity syndrome is rarely seen until the serum viscosity exceeds 4.0-cp units, relative to normal saline, and it is usually manifested by the occurrence of neurologic findings and by spontaneous bleeding phenomena in the absence of thrombocytopenia. In other instances, an M-component exhibits antibody activity-leading clinical syndromes such as acquired deficiency of factor VIII,[163] with bleeding phenomena, and hyperlipidemia.[164,165]

GROWTH KINETICS AND TUMOR BURDEN

Myeloma is a low-growth fraction tumor, with only a small percentage of tumor cells in cycle at any given time. It is considered to arise from a single transformed cell (10^0 cell). Tritiated thymidine-labeling indices for myeloma cells in active disease patients generally are in the range of 1% to 3%.[136] Studies of the generation time indicate that the cell cycle time of actively proliferating cells is generally about 1 to 3 days.[166,167] Total-body tumor burden in myeloma patients has been determined from M-component synthesis rates measured both in vivo with metabolic turnover studies, and in vitro on bone marrow specimens from these patients.[17] These studies have indicated that, in IgG myeloma, tumor burden ranges from 0.5×10^{12} cells in "early" asymptomatic cases to 5×10^{12} cells, or more, in patients with widespread bone destruction.[17] Studies of growth kinetics have also been carried out by measuring the doubling-time of serum M-components of patients not actively receiving treatment and by use of mathematical modeling for measurements of progressive tumor growth in patients who have had their total-body tumor burden determined.[166] The doubling-time of serum M-component levels in untreated patients usually ranges from 4 to 6 months. Given the serum M-component doubling-times, it was initially proposed, from an assumption of exponential cell growth, that the natural history of myeloma might require 20 to 30 years to evolve from a single malignant plasma cell to clinically evident disease.[168] In some instances, this model would predict that myeloma was initiated before conception! However, subsequent studies using measurements of M-component metabolism and more precise mathematical modeling techniques determined that the growth of myeloma followed gompertzian kinetics, and that the subclinical phase of malignant tumor cell proliferation was about 1 to 3 years before clinical diagnosis.[167] In this analysis, the initial doubling-times (one cell to two cells) were back-extrapolated to be 1 to 3 days,[166] thus agreeing with tritiated thymidine measurements of the myeloma cell generation time.[167] A typical myeloma growth curve is depicted in Figure 54-4. The phase of myeloma after diagnosis can be viewed as a chronic phase, not dissimilar to that present in chronic myeloid luekemia. This chronic phase in myeloma may last from 1 to 10 or more years, during which time treatment is usually beneficial. Late in the course of myeloma, the disease often becomes far more aggressive than it had been previously. The myeloma cell mass doubling-time (as determined from serum M-component levels) may progressively shorten; this may be analogous to the blast crisis phase of chronic myeloid leukemia.[169] Integration of tritiated thymidine-labeling index and tumor-burden studies has led to the definition of such patients as having high–growth-fraction, high–tumor-burden myeloma.[136] This patient group has a very poor prognosis, with rapid myeloma growth and early death.[136,170] Such patients may have residual drug sensitivity after each course of therapy, but the myeloma grows back rapidly, and sometimes more rapidly than the time required for normal hematologic recovery. Patients whose myeloma develops more rapid growth kinetics have a propensity for extramedullary tumor growth, including soft-tissue plasmacytomas and even CNS involvement. In some instances the neoplasm takes on a less-differentiated morphologic appearance, similar to that of a large-cell lymphoma,[96,171,172] with a cell surface Ig that usually corresponds with the prior serum Ig. In earlier

FIG. 54-4. Gompertzian growth curve in multiple myeloma. In this untreated patient with IgG myeloma, serial measurements of M-component production were used to extrapolate the preclinical phase of myeloma cell proliferation of approximately 1 year's duration.

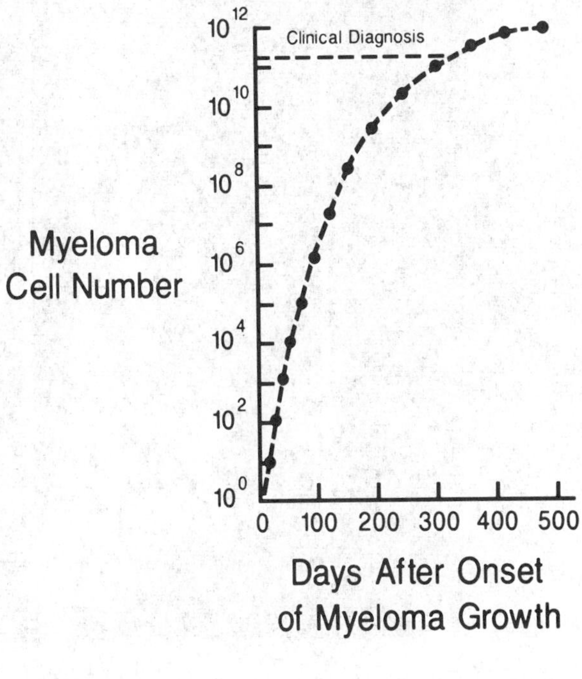

phases of disease, the quantity of M-component synthesis as determined from serum or urine measurements corresponds with the amount of tumor in the body. However, in the terminal phase, the M-component synthesis rate per tumor may decline or qualitatively change as the tumor progresses, suggesting the development of a mutant subclone. In some instances, the patients who previously have had only a serum M-component switch to primarily urinary light chains, reflecting additional biochemical abnormalities in Ig synthesis and assembly.[173] In contrast with these aggressive forms of the disease, another subset of patients have indolent or smoldering myeloma in which, despite evidence of bone lesions, the disease progresses very slowly, even in the absence of treatment. These patients previously could be identified only from their clinical course; however, the use of tritiated thymidine-labeling studies usually identifies these patients as having hypoproliferative myeloma cells, with $< 0.5\%$ of the tumor cells labeling and in a range quite similar to that of MGUS.[135,136]

DIAGNOSIS AND CLINICAL STAGING OF MYELOMA

Presenting symptoms and signs of myeloma usually include bone pain (which may be associated with compression fractures of the spine or pathologic fractures of long bones), weakness and anemia, and infection (usually due to pneumococcus or other gram-positive bacteria). Hypercalcemia, renal failure, spinal cord compression, or a mixture of these findings may be present. Punched-out osteolytic bone lesions are commonly seen on skeletal x-ray films (see Fig. 54-3). A complete skeletal x-ray series, including both the axial and appendicular skeleton, should always be obtained at the time of diagnosis. Only in this way can the number and location of lesions be identified to determine if any potentially unstable osteolytic lesions are present. Recent studies using magnetic resonance imaging (MRI) scanning suggest that this approach can provide greater detail on myelomatous abnormalities in the vertebral column than conventional radiographs (Fig. 54-5). However, this procedure is expensive, and currently it takes several hours to acquire the imaging information on the entire spine of a single patient and, therefore, this technique must be used selectively. Bone scans are of no value in the assessment of skeletal involvement in myeloma because the bone disease is almost purely osteolytic and the nuclear medicine isotopes are taken up only in areas of osteoblastic activity. Accordingly, radiographic lesions in untreated myeloma rarely, if ever, show evidence of a sclerotic margin on the lytic lesions. An increase in the number of plasma cells is usually demonstrable either in the bone marrow or in a biopsy of a plasmacytoma. A serum or urinary M-component can be demonstrated in 99% of the patients. However, in some instances, not all criteria are present, and a mixture of criteria is needed to establish a diagnosis of multiple myeloma and to distinguish it from other plasma cell disorders. Useful diagnostic criteria are summarized in Table 54-3.

A clinical-staging system for multiple myeloma was developed at the Arizona Cancer Center by Durie and Salmon[177] by analyzing the presenting clinical features of a series of patients with multiple myeloma who had their tumor burden directly measured using the foregoing metabolic techniques. On the basis of these clinical correlations, multiple myeloma was divided into three tumor burden groups: Stage I (low), II (intermediate), and III (high). Tumor mass stage alone was predictive of survival. However, an additional prognostic factor, renal function, independently impinged on survival and was, therefore, included in the staging system, with normal renal function (serum creatinine < 2.0 or blood urea

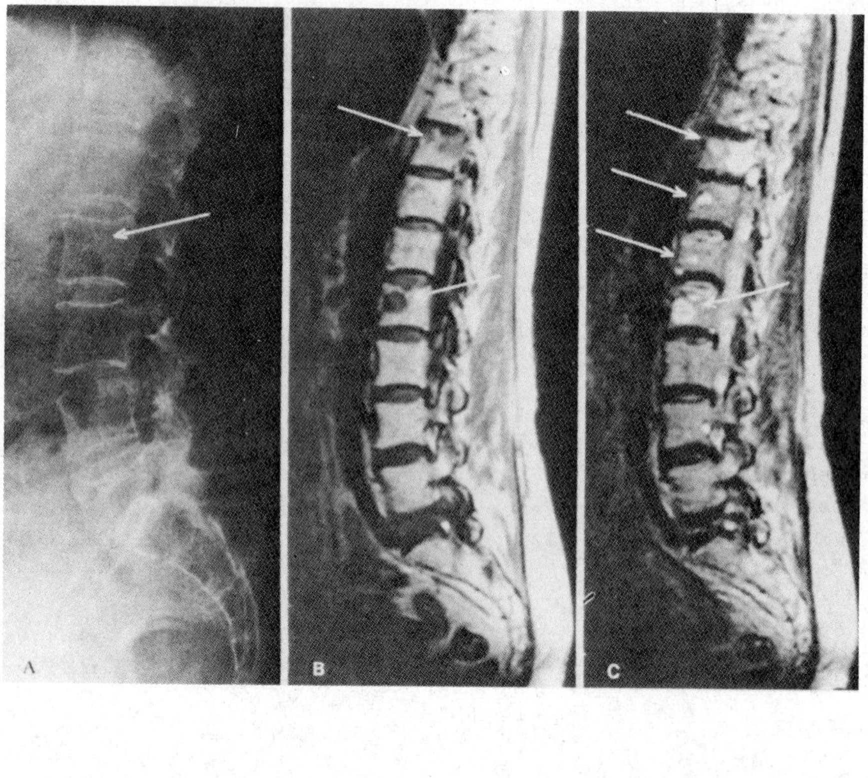

FIG. 54-5. Radiograph of lower spine (**A**) compared to magnetic resonance images (**B** and **C**). Note that the osteolytic lesions in the vertebral bodies of T10-12 and L1 that were poorly visualized on plain films were much more visible in T_1 weighted (**B**) and especially T_2 weighted (**C**) MR images. (Ludwig M, Tscholakoff D, Neuhold A, et al: Magnetic resonance imaging of the spine in multiple melanoma. Lancet 2:364–366, 1987)

TABLE 54-3. Diagnostic Criteria for Multiple Myeloma, Myeloma Variants, and Monoclonal Gammopathy of Unknown Significance (MGUS)

A. Multiple myeloma
  Major criteria
    I. Plasmacytoma on tissue biopsy
    II. Bone marrow plasmacytosis with >30% plasma cells
    III. Monoclonal globulin spike on serum electrophoresis exceeding 3.5 g/dl for G peaks or 2.0 g/dl for A peaks, ≥ 1.0 g/24 h of κ- or λ-light chain excretion on urine electrophoresis in the presence of amyloidosis
  Minor criteria
    a. Bone marrow plasmacytosis 10% to 30% plasma cells
    b. Monoclonal globulin spike present, but less than the level defined above
    c. Lytic bone lesions
    d. Residual normal IgM < 50 mg/dl, IgA < 100 mg/dl, or IgG < 600 mg/dl
    Diagnosis will be confirmed when any of the following features are documented in symptomatic patients with clearly progressive disease. The diagnosis of myeloma requires a minimum of one major + one minor criterion or three minor criteria that must include a + b, *i.e.*:
    1. I + b, I + c, I + d (I + a not sufficient)
    2. II + b, II + c, II + d
    3. III + a, III + c, III + d
    4. a + b + c, a + b + d
B. Indolent myeloma (same as myeloma except)
    I. No bone lesions or only limited bone lesions (≤3 lytic lesions); no compression fractures
    II. M-component levels: (a) IgG < 7 g/dl; (b) IgA < 5/dl
    III. No symptoms or associated disease features, *i.e.*:
      a. Performance status > 70%
      b. Hemoglobin > 10 g/dl
      c. Serum calcium normal
      d. Serum creatinine < 2.0 mg/dl
      e. No infections
C. Smoldering myeloma (same as indolent myeloma except)
    I. No bone lesions
    II. Bone marrow plasma cells ≤ 30%
D. MGUS
    I. Monoclonal gammopathy
    II. M-component level
      IgG ≤ 3.5 g/dl
      IgA ≤ 2.0 g/dl
      BJ protein ≤ 1.0 g/24 h
    III. Bone marrow plasma cells < 10%
    IV. No bone lesions
    V. No symptoms

See Refs. 135, 157, 175, 176. IgA, immunoglobulin A; IgG, immunoglobulin G; IgM, immunoglobulin M; BJ, Bence Jones light chain.

nitrogen < 30) as substage A, and higher values as substage B (Table 54-4).

A number of other investigative groups have now applied the Durie–Salmon myeloma-staging system to evaluate survival by stage in myeloma (Table 54-5).

This same patient group had follow-up data on response to treatment and survival, and the clinical features that correlated with a given stage in terms of tumor burden were predictive of survival both in the original patient set and in subsequent reports by other investigative groups.[179,185,186] Figure 54-6 depicts the influence of clinical stage and renal function on the survival of patients with multiple myeloma. In the original study used in developing the Durie–Salmon myeloma-staging system, the percentage of bone marrow plasma cells was an important factor; however, it was not included in the staging system because it could be replaced by other clinical features and was potentially susceptible to sampling errors. Bone marrow involvement was also deleted from the staging criteria after consideration of the potential difficulties that might be encountered in accurately and reproducibly counting plasma cells in the bone marrow differential at different centers. Patients with Bence-Jones-only myeloma have more recently been assessed for measured tumor cell burden, and they appear to represent a higher-risk subgroup with a higher tumor cell mass and shorter survival.[188]

DIFFERENTIAL DIAGNOSIS

The criteria shown in Table 54-3 provide the basis for differentially diagnosing myeloma from other major plasma cell disorders with M-component secretions other than IgM. The IgM M-components are usually attributable to Waldenström's macroglobulinemia, and occasionally to MGUS or other entities. Multiple myeloma with IgM secretion has rarely been reported, and it should be diagnosed only if the patient has multiple osteolytic bone lesions that contain monoclonal plasma cells.[96] Marrow plasmacytosis is observed in a number of chronic infectious or inflammatory diseases as well as in hypersensitivity reactions, autoimmune disease, unrelated neoplasms and, occasionally, with other conditions; it is not associated with secretion of an M-component but, rather, with polyclonal hyperglobulinemia. The major differential diagnosis is usually between myeloma and MGUS. There is an overlap between presenting findings in patients with MGUS and those with Stage I myeloma (or macroglobulinemia) that can often be recognized only by serial follow-up of the patient for at least 1 year without any form of treatment. In MGUS, the M-component level remains constant over many years, whereas in the malignant plasma cell disorders, the M-component gradually rises, and other symptoms and signs of the disease develop. A policy of watch and wait is completely justifiable because there is no evidence that treatment improves the outcome in either Stage I myeloma or MGUS, and the use of chemotherapy has potential hazards that should be avoided if the patient does not have an invasive, progressive plasma cell malignancy. If, after a year's follow-up of the patient's M-component and symptoms and signs at 1 to 2 month intervals, there is no evidence of progression, then the most likely diagnosis is MGUS, and follow-up can be at least annual because about 2% of these patients will progress to a diagnosis of B-cell neoplasm each year.[1] Patients presenting with only Bence Jones proteinuria usually have myeloma alone or with amyloidosis,[189,190] and it has been stated that its excretion has "sinister significance."[191] However, Bence Jones MGUS has been reported and followed without specific therapy for a number of years in a few patients.[157,192] It is, nonetheless, reasonable to have a higher index of suspcicion when patients present with idiopathic Bence Jones proteinuria, because it usually progresses within 6 months to 1 year to clearly diagnosed myeloma, which then should be treated appropriately. Patients with unrelated metastatic neoplasms occasionally also have MGUS, and a series of diagnostic studies and biopsies are required to establish that the patient

TABLE 54-4. Myeloma Staging System

Criteria	Measured Myeloma Cell Mass (Cells × $10^{12}/m^2$)
Stage I	
All of the following:	
Hemoglobin value > 10 g/dl	
Serum calcium value normal (<12 mg/dl)	
On roentgenogram, normal bone structure (scale 0) or solitary bone plasmacytoma only	
Low M-component production rates	<0.6 (low)
IgG value < 5 g/dl	
IgA value < 3 g/dl	
Urine light chain M-component on electrophoresis < 4g/24 h	
Stage II	
Overall data not as minimally abnormal as shown for stage I and no single value as abnormal as defined for stage III.	0.6 – 1.20 (intermediate)
Stage III	
One or more of the following	
Hemoglobin value < 8.5 g/dl	
Serum calcium value > 12 mg/dl	
Advanced lytic bone lesions (scale 3)	
High M-component production rates	>1.20 (high)
IgG value > 7 g/dl	
IgA value > 5 g/dl	
Urine light chain M-component on electrophoresis > 12 g/24 h	
Subclassification	
A = relatively normal renal function (serum creatinine value > 2.0 mg/dl)	
B = abnormal renal function (serum creatinine value ≥ 2.0 mg/dl)	
Examples	
Stage IA = low cell mass with normal renal function	
Stage IIIB = high cell mass with abnormal renal function	

Modified from Ref. 178. IgA, immunoglobulin A; IgG, immunoglobulin G.

does not have myeloma. Myeloma and an unrelated metastatic neoplasm may, of course, also be diagnosed.

β_2-MICROGLOBULIN

β_2-microglobulin (β-2M) has been identified as an important prognostic factor in multiple myeloma.[193] β_2-Microglobulin is a low molecular mass protein, which is the light chain of the HLA-antigen, and is synthesized by all nucleated cells.[194] It also falls in the class of tubular proteins that pass the glomerulus and are excreted in the urine. Therefore, renal functional impairment also leads to an elevation in the serum level of β-2M. Measurements of β-2M can be carried out simply by radioimmunoassay. A series of studies have shown that, when corrected for renal function, serum β-2M levels correlate strongly with tumor burden in multiple myeloma.[193,195–199] Inasmuch as the β2M levels in the serum are a function of both myeloma cell mass and renal function, measurement of β-2M may provide an alternative to clinical staging to predict survival.[200] The relationship of β-2M to survival in myeloma is depicted in Figure 54-7. One potential advantage of β-2M is in application as a pretreatment prognostic factor in clinical trials because it permits a more direct comparison of risk factors in the various cooperative groups and institutions interested in myeloma therapy. Although it has been proposed that β-2M can be used to distin-

TABLE 54-5. Median Survival in Relation to Stage at Diagnosis

		Median Survival (mo)				
				Stage		
Series (Ref)	*No. of Cases*	*I*	*II*	*III*	*A*	*B*
Durie and Salmon[177]	71	>60	50	26		
Alexanian et al[178]	343	39	27	17		
Woodruff et al[179]	237	64	32	6	21	2
Merlini et al[180]	123	76	41	12		
Belpomme et al[181]	118	>60	28	7	>60	12
Gobbi et al[182]	91	>79	51	33		
Santoro et al[183]	81	48	41	23	35	7
Bergsagel et al[184]	364	46	32	23	32	11
Summary	1428	>60	41	23		

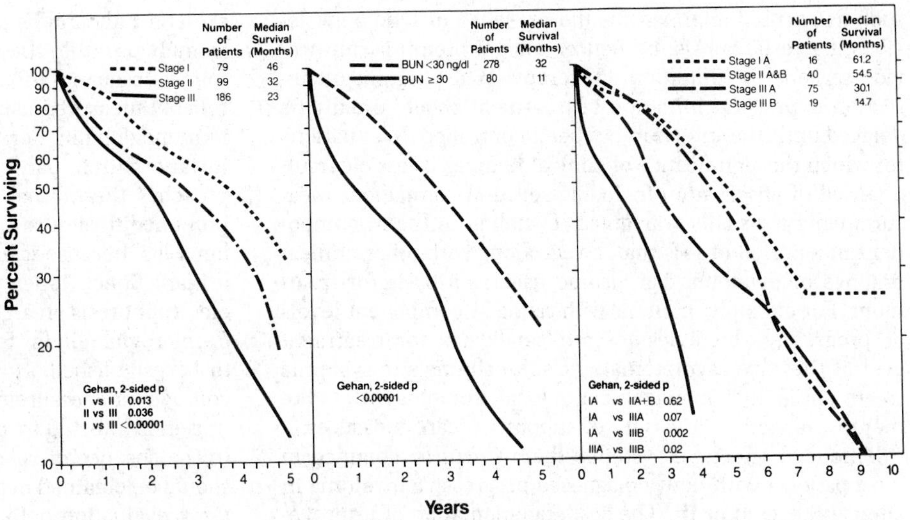

FIG. 54-6. Influence of clinical stage and renal function on survival in patients with plasma cell myeloma as redrawn from published illustrations. The left two panels are from a Canadian NCI study[185] and show the separate effects of clinical stage and renal function, respectively. The right-hand panel depicts an Arizona Cancer Center study[187] wherein the survival curves are shown with clinical stage and renal function integrated with the use of the clinical staging system shown in Table 54-4. Statistical comparisons of survival outcome in the various stages and risk groups in the studies appear in each panel.

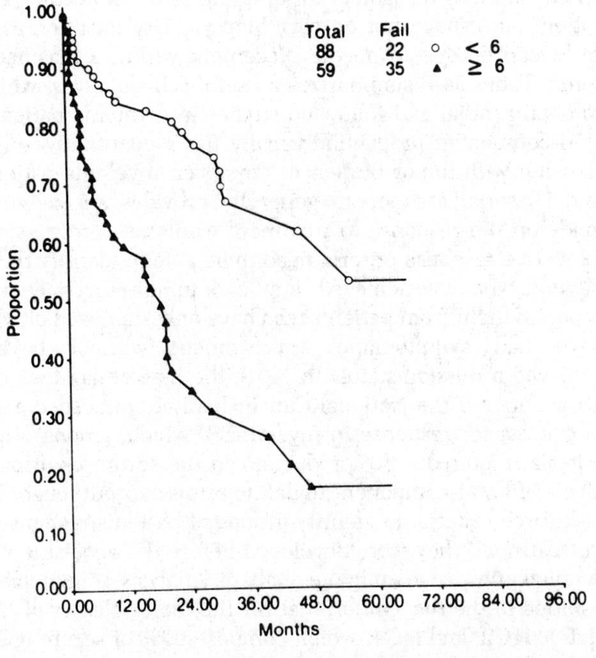

FIG. 54-7. Life table survival curves in multiple myeloma in relation to serum β-2 microglobulin (β2M) concentration. The upper curve (○----○) is for 88 patients with a serum βM) of less than 6 μg/ml. The lower curve (<---->) is for 59 patients with β2M values of 6 μg/ml or greater. The difference between the curves is highly significant (p <0.001). (Bataille R, Durie BGM, Grenier J, et al: Prognostic factors and staging in multiple myeloma: A reappraisal. J Clin Oncol 4:80–87, 1986)

guish between MGUS and myeloma, there is significant overlap, and it is not a sufficient discriminant.[193,196,201] Preliminary data suggest that β-2M also may have some use as a marker with which to follow response to treatment. However, it is uncertain whether or not it will be as useful as M-component measurements because it is influenced by renal function as well as tumor burden. In our own experience, it has not proved useful in patients lacking an M-component (nonsecretory myeloma).

TREATMENT

GENERAL COMMENTS

It is important to remember that the diagnosis of a monoclonal gammopathy does not represent an immediate mandate for treatment and that patients with MGUS, Stage I myeloma, as well as indolent or smoldering myeloma, are often best followed without treatment until such time as it is warranted by the development of clearcut progression of the disease. Inasmuch as multiple myeloma is a disseminated plasma cell neoplasm, the primary approach to treatment is with systemic antineoplastic therapy. Symptoms and signs that warrant immediate institution of therapy include the development of bone pain, hypercalcemia, renal failure, severe suppression of bone marrow functions, or spinal cord compression. When spinal cord compression is present, completion of local therapy (almost always with radiation therapy) should normally precede the initiation of systemic chemotherapy unless other serious complications mandate simultaneous systemic treatment and radiation therapy. Patients presenting with long-bone fractures should have them internally fixed orthopedically before the initiation of chemotherapy. Presentation with constellations of findings, such as marked anemia plus the presence of lytic bone lesions, bacterial sepsis, or Bence Jones proteinuria, all provide reasons for initiation of therapy. When significant infection is present, initiation of treatment should usually be delayed until the infection has been controlled. In situations for which the significance of clinical findings is less clearcut, a period of observation including serial M-component measurements is usually warranted. Doubling in the M-component in a period of less than a year along with other clinical findings of myeloma can also be used as a basis for treatment. For example, patients with rising M-component levels or progressive bone lesions are candidates for treatment even if they are asymptomatic. Useful adjuncts to systemic treatment include management of local problems with radiotherapy as well as a variety of supportive care measures.

Beneficial effects of systemic therapy can be obtained in most patients with newly diagnosed progressive myeloma in clinical Stages II or III. The best documentation of improvement in survival of patients with myeloma has been obtained in Stage III patients. Clinical phases of myeloma under treatment can be considered to include an initial drug sensitive phase, which is observed in most patients; a "plateau phase," during which tumor burden as assessed clinically appears to be stable during maintained or unmaintained remission;[202] and an eventual drug-resistant phase, during which the neoplasm may exhibit altered growth kinetics as well as resistance to conventional cytotoxic drugs.[2] About 15% to 20% of patients manifest resistance even to aggressive parenteral chemotherapy at the time of initial presentation with progressive myeloma. Systemic therapy usually relieves bone pain relatively promptly, whereas many other aspects of the disease improve more gradually and may require other supportive measures initially. Even with prompt institution of systemic treatment, the drug-sensitive phase of disease usually lasts only 2 to 3 years for most patients before drug resistance is manifest. Although the median survival before the era of effective systemic therapy was less than a year, it is now in the range of 3 to 4 years in many studies. In a few patients, sensitivity to systemic therapy may persist for 5 to 10 years, and occasionally longer.

Specific details of therapy will be discussed later; however, general aspects of care that should not be neglected include maximum efforts to relieve pain, hypercalcemia, severe anemia, and various local complications promptly to keep the patient from being bedridden and, thereby, minimize further bone demineralization and superinfections. Patients should be encouraged to drink several liters of fluid daily to avoid dehydration and enhance urinary excretion of light chains and calcium.

EVALUATION OF RESPONSE TO TREATMENT

Inasmuch as myeloma has a variety of clinical manifestations, a series of initial and follow-up studies are needed to assess the response to systemic treatment. These include clinical assessment of history and physical examination as well as following laboratory studies that include the complete blood count with differential and platelet counts; M-component levels in the serum or in 24-h urine or both; serum calcium, creatinine, or blood urea nitrogen levels; and skeletal radiographs. Although serum electrophoresis is extremely useful in the initial diagnostic workup, baseline and follow-up quantitation of the serum M-components is most reliably measured using laser nephalometry of the involved immunoglobulin. Serum electrophoresis is sometimes a useful alternative, particularly as the M-component level approaches the normal range for the involved Ig. The radial immunodiffusion test should not be used to measure myeloma Igs, because it has not proved reliable. Quantitation of urinary Bence Jones protein is best determined by protein electrophoresis on a 24-hr concentrate. The relative value of β_2-microglobulin for following the course of myeloma has yet to be established. However, β-2M is not as specific as M-component measurements, inasmuch as its serum concentration is affected by both tumor burden and renal function. In the absence of specific symptoms, follow-up radiographs should be obtained every 6 to 12 months. The initial skeletal x-ray evaluation before therapy should include a complete metastatic x-ray survey, as myelomatous involvement can be located in any area of the axial or appendicular skeleton. Isotopic bone scans are of little-to-no value in most myeloma patients and are, therefore, not recommended. Bone marrow involvement should be assessed initially, including both an aspirate and a core bone marrow biopsy. Caution is needed to avoid excessive pressure on the needle when the needle is inserted because in some myeloma patients the bone matrix is extremely fragile. Follow-up bone marrow specimens are obtained to confirm remission status after therapy as well as to explain an unexpected pancytopenia. Marrow involvement with myeloma is usually diffuse but, occasionally, it is spotty and may be subject to sampling error on needle aspiration, but usually not on core biopsy. "Dry taps" on aspirates can be due to needle placement within a plasmacytoma. Table 54-6 summarizes a useful schedule with which to obtain initial and follow-up studies in myeloma patients.

M-component production usually has a quantitative relationship with tumor burden in any given myeloma patient, and its serial assessment generally provides an excellent guide on the response to treatment or disease progression. Objective response criteria need to be able to identify those patients who have achieved significant tumor regression and separate them from patients who have only stabilized or who have had symptomatic improvement without having achieved remission status. In 1973, the Leukemia-Myeloma Task Force of the National Cancer Institute published a set of criteria for response in myeloma[203] which, among other criteria, required a 50% reduction in the serum or urinary levels of an M-component to define remission. Although the task force criteria do identify groups of patients responsive to treatment, they were developed before the acquisition of detailed knowledge on Ig metabolism. Analysis of Ig metabolism led to the recognition that for the major classes of IgG (IgG1, IgG2, and IgG4, which compose 90% of serum IgG), metabolism is not linear with the serum concentration.[204] With a relatively high serum IgG M-component value, the half-life of IgG may be as short as 8 to 10 days, whereas with a low value, the half-life may be as long as 40 days or longer. This concentration-dependent phenomenon applies to IgG M-component levels in 90% of patients with IgG myeloma, which in turn comprises approximately 50% of all myeloma

TABLE 54-6. Checklist of Laboratory Studies for Patients with Multiple Myeloma

Routine Pretreatment Evaluation
Complete blood count, differential, and platelets
Serum protein electrophoresis
Serum immunoglobulins (nephalometry)
Serum β_2-microglobulin
24-h urine for total protein and electrophoresis
Antigenic typing of serum and urine monoclonal Igs by immunofixation or immunoelectrophoresis
Bone marrow aspiration and biopsy
Serum creatinine
Serum calcium
Serum electrolytes
Serum uric acid
Liver functions
Chest x-ray
Skeletal x-ray survey (entire skeleton)
Electrocardiogram
Specialized Studies for Selected Patients (when indicated)
Abdominal fat pad or rectal biopsy for amyloid (also tap joint effusions for amyloid)
Solitary lytic lesion, soft-tissue or lymph node biopsy
Serum viscosity if IgM component present or if any serum M-component > 7.0 g/dl
Plasma volume if serum relative viscosity > 4.0
Myelogram (or in some instances MRI) if paraspinal mass or symptoms and signs of spinal cord or nerve root compression. (Spinal fluid should be sent for cell count, cytospin differential, glucose, and protein.)
Routine Follow-up Studies
Before every course of treatment
CBC, differential, platelets (should be repeated to check nadirs on first few courses)
At least every 3 months (and on completion of induction or change to alternative therapy for refractory patients)
Serum monoclonal Ig by nephalometry or electrophoresis
24-hr urine protein electrophoresis (when BJP present)
Serum chemistry panel
At least annually
Skeletal x-ray survey (entire skeleton) chest x-ray serum β^2-microglobulin
Bone marrow aspiration if any significant abnormality in blood counts, Igs, or new symptoms
Serum Igs (nephalometry)

cases. Thus, mere comparisons of serum levels in such cases underestimate the degree of change to a varying extent, depending on the specific patient's initial and follow-up serum M-protein values.[2] Correction can be made for changes in the metabolic rate for IgG through the calculation of a synthetic index from the serum values. A useful nomogram for this purpose has been derived from the metabolic equations.[2] A nomogram with an extended scale for IgG values appears in Figure 54-8.

Assessment of urinary light chain excretion is affected significantly by the degree of catabolism that takes place in the kidney, which is a function of the absolute levels of light chains passing the glomerulus and the degree of renal functional impairment.[188] To avoid such difficulties in assessment, criteria for improvement in Bence Jones proteinuria also need to be quite stringent. The response criteria adopted by the Southwest Oncology Group (SWOG) are summarized in Table 54-7. Response in accord with their SWOG criteria is strongly correlated with improvement in survival. When

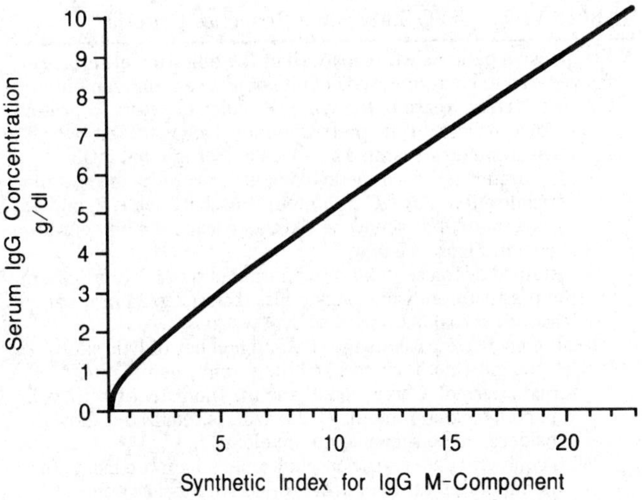

FIG. 54-8. Nomogram for determining the synthetic index for IgG M components of subclasses IgG1, IgG2, and IgG4 (which comprise 90% of IgG myelomas). Using the patient's initial serum IgG concentration (g/dl) on the vertical axis, read down from the line to the horizontal axis to determine the synthetic index for that IgG value (Syn1). The same procedure is followed for the follow-up value (Syn2). Syn2/Syn1 × 100 = % of baseline synthetic index and tumor burden. This nomogram corrects for concentration-dependent changes in M-component synthesis and myeloma cell mass and gives a more accurate assessment of changes in tumor burden in IgG myeloma than can be calculated directly from the serum levels. The nomogram is not required for IgG3, IgA, IgD, or IgM serum M-components, and changes in serum values for these Igs can be used directly to determine the percent change in tumor burden. The equation used to develop this nomogram has also been incorporated into a program for a pocket calculator to calculate tumor cell mass.[205]

these criteria are applied, reduction in the synthetic index of serum M-proteins to less than 10% of control is associated with a better survival than when reduction is to 10% to 24% of control, which in turn is better than reduction to 24% to 50% of control. Lesser degrees of reduction in tumor burden are not associated with improvement in survival. Patients whose hemoglobin, renal function, and albumin levels also improve have a better outcome than when these clinical variables remain unchanged or worsen. Responsive patients also have improvement in general well-being, in ambulation, and have marked relief of symptoms of bone pain. However, recalcification of osteolytic bone lesions is observed in less than 5% of patients who respond to chemotherapy.

A recent retrospective analysis on 69 Stage II and 80 Stage III myeloma patients treated at a single institution has been evaluated with both Myeloma Task Force and SWOG response criteria.[206] In carrying out this analysis, two Stage II patients and nine Stage III patients who failed to live 3 months were also censored to minimize the "guarantee time" inherent in including early deaths as nonresponders by usual statistical methods. The authors concluded from this analysis of a relatively small series of patients that the Myeloma Task Force criteria of response may have similar predictive value to those of the SWOG for Stage II cases. They also found that the SWOG criteria had greater predictive value for Stage III cases but believed that the latter difference was of questionable significance. In view of the limited

TABLE 54-7. SWOG Myeloma Response Criteria

A. Responsive patients who satisfy all of the following criteria are considered to have achieved definite objective improvement.
  A sustained decrease in the synthesis index of serum M protein to 25%, or less, of the pretreatment value on at least two measurements separated by 4 weeks. For IgA and IgG3 M = proteins, the synthetic index is the same as the serum concentration. For IgG M-proteins of subclasses 1, 2, and 4, the synthetic index must be estimated using the nomogram shown in Figure 47-6.
  A sustained decrease in 24-hr urine globulin to 10%, or less, of the pretreatment value, and to less than 0.2 g/24 hr on at least two occasions separated by 4 weeks.
  In all responsive patients the size and number of lytic skull lesions must not increase, and the serum calcium must remain normal. Correction of anemia (hematocrit > 27 vol. %) and hypoalbuminemia (>3.0 g/dl) is required if they are considered to be secondary to myeloma.
  With equivocal data (*e.g.*, nonsecretors, L chain producers for whom the pretreatment urine collection was lost), the following support the conclusion that an objective response has occurred:
    Recalcification of lytic skull lesions.
    Significant increments in depressed normal immunoglobulins (*e.g.*, increments >200 mg/dl IgM, >400 mg/dl IgA, and >4000 mg/dl IgG).

B. Improved patients show a decline in the serum M-protein synthesis rate to less than 50%, but not less than 25% of the pretreatment value.

C. Unresponsive patients fail to satisfy the criteria for responsive or improved patients.

Reprinted from Ref. 24.

sample size of this recent comparison, it remains our preference to apply SWOG response criteria in myeloma because they are based on scientifically established observations relevant to M-component metabolism, whereas the task force criteria are not. Further analysis of significantly larger patient populations is warranted to shed additional light on this issue.

SYSTEMIC CHEMOTHERAPY

The initial approach to treatment for most patients with symptoms and signs of progressive disease is with systemic chemotherapy. Cycle-nonspecific cytotoxic drugs (particularly alkylating agents) represent the current mainstay of standard therapy.

Major Agents

Bifunctional alkylating agents [particularly melphalan (M) and cyclophosphamide], nitrosoureas [including both carmustine (BCNU) and lomustine (CCNU)],[26] doxorubicin,[27] as well as glucocorticoids,[23,207] represent the major active agents used in systemic therapy for multiple myeloma.[208] Vincristine has been used in a number of treatment programs as well; although there is evidence it can reduce tumor burden somewhat,[209,210] there is now no indication that its addition to other regimes increases survival.[211] Interferon-α (INF-α) also has antitumor activity in myeloma[212-216] and is currently under investigation to determine whether or not it will play a role along with other systemic agents in the drug-sensitive phase of disease.[217] All of the foregoing agents have been subjected to clinical trials as single agents in myeloma and have also been incorporated into various drug combinations for evaluation in previously untreated patients.

RADIATION THERAPY FOR PALLIATION OF BONE PAIN

Radiation therapy has been recognized for many years as a rapid and highly effective palliative agent in the treatment of multiple myeloma.[218-222] Despite advances in the systemic treatment of this disease, this role for radiation therapy continues to be of significant importance.

Treatment of painful, disabling bony sites is usually rapidly successful because of the radioresponsive nature of myeloma and results in many positive benefits. In addition to rapid relief of pain, with accompanying decrease in narcotic requirements, pain relief allows patients to maintain much more normal activity and, thereby, reduces additional structural weakness in bone caused by calcium loss from bed rest.

As treatment is often rapidly effective at relatively modest doses of irradiation, irradiation can arrest local tumor progression in bone and prevent pathologic fractures, thereby further minimizing the morbidity of more invasive therapeutic interventions for these patients. All of these positive features are well recognized and make possible a much more normal functional existence for patients.[218-221]

Myeloma is usually quite responsive to irradiation and tumor doses of approximately 2000 to 2400 rad in five to seven fractions over 1 to 1.5 weeks are nearly always sufficient.[219,221] Unless solitary disease is present (see later discussion), higher doses have not been shown to be advantageous and, given the generalized nature of the disease and its relatively long natural history, may preclude a necessary second course of treatment to a site caused by tumor reseeding, extension, or regrowth.

Careful treatment planning is necessary to assure inclusion of the entire lesion(s) responsible to the localized problem requiring treatment, and imaging studies such as computed tomography (CT) scans may be helpful in delineation of the full extent of tumor.

Judgment and experience are necessary in determining when radiation therapy is appropriate (versus systemic treatment), especially early in the course of this often chronic condition. Although irradiation will result in relief of the most disabling symptom(s), a similar result often can also be achieved by chemotherapy, especially early in the course of myeloma, with no resultant potential compromise in future delivery of chemotherapy because of myelosuppression. This is particularly true in the treatment of sites containing considerable bone marrow such as the pelvis. Ideal management, therefore requires close coordination with the physician managing the patient's systemic chemotherapy.

Finally, structural changes brought about by tumor involvement may, by nerve compression or orthopedic instability, be responsible for a substantial portion of a patient's pain. It is, therefore, generally a mistake to treat a patient with multiple myeloma to progressively higher doses than those previously noted if some level of pain persists, assuming that careful prior imaging studies and treatment planning have been accomplished.

Special Indications for Radiation Therapy

A number of other localized manifestations of myeloma may be indications for palliative irradiation, especially in the patient who has proved resistant to most conventional systemic agents. Included are patients who present with proptosis caused by sphenoid or orbital bone involvement, those who present with dental or facial abnormalities caused by maxillary or mandibular involvement or, rarely, those who present with CNS symptoms caused by extensive calvarial or base of skull involvement. A treatment philosophy and approach similar to that noted in the section on palliation of bone pain is appropriate in these patients.

REMISSION-INDUCTION CHEMOTHERAPY

Alkylating Agents with or Without Prednisone

A variety of simple alkylating agent–prednisone combinations, as well as more complex regimens, have been used for remission-induction chemotherapy for patients with multiple myeloma. Overall objective response rates in various series with use of single alkylating agents alone or in combination with prednisone generally run between 20% to 70% and are influenced by the response criteria used and the aggressiveness with which the regimens are administered in relation to their myelosuppressive effects. Prednisone as well as other glucocorticoids have been combined with alkylating agents because of their single-agent activity, lack of overlapping toxicity, and the suggestion that they may potentiate the action of other agents. In most instances, patients in these trials received maintenance chemotherapy after remission induction. A substantial number of studies have been carried out that use a variety of schedules of oral administration of melphalan or cyclophosphamide alone or in combination with prednisone, with generally similar therapeutic results. Useful dosage schedules for the commonly used alkylating agents appear in Table 54-8. Dosage adjustments for myelosuppression are commonly employed; however, dose escalation in the absence of myelosuppression is, unfortunately, not usually followed satisfactorily. Lack of dose escalation (particularly with melphalan) in the absence of myelosuppression can lead to patients being significantly underdosed because melphalan has a quite variable absorption by the oral route.[223] Although oral absorption is not usually a problem with oral cyclophosphamide or CCNU, such regular monitoring of the white blood count and differential can also detect patients with compliance problems for self-administration of oral agents. Nadir absolute granulocyte counts below 2000/μl should be achieved between intermittent courses of therapy, whereas with continuous courses, the dosage should be adjusted to maintain the leukocyte count between 2000 and 3500/μl. Although intravenous schedules provide more predictable dose delivery, the largest experience has been with oral regimens.

TABLE 54-8. Selected Schedules Using Intermittent or Continuous Schedules of Alkylating Agents for Treatment of Myeloma (Alone or in Combination with Prednisone)

Intermittent Schedules		
Alkylating agent		
Cyclophosphamide		
	IV	1000 mg/m^2 (27 mg/kg) q 3 weeks
	Note:	Significantly higher doses now being evaluated. See text.
	Oral	250 mg/m^2 per d $\times$ 4d q 3 wk
Melphalan		
	IV	16 mg/m^2 q 2 wk $\times$ 4 then q 4 wk. Reduce initial dosing by 50% if serum creatinine >2.0 mg/dl (BUN > 30 mg/dl)
	Oral	8 mg/m^2 q 3 wk or 9 mg/m^2 q 4 wk
	Note:	Because of varying bioavailability of oral melphalan, the dose must be increased to induce hematologic toxicity or significant underdosing may occur.
Carmustine (BCNU)		
	IV	100–150 mg/m^2 q 4–6 wk
Lomustine (CCNU)		
	Oral	130 mg/m^2 q 4–6 wk

Irrespective of dosage schedules (daily or intermittent) or reported objective response rates, in major clinical trials reported between 1964 and 1980, the median survival time in patients receiving either oral melphalan or cyclophosphamide alone or in combination with prednisone have ranged from 18 to 35 months, with an overall median of about 24 months (Table 54-9).

Reported "response rates" have varied, at least partly, because differing criteria were used to determine objective response in the reported studies. Similar results have been observed with the nitrosoureas, although these agents have not been studied extensively.[26] The survival outcome in myeloma patients is now clearly superior to that observed before the introduction of alkylating agents, when median survival times from diagnosis were reported for various studies to be in the range of 3.5 to 11.5 months.[19,22,224–226] It is generally concluded that the improvement in survival that occurred in myeloma after the introduction of the alkylating agents is due to these drugs, rather than to changes in earlier diagnosis or changes in supportive care. Equivalent therapeutic effects have been reported with both intermittent and continuous schedules. Similarly, an initial loading dose followed by a subsequent continuous dose, as used by the Cancer and Leukemia Group B (CALGB), also produced similar results.[25] Intermittent schedules may have advantages in terms of assuring regular monitoring of the patient's progress and avoiding cumulative toxicity.

Multiagent Combination Chemotherapy

An area of continuing controversy for myeloma therapy relates to the comparative effectiveness of the simple oral melphalan–prednisone (MP) or cyclophosphamide–prednisone (CP) combinations with more complex regimens. A number of institutions and cooperative groups have explored a variety of multiagent combinations, with a subset of these studies reporting significantly better survival results than have been observed with the simple combinations; however, this is far from uniform. The rationale for use of the multiagent combinations is based on the objective of incor-

TABLE 54-9. Effects of Some Major Trials of Single Alkylating Agents Alone or in Combination with Prednisone on Survival in Multiple Myeloma

Author (Ref.)	*Treatment (Alkylating Agent Scheduled)*	*No. of Patients*	*Response Rate*	*Median Survival from Start of Rx (Mo)*
Alexanian et al[227]	Melphalan (i)	82	49–59	23
Alexanian et al[228]	Melphalan (d)	35	17–19	18
	Melphalan Prednisone (i)	79	~65	24
Bergsagel et al[21]	Melphalan (d)	165	14	25
Bergsagel et al[185]	Melphalan Prednisone (i)	100	72	28
Costa et al[25]	Melphalan (d)	60	~25	26
	Melphalan Prednisone (d)	71	~48	35
	Melphalan Prednisone + Testosterone (d)	58	~54	24
Hoogstraten et al[229]	Melphalan (d)	64	45	23
Hoogstraten et al[230]	Melphalan (i)	48	45	26
Korst et al[22]	Cyclophosphamide (d)	165	~48	24.5
McArthur et al[226]	Melphalan (d)	39	41	28
MRC 1st study[231]	Melphalan (d)	133	NR	18
	Cyclophosphamide (d)	141	NR	18
MRC 2nd study[232]	Melphalan Prednisone (d)	128	NR	20
	Cyclophosphamide (d)	124	NR	20
MRC 3rd study[233]	Melphalan (i)	179	NR	20
	Cyclophosphamide (i) (intravenous)	174	NR	26

d = daily, i = intermittent, NR = not reported.
Response rates shown with Myeloma Task Force Criteria or approximated from published data.

porating agents with different mechanisms of action and lack of cross-resistance as well as reduced overlapping toxicities and, it is hoped, greater cytoreductive effects against the myeloma cell burden. Some experimental evidence suggests that combinations of alkylating agents may also be potentiating because there are different mechanisms of membrane uptake as well as other potential differences in their mode of action and cellular cytotoxicity.[234] Some of the most widely used multiagent combinations include the M2 protocol developed at Memorial Hospital[235] and the alternating combination chemotherapy regimens developed by SWOG.[186] In the initial SWOG report of the alternating combinations, vincristine–melphalan–carmustine–prednisone (VMCP) was alternated with either vincristine–carmustine–doxorubicin–prednisone (VBAP) or vincristine–cyclophosphamide–doxorubicin–prednisone (VCAP);[186] however in subsequent trials, the alternation has been limited to VMCP and VBAP because VBAP has been shown to be capable to reinducing remission in myeloma patients who have previously responded and relapsed from therapy with melphalan or cyclophosphamide combinations.[236] The dosage schedules for these Memorial and SWOG combination programs are summarized in Table 54-10. The MRC5 trial[237] of alternating combination chemotherapy used drug dosages that were essentially identical with that of SWOG with the deletion of vincristine and prednisone (see Table 54-10).

Slight changes in dosages of the M2 regimen have been used in various series and have recently been summarized.[208] With the M2 regimen, improved survival has been reported in a nonrandomized study, wherein survival was calculated from the date of diagnosis rather than from the onset of therapy.[235] Subsequent cooperative group randomized studies carried out by the Eastern Cooperative Group (ECOG) in the United States and by a multihospital group from Denmark compared the M2 regimen to melphalan–prednisone.[238,239] Both studies failed to show a survival ad-

TABLE 54-10. Dosage Schedules for the M2 and the VMCP–VBAP Regimens

Drug Regimen (Ref.)	*Vincristine*	*Melphalan*	*Cyclophosphamide*	*BCNU*	*Doxorubicin*	*Prednisone*
M2 regimen[235]	0.03 mg/kg day 1	0.25 mg/kg days 1–7	10 mg/kg day 1	0.5 mg/kg day 1		1 mg/kg days 1–7
VMCP[186]	1.0 mg day 1	6 mg/m^2/d days 1–4	125 mg/m^2/d days 1–4			60 mg/m^2/d days 1–4
VBAP[186]	1.0 mg day 1			30 mg/m^2 day 1	30 mg/m^2 day 1	days 1–4

Note: As currently used, the M2 protocol is usually repeated at 4- to 5-wk intervals. The VMCP–VBAP program repeats courses of chemotherapy in 21-day cycles using either a direct alternation of the two regimens or a syncopated alternation wherein VMCP is used for three cycles followed by VBAP for three cycles with similar therapeutic results by either of these schedules. Currently an every-3-week alternation is utilized. The MRC has used a schedule virtually identical with VMCP–VBAP in their alternating program with the exception being that vincristine and prednisone have been deleted. Alternations are also at 3-wk intervals in the MRC schedule.

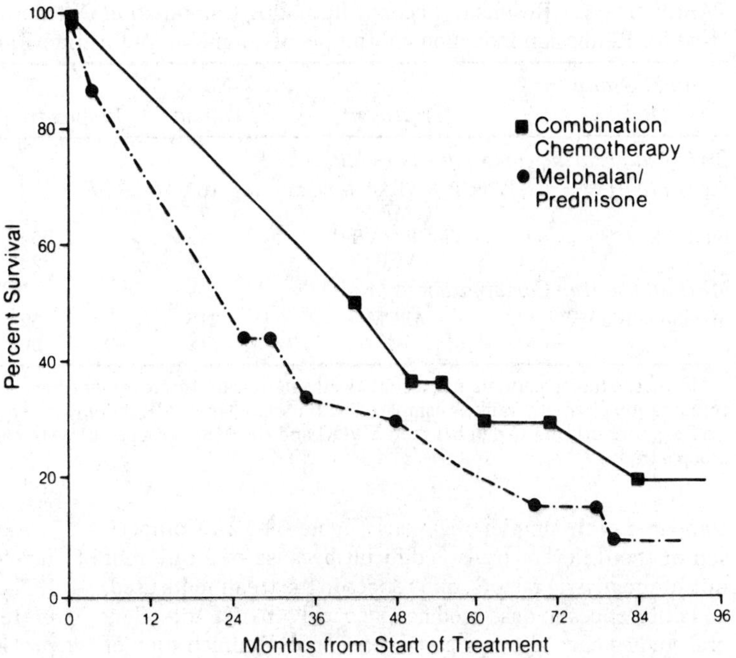

FIG. 54-9. Long-term follow-up on a randomized trial comparing alternating combination chemotherapy to melphalan and prednisone in a Southwest Oncology Group Study initiated in 1977. Therapy was administered at 3-week intervals. The alternating combinations used (VMCP–VBAP or VMCP–VCAP) yielded a superior survival outcome to that achieved with melphalan and prednisone ($p = 0.021$). The median survival with the alternating combinations was 42 months, whereas with melphalan and prednisone it was only 24 months and similar to historical controls. (Durie BGM, Dixon B, Carter S, et al: Improved survival duration with combination chemotherapy induction for multiple myeloma: A Southwest Oncology Group Study. J Clin Oncol 4:1127–1237, 1986)

vantage with the M2 regimen, although good risk subsets in the ECOG study had improved survival,[238] recent update on the ECOG study has reported improved survival for Stage III patients.[236] Two successive studies carried out by SWOG compared the alternating combination regimens to a simpler regimen [MP or vincristine–cyclophosphamide–prednisone (VCP)]. In both studies (evaluated by different study coordinators) quite similar advantages in terms of improved response rate and improved median survival were observed with the alternating combinations when compared with the simpler regimen.[186,240] Results of the first of these studies[186] were reanalyzed in 1985,[240] and the patient survival rate replotted, again demonstrating a survival advantage of alternating combination chemotherapy versus MP (Fig. 54-9). With shorter follow-up, the second of SWOG's evaluations of alternating combinations demonstrated remarkably similar survival plots for the VMCP plus VBAP versus the simpler VCP regimen. Analysis of pretreatment prognostic factors showed that the treatment groups were quite comparable. Despite identical guidelines for dose escalation in relation to blood counts for the alternating combination and simpler regimens, greater degrees of myelosuppressive toxicity were observed with the alternating combinations, compared with the simpler regimens in both studies, suggesting more consistent drug delivery with the multiagent combinations. Of interest, despite the higher overall response rates and improved survival with the alternating combinations, the overall duration of remissions was not improved in patients responsive to the alternating combinations when compared with those responsive to MP or VCP. Inasmuch as a significantly larger proportion of patients responded to the alternating combinations, this suggests that the additional responsive patients may have required combination therapy to reach remission status and could be anticipated to have had a poorer prognosis and less-than-average remission duration. Analysis of the data on high-risk Stage III patients supports this interpretation and is consistent with the overall remission duration in the VMCP–VBAP group being diluted with the addition of poor-risk patients "recruited into" the responsive category with the aggressive combinations who would not have achieved remission with the simple regimens.[235] A similar interpretation might apply to studies from ECOG and the CALGB, who found improved response rates or survival time, or both, in specific subsets of patients with their multiagent combinations when compared with the MP regimen.[238,242] In these two studies, overall survival for all patients was not improved, suggesting that the increased toxicity of the aggressive regimens may have a detrimental effect on survival subsets of patients. Finally, a recently presented result in the fifth Medical Research Council (MRC) study made a very similar observation to that obtained by SWOG. In the MRC study, 627 patients were randomized to receive almost identical schedules of the cytotoxic agents used in the SWOG VMCP–VBAP studies, with the exception that vincristine and prednisone were omitted. Thus, the MRC study compared alternating MC/BA to M in a study begun in 1982 and closed in 1986. In the MRC's most recent public report[237] the survival advantage for the 315 patients receiving the alternating combinations was significantly superior ($p = 0.0004$) to that obtained with M alone. Curves for the MRC5 study are almost superimposable with SWOG results. A summary of results from the recent SWOG and MRC5 studies appear in Table 54-11. The data from these studies suggest that the aggressive multidrug programs have their greatest current application to Stage III myeloma patients who need to achieve remission quickly before adverse disease-related complications result in premature death. On the other hand, other recent multicenter randomized trials using variants of the M2 protocol (VBMCP) have failed to show improvement with such combinations when

TABLE 54-11. Results of Recent Alternating Combination Chemotherapy Regimens Used for Remission Induction in Multiple Myeloma in Multicenter Randomized Trials *

Study Group (Ref.)	*Treatment*	*No. of Patients*	*% Responding*† (mo)	*Median* Survival
SWOG alternating combinations vs MP or VCP				
Study 7704[186,240]	VMCP + VBAP or VCAP	160	54	42
	MP	77	32	23
Study 7927[240]	VMCP + VBAP	93	54	48
	VCP	107	28	29
MRC Alternating Combination vs M				
Myelomatosis V[237]	ABCM	315	62	~34
	M	312	50	~23

*In these studies patients had a statistically significant improvement in survival with alternating combination chemotherapy as compared with melphalan or MP therapy.

†Response criteria varied between SWOG and the MRC groups but were consistent within each group's trial.

compared with simpler regimens (Table 54-12). Comparison of the different trials is difficult because of a different mix of prognostic factors, differences in the treatments used, and differences in dose modifications and other factors. Several studies have also compared sequential administration of various alkylating agents with simultaneous combinations or MP (data not shown). These studies showed either inferiority or no advantage for the sequential regimens.[184,242]

Thus, optimal chemotherapy for myeloma now appears to be with the alternating combination regimens as used by SWOG and the MRC and not with variants of the M2 combination. At best, however, the SWOG and MRC study results represent a modest incremental advance in therapy and newer or alternative approaches need to be investigated for remission-induction therapy.

Although interferon-α is known to have some activity in myeloma patients in relapse,[212–215,248–250] the recombinant IFN-αs have thus far had only limited study in previously untreated patients. In an initial report, 7 of 14 patients with previously untreated myeloma with Stages I–II myeloma responded to treatment.[216] Interestingly, response was associated with an increase in residual polyclonal Igs. However, two randomized trials comparing initial therapy and IFN-α to chemotherapy have shown IFN-α monotherapy to be less active than standard chemotherapy.[251,252] Of perhaps greater interest will be the integration of recombinant IFN-α into combination chemotherapy with alkylating agent–prednisone combinations.[217] On the basis of the initial experience with this approach, the CALGB has initiated a randomized trial comparing the effectiveness of MP to MP plus

TABLE 54-12. Results with Combination Chemotherapy Regimens Used for Remission Induction in Multiple Myeloma in Multicenter Randomized Trials That Failed to Show a Survival Advantage with Multiagent Chemotherapy Compared with Simple Alkylating Agent Regimens

Study Group (Ref.)	*Treatment*	*No. of Patients*	*% Response (mo)*	*Median Survival*
Argentine[244]	MeCCMVP	105	46	41
	MP	129	38	39
CALGB[243]	MCBP (iv)	156	56	29
	MCBPA (iv)	157	44	26
	MP (iv)	146	47	33
Canadian[185]	MCBP	116	47*	31
	MP	125	31*	28
Danish[239]	M2	31	45	21
	VMP	32	73	30
	MP	33	58	21
ECOG[245]	M2	134	74	~31
	MP	131	53	~30
Finnish[246]	MOCCA	64	75	41
	MP	66	54	45
Norwegian[247]	M2	33	74	33
	MP	34	67	33
SECSG[245]	BCP	186	49	36
	MP	187	52	36

MeC = methyl-CCNU, B = BCNU, C = cyclophosphamide, V = vincristine, P = prednisone, A = doxorubicin (Adramycin; MOCCA = melphalan, vincristine, CCNU, cyclophosphamide, doxorubicin).

*SWOG response criteria (all others reported by Myeloma Task Force Criteria).

recombinant IFN-α_2.[250] Inasmuch as current systemic therapy is not curative in myeloma, there appears to be no advantage to using aggressive regimens in treatment of Stage I patients. The major issue related to this patient population is, rather, if any therapy at all should be employed until clear evidence of symptomatic disease progression occurs. Application of additional prognostic factors, such as the pretreatment β_2-microglobulin, may assist in better identifying the patient groups most likely to benefit from aggressive systemic therapy for myeloma.

Magnitude of Myeloma Cell Kill with Induction Chemotherapy

For the various foregoing chemotherapy regimens, the magnitude of tumor cell reduction with chemotherapy can be assessed using the quantitative methods to determine response in terms of the degree of cytoreduction achieved. This was first achieved in myeloma by using a computer-based method in which serial measurements of the amount of M-component produced per cell in vitro, intravascular mass of M-component, and catabolic rate were integrated.[2,166] Similar estimates of cytoreduction can be obtained by using the nomogram and response criteria utilized by SWOG. Irrespective of the treatment regimen, with the current standard treatment programs and magnitude of cell kill as determined from such M-component-derived measurements, the maximum degree of total tumor cell kill observed in responsive patients rarely exceeds 90% to 99%. Despite continued treatment, tumor burden appears to "plateau" in most cases.[166] Kinetic analysis of the plateau-phase population suggests that the residual tumor cells behave differently from those present before treatment, and by comparison they are hypoproliferative and perhaps less responsive to cytotoxic chemotherapy.[202] With a total tumor burden in most patients in the range of 10^{12} myeloma cells or more, it is perhaps not surprising that there is not a strong correlation between the exact magnitude of cytoreduction (*e.g.*, 75%, 90%, 99%) and overall survival. On the other hand, remission durations after induction chemotherapy can vary substantially in comparably staged patients with similar degrees of apparent cytoreduction and the presence of a clearly measurable residual M-component peak in the serum. Although the median duration of unmaintained remission is 11 months,[253] in some instances, unmaintained remissions after induction chemotherapy in patients with Stage III myeloma may last for 5 years or longer.[254] This suggests that in some cases there is an alteration in the residual myeloma cell population or in the tumor–host relationship. Such observations provide the basis to seriously question whether or not the residual cell mass determined from M-component levels in remission reflects the initial population of malignant plasma cells or a less malignant population more akin to that present in patients with MGUS. However, patients regularly do relapse with overt myeloma from unmaintained remissions, so that an underlying highly malignant monoclone persists but may be "submerged" under a population of less highly proliferative M–component-secreting cells. Analysis of the myeloma regrowth rate based on M-component doubling-times has been carried out on individual patients studied sequentially after a series of unmaintained remissions.[169] Of interest, even in the presence of continued chemosensitivity (as reflected by cytoreduction after reinstitution of chemotherapy), most patients studied developed a progressive shortening of the M-component doubling-time during subsequent unmaintained remissions. Such observations suggest progressive loss of growth control with the emergence of a kinetically more aggressive tumor cell population.

REMISSION MAINTENANCE VERSUS UNMAINTAINED REMISSION

Therapeutic approaches in myeloma have generally been developed in an analogous fashion to those for other advanced neoplasms and have included both remission-induction phase and remission-maintenance phase treatments. Thus, those myeloma patients who exhibit drug sensitivity and achieve remission usually have been maintained on a similar form of chemotherapy until the time of relapse. The usefulness of maintenance therapy with cytotoxic drugs was first addressed by the SWOG.[253,255] In that SWOG study, patients who achieved remission with chemotherapy were randomized to maintenance chemotherapy with MP versus no maintenance. Patients randomized to no maintenance received alkylating agent chemotherapy again at the earliest evidence of relapse as manifest by a rise in M-component or recurrent symptoms and signs of active myeloma. Of interest, there was no overall survival advantage for those patients receiving maintenance treatment, and the authors felt that there were more infections and other complications in those patients who were receiving continued chemotherapy.[253] The lack of efficacy of maintenance chemotherapy was subsequently confirmed in several studies by other cooperative groups.[256,257] These findings are consistent with the change in tumor growth behavior observed during the plateau phase of myeloma and the varying times to relapse from unmaintained remission discussed earlier. Thus, continuation of conventional alkylating agent therapy for patients achieving remission appears to offer no obvious advantage over unmaintained remission, as long as patients are followed closely and have treatment reinstituted when there is laboratory or clinical evidence of reactivation of myeloma. In general, patients followed in unmaintained remission should be followed monthly, with regular monitoring of serum and urine M-components to detect the first signs of relapse. Patients presenting initially with Stage III myeloma with heavy Bence Jones proteinuria or amyloidosis must be followed very closely because fulminant relapse from unmaintained remission can potentially lead to irreversible complications unless treatment is reinstituted promptly at the first sign of disease reactivation. An alternative approach to remission maintenance using recombinant IFN-α has recently been reported by the Italian Multiple Myeloma Study Group.[258,259] In this study, 70 patients with remissions induced with either MP or VMCP–VBAP (on a randomized induction) were re-randomized to maintenance therapy with recombinant IFN-α_2, or no treatment. The IFN-α_2 was administered at a dosage of 3×10^6 IU/m^2 subcutaneously three times weekly. After 27 months of follow-up, 8 of 33 (24%) of evaluable patients receiving IFN-α_2 and 22 of 37 patients with no maintenance (59%) had relapsed with a significant difference ($p < 0.01$) in the actuarial curves of remission duration in the two groups.[259] Further follow-up will be required to assess the impact of maintenance IFN-α therapy on overall survival. This initial observation suggests a potentially new approach to maintenance therapy for myeloma and, therefore, warrants expanded study with confirmation by other cooperative study groups. One such study is now underway by the SWOG.

SOLITARY PLASMACYTOMA OF BONE AND EXTRAMEDULLARY PLASMACYTOMA

A small fraction (~7%) of all patients who present with plasma cell malignancies will present with solitary lesions in bone or soft tissues, with bone marrow examinations demonstrating less than 5% plasmacytes. Several differences (in addition to survival characteristics) distinguish patients with solitary lesions from those with multiple myeloma.

Age at presentation tends to be younger and a higher percentage are male (~70% versus 55%). A smaller fraction (~30% versus 97%) present with serum or urinary M-component.

The demonstration that an elevated in M-component may persist after high-dose local irradiation, but after nonradical surgical excision of Waldeyer's ring material, may return to normal with subsequent long-term disease-free survival suggests two alternative possibilities for the response of certain malignant plasma cells to radiation.

One alternative is that a substantial population of cells in certain patients is highly resistant to radiation. However, several factors mitigate against this explanation—most notably the long disease-free survival after a less-than-radical surgical approach. In addition, given the monoclonal nature of the disease in these patients and their generally excellent response to radiation, it seems more likely that these persistent cells represent clonogenically nonviable foci that fail to manifest radiation damage as they divide very slowly, or not at all. Such behavior is somewhat analogous to functioning pituitary adenomas in which elevated hormone levels may be observed for months, and even years, after radiation therapy without evidence of ultimate progression.

Several studies have shown the relatively favorable course for both these groups of patients. However, many long-term studies have demonstrated the distinct difference in ultimate prognosis between patients with solitary lesions in bone and those with extramedullary lesions.[260-263,265]

Although they experience significantly longer survivals, on average, than patients with classic multiple myeloma, virtually all patients with solitary bone lesions will develop systemic disease if followed for sufficient periods.[260-263] In one study, although nearly 35% of patients were progression-free at 10 years, by 13 years, more than 90% of patients experienced widespread evidence of disease.[262] The report by Chak and co-workers is slightly more optimistic.[264] In contrast, more than 80% of patients treated for extramedullary lesions are progression-free at periods exceeding 10 years after treatment.[260-262,265]

Despite this difference in ultimate prognosis, long-term survival is observed in substantial numbers in both groups and suggests the desirability for long-term local control. Radiation doses of 3500 to 5000 rad have been proposed, with doses at the lower end of this spectrum generally being applied with shortened treatment times and altered (increased) daily radiation fractions. We favor a total dose of 4500 to 5000 rad in 4.5 to 5 weeks, utilizing megavoltage fields that adequately encompass necessary soft-tissue and bony structures. In primary bony lesions, the entire medullary cavity of the bone must be encompassed, as in patients with Ewing's tumor, because of the possibility of medullary cavity spread.

Few data are available on the probability of regional lymph node spread, and treatment of nodal sites, in addition to adequate encompassing of the primary lesion, generally is not recommended. The report of Knowling and associates suggests, however, that treatment may be of value in selected patients.[261]

Typical survival curves after radiation treatment for these two groups of patients appear in Figure 54-10.[262,264]

IN VITRO TESTING OF CLONOGENIC MYELOMA CELLS

In vitro soft agar methods have been developed to support the growth of colony-forming neoplastic plasma cells from the bone marrows of some patients with multiple myeloma[61,266,267] and to assess the response of the clonogenic or myeloma stem cells to a variety of anticancer drugs.[268,269] By using a visual endpoint for colony formation, clonogenic growth of myeloma cells has been applied to in vitro drug testing by several laboratories.[266,267,270] A series of technical problems has been identified with human tumor clonogenic assays, and most of these have been resolved satisfactorily.[271] In the absence of specific growth stimulants, myeloma colony formation can be detected visually in only a few

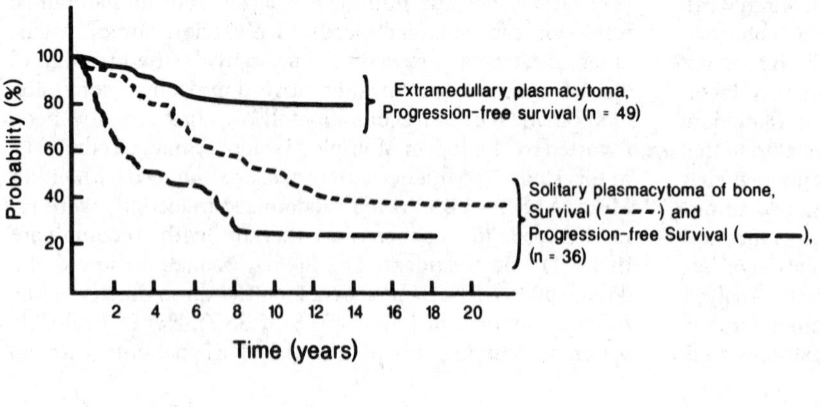

FIG. 54-10. Survival and disease-free survival in patients with solitary plasmacytoma of bone and disease-free survival of those with solitary soft-tissue disease.[260-262, 264, 265] Note significant advantage for those with soft tissue disease and low disease-free survival (in time) for those with bone disease.

patients studied (particularly those with high tritiated thymidine-labeling indices of plasma cells).[136] From our own center, we have reported on a total of 63 correlative clinical trials in 31 patients with multiple myeloma who were tested in vitro and treated clinically with agents to which their cells were tested.[269] True-positive correlations between in vitro sensitivity and clinical response were obtained in 22 of 28 instances wherein in vitro sensitivity was observed (79%), and true-negative correlation with in vitro drug resistance was observed in 35 of 37 instances (99%). Although such findings would suggest that this assay might have potentially broad application, it is still applicable to only a few of the patients tested, owing to inadequate visual colony growth, in many instances. Thus, it is currently impractical to routinely test patients' myeloma cells for drug sensitivity and select treatments for most myeloma patients. However, in the research setting we continue to find this approach to be of interest for aiding in the discovery of new drugs with activity against myeloma cells as well as in identifying potentially active drugs for a selected subset of patients whose cells can be cultivated in vitro. New information on cytokines that supports the growth of plasmacytoma cells,[63,65,272,273] as well as use of more sensitive nonvisual endpoints for the cloning assay,[274] may increase the applicability of this approach to myeloma in the future.

TREATMENT OF REFRACTORY MYELOMA

Patients who relapse after unmaintained remission can often be reinduced into remission with a regimen similar to that used initially for the patient[253,275] and are not considered to be refractory to therapy unless they fail to achieve remission on reinduction. However, at least one-third of patients with multiple myeloma fail to respond to induction chemotherapy, and those who initially achieve remission eventually relapse and require additional treatment. Both standard and new agents and approaches have been evaluated in such refractory patients and have been reviewed recently.[276,277] Therapeutic agents used for treatment of refractory patients usually include the same drugs used in initial remission-induction therapy (*e.g.*, anthracyclines, glucocorticoids, vinca alkaloids, alkylating agents, and nitrosoureas), with these various agents often in alternative dosages, schedules, and combinations to those used initially. Interferon-α has been shown to have clear activity as a Phase II agent;[214,215,278–280] however, remissions are usually short, and IFN-α has yet to be integrated effectively into combination therapy for second-line therapy.

It is important to distinguish between the two subsets of patients who are generally classified as refractory, because their prognosis differs substantially. Patients who fail to respond to induction chemotherapy and are drug-*resistant* have the poorest overall prognosis, and only a few such patients respond to alternative treatments. The second major category comprises *relapsing* patients who respond to induction chemotherapy but then relapse while still receiving chemotherapy or within a few months thereafter. Such patients have a higher probability of responding to second-line therapy than do the drug-resistant patients. For simplicity, refractory myeloma patients are usually divided dichotomously into drug-resistant and relapsing groups.

High-Dose Glucocorticoids

The antitumor activity of single-agent prednisone for a high-dose, alternate-day schedule for resistant and relapsing patients was first reported over 20 years ago.[23] This single-agent activity of high doses of glucocorticoids has been confirmed and extended using both prednisone and dexamethasone in alternate-day or pulse schedules.[207,276,281] Recently a *p*-glycoprotein-expressing multidrug-resistant myeloma cell line was reported to develop collateral sensitivity to glucocorticoids, suggesting that there may be some specificity of steroids for drug-resistant cells.[282] Overall, about 40% of both resistant and relapsing myeloma patients achieve second remissions with glucocorticoids. Inasmuch as glucocorticoids are nonmyelosuppresive, they are particularly useful in refractory patients with poor bone marrow reserve. In our experience, some pancytopenic patients will have remissions myeloma for several years' duration with alternate-day prednisone alone. Recently, efforts have been made to quantitate glucocorticoid receptors in myeloma;[243] such measurements may aid in identifying patients potentially sensitive to glucocorticoids.

Combination Chemotherapy Regimens

Although there were a few initial favorable reports on combination regimens that comprised primarily alkylating agents,[235,284] most reports have been less promising,[285–290] with response rates in the range of 8% for resistant and 22% for refractory patients. As mentioned earlier, such regimens are far more active for reinducing remissions in patients who have disease reactivation from unmaintained remission.[253,275,291–293]

More favorable results have been obtained with doxorubicin-based combinations. Although doxorubicin alone exhibits activity in only 10% of patients,[27] when combined with carmustine (BCNU),[294] or these two drugs plus vincristine and prednisone (VBAP)[295,296] or cyclophosphamide instead of vincristine,[297,298] somewhat better results are obtained. Overall, about 30% of relapsing patients respond to these regimens, but only 10% of resistant patients respond. Although not all studies report remission duration of responders or overall survival, the remission duration of responders is generally less than 1 year. Significantly better results have been obtained by using the vincristine–doxorubicin–dexamethasone (VAD) regime developed at M. D. Anderson Hospital.[299] In this program, vincristine and doxorubicin are administered by continuous infusion over 4 days through an indwelling venous catheter, along with oral dexamethasone (Table 54-13).

In the initial report on VAD, 14 of 20 patients (70%) with refractory myeloma responded to VAD, with a projected survival in excess of 1 year for responders.[299] Although granulocytopenia was only moderate, infection represented the most frequent complication, perhaps because of the large doses of dexamethasone used. In a follow-up report,[207] either VAD or dexamethasone were administered on a nonrandom basis to

TABLE 54-13. Dosage Schedule for VAD Regimen

Vincristine	0.4 mg/d IV for 4 d
Doxorubicin	9 mg/m²/d IV for 4 d (Note: both drugs may be mixed in IV bag)
Dexamethasone	40 mg/d orally for 4 d beginning on days 1, 9, and 17 of the first 28-d cycle and on alternate cycles thereafter. On the other cycles dexamethasone is given only on days 1–4.
All patients also received cimetidine for antacid prophylaxis and trimethoprim–sulfamethoxazole as anti-infective prophylaxis.	

See Ref. 299.

85 refractory patients.[207] Among relapsing patients, 65% responded to VAD, whereas only 21% responded to dexamethasone alone. In contrast, among resistant patients only 32% responded to VAD, a result quite similar to the 27% response rate observed with dexamethasone alone. This suggests that response to the VAD regimen in initially unresponsive patients is primarily due to the glucocorticoid in the regimen.[207] Similar therapeutic results have been confirmed with the VAD regimen by other investigators.[300–302] Toxicity has been the major limitation of the VAD regimen, with serious infection attributed primarily to the steroid program. Serious gastrointestinal toxicity, including gastric perforations, as well as steroid psychoses have been observed. Overall, about one-third of patients receiving VAD develop moderate to severe toxicity. Nonetheless, at the present time it appears to be the most effective treatment for myeloma in relapse. For patients with primary drug resistance, steroid alone is preferable to VAD. Recently, a novel means for potentially reversing resistance to VAD has been reported for relapsing patients who previously responded to the VAD regimen and subsequently developed multidrug resistance associated with expression of the *p*-glycoprotein.[303] In this study, the presence of *p*-glycoprotein was detected using a murine monoclonal antibody and by mRNA dot blot analysis. Five refractory myeloma patients were first treated with the VAD regimen, and at the time of relapse or failure to respond to VAD, the calcium channel blocker verapamil was administered at high dosage by continuous infusion along with VAD. Resistance was at least partially reversed in two patients, with improvement in M-component and hematologic values. In one patient whose myeloma cells were tested in vitro, verapamil exposure significantly increased intracellular accumulation of doxorubicin, suggesting a possible mechanism by which the verapamil effect was mediated. Further exploration of calcium channel blockers along with VAD appears warranted for patients who acquire resistance to VAD alone.

SYSTEMIC RADIATION THERAPY

Rider, Bergsagel, and colleagues have been instrumental in pioneering a wide-field or half-body irradiation approach to this systemic illness.[304,305] A variety of treatment schemes have been used; however, in most, a radiation dose of 750 to 850 rad in 150-rad fractions (dose rate ≥ 50 rad/min) is given to the hemibody (umbilicus used as midpoint) after pretreatment preparation with corticosteroids and antiemetics. Patients have nearly always been an adversely selected group with Stage III disease,[306] who have usually relapsed with first-line chemotherapy. In the great majority of reported patients, the lower half body has been treated initially. Approximately 50% to 75% of patients complete treatment to both half-body segments in most series.[304,305,307–312]

Because of a definite incidence of radiation pneumonitis in patients treated initially, cumulative lung doses have been reduced to 600 to 650 rad (generally not corrected for air transmission) in more recently treated patients.[313] Although definite laboratory evidence of hematologic toxicity has been noted in most patients who have received treatment to the whole body, with some patients requiring platelet or red cell transfusions, major clinical morbidity from hematologic toxicity has been no more than moderate. In some instances it can be prolonged.

By using this general irradiation approach, approximately half of all treated patients have experienced a significant subjective relief.

Median survivals in irradiated patients have averaged 6 months, with mean survival times averaging approximately 12 months. Only occasional patients have survived more than 18 months in this adversely selected group.

In an attempt to use this treatment modality with more favorable patients, the SWOG is carrying out a Phase III prospectively randomized trial (SWOG 8229/8230) in which previously untreated patients who are receiving initial combination chemotherapy and have obtained a "complete response" (≥75% tumor mass regression) have been randomized to either maintenance chemotherapy or to sequential hemibody irradiation (750 rad per five fields for 1 week) with 4 to 6 weeks or more elapsing between the two irradiation courses (depending on the severity and duration of hematologic toxicity).[306]

In a recent report on this SWOG study, the survival outcome for patients receiving hemibody irradiation proved to be inferior to that of patients receiving maintenance chemotherapy. The difference in survival could be attributed to a shorter relapse-free survival with irradiation. Survival from relapse to death was identical in both groups.[306] Additionally, myelosuppression has been significantly more severe in those patients receiving hemibody radiation therapy than those receiving maintenance chemotherapy. The primary toxicity has been prolonged thrombocytopenia. These findings indicate that chemotherapy maintenance is more effective than hemibody radiation for remission consolidation in myeloma patients who respond to induction chemotherapy.

HIGH-DOSE CHEMOTHERAPY ALONE OR WITH BONE MARROW TRANSPLANTATION

A series of more aggressive approaches to the therapy of multiple myeloma are currently being explored that utilize high-dose chemotherapy alone, or high-dose chemotherapy with autologous or allogeneic bone marrow transplantation, in an attempt to overcome drug resistance to conventional-dose therapy.[314–328] The drug most commonly used in high doses has been melphalan, administered intravenously in doses ranging from 80 to 140 mg/m², either without or with autologous bone marrow transplantation. With high-dose melphalan alone, a high response rate is observed including complete remissions associated with complete disappearance of the M-component and normalization of the bone marrow.[320] Unfortunately, the responses to high-dose melphalan alone, thus far reported for relapse patients, have usually been relatively short-lived (approximately 3 months to 1 year). Toxicity has included profound myelosuppression, mucositis, diarrhea, nausea, and vomiting. Treatment-related deaths are not uncommon and are associated with host failure and very severe hematologic toxicity. However, inasmuch as the use of high-dose melphalan is still relatively new, further experience may provide a means to enhance efficacy and reduce toxicity (*e.g.*, with the use of myeloid colony-stimulating factors or by limitation of high-dose melphalan administration to good-performance status patients). The addition of autologous bone marrow transplantation (without purging) has reduced the severity of myelosuppression. When total-body irradiation was combined with high-dose melphalan and autologous bone marrow transplantation, significantly longer remissions were observed.[321] In many instances when such techniques are used, evidence of a residual M-component can still be detected with immunofixation. Efforts to develop purging techniques to remove residual myeloma from the marrow are being attempted to enhance the potential of autologous transplantation;[329] however, the main limitation, at present, appears to be the difficulty of eradicating myeloma with the available preparative regimens for transplantation. Published data on allogeneic transplantation are quite limited, in part a result of the exclusion of many patients because of age or renal complications. However, a study has recently been published by the European Cooperative Group for Bone Marrow Transplantation.[324] Of 14 patients treated (including 2 who were resistant to induction chemotherapy) 5 were reported as being alive without signs of active myeloma for 9 to 34 months after allogeneic transplantation. Four additional patients are clinically well but have evidence of persistent myeloma as reflected by serum or urinary M-component or bone marrow plasma cells. Currently, allogeneic transplantation should be considered primarily as third- or fourth-line therapy for the occasional patient under the age of 40, with a suitably matched sibling donor.

ACTIVITY OF OTHER AGENTS IN PHASE II TRIALS

A limited number of other antitumor agents has been found to induce remissions in 10% or more of myeloma patients in relapse in Phase II trials. These include deoxycoformycin (pentostatin),[330,331] epirubicin,[332] poly (I,C)-LC (an interferon inducer),[333] peptichemio,[334] and teniposide.[335] These agents [aside from poly (I,C)-LC which is an interferon inducer] warrant additional investigation in refractory cases to better define their activity.

Other chemotherapeutic agents that have been subjected to Phase II clinical trials in myeloma and found to have minimal activity (with less than a 10% response rate in refractory patients) include aclarubicin,[336] acronine,[337] amsacrine (*m*-AMSA),[338] bleomycin,[339,340] cisplatin,[341] chlorozotocin,[342,343] cytarabine,[344] diaziquone,[345,346] etoposide,[347] methenamine (hexamethylmelamine),[348] mitoxantrone,[349] prednimustine,[350] procarbazine,[351] pyrazofurin,[352] urethane,[19] vindesine.[353] Although hexamethylmelamine appeared to exhibit greater than 10% activity, this likely was attributable to the concomitant use of glucocorticoids in the protocol.[354]

MANAGEMENT OF COMPLICATIONS AND SPECIAL PROBLEMS

RENAL FAILURE

In most studies, about 20% of patients with multiple myeloma present with renal failure, and this complication has a major adverse impact on survival. In one recent report, patients who had stage IIIB myeloma had a median survival of only 4 months.[355] For patients who have normal or minimally impaired renal function, it is important to take those actions that can minimize the likelihood of subsequent development of renal failure. Myeloma patients should have a high fluid intake (*e.g.*, at least 2 liters/day) to facilitate the excretion of calcium, Bence Jones proteins, uric acid, and other excretory products. Patients with Bence Jones proteinuria and evidence of advanced or progressive myeloma should promptly be started on a chemotherapy regimen. Administration of allopurinol along with chemotherapy is a worthwhile precaution in Stage III patients (at least for the first few courses of therapy). Patients with known myeloma should not be dehydrated for intravenous pyelography, and both hypercalcemia and urinary tract infections should be treated promptly. The use of antibiotics with known nephrotoxicity (*e.g.*, the aminoglycosides) should be avoided whenever possible. When melphalan is administered intravenously to patients in renal failure, increased myelosuppression has been observed.[356] Pharmacokinetic studies in dogs with use of intravenous melphalan,[357] and oral studies in myeloma patients[358] have established that melphalan elimination is reduced in the presence of renal insufficiency. Dose reductions are, therefore, often needed for melphalan when it is administered intravenously; however, because of the varying bioavailability of oral melphalan, dose reductions for renal failure may further compromise its therapeutic activity.

In the fourth myeloma chemotherapy trial of the MRC in England, management of renal failure was studied prospectively.[359] Of the 522 patients admitted to the trial, 80 had evidence of renal failure which persisted after an initial 24-hr period of rehydration. Seventy-three of the 80 patients who had renal failure were maintained with a fluid intake of at least 3 liters/day in addition to receiving chemotherapy. These patients were also randomized to receive either sodium bicarbonate or no supplement to render their urine pH neutral. The remaining seven patients either had congestive heart failure or required continued dialysis for oliguric renal failure and, therefore, were not eligible for evaluation of oral fluid supplementation. Of 49 patients who survived more than 100 days, 39 achieved reversal of renal failure (18 complete, 21 partial). In 14 of the patients, death was directly attributable to renal failure rather than other complications or manifestations of myeloma. Patients who received bicarbonate did marginally better than those who did not. The survival outcome of patients with renal failure in the MRC's third myeloma trial appeared to be inferior to that obtained in the fourth trial wherein high fluid intake was mandated.

This study showed that, in many cases, renal failure in myeloma can be reversed, either completely or partially, by simple fluid administration, whereas in oliguric renal failure of myeloma the glomeruli may open up after a period of dialysis. A number of the patients who had improvement in renal function with these measures were subsequently able to lead a more active life. However, prolonged survival is not likely unless renal failure can be reversed rapidly.[360] For patients who have myeloma and signs of acute renal failure, dialysis is indicated.[361] Both peritoneal and hemodialysis have been used successfully in this setting; however, continued dialysis is not indicated in patients who have clear evidence of progressive myeloma while receiving chemotherapy. Plasmapheresis is an additional urgent measure that can be of temporary benefit to myeloma patients who develop acute renal failure because of an inability to adequately excrete light chains. Plasmapheresis is tenfold more effective than peritoneal dialysis for this acute complication.[362-365] Renal transplantation has been carried out successfully for a patient responsive to chemotherapy.[366] Before considering renal transplantation, the patient's presenting stage, age, response to treatment, and prognosis must be considered in detail in view of the eventual fatal outcome of the disease and the added morbidity and complexities of management associated with transplantation.

HYPERCALCEMIA

About one-fourth of multiple myeloma patients have hypercalcemia with a serum calcium concentration in excess of 11.5 mg/dl (after correction for the serum albumin),[367] and a significant fraction of patients develop it in the refractory phase of myeloma. The serum calcium concentration should be measured routinely as part of staging evaluation in the initial workup of all patients with myeloma. There is a high index of suspicion for hypercalcemia if the patient develops complaints of polyuria, constipation, nausea or vomiting, lethargy or mental confusion, or has signs of dehydration or coma. The symptoms and signs of hypercalcemia correlate well with the level of ionized calcium rather than with the total calcium level, although the ionized level usually cannot be conveniently measured. Patients with bone pain or fractures who are bedridden or immobilized are also prone to hypercalcemia, and every effort should be made to mobilize them as quickly as possible. As in other settings of malignant disease in which hypercalcemia occurs, vigorous hydration and diuresis should be used as soon as hypercalcemia is recognized and, additionally, the patient should be started promptly on corticosteroid therapy (*e.g.*, 50–100 mg of prednisone per day) because steroids have a direct role in blocking osteoclastic activity in myeloma and reducing negative calcium balance. Hypercalcemia in newly diagnosed patients and those relapsing from unmaintained remission usually comes promptly under control with institution of systemic chemotherapy for myeloma. Additional useful agents to control severe hypercalcemia (*i.e.*, serum calcium > 13.5 mg/dl) or in patients in whom fluids, diuretics, and steroids prove inadequate over several days include parenteral mithramycin, etidronate[368,369] or other diphosphonates, and calcitonin. Etidronate is administered intravenously at a dosage of 7.5 mg/kg in 250 ml of saline daily for 3 days. For chronic hypercalcemia, oral phosphates are usually administered in a dosage of 1 to 3 g/day. Phosphate enemas can be used as an alternative to oral phosphate for patients with nausea and vomiting. Phosphates should not be used in patients in renal failure with an elevated serum phosphorus level. When needed, these supplementary agents represent additions to, rather than replacement of, hydration and steroid therapy. When treatment is effective at normalizing the serum calcium, patients usually experience reduction in bone pain as well as in hypercalciuria and hydroxyproline excretion. (Additional discussion of hypercalcemia and its management appears in Chap. 58, sect.3.)

Although calcium-binding is primarily attributable to serum albumin, in occasional myeloma patients, the M-component firmly binds calcium, leading to an asymptomatic elevation in the serum calcium concentration without an increase in the ionized calcium level.[370-372] Myeloma patients who are asymptomatic but have a chronically elevated serum calcium concentration should have the serum level of ionized calcium determined by a reference laboratory.

BONE PAIN

Bone pain is the most common symptom of myeloma and usually results from pathologic fractures. As described previously (see Pathophysiology), bone disease in myeloma is the result of increased bone resorption associated with myeloma cell infiltration and osteoclast activation. Skeletal damage in myeloma is manifest either as generalized osteoporosis or as focal punched-out osteolytic lesions without the rim of new bone formation often observed with metastatic carcinomas. One common bone manifestation of myeloma consists of compression fractures in the thoracic or lumbar spine. Bone density is reduced, resulting in gradual or sudden compression of the vertebral plates that often results in a "fish-mouth" deformity. Pain is often radicular and lancinating to one or both sides, is aggravated by movement, and likely is related to instability of the weak bone substance. Such symptoms usually subside within days to weeks after initiation of systemic chemotherapy. Opiates are often useful for pain control. Nonsteroidal anti-inflammatory agents may also relieve pain but are associated with a higher prevalence of renal failure in myeloma patients.[373] For persistent pain despite chemotherapy, localized radiation therapy may be required. Orthopedic back braces are generally poorly tolerated; however, the newer lightweight braces with Velcro fasteners are useful for some severely debilitated patients. The osteolytic lesions commonly observed in the skull, although pathognomonic for myeloma, are usually asymptomatic and normally do not require treatment. Typical examples of bone destruction in myeloma appear in Figure 54-4. Lytic lesions in major long bones should be irradiated if the lesion's diameter is one-third to one-half of the bone's diameter or involves a significant component of the cortex and the risk of pathologic fracture is considered to be high. Systemic chemotherapy infrequently leads to significant recalcification of such large lesions, and they remain susceptible to pathologic fracture, even after achieving remission with systemic therapy.

Skeletal strength is enhanced by ambulation, and this should be encouraged as soon as it is feasible. Accordingly, internal fixation of a pathologic fracture of the femur should be carried out promptly, as the myeloma patient's general condition usually deteriorates rapidly if they are put at bed rest in skeletal traction. Intramedullary fixation of fractures of long bones should be followed with local radiotherapy. There is evidence that administration of sodium fluoride (50 mg twice daily) along with calcium carbonate (1.0 g four times daily) can enhance bone density as determined by quantitative studies on bone biopsies.[374] The addition of 50,000 units of vitamin D twice weekly[375] and of androgens[376] may also be of benefit. However, in a large randomized chemotherapy trial, fluoride, calcium, and vitamin D were reported not to significantly improve outcome after trial of chemotherapy alone, but conversely they were thought to contribute to morbidity.[247] Several of the newer diphosphonate derivatives may also enhance bone density, but these are not yet generally available.

SPINAL CORD COMPRESSION AND OTHER NEUROLOGIC SYNDROMES

Spinal cord compression is a serious complication of multiple myeloma that occurs in 10% to 15% of patients and is usually observed early in the patient's course or in the late relapse phase of disease. As with other neoplastic causes of spinal cord compression, back pain is usually present as the initial symptom. The presence of a paraspinal mass also suggests that this complication may be imminent. Compression of the spinal cord usually results from either ingrowth of the tumor through an intervertebral foramina or by direct extension from a heavily involved vertebra. If initial skeletal x-ray studies obtained for staging indicate the presence of a paraspinal mass, follow-up evaluation with an MRI scan or CT scan is warranted to exclude invasion of the spinal canal. The earliest symptom of spinal cord compression often is radicular pain that is accentuated by coughing or sneezing, whereas motor or sensory loss or abnormality in bowel or bladder function are signs of more extensive compression. Paraplegia is a late, and usually irreversible, finding. Given any of the symptoms or signs, imaging of the spinal cord by MRI or CT scanning or myelography is indicated. We continue to be impressed with the value and accuracy of myelography even though both lumbar and cisternal introduction of contrast are frequently necessary. Currently available data suggest that, in some instances, MRI scanning, which is noninvasive, may provide information that is equally useful. However, in some instances MRI fails to provide the needed information. Controlled studies comparing myelography, CT, and MRI are currently underway. If permanent cord damage has not yet occurred, initiation of emergency radiation therapy and high-dose steroid therapy usually results in marked improvement or complete resolution of the patient's symptoms. On the other hand, if paralysis has occurred, at best, emergency treatment usually only prevents further worsening of the patient's disability. If myelography is performed and demonstrates a partial or complete block, the contrast medium should be left in place to assist in treatment planning and for following the response to treatment. Steroid dosage for myeloma patients with spinal cord compression should initially be in the range of 16 mg/day of dexamethasone in divided dosage, with tapering starting after the completion of radiation therapy. For radiation therapy, wide margins are necessary to encompass the disease, but treatment of the entire vertebral column is rarely indicated because of the palliative treatment philosophy and the need to resume myelosuppressive chemotherapy. Decompression laminectomy is generally not required in the diagnosis or treatment of spinal cord compression syndromes in myeloma because plasma cell tumors are usually quite radiation-sensitive. In addition, the acute debilitation resulting from this form of surgery presents a special problem for myeloma patients because of the protracted period of complete bed rest after surgery, which further increases the likelihood of developing infection or hypercalcemia. Nerve root compression sydromes and the occasional instance of notable cerebral compression by a cranial or dural plasmacytoma[377–384] can usually also be treated successfully with radiation therapy. Because plasmacytomas in the skull are normally quite chemosensitive and only rarely cause substantial cerebral compression, specialized imaging studies and radiation therapy are normally indicated only if the patient develops localized CNS symptoms and signs of involvement during the course of systemic treatment.

Other neurologic syndromes that are not infrequently encountered in myeloma patients include an acute encephalopathy in association with hypercalcemia, hyperviscosity, uremia, or meningitis. A variety of peripheral neuropathies are also encountered, most commonly caused by amyloidosis.[385] Additionally, in less than 1% of patients, a mixed sensory–motor neuropathy (particularly involving the extremities) develops. It does not appear to be the result of either amyloid or direct tumor infiltrate and usually improves after initiation of chemotherapy.[386–391] The neuropathy can be both painful and debilitating. In some instances, the neuropathy may be the result of a direct binding between the M-component and peripheral nerve constituents. It has most commonly been reported in patients with macroglobulinemia, but it has also been observed in patients with multiple myeloma, including in some patients with osteosclerotic myeloma.[387,392–396] The antigen binding in sural nerve biopsies has been seen with myelin-associated glycoprotein and associated with demyelination and, in other cases, with binding to endoneurial constituents.[397] Nerve binding of IgM in such patients has been passively transferred to mice with purified IgM fractions, with evidence of specificity.[398]

HEMATOLOGIC COMPLICATIONS

Anemia

Anemia is the most common hematologic complication of myeloma, with a hemoglobin level of less than 12 g/dl in 62% of patients at the time of presentation.[399] Severe anemia with a hemoglobin level of less than 8.5 g/dl and a marked reduction in red cell mass is observed in about 25% of patients. The degree of anemia correlates with total body tumor burden.[177] In patients with the hyperviscosity syndrome (discussed later), expansion of the plasma volume and its resulting hemodilution can exaggerate the reduction in hemoglobin out of proportion to the reduction in red cell mass. The anemia of myeloma usually improves significantly in association with response to chemotherapy unless the patient has persistent renal failure. Severe anemia, when symptomatic, requires transfusion of packed red blood cells because the recovery of adequate hemoglobin values usually does not occur until the patient has been receiving chemotherapy for at least 3 months. Recovery of an adequate circulating red cell mass is not enhanced by administration of folic acid, vitamin B_{12}, or iron unless a factor deficiency can be documented. In some instances, folate deficiency may be due to excessive folate utilization by the myeloma cells.[400] Some patients whose hemoglobin level does not improve sufficiently with chemotherapy have further improvement in this level after receiving a potent androgen (*e.g.*, testosterone enanthate, 600 mg IM q 4–6 weeks or fluoxymesterone 15–30 mg daily p.o.). When utilized, androgen therapy often needs to be continued for 3 to 6 months to see benefit. Recombinant human erythropoietin has only recently entered clinical trial in anemias associated with cancer; however, it has already shown substantial effect on increasing the red cell mass in noncancer patients with the anemia of chronic renal failure.[401,402] On the basis of the renal studies, erythropoietin may prove useful therapeutically in some patients with anemia resulting from the renal failure secondary to myeloma (and perhaps in the disease-associated anemia in other myeloma patients as well). The dosage of recombinant human erythropoietin, as established in renal failure patients, is 150 U/kg IV three times weekly.[402]

Granulocytopenia and Thrombocytopenia

Although mild granulocytopenia (< 3000 granulocytes/μl) is common in myeloma, moderate to severe granulocytopenia or thrombocytopenia is uncommon, but when present it is usually attributable to extensive bone marrow involvement with myeloma. When present at the time of diagnosis, marked granulocytopenia or thrombocytopenia should not lead to reduction in the dosage of induction chemotherapy. Rather, patients should be treated aggressively with myeloma chemotherapy as well as blood components and other supportive care elements in a fasion analogous to the management of acute leukemia. In my recent experience, recombinant granulocyte–macrophage-stimulating factor can be of value for normalizing the absolute granulocyte count in neutropenic myeloma patients.[403]

Acute Leukemia and Myelodysplastic Syndromes

An association between multiple myeloma and acute leukemia was first reported in 1965,[404,405] and has been confirmed extensively since that time. For example, in the first myeloma trial conducted by the Clinical Trials Group of the NCI of Canada, 15 cases of acute leukemia were observed among 365 myeloma patients treated with combinations of alkylating agents and prednisone.[185,404] The incidence of leukemia noted in that study was 230 times higher than that expected.[404] On an actuarial basis, the risk of acute leukemia was projected to be 19.6% at 50 months after the start of treatment. Although it appears that acute leukemia was a more frequent complication in this study than in other reported myeloma trials, it nonetheless underscores the importance of this potential complication, although the actual number of cases is significantly less than the actuarial incidence predicted. There has been much speculation over the cause of acute leukemia in myeloma patients, with the predominant view being that this was a complication of the use of alkylating agents or of radiotherapy.[405,406] However, there also are reports of acute leukemia in patients with myeloma prior to the general use of alkylating agents for treatment,[407] and myelodysplastic changes have occasionally been observed in the marrow of myeloma patients before treatment.[408] Acute leukemia has also been observed in untreated patients with macroglobulinemia or MGUS. Although the actual incidence of acute nonlymphocytic leukemia in untreated myeloma patients is not known, some authors have speculated that there may be an intrinsic increased susceptibility to acute leukemia in patients with plasma cell neoplasia.[404] On the other hand, recent analyses of incidence of acute leukemia in cancer trials for myeloma or ovarian cancer, wherein patients received either melphalan or cyclophosphamide therapy, strongly incriminate melphalan as a leukemogenic agent. In the MRC's first two trials for myeloma, 12 of 648 patients developed either a myelodysplastic syndrome (considered to be preleukemic) or acute leukemia.[409] This corresponds to a 5-year actuarial prevalence of 3% and an 8-year prevalence of 10%. In these two MRC studies, patients were randomized to receive either melphalan or cyclophosphamide as treatment. A significant relationship was found with the length of melphalan treatment ($p = 0.0001$), but no relationship whatsoever to cyclophosphamide. In this analysis the authors estimated that the risk of a secondary hematopoietic neoplasm in myeloma patients after 10 years of follow-up is about 3% for each year of melphalan treatment with much of the risk occurring within 3 years of the last melphalan treatment.[409] Furthermore, it was their view that if there was an intrinsic element of increased risk for secondary hematologic neoplasms in myeloma, it would be difficult to explain the clear relationship they found with melphalan exposure. A similar conclusion about the leukomogenicity of melphalan was reached in a recently reported analysis of 1794 1-year survivors with ovarian cancer treated with chemotherapy.[410] In the ovarian cancer study there was a 93-fold increase in the incidence of acute nonlymphocytic leukemia overall, with the greatest risk in the first 5 years after chemotherapy. Among the various treatments administered, the 10-year accumulated risk of acquiring leukemia was 11.2% after receiving melphalan and 5.4% after cyclophosphamide. Moreover, there was a definite dose–response relationship after melphalan therapy, and women receiving melphalan were two to three times more likely to develop leukemia than those receiving cyclophosphamide.[410] The results of these two studies indicate that the choice of alkylating agent and dose administered may significantly influence the risk for late complications of chemotherapy in myeloma. The effect of melphalan dosage in these studies also suggests that the current trials using high-dose intravenous melphalan in myeloma may be associated with a significant incidence of leukemia as a therapy-related complication.

The acute nonlymphocytic leukemias that evolve in myeloma patients often evolve after a prior period of bone marrow injury with an associated pancytopenia or morphologic evidence of myelodysplasia. As in the situation with other secondary acute leukemias (*e.g.*, in Hodgkin's disease), treatment of the leukemia is difficult because of the preexisting impaired bone marrow reserve resulting from disease or treatment. In myeloma, advanced age, immunodeficiency, and impaired renal function may also further compromise the treatment of acute leukemia. Nonetheless, worthwhile hematologic remissions of secondary leukemia are sometimes achieved in myeloma patients using standard induction chemotherapy regimens incorporating an anthracycline and cytarabine (cytosine arabinoside).

Coagulopathy

Coagulation disorders in the absence of thrombocytopenia occur fairly frequently in patients with macroglobulinemia or cryoglobulinemia, and somewhat less often in patients with myeloma. Purpura, epistaxis, and ecchymosis, as well as retinal hemorrhages or mucosal bleeding caused by coagulopathies, all may be observed in patients with monoclonal gammopathy. In the syndromes discussed in the following section, the functional abnormality of the bleeding disorder appears related to the presence of the M-component. There is a wide variety of mechanisms of coagulopathy in patients with M-components. In a variety of specific case reports, inhibitors of individual coagulation factors have been observed,[411] including inhibitors of factors V, VII, VIII, and X, and of the prothrombin complex. In some instances, patients have reductions in multiple coagulation factors including factors II, V, VII, VIII, and fibrinogen. The mechanism of multiple-factor depression is obscure; however, it has been suggested that the M-component either binds to or coprecipitates with coagulation complexes.[412] In macroglobulinemia, specific M-components appear to interact with or bind to fibrin during the clotting process and inhibit the polymerization of the fibrin monomer. This can be detected as a prolongation in the thrombin time.[413] However, this abnormality usually does not cause clinical bleeding, unless platelet function is also impaired. In some instances, the hemostatic defect is associated with impaired platelet function. Prolonged bleeding time, impaired clot retraction, prolongation of the thromboplastin generation time with the patient's platelets, and defective platelet aggregation are all indicators of impaired platelet function.[414,415] In some instances, the M-component appears to coat the platelets, leading to the release of platelet factor 3 and impaired aggregation.[416–418] A patient with plasma cell leukemia has also been reported with a circulating heparin sulfate proteoglycan anticoagulant.[419] Fibrinolysis with severe bleeding was recently reported in a patient with myeloma and amyloidosis who had an associated deficiency of α_2-plasmin inhibitor. Treatment with ϵ-aminocaproic acid reduced bleeding and was associated with recovery of the plasmin inhibitor level.[420]

SYNDROMES RESULTING FROM PHYSICOCHEMICAL PROPERTIES OF M-COMPONENTS

Hyperviscosity

The hyperviscosity syndrome occurs in about 50% of patients with macroglobulinemia[421–427] but in fewer than 5% of patients with multiple myeloma. Hyperviscosity results from protein–protein interactions of either very large, long molecules with high intrinsic viscosity (*e.g.*, IgM M-components) or when high concentrations are present of specific IgG or IgA M-components, which have a tendency to form multimolecular aggregates.[421–426] It rarely or ever occurs in patients with light-chain-only myeloma because of the small molecular size of Bence Jones proteins. Although plasma viscosity rises with increasing concentration of an M-component, beyond a critical point, viscosity rises much more steeply even with relatively small additional increments in serum M-component concentration. Additionally, patient-to-patient variations in the relation of M-component concentration to viscosity make prediction of plasma viscosity difficult without direct measurement.[428] As a result of poorly understood homeostatic mechanisms, increases in plasma viscosity lead to expansion of the plasma volume.[429] The hemodilution resulting from plasma volume expansion can cause sufficient dilution of the circulating red blood cell mass to give the appearance of an anemia that is more apparent than real. To clarify this situation, use of nuclear medicine techniques to directly measure the plasma volume (with radioiodinated albumin) and the red blood cell mass (with radiochromate-labeled red blood cells) are of value. The intrinsic viscosity of serum or plasma can be measured simply by noting the time necessary for a given volume of serum to pass a constriction in a glass tube (Ostwald viscometer or a white-cell pipette) and relating the time to that of a normal saline control. Symptoms and signs of the hyperviscosity syndrome are generally not seen unless the serum relative viscosity is greater than 4.0, and the full-blown classic syndrome is usually not seen unless the viscosity is greater than 5.0 (normal human serum relative viscosity is in the range of 1.4–1.8). Clinical symptoms and signs of the hyperviscosity syndrome include bleeding disorders, retinopathy, neurologic findings, and evidence of hypervolemia. Hemorrhagic complications include bruising, purpura, and mucosal bleeding that is often manifest as severe or recurrent bleeding from the nose or uterus. Characteristic ocular findings include marked dilatation and segmentation of the retinal veins (giving the appearance of a line of box-cars or sausage-links), retinal hemorrhages and, in some instances, papilledema. Neurologic abnormalities range from fatigue, weakness, headache, vertigo, nystagmus, and confusion, to transient paralysis and, in some instances, to frank coma. Findings of hypervolemia include distension of peripheral blood vessels and symptoms and signs of heart failure.

Therapeutically, the initial approach to patients with the hyperviscosity syndrome is to perform plasmapheresis (apheresis). Plasmapheresis is performed most effectively with a continuous or a discontinuous flow blood cell separator. An alternative high-efficiency method uses plasma cascade filtration through a cellulose diacetate membrane that selectively removes the high-molecular mass M-component while permitting return of the patient's albumin with reasonable efficiency.[429-431] However, if the needed equipment for high-efficiency plasmapheresis or filtration is not available, conventional double-double plasma separation packs can be used with centrifugation.[432] Patients who have acute hyperviscosity usually need to be plasmapheresed at least 2 to 3 liters daily for 4 to 5 days, or as long as needed until the viscosity falls below 4.0. Although plasmapheresis relieves the hyperviscosity syndrome on a temporary basis, for long-term control, systemic chemotherapy, as used for multiple myeloma or macroglobulinemia, should then be initiated to reduce M-component production as well as tumor burden. In occasional drug-resistant cases of macroglobulinemia, satisfactory long-term control of hyperviscosity can be maintained with intermittent plasmapheresis alone at 2- to 3-week intervals.

Cryoglobulinemia

Cryoglobulinemia should be suspected in patients with acrocyanosis or Raynaud's phenomenon alone or in association with purpura, particularly after cold exposure. Cryoglobulins in macroglobulinemia or myeloma are M-components with low thermal amplitude, which can be readily demonstrated by drawing blood in a warm syringe and allowing it to clot and retract in a 37°C water bath. The serum is then transferred to a clean tube and placed in a refrigerator for 1 to 2 days, by which time the cryoglobulin has either formed a flocculant white precipitate or a gel in the bottom of the tube. Cryoglobulins can usually be quantitated simply by carrying out the cold exposure in hematocrit tubes and then centrifuging them to determine a "cryocrit." Cryoglobulins in B-cell neoplasms are usually IgM or IgG M-components; however, IgA M-components and mixed cryoglobulins have also been reported.[433-437] Treatment with alkylating agents and steroids usually relieves most symptoms of cryoglobulinemia, although some patients continue to need gloves and earmuffs or a move to a warmer climate in the winter. Patients with cryoglobulinemia who present with purpura and other bleeding manifestations or evidence of renal failure should be treated initially with plasmapheresis before the start of chemotherapy.

Anomalous Serum Chemistries

Several abnormalities in serum chemistries are commonly observed in myeloma patients who have high concentrations of serum M-components. These can be confused with abnormalities of clinical significance; however, generally, they are of little or no clinical importance. These include apparent hyponatremia[438] and hypoglycemia, as well as the "anion gap."[439,440] The apparent reductions in serum sodium and glucose are attributed to the displacement of the water-based solutes and electrolytes in serum by the large physical mass of the M-component solute, which does not contain either sodium or glucose and displaces water in the serum. For the reduced serum sodium, this has been described as "isotonic hyponatremia.[441] An apparent low anion gap has been attributed to the fact that M-components are cationic (with a net positive charge). Accordingly, to balance such unmeasured protein cations, both chloride and bicarbonate are retained to neutralize the protein's charge. A low anion gap has also been observed in MGUS.[442] The finding of a low anion gap in a patient not known to have an M-component should, therefore, lead the physician to order appropriate diagnostic studies to look for a monoclonal protein. It is also important that physicians recognize that in patients with known monoclonal gammopathies, saline infusions should not be given for hyponatremia unless there is additional documentation that the patient is sodium and volume depleted. Hyponatremia associated with inappropriate secretion of antidiuretic hormone has been reported in macroglobulinemia.[441]

BACTERIAL SEPSIS

Humoral immunodeficiency, as detailed earlier (in the pathophysiology section), is the principal underlying cause for bacterial sepsis in patients with myeloma.[443-448] *Streptococcus pneumoniae* and *Haemophilus influenzae* are the most common pathogens in previously untreated myeloma patients as well as those nonneutropenic patients responding to chemotherapy. However, in neutropenic patients and in those with refractory disease, *Staphylococcus aureus* and gram-negative bacteria are the preponderant organisms.[449] Patients with fever, with productive cough, or with other symptoms of bacterial infection should have bacterial culture and appropriate x-ray studies obtained as quickly as possible, and bactericidal antibiotic therapy should be started. When patients present with signs of sinopulmonary infection, and are in suitable condition to be treated on an outpatient basis, the combination of product consisting of amoxicillin and clavulanate usually suffices because its spectrum is broad enough to cover most common organisms. For neutropenic patients or for those whose overall condition requires hospitalization, the use of vancomycin plus a third-generation cephalosporin (*e.g.*, ceftazidime) or an aminoglycoside plus an antipseudomonal penicillin (*e.g.*, ticarcillin) is usually indicated. If an aminoglycoside regimen is used, special attention must be paid to renal function, and the frequency of follow-up doses of the aminoglycoside should be judged based on serum assays and renal function. Patients who have repeated episodes of sinopulmonary infections often benefit from being provided with a supply of a suitable oral cephalosporin (*e.g.*, cefaclor) or the amoxicillin–clavulanate combination so that they can start therapy at the time of initial symptoms. For patients who have difficulties with compliance, prophylactic treatment with benzathine pencillin G should be considered if there has been a history of recent prior pneumococcal or meningococcal infection. In a controlled study, intramuscular injection of 20 ml of gamma globulin every 2 weeks did not reduce the frequency of bacterial infections and, therefore, it is not indicated for infection prophylaxis in myeloma.[450] Use of pneumococcoal vaccination may be worth trying;[451] however, most myeloma patients respond poorly to bacterial antigenic stimulation. Vaccines containing live organisms (*e.g.*, varicella) are contraindicated in patients with myeloma because their immunodeficiencies permit infection to disseminate.

AMYLOIDOSIS

Systematic amyloidosis is a complication that occurs in about 15% of patients with multiple myeloma. The fibrilar amyloid protein deposited in myeloma has a pattern of tissue distribution characteristically observed in "primary amyloidosis" (in which patients generally have bone marrow plasmacytosis, Bence Jones proteinuria, or a serum M-component but no osteolytic bone lesions). Differentiation between the amyloid associated with myeloma and that of primary amyloidosis is artificial because the amyloid in both entities is of similar genesis and tissue distribution, and they are more appropriately considered to be parts of the spectrum of the same basic disease process. There is a clear structural relationship between amyloid fibril deposits and Bence Jones proteins. Amyloid fibrils from primary amyloidosis and amyloidosis associated with myeloma are homogeneous and homologous to the variable region fragment of either κ or λ light chains, as defined by amino acid sequence analysis of purified amyloid proteins.[452,453] Primary amyloidosis, and the amyloidosis associated with myeloma, other monoclonal gammopathies, and agammaglobulinemia, have been found to have immunoglobulin amyloid fibrils or amyloid L-chain proteins (AL). These conditions have also been called immunocytic amyloidosis.[453] Most monoclonal L chains do not appear to be "amyloidogenic," suggesting that specific structural properties must be present to undergo fibrillar deposition. Although κ-type L chains are more frequent than the λ-type L chains on M-components or as Bence Jones proteins, amyloidogenic L chains of the λ-type are significantly more frequent than those of the κ-type.[454] Amyloid fibrils are at best sparingly soluble in physiologic saline or plasma, but they can be solubilized in distilled water or low ionic strength media; therefore, it is perhaps not surprising that they tend to deposit in tissues.

The presenting symptoms of amyloidosis (with or without myeloma) include weakness, weight loss, ankle edema, dyspnea, paresthesias, light-headedness, or syncope.[455] Aching in the hands (particularly at night) can be symptomatic of median nerve compression associated with the carpal tunnel syndrome caused by amyloid infiltration of the transverse carpal ligament. Physical findings include enlargement of the tongue and liver, purpura, and ankle edema. Ankle edema is generally due to congestive heart failure or a nephrotic syndrome. A peripheral neuropathy may also be present.[385] Macroglossia occurs in about 20% of patients. The tongue frequently shows indentations from the teeth and may prevent closure of the mouth. Splenomegaly (usually slight) is present in fewer than 10% of patients. The tissues most subject to amyloid deposition in myeloma include the tongue, gastrointestinal tract, heart, skin, and skeletal muscle. Although the presence of macroglossia or periorbital purpura in a myeloma patient should suggest the diagnosis, in most instances a high index of suspicion is needed. Purpura of the eyelids is characteristic of amyloid, and unilateral or bilateral periorbital purpura ("raccoon eyes") may appear suddenly after placing the head in a dependent position, as during proctoscopy, and it has been termed postproctoscopic purpura or PPP.[456] Other skin manifestations include plaques, papules, or nodules. Joint involvement with amyloid can result in an appearance similar to rheumatoid arthritis.[457] Involvement of the glenohumoral joints can give a "shoulder pad" appearance. Low voltage on ECG can be suggestive of cardiac involvement. More specific is two-dimensional echocardiographic evidence of amyloidosis involving the heart, with thickening of ventricular walls, septum, papillary muscles, and pericardial effusion, as well as a characteristic "granular sparkling" appearance of the thickened cardiac walls.[458]

A rectal biopsy has been the classic method of establishing the diagnosis of amyloidosis, and it is positive in more than 60% of patients.[455] A more recent study, however, has shown that abdominal fat aspiration, using a 19-gauge needle, can yield positive results in over 70% of patients. This procedure can be done at the bedside and is probably the simplest way to diagnose amyloidosis.[140] Resected carpal ligaments should always be examined for the presence of amyloid, and the specimens can also be evaluated retrospectively from tissue blocks from previously resected ligaments. Amyloid can also be demonstrated in needle biopsies of the liver or kidney, but these procedures are more hazardous in amyloid patients because of their increased risk of bleeding from vascular wall involvement or from deficiency of factor X. Cracking or rupture of the liver after biopsy has been observed when there is heavy infiltration with amyloid. Amyloid stains pink with hematoxylin and eosin, and has metachromatic staining properties with methyl or crystal violet. Congo red stain produces an apple-green birefringence under polarized light and is the most specific stain for amyloid under the light microscope. Electron microscopy may be somewhat more sensitive and has shown the presence of amyloid fibrils even when Congo red staining has not revealed amyloid.[455]

Treatment for amyloidosis with myeloma is essentially the same as the treatment for multiple myeloma, but it usually does not have as great an impact in resolving amyloid deposits as it does in causing tumor regression. However, treatment may stop or slow further amyloid deposition,[459] and this can be important for patients with early cardiac involvement. Authors of a recent retrospective analysis concluded that a trial of chemotherapy was warranted in patients with myeloma and amyloidosis, and that patients with objective response of the myeloma had a better survival than those that did not. Although there were no absolute predictors of response, patients who achieved remission were much less likely to have cardiac amyloid but were more likely to have very high β_2-microglobulin or κ L-chain M-component levels.[460] In a double-blind study of primary amyloidosis (without overt myeloma), patients given melphalan–prednisone were able to continue treatment longer than those given placebo, and improvement in nephrotic syndrome or proteinuria was observed, but survival did not differ significantly between the two groups.[461] Colchicine, dimethylsulfoxide, and penicillamine, all have been tried in AL amyloid without success. Congestive heart failure caused by amyloid represents a very poor prognostic feature of the disease and usually does not respond to cardiac glycosides.[462] Diuretics are useful for relief of edema.

TABLE 54-14. Clinical Manifestations in 260 Patients with Macroglobulinemia

Mean age (yr)	
At onset of symptoms	63
At diagnosis	65 (range 18–92)
Symptoms, % of pts with	
Severe fatigue	85
Bleeding	60
Neurologic	17
Bone pain	10
Signs, % of pts with	
Lymphadenopathy	40
Hepatomegaly	30
Splenomegaly	30
Hepatosplenomegaly	25

Modified from Ref. 480.

OTHER PLASMA CELL NEOPLASMS

MACROGLOBULINEMIA

In 1944, Waldenström first raised the question of whether or not a new syndrome that differed from multiple myeloma could be identified in the setting of a high-molecular-mass M-component and a bleeding syndrome of the type that is associated with hyperviscosity.[463] The subsequent development of immunodiagnostic techniques; such as immunoelectrophoresis, led to the recognition that the presence of a serum IgM M-component was a common feature in patients with the syndrome described by Waldenström.[464] Although the disease was initially thought to occur predominantly in males, more recent reports suggest an approximately equal sex prevalence.[427,465–468] Macroglobulinemia is far less common than multiple myeloma.[108,469–471] Pathogenetic mechanisms similar to those in myeloma may be involved; however, there is considerable literature indicating an element of familial susceptibility that is more significant than that for myeloma, including families with multiple cases of either macroglobulinemia or IgM MGUS within first-degree relatives.[91,472–474] Macroglobulinemia in a pair of monozygotic twins was also reported recently.[475] The case for environmental factors was recently made for a canary breeder who developed pulmonary symptoms and was found to have a pulmonary infiltrate with IgM-containing cells as well as Waldenström's macroglobulinemia and had an M-component that exhibited antibody activity against an antigen in canary droppings.[476]

Patients with macroglobulinemia are usually first seen with findings analogous to those present in advanced non-Hodgkin's lymphomas, namely, hepatosplenomegaly and lymphadenopathy, and they often develop the hyperviscosity syndrome, with attendant bleeding manifestations (Table 54-14). The fundi of patients with macroglobulinemia should be examined routinely with an ophthalmoscope for evidence of hyperviscosity. The fundic changes can revert rapidly in response to plasmapheresis.

The presence of a serum IgM M-component is not tantamount to a diagnosis of macroglobulinemia because there are other B-cell neoplasms in which serum IgM M-components are present but, with the exception of macroglobulinemia and myeloma, the levels are generally lower than 1.0 g/dl and almost always lower than 2.0 g/dl. Only 25% of patients with IgM M-components have Waldenström's macroglobulinemia; other entities with IgM secretion include subsets of patients with chronic lymphocytic leukemia, non-Hodgkin's lymphomas, the cold hemagglutinin syndrome, and MGUS. Patients with osteolytic bone lesions, in addition to an IgM serum M-component, are very rare, but they are generally classified as having IgM multiple myeloma, rather than macroglobulinemia.[477] Lacking definitive causal agents or other markers to distinguish these entities, this spectrum of neoplasms should be considered as representing varying expressions of B-cell lymphoplasmacytic tumors, with their morphology "frozen" at differing degrees of differentiation, and with clinical manifestations that vary as a function of M-component production, tumor cell proliferation, and invasiveness.[96] Supporting that concept is the recent report on the cytogenetics in a case of Waldenström's macroglobulinemia with an 8:14 translocation with breakpoints (q24;p32) similar to those found in Burkitt's lymphoma.[478]

Hematologic manifestations of macroglobulinemia include anemia in at least 70% of patients (in many instances this at least partially dilutional because of the expanded plasma volume) and some degree of thrombocytopenia in about 30% of patients. Bone marrow involvement is common in macroglobulinemia and the morphologic appearance of the plasma cells is quite pleomorphic with a range of light microscopic appearances from small lymphoid cells to mature plasma cells. Immunofluorescent studies have shown that most of the lymphoid cells have cell surface IgM but lack cytoplasmic Ig, whereas the plasma cells contain cytoplasmic IgM. In a recent study that used flow cytometry, patients with macroglobulinemia usually had circulating lymphoid cells that contained intracytoplasmic μ chains as well as cell surface expression of the B-cell specific antigens B1, B2, and B4, as well as the plasma cell antigen PCA-1.[479]

As with myeloma, quantitation of the IgM M-component should be performed either by laser nephalometry or electrophoresis and not with immunodiffusion methods. Serum viscosity determinations should be performed in all patients at the time of diagnosis and serially in patients who have a serum relative viscosity higher than 3.0. Residual normal immunoglobulins are often depressed, but perhaps less severely than in myeloma.[480] In contrast to the high percentage of myeloma patients with urinary light chain excretion, only about 10% of macroglobulinemic patients have Bence Jones proteins detectable in the urine by standard techniques, and tubular casts are absent.[481] Renal disease is seen only infrequently in macroglobulinemia and is markedly different from that seen in myeloma, taking on the appearance of an immunologically mediated glomerulonephritis or nephrotic syndrome.[481-484]

Neurologic syndromes observed in patients with macroglobulinemia include those neurologic entities discussed under the myeloma section as "complications," and are generally due to either the hyperviscosity syndrome or present as peripheral neuropathies. Peripheral neuropathies are seen in about 20% of patients with macroglobulinemia.

The treatment of macroglobulinemia is, in general, similar to that of other indolent B-cell neoplasms. Oral alkylating agents (chlorambucil, melphalan, or cyclophosphamide) are the mainstays of therapy[465,467,468,485-490] and are generally used alone or in combination with prednisone, with the same dosage schedules as those used in multiple myeloma or chronic lymphocytic leukemia. Additionally, plasmapheresis is often needed initially in management, as discussed under the section of this chapter on the hyperviscosity syndrome. Systemic treatment is normally continued until the serum IgM level plateaus. At that point treatment can be discontinued until there is evidence of a rising serum viscosity or other evidence of relapse. Although complete remission is rarely, if ever, achieved, responsive patients have been reported to have median survivals in the range of 50 months,[427,468] whereas nonresponsive patients have survivals about half that long.[427] Some patients have very indolent macroglobulinemia (analogous to indolent myeloma) with survivals of more than 2 decades. A case has also been made for continuing the use of plasmapheresis, along with cytotoxic agents, so that the dose required of the cytotoxic agent or the frequency of plasma exchange can be reduced.[491] Sequential hemibody irradiation has also been used with apparently some benefit; however, it did not eliminate the patient's requirement for intermittent plasmapheresis.[492] Because of the relative rarity of the disease, comparative evaluations of treatment programs for macroglobulinemia have not been reported, and it is, therefore, best to use one of the standard regimens for CLL or myeloma. Patients who develop refractoriness to alkylating agents can be maintained effectively on long-term plasmapheresis, as long as the IgM production rate is not too high. In personal observations, one macroglobulinemic patient with alkylating agent resistance has been maintained on plasmapheresis every 2 weeks for the past 12 years. On the basis of our own experience and unpublished and published reports by others, patients with refractory macroglobulinemia may achieve drug-induced remissions with doxorubicin,[493] the M2 protocol,[494] VBAP, interferon-α, or pentostatin.[495] Patients with macroglobulinemia treated with alkylating agents have also developed acute leukemia[486,495-499] in a fashion analogous to that seen after treatment with melphalan or chlorambucil in myeloma or polycythemia vera.

LICHEN MYXEDEMATOSUS

Lichen myxedematosus (also known as papular mucinosis or scleromyxedema) is a rare skin disorder that is usually associated with the presence of a serum IgGλ M-component that is very basic and has a marked cathodal electrophoretic mobility.[500] Occasional cases have also been reported with IgA or IgM M-components, usually also with λ L chains. However, osteolytic bone lesions, marrow plasmacytosis, or Bence Jones proteinuria are found only rarely.[501] This dermatologic condition is manifest as raised papules or plaques containing a mucinous material mainly composed of hyaluronic acid. Skin fibroblasts from a patient with typical skin lesions and an IgGμ M-component grew to a lower cell density in culture but produced more glycosaminoglycans (with a higher ratio of hyaluronic acid/sulfated glucosaminoglycans) and less collagen than did normal fibroblasts.[502] Additionally, in comparison with the effect of normal serum, serum from a patient with lichen myxedematosus was found to stimulate hyaluronic acid and prostaglandin E production by normal foreskin or synovial fibroblasts.[503] These data suggest that the serum M-component is acting directly on the skin fibroblasts, altering their metabolism and inducing the skin lesions. Striking cutaneous and systemic improvements have been observed when patients have been treated with melphalan[504,505] or cyclophosphamide.[506] Both the presence of the monoclonal M-component and the response to alkylating agent therapy suggest that lichen myxedematosus is an unusual plasma cell neoplasm.

HEAVY-CHAIN DISEASES

The heavy-chain diseases are rare lymphoplasmacytic neoplasms in which a fragment of an Ig heavy chain is secreted by the tumor cells and is detected in the serum or in the urine. The heavy-chain fragments have an intact Fc portion but a deletion in the Fd region. The first report on a heavy-chain disease was on γ-heavy-chain disease by Franklin and associates in 1964 who, in their initial case report, predicted that α- and μ-chain diseases would also be discovered.[507] This prediction was validated with the subsequent identification of unique syndromes associated with α- and μ-chain fragment secretion. Analysis of the structure of fragments secreted in the heavy-chain diseases has shed some light on normal Ig structure and immunogenetics.[508-511]

γ-Heavy-Chain Disease

Since the initial description of γ-heavy-chain disease (γ-HCD), more than 70 additional cases have been reported, mostly as individual case reports, 65 of which were summarized in a review in 1981.[512] In most cases, the clinical description is similar to that of a non-Hodgkin's lymphoma, with nodal or external involvement and, in four cases, a picture somewhat more like that of multiple myeloma, with osteolytic bone lesions.[513] Thus γ-HCD is not a specific pathologic process but, rather, a mutant molecular expression in the spectrum of B-cell neoplasia. In four cases, chromosome abnormalities have been reported, but a unique abnormality has yet to be identified.[514] The median age at diagnosis of γ-HCD is 60, but it appears in some patients before the age of 20, and the disease is slightly more common in males.[515] Most patients have first been seen with fever, anemia, weakness, and lymphadenopathy, often accompanied with hepatosplenomegaly. Involvement of Waldeyer's ring is relatively common in γ-HCD. In addition to anemia, leukopenia, eosinophilia, and thrombocytopenia are often present, and atypical lymphocytes and plasma cells may be found in the blood smears. The bone marrow aspirate and biopsy specimens usually show an increase in the lymphoplasmacytic series and occasionally some degree of eosinophilia. Immunofluorescent studies have shown that the cells throughout the lymphoplasmacytic spectrum contain γ chains.[516] However, in some instances, the bone marrow findings are normal.

The γ chain in γ-HCD is incomplete, with major deletions being sufficiently large that the molecular mass of the protein is between one-half and three-quarters that of a normal γ chain.[517] The pattern on serum protein electrophoresis is variable, with either broad-based increases in γ-globulin, a discrete M-component spike, or a normal or hypogammaglobulinemic pattern. Immunoelectrophoresis has been used to identify most γ-HCD cases, and it is therefore likely that the frequency of this disorder might be underreported because the test is not routinely used in the workup of patients with diffuse lymphomas. Proteinuria may be undetectable or may range up to 20 g/day. Electrophoresis usually shows the presence of an M-component or γ-globulin band that is negative on the heat test for Bence Jones proteins and can be demonstrated antigenically to have γ-H chain characteristics but is totally devoid of L chain antigens. Most patients have less than 1 g/day of urinary protein excretion, and renal failure is uncommon.[507,515,518]

The clinical course of γ-HCD is highly variable, with some patients succumbing to a rapidly progressing neoplasm within weeks[519,520] to others who are very indolent with a survival of 5 years or more.[521] The median survival in 49 cases for whom data was available was 12 months (range 1–264 months).[515] Given the diffuse nature of the disease, most patients are currently treated with programs similar to those used for patients with non-Hodgkin's lymphomas (*e.g.*, CVP, CHOP). Additionally, local radiotherapy may be useful for symptomatic relief of palatal edema and respiratory distress in patients with Waldeyer's ring involvement.

α-Heavy-Chain Disease

α-Heavy-chain disease (α-HCD) was first described by Seligmann and associates[522] in an Arab woman with a severe malabsorption syndrome resulting from a lymphoplasmacytic infiltrate in the small bowel and monoclonal α chains in the serum. This disease is the most frequent of the heavy-chain diseases and there were more than 150 cases in the literature, as of 1987, including several detailed reviews of this syndrome.[523–528] α-Heavy chain disease is also known as Mediterranean lymphoma (MTL) and immunoproliferative small intestinal disease (IPSID), with a number of publications appearing in the gastroenterologic as well as the oncologic literature. Most reports on α-HCD have been on Arab or Jewish patients from the Mediterranean area, including North Africa and the Middle East. However, the disease is by no means limited to Semitic peoples or to a given geographic area; for example, a case was recently reported from Taiwan.[529] In some instances, α-HCD appears to be premalignant, with a complete reversal of the syndrome with antibiotic therapy.[530–533] However, in many instances the disease relapses despite antibiotics and takes on a more malignant form.[534] The prevalence is slightly higher in males than in females, and the age incidence is distinctly lower than that in myeloma or macroglobulinemia, with most patients appearing in their 20s or 30s but, occasionally, in children as young as 10 years of age.[535] Most patients with α-HCD are from undernourished populations with poor hygiene and infestation with intestinal parasites. In comparison with normal donors and patients with other malabsorption syndromes, patients with α-HCD have a greater association of HLA-AW19 and HLA-B12 antigens, suggesting a genetic element in the disease.[536]

Characteristic symptoms of α-HCD include diarrhea, steatorrhea, weight loss, and abdominal pain. Abdominal masses may be palpable, although hepatosplenomegaly and peripheral lymphadenopathy are uncommon.[537] Clubbing of the fingers as well as growth retardation (including secondary sex characteristics) may occur.[538] Hypocalcemia and other electrolyte disturbances occur as a result of the diarrhea in this syndrome. Both x-ray studies and intestinal biopsy specimens demonstrate extensive infiltration and thickening of the mucosa with tumor. On biopsy, the infiltrate is lymphoplasmacytic, and the neoplastic cells usually contain α chains. The lamina propria is infiltrated with plasma cells and the infiltrate may involve the submucosa and the mesenteric lymph nodes. Chromosomal analysis of mesenteric lymph nodes was recently reported in four cases of α-HCD, of which abnormalities were found in three of the patients.[539] In two of these patients, there were rearrangements of chromosome 14 (band q32) resulting from translocations that differ from those observed in most other non-Hodgkin's lymphomas. Additionally, in one prior case, a closely related abnormality in chromosome 14 (14q+) was also reported in a patient with α-HCD.[540]

Unlike other monoclonal gammopathies, an M-component "spike" is normally not seen on electrophoresis in α-HCD. In about one-half of the cases, a diffusely increased band is seen in the α_2- or β-globulin zones, whereas in the remaining cases there was no overt abnormality on serum electrophoresis. Presumptive diagnosis of α-HCD based on serum protein analysis requires that the α-H chain be identified with anti-α-chain antisera on immunoelectrophoresis or immunofixation without a reaction to anti-L chain antisera. However, inasmuch as not all L chain antisera detect L chains on IgA globulins, definitive diagnosis requires isolation and purification of the protein, followed by reduction and alkylation and demonstration that the reduced monoclonal protein constitutents do not contain light chains.[541] The reported cases of α-HCD have all been of the α_1 subtype of α chains rather than the α_2 subtype. The molecular mass of the α-HCD proteins is about one-half to three-quarters that of the intact α chain and appears to result from an internal deletion of most of the variable region in the H chain as well as the C1α domains.[515] The α chains have a tendency to polymerize to varyingly sized molecules with differing net charge; this property likely accounts for the presence of a diffuse band rather than a characteristic monoclonal spike on electrophoresis. The abnormal α chains have also been found in modest quantities in the patients' urine, again in the absence of Bence Jones proteinuria.

As mentioned earlier, treatment of some patients with

antibiotics alone (*e.g.*, tetracycline) has resulted in resolution of the syndrome, and α-HCD has, therefore, been considered as a potential example of "immune escalation" from benign monoclonal immunoproliferation to frank neoplastic transformation.[96] In most patients, aggressive therapy with melphalan or cyclophosphamide plus prednisone[542] or multiagent combinations has been required. In occasional patients complete remissions have been obtained,[541] primarily in patients with "stage A" disease (mature plasmacytic or lymphoplasmacytic infiltration limited to the lamina propria).[543] However, usually the tumor is at a more advanced stage, with involvement of the submucosa or muscularis (stage B), or has undergone conversion to an immunoblastic sarcoma with involvement of the mesenteric nodes and bowel (stage C), in which circumstances remissions are only transient and the disease progresses to a fatal outcome associated with cachexia or sepsis.

μ-Heavy-Chain Disease

The first patient with μ-heavy-chain disease (μ-HCD) was reported by several groups in 1970[544,545] and had a clinical picture of chronic lymphocytic leukemia (CLL). In 1975, Franklin reported a series of seven cases, all but one of whom had CLL.[546] Since that time, additional reports on cases of μ-HCD have almost all been of patients with CLL. Almost all of the patients with μ-HCD have a clinical picture of CLL; however, there is one clearly documented case with a clinical syndrome of myeloma with amyloid and osteolytic bone lesions with a μ-H chain in the serum,[547] and one patient with an apparent μ chain MGUS has also been identified.[515] Whereas μ-HCD patients usually have a CLL-like picture, the converse is not true. In a detailed immunologic analysis of 120 patients with CLL, none proved to have μ-HCD.[548] A common finding in the bone marrow of patients with μ-HCD is the presence of vacuolated plasma cells, and this finding should lead to a search for this entity. The diagnosis is established by demonstrating the presence of a μ-heavy chain in the serum by immunoelectrophoresis or immunofixation. Of interest, about two-thirds of patients with μ-HCD do have free L chains in the urine (Bence Jones proteins),[548] in most instances of the κ-type.

Molecular studies of the purified μ chains from such patients have been difficult because of the small amounts usually present and difficulty in isolation but, as with γ- and α-heavy-chain diseases, μ chains in μ-HCD commonly have large deletions in the variable region.[549] In one patient studied recently with a leukemic picture and μ-HCD and free L chain production, the tumor cells produced a shortened μ chain that lacked the entire variable region.[510] The deletion was further localized at the genetic level to a defect at the level of the Ig gene structure/assembly that deletes coding information and results in aberrant RNA processing that yields a truncated μ-chain protein that lacks a variable region and that cannot assemble with light chains.[511]

The clinical course of patients with μ-HCD is varied but generally follows the course of CLL. When treatment is indicated, patients are usually treated with alkylating agents and prednisone in a fashion similar to that used in the treatment of CLL, and with some benefit.

δ-Heavy-Chain Disease

A single patient who presented with osteolytic bone lesions and renal failure has been reported in whom the serum M-component was reported to comprise closed tetramers of δ chains.[550] Monoclonal L chains were not detected with standard immunologic techniques. At autopsy, the patient also had subendothelial deposits on the basement membranes of the renal glomeruli, and the patient was reported as having δ-HCD.[551] In this instance the patient's clinical syndrome was consistent with multiple myeloma.

PERSPECTIVE

There has been a substantial advancement in our understanding of multiple myeloma and related plasma cell neoplasms since 1970. This has been the result of increased research efforts in both the basic and clinical areas and the major impact of advances in immunobiology. At the clinical level, the development of a useful staging system, the identification of serum β_2-microglobulin as a major pretreatment prognostic factor, and the incorporation of anthracyclines into combination treatment regimens for remission induction in advanced stage as well as refractory patients represent definite evidence of progress. Current combination chemotherapy regimens for patients with active disease appear to have made some incremental improvement over the simpler regimens brought into use in the 1960s. However, in addition to the typical presentation with high tumor burden in myeloma, intrinsic drug sensitivity in plasma cell neoplasms is not as marked as in some of the less well-differentiated B-cell neoplasms (*e.g.*, large-cell lymphomas), and both kinetic and drug-resistance phenomena appear responsible for the inability to achieve true complete remissions. Higher-dosage alkylating agent regimens with myeloid growth factor support or with bone marrow transplantation may change this picture in good-risk patients. The potential role of interferon-α for remission maintenance after cytoreduction will require close scrutiny during the coming years but, currently, it looks promising. Inasmuch as there is now substantial clinical, as well as preclinical, evidence that melphalan is more leukemogenic than cyclophosphamide, selection among alkylating agents for use in myeloma and related disorders can now be undertaken with a view to reducing the frequency of late side effects of treatment. The use of monoclonal antibodies for identification of plasma cell and B-cell-associated cell surface antigens provides not only a new approach to classification of patients with plasma cell neoplasms, but they may also provide the basis for developing new therapeutic agents capable of purging marrow of myeloma cells for autologous transplantation, as well as for targeted cytotoxic destruction of residual myeloma-associated antigen-bearing cells in remission patients. As with many other metastatic neoplasms, the role of drug-resistance mechanisms in blunting the effectiveness of chemotherapy is only now beginning to be understood at a cellular and molecular level in myeloma. With the more complete understanding of the molecular mechanisms of drug resistance, development of pharmacologic means to abrogate drug resistance now appears to be a realistic possibility that may have a major impact on future management of multiple myeloma. Additionally, the introduction into the clinic of recombinant growth factors that stimulate the proliferation of normal progenitor populations in the bone marrow offers the promise that both the anemia of myeloma and the granulocytopenia associated with its treatment may prove amenable to major reduction in severity in patients entering the next generation of clinical trials. Finally, the recent identification of IL-6 as the major plasmacytoma growth factor may permit the development of new avenues for therapeutic approach to multiple myeloma through the development of agents to inhibit the production of IL-6 or to block its receptor-mediated effects on myeloma progenitor cells.

REFERENCES

1. Kyle RA: Monoclonal gammopathy of undetermined significance (MGUS): A review. In Hoffbrand AV, Lasch HG, Nathan DG et al. (eds), Salmon SE (guest ed): Clin Haematol 11:123–150. Eastbourne, WB Saunders, 1982
2. Salmon SE: Immunoglobulin synthesis and tumor kinetics of multiple myeloma. Semin Hematol 10:136–147, 1973
3. Salmon SE: Plasma cell disorders. In Wingaarden JB, Smith LH Jr (eds): Cecil Textbook of Medicine, 18th ed, pp 1026–1036, 1988
4. Macintyre W: Case of mollities and fragilitas ossium, accompanied with urine strongly charged with animal matter. Med Chir Trans Lon 33:211, 1850
5. Bence Jones H: On a new substance occurring in the urine of a patient with mollities and fragilitas ossium. Phil Trans R Soc Lond 55, 1848
6. Dalrymple J: On the microscopical character of mollities ossium. Dublin Q J Med Sci 2:85, 1846
7. Rustizky J: Multiple myeloma. Deutsch Z Chir 3:162–172, 1873
8. Kahler O: Zur Symptomatologie des multiplen Myeloma: Beobachtung von Albumosurie. Prog Med Wochnschr 14:33–45, 1889
9. Ellinger A. Das Vorkommen des Bence Jones'schen Korpers in Harn bei Tumoren des Knochenmarks und seine diagnostische Bedeutung. Deutsch Arch Klin Med 62:266–278, 1899
10. Wright JH: A case of multiple myeloma. Bull Johns Hopkins Hosp 52:156, 1933
11. Arinkin MI: Die intravitale Untersuchungs—Methodik des Knochenmarks. Folia Haematol (Leipz) 38:233, 1929
12. Tiselius A: Electrophoresis of serum globulin. II. Electrophoretic analysis of normal and immune sera. Biochem J 31:1464, 1937
13. Longsworth LG, Shedlovsky T, MacInnes DA: Electrophoretic patterns of normal and pathological human blood serum and plasma. J Exp Med 70:399, 1939
14. Magnus-Levy A: Multiple myeloma. Acta Med Scand 95:217–280, 1938
15. Grabar P, Williams CA: Methode permettant l'etude conjugee des proprietes electrophoretiques et immunochimiques d'un melange de proteines. Application au serum sanguin. Biochim Biophys Acta 10:193, 1953
16. Glenner GG, Terry W, Harada M et al: Amyloid fibril proteins: Proof of homology with immunoglobulin light chains by sequence analysis. Science 172:1150–1151, 1971
17. Salmon SE, Smith BA: Immunoglobulin synthesis and total body tumor cell number in IgG multiple myeloma. J Clin Invest 49:1114, 1970
18. Alwall N: Urethane and stilbamidine in multiple myeloma: Report on 2 cases. Lancet 2:388–389, 1947
19. Holland JF, Hosley H, Scharlau C, et al: A controlled trial of urethane treatment in myeloma. Blood 27:328–342, 1966
20. Bergsagel DE, Griffith KM, Haut A et al: The treatment of plasma cell myeloma. Adv Cancer Res 10:311–359, 1967
21. Bergsagel DE, Sprague CC, Austin C et al: Evaluation of new chemotherapeutic agents in the treatment of multiple myeloma. IV. L-phenylalanine mustard (NSC-8806). Cancer Chemother Rep 21:87–99, 1962
22. Korst DR, Clifford GO, Fowler WM et al: Multiple myeloma. II. Analysis of cyclophosphamide in 165 patients. JAMA 189:758–762, 1964
23. Salmon SE, Shadduck RK, Schilling A: Intermittent high-dose prednisone therapy for multiple myeloma. Cancer Chemother Rep 51:179, 1967
24. Alexanian R, Bonnet J, Gehan E et al: Combination chemotherapy for multiple myeloma. Cancer 30:382–389, 1972
25. Costa G, Engle RL, Jr, Schilling A et al: Melphalan and prednisone: An effective combination for the treatment of multiple myeloma. Am J Med 54:589–599, 1973
26. Salmon SE: Nitrosoureas in multiple myeloma. Cancer Treat Rep 60:789–794, 1976
27. Alberts DS, Salmon SE: Adriamycin (NSC-123127) in the treatment of alkylator-resistant multiple myeloma: A pilot study. Cancer Chemother Rep 59:345–350, 1975
28. Mellstedt A, Aahre A, Bjorkholm M et al: Interferon therapy in myelomatosis. Lancet 1:245–247, 1979
29. Young JL, Percy CL, Asire AJ: Surveillance, epidemiology, and end results: Incidence and mortality data, 1973–1977. National Cancer Institute Monograph 57, Department of Health and Human Services Publication (National Institutes of Health) 81-2330, 1981
30. Devesa SS, Silverman DT, Young JL Jr et al: Cancer incidence and mortality trends among whites in the United States, 1947–84. J Natl Cancer Inst 79:701–770, 1987
31. Martin NH: The incidence of myelomatosis. Lancet 1:237–239, 1961
32. Malignant neoplasms of lymphatic and haematopoietic tissues: Multiple myeloma. WHO Epidemiol Vital Stat Rep 18:414–415, 1965
33. Hewell GM, Alexanian R: Myeloma in young persons. Ann Intern Med 84:441–443, 1976
34. Blattner WA, Blair A, Mason TJ: Multiple myeloma in the United States, 1950–75. Cancer 48:2547, 1981
35. Linos A, Kyle RA, O'Fallon MW et al: Incidence and secular trend of multiple myeloma in Olmstead County, Minnesota: 1965–77. J Natl Cancer Inst 66:17, 1981
36. Blattner WA: Multiple myeloma and macroglobulinemia. In Schottenfeld D, Fraumeni JF Jr (eds): Cancer Epidemiology and Prevention, p. 722. Philadelphia, WB Saunders, 1982
37. Axelsson U, Bachmann R, Hallen J: Frequency of pathological proteins (M-components) in 6995 sera from an adult population. Acta Med Scand 179:235–247, 1966
38. Englisova M, Englis M, Kyral V, et al: Changes of immunoglobulin synthesis in old people. Exp Gerontol 3:125–127, 1968
39. Bazin H, Deckers C, Beckers A et al: Transplantable immunoglobulin-secreting tumors in rats. I. General features of Lou/Wsl strain rat immunocytomas and their monoclonal proteins. Int J Cancer 10:568–580, 1972
40. Bazin H, Beckers A, Deckers C et al: Transplantable immunoglobulin-secreting tumors in rats. V. Monoclonal immunoglobulins secreted by 250 ileocecal immunocytomas in Lou/Wsl rats. J Natl Cancer Inst 51:1359–1361, 1973
41. Cotran RS, Fortner JG: Serum-protein abnormality in a transplantable plasmacytoma of the Syrian golden hamster. J Natl Cancer Inst 28:1193–1205, 1962
42. Farrow BRH, Penny R: Multiple myeloma in a cat. J Am Vet Assoc 158:606–611, 1971
43. Kehoe JM, Hurvitz AI, Capra JD: Characterization of three feline paraproteins. J Immunol 109:511–516, 1972
44. Osborne CA, Perman V, Sautter JH et al: Multiple myeloma in the dog. J Am Vet Assoc 153:1300–1319, 1968
45. Hurvitz AI: Animal model for human disease: Canine monoclonal gammopathies/immunoglobulins. Comp Pathol Bull 3:4, 1971
46. Payne GS, Bishop JM, Varmus HE: Multiple arrangements of viral DNA and an activated host oncogene in bursal lymphomas. Nature 295:209, 1982
47. Cooper MD, Paylle LD, Dent PB et al: Pathogenesis of avian lymphoid leukosis. I. Histogenesis. J Natl Cancer Inst 41:373, 1968
48. Salahuddin SZ, Ablashi DV, Markham PD et al: Isolation of a new virus HBLV in patients with lymphoproliferative disorders. Science 234:596–601, 1986
49. Potter M: Concepts of pathogenesis and experimental models of immunoglobulin-secreting tumors in animals. In Weirnick PH, Canellos GP, Kyle RA, Schiffer CA (eds): Neoplastic Diseases of the Blood, Vol. 1, pp 393–412. New York, Churchill-Livingstone, 1985
50. Radl J, Hollander CF, VanDenBerg P et al: Idiopathic paraproteinemia. I. Studies in an animal model—the aging C57BL/KaLWRij mouse. Clin Exp Immunol 33:395, 1978
51. Dunn TB: Plasma cell neoplasms beginning in the ileocecal area in strain 3CH mice. J Natl Cancer Inst 19:371, 1957
52. Potter M, Wax JS: Genetics of susceptibility to pristane induced plasmacytomas in BALB/cAN: Reduced susceptibility in BALB/cJ with a brief description of pristane-induced arthritis. J Immunol 127:1591, 1981
53. Potter M, Wax JS: Peritoneal plasmacytomas—genesis in mice. A comparison of three pristane dose regimens. J Natl Cancer Inst 71:391, 1983
54. Potter M, Pumphrey JG, Bailey DW: Genetics of susceptibility of plasmacytoma induction. I. BALB/cAnN(C), C57BL/6N(B6), C57BL/Ka(BK), $(C \times B6)F_1$ $(C \times BK)F_1$ and $C \times B$ recombinant inbred strains. J Natl Cancer Inst 54:1413, 1975
55. Potter M: Pathogenesis of plasmacytomas in mice. In Becker FF (ed): Cancer: A Comprehensive Treatise, New York, Plenum Press, 1982
56. Potter M, Boyce C: Induction of plasma cell neoplasms in strain BALB/c mice with mineral oil and mineral oil adjuvants. Nature 193:1086, 1962
57. Merwin RM, Redman LW: Induction of plasma cell tumors and sarcomas in mice by diffusion chambers placed in the peritoneal cavity. J Natl Cancer Inst 31:998–1007, 1963
58. Anderson PN: Plasma cell tumor induction in BALB/c mice (abstr). Proc Am Assoc Cancer Res 11:3, 1970
59. Potter M, Pumphrey JG, Walters JL: Brief communication: Growth of primary plasmacytomas in the mineral oil-conditioned environment. J Natl Cancer Inst 49:305–308, 1972
60. Potter M, Walters JL: Effect of intraperitoneal pristane on established immunity to the Adj-PC-5 plasmacytoma. J Natl Cancer Inst 51:875–881, 1973
61. Hamburger AW, Salmon SE: Primary bioassay of human myeloma stem cell. J Clin Invest 60:846–854, 1977
62. Namb Y, Hanaoka M: Immunocytology of cultured IgM-forming cells of mouse. I. Requirement of phagocytic cell factor for the growth of IgM-forming tumor cells in tissue culture. J Immunol 109:1193–1200, 1972
63. Nordan RP, Potter M: A macrophage-derived factor required by plasmacytomas for survival and proliferation in vitro. Science 233:566–568, 1986

64. Metcalf D: The serum factor stimulating colony formation in vitro by murine plasmacytoma cells: Response to antigens and mineral oil. J Immunol 113:235–243, 1974
65. Tosato G, Seamon KB, Goldman ND et al: Monocyte-derived human B-cell growth factor identified as interferon-β_2 (BSF-2, IL-6). Science 239:502–504, 1988
66. Hamburger AW: Inhibition of B lymphocyte clonal proliferation by spleen cells from plasmacytoma-bearing mice. J Natl Cancer Inst 65:1337–1343, 1980
67. McIntire KR, Princler GL: Prolonged adjuvant stimulation in germfree BALB/c mice: Development of plasma cell neoplasia. Immunology 17:481–487, 1969
68. Dalton AJ, Potter M, Merwin RM: Some ultrastructural characteristics of a series of primary and transplanted plasma cell tumors of the mouse. J Natl Cancer Inst 26:1221–1267, 1961
69. Kuff EL, Smith LA, Lueders KK: Intracisternal A particle genes in *Mus musculus*. A conserved family of retrovirus-like elements. Mol Cell Biol 1:216, 1981
70. Shepard JS, Pettengill OS, Wurster-Hill DH et al: A specific chromosome breakpoint associated with mouse plasmacytomas. J Natl Cancer Inst 61:225, 1978
71. Yosida MC, Moriwaki K, Migita S: Specificity of the deletion of chromosome no. 15 in mouse plasmacytoma. J Natl Cancer Inst 60:235–238, 1978
72. Dickman SH, Goldstein M, Kahn T et al: Amyloidosis: An unusual complication of Gaucher's disease. Arch Pathol Lab Med 102:460–462, 1978
73. Selvaney P, Block M, Narni R et al: Alteration and abnormal expression of the c-*myc* oncogene in human multiple myeloma. Blood 71:30–35, 1988
74. Meltzer P, Shadle K, Durie B: Somatic mutation alters a critical region of the c-*myc* gene in multiple myeloma (abstr). Blood (Suppl 1)70:282a, 1987
75. MacMahon B, Clark DW: The incidence of multiple myeloma. J Chron Dis 4:508–515, 1956
76. McPhedran P, Heath CW Jr, Garcia J: Multiple myeloma incidence in metropolitan Atlanta, Georgia: Racial and seasonal variations. Blood 39:866, 1972
77. Bertrams J, Kuwert E, Bohme U et al: HL-A antigens in Hodgkin's disease and multiple myeloma—increased frequency of W18 in both diseases. Tissue Antigens 2:41, 1972
78. Jeannet M, Magnin C: HL-A antigens in haematological malignant diseases. Eur J Clin Invest 2:39, 1971
79. Mason DY, Cullen P: HL-A antigen frequencies in myeloma. Tissue Antigens 5:238, 1975
80. McDevitt HO, Bodner WF: Histocompatibility antigens, immune responsiveness and susceptibility to disease. Am J Med 52:1, 1972
81. Maldonado JE, Kyle RA: Familial myeloma. Report of eight families and a study of serum proteins in their relatives. Am J Med 57:875–884, 1974
82. Blattner WA: Epidemiology of multiple myeloma and related plasma cell disorders: An analytic review. In Potter M (ed): Progress in Myeloma: Biology of Myeloma, p 1. New York, Elsevier North-Holland, 1980
83. Kyle RA, Heath CW Jr, Carbone P: Multiple myeloma in spouses. Arch Intern Med 127:944–946, 1971
84. Pietruszka M, Rabin BS, Srodes G: Multiple myeloma in husband and wife. Lancet 1:314, 1976
85. Kyle RA: Monoclonal gammopathy of undetermined significance: Natural history in 241 cases. Am J Med 64:814, 1978
86. Meijers KAE, Leeuw B, Voormolen-Kalova M: The multiple occurrence of myeloma and asymptomatic paraproteinaemia within one family. Clin Exp Immunol 12:185, 1972
87. Youinou P: Genetic propensity to benignity in monoclonal gammopathy. Acta Haematol (Basel) 62:173, 1979
88. Axelsson U, Hallen J: Familial occurrence of pathological serum proteins of different gammaglobulin groups. Lancet 2:369, 1965
89. Williams RC, Erickson JL, Polesky HF et al: Studies of monoclonal immunoglobulins (M-components) in various kindreds. Ann Intern Med 67:309, 1967
90. Blattner WA, Garber J, Mann DL et al: Waldenström's macroglobulinemia and autoimmune disease in a family. Ann Intern Med 93:830, 1980
91. Bjornsson OG, Arnason A, Gudmundsson S et al: Macroglobulinema in an Icelandic family. Acta Med Scand 203:283, 1978
92. Fine JM, Lambin P, Valentin L et al: IgG monoclonal gammopathy in the sister of a patient with Waldenström's macroglobulinemia. Biomedicine 19:117, 1973
93. Fraumeni JF Jr, Wertelecki W, Blattner WA et al: Varied manifestations of a familial lymphoproliferative disorder. Am J Med 59:145, 1975
94. Kalff MW, Hijmans W: Immunoglobulin analysis in families of macroglobulinemia patients. Clin Exp Immunol 5:479, 1969
95. Seligmann M, Sassy C, Chevalier A: A human IgG myeloma protein with anti-alpha 2 macroglobulin antibody activity. J Immunol 110:85, 1973
96. Salmon SE, Seligmann M: B-cell neoplasia in man. Lancet 2:1230, 1974
97. Linet MS, Sioban DH, McLaughlin JK: A case-control study of multiple myeloma in whites: Chronic antigenic stimulation, occupation and drug use. Cancer Res 47:2978–2981, 1987
98. Hamaker WR, Lindell ME, Gomez AC: Plasmacytoma arising in a pacemaker pocket. Ann Thorac Surg 21:354, 1976
99. Gerber MA: Asbestosis and neoplastic disorders of the hematopoietic system. Am J Clin Pathol 53:204–208, 1970
100. Kagan E, Jacobson RJ, Yeung K-Y et al: Asbestosis-associated neoplasms of B cell lineage. Am J Med 67:325–330, 1979
101. Osserman EF, Takatsuki L: Considerations regarding the pathogenesis of the plasmacytic dyscrasias. Ser Hematol 4:28–49, 1965
102. Pratt PW, Estren S, Kochwa S: Immunoglobulin abnormalities in Gaucher's disease: Report of 16 cases. Blood 31:633–640, 1968
103. Wolf P: Monoclonal gammopathy in Gaucher's disease. Lab Med 4:28–29, 1973
104. MacDonald M, McCathie M, Faed MJW et al: Gaucher's disease with bronchial gammopathy. J Clin Pathol 28:757, 1975
105. Turesson I, Rausing A: Gaucher's disease and benign monoclonal gammopathy. Acta Med Scand 197:507–512, 1975
106. Penny R, Hughes S: Repeated stimulation of the reticuloendothelial system and the development of plasma cell dyscrasias. Lancet 1:77–78, 1970
107. Rosenblatt J, Hall CA: Plasma-cell dyscrasia following prolonged stimulation of reticuloendothelial system. Lancet 1:301–302, 1970
108. Isobe T, Osserman EF: Pathologic conditions associated with plasma cell dyscrasias: A study of 806 cases. Ann NY Acad Sci 90:507–518, 1971
109. Goldenberg GJ, Paraskevas F, Israels LG: The association of rheumatoid arthritis with plasma cell and lymphocytic neoplasms. Arthritis Rheum 12:569–579, 1969
110. Wegelius O, Skrifvars B: Rheumatoid arthritis terminating in plasmacytoma. Acta Med Scand 187:133–138, 1970
111. Wohlenberg H: Osteomyelitis and plasmacytoma. N Engl J Med 283:822–823, 1970
112. Isomaki HA, Hakulmen T, Joutsenlahti U: Excess risk of lymphomas, leukemias and myelomas in patients with rheumatoid arthritis. J Chron Dis 31:691–699, 1978
113. Imahori S, Moore GE: Multiple myeloma and prolonged stimulation of reticuloendothelial system. NY State J Med 72:1625, 1972
114. Jancelewicz Z, Takatsuki K, Sugai S et al: IgD multiple myeloma. Review of 133 cases. Arch Intern Med 135:87, 1975
115. Schafer AI, Miller JB: Association of IgA multiple myeloma with preexisting disease. Br J Haematol 41:19–24, 1979
116. Schafer AI, Miller JB, Lester EP et al: Monoclonal gammopathy in hereditary spherocytosis: A possible pathogenetic relation. Ann Intern Med 88:45–46, 1978
117. Waldbaum B, Gelfand M: Myelomatosis in the Rhodesian African. Trop Geogr Med 26:26, 1974
118. Krause RM: Factors controlling the occurrence of antibodies with uniform properties. Fed Proc 29:59, 1970
119. Ichimaru M, Ishimaru T, Mikami M et al: Multiple myeloma among atomic bomb survivors, Hiroshima and Nagasaki, 1950–1976. Radiation Effects Research Foundation Technical Report No 9-79. Hiroshima, Radiation Effects Research Foundation, 1979
120. Cuzik J: Radiation-induced myelomatosis. N Engl J Med 304:204–210, 1981
121. Lewis EB: Leukemia, multiple myeloma, and aplastic anemia in American radiologists. Science 142:1492, 1963
122. Matanoski GM: Risk of cancer associated with occupational exposure in radiologists and other radiation workers. In Burchenal JH, Oettgen HF (eds): Cancer, Achievements, Challenges, and Prospects for the 1980's, p 241. New York, Grune & Stratton, 1982
123. Matanoski GM, Seltzer R, Santwell RE et al: The current mortality rates of radiologists and other physician specialists: Specific causes of death. Am J Epidemiol 101:199, 1975
124. Mancuso TE, Stewart A, Kneale G: Radiation exposures of Hanford workers dying from cancer and other causes. Health Phys 33:369, 1977
125. Hayhoe FGJ, Neuman Z: Cytology of myeloma cells. J Clin Pathol 29:916, 1976
126. Paraskevas F, Heremans J, Waldenström J: Cytology and electrophoretic pattern in γ_1A (B_2A) myeloma. Acta Med Scand 170:575–589, 1961
127. Maldonado JE, Bayrd ED, Brown AL: The flaming cell in multiple myeloma: A light and electron microscopy study. Am J Clin Pathol 44:605, 1965
128. Farquhar MG, Palade GE: The Golgi apparatus (1954–1981) from artifact to center stage. J Cell Biol (Suppl.) 91:77–103, 1981
129. Blom J, Mansa B, Wiik A: A study of Russell bodies in human monoclonal plasma cell by means of immunofluorescence and electron microscopy. Acta Pathol Microbiol Scand Sect A 84:335, 1976
130. Durie B, Grogan T: CALLA positive myeloma an aggressive subtype with poor survival. Blood 66:229–232, 1985
131. Grogan TM, Durie BGM, Lomen C et al: Delineation of a novel pre-B cell component in plasma cell myeloma: Immunochemical, immunophenotypic, genotypic, cytologic, cell culture, and kinetic features. Blood 70:932–942, 1987
132. Bataille R, Durie BGM, Sany J, Salmon SE: Myeloma bone marrow acid phosphatase staining: A correlative study of 38 patients. Blood 55:802, 1980
133. Cassuto JP, Hammou JC, Pastorelli E et al: Plasma acid cell phosphatase, a discriminative test for benign and malignant monoclonal gammopathies. Biomedicine 27:197, 1977
134. Tortarolo M, Cantore N, Grande M, et al: Plasma cell acid phosphatase an adjunct in the differential diagnosis of monoclonal immunoglobulinemias. Acta Haematol 65:103, 1981
135. Kyle KA, Greipp PR: Smoldering multiple myleoma. N Engl J Med 302:1347–1349, 1980
136. Durie BGM, Salmon SE, Moon TE: Pretreatment tumor mass, cell kinetics, and prognosis in multiple myeloma. Blood 55:364–372, 1980
137. Greipp PR, Witzig TE, Gonchoroff NJ et al: Immunofluorescence labeling indices in myeloma and related monoclonal gammopathies. Mayo Clin Proc 62:969–977, 1987
138. Barlogie B, Latreille J, Alexanian R et al: Quantitative cytology in myeloma research. In Hoffbrand AV, Lasch HG, Nathan DG et al. (eds), Salmon SE (guest ed): Clin Haematol 11:19–46. Eastbourne, WB Saunders, 1982
139. Seigneurin D, David J, Sotto JJ et al: β-Glucuronidases plasmocytaires dans les dysglobulinemias. Interet diagnostique de leur mise en evidence. Pathol Biol 27:467, 1979
140. Duston MA, Skinner M, Shirahama T et al: Diagnosis of amyloidosis by abdominal fat aspiration. Am J Med 82:412–414, 1987

141. Mundy GR, Raisz LG, Cooper RA et al: Evidence for the secretion of an osteoclast stimulating factor in myeloma. N Engl J Med 291:1041–1046, 1974
142. Valentin-Opran A, Charhon SA, Meunier PJ et al: Quantitative histology of myeloma-induced bone changes. Br J Haematol 52:602–610, 1982
143. Durie BGM, Salmon SE, Mundy GR: Relation of osteoclast activating factor production to the extent of bone disease in multiple myeloma. Br J Haematol 47:21–30, 1981
144. Garret IR, Durie BGM, Nedwin GE et al: Production of lymphotoxin, a bone-resorbing cytokine by cultured human myeloma cells. N Engl J Med 317:526–532, 1987
145. Solomon A, Waldmann TA, Fahey JL et al: Metabolism of Bence Jones proteins. J Clin Invest 43:103–117, 1964
146. Waldmann TA, Strober W, Mogielnicki RP: The renal handling of low molecular weight proteins. II Disorders of serum protein catabolism in patients with tubular proteinuria, the nephrotic syndrome, or uremia. J Clin Invest 51:2162–2174, 1964
147. Wochner RD, Strober W, Waldmann TA: The role of catabolism of Bence Jones proteins and immunoglobulin fragments. J Exp Med 126:207–221, 1967
148. Hill GS, Morel-Maroger L, Mery J-P et al: Renal lesions in multiple myeloma: Their relationship to associated protein abnormalities. Am J Kidney Dis 11:423–438, 1983
149. Levi DF, Williams RC Jr, Lindstrom FD: Immunofluorescent studies of the myeloma kidney with special reference to light chain disease. Am J Med 33:92–933, 1968
150. Costanza DJ, Smoller M: Multiple myeloma with the Fanconi syndrome. Study of a case, with electron microscopy of the kidney. Am J Med 34:125–133, 1963
151. Engle RL Jr, Wallis LA: Multiple myeloma and the adult Fanconi syndrome. I. Report of a case with crystal-like deposits in the tumor cells and in the epithelial cells of the kidney. Am J Med 22:5–12, 1957
152. Finkel PN, Kronenberg K, Pesce AJ et al: Adult Fanconi syndrome, amyloidosis, and marked kappa light chain proteinuria. Nephron 10:1–24, 1973
153. Sirtoa JH, Hamerman D: Renal function studies in an adult subject with the Fanconi syndrome. Am J Med 16:138–152, 1954
154. Preuss HG, Hammack WJ, Murdaugh HV: The effect of Bence Jones protein on the in vitro function of rabbit renal cortex. Nephron 5:210–216, 1967
155. Preuss HG, Weiss FR, Iammarino RM et al: Effect on rat kidney slice functiion in vitro of proteins from the urines of patients with myelomatosis and nephrosis. Clin Sci Mol Med 46:283–294, 1974
156. Maldonado JE, Velosa JA, Kyle RA et al: Fanconi syndrome in adults. A manifestation of a latent form of myeloma. Am J Med 58:354–364, 1975
157. Kyle RA, Greipp PR: "Idiopathic" Bence Jones proteinuria. Long-term followup in seven patients. N Engl J Med 306:564–567, 1982
158. Pruzanski W, Ogryzlo MA: Abnormal proteinuria in malignant diseases. Adv Clin Chem 13:335–382, 1970
159. Pruzanski W, Gidon MS, Roy A: Suppression of polyclonal immunoglobulins in multiple myeloma: Relationship to the staging and other manifestations at diagnosis. Clin Immunol Immunopathol 17:280, 1980
160. Ullrich S, Zolla-Pazner S: Immunoregulatory circuits in myeloma. In Hoffbrand AV, Lasch HG, Nathan DG et al (eds), Salmon SE (guest ed): Clin Haematol 11:87–111, Eastbourne, WB Saunders, 1982
161. Broder S, Humphrey R, Durm M et al: Impaired synthesis of polyclonal (non-paraprotein) immunoglobulin by circulating lymphocytes from patients with multiple myeloma: Role of suppressor cells. N Engl J Med 293:887–892, 1975
162. Salmon SE: Paraneoplastic syndromes associated with monoclonal lymphocyte and plasma cell proliferation. Ann NY Acad Sci 230:228–239, 1974
163. Bovill EG, Ershler WB, Golden EA et al: A human myeloma-produced monoclonal protein directed against the active subpopulation von Willebrand factor. Am J Clin Pathol 85:115–123, 1986
164. Merlini G, Farhangi M, Osserman EF: Monoclonal immunoglobulins with antibody activity in myeloma, macroglobulinemia and related plasma cell dyscrasias. Semin Oncol 13:350–365, 1986
165. Kilgore LL, Patterson BW, Parenti DM et al: Immune complex hyperlipidemia induced by an apolipoprotein-reactive immunoglobulin A paraprotein from a patient with multiple myeloma. J Clin Invest 76:225–232, 1985
166. Sullivan PW, Salmon SE: Kinetics of tumor growth and regression in IgG myeloma. J Clin Invest 51:1597, 1972
167. Drewinko B, Alexanian R, Boyer H et al: The growth fraction of human myeloma cells. Blood 57:333, 1981
168. Hobbs JR: Growth rates and response to treatment in human myelomatosis. Br J Haematol 16:607, 1969
169. Bergsagel DE: Assessment of the response of mouse and human myeloma to chemotherapy and radiotherapy. In Drewinko B, Humphreya RM (eds): Growth Kinetics and Biochemical Regulation of Normal and Malignant Cells. University of Texas Cancer Center, M.D. Anderson Hospital and Tumor Institute, 29th Annual Symposium on Fundamental Cancer Research, pp 705-717. Baltimore, Williams & Wilkins, 1977
170. Bergsagel DE, Pruzanski W: Treatment of plasma cell myeloma with cytotoxic agents. Arch Intern Med 135:172–176, 1975
171. Suchman AL, Coleman M, Mouradian JA et al: Aggressive plasma cell myeloma: A terminal phase. Arch Intern Med 141:1315–1320, 1981
172. Falini B, DeSolas I, Levine AM et al: Emergence of B-immunoblastic sarcoma in patients with multiple myeloma: A clinicopathologic study of 10 cases. Blood 59:923–933, 1982
173. Hobbs JR: Immunocytoma o' mice an' men. Br Med J 2:67, 1971
174. Ludwig H, Tscholakoff D, Neuhold et al: Magnetic resonance imaging of the spine in multiple myeloma. Lancet 2:364–366, 1987
175. Alexanian R: Localized and indolent myeloma. Blood 56:521, 1980
176. Durie BGM, Salmon SE: Multiple myeloma, macroglobulinaemia and monoclonal gammopathies. In Hoffbrand AV, Brain MC, Hirsh J (eds): Recent Advances in Haematology, p 243. Edinburgh, Churchill-Livingstone, 1977
177. Durie BGM, Salmon SE: A clinical staging system for multiple myeloma. Correlation of measured myeloma cell mass with presenting clinical features, response to treatment and survival. Cancer 36:842–852, 1975
178. Alexanian R, Balcerzak S, Bonnet JD et al: Prognostic factors in multiple myeloma. Cancer 36:1192–1201, 1975
179. Woodruff RK, Wadworth J, Malpas JS et al: Clinical staging in multiple myeloma. Br J Haematol 42:199–205, 1979
180. Merlini G, Waldenström JC, Jayakar SD: A new improved clinical staging system for multiple myeloma based on analysis of 123 treated patients. Blood 55:1011–1019, 1980
181. Belpomme D, Simon F, Pouillart P et al: Prognostic factors and treatment of multiple myeloma: Interest of a cyclic sequential chemohormonotherapy combining cyclophosphamide, melphalan and prednisone. Recent Results Cancer Res 65:28–40, 1978
182. Gobbi M, Cavo M, Savelli G et al: Prognostic factors and survival in multiple myeloma. Analysis of 91 cases treated by melphalan and prednisone. Haematology 65:437–445, 1980
183. Santoro A, Schieppati G, Franchi F et al: Clinical staging and therapeutic results in multiple myeloma. Eur J Cancer Clin Oncol 19:1353–1359, 1983
184. Bergsagel DE, Phil D, Bailey AJ et al: The chemotherapy of plasma cell myeloma and the incidence of acute leukemia. N Engl J Med 301:743, 1979
185. Bergsagel DE, Bailey AJ, Langley GR et al: The chemotherapy of plasma cell myeloma and the incidence of acute leukemia. N Engl J Med 301:743, 1979
186. Salmon SE, Haut A, Bonnet J et al: Alternating combination chemotherapy improves survival in multiple myeloma. A Southwest Oncology Group study. J Clin Oncol 1:453, 1983
187. Durie BGM: Staging and kinetics of multiple myeloma. In Hoffbrand AV, Lasch HG, Nathan DG et al (eds), Salmon SE (guest ed): Clin Haematol 11:3–18. Eastbourne, WB Saunders, 1982
188. Durie BGM, Cole PW, Chen HSG et al: Synthesis and metabolism of Bence Jones protein and calculation of tumour burden in patients with Bence Jones myeloma. Br J Haematol 47:7, 1981
189. Waldenström J: Diagnosis and Treatment of Multiple Myeloma. New York, Grune & Stratton, 1970
190. Seligmann M, Basch A: The clinical significance of pathological immunoglobulins. In XII International Congress of Hematology (Plenary Session Papers), pp 21–31. New York, International Society of Hematology, 1968
191. Hobbs JR: Paraproteins, benign or malignant? Br Med J 3:699–704, 1967
192. Kyle RA, Maldonado JE, Bayrd ED: Idiopathic Bence Jones proteinuria—a distinct entity? Am J Med 55:222–226, 1973
193. Norfolk D, Child JA, Cooper EH et al: Serum β_2 microglobulin in myelomatosis: Potential value in stratification and monitoring. Br J Cancer 42:510–515, 1980
194. Karlsson FA, Groth T, Sege K, et al: Turnover in humans of β_2 microglobulin: The constant chain of HLA-antigens. Eur J Clin Invest 10:293–300, 1980
195. Cassuto JP, Krebs BJ, Viot G et al: β_2 microglobulin, a tumour marker of lymphoproliferative disorders. Lancet 2:108, 1978
196. Bataille R, Magullo M, Greinier J, et al: Serum beta-2-microglobulin in multiple myeloma: Relation to presenting factors and clinical status. Eur J Cancer Clin Oncol 18:59–66, 1982
197. Scarffe JH, Anderson H, Palmer MK et al: Prognostic significant of pretreatment serum β-2-microglobulin levels in multiple myeloma. Eur J Cancer Clin Oncol 19:1361–1364, 1983
198. Bataille R, Magulo M, Greinier J et al: Serum beta-2-microglobulin in multiple myeloma: A simple, reliable marker for staging. Br J Haematol 55:439, 1983
199. Bataille R, Grenier J: Serum beta-2 microglobulin in multiple myeloma—a critical review. Eur J Cancer 23:1829–1832, 1987
200. Bataille R, Durie BGM, Grenier J et al: Prognostic factors and staging in multiple myeloma: A reappraisal. J Clin Oncol 4:80–87, 1986
201. Karlsson FA, Wibell L, Evrin PE: β_2 microglobulin in clinical medicine. Scand J Clin Lab Invest (Suppl 154)40:27, 1980
202. Durie BGM, Russell DH, Salmon SE: Reappraisal of plateau phase in myeloma. Lancet 2:65–68, 1980
203. Chronic Leukemia-Myeloma Task Force, National Cancer Institute. Proposed guidelines for protocol studies. II. Plasma cell myeloma. Cancer Chemother Rep 4:145–158, 1973
204. Waldmann TA, Strober W: Metabolism of immunoglobulins. Prog Allergy 13:1, 1969
205. Salmon SE, Wampler SE: Multiple myeloma: Quantitative staging and assessment of response with a programmable pocket calculator. Blood 49:379–389, 1977
206. Palmer M, Belch A, Brox L et al: Are the current criteria for response useful in the management of multiple myeloma? J Clin Oncol 5:1373–1377, 1987
207. Alexanian R, Barlogie B, Dixon D: High-dose glucocorticoid treatment of resistant myeloma. Ann Intern Med 105:8–11, 1983
208. Sporn JR, McIntyre OR: Chemotherapy of previously untreated multiple myeloma patients: An analysis of recent treatment results. Semin Oncol 13:318–325, 1986
209. Salmon SE: Expansion of the growth fraction in multiple myeloma with alkylating agents. Blood 45:119–129, 1975
210. Jackson DV, Case LD, Pope EK et al: Single agent vincristine by infusion in refractory multiple myeloma. J Clin Oncol 3:1508–1512, 1985
211. MacLennan IC, Cusick J: Objective evaluation of the role of vincristine in induction

and maintenance therapy for myelomatosis. Medical Research Council Working Party on Leukaemia in Adults. Br J Cancer 52:153–158, 1985
212. Mellstedt H, Bjorkholm M, Johansson B: Interferon therapy in myelomatosis. Lancet 1:245–248, 1979
213. Gutterman JU, Blumenschein GR, Alexanian R: Leucocyte interferon-induced tumor regression in human metastatic breast cancer, multiple myeloma, and malignant lymphoma. Ann Intern Med 93:399–406, 1980
214. Costanzi JJ, Cooper MR, Scarffe JH et al: Phase II study of recombinant alpha-2 interferon in resistant multiple myeloma. J Clin Oncol 3:654–659, 1985
215. Oken MM, Kyle RA, Kay NE et al: A Phase II trial of interferon $alpha_2$ ($rIFN_2$) in the treatment of resistant multiple myeloma (abstract 837). Proc Am Soc Clin Oncol 4:215, 1985
216. Quesada JR, Alexanian R, Hawkins M et al: Treatment of multiple myeloma with recombinant α-interferon. Blood 67:275–278, 1986
217. Cooper MR, Fefer A, Thompson J et al: Alpha-2-interferon/melphalan/prednisone in previously untreated patients with multiple myeloma: A Phase I-II trial. Cancer Treat Rep 70:473–476, 1986
218. Benson WJ, Scarffe JH, Todd IDH et al: Spinal cord compression in myeloma. Br Med J 1:1541–1544, 1979
219. Mill WB, Griffith R: The role of radiation therapy in the management of plasma cell tumors. Cancer 45:647–652, 1980
220. Mill WB: Radiation therapy in multiple myeloma. Radiology 115:175–178, 1975
221. Garrett MJ: Spinal myeloma and cord compression—diagnosis and management. Clin Radiol 21:42–46, 1970
222. Garland LH, Kennedy BR: Roentgen treatment of multiple myeloma. Radiology 50:297–316, 1948
223. Alberts DS, Chang FY, Chen HSG et al: Oral melphalan kinetics. Clin Pharm Ther 6:737–745, 1979
224. Feinleib M, MacMahon B: Duration of survival in multiple myeloma. J Natl Cancer Inst 24:1259–1269, 1960
225. Osgood EE: The survival time of patients with plasmocytic myeloma. Cancer Chemother Rep 9:1–10, 1960
226. McArthur JR, Athens JW, Wintrobe MM et al: Melphalan and myeloma. Experience with a low-dose continuous regimen. Ann Intern Med 72:665–670, 1970
227. Alexanian R, Bergsagel DE, Migliore PJ et al: Melphalan therapy for plasma cell myeloma. Blood 31:1–10, 1968
228. Alexanian R, Haut A, Khan AU et al: Treatment for multiple myeloma. JAMA 208:1680–1685, 1969
229. Hoogstraten B, Sheehe PR, Cuttner J, et al: Melphalan in multiple myeloma. Blood 30:74–83, 1967
230. Hoogstraten B, Costa J: Intermittent melphalan therapy in multiple myeloma. JAMA 209:251–253, 1969
231. Medical Research Council: Myelomatosis: Comparison of melphalan and cyclophosphamide therapy. Br Med J 1:640–641, 1971
232. Medical Research Council: Report on the second myelomatosis trial after five years of follow up. Br J Cancer 42:813–822, 1980
233. Medical Research Council: Treatment comparisons in the third MRC myelomatosis trial. Br J Cancer 42:823–830, 1980
234. Ogawa M, Bergsagel D, McCulloch E: Chemotherapy of mouse myeloma: Quantitative cell cultures predictive of response in vivo. Blood 41:7–15, 1973
235. Case DC, Lee BJ III, Clarkson BD: Improved survival times in multiple myeloma treated with melphalan, prednisone, cyclophosphamide, vincristine and BCNU: M2 protocol. Am J Med 63:897–903, 1977
236. Bonnet J, Alexanian R, Salmon S et al: Vincristine–BCNU–Adriamycin–prednisone (VBAP) combination in the treatment of relapsing or resistant multiple myeloma. A Southwest Oncology Group study. Cancer Treat Rep 66:1267–1271, 1982
237. MacLennon ICM, Kelly Krys RA, Crockson EH et al: Results of the MRC myelomatosis trials for patients entered since 1980. In Proceedings of British Multiple Myeloma Workshop, Blenheim Palace, London, England, October 14–16, 1987
238. Oken MM, Tsiatis A, Abramson N et al: Comparison of MP wiith intensive VBMCP therapy for the treatment of multiple myeloma (MM) (abstr). Proc Am Soc Clin Oncol 3:270, 1984
239. Hansen OP, Clausen NT, Drivsholm A et al: Phase II study of intermittent 5-drug regimen (VBCMP) versus intermittent 3-drug regimen (VMP), versus intermittent melphalan and prednisone (MP) in myelomatosis. Scand J Haematol 35:518–524, 1985
240. Durie BGM, Dixon B, Carter S et al: Improved survival duration with combination chemotherapy induction for multiple myeloma: A Southwest Oncology Group study. J Clin Oncol 4:1127–1237, 1986
241. Durie BGM, Dixon B, Carter S et al: Improved survival duration with combination chemotherapy induction for multiple myeloma: A Southwest Oncology Group study. J Clin Oncol 4:1127–1237, 1986
242. Harley JB, Pajak TF, McIntyre OR et al: Improved survival of increased-risk myeloma patients on combined triple alkylating agent therapy: A study of the CALGB. Blood 54:13–22, 1979
243. Cooper MR, McIntyre OR, Propert KJ et al: Single, sequential, and multiple alkylating agent therapy for multiple myeloma: A CALGB study. J Clin Oncol 4:1331–1339, 1986
244. Pavlovsky S, Saslavsky J, Tezanos Pinto M et al: A randomized trial of melphalan and prednisone versus melphalan, prednisone, cyclophosphamide, MeCCNU, and vincristine in untreated multiple myeloma. J Clin Oncol 2:836–840, 1984
245. Palva IP, Ahrenberg A, Almquist K et al: Aggressive combination chemotherapy in multiple myeloma. A multicentre trial. Scand J Haematol. 35:205–209, 1985
246. Kildahl-Anderson P, Bjark P, Bondevik A et al: Multiple myeloma in central Norway 1981–1982: A randomized clinical trial of 5-drug combination therapy versus standard therapy. Scand J Haematol 37:243–248, 1986
247. Cohen HJ, Silberman HR, Tornyos K et al: Comparison of two long-term chemotherapy regimens, with or without agents to modify skeletal repair, in multiple myeloma. Blood 63:639–648, 1984
248. Mettstedt H, Aahre A, Bjorkholm M: Interferon therapy of patients with myeloma. In Terry WD, Rosenberg SA (eds): Immunotherapy of Human Cancer, pp 387–391. New York, Elsevier, 1982
249. Case DC, Sonneborn HL, Paul SD et al: Phase II study of rDNA alpha-2 interferon (INTRON A) in patients with multiple myeloma utilizing an escalating induction phase. Cancer Treat Rep 70:1251–1254, 1986
250. Cooper MR, Welander CE: Interferons in the treatment of multiple myeloma. Semin Oncol 13:334–340, 1986
251. Ludwig H, Cortelezzi A, Van Camp BGK et al: Treatment with recombinant-alpha-2C: Multiple myeloma and thrombocythaemia in myeloproliferative diseases. Oncology (Suppl 1) 42:19–25, 1985
252. Ahre A, Bjorkholm M, Mellstedt H et al: Human leukocyte interferon and intermittent high-dose melphalan–prednisone administration in the treatment of multiple myeloma: A randomized clinical trial from the Myeloma Group of Central Sweden. Cancer Treat Rep 68:1331–1338, 1984
253. Alexanian R, Gehan E, Haut A et al: Unmaintained remissions in multiple myeloma. Blood 51:1005–1011, 1978
254. Alexanian R: Long unmaintained remission in multiple myeloma. Am J Clin Oncol 9:458–460, 1986
255. Southwest Oncology Group Study: Remission maintenance therapy for multiple myeloma. Arch Intern Med 135:147, 1975
256. Belch A, White D, Bergsagel D et al: The role of maintenance chemotherapy for multiple myeloma (abstr c1050). Proc Am Soc Clin Oncol 3:268 1984
257. Cohen JH, Bartolucci AA, Forman WB et al: Consolidation and maintenance therapy in multiple myeloma: Randomized comparison of a new approach to therapy after initial response to treatment. J Clin Oncol 5:888–899, 1986
258. Tribalto M, Mandelli F, Cantonetti M et al: New Trends in the Therapy of Leukemia and Lymphoma 2:61–68, 1987 (Bernasconi C ed) Edizione Medic Scientifiche, Pavia, Italy
259. Mandell F, Tribalto M, Cantonetti M et al: Recombinant alpha 2_β interferon as maintenance therapy in responding multiple myeloma patients. Blood (Suppl 1) 70:247a, 1987
260. Crowin J, Lindberg RD: Solitary plasmacytoma of bone vs extramedullary plasmacytoma and their relationship to multiple myeloma. Cancer 43:1007–1013, 1979
261. Knowling M, Harwood A, Bergsagel DE: A comparison of extramedullary plasmacytoma with multiple and solitary plasma cell tumors of bone. J Clin Oncol 1:255–262, 1983
262. Wiltshaw E: The natural history of extramedullary plasmacytoma and its relation to solitary myeloma of bone and myelomatosis. Medicine 55:217–238, 1976
263. Woodruff RK, Malpas JS, White FE: Solitary plasmacytoma. II. Solitary plasmacytoma of bone. Cancer 43:2344–2347, 1979
264. Chak LY, Cox S, Bostwick DG et al: Solitary plasmacytoma of bone: Treatment, progression, and survival. J Clin Oncol 5:1811–1815, 1987
265. Woodruff RK, Whittle JM, Malpas JS: Solitary plasmacytoma. I. Extramedullary soft tissue plasmacytoma. Cancer 43:2340–2343, 1979
266. Hamburger AW, Salmon SE: Primary bioassay of human tumor stem cells. Science 197:461–463, 1977
267. Otsuka T, Okamura S, Niho Y: Colony assay in patients with multiple myeloma—relationship between colony growth and clinical stage. Acta Haematol Jpn 49:1792–1799, 1986
268. Salmon SE, Hamburger AW, Soehnlen BJ et al: Quantitation of differential sensitivity of human tumor stem cells to anticancer drugs. N Engl J Med 298:1321–1327, 1978
269. Salmon SE, In vitro cloning and chemosensitivity of human myeloma stem cells. In Hoffbrand AV, Lasch HG, Nathan DG et al (eds), Salmon SE (guest ed): Clin Haematol 11:47–64. Eastbourne, WB Saunders, 1982
270. Ludwig H, Fritz E: Individualized chemotherapy in multiple myeloma by cytostatic drug sensitivity testing of colony-forming stem cells. Anticancer Res 1:329–334, 1981
271. Hanauske AR, Hanauske U, Von Hoff DD: Recent improvements in the human cloning assay for sensitivity testing of antineoplastic agents. Eur J Cancer Clin Oncol 23:603–605, 1987
272. Nordan RP, Pumphrey JG, Rudikoff S: Purification and NH_2-terminal sequence of a plasmacytoma growth factor derived from the murine macrophage cell line P388D1. J Immunol 139:813–817, 1987
273. Van Snick J, Cayphas S, Vink A et al: Purification and NH_2-terminal amino acid sequence of a T-cell derived lymphokine with growth factor activity for B-cell hybridomas. Proc Natl Acad Sci USA 83:9679–9683, 1986
274. Tanigawa N, Kern DH, Hikasa Y et al: Rapid assay for evaluating the chemosensitivity of human tumors in soft agar culture. Cancer Res 42:2159–2164, 1982
275. Alexanian R, Salmon S, Gutterman J et al: Chemoimmunotherapy of multiple myeloma. Cancer 47:1923–1929, 1981
276. Buzaid AC, Durie BGM: Management of refractory myeloma: A review. J Clin Oncol, 6:889–905, 1988
277. Kyle RA, Greipp PR, Gertz MA: Treatment of refractory multiple myeloma and considerations for future therapy. Semin Oncol 13:326–333, 1986

278. Medenica R, Slack N: Clinical results of leucocyte interferon-induced tumor regression in resistant human metastatic cancer resistant to chemotherapy and/or radiotherapy-pulse therapy schedule. Cancer Drug Deliv 2:53–76, 1985
279. Wagstaff A, Loynds R, Scarffe JH: Phase II study of rDNA human alpha-2 interferon in multiple myeloma. Cancer Treat Rep 69:495–498, 1985
280. Ohno R, Kimura K, Amaki I et al: Treatment of multiple myeloma with recombinant human leucocyte α interferon. Cancer Treat Rep 69:1433–1435, 1985
281. Alexanian R, Yap BS, Bodey GP: Prednisone pulse therapy for refractory myeloma. Blood 62:572–577, 1983
282. Dalton WS, Durie BGM, Alberts DS et al: Characterization of a new drug resistant human myeloma cell line which expresses *p*-glycoprotein. Cancer Res 45:5125–5130, 1986
283. Murakami T, Togawa A, Satch H et al: Glucocorticoid receptor in myeloma. Eur J Haematol 39:54–59, 1987
284. Bergsagel DE, Cowan DH, Hasselbach R: Plasma cell myeloma: Response of melphalan-resistant patients to high-dose intermittent cyclophosphamide. Can Med Assoc J 107:851–855, 1972
285. Kyle RA, Sligman BR, Wallace J et al: Multiple myeloma resistant to melphalan (NSC-8806) treated with cyclophosphamide (NSC-26271), prednisone (NSC-10023), and chloroquine (NSC-187208). Cancer Chemother Rep 59:557–562, 1975
286. Tornyos K, Silberman H, Soloman A: Phase II study of oral methyl-CCNU and prednisone in previously treated alkylating agent-resistant multiple myeloma. Cancer Treat Rep 61:785–787, 1977
287. Buonanno G, Tortarolo M, Valente A et al: Drug-resistant multiple myeloma. A trial with the M_2 cyclic alkylating agent polychemotherapy. Haematologica (Pavia) 63:45–55, 1978
288. Kyle RA, Gailani S, Seligman BR et al: Multiple myeloma resistant to melphalan: Treatment with cyclophosphamide, prednisone, and BCNU. Cancer Treat Rep 63:1265–1269, 1979
289. Blade J, Feliu E, Rozman C et al: Cross-resistance to alkylating agents in multiple myeloma. Cancer 52:786–789, 1983
290. Steinke B, Busch FW, Becherer C et al: Cancer Chemother Pharmacol 14:279–281, 1985
291. Paccagnella A, Salvagno L, Bolzonella S et al: Second and third response to M_2 (BCNU, VCR, CTX, PRED) in multiple myeloma (abstr). Am Soc Clin Oncol 4:217, 1985
292. Paccagnella A, Cartel G, Fosser V et al: Treatment of multiple myeloma with M_2 protocol and without maintenance therapy. Eur J Cancer Clin Oncol 19:1345–1351, 1982
293. Belch A, Shelley W, Bergsagel D et al: A randomized trial of maintenance versus no maintenance melphalan and prednisone in responding multiple myeloma patients (abstr). Proc Am Soc Cancer Oncol, 1987
294. Alberts DS, Durie BGM, Salmon SE: Doxorubicin/BCNU chemotherapy for multiple myeloma in relapse. Lancet 1:926–928, 1976
295. Bonnet JD, Alexanian R, Salmon SE et al: Addition of cisplatin and bleomycin to vincristine–doxorubicin–prednisone (VBAP) combination in the treatment of relapsing or resistant multiple myeloma: A Southwest Oncology Group Study. Cancer Treat Rep 68:481–485, 1984
296. Blade J, Rozman C, Montserrat E et al: Treatment of alkylating resistant multiple myeloma with vincristine, BCNU, doxorubicin and prednisone (VBAP). Eur J Cancer Clin Oncol 22:1193–1197, 1986
297. Present CA, Klahr C: Adriamycin, 1,3-bis (2-chloroethyl)-1-nitrosourea (BCNU, NSC #409962), cyclophosphamide plus prednisone (ABC-P) in melphalan-resistant multiple myeloma. Cancer 42:1222–1227, 1978
298. Kyle RA, Pajak TF, Henderson ES et al: Multiple myeloma resistant to melphalan: Treatment with doxorubicin, cyclophosphamide, carmustine (BCNU), and prednisone. Cancer Treat Rep 66:451–456, 1982
299. Barlogie B, Smith L, Alexanian R: Effective treatment of advanced multiple myeloma refractory to alkylating agents. N Engl J Med 310:1353–1356, 1984
300. Sheehan T, Judge M, Parker AC: The efficacy and toxicity of VAD in the treatment of myeloma and related disorders. Scand J Hematol 37:425–428, 1986
301. Monconduit M, Le Loet X, Bernard JF et al: Combination chemotherapy with vincristine, doxorubicin, dexamethasone for refractory or relapsing multiple myeloma. Br J Haematol 63:599–601, 1986
302. Monconduit M, Bauters F, Najman A: Evaluation of the association vincristine–Adriamycin plus high-dose dexamethasone (VAD) in severe previously treated myeloma. (Suppl 1) Blood 68:240a, 1986
303. Dalton WS, Durie BGM, Salmon SE et al: Resistance in multiple myeloma and non-Hodgkin's lymphoma: Detection of P-glycoprotein and potential circumvention by addition of verapamil to chemotherapy. J Clin Oncol (in press, April 1989)
304. Fitzpatrick PJ, Rider WD: Half-body radiotherapy. Int J Radiat Oncol Biol Phys 1:197–207, 1976
305. Rider WB: Half-body radiotherapy, an update. Int J Radiat Oncol Biol Phys (Suppl 2) 4:69–70, 1978
306. Salmon S, Tesh D, Crowley J et al: Combination chemotherapy is superior to hemibody irradiation (HXRT) for remission consolidation in multiple myeloma (MM): A Southwest Oncology Group (SWOG) Study (abstr). Proc Am Soc Clin Oncol, 1989
307. Jaffe JP, Bosch A, Raich PC: Sequential hemi-body radiotherapy in advanced multiple myeloma. Cancer 43:124–128, 1979
308. Qasim MM: Techniques and results of half-body irradiation (HBI) in metastatic carcinoma and myeloma. Clin Oncol 5:65–68, 1979
309. Rowland CG, Garrett MJ, Crowley et al: Half-body radiation in plasma cell myeloma. Clin Radiol 34:507–510, 1983
310. Coleman M, Soletan S, Wolf D et al: Whole bone marrow irradiation for the treatment of multiple myeloma. Cancer 49:1328–1333, 1982
311. Richards JDM, Coates PB, Closs SP et al: Case of macroglobulinemia treated with hemibody irradiation (letter). Lancet 2:844, 1983
312. Tobias JS, Richards JDM, Blackman GM, et al: Hemibody irradiation in multiple myeloma. Radiother Oncol 3:11–16, 1985
313. Prato FS, Kurdyak R, Saibil EA et al: The incidence of radiation pneumonitis as a result of single fraction, upper half-body irradiation. Cancer 39:71–78, 1976
314. Perren TJ, Selby PJ, Mbidde EK et al: High dose chemotherapy of multiple myeloma (MM) with melphalan (HDM) and with methylprednisolone (HDMP) (abstr). Am Soc Clin Oncol 5:158, 1986
315. McElwain TJ, Powles RL: High-dose intravenous melphalan for plasma-cell leukaemia and myeloma. Lancet 2:822–824, 1983
316. Lenhard RE, Oken MM, Barnes JM et al: High-dose cyclophosphamide. An effective treatment for advanced refractory multiple myeloma. Cancer 53:1456–1460, 1984
317. Lenhard RE, Tsiatis AA, Oken MM et al: Time sequential high-dose cyclophosphamide (CY) and vincristine (VCR) treatment of multiple myeloma (MM) (abstr). Proc Am Soc Clin Oncol 4:217, 1985
318. Barlogie B, Hall R, Zander A et al: High-dose melphalan with autologous bone marrow transplantation for multiple myeloma. Blood 67:1298–1301, 1986
319. Barlogie B, Alexanian R, Dicke KA et al: High-dose melphalan (HDM) + total body irradiation (TBI) and bone marrow transplantation (BMT) for refractory myeloma. (Suppl 1) Blood 68:240a, 1986
320. Selby PJ, McElwain TJ, Nandi AC et al: Multiple myeloma treated with high dose intravenous melphalan. Br J Haematol 66:55–62, 1987
321. Barlogie B, Alexanian R, Dicke K et al: High-dose chemoradiotherapy and autologous bone marrow transplantation for resistant myeloma. Blood 70:869–872, 1987
322. Osserman EF, DiRe LB, DiRe J et al: Identical twin marrow transplantation in multiple myeloma. Acta Haematol (Basel) 68:215–223, 1982
323. Ozer H, Han T, Nussbaum-Blumenson A, et al: Allogenic bone marrow transplantation and idiotype (ID) monitoring in multiple myeloma (abstr). Clin Invest 25:161, 1984
324. Gahrton G, Tura S, Flesch M et al: Bone marrow transplantation in multiple myeloma: Report from the European Cooperative Group for Bone Marrow Transplantation. Blood 69:1262–1264, 1987
325. Gallamini A, Buffa F, Bacigalupo A et al: Allogeneic bone marrow transplantation in multiple myeloma. Acta Haematol 77:111–114, 1987
326. Feffer A: Personal communication, 1987
327. Tura S: Bone marrow transplantation in multiple myeloma: Current status and future perspectives. Bone Marrow Transplantation 1:17–20, 1986
328. Gahrton G, Ringden O, Lonnqvist: Bone marrow transplantation in multiple myeloma. Acta Med Scand 219:433–434, 1986
329. Tong AM, Lee JC, Fay JW et al: Elimination of clonogenic stem-cells from human multiple myeloma cell lines by a plasma cell-reactive monoclonal antibody and complement. Blood 70:1482–1489, 1987
330. Belch AR, Henderson JF, Brox LW: Treatment of multiple myeloma with deoxycoformycin. Cancer Chemother Pharmacol 14:49–52, 1985
331. Grever MR, McGee RA, Kraut ER, et al: Deoxycoformycin in refractory myeloma. (Suppl 1) Blood 70:246a, 1987
332. Case DC Jr, Oldham F, Ervin T et al: Phase I-II study of epirubicin in multiple myeloma (abstr). Am Soc Clin Oncol 6:146, 1987
333. Durie BGM, Levy HB, Voakes J et al: Poly (I,C)-LC as an interferon inducer in refractory multiple myeloma. J Biol Response Mod 4:518–524, 1985
334. Paccagnella A, Salvagno L, Chiarion-Sileni V et al: Peptichemio in pretreated patient with plasma cell neoplasms. Eur J Cancer Clin Oncol 22:1053–1058, 1986
335. Tirelli U, Carbone A, Zagonei V et al: Phase II study of teniposide (VM-26) in multiple myeloma. Am J Clin Oncol 8:329–331, 1985
336. Gockerman JP, Silberman H, Bartolucci AA: Phase II evaluation of aclarubicin in refractory multiple myeloma: A Southeastern Cancer Study Group Trial. Cancer Treat Rep 71:773–774, 1987
337. Scarffe JH, Beaumont AR, Crowther D: Phase I–II evaluation of acronine in patients with multiple myeloma. Cancer Treat Rep 67:93–94, 1983
338. Ahmann FR, Meyskens FL, Jones SE et al: Phase II evaluation of amsacrine (*m*-AMSA) in solid tumors, myeloma, and lymphoma: A University of Arizona and Southwest Oncology Group study. Cancer Treat Rep 67:697–700, 1983
339. Blum RH, Carter SK, Agre K: A clinical review of bleomycin, a new anti-neoplastic agent. Cancer 31:903–913, 1973
340. Bennett JM, Silber R, Ezdinli E et al: Phase II study of Adriamycin and bleomycin in patients with multiple myeloma. Cancer Treat Rep 62:1367–1369, 1978
341. Corder MP, Elliot TE, Bell SJ: Dose limiting myelotoxicity and absence of significant nephrotoxicity with the weekly outpatient schedule of cis-platinum (II) diamminedichloride. J Clin Hematol Oncol 7:645–651, 1977
342. Cornell CJ Jr, Pajak TF, McIntyre OR: Chlorozotocin: Phase II evaluation in patients with myeloma. Cancer Treat Rep 68:685–686, 1984
343. Forman WB, Cohen HJ, Bartolucci AA et al: Phase II evaluation of chlorozotocin in refractory multiple myeloma. Cancer Treat Rep 68:1409–1410, 1984
344. Kantarjian H, Dreicer R, Barlogie B et al: High-dose cytosine arabinoside in multiple myeloma. Eur J Cancer Clin Oncol 20:227–231, 1984
345. Vinciguerra V, Anderson K, McIntyre OR: Diaziquone for resistant multiple myeloma. Cancer Treat Rep 69:331–332, 1985

346. Stuckey WJ, Crowley J, Baker LH et al: Phase II trial of diaziquone in patients with refractory and relapsing multiple myeloma: A Southwest Oncology Group study. Cancer Treat Rep 71:1095–1096, 1987
347. Gockerman JP, Bartolucci AA, Nelson MO et al: Phase II evaluation of etoposide in refractory multiple myeloma: A Southeastern Cancer Study Group Trial. Cancer Treat Rep 70:801–802, 1986
348. Cohen HJ, Bartolucci AA: Hexamethylmelamine and prednisone in the treatment of refractory multiple myeloma. Am J Clin Oncol 5:21–27, 1982
349. Alberts DS, Balcerzak SP, Bonnet JP et al: Phase II trials of mitoxantrone in multiple myeloma: A Southwest Oncology Group study. Cancer Treat Rep 69:1321–1323, 1985
350. Tirelli U, Sorio R, Magri MD et al: Prednimustine in elderly patients with multiple myeloma: A Phase II study. Cancer Treat Rep 70:537–538, 1986
351. Moon JH, Edmonson JH: Procarbazine (NSC-77213) and multiple myeloma. Cancer Chemother Rep 54:245–248, 1970
352. Lake-Lewin D, Myers J, Lee BL et al: Phase II trial of pyrazofurin in patients with multiple myeloma refractory to standard cytotoxic therapy. Cancer Treat Rep 63:1403–1404, 1979
353. Houwen B, Ockhuizen T, Marrink J et al: Vindesine therapy in melphalan-resistant myeloma. Eur J Cancer 17:227–232, 1981
354. Oken MM, Lenhard RE, Tslatis AA et al: Contribution of prednisone to the effectiveness of hexamethylmelamine in multiple myeloma. Cancer Treat Rep 71:807–811, 1987
355. Cavo M, Baccarani M, Galieni P et al: Renal failure in multiple myeloma. A study of the presenting findings, response to treatment and prognosis in 26 patients. Nouv Rev Fr Hematol 28:147–152, 1986
356. Cornwell CG, Pajak TF, McIntyre OR et al: Influence of renal failure on the myelosuppressive effects of melphalan: Cancer and Leukemia Group B experience. Cancer Treat Rep 66:475–481, 1982
357. Alberts DS, Chen H-SY, Berg D et al: Effects of renal dysfunction in dogs on the disposition and marrow toxicity of melphalan. Br J Cancer 43:330–334, 1981
358. Adair CG, Bridges JM, Desai ZR: Renal function in the elimination of oral mephalan in patients with multiple myeloma. Cancer Chemother Pharmacol 17:185–188, 1986
359. MRC Working Party on Leukemia in Adults: Analysis and management of renal failure in fourth MRC myelomatosis trial. Br Med J 288:1411–1416, 1984
360. Bernstein SP, Humes DH: Reversible renal insufficiency in multiple myeloma. Arch Intern Med 142:2083–2086, 1982
361. Coward RA, Mallick NP, Delamore IW: Should patients with acute renal failure associated with myeloma be dialysed? Br Med J 287:1575–1578, 1983
362. Russell JA, Fitzharris BM, Corringham R et al: Plasma exchange vs peritoneal dialysis for removing Bence Jones protein. Br J Med 2:1397, 1978
363. Feest TG, Burge PS, Cohen SL: Successful treatment of myeloma kidney by diuresis and plasmapheresis. Br J Med 1:503–505, 1976
364. Misiani R, Remuzzi G, Bertani T et al: Plasmapheresis is the treatment of acute renal failure in multiple myeloma. Am J Med 66:684–688, 1979
365. Pasquali S, Cagnoli L, Rovinetti C et al: Plasma exchange therapy in rapidly progressive renal failure due to multiple myeloma. Int J Artif Organs 8:27–30, 1984
366. Humphrey RL, Wright JR, Zachary JB et al: Renal transplantation in multiple myeloma. A case report. Ann Intern Med 83:651–653, 1975
367. Payne R, Little A, Williams R et al: Interpretation of serum calcium in patients with abnormal serum proteins. Br Med J 4:643, 1973
368. Hasling C, Charles P, Mosekilde L: Etidronate disodium for treating hypercalcaemia of malignancy: A double blind, placebo-controlled study. Eur J Clin Invest 16:433–437, 1986
369. Jacobs TP, Gordon AC, Silverberg SH et al: Neoplastic hypercalcemia: Physiologic response to intravenous etidronate disodium. Am J Med (Suppl 2A) 82:42–50, 1987
370. Lingarde F, Zettervall O: Hypercalcemia and normal ionized serum calcium in a case of myelomatosis. Ann Intern Med 78:396–399, 1973
371. Soria J, Soria C, Dao C: Immunoglobulin bound calcium and ultrafilterable serum calcium in myeloma. Br J Haematol 34:343–344, 1976
372. Jaffe JP, Mosher DF: Calcium binding in a myeloma protein. Am J Med 67:343–346, 1979
373. Rota S, Mougenot B, Baudouin B et al: Multiple myeloma and severe renal failure: A clinicopathologic study of outcome and prognosis in 34 patients. Medicine 66:126–137, 1987
374. Kyle RA, Jowsey J, Kelly PJ et al: Multiple myeloma bone disease. The comparative effect of sodium fluoride and calcium carbonate or placebo. N Engl J Med 293:1334–1338, 1975
375. Kyle RA, Jowsey J: Effect of sodium fluoride, calcium carbonate, and vitamin D on the skeleton in multiple myeloma. Cancer 45:1669–1674, 1980
376. Gardner FH: Fluorides for multiple myeloma. N Engl J Med 287:1252–1253, 1972
377. Jakubowski J, Kendall BE, Symon L: Primary plasmacytoma of the cranial vault. Acta Neurochir 55:117–134, 1980
378. Stark RJ, Henson RA: Cerebral compression by myeloma. J Neurol Neurosurg Psychiatry 44:833–836, 1981
379. Kohli CM, Kawazu T: Solitary intracranial plasmacytoma. Surg Neurol 17:307–312, 1982
380. Atweh GF, Jabbour M: Intracranial solitary extraskeletal plasmacytoma resembling meningioma. Arch Neurol 39:57–59, 1982
381. Soffer D, Siegal T: Solitary dural plasmacytoma with conspicuous cytoplasmic inclusions. Cancer 49:2500–2504, 1982
382. Mancardi GL, Mandybur TI: Solitary intracranial plasmacytoma. Cancer 51:2226–2233, 1983
383. Coppeto JR, Monteiro MLR, Collias J et al: Foster-Kennedy syndrome caused by solitary intracranial plasmacytoma. Surg Neurol 19:267–272, 1983
384. Pritchard PB III, Martinez RA, Hungerford GD et al: Dural plasmacytoma. Neurosurgery 12:576–579, 1983
385. Benson MD, Brandt KD, Cohen AS et al: Neuropathy, M components and amyloid. Lancet 1:10–12, 1975
386. Davis LE, Drachman DB: Myeloma neuropathy. Successful treatment of two patients and review of cases. Arch Neurol 27:507–511, 1972
387. Driedger H, Pruzanski W: Plasma cell neoplasia with peripheral neuropathy. A study of five cases and a review of the literature. Medicine 59:301–310, 1980
388. Reitan JB, Pape E, Fossa SD et al: Osteosclerotic myeloma with polyneuropathy. Acta Med Scand 208:137–144, 1980
389. Delauche MC, Clauvel JP, Seligmann M: Peripheral neuropathy and plasma cell neoplasias: A report of 10 cases. Br J Haematol 48:384–392, 1981
390. Osby E, Noring L, Hast R et al: Benign monoclonal gammopathy and peripheral neuropathy. Br J Haematol 51:531–539, 1982
391. Kelly JJ Jr, Kyle RA, Miles JM et al: Osteosclerotic myeloma and peripheral neuropathy. Neurology 33:202–210, 1983
392. Besinger UA, Toyka KV, Anzil AP et al: Myeloma neuropathy: Passive transfer from man to mouse. Science 213:1027–1039, 1981
393. Lator N, Sherman WH, Nemni R et al: Plasma cell dyscrasia and peripheral nerve myelin. N Engl J Med 303:618–621, 1980
394. Lamarca J, Casquero P, Pou A: Mononeuritis multiplex in Waldenström's macroglobulinemia. Ann Neurol 22:268–272, 1987
395. Vital C, Deminiere C, Bourgouin B et al: Waldenström's macroglobulinemia and peripheral neuropathy: Deposition of M-component and kappa light chain in the endoneurium. Neurology 35:603–606, 1985
396. Ohi T, Kyle RA, Dyck PJ: Axonal attenuation and secondary segmental demyelination in myeloma neuropathies. Ann Neurol 17:255–261, 1985
397. Nobile-Orazio E, Marmiroli P, Baldini L et al: Peripheral neuropathy in macroglobulinemia: Incidence and antigen-specificity of M-proteins. Neurology 37:1506–1514, 1987
398. Hoppe U, Drager HS, Patzold U et al: Polyneuropathy in Waldenström's macroglobulinaemia. Passive transfer from man to mouse. Acta Neurol Scand 75:112–116, 1987
399. Kyle RA: Multiple myeloma. Review of 869 cases. Mayo Clin Proc 50:29–40, 1975
400. Hoffbrand AV, Hobbs JR, Kremenchuzky S et al: Incidence and pathogenesis of megaloblastic erythropoiesis in multiple myeloma. J Clin Pathol 20:699–705, 1967
401. Winearls CG, Pippard MJ, Downing MR et al: Effect of human erythropoietin derived from recombinant DNA on the anaemia of patients maintained by chronic haemodialysis. Lancet 2:1175–1177, 1986
402. Eschbach JW, Egrie JC, Downing MR et al: Correction of the anemia of end-stage renal disease with recombinant human erythropoietin. Results of a combined Phase I and II clinical trial. N Engl J Med 316:73–78, 1987
403. Rifkin RM, Hersh EM, Salmon SE: A Phase I study of therapy with recombinant granulocyte-macrophage colony-stimulating factor administered by IV bolus or continuous infusion. In Seiler FR, Schwick HG (eds): Proceedings of Behring Institute, International Symposium on Colony Stimulating Factors, West Germany, May 1988
404. Bergsagel DE: Plasma cell neoplasms and acute leukaemia. In Hoffbrand AV, Lasch HG, Nathan DG (eds), Salmon SE (guest ed): Clin Haematol 11:221–234, Eastbourne, WB Saunders, 1982
405. Holland D, Muller JM, Leger J et al: Association myeloma, leucose myeloide et lymphosarcome. Reflexions nosologiques. Lyon Med 213:967–974, 1965
406. Kyle RA, Robert MD, Pierre RV et al: Multiple myeloma and acute myelomonocytic leukemia. N Engl J Med. 283:1121–1125, 1970
407. Nordenson NG: Myelomatosis: A clinical review of 30 cases. Acta Med Scand (Suppl) 445:178–186, 1966
408. Mufti GJ, Hamblin TJ, Clein GP et al: Coexistent myelodysplasia and plasma cell neoplasia. Br J Haematol 54:91–96, 1983
409. Cuzick J, Erskine S, Edelman D et al: A comparison of the incidence of the myelodysplastic syndrome and acute myeloid leukaemia following melphalan and cyclophosphamide treatment for myelomatosis. Br J Cancer 55:523–529, 1987
410. Green MH, Harris EL, Gershensen DM et al: Melphalan may be a more potent leukemogen than cyclophosphamide. Ann Intern Med 105:360–367, 1986
411. Lackner H: Hemostatic abnormalities associated with dysproteinemias. Semin Hematol 10:125–133, 1973
412. Henstell HH, Kligerman M: A new theory of interference with the clotting mechanism: The complexing of euglobulin with factor V, factor VII, and prothrombin. Ann Intern Med 49:371–387, 1958
413. Lackner H: Hemostatic abnormalities associated with dysproteinemias. Semin Hematol 10:125–133, 1973
414. Godal HC, Borchgrevink CF: The effect of plasmapheresis on the hemostatic function in patients with macroglobulinemia Waldenström and multiple myeloma. Scand J Clin Lab Invest (Suppl 84) 17:133–137, 1965
415. Doumenc J, Prost RJ, Samama M et al: Anomalie de l'agregation plaquettaire au cours de la maladie de Waldenström (a propos de 3 cas). Nouv Rev Fr Hematol 6:734–738, 1966
416. Penny R, Castaldi PA, Whitsed HM: Inflammation and hemostasis in paraproteinemias. Br J Haematol 20:35–44, 1971
417. Pachter MR, Johnson SA, Neblett TR et al: Bleeding, platelets, and macroglobulinemia. Am J Clin Pathol 31:467–482, 1959

418. Pachter MR, Johnson SA, Basinski DH: The effect of macroglobulins and their dissociation units on release of platelet factor 3. Thromb Diath Haemorrh 3:501–509, 1959
419. Khoory MS, Nesheim ME, Bowie EJW et al: Circulating heparin sulfate proteoglycan anticoagulant from a patient with a plasma cell disorder. J Clin Invest 65:666–674, 1980
420. Meyer K, Williams EC: Fibrinolysis and acquired alpha-2 plasmin inhibitor deficiency in amyloidosis. Am J Med 79:394–396, 1985
421. Somer T: Hyperviscosity syndrome in plasma cell dyscracias. Adv Microcirc 6:1–55, 1975
422. Fahey JL: Serum protein disorders causing clinical symptoms in malignant neoplastic disease. J Chron Dis 16:703–712, 1963
423. Fahey JL, Barth WF, Soloman A: Serum hyperviscosity syndrome. JAMA 192:464–467, 1965
424. Bloch KJ, Maki DG: Hyperviscosity syndromes associated with immunoglobulin abnormalities. Semin Hematol 10:113–124, 1973
425. McGrath MA, Penny R: Paraproteinemia: Blood hyperviscosity and clinical manifestations. J Clin Invest 58:1158–1162, 1976
426. MacKenzie MR, Lee TK: Blood viscosity in Waldenström macroglobulinemia. Blood 49:507–510, 1977
427. MacKenzie MR, Fudenberg HH: Macroglobulinemia: An analysis for forty patients. Blood 39:874, 1972
428. Crawford J, Cox EB, Cohen HJ: Evaluation of hyperviscosity in monoclonal gammopathies. Am J Med 79:13–22, 1985
429. MacKenzie MR, Brown E, Fudenberg HH et al: Waldenström's macroglobulinemia correlation between expanded plasma volume and increased serum viscosity. Blood 35:934, 1970
430. Valbonesi M, Tarantino M, Montani F et al: Biochemical and clinical evaluation of a new cellulose diacetate secondary filter for cascade filtration. Int J Artif Organs 8:105–108, 1985
431. Valbonesi M, Monani F, Guzzini F et al: Efficacy of discontinuous flow centrifugation compared with cascade filtration in Waldenström's macroglobulinemia: A pilot study. Int J Artif Organs 8:165–168, 1985
432. Avnstorp C, Nielson H, Drachman O et al: Plasmapheresis in hyperviscosity syndrome. Acta Med Scand 217:133–137, 1985
433. Whittaker JA, Tuddenham EGD, Bradley J: Hyperviscosity syndrome in IgA multiple myeloma. Lancet 2:572, 1973
434. Pruzanski W, Jancelewicz Z, Underdown B: Immunological and physiochemical studies of IgAL (λ) cryogelglobulinemia. Clin Exp Immunol 15:181–191, 1973
435. Meltzer M, Franklin EC: Cryoglobulinemia: A study of twenty-nine patients. I. IgG and IgM cryoglobulins and factors affecting cryoprecipitability. Am J Med 40:828–836, 1966
436. MacKay IR, Erikson N, Motulsky AG et al: Cryo- and macroglobulinemia: Electrophoretic, ultracentrifugal, and clinical studies. Am J Med 20:564–587, 1956
437. Liss M, Fudenberg HH, Kritzman J: A Bence Jones cryoglobulin: Clinical, physical, and immunological properties. Clin Exp Immunol 2:467–475, 1967
438. Bloth B, Christensson T, Mellstedt H: Extreme hyponatremia in patients with myelomatosis. An effect of cationic paraproteins. Acta Med Scand 203:273–275, 1978
439. Emmett ME, Narins RG: Clinical use of the anion gap. Medicine 56:38–54, 1977
440. Murray T, Long W, Narins RG: Multiple myeloma and the anion gap. N Engl J Med 292:574–575, 1976
441. Braden GL, Mikolich DJ, White CF et al: Syndrome of inappropriate antidiuresis in Waldenström's macroglobulinemia. Am J Med 80:1242–1244, 1986
442. Schnur MJ, Appel GB, Karp G et al: The anion gap in asymptomatic plasma cell dyscrasia. Ann Intern Med 86:304–305, 1977
443. Jacobson DR, Zolla-Pazner S: Immunosuppression and infection in multiple myeloma. Semin Oncol 13:282–290, 1986
444. Zinneman HH, Wall WH: Recurrent pneumonia in multiple myeloma and some observations on immunologic response. Ann Intern Med 41:1152–1163, 1954
445. Fahey JR, Scoggins R, Utz JP et al: Infections, antibody response and γ globulin components in multiple myeloma and macroglobulinemia. Am J Med 35:698–707, 1963
446. Meyers BR, Hirschman SZ, Axelrod JA: Current patterns of infection in multiple myeloma. Am J Med 52:87–92, 1972
447. Twomey JJ: Infections complicating multiple myeloma and chronic lymphocytic leukemia. Arch Intern Med 132:562–565, 1973
448. Norden CW: Editorial: Infections in patients with multiple myeloma. Arch Intern Med 140:1150–1151, 1980
449. Savage DG, Lindenbaum J, Garret TJ: Biphasic pattern of bacterial infection in multiple myeloma. Ann Intern Med 96:47–50, 1982
450. Salmon SE, Samai BA, Hayes DM et al: Role of gamma globulin for immunoprophylaxis in multiple myeloma. N Engl J Med 227:1336–1340, 1967
451. Nolan CM, Baxley PJ, Frasch CE: Antibody response to infection in multiple myeloma. Implications for vaccination. Am J Med 67:331–334, 1979
452. Glenner GG, Ein D, Eanes ED et al: The creation of "amyloid" fibrils from Bence Jones protein in vitro. Science 174:712–714, 1971
453. Glenner GG: Amyloid deposits and amyloidosis: The β-fibrilloses. N Engl J Med 302:1283–1292, 1980
454. Cathcart ES, Ritchie RF, Cohen AS et al: Immunoglobulins and amyloidosis. An immunologic study of sixty-two patients with biopsy-proven disease. Am J Med 52:93–101, 1972
455. Kyle RA: Amyloidosis. In Hoffbrand AV, Lasch HG, Nathan DG (eds), Salmon SE (guest ed): Clin Hematol 11:151–180, Eastbourne, WB Saunders, 1982
456. Kyle RA, Bayrd ED: Amyloidosis: Review of 236 cases. Medicine 54:271–299, 1975
457. Gordon DA, Pruzanski W, Ogryzlo MA et al: Amyloid arthritis simulating rheumatoid disease in five patients with multiple myeloma. Am J Med 55:142–154, 1973
458. Siqueria-Filho AG, Cunha CLP, Tajik AJ et al: M-mode and two dimensional echocardiographic features in cardiac amyloidosis. Circulation 63:188–196, 1981
459. Buxbaum JN, Hurley ME, Chuba J, Spira T: Amyloidosis of the AL type: Clinical, morphologic, and biochemical aspects of the response to therapy with alkylating agents and prednisone. Am J Med 67:867–878, 1979
460. Fielder K, Durie BG: Primary amyoloidosis associated with multiple myeloma. Predictors of successful therapy. Am J Med 80:413–419, 1986
461. Kyle RA, Greipp PR: Primary systemic amyloidosis: Comparison of melphalan and prednisone versus placebo. Blood 52:818–827, 1978
462. Kyle RA, Greipp PR, O'Fallon WM: Primary systemic amyloidosis: Multivariate analysis for prognostic factors in 168 cases. Blood 68:220–224, 1986
463. Waldenström J: Incipient myelomatosis or "essential" hyperglobulinemia with fibrogenopenia—A new syndrome? Acta Med Scand 117:216–222, 1944
464. Waldenström J: Macroglobulinemia. Adv Metab Dis 2:115, 1965
465. Carter P, Koval JJ, Hobbs JR: The relation of clinical and laboratory findings to the survival of patients with macroglobulinanemia. Clin Exp Immunol 28:241–249, 1977
466. Stein RS, Ellman L, Bloch KJ: The clinical correlates of IgM M-components: An analysis of thirty-four patients. Am J Med Sci 269:209–216, 1975
467. McCallister BD, Bayrd ED, Harrison EG Jr et al: Primary macroglobulinemia. Review with a report on thirty-one cases and notes on the value of continuous chlorambucil therapy. Am J Med 43:394–434, 1967
468. Krajny M, Pruzanski W: Waldenström's macroglobulinemia: Review of 45 cases. Can Med Assoc J 114:899–905, 1976
469. Ameis A, Ko HS, Pruzanski W: M components: A review of 1242 cases. Can Med Assoc J 114:889, 1976
470. Benbassat J, Fluman N, Zlotnick A: Monoclonal immunoglobulin disorders: A report of 154 cases. Am J Med Sci 271:325, 1976
471. Peltonen S, Wasastjerna C, Wager O: Clinical features of patients with a serum M component. Acta Med Scand 203:257, 1978
472. Massari R, Find JM, Metais R: Waldenström's macroglobulinaemia observed in two brothers. Nature 196:176, 1962
473. Seligmann M: A genetic predisposition to Waldenström's macroglobulinaemia. Acta Med Scand 445:140, 1966
474. Fine JM, Lambin P, Massari M et al: Malignant evolution of asymptomatic monoclonal IgM after seven and fifteen years in two siblings of a patients with Waldenström's macroglobulinaemia. Acta Med Scand 211:237, 1982
475. Fine JM, Muller JY, Rochu D et al: Waldenström's macroglobulinemia in monozygotic twins. Acta Med Scand 220:368–373, 1986
476. James JM, Brouet JC, Orvoenfrija E et al: Waldenström's macroglobulinemia in a bird breeder: A case history with pulmonary involvement and antibody activity of the monoclonal IgM to canary's droppings. Clin Exp Immunol 68:397–401, 1987
477. Takahashi K, Yamamura F, Motoyama H: IgM multiple myeloma—its distinction from Waldenström's macroglobulinemia. Acta Pathol Jpn 36:1553–1563, 1986
478. San Roman C, Ferro T, Guzman M et al: Clonal abnormalities in patients with Waldenström's macroglobulinemia with special reference to a Burkitt-type t(8;14). Cancer Genet Gytogenet 18:155–158, 1985
479. Kucharska-Pulczynska M, Ellegaard J, Hokland P: Analysis of leukocyte differentiation antigens in blood and bone marrow from patients with Waldenström's macroglobulinemia. Br J Haematol 65:395–399, 1987
480. MacKenzie MR: Macroglobulinemia. In Wiernik PH, Canelloa GP, Kyle RA, Schiffer CA (eds): Neoplastic Diseases of the Blood, Vol. 2, pp 575–592. New York, Churchill-Livingstone, 1985
481. Morel-Maroger L, Basch A, Danon F et al: Pathology of the kidney in Waldenström's macroglobulinemia: Study of 16 cases. N Engl J Med 283:123–129, 1970
482. Martelo OJ, Schultz DR, Pardo V et al: Immunologically-mediated renal disease in Waldenström's macroglobulinemia. Am J Med 58:567–575, 1975
483. Lindstrome FD, Hed J, Enestrom S: Renal pathology of Waldenström's macroglobulinemia with monoclonal antiglomerular antibodies and the nephrotic syndrome. Clin Exp Immunol 41:196–204, 1980
484. Hory B, Saunier F, Wolff R et al: Waldenström's macroglobulinemia and nephrotic syndrome with minimal change lesion. Nephron 45:68–70, 1987
485. Bayrd ED: Continuous chlorambucil therapy in primary macroglobulinemia of Waldenström: Report of 4 cases. Proc Mayo Clin 36:40, 1963
486. Bierling P, Rochant H, Brum B et al: Macroglobulinemie de Waldenström a forme pancytopenique. Remission complete apres polychimiotherapie avec recul de 26 mois. Ann Med Interne 130:443, 1979
487. Cass RM, Anderson BR, Vaughan JH: Waldenström's macroglobulinemia with increased serum IgG levels treated with low doses of cyclophosphamide. Ann Intern Med 71:971, 1969
488. Cohen RJ, Bohannon RA, Wallerstein RO: Waldenström's macroglobulinemia: A study of ten cases. Am J Med 41:274, 1966
489. Heading RC, Girdwood RH, Eastwood MA: Macroglobulinemia treated with prednisone, azathioprine, and folic acid. Br Med J 3:750, 1970
490. Sokalova A, Gazova A, Hrubisko M et al: Clinical utilization of plasmapheresis and cyclophosphamide in the treatment of malignant lymphoproliferative processes. Neoplasma 20:335, 1973
491. Busnach G, Dal Col A, Brando B et al: Efficacy of a combined treatment with plasma exchange and cytostatics in macroglobulinemia. J Artif Organs 9:267–270, 1986
492. Jacobs P, Wood L, Le Roux I et al: Waldenström's macroglobulinemia treated with sequential hemibody irradiation. J Clin Apheresis 3:181–184, 1987

493. Clamon GH, Corder MP, Burns CP: Successful doxorubicin therapy of primary macroglobulinemia resistant to alkylating agents. Am J Hematol 9:21, 1980
494. Case DC Jr: Combination chemotherapy (M-2 protocol) (BCNU, cyclophosphamide, vincristine, melphalan and prednisone) for Waldenström's macroglobulinemia. Blood 59:934, 1982
495. Riddell S, Johnston JB, Rayner HL et al: Response of Waldenström's macroglobulinemia to pentostatin (2'deoxycoformycin) Cancer Treat Rep 70:546–548, 1986
496. Allen EL, Metz EN, Balcerzak SP: Acute myelomonocytic leukemia with macroglobulinemia, Bence Jones proteinuria, and hypercalcemia. Cancer 32:121, 1973
497. Martelli MF, Falini B, Firenze A et al: Acute leukemia complicating Waldenström's macroglobulinemia. Haematologica 66:303, 1981
498. Rosner F, Grunwald HW: Multiple myeloma and Waldenström's macroglobulinemia terminating in acute leukemia. NY State J Med 80:558, 1980
499. Sondergaard Peterson H: Erythroleukaemia in a melphalan-treated patients with primary macroglobulinaemia. Scand J Haematol 10:5, 1973
500. James K, Fudenberg H, Epstein WL et al: Studies on a unique diagnostic serum globulin in papular mucinosis (lichen myxedematosus). Clin Exp Immunol 2:153, 1967
501. Cream JJ: Pyoderma gangrenosum with a monoclonal IgM red cell agglomerating factor. Br J Dermatol 84:223–226, 1971
502. Turakainen H, Valimaki M, Penttinen R: Synthesis of glycosaminoglycans and collagen in skin fibroblasts cultured from a patient with lichen myxedematosus. Arch Dermatol Res 277:55–59, 1985
503. Yaron M, Yaron I, Yust I et al: Lichen myxedematosus (scleromyxedema) serum stimulates hyaluronic acid and prostaglandin E production by human fibroblasts. J Rheumatol 12:171–175, 1985
504. Feldman P, Shapiro L, Pick AI et al: Scleromyxedema. A dramatic response to melphalan. Arch Dermatol 99:51–56, 1969
505. Degos R, Civatte J, Clauvel JP et al: Anomalies globuliniques dans les mucinoses cutanees. Bull Soc Fr Dermatol Syphiligr 77:579–591, 1970
506. Truhan AP, Roenigk HH Jr: Lichen myxedematosus. An unusual case with rapid progression and possible internal involvement. Int J Dermatol 26:91–95, 1987
507. Franklin EC, Lowenstein J, Bigelow B et al: Heavy chain disease: A new disorder of serum γ-globulins. Report of the first case. Am J Med 37:332–350, 1964
508. Frangione B, Franklin EC: Heavy-chain diseases: Clinical features and molecular significance of the disordered immunoglobulin structure. Semin Hematol 10:53–64, 1973
509. Franklin EC, Kyle R, Seligmann M: Correlation of protein structure and immunoglobulin gene organization in the light of two new deleted heavy chain disease proteins. Mol Immunol 16:919, 1979
510. Bakhshi A, Guglielmi P, Coligan JE: A pre-translational defect in a case of human mu heavy chain disease. Mol Immunol 23:725–732, 1986
511. Bakhshi A, Guglielmi P, Siebenlist U et al: A DNA insertion/deletion necessitates an aberrant RNA splice accounting for a mu heavy chain disease protein. Proc Natl Acad Sci USA 83:2689–2693, 1986
512. Kyle RA, Greipp PR, Banks PM: The diverse picture of gamma heavy-chain disease: Report of seven cases and review of literature. Mayo Clin Proc 56:439, 1981
513. Kanoh T, Nakasato H: Osteolytic gamma chain disease. Eur J Haematol 39:60–65, 1987
514. O'Connor GT Jr, Wrandt HE, Innes DJ et al: Gamma heavy chain disease: Report of a case associated with a trisomy of chromosome 7. Cancer Genet Cytogenet 15:1–5, 1985
515. Kyle RA: The heavy-chain diseases. In Wiernik PH, Canelloa GP, Kyle RA, Schiffer CA (eds): Neoplastic Diseases of the Blood, Vol. 2, pp 593–605. New York, Churchill-Livingstone, 1985
516. Buxbaum JN, Preud'homme JL: Alpha and gamma heavy chain diseases in man: Intracellular origin of the aberrant polypeptides. J Immunol 109:1131, 1972
517. Seligmann M, Mihaesco E, Preud'homme JL et al: Heavy chain diseases: Current findings and concepts. Immunol Rev 48:145–167, 1979
518. Zamadzki ZA, Benedek TG, Ein D et al: Rheumatoid arthritis terminating in heavy-chain disease. Ann Intern Med 70:335, 1969
519. Block KJ, Lee L, Mills JA et al: Gamma heavy chain disease—an expanding clinical and laboratory spectrum. Am J Med 55:61, 1973
520. Shirakura T, Kobayshi Y, Murai Y et al: A case of gamma heavy chain disease associated with autoimmune haemolytic anaemia: Clinical haematological, immunological and pathological details. Scand J Haematol 16:387, 1976
521. Westin J, Eyrich R, Falsen et al: Gamma heavy chain disease: Reports of three patients. Acta Med Scand 192:281, 1972
522. Seligmann M, Danon F, Hurez D et al: Alpha-chain disease: A new immunoglobulin abnormality. Science 162:1396, 1968
523. Rambaud JC, Galian A, Matuchansky C et al: Natural history of alpha-chain disease and the so-called Mediterranean lymphoma. Recent Results Cancer Res 64:271, 1978
524. Roth S, Riecken EO: Alpha-chain disease: Mediterranean lymphoma and primary intestinal lymphoma in Western countries; a review of the cases in the literature. Ergeb Inn Med Kinderheilkd 39:79, 1977
525. Seligmann M: Immunobiology and pathogenesis of alpha chain disease. Ciba Found Symp 46:263, 1977
526. Selzer G, Sherman G, Callihan TR et al: Primary small intestinal lymphomas and α-heavy-chain disease: A study of 43 cases from a pathology department of Israel. Isr J Med Sci 15:111, 1979
527. Haghighi P, Wolf PL: Alpha-heavy chain disease. Clin Lab Med 6:477–489, 1986
528. Isaacson PG: Middle Eastern intestinal lymphoma. Semin Diagn Pathol 2:210–223, 1985
529. Shi LY, Liaw SJ, Hsueh S et al: Alpha-chain disease. Report of a case from Taiwan. Cancer 59:545–548, 1987
530. Monges H, Aubert L, Chamlian A et al: Maladie des chaines alpha a forme intestinale: Preventation d'un cas traite par antibiotherapie avec remission clinique, histologique et immunologique. Arch Fr Mal Appar Dig 64:223, 1975
531. Roge J, Druet P, Marche C: Lymphome Mediterranean avec maladie des chaines alpha: Triple remission clinique, anatomique et immunologique. Pathol Biol (Paris) 18:851, 1970
532. Roge J, Druet P, Marche C et al: Letter: Alpha-chain disease cured with antibiotics. Br Med J 4:225, 1975
533. Coulbois J, Galian P, Galian A et al: Gastric form of alpha chain disease. Gut 27:719–725, 1986
534. Mir-Madjlessi SH, Mir-Ahmadian M: Alpha-chain disease—A report of eleven patients from Iran. J Trop Med Hyg 82:229, 1979
535. Savilahi E, Brandtzaeg P, Kuitunen P: Atypical intestinal alpha-chain disease evolving into selective immunoglobulin: A deficiency in a Finnish boy. Gastroenterology 79:1303, 1980
536. Nikbin B, Banisadre M, Ala F et al: HLA AW19, B12 in immunoproliferative small intestinal disease. Gut 20:226, 1976
537. Al-Bahrani Z, Al-Saleem T, Al-Mondiry M et al: Alpha heavy chain disease (report of 18 cases from Iraq). Gut 19:627, 1978
538. Tabbane S, Tabbane F, Cammoun M et al: Mediterranean lymphomas with alpha heavy chain monoclonal gammopathy. Cancer 38:1989, 1976
539. Berger R, Bernheim A, Tsapis A et al: Cytogenetic studies in four cases of alpha chain disease. Cancer Genet Cytogenet 22:219–223, 1986
540. Gafter U, Kessler E, Shabtay F et al: Abnormal chromosomal marker ($D_{14q}+$) in a patient with alpha heavy chain disease. J Clin Pathol 33:136, 1980
541. Seligmann M: Immunochemical, clinical, and pathological features of α-heavy chain disease. Arch Intern Med 135:78–82, 1975
542. Doe WF: Alpha chain disease: Clinicopathological features and relationship to so-called Mediterranean lymphoma. Br J Cancer (Suppl 2) 31:350, 1975
543. Galian A, Lecestre M-J, Scotto J et al: Pathological study of alpha-chain disease with special emphasis on evolution. Cancer 39:2081, 1977
544. Ballard HS, Hamilton LM, Marcus AJ et al: A new variant of heavy-chain disease (μ-chain disease). N Engl J Med 282:1060, 1970
545. Forte FA, Prelli F, Yount WJ et al: Heavy chain disease of the μ (γM) type: Report of the first case. Blood 36:137, 1970
546. Franklin EC: μ-Chain disease. Arch Intern Med 135:71, 1975
547. Pruzanski W, Hasselback R, Ratz A et al: Multiple myeloma (light chain disease) with rheumatoid-like amyloid arthropathy and μ-heavy chain fragment in the serum. Am J Med 65:334, 1978
548. Brouet J-C, Seligmann M, Danon F et al: μ-Chain disease: Report of two new cases. Arch Intern Med 139:672, 1979
549. Levo Y, Recht B, Michaelsen T et al: The interaction of immunoglobulin heavy and light chains in the absence of the V_H domain. J Immunol 119:635, 1977
550. Vilpo JA, Irjala K, Viljanen MK et al: δ-Heavy chain disease: A study of a case. Clin Immunol Immunopathol 17:584, 1980
551. Vilpo JA, Irjala K, Viljanen MK et al: δ-Heavy chain disease: A study of a case. Clin Immunol Immunopathol 17:584, 1980

PAUL A. BUNN, JR.
E. CHESTER RIDGWAY

CHAPTER 55 *Paraneoplastic Syndromes*

Tumors produce signs and symptoms in the patient by invasion, obstruction, and bulk mass at the primary tumor site and in regional and distant deposits. In addition, tumors can produce signs and symptoms at a distance from the tumor or its metastases. These are collectively referred to as "paraneoplastic syndromes" or "remote effects" of malignancy.[1-4] By definition, these syndromes should not be produced as a direct effect of the tumor or its metastases. The best characterized paraneoplastic syndromes are those produced by tumors secreting a polypeptide hormone [*e.g.*, adrenocorticotropin (ACTH) or parathormone (PTH)] that is distributed by the circulation and acts on target organ(s) at a distance from the tumor. In these instances it can be expected that the course of the paraneoplastic syndrome will run parallel to the course of the underlying malignancy because removal or destruction of the tumor will halt production of the hormone. A thorough review of the response of paraneoplastic syndromes to various therapies was published recently.[5]

Various nonendocrine paraneoplastic syndromes were felt to be produced by unidentified tumor-secreted proteins. Over the past decade many of these new tumor-secreted proteins have been described. Previously described paraneoplastic syndromes can be attributed to these proteins, and new syndromes are being recognized. Newly described tumor-derived proteins responsible for paraneoplastic syndromes include growth factors, cytokines, and others. For example, many of the hematologic paraneoplastic syndromes are caused by tumor secretion of colony-stimulating factors.[6,7] Tumor secretion of α transforming growth factor (and possibly epidermal growth factor) by malignant melanoma cells was shown to produce acanthosis nigricans, the sign of Leser–Trelat, and multiple acrochordons.[8]

Paraneoplastic syndromes may also be caused by proteins produced by normal cells in response to the tumor. Molecular studies demonstrated that the monokines, tumor necrosis factor, and cachectin, are identical proteins.[9-11] Cachectin may be responsible for the cachexia syndrome in some patients with malignancy. Antibodies produced in response to malignancy were recently shown to be responsible for many of the neurologic paraneoplastic syndromes including cerebellar degeneration, the Eaton–Lambert syndrome, paraneoplastic retinopathy, and sensory neuronopathy.[12-15] There still remain many paraneoplastic syndromes of unknown etiology that may be produced by tumor-secreted proteins that remain to be identified. In some cases, these syndromes may be caused by other factors that are nonparaneoplastic.

For example, progressive multifocal leukoencephalopathy (PML) was initially described as a neurologic paraneoplastic syndrome.[16] More recently, it has been appreciated that PML is caused by a virus, and although patients with malignancy may be prone to develop this viral syndrome, PML is not truly "paraneoplastic."[17]

Endocrine tumors also can be functional, and their hormonal products (polypeptide, catecholamines, iodothyronine, or steroidal) give symptoms at a distance from the primary tumor (and thus are "paraneoplastic"). However, for practical purposes, this chapter will deal only with syndromes produced by tumors arising in sites other than the pituitary, adrenals, endocrine pancreas, endocrine cells of the gastrointestinal tract, and endocrine cells of the ovaries and testes, as well as all forms of the carcinoid syndrome. These are covered in detail in other chapters.

Although not rare, paraneoplastic syndromes develop in a minority of cancer patients. Their exact frequency is difficult to determine for a variety of reasons, including varying definitions, unknown etiologies, and, most importantly, lack of systematic case-controlled studies. For example, in an uncontrolled study, Croft and Wilkinson reported that 7% of cancer patients have neurologic paraneoplastic syndromes, whereas in a case-controlled study, Brody found no difference in the frequency of neurologic syndromes in patients with lung cancer and controls with benign chronic lung disease.[18,19] The frequency figures given in this chapter are, in nearly all cases, from uncontrolled studies.

The importance of the paraneoplastic syndromes (including hormones detected by immunoassay) and the elucidation of their mechanisms are important for many reasons.

1. Their appearance may be the first sign of a malignancy, which allows its early detection in a curable state.
2. They may simulate metastatic disease and thus prevent patients from having curative therapy.
3. Conversely, treatable complications of malignancy (metastatic disease, infection) may be ascribed to a paraneoplastic syndrome, leading to the withholding of appropriate therapy.
4. They can be used as tumor markers in previously treated patients to detect early recurrence or in patients undergoing adjuvant therapy to guide further therapy.
5. In patients with metastatic disease, their syndromes can be disabling and appropriate treatment of the paraneoplasia may be the best means of palliating patients.
6. The hormones released by tumors may be required for tumor growth (*i.e.*, the tumor may produce its own growth factors and "autostimulate"); thus, appropriate identification of such hormones may allow a new rational therapeutic approach to treatment of the neoplasms as well.[20]

Because of their importance, numerous articles describing paraneoplastic syndromes have been published in the past 20 years. For the interested reader, excellent detailed reviews are available.[1–4,21,22]

ETIOLOGY AND PATHOGENESIS OF PARANEOPLASTIC SYNDROMES

Paraneoplastic syndromes can arise by the following means:

1. Tumor-produced biologically active proteins or polypeptides, including peptide hormones, their precursors, growth factors, interleukins, cytokines, prostaglandins, fetal proteins such as carcinoembryonic antigen (CEA) or α-fetoprotein (AFP), other proteins such as immunoglobulins, and enzymes produced and released by tumors
2. Autoimmunity or immune complex production and immune suppression
3. "Ectopic receptor" production or a competitive blockade of normal hormone action by tumor-produced biologically inactive hormones
4. "Forbidden contact" in which there is release of enzymes (*e.g.*, placental alkaline phosphatase) or other products that normally are not circulated but that takes place because of abnormal tumor vasculature or disrupted basement membranes allowing antigenic reactions, inappropriate initiation of normal physiologic functions, and other toxic manifestations to occur
5. Unknown causes

DIFFERENTIAL DIAGNOSIS

The importance and frequency of paraneoplastic syndromes make it imperative that the appropriate diagnosis be established. In instances in which the etiology of the paraneoplastic syndrome is unknown, this may mean excluding all other known causes of the syndrome. Each section of this chapter includes a listing of the differential diagnosis because of its central importance. In general, paraneoplastic syndromes must be distinguished from

1. Direct invasion by the primary tumor or its metastases
2. Obstruction caused by tumor or tumor products
3. Vascular abnormalities
4. Infections
5. Fluid and electrolyte abnormalities
6. Toxicity of cancer therapy, including cytotoxic chemotherapy, radiation therapy, immunotherapy, or antibiotic therapy

ENDOCRINOLOGIC MANIFESTATIONS OF MALIGNANCY

Paraneoplastic syndromes caused by the production of polypeptide hormones are the most frequent and best understood paraneoplastic syndromes and consequently will be considered in the most detail. To establish a paraneoplastic cause for alterations in hormone production, conclusive evidence that the hormone is produced by the tumor must be established. The differential diagnosis of endocrinologic abnormalities in the cancer patient is shown in Table 55-1.

The laboratory evaluation begins after a complete history and physical examination. Abnormal levels of the hormone in question should be documented, usually by radioimmunoassay. Paraneoplastic hormone production usually will be independent of the normal regulatory mechanisms. Besides

TABLE 55-1. Endocrinologic Manifestations of Malignancy: Differential Diagnosis

1. Hormone production by benign cells (*e.g.*, parathyroid adenoma)
2. Hormone production by a malignancy of an endocrine organ (*e.g.*, MEA)
3. Alterations in hormone production as a direct result of infiltration of an endocrine gland by a primary tumor or its metastases
4. Alterations in hormone production by therapy
5. Alterations in hormone production by infection
6. Paraneoplastic

TABLE 55-2. Categories of Mammalian Brain Peptides Producing Proven or Potential Paraneoplastic Syndromes

Hypothalamic-releasing hormones
Thyrotropin-releasing hormone
Gonadotropin-releasing hormone
Somatostatin
Corticotropin-releasing hormone
Growth hormone-releasing hormone
Neurohypophyseal hormones
Vasopressin*†
Oxytocin
Neurophysin(s)†
Pituitary peptides
Adrenocorticotropic hormone*†
β-Endorphin†
Melanocyte-stimulating hormone*†
Prolactin
Luteinizing hormone
Growth hormone†
Thyrotropin
Invertebrate peptides
FM RT amide
Hydra head activator
Nonbrain hormones
Parathormone*†
β-hCG*†
T_3
Gastrointestinal peptides
Vasoactive intestinal peptide*†
Cholecystokinin
Gastrin
Substance P
Neurotensin†
Mete-enkephalin
Leu-enkephalin
Insulin
Glucagon†
Bombesin†
Gastrin-releasing peptide†
Secretin
Somatostatin†
TRH
Motilin
Others
Angiotensin II
Bradykinin
Carosine
Sleep peptide(s)
Calcitonin†
CGRP
Neuropeptide Y
Physalaemin†
Neuron-specific enolase†

Data from Refs. 24 and 25.
* Produces a proven paraneoplastic syndrome.
† Produced by small-cell lung cancer or carcinoid tumors.

elevated hormone levels, independent of the normal control mechanisms, other direct evidence that a tumor produces a hormone causing the paraneoplastic syndrome includes the following:

1. Fall in hormone levels after removal or treatment of the tumor
2. Maintenance of elevated hormone levels after extirpation of the "normal" gland of origin of the hormone
3. Demonstration of an arteriovenous gradient of hormone levels across the tumor
4. Demonstration of synthesis and secretion of the hormone by tumor tissue in vitro
5. Ultimately, demonstration of such synthesis and secretion by in vitro clonal tissue culture isolates of the tumor cells

Secretion of polypeptide hormones by tumors has been known for most of this century to cause recognized paraneoplastic syndromes. However, in the past 10 years many previously unknown polypeptide hormones have been discovered. Most of these recently described peptides have been identified within the CNS or the gastrointestinal tract.[24,25] Table 55-2 lists the categories of mammalian polypeptide hormones, whether they cause a known paraneoplastic syndrome, and whether they have been shown to be produced by human tumor cells. The function of many of the recently described hormones, such as neurophysin, bombesin, and physalaemin, is unknown. However, these have been shown to be produced by human tumors such as small-cell lung cancer.[26–28] Some of the paraneoplastic syndromes of unknown etiology, and perhaps some unrecognized paraneoplastic syndromes, probably will be ascribed to these hormones when more is learned of their function.

The endocrine paraneoplastic syndromes, the responsible hormone, the most frequently associated tumor types, and incidence are shown in Table 55-3.[23,29] With the development of radioimmunoassays and screening of cancer patients, it was found that hormone production in cancer patients (and presumably from their tumors) was much more frequent than previously realized.[3,23] Table 55-4 lists screening studies of lung cancer patients or tumor extracts for the presence of various hormones using radioimmunoassays.[30–35] These frequencies are much higher than those of the clinically recognized paraneoplastic syndromes related to these hormones because the large molecular weight hormone precursors, fragments, or subunits secreted by tumors are often biologically inactive. Other factors that also obscure the true frequency of hormone secretion by tumors include inadequate clinical follow-up (*e.g.*, spot-checks of patients rather than observation throughout the clinical course); production of a hormone that does not have easily recognizable clinical effect [such as development of the acromegalic effects of growth hormone (GH), which may take years to become manifest]; operation of normal physiologic feedback mechanisms, which suppress normal hormone production; secretion of multiple hormones [*e.g.*, secretion of ACTH obscuring the clinical effect of simultaneous arginine vasopressin (AVP) secretion]; and finally, investigator and available laboratory facility bias.

ACTH/CUSHING'S SYNDROME

Evidence[36–38] from analysis of cultured tumor cells, pituitary extracts, and recombinant DNA work demonstrates that the prohormone ("stem hormone") molecule of ACTH contains

TABLE 55-3. Endocrine Paraneoplastic Syndromes

Syndrome	*Hormone*	*Tumor*	*Incidence (%)*
Cushing's syndrome	ACTH	Lung cancer—all types	0–2.0
		Small-cell lung cancer	6
Inappropriate antidiuresis	AVP	Lung cancer—all types	0.9–2.0
	ANP	Small-cell lung cancer	9
Nonmetastatic hypercalcemia	PTH	Lung cancer—all types	1.0–7.5
		Squamous cell lung cancer	15
		Other tumors	14
Gynecomastia		Lung cancer—all types	0.5–0.9
		Small-cell lung cancer	2.0
Hyperthyroidism		Lung cancer	0–1.4
Calcitonin		Medullary carcinoma of the thyroid	
		Small-cell lung cancer	
		Other lung cancer types	
		Breast cancer	
Acromegaly	GHRH	Carcinoids, pheochomocytoma—rare	
		Pancreatic cancer	

Data from Refs. 23 and 29.

the following in sequence from the NH_2-terminal to the COOH-terminal end (Fig. 55-1).[24,25]

1. A putative signal peptide (amino acid position −141 to −110)
2. A NH_2-terminal region with unknown function (position −110 to −53)
3. γ-MSH (position −53 to −48)
4. A region with unknown function (position −48 to −1)
5. ACTH (position 1 to 39) = "classic" ACTH, which contains within it α-MSH (position 1 to 13) and corticotropin-like intermediate lobe peptide, CLIP (position 18 to 39)
6. β-lipotropin, β-LPH (position 42 to 134), which contains within it γ-LPH (position 42 to 101) and β-MSH (position 84 to 101)
7. Met-enkephalin (position 104 to 108)
8. β-Endorphin (position 104 to 134)

The prohormone molecule has been called "big ACTH" or pro-opiocortin and contains four repetitive sequences based on the ACTH/MSH core, with these sequences separated by paired basic residues. The importance of the promolecule is that it can be split up into many biologically active fragments. These activities include adrenal gland stimulation to make corticosteroids and androgens (*e.g.*, by ACTH); melanocyte stimulation–hyperpigmentation activity (by MSH-containing peptides); and opiate-like activity (β-LPH, β-endorphin, and met-enkephalin). There has been an explosion of knowledge concerning the biologic activity of fragments of this molecule, particularly the opioid peptides (β-LPH, β-endorphin, met-enkephalin), which mimic morphine in their action.[39–41] The paired basic residues flank the biologically active sequences. At these sites proteolytic processing takes place that determines the biologic activity (and thus the paraneoplastic syndrome) seen in humans. Thus, the regulation of cleavage of the promolecule in neoplastic states is important. The cleavage patterns change during development and may be different in tumors than in adult pituitary tissue.[41] In addition, pro-opiocortin is a glycosylated peptide, and glycosylation may play an important role in proteolysis,

TABLE 55-4. Frequency of Peptide Hormone Elevation in the Blood of Lung Cancer Patients*

	% of Patients with Significantly Elevated Levels			
Hormone	*Small-Cell*	*Epidermoid*	*Adenocarcinoma*	*Large-Cell*
ACTH	30–69	0–80	17–75	26
LPH	54	33	20	Not done
Calcitonin	48–64	9	0	11
ADH	32			
PTH	27	32	0	17
β-hCG	1–32	19	17	26
GH	0	3	0	0
GRP	74	17	20	7
SLI	27	11	Not done	Not done
NSE	69	Not done	Not done	Not done
NEUROPHYSINS	65	14	29	20

See Refs. 30–35 for details.
* Not all studies were done in all patients.

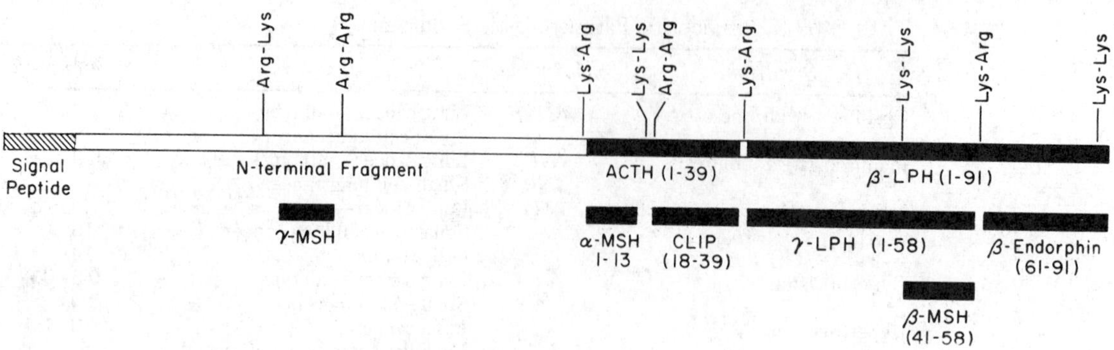

FIG. 55-1. Schematic representation of the bovine pro-opiomelanocortin molecule. See text for discussion. (Krieger DT, Martin JB: Brain peptides. N Engl J Med 304:876–885, 1981)

packaging, and storage. Although, classically, ectopic ACTH production is thought to be unregulated, some tumor tissues studied in vitro continue to show some control over ACTH secretion by way of a cyclic AMP-dependent mechanism.[42]

Clinical Features of "Ectopic" Pro-opiocortin (ACTH/LPH) Excess

The clinical features of the ectopic ACTH syndrome include hypokalemia, hyperglycemia, edema, muscle weakness or atrophy, hypertension, and weight loss. Other features seen in pituitary Cushing's disease or exogenous corticosteroid excess (centripital obesity, cutaneous striae, moon facies, buffalo hump, and pigmentation) are uncommonly seen in highly malignant tumors (oat-cell lung cancer) but are more frequent in the indolent carcinoids, thymomas, and pheochromocytomas. Although the cases first reported involved men, the increased prevalence of lung cancer in women may be associated with more cases in women, including hirsutism, which was seen in Brown's original patient.[43]

FREQUENCY OF ECTOPIC PRO-OPIOCORTIN (ACTH) PRODUCTION BY TUMORS. The major clinical association of ectopic ACTH production is with lung cancer, particularly of the small-cell carcinoma histologic type.[3,23,38] Clinically apparent Cushing's syndrome is found in 0.4% to 2% of patients with lung cancer of all histologic types (see Table 55-3).[23,29,44,45] In small-cell lung cancer, 5.5% of 473 patients in several large series had clinical manifestations of Cushing's syndrome.[46–48] Lung cancer represents over 50% of the clinically obvious cases, carcinoids and neural crest tumors (pheochromocytomas, neuroblastomas, medullary carcinomas of the thyroid) amount to 15% each, and bronchial carcinoid and thymomas represent 10% each. The frequency of significantly elevated levels of ACTH by radioimmunoassay (RIA) in the blood and tumor extracts of lung cancer patients (Table 55-5) is much higher than the frequency of the ectopic Cushing's syndrome.[49–57] Similarly, the frequency of increased fasting a.m. cortisol levels with dexamethasone suppression (49%–71%) or without dexamethasone suppression (38%) is higher than the frequency of the ectopic syndrome.[23,31,57–59] Although these differences

TABLE 55-5. Frequency of ACTH Elevation in Blood and Tumor Extracts as Detected by RIA in Lung Cancer Patients Without Clinically Evident Ectopic ACTH Syndrome

Source of Material *Tumor Type*	*Patients* (*n*)	*% Positive* (*%*)	*References*
Patient's blood			
All histologic types	290	19,41,42,88	49,50,51,52
Epidermoid	88	0–50	49,51
Adenocarcinoma	25	17–26	49,51
Large-cell carcinoma	28	26–49	49,51
Small-cell carcinoma	49,51	11, 29–30	49,51
Chronic obstructive pulmonary disease	101	25*	49,52
Tumor extracts (surgical specimens)			
All histologic types	127	31,58,93,100	49,50,53,54
Epidermoid	49	49	49
Adenocarcinoma	17	6	49
Large-cell carcinoma	8	25	49
Small-cell carcinoma-carcinoid	12	100	55,56

Data from Refs. 49–57.

*Seventeen percent of patients with elevated ACTH levels were subsequently shown to develop lung cancer within 2 years.[50,52]

could be due to the presence of inactive "big" ACTH or stress, Bondy and Gilby suggest that the tumors secrete only small amounts of excess hormone.[57] The ectopic ACTH is not secreted under feedback control, enters the plasma without normal diurnal variations and is not suppressed normally by exogenous dexamethasone. Yet it is not sufficient to cause clinical abnormalities. Thus, the clinical syndrome occurs only in the uncommon tumors that secrete large excesses of active hormone. Nearly all extracts of small-cell lung cancer tumors have increased levels of ACTH and LPH detected by RIA. The other histologic types vary in positivity between 6% and 40%. Although non–small-cell lung cancer types have increased cortisol levels, the mechanism of this is not known.[22,23,49] Likewise, the frequency of ectopic ACTH-associated clinical syndromes and adrenal function is not well described for other tumor types.[38]

HISTOLOGY OF ACTH-PRODUCING TUMORS. Azzopardi and Williams reviewed the world's literature on the ectopic syndrome and found that 112 of 130 cases arose in the lung, pancreas, or thymus.[60] The most frequent histologic finding was a small-cell cancer or a carcinoid structure. Other tumors included pheochromocytomas, related tumors, and certain ovarian tumors. Ten years later, Skrabanek and Powell continued the literature review of cases with ectopic ACTH and Cushing's syndrome and found that all such tumors with clinically apparent ACTH excess could be grouped into a carcinoid–oat cell (small-cell) group and a pheochromocytoma–neuroblastoma class based on histologic appearance.[61] They believed that tumors found in other organs besides the lung (*e.g.*, thymus, all thymic carcinoids rather than epithelial thymoma), thyroid (medullary carcinoma), esophagus, stomach, pancreas, small intestine, appendix, salivary gland, ovary, testis, uterine cervix, and prostate had either a carcinoid or a small-cell lung cancer-type tissue structure.[62,63] They, and others, postulated that these tumors arose only where normal Kulchitsky-type cells occur and hence could potentially have a common origin.

Thus, whenever it is suggested that a histologic type other than one of these is present (*e.g.*, adenocarcinoma), this should be viewed with skepticism and carefully documented. The histologic material should be reviewed and more obtained, if necessary. At present, the extrapulmonary cancers with small–cell-like tissue structure should be treated as if they were small-cell carcinoma of the lung, whereas those with a carcinoid tissue structure should be dealt with as carcinoids (see Chap. 39).[64,65] It will be important to obtain more studies on the efficacy of chemotherapy on tumors producing ACTH that do not have typical small-cell or carcinoid tissues.

DIAGNOSIS OF ECTOPIC CUSHING'S SYNDROME. About 40% of patients presenting with overt Cushing's syndrome have pituitary Cushing's with an obvious tumor, 28% have pituitary Cushing's syndrome without tumors (and both of these usually occur in women of childbearing age), 17% have adrenal Cushing's (usually presenting in children), whereas 15% have the ectopic Cushing's syndrome (which usually appears in adult men). Although the production of pro-opiocorticoid molecule may have hitherto unrecognized clinical effects, the diagnosis of clinically significant ectopic ACTH excess begins with thinking about the possibility in the appropriate clinical setting, such as an older man with small-cell lung cancer or a patient with unexplained hypokalemic alkalosis, particularly if it is accompanied by edema, hypertension, profound muscular weakness or atrophy, mental changes, or glucose intolerance. Patients with ectopic ACTH from thymic tumors and bronchial carcinoids are usually younger and present with more classic features of Cushing's syndrome, primarily because of the more indolent course of the neoplasms. When clinical features are present, a plasma ACTH value of over 200 pg/ml is suggestive of ectopic ACTH production. The biochemical diagnosis of Cushing's syndrome that results from ectopic ACTH production involves the demonstration of excessive cortisol production by a 24-hr urine free-cortisol evaluation. Abnormal values are higher than 100 μg/day and values as high as 1000 μg/day may be seen. Abnormal suppression of elevated cortisol production is documented by showing that plasma cortisol levels do not suppress after administering dexamethasone, 2 mg every 6 hr for 48 hr, or after giving a single 8-mg dose of dexamethasone at midnight before obtaining a sample to test the plasma cortisol level at 8 a.m. the next morning. Elevations in cortisol production, abnormal dexamethasone suppressibility, and plasma ACTH concentration higher than 200 pg/ml are highly suggestive of the ectopic ACTH syndrome. The same tests can be applied if the patient presents with Cushing's syndrome without an obvious tumor. If the results are consistent with ectopic ACTH secretion, then a careful evaluation for occult tumor should proceed and be rigorously continued until the source of the ACTH is identified. With benign or malignant adrenal tumors, the ACTH levels will be low (suppression of normal pituitary ACTH) even if the cortisol levels do not suppress with dexamethasone. Most pituitary tumors will suppress with the high-dose dexamethasone, and the ACTH levels usually are between 20 and 200 pg/ml. It is important to remember that half of the patients with ectopic ACTH produced by carcinoids may suppress, and occasionally a tumor may secrete in a cyclic fashion.[66,67] Furthermore, baseline ACTH levels may be between 20 and 200 pg/ml in carcinoid tumors. In difficult cases (*e.g.*, distinguishing a small pulmonary carcinoid that suppresses with dexamethasone from a pituitary lesion), the question can be resolved by selective venous catheterization with ACTH determinations.[68,69] Other sources of difficulty in initial recognition can occur in the simultaneous production of two hormones (such as ACTH and AVP) or of a peptide hormone and amine product.[23,70] However, the very occurrence of multiple hormone secretion indicates the presence of a nonpituitary tumor. Other cases of dexamethasone suppression of ectopic ACTH production have been postulated to be related to secretion of a corticotropin-releasing hormone (CRF) by the tumor.[71,72] Recently, well-defined cases of Cushing's syndrome resulting from tumor production of CRF have been documented.[73–75] The CRF is postulated to act either on the pituitary to stimulate pituitary ACTH release or at the tumor level to stimulate tumor cell ACTH production.

Treatment of Ectopic ACTH and Related Syndromes

The treatment of ectopic pro-opiocorticoid syndromes should be directed primarily at the tumor. In carcinoids, this can involve surgery, and with thymomas, surgery or radiotherapy. With appropriate therapy, the syndrome is usually cured and high levels of ACTH reduced in the majority of these patients.[76] Although previous reviews have stated that a bad prognosis of less than 4 months is expected for the ectopic ACTH syndrome with small-cell lung cancer, these were before the substantial gains in treatment and potential cure of some patients with small-cell carcinoma had been made. (The principles of the treatment of small-cell lung carcinomas with combination chemotherapy is discussed in detail in Chap. 22). If the histologic appearance of any mediastinal or extrathoracic tumor is compatible with a small-cell tumor, we would favor treating this patient as though he had small-cell lung cancer. The data on response to therapy of Cushing's syndrome in small-cell cancer patients are anecdotal, but reports of fall in ACTH levels with combination chemotherapy, with or without radiotherapy, have appeared.[30,48] If treatment of the tumor fails, drugs that inhibit adrenal corticoid production may be used, such as aminoglutethimide, metyrapone, or mitotane ($0, p' =$ DDD).[68,77–79] (The reader should review appropriate endocrinology sources for directions in using these adrenal suppressants). Obviously, after such drug treatment, patients would have to be treated with supplemental steroids to avoid hypoadrenalism. Because of the increasing use of aminoglutethimide in breast cancer patients, this drug is probably the first choice. Another possibility includes combining aminoglutethimide and metyrapone to lower the dose-related toxicity of both agents along with dexamethasone and fludrocortisone.[80] In rare cases, with chronic ectopic ACTH excess and indolent tumors, bilateral adrenalectomy can be considered.

Use of proACTH/LPH for Early Cancer Detection

Odell and co-workers have found significant blood elevations of proACTH/LPH in 92% of pancreatic cancers, 72% of lung cancers, 54% of gastric or esophagus cancers, 41% of breast cancers, and 27% of colon cancers, whereas corresponding values for elevated LPH were 25%, 36%, 14%, 0, and 10%, respectively, for these tumor types.[32] In general, the quantitative levels of proACTH/ACTH and LPH were correlated. Some 20% of patients with chronic obstructive pulmonary disease (COPD) had blood elevations of proACTH, whereas 13% had elevations of LPH. Other studies also have found proACTH elevations in chronic lung disease, suggesting that the lung may produce or bind proACTH or LPH in response to injury.[50–52] Some of the patients (5 of 20) with elevated proACTH in COPD eventually developed lung cancer, whereas only 2 of 81 COPD patients with normal plasma levels of ACTH developed lung cancer.[45]

When ACTH, calcitonin, and HCG were measured simultaneously, significant elevated levels were found in 65% of 109 lung cancer patients and 78% of small-cell cancer patients, suggesting the usefulness of several markers in concert to detect lung cancer.[31] More studies are needed to know if the proACTH/LPH or other peptide hormone assays are predictors of the development of lung cancer and if they will be useful in following the course of the disease. Extracts of other tumors besides lung cancer showed significant elevations (more than 1 ng/g tissue) of proACTH or LPH, 6 of 16 colon cancers, 3 of 4 breast cancers, and 22 of 31 miscellaneous tumors and metastatic lesions. However, although elevated levels of immunoreactive material were found, there is no direct evidence that the tumors themselves produced the peptides. Many tumors may make the preopiocorticoid, but only some have the ability to cleave it appropriately into biologically active forms. Thus, the expression of the syndromes may depend more on the promolecule processing than the presence of the ectopic prohormone itself.[2]

With the development and use of RIAs for measuring lipotropin and β-endorphin and receptor assays for measuring endogenous opiate peptides in human cerebrospinal fluid and plasma, it may become possible to relate unusual neurologic syndromes and mental behavior directly to fragments derived from the proopiocorticoid molecule.[32,39,81] It is certainly now reasonable to start applying these assays to patients with such symptoms and appropriate tumor settings (such as lung cancer). Recently, circulating immune complexes of ACTH and human immunoglobulins have been reported.[82] Thus, ACTH also may be involved in an immune complex paraneoplastic syndrome. A portion of the ACTH promolecule with opioid activity undergoes a striking increase in the pituitary of newborn monkeys. This increase in endogenous opioid may help the fetus withstand the stress of parturition.[41] Likewise, tumor production of an analgesic-like material such as β-endorphin may allow the cancer patient a measure of relief from tumor-related symptoms. Further work quantitating the amount and nature of such endogenous analgesics is necessary.

SYNDROME OF "INAPPROPRIATE" SECRETION OF ANTIDIURETIC HORMONE

The association of hyponatremia and lung cancer was noted in 1938; the syndrome of "inappropriate secretion" of antidiuretic hormone [SIADH; (ADH; arginine vasopressin (AVP))] was postulated by Schwartz and co-workers in 1957 to be caused by stimulation of the posterior pituitary to secrete AVP by the presence of the thoracic tumor.[83,84] It was then demonstrated by Amatruda and co-workers in 1963 to be related to tumor production of AVP.[85] Arginine vasopressin, oxytocin, and neurophysins have been found by RIA in tumors, and the AVP is bioactive as well as immunoreactive.[23,86] The neurophysins normally are synthesized, stored, and secreted in parallel with AVP and oxytocin.[87] These polypeptides function as binding proteins for AVP and oxytocin; there are different neurophysins for AVP and oxytocin.[88] Whether AVP and oxytocin actually form a promolecule with their respective neurophysins is under investigation.[23] At present, there are no recognized syndromes related to tumor production of neurophysins or oxytocin, whereas tumor production of AVP results in hyponatremia.

Clinical Findings and Pathophysiology of SIADH

Continuous tumor production, exogenous administration, and posterior pituitary production of AVP all result in a syndrome of hyponatremia, urine inappropriately higher in osmolality than the plasma, and high urinary sodium concentrations in the face of serum hyponatremia.[2,3,23] This is thought to result from the action of AVP on the renal tubule with resultant water retention. The hyponatremia comes from both renal sodium loss and dilution by water retention. The mechanism of the natriuresis is not defined but could include an increased filtered sodium load, a decreased aldosterone secretion, or a decreased tubular reabsorption of sodium. The major clinical symptomatology comes from water intoxication (hypo-osmality and hyponatremia) and is manifested by altered mental status, confusion, lethargy, psychotic behavior, seizures, coma, and occasionally death.[2,3,23,89] Focal neurologic findings can be associated with water intoxication from SIADH alone without brain metastases.[89] Because of the predominant occurrence of SIADH with small-cell lung cancer and the frequent presence of brain metastases in this cancer, all patients with neurologic syndromes in small-cell lung cancer should have serum sodium levels checked for the presence of hyponatremia, and all small-cell cancer patients with hyponatremia and neurologic syndromes also should be evaluated for brain metastases.

Diagnosis of Ectopic AVP Production and the SIADH Syndrome

Hyponatremia is the usual mode of presentation of SIADH because of the routine use of serum electrolytes in patient evaluation (Table 55-6). Occasionally patients present with neurologic symptoms. The first major problem is to differentiate SIADH from the multiple other causes of hyponatremia (such as diuretic use, cardiac, hepatic, and renal failure; dilutional causes; and diminished function of adrenals, anterior pituitary, or thyroid). In addition, various drugs can impair free water excretion either by acting on the renal tubule or by inducing pituitary AVP, including chlorpropamide, thiazide diuretics and, most importantly for cancer patients, cyclophosphamide, vincristine, and morphine.[90-92] To separate these causes of hyponatremia from SIADH, it is mandatory to demonstrate the following:

1. Hypo-osmolality (usually less than 280 mOsm/kg)
2. Urinary osmolality greater than the plasma (usually about 500 mOsm/kg or higher)
3. Continued urinary excretion of sodium (usually greater than 20 mEq/liter) when taking no diuretics
4. Absence of signs of volume depletion
5. Normal renal function
6. Normal adrenal and thyroid function

TABLE 55-6. Differential Diagnosis in SIADH

Tumors
Small-cell lung cancer
Other types
Pulmonary, Chest Conditions
Infection (tuberculosis, abscess, pneumonia—viral or bacterial), mitral stenosis (s/p surgical correction)
Central Nervous System
Trauma (skull fracture, subdural, concussion, subarachnoid hemorrhage, thrombosis)
Intracranial space-occupying lesions (primary and metastatic tumors)
Infections (meningitis, encephalitis, lues)
Vasculitis (lupus)
Guillian-Barré
Acute intermittent porphyria
Pain and emotional stress
Drugs
Chlorpropamide
Morphine
Nicotine
Ethanol
Cyclophosphamide
Vincristine
"Idiopathic"

Fichman and Bethune studied 86 patients with SIADH and found serum sodium levels of 88 to 126 mEq/liter, urine sodium levels of 35 to 175 mEq/24 hr, serum osmolalities of 190 to 273 mOsm/kg, and urine osmolalities of 332 to 780 mOsm/kg.[92] The most common mistake in diagnosis of SIADH is failing to notice the previous administration of a diuretic or of occult volume depletion with resulting dilutional hyponatremia. Usually, repeat clinical examinations can exclude these causes. Although AVP can be measured by RIA, this is not routinely available, and many conditions can be associated with both the "appropriate" and the "inappropriate" secretion of AVP.

The most common disorders associated with SIADH besides small-cell lung cancer include CNS diseases (*e.g.*, CNS infection, head trauma, intracranial space-occupying lesions, subarachnoid hemorrhage, acute intermittent prophyria, pain, and emotional stress) and pulmonary infections (see Table 55-6). Clearly, if any of these factors are present in patients with SIADH and malignant disease (including small-cell cancer), they should be treated in an effort to control the SIADH. Water loading can elicit clinically occult SIADH but can be very dangerous in patients with hyponatremia and probably should not be done if the serum sodium concentration is 125 mEq/liter or less.[90]

In studies of lung cancer patients with SIADH and high levels of AVP by RIA, fluid restriction further increased the already elevated AVP level. This probably resulted from stimulation of the pituitary to release AVP.[93] The other causes of SIADH (particularly drugs) could account for some of the SIADH seen in tumor patients without small-cell lung cancer or carcinoid histologic findings and stress the need for biosynthetic studies of AVP by cultured tumor cells to prove the source of the AVP. In any event, these other complications (*e.g.*, pneumonia) usually occur because of the cancer, and the development of SIADH from them represents a "secondary" paraneoplastic syndrome. For example, cyclophosphamide and vincristine are both used to treat small-cell lung cancer. When cyclophosphamide is given in high doses and the patient is hydrated to prevent cystitis, the combined effect of cyclophosphamide to decrease free water clearance and the water load can lead to the SIADH.[92,94,95]

Whether this represents release of pituitary AVP or a direct effect of cyclophosphamide metabolites on the renal tubules is not known.[94]

If the histologic structure of the tumor associated with SIADH is that of small-cell cancer, the cancer will be treated along with any other causes, and correlation can be made between the tumor response and the SIADH. If the tumor histologic structure is other than small cell or carcinoid, one should be skeptical about tumor production of AVP until all causes of the SIADH are sought. If no other causes of SIADH are apparent, thought should be given to obtaining more tumor tissue because a component of small-cell carcinoma may be present. This would dictate a more aggressive chemoradiotherapy approach than that taken for an "unresponsive" non–small-cell tumor type.

If a patient presents with "idiopathic" SIADH, a careful search and follow-up for small-cell tumor must be maintained; although cases like this are uncommon, the workup probably should include a full staging evaluation for small-cell cancer, including fiberoptic bronchoscopy and computed tomography (CT) scans of the chest and abdomen to locate small tumor masses. The tumor should declare itself within a few months. In comparing tumor-related SIADH and SIADH resulting from other causes, serum and urinary sodium levels, osmolality, blood urea nitrogen, plasma AVP, and renin levels all failed to distinguish neoplastic from nonneoplastic causes.[94] The speed of rise in serum sodium concentration with water restriction supposedly is faster (occurring in 3 days compared with 7–10 days) in nonneoplastic causes compared with neoplastic causes of SIADH.[96] However, this distinction may not be clear enough to be useful clinically.

Frequency and Tumor Types

Almost all of the tumors that produce AVP are small-cell carcinomas of the lung.[2,3,23,29] However, SIADH has been seen with other tumor types, including carcinomas of the prostate, adrenal cortex, esophagus, pancreas, duodenum, colon, bronchial carcinoids, thymomas, head and neck, Hodgkin's disease, and non-Hodgkin's lymphomas.[2,3,23] At least some of these may have had a nonpulmonary small-cell or carcinoid histologic structure. Small-cell lung cancer lines grown in tissue culture make immunologically detectable AVP.[97,98] However, there have been no clear biosynthetic studies of cultured tumor cells of other histologic types.

Collected series show that 9% of 523 small-cell lung cancer patients have clinically evident SIADH with hyponatremia.[23,46,59,99,100] Similarly to ACTH, measurement of blood AVP by RIA has shown significant elevations in an even larger fraction of cases (32%–44%).[31,100] In addition, evidence of SIADH by water loading of patients showed that 53% to 68% had subclinical but evocable SIADH.[31,100] Odell and co-workers found 41% of lung cancer patients of all histologic types and 43% of colon cancer patients to have significantly elevated blood AVP levels without clinically evident SIADH.[2] North's group has studied neurophysins in 72 small-cell cancer patients and found significantly elevated levels of either one or both (AVP or oxytocin) neurophysins in 65%.[88]

Treatment of SIADH

The fundamental principle of the treatment of tumor-associated SIADH involves successful treatment of the underlying cancer.[99] Because nearly all cases involved lung cancer, and small-cell cancer in particular, the reader is referred to Chapter 22 for tumor treatment principles. If chemotherapy is not effective, then radiotherapy of bulk tumor mass or, in selected cases of non–small-cell lung cancer limited to the chest, surgical removal of the tumor may be considered. The major decisions following those of antitumor treatment involve:

1. The problem of water restriction and high-dose chemotherapy
2. Management of severely symptomatic hyponatremia
3. The problem of distinguishing SIADH that develops during treatment from other causes and true tumor relapse
4. Treatment of recurrent SIADH with tumor progression on primary therapy

For symptomatic hyponatremia and serum sodium levels of less than 130 mEq/liter, fluid restriction to less than 500 ml/24 hr will allow patients to increase their plasma osmolality slowly over 7 to 10 days. If chemotherapy requires hydration and the chemotherapy could induce more hyponatremia (cyclophosphamide in high doses being an example of both), this usually can be handled by careful monitoring of body weight, input and output, daily or more frequent serum sodium determinations, urine sodium and potassium measurements while giving normal saline with furosemide diuretics and electrolyte replacement.[95,101,102] If the patient is severely hyponatremic or symptomatic (*e.g.*, serum sodium level less than 125 mEq/liter), correction of this over several days may be required before instituting chemotherapy. An excellent correlation of antitumor response to chemoradiotherapy and disappearance of SIADH has been reported by the NCI group in seven of seven patients and by the Vanderbilt group in 16 of 17 newly diagnosed small-cell cancer patients.[102] North and co-workers studied 18 patients with elevated neurophysins by RIA (some of which represent elevated AVP) and found complete agreement between tumor and neurophysin levels and response to chemotherapy (reduction of neurophysin levels in 12 patients with complete or partial remissions and rise in six patients with progressive tumor).[103] Because these latter markers are present in 65% of small-cell cancer patients initially, the neurophysins may prove to be excellent tumor markers.

When a patient presents severely symptomatic from SIADH (*e.g.*, comatose), more acute measures are needed. The procedure of Hantman and co-workers involves using 3% hypertonic saline and IV furosemide to increase the net free water clearance.[104] Furosemide (1 mg/kg body weight) is given IV and subsequent doses are given as needed to obtain the desired negative fluid balance. Besides routine vital signs, urinary losses of sodium and potassium are measured hourly and replaced by an infusion of appropriate amounts of hypertonic sodium chloride solution, to which appropriate amounts of potassium chloride are added. Using an estimated total body water content of 60% of body weight in females and 70% of body weight in males, the negative fluid balance necessary to raise the plasma osmolality to 270 mOsm/kg water is calculated for an individual patient by the following formula:

Desired negative water balance in liters
= total body water (TBW
= weight in kg

$$\times 0.6 \text{ or } 0.7) \text{ minus } \frac{\text{TBW} \times \text{plasma osmolality}^{104}}{270}$$

This approach resulted in the serum sodium concentrations rising from 120 to 133 mEq/liter in 6 to 8 hr.[104] Although none of these patients had small-cell carcinoma, the Johns Hopkins group has used this regimen successfully in small-cell cancer.[89] This procedure also could be used to prepare patients for chemotherapy.

In patients who have relapsed and who have recurrent SIADH with no, or only minimally effective, chemotherapy available, therapy with demeclocyline or urea can be tried. Demeclocycline has been shown to be more effective in treating SIADH than is lithium carbonate, another agent previously used to treat this condition.[105-107] Demeclocycline blocks AVP action at the level of the renal tubule (by inhibiting AVP-induced cyclic-AMP formation and blocking the effect of any cyclic-AMP generated) with more reproducibility than lithium carbonate. Recently, a positive correlation between serum sodium and blood urea was noted in patients with SIADH, suggesting the use of urea therapy to correct SIADH. Urea given in dosages of 30 g/day corrected the salt-losing tendency of SIADH in two patients with small-cell cancer and in normal persons given exogenous AVP.[108] Because it induces an osmotic diuresis, urea therapy allows a normal daily intake of water despite continued SIADH. Urea (99% pure crystalline material), 30 g, is dissolved in 100 ml of water with 15 g of magnesium and aluminum hydroxide (Maalox) and is taken at noon; this has been maintained for up to 11 weeks without water restriction.[108] The urea is taken orally because of good gastrointestinal absorption and because cells are freely permeable to urea. There is no risk of cardiac failure from rapid shifts of water, as is possible in a mannitol-induced diuresis.

Although hyponatremia and SIADH are the classic presenting features of tumor secretion of AVP, other paraneoplastic syndromes may occur because at much higher concentrations AVP acts on the cardiovascular system and other smooth muscles throughout the body.[91]

Hyponatremia Secondary to Ecotopic Atrial Natriuretic Peptide Secretion

Atrial natriuretic peptide (ANP), produced by human atrial tissue has potent natriuretic activity. Several series demonstrated that it may be a circulating hormone producing hyponatremia and SIADH.[109] Recently, Kamoi and co-workers described a patient with small-cell lung cancer and hyponatremia who had sustained high plasma levels of ANP, but normal levels of AVP, suggesting the ANP produced the hyponatremia.[110] In this case, evaluation of tumor tissue showed no ANP, indicating an increased secretion by atrial tissue. The overall frequency of ANP-induced hyponatremia in cancer patients is unknown.

HYPERCALCEMIA

Hypercalcemia is common in cancer patients; about 10% of patients with cancer will have hypercalcemia, and 10% to 15% of these will not have associated bone metastases.[111,112] The most common tumor types associated with hypercalcemia are breast cancer (15% of cases but usually associated with bone metastases), lung cancer (10%), and multiple myeloma (> 50% but usually associated with bone involvement). Although most breast cancer patients with hypercalcemia have bone metastases, a recent prospective series showed that 24% had no bone metastases and a purely hormonal mechanism was postulated.[113] Patients with squamous cell carcinomas, especially of lung, head and neck, and esophagus have a high frequency of paraneoplastic hypercalcemia.[114,115] This is rare in small-cell lung cancer. Hypercalcemia with or without bone metastases is seen in the majority of patients with adult T-cell leukemia,[116] and it is seen in lower frequency in other lymphomas. There are several documented mechanisms of hypercalcemia in cancer patients, including bone metastases, the simultaneous occurrence of primary hyperparathyroidism, ectopic-tumor-produced parathormone-like substances, tumor-produced prostaglandins (PGE_1,PGE_2), tumor-produced osteoclast-activating factor (OAF), α-TGF, 1,25-dihydroxyvitamin D, and potentially other osteolytic factors.[23,111,115,117,118,119] In normal persons, calcium is maintained by a series of control mechanisms that govern bone resorption and osteolysis, which are stimulated by PGE, PTH, OAF, thyroxine (T_4), and a monocyte-derived osteolytic factor, and are inhibited by calcitonin and estrogen. Absorption of calcium from the gastrointestinal and renal tubular tracts is stimulated by PTH, growth hormone, and vitamin D.[111] Thus, production by tumors of any of these materials could cause hypercalcemia. Whereas paraneoplastic syndromes usually are considered to be those humorally mediated at a distance from the primary tumor or its metastases, in hypercalcemia the mediators released by the tumor cells may act locally (as with PGE and OAF).

The most frequent cause of paraneoplastic hypercalcemia is tumor secretion of an immunoreactive parathyroid hormone (iPTH)-like substance. This is reported most often in squamous carcinomas, but is also observed in various adenocarcinomas. These patients have increased levels of cyclic AMP (cAMP), low levels of serum phosphorous and variable levels of immunoreactive PTH depending on the specificity of the assay used.[111,112,119] Patients with primary hyperparathyroidism have higher levels of iPTH. Recent studies demonstrated that the tumor-secreted protein is *not* PTH, but is a "PTH-like peptide" in which 8 of the first 13 amino acids are the same as human PTH, with variability in the remaining amino acids.[119-122] The entire molecule comprises 141 amino acids compared with 84 amino acids for PTH.

The hypercalcemia in multiple myeloma and lymphomas is usually ascribed to osteoclast-activating factor(s) (OAF).[116,123-127] These cases have normal or low levels of iPTH, cAMP, 1,25-dihydroxyvitamin D, and evidence of osteoclast activation on bone biopsy. The OAF appears to be a locally secreted lymphokine. It is not clear whether the lymphokine is the same or is different in various lymphomas and myelomas. Interleukin-1β (IL-1β) may also be a bone-resorbing lymphokine secreted by some of the lymphoproliferative malignancies.

Tumor secretion of PGE is rare and is associated with normal or low PTH, cAMP, and vitamin D levels. Such secretion has been reported in hypernephomas and, rarely, in other tumor types.[117,118,128–133] It is important to recognize because postaglandin inhibitors [such as indomethacin (Indocin)] may be successful therapeutically.

Active metabolites of vitamin D have also been produced by some malignancies including lymphoma, small-cell lung cancer, and melanoma. In general, these cases show hypercalcemia, elevated 1,25-dihydroxyvitamin D levels, low iPTH, and low urinary and AMP excretion.[134–136] Treatment of the tumors surgically or by chemotherapy usually reverses the chemical abnormalities. In some instances, vitamin D metabolites have either been purified from tumor cells or shown to be synthesized in vitro by the tumor cells.

Transforming growth factors α and β have also been associated with hypercalcemia of malignancy.[120] Transforming growth factor α has been isolated from squamous cell carcinomas of the lung, head and neck, kidney, and breast. It is a 5000 Da protein with 50 amino acids. It mediates its effect predominantly through the EGF receptor and antibodies; thus, the EGF receptors can block the bone-resorbing activity.

All of the mechanisms of hypercalcemia should be considered in cancer patients, and determining the cause of the hypercalcemia is important because of the therapeutic implications. The pathophysiology, clinical manifestations, and treatment are discussed in Chapter 58.

HYPOCALCEMIA

In patients with bone metastases, hypocalcemia occurs in 16% and hypercalcemia only in 9%.[137–140] Not infrequently hypocalcemia occurs with osteoblastic metastases of the breast, prostate, and lung.[138,141] Only rarely is tetanic hypocalcemia seen with these osteoblastic metastases.[142] However, with more refined studies of nerve, muscle, or other physiologic function testing, the hypocalcemia may be found to impair a patient's neuromuscular function. Hypocalcemia may be mediated by way of tumor-secreted calcitonin, although there now is no direct evidence for this. No specific therapy is indicated, except in the rare case of tetany, for which calcium can be given.

HYPOPHOSPHATEMIC OSTEOMALACIA ASSOCIATED WITH BENIGN MESENCHYMAL TUMORS ("TUMORAL OSTEOMALACIA" OR "ONCOGENIC OSTEOMALACIA")

An acquired, adult-onset, vitamin–D-resistant rickets with bone pain, severe phosphaturia, renal glycosuria, hypophosphatemia, normocalcemia, (normal PTH levels), low 1,25-dihydroxyvitamin D levels, and increased alkaline phosphatase levels is seen in association with benign mesenchymal tumors that occur in soft tissues or bone.[143–146] They are also called ossifying mesenchymal tumors, giant-cell tumors of bone, sclerosing hemangioma, cavernous hemangioma, or reparative giant-cell granuloma.[147] Often the syndrome precedes the discovery of the tumor by several years.[25] The basis of treatment is resection of the mesenchymal tumor, which results in resolution of the syndrome.[143,144,148] Otherwise, treatment requires large doses of vitamin D and phosphate. The proposed mechanisms include inhibition of the conversion of 25-hydroxyvitamin D to 1,25-dihydroxyvitamin D and a tumor-secreted "phosphaturic substance." It is possible that a single protein produces both of these effects. Active osteoclastic bone resorption has also been reported. Rarely, this syndrome has been reported with lung and prostate cancers.[149,150] The importance of recognizing this syndrome is its cure with surgical resection. Sometimes multiple osteolytic lesions or osteoblastic-like lesions are seen in sclerosing hemangiomas of bone. These require treatment with oral phosphate and vitamin D and give relief of bone pain and weakness.[145] These bone lesions can resemble diffuse metastases on roentgenogram, and thus careful pathologic examination is required.

CALCITONIN PRODUCTION BY TUMORS

The polypeptide hormone calcitonin normally is produced by the C cells of the thyroid. It prevents calcium release from bone and causes an increase in renal excretion of calcium, sodium, and phosphate.[151] However, no described clinical syndromes are associated with tumor production of calcitonin at present, although one small-cell cancer patient with high calcitonin levels had hypocalcemia.[30] The major clinical use of calcitonin assay is in monitoring patients with medullary carcinoma of the thyroid. This tumor produces large amounts of calcitonin without clinical signs or symptoms.[151] Calcitonin is an extremely sensitive indicator of residual tumor after surgery.[89] It also is useful in identifying patients with multiple endocrine neoplasia, type II, a familial disorder involving an association of medullary carcinoma of the thyroid, pheochromocytoma, and parathyroid adenomas. These are described in detail in Chapter 39. Because of the excellent clinical correlation of calcitonin with medullary thyroid cancer, the hormone has been studied in other tumor types.

Elevated plasma calcitonin levels consistently have been found in 48% to 64% of patients with small-cell lung cancer and in variable frequency with the other lung cancer cell types (see Table 55-3).[22,30,31,152] Urine calcitonin is elevated in 75% of lung cancer patients (53% of epidermoid, 45% of adenocarcinomas, 20% of large-cell cancers, but surprisingly only 17% of small-cell cancers).[153] When antiserum detecting both the COOH-terminal and midportion of the calcitonin molecule was used on both serum and urine samples, more than 90% of lung cancer patients had abnormal values.[153] Calcitonin levels mirrored clinical tumor status 67% of the time in lung cancer patients, but selective venous sampling showed both tumoral and thyroidal production of the elevated calcitonin levels.[152] Thus, its usefulness as a marker of lung cancer is not yet established. Other tumor types associated with increased plasma calcitonin levels include carcinoids, breast cancer (in some studies up to 100%), colon cancer (24%), and gastric cancer (38%). High calcitonin levels do not correlate with bone metastases.[152] However, a variety of nonneoplastic conditions are associated with elevated calcitonin levels, including hypercalcemia, chronic renal failure, pregnancy, pernicious anemia, Zollinger–Ellison syndrome, and pancreatitis.[22,152] Thus, its use as a screen for the early detection of cancer is problematic.

Because of the several possible sources of calcitonin, biosynthetic studies would be very useful. Immunoreactive calcitonin has been found in many tumor extracts, including small-cell cancer, pheochromocytomas, malignant carcinoids, other types of lung cancer, breast, melanoma, colon, gastric, esophagus, and pancreatic cancer.[97,154,155] These studies failed to show that calcitonin and ACTH were on a common precursor molecule, as predicted by some, but they did show a high-molecular-mass form of calcitonin.[156,157] The nature of the calcitonin precursor molecule is unknown. In summary, calcitonin is a polypeptide hormone, apparently produced by many cancers, waiting for definition of a clinically evident paraneoplastic syndrome and prospective documentation as a marker of response to therapy.

CHROMOGRANIN A PRODUCED BY TUMORS

Chromogranin A is an acidic glycoprotein, with a molecular mass of 48,000 Da, that may account for as much as 10% of the weight of cells of the neuroendocrine system.[158] It is secreted by several neuroendocrine tumors, especially small-cell lung cancer.[158–160] It is stored in vesicles of chromoaffin cells and released with catecholamines after splanchnic stimulation. It may act in neuroendocrine secretion by binding intravesicular calcium. Its sequence is nearly identical with pancreastatin, which inhibits insulin and somatostatin secretion from the pancreas.[161,162] Pancreastatin may be generated from chromogranin A or from a chromogranin A-like precursor. Like calcitonin, it is unknown whether or not there is an associated paraneoplastic syndrome.

HUMAN PLACENTAL AND PITUITARY GLYCOPROTEIN HORMONES AND THEIR SUBUNITS PRODUCED BY TUMORS

Gonadotropins

Precocious puberty in children, gynecomastia in men, and oligomenorrhea in premenopausal women may result from excessive gonadotropin production by tumors.[2,3,23,163] In addition, very high levels of gonadotropin secretion may result in thyroid stimulation and hyperthyroidism.[164,165] Gonadotropin secretion may occur in pituitary tumors, gestational trophoblastic tumors (choriocarcinoma and hydatidiform mole), germ cell tumors of testis and ovary, germ cell tumors arising or presenting in extragonadal primary sites, and less commonly as tumors in other sites, including hepatoblastomas in children and large-cell and adenocarcinoma of the lung in adults.[2,3,23,163,166,167]

The tumors arising in gestational tissue, testis, ovary, and endocrine organs are discussed in other chapters in which the great value of gonadotropin measurement as a marker in the treatment of gestational trophoblastic tumors and testicular cancer is discussed.[168,169] Their usefulness as a marker in these tumors stimulated intense study of gonadotropin expression in other tumors to see if they could be used as markers for early diagnosis or monitoring of subsequent treatment.[170]

The human hormones with gonadotrophic properties are follicle stimulating hormone (FSH), luteinizing hormone (LH), and human chorionic gonadotropin (hCG).[163] These three hormones are composed of two polypeptide chains, an α- and a β-subunit. The α-subunit is common to all the hormones, whereas the β-subunit confers immunologic and biologic specificity. However, both subunits together are required for bioactivity.[163] Radioimmunoassay allows distinction between the various types of β-subunits.[163] In normal persons, FSH and LH are produced by the pituitary and are normally present in serum, whereas biologically active hCG is produced by the placenta and thus usually is found only in pregnant women. Because levels of FSH and LH vary widely under normal physiologic conditions, the assay for β-hCG is theoretically the best to use for following patients with suspected paraneoplastic production of gonadotropin excess. Recently an hCG-like material has been found in extracts of all normal tissue by RIA and radioreceptor assay, calling into question the use of hCG in cancer patients. However, this hCG is carbohydrate-free, whereas that produced by the placenta and many tumors contains carbohydrate. Carbohydrate-free hCG is cleared rapidly from the circulation and has marked loss of bioactivity.[163,171]

Many studies have looked at "elevations" of hCG, the β-subunit of hCG (CGβ), and the common α-subunit (Table 55-7). Interestingly, many of the common tumors (*e.g.*, lung, colorectal, and breast) had frequent elevations of these markers. However, 5% to 10% of patients with nonmalignant chronic disease also had hormone elevations, calling the specificity of the findings in tumor patients into doubt. In pursuing this, Blackman and co-workers have conducted a detailed study of human placental and pituitary glycopeptide hormones and their subunits in the sera of patients with lung cancer, gastrointestinal cancer, malignant carcinoid, and malignant islet cell tumors and compared their results to 579 appropriately matched control subjects (Table 55-8)[170] Values for the α-subunit and the β-subunit of chorionic gonadotropin (CGβ) were significantly higher in the cancer patients, whereas elevations of FSHβ, TSHβ, and LHβ were not observed. In addition, the sensitivity of detection of cancer patients increased by combining the results from the two tests. They and others also found differences in the ratio of CGα/CGβ positivity between sexes and among cancer groups, a finding that is unexplained.

Because of the frequency of elevation in common tumors, such as lung and gastrointestinal, and because of the correlation with response in trophoblastic disease and testicular tumors, it will be important to test prospectively the role of CGα and CGβ in monitoring the therapy of common tumors. In some nontrophoblastic tumors these markers have proved of value in monitoring therapy.[172,176] However, these reports are still anecdotal. For example, Broder and co-workers re-

TABLE 55-7. Elevations of Human Chorionic Gonadotropin (hCG), the β-Subunit of hCG (CGβ) or the α-Subunit of Placental and Pituitary Glycoprotein Hormones in Various Tumors*

Tumor Type	% Elevated	
	hCG or CGβ	*α-Subunit*
Lung†	0–12	3–30
Colorectal	0–20	20–26
Breast	7–50	30
Pancreatic adenocarcinoma	11–50	
Gastric carcinoma	0–24	
Prostate cancer	1	0
Islet cell carcinoma	22–50	52
Carcinoid of gut and lung		16
Small intestine	13	
Hepatoma	17–20	
Nonmalignant lung disease	7	
Nonmalignant GI disease	9	
Nonmalignant breast disease	4	

*References for the multiple studies—83 and 96.

†Within lung there were 32% epidermoid cancers; 27% small-cell lung cancers; 13% large-cell lung cancers; 11% adenocarcinoma; and 17% miscellaneous and undetermined histologic malignant diseases. Within GI cancer there were 13% pancreatic adenocarcinomas; 8% gastric cancers; 4% hepatomas; 10% other types of upper GI cancer; and 65% lower GI cancer. Carcinoid lesions included 80% of GI origin; malignant islet cell neoplasms included 28% insulinomas, and 40% gastrinomas. Normal controls included 299 healthy subjects, 123 patients with chronic lung disease, 110 with benign GI disease, and 47 with benign endocrine diseases.

ported on a patient with prostatic cancer and elevation of hCG whose serum hCG levels mirrored the clinical course more reliably than did concomitant acid phosphatase levels.[175] Muggia and co-workers reported on four patients with metastatic cancer, and in seven of nine episodes, clinical remission was associated with marker decrease or exacerbation associated with marker increase.[172] Metz and co-workers reported on a patient with an hCG-secreting large-cell carcinoma of the lung with painful gynecomastia and testicular atrophy.[176] Investigation revealed elevated levels of CGβ subunits and elevated α-subunits, normal estradiol levels, low-normal testosterone levels, and abnormal (delayed) pituitary response to LHRH. These abnormal findings reverted to normal after surgical resection of the tumor (shown to contain high levels of hCG), recurred with tumor regrowth, and then regressed again with the addition of combination chemotherapy, which obtained a complete clinical remission of the tumor and the biochemical parameters.[176] The CGβ level was more sensitive than gynecomastia in predicting recurrence. This was an important case because it demonstrated the usefulness of the CGβ marker in a common solid tumor to monitor therapy and achieve potential cure with the use of chemotherapy in a semiadjuvant setting.

Studies of tumor lines in vitro agree with these studies of serum samples. The CGβ- and α-subunits have been shown to be produced by human tumor cell lines in vitro.[170,177,178] Unbalanced synthesis of α- and β-subunits is seen, but no evidence of production of FSHβ, TSHβ and, only rarely (and at low levels), LHβ was found.

Although tumor-produced α-subunit and CGβ are found frequently, there are no definitive reports of tumor-produced FSH, TSH, or LH.[3,23] Thus, any potential patients with suspected tumor production of these hormones should be carefully documented and reported. Some elevations of LH and FSH may occur in cancer patients, probably as the result of gonadal failure related to age, stress, chronic illness, or treatment.[170] Blackman and associates have recently shown that 50% to 59% of men with malignant lung disease, 28% to 32% of men with benign lung disease, but only 10% of normal persons had evidence of hypogonadism when assessed with serum testosterone, LH, and FSH.[179] Obviously other causes of elevated hormones, such as those seen in physiologic causes of hypergonadotropinemia, hyperthyrotropinemia, pituitary adenomas, pregnancy, and uremia, have to be excluded.[170]

TABLE 55-8. Elevations of the β-Subunits of Chorionic Gonadotropin (CGβ) or the α-Subunit of Glycoprotein Hormones in Patients with Lung and Gastrointestinal Cancer

Tumor Type*	% of Tumor Patients with Hormone Elevations Over 95th Percentile of Normal Controls			
	Patients (n)	*α*	*CGβ*	*α-Subunit CGβ*
Lung cancer				
Men	269	11	41	45
Women	31	16	16	29
GI cancer				
Men	92	32	28	48
Women	71	18	34	41
Carcinoid				
Men	25	50	0	50
Women		13	50	50
Malignant islet cell				
Men	40	61	6	61
Women		38	19	43

Data summarized from Ref. 170.

*Within lung cancer 32% were epidermoid.

DIFFERENTIAL DIAGNOSIS. The exact frequency of symptoms associated with tumor-produced gonadotropin is not known, although both an intact hormone (both subunits) and an appropriate host (child for precocious puberty, man for gynecomastia, premenopausal women for oligomenorrhea) are required simultaneously for clinical expression. A detailed discussion of the differential diagnosis of these conditions is beyond the scope of this chapter. However, the most common problem is a male patient presenting with unexplained gynecomastia. In this situation, a CGβ determination should be performed as well as a careful examination of the testes and radiographic examination of the chest and mediastinum. It is important to use an RIA, as routine urinary pregnancy tests are not sensitive enough to detect many hCG secretory neoplasms.[176] Germ cell tumors of the testis or extragonadal sites and lung cancers are the most frequent cause of the combination of gynecomastia and hCG elevation, and such men should then be persistently and thoroughly evaluated, because this syndrome can present before a clinically evident cancer is found.[179a]

In fact, other tumors associated with biologically active hCG (*e.g.*, gynecomastia and precocious puberty) are rather rare. Skrabanek and associates found only 44 extragonadal cases in the world's literature, and these involved the lung, adrenal gland, liver, gastrointestinal tract, and nongonadal portions of the genitourinary tract.[180] Analysis of the histologic specimens revealed that all contained syncytial giant cells or frankly choriocarcinomatous elements similar to classic trophoblastic germ cell tumors. Greco and coworkers found that 40% of patients with extragonadal germ cell tumors, "masquerading" as poorly differentiated carcinomas, had immunochemical tumor staining for CGβ and AFP without serum elevations of the markers.[181] Many patients responded to combination chemotherapy. These results suggest that in poorly differentiated midline carcinomas in young adults, immunohistochemistry and a chemotherapy approach similar to that for histologically classic germ cell tumors are now warranted in these potentially curable lesions.

Precocious puberty has been found in children with hepatoma or hepatoblastomas. In these children, secondary sexual characteristics were developed prematurely, along with advanced skeletal maturation and hyperplasia of prostatic and testicular interstitial cells.[23,182–184] Abnormal endocrine manifestations consisting of precocious puberty, irregular bleeding, amenorrhea, and hirsutism were present in 9 of 15 patients (60%) with tumors of the ovary, and biopsy specimens stained immunohistochemically for hCG (in syncytiotrophoblast-like cells) and for α-fetoprotein (in embryonal carcinoma cells).[185]

TUMOR-PRODUCED HUMAN PLACENTAL LACTOGEN, GROWTH HORMONE, GROWTH HORMONE-RELEASING HORMONE, PROLACTIN, AND THYROTROPIC SUBSTANCE

Human placental lactogen (hPL) was detected in the sera of 5% to 8% of patients with nontrophoblastic nongonadal tumors.[186,187] Many of these patients with elevated hPL also had elevated levels of estrogens and had gynecomastia. Apparently, some of these patients also have elevated hCG levels. When hPL is found in nonpregnant women, it is a very specific indication of malignancy.[187]

Elevated growth hormone (GH) levels have been reported in patients with lung cancer and gastric cancer, but that may be uncommon. Although patients with these neoplasms may not live long enough to develop acromegaly, it has been speculated that GH may cause hypertrophic pulmonary osteoarthropathy, and the syndrome has been reversed by resection of lung tumors.[187a] However, a study of patients with and without osteoarthropathy failed to reveal any relationship between the syndrome and elevated plasma growth hormone levels, and none were acromegalic.[188]

Acromegaly has also been produced by tumor secretion of growth hormone-releasing hormone (GHRH).[189–193] The GHRH is a 44-amino acid peptide that has been isolated from two GHRH-secreting pancreatic tumors. A GHRH-induced acromegaly was also reported with bronchial carcinoids. The clinical symptoms of acromegaly decreased after surgical resection. The secretion of GHRH can also be controlled by administration of long-acting somatostatin analogues.

Three patients with elevated prolactin levels have been found (undifferentiated lung cancer, small-cell lung cancer, and hypernephroma), only one of whom had associated galactorrhea.[3,23] Resection or irradiation resulted in the fall of prolactin in all patients. Thus, cases of nonpituitary prolactin-secreting tumors are rare, and any suspected cases should be distinguished carefully from pituitary lesions and reported.

Cancer patients frequently have a "hypermetabolic state" that may resemble hyperthyroidism, and 1.4% of lung cancer patients reportedly are hyperthyroid, but documentation of tumor-caused syndromes is uncommon.[194] Four potential substances that could stimulate the thyroid gland are pituitary-like TSH, chorionic thyrotropin, hCG, and long-activating thyroid-stimulating substances (LATS). Documented examples of hyperthyroidism produced by TSH, LATS, and chorionic thyrotropin probably do not exist. Isolated reports of tumor-associated TSH without thyrotoxicosis have been made.[195] However, a definite association is found between hyperthyroidism and gestational trophoblastic disease (choriocarcinoma and hydatidiform mole), in which 8% of cases can have biochemical evidence of hyperthyroidism. This is also seen in testicular tumors.[23,196] In all such cases, the relationship seems to be between trophoblastic tumors and very high levels of hCG, in which the thyroid-stimulating substance occasionally has been shown to be hCG.[164,165,197]

HYPOGLYCEMIA

Hypoglycemia frequently is caused by insulinomas. Hypoglycemia associated with non–islet-cell tumors is an uncommon and not well-characterized paraneoplastic syndrome. The other types of neoplasms associated with hypoglycemia are

1. Mesenchymal in 64% (including mesothelioma, fibrosarcoma, neurofibrosarcoma, hemangiopericytoma)
2. Hepatoma in 21%
3. Adrenal carcinomas in 6%

4. Gastrointestinal in 5%
5. Miscellaneous in 5% (including anaplastic carcinomas of unknown primary, pseudomyxoma, hypernephromas, lymphomas, pheochromocytomas)[2,3,78,198]

The tumors usually are quite large (1–10 kg, with an average weight of 2.4 kg), often invade the liver, and often have protracted courses over many years.[2,3] However, hypoglycemia as the presenting symptom of a tumor also may occur.[2] Mesotheliomas are the most common cause of hypoglycemia and about 50% of these occur in the abdomen, the remainder in the chest. The signs and symptoms are those of hypoglycemia with neurologic findings (stupor, coma, and occasionally focal findings and agitated behavior), predominating until the hypoglycemia is discovered.[89]

There are multiple potential ways tumors could cause hypoglycemia.

1. Ectopic insulin production
2. Production of nonsuppressible insulin-like activity (NSILA)/insulin-like growth factors I and II
3. Overutilization of glucose by the tumor
4. Tumor production of a material stimulating ectopic insulin release
5. Massive infiltration of the liver by tumor or tumor production of an inhibitor of hepatic glucose output
6. Insulin binding by an M-protein in myeloma[199]
7. Insulin receptor proliferation[200]

Tumor utilization of glucose to a degree that causes hypoglycemia has not yet been substantiated, and only rarely is liver infiltration by tumor massive enough to cause hypoglycemia.[2,3,201] There are rare reports of insulin production by non–islet-cell tumors but no definitive biosynthetic studies to prove this.[202] A massive thoracic mesothelioma associated with hypoglycemia and very low glucagon levels was postulated as making a factor that suppresses glucagon secretion.[203] Artifactual hypoglycemia may occur in acute leukemia when the high number of circulating leukemia cells metabolizes the plasma glucose while standing in the collection tube.[204]

Currently, the most likely, although far-from-established, mechanism is tumor production of somatomedins, also called NSILA[2,3,89] and insulin-like growth factors.[205–207] Somatomedins are a family of peptide hormones normally produced by the liver under growth hormone regulation.[208] By current definitions, substances with identical bioassay properties of insulin (in the rat diaphragm or epididymal fat pad) and that also react in insulin radioreceptor assays (RRA) but do not react in insulin RIA, are *somatomedins*. Approximately half of the 200 μU of biologically active insulin and insulin-like activity in normal human serum is related to NSILA–somatomedin activity.[209] Hypoglycemia associated with cancer generally occurs after fasting and physical exertion, whereas reactive postprandial hypoglycemia usually is not part of the paraneoplastic syndrome.[89] Some cancer patients with hypoglycemia have elevated tumor extract levels of biologically active insulin-like activity that is not suppressed or reactive with anti-insulin antibodies but is reactive in the RRA.[209,210] These patients appear to have tumors producing NSILA, and it will be important to study tissue culture lines of tumors from such patients to see if they produce this substance. At present, the evaluation of such patients is experimental after the common causes of severe hypoglycemia (exogenous insulin or sulfonylureas, insulinoma, islet cell tumor, adrenal or pituitary insufficiency, ethanol abuse, and poor nutrition) have been excluded.

Initially, the treatment of paraneoplastic hypoglycemia involves glucose infusion to control the acute symptoms. Reduction of tumor bulk, usually by surgical resection, should then be carried out, if possible. However, there are no good data on the long-term effectiveness of any surgical, radiotherapy, or chemotherapy treatment approach. If tumor treatment is not possible or is inadequate, other possibilities include the use of glucagon (intermittent subcutaneous or long-acting glucagon given IM) or high-dose corticosteroids.[89] However, there are few data on the long-term effectiveness of these agents in controlling the hypoglycemia.

NEUROGASTROINTESTINAL PEPTIDES UNASSOCIATED WITH KNOWN PARANEOPLASTIC SYNDROMES

Neurogastrointestinal peptides are known to have important roles in the perception of pain; in memory, learning, and behavior, in psychiatric diseases; and in temperature and blood pressure regulation.[24,25] Changes in levels of somatostatin, cholecystokinin, substance P, VIP, and enkephalin have been reported in two major idiopathic neurologic diseases: Alzheimer's disease and Huntington's disease.[211,215] In a patient with subacute necrotizing encephalopathy, naloxone administration reversed the symptoms of apnea, unconsciousness, hypothermia, and restlessness.[216] Analysis of spinal fluid showed an increased level of an uncharacterized opioid-like activity, and autopsy examination revealed increased concentrations of met- and leu-enkephalin in the cortex. Thus, ectopic tumor production of these hormones may produce previously described neurologic paraneoplastic syndromes of unknown etiology such as limbic encephalitis (see later discussion) or other previously undescribed syndromes.

NEUROLOGIC MANIFESTATIONS OF MALIGNANCY

Neurologic problems occur frequently in patients with cancer. In the experiences of Posner and coworkers at Memorial Hospital, 17% of all patients at admission have neurologic symptoms and signs requiring neurologic consultation.[217] In patients with established cancer, true paraneoplastic syndromes account for a minority of neurologic problems, and the diagnosis of paraneoplastic syndrome can be established only after other diagnoses are excluded. The differential diagnosis of the cancer patient with neurologic signs and symptoms is provided in Table 55-9. Most frequently, neurologic complications are caused directly by the tumor or its metastases. For example, 40% to 65% of lung cancers metastasize to the brain, and overall Posner and Chernick reported that intracranial metastases were found

TABLE 55-9. Differential Diagnosis of Neurologic Syndromes

Syndromes that are due to effects of primary or metastatic tumor
Syndromes that are due to endocrine or metabolic tumor products (*e.g.*, ADH, calcium, glucose, electrolytes)
Syndromes that are due to cerebral and spinal vascular disease
Syndromes that are due to toxicity of primary treatment (chemotherapy, radiotherapy)
Syndromes that are due to CNS infections
Paraneoplastic syndromes associated with malignancy with unknown mechanisms

in 24% of autopsies at Memorial Sloan–Kettering Cancer Center.[219–220]

Neurologic syndromes caused by endocrine and fluid and electrolyte abnormalities are the second most common cause of neurologic symptoms and signs in cancer patients. Hepatic encephalopathy and hypercalcemia are the most frequent of these. Cerebral and spinal vascular disease are common in cancer patients and are found in 13% of autopsied cancer patients.[217] The etiologies of the vascular problems in these autopsied patients are shown in Table 55-10. Clearly the causes of stroke in these patients are strikingly dissimilar from those in the general population. Marantic and septic emboli, disseminated intravascular coagulation, tumor-related hemorrhage, superior sagittal sinus occlusion, and many of the cases of subarachnoid hemorrhage were directly tumor related and account for more than 50% of strokes.[220–224] Risk factors for the general population, including hypertension, atherosclerotic heart disease, and diabetes, are less important in the cancer patient. Several associations of cancer and neurologic vascular disease are noteworthy. Marantic endocarditis with emboli (nonbacterial thrombotic endocarditis) occurs predominantly in patients with adenocarcinoma, especially of the lung, and may present neurologically as multifocal abnormalities, focal abnormalities or progressive encephalopathy without any focal deficits.[221,224] Hemorrhage is seen most often in the leukemias, especially acute nonlymphocytic leukemia.[222] Fungi

TABLE 55-10. Etiology of Stroke in Cancer Patients

Etiology	*Frequency*	*(%)*
Embolic infarction	27	
Septic		13
Marantic		12
Tumor		2
Thrombotic infarction	19	
Atherosclerotic		10
Disseminated intravascular coagulation		9
Miscellaneous infarction	6	
Intraparenchymal hemorrhage	32.5	
Spontaneous		13
Tumor related		13
Hypertension		5
Unknown		1.5
Subdural hemorrhage	8.5	
Subarachnoid hemorrhage	3	
Superior sagittal sinus occlusion	4	
Total	100	

From studies by Allen,[217] Rosen,[221] Collins,[222] and Sigsbee.[223]

are the most frequent cause of septic emboli. Paraneoplastic thrombosis of cerebral venous structures, a part of the hypercoagulable state associated with malignancy (see later discussion), produces headaches, followed by the abrupt onset of central nervous system dysfunction.[225] This may include motor abnormalities, sensory complaints, vision and speech abnormalities, rapid mental deterioration, and seizures. The diagnosis is made by angiography. Angioendotheliosis may be another neurologic paraneoplastic syndrome associated with vascular disease produced by endothelial cell proliferation and causing silent strokes and dementia.[226–229]

Paraneoplastic syndromes or "remote effects" of tumors on the CNS are uncommon although the incidence varies considerably in different reports. For example, Croft and Wilkinson found neuromyopathies in 7% of 1476 cancer patients; lung cancers were the most frequent.[18] Brody, however, found no difference in the frequency of neurologic syndromes between patients with lung cancer and controls with chronic lung disease.[19] Clearly some specific neurologic syndromes occur exclusively or with much higher frequency in cancer patients. The patient with no known cancer who develops one of these syndromes should lead one to suspect an occult cancer, and a full evaluation for cancer is warranted. These syndromes include subacute cerebellar degeneration, subacute motor neuropathy, dermatomyositis in older men, Eaton–Lambert syndrome, and dorsal root ganglionitis. If a patient not known to have cancer develops a neurologic syndrome less often associated with malignancy, a careful history and physical examination should be performed, but an exhaustive laboratory and radiologic search for tumor is not indicated (Table 55-11). In these instances and in instances with a highly suspect syndrome with negative evaluation, careful patient follow-up is required.

Most paraneoplastic syndromes run a course parallel to the underlying tumor. This is less often the case in neurologic paraneoplastic syndrome, in which the course of the neurologic abnormalities is frequently independent of the underlying tumor. In many instances, this can be attributed to the inability of the nervous tissue to divide and repair damage. In some instances, such as the myasthenic syndrome and polymyositis, however, cases of a parallel course of tumor and syndrome have been documented. Many neurologic paraneoplastic syndromes were recently found to be produced by "autoimmune" immunologic reactions where the tumor shares antigens with normal nervous tissue.[230–232] The host immune response to the tumor then produces immunologic damage of the nervous system. Recent evidence suggests that subacute cerebellar degeneration,[12,238] optic neuritis,[13,245] sensory carcinomatous neuropathy,[14,233] and the Eaton-Lambert syndrome[15,272] may be caused by such cross immunological reactions.

Numerous neurologic syndromes have been described. For convenience they are listed in Table 55-11, which is divided by area within the nervous system.

"REMOTE EFFECTS" ON THE CEREBRUM AND CRANIAL NERVES

Remote paraneoplastic syndromes involving the brain and cranial nerves are less common than those involving other

TABLE 55-11. Paraneoplastic Syndromes of the Nervous System

Site	Syndrome	Reference	Clinical Features	Associated Neoplasms	Comments
I. Cerebral	Subacute cerebellar degeneration*	Brain[234] Paone[235] Victor[236] Steven[237] Greenlee[12] Dropcho[238]	Subacute, progressive, bilateral, symmetric, cerebellar failure often with dementia, dysarthria, CSF lymphocytosis, and elevated protein	Lung Prostate Colorectal Ovary Cervix Other	Some reports of improvements with removal of primary tumor; no other known treatment
	Dementia	Shapiro[239] Dorfman[240]	Variable presentation, acute to slowly progressive; often associated with abnormalities in other areas of the neuraxis; EEG shows slowing; CSF pleocytosis sometimes seen.	Lung	Relatively common (30–40%)
	Limbic encephalitis	Corsellis[241] Dorfman[240] Brennan[242] Carr[293]	Dementia with degenerative changes in the hippocampus and amygdaloid nuclei; often associated with inflammatory and degenerative lesions in other areas of the neuraxis	Lung Hodgkin's Other	May or may not improve with removal of primary tumor (Ophelia syndrome)
	Optic neuritis/visual retinopathy	Sawyer[244] Grunwald[13,245] Pillay[246]	Decrease in vision, papilledema; unilateral or bilateral	Small-cell lung cancer	Rare; produced by antiretinal antibodies
	Progressive multifocal leukoencephalopathy	Padgett[247] Richardson[16] Weiner[17]	Dementia, paralysis, aphasia, ataxia, dysarthria, visual field defects, blindness, coma, seizures; demyelination of white matter; CSF often normal; death usually rapid	Leukemias, lymphomas, sarcomas, other	Caused by papova viruses of 2 types: JC virus or SV-40-like virus
	Angioendotheliosis	Petito[227] Person[226] Gallego[228] Folkman[229]	Rapid onset of multiple infarct dementia; CT/MRI findings consistent with multiple strokes	Lymphomas, other	Not proved; may be caused by angiogenic peptides
II. Spinal cord	Amyotropic lateral sclerosis (ALS)	Norris and Engel[248]	Upper and lower motoneuron disease with spasticity, extensor plantar responses, wasting, and fasciculations		Syndrome similar to that in patients without cancer but sometimes progresses more slowly; cancer found in 10% of ALS patients in one report, but others find cancer less frequently
	Subacute necrotic myelopathy	Mancall[249] Handforth[250]	Rapid ascending motor and sensory paralysis to thoracic level; elevated CSF protein	Lung Kidney	Severe tissue destruction of grey and white matter
	Subacute motor neuropathy*	Walton[251]	Slowly developing lower motoneuron weakness without	Lymphoma	No known treatment; occasional spontaneous

(continued)

TABLE 55-11. Paraneoplastic Syndromes of the Nervous System (*continued*)

Site	*Syndrome*	*Reference*	*Clinical Features*	*Associated Neoplasms*	*Comments*
			sensory changes; most often in irradiated patients with lymphoma		recovery; ? viral origin
III. Peripheral nerves	Sensory neuropathy*	Horwich[252] Henson[253] Graus[14]	Subacute onset of sensory loss including deep tendon reflexes, with normal strength and normal motor conduction velocity; elevated CSF protein	Lung Other	Uncommon, also called dorsal root ganglionitis may be caused by antineuronal antibody
	Sensorimotor peripheral neuropathy	Croft[254] Dayan[255] Newman[256] Victor[257]	Distal weakness and wasting, areflexia, distal sensory loss; elevated CSF protein	Lung GI Breast Other	Quite common; recovery rare even with removal of primary tumor
	Ascending acute polyneuropathy (Guillain–Barré)	Lisak[258]	Bilateral, usually symmetric weakness (flaccid), usually beginning in lower extremities and ascending; sensory symptoms and signs usually develop as well; elevated CSF protein	Lymphoma	Association not definite
	Autonomic and gastrointestinal neuropathy	Schuffer[259] Siemsen[260] Park[261] Ahmed[262] Ogilvie[263]	Orthostatic hypotension; neurogenic bladder; intestinal pseudo-obstruction	Lung (small-cell)	Many cases of Ogilvie's syndrome (colonic pseudo-obstruction) may be paraneoplastic
IV. Muscle and neuro-muscular junction	Dermatomyositis and polymyositis*	DeVere[264] Barnes[265] Williams[266]	Progressive muscle weakness developing gradually over weeks to months (proximal > distal); usually not disabling; elevated muscle enzymes and sedimentation rate	Lung Stomach Ovary Other	Stringent association in older males; less frequent in colorectal tumors
	Myasthenic syndrome* (Eaton–Lambert syndrome)	Lambert[267,268] Simpson[269] Cherrington[270] Jenkyn[271] Fukunaga[15] Login[272]	Weakness and fatigability of proximal muscles, especially pelvic girdle and thigh; dryness of mouth, dysphagia, dysarthria, and peripheral paresthesias common; EMGs show a facilitated response in active muscles	Lung (small-cell) Stomach Ovary Other	Poor response to Tensilon; should respond to therapy of primary tumor; guanidine may also be useful
	Myasthenia gravis	Tyler[273]	Weakness with predilection for ocular and cranial muscles, tendency for fluctuation and partial reversibility by cholinergic drugs	Thymoma Lymphomas Breast Other	Except for thymoma, association not proved

*These syndromes are so strongly associated with malignancy that a thorough investigation for malignancy is indicated when they develop in patients not known to have cancer.

areas of the neuraxis. In one large series involving 1476 cancer patients, only 162 had neurologic abnormalities, and, of these, only 15 had lesions of the brain.[18] These 15 all had subacute cerebellar degeneration, which is one of the syndromes with a strong association with malignancy.

Subacute cerebellar degeneration occurs most commonly in association with lung cancer, but many other tumor types have been described. It is characterized by a subacute and progressive, bilateral, symmetric cerebellar failure with ataxia, dysarthria, hypotonia, and pendular reflexes.[234–238] Dementia may occur. Frequently present are a cerebrospinal fluid (CSF) lymphocytosis and elevated protein levels. Pathologically, there is atrophy with loss of Purkinje cells. In several instances the syndrome was produced by synthesis of anticerebellar antibodies both systematically and within the central nervous system.[12] The use of such an autoantibody allowed the cloning of a gene whose peptide was expressed in brain and cell lines derived from cancers of neuroectodermal, kidney, and lung origin.[238] Improvement in the syndrome has been noted following removal of the primary tumor, corticosteroid administration, and plasmapheresis.

Dementia is probably the most frequent cerebral abnormality in cancer patients. Because it is also frequent in the general population, its association with malignancy is less strong. Dementia is often associated with abnormalities in other areas of the nervous system. The EEG shows generalized slowing and a CSF pleocytosis sometimes is present. In some instances, rapid-onset dementia may be caused by angioendotheliomatosis. This syndrome is a proliferative disorder of endothelial cells of blood vessels and may produce a clinical picture of multiple infarct dementia with edema.[226–228] It has been described as a primary endothelial disorder, perhaps even malignant. More likely, it is produced by tumor secretion of one of several angiogenic peptides.[228,229] Angiogenic peptides include fibroblast growth factors (acidic and basic), tumor necrosis factor, transforming growth factors α and β and interleukin-1β (IL-1β). Acidic fibroblast growth factor and IL-1β are quite homologous. The syndrome has responded to high-dose steroids, chemotherapeutic agents, and radiation.

Limbic encephalitis is characterized by a progressive dementia associated with degenerative changes in the hippocampus and amygdaloid nuclei. Pathologically, there are inflammatory as well as degenerative changes. The CSF may be normal or show a pleocytosis. The syndrome does not appear to improve with removal of the primary tumor and did not improve after resection of primary lung tumors; it has, however, been reported to improve after successful chemotherapy for small-cell lung cancer and Hodgkin's disease.[241–243] The etiology is unknown, although a viral cause has been postulated.

Optic neuritis is characterized by scotomas, decreased vision, and papilledema, which may be unilateral or bilateral. Pathologically, demyelination is found. This syndrome is related to the visual paraneoplastic syndrome characterized by binocular loss of vision in patients with small-cell lung cancer.[13,245,246] There is specific loss of retinal ganglion cells and their processes due to immune deposits of antibodies that react with antigens shared by normal retinal and small-cell lung cancer cells.

Progressive multifocal leukoencephalopathy is included in this section, even though multiple areas of the neuraxis are involved and it is not a true paraneoplastic syndrome, since a viral cause has been quite well established in recent years. The syndrome is characterized by dementia, paralysis, aphasia, ataxia, dysarthria, visual field defects, blindness, and sometimes coma or seizures. It usually is rapidly progressive, with death occurring within 6 months. The CSF is usually normal. This syndrome occurs most often in malignancies associated with impaired immunity (leukemias and lymphomas) but also occurs in many benign conditions with altered immunity (sarcoidosis or steroid therapy). Pathologically, demyelination of white matter is found throughout the nervous system. Recent evidence suggests the illness is caused by one or two types of papovavirus.[17,247]

REMOTE EFFECTS INVOLVING THE SPINAL CORD

In the large series of Croft and Wilkinson, paraneoplastic syndromes primarily involving the spinal cord accounted for only 9% of all nervous system syndromes.[18] From a different perspective, Norris and Engel reported that 10% of 130 patients with amyotrophic lateral sclerosis had an underlying malignancy.[248]

Amyotrophic lateral sclerosis (ALS) is characterized by widespread lower motor neuron muscle weakness, atrophy, spasticity, hyperreflexia, extensor plantar responses, and fasciculations. When associated with cancer, the sex distribution is predominantly male and the age is older. The course of ALS may progress more slowly in cancer patients. Despite the report of Norris and Engel, many observers feel that far fewer than 10% of ALS patients have an underlying cancer.[248]

Subacute necrotic myelopathy is characterized by a rapidly ascending motor and sensory paralysis, which is most severe in the thoracic region. It usually terminates in death in a matter of days or weeks. There are often degenerative lesions in other areas of gray and white matter as well. The CSF protein level usually is elevated. The syndrome most often is reported in association with lung cancer, but other tumors have been reported as well.

Subacute motor neuropathy has a strong association with malignancy, particularly with the lymphomas. It is characterized by slowly developing but progressive lower motor weakness without sensory changes. It occurs most often in irradiated patients. Although the course often progresses slowly, it may wax and wane, and there may be spontaneous recovery. A viral cause has been speculated.

REMOTE EFFECTS ON THE PERIPHERAL NERVOUS SYSTEM

Paraneoplastic syndromes involving the peripheral nerves are the most frequent site in the nervous system. The association was first reported in the late 1800s, and a number of reports appeared in the late 1940s and early 1950s. A large series was reported by Croft and Wilkinson in 1965, who divided these neuropathies into two groups: a symmetrical sensory peripheral neuropathy that usually developed late in the course of the neoplasm, and an acute or subacute severe sensory motor neuropathy that often progresses to paralysis before other signs of malignancy.[18] The CSF protein often is elevated in these syndromes. The neurologic abnormalities may wax and wane, and steroids are occasionally associated with clinical improvement. However, surgical removal of the tumor rarely leads to improvement. The syndrome has been reported with a wide variety of neoplasms, most commonly lung cancer.[273]

Pure sensory neuropathy associated with degeneration of dorsal root ganglia (dorsal root ganglionitis) is strongly associated with malignancy. In most instances, the tumor is located in the chest (lung cancer, thymoma, lymphomas, involving the mediastinum, laryngeal or esophageal carcinomas). The syndrome is characterized by the subacute development of distal sensory loss, especially proprioception, and loss of deep tendon reflexes with normal muscle strength. Motor nerve conduction velocities are normal. The CSF protein often is elevated. The illness usually precedes the development of cancer, leaves the patient severely disabled, and rarely improves. An immunologic mechanism has been postulated for these sensory neuropathies because organ-specific antibrain antibodies have been reported in sera and CSF.[14] In one patient with a plasma cell dyscrasia and peripheral neuropathy, pathologic and immunologic studies indicated that an IgM kappa-antibody directed against peripheral nerve myelin produced the neuropathy.[274]

Ascending acute polyneuropathy (Guillain–Barré syndrome) has been reported in some patients with malignancy, particularly Hodgkin's disease and malignant lymphomas.[233] The syndrome has been clinically similar to that found in patients without malignancy. Because both are relatively common and parallel clinical courses have not been demonstrated, the association may be coincidental. Autonomic neuropathy has been associated most commonly with lung cancer (generally small-cell lung cancer).[259,263] The most frequently reported syndrome has been orthostatic hypotension. Neurogenic bladder, disordered peristalsis of the esophagus, stomach, and intestine, and intestinal pseudo-obstruction (Ogilvie's syndrome) also have been reported. The neuropathologic findings in these cases have resembled those in other neurologic paraneoplastic syndromes with neuronal and axonal degeneration in association with infiltration by lymphocytes, plasma cells, and histiocytes.[259]

Peripheral nerve abnormalities also may be found as a result of other phenomena associated with the cancer. For example, patients with multiple myeloma may have neuropathies secondary to amyloid deposition. Johnson and co-workers reported three patients who developed peripheral neuropathy (mononeuritis multiplex) as a result of tumor-related vasculitis limited to the peripheral nervous system.[275] Neuropathies secondary to hemorrhage into the nerves also have been reported in leukemic patients.

REMOTE EFFECTS ON MUSCLE AND NEUROMUSCULAR FUNCTION

Dermatomyositis and Polymyositis

In large series, 7% to 34% of patients with dermatomyositis or polymyositis have been reported to have cancer. Thus, the patients with these disorders have five to seven times the incidence of malignancy as the general population.[264,266] These estimates are based on compilations of uncontrolled single institution studies lacking strict comparisons with the general population. In addition, a parallel clinical course has been reported in only a few patients.[265] It does appear from these retrospective series that the association is most striking in males over 50, of whom more than 70% have developed cancer.

Clinically, the syndrome is characterized by gradually progressive muscle weakness over a period of weeks to months. The weakness eventually stabilizes and usually is not disabling. The weakness involves the proximal musculature. Reflexes usually are present but diminished. Muscle enzymes and sedimentation rate usually are elevated. The electromyogram (EMG) tracing is abnormal, and muscle biopsies show muscle fiber necrosis with minimal inflammatory changes.

In most instances, the myopathy and cancer appear within 1 year of each other. There have been no long-term follow-up studies to determine whether patients with dermatomyositis who do not develop cancer within 1 year continue at high risk for developing cancer. Most reported cases do not relate the temporal cause of the tumor and the dermatomyositis. Barnes was able to find 29 reports of improvement in both tumor and dermatomyositis and seven reports of worsening of both in a review of 258 cases.[265] Steroids have been reported to be useful by some observers, although this is controversial and there are no well-controlled therapeutic studies.

Myasthenic (Eaton–Lambert) Syndrome

The myasthenic syndrome is uncommon but strongly associated with small-cell undifferentiated bronchogenic carcinoma. The syndrome is characterized by muscle weakness and fatigue, which are most pronounced in the pelvic girdle and thigh, making it difficult to climb stairs or get out of a chair. Other features include dryness of mouth, dysarthria, dysphagia, blurred vision or diplopia, ptosis, paresthesias, and muscle pain. In contrast to true myasthenia gravis, muscle strength improves with exercise and there is poor response to edrophonium (Tensilon). The EMG confirms the increase in muscle action potential with repeated nerve stimulation at rates faster than 10 per second. Most patients have lung cancer, particularly small-cell lung cancer. Lambert and co-workers reported that fewer than 1% of all lung cancer patients, but 6% of all small-cell lung cancer patients, have this syndrome.[267,268] In the authors' experience, these syndromes are infrequent in lung cancer patients. There are a few reports of the relationship between response to antitumor therapy and improvement in the syndrome.[271] Recovery from the syndrome has been noted in patients with small-cell lung cancer treated with combination chemotherapy. Because more than 90% of patients with small-cell lung cancer respond to combination chemotherapy, this should be tried as a first measure. For patients failing chemotherapy or having no improvement in muscle strength with response to chemotherapy, guanidine has been reported to be useful.[270] There are accumulating data that the Eaton–Lambert syndrome is also "autoimmune." This is supported by the ability to transfer the syndrome to mice by the administration of immunoglobulin or purified IgG from patients' serum.[15] Recent studies suggest that the IgG autoantibody inhibits acetylcholine release through a functional blockade of calcium channels.[272] Alternatively, the autoantibodies may induce excess production of acetylcholinesterase.[269]

Myasthenia Gravis

The association of myasthenia gravis and thymoma is well established. A number of tumors including lymphomas, pancreas, breast, prostate, ovary, thyroid, cervix, kidney, rectum, and palate have been reported in association with myasthenia gravis, but many authors conclude that the incidence is no greater than that expected in the normal population.[273]

HEMATOLOGIC MANIFESTATIONS OF MALIGNANCY

Abnormalities in all the hematopoietic cell lines, as well as in the clotting proteins, have been reported in cancer patients. As with the other paraneoplastic syndromes, these abnormalities are most often produced as a direct result of marrow infiltration by the tumor or its metastases. Infection and toxicity from cancer therapies are also more common than true paraneoplastic effects. As our understanding of hormones and protein factors regulating hematopoiesis has increased in recent years with newer in vitro cell culture techniques, the mechanisms for hematologic paraneoplastic syndromes, particularly increases in cell numbers, appear to be caused by aberrant production of hematopoietic colony-stimulating factors.[6,7,270,276]

ERYTHROCYTOSIS

Tumor-associated erythrocytosis is well documented in the literature. In a review of 340 cases of tumor-associated erythrocytosis, 35% were hypernephromas, 14% were benign renal problems (cystic kidneys or hydronephrosis), 3% were other tumors involving the kidney (Wilms', hemangioma, adenomas, and sarcomas), 19% were hepatomas, 15% were cerebellar hemangioblastomas, 7% were uterine fibroids (often aldosterone-secreting adenomas), 3% were adrenal (often aldosterone-secreting adenomas) tumors and pheochromocytomas, and 3% were miscellaneous tumors (ovary, lung, thymus).[277] Overall, 53% of cases had some renal involvement. About 1% to 5% of patients with renal tumors and 9% to 20% of patients with cerebellar hemangioblastomas have erythrocytosis.[278] The erythrocytosis usually regresses with removal of the primary tumor and recurs with tumor progression.[277] Increased erythropoietin levels were found in 64% of the tumor extracts or cystic fluids tested, but no erythropoietin was detected in normal tissues. Elevated serum erythropoietin levels were found in 53% of patients. Although Wilms' tumor usually is not associated with erythrocytosis, elevated plasma erythropoietin levels have been found in patients without erythrocytosis, but the exact frequency of this is unknown.[277] All of this suggests that about half of certain tumors associated with erythrocytosis make erythropoietin.[277]

Erythropoietin normally is produced by the kidney but also may be produced by the liver in anephric persons.[23] Thus, it is not surprising that certain renal and liver tumors may produce erythropoietin. Direct production of erythropoietin activity by human renal cell carcinomas in vitro has been demonstrated.[279] There are various mechanisms by which tumors could cause elevated erythropoietin levels.

1. Tumor production of erythropoietin
2. Induction of either local kidney or systemic hypoxia by tumor mass effect, vascular obstruction, or hypoxia
3. Secretion by the tumor of a factor that stimulates the release of ectopic erythropoietin
4. Change in the metabolism of erythropoietin by the tumor[277]

With renal cysts, local renal hypoxia is a likely cause,[277] whereas most cases are probably a result of tumor production of erythropoietin.

Other Mechanisms Generating Erythrocytosis in Cancer Patients

Because not all cancer patients with erythrocytosis had elevated tumor levels of erythropoietin, other mechanisms that cause erythrocytosis must exist. Adrenal cortical tumors and virilizing ovarian tumors can produce androgenic hormones with erythropoietic effects.[23] This may be the mechanism of erythrocytosis associated with Cushing's syndrome. Although pheochromocytomas and aldosterone-producing adrenal adenomas also may cause erythrocytosis by this mechanism, the exact hormonal basis has not yet been defined.[277]

Another possible mechanism would be by way of tumor-produced prostaglandins, because prostaglandins will enhance the effects of erythropoietin on erythroid differentiation.[23] This is likely because elevated prostaglandin levels associated with hypercalcemia usually were found in patients with renal tumors.[129,130] Because of this it would be extremely interesting to consider a trial of indomethacin in cancer-associated erythrocytosis in patients without elevated erythropoietin levels.

By convention, erythrocytosis is diagnosed when there is increased red cell mass, usually associated with a hematocrit values over 55% for a man and over 50% for a woman.[280] Obviously, elevated but lower hematocrits in the setting of appropriate tumors (*e.g.*, hypernephromas, hepatomas, or CNS tumors) should alert clinical suspicion of a paraneoplastic syndrome. The differential diagnosis of erythrocytosis is between the panmyelosis (all blood elements) and splenomegaly of polycythemia vera, stress polycythemia, arterial unsaturation from many causes, a hemoglobinopathy with aberrant oxygen-binding features, and dehydration with hemoconcentration.[280] A physical examination, arterial P_{O_2} determination, a hemoglobin electrophoresis, and family history will resolve most of these. Demonstration of elevated erythropoietin in the blood would confirm the diagnosis, but this test is usually not performed because of the difficulty bioassay. If a tumor is evident, it is still probably wise to rule out other causes of erythrocytosis; an intravenous pyelogram (looking for cysts or other benign abnormalities), careful pelvic examination (looking for fibroids), and neurologic examination for cerebellar signs should always be performed.

The erythrocytosis per se usually does not need treatment, and phlebotomy is rarely used.[277] Tumor resection is successful in controlling the erythrocytosis in more than 97% of resectable cases; this should be the primary approach.[277] There are no good data on the response of erythrocytosis to chemotherapy (*e.g.*, of a hepatoma). Because only half of the patients with resectable tumors had increased serum or tumor extract erythropoietin levels before surgery and because the erythrocytosis corrected with resection, non-erythropoietin-mediated tumor erythrocytosis also should be treated primarily with resection, if possible.

ANEMIA ASSOCIATED WITH CANCER

Anemia occurs frequently in cancer patients, and various mechanisms may explain the anemias, including the anemia of "chronic disease"; bone marrow invasion; blood loss; marrow suppression by chemoradiotherapy; hypersplenism; immune hemolysis of both warm and cold antibody types; megaloblastic anemia; vitamin and iron deficiency; microangiopathic hemolytic anemia; and "pure red cell aplasia."[281-303] The reader is referred to other general hematologic sources for the general evaluation of anemia in cancer patients. However, the mechanisms of anemia associated with cancer usually have not been elucidated.[281,282] For example, anemia found in leukemias probably is not explained by "crowding out" of normal marrow.[281] In many patients a good explanation of anemia cannot be found, and the diagnosis of anemia of "chronic disease" is given. Although this is easy to treat with transfusions, the cause is unknown and probably represents a remote effect of the tumor on bone marrow function, red cell metabolism, or kinetics. The anemia of "chronic malignancy" has no associated cancer types and is usually normocytic and normochromic or hypochromic, with normal iron stores (but low serum iron levels and low total iron-binding capacity), normal reticulocyte count, normal red cell maturation, moderately increased erythropoiesis, and slightly shorter red cell survival.[281,283,284] New approaches to finding the mechanisms would include study of red cell production in nude mice bearing human tumors associated with malignancy or cocultivation of in vitro erythropoiesis systems with human tumor cells.

Pure red aplasia with a severe anemia is found in association with a variety of tumors, with about one-half having thymomas.[285-287] A selective absence of marrow erythropoiesis occurs, and hypogammaglobulinemia may occur.[285,286] Reports of pure red cell aplasia associated with carcinomas have included gastric and breast adenocarcinomas, adenocarcinomas of unknown primary, lung and skin squamous cell carcinomas, anaplastic lung cancers, and T-gamma lymphoproliferative diseases.[288] In the latter cases, T-cell-mediated suppression of erythropoiesis was demonstrated, and the anemia improved after cylophosphamide therapy. Many patients with and without thymomas have also responded to cyclophosphamide therapy, and the mechanism of the aplasia may be through some T-lymphocyte-mediated system.

Megaloblastic anemia without folate or vitamin B_{12} deficiency is seen in the bone marrow of cancer patients before chemotherapy; this is unexplained. A macrocytic anemia of unknown origin occasionally is seen in association with multiple myeloma. The marrow is megaloblastic, and the serum vitamin B_{12} levels low, but the patients fail to respond to B_{12}.[289]

Hypersplenic anemia with shortened red cell survival probably is not a paraneoplastic syndrome because it nearly always occurs with myelofibrosis or, rarely, with a chronic granulocytic leukemia.[280] However, the cause of the fibrosis in the marrow and the spleen may be a humoral factor.

Autoimmune hemolytic anemias (AHA) associated with tumors usually are found with B-cell lymphoproliferative neoplasms.[290,292] The mechanisms by which the B-cell neoplasms upset the normal immunoregulatory circuits remain to be identified. However, the monoclonal immunoglobulins produced by the B-cell neoplasms on their surface membranes probably are not themselves responsible for the hemolysis.

Rarely, AHA is found associated with solid tumors. In a review of a large series of patients with AHA, only 2% had associated solid tumors.[296-298] In these cases, the mean age is 10 years older than in patients presenting with idiopathic AHA.[295] Thus, when AHA presents in the elderly, it is important to consider the possibility of an underlying carcinoma. A wide variety of tumor types are reported to be associated with AHA, including lung cancer of all histologic types, hypernephromas, ovarian, breast, stomach, uterine cervix, colon, and cecal cancer, seminoma, dermoid cysts of the ovary, and microcysts in adenomas of the pancreas.

In tumor-associated AHA, anemia is often the presenting symptom, with mean hemoglobin levels of 7.4 g/dl and frequent reticulocytosis. Splenomegaly also is common. Response to corticosteroids is infrequent, in contrast with the high response seen in idiopathic AHA. However, successful treatment of the primary tumor with resection, radiation therapy, or chemotherapy usually leads to improvement or cure of the AHA.[295,300] In some cases, recurrent tumor was associated with recurrent AHA. Thus, definitive tumor treatment should be the first approach, rather than corticosteroids or splenectomy. If this fails, splenectomy can be tried and does work in some patients. Although the etiology is not known, the two most likely causes are immune response to antigens shared by the tumor with erythrocytes (but exposed on the erythrocyte in a nonstimulating form) or attachment of immune complexes to red cells. Evans' syndrome is characterized by the simultaneous occurrence of AHA and immune thrombocytopenia (ITP).[298,299] It occurs less often than AHA or ITP alone and has been observed with various carcinomas and lymphomas. The syndrome could be caused by cross-reacting antibodies, tumor production of autoantibodies, or tumor production of a substance altering red cells and platelets, rendering them immunogenic to the host immune system.

Microangiopathic hemolytic anemia (MAHA) has been reported in association with 55 cancer patients in a comprehensive review.[301] By definition, the peripheral blood smear in MAHA contains fragmented red blood cell (RBC) forms.[302] Severe MAHA is rare in cancer patients, in one series occurring in only 8 of 3200 patients.[303] However, Antman and associates postulate that a careful search of the peripheral blood film for signs of microangiopathy (schistocytosis) may uncover many more cases of a milder nature.[301] In the reported MAHA patients, the hemolysis was abrupt and severe, requiring several units of transfused blood daily to maintain a 20% hematocrit. The mean hemoglobin level was 7 g/dl, the mean number of nucleated red blood cells was 30%, elevated bilirubin levels were found in 93%, and a leukoerythroblastic blood film was found in 35% of patients. The mean number of days from diagnosis of MAHA to death was 21 (range, 2–90 days). The Coombs' test result was always negative. Associated laboratory findings of disseminated intravascular coagulation (DIC) were found in 50% to 60%, and some of the patients had migratory thrombophlebitis. However, some of the patients with MAHA did not have signs of DIC.

Most of the tumors were mucin-producing adenocarcinomas; 55% were gastric cancer, 10% were of unknown primary (possibly gastric), and breast and lung accounted for 13% and 7%, respectively. The remainder were divided between prostate, ovary, pancreas, colon, hepatoma, cholangiocarcinoma, and seminal vesicle.[301] Of interest, several of the gastric primaries were occult and found only at autopsy.

MAHA is easily diagnosed by the presence of a severe hemolytic anemia, with fragmented RBC forms on the peripheral blood smear and a negative Coombs' test result. The causes of the MAHA syndrome represent various diseases associated with lesions of small blood vessels, including thrombotic thrombocytopenic purpura (TTP); congenital vascular abnormalities such as the Kasabach–Merritt syndrome; hemolytic–uremic syndrome; DIC; malfunction at an aortic valve prosthesis; and neoplastic disease. The differential diagnosis of MAHA caused by neoplastic diseases from TTP or DIC may be impossible because TTP and DIC have been reported in association with malignancy.[304,305] The renal function of patients with MAHA associated with malignancy was not indicated but supposedly was not unusual.

Although heparin has been used to treat other causes of MAHA, particularly the hemolytic uremic syndrome, it appears ineffective when given alone in MAHA of neoplastic disease. In contrast, in seven of nine patients, the MAHA syndrome responded to hormonal anticancer therapy (for breast and prostate cancer) or chemotherapy.[301] However, if DIC is associated with MAHA, it would appear reasonable to treat with heparin to control the immediate DIC problem while instituting appropriate anticancer therapy, as is done in acute promyelocytic leukemia.[305]

The pathophysiology of MAHA associated with cancer may represent various causes of RBC shearing, including fibrin strands from DIC; pulmonary intraluminal tumor emboli (found in 31% of MAHA patients); and narrowing of pulmonary arterioles by intimal proliferation or a side-effect of chemotherapy.[301] The presence of tumor emboli diffusely involving pulmonary arterioles occurs in about 1% of cancer patients.[301] Association of MAHA with gastric cancer may be explained by its tendency for widespread vascular metastasis and mucin production. Mucin can act as a procoagulant and potentially cause DIC. The occurrence of intimal proliferation is postulated to give pulmonary hypertension and increase the shearing force on the RBC.[301]

GRANULOCYTOSIS ASSOCIATED WITH NONHEMATOLOGIC MALIGNANCIES

Elevation in the peripheral granulocyte count to more than 20,000/μl without overt infection or leukemia occurs in association with several neoplasms.[6,280,306–309] Similarly, monocyte elevation also may be seen.[310] Neoplasms associated with a granulocytosis syndrome are gastric, lung, pancreas, melanoma, brain tumors, Hodgkin's disease, and diffuse histiocytic lymphoma ("reticulum cell sarcoma").[280,311] The exact frequency in each histologic type is not known, but many cases have been reported over the past 50 years.[280] The granulocytosis usually is asymptomatic and consists of mature neutrophils.[282]

Although there are many potential causes of neutrophilia in cancer patients (including infection, inflammatory disorders, drugs, metabolic disorders, physical and emotional stimuli), the major differential diagnostic problem for a persistently high neutrophil count is to distinguish it from coexistent chronic myelogenous leukemia (CML).[280] The major features distinguishing a paraneoplastic "leukemoid reaction" in the cancer patient from CML are a white blood count less than 100,000/μl; no left shift to blast or progranulocytic forms; normal platelet and basophil levels; absent splenomegaly; elevated leukocyte alkaline phosphatase levels; normal serum B_{12} levels; and, of course, an absent Philadelphia chromosome.[282] Once other disorders and coexistent CML are ruled out in cancer patients, a paraneoplastic granulocytosis is likely. The mechanism behind tumor-associated granulocytosis is most often tumor production of a colony-stimulating factor (CSF). The colony-stimulating factors include granulocyte CSF (G-CSF), granulocyte–macrophage CSF (GM–CSF), macrophage CSF (M-CSF; CSF-1), interleukin-3 (IL-3), and interleukin-1 (IL-1).[276] The gene for these proteins has been cloned, probes for DNA and RNA expression are available, as are antibodies to the factors. Thus, future studies will establish exactly which protein is responsible for these syndromes. Prior studies were concluded before these tools were available. For example, Robinson tested the serum and urine of 12 patients with cancer and unexplained, sustained granulocytosis for CSF activity using in vitro bone marrow culture assays.[306] Of interest, in his series there were five lung cancers (type unspecified), two melanomas, and two adrenal cancers, as well as an unknown primary, hepatoma, and multiple myeloma. He found elevated CSF levels in all of these patients, and the levels correlated with the degree of elevation of the peripheral neutrophil count. The two adrenal tumors did not make CSF in culture; the other tumors were not tested. Recently, several laboratories have reported on establishing human tumor tissue culture cell lines of lung cancer (squamous),[312] oral cavity (squamous),[313] and fibrous histiocytoma,[314] which produce large amounts of a CSF-like factor. The activity can be demonstrated in marrow cultures in vitro and, interestingly, when the human tumors are heterotransplanted, they cause neutrophilia in athymic nude mice.[312,313] Neutrophilia is also frequent in Sweet's syndrome characterized by pyrexia, neutrophilia, and painful cutaneous plaques (described under cutaneous paraneoplastic syndromes).[315] It is likely that this syndrome is also caused by tumor production of a CSF, perhaps IL-1. There is no specific therapy for the granulocytosis other than to treat the underlying malignancy.[282]

GRANULOCYTOPENIA AS A PARANEOPLASTIC SYNDROME

Granulocytopenia associated with cancer usually is the result of chemotherapy, radiotherapy, other drugs, or severe infection.[311] Granulocytopenia rarely has been reported with thymomas and may have the same immunologic basis as pure red cell aplasia.[311] Neutropenia alone may develop with marrow involvement by carcinoma, lymphoma, myeloma, or leukemia, but a pancytopenia is more common.[371] With the exception of leukemia, the neutropenia usually is not life-threatening. Despite the frequent involvement of the bone marrow with cancer, significant granulocytopenia unrelated to therapy must be uncommon in cancer patients. However, recent experimental evidence suggests that a paraneoplastic syndrome involving granulopoiesis may exist. When 10^5 normal bone marrow cells are plated in semisolid medium with CSF, 20 to 100 hematopoietic colonies (containing 40 or more cells) and 5 to 10 times that number of "cluster" (aggregates of 3–40 cells) are found.[316] In contrast, when marrow from patients with acute leukemia, preleukemic states, and CML in blast transformation are plated, mainly clusters and only rare colonies are found, suggesting that the leukemic process may inhibit the activity of the exogenously added CSF in some unknown way. Similar findings also occur with solid tumors. McCarthy and co-workers studied nine small-cell lung cancer patients for bone marrow colony formation with CSF.[316] The marrows of two of these patients (one with and one without small-cell cancer marrow involvement) were not able to form colonies in agar but had large numbers of clusters with or without CSF. Of interest, the patient with marrow involvement had neutrophilia, whereas the one without had neutropenia.[316] Thus, it is likely that some tumors may suppress granulopoiesis by interfering with the action of CSF on marrow progenitor cells. Neutropenia is also associated with T-gamma lymphoproliferative diseases.[317] In these instances, it is believed that the abnormal T cells interfere directly with granulocyte production. Corticosteroids and alkylating agents have led to improvement in some patients.

EOSINOPHILIA AND BASOPHILIA ASSOCIATED WITH NEOPLASMS

Eosinophilia also is associated with nonleukemic neoplasms, particularly Hodgkin's disease (in up to 20% of cases) and mycosis fungoides, but also it has been found with other lymphomas, melanoma, brain tumors, and other cancer. The exact frequency in these tumors is not documented.[280,311,318]

It is possible that the eosinophilia itself could be symptomatic if the cell count were sufficiently high and an allergic or Loeffler's-like syndrome (fleeting nodular pulmonary infiltrates with eosinophilia, the PIE syndrome, with mild cough, lassitude, and low-grade fever) were produced in cancer patients. A small peptide that acts as an eosinophilopoietin has been described, and the tumor cells may be producing or stimulating the secretion of this factor.[319] Slungaard and associates found that serum and tumor extracts from a patient with large-cell bronchogenic carcinoma and eosinophilia markedly stimulated the growth of eosinophil colonies from human bone marrow.[320] The tumor-associated eosinophilopoietic factor was found to be a glycoprotein of M_r 45,000 Da.

Therapy should be directed against the tumor, particularly in cases of the malignant lymphomas that are potentially curable. If this does not work or if pulmonary symptoms are troublesome, a trial of corticosteroids could be given because this sometimes gives dramatic results in other forms of the PIE syndrome, but data in cancer patients are lacking.[318]

Eosinopenia as a tertiary result of tumor secretion of ACTH or other hormones is possible but should give no clinical symptoms. Basophilia commonly is associated with CML, myelofibrosis, and polycythemia vera, but it has not yet been reported with other malignancies, and there now is no recognized basophilic paraneoplastic syndrome.[280]

THROMBOCYTOSIS ASSOCIATED WITH CANCER

Thrombocytosis (platelet count above 400,000/μl) is said to occur in up to 30% to 40% of cancer patients.[321,323] The differential diagnosis of thrombocytosis in the cancer patient includes myeloproliferative disorders (which may represent a paraneoplastic syndrome); acute and chronic inflammatory disorders; acute hemorrhage, iron deficiency; hemolytic anemias; postsplenectomy and other surgical procedures; and as a response to vincristine or epinephrine.[321] Thrombocytosis has been seen with carcinomas, leukemias, Hodgkin's disease, and non-Hodgkin's lymphomas; a fall in the platelet count is associated with a response to therapy.[282] Although not characterized yet, there is a "thrombopoietin" that regulates normal megakaryocyte production and maturation.[324] Thus, patients with neoplasms and thrombocytosis will have to have serum and tumor levels of thrombopoietin assayed. Although platelet counts above 1 million/μl may lead to thrombosis or hemorrhage, these are rarely seen associated with malignancy, and such symptoms do not appear to occur with any regularity with the thrombocytosis of malignancy. As of now, no specific treatment of the thrombocytosis is indicated except to treat the underlying malignancy.

UNEXPLAINED THROMBOCYTOPENIA IN CANCER PATIENTS

Thrombocytopenia commonly is seen in cancer patients and usually is related to chemotherapy, radiotherapy, acute leukemia, or DIC. A syndrome resembling idiopathic thrombocytopenic purpura (ITP) occasionally is seen associated with malignancy.[325–330] This association is uncommon, and in one study of ITP, it represented 4% of 381 patients with otherwise unexplained thrombocytopenia; all of these patients had lymphomas.[326] In another evaluation of patients with ITP, 9 of 52 had cancer.[325]

The diagnosis of an "ITP-like" syndrome is made by finding thrombocytopenia without anemia and with normal or increased numbers of normal red cells on a peripheral smear; no evidence of DIC; and no evidence of a drug-induced thrombocytopenia.[325] The types of neoplasms reported in the literature associated with this syndrome are Hodgkin's disease; chronic lymphocytic leukemia; non-Hodgkin's lymphoma; acute lymphoblastic leukemia; immunoblastic sarcomas; and carcinomas of the lung, breast, rectum, gallbladder, and testis.[283,284] The association with CLL and Hodgkin's disease is widely known, and the syndrome occurs in approximately 30% of patients with immunoblastic lymphadenopathy.[328–330] However, the association with other tumors is less widely recognized. The mean age of patients is older (54 years) than the mean age of patients with ITP alone. About 80% of patients are symptomatic, with bleeding, petechiae, or purpura. Most have platelet counts under 30,000/μl.[325] Response of platelet counts to high-dose (60 mg/day) prednisone is common but transient. However, six of ten patients had a complete and apparently permanent response to splenectomy.[325]

The syndrome is called ITP-like because the course is very much like classic ITP, but an immune mechanism has not been demonstrated. In the future, studies of antiplatelet antibodies will have to be done, as well as tests of antibody cross-reactivity with tumor cells. Nearly all patients have been treated with splenectomy in addition to various antineoplastic therapies; thus, the effect of tumor treatment alone on the thrombocytopenia is currently unknown.[325] Obviously, other causes of thrombocytopenia need to be excluded, particularly the use of thiazide diuretics and quinidine or the presence of DIC or severe infection. In thrombocytopenic patients receiving antineoplastic therapy, ITP-like syndromes should be considered. The clues are thrombocytopenia disproportionate to granulocytopenia, normal or increased numbers of marrow megakaryocytes, and a rapid fall in transfused platelets. This diagnosis should be remembered particularly in lymphoproliferative disorders. Therapy will consist of platelet transfusions, initial corticosteroids, then splenectomy. At present, because of the poor response to steroids and inconsistent response to treatment of the underlying malignancy, a reasonable approach is to take the patient directly to splenectomy after other causes of thrombocytopenia have been excluded.

Abnormalities of platelet function sometimes are seen associated with plasma cell dyscrasias and are believed to result from the interference of the monoclonal protein with platelet function.[292]

THE HYPERCOAGULABLE STATE IN CANCER: MIGRATORY THROMBOPHLEBITIS, DISSEMINATED INTRAVASCULAR COAGULATION (DIC), AND NONBACTERIAL THROMBOTIC ENDOCARDITIS

Hemorrhage, thrombotic, and embolic complications occur frequently in cancer patients.[304,305,331] These may arise from a variety of specific mechanisms, including treatment-related thrombocytopenia, local tissue disruption from tumor or therapy, infection, vitamin deficiency, liver disease, circulating anticoagulants, and DIC. Usually, however, there is no specific cause, and successful therapy of the underlying malignancy alleviates the problem. The clinical association between cancer and thrombophlebitis was first noted by Trousseau.[332] In 1949, Marder and colleagues reported afibrinogenemia in metastatic prostate cancer.[333] Other abnormalities in clotting characteristics, frank DIC, and nonbacterial thrombotic endocarditis (NBTE) were later recognized to occur with greater-than-expected frequency in patients with cancer.[334–352] Sack and co-workers recognized that thrombophlebitis, DIC, coagulation abnormalities, and NBTE often occurred in the same patient and that each was part of a spectrum of the hypercoagulable state in cancer.[304] Many theories on mechanisms of activation of the coagulation system have been postulated and are reviewed by Rickles and Edwards.[349]

Thrombophlebitis

The incidence of clinical episodes of thrombophlebitis in cancer patients has varied from 1% to 11% and the incidence has been even higher in autopsy studies.[334] Many years ago Trousseau recognized that cancer patients frequently have multiple episodes of thrombophlebitis and that these often occurred in veins in which deep venous thromboses were uncommon.[332] This syndrome of migratory thrombophlebitis is referred to as Trousseau's syndrome, a syndrome that he developed after its description. Migratory thrombophlebitis may occur before or after malignancy is documented. Like many paraneoplastic syndromes, its presence should lead to an investigation for occult cancer. For patients presenting with a deep venous thrombosis, a recent series showed that patients subsequently shown to have cancer were older, had lower hemoglobin levels and higher eosinophil counts than patients who did not develop cancer.[352] Thus, these factors can be used to select patients for a workup for occult cancer.

Mucin-secreting adenocarcinomas of the gastrointestinal tract most frequently are associated with migratory thrombophlebitis, but lung, breast, ovarian, prostate, and other tumors also are associated.[349] Although the greatest risk may be associated with pancreatic cancer (a prevalence of up to 57%, or 50 times higher than control subjects with chronic pancreatitis), lung cancer is the most common association because of its greater prevalence. The treatment of migratory thrombophlebitis usually is difficult; acute episodes require heparin therapy. Long-term therapy with warfarin generally is unsuccessful, and extended subcutaneous heparin therapy has met with only limited success.[304,353] Treatment of the underlying malignancy is the mainstay of treatment.

Coagulation Abnormalities and DIC

Disseminated intravascular coagulation may present as a chronic coagulation disorder, usually of a thrombotic nature, as an acute hemorrhage diathesis, or as a coagulation abnormality detected by laboratory tests alone (Table 55-12).[304,305,331–342] Abnormalities of routine blood coagulation tests have been reported in as many as 92% of cancer patients.[349] The most common abnormalities are elevated levels of fibrin/fibrinogen degradation products, thrombocytosis, and hyperfibrinogenemia.[349] These abnormalities are

TABLE 55-12. Frequency of Different Cancer Types Associated with DIC in Various Studies*

Tumor Type	Chronic DIC (n = 213)[304]	% of Tumors Making Up Various DIC Series: Bleeding Disorder (n = 134)[305]	Coagulation Abnormality (n = 86)[354]
Pancreas	24	2	0
Lung	20	1.5	12
Prostate	13	18	8
Stomach	12	4	0
Acute leukemia	9	64	19
Colon	5	0.7	6
Unknown primary	5	0	0
Ovary	4	0.7	1
Gallbladder (Cholangiocarcinoma)	4	0.7	2
Lymphomas	1	1.5	16
Breast	0.5	0	10
Melanomas	0.5	0	3
Miscellaneous others	3	3	10

* Some of the cases in Refs. 304 and 305 may overlap. The data in Ref. 304 were obtained from a literature review from 1960–1970 looking for the association of malignancy and thrombophlebitis, hemorrhagic diathesis, DIC, arterial embolism, or nonbacterial thrombotic endocarditis. The data in Ref. 305 are based on a literature review to find cases to permit a tentative diagnosis of DIC. The data in Ref. 354 come from review of the coagulation laboratory and medical records from 1971–1974 at the Memorial Sloan–Kettering Cancer Center looking for laboratory evidence of DIC.

consistent with overcompensated intravascular coagulation with fibrinolysis. The low-grade coagulation with accelerated factor utilization may be accompanied by increased synthesis rates for fibrinogen, clotting factors, and platelets, resulting in actual increases in their circulating levels. In contrast, overt DIC with consumption of platelets and clotting factors and resultant bleeding is rare. The most commonly associated neoplasms are acute promyelocytic leukemia and adenocarcinomas.[349] The DIC may be exacerbated in patients with acute promyelocytic leukemia after treatment with cytotoxic agents.

In cancer patients suspected of having DIC or other thrombotic or hemorrhagic phenomena, Sack and co-workers stressed the need for sequential monitoring of coagulation tests and the striking decreases that occurred in fibrinogen and platelet levels associated with the acute vascular events.[304] They postulated that this was due to a shift from a "compensated" to a "decompensated" coagulation status engendered by the tumor.[304] Although the thrombotic events of chronic DIC are clearly related to the coagulation disorder, the relationship is not so clear for the multiple organ system dysfunction seen in acute (often hemorrhagic) DIC.[305] The situations that appear most related to DIC are the adult respiratory distress syndrome; oliguric renal insufficiency with gram-negative sepsis and the hemolytic–uremic syndrome; neurologic syndromes related to intracranial bleeding and thrombosis; pulmonary hemorrhage syndrome; and the infarcted skin of purpura fulminans.[305] In any event, autopsy studies show DIC usually contributes strongly to patient morbidity and mortality, particularly with thrombosis or bleeding in the lung, CNS, or gastrointestinal tract.[305]

Management of DIC in Malignancy

There is universal agreement that identification and treatment of all precipitating factors is the keystone to DIC management.[260,293] This should include not only treatment of cancer, but also evaluation of patients with DIC for other precipitating factors (*e.g.*, sepsis, volume deficit, hypotension, hypoxemia, acidosis, fungus infection, transfusion reactions, and vessel manipulation). In addition, identification and correction of other hemostatic deficits should take place. A response of the malignancy to tumor treatment often is associated with response of the DIC, and thus the long-term goal is appropriate antineoplastic therapy.[304,347]

A major controversy is whether or not heparin should be used.[305,335] There is a tendency to use heparin more in DIC with thrombotic, thromboembolic, or necrotizing complications, as is often seen in the chronic DIC of malignancy.[305,306] However, randomized trials of heparin therapy in the DIC of malignancy have not been conducted. After the association between DIC and acute promyelocytic leukemia (APL) was established, Gralnick and associates showed that heparin could improve the coagulation abnormalities.[336] Subsequently, nonrandomized trials suggested that heparin should be used prophylactically in all APL patients.[341,342] More recent studies suggest heparin need not be given to all patients.[343] The liberal use of fresh-frozen plasma and platelets was suggested by these authors. Until randomized trials are conducted, coagulation values should be monitored closely in APL patients. Heparin should be considered if there is overt bleeding or a change in laboratory evaluations.

Sack and associates,[304] in their literature review of chronic DIC in malignancy, found positive responses to anticoagu-

TABLE 55-13. Treatment of Chronic DIC Malignancy*

Treatment Given			*% Response*	
Antineoplastic	*Anticoagulant*†	*Patients (n)*	*Short-Term*	*Long-Term*
+	+	27	52	15
+	−	22	55	18
−	+	48	60	10
+	+	12‡	75	?

*Data from Ref. 304. Response is defined as cessation of signs or symptoms of thrombophlebitis, hemorrhage, or arterial emboli. Long-term indicates for over 250 days or until death.

†In nearly all cases the anticoagulant therapy was heparin (81 of 87 patients reported for anticoagulant response received heparin).

‡Patients with recurrent DIC after stopping heparin therapy were again given heparin.

lant therapy (defined as cessation of signs or symptoms of thrombophlebitis, hemorrhage, or arterial emboli) in 65% of 55 patients treated with heparin initially and 33% of 26 patients treated with heparin after failing warfarin therapy. In contrast, only 19% of 32 patients treated with warfarin alone responded. In addition, 53% of 36 patients had recurrence of symptoms of the thrombotic–hemorrhage disorder after the heparin was stopped, suggesting a therapeutic role of heparin in control of the DIC. Table 55-13 summarizes the results of anticoagulant and antineoplastic therapy in the treatment of the chronic DIC of malignancy. Clearly, all combinations of antineoplastic and anticoagulant therapy were associated with response of the DIC symptoms in more than half of the cases, but only 10% to 20% of patients had long-term control, presumably reflecting the lack of control of the underlying tumor. Although in many patients the temporal correlation of heparin therapy with cessation of DIC is persuasive, spontaneous remission of DIC occurring with persistent cancer has been reported.[348]

At present, once DIC associated with malignancy is diagnosed and other factors corrected, it is wise to establish the tempo of the DIC. If the DIC is acute and symptoms life-threatening (*e.g.*, uncontrolled bleeding), or if it is chronic and the symptoms debilitating (*e.g.*, recurrent thromboembolic lesions), a trial of heparin therapy should be given. The doses used in the literature range from 300 to 600 U/kg per 24 hr. Bell and co-workers showed that heparin prevented thrombotic events in several patients and that sudden catastrophic events occurred when it was discontinued.[353] They recommended continuous intravenous heparin (administered by an external pump connected to an indwelling catheter) if the heparin requirements (to maintain the PTT at 1.5 to 2 times normal) exceed 40,000 U/day. Otherwise, intermittent subcutaneous or intravenous (every 6–8 hr) heparin was satisfactory. Once heparin therapy has begun, the repletion of coagulation factors with platelets, cryoprecipitates, and whole blood can be used, particularly in highly symptomatic, hemorrhagic, acute DIC.[305] It should be reemphasized that although heparin treatment may be maintained for weeks, it is only a temporary measure, and control of the underlying malignancy will afford the only long-term control of chronic DIC.

Nonbacterial Thrombotic Endocarditis

Another cause of thrombotic or hemorrhagic complications, nonbacterial thrombotic endocarditis (NBTE), may occur with or without DIC and is characterized by the presence of sterile verrucous, bland, fibrin–platelet lesions in the left-side heart valves.[221,304,344–346] Clinically, patients often present with emboli to the brain as well as to other organs. The brain emboli may have either an abrupt or a gradual onset of neurologic symptoms with development of either focal neurologic deficits or diffuse abnormalities such as confusion, disorientation, generalized seizure, or disturbances in consciousness. Neurologic signs are often the only evidence of thromboembolism.[224] For these patients cerebral angiography showing multiple arterial occlusions is the definitive diagnostic test.[224] Only one-third or fewer patients have heart murmurs, usually systolic. Patients are usually afebrile; however, all patients should have blood cultures if emboli are suspected. Echocardiography may be of diagnostic use for vegetations larger than 2 mm, but most lesions are smaller and, therefore, are not detected by echocardiography. Arterial emboli can go to the CNS, heart, spleen, kidneys, and peripheral sites. Occlusion of both large and small vessels is seen pathologically in the brain. Myocardial infarction can result from emboli to coronary arteries.[344,345] Of import, paraneoplastic endocarditis can present with early malignancy as well as at later stages and thus does not mean incurability.[346] In Rosen's series the autopsy incidence of NBTE in patients with adenocarcinoma of the lung (7.5%) was twice that of adenocarcinomas of the prostate or pancreas (3%–4%) and more than seven times that of other solid tumors, lymphomas, or leukemias.[350] In Goodnight's review of NBTE, bleeding frequently was found in the skin (77%–100%), CNS (22%–49%), genitourinary tract (38%–42%), eye, ear, nose, mouth (31%–47%), and gastrointestinal (24%–56%) and respiratory (20%–31%) tracts in leukemias and solid tumor patients, respectively.[334] Of both the leukemias and solid tumor patients, 37% had autopsy evidence of fibrin thrombi, but only 1% had evidence of NBTE. The principles of treating NBTE are similar to those in treating other aspects of the hypercoagulable state. Treatment of the underlying malignancy is the primary therapy.

In anecdotal cases, warfarin has been unsuccessful; heparin has been used with limited success. There are no studies reporting the use of antiplatelet drugs or fibrinolytic agents.

RENAL MANIFESTATIONS OF MALIGNANCY

Numerous problems involving the kidneys develop in patients with malignancies. The etiology of these complications is listed in Table 55-14. This table demonstrates that in most instances the renal abnormalities are not paraneoplastic in origin. Only the glomerular lesions and obstruction by tumor products can be considered to be true paraneoplastic syndromes.

GLOMERULAR LESIONS OF INDIRECT CAUSE

Massive proteinuria with the nephrotic syndrome is the major consequence of these paraneoplastic glomerular lesions, although renal failure may develop later. In patients with malignancy, the nephrotic syndrome may develop as a result of neoplastic infiltration of the kidneys, renal vein thrombosis, or amyloid infiltration. Besides these established causes of the nephrotic syndrome, there does seem to be a true paraneoplastic syndrome. Until 1966, there were only a few scattered case reports of an association between idiopathic nephrotic syndrome and malignancy. In 1966, Lee and associates reported that among 101 patients with the nephrotic syndrome of unknown etiology, 11 were found to have cancer.[355] The neoplastic syndrome preceded discovery of the cancer in 7 of these 11 patients, who were all over the age of 40. Since that time, the nephrotic syndrome has been reported in association with a number of cancers, although recent studies suggest the incidence is lower than that reported by Lee and associates.[356]

Clinical and immunologic evidence supports the true paraneoplastic nature of this syndrome.[355–362] The nephrotic syndrome may precede the development of neoplastic disease.[358] Surgical removal of tumor or response to radiotherapy or chemotherapy usually is associated with dramatic diminution in proteinuria, whereas recurrence of the neoplasm is followed by increased proteinuria.[357,359,360] Tumor-specific antigens and antibodies and carcinoembryonic antigen have been found in the glomeruli of some patients.[361–363]

TABLE 55-14. Differential Diagnosis of Renal Abnormalities in Patients with Malignancy

Direct infiltration of the kidney by tumor
Obstruction of the urinary tract by tumor
Electrolyte imbalances, many of which are caused by the tumor or its treatment (*e.g.*, calcium, uric acid, potassium)
Fluid imbalances induced by the tumor or its treatment (prerenal)
Infection
Toxicity of therapy (chemotherapy, radiotherapy, immunotherapy, antibiotics)
Glomerular lesions of uncertain etiology (usually associated with nephrotic syndrome), paraneoplastic
Obstruction by tumor products

The most frequently reported associated neoplasm has been Hodgkin's disease.[357,358,360,364–366] In patients with Hodgkin's disease, the most common renal lesion is lipoid nephrosis (minimal glomerular changes), which occurs in about 80% of cases.[364–367] In most of these instances, the renal findings have been similar to those seen in idiopathic lipoid nephrosis, including an absence of electron-dense deposits on electron microscopy and an absence of immunoglobulin deposits.[364] In the remaining 20% of cases, lesions typical of membranous glomerulopathy, focal sclerosis, or a membranoproliferative glomerulonephritis have been observed.[357,360,365]

In the non-Hodgkin's lymphomas (Burkitt's lymphomas, lymphocytic, and histiocytic lymphoma), the frequency of the nephrotic syndrome appears to be lower than that in Hodgkin's disease and some other carcinomas, although there are numerous case reports.[369,374] In 35 patients in the literature, five had minimal-change lesions, seven had membranous, and seven had membranoproliferative lesions.[369] In several of the patients with non-Hodgkin's lymphomas, immunoglobulin deposits have been identified, suggesting an immune complex cause of the syndrome.[373,374]

There is a striking difference in the type of renal lesions described in patients with carcinomas when compared with Hodgkin's disease. The most frequently observed glomerular lesion in patients with carcinomas is membranous glomerulonephritis.[368,370–372,375,376] Membranous glomerulonephritis is characterized by subepithelial electron-dense deposits and granular peripheral capillary deposits of IgG with or without C3.[357] It is present in 80% to 90% of patients with carcinoma and nephrotic syndrome. The remaining patients have lipoid nephrosis or proliferative glomerulonephritis.[357,368,372] When considering all patients with membranous glomerulonephritis, patients with neoplasia have accounted for 5% to 10% of cases.[377,378]

There is a similarity between the immunopathologic features of the membranous glomerulonephritis associated with carcinomas and experimentally induced immune complex nephritis in animals. It has been suggested that there is a common pathophysiologic mechanism with glomerular deposition of circulating antigen–antibody complexes.[357,370] Tumor-specific antibodies have been eluted from the kidneys of two patients with lung cancer and the nephrotic syndrome, and a tumor-specific antigen was demonstrated in the glomeruli of a patient with colonic carcinoma.[357,362,370] In another patient with colon cancer, carcinoembryonic antigen–antibody complexes were found in the glomeruli.[363]

The pathogenesis of lipoid nephrosis in patients with Hodgkin's disease seems to have a different mechanism. There is some evidence that lipoid nephrosis may be a result of deficient T-cell function, and abnormalities of T-cell function are common in Hodgkin's disease.[379]

Other renal abnormalities caused directly or indirectly by tumor products include renal dysfunction in patients with multiple myeloma amyloidosis; renal potassium wasting and hypocalcemia related to lysozyme in acute monocytic or myelomonocytic leukemia; intrarenal obstruction by mucoprotein in pancreatic carcinoma; and nephrogenic diabetes insipidus with leiomyosarcoma.[380–398]

The renal problems of myeloma are discussed in Chapter 58.

PARANEOPLASTIC LESIONS INVOLVING THE SKIN

A long list of fascinating cutaneous syndromes have been reported with malignancies. The salient features of these syndromes are outlined in Tables 55-15 through 55-20. There is great variation in the relationships between the cutaneous lesions and the malignancy. In some instances (*e.g.*, acanthosis nigricans and erythema gyratum repens) the cutaneous syndrome is uncommon but almost always associated with cancer. In other instances the cutaneous lesions may be common (*e.g.*, bullous lesions, exfoliative dermatitis, erythema multiforme) and have an association with various benign disorders as well as cancers. In some instances (*e.g.*, bullous lesions, pemphygoid), the association of the skin lesion and cancer may not be proved. The cutaneous syndrome may always be associated with a particular tumor (*e.g.*, esophageal cancer and tylosis), or the cutaneous lesions may be associated with various neoplasms (*e.g.*, dermatomyositis). The cause of the cutaneous lesion is well-known in some instances (*e.g.*, hirsutism in adrenal or ovarian tumors or flushing in carcinoid tumors), whereas in most the mechanism is unknown. Because many cutaneous paraneoplastic syndromes are proliferative, a causal role for tumor-secreted growth factors has been suggested. Recently, Ellis and co-workers demonstrated that malignant melanoma cells secreted transforming growth factor α (TGFα). This growth factor then bound to normal EGF receptor-bearing epidermal cells producing acanthosis nigricans, the sign of Leser–Trelet, and multiple acrochordons.[8]

EVALUATION OF PATIENTS WITH SUSPECTED PARANEOPLASTIC SKIN LESIONS

The evaluation of cutaneous lesions suspected of being paraneoplastic begins with the clinical history, with particular emphasis on drug and other exposures, associated medical conditions, and family history. An evaluation for an underlying cancer should be undertaken only if there is no evidence of drug exposure. Many of the cutaneous syndromes are hereditary. The onset of symptoms in the paraneoplastic cutaneous lesions often is more rapid than in other benign conditions (*e.g.*, dermatomyositis, malignant down, or erythema gyratum repens). The physical examination also is of critical importance. For example, while café au lait spots are not always associated with von Recklinghausen's disease, the finding of six or more café au lait spots greater than 1.5 cm in diameter or the presence of axillary freckling are diagnostic aids for the earlier recognition of neurofibromatosis.[402]

Laboratory evaluations are most helpful for cutaneous lesions suspected of being metabolic (*e.g.*, hyperpigmentation in Cushing's and Addison's disease). Skin biopsy is the most important procedure for establishing the correct diagnosis and should be performed in most instances; it may provide important information. For example, exfoliative dermatitis in patients with mycosis fungoides may be associated with infiltration of the skin, as in the Sézary syndrome, but may occur in patients with uninvolved skin areas. It also may occur in these patients as a result of treatment with chemotherapy or electron beam radiotherapy.

The differential diagnosis for cutaneous lesions of possible paraneoplastic origin includes benign, nonrelated skin conditions, cutaneous lesions resulting from a primary tumor or its metastases, cutaneous infections, and toxicity from anticancer therapy (particularly cytotoxic chemotherapy or radiotherapy). Numerous cytotoxic chemotherapeutic agents have mucocutaneous toxicities. Although a detailed discussion is beyond the scope of this chapter, an excellent review is available.[403]

Pigmented Lesions

Of special interest is acanthosis nigricans.[8,404–406] This skin lesion is characterized by the presence of symmetric brown areas of hyperpigmentation with hyperkeratosis, exaggerated skin markings, and warty lesions, particularly in the intertriginous and flexural areas such as the axilla, neck, anogenital region, umbilicus, and areola. The salient features are shown in Table 55-15. The lesions of Leser–Trelat with multiple seborrheic keratoses also have been described in patients with acanthosis nigricans (see Table 55-15),[8,407] and both may be produced by tumor secretion of TGF-α.[8] There is a strong association between acanthosis nigricans and malignancy, with more than half of all reported cases having cancer. However, the acanthosis nigricans may precede, occur simultaneously with, or occur after the diagnosis of malignancy has been made. There are several documented cases of regression following surgical tumor removal. The most frequent association is with adenocarcinomas of the gastrointestinal tract (92%), particularly of the stomach (50%–60%). However, the lesions have been reported in a variety of other tumors, including breast cancer, lymphomas, and squamous carcinomas.[404,405]

The most important part of the differential diagnosis is to distinguish between true acanthosis nigricans associated with malignancy, benign acanthosis, and pseudoacanthosis. Benign acanthosis is a nevoid condition present at birth or beginning in childhood and associated with a number of benign syndromes. Pseudoacanthosis occurs in obsese persons, especially those with a dark complexion. It may occur in patients with gigantism, acromegaly, Stein–Leventhal syndrome, or diabetes mellitus. It also may develop after prolonged administration of corticosteroids, diethylstilbestrol (DES), or nicotinic acid. Insulin resistance is common in these patients. However, insulin resistance caused by the development of antibodies against the insulin receptor has also been reported in acanthosis nigricans associated with malignancy (pheochromocytoma).[406] Because of the strong association of acanthosis and cancer, patients developing true acanthosis nigricans after the age of 40 should be evaluated for malignancy, including a thorough evaluation of the gastrointestinal tract, lymph nodes, and breasts.

Although more rare than acanthosis nigricans, the sudden development and rapid increase in size of seborrheic kera-

TABLE 55-15. Pigmented Lesions—Keratoses

Disorder	Reference	Description	Predominant Malignancy	Etiology	Comments
Acanthosis nigricans*	Brown[404] Curth[405] Ellis[8] Matsuoka[406]	Hyperkeratosis and pigmentation, especially of axillae, neck, flexures, and anogenital region	Gastric 60%; abdominal 90%; other	Unknown	Most important to distinguish benign forms present from birth and benign forms associated with various syndromes
Leser—Trelat*	Dantzig[408] Ronchese[409] Snedden[407] Holdiness[410] Curry[411]	Sudden showing of large numbers of seborrheic (wartlike) keratoses	NHL; miscellaneous GI adenocarcinomas	Unknown	Must be distinguished from multiple seborrheic keratoses, which are common and may not be associated with malignancy; occasionally associated with acanthosis nigricans
Bowen's disease	Graham[412] Anderson[413]	A persistent, progressive, nonelevated red, scaly, or crusted plaque caused by an intraepidermal neoplasm	Lung; GI; GU; skin	Generally unknown; arsenic exposure in some cases	25% developed systemic cancers an average of 5 years after initial skin lesions, but significance of association has been questioned
Chronic arsenism	Minkowsky[414]	A corn-like, punctate keratosis more profuse on the extremities and characteristically affecting the palms and feet	Lung; miscellaneous	Chronic exposure to arsenic	Not a true paraneoplastic lesion
Generalized melanosis	Fitzpatrick[415] Helm[400]	A diffuse darkening of the skin with a ruddy gray color secondary to chronic liver disease. Generalized blue-gray appearance	Lymphoma; hepatoma; metastatic liver tumors, melanoma	Melanin deposits in dermis	Also seen in a variety of benign conditions; may be rapid at onset
Paget's disease	Ashikari[416]	Erythematous keratotic patch over areola, nipple, or accessory breast tissue	Breast	Paget cells are either migrants from the carcinoma or Langerhans' cells	Occurs in less than 3% of breast cancers
Bazex's disease*	Braverman[401] Witkowski[417] Wishart[418]	Erythema hyperkeratosis with scales and pruritus predominantly on palms and soles.	Head and neck, GI, lung	Unknown	Males only. Responds to removal of primary tumor may respond to etretinate (Tegason)
Sweet's syndrome*	Cohen[315]	Fever, neutrophilia, multiple painful cutaneous plaques and neutrophilic dermal infiltrate	Hematologic malignancies, various carcinomas	? section of a lymphokine such as IL-1.	Rapid response to steroids; 10–15% associated with cancer

*True paraneoplastic syndromes.[315]

toses (sign of Leser–Trelat) are strongly associated with malignancy, particularly of the gastrointestinal tract.[407,408] As with many cutaneous paraneoplastic syndromes, the most important feature is the rapid change, because multiple seborrheic keratoses may be common, especially in older age groups.

Salient features of other pigmented or proliferative lesions are summarized in Table 55-15.

Erythemas

The major features of erythemas associated with malignancy are summarized in Table 55-16. Of note, erythema gyratum repens is nearly always associated with malignancy, and necrolytic migratory erythema is pathognomonic of glucagonoma. Exfoliative dermatitis can be caused by a variety of malignancies, drug reactions, or unknown causes.[400,427,428]

TABLE 55-16. Erythemas

Disorder	*Reference*	*Description*	*Predominant Malignancy*	*Etiology*	*Comments*
Erythema gyratum repens*	Purdy[420] Gammell[419] Summerly[421]	Rapidly changing and advancing gyri with scaling and pruritus	Breast, lung, other	Unknown	Almost always associated with malignancy
Erythema annulare centrifugum	Lazar[422]	Slowly migrating annular and configurate erythematous lesions	Prostate, myeloma, other	Unknown	Occurs also with infections and other disorders
Necrolytic migratory erythema (glucagonoma)*	Wilkinson[423] Church[424]	Circinate and gyrate areas of blistering and erosive erythema on limbs; stomatitis	Islet cell on pancreas	Glucagonoma or other metabolic product	See chapter on islet cell tumors
Flushing*	Sjoerdsma[425]1 Mason[426]	Episodic flushing of face and neck	Carcinoids, medullary carcinoma of thyroid	Serotonin or other vasoactive peptides	See chapter on carcinoids
Exfoliative dermatitis*	Abrahams[427] Nicolis[428] Helm[400]	Progressive erythema followed by scaling	Cutaneous T-cell lymphomas, NHL, Hodgkin's disease, non-Hodgkin's lymphoma	Unknown	Account for 10%–20% of all exfoliative dermatitis
Erythema multiforme	Elias[429]	Distinctive target lesions in symmetric distribution, sometimes with plaques or bullae			

*True paraneoplastic syndromes.
†True neoplastic syndrome only in some instances.

TABLE 55-17. Endocrine and Metabolic Lesions

Disorder	*Reference*	*Description*	*Predominant Malignancy*	*Etiology*	*Comments*
Systemic nodular panniculitis* (nodular relapsinig fat necrosis; Weber–Christian disease*)	Fitzpatrick[430]	Recurrent crops of tender erythematous subcutaneous nodules; may be accompanied by abdominal pain, fat necrosis in bone marrow, lungs, and other organs	Adenocarcinoma of pancreas	Effect of pancreatic enzymes released into circulation on fatty tissues	Usually associated with pancreatic disease but may be benign pancreatic disease
Porphyria cutanea tarda*	Weddington[431] Thompson[432]	Photosensitive skin lesions, often painful or pruritic	Liver	Increased porphyrins in skin tissues	Rare
Cushing's syndrome		Broad purple striae, atrophy, hyperpigmentation (uncommon), plethora, telangiectasia, mild hirsutism	Ectopic lung (small-cell), thyroid, testes, ovary, adrenal tumors; pancreatic islet cell, pituitary, other	Increased ACTH	
Addison's syndrome		Generalized hyperpigmentation, especially scars, pressure points, points of friction; increased amounts of hair	Adrenal gland invasion, lymphomas or carcinomas	Decreased glucocorticoids	Rarely caused by tumors invading the adrenal
Hirsutism			Adrenal tumors, ovarian tumors	Increased glucocorticoid, increased testosterone	Associated with virilism

*True paraneoplastic syndrome.

TABLE 55-18. Bullous and Urticarial Lesions

Disorders	Reference	Description	Predominant Malignancy	Etiology	Comments
Pemphigoid	Stone[433]	Large tense bullae with histologically absent acantholysis	Miscellaneous	Unknown	Although the clinical association of bullous pemphigoid and malignancy was once accepted, recent age-matched studies have failed to support the association
Dermatitis herpetiformis	Tobias[434] Helm[400]	Pleomorphic symmetric subepidermal bullae particularly with scarring	Lymphomas, miscellaneous	Related to autoantibodies	

Various studies report that 10% to 20% of cases may be associated with malignancy, particularly lymphomas. In some instances, the skin lesions are not paraneoplastic, as cutaneous infiltration of the skin can be documented by skin biopsy. In some instances, there is no demonstrable cutaneous tumor, and the condition may improve after therapy. In these instances the skin condition appears to be a true paraneoplastic syndrome. Although the mechanism in these cases is unknown, some have speculated that there is an immunologic response to some antigenic material derived from the tumor.[400]

Endocrine and Metabolic Lesions (Table 55-17) and Bullous and Urticarial Lesions (Table 55-18)

Important skin lesions associated with endocrine and metabolic tumors are systemic nodular panniculitus, with adenocarcinoma of the pancreas, and porphyria cutanea tarda, with hepatomas. The associations of malignancy with bullous and urticarial lesions are as yet unproved (Table 55-18).

Miscellaneous Lesions (Table 55-19)

The cutaneous lesions in dermatomyositis are characterized by purplish pink heliotrope erythema of the face with edema of the eyelids, with spread to the neck and arms. Erythematous purplish papules and plaques over the knuckles and interphalangeal joints (Grotton's sign) may be characteristic but usually occur late. All types of malignancies have been reported.[264–266,435] Overall, cancers are reported in 7% to 52% of patients with dermatomyositis. There are reports of dramatic improvement in dermatomyositis after antitumor therapy, supporting the concept of a true paraneoplastic syndrome.[266,435]

An important feature of paraneoplastic acquired ichthyosis is the rapid development of the lesions. The lesions are

TABLE 55-19. Miscellaneous Lesions

Disorder	Reference	Description	Predominant Malignancy	Etiology	Comments
Dermatomyositis*	Williams[466] Arundell[435] DeVere[264] Barnes[265]	Purplish pink erythema, especially of eyelids, neck, and hands	Miscellaneous	Unknown	Malignant disease reported in 7%–50%; precedes carcinoma by days–years with an average of 6 mo
Hypertrichosis languginosa* (malignant down)	Lyell[436] Hegedus[437]	Rapid development of fine, long, silky hair, especially on ears and forehead and may involve the entire body	Lung, colon, bladder, uterus, gall bladder	Unknown	High association with cancer
Acquired ichthyosis*	VanDijk[438] Flint[439]	Generalized dry, crackling skin, hyperkeratotic palms and soles, rhomboidal scales	Hodgkin's disease, other lymphomas, multiple myeloma, other	Unknown	Should be distinguished from hereditary form, which occurs before age 20

(continued)

TABLE 55-19. Miscellaneous Lesions (*continued*)

Disorder	*Reference*	*Description*	*Predominant Malignancy*	*Etiology*	*Comments*
Pachydermoperiostosis*	Vogl[440]	Thickening of skin and creation of new folds; thickened lips, ears, and lids; macroglossia; thick forehead and scalp; clubbing; excessive sweating	Lung (uterus)	Unknown	Occurs also in lung abscess and benign tumors
Pruritus*	Rajka[441] Cormia[442]	Failure to determine an overt or covert cutaneous cause of generalized pruritus necessitates evaluation for a possible underlying systemic disease.	Lymphomas, leukemias, multiple myelomas, CNS tumors, abdominal tumors	Unknown	Also associated with many benign diseases
Amyloid deposits		Macroglossia, pinch purpura, superficial waxy yellow and pink elevated nodules	Multiple myeloma, Waldenström's macro-globulinemia	Amyloid deposition in blood vessels and dermis	Also associated with primary systemic amyloid and other benign conditions
Herpes zoster	Schimpff[443] Dolin[444] Huberman[445]	Vesicular eruption in a dermatomal distribution	Hodgkin's disease, non-Hodgkin's lymphomas, chronic lymphocytic leukemia, small cell lung cancer	Immunosuppression	Increased incidence in cancers associated with immunosuppression and following severely immunosuppressive therapy
Caput medusa					
Thrombophlebitis					
Gynecomastia					

*True paraneoplastic syndrome.

characterized by generalized dry cracking skin with hyperkeratotic palms and soles. The acquired forms are associated most often with Hodgkin's disease and other malignant lymphomas, although associations with other solid tumors have been reported.[438,439] The acquired forms can be distinguished from genetic forms by the fact that the latter arise almost always before the age of 20. A parallel course of the malignant lymphoma and acquired ichthyosis has been reported in many patients.[439]

Hereditary Disorders

A large number of hereditary disorders associated with malignant disease and skin lesions of presumed paraneoplastic nature are summarized in Table 55-20.

GASTROINTESTINAL PARANEOPLASTIC SYNDROMES

The Zollinger–Ellison, carcinoid, and other syndromes resulting from hormone-producing endocrine tumors are discussed in Chapter 39. One of the most frequent of all the paraneoplastic syndromes is the malignancy associated anorexia and cachexia. The etiology for this syndrome was unidentified until recent studies suggest it may be caused by a tumor-secreted cytokine, tumor necrosis factor-α (TNFA; also known as cachectin).[8–11]

PROTEIN-LOSING ENTEROPATHIES ASSOCIATED WITH MALIGNANCY

More than 90% of cancer patients have low serum albumin levels.[412] Metabolic studies show that this can be due to decreased albumin synthesis; abnormal distribution of albumin in effusions; or increased loss of protein into the gastrointestinal tract (protein-losing enteropathy).[460] The most common mechanism is decreased albumin synthesis, but why this is so is not known.[460] Although patients usually either present with other signs of malignancy, unexplained edema and hypoproteinemia were the initial manifestations of malignancy in a few patients. The mechanisms of protein-losing enteropathy include inflammation and ulceration of the gastrointestinal mucosa and exudative loss of proteins; disorders of the intestinal lymphatic channels from neoplastic obstruction (seen with lymphomas); congestive failure (seen in patients with carcinoid or pericardial constriction) with resultant loss of protein and lymphocytes rich in lymph

TABLE 55-20. Hereditary Disorders

Disorders	*Reference*	*Description*	*Predominant Malignancy*	*Heredity*	*Comments*
Gardner's syndrome	Gardner[446] Bussey[447] Jones[448]	Epidermal cysts, sebaceous cysts, dermoid tumors, lipomas, fibromas	Adenocarcinoma of large or small bowel	Autosomal-dominant	Associated with polyposis of colon and bony exostoses
Peutz–Jeghers syndrome	Jeghers[449] Riley[450]	Pigmentation of lips, face, oral mucosa, and digits	GI adenocarcinomas	Autosomal-dominant	Low (2–3%) incidence
Tylosis (palmaris and plantaris)	Howel–Evans[451]	Hyperkeratosis of palms and soles after age 10	Esophageal carcinoma	Autosomal-dominant	95% incidence of carcinoma by age 65
Multiple mucosal neuromas	Williams[452]	Neuromas of eyelids, lips, tongue, and oral mucosa	Pheochromocytoma, medullary carcinoma of thyroid (MEA II)	Autosomal-dominant	Parathyroid adenomas, hypertension common
Cowden's disease—multiple hamartoma syndrome	Lloyd[435]	Fibromas of oral mucosa, acral venucous papulas, trichilemmomas of the face	Thyroid, breast carcinomas	Autosomal-dominant	Associated with multiple hamartomas, lipomas, neuromas, hemangiomas, thyroid adenomas
Multiple basal cell neuromas syndrome	Solomon[454]	Multiple basal cell carcinomas, pits on soles and palms	Medulloblastoma, fibrosarcoma (jaw)	Autosomal-dominant	Infrequent association with internal malignancy
Phakomatoses					
Neurofibromatosis (von Reck-linghausen)	Crowe[402]	Neurofibromas, café au lait	Pheochromocytoma	Autosomal-dominant	Malignancies develop in a minority of patients
Tuberous sclerosis (Bourneville)	Butterworth[455]	Lipopigmented macules, adenomas, fibromas	Neurologic malignancies	Autosomal-dominant	Malignancies develop in a minority of patients
Cerebelloretinal hemangioblastoma (von Hippel–Lindau)	Christoferson[456]	Retinal malformation, papilledema	Neurologic malignancies	Autosomal-dominant	Malignancies develop in a minority of patients
Encephalotrigeminal syndrome (Sturge–Weber)	Doll[457]	Capillary or cavernous hemangiomas within the cutaneous distribution of the trigeminal nerve	Neurologic malignancies	Autosomal-dominant	Malignancies develop in a minority of patients
Ataxia telangiectasia	Doll[457] Frizzera[458]	Telangiectasias	Lymphomas, leukemias	Autosomal-recessive	IgA ± IgE deficiency; Sinopulmonary infections, tumors in < 10%
Bloom's syndrome	Helm[402]	Photosensitivity, telangiectasias, erythema of face	Leukemia	Autosomal-recessive	Stunted growth, high incidence
Fanconi's anemia	Helm[400]	Patchy hyper-pigmentation	Leukemias	Autosomal-recessive	High incidence
Chédiak–Higashi syndrome	Doll[456]	Recurrent pyoderma, giant melanosomes, dilution of skin and hair color	Lymphomas	Autosomal-recessive	High incidence
Werner's syndrome (adult progeria)	Epstein[459]	Scleroderma-like changes, premature aging, leg ulcers, short stature	Sarcomas, meningiomas, others	Autosomal-recessive	Cancers in about 10%
Wiskott–Aldrich syndrome	Doll[457] Frizzeria[458]	Eczematous dermatitis, pyroderma	Lymphomas	Sex-linked, (males)	>10% incidence
Bruton's sex-linked agammaglobulinemia	Helm[400]	Recurrent infections	Lymphoma, leukemias	Sex-linked	>5% incidence

into the gastrointestinal lumen; and a group of undefined mechanisms. The resulting hypoalbuminemia leads to edema, and the lymphopenia gives decreased cellular immunity with impaired skin test reactivity.[460] Although these syndromes may not fulfill all of the criteria for paraneoplastia (that is, acting at a distance from the tumor), anecdotal case reports indicate that protein-losing enteropathy can be reversed by appropriate treatment of the underlying tumor. Profuse watery diarrhea, hypokalemia, and hypochlorhydria usually are associated with pancreatic non-β-islet cell tumors or villous adenomas of the rectum. In addition, this syndrome can be found in patients with lung cancer; however, the mechanism is unknown.[461]

Malabsorption

Malabsorption syndromes for several or specific substances may occur by a variety of mechanisms in cancer patients, including side-effects of surgery, irradiation, and chemotherapy. Malabsorption often is associated with lymphoma involving the small bowel or with gastric, hepatic, or biliary tract tumors, particularly if biliary obstruction is present. These examples are not "remote effects" of the tumor. However, some malabsorption syndromes may be paraneoplastic, as suggested by finding histologic abnormalities of the small bowel in up to 62% of various cancers in some studies.[462–464] Although the exact frequency of various histologic types is unknown, the histologic abnormalities include "flat" mucosa with simple or partial villous atrophy. Subtotal villous atrophy is less common. However, the severity of associated malabsorption does not correlate with the severity of the small-bowel histologic changes.[462] The tumors associated with small-bowel abnormalities have been colon, lung, prostate, pancreas, and lymphomas, as well as other tumors. The mechanisms behind the loss of villous height are unknown. Treatment should be directed at the underlying tumor, plus administration of exogenous nutrients and vitamins to bypass the malabsorption.

HEPATOPATHY AS A PARANEOPLASTIC SYNDROME

An elevated hepatic alkaline phosphatase level has occurred with a malignant schwannoma and disappeared with surgical resection.[465] This also can be seen in hypernephroma, in which there can be reversible abnormalities of liver function not associated with liver metastases.[465–468] Decreased albumin synthesis will rise to normal after resection of the renal tumor. Biochemical abnormalities, such as elevated alkaline phosphatase levels or hyperglobulinemia, hypocholesterolemia, and prolonged prothrombin time, as well as hepatosplenomegaly, have disappeared after primary tumor removal in four of six patients.[466,468] The mechanisms for the hepatopathy associated with hypernephroma are unknown, but that may include hepatic amyloid or be related to either the generalized hepatic hypervascularity seen on angiography or the nonspecific focal periportal inflammation seen on biopsy.[466,467,469] It is important to recognize the hepatopathy syndrome so that these signs will not be confused with metastases to the liver. Thus, biopsy confirmation of liver metastases from renal carcinoma is highly desirable if this metastatic site alone would preclude resection of the primary renal tumor for cure.

ANOREXIA, CACHEXIA, AND TASTE ABNORMALITIES AS PARANEOPLASTIC MANIFESTATIONS

Problems with anorexia, taste, weight loss, and cachexia are common in cancer patients.[470,476] One-third or more of cancer patients are in negative nitrogen balance; they can even be in positive nitrogen balance and still maintain a caloric deficit.[472] The syndrome comprises anorexia, cachexia, asthenia, loss of body tissue, and inability to conserve normal regulatory functions of metabolism and bears no correlation to the amount, type, or site of neoplastic tissue.[473] It can occur as an early symptom of disease or appear in the presence of bulk neoplasms. The best evidence of the paraneoplastic nature of the anorexia–cachexia syndrome comes when it appears before the malignancy is discovered and disappears with the resection or control of the tumor.[472] Obviously, cancer patients can have these symptoms as a result of therapy toxicity, gross invasion, or obstruction of structures by tumor. Cachexia may result from decreased caloric intake, malabsorption, loss of material from the body (*e.g.*, from effusions, hemorrhage, ulcers), or a change in the body metabolism. Anorexia and taste changes may result in decreased caloric intake. However, a variety of experimental evidence suggests that malnutrition alone cannot explain the cachexia of malignancy.[472] Thus, in malignancy and cachexia, the caloric expenditure remains high, and the basal metabolic rate is increased despite the reduced dietary intake, indicating a profound systemic derangement of host metabolism.[472] These findings are in contrast to the lower metabolic rates and adaptation that normal subjects make after starvation.[473] In normal subjects with starvation, the caloric expenditure is lowered, amino acids cease being used for gluconeogenesis, and exogenous glucose is readily oxidized, whereas it is not in malignancy. In addition, protein synthesis is maintained in malignancy rather than reduced as in starvation.

Recent experimental studies demonstrated that circulatory factors could produce cancer anorexia–cachexia.[474] Other studies demonstrated that the cytokines, TNFα and IL-1β, could produce a similar syndrome in experimental animals.[475] Tumor necrosis factor-α was shown to be identical with cachectin.[8–11] This cytokine inhibits lipoprotein lipase activity in peripheral tissues and may orchestrate the metabolic changes leading to tumor cachexia–anorexia. Aversion to meats and other protein-containing food frequently occurs in cancer patients. DeWys found that 16 of 50 cancer patients of various types had an aversion to meat; this was correlated with a lowered threshold for bitter taste (urea).[471] In addition, these patients had elevated thresholds for sweet (sucrose) substances. The taste abnormalities were correlated with a patient's body burden of tumor and then normalized after response to treatment.[471]

In addition to taste, the regulation of hunger and satiety is complex and involves a CNS "satiety" center in the ventromedial nuclei of the hypothalmus and a "feeding" center in the lateral hypothalamic nuclei.[472] Also, alimentary tract regulation; glucostatic, lipostatic, thermostatic, and osmotic regulation; hormone regulation by insulin; regulation of growth hormone, glucagon, enterogastrone, adrenal corticosteroids, amino acid levels, and of an as yet unidentified anorexigenic pituitary polypeptides take place.[479] Thus, it appears likely that mechanisms underlying the paraneoplastic anorexia–cachexia syndrome involve molecules produced by the tumor that then impinge on one or more of the regulatory mechanisms of hunger, satiety, metabolism, or taste and cause the organism to falsely disrupt these patterns and thus enter into a metabolic "chaotic" state.[472] The treatment of the underlying tumor appears to be the best general approach to reversing the state of cancer cachexia.

MISCELLANEOUS PARANEOPLASTIC SYNDROMES

FEVER AS A PARANEOPLASTIC SYNDROME

Fever occurs frequently in cancer patients and usually is caused by infection. Although other noninfectious causes (such as drug toxicity and adrenal insufficiency) exist, certain tumors are associated with fever.[477] Of 351 cancer patients, Petersdorf found that 30% developed fever and 5% had fever that could be related only to their cancer.[494] The major associations are with Hodgkin's disease, myxomas, hypernephromas, osteogenic sarcomas, and a variety of other tumors.[478,479] Tumor-associated fever usually is defined as unexplained fever that coincides with tumor growth, disappears promptly on tumor removal or control, and reappears with tumor regrowth. Alternatively, when the fever persists with uncontrolled tumor without any other reasonable cause, the tumor is a likely cause of the fever.[477] In Hodgkin's disease, fever as a systemic symptom suggests a worse prognosis stage-by-stage, and its disappearance is required to document remission of tumor and subsequent cure (see Chap. 49). There are no data about the influence on prognosis of fever associated with other tumors.

The etiology of the tumor-associated fever could come from release of pyrogen from tumor cells, normal leukocytes, or a variety of other normal cells that have been demonstrated to have "endogenous" pyrogen. For example, the Kupffer cells of the liver contain endogenous pyrogen that could cause fever with hepatoma or with metastases to the liver from other tumors.[480] The pyrogen acts on the hypothalamus to cause some reset of temperature regulation. Tumor cells can produce pyrogen as well. Bodel showed that five of six hypernephromas placed in vitro released pyrogen into the supernatant medium (detected by injection into a rabbit).[477] Similarly, spleen and lymph node tissue from Hodgkin's disease patients produced pyrogen when cultured into the medium in vitro. However, pyrogen production, although correlated with lymph node involvement, did not correlate with histologic involvement of the spleen or with fever in the patient.[477] It is still unknown whether tumor cells themselves or other normal cells mixed in the incubated specimens produce the pyrogen. Treatment should be directed at the underlying tumor, and the most dramatic remissions of paraneoplastic fever come in successfully treated patients with Hodgkin's disease or hypernephroma.

LACTIC ACIDOSIS

Lactic acidosis usually is associated with acute lymphatic or myelogenous leukemia, Hodgkin's disease, and other lymphomas and responds in parallel with tumor regression to therapy.[481–483] Often bicarbonate therapy is also needed.

HYPERLIPIDEMIA

Hyperlipidemia frequently is seen in lymphoma-bearing hamsters and normalizes after tumor treatment.[480] Hyperlipidemias also have been seen in multiple myeloma, hepatoma, and color cancer.[484–486] Total lipid levels of 2 g/dl, cholesterol levels above 500 mg/dl, and triglyceride levels of 580 mg/dl have been found. However, no associated vascular abnormalities have been reported. With myeloma, monoclonal proteins sometimes have reacted with α- or β-lipoproteins or with lipolytic enzymes. The mechanism in the other tumor types is obscure but could involve invasion by tumor.

HYPERTENSION–HYPOTENSION

Malignant hypertension and hypokalemia associated with apparent tumor production of renin have been reported with lung cancer, hypernephroma, and Wilms' tumor.[487–490] Hypertension recedes with control of the tumor.

An antihypertension syndrome has been seen with a prostaglandin–A-secreting renal cell tumor, and abnormally low baroreceptor pressure responses have been seen with intrathoracic carcinomas.[491,492] The latter syndrome appears related to interference of transmission of impulses from intrathoracic stretch receptors, resulting in orthostatic hypotension and abnormalities of sodium excretion.

AMYLASE ELEVATION

Synthesis and secretion of amylase by tumors are uncommon; the tumors have all been lung cancer, usually of the adenocarcinoma variety.[493] These tumors make the salivary type of amylase, which allows distinction from a pancreatic source of the amylase elevation. The amylase itself apparently does not cause symptoms, but its appearance can lead to great concern and medical evaluation for the presence of pancreatitis or various types of pancreatic fistulas, when in reality the amylase is produced by the tumor cells.[493]

HYPERTROPHIC PULMONARY OSTEOARTHROPATHY

Hypertrophic pulmonary osteoarthropathy (HPO) is a paraneoplastic syndrome comprising clubbing of the fingers and toes, periostitis of the long bones, and sometimes a polyarthritis resembling rheumatoid arthritis.[494–497] Periostitis–arthritis produces joint pains in the knees, wrists, and ankles with pain, tenderness, and swelling of the affected bones. Involved bones usually include the distal ends of the tibia, fibula, humerus, radius, or ulna. Hyperemia of the affected joints or hands and feet is also seen.[494] The syndrome may precede the discovery of the neoplasm by several months and usually has a fairly defined onset. Often patients do not present with clubbing but appear with joint pain or polyarthritis, and in adult patients presenting with unexplained polyarthritis or joint pain, the HPO syndrome should be kept in mind.[494] Pathologic examination of the joints may show pannus formation; however, most joints show only hyperemia.[494] If polyarthritis is present, joint effusions, particularly of the knees, with noninflammatory synovial fluid and good mucin clot are present. Ossifying periostitis is seen on roentgenogram at the distal end of the shafts of long bones as a thin opaque line of new bone formation, separated from the underlying denser cortex by a narrow radiolucent band. Radionuclide bone scans often are positive over the bones involved with periostitis before the other radiologic changes appear.[498] In advanced cases, other bones (*e.g.*, the ribs, clavicle, iliac crests, and vertebral column) may be involved.

Hypertrophic pulmonary osteoarthropathy is encountered most frequently in lung cancer, occurring in 12% of patients with adenocarcinoma and less frequently in other cell types; HPO is almost nonexistent in small-cell lung cancer.[499,500] Of interest, the HPO syndrome occurs often with benign mesothelioma and the rare neurolemmomas of the diaphragm, whereas malignant mesotheliomas are said never to produce HPO.[494] Other tumors metastatic to the chest can cause HPO, including metastases from renal cancer, thymoma, leiomyoma of the esophagus, intrathoracic Hodgkin's disease, osteogenic sarcoma, fibrosarcoma, and the undifferentiated nasopharyngeal tumors of young people when the tumors metastasize to mediastinal lymph nodes.[501-507]

The diagnosis is made by physical findings, radionuclide bone scan, and radiographic appearance of the bones. Although benign causes have to be considered, the bone changes of hyperparathyroidism can simulate HPO and should be ruled out, although it is possible for HPO and ectopic PTH to coexist. The etiology is unknown, although estrogens, circulatory factors, neurogenic factors, and growth hormone have been postulated to play a role.[452,457,508-510]

AMYLOIDOSIS (PARANEOPLASTIC β-FIBRILS)

Amyloid deposition is a pathologic process whose manifestations depend on the formation of a specific, unique protein conformation—the twisted β-pleated sheet fibril.[511] Histochemically, these fibrils have green polarization color after Congo red staining. This structure normally is not found in mammalian tissues and can occur with a variety of proteins produced by several different pathogenic mechanisms. Immunoglobulin fragments produced by plasma cell dyscrasias are the most common neoplastic mechanism. Because of the β-pleated structure, the fibrils are very resistant to normal proteolytic digestion under physiologic conditions and thus accumulate as inert fibriils in tissues. This results in pressure atrophy, morbidity, and death from interference of normal physiologic processes of the affected vital organs (heart, kidneys, nerves, joints).

Although amyloidosis may have several nonmalignant causes, 15% of cases occur with malignant disease, including multiple myeloma, lymphomas, and carcinomas.[511,513] Amyloid occurs in 6% to 15% of multiple myeloma and Waldenström's macroglobulinemia, in 4% of Hodgkin's disease, and 1% of other lymphomas, and probably all B-cell lymphomas can give rise to amyloidosis. Carcinomas associated with amyloidosis are hypernephromas, bladder and renal pelvic cancer, uterine cervix cancer, and biliary tract cancer.[512] Hypernephroma is reported to represent more than 25% of all tumors associated with amyloidosis, but the nature of the protein in the amyloid deposit of hypernephromas is unknown.[511,512]

The "amyloidogenic" protein can be monoclonal light chains (designated AL) or other proteins (designated AA).[511] Amyloid fibrils from medullary carcinoma of the thyroid contain part of the calcitonin molecule; thus peptides produced by several tumors, if they contain sequences that can form β-pleated sheets, may cause amyloid.[511] In amyloidosis with multiple myeloma, usually Bence Jones proteinuria is present, and the occurrence is higher in free light-chain myeloma.[511]

The signs and symptoms of amyloidosis of malignancy, particularly with myeloma, are a peripheral neuropathy (painful stocking-glove), autonomic nervous symptoms of sexual impotence, gastrointestinal motility disturbances, orthostatic hypotension, and dyshidrosis.[511] Motor function is impaired from median nerve entrapment, and weight loss is frequent. A restrictive cardiomyopathy, with signs and symptoms of right heart failure with only minimal radiographic evidence of cardiomegaly, occurs. Low voltage ECG changes, arrhythmias, conduction disturbances, and ECG pattern-simulating myocardial infarction may occur. The patients are extremely sensitive to digitalis, and several toxic deaths from this have been reported. Pinch purpura, periorbital purpura after procedures, macroglossia, waxy cutaneous papules, subcutaneous nodules, alopecia, and scleroderma-like skin infiltration may occur. Joint infiltration often gives painless limitation of range of motion. The large joints are affected in amyloid arthropathy, and the "shoulder pad" sign develops, with massive infiltration of the glenohumeral articulation. Carpal and tarsal tunnel syndromes occur with infiltration of these regions.

The diagnosis of amyloid is made by the demonstration of the characteristic emerald-green birefringence of tissue specimens stained by Congo red and examined by polarization microscopy.[511] Biopsies of infiltrated lesions, gingiva, skin, bone marrow, or rectum can be used. The prognosis of clinically evident amyloidosis with malignancy is poor and, in myeloma, median survival from diagnosis is 14 months or less.[511] This is not good evidence that treatment of myeloma or other neoplastic disorders will reverse the amyloid already deposited, but it probably will halt amyloid progression. Supportive care problems abound as the congestive heart failure from amyloid does not respond to digitalis. (It is said that all amyloid patients when being started on digitalis therapy, should be hospitalized because of potential toxicity.) Diuretics can cause dehydration and cardiovascular collapse because of concurrent renal damage, postural hypotension, adrenal insufficiency, autonomic neuropathy, and low cardiac output. Mineralocorticoids, elastic stockings, broad-spectrum antibiotics for bacterial overgrowth in bowel with disturbed motility, gastrostomy and tracheostomy for macroglossia, hemodialysis, and surgical decompression of carpal tunnel syndrome have all been used.[511]

PALMAR FASCIITIS AND ARTHRITIS (REFLEX SYMPATHETIC DYSTROPHY/SHOULDER-HAND SYNDROME)

The shoulder-hand syndrome, a variant of reflex sympathetic dystrophy has been reported with malignancy.[514-516] Brain and lung cancers were reported most often, although cancers of the bladder, uterus, breast, and esophagus were also described. Palmar fasciitis and arthritis associated with ovarian carcinoma have more dramatic and progressive findings with complete loss of upper extremity function and contracture. The severe syndrome has been reported in patients with small-cell lung cancer, adenocarcinoma of the pancreas, CML, and Hodgkin's disease. The etiology is unknown but immunoglobulin deposits were found in the fascial tissue of one patient, suggesting an immunologic cause. The syndrome often preceded the diagnosis of malignancy and improved after successful antitumor therapy.

ARTHRITIS, POLYMYALGIA RHEUMATICA, SYSTEMIC LUPUS ERYTHEMATOSUS

Rheumatoid arthritis, or an asymmetric polyarthritis, may occur with malignancy or may be related by chance.[4,517-519] Joint manifestations are said to regress on removal or control of the underlying malignancy in 48% of patients. Some 80% of female patients with asymmetric polyarthritis and malignancy had breast cancer. Some 83% of patients with polymyalgia rheumatica are said to develop a malignancy within 3 months, and some of these cases may represent arterial emboli to muscle from nonbacterial thrombotic endocarditis. Lymphomas may be associated with systemic rheumatic disease.[519,520] In Sjögren's syndrome, a spectrum of benign to malignant lymphoproliferation can be seen, but whether this is "at a distance from the tumor" remains to be determined.[521] It is also important to remember that metastases to joints can simulate rheumatoid arthritis, and cytologic studies should be done on joint effusions in cancer patients.[522,523] Systemic lupus erythematosus (SLE) is associated with lymphomas, lymphoblastic leukemia, thymomas, testicular and ovarian tumors, and lung cancer, and remission of the SLE is said to occur with tumor treatment.[521,524]

REFERENCES

1. Hall TC (ed): Paraneoplastic syndromes. Ann NY Acad Sci 230:1-577, 1974
2. Odell WD, Wolfsen AR: Humoral syndromes associated with cancer. Ann Rev Med 29:379-406, 1978
3. Blackman MR, Rosen SW, Weintraub BD: Ectopic hormones. Adv Intern Med 23:85-113, 1978
4. Shneider BS, Manalo A: Paraneoplastic syndromes. Unusual manifestations of malignant disease. DM Feb: 1-60, 1979
5. Markman M: Response of paraneoplastic syndromes to antineoplastic therapy. West J Med 144:580-585, 1986
6. Ascensao JL, Oken MM, Ewing SL et al: Leukocytosis and large cell lung cancer. A frequent association. Cancer 60:903-905, 1987
7. Hocking W, Goodman J, Golde D: Granulocytosis associated with tumor cell production of colony stimulating activity. Blood 61:600-603, 1983
8. Ellis DL, Kafka SP, Chow JC et al: Melanoma, growth factors, acanthosis nigricans, the sign of Leser-Trelat, and multiple acrochordons. A possible role of alpha-transforming growth factor in cutaneous paraneoplastic syndromes. N Engl J Med 317:1582-1587, 1987
9. Beutler B, Greenwald D, Hulmes JD et al: Identity of tumor necrosis factor and the macrophage-secreted factor cachectin. Nature 316:552-554, 1985
10. Torti FM, Dieckmann B, Beutler B et al: A macrophage factor inhibits adipocyte gene expression: An in vitro model of cachexia. Science 229:867-870, 1985
11. Theologides A: Anorexins, asthenins, and cachectins in cancer. Am J Med 81:696-698, 1986
12. Greenlee JE, Lipton HL: Anticerebellar antibodies in serum and cerebrospinal fluid of a patient with oat cell carcinoma of the lung and paraneoplastic cerebellar degeneration. Ann Neurol 19:82-85, 1986
13. Grunwald GB, Kornguth SE, Towfighi J et al: Autoimmune basis for visual paraneoplastic syndrome in patients with small cell lung carcinoma. Cancer 60:780-786, 1987
14. Graus F, Elkon KB, Cordon-Cardo C, Posner J: Sensory neuronopathy and small cell lung cancer. Antineuronal antibody that also reacts with the tumor. Am J Med 80:45-52, 1986
15. Fukunaga H, Engel AG, Lang B et al: Passive transfer of Eaton-Lambert myasthenic syndrome with IgG from man to mouse depletes the presynaptic membrane active zones. Proc Natl Acad Sci USA 80:7636-7640, 1983
16. Richardson EP: Progressive multifocal leukoencephalopathy. In Vinken PJ, Bruryn GW (eds): Handbook of Clinical Neurology, pp 485-499. Amsterdam, North-Holland, 1970
17. Wiener LP, Henden RM, Narayan O et al: Virus related to SV40 in patients with progressive multifocal leukoencephalopathy. N Engl J Med 286:385-390, 1972
18. Croft P, Wilkinson M: The incidence of carcinomatous neuromyopathy in patients with various types of carcinoma. Brain 88:427-434, 1965
19. Wilner EC, Brody JA: An evaluation of the remote effects of cancer on the nervous system. Neurology 18:1120-1124, 1967
20. DeLarco JE, Todaro GJ: Growth factors from murine sarcoma virus-transformed cells. Proc Natl Acad Sci USA 75:4001-4005, 1978
21. Waldenström JG: Paraneoplasia, Biological Signals in Diagnosis of Cancer. New York, John Wiley & Sons, 1978
22. Odell WD, Wolfsen AR: Hormones from tumors: Are they ubiquitous? Am J Med 68:317-318, 1980
23. Lees LH: The biosynthesis of hormones by nonendocrine tumours-a review. J Endocrinol 67:143-175, 1975
24. Kreiger DT, Martin JB: Brain peptides. N Engl J Med 304:876-885, 1981
25. Kreiger DT: Brain peptides: What, where, and why? Science 222:975-985, 1983
26. Moody TW, Pert CS, Gazdar AF et al: High levels of intracellular bombesin characterize human small-cell lung carcinoma. Science 214:1246-1248, 1981
27. Maurer LH, O'Donnell JF, Kennedy S et al: Human neurophysins in carcinoma of the lung. Relation to histology, disease stage, response rate, survival and syndrome of inappropriate antidiuretic hormone secretion. Cancer Treat Rep 67:971-976, 1983
28. Lazarus LH, DiAugustine RP, Jahnke CD, Hernandez O: Physalaemin: An amphibian tachykinin in human lung small cell carcinoma. Science 219:79-81, 1983
29. Richardson RL, Greco FA, Oldhan RK, Liddle GW: Tumor products and potential markers in small cell lung cancer. Semin Oncol 5:253-262, 1978
30. Gropp C, Havemann K, Scheuer A: Ectopic hormones in lung cancer patients at diagnosis and during therapy. Cancer 46:347-354, 1980
31. Hansen M, Hansen HH, Hirsch FR et al: Hormonal polypeptides and amine metabolites in small cell carcinoma of the lung, with special reference to stage and subtypes. Cancer 45:1432-1437, 1980
32. Odell WD: Wolfsen AR, Bachelot I, Hirose FM: Ectopic production of lipotropin by cancer. Am J Med 66:631-638, 1979
33. Roos BA, Lindall AW, Ells J et al: Increased plasma and tumor somatostatin-like immunoreactivity in medullary thyroid carcinoma and small cell lung cancer. J Clin Endocrinol Metab 52:187-194, 1981
34. Yamaguchi K, Abe K, Kameya T et al: Production and molecular size heterogeneity of immunoreactive gastrin-releasing peptide in fetal and adult lungs and primary lung tumors. Cancer Res 43:3932-3939, 1983
35. Carney DN, Ihde DC, Cohen MH et al: Serum neuron-specific enolase: A marker for disease extent and response to therapy of small cell lung cancer. Lancet 1:583-585, 1982
36. Nakanishi S, Inoue A, Kita T et al: Nucleotide sequence of cloned cDNA for bovine corticotropin-β-lipotropin precursor. Nature 278:423-427, 1979
37. Bertagna XY, Nicholson WE, Pettengill OS et al: Corticotropin, lipotropin, and β-endophin production by a human nonpituitary tumor in culture: Evidence for a common precursor. Proc Natl Acad Sci USA 75:5160-5164, 1978
38. Jeffcoate WJ, Rees LH: Adrenocorticotropin and related peptides in nonendocrine tumors. Curr Top Exp Endocrinol 3:57-74, 1978
39. Guillemin R: Endorphins, brain peptides that act like opiates. N Engl J Med 296:226-228, 1977
40. Huges J: Opioid peptides and their relatives. Nature 278:394-395, 1979
41. Silman RE, Holland D, Chard T et al: The ACTH "family tree" of the rheusus monkey changes with development. Nature 276:526-528, 1978
42. Hirata Y, Yamamoto H, Matsukura S, Imura H: In vitro release and biosynthesis of tumor ACTH in ectopic ACTH producing tumors. J Clin Endocrinol Metab 41:106-114, 1975
43. Brown WH: A case of pluriglandular syndrome: Diabetes of bearded women. Lancet 2:1022-1023, 1928
44. Rassam JW, Anderson G: Incidence of paramalignant disorders in bronchogenic carcinoma. Thorax 30:86-90, 1975
45. Ross EJ: Endocrine syndromes of non-endocrine origin: Cancer and the adrenal cortex. Proc R Soc Med 59:335-338, 1966
46. Lokich JJ: The frequency and clinical biology of the ectopic hormone syndromes of small cell carcinoma. Cancer 50:2111-2114, 1982

47. Singer W, Kovacs K, Ryan N, Horvath E: Ectopic ACTH syndrome. Clinicopathological correlation. J Clin Pathol 31:591–598, 1978
48. Abeloff MD, Trump DL, Baylin SB: Ectopic adrenocorticotrophic (ACTH) syndrome and small cell carcinoma of the lung: Assessment of clinical implications in patients on combination chemotherapy. Cancer 48:1082–1087, 1981
49. Yallow RS, Eastridge CE, Higgins G Jr, Wolf J: Plasma and tumor ACTH in carcinoma of the lung. Cancer 44:1789–1792, 1979
50. Wolfsen AR, Odell WD: ProACTH: Use for early detection of lung cancer. Am J Med 66:765–772, 1979
51. Liddle GW, Island D, Meador CK: Normal and abnormal regulation of corticotropin secretion in man. Recent Prog Horm Res 18:125–166, 1962
52. Ayvazian LF, Schneider B, Gewirtz G, Yalow RS: Ectopic production of big ACTH in carcinoma of the lung. Its clinical usefulness as a biologic marker. Am Rev Respir Dis 3:279–287, 1975
53. Ratcliff JG, Knight RA, Besser GM: Tumour and plasma ACTH concentrations in patients with and without the ectopic ACTH syndrome. Clin Endocrinol 1:27–44, 1972
54. Gewirtz G, Yalow RS: Ectopic ACTH production in carcinoma of the lung. J Clin Invest 53:1022–1032, 1974
55. Abe K, Adachi I, Miyakawa S et al: Production of calcitonin, adrenocorticotropic hormone, and β-melanocyte stimulating hormone in tumors derived from amine precursors uptake and decarboxylation cells. Cancer Res 37:4100–4194, 1977
56. Bloomfield GA, Holdaway IM, Corrin B et al: Lung tumours and ACTH production. Clin Endocrinol 6:95–104, 1977
57. Gilby ED, Rees LH, Bondy PK: Ectopic hormones as markers of response to therapy in cancer. In Proceedings of the Sixth International Symposium of Biological Characterizations of Human Tumors, pp 132–138. Amsterdam, American Elsevier, 1976
58. Amatruda TT, Upton GV: Hyperadrenocorticism and ACTH-releasing factor. Ann NY Acad Sci 230:168–180, 1974
59. Eagan RT, Maurer LH, Forcier RJ, Tulloh M: Small cell carcinoma of the lung: Staging, paraneoplastic syndromes, treatment and survival. Cancer 33:527–532, 1974
60. Azzopardi JG, Williams ED: Pathology of "nonendocrine" tumors associated with Cushing's syndrome. Cancer 22:273–286, 1968
61. Skrabanek P, Powell D: Unifying concept of non-pituitary ACTH secreting tumors: Evidence of common origin of neural-crest tumors, carcinoids, and oat-cell carcinomas. Cancer 42:1263–1269, 1978
62. Lojek MA, Fer MF, Kasselberg AG et al: Cushing's syndrome with small cell carcinoma of the uterine cervix. Am J Med 69:140–144, 1980
63. Matsuyama M, Inoue T, Ariyoshi Y et al: Argyrophil cell carcinoma of the uterine cervix with ectopic production of ACTH, β-MSH, serotonin, histamine, and amylase. Cancer 44:1813–1823, 1979
64. Levenson RM, Ihde DC, Matthews MJ et al: Small cell carcinoma arising in extrapulmonary sites: Response to chemotherapy. Proc AACR–ASCO 21:143, 1980
65. Fer MF, Oldham RK, Richardson RL et al: Extrapulmonary small cell carcinoma. Proc AACR–ASCO 21:475, 1980
66. Rees LH, Ratcliffe JG: Ectopic hormone production by nonendocrine tumors. Clin Endocrinol 3:263–299, 1974
67. Bailey RE: Periodic "hormonogenesis"—a new phenomenon. Periodicity in function of a hormone-producing tumor in man. Clin Endocrinol 32:317–327, 1971
68. Gold EM: The Cushing syndromes: Changing views of diagnosis and treatment. Ann Intern Med 90:829–844, 1979
69. Howlett TA, Perry L, Rees LH et al: Diagnosis and management of ACTH dependent Cushing's syndrome: Comparison of the features in ectopic and pituitary ACTH production. Clin Endocrinol 24:699–713, 1986
70. Hattori M, Imura H, Matsukura S et al: Multiple hormone-producing lung carcinoma. Cancer 43:2429–2437, 1979
71. Mason AMS, Ratcliffe JA, Buckly RM, Mason AS: ACTH secretion by bronchial carcinoid tumors. Clin Endocrinol 1:3–25, 1972
72. Imura H, Matsukura S, Yamamoto H et al: Studies on ectopic ACTH-producing tumors. II. Clinical and biochemical features of 30 cases. Cancer 35:1430–1437, 1975
73. Corey RM, Varma SK, Drake CR et al: Ectopic secretion of corticotropin-releasing factor as a cause of Cushing's syndrome. A clinical, morphologic and biochemical study. N Engl J Med 311:13, 1984
74. Belsky JL, Cuello B, Swanson LW et al: Cushing's syndrome due to ectopic production of corticotropin-releasing factor. J Clin Endocrinol Metab 60:496, 1985
75. Schleingart DE, Lloyd RV, Akil H et al: Cushing's syndrome secondary to ectopic corticotropin-releasing hormone—adrenocorticotropin secretion. J Clin Endocrinol Metab 63:770, 1986
76. Orth DN, Liddle GW: Results of treatment of 108 patients with Cushing's syndrome. N Engl J Med 285:243–247, 1971
77. Gordon P, Becker CE, Levey GS, Roth J: Efficacy of aminoglutethimide in the ectopic ACTH syndrome. J Clin Endocrinol Metab 28:921–923, 1968
78. Carey RM, Orth DN, Hartmann WH: Malignant melanoma with ectopic production of adrenocorticotrophic hormone: Palliative treatment with inhibitors of adrenal steroid biosynthesis. J Clin Endocrinol Metab 36:482–487, 1973
79. Vaughn CB, Pearson S, Chapman J et al: The treatment of ACTH paraneoplastic syndrome with aminoglutethimide. J Natl Med Assoc 71:21–23, 1979
80. Child DF, Burke CW, Burley DM et al: Drug control of Cushing's syndrome. Combined aminoglutethiamide and metapyrone therapy. Acta Endocrinol 82:330–341, 1976
81. Naber D, Pickar D, Dionne RA et al: Assay of endogenous opiate receptor ligands in human CSF and plasma. Subst Alcohol Actions–Misuse 1:83–91, 1980
82. Gropp C, Havemann K, Scharfe T, Ax W: Incidence of circulating immune complexes in patients with lung cancer and their effect on antibody dependent cytotoxicity. Oncology 37:71–76, 1980
83. Winkler WA, Crankshaw OF: Chloride depletion in conditions other than Addison's disease. J Clin Invest 17:1–6, 1938
84. Schwartz WDF, Bennett W, Curelop S, Bartter F: A syndrome of renal sodium loss and hyponatremia probably resulting from inappropriate secretion of antidiuretic hormone. Am J Med 23:529–542, 1957
85. Amatruda TT, Mulrow PJ, Gallagher JC, Sawyer WH: Carcinoma of the lung with inappropriate antidiuresis. N Engl J Med 269:544–549, 1963
86. Hamilton BPM, Upton GV, Amatruda TT: Evidence for the presence of neurophysins in tumors producing the syndrome of inappropriate antidiuresis. J Clin Endocrinol Metab 35:764–767, 1972
87. Cheng KW, Friesen HG: Physiological factors regulating secretion of neurophysin. Metabolism 19:876–890, 1970
88. Kennedy SS, Maurer LH, O'Donnell JF, North WG: Human neurophysins in small cell cancer of the lung. Proc AACR–ASCO 21:324, 1980
89. Trump DL, Baylin SB: Ectopic hormone syndromes. In Abeloff MD (ed): Complications of Cancer: Diagnosis and Management, pp 211–241. Baltimore, Johns Hopkins University Press 1979
90. Moses AM, Miller M, Streeten DHP: Pathophysiologic and pharmacologic alterations in the release and action of ADH. Metabolism 25:697–721, 1976
91. Goodman LS, Gilman A, Gilman AG, Koelle GB: The Pharmacological Basis Of Therapeutics, 5th ed. New York, Toronto, London, MacMillan, 1975
92. Fichman M, Bethune J: Effects of neoplasms on renal electrolyte function. Ann NY Acad Sci 230:448–472, 1974
93. Padfield PL, Morton JJ, Brown JJ et al: Plasma arginine vasopressin in the syndrome of antidiuretic hormone excess associated with bronchogenic carcinoma. Am J Med 61:825–831, 1976
94. Harlow PJ, DeClerck YA, Shore NA et al: A fatal case of inappropriate ADH secretion induced by cyclophosphamide therapy. Cancer 44:896–898, 1979
95. DeFronzo RA, Braine H, Colvin OM, Davis PJ: Water intoxication in man after cyclophosphamide therapy: Time course and relation to drug activation. Ann Intern Med 78:861–869, 1973
96. Thomas TH, Morgan DB, Swaminathan R et al: Severe hyponatremia. Lancet 1:621–624, 1978
97. Radice PA, Dermody WC: Clonal heterogeneity of hormone produced by continuous cultures of small cell carcinoma of the lung. Proc AACR–ASCO 21:41, 1980
98. Pettengill OS, Caulkner CS, Wurster-Hill DH et al: Isolation and characterization of a hormone-producing cell line from human small cell anaplastic carcinoma of the lung. J Natl Cancer Inst 58:511–518, 1977
99. Hainsworth JD, Workman R, Greco FA: Management of the syndrome of inappropriate antidiuretic hormone secretion in small cell lung cancer. Cancer 51:161–165, 1983
100. Comis RL, Miller M, Ginsberg SJ: Abnormalities in water homeostasis in small cell anaplastic lung cancer. Cancer 45:2414–2421, 1980
101. Munro AHG, Crompton GK: Inappropriate antidiuretic hormone secretion in oat cell carcinoma of bronchus: Aggravation of hyponatremia by intravenous cyclophosphamide. Thorax 27:640–642, 1972
102. Cohen MH, Bunn PA Jr, Ihde DC et al: Chemotherapy rather than demeclocycline for inappropriate secretion of antiuiretic hormone. N Engl J Med 298:1423, 1978
103. North WG, Maurer H, O'Donnell JF: Human neurophysins and small cell carcinoma. Clin Res 27:390A, 1979
104. Hantman D, Rossier B, Zohlman R, Schrier R: Rapid correction of hyponatremia in the syndrome of inappropriate secretion of antidiuretic hormone. An alternative treatment to hypertonic saline. Ann Intern Med 78:870–875, 1973
105. Forrest JN Jr, Cox M, Hong C et al: Superiority of demeclocycline over lithium in the treatment of chronic syndrome of inappropriate secretion of antidiuretic hormone. N Engl J Med 298:173–177, 1978
106. DeTroyer A: Demeclocycline treatment for syndrome of inappropriate antidiuretic hormone secretion. JAMA 237:2823–2826, 1977
107. White MG, Fetner DC: Treatment of the syndrome of inappropriate secretion of antidiuretic hormone with lithium carbonate. N Engl J Med 292:390–392, 1975
108. Decaux G, Brimioulle S, Genette F, Mockel J: Treatment of the syndrome of inappropriate secretion of antidiuretic hormone by urea. Am J Med 69:99–106, 1980
109. Cogan E, Debieve M-F, Philipart I et al: High plasma levels of atrial natriuretic factor in SIADH. Lancet 2:1258–1259, 1986
110. Kamoi K, Ebe T, Hasegawa A et al: Hyponatremia in small cell lung cancer. Mechanisms not involving inappropriate ADH secretion. Cancer 60:1089–1093, 1987
111. Trump DL: Abnormalities of bone and mineral metabolism. In Abeloff MD (ed): Complications of Cancer. Diagnosis and Management, pp 263–281. Baltimore, Johns Hopkins University Press, 1979
112. Myers WPL: Differential diagnosis of hypercalcemia and cancer. CA 27:258–272, 1977
113. Isales C, Carcangiu ML, Stewart AF: Hypercalcemia in breast cancer. Reassessment of the mechanism. Am J Med 82:1143–1147, 1987
114. Holtz G, Johnson TR Jr, Schrock ME: Paraneoplsatic hypercalcemia in ovarian tumors. Obstet Gynecol 54:483–487, 1979
115. Cryer PE, Kissane JM: Clinicopathologic conference. Malignant hypercalcemia. Am J Med 65:486–494, 1979

116. Bunn PA, Schechter GP, Blayney DP et al: Clinical course of retrovirus-associated adult T-cell lymphoma in the United States. N Engl J Med 309:257–262, 1983
117. Moseley JM, Kubota M, Diefenbach-Jagger H et al: Parathyroid hormone related protein purified from a human lung cancer cell line. Proc Natl Acad Sci USA 84:5048–5052, 1987
118. Tashjian AH, Voelkel EF, Levine L: Evidence that the bone resorption-stimulating factor produced by mouse fibrosarcoma cells is prostaglandin E_2: A new model for the hypercalcemia of cancer. J Exp Med 135:1329–1343, 1972
119. Voelkel EF, Tashjian AH Jr, Franklin R et al: Hypercalcemia and tumor-prostaglandins: The VX2 carcinoma model in the rabbit. Metabolism 24:973–986, 1975
120. Mundy GR: The hypercalcemia of malignancy. Kidney Int 31:142–155, 1987
121. Strewler GJ, Nissensen RA: Nonparathyroid hypercalcemia. Adv Intern Med 32:235–258, 1987
122. Stewart AF: The relative potency of a human tumor derived PTH-like adenylate cyclase-stimulating preparation in three bioassays. J Bone Miner Res 2:37–42, 1987
123. Horton JE, Raisz LG, Simmons HA et al: Bone resorbing activity in supernatant fluid from cultured human peripheral blood leukocytes. Science 177:793–795, 1972
124. Luben RA, Mundy GR, Trummel CL, Raisz LG: Partial purification of osteoclast-activating factor from phytohemagglutinin-stimulated human leukocytes. J Clin Invest 53:1473–1480, 1974
125. Mundy GR, Raisz LG, Cooper RA et al: Evidence for the secretion of an osteoclast stimulating factor in myeloma. N Engl J Med 291:1041–1046, 1974
126. Elion G, Mundy GR: Direct resorption of bone by human breast cancer cells in vitro. Nature 276:726–728, 1978
127. Koeffler HP, Mundy GR, Golde DW, Cline MJ: Production of bone-resorbing activity in poorly differentiated monocytic malignancy. Cancer 41:2438–2443, 1978
128. Seyberth HW: Prostaglandin-mediated hypercalcemia: A paraneoplastic syndrome. Klin Wochenscher 56:373–387, 1978
129. Brereton HD, Halushka PV, Alexander RW et al: Indomethacin-responsive hypercalcemia in a patient with renal-cell adenocarcinoma. N Engl J Med 29:83–85, 1975
130. Robertson RP, Baylink DJ, Marini JJ, Adkison HW: Elevated prostaglandins and suppressed parathyroid hormone associated with hypercalcemia and renal cell carcinoma. J Clin Endocrinol Metab 41:164–167, 1975
131. Ito H, Sanada T, Katayama T, Shimazaki J: Indomethacin-responsive hypercalcemia. N Engl J Med 293:558–559, 1975
132. Seyberth HW, Segre GV, Morgan JL et al: Prostaglandins as mediators of hypercalcemia associated wiith certain types of cancer. N Engl J Med 293:1278–1283, 1975
133. Tashjian AH Jr: Prostaglandins, hypercalcemia and cancer. N Engl J Med 293:1317–1318, 1975
134. Shigeno C, Yamamoto I, Dokoh S et al: Identification of 1,24-dihydroxyvitamin D_3-like bone-resorbing lipid in a patient with cancer-associated hypercalcemia. J Clin Endocrinol Metab 61:761–768, 1985
135. Rosenthal N, Insogua KL, Godsall JW et al: Elevations in circulating 1,25-dihydroxyvitamin D in three patients with lymphoma-associated hypercalcemia. J Clin Endocrinol Metab 60:29–33, 1985
136. Frankel TL, Mason RS, Hersey P et al: The synthesis of vitamin D metabolites by human melanoma cells. J Clin Endocrinol Metab 57:627–630, 1983
137. Raskin P, McClain CJ, Medsger TA: Hypocalcemia associated with metastatic bone disease. Arch Intern Med 132:539–543, 1973
138. Sackner MA, Spivak AP, Balian LJ: Hypocalcemia in the presence of osteoblastic metastases. N Engl J Med 262:173–176, 1960
139. Hall TC, Griffiths CT, Petranek JR: Hypocalcemia: An unusual metabolic complication of breast cancer. N Engl J Med 275:1474–1477, 1966
140. Jackson HJ, Taylor FHL: Calcium, potassium, and inorganic phosphate content of the serum in cancer patients. Effect of roentgen ray radiation on the level of these substances in the blood of cancer patients. Am J Cancer 19:379–388, 1933
141. Ehrlich M, Goldsten M, Heinemann HO: Hypocalcemia, hypoparathyroidism and osteoblastic metastases. Metabolism 12:516–526, 1963
142. Gordon GS: Hyper- and hypocalcemia: Pathogenesis and treatments. Ann NY Acad Sci 230:181–186, 1974
143. Salassa RM, Jowsey J, Arnaud C: Hypophosphatemia osteomalacia associated with "nonendocrine" tumors. N Engl J Med 283:65–69, 1970
144. Stanbury W: Tumor-associated hypophosphatemia, osteomalacia and rickets. Clin Endocrinol Metabol 1:256–259, 1972
145. Daniels RA, Weisenfeld I: Tumorous phosphaturic osteomalacia. Report of a case associated with multiple hemangiomas of bone. Am J Med 67:155–159, 1979
146. Siris ES, Clemens TL, Dempster DW et al: Tumor-induced osteomalacia. Kinetics of calcium, phosphorus, and vitamin D metabolism and characteristics of bone histomorphometry. Am J Med 82:307–312, 1987
147. Olefsky J, Compson R, Jones H, Reaven G: "Tertiary" hyperparathyroidism, and apparent "cure" of vitamin D resistant rickets after removal of an ossifying mesenchymal tumor of the pharynx. N Engl J Med 286:740–746, 1972
148. Evans DJ, Azzopardi JG: Distinctine tumours of bone and soft tissue causing acquired vitamin-D-resistant osteomalacia. Lancet 1:353–354, 1972
149. Taylor HC, Velasco ME, Fallan MD: Oncogenic osteomalacia and inappropriate anti-diuretic hormone secretion due to oat cell carcinoma. Ann Intern Med 101:786–788, 1984
150. Ryan EA, Reiss E: Oncogenous ostoemalacia. Review of the world literature of 42 cases and report of two new cases. Am J Med 77:501–512, 1984
151. Tashjian AH, Wolfe HJ, Voelkel EF: Human calcitonin: Immunologic assay, cytologic localization and studies of medullary thyroid carcinoma. Am J Med 56:840–849, 1974
152. Silva OL, Broder LE, Doppman JL et al: Cohen MH, Becker KL: Calcitonin as a marker for bronchogenic cancer: A prospective study. Cancer 44:680–684, 1979
153. Becker KL, Nash DR, Silva OL et al: Urine calcitonin levels in patients with bronchogenic carcinoma. JAMA 243:670–672, 1980
154. Ellison M, Woodhouse D, Hillyard C et al: Immunoreactive calcitonin production by human lung carcinoma cells in culture. Br J Cancer 32:373–379, 1975
155. Bertagna XY, Nicholson WE, Pettengill OS et al: Ectopic production of high molecular weight calcitonin and corticotropin by human small cell carcinoma cells in tissue culture: Evidence for separate precursors. J Clin Endocrinol Metab 47:1390–1393, 1978
156. Lips CJ, Vander Sluys V, Van Der Donk JA, Van Dam RH: Common precursor molecule as origin for the ectopic-hormone-producing tumor syndrome. Lancet 1:16–18, 1978
157. Hillyard V, Coombes RC, Greenberg PB et al: Calcitonin in breast and lung cancer. Clin Endocrinol 5:1–8, 1976
158. Iacangelo A, Affolter HV, Eiden LE et al: Bovine chromogranin A sequence and distribution of its messenger RNA in endocrine tissues. Nature 323:82–86, 1986
159. Sobol RE, O'Connor DT, Addison J et al: Elevated serum chromogranin A concentrations in small cell lung cancer. Ann Intern Med 105:698–700, 1986
160. O'Connor DT, Deftos LI: Secretion of chromogranin A by peptide producing endocrine neoplasms. N Engl J Med 314:1145–1151, 1986
161. Huttner WB, Benedum UM: Chromogranin A and pancreastatin. Nature 325:305, 1987
162. Eiden LE: Is chromogranin a prohormone? Nature 325:301, 1987
163. Vaitukaitis JL, Ross GT, Braunstein GD, Rayford PL: Gonadotropins and their subunits: Basic and clinical studies. Recent Prog Horm Res 32:289–321, 1976
164. Kenimer JG, Hershman JM, Higgins HP: The thyrotropin in hydatidiform moles is human chorionic gonadotropin. J Clin Endocrinol Metab 40:481–491, 1975
165. Nisula BC, Ketelslegers JM: Thyroid-stimulating activity and chorionic gonadotropin. J Clin Invest 54:494–499, 1974
166. Faiman C, Colwell JA, Ryan RJ et al: Gonadotropin secretion from a bronchogenic carcinoma. N Engl J Med 277:1395–1399, 1967
167. Fusco FD, Rosen SW: Gonadotropin-producing anaplastic large-cell carcinomas of the lung. N Engl J Med 275:507–515, 1966
168. Anderson T, Waldmann TA, Javadpour N, Glatstein E: Testicular germ-cell neoplasms: Recent advances in diagnosis and therapy. Ann Intern Med 90:373–385, 1979
169. Lewis JL: Chemotherapy of gestational choriocarcinoma. Cancer 30:1517–1521, 1972
170. Blackman MR, Weintraub BD, Rosen SW et al: Human placental and pituitary glycoprotein hormones and their subunits as tumor markers: A quantitative assessment. J Natl Cancer Inst 65:81–93, 1980
171. Tsuruhara T, Dufau ML, Hickman J, Catt KJ: Biological properties of hCG after removal of terminal sialic acid and galactose residues. Endocrinology 91:296–301, 1972
172. Muggia FM, Rosen SW, Weintraub BD, Hansen HH: Ectopic placental proteins in nontrophoblastic tumors: Serial measurements following chemotherapy. Cnacer 36:1327–1337, 1975
173. Kahn CR, Rosen SW, Weintraub BD et al: Ecotpic production of chorionic gonadotropin and its subunits by islet cell tumors: A specific marker for malignancy. N Engl J Med 197:565–569, 1977
174. Bender RA, Weintraub BD, Rosen SW: Prospective evaluation of two tumor-associated proteins in pancreatic adenocarcinoma. Cancer 45:591–595, 1979
175. Broder LE, Weintraub BD, Rosen SW et al: Placental proteins and their subunits as tumor markers in prostatic carcinoma. Cancer 40:211–216, 1977
176. Metz SA, Weintraub B, Rosen SW et al: Ectopic secretion of chorionic gonadotropin by a lung carcinoma. Pituitary gonadotropin and subunit secretion and prolonged chemotherapeutic remission. Am J Med 65:325–333, 1978
177. Tashjian AH Jr, Weintraub BD, Barowksy NJ et al: Subunits of human chorionic gonadotropin: Unbalanced synthesis and secretion by clonal cell strains derived from a bronchogenic carcinoma. Proc Natl Acad Sci USA 70:1419–1422, 1973
178. Rosen SW, Weintraub BD, Aaronson SA: Nonrandom ecotpic protein production by malignant cells: Direct evidence in vitro. J Clin Endocrinol Metab 50:834–841, 1980
179. Blackman MR, Weintraub BD, Rosen SW, Harmen SM: Comparison of the effects of lung cancer, benign lung disease, and normal aging on pituitary–gonadal function in men. J Clin Endocrinol Metab 66:88–95, 1988
179a. Rudnick P, Odell WD: In serach of a cancer. N Engl J Med 284:405–408, 1971
180. Skrabanek P, Kirrane J, Powell D: A unifying concept of chorionic gonadotropin production in maligancy. Invest Cell Pathol 2:75–85, 1979
181. Greco FA, Fer MF, Oldham RD et al: Intracytoplasmic localization of ectopic β-human chorionic gonadotropin and α-fetoprotein in suspected extragonadal germ cell cancers by immunohistochemical methods. Clin Res 28:415A, 1980
182. Novarro C, Sancho A, Morales L et al: Paraneoplastic precocious puberty. Report of a new case with hepatoblastoma and review of the literature. Cancer 56:1725–1729, 1985
183. Root AW, Bongiovanni AM, Eberlein WR: A testicular-interstitial-cell stimulating gonadotropin in a child with hepatoblastoma and sexual precocity. J Clin Endocrin Metab 28:1317–1322, 1968
184. McArthur J, Toll GD, Russfield AB et al: Sexual precocity attributable to ectopic gonadtropin secretion by hepatoblastoma. Am J Med 54:390–403, 1973
185. Kurman RJ, Norris HJ: Embryonal carcinoma of the ovary: A clinicopathologic

entity distinct from endodermal sinus tumor resembling embryonal carcinoma of the adult testes. Cancer 38:2420–2433, 1976
186. Weintraub BD, Rosen SW: Ectopic production of human chorionic somatomammotrophin by nontrophoblastic cancers. J Clin Endocrin Metab 32:94–101, 1971
187. Rosen SW, Weintraub BD, Vaitukaitis JL et al: Placental proteins and their subunits as tumor markers. Ann Intern Med 82:71–83, 1975
187a. Steiner H, Dahlback O, Waldenstrom J: Ecotpic growth-hormone production and osteoarthropathy in carcinoma of the bronchus. Lancet 1:783–785, 1968
188. Ennis CG, Cameron DP, Burger HG: On the etiology of hypertrophic pulmonary osteoarthropathy in bronchogenic carcinoma: Lack of relationship to elevated growth hormone levels. Aust NZ J Med 3:157–161, 1973
189. Sonksen PH, Ayres AB, Braimbridge M et al: Acromegaly caused by pulmonary carcinoid tumors. Clin Endocrinol 5:505–513, 1976
190. Scheithauer BW, Bloch B, Carpenter PC, Brazeau P: Ectopic secretion of a growth hormone-releasing factor. Report of a case of acromegaly with bronchical carcinoid tumor. Am J Med 76:605–616, 1984
191. Thorner MO, Vance ML, Kovacs K: Ectopic growth hormone-releasing hormone (GHRH) syndrome and significance. Proc Int Chemother Cong Abstr 5051, 1986
192. Boizel R, Labat F, Bachelot I et al: Acromegaly due to a growth hormone releasing hormone secreting bronchial carcinoid tumor. Further information on the abnormal responsiveness of the somatotroph cells and their recovery after successful treatment. J Clin Endocrinol Metab 64:304–308, 1987
193. Roth KA, Eberwine J, Kovacs K et al: Acromegaly and pheochromocytoma: A multiple endocrine syndrome caused by a plurihormonal adrenal medullary tumor. J Clin Endocrinol Metab 63:1421–1426, 1986
194. Anderson G: The incidence of paramalignant syndromes. In Anderson G (ed): Paramalignant Syndromes in Lung Cancer, p 4. London, William Heinemann, 1973
195. Hennen G: Characterization of a thyroid-stimulating factor in human cancer tissue. J Clin Endocrin Metab 27:610–614, 1967
196. Odell WD, Bates RW, Rivlin RS et al: Increased thyroid function without clinical hyperthyroidism in patients with choriocarcinoma. J Clin Endocrinol Metab 23:658–668, 1963
197. Cave WT Jr, Dunn JT: Choriocarcinoma with hyperthyroidism: Probable identity of the thyrotropin with human chorionic gonadtropin. Ann Intern Med 85:60–63, 1976
198. Bommer G, Altenahr E, Kuhnau J Jr, Kloppel G: Ultrastructure of hemangiopericytoma associated with paraneoplastic hypoglycemia. Z Krebsforsh 85:231–241, 1976
199. Sluiter WJ, Marrink J, Houwen B: Monoclonal gammopathy with an insulin binding IgG(κ) M-component associated with severe hypoglycemia. Br J Haematol 62:679–687, 1986
200. Stuart CA, Prince MJ, Peters EJ et al: Insulin receptor proliferation: A mechanism for tumor-associated hypoglycemia. J Clin Endocrinol Metab 63:879–885, 1986
201. Younus S, Soterakis J, Sossi AJ et al: Hypoglycemia secondary to metastases to the liver. A case report and review of the literature. Gastroenterology 72:334–337, 1977
202. Kiang DT, Bauer GE, Kennedy BJ: Immunoassayable insulin in carcinoma of the cervix associated with hypoglycemia. Cancer 31:801–805, 1973
203. Silvert CK, Rossini AA: Ghazvinian S et al: Tumor hypoglycemia: Deficient splanchnic glucose output and deficient glucagon secretion. Diabetes 25:202–206, 1976
204. Solomon J: Case report: Spurious hypoglycemia and hypperkalemia in myelomonocytic leukemia. Am J Med Sci 267:359–363, 1974
205. Zapf J, Walter H, Froesch ER: Radioimmunological determination of insulin-like growth factors I and II in normal subjects and in patients with growth disorders and extrapancreatic tumor hypoglycemia. J Clin Invest 68:1321–1330, 1981
206. Gorden P, Hendricks CM, Kahn CR et al: Hypoglycemia associated with non-islet cell tumor and insulin like growth factors. N Engl J Med 305:1452–1455, 1981
207. Li TCM, Reed C, Stubenbard WT et al: Surgical cure of hypoglycemia associated with cystosarcoma phylloides and elevated NSILP. Am J Med 74:1080–1084, 1983
208. Van Wyk JJ, Underwood LE, Hintz RL et al: The somatomedins: A family of insulin-like hormones under growth hormone control. Recent Prog Horm Res 30:259–318, 1974
209. Chandalia HB, Boshell BR: Hypoglycemia in association with extrapancreatic tumors. Arch Intern Med 129:447–456, 1972
210. Megyesi K, Kahn CR, Roth J, Gordon P: Hypoglycemia in association with extrapancreatic tumors: Demonstration of elevated plasma NSILA-S by a new radioreceptor assay. J Clin Endocrinol Metab 38:931–934, 1974
211. Farsang C, Ramirez-Gonzalez MD, Mucci L, Kunos G: Possible role of an endogenous opiate in the cardiovascular effects of central α-adrenoceptor stimulation in spontaneously hypertensive rats. J Pharmacol Exp Ther 214:203–208, 1980
212. Davies P, Joseph J, Thompson A: Anterior to posterior variations in the concentration of somatostatin-like immunoreactivity in human basal ganglia. Brain Res Bull 7:365–368, 1981
213. Perry RH, Dockray GJ, Dimaline R et al: Neuropeptides in Alzheimer's disease, depression and schizophrenia. J Neurol Sci 51:465–472, 1981
214. Emson PC, Arregui A, Clement-Jones V et al: Regional distribution of methionine-enkephalin and substance P-like immunoreactivity in normal brain and in Huntington's disease. Brain Res 199:147–160, 1980
215. Aronin N, Cooper PE, Lorenz LJ et al: Somastostatin is increased in the basal ganglia in Huntington disease. Ann Neurol 13:519–526, 1983
216. Brandt NJ, Teremius L, Jacobsen BB et al: Hyper-endorphin syndrome in a child with necrotizing encephalomyelopathy. N Engl J Med 303:914–916, 1980
217. Allen JC, Deck MDF, Foley FM et al: Neuro-oncology: II. Dept. of Neurology, Memorial Sloan–Kettering Cancer Center, NY, 1979
218. Newman SJ, Hansen HH: Frequency, diagnosis, and treatment of brain metastases in 247 consecutive patients with bronchogenic carcinoma. Cancer 33:492–496, 1974
219. Nugent JL, Bunn PA Jr, Matthews MJ et al: CNS metastases in small cell bronchogenic carcinoma. Increasing frequency and changing pattern with lengthening survival. Cancer 44:1855–1893, 1979
220. Posner JB, Chernik NL: Intracranial metastasis from systemic cancer. Adv Neurol 19:575–587, 1978
221. Rosen P, Armstrong D: Nonbacterial thrombotic endocarditis in patients with malignant neoplastic disease. Am J Med 54:23–29, 1973
222. Collins RC, Al-mondhiry H, Chernik NL, Posner JB: Neurologic manifestations of intravascular coagulation in patients with cancer: A clinical-pathological analysis of 12 cases. Neurology 25:795–806, 1975
223. Sigsbee B, Deck MDF, Posner JB: Non-metastatic superior saggital sinus thrombosis complicating systemic cancer. Neurology 29:139–146, 1979
224. Rogers LR, Cho ES, Kempin S, Posner JB: Cerebral infarction from nonbacterial thrombotic endocarditis. Clinical and pathologic study including effects of anticoagulation. Am J Med 83:746–756, 1987
225. Hickey WF, Garnick MB, Henderson IC, Dawson DM: Primary cerebral venous thrombosis in patients with cancer—a rarely diagnosed paraneoplastic syndrome. Am J Med 73:740–750, 1982
226. Persen JR: Systemic angioendotheliosis: A possible disorder of a circulating angiogenic factor. Br J Dermatol 96:329–331, 1977
227. Petito CK, Gottlieb GJ, Dougherty JH, Petito FH: Neoplastic angioendotheliosis: Ultrastructural study and review of the literature. Ann Neurol 3:393–399, 1978
228. Gimenez-Gallego G, Rodkey J, Bennett C et al: Brain derived acidic fibroblast growth factor: Complete amino acid sequence and homologies. Science 1385–1833, 1985
229. Folkman J: A family of angiogenic peptides. Nature 329:671–672, 1987
230. Bell CE Jr, Seetharam S: Expression of endodermally derived and neural crest-derived differentiation antigens by human lung and colon tumors. Cancer 44:12–18, 1979
231. Bunn PA, Gazdar AF, Carney DN, Minna JD: Small cell lung carcinoma and natural killer cells share an antigen determinant, Leu 7. Clin Res 32:413A, 1984
232. Schuller-Petrovic S, Gebhart W, Lassmann H, Rumpold H, Kraft D: A shared antigenic determinant between natural killer cells and nervous tissue. Nature 306:179–181, 1983
233. Wilkinson PC, Zeroniski J: Immunofluorescent detection of antibodies against neurones in sensory carcinomatoms neuropathy. Brain 88:529–538, 1965
234. Brain WR, Wilkinson M: Subacute cerebellar degeneration associated with neoplasms. Brain 88:465, 1965
235. Paone JF, Jeyasingham K: Remission of cerebellar dysfunction after pneumonectomy for bronchogenic carcinoma. N Engl J Med 302:156–157, 1980
236. Victor M, Adams RD, Mancall EL: A restricted form of cerebellar cortical degeneration occurring in alcoholic patients. Arch Neurol 1:579–688, 1959
237. Steven MM, Carnegie PR, Mackay IR et al: Cerebellar cortical degeneration with ovarian carcinoma. Postgrad Med J 58:47–51, 1982
238. Dropcho EJ, Chen Y-T, Posner JB, Old LB: Cloning of a brain protein identified by autoantibodies from a patient with paraneoplastic cerebellar degeneration. Proc Natl Acad Sci USA 84:4552–4556, 1987
239. Shapiro WR: Remote effects of neoplasm on the central nervous system: Encephalopathy. Adv Neurol 15:101–117, 1976
240. Dorfman LH, Forno LS: Paraneoplastic encephalomyelitis. Acta Neurol Scand 48:556–574, 1972
241. Corsellis JAN, Goldberg GJ, Norton AR: "Limbic encephalitis" and its association with carcinoma. Brain 91:481–497, 1968
242. Brennan LV, Craddock PR: Limbic encephalopathy as a nonmetastatic complication of oat cell lung cancer. Am J Med 75:518–520, 1983
243. Carr I: The Ophelia syndrome: Memory loss in Hodgkin's disease. Lancet 1:844–845, 1982
244. Sawyer RA: Blindness caused by photoreceptor degeneration as a remote effect of cancer. Am J Ophthalmol 81:606–613, 1976
245. Grunwald GB, Simmonds MA, Klein R, Kornguth SE: Autoimmune basis for visual paraneoplastic syndrome in patients with small cell lung carcinoma. Lancet 1:658–661, 1985
246. Pillary N, Ebers GC, Gilbert JJ, Brown JD: Internuclear opthalmoplegia and "optic neuritis": Paraneoplastic effects of bronchial carcinoma. Neurology 34:788–791, 1984
247. Padgett BL: JC papovavirus in progressive multifocal leukoencephalopathy. J Infect Dis 133:686–690, 1976
248. Norris FH Jr, Engel WK: Carcinomatous amyotrophic lateral sclerosis. In Brain WR, Norris FH Jr (eds): The Remote Effects of Cancer on the Nervous System. New York, Grune & Stratton, 1965
249. Mancall EL, Rosales RK: Necrotizing myelopathy associated with visceral carcinoma. Brain 87:636–639, 1964
250. Handforth A, Nag S, Sharp D, Robertson DM: Paraneoplastic subacute necrotic myelopathy. Can J Neurol Sci 10:204–207, 1983
251. Walton JN, Tomlinson BE, Pearce GW: Subacute "poliomyelitis" and Hodgkin's disease. J Neurol Sci 6:435–445, 1968
252. Horwich MS, Cho L, Porro RS, Posner JB: Subacute sensory neuropathy: A remote effect of carcinoma. Ann Neurol 1:7–19, 1977
253. Henson RA, Hoffman HL, Urich H: Encephalomyelitis with carcinoma. Brain 88:449–464, 1965

254. Croft PB, Urich H, Wilkinson M: Peripheral neuropathy of sensorimotor type associated with malignant disease. Brain 90:31–66, 1967
255. Dayan AD, Croft PB, Wilkinson M: Association of carcinomatous neuromyopathy with different histological types of carcinoma of the lung. Brain 88:435–448, 1965
256. Newman MK, Gugino RJ: Neuropathies amd myopathies associated with occult malignancies. JAMA 190:575–577, 1964
257. Victor M, Banker BQ, Adams RD: The neuropathy of multiple myeloma. J Neurol Neurosurg Psychiatry 21:73–88, 1958
258. Lisak RP: Gullain–Barre syndrome and Hodgkin's disease: Three cases with immunological studies. Ann Neurol 1:72–78, 1977
259. Schuffer MD, Baird HW, Fleming CR et al: Intestinal pseudo-obstruction as the presenting manifestation of small cell carcinoma of the lung. Ann Intern Med 98:129–134, 1983
260. Siemsen JK, Meister L: Bronchogenic carcinoma associated with severe orthostatic hypotension. Ann Intern Med 58:669–676, 1963
261. Park DM, Johnson RH, Crean GP, Robinson JF: Orthostatic hypotension in bronchial carcinoma. Br Med J 3:510–511, 1972
262. Ahmed MN, Carpenter S: Autonomic neuropathy and carcinoma of the lung. Can Med Assoc J 113:410–412, 1975
263. Ogilvie H: Large intestine colic due to sympathetic deprivation. Br Med J 2:671–673, 1948
264. DeVere R, Bradley WG: Polymyositis: Its presentation, morbidity and mortality. Brain 98:637–666, 1976
265. Barnes BE: Dermatomyositis and malignancy. A review of the literature. Ann Intern Med 84:68–76, 1976
266. Williams RC Jr: Dermatomyositis and malignancy: A review of the literature. Ann Intern Med 50:1174–1181, 1959
267. Lambert EH, Eaton LM, Rooke ED: Defect of neuromuscular conduction associated with malignant neoplasms. Am J Physiol 187:612, 1956
268. Lambert EH, Rooke ED: Myasthenic state and lung cancer. In Brain WR, Norris FH Jr (eds): The Remote Effects of Cancer on the Nervous System, pp 67–80. New York, Grune & Stratton, 1965
269. Simpson JA: The myasthenic (Eaton-Lambert) syndrome associated with carcinoma: Enzyme induction as a possible mechanism of paraneoplastic syndromes. Scott Med J 27:220–228, 1982
270. Cherington M: Guanidine and germine in Eaton–Lambert syndrome. Neurology 26:944–946, 1976
271. Jenkyn LR, Brooks PL, Forcier RJ et al: Remission of the Lambert–Eaton syndrome and small cell anaplastic carcinoma of the lung induced by chemotherapy and radiotherapy. Cancer 46:1123–1127, 1980
272. Login IS, Kim YI, Judd AM et al: Immunoglobulins of Lambert–Eaton myasthenic syndrome inhibit rat pituitary hormone release. Ann Neurol 22:610–614, 1987
273. Tyler HR: Paraneoplastic syndromes of nerve, muscle, and neuromuscular junction. Ann NY Acad Sci 230:348–357, 1974
274. Latov N, Sherman WH, Nemni R et al: Plasma cell dyscrasia and peripheral neuropathy with a monoclonal antibody to peripheral-nerve myelin. N Engl J Med 303:618–621, 1980
275. Johnson PC, Rolak LA, Hamilton RH, Laguna JF: Paraneoplastic vasculitis of nerve: A remote effect of cancer. Ann Neurol 5:437–444, 1979
276. Clark SC, Kamen R: The human hematopoietic colony stimulating factors. Science 236:1229–1237, 1987
277. Hammond D, Winnick S: Paraneoplastic erythrocytosis and ectopic erythropoietins. Ann NY Acad Sci 230:219–227, 1974
278. Valentine WN, Hennessy TG, Lang E et al: Polycythemia: Erythrocytosis and erythremia. Ann Intern Med 69:587–606, 1968
279. Sytkowski AJ, Richie JP, Bicknell KA: New human renal carcinoma cell line established from a patient with erythrocytosis. Cancer Res 43:1415–1419, 1983
280. Williams WJ, Beutler E, Erslev AJ, Rundles RW: Hematology, 2nd ed. New York, McGraw-Hill, 1977
281. Berlin NI: Anemia of cancer. Ann NY Acad Sci 230:209–211, 1974
282. Waterbury L: Hematologic problems. In Abeloff MD (ed): Complications of Cancer. Diagnosis and Management, pp 121–145. Baltimore, Johns Hopkins Press, 1979
283. Cartwright GE, Lee GR: The anemia of chronic disorders. Br J Haematol 21:147–152, 1971
284. Crowthers D, Bateman CJT: Hematological aspects of systemic disease-malignant disease. Clin Haematol 1:447–455, 1972
285. Jacobs EM, Hutter RVP, Pool JL, Ley AB: Benign thymoma and selective erythroid aplasia of the bone marrow. Cancer 12:47–57, 1959
286. Vasavada PJ, Bournigal LJ, Reynolds RW: Thymoma associated with pure red cell aplasia and hypogammaglobulinemias. Postgrad Med 54(6):93–98, 1973
287. Guthrie TH, Thornton RM: Pure red cell aplasia obscured by a diagnosis of carcinoma. South Med J 76:632–634, 1983
288. Akard LP, Brandt J, Lee L et al: Chronic T cell lymphoproliferative disorder and pure red cell aplasia. Am J Med 83:1069–1074, 1987
289. Hoffbrand AV, Hobbs JR, Kremenchuzky S, Mallin DL: Incidence and pathogenesis of megaloblastic erythropoiesis in multiple myeloma. J Clin Pathol 20:699–705, 1967
290. Pirofsky B: Clinical aspects of autoimmune hemolytic anemia. Semin Hematol 13:251–265, 1976
291. Ludwin D, Sacks P, Lynch S et al: Autoimmune hematological complications occurring during the treatment of malignant lymphoproliferative diseases. S Afr Med J 48:2143–2145, 1974
292. Lackner H: Hemostatic abnormalities associated with dysproteinemias. Semin Hematol 10:125–133, 1973
293. Burkert L, Becker G, Pisciotta AV: Ovarian malignancy and hemolytic anemia. Ann Intern Med 73:91–93, 1970
294. Dawson MA, Tolbert W, Yarbro JW: Hemolytic anemia associated with an ovarian tumor. Ann J Med 50:552–556, 1971
295. Spira MA, Lynch EC: Autoimmune hemolytic anemia and carcinoma: An unusual association. Am J Med 67:753–758, 1979
296. Dacie JV: The Hemolytic Anemias: Congenital and Acquired Part III. Secondary and Symptomatic Hemolytic Anemias. New York, Grune & Stratton, 1967
297. Pirofsky B: Autoimmunization and the Autoimmune Hemolytic Anemias, Baltimore, Williams & Wilkins, 1968
298. Evans RS, Takahasi K, Duane RT et al: Primary thrombocytopenic purpura and acquired hemolytic anemia. Evidence for a common etiology. Arch Intern Med 87:48–65, 1957
299. Doll DC, List AF, Yarbro JW: Evans' syndrome associated with microcystic adenoma of the pancreas. Cancer 59:1366–1368, 1987
300. Barry KG, Crosby WH: Autoimmune hemolytic anemia arrested by removal of an ovarian teratoma: Review of the literature and report of a case. Ann Intern Med 47:1002–1007, 1957
301. Antman KH, Skarin AT, Mayer RJ et al: Microangiopathic hemolytic anemia and cancer: A review. Medicine 58:377–384, 1979
302. Brain MC, Dacie JV, Hourihane OB: Microangiopathic hemolytic anemia: The possible role of vascular lesions in pathogenesis. Br J Haematol 8:358–374, 1962
303. Lohrmann HP, Adam W, Heymer B, Kubanek B: Microangiopathic hemolytic anemia in metastatic carcinoma: Report of eight cases. Ann Intern Med 79:368–375, 1973
304. Sack GH, Levin J, Bell WR: Trousseau's syndrome and other manifestations of chronic disseminate coagulopathy in patients with neoplasms. Medicine 56:1–37, 1977
305. Colman RW, Robboy SJ, Minna JD: Disseminated intravascular coagulation: A reappraisal. Ann Rev Med 30:359–374, 1979
306. Robinson WA: Granulocytosis in neoplasia. Ann NY Acad Sci 230:212–218, 1974
307. Meyer LM, Rotter SD: Leukemoid reaction (hyperleukocytosis) in malignancy. Am J Clin Pathol 12:218–222, 1942
308. Fahey RJ: Unusual leukocyte response in primary carcinoma of the lung. Cancer 4:930–935, 1951
309. Hughes WF, Highley CS: Marked leuckocytosis resulting from carcinomatosis. Ann Intern Med 37:1095–1098, 1952
310. Barrett O Jr: Monocytosis in malignant disease. Ann Intern Med 73:991–992, 1970
311. Finch SC: Granulocytopenia and granulocytosis. In Williams WJ, Beutler E, Erslev AJ, Rundles RW (eds): Hematology, 2nd ed. New York, McGraw-Hill, 1977
312. Asano S, Urabe A, Okabe T et al: Demonstration of granulopoietic factor(s) in the plasma of nude mice transplanted with a human lung cancer and in the tumor tissue. Blood 49:845–852, 1977
313. Okabe T, Sato N, Kondo Y, Asano S, Ohsawa N, Kosaka K, Ueyama Y: Establishment and characterization of a human cancer cell line that produces human colony-stimulating factor. Cancer Res 38:3910–3917, 1978
314. DiPersio JF, Brennan JK, Lichtman MA, Speiser BL: Human cell lines that elaborate colony-stimulating activity for the marrow cells of man and other species. Blood 51:507–519, 1978
315. Cohen PR, Kurzrock R: Sweet's syndrome and malignancy. Am J Med 82:1220–1226, 1987
316. McCarthy JH, Sullivan JR, Ungar B, Metcalf D: Two cases of carcinoma of the lung characterized by a bone marrow agar culture pattern resembling acute myeloid leukemia. Blood 54:530–533, 1979
317. Aisenberg AC, Wilkes BM, Harris N et al: Chronic T-cell lymphocytosis with neutropenia: Report of a case studied with monoclonal antibody. Blood 58:818–823, 1981
318. Knowles JH: Miscellaneous disorders of the lung. In Harrison TR, Adams RD, Bennett IL et al (eds): Harrison's Principles of Internal Medicine, 5th ed, pp 955–957, New York, McGraw-Hill, 1966
319. Liddle GW, Nicholson WE, Island DP et al: Clinical and laboratory studies of ecotopic humoral syndromes. Recent Prog Horm Res 25:283–314, 1969
320. Slungaard A, Ascensao J, Zanjani E, Jacob HS: Pulmonary carcinoma with eosinophilia: Demonstration of a tumor-derived eosinophilopoietic factor. N Engl J Med 309:778–781, 1983
321. Williams WJ: Thrombocytosis. In Williams WJ, Beutler E, Erslev AJ, Rundles RW (eds): Hematology, 2nd ed. New York, McGraw-Hill, 1977
322. Levin J, Conley CL: Thrombocytosis associated with malignant disease. Arch Intern Med 114:497–500, 1964
323. Davis RB, Theologides A, Kennedy BJ: Comparative studies of blood coagulation and platelet aggregation in patients with cancer and nonmalignant disease. Ann Intern Med 71:67–80, 1967
324. Aster RH: Control of platelet production. In Williams WJ, Beutler E, Erslev AJ, Rundles RW (eds): Hematology, 2nd ed. New York, McGraw-Hill, 1977
325. Kim HD, Boggs DR: A syndrome resembling idiopathic thrombocytopenic purpura in 10 patients with diverse forms of cancer. Am J Med 67:371–377, 1979
326. Doan C, Bouroncle BA, Wiseman BK: Idiopathic and secondary thrombocytopenic purpura. Clinical study and evaluation of 381 cases over a periiod of 28 years. Ann Intern Med 53:861–876, 1960
327. Bellone JD, Kunicki TS, Aster RH: Immune thrombocytopenia associated with carcinoma. Ann Intern Med 99:470–472, 1983

328. Kaden BR, Rosse WF, Hauch TW: Immune thrombocytopenia in lympho proliferative diseases. Blood 53:545–551, 1979
329. Khilanani P, Al-Sarraf M: The association of autoimmune thrombocytopenia and Hodgkin's disease. Oncology 28:238–245, 1973
330. Jones SE: Autoimmune disorders and malignant lymphoma. Cancer 31:1092–1098, 1973
331. Bowie EJW, Owen CA Jr: Hemostatic failure in clinical medicine. Semin Hematol 14:341–364, 1977
332. Trousseau A: Phlegmasia alba dolens. Clinique medicale de l'Hotel-Dieu de Paris. London. The New Sydenham Society 3:94, 1865
333. Marder M, Weiner M, Shulman P, Shapiro S: Afibrinogenemia occurring in a case of malignancy of the prostate with bone metastases. NY State J Med 49:1197–1198, 1949
334. Goodnight SH Jr: Bleeding and intravascular clotting in malignancy: A review. Ann NY Acad Sci 230:271–288, 1974
335. Sharp AA: Diagnosis and management of disseminated intravascular coagulation. Br Med Bull 33:265–272, 1977
336. Gralnick HR, Abrell E: Studies of the procoagulant and fibrinolytic activity of promyelocytes in acute promyelocytic leukemia. Br J Hematol 24:59–99, 1973
337. Colman RW, Robby SJ, Minna JD: Disseminated intravascular coagulation (DIC): An approach. Am J Med 52:679–689, 1972
338. Siegal T, Seligsohn U, Aghai E, Modan M: Clinical and laboratory aspects of disseminated intravascular coagulation (DIC): A study of 118 cases. Thrombos Haemostas 39:122–134, 1978
339. Merskey C, Johnson AJ, Kleiner GJ, Wohl H: The defibrination syndrome: Clinical features and laboratory diagnosis. Br J Haematol 13:528–549, 1967
340. Owen CA Jr, Bowie EJ: Chronic intravascular coagulation syndromes: A summary. Mayo Clin Proc 49:673–679, 1974
341. Drapkin RL, Gee TS, Dowling MD et al: Prophylactic heparin therapy in acute promyelocytic leukemia. Cancer 41:2484–2490, 1978
342. Gralnick HR, Sultan C: Acute prolmyelocytic leukemia: Haemorrhagic manifestation and morphologic criteria. Br J Haematol 29:333–336, 1975
343. Goldberg MA, Ginsberg D, Mayer RJ et al: Is heparin administration necessary during induction chemotherapy for patients with acute promyelocytic leukemia? Blood 69:187–191, 1987
344. Fayemi AO, Deppisch LM: Nonbacterial thrombotic endocarditis and myocardial infarction. Am Heart J 97:405–406, 1979
345. MacDonald RA, Robbins SL: The significance of nonbacterial thrombotic endocarditis: Autopsy and clinical study of 78 patients. Ann Intern Med 46:255–273, 1957
346. Studdy P, Wiloughby JMT: Non-bacterial thrombotic endocarditis in early cancer. Br J Med 1:752, 1976
347. Susens GP, Hendrickson C, Barto DA, Sams BJ: Disseminated intravascular coagulation syndrome with metastatic melanoma: Remission after treatment with 5-(3,3-dimethyl-l-traizeno) imidazole-4-carboxamide (DTIC). Ann Intern Med 84:175, 1976
348. Alving BM, Abeloff MD, Bell W: Spontaneous remission of recurring disseminated intravascular coagulation associated with prostatic carcinoma. Cancer 37:928–930, 1976
349. Rickles FR, Edwards RL: Activation of blood coagulation in cancer: Trousseau's syndrome revisited. Blood 63:14–31, 1983
350. Rosen P, Armstrong D: Nonbacterial thrombotic endocarditis in patients with malignant neoplastic disease. Am J Med 54:23–29, 1973
351. Sun NC, McAfee WM, Hum GJ, Weiner JM: Hemostatic abnormalities in malignancy: A prospective study in one hundred eight patients: I. Coagulation studies. Am J Clin Pathol 71:10–16, 1979
352. Aderka D, Brown A, Zelikovski A, Pinkhas J: Idiopathic deep vein thrombosis in an apparently healthy patient as a premonitory sign of occult cancer. Cancer 57:1846–1849, 1986
353. Bell WR, Starksen NF, Tang S, Porterfield JK: Trousseau's syndrome. Devastating coagulopathy in the absence of heparin. Am J Med 79:423–430, 1985
354. Al-Mondhiry H: Disseminated intravascular coagulation: Experience in a major cancer center. Thrombos Diathes Haemorrh 34:181–193, 1975
355. Lee JC, Yamuchi H, Hopper J Jr: The association of cancer and the nephrotic syndrome. Ann Intern Med 64:51–51, 1966
356. Alpers CE, Cotran RS: Neoplasia and glomerular injury. Kidney Int 30:465–473, 1986
357. Glassock RJ, Friedler RM, Massry SG: Kidney and electrolyte disturbances in neoplastic diseases. Contrib Nephrol 7:2–41, 1977
358. Ghosh L, Meuhrhe RC: The nephrotic syndrome: A prodrome to lymphoma. Ann Intern Med 72:379–382, 1970
359. Cantrell EG: Nephrotic syndrome cured by removal of gastric carcinoma. Br Med J 2:739, 1969
360. Plager J, Stutzman L: Acute nephrotic syndrome as a manifestation of active Hodgkin's disease. Am J Med 50:56–66, 1971
361. Lewis MG, Loughridge LW, Phillips TM: Immunological studies in nephrotic syndrome associated with extrarenal malignant disease. Lancet 2:134–185, 1971
362. Couser WG, Wagonfeld JB, Spargo BH, Lewis EJ: Glomerular deposition of tumor antigen in membranous nephropathy associated with colonic carcinoma. Am J Med 57:962–970, 1974
363. Costanza ME, Perin V, Schwartz RS, Nathansen L: Carcinoembryonic antigen–antibody complexes in a patient with colonic carcinoma and nephrotic syndrome. N Engl J Med 289:520–522, 1973
364. Sherman RL, Susin M, Weksler ME, Becker EL: Lipoid nephrosis in Hodgkin's disease. Am J Med 52:699–706, 1972
365. Lokich JJ, Galvanek EG, Moloney WC: Nephrosis of Hodgkin's disease. Arch Intern Med 132:597–600, 1973
366. Moorthy AV, Zimmerman SW, Burkholder PM: Nephrotic syndrome in Hodgkin's disease. Am J Med 61:471–477, 1976
367. Carpenter CB: Case records of the Massachusetts General Hospital. N Engl J Med 289:1241–1247, 1973
368. Richard-Mendes da Costa C, Dupont E, Hamers R et al: Nephrotic syndrome in bronchogenic carcinoma: Report of two cases with immunochemical studies. Clin Nephrol 2:245–251, 1974
369. Dobbs DJ, Striker LM, Mignon F, Striker G: Glomerular lesions in lymphomas and leukemias. Am J Med 80:63–70, 1986
370. Gagliano RG, Costanzi JJ, Beathard GA et al: The nephrotic syndrome associated with neoplasia: An unusual paraneoplastic syndrome: Report of a case and review of the literature. Am J Med 60:1026–1031, 1976
371. Moorthy AV: Minimal change glomerular disease: A paraneoplastic syndrome in 2 patients with bronchogenic carcinoma. Am J Kidney Dis 3:58–62, 1983
372. Jermanovich NB, Glammarco R, Ginsberg SJ et al: Small cell anaplastic carcinoma of the lung with mesangial proliferative glomerulonephritis. Arch Intern Med 142:397–399, 1982
373. Cameron JS: Nephrotic syndrome in chronic lymphatic leukemia. Br Med J 4:164–167, 1974
374. Hyman LR, Burkholder PM, Joo PA, Segar WE: Malignant lymphoma and the nephrotic syndrome: A clinicopathologic analysis with light immunofluorescence and electron microscopy of the renal lesions. J Pediatr 82:207–217, 1973
375. Higgins MR, Randall RE, Still WJS: Nephrotic syndrome with oat-cell carcinoma. Br Med J 3:450, 1974
376. Karpen HO, Bhat JG, Feiner HD, Baldwin DS: Membranous nephropathy associated with renal cell carcinoma: Evidence against a role of renal tubular or tumor antibodies in pathogenesis. Am J Med 64:864–867, 1978
377. Hopper JH Jr: Tumor related renal lesions. Ann Intern Med 81:550–551, 1974
378. Row PG, Cameron JS, Turner DR et al: Membranous nephropathy: Long-term followup and association with neoplasia. Q J Med 44:207–239, 1975
379. Shalhoub RJ: Pathogenesis of lipoid nephrosis: A disorder of T-cell function. Lancet 2:556–558, 1974
380. Osserman EF, Lawlor DP: Serum and urinary lysozyme (muramidase) in monocyte and monomyelocytic leukemia. J Exp Med 124:921–951, 1966
381. Pruzanki W, Platts MF: Serum and urinary proteins, lysozyme (muramidase) and renal dysfunction in mono- and myelomonocytic leukemia. J Clin Invest 49:1694–1707, 1970
382. Hobbs JR, Evans DJ, Wrong OM: Renal tubular obstruction by mucoprotein from adenocarcinoma of pancreas. Br Med J 2:87–89, 1974
383. Freibusch J, Barbosa-Saldivar JL, Bernstein RS, Robertson GL: Tumor-associated nephrogenic diabetes insipidus. Ann Intern Med 92:797–798, 1980
384. Kyle RA: Multiple myeloma: Review of 869 cases. Mayo Clin Proc 50:29–40, 1975
385. DeFronzo RA, Cooke CR, Wright JR, Humphrey RL: Renal function in patients with multiple myeloma. Medicine 57:151–161, 1978
386. Zlotnick A, Rosenmann E: Renal pathologic findings associated with monoclonal gammopathies. Arch Intern Med 135:40–45, 1975
387. Schubert GE, Viegel J, Lennert K: Structure and function of the kidney in multiple myeloma. Virchow Arch Abt A Pathol Anat 355:135–137, 1972
388. Brown WW, Herbert LA, Piering WF et al: Reversal of chronic and stage renal failure due to myeloma kidney. Ann Intern Med 90:793–794, 1979
389. Leech SH, Polesky HF, Shapiro FL: Chronic hemodialysis in myelomatosis. Ann Intern Med 77:239–242, 1972
390. Richmond J, Sherman RS, Diamond HD, Craver LF: Renal lesions associated with malignant lymphomas. Am J Med 32:184–207, 1962
391. Martinez-Maldonado M, Ramirez de Arellano GA: Renal involvement in malignant lymphomas: A survey of 49 cases. J Urol 95:485–488, 1966
392. Matthews MJ: Problems in morphology and behavior of monchopulmonary malignant disease. In Israel L, Chanimian P (eds): Lung Cancer, Facts, Problems and Perspectives, pp 23–62. New York, Academic Press, 1976
393. Brin EN, Schiff M Jr, Weiss RM: Palliative urinary diversion for malignancy. J Urol 113:619–622, 1975
394. Fichman M, Bethune J: Effects of neoplasms on renal electrolyte function in paraneoplastic syndromes. Ann NY Acad Sci 230:448–472, 1974
395. Garnic MB, Mayer RJ: Acute renal failure associated with neoplastic disease and its treatment. Semin Oncol 5:155–165, 1976
396. Keane WF, Crosson JT, Staley NA et al: Radiation-induced renal disease: A clinicopathologic study. Am J Med 60:127–137, 1967
397. Dosik GM, Gutterman JE, Hersh EM et al: Nephrotoxicity from cancer immunotherapy. Ann Intern Med 89:41–46, 1978
398. Bennett WM, Muther RS, Parker RA et al: Drug therapy in renal failure: Dosing guidelines for adults. Ann Inter Med 93:286–325, 1980
399. Kierland RR: Cutaneous signs of internal malignancy. South Med J 65:563–568, 1972
400. Helm F, Helm J: Cutaneous markers of internal malignancies. In Helm F (ed): Cancer Dermatology, pp 247–283. Philadelphia, Lea & Febiger, 1979
401. Braverman IM: Skin Signs of Systemic Disease. Philadelphia, WB Saunders, 1970
402. Crowe FW: Axillary freckling as a diagnositc aid in neurofibromatosis. Ann Intern Med 61:1142–1143, 1964
403. Levine N, Greenwald ES: Mucocutaneous side effects of cancer chemotherapy. Cancer Treat Rev 5:67–84, 1978

404. Brown J, Winkelmann RK: Acanthosis nigricans: A study of 90 cases. Medicine 47:33–51, 1968
405. Curth HO: Classification of acanthosis nigricans. Int J Dermatol 15:592, 1976
406. Matsuoka MY, Goldman J, Wortsman J et al: Antibodies against the insulin receptor in paraneoplastic acanthosis nigricans. Am J Med 82:1253–1256, 1987
407. Sneddon IB, Roberts JBM: An incomplete form of acanthosis nigricans. Gut 3:269–272, 1962
408. Dantzig PI: Sign of Leser-Trelat. Arch Dermatol 108:700–701, 1973
409. Ronchese F: Keratoses, cancer and "the sign of Leser-Trelat." Cancer 18:1003–1006, 1965
410. Holdiness MR: The sign of Leser–Trelat. Int J Dematol 25:564–572, 1986
411. Curry SS, King LE: The sign of Leser–Trelat. Arch Dermatol 116:1059–1060, 1980
412. Graham JH, Helwig EB: Bowen's disease and its relationship to systemic cancer. Arch Dermatol 83:738–758, 1961
413. Anderson SL, Nielsen A, Reymann F: Relationship between Bowen's disease and internal malignancy. Arch Dermatol 108:367–370, 1973
414. Minkowsky S: Multiple carcinomata following the ingestion of medicinal arsenic. Ann Intern Med 61:296–299, 1964
415. Fitzpatrick TB, Montgomery H, Lerner AB: Pathogenesis of generalized dermal pigmentation secondary to malignant melanoma and melanuria. J Invest Dermatol 22:163–172, 1954
416. Ashikari R, Park K, Huvos AG, Urban JA: Paget's disease of the breast. Cancer 26:680–685, 1970
417. Witkowski JA, Parish LC: Bazex's syndrome: Paraneoplastic acrokeratosis. JAMA 248:2883–2884, 1983
418. Wishart JM: Bazex paraneoplastic acrokeratosis: A case report and response to Tagason. Br J Dermatol 115:595–599, 1986
419. Gammel JA: Erythema gyratum repens: Skin manifestations of patients with carcinoma of breast. Arch Dermatol 66:494–505, 1952
420. Purdy MJ: Erythema gyratum repens: Report of a case. Arch Dermatol 80:590–591, 1959
421. Summerly R: The figurate erythemas and neoplasia. Br J Dermatol 80:370–373, 1964
422. Lazar P: Cancer, erythema annulare centrifugum and autoimmunity. Arch Dermatol 87:246–253, 1963
423. Wilkinson DS: Necrolytic migrating erythema with pancreatic carcinoma. Proc R Soc Med 64:1197–1198, 1971
424. Church RE, Crane WAJ: A cutaneous syndrome associated with islet cell carcinoma of the pancreas. Br J Dermatol 79:284–286, 1967
425. Sjoerdsma A, Weissbach H, Udenfriend S: A clinical, physiologic, and biochemical study of patients with malignant carcinoid (argentaffinoma). Am J Med 21:520–532, 1956
426. Mason DT, Melmon KL: New understanding of the mechanism of the carcinoid flush. Ann Intern Med 65:1334–1339, 1966
427. Abrahams F, McCarthy JT, Sanders SL: 101 cases of exfoliative dermatitis. Arch Dermatol 87:96–103, 1963
428. Nicolis GD, Helwig EB: Exfoliative dermatitis: A clinicopathologic study of 135 cases. Arch Dermatol 108:788–979, 1973
429. Elias PM, Fritsch PO: Erythema multiforme. In Fitzpatrick TB, Eisen AZ, Wolf K et al (eds): Dermatology in General Medicine, 2nd ed, pp 295–303. New York, McGraw-Hill, 1979
430. Fitzpatrick TB, Clark WH Jr: Recurrent attacks of abdominal pain and cutaneous lesions. N Engl J Med 270:1248–1251, 1964
431. Waddington RT: A case of primary liver tumor associated with porphyria. Br J Surg 59:653–654, 1972
432. Thompson RPH, Nicholson DC, Farman T et al: Cutaneous porphyria due to a malignant primary hepatoma. Gastroenterology 59:779–783, 1970
433. Stone SP, Schroeder AL: Bullous pemphigoid and associated malignant neoplasms. Arch Dermatol 111:991–994, 1975
434. Tobias N: Dermatitis herpetiformis associated with visceral malignancy. Urol Cutan Rev 55:352, 1951
435. Arundell FD, Wilkinson RD, Haserick Jr: Dermatomyositis and malignant neoplasm in adults. Arch Dermatol 82:772–775, 1960
436. Lyell A, Whittle CH: Hypertrichosis languginosa acquired type. Br J Dermatol 63:411–413, 1951
437. Hegedus SI, Schorr WF: Acquired hypertrichosis lanquinosa and malignancy. Arch Dermatol 106:84–88, 1972
438. Van Dijk E: Ichthyosiform atrophy of the skin with internal malignant diseases. Dermatologica 127:413–428, 1963
439. Flint GL, Flam M, Soter NA: Acquired ichthyosis. Arch Dermatol 111:1446–1447, 1975
440. Vogl A, Goldfischer S: Pachydermoperiostosis. Primary or idiopathic hypertrophic osteoarthopathy. Am J Med 33:166–187, 1962
441. Rajka G: Investigation of patients suffering from generalized pruritus, with special references to systemic diseases. Acta Dermato-Venereol 46:190–194, 1966
442. Cormia FE: Pruritus, an uncommon but important symptom of systemic cancer. Arch Dermatol 92:36–39, 1965
443. Schimpff S, Serpick A, Stoler B et al: Varicella-zoster infection in patients with cancer. Ann Intern Med 76:241–254, 1972
444. Dolin R, Reichman RC, Mazur MH, Whitley RJ: Herpes zoster–varicella infections in immunosuppressed patients. Ann Intern Med 89:375–388, 1978
445. Huberman M, Fossieck BE Jr, Bunn PA Jr et al: Herpes zoster and small cell bronchogenic carcinoma. Am J Med 68:214–218, 1980
446. Gardner EJ: Follow-up study of a family group exhibiting dominant inheritance for a syndrome including intestinal polyps, osteomas, fibromas, and epidermal cysts. Am J Hum Genet 16:376–390, 1962
447. Bussey HJR: Gastrointestinal polyposis. Gut 11:970–978, 1970
448. Jones EL, Cornell WP: Garnder's syndrome: Review of the literature and report on a family. Arch Surg 92:287–300, 1966
449. Jeghers H, McKusick VA, Katz KH: Generalized intestinal polyposis and melanin spots of the oral mucosa, lips and digits: A syndrome of diagnostic significance. N Engl J Med 241:933–1005, 1031–1036, 1949
450. Riley E, Swift M: A family with Peutz-Jeghers syndrome and bilateral breast cancer. Cancer 46:815–817, 1980
451. Howel-Evans W, McConnell RR, Clarke CA, Sheppard PM: Carcinoma of the esophagus with keratosis palmaris et plantaris (tylosis). Q J Med 27:413–429, 1958
452. Williams ED, Pollock DJ: Multiple mucosal neuromata with endocrine tumors: A syndrome allied to Von Recklinghausen's disease. J Pathol Bacteriol 91:71–80, 1966
453. Lloyd KM, Dennis M: Cowden's disease, a possible new symptom complex with multiple system involvement. Ann Intern Med 58:136–142, 1963
454. Solomon LM, Fretzin DF, Dewald RL: The epidermal nevus syndrome. Arch Dermatol 97:273–285, 1968
455. Butterworth T, Wilson M Jr: Dermatologic aspects of tuberous sclerosis. Arch Dermatol Syph 43:1–41, 1941
456. Christoferson LA, Gustafson MB, Petersen AG: Von Hippel–Lindau's disease. JAMA 178:280–282, 1961
457. Doll R, Kinlen L: Immunosurveillance and cancer: Epidemiologic evidence. Br Med J 4:420–422, 1970
458. Frizzera G, Rosai J, Dehner LP et al: Lymphoreticular disorders in primary immunodeficiencies: New findings based on an up-to-date histologic classification of 35 cases. Cancer 46:692–699, 1980
459. Epstein CJ, Martin GM, Schultz AL, Motulsky AG: Werner's syndrome: A review of the symptomatology, natural history, pathologic features, genetics, and relationship to the natural aging process. Medicine 45:177–221, 1966
460. Waldman TA, Broder S, Strober W: Protein-losing enteropathies in malignancy. Ann NY Acad Sci 230:306–317, 1974
461. Watery diarrhoea (WDHA) syndrome associated with carcinoma of the lung. Aust NZ J Med 6:490–491, 1976
462. Troncale FJ: Distant manifestations of colonic carcinoma. Ann NY Acad Sci 230:332–347, 1974
463. Klipstein FA, Smorth G: Intestinal structure and function in neoplastic disease. Am J Dig Dis 14:887–889, 1969
464. Gilat T, Fischel B, Danon J, Lowewnthal M: Morphology of small bowel mucosa and malignancy. Digestion 12:147–155, 1972
465. Henderson AR, Grace DM: Liver-originating isoenzymes of alkaline phosphatase in the serum: A paraneoplastic manifestation of a malignant schwannoma of the sciatic nerve. J Clin Pathol 29:237–240, 1976
466. Walsh PN, Kissane JM: Nonmetastatic hypernephroma with reversible hepatic dysfunction. Arch Intern Med 122:214–222, 1968
467. Utz DC, Warren MM, Gregg JA et al: Reversible hepatic dysfunction associated with hypernephroma. Mayo Clin Proc 45:161–169, 1970
468. Cronin RE, Kaehny WD, Miller PD et al: Renal cell carcinoma: Unusual systemic manifestations. Medicine 55:291–311, 1976
469. Mena E, Bull FE, Bookstein JJ et al: Angiography of the nephrogenic hepatic dysfunction syndrome. Radiology 111:65–68, 1974
470. DeWys WD: Working conference on anorexia and cachexia of neoplastic disease. Cancer Res 30:2816–2818, 1970
471. DeWys WD: Abnormalities of taste as a remote effect of a neoplasm. Ann NY Acad Sci 230:427–434, 1974
472. Theologides A: The anorexia-cachexia syndrome: A new hypothesis. Ann NY Acad Sci 230:14–22, 1974
473. Waterhouse C: How tumors affect host metabolism. Ann NY Acad Sci 230:86–93, 1974
474. Beck SA, Tisdale MJ: Production of lipolytic and proteolytic factors by a murine tumor producing cachexia in the host. Cancer Res 47:5919–5923, 1987
475. Ternell M, Moldawer LC, Lonnroth C et al: Plasma protein synthesis in experimental cancer compared to paraneoplastic conditions, including monokine administration. Cancer Res 47:5825–5830, 1987
476. Gold J: Cancer cachexia and gluconeogenesis. Ann NY Acad Sci 230:103–110, 1974
477. Bodel P: Tumors and fever. Ann NY Acad Sci 230:6–13, 1974
478. Petersdorf RG: Fever and cancer. Hosp Med 1:2–10, 1965
479. Lobell M, Boggs DR, Wintrobe MM: The clinical significance of fever in Hodgkin's disease. Arch Intern Med 117:335–342, 1966
480. Gluckman JB, Turner MD: Systemic manifestations of tumors of the small gut and liver. Ann NY Acad Sci 230:318–331, 1974
481. Block JB: Lactic acidosis in malignancy and observations on its possible pathogenesis. Ann NY Acad Sci 230:94–102, 1974
482. Nadiminti Y, Wang JC, Chou S et al: Lactic acidosis associated with Hodgkin's disease: Response of chemotherapy. N Engl J Med 303:15–17, 1980
483. Spechler SJ, Esposito AL, Koff RS, Hong WK: Lactic acidosis in oat cell carcinoma with extensive hepatic metastases. Arch Intern Med 138:1663–1664, 1978
484. Eridani S, Burdick L, Periti M, Arosio A, Libretti A: Primary carcinoma of the colon and hyperlipemia: A paraneoplastic syndrome. Biomedicine 25:324–326, 1976
485. Glueck HL, MacKenzie M, Glueck CJ: Crystalline IgG protein in multiple myeloma:

Identification of effects on coagulation and on lipoprotein metabolism. J Lab Clin Med 79:731–744, 1972
486. Santer MA, Waldmann TA, Fallon HJ: Erythrocytosis and hyperlipemia as manifestations of hepatic carcinoma. Arch Intern Med 120:735–739, 1967
487. Gangulu A, Gribble J, Tune B et al: Renin-secreting Wilms' tumor with severe hypertension: Report of a case and brief review of renin-secreting tumors. Ann Intern Med 79:835–837, 1973
488. Genest J, Rojo-Ortega JM, Kuchel O et al: Malignant hypertension with hypokalemia in a patient with renin-producing pulmonary carcinoma. Trans Assoc Am Physicians 88:192–201, 1975
489. Aurell M, Rudin A, Tisell LE et al: Captopril effort on hypertension in patient with renin-producing tumor. Lancet 2:149–150, 1979
490. Hollifield JW, Page DL, Smith C et al: Renin-secreting clear cell carcinoma of the kidney. Arch Intern Med 135:859–864, 1975
491. Zusman RM, Snider JJ, Cline A et al: Antihypertensive function of renal-cell carcinoma: Evidence for a prostaglandin A secreting tumor. N Engl J Med 290:43–845, 1974
492. Boasberg PD, Henry JP, Rosenbloom AA et al: Case reports and studies of paraneoplastic hypotension: Abnormal low pressure baroreceptor responses. Med Pediatr Oncol 3:59–66, 1977
493. Braganza JM, Butler EB, Fox H et al: Ectopic production of salivary type amylase by a pseudomesotheliomatous carcinoma of the lung. Cancer 41:1522–1525, 1978
494. Mills JA: A spectrum of organ systems that respond to cancer: The joints and connective tissue. Ann NY Acad Sci 230:443–447, 1974
495. Greenfield GB, Schorsch HA, Shkolnik A: The various roentgen appearance of pulmonary hypertrophic osteoarthropathy. Am J Roentgenol Radium Ther Nucl Med 101:927–931, 1967
496. LeRoux BT: Bronchial carcinoma with hypertrophic pulmonary osteoarthropathy. S Afr Med J 42:1074–1075, 1968
497. Jao JY, Barlow JJ, Krant MKJ: Pulmonary hypertrophic osteoarthropathy, spider angiomata and estrogen hypersecretion in neoplasms. Ann Intern Med 70:580–584, 1969
498. Donnelly B, Johnson PM: Detection of hypertrophic pulmonary osteoarthropathy by skeletal imaging with ^{99m}Tc-labeled diphosphonate. Radiology 114:389–391, 1975
499. Green N, Kurohara SS, George FW III, Crews QE Jr: The biologic behavior of lung cancer according to histologic type. Radiol Clin Biol 41:160–170, 1972
500. Yesner R: Spectrum of lung cancer and ectopic hormones. In Sommers SC, Rosen PP (eds): Pathology Annual, Vol 12 (part 1), pp 217–240. New York, Appleton-Century-Crofts, 1978
501. Goldstraw P, Walbraun PR: Hypertrophic pulmonary osteoarthropathy and its occurrence with pulmonary metastases from renal carcinoma. Thorax 31:205–211, 1976
502. Miller ER: Carcinoma of the thymus with marked pulmonary osteoarthropathy. Radiology 32:651–660, 1939
503. Ullal SR: Hypertrophic osteoarthropathy and leiomyoma of the oesophagus. Am J Surg 123:356–358, 1972
504. Shapiro RF, Zvaifler NJ: Concurrent intrathoracic Hodgkin's disease and hypertrophic osteoarthropathy. Chest 63:912–916, 1973
505. Howard CP, Telander RL, Hoffman AD, Burgert EO Jr: Hypertrophic osteoarthropathy in association with pulmonary metastasis from osteogenic sarcoma. Mayo Clin Proc 53:538–541, 1978
506. Papavasiliou C, Pavlatou M, Pappas J: Nasopharyngeal cancer in patients under the age of thirty years. Cancer 40:2312–2316, 1977
507. Ellouz R, Cammoun M, Attia RB, Bahi J: Clinical aspects: Nasopharyngeal carcinoma in children and adolescents in Tunisia: Clinical aspects and the paraneoplastic syndrome. IARC Sci Pub 20:115–129, 1978
508. Cudkowicz L, Armstrong, JB: Finger clubbing and changes in the bronchial circulation: Arterio-venous shunts in hypertrophic pulmonary osteoarthropathy. Br J Tuberc 47:227–232, 1953
509. Carroll KB, Doyle L: A common factor in hypertrophic osteoarthropathy. Thorax 29:262–264, 1974
510. Riyami AM, Anderson EG: Hypertrophic pulmonary osteoarthropathy: A clinical and biochemical study. Br J Dis Chest 68:193–196, 1974
511. Glenner GC: Amyloid deposits and amyloidosis: The β-fibriloses. N Engl J Med 303:1283–1292, 1333–1347, 1980
512. Azzopardi JG, Lehner T: Systemic amyloidosis and malignant disease. J Clin Pathol 19:539–548, 1966
513. Kyle RA, Bayrd ED: Amyloidosis: Review of 236 cases. Medicine 54:271–547, 1975
514. Shiel WC, Prete PE, Jason M, Andrews BS: Palmar fasciitis and arthritis with ovarian and non-ovarian carcinomas. Am J Med 79:640–644, 1985
515. Pfinsgraff J, Buckingham RB, Killian PJ et al: Palmar fasciitis and arthritis with malignant neoplasms: A paraneoplastic syndrome. Semin Arthritis Rheum 16:118–125, 1986
516. Michaels RM, Sorber JA: Reflex sympathetic dystrophy as a probable paraneoplastic syndrome: Case report and literature review. Arthritis Rheum 27:1183–1185, 1984
517. Mills JA: Connective tissue disease associated with malignant neoplastic disease. J Chronic Disi 16:797–811, 1963
518. Calabro J: Cancer and arthritis. Arthritis Rheum 10:553–567, 1967
519. Cammarata R, Rodnan GP, Jensen WM: Systemic rheumatic disease and malignant lymphoma. Arch Intern Med 111:112–119, 1963
520. Miller D: The association of immune disease and malignant lymphoma. Ann Intern Med 66:507–521, 1967
521. Anderson LG, Talal N: The spectrum of benign to malignant lymphoproliferation in Sjögrens syndrome. Clin Exp Immunol 9:199–221, 1971
522. Murray GC, Persellin RH: Metastatic carcinoma presenting as monarticular arthritis: A case report and review of the literature. Arthritis Rheum 23:95–100, 1980
523. Karten I, Bartfield H: Bronchogenic carcinoma simulating early rheumatoid arthritis. JAMA 179:160–161, 1962
524. Tumulty PA: Systemic lupus erythematosus. In Winthrobe, Thorn, Adams et al (eds): Harrison's Principles of Internal Medicine, 6th ed. pp 1962–1967. New York, McGraw-Hill, 1971

JOHN E. ULTMANN

THEODORE L. PHILLIPS

CHAPTER 56 *Cancer of Unknown Primary Site*

The patient with histologically documented cancer with no obvious primary site presents a difficult but not uncommon problem for the practicing physician. Between 0.5% and 9% of cancer patients have an occult primary site, depending on the thoroughness of the investigation undertaken to find the primary site and the population studied. Two questions are foremost in the mind of the clinician treating the patient with a malignancy of unknown primary site: [1] Which diagnostic studies should be undertaken to locate the primary site? [2] What treatment if any, is indicated when the primary site is not found after an appropriate investigation? This chapter will discuss these questions in detail and provide a guide for patient management.

A critical analysis of the literature concerning the patient with cancer of unknown origin is difficult. All studies have been retrospective. Comparisons between individual studies usually are not valid because the patient populations studied differ and the criteria used to define the patient with an unknown primary site vary. Patient cohorts may involve all patients in a hospital tumor registry or only those patients referred to a special oncology unit. Some physicians consider a patient to have an unknown primary site if the history, physical examination, and chest films are unrevealing; others require the patient to have undergone more extensive testing which includes additional biopsies. A few physicians exclude any patient for whom the diagnosis was suspected during life or eventually known, no matter how late during the clinical course it occurred. A further point of variation among studies concerns the evidence needed to establish the primary site. Is one radiologic study adequate? Should two positive clinical tests be required? Is a biopsy of the suspected primary site necessary? Despite these difficulties, sufficient clinical information is now available to form a rational basis for the management of these patients, provided physicians precisely define the patient population of interest.

OCCULT PRIMARY MALIGNANCY

For clarity of discussion, a patient will be said to have a possible *occult primary malignancy* (OPM) if [1] he has a biopsy-proven malignancy; and [2] a history, physical examination, chest film, complete blood count, urinalysis, and stool test for blood are not indicative of a primary site. Histologic study of the biopsy must demonstrate unequivocal malignancy and must be inconsistent with a primary tumor at the biopsy site. In most cancer patients, the localization of the primary site is not difficult. If after all clues from a thorough history, a complete physical examination, and the foregoing screening laboratory studies, as well as **indicated additional diagnostic studies**, have been investigated, the primary site is not found, it is concluded that the patient has an OPM. For example, the patient presenting with squamous cell carcinoma in a high cervical node is not classified as having an OPM until he has received a meticulous ear, nose, and throat examination by a specialist, computed tomography (CT) and magnetic resonance imaging (MRI) scans have been obtained, and directed biopsies of oral and pharyngeal areas are negative.

DIAGNOSTIC EVALUATION IN OCCULT PRIMARY MALIGNANCY

In many hospitals, patients with an OPM undergo extensive diagnostic studies based on the belief that optimal management depends on identification of the primary site. The usefulness of such an approach has been questioned by many investigators.[1-3] Median survival for OPM patients is poor, usually only 3 to 4 months. Survival curves from three publications show that fewer than 25% of patients are alive at 1-year and fewer than 10% at 5-year follow-up (Fig. 56-1).[4-6] Patients with poor performance status and disease in multiple organs have a median survival of 1 month, and 87% are dead within 3 months.[7] As a group, patient survival is unchanged by treatment, with the major exception of patients with cervical lymph node metastases, who may have occult head and neck cancer; patients with probable lymphoma or germ cell neoplasms; and a few others. Hence, the cost and discomfort of elaborate diagnostic studies (which may consume a substantial part of a patient's life expectancy) need to be weighed carefully.[8-10] In most OPM patients, a primary site will not be located during their lifetimes. Even after postmortem examination, the primary site will not be identified in 15% of these patients. Chemotherapy of OPM patients before the advent of doxorubicin (Adriamycin) was also uniformly unsuccessful, with a response rate of 15% or less.

Table 56-1 lists the primary sites identified by Nystrom and co-workers, either during life or at autopsy.[11,12] The distribution of primary sites eventually found in their OPM patients and in the literature is quite different from the overall incidence of primary cancers reported from the End Results Group. The lungs were the most common primary site in patients with supradiaphragmatic metastases, whereas the pancreas was the most common primary site in patients with subdiaphragmatic metastases. The value of systemic therapy for most primary sites ultimately detected is in question.[2,3]

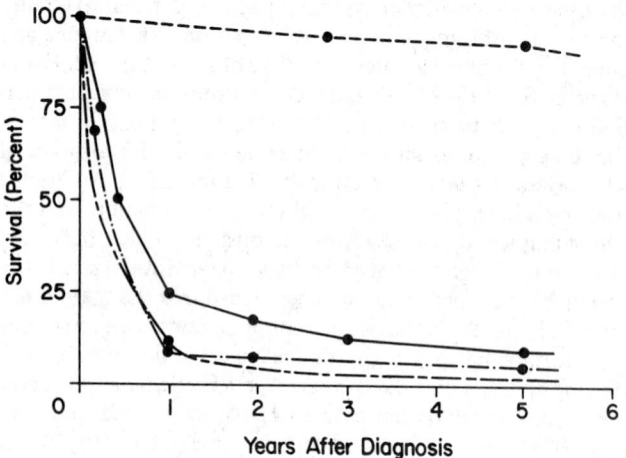

FIG. 56-1. Survival curve of patients with metastatic cancer with an unknown primary site. (•—• Smith PE, Krementz ET, Chapman W: Metastatic cancer without a detectable primary site. J Surg 113:633–637, 1967; •-–-• Holmes FF, Fouts TL: Metastatic cancer of unknown primary site. Cancer 26:816–820, 1970; •-—• Richardson RG, Parker RG: Metastases from undetected primary cancers—Clinical experience at a radiation oncology center (Medical Information). West J Med 123:337–339, 1975; •---• Survival of age-adjusted normal controls.

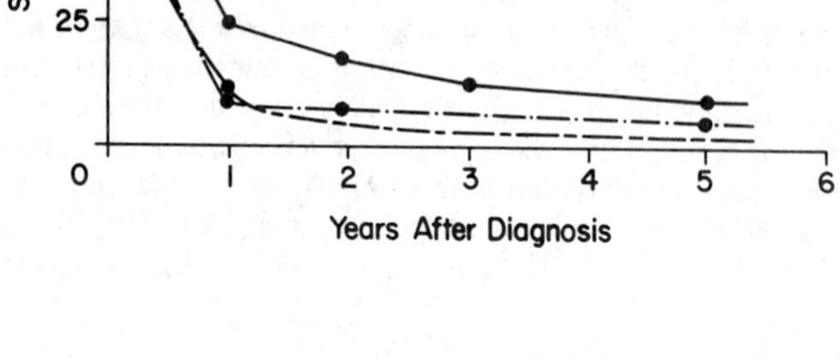

The search for a primary site is difficult because the pattern of metastases may be atypical when compared with the metastatic spread of a clinically obvious primary site presenting in the traditional manner.[11] Table 56-2 compares the pattern of metastatic involvement in patients with an OPM, in whom a primary site was eventually proved, with published values for patterns of metastases of patients with obvious primary sites. For example, 30% to 50% of patients with metastatic lung cancer can be expected to have bone involvement, but only 4% of patients with an OPM, later proved to be lung cancer, had bone metastases. The normal relative frequency of metastases from known primary sites is, therefore, not useful in making a diagnosis. Several common tumors, such as breast and prostate, are detectable by simple means, and thus they rarely present as OPM.

Patients with OPM have a different pattern of metastatic spread, as well as a different frequency of ultimately proven primary sites when compared with patients with metastatic malignancies and obvious primary sites. The statistics cited in Tables 56-1 and 56-2 describe the distribution of primary cancer sites and the patterns of metastatic involvement. The biologic reasons for these observations have not yet been elucidated; however, Holmes and Fouts have cited four reasons for metastatic cancer remaining undiagnosed for the primary origin. [1] Present clinical tools are inadequate; [2] the primary may remain inapparent despite autopsy because standard sampling and lack of serial sections may not constitute a sufficient search; [3] the primary may have been removed by excision or fulguration (*e.g.*, melanoma), by dilatation and curettage (*e.g.*, endometrial cancer), or by sloughing of the necrotic tumor from skin or the gastrointestinal tract; and [4] a spontaneous regression of the primary may have occurred.[5]

In the patients in whom primary sites are ultimately detected the primary sites are smaller than tumors whose metastases have occurred from easily detectable sites. Often the histologic appearance of the metastasis, or of the later-discovered primary, is undifferentiated or a poorly differentiated carcinoma; lymphoma, or sarcoma. Apparently, these tumors metastasize early, and the metastases have a tendency to proliferate more rapidly than does the primary tumor. The response to therapy and survival are poor. Fer and associates have pointed out that, within a given tumor, certain cells have a high metastatic potential, and others do not. Variations in immunogenicity and antigen content of these tumor cells may determine host responses of different intensity as well as preferential spread to specific sites.[13] Current studies on the amplification of oncogene expression may provide clues to the aforementioned observations.

Further difficulty arises because clinical studies are often incorrect, with both false-positive and false-negative results. Even chest roentgenographic patterns normally considered diagnostic of primary lung tumors may be erroneous when metastatic disease is present. The relatively low sensitivity

TABLE 56-1. Distribution of Primary Cancer Sites: Comparison with Literature and End Results Group

Primary Site	*Present Series* *n*	%	*Literature* %	*End Results Group* %
Above diaphragm				
Lung	28	18	17	10
Breast	3	2	3	26
Thyroid	2	1	5	1
Parotid	1	<1		<1
Subtotal	34			
Below diaphragm				
Pancreas	30	20	21	1.5
Liver	16	11	10	1.5
Colorectal	15	10	7	14
Gastric	12	8	10	5
Renal	9	6	3	2
Ovary	4	4	2	5
Prostate	4	3	3	17
Adrenal	1	<1	2	
Subtotal	91			
Other	4	2		
Not classified	23	15	15	
Total	152			

Nystrom JS, Weiner JM, Heffelfinger–Juttner J et al: Metastatic and histologic presentations in unknown primary cancer. Semin Oncol 4:53–58, 1977.

and very poor selectivity of three commonly employed contrast studies in patients with an OPM have been emphasized by a number of authors [*i.e.*, upper GI films (64% and 50%, respectively), barium enema (62% and 54%, respectively), and intravenous pyelogram (IVP; 41% and 27% respectively)]. The roles of CT and MRI scans have not yet been fully assessed.[1,9,14] Tentative diagnoses are often not confirmed at autopsy. One clinical study alone should not be considered diagnostic.

Although the foregoing data would seem to suggest that no evaluation is justified for the patient with OPM, this is not true. About 10% or 15% of patients with an OPM will ultimately be proved to have tumors for which *effective local or systemic therapy* is available, although, unfortunately, not all of these patients will be identifiable before death. For example, a group of female patients present with axillary lymph node and distant metastases. They are found to have breast cancer effectively controllable by combination chemotherapy. A search for these primary tumors is indicated, for their identification will select those patients who will benefit greatly from specific therapy. A list of these tumors appears in Table 56-3 and includes tumors for which there is highly effective therapy; moderately effective but quite specific therapy; or therapy with no toxicity. Table 56-3 lists the number and types of potentially treatable malignancies found in patients with OPM.[14]

A second reason for diagnostic studies is the prevention of local catastrophes. For example, if searching for an OPM of

TABLE 56-2. Pattern of Metastatic Involvement: Comparison of Clinically Overt Primaries (B) and Primaries Presenting as OPM (A)

Primary Site	*Bone* A	*Bone* B	*Lung* A	*Lung* B	*Liver* A	*Liver* B	*Brain* A	*Brain* B
Lung	4	30–50	90	34	36	30–50	21	15–30
Breast	33	50–85	66	60	66	45–60	33	15–25
Thyroid	0	39	100	65	50	60	0	1
Pancreas	28	5–10	31	25–40	72	50–70	3	1–4
Liver	31	8	19	20	100		6	0
Colorectal	13	5–10	40	25–40	87	71	0	1
Gastric	9	5–10	18	20–30	36	35–50	9	1–4
Renal	66	30–50	77	50–75	33	35–40	0	7–8
Ovary	0	2–6	25	10	25	10–15	0	1
Prostate	25	50–75	75	13–53	50	13	25	2

(% Metastatic Involvement)

Nystrom JS, Weiner JM, Heffelfinger–Juttner J et al: Metastatic and histologic presentations in unknown primary cancer. Semin Oncol 4:53–58, 1977.

TABLE 56-3. Tumors for Which Effective Local or Systemic Treatment Is Available

Cure possible by local therapy
Radiotherapy: head and neck cancer
Radical surgery: melanoma
Cure possible by systemic therapy
Germ cell tumors
Hodgkin's disease
Non-Hodgkin's lymphoma
Trophoblastic tumors
"Nontoxic" hormonal treatment
Breast cancer
Prostatic cancer
Endometrial cancer
Highly effective chemotherapy (response ≥ 50%)
Breast cancer
Ovarian cancer
Oat cell carcinoma of lung
Head and neck cancer

a poorly differentiated adenocarcinoma leads to the detection of a primary lesion in the colon, local resection of the primary colon carcinoma may be justified to prevent an impending bowel obstruction. Similarly, a search for bone metastases in weight-bearing bones or an investigation of back pain to detect impending spinal cord compression is indicated because local therapy can prevent debilitating complications.[3]

ORGANIZATION OF THE DIAGNOSTIC EVALUATION

As described previously, the diagnostic evaluation of the patient with an OPM has two goals: the identification of any tumor for which effective, or at least specific, therapy is available and the identification of any imminent local complication for which local therapy is required. These are best pursued using a systematic approach. Only those studies that result in data that would potentially alter therapy are useful.[10,14] For example, the measurement of acid phosphatase levels, which may lead to the diagnosis of prostate carcinoma, is useful because there is specific therapy available for the tumor. However, the measurement of a carcinoembryonic antigen level, which is elevated in many tumors and nonmalignant states, is useless. To distinguish between primary tumors for which there is only minimally effective systemic therapy is of no value because the patient's management will be unchanged. Therefore, before any diagnostic test is ordered, the physician should ask, "Will the results affect patient management?" If the answer is no, the tests should not be ordered.[10]

Diagnostic studies must be selected carefully to ensure that the most information is obtained at the least cost to the patient in terms of money, time, and discomfort, and at the lowest risk of morbidity or mortality. Studies directed by signs of symptoms are more likely to be fruitful than those that are not. Careful attention must be directed to evaluating biopsy material for precise histologic classification.[15-17] The presenting anatomic site must be analyzed for clues to the origin of the OPM. A repeat history and physical examination may yield clues that were missed earlier. In addition, careful attention must be paid to smoking history, pains (particularly in the epigastrium), change in bowel habits or voiding pattern, vaginal or other bleeding, and pelvic discomfort. The examination must include pelvic and rectal examinations. Specific studies should be undertaken to search systematically for those primary sites for which therapeutic options are available and useful.

The optimal sequence of steps when evaluating the patient with an OPM concentrates on the reevaluation of the biopsy material. Note that this differs from the traditional order of inquiry (history, physical examination, laboratory studies) used to delineate other clinical problems. The biopsy should be reviewed first because a history and physical examination are usually unrevealing. Any clues that the biopsy specimen provides will facilitate a directed history and a physical examination with emphasis on specific areas of interest.

Data from Biopsy Specimens

The first step in the evaluation of the patient with an OPM is to review the biopsy material with an experienced pathologist. Subtle features in the histologic appearance may well give an indication of likely primary sites.[15-17] If there is any question about the adequacy of the original biopsy material and if an easily accessible site is available, a second biopsy should be done. Note that careful planning is necessary to ensure that the surgical specimen is properly divided for any desired special studies *before* it is put into a routine fixative. Many of the antigens that are particularly useful for diagnostic purposes are not preserved in formalin-fixed, paraffin-embedded tissue. Thus, it is necessary, for the routine processing of tumors of unknown origin, that samples of tissues should be fixed in glutaraldehyde for electron microscopy, frozen for immunohistochemical and gene arrangement studies, and then fixed for standard light-microscopic examination.

Sometimes special stains are useful. Some tumors appear totally undifferentiated on hematoxylin–eosin-stained sections. In adults, the most common of these are poorly differentiated squamous cell carcinoma, poorly differentiated adenocarcinoma, diffuse large-cell or undifferentiated lymphoma, poorly differentiated sarcoma, amelanotic melanoma, and undifferentiated germ cell cancer (Table 56-4). Intracellular mucin, detected with a mucicarmine stain, would identify an adenocarcinoma; diastase-resistant, periodic acid–Schiff (PAS) positivity of such an adenocarcinoma would point to a gastric carcinoma. However, electron microscopy is often much more useful.[18,19] For example, premelanosomes are diagnostic of melanomas, whereas desmosomes identify poorly differentiated carcinomas. In females, the measurement of estrogen receptors is helpful.[20] These are found classically in breast carcinoma, but they may also be present in ovarian and endometrial carcinomas and melanomas. An axillary metastasis in a woman with positive estrogen receptors should be considered diagnostic of breast carcinoma, despite a physical examination of the breast that showed no abnormalities and a normal mammogram.

Recent progress in immunocytochemistry, including immunoperoxidase techniques, has led to the development of

TABLE 56-4. Examples of the Usefulness of Electron Microscopy, Histochemistry, Immunologic Surface Markers, and Hormone Receptors in the Classification of OPM

	Electron Microscopy	*Histochemistry*	*Immune Markers*	*Hormone Receptors*
Poorly differentiated squamous cell carcinoma	Intercellular bridges, tonofilaments, desmosomes			
Poorly differentiated adenocarcinoma	Junctional complex, tight junction, intermediate junction, desmosome	Mucicarmin, diastase-resistant PAS		Estrogen receptor, progesterone receptor
Diffuse histiocytic or undifferentiated lymphoma	Polyribosomes, absence of junctions	PAS MGP	EAO rosettes, E rosettes, surface Ig	Steroid receptor
Poorly differentiated sarcoma	Myofibrils, dilated rough endoplasmic reticulum, or extracellular osteoid	Trichrome stain	Monoclonal antibodies to leukocyte differentiation antigens	
Amelanotic melanoma	Premelanosomes	Fontana-Mason argyrophil stain		Estrogen receptor
Undifferentiated germ cell carcinoma				Estrogen receptor
Neuroectoderm-derived tumors	Dense secretory granules			

probes to search for enzymes, hormones, oncofetal antigens, serum proteins, and other products useful in classifying neoplasms (Table 56-5).[16,17,20–24]

Recent developments in molecular biology have demonstrated that lymphoproliferative disorders may be definitively detected and assigned to B-cell or T-cell lineages by determination of lineage-specific gene rearrangements. The usefulness of these techniques in studies of OPMs has not yet been reported.

Data from the Anatomical Location

For practical purposes, patients with OPM can be divided into two major categories according to anatomical presentation—those with metastatic disease above the diaphragm, and those with metastatic disease below the diaphragm. In addition, those patients with involvement of only the cervical lymph nodes or axillary lymph nodes deserve special consideration (Table 56-6).

CERVICAL LYMPH NODES. Despite the dismal prognosis, patients with OPM shown in only cervical nodes are greatly benefited by local and regional therapy.[25] The 3-year survival after radical irradiation, radical surgery, or both, ranges from 30% to 60%. An OPM in a cervical node most often is due to regional spread from a clinically inapparent primary lesion in the head and neck.[25–30] A CT scan[29] or an MRI scan[31] may be particularly useful in detecting the inapparent primary source. About 78% of the primary sites that became apparent after therapy were, in fact, in the head and neck. High cervical nodes are more likely to have a head and neck primary site in Waldeyer's ring than are low cervical nodes. Consequently, high cervical nodes indicate a better prognosis.[25–28, 30]

SUPRACLAVICULAR LYMPH NODES. Patients with OPM in the supraclavicular nodes have a much poorer prognosis. These most often represent widely metastatic disease from a distant primary lesion. On the right side, the most likely primary sites are lung and breast. On the left side, spread from intra-abdominal malignancies by way of the thoracic duct is probable and needs to be considered (*i.e.*, Virchow's node), but a lung cancer is still the most likely source.[28,30] The small number of long-term survivors with radical irradiation (12%) is probably due to primary sites in the head and neck.

AXILLARY LYMPH NODES. Among patients with OPM above the diaphragm, those with an isolated axillary node have unique clinical features. Most of these tumors are adenocarcinomas and occur in women.[30,32] The prognosis for patients who have an isolated axillary node is somewhat better than for OPM in general.[32] In a report from M. D. Anderson Hospital, 18 of 37 females who had a malignant axillary node and a normal breast examination result were ultimately shown to have breast carcinoma.[33] Mammography was normal in 9 of the 17 patients in whom the study was performed. Thus, normal physical examination and mammography results do not completely rule out breast carcinoma. In addition, 9 of 60 patients in another study from the M. D. Anderson Hospital remained disease-free for 2 to 10 years after diagnosis. Therapy consisted of only local excision or axillary dissection. Two patients who died of other causes had no evidence of malignancy at postmortem examination. No primary site was identified in any of these patients. Feigenberg and co-workers reported eight patients with axillary lymph node metastases. The primary growth in three of these patients was ultimately found in the ipsilateral breast.[34] The investigators advocated conservative sector mastectomy of the upper-outer quadrant as a diagnostic pro-

TABLE 56-5. Tumor Markers Most Commonly Used to Classify Neoplasms of Unknown Origin

Tissue Marker	Diagnostic Application
Enzymes	
Prostatic acid phosphatase	Identification of metastatic carcinomas of prostate
Muramidase (lysozyme)	Differentiation of true histiocytic lymphoma. Myelomonocytic leukemias
Histaminase	Medullary thyroid carcinoma. Undifferentiated small (oat)-cell carcinoma of the lung
Placental alkaline phosphatase	Germ cell tumor
Hormones	
Anterior pituitary hormones (ACTH, prolactin, TSH, LH)	Functional classification of pituitary tumors. Differentiation of pituitary tumors from poorly differentiated neoplasms originating from the ethmoidal and sphenoidal sinuses
Calcitonin	Medullary carcinoma of thyroid. C-cell hyperplasia
Thyroglobulin, T_3, T_4	Metastatic thyroid carcinoma
Pancreatic islet cell and gastrointestinal hormones (insulin, glucagon, gastrin)	Functional classification of pancreatic islet cell and carcinoid tumors
Human chorionic gonadotropin (hCG)	Identification of trophoblastic elements in gonadal germ cell tumors; other neoplasms
Testosterone	Sertoli-Leydig tumors
Estradiol	Granulosa and theca cell tumors
Intermediate filaments	
Keratins	Classification of poorly differentiated squamous carcinomas, some adenocarcinomas, mesotheliomas, thymomas, epithelial–synovial, sarcoma, nonseminomatous germ cell tumors
Desmin	Tumors of muscle origin, rhabdomyosarcoma
Vimentin	Tumors of mesenchymal origin
Glial fibrillary acidic protein	Differentiation of gliomas from other tumors
Neurofilament	Tumors of neural origin, neuroblastoma, neuroendocrine tumors
Leukocyte differentiation antigens	
Leukocyte common antigen (CD45, T200, LCA)	Hematopoietic neoplasms, especially large-cell lymphoma
Ki 1 (CD30)	Hodgkin's disease, Ki 1 lymphoma
Leu M1 (CD15, X-hapten)	Differentiation of carcinoma from mesothelioma
Oncofetal antigens	
α-Fetoprotein (AFP)	Differential diagnosis and classification of gonadal and extragonadal germ cell tumors; hepatocellular carcinoma, other tumors
Carcinoembryonic antigen (CEA)	Adenocarcinoma of colon, other tumors; differentiation of carcinoma from mesothelioma
Serum proteins	
Immunoglobulins	Differentiation of large (B)-cell lymphomas from poorly differentiated carcinomas; differentiation of atypical lymphocytic proliferations from lymphomas; characterization of multiple myeloma
α-1-Antitrypsin	Hepatocellular carcinoma, gonadal and extragonadal germ cell tumors, other neoplasms
Other products	
α-Lactalbumin, casein	Metastatic breast carcinoma; differentiation of extramammary Paget's disease from other tumors
Myoglobin	Tumors derived from skeletal muscle
Actin, myosin	Tumors derived from smooth and skeletal muscle, other neoplasms
Factor VIII-related antigen	Tumors derived from endothelial cells
Prostate-specific antigen (PSA)	Prostate carcinoma

(continued)

TABLE 56-5. Tumor Markers Most Commonly Used to Classify Neoplasms of Unknown Origin—(*continued*)

Tissue Marker	*Diagnostic Application*
Estrogen receptor, progesterone receptor	Breast, ovary carcinoma, germ cell carcinoma, melanoma
Protein S100	Amelanotic melanoma, schwannoma, granular cell tumor, chordoma, and cartilaginous tumors
Milk-fat globule-derived antigen (MFGDA)	Mesothelioma, carcinoma
Chromogranin, Leu 7, NKH1	Neuroendocrine tumors

Modified from Mackay B, Ordonez NG: The role of the pathologist in the evaluation of poorly differentiated tumors. Semin Oncol 9:396–415, 1982; and Battifora H: Recent progress in the immunochemistry of solid tumors. Semin Diagn Pathol 1:251–271, 1984.

cedure and radiotherapy to the affected axilla and, if breast cancer was proved, to the residual breast as well. Others have reported similar approaches.[35,36]

The ready availability of estrogen (ER) and progesterone (PR) receptor tests and an immunohistochemical marker for α-lactalbumin changes the strategy of the workup of an isolated axillary mass. Therefore, the initial biopsy in all female patients should be processed for receptor activity and α-lactalbumin. Carcinoma of the breast can be presumed to be the primary (even if no primary lesion is demonstrable) if an ER+ or PR+ adenocarcinoma is found in axillary lymph nodes. Such patients may also benefit from hormonal therapy.[30] If ER and PR results were negative or not obtained, it is best to treat the most treatable cancer for the particular region. Thus, if the patient is a 48-year-old woman who has axillary involvement and no primary lesion is found, the best way to manage her disease would be to treat it as if it were carcinoma of the breast. This should be done whether or not estrogen receptor sites are found.

TABLE 56-6. Anatomical Analysis of OPM

Anatomical Location	*Primary Source to be Considered*
Above diaphragm	
High cervical lymph nodes	Head and neck, (nasopharynx, oropharynx) Thyroid Lungs
Low cervical supraclavicular lymph nodes	Head and neck Thyroid Left or right lung Left > right gastrointestinal
Axillary lymph nodes	Breast Left or right lung Left > right gastrointestinal
All presentations above diaphragm	Lungs
Below diaphragm	
Umbilical mass (Sister Mary Joseph's nodule)	Gastrointestinal (stomach > others) Ovarian Uterine
Groin mass/lymph nodes	Anus and rectum Prostate Vulva Testicle (after testicular biopsy or repair of hernia)
All presentations below diaphragm	Pancreas

Malignant melanoma may present as an OPM in the axillary (or inguinal) lymph nodes, following the pattern of spread for melanoma reported for women and men, and it should be managed as Stage II melanoma, with radical lymph node dissection.[37-39]

With the exceptions already discussed (*i.e.*, high cervical axillary and left supraclavicular lymph node presentations), lung cancer remains the most common primary site for OPM presenting *above* the diaphragm.[11]

In analyses of OPM that appears as metastases *below* the diaphragm, carcinoma of the pancreas is the most common primary site ultimately detected.[11] However, two other areas deserve special consideration—an umbilical mass and a groin mass or lymph nodes.

UMBILICAL MASS. Primary carcinoma of the umbilicus is rare and is usually epidermoid. Adenocarcinomas detected in the umbilicus are likely to be metastatic (35 of 36 cases), and the most common primary source is carcinoma of the stomach. Occasionally, carcinoma of the gallbladder, colon, appendix, ovary, or uterus is the primary lesion. In 18 of 40 patients with umbilical masses, the umbilical lesion was the only reason for seeking medical attention. The finding of the mass (referred to as Sister Mary Joseph's nodule) initiated the appropriate workup for the OPM.[40-44]

GROIN MASS. Groin masses or lymph nodes showing metastatic cancer most commonly point to a primary site in the lower extremities, the vulva–anorectal region, or prostate.[30,45] Infrequently, ovarian or testicular cancers will metastasize to this region. In the latter, this may occur after a transscrotal biopsy of the testis or after hernia repair when the lymphatics are interrupted.

SKIN. When an OPM is detected in the skin, consideration must be given to malignant tumors that spread by the hematogenous route; among these are melanomas and carcinomas of the lung, breast, kidney, and ovary.[30] A previous history of skin fulguration may point to a metastasis from a melanoma. If no distant primary lesion is detectable, further consideration must be given to the primary site in the skin or its appendages. Occasionally, lymphoma, particularly diffuse large-cell lymphoma, arises in the skin. Then the OPM may, in fact, represent the primary lesion.

LUNG. Major mass lesions detected on chest roentgenograms are most likely lung cancer. Weber and associates reported that 18 of 94 patients with confirmed carcinoma of the pancreas had an initial diagnosis of primary carcinoma of the bronchus that had been based on clinical signs, results of radiologic examinations, lung scanning, and bronchoscopy, with histologic or cytologic examination.[46] Other metastatic tumors also may mimic mass lesions of primary lung cancer.

When a single atypical lesion is seen on the chest roentgenogram, the most likely diagnosis is primary lung cancer.[30] If the lesion is a metastasis, it is still most likely to originate from a primary lesion in the lung, particularly if the histologic appearance is that of a squamous cell carcinoma.[30] If an adenocarcinoma is demonstrated, the source may be lung, pancreas, and other sites in the gastrointestinal tract or breast. Solitary nodules in the lung frequently arise from kidney or primary liver cancer. In addition, undifferentiated tumors may originate from occult amelanotic melanoma, testis cancer, sarcoma, choriocarcinoma, or kidney, thyroid, or breast cancer.[30] The role of CT and MRI scans in the work-up of OPM in the lung remains to be defined.[47]

LIVER. The suspicion of an OPM in the liver arises in patients presenting with cachexia, fever, or jaundice, with or without hepatomegaly. The serum alkaline phosphatase (hepatic isozyme) level usually is elevated, and a liver scan may be abnormal. If stool is positive for blood, a workup of the gastrointestinal tract is indicated, and a search for a primary lesion may be fruitful. A CT scan of the abdomen is usually indicated when OPM and liver metastases are present.[48] If a diagnosis is not achieved, a liver biopsy is indicated; it is preferable to perform such a procedure by laparoscopy or laparotomy, rather than by closed-needle biopsy, because hemorrhage from a vascular tumor is a real risk. Fine-needle aspiration (FNA) performed under CT guidance is an alternative. In addition to the gastrointestinal tract (including the pancreas), the lung or breast may be the primary site of metastases. In some cases, it is difficult to separate poorly differentiated hepatocellular carcinomas and biliary carcinomas from OPM to the liver.[30,49]

BONE. Patients presenting with pain in a bone or an unexplained fracture may have an OPM. Bone scans may be positive in 47% of asymptomatic and 88% of symptomatic patients with OPM.[9] If a fracture is present, open reduction will yield tissue that may give clues to tumor origin. Often the serum alkaline phosphatase (bone isozyme) level is elevated. A serum protein electrophoresis can establish the diagnosis of multiple myeloma. An elevated serum acid phosphatase value can point to prostatic carcinoma, which also is characterized by purely blastic lesions on radiologic examination of the skeleton. Blastic lesions also may be seen in ovarian cancer, carcinoid, Hodgkin's disease and, very infrequently, in oat cell cancer. A mixed blastic and lytic picture often is seen in breast cancer, whereas punched-out purely lytic lesions are characteristic of multiple myeloma. In addition to lung, breast, prostate, and ovarian cancer, cancer of the kidney and gastrointestinal tract must be considered when evaluating OPM in bone.[30]

HEMATOLOGIC ABNORMALITIES. Unexplained increases or decreases in the formed elements of the blood may suggest that a workup be initiated and, hence, lead to the discovery of an OPM. Erythrocytosis resulting from excess erythropoietin usually is associated with kidney tumors but also may occur in infratentorial hemangioblastoma and hepatic carcinoma. Thrombocytosis, without other hematologic abnormalities, has been described in a number of tumors including ovarian, lung, and pancreatic carcinoma and Hodgkin's disease. Anemia, leukopenia, and thrombocytopenia should suggest a hematologic workup, including a bone marrow aspiration and bone core biopsy that could reveal a tumor.[50] Almost any primary tumor may be the source of these metastases, but the lung, breast, gastrointestinal tract, and pancreas are the most common sources. A characteristic hematologic picture, referred to as leukoerythroblastic anemia, most frequently is seen in association with widespread bone marrow invasion from breast cancer; other primary sources, including lung, also may be found.

BRAIN. Although the routine preoperative workup for a brain tumor includes search for OPM with emphasis on lung, breast, and prostate, it is not uncommon at craniotomy to find an unsuspected metastatic tumor. For practical purposes carcinomas of the lung, breast, prostate, and pancreas, and melanomas are the most common sources of OPM. Carcinoma of the nasopharynx or pterygoid area may present as a temporal fossa mass. For these, surgical resection and postoperative radiotherapy are indicated. However, surgical resection is not required if other metastases are demonstrated. Survival is improved when surgical resection of a solitary brain metastasis is performed, followed by radiotherapy. The type of radiotherapy (whole brain versus whole brain with local boost) will depend on the preoperative findings, including CT, MRI, as well as the operative findings. If the primary lesion can be detected, appropriate chemotherapy can be selected. Often, a brain metastasis is the presenting sign of a primary lung lesion. Patients in whom this sign is detected benefit from treatment to both the brain and the primary lung lesion.[30,51,52]

SPINAL CORD. The dramatic events that suggest impending cord compression often lead to surgical intervention, which results in decompression and the diagnosis of an OPM. High (thoracic) spinal cord lesions most commonly originate from cancer of the lung or breast, whereas low (thoracolumbar) spinal cord lesions usually can be traced to retroperitoneal lymphomas or prostatic cancer. In any event, vigorous postoperative management with radiotherapy, chemotherapy, or both, is indicated.

MALIGNANT EFFUSIONS. Infrequently, the first sign and symptom of a malignant tumor is pleural effusion or ascites. The demonstration of malignant cells not only proves the nature of the effusion but also could give clues about the origin of the tumor. Both cytologic analysis and study of cell blocks should be undertaken.[19] Malignant pleural effusions with positive cytology most frequently originate in the lung, breast, ovary,[30] gastrointestinal tract, or pancreas; malignant ascites most frequently originates in the ovary, pancreas, stomach, or colon. Pericardial effusions of OPM occur infrequently and are usually associated with lung cancer.[30]

PAIN. Pain may be the first sign of a primary cancer as well as of a tumor presenting as an OPM. Obvious examples are bone pain leading to the discovery of a bone metastasis and long tract signs leading to the detection of an intrathecal tumor. Occasionally the pain problem is related to nerve or nerve root involvement, as in Pancoast tumors, pancreatic cancer, or mesothelioma.

MIGRATORY THROMBOPHLEBITIS. Recurrent episodes of thrombophlebitis in multiple locations (migratory thrombophlebitis) that are not readily explained by the usual antecedent factors are likely to be associated with an OPM. Without trauma, an episode of thrombophlebitis in the upper extremity suggests cancer. Cancer of the pancreas is the most common primary site associated with migratory thrombophlebitis, but lung cancer, gastrointestinal cancers, and other malignancies have been described.

PARANEOPLASTIC SYNDROMES. The appearance of any syndrome suggestive of one of the many manifestations of paraneoplastic syndromes (endocrine, neurologic, hematologic, renal, dermatologic, or collagen–vascular) may be the first clue leading to the subsequent discovery of an OPM.

HISTORICAL APPROACH

The discovery of an OPM should prompt a thorough historical review to detect clues about the origin of the metastatic tumor. In general, this approach is less rewarding than the histologic and anatomic approaches already discussed. Most importantly, patients should be questioned about fulgurations or biopsies of "harmless" skin lesions, removal of benign polyps of the colon, dilatation and curettage (or conization) procedures that revealed "no cancer," biopsies of the prostate that showed "only prostatic hypertrophy," and any other surgical procedures in which tissue was removed. Occasionally, this line of questioning reveals that the tissue that was removed and considered benign may well have been the location of the primary malignancy that now is manifest as a metastasis. The opportunity to perform a second biopsy allows the pathologist to perform "directed" procedures to support a diagnosis suspected from history.

The family history rarely is helpful because most familial and hereditary cancers are obvious for primary site. However, the geographic or racial history occasionally may offer clues, because it is known that in certain regions particular cancers have a high incidence (*e.g.*, the prevalence of skin cancer in Sunbelt residents, stomach cancer among the Japanese, or nasopharyngeal cancer in Chinese populations).

Knowledge of age and sex differences in cancer incidence may be of some help in planning the strategy for the OPM patient workup. Risk factors, including knowledge of occupational exposure, may offer subtle clues that assist in planning a directed search for the primary tumor.

BASIC SCREENING STUDIES

In the strategy for evaluating an OPM the laboratory and radiology studies must be selected carefully, based on data obtained from various clues. The usefulness of the radiologic examination of the chest, urinalysis for detection of blood, and stool examination for blood, has already been mentioned. In addition, serum chemistries, with particular emphasis on calcium and uric acid concentrations and liver function, should be performed. In most instances, these tests are done on admission to the hospital and should pass scrutiny. However, a reexamination of these simple tests is in order to detect abnormalities that might have major impact on the strategy of further workup.

SPECIFIC STUDIES

Kennedy and Luedke have outlined a strategy for undertaking the workup of an OPM:

> If no clues are forthcoming from the basic screening studies, the physician faces the challenging question of how far to proceed with a low-yield diagnostic workup on a patient with a short life expectancy. The benefits of an established diagnosis must outweigh the expense, time, and risk to the patient involved in making the diagnosis. Ultimately, the extent of disease, the organ involvement, and the age, social situation, and performance level of the patient should dictate the extent of the diagnostic workup. A critically ill patient with rapidly progressive tumor requires therapeutic intervention rather than an extensive diagnostic evaluation. However, in patients able to undergo additional studies, strong consideration should be given to systematic assessment of the sites of common primary tumors which metastasize widely (lung, breast, pancreas, kidney) and of those that are most amenable to treatment (breast, prostate, ovary).[53]

The cost in time and money needed to perform tests to detect the primary site from which an OPM may have originated is substantial.[10] The armamentarium available for the diagnostic workup of an OPM spans the entire repertoire of radiologic, radioisotopic, chemical, and immunologic tests. Some tests are simple, atraumatic for the patient, and need little justification (*e.g.*, mammogram, ultrasound, bone scan, upper GI series); others are more complex and may be very expensive (*e.g.*, CT scan, PTH assay, MRI scan, ^{67}Ga scans); still other tests are complex and expensive and may cause significant complications, thus requiring the physician to weigh the cost/benefit ratio (*e.g.*, bronchoscopy, ERCP, arteriography) carefully. The guiding rule should be selectivity, keeping effectiveness in mind in terms of therapeutic decision-making, complication rate, cost, and time.[10] Some costly tests may actually save time and money.[29,31,47,48,54–58] For example, a CT scan of the abdomen can, in many instances, replace upper GI series, IVP, barium enema, and liver scan.[9,54] A high-quality MRI scan obtained in the CNS and head and neck area can replace CT, sinus films, and extensive surgical procedures.

TREATMENT

Local metastases, if symptomatic, are treated with local radiotherapy. When selective workup reveals the primary site with a high degree of certainty, appropriate specific therapy is initiated.

For squamous cell cancers presenting with high cervical lymph nodes, an aggressive approach, similar to that used in proven head and neck cancers, using radiation therapy or surgery with neoadjuvant and adjuvant chemotherapy is indicated, even if a primary site cannot be determined. Data have already been summarized that demonstrate a 3-year survival in up to 60% of cases with this approach. An appropriate radiation port can be designed to cover most potential head and neck primary sites at the same time the cervical nodes are irradiated. Generally, ports typical for the nasopharynx, base of tongue, and tonsils are used for nodes along the jugular vein in the midneck or posterior neck region. Nodes in the submaxillary or subdigastric areas require oral cavity irradiation. Treatment of patients with radical neck dissection rather than with radiation results in a higher incidence of primary site relapses. However, it has not been fully established whether or not these relapses can be salvaged successfully by additional local resection and radiotherapy. Well-differentiated squamous cell carcinoma in upper anterior nodes is surgically treatable; lower nodes should receive radiation. Neoadjuvant or adjuvant multidrug chemotherapy, now developed for the treatment of head and neck cancers, has not been tested in OPM presenting in cervical nodes, but its use appears to be rational and promisiing. For patients with tumors of the head and neck, squamous and anaplastic carcinoma have the best prognosis. Long-term survivors with adenocarcinoma are rare.[25–30]

Patients with symptoms suggestive of malignant melanoma to cervical, parotid, axillary, or inguinal lymph nodes should be managed with appropriate radical lymph node dissection, with or without additional regional chemotherapy.[37–39,59–62] Metastatic inguinal lymph nodes from an OPM may respond significantly to radiotherapy without radical surgery.[45]

In general, we believe that systemic treatment should be applied *only* when a patient becomes symptomatic, except under the circumstances when the presumed treatable lesion is one that is known to be curable with systemic therapy. For the tumors listed in Table 56-3, specific, effective systemic therapy is available and should be initiated with intent to offer cure or maximum palliation.

For patients with advanced, poorly differentiated carcinoma of unknown primary site, new treatment strategies have recently been proposed based on recognition of a treatable syndrome.[63,64] For men under 50 years of age, with or without serologic or histologic evidence of germ cell tumor, intensive, usually cisplatin-based[63,64] chemotherapy should be employed with curative intent.[63–65] Predictors of response to therapy and survival are listed in Table 56-7. The results with this approach[64] are summarized in Table 56-8 and indicate significant curability (25%) in a heretofore hopeless situation. Estimating that 4000 to 5000 patients a year may have this newly described syndrome, this approach may render 1000 to 1200 patients free of disease for a prolonged period.

TABLE 56-7. Predictors of Response to Therapy and Survival for Patients with Poorly Differentiated Carcinoma or Adenocarcinoma

Predictive Factors	*Response*
Tumor location	
Mediastinum	+
Retroperitoneum	+
Other lymph node areas	+
Organ involvement	–
Age	
Under 50	+
Over 50	+/–
Smoking history	
Nonsmoker	+
Smoker	–
Histologic diagnosis	
Poorly differentiated carcinoma	+
Poorly differentiated adenocarcinoma	+/–
Other	
Sex	–
Tumor marker status	–

Adapted from Greco FA, Vaughn WK, Hainsworth JD: Advanced poorly differentiated carcinoma of unknown primary site: Recognition of a treatable syndrome. Ann Intern Med 104:547–553, 1986.

Patients believed to have Hodgkin's disease, large-cell lymphoma, or trophoblastic tumors should receive appropriate chemotherapy.

For women presumed to have OPM from breast cancer, chemotherapy with or without hormonal management is indicated.[66–68] Men whose symptoms suggest prostatic cancer[23] may benefit from diethylstilbestrol or leuprolide.[69] Women whose symptoms suggest ovarian cancer should be treated with cyclophosphamide, doxorubicin, and cisplatin.[70]

In a significant number of patients, an OPM will remain with no clues about the site of origin of the tumor. The literature offers little help concerning useful approaches in selecting combinations of agents likely to be effective in

TABLE 56-8. Response to Treatment and Survival in 68 Patients with Poorly Differentiated Carcinoma or Adenocarcinoma of Unknown Primary Site

	n	%
Patients receiving therapy	68	100
Major responses	38	56
Complete response (CR)	15*	22
Partial response	23	34

Adapted from Greco FA, Vaughn WK, Hainsworth JD: Advanced poorly differentiated carcinoma of unknown primary site: Recognition of a treatable syndrome. Ann Intern Med 104:547–553, 1986.

*Nine of 15 patients with CR had a disease-free state of 36 to 67 months.

such situations.[10,53,71-73] The response rate to chemotherapy of cancer of the lung (other than oat cell), pancreas, stomach, colon, and kidney, of amelanotic melanomas, or of undifferentiated sarcoma may be as high as 40% to 60%, but these responses generally are short, and survival is not extended.

A number of published reports on the management of patients with an adenocarcinoma of OPM describe the use of doxorubicin (Adriamycin).[71-74] Wood and co-workers describe a randomized treatment study of symptomatic patients with metastatic adenocarcinomas of unknown primary origin using two combination chemotherapy regimens.[74] One regimen combined doxorubicin and mitomycin C; the other consisted of cyclophosphamide, methotrexate, and 5-fluorouracil. Although both regimens demonstrated a wide range of antitumor activity, the regimen containing doxorubicin and mitomycin C was found to be superior. However, these results have been questioned.[75] The spectrum of usefulness of doxorubicin, alone or in combination, should lead to a reassessment of treatment programs for patients with an OPM.[2] Regimens not employing doxorubicin have been described.[2,74,76]

Our current approach takes these observations into account, and our program for patients with an OPM includes doxorubicin, cyclophosphamide, vincristine, and methotrexate, with or without leucovorin rescue. Clearly, further studies are needed to develop data demonstrating that such an aggressive approach for patients with an OPM is useful.

REFERENCES

1. Nystrom JS, Weiner JM, Wolf RM et al: Identifying the primary site in metastatic cancer of unkown origin: Inadequacy of roentgenographic procedures. JAMA 241:381–383, 1979
2. Markman M: Metastatic adenocarcinoma of unknown primary site: Analysis of 245 patients seen at the Johns Hopkins Hospital from 1965–1979. Med Pediatr Oncol 10:569–574, 1982
3. Altman E, Cadman E: An analysis of 1539 patients with cancer of unknown primary site. Cancer 57:120–124, 1986
4. Smith PE, Krementz ET, Chapman W: Metastatic cancer without a detectable primary site. J Surg 113:633–637, 1967
5. Holmes FF, Fouts TL: Metastatic cancer of unknown primary site. Cancer 26:816–820, 1970
6. Richardson RG, Parker RG: Metastases from undetected primary cancers—Clinical experience at a radiation oncology center (Medical Information). West J Med 123:337–339, 1975
7. Snee MP, Vyramuthu N: Metastatic carcinoma from unknown primary site: The experience of a large oncology centre. Br J Radiol 58:1091–1095, 1985
8. Steckel RJ, Kagan AR: Diagnostic persistence in working up metastatic cancer with an unknown primary site. Radiology 134:367–369, 1980
9. Gaber AO, Rice P, Eaton C et al: Metastatic malignant disease of unknown origin. Am J Surg 145:493–497, 1983
10. Levine MN, Drummond MF, Labelle RJ: Cost-effectiveness in the diagnosis and treatment of carcinoma of unknown primary origin. Can Med Assoc J 133:977–978, 1985
11. Nystrom JS, Weiner JM, Heffelfinger-Juttner J et al: Metastatic and histologic presentations in unknown primary cancer. Semin Oncol 4:53–58, 1977
12. Neumann KH, Nystrom JS: Metastatic cancer of unknown origin: Nonsquamous cell type. Semin Oncol 9:427–434, 1982
13. Fer MF, Greco FA, Oldham RK: Poorly differentiated neoplasms and tumors of unknown origin: Introduction. Semin Oncol 9:393–395, 1982
14. Kelley SL, Meyer TJ: Carcinoma of unknown primary site: A prudent approach. Postgrad Med 74:269–280, 1983
15. Kern WH, Abbott M: The determination of unknown primary sites based upon the histologic appearance of metastases. Surg Gynecol Obstet 151:73–76, 1980
16. Mackay B, Ordonez NG: The role of the pathologist in the evaluation of poorly differentiated tumors. Semin Oncol 9:396–415, 1982
17. Battifora H: Recent progress in the immunochemistry of solid tumors. Semin Diagn Pathol 1:251–271, 1984
18. Herrera GA, Reimann BEF: Electron microscopy in determining origin of metastatic adenocarcinomas. South Med J 77:1557–1566, 1984
19. Hanna W, Kahn HJ: The ultrastructure of metastatic adenocarcinoma in serous fluids: An aid in identification of the primary site of the neoplasm. Acta Cytol 29:206–210, 1985
20. Holt JA, Bolanos J: Enzyme-linked immunochemical measurement of estrogen receptor in gynecologic tumors, and an overview of steroid receptors in ovarian carcinoma. Clin Chem 32:1836–1843, 1986
21. Ruddon RW: Tumor markers in the recognition and management of poorly differentiated neoplasms and cancers of unknown primary. Semin Oncol 9:416–426, 1982
22. Stein BS, Vangore S, Petersen RO et al: Immunoperoxidase localization of prostate-specific antigen. Am J Surg Pathol 6:553–557, 1982
23. Yam LT, Winkler CF, Janckila AJ et al: Prostatic cancer presenting as metastatic adenocarcinoma of undetermined origin: Immunodiagnosis by prostatic acid phosphatase. Cancer 51:283–287, 1983
24. Lee AK, De Lellis RA, Rosen PP et al: Alpha-lactalbumin as an immunohistochemical marker for metastatic breast carcinomas. Am J Surg Pathol 8:93–100, 1984
25. De Santo LW, Neel HB III: Squamous cell carcinoma: Metastasis to the neck from an unknown or undiscovered primary. Otolaryngol Clin North Am 18:505–513, 1985
26. Silverman CL, Marks JE, Lee F et al: Treatment of epidermoid and undifferentiated carcinomas from occult primaries presenting in cervical lymph nodes. Laryngoscope 93:645–648, 1983
27. Spiro RH, DeRose G, Strong EW: Cervical node metastases of occult origin. Am J Surg 146:441–446, 1983
28. Silverman C, Marks JE: Metastatic cancer of unknown origin: Epidermoid and undifferentiated carcinomas. Semin Oncol 9:435–441, 1982
29. Muraki AS, Mancuso AA, Harnsberger HR: Metastatic cervical adenopathy from tumors of unknown origin: The role of CT. Radiology 152:749–753, 1984
30. Ringenberg QS: Tumors of unknown origin. Med Pediatr Oncol 13:301–306, 1985
31. Harnsberger HR, Dillon WP: Imaging tumors of the central nervous system and extracranial head and neck. CA 37:225–238, 1987
32. Haupt HM, Rosen PP, Kinne DW: Breast carcinoma presenting with axillary lymph node metastases: An analysis of specific histopathologic features. Am J Surg Pathol 9:165–175, 1985
33. Copeland BM, McBride OM: Axillary metastases from unknown primary sites. Ann Surg 178:25–27, 1973
34. Feigenberg Z, Zer M, Dintsman M: Axillary metastases from an unknown primary source: A diagnostic and therapeutic approach. Isr J Med Sci 12:1153–1158, 1976
35. Patel J, Nemoto T, Rosner D et al: Axillary lymph node metastasis from an occult breast cancer. Cancer 47:2923–2927, 1981
36. Inglehart JD, Ferguson BJ, Shingleton WW et al: An ultrastructural analysis of breast carcinoma presenting as isolated axillary adenopathy. Ann Surg 196:8–13, 1982
37. Giuliano AE, Cochran AJ, Morton DL: Melanoma from unknown primary site and amelanotic melanoma. Semin Oncol 9:442–445, 1982
38. Panagopoulos E, Murray D: Metastatic malignant melanoma of unknown primary origin: A study of 30 cases. J Surg Oncol 23:8–10, 1983
39. Reintgen DS, McCarty KS, Woodard B et al: Metastatic malignant melanoma with an unknown primary. Surg Gynecol Obstet 156:335–340, 1983
40. Key JD, Shephard DAE, Walters W: Sister Mary Joseph's nodule and its relationship to diagnosis of carcinoma of the umbilicus. Minn Med 59:561, 1976
41. Samitz MH: Umbilical metastases from carcinoma of the stomach: Sister Mary Joseph's nodule. Arch Dermatol 111:1478–1479, 1975
42. Scarpa FJ, Dineen JP, Boltax RS: Visceral neoplasia presenting at the umbilicus. J Surg Oncol 11:351–359, 1979
43. Jager RM, Max MH: Umbilical metastasis as the presenting symptom of cecal carcinoma. J Surg Oncol 12:41–45, 1979
44. Steck WD, Helwig EB: Tumors of the umbilicus. Cancer 18:907–915, 1965
45. Guarischi A, Keane TJ, Elhakim T: Metastatic inguinal nodes from an unknown primary neoplasm: A review of 56 cases. Cancer 59:572–577, 1987
46. Weber P, Troger J, Ernst H: Das pankreaskarzinom klinisch als zentrales Brouchuskarzinom maskiert. Dtsch Med Wochenschr 98:1389–1391, 1973
47. Chasen MH: Imaging primary lung cancers, pleural cancers, and metastatic disease. CA 37:194–210, 1987
48. Thompson WM: Imaging strategies for tumors of the gastrointestinal system. CA 37:165–185, 1987
49. Jordan WE III, Shildt RA: Adenocarcinoma of unknown primary site: The Brooke Army Medical Center experience. Cancer 55:857–860, 1985
50. Ringenberg QS, Doll DC, Yarbro JW et al: Tumors of unknown origin in the bone marrow. Arch Intern Med 146:2027–2028, 1986
51. Dhopesh VP, Yagnik PM: Brain metastasis: Analysis of patients without known cancer. South Med J 78:171–172, 1985
52. Le Chevalier T, Smith FP, Caille P: Sites of primary malignancies in patients presenting with cerebral metastases: A review of 120 cases. Cancer 56:880–882, 1985
53. Kennedy PS, Luedke DW: Adenocarcinoma of unknown origin: A rational approach to a diagnostic puzzle. Postgrad Med 65:151–160, 1979
54. McMillan JH, Levine E, Stephens RH: Computed tomography in the evaluation of metastatic adenocarcinoma from an unknown primary site: A retrospective study. Radiology 143:143–146, 1982
55. Karsell PR, Sheedy PF II, O'Connell MJ: Computed tomography in search of cancer of unknown origin. JAMA 248:340–343, 1982
56. Paulus DD: Imaging in breast cancer. CA 37:133–150, 1987
57. Davidson AJ, Hartman DS: Imaging strategies for tumors of the kidney, adrenal gland, and retroperitoneum. CA 37:151–164, 1987
58. Edeiken J, Karasick D: Imaging in bone cancer. CA 37:239–245, 1987

59. Lopez R, Holyoke ED, Moore RH et al: Malignant melanoma with unknown primary site. J Surg Oncol 19:151–154, 1982
60. Klausner JM, Gutman M, Inbar M et al: Unknown primary melanoma. J Surg Oncol 24:129–131, 1983
61. Santini H, Byers RM, Wolf PF: Melanoma metastatic to cervical and parotid nodes from an unknown primary site. Am J Surg 150:510–512, 1985
62. Muchmore JH, Krementz ET, Carter RD et al: Isolated perfusion of extremities for metastatic melanoma from an unknown primary lesion. South Med J 79:288–290, 1986
63. Williams S, Einhorn L, Greco A et al: Disseminated germ cell tumors: A comparison of cisplatin plus bleomycin plus either vinblastine (PVB) of VP-16 (BEP). Proc Am Soc Clin Oncol 4:100, 1985
64. Greco FA, Vaughn WK, Hainsworth JD: Advanced poorly differentiated carcinoma of unknown primary site: Recognition of a treatable syndrome. Ann Intern Med 104:547–553, 1986
65. Bosl GJ, Gluckman R, Geller NL et al: VAB-6: An effective chemotherapy regimen for patients with germ-cell tumors. J Clin Oncol 4:1493–1499, 1986
66. Glucksberg H, Rivkin SE, Rasmussen S et al: Combination chemotherapy (CMFVP) versus L-phenylalanine mustard (L-PAM) for operable breast cancer with positive axillary nodes: A Southwest Oncology Group study. Cancer 50:423–434, 1982
67. Tancini G, Bonadonna G, Valagussa P et al: Adjuvant CMF in breast cancer: Comparative 5-year results of 12 versus 6 cycles. J Clin Oncol 1:2–10, 1983
68. Fisher B, Redmond C, Brown A et al: Influence of tumor estrogen and progesterone receptor levels on the response to tamoxifen and chemotherapy in primary breast cancer. J Clin Oncol 1:227–241, 1983
69. The Leuprolide Study Group: Leuprolide versus diethylstilbestrol for metastatic prostate cancer. N Engl J Med 311:1281–1286, 1984
70. Omura G, Blessing JA, Ehrlich CE et al: A randomized trial of cyclophosphamide and doxorubicin with or without cisplatin in advanced ovarian carcinoma: A gynecologic oncology group study. Cancer 57:1725–1730, 1986
71. Indupalli SR, Bedikian AY, Bodey GP: Adenocarcinoma of unknown primary origin: Impact of chemotherapy on survival. South Med J 74:1431–1435, 1981
72. Nissenblatt MJ: The CUP syndrome (carcinoma unknown primary). Cancer Treat Rev 8:211–224, 1981
73. Anderson H, Thatcher N, Rankin E et al: VAC (vincristine, Adriamycin, cyclophosphamide) chemotherapy for metastatic carcinoma from an unknown primary site. Eur J Cancer Clin Oncol 19:49–52, 1983
74. Wood RL, Fox RM, Tattersall MHN et al: Metastatic adenocarcinomas of unknown primary site: A randomized study of two combination chemotherapy regimens. N Engl J Med 303:87–89, 1980
75. Nelson RB: Chemotherapy of metastatic adenocarcinoma of unknown origin. N Engl J Med 303:1478, 1980
76. Walach N, Horn Y: Combination chemotherapy in the treatment of adenocarcinoma of unknown primary origin. Cancer Treat Rep 71:605–607, 1987

JEROME E. GROOPMAN
SAMUEL BRODER

CHAPTER 57 *Cancer in AIDS and Other Immunodeficiency States*

The medical oncologist should be aware of the strong relation between certain immunodeficiency states and neoplastic disease. An improved understanding of the pathogenesis of certain malignancies and selective immune defects may provide insights into innovative therapeutic approaches to cancer. Immunodeficiency produced in experimental animals often brings about an increased risk of cancer, and the animal model served an important role in identifying interleukin-2 as a potential agent for cancer therapy.[1,2]

In humans various conditions characterized by impaired immune function are associated with a higher frequency of certain cancers than occur in age-matched controls.[3,4] We shall review certain genetically determined immunodeficiency states and discuss their relation to cancer. The features of the major immunodeficiency diseases are important because of their practical clinical importance and the research opportunities that they provide. Certain immunodeficiency states have been mapped to different loci, on chromosome X, opening new possibilities for genetic counseling and an understanding of specific genes that control immune functions.[5,7] Other immunodeficiency states (in particular ataxia telangiectasia) serve as "experiments of nature" in establishing the concept of preferred chromosomal breakpoints in the pathogenesis of lymphoid malignancies.[8]

CANCER IN ALLOTRANSPLANT RECIPIENTS

There is about a 6% incidence of de novo cancer in organ allotransplant recipients who receive immunosuppressive therapy. This frequency of cancer represents at least a 100-fold (and possibly higher) increase in risk compared with that of an age-corrected general population.[9,11] Most of these cancers occur in young adults, and the average time of tumor appearance is 28 months after transplantation. The increased incidence does not represent a generalized risk for all histologic forms of cancer. A high percentage of these malignancies are lymphoreticular in origin, and there is a striking predisposition to central nervous system lymphoma. There is also an increased risk for the development of Kaposi's sarcoma in allograft recipients. There also is an increase in epithelial cancers that involve skin.

GENERALIZATION ABOUT CANCER IN PATIENTS WITH INHERENT ABNORMALITIES OF THE IMMUNE SYSTEM

Clinical investigation of genetically determined immunodeficiency diseases has been under way for several years, and considerable progress has been made in certain areas (*e.g.*, in developing an awareness of immunoregulatory cell network in the context of immunodeficiency and cancer).[12] Certain clinical observations are striking. In some immunodeficiency diseases with short life spans, for example, there may be a 100-fold increase in the risk of developing a lymphoma, reminiscent of the risk in organ transplantation discussed above. Investigators at the University of Minnesota complied data from the Immunodeficiency-Cancer Registry (ICR), which was established to monitor the cancer incidence in patients with defined immunodeficiency diseases both within the United States and abroad.[13,14] Attempts to analyze the true incidence of cancer in patients with abnormalities of immunity are complicated by at least three potential sources of error: (1) certain kinds of immunodeficiency disease may be underreported; (2) certain histologic forms of cancer may be seriously overreported; and (3) the histopathologic classification of neoplasms, especially non-Hodgkin's lymphoma, has changed in the years since the Registry patients were diagnosed. Nonetheless, much useful information is available, and Spector and colleagues[13] have used the data from the Registry to formulate three generalizations.

1. Children with inherited immunodeficiency diseases who develop cancer tend to have a non-Hodgkin's lymphoma. Adults with immunodeficiency diseases tend to develop both non-Hodgkin's lymphoma and carcinomas. In the published literature the most common single histologic type of non-Hodgkin's lymphoma is "histiocytic" lymphoma. This pathologic type is now known to represent a large-cell lymphoma and should not be taken to mean a neoplasm of macrophage origin.
2. Certain immunodeficiency states have an association with a particular type or pattern of neoplastic disease. There appears, for example, to be a disproportionate association between the Wiskott–Aldrich syndrome and myelogenous leukemia. This syndrome has other noteworthy associations, which are discussed later.
3. The stomach is a common target organ for carcinomas in adult patients with one recognized acquired immunodeficiency disease, common variable immunodeficiency disease.

SEVERE COMBINED IMMUNODEFICIENCY

Severe combined immunodeficiency (SCID) represents a fundamental defect of both B-cell and T-cell development. A defect at the stem cell level or, in some cases, a profound defect of T cells, including a severe deficit of helper T cells necessary for adequate B-cell function, could account for the clinical syndrome observed. Three modes of inheritance for this entity give rise to the same ultimate catastrophe of immune system dysfunction: sporadic, autosomal recessive, and sex-linked. There also is an association with deficiency of adenosine deaminase in the subset of patients who have SCID, and there is a variant of the syndrome associated with dysostosis.

Patients with SCID lack both humoral and cellular immune responses. Profound lymphocytopenia is common. Clinically, SCID becomes evident soon after birth and is marked by repeated infections with bacteria, fungi (candidal infections of the skin and mucous membranes are almost always present), viruses, and protozoa (*Pneumocystis carinii*). Nearly all of these patients have significant diarrhea, and even though *Salmonella* and pathogenic strains of *Escherichia coli* are identified in certain patients, it is common for the cause of the diarrhea to remain undiagnosed. Such patients are at risk of graft-versus-host reactions if they receive transfusions of unirradiated blood components containing immunocompetent cells. Patients with SCID disease can, in principle, be immunologically reconstituted with HLA-matched stem cells given in the form of bone marrow transplantation. As a practical matter, however, the prognosis for these patients is quite poor.

The percentage of cancer observed in patients with this disease is about 1.5%, with 0.9 years as the median age at diagnosis of malignancy.[13] The incidence of lymphoreticular cancer, including leukemia, Hodgkin's disease, and non-Hodgkin's lymphoma, is especially noteworthy. Solid lymphoid malignancies are rare in infants, and it might be assumed that the lymphomas do not occur by chance alone in this patient population. The true risk of acquiring lymphoma is not defined.

ATAXIA TELANGIECTASIA

Ataxia telangiectasia is an autosomal recessive multisystem disorder characterized by serious degenerative changes in the central nervous system (CNS), especially within the cerebellum, oculocutaneous telangiectasias, recurrent sinopulmonary infections, a high incidence of cancer, and a complex immunodeficiency state.[15–17] Progressive neurologic abnormalities dominated by cerebellular ataxia usually are recognized very early in childhood. However, the characteristic telangiectasias consisting of dilated venules usually appear between the ages of 2 years and 8 years, most often appearing on the conjunctivae and exposed areas of the skin. This may make the correct diagnosis extremely difficult on clinical grounds alone before 2 years of age. Other integumental abnormalities include vitiligo, café au lait spots, sclerodermoid changes, and gray hair. These patients frequently have significant retardation of growth. Abnormalities of endocrine function have been described, including abnormalities of ovarian histology in some patients or absence of ovaries in others. More than half the patients have an abnormality of carbohydrate metabolism consisting of glucose intolerance and increased plasma insulin levels.[18] Anti-insulin receptor antibodies have been demonstrated in certain patients with ataxia telangiectasis and insulin resistance.

Using a sensitive double-antibody radioimmunoassay that can detect nanogram-per-milliliter concentrations, Waldmann and McIntire[19] have demonstrated that essentially all patients with ataxia telangiectasia have elevated serum levels of alpha-fetoprotein. This observation has provided an invaluable tool in diagnosing this disorder, especially in atypical cases. Normally only fetal liver cells or regenerating liver cells secrete significant amounts of alpha-fetoprotein. Certain neoplasms that have a hepatic or germ cell origin also release substantial amounts of this protein. Elevated levels of alpha-fetoprotein appear to be a distinctive feature of ataxia telangiectasia that is characteristically not found in other immunodeficiency states. The reasons for the association between ataxia telangiectasia and elevated levels of this oncofetal marker are unknown.

Patients with ataxia telangiectasia exhibit a complex series of immunologic impairments that involve both cellular and humoral immune responses. The full extent of these impairments varies from patient to patient, and even varies at different times in any given patient's clinical course. With respect to humoral immune function, about 75% of the patients have depressed levels of serum IgA, often with no IgA detectable by conventional quantitative immunodiffusion techniques. This deficiency of IgA is seen in respiratory and intestinal secretions as well. IgE also is undetectable or reduced in a large percentage of the patients studied.[20,21] Serum IgG levels usually are normal, whereas serum IgM levels often are estimated to be high in radial diffusion assays. However, these high estimates for serum IgM often reflect the unusual presence of a low molecular (monomeric) form of IgM in a large number of patients with ataxia telangiectasia. Such low-molecular-weight IgM molecules diffuse more rapidly in immunodiffusion plates than do the standard (pentameric) IgM molecules, giving falsely high values.

Most of the patients tested can mount an antibody response to blood group substance, the Vi antigen of *E. coli*, and the tularemia antigen, although the antibody titers achieved are significantly less than normal. Serum antibody responses in the IgA class appear deficient even in those patients whose serum contains circulating IgA. Moreover, patients with ataxia telangiectasia have relatively poor antibody responses to viral agents, such as poliomyelitis and influenza virus. Local secretory antibody responses usually are poor. This apparently leads to recurrent infection, particularly involving the sinopulmonary tree. In a large percentage of patients chronic infections result in structural lung damage and respiratory insufficiency.

Patients with ataxia telangiectasia have a variable impairment of cellular immunity.[17–22] A large number of patients with this disorder are cutaneously anergic to a battery of common skin test antigens. In an era in which skin transplantation across histocompatibility barriers was used as a standard test of clinical immune function, a number of patients exhibited delayed rejection of skin allografts. It appears that the critical combination of severe cellular and humoral immune defects is a key factor in the predisposition to infection seen in this disease.

The clinical deficiency of cellular and humoral immunity already discussed is reflected in the microscopic architecture of lymphoid tissues. It is common to observe very small lymph nodes with severe lymphocyte depletion. Perhaps one of the most striking histopathologic features is the significant abnormality of thymic structure seen in many patients with this disease. The thymus gland may be absent or very small. It often has an embryonic appearance. The number of thymic lymphocytes is decreased, and the predominant cell type has a reticuloendothelial–stromal origin. Typically, no differentiation between thymic cortex and medulla is observed. Moreover, Hassall's corpuscles are generally not seen. It is probably not accurate to characterize the thymus of patients with this disease as truly atrophic; rather, the thymus glands in this disease can be best characterized as immature or underdeveloped.

Although more research is needed, published data suggest that patients with ataxia telangiectasia have a defect of deoxyribonucleic acid (DNA) repair mechanisms; the precise nature of the defect is not understood. Patients with this disorder tend to be extremely sensitive to x-ray photons.[23,24] Fibroblasts from these patients exhibit defective DNA repair after exposure to x-irradiation. (However, unlike patients with xeroderma pigmentosum, patients with ataxia telangiectasia do not appear to have an unusual sensitivity to ultraviolet photons.) A number of patients who have undergone ionizing radiotherapy for an underlying malignancy have developed severe reactions; therefore, dosing and fractionation schedules require special attention. The lymphocytes of some patients have a high frequency of spontaneous breaks in their chromosomes,[8,25] and we will return to this point again.

Patients with ataxia telangiectasia have a high cancer incidence. The precise percentage of malignancies is estimated to be about 12%, with 9 years as the median age at the time of diagnosis.[13] Morrell and co-workers estimate[26] a 61-fold cancer excess for white probands and a 184-fold excess for blacks. A large number of malignancies observed are leukemias or lymphomas, of both B-cell and T-cell origins. These patients, however, appear to have an increased risk of other malignancies as well. Some estimates suggest that 40% of patients develop a malignancy. Cases of gastric, hepatic, central nervous system, ovarian, and cutaneous cancer have all been reported. Malignancies with different histologic patterns have occurred sequentially in the same individuals.

Neoplasms have occurred in siblings with ataxia telangiectasia but not in other siblings without the phenotypic expression of this disease. This could be viewed as yet another indication that the occurrence of these neoplasms is not a mere chance phenomenon.

Hecht and Hecht[8] have used ataxia telangiectasia to provide a paradigm for the role that recombination between an oncogene and an immunoglobulin gene and a T-cell receptor gene may play in the emergence of malignant lymphocytes. Several kinds of tumor are characterized by specific patterns of chromosomal rearrangements, which are discussed in other chapters of this book. One of the most important and informative patterns of chromosomal translocation is found in Burkitt's lymphoma, a tumor that occurs in several clinical settings, including acquired immunodeficiency syndrome (AIDS). The chromosomal abnormalities in this B-cell malignancy involve the translocation and juxtaposition of the

TABLE 57-1. Breakpoints for Chromosomal Abnormalities in Burkitt's Lymphomas*

Breakpoint	*Genetic Region Affected*
2p12	Immunoglobulin kappa light chain
8q24	c-*myc* (proto)-oncogene
14q32.3	Immunoglobulin heavy chain
22q11	Immunoglobulin lambda light chain

c-*myc* oncogene and an immunoglobulin gene, most commonly affecting chromosomes 8 and 14. This is summarized in Table 57-1.

The lymphocytes of patients with ataxia telangiectasia provide an interesting profile of cytogenetic abnormalities. Such patients exhibit a phenomenon of preferential chromosomal instability in their lymphoid cells, which facilitates the emergence of lymphocyte clones with nonrandom chromosomal translocations and inversions (particularly affecting chromosome 14). These rearrangements in turn may give rise to leukemias and lymphomas. The preferred chromosomal breakpoints in ataxia telangiectasia involve genetic loci that are within the immunoglobulin supergene family (see Table 57-2). These preferred breakpoints are likely to contain genetic sequences that, in the setting of a translocation, have the properties of oncogenes.

In effect, the predilection for cytogenetic abnormalities in ataxia telangiectasia can be viewed as an amplification of a spontaneous process of chromosomal rearrangement occasionally observed in normal lymphocytes. There is a rare subset of T cells from normal individuals that express chromosomal rearrangements similar to those seen in ataxia telangiectasia. One can speculate that the rarity of these cytogenetic changes and a normal immune surveillance mechanism limit the development of a lymphoid malignancy in normal individuals. On the other hand, in ataxia telangiectasia the genetic deficiency could permit the emergence of lymphocyte clones with oncogenic chromosomal translocations.

Basic scientists can influence clinicians and clinicians can influence basic scientists to generate knowledge that neither could attain alone. Ataxia telangiectasia has provided, and will continue to provide, a dramatic reminder of this fact.

TABLE 57-2. Common Breakpoints Seen in Lymphocytes from Patients with Ataxia Telangiectasia

Breakpoint(s)	*Genetic Region Affected*
7p14-15	Gamma chain of the T-cell antigen receptor
7q33-35	Beta chain of the T-cell antigen receptor
14q11	Alpha chain of the T-cell antigen receptor
14q32.1–14q32.3	Immunoglobulin heavy chain

Modified from Hecht F, Hecht BKM: Chromosome changes connect immunodeficiency and cancer in ataxia-telangiectasia. Am Pediatr Hematol Oncol 9:185, 1987.

WISKOTT–ALDRICH SYNDROME

The Wiskott–Aldrich syndrome encompasses a sex-linked disorder characterized clinically by the triad of thrombocytopenia, eczema, and recurrent infections with all classes of microorganisms. The genetic locus responsible for the disease has been mapped to the pericentric or proximal short arm of chromosome X.[6] In certain respects it is one of the most devastating immunodeficiency diseases. This disease was described in the German literature more than 40 years ago but was not widely recognized until Aldrich and coworkers described affected males in a large family pedigree.[17,26]

Infection, bleeding that requires platelet support, and, as discussed later in more detail, malignancies are significant problems in this syndrome. Previously, few patients survived into the second decade, but one should expect longer survivals in the era of modern antibiotics and platelet support. Patients with this syndrome have profound abnormalities of both the humoral and cellular immune systems.[4,28] In addition, they have functional defects of cells belonging to the monocyte–macrophage series.[29] The constellation of abnormalities seen in this disorder is strikingly different from all other recognized immunodeficiency diseases. Currently, bone marrow transplantation represents the only successful mode of clinical reconstitution, provided that a suitable donor is available.

Marked abnormalities in immunoglobulin production occur. These patients may have extremely elevated IgA and IgE serum levels. Using data collected from metabolic turnover studies, it is known that the in vivo synthetic rate for IgG is high. However, for reasons not fully understood, these patients have an excessive fractional catabolic rate that masks the elevated synthetic rate and leads to an apparently normal serum IgG concentration.[4] Patients with Wiskott–Aldrich syndrome have a marked predilection for developing monoclonal immunoglobulin spikes.[30] These patients generally have very low IgM levels in their serum. Even when these boys synthesize normal or elevated levels of total immunoglobulin, they have decreased titers of various natural antibodies. Patients with this disease characteristically have poor antibody responses after immunization, and antibody responses to polysaccharide antigens are especially poor. This may be one factor for the known risk of patients with this disease to develop recurrent episodes of pneumococcal sepsis.

Marked abnormalities of delayed cutaneous hypersensitivity (one measure of cellular immunity) are associated with this syndrome. Typically, patients with Wiskott–Aldrich syndrome have poor or absent delayed reactions in recall skin testing to such agents as *Candida*, purified, protein derivative, *Trichophyton*, mumps, diphtheria, and tetanus toxoid. Patients with this syndrome also have defective delayed hypersensitivity reactions on primary exposure to new antigens. Moreover, in the era in which skin allografts was used clinically in the immune elevation of patients, it was learned that these patients had defective allograft rejection.

Patients with Wiskott–Aldrich syndrome have a somewhat unusual profile of in vitro function cellular immunity. Typically, patients with the Wiskott–Aldrich syndrome have an adequate number of peripheral T cells. Lymphocytes from these patients have normal (or supranormal) proliferative response when exposed to nonspecific mitogens, such as phytohemagglutinin.[4] However, when lymphocytes are exposed to specific antigenic stimuli in vitro, defective proliferation is observed. The patients' lymphocytes respond poorly to such specific recall antigens as diphtheria, or tetanus toxoid, and they generally serve as poor responder cells in one-way mixed leukocyte reaction cultures. Although there is no question about the severity or clinical significance of the immune abnormalities seen in the Wiskott–Aldrich syndrome, it is difficult to provide a simple classification of the immunodeficiency. There are no satisfactory animal models for this disease, although sex-linked, B-cell dysfunction exists in mice. It is worth re-emphasizing that the Wiskott–Aldrich syndrome represents a multisystem abnormality of immunity involving T-cell, B-cell, and monocyte function. This syndrome may represent a disorder of antigen processing or recognition, with a preservation of immune effector function at a polyclonal level.[28] A resolution of the basic defects in this disease will have far-reaching clinical and theoretical implications for AIDS research. It is important to gather more data about the role of bone marrow transplantation in treating or preventing neoplasms in patients with the Wiskott–Aldrich syndrome.[33,34]

One of the most impressive features of the Wiskott–Aldrich syndrome is its high association with malignant disease.[13] The overall relative risk for certain malignancies is probably 100 times that of the general population and worsens with increasing age.[31,32,35] Many of these malignancies are large-cell immunoblastic reticuloendothelial tumors, and it has not been possible to find reliable criteria to designate the lymphomas as T, B, or true macrophage in origin.[36] Infiltration of visceral organs is common, but there is a paradoxical dearth of peripheral lymph node involvement.[36] Moreover, patients with the Wiskott–Aldrich syndrome have a marked tendency to develop lymphomatous infiltration of the brain, sometimes as the primary, or only, site of their neoplasm. This is reminiscent of the cancer pattern seen in organ allotransplant patients and in certain AIDS patients. As already mentioned, there appears to be a predisposition for the development of myelogenous leukemias in these boys.

The clinical course of neoplasms in patients with this disorder is capricious and demands the physician's highest acumen. Patients may develop variable aggressive lymphomas at unusual sites and without warning. Any patient with this syndrome who develops unexplained headaches, nausea, or vomiting should be considered at risk for a neoplasm of the CNS. One patient at the Metabolism Branch of the National Cancer Institute (NCI) underwent laparotomy and resection of a Stage I malignant lymphoma of the jejunum, without additional chemotherapy or radiotherapy.[1] The patient died nearly 5 months after surgical resection from an intracerebral bleed, and postmortem examination did not reveal residual lymphoma. There also has been a report of a patient with primary reticulum cell sarcoma of the brain treated with cobalt radiotherapy and intravenous vinblastine.[32] About 4 months after diagnosis the patient died of bronchopneumonia and had no evidence of viable reticulum cell sarcoma at autopsy.

Patients with the Wiskott–Aldrich syndrome who develop neoplasms may present difficult therapeutic challenges. Essentially all patients have thrombocytopenia. A number of patients have almost continuous bacterial or viral infections. Chronic herpes infections are a common problem, and *P. carinii* pneumonia is a concern even before chemotherapy. These conditions significantly magnify the risk of therapy-related complications and make it more difficult to deliver full doses of cytotoxic chemotherapy.

Allogeneic bone marrow transplantation represents an important modality that can restore immunocompetence to certain patients with the Wiskott–Aldrich syndrome.[33,34] This approach may theoretically lower the risk of neoplastic disease in some of these patients and may be useful in some patients as part of a combined modality approach once a neoplasm has arisen.

SEX-LINKED/EPSTEIN–BARR VIRUS–ASSOCIATED LYMPHOPROLIFERATIVE SYNDROME

One unique disorder is associated with a severe infectious mononucleosis–like disorder, immunodeficiency, and lymphoproliferative disease.[37–39] This appears to be sex-linked and characterized by a susceptibility to fulminant infection with Epstein–Barr virus that may be promptly lethal or may lead to unusual sequelae, including hypogammaglobulinemia, massive hepatic necrosis, aplastic anemia, and a variety of malignant lymphoproliferative disorders. The patients may appear well and have normal cellular and humoral immune responses until they encounter the Epstein–Barr virus. The malignant lymphoproliferative sequelae often represent an expansion of B cells, which contain the Epstein–Barr virus genome. The pathogenesis of this syndrome (or group of syndromes) is unknown, but it is thought that there is defective natural killer (NK) function. This disorder focuses attention on the role of sex-linked genes in the expression of immunodeficiency states and certain neoplasms in the setting of infection by a DNA virus such as the Epstein–Barr virus. Research defining the genetic locus for this disease is under way, and the relevant region is in a different segment of chromosome X than the one containing the Wiskott–Aldrich gene or infantile sex-linked hypogammaglobulinemia (see below).[7]

INFANTILE SEX-LINKED HYPOGAMMAGLOBULINEMIA (BRUTON TYPE)

In Bruton-type hypogammaglobulinemia the B-cell limb of immune cell development is impaired. This sex-linked immunodeficiency disease is characterized by defective B-cell function and intact T-cell function. The gene responsible for this disease has been mapped to the proximate region of the lone arm of chromosome X.[5] It has been thought that this disease results from a defect in the bursal-equivalent microenvironment necessary for B-cell maturation. Surgical or pharmacologic bursectomy in chickens produces a similar immune deficit.

Patients with this form of immunodeficiency lack tonsils and generally lack plasma cells in germinal centers, whereas thymic histology is normal. Most totally lack mature B cells in their circulation. These patients have very low concentrations of serum immunoglobulins and have few or no specific antibodies in response to antigenic challenge. Clinically, patients with infantile sex-linked hypogammaglobulinemia are subject to recurrent infections with high-grade pathogens, such as *Haemophilus influenzae* or *Streptococcus pneumoniae*. The sinopulmonary tree is a key target of these infections, and crippling lung damage may occur. Intramuscular or intravenous gammaglobulin preparations may significantly improve the clinical course of these patients.

Several cases of malignancy have been described in patients with infantile sex-linked hypogammaglobulinemia. In what might have been the earliest description, Page and associates reported a child with agammaglobulinemia and dermatomyositis who was found to have a lymphoma involving lymph nodes, liver, and kidneys at autopsy.[40] The same report described a child with agammaglobulinemia who was noted to have acute lymphoblastic leukemia at about 4 years of age. Several other cases of leukemia, one in association with a thymoma, have been described.[3]

At one time the risk of malignancy in patients with infantile sex-linked hypogammaglobulinemia was estimated to be about 6%. In a more recent report from the ICR, including a period from the fall of 1975 to the spring of 1977, the percentage of patients with cancer was 0.7%. The true risk of cancer in this disease requires further research.

COMMON VARIABLE IMMUNODEFICIENCY

Common variable immunodeficiency disease represents a heterogeneous group of disorders in which the immunodeficiency state may arise after a period of apparently normal immunologic function. Unfortunately this diagnosis may mean different things to different physicians. Certain cases of what once was termed acquired hypogammaglobulinemia would now be classified as common variable immunodeficiency. As with Bruton-type immunodeficiency, these patients have depressed serum immunoglobulin levels. They generally have little or no specific antibody in response to antigenic challenge and replacement gammaglobulin therapy is necessary. Near-relatives of patients with common variable immunodeficiency have a high incidence of dysgammaglobulinemia and autoimmune phenomena. A large percentage of patients with common variable immunodeficiency also have significant abnormalities of in vivo or in vitro assays of cellular immune function. Thus this disease is often associated with significant T-cell dysfunction. In a large subset of patients circulating B cells can be detected. Data indicate that perhaps one factor in the cause of perpetuation of this disease is the presence of abnormal suppressor T cells that can act to inhibit the terminal maturation of B cells into immunoglobulin-synthesizing and -secreting plasma cells.[41]

Patients with common variable immunodeficiency referred to the Metabolism Branch of the NCI have presented with a constellation of symptoms. Perhaps the most common presenting symptoms are related to sinopulmonary infections reminiscent of Bruton-type immunodeficiency. Patients often have recurrent sinusitis, mastoiditis, and otitis media. Even while receiving replacement gammaglobulin therapy a number of patients develop recurrent pulmonary infections in the form of severe bronchitis and pneumonia, which may lead to bronchiectasis. One problem is that many patients already have significant pulmonary damage by the time their immunodeficiency is diagnosed, and the structurally damaged lung per se is a risk factor for recurrent infections. The pathogens for these infections, at least early in the disease's course, tend to be encapsulated bacteria such as *S. pneumoniae* and *H. influenzae*.

A large number of patients with common variable immunodeficiency also may have serious gastrointestinal problems, especially diarrhea and malabsorption. In a small number of patients gastrointestinal symptoms represent the major manifestations of this disease complex. Some patients with common variable immunodeficiency have giardiasis, frequently in association with nodular lymphoid hyperplasia of the gastrointestinal tract. There also is a subset of patients who develop gastrointestinal bacterial overgrowth, which may be accompanied by partial villous atrophy of the small intestine.

For unknown reasons, in some series 10% to 15% of patients with common variable immunodeficiency may have atrophic gastritis in association with pernicious anemia. These patients have positive Schilling's tests and show both hematologic and neurologic sequelae of vitamin B_{12} deficiency if left untreated. Other unexplained features of this syndrome are splenomegaly and idiopathic noncaseating granulomas of visceral organs, including the liver. Some patients with common variable immunodeficiency suffer the paradoxical development of autoimmune hemolysis and may have Coombs'-positive hemolytic anemias. Thus simply because a patient has a humoral immune impairment, it is not justifiable to dismiss the possibility of autoimmune disease. To further emphasize this, a number of patients have arthralgias and arthritis, primarily of smaller joints, although true erosive changes are not common. Some patients have a syndrome that resembles overt rheumatoid arthritis. Also, serous dermatomyositis and vasculitis-type syndromes may complicate the course of patients with common variable immunodeficiency.

The incidence of malignancy among patients with common variable immunodeficiency is higher than that found in the general population. In one series, for those patients in whom the onset of the immunodeficiency appeared before 16 years of age, the percentage of cancer observed was about 2.5%.[13] In those patients in whom the onset of immunodeficiency took place at age 16 or older, the percentage of cancer observed is 8.5%. Patients with selective absence of certain immunoglobulin classes (especially IgM) who do not readily fit the diagnosis of common variable immunodeficiency also may be at increased risk of neoplasia. Kinlen and co-workers in a prospective study reported a 47-fold excess of gastric cancer and a 30-fold excess of lymphomas in patients with hypogammaglobulinemia, most of whom had common variable immunodeficiency.[42]

Because gastric carcinomas constitute a substantial proportion of the neoplasms seen in this patient population (perhaps owing to the known tendency for certain patients to develop atrophic gastritis), careful monitoring of adult patients, especially those with atrophic gastritis, for the development of stomach cancer is essential.

Early and aggressive surgical intervention may be worthwhile in these patients.[42] Also, one can argue that patients with common variable immunodeficiency plus achlorhydria should receive regular endoscopic screening. Aggressive therapeutic interventions may also be of value in the therapy of the lymphomas that arise in these patients.[43]

CANCER AND THE ACQUIRED IMMUNODEFICIENCY SYNDROME

Associated with AIDS as well as with other acquired and congenital immunodeficiency disorders is a wide spectrum of neoplasms. Foremost among these cancers are aggressive forms of Kaposi's sarcoma or B-cell lymphoma. Hodgkin's disease may also occur at an increased frequency, and with a different clinical manifestation, compared with Hodgkin's disease arising in the otherwise immunocompetent host. The pathogenesis of these neoplasms is an area of intense study, which may yield insights into more general mechanisms in the development of cancers. Although a decade ago these cancers were relatively unusual and seen mainly in children with congenital immunodeficiency disorders and in the setting of organ transplantation, the explosive increase in cases of AIDS in the United States now makes it imperative for the clinician to have a detailed and competent diagnostic and therapeutic approach to Kaposi's sarcoma and B-cell lymphoma. We will synthesize the current hypotheses offered to explain the pathogenesis of these neoplasms in this immunodeficient host, provide data on clinical presentation and staging, present therapeutic options, and discuss infectious complications that may occur during chemotherapy and radiation therapy.

EPIDEMIOLOGY AND PATHOPHYSIOLOGY OF KAPOSI'S SARCOMA

AIDS was initially recognized in 1980 in the United States in part due to the unusual occurrence of an aggressive form of Kaposi's sarcoma among young male homosexuals.[44] Kaposi's sarcoma, first described by Moricz Kaposi as "idiopathic, multiple, pigmented sarcomas of the skin," eventually merged as a neoplasm bearing this dermatologist's name and was recognized as an unusual tumor primarily affecting elderly males of Mediterranean or Ashkenazic Jewish origin.[45,46] An African form of Kaposi's sarcoma was recognized three decades ago and appeared to occur in relatively well defined areas of Central Africa, accounting for approximately 10% of all neoplasms in Kenya, Tanzania, and the Congo.[46–48] Kaposi's sarcoma was also recognized to occur among organ transplant recipients who received immunosuppressive therapy, which, when discontinued, was occasionally associated with spontaneous regression of Kaposi's sarcoma lesions.[49,50] These anecdotal observations among the organ transplant population led to the hypothesis that the pathogenesis of the neoplasm was associated with loss of integrity of the cellular immune system. Epidemic Kaposi's sarcoma occurring in association with AIDS clearly rises on the basis of human immunodeficiency virus (HIV)-mediated suppression of cellular immunity.

As discussed earlier, there are accumulating data to support the hypothesis that certain neoplasms arise because of impairment in the cellular or humoral immune system in humans. Immunodeficient lower animals, such as athymic nude mice, have long been recognized to be convenient models for the propagation of a number of murine and human cancers. This has lead to the model of "immune surveillance" whereby it is postulated that neoplastic events occur during life and that an intact immune system is capable of recognizing and eliminating the oncogenically transformed cells. Such mechanisms of recognition and elimination are believed to occur because of antigenic changes on the surface of malignant cells compared with their normal counterparts. These antigenic changes then identify the cell to the host's immune system, as being different from "self," with antibody-mediated or direct cellular cytotoxicity resulting in destruction of the transformed cells. There are few data to support such a hypothesis for most cancers. Nonetheless, the unique occurrence of certain types of neoplasms in the setting of AIDS as well as other acquired and congenital immunodeficiency disorders provides the opportunity to investigate the interplay of viral or environmental carcinogens, the function of immune effector cells such as T and B lymphocyte, monocyte–macrophages, and NK cells. It is clear that certain neoplasms such as Kaposi's sarcoma and non-Hodgkin's lymphoma arise at an increased frequency and have different clinical behavior in immunocompromised hosts compared with immunocompetent hosts. Other neoplasms such as Hodgkin's disease and squamous carcinoma of the head and neck or anus may or may not occur at an increased rate in immunocompromised patients, but do appear to have a more aggressive natural history and are more difficult to effectively treat. Because our understanding of the pathogenesis and therapy of neoplasms in the immunocompromised host is in a dynamic, evolving process, the clinician is uniquely positioned to contribute to the research effort in this area. Careful clinical study and reporting of the appearance of these and other neoplasms in immunocompromised hosts may allow for new avenues of research in the laboratory to better identify the causative mechanisms involved and more effective forms of treatment. Kaposi's sarcoma in the setting of AIDS is a prototype for our understanding of the epidemiology, pathophysiology, clinical behavior, and therapeutic interventions in cancer arising in the immunodeficient host. For that reason, and because it is certainly the most frequently encountered neoplasm in the United States for the practicing physician caring for AIDS patients, we shall discuss these aspects in depth.

EPIDEMIOLOGY AND PATHOPHYSIOLOGY OF EPIDEMIC KAPOSI'S SARCOMA

Initially described by Moricz Kaposi as "idiopathic, multiple pigmented sarcomas of the skin," this neoplasm later became identified as Kaposi's sarcoma among elderly men of

Mediterranean or Ashkenazic Jewish origin in the West.[45,46] It was a rare neoplasm with an indolent clinical course, commonly effecting the lower extremities and only occasionally requiring therapeutic intervention with local radiation therapy or single-agent chemotherapy. An endemic form of Kaposi's sarcoma was recognized in Central Africa.[47,48] It occurred in fairly well defined areas of Africa, constituting approximately 10% of all neoplasms in Kenya, Tanzania, and Zaire. Again, there appears to be a strong male predominance for endemic Kaposi's sarcoma in Central Africa, with male-female ratios of about 10:1. The neoplasm in Central Africa generally occurs in the 25-to-40 age group with a spectrum of clinical severity ranging from localized nodular lesions to large aggressive exophytic tumors. Among Central African children the male-female ratio is less marked, approximately 3:1, and the neoplasm is generally rapidly progressive and fatal. The initial clue that Kaposi's sarcoma may be associated with cellular immunodeficiency came from its sporadic occurrence among organ transplant recipients.[49–51]

Iatrogenically immunosuppressed patients treated with corticosteroids, azathioprine, or cyclosporine manifested Kaposi's sarcoma at an increased rate, with a male-female ratio of about 2:1. The neoplasm can be indolent or rapidly progressive, localized or widespread; anecdotal cases have reported regression of the neoplasm when immunosuppressive therapy is discontinued. Similarly, patients with primary neoplasms that are associated with immunodeficiency, such as non-Hodgkin's lymphoma, Hodgkin's disease, and multiple myeloma, have been reported to develop Kaposi's sarcoma as a second neoplasm.[51,52]

The epidemic form of Kaposi's sarcoma that occurs in association with AIDS was initially recognized in 1980 among male homosexuals in the United States.[53,54] It is intriguing that Kaposi's sarcoma occurs among approximately 40% of male homosexual AIDS cases but only about 8% of heterosexual AIDS cases.[55,56] This has lead to considerable search for a viral or environmental factor present in the male homosexual community in the United States that might potentiate the development of Kaposi's sarcoma. Initial studies suggested that there may be an increased frequency of human leukocyte antigen DR5 (HLA-DR5) among Italian and Jewish Kaposi's sarcoma patients.[57] HLA-DR2 appeared to be increased in patients of northern European background with AIDS-associated Kaposi's sarcoma. However, evaluation of larger cohorts of AIDS patients with Kaposi's sarcoma has failed to substantiate this initial observation of an association with HLA type.[58] It is thus unclear whether genetic factors are operative in the pathogenesis of epidemic Kaposi's sarcoma. Similarly, recreational drugs such as amyl and butyl nitrite, which were popular in the male homosexual community, have been associated in some studies with epidemic Kaposi's sarcoma.[55,58] Again, these data are hard to reproduce in other epidemiologic studies. Furthermore, because substantial numbers of heterosexual patients with epidemic Kaposi's sarcoma, as well as homosexual AIDS cases with the neoplasm, have had no exposure to these volatile nitrites, it is unclear what role, if any, they play in the pathogenesis of the neoplasm.

A number of studies of classic Kaposi's sarcoma suggested an association between cytomegalovirus (CMV) infection and the neoplasm. Giraldo and co-workers initially reported an increased prevalence of antibody to CMV among elderly men in Europe with classic Kaposi's sarcoma compared with controls.[59] Further studies using molecular probes to CMV reported a moderate degree of hybridization between CMV, DNA, reportedly detected in Kaposi's sarcoma lesions compared with normal skin.[60] A hypothesis emerged that Kaposi's sarcoma may have an important viral etiology based on these studies a decade ago. Unfortunately more recent studies on epidemic Kaposi's sarcoma have failed to confirm these reported observations in classic Kaposi's sarcoma.[61] No difference in serologic prevalence or titer to CMV among AIDS patients with Kaposi's sarcoma versus case controls has been observed.[55] Similarly, concern has been raised that the early probes used to detect CMV may have been relatively nonspecific and would hybridize with normal elements within human DNA.[61] More specific probes for CMV have failed to consistently detect viral sequences within Kaposi's sarcoma lesions. A critical assessment of the current data fails to support a role for CMV in a pathogenesis of epidemic Kaposi's sarcoma. Another obvious question is whether HIV might directly infect and oncogenically transform cells that give rise to Kaposi's sarcoma. Again, molecular studies of Kaposi's sarcoma lesions have failed to identify HIV sequences within the tumor.[61] Perhaps the most detailed and intriguing molecular studies on the pathogenesis of Kaposi's sarcoma have been done by Giacarlo. His group has recently reported rearrangements in cellular oncogenes in Kaposi's sarcoma lesions as well as a putative, previously undescribed oncogene that may code for a protein with fibroblast growth factor–like activity.[62,63] A hypothesis emerging from these studies postulates that overexpression of this oncogene product leads to an autocrine model whereby the growth factor

TABLE 57-3. Taylor Classification of Kaposi's Sarcoma

Clinical Type	*Behavior*	*Age Group (yr)*	*Bone Involvement*	*Lymph Node Involvement*	*Predominant Skin Tumor*
Nodular	Indolent	>25	Rare	Rare	Nodules, plaques
Florid	Locally aggressive	>25	Often	Rare	Fungating (exophytic)
Infiltrative	Locally aggressive	>25	Always	Rare	Diffuse infiltration
Lymphadenopathic	Disseminated aggressive	<25	Rare	Always	Nodules

Taylor et al: Kaposi's sarcoma in Uganda: A clinico-pathologic study. Int J Cancer 8:122, 1971.

produced by the tumor cells feeds back on the tumor and promotes increased growth.

Indeed, it is still unclear whether Kaposi's sarcoma should be classified as a true cancer, that is, a monoclonal proliferation of cells derived from a single oncogenically transformed progenitor, or whether the neoplasm is polyclonal. As will be discussed below, the neoplasm does not appear to spread in many cases in a clearly contiguous or metastatic manner, but may appear at multiple and apparently differing primary sites contemporaneously.[61] Furthermore, among homosexual men, there may be a predilection for appearance of the neoplasm within the oral cavity and head neck and within the anus and rectum, suggesting inoculation of susceptible tissue by a transmissible agent during oral or anal sex. Kaposi's sarcoma associated with AIDS is thus a fertile opportunity for epidemiologic and molecular studies to better define the pathogenesis in nature of the neoplasm.

HISTOPATHOLOGY

Histopathologically, classic Kaposi's sarcoma, endemic Kaposi's sarcoma in Africa, and epidemic Kaposi's sarcoma associated with AIDS are quite similar.[51,61] Generally, the lesions show interlacing bands of spindle cells, with vascular structures in a network of reticular and collagen fibers. The vascular structures form cleft-like spaces with extravasated erythrocytes, and lymphatics and blood vessels extend to the periphery of the lesions. A wide range of nuclear pleomorphism may be seen in the spindle cells. Between the spindle cells one generally finds hemosiderin deposits and extravasated erythrocytes. Macrophages within the lesions may phagocytose the hemosiderin. Often the lesions have an inflammatory infiltrate consisting of histiocytes, lymphocytes, and plasma cells. Less frequently the lesions may have globules of a hyaline eosinophilic material contained within the macrophages of spindle cells or deposited in extracellular locations.

Histopathologic diagnosis may be difficult, particularly during the earlier macular stage of the lesions. The dermatologic changes may be quite subtle, and microscopically, the pathologist may note only abnormal dilated vessels around a normal superficial vasculature. At this stage, pathologically, the inflammatory infiltrate may be sparse, and the nuclear pleomorphism restricted to occasional mitoses and nuclear atypia. Later, in the plaque formation stage, the Kaposi's sarcoma lesions show more extensive neoplastic involvement with proliferation from the superficial to the deep dermis and, occasionally, invasion into underlying adipose layers. The inflammatory infiltrate becomes more marked in the plaque stage with increased numbers of spindle cells and greater extravasation of erythrocytes. The hemosiderin deposition is more prominent, although nuclear pleomorphism may still be somewhat mild. In the advanced nodular lesions the spindle cell population is dense and there is considerable reticulum deposition. These histopathologic features, particularly in the early stages of lesion development, may be difficult to distinguish from inflammatory processes or granulation tissue.

The cell of origin of Kaposi's sarcoma is controversial, with various cell types proposed in different histopathologic studies.[58,64–66] Histochemical studies have suggested the Schwann cell (a multipotential primitive mesenchymal cell), the endothelial or perithelial cell of small vessels, or transformed vascular cells. The spindle cells of Kaposi's sarcoma demonstrate a different staining pattern than the perivascular cells, with the former positive for acid phosphatase and the latter negative. The reverse is true for histochemical staining for alkaline phosphatase. Electron microscopic studies demonstrate a morphologic appearance suggestive of a vascular cell origin, as do immunohistochemical studies that demonstrate factor VIII–related antigens in Kaposi's sarcoma specimens.[65,66] Unfortunately the factor VIII–positive cells are generally those within the proliferating vessels, while the spindle cells are only faintly positive. A specific type of endothelial cell, that associated with lymphatic endothelium, has also been suggested as the cell of origin. At this time none of these studies convincingly demonstrates the cell of origin because the factor VIII–related antigen may simply be seen in the nonmalignant endothelial cells that form the interior of the proliferating vascular structures and others secondary to the malignant process.

CLINICAL MANIFESTATIONS OF EPIDEMIC KAPOSI'S SARCOMA

Although epidemic Kaposi's sarcoma may occasionally present as a solitary lesion, a multifocal presentation is more common, with multiple red to purple macules, nodules, or papules.[53,58,61] These lesions may progress to the plaque and nodular stage, coalesce, and ultimately develop into large and erosive ulcerating or fungating lesions. Generally the cutaneous lesions of epidemic Kaposi's sarcoma are smaller than those of classic Kaposi's sarcoma during the initial presentation, and are more often located in the mouth, head and neck, and upper trunk, whereas classic Kaposi's sarcoma occurs in the lower extremities in approximately three-fourths of cases.[6] AIDS-associated Kaposi's sarcoma frequently effects the mucosa of the mouth and anus, lymph nodes, and gastrointestinal tract. More than 50% of patients will have visceral lesions, particularly in the gastrointestinal tract, at the time of initial presentation. At autopsy Kaposi's sarcoma lesions in AIDS patients have been noted in virtually any and every organ, including the lung, liver, pancreas, spleen, adrenals, brain, and testes. These visceral lesions are usually asymptomatic, although the gastrointestinal lesions may occasionally result in hemorrhage and malabsorption. Pulmonary involvement is particularly ominous and may present with insidious dyspnea or hemoptysis, or both. The cutaneous lesions are nonblanching, pink to red to purple, nontender, and generally not pruritic. As the lesions progress and coalesce they may obstruct lymphatic drainage from the area and result in significant lymphedema, particularly in the lower extremities and head and neck.

CLINICAL STAGING

Before the recognition of epidemic Kaposi's sarcoma associated with AIDS, a widely used classification system for Kaposi's sarcoma was developed by Taylor (Table 57-3).[48] The basis of the staging system was the nature of clinical

TABLE 57-4. Staging of Epidemic Kaposi's Sarcoma

	*NYU Staging System**	*Mitsuyasu Staging System†*
Stage		
I	Cutaneous, locally indolent	Limited cutaneous (<10 lesions or one anatomical area)
II	Cutaneous, locally aggressive with or without regional lymph nodes	Disseminated cutaneous (>10 lesions or more than one anatomical area)
III	Generalized mucocutaneous and/or lymph node involvement‡	Visceral only (GI, lymph node)
IV	Visceral	Cutaneous and visceral, or pulmonary KS
Subtype		
A	No systemic signs or symptoms	No systemic signs or symptoms
B	Systemic signs; weight loss (10%) or fever (>100°F orally, unrelated to an identifiable source of infection lasting >2 weeks)	Fevers >37.8°C unrelated to identifiable infection lasting >2 weeks, or weight loss >10% of body weight

*Krigel RL et al: Kaposi's sarcoma: A new staging classification. Cancer Treat Rep 67:531, 1983.

†Mitsuyasu RT, Groopman JE: Biology and therapy of Kaposi's sarcoma. Semin Oncol 11:53, 1984.

‡Generalized = more than upper or lower extremities alone; includes minimal GI disease defined as <5 lesions and <2 cm in combined diameters.

presentation of the predominant lesions and the progression of the tumor. Four major types of classic Kaposi's sarcoma were recognized. An indolent nodular variety was generally manifest as plaque-like or nodular cutaneous lesions with rare involvement of lymph nodes or bone. The florid type was locally aggressive with cutaneous lesions that frequently were fungating and exophytic. Again, lymph node involvement was rare. Infiltrative Kaposi's sarcoma uniformly invaded bone by way of penetration from the overlying soft tissue but did not involve lymph nodes. The lymphadenopathic type was disseminated and acted aggressively with frequent involvement of viscera and nodes.

Unfortunately the clinical staging system that was applicable to classic Kaposi's sarcoma breaks down in the case of epidemic Kaposi's sarcoma. A clinical staging system should have prognostic as well as clinical significance. In the case of epidemic Kaposi's sarcoma associated with AIDS, the clinical outcome for the patient may often be determined by infectious complications of the underlying immunodeficiency as opposed to morbidity and mortality associated with the neoplasm.

Despite several proposed classification systems for AIDS-associated Kaposi's sarcoma, none has emerged as a generally accepted scheme. Krigel and co-workers proposed that AIDS-associated Kaposi's sarcoma can be divided into four stages, depending on the predominant type of lesion and the degree of involvement and presentation.[67] They observed that patients frequently presented with cutaneous lesions as well as lesions in lymph nodes and viscera. The extent of dermal involvement by the skin lesions also ranged from macules and relatively thin plaques measuring a few millimeters to elevated nodules. Approximately 10% of the 49 patients studied by Krigel and associates had no cutaneous lesions on presentation, 25% had fewer than five localized skin lesions, two-thirds had many widely distributed cutaneous lesions, and 2% had a locally aggressive exophytic lesion. Nearly two-thirds had generalized lymphadenopathy on presentation, with pathologic confirmation of Kaposi's sarcoma within the lymph nodes in 80%. The four patients without skin involvement on presentation had generalized lymphadenopathy, with biopsy-proven Kaposi's sarcoma restricted to the lymph nodes. About half of their patients had involvement of the gastrointestinal tract, with most of these also having cutaneous lesions. The patients with gastrointestinal Kaposi's sarcoma did not appear clinically different from those with lesions restricted to the integuments. About two-thirds of the patients had constitutional symptoms on presentation, including unexplained fever and weight loss. These clinical and pathologic observations led this group to propose a staging system as follows: Stage I, cutaneous, locally indolent; Stage II, cutaneous, locally aggressive with or without regional lymph node involvement; Stage III, generalized mucocutaneous or lymph node involvement, or both; and Stage IV, visceral (Table 57-4). The subtypes A, no systemic signs or symptoms, and B, systemic signs such as greater than 10% weight loss and fever unrelated to an identifiable infection, would subdivide each stage. Their staging system reflects in part the presentation and clinical behavior of the different types of classic Kaposi's sarcoma, whereby Stage I represents the typical elderly Mediterranean or Ashkenazic Jewish patient with Kaposi's sarcoma, Stage II, the locally invasive African Kaposi's sarcoma; and Stages III and Stage IV, the aggressive disseminated Kaposi's sarcoma seen in African children and in certain iatrogenically immunocompromised patients. Unfortunately it may be difficult to predict progression of disease or survival based on clinical stage. For that reason, Mitsuyasu and Groopman proposed an alternative staging system that appears to encompass most

TABLE 57-5. Therapy of AIDS-Associated Kaposi's Sarcoma

Disease Characteristic	*Options*
Minimal tumor	
No B symptoms	Observe; alpha interferon; vinca alkaloids
B symptoms	Single-agent chemotherapy (*e.g.*, vinblastine, vincristine)
Extensive tumor	
No B symptoms	Alpha interferon; etoposide; vinblastine; vincristine, bleomycin
B symptoms and/or rapid growth	Doxorubicin; etoposide
Painful or disfiguring lesions	Radiation therapy

patients with epidemic Kaposi's sarcoma (Table 57-5).[68] In that staging system, patients with ten or fewer cutaneous lesions or lesions restricted to a single anatomical region (such as one extremity) are classified as Stage I; patients with more than ten cutaneous lesions or involvement beyond a single anatomical site are Stage II; those with visceral involvement without lesions on the integument (usually involving lymph nodes or gastrointestinal tract, or both) are grouped as Stage III; and those with both visceral and cutaneous lesions constitute Stage IV. Patients with pulmonary Kaposi's sarcoma are classified as Stage IV. The rationale of this staging system is to subdivide the Stages II, III, and IV of Krigel and co-workers into four distinct stages that approximately reflect the bulk of tumor. Because approximately half of all patients with AIDS-associated Kaposi's sarcoma have visceral disease, they would be classified as Stage III or IV by the Mitsuyasu and Groopman classification system. Similar to Krigel and associates' system patients are subdivided within a stage according to clinical symptoms of fever, unexplained weight loss, night sweats, and diarrhea as subclass B, while asymptomatic patients are subclass A. Patients with a history of opportunistic infection but not currently manifesting constitutional symptoms are nonetheless classified as subtype B.

This classification system was applied in a retrospective study of the clinical course and response to treatment of 96 consecutive AIDS patients with biopsy-proven Kaposi's sarcoma.[69] In this analysis Mitsuyasu and co-workers demonstrated that stage was of prognostic importance but did not appear to correlate with response to therapy. In their series 23 of 96 patients were Stage I, 40 were Stage II, 9 were Stage III, and 24 were Stage IV. Thirty-three patients were classified as subtype B, while 63 patients were asymptomatic. Fifteen of 96 patients had prior or concurrent opportunistic infections. Survival plotted according to the method of Kaplan–Meier by tumor stage for the cohort of 96 patients showed a statistically significant survival advantage for patients with Stage I or III compared with those with Stage II or IV. The response to treatment, specifically recombinant interferon alpha A, was not correlated with tumor stage but did appear to correlate with subtype A (36% response rate) compared with subtype B (12%) response rate. Interestingly, visceral disease was not an independent variable that affected response to treatment or survival, with similar treatment responses in patients with low tumor bulk in Stage III compared with nonvisceral disease in Stage I. This is contrary to the general impression of a negative prognostic significance associated with visceral disease in most neoplasms.

The major parameters that strongly correlated with survival were lack of history of opportunistic infection and absence of concurrent constitutional symptoms. A large number of immunologic studies done on these patients revealed that the total number of CD4-positive cells and the CD4-CD8 ratio were also of prognostic value. In this study all patients were male homosexuals with serologic evidence of HIV infection. No correlation with survival was found with total leukocyte count, HLA-DR type, proliferative response to mitogen such as phytohemagglutinin level of NK cell activity, skin test reactivity to recall antigens, presence of circulating immunocomplexes, and level and distribution of the serum immunoglobulins IgG, IgA, and IgM. This study comprises the most detailed data based on consecutive patients with Kaposi's sarcoma from time of presentation to death. As expected, the limitation of the analysis may be related to different forms of therapy that these patients received. Thus, although patients treated with recombinant interferon alpha 2 (35 of 96 patients in this study) did not differ from others in terms of age, clinical stage, or immunologic parameters, it would be difficult to dissect out the multiple and intermittent treatment approaches as to effects on the survival curve. As for AIDS patients not manifesting Kaposi's sarcoma, the major prognostic parameters are those that predict for life-threatening opportunistic infections.[61] Such infections are believed to develop on the basis of progressive deterioration of cellular immunity. Constitutional symptoms such as fever, night sweats, or weight loss among patients with epidemic Kaposi's sarcoma are clearly correlated with poor survival; some symptoms may reflect an undiagnosed opportunistic infection and/or a systemic response to activity of HIV itself. A total number of CD4-positive lymphocytes less than 200 with a ratio of CD4 to CD8 cells of less than 0.5 bespeaks a particularly impaired cellular immune state and a high degree of susceptibility to opportunistic infections in the population with epidemic Kaposi's sarcoma.

Vadhan–Raj and colleagues, in a multivaried analysis of 70 patients with epidemic Kaposi's sarcoma treated with interferon alpha 2A, found that impaired delayed hypersensitivity response to one or more recall antigens and a high proliferative response to *E. coli* antigen significantly predicted poor outcome. In addition, these workers found that the presence of endogenous serum interferon activity before any treatment intervention, particularly an acid-labile alpha interferon species, had a negative predictive value. The studies of Mitsuyasu and colleagues and Vadhan–Raj and associates emphasize the underlying immunologic problem faced by AIDS patients with Kaposi's sarcoma. Integration of such immunologic parameters into a staging system for Kaposi's sarcoma is a current endeavor and may be particularly useful in planning therapeutic modalities for these patients. Furthermore, since opportunistic infection is the major cause of death in these patients, prophylaxis with oral or inhaled antibiotics may be applicable to that groups of AIDS-associated Kaposi's sarcoma patients with poor prognostic parameters that predict subsequent infections.

THERAPEUTIC MODALITIES IN EPIDEMIC KAPOSI'S SARCOMA

The major therapeutic interventions for patients with AIDS-associated Kaposi's sarcoma are observation without treatment, recombinant interferons, single-agent or multiagent chemotherapy, and radiation therapy.[61] Because of the variable natural history of epidemic Kaposi's sarcoma, the complicating factor of significant immunosuppression with death generally caused by opportunistic infection, and the absence of any placebo controlled trials, it is difficult to critically assess the indications for each therapeutic modality as well as an objective response rate. Moreover, gauging response of lesions may be quite difficult because many patients have multiple lesions that are difficult to follow accurately, and changes in nodularity or color of lesion may indicate some effect of the treatment intervention but would not necessarily be reflected in the classic oncologic criterion of shrinkage of lesion diameter. Finally, assessment of benefit of treatment needs to take into account the effects of this treatment on the underlying immunodeficiency. Despite these formidable difficulties in analyzing outcome of several treatment studies of epidemic Kaposi's sarcoma, certain clinical guidelines can be suggested for optimal management (Table 57-5). Because epidemic Kaposi's sarcoma is still an evolving problem with a limited data base, patients who are appropriate for research protocols should be entered onto such protocols in order to increase the scientific information available regarding their prognosis and management.
able regarding their prognosis and management.

Recombinant and natural interferons have been extensively studied in epidemic Kaposi's sarcoma.[71–82] The rationale for using interferon in the treatment of this neoplasm included its properties as an immunomodulator, an antineoplastic agent, and an antiviral. The interferons had been recognized to augment T-cell–mediated cytotoxicity, NK cell activity, and certain macrophage functions. The results of various treatment trials with different, highly purified alpha interferon species, including recombinant interferon alpha 2A, recombinant interferon alpha 2B, and interferon alpha N1 (from human lymphoblastoid cells), are summarized in Table 57-6. The initial observations of efficacy of interferon in AIDS-associated Kaposi's sarcoma was made during a Phase I trial of interferon alpha 2A.[71] Serendipitously the patients with epidemic Kaposi's sarcoma who were entered on this Phase I program received interferon in amounts that matched or exceeded the maximum tolerated dose. The results of that Phase I trial were objective responses (complete or partial tumor regression) in 5 of 12 evaluable patients. These preliminary data were later confirmed in larger studies with interferon alpha 2A as well as with interferon alpha 2B and interferon alpha N1 at doses of greater than 20 million U/m^2 of body surface area. The average objective response rate has consistently ranged between 25% and 40%.[72–82]

A program of gradual dose escalation of interferon has been explored. It appears that some of the acute toxicity associated with high-dose interferon therapy, such as fever and chills, can be ameliorated with this program. It appears that low doses of interferon lead only to occasional response rates of 5% to 10%. The mechanism of action of interferon in epidemic Kaposi's sarcoma may be antineoplastic, as suggested by the significantly higher response rate with higher doses of drug. Nonetheless, it is also possible that the antiviral effect of interferon on HIV requires such higher doses.[83] There has not been a clearly discernible immunologic effect in Kaposi's sarcoma patients treated with interferons.

Phase I studies have recently been initiated to evaluate the combination of interferon alpha with other therapeutic agents for epidemic Kaposi's sarcoma. Combinations include interferon alpha plus vinca alkaloids such as vinblastine. Although two initial trials suggested that the combination of interferon alpha and vinblastine has substantial activity against AIDS-associated Kaposi's sarcoma,[81,82] a randomized study of interferon alpha 2A alone versus interferon alpha 2A plus vinblastine revealed no significant difference in response rates (24% versus 30%), but the combination induced a significantly higher rate of major constitutional and hematologic toxicities.[75] Similarly, a study of sequential concurrent therapy with interferon alpha 2B and etoposide (VP-16) revealed little likely benefit from the combination.[79] Most recently interferon alpha 2A or interferon alpha

TABLE 57-6. Responses to Interferon by Tumor Stage, Symptoms, or Prior Opportunistic Infections

	Responders/Total (%)	*Statistical Significance*
Stage		
I	2/11 (18)	NS
II	10/41 (24)	NS
III	1/4 (25)	NS
IV	6/19 (31)	NS
Subcategory		
A	15/41 (36)	$p < 0.01$
B	4/34 (12)	
Opportunistic Infection		
With	0/14 (0)	$p < 0.001$
Without	19/61 (31)	

Mitsuyasu RT, Groopman JE: Biology and therapy of Kaposi's sarcoma. Semin Oncol 11:53, 1984.

N1 has been combined with azidothymidine, a recognized antiretroviral nucleoside derivative with activity in AIDS. The results of these studies are not yet sufficiently mature to determine benefit, although hematologic toxicity has been a formidable obstacle in most patients.

Analysis of response to interferon alpha by Krown and associates with respect to prognostic features of epidemic Kaposi's sarcoma suggests that there is no association between responsiveness and either tumor burden or the presence of gastrointestinal lesions.[71-74] Thus, contrary to the usual situation in oncology, tumor burden is not necessarily associated with poor response. The clinical parameters most clearly associated with a poor response to interferon include a history of opportunistic infection and the presence of B symptoms such as fever, night sweats, and weight loss.[73,78,80] Because this prognostic variable is so major in virtually all prior studies, patients with B symptoms or prior opportunistic infection are currently excluded from most studies of interferon. Such clinical variables are associated with certain immunologic parameters such as total lymphocyte count, absolute number of CD4-positive circulating lymphocytes, the CD4-CD8 lymphocyte ratio, delayed hypersensitivity, or lymphoproliferative responses to various stimuli. Furthermore, certain studies suggested that the presence of acid-labile alpha interferon in the circulation was associated with unresponsiveness to interferon therapy.[70] It is difficult to conclude from such analyses that interferon may be working through effects on a more intact immune system.

The lack of randomized, prospective, and placebo controlled studies makes it impossible to determine if interferon therapy, or any other therapy, improves quality of life or survival in AIDS-related Kaposi's sarcoma. It is likely that because of the progressive nature of the neoplasm and the desire of Kaposi's sarcoma patients for nonplacebo therapy that such randomized and placebo controlled trials will not be done in this disease.

Interferon gamma has also been explored for the therapy of epidemic Kaposi's sarcoma.[81,82] The rationale for this included the frequent occurrence of opportunistic infections that are handled in part by the monocyte–macrophage system and the known activating effects of interferon gamma on monocyte–macrophages. Initial studies of partially purified and highly purified recombinant interferon gamma in patients with epidemic Kaposi's sarcoma failed to demonstrate significant antitumor activity.

It is still controversial whether interferon suppresses HIV replication in vivo in patients with Kaposi's sarcoma. It has been difficult to accurately assess viral activity in patients. Nonetheless, preliminary studies have demonstrated that patients in complete remission on interferon alpha became virus culture negative; with subsequent discontinuation of treatment, cultures turned positive.[86] This, of course, could be related to factors other than interferon therapy that would be operative in these patients.

Chemotherapy clearly has a role in the therapy for epidemic Kaposi's sarcoma. As with evaluation of other treatment modalities, the lack of a uniform staging system and the difficulty in performing randomized prospective trials make it difficult to strongly support the comparative advantage of any one approach over another. The initial studies of chemotherapy for AIDS-related Kaposi's sarcoma utilized the prior experience in the management of Kaposi's sarcoma in Central Africans or in elderly European men with the classic form.[87-89] In classic Kaposi's sarcoma a fairly uniform response rate of 90% to 95% was observed with vinca alkaloids, particularly vinblastine. The duration of response generally lasted for less than 8 to 12 months, and no clear survival advantage had been identified. African trials using combination chemotherapy, particularly bleomycin, BCNU, vinca alkaloids, actinomycin D, and DTIC, confirmed the chemoresponsiveness of Kaposi's sarcoma occurring in an aggressive form in this population. Both single-agent and combination chemotherapy has been studied in AIDS-related Kaposi's sarcoma.[90-96] Again, drawing on the experience in the classic European and African forms, vinca drugs, as well as etoposide (VP-16), have been most extensively utilized. In addition, combination regimens with vinblastine or vincristine, bleomycin, and doxorubicin have been explored.

The most extensive studies have been done by Volberding and co-workers.[90,93,97] Using relatively low doses of vinblastine, 4 to 8 mg intravenously on a weekly basis, 38 patients were studied. The dose was titrated according to the leukocyte count, with the initial dose of 4 mg increased weekly to titrate the total leukocyte count above 2500 cells/μl. The median weekly dose was 6 mg and the median duration of therapy spanned 20 weeks. A complete response was observed in 1 of the 38 patients with 9 partial responses and stable disease in 19. The median time to response was 5 weeks and the median duration of response for all patients was 13 weeks. The regimen was well tolerated, with the major toxicity being leukopenia. The median nadir leukocyte count was 2600 cells/μl. There was no significant effect on hemoglobin or T-cell populations. Four patients had mild distal paresthesia but no severe neurologic toxicity. Thus, using these regimens, disease can be controlled in approximately one-third of patients and the tumor progression arrested in approximately one-half. Laubenstein used etoposide as a single-agent chemotherapy.[91] The response rate in this study was as high as 80% in patients receiving a dose of 150 mg/m^2 body surface intravenously 3 days every 4 weeks. In patients who did not have B symptoms the response rate to etoposide approached 90%. The drug was moderately well tolerated, although there was hematologic toxicity as well as significant alopecia.

In order to improve response duration as well as response rate, combination therapies have been developed. The group at San Francisco General Hospital has used vincristine and vinblastine in alternating cycles.[93] Twenty-four patients with epidemic Kaposi's sarcoma received vincristine, 2 mg intravenously, on alternate weeks with vinblastine, 0.1 mg/kg intravenously, on the subsequent week. The dosage of vinblastine was reduced for a leukocyte count below 3000/μl or platelet count below 50,000. Vincristine was withdrawn if muscle weakness or severe paresthesia developed. Of 21 evaluable patients, 1 (5%) achieved a complete response, while 8 (38%) had disease stabilization and 5 (24%) had disease progression. The median destination of response was 13 weeks. Two patients developed major opportunistic infections during the first month of treatment and a third was lost to follow-up. The major observed toxicity was neurologic, with muscle weakness detected in three patients and mild paresthesias (not requiring dose reduction) in six patients. Only two patients had episodes of severe granulocytopenia, none of which was complicated by fever. The platelet count and hemoglobin were well sustained. The investigators were able to administer 86% of the planned total vinblastine doses and 90% of the planned vincristine doses. These preliminary data suggested that this alternating vincristine–vinblastine regimen might reduce the toxicity of each drug without compromising overall efficacy.

Other combination regimens have been reported. Minor and Brayer reported results in 24 patients with a vinblastine and methotrexate combination regimen using leucovorin rescue.[94] A response rate of 77% was observed with three complete responses and four partial responses. Although no increase in opportunistic infections was observed, neutropenia and mucositis were common. The response duration, as in other studies, was relatively short, approximately 8 months. Glaspy and co-workers reported that vincristine and bleomycin, two nonmyelosuppressive agents with efficacy in epidemic Kaposi's sarcoma, yielded four minimal responses in eight evaluable patients.[95] Median time to response was 3 months from the start of therapy. Two patients developed fever possibly related to bleomycin and two others showed signs of peripheral neuropathy.

A study of Wernz and associates using bleomycin and vinblastine found the combination to be well tolerated and to produce a high response rate.[96] Thirty-one patients were treated with vinblastine at 4 mg/m^2 intravenously alternating weekly with bleomycin, 15 U/m^2 intravenously. Twenty-four partial responses (62%) were observed with disease stabilization in four patients and no response in two patients. During the study 15 patients developed a first opportunistic infection, and of these 10 patients developed *P. carinii* pneumonia.

The major concern about chemotherapy in AIDS-related epidemic Kaposi's sarcoma is whether cytotoxic treatment will further immunosuppress the patient. It is unclear at this time whether this occurs. It does appear that doxorubicin is one of the most effective single agents for Kaposi's sarcoma, and this is being explored alone and in combination with bleomycin and vincristine in a recently initiated cooperative group (ATEU) study. The indications for treatment with chemotherapy generally include rapidly progressive disease, morbidity associated with lymphedema of the extremities or face, and pulmonary involvement. Because of the goal of rapid diminution in bulk disease in such settings, patients are generally not candidates for interferon, since the median time to response is 8 to 12 weeks with that agent. Responses to chemotherapy may be seen within the first 2 to 3 weeks of treatment, particularly in regimens that use anthracyclines.

Consideration is also being given to the role of azidothymidine (Retrovir) in epidemic Kaposi's sarcoma. Azidothymidine has recently been demonstrated to have clinical efficacy in prolonging survival and reducing the incidence of recurrent opportunistic infections and/or neoplasms in AIDS patients' status post first episode of *P. carinii* pneumonia.[98,99] Used as a single agent, azidothymidine does not appear to have a major antineoplastic effect. For that reason it is being studied in combination with nonmyelosuppressive chemotherapy, such as bleomycin and vincristine. Finally, programs have been proposed to utilize recombinant granulocyte–macrophage colony-stimulating factor to attenuate the leukopenia seen in myelosuppressive chemotherapy of epidemic Kaposi's sarcoma.[100]

Finally, radiation therapy has a clear role in some patients with AIDS-associated Kaposi's sarcoma.[101] The neoplasm is radiosensitive, similar to classic and African Kaposi's sarcoma.[102,103] Because palliation is a major goal, and Kaposi's sarcoma is often associated with disfigurement of the AIDS patients, cosmesis can be achieved with this treatment modality. Indeed, the radiosensitivity of Kaposi's sarcoma is exquisite.[101,104,105] In classic Kaposi's sarcoma, treatment approaches have ranged from encompassing limited lesions with small treatment fields in a fractionated way over a long period of time to larger fields treated in a single fraction. In nearly all cases there was excellent control of local disease. Other radiation therapy approaches in Kaposi's sarcoma included extended-field radiation, hemibody treatment, and electron beam. The overall response rate approached 90% to 100% with dose-fractionated methods.

In epidemic Kaposi's sarcoma single doses of 800 cGy or the equivalent in fractionated doses can produce regression. Harris and Reed proposed fractionating therapy of foot, eye, or oral cavity lesions over 2 to 4 weeks to reduce morbidity, with single high-dose therapy used for lesions on the extremities.[101] These recommendations were based on a retrospective review of 32 AIDS patients treated at the University of California, San Francisco. A large cohort of 182 homosexual men with epidemic Kaposi's sarcoma seen at the New York University Medical Center had a subset of 15 patients who were selected for management with low to moderate doses of ionizing radiation.[104] Seven had had opportunistic infection in addition to their neoplasm. Patients were selected for primary management with radiation therapy if they had limited, Stage I disease (by Krigel classification) and if lesions were readily accommodated within a single radiation portal. Another indication for radiation therapy was amelioration of painful lesions or cosmetically or functionally disturbing lesions. Superficial lesions were treated with doses of 1800 to 3000 cGy, and field sizes range from 3.5×3.5 cm to 27.5×29.0 cm. The overall results were positive in that partial regression of all cutaneous lesions was achieved in 15 patients with nearly no morbidity. Nine patients demonstrated complete remission and three had regression of lesions that left little residual discoloration. Three patients had partial responses. Pain relief was complete or substantial in all cases.

A study from Memorial-Sloan Kettering Cancer Center utilized subtotal skin electron beam therapy.[105] Thirty-eight patients who had previously received chemotherapy or hormonal therapy were treated to localize fields for palliation. Twelve patients underwent radiotherapy of the oral cavity, while 5 received treatment to the orbit. Significant palliation was achieved for periorbital edema, bony metastases, and ulcerated nephrotic anal or rectal lesions. Treatment of mucocutaneous lesions had to be discontinued at relatively low doses because of significant mucositis or appearance of opportunistic infections. It has been the experience from this study and others that the mucosa of the oral pharynx tolerates radiation therapy poorly, possibly because lesions become colonized with *Candida albicans*.

High-dose hemibody radiation was used at the University of California, Los Angeles, in four patients with extensive Kaposi's sarcoma.[68] Each patient responded to 600 to 800 cGy of treatment with partial regression of lesions and minimal immunologic pulmonary toxicity.

It can be concluded from these studies that epidemic Kaposi's sarcoma is as radiosensitive as the classic form of the neoplasm. Radiation therapy forms an important component in the therapeutic armamentarium, specifically for palliation and reduction of morbidity of lesions.[106] Consideration should be given to radiation treatment of disfiguring lesions in the head and neck and obstructive lesions in the extremities or anus and rectum.

Patients with AIDS are predisposed to neoplasms other than Kaposi's sarcoma. Indeed, one would predict based on the increased incidence of certain cancers and in patients with inherited immunodeficiency disorders.

LYMPHOMA AND OTHER NEOPLASMS

Safai and co-workers have reported an interesting observation of second malignancies that occur in elderly men with classic Kaposi's sarcoma, frequently lymphoma.[107] Similarly, in renal transplant patients who subsequently developed Kaposi's sarcoma, B-cell lymphomas occurred in some cases after an average interval of 12 to 16 months.[108] It appears from these immunosuppressed patients that Kaposi's sarcoma and B-cell lymphoma are linked, probably not in terms of cause, but in terms of likelihood of development given in certain constellation of defects in immunity.

In 1984 it was noted that homosexual men at risk for AIDS had a high incidence of aggressive B-cell lymphoma.[109,110] Subsequently such lymphomas were recognized in other risk groups for AIDS, specifically intravenous drug addicts and hemophiliacs who had received factor VIII concentrates.[111,112] Currently, non-Hodgkin's lymphoma occurs in 5% to 10% of AIDS patients. It is generally pathologically an aggressive type, including B-cell neoplasms of small non-cleaved (Burkitt's or Burkitt's-like) cells or immunoblastic sarcoma. Although case reports of HIV-infected patients with low-grade B-cell lymphoma or B-cell acute lymphoblastic leukemia have been reported, these neoplasms may be coincidental and are not clearly related to the immunodeficiency.

A large multicenter study by Ziegler and co-workers of 90 male homosexuals with non-Hodgkin's lymphoma revealed that 42 (47%) had a prior diagnosis of AIDS, while 33 (37%) had AIDS-related complex.[109] Extranodal involvement was frequent, occurring in 80 (89%) patients, with 38 (42%) involving the CNS, 30 (33%) in the bone marrow, and 15 (17%) in the gastrointestinal tract. High-grade histology was noted in 56 cases (62%), intermediate-grade in 26 (29%), low-grade in 6 (7%), and 2 were unclassified.

B-cell lymphoma in the HIV-infected patient may present as hectic fevers, weight loss, malaise, or night sweats, or with neurologic symptoms. Frequently there is rapid growth of a lymph node or appearance of an extranodal mass. Occasionally the neurologic presentation of CNS lymphoma may be dramatic with seizure, but more often patients manifest dementia or frontal lobe signs.[113]

B-cell neoplasia arising in the setting of HIV infection provides an important opportunity to better understand mechanisms of oncogenesis. Considerable attention has focused on the role of the Epstein–Barr virus in AIDS-related lymphoma.[115,116] Previously the Epstein–Barr virus has been linked with African Burkitt's lymphoma and nasopharyngeal carcinoma.[117] It is a very frequent herpesvirus infection among risk groups for HIV, particularly homosexual men, intravenous drug addicts, and hemophiliacs. Because the Epstein–Barr virus can activate B cells in a polyclonal manner, it has been postulated that with sustained B-cell proliferation, an abnormal clone may arise, particularly if cell-mediated immunity is impaired. It is further hypothesized that normally T cells would limit proliferation of such Epstein–Barr virus–driven B cells. In the setting of T-cell impairment consequent to HIV infection, the abnormal clone of B cells is capable of unchecked proliferation and ultimately emerges as an aggressive lymphoma.[112] Chromosomal abnormalities have been noted in the majority of AIDS-related lymphomas.[115,116] Translocations involving chromosomes 8 and 14 or 8 and 22, with consequent translocation of the c-*myc* onocgene from the long arm of chromosome 8 to the region of the immunoglobulin gene for the heavy chain (on chromosome 14) or the lambda light chain (on chromosome 22), are frequent. The Epstein–Barr virus genome has been identified in the B-cell lymphoma DNA in patients with AIDS. Despite these intriguing circumstantial data, a direct role for the Epstein–Barr virus or the c-*myc* oncogene product, or both, in B-cell neoplasia is still not apparent. The molecular phenotype of the AIDS-related lymphoma with these chromosomal translocations and overexpression of the c-*myc* oncogene are similar to those seen in B-cell neoplasms not associated with AIDS.

The clinical behavior of AIDS-associated lymphoma is quite striking. Patients may have very rapid growth of the tumor, with tumor doubling times occasionally measured in days. Although Ziegler and co-workers reported a 53% complete remission regimen with cyclophosphamide, doxorubicin, vincristine, and prednisone with cycles of bleomycin, methotrexate, and/or radiation therapy in some patients, these responses were of very limited duration.[109] The prognosis for CNS lymphoma appears even worse than that for systemic lymphoma, with a mortality rate of between 98% and 100% over 12 to 18 months.[113] Gill and co-workers reported results of intensive-treatment high-dose cytosine arabinoside, high-dose methotrexate with leucovorin rescue, and high-dose cyclophosphamide with other agents.[118,119] This aggressive regimen was poorly tolerated, and nearly 80% of the patients developed opportunistic infections during treatment. These infections were fatal in many cases. Lymphoma was evident at autopsy in many patients despite this aggressive therapy. We have had similar results in 30 patients with B-cell lymphoma and AIDS seen at the New England Deaconess Hospital over the preceding 2 years. Only two patients have been in continuous complete remission for more than 12 months, one treated with COMLA and the second with M-BACO. The first patient had bone marrow involvement but no evident CNS lymphoma and was treated prophylactically with cranial irradiation and intrathecal methotrexate. The second patient did not receive CNS prophylaxis. The remaining 28 patients had relapse, frequently at the site of primary disease as well as within the CNS, despite M-BACO therapy. Opportunistic infections frequently complicated therapy, and prolonged pancytopenia was seen in nearly all patients, requiring adjustment of doses.

It would appear from the experience accrued to date that therapy for lymphoma in AIDS patients is difficult. Because of the severe immune compromise, as well as the generally poor tolerance of the bone marrow to cytotoxic chemotherapy, patients may die of opportunistic infections and/or bacterial sepsis during chemotherapy. The high incidence of CNS involvement and the poor response of CNS lymphoma to treatment further complicate the picture. CNS lymphoma is generally managed by corticosteroids such as dexamethasone and by radiation. Because the response duration is measured in several months, some patients elect not to be treated. Consideration is being given to palliative therapy with less intensive regimens for systemic lymphoma to see if the high mortality rate observed with aggressive combination chemotherapy can be reduced.

Hodgkin's disease has also been observed in homosexual men at risk for AIDS.[120–125] Because this neoplasm occurs in men of this age group, it was not clear that the incidence of Hodgkin's disease is increased in HIV-infected patients. A case report from Mitsuyasu and co-workers on the simultaneous occurrence of Hodgkin's disease and Kaposi's sarcoma in the same lymph node in a 31-year-old homosexual man with AIDS is of interest.[120] We also have observed Kaposi's sarcoma that developed several months after the diagnosis of untreated Hodgkin's disease in an HIV-infected patient. The pathology noted in these small series of HIV infection and Hodgkin's disease is generally nodular sclerosis or mixed cellularity. The neoplasm may have an unusual, indeed atypical, presentation or distribution with reports of primary bone marrow, skin, pulmonary, and brain involvement. Few data exist on optimal management, but it appears that, as with B-cell lymphoma, combination chemotherapy regimens frequently result in opportunistic infections. We have chosen to treat HIV-infected patients with Hodgkin's disease in a palliative manner with vinca alkaloids, cyclophosphamide, or low doses of doxorubicin, or a combination of these. Because the average survival for an AIDS patient who has had an opportunistic infection is about 12 to 14 months, it is difficult to justify aggressive chemotherapy for a secondary neoplasm such as Hodgkin's disease, particularly if such therapy may reduce an already short life span.

It is of interest that other secondary neoplasms, including squamous cell carcinoma of the head and neck, squamous cell of the oral cavity, and colacogenic and rectal carcinomas, have been noted among HIV-infected male homosexuals.[124,126,127] It is unclear if these are sporadic cases occurring among HIV-infected patients or whether they may occur at increased frequency. Both papilloma viruses and herpes simplex viruses have been implicated in the pathogenesis of such squamous cancers, and it is possible that these viruses have a greater malignant potential in the setting of cellular immunodeficiency.

REFERENCES

1. Krueger CRF, Malmgren RA, Berard CW: Malignant lymphomas and plasmacytosis in mice under prolonged immunosuppression and persistent antigenic stimulation. Transplantation 11:138, 1971
2. Kersey J, Spector B, Good RA: Immunodeficiency and cancer. Adv Cancer Res 18:211, 1973
3. Gatti RA, Good RA: Occurrence of malignancy in immunodeficiency diseases. Cancer 28:89, 1971
4. Waldmann TA, Strober W, Blaese RM: Immunodeficiency disease and malignancy: Various immunologic deficiencies of man and the role of immune processes in the control of malignant disease. Ann Intern Med 77:605, 1972
5. Kwan S-P, Kunkel L, Bruns G et al: Mapping of the X-linked agammaglobulinemia locus by use of restriction fragment-length polymorphism. J Clin Invest 77:649, 1986
6. Peacocke M, Siminovitch KA: Linkage of the Wiskott–Aldrich syndrome with polymorphic DNA sequences from the human X chromosome. Proc Natl Acad Sci USA 84:3430, 1987
7. Skare JC, Milunsky A, Byron KS et al: Mapping the X-linked lymphoproliferative syndrome. Proc Natl Acad Sci USA 84:2015, 1987
8. Hecht F, Hecht BKM: Chromosome changes connect immunodeficiency and cancer in ataxia-telangiectasia. Am J Pediatr Hematol Oncol 9:185, 1987
9. Penn I: Occurrence of cancer in immune deficiencies. Cancer 34:858, 1974
10. Penn I: Second malignant neoplasma associated with immunosuppressive medications. Cancer 37:1024, 1976
11. Penn I: Kaposi's sarcoma in organ transplant recipients. Transplantation 27:8, 1979
12. Broder S, Waldmann TA: The suppressor-cell network in cancer. N Engl J Med 299:1281, 1978
13. Spector BD, Perry GS III, Kersey JH: Genetically determined immunodeficiency diseases (GDID) and malignancy: Report from The Immunodeficiency-Cancer Registry. Clin Immunol Immunopathol 11:12, 1978
14. Filipovich AH, Heinitz, KJ, Robison LL et al: The Immunodeficiency Cancer Registry: A research resource. Am J Pediatr Hematol Oncol 9:183, 1987
15. Boder E: Ataxia-telangiectasia: Some historic, clinical and pathologic observations. In Bergsma D, Good RA, Finstad J et al (eds): Immunodeficiency in Man and Animals, p 255. Sunderland, Mass, Sinauer, 1975
16. Boder E, Sedgwick RP: Ataxia-telangiectasia. A familial syndrome of progressive cerebellar ataxia, oculocutaneous telangiectasia and frequent pulmonary infection. Pediatrics 21:526, 1958
17. McFarlin DE, Strober W, Waldmann TA: Ataxia telangiectasia. Medicine (Baltimore) 51:281, 1972
18. Bar RS, Levis WR, Rechler MM et al: Extreme insulin resistance in ataxia telangiectasia; defect in affinity of insulin receptors. N Engl J Med 298:1164, 1978
19. Waldmann TA, McIntire KR: Serum-alpha-fetoprotein levels in patients with ataxia-telangiectasia. Lancet 2:1112, 1972
20. Buckley RH: Clinical and immunologic features of selective IgA deficiency. In Bergsma D, Good RA, Finstad J et al (eds): Immunodeficiency in Man and Animals, p 133. Sunderland, Mass, Sinauer, 1975
21. Polmar SH, Waldmann TA, Balestra JT et al: Immunoglobulin E in immunologic deficiency diseases: I. Relation of IgE and IgA to respiratory tract disease in isolated IgE deficiency, IgA deficiency and ataxia telangiectasia. J Clin Invest 51:326, 1972
22. Biggar WD, Good RA: Immunodeficiency in ataxia-telangiectasia. In Bergsma D, Good RA, Finstad J et al (eds): Immunodeficiency in Man and Animals, p 171. Sunderland, Mass, Sinauer, 1975
23. Kraemer KH: Progressive degenerative diseases associated with defective DNA repair: Xeroderma pigmentosum and ataxia telangiectasia. In Nichols WW, Murphy DG (eds): DNA Repair Processes, p 37. Miami, Symposia Specialists, 1977
24. Taylor AMR, Harnden DG, Arlett CF et al: Ataxia telangiectasia: A human mutation with abnormal radiation sensitivity. Nature 258:427, 1975
25. Webb I, Harnden DG, Harding M: The chromosome analysis and susceptibility to transformation by Simian virus 40 of fibroblasts from ataxia-telangiectasia. Cancer Res 37:997, 1977
26. Morrell D, Cromarie E, Swift M: Mortality and cancer incidence in 263 patients with ataxia telangiectasia. J Natl Cancer Inst 77:89, 1986
27. Wiskott A: A familiarer, angeoborener morbus werlhofli? Monatsschr Kinderheilkd 68:212, 1937
28. Aldrich RA, Steinberg AG, Campbell DC: Pedigree demonstrating a sex-linked recessive condition characterized by draining ears, eczematoid dermatitis and blood diarrhea. Pediatrics 13:133, 1954
29. Blaese RM, Strober W, Brown RS et al: The Wiskott–Aldrich syndrome: A disorder with a possible defect in antigen processing or recognition. Lancet 1:1056, 1968
30. Poplack DG, Bonnard GD, Holiman BJ et al: Monocyte-mediated antibody-dependent cellular cytotoxicity: A clinical test of monocyte function. Blood 48:809, 1976
31. Bruce RM, Blaese RM: Monoclonal gammopathy in the Wiskott–Aldrich syndrome. J Pediatr 85:204, 1974
32. Faraci RP, Hoffstrand HJ, Witebsky FG et al: Malignant lymphoma of the jejunum in a patient with Wiskott–Aldrich syndrome. Surgical treatment. Arch Surg 110:218, 1975
33. Heidelberger KP, LeGolvan DP: Wiskott–Aldrich syndrome and cerebral neoplasia: Report of a case with localized reticulum cell sarcoma. Cancer 33:280, 1974
34. Parkman R, Rappeport J, Geha R et al: Complete correction of the Wiskott–Aldrich syndrome by allogeneic bone-marrow transplantation. N Engl J Med 298:921, 1978
35. Kapoor N, Kirkpatrick D, Blaese RM et al: Reconstitution of normal megakaryocytopoiesis and immunologic functions in Wiskott–Aldrich syndrome by marrow transplantation following myeloablation and immunosuppression with busulfan and cyclophosphamide. Blood 57:692, 1981
36. Perry GS, Spector BD, Schuman LM et al: The Wiskott–Aldrich syndrome in the United States and Canada. J Pediatr 97:72, 1980

37. Cotelingam JD, Witebsky FG, Hsu SM et al: Malignant lymphoma in patients with the Wiskott–Aldrich syndrome. Cancer Invest 3:515, 1985
38. Provisor AJ, Iacuone JJ, Chilcote RR et al: Acquired agammaglobulinemia after a life-threatening illness with clinical and laboratory features of infectious mononucleosis in three related male children. N Engl J Med 293:62, 1975
39. Purtilo DT: Opportunistic non-Hodgkin's lymphoma in X-linked recessive immunodeficiency and lymphoproliferative syndrome. Semin Oncol 4:335, 1977
40. Purtilo DT, Sakamoto K, Barnabei V et al: Epstein–Barr virus–induced diseases in boys with the X-linked lymphoproliferative syndrome (XLP). Am J Med 73:49, 1982
41. Page AR, Hansen AE, Good RA: Occurrence of leukemia and lymphoma in patients with agammaglobulinemia. Blood 21:197, 1963
42. Waldmann TA, Broder S: Suppressor cells in the regulation of the immune response. Prog Clin Immunol 3:155, 1977
43. Kinlen LJ, Webster ADB, Bird AG et al: Prospective study of cancer in patients with hypogammaglobulinemia. Lancet 1:263, 1985
44. Gelmann E, Anderson I, Jaffe E et al: Chemotherapy for lymphoma in a patient with common variable immunodeficiency: Case report, literature review, and recommendations for chemotherapy in immunodeficient patients. Arch Intern Med 142:90, 1982
45. Centers for Disease Control: Kaposi's sarcoma and *Pneumocystis* pneumonia among homosexual men—New York City and California. MMWR 30:305, 1981
46. Kaposi M: Idiopathisches multiples Pigmentsarkom der Haut. Arch Dermatol Syph 4:265, 1872
47. Safai B, Good RA: Kaposi's sarcoma: A review and recent developments. Clin Bull 10:62, 1980
48. Smith EC, Elmes BGT: Malignant disease in the natives of Nigeria. An analysis of 500 tumors. Ann Trop Med Parasitol 28:641, 1934
49. Taylor JF, Templeton AC, Vogel CL et al: Kaposi's sarcoma in Uganda: A clinico-pathological study. Int J Cancer 8:122, 1971
50. Penn I: Kaposi's sarcoma in organ transplant recipients: Report of 20 cases. Transplantation 27:8, 1979
51. Harwood AR, Osoba D, Hofstader SL et al: Kaposi's sarcoma in recipients of renal transplants. Am J Med 67:759, 1979
52. Safai B: Kaposi's sarcoma: A review of classical and epidemic forms. Ann NY Acad Sci 437:373, 1984
53. Safai B, Mike G, Giraldo G et al: Association of Kaposi's sarcoma with second primary malignancies: Possible etiopathogenic implications. Cancer 45:1472, 1980
54. Friedman–Kien AE: Disseminated Kaposi's sarcoma syndrome in young homosexual men. J Am Acad Dermatol 5:468, 1981
55. Urmacher C, Myskowski P, Ochoa M et al: Outbreak of Kaposi's sarcoma in young homosexual men. Am J Med 72:569, 1982
56. Haverkos HW, Curran JW: The current outbreak of Kaposi's sarcoma and opportunistic infections. CA 32:330, 1982
57. Curran JW, Morgan WM, Hardy AM et al: The epidemiology of AIDS: Current status and future prospects. Science 229:1352, 1985
58. Pollack M, Safai B, Dupont B: HLA-DR5 and DR2 are susceptibility factors for acquired immunodeficiency syndrome with Kaposi's sarcoma in different ethnic populations. Disease Markers 1:135, 1983
59. Safai B: Pathophysiology and epidemiology of epidemic Kaposi's sarcoma. Semin Oncol 14(suppl):7, 1987
60. Giraldo G, Beth E, Lourilsky F et al: Antibody patterns to herpes viruses in Kaposi's sarcoma: Serological association of European Kaposi's sarcoma with cytomegalovirus. Int J Cancer 15:839, 1975
61. Giraldo G, Beth E, Huang E: Kaposi's sarcoma and its relationship to cytomegalovirus. III. CMV, DNA and CMV early antigens in Kaposi's sarcoma. Am J Cancer 26:23, 1980
62. Groopman JE: Biology and therapy of epidemic Kaposi's sarcoma. Cancer 59:633, 1987
63. Bovi PD, Basilico C: Isolation of a rearranged human transforming gene following transfection of Kaposi's sarcoma DNA. Proc Nat Acad Sci USA 84:5660, 1987
64. Bovi PD, Curatola AM, Kern FG et al: An oncogene isolated by transfection of Kaposi's sarcoma DNA encodes a growth factor that is a member of the FGF family. Cell 50:729, 1987
65. Dorfman RF: Kaposi's sarcoma: The contribution of enzyme histochemistry to the identification of cell types. Acta Un Int Cancer 18:464, 1962
66. Nadji MD, Morales AR, Aiegler–Weissman J et al: Kaposi's sarcoma: Immunologic evidence for an endothelial origin. Arch Pathol Lab Med 105:274, 1981
67. Guarda LG, Silva EG, Ordonez NG et al: Factor VIII in Kaposi's sarcoma. Am J Clin Pathol 76:197, 1981
68. Krigel RL, Laubenstein LJ, Muggia FM: Kaposi's sarcoma: A new staging classification. Cancer Treat Rep 67:531, 1983
69. Mitsuyasu RT, Groopman JE: Biology and therapy of Kaposi's sarcoma. Semin Oncol 11:53, 1984
70. Mitsuyasu RT, Taylor MG, Glaspy J et al: Heterogeneity of epidemic Kaposi's sarcoma. Cancer 57:1657, 1986
71. Vadhan–Raj S, Wong G, Gnecco C et al: Immunological variables as predictors of prognosis in patients with Kaposi's sarcoma and the acquired immunodeficiency syndrome. Cancer Res 46:417, 1986
72. Krown SE, Real FX, Cunningham–Rundles S et al: Preliminary observations on the effect of recombinant leukocyte A interferon in homosexual men with Kaposi's sarcoma. N Engl J Med 308:1071, 1983
73. Krown SE, Real FX, Krim M et al: Recombinant leukocyte A interferon in Kaposi's sarcoma. Ann NY Acad Sci 437:431, 1984
74. Real FX, Oettgen HF, Krown SE: Kaposi's sarcoma and the acquired immunodeficiency syndrome: Treatment with high and low doses of recombinant leukocyte A interferon. J Clin Oncol 4:544, 1986
75. Krown SE, Real FX, Gold JWM et al: Therapeutic trials of interferon alfa-2a (IFN-a2a) in AIDS-related Kaposi's sarcoma (KS/AIDS). Proceedings, International Conference on AIDS, Paris, France, June 23–25, 1986 (abstrS14F). Communication 88:35, 1986
76. Krown SE, Gold JWM, Real FX et al: Interferon alfa-2a ± vinblastine (VLB) in AIDS-associated Kaposi's sarcoma (KS/AIDS): Therapeutic activity, toxicity and effects on HTLV-III/LAV viremia (abstr). J Interferon Res 6(suppl 1):3, 1986
77. Groopman JE, Gottlieb MS, Goodman J et al: Recombinant alpha-2 interferon therapy for Kaposi's sarcoma associated with acquired immunodeficiency syndrome. Ann Intern Med 100:671, 1984
78. Volberding PA, Valera R, Rothman J et al: Alpha interferon therapy of Kaposi's sarcoma in AIDS. Ann NY Acad Sci 437:439, 1984
79. Mitsuyasu RT, Volberding P, Jacobs A et al: High-dose alpha-2 recombinant interferon in the therapy of epidemic Kaposi's sarcoma (KS) in acquired immunodeficiency (AIDS) (abstr). Proc Am Soc Clin Oncol 3:51, 1984
80. Lonberg M, Odajnyk C, Krigel R et al: Sequential and simultaneous alpha 2 interferon (IFN) and VP16 in epidemic Kaposi's sarcoma (abstr). Proc Am Soc Clin Oncol 4:2, 1985
81. Gelmann EP, Preble OT, Steis R et al: Human lymphoblastoid interferon treatment of Kaposi's sarcoma in the acquired immune deficiency syndrome. Clinical response and prognostic parameters. Am J Med 78:737, 1985
82. Rios A, Mansell PWA, Newell GA et al: Treatment of acquired immunodeficiency syndrome-related Kaposi's sarcoma with lymphoblastoid interferon. J Clin Oncol 3:506, 1985
83. Fischl M, Lucas S, Gorowski E et al: Interferon alfa-N1 Wellferon (WFN) in Kaposi's sarcoma: Single agent or combination with vinblastine (VLB) (abstr). J Interferon Res 6(suppl 1):4, 1986
84. Ho DD, Hartshorn KL, Rota TR et al: Recombinant human interferon alfa-A suppresses HTLV-III replication in vitro. Lancet 1:602, 1985
85. Odajnyk C, Laubenstein L, Friedman–Kien A et al: Therapeutic trial of human gamma-interferon (IFN) in patients with epidemic Kaposi's sarcoma (EKS) (abstr). Proc Am Soc Clin Oncol 3:61, 1984
86. Vadhan–Raj S, Al-Katib A, Pelus L et al: Phase I trial of recombinant interferon gamma in cancer patients. J Clin Oncol 4:137, 1986
87. Krown SE: Therapeutic trials of interferon alfa-2a (IFN-a2a) in AIDS-related Kaposi's sarcoma (KS/AIDS). Presented at the Second International Conference on AIDS. Paris, France, June 24, 1986
88. Vogel CL, Clements D, Wanume AK et al: Phase II clinical trials of 1, BIS (2-chlorethyl-1-nitrosurea), BCNU, (NSC 4099621) and bleomycin (NSC 125066) in Kaposi's sarcoma. Cancer Chemother Rep 57:325, 1973
89. Olweny CLM, Masaba JP, Sikyewunda W et al: Treatment of Kaposi's sarcoma with IRCF (NSC 129943). Cancer Chemother Rep 60:111, 1976
90. Vogel CL, Templeton CJ, Templeton AC et al: Treatment of Kaposi's sarcoma with actinomycin-D and cyclophosphamide. Results of a randomized clinical trial. Int J Cancer 8:136, 1971
91. Volberding PA, Abrams DI, Conant M et al: Vinblastine therapy for Kaposi's sarcoma in the acquired immunodeficiency syndrome. Ann Intern Med 103:335, 1985
92. Laubenstein L: Post-graduate course on epidemic Kaposi's sarcoma and opportunistic infections in homosexual men—NYU Medical Center, March 1983. New York, Masson, 1984
93. Krigel RL: The natural history and treatment of epidemic Kaposi's sarcoma. Ann NY Acad Sci 437:447, 1984
94. Kaplan L, Abrams D, Volberding P: Treatment of Kaposi's sarcoma in acquired immunodeficiency syndrome with an alternating vincristine-vinblastine regimen. Cancer Treat Rep 70:1121, 1986
95. Minor DR, Brayer T: Velban and methotrexate (MTX) combination chemotherapy for epidemic Kaposi's sarcoma (abstr). Proc Am Soc Clin Oncol 5:1, 1986
96. Glaspy J, Miles S, McCarthy S et al: Treatment of advanced stage Kaposi's sarcoma with vincristine and bleomycin (abstr). Proc Am Soc Clin Oncol 5:3, 1986
97. Wernz J, Laubenstein L, Hymes K et al: Chemotherapy and assessment of response in epidemic Kaposi's sarcoma (EKS) with bleomycin (B)/Velban (V) (abstr). Proc Am Soc Clin Oncol 5:4, 1986
98. Volberding P: The role of chemotherapy for epidemic Kaposi's sarcoma. Semin Oncol 14:23, 1987
99. Mitsuya H, Broder S: Strategies for antiviral therapy in AIDS. Nature 325:773, 1987
100. Fischl MA, Richman DD, Grieco MH et al: The efficacy of azidothymidine (AZT) in the treatment of patients with AIDS and AIDS-related complex: A double-blind placebo-controlled trial. N Engl J Med 317:185, 1987
101. Groopman JE, Mitsuyasu RT, DeLeo MJ et al: Effect of recombinant human granulocyte-macrophage colony-stimulating factor on myelopoiesis in the acquired immunodeficiency syndrome. N Engl J Med 317:593, 1987
102. Harris JW, Reed TA: Kaposi's sarcoma in AIDS: The role of radiation therapy. Front Radiat Ther Oncol 19:126, 1985
103. Holecek MJ, Harwood AR: Radiotherapy of Kaposi's sarcoma. Cancer 41:1733, 1978
104. Nisce LZ, Safai B, Poussin–Rosillo H: Once weekly total and subtotal skin electron beam therapy for Kaposi's sarcoma. Cancer 47:640, 1981
105. Cooper JS, Fried PR, Laubenstein LJ: Initial observations of the effect of radiotherapy on epidemic Kaposi's sarcoma. JAMA 252:934, 1984
106. Nisce LZ, Safai B: Radiation therapy of Kaposi's sarcoma in AIDS. Front Radiat Ther Oncol 19:133, 1985

107. Hill DR: The role of radiotherapy for epidemic Kaposi's sarcoma. Semin Oncol 14:19, 1987
108. Safai B, Mike V, Giraldo B et al: Association of Kaposi's sarcoma with second malignancies, possible etiopathogenic mechanisms. Cancer 45:1472, 1980
109. Penn I: Kaposi's sarcoma in immunosuppressed patients. J Clin Lab Immunol 12:1, 1983
110. Ziegler JL, Beckstead JA, Volberding PA et al: Non-Hodgkin's lymphoma in 90 homosexual men. N Engl J Med 311:565, 1984
111. Levine AM, Meyer PR, Begandy MK et al: Development of B-cell lymphoma in homosexual men. Ann Intern Med 100:7, 1984
112. Gill PS, Meyer PR, Pavlova Z et al: B-cell ALL in adults: Clinical morphologic and immunologic findings. J Clin Oncol 4:737, 1986
113. Fauci AS, Macher AM, Longo DL et al: Acquired immunodeficiency syndrome: Epidemiologic, clinical, immunologic, and therapeutic considerations. Ann Intern Med 100:92, 1984
114. Gill PS, Levine AM, Meyer PR et al: Primary central nervous system lymphoma in homosexual men. Clinical, immunologic and pathologic features. Am J Med 78:742, 1985
115. Kalter SP, Riggs SA, Cabanillas F et al: Aggressive non-Hodgkin's lymphoma in immunocompromised homosexual males. Blood 66:655, 1985
116. Groopman JE, Sullivan JL, Mulder C et al: Pathogenesis of B cell lymphoma in a patient with AIDS. Blood 67:612, 1986
117. Chaganti RSK, Jhanwar SC, Koziner B et al: Specific translocations characterize Burkitt's-like lymphoma of homosexual men with the acquired immunodeficiency syndrome. Blood 61:1265, 1983
118. Andiman W, Gradoville L, Heston L et al: Use of cloned probes to detect Epstein-Barr viral DNA in tissues of patients with neoplastic and lymphoproliferative diseases. J Infect Dis 148:967, 1983
119. Gill PS, Rarick M, Deyton L et al: Malignant non-Hodgkin's lymphoma in AIDS: Results of prospective treatment trials (abstr). Blood 68:126a, 1986
120. Gill PS, Levine AM, Krailo M et al: AIDS-related malignant lymphoma: Results of prospective treatment trials. J Clin Oncol (in press)
121. Mitsuyasu RT, Colman MF, Sun NCJ: Simultaneous occurrence of Hodgkin's disease and Kaposi's sarcoma in a patient with the acquired immune deficiency syndrome. Am J Med 80:954, 1986
122. Dancis A, Odajnyk C, Kritgel RL et al: Association of Hodgkin's and non-Hodgkin's lymphomas with the acquired immunodeficiency syndrome (AIDS) (abstr C-236). Proc Am Soc Clin Oncol 3:61, 1984
123. Robert NJ, Schneiderman H: Hodgkin's disease and the acquired immunodeficiency syndrome. Ann Intern Med 101:142, 1984
124. Schoeppel SL, Hoppe RT, Dorfman RF et al: AIDS and Hodgkin's disease. Front Radiat Ther Oncol 19:66, 1985
125. Groopman JE, Mayer K, Zipoli T et al: Unusual neoplasms associated with HTLV-III infection (abstr 14). Proc Am Soc Clin Oncol 5:4, 1986
126. Schoeppel SL, Hoppe RT, Abrams DI et al: Hodgkin's disease (HD) in homosexual men: The San Francisco Bay Area experience (abstr 9). Proc Am Soc Clin Oncol 5:3, 1986
127. Conant MA, Volberding PA, Fletcher V et al: Squamous cell carcinoma in sexual partner of Kaposi's sarcoma patients. Lancet 1:286, 1982
128. Croxson T, Chabon AB, Rorat E et al: Intraepithelial carcinoma of the anus in homosexual men. Dis Colon Rectum 27:325, 1984

CHAPTER 58 *Oncologic Emergencies*

SECTION 1

JOACHIM YAHALOM

Superior Vena Cava Syndrome

Superior vena cava syndrome (SVCS) is the clinical expression of obstruction to the blood flow through the superior vena cava (SVC). Characteristic symptoms and signs may develop quickly or gradually when this thin-walled vessel is compressed, invaded, or thrombosed by processes in the superior mediastinum. The first pathologic description of SVC obstruction appeared in 1757, in a patient with syphilitic aortic aneurysm.[1] In 1954, Schechter [2] reviewed 274 well-documented cases of SVCS reported in the literature until that time; 40% of them were due to syphilitic aneurysms or tuberculous mediastinitis. These entities have since virtually disappeared and, currently, cancer of the lung is the underlying process in approximately 70% of the patients with SVCS.

ANATOMY AND PATHOPHYSIOLOGY

The SVC is the major vessel for drainage of venous blood from the head, neck, upper extremities, and upper thorax. It is located in the middle mediastinum and is surrounded by relatively rigid structures such as the sternum, trachea, right bronchus, aorta, pulmonary artery, and the perihilar and paratracheal lymph nodes. The SVC extends from the junction of the right and left innominate veins to the right atrium, for a distance of 6 to 8 cm. The distal 2 cm of the SVC is within the pericardial sac with a point of relative fixation of the vena cava at the pericardial reflection. The azygos vein, the main auxiliary vessel, enters the SVC posteriorly, just above the pericardial reflection. The SVC maintains blood at a low pressure. It is large, but thin-walled, compliant, and easily compressible. Therefore, it is vulnerable to any space-occupying process in its vicinity. The SVC is completely encircled by chains of lymph nodes that drain all the structures of the right thoracic cavity and the lower part of the left thorax. The auxiliary azygos vein is also threatened by enlargement of paratracheal nodes. Other critical structures in the mediastinum, such as the main bronchi, esophagus, and the spinal cord, may be involved by the same process that led to obstruction of the SVC.[3-5]

When the SVC is fully or partially obstructed, an extensive venous collateral circulation may develop. The azygos venous system is the most important alternative pathway. Carlson[6] found that dogs could not survive sudden ligation of the SVC below the level of the azygos vein, but they tolerated well ligation of the SVC above it. He could, however, successfully obstruct the SVC and the azygos vein in operations performed in two stages presumably by allowing time for collaterals to form . In addition to the azygos venous system, other collateral systems are the internal mammary veins, lateral thoracic veins, paraspinous veins, and the esophageal venous network. The subcutaneous veins are important pathways, and their engorgement in the neck and thorax is a typical physical finding in SVCS. In spite of these collateral pathways, venous pressure is almost always elevated in the upper compartment when there is obstruction of the SVC. Venous pressures have been recorded as high as 200–500 cm H_2O in severe SVCS.[7]

TABLE 58-1. SVCS: Common Symptoms and Physical Findings

Symptoms	%	*Physical Findings*	%
Dyspnea	63	Venous distension of neck	66
Facial swelling/head fullness	50	Venous distension of chest wall	54
Cough	24	Facial edema	46
Arm swelling	18	Cyanosis	20
Chest pain	15	Plethora of face	19
Dysphagia	9	Edema of arms	14

Analysis based on data from 370 patients from Refs. 8–10.

CLINICAL PICTURE

The syndrome usually has an insidious onset and progresses to develop typical symptoms and signs. Review of the data from three recent series[8–10] (Table 58-1), shows dyspnea to be the most common symptom. Dyspnea was present in 63% of the patients with SVCS. A sensation of fullness in the head and facial swelling was reported by 50% of the patients. Other complaints were cough (24%), arm swelling (18%), chest pain (15%), and dysphagia (9%). The characteristic physical findings were venous distension of the neck (66%) and chest wall (54%), facial edema (46%), plethora (19%), and cyanosis (19%). These symptoms and signs may be aggravated by bending forward, stooping, or by lying down.

ETIOLOGY

Malignant disease is the most common cause of SVCS. The percentage of patients in different series with a confirmed diagnosis of malignancy varies from 78% to 86%[3,9,10] (Table 58-2). Lung cancer was diagnosed in 68% of 352 patients analyzed in these series.[3,9,10] Armstrong and Perez[8] did a retrospective review of 4100 cases treated for bronchogenic carcinoma between 1965 and 1984, and identified 99 patients (2.4%) with SVCS. Salsali[11] observed SVCS in 4.2% of 4960 patients with lung cancer; 80% of the tumors inducing SVCS were of the right lung. Small-cell lung cancer is the most common histologic subtype (Table 58-3), and it was found in 41% of the patients who had lung cancer and SVCS. Among 225 consecutive patients with small-cell cancer, 26 (11.5%) had SVCS when the malignancy was diagnosed.[12] The second most common histologic subtype is squamous cell carcinoma, found in 27% of lung cancer patients with SVCS.

Lymphoma involving the mediastinum was the cause of SVCS in 6% of the patients reported in the series (see Table 58-2). Armstrong and Perez[8] found SVCS in 1.9% of 952 lymphoma patients. Perez-Soler[13] identified 36 cases (4%) of SVCS among 915 patients with non-Hodgkin's lymphoma treated in M. D. Anderson Hospital. Twenty-three patients (64%) had diffuse large-cell lymphoma, 12 (33%) had lymphoblastic lymphoma, and one patient had follicular large-cell lymphoma. Of their patients with diffuse large-cell lymphoma and lymphoblastic lymphoma, 7% and 21% had SVCS, respectively. Hodgkin's lymphoma commonly involves the mediastinum, but rarely causes SVCS. Other primary mediastinal malignancies found to cause SVCS are thymoma, and germ cell tumors.[3,9] Breast cancer is the most common metastatic disease to cause SVCS.[3,9]

Nonmalignant conditions causing SVCS are not as rare as previously reported.[8,14] When the data were collected from general hospitals, up to 22% of the cases had a noncancerous etiology for SVCS.[3,9] Parish[9] reported 19 patients with benign causes of SVCS, and Schraufnagel[3] included 16 such patients in his series. Fifty percent of the patients in both reports had a diagnosis of mediastinal fibrosis, which was probably due to histoplasmosis. Parish[9] reported six patients with thrombosis of SVC, and in five of these cases the thrombosis developed in the presence of central vein catheters or pacemakers. Sculier[15] reviewed 24 cases of central venous catheter-induced SVCS. Of these, 18 were caused by pacemaker catheters. LeVeen shunts, Swan-Ganz and hyperalimentation catheters were the other types of catheters involved. The increasing use of these devices for the delivery of chemotherapy agents or for hyperalimentation contributes an additional factor for the development of SVCS in the cancer patient.[16]

Obstruction of SVC in the pediatric age group is rare and has a different etiologic spectrum. The causing factors are

TABLE 58-2. SVCS: Primary Pathologic Diagnoses

	Bell[10] 159 Cases (%)	*Schraufnagel[3] 107 Cases (%)*	*Parish[9] 86 Cases (%)*	*Total 352 Cases (%)*
Histologic diagnosis				
Lung cancer	129 (81)	67 (63)	45 (52)	241 (68)
Lymphoma	3 (2)	10 (9)	8 (9)	21 (6)
Other malignancies (primary or metastatic)	4 (3)	14 (13)	14 (16)	32 (9)
Non-neoplastic	2 (1)	16 (15)	19 (22)	39 (11)
Undiagnosed	21 (13)			21 (6)

TABLE 58-3. SVCS: Lung Cancer Subtypes

Histology	*n*	*%*
Small cell	138	41
Squamous cell	91	27
Adenocarcinoma	46	14
Large cell	43	13
Unclassified	22	6
Total	340	100

Data from Refs. 3, 8–10.

mainly iatrogenic,[17] secondary to cardiovascular surgery for congenital heart disease, ventriculoatrial shunt for hydrocephalus, and SVC catheterization for parenteral nutrition. In a report of 175 children with SVCS, 70% were iatrogenic. Of the remaining 53 cases, 37 (70%) were caused by mediastinal tumors, 8 (15%) were caused by benign granuloma, and 4 (7.5%) by congenital anomalies of the cardiovascular system. Two-thirds of the tumors causing SVCS in childhood are non-Hodgkin's lymphomas.[17,18] Issa[18] reported that mediastinal fibrosis secondary to histoplasmosis caused SVCS in seven (5%) of the 150 patients reviewed.

DIAGNOSTIC PROCEDURES

The superior vena cava syndrome has long been considered to be a potentially life-threatening medical emergency.[4,14,19] It was common practice to immediately apply radiation therapy with initial high-dose fractions, sometimes, even before the histologic diagnosis of the primary lesion was established.[14,19,20] Diagnostic procedures, such as bronchoscopy, mediastinoscopy, thoracotomy, or supraclavicular lymph node biopsy, were often avoided because they were considered to be hazardous in the presence of SVCS.[4,14] The traditional therapeutic philosophy was recently challenged.[3,21,22] The reported clinical experience was reassessed, and both the safety and importance of diagnostic procedures were reevaluated. Multidrug chemotherapy, sometimes combined with radiation therapy, is potentially curative for small-cell carcinoma of the lung and non-Hodgkin's lymphoma even when presented as SVCS.[12,13] The current practice of using different modalities for different primary causes of SVCS makes the accurate histologic diagnosis of SVCS invaluable.

TABLE 58-4. SVCS: Findings on Chest Roentgenogram in 86 Patients

	Patients	
Finding	*n*	*%*
Superior mediastinal widening	55	64
Pleural effusion	22	26
Right hilar mass	10	12
Bilateral diffuse infiltrates	6	7
Cardiomegaly	5	6
Calcified paratracheal nodes	4	5
Mediastinal (anterior) mass	3	3
Normal	14	16

Parish JM et al: Etiologic considerations in SVCS. Mayo Clin Proc 56:407–413, 1981.

The clinical identification of SVCS is simple, as the symptoms and signs are typical and unmistakable. The chest film will show a mass in most patients. Only 16% of the patients studied by Parish had a normal chest film.[9] The most common radiographic abnormalities are superior mediastinal widening and pleural effusion (Table 58-4). A computed tomography (CT) scan will provide more detailed information about the SVC and its tributaries, as well as information about other critical structures such as the bronchi and the cord. This additional information is necessary because the involvement of these structures will require prompt action for relief of pressure. Moncada [23] outlined the advantages of combining a CT scan with CT digital phlebography in SVCS: [1] detailed resolution of the intrathoracic structures and musculoskeletal anatomy; [2] accurate identification of the site and extent of obstructing thrombus in the SVC, as well as of any external compression or invasion by mediastinal mass; [3] contrast opacification of the venous trunks and collateral circulation sufficient to make confident surgical decisions and to determine late graft patency; [4] accurate guidance for percutaneous biopsy techniques; [5] guide planning of radiation therapy to be sure that radiation ports fully encompass the disease; and [6] monitoring the effect of therapy.

The importance of contrast venography is controversial.[14,24] On the one hand, it provides important information to determine if the vena cava is completely obstructed or remains patent and extrinsically compressed.[24] Dyet and Moghissi[25] have shown by venography that 41% of patients with SVCS will have a patent SVC that is displaced or involved but not obstructed by a tumor. Another 19% will have SVC obstruction below the azygos vein, thus collateral venous decompression should be adequate. Venography is of great value when surgical bypass is considered for the obstructed vena cava.[26] Alternatively, Lokich [14] stated that venograms are relatively contraindicated because the interruption of the integrity of the vessel wall, in the presence of increased intraluminal pressures, may result in excessive bleeding from the puncture site. However, there is no recorded evidence for this complication. Although a venography would confirm the clinical diagnosis and outline the anatomy, priority should still be given to procedures that will help establish the histologic diagnosis. Radionuclide technetium-99m venography is an alternative, minimally invasive method of imaging the venous system.[27,28] Although images that are obtained by this method are not as well defined as those that are achieved with contrast venography, they still will demonstrate patency and flow patterns. Collateral circulation can be evaluated in a general manner and quantified to some degree by radionuclide venography.

In 58% of 107 patients reported by Shraufnagel,[3] the SVCS developed before the primary diagnosis was established. The diagnostic procedures that were employed in different studies to obtain the histologic diagnosis are summarized in Table 58-5. Sputum cytology established the diagnosis in almost half of the patients. Cytologic diagnosis is as accurate as tissue diagnosis in small-cell lung carci-

TABLE 58-5. SVCS: Positive Yield of Diagnostic Procedures

	No. of Procedures	*No. Positive*	*% Positive*
Sputum cytology	59	29	49
Thoracocentesis	11	8	73
Bone marrow biopsy	13	3	23
Lymph node biopsy	88	59	67
Bronchoscopy	111	57	51
Mediastinoscopy	39	30	77
Thoracotomy	48	47	98

Data from Refs. 3, 8, 29.

noma.[30] Bronchoscopy will supply the malignant cells for cytologic evaluation in most cases with a small-cell histologic diagnosis.[30] In the presence of pleural effusion, thoracocentesis established the diagnosis of malignancy in 73% of the patients. Biopsy of a supraclavicular node, especially when there was a suspicious palpatory finding, was rewarding in two-thirds of the reported attempts. Small-cell carcinoma of the lung and non-Hodgkin's lymphoma often involve the bone marrow. A biopsy of the bone marrow may provide diagnosis and stage in these patients. Mediastinoscopy has a high yield in obtaining the diagnosis. However, Painter[29] reported complications in five of the nine procedures attempted. In two patients, the procedure had to be terminated before completion. In three patients, complications occurred after the mediastinoscopy, but these complications were managed successfully, and the procedure was diagnostic in each case. Lewis and associates[32] reported their experience in performing cervical mediastinoscopies in 15 patients with SVCS. All mediastinoscopies were diagnostic, and no complications were observed. A thoracotomy is diagnostic when all other procedures have failed.

Ahmann[20] examined the traditional opinion that diagnostic procedures carry with them significant hazard, primarily for excessive bleeding.[14,19] He reviewed 843 invasive and semi-invasive diagnostic procedures and found only 10 reported complications, none of them fatal. Ahmann and others [3,22] demonstrated that there appears to be minimal evidence to suggest that diagnostic procedures such as venographies, thoracotomies, bronchoscopies, mediastinoscopies, and lymph node biopsies carry an excessive risk in patients with SVCS.

TREATMENT

The goals of treatment of SVCS are not only to relieve the symptoms, but also to attempt the cure of the primary malignant process. Small-cell carcinoma of the lung, non-Hodgkin's lymphoma, and germ cell tumors constitute nearly half of the malignant causes of SVCS. These disorders are potentially curable, even in the presence of SVCS. The treatment of SVCS should be selected according to the histologic disorder and stage of the primary process. The prognosis of patients with SVCS strongly correlates with the prognosis of the underlying disease.

SMALL-CELL LUNG CANCER

Combination chemotherapy alone or in conjunction with radiation therapy is considered to be the standard treatment for small-cell lung cancer. Dombernowsky[12] reported the results of the treatment of 26 patients with small-cell carcinoma of the lung presenting with SVCS. Of these 26 patients, 22 were initially treated with combination chemotherapy alone and, in all these patients, the resolution of the SVCS was prompt within a median of 7 days. Maddox[33] reported on 56 patients with small-cell lung cancer who presented with SVCS. Correction of SVCS was obtained in 64% (9 of 16) of patients treated with radiation alone, in 100% (23 of 23) of those given chemotherapy, and in 83% (5 of 6) of patients receiving combined therapy. The type of treatment did not substantially influence survival. Among 643 patients with small-cell lung cancer, Sculier[34] identified 55 patients (8.5%) with SVCS. One-half of the patients developed the manifestations of SVCS before the histologic diagnosis was established. In the rest of the patients, the syndrome developed after the pathologic diagnosis of small-cell lung cancer was made, but before a specific treatment was started. Symptomatic relief of SVCS was obtained in 35 of 48 (73%) patients initially treated with chemotherapy and in three of seven (43%) patients who were initially treated with radiation. Relief of SVCS occurred promptly within 7 to 10 days after initiation of therapy. Fourteen patients had a recurrence of SVCS after initial treatment. Improvement of recurrent SVCS was obtained in 8 of 12 patients treated with radiation, one of two patients treated with chemotherapy, and three of four patients treated with combined modality. Spiro[35] analyzed 37 patients with SVCS who, after initial chemotherapy for small-cell lung cancer, were randomized to receive chemotherapy alone or radiation therapy followed by more chemotherapy. In this study the addition of a radiation dose of 40 Gy to the mediastinum did not increase the protection from local recurrence or improve the survival. In several reports[12,34–36] the presence of SVCS was not found to be an adverse prognostic for patients with small-cell lung cancer. Three randomized trials[37–39] have shown that when compared with chemotherapy alone, there is an advantage for combining radiation therapy with chemotherapy in the treatment of limited-disease small-cell cancer of the lung. The optimal sequence of the two modalities, as well as the dose and fractionation of radiotherapy, have not yet been established. However, the use of combination chemotherapy as the initial modality, with subsequent rapid shrinkage of the tumor, may eliminate the necessity to irradiate a large volume of lung tissue. When chemotherapy is administered, the arm veins should be avoided. Veins of the lower extremities will provide an alternative simple venous access.

NON-HODGKIN'S LYMPHOMA

The most extensive experience of treating SVCS secondary to non-Hodgkin's lymphoma is reported from the M. D. Anderson Hospital.[13] Twenty-two patients with diffuse large-cell lymphoma and eight patients with lymphoblastic lymphoma could be evaluated for results of treatment. The patients were treated with chemotherapy alone, chemotherapy combined with radiation, and with radiotherapy alone. All patients achieved a complete relief of SVCS symptoms within 2 weeks of the onset of treatment with any one of the three choices of treatment. No single treatment modality appeared to be superior in achieving clinical improvement. The presence of either dysphagia, hoarseness, or stridor was a major adverse prognostic factor in patients with lymphoma presenting with SVCS. Eighteen (81%) of 22 patients with large-cell lymphoma achieved complete response. Relapse occurred in all six patients treated with radiation alone, in four of seven patients treated with chemotherapy alone, and in five of nine patients treated with chemotherapy and radiotherapy. Median survival was 21 months. All eight patients with lymphoblastic lymphoma achieved complete response. Six relapses occurred in this group and all were exclusively systemic in sites not initially involved. Median survival was 19 months. From these results, the authors concluded that SVCS secondary to lymphoma is rarely an emergency that requires treatment before a histologic diagnosis is made. They recommended that the choice of treatment will be based on the specific histologic diagnosis and that the patients should undergo, if possible, a complete staging workup before therapy. However, lymphangiography should be avoided to prevent embolization of contrast material that could result in respiratory failure. The authors advocated chemotherapy as the treatment of choice because it provides both local and systemic therapeutic activity. They suggested that local consolidation with radiation therapy may be beneficial in patients with large-cell lymphoma with mediastinal masses larger than 10 cm.

NONMALIGNANT ETIOLOGY

Patients with nonmalignant causes of SVCS differ significantly from patients with malignant disease. When the cause is not malignant the patients often have symptoms long before they seek medical advice, it takes more time to establish the diagnosis, and their survival is markedly longer.[3] Schraufnagel[3] reported that when the primary process is benign, the average survival was 9 years, compared with an average survival of 5 months for patients with lung cancer. Mahajan[40] reviewed the literature of benign SVCS and reported 16 new cases. Twelve of these 16 patients (75%) had a mediastinal granuloma that was attributed to histoplasmosis. Most patients had an insidious onset of SVCS and were relatively young. Ten patients who were available for a follow-up of 1 to 11 years were all doing well at the time of the report. It was suggested that the good prognosis of patients with benign SVCS caused by fibrosing mediastinitis does not leave a role for SVC bypass surgery.[40,41] However, Nieto and Doty[24] advocated surgery for SVCS caused by benign disorders, when the syndrome develops suddenly, progresses, or persists after 6 to 12 months of observation for possible collaterals' development.

CATHETER-INDUCED SVCS

In catheter-induced SVCS, the mechanism of obstruction is usually thrombosis. Streptokinase or urokinase may cause lysis of the thrombus early in its formation.[15,45] Heparin and oral anticoagulants may reduce the extent of the thrombus and prevent its progression. Removal of the catheter, when possible, is another option and should be combined with anticoagulation to avoid embolization. In patients for whom electrodes of a pacemaker have to be changed, the broken wire should be removed to prevent the risk of developing SVCS.[15]

RADIATION THERAPY

In patients with SVCS as a result of non–small-cell carcinoma of the lung, radiotherapy is the primary treatment. The likelihood of relieving the symptoms and signs of SVCS is high,[4,8] but the overall prognosis for these patients is poor.[3,8,21] In Armstrong's[8] series, the 1-year survival for these patients was 17% and the survival at 2 years declined to 2%. Radiotherapy has been advocated to be the standard treatment for most patients with SVCS.[14,19,20] It is employed as the initial treatment when a histologic diagnosis cannot be established, and the clinical status of the patient is deteriorating. However, recent reviews suggest that SVC obstruction alone will rarely represent an absolute emergency that will require treatment without a specific diagnosis.[3,21,22] The syndrome may be the earliest manifestation of invasive involvement of additional critical structures in the thorax (Table 58-6), such as the bronchi. Under such circumstances, prompt treatment with radiation may be required without any delay.

The fractionation schedule of radiation usually includes two to four large initial fractions of 300 cGy to 400 cGy, followed by conventional fractionation to a total dose of 3000 to 5000 cGy.[4,14,19] Patients treated with initial high-dose fractions showed a slightly faster symptomatic improvement in comparison with patients receiving conventional-dose radiation.[8] Improvement within 2 weeks or less was observed in 70% of those patients treated with initial high-dose fractions in contrast with 56% of patients receiving conventional-dose radiation therapy. This difference was not statistically significant. Serial venograms and autopsies[21] suggest that the symptomatic improvement achieved by radiotherapy is not always due to improvement of flow through the SVC, but it is probably also due to development of collaterals, once the pressure in the mediastinum is eased. The field of radiation in SVCS induced by lung cancer should encompass

TABLE 58-6. SVCS: Complications Recorded at Any Time During Course

Complication	No. of Patients* (%)
Esophagus	
Symptoms of dysphagia or esophageal dysfunction	26 (24)
Anatomical evidence of esophageal invasion	6 (6)
Trachea	
Displaced on examination or roentgenogram	7 (7)
Compressed or invaded by lesion	14 (13)
Vocal cord paralysis	
Unilateral	6 (6)
Bilateral	3 (3)
Pericardium	
Tamponade	3 (3)
Neoplastic invasion at necropsy	6 (6)

Data from Schraufnagel DE et al: Superior vena caval obstruction. Am J Med 70:1169–1174, 1981.

* Some patients may have had more than one complication.

the gross tumors with appropriate margins, the mediastinal, hilar, and supraclavicular lymph nodes. In Armstrong's series,[8] supraclavicular failures occurred in 8 of 91 (9%) patients receiving radiation therapy to the supraclavicular fossae, whereas two of six (33%) patients not receiving therapy to these lymph nodes failed at this site.

SURGERY

The experience with successful direct bypass graft for SVC obstruction is quite limited. It was recommended that autologous grafts of nearly the same size as the SVC will be used.[42] Doty[43] used a composite spiral graft, which was constructed from the patient's saphenous vein. He reported 6 years experience with this procedure in ten patients with benign and malignant obstruction of SVC, with all grafts patent and all patients relieved of symptoms of SVCS. Avashti[44] reported successful bypass of an obstructed SVC in four patients using a Dacron prothesis. The preferred bypass route is between the innominate or jugular vein on the left side and the right atrial appendage, using an end-to-end anastomosis.[24] In the patient with malignant etiology for SVCS, surgical intervention should be considered only after other therapeutic maneuvers with radiation and chemotherapy have been exhausted. Most patients with SVCS of benign etiology will have a long survival without surgical intervention.[40,41] However, when the process is rapidly progressing, or in cases such as retrosternal goiter or aortic aneurysm, surgical intervention may relieve the obstruction.

GENERAL MEASURES

Medical measures other than specific chemotherapy may be beneficial in temporarily relieving the symptoms of SVCS. Bed rest with the head elevated and oxygen administration will reduce the cardiac output and venous pressure. Diuretic therapy and reduced salt diet to reduce edema may have an immediate palliative effect. However, the risk of thrombosis enhanced by dehydration should not be ignored. Steroids are commonly used, but their effectiveness has never been properly evaluated. They may improve obstruction by decreasing a possible inflammatory reaction associated with tumor or with radiation. However, Green and Rubin[46] have demonstrated the lack of inflammatory reaction and edema following radiotherapy for experimental SVCS. Anticoagulants have been employed frequently in SVCS, but actual documentation of their effectiveness in a controlled fashion is lacking. Thrombolytic therapy with urokinase and streptokinase was found to be effective in SVCS induced by indwelling catheters.[45]

MANAGEMENT RECOMMENDATIONS

In patients without a clear cause of SVCS, an efficient diagnostic effort should be attempted before any specific treatment. Three deep-cough sputum specimens should be obtained for cytologic analysis. A positive cytologic evaluation provides reliable pathologic information, particularly in the diagnosis of small-cell lung carcinoma.[30] If pleural effusion is present, thoracocentesis should be performed, and the centrifuge-prepared specimen examined for the presence of malignant cells. When a suspicious lymph node is palpable, particularly in the supraclavicular area, a needle or an open biopsy should be the next diagnostic step. In the absence of positive sputum results, pleural effusion, or accessible suspicious lymph node analysis, a bronchoscopy should be performed and brushing, washing, and biopsy samples should be obtained for cytologic and histologic analysis. When these efforts do not provide the histologic diagnosis of the primary process, percutaneous transthoracic fine-needle biopsy under CT or fluoroscopic guidance is safe and highly rewarding.[47] In the rare patient for whom less-invasive procedures have failed to establish the diagnosis, the location of the suspicious lesion in the chest and the experience of the surgical team should determine whether mediastinoscopy or thoracotomy be performed.

During the diagnostic process the patient will benefit from bed rest with the head elevated and with oxygen administration. Some clinicians advocate the use of diuretics and steroids (*e.g.*, dexamethasone 6–10 mg p.o. or IV q6h) as a temporary palliative measure if the patient is uncomfortably symptomatic. Anticoagulation is of no proven benefit and may interfere with diagnostic procedures. Once the cause of SVCS has been established, treatment of the primary process should promptly follow. Combination chemotherapy with an appropriate regimen is the treatment of choice for small-cell lung cancer and non-Hodgkin's lymphoma. Radiation therapy of the lesion and adjacent lymph node-bearing areas may enhance control after initial response to chemotherapy. Non–small-cell lung cancer causing SVCS is best treated with radiation therapy. The incorporation of CT scan information into a carefully designed treatment plan may enable the administration of a total radiation dose above 5000 cGy, which may provide long-term local control for some patients. Most patients with nonmalignant causes for SVCS have an indolent course and a good prognosis. Surgery is indicated only when the process is rapidly progressing or caused by a retrosternal goiter or an aortic aneurysm. When

SVCS is induced by a catheter, the catheter should be removed if possible. Heparin should be administered during removal of the catheter to prevent embolization. In catheter-induced SVCS, streptokinase or urokinase are of value when used early in the thrombotic process.

The clinical course of SVCS will rarely represent an absolute emergency. In these situations the bronchus is likely to be obstructed by the same basic process, and radiation may have to be started immediately, even before the histologic diagnosis is established.

REFERENCES

1. Hunter W: The history of an aneurysm of the aorta, with some remarks on aneurysms in general. Med Obser Inq 1:323–357, 1757
2. Schechter MM: The superior vena cava syndrome. Am J Med Sci 227:46–56, 1954
3. Schraufnagel DE, Hill R, Leech JA, Pare JAP: Superior vena caval obstruction. Is it an emergency? Am J Med 70:1169–1174, 1981
4. Davenport D, Ferree C, Blake D, Raben M: Radiation therapy in the treatment of superior vena caval obstruction. Cancer 42:2600–2603, 1978
5. Rubin P, Hicks GL: Biassociation of superior vena caval obstruction and spinal-cord compression. NY State J Med 73:2176–2182, 1973
6. Carlson HA: Obstruction of the superior vena cava: An experimental study. Arch Surg 29:669–677, 1934
7. Roswit B, Kaplan G, Jacobson HG: The superior vena cava obstruction syndrome in bronchogenic carcinoma. Radiology 61:722–737, 1953
8. Armstrong BA, Perez CA, Simpson JR, Hederman MA: Role of irradiation in the management of superior vena cava syndrome. Int J Radiat Oncol Biol Phys 13:531–539, 1987
9. Parish JM, Marschke RF, Dines DE, Lee RE: Etiologic considerations in superior vena cava syndrome. Mayo Clin Proc 56:407–413, 1981
10. Bell DR, Woods RL, Levi JA: Superior vena caval obstruction: A 10-year experience. Med J Aust 145:566–568, 1986
11. Salsali M, Cliffton EE: Superior vena caval obstruction in carcinoma of lung. NY State J Med 69:2875–2880, 1969
12. Dombernowsky P, Hansen HH: Combination chemotherapy in the management of superior vena caval obstruction in small-cell anaplastic carcinoma of the lung. Acta Med Scand 204:513–516, 1978
13. Perez-Soler R, McLaughlin P, Velasquez WS et al: Clinical features and results of management of superior vena cava syndrome secondary to lymphoma. J Clin Oncol 2:260–266, 1984
14. Lokich JJ, Goodman R: Superior vena cava syndrome: Clinical management. JAMA 231:58–61, 1975
15. Sculier JP, Feld R: Superior vena cava obstruction syndrome: Recommendation for management. Cancer Treat Rev 12:209–218, 1985
16. Bertrand M, Presant CA, Klein L, Scott E: Iatrogenic superior vena cava syndrome. A new entity. Cancer 54:376–378, 1984
17. Janin Y, Becker J, Wise L et al: Superior vena cava syndrome in childhood and adolescence: A review of the literature and report of three cases. J Pediatr Surg 17:290–295, 1982
18. Issa PY, Brihi ER, Janin Y, Slim MS. Superior vena cava syndrome in childhood: Report of ten cases and review of the literature. Pediatrics 71:337–341, 1983
19. Perez CA, Presant CA, Van Amburg AL III: Management of superior vena cava syndrome. Semin Oncol 5:123–134, 1978
20. Scarantino C, Salazar OM, Rubin R et al: The optimum radiation schedule in the treatment of superior vena caval obstruction: Importance of ^{99m}Tc scintinangiograms. Int J Radiat Oncol Biol Phys 5:1987–1995, 1979
21. Ahmann FR: A reassessment of the clinical implications of the superior vena cava syndrome. J Clin Oncol 2:961–969, 1984
22. Shimm DS, Lugue GL, Tigsby LC: Evaluating the superior vena cava syndrome. JAMA 245:951–953, 1981
23. Moncada R, Cardella R, Demos TC et al: Evaluation of superior vena cava snydrome by axial CT and CT phlebography. AJR 143:731–736, 1984
24. Nieto AF, Doty DB: Superior vena cava obstruction: Clinical syndrome, etiology and treatment. Curr Prob Cancer 10:442–484, 1986
25. Dyet JF, Moghissi K: Role of venography in assessing patients with superior vena cava obstruction caused by bronchial carcinoma for bypass operations. Thorax 35:628–630, 1980
26. Stanford W, Jolles H, Ell S, Chiu LC: Superior vena cava obstruction: A venographic classification. AJR 148:259–262, 1987
27. Son YH, Wetzel RA, Wilson WA: ^{99m}Tc Pertechnetate scintiphotography as diagnostic and follow-up aids in major vascular obstruction due to malignant neoplasm. Radiology 91:349–375, 1968
28. Van Houtte P, Fruhling J: Radionuclide venography in the evaluation of superior vena cava syndrome. Clin Nucl Med 6:177–183, 1981
29. Painter TD, Karpf M: Superior vena cava syndrome: Diagnostic procedures. Am J Med Sci 285:2–6, 1983
30. Yesner R, Gersti B, Auerbach O: Application of the World Health Organization classification of lung carcinoma to biopsy material. Ann Thorac Surg 1:33–49, 1965
31. Ihde DC, Cohen MH, Bernath AM et al: Serial fiberoptic bronchoscopy during chemotherapy of small cell carcinoma of the lung. Chest 74:531–536, 1978
32. Lewis RJ, Sisler GE, Mackenzie JW: Mediastinoscopy in advanced superior vena cava obstruction. Ann Thorac Surg 32:458–462, 1981
33. Maddox AM, Valdivieso M, Lukeman J et al: Superior vena cava obstruction in small cell bronchogenic carcinoma. Cancer 52:2165–2172, 1983
34. Sculier JP, Evans WK, Feld R et al: Superior vena caval obstruction in small cell lung cancer. Cancer 57:847–851, 1986
35. Spiro SG, Shah S. Harper PG et al: Treatment of obstruction of the superior vena cava by combination chemotherapy with and without irradiation in small-cell carcinoma of the bronchus. Thorax 38:501–505, 1983
36. Van Houtte P, De Jager R, Lustman-Marechal J, Kenis Y: Prognostic value of the superior vena cava syndrome as the presenting sign of small-cell anaplastic carcinoma of the lung. Eur J Cancer 16:1447–1450, 1980
37. Perez CA, Einhorn LH, Oldham RK, et al: Randomized trial of radiotherapy to the thorax in limited small cell carcinoma of the lung treated with multiagent chemotherapy and elective brain irradiation: A preliminary report. J Clin Oncol 2:1200–1208, 1984
38. Perry MC, Eaton WL, Chahinian P et al: Chemotherapy with or without radiation therapy in limited small cell cancer of the lung. Proc Am Soc Clin Oncol 5:173, 1986
39. Bunn P, Cohen M, Lichter A et al: Randomized trial of chemotherapy versus chemotherapy plus radiotherapy in limited stage small cell lung cancer. Proc Am Soc Clin Oncol 2:200, 1983
40. Mahajan V, Strimlan V, Van Ordstrand HS, Loop FD: Benign superior vena cava syndrome. Chest 68:32–35, 1975
41. Effler DB, Groves LK: Superior vena caval obstruction. J Thorac Cardiovas Surg 43:574–584, 1962
42. Scherck JP, Kerstein MD, Stansel HC: The current status of vena caval replacement. Surgery 76:209–233, 1974
43. Doty DB: Bypass of superior vena cava. J Thorac Cardiovasc Surg 83:326–338, 1982
44. Avashti RB, Moghissi K: Malignant obstruction of the superior vena cava and its palliation. J Thorac Cardiovasc Surg 74:244–248, 1977
45. Katz PO, Hackshaw BT, Barish CF, Powell BL: Thrombosis as a cause of superior vena cava syndrome. Rapid response to streptokinase. Arch Intern Med 143:1050–1053, 1983
46. Green J, Rubin P, Holzwasser G: The experimental production of superior vena cava obstruction. Radiology 81:406–414, 1963
47. Sinner WN: Pulmonary neoplasms diagnosed with transthoracic needle biopsy. Cancer 43:1533–1540, 1979

SECTION 2

THOMAS F. DELANEY
EDWARD H. OLDFIELD

Spinal Cord Compression

Spinal cord or cauda equina compression frequently complicates uncontrolled cancer. At autopsy, its occurrence is documented in approximately 5% of patients with malignancy.[1] Black[2] estimated an annual incidence of 18,000 new cases in the United States. Spinal cord compression is a medical emergency because delay in treatment often results in irreversible paralysis and loss of sphincter control.

The neurologic status at initiation of treatment is the most important factor influencing the neurologic outcome. This is so irrespective of the tumor type, level of spinal axis involved, degree of systemic tumor involvement, or treatment by radiotherapy or by surgery and radiotherapy. Because successful treatment is much more likely in ambulatory patients who retain intact bowel and bladder control at the start of treatment, early recognition of the problem and initiation of therapy is extremely important.[3] Fortunately, most patients with spinal metastasis have pain and characteristic physical and diagnostic findings that can lead to early diagnosis by the astute clinician before significant and irreversible loss of neurologic function occurs and, thereby, improve the chances for a successful outcome.

PATHOPHYSIOLOGY

Although compression of the spinal cord or the cauda equina can arise from intradural metastases, the spinal involvement is almost always extradural.[4,5] Compression usually results from tumor involvement of the vertebral column, either affecting a vertebral body or a neural arch. Most often, tumor in the vertebral body presses on the anterior aspect of the dural sac. Progressive tumor expansion posteriorly compresses the spinal cord (or the cauda equina in the case of lesions below the L1–L2 vertebral level) and produces neurologic impairment. A tumor occasionally metastasizes to the epidural space without bone involvement.[6] In addition, paraspinal tumors, such as malignant lymphoma or neuroblastoma, may invade through the intervertebral foramen and compress the cord without manifest bony involvement. No difference in treatment or functional outcome has been reported for lesions involving the cauda equina, so they will be discussed together with spinal cord compression.[6]

Several experimental models have been used to provide insights into the pathophysiology of neurologic dysfunction from compression of the spinal cord by tumor. Tarlov[7–9] related neurologic recovery after release of mechanically induced cord compression in dogs to the rate of induction and the duration of compression. After gradual induction, decompression could be delayed and neurologic function still return. In contrast, rapid compression required rapid decompression if paralysis was to be reversed. Furthermore, with incomplete cord compression, the recovery of neurologic function was greatly enhanced. Ushio and co-workers[10] induced experimental spinal cord compression by transplanting Walker 256 carcinoma into the perivertebral area of rats. They noted vasogenic edema in the compressed cord, as well as histologic evidence of neuronal injury. Both spinal cord edema and clinical symptoms were transiently improved by treating symptomatic animals with dexamethasone.

CLINICAL PRESENTATION

The most common tumors causing spinal cord compression are listed in Table 58-7.[11] A surprisingly large proportion of patients have spinal cord compression as the initial clinical manifestation of malignancy. Depending on the institution, this proportion ranges from 8% to 47%.[1,3,4] More commonly, spinal cord compression occurs in patients with previously diagnosed cancer. The interval from primary diagnosis to epidural cord compression from metastatic disease varies widely with different tumors. Patients with lung cancer usually develop epidural cord compression within a few months after the diagnosis of their primary lesion (average of 6 months).[4] Patients with breast cancer, on the other hand, often manifest spinal cord compression years after presentation of their primary tumor (as long as 20 years and with an average of 4 years).[3]

The segment of spine involved, approximately 10% cervical, 70% thoracic, and 20% lumbosacral,[1,11–13] reflects the number and volume of vertebral bodies in each anatomic segment.[3] Epidural cord compression at one site frequently accompanies spinal involvement elsewhere that may also threaten the cord. This is particularly true with widely disseminated breast and prostate cancer, as well as myeloma.

Over 90% of patients present with pain, often localized to the spine.[6] Pain, which is usually from involved bone, may be exacerbated by movement, recumbency, cough, sneeze, or strain. The distribution of pain may also be radicular.[3] Radicular pain localizes the lesion to within one or two vertebral segments. Most patients have pain for weeks to months be-

TABLE 58-7. Incidence of Spinal Cord Compression by Site of Tumor

	Lung	*Breast*	*Unknown Primary*	*Lymphoma*	*Myeloma*	*Sarcoma*	*Prostate*	*Kidney*	*GI*	*Thyroid*	*Miscellaneous*
Number of patients	129	94	91	86	68	65	52	44	34	24	116
Percent	16	12	11	11	9	8	7	6	4	3	15

Adapted from Bruckman JE, Bloomer WD: Management of spinal cord compression. Semin Oncol 5:135–140, 1978.

fore the onset of neurologic symptoms. Hence, the development of neck or back pain in a patient with cancer should be considered an ominous symptom that requires investigation. Without treatment, the next symptom is usually weakness. This is often accompanied, or occasionally preceded, by sensory loss. Numbness usually begins in the toes and gradually ascends to the level of cord compression. Weakness combined with sensory loss, particularly loss of proprioception, may produce ataxia. Autonomic dysfunction with urinary retention and constipation usually appears late. Pain almost always precedes the other symptoms by days or weeks, but once sensory, motor, or autonomic symptoms or signs develop, progression is usually rapid, and without treatment complete and irreversible paraplegia often develops over hours to days. Examination usually establishes the level of cord compression, and in a cancer patient, the likely diagnosis.

Signs include tenderness to percussion over the involved spine. Neck flexion or straight-leg raising may produce pain over the involved vertebra or in the distribution of an involved nerve root. Motor findings include weakness, spasticity, abnormal muscle stretch reflexes, and extensor plantar responses. Sensory loss occurs below the involved cord segment and is usually most marked distally. If present, a "level" of decreased sensation in the trunk indicates the site of cord compression. In patients with autonomic dysfunction, a palpable bladder, large postvoid urinary residual, or diminished anal tone may be present.

DIAGNOSTIC EVALUATION

The patient's neurologic status influences the nature and tempo of the diagnostic evaluation. Patients with signs or symptoms of spinal cord compression, such as motor impairment, urinary urgency or retention, or ascending numbness, require emergent evaluation and treatment. Patients should be seen by the oncologist, neurologist, radiotherapist, and neurosurgeon. Dexamethasone should be administered immediately after a history and neurologic examination suggest cord compression.[14] High-dose intravenous dexamethasone, 10 mg intravenously followed by 4 mg every 6 hrs may produce rapid relief of pain[3] and improvement in function.[13] Animal studies demonstrate reduction in cord edema and a diminished rate of neurologic function loss by high-dose steroids.[15] The steroid dosage is tapered after radiation therapy or after surgery, as clinical circumstances permit. The serious complications of high-dose steroids (e.g., infection myopathy, ulcer) can be avoided if the duration of use is not prolonged.[16]

More than two-thirds of patients with cord compression have bony abnormalities on plain radiographs of the spine.[12,17–19] Spine radiographs are accurate in predicting the presence or absence of spinal epidural metastases in 83% of patients with back pain.[20] Findings diagnostic of spinal tumor include erosion and loss of pedicles, partial or complete collapse of vertebral bodies, and paraspinous soft tissue masses. Normal spine films, however, do not exclude epidural metastases. In patients with lymphoma, more than 60% of patients with epidural tumor may have normal spine radiographs.[20]

The standard for diagnosis and localization of epidural cord compression, the myelogram,[14,20–22] has been supplemented in recent years by computed tomography (CT)[22] and, more recently, by magnetic resonance (MRI).[23,24] Oil-based iodinated contrast agents were used extensively for myelograms until the development of metrizamide (Amipaque), a nonirritative water-soluble agent. Metrizamide, because of its lower viscosity and water solubility, mixes more readily with cerebrospinal fluid, travels more freely in the subarachnoid space, and provides homogeneous diffusion in the cerebrospinal fluid that can be used for CT imaging of the spine after conventional myelography. However, unlike oil-based contrast, which can be left in the subarachnoid space for delayed reassessment of the resolution of a myelographic block after treatment, water-soluble agents are fully resorbed from the cerebrospinal fluid. A spinal needle with a small diameter, 22-gauge or smaller, is used for myelography. Just before instillation of the contrast agent, a small CSF sample (<2 ml) should be drawn for cytologic, protein, and glucose evaluation.

In patients with a complete myelographic block, routine myelography after lumbar injection fails to demonstrate the upper extent of the lesion, and additional rostral lesions that compromise the subarachnoid space are present in about 15% of patients. Because such information is important for treatment planning, contrast may also be introduced in such patients through a C1-2 puncture to demarcate the upper border of the myelographic block and define any other lesions. An alternative approach is CT after metrizamide myelography to define the extent of epidural compression in patients with complete block.[22] Although this approach is less uncomfortable than performing a C1-2 puncture,[25] it is often less satisfactory in the patient with another spinal lesion above the block.

In patients with back pain, but no neurologic signs, the diagnostic evaluation can be performed as an outpatient, but in an expedient manner. Patients with abnormalities on plain films should undergo myelography because as many as 81% of such patients have epidural tumor.[20] If bone films are normal, bone scintigraphy is indicated because it is more sensitive than plain films in detecting bony involvement by tumor. Although epidural metastases are uncommon with an abnormal bone scan and normal plain radiographs,[20] the information that the bone scan provides about other bony areas involved by the tumor will be helpful in planning and assessing the results of treatment.

Magnetic resonance imaging is increasingly used to evaluate patients with spinal diseases.[23,26] The technique is noninvasive, images the entire spine with sagittal and parasagittal images, and provides transverse images of selected areas (Fig. 58-1). It also distinguishes extradural, intradural, extramedullary, and intramedullary lesions. Magnetic resonance imaging avoids the risk of neurologic deterioration after lumbar puncture, which occurs in as many as 14% of patients with complete myelograph block.[27] The indications for use of MRI done in this setting, however, are still being defined.

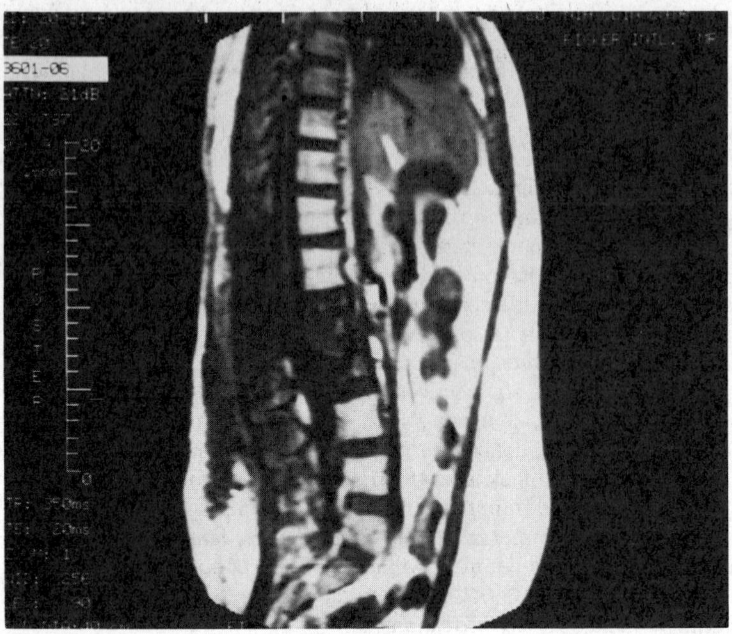

FIG. 58-1. T1-weighted, sagittal magnetic resonance image (MRI) of a 21-year-old woman with a Ewing's sarcoma involving the first and second lumbar vertebrae, which appear darker than the uninvolved spine. Tumor has produced structural deformities in the involved vertebral bodies and is compressing the dural sac.

TREATMENT

The goals of therapy of patients with epidural spinal neoplasms are recovery or preservation of normal neural function, local tumor control, spinal stability, and pain relief. Because cure is not yet possible for most patients with advanced cancer, palliation is a reasonable objective in the management of spinal metastases.

Several important points about the anticipated response to treatment merit emphasis. Approximately 40% to 60% of all patients treated for epidural cord compression by radiotherapy alone or combined laminectomy and radiation will be ambulatory after treatment.[3,13,16–19,28,29] The outcome after treatment closely correlates with the degree of neurologic impairment before therapy (Table 58-8). Almost all ambulatory patients treated with either radiation alone or decompressive laminectomy followed by postoperative radiation remain ambulatory after treatment.[16] In contrast, only 25% of patients who are nonambulatory, but who have some residual motor function, become ambulatory after therapy.[16] Paraplegia is a grave prognostic feature; fewer than 10% of patients with no voluntary movement in their lower extremities will become ambulatory after treatment.[16,18,19] The importance of early diagnosis and initiation of treatment is clear.

For many years, treatment for spinal metastases implied decompressive laminectomy. Laminectomy entails removal of the spinous processes and laminae overlying and one level above and below the site of cord compression (Fig. 58-2). If the tumor involves the posterior bony elements, or if the tumor is visible in the spinal canal, it is removed. The theoretical basis of the universal application of this procedure, regardless of whether the patient had tumor anterior or posterior to the spinal cord, was that it permitted the cord to move dorsally away from compression by anterior lesions, or it allowed removal of the offending tumor mass with lesions located posteriorly. However, the results of laminectomy were disappointing. Only about 30% of patients were improved (ambulatory after treatment) and operative mortality averaged 9%, 11% had nonfatal complications, and 12% were worse after surgery.[2] (Table 58-9).

By the early 1980s, several retrospective reviews that compared laminectomy with radiation therapy had demonstrated that radiation alone produces similar or superior results and less morbidity and mortality than treatments that included laminectomy.[2,3,28,30,31] If all patients are considered (i.e., without consideration of tumor type) radiotherapy was shown by Gilbert and associates[3] and by Black[2] (in a review of reports before 1979) to provide benefit comparable with surgery plus radiation therapy, and both radiation alone and

TABLE 58-8. Effect of Pretreatment Motor Function on Treatment Outcome

	Laminectomy and Radiation		*Radiation Only*	
Pretreatment Condition	*Ambulatory/Treated (n)*	*Ambulatory (%)*	*Ambulatory/Treated (n)*	*Ambulatory (%)*
Ambulatory	14/22	64	46/58	79
Paraparetic	15/33	45	37/83	45
Paraplegic	1/10	10	1/29	3

Adapted from Gilbert RW, Kim JH, Posner, JB: Epidural spinal cord compression from metastatic tumor: Diagnosis and treatment. Ann Neurol 3:40–51, 1978.

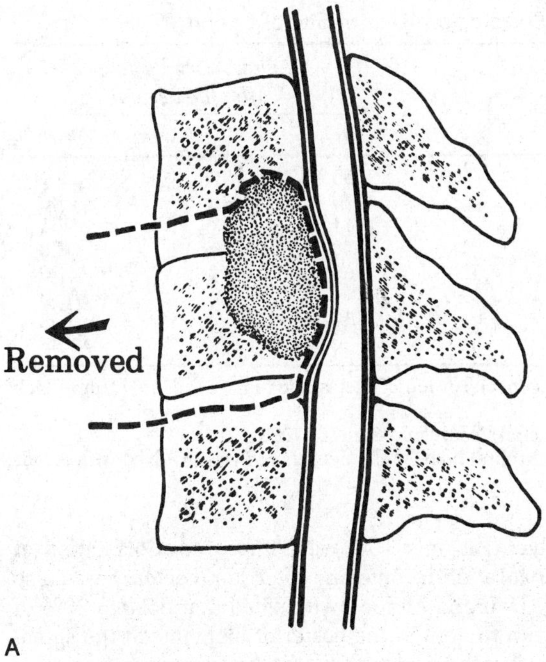

FIG. 58-2. **A.** Most spinal metastases occur in the vertebral column anterior to the spinal canal. When surgery is indicated for tumors anterior to the spinal canal, surgical excision of the tumor and involved vertebral body with immediate stabilization of the spinal column effectively reverses compression of the spinal cord. **B,C.** Cord compression by tumors posterior to the spinal canal can be successfully relieved by laminectomy (removal of the laminae and spinous processes one level above and one level below the site of tumor) and tumor excision.

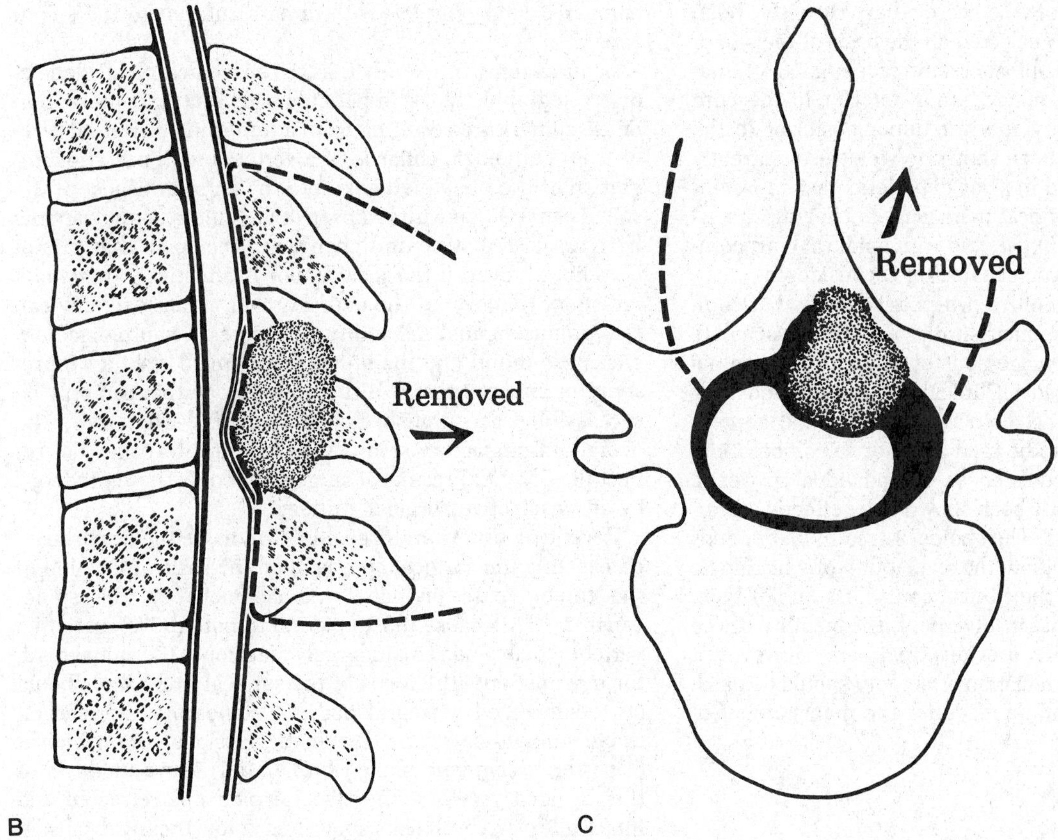

surgery followed by radiation were superior to surgery alone (see Table 58-9). This also applied when patients were analyzed according to the degree of neurologic deficit before treatment. As has been the experience of all authors, the better the neurologic status of the patient before treatment, the better the outcome, irrespective of the treatment used (see Table 58-8).

As a result of these studies, radiation therapy combined with steroids became the treatment used for most patients. Surgery was recommended only for those patients with no

TABLE 58-9. Results of Radiation Therapy, Laminectomy, and Surgery Selected on Basis of Site of Lesion

Treatment	*No. of Patients*	*Ambulatory Patients After Treatment*	
		n	*Mean %*
Laminectomy*	275	85	31
Radiotherapy*	387	176	45
Laminectomy plus radiotherapy*	216	111	51
Vertebral body resection†	101	78	78
Selective surgery‡	86	66	76
Vertebral body resection for anterior tumor	61	57	93
Laminectomy for posterior tumor	25	9	35

*Cumulative data from several published series. Each series consisted of a heterogeneous group of metastatic tumors (adapted from Black P. Neurosurgery 5:726, 1979).

†Includes only patients with vertebral body involvement with tumor (Sundaresan et al. Neurosurg 63:676, 1985).

‡Treatment selected on basis of site of spinal involvement, that is, whether the vertebral body or the neural arch was involved with tumor (Siegal T, Siegal T: Neurosurgery 17:424, 1985).

previous tissue diagnosis, progressive neurologic dysfunction during radiation, or recurrent cord compression after previous radiation therapy. However, that surgical management should be limited only to decompressive laminectomy to relieve cord compression, regardless of the site of pressure at the circumference of the cord, has recently been questioned.[24,32–34] Surgery selected on the basis of the site of tumor involvement in the spinal column (see Fig. 58-2), that is, vertebral body resection for tumor anterior to the cord and posterior laminectomy only for tumor posterior to the cord,[23,32–34] has recently been shown to yield results greatly superior to those obtained in prior experience, when laminectomy alone was the surgical management. For these reasons, the role of surgery in patients with epidural cord compression and metastatic tumor is being reconsidered.

Because there is no definitive prospective study that compares current treatments under similar conditions, absolute recommendations for management of patients with spinal metastases cannot be made. Clinical experience and published reports indicate that both radiotherapy and surgery are effective treatments to be used alone or in combination, as required by the circumstances of individual patients. Chemotherapy has recently been shown to be effective treatment for selected patients. The choice of treatment depends upon the clinical presentation, the availability of a histologic diagnosis, the rapidity of the clinical course, the tumor type, if known, the site of spinal involvement, the stability of the spine, and the nature of any previous treatment. However, it is reasonably clear when radiation or surgery should be used, and recommendations can be made for the management of most patients.

SURGERY

Although epidural tumors located lateral or posterior to the spinal canal, in the laminae or pedicles, can be readily removed by laminectomy, tumor involvement of the vertebral body limits the potential for improvement after laminectomy. This was observed by Wright as early as 1963.[18] In 81 patients with metastatic spinal tumor treated with laminectomy, 38% of the patients with lateral or posterior compartment tumor had a satisfactory outcome, whereas with vertebral involvement only 19% were improved. Correlation of the tumor location to outcome after laminectomy was also studied by Hall and McKay, who noted that 35% to 39% of patients with tumors in the posterior elements of the spinal canal and, therefore, removable by laminectomy, improved compared with only 9% with tumors anterior to the spinal canal.[35]

Laminectomy frequently fails to relieve neurologic deficits or myelographic block in patients with ventral compression of the spinal cord resulting from a tumor in a vertebral body or from pathologic collapse of a vertebra with posterior migration of the bony elements into the anterior aspect of the spinal canal. Even with radiosensitive tumors, many patients have associated structural changes in the spine that cannot be relieved, even if the local tumor is effectively treated by radiation. Removal of the neural arches at laminectomy can also produce spinal instability and increase neurologic deficits. Restoration and maintenance of spinal stability represents an important goal of therapy and one that can only be successfully accomplished with surgery. Therefore, the overall unsatisfactory results with laminectomy may not reflect the potential results of surgery, but only those produced by an unselective surgical strategy.

Recent reports from three clinics indicate the importance of selecting the surgical approach on the basis of location of the tumor mass or bone encroachment on the spinal canal.[24,32–34] Because most epidural tumors (85%) arise in a vertebral body and remain largely anterior to the spinal cord, for most patients the focus of the surgical procedure should be the involved vertebral body. A standard posterolateral thoracotomy is performed for thoracic lesions. After removal of posterior segment of the rib (4–5 cm) above the level of the involved vertebra, the visceral pleura is retracted and intact intervertebral disks above and below the involved segments are isolated.[24,32–34] With cervical and lumbar lesions, a more direct anterior approach is used. The intervertebral disks and the vertebral body are removed. All tumor and devitalized bone are removed down to the dura. Steinman pins, or spinal hooks on an intervening rod, are placed between the vertebral bodies above and below to straddle the space between the healthy vertebrae and, after covering the dura with Gelfoam or fat, fixation of the involved spinal segment is achieved by filling the space left after vertebral body resection by injection of methylmethacrylate into the cavity.[24,32–34]

Sudaresan and co-workers treated 101 consecutive patients with epidural cord compression by vertebral body resection, tumor excision, and immediate stabilization.[34] Patients received surgery who had a pathologic compression fracture as the presenting feature of malignancy, a solitary site of tumor relapse, destruction of the spine by a paraspinous tumor, a known radioresistant tumor (melanoma, sarcoma, or kidney tumor), a structural abnormality of the spine producing compression of the spinal cord, or segmental instability of the spine following previous local treatment with radiation. Of the 101 patients, 78 (78%) left the hospital walking (including 51 patients who had local tumor relapse after a full course of radiation). Thirty-two of 46 patients (70%), nonambulatory before treatment, were ambulatory, with or without support, at hospital discharge. In addition, pain relief occurred in 85% of the patients with major back or radicular pain. The incidence of complications (eight patients died within 30 days and 10% had nonfatal complications) was considered acceptable. The median survival of all patients was 8 months, and 37% lived 1 year after treatment. Similar results have been reported by Harrington.[32]

Siegal and Siegal treated 167 episodes of cord compression prospectively by a standard protocol in which the selection of the surgical approach, when surgery was indicated, was dependent on the tumor location.[33] This was the first study in which selection of the appropriate surgical approach (anterior versus posterior) in neoplastic cord compression was carried out according to strict criteria. Because most tumors arise anteriorly, most patients received vertebral body resection. Radiation was the primary therapy for patients who were in very poor general medical status, had multiple myelographic blocks, were paraplegic for over 72 hrs, or had previously diagnosed radiosensitive tumors without previous radiation treatment. Of the 18 patients with radiosensitive tumors who were treated only with radiation, 13 (72%) were ambulatory after treatment. Surgical treatment was assigned primarily to 86 patients who had no previous histologic diagnosis of their tumor, received previous treatment with radiation at the involved site, had a known radioresistant tumor (osteogenic sarcoma, melanoma, giant-cell tumor of bone), or developed neurologic deterioration during radiation treatment. Twenty-five patients had posterior or posterolateral tumor and received laminectomy for tumor removal, decompression of the spinal cord and, when instability was judged to be present, spinal fixation with spinal rods and bone cement. Although 25% of this group deteriorated as a direct result of surgery, 40% were ambulatory after surgery (92% of this group were nonambulatory before surgery) and normal sphincter control was achieved in 57% (76% were incontinent before surgery).

Sixty-one patients had anterior tumor and received vertebral body resection; 55 of the 61 (91%) had spinal instability and received immediate internal spinal fixation using acrylic replacement of the involved vertebral body. The 30-day mortality in this group was 7%, 80% were ambulatory within 30 days (72% of this group were nonambulatory before surgery), 93% had normal sphincter control (41% were incontinent preoperatively), and although 97% had persistent pain before treatment, complete pain relief was obtained in 56% after surgery. The median survival of these patients was 16 months. The overall ambulation rate, which was superior to that generally reported for radiation alone, occurred even though over half of the patients treated by vertebral body resection had relapsed after receiving previous radiation.

These studies indicate that proper patient selection and the choice of surgical approach based on the tumor location are prerequisites for successful surgery. The generally accepted surgical approach to the treatment of metastatic epidural mass lesions—laminectomy—is ineffective and can be harmful when the pathologic process is anterior to the spinal cord. The outcome of a selective surgical approach (80% ambulation and 93% sphincter control) is superior to results obtained by radiation alone or radiation combined with laminectomy (see Table 58-8). It remains to be determined if similar results can be achieved at most general hospitals, at which most patients are treated.

If surgical decompression is to be used, adequate decompression of the spinal cord and correction of any serious spinal deformity must be accomplished. To ensure decompression at the site of direct pressure on the spinal cord, posterior lesions are approached posteriorly through a wide laminectomy and anterior and anterolateral lesions are excised by vertebral body resection. With instability of the spine, fusion should be performed during the same procedure by instrumentation and methylmethacrylate reconstruction, which produce immediate stability. Neurologic improvement is not only due to correctly directed and efficient decompression of the spinal cord but also to immediate stabilization of the spinal column. Local pain in patients with spinal metastases results from segmental spinal instability. This is suggested by demonstration of a collapsed vertebra, and pain that is relieved by immobilization, bed rest, or traction. Immediate spinal stability enhances rehabilitation by permitting immediate ambulation, if neurologic recovery allows, and eliminates pain from segmental instability.

RADIATION THERAPY

Response to treatment with radiation alone is now well established. An early report by Mones and associates described a favorable response, defined as the ability to ambulate, in 14 of 41 patients (34%) with epidural cord compression treated only with radiation therapy.[30] Response to treatment was excellent in their patients with radioresponsive tumors such as lymphoma, Ewing's sarcoma, and neuroblastoma, less satisfactory in patients with metastatic breast cancer, and poor in patients with lung cancer.[30] Complete or partial reversal of neurologic deficits occurred in 41% of 82 additional patients treated similarly at the same hospital.[36] Paraplegic patients had limited response, with only 16% improved compared with 58% of patients with some motor function.

Gilbert and co-workers[3] at Memorial Hospital retrospectively reviewed the clinical findings and results of treatment in 130 consecutive patients who were treated for epidural spinal cord compression by radiation alone or laminectomy followed by radiation. No significant differences in treatment outcome were seen. After treatment, 49% of patients who received irradiation only walked, compared with 46% of those who received both surgery and postoperative radiation. The duration of improvement in the two treatment groups was similar, with approximately 75% of patients ambulatory after treatment remaining so for 6 months or longer. Patients with radioresponsive tumors generally received radiation, as did most who were paraplegic at presentation and believed to have little chance to recover after laminectomy. Patients without prior tissue diagnosis, those who had previously received spinal irradiation, and patients with rapidly progressing tumors generally received surgery. Regardless of treatment chosen, 73% of ambulatory patients remained so, 36% of the paraparetic patients (nonambulatory but able to lift the legs) regained ambulation, whereas only 1 of 39 paraplegic patients improved. Tumors considered radioresponsive (i.e., seminoma, lymphoma myeloma, Ewing's sarcoma, and neuroblastoma) responded better to either therapy than less radioresponsive tumors such as carcinomas, melanoma, and soft-tissue sarcomas. Patients with rapid progression of spinal cord dysfunction, formerly considered an indication for surgery, improved more often with radiation alone than with decompressive laminectomy followed by radiation. Of the nine patients with weakness that developed over less than 48 hrs who underwent surgical decompression, none improved, whereas 7 of 13 patients irradiated without surgery improved. Autonomic dysfunction predisposed to a worse outcome after treatment. Of 65 patients with urinary incontinence or retention before treatment, 43 (66%) either were, or became, nonambulatory, whereas inability to walk occurred in fewer than 50% of patients without autonomic dysfunction.

Greenberg and associates[13] administered high-dose dexamethasone (100 mg) at diagnosis and began radiation within several hours. After daily doses of 500 rad for the first 3 days of treatment, 300 rad/day were given to a total dose of 3000 rad. Dexamethasone was continued at 96 mg daily in divided doses for 3 days and then tapered during the course of radiation if symptoms permitted. They compared their results with those from the same institution by Gilbert and coworkers[3] and reported no differences in outcome with the new treatment program. They did, however, note a substantial reduction in pain in 64% of patients in the first day of treatment, which they attributed to dexamethasone because improvement occurred even before the initiation of radiation in six patients.

Cobb and associates[28] reported the retrospective analysis of 44 patients with epidural cord compression from metastatic breast cancer, 26 of whom received initial laminectomy and the remainder initial radiotherapy. No significant difference in treatment outcome occurred, with 75% of ambulatory patients remaining so. Deterioration of neurologic function developed in six patients undergoing initial radiation therapy. Two of these patients underwent decompressive laminectomy, with a favorable outcome in one. The authors highlight the need for close neurologic examination during radiotherapy and recommend surgery in patients who show evidence of neurologic deterioration during radiation therapy.

Although the number of patients is small, one randomized, prospective study compares the outcome in 16 patients who underwent decompressive laminectomy plus radiotherapy with 13 patients who had just received radiation therapy.[31] There were no significant differences in outcome between the two groups.

The effect of the type of tumor on outcome of treatment with radiation is difficult to assess because of the relatively small numbers of patients with each specific histologic diagnosis in any single series. Pooled data may not account for difference in ambulatory status, treatment techniques, and dose. Nevertheless, the results reported suggest excellent outcomes after radiation with lymphomas and myelomas, good results in patients with prostate, breast, and renal cancers, and generally disappointing results in patients with lung carcinomas.[3,11,13,16,28,29,31,37,38]

Radiation therapy portals are designed using information from the history and physical examination, spine radiographs, myelogram, bone scan if available, and CT or MRI scans where indicated. A myelogram is mandatory for radiation therapy planning for patients with neurologic symptoms or signs. Calkins and coworkers[21] showed that myelography influenced field size in 69% of patients. Even in patients with discrete bony lesions, results of myelography affect treatment 45% of the time. Whether or not MRI will provide a noninvasive substitute for myelography awaits further trials.

Upon the diagnosis of spinal cord compression, high-dose steroid therapy should be started. Patients who are to undergo radiation should start treatment immediately after diagnosis. The radiation portal includes the site of the myelographic block and generally extends two vertebral bodies above and below the block.[39] Modification may be necessary depending on previous radiation portals and other sites of tumor seen on bone radiographs or scans. For cervical spine lesions, parallel-opposed lateral portals are usually employed. Most thoracic lesions are most appropriately treated with a single posterior field, generally prescribing to a depth of 6 cm. Because the anterior edge of the lumbar spine is nearly at midline, lesions of the lumbar spine generally require parallel-opposed anteroposterior fields. This technique will avoid overdosage to the spinal cord from a single posterior field.

The optimum radiation dose and fractionation scheme have not been definitively established. Several guidelines, however, are available. Clearly, spinal cord tolerance to radiation cannot be exceeded. The radiation should be delivered such that the rapidity of tumor regression and the probability of disease control in the irradiated volume are maximized. Friedman and associates[40] demonstrated a good response in 71% of patients who received greater than 2500 rad for epidural cord compression from malignant lymphoma compared with 34% in the group that received 2500 rad or less. No clear dose–response relationship has been demonstrated for other histologic types, although higher doses (time–dose fraction >60.5) appear to reduce the rate of recurrence within the original treatment field.[41] Commonly employed doses are 3000 to 4000 rad over 2 to 4 weeks.[39]

Experimental data in rats with epidural cord compression secondary to lymphoma[42] or carcinoma[15] demonstrate more rapid neurologic recovery after large daily fractions of radiation (500 rad) than after smaller daily doses (100–200 rad). Fractionated radiation provides more prolonged functional improvement than large single-dose treatment in the rat model.[15] Hence, large initial fractions (400–500 rad) are advocated for the first 3 days of therapy,[13,43] which are followed by smaller daily doses (150–300 rad). Despite theoretical concern about radiation-induced edema from large fractions, experimental evidence fails to confirm its development.[42,44]

CHEMOTHERAPY

Several reports describe successful chemotherapy for epidural cord compression for tumors known to be responsive to chemotherapy such as lymphoma,[46] germ cell neoplasm,[47,48] neuroblastoma,[45] and Ewing's sarcoma.[45] Experiments with the Walker 256 carcinoma in the rat show cyclophosphamide is more effective in relieving the neurologic signs of cord compression than either laminectomy or 1500 rad of irradiation delivered in three fractions.[15] Hayes and colleagues[45] reported on nine children with neuroblastoma and five children with Ewing's sarcoma who had epidural cord compression by the tumor. Five children received laminectomy before referral, but only one had neurologic recovery. The other nine patients did not undergo surgery. All 14 patients received chemotherapy with rapid regression of tumor and neurologic deficits. Therefore, chemotherapy is a feasible alternative to laminectomy and radiation in the management of certain types of epidural tumors. In infants and children, where growth inhibition from radiation may be significant, it seems reasonable to consider chemotherapy in sensitive tumors, as long as the patients are closely monitored by the oncologist, radiation therapist, and neurosurgeon so that other interventions may be quickly undertaken if needed. Friedman and associates[47] reported on two adult patients with testicular cancers who had neurologic recovery after successful decompression of an epidural cord compression by chemotherapy with cyclophosphamide, bleomycin, vinblastine, and cisplatin. In the adult patient with epidural cord compression from metastatic tumor that is responsive to chemotherapy, one should consider adding chemotherapy to surgery/radiation or using chemotherapy if surgery or radiation are not tenable.

CONCLUSION

Epidural spinal cord compression is an oncologic emergency that requires prompt evaluation and treatment. Because the best results are obtained when there has been minimal loss of neurologic function, early diagnosis and treatment are the most important elements of successful treatment. Evaluation should include a careful physical examination, complete spinal radiographs, complete myelography (including cervical myelography in cases of complete block) and, where indicated, bone scintigraphy, CT, or MRI. Patients should be assessed at presentation by the medical or pediatric oncologist, neurologist, radiation oncologist, and neurosurgeon.

TABLE 58-10. Recommendations for Management of Patients with Spinal Metastases

*Radiation therapy only**
Known radiation-sensitive tumor and no spinal instability (regardless of rate of progression or neurologic condition)
Spinal involvement without spinal instability or neurologic deficit
*Surgery followed by radiation**†
Pathologic fracture with spinal instability or compression of the spinal cord by bone
Radiation-resistant tumor with neurologic deficit
Unknown tissue diagnosis
*Surgery only**†
Relapse at the site of previous radiation
Failure to respond to radiation
Chemotherapy
Pediatric patients with responsive tumors
Adjuvant treatment in adult patients with responsive tumors
Relapse of responsive tumor at site of previous radiation and surgery

*Steroid therapy should be used in the early phases of therapy with radiation or surgery.

†Surgery should be based on the site of tumor (anterior versus posterior).

Corticosteroid therapy should be started when the diagnosis has been established.

Although there is no definitive prospective study that compares current treatments under similar conditions, it is reasonably clear when radiation or surgery should be used and recommendations can be made for the management of most patients as outlined in Table 58-10. Radiation therapy is recommended as initial treatment for patients with cord compression who have radiation-sensitive tumors that are not associated with spinal instability. Patients who have spinal involvement by tumor that is not causing neurologic symptoms or spinal instability should also undergo radiation therapy as initial treatment. Patients whose neurologic status deteriorates during radiation therapy and patients who relapse at the site of previous radiation should undergo surgery. Surgery should be the initial treatment in patients with a pathologic fracture resulting in spinal instability or compression of the spinal cord by bone, in patients with radiation-resistant tumors (e.g., osteosarcoma), and in patients without a previous tissue diagnosis. If surgery is indicated, the surgical procedure should be based on the site of tumor involvement by using the appropriate anterior or posterior approach. Because of the difficulty of completely resecting tumor adjacent to the spinal cord, surgery should be followed by postoperative radiation therapy in these patients if spinal cord radiation tolerance will not be exceeded.

Chemotherapy may be used as an adjuvant in adult patients with tumors responsive to chemotherapy or as primary therapy if radiation or surgery are not tenable. In selected pediatric patients with tumors sensitive to chemotherapy, chemotherapy may be considered for initial treatment if patients are closely monitored for any signs of progressive neurologic dysfunction during chemotherapy. It is to be emphasized thatt the most appropriate treatment in each case will also be the most effective, if instituted before major neurologic dysfunction develops.

REFERENCES

1. Barrons KD, Hirano A, Araki S, Terry RD: Experiences with metastic neoplasms involving the spinal cord. Neurology 9:91, 1959
2. Black P: Spinal metastasis: Current status and recommended guidelines for management. Neurosurgery 5:726, 1979
3. Gilbert RW, Kim JH, Posner JB: Epidural spinal cord compression from metastatic tumor: Diagnosis and treatment. Ann Neurol 3:40, 1978
4. Stark, RJ, Henson RA, Evans SJW: Spinal metastases. A restrospective survey from a general hospital. Brain 105:189, 1982
5. Meyer PC, Reah TG: Secondary neoplasms of the central nervous system and meninges. Br J Cancer 7:438, 1953
6. Posner JB: Spinal cord compression: A neurologic emergency. Clin Bull 1:65, 1971
7. Tarlov IM, Klinger H, Vitale S: Spinal cord compression studies. I. Experimental techniques to produce acute and gradual compression. Arch Neurol Psychiatry 70:813, 1957
8. Tarlov IM, Klinger H: Spinal cord compression studies. II. Time limits for recovery after acute compression in dogs. Arch Neurol Psychiatry 71:271, 1954
9. Tarlov IM: Spinal cord compression studies. III. Time limits for recovery after gradual compression in dogs. Arch Neurol Psychiatry 71:588, 1954
10. Ushio Y, Posner R, Posner JB, Shapiro WR: Experimental spinal cord compression by epidural neoplasms. Neurology 27:422, 1977
11. Bruckman JE, Bloomer WD: Management of spinal cord compression. Semin Oncol 5:135, 1978
12. Torma T: Malignant tumors of the spine and the spinal epidural space. A study based on 250 histologically verified cases. Acta Chir Scand 225:1, 1957
13. Greenberg HS, Kim JH, Posner JB: Epidural spinal cord compression from metastatic tumor: Results with a new treatment protocol. Ann Neurol 8:361, 1980
14. Portenoy RK, Lipton RB, Foley KM: Back pain in the cancer patient: An algorithm for evaluation and management. Neurology 37:134, 1987
15. Ushio Y., Posner R, Kim J et al: Treatment of experimental spinal cord compression caused by extradural neoplasms. J Neurosurg 47:380, 1977
16. Martenson JA Jr., Evans RG, Lie MR et al: Treatment outcome and complications in patients treated for malignant epidural spinal cord compression (SCC). J Neurooncol 3:77, 1985
17. Wild WO, Portner RW: Metastatic epidural tumor of the spine. A study of 45 cases. Arch Surg 87:137, 1963
18. Wright RL: Malignant tumors in the spinal extradural space: Results of surgical treatment. Ann Surg 147:227, 1963
19. White WA, Patterson RH, Bergland RM: Role of surgery in the treatment of spinal cord compression by metastatic neoplasm. Cancer 27:558, 1971
20. Rodichok LD, Harper GR, Ruckdeschel JC et al: Early diagnosis of spinal epidural metastases. Am J Med 70:1181, 1981
21. Calkins AR, Olson MA, Ellis JH: Impact of myelography on the radiotherapeutic management of malignant spinal cord compression. Neurosurgery 19:614, 1986
22. Fink IJ, Garra BS, Zabell A, Doppman JL: Computed tomography with metrizamide myelography to define the extent of spinal canal block due to tumor. J Comput Assist Tomogr 8:1072, 1984
23. Aichner F, Poewe W, Rogalsky W et al: Magnetic resonance imaging in the diagnosis of spinal cord diseases. J Neurol Neurosurg Psychiatry 48:1220, 1985
24. Bosley TM, Cohen DA, Schatz NJ et al: Comparison of metrizamide computed tomography and magnetic resonance imaging in the evaluation of lesions at the cervicomedullary junction. Neurology 35:485, 1985
25. Johansen JG, Orrison WW, Amundsen P: Lateral C1-2 puncture for cervical myelography. Part I: Report of a complication. Radiology 146:391, 1983
26. Sarpel S, Sarpel G. Yu E et al: Early diagnosis of spinal–epidural metastasis by magnetic resonance imaging. Cancer 59:1112, 1987
27. Hollis PH, Malis LI, Zappullo RA: Neurological deterioration after lumbar puncture below complete spinal subarachnoid block. J Neurosurg 64:253, 1986
28. Cobb CA III, Leavens ME, Eckles N: Indications for nonoperative treatment of spinal cord compression due to breast cancer. J Neurosurg 47:653, 1977
29. Raichle ME, Posner JB: The treatment of extradural spinal cord compression. Neurology 20:391, 1970
30. Mones RJ, Dozier D, Berrett A: Analysis of medical treatment of malignant extradural spinal cord tumors. Cancer 19:1842, 1966
31. Young RF, Post EM, King GA: Treatment of spinal epidural metastases: Randomized prospective comparison of laminectomy and radiotherapy. J Neurosurg 53:741, 1980
32. Harrington KD: Anterior cord decompression and spinal stablization for patients with metastatic lesions of the spine. J Neurosurg 61:107, 1984
33. Siegal T, Siegal T: Surgical decompression of anterior and posterior malignant epidural tumors compressing the spinal cord: A prospective study. Neurosurgery 17:424, 1985
34. Sundaresan N, Galicich JH, Lane JM, et al: Treatment of neoplastic epidural cord compression by vertebral body resection and stabilization. J Neurosurg 63:676, 1985
35. Hall AJ, MacKay NNS: The results of laminectomy for compression of the cord and cauda equina by extradural malignant tumor. J Bone Joint Surg 55:497, 1973
36. Zevallos M, Chan PYM, Munoz L et al: Epidural spinal cord compression from metastatic tumor. Int J Radiat Oncol Biol Phys 13:875, 1981
37. Haddad P, Thaell JF. Kiely JM et al: Lymphoma of the spinal extradural space. Cancer 38:1862, 1976
38. Khan FR, Glicksman AS, Chu FCH, Nickson JJ: Treatment by radiotherapy of spinal cord compression due to extradural metastases. Radiology 89:495, 1967
39. Kornblith PL, Cassady JR: Central nervous system emergencies. In DeVita VT, Hellman S, Rosenberg SA (eds): Principles and Practice of Oncology, 2nd ed, p 1960. Philadelphia, JB Lippincott, 1985
40. Friedman M, Kim TM, Panahon AM: Spinal cord compression in malignant lymphoma. Cancer 37:1485, 1976
41. Loeffler JS, Glicksman AS, Tefft M, Gelch M: Treatment of spinal cord compression: A retrospective analysis. Med Pediatr Oncol 11:347, 1983
42. Rubin P: Extradural spinal cord compression by tumor. Part I: Experimental production and treatment trials. Radiology 93:1243, 1969
43. Rubin P, Mayer E. Poutter C: Extradural spinal cord compression by tumor. Part II: High daily dose experience without laminectomy. Radiology 93:1243, 1969
44. Redmond H: Effects of whole-brain irradiation. Presented at the Work in Progress Session of the 52nd Scientific Assembly and Meeting of the Radiological Society of North America, Chicago, 1966
45. Hayes FA, Thompson EL, Avizdala E et al: Chemotherapy as an alternative to laminectomy and radiation in the management of epidural tumor. J Pediar 104:221, 1984
46. Silverberg IJ, Jacobs EM: Treatment of spinal cord compression in Hodgkin's disease. Cancer 27:308, 1971
47. Friedman HM, Sheetz S, Levine HC et al: Combination chemotherapy and radiation therapy. The medical management of epidural spinal cord compression from testicular cancer. Arch Intern Med 146:509, 1986
48. Gale GB, O'Connor DM, Chu J-Y et al: Successful chemotherapeutic decompression of epidural malignant germ cell tumor. Med Pediatr Oncol 14:97, 1986

SECTION 3

RAYMOND P. WARRELL, JR
RICHARD S. BOCKMAN

Metabolic Emergencies

Patients with cancer present a microcosm of metabolic and endocrinologic problems encountered in internal medicine, albeit frequently to an extreme degree. Grouped among the "paraneoplastic syndromes" are disorders of metabolism that are associated with the underlying cancer or that are complications of anticancer therapy. This chapter discusses acute metabolic disorders that require urgent medical therapy for treatment or prevention. Other disorders, such as the syndrome of inappropriate secretion of antidiuretic hormone (SIADH) are discussed in Chapter 55.

HYPERCALCEMIA

EPIDEMIOLOGY

Hypercalcemia is the most common life-threatening metabolic disorder associated with cancer. The precise incidence of this disorder is difficult to assess. Surveys of hospitalized patients tend to overstate its prevalence. Because fewer asymptomatic persons with cancer are included in ambulatory screening programs, surveys of the general population tend to understate the problem.[1,2] However, a reasonable estimate of the prevalence of hypercalcemia due to cancer in the United States and Western Europe is approximately 15 to 20 cases per 100,000 persons. The ratio of hypercalcemic patients with primary hyperparathyroidism relative to those with cancer is approximately 1.5:1.

The incidence of hypercalcemia varies with the underlying cancer diagnosis. The incidence is highest in multiple myeloma and breast cancer wherein 40% to 50% of patients develop an elevated serum calcium level at some point in their course.[3-5] Hypercalcemia occurs in 12.5% of patients with lung cancer,[6,7] although the prevalence is higher in patients with epidermoid cancers and lower in those with small cell tumors.[8] By contrast, only exceptional patients with carcinoma of the colon develop hypercalcemia.

DIFFERENTIAL DIAGNOSIS

Hypercalcemia is associated with a wide variety of pathologic states (Table 58-11). Several excellent reviews have recently discussed the diagnostic evaluation and differential diagnosis of patients with hypercalcemia.[9-11] Primary hyperparathyroidism and cancer are the most common causes of hypercalcemia, and both diseases are prevalent.[12] Although certain reports[13-16] suggested that primary hyperparathyroidism occurred more frequently than expected in patients with breast cancer, a recent study demonstrated that the coincidental occurrence of these two diseases is not different from that expected.[17]

Although the differential diagnosis of hypercalcemia in cancer and hyperparathyroidism has been linked to changes in serum chloride concentration,[18] phosphorus, nephrogenous cyclic adenosine monophosphate, immunoreactive parathyroid hormone (PTH),[19] and results of steroid suppression tests,[20,21] none of these tests individually distinguish the two diseases.[11] An accurate history is extremely valuable because patients who have a recent onset of symptomatic hypercalcemia and weight loss are more likely to have a malignant disorder. A survey of hospitalized patients with hypercalcemia found that cancer had been previously diagnosed or was readily apparent after minimal diagnostic evaluation in more than 98% of the patients.[1] By contrast, asymptomatic hypercalcemia and chronic symptoms are the most common presentations of primary hyperparathyroidism.[2] A low or normal serum immunoreactive PTH level using a double-antibody method can usually exclude the diagnosis of primary hyperparathyroidism.

TABLE 58-11. Diseases Associated with Hypercalcemia

Endocrine/metabolic diseases
Primary hyperparathyroidism
Hyperthyroidism
Pheochromocytoma
Osteopetrosis
Infantile hyperphosphatasia
Familial hypercalcemia with hypercalciuria
Cancer
Infectious diseases
Tuberculosis
Coccidioidomycosis
HIV infection (AIDS)
Renal insufficiency
Granulomatous diseases
Sarcoidosis
Berylliosis
Dietary/drug-related
Vitamin D intoxication
Vitamin A intoxication
Calcium supplements
Lithium
Milk–alkali (Burnett's) syndrome

Because serum calcium is highly bound to albumin, measurements of total serum calcium fluctuate with changes in serum protein concentrations. Thus, measurements of ionized calcium by use of an ion-specific electrode are often helpful. Occasionally, patients with myeloma may have striking elevations of total serum calcium solely because of an increase in serum proteins that bind calcium.[22,23] However, an approximate estimate of the severity of hypercalcemia can be made by using one of several formulas that adjusts serum calcium levels for serum concentrations of albumin, as follows:

Corrected [calcium] (mg/dl)* = measured [calcium] (mg/dl) − [albumin] (g/dl) + 4.0.[24]

TABLE 58-12. Clinical Presentations of Cancer-Related Hypercalcemia

General: dehydration, weight loss, anorexia, pruritus, polydipsia
Neuromuscular: fatigue, lethargy, muscle weakness, hyporeflexia, confusion, psychosis, seizure, obtundation, coma
Gastrointestinal: nausea, vomiting, constipation, obstipation, ileus
Genitorenal: polyuria, renal insufficiency
Cardiac: bradycardia, prolonged P-R interval, shortened Q-T interval, wide T-wave, atrial or ventricular arrhythmias

CLINICAL MANIFESTATIONS

Because calcium is a critical regulator of many cellular functions, patients with hypercalcemia can have a wide variety of symptoms affecting multiple organ systems (Table 58-12). The severity of the presentation is not exclusively related to the degree of elevation in the serum calcium value. Patients with a slight to moderate elevation (11–12 mg/dl) may present in an obtunded state if the increase has occurred suddenly. Conversely, patients with long-standing hypercalcemia (such as those with parathyroid carcinoma) may tolerate a serum calcium level > 13 mg/dl, with few symptoms. Other factors, including age, performance status, sites of metastases, and hepatic or renal dysfunction, will also contribute to the severity of symptoms.

In patients with evolving hypercalcemia, fatigue, lethargy, constipation, nausea, and polyuria are the most common initial complaints. It is important to evaluate the serum calcium level in patients who have these relatively nonspecific complaints because the combination of polyuria and nausea can lead to rapid dehydration and substantial worsening of the hypercalcemic state. Patients in late stages may present in stupor or coma and are easily mistaken for persons with diabetic ketoacidosis or drug overdose.

*(Concentrations in mg/dl can be converted to SI units by multiplication by 0.2495, yielding concentration expressed in mmol/liter.)

TABLE 58-13. Etiologic Factors Associated with Cancer-Related Hypercalcemia

Circulating Humoral Factors or Factors Locally Active Within Bone
Parathyroid hormone (PTH; rare except in parathyroid carcinoma)
PTH-like factors
Transforming growth factors (TGFα, TGFβ)
Prostaglandins (PGE)
Interleukin-1
Tumor necrosis factors [TNFα, TNFβ (lymphotoxin)]
Platelet-derived growth factor (PDGF)
Colony-stimulating factors (GM-CSF, G-CSF)
Vitamin D (1,25-$(OH)_2$-vitamin D_3)
Other causes
Direct bone resorption by tumor cells (rare)
Increased gastrointestinal absorption of calcium (rare)
Increased renal reabsorption of calcium (amplifies other causes)

PATHOPHYSIOLOGY

Theoretically, hypercalcemia can result from increased calcium absorption from the gastrointestinal tract, decreased excretion of calcium into urine, and increased calcium resorption from bone (Table 58-13). Although an animal model of hypercalcemia (VX_2 carcinoma) has been associated with increased gastrointestinal absorption of calcium,[25] most clinical studies have shown that intestinal absorption of calcium is actually decreased in hypercalcemic patients with cancer.[26] Therefore, dietary factors are not believed to have substantial causal importance in cancer-related hypercalcemia.

The contribution of renal mechanisms to the hypercalcemia of patients with cancer is less well characterized. In myeloma, hypercalcemia is often accompanied by renal insufficiency,[27] and circulating factors with "PTH-like" activities (discussed later) may induce phosphaturia and increase calcium reabsorption from the renal tubules. Although decreased filtration and increased reabsorption of calcium because of volume contraction aggravate hypercalcemia induced by osteolysis, renal mechanisms, by themselves, probably have only a secondary role in the development of hypercalcemia.

Traditionally, cancer-related hypercalcemia has been categorized according to the presence or absence of bone involvement. Hypercalcemia in the former group was believed to be associated with direct bone destruction by cancer cells, and the second group was characterized by various "humorally mediated" mechanisms. This distinction explained several observations. For example, breast cancer was known to be osteotropic (*i.e.*, to preferentially metastasize to bone) and was usually associated with lytic bone lesions. Furthermore, certain breast cancer cells could be shown to directly resorb bone in vitro, independently of osteoclasts.[28]

However, the distinction based on bone involvement failed to account for certain discrepancies. First, the frequency and severity of bone involvement bears little relation to the frequency and severity of hypercalcemia.[28] Second, many hypercalcemic patients with bone metastases also have features that are consistent with "ectopic" or "pseudo"-hyperparathyroidism.[29] Third, malignant cells from most tumor types that are clinically associated with hypercalcemia cannot resorb devitalized bone matrix. Histologic examination of bone from patients with metastases has also indicated that bone resorption is mediated by normal osteoclasts and not directly by tumor cells. These data imply that even for osteotropic tumors, local factors that activate normal osteoclasts are probably critical for initiating osteolysis.

Recent research has provided important insights into the pathogenesis of bone loss resulting from cancer. Hypercalcemia—even in patients with extensive osteolysis—is probably mediated by factors released from, or induced by, malignant cells that ultimately act to resorb calcium from bone.

"Ectopic Hyperparathyroidism"

Albright first suggested that tumors could cause hypercalcemia by the ectopic production of PTH.[31] More recent studies have confirmed that some patients with cancer-related hypercalcemia have biochemical characteristics that suggest PTH stimulation, including increased tubular reabsorption of calcium,[32] hypophosphatemia with phosphaturia, and elevated levels of "nephrogenous" CAMP.[33,34]

Inappropriately elevated PTH levels have been detected in varying proportions of patients with cancer-related hypercalcemia, depending upon the radioimmunoassay.[35,36] However, virtually all reported cases of ectopic hyperparathyroidism have been based upon measurements of immunoreactive material, and none entirely satisfy the criteria necessary to prove ectopic hormone production.[37] Studies looking for PTH-specific mRNA in tumors have confirmed that ectopic PTH production cannot be a frequent cause of cancer-related hypercalcemia.[38] Recently, studies examining translation of mRNA have shown that proteins with PTH-like activity are produced by certain tumors,[39] and a variety of humoral factors functionally similar to PTH have now been described. Such factors bind to PTH receptors[40] and are capable of activating PTH-dependent adenylate cyclase;[41–43] however, most do not cross-react with PTH-specific antibodies.[19,40]

The PTH-like factors produced by tumors have been partially characterized.[44–46] Partial homology between these factors and authentic human PTH has been shown in the first 15 amino acids of the NH_2-terminal portion. However, these substances have molecular masses that range from 6000 to 18,000, which clearly distinguish them from native PTH. Genes that encode for PTH-like proteins are not solely expressed in malignant cells because expression of these factors has also been found in normal keratinocytes.[47]

In the future, it may be important to prospectively identify patients who secrete PTH-like factors. Because these factors presumably mediate their effects through PTH receptors, agents that block receptor binding of PTH could be used as specific treatment for hypercalcemia in such patients.[48,49]

Prostaglandins

Prostaglandins have long been implicated as circulating mediators of cancer-related hypercalcemia.[50,51] Malignant cells are known to secrete or induce the endogenous release of prostaglandins.[52–56] Certain prostaglandins, notably of the E series, have potent bone-resorptive activity in vitro.[57–59] Hormonally induced "flares" of hypercalcemia in breast cancer[60] have been linked to the release of prostaglandins.[61] Despite this circumstantial evidence, cancer-related hypercalcemia rarely responds to cyclooxygenase inhibition,[62,63] and circulating levels of prostaglandin E (PGE) in hypercalcemic patients are far too low to account for the observed degree of accelerated bone resorption.[55,56]

Prostaglandins probably have an important (but time-dependent and highly local) role in cancer-related osteolysis. Although circulating prostaglandins no longer appear to be primary effectors of clinical hypercalcemia, local release of these compounds within bone[64-66] may amplify the activation of osteoclasts[67] and induce the release of bone-resorbing enzymes.[68] Locally active prostaglandins are probably derived from endogenous production by bone cells that have been stimulated by tumor-derived factors.[69]

Cytokines

Osteoclast-activating factors (so-called OAF's) were originally isolated from lymphoid cells. These substances, which stimulate osteoclast-mediated bone resorption,[70,71] comprise a variety of cytokines.

From an etiologic standpoint, the transforming growth factors (TGFs) may be important regulatory factors for cancer-related hypercalcemia. These factors are released in an autocrine manner by a variety of cancer cells.[72] Both TGFα and TGFβ are potent inducers of bone resorption in vitro.[73-76] The TGFα shares partial similarity of amino acid sequence with epidermal growth factor (EGF) and binds to the EGF receptor.[77] Antisera against EGF receptor blocks bone resorbing activity in a rat model of hypercalcemia (Leydig cell carcinoma).[78] A recent study has shown that TGFβ shares certain PTH-like activities described earlier.[79]

A variety of other cytokines also have bone resorptive activities. Interleukin-1 (IL-1), derived from monocytes, has potent OAF activity.[80-82] Tumor-derived hematopoietic colony-stimulating factors (CSFs) also stimulate bone resorption.[83-85] The product of the oncogene v-*sis* is a protein similar to platelet-derived growth factor (PDGF).[86] Although there are conflicting reports on the independent effects of PDGF on bone resorption in vitro,[87,88] it has been proposed that PDGF potentiates the effects of TGFs on bone resorption.[89]

Tumor necrosis factors (TNFs), in particular TNFβ (lymphotoxin), are highly potent inducers of bone resorption in vitro.[90,91] Tumor necrosis factor also induces the synthesis of IL-1.[92] Conversely, interferon-γ inhibits both the formation and function of osteoclasts.[93-95] The interaction of each of these factors in vivo is undoubtedly complex, and a clear understanding of their role in the pathogenesis of cancer-related hypercalcemia remains to be established.

Vitamin D

Although hypercalcemia is uncommon in patients with malignant lymphoma, some patients with T-cell non-Hodgkin's lymphoma[96] have increased circulating levels of 1,25-dihydroxyvitamin D (calcitriol).[97] Elevated vitamin D levels have also been reported in patients with Hodgkin's disease,[98] myeloma,[99] as well as rare patients with solid tumors.[100] This effect may result from increased conversion of 25-hydroxyvitamin D to 1,25-dihydroxyvitamin D by an enzyme with 1-α-vitamin D hydroxylase activity, similar to patients with granulomatous disease. However, lymphocytes infected with human T-cell lymphotropic virus type I (HTLV-1) in vitro synthesize increased quantities of vitamin D[101] and patients with acquired immunodeficiency syndrome (AIDS)-related lymphoma and human immunodeficiency virus (HIV; HTLV-3/LAV) infection also have increased circulating levels of vitamin D.[102] Because HTLV-1-infected cells produce a variety of bone-resorbing factors,[103,104] these observations do not prove an etiologic association. Decrease in serum vitamin D and resolution of hypercalcemia occurs with control of the underlying disease.

SUMMARY. Owing to the aforementioned complexities, a unifying hypothesis for the etiology of cancer-related hypercalcemia is lacking. Breast cancer and other osteotropic tumors appear to require proximity to bone to effect hypercalcemia. These observations strongly implicate the release of locally active substances such as prostaglandins. Similarly, multiple myeloma is characterized by extensive osteolysis and locally increased production of cytokines that accelerate bone resorption by normal osteoclasts. Epidermoid carcinomas may elaborate circulating factors with biologic activities similar to PTH. Release of TGFs may be important for other patients who present with hypercalcemia in the absence of substantial bone involvement. Because a large number of patients with cancer have obvious lytic bone disease, but only a small proportion develop hypercalcemia, interaction of these factors and amplification of the pathophysiology (presumably at the renal level) must also occur.

TREATMENT OF CANCER-RELATED HYPERCALCEMIA

General Measures

Although the best treatment for cancer-related hypercalcemia is therapy directed at the underlying disease, hypercalcemia most commonly occurs in patients with advanced disease who have failed prior therapy. Despite advances in understanding the pathogenesis of hypercalcemia, treatment of specific causes in individual patients has not evolved.

Usual therapies for hypercalcemia are nonspecific and are often directed at decreasing the serum calcium concentration by increasing urinary calcium excretion or causing lethal toxicity to normal bone cells. In principle, such maneuvers accelerate calcium loss from bone, aggravate osteopenia, and lead to further skeletal dysfunction (pain and fractures). Although these considerations have minor importance in emergency situations, such treatment broadly applied is ultimately detrimental, and specific therapies that reduce accelerated bone resorption would be preferred.

Numerous dietary restrictions have been placed upon patients to achieve a low calcium intake. For practical purposes, increased intestinal absorption of calcium does not make an important contribution to hypercalcemia in patients with cancer. Low-calcium diets are distinctly unpalatable, impractical for long-term use, and exacerbate chronic malnutrition.

TABLE 58-14. Drugs Available for Treatment of Cancer-Related Hypercalcemia

	Normal Saline	*Furosemide*	*Oral Phosphorus*	*Intravenous Phosphorus*	*Corticosteroids*
Dose	200–400(+) ml/h	20–80(+) mg IV (as needed)	1–3 g/day orally, divided doses	50 mmol (1.5 g) by IV infusion over 6 h	40–100 mg/day prednisone (or equivalent)
Indications	Hypovolemia, dehydration	Fluid overload, diuresis	Mild-moderate hypercalcemia; hypophosphatemia	Severe, intractable hypercalcemia with normal renal function, established urinary output.	Hypercalcemia from myeloma, lymphoma, "flare" from hormonal treatment of breast cancer
Onset of action	12–24 h		24 h	<1 h	3–5 days
Relative* potency	20%		30%	80%	0–40% (depends on disease)
Advantages	Corrects dehydration	Increases calciuresis (?)	Orally available; minimal toxicity	Highly effective	Orally available
Disadvantages/toxicity	Fluid overload, hypernatremia	Hypokalemia, hypomagnesemia, hypovolemia	Nausea, diarrhea, extraosseous calcification	Highly toxic; hypotension, renal failure, extraosseous calcification	Hyperglycemia, gastritis, osteopenia, Cushing's syndrome

*Estimated proportion of patients with serum calcium ≥ 120 mg/dl who achieve normocalcemia after one course of treatment

Where possible, immobilization should be minimized because inactivity tends to aggravate hypercalcemia. All medications should be carefully reviewed. Thiazides increase renal calcium reabsorption[105] and should be discontinued. Patients with bone metastases may be ingesting analgesic, nonsteroidal anti-inflammatory drugs or H_2-receptor antagonists (cimetidine or ranitidine), that decrease renal blood flow. These drugs should be avoided if possible, especially during acute phases of hypercalcemia. The patient should be carefully interviewed with respect to dietary aberrations and vitamin ingestion. Preparations containing calcium or vitamin D should obviously be eliminated.[106] Large doses of vitamin A and retinoids have been associated with hypercalcemia[107,108] and should also be discontinued.

Specific Measures

The literature on the treatment of cancer-related hypercalcemia contains very few controlled studies. Therefore, most current recommendations for treatment are based largely on personal experiences from uncontrolled series. Interpretation of results from clinical trials is further confounded by tremendous variability in patient selection, underlying diagnoses, severity of hypercalcemia, and method of reporting results. Table 58-14 summarizes current treatment recommendations and provides an estimate of the relative potency of particular therapies. For this discussion, potency is defined as the expected proportion of patients with serum calcium ≥ 12.0 mg/dl (corrected for albumin) who will achieve normocalcemia after a single course of treatment.

INTRAVENOUS FLUIDS. Hypercalcemic patients frequently present with dehydration. Loss of intravascular volume is caused by an obligate water loss associated with calciuresis, along with added loss of fluids from vomiting. Intravenous hydration is the mainstay of acute therapy for hypercalcemia. Isotonic saline is preferred to avoid dilutional hyponatremia. Volume expansion and natriuresis increase renal blood flow and enhance calcium excretion because of ionic exchange of calcium for sodium in the distal tubule.[109–112]

The rate of fluid administration depends upon a clinical estimate of the extent of dehydration, upon an estimation of cardiovascular function, and upon the renal excretory capacity. Assuming renal function has previously been normal and cardiac reserves are adequate, saline infusion at a rate of 300 to 400 + ml/hr is recommended for 3 to 4 hr. Slower hydration is indicated for less severe metabolic disturbances or in the settings of oliguric renal failure or congestive heart failure. After several hours, the patient should be thoroughly reassessed. Serum calcium, creatinine, and electrolyte concentrations should be checked, along with measurement of urinary output and evaluation of cardiac status, with particular attention to evidence of congestive heart failure. Potassium and magnesium losses frequently occur with saline hydration and may be exacerbated by diuretics.[113]

The effectiveness of hydration (with or without loop diuretics) for correction of hypercalcemia remains uncertain. A recent report noted that a "majority of patients" achieved normocalcemia with rehydration alone.[5] However, this observation presumably included patients with trivial elevations of serum calcium values. In a prospective study of patients with a serum calcium concentration of ≥ 13.0 mg/dl (3.25 mmol/liter), Hosking and co-workers reported that 5 of 16 patients (31%) achieved normocalcemia with normal saline (4000 ml/day × 2 days).[114] In a recent study of patients hospitalized at Memorial Sloan-Kettering with serum calcium values of ≥ 12.0 mg/dl, the serum calcium concentration was lowered below 12.0 mg/dl in 34 of 198 (17%) patients after 2 days of hydration.[115] A higher propor-

TABLE 58-14. *(continued)*

Calcitonin	*Disodium Etidronate*	*Mithramycin*	*Gallium Nitrate*	*Aminohydroxypropylidene Diphosphonate (APD)*
2–8 units/kg SC or IM every 6–12 h	7.5 mg/kg IV over 4 h daily for 3 days	10–50 (usually 25) μg/kg IV by injection or 2–4 h infusion	100–200 mg/m² IV by continuous infusion × 5 days	60 mg IV by infusion over 24 hr
Mild-moderate hypercalcemia; acute control	Mild-moderate hypercalcemia	Moderate-severe hypercalcemia	Moderate-severe hypercalcemia	Moderate-severe hypercalcemia
1–4 h	48 h	24–48 h	24–48 h	48 h
30%	30%	80%	80%	60%
Minimal toxicity	Usually well tolerated; decreases bone resorption	Highly effective	Highly effective; decreases bone resorption	Decreases bone resorption
Nausea, hypersensitivity	Occasional nephrotoxicity	Toxic: nausea, nephrotoxicity, hepatoxicity, thrombocytopenia, coagulopathy; toxic to bone cells	Must be given by prolonged infusion; nephrotoxicity; hypophosphatemia; (investigational)	Nausea, fever, hypophosphatemia (investigational)

tion of patients with less extreme elevations of serum calcium values (*i.e.*, 10.5–12.0 mg/dl) would be expected to improve.

DIURETICS. Although it is common practice to administer loop diuretics such as furosemide with normal saline, there is little evidence that these agents add substantial benefit. In theory, furosemide-induced natriuresis should enhance urinary calcium excretion.[113] However, no controlled clinical studies have been performed to indicate that hypercalcemic patients benefit from routine treatment with furosemide. The drug increases the risk of developing hypovolemia, and the resultant decrease in glomerular filtration may then stimulate renal calcium reabsorption.[116] Furosemide also induces hypokalemia, alkalosis, and hypomagnesemia. Obtunded patients with hypercalcemia may develop marked hypernatremia and a hyperosmolar state when treated with vigorous saline hydration.[5] Management of this complication depends upon prompt recognition and substitution of hypotonic fluids for normal saline.

Suki and co-workers[117] treated eight patients with extremely large amounts of intravenous saline (10 liters/24 hr) along with high doses of furosemide (mean of 1240 mg/patient). By using this method, they achieved a mean urine output of 727 ml/hr; however, only three of eight patients actually achieved a normal serum calcium concentration. With the current availability of other therapy, this heroic degree of hydration and forced diuresis is no longer indicated.

PHOSPHATES. The action of phosphates is complex. Orally administered phosphorus may decrease gastrointestinal absorption of calcium through the formation of insoluble calcium-phosphate complexes in the gut.[118,119] An increase in serum phosphorus decreases secretion of PTH which results in decreased formation of 1,25$(OH)_2$-vitamin D_3 and decreased intestinal absorption of calcium. Because "hyperabsorption" is not an important cause of cancer-related hypercalcemia, it is unlikely that the gastrointestinal effects of phosphates contribute substantially to their effectiveness. An increase in serum phosphorus concentrations leads to an inhibition of calcium resorption from bone[120–122] and a significant reduction in urinary calcium excretion.[121] However, phosphate also shifts calcium from blood to other tissues,[123] and this shift can result in severe toxicity. Renal failure from intrarenal precipitation of calcium phosphate is a common occurrence after intravenous phosphate therapy.[124] The effect has also been seen with the long-term use of oral phosphate. Widespread extraosseous deposition of calcium can occur, leading to calcifications in muscle, eye, heart, and lungs.[125–127]

Phosphates can be administered orally in divided dosages of 0.5 to 3 g/day. Oral phosphate may be highly effective, particularly in mild forms of hypercalcemia.[129–131] Principal side effects are diarrhea and nausea, which may lead to noncompliance. For patients with nausea or impaired mental status, phosphate can be administered rectally by retention enema at a dosage of 1.5 g twice a day. Serum phosphorus concentrations should be monitored in all patients who receive oral phosphorus, especially patients with decreased renal function.[128] Phosphates should not be used if the serum phosphorus concentration is elevated. Serum creatinine levels should be regularly monitored to avoid renal insufficiency.

Intravenous phosphate is highly effective and the onset of hypocalcemic action occurs more rapidly than with any other hypocalcemic therapy.[132–134] However, the benefit of rapid action is outweighed by excessive toxicity. Renal failure, hypotension, extraskeletal calcification, and severe hypocalcemia are common sequelae of parenteral phosphate therapy.[135] Accordingly, the use of intravenous phosphate has largely been abandoned. This treatment should be considered only for patients in exceptional circumstances who must achieve rapid lowering of serum calcium concentration. (An example of this condition would be a patient resistant to mithramycin with a serum calcium value of > 16.0 mg/dl and serious ventricular arrhythmia.) Intravenous phosphate is preferably administered in an intensive care setting with close monitoring of cardiac, renal, and electrolyte status.

A dose-related reduction in serum calcium occurs with increasing doses of IV phosphate. Fulmer and colleagues[136] found that increasing doses of phosphate (ranging from 25, 50, and 75 mmol) caused reduction in serum calcium by 1.1, 2.4, and 4.1 mg/dl, respectively. In general, a dose of 1.5 g (50 mmol of elemental phosphorus diluted in 1000 ml) can be administered over 6 to 8 hr. If necessary, treatment can be repeated once after 24 hr of observation.

PROSTAGLANDIN INHIBITORS. Several early reports noted that inhibitors of prostaglandin synthesis caused a reduction of serum calcium levels in selected patients with cancer-related hypercalcemia.[50,137] Seyberth and associates[137] found that certain patients (particularly those with epidermoid lung cancer) had elevated urinary levels of PGE-M and that these patients responded to treatment with salicylates.

In actual practice, responding patients are difficult to identify prospectively, and most clinical laboratories lack the facility to readily measure prostaglandin metabolites. Fewer than 5% of unselected patients with cancer-related hypercalcemia respond to any prostaglandin inhibitor, and it is generally not possible to predict which patients will respond based on clinical findings.[139,140] Indomethacin, 25 mg orally three times per day, or ibuprofen, 200 to 400 mg orally every 6 to 8 hr, can be attempted as a clinical trial in ambulatory patients. Because most nonsteroidal anti-inflammatory drugs decrease renal blood flow, the use of these drugs for treatment of hospitalized patients or those who have compromised renal function is not recommended.

SULFATE, CITRATE, EDTA. Sodium sulfate has been used to increase natriuresis because of its high sodium content and also because calcium sulfate complexes are formed in urine.[141] Sodium citrate has been used for similar reasons. However, these therapies are associated with substantial risks, including hypervolemia, congestive heart failure, pulmonary edema, and renal failure.[142,143] Ethylene diaminetetraacetate (EDTA) is a calcium-chelating agent that also has been associated with a particularly high frequency of renal failure when used in patients with hypercalcemia.[144] These agents are of historical interest only, and their use is no longer recommended.

CORTICOSTEROIDS. Glucocorticoids are widely used for the treatment of cancer-related hypercalcemia; however, their utility and efficacy are not clearly established. Steroids rapidly inhibit bone resorption by osteoclasts in vitro[145,146] and decrease calcium resorption from the gastrointestinal tract.[147,148]

Corticosteroids are most beneficial in patients whose underlying tumor may be responsive to the cytostatic action of these drugs. This includes patients with myeloma, lymphoma, leukemia, and occasional patients with carcinoma of the breast,[149,150] particularly those who have a hypercalcemic "flare" caused by treatment with hormones. Steroids do not have consistent hypocalcemic activity in other diseases.[151-153] The use of steroids in patients with cancer is associated with a variety of undesirable consequences. Steroid-induced hyperglycemia may exacerbate hypovolemia and contribute to a hyperosmolar state. Acute and chronic upper gastrointestinal bleeding may occur. Chronic use is associated with osteopenia that further compromises skeletal integrity in patients with bone metastases.

Prednisone in dosages of 40 to 100 mg/day (or equivalent) is usually effective in controlling hypercalcemia caused by hematologic cancers. Lower dosages (15–30 mg/day) may be useful for patients with hypercalcemic flares caused by breast cancer.

CALCITONIN. Calcitonin is secreted by parafollicular cells of the thyroid gland. Although the physiologic role of this hormone in normal calcium homeostasis is uncertain,[154] pharmacologic doses of calcitonin can reduce serum calcium by increasing renal calcium excretion and inhibiting bone resorption.[155-157] Calcitonin is especially advantageous because it is devoid of serious toxicity (other than rare hypersensitivity reactions). Given its lack of myelosuppression, the drug does not interfere with concurrent cytotoxic therapy. The onset of action occurs within 2 to 4 hr.[158-161] The hypocalcemic effect of calcitonin is relatively weak and rapidly wears off (so-called escape).[162,163] As shown in Figures 58-3 and 58-4, response to calcitonin peaks at 48 hr, with loss of the effect thereafter, despite continued treatment. Approximately 30% of hypercalcemic patients treated with calcitonin will achieve a normal serum calcium value. Maximally recommended doses of calcitonin (8 IU/kg every 6 hr) should be employed for short-term treatment of hypercalcemia, and the drug should be administered intramuscularly, rather than subcutaneously, to ensure complete absorption. For extended use, lower doses (4 IU/kg) can be injected subcutaneously once or twice each day on an ambulatory basis.

It is widely believed that the addition of corticosteroids enhances the effect of calcitonin. This belief is based on limited in vitro data,[162] an anecdotal report in parathyroid carcinoma,[164] and an uncontrolled clinical study wherein most patients had myeloma or lymphoma.[165] A more recent study has failed to show that patients treated with calcitonin plus steroids fared better than patients who received calcitonin alone.[115] Use of the combination should rest with the expectation that the patient's underlying disease will respond to steroids. As previously noted, this expectation is limited to patients with myeloma, lymphoma, leukemia, and certain patients with breast cancer.

DIPHOSPHONATES. Diphosphonates (or bisphosphonates) are chemical analogues of pyrophosphate. The compounds are not susceptible to hydrolysis by pyrophosphatase and thus are stable for long periods in vivo. Diphosphonates adsorb to the surface of crystalline hydroxyapatite and di-

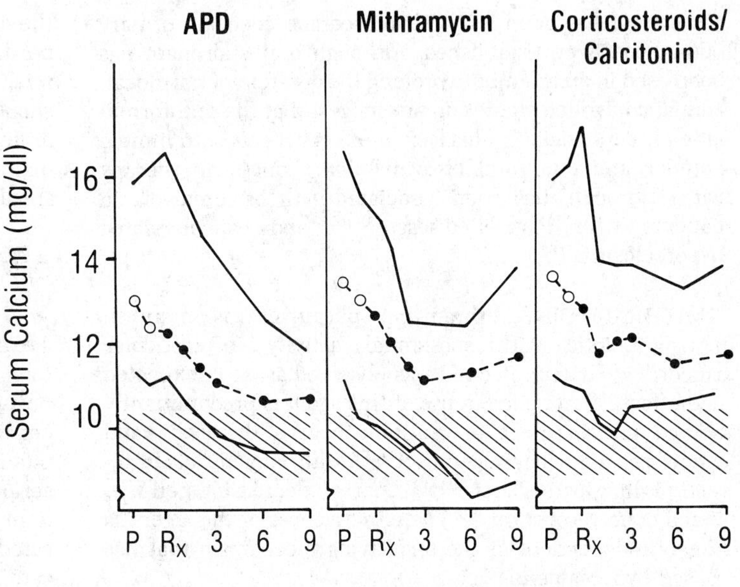

FIG. 58-3. Relative hypocalcemic effects of aminohydroxypropylidene diphosphonate (*APD*), mithramycin, and a combination of calcitonin plus corticosteroids. Data points represent the mean daily concentration of total serum calcium. Solid lines indicate the range of values. Shaded areas indicate the normal range for serum calcium concentration. (Adapted from Ralston SH, Gardner MD, Dryburgh FJ et al: Comparison of aminohydroxypropylidene diphosphonate, mithramycin, and corticosteroids/calcitonin in treatment of cancer-associated hypercalcemia. Lancet 2:907–910, 1985)

rectly inhibit calcium release from bone.[166,167] The main compounds in clinical use are ethane-1-hydroxydiphosphonate (EHDP; disodium etidronate), dichloromethylene diphosphonate (Cl_2MDP; clodronate), aminohydroxypropylidene diphosphonate (APD, and aminohydroxybutylidene biphosphate (AHButBP). The mechanism of action for each of these compounds appears to be different. Although all diphosphonates inhibit the growth and dissolution of hydroxyapatite crystals in vitro, the primary effect of Cl_2MDP appears to result from cytotoxicity to bone cells. Conversely, APD is toxic to osteoclasts only at suprapharmacologic concentrations. These agents do not affect the attachment of bone cells to matrix or decrease the solubility of bone mineral.[167]

Clinical investigations with clodronate[168-171] were suspended following reports of a potential association with acute leukemia; APD and AHButBP (still investigational) are the most potent diphosphonates currently in clinical trials.[172-174] In an open study, daily infusions of APD (up to 9 days) caused a delayed but sustained decrease in serum calcium (see Figure 58-4); however, approximately half of the patients remained persistently hypercalcemic.[175]

Only etidronate is commercially available. Reports of the effectiveness of etidronate have varied.[176,177] In a randomized study against saline placebo, a normal serum calcium level (corrected for albumin) was achieved in 27% of patients treated with intravenous etidronate.[178] This degree of potency is thus comparable with calcitonin.[115] Etidronate is administered intravenously at a maximum dosage of 7.5 mg/kg per day. The drug should be given as a slow infusion over 4–6 hr because acute renal failure has occurred with more rapid infusions.[179] The drug should not be given until

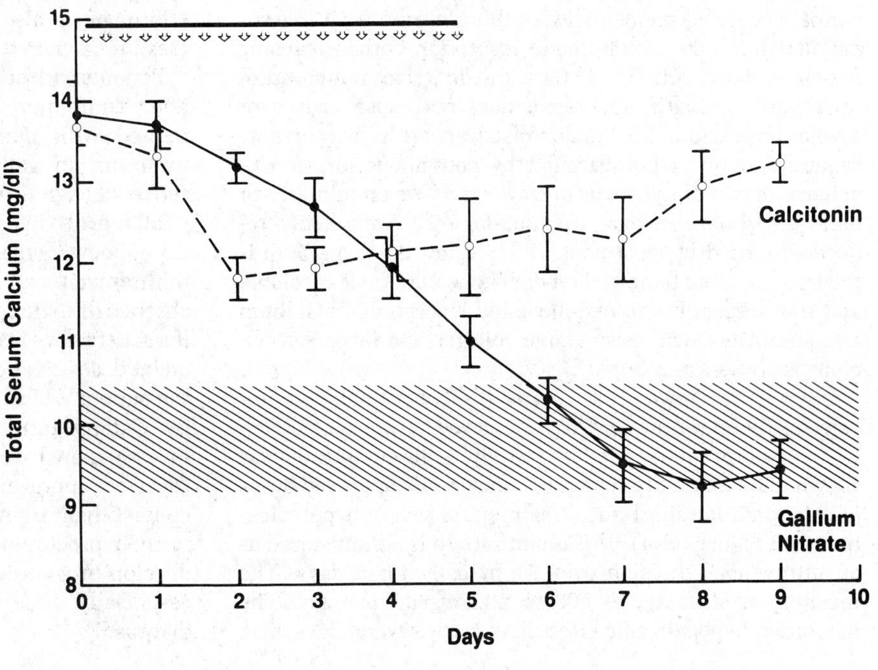

FIG. 58-4. Relative hypocalcemic effects of gallium nitrate and calcitonin. Solid line and closed data points represent mean daily concentrations (± SE) of serum calcium for patients receiving gallium nitrate; dashed line and open data points represent calcium concentrations for patients receiving calcitonin. Open arrows and solid bar at top indicate duration and frequency of calcitonin injections and gallium nitrate infusion, respectively. Normal range for total serum calcium is indicated by the shaded area. (Adapted from Warrell RP Jr, Israel R, Frisone M, et al: Gallium nitrate for acute treatment of cancer-related hypercalcemia: A randomized double-blind comparison to calcitonin. Ann Intern Med 108:669–674, 1988.)

the patient has been fully rehydrated and adequate urinary output has been established. Although oral etidronate has been used in an attempt to prolong the duration of normocalcemia, controlled studies do not suggest that the oral formulation is beneficial.[180] This lack of effect reflects both limited potency and poor oral bioavailability. Long-term therapy with etidronate has been associated with osteomalacia in patients with Paget's disease[181,182] and cancer-related hypercalcemia.[183]

MITHRAMYCIN. Mithramycin (plicamycin) is an antitumor antibiotic with substantial activity in testicular cancer.[184,185] Hypocalcemia was observed as an unexpected side-effect,[186] and current use of this agent is predominantly limited to treatment of resistant Paget's disease[187] and cancer-related hypercalcemia.[188-192] Mithramycin acts by directly killing osteoclasts,[193-197] thereby decreasing cell-mediated bone resorption.[198] The effectiveness of this agent is largely independent of the underlying mechanism that has caused hypercalcemia.

Mithramycin is administered at doses ranging from 10 to 50 μg/kg of body weight. (The usual dose is 25 μg/kg or 1.5–2.0 mg, total dose.) The drug can be administered as a bolus injection or as an infusion over 2 to 4 hr. The infusion may decrease the severity of nausea but does not otherwise improve tolerance or potency. Because the onset of action occurs after 24 to 48 hr, doses should not be repeated more frequently than every 2 days. Although a single injection is generally well tolerated, toxicity from mithramycin increases markedly with multiple injections. Cumulative renal toxicity and hepatotoxicity have occurred, even after relatively small doses.[199] Thrombocytopenia is a common side-effect and may interfere with the administration of other anticancer treatment. Less commonly, a poorly characterized bleeding diathesis has been observed— the incidence of which is increased in the presence of renal insufficiency.

GALLIUM NITRATE. Like mithramycin, gallium nitrate was originally developed as an anticancer agent and hypocalcemia was noted incidentally. Gallium nitrate (still investigational) directly inhibits bone resorption without causing toxicity to bone cells;[200-202] thus, the drug does not compromise bone strength. The agent does not cause nausea or myelosuppression. The major disadvantage is a (current) requirement for administration by continuous infusion to achieve maximal hypocalcemic effects.[203] As an inhibitor of bone resorption, urinary calcium losses are markedly reduced during drug treatment.[204-206] At low doses, gallium is incorporated into bone and renders bone mineral less soluble and less susceptible to cell-mediated resorption.[206] Gallium also stimulates synthesis of bone collagen and increases calcium accretion into bone.[207]

Open trials showed that 75% to 85% of patients who received gallium nitrate for 5 days achieved normocalcemia.[203] In a randomized double-blind study, gallium nitrate was shown to be markedly superior to maximally approved doses of calcitonin for short-term treatment of severe hypercalcemia (see Figure 58-4).[115] Gallium nitrate is administered as an intravenous infusion over 24 hr daily for 5 days. The recommended dosage is 100 to 200 mg/m^2 per day. The maximum hypocalcemic effect may occur several days after the drug has been discontinued. Thus, the drug infusion can be discontinued after patients have achieved normocalcemia. Nephrotoxicity is the major side-effect. The drug should be administered after the patient has been rehydrated, and a daily urinary output of 2000 ml should be maintained during the infusion. Aminoglycoside antibiotics should not be administered concomitantly.

GENERAL APPROACH TO TREATMENT OF HYPERCALCEMIA

Treatment of patients with hypercalcemia can be divided into two groups: those who require urgent therapy in the hospital, and patients for whom outpatient therapy can be considered. Table 58-15 lists treatment considerations. Hospitalization should be considered for any patient with a serum calcium level higher than 12.0 mg/dl or for any patient who is symptomatic. Hospitalization is especially indicated for patients who are dehydrated or who have a significant degree of nausea that precludes increased oral hydration. Hypercalcemia that has evolved slowly can rapidly progress when a patient develops vomiting or when cognition is impaired.

Emergency Treatment of Hospitalized Patients

Intravenous hydration is the initial treatment of choice for all patients who require hospitalization. Furosemide should be given if diuresis is inadequate or to avoid symptoms related to fluid retention. The only other therapy that can be safely administered close to the time of presentation is calcitonin. Large doses of calcitonin (4–8 units/kg as an intramuscular injection every 6–8 hr) can be given; however, the hypocalcemic effects of calcitonin are limited to the first 48 hr (see Figs 58-3 and 58-4) and are not enhanced by the routine administration of corticosteroids. Corticosteroids are distinctly beneficial if the primary disease is steroid responsive. Prednisone (or equivalent) should be administered at dosages of 40 to 100 mg/day for up to 7 days. Intravenous etidronate is also useful for mild forms of hypercalcemia (serum calcium ≤ 12.0 mg/dl).

Patients with severe hypercalcemia that has not responded after a minimum of 24 hr of vigorous hydration should be treated with more potent hypocalcemic drugs, such as mithramycin, gallium nitrate, APD, or AHButBP. In the absence of significant renal insufficiency (serum creatinine <2.0 mg/dl), hepatic dysfunction (bilirubin < 2.5 mg/dl), or thrombocytopenia (platelet count > 75,000 cells/mm^3), mithramycin can be administered at a dose of 25 μg/kg. In absence of toxic reactions, the dose can be repeated in 48 hr if a satisfactory hypocalcemic response is not evident. Subsequent doses can be repeated every 48 to 72 hr providing that the patient is closely monitored for signs of cumulative toxicity. Gallium nitrate, APD, and AHButBP are available on an investigational basis in the United States. Until they have received approval for general distribution, clinicians can contact the National Cancer Institute for information related to their procurement on an emergency basis. Patients who develop progressive renal insufficiency with hypercalcemia (especially those with myeloma) should be considered for dialysis.[208]

TABLE 58-15. Approach to the Management of Patients with Cancer-Related Hypercalcemia

Criteria to Ascertain Level of Care	
Outpatient	**Inpatient**
Serum calcium <12.0 mg/dl	Serum calcium ≥12.0 mg/dl
No significant nausea	Nausea or vomiting
Able to ingest fluids	Dehydration
Fatigue	Altered mental status
Normal renal function	Renal insufficiency
Stable cardiac rhythm	Cardiac arrhythmia
Mild constipation	Obstipation, ileus
Companion for supervision	Lives alone
Access to emergency care	Limited access to medical care
Medical Management	
Outpatient	**Inpatient**
LEVEL 1	
Increase oral hydration	Fluids IV (normal saline (200–400+ ml/hr)
Eliminate drugs	Electrolyte replacement as needed
Reduce dietary factors (*e.g.*, calcium, vitamins)	Monitor intake/output
Cytotoxic chemotherapy	
LEVEL 2	
Oral phosphates	Calcitonin
Corticosteroids (myeloma, lymphoma, breast)	Corticosteroids
Nonsteroidal anti-inflammatory drugs	Etidronate (IV)
LEVEL 3	
Calcitonin	Mithramycin
Mithramycin (10–25 μg/kg IV 1–2 × /wk)	Gallium nitrate
	APD
LEVEL 4	
Hospitalization	Renal dialysis

Ambulatory Management of Hypercalcemic Patients

Treatment of ambulatory patients is preferably undertaken in conjunction with specific cytotoxic therapy, such as radiation or chemotherapy. Certain anticancer drugs may have hypocalcemic actions independent of demonstrable effects on the primary tumor. Noteworthy are actinomycin D, doxorubicin, and cisplatin (in lung cancer).[209] The hypocalcemic mechanism appears to be the same as with mithramycin, namely direct cytotoxicity to bone cells.[210]

Ambulatory patients must receive clear instructions about increased oral fluid intake. The amount of fluid should be stated in terms the patient and family will understand. It is imperative that a family member or companion attend the patient to ensure that nausea resulting from worsening hypercalcemia does not lead to further dehydration. Diuretics such as furosemide generally should not be added because the risk of dehydration outweighs theoretical benefits in ambulatory patients who are not edematous. Oral phosphates can be extremely useful adjuncts. One to three g of oral neutral phosphorus per day in divided doses are usually well tolerated. Patients who receive phosphorus should not have preexisting hyperphosphatemia nor any significant degree of renal impairment (*i.e.*, creatinine clearance < 30 ml/min). Cortico-steroids are helpful where the underlying disease may be responsive. Subcutaneous injections of calcitonin (100–200 units/day) may be useful for mild forms of hypercalcemia. Oral etidronate, the only diphosphonate currently available, is not useful for long-term treatment. Newer diphosphonates have greater promise and are available on an investigational basis. Gallium nitrate can be administered subcutaneously, and an oral formulation of gallium may become available; however, maintenance of normocalcemia by continuing administration has not been rigorously evaluated. Finally, mithramycin can be administered in doses of 10 to 25 μg/kg once or twice per week. Patients who receive mithramycin therapy as outpatients must be closely monitored for evidence of myelosuppression and for changes in renal or hepatic function.

HYPERURICEMIA

Clinical syndromes caused by hyperuricemia present with extreme elevations of serum uric acid that develop rapidly or, with lower elevations they may be of longer duration. Renal complications are the only important consequences of hyperuricemia,[211–214] although acute attacks of gouty arthritis have occasionally been observed.[215]

Hyperuricemia occurs most commonly in hematologic disorders, particularly the leukemias (both acute and chronic),[215] high-grade lymphomas (especially Burkitt's-type),[211,216,217] and myeloproliferative diseases such as polycythemia vera.[218] Acute urate nephropathy has also been reported after chemotherapy for solid tumors.[215,219] Patients with extensive, anaplastic, and rapidly proliferating tumors appear to be at highest risk. Hyperuricemia is also a specific side-effect of certain cytotoxic agents, notably tiazofurin[220] and the aminothiadiazoles.[221]

PATHOPHYSIOLOGY

Uric acid is formed as a result of the sequential catalysis of hypoxanthine and xanthine by the enzyme xanthine oxidase. Renal insufficiency develops when urine becomes supersaturated with urate, and crystals of uric acid form in the renal tubules and distal collecting system.[212,222-224] Uric acid stones may also develop, although this presentation is more commonly associated with chronic hyperuricemia.[225]

A variety of drugs can contribute to hyperuricemia, either by increasing production or by decreasing excretion.[221] Although diuretics (such as thiazides, furosemide, and ethacrynic acid) cause an acute uricosuria, hyperuricemia may occur as a result of volume contraction.[222] Drugs used for the treatment of tuberculosis (pyrizinamide, ethambutol, and nicotinic acid) are also commonly associated with hyperuricemia.

Acute renal failure is the most serious consequence of hyperuricemia, and major therapeutic effort should be undertaken to prevent this outcome. Recognition of patients at risk is essential for proper therapy. Patients at highest risk include those with bulky lymphomas (especially high-grade),[216] and patients undergoing remission-induction chemotherapy for acute leukemia. Patients with chronic myelocytic leukemia (especially those in accelerated or blastic phase) and patients with chronic lymphocytic leukemia who have extremely high leukocyte counts ($> 100{,}000/mm^3$) are also at risk. Individuals with preexisting renal impairment (especially those with ureteral obstruction caused by abdominal lymphoma) are likewise at high risk.

TREATMENT

It is essential that prophylactic measures be undertaken *before* cytotoxic therapy is initiated. Drugs that tend to elevate serum urate[212] or that produce an acidic urine should be withdrawn (especially thiazides and salicylates). All patients should receive intravenous hydration to correct preexisting deficits of intravascular volume and to ensure continued urinary output. Increased urinary volume decreases the concentration of urate in urine and thus minimizes problems with respect to urate solubility.[227] Potent diuretics such as furosemide may be used as needed to maintain satisfactory urine output as long as urine volume and electrolytes are carefully monitored and replaced as needed. Although furosemide theoretically promotes increased tubular urate reabsorption, this effect is outweighed by its diuretic action in the acute setting.

Alkalization of the urine should also be initiated to maintain a urine pH ≥ 7.0. In principle, oral sodium bicarbonate can be used. However, to ensure compliance, it is simpler to add sodium bicarbonate solution (50–100 mmol/liter) to intravenous fluids and to then adjust the concentrations so that an alkaline urine pH is maintained. Acetazolamide (an inhibitor of carbonic anhydrase) can also be used to increase the effects of alkalization. It should be recognized that alkalization is secondary to the overall goal of decreasing urinary uric acid concentration by increasing urinary volume.[227]

The mainstay of current drug therapy is allopurinol.[228-230] Initially developed as a method of cancer treatment,[231] allopurinol was found to cause hypouricemia,[232] and this indication represents its major current use. Allopurinol inhibits xanthine oxidase, which is responsible for the enzymatic conversion of hypoxanthine to xanthine and of xanthine to uric acid. As a consequence, plasma and urinary concentrations of xanthine and hypoxanthine are increased. Although xanthine is somewhat more soluble than uric acid, allopurinol has occasionally been associated with renal failure because of xanthine nephropathy.[233-236] Administration of allopurinol is also associated with increases in the urinary concentrations of orotidine and orotic acid,[237] as well as depletion of intraerythrocytic phosphoribosylpyrophosphate (PRPP).[238]

Allopurinol is generally well tolerated. The most common adverse reaction is a blanching, erythematous skin rash, which indicates hypersensitivity. The onset of this reaction is usually delayed for several days after initial administration. The drug can usually be given throughout the period of greatest need in patients who have not had prior exposure. In acute situations, the drug is administered orally once or twice a day in daily dosages ranging from 300 to 900 mg. Intravenous allopurinol is available on an investigational basis.[239] The dose of certain drugs that are metabolized by xanthine oxidase (*e.g.*, 6-mercaptopurine) must be substantially reduced during treatment with allopurinol.

Patients in renal failure and those individuals who have previously received allopurinol and developed hypersensitivity, vasculitis, or blood dyscrasias represent uncommon but difficult management problems.[240] Apazone (azapropazone)[241,242] and benzbromarone are effective hypouricemic drugs that are available on an investigational basis. Merbarone, a nonsedating thiobarbiturate, is a newly developed inhibitor of xanthine oxidase that is also uricosuric.[243] This agent may be useful in patients who are intolerant of or resistant to allopurinol. The IV administration of uricase has also been useful in circumstances in which allopurinol was not available.[244]

In the face of acute oliguria, ureteral obstruction by urate calculi should be evaluated by ultrasonography or CT scanning. Administration of intravenous contrast agents for pyelography should be avoided because of an increased risk of acute tubular necrosis.[245] Peritoneal or hemodialysis has been quite effective in reversing renal failure caused by urate deposition.[214,246]

TUMOR LYSIS SYNDROME

The tumor lysis syndrome occurs as a result of the rapid release of intracellular contents into the bloodstream which then increase to life-threatening concentrations. The syndrome is characterized by hyperuricemia, hyperkalemia, hyperphosphatemia, and hypocalcemia. The consequences of hyperuricemia are detailed in the preceding section. Lethal cardiac arrhythmias are the most serious consequences of hyperkalemia. Hyperphosphatemia may result in acute renal failure.[247-249] Elevated serum phosphorus may decrease renal function which leads to further reductions in urinary excretion of potassium and phosphate. Hypocalemia—a result of hyperphosphatemia—may cause muscle cramps, cardiac arrhythmias, and tetany.

The tumor lysis syndrome occurs most commonly in diseases with large tumor burdens and high proliferative fractions that are exquisitely sensitive to cytotoxic treatment.

These disorders include high-grade lymphomas,[216,250–253] leukemias with high leukocyte counts,[249,254–256] and, less commonly, solid tumors.[257–259] The syndrome has occurred with investigational drugs, not only with agents that have potent myelosuppressive activity (such as amsacrine,[260] homoharringtonine,[261] and etoposide [VP-16-213][262]), but also with drugs generally thought to have marginal bone marrow toxicity, such as interferon-α[263] and tamoxifen.[264] Although technically not related to tumor lysis, severe hypocalcemia has been associated with cisplatin treatment,[265] estrogenic treatment of prostate cancer,[266] and with accelerated bone formation in patients with leukemia.[267]

TREATMENT

Recognition of risk and prevention are essential to the management of this disorder. Patients at risk should be identified before the initiation of chemotherapy. Intravenous hydration should be started 48 hr before the administration of chemotherapy. Any acid–base or electrolyte disorders should be corrected, although intravenous administration of sodium bicarbonate may aggravate symptoms of hypocalcemia. Treatment with allopurinol should be undertaken along with other measures to minimize hyperuricemia as described earlier. Serum electrolytes, uric acid, phosphorus, calcium, and creatinine levels should be checked repeatedly for 3 to 4 days after initiating cytotoxic treatment. The frequency of monitoring should depend on the clinical condition of the patient. If hyperkalemia or hypocalcemia become evident, an electrocardiogram should be obtained, and the cardiac rhythm should be monitored while these abnormalities are corrected. Hypocalcemia can be corrected with intravenous administration of calcium gluconate; however, hypocalcemia may persist for several days despite continued therapy. Hyperkalemia (serum $K^+ \geq 5.0$ mg/dl) should be treated with an oral sodium–potassium exchange resin (*e.g.*, Kayexalate 15 g orally every 6 hr).

In the face of acutely worsening renal function after administration of chemotherapy, consideration should be given to the *early* initiation of renal dialysis to rapidly control serum concentrations of potassium, calcium, phosphate, and uric acid, as well as other problems related to uremia.[215] The dose of many drugs, especially antineoplastics, requires substantial modification in the presence of renal insufficiency.[268]

HYPOGLYCEMIA

Insulin-producing islet cell tumors are the most frequent cause of hypoglycemia in patients with cancer. However, more than 250 cases of hypoglycemia associated with non-islet cell tumors have also been reported.[269,270] In contrast with islet cell tumors, malignant tumors associated with hypoglycemia tend to be large. In such patients, mesenchymal tumors (fibrosarcomas, leiomyomas, rhabdomyosarcomas, liposarcomas, and mesotheliomas) compose approximately 50% of cases, with hepatomas making up an additional 25%.[269]

Classic symptoms of hypoglycemia (*e.g.*, weakness, dizziness, diaphoresis, nausea) are nonspecific and may develop slowly. In the initial phases, symptoms tend to be worse in the early morning (a result of fasting overnight), with improvement after ingestion of food. However, patients may also have focal and diffuse neurologic deficits, seizures, or coma.

PATHOPHYSIOLOGY

Several etiologic mechanisms for cancer-related hypoglycemia have been proposed: [1] secretion of "insulin-like" substances, [2] excessive glucose utilization by the tumor which exceeds hepatic production, and [3] failure of counterregulatory mechanisms that usually prevent hypoglycemia.

Substances with nonsuppressible insulin-like activities (NSILAs) have been detected in serum from patients with hypoglycemia. These factors comprise two general classes. The first group includes compounds of low molecular weight that are soluble in acid–ethanol.[271–273] The second group includes high-molecular-weight substances that are precipitated by acid–ethanol. The low-molecular-weight compounds consist of four peptides that are insulin-like growth factors (IGF-I, IGF-II, somatomedin A, and somatomedin C).[274,275] Both IGF-I and II share a high degree of amino acid similarity with proinsulin, but they do not react with anti-insulin antibodies. Like insulin, both of these IGFs promote growth and increase sulfate incorporation into cartilage, but they have only 1% to 2% of the specific metabolic activity of insulin. The NSILAs with high molecular weights are not well characterized.

By use of a radioreceptor assay, approximately 40% of cancer patients with symptomatic hypoglycemia have been shown to have elevated plasma levels of low-molecular-weight NSILAs.[270,276] These observations have suggested that humoral mechanisms (*i.e.*, tumor production of IGFs) might be responsible for hypoglycemia in a large proportion of patients.

Accelerated glucose catabolism by large tumors could also account for cancer-related hypoglycemia.[277] It has been estimated that a 1-kg tumor may catabolize from 50 to 200 g of glucose per day.[277] Because the liver can produce approximately 700 g of glucose per day, hepatic production should theoretically be sufficient to prevent hypoglycemia. However, many patients with hypoglycemia have tumors with weights of several kilograms, along with extensive hepatic metastases. This, the combination of accelerated glucose catabolism with impaired production, may lead to hypoglycemia.

Finally, a failure of the usual counterregulatory mechanisms in patients with large tumors may also induce hypoglycemia. Impaired liver function can decrease glycogenolysis and gluconeogenesis. Certain patients with cancer have a depressed hyperglycemic response to the administration of glucagon, and depressed secretion of counterregulatory hormones such as glucagon, ACTH, glucocorticoids, and growth hormone has also been noted. However, insufficient data currently exist to establish the importance of these mechanisms as independent causes of hypoglycemia.

THERAPY

Therapy of hypoglycemia should match the severity of the condition. As with most paraneoplastic syndromes, specific antitumor therapy is the preferred method of treatment. To date, chemotherapeutic agents that are cytotoxic for islet cells or that block insulin release or activity have had no effect on production, release, or activity of NSILAs.

Mild hypoglycemia can usually be managed by increasing the frequency of feedings. In patients with more severe or unpredictable symptoms, the administration of corticosteroids and glucagon may afford symptomatic relief. Intravenous infusions of glucose provide temporary support while other specific treatment is administered (*i.e.*, surgery, chemotherapy, or radiation). Under certain circumstances, continuous infusions of glucagon with portable pumps have been used with some success.[279]

ADRENAL FAILURE

Symptomatic adrenocortical insufficiency caused by destruction of cortical tissue by metastatic carcinoma is uncommon. However, technical improvements in CT and magnetic resonance imaging (MRI) have increased the likelihood of making an antemortem diagnosis of this condition. In a recent study, 19% of patients with metastatic cancer and enlargement of the adrenal glands by CT scans developed symptoms of adrenal insufficiency.[280] In a separate study wherein 15 patients with metastatic cancer and adrenal enlargement on CT scan were evaluated by ACTH (cosyntropin) stimulation, one-third were judged to have adrenal insufficiency. Further clinical study revealed symptoms of nausea, anorexia, and orthostatic hypotension in all of these patients.[281] Adrenal insufficiency may thus develop insidiously in patients with adrenal metastasis, and CT scans and ACTH testing may be useful diagnostic tools.

Iatrogenic causes of adrenal insufficiency are particularly common. Surgical adrenalectomy for breast cancer results in total adrenal insufficiency. The administration of mitotane (*o-p′*-DDD) and inhibitors of steroid synthesis, such as aminoglutethimide, can produce adrenal insufficiency in a dose-dependent fashion. However, current use of aminoglutethimide (*i.e.*, $\leq$ 1.0 g/day) can effect a reduction in adrenal sex steroids without a high frequency of glucocorticoid or mineralocorticoid insufficiency.[282] Short courses of high-dose glucocorticoid treatment in patients with malignant lymphoma can cause biochemical evidence of impaired adrenal function.[284] However, such therapy is rarely associated with symptoms and does not require routine endocrinologic investigation. Prolonged use of glucocorticoids at supraphysiologic levels can lead to suppression of the pituitary–adrenal axis. Therefore, the dose of steroids should be tapered slowly and the integrity of this axis evaluated when chronic steroid therapy is abruptly discontinued.

CLINICAL MANIFESTATIONS

Classic signs and symptoms of adrenal insufficiency include weakness, weight loss, anorexia, hyperpigmentation of skin and mucous membranes, and postural hypotension. One or more of these symptoms are evident in almost all patients. The onset of symptoms is insidious. Severe circulatory collapse and shock are uncommon but may develop with the onset of infection. Biochemical evaluation frequently reveals a mild acidosis without an anion gap, hyponatremia, and hypokalemia.

EVALUATION AND TREATMENT

As an ACTH-stimulation test is a benign procedure, this test is recommended when symptoms suggestive of adrenal insufficiency are evident. Typically, patients receive cosyntropin 0.25 mg IV and serum cortisol is monitored at baseline, 30 min, and 1 hr. An increase in serum cortisol of 5 to 7 μg/dl over baseline levels (to a minimum of 15 μg/dl) is considered a normal response. If adrenal insufficiency is strongly suspected on clinical grounds, steroid replacement therapy (or stress doses of steroids) should be started immediately. Therapy can subsequently be reevaluated when results of the ACTH test become available.

Physiologic glucocorticoid replacement is attained by administration of cortisone acetate 25 mg in the morning with an additional 12.5 mg in the early evening. During periods of stress (*e.g.*, operative procedures or infection), these doses may need to be doubled or tripled. Occasionally, mineralocorticoid replacement with 0.05 to 0.1 mg of fludrocortisone is required in addition to cortisone acetate. In patients with no adrenocortical function whatsoever, maintenance doses of dexamethasone or prednisone do not provide adequate mineralocorticoid coverage, and fludrocortisone must be given. Pharmacologic doses of parenteral glucocorticoids are required in the setting of acute adrenal failure and circulatory collapse. Typically, aqueous-soluble forms of hydrocortisone (*e.g.*, sodium succinate salt) at dosages of 100 mg IV every 8 hr are required. Thereafter, the patient should be monitored for evidence of hyperglycemia, hypokalemia, or hypernatremia.

LACTIC ACIDOSIS

Lactic acidosis is a rare, but potentially severe, metabolic complication in patients with cancer. Type A lactic acidosis is due to impaired delivery of oxygen to peripheral tissue and is commonly seen with shock and septicemia (Table 58-16). Type B lactic acidosis is associated with a variety of diseases (including diabetes, renal failure, liver disease, infection, and cancer) as well as drugs, toxins, and hereditary diseases.

Lactic acidosis presents with a decreased arterial pH ($<$ 7.37) secondary to accumulation of blood lactate ($>$ 2 mEq/liter). The disorder is a consequence of both increased lactate production and impaired catabolism. Lactate is a metabolite of pyruvate and is produced in a cytosolic reaction catalyzed by lactic dehydrogenase. The enzyme has an absolute requirement for nicotinamide adenine dinucleotide (NAD). Consequently, the concentrations of pyruvate, hydrogen ion, and NAD regulate lactate metabolism. Accelerated glycogenolysis increases pyruvate production and decreases tissue oxygen, which in turn decreases levels of NAD. As NAD is depleted, gluconeogenesis is halted and

TABLE 58-16. Classification and Causes of Lactic Acidosis

Type A: Tissue hypoxia	*Type B*
Shock	Diseases
Cardiogenic	Cancer
Endotoxic	Infection
Hypovolemic	Hepatic failure
Severe anemia	Renal insufficiency
Congestive heart failure	Diabetes mellitus
Asphyxia	Drugs/toxins
Carbon monoxide poisoning	Biguanides
	Salicylates
	Ethanol
	Methanol
	Fructose
	Sorbitol
	Xylitol
	Ethylene glycol
	Hereditary diseases
	Glucose-6-phosphate deficiency
	Fructose-1-6-diphosphatase deficiency
	Pyruvate dehydrogenase and carboxylase deficiency
	Defective oxidative phosphorylation deficiency

Adapted from Frommer.[286]

pyruvate increases. Anaerobic metabolism of pyruvate to lactate is increased, which also leads to accumulation of NADH and hydrogen ion.[285-288]

Sculier and associates recently reviewed 25 cases of lactic acidosis in which the underlying tumor was believed to represent the primary causal factor.[289] More than two-thirds of these cases were associated with leukemia or lymphoma, with the remainder in various solid tumors. The development of lactic acidosis coincided with the onset of progressive disease, and most patients with solid tumors had extensive liver metastases.

Typically, the patient with lactic acidosis presents with hyperventilation and hypotension. Nonspecific clinical symptoms such as tachycardia, weakness, nausea, and stupor may proceed to frank shock as the acidosis worsens. Laboratory studies show decreased blood pH, a widened anion gap, and low serum bicarbonate.

The prognosis for patients with a serum lactate concentration greater than 4 mEq/liter is exceedingly poor. Symptomatic treatment is usually unsuccessful. Several reports have suggested that administration of sodium bicarbonate increases production of lactate and CO_2 and impairs oxygen delivery, without improving survival.[290-292] However, prognosis is largely determined by the underlying disease, not the acidosis. Detrimental effects of severe acidemia on cardiovascular function[293,294] can probably be ameliorated by bicarbonate administration, and this temporizing measure may be useful while effective anticancer therapy is attempted.[295,296]

REFERENCES

1. Fisken RA, Heath DA, Bold AM: Hypercalcemia—a hospital survey. QJ Med 49:405–418, 1980
2. Mundy GR: Primary hyperparathyroidism: Changes in the pattern of clinical presentation. Lancet 1:1317–1320, 1980
3. Hicker RC, Samaan NA, Jackson GL et al: Hypercalcemia in patients with breast cancer. Arch Surg 116:545–552, 1981
4. Mundy GR, Bertolini DR: Bone destruction and hypercalcemia in plasma cell myeloma. Semin Oncol 13:291–299, 1986
5. Mundy GR, Martin TJ: The hypercalcemia of malignancy: Pathogenesis and management. Metabolism 31:1247–1277, 1982
6. Bender RA, Hanson H: Hypercalcemia in bronchogenic carcinoma: A prospective study of 200 patients. Ann Intern Med 80:205–208, 1974
7. Coggeshall J, Merrill W, Hande K, Des Prez R: Implications of hypercalcemia with respect to diagnosis and treatment of lung cancer. Am J Med 80:325–328, 1986
8. Hayward ML Jr, Howell DA, O'Donnell JF, Maurer LH: Hypercalcemia complicating small cell carcinoma. Cancer 48:1643–1646, 1981
9. Strewler GJ, Nissenson RA: Nonparathyroid hypercalcemia. Adv Intern Med 32:235–258, 1987
10. Insogna KL, Broadus AE: Hypercalcemia of malignancy. Annu Rev Med 38:241–256, 1987
11. Boyd JC, Ladenson JH: Value of laboratory tests in the differential diagnosis of hypercalcemia. Am J Med 77:863–872, 1984
12. Heath HH III, Hodgson SF, Kenedy MA: Primary hyperparathyroidism; incidence, morbidity, and potential economic impact on the community. N Engl J Med 302:189–193, 1980
13. Monsaingon A, Ridoux G, Thomas J et al: Cancer du sein metastique et hyperparathyroidie. Chiurgie 104:804–811, 1978
14. Katz AK, Kaplan L, Massry SG et al: Primary hyperparathyroidism in patients with breast carcinoma. Arch Surg 101:582–585, 1970
15. Vichayanrat A, Avraamides A, Gardner B et al: Primary hyperparathyroidism and breast cancer. Am J Med 61:136–139, 1976
16. Farr HW, Fahey TJ Jr, Nash AG et al: Primary hyperparathyroidism and cancer. Am J Surg 126:539–543, 1973
17. Axelrod DM, Bockman RS, Wong GY et al: Distinguishing features of primary hyperparathyroidism in patients with breast cancer. Cancer 60:1620–1624, 1987
18. Wills MR: Value of plasma chloride concentration and acid–base status in the differential diagnosis of hyperparathyroidism from other causes of hypercalcaemia. J Clin Pathol 24:219–227, 1971
19. Lufkin EG, Kao PC, Heath H: Parathyroid hormone radioimmunoassays in the differential diagnosis of hypercalcemia due to primary hyperparathyroidism or malignancy. Ann Intern Med 106:559–560, 1987
20. Kvetny J, Orthman-Brask H, Frederiksen PK et al: Hypercalcemia due to primary hyperparathyroidism or malignant disease. Evaluated by means of biochemical tests and the steroid suppression test. Acta Med Scand 212:163–166, 1982
21. Watson L, Moxham J, Fraser P: Hydrocortisone suppression test and discriminant analysis in differential diagnosis of hypercalcemia. Lancet 1:1320–1325, 1980
22. Hazani A, Silvian I, Tatarsky I, Spira G: Non-symptomatic hypercalcemia in a myeloma patient. Am J Med Sci 283:169–273, 1982
23. Annesley TM, Burritt MF, Kyle RA: Artifactual hypercalcemia in multiple myeloma. Mayo Clin Proc 57:572–575, 1982
24. Payne RB, Carver ME, Morgan DB: Interpretation of serum total calcium: Effects of adjustment for albumin concentration on frequency of abnormal values and on detection of change in the individual. J Clin Pathol 32:56–60, 1979

25. Doppelt SH, Slovik DM, Neer RM et al: Gut-mediated hypercalcemia in rabbits bearing VX_2 carcinoma: New mechanism for tumor-induced hypercalcemia. Proc Nat Acad Sci USA 79:640-644, 1982
26. Coombes RC, Ward MK, Greenberg PB et al: Calcium metabolism in cancer: Studies using calcium isotopes and immunoassays for parathyroid hormone and calcitonin. Cancer 38:2111-2120, 1976
27. Heyburn PJ, Child JA, Peacock M: Relative importance of renal failure and increased bone resorption in the hypercalcemia of myelomatosis. J Clin Pathol 334:54-57, 1981
28. Elion G, Mundy GR: Direct resorption of bone by human breast cancer cells in vitro. Nature 276:726-728, 1978
29. Ralston S, Fogelman I, Gardner MD, Boyle IT: Hypercalcaemia and metastatic bone disease: Is there a causal link? Lancet 2:903-905, 1982
30. Ralston SH, Fogelman I, Gardner MD, Boyle IT: Relative contribution of humoral and metastatic factors to the pathogenesis of hypercalcaemia of malignancy. Br Med J 288:1405-1408, 1984
31. Albright F: Case Records of the Massachusetts General Hospital (#39061) N Engl J Med 225:789-791, 1941
32. Rizzoli R, Caverzasia J, Fleisch H, Bonjour JP: Parathyroid hormone-like changes in renal calcium and phosphate reabsorption induced by Leydig cell tumor in thyroparathyroidectomized rats. Endocrinology 119:1004-1009, 1986
33. Stewart AF, Horst R, Deftos LJ et al: Biochemical evaluation of patients with cancer-associated hypercalcemia: Evidence for humoral and non-humoral groups. N Engl J Med 303:1377-1383, 1980
34. Kukreja SC, Shemerdiak WP, Lad TE et al: Elevated nephrogenous cyclic AMP with normal serum parathyroid hormone levels in patients with lung cancer. J Clin Endocrinol Metab 52:765-771, 1980
35. Berson SA, Yalow RS: Parathyroid hormone in plasma in adenomatous hyperparathyroidism, uremia, and bronchogenic carcinoma. Science 154:907-909, 1966
36. Benson RC, Riggs BL, Pickard BM et al: Immunoreactive forms of circulating parathyroid hormone in primary and ectopic hyperparathyroidism. J Clin Invest 54:175-181, 1979
37. Skrabanek P, McPartlin J, Powell D: Tumor hypercalcemia and "ectopic hyperparathyroidism." Medicine 59:262-282, 1980
38. Simpson EL, Mundy GR, D'Souza SM et al: Absence of parathyroid messenger RNA in nonparathyroid tumors associated with hypercalcemia. N Engl J Med 309:325-330, 1983
39. Broadus AC, Goltzman D, Webb AC, Kronenberg HM: Messenger ribonucleic acid from tumors associated with humoral hypercalcemia of malignancy directs the synthesis of a secretory parathyroid hormone-like peptide. Endocrinology. 117:1661-1666, 1985
40. Strewler GJ, Williams RJ, Nissenson RA: Human renal carcinoma cells produce hypercalcemia in the nude mouse and a novel protein recognized by parathyroid hormone receptors. J Clin Invest 71:769-774, 1983
41. Stewart AF, Insogna KL, Goltzman D, Broadus AE: Identification of adenylate cyclase-stimulating activity and cytochemical glucose-6-phosphate dehydrogenase-stimulating acitivity in extracts of tumors from patients with humoral hypercalcemia of malignancy. Proc Natl Acad Sci USA 80:1454-1458, 1983
42. Stewart AF, Wu T, Burtis WJ et al: The relative potency of a human tumor-derived PTH-like adenylate cyclase-stimulating preparation in three bioassays. J Bone Miner Res 2:37-43, 1987
43. Rodan SB, Insogna KL, Vignery M-C et al: Factors associated with humoral hypercalcemia of malignancy stimulate adenlyate cyclase in osteoblastic cells. J Clin Invest 72:1511-1515, 1983
44. Moseley JM, Kubota M, Dieffenbach-Jagger H et al: Parathyroid hormone-related protein purified from a human lung cancer cell line. Proc Natl Acad Sci USA 84:5048-5052, 1987
45. Suva LJ, Winslow GA, Wettenhall REH et al: A parathyroid hormone-related protein implicated in malignant hypercalcemia: Cloning and expression. Science 237:894-897, 1987
46. Burtis WJ, Wu T, Bunch C et al: Identification of a novel 17,000-dalton parathyroid hormone-like adenylate cyclase-stimulating protein from a tumor associated with humoral hypercalcemia of malignancy. J Biol Chem 262:7151-7156, 1987
47. Merendino JJ Jr, Insogna KL, Milstone LM et al: A parathyroid hormone-like protein from cultured human keratinocytes. Science 231:288-290, 1986
48. Horiuchi N, Hlick MF, Potts JT Jr, Rosenblatt M: A parathyroid inhibitor in vivo: Design and biological evaluation of a hormone analog. Science 220:1053-1055, 1983
49. D'Souza SM, Ibbotson JH, Mundy GR: Failure of parrathyroid hormone antagonists to inhibit in vitro bone resorbing activity produced by two animal models of the humoral hypercalcemia of malignancy. J Clin Invest 74:1104-1107, 1984
50. Brereton HD, Halushka PV, Alexander RW et al: Indomethacin-responsive hypercalcemia in a patient with renal-cell adenocarcinoma. N Engl J Med 291:83-85, 1974
51. Seyberth HW, Segre GV, Morgan JL et al: Prostaglandins as mediators of hypercalcemia associated with certain types of cancer. N Engl J Med 293:1278-1283, 1975
52. Atkins D, Ibbotson KJ, Hillier K et al: Secretion of prostaglandins as bone resorbing agents by renal cortical carcinoma in culture. Br J Cancer 36:601-607, 1977
53. Greaves M, Ibbotson KJ, Atkins D et al: Prostaglandins as mediators of bone resorption in renal and breast tumors. Clin Sci 58:201-210, 1980
54. Tashjian AH Jr: Prostaglandins, hypercalcemia and cancer. N Engl J Med 293:1317-1318, 1975
55. Robertson RB, Baylink DJ, Metz SA, Cummings KB: Plasma prostaglandin E in patients with cancer with and without hypercalcemia. J Clin Endocrinol Metab 43:1330-1335, 1976
56. Demers LM, Allegra JC, Harvey HA et al: Plasma prostaglandins in hypercalcemic patients with neoplastic disease. Cancer 39:1559-1562, 1977
57. Tashjian AH Jr, Tice JE, Sides R: Biological activities of prostaglandin analogues and metabolites on bone resorption in vitro. Nature 266:645-647, 1977
58. Raisz LG, Dietrich JW, Simmons HA et al: Effects of prostaglandin endoperoxides and metabolites on bone resorption in vitro. Nature 267:532-535, 1977
59. Klein DC, Raisz LG: Prostaglandins: Stimulation of bone resorption in tissue culture. Endocrinology 85:657-661, 1970
60. Legha SA, Powell K, Buzdar AU et al: Tamoxifen-induced hypercalcemia in breast cancer. Cancer 47:2803-2806, 1981
61. Valentin-Opran A, Eilon G, Saez S et al: Estrogens and antiestrogens stimulate release of bone-resorbing activity by cultured human breast cancer cells. J Clin Invest 75:726, 1985
62. Brenner BE, Harvey HA, Lipton A, Demers L: A study of prostaglandin E_2, parathormone, and response to indomethacin in patients with hypercalcemia of malignancy. Cancer 49:556-561, 1982
63. Metz SA, McRae JR, Robertson RP: Prostaglandins as mediators of paraneoplastic syndromes: Review and update. Metabolism 30:299-316, 1981
64. Gebhardt MC, Lippiello L, Bringhurst FR, Mankin HJ: Prostaglandin E_2 synthesis by human primary and metastatic bone tumors in culture. Clin Orthop 186:300-305, 1985
65. Lau K-HW, Lee MY, Linkhart TA et al: A mouse tumor-derived osteolytic factor stimulates bone resorption by a mechanism involving local prostaglandins production in bone. Biochim Biophys Acta 840:56-68, 1985
66. Bringhurst FR, Bierer BE, Godeau F et al: Humoral hypercalcemia of malignancy: Release of a prostaglandin-stimulating bone-resorbing factor in vitro by human transitional-cell carcinoma cells. J Clin Invest 77:456-464, 1986
67. Yoneda T, Mundy GR: Prostaglandins are necessary for osteoclast activating factor production in activated peripheral blood leukocytes. J Exp Med 149:279-283, 1979
68. Wahl LM, Olsen CE, Sandberg AL, Mergenhage SE: Prostaglandins regulation of macrophage collagenase production. Proc Natl Acad Sci USA, 74:4955-4958, 1977
69. Tashjian AH, Voelkel EF, Lazzaro M et al: Alpha and beta transforming growth factors stimulate prostaglandin production and bone resorption in cultured mouse calvaria. Proc Natl Acad Sci USA 82:4535-4538, 1985
70. Mundy RR, Raisz LG, Cooper RA et al: Evidence for the secretion of an osteoclast stimulating factor in myeloma. N Engl J Med 291:1041-1046, 1974
71. Mundy GR, Luben RA, Raisz LG et al: Bone-resorbing activity in supernatants from lymphoid cell lines. N Engl J Med 290:867-871, 1974
72. Sporn MB, Roberts AB: Autocrine growth factors and cancer. Nature 313:745-747, 1985
73. Ibbotson KJ, Twardzik DR, D'Souza SM et al: Stimulation of bone resorption in vitro by synthetic transforming growth factor-alpha. Science 228:1007-1009, 1985
74. Mundy GR, Ibbotson, KJ, D'Souza SM et al: Evidence that transforming growth factor alpha production causes bone resorption and hypercalcemia in squamous cell carcinoma of the lung. Clin Res 573A, 1985
75. Stern PH, Krieger NS, Nissenson RA et al: Human transforming growth factor-alpha stimulates bone resorption in vitro. J Clin Invest 76:2016-2019, 1985
76. Ibbotson KJ, D'Souza SM, Ng KW et al: Tumor derived growth factor increases bone resorption in a tumor associated with humoral hypercalcemia of malignancy. Science 221:1292-1294, 1983
77. Todaro GJ, Fryling C, De Larco JE: Transforming growth factors produced by certain human tumor cells: Polypeptides that interact with epidermal growth factor receptors. Proc Natl Acad Sci USA 77:5258-5262, 1980
78. Ibbotson KJ, D'Souza SM, Smith DD et al: EGF receptor antiserum inhibits bone resorbing activity produced by a rat Leydig cell tumor associated with the humoral hypercalcemia of malignancy. Endocrinology 116:469-471, 1985
79. Insogna KL, Weir EC, Wu TL et al: Co-purification of transforming growth factor beta-like activity with PTH-like and bone-resorbing activities from a tumor associated with humoral hypercalcemia of malignancy. Endocrinology 120:2183-2185, 1987
80. Gowen G, Wood DD, Ihrie EJ et al: An interleukin 1-like factor stimulates bone resorption in vitro. Nature 306:378-380, 1983
81. Dewhirst FE, Stashenko PP, Mole JE et al: Purification and partial sequence of human osteoclast activating factor: Identity with interleukin-1 beta. J Immunol 135:2562-2568, 1985
82. Stashenko P, Dewhirst FE, Peros WJ et al: Synergistic interactions between interleukin 1, tumor necrosis factor, and lymphotoxin in bone resorption. J Immunol 138:1464-1468, 1987
83. Kondo Y, Sato K, Ohkawa H et al: Association of hypercalcemia with tumors producing colony-stimulating factor(s). Cancer Res 43:2368-2374, 1983
84. Lee MY, Liu CC, Lottsfeldt JL et al: Production of granulocyte-stimulating and bone cell-modulating activities from a neutrophilia hypercalcemia-inducing murine mammary cell line. Cancer Res 47:4059-4065, 1987
85. Sato K, Mimura H, Han DC et al: Production of bone-resorbing activity and colony-stimulating activity in vivo and in vitro by a human squamous cell carcinoma associated with hypercalcemia and leukocytosis J Clin Invest 78:145-154, 1986
86. Deuel TF, Huang JS, Huang SS et al: Expression of a platelet-derived growth factor-like protein in simian sarcoma virus transformed cells. Science 221:1348-1350, 1983
87. Tashjian AH Jr, Hohmann EL, Antoniades HN, Levine L: Platelet derived growth factor stimulates bone resorption via a prostaglandin mediated mechanism. Endocrinology 111:118-124, 1982
88. Mundy GR: Pathogenesis of hypercalcemia of malignancy. Clin Endocrinol 23:705-714, 1985

89. Mundy GR, Ibbotson KJ, D'Souza DM: Tumor products and the hypercalcemia of malignancy. J Clin Invest 76:391–394, 1985
90. Bertolini DR, Nedwin GE, Bringman TS et al: Stimulation of bone resorption and inhibition of bone formation in vitro by human tumor necrosis factors. Nature 319:516–518, 1986
91. Garrett IR, Durie BGM, Nedwin GE et al: Production of lymphotoxin, a bone-resorbing cytokine, by cultured human myeloma cells. N Engl J Med 317:526–532, 1987
92. Dinarello CA, Cannon JG, Wolf SM et al: Tumor necrosis factor (cachectin) is an endogenous pyrogen and induces production of interleukin-1. J Exp Med 163:1433–1450, 1986
93. Gowen M, Nedwin G, Mundy GR: Preferential inhibiton of cytokine-stimulated bone resorption by recombinant interferon gamma. J Bone Miner Res 1:469–474, 1986
94. Takahashi N, Mundy GR, Roodman GD: Recombinant human interferon gamma inhibits formation of human osteoclast-like cells. J Immunol 137:3544–3549, 1986
95. Gowen M, Mundy GR: Actions of recombinant interleukin 1, interleukin 2, and interferon gamma on bone resorption in vitro. J Immunol 132:2478–2482, 1986
96. Bunn PA, Schechter GP, Jaffe E et al: Clinical course of retrovirus-associated adult T-cell lymphoma in the United States. N Engl J Med 309:257–264, 1983
97. Breslau NA, McGuire JL, Zerwekh JE et al: Hypercalcemia associated with increased serum calcitriol levels in three patients with lymphoma. Ann Intern Med 100:1–7, 1984
98. Davies M, Mawer EB, Hayes ME, Lumb GA: Abnormal vitamin D metabolism in Hodgkin's lymphoma. Lancet 1:1186–1188, 1985
99. Helikson MA, Harvey AD, Zerwekh JE et al: Plasma cell granuloma producing calcitriol and hypercalcemia. Ann Intern Med 105:379–381, 1986
100. Shigeno H, Yamamoto I, Dokoh S et al: Identification of 1,24 (R)-dihydroxyvitamin D_3-like bone-resorbing lipid in a patient with cancer-associated hypercalcemia. J Clin Endocrinol Metab 61:761–768, 1985
101. Fetchik DA, Bertolini DR, Sarin PS et al: Production of 1,25 dihydroxyvitamin D_3 by human T cell lymphotropic virus-I-transformed lymphocytes. J Clin Invest 78:592–596, 1986
102. Adams JS, Fernandez M, Gacad MA et al: Hypercalcemia and hypercalciuria associated elevated serum 1,25-dihydroxyvitamin D concentrations in patients with AIDS and non-AIDS-related lymphoma. Blood (in press)
103. Salahuddin SZ, Markham PD, Lindner SG et al: Lymphokine production by cultured human T cells transformed by human T-cell leukemia lymphoma virus-1. Science 223:703–707, 1984
104. Bertolini DR, Sarin P, Mundy GR: Production of macromolecular bone resorbing activity by human T-cell leukemia virus (HTLV) transformed cell lines (abstr). Calcif Tissue Int 34:452, 1984
105. Stote RM, Smith LH, Wilson DM et al: Hydrochlorothiazide effects on serum calcium and immunoreactive parathyroid hormone concentration: Studies in normal subjects. Ann Intern Med 77:587–591, 1972
106. Mawer EB, Hann JT, Berry JL et al: Vitamin D metabolism in patients intoxicated with ergocalciferol. Clin Sci 68:135–141, 1985
107. Katz CM, Tzagounis M: Chronic adult hypervitaminosis A with hypercalcemia. Metabolism 21:1171–1176, 1972
108. Valentic JP, Elias AN, Weinstein GD: Hypercalcemia associated with oral isotretinoin in the treatment of severe acne. J Am Med Assoc 250:1899–1900, 1983
109. Blythe WB, Gitelman HJ, Welt LG: Effect of expansion of the extracellular space on the rate of urinary excretion of calcium. Am J Physiol 214:52–57, 1968
110. Massry SG, Coburn JW, Chapman LW et al: Effect of NaCl infusions on urinary Ca^{++} and Mg^{++} during reduction in their filtered loads. Am J Physiol 213:1218–1224, 1967
111. Massry SG, Friedler RM, Coburn JW: Excretion of phosphate and calcium: Physiology of their renal handling and relation to clinical medicine. Arch Intern Med 131:828–836, 1973
112. Wasler M: Calcium clearance is a function of saline clearance in the dog. Am J Physiol 200:1009–1104, 1961
113. Eknoyan G, Suki WN, Martinez-Maldonado M: Effects of diuretics on urinary excretion of phosphate, calcium, and magnesium in thyroparathyroidectomized dogs. J Lab Clin Med 76:257–268, 1970
114. Hosking DJ, Cowley A, Bucknall CA: Rehydration in the treatment of severe hypercalcemia. Q J Med 200:473–481, 1981
115. Warrell RP Jr, Isarel R, Frisone M et al: Gallium nitrate for acute treatment of cancer-related hypercalcemia: A randomized double-blind comparison to calcitonin. Ann Intern Med 108:669–674, 1988
116. Suki WN, Hull HR, Rector FC Jr et al: Mechanism of the effect of thiazide diuretics on calcium and uric acid. J Clin Invest 46:1121, 1967
117. Suki WN, Yium JJ, Von Minden M et al: Acute treatment of hypercalcemia with furosemide. N Engl J Med 283:836–840, 1970
118. Raisz LG: Physiologic and pharmacologic regulation of bone resorption N Engl J Med 282:909–916, 1970
119. Avioli LV, Raisz LG: Bone metabolism and disease. In Bondy K, Rosenberg LE (eds): Metabolic Control and Disease, 8th ed, pp 1709–1814. Philadelphia, WB Saunders, 1980
120. Raisz LG, Niemann I: Effect of phosphate, calcium, and magnesium on bone resorption and hormonal responses in tissue culture. Endocrinology 85:446–452, 1969
121. Herbery LA, Lemann J, Peterson JR et al: Studies of the mechanism by which phosphate infusion lowers serum calcium concentration. J Clin Invest 45:1886–1894, 1966
122. Eisenberg E: Effect of intravenous phosphate on serum strontium and calcium. N Engl J Med 282:889–892, 1970
123. Spaulding SW, Walser M: Treatment of experimental hypercalcemia with oral phosphate. J Clin Endrocrinol 31:531–538, 1970
124. Shackney S, Hasson J: Precipitous fall in serum calcium, hypotension, and acute renal failure after intravenous phosphate therapy for hypercalcemia: Report of two cases. Ann Intern Med 66:906–916, 1967
125. Carey RW, Schmott GW, Kopald HH et al: Massive extraskeletal calcification during phosphate treatment of hypercalcemia. Arch Intern Med 122:150–155, 1968
126. Dudley FJ, Blackburn CRB: Extraskeletal calcification complicating oral neutral phosphate therapy. Lancet 2:628–630, 1970
127. Laflamme GH, Jowsey J: Bone and soft tissue changes with oral phosphate supplements. J Clin Invest 51:2834–2840, 1972
128. Ayala G, Chertow BS, Shah JH et al: Acute hyperphosphatemia and acute persistent renal insufficiency induced by oral phosphate therapy. Ann Intern Med 83:520–521, 1975
129. Mundy GR, Wilkinson R, Heath DA: Comparative study of available medical therapy for hypercalcemia of malignancy. Am J Med 74:421–432, 1983
130. Heath DA: The use of inorganic phosphate in the management of hypercalcemia. Metab Bone Dis Relat Res 2:213–215, 1980
131. Thalassinos N, Joplin GF: Phosphate treatment of hypercalcemia due to carcinoma. Br Med J 4:14–19, 1968
132. Goldsmith RS, Ingbar SH: Phosphate, sulphate, and hypercalcemia. Ann Intern Med 67:463–464, 1967
133. Goldsmith RS, Ingbar SH: Inorganic phosphate in the treatment of hypercalcemia of diverse etiologies. N Engl J Med 274:1–7, 1966
134. Massry SG, Mueller E, Silverman AG et al: Inorganic phosphate treatment of hypercalcemia. Arch Intern Med 121:307–312, 1968
135. Breuer RI, LeBauer J: Caution in the use of phosphates in the treatment of severe hypercalcemia. J Clin Endocrinol Metab 27:695–698, 1967
136. Fulmer DH, Dimich AB, Rothschild EO et al: Treatment of hypercalcemia: Comparison of intravenously adminstered phosphate, sulphate, and hydrocortisone. Arch Intern Med 129:923–930, 1972
137. Seyberth HW, Segre GV, Hamet P et al: Characterization of the group of patients with the hypercalcemia of cancer who respond to treatment with prostaglandin synthesis inhibitors. Trans Assoc Am Physicians 89:92–104, 1976
138. Bockman RS, Repo MA: Lymphokine-mediated bone resorption requires endogenous prostaglandin synthesis. J Exp Med 154:529–534, 1981
139. Brenner DE, Harvey HA, Lipton A: A study of prostaglandin E_2, parathormone, and response to indomethacin in patients with hypercalcemia. Cancer 49:556–561, 1982
140. Coombes RC, Neville AM, Bondy PK et al: Failure of indomethacin to reduce hydroxyproline excretion or hypercalcemia in patients with breast cancer. Prostaglandins 12:1027–1035, 1976
141. Chakmajian ZH, Bethune JE: Sodium sulfate treatment of hypercalcemia. N Engl J Med 275:862–869, 1966
142. Heckman BA, Walsh JH: Hypernatremia complicating sodium sulfate therapy for hypercalcemic crisis. N Engl J Med 276:1082–1083, 1967
143. Kahill M, Orman B, Gyorkey F, Brown H: Hypercalcemia—experience with phosphate and sulphate therapy. JAMA 201:721–724, 1967
144. Spencer H, Greenberg J, Berger E et al: Studies on the effect of ethylenediaminetetraacetic acid in hypercalcemia. J Lab Clin Med 47:29–41, 1956
145. Raisz LG, Trummel CL, Wener JA et al: Effect of glucocorticoids on bone resorption in tissue culture. Endrocrinology 90:961–967, 1972
146. Storey E: Cortisone-induced bone resorption in the rabbit. Endocrinology 68:533–542, 1961
147. Bentzel CJ, Carbone PP, Rosenberg L: The effect of prednisone on calcium metabolism and ^{47}Ca kinetics in patients with multiple myeloma and hypercalcemia. J Clin Invest 43:2132–2145, 1964
148. Kimberg DB, Baerg RD, Gershon E et al: Effect of cortisone treatment on the active transport of calcium by the small intestine. J Clin Invest 50:1309–1321, 1971
149. Muggia FM, Heinemann HO: Hypercalcemia associated with malignant disease. Ann Intern Med 73:281–290, 1970
150. Myers WPL: Cortisone in the treatment of hypercalcemia in neoplastic disease. Cancer 11:83–88, 1958
151. Percival RC, Yates AJP, Grey RES et al: Role of glucocorticoids in the management of malignant hypercalcemia. Br Med J 289:297, 1984
152. Ashkar FS, Miller R, Katins RB: Effect of corticosteroids on the hypercalcemia of malignant disease. Lancet 1:41, 1971
153. Thalassinos NC, Joplin G: Failure of corticosteroid therapy to direct the hypercalcemia of malignant disease. Lancet 2:537–538, 1970
154. Austin LA, Heath H III: Calcitonin: Physiology and pathophysiology. N Engl J Med 304:269–278, 1981
155. Krane SM, Harris ED Jr, Singer FR et al: Acute effects of calcitonin on bone formation in man. Metabolism 22:51–58, 1973
156. Hirsch PF, Munson PL: Thyrocalcitonin. Physiol Rev 49:548–622, 1969
157. Friedman JL, Au WYW, Raisz LG: Responses of fetal rat bone to thyrocalcitonin in tissue culture. Endocrinology 82:149–156, 1968
158. Vaughn CB, Vaitkevicius K: The effects of calcitonin in hypercalcemia in patients with malignancy. Cancer 34:1268–1271, 1974
159. Silva O, Becker KL: Salmon calcitonin in the treatment of hypercalcemia. Arch Intern Med 132:337–339, 1973
160. Hosking DJ: Treatment of severe hypercalcemia with calcitonin. Metab Bone Dis Relat Res 2:207–212, 1980
161. Wisnecki LA, Groom WP, Silva DL, Becker KL: Salmon calcitonin in hypercalcemia. Clin Pharmacol Ther 23:219–222, 1978

162. Wener JA, Gorton SJ, Raisz LG: Escape from inhibition of resorption in cultures of fetal bone treated with calcitonin and parathyroid hormone. Endocrinology 90:752–759, 1978
163. Tashjian AH Jr, Wright DR, Ivey JL et al: Calcitonin binding sites in the dog. Relationships to biological response and escape. Recent Prog Horm Res 34:285–334, 1978
164. Au WYN: Calcitonin treatment of hypercalcemia due to parathyroid carcinoma: Synergistic effect of prednisone on long-term treatment of hypercalcemia. Arch Intern Med 135:1594–1597, 1975
165. Binstock ML, Mundy GR: Effect of calcitonin and glucocorticoids in combination on the hypercalcemia of malignancy. Ann Intern Med 93:269–272, 1980
166. Shinoda H, Adamek G, Felix R et al: Structure–activity relationships of various biphosphonates. Calcif Tissue Int 35:87–99, 1983
167. Reitsma PH, Teitelbaum SL, Bijvoet OLM, Kahn AJ: Differential action of the biphosphonates (3-amino-1-hydroxypropylidene)-1,1-biphosphonate (APD) and disodium dichloromethylidene biphosphonate (Cl_2MDP) on rat macrophage-mediated bone resorption in vitro. J Clin Invest 70:927–933, 1982
168. Jacobs TP, Siris ES, Bilezikian JP et al: Hypercalcemia of malignancy: Treatment with intravenous dichloromethylene diphosphonate. Ann Intern Med 94:312–316, 1981
169. Rastad J, Benson L, Johansson H et al: Clodronate treatment in patients with malignancy-associated hypercalcemia. Acta Med Scand 221:489–494, 1987
170. Chapuy MC, Meunier PJ, Alexandre CM et al: Effects of disodium dichloromethylene diphosphonate on hypercalcemia due to bone metastases. J Clin Invest 65:1243–1247, 1980
171. Paterson AD, Kanis JA, Cameron EC et al: The use of dichloromethylene diphosphonate for the management of hypercalcemia in multiple myeloma. Br J Haematol 54:121–132, 1983
172. Body JJ, Pot M, Borkowski A et al: Dose-response study of aminohydroxypropylidene bisphosphonate in tumor-associated hypercalcemia. Am J Med 82:957–963, 1987
173. Body JJ, Borkowski A, Cleeren A, Bijvoet OLM: Treatment of malignancy-associated hypercalcemia with intravenous aminohydroxypropylidene diphosphonate. J Clin Oncol 4:1177–1183, 1986
174. Sleeboom HP, Bijvoet OLM, Van Oosterom AT et al: Comparison of intravenous (3-amino-1-hydroxypropylidene)-1,1-biphosphonate and volume repletion in tumor-induced hypercalcemia. Lancet 2:239–243, 1983
175. Ralston SH, Gardner MD, Dryburg FJ et al: Comparison of aminohydroxypropylidene diphosphonate, mithramycin, and corticosteroids/calcitonin in treatment of cancer-associated hypercalcemia. Lancet 2:907–910, 1985
176. Hasling C,Charles P, Mosekilde L: Etidronate disodium for treating hypercalcaemia of malignancy: A double blind, placebo-controlled study. Eur J Clin Invest 16:433–437, 1986
177. Ryzen E, Martodam RR, Troxell M et al: Intravenous etidronate in the management of malignant hypercalcemia. Arch Intern Med 145:449–452, 1985
178. Didronel (etidronate disodium) Package Insert; Norwich-Eaton Pharmaceuticals Inc., 1987
179. Bounameaux HM, Schifferli J, Monatni JP, Chatelanat F: Renal failure associated with intravenous diphosphonates. Lancet 1:471, 1983
180. Schiller JM, Rasmussen P, Benson AD et al: Maintenance etidronate in the prevention of malignancy-associated hypercalcemia. Arch Intern Med 147:963–966, 1987
181. Boyce BF, Smith L, Fogelman I et al: Focal osteomalacia due to low-dose diphosphonate therapy in Paget's disease. Lancet 1:821–824, 1984
182. Ralston SH, Boyce BF, Cowan RA et al: The effect of 1 alpha-hydroxyvitamin D_3 on the mineralization defect in disodium etidronate-treated Paget's disease–a double-blind randomized clinical study. J Bone Miner Res 2:5–12, 1987
183. Meunier PJ, Chapuy MC, Delmas P et al: Intravenous disodium etidronate therapy in Paget's disease of bone and hypercalcemia of malignancy: Effects on biochemical parameters and bone histomorphometry. Am J Med (Suppl 2A) 82:71–78, 1987
184. Kennedy BJ: Mithramycin therapy in advanced testicular neoplasms. Cancer 26:755–766, 1970
185. Brown, JH, Kennedy BJ: Mithramycin in the treatment of disseminated testicular neoplasms. N Engl J Med 272:111–118, 1965
186. Kennedy BJ: Metabolic and toxic effects during mithramycin therapy. Am J Med 49:494–503, 1970
187. Lebbin D, Ryan WG, Schwartz TB: Outpatient treatment of Paget's disease of bone with mithramycin. Ann Intern Med 81:635–637, 1974
188. Singer FR, Neer RM, Murray TM et al: Mithramycin treatment of intractable hypercalcemia due to parathyroid carcinoma. N Engl J Med 283:634–636, 1970
189. Perlia CP, Gubisch NJ, Wolter J et al: Mithramycin treatment of hypercalcemia. Cancer 25:389–394, 1970
190. Elias EG, Evans JT: Hypercalcemic crisis in neoplastic diseases: Management with mithramycin. Surgery 71:631–635, 1972
191. Stapleton FB, Linshaw MA: Treatment of hypercalcemia associated with osseous metastases. J Pediatr 89:1029–1030, 1976
192. Coombes RC, Dady P, Parsons C et al: Mithramycin therapy: An adjunct to conventional treatment of hypercalcemia and bone metastases in breast cancer. Metab Bone Dis Relat Res 2:199–202, 1980
193. Yarbro JW, Kennedy BJ, Barnum CP: Mithramycin inhibition of ribonucleic acid synthesis. Cancer Res 26:36–39, 1966
194. Wolheim MS, Yarbro JW, Kennedy BJ: Effect of mithramycin on HeLa cells. Cancer 21:22–25, 1968
195. Kiang DT, Loken MK, Kennedy BJ: Mechanism of the hypocalcemic effect of mithramycin. J Clin Endocrinol Metab 48:341–344, 1979
196. Northrop G, Taylor SG III: Biochemical effects of mithramycin on cultured cells. Cancer Res 29:1916–1919, 1969
197. Minkin C: Inhibition of parathyroid hormone stimulated bone resorption in vitro by the antibiotic mithramycin. Calcif Tissue Res 13:249–257, 1973
198. Parsons DM, Baum M, Self M: Effect of mithramycin on calcium and hydroxyproline metabolism in patients with malignant disease. Br Med J 1:474–477, 1967
199. Green L, Donehower RC: Hepatic toxicity of low doses of mithramycin in hypercalcemia. Cancer Treat Rep 68:1379–1381, 1984
200. Warrell RP Jr, Bockman RS, Coonley CJ et al: Gallium nitrate inhibits calcium resorption from bone and is effective treatment for cancer-related hypercalcemia. J Clin Invest 73:1487–1490, 1984
201. Bockman RS, Boskey A, Alcock N et al: Gallium nitrate inhibits bone resorption, increases bone calcium content, but is not cytotoxic to bone cells. Bone Miner Res 1:65, 1985
202. Cournot-Witmer G, Bourdeau A, Lieberherr M et al: Bone modeling in gallium nitrate-treated rats. Calcif Tissue Int 40:270–275, 1987
203. Warrell RP Jr, Skelos A, Alcock NW, Bockman RS: Gallium nitrate for acute treatment of cancer-related hypercalcemia: Clinicopharmacologic and dose-response analysis. Cancer Res 46:4208–4212, 1986
204. Warrell RP Jr, Issacs M, Coonley CJ et al: Metabolic effects of gallium nitrate administered by prolonged infusion. Cancer Treat Rep 69:653–655, 1985
205. Warrel RP Jr, Alcock NW, Skelos A, Bockman RS: Gallium nitrate inhibits accelerated bone turnover in patients with bone metastases. J Clin Oncol 5:292–298, 1987
206. Bockman RS, Bosley A, Blumenthal NC et al: Gallium increases bone calcium and crystallite perfection of hydroxyapatite. Calcif Tissue Int 39:376–381, 1986
207. Bockman RS, Israel R, Alcock N et al: Gallium nitrate stimulates bone collagen synthesis. Clin Res 35:620A, 1987
208. Miach PH, Dawborn JK, Martin TJ et al: Management of the hypercalcemia of malignancy by peritoneal dialysis. Med J. Aust 1:782–784, 1975
209. Lad TE, Mishoulam HM, Shevrin DH et al: Treatment of cancerassociated hypercalcemia with cisplatin. Arch Intern Med 147:329–332, 1987
210. Bockman RS, Bohnsack R, Warrell RP: Effect of metal-based compounds on bone resorption. Clin Res 34:390A, 1986
211. Robinson RR, Yarger WE: Acute uric acid nephropathy. Arch Intern Med 137:839–840, 1977
212. Klinenberg JR, Kippen I, Bluestone R: Hyperuricemic nephropathy: Pathophysiologic features and factors influencing urate deposition. Nephron 14:88–98, 1975
213. Crittendon DR, Ackerman GL: Hyperuricemic acute renal failure in disseminated carcinoma. Arch Intern Med 137:97–99, 1977
214. Kjellstrand CM, Campbell DC, Von Hartizsch B et al: Hyperuricemic acute renal failure. Arch Intern Med 133:349–359, 1974
215. Maidemont CG, Greaves MF, Black AJ: T-cell leukemia presenting with hyperuricaemia, acute renal failure, and gout. Clin Lab Haematol 5:423–426, 1983
216. Cohen LF, Balow JE, Magrath IT et al: Acute tumor lysis syndrome. A review of 37 patients with Burkitt's lymphoma. Am J Med 68:486–491, 1980
217. Garnick MB, Mayer RB: Acute renal failure associated with neoplastic disease and its treatment. Semin Oncol 5:155–165, 1978
218. Yu T-F: Secondary gout associated with myeloproliferative diseases. Arthritis Rheum 8:765–771, 1965
219. Ultmann J: Hyperuricemia in disseminated neoplastic disease other than lymphomas or leukemias. Cancer 15:122–129, 1962
220. Melink TJ, Von Hoff DD, Kuhn JG et al: Phase I evaluation and pharmacokinetics of tiazofurin (2-beta-D-ribofuranosylthiazole-4-carboxamide, NSC 286193). Cancer Res 45:2859–2865, 1985
221. Hill DL: Aminothiadiazoles. Cancer Chemother Pharmacol 4:215–220, 1980
222. Wyngaarden JB, Kelley WN: Gout. In Stanbury JB, Wyngaarden JB, Fredrickson DS, Goldstein JL, Brown MS (eds): The Metabolic Basis of Inherited Disease, pp. 1043–1114. New York, McGraw-Hill, 1983
223. Boss GR, Seegmiller JE: Hyperuricemia and gout: Classification, complications, and management. N Engl J Med 300:1459–1468, 1979
224. Kanwar YS, Manaligod JR: Leukemic urate nephropathy. Arch Pathol 99:467–472, 1975
225. Yu T-F: Urolithiasis in hyperuricemia and gout. J Urol 126:424–430, 1981
226. German DG, Holmes EW: Hyperuricemia and gout. Med Clin North Am 70:419–436, 1986
227. Conger JD, Falk SA: Intrarenal dynamics in the pathogenesis and prevention of acute urate nephropathy. J Clin Invest 59:786–793, 1977
228. Muggia FM, Ball TJ Jr, Ultmann JE: Allopurinol in the treatment of neoplastic disease complicted by hyperuricemia. Arch Intern Med 120:12–18, 1967
229. Krakoff IH, Meyer RL: Prevention of hyperuricemia in leukemia and lymphoma. JAMA 193:1–6, 1965
230. Yu T-F, Gutman AB: Effect of allopurinol (4-hydroxypyrazolo-[3,4-d]pyrimidine) on serum and urinary uric acid in primary and secondary gout. Am J Med 37:885–898, 1964
231. Skipper HE, Robins RK, Thomson JR et al: Structure–activity relationships observed on screening a series of pyrazolopyrimidines against experimental neoplasms. Cancer Res 17:579–596, 1957
232. Rundles RW, Wyngaarden JB, Hithcings GH et al: Effects of a xanthine oxidase inhibitor on thiopurine metabolism, hyperuricemia, and gout. Trans Assoc Am Physicians 76:126–140, 1963
233. Band PR, Silverberg DS, Henderson JF et al: Xanthine neophropathy in a patient with lymphosarcoma treated with allopurinol. N Engl J Med 283:354–357, 1970
234. Ablin A, Stephens BG, Hirata T et al: Nephropathy, xanthinuria, and orotic aciduria

complicating Burkitt's lymphoma treated with allopurinol. Metabolism 21:771–778, 1972
235. Andreoli SP, Clark JH, McGuire WA, Bergstein JM: Purine excretion during tumor lysis in children with acute lymphocytic leukemia receiving allopurinol: Relationship to acute renal failure. J Pediatr 109:292–298, 1986
236. Hande KR, Hixson CV, Chabner BA: Postchemotherapy purine excretion in lymphoma patients receiving allopurinol. Cancer Res 41:2273–2279, 1981
237. Kelly WN, Beardmore TD: Allopurinol: Alteration in pyrimidine metabolism in man. Science 169:388–390, 1970
238. Fox IH, Wyngaarden JB, Kelley WN: Depletion of erythrocyte phosphoribosylpyrophosphate in man: A newly discovered effect of allopurinol. N Engl J Med 283:1177–1182, 1970
239. Ortega JA, Ruccione K, Weinberg K et al: Use of an investigational form of intravenous (IV) allopurinol for the treatment of hyperuricemia in children with malignancy. Proc Am Soc Clin Oncol 4:257, 1985
240. Simmonds HA, Cameron JS, Morris GS, Davies PM: Allopurinol in renal failure and the tumor lysis syndrome. Clin Chim Acta 160:189–195, 1986
241. Templeton JS: Azapropazone or allopurinol in the treatment of chronic gout and/or hyperuricemia. A preliminary report. BR J Clin Pract 36:353–358, 1982
242. Gibson T, Simmonds HA, Armstrong RD et al: Azapropazone—a treatment for hyperuricaemia and gout? Br J Rheumatol 23:44–51, 1984
243. Warrell RP Jr: Induction of profound hypouricemia by a non-sedating C-5 monosubstituted thiobarbiturate. Clin Res 35:805A, 1987
244. Jankovic M, Zurlo MG, Rossi E et al: Urate-oxidase as hypouricemic agent in a case of acute tumor lysis syndrome. Am J Pediatr Hematol Oncol 7:202–204, 1985
245. Mandell GA, Swacus JR, Rosenstock J, Buck BE: Danger of urography in hyperuricemic children with Burkitt's lymphoma. J Can Assoc Radiol 34:273–277, 1983
246. Steinberg SM, Galen MA, Lazarus JM: Hemodialysis for acute uric acid nephropathy. Am J Dis Child 129:956–958, 1975
247. Monballyou J, Zachee P, Verherckmoes R, Boogaerts MA: Transient acute renal failure due to tumor lysis-induced severe phosphate load in a patient with Burkitt's lymphoma. Clin Nephrol 22:47–50, 1984
248. Wollner A, Shalit M, Brezis M: Tumor genesis syndrome. Hypophosphatemia accompanying Burkitt's lymphoma cell leukemia. Miner Electrolyte Metab 12:173–175, 1986
249. Boles JM, Dutel JL, Briere J et al: Acute renal failure caused by extreme hyperphosphatemia after chemotherapy of an acute lymphoblastic leukemia. Cancer 53:2425–2429, 1984
250. Tsokos GC, Balow JE, Speigel RJ et al: Renal and metabolic complications of undifferentiated and lymphoblastic lymphomas. Medicine 60:218–229, 1981
251. Cervantes F, Ribera JM, Granena A et al: Tumor lysis syndrome with hypocalcemia in chronic granulocytic leukemia. Acta Haematol 68:157–159, 1982
252. Anger B, Bunjes D, Carbonell F et al: Treatment results of nine patients with Burkitt's lymphoma. Blut 53:279–286, 1986
253. Boccia RV, Longo DL, Lieher ML et al: Multiple recurrences of acute tumor lysis syndrome in an indolent non-Hodgkin's lymphoma. Cancer 56:2295–2297, 1985
254. Zusman J, Brown DM, Nesbit ME: Hyperphosphatemia, hyperphosphaturia, and hypocalcemia in acute lymphoblastic leukemia. N Engl J Med 289:1335–1340, 1973
255. Ettinger DS, Harker WG, Gerry HW et al: Hyperphosphatemia, hypocalcemia, and transient renal failure: Results of cytotoxic treatment of acute lymphoblastic leukemia. JAMA 239:2472–2474, 1978
256. Gomez GA, Han T: Acute tumor lysis syndrome in prolymphocytic leukemia. Arch Intern Med 147:375–376, 1987
257. Vogelzang NJ, Nelimark RA, Nath KA: Tumor lysis syndrome after induction chemotherapy of small cell bronchogenic carcinoma. JAMA 249:513–514, 1983
258. Tomlinson GC, Solberg LA Jr: Acute tumor lysis syndrome with metastatic medulloblastoma. Cancer 53:1783–1785, 1984
259. Stark ME, Dyer MC, Coonley CJ: Fatal acute tumor lysis syndrome with metastatic breast carcinoma. Cancer 60:762–764, 1987
260. Vogler WR, Morris JG, Winton EF: Acute tumor lysis in T-cell leukemia induced by amsacrine. Arch Intern Med 143:165–166, 1983
261. Warrell RP Jr, Coonley CJ, Gee TS: Homoharringtonine: An effective new drug for remission induction in refactory nonlymphoblastic leukemia. J Clin Oncol 3:617–621, 1985
262. Thomas MR, Robinson WA, Mughal TI, Glode LM: Tumor lysis syndrome following VP-16-213 in chronic myeloid leukemia in blast crisis. Am J Hematol 16:185–188, 1984
263. Fer MF, Bottino GC, Sherwin SA et al: Atypical tumor lysis syndrome in a patient with T-cell lymphoma treated with recombinant leukocyte interferon. Am J Med 77:953–956, 1984
264. Cech P, Block JB, Cone IA, Stone R: Tumor lysis syndrome after tamoxifen flare. N Engl J Med 315:263–264, 1986
265. Gonzalez C, Villasanta U: Life-threatening hypocalcemia and hypomagnesemia associated with cisplatin chemotherapy. Obstet Gynecol 59:732–734, 1982
266. Harley HA, Mason R, Phillips PJ: Profound hypocalcemia associated with oestrogen treatment of carcinoma of the prostate. Med J Aust 2:41–41, 1983
267. Schenkein DP, O'Neill WC, Shapiro J, Miller KB: Accelerated bone formation causing profound hypocalcemia in acute leukemia. Ann Intern Med 105:375–378, 1986
268. Schilsky RL: Renal and metabolic complications of cancer chemotherapy. Semin Oncol 9:75–83, 1982
269. Papaioannou AN: Tumors other than insulinoma associated with hypoglycemia. Surg Gynecol Obstet 123:1093–1109, 1966

SECTION 4

RICHARD E. WILSON

Surgical Emergencies

Acute abdominal complications are common in patients with malignant disease. They may be the result of the primary tumor itself or may occur during or after treatment of the malignancy. This section will define the problems in both general and specific terms and discuss the appropriate methods of management.

GENERAL ASPECTS OF SURGICAL EMERGENCIES

DEFINITIONS

The primary decision required in treating abdominal problems is whether or not surgical intervention is necessary.[1] The acute nature of the problem determines the timing of the decision and potential intervention. The frequency of observation of the patient and the continuous balance between the decision for intervention versus nonintervention are the critical judgment factors. This decision is most difficult in patients with malignant disease and its complications because the usual responses and criteria for decision-making are altered, and specific expertise is necessary.

SYMPTOMS

Pain remains the most important indicator of acute abdominal disease, even in patients with muted responses. The complaints of oncologic patients must be evaluated and investigated even more carefully because these complaints frequently seem less important to the inexperienced physician. Necessary aspects of the definition of pain are location, timing, radiation, description, relationship to normal function (*e.g.*, eating, defecation, and urination), and what makes the pain better or worse.

Nausea and vomiting also may be important complaints but, along with diarrhea and constipation, they represent abnormalities of gastrointestinal (GI) function, so frequently a complication of treatment of malignancy as to be especially confounding. The presence or absence of blood in the stool or vomitus, and the timing of the complaints in relationship to other signs and symptoms, are particularly critical. Other abdominal complaints, such as distention, cramps, lack of passage of flatus, or anorexia, also should be identified. Chills and fever are important constitutional symptoms that may be the only markers of acute abdominal disease in these patients. The timing of fever—particularly when patients are receiving chemotherapy—is important. Previous history, presence or absence of positive blood cultures, or accompanying findings such as jaundice, localized pain, or other physical signs may be needed to place the complaint in proper perspective.

SIGNS

Nowhere in the body is the use of the four hallmarks of physical diagnosis—inspection, percussion, palpation, and auscultation—more valuable than for the acute abdomen. The physician must look for abnormalities of skin color and tone, distention, abdominal venous patterns, disproportionate swelling or edema, and finally, how the patient tries to protect himself from discomfort. Percussion performed in a most gentle manner can localize pain without alarming or hurting the patient. A cooperative patient is essential for accurate physical examination. Absence of liver dullness may indicate free abdominal air, whereas a resonant epigastric region may define acute gastric dilation. The identification of acute urinary retention and shifting dullness also depends on accurate percussion. Palpation should define localized muscle spasm, organomegaly, abdominal masses, and areas of specific point tenderness. Like percussion, palpation should be gentle; otherwise, false impressions of pain will be assumed or masses can be missed. Auscultation should be directed at identifying the presence and quality of bowel sounds, a succession splash in the dilated stomach, or unusual bruits. Both the pelvic and the rectal examinations should be a direct part of the abdominal examination, and not deferred or delayed because they provide the most critical information for lower abdominal complaints. Not only can one palpate masses or tumor nodules, but also one can find evidence of peritoneal irritation, dilated bowel loops, pelvic wall disproportions, evidence of fistulous drainage, and insidious abscesses in the perirectal tissues. Great care must be taken with proper comfort and positioning of the patient. Rectal examinations should always be performed with patients of both sexes in the lithotomy position to maximize the definition of pelvic disease. Examination of the pelvis often requires both right- and left-handed examination to palpate each side accurately. Careful anal and perirectal examination will require having the patient turn to the lateral position as well. Anoscopy and sigmoidoscopy should be almost routine accompaniments to the rectal examination, even without prior bowel preparation. Anoscopy is performed best in the lateral position, whereas sigmoidoscopy is accomplished best in the knee–chest position. If inadequate information is obtained, repeat the anoscopy and sigmoidoscopy after an enema, but frequently this is unnecessary. Important observations include the presence or absence of fissures, fistulas, and perianal abscesses, the status of the intestinal mucosa, the level of positive guaiac stool, and the identification of rectal lesions as being either intraluminal or extraluminal. Gastric aspiration can also be an important extension of the physical examination of the abdomen, as is catheterization of the bladder, or paracentesis if a pelvic mass is difficult to define.

LABORATORY AIDS

In the patient with malignancy, a situation in which complex problems are frequent, the use of more sophisticated laboratory studies may be critical in defining and following acute abdominal problems. These studies cannot, however, supplant a careful physical examination and history; rather, as in all other aspects of medicine, these basic elements lead the physician to the appropriate studies. In addition to routine complete blood counts and SMA-20 examinations, consideration of standard enzyme determinations such as serum amylase or unique enzyme measurements, and serial determination of special tumor markers such as hormone and carcinoembryonic antigen (CEA) assays, may be particularly important.[2] Frequent blood cultures are essential in febrile patients, as is the determination of antibiotic and other drug levels in the serum. Radiologic examinations have grown in sophistication and value and include routine plain films of the abdomen, nuclide scans, ultrasound evaluation, and contrast studies of the gastrointestinal tract, urinary tract, pancreaticobiliary ducts, and fistulae. Ultrasound-guided biopsies and contrast studies now are also available.[3] Angiography to define vascular anatomy may be particularly useful for the surgeon once he has decided that operative intervention is necessary. Computed tomography (CT) scan has opened up whole new areas of noninvasive evaluation, particularly of the liver, pelvis, and retroperitoneum. The specific roles of these various techniques will be discussed as individual problems are reviewed.

COMPLICATING FEATURES OF ONCOLOGIC PATIENTS

Because the malignant disease and its treatment may confuse and confound the acute abdominal problem, it is essential that the examiner obtain the most complete history possible. This may require questioning the family and other involved physicians, as well as the patient. A thorough understanding of previous operative procedures, forms of radiation and chemotherapy, and previous abnormal findings are necessary for the correct management of acute abdominal complaints. The patient's symptoms, such as pain and fever, may be suppressed by corticosteroids or opiates, whereas ongoing radiation or chemotherapy can cause nausea, vomiting, or diarrhea. Jaundice, gastrointestinal mucosal bleeding, or anemia may be drug- or disease-induced. Generalized serositis, with its full gamut of acute peritoneal signs, may result from drug therapy, diffuse tumor infiltrates, or local perforative lesions. Pneumonia or pulmonary embolism, both frequent in cancer patients, may appear to the physician as an acute abdominal condition. Immunologic anergy is well-known in Hodgkin's disease and in patients with advanced malignancy.[4,5] Normal immune responses, including those of inflammation, can be lacking in these patients. In addition, pancytopenia may result from drug or radiation therapy or from marrow involvement with the tumor itself.[6] The lack of white blood cell response to acute disease also may be misleading in some cancer patients.

If marrow response is blunted, the expected leukocytosis will not occur to indicate a complicating infectious process. On the other hand, collections of pus may not develop and abscesses cannot form in the usual sense. This is particularly true in extraperitoneal invasive sepsis of the perineum or abdominal wall. Ubiquitous infections with viral or fungal organisms in immunosuppressed patients may induce lymphocytosis rather than leukocytosis, further confusing diagnostic decisions. Bleeding and clotting factors may be totally disturbed; bleeding from mucosal surfaces into the retroperitoneum or into a necrotic tumorous lesion is common and may be the cause of abdominal complaints. Febrile reactions may be the result of host–tumor interactions or a new complicating illness. Frequent transfusion requirements, daily alteration in bone marrow function, and infection with unique bacteria, viruses, and fungi complete the picture of diagnostic and therapeutic confusion.[7] This is why the need for a multidisciplinary approach to all problems of cancer patients is so essential.

SURGICAL PROCEDURES AND LOGISTICS

The armamentarium of surgical procedures for dealing with acute abdominal problems is broad, but in cancer patients, certain special considerations are necessary. Because of the many aforementioned complicating features, the diagnosis may be unusually obscure, even when laparotomy is performed. Previous abdominal surgery and abnormal wound repair make the surgical decisions especially critical. Staging of operative procedures may become necessary even when this is not the usual practice. Poor host "reserve" may make earlier surgical intervention essential, even though apparent risks are greater and diagnosis may be less certain.

Modern techniques allow better preparation of patients with leukopenia and thrombocytopenia for surgical procedures. In general, white cell transfusions are not necessary before surgical exploration for drainage of a septic process. Identification of the offending organism, appropriate antibiotics, and adequate drainage usually suffice. Frequently, white blood cell counts will rise spontaneously if successful drainage occurs. If no operable focus can be identified or if the predicted response is not achieved, then white blood cell transfusions are indicated. On the other hand, platelet transfusions can be critical for a successful operative procedure. Usually, 6 to 12 units of platelets is given during induction of anesthesia. The surgeon must take special pains to control every possible bleeding point, and then platelet transfusions, 6 units at a time, may be administered postoperatively only if bleeding is a problem.

Peritoneal tap and lavage may be useful, combined with laparoscopy for more accurate diagnosis.[8] Surgeons dealing with cancer patients should become expert in this latter technique. Exploratory laparotomy may be the only way to be certain of the abdominal status of a given patient, despite the lack of more specific operative indications. The simplest operative concepts of diversion, drainage, and decompression may be the only procedures to be performed; complicated resectional or anastomotic operations may fail because of the underlying nature of the disease or the patient's status.[9]

INFLAMMATORY LESIONS

Inflammatory lesions causing acute abdominal disease may be divided into perforative and nonperforative problems. Obviously, many of the nonperforative lesions may progress to perforation, and this must be considered in their management. For this reason, nonperforative lesions will be discussed first.

NONPERFORATIVE LESIONS

Inflammatory lesions may involve the entire gastrointestinal tract and its accessory organs, as well as the genitourinary system. They are, by far, the most common cause of acute abdominal complaints in oncologic cancer patients. Identifying and differentiating them from those lesions that require immediate surgical intervention often are difficult, particularly in this patient population.

Esophagitis

Esophagitis may occur from prolonged nasogastric intubation, specific drug therapy, radiation, or bacterial, fungal, or candidal infection. Intraoral ulceration often may accompany esophagitis and aid in the diagnosis. Perforation is rare, but transmural penetration with mediastinitis may occur. Endoscopy is the best technique for diagnosis; acute abdominal pain and dysphagia may be the primary complaints. Treatment must be based on the diagnosis of the specific cause of the esophagitis. Very rarely, prolonged vomiting and retching may lead to spontaneous perforation of the esophagus, which occurs in the distal third just above the hiatus.[10]

Gastritis and Duodenitis

Epigastric pain, nausea and vomiting, hematemesis, gastric dilation, and discrete or diffuse ulceration may be present. Again, endoscopic examination is the best diagnostic tool, although an upper GI series sometimes may be helpful, particularly for identifying discrete ulcers or obstruction. Bleeding points also are best seen by endoscopy or angiography. The treatment of choice is the combination of decompression and, where possible, the removal of the offending agents. Modern drug therapy includes the addition of H_2-blocking agents, administered intravenously. Antacid drip therapy is useful in acid–peptic gastritis and steroid-induced ulcerations. Conservative management is best except for complications of the gastritis.

Cholecystitis

Localized right upper quadrant pain, jaundice, and the identification of gallstones classically define cholecystitis; however, unexplained fever may be the only finding in cancer patients. Ultrasound examinations for gallstones or CT scan may be useful in the acute situation in which an oral cholecystogram fails to provide critical information.[11] A history of stones and fatty food intolerance is most valuable. Treatment will depend on the status of the patients; cholecystostomy under local anesthetic or cholecystectomy under general anesthetic both may provide definitive management if the attack fails to subside. The need for common duct exploration in the presence of jaundice and sepsis may be essential, regardless of the cholangiographic findings or the status of the common duct at surgical inspection.

Pancreatitis

Pancreatitis may be an insidious lesion in patients with other abdominal disease.[12] It may produce pain disproportionate to the abdominal findings and may be associated with sudden development of generalized ileus, nausea and vomiting, and unexplained fever. Any sudden plasma volume deficit, indicated by a rising hematocrit, reduced urine output, hypovolemia, or hypotension may be the clue to this diagnosis. Serum or urine amylase elevation, falling serum calcium level, serum lipase elevation, or urinary amylase/creatinine ratio measurements confirm the diagnosis. Treatment is conservative, directed toward suppression of pancreatic secretions because this primarily is an obstructive disease. Both cholangitis and pancreatitis are more common in patients who have fasted and then have begun later to eat, a pattern frequently seen in cancer patients, particularly those receiving chemotherapy. Operative intervention in pancreatitis is for its complications only—persistent pseudocyst, fistula, or abscess. Common duct obstruction may result from recurrent pancreatitis and may be impossible to differentiate from primary of metastatic carcinoma.[13] Ultrasound examination of the pancreas, as well as CT scanning, may be extremely useful but not always accurate. Endoscopic retrograde dye studies of the common and pancreatic ducts may also be valuable.

Enterocolitis

Enterocolitis frequently may result from radiation therapy to the abdomen or from chemotherapy. With chemotherapy, enterocolitis usually can be related temporarily to the treatment pattern, frequently occurring right after treatment, when reflex diarrhea or vomiting ensue, or at the time of the white cell nadir, when mucosal damage to the bowel is associated with local inflammation. Antibiotic therapy also may produce mucosal inflammation, vasculitis, and pseudomembranous colitis.[14] Mucosal bleeding with intramural hemorrhage may occur in these patients as well. Radiation effects tend to be later, usually 2 years to 10 years after treatment, although early edematous and inflammatory reaction may produce acute symptoms.

Appendicitis

The localizing symptoms of acute appendicitis frequently are more difficult to identify in debilitated patients. Constipation and other alterations of acute illness probably make appendicitis a greater risk because this disease starts as an obstructive phenomenon in the appendiceal lumen. Smoldering local sepsis, with eventual abscess formation, is a serious risk. The surgeon must look for reproducible localizing abdominal signs as the best index of appendicitis in patients with abdominal pain. Laboratory studies are unreliable, with fever and leukocytosis often not apparent. In this patient population, newer studies with ultrasound and CT scans may be particularly useful. Operative treatment remains the same, namely, appendectomy, with drainage only if there is a localized abscess. As with other surgical procedures in this patient population, prophylactic antibodies during the acute operative period in short, high-dose courses definitely are indicated.

Diverticulitis

Diverticular disease is much more common in patients with chronic illness, inactivity, dehydration, constipation, and poor immune responses. Instead of a walled-off inflammation of the diverticular microabscess, which normally produces some crampy pain, low-grade fever, and a tender sigmoid, with or without a mass, diverticulitis in this patient group has a high incidence of free perforation, fecal peritonitis, and death.[15] This often occurs with the most minimal signs and symptoms, sometimes acute left lower quadrant abdominal pain, groin pain, diarrhea, or fever. Obtain limited emergency barium or Gastrografin enema examinations in these patients at the least provocation. Early diagnosis, rapid operation, and sigmoid resection with double-end colostomies are the steps needed for salvage. This has been a highly successful method of effective management.

Proctitis and Perirectal Inflammation

Proctitis is a common consequence of pelvic radiation; pain, tenderness, rectal bleeding, and mucosal discharge are the most common findings. Proctitis also may result from chemotherapy, especially if diarrhea is present as well. It must be distinguished from perirectal abscess, fistula-in-ano, cryptitis, and fistulas. The perirectal and perianal lesions are more localized and may require surgical treatment. They may occur with proctitis, however, and careful anoscopic and sigmoidoscopic examinations are necessary. Local pain may be so great that anesthetic is required for adequate evaluation of the area. With severe neutropenia, perirectal abscess may be devoid of pus and, instead, may appear as an area of dense and painful cellulitis. High-dose antibiotics for gram-negative bowel organisms, covering both aerobes and anaerobes, as well as sitz baths, stool softeners, and bed rest, should precede any plans for surgical drainage. As white blood cells return, the local condition often improves; white blood cell or platelet transfusions may be very helpful because some of these lesions start as intramural hematomas related to constipation. Careful and frequent examination is necessary for the proper decision, especially if fever and septicemia are present. If drainage is necessary in the patient with pancytopenia, small incisions with packs sewn into the cavity will reduce bleeding and local pain.

Prostatitis and Pyelonephritis

Male patients requiring prolonged or frequent urinary catheterization are at high risk for these complicating infections. A patient with prostatitis presents with fever, urinary retention, deep pelvic pain, and a boggy, tender prostate on rectal examination. Appropriate high-dose antibiotics followed by chronic suppressive therapy is the treatment of choice, with urinary catheterization used only for retention. Pyelonephritis, particularly if there is a history, is a risk when pancytopenia is present. This can be another source of septicemia in a debilitated patient population; urinary cultures frequently will define the organism and its sensitivity. Abdominal and flank pain with fever, sometimes associated with reflex nausea and vomiting, will lead to the diagnosis.

PERFORATIVE LESIONS

Although some of the potentially perforative lesions, such as appendicitis and diverticulitis, have been referred to in the preceding section, there are some circumstances that particularly present as gastrointestinal perforations. Many of these are related to the primary malignancy itself.

Gastroduodenal

Gastric carcinoma frequently may present with perforation as the initial complaint, as can acid–peptic gastric and duodenal ulcers. Acute upper abdominal pain, muscle rigidity, and free air in the abdomen on plain abdominal upright films represent the most common triad of findings. The presence of anemia, guaiac-positive stool, or a history of weight loss and obstructive symptoms frequently will suggest that the lesion is malignant rather than benign. Early laparotomy is the treatment of choice. If the perforation is beyond the pylorus, simple plication remains the best treatment unless the patient has a long history of peptic ulcer disease.[16] For lesions in the stomach, frozen section is essential to be certain that one is not dealing with a perforated carcinoma. With local inflammation and edema, it is not always possible to identify a gastric carcinoma by palpation, and identification by frozen section may be difficult as well. That is why the history and complete physical examination are important. Existence of cancer throughout the gastric wall may be accompanied by supraclavicular (Virchow) nodes, rectal shelf, celiac lymph node involvement, or liver metastases, and the surgeon should look for these. Gastric resection is the treatment of choice—routine or extended subtotal gastrectomy with omentectomy. Gastric resection should be done even in the presence of proven distant metastases because the best possible palliation and opportunity for chemotherapy will result. If uncertain about the benign or malignant nature of a gastric ulcer, perform gastric resection because that is the most efficient treatment for benign gastric ulcer as well.[17]

Small Intestine

Small-bowel perforation is rare and results from strangulating obstruction, vasculitis, or tumor perforation. It may occur during treatment of intestinal lymphomas. The treatment is always surgical and is difficult to differentiate from gastroduodenal perforation unless there is known enteric disease. It is most unusual for small-intestinal obstruction secondary to extrinsic tumors to strangulate, but obstruction in cancer patients may be benign. Tumor of the small intestine usually presents with obstruction rather than perforation. Vasculitis from drugs or in collagen disease is on the antimesenteric surface and can be mimicked by intraluminal hemorrhage and necrosis in the thrombocytopenic patient. The signs and symptoms of small-bowel perforation are those of diffuse peritonitis—usually of sudden onset, with pain, rigidity, lack of bowel sounds, and free abdominal air. Immediate laparotomy is indicated, and resection of the perforation should be performed. If there is extensive soilage so that primary enteric anastomosis is deemed unwise, temporary end-enterostomy and mucous fistula for the divided bowel loops are far safer.

Appendix and Colon

Although the diagnostic criteria for acute appendicitis in this patient population have been discussed, it should be stressed that perforation, particularly with free peritonitis, is far more frequent; thus early decision for operation is required, usually with fewer diagnostic findings.

Colonic perforations usually are either at or just proximal to the obstructing tumor or at the cecum.[18] Encircling colonic tumors in the rectosigmoid region may produce local perforation and abscess formation, but far more frequently are responsible for colonic obstruction in a closed loop limited by the ileocecal valve. The cecum is the most distensible portion of the colon and likewise has the thinnest wall. Free perforation and varying degrees of necrosis of the cecal wall are the usual consequences of colonic obstruction. Generalized peritonitis results, with dangerous fecal soilage. Obstructive symptoms will be discussed later, but they may be amazingly minimal. A history of progressive constipation, some cramps and fullness, and sometimes blood in the stool usually may be elicited. The simplest diagnostic workup is usually all that is necessary or justified. Complete blood count shows an elevated hematocrit and a leukocytosis. The hematocrit rise is associated with plasma loss and outpouring of peritoneal fluid. The acute onset of the perforation rarely is associated with any other serum abnormality, and abdominal plain films confirm the clinical diagnosis.

Immediate operation with resection of the right colon, temporary end-ileostomy, and mucous fistula for the transverse colon is the treatment of choice. Extensive irrigation, wide drainage, and aggressive antibiotic therapy usually are successful, although septic shock and death may occur. Subsequent resection of the primary cancer and closure of the diverted limbs of bowel provide colonic continuity. Local perforation of the tumor is treated best by primary resection of the lesion, drainage of the abscess, if such is present, and either direct or delayed colonic anastomosis, depending on the state of the bowel and the surrounding peritoneal surfaces. Diversion and drainage alone are not the preferred treatment. If the lesion is too low in the pelvis to permit distal mucous fistula, then a Hartmann turn-in at the pelvic floor can be used with a proximal end-sigmoid colostomy. Although the cancer prognosis in patients with colonic perforation usually is not as good as that in patients with nonperforated lesions, aggressive surgical management clearly is justified because the end results may be surprisingly good.[18]

OBSTRUCTIVE DISEASE

Obstruction of the gastrointestinal tract constitutes a common and serious abdominal problem in cancer patients. Essentially, there are two types of obstructive situations: those caused by malignant tumor and those resulting from benign lesions that accompany some form of malignant process. Even in patients with known previous cancer, it cannot be assumed that all obstruction results from tumor recurrence, nor need it be treated by operative intervention.

Because intestinal obstruction results in a severe metabolic deficit, it is important that extrarenal fluid and electrolyte losses be replaced promptly. In addition, nutritional support in the form of either peripheral or central hyperalimentation can proceed while either operative or nonoperative treatment is considered.[19] High intestinal obstruction results in greater risk for metabolic alkalosis because of the relatively high levels of gastric fluid losses and its disproportionate hydrogen ion concentration. Vomiting and distention are the key features for all sites of intestinal obstruction. Crampy abdominal pain, particularly coming in waves, associated with high-pitched peristalsis, lack of flatus, and no specific site of tenderness, is the typical finding of lower small-bowel or large-intestinal obstruction. When large-bowel obstruction is associated with an incompetent ileocecal valve, it is more difficult to distinguish from small bowel obstruction (Fig. 58-5). The closed loop form of colonic obstruction, mentioned earlier, is far more likely to rupture the cecum.

The initial investigation of all forms of intestinal obstruction should be the flat and upright plain films of the abdomen. Serial examinations will serve to document progression or improvement of obstruction if conservative treatment is chosen. The barium enema is a valuable and very safe examination and can identify unrecognized colonic obstruction; upper GI series is contraindicated except for esophageal or gastric lesions. In general, the treatment of all forms of mechanical intestinal obstructions should be surgical. Early postoperative obstruction, associated with new adhesive bands and partially functioning small-bowel loops, may respond to nasogastric or small-intestinal intubation and decompression. Experience at the Brigham and Women's Hospital with intestinal obstruction in cancer patients reveals that one third had a benign cause.[20] Obstruction was more likely to be caused by a malignant process if the patient had known metastatic carcinoma, the primary tumor was an advanced stage, colorectal cancer had been the primary lesion, or the free interval from the time of initial treatment was short. Relief of obstruction with nasogastric suction alone occurred in 24% of the episodes in these patients and always was seen within 3 days of admission. Of those patients achieving relief by conservative means, however, 41% eventually were readmitted and required surgical decompression.

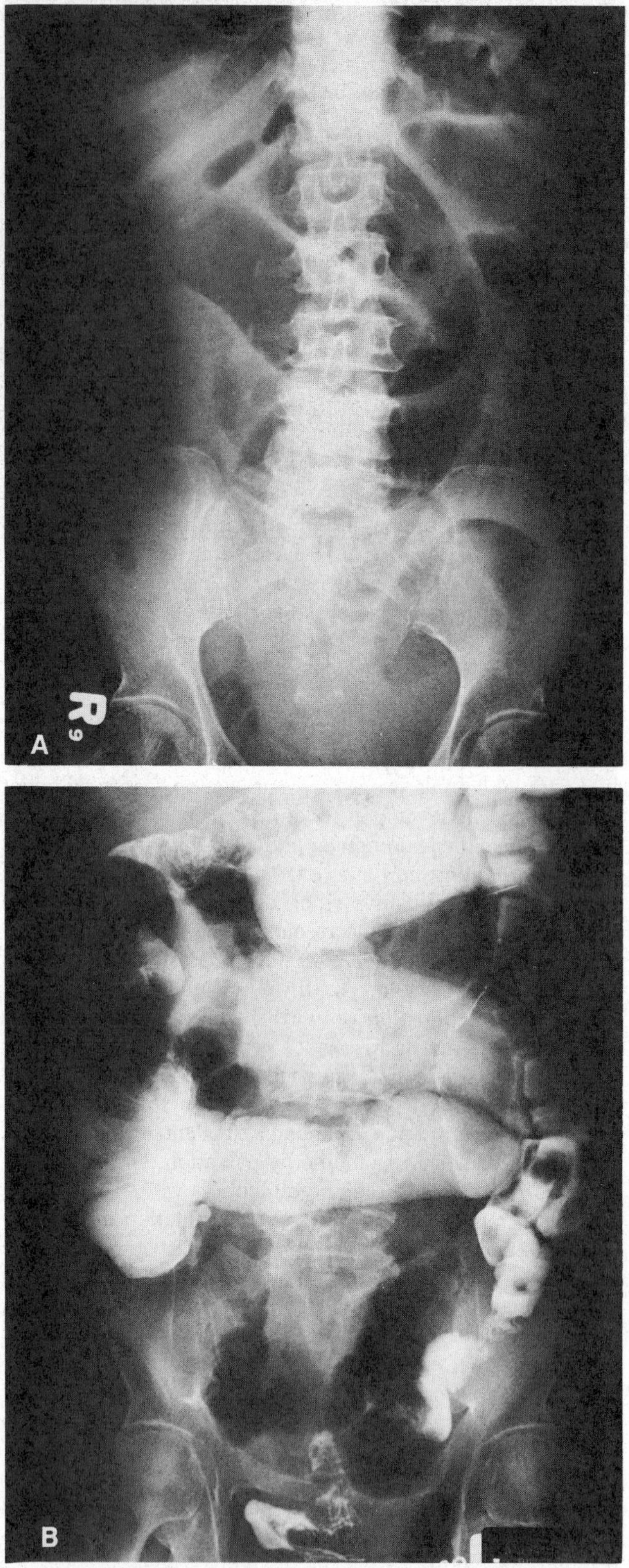

FIG. 58-5. Mechanical small bowel obstruction secondary to right colon carcinoma. **A.** Plain film of the abdomen shows small bowel obstructive pattern involving the entire jejunum and ileum. **B.** Barium enema demonstrates the responsible lesion—an annular carcinoma of the ascending colon. Barium enema is the diagnostic study of choice for patients with small bowel obstruction.

Specific aspects of obstruction lesions at different locations in the intestinal tract will be discussed from the standpoint of diagnosis and treatment.

ESOPHAGUS

Esophageal obstruction as a result of tumor or inflammatory reaction related to infection, radiation, or ulceration secondary to chemotherapy rarely presents as an acute complaint. The symptoms of dysphagia and local pain usually are progressive. However, perforation may occur, with acute epigastric complaints, and the acute pain of an obstructing ulcer may be severe. The diagnosis is best made with endoscopy so that biopsy can be obtained. Treatment is expectant and symptomatic.

GASTRIC

Gastric outlet obstruction is either the result of a benign peptic ulcer in the duodenum or pyloric channel or a gastric carcinoma of the antrum. It is rare for duodenal ulcers to obstruct without a significant history. Acute ulcers often perforate or bleed but rarely obstruct. Hydrogen ion concentration is always high so that a metabolic alkalosis is usually present by the time the diagnosis is made.[21] Pyloric channel ulcers obstruct most frequently, even when they heal. Duodenal ulcer disease can develop or become aggravated as a result of corticosteroid therapy, operative procedures, and the general anxiety state surrounding cancer management. Although conservative treatment with gastric decompression, H_2-blocking agents, and fluid and electrolyte replacement is necessary as the initial therapy, an obstructing duodenal ulcer almost uniformly requires operative therapy. Pyloroplasty with vagotomy is the treatment of choice. This is a particularly safe operation for patients with a debilitating disease (*e.g.*, malignancy) or during the course of chemotherapy because there is no circumferential anastomosis, and tissue healing is excellent.

Obstructing gastric carcinoma or obstruction of the gastric outlet by extension of pancreatic carcinoma or other metastatic malignancy requires a different approach (Fig. 58-6). Obstruction by gastric carcinoma need not be a late-stage or an antral carcinoma; thus, a radical subtotal gastrectomy is indicated if operative findings warrant it. Even if there is evidence of metastatic disease to the liver, celiac nodes, or pelvis, palliation is best achieved by a gastric resection, albeit more limited. Obstruction of the stomach by a diffuse gastric carcinoma, such as linitis plastica, which extends from the esophagus to duodenum and is spread to local lymph nodes, carries a graver prognosis, and deciding whether a total gastrectomy should be performed in such a patient depends on the age and general status of the patient, as well as on the availability of radiation and chemotherapy programs to follow.

Gastric outlet obstruction by extension of pancreatic or biliary tract carcinoma or as a result of metastatic lesions (*e.g.*, carcinoma of the cervix, colon, and ovary), is best treated by gastrojejunostomy (side-to-side). Retrocolic posterior gastroenterostomy is sometimes easier if there is extensive omental involvement with tumor, making access to the anterior gastric surface difficult. It is essential to anastomose the jejunum to uninvolved stomach; otherwise, peristaltic activity will be ineffective, and the procedure will fail to provide gastric emptying.

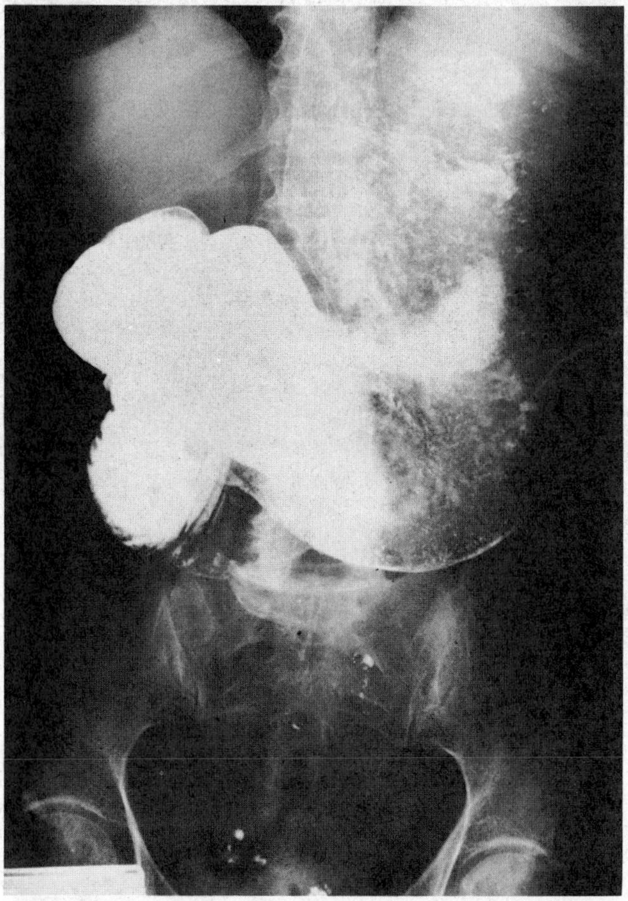

FIG. 58-6. Gastric outlet obstruction. Upper GI series demonstrates massive gastric dilatation with duodenal obstruction. The obstruction was produced by metastatic carcinoma of the breast involving the retroperitoneum in the vicinity of the duodenum and the ligaments of Treitz.

SMALL INTESTINE

Most small-bowel obstruction in cancer patients with previous abdominal malignancy is the result of neoplastic implants. Because many of these patients have multiple foci of involvement and the obstruction may not be complete, as a general rule conservative management with intubation is appropriate as the initial step (Figs. 58-7 and 58-8). This is particularly true if a previous operation for malignant obstruction has taken place. It is rare for multiple surgical attempts to be successful when treating intestinal obstruction owing to malignant bowel involvement. An initial operative procedure is always justified if decompression fails to reverse the situation. Sometimes preoperative passage of a Miller–Abbott or other long intestinal tube will permit better identification of both the site of obstruction and the proximal and distal limbs of an obstructive bowel. These features may be obscured completely by extensive peritoneal carcinoma-

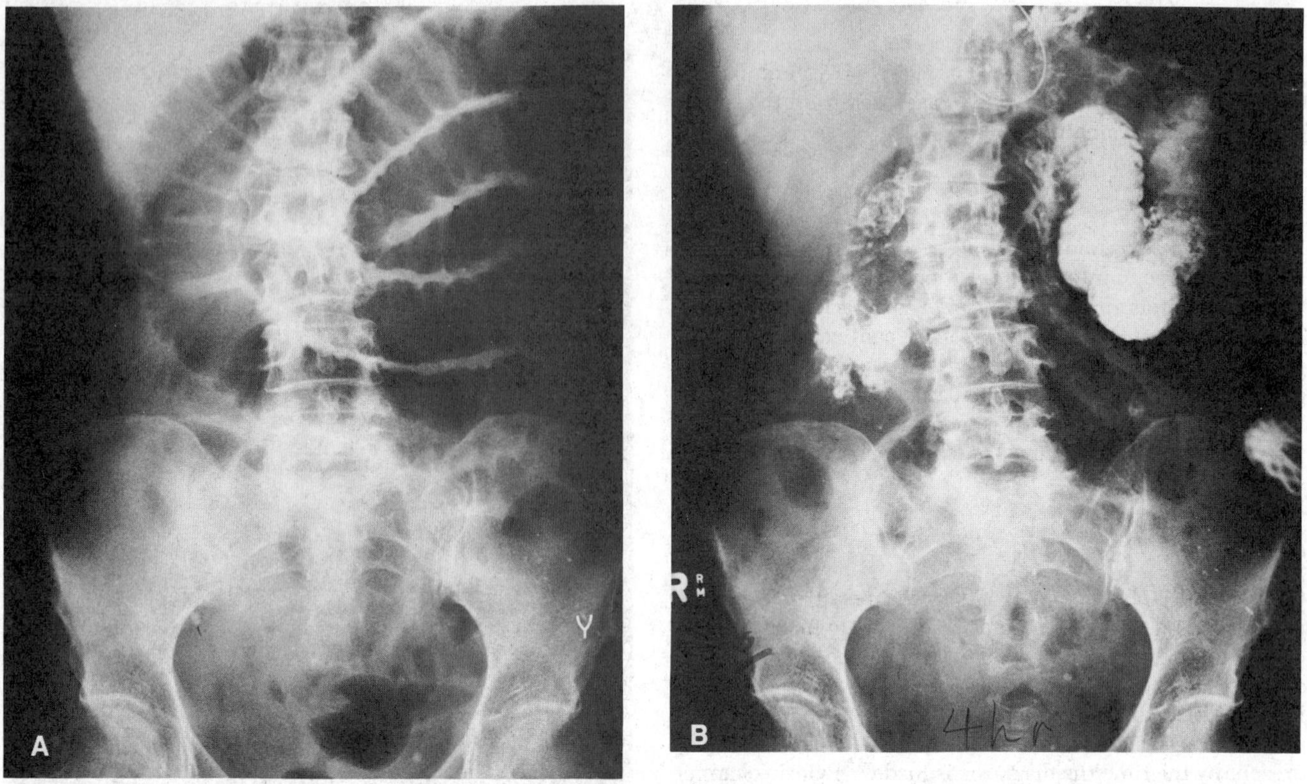

FIG. 58-7. Small bowel obstruction due to postirradiation enteritis and metastatic endometrial carcinoma. **A**. Plain film of the abdomen shows small bowel dilatation, thickened intestinal wall, and some air in the distal colon. **B**. History was that of intermittent obstruction, confirmed by upper GI series that demonstrated moderate dilatation and poor motility. Upper GI series is indicated in this type of patient when the obstructive pattern is much less clear.

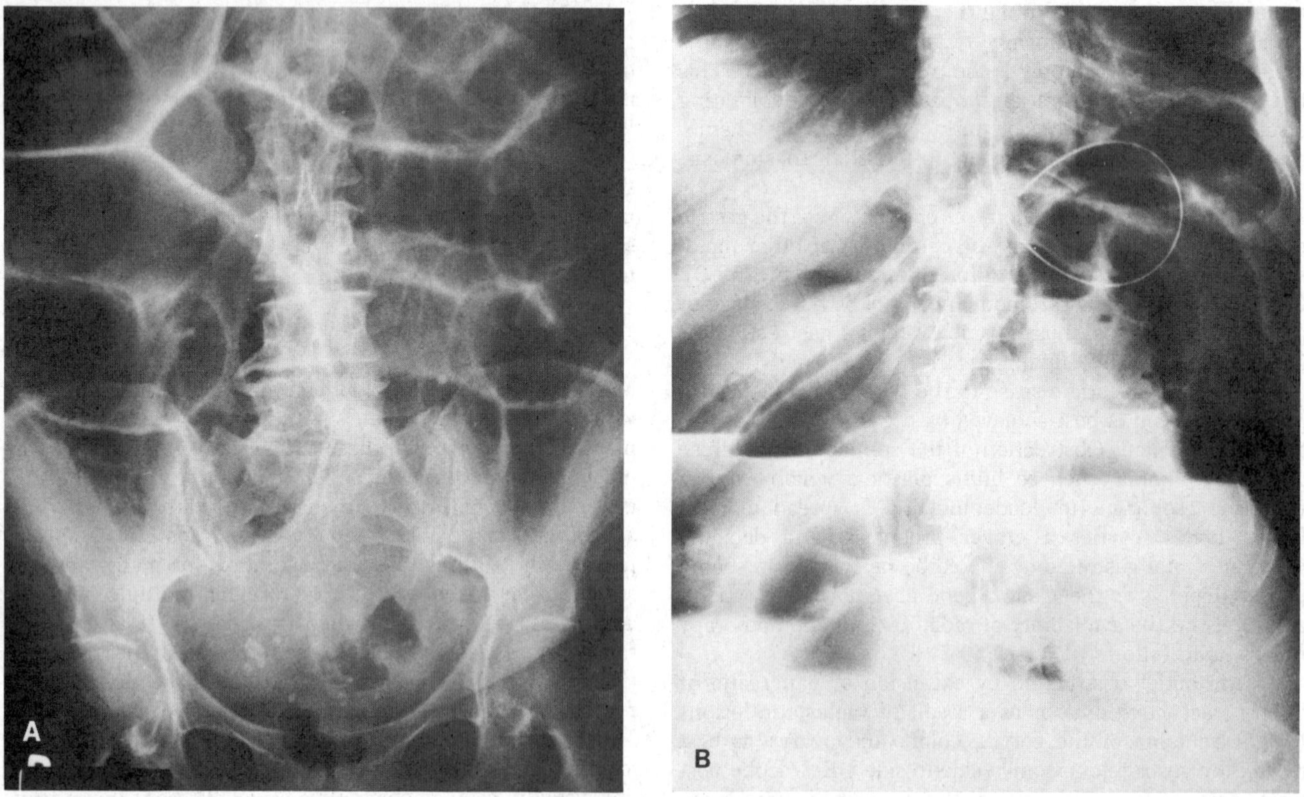

FIG. 58-8. Mechanical small bowel obstruction secondary to metastatic carcinoma of the cervix. **A**. Obstruction is complete and acute with thin bowel wall, large air-fluid filled loops of bowel, and minimal large intestinal gas. **B**. Upright film shows the air–fluid levels most dramatically. The site of obstruction was in the terminal ileum.

tosis, the most common type of metastatic disease that produces obstruction. Pancreatic, ovarian, colonic, and gastric carcinomas are the most common offenders. No aggressive attempts at freeing up loops of involved bowel or resection should be made; it is preferable to perform the simplest side-to-side bypass anastomosis possible. Frequently, the transverse colon is the most identifiable distal bowel. The second choice is the terminal ileum. The risk of small-bowel fistula is very high if dissection of tumor-involved bowel is attempted, and that is a dire complication. If the intestinal lumen is accidentally opened where tumor is present, it is wise either to resect or to bypass that site. Abdominal cavity drainage and enterostomy catheters should be avoided because of the high incidence of tumor growth along the tracts.

If the cancer patient presenting with small-bowel obstruction is fortunate enough to have a benign cause, such as adhesive bands or internal hernia, standard treatment should be used. More attention should be paid to wound management and to early nutritional support because the patient may be significantly depleted of calories and protein, even before the onset of the obstruction. The diagnosis may be somewhat obscured in patients receiving chemotherapy or radiation because of the high incidence of gastrointestinal symptoms associated with these treatments. Therefore, one must be certain that patients receiving chemotherapy who have persistent vomiting also do not have crampy abdominal pain or lack passage of flatus.

COLONIC

Presentation of the problem of colonic obstruction has been discussed partially in the section on colonic perforation. The symptoms may be insidious or very acute. The end result, however, is dilated bowel, vomiting, crampy pain, and lack of flatus or stool passage (Fig. 58-9). It is rare for the right colon to be obstructed by tumor, but in the rest of the colon, except the rectum, it is not an uncommon occurrence. Prompt treatment is required to avoid perforation. No attempts should be made to resect the obstructing lesion in an unprepared colon. It is far safer to perform a diverting colostomy, usually right transverse or, if necessary, an end-ileostomy or cecostomy for hepatic flexure lesions. This diverting procedure usually can be performed while the patient is under local anesthesia, with or without intercostal block, and avoids the dangers of using a general anesthetic in a sick, distended, depleted, and frequently uncompensated patient. Rapid restoration of homeostasis and thorough workup usually can be followed by a safe, elective bowel resection in 10 to 14 days. Barium enema is the x-ray study of choice once the plain films have defined the problem. No preparation is necessary, and the radiologist should use minimal pressure.

Rectal cancers that obstruct are rare and generally are locally advanced lesions. A rectal examination usually will reveal a large, fungating tumor with extension to the adjacent organs of the pelvis or the pelvic wall. Most patients with this form of obstructing rectal carcinoma will require radiation therapy, with a diverting colostomy, before an attempt is made to resect the primary. Resection should be performed, however, because radiation alone rarely achieves good palliation. With no evidence of distant metastases, after

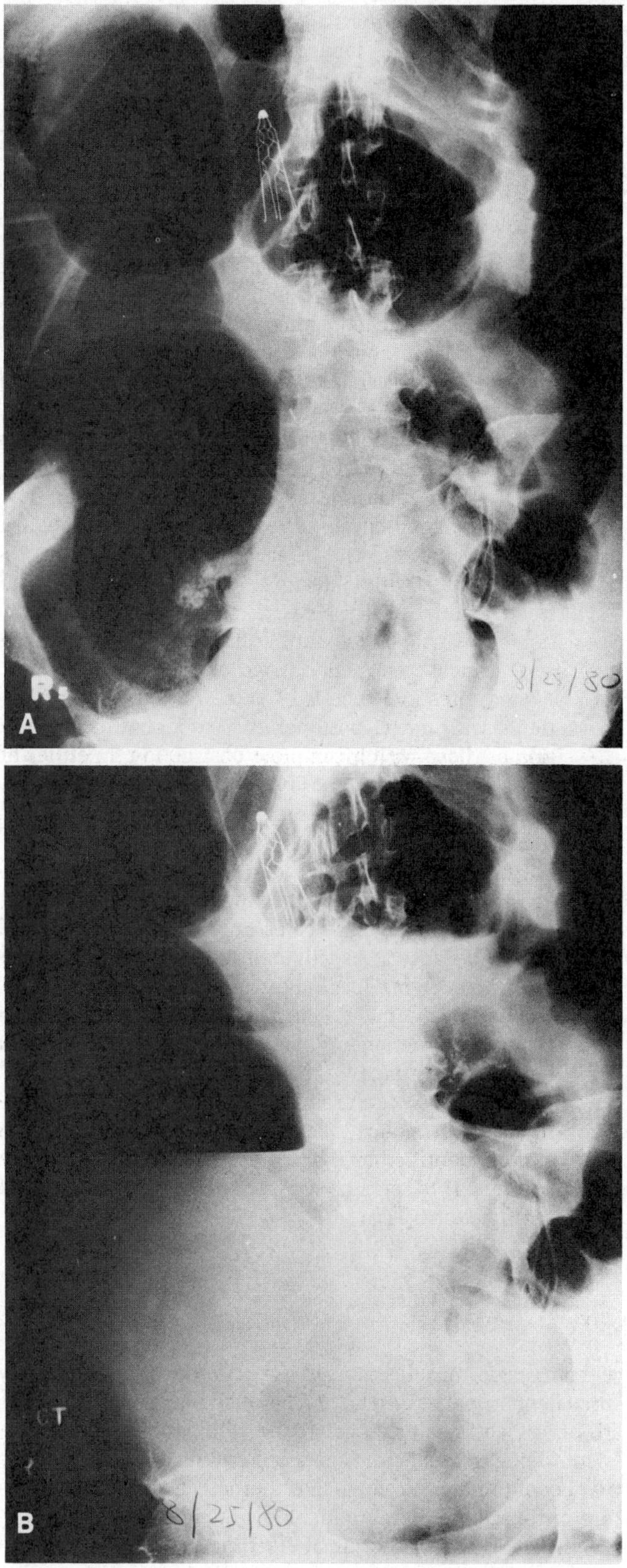

FIG. 58-9. Colonic obstruction with competent ileocecal valve produced by an intra-abdominal sarcoma. **A**. Obstruction was at the level of the sigmoid colon where the gas pattern ends. **B**. The cecum is critically dilated, requiring emergency transverse colostomy. No small bowel dilatation is seen—evidence of the close loop obstruction. A caval umbrella is present in the right upper quadrant.

a thorough evaluation, particularly of the liver, exenterative procedures are justified for locally extensive rectal cancer.

STRATEGIES FOR MANAGING INTESTINAL OBSTRUCTION

A practical summary for managing various forms of intestinal obstruction follows:

1. The diagnosis of the site of obstruction is critical for treatment.
2. Plain films of the abdomen may separate gastric, small bowel, or large bowel obstruction rapidly.
3. Upper GI series should be obtained only in patients with gastric or duodenal obstruction.
4. Barium enema should be performed for patients with large- or small-bowel obstructions.
5. Patients with incomplete small-bowel obstruction may require a small-bowel series by mouth or through a tube to define the site of disease.
6. All patients with intestinal obstruction should be treated initially with a nasogastric tube. For most patients this will suffice until a diagnosis has been made and surgical treatment carried out.
7. A long intestinal tube is of value only in treating patients with early, postoperative small-bowel obstruction or those with incomplete obstruction. In either of these two situations, the obstruction may be reversible, which is the prime indication for small-bowel intubation.
8. Large bowel obstruction requires early surgical decompression, particularly if the ileocecal valve is competent. Right transverse colostomy is the treatment of choice because it usually can be performed with the patient receiving local anesthetic and does not interfere with subsequent cancer resection.
9. Gastric obstruction and small-bowel obstruction should be treated surgically unless a brief period of decompression reverses the situation. Nonoperative management is particularly justified if no obstructing lesion can be identified or if acute gastric dilation or ileus is presumed to be the cause of the gastrointestinal malfunction.

HEMORRHAGE

Hemorrhagic complications in the abdomen are particularly prevalent in patients with malignancy because of the high risk of mucosal damage, combined with pancytopenia in patients being treated with aggressive multimodal therapy for a variety of tumors. Although most hemorrhagic complications are intraluminal, extraluminal bleeding likewise may occur. Prompt diagnosis of the site of bleeding is even more critical in this patient population because treatment decisions may be particularly complex. The critical factor is always whether or not bleeding is sufficiently massive for emergency operation to be performed. This decision is often difficult, even in people without malignant disease or complicating treatment plans. Three important considerations include the following: Are the causes of bleeding correctable—short of surgery; How effectively can a surgical procedure control the bleeding; How disabling is the surgery? The final decision for or against a surgical procedure must answer these questions.

INTRALUMINAL BLEEDING

Esophagus

Esophageal varices can be a complication of primary hepatic tumors, liver metastases, or myeloproliferative disorders, with either liver involvement or intrahepatic hematopoiesis. Obviously, the degree of portal hypertension and associated trauma or ulceration will be responsible for variceal bleeding. Emergency portacaval shunt may be required for such variceal bleeding if it becomes exsanguinating and cannot be controlled by either a Sengstaken–Blakemore tube or vasopressin. All patients with variceal bleeding may be treated initially with intravenous vasopressin, but, should this fail, intra-arterial vasopressin should be administered through the left gastric artery. The dosage for intra-arterial vasopressin is between 0.2 U/min and 0.4 U/min. If the patient is relatively stable and not bleeding too vigorously, then 0.2 U/min is the starting dosage. Rapid bleeding requires initiation of the dosage at 0.4 U/min. Dosages above that level usually are not any more effective and do have a greater complication rate from systemic effects of vasopressin. Older patients will have complications, particularly in the form of arrhythmias, even at the 0.2 to 0.4 U/min level. The usual length of intra-arterial vasopressin therapy is 12 hr. If successful cessation of bleeding occurs, then the dosage should be tapered, with reduction at the rate of 0.1 U/12 hr. The catheter is left in place for 12 hr after vasopressin therapy has been discontinued before it is removed. As with treatment of gastrointestinal bleeding in other sites, failure of response to vasopressin indicates the possibility of using autogenous embolization to the varices, and, if that fails, surgical treatment is the choice.

Patients with hiatal hernia and reflux esophagitis can develop significant gastrointestinal bleeding with ulceration, particularly during corticosteroid therapy or if vomiting is prolonged. Usually antacid therapy with dietary management is sufficient for control, but on occasion an antireflux procedure, such as the Nissen fundoplication, is required.[22]

Stomach

Massive life-threatening bleeding may occur from gastritis, benign ulcers, or gastric carcinoma. Gastritis is common in patients with malignancy; pain medications, so frequently taken, often are irritating to the gastric muscosa. Likewise, specific forms of chemotherapy either may damage the gastric mucosa or certainly be associated with gastric irritation, dilatation, and vomiting. Septic episodes may invoke gastritis and shallow gastric ulcers, as may corticosteroid ingestion. Thrombocytopenia, uremia, and hepatic dysfunction will aggravate the problem. The diagnosis is best made by endoscopy, but selective angiography may be effective not only in defining the bleeding point but also in permitting control with either vasopressin or autogenous clots. Bleeding must be sufficiently vigorous from a site in the gastrointestinal tract to identify the bleeding point by this technique; thus, it has limited usefulness. Treatment of gastritis-induced bleeding should be conservative at first; gastric decompression, lavage with cold saline to reduce mucosal flow, irrigation with antacids for acid neutralization and H_2-blocking therapy all should be attempted. If, after adequate blood replacement, correction of clotting and bleeding abnormalities, and sufficient vasopressin administration by intra-arterial infusion (see foregoing schedule), the bleeding persists, then surgical control will be required.[23] The surgical treatment of choice is a radical subtotal gastrectomy. Even though the entire mucosa appears to be the source of bleeding, it is rarely necessary to perform a total gastric resection for gastritis. Even preserving a small gastric cuff reduces the frequency of anastomotic disruption and postoperative difficulties.

Benign gastric ulcers rarely result in major bleeding; pain or perforation is more common. Occasionally, however, they will bleed massively, so that emergency gastric resection is required. Upper GI series or endoscopy is the method of diagnosis. It is difficult to distinguish a benign ulcer from carcinoma, particularly when bleeding occurs. Persistent gastric ulcers that do not heal promptly require surgical resection anyway, so that subtotal gastrectomy produces the most effective treatment. Older patients with arteriosclerotic vessels and those with abnormal clotting factors will bleed more persistently and will require more prompt resection. As we stated before, in the emergency treatment of gastric carcinoma, whether it is perforated, obstructing, or bleeding, radical subtotal gastrectomy is the operation of choice. Extensive carcinomas of the entire gastric lumen will require total gastrectomy for bleeding control, contrary to the experience with diffuse gastritis.

Other malignant lesions that may produce major gastric bleeding are leiomyosarcoma of the stomach, carcinoid tumors of the stomach, gastric lymphoma, and metastatic tumor, particularly melanoma. The latter, on GI series, produces a typical "doughnut" ulcer in the stomach, a metastatic focus with a necrotic center that bleeds. Leiomyosarcomas of the stomach commonly present with bleeding when the mucosa over the tumor becomes eroded. The treatment of choice for all these lesions is gastric resection, with an attempt to leave some normal proximal or distal stomach. Any proximal resection should be accompanied by a pyloroplasty because of vagal nerve resection and gastric atony.

Small Intestine

The most common bleeding point in the small intestine is in the duodenum. Acute duodenal ulcer with bleeding may occur after any surgical operation, after major injury, as a complication of corticosteroid or other drug therapy, or after major septic episodes. A history of duodenal ulcer also makes it more likely, and bleeding will be more frequent in the pancytopenic patient. Treatment should be conservative at the start, with cimetidine or other H_2-receptor antagonists, antacids, decompression if vomiting is present, and correction of bleeding problems. Bleeding from duodenal and some gastric ulcers may be controlled successfully by embolization of the artery from which the bleeding is identified by angiography. Embolization, rather than intra-arterial vasopressin, is the treatment of choice for specific ulcers in either duodenum or the stomach.[24] If bleeding cannot be controlled, prompt surgical attack should be made before problems of coagulation and pneumonia develop. The combination of pyloroplasty, suture ligation of the bleeding point with nonabsorbable material, and vagotomy is the treatment of choice. Massive hemorrhage usually will not occur from a duodenal ulcer unless the gastroduodenal artery or one of its branches is eroded. Duodenitis will not produce that degree of bleeding. Occasionally, the use of radiolabled red blood cells for a nucleotide scan may identify the site of bleeding within the small or large intestine in a much less invasive manner than that required for angiography.

Major bleeding is rare from metastases to the small intestine. Ovarian metastases may not even extend through the serosa, but most other tumors can invade into the mucosa and produce hemorrhage. Likewise, effective treatment of lymphomatous nodules in the small intestine may produce tumor necrosis and bleeding. Lymphoma and large mesenteric lymph nodes can extend into the intestinal wall and produce bleeding when necrosis ensues. Intestinal fistula from neoplastic growth may also bleed extensively. The diagnosis of these lesions usually is made by small-intestinal barium study, but sometimes not until laparotomy is performed. The treatment of small-intestinal tumors is important because loss of enteric continuity in a cancer patient results in severe nutritional consequences. The large intestine serves no digestive function and can always be partially or totally bypassed.

Colorectum

Major bleeding from the colon and the rectum is not common in patients with malignant disease, unless there are serious bleeding abnormalities. Primary tumors usually bleed slowly and insidiously. Polypoid tumors, particularly of the rectum, may bleed sufficiently so that rectal bleeding is the cause for the patient to visit the physician. Any other causes of major colonic bleeding, such as diverticular disease, colitis, or proctitis can be treated expectantly, assuming attempts are made to correct any defects and clotting factors. Angiographic identification and arterial infusion of vasopressin are most effective for colonic bleeding and should be attempted before any surgical attack is considered (Fig. 58-10).[25] Large villous adenomas in the rectum can be fulgurated directly or excised transrectally to control bleeding.[26] As with all chronically ill patients, stool softeners and adequate hydration will minimize the risk of anorectal bleeding and other complications.

EXTRALUMINAL BLEEDING

Abdominal bleeding outside the intestinal lumen most frequently is in the retroperitoneum and mesentery or in other

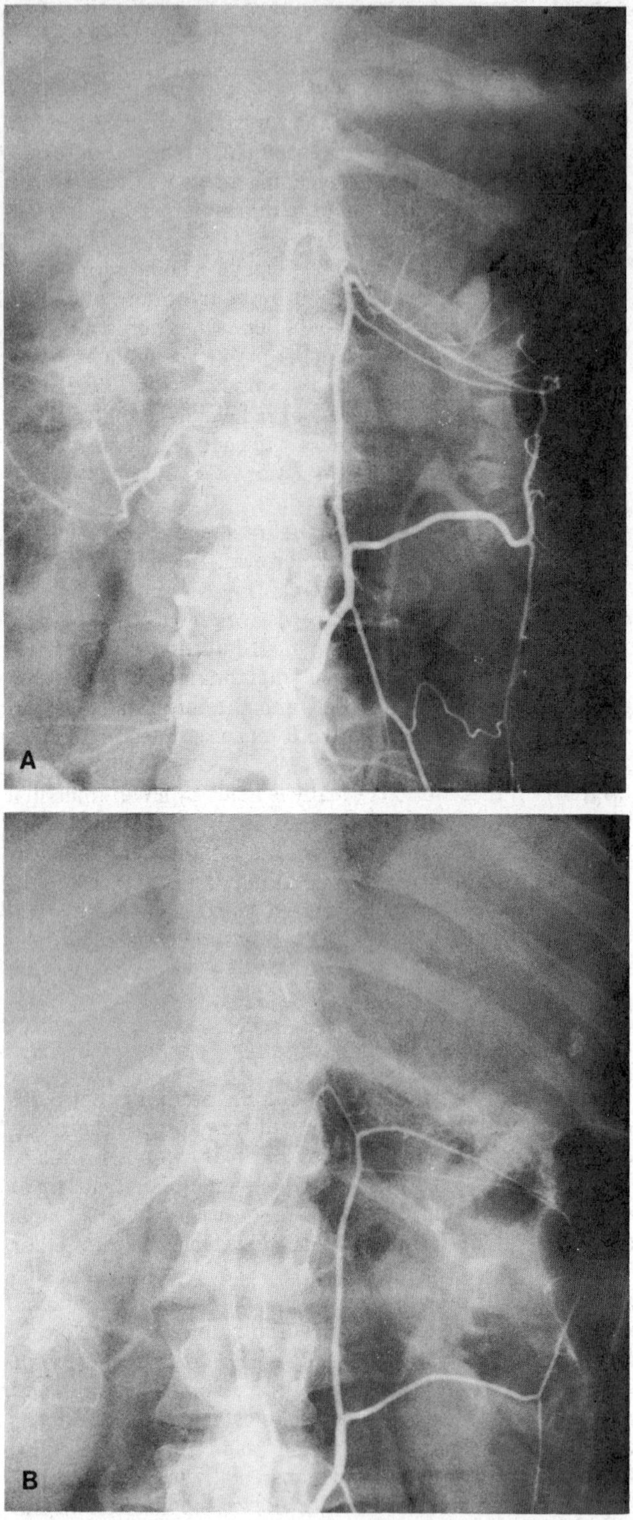

FIG. 58-10. Angiographic technique for controlling GI bleeding. **A**. Intraluminal bleeding point identified in transverse colon (*arrow*) by infusion of middle colic artery with contrast. **B**. Bleeding controlled by infusion of vasopressin at 0.3 U/min by way of *both* superior mesenteric and inferior mesenteric arteries. Infusion of either artery alone failed to control the bleeding. No surgical treatment was needed for this patient.

abnormal organs. The diagnosis of bleeding rarely is made as early or as accurately as it is with intraluminal bleeding, and the treatment is more varied.

Retroperitoneal bleeding usually is the result of thrombocytopenia or some other coagulopathy. For the most part, it is spontaneous and controlled by restoration of the clotting defect and retransfusion. Surgery should not be considered for this problem. Extension of bleeding into the mesentery is common and similarly should be treated conservatively. The diagnosis usually is made when bulging of the flanks of the abdomen is identified, frequently with ecchymosis and sometimes accompanied by tenderness. Hypovolemia, falling hematocrit, and unexplained hypotension without evidence of intraluminal bleeding are the usual observations.

Bleeding into the spleen may occur suddenly. The spleen in this case is enlarged, usually from either infarct or trauma. Numerous forms of malignancy are associated with splenomegaly, and such spleens are at greater risk for rupture, usually with subscapular tears but, sometimes, with free perforations and rapid hypovolemic shock. Pain, either referred to the left shoulder or the left flank, is the most common specific complaint. With trauma, the history of the type and direction of injury is valuable. The presence of fractured ribs in the left lower rib cage also is important evidence leading to a diagnosis. Plain films showing shift of the gastric air bubble and the splenic flexure or abnormalities on either nuclide or CT scan are helpful in showing splenic infarcts or fracture. An angiogram, with placement of autogenous clots in the splenic artery, occasionally may prevent emergency splenectomy in selected patients in whom this is contraindicated. When free perforation has occurred, a peritoneal tap will demonstrate free blood. Splenectomy is the treatment of choice for splenic bleeding and usually can be performed safely. Splenorrhaphy can be attempted for smaller splenic injuries.

Hepatic bleeding most frequently results from primary hepatomas, liver cell adenoma, or focal nodular hyperplasia. It is a rare finding for patients with focal nodular hyperplasia, but is very commonly seen in primary hepatomas and liver cell adenoma patients. This is particularly true for liver cell adenomas in which, aside from the presence of a mass, retroperitoneal bleeding is the most common method of presentation.[27] Bleeding from both hepatoma and liver cell adenomas can be massive and exsanguinating. Evaluation of hepatic lesions with angiography, CT, and ultrasound scans, as well as nuclide scans, should provide useful evidence of the location and the resectability of primary hepatic tumors, but generally, laparotomy is necessary for the ultimate decision. Metastatic hepatic tumors rarely produce bleeding.

In the female patient, significant menorrhagia can occur with thrombocytopenia. It may be necessary to suppress menstrual cycles with hormone therapy, or rarely, perform hysterectomy to control this.

Another important cause of extraluminal bleeding is from abdominal aortic aneurysms. Although this would be considered only a coincidental problem in cancer patients, they can coexist. Because this is such a treatable condition, it must be considered in the differential diagnosis of any major abdominal catastrophy, even in patients with malignant disease.

SPECIAL ABDOMINAL PROBLEMS IN POSTOPERATIVE PATIENTS

Certain acute abdominal conditions may occur after major surgical procedures in any part of the body. These include acute pancreatitis, acute cholecystitis, mesenteric vascular accident, and pulmonary embolism with infarction on the diaphragmatic surface. After abdominal surgery, a variety of complications can present as acute abdominal problems, including bleeding, anastomotic leak, abscess formation, and diffuse peritonitis. Most patients with malignant disease are more prone to develop problems of tissue healing and control of sepsis, so much a part of the normal recovery process after surgery.

Because of usual problems after major surgery, such as incisional pain, tachycardia, and low-grade fever, acute abdominal complications often are more difficult to diagnose than they might be in their usual setting. The nutritionally depleted patient with extensive abdominal surgery, a description that often characterizes the cancer patient, makes concern for the type and form of anastomosis critical and consideration of diversion and staging of procedures important. The surgeon must be alert to the postoperative circumstances of unexplained or prolonged ileus, pleural effusion, jaundice, unusual pain, tachycardia, and hypotension. These findings may be the only indicators that the patient's course is not proceeding normally after surgery. Frequent observation and the possibility of reexploration must always be considered if these findings persist.

FIG. 58-11. Pelvic abscess defined by ^{67}Ga citrate imaging. Posterior view of the abdomen and pelvis in a 77-year-old woman with fever 1 week after an anterior resection with Hartmann turn-in of the distal sigmoid colon. A large extraperitoneal pelvic abscess was defined by this scan. There is a prominent ring-shaped accumulation of the isotope in the abscess cavity around the rectum.

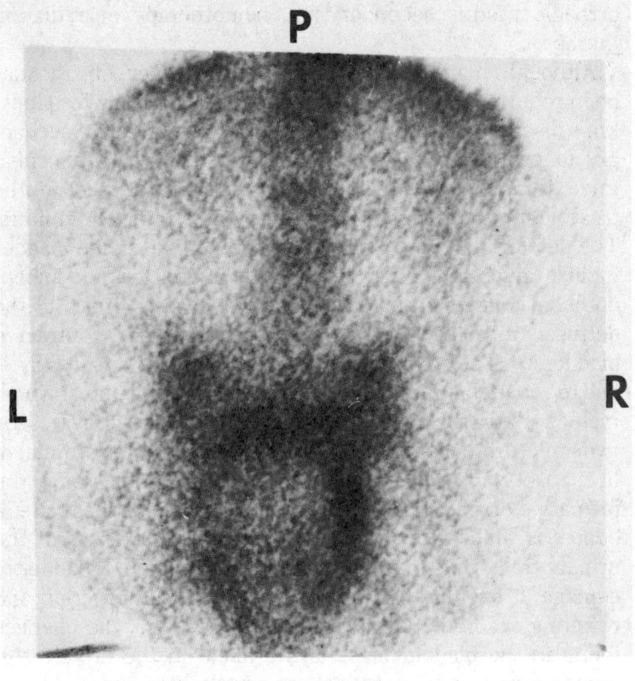

Ultrasound examination can be particularly useful in identifying postoperative abscess, biliary stones in acutely jaundiced patients, and evidence of pancreatitis. Intra-abdominal abscess formation may be particularly insidious and difficult to define. Recently, McNeil and co-workers reported a prospective study comparing CT scans, ultrasound, and^{67} Gacitrate imaging in patients suspected of having a focal source of sepsis (Fig. 58-11).[28–30] These authors found that if any two of these three examinations were used and if the result of either examination was abnormal, the sensitivity of the evaluation increased from 60% to nearly 90%, but the false-positive rate increased from 15% to 25%. On the other hand, if focal sepsis was diagnosed only when the results of two examinations were abnormal, the false-positive rate dropped to near zero, but the sensitivity dropped to under 40%. McNeil and co-workers concluded that all three modalities seemed similar in their ability to detect focal sources of sepsis and that is was more advisable to use multiple methods of evaluation rather than a single study. One of the disadvantages of gallium citrate imaging is the 48- to 72-hr delay necessary for the most favorable type of study, whereas ultrasound and computerized tomography can provide immediate information.

Contrast studies will identify anastomotic leaks, usually with Gastrografin to minimize barium staining. Wound dehiscence often will result from sepsis, pancreatitis, or anastomotic leakage, depending on the time of occurrence after operation. The surgeon caring for patients with malignant disease must use special diagnostic and therapeutic expertise to reduce the risk of complications and to achieve the best possible results.

REFERENCES

1. Botsford TW, Wilson RE: The Acute Abdomen: An Approach to Diagnosis and Management, 2nd ed. Philadelphia, WB Saunders, 1977
2. Steele G Jr, Sonis S, Stelos P et al: Circulating immune complexes in patients following clinically curative resection of colorectal cancer. Surgery 83:648–654, 1978
3. Rainer P, Deyhle P: Guided puncture under real-time sonographic control. Radiology 134:784–785, 1980
4. Kelly WD, Good RA: Immunologic deficiency in Hodgkin's disease. In Good RA, Bergsma D (eds): Immunologic Deficiency Diseases in Man. Birth Defects Original Article Series, Vol IV, pp 349–356. New York, National Foundation Press, 1968
5. Rosenberg SA: Cancer immunology. In Munster AM (ed): Surgical Immunology, pp 231–281. New York, Grune & Stratton, 1976
6. Sugarbaker PH, Skarin AT, Wilson RE: Thrombocytopenia from metastatic carcinoma of the breast: Effective managements of patients with this complication. Arch Surg 107:523–527, 1973
7. Gantz NM, Myerowitz RL, Medeiros AA et al: Listeriosis in immunosuppressed patients: A cluster of eight cases. Am J Med 58:637–643, 1975
8. Sugarbaker PH, Wilson RE: Using celioscopy to determine stages of intra–abdominal malignant neoplasms. Arch Surg 111:41–44, 1976
9. Wilson RE: Surgical problems in immunodepressed patients. In Major Problems in Clinical Surgery, Vol 30. Philadelphia, WB Saunders, 1984
10. Rosoff L, White EJ: Perforation of the esophagus. Am J Surg 128:207–218, 1974
11. McIntosh DMF, Penney HF: Gray-scale ultrasonography as a screening procedure in the detection of gallbladder disease. Radiology 136:725–727, 1980
12. Peterson LM. Collins JJ Jr, Wilson RE: Acute pancreatitis occurring after operation. Surg Gynecol Obstet 127:23–28, 1968
13. Sidel VW, Wilson RE, Shipp JC: Pseudocyst formation in chronic pancreatitis: A cause of obstructive jaundice. Arch Surg 77:933–937, 1958
14. Bartlett JG, Chang TW, Gurwith M et al: Antibiotic associated pseudomembranous colitis due to toxin-producing clostridia. N Engl J Med 298:531–534, 1978
15. Misra MK, Pinkus GS, Birtch AG et al: Major colonic diseases complicating renal transplantation. Surgery 73:942, 948, 1973

16. Sawyers JL, Herrington JL Jr, Mulherin JO et al: Acute perforated duodenal ulcer: An evaluation of surgical management. Arch Surg 110:527-536, 1975
17. Grossman MI: Resume and comment. In The Veterans Administration Cooperative Study on Gastric Ulcer Gastroenterology 61:635-638, 1971
18. Miller LD, Boruchow IB, Fitts WT Jr: An analysis of 284 patients with perforative carcinoma of the colon. Surg Gynecol Obstet 123:1212-1218, 1966
19. Dudrick SJ, Wilmore DW, Vars HM et al: Can intravenous feeding as the sole means of nutrition support growth in the child and restore weight loss in an adult? An affirmative answer. Ann Surg 169:974-984, 1969
20. Osteen RT, Guyton S. Steele G et al: Malignant intestinal obstruction. Surgery 87:611-615, 1980
21. Harken AH, Gabel RA, Fencl V et al: Hydrocholoric acid in the correction of metabolic alkalosis. Arch Surg 110:819-821, 1975
22. Demeester TR, Johnson LF, Kent AH: Evaluation of current operations for the prevention of gastroesophageal reflux. Ann Surg 180:511-525, 1974
23. Athanasoulis CA, Baum S, Waltman AC et al: Control of acute gastric mucosal hemorrhage: Intra-arterial infusion of posterior pituitary extracts. N Engl J Med 290:597-603, 1974
24. Rosch J, Dotter CT, Brown MJ: Selective arterial embolization. A new method for control of acute gastrointestional bleeding. Radiology 102:303-306, 1972
25. Baus S, Athanasoulis CA, Waltman AC et al: Angiographic diagnosis and control of gastrointestinal bleeding. In Welch C (ed): Advances in Surgery, Vol 7, pp 149-198. Chicago. Year Book Medical Publishers, 1973
26. Wlech CE: Practical consideration in treatment of polypoid lesions of colon and rectum. In Dunphy JE (ed): Polypoid Lesions of the Gastrointestinal Tract, pp 98-122. Philadelphia, WB Saunders, 1964
27. Foster JH, Berman MM: The benign lesions: Ademona and focal nodular hyperplasia. In Ebert PA (ed): Solid Liver Tumors, pp 138-178. Philadelphia, WB Saunders, 1977
28. McNeil BJ, Sanders R, Alderson PO et al: A prospective study of computed tomography ultrasound, and gallium imaging in patients with fever. Radiology 139:647, 1981
29. Kumar B, Alderson PO, Geisse G: The role of Ga-67 citrate imaging and diagnostic ultrasound in patients with suspected abdominal abcesses. J Nucl Med 18:534-537, 1977
30. Levitt RG, Biello DR, Sagel SS et al: Computed tomography and ^{67}Ga citrated radionuclide imagery for evaluating suspected abdominal abscess. Am J Roentgenol 132:529-534, 1979

SECTION 5 WILLIAM R. FAIR

Urologic Emergencies

Most urologic emergencies in cancer patients arise as a consequence of hemorrhage, uremia secondary to obstructive uropathy, or infection—with or without superimposed obstructions. The clinical presentation may include disturbances of urination, hematuria, a marked decrease or absence of urine output, pain, fever, and clinical signs of azotemia. Urinary tract infection in the presence of obstruction can rapidly lead to sepsis and, if untreated, to death. A patient with an already compromised immune system secondary to massive tumor burden and the effects of chemotherapy or radiation therapy may be especially susceptible.

The physician must be aware of these potential problems in treating cancer patients and must be prepared to act quickly and decisively when these complications are encountered. This chapter section will briefly discuss the diagnosis and management of urologic emergencies in the cancer patient.

HEMATURIA

Serious and, at times, life-threatening hematuria in the cancer patient usually is the result of recurrent tumor in the urinary tract, hemorrhagic cystitis as a sequelae of either chemotherapy or radiation treatment and, rarely, evidence of systemic bleeding secondary to disseminated intravascular coagulation or other defects in the coagulation system. The character of hematuria often suggests the site of origin.

Initial hematuria that clears toward the end of the urinary stream most commonly is associated with lesions in the urethra, whereas terminal hematuria suggests a source of bleeding from the bladder or the kidney. Total hematuria, the most common presentation, may occur with lesions anywhere in the urinary tract. Pain (or lack of pain) on urination is often a useful clinical clue to the cause of the bleeding. Urinary tract infections sufficient to cause gross hematuria often present with pain on urination, frequency of urination, nocturia, suprapubic tenderness or pressure and, occasionally, fever. Control of the infection will control the hematuria. In patients with painless hematuria the likelihood of a cause other than infection is great, and additional investigative and diagnostic approaches should be considered. Steps to determine the etiology of hematuria in a cancer patient include a careful physical examination, x-ray studies (excretory urogram, CT scan), and endoscopic examination, preferably during active bleeding, to localize the source. Endoscopic examinations should be considered with caution until infection has been ruled out as a cause of the hematuria, because instrumentation in the presence of grossly infected urine may increase the likelihood of sepsis.

CHEMOTHERAPY-INDUCED HEMATURIA

One of the more common, challenging, and frustrating problems confronting the physician dealing with the cancer patient with urologic complications is the occurrence of hemorrhagic cystitis secondary to chemotherapy or radiation therapy.

Although hemorrhagic cystitis and bladder fibrosis has been reported in patients receiving MOPP therapy for Hodgkin's disease, most cases of hemorrhagic cystitis are secondary to cyclophosphamide administration.[1,2] Cyclophosphamide is a cytotoxic alkylating agent widely used in the treatment of leukemia, lymphoma, and certain solid tumors. The deleterious effects of cyclophosphamide on the bladder include mucosal edema, hemorrhage and ulceration, subendothelial telangiectasia and, in severe cases, fibrosis of the detrusor muscle, resulting in a permanently contracted bladder.[3-8] The toxicity of cyclophosphamide apparently is due to the metabolites of the drug. These metabolites, which include chlorethylazairidine and acrolein, are activated by liver microsomes and excreted in the urine. These metabolites react with the urothelium. Because the bladder is the primary storage organ for urine, the content of these metabolites is higher in the bladder than in other areas of the urinary tract, thus increasing the sensitivity of the bladder to damage. It should be emphasized that with obstruction and resulting accumulation of urine in the ureters, the changes found in the bladder also can be found in the ureters. Although direct contact with these metabolites appears to be the primary cause of bladder irritation, dogs that have ileal conduits and are receiving intravenous cyclophosphamide also exhibit a small amount of bladder toxicity. This finding indicates that the hematogenous route also may be responsible for some of the cyclophosphamide-induced bladder toxicity.[2]

Long-term cyclophosphamide therapy may produce either an acute hemorrhagic cystitis or chronic bladder fibrosis. Massive telangiectasia and ulceration may lead to severe, life-threatening bleeding from the bladder, requiring emergency treatment. Although the exact prevalence is unknown, acute hemorrhagic cystitis has been observed in 7% to 12% of patients receiving high-dose cyclophosphamide therapy.[2] Some authors report an occurrence of hemorrhagic cystitis in up to 40% of patients[9] with a frequency of 68% with high-dose administration in patients receiving allogeneic bone marrow transplantation.[10]

The histopathologic changes in cyclophosphamide-induced hemorrhagic cystitis have been well established. Grossly, the mucosa appears edematous and hyperemic, with multiple punctate hemorrhagic areas. With bladder distension, a diffuse capillary ooze is observed. Mucosal sloughing and erosions frequently are observed, which may extend through the bladder wall. Microscopically, granulation tissue and reactive fibroblasts, many of which are multinuclear, may be found beneath the mucosal surface; in long-standing cases, fibrosis and contraction of the bladder musculature have been observed.

The bladder toxicity does not necessarily occur during the active administration of the drug and may occur months after therapy has been discontinued.[11,12] Although controlled studies are lacking, it is the clinical impression of some oncologists that prolonged maintenance therapy with oral cyclophosphamide (Cytoxan) is associated with a higher incidence of hemorrhagic complications than is intermittent intravenous administration. At least in children, severe toxicity appears to be dose related.[13]

The treatment of cyclophosphamide-induced cystitis should first include conservative measures such as discontinuing the drug and encouraging adequate hydration to reduce the urinary concentration of cyclophosphamide metabolites and minimize the effects on the urothelium.

The use of a urethral catheter at this stage is controversial. Proponents of this approach argue that catheterization to drain the bladder and put it at rest is beneficial; however, in some patients, the occurrence of bladder spasms secondary to the Foley balloon may aggravate the cystitis. In addition, patients are able to urinate larger blood clots than will pass through a urethral catheter. In a patient with active bleeding, plugging of the catheter by large blood clots may be a common problem. Continuous bladder irrigation may aid in keeping the catheter open, but it does little to treat the underlying abnormality. If the hematuria persists after these simple measures, endoscopy should be performed and an attempt should be made to cauterize the bleeding areas. This is best done with a ball-tip electrode and a light coagulation current.

The occurrence of cyclophosphamide-induced hemorrhagic cystitis can be greatly reduced by careful attention to measures designed to decrease the concentration of metabolites in contact with the bladder mucosa and to minimize the time of such contact. Droller and associates used a regimen of diuresis and frequent voiding or catheter drainage in patients at risk for the development of hemorrhage.[14] Before this regimen, 95% of patients experienced massive clot-producing hemorrhage; 75% of these patients died as the result of such hemorrhage. The incidence of clot-producing hemorrhage fell to less than 1% subsequent to the use of this regimen.

In some patients, there appears to be a direct tubular toxicity of cyclophosphamide. DeFronzo and colleagues described the syndrome of impaired water excretion, weight gain, hyponatremia, and inappropriately concentrated urine in patients treated with cyclophosphamide.[15,16] This condition appeared to result from a direct effect of the cyclophosphamide metabolites on the distal tubular cells. These authors recommended that cyclophosphamide be given in the early part of the day to avoid pooling of toxic metabolites in the bladder urine overnight. The renal tubular toxicity suggests that diuretics may be more appropriate than hydration in maintaining diuresis.[16]

If conservative measures are not successful, additional treatment is indicated. Intravesical administration of compounds that contain sulfhydryl groups may be warranted, in an attempt to bind the acrolein and other metabolites. One such agent, *N*-acetylcysteine has been effective in a few patients.[17,18] Alum irrigation may also be effective in some patients,[19] because agents containing this substance can be administered in the unanesthetized patients. They are often tried before formalin instillations. When severe hemorrhage persists, intravesical instillation of a dilute formalin solution is often required.

In 1968, Brown reported the use of 10% formalin instillation for control of massive hemorrhage of the bladder in patients with inoperable carcinoma.[20,21] In 1972, Fair reported preliminary results with this method in the treatment of hemorrhagic cystitis secondary to irradiation or cyclophosphamide. The bleeding stopped in all four patients treated with 10% formalin solution, but three of the four patients developed serious complications. Two of these had markedly reduced bladder capacity with the subsequent development of a moderate amount of hydroureteronephrosis. In another patient with unrecognized right ureteral reflux, the instillation of 10% formalin led to fibrosis of the right ureter, which subsequently required urinary diversion. Shah and Albert instilled a 4% solution of formalin and left it in place for 30 min.[22] Our subsequent experience using 1% to 2% formalin solution passively irrigated in and out of the bladder for 10 min proved extremely successful without the complications encountered with the 10% solution.[23] In 1976, Shrom and co-workers reported success in 14 of 16 patients treated with 4% or weaker formalin solutions.[13] In a literature review, 91 of 106 patients (86%), had cessation of the bleeding after a single treatment.

The technique currently employed in the treatment of hemorrhagic cystitis is as follows:

1. Instill formalin, with the patient under general or regional anesthesia because there is discomfort accompanying instillation without anesthesia.

2. Evacuate all clots from the bladder by thorough irrigation.
3. Inspect the bladder carefully, and fulgurate any large bleeding vessels. (Usually no large bleeders are found, and the bladder is diffusely irritated if there is evidence of multiple capillary oozing.)
4. Insert an 18-French straight Robinson catheter into the bladder.
5. From 500 to 1000 ml of 1% formalin solution in water is passively irrigated in and out of the bladder for a total of 10 min. For this procedure the bottom half of an Asepto syringe is attached to the catheter with the syringe held no higher than 15 cm above the pubis. In those patients in whom a previous cystogram reveals reflux, elevate the patient's head in the Fowler position to keep the level of the kidneys higher than the level of the formalin irrigation. Fill the bladder to capacity and allow the formalin to stay in the bladder for a few minutes, then empty through the catheter. At no time is the catheter clamped. Holding the syringe no higher than 15 cm above the bladder will ensure that the intravesical pressure will not increase above that level. Avoid clamping the catheter, because if the patient strains or attempts to urinate while the catheter is clamped, the intravesical pressure may rise high enough to force the formalin solution up to the kidneys or into the systemic circulation.
6. After instillation of the formalin for 10 min, wash the bladder with at least 1 liter of distilled water irrigating solution.
7. A 14-French catheter with a 5-ml bag is left in place from 12 to 24 hr.

The severe complications of formalin therapy have included the development of a severely contracted bladder, ureterovesical obstruction with hydronephrosis, anuria, papillary necrosis, uterofibrosis, and intraperitoneal extravasation following formalin instillation after a bladder biopsy. All of these complications appear to have been associated with the 10% solution; the use of more dilute formalin has led to equal success with far fewer complications.[13,22–27] There appears to be no additional therapeutic value in using solutions of formalin more concentrated than 4%.

The use of 1% to 4% formalin appears to provide a safe approach for the control of massive intravesical bleeding in those patients who might otherwise be considered for major surgical procedures such as cystectomy. Although the overall results have been quite satisfactory, observe the following general precautions when using the chemical:

1. Formalin (37% solution of formaldehyde) should be diluted with sufficient sterile distilled water to make a 1% formalin solution. This represents a concentration of 0.37% formaldehyde. One must be explicit in ordering this solution lest a 1% formaldehyde solution be prepared.
2. The bladder should be free of clots, and any large bleeding vessels should be fulgurated before instilling formalin to minimize the risk of intravascular absorption of formalin.
3. A cystogram should always be done before using the formalin. If refulx is present, place the patient in the reverse Trendelenburg position while the irrigation is being done. If the patient is under low regional anesthesia and experiences flank pain, discontinue the irrigation immediately.
4. Instillation should begin with a solution of no higher concentration than 1% formalin. In those patients who do not respond to the initial treatment, we consider repeating the 1% treatment or cautiously increasing the concentration of the agent; however, there seems to be a marked risk in using solutions of formalin more concentrated than 4%. Higher concentrations have been no more effective in controlling bleeding than has the 4% solution.

Other techniques have been used in an attempt to minimize upper tract damage in the presence of ureterovesical reflux. Bilateral occlusion of the ureters with Fogarty catheters before the instillation of formalin has been advocated, but rarely required.[28]

In the past, failure to control massive bladder hemorrhage by evacuation of the clots and coagulation frequently was followed by more aggressive attempts at therapy, including bilateral ligation of the hypogastric arteries and urinary diversion with or without cystectomy. The recent introduction of formalin bladder irrigation has been a major advance in the control of life-threatening hemorrhagic cystitis secondary to cyclophosphamide or radiation therapy.

Prevention of cyclophosphamide hemorrhagic cystitis is often more effective than treatment once it has developed. Careful attention to the total cyclophosphamide dose and adequate hydration of the patient during and following administration may be helpful.

Particularly encouraging have been the reports of the apparent effectiveness of the prophylactic administration of sodium 2-mercaptoethanesulfonate (Mesna) in children or adults receiving high-dose cyclophosphamide chemotherapy.[29–31] Sodium mercaptoethanesulfonate appears to be effective through a dual mechanism. It prevents the formation of acrolein from the breakdown of the oxazaphosphorine ring of cyclophosphamide, as well as binding to the acrolein that is formed, thus preventing its interaction with the urothelium. In a small number of patients treated to date, it appears that this agent is effective in reducing the incidence of cyclophosphamide-induced hematuria without interfering with the efficacy of cyclophosphamide.[29,30]

The daily dose of Mesna administered was 160% of the total cyclophosphamide given. The first dose was administered intravenously just before, or concurrently with, the cyclophosphamide and repeated at 3, 6, and 9 hr after the chemotherapeutic agent. Mesna appears to eliminate totally the need for bladder catheterization and irrigation, thus minimizing additional morbidity related to an indwelling catheter.

RADIATION CYSTITIS

The cystoscopic findings and histopathologic changes described for cyclophosphamide cystitis can also be found with severe radiation cystitis. Typically, the irradiated bladder

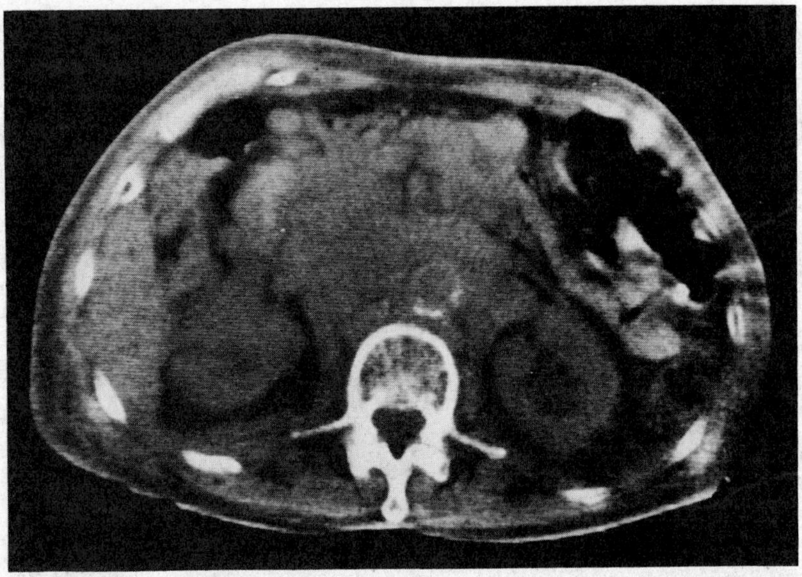

FIG. 58-12. CT scan of a patient with a malignant lymphoma showing massive retroperitoneal lymphadenopathy and marked left hydronephrosis.

mucosa has a pale appearance and bleeds easily on catheterization or endoscopic examination.

As with cyclophosphamide cystitis, the initial treatment of severe radiation cystitis consists of thorough irrigation of the bladder to remove all clots and coagulation of any obvious bleeding areas.

Other agents and procedures used intravesically such as silver nitrate,[32] alum,[19] hydrostatic dilatation,[33] and bilateral hypogastric artery occlusion have been employed as required.

Recently, the successful treatment of radiation-induced cystitis in three patients, by using a hyperbaric oxygen chamber, has been described and appears to merit further consideration.[34] As with cyclophosphamide cystitis, the use of intravesical formalin, as described earlier, has obviated the need for more aggressive surgical approaches in virtually all patients.

Prevention of radiation cystitis is of primary importance. Adequate hydration of the patient is essential. Every attempt should be made to avoid an indwelling urethral catheter during the administration of radiation therapy. Patients receiving irradiation to the bladder or prostate who also require urinary drainage should be treated with a suprapubic cystotomy, rather than a urethral catheter, to minimize bladder irritability and subsequent hemorrhage.

OBSTRUCTIVE UROPATHY

UPPER TRACT OBSTRUCTION

Upper tract obstruction may be either unilateral or bilateral, partial or complete. Bilateral complete obstruction is obviously the most life-threatening condition, resulting in acute anuria and, if unrelieved, uremia and death. Obstruction to the free flow of urine may lead eventually to significant hydronephrotic atrophy of the kidney proximal to the obstruction. The clinical features of obstruction vary with the degree and extent of the obstructive lesion. A patient with acute unilateral obstruction may have severe colic such as accompanies a ureteral calculus. Conversely, slowly progressive bilateral obstruction may lead to total anuria with a minimum of preceding symptoms. In the presence of infection, frequency of urination, dysuria, nocturia, fever, chills, and flank pain are common findings.

The cause of upper tract obstruction may be the result of recurrent tumor or the sequelae of tumor therapy. The most common primary tumors causing ureteral obstruction are cancer of the cervix, ovary, bladder, prostate, and rectum. Nonmalignant conditions leading to upper tract urinary obstruction may result from scarring secondary to previous

FIG. 58-13. Technique of percutaneous nephrostomy drainage with fluoroscopic or sonographic guidance.

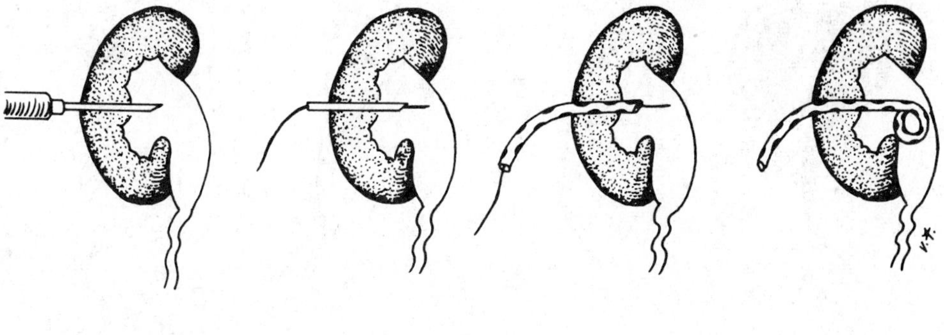

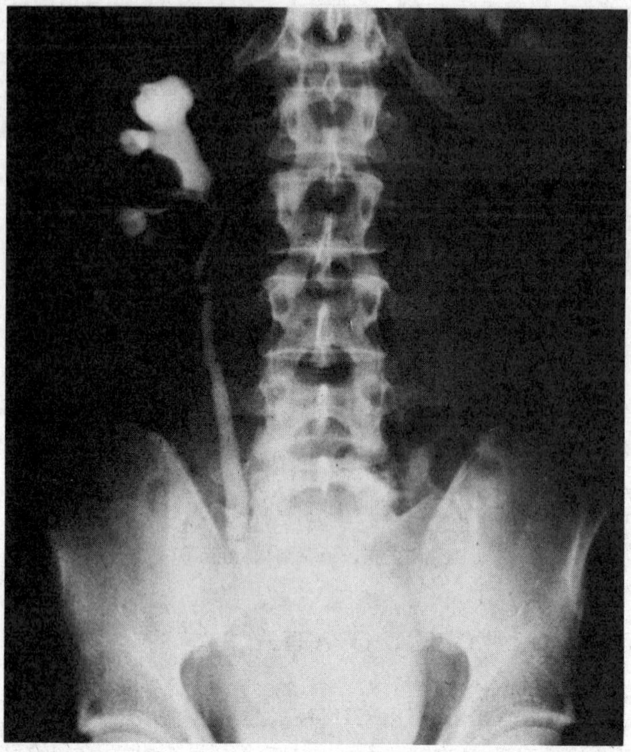

FIG. 58-14. Antegrade pyelogram in a patient with pelvic sarcoma showing obstruction at the ureterovesical area.

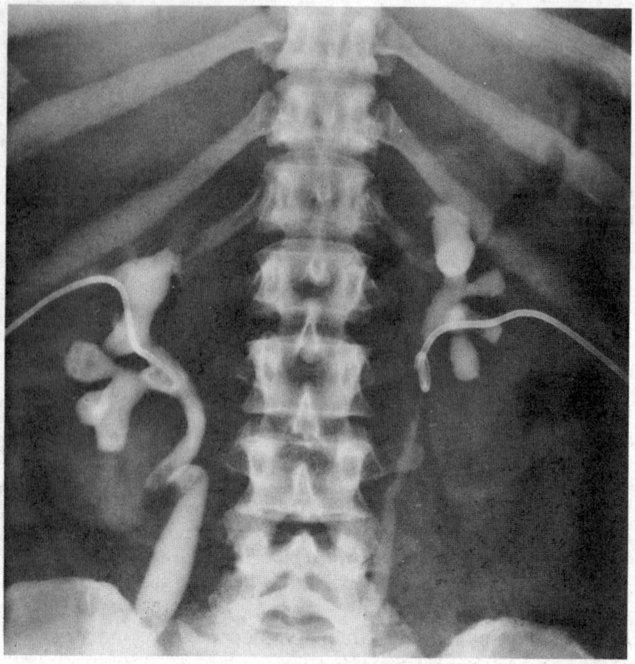

FIG. 58-15. Bilateral percutaneous nephrostomies in a patient with pelvic malignant sarcoma causing bilateral hydronephrosis. Note two No. 8 "pigtail" catheters in both renal pelves.

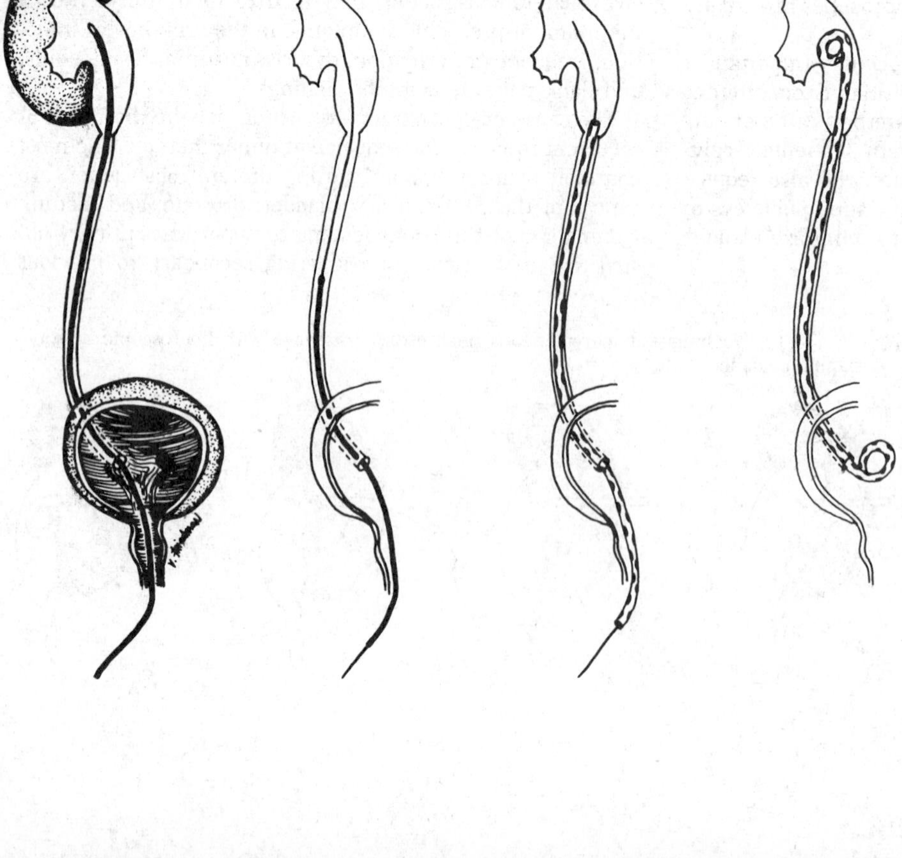

FIG. 58-16. Technique of inserting self-retaining ureteral stents over guidewire.

surgery, radiation therapy, chemotherapy, or idiopathic retroperitoneal fibrosis.

The diagnosis of upper tract obstruction is most quickly and effectively made by renal ultrasonography. In the azotemic patient, the administration of a contrast medium should be minimized. Ultrasound is preferable to the excretory urogram in establishing a diagnosis of hydronephrosis. The CT scan, with or without contrast, is often particularly helpful for establishing the level of obstruction, as well as for visualizing retroperitoneal lymph nodes or other masses that may be the cause of the obstruction. (Fig. 58-12). Other techniques, such as retrograde ureterograms and ileoureterograms in patients with cutaneous urinary diversions, are often very helpful and may be used safely in the azotemic patient without increasing the risk of further renal damage resulting from intravenous administration of contrast medium. Once the diagnosis of obstruction has been established, percutaneous nephrostomy with antegrade pyelograms may be of great value in elucidating the site and nature of the obstruction, as well as providing drainage of the obstructed kidney (Fig. 58-13).

THERAPY

Temporary

Unilateral or bilateral percutaneous nephrostomy will provide prompt relief of obstruction and allow for the performance of antegrade contrast studies to determine the level and nature of the obstruction (Fig. 58-14). After the patient has stabilized and renal function has improved, the percutaneous tract may provide a means of dilating the obstructed renal pelvis ureter by antegrade passage of successively larger catheters.

Permanent

Bilateral percutaneous nephrostomy tubes will provide adequate relief of urinary obstruction (Fig. 58-15), but if possible, it should not be considered as a permanent form of drainage because of the difficulty in maintaining the tubes and the discomfort occasioned by patient's attempting to lie comfortably with a tube positioned in each flank. Permanent indwelling ureteral stents are best positioned by retrograde ureteral catheterization over a guide wire as demonstrated in Figure 58-16. The antegrade insertion of ureteral stents in patients with ileal or colonic conduits provides a permanent internal stent that is well tolerated by the patient (Fig. 58-17). The stents are generally replaced every 3 months to minimize the accumulation of encrustations on the tubes, although in some patients, the stents may remain in place indefinitely without difficulty. Other measures employed in the relief of supravesical obstruction include simple lysis of ureteral adhesions, transureteroureterostomy in unilateral obstruction, and unilateral or bilateral ileal substitution in patients in whom ureteral replacement is required (Fig. 58-18).

Permanent external urinary diversion may be considered in those patients with pelvic malignancies or in those in whom the bladder capacity is no longer adequate to function as a urinary reservoir. The use of an indwelling catheter to effect upper tract drainage is, in general, much less desirable than an ileal or colonic cutaneous diversion (Fig. 58-19). Tubeless cutaneous ureterostomy, which has the advantage of requiring substantially less surgery than intestinal diversion, rarely is indicated because subsequent stomal stenosis at the ureterocutaneous junction will, usually, lead to recurrence of the upper tract obstruction.

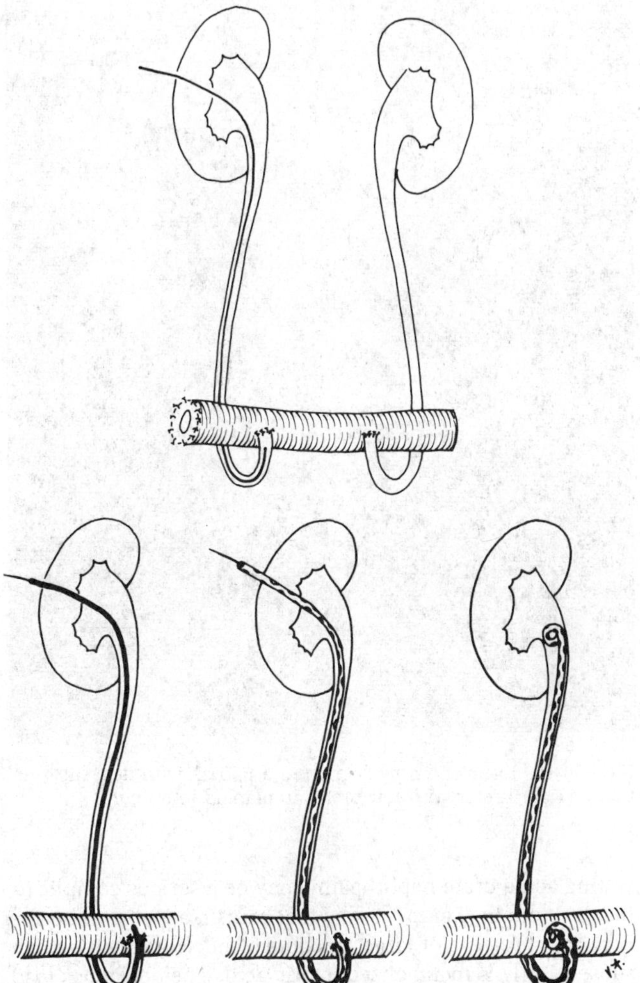

FIG. 58-17. Technique of percutaneous antegrade insertion of self-retaining ureteral stents in patients with urinary diversion.

URIC ACID NEPHROPATHY

Urate nephropathy has long been a recognized complication in patients with chronic myeloproliferative disorders. The physiologic abnormality in these conditions appears to be related to excessive urate production resulting from nucleoprotein metabolism accompanying the accelerated turnover of myeloid cells. With effective chemotherapy or radiation therapy in the treatment of certain leukemias and lymphomas, acute episodes of excess urate production with re-

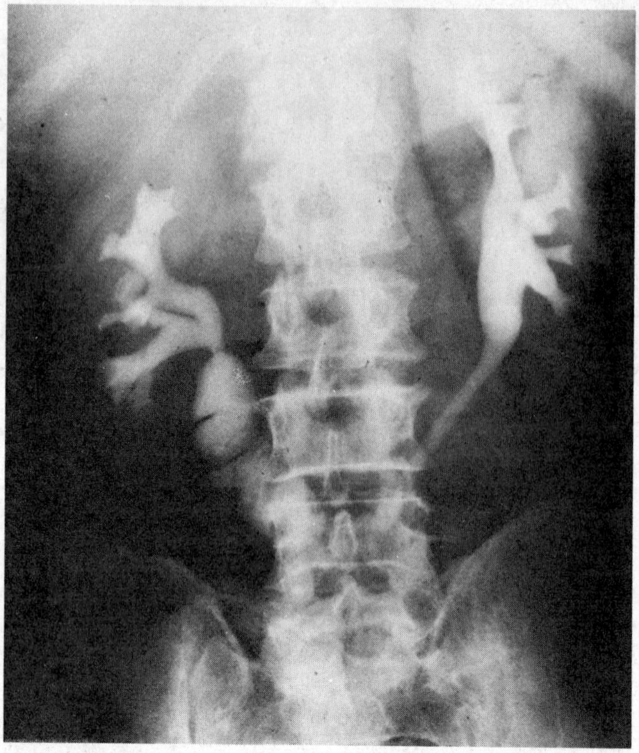

FIG. 58-18. Intravenous pyelogram in a patient with ileal substitution of right ureter with left ureter implanted into ileum.

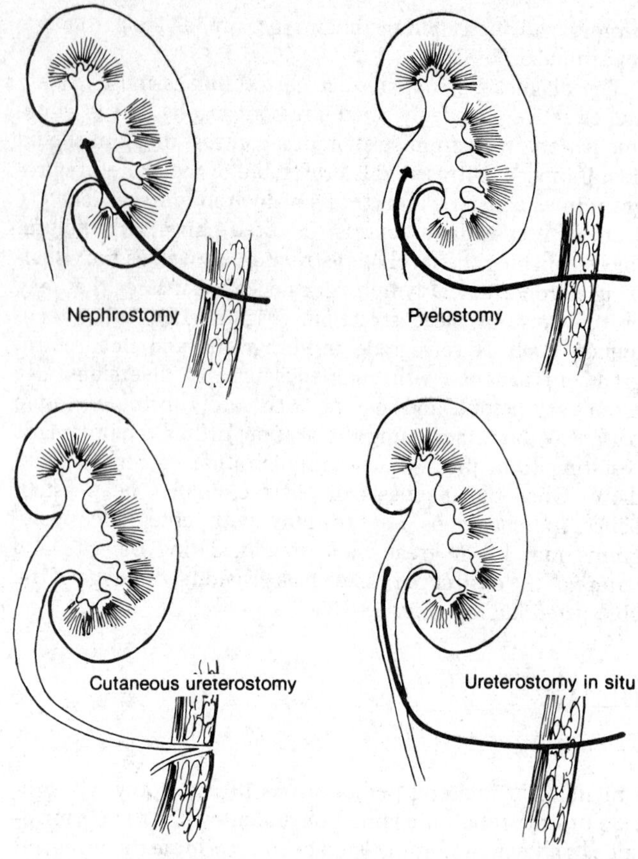

FIG. 58-19. Methods of supervesicular urinary diversions for relieving the obstruction of the upper urinary tract.

sulting acute urate nephropathy may be a serious complicating problem in therapy.[35] The mechanism appears to be the very rapid release of large amounts of nucleoprotein, which subsequently is metabolized to uric acid. The enormous load of uric acid simply exceeds the capacity of the kidney to maintain its excretion, and extreme degrees of hyperuricemia may develop.

The pathologic findings in the kidney consist of urate crystals in the collecting system and in the renal pyramids, frequently leading to acute renal shutdown. Intravenous pyelography will demonstrate nonfunction of the kidneys, and ultrasound or retrograde pyelograms will confirm the absence of hydronephrosis and extrarenal obstruction.

Prevention is paramount in this condition; if anuria occurs, these patients, in general, do very poorly. Adequate hydration is essential; administration of carbonic anhydrase inhibitors and intravenous bicarbonate to alkalize the urine and dissolve the urate crystals may prevent or reverse the process. Large doses of allopurinol should also be administered simultaneously.[35]

Preventive measures include the measurement of serum and, if necessary, urine uric acid levels in patients with myeloproliferative disorders before therapy is instituted. High-normal or elevated levels may reflect marked urate overproduction. In these patients, urinary output of at least 1500 ml/day should be maintained, and the administration of a carbonic anhydrase inhibitor or bicarbonate, along with allopurinol, before the initiation of antitumor therapy should be considered.[36,37]

The differential diagnosis between uric acid nephropathy and obstructive uropathy in thee cancer patient can be determined most readily and accurately by the performance of a renal ultrasound scan and, if any urine is available, a careful urinalysis. An acidic urinary pH and the finding of uric acid crystals microscopically, with ultrasonic evidence of an unobstructed collecting system, should be adequate to begin aggressive therapy of uric acid nephropathy.

LOWER TRACT OBSTRUCTION

Conditions causing lower tract obstruction usually arise from neoplasm, stricture, or a fibrotic contracted bladder. Large bladder tumors may cause obstruction from either a space-occupying mass in the bladder or by obstruction of the ureteral orifice. A patient with a thick-walled fibrotic bladder, resulting from radiation contracture or an infiltrating neoplasm within the bladder wall, may present with symptoms of acute lower tract obstruction.

Conditions causing intravesical urinary tract obstruction include prostatic tumors, urethral strictures, and ureteral tumors (Figs. 58-20A,B). The symptoms of lower tract obstruction may be indistinguishable from those resulting from obstruction of the upper tract. If, on physical examination, one finds a large bladder by palpation or abdominal percus-

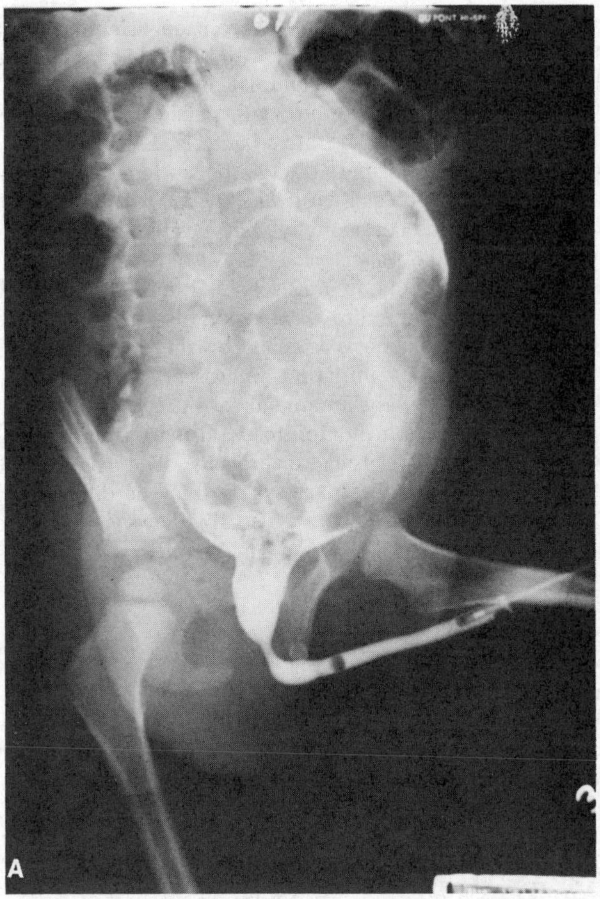

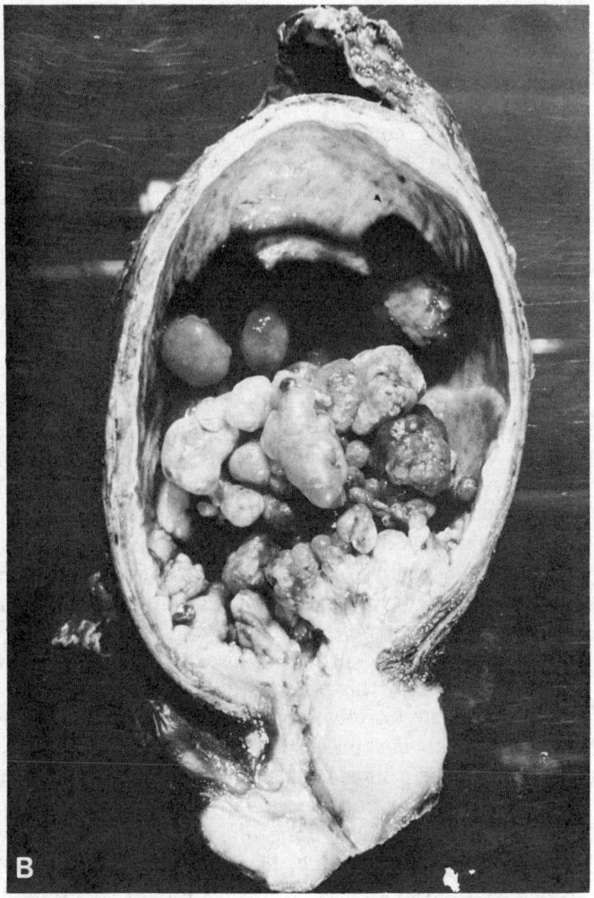

FIG. 58-20. **A**. Rhabdomyosarcoma of prostate in a child presenting with obstructive uropathy. **B**. Gross pathology of above case.

sion, this is strong clinical evidence for a lower tract site of obstruction. Other physical findings that indicate a lower tract obstruction are a large mass on rectal examination or the inability to pass a urethral catheter.

The steps in diagnosis should first include a careful physical examination and the passage of a small (14-French) urethral catheter. If the obstruction appears to be at the level of the prostate or the bladder neck, a coudé tip catheter may make it possible to negotiate the catheter into the bladder. Urethral strictures may be suggested by an inability to pass the catheter beyond the membranous urethra. The use of filiforms and followers, or the passage of a filiform directly through the strictures observed at urethroscopy, may be necessary to provide adequate drainage.

If catheterization through the urethra is not possible, a suprapubic cystostomy or cutaneous vesicostomy may be necessary (Fig. 58-21). In adults, a cutaneous vesicostomy rarely is indicated, although in children it may provide an ideal way for long-term bladder drainage without the need of an indwelling catheter. A percutaneous suprapubic puncture in a patient with a palpably distended bladder is a simple procedure and an excellent way to drain the bladder. It possesses several advantages over the indwelling Foley catheter: ease of passage, particularly in men with a dense urethral stricture; greater patient confort; and fewer infections (this is particularly true in men in whom the incidence of epididymitis seems to be markedly lessened in patients with a percutaneous cystotomy compared with long-term indwelling catheter drainage). The suprapubic catheter also provides the ability to give the patient a voiding trial simply by clamping the tube intermittently, thus obviating the need for repeated urethral catheterization. In acute urinary retention, secondary to prostatic obstruction or inflammation, suprapubic drainage will tend to minimize the prostatic edema that

FIG. 58-21. Methods of urinary diversion from the bladder with or without tubes.

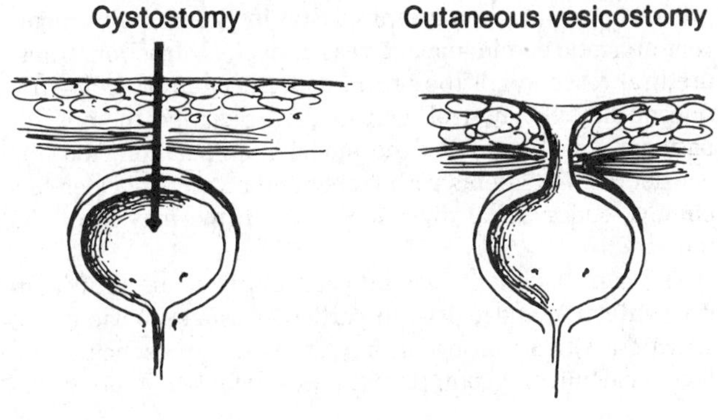

often accompanies urethral catheterization. A suprapubic tube also eliminates the risk of an urethrocutaneous fistula, which is a potential hazard in patients with an indwelling Foley catheter; the development of urethral stricture is also minimized. A considerable controversy exists over the proper length of time to leave a suprapubic tube or nephrostomy tube in place. Before the introduction of silicone catheters, it was usually customary to change these tubes monthly to prevent the buildup of calculi on the surface of the tube. Since the introduction of the silicone catheter, the period of change can be greatly lengthened. In fact, there is no real reason to change the catheter unless it appears that encrustations are developing on the tube. Certainly, many people can go 6 months or longer with a silicone suprapubic or nephrostomy tube before requiring a change.

The use of agressive antimicrobial therapy in asymptomatic patients with indwelling tubes in any site of the urinary tract should be discouraged. Our practice is to culture the urine frequently. If the tube is freely draining, no antibacterial therapy is given in the presence of infected urine unless the organisms recovered are urease-producing bacteria. These organisms, most commonly *Proteus mirabilis*, will produce an alkaline urine because of their ability to split urea, resulting in the precipitation of magnesium ammonium phosphate (strutive) calculi. In those patients in whom a urease-positive bacterial infection is diagnosed, the patient should be given a short course of an appropriate antibiotic to sterilize the urine, and then the antibiotic should be discontinued. Intensive and prolonged antibacterial therapy in patients with a tube draining the urinary tract will invariably lead to a bacterial infection with an antibiotic-resistant, urea-splitting organism. For this reason, no effort should be made to treat freely draining urine if infected with non–urea-splitting bacteria.

The indications for urinary diversion or bladder augmentation are pelvic malignancies and a fibrotic contracted bladder secondary to chemotherapy or radiation therapy. Hydraulic dilation, with the patient under general or regional anesthesia, may be successful in increasing the size of some fibrotic bladders, but often augmentation with an intestinal patch or an ileocecocystoplasty may be required to increase the bladder capacity permanently. In some patients, permanent urinary diversion by means of an ileal or colonic conduit is the only solution to dealing with a small, scarred, contracted bladder.

The treatment of urethral obstruction obviously depends on its cause. With urethral stricture disease, urethral dilatation or internal urethrotomy generally is considered before proceeding to an open urethroplasty. In patients with recurrent prostatic carcinoma and vesical neck obstruction, transurethral resection of the prostate, orchiectomy, administration of diethylstilbestrol, or palliative radiation therapy for patients who have failed hormonal manipulation, may be considered. In patients with inoperable invasive bladder carcinoma, supravesical diversion of the urine may rarely be indicated.

The cancer patient may be particularly prone to urinary tract infection and sepsis, in particular as a sequelae of obstruction with resulting urinary stasis, the presence of infected calculi, and compromised host defenses. Acute infection usually presents as pain on urination or frequency of urination, occasionally with hematuria, chills, fever, and gastrointestinal or abdominal manifestations.

The most common pathogens causing urinary tract infection are gram-negative bacteria. *Escherichia coli* is the predominant urinary tract pathogen found, although other organisms such as *Klebsiella, Pseudomonas, Proteus, Enterobacter* spp., and occasionally gram-positive cocci (*e.g., Staphylococcus* and *Streptococcus*) may also be pathogenic. Most urinary tract infections are ascending, but hematogenous, lymphogenous, and direct extension also may be routes of spread.

The diagnosis is made by the characteristic findings on physical examination, microscopic examination, culture of the urine, and microbial sensitivity.

Abscess formation in the urinary tract generally presents as renal, perirenal, or prostatic. The diagnosis of an abscess in the genitourinary system may be difficult to make. The laboratory evaluation usually shows a leukocytosis, with a

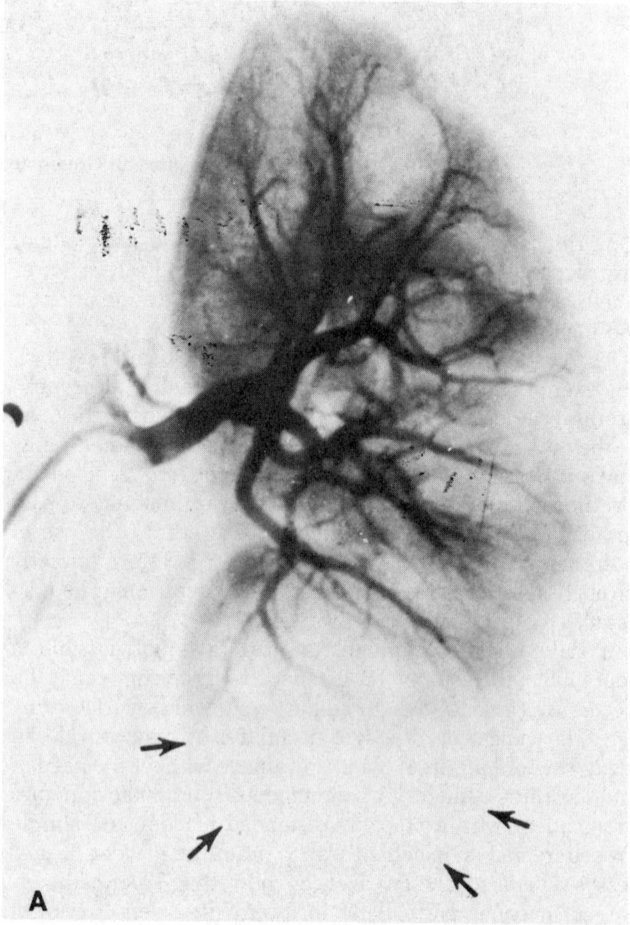

FIG. 58-22. (*Legend on facing page.*)

shift to the left, and an elevated sedimentation rate. With a prostatic abscess, the patient is exquisitely tender on rectal examination, and vigorous prostatic manipulation should be avoided. The diagnosis of renal and perirenal abscess may require, in addition to the excretory urogram, the use of angiography, CT scan, ultrasonography, or gallium scan (Fig. 58-22). The excretory urogram may show evidence of a mass and the physical examination reveal exquisite costovertebral angle tenderness or a mass in the flank. The ultrasound finding is typically a "mixed" echo pattern or a pattern suggestive of a cystic mass. The gallium scan may be helpful in localizing the abscess, but the time required for the performance of the scan may limit its value in an acutely septic patient. The clinical course, plus the physical examination and the results of x-ray and ultrasonography, will often provide the surgeon with enough evidence to consider exploration and drainage. The immediate management of a renal or perirenal abscess is to provide adequate drainage of the abscess and the institution of prompt antimicrobial therapy. While cultures are pending, broad-spectrum coverage should be provided by the administration of an aminoglycoside antibiotic together with a semisynthetic penicillin. When bacterial suspectibility results are known, therapy should be changed, if indicated, to the appropriate specific antibacterial agent. Prompt and adequate drainage is the primary treatment of renal or perirenal abscess. Reliance on antibiotic coverage alone will not eradicate the infection in the presence of obstruction or calculi.[38] The use of percutaneous drainage may be considered in those patients whose medical condition will not permit surgical exploration. The best treatment of an abscess is adequate drainage and debridement of infected tissue. However, such drainage is often not possible through a small percutaneous tube; thus, when possible, these conditions should be treated with surgical drainage.

Acute epididymitis occasionally presents in the cancer pa-

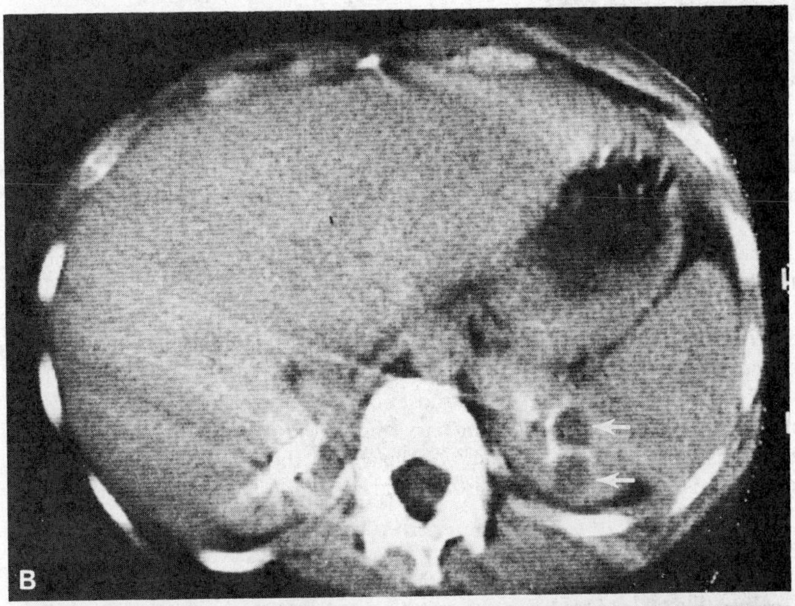

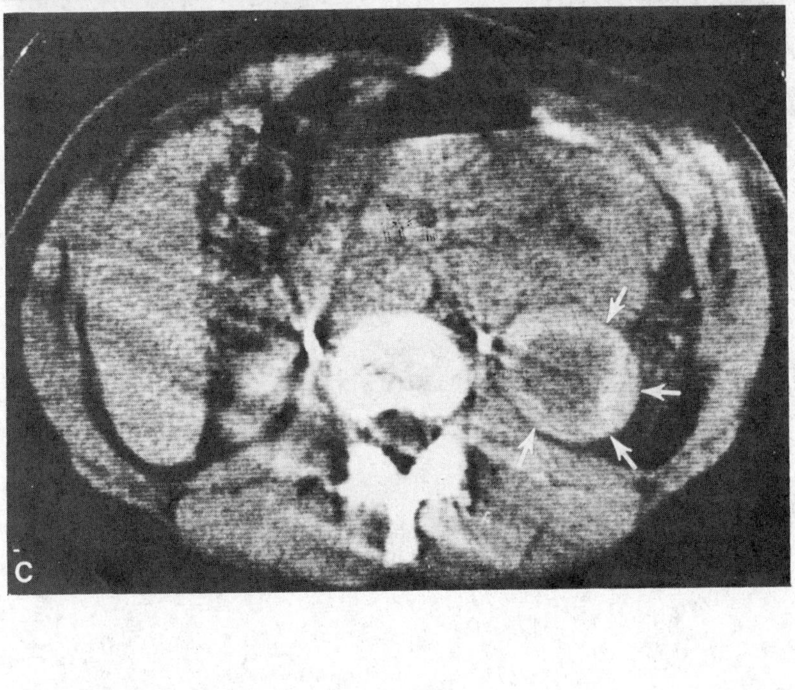

FIG. 58-22. Twenty-three-year-old woman with hematuria, left flank pain, and urinary tract infection. IVP showed mass in left lower pole. **A**. Angiogram shows avascular mass (*black arrows*). Two small avascular masses are seen in left upper pole. **B**. CT scan after intravenous contrast through left upper pole shows small cysts (*white arrows*). **C**. Scan through left lower pole shows thick-walled mass (*arrows*) with enhancing rim and central area of decreased density characteristic of renal abscess.

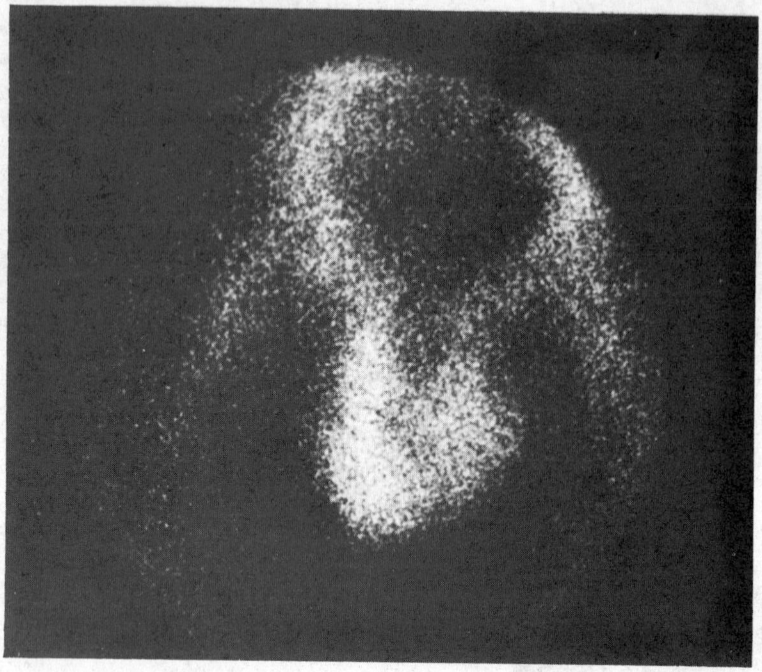

FIG. 58-23. Radionuclide scan of testes showing increased uptake of technetium by the right scrotal structures in a patient with right epididymo-orchitis.

tient as a result of hematogenous ascending or descending infection along the urethra. The symptoms are pain, swelling of the epididymis and testicle, scrotal edema, and fever. The diagnosis is confirmed by the finding of a markedly swollen and tender epididymis; in severe cases the inflammation can involve a testicle causing an epididymo-orchitis. Clinically, the diagnosis may be suggested if the patient notes that the pain is lessened when the examiner's hand elevates the testicle. In young men, the clinical differentiation between an epididymo-orchitis and testicular torsion can be made most accurately by a radionuclide testicular scan. The increased vascularity noted on the scan in patients with epididymitis (Fig. 58-23) contrasts with the lack of isotope uptake in testicular torsion (Fig. 58-24). Acute epididymitis is often found in patients with long-term indwelling urethral catheters. The treatment consists of bed rest, scrotal support, analgesics, and in the presence of a scrotal abscess, incision and drainage of the abscess.

The infecting agent in acute epididymitis varies with the age of patient. In men under the age of 35, infection with *Chlamydia* is the most common cause; in men over this age, gram-negative urinary tract pathogens are the most common inciting agents.[39] Antibacterial therapy should be based on appropriate cultures and susceptibility results in those pa-

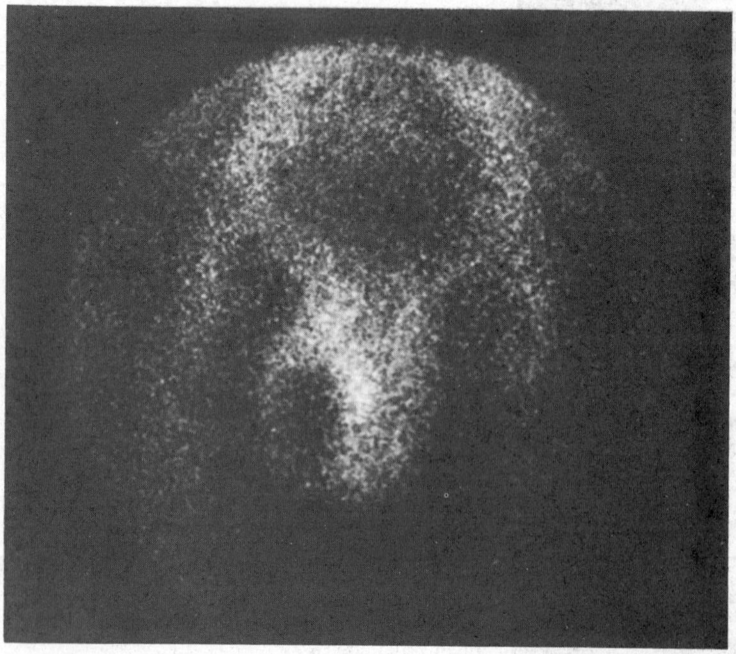

FIG. 58-24. Radionuclide scan of testes in a patient with right testicular torsion. Note area of avascularity manifested by decreased isotope uptake on the right side.

tients with an associated urinary tract infection. In younger patients with sterile urine, tetracycline or erythromycin should be given empirically to treat presumed chlamydial infections.

Acute phimosis and paraphimosis are seen not infrequently in patients receiving radiotherapy or in those with local pelvic lymphatic obstruction. The proper treatment consists of a dorsal slit of the foreskin, or circumcision in those patients in whom urinary obstruction is associated. A urethral or suprapubic catheter also may be indicated.

STONES

Acute urinary calculi in the cancer patient should be treated in the same manner as those occurring in the patient without cancer. Of particular interest are the infection stones formed in the presence of urea-splitting bacteria in the urine. The presence of urea-splitting organisms in the urinary tract of a patient with a urinary diversion is an ominous finding, and careful follow-up is indicated to detect or prevent stone formation. *Proteus mirabilis* is the most common urinary tract pathogen producing urease, but any organism that splits urea may lead to the formation of struvite calculi. Other members of the genus *Proteus* will also split urea, but they cause urinary tract infections less frequently. *Klebsiella* species and *Staphylococcus albus* occasionally are found to produce struvite calculi. *Escherichia coli*, the most common urinary tract pathogen, does not produce urease. Although some strains of *Pseudomonas* do produce urease, most do not.

Periodic urine cultures are important in following patients with urinary tract diversion. When the culture returns positive results for a urinary tract infection with a urea-splitting organism, appropriate antimicrobial therapy should be given for a short period, no longer than 7 to 10 days, to sterilize the urine and to eradicate the bacteria. Follow-up cultures should document that the urea-splitting organism has been eradicated. If the urine remains sterile or becomes infected with a non–urease-producing organism and no obstruction is demonstrated in the urinary system, no additional therapy should be given. The presence of an acute obstruction behind an infected ureteral calculus is a urologic emergency and, unless promptly treated, can lead to overwhelming sepsis and death. Treatment consists of establishing drainage. In the patient with an intact urinary system, this may be achieved best by the passage of a retrograde ureteral catheter. In those patients in whom a cutaneous urinary diversion is in place, a percutaneous nephrostomy to establish drainage and relieve the impaired kidney function may be required as a temporary measure to stabilize the patient until the stone is removed.

MISCELLANEOUS CONDITIONS

Priapism, which is defined as a prolonged, painful erection, may occur in patients with leukemia, lymphoma, and polycythemia. The therapy usually is directed toward the treatment of the underlying malignancy, although in some patients improved drainage from the penis by the establishment of a cavernosapongiosa shunt may be effective in relieving the pain and treating the priapism. Prompt correction of the condition may lessen the frequence of postpriapism impotence.

REFERENCES

1. Royal JE, Seeler RA: Hemorrhagic cystitis with MOPP therapy. Cancer 41:1261, 1978
2. Javadpour N: Urologic emergencies In DeVita VT Jr, Hellman S, Rosenberg SA (eds): Cancer: Principles and Practice of Oncology, pp 1616–1627. Philadelphia, JB Lippincott, 1982
3. Javadpour N, Barakat HA: Bladder toxicity due to cyclophosphamide. Urology 2:634, 1973
4. Johnson WW, Meadows DC: Urinary-bladder fibrosis and telangiectasia associated with long-term cyclophosphamide therapy. N Engl J Med 284:290, 1971
5. Duckett JW Jr, Peters PC, Donaldson MH: Severe cyclophosphamide hemorrhagic cystitis controlled with phenol. J Pediatr Surg 8:55, 1973
6. Blue KG, Blume KG, Beuter E et al: Bone-marrow ablation and allogeneic marrow transplantation in acute leukemia. N Engl J Med 302:1041–1046, 1980
7. Ershler WB, Gilchrist KW, Citrin DL: Adriamycin enhancement of cyclophosphamide-induced bladder injury. J Urol 123:1212, 1980
8. Bischel MD: Cyclophosphamide hemorrhagic cystitis following prolonged low dose therapy. JAMA 20:238, 1979
9. Watson NA, Notley RG: Urologic complications of cyclophosphamide. Br J Urol 45:606, 1973
10. Texter JH Jr, Koontz WW Jr, McWilliams NB: Hemorrhagic cystitis as a complication of the management of pediatric neoplasm. Urol Surv 29:47, 1979
11. Hutter AN Jr, Bauman AW, Frank IN: Cyclophosphamide and severe hemorrhage cystitis. NY State J Med 69:305–309, 1969
12. Rubin JS, Rubin RT: Cyclophosphamide hemorrhagic cystitis. J Urol 96:313–316, 1966
13. Shrom SH, Donaldson MH, Duckett JW et al: Formalin treatment for intractable hemorrhagic cystitis. Cancer 38:1785–1789, 1976
14. Droller MJ, Saral R, Santos G: Prevention of cyclophosphamide-induced hemorrhagic cystitis. Urology 20:256–258, 1982
15. DeFronzo RA, Braine H, Colvin OM et al: Water intoxication in man after cyclophosphamide therapy—time course in relation to drug activity. Ann Intern Med 78:861–869, 1973
16. DeFronzo RA, Colvin OM, Braine H et al: Cyclophosphamide in the kidney. Cancer 33:483–491, 1974
17. Primack A: Amelioration of cyclophosphamide-induced cystitis J Natl Cancer Inst 47:223, 1971
18. Tolley DA: The effect of *N*-acetylcysteine on cyclophosphamide cystitis. Br J Urol 49:649, 1977
19. Reference deleted
20. Brown RB: A method of management in inoperative carcinoma of the bladder. Br J Urol 40:489, 1968
21. Brown RB: A method of management of inoperative carcinoma of the bladder. Med J Aust 1:23–24, 1969
22. Shah BC, Albert DJ: Intravesical instillation of formalin for the management of intractable hematuria. J Urol 110:519–520, 1973
23. Fair WR: Formalin in the treatment of massive bladder hemorrhage: Techniques, results, and complications. Urology 3:573–576, 1974
24. Firlit CF: Intractable hemorrhagic cystitis secondary to extensive carcinomatosis: Management with formalin solution. J Urol 110:57–58, 1973
25. Kalish M, Silber SJ, Herwig KR: Papillary necrosis: Result of intravesical instillation of formalin. Urology 2:315–317, 1973
26. McGuire EJ, Weiss RM, Schiff M, Lytton B: Hemorrhagic radiation cystitis. Urology 3:204–208, 1974
27. Spiro LH, Hecht H, Horowitz A et al: Formalin treatment for massive bladder hemorrhage. Urology 2:699–671, 1983
28. Bergman S, Javadpour N: Massive intractable hematuria secondary to cyclophosphamide: Intravesical instillation of formaldehyde in patients with vesicoureteral reflux. Urology 10:256, 1977
29. Scheef W, Klein HO, Brock N et al: Controlled clinical studies with an antidote against urotoxicity of oxazaphophorines: Preliminary result. Cancer Treat Rep 63:501–505, 1979
30. Ehrlich R: Sodium agent said to prevent cyclophosphamide cystitis. Urology Times 12:1, 1974
31. Ehrlich RM, Freedman A, Goldsobel AB et al: The use of sodium 2-mercaptoethane sulfonate to prevent cyclophosphamide cystitis. J Urol 131:960–962, 1984
32. Kumar APN, Wrenn EL Jr, Jayalakshmamma B et al: Silver nitrate irrigation to control bladder hemorrhage in children receiving cancer therapy. J Urol 116:85, 1976

33. Hansen RI, Djurhuus JC, Nerstrom B: Hydrostatic pressure treatment for carcinoma of the bladder. A clinical and urodymanic evaluation of the effect on bladder hemorrhage and fibrosis in irradiated patients. Scand J Urol Nephol 10:209, 1976
34. Weiss JP, Boland FP, Mori H et al: Treatment of radiation induced cystitis with hyperbaric oxygen. J Urol 134:352–354, 1986
35. Tyler FH: Urate nephropathy. In Stauss MB, Welt LG (eds): Diseases of the Kidney, pp 899. Boston, Little, Brown & Company, 1971
36. Barlow KA: Hyperlipidemia in primary gout. Metabolism 17:289–299, 1968
37. Muggia FM, Ball TJ, Ultmann JE: Allopurinol in the treatment of neoplastic disease, complicated by hyperuricemia. Arch Intern Med 120:12–18, 1967
38. Grabstald H: Life-threatening complication in cancer patients: Urinary tract emergencies in the cancer patient. Part II. Curr Prob Cancer 4:27–29, 1979–1980
39. Berger RE, Alexander ER, Harnisch JP et al: Etiology, manifestations and therapy of acute epididymitis: Prospective study of 50 cases. J Urol 121:750–754, 1979

CHAPTER 59 *Supportive Care of the Cancer Patient*

MOSHE SHIKE
MURRAY F. BRENNAN

SECTION 1

Nutritional Support

Malnutrition and cachexia are frequent manifestations of cancer and are major contributors to morbidity and mortality from the disease. Weight loss is often a presenting symptom of cancer or frequently develops during the course of the disease. The important role of nutritional status in the outcome of cancer has been recognized for many years. In a paper published in 1932, based on data from autopsies, Warren concluded that cachexia was the most common cause of death in cancer patients.[1] Weight loss is an independent factor affecting morbidity and mortality of patients with tumors.[2] Recent developments in nutritional support modalities, particularly in enteral and parenteral nutrition, make it possible to nourish almost any cancer patient, both in the hospital and at home. No patient need now be subjected to the ravages of malnutrition due to inadequate intake. In selected groups of cancer patients, aggressive nutritional support is clearly beneficial. However, the impact of nutritional therapy on the ultimate outcome in many cancer patients is still under scrutiny.

PREVALENCE OF MALNUTRITION

The prevalence of malnutrition in cancer patients varies with the type of tumor, stage of the disease, the response to therapy, and the definition of malnutrition. Most commonly, malnutrition refers to protein–calorie deficiencies manifested as weight loss. Deficiencies of other nutrients can occur singularly or in combination with protein–calorie malnutrition. Studies in hospitalized adult patients demonstrated that cancer patients had higher rates of malnutrition than patients with other diseases.[3] In children, the incidence of malnutrition at the time of cancer diagnosis is not different from that of children admitted with benign diseases to the same institution.[4,5] Data from 3047 adult cancer patients enrolled in 12 chemotherapy protocols for advanced diseases indicated the frequency of pretreatment weight in a variety of tumors.[2] The group of patients with the lowest frequency of weight loss (31–40%) included those with breast cancer, acute nonlymphocytic leukemia, sarcomas, and non-Hodgkin's lymphoma. Intermediate frequency of weight loss (48–61%) was seen in colon, prostate, and lung cancers, and the highest frequency (83–87%) was seen in patients with pancreatic and gastric cancers. There was no correlation between the tumor extent and weight loss in eight types of cancer, but for breast cancer a correlation existed.

A survey of 457 adult patients with various tumors done at

the time of admission to Memorial Sloan-Kettering Cancer Center showed that 24.7% of the patients had lost more than 10% of pre-illness body weight, and in 17.5%, the weight loss equated or exceeded 20%.[6] About a third of all assessed patients were judged to have nutritional problems severe enough to require nutritional therapy. Continued follow-up in the hospital indicated that in a substantial portion of patients, the nutritional status worsened during hospitalization when no nutritional therapy was employed. This is not surprising, considering that patients may be kept NPO (for tests, surgery); develop nausea, vomiting and diarrhea as side-effects of chemotherapy or radiation therapy; or may be in a relative "hypermetabolic state" due to infection, surgical stress, or tumor burden.

Outpatient cancer therapy can also be associated with weight loss. Among 186 patients with various tumors treated with chemotherapy in the outpatient clinics at Memorial Sloan-Kettering Cancer Center, 25% had significant weight loss (>5% of body weight) during treatment.

Causes of Malnutrition

Etiologic factors implicated in cancer-induced malnutrition are outlined in Table 59-1. The most obvious and common cause is anorexia with diminished intake. The cause of the anorexia remains unclear.[7] Abnormalities of central control of food intake have been suggested, but there is only minimal evidence that the hypothalamic center is altered to any marked degree in the patient or the animal with malignancy.[8] An attempt has been made to associate cancer anorexia with central effects of specific circulating amino acids, particularly plasma tryptophan.[9] Von Meyenfeldt has suggested that increases in tryptophan and serotonin can be observed in two different lines of anorexia-producing tumors, but these effects are not reversed when serotonin is depleted using analogues such as parchloroamphetamine.[10,11] This attractive hypothesis seems to have minimal current evidence.

Abnormalities of taste and smell do occur in the patient with malignancy and may contribute to the diminished food intake.[12] The obvious cause of diminished intake is an obstructing malignancy of the gastrointestinal tract (GI) which can be compounded by progressive malaise, weakness, depression, and the consequences of antineoplastic therapy.

The effects of cancer therapy have often been underappreciated in the etiology of malnutrition. Surgical resection, particularly of the oropharynx and esophagus, can prohibit intake and induce inanition unless circumvented by enteral or parenteral feeding. Conversely, resections of the distal bowel, such as colectomy, have minimal effect as causes of malnutrition.[13,14]

Antineoplastic chemotherapy can be a major factor in the genesis of malnutrition. It can cause diminished intake, anorexia, nausea, vomiting, and depression, or in a more specific way, it can disrupt the absorptive intestine, as with methotrexate and 5-fluorouracil. The effects of antineoplas-

TABLE 59-1. Etiology of Cancer Malnutrition

First Degree	*Second Degree*	*Third Degree*
Diminished nutrient intake	Anorexia	Taste, smell abnormality Malaise, weakness Loss of central anticipatory stimuli
	Malfunction of gastrointestinal tract	Nausea, vomiting, diarrhea Obstruction, ileus Mucositis, esophagitis
	Increased nutrient demand	Catabolic consequences of therapy, including fever Effect of tumor on intestinal absorption
Tumor consumption of nutrient	Metabolic "activity" of the tumor	Anaerobic glycolysis and lactate production
Remote metabolic effects of tumor on the host	Hormonal production by the tumor	Tumor-induced hypoglycemia
	Inability of host to adapt to diminished intake	Diarrhea syndromes Failure to use fat for energy Loss of substrate-hormonal feedback
	Increase in host lean tissue dissolution	Gluconeogenesis for tumor consumption Increase in recycling of lactate Use of wasteful energy cycles Alteration in tissue lysozymal content
	Increase in energy expenditure	Catabolic hormonal milieu
	Increase in protein turnover	Protein breakdown exceeds synthesis

TABLE 59-2. Intestinal Response to Antineoplastic Agents

Drug	*Effects*
Agents Associated with Severe Nausea and Vomiting	
Nitrogen mustard	Occurs in virtually all patients. May be severe but usually subsides within 24 hours.
Chloroethyl nitrosoureas	Variable but may be severe.
Streptozotocin	Occurs in nearly all patients. Tolerance improves with each succeeding dose on a 5-day schedule.
Cisplatin	May be very severe. Tolerance improved with intravenous hydration and continued 5-day infusions. Nausea may persist for several days.
Imidazole carboxamide (DTIC)	Occurs in most patients. Tolerance improves with each succeeding dose on a 5-day schedule.
Agents Associated with Mucositis	
Methotrexate	May be quite severe with prolonged infusions or compromised renal function. Severity is enhanced by irradiation. May be prevented with adequate citrovorum rescue.
5-Fluorouracil	More severe with higher doses, frequent schedule, and arterial infusions.
Dactinomycin	Very common and may prevent oral alimentation. Severity enhanced by irradiation.
Adriamycin (doxorubicin)	May be severe and ulcerative. Increased severity with liver disease or irradiation.
Bleomycin	May be severe and ulcerative.
Vinblastine	Frequently ulcerative.

tic agents on intestinal function are summarized in Table 59-2.[15] Radiotherapy can also affect the GI tract both acutely and chronically (Table 59-3).[16] Small intestine absorption is minimally affected by malignancy, with the single exception of small intestine lymphoma.[17]

Substrate consumption by the tumor has been suggested as a cause of malnutrition. Calculations of glucose consumption by human tumors are based on the assumption that a metabolically active tumor and the human brain have similar glucose consumption. It is unlikely that the commonly sized tumors (100–500g) could consume more than approximately 5% of the daily caloric intake of the normal cancer-bearing host. Only metabolically active, extremely large tumors (> 1.4 kg, the approximate size of the human brain) could consume a significant percentage (15–30%) of the daily caloric intake of some cancer patients.

The patient with malignancy may have an increased energy expenditure. In a heterogeneous population of hospitalized cancer patients, Knox and co-workers did not show a uniform increase in whole-body energy expenditure, but rather a wide spectrum of abnormalities, including the hypometabolic, normal, and hypermetabolic states.[18] There were no correlations, with age, height, weight, sex, nutritional status, tumor burden, or liver metastasis. The only factor that appeared to correlate with increased whole-body energy expenditure was the presence of malignancy. Conversely, studies in well-defined patients with uniform tumors suggested a relative increase in the metabolic rate compared with similarly malnourished, hospitalized cancer patients or normals. A study in patients with small cell lung cancer demonstrated that the mean energy expenditure was 37% above the expected rate in comparable normals.[19] The increase was the same in patients with metastatic disease and in those with disease limited to the lungs. Patients who had a complete response to chemotherapy showed a significant decrease in energy expenditure, but the nonresponders had no change. Schersten, Warnold, and Arbeit have also suggested that defined groups of patients do show increases in energy expenditure, compared with the appropriate controls, and that this can be reversed by resection of the tumor.[20–22]

Many abnormalities of protein, fat, and carbohydrate metabolism have been suggested in the cancer patient (Table 59-4).[23] The major functional abnormality seems to be the increase in the energy-wasteful Cori cycle, resulting in an increase in recycling of lactate. Specificity of this observation in cancer patients remains a matter of great debate.

TABLE 59-3. Radiotherapy-Induced Nutritional Sequelae

Region	*Early*	*Late*
Head and Neck	Odynophagia Xerostomia Mucositis Anorexia Dysosmia Hypogeusia	Ulcer Xerostomia Dental caries Osteoradionecrosis Trismus Hypogeusia
Thorax	Dysphagia	Fibrosis Stenosis Fistula
Abdomen and pelvis	Anorexia Nausea Vomiting Diarrhea Acute enteritis Acute colitis	Ulcer Malabsorption Diarrhea Chronic enteritis Chronic colitis

Donaldson SS, Lenon RA: Alterations of nutritional status: Impact of chemotherapy and radiation therapy. Cancer 43:2036, 1979.

TABLE 59-4. Nutritional and Metabolic Comparison of Starvation, Injury, and Tumor Bearing

Category	*Starvation**	*Injury*	*Tumor Bearing*
Anorexia	+ (24)	+ (25)	+ (26)
Weight	↓ (27)	↓ (28)	↓ (29)
Basal metabolic rate	↓ (30)	↑ (31)	↑ (19,21), ± (22)
Blood glucose	↓ (27)	↑ (32)	± (33)
Blood lactate	± (34)	↑ (35)	↑ (36)
Serum insulin	↓ (27)	↓ (32)	± (37)
Plasma glucagon	↑ (38)	↑ (32)	± (39)
Total plasma amino acids	↓ (40)	↑ (41)	↓ (42)
Urinary nitrogen excretion	↓ (27)	↑ (43)	± (44)
Glucose tolerance	↓ (27)	↓ (41)	↓ (33)
Whole-body glucose turnover rate	↓ (45)	↑ (46)	↑ (39)
Whole-body glucose recycling (%)	↑ (45)	± (46)	± (39)
Whole-body glucose recycling	± (45)	↑ (47)	↑ (36)
Whole-body protein turnover	↓ (48)	↑ (49)	± (50)
Whole-body protein synthesis	↓ (48)	↑ (49)	± (50)
Whole-body protein catabolism	± (48)	↑ (49)	↑ (50)
Gluconeogenesis from alanine	↑ (51)	↑ (52)	↑ (53)
Whole-body fat turnover	↑ (54)	↑ (54)	± (54)
Glycerol turnover	↑ (55)	↑ (55)	± (55)

Adapted and expanded from Brennan MF: Total parenteral nutrition in the cancer patient. N Engl J Med 305:375, 1981.

* The ↑ indicates a significant increase, ↓ a significant decrease, and ± either no change or a nonsignificant trend. For anorexia, + denotes its presence. The figures in parentheses are reference numbers.

Many patients show abnormalities that can be due to other stress factors, such as infection and fever. We have reported a marked increase in whole-body fat turnover that is unresponsive to the addition of intravenous glucose at 87% to 90% of the energy intake.[54,55] This has also been shown with increased glycerol turnover in these patients.[56]

There has been a search for various mediators of a distant tumor effect on the metabolic and nutritional status of the cancer-bearing host. In a model reported by Strain,[57] a renal cell neoplasm was removed from a patient who had lost 30 kg in the 2 months before the operation. The tumor was then grown as a nonmetastasizing, transplantable xenograft in immuno-suppressed mice. The tumor produced marked weight loss in the animal model at a time when the tumor itself was extremely small. This weight loss could not be explained by a decrease in energy intake. Other models are much less realistic, with tumors making up 15% to 20% of the animal's body weight when anorexia begins. A tumor weighing 10 to 15 kg occurring in man is rare, and these models are mostly irrelevant.

Paraneoplastic syndromes have been described and are important causes of malnutrition in selected patients with malignancy. These, however, are rare and cannot be widely applied to the overall cause of malnutrition in the vast majority of cancer patients.

Hormonal consequences of malignancy are a powerful possibility for explaining many of the changes associated with malnutrition in cancer patients. Clearly, glucagon and epinephrine can decrease appetite and cause insulin resistance and increased whole-body protein catabolism. However, only modestly elevated glucagon concentrations have been observed in cancer patients, not too different from patients with mild degrees of stress.

Perhaps the best support for humoral effects are parabiotic experiments, showing that cross-circulation of 1% to 2% of blood volume per minute can result in marked anorexia of the parabiotic pair.[58]

Recently interest has focused on the ability of various monokines, such as tumor necrosis factor (TNF) and interleukin-1 (IL-1), to reproduce the metabolic abnormalities associated with malignancy.[59,60] Administration of TNF in doses that cause fever can result in accelerated whole-body protein turnover and some inhibition of whole-body protein synthesis. This is associated with increased glycerol turnover in some patients. Unlike stress states that would be expected to lead to whole-body protein dissolution, whole-body catabolism was not accelerated.

The suggestion that a macrophage-derived protein, "cachectin," which suppresses the synthesis of lipoprotein lipase in adipocytes, may be the cause of the cachectic state in endotoxin-treated animals is a very attractive hypothesis.[61-63] Murine cachectin appears to be identical to TNF, but the ability to reproduce the metabolic consequences of advanced malignancy has not been replicated by administration of TNF to patients.

CONSEQUENCES OF MALNUTRITION

The consequences of malnutrition in the cancer patient can be broadly defined as alterations in body composition and impairment of various functions from generalized protein–calorie malnutrition and from depletion of specific nutrients.

Body energy reserves in normal persons are retained mainly as fat (Fig. 59-1). The limiting factor in survival in the absence of any food intake are the protein reserves.

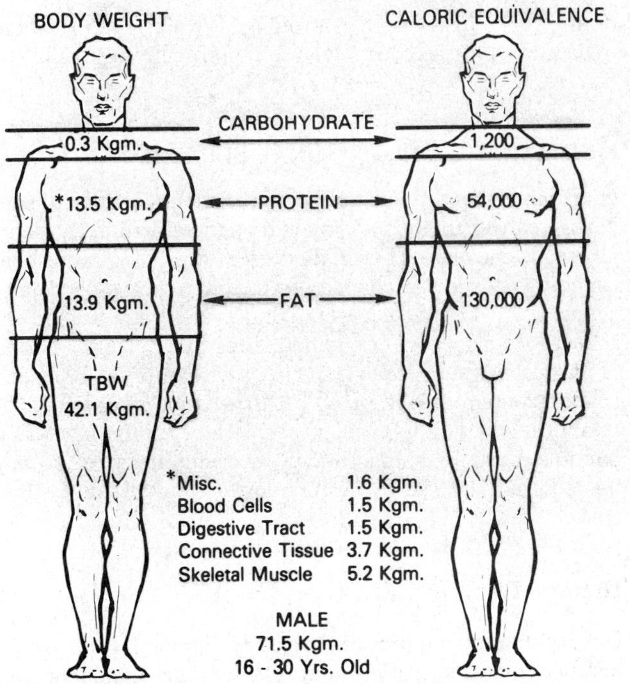

FIG. 59-1. Body composition of a healthy, well-developed young man, expressed as caloric equivalence. (Brennan MF: Metabolic response to surgery in the cancer patient. Consequences of aggressive multimodality therapy. Cancer 43:2053, 1979)

Normal man, in situations of simple fasting, progressively adapts to conserve protein. This progressive adaptation is done by tissues that are obligatory glucose users, such as the brain, by switching to the use of the products of fat breakdown, especially acetoacetate and beta-hydroxybuturate.[24,64] The amount of lean tissue reserves that exist in normal patients can be calculated. Depletion times for varying catabolic rates can be calculated as can the time to lose approximately 50% of lean tissue mass, a figure usually thought of as incompatible with survival (Table 59-5). These calculations have been validated by self-imposed fasting in criminal and political detainees for whom survival was approximately 60 days.

Rarely is the cancer-bearing host in an uncomplicated, adapted, semistarved state. Often other factors, such as associated infection or antineoplastic treatment, produce a superimposed mild to severe hypercatabolic state. The time then taken to lose 50% of the body cell mass is rapidly accelerated, inducing a quick depletion of protein stores.

The loss of lean body tissue is not necessarily associated with a decrease in circulating proteins. Total serum proteins and serum albumin levels were normal in patients with small cell lung cancer who were suffering from malnutrition, as assessed by weight loss, creatinine–height index, and decreases in total-body nitrogen, potassium, and fat.[65] Other reports have suggested that the changes in body composition are reflected in changes in serum albumin.

Some body composition studies have emphasized the loss of body fat that occurs in untreated malnourished cancer patients, and others have emphasized the major loss of protein.[66,67] The losses of body proteina are not all-encompassing but appear to be mainly from peripheral muscle tissue rather than the central, visceral fraction. Nonmuscle tissue can actually increase relatively in the malnutrition of cancer. Other studies by Cohn and Shike have suggested that changes in body composition are not limited to one component and do include loss of fat and water in addition to the loss of nitrogen.[65,68]

TABLE 59-5. Body Substrate Reserves: Depletion Times for Varying Catabolic Rates

Cause	*Nitrogen Loss Each Day (g)*	*Equivalent Lean Tissue Loss (g)*	*Days to Lose 50% of BCM**
Acute fasting	10	280	69
Chronic fasting	3	84	232
Major infection or injury	20	560	34
Month prior starvation and sepsis	15	420	35

Modified from Brennan MF: Uncomplicated starvation versus cancer cachexia. Cancer Res 37:2359, 1977.
* BCM = body cell mass.

NUTRITIONAL THERAPY

INDICATIONS

Nutritional support in cancer is indicated for malnourished patients or for those expected to become malnourished during the course of their disease. The benefits of the nutritional support should be proven or self-evident. Although these guidelines seem obvious, specific formulations as to which cancer patient should receive nutrition support are complicated by lack of a precise definition of clinical malnutrition, lack of knowledge about the efficacy of nutritional therapy, lack of rigorous scientific evaluation and ethical issues.[69]

Nutritional assessment has to be a part of the general medical examination of any cancer patient. Indicators of the nutritional status used clinically and as research tools are outlined in Table 59-6. Various combinations of these parameters have been proposed as nutritional indices that can predict complications of malnutrition and guide nutritional therapy.[70,71] However, these are controversial, and their usefulness in the clinical setting is questionable. In the management of the individual patient, the history and physical examination remain the best indicators of the nutritional status and the need for nutritional therapy.[72] History of weight loss in excess of 5% of body weight, markedly diminished food intake, history of severe malabsorption, and anticipated prolonged gastrointestinal dysfunction (*e.g.*, bone marrow transplantation, major abdominal surgery, or chemotherapy with severe side-effects) are indications for nutritional support. Laboratory data, such as serum albumin, blood levels of minerals (Ca, Mg, P), trace elements (Zn), and vitamins, can also indicate the need for nutritional therapy.

Once a decision is reached that the patient requires nutritional therapy, there are three main options: oral dietary therapy, enteral nutrition, and parenteral nutrition.

TABLE 59-6. Nutritional Assessment

History and physical examination
Weight loss
Decrease in regular food intake
History of malabsorption
Weakness
Muscle wasting
Findings suggestive of specific nutrients deficiencies
Anthropometric parameters
Triceps skin folds (measure of body fat)
Midarm muscle circumference (measure of skeletal muscle)
Percentage of ideal body weight
Laboratory parameters
Creatinine–height index (measure of skeletal muscle reserve)
Serum proteins: albumin, prealbumin, transferrin
Blood levels of nutrients (trace elements, vitamins, minerals)
Body composition
Total-body potassium (whole-body counter)
Total-body nitrogen (neutron activation)
Total-body water (^3H or ^2H dilution)
Bone content of calcium (photon absorptometry, neutron activation analysis)
CT indices of muscle, fat, bone
Immunologic parameters
Reactivity to skin tests
Total lymphocytes count
Serum immunoglobulins
Nutrient balance studies
Nitrogen balance
Trace element and mineral balance
Energy expenditure
Functional tests
Muscle function testing (voluntary or by nerve stimulation)
Protein turnover (stable isotopic enrichment)
Fat turnover (^{14}C-palmitate turnover)
Carbohydrate turnover (^{14}C or $^3H_2$ glucose)
Gluconeogenesis (^{14}C or ^{13}C glucose)
Glycerol turnover (2-stage glycerol infusion)
Enzyme activity (*e.g.*, glutathion peroxidase activity reflects selenium status)

Oral dietary therapy is indicated in any patient who is able to ingest sufficient nutrients but whose physiologic status requires a specific dietary regimen. Included in this group are cancer patients who have had operations on the GI tract (including oropharynx) and patients with mild or moderate chronic radiation-induced enteritis and pancreatic insufficiency.

Enteral feeding is indicated in patients who are unable to ingest sufficient nutrients but whose GI function is adequate for digestion and absorption of the required nutrients. This group includes patients with radical surgery in the oropharyngeal area, partial GI obstruction, mild or moderate malabsorption, short bowel syndrome, unconsciousness, and anorexia. Our surveys in hospitalized patients indicate that the provision of oral nutritional supplements to these patients is ineffective and cannot be used as a substitute for enteral feeding. The intake from supplements does not adequately replace the deficient nutrients.

Parenteral feeding is indicated in patients in whom the GI tract cannot be used for adequate feeding. Included in this category are patients with prolonged ileus (*e.g.*, after surgery, drug-induced), extreme short bowel syndrome, obstruction of the GI tract, diffuse mucositis caused by medications or irradiation, prolonged diarrhea, severe malabsorption, recurrent nausea and vomiting, and GI fistulae.

MODALITIES OF NUTRITIONAL SUPPORT

Nutritional support constitutes one of the modalities of supportive cancer therapy and should be integrated in the overall treatment plan. The method used to provide nutritional support may require changes to fit the patient's needs and status. For instance, severely malnourished patients who are scheduled for surgery or chemotherapy may require a period of nutritional support prior to those treatments. For such support, enteral feeding may be the method of choice prior to antitumor therapy. In the postoperative period or during administration of chemotherapy, parenteral nutrition may be required because of dysfunction of the gastrointestinal tract.

Dietary Therapy

Dietary therapy requires appropriate, thorough, and specific instructions to the patient and to the family members who are involved in food preparation. The prescribed diet reflects the pathophysiology of the patient's medical condition. Dietary therapies commonly used in cancer patients are outlined in Table 59-7. The choice of diet must be converted into instructions regarding the actual types of food and size and frequency of meals. This can best be done by a dietitian who, using the prescribed diet, can plan meals that adequately provide the patient's nutritional requirements and meet the appropriate restrictions. Occasionally, specific

TABLE 59-7. Diets Commonly Prescribed for Cancer Patients

Patient's Condition	*Diet*
Gastric resection	5–6 small meals Separation of liquids from solids Restriction of monocarbohydrates Restriction of lactose-containing foods Iron supplementation Parenteral vitamin B_{12}
Short bowel	Frequent small meals Low-fiber, low-fat diet Restriction of monocarbohydrates Restriction of lactose-containing foods Calcium, magnesium, zinc supplementation Parenteral vitamin B_{12} if terminal ileum was resected
Pancreatic insufficiency	Low-fat diet Pancreatic enzymes supplementation Medium-chain triglycerides
Chronic radiation enteritis	Diet low in fiber, fat, and lactose
Esophageal strictures	Soft diet, emphasis on liquids or high caloric nutritional supplements
Postsupraglottic laryngectomy	Solids and soft foods Avoid liquids

nutrients such as magnesium, phosphorous, potassium, zinc, or various vitamins have to be prescribed. A successful outcome of dietary management requires consistent follow-up of the patient by both the dietitian and the physician.

Enteral Feeding

ENTERAL FEEDING ROUTES. Enteral feeding can be provided through a variety of tubes; the most commonly used are nasogastric tubes. There are many commercial tubes, most of which are made from silicon or polyurethane. Their lengths range between 30 and 43 inches, with diameters ranging from 5 to 16 French. A list of available feeding tubes and the companies that produce them has been published.[73] These nasogastric tubes are suitable for short-term enteral feeding, usually in the hospital. If prolonged enteral feeding is required, gastrostomy or jejunostomy tubes are preferable. The recent development of endoscopic percutaneous techniques for placement of these tubes has facilitated enteral feeding in cancer patients. The percutaneous endoscopic gastrostomy can be placed safely using mild sedation and local anesthetic. It does not require an operating room and can be done on an outpatient basis. In our experience with the first 153 endoscopic gastrostomies in cancer patients, the complication rate was 8.3%, with no mortality.[74] The results compare favorably with the complication rate of surgically placed gastrostomies, which range between 6% and 75%.[75,76] They also compare favorably with the results of endoscopic gastrostomies in patients with nonmalignant diseases,[77] indicating that the cancer patient is not at increased risk from the procedure.

For long-term enteral feeding, the advantages of a feeding gastrostomy over a nasogastric tube are evident. The diameter of the gastrostomy tube is 16 to 20 French, about twice that of the nasogastric tube, and does not tend to clog. It is more esthetically acceptable and less irritating to the patient. It cannot be accidentally pulled out or dislodged, as in the case of the nasogastric tube. Tube dislodgement often limits provision of nutrients through a nasogastric tube. We used a button gastrostomy to replace the normal gastrostomy tube (Fig. 59-2). The button is more convenient and esthetically more acceptable to the patient. It is particularly useful for patients who are well and active but require long-term enteral feeding. When the gastrostomy tube is no longer required, it can be removed easily and the gastrocutaneous fistula closes within 2 to 3 days.

FIG. 59-2. A button gastrostomy in a patient requiring long-term enteral feeding.

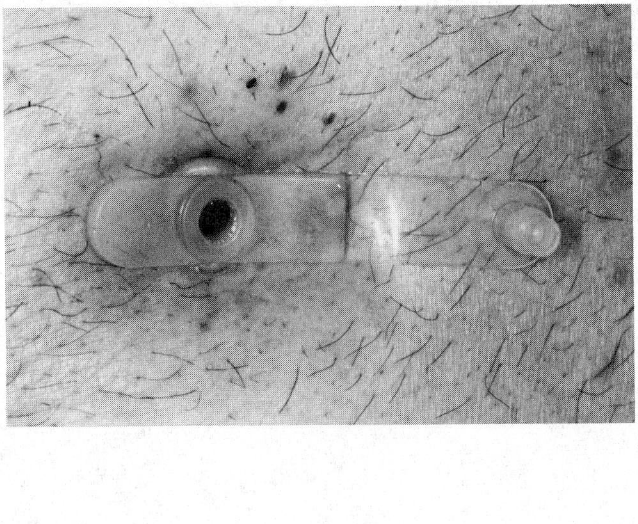

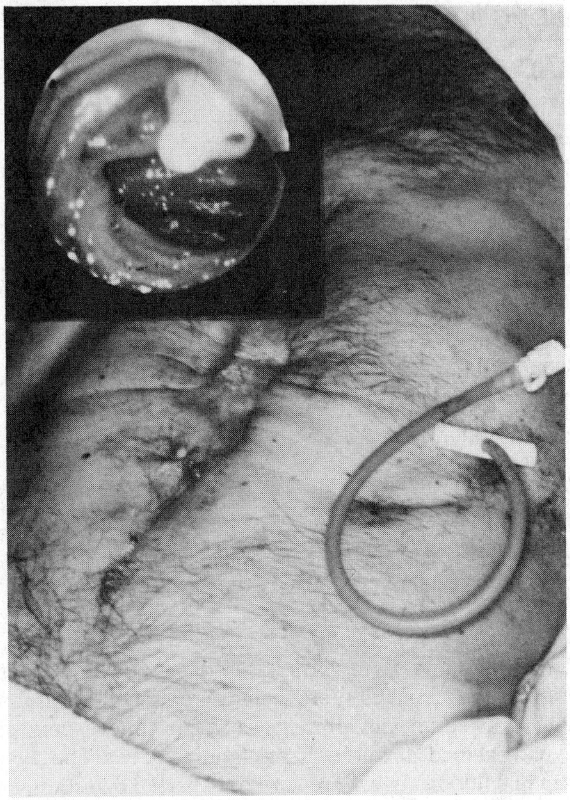

FIG. 59-3. A percutaneous endoscopic jejunostomy in a patient with total gastrectomy. **Insert**. Endoscopic view of the intrajejunal part of the tube.

We have also developed a method for placement of percutaneous endoscopic jejunostomies in patients who have had previous gastrectomies, which precludes the placement of endoscopic gastrostomies (Fig. 59-3).[78] In these patients, endoscopic percutaneous feeding jejunostomies can be placed in the efferent loop of the jejunum. Although the procedure is more elaborate, the complication rate is the same as that for the endoscopic gastrostomy.

ENTERAL FEEDING SOLUTIONS. There are over 70 commercial enteral feeding solutions, and a comprehensive table listing the solutions and their compositions has been published.[79] The solutions vary in the degree of predigestion of the protein, the content of fat, carbohydrates, lactose, caloric density, and osmolality. Almost all solutions contain sufficient minerals, trace elements, and vitamins.

Based on their composition, enteral feeding solutions can be divided into two groups: those requiring full digestion (Table 59-8) and those requiring partial digestion (Table 59-9). Formulas included in the first group contain whole proteins, significant amounts of fat in the form of triglycerides, and long-chain carbohydrates. In most, the caloric density is around 1 cal/ml, although in some cases the density is

TABLE 59-8. Enteral Feeding Solutions Requiring Full Digestion*

Content per 1000 kcal	*Isocal*	*Isocal HCN*	*Ensure*	*Isotein HN*	*Magnacal*	*Osmolites*	*Sustacal Liquid*
	(Mead Johnson)	*(Mead Johnson)*	*(Rose)*	*(Sandoz)*	*(Sherwood Medical)*	*(Ross)*	*(Mead Johnson)*
Protein (g)	32.5	37.5	35.2	57.1	35.0	35.2	60.1
% of total calories	13	15	14	23	14	14	24
Fat (g)	42.0	51.0	35.2	28.6	40.0	36.4	23.1
% of total calories	37	45	31	25	36	31	21
Carbohydrate (g)	126.0	100.0	137.2	131.4	125.0	137.2	137.8
% of total calories	50	40	55	53	51	55	55
Volume (ml)	1000	500	996	843	500	946	980
Osmolality (mOsm/kg)	300	690	450	300	590	300	320
Sodium (mEq)	21.5	17.5	34.8	22.8	21.8	26.0	39.8
Potassium (mEq)	32.1	21.5	37.8	23.2	16.0	24.4	51.9
Phosphorus (mg)	500	500	520	476.2	500	498.1	925.9
Calcium (mg)	600	500	520	476.2	500	498.1	1000

This is a partial list adapted from Block AS, Shils ME: Appendix Tables A40b and A40c. In Shils ME, Young V (eds): Modern Nutrition in Health and Disease, 7th ed. Philadelphia, Lea & Febiger, 1987.
* Solutions contain intact proteins, fat, and carbohydrates; all are lactose free and low residue.

to 2 cal/ml. Some of the formulas in this group are prepared from natural foods; others contain extracts of proteins (mainly casein and soy proteins) and fats (mostly corn oil). The natural foods formulas have higher residues. The second group of solutions, which require only partial digestion, contain prehydrolyzed proteins or amino acids. The fat content is minimal and is mostly in the form of medium-chain triglycerides. The osmolality of the group 1 solutions tends to be lower than that of the group 2 solutions.

Patients with an intact GI tract (*e.g.*, head and neck cancer, esophageal obstruction, unconsciousness) tolerate the solutions from group 1 quite well. Patients with maldigestion (*e.g.*, pancreatic insufficiency), malabsorption (*e.g.*, chronic radiation enteritis), or rapid GI transit (*e.g.*, gastrectomy, gastrojejunostomy, short bowel) benefit from the partially digested formulae.

The rate of administration of enteral feedings has to be determined according to the patient's status. Patients with head and neck cancer whose GI tract is intact can be fed by bolus of 300 to 500 ml a few times a day.[80] Patients after gastrectomies require a slow drip of no more than 200 ml/hour; those with short bowel, malabsorption, or radiation-induced enteritis may not be able to tolerate more than 100 ml/hour. If beginning enteral feeding by a drip, it is not necessary to use "starter regimens" with diluted solutions or rates below 50 to 100 ml/hour, because they result in decreased nutrients delivery and do not improve tolerance to enteral feeding.[81,82]

Complications from enteral feeding can be avoided by monitoring the patient. If a nasogastric feeding tube is used, it is essential to ensure that the tip of the tube is placed in the antrum of the stomach or more distally to avoid aspiration. Diarrhea can be avoided by choice of appropriate solutions and by adjustment of the infusion rate. Antidiarrheal agents should not be used as a means of increasing tolerance to enteral feeding. Monitoring of blood glucose, BUN electrolytes, calcium, magnesium, and phosphorus should be done initially on a daily basis, until the patient's metabolic status is

TABLE 59-9. Enteral Feeding Solutions Requiring Partial Digestion

Content per 1000 kcal	*Criticare HN*	*Vital HN*	*Vivonex*
	(Mead Johnson)	*(Ross)*	*(Norwich-Eaton)*
Protein (g)	36.0	41.7	21.8
% of total calories	14	17	9
Fat (g)	3.0	10.8	1.4
% of total calories	3	8	1
Carbohydrates (g)	210.0	188.3	230.9
% of total calories	83	75	90
Volume (ml)	946	1000	1000
Osmolality (mOsm/kg)	650	460	550
Sodium (mEq)	26.0	16.7	20.4
Potassium (mEq)	32.0	29.8	30.0
Phosphorous (mg)	500.0	667.0	550.0
Calcium (mg)	500.0	667.0	550.0

* Solutions contain hydrolyzed protein or amino acids and small amounts of fat.

stable while receiving the prescribed nutritional regimen. After this is accomplished, metabolic monitoring can be done less frequently. Occasionally, supplements of specific nutrients, particularly phosphorus, have to be given to maintain normal blood levels. These should be administered separately from the enteral feedings to prevent precipitation and malabsorption.

Parenteral Nutrition

VENOUS ACCESS. Parenteral nutritional support requires a durable, reliable source of central venous access. Access sites are often required for the administration of chemotherapeutic drugs and for obtaining blood for metabolic monitoring. The common and widely used access is the percutaneous infraclavicular subclavian catheter, which has stood the test of time and is the primary method of access in the acute or short-term situation.

There has been progress in the quality of long-term venous access. Current preference is for the double lumen (cuffed Silastic) type of device, which can usually be placed into the external jugular vein by a small supraclavicular incision and brought out subcutaneously on the chest wall. This provides a reliable, durable access site for delivery of chemotherapy, for monitoring, and for long-term parenteral nutrition.

Subcutaneously placed access devices (*e.g.*, infus-a-port, mediport) are alternatives that allow the isolation of the catheter access site from the external environment. These are excellent for safe percutaneous delivery of chemotherapeutic agents, but have been only minimally employed for nutritional support.

SOLUTIONS. Parenteral nutrition solutions are designed to provide all the nutrients known to be essential to humans. Solutions currently in clinical use include amino acids, glucose, fat emulsions, minerals, trace elements, vitamins, and fluids. Whether other nutrients such as carnitine and choline need to be added to total parenteral nutrition (TPN) solutions is currently under investigation.[83,84] Parenteral nutrition solutions are prepared by mixing appropriate amounts of the component nutrients. The infused nutrients must provide the individual requirements of the patient. Standard solutions can be designed for use in patients with standard nutritional requirements (Table 59-10). However, many cancer patients require individual prescriptions because of special nutritional requirements due to prior malnutrition, glucose intolerance, specific nutrient deficiencies, organ failure, or changing therapies. The advent of efficient, computerized automatic mixing devices in the TPN pharmacy facilitated the use of individual formulas.

PROTEIN. The protein source in parenteral nutrition formulas is in the form of synthetic amino acids. Protein hydrolysates have been abandoned. The synthetic amino acid solutions contain all the essential amino acids, which constitute between 35% and 45% of the total amino acids in the solutions. Most of the commercial solutions contain nonessential amino acids, which were found to have an important role in intravenous feeding.[85] Early work demonstrated that the nutritional value of intravenous amino acids is similar to that of

TABLE 59-10. Proposed Standard TPN Formula for Infusion Through a Central Vein

Content	*Amount*
Amino acids	70 g
Non-protein calories*	2400 kcal
Fluids	2000 ml
Minerals†	
Sodium	80–120 mEq
Chlorine	150–200 mEq
Potassium	60–100 mEq
Calcium	300–400 mg
Phosphorus	500–1000 mg
Magnesium	20 mEq
Acetate	as needed
Iron	as needed
Trace elements	
Zinc	3.0–6.0 mg
Copper	0.3 mg
Chromium	15 μg
Selenium	20 μg
Manganese	0.1 mg
Vitamins	
AMA–FDA formula‡	

* The percentage of fat calories can range between 0 and 50%. If fat is not used as a caloric source, 500 ml of fat emulsions should be administered twice a week as a source of essential fatty acids.

† The doses may require adjustments in the case of organ failure, such as heart failure or renal insufficiency. Medications commonly prescribed for cancer patients may significantly affect the minerals required in TPN solutions.

‡ See Table 59-11.

oral ingestion of comparable amounts of protein.[86] It has been proposed that dipeptides can be used efficiently in parenteral nutrition, that they are well tolerated, appropriately broken down to the component amino acids, and have the advantage of decreasing the osmolar loads and fluid requirements in parenteral nutrition.[87] These solutions are under investigation and are not in clinical use. The maintenance requirements for amino acids in the average adult patient are between 0.75 and 1.0 g/kg of body weight in a TPN solution. If protein losses are extensive, such as in patients with protein-losing enteropathy, nephrotic syndrome, or large burns, the dose has to be increased up to 2 g/kg of body weight. The amino acid doses required in infants and children are higher than those in adults, amounting to 2 g/kg in infants and 1.5 g/kg in small children.

Amino acid preparations specially formulated for the cancer patient do not exist. Defined formulations for renal failure have shown a decrease in the need for dialysis, but they have had minimal effect on survival.[88] The defined formula solution for liver failure (*i.e.*, high-branched-chain, low-aromatic amino acids) has shown dramatic metabolic changes, and a randomized study suggested clinical benefit in encephalopathic patients and a decrease in the hospital mortality.[89] A recent review of high-branched-chain amino acid solutions for use in infection and injury concluded that the solutions should be used as investigative agents and have limited metabolic advantage.[90]

CALORIES. Glucose and fat emulsions can both be used as caloric sources in TPN. Carbohydrates other than glucose have been tried as substitutes for glucose, particularly because they do not require insulin and thus alleviate the problem of glucose intolerance.[91] However, they were found to have unacceptable clinical or metabolic side-effects (*e.g.*, fructose induces lactic acidosis; xylitol is highly toxic to liver, kidney, and brain; and maltose is lost through the urine in large amounts). In commercial dextrose solutions, glucose is present as glucose-monohydrate and provides 3.4 kcal/g of glucose. Fat emulsions provide 1.1 kcal/ml or 2 kcal/ml when the concentrations are 10% or 20%, respectively. Commercial fat emulsions contain vegetable oil (*e.g.*, soybean or safflower) as a source of triglycerides. Egg phospholipids are added as emulsifiers, and glycerol is added to achieve isotonicity with plasma; α-tochopherol is also present in small amounts to prevent lipid peroxidation. Of the total triglycerides in fat emulsions, 50% or more are in the form of linoleic acid, which is an essential nutrient in humans. Linolenic acid, is also present in adequate amounts in fat emulsions.

The issue of what fraction of TPN calories should be given as fat has been the subject of numerous studies, most of which concluded that in the majority of patients, the effect of fat on nitrogen metabolism is comparable whether the TPN solutions contained 100% of the non-protein calories as glucose or whether various combinations of fat and glucose provided the calories. Therefore, considerations other than the effect on nitrogen metabolism may be relevant in choosing the caloric source. In patients with glucose intolerance or with fluid restrictions, provision of up to 50% of the calories from fat can facilitate management; in hyperlipidemic patients, fat calories should be avoided. In patients given peripheral parenteral feeding, the use of as many as 70% of the calories from fat emulsions decreases the osmotic load of the solutions, and this can decrease the incidence of phlebitis in the peripheral veins used.

In addition to their roles in promoting nitrogen accretion and as sources of calories, glucose and triglycerides fulfill essential metabolic roles, and minimal amounts of both must be given. Fat emulsions provide linoleic and linolenic acids, which are required to prevent essential fatty acids deficiency.[92] Linoleic acid is the precursor of arachidonic acid from which prostaglandins are synthesized. If given orally, 15% of calories need be fat; if given intravenously, 3.2% of total calories need be fat to avoid essential fatty acids deficiency.[93] Although glucose can be synthesized in the liver de novo, a minimum of about 100 g/day are necessary to prevent increased protein breakdown and to suppress gluconeogenesis. Glucose is the preferred energy source in some tissues, including the brain, the kidney medulla, and red blood cells.

The hormone-substrate profile of the patient receiving TPN reflects the energy sources used.[94] When glucose is the only energy source, the substrate hormone profile in the plasma is characterized by high glucose, pyruvate, insulin, and to a certain extent, lactate. When a major portion of calories are given as fat, there is an increase in plasma ketone bodies and circulating free fatty acids and triglycerides, with low levels of insulin.

The total nonprotein calories required in most patients to ensure weight maintenance and optimal nitrogen balance range between 30 and 40 kcal/kg. Some types of tumors, such as small cell lung cancer, induce a state of increased energy expenditure, and increased amounts of calories may be required in patients with such tumors.[19]

MINERALS. Current TPN solutions contain minerals as outlined in Table 59-10. The amounts given have to be adjusted to the patient's needs. Increased losses of minerals from diarrhea, vomiting, GI fistulas, and urine have to be replaced. Drugs commonly used in cancer patients such as cisplatin and amphothercin B can induce large urinary losses of magnesium and potassium. Patients with diarrhea and vomiting tend to lose large amounts of zinc and potassium, and fat malabsorption induces losses of large amounts of magnesium and calcium. In calculating the amounts of sodium in TPN solutions, other sources of sodium intake, particularly antibiotics, have to be considered.

TRACE ELEMENTS. Trace elements fulfill a critical role in human nutrition and metabolism. Deficiency states with severe clinical and biochemical manifestations can result from administration of TPN without added trace elements.[95] Trace elements currently recommended for addition to TPN solutions include zinc, copper, manganese, chromium, and selenium. The standard dosages are outlined in Table 59-10. Between 1 and 12.5 mg of iron can be added to TPN solutions.[96] Appropriate precautions have to be taken because of the potential of anaphylaxis from intravenous iron. Patients with iron deficiency who are maintained on TPN require intravenous iron to restore normal iron status. These amounts should be infused separately from the TPN solutions.

We have found that commonly used parenteral nutrition solutions contain ultra trace elements as contaminants. These include molybdenum, vanadium, boron, nickel, and others.[97] It is thought that some of these trace elements may fulfill an important role in human nutrition.

VITAMINS. There are various commercial preparations that combine 12 vitamins in adult and pediatric daily doses (Table 59-11). The composition of these preparations is based on the recommendations of the Nutrition Advisory

TABLE 59-11. Daily Vitamin Supplementation

Vitamin	*Adult*	*Pediatric*
Ascorbic acid (mg)	100	80
Vitamin A (IU)	3300	2300
Vitamin D (IU)	200	400
Thiamine (mg)	3.0	1.2
Riboflavin (mg)	3.6	1.4
Pyroxidine (mg)	4.0	1.0
Niacin (mg)	40.0	17.0
Pantothenic acid (mg)	15.0	5.0
Vitamin E (IU)	10	7
Biotin (μg)	60	20
Vitamin B_{12} (μg)	5	1
Folic acid (μg)	400	140
Vitamin K* (mg)		200

* Not present in adult multivitamin formulas and must be added separately.

Group of the Department of Foods and Nutrition of the American Medical Association.[98] Studies in stable adult long term TPN patients demonstrated the adequacy of the commercial preparation in maintaining normal blood levels of the vitamins.[99] In cancer patients receiving in hospital parenteral nutrition for short periods, administration of the AMA-FDA recommended vitamin preparation resulted in normal blood levels of vitamin C and pantothenic acid in all patients, but low levels of thiamin, riboflavin, and pyroxidine in 4% to 40% of the patients.[100] In adult hospitalized surgical patients, it was found that the preparation maintained the pretreatment vitamins blood levels, but it did not correct pretreatment low levels, which were frequent.[101]

In determining the adequacy of vitamins, it is essential to examine functional adequacy rather than blood levels, because these levels may not reflect tissue activity of the vitamins. Determination of the activity of vitamin-dependent enzymes or activity in target organs is preferable to determination of blood levels of vitamins. Data are lacking for most of the vitamins. Until more knowledge is gained about vitamin requirements and metabolism in TPN, the current commercial formulas based on the AMA-FDA recommendations are reasonable for most patients. Vitamin preparations should be added to the TPN solution just before infusion, because of the tendency of vitamin A to be absorbed to the container and that of vitamin C to lose activity in solutions.

METABOLIC COMPLICATIONS AND MONITORING. Parenteral nutrition is a prescription of up to 30 nutrients and fluids given intravenously. Quite often, particularly in the hospitalized cancer patient, TPN is administered to patients with unstable functions of the kidneys, liver, or heart, in conjunction with major drugs, or in situations with changing requirements for fluids and minerals. It is essential that the staff administering TPN is well trained. Preferably, TPN should be administered and supervised by a nutrition support team. Parenteral nutrition can be administered safely and with minimal complications if the formula is a priori adjusted to the physiologic state of the patient and appropriate monitoring is performed. Thus, a patient with progressive renal failure requires adjustments in the dosages of potassium, magnesium, phosphorus, and protein; in states of vomiting, diarrhea or mineral-losing nephropathy, additional minerals may be required. In liver failure or heart failure, adjustments are required in the amounts of amino acids or fluids and sodium, respectively.

Stable patients receiving TPN require little monitoring after the initial periods of adjustment. In the Memorial Sloan-Kettering Cancer Center home TPN patients, 1 year follow-up of the mineral requirements demonstrated the ratio of minimal to maximal amounts: Na, 98 ± 2%; K, 95 ± 3%; Ca, 100 ± 0%; P, 100 ± 0%; Mg, 97 ± 3%, indicating very little change in the requirements.[102] This contrasts with the hospitalized cancer patients undergoing chemotherapy, in whom the requirements varied widely, with the minimal to maximal ratio of Na, 62 ± 7%; K, 52 ± 5%; Ca, 85 ± 5%; P, 37 ± 6%; and Mg, 68 ± 5%.[102] The most important factor in dictating these changes was the variability in renal function, mostly caused by chemotherapeutic agents and antibiotics.

TPN solutions contain large amounts of glucose, particularly when glucose is the sole source of nonprotein calories. In our experience, 5% to 10% of hospitalized cancer patients receiving TPN develop glucose intolerance of a magnitude that requires insulin therapy. In most patients, addition of insulin to the TPN bags, with appropriate adjustments of the dose, resolves the hyperglycemia. When control of hyperglycemia proves to be difficult, use of fat emulsions as a nonprotein caloric source can reduce glucose intolerance.

Liver function abnormalities occur frequently in hospitalized cancer patients receiving TPN.[103] TPN-induced liver dysfunction usually occurs within days after beginning TPN and is manifested primarily as a mild increase in the serum SGOT, SGPT, and alkaline phosphatase, with no rise in the serum bilirubin. Severe liver dysfunction due to TPN is uncommon and rarely is a reason to discontinue TPN. Cancer patients have many causes for abnormal liver function tests, and these should not be immediately attributed to TPN.

EFFICACY OF NUTRITIONAL SUPPORT

Nutritional efficacy is the ability of the provided nutritional support to reverse the previous nutritional deficits from both structural and functional points of view. We chose to evaluate clinical efficacy by examination of tolerance of anticancer therapy and by clinical outcome in clinical trials (Tables 59-12, 59-13, and 59-14).

Metabolic efficacy describes the ability of nutritional support to reverse the metabolic defects, such as negative nitrogen balance, in the patient with cancer. Nitrogen balance is dependent on disease state and concomitant illness, such as sepsis, and therefore, improving the balance may be quite difficult. In some patients, it is relatively easy to reverse deficits of trace metals, such as zinc and copper, by replacement of necessary quantities. We performed several studies to identify the requirements for reversing the deficiencies of such trace metals.[128,129] Replacement readily reverses the abnormality, as determined by the plasma concentration and balance studies.

Studies have determined the requirements for reversing nutritional deficiencies of fat and water-soluble vitamins.[130,131] It is relatively easy to calculate, predict, and then resolve the issue of adequacy of a vitamin replacement regimen that will reverse serum or plasma deficits of these nutrients. However, very few data exist to settle conclusively whether the functional consequences are reversed simply by maintaining the plasma levels. Rare tissue comparisons have shown that the restoration of the normal serum values will restore the tissue availability for some nutrients.[132]

Other nutritional parameters commonly measured, such as serum albumin, are poor indicators of efficacy of nutritional support. It is quite difficult to restore serum albumin in the cancer patient, even with prolonged intravenous nutritional support, unless the primary underlying malignancy has been treated and there is a documented therapeutic response. Although body weight is readily replaced, individual constituents of body composition are not restored easily in the cancer patient, compared with the noncancer bearing host.[65,133] It is easy to restore both fat and water to the

TABLE 59-12. Results of Randomized Trials of TPN in Patients Undergoing Surgery for Malignancies

Cancer (Reference)	TPN in Relation to Operation (days)	Length of TPN (days)	No. of Patients		Major Postoperative Complication		Postoperative Wound Infection		Postoperative Mortality (%)	
			TPN	Control	TPN	Control	TPN	Control	TPN	Control
Gastrointestinal										
(104, 105)	2–3 before 10 after	12–13	30	26	13	19			7	8
(106)	5–14 before Variable	5–14	12	9	17	11	17	22	0	0
(107)	10 before Variable after	10	66	59	16	32*	21	25	5	19*
Esophageal										
(108)	5–7 before	13–41	10	5			0	20		
(109)	Perioperative	28	10	10	40	10	30	50	10	20
Esophageal/gastric										
(110)	7–10 before 7–10 after	7–10	10	10					0	10
(111)	7–10 before	7–10	38	36			8	31*	16	22
(112)	10 before Variable after	10	58	55	8	17*	6	9	4	11

* p = 0.05, versus TPN group.

cancer-bearing patient receiving parenteral support, but rebuilding protein reserves is difficult.[65]

The impact of additional events, such as exercise, are unclear. We originally showed in an animal model that exercise could overcome some of the muscle-wasting effects of the tumor-bearing state.[134] Recently, careful attempts to quantify the ability of exercise to reverse weight loss more efficiently, after superimposed starvation in man, have been less convincing.[135] After a 10-day fast, exercise was randomly added for one of two groups of normal volunteers undergoing nutritional replenishment by the intravenous route. Submaximal stationary bicycle exercise (51% of VO_2 max) was performed daily but did not significantly improve urinary nitrogen balance, resting energy expenditure, extremity amino acid flux, or maximal oxygen consumption. It would appear, therefore, that exercise alone is not a sufficient anabolic stimulus for the nutritionally depleted patient with cancer.

Patients who are malnourished have deficits in immunologic response. These, in the absence of malignancy, can be

TABLE 59-13. Results of Randomized Trials of TPN in Patients Receiving Radiation Therapy

Cancer (Reference)	Number of Patients		Length of TPN (days)	% of Planned Dose Given		Median Mortality (%)		Survival (wk)	
	TPN	Control		TPN	Control	TPN	Control	TPN	Control
Ovarian carcinoma (113)	42	39						39	36
Pelvic carcinoma (114)	11	9		92	101	45	33		
Pediatric abdomen or pelvic (115)	11	14	44	100	100	0	0		
Pelvic curative palliative	8	10	~35	100	90			100	80*
(116)	9	5	~35	55	60	66	60	11	0†

* At a median of 16 months.
† p = 0.03 in favor of TPN in those who also received chemotherapy.

TABLE 59-14. Results of Randomized Trials of TPN in Patients Receiving Chemotherapy

Cancer (Reference)	*Number of Patients*		*Length of TPN (days)*	*Percent of Planned Dose Given*		*Complete Response (%)*		*Partial Response (%)*		*WBC Nadir ($\times 10^3$)*		*Mortality (%)*		*Median Survival (wk)*	
	TPN	Control		TPN	Control	TPN	Control	TPN	Control	TPN	Control	TPN	Control	TPN	Control
Acute leukemia (117)	11	12	30–70												
Diffuse lymphoma (118,119)	17	19	14–16	88	85				−2.3	2.0				ND*	
Lung, squamous (120)	13	13	31			0	0	31	8	2.5	1.5†				
Lung, non-oat cell (121)	14	13	14–19			0	0	14	23					11	12
Lung, small cell (122)	21	28	42			85	59	15	41	0	0	24	32	ND	
Lung, small cell (123)	10	9				83	80			0.6	0.8				
Colon, metastatic (124)	20	25	24											11	44
Testis, Stage III (125)	16	14	18–48			63	79	25	14	0.9	0.9		−4	60	60
Adenocarcinoma, lung (126)	19	24	25			0	11	15	28	1.7	1.5	11	4	22	40
Metastatic sarcoma (127)	14	18									ND	0	27		

* ND = no difference.
† $p < 0.05$, compared with TPN group.

restored by nutritional support. Probably some of the immunologic defects in the cancer patient are due to malnutrition or compounded by it. At least some of these can be reversed by appropriate nutritional support, although the data to show that severe anergy can be restored by nutritional support alone are somewhat limited. In one study, patients for whom surgery for tumor resection was not feasible underwent nutritional support. Some benefit was shown in the restoration of skin test anergy.[136]

Clinical efficacy is a difficult determinant. Clearly, patients undergoing nutritional support after chronic malnutrition often have restoration of a sense of well-being and become more physically functional. Whether this support results in long-term clinical benefits is difficult to evaluate. The various prospective randomized trials that have been performed in different disease categories and with different treatment modalitites are summarized in Tables 59-12, 59-13, and 59-14. There are many deficiencies in these studies, especially the small number of patients in each study. From the available information, it appears that routine application of nutritional support to all patients undergoing treatment for malignancy is not justified.[137] In patients with no effective antineoplastic therapy, nutritional support, particularly TPN, may be harmful. It appears that the primary indication for nutritional support is for the malnourished patient undergoing a major operation for upper GI malignancy and for the chemotherapy patient with severe gastrointestinal dysfunction. These issues will not be resolved without a large-scale clinical trial.

HOME NUTRITIONAL SUPPORT

Home nutritional support is required in patients who cannot take sufficient oral nutrition and depend on enteral or parenteral nutrition to provide the required nutrients. These patients can be divided into two groups. In one group are included those who have been cured of their cancer or have a good prognosis. The other group includes terminal patients for whom home nutritional support allows them to be nursed at home or in terminal care institutions. The main thrust of home nutrition in cancer patients should be directed at patients in the first group, which includes patients with severe radiation-induced enteritis, short bowel syndrome, severe mucositis, and severe dysphagia (*e.g.*, patients with head and neck cancer). The choice between home enteral or parenteral nutrition is based on the principles discussed earlier, that the GI tract should be used for enteral feeding whenever possible and that TPN should be reserved only for patients with severe malabsorption who cannot tolerate enteral feeding.

Home enteral feeding requires a convenient route of administration. The placement of percutaneous endoscopic gastrostomies, percutaneous endoscopic jejunostomies, and gastrostomy buttons has facilitated long-term enteral feeding in the home. These tubes are easy for patients to handle, do not constitute an esthetic problem, do not become clogged, and are better tolerated than the nasogastric tubes. Patients maintained on this form of therapy can infuse nutrient solutions in the home. Enteral feeding at home is simple, and the patient or a family member can be taught in 1 hour to perform it. Our experience with 153 patients maintained for prolonged periods on this system demonstrates that it can provide the nutritional requirements and induce nutritional rehabilitation in those patients whose prognosis is good but cannot ingest sufficient nutrients.[74] In terminal patients, this mode of nutritional therapy can provide sufficient fluids to prevent rehospitalization for dehydration and give psychological comfort to the patient and to the family.[74]

In patients requiring parenteral feeding, a tunneled central venous catheter has to be placed. The patient or a family member has to be trained in handling the system and in monitoring problems. Self-management of home TPN requires a few days' admission to the hospital, during which time the central venous catheter is placed and instructions in aseptic techniques are given to the patient and a family member. The TPN solution can be formulated and adjusted to the patient's nutritional and metabolic requirements during the admission. Home TPN requires a metabolically stable patient.

The nutrient solutions and all necessary equipment (*e.g.*, pump, solutions, tubing) can be provided by commercial companies that deliver the items to the patient's home. Patients have to be monitored by a nutrition team or a physician to assure success of the program.

A nutrition survey performed in 1985 by the Oley Foundation revealed that there were 1477 patients in 74 home nutritional programs throughout the United States and Canada.[138] Of these, 1141 were receiving home parenteral nutrition, and the rest received enteral feeding. These numbers refer only to programs registered with the foundation and under-report the number of patients receiving home nutritional support. Of all reported patients, cancer patients constituted the second largest group, totaling 24.2%; in 1978, cancer patients constituted only 17%.

Home nutritional support can be remarkably safe. The use of percutaneous endoscopic gastrostomies and appropriate training has almost eliminated the problems of aspiration in enteral nutritional support. Diarrhea and metabolic complications are also rare after the patient is stabilized on the appropriate regimen and formulation. Home TPN also has a good safety record. Mild liver dysfunction is common, but progressive liver dysfunction occurs only in a minority of patients, particularly in children. Metabolic bone abnormalities are commonly seen in patients receiving prolonged TPN, but they rarely lead to severe bone disease.[139–141] The Oley Foundation's 1985 survey shows that 41% of the home TPN patients had no reported hospitalizations. Of all hospitalizations, 45% were related to TPN complications, 45% to the underlying disease, and 10% to other medical problems. Of all TPN-related hospitalizations, 46% were because of sepsis, 32% because of catheter-related problems, and the rest for a variety of other reasons.

It is our view that home TPN for cancer patients should be employed in those patients who have a reasonable prognosis or are undergoing antitumor therapy. The lack of demonstrable benefit of TPN and the complexity of the system argue against its use in terminal patients.

ETHICAL AND MORAL CONSIDERATIONS

Nutritional support should be provided if indicated, and no patient should suffer or die of starvation because of inability to ingest, digest, or absorb food. The responsibility of the medical profession for provision of nutrition as a component of overall medical treatment has been emphasized in the medical literature and has been echoed in court decisions and the lay literature.[142–144] It has even been argued that nutrition is a fundamental right and should not be subjected to the usual scientific criteria that form the bases of the practice of medicine.[69]

We believe that nutritional therapy should be provided to all patients in whom it is indicated. However, in terminal patients with no antitumor therapeutic options, intravenous parenteral nutrition should not be used routinely. On some occasions, nutritional support may allow social and psychologic comfort to the patient and family. In such cases an effort should be made to use enteral feeding.[74]

COST EFFECTIVENESS

It is difficult not to examine the cost effectiveness of nutritional support in the current socioeconomic environment. The opportunity to be provided with nutrition is a right held by all. The issue of cost effectiveness occurs only when the extremely expensive modality of TPN is examined. Very few studies address this issue.

A study examining the cost effectiveness of TPN in the period after GI surgery for malignancy developed a hypothetic model of 100 patients who would receive preoperative TPN before undergoing a GI cancer operation.[145] Based on a prior randomized study of the ability of therapy to decrease mortality and morbidity,[107] the authors calculated a savings of $1,700 by the provision of preoperative parenteral nutrition. These figures depend on relative costs within the state and the environment in which TPN is delivered.

As nutritional support is defined as being effective or noneffective in a routine sense, cost-effective analyses will have to be performed, and decisions about availability and utilization will be made, not only by the physician, but by society as well.

REFERENCES

1. Warren S: The immediate causes of death in cancer. Am J Med Sci 184:610, 1932
2. DeWys WD, Begg C, Lavin PT et al: Prognostic effect of weight loss prior to chemotherapy in cancer patients. Am J Med 69:491, 1980
3. Bistrian BR, Blackburn GL, Vitale J et al: Prevalence of malnutrition in general medical patients. JAMA 235:1567, 1976
4. Donaldson SS, Wesley MN, DeWys WD et al: A study of the nutritional status of pediatric cancer patients. Am J Dis Child 135:1107, 1981
5. Carter P, Carr D, vay Eys J et al: Nutritional parameters in children with cancer. J Am Diet Assoc 82:616, 1983
6. Shils ME, Coiso D: Report to the medical board on nutritional assessment of hospitalized adult patients in Memorial Hospital. 1979
7. DeWys WD: Anorexia as a general effect of cancer. Cancer 43:2013, 1979
8. Morrison SD: Anorexia and the cancer patient. In van Eys J, Nichols BL, Seelig MS (eds): Nutrition and Cancer 3, p 31. New York, SP Scientific and Medical Books, 1979
9. Krause R, James JH, Ziparo V et al: Brain tryptophan and the neoplastic anorexia/cachexia syndrome. Cancer 44:1003, 1979

10. von Meyenfeldt M, Chance WT, Fischer JE: Correlation of changes in brain indoleamine metabolism with onset of anorexia in rats. Am J Surg 143:133, 1982
11. Chance WT, von Meyenfeldt M, Fischer JE: Serotonin depletion by 5,7-dihydroxytryptamine or para-chloroamphetamine does not affect cancer anorexia. Pharmacol Biochem Behav 18:115, 1983
12. DeWys WD: Changes in taste sensation and feeding behavior in cancer patients. A review. J Hum Nutr 32:447, 1978
13. Lawrence W Jr: Nutritional consequences of surgical resection of the gastrointestinal tract for cancer. Cancer Res 37:2379, 1977
14. Shils ME: Effects on nutrition of surgery of the liver, pancreas and genitourinary tract. Cancer Res 37:2387, 1977
15. Mitchell EP, Schein PS: Gastrointestinal toxicity of chemotherapeutic agents. Semin Oncol 9:52, 1982
16. Donaldson SS, Lenon RA: Alterations of nutritional status: Impact of chemotherapy and radiation therapy. Cancer 43:2036, 1979
17. Rappaport H, Ramot B, Hulu N et al: The pathology of so-called Mediterranean abdominal lymphoma with malabsorption. Cancer 29:1502, 1972
18. Knox LS, Crosby LO, Feurer ID et al: Energy expenditure in malnourished cancer patients. Ann Surg 197:152, 1983
19. Russell D, Shike M, Marliss ED et al: Effects of total parenteral nutrition and chemotherapy on the metabolic derangements in small cell lung cancer. Cancer Res 44:1706, 1984
20. Schersten T, Lundholm K, Eden E et al: Energy metabolism in cancer. Acta Chir Scand (Suppl) 498:130, 1980
21. Warnold I, Lundholm K, Schersten T: Energy balance and body composition in cancer patients. Cancer Res 38:1801, 1978
22. Arbeit JM, Lees DE, Corsey R et al: Resting energy expenditure in controls and cancer patients with localized and diffuse disease. Ann Surg 199:292, 1984
23. Brennan MF: Total parenteral nutrition in the cancer patient. N Engl J Med 305:373, 1981
24. Cahill GF Jr: Starvation in man. N Engl J Med 282:668, 1970
25. Warnold I, Falkheden T, Hulten B et al: Energy intake and expenditure in selected groups of hospital patients. Am J Clin Nutr 31:742, 1978
26. DeWys WD, Walters K: Abnormalities of taste sensation in cancer patients. Cancer 36:1888, 1975
27. Cahill GF Jr, Herrera Mg, Morgan AP et al: Hormone-fuel interrelationships during fasting. J Clin Invest 45:1751, 1966
28. Kinney JM, Duke JH, Long CL: Tissue fuel and weight loss after injury. J Clin Pathol (Suppl) 23:65, 1970
29. DeWys WD, Begg C, Lavin PT et al: Prognostic effect of weight loss prior to chemotherapy in cancer patients. Am J Med 69:491, 1980
30. Benedict FG: A study of prolonged fasting. Carnegie Institute of Washington, publication no 203. Washington, DC, Carnegie Institute, 1915
31. Long CL, Schaffel N, Geiger JW et al: Metabolic response to injury and illness: Estimation of energy and protein needs from indirect calorimetry and nitrogen balance. JPEN 3:452, 1979
32. Meguid MM, Brennan MF, Aoki TT et al: Hormone-substrate interrelationships following trauma. Arch Surg 109:776, 1974
33. Marks PA, Bishop JS: The glucose metabolism of patients with malignant disease and of normal subjects as studied by means of an intravenous glucose tolerance test. J Clin Invest 36:254, 1957
34. Owen OE, Reichard GA Jr: Human forearm metabolism during progressive starvation. J Clin Invest 50:1536, 1971
35. Harken AH: Lactic acidosis. Surg Gynecol Obstet 142:593, 1976
36. Waterhouse C: Lactate metabolism in patients with cancer. Cancer 33:66, 1974
37. Lundholm K, Holm G, Schersten T: Insulin resistance in patients with cancer. Cancer Res 38:4665, 1978
38. Marliss EB, Aoki TT, Unger RH et al: Glucagon levels and metabolic effects in fasting man. J Clin Invest 49:2256, 1970
39. Burt ME, Gorschboth C, Brennan MF: A controlled prospective randomized trial evaluating the metabolic effects of enteral and parenteral nutrition in the cancer patient. Cancer 49:1249, 1982
40. Felig P, Owen OE, Wahren J et al: Amino acid metabolism during prolonged starvation. J Clin Invest 48:584, 1969
41. Dahn M, Kirkpatrick JR, Bouwman D: Sepsis, glucose intolerance and protein malnutrition: A metabolic paradox. Arch Surg 115:1415, 1980
42. Rudman D, Vogler WR, Howaard CH et al: Observations on the plasma amino acids of patients with acute leukemia. Cancer Res 31:1159, 1971
43. Moore FD: Metabolic Care of the Surgical Patient. Philadelphia, WB Saunders, 1959
44. Mider GB: Some aspects of nitrogen and energy metabolism in cancerous subjects: A review. Cancer Res 11:821, 1951
45. Streja DA, Steiner G, Marliss EB et al: Turnover and recycling of glucose in man during prolonged fasting. Metabolism 26:1089, 1977
46. Wolfe RR, Durkot MJ, Allsop JR et al: Glucose metabolism in severely burned patients. Metabolism 28:1031, 1979
47. Wilmore DW, Aulick HL, Goodwin CW: Glucose metabolism following severe injury. Acta Chir Scand (Suppl) 498:43, 1980
48. Winterer J, Bistrian BR, Bilmazes C et al: Whole body protein turnover, studied with ^{15}N-glycine, and muscle protein breakdown in mildly obese subjects during a protein-sparing diet and a brief total fast. Metabolism 29:575, 1980
49. Birkhahn RH, Long CL, Fitkin D et al: Effects of major skeletal trauma on whole body protein turnover in man measured by L-(1,^{14}C)-leucine. Surgery 88:294, 1980
50. Norton JA, Stein TP, Brennan MF: Whole body protein turnover studies in normal humans and malnourished patients with and without cancer. Surg Forum 31:94, 1980
51. Felig P, Pozefsky T, Marliss E et al: Alanine: Key role in gluconeogenesis. Science 167:1003, 1970
52. Long CL, Kinney JM, Geiger JW: Nonsuppressability of gluconeogenesis by glucose in septic patients. Metabolism 25:193, 1976
53. Waterhouse C, Jeanpretre N, Keilson J: Gluconeogenesis from alanine in patients with progressive malignant disease. Cancer Res 39:1968, 1979
54. Sauerwein HP, Pesola GR, Levinson MR et al: Free fatty acid kinetics in septic cancer bearing patients: The influence of insulin. J Clin Invest (submitted)
55. Levinson MR, Groeger JS, Jeevanandam M et al: Free fatty acid turnover and lipolysis in septic mechanically ventilated cancer bearing man. Metabolism (submitted)
56. Eden E, Edstrom S, Bennegard K et al: Glucose flux in relation to energy expenditure in malnourished patients with and without cancer during periods of fasting and feeding. Cancer Res 44:1718, 1984
57. Strain AJ, Easty GC, Neville AM: A new experimental model of human cachexia. Invest Cell Pathol 2:87, 1979
58. Norton JA, Moley JF, Green MV et al: Parabiotic transfer of cancer anorexia/cachexia in male rats. Cancer Res 45:5547, 1985
59. Warren RS, Starnes HF Jr, Gabrilove JL et al: The acute metabolic effects of tumor necrosis factor administration in man. Arch Surg (in press)
60. Warren RS, Donner DB, Starnes HF et al: Modulation of endogenous hormone action by recombainant human tumor necrosis factor. Proc Natl Acad Sci USA (in press)
61. Beutler B, Cerami A: Cachectin and tumour necrosis factor as two sides of the same biological coin. Nature 320:584, 1986
62. Kawakami M, Pekala PH, Lane MD et al: Lipoprotein lipase suppression in 3T3-L1 cells by an endotoxin-induced mediator from exudate cells. Proc Natl Acad Sci USA 79:912, 1982
63. Torti FM, Dieckermann B, Beutler B et al: A macrophage factor inhibits adipocyte gene expression: An in vitro model of cachexia. Science 229:867, 1985
64. Brennan MF: Uncomplicated starvation versus cancer cachexia. Cancer Res 37:2359, 1977
65. Shike M, Russell DM, Detsky AS et al: Changes in body composition in patients with small cell lung cancer: The effect of TPN as an adjunct for chemotherapy. Ann Intern Med 101:303, 1984
66. Eden E, Edstrom S, Bennegard K et al: Glycerol dynamics in weight-losing cancer patients. Surgery 97:176, 1985
67. Cohn SH, Gartenhaus W, Sawitsky A et al: Compartmental body composition of cancer patients by measurement of total body nitrogen, potassium and water. Metabolism 30:222, 1981
68. Cohn SH, Gartenhaus W, Vartsky D et al: Body composition and dietary intake in neoplastic disease. Am J Clin Nutr 34:1997, 1981
69. Childress JF: When is it morally justifiable to discontinue medical nutrition and hydration? In Lynn J (ed): By No Extraordinary Means, p 67. Bloomington, Indiana University Press, 1986
70. Harvey KB, Moldawer LL, Bistrian RR et al: Biological measures for the formulation of a hospital prognostic index. Am J Clin Nutr 34:2013, 1981
71. Mullen JL, Buzby GP, Matthews DC et al: Reduction of operative morbidity and mortality by combined preoperative and postoperative nutritional support. Ann Surg 192:604, 1980
72. Baker JP, Detsky AS, Wesson DE: Nutritional assessment. A comparison of clinical Judgment and objective measurements. N Engl J Med 306:969, 1982
73. Fagerman KE: Enteral feeding tubes: A comparison and history. Nutr Support Serv 7:10, 1987
74. Berner Y, Schroy P, Herrman-Zaidans M et al: Long term enteral feeding with percutaneous endoscopic gastrostomy (PEG) in cancer patients (abstr). JPEN 12(supp):1988
75. Wasilijew BK, Ujiki GT, Beal JM: Feeding gastrostomy: Complications and mortality. Am J Surg 143:194, 1982
76. Wilkinson WA, Pickelman J: Feeding gastrostomy: A reappraisal. Am Surg 48:273, 1982
77. Larson DE, Burton DD, Schroeder KW et al: Percutaneous endoscopic gastrostomy: Indications, success, complications and mortality in 314 consecutive patients. Gastroenterology 93:48, 1987
78. Shike M, Schroy P, Ritchie MA et al: Percutaneous endoscopic jejunostomy in cancer patients with previous gastric resection. Gastrointest Endosc 33:372, 1987
79. Block AS, Shils ME: Appendix Tables A40b and A40c. In Shils ME, Young V (eds): Modern Nutrition in Health and Disease, 7th ed. Philadelphia, Lea & Febiger, 1987
80. Shike M, Berner YN, Gerdes H, et al: Percutaneous endoscopic gastrostomy and jejunostomy for long term enteral feeding in patients with cancer of the head and neck. Otolaryngol Head Neck Surg, 1989 (in press).
81. Keohane PP, Altrill H, Love M et al: Relation between osmolality of diet and gastorintestinal side effects in enteral nutrition. Br Med J 288:678, 1984
82. Rees RGP, Keohane PP, Grimble GK et al: Elemental diet administered nasogastrically without starter regimens to patients with inflammatory bowel disease. JPEN 10:258, 1986
83. Burt ME, Hanin I, Brennan MF: Choline deficiency associated with total parenteral nutrition. Lancet 2:638, 1980

84. Larchian W, Shike M, Arbeit J et al: Carnitine supplementation of TPN: A prospective trial in man (abstr). JPEN 12, 21S, 1988
85. Shenkin A, Wretlind A: Complete parenteral nutrition and its use in diseases of the alimentary tract. Prog Food Nutr Sci 3:191, 1979
86. Anderson GH, Patel DG, Jeejeebhoy KN: Design and evaluation by nitrogen balance and blood aminogram of an amino acid mixture for total parenteral nutrition of adults with gastrointestinal disease. J Clin Invest 53:904:1974
87. Adibi SA: Experimental basis for use of peptides as substrates for parenteral nutrition: A review. Metabolism 36:1001, 1987
88. Abel RM, Beck CH, Abbott WM: Acute renal failure treatment with intravenous amino acids and glucose. N Engl J Med 288:695, 1973
89. Cerra FB, Cheung NK, Fisher JE et al: A multicenter trial of branched chain enriched amino acid infusion (F080) in hepatic encephalopathy (HE). JPEN 9:288, 1985
90. Brennan MF, Cerra F, Daly JM et al: Report of a research workshop: Branched chain amino acids in stress and injury. JPEN 10:446, 1986
91. Shenkin A, Wretlind A: Parenteral nutrition. World Rev Nutr Diet 28:37, 1978
92. Goodgame JT, Lowry SF, Brennan MF: Essential fatty acid deficiency in total parenteral nutrition: Time course of development and suggestions for therapy. Surgery 84:271, 1978
93. Barr LH, Dunn GD, Brennan MF: Essential fatty acid deficiency during total parenteral nutrition. Ann Surg 193:304, 1981
94. Jeejeebhoy KN, Anderson GH, Nakhooda AF et al: Metabolic studies during total parenteral nutrition. J Clin Invest 75:125, 1976
95. Shike M: Trace elements in parenteral and enteral nutrition. Curr Concepts Nutr 3:1, 1984
96. Norton JA, Peters ML, Wesley R et al: Iron supplementation of total parenteral nutrition: A prospective study. JPEN 7:457, 1983
97. Berner YN, Shuler TR, Nielsen FH, et al: The content of ultratrace elements in total parenteral nutrition solutions. Am J Clin Nutr, 1989 (in press)
98. Nutrition Advisory Group: Multivitamin preparations for parenteral nutrition. JPEN 3:258, 1979
99. Shils ME, Backer H, Frank O: Blood vitamin levels of long-term adult home total parenteral nutrition patients: The efficacy of the AMA-FAD parenteral multivitamin formulation. JPEN 9:179, 1985
100. Inculet RI, Norton JA, Nichoalds GE et al: Water-soluble vitamins in cancer patients on parenteral nutrition: A prospective study. JPEN 11:243, 1987
101. Dempsey DT, Mullen JL, Rombeau JL et al: Treatment effects of parenteral vitamins in total parenteral nutrition patients. JPEN 11:229, 1987
102. Ito YMB, Flombaum C: Electrolyte disturbances and requirements in cancer patients receiving total parenteral nutrition (abstr). JPEN 12, 11S, 1988
103. Wagman LD, Burt ME, Brennan MF: The impact of total parenteral nutrition on liver function tests in patients with cancer. Cancer 49:1249, 1982
104. Holter AR, Rosen HM, Fischer JE: The effects of hyperalimentation on major surgery in patients with malignant disease: A prospective study. Acta Chir Scand (Suppl) 466:86, 1976
105. Holter AR, Fischer JE: The effects of perioperative hyperalimentation on complications in patients with carcinoma and weight loss. J Surg Res 23:31, 1977
106. Thompson BR, Julian TB, Stremple JF: Preoperative total parenteral nutrition in patients with gastrointestinal cancer. J Surg Res 30:497, 1981
107. Mueller JM, Brenner U, Dienst C et al: Preoperative parenteral feeding in patients with gastrointestinal carcinoma. Lancet 1:68, 1982
108. Moghissi K, Hornshaw J, Teasdale PR et al: Parenteral nutrition in carcinoma of the esophagus treated by surgery: Nitrogen balance and clinical studies. Br J Surg 64:125, 1977
109. Donaldson SS, Wesley MN, Ghavimi F et al: A prospective randomized clinical trial of total parenteral nutrition in children with cancer. Med Pediatr Oncol 10:129, 1982
110. Simms JM, Oliver E, Smith JAR: A study of total parenteral nutrition (TPN) in major gastric and esophageal resection for neoplasia. JPEN 4:422, 1980
111. Heatley RV, Williams RHP, Lewis MH: Preoperative intravenous feeding-controlled trial. Postgrad Med J 55:541, 1979
112. Muller JM, Keller HW, Brenner U et al: Indications and effects of preoperative parenteral nutrition. World J Surg 10:53, 1986
113. Solassol C, Joyeuz H, DuBois JB: Total parenteral nutrition (TPN) with complete nutritive mixtures. An artificial gut in cancer patients. Nutr Cancer 1:13, 1979
114. Valerio D, Overett MT, Malcolm A et al: Nutritional support for cancer patients receiving abdominal and pelvic radiotherapy: A randomized, prospective, clinical experiment of intravenous vs oral feeding. Surg Forum 29:145, 1978
115. Ghavimi F, Shils ME, Scott BF et al: Comparison of morbidity in children requiring abdominal radiation and chemotherapy with and without total parenteral nutrition. J Pediatr 4:530, 1982
116. Kinsella TJ, Malcolm A, Bothe A et al: Prospective study of nutritional support during pelvic irradiation. Int J Radiat Oncol Biol Phys 7:543, 1986
117. Jordan WM, Valdevieso M, Frankman C et al: Treatment of advanced adenocarcinoma of the lung with florofur, doxorubicin, cyclophosphamide, and cis-platinum and intensive IV hyperalimentation. Cancer Treat Rep 64:197, 1981
118. Waterhouse C, Kemperman JH: Carbohydrate metabolism in subjects with cancer. Cancer Res 31:1273, 1971
119. Popp MB, Fisher RI, Wesley R et al: A prospective randomized study of adjuvant parenteral nutrition in the treatment of advanced diffuse lymphoma. Influence on survival. Surgery 90:195, 1981
120. Issell BF, Valdivieso M, Zaren HA et al: Protection against chemotherapy toxicity by IV hyperalimentation. Cancer Treat Rep 59:437, 1978
121. Lanzotti V, Copeland EM, Bhuchar V et al: A randomized trial of total parenteral nutrition (TPN) with chemotherapy for non-oat cell cancer (NOCLC) (abstr). Am Soc Clin Oncol C:277, 1980
122. Valdivieso M, Bodney GP, Benjamin RS et al: Role of intravenous hyperalimentation as an adjunct to intensive therapy for small ceil bronchogenic carcinoma: Preliminary observations. Cancer Treat Rep (Suppl 5) 65:145, 1981
123. Serrou B, Cupissol D, Plagne R et al: Parenteral intravenous nutrition (PNN) as an adjunct to chemotherapy in small cell anaplastic lung carcinoma. Cancer Treat Rep (Suppl 5) 65:151, 1981
124. Nixon D, Moffitt S, Lawson DH et al: Total parenteral nutrition as an adjunct to chemotherapy of metastatic colorectal cancer. Cancer Treat Rep (Suppl 5) 65:137, 1981
125. Samuels ML, Selig DE, Ogden S et al: IV hyperalimentation and chemotherapy for stage III testicular cancer: A randomized study. Cancer Treat Rep 65:615, 1981
126. Van Eys J, Copeland EM, Cangir A et al: A randomized, controlled clinical trial of hyperalimentation in children with metastatic malignancies. Med Pediatr Oncol 8:63, 1980
127. Shamberger RC, Pizzo PA, Goodgame JT et al: The effect of total parenteral nutrition on chemotherapy induced myelosuppression: A randomized study. Am J Med 74:40, 1983
128. Lowry SF, Smith JC, Brennan MF: Zinc and copper replacement during total parenteral nutrition. Am J Clin Nutr 34:1853, 1981
129. Shike M, Roulet M, Kurian R et al: Copper metabolism and requirements in total parenteral nutrition. Gastroenterology 81:290, 1981
130. Lowry SF, Goodgame JT Jr, Maher MM et al: Parenteral vitamin requirements during intravenous feeding. Am J Clin Nutr 31:2149, 1978
131. Kirkemo AK, Burt ME, Brennan MF: Serum vitamin level maintenance in cancer patients on TPN. Am J Clin Nutr 35:1003, 1982
132. Arbeit JM, Yoshimura N, Nicora R et al: A prospective randomized study of the effect of carnitine supplementation on the liver function of cancer patients receiving TPN. JPEN (submitted)
133. Nixon DW, Heymsfield SB, Cohen AE et al: Protein calorie undernutrition in hospitalized cancer patients. Am J Med 68:683, 1980
134. Norton JA, Lowry SF, Brennan MF: Effect of work-induced hypertrophy on skeletal muscle of tumor and non-tumor bearing rats. J Appl Physiol 46:654, 1979
135. Fong Y, Hesse D, Tracey KJ et al: Submaximal exercise during intravenous hyperalimentation on depleted subjects. Ann Surg (in press)
136. Daly JM, Dudrick SJ, Copeland EM III: Intravenous hyperalimentation: Effect on delayed cutaneous hypersensitivity in cancer patients. Ann Surg 192:587, 1980
137. Detsky AS, Baker JP, O'Rourke K et al: Perioperative parenteral nutrition: A meta-analysis. Ann Intern Med 107:195, 1987
138. OASIS, Oley Foundation: Preliminary home nutritional support patient registry data, 1985. Albany, Albany Medical Center, 1985
139. Shike M, Harrison JE, Strutridge WE et al: Metabolic bone disease in patients receiving long term total parenteral nutrition. Ann Intern Med 92:343, 1980
140. Klein GL, Ament ME, Bluestone R et al: Bone disease associated with total parenteral nutrition. Lancet 2:1041, 1980
141. Shike M, Shils ME, Heller A et al: Bone disease in prolonged parenteral nutrition: Osteopenia without mineralization defect. Am J Clin Nutr 44:89, 1986
142. ATLA L. Rep. 525, November 1982
143. ATLA L. Rep. 285, August 1984
144. Teitelman R: Skeleton in the closet. Forbes 133:156, 1984
145. Twomey LP, Patching SC: Cost effectiveness of nutritional support. JPEN 9:3, 1985

SECTION 2

ALBERT DEISSEROTH
RALPH WALLERSTEIN, JR.

Use of Blood and Blood Products

Cancer patients often require hematopoietic and hematologic supportive care. Decisions about therapeutic options require careful consideration of the patient's condition and of the techniques that are available. Because transfusion of whole blood is rarely indicated, this section addresses current use of blood component therapy.

ERYTHROCYTE TRANSFUSION

The indications for erythrocyte transfusions depend on the physiologic status of the host, the cause of the anemia, and the rate of development of the anemia. Before ordering a transfusion, it is useful to recall that anemia is not a diagnosis, but a laboratory finding (hemoglobin <2 SD below normal) for which an explanation should be sought. It is not sufficient to attribute the anemia to cancer. A minimal examination should include the mean corpuscular volume, reticulocyte count, and peripheral smear. A systematic approach to the laboratory evaluation of anemia ensures appropriate specific therapy and prevent serious morbidity due to delayed diagnosis (*e.g.*, Coombs'-positive hemolytic anemia in lymphoma or mitomycin-induced hemolytic uremic syndrome).[1] Most patients tolerate a hemoglobin level as low as 10 g/dl. Young patients without cardiopulmonary, renal, hepatic, or cerebral vascular disease may tolerate a hemoglobin as low as 6 or 7. Because cardiac output begins to increase below a hemoglobin of 10, most patients with cancer should be transfused to maintain a hemoglobin level between 9 and 10.

For most transfusions, one should order packed erythrocytes. Specific erythrocyte component therapy limits the volume of the transfusion and allows the plasma and platelets to be used for other patients. Even for massive bleeding, one can order crystalloid, packed erythrocytes, platelets, and fresh-frozen plasma as needed. Each unit of packed cells contains 100% of the erythrocytes, 100% of the leukocytes, and 20% of the plasma originally present in the donated unit of whole blood. The leukocytes may cause reactions if the recipient has antileukocyte antibodies. These antibodies, probably directed at granulocyte-specific non-HLA antigens, occur in approximately 20% of multiparous females and will develop in as many as 79% of multiply transfused patients. Transfusions of packed erythrocytes or platelets in these alloimmunized patients may cause chills and fever. Although these reactions can be treated or in some cases prevented by the use of acetaminophen before transfusion, some patients still experience recurrent severe chills and fever with the use of packed erythrocytes. For these patients, the use of leukocyte-poor packed cells is indicated.

Several methods are used to prepare leukocyte-poor packed cells, including differential centrifugation, filters, or washing.[2] Standards for leukocyte removal in the past required removal of at least 70% of the leukocytes while retaining 70% of the erythrocytes. However, because there is significant variation in the leukocyte count of donated blood, and because it is probably the absolute number of residual leukocytes that cause febrile reactions, some centers require leukocyte-poor packed cells to contain fewer than 0.5 to 1.0×10^9 residual leukocytes, which will not cause febrile reactions in most alloimmunized patients.[3]

Differential centrifugation has been the most widely used means for producing leukocyte-poor erythrocytes, but this technique results in significant loss of erythrocytes. A new leukocyte removal filter (Sepacell R-500, Fenwall Laboratories, Deerfield, IL), which can be used at the bedside, results in 99.8% removal, with an absolute residual of 6.1×10^6 and in an acceptable erythrocyte loss of 13% if 2 units of red cells are transfused per filter.[4,5] Another new method for preparing leukocyte-poor erythrocytes is the use of a leukocyte filter within the Leukotrap Closed Bag Red Cell Storage System (Cutter) used for procurement. Its use results in 2.3×10^8 absolute residual leukocytes, with 90% erythrocyte recovery.[6] A theoretic attraction of removing the leukocytes before storage is that enzyme, surface protein, and membrane shedding are prevented and that microaggregate formation is decreased.

The major indication for leukocyte-poor blood products is for patients who have had prior febrile nonhemolytic transfusion reactions. However, it is possible that the use of leukopoor-blood products for patients who require recurrent platelet transfusions may significantly delay the development of alloimmunization and refractoriness to random donor platelets.[7] Leukocyte depletion may decrease the risk of transmission of cytomegalovirus (CMV).

Allergic reactions, including urticaria and hives, may occur in 3% to 5% of transfused patients. Some of these reactions are due to recipient antibodies against immunoglobulin components or other soluble proteins in the plasma.[8] The most well-defined of these reactions occurs in patients with congenital deficiency of IgA. Some patients with congenital IgA deficiencies develop anti-IgA antibodies, and when transfused with plasma or packed erythrocytes with admixed plasma containing IgA, these patients may have a severe allergic or, rarely, fatal anaphylactic reactions. Most urticarial reactions which occur in non-IgA-deficient patients, are rarely serious or life threatening, and can be easily prevented or treated with antihistamines (*e.g.*, diphenhydramine). For patients with severe or recurrent urticarial reactions or for patients known to be IgA deficient and for whom blood from an IgA-deficient donor is not available, the physician should order washed erythrocytes in which all of the plasma has been removed.

Frozen-thawed deglycerolized erythrocytes, which are used for maintaining a supply of rare blood types and occasionally for autologous donation, contain very few leukocytes and virtually no plasma because of the extensive washing used to perform deglycerolization. Washed, frozen erythrocytes should be used for those patients who continue to have febrile transfusion reactions with other leukocyte-poor products.

The most common reactions after a transfusion of erythro-

TABLE 59-15. Differential Diagnosis of Acute Transfusion Reactions

Fever and chills	Major hemolytic transfusion reaction
	Reaction to foreign HLA and granulocyte-specific antigens on transfused leukocytes and platelets
	Contaminated blood
Dyspnea	Fluid overload
	Major hemolytic transfusion reaction
	Contaminated blood
	Air embolism
	Anaphylactic reaction due to transfusion of IgA-containing plasma to IgA-deficient recipient with anti-IgA
	Pulmonary leukoagglutin
Bleeding	Disseminated intravascular coagulation due to major hemolytic transfusion reaction or contaminated blood
	Thrombocytopenia due to massive transfusion of packed erythrocytes
	Washout of coagulation factors due to massive transfusion of packed erythrocytes
Arrhythmia	Circulatory overload
	Hyperkalemia
	Hypothermia
	Hypocalcemia
	Major hemolytic transfusion reaction
	Contaminated blood
	Air embolism
Hypotension	Major hemolytic transfusion reaction
	Contaminated blood
	Anaphylaxis due to IgA deficiency
Hemoglobinuria	Major hemolytic transfusion reaction
	Excessive infusion pressure through small-bore needle
	Overheating with blood warmer
	Contaminated blood

cytes are fever and chills. There are also the possibilities of a major hemolytic transfusion reaction and of contaminated blood (Table 59-15). Transfusion of ABO-incompatible blood is the most dangerous complication of transfusion because the naturally occurring IgM antibodies fix complement, resulting in rapid intravascular hemolysis. In severe reactions this may be followed by disseminated intravascular coagulation (DIC), acute renal failure, and death. Chills and fever that occur very early in the transfusion or that occur in a nulliparous patient or one who never has been transfused should raise the possibility of a hemolytic transfusion reaction. Associated symptoms include low-back pain, chest pain, restlessness, dyspnea, and pain at the site of transfusion. Signs include tachycardia, hypotension, oliguria, hemoglobinuria, tachypnea, and generalized bleeding if DIC has developed.

Bacterial contamination of packed erythrocytes is very rare because rigorous antiseptic techniques are used in blood collection, the blood is stored at 4°C, and the blood itself has natural antibacterial properties. Bacterial contamination is more of a problem with platelet transfusions because platelets are stored at 22°C. If platelets are stored for longer than 3 to 5 days, the risk of bacterial contamination increases significantly, and all febrile transfusion reactions to platelet concentrates should be thoroughly evaluated for possible bacterial contamination.

Although transfusion of erythrocytes or other blood components is capable of transmitting many infections, non-A, non-B hepatitis and retrovirus transmission are the major concerns. The incidence of post-transfusion non-A, non-B hepatitis depends on the effort taken to detect hepatitis, the adequacy of follow-up of patients, and the prevalence of the disease in the donor population. Although post-transfusion hepatitis is usually anicteric and asymptomatic, it is a serious problem because approximately 50% to 60% of infected patients develop chronic, active hepatitis, and 10% to 20% develop cirrhosis.[9] The peak incidence of non-A, non-B hepatitis occurs at 7 to 8 weeks but may occur 2 weeks to 6 months after transfusion. It is unclear whether the degree of hepatic dysfunction with associated portal hypertension, bleeding, and encephalopathy that occurs in cirrhosis after hepatitis B will occur in these cases of post-transfusion non-A, non-B hepatitis.[10]

Before the summer and fall of 1986, it was estimated that the incidence of post-transfusion hepatitis was 5% to 20%. At that time, many blood banks instituted a new policy of "surrogate" testing of donated blood in order to decrease the incidence of non-A, non-B hepatitis. Surrogate testing involves the use of elevated alanine aminotransferase (ALT) and hepatitis B core antibody as markers in the donated blood, which are associated with an increased risk of coexisting non-A, non-B hepatitis infection.[11] Data from the transfusion-transmitted virus study (TTV) indicate that discarding donor units with ALT levels greater than 45 international units/liter would result in a 47.4% reduction in post-transfusion non-A, non-B hepatitis.[12] Discarding donor units with anti-hepatitis B core antibody would eliminate 33%. The TTV data predict that testing for both surrogate markers together could eliminate 61.2% of post-transfusion hepatitis. A review on January 20, 1987, by the Office of Biologic Research and Review of the Food and Drug Administration supported the conclusion that surrogate testing would be effective in reducing non-A, non-B hepatitis after transfusion.[12] Until specific tests for the agent or agents of non-A, non-B hepatitis become available, surrogate testing will probably continue. Since the institution of surrogate testing, the incidence of post-transfusion hepatitis is estimated to be about 1% to 2% of recipients, although reliable prospective data are not yet available.

The risk of human immunodeficiency virus (HIV) infection in a recipient of blood from an infected donor is substantial. Perkins and colleagues identified patients with newly diagnosed acquired immune deficiency syndrome (AIDS) reported to the San Francisco Public Health Department who had donated blood before the diagnosis of AIDS.[13] Sixty-two percent of the recipients showed evidence of infection, including recipients of whole blood, erythrocytes, platelet concentrates, and fresh-frozen plasma. The closer the donation was given before the diagnosis of AIDS in the donor, the higher the risk of infection. Nine of ten recipients from donations in the year before AIDS diagnosis became infected. Recipients younger than age 11 or older than age 79 were more likely to have developed AIDS or AIDS-related complex (ARC) at the time of follow-up.[14] Other investigators reported an 89% incidence of infection after transfusion of HIV-seropositive blood. A recent projection by Medley suggests that the mean incubation period for transfusion as-

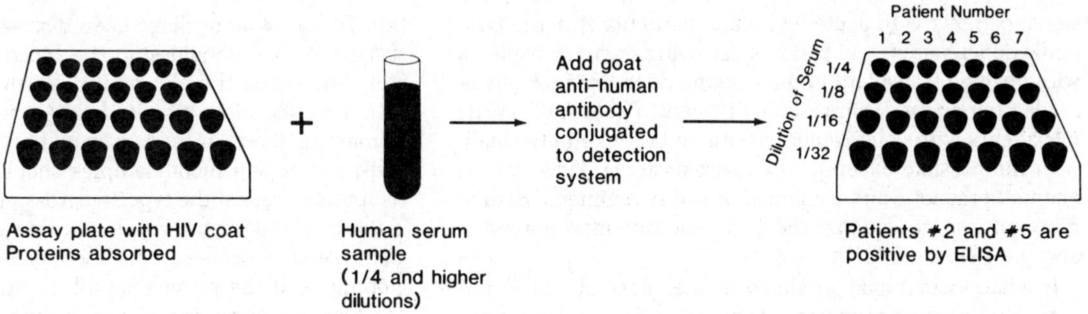

FIG. 59-4. ELISA assay for HIV antibodies in man.

sociated with AIDS will be 1.97 years for children younger than 5 and 8.23 years for persons 5 to 59 years old.[15]

The majority of severe hemophiliacs who received factor VIII or IX in significant quantities before screening for HIV antibody and heat inactivation of the virus HIV-antibody-positive. In one study of hemophiliacs in which the dates of seroconversion were known, 32% of those seropositive for 5 or more years had developed AIDS.[16] Data are not yet available to compare the natural history of transfusion HIV infection among homosexuals, IV drug abusers, and hemophiliacs, in whom co-infection with other viruses are common.

HIV infection from blood transfusion has been significantly reduced since blood banks excluded high-risk groups from donating in March 1983, and began screening donated blood for antibody to HIV in the spring of 1985. The physician must be alert for the development of HIV-related disorders in patients transfused between 1976 and 1985. Because some donors acutely infected with HIV may not develop an antibody response for a few weeks or months, the risk of acquiring HIV infection from blood products, although quite small, is not zero.[17]

Several recently developed methods may improve the ability to detect viral infection. An enzyme-linked immunosorbent assay (ELISA), as shown in Figure 59-4, for the p24 core protein antigen of HIV can detect antigenemia within the first few weeks of infection before the development of antibody.[18] After attachment to the CD4 molecule on T4 cells and internalization, the HIV genomic RNA is transcribed to DNA by reverse transcriptase.

The proviral DNA may remain unintegrated or be integrated into the host DNA.[19] Peripheral-blood mononuclear cells can be induced by the polymerase chain reaction (PCR) technology to amplify specific sequences of HIV DNA (*e.g.,* LTR, *gag, env* regions), and if present, probes can locate these sequences.[20] Remarkably, this complex process can be completed in 3 days, and a positive result indicates HIV DNA is present as the free episomal form or integrated into the host DNA. Thus, PCR technology may be used to identify infected patients who lack circulating antigen or antibody. It should be able to identify persons who are only passively antibody-positive and not truly infected (*e.g.,* after intravenous immuno-globulin or some newborn children of antibody-positive mothers). DNA amplification using PCR technology and probing for HIV sequences should be able to detect intracellular virus.

After integration, the virus may have a latent phase. A third new method for detecting HIV infection, even in antibody-negative patients, also indicates whether the virus is latent or actively replicating. If it is actively replicating, HIV produces a 14-kilodalton, 86-amino-acid transactivator or tat protein that interacts with the long terminal repeat (LTR) region of the virus to increase steady-state viral mRNA levels tenfold and the protein product of the mRNA 500-fold. By constructing a human indicator lymphoid cell line containing integrated copies of HIV-1 LTR ligated to the chloramphenicol acetyltransferase (CAT) gene, Felber and Pavlakis[21] were able to detect as few as ten HIV-infected lymphoid cells by infection of the indicator cell lines and the CAT protein expression. This transactivation assay may also prove useful for determining the activity or latency of HIV and for assessing the effects of anti-HIV drug therapy.

Human T-lymphotropic virus (HTLV-1) is a retrovirus that causes adult T-cell leukemia or lymphoma and a degenerative neurologic disorder called tropical spastic paraparesis (TSP) or HTLV-1-associated myelopathy (HAM). The virus is endemic in parts of Japan, Africa, and the Caribbean. Blood transfusion is an effective means of transmission, with 70% of recipients of seropositive blood developing seroconversion in one study.[22] Since the introduction of screening donor blood in Japan for antibody to HTLV-1, the seroconversion rate has decreased from 9% to 0.1%.[22]

In areas of the United States where HTLV-1 has become endemic (*e.g.,* among IV drug addicts in New York City and the southeastern United States), the risk of acquiring HTLV-1 infection from blood products has become a concern. The availability of an ELISA test for antibody to HTLV-1 makes routine blood bank testing for this retrovirus possible, and this may soon be required by blood bank regulatory agencies.

Graft-versus-host disease (GVHD) is a potential complication of blood cell transfusion. It occurs when immunocompetent lymphocytes from the donor are transfused into an immunocompromised recipient. Patients at highest risk for this problem are those with congenital immune deficiency syndromes (*e.g.,* Wiskott-Aldrich syndrome), patients receiving bone marrow transplants, and rarely, patients with Hodgkin's and non-Hodgkin's lymphoma undergoing combined chemotherapy and radiation. Neonatal patients receiving intrauterine transfusions followed by exchange transfusions, premature babies or infants receiving exchange transfusions, patients with acute leukemia, particularly acute lymphocytic leukemia, and patients receiving organ transplants with ongoing transplant immunosuppression are probably at moderate risk for donor cell engraftment. The risk of GVHD in patients with solid tumors seems to be extremely small, with the possible exception of neuroblastoma. However, as chemotherapeutic and combined modality regimens become more intense, so also may the degree of immunosuppression and the risk for GVHD.

Irradiation of blood products is the most effective and probably the most economic means to prevent post-transfusion GVHD.[23] Lymphocyte proliferation in response to allogeneic cells is completely abolished after 500 rad. After 1500 rad, there was a 90% reduction in mitogen-stimulated ^{14}C-thymidine incorporation in one study and an 85% reduction in mitogen-induced blast transformation in another. A dose of 5000 rads decreased these to 97% and 98.5%, respectively.

Other cells are less sensitive than lymphocytes to irradiation. Erythrocytes are unaffected by doses up to 20,000 rad. Platelets, however, may suffer after exposure to 5000 rad. Granulocyte function may be affected above 2000 to 5000 rad. Although 500 rad may be sufficient to inhibit some lymphocyte functions, a dose of 1500 rad provides a safe and effective dose, and there have been no documented transfusion-related GVHD cases reported from large centers using this dose. Although there have been no adverse reactions reported from the use of irradiated blood products, their use is associated with additional expense because the cost of the irradiator and the radiation source is $30,000 to $50,000. In addition, irradiated pleuripotent stem cells may survive with sublethal damage, which may allow mutated stem cells to survive. Although the likelihood of harm is remote, because of theoretical concerns and real cost concerns, irradiated blood products should only be used for the specific indications mentioned.

Other possible complications of transfusion are listed in Table 59-16. The signs and symptoms of a major hemolytic transfusion reaction have been discussed. If the reaction is suspected, one should stop the blood transfusion immediately and notify the blood bank. Verification of the identification on the blood unit and the patient should be sought. Remaining blood in the bag should be returned to the blood bank and repeat blood samples should be drawn from the recipient to repeat the type and crossmatch and to determine if there is pink or brown plasma that would indicate hemoglobinemia. A urine sample should also be tested for hemoglobinuria. If the plasma is pink or brown suggesting intravascular hemolysis has occurred, the physician should order a "DIC screen" (including partial thromboplastin time [PTT], platelet count, fibrinogen, fibrin monomer, and fibrin-split products). If the patient is bleeding and has DIC, replace clotting factors and platelets if a significant deficiency is documented. Blood pressure should be maintained with intravenous fluids and pressors, and a urine output greater than 100 ml/hour should be maintained with intravenous fluids. If needed, mannitol or Lasix should be used to prevent oliguric ATN. The physician should monitor input, output, and serum electrolytes, blood urea nitrogen (BUN), and creatinine. A nephrologist should be consulted if renal failure occurs. Most major hemolytic transfusion reactions are due to a clerical error, which occurs at the time the initial blood type and crossmatch is drawn and labeled.

TABLE 59-16. Complications of Transfusion

- Fever, chills
- Allergy
  - urticaria
  - anaphylaxis
- Infection
  - non-A, non-B hepatitis
  - retrovirus
  - cytomylavirus
  - bacterial contamination
  - other
- Volume overload
- Major hemolytic transfusion reaction
- Delayed hemolytic transfusion reaction
- Graft-versus-host disease
- Post-transfusion purpura
- Hypocalcemia
- Hyperkalemia
- Hypothermia
- Respiratory distress
- Iron overload
- Air embolism
- Alloimmunization

Delayed hemolytic transfusion reactions occur if the recipient has a titer of alloantibody that is too low to be detected in the antibody screen and crossmatching procedure. The recipient develops an anamnestic response, with a subsequent fall in hemoglobin that is associated with a rise in bilirubin and lactate dehydropenase (LDH) 5 to 10 days after transfusion. This is particularly common for alloantibodies to antigens of the Kidd blood group system.[24]

Patients who develop profound thrombocytopenia 5 to 8 days after transfusion should be suspected of having post-transfusion purpura. Two percent of people lack the platelet antigen $P1^{A1}$. $P1^{A1}$-negative patients, when transfused with blood containing platelets or soluble platelet antigen, particularly if they have been previously immunized by prior transplacental contamination from a $P1^{A1}$-positive fetus or by prior transfusion, may develop severe thrombocytopenia. The intriguing aspect of this is that the transfused $P1^{A1}$-positive platelets are destroyed and the patient's own platelets are destroyed as well, a process that may continue for several weeks if untreated. Suspected cases of post-transfusion purpura are confirmed by measuring antibody to $P1^{A1}$ in the recipient's serum. Plasmapheresis is the treatment of choice for this problem. The cause of the destruction of the patient's own platelets is unclear. Some investigators suspect that the $P1^{A1}$ antigen is soluble and circulates and binds to the patient's platelets, causing their destruction. Other investigators feel that the development of the alloantibody to $P1^{A1}$ causes the simultaneous development of an autoantibody.

Although massive transfusions ($>$10 units in 1–6 hours) have been associated with hypocalcemia, hyperkalemia, hypothermia, and bleeding due to coagulation factor and platelet washout, these reactions are relatively uncommon in patients with cancer. Low levels of ionized calcium are due to the citrate in the anticoagulated packed erythrocytes. Except in severe liver dysfunction, citrate usually is rapidly metabolized. Although stored erythrocytes progressively increase the extracellular potassium concentration, it is quite unusual to see clinical hyperkalemia, except with renal failure. Coagulation factor washout has occurred in patients with trauma, in whom accelerated consumption due to DIC is probably more of a factor than dilution. Prophylactic transfusion of fresh-frozen plasma is not indicated, but should be guided by the PT and activated PTT. Platelet washout, however, is a potential problem with massive transfusion, but the physician should follow the specific platelet count as a guide to platelet repletion.

PLATELET TRANSFUSIONS

Platelet transfusions are indicated for prophylaxis or treatment of bleeding due to decreased number or function of platelets. As with anemia, it is important to have a systematic method for the laboratory evaluation of the bleeding patient in order to direct specific therapy and avoid missing factors contributing to the bleeding.[25]

The bleeding time increases linearly as the platelet count falls from 100,000 to 10,000, below which it tends to be prolonged indefinitely.[26] If the platelet count is greater than 100,000 and the bleeding time is prolonged, the patient either has von Willebrand's disease or a qualitative platelet defect.[27,28] If von Willebrand's disease has been excluded by normal factor VIII antigen, factor VIII activity, ristocetin cofactor activity, and multimer analysis, the patient has a qualitative platelet defect. Patients with life-threatening bleeding due to a qualitative platelet defect should be given a platelet transfusion. For patients with qualitative platelet dysfunction due to uremia, however, transfused platelets will acquire the same qualitative defect, and the treatment of choice is vigorous hemodialysis. For patients already being dialyzed, 1-deamino-8-D-arginine vasopressin (DDAVP) or cryoprecipitate may be useful. For patients with other than life-threatening bleeding due to qualitative platelet dysfunction, a trial of DDAVP is indicated because it is not associated with the risk of viral infection seen with cryoprecipitate and platelets.[29]

In 1962, Gaydos and co-workers documented a quantitative relationship between platelet counts and hemorrhages in patients with acute leukemia (Fig. 59-5).[30] In these patients, the incidence of hemorrhage of any kind, including gross hemorrhage, rose dramatically as platelet counts declined, especially to levels less than 20,000/mm^3. They also observed that bleeding episodes associated with thrombocytopenia frequently follow a decline in platelet count. They reported that of eight patients with intracranial hemorrhage unassociated with high blast counts and intracerebral leukostasis, seven patients had platelet counts of less than 5000/mm^3. No intracranial bleeding was observed at a platelet count of 10,000/mm^3 or more.

Both retrospective and prospective studies have shown a decreased incidence of bleeding episodes when platelets were transfused prophylactically for patients with platelet counts less than 20,000 to 30,000/mm^3.[31] In patients who are severely thrombocytopenic (<10,000/mm^3), particularly if due to decreased production, platelet transfusions are given prophylactically because the first site of bleeding may be intracranial and fatal before therapeutic platelet transfusions can be given.

At any given level, patients with thrombocytopenia due to decreased platelet production have a more prolonged bleeding time than patients with thrombocytopenia due to increased destruction. This is presumably due to the fact that with accelerated destruction, the platelets that are in the peripheral blood are young, vigorous platelets, which are more hemostatically effective than the older circulating platelets in the case of decreased production.

The benefit of preventing bleeding by prophylactic platelet transfusions must be balanced against the risk that the patient will develop alloantibodies to the transfused platelets and that, if bleeding occurs in the future, transfused platelets may be less effective. In practice, when thrombocytopenia is expected to be limited (*e.g.*, in induction chemotherapy for acute leukemia), sustain the patient with regular platelet transfusions to keep the platelet count above 10,000 to 20,000/mm^3. For chronic thrombocytopenia (*e.g.*, aplastic anemia or myelodysplasia after prolonged chemotherapy),

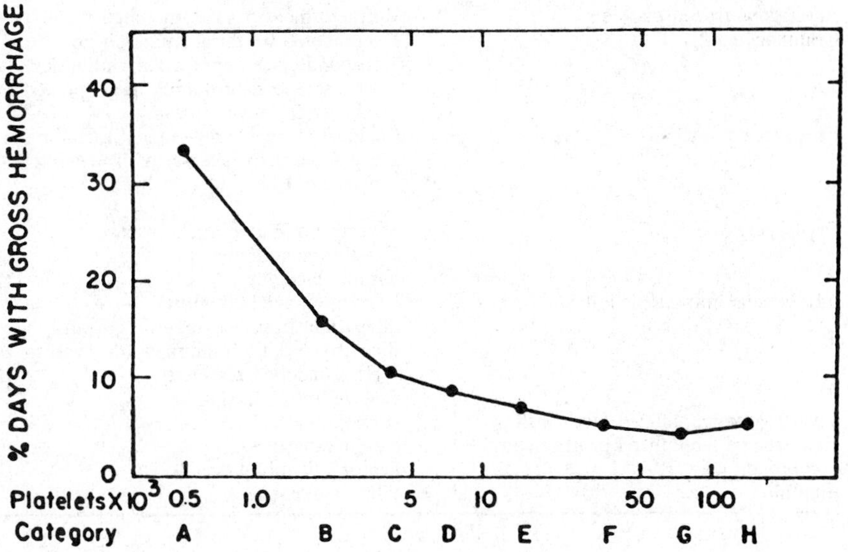

FIG. 59-5. Relationship between platelet count and the number of days patients had grossly visible hemorrhage. Capital letters along the abscissa refer to the following categories of platelet counts: A = less than 1000/mm^3; B = 1000–3000/mm^3; C = 3000–5000/mm^3; D = 5000–10,000/mm^3; E = 10,000–20,000/mm^3; F = 20,000–50,000/mm^3; G = 50,000–100,000/mm^3; and H = greater than 100,000/mm^3.

prophylactic platelet transfusions are not indicated, and most clinicians reserve platelet transfusions for bleeding episodes.

Platelets are prepared from differential centrifugation of donated whole blood or from platelet pheresis of single donors. Platelet concentrates can be administered through a standard blood bank filter (170 micropore size) during 10 to 20 minutes. Platelets in whole blood stored at 4°C are viable only for 12 to 18 hours. Therefore, platelets, whether obtained from multiple donors or from a single donor by platelet pheresis, are stored at 22°C ± 2°. Even small decreases in the storage temperature from 21° to 19° or 18° may result in a drop in the lifespan of transfused platelets from 8.12 days to 5.21 and 1.85 days, respectively.[32] The development of thinner plastic film bags with a greater surface area has allowed more oxygen to enter the bags and greater amounts of carbon dioxide to escape, resulting in a higher pH, which has improved platelet viability and permitted storage for up to 7 days.[33] But, because the platelets are stored at room temperature, small amounts of contaminating microorganisms present on day 1 may reach high titers by days 5 to 7.[34] At some major centers, platelet concentrates became the

TABLE 59-17. Blood Component Therapy Indications and Complications

Component	*Indications*	*Complications*
Packed erythrocytes	Anemia	Fever Volume overload Hepatitis and other infections Urticaria Hemolytic transfusion reaction Increased viscosity
Leukocyte-poor packed erythrocytes	Prior febrile reactions to packed erythrocytes May delay alloimmunization	
Washed or plasma-poor packed erythrocytes	Prior urticarial reactions IgA deficiency Need to avoid complement transfusion	
Frozen packed erythrocytes	Rare blood types Autologous donations Process also removes leukocytes and plasma	
Whole blood	None	
Random-donor platelets	Bleeding with platelet count <100,000/mm³ Bleeding and qualitative platelet dysfunction Elective surgery and thrombocytopenia Prophylactic for platelets <10,000–20,000/mm³	Fever Urticaria Hepatitis Bacterial contamination
Single-donor platelets	May delay alloimmunization Lower risk of infection because exposed to one donor	
Leukocyte-poor platelets	Prior febrile reactions to packed erythrocytes or platelets May delay alloimmunization	
HLA-matched single-door platelets	Poor response to platelet transfusion due to alloimmunization	
Autologous frozen platelets	Refractoriness to HLA-matched platelets	
Granulocytes	Documented bacterial infection not responding to appropriate antibiotics, with severe neutropenia not expected to recover for several days.	Fever Respiratory distress Alloimmunization
Fresh-frozen plasma	Coagulation factor deficiency, including rapid warfarin reversal with plasmapheresis for TTP	Volume overload Hepatitis and other infections Hypernatremia Hypocalcemia
Cryoprecipitate	Severe von Willebrand's disease Hypofibrinogenemia Uremic bleeding	Hepatitis and other infections
Intravenous immunoglobulin	Hypogammaglobulinemia Idiopathic thrombocytopenic purpura Bleeding and alloimmunization, even to HLA-matched platelets Passive immunization	Systemic reactions Local venous reaction Anaphylaxis
Heat-treated lyophilized factor VIII	Hemophilia A	Non A, non B hepatitis
Heat-treated lyophilized prothrombin complex	Hemophilia B Factor VIII inhibitor	Non A, non B hepatitis Thrombosis
Albumin	Volume expansion	

major source for transfusion-induced sepsis, and storage of platelets beyond 5 days is no longer permitted.[35]

In addition to the risk of viral infection associated with the transfusion of all blood products, the major complication of platelet transfusion is the development of alloimmunization. There are many determinants of alloimmunization. Because of the immunosuppressive effects of their diseases and treatments, patients with acute leukemia or lymphoma are less likely to develop alloantibodies to transfused platelets, than patients with aplastic anemia.[36] There also must be individual variations in developing alloimmunization, because not all studies have shown a direct correlation between the number of transfused platelets and the rate of alloantibody formation.[37] The rate of alloantibody formation may be a function of the number of contaminating leukocytes present.[38,39]

Because the efficacy of platelet transfusion appears to be directly related to the increment in platelet count after transfusion, 1-hour and 24-hour post-transfusion platelet counts should be checked. A poor 1-hour post-transfusion increment suggests alloimmunization.[40] Poor increments at 24 hours occur with alloimmunization but also occur with bleeding, fever, infection, drug or autoimmune destruction, hypersplenism, and DIC.[41]

When platelet transfusions are indicated, 1 unit/10 kg of body weight is given, which should result in an increment of 6,000 to 10,000 platelets/mm^3 per unit. After platelet transfusion, approximately a third of the platelets accumulate in the spleen; 90% of the platelets can be recovered in an asplenic individual, 65% in a normal individual, and <65% or no increment in patients with hypersplenism. The half-life of the transfused platelets is 2 to 7 days, depending on the age and condition of the transfused platelets, consumption, and alloimmunization. For patients who show a poor increment in response (<4000/unit), HLA-matched, single-donor platelets should be used (Table 59-17). Although HLA-identical sibling donors are preferred, platelets from donors whose HLA antigens are serologically similar are almost as effective.[31] The use of HLA-matched platelets may permit prolonged support of severely thrombocytopenic patients after they have become alloimmunized. However, even with HLA-matched platelets, approximately 20% of platelet transfusions are not successful. These cases may reflect alloimmunization to platelet-specific antigens or possibly other causes of accelerated platelet destruction.

For patients who are refractory to HLA-matched platelet transfusions, consider using platelet crossmatching techniques or high-dose intravenous immunoglobulin. Platelet crossmatching is an investigational procedure, but 17 (31%) of 54 patients with a positive crossmatch (recipient antibody bonding to donor platelets in vitro) had adequate increments in platelet count after transfusion, and 95 (57%) of 168 of those with negative crossmatches had such increments ($p < 0.001$).[42] Despite the fact that the difference between these results is statistically significant, the 43% of patients with a negative crossmatches and poor increments are disappointing compared with early optimistic reports. The administration of intravenous immunoglobulin, which is effective in some cases of refractory idiopathic thrombocyto-

TABLE 59-18. Transfusion Guidelines for Commonly Encountered Hematologic Problems

Chronic anemia
- No significant cardiopulmonary compromise; stable patient.
  - No absolute indication for transfusion if hemoglobin is above 6 to 7 g/100 mg.
  - Consider transfusion in the presence of otherwise unexplained lassitude, malaise, tachycardia, dyspnea in association with hemoglobin less than 9 to 10 g/100 ml.
  - Cardiopulmonary disease; fever; surgery. Maintain hemoglobin level at 10 g/100 ml.
  - If management protracted (years), monitor for evidence of iron overload (secondary hemochromatosis).

Thrombocytopenia
- Thrombocytopenia due to failure of platelet production.
  - Platelet count >20,000/mm^3; stable patient without retinal hemorrhages: Platelet transfusion probably not necessary.
  - Platelet count <20,000/mm^3; patient not bleeding: Provide prophylactic platelet transfusion unless thrombocytopenia expected to be chronic, in which case transfuse only for bleeding.
  - Platelet count <50,000/mm^3; patient bleeding or surgery anticipated: Use local measures to control bleeding; look for defects in coagulation pathways; maintain platelet counts at 50,000/mm^3 or above with transfusion every 12 to 24 hours.
  - Platelet count <20,000/mm^3; patient refractory to random platelet transfusion: Consider transfusion for evidence of bleeding, if retinal hemorrhages noted, or if platelet count is <10,000/mm^3; use HLA-matched platelets.

Granulocytopenia
- Patient candidate for aggressive supportive care.
  - Granulocytes <500/mm^3; afebrile, stable patient: No established indication for granulocyte transfusion.
  - Granulocytes <500/mm^3; patient febrile, but cultures negative and no clinical evidence of infected area or tissue: No established indication for granulocyte transfusion.
  - Documented bacterial infection not improving after 48 hours of antibiotics to which the organism is sensitive in a patient with <500 neutrophils/mm^3 and who is expected to have marrow aplasia for more than 1 week: Granulocyte transfusion indicated.

penic purpura (ITP), has been reported anecdotally to be useful for patients refractory to HLA-matched platelet transfusions (Table 59-18).[43-46]

For patients with bleeding and severe thrombocytopenia who are refractory to random donor and HLA-matched, single-donor platelets, there are few options and little to lose from using platelet crossmatching or high-dose intravenous immunoglobulin. For patients with acute leukemia refractory to HLA-matched platelets and who enter complete remission, autologous platelets can be frozen for subsequent cycles of consolidation therapy.[47] Although half of the frozen platelets are rendered nonfunctional by freeze-thaw damage, the other half are unharmed and function normally in vitro and in vivo.[48]

Several strategies have been suggested to delay or prevent the development of alloimmunization. Both theoretical and clinical data suggest that alloimmunization can be delayed or prevented by leukocyte depletion. Platelets have Class I histocompatibility antigens (HLA-A, B, and C) but not Class II antigens (HLA-DR). In rats, pure platelet preparations are nonimmunogenic. It has been suggested that viable lymphocytes bearing Class II antigens are required to stimulate an immune response to the Class I antigens on platelets. Murphy and colleagues were able to reduce the incidence of refractoriness to random-donor platelet transfusion from 23% to 5% using leukocyte-poor erythrocyte and platelet transfusions.

A simple means for preparing leukocyte-depleted platelets (Leukotrap Platelet Pooling System, Cutter) uses a special bag with a pouch at the bottom and a centrifuge cup with a slit, through which the pouch protrudes.[49,50] After pooling of the random-donor bags into the Leukotrap bag, a simple centrifugation pools the leukocytes and erythrocytes in the pouch, which is then clamped. This system removes up to 96% of contaminating leukocytes and erythrocytes, with less than a 5% platelet loss. After transfusion, platelet count increments are normal, and febrile reactions are greatly reduced.

Clinical trials are in progress to confirm that the use of leukocyte-poor erythrocytes and platelets decreases or eliminates alloimmunization and refractoriness to random-donor platelets. In addition to the exclusive use of leukocyte-poor blood products, some have advocated the use of single-donor platelets. Because of the more restricted exposure to foreign HLA antigens, theoretically there may be less alloimmunization.[51,52] This area remains controversial, and because of the additional expense of single-donor platelets, their routine use to prevent alloimmunization is not indicated.[53]

There are two other problems with platelet transfusion. If possible, ABO-compatible platelets should be transfused, because they appear to have a better survival rate after transfusion. However, if ABO-matched platelets are not available, unmatched platelets provide good hemostatic results. If the admixed plasma contains anti-A or anti-B IgM, a small amount of isoimmune hemolysis may occur in the recipient. A Rh-negative woman of childbearing age should be given platelets from an Rh-negative donor, because the admixed erythrocytes, if they contain the Rh antigen, may immunize her, causing fetal death in an Rh-positive baby. If there is no alternative, the platelets from the Rh-positive donor may be given, but the woman should be treated simultaneously with an injection of Rh_0 immunoglobulin to prevent sensitization.

GRANULOCYTE TRANSFUSION

The frequency and severity of infection is inversely related to the number of circulating neutrophils and the duration of neutropenia. In 1966, Bodie and co-workers showed that, for patients with acute leukemia, the incidence of infection began to increase as the absolute neutrophil count fell below $1000/mm^3$.[54] For patients with breast cancer undergoing chemotherapy, the incidence of infection appears to increase below an absolute neutrophil count of $500/mm^3$.[55] It is likely that these differences are related to the immunosuppressive effect of the disease and to the concomitant mucositis often seen with induction therapy of acute leukemia, which increases the likelihood that intestinal bacteria will invade the bloodstream.

With platelet transfusions to prevent death due to bleeding during nadir pancytopenia from chemotherapy, death from infection became the major cause of chemotherapy-related mortality, particularly in patients treated for acute leukemia, for whom pancytopenia lasts for several weeks.[56] Because of the clear-cut relationship between the absolute neutrophil count and the incidence of infection, it was logical to try granulocyte transfusions to treat and prevent serious infections. Several prospective, randomized studies showed increased survival for patients who received therapeutic granulocyte transfusions to treat established infections. At least six randomized, prospective trials of prophylactic granulocyte transfusions to prevent infection showed a decreased incidence of infection in the granulocyte transfusion recipients, but no ultimate survival advantage. Several reviews of these studies have appeared.[57-59] There has been a marked reduction in the use of granulocyte transfusions, primarily for two reasons. First, the ability to prevent and control infection without granulocyte transfusions has improved significantly. The importance of immediate, empiric broad-spectrum antibiotic coverage for the febrile neutropenic host has been widely accepted. More potent antibiotics have become available, and policies on when to add and how long to continue antibiotics have been established. Improved induction therapy, particularly for acute leukemia, has increased the complete response rate to initial therapy, avoiding immediate reinduction with its prolonged neutropenia. In fact, the most recent prospective study of therapeutic granulocyte transfusions by Winston and colleagues was unable to confirm the benefit of granulocyte transfusion found in earlier studies.[60]

Second, disillusionment with the toxicities of granulocyte transfusions led many clinicians to abandon the use of this blood product. Significant advances, however, have occurred in our understanding of the nature of these toxic reactions and the ways in which the granulocytes should be procured, stored, and delivered in order to diminish toxicity.

Most granulocytes are obtained by the use of a continuous-flow cell separator. Filtration leukapheresis, in which blood was passed over nylon filters, resulting in the adherence of granulocytes that can be eluted, has largely been abandoned due to the damage to neutrophils. Not only is the efficacy of these damaged granulocytes suspect, but this method was also associated with unacceptable toxicity to both donor and recipient. Many pulmonary complications of granulocyte transfusions probably were caused by partially damaged granulocytes, especially in alloimmunized recipients.

The normal granulocyte production in an adult is approximately 10^{11} cells each day. In response to infection, this daily production is increased several fold. Most investigators think that a total granulocyte dose of greater than 10^{10} cells per transfusion is desirable. To achieve this dose, agents are added to facilitate the separation of the granulocytes from the leukocytes, and many donors have been pretreated with steroids. Most centers use hydroxyethyl starch (HES) as an erythrocyte sedimenting agent.

A low-molecular-weight starch called pentastarch has been developed.[61] Pentastarch is structurally similar to hetastarch, but it has a lower molecular weight and a more rapid urinary excretion, such that 90% is cleared within 24 hours, and virtually 100% is cleared within 96 hours. Concern had been raised about the long circulating time of hetastarch and the possible effects on donors, particularly if they were repeatedly leukapheresed. These problems include volume expansion and a mild bleeding diathesis. Using pentastarch alone in a continuous cell separator produces approximately 16×10^9 leukocytes and 8×10^9 neutrophils during a single leukapheresis procedure in which 8 liters of blood are processed.

By pretreating the donors with steroids several hours before the leukapheresis (*e.g.*, Decadron, 3–8 mg/m^2 orally, 12 and sometimes 3 hours before leukapheresis), the yield from a single session can be increased to 30×10^9 leukocytes and 27×10^9 neutrophils. The toxic effects are mild, with adverse reactions occurring in approximately 8.9% of the procedures.[62] The most common side-effects of apheresis are chilling and other citrate effects, including paresthesias, circumoral tingling, nausea, and abdominal cramps. The hetastarch causes mild fluid overload, leading to edema and headache and may cause dermatitis after repeated exposures.

Even with the pentastarch sedimenting agent and steroid premedication of donors, the maximum yield from leukapheresis is still only 20 to 30×10^9 neutrophils, which is 20% to 33% of the normal daily granulocyte production. The premedication of the donors with granulocyte colony-stimulating factor (G-CSF) or granulocyte-macrophage colony-stimulating factor (GM-CSF) may increase the yield.

The granulocytes are maintained at $22°C \pm 2°$. Unlike platelets, granulocytes begin to lose function after 24 to 48 hours of storage, ideally, they should be used within a few hours of pheresis, but they must be transfused within 24 hours.[63]

Because granulocyte transfusions contain lymphocytes capable of engraftment, which could result in GVHD in a severely immunosuppressed host, the indications for irradiation should be the same as for irradiation of other blood products. Irradiation with 1500 rad does not appear to decrease granulocyte function. Leukapheresis removes mature lymphocytes, and repeated leukapheresis results in a decrease in B-lymphocyte count in the donor.[64] The number of total lymphocytes, T lymphocytes, and T_4 lymphocytes is unchanged. Surprisingly, the suppressor T_8 lymphocytes are increased. This has been reported for patients receiving plasmapheresis, and it is probably related to the apheresis procedure, although it is also possible that repeated exposure to the sedimenting agent is involved. Despite this reduction in B-lymphocyte counts and increase in suppressor T-lymphocytes, there have been no increased incidence of infection or other immune complications observed in the leukapheresis donors.

In addition to the risk of viral transmission, granulocyte transfusions carry a significant risk of CMV infection. This is limited to the use of granulocytes from a CMV-seropositive donor to a CMV-seronegative recipient, particularly an immunosuppressed recipient like a bone marrow transplantation patient. For seronegative bone marrow transplant recipients not treated with granulocyte transfusions, the incidence of CMV seroconversion, virus excretion, or culture-positive infection in one study was 33%. If they received prophylactic granulocyte transfusions from a seronegative donor, the rate of CMV infection was 35%, but if the donor was seropositive, the rate of infection increased to 75%.[65] Because of the possible relationship between CMV infection and interstitial pneumonia, it is prudent to avoid seropositive donors for seronegative recipients who have been immunosuppressed for a bone marrow transplant.

A major difficulty in the clinical use of granulocytes is alloimmunization in the recipient. Granulocytes have HLA antigens and granulocyte-specific antigens on their surface. Both anti-HLA antibodies and antigranulocyte antibodies can cause reactions in the recipient, primarily acute chills and fever. In animal and human studies, if ^{111}In-oxine-labeled granulocytes are transfused, scans over areas of infection detect the transfused granulocytes exiting from the circulation and migrating to the site of infection. Using labeled random-donor granulocytes in nonalloimmunized patients, 20 of 20 scans in one institution were positive at known sites of infection, indicating granulocyte migration after infusion. However, in a group of alloimmunized patients, only 3 of 14 scans were positive, indicating a lack of random-donor granulocyte migration to sites of infection.[66]

In addition to febrile reactions and lack of efficacy, the use of random-donor granulocytes in alloimmunized recipients may increase the incidence of pulmonary toxic effects. Wright and co-workers reported that the concurrent administration of amphotericin B and granulocyte transfusions obtained by leukofiltration may be associated with severe pulmonary reactions.[67] Buckner and Clift, using HLA-matched granulocytes obtained with a cell separator, found no evidence of pulmonary toxicity related to granulocytes or granulocytes plus amphotericin B, although the number of pulmonary events was small.[57]

Dana and colleagues failed to find significant pulmonary toxicity with concomitant administration of granulocyte transfusions and amphotericin B.[68] As reviewed by Schiffer, the explanation for the divergent findings may be that the in vivo and in vitro animal data suggest an effect of amphotericin B on previously damaged granulocytes (*e.g.*, obtained by leukofiltration rather than leukapheresis).[69]

Efficacy may be improved and toxicity decreased if only

matched granulocytes are used. Unfortunately, no method exists for crossmatching granulocytes for granulocyte-specific antigens, and it is not clear if all of the reactions are related to the granulocyte-specific antigens or if HLA antigens contribute. It is wise to use HLA-matched siblings whose platelets produce a good increment when transfused into the recipient.[70] If there is no suitable family donor, serologically matched HLA-compatible donors can be used, using the increment in platelet count as a surrogate marker for alloimmunization. If significant transfusion reactions occur, new donors should be selected.

There are no data that justify the use of prophylactic granulocyte transfusions. Several prospective, randomized studies showed an increase in survival rates after therapeutic granulocyte transfusions, particularly when antibiotics were less effective, but the availability of more potent antibiotics and the knowledge of how to use them have markedly diminished the need for granulocyte transfusions. However, for the severely neutropenic patient ($<200/mm^3$), not expected to recover neutrophil counts for 1 week and with a documented bacterial or fungal infection not responding to appropriate antibiotics, granulocyte transfusions are still indicated. For alloimmunized recipients, HLA-matched and granulocyte-compatible donors should be found. CMV-seronegative donors should be used for seronegative recipients.[71] The granulocytes should be irradiated for severely immunosuppressed patients. The donor should be pretreated with steroids or hematopoietic growth factors, and a sedimenting agent like pentastarch should be used. The granulocytes should be leukapheresed daily by a continuous cell separator and transfused promptly. This should be repeated daily until the patient's granulocyte count recovers or the patient is off antibiotics and a febrile for 48 to 72 hours.[72,73]

IMMUNOGLOBULIN

Historically, the use of intramuscular gammaglobulin to prevent or treat infections in patients with hypogammaglobulinemia due to low-grade B-cell neoplasms had never been effective. With the introduction of intravenous immunoglobulin in 1981, interest was rekindled. A prospective, randomized, double-blind, placebo-controlled trial for patients with advanced chronic lymphocytic leukemia (CLL) is being conducted by an international collaborative group. Entry requirements were moderate or severe hypogammaglobulinemia, with a history of serious infection and lack of response to immunizing Influenza and Pneumococcal vaccine. Patients received 400 mg/kg/day of intravenous IgG every 3 weeks for 1 year or placebo. The randomization has not been broken, but one of the groups is showing a statistically significant reduction in overall infections, particularly bacterial infections.[45] When the results of this trial are known, it is very likely that intravenous immunoglobulin will be used for patients with multiple myeloma and CLL who experience recurrent bacterial infections. Because of the extremely high cost of this product, it is unlikely that it will be used prophylactically for patients, unless they are experiencing recurrent infections.

For patients with severe bacterial infection not responding to the appropriate antibiotics, the physician may consider using intravenous immunoglobulin. One caveat has been raised. In animal models, in some cases the concurrent administration of antibiotics with immunoblobulin significantly increased the mortality, compared with antibiotics alone, apparently due to reticuloendothelial blockade by the intravenous immunoglobulin, resulting in impaired clearance of the antibody–bacteria complexes. Three human cases have been recorded that, although not proving a similar mechanism, suggest that this very expensive product should not be used indiscriminately without controlled trials.

Intravenous immunoglobulin or specific CMV hyperimmunoglobulin have decreased the incidence of CMV infection in bone marrow transplant recipients and significantly reduced the incidence of CMV pneumonia. The product may prevent infection in some cases or modify the course of infection in others. Winston and co-workers performed a randomized, controlled trial of prophylactic intravenous immunoglobulin in patients undergoing allogeneic bone marrow transplantation for acute leukemia or aplastic anemia.[74] The incidence of symptomatic CMV infection was 21% in the intravenous immunoglobulin, compared with 46% in the controls ($p = 0.03$), and the incidence of interstitial pneumonia was 18%, compared with 46% in the controls ($p = 0.02$). The incidence of GVHD was only 34%, compared with 65% in controls ($p = 0.01$).

Administration of intravenous immunoglobulin or specific antivaricella-zoster hyperimmunoglobulin may be used in immunosuppressed patients after inadvertent exposure to *Varicella-Zoster* virus. There is no convincing evidence that intravenous immunoglobulin is useful in treating established CMV or varicella-zoster infection.

High-dose intravenous immunoglobulin (400 mg/kg/day for 5 days) has been advocated as a salvage regimen for patients who are bleeding from thrombocytopenia and who are alloimmunized to HLA-matched platelets. The current intravenous immunoglobulins are derived from human plasma selected for providing acceptable antibody titers. Specific hyperimmunoglobulins are available by selecting specific donors or by immunizing donors. After plasmapheresis, a primary purification process is used to isolate the IgG from the plasma. This is usually done by cold ethanol precipitation. A second process modifies the IgG to render it suitable for intravenous infusion. Without alteration, the IgG in gammaglobulin undergoes in vitro aggregation and activates complement after infusion. Many approaches are used, including alkylating agents to modify surface hydroxyl groups, enzymatic modification of the molecule, and processing to remove and prevent aggregates. Studies involving deliberate spiking of the raw plasma with HIV virus have shown that the process used to isolate and purify the IgG completely inactivates and removes the virus.[75]

These newer intravenous preparations are well-tolerated with minor side-effects in the range of 3% to 12%, primarily related to the rate of infusion. Symptoms include chest tightness, a sense of tachycardia (pulse was 84), a burning sensation in the head, chills, nausea, flushing, abdominal pain, dizziness, and joint pain. Most can be prevented or aborted by slowing the infusion rate. Anaphylaxis has occurred in patients with congenital IgA deficiency who have preformed anti-IgA antibody. Although non-A, non-B hepatitis has occurred with use of intravenous immunoglobulin prepared in Europe, the product used in the United States is prepared by Cohn methods 6 and 9, and there is no evidence that the immunoglobulin preparation in the United States can transmit non-A, non-B hepatitis.

APHERESIS

Apheresis, using the current generation of cell separators, has a limited but specific role to play in the management of malignant disease. Apheresis is the general term for all of the procedures for which these separators can be used, including plasmapheresis, thrombocytopheresis, and leukapheresis.

Plasmapheresis is a rapid and efficient means for reducing IgM levels if Waldenstrom's macroglobulinemia is complicated by the development of hyperviscosity. A single plasmapheresis of 1.5 times the patient's plasma volume (plasma volume = 40 mg/kg) should decrease the IgM level by 50% to 80%, which should reduce the serum viscosity below the symptomatic level.[76] When plasmapheresis is begun, chemotherapy is instituted to provide long-term, less-expensive control. For patients who are unable to tolerate chemotherapy, plasmapheresis can be used every 2 to 3 months to maintain IgM levels in a range that will prevent hyperviscosity, but this will not accomplish any cytoreduction of the plasmacytoid lymphocyte infiltration of marrow, lymph nodes, liver, and spleen.

Plasmapheresis may be used when hyperviscosity complicates multiple myeloma, particularly in IgA myeloma and the rare IgM myeloma. Plasmapheresis has been used when neuropathy complicates myeloma because some cases of myeloma-induced neuropathy have been associated with an antimyelin specificity of the monoclonal protein.

Leukapheresis has been used for patients with acute myelogenous (AML) or acute lymphocytic leukemia (ALL) with very high blast counts. When the blast count is greater than 100,000 in AML, a patient may have life-threatening pulmonary and central nervous system leukostasis. Prompt reduction in the blast counts is clearly indicated, which may be accomplished rapidly with leukapheresis. Although prompt cytoreduction may be accomplished with chemotherapy, the physical removal of the blasts from the blood prevents tumor lysis syndrome and DIC, which may occur with rapid cytolysis of the myeloblasts. Plasma exchange may be employed in acute promyelocytic leukemia patients undergoing induction therapy if severe DIC develops after heparin administration. DIC, pulmonary and CNS leukostasis, and intracerebral hemorrhage are less common in ALL than in AML at equivalent blast counts, and there is probably a higher threshold for using leukapheresis in ALL than in AML.[77]

For patients with extremely high platelet counts due to essential thrombocytosis or polycythemia vera who develop bleeding or thrombotic complications, the platelet count can be lowered rapidly with plateletpheresis, which lowers the platelet count more quickly than hydroxyurea.

Apheresis may be used as a nonmyelosuppressive and nonmutagenic form of cytoreduction. In patients who have CLL with bone marrow failure from chemotherapy or who have become refractory to chemotherapy, leukapheresis permits short-term support of the patient and allows the platelet count to increase.[78] In hairy cell leukemia, leukapheresis has been used with some good results.[79] However, with the availability of alpha-interferon and deoxycoformycin, the need for this expensive and inconvenient means of support has diminished.[80] Leukapheresis has been used in CML occurring during pregnancy to keep the granulocyte count under control but avoid the possible teratogenic effects of chemotherapy.[81] Leukapheresis does not represent a primary form of therapy for any of these diseases, but it does give a nonmyelosuppressive option for specific cases.

Apheresis is used to collect specific cell fractions for in vitro activation, treatment, or manipulation before reinfusion. Leukapheresis, followed by Ficoll-Hypaque density-gradient isolation of the mononuclear fraction and incubation with interleukin-2, has been used to generate lymphokine-activated killer cells (LAK), which are reinfused with systemic interleukin-2.[82]

Another in vitro treatment involved the oral administration of 8-methoxypsoralen to 37 patients with resistant cutaneous T-cell lymphoma.[83] Methoxypsoralen transiently intercalates into DNA, but it is almost completely excreted with 24 hours, unless it is activated by ultraviolet A and covalently cross-links the DNA. After ingesting methoxypsoralen, the patients underwent leukapheresis with extracorporeal ultraviolet A irradiation of the leukocytes, which were then returned to the patients. Twenty-seven of 37 patients responded, with an average 64% decrease in cutaneous involvement and with minimal toxicity. Two patients with particularly severe skin involvement remained free of symptoms for 21 and 29 months, respectively, after discontinuing treatment. This prolonged response suggests a possible immunologic response to the reinfused damaged lymphocytes.

Circulating peripheral stem cells can be harvested by apheresis for use in autologous bone marrow transplantation. Plasmapheresis with perfusion over a Staphylococcal protein A column has been used investigationally in the treatment of solid tumors[84,85,86] and has been recommended by some as the treatment of choice for mitomycin-induced hemolytic uremic syndrome.[87,88]

In experienced hands, apheresis is a relatively safe procedure with minimal morbidity. Because citrate is used as an anticoagulant, hypocalcemia can develop, which usually manifests as paresthesias but can result in tetany or arrhythmias. Vasovagal reactions can result in hypotension, and this usually responds to volume infusion. If fresh-frozen plasma is used (*e.g.*, in the treatment of TTP), patients can have allergic reactions to the plasma and may acquire viral infections. Because of the vascular access, complications may include thrombosis, bleeding, and infection. Overall, the incidence of minor morbidity is approximately 10%. However, because at least 10 deaths have been reported with cytopheresis and more than 50 with plasmapheresis, this procedure should be reserved for specific, appropriate indications and only performed under the direction of physicians skilled in the use of this technique.[89,90]

AUTOLOGOUS BONE MARROW TRANSPLANTATION

The most sophisticated form of supportive care using blood products is the infusion of pleuripotent stem cells to repopulate the bone marrow after high-dose chemotherapy or radiation. These stem cells may be syngeneic, allogeneic, or autologous. The appeal of autologous bone marrow transplant is the universal availability of donors and the lack of GVHD. The only drawback to autologous transplant is the possibility that the marrow is contaminated with malignant cells.

Pleuripotent stem cells for autologous bone marrow transplant are obtained by two means. The standard approach has been marrow collection as described by Thomas and Storb in 1970.[91,92] In the operating room under general or spinal anesthesia, 600 to 1000 ml of marrow is aspirated through the anterior or posterior iliac crests. The aspirated marrow is filtered and then placed into tissue culture medium with heparin. If in vitro purging is attempted, an additional 300 to 500 ml may be harvested to use as a backup if the purging method damages the pleuripotent stem cells and hematopoietic recovery does not occur. In many institutions, the stem cell population is purified by isolating the mononuclear cell fraction using a cell separator or Ficoll-Hypaque gradient.

The other method takes advantage of the fact that peripheral blood contains stem cells.[93] The concentration of granulocyte-macrophage colony forming units in the circulation is increased during rebound from chemotherapy.[94,95] In the future, hematopoietic growth factors (*e.g.*, IL-3 or GM-CSF) may increase the number of stem cells in the peripheral blood or in the bone marrow. A comparable number of stem cells can be obtained by using a cell separator to remove the leukocyte fraction from 17 liters of whole blood. The mononuclear fraction often is isolated from the leukocytes that are removed. After the mononuclear fractions are obtained, additional processing is comparable to the purification of mononuclear cells from bone marrow aspirate.

In most cases the mononuclear cell fraction is frozen using glycerol or DMSO as a cryoprotective agent with a carefully controlled rate of freezing and stored in liquid nitrogen. Stiff and colleagues questioned the need for rate-controlled freezing and liquid-nitrogen storage.[96] A simplified method, using DMSO and hydroxyethyl starch as cryoprotectants and simple placement of the autologous marrow into a −80°C freezer, produced equivalent hematopoietic reconstitution, and it was simple, rapid, and inexpensive. Thawing should be accomplished by very rapid rewarming. Aliquots of the autologous marrow are studied in tissue culture to ensure that an engrafting dose of viable stem cells exist ($0.05-2 \times 10^8$/kg).

The theoretical attraction of high-dose chemotherapy or radiation followed by autologous rescue is based on the steep dose-response curve for most chemotherapeutic agents and the fact that myelosuppression is the dose-limiting toxicity for many agents. However, even using autologous rescue to avoid myelosuppression, the ability to escalate single agents is limited by nonhematologic dose-limiting toxicity.[97] In Phase I dose-escalation studies using single agents with autologous marrow support, cardiac toxicity limits the maximum dose of Cytoxan to 200 mg/kg. Pulmonary toxicity is limiting for dose escalation with total-body irradiation or BCNU. Hepatic toxicity is limiting for BCNU, busulfan, and mitomycin. Mucositis and gastrointestinal toxic effects limit dose escalation for melphalan and VP-16. Thiotepa and nitrogen mustard are limited by neurotoxicity. For some drugs, such as Cytoxan and VP-16, it appears that, at the maximally tolerated dose that produces nonhematologic toxicity, the period of pancytopenia with autologous rescue is probably not significantly shorter than without rescue.

Even with the less than one order of magnitude increase in dose that can be achieved using autologous rescue, the response rates of many tumors are increased. If different drugs are selected, each with a different mechanism of resistance and different nonmarrow dose-limiting toxicities, combinations of chemotherapeutic agents can be assembled much as standard combination chemotherapy is designed. A number of such combinations have been tested to date against a wide variety of tumors.[98–102] For most solid tumors, high-dose chemotherapy with autologous rescue, even for patients with grossly relapsed disease, produces a significant response rate. These responses, however, are very short and not worth the expense and toxicity. The chemotherapeutic regimens, even in high doses, are unable to eradicate grossly relapsed, chemotherapy-resistant cancer.

Current efforts have shifted to identifying early those patients with a poor prognosis with conventional treatment. These patients are first exposed to conventional treatment, then treated intensively with autologous rescue while the tumor burden is minimal. In order to justify such aggressive treatment for patients with minimal body tumor burden, clear definition of prognostic variables is essential.

For patients in frank relapse, the duration of response is currently so poor that failure is probably due to inability to eradicate resistant disease rather than to the reinfusion of tumor cells, which may be contaminating the autologous marrow infusions. In the future, however, avoiding reinfusion of tumor cells is likely to be more important.

There are several ways to prevent reinfusion of malignant cells. One of the first methods used were monoclonal antibodies specific for antigens on the tumor cells but not on the pleuripotent stem cells. These monoclonal antibodies (*e.g.*, anti-calla or anti-B-1) are incubated with the autologous marrow in vitro. In some cases, complement is added to cause cytolysis of the malignant cells. In other cases, the monoclonal antibody has been coupled to ricin or to magnetic spheres.

Another strategy involves the in vitro incubation of the marrow with chemotherapy. Investigators at Johns Hopkins have studied the use of 4-hydroperoxycyclophosphamide to treat autologous marrow in vitro. Preclinical studies showed that this agent was able to eradicate leukemic cells in animals.

In a Phase II study, 25 patients with acute nonlymphocytic leukemia in second or third remission were prepared with busulfan and Cytoxan or Cytoxan and total body irradiation (TBI), followed by reinfusion of autologous marrow that had been treated in vitro with the 4-hydroperoxycyclophosphamide.[103] Recovery of neutrophil and platelet counts was delayed until days 29 and 57, respectively. Four patients died from bacterial or fungal sepsis within the first month after transplantation, and one patient did not recover marrow function. The remaining 20 patients all had marrow recovery, and 11 of the 25 patients remained in remission at a median of more than 400 days after transplantation. Although the incidence of leukemia relapse in these patients after autologous transplantation (35%) is significantly higher than that after allogeneic transplant in similar patients (5%), the overall disease-free survival rate of 43% is clearly superior to a 5% disease-free survival that could be achieved with chemotherapy alone at this stage.[104] In addition, there were no deaths due to GVHD. The follow-up is not long enough to compare the overall survival rate after autologous transplant and the overall survival rate after allogeneic transplant.

A third method for avoiding reinfusion of malignant cells has been developed by Chang and co-workers from the Christie Hospital.[105] When autologous marrow is placed into long-term marrow culture for 10 to 14 days under appropriate conditions, the leukemia population is replaced by apparently normal hematopoiesis, with conversion occurring between days 7 and 14. It appears that under the right conditions, the leukemia cells have a growth disadvantage. One patient in florid relapse, who was conditioned with TBI and autotransplanted with his own marrow after growth in long-term bone marrow culture, achieved complete remission that lasted 9 months. A second patient transplanted in relapse achieved complete remission, but he has been followed only for 2 months. Three patients transplanted in this fashion during first remission of AML are without evidence of disease 9 to 26 months after transplantation. Two patients whose marrows did not convert in vitro did not achieve complete remissions.

A fourth approach being explored by several investigators is the identification, "positive selection," and specific reinfusion of the normal pleuripotent stem cells, leaving the malignant marrow behind.[106] CD34 is an antigen present on 1% to 4% of human marrow cells, including virtually all hematopoietic progenitors detectable by in vitro assays. Many monoclonal antibodies have been made to different epitopes of this antigen. Using one such antibody (12-8), which reacts with CD34 in humans and monkeys, Berenson and colleagues were able to show in monkeys that the CD34-positive cells removed from autologous marrow produced engraftment, but marrow depleted by CD34 was not.[107] Because most or all solid tumors lack CD34 antigen, they have started a Phase I trial of autologous bone marrow transplantation using only the CD34-positive cells.

Some investigators question whether purging is necessary, because it is not clear that phenotypically malignant cells in vitro are capable of engraftment and self-renewal. It has not yet been demonstrated that some patients relapsed due to infusion of malignant cells, which contaminate normal hematopoietic cells in the marrow. One opportunity for testing is to compare the results of syngeneic transplants with those of autologous transplants in patients with similar stages of disease, because neither would be expected to develop GVHD, but only the autologous transplants would contain malignant cells.

The largest experience and greatest success using autologous bone marrow transplants has been in the treatment of relapsed high-grade Hodgkin's and non-Hodgkin's lymphomas, childhood neuroblastoma, and acute leukemia. Takvorian and co-workers selected 49 patients with relapsed or poor-prognosis non-Hodgkin's lymphoma who were still responsive to conventional-dose chemotherapy, who had minimal disease status (*i.e.*, nodal disease <2 cm and bone marrow involvement <5% on histologic examination), and whose tumor expressed the B-1 antigen.[108] These selected patients were prepared with Cytoxan and total-body irradiation and then rescued with their autologous bone marrow that had been incubated in vitro with anti-B-1 monoclonal antibody and complement. All patients achieved hematologic and immunologic engraftment. There were two treatment-related deaths, one from veno-occlusive disease of the liver and one from intercerebral hemorrhage. At a median follow-up of more than 11 months, 34 patients are disease-free without maintenance chemotherapy 2 to 52 months after diagnosis.

In a multicenter study, 100 patients with intermediate or high-grade non-Hodgkin's lymphoma with refractory or relapsed disease were treated with high-dose chemotherapy or chemotherapy plus irradiation and autologous bone marrow transplants.[109] For patients not responding to primary therapy, the 3-year disease-free survival rate was zero. For patients who had initially responded to chemotherapy but then relapsed and were unresponsive to salvage treatment, there was a 14% 3-year survival rate. For patients who had originally responded, then relapsed, and were responding to salvage treatment (a subset similar to the group studied by Takvorian), there was a 36% 3-year disease-free survival rate. The authors concluded that patients who never have a complete remission and whose disease is progressing before high-dose chemotherapy and autologous transplant can still have complete responses, but these remissions are not durable, and in view of the massive treatment regimen, the authors thought that treatment was inappropriate. However, for patients relapsing from complete remissions, this approach is indicated and offers the best prognosis for those who are responding to salvage treatment.

For patients with AML in first relapse or patients with ALL in second relapse, it appears that no form of intensive chemotherapy will be curative. For these relapsed patients younger than 40 years old with an HLA-matched sibling, allogeneic bone marrow transplantation appears to be the treatment of choice.[110,111] For patients older than 40, the risk of GVHD increases. For patients younger than 40 who do not have HLA-matched siblings, allogeneic transplants from a partially matched family donor or a matched unrelated donor can be undertaken at centers in which experience with unmatched transplants has been accumulated. In these cases, the incidence of GVHD increases. For relapsed patients older than 40 or younger than 40 but without an HLA-matched sibling, an autologous transplant may avoid the risk of GVHD. Allogeneic transplant, however, has the advantage of not infusing malignant cells and of achieving a graft-versus-leukemia effect. The risk of serious morbidity or death due to GVHD must be weighed against the increased risk of relapsed leukemia with an autologous transplant, but data are insufficient to favor either approach.

A number of centers have reported prolonged disease-free survival in some children with relapsed neuroblastoma.[112] Children's Hospital in Philadelphia has reported a 36% survival rate at 12 months in a group of relapsed children who responded to salvage irradiation. Based on these successes in relapsed patients, a number of groups have begun to study the use of high-dose chemotherapy with autologous rescue for children with bad prognoses. Specifically, 90% of children with Stage IV neuroblastoma will die of this disease, and it is reasonable to attempt consolidation therapy for these children when in first remission. Hartmann and colleagues treated 62 children 1 year of age and older with Stage IV neuroblastoma with conventional chemotherapy, and 33 of them had complete remissions or good partial remissions and were treated with high-dose chemotherapy using BCNU, VM-26, and melphalan, followed by rescue with autologous bone marrow that had been purged in vitro with the chemotherapeutic agent Asta-Z 7557.[113] At a median follow-up of 28 months, 16 of the 33 grafted children are alive in continuous complete remission.

The results of high-dose chemotherapy or chemotherapy and radiation therapy with autologous rescue for other relapsed solid tumors have been disappointing, with higher response rates than can be achieved with standard chemotherapy but with short responses. The agents used include Cytoxan, cisplatin, BCNU, melphalan, thiotepa, VP-16, and ara-C. In some cases, they have been combined with total-body irradiation. The tumors most studied include relapsed testicular and germ cell, small cell lung, breast, brain, ovary, melanoma, childhood sarcomas, and colon. The prospects for autologous bone marrow transplantation are quite promising.

Although the availability of the hematopoietic growth factors is likely to shorten the period of pancytopenia after chemotherapy and obviate the need for autologous rescue in some patients, they probably will make autologous rescue more feasible. Hematopoietic growth factors can increase the yield of pleuripotent stem cells from the bone marrow and peripheral blood, and it is conceivable that these growth factors may be used in vitro to expand the number of stem cells or allow the stem cells to be separated from the malignant cells by growth advantage. After infusion of the autologous transplant, the growth factors may be used to expedite recovery of peripheral blood counts.

The use of monoclonal and molecular markers to identify patients with poor prognoses at diagnosis, who are likely to fail conventional therapy, will permit autologous transplants as induction or as early consolidation therapy. Theoretically, the preparative regimens for autologous transplants have more efficacy when the tumor burden is smallest and there are fewer chemotherapy-resistant cell lines. For patients in frank relapse, better systemic preparative regimens are necessary. As patients are transplanted earlier in the course of their disease with better curative potential or as better preparative regimens are developed, the need for purging of the autologous marrow will become more important.

REFERENCES

1. Wallerstein R Jr: Laboratory evaluation of anemia. West J Med 146:443–451, 1987
2. Meryman HT, Hornblower M: The preparation of red cells depleted of leukocytes. Transfusion 26:101–106, 1986
3. Perkins HA, Payne R, Ferguson J et al: Nonhemolytic febrile transfusion reactions. Quantitative effects of blood components with emphasis on isoantigenic incompatibility of leukocytes. Vox Sang 11:578–600, 1966
4. Sirchia G, Rebulla P, Parravicini A et al: Leukocyte depletion of red cell units at the bedside by transfusion through a new filter. Transfusion 27:402–405, 1987
5. Domen RE, Williams L, Gilbert DM: Preparation of leukocyte-depleted red cells by filtration. Transfusion 27:504, 1987
6. Leng B, Chong C, Lovric VA et al: Simple and economical preparation of leukocyte-poor red cells (abstr). Transfusion 24:419, 1984
7. Murphy MF, Metcalfe H, Thomas J et al: Use of leukocyte-poor blood components and HLA-matched platelet donors to prevent HLA alloimmunization. Br J Hematol 62:529–534, 1986
8. Barton JC: Nonhemolytic, noninfectious transfusion reactions. Semin Hematol 18:95–121, 1981
9. Bove JR: Transfusion-transmitted diseases: Current problems and challenges. Prog Hematol 14:123–147, 1986
10. Wick MR, Moore S, Taswell HF: Non-A, non-B hepatitis associated with blood transfusion. Transfusion 25:93–101, 1985
11. Koziol DE, Holland PV, Alling DW et al: Antibody to hepatitis B core antigen as a paradoxical marker for non-A, non-B hepatitis agents in donated blood. Ann Intern Med 104:488–495, 1986
12. Zuck TF, Sherwood WC, Bove JR: A review of recent events related to surrogate testing of blood to prevent non-A, non-B posttransfusion hepatitis. Transfusion 27:203, 1987
13. Perkins HA, Samson S, Garner J et al: Risk of AIDS for recipients of blood components from donors who subsequently developed AIDS. Blood 70:1604–1610, 1987
14. Curran JW, Jaffe HW, Hardy AM et al: Epidemiology of HIV infection and AIDS in the United States. Science 239:610–616, 1988
15. Medley GF, Anderson RM, Cox DR et al: Incubation period of AIDS in patients infected via blood transfusion. Nature 328:719–721, 1987
16. Ragni MV, Winkelstein A, Kingsley L et al: 1986 update of HIV seroprevalence, seroconversion, AIDS incidence, and immunologic correlates of HIV infection in patients with hemophilia A and B. Blood 70:786–790, 1987
17. Bove JR: Transfusion-associated hepatitis and AIDS, what is the risk. N Engl J Med 317:242–244, 1987
18. von Sydow M, Gaines H, Sönnerborg A et al: Antigen detection in primary HIV infection. Br Med J 296:238–240, 1988
19. Fauci A: The human immunodeficiency virus: Infectivity and mechanisms of pathogenesis. Science 239:617–622, 1988
20. Ou C-Y, Kwok S, Mitchell SW et al: DNA amplification for direct detection of HIV-1 in DNA of peripheral blood mononuclear cells. Science 239:295–297, 1988
21. Felber BK, Pavlakis GN: A quantitative bioassay for HIV-1 based on trans-activation. Science 239:184–187, 1988
22. Editorial: 91: HTLV-1 comes of age. Lancet 1:217–219, 1988
23. Leitman SF, Holland PV: Irradiation of blood products. Transfusion 25:293–303, 1985
24. Mollison PL: Blood Transfusion in Clinical Medicine, 6 ed, pp 578–583. Oxford, Blackwell Scientific, 1979
25. Wallerstein R Jr: Laboratory evaluation of the bleeding patient. West J Med (in press)
26. Harker LA, Slichter SJ: The bleeding time as a screening test for evaluation of platelet function. N Engl J Med 287:155–159, 1972
27. Malpass TW, Harker LA: Acquired disorders of platelet function. Semin Hematol 17:242–258, 1980
28. Day HJ, Rao AK: Platelets and megakaryocytes. V. Semin Hematol 23:89–101, 1986
29. Kobrinsky NL, Gerrard JM, Watson CM et al: Shortening of bleeding time by 1-deamino-8-D-arginine vasopressin in various bleeding disorders. Lancet 1:1145–1148, 1984
30. Gaydos LS, Freireich EJ, Mantel N: The quantitative relation between platelet count and hemorrhage in patients with acute leukemia. N Engl J Med 266:905–909, 1962
31. Menitove JE, Aster RH: Transfusion of platelets and plasma products. Clin Haematol 12:239–266, 1983
32. Gottschall 1JL, Rzad L, Aster RH: Studies of the minimum temperature at which human platelets can be stored with full maintenance of viability. Transfusion 26:460–462, 1986
33. Simon TL, Nelson EJ, Murphy S: Extension of platelet concentrate storage to 7 days in second-generation bags. Transfusion 27:6–9, 1987
34. Heal JM, Singal S, Sardisco E et al: Bacterial proliferation in platelet concentrates. Transfusion 26:388–90, 1986
35. Braine HG, Kickler TS, Charache P et al: Bacterial sepsis secondary to platelet transfusion: An adverse effect of extended storage at room temperature. Transfusion 268:391–393,1986
36. Holohan TV, Terasaki P, Deisseroth A: Suppression of transfusion-related alloimmunization in intensively treated cancer patients. Blood 58:122–128, 1981
37. Dutcher JP, Schiffer CA, Aisner J et al: Alloimmunization following platelet transfusion: The absence of a dose-response relationship. Blood 57:395, 1981
38. Claas FHJ, Smeenk RJT, Schmidt R et al: Alloimmunization against the MHC antigens after platelet transfusions is due to contaminating leukocytes in the platelet suspension. Exp Hematol 9:84–9, 1981
39. Eernisee JG, Brand A: Prevention of platelet refractoriness due to HLA antibodies by administration of leukocyte-poor blood components. Exp Hematol 9:77–83, 1981
40. Daly PA, Schiffer CA, Aisner J et al: Platelet transfusion therapy. One-hour posttransfusion increments are valuable in predicting the need for HLA-matched preparations. JAMA 243:435–438, 1980
41. Bishop JF, McGrath K, Wolf MM et al: Clinical factors influencing the efficacy of pooled platelet transfusion. Blood 71:383–387, 1988
42. Heal JM, Blumberg N, Masel D: An evaluation of crossmatching, HLA, and ABO matching for platelet transfusions to refractory patients. Blood 70:23–30, 1987
43. Junghans RP, Ahn YS: High-dose intravenous gamma globulin to suppress alloimmune destruction of donor platelets. Am J Med 76:204–208, 1984

44. Schiffer CA, Hogge DE, Aisner J et al: High-dose intravenous gamma globulin in alloimmunized platelet transfusion recipients. Blood 64:937–940, 1984
45. Lee EJ, Norris D, Schiffer CA: Intravenous immune globulin for patients alloimmunized to random donor platelet transfusion. Transfusion 27:245–247, 1987
46. Stiehm ER, Ashida IE, Kim KW et al: Intravenous immunoglobulins as therapeutic agents. Ann Intern Med 107:367–382, 1987
47. Schiffer CA, Aisner J, Wiernik PH: Frozen autologous platelet transfusion for patients with leukemia. N Engl J Med 299:7–12, 1978
48. Dullemond-Westland AC, van Prooijen HC, Riemens MI et al: Cryopreservation disturbs stimulus-response coupling in a platelet subpopulation. Br J Haematol 67:325–333, 1987
49. Schiffer CA, Patten E, Reilly J et al: Effective leukocyte removal from platelet preparations by centrifugation in a new pooling bag. Transfusion 27:162–164, 1987
50. Kalmin ND, Orrell JE, Villarreal IG: An effective method for the preparation of leukocyte-poor platelets. Transfusion 27:281–283, 1978
51. Gmur J, von Felton A, Osterwalder B et al: Delayed alloimmunization using random single donor platelet transfusion: A prospective study in thrombocytopenic patients with acute leukemia. Blood 62:473–479, 1983
52. Sintincolas K, Sizoo W, Haije WG et al: Delayed alloimmunization by random single donor platelet transfusion. Lancet 1:750–759, 1981
53. Eisenstaedt R: Blood component therapy in the treatment of platelet disorders. Semin Hematol 23:1–7, 1986
54. Bodey GP, Buckley M, Sathe YS et al: Quantitative relationships between circulating leukocytes and infection in patients with acute leukemia. Ann Intern Med 64:328–340, 1966
55. Esparza L, Yap HY, Smith T et al: Quantitative relationship between degree of myelosuppression and infection in patients with metastatic breast cancer (MBC) (abstr C-348). Proc Am Soc Clin Oncol 2:89, 1983
56. Bodey GP: Infection in cancer patients: A continuing association. Am J Med 81:11–26, 1986
57. Clift RA, Buckner CD: Granulocyte transfusions. Am J Med 76:631–636, 1984
58. Wright DG: Leukocyte transfusions: Thinking twice. Am J Med 76:637–44, 1984
59. Young LS: The role of granulocyte transfusions in treating and preventing infection. Cancer Treat Rep 67:109–11, 1983
60. Winston DJ, Ho WG, Gale RP: Therapeutic granulocyte transfusions for documented infections. Ann Intern Med 97:509–515, 1982
61. Strauss RG, Hester JP, Vogler WR et al: A multicenter trial to document the efficacy and safety of a rapidly excreted analog of hydroxyethyl starch for leukapheresis with a note on steroid stimulation of granulocyte donors. Transfusion 26:258–264, 1986
62. Strauss RG, Goeken JA, Eckermann I et al: Effects of intensive granulocyte donation on donors and yields. Transfusion 26:441–445, 1986
63. Robinson EAE: Single donor granulocytes and platelets. Clin Haematol 13:185–216, 1984
64. Strauss RG, Goeken JA, Imig KM: Effects on immunity of multiple leukapheresis using a rapidly excreted analog of hydroxyethyl starch. Transfusion 26:265–268, 1986
65. Hersman J, Meyers JD, Thomas Ed et al: The effect of granulocyte transfusions upon the incidence of cytomegalovirus infection after allogeneic marrow transplantation. Ann Intern Med 96:149–152, 1982
66. Dutcher JP, Schiffer CA, Johnston GS et al: Alloimmunization prevents the migration of transfused indium-III-labeled granulocytes to sites of infection. Blood 62:354–60, 1983
67. Wright DG, Robichaum KJ, Pizzo PA et al: Lethal pulmonary reactions associated with the combined use of amphotericin B and leukocyte transfusions. N Engl J Med 304:1185–1189, 1981
68. Dana BW, Durie BGM, White RF et al: Concomitant administration of granulocyte transfusions and amphotericin B in neutropenic patients: Absence of significant pulmonary toxicity. Blood 57:90–94, 1981
69. Schiffer CA: Granulocyte transfusion therapy. Cancer Treat Rep 67:113–119, 1983
70. Buckner CD, Clift RA: Prophylaxis and treatment of infection of the immunocompromised host by granulocyte transfusions. Clin Haematol 13:557–72, 1984
71. Bowden RA, Sayers M, Flournoy N et al: Cytomegalovirus immune globulin and seronegative blood products to prevent primary cytomegalovirus infection after marrow transplantation. N Engl J Med 314:1006–10, 1986
72. Herzig RH, Herzig GP, Graw RG et al: Successful granulocyte transfusion therapy from gram-negative septicemia. N Engl J Med 296:701–705, 1977
73. Alavi JB, Root RK, Djerassi I et al: A randomized clinical trial of granulocyte transfusions for infection in acute leukemia. N Engl J Med 296:706–711, 1977
74. Winston DJ, Ho WG, Lin CH et al: Intravenous immune globulin for prevention of cytomegalovirus infection and interstitial pneumonia after bone marrow transplantation. Ann Intern Med 106:12–18, 1987
75. Mitra C, Wong MF, Mozen MM et al: Elimination of infectious retroviruses during preparation of immunoglobulins. Transfusion 26:394–397, 1986
76. Linker CL: Plasmapheresis in clinical medicine. West J Med 138:60–69, 1983
77. Bunin NJ, Pui CH: Differing complications of hyperleukocytosis in children with acute lymphoblastic or acute nonlymphoblastic leukemia. J Clin Oncol 3:1590–1595, 1985
78. Gale RP, Foon KA: Chronic lymphocytic leukemia. Ann Intern Med 103:101–120, 1985
79. Yam LT, Klock JC, Mielke CH: Therapeutic leukapheresis in hairy cell leukemia: Review of literature and personal experience. Semin Oncol 11:493–501, 1984
80. Golomb HM: The treatment of hairy cell leukemia. Blood 69:979–983, 1987
81. Fitzgerald D, Rowe JM, Heal J: Leukapheresis for control of chronic myelogenous leukemia during pregnancy. Am J Hematol 22:213–218, 1986
82. Rosenberg SA, Lotze MT, Muul LM et al: A progress report on the treatment of 157 patients with advanced cancer using lymphokine-activated killer cells and interleukin-2 or high-dose interleukin-2 alone. N Engl J Med 316:889–97, 1987
83. Edelson R, Berger C, Gasparro F et al: Treatment of cutaneous T-cell lymphoma by extracorporeal photochemotherapy. N Engl J Med 316:297–303, 1987
84. Ventura GJ, Buzdar AU, Kau S et al: Clinical trial of plasma perfusion over immobilized staphylococcal protein A in metastatic breast cancer. Cancer Treat Rep 71:411–413, 1987
85. MacKintosh FR, Bennett K, Schiff S et al: Treatment of advanced malignancy with plasma perfused over staphylococcal protein A. West J Med 139:36–40, 1983
86. Messerschmidt GL, Henry DH, Snyder HW et al: Protein A immunoadsorption in the treatment of malignant disease. J Clin Oncol 6:203–212, 1988
87. Murgo AJ: Thrombotic microangiopathy in the cancer patient including those induced by chemotherapeutic agents. Semin Hematol 24:161–177, 1987
88. Korec S, Schein PS, Smith FP et al: Treatment of cancer-associated hemolytic syndrome with staphylococcal protein A immunoperfusion. J Clin Oncol 4:210–215, 1986
89. Hazards of apheresis. Lancet 2:1025–1026, 1982
90. Council on Scientific Affairs: Current status of therapeutic plasmapheresis and related techniques: Report of the AMA panel on therapeutic plasmapheresis. JAMA 253:819–825, 1985
91. Thomas ED, Storb R: Technique for human marrow grafting. Blood 36:507–515, 1970
92. Gorin NC: Collection, manipulation and freezing of haemopoietic stem cells. Clin Haematol 15:19–48, 1986
93. Abrams RA, Glaubiger D, Appelbaum FR et al: Result of attempted hematopoietic reconstitution using isologous, peripheral blood mononuclear cells: A case report. Blood 56:516–520, 1980
94. Abrams RA, McCormach K, Bowles C et al: Cyclophosphamide treatment expands the circulating hematopoietic stem cell pool in dogs. J Clin Invest 67:1392–1399, 1981
95. Abrams RA, Johnston-Early A, Kramer C et al: Amplification of circulating granulocyte-monocyte stem cells numbers following chemotherapy in patients with extensive small cell carcinoma of the lung. Cancer Res 41:35–41, 1981
96. Stiff PJ, Koester AR, Weidner MK et al: Autologous bone marrow transplantation using unfractionated cells cryopreserved in dimethysulfoxide and hydroxyethyl starch without controlled-rate freezing. Blood 70:974–978, 1987
97. Appelbaum FR, Buckner CD: Overview of the clinical relevance of autologous bone marrow transplantation. Clin Haematol 15:1–18, 1986
98. Souhami R, Peters W: High dose chemotherapy in solid tumours in adults. Clin Haematol 15:219–234, 1986
99. Antman K, Eder JP, Ellas A et al: High-dose combination alkylating agent preparative regimen with autologous bone marrow support: The Dana-Farber Cancer Institute/Beth Israel Hospital Experience. Cancer Treat Rep 71:119–125, 1987
100. Dicke KA, Jagannath S, Spitzer G et al: The role of autologous bone marrow transplantation in various malignancies. Semin Haematol 21:109–122, 1984
101. Verdonck LF, Dekker AW, Vendrick PJ et al: Intensive cytoreductive therapy followed by autologous bone marrow transplantation for patients with hematologic malignancies or solid tumors. Cancer 60:289–295, 1987
102. Antman K, Eder JP, Frei E: High-dose chemotherapy with bone marrow support for solid tumors. In DeVita VT, Hellman S, Rosenberg SA (eds): Important Advances in Oncology, 1987, pp 221–235. Philadelphia, JB Lippincott, 1987
103. Yaeger AM, Kaizer H, Santos GW et al: Autologous bone marrow transplantation in patients with acute nonlymphocytic leukemia, using ex vivo marrow treatment with 4-hydroperoxycyclophosphamide. N Engl J Med 315:141–147, 1986
104. O'Reilly RJ: New promise for autologous marrow transplants in leukemia. N Engl J Med 315:186–188, 1986
105. Chang JG, Continho L, Testa N et al: The clinical use of bone marrow cells grown in long-term culture for autologous transplantation (abstr). Fourth Terry Fox Cancer Conference.
106. Berenson RJ, Bensinger WI, Kalamasz D: Positive selection of viable cell populations using avidinbiotin immunoadsorption. J Immunol Methods 91:11–19, 1986
107. Berenson RJ, Bensinger WI, Andrews RG et al: Hematopoietic stem cell transplants. In Gale RP, Golde DW (eds): Recent Advances in Leukemia and Lymphoma—UCLA Symposia on Molecular and Cellular Biology, Vol 61. New York, Alan R. Liss, 1987
108. Takvorian T, Canellos GP, Ritz J et al: Prolonged disease-free survival after autologous bone marrow transplantation in patients with non-Hodgkin's lymphoma with a poor prognosis. N Engl J Med 316:1499–1505, 1987
109. Philip T, Armitage JO, Spitzer G et al: High-dose therapy and autologous bone marrow transplantation after failure of conventional chemotherapy in adults with intermediate-grade or high-grade non-Hodgkin's lymphoma. N Engl J Med 316:1493–1498, 1987
110. Champlin R, Gale RP: Bone marrow transplantation for acute leukemia: Recent advances and comparison with alternative therapies. Semin Haematol 24:55–67, 1987
111. Champlin R, Gale RP: Acute myelogenous leukemia: Recent advances in therapy. Blood 69:1551–1562, 1987
112. Pinkerton R, Philip T, Bouffet E et al: Autologous bone marrow transplantation in paediatric solid tumors. Clin Haematol 15:187–203, 1986
113. Hartmann O, Benhamou E, Beaujean F et al: Repeated high-dose chemotherapy followed by purged autologous bone marrow transplantation as consolidation therapy in metastatic neuroblastoma. J Clin Oncol 5:1205–1211, 1987

SECTION 3

ALBERT DEISSEROTH
RALPH WALLERSTEIN JR.

Use of Hematopoietic Growth Factors

Purified human recombinant hematopoietic growth factors or colony-stimulating factors (CSF) have become available for clinical investigation. These glycoprotein hormones will have a major impact on the clinical practice of hematology and oncology and will significantly alter the practice of supportive care. The term "colony-stimulating factor" derives from the observation that bone marrow cells in tissue culture require serum factors to survive, proliferate, and differentiate. These factors appear to regulate the progression from pleuripotent stem cells to mature differentiated cells and to influence the function of mature cells (Fig. 59-6). Excellent reviews have been published.[1-3]

Multi-CSF, which is also called interleukin-3 (IL-3), is a small glycoprotein coded for on the long arm of chromosome 5.[4,5] This same region contains the genes coding for granulocyte-macrophage CSF (GM-CSF), M-CSF, the proto-oncogene c-*fms* (which may code for the receptor for M-CSF), and the genes for several other growth factors and their receptors. Deletions of the long arm of chromosome 5 result in myelodysplastic syndromes (*i.e.*, the 5q⁻syndrome).[6] IL-3 stimulates the pleuripotent stem cell to produce the committed multipotential colony-forming units granulocyte, erythrocyte, monocyte, megakaryocyte (CFU-GEMM). It also increases megakaryocyte colony formation, either alone or in concert with the as yet poorly characterized megakaryocytic colony-stimulating activity (MK-CSA). It may also act in concert with other colony-stimulating factors upon committed progenitor cells (*e.g.*, with erythropoietin to produce [BFU-E]). IL-3 is produced by activated T-cells; it is unclear whether IL-3 is produced in small amounts in normal marrow by nonactivated cells.

GM-CSF was named for its ability in vitro to produce colonies of granulocytes and macrophages from pleuripotent lymphoblast-like cells. Purified recombinant human GM-CSF stimulates granulocyte and macrophage colony formation and eosinophil colony formation.[7] Like IL-3, but to a lesser extent, GM-CSF induces multipotential CFU-GEMM colony formation and acts in concert with erythropoietin to induce BFU-E colony formation and with MK-CSA to induce megakaryocyte colony formation.[7-9]

GM-CSF has several effects on mature cells. In granulocytes, GM-CSF inhibits migration, enhances granulocyte adhesion, increases bacterial phagocytosis, and alters surface membrane antigen expression.[10,11] GM-CSF also stimulates peripheral blood monocytes to become cytotoxic for a number of tumor cells.[12] It increases antibody-dependent killing of tumor cells by mature human neutrophils and eosinophils.[7] GM-CSF can be produced by a variety of cells, including T lymphocytes, endothelial cells, and fibroblasts. Both IL-1 and tumor necrosis factor can stimulate the release of GM-CSF, but the exact pathways of normal hematopoietic regulation are uncertain.[13-16]

After in vitro and in vivo tests in primates, in which GM-CSF increased neutrophil and eosinophil counts, GM-CSF was tested in patients with leukopenia due to AIDS, myelodysplasia, chemotherapy, or aplastic anemia (Table 59-19).

In the first 16 patients with AIDS treated with a bolus followed by a 14-day continuous intravenous infusion of GM-CSF, dose-dependent increases in total leukocyte, neutrophil, eosinophil, and monocyte counts were observed.[17] Six hours after the single intravenous bolus, the circulating leukocyte count increased transiently and decreased to baseline levels within 48 hours. With continuous infusion, there was an immediate, rapid increase, followed by a more gradual increase in counts. After discontinuing the infusion, the counts returned to baseline within 3 to 9 days. Although there were several mild toxic effects, it was difficult to link the toxicities to the drug because of the systemic infections in several of the patients. Four of the 16 patients developed phlebitis after the drug was administered by a peripheral vein.

Gutterman and colleagues at M.D. Anderson treated 8 patients who had myelodysplasia in varying degrees of leukemic transformation in a Phase I study of escalating doses of continuous 14-day intravenous infusions of GM-CSF.[18] Over the entire dosage range tested (30 $\mu g/m^2$ to 500 $\mu g/m^2$), all 8

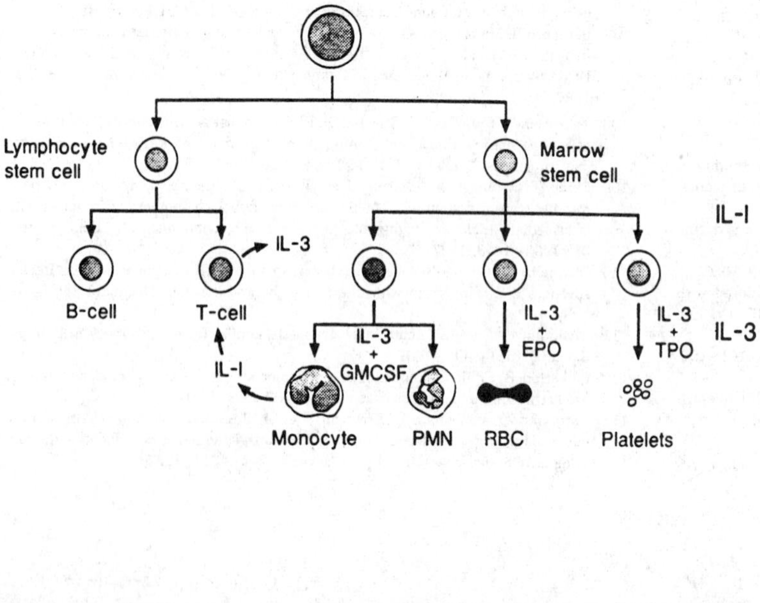

FIG. 59-6. Hematopoiesis of normal marrow. IL-3 acts along with lineage specific factors at the late progenitor stage as well as at the earlier progenitor stage by itself. IL-1 acts, at a much earlier progenitor stage.

TABLE 59-19. Clinical Trials of GM-CSF

Dose Level (Reference)	*Baseline*	*2 Weeks*
	AIDS (17)	
1.3×10^3 units/kg/day [≈7 μg/m^2]		
Leukocytes	1850	4575
Neutrophils	1248	3327
2.6×10^3 (0.15 μg/m^2)		
Leukocytes	2675	8875
Neutrophils	1576	3603
5.2×10^3 (30 μg/m^2)		
Leukocytes	2250	8625
Neutrophils	1555	5209
1.0×10^4 (~60 μg/m^2)		
Leukocytes	2300	15,267
Neutrophils	1592	9095
2.0×10^4 (~120 μg/m^2)		
Leukocytes	1600	48,700
Neutrophils	864	35,064
	Myelodysplasia (18)	
30 μg/m^2		
Leukocytes	1400	7000
Neutrophils	260	4600
60 μg/m^2		
Leukocytes	2100	9500
Neutrophils	965	5950
120 μg/m^2		
Leukocytes	2000	28,750
Neutrophils	830	17,000
250 μg/m^2		
Leukocytes	1750	61,200
Neutrophils	110	37,800
500 μg/m^2		
Leukocytes	1500	106,000
Neutrophils	630	66,800
	Mean Maximum Increase in Neutrophils and Bands (%)	
	Myelodysplasia (19)	
15 μg/m^2 as 1-h infusion × 7 days	42	
30 μg/m^2	156	
60 μg/m^2	190	
	Aplastic Anemia (19)	
15 μg/m^2	61	
30 μg/m^2	96	
60 μg/m^2	127	
	MAID chemotherapy for sarcoma (20)	
	With GM-CSF	*Without*
4 μg/kg/day		
Leukocyte nadir	1400	530
Neutrophil nadir	499	110
8 μg/kg/day		
Leukocyte nadir	1000	400
Neutrophil nadir	200	160
	Autologous bone marrow transplant (21)	
	Mean WBC, Day 14	
Control	804	
2 μg/kg/day	1511	
4 μg/kg/day	1511	
8 μg/kg/day	1511	
16 μg/kg/day	2575	
32 μg/kg/day	3120	

patients developed marked increases in total leukocyte and granulocyte counts. The absolute number of monocytes, eosinophils, and lymphocytes increased as well. Surprisingly, 3 of the 8 patients had a significant increase in platelet count and erythropoiesis, as evidenced by an increase in reticulocyte count and hematocrit and no need for erythrocyte transfusion. No acceleration of the transformation to acute leukemia was observed during the study. Mild or moderate bone pain was the most common side-effect. Two patients who developed marked leukocytosis (96,500/mm^3 and 106,000/mm^3) at the highest dose levels tested (250 μg/m^2 and 500 μg/m^2, respectively) experienced severe bone pain requiring treatment cessation, and they were subsequently retreated at 30 μg/m^2 with minimal toxicity but retained biologic effect.

Antin and colleagues gave 1-hour intravenous infusions of GM-CSF daily for 7 days to 6 patients with severe aplastic anemia and 3 patients with myelodysplasia.[19] Four of 6 aplastic patients and 2 of 3 myelodysplastic patients had at least a doubling of pretreatment neutrophil counts. Neutrophil counts returned to baseline levels in all patients after discontinuing the infusion. A transient decrease in counts during the first few days was seen in 6 patients. Toxicity at these doses was minimal, with transient low-back pain in 2 patients and low-grade fever in 3 patients.

Antman and colleagues studied the ability of GM-CSF to attenuate the neutrophil nadir in 8 adults receiving doxorubicin, ifosfamide with MESNA, and dacarbazine (MAID) for inoperable primary or metastatic sarcoma. Patients initially received a continuous infusion of GM-CSF for 3 to 7 days until the leukocyte count was greater than 20,000/μl.[20] After 1 week off therapy, the combination chemotherapy was given and a GM-CSF infusion was begun and continued through the expected nadir. Cycle 2 of MAID was given without GM-CSF, and the nadirs were compared. GM-CSF infusion resulted in a significantly higher leucocyte ($p = 0.02$) and neutrophil ($p = 0.05$) nadir and fewer days ($p = 0.02$) with less than 500 polymorphonuclear leucocytes/μl.

Brandt and co-workers studied 19 patients undergoing autologous bone marrow transplant for metastatic breast cancer or melanoma.[21] The patients were treated with cyclophosphamide, cisplatin, and carmustine, followed 3 days later with autologous rescue. GM-CSF was given as a continuous infusion for 14 days, starting 3 hours after bone marrow infusion. There was a dose-dependent acceleration in total leukocyte and neutrophil recovery, with significantly increased day 14 counts compared with historical controls. No consistent influence on platelet or reticulocyte counts was observed. Toxicity (*e.g.*, myalgias, rash, edema) was not dose-related at doses of 2 to 16 μg/kg/day, but at 32 μg/kg/day, all patients had edema, weight gain, and myalgias, and 2 patients had capillary leak syndromes. Despite apparent accelerated recovery, counts declined rapidly when the GM-CSF infusion was stopped on day 14.

Limited clinical experience with GM-CSF at doses of 15 to 60 μg/m^2, either as a 1-hour or continuous 24-hour infusion daily for 7 to 14 days, appear to improve the total leukocyte and neutrophil counts in some patients with myelodysplasia and aplastic anemia. These doses appear to be tolerated well, with minimal myalgia and occasional low-grade fever, rash, edema, headache, anorexia, nausea, and phlebitis, if given by peripheral vein. At doses of 250 to 500 μg/m^2/day, severe bone or muscle pain can occur, and at 32 μg/kg/day (*i.e.*, >1000 μg/m^2), a capillary leak syndrome may occur. Doses of 4 to 16 μg/kg/day (140–560 μg/m^2) can attenuate the nadir of myelosuppressive chemotherapy and of accelerating neutrophil recovery after autologous bone marrow transplant.

Baldwin and colleagues reported that small cell carcinoma cell lines specifically bind and respond to GM-CSF in colony growth assays.[22] It has been shown that GM-CSF can stimulate the proliferation of blast cells in acute leukemia.[23,24] Thus, it will be important to assess the effects of GM-CSF and other hematopoietic growth factors on tumor cell lines before routinely applying these factors to attenuate nadirs or accelerate bone marrow recovery after autologous transplantation.

Granulocyte colony-stimulating factor (G-CSF) is a lineage-specific growth factor that causes proliferation of neutrophil colonies from the committed CFU-GEMM and CFU-GM.[25] Like GM-CSF, the G-CSF appears to activate mature neutrophils. The gene coding for G-CSF is located on chromosome 17, and the 15:17 translocation in acute promyelocytic leukemia may affect this gene. Administration of recombinant human G-CSF to normal monkeys increases overall leucocyte count, neutrophil count, and neutrophil function. After Cytoxan or high-dose chemotherapy with bone marrow rescue, monkeys given G-CSF experienced significantly shortened periods of neutropenia.[26]

Gabrilove and co-workers studied the effects of G-CSF on 22 patients with transitional cell carcinoma of the genitourinary tract before MVAC chemotherapy.[27] Doses of G-CSF from 1 to 60 μg/kg were given as a 30-minute intravenous infusion daily for 6 days. At the lowest doses, there was a gradual increase in mature neutrophils, plateauing by day 3 without an increase in the bone marrow M:E ratio or cellularity. At higher doses, the neutrophil count increased rapidly and continued to rise throughout the infusion without reaching a plateau. At these higher doses, there was also a shift to earlier myeloid forms in the peripheral blood, an increase in marrow cellularity and M:E ratio, and the appearance in the peripheral blood of Dohle bodies, toxic granulation, and decreased nuclear lobulation. Eosinophil, basophil, erythocyte, and platelet counts were unchanged. A ten-fold increase in monocytes was noticed at higher doses. After discontinuing the G-CSF, the total leukocyte count and absolute neutrophil count decreased by half within the first 48 hours, returning to normal by 2 to 4 days at the lower doses and by 4 to 7 days at higher doses. Toxicity was mild, consisting primarily of bone pain in the low back, sternum, and pelvis.

The study evaluated the ability of G-CSF to attenuate the MVAC chemotherapy-induced grannlocyte nadir in 24 patients with transitional cell carcinoma.[28] Eighteen of the 24 were chosen from the original study of 22 with G-CSF alone, and they received G-CSF in doses from 3 to 160 μg/kg/day as a half-hour intravenous infusion on days 4 through 11 with methotrexate (30 mg/m^2) on days 1, 14, and 21; doxorubicin (30 mg/m^2) on day 2; vinblastine (3 mg/m^2) on days 2, 14, and 21; and cisplatin (70 mg/m^2) on day 2. During the second cycle of MVAC, G-CSF was not given. Six patients not previously tested with G-CSF received MVAC alone for their first cycle and MVAC with G-CSF during their second cycle. In 12 (67%) of 18 patients receiving G-CSF, the absolute neutrophil count never fell below 1000. Four of the 18 who experienced neutrophil nadirs below 1000 had received prior pelvic irradiation. In fact, 2 of these 4 patients experienced lower nadirs during cycle 1 with G-CSF than during cycle 2 without G-CSF.

For all of the patients receiving G-CSF, the pattern of fall of total leucocytes and neutrophils was altered. Without G-CSF, counts declined slowly, starting about day 7, with a nadir about day 14. With G-CSF, starting day 4, the counts increased on day 5 and then declined sharply to nadir on day 9 or 10; counts returned to normal by day 12. Thus, 100% of the G-CSF treated patients were able to receive day 14 chemotherapy, compared with only 29% of the controls. The G-CSF-treated patients had 91% fewer days with less than 1000 neutrophils than the controls. There was a significant decrease in the incidence of mucositis during the first cycle of MVAC in the G-CSF-treated patients (2 of 18), compared with controls (3 of 6), due to decreased neutropenia or possibly an effect of G-CSF on the oral epithelium.

This preliminary experience is quite encouraging for the ability of G-CSF to diminish and shorten the neutrophil nadir and accelerate recovery following chemotherapy. There was no effect on erythrocyte or platelet counts, and toxicity was mild and consisted of bone pain in 3 of 18 patients. The biphasic neutrophil response seen in all patients and exaggerated in those receiving prior pelvic irradiation may be due to the ability of G-CSF to increase marrow cellularity and M:E ratio and to accelerate marrow release. If the G-CSF continued to cause accelerated release when chemotherapy was causing a decline in the myeloid progenitors upon which G-CSF acts, a transient depletion of mature marrow myeloid cells could develop, which would be expressed as an earlier nadir, possibly exaggerated by stem cell depletion due to irradiation. This somewhat unexpected clinical finding serves to emphasize the importance of continued well-designed clinical trials to refine the optimal use of these exciting new agents.

Recombinant human M-CSF is perhaps the least-well characterized of the colony-stimulating factors. Although human M-CSF can stimulate murine macrophage colony formation, it has been less active in human tissue culture. However, it appears to be a potentiator of human macrophage cytotoxicity, and there is a great deal of interest in using M-CSF or GM-CSF to stimulate macrophage tumoricidal activity, possibly in association with monoclonal antibodies or immunotoxin. The protein that functions as the receptor for M-CSF is the product of the c-*fms* proto-oncogene. Because this protein exhibits tyrosine kinase activity, which is known to regulate cell function, it is possible that overexpression of the c-*fms* oncogene protein renders the cell more sensitive to growth factors or that production of an altered protein allows cell proliferation to occur in the absence of a regulatory growth factor.

Although the existence of erythropoietin has been known for some time, quantities isolated from plasma and urine have never permitted clinical trials. The isolation and purification in 1977 of erythropoietin led to the generation of DNA probes to isolate the erythropoietin gene. Erythropoietin has 166 amino acids, with a molecular weight between 34,000 and 39,000 daltons and with heavy glycosylation. The gene has been localized to chromosome 7q11-q22.

The recombinant and the natural erythropoietins stimulate the proliferation of mature BFU-E and the proliferation and terminal differentiation of CFU-E. Human recombinant erythropoietin must be generated in animal cells, rather than in bacteria, because heavy glycosylation is necessary for function.

In patients with end-stage renal disease on dialysis three times a week, recombinant erythropoietin produces a dose-dependent rise in hemoglobin.[29,30] Increases in the hematocrit by as much as 10% in 3 weeks are possible, and the majority of patients who previously had been transfusion-dependent no longer needed them.

There were a few complications of erythropoietin treatment. Most are probably related to the efficacy of the treatment rather than the toxicity of the agent itself. A number of patients experienced a rise in blood pressure as the hemoglobin increased. In addition, predialysis creatinine, blood urea, nitrogen, and potassium levels increased as the hemoglobin increased. This was attributed to decreased dialysis clearances and increased food intake. Hyperkalemia was fatal in one patient. Several patients developed iron deficiency, which caused a plateauing of the effect of erythropoietin. Additional therapeutic benefit of erythropoietin was observed after iron replacement.

Six patients who initially had a serum ferritin levels between 2000 and 5700 ng/ml had a significant decrease in their ferritin levels (approximately 90 ng/ml/week). It has been suggested that erythropoietin could be used to increase the efficacy of phlebotomy in the treatment of hemochromatosis. In another study, an improved sense of well-being, including increased exercise tolerance, was described by 9 of 10 patients with end-stage renal disease on dialysis after treatment with erythropoietin. Four patients, however, experienced several episodes of aching in the limbs and pelvis 2 hours after injections of erythropoietin, which was accompanied by a feeling of cold and then sweating, but no fever. The episodes lasted no longer than 12 hours and were not regarded as significant toxic effects by the patients. After ending the erythropoietin, the hemoglobin returned to pretreatment values within 3 weeks.

Multi-CSF or IL-3 appears to be necessary for the erythropoietin-induced generation of BFU-E from the CFU-GEMM.

Means and colleagues treated two anemic patients with rheumatoid arthritis with erythropoietin in intravenous doses of 100 to 200 units/kg 3 times a week for 5 months.[31] Both patients showed increases in hematocrit (27–43% and 30–39%), suggesting that erythropoietin may correct some cases of anemia of chronic disease.

The availability of purified recombinant human hematopoietic growth factors undoubtedly opens an exciting chapter in clinical investigation. Multi-CSF, GM-CSF, and G-CSF are already undergoing trials in humans for their ability to shorten the leukocyte nadir from chemotherapy. If this is successful, it will probably lead to trials of increased chemotherapeutic doses as myelosuppression ceases to be the dose-limiting toxicity. These agents may shorten the duration of pancytopenia after autologous and allogeneic bone marrow transplantation. Because infection is the major cause of death with these procedures, if the colony-stimulating factors are successful, increased use of these procedures may follow.

Because continuous GM-CSF appears to be necessary and because phlebitis is associated with the peripheral venous route of administration, it is likely that these agents will be tried by intermittent or continuous subcutaneous injection. GM-CSF and M-CSF will undoubtedly be tried to augment cell-mediated cytotoxicity and antibody-dependent, cell-mediated tumor cell killing, either alone or in association with chemotherapy or monoclonal antibodies conjugated to immunotoxins, chemotherapeutic agents, or isotopes. Erythropoietin already seems to be highly effective in improving the quality of life of patients on renal dialysis. It may also broaden the applicability of autologous erythrocyte transfusion preoperatively by decreasing the time during which the blood can be donated. Erythropoietin may be able to correct the anemia seen in patients with malignancies.

The clinical use of these agents may result in observations that will generate new ideas about the mechanisms by which alterations of growth factors and their receptors function in hematologic and solid tumor malignancies.

REFERENCES

1. Sieff CA: Hematopoietic growth factors. J Clin Invest 79:1549–1557, 1987
2. Clark SC, Kamen R: The human hematopoietic colony-stimulating factors. Science 236:1229–1237, 1987
3. Metcalf D: The granulocyte-macrophage colony-stimulating factors. Science 229:16–22, 1985
4. Welte KE, Platzer E, Lu L, et al: Purification and biochemical characterization of human pleuripotent hematopoietic colony-stimulating factor. Proc Natl Acad Sci USA 82:1526–1530, 1985
5. Yang Y, Ciarletta AB, Temple PA et al: Human IL-3 (multi-CSF): Identification by expression cloning of a novel hematopoietic growth factor related to murine H-3. Cell 47:3–10, 1986
6. LeBeau MM, Westbrook CA, Diaz MO et al: Evidence for the involvement of GM-CSF and FMS in the deletion (5q) in myeloid disorders. Science 231:984–987, 1986
7. Metcalf D, Begley CG, John GR et al: Biologic properties in vitro of a recombinant human granulocyte-macrophage colony-stimulating factor. Blood 67:37–45, 1986
8. Emerson SG, Wang YC, Clark SC et al: Human recombinant IL-3 and GM-CSF have distinct but overlapping hematopoietic activities. Blood (Suppl) 70:171a, 1987
9. Dessypris EN, Armstrong OL: Effects of recombinant human granulocyte-macrophage colony stimulating factor on the growth of human megakaryocyte colony forming units in vitro. Blood (Suppl) 70:170a, 1987
10. Arnaout MA, Wang EA, Clark SC et al: Human recombinant granulocyte-macrophage colony-stimulating factor increases cell-to-cell adhesion and surface expression of adhesion-promoting surface glycoproteins on mature granulocytes. J Clin Invest 78:597–601, 1986
11. Fleischmann J, Golde DW, Weisbart RH et al: Granulocyte-macrophage colony-stimulating factor enhances phagocytosis of bacteria by human neutrophils. Blood 86:708–711, 1986
12. Grabstein KH, Urdal DL, Tushiniski RJ et al: Induction of macrophage tumoricidal activity by granulocyte-macrophage colony-stimulating factor. Science 232:506–508, 1986
13. Zsebo K, Yuschenkoff VN, Schiffer S et al: Vascular endothelial cells and granulopoiesis: Interleukin-1 stimulates release of G-CSF and GM-CSF. Blood 70:99–103, 1988
14. Fibbe WE, van Damme J, Billiau A et al: Interleukin 1 induces human marrow stromal cells in long-term culture to produce granulocyte colony-stimulating factor and macrophage colony-stimulating factor. Blood 70:430–435, 1988
15. Munker R, Gasson J, Ogawa M et al: Recombinant human TNF induces production of granulocyte-monocyte colony-stimulating factor. Nature 323:79, 1986
16. Broudy VC, Kaushansky K, Segal GM et al: Tumor necrosis factor type alpha stimulates human endothelial cells to produce granulocyte/macrophage colony-stimulating factor. Proc Natl Acad Sci USA 83:7467, 1986
17. Groopman JE, Mitsuyasu RT, DeLeo MJ et al: Effect of recombinant human granulocyte-macrophage colony-stimulating factor on myelopoiesis in the acquired immunodeficiency syndrome. N Engl J Med 317:593–598, 1987
18. Vadhan-Raj S, Keating M, LeMaistre A et al: Effects of recombinant human granulocyte-macrophage colony-stimulating factor in patients with myelodysplastic syndromes. N Engl J Med 317:1545–1552, 1987
19. Antin JH, Smith BR, Rosenthal DS et al: Phase I/II study of recombinant human granulocyte-macrophage colony-stimulating factor (GM-CSF) in bone marrow failure. Blood (Suppl) 70:129a, 1987
20. Antman K, Griffin J, Elias A et al: Use of rGM-CSF to ameliorate chemotherapy induced myelosuppression in sarcoma patients. Blood (Suppl) 70:129a, 1987
21. Brandt SJ, Kurtzberg J, Atwater SK et al: Effect of recombinant human granulocyte-macrophage colony-stimulating factor (rHuGM-CSF) on hematopoietic reconstitution following high-dose chemotherapy and autologous bone marrow transplantation (ABMT). Blood (Suppl) 70:131a, 1987
22. Baldwin GC, DiPersio J, Kaufman SE et al: Characterization of human GM-CSF receptors on nonhematopoietic cells. Blood (Suppl) 70:166a, 1987
23. Griffin JD, Young D, Herrmann F et al. Effects of recombinant human GM-CSF on proliferation of clonogenic cells in acute myeloblastic leukemia. Blood 67:1448–1453, 1986
24. Miyauchi J, Kelleher CA, Yang YC et al: The effects of three recombinant growth factors, IL-3, GM-CSF, and G-CSF, on the blast cells of acute myeloblastic leukemia maintained in short-term suspension culture. Blood 70:657–663, 1987
25. Souza LM, Boone TC, Gabrilove J et al. Recombinant human granulocyte colony-stimulating factor; effects on normal and leukemia myeloid cells. Science 232:61–65, 1986
26. Welte K, Bonilla MA, Gillio AP et al: Recombinant human granulocyte colony-stimulating factor. Effects on hematopoiesis in normal and cyclophosphamide-treated primates. J Exp Med 165:941–948, 1987
27. Gabrilove J, Jakubowski A, Fain K et al: A study of recombinant granulocyte colony-stimulating factor in patients with transitional cell carcinoma (submitted, NEJAM)
28. Gabrilove JL, Jakubowski A, Scher H et al: A study of recombinant human granulocyte colony-stimulating factor in cancer patients at risk for chemotherapy-induced neutropenia. N Engl J Med (in press)
29. Eschbach JW, Egrie JC, Downing MR et al: Correction of the anemia of end-stage renal disease with recombinant human erythropoietin. N Engl J Med 316:73–78, 1987
30. Winearls CG, Oliver DO, Pippard MJ et al: Effect of human erythropoietin derived from recombinant DNA on the anaemia of patients maintained by chronic haemodialysis. Lancet 2:8517, 1986
31. Means RT, Olsen NJ, Krantz SB et al: Treatment of the anemia of rheumatoid arthritis with recombinant human erythropoietin: Clinical and in vitro results. Blood (Suppl) 70:139a, 1987

SECTION 4

KATHLEEN M. FOLEY
EHUD ARBIT

Management of Cancer Pain

For the patient with cancer, pain is one of the most feared consequences.[1] For the clinician, pain is a difficult diagnostic and therapeutic medical problem. Advances in the diagnosis and treatment of cancer, coupled with recent advances in our understanding of the anatomy, physiology, pharmacology, and psychology of pain perception, have led to improved care of the patient with pain of malignant origin.[2] Specialized methods of cancer diagnosis and treatment provide the most direct approach to treating cancer pain by treating the cause of the pain. However, if treatment of the cause of the pain has failed or if injury to bone, soft tissue, or nerve has occurred as a result of therapy, appropriate management of pain is essential.[3] Patients with cancer are managed most effectively with a multidisciplinary approach that includes the expertise of a wide range of medical personnel.[4]

The goal of pain therapy for patients receiving active treatment is to provide them with sufficient relief to tolerate the diagnostic and therapeutic approaches required to treat their cancer. For patients with advanced disease, pain control should allow them to function at a level they choose and to die relatively free of pain. Critical to the management of cancer pain is establishing a trusting relationship between the patient and physician, who respects the pain complaint.

EPIDEMIOLOGY

Although large-scale national epidemiologic studies of the incidence and severity of cancer pain are lacking, existing studies suggest that moderate or severe pain is experienced by a third of cancer patients receiving active therapy and by 60% to 90% of patients with advanced cancer. These data have been generated from several surveys of small groups of patients in specific medical care settings and provide a biased view of the problem.[5-14] Patients with cancer frequently have many causes of pain, and 15% of patients with nonmetastastic cancer have pain.[15,16] From data collected by the Cancer Unit of the World Health Organization (WHO), it is postulated that 25% of all patients with cancer throughout the world die without relief from severe pain.[17] To remedy this situation and as part of a broader cancer program, WHO has formulated a Cancer Pain Relief Program to conduct epidemiologic studies of cancer pain in developed and developing countries, to provide guidelines for pain management, particularly in patients with advanced disease, and to encourage national governments to make therapeutic approaches, specifically oral opioid therapy available.[18,19]

DEFINITION OF PAIN

For this discussion, the definition of pain proposed by the International Association for the Study of Pain is "an unpleasant sensory and emotional experience associated with actual or potential tissue damage or described in terms of such damage."[20] Pain is always subjective. There is no definitive way to distinguish pain occurring without tissue damage from pain resulting from damaged tissue. Pain as a somatic delusion or a masked depression is very rare in cancer patients, and it usually implies a pathologic process.

MODULATION OF PAIN

Extensive investigations during the last 17 years have refined and expanded our knowledge of ascending and descending central nervous system pathways that process and modulate nociceptive information. These advances in pain research provide a scientific rationale for the use of new and improved methods of treatment.[21,22] A brief review of pain modulation provides a background for the later descriptions of specific drug, anesthetic, and neurosurgical approaches.

Pain results from the activation of peripheral receptors by mechanical and chemical stimuli that excite afferent discharges in two types of nerve fibers: thinly myelinated A-delta fibers and unmyelinated C fibers. These primary sensory afferents have their cell bodies in the dorsal root ganglion, and their axons enter the spinal cord by way of the dorsal root. They ascend or descend from one or two segments in Lissauer's tracts and synapse in specific lamina in the dorsal horn.

The dorsal horn is an important site for modulating sensory input. Several ascending pathways arise from second-order neurons and decussate in the central gray spinal cord to become the neospinothalamic and paleospinothalamic tracts. These tracts project to discrete regions of the thalamus and cortex. The neospinothalamic pathways subserve pain intensity and localization, and the phylogenetically older paleospinothalamic pathways subserve the arousal and emotional components of pain. Descending pathways, the most important of which originate from the periaqueductal gray nuclei of the midbrain, synapse in the raphae magnus nucleus of the medulla. From this nucleus, a medial pathway, the dorsal longitudinal fasciculus, projects to the dorsal horn to modulate pain transmission. This pathway represents an important descending inhibitory pathway. There is a more laterally placed descending pathway from the locus ceruleus to dorsal horn, which also plays a role in pain modulation at the spinal cord level.

Neurotransmitters play a significant role in this modulatory system. Dopamine, serotonin, norepinephrine, and the endogenous opioid peptides (*i.e.*, enkephalin, beta-endorphin, and dynorphin) modulate pain at spinal and supraspinal sites. Attempts to enhance and mimic the role of these neurotransmitters in pain modulation have led to a series of clinical analgesic studies of amitriptyline and other adjuvant drugs. Amitriptyline has analgesic properties independent of its antidepressant effects.[23,24] It appears to work by enhancing serotonin activity centrally by presynaptic inhibition of its reuptake and by activation of the descending inhibitory pain system.

Opiate receptors, stereospecific binding sites on the end of free nerve endings that bind endogenous and exogenous opioids, are localized in the ascending and descending pain pathways. These receptors mediate the multiple pharmacologic effects of the opioid analgesics. Subpopulations of opioid receptors, including high-affinity and low-affinity mu receptors and delta, kappa, sigma, and epsilon receptors, are the subjects of intense investigation.[25] The identification of subclasses of receptors that mediate different pharmacologic effects and that are located in specific cerebral and spinal sites offers the possibility of developing new analgesics targeted for specific receptors. The periaqueductal gray (PAG) region in the midbrain and the dorsal horn in the spinal cord are rich in opioid receptors and represent the supraspinal and spinal sites that mediate opioid analgesia. Identification of these areas as selective sites of analgesia has resulted from studies in animals and humans that showed that electric stimulation in the PAG region produces total-body analgesia, without motor or sensory changes. Administration of opioids directly into the PAG region inhibits pain transmission at the level of the spinal cord by activating this medial descending inhibitory pathway. The use of brain-stem stimulation and the administration of the opioid analgesics directly into the cerebrospinal fluid bathing these selective sites in animals and cancer patients with pain are procedures based on this research. Pain transmission at the spinal cord level can be inhibited by the direct application of morphine, and these studies have led to the use of spinal opioid analgesia in clinical pain states.[26,27] These advances in our understanding of pain modulatory systems and their neuropharmacologic correlates have had a major impact on the management of patients with pain.

DIFFERENT TYPES OF PAIN

Cancer patients have both acute and chronic pain. This division is based on an understanding of pain mechanisms and on the recognition that the central modulation for these types of pain may be different and that the clinical management of and response to treatment is different.

Acute pain is characterized by a well-defined temporal pattern of pain onset, generally associated with subjective and objective physical signs and with hyperactivity of the autonomic nervous system. These signs provide the physician with objective evidence that substantiates the patient's complaint of pain. Acute pain is usually self-limited and responds to treatment with analgesic drug therapy and to treatment of its precipitating cause.

Chronic pain is the persistence of pain for more than 3 months, with a less-well-defined temporal onset. Adaptation of the autonomic nervous system occurs, and chronic pain patients lack the objective signs common to acute pain. Chronic pain leads to significant changes in personality, lifestyle, and functional ability: These patients require a management approach that encompasses the treatment of the cause of the pain and the treatment of the complications affecting their functional status, their social lives, and their personalities.[28] It is this particular group of patients that challenges physicians in the management of pain. It is also this group of patients that colors physicians' attitudes toward the management of acute pain problems. Treatment of chronic pain in the cancer patient is especially challenging, because it requires careful assessment of the intensity of the pain and the degree of suffering characterized by changes in mood.[29]

PATHOPHYSIOLOGIC MECHANISMS OF PAIN

The pathophysiologic mechanisms of cancer pain include a series of neurophysiologic and neuropharmacologic changes that occur in the peripheral and central nervous system.[22] Three categories of pain have been described, based on physiologic mechanisms. These are somatic, visceral, and deafferentation pain. Common to each of these categories is the fact that they result from either activation and sensitization of nociceptors and mechanoreceptors in the periphery by mechanical (*e.g.*, tumor compression or infiltration) and chemical (*e.g.*, epinephrine, serotonin, bradykinin, prostagladins, histamine) stimuli. When nociceptors are activated in cutaneous or deep tissues, somatic pain results and is typically characterized as dull, or aching, but well localized. Metastatic bone pain, postsurgical incision pain, and myofascial and musculoskeletal pain are common examples of somatic pain.

Visceral pain results from activation of nociceptors caused by infiltration, compression, distention, or stretching of thoracic and abdominal viscera, as typically occurs with bone metastases and pancreatic cancer. This type of pain is poorly localized, often described as deep squeezing and pressure-like, and when acute, it is associated with significant autonomic dysfunction, including nausea, vomiting, and diaphoresis. Visceral pain is often referred to cutaneous sites that may be remote from the site of the lesion (*e.g.*, shoulder pain with diaphragmatic irritation) and may be associated with tenderness in the referred cutaneous site.

Deafferentation pain results from injury to the peripheral and or central nervous system as a consequence of tumor compression, infiltration of peripheral nerves or the spinal cord, or the trauma or chemical injury to peripheral nerves caused by surgery, irradiation, or chemotherapy for cancer. Examples include metastatic or radiation-induced brachial and lumbosacral plexopathies, postherpetic neuralgia, and vincristine or cisplatin neuropathy. Pain from nerve injury is often severe and described as burning or dysesthetic with a vise-like quality, and it is often referred to as causalgic pain. Intermittently, patients complain of paroxysms of burning or electric shock-like sensations.

These different categories of pain may occur in the same patient and account for differences in responses to drug and nondrug approaches. For example, the nonsteroidal anti-inflammatory drugs reduce the chemical activation of nociceptors peripherally (*e.g.*, bone pain), but anesthetic approaches suppress pain transmission in the peripheral nerves. Management of the deafferentation component of cancer pain is the most challenging, and treatment approaches are only partially effective.

CLASSIFICATION OF PATIENTS WITH PAIN

Five different types of patients with cancer pain can be identified (Table 59-20).[3] Although these categories are artificial, they serve as a useful preamble for discussion of the specific therapeutic approaches to the management of patients with cancer pain.

Group I: Acute Cancer-Related Pain

Group I includes patients with acute cancer-related pain. This group can be subdivided further according to the cause of the pain.

GROUP IA: TUMOR-ASSOCIATED PAIN. Group IA includes patients with tumor-associated pain. For these patients, pain is the major symptom prompting medical consultation and the diagnosis of cancer. In addition, pain has a

TABLE 59-20. Types of Patients with Pain from Cancer

Patients with acute cancer-related pain
Associated with the diagnosis of cancer
Associated with surgery, chemotherapy, or irradiation
Patients with chronic cancer-related pain
Associated with cancer progression
Associated with surgery, chemotherapy, or irradiation
Patients with preexisting chronic pain and cancer-related pain
Patients with a history of drug addiction and cancer-related pain
Actively involved in illicit drug use
In methadone maintenance program
With a history of drug abuse
Dying patients with cancer-related pain

special significance as the harbinger of their illness. Recurrent pain during the course of the illness or after successful therapy has the immediate implication of recurrent disease. Defining the cause of the pain may be a diagnostic problem, but effective treatment of its cause (*e.g.*, radiation therapy for bone metastases) usually is associated with dramatic pain relief in most patients.

GROUP IB: PAIN ASSOCIATED WITH CANCER THERAPY. In the second group of patients with acute cancer-related pain, the pain is associated with the cancer therapy. These are patients with postoperative pain (*e.g.*, pain caused by oral ulceration from chemotherapy or myalgias secondary to steroid withdrawal). The cause of the pain is readily identifiable, and its course is predictable and self-limiting. These patients do not represent difficult diagnostic problems. Pain treatment directed at the cause of the pain is used to manage the transient symptoms. These patients endure significant pain for the promise of a successful outcome.

Group II: Chronic Cancer-Related Pain

Group II comprises patients with chronic cancer-related pain. In contrast to patients with acute pain, these patients represent difficult diagnostic and therapeutic problems. They can be divided into two groups: patients with chronic pain from tumor progression and patients with chronic pain related to cancer treatment. Both of these groups share the characteristic of pain that has persisted for more than 3 months.

GROUP IIA: CHRONIC PAIN FROM TUMOR PROGRESSION. In patients with chronic pain associated with progression of disease (*e.g.*, patients with carcinoma of the pancreas, metastatic melanoma to bone, or Pancoast syndrome), the pain escalates in intensity after tumor infiltration of adjacent bone, nerve, or soft tissue. Combinations of antitumor therapy, analgesic drug therapy, anesthetic blocks, and behavioral approaches to pain control are all applied with varying degrees of success. Psychological factors play a significant role in this group of patients, in whom palliative therapy may be of little value and is physically debilitating. The sense of hopelessness and fear of impending death may exaggerate the pain complaint. Pain then becomes an aspect of the global "suffering" component. Identifying both the pain and the suffering component is essential to developing adequate therapy for this group of patients. The chronicity of the pain is associated with a series of psychological symptoms and signs, including disturbances in sleep, reduction in appetite, impaired concentration, or irritability, mimicking a depressive disorder. This syndrome has been well-described in patients with chronic nonmalignant pain.[28] Management must be directed at controlling the pain, recognizing that antitumor therapy has failed. Analgesic therapy combined with a wide range of alternative approaches is necessary to provide adequate analgesia.

GROUP IIB: CHRONIC PAIN ASSOCIATED WITH CANCER THERAPY. Group IIB includes patients with chronic pain associated with cancer therapy (*e.g.*, patients who develop pain after mastectomy, limb amputation, or thoracotomy). The pain in this group of patients is caused by nerve injury, with the development of a traumatic neuroma. Treatment of the pain for this group of patients is limited by the lack of available methods to remove the cause of the pain. Treatment is directed at the symptoms, not at the cause. This group of patients closely parallels those in the general population with chronic, intractable pain syndromes.

Psychological factors play a significant role in how these patients adapt to and function with chronic pain. Identification of the cause of the pain as not directly related to tumor markedly alters the patient's therapy, prognosis, and psychological state. Each of the primary modalities of cancer therapy is associated with a series of specific chronic pain syndromes with characteristic pain patterns and clinical presentations (Table 59-21). Although it is consoling to the patient and the physician to realize that the pain does not represent recurrent or progressive disease, the persistence of the pain is a constant reminder of the previous diagnosis of cancer. All approaches aimed at maintaining the functional status of the patient should be used. Alternative methods of therapy represent the major management approach. This group of patients is increasing in number and accounts for 25% of patients referred to a medical pain clinic.[30]

Group III: Preexisting Chronic Pain and Cancer-Related Pain

Group III includes those patients with a history of chronic, nonmalignant pain who develop cancer pain. Psychological factors play a significant role in this group of patients, whose psychological and functional status is already compromised by their chronic nonmalignant pain.[28] These patients are at high risk for developing additional functional incapacity and escalating chronic pain symptoms. However, their history should not be used in a punitive way to minimize or deny their complaints. Identifying this group of patients as a high-risk group improves their psychological assessment and intervention.

Group IV: Patient with History of Drug Addiction and Pain

Group IV includes patients with a history of drug addiction who have cancer-related pain. Three subgroups can be identified: patients actively involved in illicit drug use and drug-seeking behavior; those receiving methadone in a maintenance program; and those who have not used drugs for several years. Undertreatment with analgesic drugs occurs most commonly in this group of patients. Assessment of reported pain by physicians and nurses is colored by the fact that the pain symptoms are confused with drug-seeking behavior. Attention to the medical and psychological needs of these patients requires individualized assessment and consultation with experts in drug-related problems. The first subgroup represents a major management problem, straining the most tolerant of medical care systems. Pain in the other two subgroups is readily managed, with the recognition that the psychological stresses from the pain and cancer may place the patient at high risk for recidivism.

TABLE 59-21. Pain Syndromes in Patients with Cancer

Pain Syndromes	*Reference*
Pain Associated with Direct Tumor Involvement	
Tumor infiltration of bone	
Metastases to the cranial vault	44
Metastases to the base of skull	45
Jugular foramen syndrome	
Clivus metastases	
Sphenoid sinus metastases	
Vertebral body syndromes	38,46
Fracture of the odontoid	47
C7–T1 metastases	32
L1 metastases	48
Sacral syndrome	49
Tumor infiltration of nerve	
Peripheral nerve	
Peripheral neuropathy	35
Intercostal neuropathy	35
Plexus	
Brachial plexopathy	36,50
Lumbosacral plexopathy	48,49,51
Root	
Radiculopathy	38
Leptomeningeal metastases	52
Spinal cord	
Epidural spinal cord compression	38,46
Brain	
Intracranial metastases	44
Postsurgical Pain Syndromes	
Acute	
Postoperative pain	
Chronic	
Post-thoracotomy syndrome	43
Postmastectomy syndrome	42
Postradical neck syndrome	35
Phantom limb syndrome	53
Postchemotherapy Pain Syndromes	
Acute	
Oral mucositis	54
Bladder spasms	55
Chronic	
Peripheral neuropathy	56
Aseptic necrosis of the femoral head	57
Steroid pseudo rheumatism	58
Postherpetic neuralgia	24,59
Postradiation Pain Syndromes	
Acute	
Oral mucositis, esophagitis	60
Skin burns	60
Chronic	
Radiation fibrosis of brachial and lumbar plexus	36,51
Radiation myelopathy	61
Radiation-induced second primary tumor	62,63

Group V: Dying Patients with Pain

In Group V patients, diagnostic and therapeutic considerations are directed at maintaining the comfort of the patient. This group is identified separately from Group II patients, because the psycholcgical factors compound adequate pain management. The issues of hopelessness, death, and dying become more prominent, and the suffering component must be addressed.

Inadequate control of pain in the dying patient exacerbates the suffering component and demoralizes the family and the caregivers who feel that they have failed in treating the patient's pain at a time when adequate treatment may have mattered most. Rapid escalation of analgesic drug therapy, usually by the intravenous route, and attempts to ameliorate the psychological symptoms should be made.

The risk-to-benefit ratios in analgesic approaches become less of an issue when the goal of pain therapy is the comfort of the patient. These patients emphasize the need to understand the temporal setting of pain in assessing the indication for and usefulness of various therapeutic approaches.

MEASUREMENT OF CANCER PAIN

To measure clinical pain appropriately, it is necessary to measure separately three related dimensions: pain intensity, pain relief, and psychological distress. Although these dimensions are not usually distinguished by patients as aspects of their global pain experience, they are independent subjective judgements that interact in a complex way to determine the experience and expression of cancer pain. A wide variety of assessment instruments have been developed but have not been used clinically.

To provide a simple, efficient, and valid assessment instrument to rapidly evaluate the major aspects of the pain experienced by cancer patients, the Memorial Pain Assessment Card (MPAC) has been introduced for use in clinical trials.[29] The card is a simple self-rating instrument. On this 8.5-inch by 11-inch card are printed a verbal pain rating scale and three visual analogue scales that measure pain intensity, pain relief, and mood (Fig. 59-7). Experienced patients can complete the MPAC in less than 20 seconds with very little effort, and it can be administered as often as necessary to obtain an ongoing record of the patient's response to therapy. The particular combination and arrangement of scales as presented together on the MPAC can provide rapid and valid multidimensional assessment of pain in cancer patients. This assessment can be practically equivalent to the assessment provided by a combination of lengthy and more sophisticated instruments. The MPAC facilitates communications about pain and suffering and provides the clinician with a simple tool to assess pain symptoms.

COMMON PAIN SYNDROMES

Careful analysis of patients with cancer and pain reveals a series of relatively common, specific pain syndromes unique to this disease process that are often misdiagnosed because they are unfamiliar to general physicians. The pain syndromes that occur in patients with cancer can be divided into three major categories. A detailed discussion of these syndromes is beyond the scope of this chapter but appropriate references are cited in Table 59-21.

Pain Associated with Direct Tumor Involvement

The first and most important category is pain associated with direct tumor involvement. Seventy-eight percent of persons in an inpatient cancer pain population and 65% in an outpatient pain clinic were in this category.[6,30] Metastatic bone

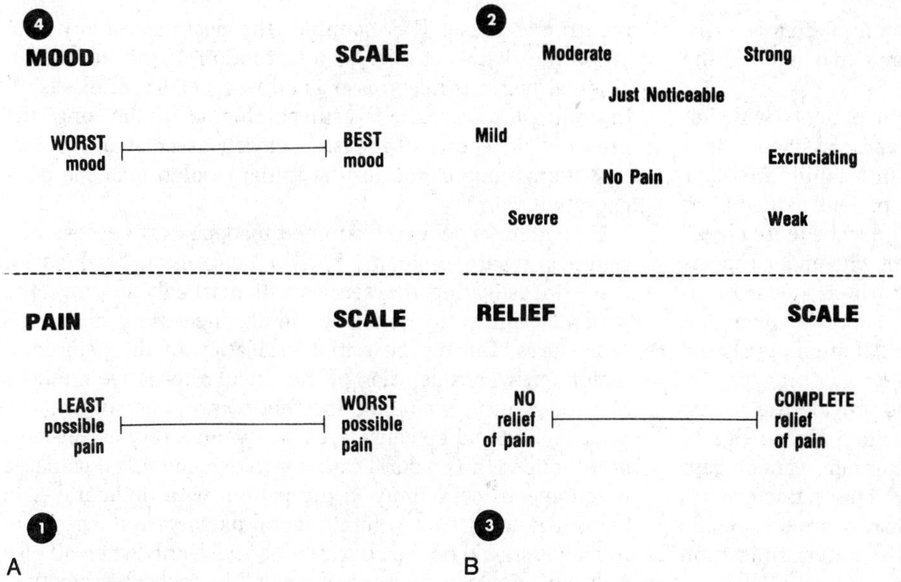

FIG. 59-7. Front (*1* and *4*) and back (*2* and *3*) sides of the Memorial Pain Assessment Card. The card is folded along the broken line, and each measure is presented to the patient separately, in the numbered order: (1) Visual Analog Scale (VAS) Pain Intensity; (2) Modified Tursky Pain Descriptors Scale; (3) VAS Pain Relief; (4) VAS Mood. (Fishman B, Pasternak S, Wallenstein SL, et al: The Memorial Pain Assessment Card: A valid instrument for the evaluation of cancer pain. Cancer 60:1151–1158, 1987)

disease, nerve compression or infiltration, and hollow viscus involvement are the most common causes of pain from direct tumor involvement.

Pain Associated with Cancer Therapy

The second category includes those pain syndromes associated with cancer therapy. Approximately 19% of patients in an inpatient population and 25% of those in an outpatient population belonged to this group.[6,30] The group includes those patients in whom pain occurred during the therapeutic course or as a result of chemotherapy, surgery, or radiation therapy. Each of these primary therapy modalities is associated with a series of specific pain syndromes with characteristic pain patterns and clinical presentations.

Pain Unrelated to the Cancer or the Cancer Therapy

The third major category of pain syndromes includes those unrelated to the cancer and the cancer therapy. Approximately 3% of inpatients have pain unrelated to their cancer or cancer therapy; this figure increases to 10% in outpatient cancer populations.[6,30] Accurate diagnosis in this group of patients clearly alters both therapy and prognosis.

CLINICAL ASSESSMENT OF PAIN

Certain general principles should be adhered to in evaluating all cancer patients who complain of pain. Lack of attention to these general principles, listed below, is the major cause for misdiagnosis of a specific pain syndrome.

- Believe the patient's complaint
- Take a careful history
- Assess the psychosocial status of the patient
- Perform a careful medical and neurologic examination
- Evaluate the patient's extent of disease
- Treat the pain to facilitate the diagnostic workup
- Consider alternative methods of pain control during the initial evaluation
- Reassess the pain complaint during the prescribed therapy
- Use pain measurement scales

Critical to the management of the patient with cancer pain is the establishment of a trusting relationship with the physician. The complaint of pain is a symptom, not a diagnosis. Pain perception is not simply a function of the amount of physical injury sustained by the patient, but a complex state determined by many factors, including age, sex, cultural and environmental influences, medical history, and psychological factors.

In patients with cancer, the diagnosis is not always made in the initial examination. It may take several weeks to define its nature without radiologic or pathologic verification. Superior sulcus tumor of the lung (Pancoast) is a clear example in which the reason for the pain in the majority of patients is not diagnosed for 6 to 8 months, dramatically altering the prognosis.[32]

There is no substitute for a complete history of the pain complaint. This should include the patient's description of the site of pain, its quality, exacerbating and relieving factors, temporal pattern, exact onset and associated circumstances, interference with activities of daily living, and psychological factors. The history should also include the patient's psychiatric history, current level of anxiety or depression, suicidal ideation, and degree of functional incapacity.

Several studies support the significance of psychological factors in accounting for differences in pain experiences in patients with cancer. A series of psychiatric syndromes have been described in patients with cancer, with depression occurring in as many as 25% of patients; the depression presents either as an acute stress response or as a major depression.[33] Awareness of these common psychiatric syndromes when evaluating a pain complaint may expand the physician's understanding.[34]

Multiple pain complaints, common in patients with advanced disease, need to be prioritized and classified.[15] It is also necessary to verify the history from a family member who may provide information that the patient is unable or unwilling to provide; the family member may be more objective in assessing the disability of a patient who under-reports his symptoms. Similarly, for the patient who is a poor historian, the family member may provide essential information that may alter the diagnostic approach. All attempts should be made to compile a careful history.

Medical and neurologic examinations provide the necessary data to substantiate the clinical history. Knowledge of the referral patterns of pain and the common cancer pain syndromes can direct the examination.[35] The characteristics of pain in patients with brachial plexopathy are so specific that they can help define the diagnosis of tumor infiltration of the brachial plexus or radiation-induced fibrosis.[36,37] Similarly, the commonly described pain syndromes in cancer patients must be known to the physician assessing the patient. This is best exemplified by the use of algorithms to evaluate back pain in the cancer patient.[38]

The purpose of diagnostic studies is to confirm the clinical diagnosis and to define in patients with metastatic disease the site and extent of tumor infiltration. The computed tomography (CT) scan and magnetic resonance imaging (MRI) represent the most useful diagnostic procedures in evaluating patients with pain and cancer. CT visualizes bone and soft tissue in a two-dimensional view and is useful in defining early bony changes. MRI is particularly useful in evaluating vertebral involvement, epidural spinal cord compression, and parenchymal brain metastases. CT is also useful in directing needle placement for biopsy and for anesthetic procedures, such as coeliac plexus block.

Although plain x-ray films are a useful screening procedure, they should not be used to overrule a clinical diagnosis if they are negative. They are inadequate to assess areas of the body where bone shadows overlap and in which specific pain syndromes may arise, such as the base of the skull, vertebral bodies—specifically the C2, C7, T1 areas—and the sacrum. Similarly, the bone scan, although it provides a more sensitive method for demonstrating abnormalities in bone before changes appear on plain x-ray films, does not, if positive, establish a diagnosis of metastatic disease, because patients with osteoporosis and collapsed vertebral bodies may have positive bone scans without any metastatic disease.[39] Infections and disuse atrophy are associated with positive bone scans. A negative bone scan does not rule out bony metastatic disease.[40] This is most evident in the patient with bony metastatic disease occurring in a previously irradiated site, for which the bone scan is often negative.[32] There are an increasing number of lung cancer patients wtih proven bony disease and negative bone scans.[41]

The physician, when ordering the necessary diagnostic procedures, should review them personally with the radiologist to correlate any pathologic changes with the site of pain.

Evaluation of the extent of metastatic disease may help to discern the relationship of the pain complaint to possible recurrent disease. For example, the postmastectomy pain syndrome that is caused by interruption of the intercostobrachial nerve is never associated with recurrent disease.[42] In contrast, in a patient with carcinoma of the lung, the presence of recurrent disease is closely associated with late post-thoractomy pain after the initial resolution of the postoperative pain.[43]

No patient should be examined inadequately because of a significant pain problem. Early management of the pain while investigating the source will markedly improve the patient's ability to participate in the necessary diagnostic procedures. During the initial evaluation of the pain complaint, early consideration of the use of alternative methods of pain control, including anesthetic and neurosurgical approaches, should be considered (*e.g.*, temporary use of local anesthetic via an epidural catheter to manage sacral pain or a percutaneous cordotomy in the patient with unilateral pain below the waist from a lumbosacral plexopathy). These approaches should not be considered for use only when all else fails, but should be an integral part of the early assessment of the patient with pain.

Continual reassessment of the response of the patient's pain to the prescribed therapy provides the best validation of the initial diagnosis. However, in patients in whom the response to therapy is less than predicted or in whom exacerbation of the pain occurs, reassessment of the treatment approach or a search for a new cause of the pain should be considered (*e.g.*, in the patient with epidural cord compression who develops a second block proximal to the one being irradiated).

Integrating the use of the MPAC scale to follow patients during their diagnostic and therapeutic procedures provides the opportunity to fully assess the degree of pain relief and impact on resultant moods. Successful evaluation and treatment of the pain complaint in cancer patients implies continuity of care from diagnosis to treatment.

MANAGEMENT OF CANCER PAIN

Recent advances in pain research provide the scientific rationale for using improved methods of treatment, including better and more effective use of standard drug therapy (non-narcotic, narcotic, and adjuvant analgesic drugs); the development of new drugs; the use of novel methods and routes of drug administration; and the use of selective anesthetic and neurosurgical approaches to conrol pain.[2] A series of medical and surgical approaches to the management of cancer pain are currently available. The use of certain techniques often depends on the clinical expertise in a particular center. Approaches such as drug therapy and some of the behavioral methods should be within the armamentarium of any physician or nurse who cares for patients with pain and cancer. Other approaches, such as specific anesthetic and neurosurgical techniques, require trained medical personnel who have clinical experience in managing cancer pain.

DRUG THERAPY

Analgesic drugs may be divided into three groups: Group I, the non-narcotic analgesics, such as aspirin and acetaminophen, and the nonsteroidal anti-inflammatory drugs (NSAID) that act on the peripheral mechanisms of pain; Group II, the narcotic agonist and antagonist drugs that activate opiate receptors in the central and peripheral nervous system and mediate analgesia; and Group III, the adjuvant analgesic drugs that produce analgesia in certain pain states (*e.g.*, amitriptyline in postherpetic neuralgia) or potentiate the opioid analgesics.

Group I: Non-Opioid Analgesics

The non-narcotic analgesics are the drugs of choice for mild or moderate pain. Their mechanisms of action are controversial, but they probably reduce or prevent sensitization of pain receptors to nociceptive stimuli by preventing prostaglandin release. This class of drugs consists of a heterogeneous group of substances differing in chemical structure and pharmacologic action. Many of these drugs have analgesic, anti-inflammatory, and antipyretic properties. All drugs in this class have an analgesic potency similar to or greater than that of aspirin. However, the analgesic effects of these drugs have a ceiling, and escalation of the dose beyond a cetain level does not produce additional analgesia. Experimental evidence suggests that these drugs may play a special role in the pain management of patients with bone metastases because of the documented role of prostaglandins in bone resorption in metastatic bone disease. Aspirin has been shown to have an antitumor effect in an animal bone tumor model.[64,65]

In clinical practice, this class of drugs represents the first-line approach to the management of cancer pain with analgesics, but the choice and use of the non-narcotic must be individualized. Each patient should be given an adequate trial of one non-narcotic analgesic before switching to another. The trial should include administration of the drug to maximal levels at regular intervals. The gastrointestinal and hematologic side-effects often limit their long-term use. For the patient with moderate pain, the combination of a narcotic and a non-narcotic provides additional analgesia.[64] Combinations with codeine, oxycodone, or propoxyphene are available, but these combinations often contain less than the full dose of 650 mg aspirin or acetaminophen. Prescribing each drug separately provides individualized pain control. This is particularly important when the patient requires escalation of the combination to provide analgesia and the additional dosage of the NSAID component may become excessive.

Several NSAID have been approved by the Food and Drug Administration for use as analgesics for mild or moderate pain. The drugs are listed in Table 59-22.

Group II: Opioid Analgesics

The opioid analgesics, of which morphine is the prototype, vary in potency, efficacy, and adverse effects. These drugs produce their analgesic effects by binding to discrete opiate receptors in the peripheral and central nervous systems. This group includes a series of heterogeneous substances with different chemical structures. In contrast to the non-opioid analgesics, opioid analgesics do not appear to have a ceiling; as the dose is escalated on a log scale, the increment in analgesia is linear to the point of loss of consciousness. Effective use of the opioid analgesics requires the balancing of the most desirable effects of pain relief with the undesirable effects of nausea, vomiting, mental clouding, sedation, constipation, tolerance, and physical dependence. These undesirable effects impose a practical limit on the dose useful for a particular patient.

Much of the difficulty encountered in the clinical use of these drugs arises from different responses of patients to the same drug dose. This difficulty is compounded by the lack of pharmacologic and pharmacokinetic data for many of the narcotic analgesics. This lack of information and a series of uncontrolled survey-type studies have led to several controversies in the drug management of cancer pain.[67] These include the choice of the opioid analgesic, its route and method of administration, and questions about the problems of tolerance and the risk of substance abuse. However, there is sufficient pharmacologic information and clinical experience to help resolve some of these issues. An outline for the rational use of analgesics is provided in Table 59-23.

START WITH A SPECIFIC DRUG FOR A SPECIFIC TYPE OF PAIN. The WHO Cancer Pain Relief Program has advocated the use of an analgesic ladder (Fig. 59-8).[17] This approach advocates the use of non-opioid, opioid, and adjuvant analgesics alone or in combinations titrated to the needs of the individual patient. The non-opioid drugs are the first-line approach for the patient with mild or moderate pain. If pain relief is not obtained or if the side-effects of the non-opioid are intolerable, the opioid analgesics should be used. Codeine, oxycodone, and propoxyphene are classified as "weak" opioids, but all these drugs possess a higher analgesic potential than the nonopioids. These are most often used in oral fixed-dose mixtures.

For the management of moderate or severe pain, morphine, hydromorphone, levorphanol, methadone, and oxymorphone are the drugs most commonly used. After chronic administration, meperidine produces central nervous system irritability and is not recommended for chronic cancer pain management.[69] Heroin is not available in the United States, but it is comparable to morphine in its analgesic, mood, and unwanted effects.[70] Heroin must be metabolized to morphine and 6-acetylmorphine to produce analgesic effects, and it does not bind to opiate receptors.[71] The WHO has advised that morphine should be the drug of choice by the oral route and has requested that it be part of the essential drug list worldwide.

Alternatives to morphine include hydromorphone and levorphanol, both congeners of morphine. Hydromorphone has poor oral bioavailability but a short half-life, and it is highly soluble and available in high-potency form. It is a useful alternative to morphine and to levorphanol.[72] Levorphanol has good bioavailability but a long plasma half-life (12–16 hours), and it must be used cautiously because accumulation will occur with repeated administration. Oxymorphone is only available in parenteral and suppository forms thereby limiting its wide use.

TABLE 59-22. Non-opioid and Adjuvant Analgesic Drugs in the Management of Cancer Pain

Class/Drug	*Indications*	*Starting Oral Dose (mg)/Range (24 h)*	*Comments*
NSAID			
Aspirin	Soft tissue and metastatic bone pain	650 650–1000	Used in combination with opioids, GI and hematologic effects; avoid combination with steroids
Acetaminophen	Like aspirin	650 650–1000	Fewer GI effects; no effects on platelet function; no significant anti-inflammatory effects
Ibuprofen		400 200–800	Higher analgesic potential than aspirin; fewer GI and hematologic effects than asirin
Choline magnesium Trilisate	Like aspirin	1500 1000–4000	Anti-inflammatory and analgesic effects, similar to aspirin, without hematologic effects
Fenoprofen	Like aspirin	200 200–400	Like ibuprofen
Diflunisal	Like aspirin	500 500–100	Longer duration of action than ibuprofen; higher analgesic potential than aspirin
Naproxen	Like aspirin	250 250–500	Like diflunisal
Anticonvulsants			
Phenytoin	Neuropathic pain, acute lancinating type, tic	100 100–300	Start with low dose, titrate slowly
Carbamazepine	Neuropathic pain, acute lancinating type, tic	100 200–800	Useful in paroxysmal nerve pain
Antidepressants			
Amitriptyline Imipramine	Deafferentation pain, *e.g.*, postherpetic neuralgia	10 10–150	Start at low dose and titrate slowly; has analgesic properties
Amphetamines			
Dextroamphetamine	Somatic and visceral pain, e.g., post-operative pain	2.5 2.5–10	Additive analgesia in combination with narcotics; reduces sedative effects
Antihistamines			
Hydroxyzine	Somatic and visceral pain	25 25–100	Additive analgesia in combination with narcotics; antiemetic, antianxiety properties
Phenothiazines			
Methotrimeprazine	Somatic and visceral pain; useful in narcotic-tolerant patients with GI obstruction and pain	5–15 IM	Has antianxiety and antiemetic effects; available only in IM preparation
Steroids			
Prednisone	Somatic and Deafferentation pain, *e.g.* inflammatory bone pain	5 5–60	Anti-inflammatory, anti-emetic, analgesic effects
Dexamethasone	Reflex sympathetic dystrophy; brachial, lumbar plexopathy	0.5–16	

The role of methadone in cancer pain remains the most controversial.[67,73–75] Its bioavailability is 85%, and for single-dose studies, its oral to parenteral potency ratio is 1:2. Its plasma half-life averages 24 hours, but may range from 13 to 50 hours, but its analgesia often lasts only 4 to 8 hours. Repetitive analgesic doses of methadone lead to drug accumulation because of the discrepancy between its plasma half-life and the duration of analgesia. Sedation, confusion, and even death can occur when patients are not carefully monitored. The clinical use of methadone requires sophistication, and it should be considered as a second-line drug, most useful in the patient with some prior opioid experience and a degree of tolerance. In the opioid-native patient, initial doses should be titrated carefully.

The role of the narcotic partial agonists, such as buprenorphine, and the mixed agonist antagonists, such as pentazocine, butorphanol and nalbuphine, are quite limited in cancer pain management.[76] Buprenorphine is only available

TABLE 59-23. Guidelines for the Rational Use of Analgesics in the Management of Cancer Pain

Start with a specific drug for a specific type of pain
Know the pharmacology of the drug prescribed
Relative potency of the drug
Duration of the analgesic effect
Pharmacokinetics of the drug
Equianalgesic doses for the drug and its route of administration
Administer analgesic on a regular basis
Gear the route of administration to the patient's needs
Use a combination of drugs to provide additive analgesia
Narcotic plus non-narcotic (aspirin, acetaminophen, NSAID)
Narcotic plus antihistamine (hydroxyzine)
Narcotic plus amphetamine (dexedrine)
Avoid combinations that increase the sedation only
Narcotic and benzodiazepine (diazepam)
Narcotic and phenothiazine (chlorpromazine)
Anticipate and treat side-effects
Sedation
Respiratory depression
Nausea and vomiting
Constipation
Multifocal myoclonus and seizures
Manage the tolerant patient
Use combinations of non-opioid and opioid drugs
Use combinations of drug therapy, anesthetic, and neurosurgical procedures
Switch to an alternative opioid analgesic, starting with half the equianalgesic dose
Reassess the nature of the pain
Prevent and treat acute withdrawal
Taper drugs slowly
Anticipate complications
Overdose
Psychologic dependence

in the United States in a parenteral form but available worldwide in sublingual form. It is a useful first-line drug, before the use the full agonist drugs, because its analgesic efficacy will be reduced when used in patients receiving narcotic agonist drugs. Pentazocine is the only mixed agonist–antagonist available orally, but in the United States, it is only available in combination with naloxone, aspirin, or acetaminophen. Escalation of the dose of pentazocine produces psychotomimetic effects, limiting its usefulness in chronic cancer pain management. The choice of the opioid analgesic depends on the patients prior opioid experience and physical and neurologic status; individualization is the rule.

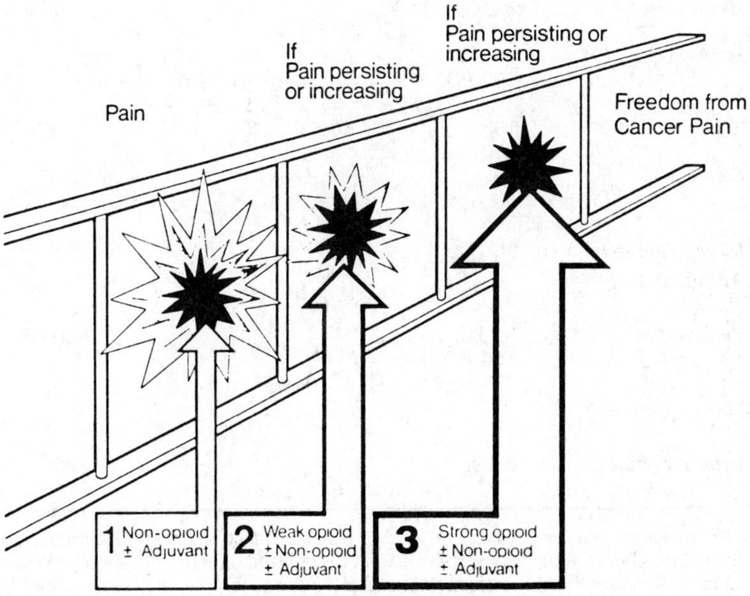

FIG. 59-8. The world health organizations's three-step ladder approach to analgesic drug therapy. (World Health Organization: Cancer Pain Relief. World Health Organization, Geneva, 1986)

KNOW THE EQUIANALGESIC DOSE AND ROUTE OF THE DRUG. Knowledge of the equianalgesic dose can ensure more appropriate drug use. Lack of attention to these differences in drug dose is the most common cause of undermedication of pain patients.[77] These doses have been derived from assessing the relative analgesic potency of a drug.[78] Relative potency is the ratio of the doses of two analgesics required to produce the same effect. Estimates of relative potency allow calculation of the equianalgesic dose, which provides the basis for selecting the appropriate dose when switching drugs or the route of administration of the same drug. The values depicted in Table 59-24 are based on studies in which 10 mg of morphine was the standard dose. The equianalgesic dose is the recommended starting dose, with the optimal dose for each patient determined by adjustment of the dose. This table can be useful, but its limitations also need to be understood (see footnote 1, Table 59-24).

One important controversy is the reported differences in relative potencies for morphine. On the basis of a series of survey studies, Twycross has suggested that the relative potency of morphine with repeated administration is 1:2 or 1:3.[13] As judged by single-dose studies in patients with acute and chronic pain, the relative potency of intramuscular to oral morphine is 1:6.[78] Relative potency may differ in single-dose and repeated-dose studies. In practice, the 1:6 relative analgesic potency ratio should be used for patients with acute pain and the 1:2 or 1:3 ratio employed in patients treated with repeated doses on a chronic basis. This controversy has confused the care of patients who are often undermedicated with morphine during the initial titration, when a 1:3 ratio is used.[79] Recent evidence suggests that morphine has an active metabolite, morphine-6-glucuronide, that accounts for this difference.

ADMINISTER ANALGESIC REGULARLY FOLLOWING INITIAL TITRATION. Medication should be administered regularly, which should include awakening the patient from sleep. The pharmacologic rationale of this approach is to

TABLE 59-24. Opioid Analgesics for Management of Cancer Pain

Drug	*Equianalgesic Dose (mg)*	*Plasma Half-Life (h)*	*Starting Oral Dose (mg)*	*Commercial Preparations*
Opioid Agonists				
Morphine	10 IM 60 PO	3–4	30–60	Oral: tablet, liquid, slow-release tab Rectal Injectable: SC, IM, IV, epidural, intrathecal
Hydromorphone	1.5 IM 7.5 PO	2–3	4–8	Oral: tablets Rectal Injectable: SC, IM, IV, 2 mg/ml and HP 10 mg/ml
Methadone	10 IM 20 PO	12–24	5–10	Oral: tablets, liquid Injectable: SC, IM, IV
Levorphanol	2 IM 4 PO	12–16	2–4	Oral: tablets Injectable: SC, IM, IV
Oxymorphone	1 IM 10 PR	2–3	NA†	Rectal: 10 mg Injectable: SC, IM, IV
Heroin	5 IM 60 PO	3–4	NA	NA
Meperidine	75 IM 300 PO	3–4 (normeperidine 12–16)	75	Oral: tablets Injectable: SC, IM, IV
Codeine	130 200	3–4	60	Oral: tablets and combination with ASA, acetaminophen, liquid
Oxycodone	15 30		5	Oral: tablets, liquid, oral formulation in combination with acetaminophen (tab, liquid) and aspirin (tab)
Mixed Agonists/ Antagonists				
Pentazocine	60 IM 180 PO		30–60	Oral: tablets only in combination with naloxone or acetaminophen Injectable: SC, IM
Partial Agonist				
Buprenorphine	0.4 sl		NA	Sublingual: NA in US Injectable: SC, IM

* For these equianalgesic IM doses, the times of peak analgesia in nontolerant patients ranges from one-half to 1 hour, and the duration from 4 to 6 hours. The peak analgesic effect is delayed, and the duration prolonged after oral administrations. These doses are recommended starting IM doses from which the optimal dose for each patient is determined by titration and the maximal dose limited by adverse effects.

† NA = not available.

maintain the plasma level of the drug above the minimal effective concentration for pain relief. In the initial titration, patients should be advised to take their medication as needed in order to determine their total 24-hour requirements. This is also the period for them to reach a steady-state level of drug, which depends on the half-life of the drug. For morphine, steady state can be reached in 24 hours, but with methadone, it may take 5 to 7 days to reach steady state. Full assessment of the analgesic efficacy of a drug regimen may take several days.

GEAR THE ROUTE OF ADMINISTRATION TO THE PATIENT'S NEEDS. The oral route is the most practical, but in the patient who requires immediate pain relief, parenteral administration subcutaneously, intramuscularly, or intravenously is the route of choice. Various methods of drug delivery of opioids have been developed in an attempt to maximize pharmacologic effects and to minimize side-effects.

A recent review of the patterns of drug use in patients with cancer pain throughout their illness demonstrates that, from the onset of pain until death, the majority of patients will require at least two routes of drug administration, and 20% of patients required as many as four approaches. These data emphasize the need for alternative routes and the development of guidelines for chronic drug management.[80]

Buccal and sublingual preparations of morphine have been clinically useful as alternatives to the oral route in patients unable to swallow.[81,82] These routes obviate the first-pass effect of liver metabolism. Recent pharmacologic studies of sublingual morphine suggests a bioavailability of only 6%.[83] Buprenorphine, a partial agonist is available outside the United States in sublingual form has been useful as a first-line drug in cancer pain management. Rectal suppositories of morphine, oxymorphone, and hydromorphone are available. Rectal oxymorphone is only 10% as potent as intramuscular oxymorphone, suggesting poor absorption from the rectum and canceling any advantage that may result from avoiding the first-pass effect by rectal administration.[84] A 10-mg rectal suppository of morphine has a comparable pharmacokinetic profile to a 10-mg oral solution, supporting the usefulness of this approach.[85]

For patients requiring chronic opioid administration, the use of continuous subcutaneous and continuous intravenous infusions offer special advantages.

Continuous Subcutaneous Infusions. This approach also avoids the presystemic clearance by the liver and is most useful in patients who cannot tolerate oral analgesics because of gastrointestinal obstruction or intractable nausea and vomiting. It is the approach of choice for the patient with gastrointestinal obstruction and pain. Many series have reported the usefulness of this technique using morphine, heroin, hydromorphone, methadone, and levorphanol. Pumps designed to infuse continuously, but with options for bolus administration, are connected to a 27-gauge butterfly needle that the patient can insert into a new subcutaneous site every third to sixth day. Limited pharmacokinetic studies suggest that morphine's bioavailability is 100%. Guidelines for this approach have been published.[86,87]

Continuous Intravenous Infusions. This approach is used as an alternative method of pain control in 13% to 20% of terminally ill patients. Infusions can be used in ambulatory and in hospitalized patients, with successful pain control in most patients. The infusion is titrated to the needs of the individual patient, with reported doses of morphine in adults ranging from 1 mg/hour to 750 mg/hour. Specific guidelines for the use of this approach have been detailed.[89] In implementing this approach, one difficulty is the inability to predict an ideal maintenance infusion rate and to accommodate for differences among patients. Rapid achievement of an optimal steady-state infusion rate is crucial, but at times difficult to obtain. The intravenous (IV) and oral relative analgesic potencies for the narcotic analgesics are not known for many of the drugs. When patients are switched to continuous IV infusions, the starting dose is calculated on the basis of morphine equivalents for a 24-hour period for the route. This dose is then halved for IV administration. The procedure is based on clinical experience, not on controlled studies.

Intermittent and Continuous Epidural and Intrathecal Opioid Infusions. These approaches are based on the demonstration of opiate receptors in the dorsal horn of the spinal cord and the ability of opioid drugs to suppress noxious stimuli at the spinal cord level.[26] Localized selective analgesia is produced without motor or sensory blockade. This approach minimizes the distribution of drugs to receptors in the brain stem and cerebral hemispheres, thereby avoiding the side-effects of systemic administration of opiates, including sedation, drowsiness, and respiratory depression.

The use of an intermittent bolus of opioid via an epidural catheter has been widely used clinically, with varying reports of its success. No studies have directly compared this approach to the other routes detailed above. The pharmacokinetics of epidural opioid administration demonstrate that there is significant systemic uptake after epidural injection, comparable to an intramuscular (IM) injection of the same drug and dose.[27] However, distribution of the drug directly into the cerebrospinal fluid is 10 to 100 times greater.

Continuous epidural and intrathecal infusions have been given using the Infusaid pump. Intrathecal administration has limited systemic uptake, making this theoretically a more useful approach. However, after both epidural and intrathecal administrations, there is significant rostral redistribution of drug in the cerebrospinal fluid, and rapid development of tolerance has been reported.[90,91] The clinical dilemma are at what point this approach should be considered in the management of cancer patients with pain and what are the risk-benefit ratios for the individual patient. There is significant cross-tolerance induced by systemic opiates, confounding the indications for this approach. Controlled analgesic studies of this approach in the long-term management of cancer patients are needed before this technique, with its potential risks of meningitis, epidural hematomas, and abscess, is fully implemented.

USE A COMBINATION OF DRUGS. The use of a combination of drugs enables the prescribing physician to increase analgesic effects for the patient without escalation of the narcotic dose. Combinations that produce additive analgesic effects include a narcotic plus a non-narcotic (*e.g.*, aspirin, acetaminophen, ibuprofen, trilisate), a narcotic plus an antihistamine (*e.g.*, 100 mg IM hydroxyzine), and a narcotic plus an amphetamine (*e.g.*, 10 mg IM dexedrine).[66,93,94] Studies demonstrating the efficacy of these combinations were single-dose studies. In clinical practice, hydroxyzine in 25-mg doses has been used regularly, with anecdotal observations that it is an effective combination. Similarly, amphetamine in 2.5-mg to 5.0-mg doses twice a day can effectively reduce the sedative effects of the narcotics in patients who are receiving adequate analgesia, but who are excessively sedated.

Certain combinations do not provide additive analgesia; these include a narcotic plus a benzodiazepine or a narcotic plus a phenothiazine.

ANTICIPATE AND TREAT SIDE-EFFECTS. The side-effects of the narcotic analgesics often limit their effective use. The most common side-effects include sedation, respiratory depression, nausea, vomiting, constipation, and multifocal myoclonus and seizures.

Sedation. Sedation and drowsiness vary with the drug and dose and may occur after single or repetitive administration. They are mediated through activation of opiate receptors in the reticular formation and diffusely throughout the cortex. Management of these effects includes reducing the individual drug dose but prescribing the drug more frequently or switching to an analgesic with a shorter plasma half-life. Amphetamines can be used to counteract these sedative effects.[94] It is important to discontinue all other drug therapy that may exacerbate the sedative effects of the narcotic analgesic, including medications such as cimetidine, barbiturates, and other anxiolytic medications.

Respiratory Depression. Respiratory depression is the most serious adverse effect of the opioid drugs. It occurs most commonly after short-term administration of the narcotic and is usually associated with other signs of central nervous system depression, including sedation and drowsiness. The narcotic agonist drugs act on brain stem respiratory centers to produce, as a function of dose, increasing respiratory depression to the point of apnea. Tolerance to this effect develops rapidly with repeated drug administration, allowing their prolonged use without significant risk of respiratory depression.

If respiratory depression occurs, it can be reversed by administering naloxone. The dose suggested is 0.4 mg/ml of naloxone. Naloxone is a short-acting, narcotic antagonist. Repeated administration, including an intravenous drip, may be necessary to prevent respiratory arrest in these patients. In patients receiving narcotics for prolonged periods who develop respiratory depression, diluted doses of naloxone (0.4 mg in 10 ml of saline) should be titrated carefully to prevent severe withdrawal symptoms while reversing the respiratory depression. In certain patients, the use of naloxone to reverse drug-induced respiratory depression can be dangerous. An endotracheal tube should be placed in the comatose patient before administering naloxone to prevent aspiration from excessive salivation and bronchial spasm induced by naloxone. In patients receiving meperidine over a longer period, naloxone may precipitate seizures by lowering the seizure threshold and by allowing the convulsant activity of the active metabolite normeperidine to become evident. If naloxone is to be used, diluted doses, slowly titrated, and appropriate seizure precautions are advised. There is insufficient clinical evidence to make more specific recommendations. If respiratory support can be effected by other means (*i.e.*, continuous stimulation to maintain the patient's wakefulness), the patient may be at less risk and clearly in less discomfort.

Nausea and Vomiting. The narcotic analgesics produce nausea and vomiting by an action limited to the medullary chemoreceptor trigger zone. The incidence of nausea and vomiting is markedly increased in ambulatory patients. Tolerance develops to these side-effects with repeated administration of the drugs. Nausea to one drug does not mean that all drugs will produce similar symptoms. Switching to alternative narcotic analgesics or using an antiemetic in combination with the narcotic analgesics can obviate this effect.[97]

Constipation. Constipation results from the action of these drugs at many sites in the gastrointestinal tract and in the spinal cord to produce a decrease in intestinal secretions and peristalsis that results in a dry stool and constipation. At the same time that narcotic analgesics are started, provisions for a regular bowel regimen, including cathartics and stool softeners, should be instituted. Several bowel regimens have been suggested because of their specific ability to counteract the effects of the narcotic drugs, but none of these has been studied in a controlled way.[98] The anecdotal surveys suggest that doses far above those used for routine bowel management are necessary and that careful attention to dietary factors when using a bowel regimen can reduce patient complaints dramatically. Tolerance to this effect develops at a relatively slow rate.

Multifocal Myoclonus and Seizures. Multifocal myoclonus may occur with high doses of all of the opioid drugs. Multifocal myoclonus with seizures have been reported in patients receiving multiple doses of meperidine, although signs and symptoms of central nervous system hyperirritability may occur with toxic doses of any narcotic analgesic. In a series of cancer patients receiving meperidine, accumulation of the active metabolite, normeperidine, is associated with these neurologic signs and symptoms.[69] However, in a similar group of cancer patients with pain, subtle mood effects were noted after meperidine administration, which suggests a spectrum of neurologic effects. Management of this hyperirritability includes discontinuing the meperidine, using intravenous valium if seizures occur, and substituting morphine to control the persistent pain. Since the half-life of normeperidine is 16 hours, it may take 2 or 3 days for hyperirritability to clear completely. Meperidine is contraindicated in patients with chronic renal disease.

MANAGE THE TOLERANT PATIENT. The earliest sign of drug tolerance is the patient's complaint that the duration of effective analgesia has decreased. For reasons not yet understood, the rate of development of tolerance varies greatly among cancer patients. Some demonstrate tolerance within days of initiating narcotic therapy, others remain controlled for many months on the same dose. Studies in an outpatient clinic population, a hospitalized population, and a home-care population revealed three patterns of drug use: those who rapidly increase their opioid requirements, those who stabilize at one dose for several weeks or months, and those who decrease or eliminate opioids.[30,80,89] The increase in opioid requirements most commonly is associated with progression of disease.

With the development of tolerance, increases in the frequency or the dose of the opioid are required to provide continued pain relief. Because the analgesic effect is a logarithmic function of the dose of opioid, a doubling of the dose may be required to restore full analgesia. There appears to be no limit to the development of tolerance, and with appropriate adjustment of dose, patients can continue to obtain pain relief. Cross-tolerance among the opioid analgesics is not complete, and it is advantageous to change to another opioid, selecting half the predicted equianalgesic dose as the starting dose. The use of analgesic combinations can reduce the amount of opioid required. Similarly, the use of bolus or continuous epidural local anesthetic in patients with perineal pain can dramatically reduce the need for systemic opioids and reverse tolerance.

Taper Drugs Slowly. The long-term administration of narcotic analgesics is associated with the development of physical dependence, a state in which the sudden cessation of the narcotic analgesic will produce signs and symptoms of withdrawal characterized by agitation, tremors, insomnia, fear, marked autonomic nervous system hyperexcitability, and exacerbation of pain. Slowly tapering the dose of the narcotic analgesic will prevent these symptoms. The appearance of abstinence symptoms from the time of drug withdrawal is related to the elimination half-life for the particular drug. The type of abstinence syndrome varies with the individual drug. For example, with morphine, withdrawal symptoms will occur within 6 to 12 hours after cessation of the drug. Reinstituting the drug in doses of approximately 25% of the previous daily dose will suppress these symptoms.

ANTICIPATE COMPLICATIONS. *Overdose.* Overdose with narcotic analgesics occurs intentionally when a patient takes an excessive amount of drug in a suicide attempt or unintentionally when the recommended dosage accidentally produces excessive sedation and respiratory depression. The complication can be treated effectively with naloxone. Intentional overdose in cancer patients occurs rarely, and concern for this is overemphasized. Overdose in patients previously stabilized on a narcotic regimen for cancer pain rarely is caused by drug intake alone. More commonly, it is the medical deterioration of the patient with a superimposed metabolic encephalopathy. Reduction of the narcotic drug dosage and careful assessment of the patient's metabolic status usually provide the differential diagnosis. Patients who develop unintentional drug overdose should be scrutinized carefully to rule out other causes of excessive sedation, confusion, or respiratory depression. A reversal of these effects with naloxone is more therapeutic than diagnostic.

Psychological Dependence. Psychological dependence or addiction has a concomitant behavioral pattern of drug abuse, characterized by craving a drug for other than pain relief and overwhelming involvement in the use and procurement of the drug. This is a state distinct from tolerance and physical dependence, which are responses to the pharmacologic effects of long-term narcotic administration. It is the profound fear of causing psychological dependence that plays a major role in a physician's reluctance to prescribe narcotic analgesics, particularly in cancer patients in the early phase of their disease.[77] This same fear is shared by patients who consistently take less analgesic drug than is effective to control their pain. From clinical experience, there is increasing evidence to suggest that cancer patients with pain can take narcotic analgesics for prolonged periods but can discontinue such drugs when adequate pain relief is achieved from other approaches. In almost all instances, dramatic escalation of drug intake is associated with progression of disease and subsequent death.[30,80,89] A very small percentage of patients with cancer and pain may become psychologically dependent on the drugs and participate in drug-seeking behaviors and illicit drug use. This concern should not be punitive to the patient with severe cancer pain.

Group III: Adjuvant Analgesics Drugs

This group of drugs has a unique place in the management of cancer pain, but knowledge about their use is empiric. This group consists of a number of heterogenous substances whose use has been to increase the analgesic effects of the opioid analgesics, to counteract opioid side-effects, or to act as analgesics themselves. Any attempt to develop guidelines for the use of these adjuvants must be prefaced with certain caveats. These drugs have been developed and released for clinical indications other than analgesia, including nausea, vomiting, anxiety, mania, depression, and delirium; these drugs are not as effective in relieving pain as are the narcotic analgesics, except for methotrimeprazine (Levoprome); there are no efficacy studies for their co-analgesic properties in cancer patients; and the choice of these drugs should be individualized, using the simplest but most potent combination of drugs. Table 59-22 summarizes the most commonly used agents, their doses, side-effects, and pertinent references.

ANTICONVULSANTS. Phenytoin and carbamazepine are anticonvulsant drugs that suppress spontaneous neuronal firing and represent the drugs of choice for treating trigeminal neuralgia and other neuropathic pains.[99] In cancer pain, carbamazepine has been useful specifically in managing the acute shock-like neuralgic pain in the cranial and cervical distribution caused by tumor infiltration or surgical injury. It also has been effective in patients with stump pain secondary to traumatic neuroma and in patients with lumbosacral plexopathy. The starting dose is 100 mg, slowly titrated to between 400 and 800 mg/day.

PHENOTHIAZINES. Of the phenothiazine drugs, methotrimeprazine has had definitive analgesic properties in single-dose studies in patients with postoperative pain and chronic cancer pain. A dose of 15 mg IM is equivalent to 15 mg of morphine IM.[100] This drug is useful in special circumstances. In the patient who is tolerant, it provides a temporary analgesia by a non-opiate receptor mechanism. In the patient with bowel obstruction and pain, it avoids the constipating effects of narcotics. In patients whose respiration is compromised, it avoids the respiratory depressant effects of narcotics, although it can produce significant sedative effects. In patients with pain and narcotic-induced nausea and vomiting, it acts as both an analgesic and an antiemetic. Long-term administration of this drug in patients with cancer pain has not been fully assessed.

BUTYROPHENONES. Haloperidol is the first-line drug in the management of the cancer patient with acute psychosis and delirium, but its role in pain management is less clear.[34] In animals, it potentiates morphine analgesia. Several authors have reported its clinical usefulness in cancer patients with pain, which suggests that it works as a co-analgesic, allowing reduction of the narcotic dose. The doses suggested to produce co-analgesic effects are lower than those used to manage psychiatric symptoms: 0.5 to 1 mg orally, two to three times daily is the suggested starting dose.

ANTIDEPRESSANTS. The tricyclic antidepressants may represent the most useful group of psychotropic drugs in pain management. Their analgesic effects are mediated by enhancement of serotonin activity. Animal studies demonstrate the direct analgesic effects of amitriptyline and its ability to enhance morphine analgesia. Amitriptyline is useful in the management of patients with migraine, postherpetic neuralgia, diabetic neuropathy, and several chronic pain states.[23,24,101] No controlled studies in patients with cancer pain have been performed, but strong anecdotal information suggests the role of these drugs in the management of patients with neuropathic pain and in the management of their pain-related sleep disturbances. The doses used for analgesia are far below those needed to produce an antidepressant effect, and the analgesic properties of these drugs occur independently of their mood-altering effects.

STEROIDS. Corticosteroids have specific and nonspecific benefits in managing acute and chronic pain. Their ability to produce euphoria, increased appetite, and weight gain contributes greatly to the sense of well-being in the cancer patient with pain. Steroids reportedly reduce bone pain of metastatic origin and are used as oncolytic agents in certain types of tumors. Several studies demonstrate prolonged survivial time and reduced narcotic doses to control pain in terminal cancer patients receiving steroids.[102] In certain cancer pain syndromes, such as epidural cord compression, 85% of patients receiving 100 mg of dexamethasone as part of a radiotherapy protocol reported significant pain relief associated with marked reduction in analgesic requirements.[46] In patients with tumor infiltration of the brachial and lumbosacral plexus, steroids provide additional analgesic effects. The antihistamines, specifically hydroxyzine, and the amphetamine dextroamphetamine were discussed previously as adjuvant analgesic drugs.

PSYCHOLOGICAL APPROACHES

Psychological approaches should be an integral part of the care of the cancer patient with pain. The major goal of these interventions is to promote an increased sense of control by reducing the sense of hopelessness and helplessness that many cancer patients with pain experience. Comparative effectiveness of any one of these techniques to medical or surgical therapy is impossible. These techniques are especially useful in three clinical situations: in the management of patients with intermittent, predictable pain, such as the pain associated with procedures; in the management of incidental pain of patients with metastatic bone disease controlled at rest but markedly exacerbated by movement; and in the management of chronic cancer pain. Focused psychological interventions can facilitate patients' coping with acute exacerbations of cancer pain and can help patients with some chronic cancer-related pain syndromes functionally adjust to living.

A specialized psychological approach called Cognitive-Behavior Therapy (CBT) has been used to treat pain disorders, including cancer pain. This approach combines a set of short-term therapeutic interventions based on both theoretically and empirically derived principles that can be adapted to the specific problems and needs of patients. It consists of a set of systematic mental and behavioral techniques designed to modify specific emotional, behavioral, and social problems and the global experiences of pain and distress. The major goal of CBT is enhancing the sense of personal control or self-efficacy. In a multidisciplinary approach to cancer pain, not every patient needs referral for CBT. It is useful, however, if all members of the pain team follow a cognitive behavioral model. Because CBT is a pragmatic, commonsense approach consisting of a set of specific techniques, it can be learned and practiced by any interested clinician, nurse, or social worker who can gain practical training in CBT techniques. The assessment of the patent for CBT is described in Table 59-25. A variety of intervention methods have been developed and are arbitrarily divided into behavioral and cognitive methods for didactic purposes.[103,104]

Behavioral techniques include methods of modifying physiologic pain reactions and pain behaviors. Relaxation training is a psychological approach that can be used by all caregivers who manage patients who have pain and cancer. The mechanism of action includes the reduction of muscle tension. It can provide the patient with a sense of improved self-control and a calming diversion of attention, breaking the associated pain–anxiety–tension cycle. Techniques include simple deep breathing exercises to more special methods of biofeedback and hypnosis. Contingency management is another type of behavioral approach designed to modify dysfunctional pain behaviors and replace them with "well" behaviors.

Cognitive techniques are a set of methods designed to modify dysfunctional mental processes or to train adaptive coping strategies. Cognitive coping and cognitive modifica-

TABLE 59-25. Assessment for Cognitive Behavioral Interventions

Pain experience	Pattern, variation in intensity, quality; precipitating factors, relieving factors. Reactive thoughts and feelings, belief about meaning, future expectation, sense of control.
Pain behaviors	Expressive, stoic, respondent, operant, verbal, nonverbal, idiosyncratic. Specific descriptions and frequencies. Secondary gains. Attitudes regarding pain behaviors. Insight about operant contingencies; sense of control.
Medication use	Type, frequency, pattern (time-contingent or pain-contingent), pain relief, distress relief, side-effects; attitudes toward medication, sense of control, beliefs about addiction.
Mood	Depression, anxiety, anger, tension, agitation, restlessness, fatigue, confusion. Positive feelings: joy, love, excitement, interest. Ability to relax.
Hopefulness	Degree of hopefulness versus hopelessness; beliefs about the meaning of life and death; "fighting spirit," fatalism, nihilism.
Perception of social support	Tangible support, sense of belongingness, trust, social esteem, commitment.
Coping skills	Attitudes, thoughts, or activities related to habits of coping with illness, stress, and pain: escape, confrontation, catastrophizing, minimizing, active, passive, planning, impulsive, information seeking/avoiding. Habits of problem management and emotion regulation.
Social skills and assertiveness	Habits of behavior in social situations, private and public. Ability to assert wishes without aggression, tendencies to manipulate, or be manipulated.
Family and social situation	Effects of illness and pain on parents, spouse, children, other relative and circle of friends. Interaction and alliance patterns in family.
Daily activities	Pattern, frequency; physical, mental, passive, active, solitary, social; hobbies, duties, work.

From Fishman B, Loscalzo M: Cognitive-behavioral interventions in management of cancer pain: principles and applications (Payne R, Foley KM [eds]). Med Clin North Am 71:271–288, 1987.

TABLE 59-26. Types of Anesthetic Procedures Commonly Used in Cancer Pain

Type of Procedure	*Most Common Indications*
Nerve block	
Peripheral	Pain in discrete dermatomes in chest and abdomen
Epidural	Unilateral lumbar or sacral pain Midline perineal pain Bilateral lumbosacral pain
Intrathecal	Midline perineal pain Bilateral lumbosacral pain
Autonomic	
Stellate ganglion	Reflex sympathetic dystrophy, *e.g.*, frozen shoulder Arm pain
Lumbar sympathetic	Reflex sympathetic dystrophy Lumbosacral plexopathy Vascular insufficiency of the lower extremity
Celiac plexus	Midabdominal pain
Continuous epidural infusion with local anesthetics	Unilateral and bilateral lumbosacral pain Midline perineal pain
Chemical hypophysectomy	Diffuse bone pain
Inhalation therapy	Generalized pain Incident pain
Trigger-point injection	Focal muscle pain

tion are approaches in which distraction, focusing, perception, and interpretation of the meaning of pain are assessed.

ANESTHETIC AND NEUROSURGICAL APPROACHES

The anesthetic and neurosurgical approaches are most effective in treating patients with well-defined localized pain. Tables 59-26 and 59-27 outline the indications for their use. Because diffuse pain problems are common in cancer patients, the role of these approaches is limited. These clinical limitations are magnified by the fact that patients, as they become more cognizant of their disease and treatment options, are hesitant to undergo neurodestructive procedures. They consider the pain an important marker for their disease and are frightened of the potential, albeit unlikely, complications of these procedures. Therefore, these procedures are performed late in a patient's illness, and full evaluation of their effectiveness and duration of action is limited by the patient's overriding medical problems. Another limitation is that these procedures are not very effective in managing deafferentation pain, the pain associated with nerve injury. They are most helpful in various types of somatic or visceral pain in which nerve injury has not occurred. The dilemma is that cancer pain includes all three types of pain. Antitumor, analgesic, and psychologic therapies represent a true multidisciplinary approach to pain management.

TABLE 59-27. Neuroablative and Neurostimulatory Procedures for Relief of Pain from Cancer

Site	*Procedure*	*Indications*
Neuroablative Procedures		
Peripheral nerve	Neurectomy	Not indicated, neurolytic blocks are the procedure of choice
Nerve root	Rhizotomy	Useful in somatic and deafferentation pain from tumor infiltration of the cranial and rarely intercostal nerves
Spinal cord	Dorsal root entry zone lesion	Useful in unilateral deafferentation pain from brachial, intercostal and lumbosacral plexopathy, and postherpetic neuralgia
	Cordotomy	Useful in unrelated pain below the waist, often combined with local neurolytic blocks in perineal and bilateral lumbosacral plexopathy
	Myelotomy	Useful in midline pain below the waist, but rarely employed because it involves extensive surgery
Brain stem	Mesencephalic tractomy	Useful in pain in the nasopharynx and trigeminal region
Thalamus	Thalamotomy	Useful in unilateral deafferentation pain in the chest and lower extremity
Cortex	Cingulumotomy Frontal lobotomy	Not used for cancer pain
Pituitary	Transsphenoidal hypophysectomy	Useful in pain control of bone metastases in endocrine-dependent tumors, breast and prostate
Neurostimulatory Procedures		
Peripheral nerve	Transcutaneous and percutaneous electrical nerve	Useful in reducing painful dysethesias from tumor infiltration of nerve or trauma, *e.g.*, neuroma
Spinal cord	Dorsal column stimulation	Of limited use in deafferentation pain in the chest, midline, and lower extremities
Brain stem	Periaqueductal stimulation	Rarely used to treat deafferentation pain in the chest, midline, or lower extremities.
Thalamus	Thalamic stimulation	Rarely used to treat deafferentation pain in the chest, midline, or lower extremity

Anesthetic Approaches

Anesthetic approaches can be divided into five types: myofascial trigger point injections, peripheral nerve blocks, autonomic nerve blocks, intrathecal nerve blocks, and the use of nitrous oxide. The techniques for each of these procedures are described in detail in standard textbooks.[105-107] Short-acting and long-acting anesthetics are used for temporary and diagnostic nerve blocks (*e.g.*, trigger point injections), but phenol, alcohol, and freezing of the nerves are the commonly used for permanent blocks. Anesthetic agents temporarily depolarize nerves by an increase in sodium permeability through membrane lipoprotein channels. Neurolytic agents product permanent conduction blocks by disrupting neural tissue. The block produced by phenol tends to be less profound and of shorter duration than that of alcohol, and phenol is more commonly used to this advantage when the risk of motor paresis or loss of bowel or bladder control is high. Local freezing of the nerve produces a functional loss in the nerve that lasts only for several weeks. In most instances, a permanent nerve block is performed only when a temporary nerve block has demonstrated some efficacy.

TRIGGER POINT INJECTIONS. The use of trigger point injections is within the scope of the practicing physician.[109] Patients with significant musculoskeletal pain will often describe specific, tender trigger point areas that, when injected with saline or local anesthetic, have significant pain relief. Effective relief of pain from trigger point injections, however, is not diagnostic of musculoskeletal pain alone, and an evaluation of the cause of the pain is still necessary to rule out the specific cause.

PERIPHERAL NERVE BLOCKS. Peripheral nerve blocks are used diagnostically to localize the nerve distribution and therapeutically to interrupt pain transmission within a determined nerve distribution. The usefulness of this technique is limited to areas of the body in which interruption of both motor and sensory function will not interfere with the patient's functional status. This approach is most commonly used with patients who have pain in the head, chest, or abdomen. This technique is also limited by the fact that each peripheral nerve subserves sensory function on many levels, and usually several nerves must be blocked to provide adequate analgesia. These techniques are most useful in patients with somatic pain. Deafferentation pain is rarely controlled by peripheral nerve blocks. Examples of successful blocks include gasserian ganglion block for craniofacial pain, intercostal blocks for chest wall infiltration from tumor, and parvertebral blocks for radicular pain.[105,109]

In those patients with somatic pain who respond to a local anesthetic block, neurolytic blockade with phenol may provide more prolonged (2–3 months) relief. Phenol acts by protein denaturation. As the susceptability of the nerves to instilled solutions is indirectly proportional to the concentration of the solution and inversely proportional to the diameter or presence of myelin, a differential block is possible. Blockade of pain and temperature sensation mediated by the unmyelinated C fibers can be done, and thicker, myelinated fibers subserving other modalities can be spared. It appears that a 5% solution of phenol produces a selective blockade of the small fibers, but higher concentrations are less selective.[110,111]

The most common peripheral nerve neurolytic block is a paravertebral block for localized intercostal pain. This is most commonly performed under fluoroscopic control.

EPIDURAL INFUSIONS AND LOCAL ANESTHETICS. Epidural and intrathecal nerve blocks have been used widely to manage cancer pain. Intermittent and continuous epidural infusions of local anesthetic have been devised to manage the difficult chronic pain associated with metastatic disease involving the sacrum or lumbosacral plexus. This method consists of the intermittent or continuous infusion of a local anesthetic into a subcutaneous infusion pump or Ommaya reservoir connected to a catheter that has been temporarily or permanently placed in the epidural space. If the amount and concentration of the anesthetic are varied, effective pain relief can be achieved without interruption of significant motor or autonomic function. The risk of infection is minimized because local anesthetics have antimicrobial effects. The use of continuous low-dose infusions of local anesthetics is associated with minimal systemic side-effects. Further studies are needed to define its place in the management of the cancer patient. Its major advantages are that the resultant analgesia is not cross-tolerant with the analgesia produced by narcotics and that temporary use of this technique allows reduction of systemic opiate drugs, partially reversing tolerance. This has been a useful preliminary approach for patients in whom the use of spinal opiate analgesia is considered, but in whom large doses of systemic opiates have induced tolerance. Tolerance develops to these analgesic effects; thus, this approach is temporary (days to weeks).[112,113]

EPIDURAL AND INTRATHECAL NEUROLYTIC BLOCKS. Epidural and intrathecal neurolytic blocks have been used primarily to manage patients with far advanced disease in whom the pain is either unilateral in the chest or abdomen or midline in the perineum. These approaches are less useful in managing upper-limb and lower-limb pain associated with brachial and lumbosacral plexopathy because of the high risk of motor weakness associated with effective neurolytic blockade. Epidural phenol blocks are useful in managing the patient with chest wall pain over several dermatomes. Such an approach obviates the need to perform multiple paravertebral injections. Phenol is injected in small increments (1–2 ml) per segment over 2 to 3 days by an epidural catheter, and preliminary data demonstrate 80% pain relief in patients with documented somatic pain.[114]

Both epidural and intrathecal phenol blocks can be used to manage perineal pain, but no studies have delineated the superiority of one approach or the other. For an intrathecal block, phenol-glycerine solution, which is viscous and hyperbaric, can be directed to the site by gravity. An 18-gauge spinal needle is used to introduce the phenol intrathecally, and the substance is injected in small increments of 0.4 ml, to a total of 1 to 1.5 ml.

Complications are rare and usually are transient. The most common complications include a meningeal syndrome, hypotension, and motor paresis. Sphincter dysfunction is common but is often transitory. However, patients should be informed of these potential risks, especially incontinence. These complications can be reduced if the procedure is done in the sitting position, if the injections are given in two separate sessions, and if the patient is kept leaning backward at a 45° angle after drug instillation. In this position, the phenol gravitates to the posterior sacral region, and only the dorsal sensory roots are immersed and the anterior motor roots are spared. In injecting the neurolytic agent, the patient is asked repeatedly about paresthesias in the soles of the feet. If they occur, involvement of the S1 roots is imminent and no further phenol should be administered.

The selection of patients for management with either epidural or intrathecal neurolytic agents should be based on the following criteria: exhaustion of the appropriate antitumor approaches; clear clinical and radiologic definition of the pain; poor candidacy for percutaneous cordotomy; failure of narcotic analgesics to produce adequate analgesia without significant side-effects; a favorable response to diagnostic or epidural or intrathecal blocks, producing at least 75% pain relief; and myelography performed before the procedure to rule out tumor infiltration.

AUTONOMIC NERVE BLOCK. Sympathetic block is effective in conditions with vasomotor or visceromotor hyperactivity. This hyperactivity accompanies many of the cancer-related pain syndromes, such as visceral pain or plexopathies. The most rewarding sympathetic block is that of the coeliac ganglion for pain due to abdominal malignancy, including cancer of the pancreas, stomach, duodenum, liver, gallbladder, adrenal gland, and colon. Nociceptive fibers of the splanchnic, sympathetic, vagal, phrenic, and somatic nerves converge upon the coeliac ganglion, which is amenable to a regional block that is 85% successful. Standardized approaches for the use of this technique have been described using CT monitoring or fluoroscopic control (Fig. 59-9).[115,116]

After placement of the needle, 25 ml of absolute alcohol mixed with local anesthetic and contrast material is injected. Bilateral needle placement has been reported to provide the best results, but anecdotal reports suggest that unilateral needle placement on the right provides comparable analgesia. The major side-effect of the procedure is transient hypotension, and patients must be well hydrated and monitored carefully during the procedures and for 4 to 6 hours after the procedure. Significant neurologic complications occur in less than 1% of patients if proper technique is used. Complications have included paraparesis, and a nephrectomy was required to treat a renal hemorrhage in one patient. The procedure should only be performed under radiologic guidance to avoid these complications.[116]

Lumbar sympathetic block may provide significant relief of intractable urogenital pain or pain due to carcinomatous invasion of local nerves and plexi. Stellate ganglion block may alleviate postherpetic neuralgia and pain from brachial plexopathies. It has also been useful in postherpetic neuralgia involving the trigeminal distribution.

NEUROADENOLYSIS OF THE PITUITARY. Chemical hypophysectomy represents a special use of a neurolytic method. Recent studies suggest that 35% to 93% of patients undergoing this therapy report pain relief, with a median duration of 6 to 7 weeks and a maximum duration of 20 weeks.[117] The mechanism by which analgesia is produced may result from alcohol tracking up the pituitary stalk into the hypothalamus, with consequent disruption of the hypothalamic-thalamic endorphinergic pain pathways. Side-effects include diabetic insipidus, cranial nerve palsies, cerebrospinal fluid leakage, and rarely, meningitis. A lack of detailed clinical data limits critical assessment of these studies.

NITROUS OXIDE. Nitrous oxide has analgesic properties and has been used in the management of patients with far-advanced disease. It is administered with oxygen through a nonrebreathing face mask with concentrations varying from 25% to 75%. Its use in combination with systemic narcotic analgesics is associated with improvement of symptoms of pain and anxiety and with a demonstrable improvement in alertness.[118] Although long-term nitrous oxide use has been associated with the development of pancytopenia, its short-term use is relatively safe.

FIG. 59-9. Cross-section of the spinal cord shows sites of neuroablative procedures for pain control.

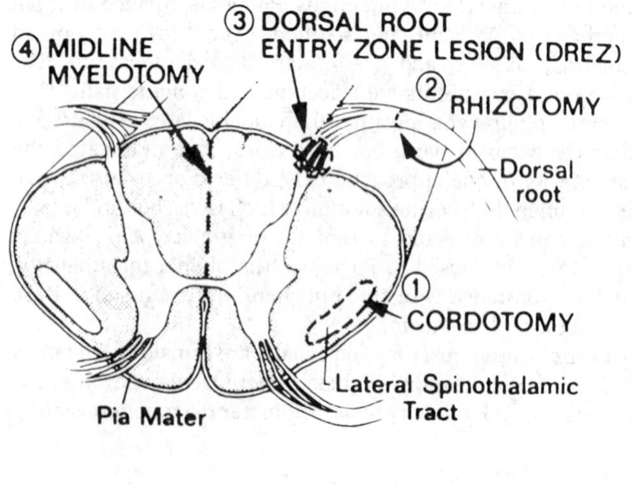

Neurosurgical Approaches

CRANIAL NERVE RHIZOTOMY. Tumors of the skull base, paranasal sinuses, or nasopharynx may be associated with significant pain, and ablative procedures through a posterior fossa craniectomy and upper cervical laminectomy can be useful. Sectioning of the sensory roots of the trigeminal nerve with the glossopharyngeal nerve, upper filaments of the vagus nerve, and the upper four cervical sensory roots may provide pain relief for selected patients with unilateral cancer pain. Interruption of the spinothalamic tract in the medulla and mesencephalon by stereotactic and by open techniques have had some degree of success. Although pain relief may be achieved after these brain stem procedures, there is a tendency for disagreeable dysesthesias to develop in the early postoperative period. Another approach is a percutaneous method guided by CT to produce a rhizotomy with

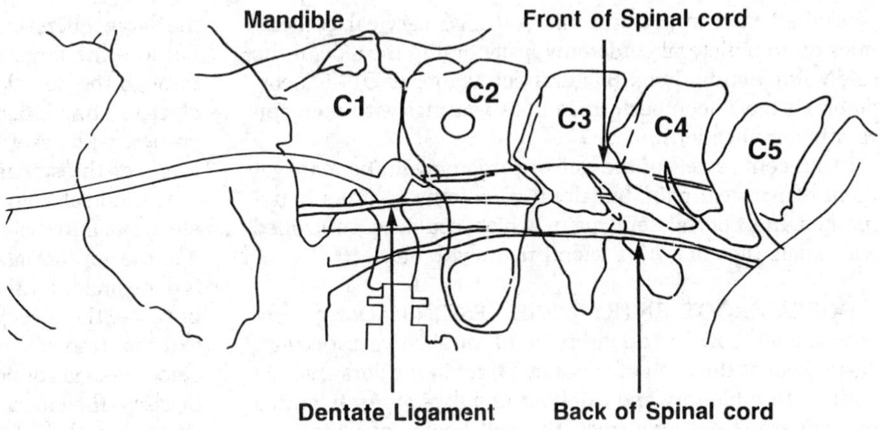

FIG. 59-10. The relationship of the dentate ligament to the anterior and posterior aspects of the spinal cord in a patient undergoing percutaneous cordotomy.[125] The dentate ligament is a reliable landmark separating the corticospinal from the spinothalamic tract (see Fig. 59-5).

radiofrequency lesioning. This technique is well-tolerated by patients and may provide for significant benefit in cases of unilateral or bilateral facial and nasopharyngeal pain.

CORDOTOMY. Cordotomy is a procedure whereby the anterolateral spinothalamic tract is ablated by surgery or by radiofrequency coagulation. The percutaneous cervical cordotomy is performed under local anesthesia with biplane fluoroscopic and impedence monitoring. Figure 59-10 provides a schematic diagram of the needle placement, and Figure 59-11 describes the neuroanatomy of the spinal cord. A miniature electrode is inserted into the anterolateral quadrant of the cervical spine, and a thermal lesion is made with a radiofrequency generator. Because the patient is awake, it is possible to test placement of the electrode and gauge the size of the lesion to the exact location of the pain. The open cordotomy is performed through a posterior laminectomy or an anterior low cervical approach. We reserve the open cordotomy for patients who are unable to lie in the supine position or who are not cooperative enough to undergo a percutaneous procedure.

The major indication for a cordotomy is unilateral somatic pain. Dysesthetic pain, deafferentation pain, and postherpetic neuralgia respond poorly to cordotomy. Significant pain relief is achieved in more than 90% of patients in the period immediately after the procedure. By 6 months, however, the success rate drops to 60%, and by 1 year, 50% of patients have recurrence of pain. Repeat cordotomy may be necessary in approximately 25% of patients as a result of an initial unsatisfactory lesion. Almost 30% of cancer patients undergoing cordotomy require bilateral procedures; in these cases, the second procedure is done at a later date.

Complications include paresis, ataxia, and bladder dysfunction. The complications are transient in most cases; however, in approximately 5%, they can be protracted and disabling. A potential late complication of cordotomy is dysesthetic pain. Fortunately, this vexing problem affects fewer than 1% of patients and is rarely seen earlier than 18 months after cordotomy.

The most serious potential complication is respiratory dysfunction, which may occur in the form of phrenic nerve paralysis or sleep-induced apnea. The paralysis is a result of interrupting ascending reticular pathways. It is, therefore,

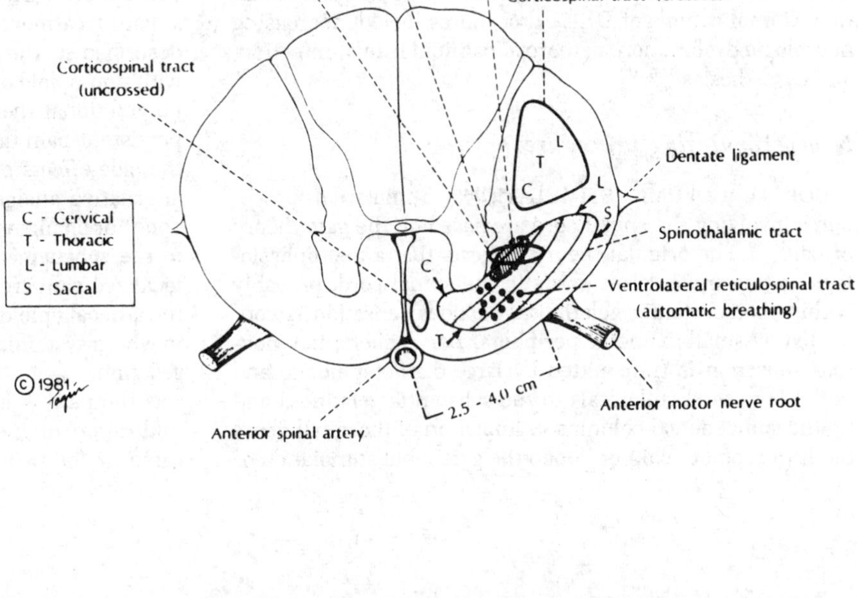

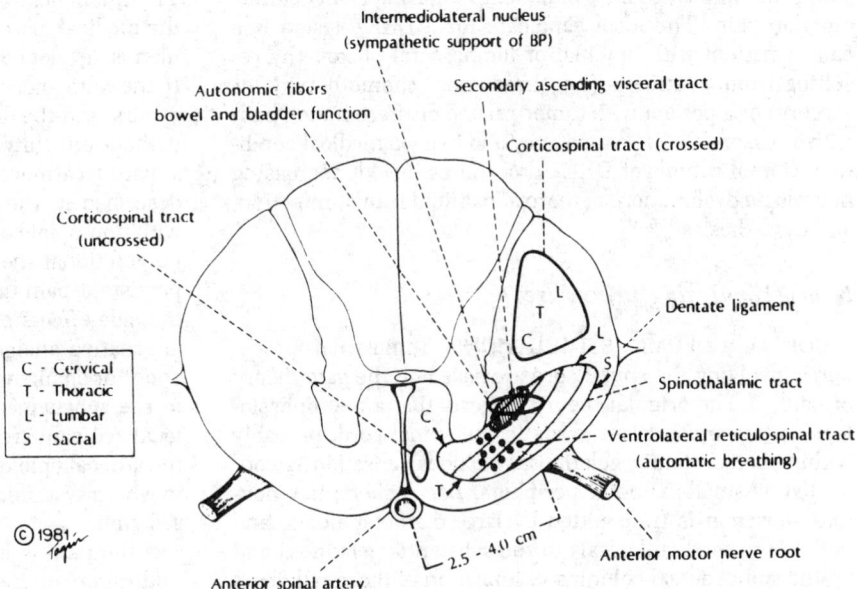

FIG. 59-11. Cross-section of the spinal cord shows the relationship of the spinothalamic tract to other motor and autonomic fibers[122] and serves as the anatomical basis for percutaneous and open cordotomy.

contraindicated to perform bilateral high cervical cordotomies or an unilateral cordotomy ipsilateral to the side of the solely functioning lung. Bilateral percutaneous C1–C2 cordotomies have been performed in two sittings with no respiratory complications.

In a recent review of the role of cordotomy in the management of perineal pain, unilateral cordotomy commonly unmasked the contralateral pain, which could be controlled with analgesics or with a sacral neurolytic block.[125]

DORSAL ROOT ENTRY ZONE LESIONS. Dorsal root entry zone (DREZ) lesions refer to an ablative procedure carried out at the level of Lissauer's tract in the dorsal spinal cord. Both inhibitory and exitatory impulses are transmitted by axons in Lissauer's tract, the cell bodies of which are located within the substantia gelatinosa of neighboring spinal cord segments. Interruption of the transmission of abnormal nociceptive impulses either in Lissauer's tract or at their origin in the substantia gelatinosa may decrease the pathologic influence these areas have on pain perception. Anatomical studies of the dorsal root spinal cord junction reveal a topographic segregation of the afferent fibers according to their size, destination, and function. A selective interruption of the small nociceptive fibers situated in the dorsal and central aspect of the DREZ can be carried out while sparing the large lemniscus fibers grouped more medially. The procedure is done under general anesthesia, and it requires a multilevel laminectomy or hemilaminectomy and exposure of the spinal cord. The cord lesion is made at the root entry zone in the dorsolateral sulcus. The lesion can be achieved by sharp instruments, laser, or radiofrequency electrodes and has to be 1 to 2 mm deep and obliquely oriented to reach Lissauer's tract.

The primary indication for a DREZ lesion is deafferentation pain.[123] The majority of DREZ procedures performed have been on patients with trauma-related deafferentation conditions. However, patients with cancer-related deafferentation pain also have responded favorably to DREZ procedures. Long-term follow-up results show good to excellent pain relief in 60% to 85% of patients suffering from deafferentation pain. The ideal candidate for a DREZ lesion is a cancer patient with brachial or lumbosacral plexopathy resulting from treatment (*e.g.*, irradiation, chemotherapy, or surgery) or a patient with tumor-related deafferentation pain with a reasonable life expectancy and in good medical condition. Complications of DREZ procedures include increasing neurologic dysfunction, cerebrospinal fluid fistula, infection, and dysesthesias.[126,127]

Neurostimulating Procedures

DORSAL COLUMN STIMULATION. Stimulation procedures involving the spinal cord are based on the gate theory of pain.[128] The original theory suggests that a neurophysiologic gating mechanism exists in the spinal cord, probably within the substantia gelatinosa. Noxious sensation is conducted by small-diameter peripheral nerve fibers; non-noxious sensation is transmitted by large-diameter fibers; and both fibers send collaterals to the substantia gelatinosa and up the spinal dorsal columns. Stimulation of the small fibers tends to promote pain or "open the gate," but stimulation of the large fibers tends to inhibit pain or "close the gate." Because the large nerve fibers ascend in a compact bundle through the dorsal columns, they are accessible to selected electric stimulation. Retrograde firing of the large fibers ensues, with resulting inhibition of pain sensation in many levels of the spinal cord below that being stimulated.

The dorsal column stimulating technique introduces an electrode into the epidural or intrathecal space and advances it to the appropriate level overlying the dorsal columns. This is done under local anesthesia and biplane fluoroscopy. Once in place, the electrode is implanted subcutaneously, and an external transmitting electrode is placed over the receiving electrode and connected to a transmitter. A trial is then done to assess the efficacy of the electrode, check its position, and determine the stimulatory parameters for the patient. Parameters that can be controlled are frequency, amplitude, and duration of stimulatory cycles. The electrode that we found most suitable is the quadripolar lead, which is a multielectrode lead that permits one to choose the pair of electrodes that produce the best response.[129,130]

The main indications for placing a dorsal column stimulator are intractable dysesthetic or deafferentation pain of the limbs or trunk, such as radiation-induced brachial or lumbosacral plexopathy.[123] This procedure is effective in 43% to 75% of patients and has a low morbidity rate. The most common complication is failure of the device itself, which occurs in approximately 10% of patients annually. Other complications include infection, cerebrospinal fluid fistula, allergic or rejection responses to the device material, and changes in stimulation over time, which may be related to cellular changes around the electrode or shifts in its position.

ALGORITHM FOR CANCER PAIN MANAGEMENT

Figure 59-12 provides an algorithm describing the integration of the previously discussed management approaches for cancer pain. It attempts to integrate assessment techniques, drug therapy, behavioral approaches, and anesthetic and neurosurgical approaches, and it stresses continuity of care. Treatment begins with a diagnostic evaluation that addresses the medical, psychological, and social components of pain. A plan is developed to treat both the cancer and the pain itself. If the anticancer treatment is effective, pain relief usually occurs, and the drugs used for analgesia can be discontinued without difficulty.

Pain treatment begins with the use of analgesic drugs as described in the analgesic ladder (see Fig. 59-8), starting with non-opioid drugs alone or in combination. If successful, no additional therapy is necessary. In patients with severe, persistent pain unresponsive to analgesic drugs or in whom the side-effects of the drugs are not tolerated, switching to alternative analgesics (*e.g.*, from oral morphine to methadone) or changing the route of administration (*e.g.*, from oral to the subcutaneous route) or performing a cordotomy for localized pain are approaches the physician should consider. Intrathecal opioids are indicated for relief of pain in patients in whom systemic analgesics produce confusion or excessive sedation.

If the pain is localized (*e.g.*, intercostal pain from tumor infiltration of the chest wall), neurolytic blocks are indicated. If the pain is unilateral and below the waist, cordot-

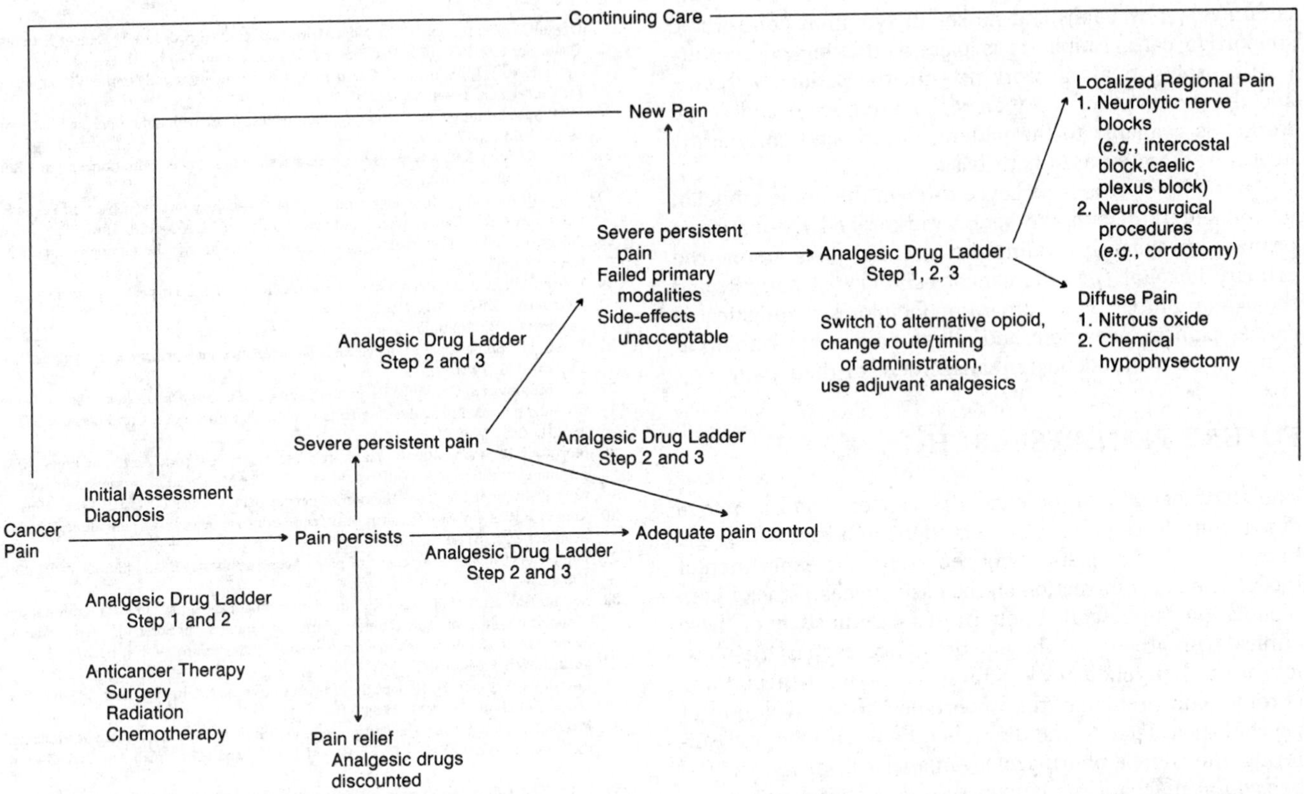

FIG. 59-12. Algorithm for the integration of management approaches to cancer pain.

omy should be considered. For diffuse pain, nitrous oxide inhalation and, rarely, chemical hypophysectomy may be tried. Cognitive-behavioral approaches need to be integrated from the onset of treatment and should be used with the medical and surgical approaches.

Whatever techniques of pain management are used, the physician is responsible for providing continuing care and for constantly reassessing the diagnosis and the treatment to achieve optimum relief of pain and suffering for patient and family. For example, in a patient with breast cancer and a brachial plexopathy, the initial treatment approach would include chemotherapy or irradiation therapy. Non-opioid analgesics, such as acetaminophen or ibuprofen, would be given on a regular basis around the clock. If pain relief did not occur, the additional use of a weak opioid, such as oxycodone or codeine, would be the next step. If there was an associated complaint of burning dysethesias, amitriptyline, starting at 10-mg doses at bedtime, would be added, and if possible, a stellate ganglion block would be considered to manage the deafferentation component of the pain. If pain control is achieved, this combination of a non-opioid, an opioid, and an adjuvant is maintained until the patient has improvement in pain relief heralded by the clinical observation that the analgesics worked for longer than the initial 3 to 4 hours. The opioid is reduced by initially extending the time interval between doses and eventually within 2 to 3 days of discontinuing the opioid.

If pain relief is not achieved by the radiation therapy or chemotherapy, switching to a strong opioid, such as oral morphine or methadone, and titrating the dose to effective analgesia is in order. If anxiety or depression are components of the pain, the early introduction of cognitive and behavioral approaches provide the patient with a mechanism to manage these symptoms and remain in control. The use of devices to reduce lymphedema and to provide mechanical support to the neurologically impaired arm can also impact the pain. Our experience with neurolytic blocks and cordotomy for pain from tumor infiltration of the brachial plexus has been disappointing, and a drug therapy approach has offered the most generally useful approach. Continuing care for these patients become paramount, particularly when all primary care approaches have been exhausted.

CONTINUITY OF CARE

The care of patients with cancer and chronic pain strains the resources of a single physician, especially after the patient's discharge from hospital. A variety of supportive-care and continuing-care programs have been developed to manage dying patients at home, where the focus shifts from care to comfort. Hospice and home-care programs represent the common approach used by community hospitals to help care for such patients.[126] Cancer centers have relied on these programs in referring patients back into the community. Recently a model of continuity of care has been developed to meet the needs of patients cared for at Memorial Sloan-Kettering Cancer Center.[127] This program is a patient-centered and family-centered, nurse-coordinated model, using a collaborative approach among a nurse, physician, and social worker. The nurse is responsible for the daily management of the patient's pain and works with the patient, family, and community physicians and nurses in symptom control and supportive care. Emphasis is placed on using community health professionals in working with the patient at home, and the expertise of the team's nurse clinician and social worker is available to the patient, family, and community health workers on a 24-hour basis.

Continuity of care is achieved through the nurse clinician in collaboration with the social worker and the patient's primary physician, providing the essential links among the primary hospital (*i.e.*, the cancer center), the patient, and the community. This program facilitates sophisticated cancer pain management and allows patients to remain at home to die with adequate management of their pain.

FUTURE PAIN RESEARCH

The study of pain in patients with cancer offers a unique opportunity to use clinical observations to advance biologic knowledge. The cancer patient represents the experimental model of pain. Information on the basic mechanisms of pain modulation can be culled only from a careful study of these clinical pain problems. These patients can teach us the physiologic and psychological differences between acute and chronic pain problems, the importance of the evolution of psychological factors, the difference between pain and suffering, the clinical pharmacology of analgesic drugs, and the behavioral mechanisms humans use to suppress pain.

The use of innovative approaches based on sound scientific principles and advances in research technology offer the opportunity to understand the complex phenomenon of pain and improve the control of pain in patients.

REFERENCES

1. Levin D, Cleeland CS, Dar R: Public attitudes toward cancer pain. Cancer 56:2337–2339, 1985
2. Payne R, Foley KM: Advances in the management of cancer pain. Cancer Treat Rep 68:173–183, 1984
3. Foley KM: The treatment of cancer pain. N Engl J Med 313:84–95, 1985
4. Payne R, Foley KM (eds): Cancer pain. Med Clin North Am 17(2), 1987
5. Cartwright A, Hockey L, Anderson ABM: Life Before Death. London, Routledge and Kegan Paul, 1973
6. Foley KM: Pain syndromes in patients with cancer. In Bonica JJ, Ventafridda V (eds): Advances in Pain Research and Therapy, Vol 2, pp 59–75. New York, Raven Press, 1979
7. Haram BJ: In Saunders CM (ed): Facts and Figures in Management of Terminal Disease, pp 12–18. London, Edward Arnold, 1978
8. Molinari R: Therapy of cancer pain in the head and neck. In Bonica JJ, Ventafridda V (eds): Advances in Pain Research and Therapy, Vol 2, pp 131–138. New York, Raven Press, 1979
9. Norton WS, Lack SA: Control of symptoms other than pain. In Twycross RG, Ventafridda V (eds): The Continuing Care of Patients with Terminal Cancer, pp 167–178. Oxford, Pergamon Press, 1980
10. Pannuti E, Rossi AP, Marraro D et al: In Twycross RG, Ventafridda V (eds): The Continuing Care of Patients with Terminal Cancer, pp 75–78. Oxford, Pergamon Press, 1980
11. Rubin R, Rogers A, Foley KM: The measurement of pain in children with cancer (in press)
12. Trotter JM, Scott R, MacBeth FR et al: Problems of the oncology outpatient: Role of the liaison health visitor. Br Med J 282:122–124, 1981
13. Twycross RG: Clinical experience with diamorphine in advanced malignant disease. Int J Clin Pharmacol Ther Toxicol 9:184–198, 1974
14. Wilkes E: Some problems in cancer management. Proc R Soc Med 67:23–27, 1974
15. Twycross RG, Fairfield S: Pain in far-advanced cancer. Pain 14:303–310, 1982
16. Daut RL, Cleeland CS: The prevalance and severity of pain in cancer. Cancer 50:1913–1918, 1982
17. World Health Organization: Cancer Pain Relief. Geneva, World Health Organization, 1986
18. Takeda F: Management of cancer pain: WHO cancer pain relief programme. In Organizing Committee of the 1984 Workshop on Quality of Life in Cancer Patients: Quality of Life in Cancer Patients, pp 61–69. Tokyo, 1985
19. Ventafridda V, Tamburini M, Caraceni A et al: A validation study of the WHO method for cancer pain relief. Cancer 59:850–856, 1987
20. IAAP Subcommittee on Taxonomy: Pain terms: A list with definitions and notes on usage. Pain 8:249–252, 1980
21. Payne R, Foley KM: Advances in the management of cancer pain. Cancer Treat Rep 68:173–183, 1984
22. Payne R: Anatomy, physiology, and neuropharmacology of cancer pain. In Payne R, Foley KM (eds): Cancer pain. Med Clin North Am 71:153–168, 1987
23. Spiegel K, Kalb R, Pasternak GW: Analgesic activity of tricyclic antidepressants. Ann Neurol 13:462–465, 1983
24. Watson CP, Evan RJ, Reed K et al: Amitriptyline vs placebo in postherpetic neuralgia. Neurology 32:671–673, 1982
25. Pasternak GW: Multiple opiate receptors. JAMA (in press)
26. Yaksh TL: Spinal opiate analgesia: Characteristics and principles of action. Pain 11:293–346, 1981
27. Max MB, Inturrisi CE, Kaiko RF et al: Epidural and intrathecal opiates: Distribution in CSF and plasma and analgesic effects in patients with cancer. Clin Pharmacol Ther 38:631–641, 1985
28. Sternbach RA: Pain Patients: Traits and Treatment. New York, Academic Press, 1974
29. Fishman B, Pasternak S, Wallenstein SL et al: The Memorial pain assessment card: A valid instrument for the evaluation of cancer pain. Cancer 60:1151–1158, 1987
30. Kanner RM, Foley KM: Patterns of narcotic drug use in a cancer pain clinic. Ann NY Acad Sci 362:161–172, 1981
31. Foley KM: Clinical assessment of pain. Acta Anesthesiol Scand [Suppl] 74:91–96, 1982
32. Kanner RM, Martini N, Foley KM: Incidence of pain and other clinical manifestations of superior pulmonary sulcus tumor (Pancoast's tumors). In Bonica JJ, Ventafridda V, Pagnis CA (eds): Advances in Pain Research and Therapy, Vol 4, pp 27–38. New York, Raven Press, 1982
33. Bukberg J, Penman D, Holland JC: Depression in hospitalized cancer patients. Psychosom Med 46:199–212, 1984
34. Massie MJ, Holland JC: The cancer patient with pain: Psychiatric complications and their management (Payne R, Foley KM [eds]). Med Clin North Am 71:243–258, 1987
35. Foley KM: Pain syndromes in patients with cancer (Payne R, Foley KM [eds]). Med Clin North Am 71:169–184, 1987
36. Kori S, Foley KM, Posner JB: Brachial plexus lesions in patients with cancer: Clinical findings in 100 cases. Neurology 31:45–50, 1981
37. Foley KM: Brachial plexopathy in patients with breast cancer. In Harris JR, Hellman S, Henderson IC et al (eds): Breast Diseases, pp 532–537. Philadelphia, Lippincott, 1987
38. Portenoy RK, Lipton RB, Foley KM: Back pain in the cancer patient: An algorithm for evaluation and management. Neurology 37:134–138, 1986
39. Kori SH, Krol G, Foley KM: Computed tomography evaluation of bone and soft tissue metastases. In Weiss L, Gilbert HA (eds): Bone Metastases, Metastases Monograph Series, Vol 3, pp 245–257. Boston, GK Hall, 1981
40. Thrupkaew A, Henken R, Quinl JL: False negative bone scans in disseminated metastatic diseases. Radiology 113:383–386, 1975
41. Kelly RJ, Cowan RJ, Ferree CB et al: Efficacy of radionuclide scanning in patients with lung cancer. JAMA 242:2855–2857, 1979
42. Granek I, Ashikari R, Foley KM: Postmastectomy pain syndrome: Clinical and anatomical correlates. Proc ASCO 3:122, 1983
43. Kanner RM, Martini N, Foley KM: Nature and incidence of post-thoracotomy pain. Proc ASCO 1:152, 1982
44. Patchell R, Posner JB: Neurologic complications of systemic cancer. Neurol Clin 3:729–750, 1985
45. Greenberg HS, Deck MD, Vikram B et al: Metastasis to the base of the skull: Clinical findings in 43 patients. Neurology 31:530–537, 1981
46. Posner JB: Back pain and epidural spinal cord compression (Payne R, Foley KM [eds]). Med Clin North Am 71:185–205, 1987
47. Sundaresan N, Galicich JH, Lane J: Treatment of odontoid fractures in cancer patients. J Neurosurg 54:468–472, 1981
48. Jaeckle KA, Young DF, Foley KM: The natural history of lumbosacral plexopathy in cancer. Neurology 35:8–15, 1985
49. Stillman MJ: Perineal pain syndromes in cancer patient (abstr). Neurology (in press)
50. Cascino TL, Kori S, Krol G et al: CT scanning of the brachial plexus in patients with cancer. Neurology 33:1553–1557, 1983
51. Thomas JE, Cascino TE, Earle JD: Differential diagnosis between radiation and tumor plexopathy of the pelvis. Neurology 35:1–7, 1985
52. Olson ME, Chirnik NL, Posner JB: Infiltration of the leptomeninges by systemic cancer. A clinical and pathological study. Arch Neurol 30:122–137, 1978
53. Sherman RA, Sherman CJ, Parker L: Chronic phantom and stump pain among American veterans. Results of a survey. Pain 18:83–95, 1984
54. Aker SN: Oral findings in the cancer patient. Cancer 43:2103–2107, 1979
55. Fair WR: Urologic emergencies. In DeVita VT Jr, Hellman S, Rosenberg SA (eds): Principles and Practice of Oncology, 2nd ed, pp 1894–1906. Philadelphia, JB Lippincott, 1985
56. Lequesne PM: Neuropathy due to drugs. In Dyck PJ, Thomas PK, Lambert EH et al (eds): Peripheral Neuropathy, Vol II, 2nd ed, pp 2126–2179. Philadelphia, WB Saunders, 1983
57. Ihde DC, Devita VT: Osteonecrosis of the femoral head in patients with lymphoma

treated with intermittent combination chemotherapy (including corticosteroids). Cancer 36:1585–1588, 1975
58. Rotstein J, Good RA: Steroid pseudorheumatism. Arch Intern Med 99:545–555, 1957
59. Portenoy RK, Duma C, Foley KM: Acute herpetic and postherpetic neuralgia: Review of clinical features and current therapy. Ann Neurol 20:651–664, 1987
60. Twycross R, Lack SA: Symptom control in far advanced cancer. In Pain Relief. London, Pitman Books, 1984
61. Jllinger K, Sturm KW: Delayed radiation myelopathy in man. J Neurol Sci 14:389–408, 1971
62. Foley KM, Woodruff JM, Ellis F et al: Radiation-induced malignant and atypical peripheral nerve sheath tumors. Ann Neurol 7:311–318, 1980
63. Payne R, Foley KM: Exploration of the brachial plexus in patients with cancer. Neurology 36:329, 1986
64. Kantor TG: Control of pain by non-steroidal anti-inflammatory drugs. Med Clin North Am 66:1053–1059, 1982
65. Galasko CSB: Mechanisms of bone destruction in the development of skeletal metastases. Nature 263:507–510, 1976
66. Beaver WT: Combination analgesics. Am J Med 77:38–53, 1985
67. Foley KM: Current controversies in opioid therapy. In Foley KM, Inturrisi CE (eds): Advances in Pain Research and Therapy: Opioid Analgesics in the Management of Clinical Pain, pp 3–11. New York, Raven Press, 1986
68. Foley KM, Inturrisi CE: Analgesic drug therapy in cancer pain: Principles and practice (Payne R, Foley KM [eds]). Med Clin North Am 71:207–232, 1987
69. Kaiko RF, Foley KM, Grabinski PY et al: Central nervous system excitatory effects of meperidine in cancer patients. Ann Neurol 13:180–185, 1983
70. Kaiko RF, Wallenstein SL, Rogers AG et al: Analgesic and mood effects of heroin and morphine in cancer patients with postoperative pain. N Engl J Med 304:1501–1505, 1981
71. Inturrisi CE, Max M, Foley KM et al: The pharmacokinetics of heroin in patients with chronic pain. N Engl J Med 310:1213–1217, 1984
72. Dixon R, Crews I, Mohacsi E et al: Levorphanol: A simplified radioimmunoassay for clinical use. Res Commun Chem Pathol Pharmacol 32:545–548, 1981
73. Brevik H, Rennemo F: Clinical evaluation of combined treatment with methadone and psychotropic drugs in cancer patients. Acta Anesthesiol Scand [Suppl] 74:135–140, 1982
74. Ventafridda V, Ripamonti C, Bianchi M et al: A randomized study on oral administration of morphine and methadone in the treatment of cancer pain. J Pain Sympt Manage 1:203–207, 1986
75. Sawe J, Hansen J, Ginsman C et al: Patient controlled dose regimen for methadone for chronic cancer pain. Br Med J 282:771–773, 1981
76. Ventafridda V, DeConno F, Guarise G et al: Chronic analgesic study on buprenorphine action in cancer pain—comparison with pentazocine. Drug Res 33:587–590, 1983
77. Marks RM, Sachar EJ: Undertreatment of medical inpatients with narcotic analgesics. Ann Intern Med 78:173–181, 1973
78. Houde RW: Methods for measuring clinical pain in humans. Acta Anaesthesiol Scand [Suppl] 74:25–29, 1982
79. Kaiko RF: Commentary: Equianalgesic dose ratio of intramuscular/oral morphine, 1:6 versus 1:3. In Foley KM, Inturrisi CE (eds): Advances in Pain Research and Therapy: Opioid Analgesics in the Management of Clinical Pain, Vol 8, pp 87–94. New York, Raven Press, 1986
80. Coyle N, Adelhardt J, Foley KM: Changing patterns in pain, drug use and routes of administration in the advanced cancer patient. Pain (Suppl 4), Fifth World Congress on Pain, IASP, S339, 1987
81. Hirsch JD: Sublingual morphine sulfate in chronic pain management. Clin Pharm 3:585–586, 1984
82. Bell MD, Mishra P, Weldon BD et al: Buccal morphine—a new route of analgesia. Lancet 1985
83. Weinberg DS, Inturrisi CE, Reidenberg B et al: Sublingual absorption of selected opioid analgesics. Clin Pharmacol Ther (in press)
84. Beaver WT, Feise GA: A comparison of the analgesic effects of oxymorphones by rectal suppository and intramuscular injection in patients with postoperative pain. J Clin Pharmacol 17:276–291, 1977
85. Pannuti F, Rossi AP, Iafellice G et al: Control of chronic pain in very advanced cancer patients with morphine hydrochloride administered by oral, rectal and sublingual route. Clinical report and preliminary results of morphine pharmacokinetics. Pharmacol Res Commun 14:369–380, 1982
86. Coyle N, Mauskop A, Maggard J et al: Continuous subcutaneous infusions of opiates in cancer patients with pain. Nurs Forum 13:53–57, 1986
87. Bruera E, Chadwick S, Brenneis C et al: Subcutaneous infusion of narcotics using a disposable portable device. Cancer Treat Rep (in press)
88. Ventafridda V, Spoldi E, Caraceni A et al: The importance of continuous subcutaneous morphine administration for cancer pain control. Pain Clin 1:47–55, 1986
89. Portenoy RK, Moulin DE, Rogers A et al: Intravenous infusion of opioids in cancer pain: Clinical review and guidelines for use. Cancer Treat Rep 70:575–581, 1985
90. Coombs DW, Saunders RL, Gaylor MS: Epidural narcotic infusion reservoir: Implantation technique and efficacy. Anesthesiology 56:469–473, 1982
91. Moulin DE, Inturrisi CE, Foley KM: Epidural and intrathecal opioids: Cerebrospinal fluid and plasma pharmacokinetics in cancer pain patients. In Foley KM, Inturrisi CE (eds): Advances in Pain Research and Therapy: Opioid Analgesics in the Management of Clinical Pain, Vol 8, pp 369–384. New York, Raven Press, 1986
92. Payne R: Role of epidural and intrathecal narcotics and peptides in the management of cancer pain (Payne R, Foley KM [eds]). Med Clin North Am 71:313–328, 1987
93. Beaver WT: Comparison of analgesic effects of morphine sulfate, hydroxyzine and other combination in patients with postoperative pain. In Bonica JJ, Ventafridda V (eds): Advances in Pain Research and Therapy, pp 553–557. New York, Raven Press, 1976
94. Forrest WH et al: Dextroamphetamine with morphine for the treatment of postoperative pain. N Engl J Med 296:712–715, 1977
95. Singh PN, Sharma P, Gupta S et al: Clinical evaluation of diazepam for relief of postoperative pain. Br J Anesth 53:831–835, 1981
96. Houde RW, Wallenstein SL: Analgesic power of chlopromazine alone and in combination with morphine (abstr). Fed Proc 14:353, 1955
97. Gralla RJ, Tyson LB, Kris MG et al: The management of chemotherapy-induced nausea and vomiting (Payne R, Foley KM [eds]): Med Clin North Am 71:289–302, 1987
98. Portenoy RK: Constipation in the cancer patient: Causes and management (Payne R, Foley KM [eds]): Med Clin North Am 71:303–310, 1987
99. Swerdlow M: Anticonvulsant drugs and chronic pain. Clin Neuropharmacol 7:51–82, 1984
100. Beaver WT, Wallenstein SL, Houde RW et al: A comparison of the analgesic effect of methotrimeprazine and morphine in patients with cancer. Clin Pharmacol Ther 7:436–446, 1983
101. Walsh TD: Antidepressants and chronic pain. Clin Neuropharmacol 6:271–295, 1983
102. Schell HW: The risk of adrenal corticosteroid therapy with far-advanced cancer. Am J Med Sci 252:641–649, 1966
103. Fishman B, Loscalzo M: Cognitive-behavioral interventions in management of cancer pain: Principles and applications (Payne R, Foley KM [eds]: Med Clin North Am 71:271–288, 1987
104. Turk D, Meichenbaum D, Genert M: Pain and Behavioral Medicine. New York, Guilford Press, 1983
105. Cousins MJ, Bridenbaugh PO (eds): Neural Blockade in Clinical Anesthesia and Management of Pain. Philadelphia, JB Lippincott, 1980
106. Bonica JJ: The Management of Pain. Philadelphia, Lea & Febiger, 1953
107. Lipton S: Persistent Pain. london, Academic Press, 1977
108. Travell JG, Simons DG: Myofascial Pain and Dysfunction: The Trigger Point Manual. Baltimore, Williams & Wilkins, 1983
109. Borzecki PR, Hilgien SE: Treatment of chronic pain by continuous blockade of peripheral nervous system. Reg Anesth: 16–17, 1979
110. Nathan PW, Sears TA, Smith MC: Effect of phenol solution on the nerve roots of the cat: An electrophysiological and histological study. J Neurol Sci 2:7–29, 1965
111. Mark VH, White JC, Zervas NT et al: Intratheal use of phenol for the relief of chronic severe pain. N Engl J Med 267:589–593, 1962
112. Pilon RN, Baker AR: Chronic pain control by means of an epidural catheter. Cancer 37:903–905, 1976
113. Raj P, Phero JC: Pain control in cancer of head and neck. In Thawley S, Panje WR (eds): Comprehensive Management in Head and Neck Tumors, pp 42–68. Philadelphia, WB Saunders, 1987
114. Jain S, Foley KM, Thomas J et al: Factors influencing efficacy of epidural neurolysis therapy for intractable cancer pain. pain (Suppl 4), Fifth World Congress on Pain, IASP, S134, 1987
115. Singler RC: An improved technique for alcohol neurolysis of the coeliac plexus. Anesthesiology 56:137–141, 1982
116. Thompson GE, Moore DC, Bridenbaugh LD et al: Abdominal pain and alcohol coeliac plexus nerve block. Anesth Analg 56:1–5, 1977
117. Waldman SD, Feldstein LS, Allen ML: Neuroadenolysis of the pituatory: Description of a modified technique. J Pain Sympt Manage: 45–49, 1987
118. Fosburg MT, Crone RK: Nitrous oxide analgesia for refractory pain in the terminally ill. JAMA 250:511–513, 1983
119. Siegfried J, Broggi G: Percutaneous thermocoagulation of the gasserian ganglion in the treatment of pain in advanced cancer. In Bonica JJ, Ventafridda V (eds): Advances in Pain Research and Therapy, Vol 2, pp 453–462. New York, Raven Press, 1979
120. Bricolo A: Medullary tractotomy for cephalic pain of malignant diseases. In Bonica JJ, Ventafridda V (eds): Advances in Pain Research and Therapy, Vol 2, pp 463–469. New York, Raven Press, 1979
121. Rosomoff HL, Carroll F, Brown J: Percutaneous radiofrequency cervical cordotomy: Technique. J Neurosurg 23:639–644, 1975
122. Poletti CE: Open cordotomy—new techniques. In Schmidek HH, Sweet WH (eds): Operative Neurosurgical Techniques: Indications, Methods and Results, Vol 2. New York, Grune & Stratton, 1982
123. Tasker RR, Tsuda T, Howrylyshyn P: Clinical neurophysiological investigation of deafferentation pain. In Bonica JJ, Ventafridda V (eds): Advances in Pain Research and Therapy, Vol 5, 691–700. New York, Raven Press, 1983
124. Nathan PW: Pain in cancer: Comparison of results of cordotomy and chemical rhizotomy. In Fusek I, King I (eds): Present Limits of Neurosurgery, pp 513–516. Amsterdam, Excerpta Medica, 1972
125. Macaluso C, Foley KM, Arbit E: Cordotomy for lumbosacral, pelvic, and lower extremity pain of malignant origin: Safety and efficacy. Neurology (Suppl) 38:110, 1988
126. Standards of a Hospice Program of Care. Washington DC, National Hospice Organization, 1979
127. Coyle N, Monzillo E, Loscalzo M et al: A model of continuity of care for cancer patients with pain and neuro-oncologic complications. Cancer Nurs 8:111–119, 1985

SECTION 5

PHILIP A. PIZZO
JOEL MEYERS

Infections in the Cancer Patient

The relationships among malignancy, immunocompromise, and infectious morbidity and mortality are established.[1-4] More intensive treatment regimens have produced more patients with cancer who are immunocompromised. The infectious complications that can occur are life-threatening and may limit the benefits of antineoplastic therapy. Therefore, the oncologist must be familiar with the risk factors contributing to infection and be knowledgeable about the infectious syndromes and the available therapies.

The patient with cancer may be immunocompromised because of the underlying malignancy or the antineoplastic therapy. Specific malignancies may be associated with immune deficits that predispose to infection with particular pathogens. For example, patients with Hodgkin's or non-Hodgkin's lymphomas tend to have abnormalities of the cellular immune system that heighten their risk for viral and fungal infections. Therapeutic modalities such as corticosteroids, cytotoxic chemotherapy, and localized or widespread irradiation result in further deficiencies of host defense. The consequence of these interrelated abnormalities of immune function is the immunocompromised cancer patient (Fig. 59-13).

IMPAIRED HOST DEFENSES OF THE CANCER PATIENT

INTEGUMENTARY AND MUCOSAL BARRIERS

The skin and mucosal surfaces constitute the primary host defense against invasion by endogenous and acquired micro-organisms. The integrity of this physical barrier can be disrupted by the patient's tumor or by its treatment. Mucosal and epithelial cells contain specific and nonspecific receptors for the attachment or adherence of micro-organisms.[5,6] These receptors can be altered by disease and by certain therapies, particularly antibiotics, permitting colonization of the immunosuppressed cancer patient with new pathogens.[6-8] Colonization is also influenced by suppression of the host's anaerobic microflora, because these organisms can resist colonization by aerobic pathogens.[9] The anaerobic flora are suppressed by many antibiotics, particularly the β-lactams. The mucosal changes provide a nidus for microbial colonization, a focus for local infection, and a portal for systemic invasion.

FIG. 59-13. Interactions of the defense matrix that delineates the compromised host. (Hathorn JW, Pizzo PA: Infectious complications in the pediatric cancer patient. In Pizzo PA, Poplock DG (eds): Principles and Practice of Pediatric Oncology, p 839. Philadelphia, JB Lippincott, 1989)

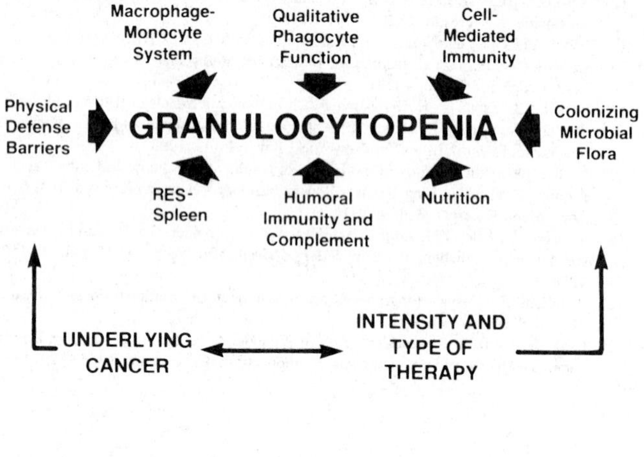

PHAGOCYTIC DEFENSES

The neutrophil and the monocyte–macrophage are the major cellular defenses against most bacteria and fungi.[10] Whether disease related or as a consequence of therapy, the degree of severe neutropenia is directly related to the risk of serious infection (Table 59-28).[11] To meet rapidly changing needs, there is normally a large bone marrow granulocyte reserve that exceeds the circulating pool of neutrophils and that is distributed equally between the blood stream and a marginating pool. The half-life of cells in the circulating granulocyte pool is 6 to 7 hours, following which these cells either marginate along the vascular endothelial surfaces or move into extravascular spaces. When granulopoiesis is depressed by disease or treatment, the granulocyte reserves are rapidly depleted, with severe granulocytopenia ensuing within 5 to 7 days.

A number of glycoprotein hormonal growth factors integral to granulopoiesis have been characterized, their genes cloned and recombinant proteins purified. It has become apparent that various cells, including T and B lymphocytes, monocytes, fibroblasts, and endothelial cells, produce cytokines that are integral to hematopoiesis. The colony stimulating factors (CSF) include the granulocyte–macrophage CSF (GM-CSF), granulocyte CSF (G-CSF), macrophage CSF (M-CSF), and multiprotein CSF (also referred to as IL-3).[12,13] These hematopoietic growth factors affect many target cells, and some (*e.g.,* IL-3, GM-CSF) stimulate several blood cell lineages. Cloned GM-CSF and G-CSF have the capacity to shorten the recovery of neutrophils after chemotherapy-induced or radiation-induced myelosuppression. For example, subhuman primates treated with total-body irradiation recovered their neutrophils to 1000/mm^3 8 to 9 days after transplant if they received GM-CSF; the process took 17 to 24 days if they did not receive GM-CSF.[14] In addition to accelerating neutrophil recovery, GM-CSF also appears to enhance phagocyte activity, including superoxide generation, phagocytosis, and antibacterial activity.[15-18]

A number of cytokines appear to be interlinked in generating GM-CSF or in initiating cell reactivity. Included among these are tumor necrosis factor (TNF or cachectin), interleukin-1, interleukin-2, and interferon.[19-28] A variety of cytokines play an integral role in host defense and cell regulation. The characterization, purification, cloning, and production of these growth factors offer new prospects for studying the biology of hematopoiesis and for bolstering host

TABLE 59-28. Percentage of Cancer Patients Who Develop Serious Infections with Granulocytopenia and the Cumulative Risk of Infection with Prolonged Granulocytopenia

Granulocyte Level (per mm³)		*Percentage of Serious Infections (Duration of Granulocytopenia in Weeks)*							
Initial	*Change*	*1*	*2*	*3*	*4*	*6*	*10*	*12*	*14*
Any level	Any fall	12							
Any level	Fall to 2000	2							
Any level	Fall to 1500	5							
Any level	Fall to 1000	10	30	45	50	65	70	85	100
Any level	Fall to 500	19							
Any level	Fall to <100	28	50	72	85	100			

Adapted from Bodey GP et al: Quantitative relationships between circulating leukocytes and infection in patients with acute leukemia. Ann Intern Med 61:328–340, 1966.

defenses that are altered in patients undergoing treatment for cancer.[29]

In addition to quantitative defects, qualitative abnormalities of neutrophil function have been described in patients with hematologic malignancies. These include defects in chemotaxis, phagocytosis, bactericidal capacity, and the absence of the respiratory burst that usually accompanies phagocytosis.[30] Although phagocytic capacity remains normal, decreased spontaneous migratory and chemotactic leukocyte functions have been described in untreated patients with lymphoma and carcinoma, suggesting the presence of a circulating inhibitor in the sera of these patients.[31,32]

Cancer chemotherapy may also produce defects of neutrophil function. Corticosteroids, for example, can decrease phagocytosis and neutrophil migration. The combination of prednisone with vincristine and asparaginase or 6-mercaptopurine and methotrexate can produce a significant decrease in the phagocytic and killing capability.[33]Although the mechanism is not clear, bactericidal activity may be transiently impaired within the 3 months after craniospinal irradiation in patients with leukemia, which may contribute to the infectious complications that occur during that period.[34] Analgesic narcotics such as morphine can also cause a dose-dependent suppression of granulocytes and can exacerbate infections in experimental animals.[35]

The mature macrophage is more resistant to cytotoxic chemotherapy than the granulocyte and hence provides some residual phagocytic capacity during periods of severe neutropenia. The activated macrophage is also an important defense against mycobacteria, *Listeria, Brucella,* and several fungi, protozoans, and viruses. Macrophages are important in the initiation of the immune responses, because they are triggered into a metabolically active state by antigenic stimuli and subsequently process and present these antigens to T and B lymphocytes. Macrophages also produce a variety of low-molecular-weight polypeptide hormones (monokines) that regulate lymphocyte function and colony-stimulating factors that are important in granulopoieses.[12,13] If macrophage function is altered, as with steroids, the primary defense against fungal pathogens is altered, further aggravating the altered host defense of the neutropenic host.[36]

CELLULAR AND HUMORAL IMMUNITY

Patients with lymphoid malignancies, especially Hodgkin's disease, may also have abnormalities of cell-mediated immunity, such as anergy and decreased phytohemagglutinin (PHA) responsiveness, which may persist even after the underlying malignancy has been treated.[37] These defects are aggravated by chemotherapy with glucocorticosteroids and by infections like disseminated histoplasmosis, making patients susceptible to viral *(Herpes zoster)* or fungal *(Cryptococcus)* infections.[38]

Cytotoxic chemotherapy adversely affects B-cell and T-cell functions, resulting in diminished opsonizing activity, inadequate agglutination and lysis of bacteria, and deficient neutralization of bacterial toxins.[39] Impaired antibody production has been described in untreated patients with chronic lymphocytic leukemia, multiple myeloma, or Hodgkin's disease.[40] Suppressor lymphocytes may also contribute to impaired antibody production in patients with multiple myeloma and Hodgkin's disease and may relate to the fungal infections that occur in some of these patients.[41] In experimental animals, the glucocorticoid-induced defects in lymphocyte function and decreased neutralizing-antibody formation contribute to the increased lethality of fungal, protozoan, and viral infections.

The importance of humoral defenses in the cancer patient has become apparent from several lines of evidence.[42–46] First, the observation that patients with defective antibody production (*e.g.*, chronic lymphocytic leukemia and multiple myeloma) have an increased frequency of pyogenic infections, even if the patients are not neutropenic. Patients with acute leukemia have lower levels of antibody to the core glycolipid of the *Enterobacteriaceae* than noncancer patients, and the antibody level falls in patients receiving cytotoxic therapy.[47] The protective role of this antibody is based on the fact that gram-negative bacteria share in common a core glycolipid composed of 2-keto-3-deoxy-octonate (KDO) and lipid A (endotoxin). A rough mutant of *Escherichia coli* 0111 exposes this core glycolipid and has been used to prepare a vaccine and antisera, known as the J-5 antisera, which has protected rabbits challenged with endotoxin and has improved survival in patients with gram-negative sepsis.[48,49]

RETICULOENDOTHELIAL SYSTEM AND SPLENECTOMY

The spleen serves as both a mechanical filter and an early source of opsonizing activity. Splenectomized patients manifest diminished antibody production when challenged with particulate antigens, are deficient in tuftsin (phagocytosis-promoting peptide), and have decreased levels of IgM and properdin.[50] Consequently, splenectomized patients are at increased risk for septicemia with encapsulated bacteria, particularly *Streptococcus pneumonia, Neisseria meningitis,* and *H. influenza,* as well as with *Babesia microti.*[51] Septicemia in these patients is characteristically fulminant, with large numbers of organisms in the blood stream. Although the incidence of postsplenectomy septicemia is especially significant in children and adolescents (1.4–20%) receiving chemotherapy, bacteremia with *S. pneumonia* or *H. influenza* can occur even when patients are not granulocytopenic, suggesting that splenectomy is an important independent risk factor for cancer patients.[52–54] Splenectomy does not appear to enhance the risk for most nonbacterial infections.[55]

NUTRITION

Malnutrition is a frequent complication of cancer, and its treatment contributes to the loss in integrity of the integumentary and mucosal barrier, to impaired phagocytic capacity, to decreased macrophage mobilization, and to depressed lymphocyte function.[56] Total parenteral nutrition to attenuate drug-induced bone marrow suppression or decrease mucosal cell damage has produced mixed results in clinical trials.[57]

EXOGENOUS AND ENDOGENOUS MICROBIAL FLORA

Unperturbed, the endogenous microbial flora exists as a carefully balanced synergistic microenvironment within the host. However, more than 80% of the infections that occur in cancer patients arise from endogenous microbial flora, nearly half of which are acquired by the patient during hospitalization. The most frequent isolates are *E. coli, K. pneumonia, Pseudomonas,* and *C. albicans.*[58–62] Numerous sources contribute to the colonization of the hospitalized patient, including transmissions from staff to patient and from patient to patient, and food, air, water, special equipment such as catheters, respirators, or humidifiers, and medical or surgical procedures (Fig. 59-14).[63,64] These inanimate reservoirs of micro-organisms require human vectors for transmission, particularly as a consequence of poor hand-washing techniques.[65] Unfortunately, fewer than 30% of physicians caring for seriously ill patients washed their hands between patient contacts.[66] This emphasizes the need for continued education and re-enforcement of this important infection-control practice.

Current technology has also provided new routes for the transmission of micro-organisms, particularly the increased use of indwelling catheters, hyperalimentation lines, and hemodynamic monitoring devices.[67,68] Even the disinfectants and antiseptics used to cleanse the skin before an invasive procedure are occasionally contaminated.

Interface of Colonization and Infection

Contact with micro-organisms does not necessarily result in colonization or infection; hospital workers or psychiatric patients rarely become colonized with gram-negative organisms. However, more than 80% of seriously ill noncancer

FIG. 59-14. Sources of nosocomial infection in high-risk patients. Interactions between colonization and infection.

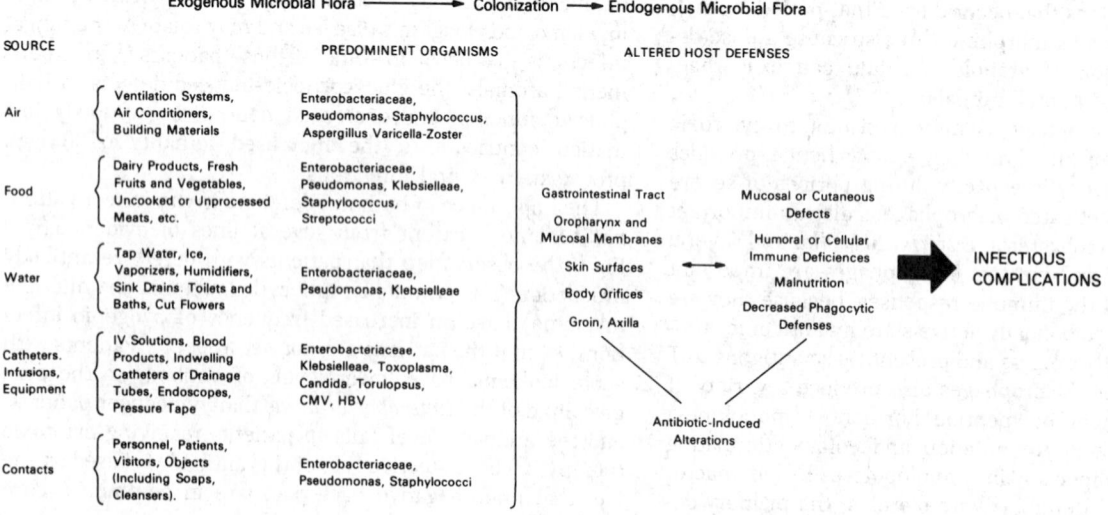

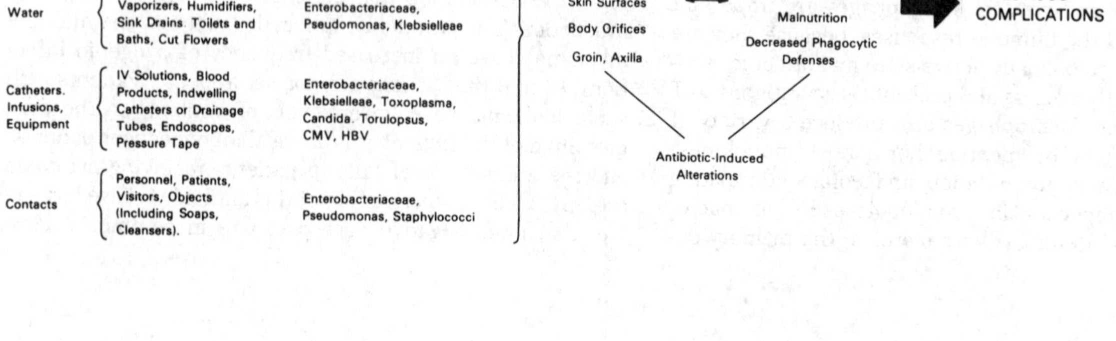

patients eventually become colonized in their oropharynx with gram-negative bacteria, presumably due to alterations in the epithelial adherence of these organisms.[5] Attachment is mediated by a specific "lock-and-key" mechanism, whereby ligand molecules (adhesions) on the surface of the microbe interact with complementary molecules (receptors) on the epithelial cell surface. The biochemical structures of adhesions are variable and have included proteins *(e.g., E. coli, Neissera gonorrhea)*, the lipid protein of a glycolipid *(e.g., S. pyogenes)*, and carbohydrates (*e.g.*, in many cariogenic streptococci). In healthy individuals, integumentary and mucosal attachment sites are populated with relatively innocuous "normal flora," consisting predominantly of aerobic gram-positive and a variety of anaerobic organisms.[5,6]

In cancer patients, a decrease in the normal aerobic gram-positive flora and colonization of the oropharynx and stool with aerobic gram-negative organisms is observed soon after hospitalization, even before the patient receives antibiotics, although antibiotics clearly enhance colonization.[8] Endogenous properties of the micro-organisms themselves are also important for both colonization and infection. For example, certain biotypes of *Enterobacteriaceae* are more capable of colonizing the host than others, and certain colonizing organisms are more likely to result in infection, presumably as a consequence of their inherent virulence.[59,60] Although *E. coli* is the most frequently isolated organism, only a minority of the patients who become colonized develop infections. In contrast, 40% to 68% of patients who are colonized with or who acquire *Pseudomonas aeruginosa* while in the hospital develop serious infections with this organism during subsequent periods of granulocytopenia.[60] This has led some investigators to propose a pathogenicity index, in which colonization with *Klebsiella, Enterobacteriaceae, Proteus,* and *Pseudomonas* is more likely to result in infection of immunocompromised patients than is colonization with other organisms, such as *E. coli.*[61]

The relationship between colonization and infection also applies to nonbacterial organisms. For example, *Candida albicans* is ubiquitous and can be cultured from the oropharynx and stool of more than 80% patients who have received broad-spectrum antibiotics.[62] Although *C. tropicalis* is less frequently isolated and causes fewer overall infections, it appears to be more pathogenic, because 14 of the 25 patients colonized by *C. tropicalis* in the series reported by Wingard and colleagues developed an infection with this organism.[70] The reservoir for organisms may also vary among institutions.

Furthermore, interactions among different components of the host's endogenous microflora (*i.e.*, viruses with bacteria or protozoa) may also result in alterations of the microenvironment and consequent infectious complications, such as synergistic gangrene of Meleney caused by combined infection with microaerophilic *Streptococcus* and *Staphylococcus aureus,* or the putative interaction of *Toxoplasma gondii* and *Pneumocystis carinii* with cytomegalovirus (CMV).[72] Viruses can also suppress or alter immune functions, which has been appreciated since the advent of the acquired immune deficiency syndrome (AIDS) and its etiologic agent, the human immunodeficiency virus (HIV). In addition to retroviruses, other human viruses, including parvoviruses and herpesviruses (*e.g., H. simplex, Epstein-Barr virus,* CMV), can also be immunosuppressive. This can result from destruction of a specific lymphocyte or macrophage target or from the release of soluble factors or activated suppressor cells that alter host immunity while responding to the viral infection.[73]

Predominant Pathogens in the Cancer Patient

The spectrum of infecting organisms has changed during the last three decades. During the 1950s and early 1960s, *S. aureus* was the most frequent bacterial isolate in immunosuppressed patients. When the β-lactamase-resistant antistaphylococcal penicillins were introduced and provided effective therapy for *S. aureus,* gram-negative bacillary organisms became the predominant bacterial pathogens (especially *E. coli, Klebsiella spp.,* and *P. aeruginosa*).[1-4] During the last decade, infections due to *P. aeruginosa* have inexplicably decreased in many institutions, a phenomenon that affects both the selection and the probable success of initial empiric antibiotics. An increase in infections due to nonaeruginosa pseudomonads *(e.g., P. maltophilia, P. cepacia, P. stuterzi)* have been observed in cancer patients, either as nosocomial infections or as a consequence of antibiotic resistance.[74] In some centers, an increase in multiply resistant gram-negative bacterial isolates *(e.g., Enterobacter spp., Citrobacter spp., Acinetobacter spp., S. marcescens)* are presumably a consequence of antibiotic use and misuse.

In most centers, gram-positive bacteria have become the most common isolates.[75] Both *S. aureus* and the coagulase-negative staphylococci represent the predominant isolates, especially in patients with indwelling intravenous catheters.[76-78] Although some centers have experienced major problems with methicillin-resistant *S. aureus* (MRSA), the majority of centers have been able to contain the spread of the isolates with careful infection control practices, especially hand washing.[79-81] During the last decade, the coagulase-negative staphylococci have become increasingly resistant to all β-lactam antibiotics, making vancomycin the drug of choice. There has been a report of a coagulase-negative staphylococcal isolate that was resistant to vancomycin.[82] Although some investigators have reported serious infectious complications, including pneumonia, endocarditis, meningitis, with coagulase-negative staphylococci, most have found this organism to be less virulent and only rarely associated with serious sequelae.[83-86]

Alpha hemolytic and viridans streptococci, as well as corynebacteria, some of which are multiply antibiotic-resistant diptheroids (CDC group JK), can result in serious infections, particularly in patients with prolonged granulocytopenia.[87-92]

Although anaerobes play a lesser role than aerobes in primary infections in cancer patients, they are responsible for approximately 5% of bacteremias and are responsible for mixed infections at body sites like the mouth and perianal area. *Clostridia perfringes* and *C. septicum* are well-described isolates, but *C. tertium,* previously considered a contaminant, also has been associated with serious infection.[93] Only half of the isolates of *C. tertium* are sensitive to standard antianaerobic agents (*e.g.*, clindamycin, metronidazole), but the majority are sensitive to vancomycin. *Bacillus spp.* also have been associated with infection in cancer patients and are difficult to eradicate in patients who have indwelling silastic catheters, unless the venous access devise is removed.[94]

Mycobacterial infections are uncommon in cancer patients, although *M. avium-intracellulare* has become a highly prevalent pathogen in patients with AIDS.[95,96] Infections with rapid growers *(e.g., M. chelonii or M. fortuitum)* have been observed in patients with indwelling catheters.[97]

Fungi are major pathogens, especially in immunosuppressed patients who have prolonged granulocytopenia and who receive protracted courses of antibiotics.[98] The predominant fungal pathogens are *Candida spp., Aspergillus spp., Cryptococcus neoformans,* and the *Phycomycetes.* There is a considerable institutional variation in the predominant fungal pathogens, although in many centers *Aspergillus* has increased in frequency in recent years.[98] Although their incidence is less common, the *Mucoraceae (Mucor, Absidia,* and *Rhizopus spp.)* can cause pulmonary disease or invade the sinuses, causing rhinocerebral syndrome. *Cryptococcus* is a noteworthy pathogen for patients with lymphoma, and it is responsible for disseminated infection in AIDS patients.[99] *Trichosporon spp.*, an arthrospore-forming yeast, can cause local skin lesions and invasive disease.[100] Infections due to *Fusarium spp., Dreschlera, Pseudoallescheria boydii,* and *Malassezia furfur* have also been described in cancer patients.[98] Although geographic mycoses such as *Histoplasma, Coccidioides,* and *Blastomyces* have not increased in frequency, there is an increase in their severity and invasiveness when infection occurs.

In addition to bacteria and fungi, parasitic and viral infections are important primary or secondary complications. *P. carinii* is an important cause of pneumonia, particularly in patients on corticosteroids or with AIDS. Viral infections represent a considerable source of morbidity in immunosuppressed hosts. The herpesviruses *H. simplex* (HSV), *Varicella-Zoster virus* (VZV), and CMV are particularly important. Rodents infected with CMV have a higher mortality when challenged with *P. aeruginosa* or *Candida sp.* than do noninfected controls; the clinical corollary of this is that patients who become infected with CMV have a higher incidence of bacterial superinfections.[101,102]

The immunosuppressed host is at risk for a staggering array of infectious complications. Often, the same patients have multiple infections, further confounding their management.

INITIAL EVALUATION AND MANAGEMENT OF THE FEBRILE CANCER PATIENT

FEVER AND GRANULOCYTOPENIA

Fever is common in cancer patients and can result from tumor necrosis, inflammation, transfusions, and chemotherapeutic or antimicrobial drugs. Although the patient's underlying malignancy can cause fever, 55% to 70% of the fevers that occur in cancer patients are caused by infections, especially if the patient is granulocytopenic defined as having fewer than 500 polymorphonuclear (PMN) leukocytes and bandforms per mm^3.[103] The molecule responsible for the production of fever, interleukin-1 (IL-1), has been cloned and sequenced.[27] The activated monocyte/macrophage is believed to be the most important source of physiologically relevant IL-1, but other phagocytic cells, including polymorphonuclear leukocytes, fixed tissue cells of the reticuloendothelial system, keratinocytes, gingival and corneal epithelial cells, renal mesangial cells, and astrocytes, are also capable of producing IL-1-like molecules.[28] IL-1 mediates an array of metabolic, endocrinologic, neurologic, and immunologic functions common to the acute-phase inflammatory response, the effect of which is a unified host response against an infectious insult. Directly or indirectly, these include the production of fever, polymorphonuclear leukocytosis, hepatic synthesis of acute-phase reactants, activation of T and B lymphocytes, and the metabolic changes (*e.g.*, mobilization of amino acids, decreased serum iron and zinc, and increased serum copper) that act to inhibit bacterial replication.

The initial evaluation and management of the febrile patient depends on the underlying malignancy and the degree of treatment-induced host compromise. For example, altered cellular immunity places the patient with Hodgkin's disease at increased risk for *H. zoster* infection or cryptococcal meningitis; patients who have undergone allogeneic bone marrow transplantation are at risk for severe interstitial pneumonia, especially with CMV.[104–106]

Although the evaluation of the nonimmunosuppressed febrile cancer patient can proceed according to general medical principles, the detection of infection and the management of the febrile granulocytopenic patient is complicated by two important factors. First, granulocytopenia markedly alters the host's inflammatory response, making it difficult to detect the presence of infection. Second, an undetected and untreated infection can be rapidly fatal in the granulocytopenic cancer patient.[107]

Because the classic signs and symptoms of infection often are missing in the granulocytopenic cancer patient (*e.g.*, pyuria may be detectable in only 11% of patients with a urinary tract infection or purulent sputum in only 8% of patients with pneumonia), the physician must take a careful history and perform a scrupulous physical examination, being especially attentive to subtle signs of inflammation.[108] The physical exam may need to be repeated frequently, especially when an initial source of infection is not discernible.

All granulocytopenic cancer patients deserve prompt empiric antibiotic management when they become febrile. Adults with solid tumors are at risk for fever when rendered neutropenic and appear to do well when treated empirically with antibiotics.[109] In a survey of 1001 consecutive episodes of fever in 324 pediatric and young adult cancer patients treated at the National Cancer Institute (NCI), 39.5% had at least one febrile episode when they were granulocytopenic.[100] There was no apparent difference in the incidence, pattern, or severity of infectious complications that occurred, regardless of the patient's underlying malignancy, once they became granulocytopenic. As a matter of practice, all granulocytopenic patients should be considered to be at risk for infection and, once febrile, should be considered as candidates for early empiric therapy.

Although some investigators recommend starting antibiotics if the granulocyte count falls below 1,000/mm^3, most define the risk to be increased when the granulocyte count is less than 500/mm^3. The incidence of bacteremia is particularly increased when the granulocyte count is less than 100/mm^3. Perhaps more important than the absolute nadir, however, is the rate at which the counts are falling.

The level of fever that should prompt therapy also has been defined arbitrarily. In general, two or three low-grade elevations above 38°C (orally) or a single elevation above 38.5°C, in concert with a granulocyte count of less than 500/mm^3, are sufficient criteria to begin empiric therapy. Fever should not be caused by blood products, cancer, or medications, and the physician should ascertain if the patient is receiving drugs that mask a febrile response (*e.g.*, steroids, antipyretic-containing analgesics). Institutional criteria for fever and granulocytopenia should be defined and rigidly adhered to. Such a policy plays an important role in reducing infection-related morbidity and mortality.

PREANTIBIOTIC EVALUATION

In a prospective evaluation of 140 febrile granulocytopenic patients, it was not possible to differentiate patients with bacteremia-induced fever from those with unexplained fever by their age, sex, underlying malignancy, or the types of therapeutic modalities or invasive diagnostic procedures they had received.[110] The absence of physical findings suggesting infection did not exclude a potentially life-threatening bacteremia, because more than half of the bacteremic patients in this study lacked any specific physical findings.

Patients about to receive empiric therapy should have a baseline chest radiograph, urinalysis, at least two sets of preantibiotic blood cultures, and aspirate or biopsy cultures from any accessible sites suggesting infection. If blood cultures are obtained from an indwelling Silastic catheter, it is important also to obtain additional cultures from a peripheral vein. In addition, it is important to obtain blood cultures from each port in patients with multilumen catheters.

Even with a comprehensive evaluation, an infectious cause is initially demonstrated in only 30% to 50% of febrile granulocytopenic patients.[111,112] Moreover, definitive diagnosis may take days, presumably because of the low microbial inoculum. This probably reflects the short period that elapses between the onset of fever and evaluation and initiation of empiric therapy. Even subtle indications of inflammation must be considered as sites of infection in the presence of granulocytopenia. For example, minimal perirectal erythema and tenderness may be the harbinger of a perirectal cellulitis. Minimal erythema and serious discharge at the site of a Hickman catheter exit may herald a tunnel or exit-site infection. Accordingly, any clinically suspicious and accessible site of infection in the neutropenic patient should be aspirated for culture and tested with Gram stain. It is generally not possible to differentiate granulocytopenic patients who have a bacteremia from those with unexplained fever (FUO).[110]

Because the patients' colonizing flora frequently can be implicated in the cause of infection, some have advocated surveillance cultures as an aid to diagnosis and antibiotic management. To assess this approach, we evaluated serial surveillance cultures of the nose, throat, urine, and stool from 271 patients at the NCI during 652 episodes of fever and neutropenia.[62] Sixty-two percent of these patients were colonized with the organism ultimately found to be responsible for the infection. However, the clinical usefulness of these surveillance cultures was limited, because there was not any one body site that was consistently predictive, and invariably other potential pathogens were also isolated, making it difficult to distinguish prospectively the true pathogen. Furthermore, by the time the results from a routine surveillance culture (stool) were known, the true pathogens had been found in pure growth in blood cultures. The cost of routine surveillance is enormous. Even knowing the colonizing flora is unlikely to have a tremendous impact on initial antibiotic management, because most clinicians routinely employ broad-spectrum antibiotics for empiric treatment of febrile granulocytopenic patients. Thus, routine surveillance cultures should not be part of the patients' evaluations. Exceptions to this may be patients in protected isolation, where stool cultures may be of use, or centers with a high incidence of *Aspergillus* infections, where nasal swabs may be helpful in identifying high-risk patients.[64]

Nuclear scanning has also been used to define occult sites of infection. Gallium citrate accumulates in inflammatory lesions because of its avid binding to lactoferrin and has been used with variable success to localize sites of occult infection in non-neutropenic FUO patients.[113] In the neutropenic cancer patient, gallium does not localize an infection in granulocytopenic patients.

As an alternative, indium-111 has been evaluated in neutropenic leukemia patients by labeling autologous or allogenic leukocytes in vitro. When transfused into animal models or surgical patients with known abdominal abscesses, these labeled leukocytes localize at the site of infection.[114] Although encouraging, the effect of alloimmunization on leukocyte trafficking is unclear, and the numbers of patients in studies to date are small.[115,116] Even when the scan is positive, microbiologic identification of the putative infection still requires additional investigation.

Although rapid diagnostic assays, such as the limulus assay for endotoxin, the enzyme-linked immunosorbent assay (ELISA), and latex particle agglutination (LPA), have been successfully employed in certain common infections, they have had little impact on the rapid diagnosis of the bacterial and fungal infections that occur in cancer patients. This is primarily a consequence of the large number of antigenically diverse pathogens that can infect the cancer patient. Because of the difficulty in diagnosing fungal infections in cancer patients, a number of nonculture-dependent, rapid diagnostic techniques have been investigated. However, measurement of circulating antigens, such as mannan or *Aspergillus fumigatus*, or serum arabinatol and creatinine clearance ratios have been hampered by limited sensitivity.[98]

EMPIRIC ANTIBIOTIC THERAPY

The prompt initiation of empiric antibiotics when the neutropenic cancer patient becomes febrile has been the single most important advance in the management of the immuno-

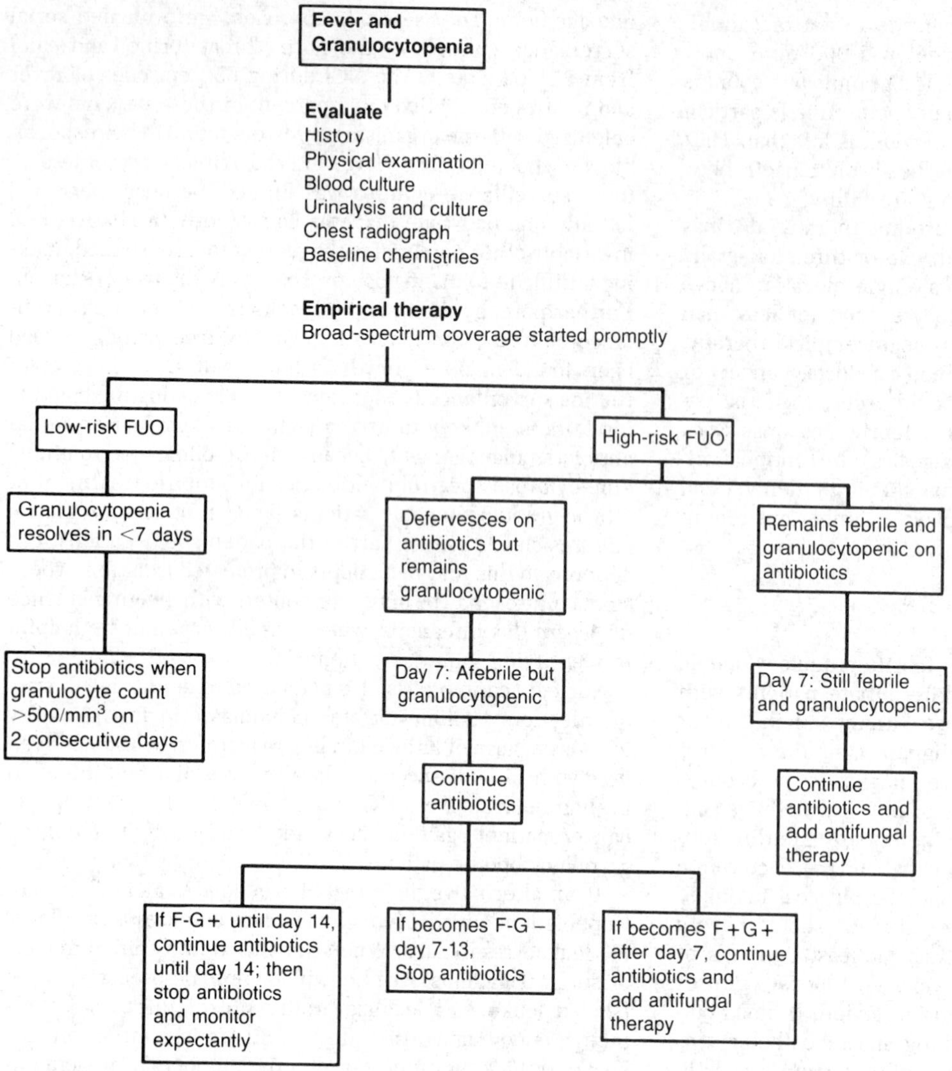

FIG. 59-15. Algorithm for the initial management of the patient who has unexplained fever and neutropenia.

compromised host (Fig. 59-15).[108] Before this policy, the mortality of gram-negative infections, especially with *P. aeruginosa, E. coli,* and *K. pneumoniae,* approached 80%.[117,118] Since the widespread use of effective empiric antibiotics, the overall survival rate is between 60% and 90%.[119,120]

What are the criteria upon which an empiric antibiotic regimen should be based? Between 85% and 90% of pathogens associated with new fevers in the immunosuppressed patients are bacteria.[110,120] However, because both gram-positive and gram-negative bacteria can be responsible for these initial infections, the empiric regimen must be broad, achieve high bactericidal levels, and be as nontoxic and as simple to administer as possible. This has usually necessitated the combination of two or more antibiotics. The availability of third-generation cephalosporins and carbapenems may offer an alternative to combination regimens, because many of these antibiotics provide, as single agents, an exceedingly broad range of activity and high bactericidal levels (Table 59-28.[121-123] Unlike the aminoglycosides, these newer β-lactam antibiotics do not require monitoring of serum levels and have minimal toxicity.

An aminoglycoside plus a β-lactam-containing regimen (*e.g.,* ceftazidine plus amikacin) is considered by many the standard of care, particularly for patients with documented gram-negative infection.[124] However, no particular combination has been shown to be clearly superior, and the regimen that is chosen at a given institution should reflect specific epidemiologic considerations (*e.g.,* "local" resistance patterns) and cost.

Despite the proven efficacy of combination therapy, the potential of a single antibiotic for the empiric management of the febrile neutropenic patient is attractive for its ease of administration, cost, and lack of toxicity. To assess the efficacy of a monotherapeutic regimen, a prospective randomized trial was initiated at the NCI that compared monotherapy with ceftazidime to combination therapy with cephalothin, carbenicillin, and gentamicin for the initial empiric management of 550 episodes of fever and neutropenia.[112] The early evaluation at 72 hours was specifically performed to assess the efficacy of the antibiotics during the period when they were truly used in an empiric manner (*i.e.,* before definitive microbiologic data). The overall evaluation

TABLE 59-29.

	No. of Episodes (%) with Indicated Therapy			
	FUO		DI	
Characteristic	Combination	Single Agent	Combination	Single Agent
Early Evaluation				
Evaluable	204	190	64	92
Afebrile at 72 h	126 (62)	114 (60)	37 (58)	54 (59)
Success without modification	197 (97)	176 (93)	41 (64)	45 (49)
Success with modification	7 (3)	13 (7)	22 (34)	45 (49)
Addition of antibiotics	7 (3)	13 (7)	15 (23)	33 (36)
Addition of antifungal agent	0	1 (0.5)	0	1 (1)
Addition of antiviral agent	0	0	1 (2)	1 (1)
Crossover	2 (1)	1 (0.5)	3 (5)	4 (4)
Change to specific therapy	0	0	3 (5)	8 (9)
Failure	0	1 (1)	1 (2)	2 (2)
Total initial successes	204 (100)	189 (99)	63 (98)	90 (98)
Overall Evaluation				
Evaluable	204	190	64	92
Success without modification	159 (78)	147 (77)	20 (31)	28 (30)
Success with modification	40 (20)	39 (21)	38 (60)	54 (59)
Addition of antibiotics	32 (16)	29 (15)	24 (38)	46 (50)
Addition of antifungal agent	23 (11)	21 (11)	12 (19)	11 (12)
Addition of antiviral agent	1 (0.5)	4 (2)	1 (2)	2 (3)
Crossover	8 (4)	14 (7)	7 (11)	15 (16)
Change to specific therapy	0	0	13 (20)	12 (13)
Failure	5 (2)	4 (2)	6 (9)	10 (11)
Total initial successes	199 (98)	186 (98)	58 (91)	82 (89)

was performed at the resolution of the neutropenic episode. The responses were categorized as "successes" (with or without modification of the initial regimen) if the patients survived the episode of neutropenia and as "failures" if the patients died while neutropenic.

There was no significant difference in terms of success for patients randomized to ceftazidime or the combination regimen among patients classified as FUO or as having a clinically or microbiologically documented infections. A significantly greater number of modifications were required, however, among the patients randomized to ceftazidime: 58 (21%) of 282 compared with 29 (11%) of 268; $p^2 = 0.002$ by chi-square (Table 59-29).[115] This increased need for antibiotic modifications at the early evaluation reflected the need for anaerobic coverage in patients randomized to ceftazidime who developed necrotizing gingivitis or perirectal cellulitis and the greater need for vancomycin in patients with documented gram-positive infections, especially those due to *S. epidermidis.*

The result at the overall evaluation demonstrated equivalent success rates for the two regimens for patients with FUO or with documented infections. The percentage of patients treated successfully without modification of the initial antimicrobial therapy was predictably less than that at the early evaluation (Table 59-30). Patients with documented infections required changes in antimicrobial therapy more often than FUO patients, but the need for modifications of the initial therapy for patients randomized to monotherapy (59%) and those randomized to combination therapy (59%). Therefore, in terms of the overall outcome and the frequency with which modifications of the initial empiric regimen were necessary, monotherapy with ceftazidime was as effective as combination therapy with keflin, carbenicillin, and gentamicin for these patients.

Despite these results and the encouraging findings of other investigators, several concerns must be raised.[125-127] First, the relative lack of activity of third-generation cephalosporins against gram-positive organisms, particularly the coagulase-negative staphylococci, has prompted investigators to advocate that vancomycin be included in the primary empiric regimen.[128,129] Second, several investigators have argued for the inclusion of an aminoglycoside in the initial regimen to maximize the activity against gram-negative pathogens and to decrease the emergence of resistant organisms.[124] However, analysis of the NCI data fails to substantiate these concerns.

Gram-positive bacteria have become increasingly problematic and were isolated in 75 (14%) of the 550 episodes in an NCI study, 53 of these 75 isolates were from the preantibiotic evaluation (*i.e.*, primary infections). The remaining 22 gram-positive isolates were responsible for secondary or "breakthrough" infections. Vancomycin was ultimately required in 26 (49%) of the 53 primary infections, but was added after the identification of a resistant isolate in 14 of 17 cases. There was no mortality nor significant morbidity associated with the addition of vancomycin after identification of an organism resistant to the initial empiric regimen. The routine inclusion of vancomycin as a component of the initial empiric therapy would have overtreated most patients, needlessly exposed them to a potentially toxic compound, and increased the cost of therapy without improving the overall clinical response. Thus, it seems more appropriate to

TABLE 59-30. Commonly Used Antimicrobial Agents in Cancer Patients

	Trade Name	*Major Indications*	*Usual Daily Dosage (IV)*	*Daily Dosage Schedule*
A. The Penicillins				
Penicillin G	Benzathin Permapen Bicillin	*S. pneumoniae, S. pyogenes, S. viridens, S. bovis, Neisseria,* most anaerobes (except *B. fragilis*)	25–500,000 units kg	q 4 h
Penicillinase Resistant				
Methicillin	Staphcillin, celbenin	*S. aureus,* streptococci	1–300 mg/kg	q 4 h
Nafcillin	Unipen		1–300 mg/kg	q 4 h
Oxacillin	Prostaphin, bactocill		1–300 mg/kg	q 4 h
Aminopencillin				
Ampicillin	Omipen Principen Polycillin Penbritin	*S. fecalis,* *L. monocytogenes,* *Hemophilus, E. coli,* *Salmonella, Proteus*	2–400 mg/kg	q 4 h
Carboxy Penicillins				
Carbenicillin	Pyopen, Geopen	*P. aeruginosa, Enterobacter, Proteus, Serraha, Acinetobacter, Providentia.*	500 mg/kg	q 4 h
Ticarcillin	Ticar	Anaerobes including some *Bacteroides sp,* some *Clostridium sp. Peptostreptococcis, Fusobacterium*	300 mg/kg	q 4 h
Extended-Spectrum Penicillins				
Mezlocillin	Mezlin	Same as carboxy penicillin plus *Klebsiella sp.*	300 mg/kg	q 4 h
Piperacillin	Pipercil	Same as mezlocillin plus increased activity against *P. aeruginosa*	300 mg/kg	q 4 h
Azlocillin	Azlin	Same as piperacillin	300 mg/kg	q 4 h
B. The Cephalosporins				
First generation:				
Cephalothin	Keflin	*E. coli. Klebsiella, Proteus, Hemophilus, S. aureus, S. epidermidis, streptococci*	170 mg/kg	q 4 h
Cefazolin	Kefzol, Ancef	Similar to cephalothin, more active against *Klebsiella, E. coli*	50 mg/kg	q 6 h
Second generation:				
Cephamandole	Mandol	More active against *Hemophilus, Klebsiella, E. coli, Enterobacter sp., Proteus;* less active against gram-positive cocci	100–200 mg/kg	q 4 h
Cefoxitin	Mefoxitin	Same as cephalothin plus *Proteus sp,* and anaerobes, including *B. fragilis*	200 mg/kg	q 4 h
Cefuroxime	Zinacef	Similar to cefamandole, penetrates into CSF	0.75–1.5 g	q 8 h
Third generation:				
Cefotaxime	Claforan	Same as cephalothin plus *Enterobacter sp,* indole positive *Proteus, H. influenza, Citrobacter sp., Serratia sp* and some *P. aeruginosa* and *Bacteroides sp.*	200 mg/kg	q 4 h
Moxalactam	Moxam	Same as cefotaxime but better anaerobe coverage (including *B. fragilis*)	200 mg/kg	q 8 h
Ceftriaxone	Rocephin	Similar to cefotaxime	1–2 g	q 12-24 h
Cefoperazone	Cefaloid	Same as moxalactam but with better *P. aeruginosa* activity	200 mg/kg	q 8
Ceftizoxime	Cefizox	Same as moxalactam	200 mg/kg	q 8
Ceftazidime	Fortaz	Same as cefoperazone but with less anaerobic activity. Most active agent against *P. aeruginosa*	100 mg/kg	q 8

Usual Maximum Adult Dose per Day	*Peak Serum Level (μg ml)*	*T½ (h)*		*Modifications for Renal Failure (Adults)*		*Additional Comments*
		Normal	*Renal Failure*	*Moderate C_{CR} 10–50 ml/min*	*Severe C_{CR} <10 ml/min*	
20 g	2	0.5	2.5	NC	1,600,000 units q 6 h	
12 g	40	0.5	4	NC	2 gm q 8 h	Rare nephritis
12 g	6	0.5	1.5	NC	NC	Rate SGOT elevation
12 g	2.6	0.5	1.0	NC	NC	Rare neutropenia, hepatotoxicity
12 g	3.5	1.0	8	NC	0.5–1 g q 8 h	Diarrhea common Synergistic with aminoglycoside for *Enterococcus*
36 g	200	1.1	15	3 g q 4 h	2 g q 8 h	Synergistic with gentamicin for *Pseudomonas* Higher sodium load (carbticar) hypokalemia
21 g	140	1.2	15	2 g q 4 h	2 g q 8 h	Rare platelet dysfunction Should never be mixed in same bottle with aminoglycosides
21 g	100–110	0.8	1.6	NC	25 mg/kg dose q 6 h	Similar to carboxy penicillins Bleeding reactions not described
21 g	100–110	1.0	3.1	NC	25 mg/kg day q 6 h	The extended-spectrum penicillins have a lower sodium content (1.8–2.0 mEq g)
21 g	100–110	0.8	4	NC	45 mg/kg dose q 12 h	They have a lower protein binding and higher biliary excretion than the carboxy penicillins.
12 g	80	0.5–0.8	2	1 g q 4–6 h	1 g q 8 h	Most gram-positive activity among cephalosporins
2–6 g	135	1.5	20–40	0.5 g q 6–12 h	0.5 g q 24–48 h	Longer half-life than cephalothin
6–12 g	36	0.9–1.5		1.2 g q 6–8 h	0.5 g q 8–12 h	Cefuroxime (Zinacef) provides comparable coverage with a slightly longer half-life
6–12 g	20–23	0.75	22	15–30 mg kg dose q 12–24 h	15 mg kg dose q 24 h	Cefoxitin can induce production of β-lactamases which can hydrolyze other β-lactam antibodies used in combination
5–9 g	100	1–2	15	0.75–1.5 g q 8–12 h	0.75–1.5 q 24 h	Cefuroxime also is dispensed in an oral formulation
12 g	125–175	1.3–1.6	27	NC	30 mg/kg q 12 h	All third generation cephalosporins have less gram-positive activity than first generation agents. None are effective against enterococci or *Listeria*. They have variable coverage against pseudomonads and anaerobes
12 g	150–200	2.3–2.7	19	15–30 mg kg dose q 8 h	7.5 mg kg dose q 12 h	Bleeding reactions including hypoprothrombinemia have been reported. Vitamin K should be given weekly Antabuse-like reactions
2 g	270	8	11.9–15.4	0.5–1 g q 12–24 h	0.5–1 g q 12–24 h	Longest half life of 3rd generation cephalosporins, permits once to bid dosing. Also has activity against *N. gonorrhea*
12 g	175–225	1.6–2.1	4.2	NC	20 mg kg dose q 12 h	Highest biliary excretion of the third generation group. Like moxalactam, it contains the methylthiotetrazole group and may cause serious bleeding
12 g 6	150–200 150–200	2.1–2.8 1.6–2.1	19.3	1 g q 12 C_{CR}31–50: 1 g q 12 h C_{CR}16–30: 1 g q 24 h	0.5 g q 24 h C_{CR}6–15: 0.5 mg q 24 h C_{CR}5: 0.5 mg q 48 h	Best activity against *P. aeruginosa*

(continued)

TABLE 59-30. Commonly Used Antimicrobial Agents in Cancer Patients *(continued)*

	Trade Name	*Major Indications*	*Usual Daily Dosage (IV)*	*Daily Dosage Schedule*
C. The Carbapenems				
Imipenem/cilastatin	Primaxin	In addition to the *Enterbacteriaceae* and *P. aeruginosa*, primaxin has efficacy against *S. aureus*, Group D streptococci, many coagulase-negative staphylococci, listeria, and anaerobes. Only *P. maltophilia* and *P. cepacia* are not covered.	50–60	q 6 h
D. The Monobactams				
Monobactems Aztreonam	Azactam	Broad gram-negative but no gram-positive coverage. Is not cross-reactive with other β-lactams so can be used in penicillin or cephalosporin allergic patients	100–150	q 6 h
Aminoglycosides				
Gentamicin	Garamycin	*P. aeruginosa*, *Enterobacteriaceae*, *Enterococcus* (with ampicillin)	3–6 mg/kg	q 6–8 h
Tobramycin	Nebicin	Similar to gentamicin (except not as active against enterococcus with ampicillin)	3–6 mg/kg	q 6–8 h
Amikacin	Amikin	*Serratia*, *Proteus*, *Pseudomonas*, *Enterobacteriaceae*, *Providentia*	15 mg/kg	q 8–12 h
Miscellaneous				
Chloramphenicol	Chloromycetin	*Hemophilus*, *B. fragilis*, *S. pneumonia*, *Neisseriae*, *Salmonella*, *Klebsiella*, most anaerobes, *Rickettsia*	50–100 mg/kg	q 6 h
Erythromycin	Ilotycin Gluceptate	*Legionella*, *Mycoplasma*	30–50 mg/kg	q 6 h
Clindamycin	Cleocin	*B. fragilis*, *Clostridia*, *S. pneumoniae*, *S. viridens*, *S. pyrogenes*, *S. aureus*	30 mg/kg	q 6 h
Vancomycin	Vancocin	*C. difficile*, *S. aureus*, *S. epidermidis*, *S. fecalis*, multiply resistant *Corynebacteria*, *S. bovis*	25–40 mg/kg	q 8–12 h
Trimethoprim-Sulfamethoxazole (1–5 ratio)	Bactrim Septra	*P. carinii*, *S. aureus* *S. pneumonia*, *S. pyogenes*, *Salmonella*, *Listeria*, *E. coli*, *Proteus*, *Serratia*, *Hemophilus*, *Neisseria*	10–20 mg/kg as trimethoprim	q 8–12 h
Ciprofloxacin	Cinoxacin	Gram negatives including Enterobacteriaceae, *P. aeruginosa*, *Hemophilus*, *Branhamella*, gonococci. Also active against Chlamydia, some mycoplasma, Legionella. Less active against gram-positive, especially streptococci	250–500 mg	q 6-12
Antiparasitics				
Pentamidine Isethionate	Lomidine	*P. carinii*	4 mg/kg IM	Once/day
Thiabendazole	Mintezol	*Strongloides*, visceral larva migrans	50 mg/kg 2 days	q 12 h
Antifungal Agents				
Amphotericin B	Fungizone	*Candida*, *Aspergillus*, *Zygomycetes*, *Torulopsis*, *Cryptococcus*, *Histoplasma*	0.5–1.0 mg/kg	Once/day
5-Fluorocytosine	Flucytosine Ancobon	*Cryptococcus*, *Candida*, *Torulopsis*, *Chromomycosis*	50–150 mg/kg	q 6 h
Clotrimazole	Lotrimin	*Candida sp*, dermatophytes	50 mg (troche)	q 6 h

Usual Maximum Adult Dose per Day	*Peak Serum Level (μg ml)*	*T½ (h)*		*Modifications for Renal Failure (Adults)*		*Additional Comments*
		Normal	*Renal Failure*	*Moderate C_{CR} 10–50 ml/min*	*Severe C_{CR} <10 ml/min*	
3–4	43–78	1	4	0.5–1 g q 6–12 h	0.5–1 g q 12–24	Can cause seizures in patients with pre-existing CNS disease or in patients with altered renal functions. Higher doses can also cause nausea and sometimes vomiting
4–6	125	1.7–2	6–8.7	0.5–2 g q 12–24 h	0.5–2 g q 12–24 h	Not cross-reactive with β-lactams and can be used in the penicillin or cephalosporin allergic patient.
	4–8	2.3	45–55	Monitor serum levels		All aminoglycosides synergistic or additive with penicillins or cephalosporins against *Pseudomonas, enterococcus* staph, strep, *Enterobacteriaceae*
	4–8	2.3	45–55	Monitor serum levels		All have renal and ototoxicity
	15–25	2.3	50–80	Monitor serum levels		
3–6 g	12	4.1	4.2	NC	NC	Both idiosyncratic and dose related bone marrow toxicity Dosage must be reduced with hepatotoxicity
6 g	0.4–1.8	1.4	5	NC	NC	Burning and phlebitis intravenously
2400 mg	10	2.4	6	NC	NC	Risk for pseudomembraneous enterocolitis (Treat with vancomycin or metranidazole)
3 g	25–50	6	9 days	1 g q 36 h	1 g q 10–14 days	Drug of choice for antibiotic (*C. difficile*) induced colitis but must be given orally (125 mg PO q 6 h). Also drug of choice for *S. epid.* and methicillin-resistant staph (IV).
960 g	1.6–3.2 trimeth-oprim)	7½	25	10 mg/kg q 12 h	5 mg/kg q 12 h	May be useful for prophylaxis against *P. carinii* May result in myelosuppression—particularly in AIDS
1.5 g	2.4	3.9	5–10	250 mg q 12–24 h	Not recommended	Both oral and parenteral formulations available. Accumulates in cartilage and not approved for children
	0.2	Very short		q 36 h	q 48 h	Very toxic: hypotension, renal damage, sterile abscesses hypo and hyperglycemia Available only through CDC
3 g		1				Rare hepatoxicity. May cause nausea, vomiting, headache, dizziness
	0.5–2.0	24	NC	NC	0.5 mg/kg q 36 h	Dose modification necessary for patients with hepatic abnormalities Major toxicities are fever, electrolyte disturbances. May be combined with 5-FC to treat cryptococcal meningitis
	30	3.4	200	12–25 mg/kg once	Not given	Rapid resistance develops when used alone Normal use is in conjunction with amphotericin Parenteral form investigational
						For topical use only (*e.g.*, oral troche). If systemically absorbed, is inactivated by hepatic enzymes

(*continued*)

TABLE 59-30. Commonly Used Antimicrobial Agents in Cancer Patients *(continued)*

	Trade Name	*Major Indications*	*Usual Daily Dosage (IV)*	*Daily Dosage Schedule*
Miconazole	Monistat	*Candida sp, Aspergillus sp, Zygomycetes, Torulopsis, Cryptococcus, Petrielldium, Blastomyces, Coccidioides, Histoplasma, Paracoccidioides, Sporothrix*	1500–3600 mg/d	
Ketoconazole	Nizoral	Similar to miconazole	2–400 mg/d	qd
Antiviral Agents				
Adenosine arabinoside	Vidarabine	*H. simplex varicella-zoster*	10–15 mg/kg/d	12 h infusion
Acycloguanosine	Acyclovir	*H simplex,* varicella-zoster	750 mg/m²/d (*H. simplex*) 1500 mg/m²/d (*VZV*)	q 8 h
Interferons (alpha, beta, gamma)		*H. simplex, VZV*	1×10^4 5×10^5 units/kg/d	qd

withhold vancomycin until the pathogen is identified.[86] However, if there is a high incidence of methicillin-resistant *S. aureus* at a given center, the initial inclusion of vancomycin in the antibiotic regimen is appropriate.

In addition to gram-positive coverage, 36 (13%) of 282 patients randomized to ceftazidime in the NCI study required an aminoglycoside at some time during the neutropenic episode.[112,130] Twenty-four (67%) of 36 patients received the aminoglycoside because of prospectively designed protocol modifications for clinical deteriorations or breakthrough bacteremias. Patients with documented infections received aminoglycosides somewhat more frequently than did patients with unexplained fevers: 16 (17%) of 92, compared with 20 (11%) of 190, respectively). However, the majority of patients (87%) never required an aminoglycoside as a component of their antimicrobial regimen, and the inclusion of an aminoglycoside as part of the initial empiric therapy would have unnecessarily exposed the patients to potentially ototoxic and nephrotoxic agents.

Ultimately, the decision regarding the appropriate empiric regimen must be individualized at each institution. Oncology centers have different patterns of microbial isolates and antibiotic resistance patterns, and this must be taken into account. Nevertheless, there is mounting evidence that the initial empiric management of a febrile, neutropenic cancer patient may be accomplished with a single antibiotic, especially with selected third-generation cephalosporins. Regardless of the empiric regimen chosen, the clinician must recognize the indications for and appropriately employ the modifications of therapy essential to ensure a successful outcome for a neutropenic patient (Table 59-30).[125]

ADJUNCTS TO ANTIBIOTIC THERAPY

In patients who have not responded to antibiotic therapy, replacement of granulocytes has been explored as adjunct therapy. Five prospectively randomized, controlled clinical trials have investigated the efficacy of daily prophylactic granulocyte transfusions for patients undergoing induction chemotherapy for acute leukemia or bone marrow transplantation.[131–135] The two trials conducted at UCLA failed to demonstrate a decrease in the frequency of infections or enhancement of remission or survival rates.[131,134] These trials, however, used a relatively low daily dose of transfused granulocytes (median, 0.5×10^{10} granulocytes/day) that had been harvested by a discontinuous flow centrifugation leukopheresis without steroid premedication of donors. More evidence is needed, but a dose-response relationship between the number of transfused leukocytes and clinical response has been demonstrated in animal models and early human trials using leukocytes collected from donors with chronic myelogenous leukemia.[136–138]

Despite conflicting data, it is probable that the daily administration of a sufficient number of properly collected leukocytes ($>10^{10}$/m²/day) would reduce the incidence of infectious complications among neutropenic patients. How-

Usual Maximum Adult Dose per Day	*Peak Serum Level (μg ml)*	*T½ (h)*		*Modifications for Renal Failure (Adults)*		*Additional Comments*
		Normal	*Renal Failure*	*Moderate C_{CR} 10–15 ml/min*	*Severe C_{CR} 10 ml/min*	
	2–8 μg	0.4, 2.1, 24.2 24.2 h (3 compartment)		NC	NC	No proven efficacy in invasive fungal infections in immunocompromised hosts Can cause hyponatremia, anemia, thrombocytosis, nausea, vomiting, cardiac arrythmias. Less than 1% excreted in urine. 50% excreted in feces
400 (higher doses are being investigated)	2–13 μg	2–8 h (biphasic)		NC	NC	No proven value in immunocompromised hosts. May cause nausea, vomiting, hepatic enzyme elevation, dizziness, gynecomastia, adrenal insufficiency. Antacids and cimetidine impede absorption
	4–8 μg ml	3–5 h		No established guidelines. Reduce by 25% in severe renal failure and monitor metabolites		No activity against CMV. Anorexia, nausea, vomiting, diarrhea. Rare myelosuppression, neurotoxicity. Excessive fluid requirements
	30–50 μM	2.2–5 h		5–10 mg/kg q12h for C_{CR} 25–50 5–10 mg/kg q 24 h for C_{CR} 10–25	2.5–5 mg/kg q 24 h	Twice-maintenance fluids necessary with higher doses to avoid renal toxicity Neurotoxicity (at high doses) Thymidine kinase resistant mutants have been described
						Local pain, fever, alopeia, fatigue, anorexia, bone marrow suppression

ever, this approach is not economically or medically feasible with our current technology, and the severity of the potential adverse effects (*e.g.*, transmission of CMV, alloimmunization, pulmonary toxicity, and donor complications) argue against their use.[139–143]

Several well-designed, prospectively randomized clinical trials have investigated the therapeutic use of transfused granulocytes.[144–149] Unfortunately, the interpretation of these trials is complicated by disparate techniques for leukocyte collection, the lack of histocompatibility information, variable numbers of transfusions and doses of transfused granulocytes, and inconsistent criteria for instituting therapy and evaluating results. Although earlier trials suggested a beneficial role for granulocyte transfusions to neutropenic patients with gram-negative bacteremias who were not expected to have a recovery of marrow function within several days, the relevance of these data has been questioned because of advances in induction regiments for patients with acute leukemia and because of the availability of more efficacious antimicrobial regimens. There has been no recent documentation that therapeutic granulocyte transfusions would further improve the short-term or long-term survival of any neutropenic patients. The cost considerations and potential for adverse reactions are similar to those cited for prophylactic granulocyte transfusions. Thus, current data do not support the use of granulocyte transfusions for neutropenic patients.[150–151]

Although it is possible that improvement in biotechnology may make the collection of leukocytes or monocytes more successful, an alternative approach is to use recombinant GM-CSF to accelerate neutrophil recovery after cytotoxic therapy. Preclinical data shows considerable promise and a number of clinical trials are currently under way.[14–18]

MANAGEMENT OF THE NEUTROPENIC PATIENT WITH UNEXPLAINED FEVER

Many neutropenic cancer patients who become febrile do not have an identifiable source for their initial fever.[110,112] Although some of these patients may become febrile in response to a medication or blood product or because of their underlying malignant process, the majority have an occult infection, but the site is undefined because of rapid evaluation and institution of effective empiric therapy. In spite of the frustration inherent in not defining the site of the infection and the prospect that early empiric antibiotics are masking infection, the reduced morbidity and mortality justify this approach.

The physician must determine how long to continue antibiotics when a site of infection has not been defined. Stopping antibiotics too early can lead to clinical deterioration in patients who remain granulocytopenic, particularly when they are persistently febrile. Patients with FUO can be divided into low-risk and high-risk groups. Low-risk FUO patients resolve their granulocytopenia within 1 week of starting antibiotics and do well if their antibiotics are continued until their granulocyte count is about 500/mm^3.[110]

The major dilemma pertains to the high-risk FUO patients, who remain neutropenic for more than 1 week. The management of these patients has been addressed in a series of prospective clinical studies, stratifying them according to whether they had defervesced after the initiation of broad-spectrum therapy or whether they remained persistently febrile in spite of empiric antibiotics (Fig. 59-15).[152–153] Within 3 days of stopping antibiotics on day 7 in patients who had defervesced on therapy but who were afebrile, 41% again became febrile; the isolate(s) obtained from the patients who became febrile again were sensitive to the antibiotics that had been discontinued. In contrast, no subsequent infections were observed in the patients who continued on antibiotics. However, these data did not define whether antibiotics should be continued until the final resolution of neutropenia or whether a defined but limited course of antibiotic therapy would suffice. Therefore, we have tried to further evaluate the appropriate duration of antibiotic therapy by continuing antibiotics for afebrile but persistently granulocytopenic FUO patients for a full 14-day treatment course, as if they had an occult infection, and then randomizing them to stop antibiotics or to continue treatment until the resolution of the granulocytopenia. After day 14, approximately a third of the patients either stopping or continuing antibiotic therapy will become febrile again. Because patients randomized to discontinue antibiotics responded to the reinstitution of therapy when a new fever developed, it seems reasonable to continue FUO patients on a standard 14-day treatment course if they remain granulocytopenic and then to stop the antibiotics, recognizing that approximately 30% of the patients will require further intervention.

EMPIRIC ANTIFUNGAL THERAPY

The situation is more complicated for patients who remain persistently febrile and granulocytopenic in spite of antibiotic therapy. In a randomized clinical trial, we observed that 56% of the FUO patients who had remained febrile after receiving empiric antibiotics developed complications within 3 days of stopping therapy. Of these, 38% became hypotensive once antibiotic therapy was stopped. However, continuing antibiotics alone in FUO patients with persistent fever and granulocytopenia was not satisfactory, because 31% of these patients eventually developed invasive fungal infections. It is not possible to determine whether these fungal infections were the cause of the patient's persistent fever or a consequence of their continued antibiotic therapy and prolonged granulocytopenia. However, patients with persistent fever and granulocytopenia did best when their antibiotics were continued and amphotericin B was added empirically (Fig. 59-16).

The rationale for the empiric use of an antifungal compound is based upon several lines of reasoning. Diagnosis of fungal disease is difficult in an immunocompromised host, and withholding antifungal therapy until the establishment of a definitive diagnosis frequently allows dissemination to occur.[154] It also appears that the outcome of a fungal infection in an immunocompromised patient is improved with the early institution of effective therapy. It is possible to identify patients who are at greatest risk for the development of invasive mycoses; neutropenic patients who remain febrile despite a 4 to 7 days of broad-spectrum antimicrobial therapy are particularly prone to fungal disease.[155,156] Empiric antifungal therapy suppresses fungal overgrowth that inevitably accompanies broad-spectrum antimicrobial therapy, and treats subclinical, localized mycotic disease.

Further support for the empiric antifungal therapy comes from several retrospective studies. Burke and co-workers used amphotericin B in patients with acute leukemia with recurrent or persistent fever despite antibiotic coverage with gentamicin and carbenicillin.[155] Stein and colleagues employed amphotericin B (0.4 mg/kg/day) for patients with persistent or recrudescent fever after a week of antimicrobial therapy during induction therapy for acute myelogenous leukemia.[156] Both of these studies reported fewer deaths due to invasive mycoses than in historic control groups.

Despite the theoretic and clinical evidence substantiating the efficacy of empiric antifungal therapy, the widespread acceptance and clinical use of this information has been hindered because of the significant toxicity associated with amphotericin B. Fever, nephrotoxicity, hepatotoxicity, chilling reactions, and electrolyte imbalances (particularly hypokalemia) are frequently associated with the administration of amphotericin B. Less toxic alternatives to amphotericin B are desirable.

The imidazoles are a new class of broad-spectrum antifungal agents that are low in toxicity and easily delivered.[157] An NCI study randomized 72 patients who remained febrile and neutropenic after 7 days of antimicrobial therapy to receive amphotericin B (0.5 mg/kg/day) or ketoconazole (800 mg/day).[158] The results were similar for the duration of fever after the antifungal randomization, the number of documented fungal infections, the number of patients requiring cross-over due to intolerance, and the overall survivals or deaths. However, after the diagnosis of an invasive fungal infection was documented, disease progression was likely unless the patient received amphotericin B.

Fainstein corroborated these findings in a study of 172 neutropenic patients who remained febrile for 72 to 96 hours after the institution of empiric antibiotic therapy and who were randomized to receive amphotericin B (0.6–1.0 mg/kg/day) or ketoconazole (200 mg orally, every 6 hours).[159] There was no difference between the two regimens in the response of patients with documented, "probable," or "possible" fungal infections. However, patients with documented infections due to *C. tropicalis* responded more often to amphotericin B (5 of 8 patients) than to ketoconazole (0 of 8 patients). Unfortunately, the unusual design and response criteria used for this study hinder its correlation with previously established data. Also, treatment failures and toxicity (*e.g.,* adrenal and testosterone suppression) have been observed with prolonged ketoconazole use.[160–161] Recently, Winegard evaluated parenteral miconazole as an empiric antifungal agent (versus a placebo) and demonstrated a significant reduction in the incidence of invasive mycoses.[162]

The optimal time for initiating antifungal therapy is unknown. The arbitrary designation of day 7 avoids the overuse of antifungal agents in patients who are slow to defervesce after empiric antibiotics or those who recover their granulocyte counts before day 7. The potential value of alternative antifungal compounds (*e.g.*, liposome-encapsulated amphotericin B, itraconazole, fluconazole) must be established by prospectively randomized clinical trials.[163-168]

Empiric antifungal therapy is indicated for patients who remain neutropenic and febrile or who recrudesce a fever despite 1 week of broad-spectrum antibiotic therapy. It appears that ketoconazole is a viable alternative to amphotericin B, but an invasive fungal infection necessitates amphotericin B. The optimal duration of empiric antifungal therapy is based upon clinical experience. For patients who remain neutropenic, antifungal therapy should be continued until the resolution of granulocytopenia. Persistence or recrudescence of fever should prompt a meticulous investigation for nonfungal infections. Patients who develop a documented fungal infection should be treated according to established clinical guidelines for the offending pathogen (generally, 2 g of amphotericin B).

MANAGEMENT OF SPECIFIC INFECTIOUS COMPLICATIONS

BACTEREMIA

Approximately 10% to 20% of febrile neutropenic cancer patients will have a bacteremia at the time of presentation. Among immunocompromised patients, the respiratory tract is the most common initial site of sepsis (25%), followed by a perianal and perioral cellulitis, the gastrointestinal tract, and the genitourinary tract (each approximately 10%). Indwelling intravascular devices have become a more common source of bacteremias.[169] Unfortunately, there is no clinically reliable method by which to prospectively identify those febrile neutropenic patients who are bacteremic.[62,110,170]

Until the late 1970s, gram-negative aerobic organisms were the most frequently isolated pathogens. The pattern of infections has shifted, and gram-positive bacteria now are isolated as often as gram-negative bacteria at most cancer centers. Among the gram-positive pathogens, *S. aureus, S. epidermidis,* and *Streptococcus spp.* (including the viridens and Group D) are the most commonly isolated. Documented septicemia with *S. bovis,* although uncommon, is important because of its close association with carcinoma of the colon and should heighten the clinician's suspicion of an undetected neoplasm.[171] Species of *Corynebacterium* (*e.g.*, CDC group JK, *C. diphtheriae,* and *C. equi*) and *Bacillus* are less frequently isolated and tend to occur in patients with prolonged episodes of granulocytopenia or indwelling vascular access devices, respectively. *E. coli, K. pneumonia,* and *P. aeruginosa* are the most frequently isolated gram-negative bacilli, although more resistant species (*e.g.*, nonaeruginosa *Pseudomonades, Serratia marcescens, Enterobacter spp., Citrobacter spp.*) are also found. Primary bacteremia due to anaerobic organisms are uncommon, accounting for less than 5% of the septicemia in cancer patients. For reasons that are unclear, the incidence of infections due to *P. aeruginosa* has been decreasing in recent years. The morbidity and mortality rates due to gram-positive bacteria, especially the coagulase-negative staphylococci, are less than those due to gram-negative pathogens.

The most important therapeutic intervention for patients ultimately shown to be bacteremic is the prompt initiation of empiric antibiotics when fever and neutropenia occur. Modifications of the regimen should be based upon the microbiologic sensitivity pattern of the bloodstream isolate (Table 59-31). The minimal duration of therapy for bacteremic patients is 10 to 14 days, although patients with persistent neutropenia or a persistent site of infection are likely to require longer treatment.

Catheter-Associated Bacteremias

Catheter-related bacteremias have become increasingly important during the past several years, largely because of the increased use of indwelling right atrial Hickman-Broviac catheters.[68,169] Although the benefit of these catheters in providing venous access to patients is enormous, the frequency of catheter-associated bacteremia and other problems is significant. Complication rates have been between 3% and 60%, which may be caused by different techniques of catheter insertion, care, and maintenance. Differences in patient populations, their therapies, degree of catheter use, and definition of catheter-related infection and complications also influence the rates of complications.[172-175]

The diagnosis of a catheter-related bacteremia is made by documenting positive blood cultures from the catheter lumen(s) and a peripheral venous site. The colony count from the lumen sample is ordinarily greater than that from the peripheral site. The majority of catheter-associated infections are caused by the coagulase-positive staphylococci, but other gram-positive bacteria (*e.g., S. aureus,* streptococci), gram-negative organisms *(Acinetobacter spp., P. aeruginosa) Bacillus spp., Corynebacterium spp.,* and *Candida* can cause infection. *Malassezia furfur* has been isolated in compromised hosts, particularly where hyperalimentation and intralipids are being delivered. Polymicrobial infections occur in rare cases. Recently, an outbreak of catheter-exit site infections due to *Aspergillus flavus* were described in association with air contamination in an operating room.[176] Local skin infection due to mycobacteria, particularly *M. fortuitum* and *M. cheloni,* also were described, although these are geographically distributed.[97]

It is important to obtain blood cultures from all ports and from peripheral sites. Careful inspection of the catheter-exit site and the subcutaneous tunnel for Hickman-Broviac catheters or the subcutaneous reservoir for implanted Port-A-Cath and Med-I-Port catheters is imperative in management of infections.

If bacteremia occurs in a patient with a foreign body, the device or catheter usually should be removed to assure eradication of the infection. However, it has become apparent that more than 80% of catheter-associated bacteremias caused by coagulase-negative staphylococci can be treated without removing the catheter if a 10-day course of vancomycin is infused through the catheter (Fig. 59-16).[177] If the patient has a multilumen catheter, the antibiotic infusion

TABLE 59-31. Modification of Therapy

Clinical Event	*Possible Modifications of Therapy*
Breakthrough bacteremia	If gram-positive isolate (*e.g., S. epidermidis*), add vancomycin. If gram-negative isolate (*i.e.*, presumably resistant), switch to regimen containing non-cross-resistant antibiotics (*e.g.*, aminoglycoside plus a carbapenem or extended-spectrum penicillin).
Catheter-associated infection	Add vancomycin (as well as gram-negative coverage if not already being given).
Severe oral mucositis or necrotizing gingivitis	Add specific antianaerobic agent (*e.g.*, clindamycin or metronidazole)
Esophagitis	Trial of oral clotrimazole, ketoconazole, or IV amphotericin B.
Pneumonitis	
Diffuse or interstitial	Trial of trimethoprim-sulfamethoxazole and erythromycin (plus broad-spectrum antibiotics if the patient is granulocytopenic).
New infiltrate in a granulocytopenic patient also receiving antibiotics	If granulocyte count is rising, watch and wait. If granulocyte count is not recovering, biopsy to establish diagnosis; if biopsy cannot be done, add amphotericin B empirically.
Perianal tenderness	If patient is already receiving broad-spectrum antibiotics, add a specific antianaerobic agent. If patient is not on antibiotics, begin broad-spectrum therapy with anaerobic coverage.
Persistent fever and neutropenia	Continue antibiotics after 1 week of persistent fever and neutropenia; add systemic antifungal therapy empirically.

should be rotated to include all ports and lumens. Both catheter and peripheral venous samples must be obtained after therapy is started. If the cultures remain positive despite 24 hours of appropriate therapy, the catheter should be removed and vancomycin continued; the possibility of endocarditis should be considered for patients with persistent positive blood cultures, and a cardiac echo should be performed. If there is evidence of tenderness or induration along the subcutaneous track of the catheter from its exit to its insertion into the subclavian or jugular vein ("tunnel infection"), the catheter should be removed because these infections are not otherwise treatable.

Not all organisms are treatable as the coagulase-negative staphylococci. For example, catheter-associated bacteremia caused by *Bacillus spp.* or by *Candida* usually necessitates catheter removal, even if the organisms are sensitive to the antibiotics being administered.[94] In order to determine if the type of catheter influences the incidence of infection or ease of the treatment, we are comparing the Hickman-Broviac type catheter to a subcutaneously implanted catheter (Port-A-Cath) in a prospective randomized trial.

The pressure of an indwelling catheter may influence the choice of antibiotics for a febrile cancer patient. Data for non-neutropenic patients with catheters are lacking, but because of the morbidity associated with untreated gram-negative infection, we recommend that these patients should have cultures obtained and then receive a 48-hour trial of antibiotics (usually vancomycin plus an aminoglycoside) until it is determined that the fever was not due to a catheter-associated infection. If the cultures are negative, the antibiotics are discontinued; if positive, a full course of treatment is administered.

If the patient is neutropenic, has a catheter, and becomes febrile, some advocate the inclusion of vancomycin in the antibiotic regimen. We have reviewed our experiences at the NCI and found that, although gram-positive and gram-negative bacteremias are more common in patients with indwelling catheters than without, there was no apparent advantage from the addition of vancomycin to the broad-spectrum regimen. Thus, we treat neutropenic patients who become febrile without empiric vancomycin, regardless of whether they have or do not have an indwelling catheter.[169]

Antibiotic Considerations for the Septicemia Patient

The optimal management of the neutropenic patient with a defined infection poses a dilemma. Should the patient continue to receive a broad-spectrum antibiotic regimen or can the antibiotics be narrowed to a pathogen-directed therapy? Continuing broad-spectrum therapy maintains antimicrobial activity against a wide range of gram-positive and gram-negative pathogens and may effectively eradicate or suppress second bacterial infections. However, this approach may allow the proliferation of resistant bacteria and fungi and

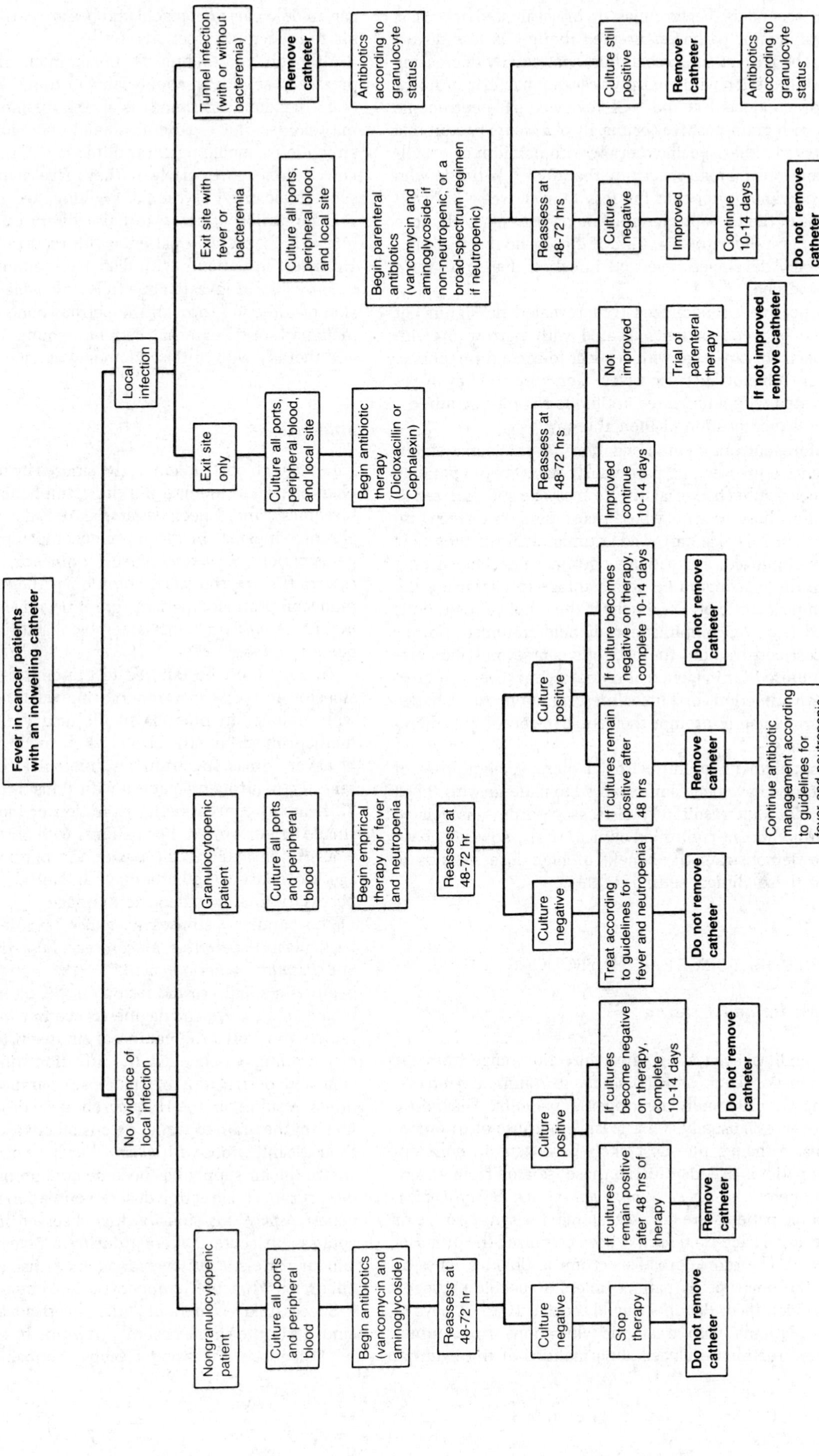

FIG. 59-16. Algorithm for the management of fever in the cancer patient with an indwelling intravenous catheter.

result in secondary bacteremias or disseminated mycoses. The advantage of pathogen-directed therapy is less disturbance of the patient's microbial flora, potentially decreasing the risk of infection with multiply-resistant bacteria or fungi.

A study conducted at the NCI reviewed 78 neutropenic patients with gram-positive (primarily *S. aureus*) bacteremia who received either specific therapy with nafcillin or oxacillin or continued broad-spectrum therapy.[178] Patients who remained granulocytopenic for less than 1 week did well regardless of the therapy chosen. Among patients with more prolonged granulocytopenia, 47% of those who received specific therapy developed a second infection due to a gram-negative aerobe.

A prospectively randomized trial revealed no significant difference between patients treated with narrow or with broad-spectrum coverage with respect to second infections, new fevers, or mortality. However, a greater number of patients treated with a narrowed antibiotic regimen required a subsequent modification of their therapy.[179]

Therefore, current recommendations for the management of immunosuppressed and particularly neutropenic patients with a documented bacterial infection can be summarized as follows: For those patients whose neutropenia is expected to last less than 7 days, a narrowed antimicrobial regimen may be safely employed. For patients with more prolonged neutropenia, there seems to be no advantage to narrowing the initial empiric antibiotic regimen. If the empiric regimen is narrowed (*e.g.*, for simplification of fluid administration or due to cost constraints), the patient's course must be carefully monitored for evidence of recrudescent fever, progression of an infection, or clinical deterioration. Any change should immediately prompt the re-expansion of antimicrobial coverage.

As a supplement to antimicrobial therapy, high doses of corticosteroid have been administered to patients with shock or with the adult respiratory distress syndrome associated with sepsis. Recent controlled clinical trials, however, have failed to demonstrate the benefit of high-dose steroids in either of these clinical settings.[180,181]

UPPER RESPIRATORY TRACT INFECTIONS

Otitis Media and Externa

Clinical findings suggesting an ear infection range from ear pain, drainage, fever, and irritability to minimal tympanic erythema in profoundly neutropenic patients. Diagnostic tympanocentesis usually is not feasible because of thrombocytopenia. Although the most likely pathogens in non-neutropenic patients are identical to those isolated from an immunocompetent host (*i.e., S. pneumoniae* and *H. influenza*), neutropenic patients are also susceptible to gram-positive or gram-negative bacteria that may have colonized the oronasopharynx.[181] Therefore, broad-spectrum antibiotics must be used in the neutropenic patient unless a specific pathogen has been identified. Patients should receive 10 to 14 days of therapy. Patients with anatomic alterations from tumor growth or treatment-induced abnormalities of the external ear, middle ear, or eustachian tubes are particularly susceptible to recurrent infections.

Although mastoiditis is uncommon, the immunosuppressed host with an abnormality or tumor of the middle ear (*e.g.*, rhabdomyosarcoma) is at risk for the development of mastoiditis. These patients should undergo appropriate examinations, including x-ray films and CT scans of the involved area, particularly if they have symptoms or signs, such as localized erythema, swelling, and tenderness.

Colonization of the external auditory canal with *P. aeruginosa* is frequent in patients with recurrent ear infections. However, in patients with diabetes mellitus or altered host defenses, local invasion due to *Pseudomonas* result in extension of infection through the petrous bone into the brain as malignant otitis externa. Patients require aggressive antibiotic therapy with antipseudomonal agents.

Sinusitis

Patients with obstruction of the sinuses by tumor (*e.g.*, nasopharyngeal carcinomas, Burkitt's lymphoma, or rhabdomyosarcomas) are especially at risk for developing acute or chronic sinusitis. In the immunocompetent or non-neutropenic patient, *S. pneumoniae, H. influenza,* and *Branhamella catarrhalis* are the most common pathogens.[182] In an immunocompromised patient, gram-negative aerobes, including *P. aeruginosa,* and anaerobic bacteria are more frequently found.[183–185]

Therapy must be tailored to the clinical situation. Acute sinusitis in a non-neutropenic individual is best managed with amoxicillin plus clavulanic acid (Augmentin) or trimethoprim-sulfamethoxazole. For neutropenic patients, however, broad-spectrum antimicrobial therapy is necessary. If a neutropenic patient with sinusitis does not improve 72 hours after treatment, aspiration or biopsy of the sinus should be performed. For patients with chronic or recurrent sinusitis, particularly those with a local tumor mass or damage secondary to radiotherapy, an"antral window" may be necessary to allow adequate drainage.

The paranasal sinuses may also be infected with fungi, particularly *Aspergillus, Mucoraceae, Fusarium, Exserohilum,* and *Pseudoalescheria boydii.*[98,186–189] Fungal sinusitis may begin as a small crusted lesion on the anterior, inferior turbinate, or adjacent cartilagineous spetum, but it can progress rapidly to involve the paranasal sinuses with consequent facial swelling. Unchecked, the infection will cause bony erosion and destruction of the nose, paranasal sinuses, and orbits, resulting in the rhinocerebral syndrome with involvement of the brain by direct extension or vascular thrombosis. Sinusitis infections with *Aspergillus* have occurred in centers where the air supply has become contaminated with spores, either from construction dust or ventilation problems. At one center *Aspergillus* sinusitis was observed in almost 20% of adults with acute leukemia during a 5-year period.[189,190] A similar pattern (but lower incidence) has been observed in children with acute lymphocytic leukemia.[191]

Successful treatment of patients with advanced *Aspergillus* sinusitis or the rhinocerebral syndrome has been disappointing. Diagnosis necessitates biopsy confirmation, and treat-

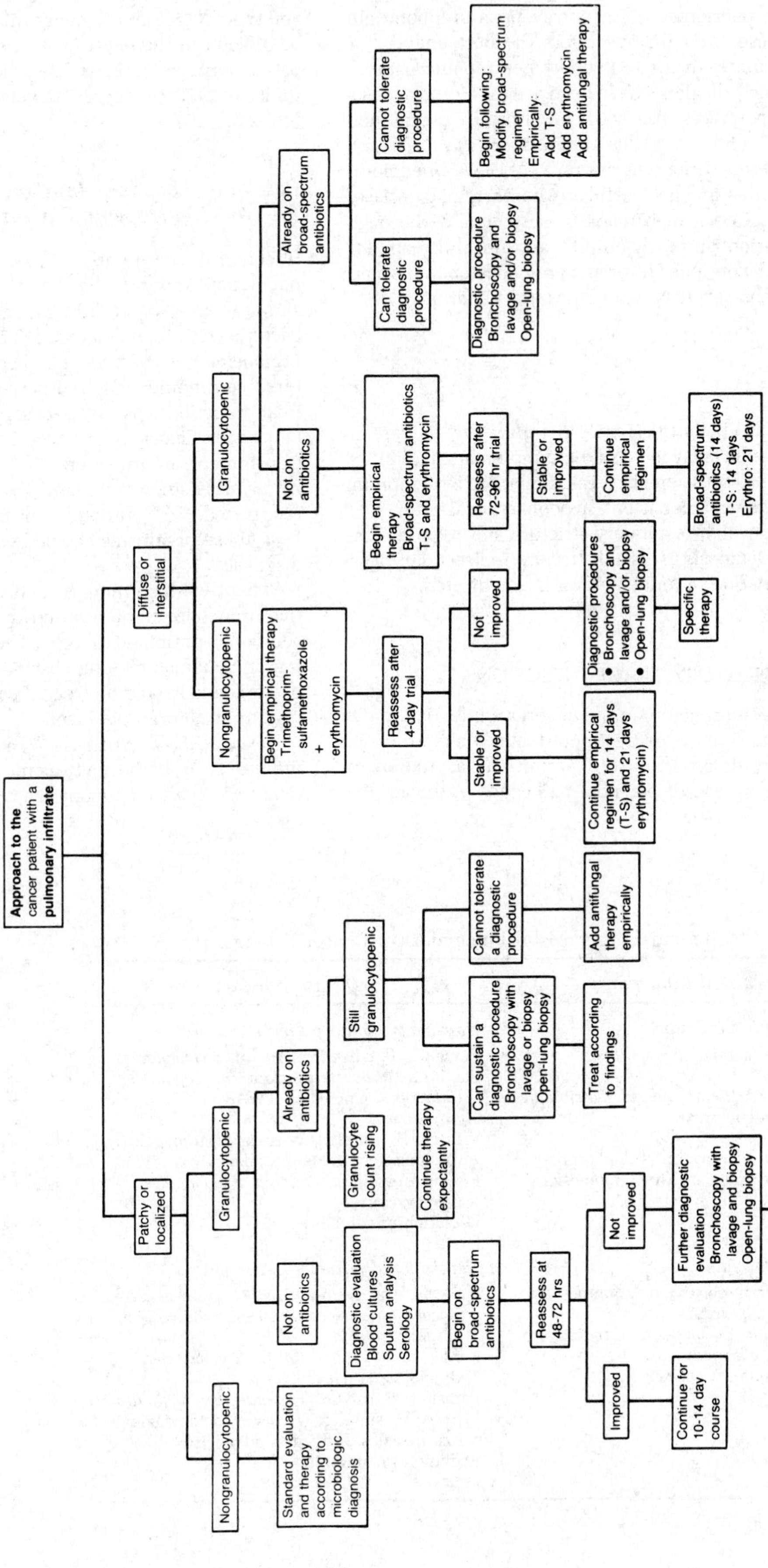

FIG. 59-17. Algorithm for the management of the cancer patient with a pulmonary infiltrate.

ment requires debridement and intravenous amphotericin B.[189-192] Because early therapy offers the best chance for control, particularly in the profoundly neutropenic patient, methods for early diagnosis have been sought. Serodiagnosis of invasive aspergillosis has not been clinically useful, and although nasal culture surveillance for *Aspergillus flavus* has been used to detect patients at risk for *Aspergillus* pneumonitis, these cultures are not useful in the early diagnosis of sinusitis. Therefore a high index of suspicion, a thorough nasal examination, and early empiric antifungal therapy for the patient with continued fever and granulocytopenia who is already on broad-spectrum antibiotics are important.

Epiglottitis

Acute bacterial epiglottitis *(e.g., H. influenzae)* is rare in adults but must be considered in the symptomatic patient.[192] *Candida* can also cause epiglottitis, hallmarked by symptoms of odynophagia and persistent hypopharyngeal pain.[193,194] Patients can develop respiratory stricture and require close monitoring. Diagnosis is established by indirect laryngoscopy, and initiation of amphotericin B is indicated.

LOWER RESPIRATORY TRACT INFECTIONS

The lung is the most common site of serious infection in the cancer patient. Disease- or treatment-induced alterations of the respiratory defense network permit the aspiration or hematogenous spread of potential pathogens. Although the ability to detect a pulmonary infiltrate radiographically may be difficult in the neutropenic patient, it is possible to place patients into one of four categories according to their type of infiltrate and the degree of neutropenia (Fig. 59-17; Table 59-32).

Patchy or Localized Infiltrate in the Non-Neutropenic Patient

Infection in these patients is similar to that in the general population and may be due to viruses (*e.g.,* RSV, herpes simplex virus, parainfluenza, adenovirus), mycoplasma, or bacteria *(e.g., S. pneumonia, H. influenza)*. In some centers, *Legionella pneumophila* has become a frequently encountered community-acquired pathogen, but in others nosocomial infection has been observed, with hospital cooling tanks, sink faucets, and showerheads being implicated in the transmission of infection.[195-197] Pneumonitis due to chlamydia and its newer variant, TWAR, have been increasingly recognized.[198,199] Although not unique to the compromised host, these organisms should be included in the differential diagnosis.

Patients with pulmonary metastases are at risk for obstructive bronchopneumonias and may require bronchoscopy in addition to antibiotic therapy. The majority of these necrotizing pneumonias or lung abscesses are caused by anaerobic bacteria and should be treated with either penicillin, clindamycin, or chloramphenicol.

Herpes simplex virus (HSV) may cause localized or focal infiltrates in both neutropenic and non-neutropenic patients.[200] Localized pneumonia is due to contiguous spread of

TABLE 59-32. Differential Diagnosis of Pneumonia in Cancer Patients

Localized Infiltrate	*Diffuse Infiltrate*
Non-neutropenic patients	*Non-neutropenic patients*
Bacteria: *S. pneumonia, Hemophilus, Myocobacteria*	Parasites: *P. carinii, T. gondii, Strongyloides*
Fungi: *Cryptococcus, Histoplasma, Coccidioides*	Bacteria: *Mycobacteria, Nocardia, Legionella, Chlamydia* (including TWAR)
Viruses: RSV, adenovirus	*Mycoplasma*
Underlying tumor	Viruses: H. simplex, V. zoster, cytomegalovirus, measles, influenza, adenovirus
Drugs: busulfan, bleomycin, cyclophosphamide, methotrexate, cytosine arabinoside	Fungi: *Aspergillus, Candida, Zygomycetes, Cryptococcus*
Radiation	Radiation pneumonitis
	Drugs
Neutropenic Patients	*Neutropenic Patients*
Bacteria: Any gram-positive or gram-negative, *Mycobacteria, Nocardia*	Bacteria: Any gram-positive or gram-negative, *Mycobacteria, Nocardia, Legionella, Chlamydia Mycoplasma*
Fungi: *Aspergillus, Zygomycetes, Candida, Cryptococcus, Histoplasma*	Fungi: *Candida, Aspergillus, Zygomycetes, Cryptococcus, Histoplasma*
Viruses: H. simplex, V. zoster	Parasites: *P. carinii, T. gondii, Strongyloides*
Drugs (see above)	Viruses: H. simplex, V. zoster, cytomegalovirus, measles, influenza, adenovirus, RSV
Radiation	Radiation pneumonitis
	Drugs

HSV from the oropharynx of patients who are intubated for other underlying pulmonary diseases or who undergo diagnostic bronchoscopy. Because the oropharynx is the source of virus, most cases are due to type 1 rather than type 2 HSV. The radiologic picture is indistinguishable from other localized pneumonias, and appropriate studies (*i.e.*, bronchoscopy and specific immunofluorescence and virus cultures performed on respiratory specimens) must be carried out to provide the specific diagnosis. Treatment is with intravenous acyclovir (500 mg/m^2 every 8 hours).

Non-neutropenic patients who are receiving immunosuppressive therapy (including corticosteroids) and patients with AIDS are at risk for tuberculosis and atypical mycobacterial disease. In recent years, infections due to *M. tuberculosis* have increased, particularly in areas where there are large numbers of patients with AIDS, such as New York City.[200] This change in the reservoir of *M. tuberculosis* may alter the incidence of infection in cancer patients. Identification of the offending organism is important because the atypical mycobacteria, particularly *M. fortuitum, M. avium-intracellulare* (MAI), and *M. kansasii,* are often resistant to available agents. Although *M. fortuitum* and *M. chelonii* can be treated with agents like cefoxitin, amikacin, tetracycline, and sulfonamides, MAI is unresponsive to conventional antibiotics and antituberculosis drugs. Although ansamycin and clofazimine have been used for MAI, data to support their efficacy are lacking.

Infection with mycobacteria most frequently becomes apparent after immunosuppressive therapy, especially after corticosteroids, suggesting a reactivated infection. The mortality of tuberculous infections ranges from 17% to 50% in cancer patients, and a high index of suspicion is important, because the pulmonary lesions may be confused with the underlying malignancy or other infections.[201,202] Sputum should be cultured, and new infiltrates may be successfully diagnosed by fiberoptic bronchoscopy and brush biopsy with minimal complications.[203] Tuberculin skin testing should be performed before chemotherapy in all patients. Reactive patients who have not been previously treated with isoniazid should be treated prophylactically for approximately 1 year. Patients with radiographic and culture evidence (positive sputum) for typical tuberculosis should be treated for 9 to 12 months with at least two drugs (usually INH and ethambutol or rifampin).

Less commonly encountered causes for a localized pulmonary infiltrate in a non-neutropenic patient include progression of an underlying malignancy, atelectatic segment of lung due to a compromised airway, and a localized reaction to a chemotherapeutic agent, particularly methotrexate, cyclophosphamide, or bleomycin. Drug reactions, however, are more commonly manifested as diffuse, interstitial pulmonary processes.

Patchy or Localized Infiltrates in the Neutropenic Patient

In addition to the pathogens causing a localized infiltrate in the non-neutropenic patient, an array of opportunistic pathogens must be considered in the differential diagnosis of a neutropenic patient with a localized infiltrate. Any gram-positive or gram-negative organism and a variety of fungal, parasitic, and viral pathogens can be responsible for a localized pneumonic process in a neutropenic patient (Table 59-32). In patients with periods of neutropenia less than 14 days, bacterial pathogens predominate. Patients with more prolonged periods of neutropenia or those with a particular clinical pattern (*e.g.*, after allogeneic bone marrow transplantation) are more prone to develop a fungal (*Candida* or *Aspergillus*) or viral infection CMV.

Unless the clinical presentation suggests otherwise, it is appropriate to initiate 48 to 72 hours of broad-spectrum antibiotic therapy before proceeding to an invasive diagnostic procedure (Fig. 59-17). If the patient has stabilized or improved by 72 hours, continuing treatment for 10 to 14 days is necessary. If the patient has not stabilized or improved after broad-spectrum antibiotics, further evaluation is mandatory to exclude other potentially treatable organisms. Although diagnostic material occasionally can be obtained with transtracheal aspiration, bronchoscopy, or percutaneous needle biopsy, the yield with these procedures rarely approaches 50%.

In recent years the bronchoalveolar lavage (BAL) has come into vogue because it has a low morbidity and can be safely performed by experienced hands in neutropenic patients with platelet counts as low as 30,000/mm^3.[204-207] A transbronchial biopsy, however, should not be performed during the BAL in patients whose platelet count is less than 50,000/mm^3.

If the diagnosis cannot be established with BAL, the next procedure to consider is the open lung biopsy. Unlike the minithoracotomy, which can be performed for the patient with a diffuse infiltrate, a more complete thoracotomy is often necessary for the patient with a localized infiltrate.[208] It is important that the biopsy be obtained from the center of the lesion and from its outer borders to decrease the chance for a false-negative biopsy. Biopsy or tissue samples, touch preps, ground material, and sections should be comprehensively analyzed microscopically by Gram stain, wet mount, toluidine blue, modified methylene blue, acid-fast, methenamine silver, Dieterle or Gimenez, and if necessary, *Legionella*-direct immunofluorescent antibody and electron microscopy. Routine aerobic, anaerobic, acid fast, fungal, and supplemented charcoal–yeast-extract cultures should be made. After a comprehensive analysis, the diagnostic yield from an open lung biopsy is very high, unless the patient is already receiving multiple antimicrobial therapies.

LEGIONELLA. Although not common at most centers, an important pathogen to consider as the cause of localized pneumonia in an immunosuppressed host is *Legionella*.[209-212] *Legionella* species are ubiquitous and usually found in water, including air conditioning cooling towers and hospital shower heads.[213,214] Aerosolization of contaminated water is probably the most common mechanism of transmission, and nosocomial infections have been described.

Although legionellosis is a multisystem disease, the lung represents the primary target organ. Incubation ranges from 2 to 10 days (median, 4 days), although immunosuppressed patients tend to have shorter incubation periods and a more abrupt onset of symptoms. The initial symptoms are generally nonspecific and include malaise, anorexia, lethargy, and headache. A nonproductive cough develops in 90% of patients, although it usually follows the initial symptoms by 2 to 3 days. Diarrhea, which occurs in approximately 50% of patients, may either proceed or follow the respiratory symptoms.

Fever is usually the initial sign of legionella and is normally unremitting until institution of effective therapy. Two-thirds of patients will manifest a pulse deficit (*i.e.*, relative bradycardia) and one-third will have some degree of neurologic dysfunction, ranging from disorientation, depression, hallucinations, and seizures to lethargy, stupor, and coma.[214-217] Physical examination may reveal either hyperreactive or hyporeactive deep tendon reflexes, nystagmus, peripheral sensory or motor neuropathies, and rarely, signs of meningeal irritation.

The initial radiographic abnormality is a patchy, alveolar infiltrate involving a single lobe. If translobar consolidation occurs, it usually involves contiguous segments.[218] Cavitary lesions or abscess formation is unusual except for *L. midadei.*

The most rapid and accurate means of diagnosis is a direct fluorescent antibody (DFA) test performed on respiratory tract secretions, pulmonary tissue from biopsy specimens, pleural fluid, or pus. However, not all serotypes are detectable and a negative DFA does not eliminate *Legionella* as a diagnostic consideration. Culturing of the organism on a charcoal–yeast-extract medium requires 2 to 7 days.

Erythromycin (40–50 mg/kg/day, with a maximum of 4 g, in 4 divided doses for 3 weeks) is the treatment of choice. Therapy should be administered intravenously for the first several days in seriously ill patients; subsequent therapy may be oral. Patients unable to tolerate erythromycin should receive doxycycline (5 mg/kg/day in 2 divided doses). Rifampin (20 mg/kg/day in 2 divided doses) may be given in addition to erythromycin or doxycycline for seriously ill patients. Response to therapy is normally prompt, with a resolution of fever and subjective improvement within 24 to 48 hours.

Nocardia asteroides and *N. brasiliensis* may also present as a localized pulmonary infiltrate, although miliary and microcavitary patterns have been described in cancer patients.[219-222] Approximately 30% of patients with a pulmonary infection due to *N. asteroides* will have associated cutaneous and CNS infection (usually brain abscesses) as well. Diagnosis depends on positive cultures or histopathologic demonstration of tissue invasion by the organisms. Microscopically, the organisms are gram-positive, irregularly stained, beaded or branching, and partially acid-fast and filamentous. Skin lesions, usually subcutaneous abscesses, are associated with *Nocardia.* Sulfonamides (sulfadiazine, 4–6 g/day for 4–6 months) provide the most effective therapy for this infection, but mortality is significant (30%) once the infection has become disseminated. Favorable responses also have been observed with ampicillin plus erythromycin or with minocycline. Trimenthoprim-sulfamethoxazole has in vitro activity and has been used clinically, although late relapses have been reported.

FUNGI. Fungal infections constitute the greatest threat for the neutropenic patient who develops a new or progressive pulmonary infiltrate while receiving broad-spectrum antibiotic therapy, often occurring as part of a disseminated infection (See Table 59-32).[222-224] We reviewed our experience with these patients and observed two distinct groups: patients who developed a new infiltrate while the granulocyte count was rising and patients who developed a new infiltrate while they were granulocytopenic.[225] Patients who developed infiltrates in conjunction with bone marrow recovery did well without therapeutic modifications. In contrast, the patients who developed a new and progressive infiltrate while on antibiotics and while still granulocytopenic were likely to have a fungal cause for their new infiltrates. Ideally an open lung biopsy should be performed in these patients to establish the diagnosis and guide the therapy. If a biopsy cannot be performed, amphotericin B should be instituted empirically, because we observed a significant survival advantage for patients who received early, empiric antifungal therapy.

Candida is the most common fungal infection. A characteristic radiographic appearance cannot be described, and the altered inflammatory response of the immunosuppressed patient may result in a false-negative chest roentgenogram or as perihilar densities or a miliary pattern.[226] The presence of *Candida* in the sputum correlates poorly with overt infection. Although a positive blood culture for *Candida* is highly correlated with invasive or disseminated infection in the immunocompromised patient, negative blood cultures are much more likely.[227] Isolation of *C. tropicalis* from multiple body sites (*e.g.*, sputum, urine, and stool) has been correlated with invasive disease.[71] In most instances, however, definitive diagnosis requires histopathologic confirmation.

Endophthalmitis, characterized by focal, white, fluffy, mound-like retinal lesions that can extend rapidly into the vitreous, has been associated with disseminated candidiasis.[228] Measurement of serum antibody or precipitins has proven unreliable, and the newer antigen tests remain relatively insensitive.

In many treatment centers, the incidence of aspergillosis in cancer patients from *A. fumigatus, A. flavus, A. niger,* and *A. terreus* has increased over the last decade. The upper airway is the most frequent route of entry of these organisms, and clusters of nosocomial aspergillosis have occurred in hospitals in which construction materials have been contaminated with *Aspergillus* spores.[179,229-232] The pathologic hallmark of aspergillosis is blood vessel invasion, with consequent thrombosis and infarction. *Aspergillus* pneumonia in the immunocompromised host is a rapidly invasive, necrotizing bronchopneumonia or a hemorrhagic infection with thrombosis of the pulmonary arteries and veins, with a possibility for life-threatening hemoptysis. Approximately half of the patients are also infected with other organisms, especially *Pseudomonas.*

A characteristic radiographic appearance for *Aspergillus* pneumonia has not been described, but the development of a new pulmonary infiltrate in a neutropenic patient who is receiving broad-spectrum antibiotics should raise suspicion.[225] Blood cultures are rarely positive, even though disseminated infection occurs in 30% of patients. Extrapulmonary sites include the sinuses, CNS, liver, kidney, skin, and heart valves. Diagnosis of aspergillosis by noninvasive measures is suboptimal, although recent reports suggest that positive sputum or BAL cultures in a patient with prolonged fever, neutropenia, and a progressive infiltrate is highly correlated with a diagnosis of *Aspergillus* pneumonia.[233] Despite initially optimistic reports, antigen and antibody methods of detection have not been as sensitive as had been hoped and are associated with too many false-negative results.[98] A definitive diagnosis still requires histologic confirmation or a positive BAL culture obtained in a clinically relevant setting. Treatment of *Aspergillus* pneumonia requires an early diagnosis and prompt intervention. Optimal therapy is amphotericin B. Although standard dosages of amphotericin B have ranged between 0.5 and 1.0 mg/kg/day, 14 patients treated with high-dose amphotericin (1–1.5 mg/kg/day) had an exceptional survival rate.[234] Controlled clinical trials are needed to test this approach and to test amphotericin B encapsulated into liposomes because of the encouraging results obtained in preclinical models and early clinical trials.[163,164] Although not proven, the addition of 100 to 150 mg/kg/day of 5-fluorocystosine (5-FC) in 3 divided dosages to amphotericin B may be helpful. If 5-FC is given, blood levels should be measured. Even with appropriate pharmacologic intervention, however, the most important prognosticator of a successful outcome is the return of adequate levels of granulocytes. Infrequently, *Aspergillus* will cause a mycetoma or fungus ball in immunocompromised patients, and resection is generally recommended.

The *Phycomycetes* (especially *Mucor* and *Rhizopus*) are the third most frequent cause of invasive fungal infection in cancer patients.[186,187] Like *Aspergillus*, the *Phycomycetes* are acquired by way of the respiratory tract and cause a necrotizing bronchopneumonia or infarction after vascular invasion and thrombosis. Dissemination to the kidney, gastrointestinal tract, CNS, liver, pancreas or heart may occur in 50% of patients with *Phycomycetes* infections. Early biopsy of suspicious lesions and aggressive therapy with amphotericin B and surgical debridement are essential.

Histoplasmosis can also cause serious pneumonia in the cancer patient, usually manifested as a military infiltrate.[235] Infection is usually disseminated, and the reticuloendothelial system is generally so heavily infected that the resultant adenopathy, hepatosplenomegaly, and bone marrow involvement can sometimes be confused with the underlying malignancy.[236] Consequently, careful histologic examination of biopsies from the nodes, liver, or bone marrow for the intracellular yeast forms, using Giemas or methenamine-silver staining, is extremely important in evaluating suspected patients or those from endemic areas.[237]

Coccidioides imitis and *Cryptococcus neoformans* can also result in serious pneumonia and disseminated infections in cancer patients.[238,239] *Torulopsis* (or *Candida*) *glabrata* has been isolated increasingly from cancer patients and associated with serious fungal infections. Infection with *T. glabrata* occurs predominantly in debilitated, neutropenic patients, but it has also been associated with a foreign body (*e.g.*, hyperalimentation catheter, urinary catheter).[240,241] The most common sites of infection are lung, kidney, and gastrointestinal tract. Fungemia with this organism may occasionally produce an endotoxin-like shock syndrome. Because of its similarity to *Candida*, diagnosis of *T. glabrata* is difficult, and differentiation rests upon its smaller size and lack of pseudomycelia. *Trichosporon spp.*, an arthrospore-forming yeast, can cause both local skin lesions and invasive disease in cancer patients.[98] *T. beigeli* is the cause of white piedra in noncompromised hosts but can involve the lungs, kidneys, skin, and eyes in immunocompromised patients. The serum from patients with trichosporonosis can react with the cryptococcal latex agglutination test due to shared antigens between *T. beigeli* and *C. neoformans*. Successful therapy depends on the early initiation of amphotericin B and, most importantly, recovery from neutropenia.[242] Although rare, serious pulmonary infection can result from *Fusarium* and *Pseudoallecheria boydii*, both of which can mimic *Aspergillus*.

Treatment options for the patient with serious fungal disease are currently limited to a small number of drugs, the most reliable of which is still amphotericin B (see Table 59-28).[157,243] Although amphotericin achieves a concentration in excess of the minimum inhibitory concentration of most major fungal pathogens, it is associated with significant acute and delayed toxicity. There is, moreover, a spectrum of sensitivity. For example, some isolates of *Candida* appear tolerant to amphotericin B, and all isolates of *Pseudoallescheria boydii* are resistant to amphotericin B, although sensitive to miconazole.

Most patients receiving amphotericin B experience fever, chills (sometimes with rigors), nausea, and vomiting. Less commonly, hypotension, bronchospasm, or seizures may occur. With continued administration, nephrotoxicity, including azotemia, elevated creatinine, renal tubular acidosis, and cylindruria, and electrolyte disturbances, especially hypokalemia, occur. A decreased erythrocyte production and thrombocytopenia may occur after 22 to 35 days of amphotericin B therapy. Because most immunosuppressed patients who become candidates for amphotericin are already receiving nephrotoxic antibiotics, the decision to initiate therapy is often difficult.

When therapy is instituted in the cancer patient, it is important to achieve an effective serum concentration of amphotericin as rapidly as possible. We initially administer a test dose of 1 mg; if tolerated, the remaining dose of 0.5 mg/kg/day is given within 2 to 4 hours. Premedication with acetaminophen and the addition of hydrocortisone sodium succinate (25–50mg) to the infusion bottle may reduce toxicity. The dose of 0.5 mg/kg (therapeutic range, 0.4–0.6 mg/kg) is administered over 2 to 3 hours daily. The infusion should not be interrupted because of fever and chills, because this is a self-limited reaction. Meperidine (or Demerol, 0.5–1 mg/kg IV) is helpful in controlling the rigors, although the mechanism of action is unknown. Potassium supplementation is important, and if toxicity is excessive, an every-other-day amphotericin schedule may help.

The total dose for disseminated infection appears to be in the range of 1.5 to 2 g (30–40 mg/kg). Recommended doses of amphotericin B are not based on controlled clinical trials and depend on the site and nature of infection. For example, a short course (5–7 days) of low-dose amphotericin B (0.1–0.3 mg/kg) may be adequate for patients with oral or esophageal mucosal candidiasis.[244] For uncomplicated candidemia, a course of 500 mg/kg (10 mg/kg total dose) is successful in treating the fungemia and preventing endophthalmitis. More protracted and higher doses of amphotericin B (*e.g.*, 5–7 g) may be necessary for the treatment of hepatic candidiasis. The combination of amphotericin B with other agents, such as rifampin or 5-FC, is frequently considered, but demonstrable efficacy with amphotericin B plus 5-FC has been shown only for the treatment of patients with cryptococcal meningitis.[245–248] The therapeutic index in experimental candidiasis was improved when amphotericin B was encapsulated into lipsomes, and preliminary reports suggest enhanced clinical efficacy, particularly in hepatic candidiasis.[163,164] Unfortunately, difficulties in formulating a standard liposomal preparation have hampered controlled clinical trials, although multicenter studies are now beginning.

5-FC is an antimetabolite that has demonstrable in vitro efficacy against most fungi.[249] It can be administered orally (150 mg/kg/day every 6 hours) and is well absorbed. The data to support its efficacy as a single agent for the treatment of serious fungal infections in humans are meager. In vivo resistance to 5-FC develops rapidly, but 5-FC may be additive or synergistic with amphotericin B.[250] Toxic effects from 5-FC include nausea, vomiting, hepatotoxicity, and bone marrow depression.

The newest antifungal drugs are the imidazoles and the azoles, a group of synthetic agents with in vitro activity against most fungi.[157,243,251] Clotrimazole has efficacy for the treatment of chronic mucocutaneous candidiasis, but it does appear to be useful for systemic therapy.[252] Clotrimazole may be useful in preventing oral *Candida* infections, and we have found it helps some patients with esophagitis.[253]

Miconazole has in vitro activity against almost all pathogenic fungi except *Mucor* and *Rhizopus.* The most extensive clinical experience with miconazole has been for patients with chronic or disseminated coccidioidomycoses. Miconazole has also shown some efficacy against paracoccidioidomycosis, South American blastomycosis, chronic mucocutaneous candidiasis, esophageal candidiasis, and petriellidosis, although frequent relapse remains a problem.

The role of miconazole in cancer patients with invasive fungal infection has been limited.[253] Jordan and colleagues reported a 41% response rate for 37 *Candida* and *Torulopsis* infections in patients with various malignancies.[254] Among patients with neutrophil counts less than 1000/mm^3, the response rate was 67%; however, only 2 of 7 patients with neutrophil counts less than 100/mm^3 were cured. None of the 8 patients with other fungal infections (4 *Aspergillus,* 2 *Penicillium,* 1 *Mucor,* and 1 *Cryptococcus*) responded.

Toxic effects with miconazole has included nausea, phlebitis, anemia, hyponatremia, and pruritus; anaphylaxis and cardiac arrhythmia have also been observed during infusion. Miconazole is poorly absorbed, necessitating parenteral administration for prolonged periods. Coupled with its limited efficacy and high relapse rate, miconazole cannot be considered a first-line antifungal drug for cancer patients.

Ketoconazole has been the imidazole receiving the widest interest for cancer patients.[157,251] In vitro testing has documented sensitivity for a variety of fungi, including *Candida sp., Paracoccidioides, Coccidioides, Cryptococcus,* and *Histoplasma.* Animal studies have shown ketoconazole to be effective against *C. albicans, Coccidioides,* and the *Dermatophytes.* Human trials have used ketoconazole has a single daily oral dose of 200 to 1200 mg and estimated the half-life range from 4 to 12 hours. However, ketoconazole is not effective against *Aspergillus* and *Mucor,* and its spectrum against *Candida spp.* is not complete. For example, *C. tropicalis* and *T. glabrata* are not covered by ketoconazole.

In spite of the advantages of an oral preparation, patients with oral mucositis or who are severely ill have difficulty swallowing ketoconazole. Moreover, absorption is diminished by antacids or H2 blockers, and co-administration of these medications can result in subtherapeutic levels of ketoconazole. Although relatively nontoxic, a range of problems includes poor intestinal absorption, nausea and vomiting, dizziness, lethargy, headache, and confusioned states. Hepatic enzyme elevation is common, and one case of fatal hepatic necrosis has been reported. Prolonged use may result in gynecomastia, azoospermia, depressed adrenal and testosterone synthesis, and decreased libido.[161]

Although ketoconazole appears useful for the treatment of patients with mucosal infections (*e.g.*, oral mucositis, esophagitis), its efficacy for immunosuppressed patients with invasive mycoses is unestablished. Studies suggest that ketoconazole should not be used for invasive mycoses and should be restricted to use in patients with superficial mycoses.[158,160] Ketoconazole has also been evaluated for antifungal prophylaxis, but its efficacy is limited. The observation in a rat model of aspergillosis that pretreatment with ketoconazole may limit the subsequent effectiveness of amphotericin, presumably by interfering with ergosteral synthesis, is disturbing and offers an additional concern about the prophylactic use of ketoconazole in cancer patients.[254]

Although only now entering clinical evaluation, the triazoles have promise as antifungal agents. Itraconazole inhibits steroid synthesis, is available with an oral formulation, and has a broad spectrum of antifungal activity that includes *Candida* and *Aspergillus.* Fluconazole has a narrower spectrum of activity that includes *Candida* and *Cryptococcus* but does not include *Aspergillus.* It has a long half-life and high bioavailability, and it crosses the blood-brain barrier avidly.[165–168] It is likely that these agents will assume important roles in the treatment or prevention of fungal infections, especially *Candida* and *Cryptococcus,* in the coming years.

Interstitial Infiltrates in the Non-Neutropenic Patient

Diffuse pulmonary infiltrates can be caused by bacterial, viral, fungal, and protozoal pathogens and are influenced by whether or not the patient is neutropenic (see Table 59-32).

PNEUMOCYSTIS PNEUMONIA. A non-neutropenic patient with diffuse pulmonary infiltrate is unlikely to have a bacterial or fungal process. Perhaps the most commonly encountered infection in this setting is *Pneumocystis carinii* pneumonia.[255] This infection is believed to result from a reactivation of latent cysts, because 100% of normal children possess detectable antibody to *P. carinii.*[256] However, patient-to-patient transmission has been suggested by reports on nosocomial clusterings of cases.[257] It is also possible that certain chemotherapeutic regimens predispose patients to interstitial infiltrates caused by *P. carinii.*[258] *For example, an increased prevalence of* P. *carinii* pneumonia was observed at the NCI in a group of non-Hodgkin's lymphoma patients receiving combination chemotherapy. Patients had been randomized to one of two treatment arms, and only in the one containing cytosine arabinoside and bleomycin, in addition to drugs shared in common in both treatment arms, was the prevalence of *P. carinii* pneumonia increased. Whether this chemotherapy regimen enhanced reactivation of latent organisms or made patients more susceptible to reinfection from ambient organisms is unclear. This problem, however, has been abrogated by the prophylactic administration of trimethoprim-sulfamethoxazole to patients receiving this treatment regimen.

The most common clinical manifestations of pneumocystis in cancer patients include fever, cough, and tachypnea, generally with intercostal retractions and the absence of detectable rales. A chest radiograph shows a hazy, bilateral alveolar infiltrate, which often begins at the hilus and spreads to the periphery. Arterial blood gases reflect a low PaO_2, normal Pa CO_2, and alkaline pH. The clinical presentation can be indolent (1–2 months) but more often is fulminant (4–5 days). The chest roentgenographic findings may occasionally be atypical (*e.g.*, lobar consolidation, effusion, and even nodular) and, in rare cases, the radiograph may appear normal despite the presence of pneumocysts on biopsy. *P. carinii* pneumonia in cancer patients differs from that in AIDS patients by having a more smoldering and indolent course; the median duration of symptoms is 28 days in AIDS patients, but 5 days for non-AIDS patients.[259]

Diagnosis of *P. carinii* pneumonia requires demonstration of cysts or trophozoites in pulmonary material from patients with a clinically compatible course; cysts have been found in asymptomatic, previously healthy individuals autopsied following traumatic deaths. In patients with AIDS, positive specimens may be obtained from sputum samples because the "cyst-burden" is high, but in cancer patients, cysts are best demonstrated by BAL or open lung biopsy. Serologic confirmation is of questionable value.

In clinical situations where the likelihood of *P. carinii* pneumonia is great, the choice is to proceed with diagnostic procedure or to administer an empiric course of therapy with trimethoprim-sulfamethoxazole (see Fig. 59-17). If BAL is readily available, it is the procedure of choice for establishing the diagnosis.[204] However, if BAL is not available or if the patient's clinical or hematologic status does not permit a BAL, an empiric trial of trimethoprim-sulfamethoxazole (20 mg/kg/day of trimethoprim) plus erythromycin (for *Legionella*) is recommended, rather than proceeding directly to open lung biopsy. This is based on the results of a randomized NCI trial demonstrating that in non-neutropenic patients with diffuse infiltrates, empiric therapy is as safe and effective an open lung biopsy.[260] However, a response may not be apparent for 4 to 5 days, although stabilization or slight improvement in alveolar air exchange generally occurs within 72 to 96 hours. Failure to improve (*e.g.*, continued fever, depressed PaO_2, progressive infiltrates) after 4 days of therapy serves as an indication to modify therapy, usually with the addition of pentamidine (4 mg/kg/day as a 1–2 hour infusion).

If a histologic diagnosis is necessary and not achievable by BAL, not all procedures, such as transtracheal aspirate, transbronchial biopsy or aspirate, or open lung biopsy, are of comparable diagnostic accuracy. Burt and colleagues examined each of 17 patients having an open lung biopsy for the diagnosis of a diffuse interstitial infiltrate with a transthoracic needle aspirate and a transbronchial brush and biopsy.[261] The patients in this unique study served as their own controls. A diagnosis was established from only 30% of the aspirates and from 59% of the transbronchial biopsy samples; it suggests that the open lung biopsy is the procedure of choice. Open lung biopsy provides the soundest guidance for patient management, especially if the patient is neutropenic and requires multiple antimicrobial agents. The role of open lung biopsy for neutropenic patients already receiving antibiotic and antifungal therapy, however, appears less defined because the diagnostic yield is low and therapeutic modifications are minimal.[262]

Because the patients who are candidates for open lung biopsy are often thrombocytopenic, appropriate hematologic preparation for surgery is vital. Elevation of the platelet count to a surgically safe level of 30,000/mm^3 or greater can usually be accomplished by the infusion of 4 to 8 units of platelet concentrates 1 hour before surgery. Maintenance of the platelet count at this level for 24 hours after surgery with additional platelet concentrates minimizes any postoperative bleeding complications.

Because of the importance the *P. carinii* has assumed in patients with AIDS, the search for new therapeutic agents has intensified. The most promising of these to date is the antifolate, trimetrexate, which has proven effective in AIDS patients who are refractory to trimethoprim-sulfamethoxazole and pentamidine.[263]

The appropriate course of treatment in the cancer patient with proved or putative *P. carinii* pneumonia is to begin with trimethoprim-sulfamethoxazole and, if the patients has not stabilized or improved by day 4 of therapy, to add pentamidine. If there is no improvement after 4 days of pentamidine, trimetrexate should be substituted.

VIRAL PNEUMONIAS. CMV has been a cause of severe interstitial pneumonia, especially among patients receiving allogeneic marrow transplants for hematologic malignancies. Renal, cardiac, and liver allograft recipients and patients with lymphoma or leukemia are also at risk, albeit at a lower incidence. Although the pathogenesis of CMV pneumonia is incompletely defined, several risk factors for CMV pneumonia after allogeneic marrow transplant have been identified.[264,265] These include being seropositive for antibody to CMV before transplant, undergoing allogeneic or autologous transplantation, receiving total-body irradiation as part of the conditioning regimen, and developing acute graft versus host disease (GVHD) after transplant.

In addition to active CMV infection, disordered immune function undoubtedly underlies the development of CMV pneumonia. For example, the lack of GVHD, which is as immunosuppressive as its treatment, is the putative explanation for the paucity of CMV pneumonia after syngeneic or autologous transplantation. However, whether it is the lack of specific immune responsiveness to CMV or an immunopathologic immune response directed at CMV antigens in pulmonary tissue is undefined.[266,267] Investigation of pulmonary immune responses may clarify the pathogenesis of this syndrome.

Depending on the presence of these various risk factors, up to 50% of marrow allograft recipients develop interstitial pneumonia, 70% of which is associated with CMV. CMV pneumonia characteristically occurs within the first 3 months after transplant, with a median onset of 50 to 70 days. Late cases developing after 100 days also occur among patients with chronic GVHD.[268] Diffuse infiltrates are most common, but localized and nodular infiltrates have been described. However, patients with apparently localized disease have diffuse involvement when other portions of lung are examined by sensitive virologic techniques.[269] Pleural effusions are rare.

CMV pneumonia is clinically indistinguishable from other causes of diffuse infiltrates in the compromised host, especially *Pseumocystis carinii,* and specific virologic studies must be done to provide the diagnosis. Rising antibody titers to CMV or excretion of virus in throat, urine, or blood are not of sufficient to obviate the need for direct examination of pulmonary specimens.[270,271] Open lung biopsy was previously considered the necessary diagnostic procedure, but BAL has shown high sensitivity among marrow transplant patients with pulmonary infiltrates.[272] Specificity and negative predictive value are of concerns, and results in marrow transplant patients cannot necessary be extrapolated to other immunocompromised patients, especially those with AIDS. If BAL is not diagnostic, open lung biopsy should be performed. Specimens obtained by open biopsy or BAL should be examined by rapid virologic techniques because conventional cultures usually do not become positive for CMV for 2 to 3 weeks, and 4 to 5 weeks is sometimes required. Direct examination of specimens by specific immunofluorescence using murine monoclonal antibodies is rapid (2–4 hours), but has a sensitivity of only about 60% depending on the quality of the specimen.[272] Inoculation of viral cultures by centrifugation followed by immunofluorescent staining for immediate or early CMV antigens (centrifugation or "shell vial" cultures) is extremely sensitive (>95%), specific, and rapid, with results available within 24 hours; some specimens may be positive as soon as 4 hours.[273] Other techniques include standard histologic staining for intranuclear inclusions and cytomegalic cells. Nucleic acid hybridization remains investigational and may not be more sensitive than centrifugation cultures.

CMV may also involve other organs, including the liver, spleen, kidney, adrenal, gastrointestinal tract, heart, CNS, and the eye. Enteritis and retinitis have been particularly common among patients with AIDS, but they also occur in organ allograft recipients. CMV has also been identified in association with other organisms including *P. carinii,* bacteria, fungi, and other viruses.

Therapy for CMV pneumonia after marrow transplant has been unsatisfactory. Treatment with a variety of antiviral agents, including vidarabine, acyclovir, interferons, and combination of these, were not successful.[274] Even use of the new acyclovir derivative, ganciclovir, did not improve outcome of CMV pneumonia in marrow transplant patients despite its dramatic effect in inhibiting CMV replication in vivo.[275,276] Ganciclovir appears to be effective in treating CMV pneumonia and other CMV syndromes (*e.g.,* retinitis, enteritis) in other immunocompromised patients, especially AIDS patients, in initial uncontrolled trials.[277] Most recently, the combination of ganciclovir and intravenous CMV immunoglobulin is promising in initial trials in marrow transplant recipients, and effective treatment of CMV pneumonia, even in marrow allograft recipients, may be available in the future.

The sole use of seronegative blood products can eliminate primary CMV infection in seronegative marrow transplant recipients who have seronegative marrow donors.[278] Similar observations have been made after cardiac and renal transplants. Although passive immunoprophylaxis with intravenous immune globulins continues to be studied in seronegative patients, results of clinical trials have been conflicting, and this modality should not be used in place of seronegative blood products.[278,279] Other approaches to prophylaxis, such as use of interferon, have not been successful after marrow transplantation.[280] It is likely that the future use of antiviral agents, such as ganciclovir, foscarnet, or acyclovir, will prevent CMV infection in patients seropositive before transplant.

Other viruses may cause severe, diffuse pneumonias. HSV may also cause diffuse pulmonary infiltrates. In this situation, pathogenesis includes viremia and involvement of other organs, including liver or brain; both type 1 and type 2 HSV have been implicated. Because of clinical similarity to other viral pneumonias like CMV, bronchoscopy or open biopsy is needed for diagnosis. Varicello-2 zoster virus (VZV) can also cause severe, diffuse pneumonia, although this is rare in the absence of cutaneous manifestations of disseminated VZV infection. Treatment of both HSV and VZV pneumonia is with intravenous acyclovir (500 mg/m^2 every 8 hours).

The measles virus can also cause severe pneumonia in immunocompromised patients. It may occur concomitantly with the initial illness with fever, coryza, and rash, or it may develop up to 6 months after initial infection.[281] Diagnosis may require open lung biopsy for specific immunofluorescence and culture. Immunosuppressed patients who have never received measles vaccine and are seronegative for antibody to measles and who have contact with measles should receive prophylactic gamma globulin (0.5 ml/kg, maximum dose of 15 ml) as soon after exposure as possible. Treatment of measles is supportive. Live virus vaccines should not be used in immunocompromised patients.[282]

Although the incidence of influenza and other common respiratory viruses (*i.e.,* parainfluenza 1 and 3, respiratory syncytial virus, rhinoviruses) does not appear to be increased in the cancer patient, infection due to these viruses may be severe. Both primary viral pneumonias and secondary bacterial infections may occur. With adenoviruses, both increased severity and an increased incidence due to reactivation of latent viruses may occur.[283] Disseminated adenovirus infection commonly involves lung, liver, and kidney, although hemorrhagic cystitis with or without nephritis may occur without other manifestations. Specific immunofluorescence performed on respiratory specimens and virus cultures are necessary for diagnosis. Respiratory syncytial virus (RSV) pneumonia in immunocompromised patients occurs in children and adults.

The synthetic nucleoside, ribavirin, given by aerosol, has been used for treatment of RSV, influenza, and parainfluenza infections.[284–286] Amantadine (or rimantidine) has prophylactic efficacy against influenza A and may have some therapeutic efficacy as well.[287] Some centers routinely use the killed influenza vaccine for cancer patients, although the antibody response to this vaccine may be diminished in patients receiving chemotherapy.[288,289]

Interstitial Infiltrate in the Neutropenic Patient

In addition to *P. carinii* and CMV, gram-positive and gram-negative bacteria and several fungi can cause interstitial infiltrates in neutropenic patients. Broad-spectrum antibiotics and trimethoprim-sulfamethoxazole are necessary for empiric therapy in these patients. Failure of the patient to improve necessitates lung biopsy and consideration of antifungal therapy.

CARDIOVASCULAR INFECTIONS

Cardiovascular infections are relatively uncommon among cancer patients, probably because of the early institution of broad-spectrum antimicrobial therapy. However, cancer patients who have predisposing factors for cardiovascular infections (*i.e.*, dental abscesses, IV drug abuse, congenital cardiac anomalies) are at risk. Guidelines for dental prophylaxis should be followed, and procedures should be avoided in patients who are neutropenic.[290] If however, dental work is essential in a patient who is neutropenic, broad-spectrum antibiotic prophylaxis should be used.

Endovascular infections are more likely with the increased use of indwelling venous access catheters. Although gram-positive bacteria (*e.g.*, enterococcus, viridans streptococci, beta-hemolytic streptococci, and *S. aureus*) most commonly cause endovascular infections, aerobic gram-negative bacilli (*e.g., P. aeruginosa*) and fungal organisms (*Candida, Aspergillus*) may also cause disease.[291] These pathogens are particularly difficult to eradicate, and morbidity and mortality are discouragingly high. Myocardial microabscesses occur more frequently (*Candida*), and myocarditis may be associated with both viruses and protozoa (*Toxoplasma*). Endocarditis may also suggest an underlying malignancy (*e.g.*, association of *S. bovis* with colon cancer).[171]

The clinical manifestations of endocarditis in the immunosuppressed patient are similar to those in an immunocompetent patient. Nonspecific complaints of fever, chills, malaise, fatigue, night sweats, and weight loss are common. Unfortunately, these complaints are not diagnostically specific. In most instances, the diagnosis of an endovascular infection in an immunocompromised patient must be made based on physical and laboratory evaluation. The numerous physical stigmata of endocarditis should be sought (*e.g.*, heart murmurs, splinter hemorrhages, Roth's spots, splenomegaly), but the diagnosis is confirmed by the isolation of an organism from multiple blood cultures. The complications of endovascular infections are similar to those described for noncancer patients. Valvular insufficiency resulting in congestive heart failure, embolic phenomenon, and renal failure are the most serious complications. Fungal endocarditis is particularly likely to cause large vessel embolization. Patients with *Candida* or *Aspergillus* endocarditis are candidates for valve replacement.

Therapy must be directed at the specific pathogen. The isolation of *S. aureus* or *S. epidermidis* from multiple blood samples, even if the patient has an indwelling catheter, is not sufficient criteria for prolonged antibiotic therapy unless confirmation of a valvular infection can be made. Standard therapy of 10 to 14 days suffices for these patients.[292]

GASTROINTESTINAL TRACT INFECTIONS

The gastrointestinal tract is a major reservoir of micro-organisms, is associated with several characteristic infectious complications, and serves as a major portal for systemic infection during periods of host compromise.

Oral Mucositis

Ulceration of the oral mucosa frequently occurs with chemotherapy. Colonization of drug-induced lessons by the indigenous aerobic or anaerobic oral flora may result in local infection and, in the neutropenic patient, may provide portal for septicemia. Mucositis, gingivitis, and other dental-related problems may occur in as many as 85% of leukemic patients during the course of their disease.

Measures have been sought to lower the risk of oral gingivitis and mucositis. Peterson and co-workers evaluated 38 febrile patients undergoing treatment for acute nonylmphocytic leukemia and found a 32% incidence of local oral infections, more than half of which were thought to cause the patients' fevers.[293] The periodontium was the most common site of infection, cultures of which usually revealed mixed flora, including many of the organisms associated with systemic infection in cancer patients (*e.g., S. aureus, S. epidermidis, C. albicans, P. aeruginosa*). In adults, pre-existing periodontitis is common (>90%) and is exacerbated with immunosuppression. The presence of marginal or necrotizing gingivitis, characterized by an erythematous periapical gingiva, is caused by mouth anaerobes and should be treated with specific antianaerobic agents (*e.g.*, clindamycin or metronidazole). The vigorous use of mouth cleansing salts and solutions (*e.g.*, equal parts of a nonirritating mouth wash, hydrogen peroxide, and water swished every 2 hours) may decrease or control the mucositis.

Unfortunately the oral mucosa is a difficult site to decontaminate fully, and several organisms, such as *C. albicans*, are especially problematic. Although oral candidiasis (thrush) is predominantly a superficial infection, in severely neutropenic patients it may serve as a portal for systemic invasion. Oral nystatin is of only minimal benefit; patients with more extensive oral candidiasis, however, usually respond to a short course of amphotericin B (0.1–0.5 mg/kg/

day for 7 days). Oral clotrimazole troches (10 mg, 5 times daily) have been used successfully for cancer patients.

In addition to bacteria and fungi, HSV may cause significant oral disease. Oral HSV infection may not manifest with typical cutaneous or intraoral vesicles and may not be distinguishable from radiation-induced or chemotherapy-induced mucositis. Viral cultures or immunofluorescence or both must be performed for diagnosis. Both intravenous acyclovir and vidarabine have demonstrated efficacy in the treatment of immunosuppressed patients with proven mucocutaneous HSV infection.[294,295] Results are better with acyclovir. Treatment with intravenous acyclovir (250mg/m^2 every 8 hours for 7 days) shortened the period of virus shedding by nearly 2 weeks and the period of healing by 1 week.[296] Orally administered acyclovir (400 mg 5 times daily for 7–10 days) appears comparable to intravenous acyclovir among patients who can comply with oral drugs.[296] Topical acyclovir ointment is beneficial, but it is only effective against external lesions and is less effective than oral or intravenous acyclovir.[297] Patients who are seropositive for antibody to HSV have a 70% to 80% incidence of HSV reactivation during leukemic induction therapy or after organ allografting.[298] Such patients may be protected against virus reactivation with either intravenous (250 mg/m^2 every 8–12 hours) or oral (400 mg 4–5 times daily or 800 mg every 12 hours) acyclovir given during the period of major risk, usually defined as the period of leukopenia.[299–302] Reduction in streptococcal superinfection and bacteremia also has been reported among patients receiving prophylaxis.[303]

Esophagitis

Clinically significant esophagitis may be the result of both infectious and noninfectious causes. For example, a syndrome clinically identical to an infectious esophagitis occurs in patients who have received extensive chest wall or mediastinal irradiation. An infectious esophagitis most commonly occurs among patients who have been granulocytopenic and receiving antibiotics for several days. Patients most often present with a subacute onset of retrosternal, burning chest pain and odynophagia. Fungal, viral, and bacterial organisms can all cause an infectious esophagitis in the immunocompromised host.[304–306]

The occurrence of an infectious esophagitis in the non-neutropenic individual is rare. In fact, in non-neutropenic patients, esophagitis is most commonly due to chemical irritation of the distal esophagus by refluxed gastric contents (*e.g.*, chemotherapy-induced emesis). These patients are best managed with judicious use of antacids or histamine antagonists. If the non-neutropenic patient has persistent esophageal discomfort, esophagoscopy with brushings for culture and a biopsy should be done. In non-neutropenic patients with AIDS, herpetic or candidal esophagitis are common.

For the neutropenic patient who is already receiving broad-spectrum antibiotic therapy, *Candida* is the most likely cause of esophagitis, but *H. simplex*, either alone or with *Candida*, and bacteria also deserve careful consideration. CMV has emerged as a frequent cause of esophagitis in AIDS patients or marrow allograft recipients. A common dilemma is whether endoscopy and biopsy should be performed to establish the diagnosis. While barium swallow or simple fiberoptic esophagoscopy can demonstrate cobblestoning or the putative "white curtain" associated with *Candida*, both are nonspecific and are associated with false-positive and false-negative results. The only definitive way to establish the diagnosis is with biopsy, culture, and histologic examination. For example, when patients with acute nonlymphocytic leukemia with symptomatic esophagitis were endoscoped, three of seven cases that appeared to be *Candida* were shown by biopsy to be nonfungal.

It is not always possible or safe to biopsy the patient with esophagitis, particularly if the patient is also profoundly thrombocytopenic. An alternative to biopsy is a short course of empiric therapy. Patients with esophageal candidiasis will generally respond within 48 hours to oral clotrimazole (10 mg troches, 5 times daily). If patients have persistence or worsening of the esophageal complaints after 48 hours of therapy, they should be given a trial of low-dose amphotericin B (0.1–0.5 mg/kg/day for 5 days). If the patient has persistent symptoms after 48 hours of intravenous amphotericin B, it is unlikely that *Candida* is the cause. Although some physicians advocate esophagoscopy at this point, a reasonable alterative is an empiric course of acyclovir (750 mg/m^2/day, at 8-hour intervals), because the second most likely pathogen (or copathogen) is *H. simplex*. If the patient responds, acyclovir should be given for 5 to 7 days.

Intra-Abdominal Infections

The clinical presentation of even common intra-abdominal processes (*e.g.*, appendicitis, infectious diarrheal syndromes) can be altered by granulocytopenia and compounded by complications of cancer or its treatment. For example, obstructive lesions may be due to primary or metastatic cancer (*e.g.*, lymphoma); cholangitis or a conjugated hyperbilirubinemia may be due to extrahepatic biliary obstruction by tumor (*e.g.*, rhabdomyosarcoma); and chronic abdominal pain or diarrheal syndromes may be caused by bowel wall infiltration by malignant disease or infection.

Intra-abdominal complaints must be expeditiously evaluated with a thorough abdominal and pulmonary examination, including a judiciously performed rectal examination. Repetitive rectal examinations must not be performed in the neutropenic patient, because bacteremia and "local" infection may result. Appropriate laboratory studies include routine hematologic and serum chemistry values, tests for amylase and total and direct bilirubin, and flat and upright abdominal radiographs. Additional diagnostic procedures (*e.g.*, abdominal or pelvic ultrasound, CT scans) should be pursued if appropriate. As a general rule, invasive diagnostic or radiographic procedures (*e.g.*, barium enema, endoscopy) should be avoided in the neutropenic patient unless absolutely required.

There are several intra-abdominal infections that are unique to the cancer patient. Foremost among these is *typhlitis* (or necrotizing enterocolitis), an inflammatory cellulitis involving the cecum.[307,308] Typhlitis most commonly occurs in association with prolonged episodes of granulocytopenia and broad-spectrum antimicrobial therapy in patients with acute leukemia, although any granulocytopenic patient is at risk. Patients normally present with subacute or acute onset of right lower quadrant abdominal pain, which frequently becomes generalized over several hours, along with fever, diarrhea, and prostration. The agents responsible for typhlitis include gram-negative bacteria, especially *P. aeruginosa.* Abdominal ultrasonography reveals bowel wall thickening and ascites and can help in the differential diagnoses.[309] Optimal management includes supportive care, adjustments of antimicrobial therapy to cover resistant gram-negative and anaerobic species, and aggressive surgical intervention to resect a necrotic bowel. Despite aggressive measures, mortality is 30% to 50%.[309]

An infrequently encountered clinical syndrome is *peritonitis* and bacteremia due to *Clostridia.* Patients with clostridial peritonitis classically have a fulminant clinical course with fever, tachycardia, abdominal wall ecchymoses and crepitance, and significant hemolysis.[311] *C. perfringens* and *C. septicum* are the two most frequently isolated organisms. Recently, however, a less fulminant bacteremic syndrome due to *C. tertium* has been described.[93] The majority of these patients have been granulocytopenic children with acute leukemia maintained on broad-spectrum antimicrobial therapy for prolonged periods (*e.g.*, 17 days). The gastrointestinal tract has most often implicated as the source of infection. The majority of patients with *C. teritum* have been relatively resistant to the penicillins, cephalosporins, and clindamycin, and require the use of vancomycin for successful therapy.

Antibiotic-associated colitis (AAC) has long been associated with the administration of clindamycin, ampicillin, and broad-spectrum β-lactam antibiotics. *Clostridium difficle* has been isolated in the majority of cases.[312] The symptomatic disease is related to toxin production by the organism.[313] In cancer patients, both antineoplastic agents and antibiotics increase the risk for AAC. Patients with AAC classically present with acute, generalized abdominal pain, fever, leukocytosis, and watery or mucoid, foul-smelling diarrhea. A high index of suspicion is necessary because of similar abdominal symptoms in cancer patients receiving chemotherapy or periabdominal radiation therapy. Cancer patients with diarrhea should be evaluated with stool cultures for *C. difficile* and with toxin assays. Toxin production, not just a positive culture for *C. difficile,* is necessary for diagnosis of ACC, because as many as 42% of hospitalized patients receiving antibiotics will be culture positive, but not toxin positive, for *C. difficile.*[314]

Treatment of documented *C. difficile*-associated colitis requires either oral vancomycin (125 mg 4 times daily for 10–14 days) or metronidazole (250 mg 4 times daily for 10 days). There is a 10% to 20% rate of relapse, although the majority of patients will respond to a second course with the same or alternative therapy. *C. difficile* may be nosocomically transmitted, and patients who are culture and toxin positive for *C. difficile* should be placed on enteric precautions.

Hyperinfection syndrome is an infrequently encountered clinical problem. It is caused by the intestinal nematode, *Strongyloides stercoralis.*[315–316] The clinical syndrome of fever, nausea, vomiting, diarrhea, and abdominal pain is caused by the invasion and ulceration of the gastrointestinal mucosa by the filariform larvae. Chemotherapy promotes the maturation of these filariform larvae from a quiescent rhabditiform stage. Polymicrobial sepsis may accompany the stage of intestinal invasion, presumably as a result of the ulcerated intestinal mucosa. Overwhelming pulmonary and meningeal involvement has been described in immunocompromised patients. Diagnosis requires demonstration of the larvae in feces or duodenal fluid and should be sought in patients who have resided in subtropical climates or endemic regions. Treatment of asymptomatic infestation is accomplished with the administration of thiabendazole (25 mg/kg twice daily for 2 days). Immunocompromised patients with the hyperinfection syndrome should be treated for 2 to 3 weeks, although the mortality is high despite long-term treatment.

Hepatitis may be caused by a variety of infectious agents, including those that infect the liver primarily (*e.g.*, hepatitis A, B, or non-A, non-B, and the delta agent) and secondarily (*H. simplex, CMV, EBV, Coxsackie B virus,* adenoviruses, toxoplasmosis).

Non-A, non-B hepatitis is now the most commonly encountered blood-transmissible hepatitis among cancer patients. Because of the widespread use of screening methods to detect hepatitis B, non-A, non-B hepatitis now accounts for 85% to 90% of all cases of post transfusion hepatitis.[317,318] Clinically, non-A, non-B hepatitis closely resembles hepatitis B, with an insidious onset and a prolonged, relapsing course. There is substantial evidence for a chronic carrier state, and chronic sequelae may occur in as many as 50% of infected individuals.[317] Alpha-interferon has been effective in patients with non-A, non-B hepatitis.[319]

Hepatitis B infection (HBV) may result in both acute and chronic infections, including chronic active, chronic persistent, and an asymptomatic carrier state. Diagnosis is aided by detection of specific viral antigens in the serum of infected patients, especially hepatitis B surface antigens (HBsAg), DNA polymerase, and the hepatitis Be antigen, all of which are present before and at the onset of clinical symptoms. HBsAg may be detected in the serum as early as 6 days after infection with HBV, although it is usually observed 29 to 43 days after parenteral exposure and 67 to 82 days after oral exposure.[320] In patients with self-limited HBV infection, the DNA polymerase titer falls early, and the HBsAg titer falls later in the clinical disease course, eventually being replaced by antibody to HBsAg and HBeAg.

HBV may result in acute infection, chronic infection, or a symptomatic carrier state, with or without hepatic disease. Although the frequency of HBsAg is approximately 0.1% in the general population of the United States, it has been detected in 10% to 20% of children or adults with cancer.[321–322] This is a consequence of multiple transfusions, although currently available sensitive screening tests have reduced this risk dramatically. Nonparenteral transmission (*e.g.*, saliva, urine, feces, semen, effusions, CSF) also constitutes an important mechanism for infection. Immunosuppressive therapy may increase the risk of hepatitis, and enhance the development of a chronic carrier state and can reactivate HBV infections in asymptomatic chronic carriers.[323–325]

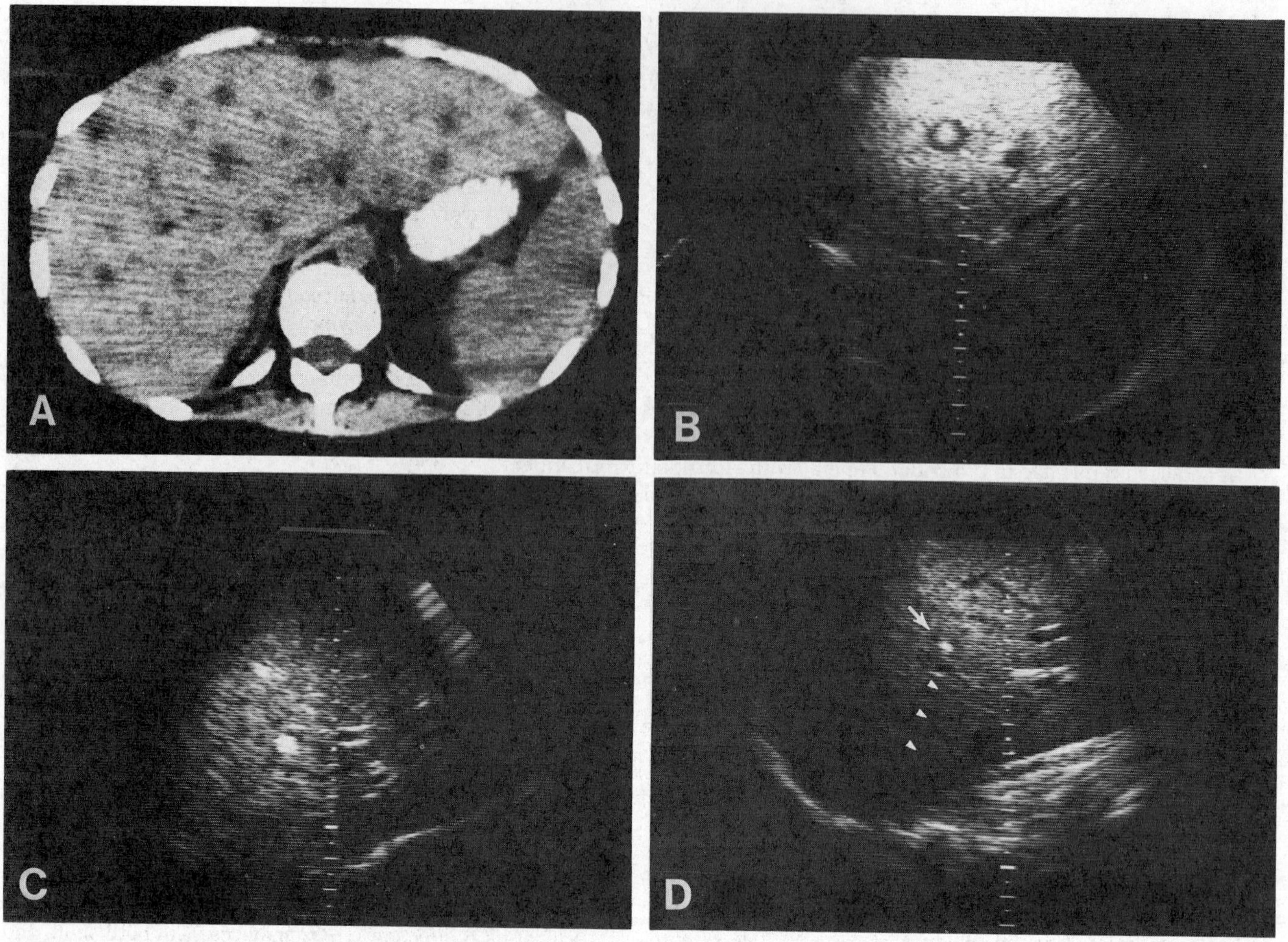

FIG. 59-18. **A.** CT scan of the liver shows numerous rounded areas of decreased attenuation compatible with the diagnosis of hepatic candidiasis. This is a nonspecific finding. **B.** Ultrasound examination in the same patient shows the typical bull's eye lesion of candidiasis characterized by a central echogenic nidus surrounded by a radiolucent halo. This is seen early in the natural history of the disease. **C.** The radiolucent halo is now less obvious than in **B**. This illustrates the variable appearances of *Candida* abscesses on ultrasound studies at different times in the same patient. **D.** Late in the course of the disease, the microabscesses become denser (*arrow*). Note the acoustical shadow posterior to the lesion caused by attenuation of the sound beam (*arrow heads*). (Thaler M, Pastakia B, Shawker TM, et al: Hepatic candidiasis in cancer patients: The evolving picture of the syndrome. Ann Intern Med 108:88–100, 1988)

Because many of the chemotherapeutic agents currently used in cancer treatment are either metabolized or excreted by the liver, altered hepatic function caused by HBV hepatitis can seriously compromise the pharmacokinetics of administered chemotherapy. This is most pronounced for patients with chronic hepatitis, in whom even reduced dosages of chemotherapy may permit the maintenance of the viral carrier state and aggravate drug-induced hepatic injury.

The delta agent, an incomplete RNA virus, requires existing or co-infection with the hepatitis B virus for clinical expression. Therefore, hepatitis due to the delta agent only occurs in three circumstances: as a superimposed infection in a patient with active hepatitis B; as an acute delta hepatitis in a chronic hepatitis B carrier; and as a chronic delta infection in a chronic hepatitis B carrier.[326] Although hepatitis due to the delta agent has been noticed among multiply-transfused patients, its incidence will presumably decrease as the prevalence of hepatitis B diminishes.

Treatment of the patient with chronic active hepatitis is controversial. The current recommendation is that immunosuppressive therapy be restricted to patients who are symptomatic and who have subacute hepatitis with multilobular necrosis and active cirrhosis. Encouraging therapeutic results have been observed using human leukocyte and fibroblast interferon for patients with chronic hepatitis.[327-330] A short course (10–14 days) of interferon leads to a decreased serum levels of DNA polymerase, HBsAg, and anti-HBsAg; HBeAg remains unchanged; and all virologic markers again become elevated following the termination of the interferon therapy. However, with 4 to 5 months of continuous interferon therapy, HBsAg may be eliminated in some patients without rebound after discontinuing therapy. Further study of the dose and schedule of interferon may enhance this therapy.

Because of the morbidity of HBV, trials using standard immune serum globulin have been compared with serum globulin containing either high titer or an intermediate titer of antibody to HBsAg for patients or medical staff who have been potentially inoculated with HBV. Although earlier studies suggested that the high-titer globulin was effective, subsequent observations suggest that it may merely delay the onset of hepatitis (up to 9 months), with the incidence of hepatitis remaining unchanged at 7%.[331,332] High-titer globulin (0.07 mg/kg) is, however, currently recommended for patients or staff who have had a significant inoculation or ingestion of HBV and who are also negative for anti-HBsAg. Hepatitis B vaccine produced by recombinant technology (Recombivax) is now commercially available and is recommended for seronegative hospital personnel at high risk for hepatitis B.

A number of viruses may secondarily effect the liver as part of a more widespread systemic infection. EBV, CMV, *H. simplex,* rubella, rubeola, mumps, adenovirus, and *Coxsackie B* virus have been associated with hepatic enzyme elevation. The hepatic dysfunction with these secondary infections is generally self-limited and less severe than that associated with primary viral hepatitis. However, fulminant hepatic necrosis, coma, and death have been described with several of these agents, especially the herpes virus group, in the immunocompromised host.

All cancer patients with clinical or biochemical evidence of hepatitis should undergo a serologic evaluation to characterize the cause. Serum tests for anti-HAV (IgM), HBsAg, and anti-HBs (IgM) will identify those patients with hepatitis A or B. Patients with a negative antibody screen will have either non-A, non-B, delta agent, or a hepatitis due to another infectious or noninfectious cause. Hepatitis enzyme elevation or hyperbilirubinemia can occur with bacterial sepsis, fungal infection of the liver (especially *Candida* or *Aspergillus*), or toxoplasmosis.

In addition to the morbidity and mortality directly attributable to the hepatitis, significant alteration in hepatic function can affect the pharmacokinetics of antineoplastic agents, especially those metabolized or excreted by the liver (*e.g.,* methotrexate, doxorubicin).

Therapy for patients with hepatitis is primarily supportive, with bed rest and avoidance of further hepatic insult. Patients with hepatitis due to *H. simplex* should receive acyclovir. Chronic non-A, non-B hepatitis can be treated with alpha-interferon.

Hepatic candidiasis has become increasingly recognized and is characterized by the presence of "bull's eye" lesions in the liver on ultrasound or CT scans (Fig. 59-18A-D).[333,334] These lesions are not apparent in patients who are neutropenic, but rather become recognizable at the time of neutrophil recovery. Patients are characterized by the persistence of fever at the time of recovery from an episode of neutropenia, frequently with right upper quadrant discomfort, nausea, and an elevated level of alkaline phosphatase. The lesions are granulomas, consisting of an inner core of central necrosis (where the yeast and pseudophyphae can be found), surrounded by a ring of inflammatory cells and an outer ring of fibrosis. These imaged lesions change over time and with treatment; on resolution, they become calcified, an important endpoint of therapy. The diagnosis requires a liver biopsy.

Hepatic candidiasis poses a therapeutic challenge because long courses of treatment are necessary, and the average dose of amphotericin B is 5 g. Experimental data suggest that the combination of amphotericin B with 5-FC is preferable.[335] Serial biopsy may be necessary to confirm the resolution of infection. Hepatic lesions may be smaller than the degree of resolution of current imaging techniques and in high-risk patients with a negative abdominal ultrasound or CT scans, a biopsy may still be necessary to confirm or rule out hepatic candidiasis. Although experience is preliminary, magnetic resonance imaging of the liver may be more sensitive than the CT or ultrasound scans. If the future, liposomal amphotericin B may permit a more rapid recovery from hepatic candidiasis.

Perirectal Cellulitis

The overall incidence of perirectal cellulitis has decreased in recent years, presumably due to the early use of empiric antibiotic therapy when granulocytopenic patients become febrile. Nonetheless, there is still a risk for perianal cellulitis, especially for patients with prolonged (>7 days) and profound degrees (<100/mm³) of granulocytopenia. Predisposing factors include perirectal mucositis due to chemotherapy or localized radiotherapy, hemorrhoids, anal fissures, and any type of rectal manipulation (*e.g.,* barium enema, anoscopy, sigmoidoscopy). Constipation should be avoided with stool softeners because passage of hard stool promotes the formation of anal fissures and increases the risk for perianal infections.

The most common pathogens in perirectal cellulitis are aerobic gram-negative bacilli (*e.g., P. aeruginosa, K. pneumoniae, E. coli*), the Group D streptococci, and bowel anaerobes.[336] Because of the involvement and anaerobic organisms, antibiotic coverage must include a specific antianaerobic agent (*e.g.,* clindamycin or metronidazole) in addition to the broad-spectrum aerobic coverage. Therapy should commence at the time of the first complaints of tenderness, and ideally before florid symptoms of cellulitis develop. Additional supportive measures include the use of sitz baths three or four times daily, stool softeners, a low bulk diet, and avoidance of unnecessary rectal manipulation, especially repetitive digital exams. Surgical intervention should be restricted to those cases that demonstrate persistence of erythema or induration or progressive involvement of ischiorectal fossa despite optimal antimicrobial therapy.[336,337]

GENITOURINARY TRACT INFECTIONS

The genitourinary tract is infrequently the source of infection in the immunocompromised child. However, local obstruction due to tumor, neurologic dysfunction mediated by spinal cord compression or medications (*e.g.*, vincristine or narcotics), and local therapeutic maneuvers (*e.g.*, radiotherapy, surgery, or bladder catheterization) can predispose cancer patients to genitourinary infection. Most commonly, gram-negative aerobic bacilli (*e.g., E. coli, Klebsiella spp., Proteus spp., P. aeruginosa*) and enterococci will be the causative agents.

An important distinction must be made between a pathogen and colonizing organism when interpreting the results of the urine cultures obtained from an immunocompromised patient. In a non-neutropenic patient, a single organism colony count of greater than 10^5/ml is considered diagnostic of a urinary tract infection in a symptomatic individual. In neutropenic patients, a colony count greater than 10^3/ml of a single organism may be considered diagnostic of a urinary tract infection if the patient is symptomatic (*i.e.*, dysuria, urgency, frequency, fever), and a colony count greater than 10^5 organisms/ml of a single organism should prompt antibiotic intervention whether or not the patient is symptomatic. Obviously, the presence of leukocytes in the urine must not be relied on as a diagnostic criterion in the neutropenic patient.

The distinction between colonization and tissue invasion is particularly difficult for fungal pathogens. Fungal colonization is especially prevalent among patients with indwelling urinary catheters or in patients receiving broad-spectrum antimicrobial therapy. Unlike the typical situation with bacterial pathogens (in which clinical signs and symptoms are present, fungal invasion of the genitourinary tract may be insidious. The repetitive isolation of a particular fungal species (usually *C. albicans, C. tropicalis,* or *T. glabrata*) in association with fever, deteriorating renal function, and rarely, flank pain, should prompt the institution of systemic amphotericin B. Heavily colonized or superficial bladder infections, manifested by the persistence of positive urine cultures despite removal of predisposing factors, may be effectively treated with instillation of amphotericin B (50 mg in 1 liter D5W daily) into the bladder.

CUTANEOUS INFECTIONS

The integrity of this primary physical defense barrier is frequently disrupted in the cancer patient (*e.g.*, needle punctures, biopsies, surgery, radiation, chemotherapy). Consequently local cutaneous infections with bacteria or fungi are common and may result in disseminated infection during periods of immunosuppression. Vigilant skin cleansing with iodophor solutions is essential before any procedure that may permit pathogens. Also, careful attention to the physical examination of the skin in febrile cancer patients may yield a lesion from which a specific diagnosis can be made.[338]

For example, the skin can become infected during bacteremia (*P. aeruginosa, A. hydrophilia, C. equi, S. marcesens*); fungemia (*Aspergillus, Candida, Mucor, C. neoformans, H. capsulatum*); or viremia (*H. simplex* and VZV). There are also noninfectious processes that mimic infection (*e.g.*, pyoderma gangrenosa or Sweet's syndrome).[339–340] Skin lesions may permit the early diagnosis of generalized infection, and fresh lesions should be aspirated or biopsied and the material cultured and examined with Gram stain, KOH, methylene blue, and modified acid-fast stain.

If a viral infection is suspected, the base of several fresh vesicles should be scrapped with a dacron swab, which should then be used to prepare microscope slides and placed into appropriate viral transport media for subsequent virus culture. The microscope slides should be examined by specific immunofluorescence for both HSV and VZV. Immunofluorescence performed on appropriately prepared slides remains the most sensitive (approximately 85%) diagnostic test for either varicella or herpes zoster.[341] Viral cultures are useful for diagnosis if immunofluorescence is negative or if the slides are not adequate for examination, although cultures may not be positive for 2 to 4 weeks in the case of VZV. Wright-Giemsa staining (Tzanck test) of the microscope slides for detection of multinucleated giant cells may also be performed, but the process will not differentiate between HSV and VZV infection.

The diagnosis of vesicular lesions in the cancer patient is important for appropriate patient management and permits the physician to decide if isolation is necessary for the protection of other patients and staff members.[342,343]

Primary varicella (chicken pox) is the most serious vesicular eruption in pediatric cancer patients, with a mortality rate of 7%. The major complication is the visceral dissemination that occurs in 32% of patients. Pneumonia occurs in 79% of patients with visceral varicella, generally developing 3 to 7 days after the onset of skin lesions, usually presenting as bilateral, "fluffy," nodular infiltrates. Other target organs during disseminated VZV infection include the liver, spleen, CNS, gastrointestinal tract, bone marrow, and lymph nodes. Secondary bacterial infections account for the additional severity of varicella dissemination. The risk for visceral dissemination is increased in patients receiving chemotherapy at the time of infection, especially if they are also lymphopenic ($<500/mm^3$).

Because of the severity of varicella infection in patients with cancer, attention has been directed at immunoprophylaxis. The most effective regimen is varicella-zoster immune globulin (VZIG), prepared from the sera of patients who have recently recovered from zoster and provided through the American Red Cross Blood Services. Administered within 72 hours of exposure, VZIG usually modifies the infection to a mild or subclinical form. If VZIG is not available, an alternative is one of the licensed intravenous immunoglobulins (4 ml/kg) or zoster immune plasma (ZIP, 10 ml/kg); the former is preferred.[344–346]

Management of the seronegative patient exposed to varicella, commonly from a household or playmate contact, should include the discontinuation of all chemotherapy and the administration of ZIG or ZIP within 72 hours of exposure.[345,346] Chemotherapy should be withheld in patients with documented exposure until the end of the average incubation period, which is 21 days. In patients who develop overt varicella, immunosuppressive therapy should not be reinstituted until all the skin lesions have dried and scabbed.

Acyclovir, vidarabine, and interferon have all been evaluated in the treatment of both varicella and herpes zoster infections in immunocompromised patients. All three have been effective when compared with placebo.[347–350] Both vidarabine (10 mg/kg/day) and intravenous acyclovir (500 mg/m^2 every 8 hours) reduced the duration of new lesion formation and fever, reduced or eliminated visceral dissemination, and eliminated mortality in children with varicella; 9% mortality was observed with interferon treatment. Acyclovir also appeared to be effective in patients who had already developed pulmonary infiltrates. Complications with vidarabine or acyclovir were infrequent. The poor solubility of vidarabine necessitates continuous infusion, usually over 12 hours, and acyclovir given at the recommended dose requires adequate hydration to avoid potential renal compromise. Although comparative trials have not been performed for varicella, acyclovir appears to be preferable to vidarabine. Orally administered acyclovir has been used for treatment of varicella in immunocompromised children, but it is poorly absorbed and produces plasma levels substantially lower than with intravenous acyclovir. Until controlled trials proving efficacy are available, oral acyclovir cannot be recommended for this purpose. Supportive management and early treatment of secondary bacterial infections are crucial for patients with established varicella.

Alpha-interferon has been compared with placebo for treatment of varicella.[350] A reduction in new lesion formation, fever, visceral dissemination, and mortality was observed in interferon recipients but the side-effects of interferon and the availability of other safer, more effective antiviral agents eliminates any role for interferon in treatment of varicella.

Because varicella is very contagious, there is a considerable risk for spread to other seronegative immunosuppressed patients. Indeed, varicella may be transmitted for 2 days before the appearance of rash. Therefore, extreme caution must be exercised in the management of potentially or overtly infected patients. Careful patient, parent, and staff education is essential. Absence from school where chicken pox has occurred may be necessary (generally for the 21-day incubation period). Parents also should be alerted not to bring their children to the clinic waiting room area if chicken pox is suspected, and if hospitalization is required, reverse isolation should be undertaken, ideally on a hospital floor where immunosuppressed patients are not located.[342] Staff members should be checked for a history of chicken pox or tested serologically using the fluorescent antibody against membrane antigen or immune adherence hemagglutination technique to further minimize the possibility of nosocomial transmission.

A live attenuated chicken pox vaccine has been developed and has been tested extensively in Japan with demonstrable protection in both normal and immunosuppressed children.[351] Although most active immunizations in patients receiving chemotherapy have been unsuccessful because of the inability to maintain effective antibody titres, current data suggest that children receiving maintenance chemotherapy can mount an antibody response if they can be vaccinated at a time when chemotherapy is stopped for 2 weeks.[352,353] Whether a similar response can be obtained in more intensively treated patients has not been established, and the consequences of administering a live vaccine to seriously immunosuppressed patients must be carefully considered.

The incidence of reactivation infection with VZV (*i.e.*, herpes zoster or shingles) among patients with previous varicella infections ranges from 5% to 10% among patients with solid tumors to 35% to 50% among patients treated for Hodgkin's disease or who have received marrow allografts.[354–359] Most cases occur within the first 2 years after treatment. Herpes zoster is due to reactivation of VZV that had been latent in dorsal root ganglia. The likelihood of reactivation increases with intensity of immunosuppression, with the suppression of cell-mediated immunity more important than humoral immunity. Local irradiation may also have a role in reactivation of virus, with disease occurring in the radiated dermatome. The most important complication of herpes zoster is dissemination outside of the original dermatome, which occurs 4 to 9 days after onset. Some patients with cutaneous dissemination will also develop manifestations of visceral dissemination, most commonly including pneumonia, hepatitis, and encephalitis. Cutaneous dissemination rates of 5% to 50% have been observed, with higher rates among those patient groups with more severe immunosuppression. Some patients develop cutaneously disseminated disease without an initial dermatome infection ("atypical disseminated zoster"), and these patients have higher mortality than patients with initial localization.[356,357] The overall mortality of herpes zoster is lower than that of primary varicella, although mortality rates as high as 10% have been observed in some series. Death is usually due to VZV pneumonia, although encephalitis due to direct invasion of the CNS may also occur.

The local morbidity of herpes zoster may also be considerable, due to acute pain, secondary bacterial infection, or neurologic complications, including peripheral neuropathies, aseptic meningitis, or myelitis. Encephalitis may occur by direct involvement of the CNS by VZV or may be postinfectious. Zoster encephalitis usually appears within 2 weeks of the rash, although it may occur from 1 week before rash to 8 weeks after.

Ophthalmic zoster is associated with involvement of the nasociliary nerve and is suggested by lesions on the tip of the nose. A unique syndrome of ophthalmic zoster with contralateral hemiplegia has been described. Herpes zoster of the ophthalmic division of the trigeminal nerve may be especially troublesome because of acute pain and corneal involvement with scarring and subsequent blindness.

Another zoster syndrome is abdominal pain occurring either before or without development of a rash; because of obvious difficulties in diagnosis, these patients may have many diagnostic procedures performed, including laparotomy, before herpes zoster becomes apparent as the cause. The most common problem is postherpetic neuralgia, particularly in older patients; it has been reported in as many as 45% of patients in some treatment trials. Pain may last for months or years in some cases. Treatment of pastherpetic neuralgia is often unsatisfactory, although some patients may derive benefit from dilantin or tegretol.

Diagnosis of varicella or herpes zoster is based on the characteristic appearance of the skin lesions, on the distribution of lesions, and on immunofluorescent staining of material from the base of the vesicles.[341] HSV can cause localized cutaneous disease and dermatomal-appearing rashes, which may be mistaken for herpes zoster. Wright-Giemsa staining of vesicle scrapings or electron microscopy will not differentiate between HSV and VZV, and specific immunofluorescence and viral cultures should be performed for diagnosis.

Local skin care and observation for secondary bacterial infections are important. Data about therapy with antiviral agents are similar to those for varicella: Although interferon, vidarabine and acyclovir have all been shown to be effective when compared to placebo, acyclovir appears to be the agent of choice.[360–362] A direct comparison of acyclovir (500 mg/m^2 every 8 hours) and vidarabine for treatment of herpes zoster, conducted primarily among marrow transplant recipients, showed acyclovir to be superior, with shorter durations of fever, new lesion formation, and acute pain and more rapid healing and elimination of cutaneous dissemination.[363] Acyclovir also appears to be effective among patients in whom cutaneous dissemination has already occurred, although initiation of treatment within 48 to 72 hours of onset is highly desirable.[361] VZV resistance to acyclovir has not been observed in vivo and continuation of new lesion formation and cutaneous dissemination occurring within the first 2 to 3 days after initiation of treatment should not be interpreted as treatment failure. Acyclovir treatment should be continued for 7 days or for 2 days after the last new lesion, whichever is longer. Because of failure to develop adequate specific immune responses, some patients who have received acyclovir treatment for herpes zoster will have "relapses" of herpes zoster within the succeeding 2 months; they should receive another treatment course.[364] Attention must be paid to adequate hydration, because renal insufficiency and other side-effects such as nausea have been observed more frequently among patients who become dehydrated during treatment.[365]

Patients with lymphomas or leukemia or who have received marrow allografts, who are at highest risk of cutaneous and visceral dissemination, should be treated with intravenous acyclovir if they develop herpes zoster. Although topical acyclovir ointment has helped local healing among immunocompromised patients in a controlled trial, it is not recommended among patients at risk of dissemination.[366] Similarly, oral acyclovir cannot be recommended until data from controlled trials are available. Interferon and vidarabine have little role in the treatment of herpes zoster, although vidarabine may be used in the rare patient with a documented acyclovir allergy. Because of the potential for spread of VZV to other immunosuppresed patients, all patients with herpes zoster should be kept in single rooms, and glove and gown precautions should be used; strict isolation may be appropriate in some circumstances or institutions.[342] Susceptible patients and hospital staff can acquire primary varicella after exposure to herpes zoster.

MUSCULOSKELETAL INFECTIONS

The musculoskeletal system is an uncommon primary site of infection in cancer patients. However, atypical infections, such as deep pyomyositis due to *S. aureus* or gram-negative organisms, or psoas muscle abscesses have been described in both neutropenic and non-neutropenic leukemic patients. Treatment includes incision and drainage and appropriate antibiotic therapy.[367–369]

Crepitance and soft tissue tenderness should suggest an anaerobic infection, either with *Clostridia* or with the toxin-producing *Bacillus cereus*. Necrotizing fascitis due to *S. pyogenes* represents a potentially life-threatening infection, rarely caused by nonsteroidal anti-inflammatory drugs.[370] Immediate intervention with debridement and antibiotics is essential, and hyperbaric oxygen may be used in some cases. Other gas-forming organisms (*e.g., E. coli*) may cause a similar clinical syndrome.

Septic arthritis or osteomyelitis in the cancer patient may be caused by gram-negative organisms (*e.g., Pseudomonas, Klebsiella, Salmonella, Eikinella*), fungi (*e.g., Candida*), or the more common gram-positive bacterial pathogens. Patients with local skeletal defects or who have undergone extensive surgery, such as amputation or soft tissue dissection, and patients with bacteremia or fungemia are considered to be at high risk. Occasionally it may be difficult to differentiate osteomyelitis from Ewing's sarcoma or radionecrosis.

CENTRAL NERVOUS SYSTEM INFECTIONS

Infections of the CNS are surprisingly infrequent in children with cancer. Nevertheless, patients who present with symptoms or signs suggesting CNS dysfunction must be expeditiously evaluated with the appropriate physical, laboratory, and radiographic examinations. Evaluation of cerebrospinal fluid from cancer patients should include aerobic culture and Gram stain, cryptococcal antigen determination, fungal culture, and cytologic examination in addition to the routine CSF tests. Potential infections include shunt (*e.g.*, Ommaya reservoir) infections, meningitis or meningoencephalitis, encephalitis, and brain abscesses.

Shunt Infections

Intraventricular shunts and Ommaya reservoirs are associated with an increased incidence of CNS infection. The responsible pathogens are most commonly those colonizing the adjacent skin: coagulase-positive and coagulase-negative

Staphylococci, Corynebacterium spp., enterococci, and gram-negative bacilli.[371,372] Patients may be totally asymptomatic, or they may have fever, headache, increased intracranial pressure, and miningismus. The majority of patients with Ommaya reservoir infections can be successfully treated without removing the device.[372]

Meningitis

Meningitis or meningoencephalitis is most frequently encountered in patients with impaired cell-mediated immunity and is typically caused by *Cryptococcus neoformans* or *Listeria monocytogens. C. neoformans* causes a meningoencephalitis that is typically indolent. The most common presenting complaints include headaches, altered mental status, low-grade, intermittent fevers, and rarely, meningismus.[373] Examination of the CSF demonstrates a mild mononuclear pleocytosis (40–400 leukocytes/mm^3) and minimally decreased CSF glucose. Only 50% of patients will have a detectable organism by an India Ink preparation, and the most reliable means of diagnosis is documentation of cryptococcal antigen in serum or CSF.[374] Therapy for *C. neoformans* meningitis or meningoencephalitis includes the combination of amphotericin B (0.3–0.5 mg/kg/day) and oral 5-FC (150 mg/kg/day every 6 hours) for 4 to 6 weeks.[246,247]

L. monocytogens is a motile, gram-positive rod that causes several distinct clinical syndromes, including meningitis. Patients with impaired cell-mediated immunity and especially those with defects of T-cell-mediated immune function are susceptible.[375] Although the organism can be isolated from soil, dust, water, sewage, and contaminated foods (especially cheese and dairy products), the exact mode transmission in most immunocompromised patients is unclear. Community outbreaks have occurred and hospital-associated clustering in immunosuppressed patients has been described.[376] The most common presentation includes a subacute course of low-grade fevers and personality changes. Focal neurologic signs are occasionally present. Laboratory findings include a mild to moderate CSF pleocytosis (6–12,000 cells/mm^3) and may include a predominance of PMN leukocytes or mononuclear cells. Protein levels are generally elevated (100–300 mg/100 ml), and CSF glucose levels are usually decreased. Diagnosis must be based on a high index of suspicion. Ampicillin or penicillin provide the optimal treatment and should be continued for 3 to 6 weeks, because relapses have been reported with shorter therapy.[377] Third-generation cephalosporins are inactive against *Listeria.*

Encephalitis

HSV, VZV, and measles are the most likely causes of sporadic viral encephalitis. HSV encephalitis, which may present as a focal or generalized process, responds to acyclovir treatment; acyclovir is also appropriate treatment for VZV encephalitis.[378,379]

Patients with encephalitis or encephalomyelitis commonly present with signs of meningeal irritation (*e.g.*, fever, headache, nuchal rigidity) and evidence of altered mentation. Confusion may progress to stupor and to coma. Focal neurologic signs and seizures are relatively common. CSF examination may demonstrate a pleocytosis (10–2000 cells/mm^3), with a predominance of mononuclear cells. An increased number of CSF red cells has been reported with *H. simplex* encephalitis. CSF protein levels are normally elevated, and the CSF glucose characteristically remains within the normal range, except for a decreased level in mumps infection.

For the cancer patient with focal neurologic deficits or altered mentation, it is important to differentiate between an infectious, metabolic, toxic, or neoplastic cause. Unfortunately, diagnosis of the specific cause of encephalitis in an immunocompromised patient is difficult. Acute and convalescent serum antibody titers should be obtained, and specific CSF antibody may be detected in cases of mumps, herpes simplex, and varicella zoster. Although definitive diagnosis of *H. simplex* encephalitis requires a brain biopsy and because the clinician's therapeutic armamentarium against most causes of encephalitis is limited, empiric administration of acyclovir (500 mg/m^2 given every 8 hours) to the cancer patient with signs and symptoms suggesting of encephalitis seems warranted.

A treatable CNS infection that can present as an encephalitis in an immunosuppressed child or as a mass lesion in the AIDS patient is due to the obligate intracellular parasite *Toxoplasma gondii.*[380] Toxoplasmosis may represent newly acquired or reactivated infection and is rarely limited to the CNS, usually occurring in concert with fever, lymphadenopathy, hepatitis, pneumonitis, myocarditis, and pericarditis. The CSF typically manifests a mononuclear pleocytosis, elevated protein levels, and a normal glucose concentration. A battery of serologic tests are available for the diagnosis of toxoplasmosis in the immunocompetent host, but most of these are limited in their applicability to the immunosuppressed patient due to suboptimal antibody responses. The definitive diagnosis requires demonstration of the parasite within tissue sections.

Treatment of active toxoplasmosis should include the combination of pyrimethamine and sulfadiazine or "triple sulfa" therapy—trisulfapyrimidines-sulfamerazine, sulfamethazine, and sulfadiazine. In immunodeficient patients, therapy should be continued for 4 to 6 weeks after the resolution of all clinical symptoms and signs. Clindamycin and pyrimethamine also benefit AIDS patients with central toxoplasmosis. Trimetrexate is being studied for the treatment of toxoplasmosis.

The important differential diagnosis in a cancer patient with evidence of a focal lesion (mass) within the CNS is between metastatic or primary malignancy and a brain abscess. Predisposing factors for brain abscesses include contiguous sites of infection (*e.g.*, otitis, sinusitis, dental abscesses), a history of penetrating cranial trauma, congenital cardiac disease, bacterial endocarditis, and pulmonary infections. In addition to the usual aerobic and anaerobic bacteria responsible for abscesses in immunocompetent patients, fungal and nocardial species are particularly prone to cause disease in an immunosuppressed patient. In patients with disseminated candidiasis, nearly half may have CNS involvement, although this is usually unrecognized.[381] In AIDS patients, CNS lesions may be caused by lymphoma or *T. gondii.*[382,383] The association of pulmonary lesions with focal neurologic findings suggests *Nocardia, Aspergillus, Mucor,* or *Candida.*

Early evaluation and specific diagnosis are crucial in the management of brain abscesses, because effective antimicrobial or neurosurgical therapy is available. Diagnosis is commonly made by radiographic demonstration of a localized CNS mass, followed by an open or closed neurosurgical procedure to aspirate or resect the localized lesion.

Dementias

One of the disconcerting sequelae of modern chemotherapy has been the occurrence of leukoencephalopathy. Many of these dementing processes can be linked to intrathecal chemotherapy, especially the combination of radiation and methotrexate.[384] However, the recent awareness that slow virus infections can produce CNS deterioration in humans has raised concern that some dementing processes may have a viral cause. Adults with lymphoma and symptoms of progressive mental and emotional deterioration, including decreased visual acuity, aphasia, and sensory and cerebellar signs, may have antibody to the human papilloma virus JC and isolation of virus from infected mononuclear cells, suggesting the diagnosis of progressive multifocal leukoencephalopathy.[385]

TABLE 59-33. Methods for Preventing Infection in Cancer Patients

Prevent Acquisition and/or Suppress or Eliminate Microbial flora	*Improve or Modify Host Defenses*
Isolation	*Immunization*
Simple or reverse isolation	Active
Isolation with HEPA air filtration	*Pseudomonas*
	Pneumococcus
Prophylactic antibiotics	*Passive*
Nonabsorbable antibiotics	J-5 Core glycolipid
Trimethoprim-sulfamethoxazole	Pooled immunoglobulins
Selective decontamination	Specific
Quinolones	
Prophylactic antivirals	*Cell-component replacement*
Acycloguonosine	Leukocyte transfusions
Amantadine	
Prophylactic antifungals	*Accelerate granulocyte recovery*
Nystatin	Lithium
Imidazoles	GM-CAF
Prophylactic antiparasitics	
Thiabendazole	
Trimethoprim-sulfamethoxazole	
Combination-comprehensive	
Total protection isolation	

PREVENTING INFECTION IN CANCER PATIENTS

Despite a multitude of clinical trials investigating the efficacy of various measures to prevent or reduce the occurrence of infection, the most important anti-infective measure identified has been the simplest—careful handwashing practices.[66] A number of approaches have been taken to decrease the acquisition of new organisms or suppress those already colonizing the cancer patient (Table 59-33). Unfortunately, no method is singularly effective, each having promise and problems (Tables 59-34 and 59-35). As new preventive strategies are evaluated, they initially appear promising, but as additional studies are conducted, their beneficial results become less convincing.[386]

PREVENTING ACQUISITION OF NEW ORGANISMS

Because it has been well documented that nearly 85% of the organisms responsible for infections among patients with cancer are derived from the endogenous flora and that nearly half of these are acquired from the hospital environment, much attention has been directed toward mechanisms to prevent the acquisition of potential pathogens.

Inanimate objects within the hospital environment (*i.e.,* faucet aerators, shower heads, respirators, plants, floors) are reservoirs of pathogenic organisms. However, most epidemiologic studies suggest that transmission from such inanimate sources usually requires a human vector.[65] Therefore, the simplest yet most efficacious intervention that can be performed is adherence to strict handwashing precautions.[66] The easiest way to enforce such a policy is to educate the child and parents to disallow contact with anyone who has neglected to wash his hands.

A second maneuver to decrease the acquisition of new organisms is to maintain a cooked diet during periods of granulocytopenia, with avoidance of fresh fruits and vegetables and nonprocessed dairy products, because these foods are naturally contaminated with gram-negative bacteria, especially *K. pneumoniae, E. coli,* and *P. aeruginosa.*[387,388]

Environmental sources can contribute to fungal (*Aspergillus spp.*) and bacterial (*Legionella*) colonization and infection. In centers where *Aspergillus* is a significant problem, special air filtration systems (*e.g.,* high-efficiency particulate air filters) or water purification systems may help.

Although the technique of reverse isolation has often been used, it does not significantly reduce the acquisition of new organisms in an environment where handwashing techniques are strictly followed.[389] Therefore, there is no compelling reason to enforce this policy.

The total protective environment (TPE) is a comprehensive anti-infective regimen designed to reduce the patient's endogenous microbial burden while preventing the acquisition of new organisms (see Table 59-34). A sterile environ-

TABLE 59-34.

	Total Protected Environment	*Nonabsorbable Antibiotics*	*Trimethoprim-Sulfamethoxazole*	*Selective Decontamination*	*Quinolones*
Exogenous sources					
Air, food, water contacts	Yes	No	No	No	No
Endogenous sources					
Nares	Yes	No	No	No	Yes
Oropharynx	Yes	+/−	No	Yes	Yes
Lower respiratory tract	+/−	No	+/−	+/−	Yes
Gastrointestinal tract	Yes	Yes	Yes	Yes	Yes
Perianal area	Yes	+/−	+/−	+/−	+/−
Skin	Yes	No	No	No	No
Central venous catheter	No	No	No	No	No
Peripheral catheters	No	No	No	No	No
Systemic effect	+/−	No	Yes	Yes	Yes

ment is created in a clean air room with constant positive air flow and is maintained by an aggressive program of surface decontamination, sterilization of all objects that enter the room, and an intensive regimen to disinfect the patient, including oral, nonabsorbable antibiotics, skin antiseptics, antibiotic sprays and ointments, and a low microbial diet. A number of studies have documented that the TPE can reduce infections in profoundly granulocytopenic individuals.[390] However, the TPE is expensive, and because of the improvement in treating established infections, it does not offer a survival advantage to patients. Thus, TPE is not necessary for the routine care of cancer patients (see Table 59-35).

An interesting application of the TPE is derived from the observation that patients with aplastic anemia undergoing allogeneic marrow transplant had a lower incidence of acute GVHD. A similar effect has been more difficult to demonstrate among patients transplanted for hematologic malignancy, and additional studies are needed.

ANTIMICROBIAL PROPHYLAXIS

Antibacterial Prophylaxis

A large number of clinical trials have been conducted to investigate the utility of prophylactic antibiotic regimens in immunocompromised patients. A number of strategies have

TABLE 59-35.

	Total Protected Environment	*Nonabsorbable Antibiotics*	*Trimethoprim-Sulfamethoxazole*	*Selective Decontamination*	*Quinolones*
Efficacy					
Reduced infection	Yes	No	+/−	+/−	Yes
Decreased in fever	Yes	No	No	No	No
Decrease or shorten need for antibiotics and antifungals	No	No	No	+/−	Yes
Contributed to survival	No	No	No	No	No
Compliance					
Well tolerated?	No	No	+/−	+/−	Yes
Impact on efficacy	Yes	Yes	Yes	+/−	No
Liabilities					
Emergency of resistant organisms	Yes	Yes	Yes	Yes	Yes
Organ side effects:					
Interference with other drugs	Yes	Yes	Yes	No	No
BM suppression	No	No	Yes	Yes	No
Specific organ toxicity	No	No	Yes	Yes	Yes
Cost					
For the drugs or regimens	Yes	Yes	No	Yes	Yes
For surveillance or monitoring	Yes	Yes	Yes	Yes	Yes
Reducing need for hospitalization or need for drugs	No	No	No	+/−	?

been explored, including systemic prophylaxis, gastrointestinal decontamination, and selective gastrointestinal decontamination (*i.e.*, maintenance of "colonization resistance"). Unfortunately, the interpretation of many of these trials is difficult due to poor study design, non-uniform patient groupings, and failure to report or document compliance with the prophylactic regimens.[391]

Because the gastrointestinal tract is the source for many of the pathogens causing microbiologically defined infections, investigators have evaluated the efficacy of reducing the endogenous gastrointestinal flora by the administration of oral, nonabsorbable antibiotics. This technique has not been especially valuable and is fraught with a number of problems. The antimicrobial agents used (*e.g.*, vancomycin, gentamicin, polymyxin B, nystatin, framycetin, and colistin) are unpalatable and are generally poorly tolerated, making compliance difficult, especially among patients receiving emetogenic chemotherapy (see Table 59-34). Equally disturbing has been the emergence of resistant bacterial strains when aminoglycoside-containing regimens have been used. Therefore, prophylactic regimens aimed solely at reducing the endogenous gastrointestinal flora cannot be recommended (see Table 59-35).

A modified technique is the "selective decontamination" of the gastrointestinal tract, employing antibiotics that preserve the anaerobic flora but reduce the aerobic bacteria. This is based on experimental data showing that the preservation of the anaerobic flora of the gastrointestinal tract provides a colonization resistance against aerobic and fungal organisms.[392,393] Although initial clinical trials provided evidence of a reduction of infections in patients undergoing induction therapy for acute leukemia, clearly defined efficacy has not been established.[394,395] The most commonly investigated agent used for selective decontamination has been trimethoprim-sulfamethoxasole. Early trials investigating this antibiotic in children and adults demonstrated a reduction in all infections and in bacteremic episodes. However, a large number of follow-up clinical trials have yielded conflicting results.[391,396–402] The reasons for the contradictory results are unclear, although factors such as variability in study design, non-uniform patient populations, and failure to properly monitor compliance have played a part. The potential for reduction in infectious morbidity and mortality must be balanced against the prolongation of granulocytopenia and emergence of resistant organisms.[403] Successful use of this approach requires close monitoring in order to properly adjust the antimicrobial regimen for resistant or newly emerging species, and this surveillance is costly in time and money.

Prophylactic antibiotic trials employing a derivative of nalidixic acid, the quinoline antibiotic norfloxacin, have shown promising results in a population of bone marrow transplant patients.[404] Additional clinical trials are needed to assess the generalized applicability of these results to other immunocompromised patients. Similar studies with fluorinated quinolines (*e.g.*, ciprofloxacin) have also shown promising results, but confirmatory studies with larger numbers of patients are necessary.[405] The quinolines cannot be used in children less than 18 years old because of putative joint toxicity.

Antifungal Prophylaxis

Because of the increasing incidence of invasive mycoses in immunocompromised hosts, antifungal prophylaxis has also been studied. The most frequently evaluated antifungal agents have included nystatin, amphotericin B, miconazole, clotrimazole, and ketoconazole. The majority of prophylactic regimens have been aimed at a reduction of invasive infections due to *Candida,* and by virtue of the antifungal activity of the agents employed, they would not be expected to have a significant impact against *Aspergillus* or *Mucormycoses.*

Interpretation of existing data is difficult, because studies suffer from variable patient criteria, disparate dosage regimens, non-uniform response criteria, and lack of appropriate controls, An added problem is the inherent difficulty in the definitive diagnosis of a fungal infection in an immunocompromised patient.

Within the context of these limitations, however, several conclusions about antifungal prophylaxis can be proffered. First, when an adequate dose of antifungal agent (*e.g.*, amphotericin B, ketoconazole, or clotrimazole) has been administered, there has been a consistent decrease in fungal colonization.[406] Decreased colonization has not clearly resulted, however, in a decreased incidence of invasive mycotic disease, although a decrease in superficial infection has been noted in some studies. Second, several studies employing prophylactic and empiric antifungal regimens have reported a shift in the colonization pattern of fungal organisms. In general, these shifts have been toward more resistant fungi. Thus, the prophylactic regimens may successfully eradicate the susceptible fungi (particularly *C. albicans*) but may permit the overgrowth and ultimate invasion by more resistant species, especially *Aspergillus.* This trend will need to be closely monitored.

Overall, the potential benefits of prophylactic antifungal therapy must be balanced against the toxicities, epidemiologic considerations, and relative efficacy of the regimen employed. Until clear benefit can be proven, widespread chemoprophylaxis against fungi should not be attempted.

Antiviral Prophylaxis

Both intravenous and oral formulations of acyclovir can prevent reactivation of HSV and resultant stomatitis among patients undergoing induction therapy for leukemia or lymphoma or marrow allografting.[299,407] Twice-daily administration of intravenous acyclovir appears to be nearly as effective as use three times daily and is more convenient and less expensive. Prophylactic acyclovir may also reduce the development of acyclovir resistance.[408] Prevention of CMV infection has been more problematic. Although primary CMV infection among seronegative patients can be prevented by use of screened seronegative blood products, use of CMV immunoglobulins or the licensed intravenous immunoglobulins remains controversial.[278,279] Alpha-interferon has been shown to have a prophylactic benefit in renal allograft patients, although this effect was not reproduced in one study among marrow allograft recipients.[280,409,410] Recent studies suggest that intravenous acyclovir may have some effect against CMV if used prophylactically; greater benefit might be anticipated with ganciclovir if marrow suppression can be circumvented or with foscarnet.

Antiparasitic Prophylaxis

In centers where *P. carinii* occurs with some frequency, the administration of trimethoprim-sulfamethoxazole has convincingly reduced the incidence of infection. However, not all children undergoing cancer treatment require prophylactic treatment. Rather, this should be influenced by the patients underlying disease (*e.g.*, leukemia or solid tumors), the intensity or immunosuppression of the therapy being delivered, and the center where treatment is being administered. Although the initial recommendations were for daily prophylactic therapy, recent studies have suggested that an intermittent (*i.e.*, twice or thrice weekly) dosage schedule is effective and less toxic.[411]

Aerosolized pentamidine has been evaluated in AIDS patients to prevent pneumocystis pneumonia. The results have been encouraging and may be applicable to patients with cancer.

ACTIVE AND PASSIVE IMMUNIZATION

As a general rule, live attenuated viral vaccines should not be administered to immunosuppressed children. Although an initial antibody response may be elicited, the concurrent administration of cytotoxic chemotherapy is associated with a rapid decline of titers. A live varicella vaccine has been successfully administered to children with acute leukemia, although only patients receiving maintenance chemotherapy received the vaccine.[412]

Trials investigating the role of active immunization have evaluated the efficacy of immunization against commonly encountered pathogens, such as the influenza virus and *Streptococcus pneumoniae.* The trials have been only partially successful because of the inability to maintain an adequate degree of protection in the face of repetitive, immunosuppressive insults.

Passive immunization with ZIG reduces the incidence of pneumonitis and encephalitis and decreases the mortality from 7% to 0.5% in immunocompromised patients with primary varicella infection. Immunosuppressed children who are seronegative or possess low-titer antivaricella antibody should receive ZIG (1 vial per 15 kg) within 72 hours after exposure to a potentially infectious source.[344–346]

A number of investigators have evaluated the efficacy of passive immunization with either high-titer antibody directed against the core glycolipid of *Enterobacteriaceae* (J-5 antisera) or pooled intravenous gammaglobulin preparations. The rationale for this approach is drawn from several observations. First, patients with defective antibody production (*e.g.*, chronic lymphocyte leukemia or multiple myeloma) are known to have an enhanced susceptibility to bacterial infection.[413] Second, antibody levels fall in patients receiving cytotoxic chemotherapy, and patients who develop gram-negative bacteremia have lower levels of antibody than patients who do not develop infections.[47] The results of early clinical trials with the J-5 antisera have been encouraging. A double-blind, randomized, placebo-controlled trial involving patients with documented gram-negative bacteremia demonstrated enhanced survival among patients receiving the antisera.[49] A second placebo-controlled study using prophylactic J-5 antisera in surgical patients at high risk for gram-negative bacteremia demonstrated a reduction in infectious complications among the J-5 recipients, but not a survival advantage.[414] Unfortunately, preparation of the antisera is time and labor-intensive and quite costly, and passive immunization with the J-5 antisera will remain an investigational approach until a clear advantage can be defined.

Pooled immunoglobulin preparations have antibody titers to a wide spectrum of potential pathogens. To test whether such preparations could reduce the incidence of fever and infection in neutropenic patients and alter the outcome of the infection that did occur, we conducted a double-blind, placebo-controlled trial in which adults and children who received chemotherapy regimens that would render them neutropenic for more than a week were randomized to receive either weekly intravenous immunoglobulin (500 mg/kg/week) until their neutropenia resolved or an albumen placebo. With more than 70 entries in this study, no difference in the incidence of fever, type of infection, or outcome has been observed between the intravenous immunoglobulin arm and the placebo control.

Other investigators are evaluating hyperimmune antisera or monoclonal antibodies to prevent or treat bacterial infections.

Perhaps the most exciting development is the recent cloning and purification of molecules that can activate neutrophils or monocytes (*e.g.*, interferons, tumor necrosis factor) or accelerate recovery from neutropenia (*e.g.*, GM-CSF).[12–29] These agents offer the prospect of abbreviating or attenuating the risk for serious infection in patients receiving cytotoxic chemotherapy. If these agents are successful in reducing serious infectious complications, they may permit the delivery of chemotherapy in schedules that could maximize tumoricidal activity and minimize toxicity.

REFERENCES

1. Bodey G: Infection in cancer patients: A continuing association. Am J Med (Suppl 1A) 81:11–26, 1986
2. Sculier JP, Weerts D, Klastersky J: Causes of death in febrile granulocytopenic cancer patients receiving empiric antibiotic therapy. Eur J Cancer Clin Oncol 20:55–60, 1984
3. Chang HY, Rodriguez V, Narbone G et al: Causes of death in adults with acute leukemia. Medicine (Baltimore) 55:259–268, 1976
4. Pizzo PA: Granulocytopenia and cancer therapy: Past problems, current solutions, future challenges. Cancer 54:2649–2661, 1984
5. Beachey EH: Bacterial adherence: Adhesin-receptor interactions mediating the attachment of bacteria to mucosal surfaces. J Infect Dis 143:325–345, 1981
6. Schoolnik GK, Lark D, O'Hanley P: Bacterial adherence and anticolonization vaccines. In Remington JS, Schwarz NM (eds): Current Clinical Topics in Infectious Diseases, Vol 6, pp 85–102. New York, McGraw Hill, 1985
7. Johanson WG, Pierce AK, Sanford JP: Changing pharyngeal flora of hospitalized patients: Emergence of gram-negative bacilli. N Engl J Med 281:1137–1140, 1969
8. Fainstain V, Rodriguez V, Turk et al: Patterns of oropharyngeal and fecal flora in patients with leukemia. J Infect Dis 144:10–18, 1981
9. van der Waaij D: Gut resistance to colonization: Clinical usefulness of selective use of orally administered antimicrobial and antifungal drugs. In Klastersky J (ed): Infection in Cancer Patients, pp 73–86. New York, Raven Press, 1982

10. Spitznagel JK, Shafer WM: Neutrophil killing of bacteria by oxygen-independent mechanism: A historical summary. Rev Infect Dis 7:398–403, 1985
11. Bodey GP, Buckley M, Sathe YS et al: Quantitative relationships between circulating leukocytes and infection in patients with acute leukemia. Ann Intern Med 64:328–340, 1966
12. Sieff CA: Hematopoietic growth factors. J Clin Invest 79:1549–1557, 1987
13. Metcalf D: The molecular biology and functions of the granulocyte-macrophage colony-stimulating factors. Blood 67:257–267, 1986
14. Nienhuis AW, Donahue RE, Karisson S et al: Recombinant human granulocyte-macrophage colony-stimulating factor (GM-CSF) shortens the period of neutropenia after autologous bone marrow transplantation in a primate model. J Clin Invest 80:573–577, 1987
15. Mayer P, Lam C, Obenaus H et al: Recombinant human GM-CSF induces leukocytosis and activates peripheral blood polymorphonuclear neutrophils in nonhuman primates. Blood 70:206–213, 1987
16. Lopez AF, Williamson D, Gamble R et al: Recombinant human granulocyte-macrophage colony-stimulating factor stimulates in vitro mature human neutrophil and eosinophil function, surface receptor expression, and survival. J Clin Invest 78:1220–1228, 1986
17. Weisbart RH, Kwan L, Golde DW et al: Human GM-CSF primes neutrophils for enhanced oxidative metabolism in response to the major physiological chemoattractants. Blood 69:18–21, 1987
18. Glasson JC, Weisbard RH, Kaufman SE et al: Purified human granulocyte-macrophage colony-stimulating factor: Direct action on neutrophils. Science 226:1339–1342, 1984
19. Beutler B, Krochin N, Milsard IW et al: Control of cachectin (tumor necrosis factor) synthesis: Mechanisms of endotoxin resistance. Science 232:977–980, 1986
20. Beutler B, Milsard IW, Cerami A: Passive immunization against cachectin/tumor necrosis factor protects mice from lethal effect of endotoxin. Science 229:869–871, 1985
21. Dinarello CA: Interleukin-1. Rev Infect Dis 6:51–59, 1984
22. Estrov Z, Roifman C, Mills G et al: The regulatory role of interleukin-2 responsive T lymphocytes on human marrow granulopoiesis. Blood 69:1161–1166, 1987
23. Cannistra SA, Rambaldi A, Spriggs DR et al: Human granulocyte-macrophage colony-stimulating factor induces expression of the tumor necrosis factor gene by the U937 cell line and by normal human monocytes. J Clin Invest 79:1720–1720, 1987
24. Zucali JR, Dinarello CA, Oblon DJ et al: Interleukin-1 stimulates fibroblasts to produce granulocyte-macrophage colony-stimulating activity and prostaglandin E_2. J Clin Invest 77:1857–1863, 1986
25. Perfect JR, Granger DL, Durack DT: Effects of antifungal agents and γ interferon on macrophage cytotoxicity for fungi and tumor cells. J Infect Dis 156:316–323, 1987
26. Wilson CB, Westall J: Activation of neonatal and adult human macrophages by alpha, beta, and gamma interferons. Infect Immun 49:351–356, 1985
27. Dinarello CA, Cannon JG, Mier JW et al: Multiple biologic activities of human recombinant interleukin-1. J Clin Invest 77:1734–1739, 1986
28. Dinarello CA, Mier JW: Lymphokines. N Engl J Med 317:940–945, 1987
29. Nathan DG: Hope for hematopoietic hormones. N Engl J Med 317:626–628, 1987
30. Curnette JT, Boxer LA: Clinically significant phagocytic cell defects. In Remington J, Swartz M (eds): Current Clinical Topics in Infectious Diseases, Vol 6, pp 103–156. New York, McGraw Hill, 1985
31. McCormack RT, Nelson RD, Bloomfield CD et al: Neutrophilic function in lymphoreticular malignancy. Cancer 44:920–926, 1979
32. Snyderman R, Seigler HF, Meadows L: Abnormalities of monocyte chemotaxis in patients with melanoma. Effects of immunotherapy and tumor removal. JNCI 58:37–41, 1977
33. Pickering LK, Ericsson CD, Kohl S: Effect of chemotherapeutic agents on metabolic and bactericidal activity of polymorphonuclear leukocytes. Cancer 42:1741–1746, 1978
34. Baehner RL, Neiburger RG, Johnson DG et al: Transient bactericidal defect of peripheral blood phagocytes from children with acute lymphoblastic leukemia receiving craniospinal irradiation. N Engl J Med 289:1209–1213, 1973
35. Tubaro E, Borelli G, Croce C et al: Effect of morphine on resistance to infection. J Infect Dis 148:656–666, 1983
36. Schaffner A, Douglas H, Braude A: Selective protection against condidia by mononuclear and against mycelia by polymorphonuclear phagocytes in resistance to aspergillus. J Clin Invest 69:617–631, 1982
37. Fisher RI, DeVita VT, Bostick F: Persistent immunologic abnormalities in long term survivors of advanced Hodgkin's disease. Ann Intern Med 92:595–599, 1980
38. Dale DC, Petersdorf RG: Corticosteroids and infectious disease. Med Clin North Am 57:1277–1287, 1973
39. Nossal GJV: Current concepts: Immunology: The basic components of the immune system. N Engl J Med 316:1320–1325, 1987
40. Fahey JL, Scoggins R, Utz JP et al: Infection, antibody response and gamma globulin components in multiple myeloma and macroglobulinemia. Am J Med 35:698–707, 1973
41. Stobo JD, Paul S, Von Scoy RE et al: Suppressor thymus-derived lymphocytes in fungal infection. J Clin Invest 57:319–328, 1976
42. Zinner SH, McCabe WR: Effect of IgM and IgG antibody in patients with bacteremia due to gram-negative bacilli. J Infect Dis 133:37–45, 1976
43. Siber GR, Weitzman SA, Aisenberg AC et al: Impaired antibody response to pneumococcal vaccine after treatment for Hodgkin's disease. N Engl J Med 299:442–448, 1978
44. Pier G, Thomas DM: Characterization of the human immune response to a polysaccharide vaccine from *Pseudomonas aeruginosa*. J Infect Dis 148:206–213, 1983
45. Schildt RA, Boyd JF, McCracken JF et al: Antibody response to pneumococcal vaccine in patients with solid tumors and lymphomas. Med Pediatr Oncol 11:305–309, 1983
46. Cooper M: B lymphocytes: Normal development and function. N Engl J Med 317:1452–1456, 1987
47. Peter G, Pizzo PA, Robichaud KR et al: Possible protective effect of circulating antibodies to the shared glycolipid of enterobacteriaceae in children with malignancy. Pediatr Res 13:466, 1979
48. Braude AI, Douglas H, Davis CE: Treatment and prevention of intravascular coagulation with antiserum to endotoxin. J Infect Dis (Suppl) 128:S157–S164, 1973
49. Ziegler EJ, McCutchan JA, Fierer S et al: Successful treatment of gram-negative bacteremia and shock with human antiserum to a UPD-GAL epimerase-deficient mutant *Escherichia coli*. N Engl J Med 307:1225–1230, 1982
50. Rosse WF: The spleen as a filter. N Engl J Med 317:705–706, 1987
51. Sun T, Tenenbaum MJ, Greenspan J et al: Morphologic and clinical observations in human infection with *Babesia microti*. J Infect Dis 148:239–248, 1983
52. Donaldson SS, Glatstein E, Vosti KL: Bacterial infections in pediatric Hodgkin's disease. Relationship to radiation, chemotherapy and splenectomy. Cancer 41:1949–1958, 1978
53. Chilcote RR, Baehner RL, Hammond D et al: Septicemia and meningitis in children splenectomized for Hodgkin's disease. N Engl J Med 295:798–800, 1976
54. Weitzman S, Aisenberg AC: Fulminant sepsis after the successful treatment of Hodgkin's disease. Am J Med 62:47–50, 1977
55. Schimpff SC, O'Connell MJ, Greene WH et al: Infections in 92 splenectomized patients with Hodgkin's disease. A clinical review. Am J Med 59:695–701, 1975
56. Keusch GT: Nutrition and infection. In Remington JS, Swartz NM (eds): Current Clinical Topics in Infectious Disease. Vol 5, pp 106–123. New York, McGraw-Hill, 1984
57. Shamberger RC, Pizzo PA, Goodgame JT et al: The effect of total parenteral nutrition on chemotherapy induced myelosuppression: A randomized study. Am J Med 74:40–48, 1983
58. Schimpff SC, Young VM, Greene WH et al: Origin of infection in acute nonlymphocytic leukemia: Significance of hospital acquisition of potential pathogens. Ann Intern Med 77:707–714, 1972
59. van der Waaij D, Tielemons-Speltie TM, de Houban-Roech AMJ: Infection by and distribution of biotypes of enterobacteriaceae species in leukaemic patients treated under ward conditions and in units for protective isolation in seven hospitals in Europe. Infection 5:3–10, 1977
60. Schimpff SC, Greene WH, Young VM et al: Significance of *Pseudomonas aeruginosa* in the patient with leukemia or lymphoma. J Infect Dis (Suppl) 130:S24–S31, 1974
61. Kurrle E, Bhaduri S, Krieger D et al: Risk factors for infections of the oropharynx and the respiratory tract in patients with acute leukemia. J Infect Dis 144:128–136, 1981
62. Kramer BK, Pizzo PA, Robichaud KJ et al: Role of serial microbiological surveillance and clinical evaluation in the management of cancer patients with fever and granulocytopenia. Am J Med 72:561–568, 1982
63. Pizzo PA, Levine AS: The utility of protected environment regimens for the compromised host: A critical assessment. In Progress in Hematology, Vol X, pp 311–332. New York, Grune & Stratton, 1977
64. Aisner J, Murillo J, Schimpff SC et al: Invasive aspergillis in acute leukemia: Correlation with nose cultures and antibiotic use. Ann Intern Med 90:4–9, 1979
65. Maki DG, Alvarado CJ, Hessewer CH et al: Relation of the inanimate hospital environment to endemic nosocomial infection. N Engl J Med 307:1562–1565, 1982
66. Albert RK, Condie F: Handwashing patterns in medical intensive care units. N Engl J Med 304:1465–1466, 1981
67. Maki D: Infections associated with intravascular lines. In Remington JS, Swartz M (eds): Current Clinical Topics in Infectious Disease, pp 309–363. New York, McGraw Hill, 1982
68. Hiemenz J, Skelton J, Pizzo PA: Perspective on the management of catheter related infections in cancer patients. Pediatr Infect Dis 5:6–11, 1986
69. Craven DE, Moody B, Connolly MG et al: Pseudobacteremia caused by poviodine-iodine solution contaminated with *Pseudomona cepacia*. N Engl J Med 305:621–623, 1981
70. Johanson WG, Pierce AK, Sanford JP et al: Nosocomial respiratory infections with gram-negative bacilli. The significance of colonization of the respiratory tract. Ann Intern Med 77:701–706, 1972
71. Wingard JR, Merz WG, Saral R: *Candida tropicalis:* A major pathogen in immunocompromised patients. Ann Intern Med 91:539–543, 1979
72. Mackowiak PA: Microbial synergism in human infections. N Engl J Med 298:21–26,83–87, 1979
73. Rouse BT, Horohov DW: Immunosuppression in viral infections. Rev Infect Dis 8:850–873, 1986
74. Todeschini G, Rubin M, Gill V et al: Non-aeruginosa bacteremias in cancer patients. Review of 10 years' experience at the National Cancer Institute. Proceedings of the 27th Interscience Conference on Antimicrobial Agents and Chemotherapy, p 265, New York, 1987
75. Pizzo PA, Ladisch SL, Gill F et al: Increasing incidence of gram-positive sepsis in cancer patients. Med Pediatr Oncol 5:241–244, 1978
76. Wade JC, Schimpff SC, Newman KA et al: *Staphylococcus epidermidis:* An increasing cause of infection in patients with granulocytopenia. Ann Intern Med 97:507–508, 1982
77. Lowder JN, Lazarus HM, Herzig RH: Bacteremias and fungemias in oncologic pa-

tients with central venous catheters. Changing spectrum of infection. Ann Intern Med 142:1456–1459, 1982
78. Winston DJ, Dudnick FV, Chapin M et al: Coagulase-negative staphylococcal bacteremia in patients receiving immunosuppressive therapy. Arch Intern Med 143:32–36, 1983
79. Myers JP, Linneman CC: Bacteremia due to methicillin-resistant *Staphylococcus aureus.* J Infect Dis 145:532–536, 1982
80. Haley RW, Hightower AW, Khabbaz RF et al: The emergence of methicillin-resistant *Staphylococcus aureus* infections in United States' hospitals. Ann Intern Med 97:297–308, 1982
81. Walsh TJ, Vlahov D, Hansen SL et al: Prospective surveillance in control of nosocomial methicillin-resistant *Staphylococcus aureus.* Infect Control 8:7–14, 1987
82. Schwabe RS, Stapleton JT, Gilligon PH: Emergence of vancomycin resistance in coagulase-negative staphylococci. N Engl J Med 316:927–931, 1987
83. Lowry FD, Hammer SM: *Staphylococcus epidermidis* infection. Ann Intern Med 99:834–839, 1983
84. Joshi J, Newman K, Tenny J et al: *Staphylococcus epidermidis* pneumonia in granulocytopenic patients with acute leukemia. Proc ASCO 2:90, 1983
85. Thaler M, Gill V, Pizzo PA: Staphylococcal bacteremias in a cancer research hospital. Proceedings of the 26th Interscience Conference on Antimicrobial Agents and Chemotherapy, New Orleans, 1986
86. Rubin M, Hathorn JW, Marshall D et al: Gram-positive infections and the use of vancomycin in 550 episodes of fever and neutropenia. Ann Intern Med 108:30–35, 1988
87. Pizzo PA, Ladish SL, Witebsky F: Alpha-hemolytic streptococci: Clinical significance in cancer patients. Med Pediatr Oncol 4:367–370, 1978
88. Cohen J, Donnelly JP, Worsley AM et al: Septicemia caused by viridans streptococci in neutropenic patients with leukaemia. Lancet 2:1452–1454, 1983
89. von Etta LL, Filica GA, Ferguson RM et al: *Corynebacterium equi:* A review of 12 cases of human infection. Rev Infect Dis 5:1012–1018, 1983
90. Hande KR, Witebsky FG, Brown MS et al: Sepsis with a new species of *Cornyebacterium.* Ann Intern Med 85:423–426, 1976
91. Berg R, Chmel H, Mayo J et al: *Corynebacterium equi* infection complicating neoplastic disease. Am J Clin Pathol 68:73–77, 1977
92. Gill VJ, Manning C, Lamson M et al: Antibiotic-resistant group JK bacteria in hospitals. J Clin Microbiol 13:472–477, 1982
93. Thaler M, Gill V, Pizzo PA: Emergence of *Clostridium tertium* as a pathogen in neutropenic patients. Am J Med 81:596–600, 1986
94. Cotton DJ, Gu V, Hiemenz J et al: Bacillus bacteremias in an immunocompromised patient population: Clinical features, therapeutic interventions, and relationship to chronic intravascular catheters in sixteen cases. J Clin Microbiol 25:672–674, 1987
95. Greene JB, Sidhu GS, Levin S et al: *Mycobacterium avium-intracellulare:* A cause of disseminated life-threatening infection in homosexuals and drug abusers. Ann Intern Med 97:539–545, 1982
96. Macher AM, Kovacs JA, Gill V et al: Bacteremia due to *Mycrobacterium avium-intracellulare* in the acquired immunodeficiency syndrome. 99:782–785, 1983
97. Hoy JF, Rolston KVI, Hopfer RL et al: *Mycobacterium fortuitum* bacteremia in patients with cancer and long-term venous catheters. Am J Med 83:213–217, 1987
98. Walsh T, Pizzo PA: Nosocomial mycoses in immunocompromised patients. Annu Rev Microbiol (in press)
99. Macher AM: Infection in the acquired immunodeficiency syndrome. In Fauci AJ (moderator): Acquired immunodeficiency syndrome: Epidemiologic, clinical, immunologic, and therapeutic considerations. Ann Intern Med 100:92–106, 1984
100. Walsh TJ, Newman KR, Moody M et al: Trichosporonosis in patients with neoplastic disease. Medicine (Baltimore) 65:268–279, 1986
101. Hamilton JR, Overall JC, Glasgow LA: Synergistic effect on mortality in mice with murine cytomegalovirus and *Pseudomonas aeruginosa, Staphylococcus aureus* or *Candida albicans* infections. Infect Immun 14:982–989, 1976
102. Rand KH, Pollard RB, Merigan TC: Increased pulmonary superinfections in cardiac transplant patients undergoing primary cytomegalovirus infection. N Engl J Med 298:951–953, 1978
103. Browder AA, Hoff JA, Petersdorf RG: The significance of fever in neoplastic disease. Ann Intern Med 55:932–942, 1961
104. Goodman R, Jaffe N, Filler R et al: Herpes zoster in children with stage I–III Hodgkin's disease. Radiology 118:429–431, 1976
105. Kaplan MS, Rosen PP, Armstrong D: Cryptococcosis in a cancer hospital. Clinical and pathological correlates in forty-six patients. Cancer 39:2265–2274, 1977
106. Winston DJ, Gale RP, Meyer DV: Infectious complications of human bone marrow transplantation. Medicine (Baltimore) 58:1–31, 1979
107. Sickles EA, Green WH, Wiernik PH: Clinical presentation of infection in granulocytopenic patients. Arch Intern Med 135:715–719, 1975
108. Schimpff SC, Satterlee W, Young VM et al: Empiric therapy with carbenicillin and gentamicin for febrile patients with cancer and granulocytopenia. N Engl J Med 284:1061–1065, 1971
109. Markman M, Abeloff M: Management of hematologic and infectious complications of intensive induction therapy for small cell carcinoma of the lung. Am J Med 74:741–746, 1983
110. Pizzo PA, Robichaud KJ, Wesley R et al: Fever in the pediatric and young adult patient with cancer. A prospective study of 1001 episodes. Medicine (Baltimore) 61:153–165, 1982
111. The EORTC International Antimicrobial Therapy Project Group: Three antibiotic regimens in the treatment of infection in febrile granulocytopenic patients with cancer. J Infect Dis 137:14–29, 1978
112. Pizzo PA, Hathorn JW, Hiemenz JW et al: A randomized trial comparing ceftazidime alone with combination antibiotic therapy in cancer patients with fever and neutropenia. N Engl J Med 315:552–558, 1986
113. Ebright JR, San JS, Manoli RS: The gallium scan. Problems and misuse in examination of patients with suspected infection. Arch Intern Med 142:246–254, 1982
114. McDougall IR: The use of white blood cell scanning techniques in infectious disease. In Remington JS, Swartz MN (eds): Current Clinical Topics in Infectious Disease, Vol 4, pp 130–152. New York, McGraw Hill, 1983
115. Anstall HB, Coleman RE: Donor-leukocyte imaging in granulocytopenic patients with suspected abscesses: Concise communication. J Nucl Med 23:319–321, 1978
116. Dutcher JP, Schiffer CA, Johnston GS: Rapid migration of ^{111}Indium-labelled granulocytes to sites of infection. N Engl J Med 304:586–589, 1981
117. McCabe WR, Jackson GG: Gram-negative bacteremia. Arch Intern Med 110:847–855, 1982
118. Bryant RE, Hood AF, Hood CE et al: Factors affecting mortality of gram-negative bacteremia. Arch Intern Med 127:120–128, 1971
119. Love LJ, Schimpff SC, Schiffer CA et al: Improved prognosis for granulocytopenic patients with gram-negative bacteremia. Am J Med 68:643–648, 1980
120. Schimpff SC: Overview of empiric antiobiotic therapy for the febrile neutropenic patient. Rev Infect Dis (Suppl 4) 7:5734–5740, 1985
121. Pizzo PA, Thaler M, Hathorn J et al: New β-lactamase antibiotics in the granulocytopenic patient: New options and new questions. Am J Med 79:75–82, 1985
122. Birnbaum J, Kaham FM, Kropp H et al: Carbapenems, a new class of beta-lactam antiobiotics. Discovery and development of Imipenem/Cilastatin. Am J Med (Suppl 6A) 78:3021, 1985
123. Neu HC: β-lactam antibiotics: Structural relationships affecting in vitro activity and pharmacologic properties. Rev Infect Dis (Suppl 3) 8:S237–S259, 1986
124. The EORTC International Antimicrobial Therapy Cooperative Group: Ceftazidime combined with a short or long course of amikacin for empirical therapy of gram-negative bacteremia in cancer patients with granulocytopenia. N Engl J Med 317:1692–1698, 1987
125. Pizzo PA: After empiric therapy. What to do until the granulocyte comes back. Rev Infect Dis 9:214–219, 1987
126. de Pauw BE, Kauw F, Muytjens H et al: Randomized study of ceftazidime versus gentamicin plus cefotaxime for infections in severely granulocytopenic patients. J Antimicrob Chemother (Suppl A) 12:593–599, 1983
127. Young L: Editorial: Empirical antimicrobial therapy in the neutropenic host. N Engl J Med 315:580–581, 1986
128. Karp JE, Dick JD, Angelopoulos C et al: Empiric use of vancomycin during prolonged treatment-induced granulocytopenia. Randomized, double-blind, placebo-controlled clinical trial in patients with acute leukemia. Am J Med 81:237–242, 1986
129. Kramer BJ, Ramphal R, Rand K: Randomized comparison between two ceftazidime containing regimens and cephalothin-gentamicin-carbenicillin in febrile granulocytopenic cancer patients. Antimicrob Agents Chemother 30:64–68, 1986
130. Hathorn JW, Rubin M, Pizzo PA: Empirical antibiotic therapy in the febrile neutropenic cancer patient: Clinical efficacy and impact of monotherapy. Antimicrob Agents Chemother 31:971–977, 1987
131. Winston DJ, Ho WG, Gal PR: Prophylactic granulocyte transfusion during chemotherapy of acute nonlymphocyte leukemia. Ann Intern Med 94:616–622, 1981
132. Strauss RG, Connett JE, Gale RP et al: A controlled trial of prophylactic granulocyte transfusions during initial induction chemotherapy for acute myelogenous leukemia. N Engl J Med 305:597–603, 1981
133. Ford JM, Cullen MH, Roberts MM et al: Prophylactic granulocyte transfusions. Results of a randomized controlled trial in patients with acute myelogenous leukemia. Transfusion 22:311–316, 1982
134. Winston DJ, Ho WG, Young LS et al: Prophylactic granulocyte transfusions during human bone marrow transplantation. Am J Med 68:893–897, 1980
135. Clift RA, Sanders JE, Thomas ED et al: Granulocyte transfusions for the prevention of infection in patients receiving bone marrow transplants. N Engl J Med 298:1052–1057, 1982
136. Applebaum FR, Bowles CA, Makuch RW et al: Granulocyte transfusion therapy of experimental *Pseudomonas* septicemia: Study of cell dose and collection techniques. Blood 52:323–331, 1978
137. Epstein RB, Chow HS: An analysis of quantitative relationships of granulocyte transfusion therapy in canines. Transfusions 21:360–362, 1981
138. Morse EE, Freirich EJ, Carbone PP et al: The transfusion of leukocytes from doners with chronic myelogenous leukemia to patients with leukopenia. Transfusion 6:183–192, 1966
139. Winston DJ, Ho WG, Howell CL et al: Cytomegalovirus infections associated with leukocyte transfusions. Ann Intern Med 93:671–675, 1980
140. Schiffer CA, Aisner J, Daly PA et al: Alloimmunization following prophylactic granulocyte transfusion. Blood 54:766–774, 1978
141. Wright DG, Robichaud KJ, Pizzo PA et al: Lethal pulmonary reactions associated with the combined use of amphotericin B and leukocyte transfusions. N Engl J Med 304:1185–1189, 1981
142. Karp DD, Ervin TJ, Tuttle S et al: Pulmonary complications during granulocyte transfusions: Incidence and clinical features. Vox Sang 42:57–61, 1982
143. Maguire LC et al: The elimination of hydroxyethyl starch from the blood of donors experiencing single or multiple intermittent-flow centrifugation leukopheresis. Transfusion 21:347–353, 1981

144. Herzig RH, Herzig GP, Graw RG et al: Granulocyte transfusion therapy for gram-negative septicemia. N Engl J Med 296:701–705, 1977
145. Higby DJ, Yates JW, Henderson ES et al: Filtration leukophoresis for granulocyte transfusion therapy: Clinical and laboratory studies. N Engl J Med 292:761–766, 1975
146. Alavi JB, Root RK, Djerassi I et al: A randomized clinical trial of granulocyte transfusions for infection in acute leukemia. N Engl J Med 296:706–711, 1977
147. Volger WR, Winston EF: The efficacy of granulocyte transfusions in neutropenic patients. Am J Med 63:548–555, 1977
148. Winston DJ, Ho WG, Gale RP: Therapeutic granulocyte transfusions for documented infections. Ann Intern Med 97:509–512, 1982
149. Schiffer CA: Granulocyte transfusion therapy. Cancer Treat Rep 67:113–119, 1983
150. Schiffer CA: Current status of granulocyte transfusion therapy. In Remington JS, Swartz MN (eds): Current Clinical Topics in Infectious Diseases, Vol 5, pp 189–209. New York, McGraw Hill, 1984
151. DiNubile MJ: Therapeutic role of granulocyte transfusions. Rev Infect Dis 7:232–243, 1985
152. Pizzo PA, Robichaud KJ, Gill FA et al: Duration of empiric antibiotic therapy in granulocytopenic cancer patients. Am J Med 67:194–200, 1979
153. Pizzo PA, Robichaud RJ, Gill FA et al: Empiric antiobiotic and antifungal therapy for cancer patients with prolonged fever and granulocytopenia. Am J Med 72:101–111, 1982
154. Pennington JE, Successful treatment of *Aspergillus* pneumonia in hematologic neoplasia. N Engl J Med 295:426–427, 1976
155. Burke PJ, Braine HG, Rathbun HK et al: The clinical significance and management of fever in acute myelocytic leukemia. Johns Hopkins Med J 139:1–12, 1976
156. Stein RS, Kayser J, Flexner J: Clinical value of empirical amphotericin B in patients with acute mylogenous leukemia. Cancer 50:2247–2251, 1982
157. Drouhet E, Dupont B: Evolution of antifungal agents: Past, present, and future. Rev Infect Dis (Suppl) 9:S4–S14, 1987
158. Hathorn JW, Gress J, Thaler M et al: Empirical antifungal therapy among febrile neutropenic cancer patients: Amphotericin B versus ketoconazole. (submitted)
159. Fainstein V, Bodey GP, Elting L et al: Amphotericin B or ketoconazole therapy of fungal infections in neutropenic cancer patients. Antimicrob Agents Chemother 31:11–15, 1987
160. Brooks J, Williams WL, Sanders CV et al: Apparent ketoconazole failure in candidal cholecystitis. Arch Intern Med 142:1934–1935, 1982
161. Best TR, Jenkins JK, Murphy FY et al: Persistent adrenal insufficiency secondary to low-dose ketoconazole therapy. Am J Med 82:676–680, 1987
162. Wingard JR, Vaughan WP, Braine HG et al: Prevention of fungal sepsis in patients with prolonged neutropenia: A randomized, double-blind, placebo-controlled trial of intravenous miconazole. Am J Med 83:1103–1110, 1987
163. Lopez-Berestein G, Hopfer RL, Mehta R et al: Liposome-encapsulated amphotericin B for treatment of disseminated candidiasis in neutropenic mice. J Infect Dis 150:278–283, 1984
164. Lopez-Berestein G, Bodey GP, Frenkel LS et al: Treatment of hepatosplenic candidiasis with liposomal-amphotericin B. J Clin Oncol 5:310–317, 1987
165. Ganer A, Arathoon E, Stevens DA: Initial experience in therapy for progressive mycoses with itraconazole, the first clinically studied triazole. Rev Infect Dis (Suppl) 9:S77–S86, 1987
166. Phillips P, Fetchick R, Weisman I et al: Tolerance to and efficacy of intraconazole in treatment of systemic mycoses: Preliminary results. Rev Infect Dis (Suppl) 9:S87–S93, 1987
167. Perfect JR, Savani DV, Durack DT: Comparison of intraconazole of fluconazole in treatment of cryptococcal meningitis and candida pyelonephritis in rabbits. Antimicrob Agents Chemother 29:579–583, 1986
168. Arndt C, Walsh TJ, McCally CL et al: Cerebrospinal fluid penetration of fluconazole. J Infect Dis 157:178–180, 1988
169. Rubin M, Todeschini G, Marshall D et al: Does the presence of an indwelling venous catheter affect the type of infections in neutropenic cancer patients? An analysis of 505 episodes. Proceedings of the 27th Interscience Conference on Antimicrobial Agents and Chemotherapy, p 264, New York, 1987
170. Rubin M, Todeschini G, Marshall D et al: Can factors that predict the need for antibiotic modification be defined in febrile neutropenic patients receiving empirical monotherapy? Proceedings of the 27th Intrascience Conference on Antimicrobial Agents and Chemotherapy, p 265, New York, 1987
171. Klein RS, Catalona MT, Edberg SC et al: *Streptococcus bovis* septicemia and carcinoma of the colon. Ann Intern Med 91:560–562, 1979
172. Lazarus HM, Lowder JN, Herzog RH: Occlusion and infection in Broviac catheters during intensive chemotherapy. Cancer 52:2342–2348, 1983
173. Abrahm J, Mullen JL, Jacobson N et al: Continuous central venous access in patients with acute leukemia. Cancer Treat Rep 63:2099–2100, 1979
174. Sanders JE, Hickman RO, Aker S et al: Experience with double lumen right atrial catheters. JPEN 6:95–99, 1982
175. Begala JE, Maher K, Cherry JD: Risk of infection associated with the use of Broviac and Hickman catheters. Am J Infect Control 10:17–23, 1981
176. Allo MD, Miller J, Townsend T et al: Primary cutaneous aspergillosis associated with Hickman intravenous catheters. N Engl J Med 317:1105–1108, 1987
177. Pizzo PA: Diagnosis and management of infectious disease problems in the child with malignant disease. In Rubin RH, Young LS (eds): Clinical Approaches to the Infections in the Compromised Host, pp 439–464. New York, Plenum Publishing, 1988
178. Pizzo PA, Ladisch SL, Robichaud K: Treatment of gram-positive septicemia in cancer patients. Cancer 45:206–207, 1980
179. Cotton D, Marshall D, Gress J et al: Pathogen-specific vs broad-spectrum antibiotics for granulocytopenic patients with proven infection. Proceedings of the 24th Interscience Conference on Antimicrobial Agents and Chemotherapy, p 158, Washington DC, 1984
180. Bone RC, Fisher CJ, Clemmer TP et al: A controlled clinical trial of high-dose methylprednisolone in the treatment of severe sepsis and septic shock. N Engl Med 317:653–658, 1987
181. Bernard GR, Luce JM, Sprung CL et al: High-dose corticosteroids in patients with the adult respiratory distress syndrome. N Engl J Med 317:1565–1570, 1987
182. Wald ER, Milmoe GJ, Bowen AD et al: Acute maxillary sinusitis in children. N Engl J Med 304:749–754, 1982
183. Frederick J, Braude AI: Anaerobic infection of the paranasal sinuses. N Engl J Med 290:135–137, 1974
184. Caplan ES, Hoyt NJ: Nosocomial sinusitis. JAMA 247:639–641, 1982
185. McGill TJ, Simpson G, Healy GB: Fulminant aspergillosis of the nose and paranasal sinuses: A new clinical entity. Laryngoscope 90:748–754, 1980
186. Meyer RD, Rosen P, Armstrong D: Phycomycosis complicating leukemia and lymphoma. Ann Intern Med 77:871–879, 1972
187. Eden OB, Santos J: Effective treatment for rhinopulmonary mucormycosis in a boy with leukemia. Arch Dis Child 54:557–559, 1979
188. Viollier AF, DeJongh C, Newman K et al: Aspergillus sinusitis in cancer patients. Proceedings of the 21st Interscience Conference on Antimicrobial Agents and Chemotherapy, p 801, 1981
189. Mahoney DH, Steuber CP, Starling KA et al: An outbreak of aspergillosis in children with acute leukemia. J Pediatr 95:70–71, 1979
190. Berkow RL, Weisman SJ, Provisor AJ et al: Invasive aspergillosis of paranasal tissues in children with malignancies. J Pediatr 103:49–53, 1983
191. Swerdlow B, Doresinski S: Development of *Aspergillus* sinusitis in a patient receiving amphotericin B. Treatment with granulocyte transfusions. Am J Med 76:162–166, 1984
192. Mayosmith MF, Hirsch PJ, Wodzinski SF et al: Acute epiglottitis in adults. An eight-year experience in the state of Rhode Island. N Engl J Med 314:1133–1139, 1986
193. Cole S, Zawin M, Lundberg B et al: *Candida* epiglottitis in an adult with acute non-lymphocytic leukemia. Am J Med 82:662–663, 1987
194. Walsh TJ, Gray W: *Candida* epiglottitis in immunocompromised patients. Chest 9:482–485, 1987
195. Arnow PM, Chou T, Weil D et al: Nosocomial Legionnaires: Disease caused by aerosolized tap water from respiratory devices. J Infect Dis 146:460–467, 1982
196. Helms CM, Massanari RM, Zeitter R et al: Legionnaires' disease associated with a hospital water system: A cluster of 24 nosocomial cases. Ann Intern Med 99:172–178, 1983
197. Grayston TJ, Kuo CC, Wong SP et al: A new *Chlamydia psittaci* strain, TWAR, isolated in acute respiratory tract infections. N Engl J Med 315:161–168, 1986
198. Marrie TJ, Grayston JT, Wong SP et al: Pneumonia associated with the TWAR strain of chlamydia. Ann Intern Med 106:507–511, 1987
199. Ramsey PG, Fife KH, Hackman RC et al: Herpes simplex virus pneumonia: Clinical, virological and pathological features in 20 patients. Ann Intern Med 97:813–820, 1982
200. Centers for Disease Control: Tuberculosis and acquired immunodeficiency syndrome: New York City. MMWR 36:785–790, 1987
201. Feld R, Bodey GP, Groschel D: Mycobacteriosis in patients with malignant disease. Arch Intern Med 136:67–70, 1976
202. Ludmerer KM, Kissnae JM: Fulminant pneumonia and death in an immunocompromised woman. Am J Med 75:1043–1052, 1983
203. Lauver GL, Hasan FM, Morgan RB et al: The usefulness of fiberoptic bronchoscopy in evaluating new pulmonary lesions in the compromised host. Am J Med 66:580–585, 1979
204. Stover DE, Zamm MB, Hajdu SI et al: Bronchoalveolar lavage in the diagnosis of diffuse pulmonary infiltrates in the immunocompromised host. Ann Intern Med 101:1–6, 1984
205. Thorpe JE, Baughman RP, Frame PT et al: Bronchoalevolar lavage for diagnosing acute bacterial pneumonia. J Infect Dis 155:855–861, 1987
206. Kahn FW, Jones JM: Diagnosing bacterial respiratory infection by bronchoalveolar lavage. J Infect Dis 155:862–869, 1987
207. Daniele RP, Elias JA, Epstein PE et al: Bronchoalveolar lavage: Role in the pathogenesis, diagnosis, and management of interstitial lung disease. Ann Intern Med 102:93–108, 1985
208. Johnson HR, Pizzo PA, Fauci AS: Thoracic mass lesions in immunocompetent patients. Chest 82:164–167, 1982
209. Meyer RD, Edelstein PH: Legionella pneumonias. In Pennington JE: Respiratory Infections: Diagnosis and Management. New York, Raven Press, 1983
210. Myerowitz RL, Pasculle AW, Dowling JN et al: Opportunistic lung infection due to "Pittsburgh Pneumonia Agent." N Engl J Med 301:953–958, 1979
211. Muldoon RL, Jaecker DL, Kiefer HK: Legionnaires' disease in children. Pediatrics 67:329–332, 1981
212. Anderson RD, Lauer BA, Frazer DQ et al: Infections with *Legionella pneumophilia* in children. J Infect Dis 143:386–390, 1981
213. Tobin J, Beare J, Dunnill MS et al: Legionnaires' disease in a transplant unit: Isolation of the causative agent from shower baths. Lancet 2:118–121, 1980
214. Kirby BD, Snyder KM, Meyer RD et al: Legionnaires' disease: Report of sixty-five

nosocomically acquired cases and review of the literature. Medicine (Baltimore) 59:188–205, 1980
215. Maskill MR, Jordan EC: Pronounced cerebellar features in Legionnaires' disease. Br Med J 283:276, 1981
216. Shetty KR, Cilyo CL, Starr BD et al: Legionnaires' disease with profound cerebellar involvement. Arch Neurol 37:379–380, 1980
217. Harris LF: Legionnaires' disease associated with acute encephalomyelitis. Arch Neurol 38:462–463, 1981
218. Kirby DB, Peck H, Meyer RD: Radiograph features of Legionnaires' disease. Chest 76:562–565, 1979
219. Young LS, Armstrong D, Blevins A et al: *Nocardia asteroides* infection complicating neoplastic disease. Am J Med 50:356–367, 1971
220. Palmer DL, Harvey RL, Wheeler JK: Diagnostic and therapeutic considerations in *Nocardia asteroides* infection. Medicine (Baltimore) 53:391–401, 1974
221. Smego RA, Gallis HA: The clinical spectrum of *Nocardia brasiliensis* infection in the United States. Rev Infect Dis 6:164–180, 1984
222. Edwards JE, Lehrer RI, Stiehm ER et al: Severe candidal infections. Clinical perspective, immune defense mechanisms and current concepts of therapy. Ann Intern Med 89:91–106, 1978
223. Young RC, Bennett JE, Vogel CL et al: Asperigillosis. The spectrum of the disease in 98 patients. Medicine (Baltimore) 49:147–173, 1970
224. Krick JA, Remington JS: Opportunistic invasive fungal infections in patients with leukemia and lymphoma. Clin Haematol 5:249–310, 1976
225. Commers JC, Robichaud K, Pizzo PA: New pulmonary infiltrates in granulocytopenic patients being treated with antibiotics. Pediatr Infect Dis 3:423–428, 1984
226. Dubois PJ, Myerowitz RL, Allen CM: Patho-radiologic correlation of pulmonary candidiasis in immunosuppressed patients. Cancer 40:1026–1036, 1977
227. Young RC, Bennett JE, Geelhoed GW et al: Fungemia with compromised host resistance. A study of 70 cases. Ann Intern Med 80:605–612, 1974
228. Edwards JE: *Candida* endophthalmitis. In Remington JS, Swartz MN (eds): Current Clinical Topics in Infectious Diseases, pp 381–397. New York, McGraw Hill, 1982
229. Meyer RD, Young LS, Armstrong D et al: Aspergillosis complicating neoplastic disease. Am J Med 54:6–15, 1973
230. Rinaldi MG: Invasive aspergillosis. Rev Infect Dis 5:1061–1077, 1983
231. Aisner J, Schimpff SC, Bennett JE et al: *Aspergillus* infection in cancer patients. Association with fireproofing materials in new hospitals. JAMA 235:411–412, 1976
232. Aisner J, Schimpff SC, Wiernik PH: Treatment of invasive aspergillosis: Relation of early diagnosis and treatment response. Ann Intern Med 86:539–543, 1977
233. Yu VL, Muder RR, Poorsattar A: Significance of isolation of *Aspergillus* from the respiratory tract in diagnosis of invasive pulmonary aspergillosis. Results from a three-year prospective study. Am J Med 81:249–251, 1986
234. Burch PA, Karp JE, Merz WG et al: Favorable outcome of invasive aspergillosis in patients with acute leukemia. J Clin Oncol 5:1985–1993, 1987
235. Kauffman CA, Israel KS, Smith JW et al: Histoplasmosis in immunosuppressed patients. Am J Med 64:923–931, 1978
236. Broduer GM, Wilber RB, Melvin SL et al: Histoplasmosis mimicking childhood non-Hodgkin's lymphoma. Med Pediatr Oncol 7:77–81, 1979
237. Davies SF, McKenna RW, Sarosi GA: Trephine biopsy of the bone marrow in disseminated histoplasmosis. Am J Med 67:617–622, 1979
238. Deresinski SC, Stevens DA: Coccidioidomycosis in compromised hosts. Experience at Stanford University Hospital. Medicine (Baltimore) 54:377–395, 1974
239. Kaplan MS, Rosen PP, Armstrong D: Cryptococcosis in a cancer hospital. Clinical and pathological correlates in forty-six patients. Cancer 39:2265–2274, 1977
240. Valdivieso M, Luna M, Bodey GP et al: Fungemia due to *Torulopsis glabrata* in the compromised host. Cancer 38:1750–1756, 1976
241. Aisner J, Schimpff SC, Sutherland JC et al: *Torulopsis glabrata* infection in patients with cancer. Increasing incidence and relationship in colonization. Am J Med 61:23–28, 1976
242. Torres-Rojas JR, Stratton CW, Sanders CV et al: *Candida* suppurative peripheral thrombophelebitis. Ann Intern Med 96:431–435, 1982
243. Drutz DJ: Newer antifungal agents and their use, including an update on amphotericin B and flucytosine. In Remington JS, Swartz MN (eds): Current Clinical Topics in Infectious Diseases, Vol 3, pp 97–135. New York, McGraw Hill, 1982
244. Medoff G: Controversial areas in antifungal chemotherapy: Short course and combination therapy with amphotericin B. Rev Infect Dis 9:403–407, 1987
245. Beggs WH, Sarosi GA, Andrews FA: Synergistic action of amphotericin B and rifampin on *Candida albicans*. Am Rev Respir Dis 110:671–673, 1974
246. Bennett JE, Dismukes WE, Duma RJ et al: Amphotericin B flucytosine in cryptococcal meningitis. N Engl J Med 301:126–131, 1979
247. Dismukes WE, Cloud G, Gallis HA et al: Treatment of cryptococcal meningitis with combination amphotericin B and flucytosine for four as compared with six weeks. N Engl J Med 317:334–341, 1987
248. Thaler M, Bacher J, O'Leary T et al: Evaluation of single-drug and combination antifungal therapy in an experimental model of candidiasis in rabbits with prolonged neutropenia. J Infect Dis (in press)
249. Bennett JF: Flucytosine. Ann Intern Med 86:319–322, 1977
250. Stiller RL, Bennett JE, Scholer HJ et al: Correlation of in vitro susceptibility test results with in vivo response: Flucytosine therapy in a systemic candidiasis model. J Infect Dis 147:1070–1077, 1983
251. Saag MS, Dismukes WE: Azole antifungal agents: Emphasis on new triazoles. Antimicrob Agents Chemother 32:1–8, 1988
252. Shechtman LB, Funaro L, Robin T et al: Clotrimazole treatment of oral candidiasis in patients with neoplastic disease. Am J Med 76:91–91, 1984
253. Jordan WM, Bodey GP, Rodriguex V et al: Miconazole therapy for report of sixty-five nosocomically required cases and review of the literature. Antimicrob Agents Chemother 8:792–797, 1979
254. Schaffner A, Frick PG: The effect of ketoconazole on amphotericin B in a model of disseminated aspergillosis. J Infect Dis 151:902–910, 1985
255. Hughes WT: *Pneumocystis carinii* pneumonia. N Engl J Med 297:1381–1383, 1977
256. Meuwissen JH, Tauber I, Leewenberg AD et al: Parasitologic and serologic observations of infection with Pneumocystis in humans. J Infect Dis 136:4349, 1977
257. Ruebush TK, Weinstein RA, Baehner RL et al: An outbreak of *Pneumocystis* pneumonia in children with acute lymphocyte leukemia. Am J Dis Child 132:143–148, 1978
258. Browne M, Hubbard SM, Longo DL et al: Excess prevalence of *Pneumocystis carinii* pneumonia in lymphoma patients with chemotherapy. Ann Intern Med 104:338–344, 1986
259. Kovacs JA, Hiemenz JW, Macher AM et al: *Pneumocystis carinii* pneumonia: A comparison of clinical features in patients with the acquired immune deficiency syndrome and patients with other immune diseases. Ann Intern Med 100:663–671, 1984
260. Browne MJ, Potter D, Gress J et al: A randomized trial of open lung biopsy versus empiric antimicrobial therapy in cancer patients with diffuse pullmonary infiltrates. (submitted)
261. Burt ME, Flye MW, Webber BL et al: Prospective evaluation of aspiration needle, cutting needle, transbronchial and open lung biopsy in patients with pulmonary infiltrates. Ann Thorac Surg 32:146–153, 1981
262. McCabe RE, Brooks RG, Mark JBD et al: Open lung biopsy in patients with acute leukemia. Am J Med 78:609–616, 1985
263. Allegra CJ, Chabner BA, Tuazon CU et al: Trimetrexate for the treatment of *Pneumocystis carinii* pneumonia in patients with the acquired immunodeficiency syndrome. N Engl J Med 317:978–985, 1987
264. Meyers JD, Flournoy N, Thomas ED: Nonbacterial pneumonia after allogeneic marrow transplantation: A review of ten years' experience. Rev Infect Dis 4:1119–1132, 1982
265. Weiner RS, Bortin MM, Gale RP et al: Interstitial pneumonitis after bone marrow transplantation. Ann Intern Med 104:168–175, 1986
266. Quinnan GV, Kirmani N, Rook AH et al: Cytotoxic T cells in cytomegalovirus infection. N Engl J Med 307:7–13, 1982
267. Grundy JE, Shanley JD, Griffiths PD: Is cytomegalovirus interstitial pneumonitis in transplant recipients an immunopathological condition? Lancet (in press)
268. Wingard JR, Santos GW, Saral R: Late onset interstitial pneumonia following allogeneic bone marrow transplantation. Transplantation 39:21–23, 1985
269. Myerson D, Hackman RC, Meyers JD: The diagnosis of cytomegalovirus pneumonia by in situ hybridization. J Infect Dis 150:272–277, 1984
270. Zaia JA, Forman SJ, Gallagher MT et al: Prolonged human cytomegalovirus viremia following bone marrow transplantation. Transplantation 37:315–317, 1984
271. Meyers JD, Flournoy N, Thomas ED: Risk factors for cytomegalovirus infection after human marrow transplantation. J Infect Dis 153:478–488, 1986
272. Crawford SW, Bowden RA, Hackman RC et al: Rapid detection of cytomegalovirus pulmonary infection by bronchoalveolar lavage and centrifugation culture. Ann Intern Med (in press)
273. Gleaves CA, Meyers JD: Rapid diagnosis of invasive cytomegalovirus infection by examination of tissue specimens in centrifugation culture. Am J Clin Pathol 88:354–358, 1987
274. Meyers JD, Flournoy N, Wade JC et al: Biology of interstitial pneumonia after marrow transplantation. In Gale RP (ed): Recent Advances in Bone Marrow Transplantation, pp 405–423. New York, Alan R. Liss, 1983
275. Shepp DH, Dandliker PS, de Miranda P et al: Activity of 9-[2-hydroxy-1-(hydroxymethyl)ethoxymethyl]guanine (BW B759U) in the treatment of cytomegalovirus pneumonia. Ann Intern Med 103:368–373, 1985
276. Reed EC, Dandliker PS, Meyers JD: Treatment of cytomegalovirus pneumonia with 9-[2-hydroxy-1-(hydroxymethyl)ethoxymethyl]guanine and high-dose corticosteroids. Ann Intern Med 105:214–215, 1986
277. Erice A, Jordan MC, Chase BA et al: Ganciclovir treatment of cytomegalovirus disease in transplant recipients and other immunocompromised hosts. JAMA 257:3082–3087, 1987
278. Bowden RA, Sayers M, Flournoy N et al: Cytomegalovirus immune globulin and seronegative blood products to prevent primary cytomegalovirus infection after marrow transplantation. N Engl J Med 314:1006–1010, 1986
279. Winston DJ, Ho WG, Lin CH et al: Intravenous immune globulin for prevention of cytomegalovirus infection and interstitial pneumonia after bone marrow transplantation. Ann Intern Med 106:12–18, 1987
280. Meyers JD, Flournoy N, Sanders JE et al: Prophylactic human leukocyte interferon after allogeneic marrow transplantation. Ann Intern Med (in press)
281. Siegel MM, Walter JK, Ablin AR: Measles pneumonia in childhood leukemia. Pediatrics 60:38–40, 1977
282. Mitus A, Halloway A, Evans AE: Attenuated measles vaccine in children with acute leukemia. Am J Dis Child 103:413–418, 1962
283. Shields AF, Hackman RC, Fife KH et al: Adenovirus infections in patients undergoing bone marrow transplantation. N Engl J Med 312:529–533, 1985
284. Knight V, McClung HW, Wilson SZ et al: Ribavirin small particle aerosol treatment of influenza. Lancet 2:945–949, 1981
285. Hall CB, McBride JT, Walsh EE et al: Aerosolized ribavirin treatment of infants with

respiratory syncytial viral infection. A randomized double-blind study. New Engl J Med 308:1442–1447, 1983
286. McClung HW, Knight V, Gilbert BE et al: Ribavirin aerosol treatment of influenza B infection. JAMA 249:2671–2674, 1983
287. Dolin R, Reichman RC, Madore HP et al: A controlled trial of amantadine and rimantadine in the prophylaxis of influenza infection. N Engl J Med 307:580–584, 1982
288. Schafer AI, Churchill WH, Ames P et al: The influence of chemotherapy on response of patients with hematologic malignancies to influenza vaccine. Cancer 43:25–30, 1979
289. Schildt RA, Luedke DW, Kasai G et al: Antibody response to influenza immunization in adult patients with malignant disease. Cancer 44:1629–1635, 1975
290. Kaye D: Prophylaxis for infective endocarditis: An update. Ann Intern Med 104:419–423, 1986
291. Howat AJ, Todd CEC, Scott CA: Two cases of endocarditis due to *Candida albicans* discovered at autopsy. J Infect Dis 147:1122–1123, 1983
292. Ladisch S, Pizzo PA: *S. aureus* sepsis in children with cancer. Pediatrics 61:231–234, 1978
293. Peterson DE, Minah GE, Overholser CD et al: Microbiology of acute periodontal infection in myelosuppressed cancer patients. J Clin Oncol 5:1461–1468, 1987
294. Meyers JD, Wade JC, Mitchell CD et al: Multicenter collaborative trial of intravenous acyclovir for the treatment of mucocutaneous herpes simplex virus infection in the immunocompromised host. Am J Med (Suppl) 73:229–235, 1982
295. Whitley RJ, Spruance S, Hayden FG et al: (NIAID Collaborative Antiviral Study Group): Vidarabine therapy for mucocutaneous herpes simplex virus infection in the immunocompromised host. J Infect Dis 149:1–8, 1984
296. Shepp DH, Newton BA, Dandliker PS et al: Oral acyclovir therapy for mucocutaneous herpes simplex virus infections in immunocompromised marrow transplant recipients. Ann Intern Med 102:783–785, 1985
297. Whitley RJ, Levin M, Barton N et al: Infections caused by herpes simplex virus in the immunocompromised host: Natural history and topical acyclovir therapy. J Infect Dis 150:323–329, 1984
298. Meyers JD, Flournoy N, Thomas ED: Infection with herpes simplex virus and cell-mediated immunity after marrow transplant. J Infect Dis 142:338–346, 1980
299. Saral R, Ambinder RF, Burns WH et al: Acyclovir prophylaxis against herpes simplex virus infection in patients with leukemia. Ann Intern Med 99:773–776, 1983
300. Shepp DH, Dandliker PS, Flournoy N et al: Sequential intravenous and twice daily oral acyclovir for extended prophylaxis of herpes simplex virus infection in marrow transplant patients. Transplantation. (in press)
301. Wade JC, Newton B, Flournoy N et al: Oral acyclovir for prevention of herpes simplex virus reactivation after marrow transplant. Ann Intern Med 100:823–828, 1984
302. Prentice HG: Use of acyclovir for prophylaxis of herpes infections in severely immunocompromised patients. J Antimicrob Chemother (Suppl B) 12:153–159, 1983
303. Ringden O, Heimdahl A, Lonnqvist B et al: Letter: Decreased incidence of viridans streptococcal septicaemia in allogeneic bone marrow transplant recipients after the introduction of acyclovir. Lancet 1:744, 1984
304. McDonald GB, Sharma P, Hackman RC et al: Esophageal infections in immunosuppressed patients after marrow transplant. Gastroenterology 88:1111–1117, 1985
305. Walsh TJ, Belitsos N, Hamiltol SR: Bacterial esophagitis in immunocompromised patients. Arch Intern Med 146:1345–1348, 1986
306. Buss DH, Scharyj M: Herpes virus infection of the esophagus and other visceral organs in adults: Indicence and clincial significance. Am J Med 66:457–462, 1979
307. Varki AP, Armitage JO, Feagler JR: Typhlitis in acute leukemia: Successful treatment by early surgical intervention. Cancer 43:695–697, 1979
308. Skibber JM, Matler GJ, Lotze MT et al: Right lower quadrant complications in young patients with leukemia: A surgical perspective. Ann Surg 206:711–716, 1987
309. Gootenberg JE, Abbondanzo SL: Rapid diagnosis of neutropenic enterocolitis (Typhlitis) by ultrasonography. Am J Pediatr Hematol Oncol 9:222–227, 1987
310. Shaked A, Shinar E, Freund H: Neutropenic typhlitis: A plea for conservation. Dis Colon Rectum 26:351–352, 1983
311. Wynne JW, Armstrong D: Clostridial septicemia. Cancer 29:215–221, 1972
312. Larson HE, Price AB, Honour P et al: *Clostridium difficile* and the aetiology of pseudomembranous colitis. Lancet 1:1063–1066, 1978
313. Bartlett JG, Chang TW, Gurwith M et al: Antibiotic associated pseudomembranous colitis due to toxin producing clostridia. N Engl J Med 298:531–534, 1978
314. Elstner CL, Lindsay AN, Book LS et al: Lack of *Clostridium difficile* to antibiotic associated diarrhea in children. Pediatr Infect Dis 2:364–366, 1983
315. Scowden EB, Schaffner W, Stone WJ: Overwhelming strongyloidiasis: An unappreciated opportunistic infection. Medicine (Baltimore) 57:527–544, 1978
316. Igra-Siegman YU, Kapila R, Sen P et al: Syndrome of hyperinfection with *Strongyloides stercoralis*. Rev Infect Dis 3:397–407, 1981
317. Dienstag JL: Non-A, non-B hepatitis. I. Recognition, epidemiology, and clinical features. Gastroenterology 85:439–462, 1983
318. Tabor E, Gerety RJ, Drucker JA et al: Transmission of non-A, non-B hepatitis from man to chimpanzee. Lancet 1:463–465, 1978
319. Hoofnagle JH, Mullen KD, Jones B et al: Treatment of chronic non-A, non-B hepatitis with recombinant human alpha interferon. A perliminary report. N Engl J Med 315:1575–1578, 1986
320. Krugman S, Overby LR, Mushawar IK et al: Viral hepatitis, type B. Studies on natural history and prevention re-examined. N Engl J Med 300:101–106, 1979
321. Tabor E, Gerety JR, Mott M et al: Prevalence of hepatitis B in a high-risk setting: A serologic study of patients and staff in a pediatric oncology unit. Pediatrics 61:711–715, 1978
322. Wade JC, Gaffey M, Wiernik PH et al: Hepatitis in patients with acute nonlymphocytic leukemia. Am J Med 75:413–422, 1983
323. Berk PD, Jones A, Plotz PH et al: Corticosteroid therapy for chronic active hepatitis. Ann Intern Med 85:523–524, 1976
324. Hoofnagle JH, Dusheiko GM, Schafer DF et al: Reactivation of chronic hepatitis B virus infection by cancer chemotherapy. Ann Intern Med 96:447–449, 1982
325. Editorial: Immunosuppressive therapy for chronic active hepatitis. Lancet 2:507–508, 1978
326. Rizzetto M, Purcell RH, Gerin JL: Epidemiology of HBV associated delta agent. Geographical distribution of anti-delta and prevalence in polytransfused HBsAg carriers. Lancet 1:1215–1218, 1980
327. Dunnick J, Galasso GJ: Clinical trials with exogenous interferon. Summary of a meeting. J Infect Dis 139:109–123, 1979
328. Greenberg HB, Pollard RB, Lutwick LI et al: Effect of leukocyte interferon on hepatitis-B virus infection in patients with chronic active hepatitis. N Engl J Med 295:517–522, 1976
329. Desmyter J, Ray MB, DeGroote J et al: Administration of human fibroblast interferon in chronic hepatitis-B infection. Lancet 2:645–647, 1976
330. Dolen JG, Carter WA, Horozewicz JS et al: Fibroblast interferon treatment of a patient with chronic active hepatitis. Increased number of circulating T lymphocytes and elimination of rosette-inhibitory factor. Am J Med 67:127–130, 1979
331. Seeff LB, Wright EC, Zimmerman HJ et al: Type B hepatitis after needle-stick exposure: Prevention with hepatitis B immune globulin. Ann Intern Med 88:285–293, 1978
332. Grady GF, Lee VA, Prince AM et al: Hepatitis B immune globulin for accidental exposures among medical personnel: Final report of a multicenter controlled trial. J Infect Dis 138:625–638, 1978
333. Haron E, Feld R, Tuffnell P et al: Hepatic candidiasis: An increasing problem in immunocompromised patients. Am J Med 83:17–26, 1987
334. Thaler M, Pastakia B, Shawker TH et al: Hepatic candidiasis in cancer patients: The evolving picture of the syndrome. Ann Intern Med 108:88–100, 1988
335. Thaler M, Pizzo PA: Empiric antifungal therapy in neutropenic cancer patients. Proceedings of the 26th Interscience Conference on Antimicrobial Agents and Chemotherapy, New Orleans, 1986
336. Glenn J, Cotton D, Wesley R et al: Anorectal infections in patients with malignant diseases. Rev Infect Dis 10:42–52, 1988
337. Barnes SG, Sattler FR, Ballard JO: Improved survival after drainage of perirectal infections in patients with acute leukemia. Ann Intern Med 100:515–518, 1984
338. Kingston ME, Mackey D: Skin clues in the diagnosis of life-threatening infections. Rev Infect Dis 8:1–11, 1986
339. Hay CRM, Messenger AG, Cotton DWK et al: Atypical bullous pyoderma gangrenosum associated with myeloid malignancies. J Clin Pathol 40:387–392, 1987
340. Kanel KT, Kroboth FJ, Swartz WM: Pyoderma gangrenosum with myelofibrosis. Am J Med 82:1031–1034, 1987
341. Drew WL, Mintz L: Rapid diagnosis of varicella-zoster virus infection by direct immunofluorescence. Am J Clin Pathol 73:699–701, 1980
342. Centers for Disease Control: CDC guidelines for isolation precautions in hospitals. In Garner JS, Simmons BP (eds): Infection Control, pp 245–325. 1983
343. Leclair JM, Zaia JA, Levin MJ et al: Airborne transmission of chickenpox in a hospital. N Engl J Med 302:450–453, 1980
344. Paryani SG, Arvin AM, Koropchak CM et al: Varicella zoster antibody titers after administration of intravenous serum globulin or varicella zoster immune globulin. Am J Med (Suppl 3A) 76:124–127, 1984
345. Gershon AA, Steinberg S, Brunnell PA: Zoster immune globulin. A further assessment. N Engl J Med 290:243–245, 1975
346. Geiser CF, Bishop Y, Myers M et al: Prophylaxis of varicella in children with neoplastic disease: Comparative results with zoster immune plasma and gamma globulin. Cancer 35:1027–1030, 1975
347. Whitley R, Hilty M, Haynes R et al: Vidarabine therapy for varicella in immunosuppressed patients. J Pediatr 101:125–131, 1982
348. Prober CG, Kirk LE, Keeney RE: Acyclovir therapy of chickenpox in immunosuppressed children—a collaborative study. J Pediatr 101:622–625, 1982
349. Arvin AM, Feldman S, Merigan TC: Human leukocyte interferon in the treatment of varicella in children with cancer in preliminary controlled trial. Antimicrob Agents Chemother 13:605–607, 1978
350. Arvin AM, Kushner JH, Feldman S et al: Human leukocyte interferon for the treatment of varicella in children with cancer. N Engl J Med 306:761–765, 1985
351. Takahashi M, Otsuka T, Okuno Y et al: Live vaccine used to prevent the spread of varicella in children in the hospital. Lancet 2:1288–1290, 1974
352. Brunell PA, Shahab Z, Geiser C et al: Administration of live varicella vaccine to children with leukaemia. Lancet 2:1069–1073, 1982
353. Gelb LD, Dohner DE, Geighon AA et al: Molecular epidemiology of live, attenuated varicella virus vaccine in children with leukemia and in normal adults. J Infect Dis 155:633–640, 1987
354. Feldman S, Hughes WT, Kim HY: Herpes zoster in children with cancer. Am J Dis Child 126:178–184, 1973
355. Reboul F, Donaldson SS, Kaplan HS: Herpes zoster and varicella infections in children with Hodgkin's disease. An analysis of contributing factors. Cancer 41:95–99, 1978
356. Locksley RM, Flournoy N, Sullivan KM et al: Varicella-zoster virus infection after

marrow transplantation. J Infect Dis 152:1172–1181, 1985
357. Schimpff S, Serpick A, Stoler B et al: Varicella-zoster infection in patients with cancer. Ann Intern Med 76:241–254, 1972
358. Feldman S, Chaudary S, Ossi M et al: A viremic phase for herpes zoster in children with cancer. J Pediatr 91:597–600, 1977
359. Myers MG: Viremia caused by varicella-zoster virus. Association with malignant progressive varicella. J Infect Dis 140:229–233, 1979
360. Whitley RJ, Soong SJ, Dolin R: Early vidarabine therapy to control the complications of herpes zoster in immunosuppressed patients. N Engl J Med 307:971–975, 1982
361. Balfour HH, Bean B, Laskin OL et al: Acyclovir halts progression of herpes zoster in immunocomprised patients. N Engl J Med 308:1448–1453, 1983
362. Merigan TC, Rand KH, Pollard RB et al: Human leukocyte interferon for the treatment of herpes zoster in patients with cancer. N Engl J Med 298:981–987, 1978
363. Shepp DH, Dandliker PS, Meyers JD: Treatment of varicella-zoster virus infection in severely immunocompromised patients: A randomized comparison of acyclovir and vidarabine. N Engl J Med 314:208–212, 1986
364. Meyers JD, Wade JC, Shepp DH et al: Acyclovir treatment of varicella-zoster virus infection in the compromised host. Transplantation 37:571–574, 1984
365. Bean B, Aeppli D: Adverse effects of high-dose intravenous acyclovir in ambulatory patients with acute herpes zoster. J Infect Dis 151:362–365, 1985
366. Levin MJ, Zaia JA, Hershey BJ et al: Topical acyclovir treatment of herpes zoster in immunocompromised patients. J Am Acad Dermatol 13:590–596, 1985
367. Lehman TJA, Quinn JJ, Siegel S et al: *Clostridium septicum* infection in childhood leukemia. Report of a case and review of the literature. Cancer 40:950–953, 1977
368. Groschel D, Burges MA, Bodey GP: Gas gangrene-like infection with *Bacillus-cereus* in a lymphoma patient. Cancer 37:988–991, 1976
369. Gordin F, Stamler C, Mills J: Pyogenic psoas abscesses: Noninvasive diagnostic techniques and review of the literature. Rev Infect Dis 5:1003–1011, 1983
370. Rimailho A: Fulminant necrotizing fasciitis and nonsteroidal anti-inflammatory drugs. J Infect Dis 155:143–146, 1987
371. Schoenbaum SC, Gardner P, Shillito J: Infections of cerebrospinal fluid shunts: Epidemiology, clinical manifestations and therapy. J Infect Dis 131:543–552, 1979
372. Browne M, Dinndorf P, Perek D et al: Infectious complications of intraventricular reservoirs in cancer patients. Pediatr Infect Dis 6:182–189, 1987
373. Kaplan MS, Rosen PP, Armstrong D: Cryptococcosis in a cancer hospital: Clinical and pathological correlates in forty-six patients. Cancer 39:2265–2274, 1977
374. Diamond RD, Bennet JE: Prognostic factors in cryptococcal meningitis: A study of 111 cases. Ann Intern Med 80:176–181, 1974
375. Lavetter A, Leedom JM, Mathies AE et al: Meningitis due to *Listeria monocytogenes*. N Engl J Med 285:598–603, 1971
376. Gantz NM, Myerwitz RL, Medieros AA et al: Listeriosis in immunosuppressed patients, a cluster of eight cases. Am J Med 58:637, 143, 1975
377. Gordon RC, Barrett FF, Yow MD: Ampicillin treatment of listeriosis. J Pediatr 77:1067–1070, 1970
378. Whitley RJ, Alford CA, Hirsch MS et al (NIAAID Collaborative Antiviral Study Group): Vidarabine versus acyclovir therapy in herpes simplex encephalitis. N Engl J Med 314:144–149, 1986
379. Whitley RJ, Soong SJ, Dolin R et al: Adenosine arabinoside therapy of biopsy proved herpes simplex encephalitis. N Engl J Med 297:289–294, 1977
380. Ruskin J, Remington JS: Toxoplasmosis in the compromised host. Ann Intern Med 84:193–199, 1976
381. Lipton SA, Hickey WF, Morris JH et al: Candidial infection in the central nervous system. Am J Med 76:101–108, 1984
382. Centers for Disease Control: Acquired immunodeficiency syndrome (AIDS). Update United States. MMWR 32:309–311, 1983
383. Wong B, Gold JWM, Brown AE: Central nervous system toxoplasmosis in homosexual men and parenteral drug abusers. Ann Intern Med 100:36–42, 1984
384. Pizzo PA, Poplack DG, Bleyer WA: The neurotoxicities of current leukemia therapy. Am J Pediatr Hematol Oncol 1:127–140, 1979
385. Houff S, Major EO, Katz DA et al: Involvement of JC virus-infected mononuclear cells from the bone marrow and spleen in the pathogenesis of progressive multifocal leukoencephalopathy. N Engl J Med 318:301–305, 1988
386. Pizzo PA: Considerations for preventing infectious complications in cancer patients. Rev Infect Dis (in press)
387. Remington JS, Schimpff SC: Please don't eat the salads. N Engl J Med 304:433–435, 1981
388. Pizzo PA, Purvis D, Waters CW: Microbiological evaluation of food items for patients undergoing gastrointestinal decontamination and protected isolation. J Am Diet Assoc 81:272–279, 1982
389. Nauseef WM, Maki DG: A study of the value of simple protective isolation in patients with granulocytopenia. N Engl J Med 304:448–453, 1981
390. Pizzo PA: Do results justify the expense of protected environments? In Wiernik P (ed): Controversies in Oncology, pp 267–277. New York, John Wiley & Sons, 1982
391. Pizzo PA: Antibiotic prophylaxis in the immunosuppressed patient with cancer. In Remington JS, Swartz MN (eds): Current Clinical Topics in Infectious Diseases, 4th ed, pp 153–167. New York, McGraw Hill, 1983
392. van der Waaij D, Berghuis de Vries JN, Lekkerkerk van der Wees JEC et al: Colonization resistance of the digestive tract in conventional and antibiotic treated mice. J Hyg (Lond) 69:405–411, 1971
393. van der Waaij D, Berghuis de Vries JN: Selective elimination of enterobacteriaciae species from the digestive tract in mice and monkeys. J Hyg (Lond) 72:205–211, 1974
394. Guiot HFL, van der Brock PJ, van der Meer JWM et al: Selective antimicrobial modulation of the intestinal flora of patients with acute nonlymphocytic leukemia. A double-blind placebo-controlled study. J Infect Dis 147:615–623, 1983
395. Sleijfer DT, Mulder NK, de Vries-Hospers HG et al: Infection prevention in granulocytopenic patients by selective decontamination of the digestive tract. Eur J Cancer 16:859–869, 1980
396. Gurwith MJ, Brunton JL, Lank BA: A prospective controlled investigation of prophylactic trimethoprim-sulfamethoxazole in hospitalized granulocytopenic patients. Am J Med 66:248–256, 1979
397. Pizzo PA, Robichaud KJ, Edwards BK et al: Oral antibiotic prophylaxis in patients with cancer: A double-blind randomized placebo-controlled trial. J Pediatr 102:125–133, 1983
398. Weiser B, Lange M, Fialkow MA et al: Prophylactic trimethoprim-sulfamethaxozole during consolidated chemotherapy for acute leukemia: A controlled trial. Ann Intern Med 95:436–438, 1981
399. Dekker A, Rozenberg-Arska M, Sixma JJ et al: Prevention of infection by trimethoprim-sulfamethoxazole plus amphotericin B in patients with acute nonlymphocytic leukemia. Ann Intern Med 95:555–559, 1981
400. Kauffman CA, Leipman MJ, Bergman AG et al: Trimethoprim-sulfamethoxazole prophylaxis in neutropenic patients: Reduction of infections and effect on bacterial and fungal flora. Am J Med 74:599–607, 1983
401. Gaultieri RJ, Donowitz GR, Kaiser CE et al: Double-blind randomized study of prophylactic trimethoprim-sulfamethoxazole in granulocytopenic patients with hematoloic malignancies. Am J Med 74:934–940, 1983
402. Wade JC, DeJongh CA, Newman KA et al: Selective antimicrobial modulation as prophylaxis against infection during granulocytopenia: Trimethoprim-sulfamethaxozole versus nalidixic acid. J Infect Dis 147:624–634, 1983
403. Wilson JM, Guinery DG: Failure of oral trimethoprim-sulfamethoxazole prophylaxis in acute leukemia: Isolation of resistant plasmids from strains of enterobacteriaceae causing bacteremia. N Engl J Med 306:16–20, 1982
404. Karp JE, Merz WG, Hendricksen C et al: Oral Norfloxacin for prevention of gram-negative bacterial infections in patients with acute leukemia and granulocytopenia. Ann Intern Med 106:1–7, 1987
405. Dekker AW, Rozenberg-Arska M, Verhoef J: Infection prophylaxis in acute leukemia; A comparison of cifrofloxacin with trimethoprim-sulfamethaxozole and colistin. Ann Intern Med 106:7–12, 1987
406. Meunier F: Prevention of mycoses in immunocompromised patients. Rev Infect Dis 9:408–416, 1987
407. Saral R, Bruns WH, Laskin OL et al: Acyclovir prophylaxis of herpes simplex virus infections: A randomized, double-blind controlled trial in bone marrow transplant recipients. N Engl J Med 305:63–67, 1981
408. Ambinder RF, Burns WH, Lietman PS et al: Prophylaxis: A strategy to minimise antiviral resistance. Lancet 1:1154–1155, 1984
409. Cheeseman SH, Rubin RH, Stewart JA et al: Controlled clinical trial of prophylactic human-leukocyte interferon in renal transplantation. Effects on cytomegalovirus and herpes simplex virus infections. N Engl J Med 300:1345–1349, 1979
410. Hirsch MS, Schooley RT, Cosimi AB et al: Effects of interferon-alpha on cytomegalovirus reactivation syndromes in renal-transplant recipients. N Engl J Med 308:1489–1493, 1983
411. Hughes WT, Rivera GK, Schell MJ et al: Successful intermittent chemoprophylaxis for *Pneumocystis carinii* pneumonitis. N Engl J Med 316:1627–1632, 1987
412. Gershon A: Liver attenuated varicella vaccine. J Pediatr 110:154–157, 1987
413. Jacobson DR, Zolla-Pazner S: Immunosuppression and infection in multiple myeloma. Semin Oncol 13:282–290, 1986
414. Baumgartner JD, Glauser MP, McCutcheon JA et al: Prevention of gram-negative shock and death in surgical patients by antibody to endotoxin core glycolipid. Lancet 2:59–63, 1985

CHAPTER 60 *Adverse Effects of Treatment*

SECTION 1

CLAUDIA A. SEIPP

Hair Loss

Alopecia is a psychologically distressing yet common side-effect of many chemotherapeutic agents and radiation therapy. As patients embark on new therapies, hair loss can induce a negative body image, alter interpersonal relationships, and arouse enough anxiety to cause some patients to reject potentially curative treatment.

Frank discussion of the problem by clinicians and oncology nurses with recognition of the patient's stress is helpful in preparing the patient to confront this loss.[1] Although current methods for the prevention of total scalp hair loss or the use of wigs after hair loss are not entirely satisfactory for all patients, care-givers can offer psychological support and some practical suggestions. Often the presence of a spouse, family member, or friend during this discussion with the patient is helpful to place the problem in perspective.

The hair loss caused by scalp irradiation is unpredictable. Epilation can begin at doses of 500 rad and generally progresses with spotty areas of baldness as the course of treatment continues. The prospects for hair regrowth diminish with increasing doses.[2] Radiation ports on extremities have been noted to be hair free 10 years after radiation therapy and may never have hair regrowth. In lower dose ranges regrowth begins 8 to 9 weeks after cessation of therapy. Patients should be cautioned that the new hair may be different in character from the pretreatment hair.[3]

The extent of body hair lost by patients in any chemotherapeutic program is both drug and dose dependent and is related to the frequency of cycle repetition. Often it is caused by more than one drug used in combination.[4] Long-term therapy may result in loss of pubic, axillary, and facial hair as well as scalp hair. It should be emphasized to patients that alopecia from chemotherapy is reversible, with hair regeneration beginning 1 to 2 months after therapy is discontinued. Alteration in color and texture of hair may occur: hair may be a lighter or darker shade, and is often curlier as it regrows.[5]

Hair loss may begin 1 to 2 weeks after a single chemotherapeutic dose and reaches maximum loss within 2 months in most drug sequences. Doxorubicin and cyclophosphamide are common cytologic agents known to cause epilation after two cycles at doses of doxorubicin above 50 mg/m^2 and cyclophosphamide above 500 mg/m^2. Although agents differ in the degree to which they cause hair loss, alopecia may be expected with other single-agent antibiotics, alkylators, nitrosoureas, and especially their combinations.[6,7]

HEAD COVERING

Most patients will choose to cover their heads during periods of hair loss. Nurses and clinicians can suggest wigs or head covering with stylish scarves, turbans, or hats. Wigs should be selected before hair loss begins so that the patient is prepared when alopecia occurs and so that hair color and style can be matched. Hairpieces are tax-deductible medical expenses and are covered by some medical insurance policies. Several small private businesses have been developed by former patients who distribute or sell head coverings of various designs. Through organizations such as the American Cancer Society, patients can be put in touch with other patients or cosmetologists who can provide useful suggestions for makeup and replacement of eyelashes and eyebrows. Some of the major cosmetic firms will also assist patients with makeup through local department store representatives.[8]

PREVENTION OF ALOPECIA

Several interventions have been proposed to prevent scalp hair loss from chemotherapy. The rationale for these procedures is to prevent drug circulation to the hair follicles by causing temporary vasoconstriction with either an occlusive scalp tourniquet or localized hypothermia. The pharmacokinetics of the drugs to be used must be understood before either of these methods is considered.[9] Occlusion of the superficial scalp veins must begin before the drugs are given and, to be effective, must be extended beyond the time of the peak plasma drug levels. Multiple drug half-lives may need to be considered when planning proper timing of these methods.

SCALP TOURNIQUET. Concern for the condition of underlying tissue has led most clinicians to discard the use of a rubberized tourniquet. More recently, uniform controlled pressures have been safely provided by a narrow sphygmomanometer cuff wrapped about the head below the hairline. If applied prior to injection and maintained at pressures 50 mmHg above systolic blood pressure during drug administration, the sphygmomanometer cuff may be safely left in place for 15 minutes after the cessation of treatment. Use of the cuff is limited to therapy with drugs that reach plasma concentration below epilation levels within maximum tolerance of the tourniquet—usually 20 minutes.[10-13] Because of the wide range of reported pressures and application times, it is difficult to compare the results of scalp tourniquet studies.[7]

SCALP HYPOTHERMIA. Scalp vasoconstriction can also be achieved for some patients through the application of commercially available ice turbans, which are capable of reducing temperatures at the scalp to 23° C to 24° C after 10 minutes. These temperatures are necessary to achieve hair preservation, and uniform conformity of the cap to the scalp is required. Some caps are disposable, minimizing the chance of infection between patients. The ice helmits are applied 10 minutes before the drug is given and are left in place for 30 minutes after the infusion is completed. The chemotherapist must be committed to carrying out the procedure and must apply the turban carefully, providing comfort measures during its use. Patients complain of cap heaviness and discomfort from the cold.[14-18]

Most reports of the use of scalp hypothermia have focused on preventing alopecia from doxorubicin, and excellent protection from hair loss has been reported when this drug is given in doses of less than 50 mg/m^2. However, the procedure has been reported not to be efficacious in patients given doxorubicin who have biochemical evidence of abnormal liver function. Markedly prolonged plasma drug concentrations were found in those patients with hepatic metastases, which may explain this observation.[17,18] Reduced efficacy of scalp cooling has been reported in patients receiving epirubicin, a new analogue of doxorubicin, when used in the presence of hepatic metastases.[19] Published studies of scalp icing show inconsistent results due to difficulties with drug and dose schedules and unreliable assessment parameters.[7]

That malignant cells may be spared exposure to chemotherapeutic agents may limit the usefulness of these preventative techniques. These methods are not recommended in patients who have a high risk of scalp metastasis from leukemia, lymphoma, or multiple myeloma, and perhaps some other solid tumors as well.[20-22]

Although these techniques have the potential for improving patient acceptance of chemotherapy, they are applicable only in highly selected, motivated patients. Limitations of safety, discomfort and cost must be weighed against the possible benefit of their use and should be factors discussed with patients seeking information about their application.

REFERENCES

1. Wagner L, Bye MG: Body image and patients experiencing alopecia as a result of cancer chemotherapy. Cancer Nurs 2(5):365–369, 1979
2. Moss WT, Brand WN, Battiford H: Radiation Oncology: Rationale, Techniques, Results, 5th ed, pp 57–58. St. Louis, CV Mosby, 1979
3. Nordstrom RE, Holsti LR: Hair transplantation in alopecia due to radiation. Plast Reconstr Surg 72:454–458, 1983
4. Middleton J, Franks D, Buchanan RB et al: Failure of scalp hypothermia to prevent hair loss when cyclophosphamide is added to doxorubicin and vincristine. Cancer Treat Rep 69:373–375, 1985
5. Editorial: Cancer, cancer therapy, and hair. Lancet 2:1177–1178, 1983
6. Lindsey AM: Building a knowledge base for practice: Part II. Alopecia, breast self-exam and other human responses. Oncol Nurs Forum 12:28–29, 1985
7. Cline BW: Prevention of chemotherapy-induced alopecia: A review of the literature. Cancer Nurs 7:221–228, 1984
8. Making 'Headliners'—An honest alternative to wigs. Cope Magazine, May 1987, pp 102–106
9. Wheelock JB, Myers MB, Krebs HB et al: Ineffectiveness of scalp hypothermia in the prevention of alopecia in patients treated with doxorubicin and cis-platin combinations. Cancer Treat Rep 68:1387–1388, 1984
10. O'Brien R, Zelson JH, Schwartz AD et al: Scalp tourniquet to lessen alopecia after vincristine. N Engl J Med 283:1469, 1970
11. Lyons A: Letter: Prevention of hair loss by headband during cytotoxic therapy. Lancet 1:354, 1974
12. Lovejoy NC: Preventing hair loss during Adriamycin therapy. Cancer Nurs 2:117–121, 1979
13. Maxwell M: Scalp tourniquets for chemotherapy-induced alopecia. Am J Nurs 80:900–903, 1980
14. Dean JC, Salmon SE, Griffith KS: Prevention of doxorubicin-induced hair loss with scalp hypothermia. N Engl J Med 301:1427–1429, 1979
15. Kennedy M, Packard R, Grant M et al: The effects of using Chemocap® on occurrence of chemotherapy-induced alopecia. Oncol Nurs Forum 10:19–24, 1983
16. Satterwaite B, Zimm S: The use of scalp hypothermia in the prevention of doxorubicin-induced hair loss. Cancer 54:34–37, 1984
17. Vendelbo JL: Scalp hypothermia in the prevention of chemotherapy-induced alopecia. Acta Radiol [Oncol] 24:113–116, 1985
18. Hunt JM, Anderson JE, Smith IE: Scalp hypothermia to prevent Adriamycin-induced hair loss. Canc Nurs 5:25–31, 1982
19. Robinson MH, Jones AC, Durrant KD: Effectiveness of scalp cooling in reducing alopecia caused by epirubicin treatment of breast cancer. Cancer Treat Rep 71:913–914, 1987
20. Presser SE: Letter: Prevention of doxorubicin-induced hair loss. N Engl J Med 302:921, 1980
21. Seipp CA: Letter: Scalp hypothermia: Indications for precaution. Oncol Nurs Forum 10:12, 1983
22. Witman G, Cadman E, Chen M: Misuse of scalp hypothermia. Cancer Treat Rep 65:507–508, 1981

SECTION 2

RICHARD J. GRALLA

Nausea and Vomiting

Antiemetics have become important agents in the practice of medical oncology. Studies over the past several years have identified the more useful agents and have outlined regimens appropriate to different clinical settings. With currently available antiemetics the control of nausea and vomiting can be improved in the majority of patients receiving chemotherapy likely to induce this side-effect. Although improved antiemetic control is now more easily achieved, familiarity with several agents and emetic problems is necessary if optimal results are to be obtained.

Current antiemetic investigations are focusing on newer agents that may help to address emetic problems not sufficiently handled by available drugs. Knowledge of the mechanisms by which chemotherapy induces emesis and of the neuropharmacology of antiemetic agents is important in planning treatment. Such knowledge, coupled with observations from clinical studies, allows rational provision of antiemetic therapy.

THE PHYSIOLOGY OF EMESIS

The studies of Borison and McCarthy established our current physiologic understanding of emesis.[1] Reflex-induced emesis is caused by stimulation of receptors in the central nervous system or in the gastrointestinal (GI) tract. Receptor areas have been identified that affect a vomiting center in the lateral reticular formation of the medulla, which then coordinates the act of vomiting. An important area also located in the medulla is the chemoreceptor trigger zone (CTZ), in the area postrema. This region has a variety of neurotransmitter receptors and is sensitive to chemical stimuli from both the blood and the cerebrospinal fluid. Additionally, the receptors in the GI tract have afferents, via the vagus nerve, to the vomiting center.

Chemotherapeutic agents, their metabolites, or another messenger may stimulate neuroreceptors in the GI tract or in the CTZ. Impulses generated in the CTZ or in the gut and transmitted to the vomiting center may then lead to the initiation of emesis.

Consideration of the types of neurotransmitter receptors present in these areas has been important in developing effective antiemetic treatment. Agents that block neuroreceptors in the CTZ, the vomiting center, or in the GI tract may be useful in preventing or controlling emesis. With the knowledge that the CTZ is located in area postrema, which has many different receptor types, including dopamine receptors, interest has centered on drugs with known antagonism to these receptors. Agents such as chlorpromazine, haloperidol, and metoclopramide exert their effects via this mechanism. In addition, some of the side-effects of these agents, such as extrapyramidal reactions, would also be expected based on this activity. A prominent area of new agent investigation is concerned with the development of drugs that antagonize serotonin receptors, specifically the 5-HT3 receptor. If these agents prove to be effective, they may be particularly useful in that they should not produce the side-effects associated with dopamine antagonists.

Several important questions about the mechanisms of chemotherapy-induced emesis remain. Is it the chemotherapeutic agent or some other substance that binds to the receptor to induce emesis? Why is there a difference in the likelihood of causing emesis and in the time of onset of emesis among various chemotherapy drugs? These differences are found even among agents that are structurally related or that have similar antitumor mechanisms of action.

DIFFERING EMETIC PROBLEMS

In the approach to the patient receiving chemotherapy likely to induce emesis, it is useful to consider three different emetic problems: (1) acute chemotherapy-induced emesis, (2) anticipatory emesis, and (3) delayed emesis. Among the types of emesis important differences are found in the cause of the problem and in the appropriate treatment. An additional concern is that patients may have emesis not directly related to chemotherapy. This may include emesis induced by analgesics, bronchodilators, other medications, or by tumor-related complications such as intestinal obstruction. In these instances, adjusting the medication or treating the complications of the tumor may be more important than selecting the proper antiemetic drug.

Because the most frequently encountered emetic problem is acute chemotherapy-induced emesis, and because the majority of antiemetic studies have addressed this difficulty, acute emesis will be the major topic of discussion. Separate sections concerning anticipatory and delayed emesis will follow.

PATIENT CHARACTERISTICS AND THE CONTROL OF EMESIS

Table 60-1 outlines important considerations in antiemetic therapy. With regard to the first of these, patient characteristics, it has become apparent that several aspects of a patient's history — emesis with past courses of chemotherapy,

TABLE 60-1. Important Factors in Antiemetic Therapy

Patient Characteristics
Emesis control during prior chemotherapy
Alcohol use history
Age
Chemotherapy
Emetic potential of drug
Dosage and schedule
Route of administration
Time of onset of emesis (especially with cyclophosphamide)
Consideration individually of each drug in combinations
Antiemetics
Dosage and schedule
Route of administration
Combination regimen

alcohol intake, and age—are relevant factors influencing emetic outcome.

PREVIOUS CHEMOTHERAPY. Poor control of emesis during an earlier course of chemotherapy predisposes a patient to unsatisfactory antiemetic results with subsequent treatment. In one trial reporting on this difficulty in which all patients received the same chemotherapy regimen and the same antiemetic agent, substantial control of emesis was three times more likely to occur in patients who had not previously received chemotherapy than in patients who had previously received chemotherapy.[2] Whether this finding is related to the development of conditioned anticipatory emesis or some other factor is not known.

HISTORY OF ALCOHOL INTAKE. Emesis is more easily controlled in patients with long histories of high alcohol intake (>100 g/day, or approximately five mixed drinks) than in those without such histories.[3,4] In a prospective evaluation of 52 patients receiving high-dose cisplatin and an appropriate combination antiemetic regimen, 93% of those with a history of high alcohol intake had no emesis, as opposed to 61% ($p < 0.01$) of patients who did not have this history.[3] This finding does not imply that alcohol is an antiemetic or that antiemetic treatment is not needed in patients with prior heavy alcohol use. It may indicate that receptor sites are less sensitive in patients with such a history, and that emesis is particularly likely to be successfully controlled if such patients are given effective antiemetics. This finding is also of importance in interpreting and planning antiemetic trials.

AGE. The patient's age does not appear to influence directly the control of emesis. Instead, it is associated with an increased incidence of acute dystonic reactions in younger patients given antiemetics that act by blocking dopamine receptors. This category of antiemetics includes such useful agents as substituted benzamides, butyrophenones, and phenothiazines. In a report summarizing the experience of nearly 500 patients receiving metoclopramide, the incidence of trismus or torticollis was only 2% in those over age 30, but in younger patients it was 27%.[5] In addition, when dopamine-blocking antiemetics are given on several consecutive days, dystonic reactions are also more common.[6] This can be of particular importance for younger patients, because several regimens for malignancies in this age group utilize chemotherapy on a daily schedule. This finding emphasizes the need for effective agents with a different mechanism of action. If the studies of the newer agents that antagonize serotonin receptors prove favorable, younger patients would particularly benefit from this approach.

CHEMOTHERAPEUTIC AGENTS AND EMESIS

Table 60-2 groups several common chemotherapeutic drugs according to their potential to induce emesis. The agents most often associated with emesis also induce the most severe emesis. It must be kept in mind that differences occur among patients and even between treatment courses in the same patient. These factors are important when planning a patient's antiemetic regimen, and are essential in the design of antiemetic studies. Such trials should enlist patients receiving the same chemotherapeutic agent and in the same dose range if the results are to be useful.

TABLE 60-2. Potential of Commonly Used Chemotherapy Agents to Induce Emesis

High Potential	*Low Potential*
Cisplatin	Etoposide
Dacarbazine	Mitomycin C
Dactinomycin	Methotrexate
Mechlorethamine	5-Fluorouracil
Cyclophosphamide	Hydroxyurea
Moderate Potential	Bleomycin
Carmustine	Vinblastine
Lomustine	Vincristine
Doxorubicin	Chlorambucil
Daunorubicin	
Cytarabine	
Procarbazine	

The drug dose and the route of administration can affect the incidence of nausea and vomiting. In patients who have not previously received chemotherapy, emesis typically begins 1 to 2 hours after chemotherapy is started. An important exception to this pattern occurs with cyclophosphamide. When cyclophosphamide is given intravenously (IV) in high doses, the onset of emesis is usually delayed until 9 to 18 hours after chemotherapy.[7] This finding brings out two important factors in the approach to the patient. First, an antiemetic regimen must consider the individual pattern and potential for causing emesis of the chemotherapeutic drug. Second, when combination chemotherapy is used, the emetic pattern of each drug must be considered individually. Thus, different regimens may be needed for the effective treatment of cisplatin-induced emesis than for the control of late-onset emesis caused by cyclophosphamide.

ANTIEMETIC AGENTS

The results of the past 10 years' of antiemetic trials have shown that several antiemetic agents are safe and effective. The doses and schedules of administration of many of these agents are given in Table 60-3. Because no single agent is ideal, and because studies indicate that appropriate combinations of agents can be more useful than a single drug, familiarity with a few of the more active agents is essential. Among the best studied of the more effective agents are those that exert their activity by blocking dopamine receptors. These include such classes and agents as (1) substituted benzamides (metoclopramide), (2) butyrophenones (haloperidol and droperidol), and (3) phenothiazines (prochlorperazine and chlorpromazine). Agents with different mechanisms of action include corticosteroids (dexamethasone and methylprednisolone), cannabinoids (nabilone and dronabinol), and benzodiazepines, which are being used as adjuncts to more active drugs. Newer antiemetics currently under investigation include agents that antagonize serotonin receptors and have the potential advantages of increased efficacy and decreased side-effects.

TABLE 60-3. Doses and Schedules of Frequently Used Antiemetic Agents

Antiemetic Agent	*Route*	*Dose Range*	*Frequency of Administration*
Substituted Benzamide:			
Metoclopramide	IV	1–3 mg/kg	Every 2 h
	Oral*	1–3 mg/kg	Every 2–4 h
Butyrophenones:			
Haloperidol	IV	1–3 mg	Every 2–6 h
	Oral	1–2 mg	Every 3–6 h
Droperidol	IV	0.5–2 mg	Every 4 h
Corticosteroids:			
Dexamethasone	IV/Oral	4–20 mg	Once only, or every 4–6 h
Methylprednisolone	IV	250–500 mg	Once only, or every 4–6 h
Phenothiazines:			
Prochlorperazine	Oral	5–10 mg	Every 2–4 h
	Rectal	25 mg	Every 4–6 h
	IM/IV	10–20 mg	Every 3–6 h
Chlorpromazine	Oral	25–50 mg	Every 3–6 h
	IM/IV	25 mg	Every 3–6 h
Benzodiazepine:			
Lorazepam	IV	1–2 mg/m^2	Every 4 h
Cannabinoids:			
THC	Oral	5–10 mg/m^2	Every 3–4 h
Nabilone	Oral	2 mg	Every 6–12 h

*Investigational use; 50-mg and 100-mg tablets.

Substituted Benzamides

Metoclopramide is the most frequently used drug of this class. Initial studies with metoclopramide given IV in high doses indicated that it could be given safely in this manner and that it was effective against the emesis induced by cisplatin.[2] Pharmacologic studies have varied in their findings, but a recent trial indicated that efficacy correlated with high blood levels (>850 ng/ml) of metoclopramide in patients receiving cisplatin.[8] Random assignment studies have shown metoclopramide to be superior, or at least equivalent, to all other antiemetic agents it has been compared with, against cisplatin-induced emesis.[9–14] In preventing emesis induced by cisplatin, or by cyclophosphamide plus doxorubicin, metoclopramide administration every 2 hours (beginning shortly before chemotherapy) appears to be the most effective schedule. Doses and schedules of metoclopramide are outlined in Tables 60-3 and 60-4.

Several reports have indicated useful activity of metoclopramide against the emesis associated with a number of chemotherapeutic agents.[15–17] This finding is important because it illustrates that effective agents are likely to have a broad range of antiemetic activity. Also important is maintenance of an adequate level of the antiemetic at the time of emetic vulnerability, depending on the chemotherapeutic agents used, through the use of an appropriate dosing schedule.

High oral doses of metoclopramide (investigational; 50-mg and 100-mg tablets) can be highly effective[18–20] and can be used to establish therapeutic blood levels. In a random assignment study comparing identical high doses and schedules of metoclopramide given either orally or IV to patients receiving cisplatin, 60 mg/m^2, similar results were observed in both arms of the study.[20] Emesis was completely controlled in half of the patients, while two thirds achieved a major response (two or fewer emetic episodes).

The side-effects commonly observed with metoclopramide include mild sedation, dystonic reactions (age-related, as previously discussed), akathisia (restlessness), and diarrhea, which more correctly may be an effect of specific chemotherapeutic agents such as cisplatin.[5,9,21] In general, the side-effects are not difficult to control or prevent. While diphenhydramine can be helpful against extrapyramidal reactions,[5,6] the results of a recent random assignment study are instructive. In that trial, 120 patients were assigned to receive metoclopramide plus dexamethasone plus either diphenhydramine or lorazepam.[22] With the regimen containing the benzodiazepine lorazepam, akathisia and acute dystonic reactions were almost completely eliminated and were significantly less than observed with the diphenhydramine-containing regimen. As will be discussed in the section on combinations of antiemetics, dexamethasone in addition to metoclopramide improves efficacy and reduces diarrhea.[23]

Butyrophenones

This class of agents includes haloperidol and droperidol. Both were shown to be active antiemetics in initial trials.[24,25] Because substantial differences have not been demonstrated between these two butyrophenones, most of the comments below refer to studies conducted with haloperidol. In a randomized study comparing haloperidol with metoclopramide in patients receiving cisplatin, both antiemetics were found to be effective, although greater antiemetic activity was seen with metoclopramide.[13] Doses of 1 mg to 3 mg of haloperidol given IV every 2 to 6 hours are the most commonly used (see

TABLE 60-4. Combination Antiemetics in Patients Receiving Specific Chemotherapy Regimens

General Approach:	*Neurotransmitter blocking agent* + *Corticosteroid* + *Benzodiazepine or antihistamine*	
Chemotherapeutic Agent	*Antiemetic Regimen*	
Cisplatin:*		
>99 mg/m²	Metoclopramide,† 3 mg/kg IV	30 min before chemotherapy and 90 min after chemotherapy
	+	
	Dexamethasone, 20 mg IV	40 min before chemotherapy
	+	
	Lorazepam, 1.5 mg/m² IV	35 min before chemotherapy
40–70 mg/m²	Metoclopramide,† 2 mg/kg IV	30 min before chemotherapy and 90 min after chemotherapy
	+	
	Dexamethasone‡ (as above)	
	+	
	Lorazepam (as above) *or* Diphenhydramine, 50 mg IV	35 min before chemotherapy
<40 mg/m²	Metoclopramide,‡ 1–2 mg/kg IV	(schedule as above)
	+	
	Dexamethasone‡	(schedule as above)
	+	
	Lorazepam *or* diphenhydramine	(schedule as above)
Cyclophosphamide + doxorubicin combinations	Metoclopramide, 2 or 3 mg/kg PO	Every 2 h × 3 doses, then every 4 h × 3 doses
	or	
	Metoclopramide, 3 mg/kg IV	Every 2 h × 2 doses, then 40 mg PO every 3 h × 4 doses
	or	
	Metoclopramide, 2 mg/kg IV	Every 2 h × 3 doses, then 40 mg PO every 3 h × 3 doses
	PLUS	
	Dexamethasone, 20 mg IV	(as for cisplatin)
	PLUS	
	Diphenhydramine, 50 mg IV or PO	with the first metoclopramide dose and then every other metoclopramide dose
Dacarbazine	(as for cisplatin, 40–70 mg/m²)	

*Cisplatin total dose given over 15 to 30 minutes in these studies. A longer time of cisplatin administration might require more antiemetic doses.

†Alternative choice: haloperidol, 3 mg IV.

‡Alternative choice: methylprednisolone, 250–500 mg IV.

Table 60-3); better results are reported with the higher doses and more frequent schedules.

Common side-effects of the butyrophenones include sedation, dystonic reactions, and akathisia; hypotension is occasionally observed.

Phenothiazines

Structure–activity studies indicate that variations of the side chain at position 10 of the phenothiazine ring affect the antiemetic properties of the phenothiazines.[26] Agents such as prochlorperazine would be predicted to have greater activity than other commonly used phenothiazines, such as chlorpromazine. This predicted difference, however, has not been established in patients receiving chemotherapy. The phenothiazines appear to be useful antiemetics in several situations not related to chemotherapy. The observation of poor efficacy with these drugs given to treat the emesis of the more difficult chemotherapeutic agents convinced investigators to work with newer drugs and with different administration schedules.

Prochlorperazine given in typical oral and intramuscular doses in random assignment trials has been found to be less active than metoclopramide[9] or dexamethasone,[27] and equivalent to or less active than tetrahydrocannabinol.[28–30] In a study in which prochlorperazine was given IV, a more encouraging result was reported.[31] Two problems with this trial must be considered: an imbalance in the arms of the study (concerning additional cyclophosphamide with the late onset of emesis), and failure to adequately evaluate the incidence of orthostatic blood pressure changes, an important side-effect of phenothiazines with major implications for outpatient use. Other side-effects are similar to those listed for haloperidol.

Corticosteroids

Although several theories have been postulated, the antiemetic mechanism of action of the corticosteroids remains unclear. Several open studies and random assignment trials have confirmed the utility of the corticosteroids as antiemetics,[10,11,27,32–34] with no therapeutic advantages of one corticosteroid over another demonstrated to date. Dexamethasone and methylprednisolone are the best-studied agents in this class. At our institution, we favor dexamethasone and administer it in a variety of forms. Dexamethasone doses have generally been in the range of 4 mg to 20 mg per dose. In most studies in which a corticosteroid was added to an effective agent of another class, an improved antiemetic efficacy for the combination resulted.

The toxic effects of short courses of dexamethasone or methylprednisolone have generally been mild. In patients with diabetes or other conditions predisposing to difficulties with steroids, additional caution must be used. There has been no indication of a lessening of chemotherapeutic effect when steroids have been used as antiemetics. With the low degree of toxicity and with a different mechanism of action from that of other agents, corticosteroids are good choices for use in combination antiemetic regimens.

Benzodiazepines

Benzodiazepines can be useful additions to antiemetic regimens. Their role appears to be primarily as adjuncts to effective antiemetics rather than as agents to be used singly. Trials with lorazepam have shown a high degree of patient acceptance and subjective benefit, but in general only a small degree of objective antiemetic activity.[35] In a recent random assignment trial, the addition of lorazepam to metoclopramide plus dexamethasone resulted in a significant decrease in akathisia and anxiety over that seen with the same two agents given with diphenhydramine.[22] The addition of lorazepam resulted in only a small increase in objective antiemetic efficacy.[22]

The IV dose of lorazepam typically varies from 1.0 to 1.5 mg/m^2.[35,36] This dose range is associated with marked sedation lasting several hours, which makes the use of lorazepam difficult in most outpatient settings. Studies are now in progress with the short-acting benzodiazepine midazolam to determine if it has the same beneficial effects and if it is more suitable in outpatient situations.

Cannabinoids

Recently, two cannabinoids have become available for clinical use. These agents are dronabinol (delta-9-tetrahydrocannabinol, or THC) and the synthetic cannabinoid nabilone. THC has been tried at many doses with differing schedules. Dosages in the range of 5 to 10 mg/m^2 given orally every 3 to 4 hours appear to be among the most useful.[12,37,38] In general, dronabinol has been found to be superior to placebo, and equivalent to or superior to oral prochlorperazine.[28,30] Similar results have been reported with nabilone.[39,40] Side-effects with cannabinoids have been frequent but are generally manageable. These have included sedation, dry mouth, orthostatic hypotension, ataxia, dizziness, a "high," and euphoria or dysphoria. The role of the cannabinoids remains unclear. Dronabinol has been advertised as an effective second-choice agent; however, there is little evidence to support this claim when the agent is compared with the more active agents that are currently available. Agents such as metoclopramide and the corticosteroids are superior and have fewer side-effects.[12,41]

Serotonin Antagonists

Perhaps the most interesting new class of agents being investigated currently are those that block serotonin receptors, specifically the 5-HT3 receptor.[42] These receptors have been identified in the gut, and some recent studies have indicated that 5-HT3 receptors may also be present in the central nervous system. When used in high doses, metoclopramide may have activity at this site, in addition to its known dopamine receptor–blocking properties.[43] Although this observation may explain part of the antiemetic activity of metoclopramide, it would be especially important to have effective agents without dopamine receptor–blocking properties, because the latter action is likely responsible for the dystonic reactions associated with many antiemetics.

The best-studied serotonin antagonist currently in antiemetic trials is ondansetron (GR C-507/75). Phase I and initial open studies have indicated effective antiemetic activity of ondansetron against a variety of chemotherapeutic drugs.[44,45] To date, akathisia and dystonic reactions have not been reported with this agent. Trials are ongoing to determine effective doses and schedules for differing clinical settings. Formal comparison studies will be needed to determine the relative efficacy of this and similar agents.

ANTIEMETIC COMBINATIONS

Antiemetic studies of single agents have indicated which are the most effective and which are the most likely to be useful when combined with other active drugs. Several considerations should be kept in mind when planning combination regimens. The agents selected should be active when used singly, and the optimal doses, route of administration, and schedules should be established. The regimen should combine agents that have different mechanisms of activity and do not have overlapping toxicities. A combination may be useful if the added agent lessens the side-effects of the regimen or if it reduces other toxic effects of the chemotherapy (see Table 60-4).

Several recent studies have compared metoclopramide with the combination of metoclopramide plus a corticosteroid. The combination of the two active antiemetics has been superior to the single agent in all of the trials.[23,46–49] In addition to improved antiemetic efficacy with the steroid plus metoclopramide, the incidence of diarrhea was significantly reduced. An open study combining a butyrophenone with a corticosteroid also reported favorable results.[50]

The preferred antiemetic regimen for patients receiving high doses of cisplatin (120 mg/m^2) at our institution has been as follows: metoclopramide, 3 mg/kg IV 30 minutes before cisplatin and 90 minutes after the start of the cisplatin, plus dexamethasone, 20 mg IV 40 minutes before cisplatin, plus lorazepam, 1.5 mg/m^2 IV 35 minutes before chemotherapy.[22] Following hydration and mannitol administration, the cisplatin is administered over 20 minutes. Complete control of emesis can be expected in more than 60% of patients, and major control (zero to two emetic episodes) in almost 90%.[22]

Table 60-4 outlines recommended regimens, and alternatives, for use with a variety of chemotherapeutic drugs. These regimens have all been tested, either in formal comparison studies or in open trials. Unless a specific agent is contraindicated for a particular patient, combinations are recommended.

Chemotherapy regimens that entail several consecutive days of treatment present a special problem in emesis control. The antiemetics that block dopamine receptors appear to result in a greater incidence of dystonic reactions when given on multiple consecutive days. Of additional interest is the observation that when agents such as cisplatin or dacarbazine are given over several days, the emesis gradually lessens. The regimen currently being investigated at our institution in patients (generally older than age 30) receiving cisplatin (25–33 mg/m^2/day for 3 to 4 days) employs gradually decreasing doses of antiemetics. Patients are given dexamethasone, 20 mg IV, 30 minutes before the start of chemotherapy each day. Metoclopramide, 2 mg/kg, is also given 30 minutes before cisplatin. On the first and second treatment days, the same dose of metoclopramide is repeated 90 minutes after cisplatin; on the third day, the metoclopramide dose is repeated but only at 1 mg/kg; and on the fourth day no repeat dose of metoclopramide is given. Diphenhydramine, 50 mg IV, is given with the first metoclopramide dose each day. The study is still in progress, but initial results are encouraging in patients in this age group. As previously discussed, the newer serotonin antagonist agents, which may not produce dystonic reactions, could prove to be ideal for the multiple-day chemotherapy setting, especially in younger patients, if these drugs are found to be sufficiently active.

ANTICIPATORY EMESIS

Anticipatory emesis is defined as nausea or vomiting, often beginning before the administration of chemotherapy, in patients with poor control of emesis during previous episodes of chemotherapy. Because it is a conditioned response, the hospital environment or other treatment-related associations may trigger the onset of emesis. The administration of the chemotherapy itself may bring on this response, not only as a chemical stimulus, but also as a psychological factor. The stronger the emetic stimulus and the poorer the control, the greater the likelihood that anticipatory emesis will develop.[51,52]

Preventing anticipatory emesis is probably a more effective strategy than treating it once it has occurred. The problem of anticipatory emesis underscore the importance of giving the most effective antiemetics with the initial course of emesis-producing chemotherapy. Reports have indicated that behavior therapy techniques can be helpful once anticipatory emesis is a problem. In one random assignment study, the efficacy of systematic desensitization was compared with counseling and with no treatment in 60 patients (20 in each group) with anticipatory emesis. The patients had a variety of malignant diseases and were receiving several different chemotherapeutic regimens. With further courses of chemotherapy, improvement was seen in the group treated with desensitization. Significant differences in the incidence, severity, and duration of anticipatory emesis were reported.[53] Relaxation techniques and hypnosis have been said to have some value for this specific problem[54,55]; however, these methods have not been compared with each other or with the administration of benzodiazepines.

DELAYED EMESIS

Delayed emesis is defined as nausea or vomiting beginning 24 hours or more after chemotherapy administration. The pathophysiology of this problem is not clear. Possibilities include residual chemotherapeutic drug or its metabolites, or coexisting conditions caused by the chemotherapy, such as gastritis. Delayed emesis is a particular problem with major causes of emesis such as high-dose cisplatin. A recent natural history study noted that delayed emesis is less severe than acute emesis but still causes significant difficulties with hydration and nutrition, as well as contributing to a lowered activity level. Although delayed emesis occurs less often in patients who have complete emetic control on the day of chemotherapy, it may occur in this group as well. The majority of patients treated with cisplatin at doses above 100 mg/m^2 experience some degree of delayed emesis, with onset most frequently 48 to 72 hours after chemotherapy; in some instances the problem may occur as late as 4 or 5 days after treatment.[56]

Favorable results from two preliminary therapeutic trials led to a recent study in which a combination of oral antiemetics was compared with a single agent and with placebo in a blinded random assignment design.[57] Over the 4-day study period, 82% of patients given placebo had at least one episode of emesis, in contrast to only 39% of patients given oral dexamethasone plus oral metoclopramide ($p < 0.02$). Results with dexamethasone as a single agent in this trial were intermediate between those of placebo and the combination.[57] The doses used for the delayed emesis regimen are given in Table 60-5. Open studies using a steroid plus prochlorperazine combination have also shown beneficial results.[58]

CONCLUSION

The control of emesis is an important area for sharing of skills and experiences by physicians and nurses who are oncology specialists. While new agents would be helpful, better application of the available techniques would likely result in major improvements in patient care. This goal requires a knowledge of the more active drugs, experience with their use in combination, and consideration of the emetic problem of each patient.

Improvements in specific areas of antiemetic treatment would be most helpful. With the predisposition to dystonic reactions in younger patients and in those receiving daily chemotherapy, control of emesis remains difficult. The newer serotonin antagonists with activity not exerted through dopamine receptors might solve these problems. Effective approaches for delayed emesis remain important considerations; the results of recently reported trials appear to show improvement in the management of this problem.

It is important that new studies be accurately interpreted. Careful and critical review of antiemetic studies is necessary. Precision in evaluation techniques is mandatory if accurate results are to be obtained. Additionally, attention to the differing patient characteristics and to specific emetic patterns of individual chemotherapeutic agents must be considered in the design and interpretation of trials.

TABLE 60-5. Antiemetic Regimen for Delayed Emesis

Days 1 & 2 after chemotherapy	Days 3 & 4 after chemotherapy
Metoclopramide: 0.5 mg/kg orally, q.i.d.	as needed only (20–40 mg orally)
+	
Dexamethasone: 8 mg orally, b.i.d.	4 mg orally, b.i.d.

REFERENCES

1. Borison HL, McCarthy LE: Neuropharmacology of chemotherapy induced emesis. Drugs 25:8–17, 1983
2. Gralla RJ, Braun TJ, Squillante A et al: Metoclopramide: Initial clinical studies of high dosage regimens in cisplatin-induced emesis. In Poster E (ed): The Treatment of Nausea and Vomiting Induced by Cancer Chemotherapy, pp 167–176. New York, Masson, 1981
3. D'Acquisto RW, Tyson LB, Gralla RJ et al: The influence of a chronic high alcohol intake on chemotherapy-induced nausea and vomiting. Proc Am Soc Clin Oncol 5:257, 1986
4. Sulivan Jr, Leyden MJ, Bell R: Decreased cisplatin induced nausea and vomiting with alcohol ingestion. N Engl J Med 309:13, 796, 1983
5. Kris MG, Tyson LB, Gralla RJ et al: Extrapyramidal reactions with high-dose metoclopramide. N Engl J Med 309:433, 1983
6. Allen JC, Gralla RJ, Reilly C et al: Metoclopramide: Dose-related toxicity and preliminary antiemetic studies in children receiving cancer chemotherapy. J Clin Oncol 3:1136–1141, 1985
7. Fetting JH, Grochow LB, Folstein MF et al: The course of nausea and vomiting after high-dose cyclophosphamide. Cancer Treat Rep 66:1487–1493, 1982
8. Meyer BR, Lewin M, Dreyer DE et al: Optimizing metoclopramide control of cisplatin-induced emesis. Ann Intern Med 100:393–395, 1984
9. Gralla RJ, Itri LM, Pisko SE et al: Antiemetic efficacy of high-dose metoclopramide: Randomized trials with placebo and prochlorperazine in patients with chemotherapy-induced nausea and vomiting. N Engl J Med 305:905–909, 1981
10. Frustaci S, Tumolo S, Tirell U et al: High-dose metoclopramide versus dexamethasone in the prevention of cisplatin induced vomiting. Proc Am Soc Clin Oncol 2:87, 1983
11. Aapro MS, Plezia PM, Alberts DS et al: Double-blind crossover study of the antiemetic efficacy of high-dose dexamethasone vs. high-dose metoclopramide. Proc Am Soc Clin Oncol 2:93, 1983
12. Gralla RJ, Tyson LB, Borden LB et al: Antiemetic therapy: A review of recent studies and a report of a random assignment trial comparing metoclopramide with delta-9-tetrahydrocannabinol. Cancer Treat Rep 68:163–172, 1984
13. Grunberg SM, Gala KV, Lampenfeld M et al: Composition of the antiemetic effect of high-dose intravenous metoclopramide and high-dose intravenous haloperidol in a randomized double-blind crossover study. J Clin Oncol 2:782–787, 1984
14. Richards PD, Flaum MA, Batemen M et al: The antiemetic efficacy of secobarbitol and chlorpromazine compared to metoclopramide, diphenhydramine, and dexamethasone: A randomized trial. Cancer 58:959–962, 1986
15. Tyson LB, Clark RA, Gralla RJ: High-dose metoclopramide: Control of dacarbazine-induced emesis in a preliminary trial. Cancer Treat Rep 66:2108, 1982
16. Strum SB, McDermed JE, Opfell RW et al: Intravenous metoclopramide: An effective antiemetic in cancer chemotherapy. JAMA 247:2683–2686, 1982
17. Tyson LB, Gralla RJ, Clark RA et al: Effective oral and intravenous antiemetic combinations using high-dose metoclopramide. In Proceedings of the 4th European Conference on Clinical Oncology and Cancer Nursing, 1987, p 280
18. Garnick MB: Oral metoclopramide and cisplatin chemotherapy. Ann Intern Med 99:127, 1983
19. Gralla RJ, Tyson LB, Clark RA et al: An all oral combination antiemetic regimen of patients receiving cytoxan + Adriamycin + vincristine (CAV). Proc Am Soc Clin Oncol 4:267, 1985
20. Anthony LB, Krozely MG, Woodward NJ et al: Antiemetic effect of oral versus intravenous metoclopramide in patients receiving cisplatin: A randomized double-blind trial. J Clin Oncol 4:94–103, 1986
21. von Hoff DD, Schilsky R, Reichert CM et al: Toxic effects of cisdichlorodiammineplatinum (II) in man. Cancer Treat Rep 63:1527–1531, 1979
22. Kris MG, Gralla RJ, Clark RA et al: Antiemetic control and prevention of side effects of anticancer therapy with lorazepam or diphenhydramine when used in combination with metoclopramide plus dexamethasone: A double-blind, randomized trial. Cancer 60:2816–2822, 1987
23. Kris MG, Gralla RJ, Tyson LB et al: Improved control of cisplatin-induced emesis with high-dose metoclopramide and with combinations of metoclopramide, dexamethasone, and diphenhydramine: Results of consecutive trials in 255 patients. Cancer 55:527–534, 1985
24. Grossman B, Lessin LS, Cohen P: Droperidol prevents nausea and vomiting from cisplatinum. N Engl J Med 301:47, 1979
25. Neidhart J, Gayen M, Metz E: Haldol is an effective antiemetic for platinum and mustard induced vomiting when other agents fail. Proc Am Soc Clin Oncol 21:365, 1980
26. Wampler G: The pharmacology and clinical effectiveness of phenothiazines and related drugs for managing chemotherapy-induced emesis. Drugs 25:31–51, 1983
27. Markman M, Sheidler V, Ettinger DS et al: Antiemetic efficacy of dexamethasone: Randomized, double-blind, crossover study with prochlorperazine in patients receiving cancer chemotherapy. N Engl J Med 311:549–552, 1984
28. Frytak S, Moertel CG, O'Fallon J et al: Delta-9-tetrahydrocannabinol as an antiemetic

in patients treated with cancer chemotherapy: A double-blind comparison with prochlorperazine and a placebo. Ann Intern Med 91:825–830, 1979
29. Orr LE, McKerman JF, Bloone B: Antiemetic effect of tetrahydrocannabinol. Arch Intern Med 140:1431–1433, 1980
30. Sallan SE, Cronin CM, Zelen M et al: Antiemetics in patients receiving chemotherapy for cancer: A randomized comparison of delta-9-tetrahydrocannabinol and prochlorperazine. N Engl J Med 302:135–138, 1980
31. Carr BI, Bertrand M, Browning S et al: A comparison of the antiemetic efficacy of prochlorperazine and metoclopramide for the treatment of cisplatin-induced emesis: A prospective randomized double-blind study. J Clin Oncol 3:1127–1132, 1985
32. Aapro MS, Plezia PM, Alberts DS et al: Double-blind crossover study of the antiemetic efficacy of high-dose dexamethasone vs high-dose metoclopramide. Proc Am Soc Clin Oncol 2:93, 1983
33. Cassileth PA, Lusk EJ, Torri S et al: Antiemetic efficacy of dexamethasone therapy in patients receiving cancer chemotherapy. Arch Intern Med 143:1347–1349, 1983
34. Lee BJ: Methylprednisolone as an antiemetic. N Engl J Med 3034:486, 1981
35. Laszlo J, Clark RA, Hanson DC et al: Lorazepam in cancer patients treated with cisplatin: A drug with antiemetic, amnesic, and anxiolytic effects. J Clin Oncol 3:864–869, 1985
36. Kris MG, Gralla RJ, Clark RA et al: Consecutive dose-finding trials adding lorazepam to the combination of metoclopramide plus dexamethasone: Improved subjective effectiveness over the combination of diphenhydramine plus metoclopramide plus dexamethasone. Cancer Treat Rep 69:1257–1262, 1985
37. Chang AE, Shiling DJ, Stillman RC et al: Delta-9-tetrahydrocannabinol as an antiemetic in patients receiving high-dose methotrexate: A prospective randomized evaluation. Ann Intern Med 91:819–824, 1979
38. Vincent BJ, McQuistion DJ, Einhorn LH et al: Review of cannabinoids and their antiemetic effectiveness. Drugs 25:52–62, 1983
39. Herman TS, Einhorn LH, Jones SE: Superiority of nabilone over prochlorperazine as an antiemetic in patients receiving cancer chemotherapy. N Engl J Med 300:1295–1297, 1979
40. Steele N, Gralla RJ, Braun DW Jr: Double-blind comparison of the anti-emetic effects of nabilone and prochlorperazine in chemotherapy-induced emesis. Cancer Treat Rep 64:219–224, 1980
41. Venner P, Bruera E, Drebit D et al: Intensive treatment scheduling of nabilone (N) plus dexamethasone (DM) vs. metoclopramide (M) plus DM in cisplatinum (CP)-induced emesis. Proc Am Soc Clin Oncol 5:253, 1986
42. Miner WD, Sanger GJ: Inhibition of cisplatin-induced vomiting by selective 5-hydroxytryptamine M-receptor antagonism. Br J Pharmacol 88:497–499, 1986
43. Fozard JR: Neuronal 5-HT receptors in the periphery. Neuropharmacology 23:1473–1486, 1984
44. Cunningham D, Poplc A, Ford I-T et al: Prevention of emesis in patients receiving cytotoxic drugs by GR38032F, a selective 5-HT3 receptor antagonist. Lancet 1:1461–1462, 1987
45. Clark RA, Gralla RJ, Kris MG et al: Phase I antiemetic trial of the serotonin antagonist GRC507175. In Proceedings of the 4th European Conference on Clinical Oncology and Cancer Nursing, 1987, p 278
46. Allan SG, Cornbleet MA, Warrington PS et al: Dexamethasone and high dose metoclopramide: Efficacy in controlling cisplatin-induced nausea and vomiting. Br Med J 289:878–879, 1984
47. Rosell R, Abad-Esteve A, Ribas-Mundo M et al: Evaluation of a combination antiemetic regimen including IV high-dose metoclopramide, dexamethasone, and diphenhydramine in cisplatin-based chemotherapy regimens. Cancer Treat Rep 69:909–910, 1985
48. Roila F, Tonato M, Basurto C et al: Antiemetic activity of high doses of metoclopramide (MTC) combined with methylprednisolone (P) vs. MTX alone in cisplatin treated cancer patients (PTS): A randomized double blind trial of the Italian Oncology Group for Clinical Research 9GOIRCO. Proc Am Soc Clin Oncol 5:263, 1986
49. Grunberg SM, Akerley WL, Baker C et al: Comparison of methoclopramide (M) and metoclopramide + dexamethasone (M + D) in complete prevention of cisplatinum induced emesis (abstr). Proc Am Soc Clin Oncol 4:262, 1985
50. Mason BA, Dambra J, Grossman B et al: Effective control of cisplatin-induced nausea using high-dose steroids and droperidol. Cancer Treat Rep 66:243–245, 1982
51. Morrow GR: Prevalence and correlates of anticipatory nausea and vomiting in chemotherapy patients. JNCI 68:585–588, 1982
52. Wilcox PM, Fetting JH, Nettesheim KM et al: Anticipatory vomiting in women receiving cyclophosphamide, methotrexate and 5-FU (CMF) adjuvant chemotherapy for breast carcinoma. Cancer Treat Rep 66:1601–1604, 1982
53. Morrow GR, Morrell C: Behavioral treatment for the anticipatory nausea and vomiting induced by cancer chemotherapy. N Engl J Med 307:1476–1480, 1982
54. Burish TG, Lyles JN: Effectiveness of relaxation training in reducing adverse reactions to cancer chemotherapy. J Behav Med 4:65–78, 1981
55. Redd WH, Andersen GV: Conditioned adversion in cancer patients. Behav Therapist 4:3–4, 1981
56. Kris MG, Gralla RJ, Clark RA et al: Incidence, course, and severity of delayed nausea and vomiting following the administration of high-dose cisplatin. J Clin Oncol 3:1379–1384, 1985
57. Tyson LB, Kris MG, Gralla RJ et al: Double-blind, randomized trial for the control of delayed emesis: Comparison of placebo vs dexamethasone vs metoclopramide plus dexamethasone (abstr). Proc Am Soc Clin Oncol 6:267, 1987
58. Strum SB, McDermed J, Abrahano-Umali R et al: Management of cisplatin (DDP)-induced delayed-onset nausea (N) and vomiting (V): Preliminary results with two drug regimens. Proc Am Soc Clin Oncol 4:263, 1985
59. Homesley HD, Gainey JM, Jobson VN et al: Double-blind placebo-controlled study of metoclopramide in cisplatin-induced emesis. N Engl J Med 307:250–251, 1982

SECTION 3 STEPHEN T. SONIS

Oral Complications of Cancer Therapy

The mouth is often a significant site of complications in the patient receiving therapy for cancer. Not only are patients with malignancies of the head and neck susceptible to such problems, but also affected are patients receiving treatment for more distant disease. Virtually all patients who receive radiation therapy to the head and neck develop oral side-effects of their treatment. Approximately 40% of patients who are treated with chemotherapy develop oral complications. This frequency is even higher for patients receiving radiation to the head or neck. Of major importance has been the demonstration that aggressive pre-cancer therapy oral evaluation and intervention to eliminate potential sources of infection or irritation, as well as preventive measures during therapy, result in a precipitous drop in the frequency of oral problems.[1] In addition to affecting adversely the patient's ability to eat, speak, and control saliva, cancer therapy may have even more significant ramifications, especially relative to sepsis. Because of the mouth's vast bacterial and fungal flora, it is an important potential portal for these organisms in the myelosuppressed host; the mouth is the most frequently identifiable source of sepsis in the granulocytopenic cancer patient. Nevertheless, many of the oral problems associated with cancer therapy can be prevented or minimized with adequate pretherapy care and with aggressive preventive techniques during treatment.

ORAL COMPLICATIONS OF RADIATION THERAPY

For the most part, oral problems due to radiation therapy are the result of local tissue changes from direct radiation. For that reason, implants tend to produce more problems than does beam radiation. Radiation results in mucosal atrophy due to decreased cell renewal; fibrosis of the salivary glands, muscles, ligaments, and blood vessels; and damage to taste buds.[2]

Mucositis is the result of atrophic changes in the epithelium because of decreased cell renewal and usually is noted at a dose level of about 2000 rad when therapy is administered at a rate of 200 rad/day. Patients complain of generalized discomfort and drying of the mucosa. Erythema is present. Any traumatized area may ulcerate. Generally, nonkeratinized epithelium of the cheeks, lips, soft palate, and ventral surface of the tongue is affected. Mucositis is extremely uncomfortable for the patient and may limit oral intake. It is self-limiting, however, and usually resolves in 2 to 3 weeks after the termination of radiation treatment.

Treatment of mucositis is palliative and aimed at minimizing mucosal trauma. Rinses are helpful (*e.g.*, Xylocaine viscous, Dyclone, or Kaopectate and Benadryl). Ice chips or Popsicles are soothing. Patients should be instructed to avoid spicy or acidic foods. Unusually sharp teeth should be smoothed or eliminated. Removal of prostheses should be used sparingly. Oral hygiene should be stressed.

Xerostomia is one of the most frequent side-effects of radiation to the head and neck and is due to changes in the salivary glands.[3] Generally, there is a direct relationship between the dose of radiation to the salivary glands and the extent of glandular changes.[4] Under 6000 rad, changes in the salivary glands induced by radiation, including edema and inflammation, are reversible. over 6000 rad, changes may be permanent, with fibrosis and glandular degeneration. Clinically, xerostomia has been reported with as little as two to three doses of 200 rad to 225 rad.[4]

Xerostomia predisposes to increases in the number of oral bacteria because saliva is no longer available to help clear bacteria from the mouth, or as a source of IgA. The patient's ability to taste is altered.

The most consistent consequence of xerostomia is the development of radiation caries, which characteristically appears in the cervical regions or incisal edges of teeth a few months after the start of radiation therapy.[2,5] Left untreated, caries and decalcification may become so severe that the integrity of the tooth is compromised and fracture occurs. The causes of radiation caries include loss of salivary buffering capacity, lowered salivary *p*H, elimination of mechanical flushing, and decreased salivary IgA.

Treatment of xerostomia has four goals:

1. Stimulation of existing salivary flow
2. Replacement of lost secretions
3. Protection of the dentition
4. Reduction of sucrose intake.

Stimulation of the patient's remaining salivary apparatus may be accomplished with sucrose-free lemon drops. Sugar-free chewing gum may satisfy the same objective; mint- or cinnamon-flavored gum is to be avoided as it may irritate the mucosa. Saliva substitutes such as Xero-lube or Salivart may be used before meals and at bedtime.[6]

Prevention of radiation-induced caries is best accomplished by the aggressive use of fluorides.[7] Customized trays should be fabricated for patients so that they may deliver home fluoride treatments on a daily basis; this may be supplemented with fluoride rinses. Generally, aciuulated fluorides are the most effective, although neutral fluorides may become necessary in patients with mucositis. Fluorides should be continued until full salivary function has returned. An alternative to fluoride-containing trays is the daily use of fluoride gel as a tooth brushing agent. Stannous fluoride 0.4% gel appears to be more effective than sodium fluoride 0.1% as it reduces detectable levels of caries-causing *Streptococcus mutans*.[8] In addition, scrupulous oral hygiene and aggressive professional maintenance are critical to minimizing the development of caries. Finally, the patient's avoidance of sucrose is to be encouraged.

Loss of taste is a common sequela of radiation therapy. It usually is noted with a cumulative dose of between 1000 rad and 2000 rad.[9] Most often, loss of the ability to differentiate sweet and salty is reported as often leading to an avoidance of foods with such tastes. Bitterness is common. Taste sensation usually returns 6 to 12 months after the completion of therapy.

The most serious local sequelae of head and neck radiation therapy are osteoradionecrosis, which occurs when there is fibrotic thickening of blood vessels, replacement of marrow with connective tissue, a subsequent lack of new bone formation, and bone death. The bone becomes susceptible to infection and its ability to heal is impaired. The reported incidence of osteoradionecrosis ranges from 4% to 35%; 90% of cases occur in the mandible.[10] Approximately 39% of cases occur spontaneously and 61% are related to trauma. The most frequent form of osteoradionecrosis-producing trauma is tooth extraction. Most spontaneous cases of osteoradionecrosis occur within the first 6 to 24 months after treatment. By contrast, trauma-related osteonecrosis has two peaks of activity, the first peak 3 months after radiation therapy and the second peak 2 to 5 years after treatment.[11]

Four major risk factors predispose to the development of osteoradionecrosis: (1) the anatomical site of the tumor, (2) the dose of radiation, (3) the dental status of the patient,[10] and (4) the type and source of radiation. Patients receiving radiation therapy to tumors anatomically related to the mandible develop osteoradionecrosis at five times the rate of patients with tumors at other sites. The risk of osteoradionecrosis is increased significantly at doses of 6000 rad or more: the risk of developing osteoradionecrosis is increased twofold for patients receiving greater than 8000 rad compared to 5000 rad to 6000 rad, and is almost five times as great as when the patient receives 4000 rad to 5000 rad. Dentulous patients are more likely to develop osteoradionecrosis than are edentulous patients. Furthermore, patients with dental disease are at twice the risk of dentulous patients without dental disease.[12] Therefore, meticulous oral hygiene, elimination of diseased teeth, aggressive prophylaxis, and follow-up should be stressed. Oral hygiene techniques for the patient receiving radiation therapy may include standard brushing and flossing. Water-irrigating devices (*i.e.*, Water-Pik) may be helpful for removal of food particles or other debris but are ineffective for the elimination of toothborne bacteria. Patients should be cautioned to use them at low pressures. Similarly, sucrose intake should be minimized and topical fluorides should be used regularly. Patients receiving external beam sources of radiation are at least twice as likely to develop osteoradionecrosis as those receiving radiation from implanted sources. Patients receiving supervoltage radiation therapy of 1 meV or more are at significantly higher risk for osteonecrosis than are patients receiving particulate neutron beam therapy.[12]

Patients with poorly fitting prostheses are also at risk for osteoradionecrosis because breaks in the epithelium and pressure on supporting bone may cause infection and necrosis.

The issue of if and when dental extractions should be performed is unresolved.[11-14] At times when low-energy radiation was used, the common protocol was to extract all teeth in the path of the primary beam before the start of therapy to eliminate potential sources of infection and osteoradionecrosis. Improvements in the type of radiation used, more selective fields of radiation, increased concern for patient function and esthetics, and the success of preventive dental protocols have modified this approach, however. An approach has evolved aimed at the elimination of actively infected teeth, with aggressive dental preventive techniques for the remaining dentition. It is important to note that sites of extractions performed prior to radiation therapy are also at increased risk for the development of osteoradionecrosis, although not at the same frequency as extraction sites created after the start of radiation therapy. Therefore, teeth demonstrating periapical pathology or active periodontal infection should be extracted as long as possible before the start of radiation therapy, with a minimum of 3 weeks. Nonrestorable teeth or teeth with deep caries and a significant risk of developing infection also should be eliminated. Teeth at marginal risk and unlikely to become infected should be retained. Where possible, extractions should be postponed until 1 year after the termination of radiation. Antibiotic prophylaxis is recommended. Endodontic therapy can be used as a temporary measure to "buy time" if a problem occurs during radiation therapy, although endodontics does not appear to have permanent efficacy in this group.[15]

ORAL COMPLICATIONS OF CANCER CHEMOTHERAPY

Of all patients receiving chemotherapy, approximately 40% will develop oral problems during each exposure to drug.[16] Although the spectrum of problems is wide, essentially all oral complications of chemotherapy occur through one of two major mechanisms: they are either a direct effect of the drug on the oral mucosa (*direct stomatoxicity*) or an indirect result of myelosuppression (*indirect stomatoxicity*) (Fig. 60-1).

Not all patients are at equal risk of developing oral problems associated with their specific chemotherapy. Factors that influence the frequency and severity of these complications may be grouped into those that are related to the patient and those that are related to the drug. Patient-related factors include the type of malignancy, patient age, and the level of oral health before and during therapy.

Patients with hematologic malignancies (*e.g.*, leukemia, lymphoma) develop oral problems at two or three times the rate of patients with solid tumors.[17,19] This is probably because these patients are functionally myelosuppressed as a consequence of the malignancies.[20,21] Young patients tend to develop oral problems more frequently than older patients: whereas 90% of patients between the ages of 1 and 20 years develop oral problems after chemotherapy, only 18% of patients over age 60 develop problems.[17] Part of the reason for this finding is attributable to the high incidence of hematolo-

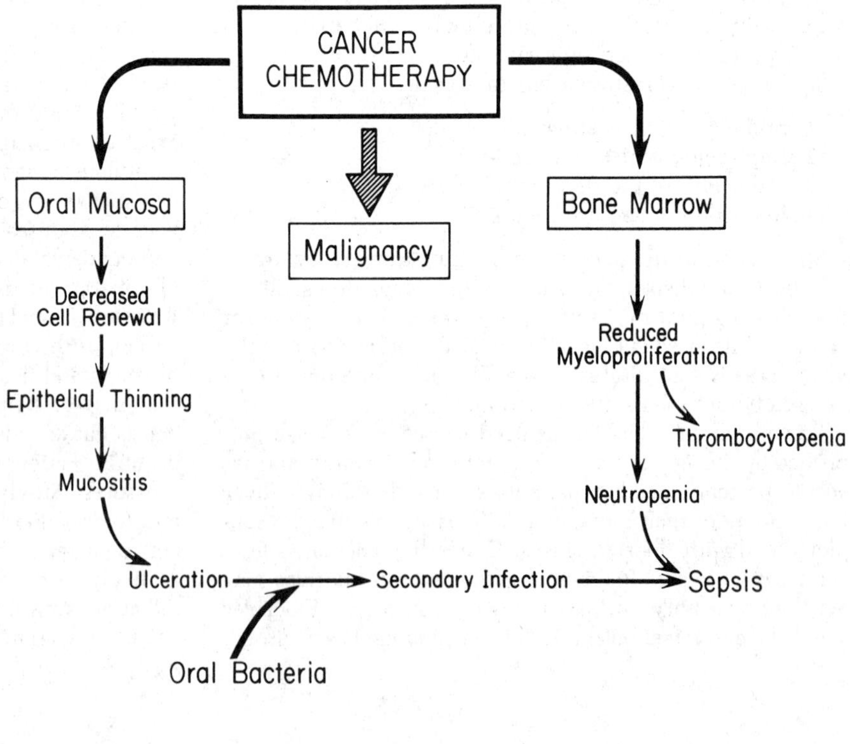

FIG. 60-1. Effects of cancer chemotherapy on both the oral basal epithelial cells and the bone marrow stem cells.

gic malignancies in the younger age group. When oral problems are evaluated in patients with the same malignancy and the same chemotherapeutic regimen, however, this finding holds up. An explanation for the above may be that cell renewal is decreased in older patients.[22] Additionally, the number of mitoses in the basal epithelium of younger patients is greater than in older patients. Patients in poor oral health, especially those with preexisting periodontal or pulpal disease, have a higher risk of developing oral infection in the face of chemotherapy-induced myelosuppression.[23-25] Similarly, patients with irritating prostheses or sharp or broken teeth are at increased risk for developing ulceration and mucositis. Patients in whom preexisting periodontal and dental disease is eliminated before therapy and who receive aggressive mouth care during treatment have a significant decrease in the frequency of oral problems associated with chemotherapy.[25-27]

Therapy-related variables also influence the frequency and severity with which patients develop problems. Probably the single most important factor in this area is choice of drug.[17,28,29] Although stomatotoxicity is a common side-effect of many forms of chemotherapy, drugs differ significantly in the extent of the stomatotoxicity they cause. In many instances, stomatotoxicity is dose related. This effect can be reduced by delivering an agent in divided doses, rather than as a bolus.[29] Finally, concomitant therapy such as radiation increases the frequency and severity with which patients develop oral problems in response to chemotherapy.

DIRECT STOMATOTOXICITY

Direct stomatotoxicity is the consequence of the nonspecific effect of a drug on cells undergoing mitosis. Cells of the mouth undergo rapid renewal over a 7- to 14-day cycle. Chemotherapy may cause a reduction in the renewal rate of the basal epithelium, which results in mucosal atrophy.[30,31] Diminished nutritional intake secondary to mucositis[32] may compound the problem because there is an overall decrease in cell migration and renewal after starvation or protein deprivation. Clinically, patients experience pain from mucositis and ulceration. Lesions are generally discrete initially, but often progress to produce confluent areas of ulceration (Fig. 60-2). Nonkeratinized mucosa is most often affected. The buccal, labial, and soft palatal mucosa, along with the ventral surface of the tongue and the floor of the mouth, are the most common sites. Lesions do not progress outside the mouth (Fig. 60-3). Direct stomatotoxicity is usually observed 5 to 7 days after the administration of the drug. Left untreated, lesions generally heal without scarring within 2 to 3 weeks in the nonmyelosuppressed patient. A wide variety of agents may produce direct stomatotoxicity (Table 60-6).

The major clinical problem associated with direct stomatotoxicity is pain, with a consequent loss of function, especially ability to eat. Patients are miserable and are often unable to sleep because of oral pain. Currently, treatment of direct stomatotoxicity is palliative (Table 60-7). A variety of agents are currently available, including Xylocaine viscous and Dyclone. A rinse of frequent benefit may be prepared by mixing equal proportions of elixir of Benadryl and Kaopectate. The use of milk of magnesia as a vehicle for the delivery of palliative agents is to be avoided because of its desiccating effect on the mucosa. In severe cases, 2.5% to 5% cocaine rinses or spray may be used. The latter is recommended only in supervised inpatient settings because of the potential for neurotoxicity. In the case of discrete ulceration, ointments, such as benzocaine in Orabase, may be applied to the affected area after it is dried with a sponge. The use of systemic pain medication is often of value. Patients often find cold soothing; ice chips, Popsicles, and cold beverages may be helpful.

Xerostomia is a common side-effect of some forms of chemotherapy and accelerates the development of mucositis.[13] Management of xerostomia is discussed elsewhere in this chapter.

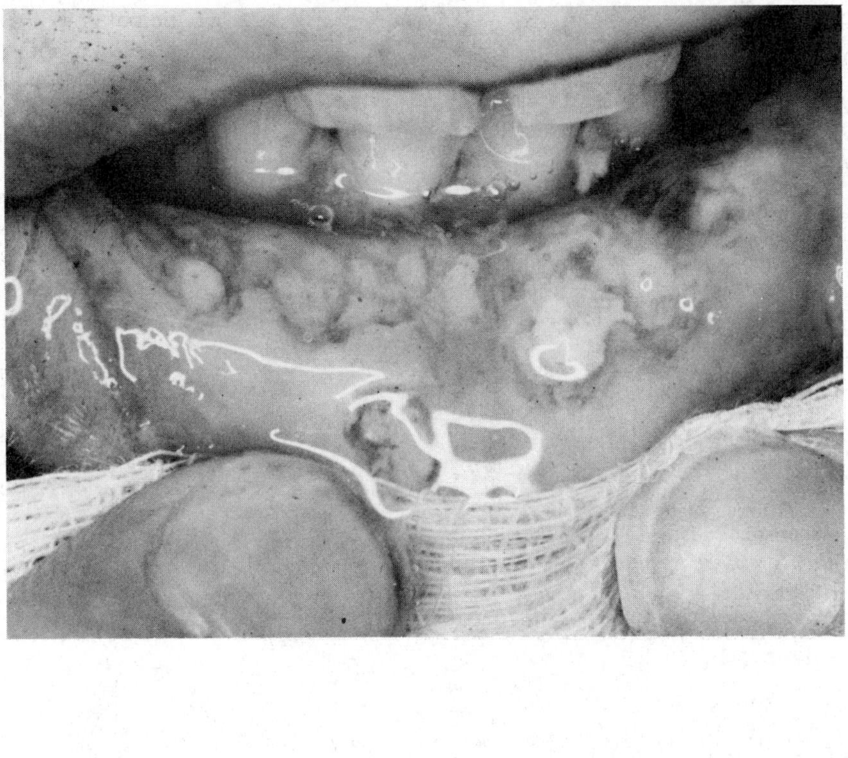

FIG. 60-2. Mucositis of the labial mucosa due to stomatotoxicity secondary to methotrexate. Note the severe disruption of epithelial integrity. (Sonis, Fazio, Fang: Principles and Practice of Oral Medicine. Philadelphia, WB Saunders, 1984)

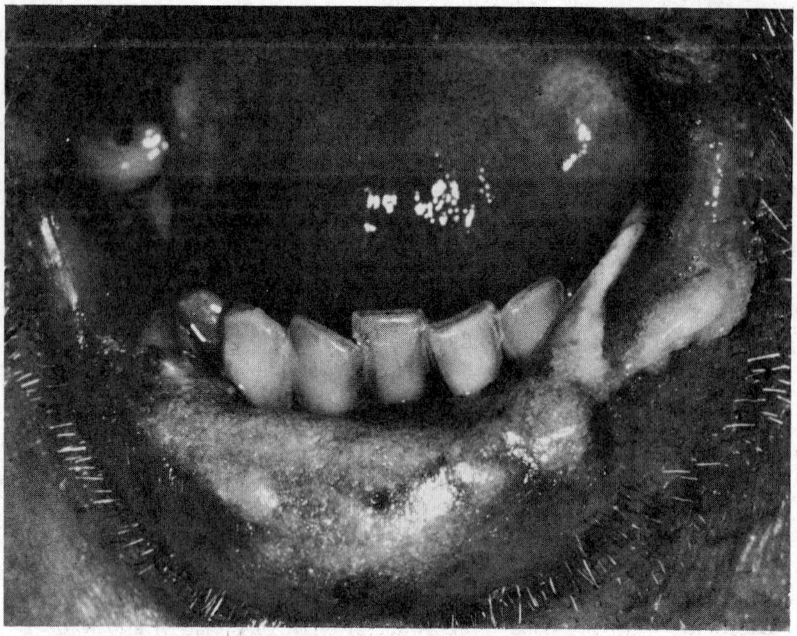

FIG. 60-3. Severe breakdown of the labial mucosa as a result of direct stomatotoxicity. Note the lack of involvement of nonmucosal surfaces. (Sonis, Fazio, Fang: Principles and Practice of Oral Medicine. Philadelphia, WB Saunders, 1984)

Plant alkaloids, particularly vincristine, may cause neurotoxicity that manifests as acute-onset dental pain, most frequently in the mandibular molar area, in the absence of odontogenic pathology.[33] The discomfort resolves after the drug is discontinued.

Recent trials have suggested that the administration of colony-stimulating factors to patients undergoing chemotherapy may reduce the incidence of mucositis. Further information on this effect of colony-stimulating factors will be forthcoming from ongoing trials.

TABLE 60-6. Cancer Chemotherapeutic Drugs That Produce Direct Stomatotoxicity

Alkylating Agents
Mechlorethamine
Antimetabolites
Cytarabine hydrochloride
Floxuridine
Fluorouracil
Mercaptopurine
Methotrexate
Thioguanine
Natural Products
Bleomycin
Dactinomycin
Daunorubicin
Doxorubicin
Mithramycin
Mitomycin
Vinblastine sulfate
Vincristine sulfate
Other Synthetic Agents
Hydroxyurea
Procarbazine hydrochloride

INDIRECT STOMATOTOXICITY

Indirect stomatotoxicity is the result of the effects of chemotherapy on a cell pool other than of the oral mucosa. The most significant target cells in this case are those of the bone marrow. Changes in the mouth that are associated with this action usually are noted at the patient's nadir, which most often occurs 12 to 14 days after drug administration.[20] The two most common forms of indirect stomatotoxicity are infection and hemorrhage.

The mouth is the most frequently identifiable source of sepsis in the granulocytopenic cancer patient.[34] Most often, oral infection is caused by bacteria, although fungal and viral infections also are relatively common. The degree and duration of granulocytopenia often determine the incidence and severity of infection. Although the normal flora is responsible for the majority of infections, during myelosuppression the oral flora changes to become primarily gram-negative (common isolated organisms include *Klebsiella*, *Serratia*, *Enterobacter*, *Escherichia coli*, *Pseudomonas*, and *Proteus*).[35] Most fungal infections are caused by *Candida albicans*.[36] Viral infections tend to be due to herpes simplex or varicella.

Bacterial infections may affect three sites in the mouth: the gingiva, the mucosa, or the teeth. Because the normal signs of inflammation and therefore infection are absent in the myelosuppressed patient, diagnosis is based on the presence of oral lesions in conjunction with fever and pain. Demonstration of a culturable local isolate in conjunction with a positive blood culture result confirms the diagnosis, although exotoxins and endotoxins from oral bacteria may produce fever in the absence of a positive blood culture.

Gingivae are a common site of infection, especially in the patient with preexisting periodontal disease.[37] Infection of this area presents as a necrotizing gingivitis that clinically resembles acute necrotizing ulcerative gingivitis (Vincent's disease). Patients develop painful necrosis of the marginal

TABLE 60-7. Formulary of Topical Medications for Specific Oral Problems

Problem	Medication	Use
General infection control	Chlorhexidine gluconate 0.12% oral rinse	Rinse twice daily after breakfast and at bedtime for 30 sec. Do not swallow.
Localized secondary topical lip infection	Neosporin	Apply to perioral lesions 2–5 times daily, depending on severity of lesion.
Prevention of caries secondary to xerostomia	Acidulated fluoride rinse	Rinse daily for 1 min with 5 ml to 10 ml. Do not swallow. Switch to neutral fluoride if mucositis is present.*†
	Neutral fluoride rinse	Rinse daily for 1 min with 5 ml. Do not swallow. Switch back to acidulated fluoride rinse when mucositis resolves.
	Stannous fluoride gel 0.4%	Brush daily for 1 min, then hold in mouth and rinse for 30 sec. Do not swallow.†
Antifungal Agents		
Prevention and treatment of oral candidiasis	Nystatin oral suspension	Rinse and swallow 300,000 units 3–4 times daily. If intolerance to swallowing, rinse only.
	Clotrimazole troche 10 mg	Dissolve 1 tablet 5 times daily. The prophylactic use of clotrimazole for the prevention of candidiasis has not been adequately studied.
Treatment of candidiasis under dentures or at corners of mouth	Mycolog ointment	Apply to affected area 2 to 3 times daily or place under denture surface.
Palliation of mucositis (generalized)	Xylocaine viscous 2% solution	Swish 15 ml for 30 sec maximum every 3 h. Expectorate.
	Dyclonine hydrochloride 0.5% or 1% solution	Swish 15 ml for 30 sec every 2 to 3 h. Expectorate.
	Benadryl and Kaopectate mix solution of 50% each.	Swish 15 ml for 30 sec every 2 to 3 h. Expectorate.
Palliation of mucositis (localized)	Benzocaine in Orabase ointment	Apply to affected dried area every 2 to 3 h. Not to be used in presence of infection.
Control of Local Bleeding		
Gingival	Topical thrombin solution	Apply to affected area with gauze sponge and hold in place with pressure for 30 min. Do not remove formed clots.
Mucosal surface bleeding	Microfibrillar collagen	Apply to dried site with dry sponge for 1 to 5 min. Do not use in closure of mucosal incisions.
Xerostomia		
Saliva substitutes	Salivart synthetic saliva spray	Spray as needed for xerostomia.
Saline may also be used	Xerolube	Rinse as needed for xerostomia.

*Fluoride gels in custom trays are preferred.
†Acidilated fluorides are contraindicated in patients with porcelain prostheses.

and papillary gingivae, usually beginning around one or two teeth and then spreading laterally. Fever and lymphadenopathy are present. The normal papillary architecture is eliminated, and a white, necrotic pseudomembrane is present. Treatment of necrotic gingivitis consists of parenteral antibiotics. Because spirochetes and fusiform organisms must be included in the spectrum of causative agents, coverage should include a penicillin as well as an agent specific for gram-negative organisms. The teeth should be gently debrided with cotton pellets soaked with 3% hydrogen peroxide. Frequent rinsing may be helpful.

Mucosal infection is usually due to secondary infection of ulcerations produced by direct stomatotoxicity or trauma (Fig. 60-4). Patients complain of pain and are febrile. Clinically, one observes ulceration, often deep, with a yellow-white necrotic center. The borders are often slightly raised and indurated. An erythematous border, usually associated with aphthous lesions, is conspicuously absent. Lesions are of variable size; it is important to remember that the size of the lesion does not always relate directly to its potential to cause sepsis. The organisms causing these infections usually are mixed; thus, isolation of organisms from the blood of septic patients is an important corroborating procedure in patients suspected of having an oral source.

It is often difficult to determine which mucosal lesions require antibiotic coverage. Patients with fever, neutropenia (WBC < 1000 cells/mm^3), and an oral lesion must be presumed to have an oral source and should be appropriately treated until the WBC count recovers, the patient is afebrile, and the lesions begin to resolve.

Odontogenic infections in the myelosuppressed patient often present with confusing signs and symptoms because of the patient's inability to mount an inflammatory response.[28,38] Tooth pain and fever may be the only signs of odontogenic infection. Thorough dental examination, including radiographs, is often necessary to make a definitive diagnosis. Because many subacute odontogenic infections become symptomatic when the patient becomes myelosuppressed, the ideal treatment is *elimination* of questionable teeth before the initiation of chemotherapy. If this is not possible and the patient develops a definite odontogenic infection, extraction to eliminate the source is the treatment of choice. This requires antibiotic and often platelet coverage. Perform extractions as atraumatically as possible, avoiding block anesthesia. Hemostatic gels should not be used because these may act as foci for bacterial infection. Primary closure of the wound with sutures is desirable.[39] Continue antibiotics for at least 1 week after extraction regardless of the patient's WBC count. Alternatively, if the patient is medically unstable, the necrotic pulp may be endodontically extricated and the tooth closed.

Oral fungal infections are common in the myelosuppressed cancer patient. These tend to be superficial infections of the oral mucosa caused by *Candida albicans*, an organism present in about 50% of the normal population. Oral infection with *Candida* produces surface necrosis, which has a wide variety of clinical manifestations. Most frequently, lesions appear as raised, white curdy areas affecting any of the oral soft tissues (Fig. 60-5). Angular cheilitis may also occur. Patients who wear removable prostheses may develop beneath their dentures infections that are broad, sensitive, erythematous macules. The major clinical significance of oral moniliasis is its potential spread to the esophagus or lungs. Patients are rarely febrile when *Candida* infections are limited to the mouth. Diagnosis is based on clinical appearance, the ability to scrape off the necrotic surface, and demonstration of the organism with potassium hydroxide smears.

The value of prophylactic antifungal medication is controversial.[40–43] One study concluded that patients whose WBC counts drop to 200 cells/mm^3 develop candidiasis despite topical medication. However, it seems that prophylactic use of topical antifungal agents begun simultaneously with chemotherapy reduces both the frequency and severity

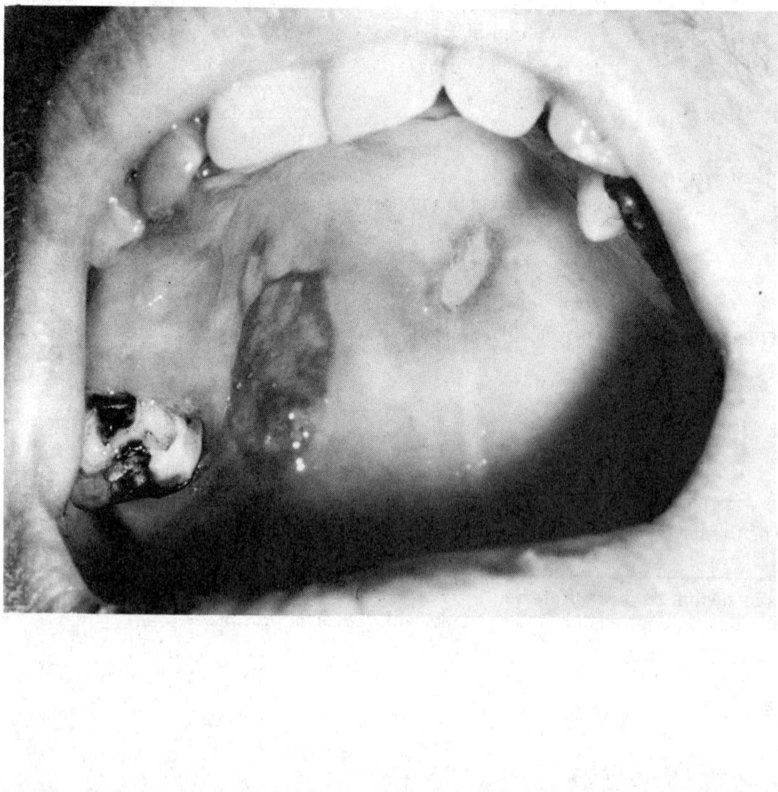

FIG. 60-4. An unusual case of localized ulcerations of the hard palate in a patient hospitalized with fever of unknown origin. At the time of admission, the larger ulcer demonstrated evidence of infection. (Lockhart PB: Dental management of patients receiving chemotherapy. In Peterson, Sonis: Oral Complications of Cancer Chemotherapy. Boston, Martinus Nijhoff, 1983)

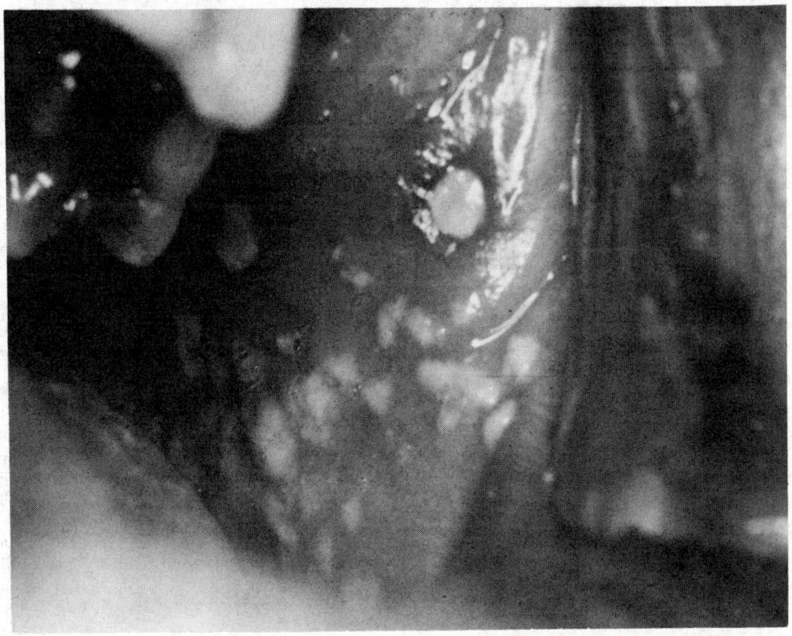

FIG. 60-5. Candidiasis of buccal mucosa in a 49-year-old woman with acute myelogenous leukemia. Note raised, white croppy areas of fungae. A small ulcer is also present.

of infection. Popsicles made of nystatin diluted in water are often soothing and provide prolonged contact with the mucosa. Gentian violet is often effective; its staining of the mucosa prohibits adequate clinical evaluation. Patients complaining of esophageal pain or dysphagia should be evaluated for spread of infection (see Chapter 59).[44] If this occurs, treat it early and aggressively with a systemic antifungal agent (*e.g.*, amphotericin B).

Other deep fungal infections may occur in the myelosuppressed patient. Fortunately, however, these are relatively rare.

The two most common viral infections affecting the mouths of myelosuppressed patients are caused by herpes simplex and varicella zoster viruses.

Herpes simplex infections may produce a primary infection in patients not previously exposed to the virus or may cause a secondary infection from reactivation of latent virus in regional nerve ganglia. Primary infection produces an oral symptom complex characterized by acute-onset gingivitis, vesicles of the mucosa, and a coated tongue. This symptom complex usually is preceded by a viral prodrome of malaise, anorexia, and fever. The mouth is extremely tender. Gingival bleeding may be noted, as well as fetor oris. Secondary herpes infection produces single or crops of vesicles, most often extraoral, at or beyond the mucocutaneous junction. Infections tend to be recurrent. Although rare in the normal person, intraoral secondary herpes infection may occur in the myelosuppressed patient and are characterized by crops of small vesicles, often on the hard palate. The vesicles frequently rupture, leaving raw, open, shallow, and painful punctate ulcers. Neutropenic patients experiencing herpes infections may be treated with acyclovir (Zovirax ointment 5%).[45] Extraoral lesions may become infected secondarily with bacteria. Healing often is helped by the presence of a lubricating ointment such as Neosporin. Lesions usually resolve within 7 to 10 days, depending on host resistance.

The frequency of herpes simplex virus infections in patients receiving chemotherapy is not well resolved; the reported incidence ranges from about 11% to 48%. The differences in reported frequency are largely dependent on the method of diagnosis. However, because of the potentially high frequency of oral herpes simplex infections, culture of suspicious lesions is recommended. In interpreting results, it must be remembered that herpes simplex virus is not an uncommon member of the normal oral flora and, in the absence of clinically detectable lesions, may not be of pathologic consequence.[46]

Recently, chlorhexidine gluconate 0.12% has been shown to be efficacious in reducing the frequency and severity of mucositis and infection associated with chemotherapy and radiation therapy for bone marrow transplants. The drug is used twice daily as a rinse. Side-effects are minimal and include occasional burning, which may be reduced by dilution with water, and brown superficial tooth staining, which can be easily polished off. Since chlorhexidine has also been shown to reduce bacterial, fungal, and viral colonization in the mouths of myelosuppressed patients, it should be considered for use prophylactically.[47]

Thrombocytopenia predisposes to oral bleeding.[48,49] Bleeding may occur anywhere in the mouth but usually is provoked by trauma or preexisting periodontal disease. Minor mucosal trauma may result in hematoma formation or frank bleeding. Generally, hematoma formation is unusual with platelet counts greater than 25,000 cells/mm.[48] When patients are more profoundly thrombocytopenic, oral hematomas form relatively easily and are of clinical significance for two major reasons: (1) hematomas can act as sites of secondary infection, especially when there are breaks in the mucosa; and (2) unchecked submucosal bleeding in the sublingual area may result in elevation of the tongue and consequent respiratory compromise.

Spontaneous gingival bleeding is unusual with platelet

counts greater than 10,000 cells/mm³. Patients with preexisting periodontal disease are more likely to demonstrate gingival hemorrhage than are patients in good gingival health. Therefore, dental prophylaxis and good oral hygiene are of significant benefit in reducing the likelihood of this problem. If gingival bleeding does occur, topical thrombin-soaked gauze held under pressure is often helpful. For open mucosal oozing, microcrystalline collagen may produce hemostasis. When local measures fail, patients may require platelet transfusion. The use of stints or surgical gingival packs is to be avoided because the pressure of these often causes necrosis. Furthermore, these appliances harbor bacteria and are irritating to the gingiva.

REFERENCES

1. Sonis ST, Kunz A: Impact of improved dental services on the frequency of oral complications of cancer therapy (in press)
2. Reynolds WR, Hickey AJ, Feldman MI: Dental management of the cancer patient receiving radiation therapy. Clin Prevent Dent 2:5–9, 1980
3. Shannon IL, Starcke EN, Wescott WB: Effect of radiotherapy on whole saliva flow. J Dent Res 56:693, 1977
4. Eneroth CM, Henrikson CO, Jakobson PA: Effects of fractionated radiotherapy on salivary gland function. Cancer 30:1147–1153, 1972
5. Karmiol M, Walsh RF: Dental caries after radiotherapy of the oral regions. J Am Dent Assoc 91:838–845, 1975
6. Shannon IL, Tordahl JN, Starcke EN: Remineralization of enamel by saliva substitute designed for use by irradiated patients. Cancer 41:1746–1750, 1978
7. Keys HM, McCasland JP: Techniques and results of a comprehensive dental care program in head and neck cancer patients. Int J Radiat Oncol Biol Phys 1:859–865, 1976
8. Keene HJ, Fleming TJ: Prevalence of caries-associated microflora after radiotherapy in patients with cancer of the head and neck. Oral Surg 64:421–426, 1987
9. MacCarthy-Leventhal EM: Postradiation mouth-blindness. Lancet 2:1138–1139, 1959
10. Murray CG, Herson J, Daly TE et al: Radiation necrosis of the mandible: A 10-year study. Part I. Factors influencing the onset of necrosis. Int J Radiat Oncol Biol Phys 6:543–548, 1980
11. Marx RE, Johnson RP: Studies in the radiobiology of osteoradionecrosis and their clinical significance. Oral Surg 64:379–390, 1987
12. Murray CG, Daly TE, Zimmerman SO: The relationship between dental disease and radiation necrosis of the mandible. Oral Surg 49:99–104, 1980
13. Murray CG, Herson J, Daly TE et al: Radiation necrosis of the mandible: A 10-year study. Part II. Dental factors: Onset, duration and management of necrosis. Int J Radiat Oncol Biol Phys 6:549–553, 1980
14. Marciani RD, Plezia RA: Management of teeth in the irradiated patient. J Am Dent Assoc 88:1021–1024, 1974
15. Markitziu A, Heling I: Endodontic treatment of patients who have undergone irradiation of the head and neck. Oral Surg 52:294–297, 1981
16. Sonis ST, Sonis AL, Lieberman A: Oral complications in patients receiving treatment for malignancies other than of the head and neck. J Am Dent Assoc 97:468–472, 1978
17. Sonis AL, Sonis ST: Oral complications of cancer chemotherapy in pediatric patients. J Pedodontics 3:122–128, 1979
18. Dreizen S, McCredie KB, Bodey GPN et al: Quantitative analysis of the oral complications of antileukemic chemotherapy. Oral Surg 62:650–653, 1986
19. Bodey GP: Oral manifestations of myeloproliferative diseases. Postgrad Med 49: 115–121, 1971
20. Lockhart PB, Sonis ST: Relationship of oral complications to peripheral blood leukocyte and platelet counts in patients receiving cancer chemotherapy. Oral Surg 48: 21–28, 1979
21. Baraket NJ, Toto PD, Choukas NC: Aging and cell renewal of oral epithelium. J Periodontol 40:599–602, 1969
22. Peterson DW, Overholser CD: Increased morbidity associated with oral infection in patients with acute leukemia. Oral Surg 53:32–36, 1982
23. Greenberg MS, Cohen SG, McKifrick, JC et al: The oral flora as a source of septicemia in patients with acute leukemia. Oral Surg 53:32–36, 1982
24. Overholser CD, Peterson DE, William SL et al: Periodontal infection in patients with acute nonlymphocytic leukemia: Prevalence of acute exacerbations. Arch Intern Med 14:551–554, 1982
25. Beck S: Impact of a systematic oral care protocol on stomatitis after chemotherapy. Cancer News 2:185–199, 1979
26. Hickey AJ, Toth BB, Lindquist SB: Effect of intravenous hyperalimentation and oral care on the development of oral stomatitis during cancer chemotherapy. J Prosthet Dent 47:188–193, 1982
27. Dreizen S, Bodey GP, Rodriquez V: Oral complications of cancer chemotherapy. Postgrad Med 58:95, 1975
28. Dreizen S: Stomatotoxic manifestations of cancer chemotherapy. J Prosthet Dent 40:650–655, 1978
29. Volger W, Huguley C, Kerr W: Toxicity and antitumor effect of divided doses of methotrexate. Arch Intern Med 115:285–293, 1965
30. Guggenheimer J, Verbin RS, Appel BN et al: Clinicopathologic effects of cancer chemotherapeutic agents on human buccal mucosa. Oral Surg 44:58–63, 1977
31. Lockhart PB, Sonis ST: Alterations in the oral mucosa caused by chemotherapeutic agents. J Dermatol Surg Oncol 7:1019–1025, 1981
32. Aker SN: Oral findings in the cancer patient. Cancer 43:2102–2107, 1979
33. Rosenthal S, Kaufman S: Vincristine neurotoxicity. Ann Intern Med 80:733–734, 1974
34. EORTC International Antimicrobial Therapy Project Group: Three antibiotic regimens in the treatment of infection in febrile granulocytopenic patients with cancer. J Infect Dis 137:14–29, 1978
35. Dreizen S, Brown LR: Oral microbial changes and infections during cancer chemotherapy. In Peterson DE, Sonis ST (eds): Oral Complications of Cancer Chemotherapy, pp 41–47. Boston, Martinus-Nijhoff, 1983
36. Bodey GP: Fungal infections complicating acute leukemia. J Chronic Dis 19:667–687, 1966
37. Peterson DE: Bacterial infections: Periodontal and dental disease. In Peterson DE, Sonis ST (eds): Oral Complications of Cancer Chemotherapy, pp 79–91. Boston, Martinus-Nijhoff, 1983
38. Lockhart PB: Dental management of patients receiving chemotherapy. In Peterson DE, Sonis ST (eds): Oral Complications of Cancer Chemotherapy, pp 113–149. Boston, Martinus-Nijhoff, 1983
39. Overholser CD, Peterson DE, Bergman SA: Dental extractions in patients with leukemia. J Oral Surg 40:296–298, 1982
40. Epstein JB, Pearsall NN, Truelove EL: Oral candidiasis: Effects of antifungal therapy upon clinical signs and symptoms, salivary antibody and mucosal adherence of *Candida albicans*. Oral Surg 51:32–36, 1981
41. Taschdjian CL, Kozinn PH, Toni EF: Opportunistic yeast infections with special reference to candidiasis. Ann NY Acad Sci 174:606–622, 1970
42. Pizzuto J et al: Nystatin prophylaxis in leukemia and lymphoma. N Engl J Med 299:661–662, 1978
43. Carpentieri U et al: Clinical experience in preventions of candidiasis by nystatin in children with acute leukemia. J Pediatr 92:593–595, 1978
44. Jones JM: Necrotizing *Candida* esophagitis: Failure of symptoms and roentgenographic findings to reflect severity. JAMA 244:2190–2191, 1980
45. Mitchell CD et al: Acyclovir therapy for mucocutaneous herpex simplex infections in immunocompromised patients. Lancet 1:1389–1392, 1981
46. Montgomery MT, Redding SW, LeMaistre CF: The incidence of oral herpes simplex virus infection in patients undergoing cancer chemotherapy. Oral Surg 61:238–242, 1986
47. Ferretti GA et al: Chlorhexidine in prophylaxis against oral infections and associated complications in patients receiving bone marrow transplantation. J Am Dent Assoc 114:292–294, 1987
48. Stafford R, Lockhart P, Sonis et al: Hemotologic parameters as predictors of oral involvement in the presentation of acute leukemia. J Oral Med 37:38–41, 1982
49. Lynch MA, Ship II: Initial oral manifestations of leukemia. J Am Dent Assoc 75: 932–940, 1977

SECTION 4

FRANK M. TORTI
BERT L. LUM

Cardiac Toxicity

The development of a number of anticancer drugs such as the anthracycline antibiotics, doxorubicin and daunorubicin, as well as the use of intensive radiation therapy for mediastinal and central pulmonary disease have brought attention to the cardiotoxic potential of these therapies. Treatment-induced cardiotoxic effects include cardiomyopathies leading to congestive heart failure, electrocardiographic (ECG) changes and life-threatening arrhythmias, pericarditis, and myocardial ischemia and infarction. However, preexisting heart disease is a more common etiology of cardiac disease in the cancer patient than the treatment for the disease. Because of the potential of these anticancer treatments to exacerbate preexisting heart disease or to produce cardiac disease on their own, the potential for treatment-induced cardiac disease should be carefully evaluated in a cancer patient presenting with cardiac symptoms. Identifying the nature of the cardiac dysfunction can prevent premature termination of therapy and excessive treatment-associated morbidity or mortality. This chapter will focus on the recognition, prevention, and management of the major cardiac problems commonly encountered with the clinical use of anticancer therapies.

ACUTE AND SUBACUTE EFFECTS OF DRUGS AND IRRADIATION

ECG CHANGES AND ARRHYTHMIAS

Anthracyclines

The most common cancer treatments associated with ECG abnormalities and arrhythmias have been the anthracycline antibiotics and the investigational drug amsacrine. Early reports of the incidence of acute doxorubicin toxicity manifested by ECG changes ranged from 0–41%.[1] The incidence of ECG changes reflect the frequency of monitoring[2] and appears to be higher in patients with abnormal pretreatment ECGs.[3,4] ECG changes can occur over a wide range of cumulative doses. The most frequent abnormalities are nonspecific ST–T-wave changes, decreased QRS voltage, sinus tachycardia, supraventricular tachyarrhythmias, premature ventricular and atrial contractions, T-wave abnormalities, and QT interval prolongation. These changes usually occur during or within a few days of drug administration and in general are reversible within a few hours after discontinuation of treatment. Reversal of ST–T-segment and T-wave abnormalities, however, may not occur for 1 or more weeks. Most of the ECG abnormalities commonly encountered with doxorubicin or daunorubicin therapy appear to be relatively benign and do not usually necessitate the discontinuation of treatment. However, rare cases of sudden death and life-threatening ventricular tachyarrhythmias during doxorubicin administration have been reported.[1]

Other Drugs

Amsacrine has been reported to cause serious, life-threatening arrhythmias in under 1% of treated patients.[5] The most common rhythm abnormality was ventricular tachycardia or fibrillation (or sudden death presumed to be due to these arrhythmias). In virtually all cases, the arrhythmias occurred during amasacrine infusion or minutes to hours after drug administration. Hypokalemia may predispose to severe amsacrine-related arrhythmias.[6,7]

Other chemotherapeutic agents have been implicated in arrhythmias, including azathioprine (atrial fibrillation),[8,9] methotrexate (extrasystoles),[10] and mechlorethamine (atrial ectopy and tachycardia)[11] at high doses. However, the relationship of azathioprine, methotrexate, and mechlorethamine to arrhythmias remains tentative, given their common use in oncology practice.

PERICARDITIS

Incidence, Etiology, and Pathophysiology

Pericarditis induced by cancer treatment is rare but well documented. More commonly, the pericarditis is due to neoplastic involvement or, in as many as 50% of patients, a nonneoplastic etiology, such as infections, autoimmune disease, trauma, idiopathic heart failure, and use of drugs such as procainamide or methysergide.[12] No clinical signs or symptoms distinguish treatment-related pericarditis from pericarditis of other causes. Idiopathic pericarditis or radiation-induced pericarditis may be managed conservatively, resulting in long-term survival, whereas neoplastic pericarditis requires more aggressive treatment and tends to have a poorer prognosis; thus, systematic evaluation of the cause of pericardial disease in these patients is important.[12]

Radiation-Induced Pericarditis

The incidence of clinical radiation-induced heart disease in a series of 318 patients treated with mediastinal irradiation for Hodgkin's disease at Stanford University Medical Center in 1970 was 6.6%.[13] The effects are dose dependent. For example, if more than 50% of the heart volume is in the radiation field, such as in the mantle field during irradiation for Hodgkin's disease, the administration of 4000 rad in 16 fractions over a 4-week period will result in radiation-induced heart disease (*e.g.*, pericarditis) in 5% of patients. Shielding techniques to lower the exposure of the heart to about 3000 rad have decreased the severity and incidence of this complication.[14,15]

There are a number of clinical presentations of radiation-induced heart disease. The most common is an acute or chronic pericarditis. Other forms include a myocardial fibrosis, accelerated coronary heart disease, and valvular dysfunction.[15–17] The acute pericarditis usually occurs within 12 months of the initiation of radiation therapy but may manifest several years later. The clinical course may be mild, but in 50% of patients a mild to severe tamponade may develop, requiring pericardiocentesis or a pericardial win-

TABLE 60-8. Cancer Treatment–Related Cardiotoxicity

Drug	*Cardiotoxicity* Acute–Subacute: *Arrhythmias*	*Pericarditis*	*Ischemia*	Chronic: *Cardiomyopathy*
Amsacrine	+		+/–	+
Bleomycin		+/–		
Azathioprine	+/–			
Cyclophosphamide		+		+
Cytarabine		+/–		
Dactinomycin		+/–		
Daunorubicin	+	+	+	+
Doxorubicin	+	+	+	+
Etoposide			+/–	
5-Fluorouracil			+	
Interleukin-2			+	
Mechlorethamine	+/–			
Methotrexate	+/–			
Radiation	+	+	+	+
Vinblastine			+	
Vincristine			+	
Vindesine			+	

Symbols: + = convincing association, +/– = limited case reports.

dow.[13] Chronic pericarditis is generally benign, with many patients having an asymptomatic enlarged pericardial silhouette on the chest roentgenogram on follow-up. An effusion may develop 2 to 5 years after treatment and clear spontaneously.[18] A constrictive pericarditis may follow an acute pericarditis or chronic effusion, appearing 6 to 30 months after radiation therapy, and may require pericardectomy.[18,19]

Chemotherapy-Induced Pericarditis

Previous irradiation of the heart appears to be a possible contributing factor to the development of a anticancer drug–induced pericarditis.

ANTHRACYCLINES. An important acute cardiac toxic effect of the anthracyclines is the development of a pericarditis–myocarditis syndrome. This syndrome occurs 1 to 23 days after the last dose of daunomycin at low cumulative doses in the range of 60 to 180 mg/m². The patients tend to be relatively young and have no prior history of heart disease. The majority of patients develop significant myocardial dysfunction as well as arrhythmias; death occurs secondary to cardiac failure.[20–22] Histopathologic assessment demonstrates an acute inflammatory process involving the pericardium and epimyocardium.[20]

CYCLOPHOSPHAMIDE. An acute lethal pericarditis–myocarditis has been observed predominantly as a consequence of high-dose cyclophosphamide–containing combination chemotherapy regimens employed in bone marrow transplantation. Probably fewer than 30 cases of cyclophosphamide-associated pericarditis–myocarditis have been re-

TABLE 60-9. Approximate Incidence of Doxorubicin Cardiotoxicity

Administration Schedule	*Cumulative Dose (mg/m²)*	*Clinical CHF (%)**	*Subclinical* *LVEF (%)†*	*Biopsy Score >1.9 (%)‡*
Every 3 weeks	200–350	1.0–2.0	15–20	41§
	400–500	2.5–5.0	28–57	62
	500–650	8.0–16	54–77	64‖
	650–800	27–42	. . .	. . .
	>800	50+	. . .	. . .
Weekly	200–350	0.3–0.5	. . .	27
	400–500	0.7–1.3	. . .	30
	500–650	1.5–4.5	. . .	33
	650–800	4.4–13	. . .	. . .
	>800	17+	. . .	. . .

Data compiled from Von Hoff et al,[84] Torti et al,[98] Ettinghausen et al,[108] Piver et al,[109] and Alexander et al.[91] Ellipses indicate limited or no data.
*Average incidence within dose range.
†Left ventricular ejection fraction (LVEF) abnormality considered to be <45% value at rest or <5% increase with exercise.
‡Significant change on endomyocardial biopsy score.
§Incidence for cumulative doses in range of 200 to 400 mg/m².
‖Incidence for cumulative doses above 500 mg/m².

ported. Most cases have occurred with doses between 135 to 270 mg/kg,[23,24] although three cases have been reported at doses of 90 to 120 mg/kg.[25] The prognosis is better if attendant myocarditis is not clinically apparent (survival 6 to 79 months for pure pericarditis *vs.* 7 to 16 days for pericarditis-myocarditis in one series[24]). Prior cardiac irradiation predisposes to this toxic effect of treatment.

OTHER DRUGS. Although cytarabine, bleomycin, and dactinomycin, have been implicated in inducing pericarditis,[26–29] the contributions of underlying disease, other chemotherapeutic agents, and irradiation make the associations uncertain.

Management

Patients developing pericardial effusion and cardiac tamponade may require pericardiocentesis to improve their hemodynamic status. In constrictive pericarditis, pericardectomy may be indicated. Cancer patients with idiopathic pericarditis have been reported to improve with the use of nonsteroidal anti-inflammatory drugs[12]; however, the role of these drugs and other drugs such as corticosteroids in drug-induced pericarditis remains to be established. Since malignant pericardial effusion, in contrast to idiopathic or radiation-induced pericarditis, may require the instillation of anticancer drugs (*e.g.*, nitrogen mustard) or sclerosing agents (such as tetracycline) for optimal management, it becomes important to define the potential etiology of the disease, as these drugs when instilled into the pericardial sac could exacerbate the condition.

MYOCARDIAL ISCHEMIA AND INFARCTION

Myocardial ischemia or infarction induced by anticancer drug therapy is a rare finding. The drugs most commonly implicated in the literature include 5-fluorouracil (5-FU), doxorubicin, and the vinca alkaloids, vinblastine and vincristine. Mediastinal irradiation has also been associated with coronary artery disease.

Chemotherapy-Induced Ischemia and Infarction

FLUOROURACIL. 5-FU-induced myocardial ischemia occurs infrequently yet can represent a major toxic effect and an impediment to treatment. 5-FU-induced ischemic heart disease has been described in over 40 patients since the initial report by Dent and McColl in 1975[30]; intra-arterial FUDR has also been implicated.[31] Although the incidence is somewhat higher in patients with preexisting heart disease (4.5% *vs.* 1.1% in one large series of 1083 patients), the ischemia has been documented in a number of patients without clinically evident underlying heart disease.[32,33] Factors such as age, sex, prior radiation therapy, concomitant use of other anticancer drugs, duration of infusion (bolus *vs.* infusion), and route of infusion do not appear to offer predictive value for the development of 5-FU-induced myocardial ischemia. Approximately one half of patients experiencing 5-FU-induced myocardial ischemia have no evidence of coronary artery disease. The anginal episodes most frequently appear about 6 hours after drug administration, but may appear minutes to a week later. Most patients experience chest pain after three to four doses of the drug with consecutive daily dosing (for 4 to 5 days) or during the third or fourth day of continuous intravenous infusion therapy. However, this is also variable: chest pain has been reported at a range of one to 13 doses, and may occur after weekly single intravenous (IV) bolus injections. There have been seven case reports of patients experiencing myocardial infarction, which constitutes approximately 17% of the reported cases of 5-FU-induced ischemia.

Some authors report that a modification in schedule from consecutive daily dosing to weekly treatment has resolved the ischemic pain.[34] In other cases, administration of nitrates has eliminated the chest pain and allowed continuation of treatment.[30,35,36] Calcium channel blockers have produced symptomatic benefit in one patient; this and other information has led to the speculation that coronary vasospasm may be associated with this disorder.[34,35,37] However, in one patient with and one patient without coronary vasodilator therapy continued treatment with 5-FU resulted in myocardial infarction.[30,36]

ANTHRACYCLINES. Daunorubicin and doxorubicin have been associated with myocardial ischemic disease and infarction in a small number of patients. Episodes usually occur within hours of drug administration. Adrenergic stimulation and vasospasm have been suggested mechanisms.[21,38,39]

VINCA ALKALOIDS AND OTHER MITOTIC INHIBITORS. The vinca alkaloids—vincristine, vinblastine, and the investigational drug vindesine—have been associated with a number of coronary artery–related toxic effects. Accelerated atherosclerosis, coronary vasospasm, angina, and myocardial infarction have been reported. Although some patients underwent cardiac irradiation and others received combination chemotherapy with bleomycin (known to cause Raynaud's syndrome and other vasospastic symptoms[40]), it appears that in a number of cases the vincas contribute to coronary toxic effects.[41–51]

OTHER DRUGS. Etoposide (VP 16-213) was associated with a myocardial infarction in a 27-year-old woman with Hodgkin's disease who had been treated with mediastinal irradiation and MOPP (mechlorethamine, vincristine, procarbazine, prednisone). Amsacrine (m-AMSA) was reported to be associated with a myocardial infarction in a 47-year-old premenopausal woman with the diagnosis of acute nonlymphoblastic leukemia.[53] Myocardial infarction has been associated with high-dose interleukin-2 therapy.[54]

Management

Myocardial ischemia or myocardial infarction associated with the use of anticancer drugs is rare. With perhaps the exception of 5-FU, where prophylaxis with nitrates and calcium channel blockers may be useful in abolishing anginal pain and allowing the continuation of treatment when the risk of continued therapy is warranted, therapy for treatment-related ischemia has not been established.

Radiation-Induced Ischemia and Infarction

High doses of radiation to the heart may damage the heart and pericardium. In animal models, the combination of radiation to the heart and a high lipid diet appears to increase the incidence and severity of coronary atherosclerosis.[55-57] In humans, radiation-associated coronary artery disease also appears to be a result of intimal thickening and atheromatous deposits.[58] Radiation-associated coronary artery disease is reported primarily in patients with Hodgkin's disease or seminomas, and to a lesser extent in those with lung and breast cancer. Overall, the incidence of severe coronary artery damage is low.[13,15,59] However, major factors that modify this incidence include the total radiation dose delivered to the heart, the fractionation schedule, the volume of cardiac tissue irradiated, and the dose of radiation delivered to the coronary arteries.

A high dose of radiation delivered to the anterior heart is associated with a high frequency of coronary artery disease. For example, in an autopsy series, of 16 patients, aged 16 to 33 years, who had received more than 3500 rad or mediastinal irradiation, six (38%) had 75% or greater narrowing of one or more coronary artery. The calculated radiation exposure to the anterior surface of the heart averaged 5592 rad, with two patients receiving over 8000 rad. Time from irradiation to death ranged from 5 to 144 months. These 16 patients were compared with a control group of 10 patients matched for age and sex. Overall, 16 (25%) of the 64 major coronary arteries in the irradiated patients were found to have 75% or greater narrowing, as compared to one (2.5%) of 40 in the control group. On histologic examination, all of the intimal lesions were found to contain fibrous tissue; in addition, 29% contained lipid and 5% had calcifications.[60] Other evidence, albeit indirect, implicating coronary artery damage from irradiation comes from functional cardiac studies of treated patients. For example, of the 45 patients treated at Freiberg between 1948 and 1975 and who underwent cardiac evaluation after irradiation, 53% had abnormal cardiac catheterization findings with exercise.[61]

Other studies support the high incidence of coronary artery disease in patients irradiated with anterior fields, particularly in the absence of a subcarinal block. In 25 patients with Hodgkin's disease treated at the NCI, the average age at evaluation was 39 years and the average time since completion of mediastinal irradiation was 10.9 years.[62] All but one patient received midplane doses of less than 4000 rad through an anterior port with no subcarinal shielding. Two patients (8%), aged 33 and 59 years, had angiographically proved coronary artery disease. The younger patient was also noted to have had a "silent" myocardial infarction on ECG. A similar incidence of coronary disease was reported in 48 patients with Hodgkin's disease who received mantle therapy by an anterior weighted technique.[63,64] The dose to the anterior portion of the heart was 4000 rad. The patients were evaluated an average of 8 years after treatment, at which time their mean age was 33 years. Six patients (12%) were found to have coronary artery disease. Five had high-grade (>75%) coronary stenosis. Two additional patients had a myocardial infarction. Other investigators have also reported cases of coronary artery stenosis or vasopasm following cardiac irradiation.[65,66] In 163 patients receiving mantle irradiation, five (18%) of 29 patients surviving 10 years or more developed coronary artery disease at an average of 13 years.[56] Three patients received coronary artery bypass grafts and two other patients died of myocardial infarctions.[67] In 28 young adults followed an average of 8.6 years after mediastinal irradiation (4250–5875 rad to the anterior heart), two patients, aged 12 and 31 years, in whom myocardial ischemia was detected on thallium exercise testing developed acute myocardial infarction. Overall, these studies suggest that the incidence of coronary artery disease and myocardial infarction in patients who receive anterior-weighted mediastinal irradiation is 5% to 18%, and that treatment-related disease usually manifests 8 to 10 years after treatment.

The use of equally weighted anterior and posterior fields, which is common practice today, reduces radiation exposure to the anterior portion of the heart severalfold when compared with the radiation exposure incurred by an anteriorly weighted field or a anterior field alone.[68] Mediastinal irradiation through equally weighted posterioanterior ports appears to be associated with lower incidence of coronary artery disease. An analysis of 377 patients with Hodgkin's disease who receive mantle irradiation at Stanford University Medical Center revealed one case of myocardial infarction. These patients received a mean midline dose of 4410 rad through opposed anteroposterior fields, with subcarinal blocks added after 2500 to 3500 rad. To be eligible for the study, there was a minimum 2-year follow-up requirement; however, many patients appeared to have been treated 5 to 10 years before the study.[14] In a study of 179 children with Hodgkin's disease, Donaldson and Kaplan found two cases of coronary artery disease, one of which was fatal.[69] Eighty percent of the patients were available for 10-year follow-up and 73% for 15-year follow-up. All patients appeared to have received high-dose (4400 rad) mantle field irradiation. Lederman et al[90] treated 58 seminoma patients with parallel-opposed mediastinal field irradiation at a median dose of 2400 cGy. The median age at treatment was 33 years. Follow-up ranged from 1 to 17 years, with a median of 6 years. Five (8.6%) of the patients had presumed coronary heart disease. There was one case of coronary artery disease requiring bypass grafting, two myocardial infarctions, and two witnessed sudden deaths. The average time to coronary artery–related disease was 8.5 years. The observed rate of cardiac disease in the group that received mediastinal irradiation was significantly different than that of the group that did not receive cardiac irradiation. However, these findings were not significantly different than those expected for a normal population, based on the Framingham study data for cardiovascular risk.

ANTHRACYCLINE CARDIOMYOPATHY

Histopathology

At least in its early stages, anthracycline cardiomyopathy is a focal disease. In the early lesions first described by Billingham et al,[71] single degenerated cells are surrounded by normal myocardium. On electron microscopy, two main types of myocyte injury are observed. The first is partial or total myofibrillar loss; the second is sarcotubular dilation with coalescence into vacuoles, with relatively intact mitochondria. These two types of degeneration may be seen together in the same cell or separately. More advanced lesions show myocyte death with mitochondrial degeneration and cristolysis and the appearance of myelin bodies. Severe lesions are accompanied by replacement fibrosis. These morphological changes form the basis for the pathologic grading system for anthracycline cardiotoxicity devised by Billingham and described in greater detail below. The degree of morphological change is dose-related, and virtually all cardiac biopsy specimens from patients treated with cumulative doxorubicin doses of 240 mg/m^2 demonstrate some change.[71,72]

Mechanisms of Action

Anthracyclines display a wide variety of cellular effects, including intercalation with DNA, disruption of RNA and protein synthesis, and interference with oxidative phosphorylation.[73] Recently, a substantial amount of evidence has accumulated which suggests that anthracycline-induced myocyte damage may be due to free radical generation. Free radical generation follows the reduction of anthracyclines by microsomal and nuclear membrane enzyme cytochrome P450 reductase to form a semiquinone radical intermediate.[74,75] This semiquinone radical can then utilize oxygen to form "secondary" free radicals such as superoxide and hydroxyl radicals.[76] Recent in vitro findings suggest that anthracyclines can chelate iron transferred from ferritin[77] and that this complex is capable of causing oxygen radical formation[78] and a marked lipid peroxidation.[78a] These free radical reactions lead to damage of mitochondrial membranes, endoplasmic reticulum, and nucleic acids.[79,80] Of note, these experimental findings correlate with the morphological findings of swelling of the sarcoplasmic reticulum and mitochondrial degeneration noted on histopathologic examination of heart tissue from doxorubicin-treated patients. Following exposure of the heart to doxorubicin, both the sarcoplasmic reticulum and mitochondria generate superoxide radicals; interestingly, glutathione peroxidase, a major protector against free radical damage, is depressed.[81-83] Since other normal cellular defenses against free radical damage, particularly catalase, are low or absent in cardiac cells, this leaves the heart particularly susceptible to free radical damage.[82,82] These findings have stimulated some of the cardiotoxicity prevention strategies discussed below. However, the in vivo mechanisms of anthracycline-mediated cardiac damage are still speculative.

Incidence and Prognosis

Cumulated data from early clinical trials suggest that the overall incidence of clinically apparent doxorubicin cardiomyopathy is in the range of 1% to 2%,[2,84] but to be highly dose dependent, rarely occurring at cumulative doses below 450 mg/m^2 body surface area but increasing along a continuum with an average incidence of 7% at 550 mg/m^2, 15% at 600 mg/m^2, and 30% to 40% at 700 mg/m^2.[84]

The onset of congestive heart failure typically occurs 30 to 60 days after the last dose[84-86] but can be variable, occurring during treatment or years later.[85-87] Daunomycin-induced congestive heart failure (CHF) has a reported incidence of 1.5% at a cumulative dose below 600 mg/m^2 and 12% in patients treated with 1000 mg/m^2.[88] The time interval between the last dose of daunorubicin and the onset of CHF is similar to that of doxorubicin.[88]

The use of clinical CHF to evaluate cardiomyopathy results in an underestimation of the incidence of this toxic effect, particularly in patients with advanced cancer, whose disease may supervene before the expression of cardiac toxicity. Evaluating patients with less extensive cancer and using more sensitive measures of cardiac dysfunction will give a more accurate estimate of the cardiotoxic potential of these drugs.

Dresdale et al[89] found that 32 (52%) of 61 asymptomatic patients with soft tissue sarcomas had radionuclide angiographic evidence of cardiomyopathy at a mean doxorubicin dose of 521 mg/m^2. Fourteen percent of the study group developed CHF. Gottdiener et al[90] reported similar results: 20 (62%) of 32 patients with soft tissue sarcomas treated with doxorubicin to a cumulative dose of 480 to 550 mg/m^2 developed radionuclide angiographic evidence of abnormalities. No patient developed clinical CHF. These studies illustrate that subclinical cardiotoxicity is a frequent finding, occurring in approximately one half of patients treated for 6 to 8 months at conventional doses; further, they illustrate the great variability in cardiac toxicity among patients: 50% of patients had no evidence of cardiotoxicity measurable by radionuclide angiography at a dose range where doxorubicin is often empirically discontinued.

Early descriptions of doxorubicin-induced CHF indicated mortality rates ranging from 33% to 70%. A recent retrospective review of 43 patients with doxorubicin-induced CHF reported that 12 (28%) died of CHF, six (14%) died primarily of progressive tumor but had CHF, and 25 (58%) recovered completely from CHF. In some[91-93] but not all[89,94,95] series, cardiac dysfunction improved during long-term assessment with radionuclide ejection fraction determinations. Patients responded to routine cardiotonic therapy consisting of digoxin, diuretics, vasodilators, and/or captopril.[86,96,97]

Risk Factors

DOSE. Total dose is the most important factor in the development of anthracycline cardiomyopathy.[84] Using a multivariate linear regression model, Torti et al[98] found dose to be the most significant variable influencing biopsy score when 160 endomyocardial biopsies were analyzed.

CARDIAC IRRADIATION. A number of investigators have reported an increased incidence of CHF in patients with a history of concurrent or prior cardiac (mediastinal) irradiation.[2,99,100] Prior mediastinal irradiation is associated with poorer endomyocardial biopsy scores for any total cumulative dose of doxorubicin.[101,102] The biopsy technique permits distinction between radiation-induced heart damage and acceleration of the cardiac damage produced by doxorubicin. Thus, there are two independent yet measurable effects when anthracyclines are combined with irradiation to the heart. The first is a poorly understood but well-documented acceleration of the typical anthracycline lesions seen at endomyocardial biopsy when patients have been previously irradiated. That is, in patients whose hearts have been previously irradiated, the amount of cardiac damage induced by any dose of anthracycline is greater, requiring more careful monitoring and earlier empirical discontinuation of the anthracycline. The second is a radiation "recall" reaction in the heart, which can be produced (rarely) by the administration of doxorubicin years after cardiac irradiation. Acute radiation effects, such as capillary endothelial cell damage, have been reported as part of this "recall" phenomenon. Additionally, a reduplication of basement membranes of venules and arterioles has been described in the myocardium of patients exposed to irradiation plus doxorubicin. This has not been observed in patients receiving doxorubicin or irradiation alone.[102]

SCHEDULE OF ADMINISTRATION. Clinical studies evaluating the incidence of CHF in doxorubicin-treated patients have suggested a strong schedule dependency for the risk of CHF.[84,103–105] Recently, more definitive evidence documenting the schedule dependency of doxorubicin cardiotoxicity has been obtained using endomyocardial biopsies.[98,106,107]

AGE. Increasing age is not an independent risk factor for the development of anthracycline-mediated cardiac damage, when the typical lesions of anthracycline damage are evaluated.[92,95] However, in older patients, other causes of cardiac injury (athersclerotic, hypertension, etc.) represent additive risks for the development of CHF in patients treated with cardiotoxic drugs. Thus, most studies that have used the clinical end point of CHF or functional measures of cardiac performance have demonstrated an increased risk of CHF with increasing age.[21,48,89,108] Some exceptions to this general observation exist, however.[91,94,109]

PREEXISTING HEART DISEASE OR HYPERTENSION. Previous heart disease and hypertension have been implicated as risk factors for the development of cardiomyopathy.[100,110] In the retrospective series reported by Von Hoff et al,[84] the probability of developing CHF appeared higher in patients with preexisting heart disease and hypertension, but was found to be not statistically significant. On multivariate linear regression analyses, these presumed risk factors have not proved to be significant in the development of a high cardiac biopsy score (*i.e.*, they were not risk factors for the myocardial lesion induced by doxorubicin).[98,101] In further support of the observation that underlying heart disease may be additive with doxorubicin-induced cardiac damage, patients with baseline radionuclide angiography abnormalities (presumed underlying cardiac dysfunction) had a higher probability of developing further ejection fraction abnormalities while receiving doxorubicin.[109]

OTHER DRUGS. Cyclophosphamide at the high doses used in bone marrow transplantation has the potential to cause a cardiomyopathy independent of doxorubicin administration.[23] However, recent investigations evaluating cardiotoxicity by (1) clinical CHF,[2,20] (2) radionuclide angiography,[91,109] or (3) endomyocardial biopsy[92,98] found no evidence for cyclophosphamide augmentation of doxorubicin cardiomyopathy. Thus, the same empirical dose limitations of doxorubicin apply when doxorubicin is administered alone or in combination with cyclophosphamide.

Clinical Assessment and Monitoring of Cardiomyopathy

The clinical signs and symptoms of doxorubicin-induced CHF are nonspecific and are typical of any type of biventricular failure. The goal of cardiac assessment and monitoring during anthracycline therapy is to identify which patients can tolerate continued drug treatment beyond traditional dose limitations (approximately 450 mg/m^2 for low-risk patients) and to predict and prevent the onset of clinical CHF.

ENDOMYOCARDIAL BIOPSY. The pathologic changes in the heart from anthracycline exposure form the basis of the histopathologic grading system developed by Billingham et al.[71,72] In this grading system, the percentage of cells showing characteristic anthracycline damage increases with increasing score, which also reflects the degree of pathologic abnormality. The biopsy specimens are obtained following catheterization and endomyocardial biopsy and are examined by electron microscopy.[99] Biopsy is the one procedure available to quantify subclinical anthracycline-induced cardiac damage and to distinguish between anthracycline-mediated and other forms of cardiac damage.

Endomyocardial biopsy with histopathologic grading appears to be the most accurate method for determining subclinical anthracycline-induced damage and for allowing continued treatment beyond traditional empirical dose limitations. the disadvantages of biopsy are its invasive nature, limited availability, and cost. Morbidity associated with this procedure in skilled hands is low. At Stanford, over 4000 biopsy procedures have been performed, with a complication rate of less than 1% and without any attendant mortality.

Bristow et al[112] defined groups with low, moderate, and high probability for developing CHF based on a combination of biopsy findings and right heart catheterization scores. With further treatment, the number of patients developing CHF within 100 mg/m^2 was one (3.2%) of 31 in the low probability group, two (12.5%) of 16 in the moderate probability group, and 14 (45%) of 31 in the high probability group.

RADIONUCLIDE ANGIOGRAPHY. Radionuclide angiography is the best readily available noninvasive procedure for identifying subclinical cardiac contractile abnormalities, and therefore for preventing overt CHF in patients treated with anthracyclines. Although the procedure is imperfect as currently employed (in a recent trial of doxorubicin in breast cancer, 18% of patients developed CHF despite monitoring with resting and exercise radionuclide left ventricular ejection fractions [LVEFs][113]), it represents a major improvement over older noninvasive tests and is currently the method of choice for routine monitoring of patients receiving anthracyclines.

McKillop et al[114] studied the sensitivity and specificity of LVEF in 37 patients receiving a mean cumulative doxorubicin dose of 412 mg/m^2. Risk was determined from a combination of endomyocardial biopsy and cardiac catheterization result. An abnormal LVEF at rest was defined as a value of 45% or less, and an exercise LVEF was considered abnormal if there was not a greater than 5% increase with maximal exercise. Of 19 patients judged to be at moderate or high risk for CHF by biopsy or catheterization criteria, only 10 had an abnormal LVEF; thus, an abnormal LVEF at rest had a sensitivity of 53% and a specificity of 75%. The addition of the exercise test in the same patients increased the sensitivity to 89% but lowered the specificity to 41%. In 12 patients at high risk for heart failure, the sensitivity of rest–exercise testing was 100%. Thirteen patients had a false positive LVEF; four received an additional mean doxorubicin and received no further doxorubicin. These data suggest that normal LVEFs on rest and exercise confer a margin of safety for additional treatment of doxorubicin over a 100 mg/m^2 dose range, obviating the need for empirical dose limitations, and that abnormal LVEFs place a patient at some risk for developing heart failure, although biopsy and catheterization would extend the dose range in 50% of these patients. These results have been confirmed, in part, by Druck et al.[115]

A large retrospective study by Schwartz et al[97] evaluated clinical outcome in 282 doxorubicin-treated patients at high risk for CHF whose LVEFs were monitored by radionuclide angiography. Clinical CHF developed in 46 (16%) of patients and resulted in one death. However, CHF occurred more frequently in patients followed without than with definite monitoring criteria (3% *vs.* 21%), suggesting that a definite monitoring strategy should be employed in following patients.

Recommendations for Cardiac Monitoring by LVEF Alone

Monitor patients according to the guidelines of Schwartz et al.[97] In patients with a normal baseline LVEF (50% or greater), the following steps should be taken. (1) a second LVEF should be determined after 250 to 300 mg/m^2. (2) In patients with risk factors heart disease, irradiation, abnormal ECG, cyclophosphamide) LVEF should again be measured at 400 mg/m^2, or at 450 mg/m^2 in those with no risk factors. (3) Sequential studies should then be performed prior to each dose. (4) Treatment should be discontinued if there is an absolute decrease in LVEF of 10% or more, or a decline to 50% or less.

In patients with an abnormal baseline LVEF (less than 50% but greater than 30%), (1) Sequential studies should be performed prior to each dose. (2) Treatment should be discontinued if there is an absolute decrease in LVEF of 10% or more and/or a final LVEF of 30% or less.

Recommendations for Cardiac Monitoring by LVEF and Cardiac Biopsy

Cardiac monitoring at Stanford University Medical Center has been outlined by McKillop et al.[116] These recommendations employ a combination of empirical dose limitations, radionuclide ejection fraction results, and endomyocardial biopsy/catheterization assessment. The suggested monitoring scheme is presented for patients with and without risk factors.

For patients with risk factors (mediastinal irradiation, hypertension, age 70 years or greater, or history of cardiac disease): (1) Measure the LVEF (with rest and exercise) before the third dose. (2) If the exercise LVEF is normal, repeat after every 100 mg/m^2. (3) If the exercise LVEF is abnormal, measure the resting LVEF every 100 mg/m^2 until 350 mg/m^2, then every 50 to 75 mg/m^2 thereafter. (4) When the resting LVEF drops by 10%, biopsy and catheterization are performed or treatment is discontinued.

Patients with no risk factors are treated to 450 mg/m^2 with no cardiac monitoring; at that dosage monitoring is begun. The LVEF is measured and the patients are monitored as in steps 2 to 4 above.

Prevention Strategies

DOSE LIMITATION. The incidence of anthracycline cardiomyopathy increases with dose. This has led to empirical limitations of 450 to 500 mg/m^2 for the cumulative doxorubicin dose, or 500 to 600 mg/m^2 for daunorubicin. These strategies are intrinsically unsatisfactory, however. Because of individual variance in sensitivity to these drugs, some patients may develop cardiomyopathic changes well below these dose levels; furthermore, in patients with other risk factors for the acceleration of the anthracycline-related cardiac lesion (*e.g.*, prior cardiac irradiation) or with other possible etiologies of cardiac dysfunction (advanced are, known preexisting cardiac disease, etc.), empirical dose limits should be reduced by approximately 150 mg/m^2. On the other hand, as many as 50% of patients may be safely treated with doses above the empirical limits, with appropriate monitoring. Thus, adequate prevention must combine empirical dose limitations with cardiac monitoring.

ALTERED SCHEDULE OF DRUG ADMINISTRATION. Weekly administration and 96-hour infusions appear to reduce but not abolish the risk of cardiotoxicity, perhaps due to decreased peak plasma drug concentrations. Torti et al[98] demonstrated that 168 mg/m^2 more doxorubicin could be delivered on a weekly schedule to produce the same amount of cardiac damage on biopsy as the three weekly schedule. Legha et al[106] reported that the maximum decreases in cardiotoxicity with continuous infusion schedules of 96 hours' duration.

ANALOGUES. Some progress has accrued in the development of anthracycline analogues. The ideal anthracycline analogue would show complete dissociation between cardiotoxicity and antitumor effect. None of the analogues tested to date fill this criterion, although a number of investigational agents show promise.[101,115,116] Numerous other anthracycline analogues are undergoing preclinical and clinical testing. The reader is directed to recent reviews on these agents.[117,118]

CARDIOPROTECTIVE AGENTS. Based primarily on postulated mechanisms of anthracycline-induced myocyte damage, a number of pharmacologic agents or chemical manipulations have been tried in hopes of blocking the deleterious effects of this class of anticancer drugs on the heart. These have included the free radical scavenger, vitamin E; coenzyme Q, an enzyme necessary for oxidative metabolism; *N*-acetylcysteine, a sulfhydryl substitute for glutathione protection from free radicals; calcium channel blockers to prevent intracellular calcium transport and cellular damage; and liposome encapsulation of the drug. While showing promise in in vitro and animal systems, none of these has demonstrated cardioprotection in man in studies with adequate cardiac assessment and patient numbers.

Recently, based on the postulated mechanism of iron doxorubicin oxygen free radical damage and lipid preoxidation described earlier, interest has grown in the ethylenediamminetetraacetic acid derivative ICRF-187. In experimental systems, this class of chelating agents exhibited synergistic cytotoxicity with doxorubicin and a cardioprotective effect.[119] In a preliminary report, it appeared that the drug conferred substantial protection against the cardiotoxicity of doxorubicin.[119]

Management

There is no specific management for anthracycline-induced cardiotoxicity. Therapy with anthracyclines should be discontinued. A major factor in effective management is early detection of cardiomyopathy, since limited functional impairment is associated with a better prognosis. Aggressive therapy of early CHF is also important. In the series of 46 patients monitored by radionuclide LVEF, 40 (87%) patients improved at least one CHF class with digoxin, diuretics, and/or vasodilators.[97] Saini et al also reported the reversibility of doxorubicin-induced left ventricular failure with aggressive therapy consisting of digoxin, diuretics, and captopril.[96]

OTHER ANTICANCER DRUGS THAT INDUCE CARDIOMYOPATHY

Cyclophosphamide cardiomyopathy is limited to a small percentage of patients receiving high doses of the drug in preparation for bone marrow transplantation. This cardiomyopathy is usually associated with a serofibrinous pericarditis. Myocardial changes show hemorrhagic areas, fibrin deposits, and multifocal necrotic areas. Electron microscopy shows changes in the nuclei and intracellular organelles.[23-25,94,120,121]

Among patients treated with amsacrine, CHF occurred in 13 (0.2%) patients previously treated with various chemotherapeutic drugs (usually anthracyclines), and there were no cases of CHF in 683 previously untreated patients. In 18 patients with cardiomyopathy, drawn from published and unpublished reports, six (43%) of 14 patients with clinical heart failure died. All of these patients developed symptoms of heart failure within 16 days of the last dose.[5]

REFERENCES

1. Wortman JE, Lucas VS, Schuster E et al: Sudden death during doxorubicin administration. Cancer 44:1588–1591, 1979
2. Praga C, Beretta G, Vigo PL et al: Adriamycin cardiotoxicity: A survey of 1273 patients. Cancer Treat Rep 63:827–834, 1979
3. Minow RA, Benjamin RS, Lee ET et al: QRS voltage change with Adriamycin administration. Cancer Treat Rep 62:931–934, 1978
4. Dindogru A, Barcos M, Henderson ES et al: Electrocardiographic changes following Adriamycin treatment. Med Pediatr Oncol 5:65–71, 1978
5. Weiss RB, Grillo-Lopez AJ, Marsoni S et al: Amsacrine-associated cardiotoxicity: An analysis of 82 cases. J Clin Oncol 4:918–928, 1986
6. Legha SS, Latreille J, McCredie KB et al: Neurologic and cardiac rhythm abnormalities associated with 4′-(9-acridinylamino) methanesulfon-m-anisidide (AMSA). Cancer Treat Rep 63:2001–2003, 1979
7. Von Hoff DD, Elson D, Polk G et al: Acute ventricular fibrillation and death during infusion of 4′-(9-acridinylamino) methanesulfon-m-anisidide (AMSA). Cancer Treat Rep 64:356–358, 1980
8. Dodd HJ, Tatnall FM, Sarkany I: Fast atrial fibrillation induced by treatment of psoriais with azathioprine. Br Med J 291:706, 1985
9. Murphy G, Fulton RA, Keegan DAJ: Fast atrial fibrillation induced by azathioprine. Br Med J 291:1049, 1985
10. Gasser AB, Tieche M, Brunner KW: Neurologic and cardiac toxicity following IV application of methotrexate. Cancer Treat Rep 66:1561–1562, 1982
11. Hartmann, 1981
12. Posner MR, Cohen GI, Skarin AT: Pericardial disease in patients with cancer. Am J Med 71:407–413, 1981
13. Stewart JR, Fajardo LF: Radiation-induced heart disease: Clinical and experimental aspects. Radiol Clin North Am 9:511–531, 1971
14. Carmel RJ, Kaplan HS: Mantle irradiation in Hodgkin's disease. Cancer 37:2813–2825, 1976
15. Fajardo LF, Berthrong M: Radiation injury in surgical pathology. Am J Surg Pathol 2:159–199, 1978
16. Fajardo LF: Radiation-induced coronary artery disease. Chest 71:563–564, 1977
17. Lancaster LD, Ewy GA: Cardiac consequences of malignancy and their treatment. Adv Intern Med 30:275–293, 1984
18. Cooper RA, Philips TL (eds): Radiation Oncology: Radiation Biology and Radiation Pathology Syllabus, pp 143–145. Chicago, American College of Radiology, 1975
19. Morton DL, Kagan AR, Roberts WC et al: Pericardiectomy for radiation-induced pericarditis with effusion. Ann Thorac Surg 8:195–208, 1969
20. Bristow MR, Billingham ME, Mason JW et al: Clinical spectrum of anthracycline antibiotic cardiotoxicity. Cancer Treat Rep 62:873–879, 1978
21. Bristow MR, Mason JW, Billingham ME et al: Doxorubicin cardiomyopathy: Evaluation by phonocardiography, endomyocardial biopsy, and cardiac catheterization. Ann Intern Med 88:168–175, 1978
22. Harrison DT, Sanders LA: Pericarditis in a case of early daunorubicin cardiomyopathy. Ann Intern Med 85:339–340, 1976
23. Appelbaum F, Strauchen JA, Graw RG et al: Acute lethal carditis caused by high-dose combination chemotherapy: A unique clinical and pathological entity. Lancet 1:58–62, 1976
24. Cazin B, Gorin NC, Laporte JP et al: Cardiac complications after bone marrow transplantation: A report on a series of 63 consecutive transplantations. Cancer 57:2061–2069, 1986
25. Trigg ME, Finlay JL, Bozdech M et al: Fatal cardiac toxicity in bone marrow transplant patients receiving cytosine arabinoside, cyclophosphamide, and total body irradiation. Cancer 59:38–42, 1987
26. Ahmed M, Slayton RE: Report on drug-induced pericarditis. Cancer Treat Rep 64:353–355, 1980
27. Corder MP, Flannery EP: Possible radiation pericarditis precipitated by actinomycin-D. Oncology 30:81–84, 1974
28. Durkin, 1976
29. Vaickus L, Letendre L: Pericarditis induced by high dose cytarabine therapy. Arch Intern Med 144:1868–1869, 1984
30. Dent RG, McColl I: 5-fluorouracil and angina. Lancet 1:347–348, 1975
31. Monk MR, Sanchez JD, Phelps CD et al: Myocardial ischemia with fluorouracil and floxuridine therapy. Clin Pharm 6:659–671, 1987
32. Labianca R, Beretta G, Clerici M et al: Cardiac toxicity of 5-fluorouracil: A study on 1083 patients. Tumori 68:505–510, 1982
33. Pottage A, Holt S, Ludgate S et al: Fluorouracil cardiotoxicity. Br Med J 1:547–548, 1978
34. Underwood DA, Groppe CW, Tsai AR et al: Coronary insufficiency and 5-fluorouracil therapy. Cleveland Clin Q 50:29–31, 1983

35. Burger AJ, Mannino S: 5-fluorouracil-induced coronary vasospasm. Am Heart J 114:433–436, 1987
36. Sanani S, Spaulding MB, Masud ARZ et al: 5-FU cardiotoxicity. Cancer Treat Rep 65:1123–1125, 1981
37. Kleiman NS, Lehane DE, Geyer CE et al: Prinzmetal's angina during 5-fluorouracil chemotherapy. Am J Med 83:566–568, 1987
38. Ippoliti G, Casirola G, Marini G et al: Daunorubicin cardiotoxicity. Lancet 1:430, 1976
39. Mancuso L, Marchi S, Canonico A: Dynamic left ventricular outflow obstruction and myocardial infarction following doxorubicin administration in a woman affected by unsuspected hypertrophic cardiomyopathy. Cancer Treat Rep 69:241–244, 1985
40. Reich SD, Crooke ST: Raynaud's phenomenon. Cancer Treat Rep 63:225–226, 1979
41. Aymard JP, Ferry R, Netter P et al: Toxicite cardiaque des alcaloides de la pervenche. Therapie 40:361–364, 1985
42. Bodensteiner DC: Fatal coronary artery fibrosis after treatment with bleomycin, vinblastine, and cis-platinum. South Med J 74:898–899, 1981
43. Edwards GS, Lane M, Smith FE: Long-term treatment with cis-dichlorodiammineplatinum (II)–vinblastine–bleomycin: Possible association with severe coronary artery disease. Cancer Treat Rep 63:551–552, 1979
44. Harris AL, Wong C: Myocardial ischemia, radiotherapy, and vinblastine. Lancet 1:787, 1981
45. Lejonc JL, Vernant JP, Macquin I et al: Myocardial infarction following vinblastine treatment. Lancet 2:692, 1980
46. Mandel EM, Lewinski U, Djaldetti M: Vincristine-indiced myocardial infarction. Cancer 36:1979–1982, 1975
47. Ricci JA, Goldstein L: Coronary artery disease in the presence of bleomycin therapy. Cancer Treat Rep 66:410, 1982
48. Somers G, Abramow M, Wittek M et al: Myocardial infarction: A complication of vincristine treatment? Lancet 2:690, 1976
49. Vogelzang NJ, Frenning DH, Kennedy BJ: Coronary artery disease after treatment with bleomycin and vinblastine. Cancer Treat Rep 64:1159–1160, 1980
50. Weinstein P, Greenwald ES, Grossman J: Unusual cardiac reaction to chemotherapy following mediastinal radiation in a patient with Hodgkin's disease. Am J Med 60:152–156, 1976
51. Yancey RS, Talpaz M: Vindesine-associated angina and ECG changes. Cancer Treat Rep 66:587–589, 1982
52. Schecter JP, Jones SE: Myocardial infarction in a 27-year-old woman: Possible complication of treatment with VP-16-213 (NSC-141540), mediastinal irradiation, or both. Cancer Chemother Rep 59:887–888, 1975
53. Lindpaintner K, Lindpaintner LS, Wentworth M et al: Acute myocardial necrosis during administration of amsacrine. Cancer 57:1284–1286, 1986
54. Nora R, Abrams J, Silverman HJ: Myocardial infarction in patients receiving high dose recombinant interleukin-2. Proc Am Soc Clin Oncol 6:245, 1987
55. Artom C, Lofland HB, Clarkson TB: Ionizing radiation, atherosclerosis, and lipid metabolism in pigeons. Radiat Res 26:165–177, 1965
56. Annest LS, Anderson RP, Li W et al: Coronary artery disease following mediastinal radiation therapy. J Thorac Cardiovasc Surg 85:257–263, 1983
57. Kirkpatrick JB: Pathogenesis of foam cell lesions in irradiated arteries. Am J Pathol 50:291–309, 1967
58. Cohn KE, Stewart JR, Fajardo LF et al: Heart disease following radiation. Medicine 46:281–298, 1967
59. Boivin J-F, Hutchinson GB: Coronary heart disease mortality after irradiation for Hodgkin's disease. Cancer 49:2470–2475, 1982
60. Brosius FC, Waller BF, Roberts WC: Radiation heart disease: Analysis of 16 young (aged 15 to 33 years) necroscopy patients who received over 3,500 rads to the heart. Am J Med 70:519–530, 1981
61. Slanina J, Musshoff K, Rahner T Stiasny R: Long-term side effects in irradiated patients with Hodgkin's disease. Int J Radiat Oncol Biol Phys 2:1–19, 1977
62. Gottdiener JS, Katin MJ, Borer JS et al: Late cardiac effects of therapeutic mediastinal irradiation. N Engl J Med 308:569–572, 1983
63. Appelfeld MM, Slawson RG, Spicer KM et al: Long term cardiovascular evaluation of patients treated by thoracic mantle radiation therapy. Cancer Treat Rep 66:1003–1013, 1982
64. Appelfeld MM, Wiernik PH: Cardiac disease after radiation therapy for Hodgkin's disease: Analysis of 48 patients. Am Heart J 51:1679–1681, 1983
65. Radwaner BA, Geringer R, Goldmann AM et al: Left main coronary artery stenosis following mediastinal irradiation. Am J Med 82:1017–1020, 1987
66. Yahalom J, Hasin Y, Fuks Z: Acute myocardial infarction with normal coronary arteriogram after mantle field radiation therapy for Hodgkin's disease. Cancer 52:637–641, 1983
67. Pohjola-Sintonen S, Totterman K-J, Salmo M et al: Late cardiac effects of mediastinal radiotherapy in patients with Hodgkin's disease. Cancer 60:31–37, 1987
68. Kinsella TJ, Fraass BA, Glatstein E: Late effects of radiation therapy in the treatment of Hodgkin's disease. Cancer Treat Rep 66:991–1001, 1982
69. Donaldson SS, Kaplan HS: Complications of treatment of Hodgkin's disease in children. Cancer Treat Rep 66:977–989, 1982
70. Lederman et al, 1987
71. Billingham ME, Mason JW, Bristow MR et al: Anthracycline cardiomyopathy monitored by morphologic changes. Cancer Treat Rep 62:865–872, 1978
72. Billingham ME, Bristow MR: Evaluation of anthracycline cardiotoxicity: Predictive ability and functional correlation of endomyocardial biopsy. Cancer Treat Symp 3:71–76, 1984
73. Unverferth DV, Magorien RD, Leier C et al: Doxorubicin cardiotoxicity. Cancer Treat Rev 9:149–164, 1982
74. Bachur NR, Gordon SL, Gee MV: Anthracycline antibiotic augmentation of microsomal electron transport and free radical formation. Mol Pharmacol 13:901–910, 1977
75. Sato S, Iwaizumi M, Handa K et al: Electron spin resonance study on the mode of generation of free radicals of daunomycin, Adriamycin, and carboquone in NAD(P)H-microsome systems. Gann 68:603–608, 1977
76. Meyers CE, Liss RH, Ifrim J et al: The role of lipid peroxidation on cardiac toxicity and tumor response. Science 197:165–167, 1977
77. Thomas CE, Aust SD: Release of iron from ferritin by cardiotoxic anthracycline antibiotics. Arch Biochem Biophys 248:684–689, 1986
78. Sugioka K, Nakano H, Noguchi T et al: Decomposition of unsaturated phospholipid by iron-ADP-Adriamycin coordination complex. Biochem Biophys Res Commun 100:1251–1258, 1981
78a. Gutteridge JMC: Lipid peroxidation and possible hydroxyl radical formation stimulated by the self-reduction of a doxorubicin-iron (III) complex. Biochem Pharmacol 33:1725–1728, 1984
79. Bachur NR, Gordon SL, Gee MV: A general mechanism for microsomal activation of quinone anticancer agents to free radicals: Cancer Res 38:1745–1750, 1978
80. Summerfield FW, Tappel AL: Determination of malonaldehyde-DNA crosslinks by fluoresence and incorporation of tritium. Anal Biochem 11:77–82, 1981
81. Doroshow JH, Locker GY, Myers CE: Enzymatic defenses of the mouse heart against reactive oxygen metabolites: Alterations produced by doxorubicin. J Clin Invest 65:128–135, 1980
82. Doroshow JH, Reeves J: Anthracycline-enhanced oxygen radical formation in the heart. Proc Am Assoc Cancer Res 21:266, 1980
83. Revis NW, Marusic N: Glutathione peroxidase activity and selenium concentration in the hearts of doxorubicin-treated rabbits. J Mol Cell Cardiol 10:945–951, 1978
84. Von Hoff DD, Layard MW, Basa P et al: Risk factors for doxorubicin-induced congestive heart failure. Ann Intern Med 91:710–717, 1979
85. Buzdar AU, Marcus C, Smith TL et al: Early and delayed clinical cardiotoxicity of doxorubicin. Cancer 55:2761–2765, 1985
86. Haq MM, Legha SS, Choski J et al: Doxorubicin-induced heart failure in adults. Cancer 56:1361–1365, 1985
87. Freter CE, Lee TC, Billingham ME et al: Doxorubicin cardiac toxicity manifesting seven years after treatment. Am J Med 80:483–485, 1986
88. Von Hoff DD, Rozencweig M, Layard M et al: Daunomycin-induced cardiotoxicity in children and adults: A review of 110 cases. Am J Med 62:200–208, 1977
89. Dresdale A, Bonow RO, Wesley R et al: Prospective evaluation of doxorubicin-induced cardiomyopathy resulting from postsurgical adjuvant treatment of patients with soft tissue sarcomas. Cancer 52:51–60, 1983
90. Gottdiener JS, Appelbaum FR, Ferrans VJ et al: Cardiotoxicity associated with high-dose cyclophosphamide therapy. Arch Intern Med 141:758–763, 1981
91. Alexander J, Dainiak N, Berger HJ et al: Serial assessment of doxorubicin cardiotoxicity with quantitative radionuclide angiocardiography. N Engl J Med 300:278–283, 1979
92. Ritchie JL, Singer JW, Thorning D et al: Anthracycline cardiotoxicity: Clinical and pathologic outcomes assessed by radionuclide ejection fraction. Cancer 46:1109–1116, 1980
93. Singer JW, Narahara KA, Richie JL et al: Time- and dose-dependent changes in ejection fraction determined by radionuclide angiography after anthracycline therapy. Cancer Treat Rep 62:945–948, 1978
94. Gottdiener JS, Mathison DJ, Borer JS et al: Doxorubicin cardiotoxicity: Assessment of late left ventricular dysfunction by radionuclide cineangiography. Ann Intern Med 94:430–435, 1981
95. Friedman MJ, Ewy GA, Jones SE et al: 1-year followup of cardiac status after Adriamycin therapy. Cancer Treat Rep 63:1809–1816, 1979
96. Saini J, Rich MW, Lyss AP: Reversibility of severe left ventricular dysfunction due to doxorubicin cardiotoxicity. Ann Intern Med 106:814–816, 1987
97. Schwartz RG, McKenzie WB, Alexander J et al: Congestive heart failure and left ventricular dysfunction complicating doxorubicin therapy: Seven-year experience using radionuclide angiocardiography. Am J Med 82:1109–1118, 1987
98. Torti FM, Bristow MR, Howes AE et al: Reduced cardiotoxicity of doxorubicin delivered on a weekly schedule: Assessment by endomyocardial biopsy. Ann Intern Med 99:745–749, 1983
99. Bristow MR, Thompson PD, Martin RP et al: Early anthracycline cardiotoxicity. Am J Med 65:823–832, 1978
100. Minow RA, Benjamin RS, Gottlieb JA: Adriamycin (NSC-123127) cardiomyopathy: An overview with determination of risk factors. Cancer Treat Rep 6:195–201, 1975
101. Torti FM, Bristow MM, Lum BL et al: Cardiotoxicity of epirubicin and doxorubicin: Assessment by endomyocardial biopsy. Cancer Res 46:3722–3727, 1986
102. Billingham ME, Bristow MR, Glatstein E et al: Adriamycin cardiotoxicity: Endomyocardial biopsy evidence of enhancement by irradiation. Am J Surg Pathol 1:17–23, 1977
103. Chlebowski RT, Paroly WS, Pugh RP et al: Adriamycin given as a weekly schedule without a loading course: Clinically effective with a reduced incidence of cardiotoxicity. Cancer Treat Rep 64:47–51, 1980
104. Weiss AJ, Manthel RW: Experience with the use of Adriamycin in combination with other cancer agents using a weekly schedule, with particular reference to lack of cardiac toxicity. Cancer 40:2046–2052, 1977
105. Weiss AJ, Metter GE, Fletcher WS et al: Studies on Adriamycin using a weekly

regimen demonstrating its clinical effectiveness and lack of cardiac toxicity. Cancer Treat Rep 60:813–822, 1976
106. Legha SS, Benjamin RS, Mackay B et al: Reduction of doxorubicin cardiotoxicity by prolonged continuous intravenous infusion. Ann Intern Med 96:133–139, 1982
107. Valdivieso M, Burgess MA, Ewer MS et al: Increased therapeutic index of weekly doxorubicin in the therapy of non-small cell lung cancer: A prospective, randomized study. J Clin Oncol 2:207–214, 1984
108. Ettinghausen SE, Bonow RO, Palmeri ST et al: Prospective study of cardiomyopathy induced by adjuvant doxorubicin therapy in patients with soft-tissue sarcomas. Arch Surg 121:1445–1451, 1986
109. Piver MS, Marchetti DL, Parthasarathy KL et al: Doxorubicin hydrochloride (Adriamycin) cardiotoxicity evaluated by sequential radionuclide angiocardiography. Cancer 56:76–80, 1985
110. Cortes, 1975
111. Fowles RE, Mason JW: Endomyocardial biopsy. Ann Intern Med 97:885–894, 1982
112. Bristow MR, Lopez MB, Mason JW et al: Efficacy and cost of cardiac monitoring in patients receiving doxorubicin. Cancer 50:32–41, 1982
113. Jain KK, Casper ES, Geller NL et al: A prospective randomized comparison of epirubucin and doxorubicin in patients with advanced breast cancer. J Clin Oncol 3:818–826, 1985
114. McKillop JH, Bristow MR, Goris ML et al: Sensitivity and specificity of radionuclide ejection fractions in doxorubicin cardiotoxicity. Am Heart J 106:1048–1056, 1983
115. Druck MN, Gulenchyn KY, Evens WK et al: Radionuclide angiography and endomyocardial biopsy in the assessment of doxorubicin cardiotoxicity. Cancer 53:1667–1674, 1984
116. Dukart G, Posner L, Henry D et al: Comparative cardiotoxicity of mitoxantrone vs doxorubicin. Proc Am Soc Clin Oncol 5:48, 1986
117. Wadler S, Fuks JZ, Wiernik PH: Phase I and II agents in cancer therapy: I. Anthracyclines and related compounds. J Clin Pharmacol 26:491–509, 1986
118. Young CW, Raymond V: Clinical assessment of the structure–activity relationship of anthracyclines and related synthetic derivatives. Cancer Treat Rep 70:51–63, 1986
119. Green MD, Speyer JL, Stacy P, et al: ICRF-187 (ICRF) prevents doxorubicin (dox) cardiotoxicity: Results of a randomized clinical trial. Proc Am Soc Clin Oncol 6:28, 1987
120. Miller, 1979
121. Steinherz LJ, Steinherz PG, Margia-Casale D et al: Cardiac changes with cyclophosphamide. Med Pediatr Oncol 9:417–422, 1981

SECTION 5

DIANE E. STOVER

Pulmonary Toxicity

Pulmonary disease can be caused by a wide spectrum of pathogens in patients with cancer. These include a variety of infectious agents and neoplastic disorders as well as pulmonary hemorrhage, pulmonary edema (cardiogenic and noncardiogenic), and leukagglutinin reactions. Pulmonary toxicity caused by antineoplastic agents is being recognized more frequently, and the number of drugs known or suspected to cause lung disease is steadily increasing. Since continuing the offending agent may cause death and withholding it can result in resolution of pulmonary toxicity, it is important to recognize radiation- and drug-induced pulmonary disease. In this chapter, parenchymal lung disease caused by irradiation and chemotherapy will be discussed. Mechanisms of lung injury, histopathologic findings, clinical and laboratory features, and diagnosis and treatment of the abnormality produced by these agents will be reviewed.

RADIATION-INDUCED PULMONARY TOXICITY

MECHANISM OF LUNG INJURY

Radiation can affect dividing and nondividing cells and can cause genetic and nongenetic damage.[1,2] In the lung, a hypothetical reconstruction of radiation injury might be as follows. Therapeutic radiation may result in nongenetic damage which is apparent in all cells, but capillary endothelial and type I epithelial cells appear most susceptible.[3] Many of these cells, whether dividing or not, undergo early necrobiosis and slough. Over time, capillaries regenerate and the alveolar epithelium is repopulated by type II cells, since type I pneumocytes do not regenerate. Some type II cells redifferentiate into type I. If the injury is severe, damage to other nondividing materials of the lung, such as proteins and polysaccharides, takes place. This can impede reconstruction of tissue architecture and result in functional derangement and scar formation. Genetic damage to dividing cells such as endothelial cells and/or type II pneumocytes can also occur. Depletion of these cells may result during successive mitoses, with loss of integrity of the pulmonary capillary and exudation of fluid into the alveoli. At the physiologic level, loss of compliance, abnormal gas exchange, and respiratory failure can occur due to leakage of plasma proteins onto the alveolar surface. This type of genetic damage also explains why pneumonitis can happen so late after radiation. One might speculate that some endothelial cells initially remain normal, but in the course of the next four cell divisions, chromosomal aberrations prevent further replication, which leads to loss of integrity of the capillary.[1]

Certain factors are critical to the development of radiation pneumonitis. In general, damage to the lungs increases as the volume of lung tissue irradiated increases. Also, the effects of radiation, as measured by symptoms and signs, roentgenologic changes, and physiologic tests, are proportionate to the amount delivered. Radiation pneumonitis seldom occurs with doses of less than 2000 rad, but it almost invariably occurs with doses in excess of 6000 rad.[4] Besides the total radiation dose, the number of fractions into which it is divided and, to a lesser extent, the span of time over which it is delivered are important factors.[5] The greater the number of fractions in which the radiation is given, the lower will be the damaging effect. It must be remembered that fractionation is different from dose rate, which refers to output of the machine during radiation therapy. Dose rate certainly has an effect on lung tolerance: radiation delivered at 5 rad per minute is less damaging than radiation delivered at 30 rad per minute, which in turn is less damaging than radiation delivered at 200 to 300 rad per minute. In summary, the incidence and severity of radiation damage to the lungs are related principally to the volume of lung tissue irradiated, the total dose, the rate of its delivery, and the quality of the radiation.

HISTOPATHOLOGY

The histopathologic changes of radiation-induced pulmonary toxicity can be divided into early, intermediate, and late stages based on the time, course, and intensity of the radiation injury.[6] Early radiation damage (0 to 2 months after radiation) is characterized by injury to the small vessels and capillaries with the development of vascular congestion and increased capillary permeability.[7] At this stage, a fibrin-rich exudate is present in the alveolar spaces. Hyaline membranes form on the alveoli, probably from condensation of the intra-alveolar fibrin. Abnormalities in the intermediate stage (2 to 9 months after irradiation) are characterized by obstruction of pulmonary capillaries by platelets, fibrin, and collagen. Alveolar lining cells (primarily type II pneumocytes) become hyperplastic and the alveolar walls become infiltrated with fibroblasts. If the radiation injury is mild, these changes may subside entirely; however, when the injury is severe, a chronic phase (9 months or more after radiation) ensues which may persist or progress for months or years. The histopathologic appearance then is dominated by dense fibrosis, thickening of the alveolar walls, vascular subintimal fibrosis, and luminal narrowing. In some instances, the lung may shrink to less than 50% of its original size with a thickened adherent pleura and scarred hilar structures.

CLINICAL FEATURES

Symptoms and Signs

The clinical syndrome of radiation pneumonitis develops in 5% to 15% of all irradiated patients. Factors that can contribute to the development of radiation pneumonitis include concomitant chemotherapy, previous radiation therapy, and withdrawal of steroids. Advanced age and underlying chronic obstructive pulmonary disease do not seem to potentiate radiation damage.

Symptoms of acute radiation pneumonitis usually become evident 2 to 3 months after the completion of therapy; rarely, they occur within the first month and occasionally as late as 6 months after irradiation. In general, early onset of symptoms implies a more serious and more protracted clinical course. The cardinal symptom of radiation pneumonitis is dyspnea.[6] It may be self-limited or it may progress to severe respiratory distress, depending on the extent and intensity of the injury. Patients may also have a nonproductive cough or cough productive of small amounts of pinkish sputum. Frank hemoptysis early in the clinical course is distinctly uncommon; however, massive hemoptysis has been reported as a late complication of therapeutic pulmonary irradiation.[8] Fever is unusual, but can be high and spiking; in severe cases, other constitutional symptoms may occur. Chest pain, which is rarely a prominent feature, may be due to fractured ribs, pleural changes, or coughing. Symptoms of airway obstruction can occur in the first few days of radiation and are usually associated with swelling of a central bronchogenic carcinoma. Severe respiratory distress can result and may be prevented by the administration of steroids a day before and several days after the initiation of radiation therapy.

On physical examination, signs of pulmonary involvement are minimal. Occasionally, moist rales, a pleural friction rub, or evidence of pleural fluid may be heard over the area of irradiation. In severe cases, tachypnea and cyanosis may be present, and occasionally evidence of acute cor pulmonale appears, usually predicting a fatal outcome. Finger clubbing due to radiation therapy is distinctly unusual, although it may be present due to the underlying malignancy. Skin changes corresponding to the ports of irradiation are often present but provide no clue as to the presence or severity of the pulmonary reaction beneath.

Although patients with acute pneumonitis may show complete resolution of signs and symptoms, most develop gradual progressive fibrosis. In some cases patients present with radiation fibrosis without a previous history of acute pneumonitis. The permanent changes of fibrosis take 6 to 24 months to evolve, but usually remain stable after 2 years. Patients with fibrosis can be asymptomatic or can have varying degrees of dyspnea. The major complications of radiation pneumonitis occur late in the disease and are secondary to persistent fibrosis of a large volume of lung. These include cor pulmonale and respiratory failure.

Chest Radiographs

Although radiographic abnormalities are invariably found at the time clinical radiation pneumonitis is present, these changes may be seen in asymptomatic patients as well. Early radiographic changes include a ground-glass opacification, diffuse haziness or indistinctness of the normal pulmonary markings over the irradiated area.[9] The chest radiograph later may show alveolar infiltrates or dense consolidation. As the pneumonitis progresses to fibrosis, the radiolographic appearance changes to that of linear streaks radiating from the area of pneumonitis and of contraction toward either the hilum, the paramediastinal, or the apical areas. Pleural effusions, if present, are usually small and are always coincident with the pneumonitis.[10] They can persist for long periods of time, but often disappear spontaneously and never increase over a period of stability unless secondary complications occur, for example, radiation-induced pericarditis. Mediastinal or hilar adenopathy and cavitation are almost always due to causes other than radiation pneumonitis.[2] Pneumothorax is occasionally associated with radiation fibrosis but not with acute pneumonitis.

One of the most characteristic features of radiation pneumonitis and fibrosis is that the radiologic changes are confined to the outlines of the field of radiation. In a few cases, extensive changes outside the field, even in the contralateral lung, have been observed. Obstruction of lymphatic flow from mediastinal irradiation,[11] hypersensitivity in response to radiation,[12] and absorption of x-rays by regions outside the irradiated ports are possible but poorly documented explanations of this phenomenon.[13]

Pulmonary Function Tests

No gross physiologic changes occur in the lung until 4 to 8 weeks after completion of irradiation, usually coincident with the period of clinical pneumonitis. Then one sees a decrease in lung volumes, which can progress.[14–17] These changes persist indefinitely, with little evidence of recovery.[17] Gas exchange abnormalities, which include a decrease in the diffusing capacity and arterial hypoxemia, especially with exercise, occur about the same time, but show some tendency toward recovery after 6 to 12 months.[15-17] A fall in compliance coincident with the clinical pneumonitis is usually seen in most subjects.[15] Accordingly, the elastic work of breathing is increased and dyspnea resulting from the increased work of breathing ensues.[15] Airflow parameters remain close to normal in most studies.[14-17]

Diagnosis

The diagnosis of radiation pneumonitis can sometimes be made clinically based on the timing of irradiation in relation to symptoms and the typical chest radiographic appearance (*i.e.*, infiltrates corresponding to the margins of the irradiated portal). Differentiation from recurrent malignancy or infection may pose a problem, and lung biopsy may be necessary. Although histopathologic changes are nonspecific for radiation pneumonitis when elements of the acute stages of radiation pneumonia (fibrin exudate in the alveoli) are seen adjacent to elements of the more chronic stages (alveolar fibrosis and subintimal sclerosis), this entity can be diagnosed with reasonable certainty.[18]

Treatment

Three modalities of therapy have been used prophylactically and therapeutically for radiation-induced pneumonitis: corticosteroids, antibiotics, and anticoagulants. Of these, corticosteroid therapy is the most important.

No controlled clinical trials in humans are available on the efficacy of steroid therapy in radiation pneumonitis. Rubin and Casarett collected data from eight studies on humans and categorized them according to whether corticosteroids were used prophylactically or therapeutically.[2] Corticosteroids given prophylactically failed to prevent radiation pneumonitis, but when they were administered as clinical pneumonitis occurred, an objective response was seen. In other reports steroid therapy failed to prevent or ameliorate severe pneumonitis. Nonetheless, it is our practice to begin prednisone (1 mg/kg) as soon as the diagnosis is reasonably certain. The dose is then maintained for several weeks and reduced cautiously and slowly. It has been our experience that if steroids are tapered too rapidly, symptoms can be exacerbated, necessitating higher doses for longer periods of time. Similarly, if corticosteroids are part of a chemotherapeutic regimen, stopping them abruptly has the potential for precipitating clinically evident radiation pneumonitis in recently treated individuals. What parameters to follow during the tapering schedule are not known, and no studies are available. Generally we follow symptoms. Most authors agree that corticosteroids have no place in the treatment of radiation fibrosis.

In both experimental and clinical reports, antibiotic administration has no effect on the course or outcome of radiation pneumonitis.[2,19] Although there is some rationale for the use of anticoagulants in view of the effects of radiation on the vascular system, both heparin injections and oral anticoagulants have not been found to be beneficial.[19]

CHEMOTHERAPY-INDUCED PULMONARY TOXICITY

There are now 19 chemotherapeutic agents reported to cause cytotoxic drug–induced lung disease (Table 60-10). An overview of the potential mechanisms of lung damage, a summary of the pathologic findings, and common clinical features of pulmonary toxicity will be discussed. Characteristics of pulmonary disease caused by some of these drugs will be presented.

MECHANISMS OF PULMONARY INJURY

Although details about the pathophysiology of specific chemotherapeutic agents are generally not known, several mechanisms of pulmonary toxicity mediated by these agents have been proposed. Certain cytotoxic drugs may induce pulmonary injury by triggering the formation of reactive oxygen metabolites, which include the superoxide anion, hydrogen peroxide, and the hydroxyl radical. These substances can produce direct toxicity through participation in redox reactions and subsequent fatty acid oxidation, which leads to membrane instability.[20] Oxidants can cause other inflammatory reactions within the lung. For example, the oxidation of arachidonic acid is an initial step in the metabolic cascade that produces immunoreactive substances, including prostaglandins and leukotrienes.[21] Cytotoxic drugs might also affect the local lung immune system. Because the lung is exposed to so many substances that can activate its immune system, there appears to be a "pulmonary immune tolerant state" to avoid unnecessary overreactions.[22] This "tolerant state" may in part be a result of effector/suppressor cell balance. Cytotoxic drugs have the potential to alter the normal effector/suppressor balance, which may cause tissue damage.[23-25] Other balance systems within the lung can be affected as well, such as the balance between collagenesis and collagenolysis.[22] Through modulation of fibroblast proliferation, excessive collagen deposition may result in severe, irreversible pulmonary fibrosis. Bleomycin is one cytotoxic agent that has this potential.[26,27] Imbalance between

TABLE 60-10. Chemotherapeutic Agents Associated with Pulmonary Parenchymal Damage

Alkylating Agents	*Nitrosoureas*
Busulfan	Carmustine (BNCU)
Cyclophosphamide	Semustine (methyl-CCNU)
Chlorambucil	Lomustine (CCNU)
Melphalan	Chlorozotozin (DCNU)
Antibiotics	*Antimetabolites*
Bleomycin	Methotrexate
Mitomycin	Azathioprine
Neocarzinostatin (Zinostatin)	Mercaptopurine
	Cytosine arabinoside
Miscellaneous	
Procarbazine	
Vinblastine	
Vindesine	
VM-26	

the protease and antiprotease system also has been implicated in a number of pulmonary disorders, including drug toxicity.[22] Bleomycin and cyclophosphamide produce substances that can inactivate the antiprotease system, enhancing the effects of proteolytic enzymes on the lung. Drugs may damage the lung through a variety of other mechanisms, and considerable investigation needs to be done to define and clarify the exact mechanism of lung injury for each chemotherapeutic drug.

HISTOPATHOLOGY

The histopathologic changes of drug-induced pulmonary toxicity show common features. Similar to radiation-induced damage, abnormalities are seen in both endothelial and epithelial cells. The vascular damage is characterized by endothelial swelling with exudation of fluid into the interstitium and the intra-alveolar spaces. There is destruction and desquamation of type I pneumocytes with delamellation and proliferation of type II pneumocytes. Mononuclear cell infiltration and fibroblast proliferation with fibrosis are common findings; the character of the inflammatory cellular infiltrate may be a feature that distinguishes the toxicity of one drug from another. Bronchoalveolar lavage studies in patients with methotrexate pulmonary toxicity have shown the presence of a helper T-cell alveolitis, while studies on some patients with bleomycin toxicity have revealed a polymorphonuclear alveolitis.[23,28] Eosinophilic infiltration has been associated with drugs causing apparent hypersensitivity reactions, for example, methotrexate,[22] procarbazine,[29] and bleomycin.[30]

CLINICAL FEATURES

Table 60-11 lists predisposing factors that have been associated with enhancement of drug-induced pneumonitis.[31–46] Since bleomycin toxicity is relatively common it deserves special mention. Although toxicity drastically increases with doses in excess of 450 to 500 mg, it can occur with much lower doses, especially when other risk factors are present. These factors include age greater than 60 years, a decrease in creatinine clearance time during the period of administration of bleomycin, simultaneous or prior radiation therapy to the lungs, and simultaneous or subsequent oxygen therapy, especially with inspired doses equal to or greater than 35%.

TABLE 60-11. Factors Associated with Increased Risk of Drug-Induced Pneumonitis

Risk Factor	*Drug(s)*
Total dose	Bleomycin,[31,32] BCNU[31]
Age	Bleomycin[32]
Oxygen therapy	Bleomycin,[33–35] cyclophosphamide,[34] mitomycin[36]
Simultaneous or prior radiation therapy to lungs	Bleomycin,[37,38] busulfan,[39] mitomycin[40]
Increased toxicity when given with other drugs	BCNU,[41] mitomycin,[42] cyclophosphamide,[43,44] bleomycin,[44,45] methotrexate[43]
Preexisting pulmonary disease	BCNU[46]

Signs and Symptoms

The cardinal symptom of drug-induced pulmonary toxicity is dyspnea. Nonproductive cough, fatigue, and malaise are other commonly associated complaints. Although symptoms usually develop over a period of several weeks to months, hypersensitivity drug-induced lung disease can develop over hours. Fever may be a common finding with this type of toxicity. Chest pain has been reported during infusion of bleomycin or immediately after therapy with methotrexate; however, it is an unusual manifestation of toxicity.[47,48] Since hemoptysis is an uncommon feature of drug-induced pulmonary toxicity, when it is present other diagnoses should be considered. Physical examination of the lungs may be normal or may reveal end-inspiratory "Velcro" rales. Finger clubbing is distinctly unusual, though it may be related to the underlying malignancy.

Chest Radiographs

The most common roentgenographic abnormality associated with drug-induced pulmonary toxicity is a reticular nodular pattern, which may be basilar or diffuse. Pleural effusions are uncommon but occasionally have been reported in association with mitomycin, busulfan, and methotrexate toxicity.[49–51] Hypersensitivity lung disease associated with methotrexate and procarbazine may present with bilateral acinar infiltrates that clear very rapidly.[52] In some instances the chest radiograph is normal, even in the presence of histologically proven pulmonary infiltration and fibrosis.[51,53] Most commonly methotrexate and BCNU toxicity have been reported with normal chest x-ray findings. Hilar adenopathy is distinctly unusual and has been reported only with methotrexate toxicity.[51]

Pulmonary Function Tests

The most common abnormalities associated with chemotherapy-induced pulmonary toxicity is a reduced diffusing capacity for carbon monoxide, accompanied by a restrictive ventilatory defect.[22] Isolated gas exchange abnormalities manifested by a decrease in the diffusing capacity and arterial hypoxemia, especially with exercise, have also been seen. Screening pulmonary function tests to predict which patients receiving chemotherapy are likely to develop toxicity would be very helpful but have not been established as yet.

Diagnosis

Although one might have a very high clinical suspicion of drug-induced pulmonary toxicity, lung biopsy is usually necessary for diagnosis. Since pathognomonic pathologic changes associated with drug-induced pneumonitis often are not present, a biopsy is necessary to eliminate other specific diagnoses, such as opportunistic infection and malignancy. Through the use of bronchoalveolar lavage, several studies now report the presence of a characteristic or predominant cell associated with particular drugs.[23,28] However, the usefulness of bronchoalveolar lavage in clinically diagnosing drug-induced toxicity has not been delineated.

Treatment

The most effective way to manage pulmonary toxicity associated with chemotherapeutic agents is to prevent it. If it occurs, withdrawal of the offending agent is the cornerstone of therapy. Although no controlled studies in humans have systematically examined the efficacy of corticosteroids, a trial of these agents is probably warranted in most cases. The optimal dose and duration of therapy are not known. However, 1 mg/kg is usually initiated with a slow and careful tapering schedule, since clinical deterioration after tapering has been reported.[54,55]

Table 60-12 lists the characteristics of pulmonary disease caused by the commonly used chemotherapeutic agents.

TABLE 60-12. Clinical and Pathologic Features of Chemotherapy-Induced Toxicity

Drug	*Mechanism of Injury*	*Histopathology*	*Clinical Features*	*Chest Roentgenogram*	*Diagnosis*	*Treatment*
Alkylating Agents:						
Busulfan[31,39,50,56–60]	No studies, but direct toxicity to epithelial lining cells is suggested.	Pneumocyte dysplasia (degeneration of type I cells; atypical hyperplastic type II cells), atypical bronchial lining cells, mononuclear cells infiltration, fibrosis.	4% incidence; no direct dose-dependent toxicity; may be threshold dose (>500 mg); radiation and alkylating agents may enhance toxicity. Insidious onset after 4 years (8 mo to 10 yr). Dyspnea, cough, weight loss, weakness, fever; crepitant basilar rales, pigementation. Prognosis: poor.	Most common bibasilar reticular pattern; rarely pleural effusion, pulmonary ossification, normal chest radiograph.	Suggested by history and bizarre pneumocytes in sputum or lavage fluid. Definitive diagnosis by open lung biopsy.	Withdrawal of the drug; anecdotal reports of improvement with high-dose steroids. Mean survival after diagnosis is 5 months.
Cyclophos-pha-mide[31,34,55,61–64]	May be toxic through production of reactive oxygen species.	Endothelial swelling, pneumocyte dysplasia, lymphocytic and histiocytic infiltration, fibrosis.	Less than 1% incidence; does not appear dose-dependent, but synergy with oxygen and other agents possible. Subacute onset 3 weeks to 8 years after initiation of therapy, up to 8 years after stopping therapy. Cough, dyspnea, fever; basilar rales.	Commonly, bibasilar reticular pattern; diffuse pulmonary edema pattern also reported.	As above.	Drug withdrawal; corticosteroids may hasten improvement, but no documented effect on mortality. Overall recovery about 65%.
Chlorambucil[22,65]	Unknown.	Similar to busulfan; fibrosis may predominate.	Rare reports; subacute onset 6 months to 3 years after therapy. Cough, dyspnea, anorexia; bibasilar rales.	Bibasilar reticular pattern; rarely, normal radiograph; alveolar infiltrates not reported.	As above.	50% of reported patients have died despite cessation of drug and administration of steroids. Anecdotal reports of response to steroids.
Melphalan[22,66,67]	Unknown.	Similar to busulfan; pneumocyte dysplasia more common than fibrosis.	Rare (five documented reports); appears 1 to 48 months after therapy. Progressive dyspnea, productive cough, fever, malaise; bibasilar rales.	Reticular and alveolar infiltrates.	As above.	Despite cessation of drug, 3 of 5 patients reported died of disease. In most cases, patients were receiving steroids for underlying disease.

(*continued*)

TABLE 60-12. Clinical and Pathologic Features of Chemotherapy-Induced Toxicity (*continued*)

Drug	*Mechanism of Injury*	*Histopathology*	*Clinical Features*	*Chest Roentgenogram*	*Diagnosis*	*Treatment*
Antibiotics:						
Bleomycin[22,26,27,68–75]	Several possible mechanisms: (*a*) direct toxicity through generation of reactive oxygen metabolites; (*b*) leukocyte influx and lung injury from release of proteases; (*c*) increased collagen synthesis and subsequent pulmonary fibrosis.	Endothelial blebbing; interstitial edema, necrosis of type I cells and metaplastic type II cells; inflammation with polymorphonuclear cells; fibroblast proliferation and fibrosis; occasionally eosinophilic infiltration.	Incidence 2% to 40%; age- and dose-related (>500 mg); synergy seen with oxygen therapy, radiation, and other agents. Occurs during and after stopping therapy. Cough, dyspnea, fever; tachypnea, rales. Hypersensitivity pneumonitis variant.	Bibasilar reticular pattern; multiple nodules similar to metastatic disease; acinar pattern, especially with hypersensitivity reaction; rarely, localized infiltrate.	Bronchoalveolar lavage might suggest diagnosis (polymorphonuclear alveolitis). Transbronchial or open lung biopsy required for diagnosis, especially to rule out other causes.	Drug withdrawal. In bleomycin hypersensitivity reactions, definite role for steroids; in other forms of bleomycin toxicity, efficacy less clear. Mortality estimated at 50%.
Mitomycin[22,40–42,49,54,76]	No studies, but probably similar to the alkylating agents.	Similar to bleomycin; in patients with microangiopathic hemolytic anemia, prominent vascular changes are present.	3% to 12% incidence; does not appear dose-related, but possible synergy with oxygen, radiotherapy, and other agents. Dry cough and dyspnea; fever not seen; bibasilar rales.	Diffuse reticular pattern; pleural effusions seen.	Lung biopsy for definitive diagnosis; no bronchoalveolar lavage studies reported.	Drug withdrawal; steroids may alter outcome. Mortality approaches 50%.
*Nitrosoureas**						
BCNU (Carmustine)[41,46,53,77–79]	Few studies; direct injury through generation of toxic oxidant molecules possible.	Similar to bleomycin; fibrosis predominates.	20% to 30% incidence; dose-related; increased risk with preexisting lung disease and tobacco use; possible synergism with other agents; can be seen after drug stopped. Dry cough, dyspnea, bibasilar rales.	Bibasilar reticular pattern; may be normal.	As above.	Early recognition and withdrawal of the drug; steroids not beneficial since most patients are on the drug for intracranial processes when toxicity develops. Mortality reported between 24% to 90%.
Antimetabolites						
Methotrexate[22,23,31,43,48,51]	Direct toxic effect may play a role but mechanism not known; hypersensitivity suggested by occurrence of eosinophils and presence of increased helper T-lymphocytes in lavage fluid.	Interstitial and alveolar infiltrate of lymphocytes, eosinophils, and plasma cells; occasional poorly formed noncaseating granuloma; fibrosis unusual.	8% incidence; synergism with other agents possible; occurs 12 days to 18 years after beginning therapy. Fever, chills, malaise, headache—a prodrome for days and weeks; cough, dyspnea, rales common. Skin rash in 17% and blood eosinophilia in 40%.	Early interstitial infiltrates; later, alveolar infiltrates; hilar and mediastinal adenopathy, pleural effusions described; chest radiography can be normal.	Clinical history suggestive; bronchoalveolar lavage might suggest diagnosis (helper T-cells in fluid), but lung biopsy required for diagnosis.	Discontinue drug, but reports of reinstitution without recurrence of the abnormality. Dramatic responses to steroids reported. Mortality 1%; outlook favorable.

(*continued*)

TABLE 60-12. Clinical and Pathologic Features of Chemotherapy-Induced Toxicity (*continued*)

Drug	*Mechanism of Injury*	*Histopathology*	*Clinical Features*	*Chest Roentgenogram*	*Diagnosis*	*Treatment*
Cytosine arabinoside[83,84]	Unknown.	Pulmonary edema; proteinaceous exudate with extravasation of red blood cells, no inflammatory cells.	If given within 30 days of death, high incidence of pulmonary edema. Abrupt onset of dyspnea; GI toxicity coexists.	Diffuse interstitial and alveolar pattern.	Clinical picture suggests diagnosis.	Supportive; no studies.
Miscellaneous						
Procarbazine[29,52,85]	Hypersensitivity.	Mononuclear cell infiltration and scattered foci of eosinophils; fibrosis in one case.	Acute onset within hours to days of first dose. Nausea, fevers, chills, arthralgias, urticaria, dry cough, and dyspnea. Blood eosinophilia common.	Interstitial infiltrates; pleural effusion.	Clinical picture highly suggestive of diagnosis.	Rapid recovery following discontinuation of drug. Role of steroids not known.
Vinca alkaloids—vinblastine and vindesine[42,54,86,87]	Unknown.	Dysplasia of alveolar lining cells; interstitial and alveolar influx of inflammatory cells; fibrosis.	Most common reports in association with mitomycin. Dyspnea and wheezing seen with vindesine. Obstructive pattern on pulmonary function testing in one patient.	Diffuse interstitial and alveolar infiltrates with combination drugs; normal chest radiograph with vinca alkaloid alone.	Clinical history suggests diagnosis.	Drug withdrawal; steroids probably beneficial. Prognosis poor if pulmonary infiltrates develop.

*Pulmonary toxicity has been reported with all other nitrosoureas, including CCNU (lomustine), methyl-CCNU (semustine), and DCNU (chlorozotocin).[80–82]

REFERENCES

1. Gross NJ: The pathogenesis of radiation-induced lung damage. Lung 159:115, 1981
2. Rubin P, Casarett GW: Clinical Radiation Pathology. Philadelphia, WB Saunders, 1968
3. Adamson ILR, Bowden DH, Wyatt JP: A pathway to pulmonary fibrosis: An ultrastructural study of mouse and rat following radiation to the whole body and hemithorax. Am J Pathol 58:481, 1970
4. Jennings FL, Arden A: Development of radiation pneumonitis: Time and dose factors. Arch Pathol 74:351, 1962
5. Wara WM, Phillips TL, Margolis LW et al: Radiation pneumonitis: A new approach to the deviation of time–dose factors. Cancer 32:547, 1973
6. Gross NJ: Pulmonary effects of radiation therapy. Ann Intern Med 86:81, 1977
7. Maisin JR: The ultrastructure of the lung of mice exposed to a supra-lethal dose of ionizing radiation on the thorax. Radiat Res 44:545, 1970
8. Isaacs RD, Wallie WJ, Wells AU et al: Massive hemoptysis as a late complication of pulmonary irradiation. Thorax 42:77, 1987
9. Bate D, Guttman RJ: Changes in lung and pleura following two-million-volt therapy for carcinoma of the breast. Radiology 73:679, 1957
10. Bachman AL, Macken K: Pleural effusions following supervoltage radiation for breast carcinoma. Radiology 72:699, 1959
11. Smith JC: Radiation pneumonitis: Case report of bilateral reaction after unilateral irradiation. Am Rev Respir Dis 89:264, 1964
12. Holt JAG: The acute radiation pneumonitis syndrome. J Coll Radiol Aust 8:40, 1964
13. Bennett DE, Million RR, Ackerman LV: Bilateral radiation pneumonitis, a complication of the radiotherapy of bronchogenic carcinoma. Cancer 23:1001, 1969
14. Brady LW, German PA, Cander L: The effects of radiation therapy on pulmonary function in carcinoma of the lung. Radiology 85:130, 1965
15. Emirgil C, Heinemann HO: Effects of radiation of chest on pulmonary function in men. J Appl Physiol 16:331, 1961
16. Prato FS, Kurdyak R, Saibil EA et al: Regional and total lung function in patients following pulmonary irradiation. Invest Radiol 12:224, 1977
17. Wohl MEB, Griscom NT, Traggis DG et al: Effects of therapeutic irradiation delivered in early childhood upon subsequent lung function. Pediatrics 55:507, 1975
18. Warren S, Spencer J: Radiation reaction in the lung. AJR 43:682, 1940
19. Moss WT, Haddy FJ, Sweany SK: Some factors altering the severity of acute radiation pneumonitis: Variation with cortisone, heparin, and antibiotics. Radiology 75:50, pneumonitis: Variation with cortisone, heparin, and antibiotics. Radiology 75:50, 1960
20. Freeman BA, Crapo JD: Biology of disease: Free radicals and tissue injury. Lab Invest 47:412, 1982
21. Lewis RA, Austen KF: The biologically active leukotrienes: Biosynthesis, metabolism, receptors, functions and pharmacology. J Clin Invest 73:889, 1984
22. Cooper JAD, White DA, Matthay RA: Drug-induced pulmonary disease: Part I. Cytotoxic drugs. Am Rev Respir Dis 133:321, 1986
23. White DA, Rankin JR, Stover DE et al: Methotrexate pneumonitis: Lavage findings suggest an immune mediated disorder. Am Rev Respir Dis (in press)
24. Askenase PW, Hayden BJ, Gershon RK: Augmentation of delayed-type hypersensitivity by doses of cyclophosphamide which do not affect antibody responses. J Exp Med 141:697, 1974
25. L'age-Stehr J, Diamanstein T: Induction of autoreactive T lymphocytes and their suppressor cells by cyclophosphamide. Nature 271:663, 1978
26. Absher M, Hildebran J, Trombley L et al: Characteristics of cultured lung fibroblasts from bleomycin-treated rats: Comparison with in vitro exposed normal fibroblasts. Am Rev Respir Dis 129:125, 1984
27. Clark JG, Kostal KM, Marino BA: Bleomycin induced pulmonary fibrosis in hamsters: An alveolar macrophage product increases fibroblast prostaglandin E2 and cyclic adenosine monophosphate and suppresses fibroblast proliferation and collagen production. J Clin Invest 72:2082, 1983
28. White DA, Kris MG, Stover DE: Bronchoalveolar lavage cell populations in bleomycin-induced pulmonary toxicity. Thorax 42:551, 1987
29. Jones SE, Moore M, Blank N et al: Hypersensitivity to procarbazine (Matulane) manifested by fever and pleuropulmonary reaction. Cancer 29:498, 1972
30. Holoye PY, Luna MA, McKay B et al: Bleomycin hypersensitivity pneumonitis. Ann Intern Med 88:47, 1978

31. Ginsberg SJ, Comis RL: The pulmonary toxicity of antineoplastic agents. Semin Oncol 9:34, 1982
32. Blum RH, Carter SK, Agre K: A clinical review of bleomycin—a new antineoplastic agent. Cancer 31:903, 1973
33. Goldiner PL, Carlon GC, Cvitkovic E et al: Factors influencing postoperative morbidity and mortality in patients treated with bleomycin. Br Med J 1:1664, 1978
34. Hakkinen PJ, Whiteley JW, Witschi HR: Hyperoxia, but not thoracic x-irradiation, potentiates bleomycin and cyclophosphamide-induced lung damage in mice. Am Rev Respir Dis 126:281, 1982
35. Tryka AF, Godleski JJ, Brian JD: Differences in effects of immediate and delayed hyperoxia exposure on bleomycin-induced pulmonary injury. Cancer Treat Rep 68:759, 1984
36. Franklin R, Buroker TR, Vaishampayan W et al: Combined therapies in esophageal squamous cell cancer (abstr). Proc Am Assoc Cancer Res 20:223, 1979
37. Einhorn L, Krause M, Hornback N et al: Enhanced pulmonary toxicity with bleomycin and radiotherapy in oat cell cancer. Cancer 37:2414, 1976
38. Samuels ML, Johnson DE, Holoye PY et al: Large-dose bleomycin therapy and pulmonary toxicity: A possible role of prior radiotherapy. JAMA 235:1117, 1976
39. Soble AR, Perry H: Fatal radiation pneumonia following subclinical busulfan injury. AJR 128:15, 1977
40. Buzdar AU, Legha SS, Luna MA et al: Pulmonary toxicity of mitomycin. Cancer 45:236, 1980
41. Durant JR, Norgard MJ, Murad TM et al: Pulmonary toxicity associated with bischloroethylnitrosourea (BCNU). Ann Intern Med 90:191, 1979
42. Luedke D, McLaughlin TT, Daughaday C et al: Mitomycin C and vindesine associated pulmonary toxicity with variable clinical expression. Cancer 55:542, 1985
43. White DA, Orenstein M, Godwin TA et al: Chemotherapy-associated pulmonary toxic reactions during treatment for breast cancer. Arch Intern Med 144:953, 1984
44. Skarin AT, Rosenthal DS, Maloney WC: The treatment of advanced non-Hodgkin's lymphoma (NHL) with bleomycin, Adriamycin, cyclophosphamide, vincristine and prednisone. Blood 49:759, 1977
45. Bauer KA, Skarin AT, Balikian JP et al: Pulmonary complications associated with combination chemotherapy programs containing bleomycin. Am J Med 74:557, 1983
46. Aronin PA, Mahaley MS, Rudnick SA et al: Prediction of BCNU pulmonary toxicity in patients with malignant gliomas: An assessment of risk factors. N Engl J Med 303:183, 1980
47. White DA, Schwartzberg L, Kris MG et al: Acute chest pain during bleomycin infusions. Cancer 59:1582, 1987
48. Walden PAM, Mitchell-Heggs PF, Coppin C et al: Pleurisy and methotrexate treatment. Br Med J 2:867, 1977
49. Orwoll ES, Kiessling P, Patterson R: Interstitial pneumonia from mitomycin. Ann Intern Med 89:352, 1978
50. Smalley RV, Wall RL: Two cases of busulfan toxicity. Ann Intern Med 64:154, 1966
51. Sostman HD, Matthay RA, Putnam CE: Methotrexate-induced pneumonitis. Medicine 55:371, 1976
52. Ecker MD, May B, Keohane MF: Procarbazine lung. AJR 131:527, 1978
53. Weiss RB, Poster DS, Penta JS: The nitrosoureas and pulmonary toxicity. Cancer Treat Rev 8:111, 1981
54. Gunstream SR, Seidenfeld JJ, Sobonya RE et al: Mitomycin-associated lung disease. Cancer Treat Rep 67:301, 1983
55. Spector JI, Zimbler H, Ross JS: Cyclophosphamide and interstitial pneumonitis. JAMA 243:1133, 1980
56. Koss LG, Melamed MR, Mayer K: The effect of busulfan on human epithelia. Am J Clin Pathol 44:385, 1965
57. Stover DE, Zaman MB, Hajdu SI et al: Bronchoalveolar lavage in the diagnosis of diffuse pulmonary infiltrates in the immunosuppressed host. Ann Intern Med 101;1, 1984
58. Kuplic JB, Higley CS, Niewoehner DE: Pulmonary ossification associated with long-term busulfan therapy in chronic myeloid leukemia. Am Rev Respir Dis 106:759, 1972
59. Heard BE, Cooke RA: Busulfan lung. Thorax 23:187, 1968
60. Burns WA, McFarland W, Matthews MJ: Busulfan-induced pulmonary disease: Report of a case and review of the literature. Am Rev Respir Dis 101:408, 1970
61. Collis CH: Lung damage from cytotoxic drugs. Cancer Chemother Pharmacol 4:17, 1980
62. Mark GJ, Lehimgar-Zadeh A, Ragsdale BD: Cyclophosphamide pneumonitis. Thorax 33:89, 1978
63. Alvarado CS, Boat TF, Newman AJ: Late-onset pulmonary fibrosis and chest deformity in two children treated with cyclophosphamide. J Pediatr 92:443, 1978
64. Maxwell I: Reversible pulmonary edema following cyclophosphamide treatment. JAMA 229:137, 1974
65. Cole SR, Myers TJ, Klatsky AU: Pulmonary disease with chlorambucil therapy. Cancer 41:455, 1978
66. Taetle R, Dickman PS, Feldman PS: Pulmonary histopathologic changes associated with melphalan therapy. Cancer 42:1239, 1978
67. Goucher G, Rowland V, Hawkins J: Melphalan-induced pulmonary interstitial fibrosis. Chest 77:805, 1980
68. Berend N: Protective effect of hypoxia on bleomycin lung toxicity in the rat. Am Rev Respir Dis 130:307, 1984
69. Frank L: Protection from O toxicity by pre-exposure to hypoxia: Lung antioxidant enzyme role. J Appl Physiol 53:475, 1982
70. Wesselius LJ, Catanzaro A, Wasserman SI: Neutrophil chemotactic activity generation by alveolar macrophages after bleomycin injury. Am Rev Respir Dis 129:485, 1984
71. Kelley J, Newman RA, Evans JN: Bleomycin-induced pulmonary fibrosis in the rat: Prevention with an inhibitor of collagen synthesis. J Lab Clin Med 96:954, 1980
72. White DA, Stover DE: Severe bleomycin-induced pneumonitis: Clinical features and response to corticosteroids. Chest 86:723, 1984
73. Luna MA, Bedrossian CWM, Lichtiger B et al: Interstitial pneumonitis associated with bleomycin therapy. J Clin Pathol 58:501, 1972
74. Glasier CM, Siegel MJ: Multiple pulmonary nodules: Unusual manifestation of bleomycin toxicity. AJR 137:155, 1981
75. DeLena M, Guzzon A, Monfardini S et al: Clinical, radiologic and histopathologic studies on pulmonary toxicity induced by treatment with bleomycin (NSC-125066). Cancer Chemother Rep 56:343, 1972
76. Jolivet J, Giroux L, Laurin S et al: Microangiopathic hemolytic anemia, renal failure, and noncardiogenic pulmonary edema: a chemotherapy-induced syndrome. Cancer Treat Rep 67:429, 1983
77. Nathan CF, Arrick BA, Murray HW et al: Tumor cell antioxidant defenses: Inhibition of the glutathione redox cycle enhances macrophage-mediated cytolysis. J Exp Med 153:766, 1981
78. Reznil-Schuller HM, Smith AC, Thenot JP et al: Pulmonary toxicity of the anticancer drug, bis-chloroethyl nitrosurea (BCNU) in rats. Toxicologist 4:29, 1984
79. Selker RG, Jacobs SA, Moore PB: BCNU (1,3-bis(2-chloroenthyl)-1-nitrosourea) induced pulmonary fibrosis. Neurosurgery 7:560, 1980
80. Cordonnier C, Vernant J-P, Mital P et al: Pulmonary fibrosis subsequent to high doses of CCNU for chronic leukemia. Cancer 51:1814, 1983
81. Lee W, Moore RP, Wampler GL: Interstitial pulmonary fibrosis as a complication of prolonged methyl-CCNU therapy. Cancer Treat Rep 62:1355, 1978
82. Sordillo EM, Sordillo PP, Stover DE et al: Chlorozotocin (DCNU)-induced pulmonary toxicity. Cancer Clin Trials 4:397, 1981
83. Haupt HM, Hutchins GM, Moore GW: Ara-C lung: Noncardiogenic pulmonary edema complicating cytosine arabinoside therapy of leukemia. Am J Med 70:256, 1981
84. Hewlett RI, Wilson AF: Adult respiratory distress syndrome (ARDS) following aggressive management of extensive acute lymphoblastic leukemia. Cancer 39:2422, 1977
85. Lokich JJ, Moloney WC: Allergic reaction to procarbazine. Clin Pharmacol Ther 13:573, 1972
86. Kris MG, Pablo D, Gralla RJ et al: Dyspnea following vinblastine or vindesine administration in patients receiving mitomycin plus vinca alkaloid combination therapy. Cancer Treat Rep 68:1029, 1984
87. Konits PH, Aisner J, Sutherland J et al: Possible pulmonary toxicity secondary to vinblastine. Cancer 50:2771, 1982

SECTION 6

RICHARD J. SHERINS
JOHN J. MULVIHILL

Gonadal Dysfunction

With the success of cytotoxic chemotherapy in the treatment of Hodgkin's disease, acute lymphocytic leukemia, germ cell testicular tumors, and other malignant and nonmalignant disorders have come new concerns for the long-term toxic effects of these therapies on normal host tissues. Although many of the acute and chronic toxic effects of antineoplastic drugs have been well defined, comparatively little attention has been paid to gonadal dysfunction resulting from antitumor therapy. In part this lack of attention has stemmed from the absence of any immediate or life-threatening symptoms resulting from gonadal injury; in part it has reflected the absence (until recently) of a group of long-term cancer survivors who are concerned about their reproductive potential.

Neoplastic disease and its treatment can potentially interfere with any of the cellular, anatomical, physiological, behavioral, or social processes that contribute to normal sexual and reproductive function. The tumor may directly involve the gonad, and cancer surgery may require incidental gonadectomy, genital mutilation, or retroperitoneal lymph node dissection, which for the male can result in failure of emission, retrograde ejaculation, loss of orgasm, and impotence (Table 60-13). Many drugs used in the treatment of cancer have profound and lasting effects on gonadal function. Both germ cell production and endocrine function may be affected. The magnitude of the effect can vary with the drug class or combination, the total dose administered, and the age and pubertal status of the patient at the time of therapy. Radiation therapy as well as chemotherapy can result in germ cell depletion and clinical hypogonadism, and potentially can induce mutagenic effects in the germ cell and teratogenic effects in the fetus. Recent evidence from rodent studies suggests that seminal transmission to the female of drugs administered to the male may have adverse effects on the developing fetus and embryo.[1]

TABLE 60-13. Reproductive Consequences of Cancer and Cancer Therapy

Tumor	Direct gonadal involvement
	Hypothalamic/pituitary involvement
Surgery	Removal of gonad
	Neurogenic dysfunction
	Failure of emission
	Retrograde ejaculation
	Loss of orgasm
	Impotence
	Genital mutilation
Therapy	Germ cell depletion
	Clinical hypogonadism
	Mutagenic changes in germ cell
	Teratogenic effects on fetus
	Seminal transmission of drug

Thus, the reproductive consequences of cancer therapy can be described as follows. They are

- drug specific,
- dose dependent,
- age related,
- sex dependent, and
- species specific.

A separate category of effects concerns social and behavioral responses to the physiological disruptions of cancer therapy. The nature of the patient's illness, the extent of necessary surgery or radiation therapy, and the patient's relationship with spouse and family all play an important role in reestablishing normal sexual interest and function following treatment for cancer. Detailed reviews of the reproductive consequences of cancer and cancer therapy are available.[2-7]

CHEMOTHERAPY EFFECTS IN ADULT MEN

CLINICAL PATHOPHYSIOLOGY

Testicular function in adult men is particularly susceptible to injury by many chemotherapeutic agents. The primary histopathologic lesion produced by the drugs studied to date is one of progressive, dose-related depletion of the germinal epithelium lining the seminiferous tubule (Fig. 60-6).[8-12] Frequently, spermatocytes and spermatogonia disappear completely and only the Sertoli cells remain lining the tubular lumen, a state described as germinal aplasia. The Leydig cells remain morphologically intact, although they may be functionally abnormal.[13]

The clinical manifestations of germinal depletion (Table 60-14) are a marked reduction in testicular volume, severe oligospermia or azoospermia, and infertility.[14,15] Because the gonad regulates gonadotropin secretion, serum follicle-stimulating hormone (FSH) and luteinizing hormone (LH) levels reflect the state of the seminiferous epithelium (Fig. 60-7). Germinal aplasia results in a fivefold increase in serum FSH levels (Fig. 60-8); and partial germinal depletion results in a lesser increase in FSH concentration, suggesting that the seminiferous tubule is the site of feedback inhibition of FSH secretion.[16] Thus, the serum FSH level serves as a marker for the presence of testicular germ cell loss. By contrast, serum LH and testosterone levels tend to remain within normal limits in the presence of germinal depletion. However, administration of LH-releasing hormone to patients with germinal aplasia results in an exaggerated LH response suggestive of subtle Leydig cell failure.[12,17-20] Furthermore, men with germinal aplasia who maintain normal plasma LH and total testosterone concentrations have a 50% reduction in both testosterone production per day and free testosterone levels (see Table 60-14).[13] These changes in Leydig cell function may account for the "selective" increase in plasma FSH level since, in steroid-replaced castrated male rats, high FSH levels but normal LH levels can be induced when testosterone production is reduced in association with high estradiol production.[21]

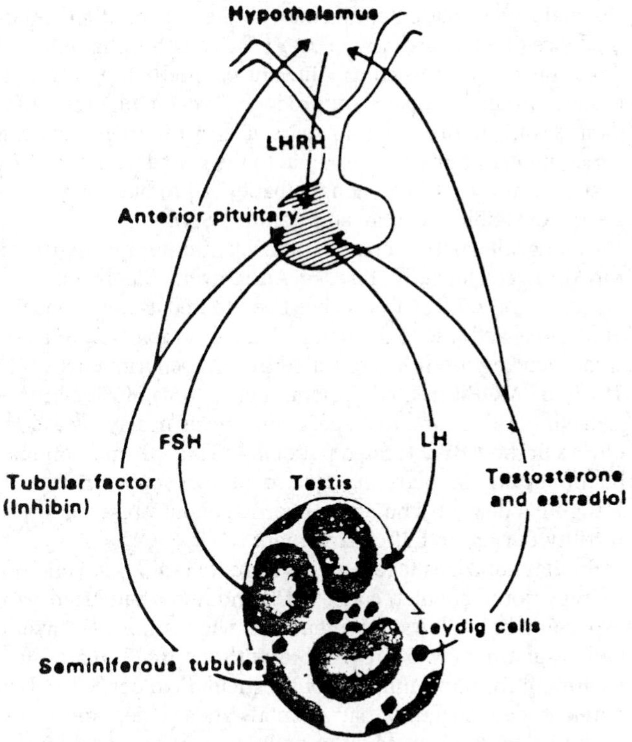

FIG. 60-6. Hypothalamic–pituitary–testicular interrelationships. Note that LH acts primarily on Leydig cells, whereas FSH primarily affects the seminiferous tubules. (Sherins RJ, Winters SJ: Management of disorders of the testis. In Melmon K, Morelli HP [eds]: Clinical Pharmacology: Basic Principles and Therapeutics, 2nd ed, p. 582. New York, Macmillan, 1978)

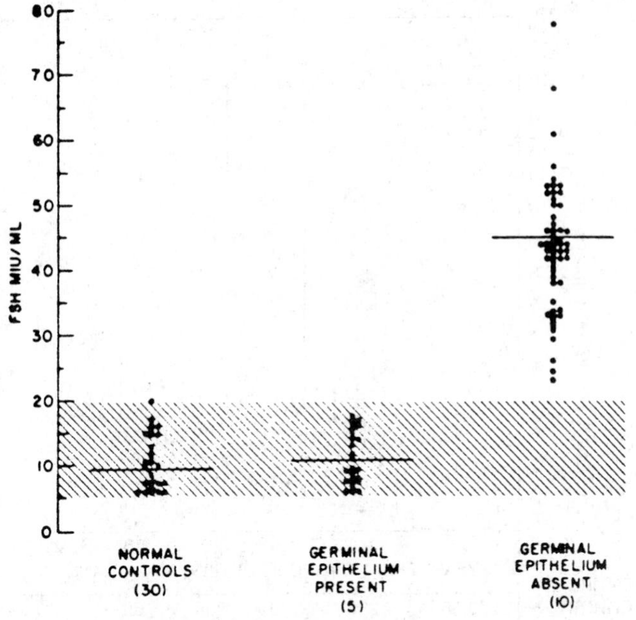

FIG. 60-7. Serum FSH levels in normal men and in men with germinal aplasia, (VanThiel DH, Sherins RJ, Myers GH et al: J Clin Invest 51:1009–1019, 1972)

SINGLE AGENTS

The anticancer agents most commonly associated with testicular germ cell depletion are listed in Table 60-15. Studies of men receiving single alkylating agents for lymphoma have been a major source of information about drug-related infertility. During alkylating agent therapy, the seminiferous epithelium is depleted in a dose-related fashion. Progressive but reversible oligospermia occurs in men receiving up to 400 mg of chlorambucil, whereas azoospermia and germinal aplasia occur in patients treated with cumulative doses in excess of 400 mg.[11] Similarly, germinal aplasia is uncommon in patients receiving less than 6 g to 10 g of cyclophosphamide.[8] Vinblastine, doxorubicin, procarbazine, and cisplatin have all been implicated as being toxic to the germinal epithelium in both animals and man,[12,22–25] although specific dose–toxicity relationships have not been established for these drugs. Further prospective evaluation of the effects of these and other single agents on testicular function is required to establish reliable data concerning the threshold drug dose above which seminiferous tubular damage becomes irreversible.

TABLE 60-14. Evaluation of Gonadal Function in Men Following Cancer Therapy

A. SEXUAL HISTORY

1. Pretreatment fertility history of both partners
2. Developmental: age of testicular descent, pubertal age, congenital anomalies of urinary tract or CNS
3. *Surgical:* orchiopexy, pelvic or retroperitoneal surgery, injury to genitals, spinal cord injury
4. *Medical:* venereal disease, mumps, renal disease, diabetes, epididymitis, tuberculosis, or other chronic illnesses
5. *Drugs:* many drugs interfere with spermatogenesis, erection, and ejaculation

B. CLINICAL AND LABORATORY FEATURES OF GERMINAL APLASIA

	Testis Size			*Hormone Profile*				
	Length × width (cm)	*Volume (cc)*	*Sperm Count (million/ml)*	*FSH (mIU/ml)*	*LH (mIU/ml)*	*Testosterone (ng/100 ml)*	*Testosterone Production Rate (mg/day)*	*Free Testosterone (ng/100 ml)*
Normal men	5.0 × 3.0	16–30	20–100	4–25	4–20	250–1200	7.5	15.3
Germinal asplasia	3.7 × 2.3	8–15	0	25–90	8–25	200–700	3.5	8.6

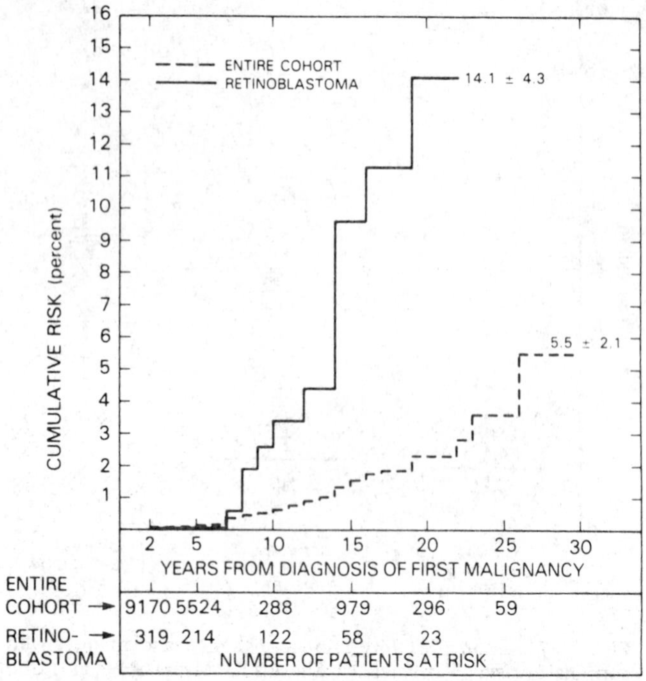

FIG. 60-8. Cumulative risk of bone cancer after treatment for childhood cancer. Mean ± SE. (Tucker MA, D'Angio DG, Boice JD et al: Bone sarcoma linked to radiotherapy and chemotherapy in children. N Engl J Med 317:588–593, 1987)

COMBINATION CHEMOTHERAPY

Combination drug regimens have a profound impact on spermatogenesis. The effects of nitrogen mustard, vincristine, procarbazine, and prednisone (MOPP) have been most carefully investigated, and it is clear that more than 80% of men receiving this regimen develop azoospermia, germinal aplasia, testicular atrophy, and elevated serum FSH levels.[19,20,26–29] Procarbazine leads to particularly long-lasting testicular damage.[30] Indeed, this drug alone induces germinal aplasia in adult male monkeys.[23]

Whereas MOPP produces irreversible germinal aplasia in the majority of patients, this may not be true of other multimodal regimens currently in use.[31,32] Cyclophosphamide and doxorubicin, when used as adjuvant chemotherapy for soft-tissue sarcoma, appear to produce irreversible testicular damage only in men over 40 years of age or in men receiving concomitant irradiation proximal to the gonads. Similar drug doses administered to younger patients produce only transient, reversible elevations of serum FSH.[32]

TABLE 60-15. Antitumor Agents Associated with Testicular Germ Cell Depletion

Degree of Risk	*Drug*
Definite	Chlorambucil Cyclophosphamide Nitrogen mustard Busulfan Procarbazine Nitrosoureas
Probable	Doxorubicin Vinblastine Cytosine arabinoside Cisplatin
Unlikely	Methotrexate 5-Fluorouracil 6-Mercaptopurine Vincristine
Unknown	Bleomycin

Among alternative combination chemotherapy regimens for advanced Hodgkin's disease, Adriamycin, bleomycin, vinblastine, and DTIC (ABVD) has been touted as being equally efficacious and less toxic than MOPP. A comparison of these treatment regimens has revealed that azoospermia occurs in 100% of MOPP-treated patients but in only 35% of those receiving ABVD, and that spermatogenesis nearly always recovers in the ABVD-treated patients.[33] This information may be important in planning treatment for young men with Hodgkin's disease who are concerned about preservation of fertility during and after treatment.

Similar concerns face patients about to embark on chemotherapy for testicular cancer. Chemotherapy-induced azoospermia that follows treatment with vinblastine, bleomycin, and cisplatin may be reversible within 2 to 3 years after treatment for nonseminomatous testicular cancer.[25,34,35] Evidence to date suggests that when a standard treatment regimen is used,[36] sperm count and semen quality recover 2 to 3 years after treatment in about half of the patients, and these individuals are capable of impregnating their partner.[25,34,35] Importantly, about 75% of men with nonseminomatous testicular cancer have a severely impaired sperm count and semen quality before chemotherapy is instituted, and in about 40% of subjects emission, ejaculation, or sexual function is compromised after retroperitoneal lymph node dissection.[37–41] These observations complicate interpretation of fertility status after therapy. In addition, some men with testicular cancer are cryptorchid, which predisposes to infertility even when testicular nondescent is unilateral.[6]

CHEMOTHERAPY EFFECTS IN ADULT WOMEN

An assessment of the impact of cancer chemotherapy on ovarian function has been hampered by the relative inaccessibility of the ovary to biopsy and the resultant inability to obtain reliable estimates of the size of the germ cell population. One must rely primarily on menstrual and reproductive history and on determinations of serum hormone levels to assess the functional status of the ovary.

CLINICAL PATHOPHYSIOLOGY

Examination of the ovaries of women who have developed chemotherapy-related ovarian failure frequently reveals arrest of follicular maturation or frank destruction of ova and follicles.[42–44] Clinically, these patients become amenorrheic and may complain of menopausal symptoms of estrogen deficiency such as "hot flashes," vaginal dryness, and dyspareunia. Abnormally low circulating estrogen levels result in marked elevation of both serum FSH and LH, a manifesta-

TABLE 60-16. Antitumor Agents Associated with Ovarian Dysfunction

Degree of Risk	*Drug*
Definite	Cyclophosphamide L-Phenylalanine mustard Busulfan Nitrogen mustard
Unlikely	Methotrexate 5-Fluorouracil 6-Mercaptopurine
Unknown	Doxorubicin Bleomycin Vinca alkaloids Cisplatin Nitrosoureas Cytosine arabinoside

tion of the loss of feedback inhibition of gonadotropin secretion consequent to drug-induced primary ovarian failure.

SINGLE AGENTS

Drugs most frequently associated with ovarian failure are shown in Table 60-16. Overall, at least 50% of women treated with single alkylating agents develop permanent ovarian failure and amenorrhea.[42-49]

Adjuvant chemotherapy in breast cancer patients may result in amenorrhea, depending on age of the patient and on the total dose administered.[50,51] Generally, patients older than 35 to 40 years of age at the time of treatment are much more likely to develop permanent amenorrhea after moderate doses of chemotherapy than younger patients. Conversely, younger patients tolerate higher total drug doses before the onset of permanent amenorrhea. In one study, amenorrhea occurred after a mean cyclophosphamide dose of 5.2 g in all patients over 40 years, whereas amenorrhea occurred in younger subjects only after a mean total dose of 9.3 g. Further, menses resumed within 6 months of discontinuing therapy in 50% of women under the age of 40 years.[52] Similar age-related phenomena have been noted following adjuvant chemotherapy with L-phenylalanine mustard.[53]

Clearly then, alkylating agent chemotherapy accelerates the onset of menopause, particularly in older patients, whereas younger patients may tolerate higher total drug doses before amenorrhea becomes irreversible. Among the antimetabolites, only high-dose methotrexate has been evaluated; appears to have no immediate ovarian toxicity.[54]

COMBINATION CHEMOTHERAPY

Most available information concerning the effects of combination chemotherapy regimens on ovarian function has come from the study of women receiving MOPP for Hodgkin's disease. Unlike the profound effects of this regimen on testicular function, MOPP produces ovarian dysfunction and amenorrhea in only 40% to 50% of treated women.[55-58] The frequency of ovarian injury clearly is related to the age of the patient at the time of treatment, with persistent amenorrhea occurring much more commonly in subjects older than 35 to 40 years of age.[55-60] Ovarian dysfunction in younger patients appears to be related to the total chemotherapy dose administered, because permanent amenorrhea occurs in women receiving the highest cumulative drug doses. Although it is impossible to predict the effect of MOPP chemotherapy on ovarian function for any individual patient, it appears unlikely that those patients treated before age 25 will experience any significant therapy-related ovarian dysfunction during the initial 5 to 10 years after completion of treatment. Continued long-term follow-up of women who maintain normal menses after chemotherapy will be necessary to determine whether these patients are still at risk for the development of premature ovarian failure and early menopause.

CHEMOTHERAPY EFFECTS IN CHILDREN

Evaluation of the effects of chemotherapy on gonadal function in children is particularly complex because of the variables introduced by the continuum of sexual development present in this patient population. Thus, knowledge of the pubertal status of the patient at the time of therapy and at the time of evaluation, along with recognition of the need to compare the results of hormonal evaluation to appropriate age-matched normal children, is required before definitive conclusions concerning drug effects can be drawn.

BOYS

Before the onset of puberty, the testicular germinal epithelium appears to be more resistant to moderate doses of alkylating agents than is the adult testis. Cyclophosphamide, in cumulative doses up to 20 g, produces only minor alterations in the testicular histology of prepubertal boys and no abnormalities in serum gonadotropins or testosterone levels.[61-63] However, at cumulative doses greater than 20 g, germinal aplasia has been documented.[64-66] Little information is available concerning the effects of other drugs on the immature testis, although recent data suggest that cytosine arabinoside and nitrosourea may be damaging to the germinal epithelium.[67,68] A commonly used antileukemic regimen (prednisone, 6-mercaptopurine, methotrexate, and vincristine), however, does not appear to cause damage to the testis in patients at any pubertal stage.[54]

Chemotherapy administered to male patients during puberty appears to have profound effects on both germ cell production and endocrine function. Following MOPP, gynecomastia, accompanied by increased serum FSH and LH levels and low normal serum testosterone levels, has been noted in many patients.[70,71] Testicular biopsy confirmed the occurrence of germinal aplasia in these patients as well. Thus, in contrast to prepubertal boys, chemotherapy administered during puberty may result in injury to both Leydig cells and the seminiferous epithelium, with gynecomastia being the clinical manifestation of this endocrine dysfunction. The reasons for the increased sensitivity to cytotoxic chemotherapy during puberty require further study.

GIRLS

Little information is available on the effects of cytotoxic drugs on the prepubertal and pubertal ovary. Postmortem studies of ovarian histology of girls treated with chemotherapy have revealed a spectrum of results ranging from normal histology to arrest of follicular maturation and frank ovarian destruction.[71,72] From clinical studies, delay in menarche or interruption of menses in girls treated with single-agent cyclophosphamide is very uncommon.[63,65,73,74] Studies of girls with acute lymphocytic leukemia treated with vincristine, methotrexate, and 6-mercaptopurine have revealed normal ovarian function in more than 80% of patients.[75] Thus, it appears that the immature ovary is relatively insensitive to cytotoxic chemotherapy; however, follow-up of these patients will be required for many years to determine accurately the long-term effects of this therapy on reproductive potential.

RADIATION THERAPY

Radiation therapy plays a major role in the management of lymphoma, sarcoma, and other malignant diseases. Sometimes it is the only therapy, but varying strategies incorporating chemotherapeutic regimens are common. In considering the potential gonadal toxicity of irradiation, one must differentiate the consequences of radiation exposure from those that accrue from the chemotherapeutic agents administered. In contrast to the growing literature describing adverse effects of chemotherapy, there is a paucity of data on the effects of radiation on gonadal function in humans. Furthermore, there are few data on the relationship of age, gender, adjunctive chemotherapy, and fractionation of the radiation dose to gonadal toxicity.

MEN

The testis is highly radiosensitive, most likely because of rapid cell division of the germinal epithelium. There has been some discussion in the literature of the effects of radiation on testicular function of men receiving radiation therapy.[76-81] Until recently, however, there have been few useful guides to the threshold for radiation damage to the human testis.[82-84] Studies of single-dose x-ray exposure to normal volunteer men demonstrate a dose-dependent depletion and recovery of the germinal epithelium.[82-84] A marked but transient suppression of sperm production is evident with doses as low as 15 rad; transient aspermia is reported with doses above 50 rad, and more prolonged periods of aspermia with higher doses. At 200 rad to 300 rad, full recovery of sperm production requires 3 years; at 400 rad to 600 rad, the interval is approximately 5 years; and above 600 rad sterility appears to be permanent. A recent assessment of the effects of conventionally fractionated irradiation on testicular function of men with Hodgkin's disease indicates that gonadal function is compromised at doses as low as 50 rad, and that at 200 rad cumulative dose, testicular dysfunction persists at least to 3 years.[85]

Techniques to shield the gonads from the radiation beam have been employed during pelvic irradiation when the chance of gonadal injury may be high, but there have been no studies that accurately assess the dose received by the gonad when the treatment beam is directed to anatomically remote sites. Radiation scatter and leakage radiation can be important contributors to gonadal toxicity. A threshold as low as 50 rad, which is less than 1% of a typical treatment dose, means that use of a gonadal shield is required if the distance between the testes and the radiation field edge is less than 30 cm.[86] A simple and practical testicular shield has now been developed for use near megavoltage radiation fields. This shield reduces testicular exposure to less than 10% of the patient's prescription dose; this effectively provides a threefold to tenfold reduction in testicular dose, depending on the distance from the field edge to the gonads.[87]

Unfortunately, there are no substantive studies of the effect of low-dose irradiation on testicular function in boys. In the few reports that appear, it is not possible to distinguish between the gonadal toxicity from chemotherapy and that caused by radiation therapy. In several recent studies, however, high doses of radiation (2400 rad) delivered directly to the testes of boys with gonadal relapse of acute lymphoblastic leukemia produced marked Leydig cell impairment with androgen deficiency, testicular atrophy, and clinical hypogonadism.[88-90]

WOMEN

The medical literature is not adequate to counsel women precisely regarding the risks of ovarian dysfunction following irradiation. At present there are only broad guidelines regarding the ovarian threshold. In comparison to men, gonadal exposure in women is complicated by the fact that the ovaries lie within the pelvis, often within the direct radiation beam, or considerably closer to major nodal areas where radiation scatter and beam leakage become critical. While successful pregnancies have been reported after fractionated ovarian doses of 650 rad, cessation of ovarian function is progressively more common with gonadal exposure above 150 rad, and at 500 rad to 600 rad most women remain persistently amenorrheic.[91] Age is a significant factor: women younger than age 20 have approximately a 70% chance of retaining regular cyclic menses after total nodal radiation, whereas by age 30 only 20% of treated women retain normal ovarian function. Older women are virtually all sterile.[92] Existing data suggest that chemotherapy plus total nodal irradiation in women with Hodgkin's disease produces additive ovarian toxicity at any age.[92]

Appropriate gonadal shielding is very difficult for the ovary because of its pelvic position. However, oophoropexy, a procedure by which the ovaries are surgically placed in the midline behind the uterus, appears to reduce ovarian exposure in approximately 50% of women receiving pelvic irradiation.[91,93] Clearly, further studies of the radiation dose received by the gonads during primary therapy to other sites are needed to determine the contribution to ovarian dysfunction, as well as to define the circumstances under which repositioning or shielding of the ovary is necessary.

TECHNIQUES TO PROTECT FERTILITY

With the recognition that cytotoxic chemotherapy, irradiation, and surgery may destroy germ cells has come increasing interest to protect the gonads from these adverse effects and to provide methods to store the germ cells for future use. The subject of suppression of germ cell proliferation to prevent gonadal toxicity associated with cancer treatment is well discussed by Redman and Bajorunas.[94] Approaches to the suppression of gonadal function have included administration of testosterone in men,[95] oral contraceptives in women,[96] and gonadotropin-releasing hormone (GnRH) analogues in both men and women.[94] Unfortunately, none of these approaches has proved effective despite encouraging preliminary results in experimental animal and human studies.[97-101] Among the numerous possible factors contributing to these discrepancies is the fact that, in the human, adequate suppression of the germinal epithelium prior to instituting cancer therapy is not feasible, owing to the urgency to treat the tumor as quickly as possible. Interspecies differences in response to pharmacologic manipulations are also well recognized.

As an alternative, pretreatment sperm banking is now a reasonable approach to preservation of reproductive potential in some men undergoing sterilizing cancer therapy.[102-106] Unlike normal fertile donors, whose semen is selected carefully for its excellent postthaw quality, pretreatment semen from cancer patients may show both reduced sperm count (less than 20 million/ml) and poor motion characteristics (less than 50% motility). Analysis of semen in men with lymphoma or testicular cancer has shown that about 50% of individuals have suboptimal semen quality (which precludes cryobanking) before treatment is begun.[37-41,102-111] Contributing factors that can impair semen quality include fever, stress, and the effects of systemic illness on pituitary gonadotropin release. In men with testicular cancer there is often secretion of human chorionic gonadotropin (hCG) from the tumor, which stimulates estrogen production, which can also adversely effect the contralateral testis. Studies of pretreatment testicular function in patients with other malignancies are not yet available to determine if such adverse effects on semen quality are commonly seen with most cancers. Cryobanking is feasible for men whose pretreatment semen has adequate numbers of reasonably motile cells; generally more than 20 million/ml with at least 40% progressive motility is required. Though data are limited, postthaw semen showing at least 30% progressive motility appears adequate for spousal insemination resulting in pregnancy.[39,102,112] For patients with low sperm counts, collection of multiple ejaculates can increase the total number of sperm available for banking, even when two or three specimens must be produced within several hours.[113]

An additional area of concern is the reproductive dysfunction that can result from cancer and cancer therapy per se.[114] Not only can tumors directly involve the gonads and the genitalia, but en bloc dissection of a tumor field may require removal of ovaries or testes as well. The psychosexual impact of mutilating surgery is not trivial, and the neuroendocrinologic residua of neoplasms near the hypothalamus and pituitary gland may, of course, impair fertility. Retroperitoneal lymph node dissection also commonly produces severe neurologic dysfunction in men, resulting in failure of emission, retrograde ejaculation, impotence, loss of orgasm, and infertility. Deliberate or inadvertent ligation of the hypogastric arteries may result in vasculogenic impotence. These factors have stimulated renewed interest in modifying surgical procedures to reduce the adverse reproductive consequences of cancer surgery without diminishing its efficacy. Sexual function can now be preserved in 70% of men undergoing radical prostatectomy for localized prostate cancer[115] and in 83% of men undergoing radical cystoprostatectomy for invasive bladder cancer[116] by placing the incision in the lateral pelvic fascia more anteriorly above the neurovascular bundle supplying the penile corpora cavernosa.

Neural injury occurs in the majority of men undergoing standard bilateral retroperitoneal lymph node dissection[117] for the staging and treatment of nonseminomatous germ cell tumors because of injury to the sympathetic innervation of the pelvic viscera. If the area surrounding the aortic bifurcation and sacral prominence is not disturbed, the final common pathways of the sympathetic innervation remain intact and no neurologic deficit results. A modified bilateral node dissection sparing the final common sympathetic pathway is feasible without missing sites of potential nodal metastases,[118] from which about 50% of men preserve ejaculatory function,[118,119] and a modified unilateral retroperitoneal lymph node dissection allows preservation of ejaculation in about 70% of men.[120,121]

Recently, the technique of electroejaculation, adopted from vast experience in veterinary practice, has been employed successfully to produce semen in neurologically impaired men.[122] From men with paraplegia[123,124] and individuals with ejaculatory failure after retroperitoneal lymph node dissection,[125] it has been possible to collect semen of sufficiently high quality to achieve pregnancies via insemination or in vitro fertilization. Advances in sperm cryopreservation enhance the feasibility of using electroejaculation to obtain semen from such patients for subsequent use as an inseminate.

GENETIC CONCERNS

The agents used to treat cancer are specifically designed to interfere with DNA and cellular metabolism, and cell division; hence, there is good reason to suspect that they may cause mutation and genetic disease in human beings.

Standard assays of the mouse at the Oak Ridge National Laboratory show a linear dose-response curve for ionizing radiation as a cause of germ cell genetic damage at several loci.[126] The Oak Ridge Laboratory has generated the experimental results used to set guidelines for radiation protection, specifically for germ cell effects in human populations. The data are based on just a few loci in a laboratory species that may not reflect directly the sensitivity of the human organism. For example, species may differ in their capacities to repair damage to germ cell DNA after environmental exposures.

Cancer treatments certainly cause genetic damage to somatic cells in human beings. After all, some modern treatments cause cancer themselves and, at the level of the cell, cancer is a genetic disease. Also, cytogenetic abnormalities are commonly seen after intensive cancer therapy. However, despite the considerable information available about somatic effects in experimental systems, some data about germ cell effects in experimental animals, and much information about somatic cell mutation in human beings, little is known about the sensitivity of the human gonad to mutagens. Dose-dependent abnormalities have been shown in meiotic chromosomes of the human testes after experimental irradiation. But to date no environmental agent has been causally linked to human germ cell mutation. Yet in genetic counseling, in the area of mutagenicity of the human gonad, the ultimate measure of concern is human hereditary disease. Does cancer treatment cause hereditary damage in human beings? Does it cause actual disease in the offspring, or mutational events without clinical significance? In theory, the effects of mutation may be neutral or even beneficial, as an essential element of biologic evolution.

The atomic bomb survivors in Japan have been extensively studied for possible genetic damage to their offspring.[127,128] The data are limited but are compatible with the interpretation that human germ cells may be much more tolerant of ionizing radiation than the standard laboratory mouse.[129] A recent evaluation of the same data suggests that the dose required to double the spontaneous mutation rate in human beings is five times greater than the dose in the mouse.[128]

PREGNANCY OUTCOMES

The actual outcomes of pregnancies in survivors of cancer are published as case reports, small series, and some 14 retrospective case series (Table 60-17).[130–143] These are patients who all had cancer as a child or young adult, mostly finished cancer treatment, and then began a pregnancy. More than 844 cancer patients or survivors, nearly four fifths of them women, initiated a total of 1761 recognized pregnancies. Of 1389 liveborn children, only 53 (about 4%) had a birth defect, a figure that resembles the rate of major malformations in the general population. The range of defects in the 14 studies included common malformations, such as congenital hip dysplasia, that may in fact represent deformity or a nongenetic extrinsic molding of fetal features. Only three of the disorders were purely genetic diseases (*i.e.*, mendelian traits or cytogenetic defects), as were also, perhaps, the two instances of multiple congenital anomalies. Pendred's syndrome (goiter and deafness) is an autosomal recessive disease. Both parents had to have contributed a mutant gene; hence, one cannot be sure that therapy caused the mutation. The other two disorders, the possible trisomy 18 syndrome and Marfan's syndrome, may represent new mutants, but one cannot be sure. Of course, all these studies were hardly comparable and included such relatively small numbers of patients (given the rarity of genetic disease in the general population) that, even in the aggregate, they have low statistical power. With only two instances of possible mutations seen in some 1400 offspring, experience is obviously limited.

A current National Cancer Institute study addressed late effects in some 2300 survivors of childhood and adolescent cancer, using siblings as controls. Only 22% had received any chemotherapy; one third had received radiation therapy. Overall, fertility was slightly depressed in men, to about 85% of the rate in male controls.[144] Fertility was only slightly depressed in women. When fertility was examined as a function of the type of treatment received in the first year after diagnosis, individuals (both men and women) who had been treated with alkylating agent chemotherapy and radiation below the diaphragm were most severely affected.

Although fertility rates differed by tumor type and therapy, each case-survivor had an average of about one child who had reached a mean age of about 11 years at the time of our interview. Seven cancers were reported in the survivors' offspring (five histologically confirmed), compared with 11 in the offspring of sibling-controls (eight histologically confirmed).[145] This represents a slight but not statistically significant excess of cancer in the offspring of case-survivors. In the first 5 years of follow-up, the children of cancer survivors had three times the number of cancers expected based on rates from the Connecticut Tumor Registry; children of sibling-controls had about half the expected numbers of cancers. After age 5 years, there was no statistically significant difference. The excess seemed attributable to some hereditary cancers (retinoblastoma, Sipple syndrome, and Wilms' tumor) and to some known syndromes of familial cancer.

In short, there does not appear to be an overall excess risk of cancer in offspring. What excess risk there was in the offspring seemed to be confined to the first 5 years of life, and could usually be attributable to a known hereditary or familial cancer. There were very few person-years of observation in the older adolescent age range, the ages when the majority of the case survivors were first diagnosed with cancer.

Cancer could be one indication of germ cell mutation. In a preliminary analysis, "genetic disease" was defined as a cytogenetic syndrome, a single gene defect, or one of 15 simple malformations tracked, for incidence, by the Centers for Disease Control, such as neural tube defects, patent ductus arteriosus, and the like.[146] "Potentially mutagenic therapy" was defined as radiation therapy below the diaphragm or above the knee, and/or chemotherapy with an alkylating agent. Finally, "sporadic" indicated that the offspring had no relative with a similar genetic disease; "familial" meant that a relative had a similar genetic disease or that the trait in the offspring was a recessive trait. The overall rate of genetic disease was 3.4% and was not different among the offspring of case-survivors compared to sibling-controls. Some possible differences in the rates of simple defects in our study groups, compared with population rates, probably arose from artifactual differences in defining the defects and differences in the length of follow-up. The case-survivors whose offspring had sporadic genetic disease received potentially mutagenic therapies no more often than did those whose offspring were normal.

TABLE 60-17. Large Series of Pregnancies in and by Survivors of Cancer

Study, Years Encompassed	Exposed Parents: Total	Exposed Parents: Females	Completed Pregnancies: Total	Fetal Loss*	Elective Abortions	Liveborns: Total	Liveborn with Defects	Type of Defects
Li and Jaffe,[131] ?–1973	45	63%	107	15	3	90	2	Hirschsprung's disease, asymptomatic heart murmur‡
Ross,[132] 1956–1973	58†	100%	96	18	?	75	3	Penrod's syndrome, tetralogy of Fallot, hemangiomata, eczema and strabismus (1 stillborn with aplasia of the anterior abdominal wall)
Holmes and Holmes,[133] 1944–1975	48	60%	93	12	3	77	6	Amblyopia, autism, scleroderma, rectal stenosis, absent fallopian tube and small uterus, slow learner and foot defect
Li et al,[134] ?–1978	146	58%	286	45	10	236	8	Possible trisomy 18 syndrome, Marfan's syndrome, deafness, pyloric stenosis, Hirschsprung's disease (same as above), cardiac, brain, and multiple malformations
Blatt et al,[135] ?–1980	30	77%	40	12	10	27	1	Congenital hip dysplasia
Horning et al,[136] 1968–1979	20	100%	28	5	5	24	0	
Marradi et al,[137] ?–1982	14	57%	23	?	?	21	2	Multiple congenital anomalies with mental and growth retardation, panhypopituitarism and cerebral atrophy, gastroschisis
Bundey and Evans,[138] ?–1973	24	83%	48	3	0	44	1	Pyloric stenosis
Andrieu et al,[139] 1972–1976	22	100%	30	9	4	21	1	Congenital hip dysplasia
Rustin et al,[140] 1958–1980	216†	100%	374	90	36	267	8	Spina bifida, tetralogy of Fallot, talipes equinovares, collapsed lung, umbilical hernia, desquamative fibrosing alveolitis (2 sibs), neonatal tachycardia, (plus 2 anencephalic stillbirths and 1 sudden infant death)
Goldstein et al,[141] 1965–1983	?†	100%	222	58	6	159	5	Not specified
Mulvihill et al,[142] 1957–1977	66	100%	87	22	12	53	6	Neurosensory deafness‡, scoliosis and slow learner‡, hydrocephalus‡, cleft lip and palate‡, hydrocephalus, tracheomalacia
Li et al,[143] 1931–1979	181	65%	246	53	32	190	5	Congenital hip dislocation (2), heart murmur, hypospadias, internal tibial torsion
Total	844	79%	1761	373	132	1389	53	(4%)

Modified with permission from Mulvihill JJ, Byrne J: Offspring of long-time survivors of childhood cancers. Clin Oncol 4:333–343, 1985.
*Fetal loss is defined as elective abortion, ectopic pregnancy, spontaneous abortion (miscarriage), or stillbirth.
†All gestational trophoblastic neoplasia.
‡Exposed to cancer treatment during gestation.
? = Uncertain.

The study of genetic disease in offspring of cancer survivors had an 87% power for detecting a twofold excess and did not, although the power is misleading because it mostly originates from the high background rate of simple birth defects, such as ventricular septal defect or cleft lip. One cannot be sure that such sporadic defects represent new mutations, because they also might be due to the polygenic or multifactoral traits that arise from parental genes interacting with environmental factors.

Apart from genetic effects, female survivors may face problems carrying a pregnancy to term. Excess rates of premature delivery and low birth weight have been documented in several studies[142,143,147] but may be confined to women who received abdominal irradiation and were incapable of maintaining a full-term, normal-weight pregnancy, perhaps because of uterine fibrosis or vascular compromise.

COUNSELING

At present, infertility must be viewed as an unfortunate complication of cancer chemotherapy and radiation therapy. Although much information has accumulated concerning the antifertility potential of alkylating agents, further study of other commonly used drugs such as doxorubicin, bleomycin, and cisplatin is required to assess fully the impact of these agents on gonadal function. As new effective antitumor agents are introduced into clinical practice, additional screening for gonadal toxicity is necessary. Furthermore, long-term prospective studies of reproductive function in patients receiving cancer chemotherapy are needed to assess accurately the magnitude and duration of gonadal dysfunction to be expected from any therapeutic regimen.

Counseling of patients facing the high probability of therapy-induced sterility is important. Several points should be considered. Although the great majority of men will become infertile after cancer chemotherapy, it is currently impossible to predict for many drugs if or when spermatogenesis may resume, and standard contraceptive practices should therefore not be abandoned for couples not desiring pregnancy. Factors such as total drug dose administered and duration of time off therapy may be important determinants of reversibility, as well as the type of drug or combination administered. Recent evidence suggests that the use of procarbazine in combination chemotherapy regimens may be associated with more long-lasting testicular damage than that seen with alkylating agents alone.[30] Certain drug regimens, such as vinblastine, bleomycin and cisplatin, appear to be associated with a high probability of reversibility.[25,34,35] Return of spermatogenesis is uncommon before 1 or 2 years off chemotherapy has elapsed but may be expected to occur within 4 years off therapy, if at all. Individual patients should be followed carefully, with testicular volume, serum FSH, and sperm count measured serially as a matter of course.

Pretreatment sperm banking may be valuable to some patients interested in having children after the completion of chemotherapy or radiation therapy. Although the technology of freezing, preserving, and thawing human sperm has advanced considerably, ultimate conception rates with cryopreserved semen remain only 50% to 60%, owing to loss of semen quality after thawing.[37-41,102-107,142,144] Unfortunately, many cancer patients may have decreased sperm counts or sperm motility prior to receiving any therapy, which militates against successful semen preservation. For example, at least 50% of patients with Hodgkin's disease and testicular cancer are oligospermic or azoospermic before receiving any therapy.[25,27,29] Indeed, it appears that only 10% to 20% of newly diagnosed cancer patients produce semen of sufficient quality to consider cryopreservation.[34,37,102-111] Nevertheless, sperm banking can be offered to patients if they are properly informed of the cost–benefit ratio of the procedure.

TABLE 60-18. Guidelines for Genetic Counseling of Couples Seeking Pregnancy after Cancer Diagnosis

1. Inquire about family history of cancer.
2. Pregnancy is contraindicated during cancer treatment; birth control should be considered.
3. Discuss risk of infertility after cancer treatment; the option of sperm banking, and the possibility of healthy children if fertility is preserved.
4. Discuss theoretical concerns about mutational damage; data in humans are limited.
5. Pregnancy probably should be monitored with ultrasound; amniocentesis should be offered for usual reasons, not just because of cancer history.
6. Existing data on pregnancy outcome do not indicate an excessive risk of congenital or genetic problems above the 4% risk of any pregnancy resulting in a baby with a major malformation.

Although women older than 40 years of age frequently develop permanent chemotherapy-induced amenorrhea, many younger women maintain normal menses throughout the treatment period or resume them shortly after therapy is discontinued.

For couples with preserved fertility, genetic counseling should be offered, as outlined in Table 60-18.[148]

REFERENCES

1. Robaire B, Hales BF: Effects of paternal exposure to anticancer drugs on pregnancy outcome: An animal model. In Mulvihill JJ, Sherins RJ (eds): Reproductive Consequences of Cancer and Cancer Therapy. New York, Raven, 1988
2. Mulvihill JJ, Sherins RJ: Reproductive Consequences of Cancer and Cancer Therapy. New York, Raven, 1988 (in press)
3. American Cancer Society: Proceedings of the Workshop on Psychosexual and Reproductive Issues Affecting Patients with Cancer—1987. Chicago, American Cancer Society publication No. 87-5M-4515, 1987
4. Fox BW, Fox M: Biochemical aspects of the actions of drugs on spermatogenesis. Pharmacol Rev 19:21–57, 1967
5. Schilsky RL, Lewis BJ, Sherins RJ et al: Gonadal dysfunction in patients receiving chemotherapy for cancer. Ann Intern Med 93:109–114, 1980
6. Sherins RJ, Howards SS: Male infertility. In Harrison JH (ed): Campbell's Urology, 4th ed, pp 715–766. Philadelphia, WB Saunders, 1978
7. Sieber SM, Adamson RH: Toxicity of antineoplastic agents in man: Chromosomal aberrations, antifertility effects, congenital malformations, and carcinogenic potential. Adv Cancer Res 22:57–155, 1975
8. Fairley KF, Barrie JU, Johnson W: Sterility and testicular atrophy related to cyclophosphamide therapy. Lancet 1:568–569, 1972
9. Kumar R, Biggart JD, McEvoy J et al: Cyclophosphamide and reproductive function. Lancet 1:1212–1213, 1972
10. Miller DG: Alkylating agents and human spermatogenesis. JAMA 217:1662–1665, 1971
11. Richter P, Calamera JC, Morgenfeld MD et al: Effect of chlorambucil on spermatogenesis in the human with malignant lymphoma. Cancer 25:1026–1030, 1970
12. Meistrich ML, Finch M, da Cunho MF et al: Damaging effects of fourteen chemotherapeutic drugs on mouse testis cells. Cancer Res 42:122–131, 1982
13. Booth JD, Merriam GR, Clark RV et al: Evidence for Leydig cell dysfunction in infertile men with a selective increase in plasma follicle stimulating hormone. J Clin Endocrinol Metab 64:1194–1198, 1987
14. Cheviakoff J, Calamera JC, Morgenfeld M et al: Recovery of spermatogenesis in patients with lymphoma after treatment with chlorambucil. J Reprod Fertil 33:155–157, 1973
15. Quershi MJA, Goldsmith HJ, Pennington HJ et al: Cyclophosphamide therapy and sterility. Lancet 2:1290–1291, 1972
16. Van Thiel DH, Sherins RJ, Myers GH et al: Evidence for a specific seminiferous tubular factor affecting follicle-stimulating hormone secretion in man. J Clin Invest 51:1009–1019, 1972
17. Chapman RM, Sutcliffe SB, Rees LH et al: Cyclical combination chemotherapy and gonadal function. Lancet 1:285–289, 1979
18. Mecklenberg RS, Sherins RJ: Gonadotropin response to luteinizing hormone releasing hormone in men with germinal aplasia. J Clin Endocrinol Metab 38:1005–1009, 1974

19. Waxman JHX, Terry YA, Wrigley PFM et al: Gonadal function in Hodgkin's disease: Long-term followup of chemotherapy. Br Med J 285:1612–1613, 1982
20. Whitehead E, Shalet SM, Blackledge G et al: The effects of Hodgkin's disease and combination chemotherapy on gonadal function in the adult male. Cancer 49:418–422, 1982
21. Sherins RJ, Patterson AP, Brightwell D et al: Alteration in the plasma testosterone/estradiol ratio: An alternative to the inhibin hypothesis. In Bardin CW, Sherins RJ (eds): The Cell Biology of the Testis. Ann NY Acad Sci 383:295–306, 1982
22. deCunha MF, Meistrich ML, Reid HL et al: Effect of chemotherapy on human sperm production. Proc Am Assoc Cancer Res 20:100, 1979
23. Sieber SM, Correa P, Dalgard DW et al: Carcinogenic and other adverse effects of procarbazine in nonhuman primates. Cancer Res 20:100, 1979
24. Vilar O: Effect of cytostatic drugs on human testicular function. In Mancini RE, Martini L (eds): Male Fertility and Sterility, pp 423–440. New York, Academic Press, 1974
25. Drasga RE, Einhorn LH, Williams SD et al: Fertility after chemotherapy for testicular cancer. J Clin Oncol 1:179–183, 1983
26. Asbjornsen G, Molne K, Kleep O et al: Testicular function after combination chemotherapy for Hodgkin's disease. Scand J Haematol 16:66–69, 1976
27. Chapman R, Sutcliffe SB, Rees L et al: Prospective study: The effects of Hodgkin's disease and nitrogen mustard, vincristine, procarbazine and prednisolone on male gonadal function. Proc Am Soc Clin Oncol 20:321, 1979
28. Sherins RJ, DeVita VT: Effects of drug treatment of lymphoma on male reproductive capacity. Ann Intern Med 79:216–220, 1973
29. Chapman RM, Sutcliffe SB, Malpas JS: Male gonadal dysfunction in Hodgkin's disease. JAMA 245:1323–1328, 1981
30. Roeser HP, Stochs AE, Smith AJ: Testicular damage due to cytotoxic drugs and recovery after cessation of therapy. Aust NZ J Med 8:250–254, 1978
31. Evenson DP, Arlin Z, Welt S et al: Male reproductive capacity may recover following drug treatment with the L-10 protocol for acute lymphocytic leukemia. Cancer 53:30–36, 1984
32. Shamberger RC, Sherins RJ, Rosenberg SA: The effects of post-operative adjuvant chemotherapy and radiotherapy on testicular function in men undergoing treatment for soft tissue sarcoma. Cancer 47:2368–2374, 1981
33. Vivani S, Santoro A, Ragri G et al: Gonadal toxicity after combination chemotherapy for Hodgkin's disease: Comparative results of MOPP vs ABVD. Eur J Cancer Clin Oncol 21:601–605, 1985
34. Berthelsen JG, Skakkebaek NE: Gonadal function in men with testicular cancer. Fertil Steril 39:68–73, 1983
35. Nijman JM, Schraffordt-Koops H, Kremer J et al: Gonadal function after surgery and chemotherapy in men with stage II and III nonseminomatous testicular tumors. J Clin Oncol 5:651–656, 1987
36. Einhorn LH, Donahue J: Cis-diammine-dichloroplatinum, vinblastine and bleomycin combination chemotherapy in disseminated testicular cancer. Ann Intern Med 87:293–298, 1977
37. Sanger WG, Armitage JO, Schmidt MA: Feasibility of semen cryopreservation in patients with malignant disease. JAMA 244:789–790, 1980
38. Rhodes EA, Hoffman DJ, Kaempfer SH: Ten years of experience with semen cryopreservation by cancer patients: Follow-up and clinical considerations. Fertil Steril 44:512–516, 1985
39. Reed E, Sanger WG, Armitage JO: Results of semen cryopreservation in young men with testicular carcinoma and lymphoma. J Clin Oncol 4:537–539, 1986
40. Carroll PR, Whitmore WF Jr, Herr HW et al: Endocrine and exocrine profiles of men with testicular tumors before orchiectomy. J Urol 137:420–423, 1987
41. Newton RA, Boyack T, Agarwal A et al: The effect of cancer on semen quality and cryopreservation of sperm. In Mulvihill JJ, Sherins RJ (eds): Reproductive Consequences of Cancer and Cancer Therapy. New York, Raven Press, 1988
42. Belohorsky B, Siracky J, Sandor L et al: Comments on the development of amenorrhea caused by myleran in cases of chronic myelosis. Neoplasma 4:397–402, rhea caused by myleran in cases of chronic myelosis. Neoplasma 4:397–402, 1060
43. Miller JJ, Williams GF, Leissring JC: Multiple late complications of therapy with cyclophosphamide including ovarian destruction. Am J Med 50:530–535, 1971
44. Sobrinho LG, Levine RA, DeConti RC: Amenorrhea in patients with Hodgkin's disease treated with antineoplastic agents. Am J Obstet Gynecol 109:135–139, 1971
45. Fosdick WM, Parsons JL, Hill DF: Long term cyclophosphamide therapy in rheumatoid arthritis. Arthritis Rheum 11:151–161, 1968
46. Galton DAG, Till M, Wiltshaw E: Busulfan: Summary of clinical results. Ann NY Acad Sci 68:967–973, 1958
47. Louis J, Limarzi LR, Best WR: Treatment of chronic granulocytic leukemia with myleran. Arch Intern Med 97:299–308, 1956
48. Uldall PR, Kerr DNS, Tacchi D: Sterility and cyclophosphamide. Lancet 1:693–694, 1972
49. Warne GL, Fairley KF, Hobbs JB et al: Cyclophosphamide-induced ovarian failure. N Engl J Med 289:1159–1162, 1973
50. Dnistrian AM, Schwartz MK, Fracchia AA et al: Endocrine consequences of CMF adjuvant therapy in premenopausal and postmenopausal breast cancer patients. Cancer 51:803–807, 1983
51. Samaan NA, DeAsis DN, Buzdar AU et al: Pituitary-ovarian function in breast cancer patients on adjuvant chemoimmunotherapy. Cancer 41:2084–2087, 1978
52. Koyama H, Wada T, Nishizawa Y et al: Cyclophosphamide-induced ovarian failure and its therapeutic significance in patients with breast cancer. Cancer 39:1403–1409, 1977
53. Fisher B, Sherman B, Rockette H et al: L-phenylalanine mustard in the management of premenopausal patients with primary breast cancer. Cancer 44:847–857, 1979
54. Shamberger RC, Rosenberg SA, Seipp CA et al: Effects of high-dose methotrexate and vincristine on ovarian and testicular function in patients undergoing postoperative adjuvant treatment of osteosarcoma. Cancer Treat Rep 65:739–746, 1981
55. Chapman RM, Sutcliffe SB, Malpas JS: Cytotoxic-induced ovarian failure in women with Hodgkin's disease: I. Hormone function. JAMA 242:1877–1881, 1979
56. Morgenfeld MC, Goldberg V, Parisier H et al: Ovarian lesions due to cytostatic agents during the treatment of Hodgkin's disease. Surg Gynecol Obstet 134:826–828, 1972
57. Sherins R, Winokur S, DeVita VT et al: Surprisingly high risk of functional castration in women receiving chemotherapy for lymphoma. Clin Res 23:343, 1975
58. Horning SJ, Hoppe RT, Kaplan HS et al: Female reproductive potential after treatment for Hodgkin's disease. N Engl J Med 304:1378–1382, 1981
59. Schilsky RL, Sherins RJ, Hubbard SM et al: Long-term followup of ovarian function in women treated with MOPP chemotherapy for Hodgkin's disease. Am J Med 71:552–556, 1981
60. Whitehead E, Shalet SM, Blackledge G et al: The effect of combination chemotherapy on ovarian function in women treated for Hodgkin's disease. Cancer 52:988–993, 1983
61. Arneil GC: Cyclophosphamide and the prepubertal testis. Lancet 2:1259–1260, 1972
62. Kirkland RT, Bongiovanni AM, Cornfeld D et al: Gonadotropin responses to luteinizing hormone releasing factor in boys treated with cyclophosphamide for nephrotic syndrome. J Pediatr 89:941–944, 1976
63. Pennisi AJ, Grushkin CM, Lieberman E: Gonadal function in children with nephrosis treated with cyclophosphamide. Am J Dis Child 129:315–318, 1975
64. Etteldorf JN, West CD, Pitcock JA et al: Gonadal function, testicular histology and meiosis following cyclophosphamide therapy in patients with nephrotic syndrome. J Pediatr 88:206–212, 1976
65. Lentz RD, Bergstein J, Steffes MW et al: Post-pubertal evaluation of gonadal function following cyclophosphamide therapy before and during puberty. J Pediatr 91:385–394, 1977
66. Rapola J, Koskimies O, Huttanen NP et al: Cyclophosphamide and the pubertal testis. Lancet 1:98–99, 1973
67. Lendon M, Hann IM, Palmer MK et al: Testicular histology after combination chemotherapy in childhood for acute lymphoblastic leukemia. Lancet 2:439–441, 1978
68. Ahmed SR, Shalet SM, Campbell RHA et al: Primary gonadal damage following treatment of brain tumors in childhood. J Pediatr 103:562–565, 1983
69. Blatt J, Poplack DG, Sherins RJ: Testicular function in boys after chemotherapy for acute lymphoblastic leukemia. N Engl J Med 304:1121–1124, 1981
70. Sherins RJ, Olweny CLM, Ziegler JL: Gynecomastia and gonadal dysfunction in adolescent boys treated with combination chemotherapy for Hodgkin's disease. N Engl J Med 299:12–16, 1978
71. Whitehead E, Shalet SM, Morris-Jones PH et al: Gonadal function after combination chemotherapy for Hodgkin's disease in childhood. Arch Dis Child 47:287–291, 1981
72. Himelstein-Braw R, Peters H, Faber M: Morphologic study of the ovaries of leukemic children. Br J Cancer 38:82–87, 1978
73. Chiu J, Drummond KN: Long-term followup of cyclophosphamide therapy in frequent relapsing minimal lesion nephrotic syndrome. J Pediatr 84:825–830, 1974
74. DeGroot GW, Faiman C, Winter JSD: Cyclophosphamide and the prepubertal gonad: A negative report. J Pediatr 84:123–125, 1974
75. Siris EJ, Leventhal BG, Vaitukaitis JL: Effects of childhood leukemia and chemotherapy on puberty and reproductive function in girls. N Engl J Med 294:1143–1146, 1976
76. Sanderman RF: The effects of irradiation on male human fertility. Br J Radiol 39:901–907, 1966
77. Ash P: The influence of radiation on fertility in man. Br J Radiol 53:271–278, 1980
78. Hahn EW, Feingold SM, Simpson L et al: Recovery from aspermia induced by low-dose radiation in seminoma patients. Cancer 50:337–340, 1982
79. Bateman JL, Bond VP: The effects of radiations of different LET on early response in the mammal. Ann NY Acad Sci 114:32–47, 1964
80. Nader S, Schultz PN, Cundiff JH et al: Endocrine profiles of patients with testicular tumors treated with radiotherapy. Int J Radiat Oncol Biol Phys 9:1723–1726, 1983
81. Tomic R, Bergman B, Damber JE et al: Effects of external radiation therapy for cancer of the prostate on the serum concentrations of testosterone, follicle stimulating hormone, luteinizing hormone and prolactin. J Urol 130:287–289, 1983
82. Rowley MJ, Leach DR, Warner GA et al: Effect of graded doses of ionizing radiation on the human testis. Radiat Res 59:665–677, 1974
83. Clifton DK, Bremner WJ: The effect of testicular x-irradiation on spermatogenesis in man: A comparison with the mouse. J Androl 4:387–492, 1983
84. Paulsen CA: The study of radiation effects on the human testis: Including histologic, chromosomal and hormonal aspects. Final Progress Report, AEC Contract AT (45-1)-225, Task Agreement 6, RLO-2225-2, 1973
85. Shapiro E, Kinsella TJ, Makoch RW et al: Effects of fractionated irradiation on endocrine aspects of testicular function. J Clin Oncol 3:1232–1239, 1985
86. Fraas BA, Kinsella TJ, Harrington FS et al: Peripheral dose to the testis: The design and use of a practical and effective gonadal shield. Int J Radiat Oncol Biol Phys 11:609–615, 1985
87. Kinsella TJ, Fraas BA, Glatstein E: Late effects of radiation therapy in the treatment of Hodgkin's disease. Cancer Treat Rep 66:991–1001, 1982
88. Brauner R, Czernichow P, Cramer P et al: Leydig cell function in children after direct testicular irradiation for acute lymphoblastic leukemia. N Engl J Med 309:25–28, 1983

89. Leiper AD, Grant DB, Chessells JM: The effect of testicular irradiation on Leydig cell function in prepubertal boys with acute lymphoblastic leukemia. Arch Dis Child 58:906–910, 1983
90. Blatt J, Sherins RJ, Niebrugge D et al: Leydig cell function in boys following testicular relapse of acute lymphocytic leukemia. J Clin Oncol 3:1227–1231, 1985
91. Thomas PRM, Winstantly D, Peckham MJ et al: Reproductive and endocrine function in patients with Hodgkin's disease: Effects of oophoropexy and irradiation. Br J Cancer 33:226–231, 1976
92. Horning SJ, Hoppe RT, Kaplan HS et al: Female reproductive potential after treatment for Hodgkin's disease. N Engl J Med 304:1377–1382, 1981
93. Ray GR, Trueblood HW, Enright LP et al: Oophoropexy: A means of preserving ovarian function following pelvic megavoltage radiotherapy for Hodgkin's disease. Radiology 96:175–180, 1970
94. Redman JR, Bajorunas DR: Suppression of germ cell proliferation to prevent gonadal toxicity associated with cancer treatment. In: Proceedings of the Workshop on Psychosexual and Reproductive Issues Affecting Patients with Cancer—1987, pp 90–94. Chicago, American Cancer Society, publication No. 87-5M-4515, 1987
95. Redman J, Davis R, Evenson D et al: Prospective, randomized trial of testosterone cypionate to prevent sterility in men treated with chemotherapy for Hodgkin's disease: Preliminary results (abstr). In: Proceedings of the 14th International Cancer Congress, Budapest, p 440. Basel, S Karger, 1986
96. Chapman RM, Sutcliffe SB: Protection of ovarian function by oral contraceptives in women receiving chemotherapy for Hodgkin's disease. Blood 58:849–851, 1981
97. Glode LM, Robinson J, Gould SF et al: Protection of spermatogenesis during chemotherapy. Drugs Exp Clin Res 8:367–378, 1982
98. da Cunha MF, Meistrich ML, Nader S: Absence of testicular protection by a gonadotropin-releasing hormone analogue against cyclophosphamide induced testicular cytotoxicity in the mouse. Cancer Res 47:1093–1097, 1987
99. Delic JI, Bush C, Peckham MJ: Protection from procarbazine-induced damage of spermatogenesis in the rat by androgen. Cancer Res 46:1909–1914, 1986
100. Lewis RN, Dowling KJ, Schally AV: D-Tryptophan-6 analog of luteinizing hormone-releasing hormone as a protective agent against testicular damage caused by cyclophosphamide in baboons. Proc Natl Acad Sci USA 82:2975–2979, 1985
101. Johnson DH, Linde R, Hainsworth JD et al: Effect of luteinizing hormone releasing hormone agonist given during combination chemotherapy on post-therapy fertility in male patients with lymphoma: Preliminary observations. Blood 65:832–836, 1985
102. Jewett MAS, Jarvi K, Zaharchuk J et al: Banking of human sperm: Techniques, success, practice. In Mulvihill JJ, Sherins RJ (eds): Reproductive Consequences of Cancer and Cancer Therapy. New York, Raven Press, 1988
103. Ansbacher R: Artificial insemination with frozen spermatozoa. Fertil Steril 29:375–379, 1978
104. Curie-Cohen M, Luttrell L, Shapiro J: Current practice of artificial insemination by donor in the United States. N Engl J Med 300:585–590, 1979
105. Sherman JK: Synopsis of the use of frozen human semen since 1964: State-of-the-art of human semen banking. Fertil Steril 24:397–412, 1973
106. Bracken RB, Smith KD: Is semen cryopreservation helpful in testicular cancer? Urology 15:581–583, 1980
107. Chlebowski RT, Heber D: Hypogonadism in male patients with metastatic cancer prior to chemotherapy. Cancer Res 42:2495–2498, 1982
108. Thacil JV, Jewett MAS, Rider WD: The effects of cancer and cancer therapy on male fertility. J Urol 126:141–145, 1981
109. Chapman RM, Sutcliffe SB, Malpas JS: Male gonadal dysfunction in Hodgkin's disease: A prospective study. JAMA 245:1323–1328, 1981
110. Vigersky RA, Chapman RM, Berenberg J et al: Testicular dysfunction in untreated Hodgkin's disease. Am J Med 73:482–486, 1982
111. Marmor D, Elefant E, Danchez C et al: Semen analysis in Hodgkin's disease before onset of treatment. Cancer 57:1986–1987, 1986
112. Scammell GD, Stedronske J, Edmonds DK et al: Cryopreservation of semen in men with testicular tumor or Hodgkin's disease: Results of artificial insemination of their partners. Lancet 2:31–32, 1985
113. Morgan BW, Rothmann SA, Baird WC: Short interval semen collection for sperm banking. In Mulvihill JJ, Sherins RJ (eds): Reproductive Consequences of Cancer and Cancer Therapy. New York, Raven Press, 1988
114. Shapiro E, Lepor H: Reproductive consequences of cancer surgery. In Mulvihill JJ, Sherins RJ (eds): Reproductive Consequences of Cancer and Cancer Therapy. New York, Raven Press, 1988
115. Walsh PC, Lepor H, Eggleston JC: Radical prostatectomy with preservation of sexual function: Anatomical and pathological considerations. Prostate 4:473–485, 1983
116. Walsh PC, Mostwin JL: Radical prostatectomy and cystoprostatectomy with preservation of potency: Results using a new nerve sparing technique. Br J Urol 56:694–697, 1984
117. Kedia KR, Markland C, Fraley EE: Sexual function following retroperitoneal lymphadenectomy. J Urol 114:237–239, 1975
118. Lange PH, Narayan P, Fraley EE: Fertility issues following therapy for testicular cancer. Semin Urol II 4:264–274, 1984
119. Narayan P, Lange PH, Fraley EE: Ejaculation and fertility after extended retroperitoneal lymph node dissection for testicular cancer. J Urol 127:685–688, 1982
120. Garnick MB, Richie JP: Toward more rational management for stage I testis cancer: Watch out for "watch and wait." J Clin Oncol 4:1021–1023, 1986
121. Pizzocaro G, Salvioni R, Zononi F: Unilateral lymphadenectomy in intraoperative stage I nonseminomatous germinal testis cancer. J Urol 134:485–489, 1985
122. Bennett CJ: Electroejaculation following retroperitoneal lymph node dissection. In Mulvihill JJ, Sherins RJ (eds): Reproductive Consequences of Cancer and Cancer Therapy. New York, Raven Press, 1988
123. Thomas RJS, McLeisch G, McDonald IA: Electroejaculation of the paraplegic male following by pregnancy. Med J Aust 2:798, 1975
124. Bennett CJ, Ayers JWT, Randolph JF et al: Electroejaculation of paraplegic males followed by pregnancies. Fertil Steril 48:1070–1072, 1987
125. Bennett CJ, Seager SWJ, McGuire EJ: Electroejaculation for recovery of semen after retroperitoneal lymph node dissection. J Urol 137:513, 1987
126. US Congress Office of Technology Assessment: Technologies for Detecting Heritable Mutations in Human Beings. Washington, DC, U.S. Government Printing Office, 1986
127. Schull WJ, Otake M, Neel JV: Genetic effects of atomic bombs: A reappraisal. Science 213:1220–1227, 1981
128. Neel JV, Reproduction and genetic effects of gonadal exposure to ionizing radiation in human beings. In Mulvihill JJ, Sherins RJ (eds): Reproductive Consequences of Cancer and Cancer Therapy. New York, Raven Press, 1988
129. Neel JV: Genetic effects of atomic bombs. Science 213:1205, 1981
130. Mulvihill JJ, Byrne J: Offspring of long-time survivors of childhood cancer. Clin Oncol 4:333–343, 1985
131. Li FP, Jaffe H: Progeny of childhood-cancer survivors. Lancet 2:707–709, 1974
132. Ross GT: Congenital anomalies among children born of mothers receiving chemotherapy for gestational trophoblastic neoplasms. Cancer 37:1043–1047, 1976
133. Holmes GE, Holmes FF: Pregnancy outcome of patients treated for Hodgkin's disease: A controlled study. Cancer 41:1317–1322, 1978
134. Li FP, Fine W, Jaffe H et al: Offspring of patients treated for cancer in childhood. JNCI 62:1193–1197, 1979
135. Blatt J, Mulvihill JJ, Ziegler JL et al: Pregnancy outcome following cancer chemotherapy. Am J Med 69:828–832, 1980
136. Horning SJ, Hippe RT, Kaplan HS et al: Female reproductive potential after treatment for Hodgkin's disease. N Engl J Med 304:1377–1382, 1981
137. Marradi P, Schaison F, Alby N et al: Les enfants nés de parents leucémiques. Nouv Rev Fr Hematol 24:75–80, 1982
138. Bundey S, Evans K: Survivors of neuroblastoma and ganglioneuroma and their families. J Med Genet 19:16–21, 1982
139. Andrieu JM, Ochoa-Molina ME: Menstrual cycle, pregnancies and offspring before and after MOPP therapy for Hodgkin's disease. Cancer 52:435–438, 1983
140. Rustin GJS, Booth M, Dent J et al: Pregnancy after cytotoxic chemotherapy for gestational trophoblastic tumours. Br Med J 288:103–106, 1984
141. Goldstein DP, Berkowitz RS, Bernstein MR: Reproductive performance after molar pregnancy and gestational trophoblastic tumors. Clin Obstet Gynecol 27:221–227, 1984
142. Mulvihill JJ, McKeen EA, Rosner F et al: Pregnancy outcome in cancer patients: Experience in a large cooperative group. Cancer 60:1143–1150, 1987
143. Li FP, Gimbrere K, Gelber RD et al: Outcome of pregnancy in survivors of Wilms' tumor. JAMA 257:216–219, 1987
144. Byrne J, Mulvihill JJ, Myers MH et al: Effects of treatment on fertility in long-term survivors of childhood and adolescent cancer. N Engl J Med 317:1315–1321, 1987
145. Mulvihill JJ, Myers MH, Connelly RR et al: Cancer in offspring of long-term survivors of childhood and adolescent cancer. Lancet 2:813–817, 1987
146. Mulvihill JJ, Byrne J, Steinhorn SA et al: Genetic disease in offspring of survivors of cancer in the young. Am J Hum Genet 39:A72, 1986
147. Byrne J, Mulvihill JJ, Myers MH et al: Reproductive problems and birth defects in survivors of Wilms' tumor and their relatives. Med Pediatr Oncol (in press)
148. Mulvihill JJ, Byrne J: Genetic counseling for the cancer survivor: Possible germ cell effects of cancer therapy. In: Proceedings of the Workshop on Psychosexual and Reproductive Issues Affecting Patients with Cancer—1987, pp 100–104. Chicago, American Cancer Society publication No. 87-5M-4515, 1987

SECTION 7

C. NORMAN COLEMAN
MARGARET A. TUCKER

Secondary Cancers

As the success of modern cancer therapy has increased the duration of survival and curability of many patients, so has the recognition of long-term complications of therapy increased. The successful treatment of first cancers has involved the use of radiation and multi-agent chemotherapy, each modality being used either as primary therapy or as an adjunct to therapy of the primary tumor, which often includes surgery. The increased use of adjuvant chemotherapy has placed a large number of patients at potential risk for developing a treatment-related malignancy.

In the past, discussion of secondary malignancies emphasized the treatments administered and the potential risk of appearance of a second tumor in relation to a specific agent. Whereas the initial reports considered single cases or small series of patients, there re now large population bases, such as patients with pediatric neoplasms, Hodgkin's disease, or breast cancer, from which a better assessment of the risk can be determined. Since most secondary tumors are rare, proper epidemiologic and statistical methods must be employed to avoid overestimating or underestimating the risk.

More recently, it has become apparent that predisposing factors beyond the treatment itself may have a major impact on the risk of developing a second tumor. One such factor is altered host immunity, such as that seen with congenital or acquired immunodeficiency states. For unknown reasons, patients with certain HLA subtypes may be at increased risk for developing certain malignancies. Advances in molecular biology techniques in the mid-1980s demonstrated that certain malignancies are related to a specific DNA lesion. Some of the seemingly anatomically unrelated malignancies have now been shown to have a common chromosomal defect.

This chapter covers the important principles relating to all of these areas, emphasizing data available within the last few years. Some topics, such as the relationship between the specific therapeutic agents and secondary cancers, were well reviewed by Li in the previous edition of this book,[1] and have been received by use elsewhere.[2,3] A discussion of late effects and secondary malignancies is possible only if the primary treatment is successful; toxic treatment should be avoided, but not at the price of cure.

INDIVIDUAL TREATMENT MODALITIES

RADIATION THERAPY

The carcinogenic effects of ionizing irradiation have been reported in individuals exposed occupationally, environmentally, in nuclear war, and in the course of medical diagnostic and therapeutic procedures.[4] With the exception of exposure associated with therapeutic irradiation, the doses have often been quite low. Extrapolation of radiation effects from high to low radiation dose ranges cannot be done with certainty.[5] In the lower dose ranges (hundreds of centigrays) the risk that a secondary tumor will develop increases with dose, although the shape of the curve relating dose to risk (*i.e.*, linear *vs.* nonlinear) has not been established with certainty. However, it is thought that at the higher dose ranges used clinically, the risk per centigray decreases, a phenomenon that has been attributed to cell killing at the higher doses.[4,5] Therapeutic radiation doses usually fall within a relatively small range, making it difficult to establish a dose–response curve between radiation dose and risk of a secondary cancer. Therefore, for a patient treated for cancer, the "risk per rad" for the development of a secondary tumor cannot be determined with certainty.[2]

Many tumor types have been associated, at least in case reports, with radiation to the tissue in which the malignancy developed—that is, there is no one "radiation-induced" tumor. The largest population studies on the carciogenicity of ionizing irradiation come from survivors of the atomic bomb explosion. The data from this population have been updated for the period 1950–1982 by Preston et al using newer statistical techniques.[6] The secondary cancers for which radiation exposure produced an increased relative risk are leukemia, multiple myeloma, and cancers of the lung, female breast, stomach, colon, esophagus, and urinary tract. The risk was of borderline significance for ovarian and liver cancer. No increased risk was observed for the lymphomas or for cancers of the gallbladder, prostate, rectum, pancreas, or uterus. Confirming previous reports was the finding that the relative risk for developing leukemia decreased with time (decreased by 10.7% per year) following the peak at 5 to 10 years. However, while the relative risk for the development of "all cancers except leukemia" increased with time, the rate of rise was small (increased by 4.8% per year). If it is possible to extrapolate from the atomic bomb data to the clinical situation, the peak risk of secondary leukemia should be highest about 5 to 10 years after treatment and should then decline, while for cancers other than leukemia the risk should rise continually to at least 30 years after radiation exposure. However, caution should be used in making such an extrapolation. In the clinical setting, secondary malignancies occur in patients who have already had one tumor, who have received a higher dose of radiation but to a localized field, and who may well have received chemotherapy. Despite the many differences between atomic bomb radiation exposure and therapeutic exposure to radiation, the clinical data, as will be illustrated in the Hodgkin's disease populations, are quite concordant with that reported by Preston et al.[6]

No one specific type of cancer is seen after therapeutic irradiation. Because secondary sarcomas have been reported by many authors,[7–13] it is of interest to review some recent data relating therapy to the development of this malignancy,[13,14] as it serves as a paradigm for the complexity in studying secondary neoplasms. Tucker et al analyzed the risk of developing bone sarcomas for patients in the Late Effects Study Group (LESG).[13] Among the 9170 patients who survived for 2 or more years, 48 cases of bone cancer occurred, compared to 0.4 expected (relative risk 133; 95% confidence interval 98–176). The relative risk by initial diagnosis was 999 for retinoblastoma, 649 for Ewing's sarcoma, 297 for rhabdomyosarcoma, 127 for Wilms' tumor, and 106 for

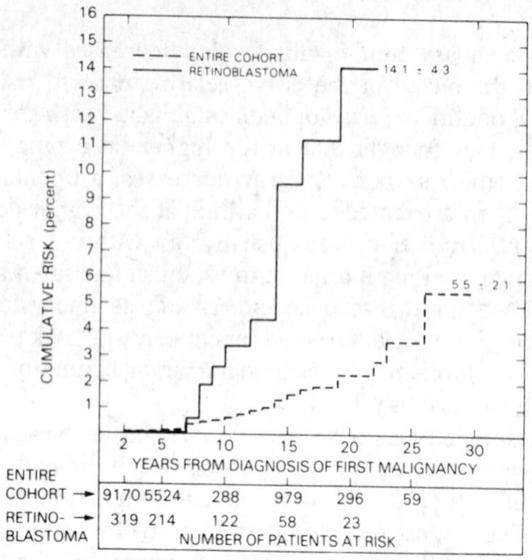

FIG. 60-9. Cumulative risk of bone cancer after treatment for childhood cancer: risk of bone cancer after all types of childhood cancer (*broken line*); risk of bone cancer after retinoblastoma (*solid line*). Value are means ±SE. (Tucker MA, D'Angio GJ, Boice JD et al: Bone sarcoma linked to radiotherapy and chemotherapy in children. N Engl J Med 317:588–593, 1987)

Hodgkin's disease. As indicated in Figure 60-9, the cumulative probability of developing secondary bone cancer at 20 years was 2.8% for the entire cohort, and 14.1% for patients with retinoblastoma.

The secondary bone sarcomas in the LESG were predominantly osteosarcomas and chondrosarcomas; 83% were within the treatment field, 9% were within 5 cm, and the remainder were more than 5 cm beyond the field. Careful radiation dosimetry was done which accounted for the absorption characteristics of bone for the different types of radiation.[2] Table 60-19 gives data on the dose-response relationship for radiation-induced sarcomas. The relative risks for radiation doses in excess of 1000 cGy are statistically significant. Of note, although the cumulative risk of developing a bone cancer after treatment is higher for patients with retinoblastoma (see Fig. 60-9), the relative risk is the same for retinoblastoma patients when compared to that of all other cancer types (see Table 60-19).

Radiation therapy was therefore a risk factor for the development of bone tumors. In addition, chemotherapy with alkylating agents also produced an increased risk, independent of radiation (relative risk 4.7; 95% confidence limits 1.0–22.3). The data in Table 60-20 indicate that the risk increased with both alkylator score (a measure of the total amount of alkylating agent received) and dose of radiation. Other drugs did not appear to be associated with the risk of developing bone cancer. Although the increased risk of developing a bone sarcoma with an alkylating agent alone is not large ($p = 0.05$), such an association had not been previously noted. That cyclophosphamide might increase the risk of radiation-induced bone tumor had been suggested by Strong et al[10] for patients with Ewing's sarcoma and by Draper et al[14] for patients with retinoblastoma. Therefore, the association between chemotherapy and the development of secondary sarcomas noted by Tucker et al[13] is consistent with prior observations.[10,14]

The association between retinoblastoma and osteosarcoma is an interesting one. In the LESG study, the actuarial risk that a patient with retinoblastoma would develop osteosarcoma was higher than the risk for patients with all other cancers, while the relative risk for the "retinoblastoma" and "other cancer" patients was the same. There is a well-known association between familial retinoblastoma and osteosarcoma,[14,15] with both tumors showing similar chromosomal abnormalities.[16] Thus, in the case of retinoblastoma, and possibly other tumors as well, the risk of developing a second tumor due to the treatment itself is in addition to an underlying predisposition for the development of a secondary tumor.[13,14]

The risk of developing bone sarcomas following therapeu-

TABLE 60-19. Risk of Bone Cancer by Radiation Dose in LESG Study*

	Radiation Dose (RAD)					
	0	*<1000*	*1000–2999*	*3000–3999*	*4000–5999*	*≥6000*
All types of cancers						
No. of cases	10	9	6	11	15	13
No. of controls†	51	70	30	18	23	12
Relative risk‡	1.0‡	0.6	6.0	16.9	21.2	38.3

	0	*<1000*	*1000–3999*	*≥4000*
Retinoblastoma				
No. of cases	4	4	7	7
No of controls	25	15	14	11
Relative risk‡	1.0‡	1.3	12.7	19.4
All other types				
No. of cases	6	5	10	21
No. of controls	26	55	34	24
Relative risk§	1.0‡	0.2	12.0	28.8

*Tucker MA, D'Angio GJ, Boice JD et al: Bone sarcoma linked to radiotherapy and chemotherapy in children. N Engl J Med 317:588–593, 1987.

†Five controls for whom the radiation dose to the site could not be estimated have been excluded from the analysis in this table.

‡Risks for radiation dose above 1000 rad are statistically significant ($P < 0.05$).

§Referent category.

TABLE 60-20. Risk of Bone Sarcoma by Radiation Dose and Alkylator Score in LESG Study*

	Alkylator Score		
Radiation Dose	*0*	*1 or 2*	*≥3*
None			
Relative risk	1.0†	4.8	8.5‡
No. cases : controls	6:44	1:4	3:3
<1000 rad			
Relative risk	1.3	0.4	1.3
No. cases : controls	5:43	1:13	3:14
≥1000 rad			
Relative risk	37.4§	14.2§	59.2§
No. cases : controls	21:45	11:26	13:12

*Tucker MA, D'Angio GJ, Boice JD et al: Bone sarcoma linked to radiotherapy and chemotherapy in children. N Engl J Med 317:588–593, 1987.

†Referent category.

‡Trend in alkylator score in subjects not exposed to radiation, $p = 0.05$.

§$p < 0.05$.

tic irradiation for other cancers is much lower than the risk following irradiation for childhood cancer. Among Hodgkin's disease patients there was a 31-fold excess of bone sarcomas, based on two osteosarcomas that developed in the radiation field in individuals who were irradiated before age 20.[17] In more than 68,000 patients with cervical cancer treated with radiation therapy the relative risk of developing bone cancer, based on 11 observed cases, was 1.9 (95% confidence interval 1.0–3.5).[18] The reason for the difference in these risks is not yet known but may include age at exposure, the use of chemotherapy as part of the treatment for the first cancer, and the immune status of the patients.

Although therapeutic radiation has been associated with an increased risk of developing secondary tumors, diagnostic radiation is much less of an offender. Linos et al did not find that the risk of developing leukemia increased after radiation doses of 0 to 3 Gy when these amounts were delivered over long periods of time as part of routine medical care.[19] Evans and co-workers concluded that only about 1% of all cases of leukemia and less than 1% of all cases of breast cancer result from diagnostic radiography.[20]

CHEMOTHERAPY

While bladder cancer has been associated with alkylating agents, particularly cyclophosphamide[1], the predominant malignancy associated with chemotherapy has been acute nonlymphocytic leukemia. Only selected publications of the large number noting this association will be mentioned.[17,21–39] The diseases in which secondary hematologic malignancies have been observed are those which are treated with alkylating agents or nitrosoureas and for which there is prolonged survival, such as Hodgkin's disease, ovarin cancer, multiple myeloma, polycythemia vera, gastrointestinal cancer, and small cell lung cancer.[21–30] However, not all treatments with alkylating agents have produced an increased incidence of secondary leukemia; the most notable exception is adjuvant treatment for breast cancer.[36–38] The relationship between the use of an alkylating agent and the development of a secondary hematologic malignancy, therefore, is not simple. As discussed below, the risk probably depends on the agent itself and on the total amount of drug given. Other factors that might be related include the drug schedule, underlying conditions such as altered immunity, and the use of other therapy such as irradiation. Animal studies have indicated that a variety of agents may be leukemogenic. However, from the clinical data available it appears that the animal studies may not always be predictive, possibly due to the high doses and prolonged schedules often used in the laboratory. An example of the discordance between animal and human studies is the drug procarbazine, which is very leukemogenic as a single agent in monkeys[40] but to date has not produced leukemias in a limited number of Hodgkin's disease patients as part of the PAVe (procarbazine, melphalan, vinblastine) regimen[17] or as part of a program using procarbazine maintenance.[41]

The alkylating agents and nitrosoureas have been considered to be the major offenders in the production of chemotherapy-related leukemia. The relative leukemogenicity of the various drugs has not been fully established, but the risk appears to be different with different drugs.[32,42] What is most important is the total amount of drug given, which almost invariably correlates with an increased duration of drug exposure.[3,24–27,32,35,39] This correlation has been observed for a variety of alkylating agents and nitrosoureas, and for a number of different disease sites—ovarian, breast, and gastrointestinal cancers, Hodgkin's disease, multiple myeloma, and non-Hodgkin's lymphoma. The time between cessation of drug treatment and the development of leukemia has also been explored; the risk of leukemia appears to be highest within a few years of completing treatment.[32,43,44]

The secondary leukemia seen is almost invariably acute nonlymphocytic leukemia; the two most common subsets are acute myelomonocytic leukemia and acute erythroleukemia. The leukemia is frequently preceded by a period of pancytopenia and may manifest as part of the spectrum of the myelodysplastic syndromes.[39] The chromosomal abnormalities encountered are not random.[45–47] Most frequently seen are deletions in chromosomes 5 and 7. As concluded by Le Beau et al, it is likely that these chromosomes contain critical genes that are involved in the pathogenesis of the secondary neoplasms.[47] The newer molecular biology techniques should help determine the specific lesion. It might then be possible to use such a chromosomal abnormality as a means of screening patients for the presence of this disorder. Early detection would be of benefit if effective therapy were available. Unfortunately, the prognosis of patients with the secondary leukemias is generally quite poor, although some authors have reported short-term success.[48,49] Patients who present with the myelodysplastic syndrome may have a prolonged survival due to the indolent nature of their disease.

SECONDARY TUMORS IN PEDIATRIC, HODGKIN'S DISEASE, AND BREAST CANCER PATIENT POPULATIONS

The two patient populations from which most of the secondary malignancy data have been derived are patients treated for pediatric malignancies and those treated for Hodgkin's disease. The spectrum of pediatric malignancy includes a number of diseases that have recently been correlated with chromosomal abnormalities, such as retinoblastoma[16,50,51] and Wilms' tumor.[52,53] The Hodgkin's disease populations treated in the "modern era" have received radiation therapy and/or chemotherapy, which are relatively "standard" among the major series. Thus, specific aspects of the treatment regimens can be studied for their carcinogenicity. However, it must be kept in mind that immunity is often impaired by Hodgkin's disease, and a further impairment of immunity is seen after treatment.[3] Despite the potential confounding factors, the excellent cure rates among these relatively young patients, coupled with long-term follow-up of large patient populations, have provided important data on the risk of developing secondary neoplasms. With the widespread use of adjuvant chemotherapy for breast cancer, there is now a third large patient population available for study of treatment-related malignancy.

PEDIATRICS—LATE EFFECTS STUDY GROUP

Although data are available from a number of investigators, the information presented will be that of the LESG, which has accumulated data from 13 major pediatric oncology centers in the United States, Canada, and western Europe.[13,54] In the most recent update from this group, Meadows et al reported 292 cases of second malignant neoplasms. The correlation between the primary malignancy and secondary neoplasm is shown in Table 60-21.[54] The primary tumors most frequently associated with second malignancies were not the most common pediatric primary tumors. Leukemias and lymphomas accounted for almost half of pediatric tumors, followed by brain tumors, neuroblastoma, Wilms' tumor, rhabdomyosarcoma, retinoblastoma, osteosarcoma, and others.[55] As noted above, the association between the first and the second neoplasm is not just a chance or purely a treatment-related event. Rather, there is a predisposition for some patients to develop a secondary malignancy, as exemplified by the association between retinoblastoma and osteosarcoma.[13-16] Of the 15 patients with Hodgkin's disease who developed secondary leukemia, all had received chemotherapy and 73% had received radiation therapy. This is consistent with the data in adults (see below), indicating that chemotherapy appears to be the major etiologic factor for secondary leukemia in patients with Hodgkin's disease. Of interest is the association between primary leukemia and secondary brain tumors noted by the LESG investigators and others.[55,56] Whether this association is related to treatment or to some predisposing factor remains to be elucidated.

Tucker and colleagues evaluated the risk of developing secondary leukemia in 9170 patients in the LESG who had survived 2 years or longer. The relative risk of 14 (95% confidence interval, 9–22) was greater than expected. As is seen in adult populations, the risk was associated with alkylating agents and increased in parallel with the alkylator score, a calculated measure of exposure to alkylating agents. Radiation therapy did not increase the risk. Therefore, the secondary leukemias in patients with childhood cancers ap-

TABLE 60-21. Correlation Between Primary and Secondary Malignant Neoplasms in LESG Study*

Secondary Neoplasm (n)	*Primary Neoplasm (No. of patients with diagnosis who developed secondary malignancy)*								
	RB (52)	*HD (40)*	*ST Sa. (40)*	*Wilms' (36)*	*Brain (31)*	*NB (28)*	*Bone Sa. (18)*	*Leuk. (13)*	*Other (34)*
Bone sa. (67)	20	5	10	6	3	6	8	1	8
ST sa. (59)	16	4	9	9	5	5	4	. . .	7
Leuk/Lym (57)	2	18	6	7	8	5	2	6	3
Brain (29)	4	1	7	3	4	1	. . .	3	6
Skin (31)	6	4	3	2	7	3	. . .	1	5
Thyroid (26)	. . .	6	2	4	2	7	. . .	. . .	5
Breast (13)	. . .	. . .	3	2	1	1	4	1	1
Other (26)	5	2	6	3	4	2	. . .	1	3

*Adapted from Meadows AT, Baum E, Bellani-Fossati F et al: Second malignant neoplasms in children: An update from the Late Effects Study Group. J Clin Oncol 3:532–538, 1985

RB = retinoblastoma, HD = Hodgkin's disease, ST Sa = soft tissue sarcoma, brain = brain tumor, NB = neuroblastoma, Leuk = leukemia, Lym = lymphoma.

pears to be related to the particular therapy, while for the development of secondary solid tumors the predisposing disease plays a very important role.

HODGKIN'S DISEASE

Many groups have published figures on the risk of development of secondary malignancies after treatment for Hodgkin's disease. This discussion will focus on the data from Stanford University,[17,23] the National Cancer Institute,[33] and Milan,[22] as these reports address the major issues. References to other series are available in these reports.[17,22,23,33,57]

Tucker et al have reported the risks of developing secondary cancers at 15 years from the Stanford series of 1507 patients.[17] Patients were divided into five treatment groups: radiation therapy alone (n = 714), adjuvant chemotherapy (n = 179), chemotherapy alone (n = 80), and radiation therapy plus colloidal gold (n = 65). The observed and expected number of secondary cancers for the entire group are given in Table 60-22. Statistically significant increases were noted for all secondary cancers as a group, leukemia, all solid tumors, lung and stomach cancers, non-Hodgkin's lymphoma, melanoma, and bone and connective tissue malignancies. Looking at the relative risk for secondary cancers by 5-year follow-up interval, Tucker et al observed the following: the risk of all secondary cancers was relatively constant, no leukemias were seen at 10^+ years, the risk of solid tumors developing rose with time and was highest at 10^+ years. Because most of the viscera are at least partly included in the radiation portals, most of the solid tumors occurred within the radiation fields. In six patients eight melanomas developed: three outside the radiation portal, three within the radiation portal, and two in unknown relationship to the portal. Five of the six patients had biopsy proven (n = 2) or family history suggestive of (n = 3) the dysplastic nevus syndrome.[58] These data suggest that immune system alterations caused by Hodgkin's disease or its treatment may be an important factor in the etiology of some secondary malignancies.

Figure 60-10 summarizes the actuarial risk of developing a secondary malignancy for the entire group. At 15 years, the actuarial risk of any second cancer (excluding nonmelanoma skin and simultaneous cancers) was 17.6% (±3.1%) compared to 2.6% (±1.0%) in the general population. The major component of the risk was due to the solid tumors, which, following a steep rise after 10 years, was 13,2% at 15 years. The risk of leukemia was 3.6%, with no new cases appearing after 9 years; the 1.6% risk of lymphoma remained relatively constant throughout the study period. The 15-year actuarial risk of leukemia by treatment group was 0.6% for radiation therapy alone, 4.9% for adjuvant chemotherapy, 1.8% for salvage chemotherapy (nongold group), and 11.5% for chemotherapy alone. For all treatment groups the observed numbers of cases were statistically significantly higher than that expected in a general population. Compared to the radiation-alone group, the risk of leukemia was significantly higher in the groups given adjuvant chemotherapy or chemotherapy alone. The extent of radiation therapy did not affect the risk of developing leukemia. Although the number of patients studied was limited, no leukemias developed among 130 patients given adjuvant PAVe, compared to 18 cases among 431 patients given adjuvant MOPP (actuarial 10-year risk, 6.2%; p = 0.06). These data suggest that while there is some risk of secondary leukemia in patients treated with radiation therapy alone, the major offender appears to be chemotherapy. As will be discussed, the specific agents used and the duration of treatment are critical to the development of secondary leukemia.

For the development of solid tumors and lymphomas the risk was about equal in the radiation-alone and in the combined modality groups. This observation suggests that it is the disease process itself and/or the radiation that is the offending agent. Of note, the secondary neoplasms seen were similar to those observed in immunosuppressed populations—non-Hodgkin's lymphoma, melanoma, nonmelanoma skin cancers, lung cancer, soft tissue sarcomas, and stomach cancers.[17] The secondary leukemias were uniformly fatal, whereas about half the patients with secondary lymphomas or solid tumors are alive after a relatively short follow-up since treatment of the second tumor.[17]

It has been consistency observed that secondary leukemias are related to chemotherapy for the first cancer. However,

TABLE 60-22. Observed and Expected Number of Secondary Malignant Tumors by Site in 1507 Patients with Hodgkin's Disease*

	Observed	*Expected*	*O/E Ratio*	*p<*
All cancers	83	15.9	5.2	0.0001
Leukemia	28	0.4	66	0.0001
All solid tumors	46	14.5	3.2	0.0001
By site				
Lung	14	1.8	7.7	0.0001
Non-Hodgkin's lymphoma	9	0.9	9.6	0.0001
Stomach	4	0.4	10	0.001
Melanoma	4	0.4	8.9	0.001
Bone	2	0.1	31	0.001
Connective tissue	2	0.1	15	0.001
Colon	4	3	3.5	NS
Breast	3	1.8	1.7	NS
Other	13	8.7	1.5	NS

*Adapted from Tucker MA, Coleman CN, Cox RS et al: Risk of second malignancies following Hodgkin's disease after 15 years. N Engl J Med 318:76–81, 1988.

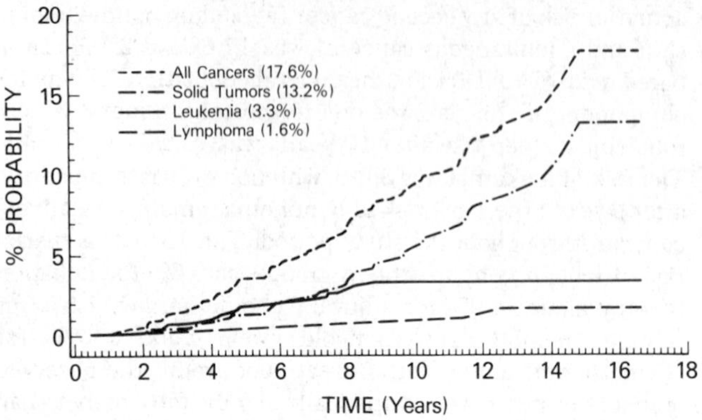

FIG. 60-10. Actuarial risk of development of secondary malignancy following Hodgkin's disease for 1507 patients treated at Stanford University Medical Center. (Tucker MA, Coleman CN, Cox RS, et al: Risk of second malignancies following Hodgkin's disease after 15 years. N Engl J Med 318:76–81, 1988)

the particular chemotherapeutic agents used have a profound influence, as noted above. In the Stanford series the PAVe regimen did not produce secondary leukemia despite the inclusion of oral melphalan. Valagussa et al from Milan reported the 12-year actuarial risk of developing leukemia by treatment group: for radiation alone it was 0%; for the combined modality regimens it was 10.2% (±5.2%) for MOPP and 0% for ABVD (Adriamycin, bleomycin, vinblastine, DTIC). The difference between the MOPP–radiation and ABVD–radiation groups is statistically at $p < 0.05$.[22] The secondary lymphoma and solid tumor data from Milan are consistent with those reported by the Stanford University group.[17] Blayney and colleagues from the National Cancer Institute reported that MOPP alone produced a 10-year actuarial risk of leukemia of less than 2%, compared with a risk of approximately 17% for patients given combined modality therapy (p value not specified).[33] Their data support previous observations that the risk of developing secondary leukemia peaks at about 5 to 8 years.[57] In their patient population no secondary leukemias occurred after 11.6 years. From these data it appears that six cycles of MOPP alone, without consolidative irradiation or without additional chemotherapy, has relatively low leukemogenic potential, which suggests that the combination of radiation therapy and chemotherapy adds to the risk. In general, the actuarial risk of developing leukemia is similar for patients given chemotherapy alone and those given combined modality therapy[57]; however, the extent of the chemotherapy has not been detailed. Additional observations from groups using primary chemotherapy alone will be needed to clarify the risk due to limited (six cycles) of chemotherapy without radiation therapy.

In summary, the occurrence of a secondary leukemia after treatment for Hodgkin's disease is related to the intensity and type of therapy. The regimens using alkylating agents, particularly the MOPP regimen, have been most commonly associated with this complication. However, it must be noted that because MOPP was the most widely used drug combination, this regimen has the longest follow-up period. Furthermore, MOPP is often used in conjunction with radiation therapy. Other drug regimens such as ABVD or PAVe appear to be less leukemogenic than MOPP (the use of only six cycles of MOPP may be less toxic than combined modality therapy). Secondary solid tumors and lymphomas occur with equal frequency in all treatment schemes, indicating that it is the disease itself and/or the radiation that is the etiologic agent. Given the increasing actuarial risk of the development of solid tumors, and the fact that about half of such tumors may be curable, careful lifelong surveillance is indicated for Hodgkin's disease patients, with special attention given to new clinical signs or symptoms. Smoking should be discouraged; and patients with the dysplastic nevus syndrome should be carefully evaluated for the potential development of malignant melanoma.[58]

BREAST CANCER

With somewhat more limited follow-up than the Hodgkin's disease populations, data are available regarding secondary neoplasms in patients given adjuvant therapy for breast cancer from the National Surgical Adjuvant Breast Project[36] and Milan[37] trials. Fisher et al observed 3 cases of leukemia among 2068 patients treated with surgery alone, 6 cases of leukemia among 1116 patients who received locoregional radiation therapy after surgery, and 27 cases of leukemia plus 7 cases of myelodysplastic syndrome in 5299 patients who received adjuvant chemotherapy containing melphalan. It is noteworthy that 2 of the 6 cases of leukemia in the radiation therapy group were CLL, which is not thought to be a radiation-related leukemia. Thus, the risk of leukemia from radiation therapy alone is an upper limit estimate. The 10-year cumulative risk of leukemia was 0.06% (±0.05%) following surgery alone for the primary tumor and 1.37% (±0.74%) following surgery plus irradiation. The 10-year risk of leukemia plus myelodysplastic was 1.54% (±0.36%) following surgery plus chemotherapy. The statistical difference between surgery and irradiation versus surgery alone was $p = 0.06$; between surgery plus chemotherapy versus surgery alone, $p = 0.002$; and between surgery plus radiation versus surgery plus chemotherapy, $p = 0.29$. Since two of the leukemias in the radiation therapy group were CLL, radiation therapy appears to carry a very small risk of inducing leukemia. The 10-year risk following chemotherapy with melphalan is relatively small, although it does represent a statistically significant increase.[36]

Valagussa et al confirmed the low risk of developing a secondary leukemia from adjuvant chemotherapy for breast cancer. With a median follow-up in excess of 10 years, no cases of leukemia were observed in 666 women treated with adjuvant CMF (cyclophosphamide, methotrexate, 5-fluorouracil). This group further observed that the risk of developing a secondary solid tumor and the risk of developing a contralateral breast cancer were not affected by the use of adjuvant CMF. Although longer follow-up is still required, the data now available indicate that current adjuvant therapy for breast cancer is associated with a minimal risk of developing a treatment-related second neoplasm. It is not surprising that the risk of leukemia following adjuvant therapy with melphalan is higher than the risk following cyclophosphamide, since a similar pattern of risks has been demonstrated after single-agent treatment for ovarian cancer.[32] The lower dose of alkylating agents delivered in the adjuvant setting may explain the lower risks than those seen following ovarian cancer treatment.

HOST-RELATED FACTORS

A number of host and environmental factors may influence the development of a secondary neoplasm.[1-3] Multiple tumors of the same organ system have been seen in patients with bladder, lung, breast, head and neck, and colon cancers, and melanoma. Multiple tumors in different organ systems are also seen when the two cancers share common risk factors, such as breast and endometrial cancers, or are caused by common exposure, such as lung and bladder cancers. In addition, single gene traits are associated with an increased risk of producing tumors that may be multiple or involve several organ systems. In the previous edition of this book Li reviewed the association between a specific disease and the development of subsequent neoplasms, including such autosomal dominant disorders as von Recklinghausen's neurofibromatosis and neural tumors and sarcomas, Gardner's syndrome with colon cancers and sarcomas, and the multiple endocrine neoplasia syndromes.[1] Chromosome instability syndromes, such as Bloom's or Fanconi's syndrome, which are both autosomal recessive traits, have been associated with the development of leukemia.[3]

There is undoubtedly an important interrelation between the immune system and the susceptibility to the development of cancer. Chakravarti et al studied the association between cases of Hodgkin's disease in multiple-case families with HLA linked and unlinked determinants of susceptibility.[59] Their analysis suggested that a recessive susceptibility gene tightly linked to the HLA complex was responsible for 60% of cases. The remaining 40% were due to environmental or other factors.[59] An association with HLA-DR5 in white populations has also been suggested for both endemic and epidemic Kaposi's sarcoma,[60] but has not been found for endemic Kaposi's sarcoma in Africa.[61]

A number of immunodeficiency states are associated with the development of neoplasms. Such associations are relevant to the study of therapy-related neoplasms, since the primary disease and treatment can lead to permanent defects in the immune system. Genetically determined immunodeficiency states associated with secondary neoplasms include ataxia-telangiectasia, the Wiskott-Aldrich syndrome,[3] and the X-linked lymphoproliferative syndrome.[62] In addition, organ transplantation[3] with iatrogenic immunodeficiency and the acquired immunodeficiency syndrome[63-65] are associated with increased risks of developing specific cancers. A common malignancy seen in these settings is intermediate- or high-grade non-Hodgkin's lymphoma. These lymphomas are almost universally of the B-cell type, similar to those seen after treatment for Hodgkin's disease.[3,57] Using molecular hybridization analysis, List and coworkers reported the association of Epstein-Barr virus genome with B-cell non-Hodgkin's lymphoma following the successful treatment for Hodgkin's disease in two patients.[66] It is postulated that due to the impaired host immunity, the Epstein-Barr virus infection is not properly controlled, perhaps leading to an expanded pool of proliferating B-lymphocytes. This process alone, possibly coupled with mutagenic effects of the therapy, could lead to the emergence of a malignant clone of B-cells.

The remarkable advances in the knowledge of the molecular aspects of neoplasia have revolutionized our thinking about primary and secondary neoplasms. The normal and abnormal functioning of oncogenes is discussed in detail elsewhere in this book. A malignant phenotype can occur as the abnormal expression of an oncogene, as the expression of an abnormal oncogene, and by the translocation of a normal gene that in its new position alters the expression of other genes.[67,68] A number of malignancies have been associated with an abnormality of an oncogene, although additional information is needed to determine if the genetic abnormality is the cause of the tumor. In some instances the abnormality detected may be a secondary effect of the malignant phenotype. Examples of diseases for which an abnormal expression of an oncogene or the expression of an abnormal oncogene have been postulated include neuroblastoma,[69,70] myelodysplastic syndrome,[71] and lung cancer.[72-74]

A cancer can develop through the loss of expression of a gene by the deletion of both alleles, at least one of which is required to prevent the development of a cancer. retinoblastoma[14-16,50,51,75] is the prototypic example of this latter mechanism, which has been proposed for other diseases as well, such as Wilms' tumor[53] and colorectal carcinoma in familial polyposis coli.[76,77]

The abnormalities in gene expression needed to produce a malignant tumor could be induced by therapy for a first malignancy. Using a technique for measuring somatic mutations in lymphocytes, Dempsy et al demonstrated that mutation frequency in lymphocytes is increased after chemotherapy and radiation therapy.[78] In a setting in which one DNA lesion is already present, it might be expected that the risk of developing a second tumor would be high, as only one additional DNA lesion would be required. Retinoblastoma and secondary osteosarcoma appear to represent such an association.[13-16,50,51,75] With further knowledge of the underlying mechanisms of carcinogenesis, the role of treatment in the production of secondary malignancies will be better defined. it may then be possible to alter the primary treatment is such a manner as to avoid this serious late effect.

METHODS OF STUDYING SECONDARY MALIGNANCIES

Several methods have been used to study second cancers. Reports of individual cases or series have been important in establishing the occurrence of second cancers but have been of limited use in quantifying risks. The more useful epidemiologic methods for studying secondary cancer risk have included both cohort and case-control studies. In cohort studies specific groups of patients are identified and observed for a number of years to determine the incidence of specific malignancies. Study groups providing large numbers of patients who may constitute a cohort include population-based tumor registries, multicenter clinical trials, and hospital-based patient groups. The group to be followed may be defined by a first cancer of interest, such as ovarian cancer or Hodgkin's disease, or by an exposure of interest, such as single-agent cyclophosphamide or interstitial radiation therapy. The person-years of observation are accrued from the start of observation to the last follow-up, death, or diagnosis of the second tumor, whichever occurs first.[79] Tumor incidence rates from the general population specific for age, sex, race, and calendar year are multiplied by the accumulated person-years to derive the number of expected tumors. The observed number is then divided by the expected number to estimate the relative risk of a second tumor. When the 95% confidence interval does not include 1.0, the excess risk is statistically significant at the $p < 0.05$ level. This method yields a risk in the cohort that is compared to the general population. The use of population-based tumor registries has some advantages, including relatively large numbers of patients, which allows the detection of even small risks (*e.g.*, the international cervical cancer study mentioned above[18]). In addition, the actual (observed) and the expected numbers of cancers come from the same reference population. Population-based registries do have some disadvantages however, including differential reporting of cancers to the registries by physicians and hospitals, variable follow-up, different autopsy rates, limited treatment data, and different diagnostic criteria for secondary cancers. Many registries record only initial therapy, and individuals may be incompletely classified if they receive additional treatment. Finally, comparisons of rates of secondary tumors in cancer patients with rates in the general population are criticized because some types of cancer may have an intrinsically increased risk of specific secondary cancers, such as the retinoblastoma–osteosarcoma association.[14-16] Despite these limitations, these studies are informative and often produce the best data available. However, they tend to give minimal estimates of risk because of the relatively incomplete follow-up.

Clinical trials are extremely valuable sources of information on risks of secondary tumors. In clinical studies, follow-up in the comparison arms of the trials is equivalent and usually as complete as possible. Individuals within each arm have received comparable treatment, and the risks of secondary tumors may be directly compared between treatment arms. This controls for any intrinsic risk of a second cancer associated with the first cancer, and also allows the comparison of risks from specific drug therapies or radiation exposure. Complete treatment information, including that administered for relapse, is usually available, so the risk of misclassification of exposure is minimized. The major disadvantage of most of the clinical trials is the relatively small number of study subjects involved. Examples of this type of analysis are the NSABP trial of adjuvant therapy for breast cancer,[36] the study of ovarian cancer that combined data from several clinical trials,[32] and the Stanford and Milan Hodgkin's disease studies.[17,22]

Another type of analysis that is useful in the cohort studies is the actuarial or life-table risk.[80] This analysis gives the cumulative risk of a particular event, such as leukemia, expressed in a percentage at a particular time period—for example, 6.2% at 10 years. To calculate this life table probability person-years of follow-up, similar to those required for the estimation of relative risk compared to the general population, are necessary. The actuarial risk of a secondary cancer occurring (see Fig. 60-10) can be compared between treatment arms using methods similar to those employed for the comparison of survival or disease-free survival.[81] The limitation of this method is that it does not account for the baseline tumor rates in the general population. An example is the comparison of acute leukemia by age category in the Stanford population.[57] Within each chemotherapy category the risk of leukemia is significantly higher among persons treated after age 50 than in persons treated at any younger age. When the relative risks are examined, which take into account the higher risk of acute leukemia in the general population over age 50, the relative risk for all age groups is essentially the same.[17]

The other major approach is the case–control study, in which exposure to chemotherapy and/or radiation therapy is compared between individuals who develop second cancers (cases) and those who do not (controls). Ideally, all therapy given to every individual treated would be reviewed. In practice, this is not usually feasible since often hundreds or thousands of individuals are involved and very few develop second cancers. In this circumstance, it is much more cost-efficient to collect the information on the cases and controls, the latter being representative of the individuals who do not develop second cancers. The selection of the appropriate controls is critical: they should be representative of the entire group. Bias in the selection of the control group can lead to spurious associations or can obscure a true association.

CONCLUSION

Secondary, treatment-related neoplasms are seen because the initial treatment is successful. Clearly, attempts should be made to reduce this complication. Indeed, most investigators studying pediatric and Hodgkin's disease populations are developing treatment strategies to reduce late complications. Changes in therapy to minimize secondary cancers are best made in the context of a carefully designed study that includes the codification of treatment and follow-up procedures. It is through such careful studies that current treatments can be made less toxic while their efficacy is maintained or improved. Practicing oncologists are encouraged to participate in such studies so that this evolutionary process can proceed as expeditiously as possible.

REFERENCES

1. Li FP: Secondary cancers. In DeVita VT Jr, Hellman S, Rosenberg SA (eds): Cancer: Principles and Practice of Oncology, 2nd ed, pp 2040–2049. Philadelphia, JB Lippincott, 1985
2. Coleman CN: Adverse effects of cancer therapy: Risk of secondary neoplasms. Am J Pediatr Hematol Oncol 4:103–111, 1982
3. Coleman CN: Secondary neoplasms in patients treated for cancer: Etiology and perspective. Radiat Res 92:188–200, 1982
4. Kohn HI, Fry RJM: Radiation carcinogenesis. N Engl J Med 310:504–511, 1984
5. National Research Council, Committee on the Biological Effects of Ionizing Radiations: The Effects on Populations of Exposure to Low Levels of Ionizing Radiation. Washington, DC, National Academy of Science, 1980
6. Preston DL, Kato H, Kopecky KJ et al: Studies of the mortality of A-bomb survivors. Radiat Res 111:151–178, 1987

7. Tountas AA, Fornasier VL, Harwood AR et al: Postradiation sarcoma of bone, a perspective. Cancer 43:182–187, 1979
8. Kim JH, Chu FC, Woodward HQ et al: Radiation-induced soft-tissue and bone sarcoma. Radiology 120:501–508, 1978
9. Doherty MA, Rodger A, Langlands AO: Sarcoma of bone following therapeutic irradiation for breast carcinoma. Int J Radiat Oncol Phys 12:103–106, 1986
10. Strong LC, Herson J, Osborne BM et al: Risk of radiation-related subsequent malignant tumors in survivors of Ewing's sarcoma. JNCI 62:1401–1406, 1979
11. Huvos AG, Woodard HW, Cahan WG et al: Postradiation osteogenic sarcoma of bone and soft tissue. Cancer 55:1244–1255, 1985
12. Boice JD, Day NE, Anderson A et al: Second cancers following radiation treatment for cervical cancer: An international collaboration among cancer registries. JNCI 74:955–975, 1985
13. Tucker MA, D'Angio GJ, Boice JD et al: Bone sarcoma linked to radiotherapy and chemotherapy in children. N Engl J Med 317:588–593, 1987
14. Draper GJ, Sanders BM, Kingston JE: Secondary primary neoplasms in patients with retinoblastoma. Br J Cancer 53:661–671, 1986
15. Abramson DH, Ellsworth RM, Kitchi FD et al: Second nonocular tumors in retinoblastoma survivors: Are they radiation-reduced? Ophthalmology 91:1351–1355, toma survivors: Are they radiation-reduced? Ophthalmology 91:1351–1355, 1984
16. Hansen FM, Koufson A, Gallie BL et al: Osteosarcoma and retinoblastoma: A shared chromosomal mechanism revealing recessive predisposition. Proc Natl Acad Sci USA 82:6216–6220, 1986
17. Tucker MA, Coleman CN, Cox RS et al: Risk of second malignancies following Hodgkin's disease after 15 years. N Engl J Med 318:76–81, 1988
18. Boice JD, Day NE, Anderson et al: Second cancer following radiation treatment for cervical cancer: An international collaboration among cancer registries. JNCI 74:955–975, 1985
19. Linos A, Gray JE, Orvis AL et al: Low-dose radiation and leukemia. N Engl J Med 302:1101–1105, 1980
20. Evans JS, Wennberg JE, McNeil BJ: The influence of diagnostic radiography on the incidence of breast cancer and leukemia. N Engl J Med 315:810–815, 1986
21. Coleman CB, Williams CJ, Flint A, et al: Hematologic neoplasia in patients treated for Hodgkin's disease. N Engl J Med 297:1249–1252, 1977
22. Valagussa P, Santoro A, Bellani-Fossati F et al: Second acute leukemia and other malignancies following treatment for Hodgkin's disease. J Clin Oncol 4:830–837, 1986
23. Coleman CN. Editorial: Second malignancy after treatment of Hodgkin's disease: An evolving picture. J Clin Oncol 4:821–824, 1986
24. Reimer RR, Hoover R, Fraumeni JF Jr et al: Acute leukemia after alkylating-agent therapy for ovarian cancer. N Engl J Med 297:177–181, 1977
25. Greene MH, Boice JD Jr, Greer BE et al: Acute nonlymphocytic leukemia after therapy with akylating gents for ovarian cancer. N Engl J Med 307:1416–1421, 1982
26. Boice JD, Greene MH, Killen JY et al: Letter: Leukemia after chemotherapy with semustine (methyl-CCNU): Evidence of a dose-response effect. N Engl J Med 314:119–120, 1986
27. Bergasagel DE, Bailey AJ, Langley GR et al: The chemotherapy for plasma-cell myeloma and the incidence of acute leukemia. N Engl J Med 301:743–748, 1979
28. Berk PD, Goldberg JD, Silverstein MN et al: Increased risk of acute leukemia in polycythemia vera associated with chlorambucil therapy. N Engl J Med 304:441–447, 1981
29. Boice JD Jr, Greene MH, Killen JY et al: Leukemia and preleukemia after adjuvant treatment of gastrointestinal cancer with semustine (methyl-CCNU). N Engl J Med 309:1079–1084, 1983
30. Chak LY, Sikic BI, Tucker MA, et al: Increased incidence of acute nonlymphocytic leukemia following therapy in patients with small cell carcinoma of the lung. J Clin Oncol 2:385–390, 1984
31. Redman JR, Vugrin D, Arlin ZA et al: Leukemia following treatment of germ cell tumors in men. J Clin Oncol 2:1080–1087, 1984
32. Greene MH, Harris EL, Gershenson DM et al: Melphalan may be a more potent leukemogen than cyclophosphamide. Ann Intern Med 105:360–367, 1986
33. Blayney DW, Longo DL, Young RC et al: Decreasing risk of leukemia with prolonged follow-up after chemotherapy and radiotherapy for Hodgkin's disease. N Engl J Med 316:710–714, 1987
34. Pederson-Bjerngaard, Ersboll J, Sorenson HM et al: Risk of acute nonlymphocytic leukemia and preleukemia in patients treated with cyclophosphamide for non-Hodgkin's lymphomas. Ann Intern Med 103:195–200, 1985
35. Greene MH, Young RC, Merrill JM et al: Evidence of a treatment dose response in acute nonlymphocytic leukemias which occur after therapy of non-Hodgkin's lymphoma. Cancer Res 43:1891–1898, 1983
36. Fisher B, Rockette H, Fisher ER et al: Leukemia in breast cancer patients following adjuvant chemotherapy or postoperative radiation: The NSABP experience. J Clin Oncol 3:1640–1658, 1985
37. Valagussa P, Tancini G, Bonadonna G: Second malignancies CMF for resectable breast cancer. J Clin Oncol 5:1138–1142, 1987
38. Henderson IC: Editorial: Second malignancies from adjuvant chemotherapy? Too soon to tell. J Clin Oncol 5:1135–1137, 1987
39. Greene MH: Epidemiologic studies of chemotherapy-related acute leukemia. In Castellani A (ed): Epidemiology and Quantitation of Environmental Risk in Humans from Radiation and Other Agents, pp 499–514. New York Plenum, 1985
40. Adamson RH, Seiber SM: Studies on the oncogenicity of procarbazine and other compounds in nonhuman primates. In Rosenberg SA, Kaplan HS (eds): Malignant Lymphomas: Etiology, Immunology, Pathology, Treatment, pp 239–257. Orlando, Fla, Academic Press, 1982
41. Henry-Amar M: Second cancer after treatment in two successive cohorts of patients with early stages of Hodgkin's disease. In Cavalli F, Bonadonna G, Rozencweig M (eds): Malignant Lymphomas and Hodgkin's Disease: Experimental and Therapeutic Advances, pp 417–428. Boston, Martinus Nijhoff, 1985
42. IARC Working Group: An evaluation of chemicals and industrial processes associated with cancer in humans based on human and animal data: IARC monographs, volumes 1 to 20. Cancer Res 40:1–12, 1980
43. Tucker MA, Meadows AT, Boice JD et al: Leukemia after therapy with alkylating agents. JNCI 78:459–464, 1987
44. Cuzik J, Erskine S, Edelman D et al: A comparison of the incidence of the myelodysplastic syndrome and acute myeloid leukemia following melphalan and cyclophosphamide treatment for myelomatosis. Br J Cancer 55:523–529, 1987
45. Rowley JD, Golomb HM, Vardiman JW: Nonrandom chromosome abnormalities in acute leukemia and dysmyeloplastic syndrome in patients with previously treated malignant disease. Blood 58:759–767, 1981
46. Pederson-Bjergaard J, Philip P, Pedersen NT et al: Acute nonlymphocytic leukemia, preleukemia, and acute myeloproliferative syndrome secondary to treatment of other malignant diseases. Cancer 54:452–462, 1984
47. Le Beau MM, Albain KS, Larson RA et al: Clinical and cytogenetic correlations in 63 patients with therapy-related myelodysplastic syndromes and acute nonlymphocytic leukemia: Further evidence for characteristic abnormalities of chromosomes No. 5 and 7. J Clin Oncol 4:325–345, 1986
48. Preisler HD, Early AP, Raza A et al: Therapy of secondary nonlymphocytic leukemia with cytarabine. N Engl J Med 308:21–23, 1983
49. Vaughan WP, Karp JE, Burke PJ: Effective chemotherapy of acute myelocytic leukemia occurring after alkylating agent or radiation therapy for prior malignancy. J Clin Oncol 1:204–207, 1983
50. Cavenee WK, Murphree AL, Shull MM et al: Prediction of familial predisposition to retinoblastoma. N Engl J Med 314:1201–1207, 1986
51. Lee W-H, Bookstein R, Hong F et al: Human retinoblastoma susceptibility gene: Cloning identification, and sequence. Science 235:1394–1399, 1987
52. Arthur DC: Genetics and cytogenetics of pediatric cancers. Cancer 58:534–540, 1986
53. Koufos A, Hansen MF, Lampkin BC et al: Loss of alleles at loci on human chromosome 11 during the genesis of Wilms' tumor. Nature 309:170–172, 1984
54. Meadows AT, Baum E, Bellani-Fossati F et al: Second malignant neoplasms in children: An update from the Late Effects Study Group. J Clin Oncol 3:532–538, 1985
55. Pizzo PA, Miser JS, Cassady JR et al: Solid tumors of childhood. In DeVita VT Jr, Hellman S, Rosenberg SA (eds): Cancer: Principles and Practice of Oncology, 2nd ed, pp 1511–1590. Philadelphia, JB Lippincott, 1985
56. Rimm IJ, Li FC, Tarbell NJ et al: Brain tumors after cranial irradiation for childhood acute lymphoblastic leukemia. Cancer 59:1506–1508, 1987
57. Coleman CN, Kaplan HS, Cox R et al: Leukemias, non-Hodgkin's lymphomas and solid tumors in patients treated for Hodgkin's disease. Cancer Surveys 1:733–744, 1982
58. Tucker MA, Misfeldt D, Coleman CN et al: Cutaneous malignant melanoma after Hodgkin's disease. Ann Intern Med 102:37–41, 1985
59. Chakravarti A, Halloran SL, Bale SJ et al: Etiological heterogeneity in Hodgkin's disease: HLA linked and unlinked determinants of susceptibility independent of histological concordance. Genet Epidemiol 3:407–415, 1986
60. Pollack MS, Falk J, Gazit E et al: Classical and AID's Kaposi sarcoma. In Histocompatibility Testing 1984, pp 403–406. New York, Springer-Verlag, Albert ED, Baur MP, Mayr WR (eds): 1984
61. Melbye M, Kestens L, Biggar RJ et al: HLA studies of endemic African Kaposi's sarcoma patients and matched controls: No association with HLA-DR5. Int J Cancer 39:182–184, 1987
62. Harrington DS, Weisenberger DD, Purtilo DT: Malignant lymphoma in the X-linked lymphoproliferative syndrome. Cancer 59:1419–1429, 1987
63. Fauci AS, Macher AM, Longo DL et al: Acquire immunodeficiency syndrome: Epidemiologic, clinical, immunologic, and therapeutic considerations. Ann Intern Med 100:92–106, 1984
64. Ziegler JL, Beckstead JA, Volberding PA et al: Non-Hodgkin's lymphoma in 90 homosexual men. N Engl J Med 311:565–570, 1984
65. Schoeppel SL, Hoppe RT, Dorfman RF et al: Hodgkin's disease in homosexual men with generalized lymphadenopathy. Ann Intern Med 102:68–70, 1985
66. List AF, Greer JP, Cousar JB et al: Non-Hodgkin's lymphoma after treatment of Hodgkin's disease: association with Epstein-Barr virus. Ann Intern Med 105:668–673, 1986
67. Goustin AS, Leof EB, Shipley GD et al: Growth factors and cancer. Cancer Res 46:1015–1029, 1986
68. Salmon DJ: Editorial: Proto-oncogenes and human cancer. N Engl J Med 317:955–956, 1987
69. Kohl NR, Gee CE, Alt FW: Activated expression of the N-*myc* gene in human neuroblastomas and related tumors. Science 226:1336–1337, 1984
70. Brodeur GM, Seeger RC, Sather H et al: Clinical implications of oncogene activation in human neuroblastomas. Cancer 58:541–545, 1986
71. Hirai H, Kobayashi Y, Mano H et al: A point mutation at codon 13 of the N-*ras* oncogene in myelodysplastic syndrome. Nature 327:430–432, 1987
72. Naylor SL, Johnson BE, Minna JD et al: Loss of heterozygosity of chromosome 3p markers in small-cell lung cancer. Nature 329:451–454, 1987
73. Wong AJ, Ruppert JM, Eggleston J et al: Gene amplification of cy-*myc* and N-*myc* in small cell carcinoma of the lung. Science 233:461–464, 1986

74. Rodenhuis S, van de Wetering ML, Moot W et al: Mutational activation of the K-*ras* oncogene. N Engl J Med 317:929–935, 1987
75. Benedict WF, Srivatsan ES, Mark C et al: Complete or partial homozygosity of chromosome 13 in primary retinoblastoma. Cancer Res 47:4189–4191, 1987
76. Solomon E, Voss R, Hall V et al: Chromosome 5 allele loss in human colorectal carcinomas. Nature 328:616–619, 1987
77. Bodmer WF, Bailey CJ, Bodmer J et al: Localization of the gene for familial adenomatous polyposis on chromosome 5. Nature 328:614–616, 1987
78. Dempsey JL, Seshadri, Morley AA: Increased mutation frequency following treatment with cancer chemotherapy. Cancer Res 42:2873–2877, 1985
79. Monson RR: Analysis of relative survival and proportional mortality. Comput Biomed Res 7:325–332, 1974
80. Kaplan EL, Meier P: Nonparametric estimation from incomplete observation. J Am Stat Assoc 53:457–481, 1958
81. Gehan EA: A generalized Wilcoxon test for comparing arbitrarily singly-censored samples. Biometrika 52:203–223, 1965

CHAPTER 61 Psychologic Aspects of Patients with Cancer

MARGUERITE S. LEDERBERG
JIMMIE C. HOLLAND
MARY JANE MASSIE

SECTION 1

Psychosocial Aspects of Patients with Cancer

HISTORICAL BACKGROUND

Cancer is a group of diseases that have struck fear in the hearts of individuals for centuries. Its previously certain fatal outcome, absence of known cause or cure, and association with pain and disfiguring lesions made it particularly frightening and loathsome. Physicians long regarded the diagnosis of cancer as too painful to reveal to patients. Consequently, family and physician conspired, often unsuccessfully, to create the illusion of a minor illness for the patient.[1] Gripping fear prevented the word cancer from appearing in the press; patients and their families kept the diagnosis a secret from all but closest acquaintances. A person who even suspected that he or she had cancer would often refuse to go to the doctor out of fatalistic resignation. The word cancer was widely used as a metaphor for an insidious, destructive force in society.[2] The fear, secrecy, and mythological elaboration contributed to making the emotional burden and social stigma much heavier to bear for patients and families.

As early as 1913, the American Cancer Society was founded to counter fears and educate the public to the fact that early diagnosis and treatment by surgery could be curative. However, negative attitudes have persisted. Only in the past four decades has a real, albeit still incomplete, change occurred in attitudes toward cancer in the United States. There is greater openness in public discussion and more candor in revealing the diagnosis to patients. Except for Scandinavia, few other countries have moved as rapidly and as far as the United States in these trends.[3]

Several factors have contributed to the change in attitudes in the United States. First, pessimism in both physicians and patients began to give way to cautious optimism, as radiation therapy and chemotherapy began to cure several common neoplasms of children and young adults.

Second, clinicians who spoke more openly with their patients observed that open disclosure was unexpectedly well tolerated. A better understanding of the rationale for treatment helped patients handle side-effects better, and truthful communications generated enhanced trust in the physician. During the 1950s, psychiatrists studying psychological reactions to cancer observed that patients given accurate facts adapted better to radical surgery.[4] It was also noted that the opportunity to prepare psychologically for the major physical changes associated with procedures such as radical mastectomy facilitated postoperative adaptation.[5]

A third factor contributing to attitudinal change was a reexamination of the care given to dying patients. Following the lead of the European hospice movement and the pioneering work of Elizabeth Kubler-Ross, it became more widely understood that terminally ill patients benefited from an opportunity to discuss not only their illness but also their feelings and fears about death.[6]

Lastly, in the 1970s advocacy of patients' rights became increasingly vocal. The right of self-determination required the physician to discuss fully all diagnostic and treatment options, so as to encourage and enable the patient to participate in decisions. Informed consent for research patients was mandated by federal guidelines. In routine clinical care, however, the patient autonomy issue overlapped with and reinforced a growing demand for greater attention to quality of life during treatment. This problem was particularly acute in oncology, where the often severe side-effects of treatment made special demands on patient trust. As physicians came to depend more on laboratory data and spent less time at the bedside, patients complained increasingly about the diminished closeness to their new, more technologically oriented doctors.

The many changes outlined above have produced a climate in which concern for the human side of cancer care has become more prominent.

An additional impetus to exploring psychosocial issues in cancer has been the recognition that psychological factors, and their resulting behaviors, are critical to the prevention and early detection of cancer. Much of the research effort in cancer prevention today, particularly that of smoking cessation, depends on the social sciences to develop ways of understanding and altering behavior. Most recently, studies of the possible role of personality factors in altering both risk and survival, through neuroendocrine and neuroimmune mechanisms, has added another important though still controversial dimension to the field.

The psychological condition of medically ill patients has been increasingly studied, in cancer patients among others.[7,8] But the developments outlined above have spurred the development of a new subspecialty in oncology, called psychosocial oncology or psycho-oncology. Seen as having little scientific interest four decades ago, it has, since the mid-1970s, rapidly established a body of information based on systematic clinical observations and scientific investigations.[9] This has occurred despite several problems: (1) the bias that psychological factors were of minor importance in cancer, (2) lack of objective psychological data on cancer patients, (3) lack of suitable assessment instruments for measuring emotional distress in physically ill patients, (4) lack of investigators trained in both social science research methods and oncology, (5) lack of collaborative research ties between social scientists and oncologists, and (6) unavailability of formal clinical and research training programs in the psychological aspects of cancer.

Despite these impediments, psycho-oncology has developed a growing body of knowledge which deals with two psychological dimensions of cancer:

1. The impact of cancer and its treatment on the psychological and social functioning of patients, their families, and the treating staff. This dimension, discussed in detail below, describes the range of normal and abnormal psychological responses to cancer and guides the oncologist in diagnosis, management, and referral.
2. The role of psychosocial factors and behaviors in cancer risk and survival. This latter dimension, reviewed only briefly, provides the basis for a burgeoning area of research in early detection, cancer prevention, and psychosocial contributions to risk and survival.

PSYCHOLOGICAL IMPACT OF CANCER

Psychological distress is to be expected as an individual confronts the implications of cancer—possible death, pain, dependence on others, disability, disfiguring changes in the body, and loss of function—which endanger his relationships to others. The initial emotional crisis is just the first of many, each requiring resiliency and rapid adaptation to new events and challenges. Most individuals cope adequately, keeping distress in a manageable range; some do not. In order to treat and prevent pathological reactions, it is important to understand their causes, which are of three kinds: societal, biomedical, and patient-related (personal and interpersonal) (Table 61-1).

SOCIETAL FACTORS

The social setting plays an immediate and important role in a patient's psychological adaptation to cancer. Yet the social determinants ambient in the milieu are seldom obvious to the patient. In the past, patients came with high hopes for

TABLE 61-1. Factors that Influence Patients' Psychological Adaptation to Cancer

Societal
Attitudes toward cancer and treatment
Stigma associated with diagnosis
Health care policy
(insurance for care, disability, and protection from job discrimination)
Medical
Tumor site, stage at diagnosis
Predicted outcome
Symptoms, functional loss(es)
Treatment(s) required
Rehabilitation available
Clinical course of illness
Associated medical conditions
Patient-Related
Personality; ability to cope with life crises
Level of maturity and ability to accept altered or unachieved life goals
Prior experiences with cancer (family members' death from cancer)
Other concurrent life crises (divorce, grief, other illness)
Support of family and others

cure, requesting little information, content to rest trust in the doctor, while also harboring a sense of shame and a need for secrecy. Today there is less shame and less secrecy, but also less simple hope, more fear of treatment, and more mistrust of the doctor and of the whole medical enterprise. For example, negative public attitudes toward the cancer research "establishment" in the 1970s pushed the National Cancer Institute to carry out a trial of laetrile in the absence of any objective evidence for its efficacy.[10] The present popularity of naturalistic alternative cancer therapies guarantees that patients will challenge the wisdom of their doctor's treatment choice, privately if not openly.

In addition, patients are deeply affected by society's provision (or nonprovision) of health insurance and other concrete supports for illness and disability. Legal protection from discrimination in the workplace is a crucial issue for returning patients. A group of cancer patients in the United States had significantly greater worries about medical expenses, decreased income, and loss of a secure future due to exhausted savings, compared with a matched group of patients in Sweden; they were also far more reluctant to reveal a history of cancer to their employers (58% *vs.* 17%).[11] This can be expected to contribute to a feeling of entitlement and anger found in many U.S. patients and families.

MEDICAL FACTORS

Once a patient receives a diagnosis of cancer, the vicissitudes of the disease and the treatment assume a central role in the patient's existence and emotional state. Issues such as the cancer site, stage, prognosis, symptoms, type of treatment, functional losses, rehabilitation available, clinical course, and psychological management by the oncologist and staff all play an important role. A few key areas are discussed below.

STAGES OF DISEASE. Adaptational needs and distress are greatest at certain crises or transition points such as diagnosis, the start of primary treatment, at the end of primary treatment when concerns about possible recurrence increase, when changing treatment modalities, at relapse, at the transition from curative to supportive treatment, and during advanced and terminal disease. The oncologist must be especially attuned to psychological distress at these junctions. For example, patients terminating an intensive course of treatment should be given an early follow-up appointment, reassured of ongoing availability of the doctor, and warned that they may go through an unexpected period of increased anxiety.

DOCTOR–PATIENT RELATIONSHIP. Any stage of illness is tolerated best by the patient whose relationship with his physicians is characterized by trust, good communication, and a sense of partnership during the medical workup. The oncologist can explore the person's emotional stability, prior ability to tolerate major crises, and previous exposure to cancer. The presence of family members during discussions allows for evaluation of the patient's social supports and prevents patient isolation. In today's social climate the doctor must balance gentleness and candor so that the patient can give as informed a consent as possible. Good communications between the referring physician and the oncologist are critical to reassure the patient about continuity of care despite referral to an unfamiliar specialist.

TERMINAL ILLNESS. In the past, terminal patients were often kept in the dark about their condition because protective families and physicians felt this was the most humane thing to do. This approach has been made obsolete by society's ethical attention to patients' rights to participate in decisions about instituting and foregoing life-sustaining measures, especially cardiopulmonary resuscitation.[12] Increasingly, institutions must have written policies to guide staff about when and under what circumstances patients may not be resuscitated. In 1984, Wanzer et al noted that both physicians and families avoided frank discussions with the fatally ill patient. However, the authors stated that practically all patients, even disturbed ones, are better off having frank discussions.[13] Concern for how the patient may react, guilt for having failed the patient, and self-consciousness about how to present the issue lead many physicians to delay and avoid the discussion. This improves with encouragement, role modeling, and practice.

ETHICAL ISSUES. The problems of informed consent and terminal care decisions are emotionally very difficult and become even more so when intertwined, as they frequently are, with ethical, legal, and psychological complications. Lederberg has explored this important interface of ethics, law, and psychiatry in oncology.[14] Frequently the initial problem is erroneously labeled and a psychiatrist is called to solve ethical problems, or an ethics committee is asked to clarify a family's emotional misunderstandings. Careful attention is required to separate the ethical, legal, and psychiatric contributions to a problem in order to arrive at the appropriate interventions. Today it is important (and in some jurisdictions mandatory) for a hospital to have an identified body, such as an Ethics Committee, which can call upon the expertise not only of oncology but also of law, psychiatry, and ethics to clarify ambiguous situations and resolve disputes.

PATIENT-RELATED FACTORS

The patient's contribution to adaptation to illness is derived from several sources (see Table 61-1). Individuals with a stable personality and no history of significant prior psychological problems can be expected to adapt well to cancer.[15] These patients confront the facts, seek available information, and actively pursue treatment. They respond to the disease as a challenge, while poorer copers often try to avoid the implications of the illness and delay the decisions required for optimal care. The best predictor of good patient adjustment is good adaptation to prior life crises.[16] However, some prior crises can make the diagnosis of cancer much more upsetting, namely cancer in a close relative or friend, especially when it involves the same site as the patient's disease. Cassileth et al have shown that older patients adapt better to a range of chronic illnesses, including cancer.[17] The coincidence of cancer with other crises such as grief, divorce, or another illness makes it much harder to bear. Without the support of close, caring individuals, many patients will unravel under the stress of cancer.[18,19] Social supports have even been found to influence mortality rates among elderly individuals.[20,21]

NORMAL PSYCHOLOGICAL RESPONSES TO CANCER

The expected range of psychological responses to cancer needs to be defined in order to recognize when a patient requires further evaluation and support. The observed response to a diagnosis of cancer is similar to that of other life-threatening illnesses or major life changes.[22,23] Initially, the person is often disbelieving. "I feel numb," "as if I am watching someone else," or "cancer couldn't happen to me" are common expressions used by patients at this time. This is a constructive attempt at dampening awareness down to tolerable levels. The next stage is one of mixed anxious and depressed feelings, preoccupation with the implications of the illness, foreboding thoughts about the future, and a sense of helplessness. Attention and concentration are impaired; sleeping and eating patterns are disrupted. These acute symptoms dissipate over a few weeks as a treatment plan is agreed upon and undertaken. During this critical time, the psychological distress and associated physiological arousal make it difficult for the person to fully comprehend the doctor's diagnosis and recommendations. The ability to process information and solve problems has been shown to be temporarily impaired, at a time when important decisions must be made.[23] Therefore, the physician should plan to repeat information several times and should not be surprised when patients appear to have poor comprehension and even poorer recall.

Although the acute response is limited to a few weeks, the overall adaptation goes on much longer.[24] Weisman and Worden described the first hundred days after diagnosis as one of continuing "existential plight," and of course some level of concern will remain indefinitely.[25] Psychologically healthy individuals use ways of coping that have worked well in the past, obtaining and processing information about the treatment, as well as help and advice from experienced others. Optimism, a sense of humor, and an interest in helping others with the same problem have also been found to be helpful.[26]

PSYCHOSOCIAL AND MEDICAL FACTORS ASSOCIATED WITH POOR ADJUSTMENT

The vulnerability factors that identify patients at increased risk of poor adjustment and psychiatric problems fall into three major categories: psychological, social, and medical factors (Table 61-2).[27] Prior psychiatric problems, alcohol or drug abuse, depression, and chronic anxiety are strong predictors for poor adjustment and for exacerbation of previous psychiatric difficulties. Evidence of unusually high initial distress that persists unusually long with high levels of anxiety and depression, especially when coupled with behavioral evidence of poor coping, is also reason for concern. A negative attitude toward doctors and treatment and low expectations for the future do not augur well. Medical factors suggesting high vulnerability are advanced disease and poorly controlled symptoms, particularly pain and insomnia. Several social factors are associated with poor adjustment: low socioeconomic status with few resources, chronic marital or family problems, perceived or actual poor support from others, and absence of affiliation with a meaningful social group, especially a religious one.

TABLE 61-2. Characteristics Associated with Poor Adjustment to Illness*

Psychological/Psychiatric
History of prior psychiatric illness
Alcoholism
Drug abuse
Depression
Anxiety disorder
Presence of:
Severe anxiety
Depression with hopelessness
Poor coping
Poor relationship to doctor
Poor expectations of treatment and of future
Medical
Advanced disease
Poorly controlled symptoms, especially pain and insomnia
Social
Low socioeconomic status with few resources
History of marital or family problems
Perceived or actual poor support from others
Absence of a social group affiliation, especially religious

*Adapted from Weisman AD: Coping with Cancer. New York, McGraw-Hill, 1979.

ABNORMAL PSYCHOLOGICAL RESPONSES TO CANCER

It is important for the oncologist to recognize when a patient's response is self-limited and when it has become pathological. The diagnosis of psychiatric disorders in cancer patients has been clouded by assumptions that severe depression and demoralization are "normal" in cancer patients. In fact, when the level and severity of physical illness are controlled for, cancer patients have the same frequency of depression as other medically ill patients.[28]

INCIDENCE OF PSYCHIATRIC DISORDERS

The actual incidence of psychiatric disorders in cancer patients has only been determined in the past decade, by assessing ambulatory and hospitalized patients in three cancer centers, using standard diagnostic criteria (Fig. 61-1).[29] Fifty-three percent of patients interviewed, though showing signs of being under stress, were coping adequately. The remaining 47% had a diagnosable psychiatric disorder. The most common by far was adjustment disorder with anxious and depressive symptoms, seen in two thirds of those with psychiatric disorders and one third of all patients interviewed. Depression was next, seen in 13% of those with a

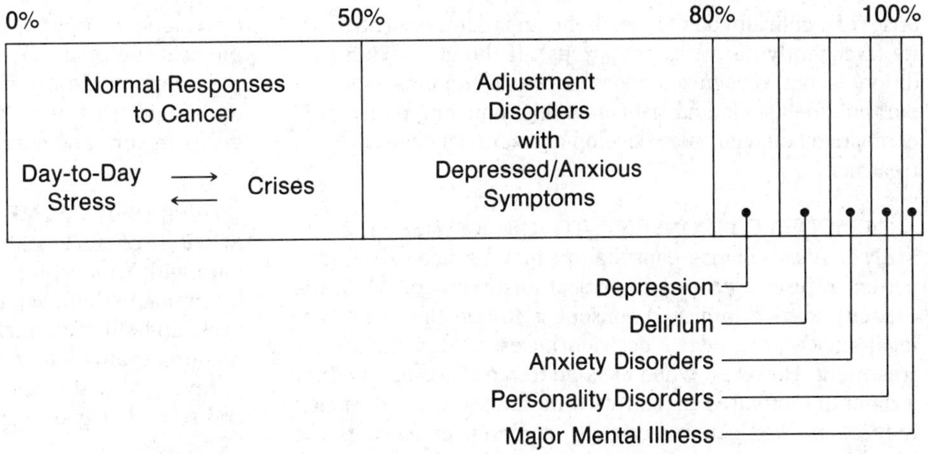

FIG. 61-1. Spectrum of psychiatric disorders in patients with cancer (derived from PSYCOG prevalence data). (Holland JC, Rowland J [eds]: Psycho-Oncology: The Psychological Care of the Patient with Cancer. New York, Oxford University Press [in press])

psychiatric diagnosis. Central nervous system complications resulting in organic mental disorders were present in 4%; prior psychiatric problems accounted for only 5% of cases.

Among hospitalized and more seriously ill patients, the frequency of major depression rises to 20%.[28] Organic mental disorders, primarily delirium, increase with worsening illness, to a frequency of 20% in hospitalized cancer patients and 80% in the terminally ill.[30,31]

INDICATIONS FOR PSYCHIATRIC EVALUATION

Many mild to moderately severe psychiatric disorders are managed successfully by the oncologist and a sensitive staff. However, from the above incidence figures it is clear that cancer patients experience a significant number of psychiatric disorders requiring accurate diagnosis for precise and effective treatment. Once treatment is outlined, management may often be carried out by the physician with help of social workers or other mental health professionals. The more severe psychiatric problems require close collaboration between the oncologist and psychiatrist.

Table 61-3 outlines the indications for psychiatric consultation, with emphasis on symptoms that require urgent psychiatric attention, as opposed to those that can be addressed more electively.

Symptoms Requiring Immediate Attention

EXPRESSION OF SUICIDAL PLANS. The patient with cancer who is depressed, feels hopeless, and announces a plan for suicide deserves an immediate psychiatric consultation. The more concretely a plan is described, the greater the risk. A concrete plan should not be confused with the verbalization of suicidal thoughts or wishes, although these also deserve eventual attention.

EXPRESSION OF WISHES OR PLANS TO HARM OTHERS. Patients under great stress, especially hospitalized ones, often are given drugs that may decrease impulse control or produce confusional states with paranoid ideation, both of which lead to disruptive behavior. Patients with a prior history of schizophrenia may have an exacerbation of their delusions and become combative during their illness. Highly stressed relatives become sleep-deprived and self-medicate with benzodiazepines for control of anxiety, both of which result in disinhibition. Frustration may lead to anger and loss of control in relatives as often as in patients themselves. Guidelines for managing violent and potentially violent individuals should be part of house staff and nursing training and orientation; a well-prepared staff working with an experienced psychiatrist can handle most situations without causing major disruption on the floor or arousing fear in other patients.

SUDDEN CHANGE IN BEHAVIOR. The previously cooperative patient who exhibits a sudden change in personality or behavior, such as becoming irritable and angry or withdrawn and apathetic, may be experiencing the insidious

TABLE 61-3. Symptoms in a Patient with Cancer for Which a Psychiatric Evaluation is Indicated

Needing immediate attention:
Expression of suicidal plans
Expression of wishes or plans to harm others
Sudden personality or behavior change (may be first evidence of underlying delirium)
Capacity to consent to or refuse treatment, including leaving against advice
Indecision about treatment
Warranting elective attention (unless severe)
Anxiety: current or history of prior phobias, panic or anxiety disorder
Depression: reactive symptoms with hopelessness, poor self-esteem
History of prior personality disorder or major mental illness
History of alcohol or drug abuse (may present as withdrawal state)
Distress about sexual dysfunction (threatened or resulting from treatment)
Significant distress resulting from conflict with family or staff

onset of a delirium due to metabolic imbalance or drug toxicity (frequently narcotics or steroids). If the underlying condition is not recognized more severe symptoms, such as paranoid delusions and hallucinations, noncompliance, and combative behavior, may develop and seriously compromise treatment.

CAPACITY TO CONSENT TO OR REFUSE TREATMENT. A psychiatric consultation may be needed when a patient refuses a procedure critical to survival or when the capacity to give informed consent is in question. Rarely is legal advice or a judge's decision necessary for emergency treatment. However, when elective treatment is planned for a mentally impaired patient with no family, court direction may be needed. An increasingly common concern is the patient who refuses a clearly life-sustaining treatment, such as dialysis, as part of a decision to forego all further treatment. Physicians and nurses often are not certain whether the patient is truly capable of assessing all the options. The presence of acute depression, which dulls mental processes and strongly biases decisions, poses a difficult and sometimes urgent reason for psychiatric consultation.

LEAVING AGAINST MEDICAL ADVICE. Requests to leave the hospital against advice are most commonly due to the presence of a confusional state secondary to illness or medication and as such often represent an acute danger to self, allowing for brief restraint and treatment following psychiatric evaluation. An acutely psychotic state or an exacerbated prior psychiatric disorder may also result in poor judgment. The cause of the behavior must be determined and a decision made as to whether the patient can be managed safely at home or whether he or she must remain in the hospital with a relative or companion. Often the severity of the patient's illness prevents safe transfer to a medical–psychiatric unit, but improvement occurs rapidly under the care of familiar medical staff, with one-to-one observation and low doses of a neuroleptic drug such as haloperidol.

INDECISION ABOUT TREATMENT. Last-minute indecision about treatment is not common but can lead to a frustrating situation for doctor and patient. Prior painful associations with cancer or acute fears of a proposed treatment can result in panic and acute fears of death. A psychiatric consultation often elicits underlying fears and helps put the experience in a more rational perspective. Usually, a little time plus support and medication enable the person to proceed.

Symptoms Requiring Elective Attention

The following problems can be electively evaluated unless the symptoms are severe.

ANXIETY SYMPTOMS WITH HISTORY OF PHOBIAS, PANIC, OR ANXIETY DISORDERS. Individuals who have a history of panic attacks, phobias, or generalized anxiety often experience exacerbations in the hospital or during treatment. Ideally, these patients should be evaluated and treated as early as possible, especially before any major intervention. Medication, behavioral, and psychotherapeutic treatments coordinated by the psychiatrist working with the medical staff can effectively minimize distress and improve management. Severe preoperative anxiety may require pharmacologic treatment in cooperation with the anesthesiologist, surgeon, and surgical nursing staff.

DEPRESSIVE SYMPTOMS WITH HOPELESSNESS AND POOR SELF-ESTEEM. Mild depressive symptoms are common with cancer; severe ones are not. Symptoms such as insomnia, withdrawal, dysphoria, self-denigration, hopelessness, and suicidal thoughts signal a major depression that requires evaluation and treatment. It responds well to supportive psychotherapy, antidepressants, cognitive therapy, and some behavioral interventions.

HISTORY OF PERSONALITY DISORDER OR MAJOR MENTAL ILLNESS. Psychiatric consultation should be routinely requested to evaluate the patient with a known history of a major psychiatric disorder (*e.g.*, schizophrenia, manic–depressive illness) or a severe personality disorder. Assessment of current emotional state and of the ability to understand treatment recommendations and comply with treatment decisions is needed and is best done prior to hospital admission, or at the start of ambulatory treatment. It is mandatory when the planned treatment (such as bone marrow transplantation) is lengthy, complex, and requires prolonged patient cooperation.

SEXUAL DYSFUNCTION. Infertility and sexual dysfunction are often unavoidable consequences of irradiation, surgery, and chemotherapy. In men, the opportunity for sperm banking before treatment can both arouse and assuage concerns about infertility. In women, psychological preparation for the premature menopause and sterility associated with chemotherapy, or the altered sexual function that results from gynecologic surgery is very useful in diminishing the inevitable adverse reactions. Soon after completion of treatment, patients are reluctant to bring up sexual problems and physicians and staff are equally reluctant to ask about them. In later follow-up visits, the burden is on the oncologist to inquire into the sexual problems common with several tumor sites: breast, testicular, gynecologic neoplasms, prostate, bladder, head and neck tumors, and Hodgkin's disease. An increasingly sophisticated literature on diagnosis and treatment is developing in this area, and is further reviewed in Section 2 of this chapter.[32–34]

SIGNIFICANT DISTRESS FROM CONFLICT WITH FAMILY OR STAFF. Sometimes a case becomes imbued with persistent conflict. This may stem from the patient's personality, but in fact it often involves the family's problems or, more rarely, the staff's inadvertent mishandling. A psychiatric consultant can provide an objective assessment that identifies and confronts the sources of the problematic behavior. Family meetings, possibly with the patient and selected staff members present, often help to ease family distress; similarly, staff conferences encourage a more concerted and effective approach to the family and patient.

TABLE 61-4. Common Psychiatric Disorders in Cancer Patients

Disorders directly related to illness
Adjustment disorders
(reactive anxiety, depression, and associated behaviors)
Major depression and suicidal risk
Delirium from CNS complications
Preexisting disorders exacerbated by illness
Anxiety disorders
Fear of needles, hospitals, enclosed spaces
Panic disorders
Agoraphobia
Generalized anxiety
Personality disorders
Paranoid, obsessive, dependent
Borderline, histrionic
Major mental illness
Schizophrenia
Manic-depressive illness

COMMON PSYCHIATRIC DISORDERS IN CANCER PATIENTS

Six psychiatric disorders occur frequently enough in cancer to warrant a description of their clinical picture. Three represent a direct reaction to the illness—adjustment disorders (reactive anxiety and depression), major depression, and delirium. The others—primary anxiety disorders, personality disorders, and major mental illness—are preexisting conditions that are often exacerbated by illness (Table 61-4).

ADJUSTMENT DISORDER WITH DEPRESSED, ANXIOUS OR MIXED FEATURES (REACTIVE ANXIETY AND DEPRESSION). This common disorder is an exaggeration of the mixed anxiety and depression seen in self-limited stress responses. The key features are unusual persistence and undue interference with functioning. When very severe, these disorders are difficult to differentiate from major depression and primary anxiety disorders, and may best be treated as if they were in the more serious category, so as to give the patient all possible treatment benefits.

Interventions are aimed at helping the individual resume successful coping by use of several modalities. Individual psychotherapy focuses on clarifying the medical situation and the meaning of illness and on reinforcing the patient's positive coping strategies. It is often desirable to include a spouse or family member to enhance support at home. Frequency of sessions should be flexible and treatment may, de facto, be intermittent. Group therapy, with a focus on illness, is often helpful, as are behavioral methods such as relaxation and hypnosis. Couple and family therapy may be helpful when interpersonal issues are prominent. The decision to prescribe a psychotropic drug requires a high level of distress and the inability to carry out daily activities. Low doses of alprazolam, lorazepam, or oxazepam control symptoms and do not cause undue daytime sedation or risk withdrawal or dependence in these psychologically healthy individuals. Alprazolam, because of its rapid onset and antidepressant action, is particularly effective at doses of 0.5 mg one to three times per day.[35] Bedtime sedation with a benzodiazepine (triazolam or temazepam) or a sedating antidepressant (such as amitriptyline) is effective and may thereby improve daytime symptoms as well.

MAJOR DEPRESSION. All depression in cancer has a strong reactive component. However, true major depressive episodes also occur and are quite responsive to treatment. Unfortunately, because it is often assumed that the person is "appropriately" depressed, major depression often is undiagnosed and untreated.

Because of the associated medical illness, diagnosis cannot depend on vegetative signs, such as lack of energy or anorexia, but rests on a constellation of psychological symptoms: dysphoric or sad mood, feelings of helplessness and hopelessness, loss of self-esteem and feelings of worthlessness, guilt, and a wish to die.[36] Psychotic depressions can occur but are rare, and usually indicate an organic syndrome. Patients at high risk for major depression are those with a history of prior depression, inadequately controlled pain, an advanced stage of illness, and disease at certain sites such as the pancreas.[37] Some of the endocrine and ectopic hormone-secreting tumors also produce depression.[38] Several drugs can produce severe depression as a part of their central nervous system toxicity; among them are interferon, steroids, BCNU, vincristine, and L-asparaginase, to mention only chemotherapeutic agents.

Depressed patients are usually treated with a combination of supportive psychotherapy and antidepressants. There are several reports of the efficacy of antidepressants in depressed patients with serious physical disorders. The antidepressants that can be considered for use in cancer patients are the tricyclics, second-generation antidepressants, monoamine oxidase inhibitors, sympathomimetic stimulants, lithium carbonate, and the benzodiazepine alprazolam. Table 61-5 lists the starting dose and range of therapeutic daily doses for these drugs.

The antidepressants most frequently used in the oncology setting are the tricyclics (*e.g.*, amitriptyline, imipramine, doxepin, nortriptyline, desipramine). They are started at low doses, such as 10 to 25 mg at bedtime, and increased by 25 mg every 1 to 2 days until a beneficial effect is observed. Depressed cancer patients often respond to much lower doses (25 to 125 mg/day) than are usually required for physically healthy patients (150 to 300 mg). The drug is usually continued for 4 to 6 months after symptoms improve, after which time the dose can be tapered under observation.

The choice of tricylic depends on the nature of the depressive symptoms, medical problems present, and expected side-effects. The depressed patient who has insomnia will benefit from a sedating drug such as amitriptyline or doxepin. Patients with psychomotor slowing will benefit from more energizing compounds such as protriptyline or desipramine. The patient who has slow intestinal mobility or urinary retention should receive desipramine or nortriptyline, which have the least anticholinergic effects.

Imipramine, amitriptyline, and doxepin are being increasingly used in the management of pain in cancer patients at a starting dose of 10 to 25 mg at bedtime. Their analgesic action is distinct from their antidepressant action and is probably centrally mediated. Tricyclic antidepressants are contraindicated in the presence of procarbazine, a chemo-

TABLE 61-5. Antidepressant Medications Used in Cancer Patients*

Generic Name	*Starting Dosage, mg/day (PO)*	*Therapeutic Dosage, mg/day (PO)*
Tricyclic antidepressants		
Amitriptyline	25	75–150
Doxepin	50	75–150
Imipramine	25	75–150
Desipramine	25	75–150
Nortriptyline	50	100–150
Second-generation antidepressants		
Trazodone	50	50–300
Maprotiline	25	50–75
Amoxapine	25	100–150
Monoamine oxidase inhibitors		
Isocarboxazid	10	20–40
Phenelzine	15	30–60
Tranylcypromine	10	20–40
Lithium carbonate	00	600–1,200
Sympathomimetic stimulants		
Dextroamphetamine	0.5 in A.M.	5–10
Methylphenidate	0.5 in A.M.	5–10
Benzodiazepine		
Alprozolam	0.25–1.00 q.d.	0.75–6.00

*Adapted from Massie MJ, Holland JC: The cancer patient with pain: Psychiatric complications and their management. Med Clin North Am 71:249, 1987.

therapeutic agent that is also a monoamine oxidase inhibitor. Caution is needed in using tricyclics in older patients and in patients receiving other anticholinergic drugs, such as atropine, scopolamine, or antipsychotics for emesis, since the incidence of anticholinergic delirium is known to increase with age and with the number of anticholinergic drugs being used.

Other treatments for depression are lithium, monoamine oxidase inhibitors, and psychostimulants. Patients who have been taking lithium prior to the diagnosis of cancer should be maintained on it throughout treatment, with close monitoring of fluid and electrolytes during the preoperative and postoperative periods. Lithium should be used with extreme caution in patients receiving cisplatin due to the potential nephrotoxicity of both drugs. Several cancer centers have explored the use of lithium to stimulate granulocyte production in neutropenic patients or to prevent leukopenia during chemotherapy; only transient effects were observed, and no mood changes were noted.[39]

The psychostimulants dextroamphetamine and methylphenidate are helpful in cancer patients whose depression produces withdrawal and apathy. They improve appetite, energy level, and well-being, in doses of 2.5 mg in the morning and at noon, to be increased as tolerance develops. Amphetamines can also be used to potentiate the analgesic effect of opiates. This class of drugs is being increasingly used for symptom control in advanced illness.[40,41] Their addictive potential is not a problem in this setting. Cancer patients rarely abuse psychotropic or narcotic medications; in fact they often reduce or stop these drugs on their own as the need diminishes, and the psychiatrist must often encourage them to take more medication for optimal relief.

SUICIDAL RISK IN CANCER PATIENTS. Thoughts of death are common in seriously ill patients. They are often born out of frustration with illness, and pain, and lead to expressions such as "I wish I were dead." However, on closer exploration, most patients describe the suicidal act as a way of maintaining ultimate control over an intolerable situation. It remains an option for "the future" or "when the time comes." Actual suicidal acts are uncommon, and studies show the incidence of suicide in cancer patients to be only slightly higher than in the general population.[42] However, the stigma of suicide leads to underreporting on death certificates, especially in terminally ill patients. Therefore, the actual incidence is probably much higher, especially in individuals with advanced disease who die from a drug overdose, as opposed to more violent and obvious means of self-destruction.

Several factors are associated with an increased risk of suicide in cancer patients:[43]

- Severe depression with hopelessness
- Chronic, poorly controlled pain
- Mild delirium (with depression and diminished impulse control)
- Emotional exhaustion and sense of helplessness
- Poor or absent family and social support
- History of alcoholism or substance abuse
- History of prior depression with suicide attempt
- Family history of depression or suicide

Most of these, especially those related to symptoms of the illness, are eminently treatable.

Chronic, poorly controlled pain frequently evokes thoughts of suicide and may even lead to a suicidal act. It is important that the doctor remain involved and optimistic about symptom control and not convey therapeutic nihilism. Untreated depression is also associated with greater risk. Patients who are depressed and mildly or intermittently confused may not be identified as a suicidal risk, yet because of their poor impulse control, they may act out a suicidal thought. Some of the organic affective states caused by steroids, interferon, and interleukin-2 can produce suicidal states. Emotional exhaustion and the sense of helplessness associated with prolonged illness are also sources of enhanced risk. Patients who have poor or absent family or social support are at greater risk for a suicidal act. A history of alcohol or drug abuse or previous depression or suicide in the patient or family should alert the physician to a high-risk situation.

Treatment of the actively suicidal patient should include (1) measures to ensure patient safety, (2) evaluation and treatment of contributing factors, and (3) treatment of depression. In the majority of cases, suicidal threats diminish when painful symptoms are treated or as the medical or personal situation improves. Even a worsening medical situation can be accommodated if the patient senses that his immediate and daily needs are met. The rare case in which a competent patient continues to threaten or ask for help in committing suicide presents difficult psychological and ethical problems. The hospitalized patient must be given ongoing support and close observation while thoughtful discussions are undertaken with him about the treatment and management options. The ambulatory patient is even more problematic. Only rarely is psychiatric hospitalization indicated and that usually in a patient with a previous history of severe depression. The decision hinges on a careful psychiatric evaluation to document the presence of a life-threatening psychiatric as opposed to a medical disorder.

DELIRIUM FROM CNS COMPLICATIONS. Delirium, the second most common psychiatric diagnosis among cancer patients, is due both to the direct effects of cancer on the central nervous system (CNS) and the indirect CNS complications of the disease and treatment. Posner has reported that 15% to 20% of hospitalized cancer patients have abnormalities of cognitive function that are not related to structural disease.[44] Approximately one fifth of all consultation requests made to a psycho-oncology service were requests for assistance in the management of symptoms of delirium. The early symptoms are often unrecognized or misdiagnosed by medical and nursing staff as symptoms of depression or "poor coping." Early recognition is important since the underlying cause may be a treatable complication of cancer.

Any patient who shows the acute onset of agitation, impaired cognitive function, altered attention span, or a fluctuating level of consciousness should be suspected of having delirium. It is usually due to one or more of seven causes: medications, electrolyte imbalance, failure of a vital organ or system, nutritional state, infections, vascular complications, or hormone-producing tumors.[45] In a study of terminally ill cancer patients, over three fourths studied developed a delirium with a multifactorial etiology.[46]

Many commonly used analgesics, such as levorphanol, morphine sulfate, and meperidine, can often cause acute confusional states. Among the more than 60 chemotherapeutic agents now available for cancer, CNS symptoms are generally not prominent. The few that have been reported to cause significant delirium are methotrexate, fluorouracil, vincristine and vinblastine, bleomycin, BCNU, cisplatin, asparaginase, procarbazine, and the glucocorticosteroids prednisone and decadron.[47]

All steroid compounds can cause symptoms ranging from minor mood disturbance to frank psychosis.[45,48] Disturbances may include affective changes (emotional lability, euphoria, depressed mood, anxiety), fears, paranoid interpretation of events and suspiciousness of others, with illusions, delusions, and hallucinations. Symptoms often develop 4 to 5 days after high-dose steroids are begun or when the dose is rapidly tapered, but they can also develop while patients are on maintenance dosages. It may be necessary to continue steroids despite psychiatric symptoms, in which case neuroleptics such as haloperidol can be used for symptom control. A steroid psychosis during one course of treatment does not predict recurrence with subsequent courses of steroids. No relationship has been shown between the development of steroid psychosis and premorbid personality or psychiatric history.

Brain radiation, combined with intrathecal methotrexate, enhances the risk of encephalopathy, which may have long-term effects on mental functioning, especially in children.[49] Prophylactic cranial irradiation in adults with small cell lung cancer also carries with it a significant risk of permanent cognitive impairment.[50]

Haloperidol is the most effective drug for prompt control of delirium and agitated or disruptive behavior. Intramuscular or intravenous injection of 0.5 to 2.0 mg reduces agitation without causing sedation or hypotension. It can be administered intravenously at 1 mg/min, if necessary, and repeated at 45- to 60-minute intervals, titrated against behavior. The patient should be changed to an oral dose of three-fourths the parenteral dose as soon as possible. For milder symptoms, 1 to 2 mg of trifluoperazine or 10 to 25 mg of thioridazine may be given orally twice a day.

ANXIETY DISORDERS: PREEXISTING PHOBIAS, PANIC ATTACKS AND GENERALIZED ANXIETY. Persistent and incapacitating anxiety symptoms in cancer patients usually represent worsening of preexisting problems. Phobias, the commonest form of abnormal fears, often revolve around physical illness, death, pain, needles, claustrophobia, or fear of solitude. Panic attacks may be precipitated, and chronic generalized anxiety syndromes are severely exacerbated. Scanning machines and magnetic resonance imaging procedures are intolerable to a significant percentage of patients, who require special handling and medication. Agoraphobic patients may be unable to tolerate the night before surgery alone in the hospital and require relaxation of rules to allow the presence of a relative. They also need longer and higher levels of preoperative sedation, with coordination between the psychiatrist and the anesthesiologist. Specific fears of needles, pain, or the sight of blood require acknowledgment and individualized management, including medication, distraction, and desensitization. Given this special care, patients are generally cooperative, grateful, and able to proceed with treatment.

Benzodiazepines are the drugs of choice for anxiety states. The most common side-effects, sedation and confusion, occur more frequently in older patients and in those with impaired liver function. Short-acting benzodiazepines, such as alprazolam, lorazepam, and oxazepam, which have no active metabolites and are excreted as glucuronides, are to be selected over longer acting drugs such as diazepam. Drug dependence and addiction in psychologically healthy cancer patients is seldom a problem when dose and length of time on medication are monitored.

PERSONALITY DISORDERS. Patients with "difficult" personalities frustrate and anger those who treat them. The stress of cancer exaggerates their normally maladaptive coping strategies and they become even more difficult than usual. The disorders are recognizable by the exaggeration of common characteristics: the paranoid person who is suspicious and constantly threatens litigation; the obsessive person whose excessive attention to details of care is accompanied by repeated criticism; the dependent person who demands care far beyond objective needs and who may be dependent on alcohol or drugs; the patient with borderline disorder who is unable to conform to rules, who manipulates, divides, and may disturb other patients as well as staff; and the histrionic person who overdramatizes symptoms and distress. Since personality disorders are not felt by the patients to be a problem, management usually depends on helping staff to understand the pattern and to contain their behavior. Many of these patients benefit from consistent limit setting, applied in a quiet, kindly manner.

MAJOR MENTAL ILLNESS. Schizophrenia and bipolar (manic–depressive) illness are rare in the general population and hence uncommon in cancer patients. However, when present, they require careful management to ensure the patient's cooperation with treatment and to prevent escalation of symptoms under stress. Previously prescribed neuroleptics should be continued, coordinating management with the anesthesiologist, when surgery is required because of potential paradoxical blood pressure reactions. Lithium should also be continued but may need to be stopped briefly during periods of fluid restriction.

The lower incidence of cancer observed in the 1960s in chronically hospitalized schizophrenics is now explained by the mildly protective effects of the hospital environment, not by any protective effect of the illness or of phenothiazines. Although reserpine and the phenothiazines increase prolactin levels, there is no evidence in humans that these drugs alter the risk of developing breast cancer or promote tumor growth. They can be safely prescribed to women with breast cancer.

THERAPEUTIC INTERVENTIONS IN CANCER

The problems outlined above are amenable to three main types of therapeutic intervention: psychological, psychopharmacologic, and behavioral. The primary indications for each are reviewed in Table 61-6. An aggressive and eclectic approach combining several modalities simultaneously is most useful.

The cornerstone is psychological support, which can take many forms, and some levels of which can be carried out by many nonpsychiatric staff. Individual sessions for both patients and families offer counseling, advice, and information about illness, treatment, and expectation of side-effects. Spiritual counseling is meaningful for many patients as they turn to their religion during the existential crisis created by cancer. The chaplain can offer not only spiritual solace but also the concrete support and services of others of the same faith. Psychotherapy usually consists of brief, crisis-oriented sessions to assist patients in regrouping their defenses and coping successfully with the problems of illness. The one-to-one visit of a veteran patient who has successfully negotiated the same experience is often very helpful.

Group interventions have also proved to be useful for cancer patients in several ways. The first is an educational function of orientation and learning what is needed to adapt to a treatment or its consequences (*e.g.*, radiation, laryngectomy, ostomy). Secondly, groups encourage emotional learning and relieve anxiety by allowing individuals to see how

TABLE 61-6. Primary Indications for Each Therapeutic Approach

Intervention	*Treatment Modality*
Psychological	
Professional crisis intervention at points of maximal stress:	
At time of diagnosis	Individual and group counseling
Prior to a new treatment	Crisis intervention
At relapse	Psychotherapy
At treatment failure	Counseling by clergy
Ongoing psychotherapy for patients with preexisting psychiatric disorders	
Nonprofessional (self-help)	
Provision of "practical" advice at times of crisis	Veteran and fellow patient counseling
Ongoing support	Self-help groups
Empowerment during chronic and survival phases	
Psychopharmacologic	
Some adjustment disorders	Antianxiety agents
Anxiety disorders	Antidepressants
Major depression	Analgesics
Delirium/dementia	Antipsychotics
Schizophrenia	
Manic–depressive illness	
Pain	
Nausea and vomiting	
Insomnia	
Behavioral interventions	
Anxiety and discomfort with procedures (bone marrow aspiration, lumbar puncture)	Relaxation
Pain (adjunct to analgesics)	Biofeedback
Nausea and vomiting (anticipatory treatment-related)	Systematic densitization
Eating disorders	Suggestion/imagery/hypnosis
Some anxiety disorders	Distraction

others are coping with the same problems and by encouraging the expression of feelings without fear of being ridiculed. Third, the advocacy provided by cancer groups often becomes a voice for more social awareness and change, while at the same time giving participants a valuable sense of strength and empowerment. These consumer groups can be effective whether led by a professional or self-directed, such as Can Surmount and I Can Cope.

Psychotropic medications have been greatly underused in cancer patients because of lack of familiarity and lack of awareness of their effectiveness. Even though antidepressants and antianxiety agents can greatly reduce patient distress during radiation therapy and chemotherapy, and depression has been diagnosed in 25% of hospitalized cancer patients, one study has shown that less than 2% of psychotropic drugs used were antidepressants.[51]

Behavioral interventions are the newest addition to patient management, with an emphasis on self-regulatory interventions. Patients like to feel they have some control over their level of distress and many use relaxation exercises, with suggestions of restful visual imagery and other self-hypnotic suggestions. These techniques, along with desensitization and distraction, are particularly effective in reducing anticipatory nausea and vomiting in patients receiving chemotherapy.[52,53]

These interventions are being actively pursued as concern for the quality of life during treatment increases. A recent study found that both anxiety and depressive symptoms were significantly reduced over a 10-day period in ambulatory chemotherapy patients who were randomly assigned to receive alprazolam, 0.5 mg three times a day, or to the use of relaxation exercises.[54] Anxiety symptoms were equally reduced with both regimens, but depression was better controlled by the drug.

An important role for the oncologist is to ensure that the patient and family have optimal access to the full range of financial, social, religious, psychological, and community resources available to them. In a large center social workers are trained to perform this function, but in more decentralized settings it behooves the oncologist to acquaint himself with a few key local resources and to use them systematically. The resulting improvement in coping benefits the patient and eases case management.

LONG-TERM SURVIVORS AND CURED PATIENTS

The increasing number of long-term survivors today is drawn largely from children and young adults, in whom the long expected life span makes the psychological consequences of cancer treatment particularly important. While early studies using crude measures, such as level of education and marriage, showed few psychological effects, investigators using more refined measures have begun to show subtle psychological changes.[55] There may be paradoxical reentry problems at the time of return to normal life. The family may remain overprotective or may push the patient into a level of "normalcy" he or she cannot yet adopt. Teachers and classmates, or employees and co-workers, may view the person as "different" and isolate him out of embarrassment, fear, or admiration. Discrimination in employment and health insurance coverage is frequent, and, coupled with the patient's fear of failure and sensitivity to the attitudes of others, can create serious difficulties in social adjustment.

Throughout their life, cancer survivors continue to have special medical concerns. Preoccupation with fears of recurrence, a sense of greater vulnerability to illness, a pervasive awareness of their mortality, a more negative view of the future, and a permanent sense of being physically inferior all remain permanently and conspire to diminish self-assurance and confidence. Concern about infertility, often submerged at the time of diagnosis and treatment, reemerges with great power when patients marry, often causing severe distress.

From a psychological perspective, there are no disabling symptoms, but levels of both anxiety and depression are significantly elevated and remain so for years. A poignant demonstration comes from a study in which some survivors of Hodgkin's disease reexperienced the anxiety and nausea and vomiting of chemotherapy when exposed to tastes and smells of treatment as long as 12 years later.[56]

Psychiatric intervention is useful at the time of reentry to prevent the development of negative behavior patterns and to assist the patient in reestablishing social and family roles. Peer support has been found especially valuable for cancer survivors, who serve each other uniquely well as advocates and emotional supports. The National Coalition of Cancer Survivorship, a newly formed organization of survivors, is an outgrowth of both the perceived need for, and the value of, peer support.

As the number of cancer survivors increases, personal and societal attitudes toward them are being examined. The problems surrounding health and life insurance policies are a prime example of an area where research is needed to delineate concrete problems and where solutions should certainly be within reach.

MANAGEMENT OF GRIEF

Grief is often encountered in cancer treatment. More particularly, the oncologist is intensely involved with families in the throes of anticipatory bereavement. This presents both an opportunity and an obligation for the oncologist and his team, since they are in a unique position to combine care and comfort for the patient with guidance of the family through the terminal illness.

Staff management during this difficult period substantially affects the nature of the bereavement process, and possibly the long-term adjustment of family survivors. The bereaved spouse or parent repeatedly recalls how the final days were handled, how the news of grave prognosis and death was conveyed, and how their final moments with the dying patient were managed. The survivor has intense but mixed feelings about the oncologist. It is normal for gratitude about the care given and closeness because of shared memories to coexist with nagging questions such as: "Was everything done?" "Could it have been prevented?" "Were mistakes made?" Oncologists should not personalize these doubts and should remember that attribution of guilt and responsibility is a common phenomenon. Relatives will tend to blame the staff or blame themselves. The oncologist must instead recognize his special meaning to the survivors and accept their reactions nonjudgmentally. A meeting held 1 to 2 months after the death serves as an important setting in which troubling questions can be discussed. Autopsy findings, if available, provide a good opportunity to clarify concerns and relieve guilt. The meeting can also be used to monitor the course of grieving. The hallmarks of normal and abnormal grief are outlined below.[57]

Even when a death is clearly anticipated, the reaction of a relative to the actual event is often one of temporary disbelief. Despite visible deterioration in a dying spouse, the surviving partner may be unable to tolerate any real emotional awareness of the death and of what life will be without the person. The available information suggests, however, that grief is tolerated better when the loss is expected and there has been some psychological preparation.

Once death has occurred, the grieving has an acute and a chronic component: acute waves of an overwhelming sense of loss, associated with crying and agitation, and usually precipitated by a reminder of the deceased, are superimposed on a chronic background of social withdrawal, preoccupation with the deceased, diminished concentration and attention, restlessness, depressed mood, anxiety, insomnia, and anorexia. The intense distress of the first few months looks like depression and may be clinically indistinguishable from it.

Over several months, the acute symptoms diminish in intensity and frequency. Reorganization of activities with resurgence of interest is seen. Preoccupation with the deceased is replaced by recall of memories associated with both pleasure and sadness. Satisfactory resolution of grief is marked by the readiness to invest deeply in new relationships and has been assumed to be usually achieved by 1 year. However, the duration of normal grieving is quite variable and often extends well beyond a year.[57] Parents, for example, are never the same again, and some never really recover. Older spouses from a long union often grieve acutely for 2 to 4 years, and some much longer.[58]

The morbidity and mortality related to grief have been actively explored in the past decade.[57] Symptoms have been described above. Bereaved individuals frequently become more dependent on smoking, alcohol, and drugs to reduce distress, if these were previously used. They visit physicians more often than nonbereaved individuals, with various physical complaints. Yet outcome studies indicate that most individuals recover with the support of only family, friends, and clergy.[58] Peer counseling through the Widow-to-Widow Programs, Compassionate Friends, or Candlelighters offers excellent support from others who have suffered a similar loss.

However, a subset of family survivors, perhaps 20%, may require special help. They can be identified early in bereavement by the presence of several risk factors, including perceived or actual poor social support, prior psychiatric history (especially alcoholism), high and intense initial distress, unanticipated death, concurrent life stresses or losses, prior high level of dependency on the deceased for primary support, and death of a child. Any one of these risk factors is sufficient reason to recommend psychiatric referral, particularly when high levels of depression and anxiety are sustained and there is little or no return to social functioning. Bereavement counseling allows the person to recount the details of the death and his subsequent feelings, to explore new ways of coping, and to try out new roles and experiences. An antidepressant to ensure sleep and reduce high levels of distress permits better daily functioning and often facilitates the exploration of painful feelings.

STRESSES ON ONCOLOGISTS

While recent studies have painted an increasingly clear picture of the emotional reaction of patients and their relatives, few studies have addressed the stresses operating on the oncologist and his staff, and the effect of these on personal and professional life.[59–61] These issues are important, both for the well-being of medical professionals and for their impact on patient care. Studies consistently show that despite recurrent criticism that medicine has become uncaring and commercial, patients still accept treatment largely because they trust their doctor and his or her recommendations.[62] They also adhere to arduous regimens for the same reason, and obtain their primary psychological support from the doctor. The harried, stressed oncologist is compromised in his or her ability to give attention to this art of medicine, yet seldom is the human aspect of care more important than in oncology.

It remains true that physicians generally tolerate work stresses well. They have the characteristics of the "hardy personality" which are known to buffer stress: a strong commitment to work, a view of daily problems as a challenge, and a sense of control of their work without letting the magnitude of the problems become overwhelming.[63]

However, physicians have other characteristics that predispose them to chronic stress. Many have personalities that lead them to work long hours and seek little recreation; they have trouble saying no to requests for added work responsibilities. The overcommitment of time results in long absences from home. Beeper and telephone intrusions into private moments strain marital relations and upset children. Socializing becomes minimal except with colleagues. Strains in the marriage and family life compound stresses at work. Conflicts with close colleagues endanger job satisfaction and performance and are especially difficult because resolution or avoidance may be impossible. The need to care for patients while pursuing research and scholarly activities adds special strains to the academic setting. Physical illness and frequent sleep loss are transient additional stressors. Chronic fatigue is more insidious.

The practice of oncology carries with it certain significant strains in addition to those outlined above: the uncertainty inherent in treatment decisions and the repeated impact of patient deaths, especially "special" patients to whom the oncologist has become attached. Some personal distress is inherent in decisions about withholding or stopping life-sustaining support measures, with all the medical, social, and ethical ambiguities that abound in the current climate. Discussing these decisions with the patient and family is difficult and painful. The two major treatment modalities, radiation therapy and chemotherapy, balance toxicity against benefits, with difficult tradeoffs of which patient and doctors are acutely aware. Some treatment regimens can be expected to result in life-threatening iatrogenic complications. The impact of patients' unrealistic expectations and the strain associated with the care of "problem" patients are additional sources of stress.[61] Care of a colleague with cancer, while recognizably a compliment, is a double burden when treatments fail, and the loss is felt as a personal as well as a medical failure. Malpractice threats and suits increase, as does paper work and outside intrusions on the ability to give the desired quality of care. It is poignantly clear that conscientious medical staff are not immune to irrational guilt, much less to ordinary sorrow. The wonder is not that symptoms of stress are observed, but rather how well doctors continue to cope.

The actual incidence of serious psychiatric problems in physicians is probably underreported. However, depression, suicide, and alcohol and drug abuse are the most common psychiatric disorders seen in physicians. The annual rate of suicide among physicians is 100 physicians per year, or the equivalent of one medical school class. When combined with the significant number who become drug or alcohol dependent, the reasons for concern become apparent, since alcoholism is estimated to occur in 7% to 10% and drug abuse at 2% to 3% of physicians. While neither of these have been examined in oncologists per se, the constant and continuing care of cancer patients, when combined with personality traits or personal problems, may provide a matrix for depression and psychological "burnout." At the extreme it may lead to the need for peer review of professional competence. New legislation places increasing attention on physician competence and encourages doctors to identify their dysfunctional colleagues at an earlier and more treatable stage. The depressed physician who continues to work is unable to provide solid emotional support, and therefore deprives his needy patient of a vital source of empathy.

What are the symptoms of emotional fatigue and burnout? The physician notices less zest and enthusiasm for work, with a sense of having to "drag in" to work. This may be coupled with feeling chronically tense, easily frustrated, and easily angered; depressed "down" moods frequently ensue. The need for a "few drinks after work" or experimentation with psychotropic drugs to "relax" are ominous signs, since the habits usually escalate.

On the physical side, insomnia is common, with either difficulty falling asleep, frequent awakening, or early morning awakening. Appetite change may lead to weight gain or loss. Feeling "exhausted," "tired all the time," headaches, and aches and pains are other indicators of distress. The tendency is to ignore the symptoms. At this point, the physician may "tune out," feel detached from patients and unable to empathize. This is an early sign of stress in house staff who say they feel less able to "care" and are cynical and pessimistic about the meaning of their work. They may begin working longer hours with a sense that "nobody can do it right but me" and "nobody works around here but me," when in fact they are less effective and efficient.

Doctors are well known to delay seeking consultation for physical symptoms; unfortunately, they delay even longer in admitting to psychiatric problems and seeking help for them. To avoid becoming identified as a psychiatric patient, doctors hide their symptoms from family and colleagues, fearing the impact on their job and practice if it should become known. The warning signs of depression, the taking of secret drinks, and surreptitious use of pills are ignored. Family, colleagues, and even patients often collude in pretending nothing is wrong. The result is a paradoxical delay in identification and treatment of the physician.

Monitoring one's self for symptoms of emotional fatigue and acknowledging one's stress is very important in oncology. "Survival" tactics must be instituted and include recognizing one's limitations, not taking oneself too seriously, accepting the inadequacies of medicine, using gallows humor to lighten the meaning of painful events, working a "normal" work day for a few weeks, stopping when others do, taking a long weekend at recurrent intervals, maintaining a regular exercise program, and lastly, bringing to these measures the same care and consistency that is given to other responsibilities. When symptoms do not remit, psychiatric consultation should be sought.

Some training programs in oncology encourage awareness of personal reactions and provide regular meetings in which difficult patients and management of personal stresses are reviewed. They have proven useful and have been well described with oncology fellows. Hospitals which have liaison psychiatrists also have a built-in mechanism for attending to staff problems, especially among nurses and house staff. However, few resources exist for practicing oncologists after leaving training, at a time when stresses may be greatest and the individual the most vulnerable. The active seeking of a supportive peer group assumes special importance.

More willingness to confront colleagues and to encourage their seeking treatment is necessary when significant symptoms are noted. Human concern for a friend should ally itself with the demands of optimal patient care, which require that doctors be strong enough to provide support and understanding to their patients. The severely distressed physician cannot meet this important human requirement of medicine, and endures much unnecessary personal suffering at the same time.

ROLE OF THE ONCOLOGIST IN HELPING OTHER MEMBERS OF THE ONCOLOGY STAFF

With the increasing complexity of therapeutic regimens, oncologists are working more and more as leaders or co-leaders of treatment teams. It has been repeatedly observed that such leaders play a critical role in maintaining group morale, thereby diminishing staff stress and improving patient care.

The main principles of good leadership include:

1. Modeling and expecting the delivery of high-quality patient care while also acknowledging realistic human limitations.
2. Exercising authority clearly and consistently where appropriate while supporting teamwork where appropriate.
3. Encouraging and respecting in others the same self-monitoring as described above.
4. Educating one's self about sources of help for one's staff, making them known, and using them.

Staff support groups have been repeatedly stated to be very effective in decreasing staff stress.[61] The oncologist may participate directly in such groups, but even if he chooses not to, his well-publicized and genuine support for such a group is a key element to its success.

PSYCHOSOCIAL AND BEHAVIORAL FACTORS IN CANCER RISK AND SURVIVAL

Psychosocial and behavioral factors in human cancer affect both the risk of developing cancer and the length of survival once cancer has developed. Patients ask many questions about these issues as they attempt to understand why they got cancer and how they can positively affect treatment outcome. Oncologists need to be familiar with the present state of research in order to respond usefully to their patients.

The psychosocial and behavioral factors that may alter cancer risk and survival fall into four areas: (1) life style and behaviors, (2) social environment and social ties, (3) personality and coping style, and (4) life events and emotional states.

LIFE STYLE AND BEHAVIORS. Individual behaviors can significantly alter exposure to carcinogens and the risk of developing many common cancers. Cancer prevention programs depend heavily on insights and techniques derived from psychology, psychiatry, and the social sciences for help in reducing smoking and alcohol intake, lowering dietary fat intake, increasing dietary fiber, and altering sexual behaviors.

In addition, much of the improvement in survival for the most common cancers, such as breast and colon cancer, depends on early detection. The complex factors that make individuals delay seeking consultation long after they have suspicious symptoms is an important area for continued research that is also anchored in psychiatry and the social sciences.

SOCIAL ENVIRONMENT AND SOCIAL TIES. It is disturbing to note the significantly poorer survival from cancer in low-income groups. Access to quality care and the preexisting state of health of the individual, as judged by nutrition, immune state and emotional well-being, are important in cancer mortality.[64,65] Social ties also influence illness incidence and mortality.[17,65]

PERSONALITY AND COPING STYLE. Data do not strongly support the theory that a particular personality style predisposes to cancer. However, two lines of psychological inquiry on cancer risk are currently promising. One study showed a small effect of chronic depression on increasing subsequent cancer risk and mortality; another is examining the possible significance of a cancer-prone personality, labeled type C, and described as cooperative, pleasant, and uncomplaining.[66,67]

Some studies of breast cancer patients have found an adverse impact on tumor progression or length of survival associated with a passive or noncomplaining personality.[68–70] These studies are difficult to interpret because the powerful medical factors affecting survival were not always adequately controlled for. Other studies that controlled extensively for medical factors have not duplicated these findings.[71–73]

LIFE EVENTS AND EMOTIONAL STATES. The contribution of grief to mortality from cancer does not appear to be as great as was previously assumed, despite indications that immune functions are perturbed following bereavement and in some other stressed states. Mortality studies of bereaved spouses and of elderly persons lacking strong social support have not found an excess of deaths from cancer.[74,75]

BODY AND MIND

The relationship between cancer and the mind is of intense interest to the general public. Its implied promises have spawned a growth industry of clinics and healers who encourage patients to use their own mental powers to fight their cancer. This is to be done with or without the help of traditional treatments. The accompanying emphasis on a healthy life style and careful attention to nutrition is commendable. However, confusion is rampant between risk and survival factors. The well-known and powerful risk factors are conflated with ambiguous and weak survival factors, while the role of personality factors is inflated far beyond the existing evidence. The intense and cultlike quality can encourage extreme hopes and beliefs, which lead to equally extreme disappointments. By placing the locus of power over cancer in the patient's mind, they play into patients' universal tendency—not to mention their families'—to feel they are to blame for their illness. It is only too common to see a nauseated, anorectic patient being badgered to eat by family members who plead with him to demonstrate his "positive attitude." Worst of all, healers let patients bear personal responsibility for failure, or blame it on their having sought traditional treatment. The hapless patient has no choice but to join the universal chorus in blaming himself or blaming "the cancer establishment." One would wish that more of the energy devoted to straining at a behavioral role in survival were devoted to more effective programs to minimize the well-recognized risk factors.

Yet there is a core of constructiveness to some of these programs. The more patients can feel energized, hopeful, and empowered to act on their own behalf, the more they maintain a healthful life style and the better their subjective sense of well-being, the more effectively they will pursue and tolerate treatment and the better will be their ongoing quality of life. If survival is improved, so much the better. If it is not, the improvement in emotional well-being is still valuable. The best traditional medical treatment has aimed for these results in patients, but perhaps not often enough and not vigorously enough.

It is to be hoped that the future will see a rapprochement between traditional cancer care and the more respectable modes of alternative care.

REFERENCES

1. Tolstoy L: The death of Ivan Illych. In Maude L, Maude A (eds): Great Short Works of Leo Tolstoy, pp 247–302. New York, Harper & Row, 1967
2. Sontag S: Illness as Metaphor. New York, Farrar, Strauss Giroux, 1977
3. Holland JC, Marchini A, Tross S: An international survey of physician attitudes and practice in regard to revealing the diagnosis of cancer. Cancer Invest 5:151–154, 1987
4. Shands HC, Finsesinger JE, Cobb S et al: Psychological mechanisms in patients with cancer. Cancer 4:1159–1170, 1951
5. Bard M, Sutherland AM: Psychological impact of cancer and its treatment: IV. Adaptation to radical mastectomy. Cancer 8:656–672, 1955
6. Kubler-Ross E: On Death and Dying. New York, Macmillan, 1969
7. Strain JJ, Grossman S (eds): Psychological Care of the Medically Ill: A Primer in Liaison Psychiatry. New York, Appleton-Century-Crofts, 1975
8. Holland JC: Psychological aspects of cancer. In Holland JF, Frei E (eds): Cancer Medicine, 2nd ed, pp 1175–1203, 2325–2331. Philadelphia, Lea & Febiger, 1982
9. Holland JC, Rowland J (eds): Psycho-oncology: The Psychological Care of the Patient with Cancer. New York, Oxford University Press (in press)
10. Whorton JC: Traditions of folk medicine in America. JAMA 257:1632–1635, 1900
11. Sullivan M. Cohen J. Bravehog I: Psychological responses to cancer in the United States and Sweden: A comparative patient and family study. In: Proceedings of the 4th European Conference on Clinical Oncology and Cancer Nursing, p 30. Satellite Symposia, European Society of Psychosocial Oncology, 1987
12. Beauchamps TL, Childress JF: The principle of autonomy: I. Conceptual foundations: An informed consent. In Abrams N, Buckner MD (eds): Medical Ethics: A Clinical Textbook and References for the Health Care Professions, pp 3–12. Cambridge, Mass, Massachusetts Institute of Technology, 1983
13. Wanzer SH, Adelstein SJ, Cransford RE et al: The physician's responsibility toward hopelessly ill patients. N Engl J Med 310:955–959, 1984
14. Lederberg MS: The interface between psychiatry, the law and ethics. In Holland JC, Rowland JH (eds): Psycho-oncology: The Psychological Care of the Patient with Cancer. New York, Oxford University Press (in press)
15. Penman DT, Bloom JR, Fotopoulos S et al: The impact of mastectomy on self concept and social function: A combined cross-sectional and longitudinal study with comparison groups. Women Health 11:101–130, 1986
16. Massie MJ, Holland JC: Psychiatry and oncology. In Grinspoon L (ed): Psychiatry Update, Vol III, pp 231–256. Washington, DC, American Psychiatric Association, 1984
17. Cassileth BR, Lusk EJ, Strouse TB et al: Psychosocial status in chronic illness: A comparative analysis of six diagnostic groups. N Engl J Med 311:506–511, 1984
18. Wortman CB: Social support and the cancer patient: Conceptual and methodological issues. Cancer [Suppl] 53:2217–2384, 1984
19. Taylor SE, Falke RL, Shaptaw SJ et al: Social support, support groups and the cancer patients. J Consult Clin Psychol 54:608–615, 1986
20. Berkman LF, Syme SL: Social networks, host resistance, and mortality: A nine-year follow-up study of Alameda County residents. Am J Epidemiol 109:186–204, 1979
21. Cohen S, Syme SL (eds): Social Support and Health. New York, Academic Press, 1985
22. Coelho G, Hamburg D, Adams J: Coping and Adaptation. New York, Basic Books, 1974
23. Scott DW: Anxiety, critical thinking and information processing during and after breast biopsy. Nurs Res 32:24–29, 1983
24. Hamburg D: Toward a conjunction of biomedical and behavioral sciences. In Williams RB Jr (ed): Perspectives on Behavioral Medicine, vol 2. Neuroendocrine Control and Behavior, pp 1–22. New York, Academic Press, 1985
25. Weisman AD, Worden JW: The existential plight in cancer: Significance of the first 100 days. Int J Psychiatry Med 7:1–17, 1976
26. Vaillant G: Adaptation and ego mechanisms of defence. Harvard Medical School Mental Health Letter 3:4–6, 1986
27. Weisman AD: Coping with Cancer. New York, McGraw-Hill, 1979
28. Bukberg J, Penman D, Holland JC: Depression in hospitalized cancer patients. Psychosom Med 46:199–212, 1984
29. Derogatis LR, Morrow GR, Fetting J et al: The prevalence of psychiatric disorders among cancer patients. JAMA 249:751–757, 1983
30. Massie MJ, Holland JC: The cancer patient with pain: Psychiatric complications and their management. Med Clin North Am 71:243–258, 1987
31. Massie MJ, Holland JC, Glass E: Delirium in terminally ill cancer patients. Am J Psychiatry 140:1048–1050, 1983
32. Anderson BL: Sexual functioning morbidity among cancer survivors: Present status and future research directions. Cancer 55:1835–1842, 1985
33. National Institutes of Health International Conference on Reproduction and Human Cancer, Bethesda, Md, May 12–14, 1987
34. Auchincloss S: Sexual dysfunction in cancer: Issues in evaluation and treatment. In Holland JC, Rowland JH (eds): Psycho-oncology: The Psychological Care of the Patient with Cancer. New York, Oxford University Press (in press)
35. Rickels K, Chung HR, Csanalosi IB et al: Alprazolam, diazepam, imipramine, and placebo in outpatients with major depression. Arch Gen Psychiatry 44:862–866, 1987
36. Plumb M, Holland JC: Comparative studies of psychological function in patients with advanced cancer: I. Self-reported depression symptoms. Psychosom Med 39:264–276, 1977
37. Holland JC, Korzun AH, Tross S et al: Comparative psychological disturbance in patients with pancreatic and gastric cancer. Am J Psychiatry 143:982–986, 1986
38. Posner JB: Neurological complications of systemic cancer. Med Clin North Am 55:625–646, 1971
39. Lyman GH, Williams CC, Preston D: The use of lithium carbonate to reduce infection and leukopenia during systemic chemotherapy. N Engl J Med 302:257–260, 1980
40. Chiarello RJ, Cole JO: The use of psychostimulants in general psychiatry: A reconsideration. Arch Gen Psychiatry 44:286–295, 1987
41. Woods SW, Tesar GE, Murray GB et al: Psychostimulant treatment of depressive disorders secondary to medical illness. J Clin Psychiatry 47:12–15, 1986
42. Breitbart W: Suicide in cancer patients. In Holland JC, Rowland JH (eds): Psycho-oncology: The Pyschological Care of the Patient with Cancer. New York, Oxford University Press (in press)
43. Breitbart W: Suicide in cancer patients. Oncology 1:44–53, 1987
44. Posner JB: Neurologic complications of systemic cancer. DM 2:7–60, 1978
45. Lipowski ZJ: Delirium: Acute brain failure in man. Springfield, Ill, Charles C Thomas, 1980
46. Moffic H, Paykel ES: Depression in medical inpatients. Br J Psychiatry 126:346–353, 1975
47. Young DF: Neurological complications of cancer chemotherapy. In Silverstein A (ed): Neurological Complications of Therapy: Selected Topics, pp 57–113. New York, Futura, 1982
48. Hall RCW, Popkin MK, Stickney SK et al: Presentation of the steroid psychosis. J Nerv Ment Dis 167:229–236, 1979
49. Rowland J, Gildewell O, Sibley R et al: Effect of different forms of central nervous prophylaxis on neuropsychologic function in childhood lymphocytic leukemia. J Clin Oncol 3:969–976, 1985
50. Maurer LH, Pajak T, Eaton W et al: Combined modality therapy with radiotherapy, chemotherapy, and immunotherapy in limited small-cell carcinoma of the lung: A phase III Cancer and Leukemia Group B Study. J Clin Oncol 3:969–976, 1985
51. Derogatis LR, Morrow GR, Fetting J et al: A survey of psychotropic drug prescriptions in an oncology population. Cancer 44:1919–1929, 1979
52. Redd WH: Behavioral control of chemotherapy side effects. In Holland JC, Rowland JH (eds): Psycho-oncology: The Psychological Care of the Patient with Cancer. New York, Oxford University Press (in press)
53. Redd WH: Behavioral intervention in pediatric oncology. In Holland JC, Rowland JH (eds): Psycho-oncology: The Psychological Care of the Patient with Cancer. New York, Oxford University Press (in press)
54. Holland JC, Morrow G, Schmale A et al: Reduction of anxiety and depression in cancer patients by alprazolam or by a behavioral technique (abstr). Proc Am Soc Clin Oncol 6:258, 1987
55. Tross S: Psychological sequelae in cancer survivors. In Holland JC, Rowland JH (eds): Psycho-oncology: The Psychological Care of the Patient with Cancer. New York, Oxford University Press (in press)
56. Cella DF, Pratt A, Holland JC: Persistent anticipatory nausea, vomiting, and anxiety in cured Hodgkin's disease patients after completion of chemotherapy. Am J Psychiatry 143:641–643, 1986
57. Osterweis M, Solomon F, Green M (eds): Bereavement: Reactions, Consequences and Care. Washington, DC, National Academy Press, 1984
58. Parkes CM, Weiss R: Recovery From Bereavement. New York, Basic Books, 1983
59. Mount BM: Dealing with our losses. J Clin Oncol 4:1127–1134, 1986
60. Kash K, Holland JC: Special problems of physicians and house staff. In Holland JC, Rowland JH (eds): Psycho-oncology: The Psychological Care of the Patient with Cancer. New York, Oxford University Press (in press)
61. Lederberg MS: Psychological problems of staff and their management. In Holland JC, Rowland JH (eds): Psycho-oncology: The Psychological Care of the Patient with Cancer. New York, Oxford University Press (in press)
62. Penman D, Holland JC, Bahna G et al: Informed consent for investigational chemotherapy: Patients' and physicians' perceptions. J Clin Oncol 2:849–855, 1984
63. Kobasa SC, Puccetti MD: Personality and social resources in stress-resistance. J Pers Soc Psychol 45:839–850, 1983
64. Lerner M: Cancer mortality differentials by income, Baltimore 1949–51 to 1979–81. In: Cancer in the Economically Disadvantaged: A Special Report, Appendix B. New York, American Cancer Society, 1986
65. Jenkins CD: Social environment and cancer mortality in men. N Engl J Med 308:395–398, 1983
66. Shekelle RB, Raynor WJ Jr, Ostfeld AM et al: Psychological depression and 17-year risk of death from cancer. Psychosom Med 43:117–125, 1981
67. Temoshok L, Heller BW: On comparing apples, oranges and fruit salad: A methodological overview of medical outcome studies in psychosocial oncology. In Cooper CL (ed): Psychosocial Stress and Cancer, pp 231–260. New York, John Wiley & Sons, 1984
68. Greer S, Watson M: Towards a psychobiological model of cancer: Psychological considerations. Soc Sci Med 20:773–777, 1985
69. Levy S, Herberman R, Lippman M et al: Correlation of stress factors with sustained depression of natural killer activity and predicted prognosis in patients with breast cancer. J Clin Oncol 5:348–353, 1987
70. Derogatis L, Abeloff M, Melisaratos N: Psychological coping mechanism and survival time in metastatic breast cancer. JAMA 242:1504–1508, 1979
71. Holland J, Korzun A, Tross S et al: Psychosocial factors and disease free survival in stage II breast carcinoma. Proc Am Soc Clin Oncol 5:C-928, 1986
72. Jamison RN, Burish TG, Wallston KA: Psychogenic factors in predicting survival of breast cancer patients. J Clin Oncol 5:768–772, 1987
73. Cassileth BR, Lusk EJ, Miller DS et al: Psychosocial correlates of survival in advanced malignant disease. N Engl J Med 312:1551–1555, 1985
74. Helsing KJ, Szklo M: Mortality after bereavement. Am J Epidemiol 114:41–52, 1981
75. Helsing KJ, Comstock G, Szklo M: Causes of death in a widowed population. Am J Epidemiol 116:524–532, 1982
76. Ader R. Psychoneuroimmunology. New York, Elsevier, 1981

LESLIE R. SCHOVER
WENDY S. SCHAIN
DROGO K. MONTAGUE

SECTION 2

Sexual Problems of Patients with Cancer

Sexual rehabilitation has become an accepted aspect of cancer treatment in the past 10 years. As an increasing number of men and women with cancer achieve long-term survival, sexual function becomes an important part of quality of life. Greater societal openness about sexuality has also allowed patients to express their need for sexual health care. Education on treating sexual problems has become more common in the training of health professionals.

We have more successful treatments to offer our patients. The discipline of sex therapy, defined by Masters and Johnson,[1] has come of age as a mental health specialty. Men with medically caused erectile dysfunction can choose among several high-technology treatments.[2,3] Postmenopausal women no longer tolerate hot flashes and vaginal atrophy as a matter of course, but instead can often benefit from new regimens of hormone replacement therapy.[4]

Some treatments for cancer work so well that they can now be modified to spare reproductive and sexual function while retaining their efficacy. Examples include nerve-sparing radical prostatectomy,[5] segmental mastectomy,[6] local excision for vulvar cancer,[7] and surveillance instead of retroperitoneal lymphadenopathy for early-stage testicular cancer.[8] This chapter summarizes current knowledge about the prevalence, assessment, and treatment of sexual problems in men and women with cancer.

SEXUAL PROBLEMS PREVALENT IN CANCER PATIENTS

Our understanding of sexual dysfunction in cancer patients has been limited by researchers' use of vague and global diagnostic categories. When rates of sexual problems have been reported after a specific cancer treatment, men have usually been categorized as "impotent" and women as sexually "inactive" or "dissatisfied." More recent studies have assessed somewhat more specific aspects of sexual function, such as the ability to have erections versus the ability to reach orgasm for men.[5] Few, however, have used the diagnostic systems based on the sexual response cycle and developed for research on sexual behavior.[9,10]

Table 61-7 presents a schema to guide clinicians in understanding the sexual response cycle. Each of its phases—desire, arousal, orgasm, and resolution—can be characterized by subjective experience, objective events that can be measured, and the physiological systems that need to be intact for these events to occur. Cancer treatments can potentially damage one or more phases of the sexual response by affecting emotions, central or peripheral components of the nervous system, the pelvic vascular system, and the hypothalamic-pituitary-gonadal axis. Consider a young woman undergoing chemotherapy for metastatic breast cancer. She may lose desire for sex because of altered body image or absence of well-being. Chemotherapy-induced menopause, combined with irritation of the vaginal mucosa, reduces vaginal lubrication and renders intercourse painful. In consequence, she may no longer be able to reach orgasm during intercourse.

TABLE 61-7. The Sexual Response Cycle

Desire
Subjective: Sexual interest or motivation
Objective: Initiating sexual activity
Physiological systems: Hormonal, central nervous system
Arousal
Subjective: Sexual excitement, pleasant genital sensations
Objective: Increased heart rate and respiration, genital vasocongestion (erection, vaginal expansion and lubrication)
Physiological systems involved: Hormonal; central nervous system; sensory, parasympathetic, sympathetic, and peptidergic peripheral nerves
Orgasm
Subjective: Sensation of orgasmic pleasure
Objective: Emission in the male, smooth muscles in both genders, rhythmic contractions of genital striated muscles
Physiological systems involved: Central nervous system, peripheral sympathetic and sensory nerves

Figure 61-2 illustrates the frequencies of a variety of sexual dysfunctions in 308 men and 76 women referred to a sexual rehabilitation program at the University of Texas System Cancer Center, M.D. Anderson Hospital and Tumor Institute.[11] Since 80% of patients were married, rates of sexual problems in their spouses were also assessed. Figure 61-2 compares sexual problems before and after cancer was diagnosed. Significant increases were seen in all sexual dysfunctions except premature ejaculation in cancer patients from before cancer diagnosis and treatment to afterwards. In contrast, husbands and wives of cancer patients did not experience an increase in sexual problems. In men with cancer, erectile dysfunction was the most common problem, whereas in women the most common problem was dyspareunia. A more detailed analysis revealed that the sexual problems were apt to be global and severe, occurring across all sexual situations.

This particular sample of cancer patients included a preponderance of men and women treated for pelvic or genital tumors. Before cancer diagnosis, sexual function was similar across patients, no matter what the site of future disease. After cancer treatment, both men and women with pelvic or genital malignancy were more likely to have arousal phase problems (erectile dysfunction or reduced vaginal expansion and lubrication). These patients also were referred for sexual counseling. Thus, Figure 61-2 should not be viewed as an estimate of sexual dysfunction in all cancer patients. Rather, it gives the reader an idea of the problems seen by a specialized service in a cancer center.

Clinicians need a clear idea of the types of problems to expect after specific cancer therapies. Since radical pelvic surgery is one of the most salient causes of sexual dysfunction in cancer patients,[11] we provide Tables 61-8 and 61-9, describing tissue removed during various operative proce-

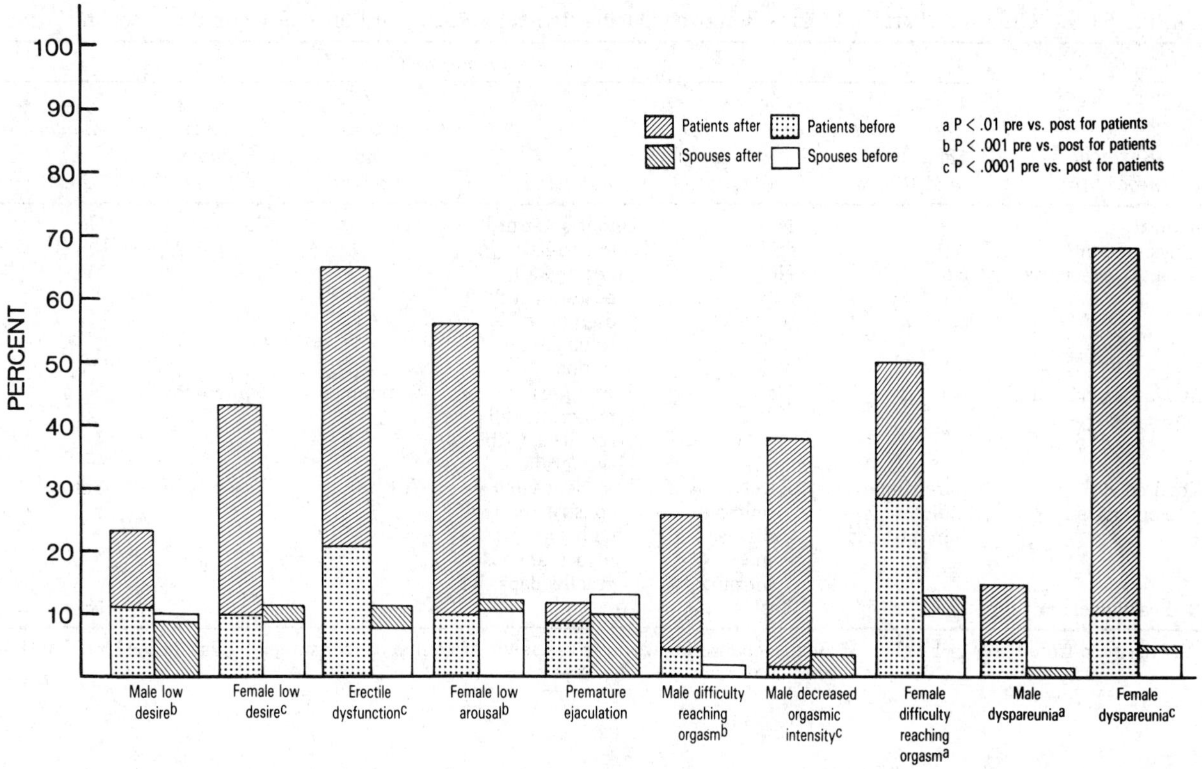

FIG. 61-2. Sexual dysfunctions in cancer patients and spouses, before and after cancer diagnosis and treatment. (Schover LR, Evans RB, von Eschenbach AC: Sexual rehabilitation in a cancer center: Diagnosis and outcome in 384 consultations. Arch Sex Behav 16: 445–461, 1987)

TABLE 61-8. Organs or Parts of Organs Removed During Radical Surgery for Pelvic or Genital Cancer in Men

Surgical Procedure	*Organ or Part*						
	Testicles	*Penis*	*Prostate*	*Vasa Deferens and Seminal Vesicles*	*Urethra*	*Bladder*	*Rectum*
Radical prostatectomy	No	No	Yes	Yes	Prostatic only	No	No
Radical cystectomy	No	No	Yes	Yes	Usually prostatic, sometimes entire	Yes	No
Abdominoperineal resection	No	No	No	No	No	No	Yes
Total pelvic exenteration	No	No	Yes	Yes	Prostatic only	Yes	Yes
Partial penectomy	No	Glans and part of shaft	No	No	Distal end only	No	No
Total penectomy	No	Corpora cavernosa, corpus spongiosum, and crus	No	No	Distal end only; perineal urethrostomy created	No	No

(Reprinted from Schover LR, Fife M: Sexual counseling with radical pelvic or genital cancer surgery. J Psychosoc Oncol 3:21–41, 1985.)

TABLE 61-9. Organs or Parts of Organs Removed During Radical Surgery for Pelvic or Genital Cancer in Women

	Organ or Part						
Surgical Procedure	*Labia Majora and Minora*	*Clitoris*	*Vagina*	*Uterus and Cervix*	*Ovaries and Fallopian Tubes*	*Bladder and Urethra*	*Rectum*
Radical hysterectomy	No	No	Upper one-third to one-half	Yes	Sometimes	No	No
Radical cystectomy	No	No	Anterior wall; posterior wall used to retubularize vagina	Yes	Yes	Yes	No
Abdominoperineal resection	No	No	Sometimes posterior wall, repaired, with skin graft	Sometimes	Sometimes	No	Yes
Total pelvic exenteration	Rarely unless disease is in introitus	Rarely, unless disease in introitus	Yes. Neovagina constructed with myocutaneous gracilis flaps	Yes	Yes	Yes	Yes
Radical vulvectomy	Yes	Yes	No	No	No	No	No

(Reprinted from Schover LR, Fife M: Sexual counseling with radical pelvic or genital cancer surgery. J Psychosoc Oncol 3:21–41, 1985.)

dures, and Table 61-10 and 61-11, detailing the consequences for the sexual response. Rather than focusing on any one cancer treatment, however, we review sexual problems by symptom picture and underlying causes.

PROBLEMS OF SEXUAL DESIRE

Most problems of sexual desire in chronically ill patients entail a global loss of interest in sex. It is rare to see increased sexual desire as a problem unless the patient is having a manic episode or perhaps has had damage to the brain resulting in disinhibition of sexual behavior.[12] Some patients with cancer, especially women, develop an aversion to sexual activity that has phobic elements.[13]

GLOBAL LOSS OF DESIRE. Low sexual desire is perhaps the most complex of all the sexual dysfunctions. Physical causes in cancer patients include central nervous system (CNS) depression, for example from generalized pain and fatigue, diffuse dementia, or pain or tranquilizing medications. Some antiemetic or opiate pain medications also elevate levels of the hormone prolactin, which can decrease sexual desire. In men, loss of sexual desire is a very common although not universal side-effect of hormonal therapy for metastatic prostate cancer that reduces circulating testosterone levels.[14] Young men treated for testicular cancer or lymphomas may also occasionally have abnormally low testosterone levels. In contrast to prostate cancer patients, these men can benefit from hormone replacement therapy.[15,16] We know that women's sexual desire is also dependent on androgens rather than on the other ovarian hormones.[17] No evidence exists thus far that any specific cancer treatment decreases women's sexual desire on a hormonal basis, but researchers have not addressed this topic.

Loss of sexual desire is also a hallmark of depression. Affective disorders are increased in prevalence in cancer patients.[18,19] In the M.D. Anderson study of sexual rehabilitation cases cited above,[11] low sexual desire was more common in men and women who were depressed and coping poorly with their cancer. Other sexual problems, except for dyspareunia, did not correlate significantly with psychological distress.

SITUATIONAL LOSS OF DESIRE. A loss of sexual desire that is situational—that is, loss of interest only in the spouse—usually signals marital conflict. Several studies suggest that a diagnosis of cancer does not produce marital distress in happy couples but may exacerbate conflict in dyads already having problems. Sexual dysfunction and marital unhappiness tend to occur in tandem.[20–23] Sometimes a spouse loses desire for the patient because the intimacy of sex is too painful, given the threat of loss through death.

AVERSION TO SEX. Aversion to sex can develop in a patient or partner if the diagnosis of cancer reactivates distress from a past sexual trauma, such as rape or incest. Cancer may be experienced as a new violation of bodily integrity. We have also seen sexual aversion in patients or partners who viewed cancer as a contamination or feared it was contagious through sexual contact.

TABLE 61-10. Effects of Surgery for Pelvic or Genital Cancer on Male Sexual Physiology

Surgical Procedure	*Hormonal Basis of Sexual Desire*	*Capacity for Pleasure with Genital Touch*	*Capacity for Erection*	*Sensation of Orgasm*	*Ejaculation*	*Dyspareunia*
Radical prostatectomy	Unchanged	Unchanged	Usually impaired.* Men younger than 60 are more likely to recover; full recovery takes 6 months	Unchanged, or mild loss of intensity	No semen produced, dry orgasm	Rare
Radical cystectomy	Unchanged	Unchanged	Usually impaired.* Men younger than 60 are more likely to recover; full recovery takes 6 months	Unchanged, or mild loss of intensity	No semen produced; dry orgasm	Rare, but is more likely after complete urethrectomy
Abdominoperineal resection	Unchanged	Unchanged	Often impaired, but recovery rates are higher than for radical prostatectomy or cystectomy	Unchanged, or mild loss of intensity	Dry orgasm is common because of damage to presacral sympathetic nerves	Rare, but some perineal pain or phantom rectal sensations
Total pelvic exenteration	Unchanged	Unchanged	Almost always permanently impaired	Unchanged, or mild loss of intensity	No semen produced; dry orgasm	Occasional
Partial penectomy	Unchanged	Erotic sensations still occur in remaining genital area	Unchanged. Penile shaft lengthens to permit coitus and (often) female orgasm	Unchanged	Unchanged	Rare; genital edema after groin dissection
Total penectomy	Unchanged	Erotic sensations still occur in remaining genital area	None	Unchanged, but need to relearn erotic zones	Unchanged, but semen is expelled through perineal urethrostomy	Occasional; genital edema after groin dissection

*With the development of new nerve-sparing surgical techniques, rates of erectile recovery are higher. However, a six-month recovery period is still necessary. Whether these procedures eradicate the cancer successfully remains controversial.

(Reprinted from Schover LR, Fife M: Sexual counseling with radical pelvic or genital cancer surgery. J Psychosoc Oncol 3:21–41, 1985.)

PROBLEMS OF SEXUAL AROUSAL

ERECTILE DYSFUNCTION. For men with cancer, problems achieving and maintaining erections are the most common reason for seeking sexual health care. Many men feel a loss of masculinity when they develop erectile dysfunction. Men treated for cancer are especially vulnerable, given their fears of losing their ability to work and take a leadership role in the family.[24] Despite changing societal values about gender roles, in clinical practice concerns about the traditional masculine role are the rule rather than the exception.

Unfortunately, cancer treatments can damage the erection reflex through a variety of mechanisms. Hormonal causes of low sexual desire, listed above, usually make it more difficult for men to get erections. Some patients, however, especially those under age 50, can achieve normal erections even with negligible levels of serum testosterone.[14] The role of testosterone in erectile function is still poorly understood.[25]

Vascular insufficiency has been highlighted in recent years as a common cause of erectile dysfunction, especially in aging men. Both pelvic arteriosclerosis[26] and leaks in the venous drainage of the penis[27,28] can interfere with erection. A tumor itself rarely impairs the vascular system of the penis, but some cancer therapies apparently can. Goldstein and colleagues[29] found evidence of reduced arterial flow to the penis after pelvic irradiation for prostate cancer. Their study was largely retrospective, however, and one small prospective case series has not confirmed their findings.[30] Further research is needed to elucidate the role of irradiation in accelerating pelvic arteriosclerosis or causing penile arterial stenosis or occlusion. Three retrospective surveys of testicular cancer patients[21,22,31] also suggest that men who receive radiation therapy to the pelvis and retroperitoneum have

TABLE 61-11. Effects of Surgery for Pelvic or Genital Cancer on Female Sexual Physiology

Surgical Procedure	*Hormonal Basis of Sexual Desire*	*Capacity for Pleasure with Genital Touch*	*Capacity for Vaginal Lubrication*	*Ease of Reaching Orgasm*	*Sensation of Orgasm*	*Dyspareunia*
Radical hysterectomy	Unchanged*	Unchanged	Unchanged†	Unchanged	Unchanged	Rare; must adjust to shallower vagina‡
Radical cystectomy	Unchanged*	Unchanged	Reduced†	Unchanged, despite loss of anterior vaginal wall	Unchanged	Frequent, but can be reduced
Abdominoperineal resection	Unchanged*	Unchanged	Unchanged†	Probably unchanged; no research available	Unchanged	Frequent but can be reduced
Total pelvic exenteration and vaginal reconstruction using myocutaneous gracilis flaps	Unchanged*	Some loss of erotic zones, vagina, and occasionally part of vulva. Erotic sensations still occur in remaining genital area. Neovagina can develop erotic sensitivity.	Lost. Must use artificial lubricants in neovagina and daily douches to reduce odor	Often must relearn how to reach orgasm	Unchanged, or mild loss of intensity	Occasional; can be reduced
Radical vulvectomy	Unchanged	Some loss of erotic zones; erotic sensations still occur in remaining genital area	Unchanged	Often must relearn how to reach orgasm	No research data available	Frequent, because of urethral irritation or stenosis of vaginal entrance. Can be reduced.

*Even if bilateral oophorectomy is included, adrenal androgens should maintain an adequate degree of desire. Some clinicians recommend a combination of androgen and estrogen replacement therapy. "Hot flashes" from estrogen deficiency may interfere with sexual pleasure.

†If bilateral oophorectomy is included, vaginal lubrication is reduced unless estrogen replacement therapy is prescribed.

‡Dyspareunia is more common when surgery is combined with pelvic irradiation, which reduces vaginal lubrication even further and can promote vaginal atrophy and stenosis.

(Reprinted from Schover LR, Fife M: Sexual counseling with radical pelvic or genital cancer surgery. J Psychosoc Oncol 3:21–41, 1985.)

increased rates of erectile dysfunction. Since the vascular impact of radiation therapy develops slowly, long-term follow-up studies are necessary. Our ability to directly measure penile circulation also is still limited despite recent advances.[32] Two European studies report that Doppler measures of arterial flow to the penis are reduced after radical cystectomy, presumably because of intraoperative ligation of arteries.[33,34]

The most common neurologic cause of erectile dysfunction related to cancer treatment is damage to the prostatic plexus during radical pelvic surgery. The anatomy of this nerve plexus has only recently been well defined.[35,36] The prostatic plexus contains both sympathetic and parasympathetic fibers. Located between the prostate and rectum, these nerves travel posterolateral to the seminal vesicles, continuing beyond the apex of the prostate to course along the bulbous urethra at the 11 and 1 o'clock position. Walsh[5] has devised a nerve-sparing procedure to minimize damage to the prostatic plexus during radical cystectomy and prostatectomy.

After abdominoperineal resection, rates of erectile dysfunction have been reported as ranging from 15% to 80% in various case series.[37–43] Tumor stage does not predict recovery of erections, but as with other radical pelvic operations,[44,45] younger men are more likely to recover fully.[38,40,41] Poor specification of the severity of erection problems in these studies make it difficult to compare findings from different centers. Patients who have undergone low anterior resection clearly have a much lower incidence of postoperative erectile dysfunction than those who have had abdominoperineal resection.[37,39,46] For example, La Monica et al[39] reported a 55% rate of erection problems after abdominoperineal resection, compared to 20% after low anterior resection. In another case series the respective rates were 67% and 30%.[42] Procedures that merely preserve the anal sphincter are not as successful in preventing sexual dysfunction, however.[40]

Other causes of neurogenic erectile dysfunction in cancer patients include autonomic neuropathy, for example after chemotherapy or immunotherapy. Although we have seen a number of cases of erectile dysfunction in men treated with interferon, Schilsky and colleagues[47] recently reported no discernible sexual side-effects of α_2-interferon in men with hairy cell leukemia. Of course, a malignancy involving the spinal cord has the potential to damage nerve centers controlling erection.

Clinicians must take care in attributing erection problems to iatrogenic effects of cancer treatment. Since cancer patients are an older group, many have had other health problems that put them at risk for erectile dysfunction. In a group of 112 men (mean age, 63 years) about to undergo radical cystectomy, noncancer health risk factors for erectile dysfunction were highly predictive of actual sexual function status.[44] Cardiovascular disease and antihypertensive medication were especially strong predictors.

Some erection problems in cancer patients also have a psychological basis. Men with cancer are just as vulnerable as healthy men, if not more so, to anxiety about sexual performance. Marital conflict, feeling stigmatized by cancer, and anxiety about sex being unhealthy during cancer treatment are common antecedents of psychogenic erectile dysfunction. Clinicians should ask carefully about the pervasiveness of the erection problem. Men who still wake from sleep with firm erections, who can masturbate with a firm erection, or who can achieve good erections with some partners or some types of sexual stimulation often have intact erectile capacity.

FEMALE AROUSAL PROBLEMS. In women, difficulty becoming sexually aroused results in less vaginal expansion in both depth and width, and reduced amounts of vaginal lubrication. A subjective lack of sexual excitement and pleasure is sometimes linked to these physical problems. If the cause is medical, however, the women may feel aroused but still have vaginal dryness.

The two major physiological causes of arousal problems in women with cancer are premature menopause and pelvic irradiation. A number of cancer treatments lead to premature menopause. If young adult women receive a dose of irradiation of 600 to 1000 rad to the ovaries, most will lose function permanently.[48] A smaller dose may suffice to destroy ovarian function in a woman in her 40s, while children can withstand somewhat higher doses and still have normal menses at puberty.[49] Cytotoxic chemotherapy, particularly with alkylating agents, also can impair production of estrogen and progesterone by the ovaries. Again, women over age 30 are more likely to experience permanent menopause after chemotherapy. Younger women who do recover menstrual function often have a shortened reproductive life before they, too, reach premature menopause. The degree of ovarian damage depends on the specific drugs used as well as dosage.[49]

The symptoms of premature and abrupt ovarian failure are often much more severe than those of natural menopause. Frequent hot flashes may interrupt a woman's sleep and embarrass her in daily life. The resulting loss of well-being can reduce her desire for sex. The most salient sexual symptom is reduced vaginal lubrication and expansion, with intercourse becoming dry and painful. Often the woman has vaginal and vulvar soreness after sexual activity. Vaginal atrophy can also be a factor in recurrent urethral irritation, a common source of dyspareunia. These symptoms are common in clinical practice, for example in young women on chemotherapy for breast cancer or Hodgkin's disease. They have been documented as very common and treatable with replacement estrogen in Hodgkin's disease patients.[50] Women with breast cancer treated with antiestrogenic agents may have particularly severe vaginal atrophy,[51] with dyspareunia that is only partially alleviated by using a water-based lubricant. Of course, women with hormone-sensitive tumors cannot take replacement estrogen and are at increased risk for osteoporosis and cardiovascular disease with aging.

Currently, a controversy exists about the mechanism underlying vaginal changes at menopause. Some researchers have documented reduced vaginal blood flow in the resting state,[52] others have been unable to observe differences from premenopausal women in vaginal blood flow during sexual arousal.[53] No physiological studies have examined women with premature menopause.

Pelvic radiation therapy has direct effects on vaginal tissue in addition to its impact on the ovaries. Even external beam irradiation to a pelvic field may result in dyspareunia because of pelvic fibrosis or because of reduced circulation of blood to the vagina due to vascular damage. Intracavitary irradiation to the vagina produces visible changes in the mucosa, which becomes thinner and more fragile.[23] A few women develop vaginal ulcers that can take months to heal. For the first several months after radiation therapy, the irritated vagina is in danger of agglutination or of developing tight, fibrous bands of scar tissue unless the woman continues to have sexual activity or uses a vaginal dilator to stretch the tissue several times a week.[54]

Conventional wisdom is that women need to use a vaginal lubricant to have comfortable intercourse after pelvic irradiation. However, our recent comparison of women undergoing radical hysterectomy versus radiation therapy for cervical cancer revealed that only about a quarter of those in either group usually needed extra lubrication by 1-year follow-up.[23]

We do not know whether autonomic neuropathy, for example after chemotherapy or immunotherapy, plays a role in women's arousal phase sexual dysfunctions as it does in erectile dysfunction. Even the role of spinal cord damage in women's sexual function is poorly understood.[55] Of course, emotional factors can reduce sexual arousal, with concomitant failure of vaginal expansion and lubrication.

PROBLEMS WITH ORGASM

One striking observation we have made over years of assessing sexual problems in cancer patients is that the orgasmic response is much harder to damage than is the arousal phase. Perhaps because orgasm depends on input from the somatic pudendal nerve, protected by fascia near the pelvic side walls, it is not as vulnerable as the arousal phase functions mediated by the fragile, centrally located pelvic autonomic nerve plexi. Even when a man's entire penis is amputated for penile or urethral cancer, orgasm can still occur with ejaculation of semen through the perineal urethrostomy.[14] Women report having orgasm even after radical vulvectomy[56,57] or total pelvic exenteration.[58]

In our case series of 384 cancer patients referred for sexual counseling, a global difficulty reaching orgasm was a complaint in 26% of men and 29% of women, whereas 61% of men and 70% of women had severe arousal phase dysfunctions.[11] After treatment for early stage cervical cancer, only 3% of women became completely inorgasmic, although 20% had trouble becoming sexually aroused.[23]

DECREASED ORGASMIC INTENSITY. One gender difference in our research is that men report decreased orgasmic intensity as a problem after cancer treatment, whereas for women the quality of orgasm rarely changes.[11,21–23,44,59] Men often, but not invariably, report that orgasm occurs with less strength and pleasure when cancer treatment has reduced semen volume, caused dry orgasm, or prevented erection.

PHASES OF MALE ORGASM. Clinicians assessing cancer patients need a clear understanding of male orgasm.[55] The first phase of orgasm, emission, consists of contractions of the prostate, seminal vesicles, and vasa deferens. Controlled by short adrenergic neurons, emission is felt subjectively as the "point of no return" just before orgasm. During emission the seminal fluid components are mixed and deposited in the prostatic urethra. The bladder neck is closed by the internal sphincter so that during the second phase of orgasm, ejaculation, semen is propelled out through the urethra. Ejaculation consists of contractions of the striated muscles at the base of the penis, mediated by the pudendal nerve. The afferent sensory impulses are experienced as the pleasure of orgasm.

Very few cancer treatments damage the ejaculation phase of orgasm, but the sympathetic nerves controlling emission are more vulnerable. A standard retroperitoneal lymphadenectomy for nonseminomatous testicular cancer usually damages the sympathetic ganglia that send input to the short adrenergic neurons.[21,60] Impaired emission is also a frequent consequence after abdominoperineal resection because of dissection in the presacral area or between the seminal vesicles and rectum.[43] Sympathetic nerve plexi also are damaged during node dissections for tumors of the sigmoid colon. The incidence of dry orgasm increases with the extent of the dissection.[61] We call the syndrome *dry orgasm* because the underlying deficit is sometimes retrograde ejaculation with simple failure of the internal sphincter and sometimes a more profound failure of the smooth muscle contractions of emission. The simplest way to differentiate the two patterns is to test for fructose and spermatozoa in urine voided after orgasm.[31]

Men who become hypogonadal after treatment or who receive pelvic irradiation[22] often notice a reduction in semen volume that can approach a totally dry orgasm. Dry orgasm can also occur after chemotherapy with neurotoxic agents.[31] Of course, men also experience dry orgasm after radical cystectomy or prostatectomy, operations in which the prostate and seminal vesicles are removed.[44]

OTHER MALE ORGASMIC PROBLEMS. Although a decreased quality of orgasm is a common complaint in men treated for cancer, a complete inability to reach orgasm is rare. In our experience, most male cancer patients who become inorgasmic after cancer treatment have simply not made much of an effort to achieve sexual arousal with prolonged stimulation. Most are experiencing erection problems and do not realize they could reach orgasm with a flaccid penis, for example with manual or oral caressing. Others resist attempting orgasm by masturbation or by noncoital stimulation from a partner because they believe that the only "normal" orgasm is one achieved intravaginally. We have also observed that cancer treatment rarely is a factor in causing premature ejaculation.[11]

ORGASM PROBLEMS IN WOMEN. Women treated for cancer often report that they can reach orgasm on occasion, but that they need more stimulation than previously. Orgasm may occur less reliably, especially during intercourse.[11,23,62] Although some have theorized that the female orgasm is a two-stage process, as in men, little physiological evidence exists for such a model.[55] The female orgasm parallels the ejaculation stage of male orgasm. It is a striated muscle event, mediated by the pudendal nerve. In addition to the clitoris, several areas of the vagina have erotic sensitivity for women,[63] but there does not seem to be one specific spot crucial for coital orgasm. Research on women after radical hysterectomy,[23] radical cystectomy,[59] and total pelvic exenteration[58,64,65] illustrates that women retain the ability to have orgasms during intercourse, even when a major part of the vagina has been removed or the entire vagina has been reconstructed.

PAIN DURING SEX

Many cancer patients experience chronic pain. Even pain at extragenital sites can interfere with sexual desire and distract from pleasurable feelings during sexual activity. Opiate pain medication not only reduces sexual desire by its CNS depressant properties, but also perhaps by elevating production of the hormone prolactin.[55] Specific genital pain that is exacerbated by sexual activity occurs fairly rarely in male cancer patients but is the most common sexual problem in female patients.[11]

MALE DYSPAREUNIA. In male patients, we have observed phantom rectal pain after abdominoperineal resection or scrotal and inguinal pain after various treatments for testicular cancer.[21] Men with Peyronie's plaques often have pain as well as curvature with erection. We have seen this syndrome several times in men who had pelvic irradiation or estrogen therapy for prostate cancer.[11] Although sexual arousal is enough to trigger the pain in some men, especially those with Peyronie's syndrome, it is more common for pain to occur during and after orgasm. Men who have had intravesical chemotherapy or who are near the end of a course of pelvic irradiation often have several weeks of pain with ejaculation because of urethral irritation.

FEMALE DYSPAREUNIA. The common causes of vaginal and vulvar pain in women treated for cancer are identical to those that interfere with sexual arousal. Often it is the loss of vaginal expansion and lubrication that makes penetration for intercourse tight and painful, causes a diffuse burning during intercourse, and leaves the vagina and vulva sore after coitus. These symptoms are even more severe when chemotherapy causes stomatitis of the vaginal mucosa. Few women are warned to expect this side-effect of many anticancer drugs.

Pain with deep thrusting is often associated with ulcers or stenosis at the vaginal apex after intracavity irradiation. Pelvic adhesions may also contribute, particularly if an ovary adheres to the vaginal cuff after hysterectomy.

Narrowing of the vaginal introitus can create dyspareunia after radical vulvectomy.[56,57] The exposure of the urethral meatus also creates painful irritation and an increased incidence of urinary tract infections after sexual activity for these women. Women who have undergone partial[59] or total vaginal reconstruction[58,65] often report pain during intercourse. Areas of scar tissue can be tender, or the entire vagina may be too narrow or too short.

Although most dyspareunia in women after cancer treatment has a physical cause, emotional factors can complicate or maintain the problem, even when sources of pain have been ameliorated. If a woman anticipates that sex will be painful, she may contract the pubococcygeal muscles without realizing it.[66] The muscular tension makes penetration more difficult and in severe cases prevents it entirely. Even during penile thrusting, muscle spasms exacerbate painful sensations.

CURRENT CONTROVERSIES IN SEXUAL REHABILITATION

Although remediating sexual problems in cancer patients is generally an area of controversy and incomplete knowledge, certain cancer treatments are receiving increased attention because they promise to reduce sexual morbidity. We highlight several cancer sites for which treatment has proved effective enough to allow modifications that seek to prevent sexual and reproductive dysfunctions.

EARLY STAGE INVASIVE CERVICAL CANCER: RADIATION THERAPY VERSUS RADICAL HYSTERECTOMY

When invasive cancer of the cervix is FIGO Stage Ia, Ib, or IIa, radical hysterectomy or combined external beam and intracavitary irradiation are equally effective therapies.[67] The choice of treatment depends on whether a woman is a good surgical candidate. Barring unusual risk factors, preservation of sexual function has become an important factor in planning therapy for this group of relatively young patients with excellent prognoses.

Unfortunately, research comparing sexual function after surgery versus radiation therapy has provided conflicting results.[23] Most studies have been retrospective, with small sample sizes and poor specification of sexual problems. Treatment parameters were also not well defined.[23,68] Although data suggest that slightly more sexual dysfunction occurs after radiation therapy, the one prospective study that randomly assigned women to treatment groups found comparable, mild rates of sexual morbidity 6 months after surgery or radiation therapy.[69]

A more recent study[23] compared 26 women treated with radical hysterectomy alone and 35 who underwent radiation therapy, with or without hysterectomy. Whether the hysterectomy group was compared to 23 women who had radiation therapy alone or to all 35 irradiated women, at 1 year after treatment women who had undergone hysterectomy alone had fewer sexual complaints and dysfunctions. Although rates of sexual activity were similar across treatment groups, women who had undergone radiation therapy had decreased sexual desire (27% *vs.* 22% for hysterectomy group), more arousal phase problems (29% *vs.* 6%), and more dyspareunia (22% *vs.* 0%). Their reports of painful intercourse correlated with gynecologists' ratings of the vaginal mucosa, vaginal size, and pain during pelvic examination. Interestingly, at 6 months after treatment both groups of women appeared to have good sexual function.[69] By 1 year, however, problems had become manifest.

Rates of sexual dysfunction at 1 year were very comparable to those observed by Andersen[70] in a mixed group of gynecologic cancer patients followed for the same interval. Andersen currently is gathering longitudinal data comparing women treated with radical hysterectomy or radiation therapy with a group having gynecologic surgery for endometriosis. Her results should further define the sexual impact of these therapies.

NEW OPTIONS IN TREATING BREAST CANCER

For more than 30 years, women undergoing radical mastectomy have been recognized as having emotional distress and sexual concerns.[71,72] Although perhaps 20% to 33% of women have significant psychological distress after mastectomy, the incidence of clinical depression is no higher than in women with malignancies at other sites.[73] Women treated for breast cancer also have reduced sexual activity and arousal compared to healthy women, though gynecologic cancer patients are more severely affected in terms of body image.[74]

With the advent of breast conservation surgery plus radiation therapy as an effective alternative to mastectomy for Stage I or II disease,[6] researchers have compared psychological adjustment after the two procedures. After mastectomy, a substantial minority of women report feeling disfigured and lopsided[75] or feeling less interested in sex, less easily aroused, and less comfortable with nudity in intimate situations.[76] Clinical observations suggested that newer treatments minimized these sources of distress. It is somewhat surprising that standardized interview or questionnaire measures of emotional distress reveal little or no difference in women who have undergone mastectomy versus conservation procedures. This finding has held true whether women actively sought a treatment of choice[77–80] or agreed to participate in a randomized study.[81,82] Even global measures of sexual satisfaction have been equivalent between treatment groups.[80,81]

Some differences have been found, however, when women are asked more detailed questions about sexual practices and body image. Steinberg and colleagues[79] found that women had overall better psychological function as well as more comfort in discussing sex, a reported enhancement rather than a decline in the husband's sexual function, and more enjoyment of breast stimulation after breast conservation procedures than after mastectomy. Another comparison found less decrement in the frequency of affection and sex in the breast conservation group.[75] In a prospective study of women in a randomized trial, mastectomy patients were more likely than the breast conservation group to have loss of sexual desire, negative feelings about their own nudity, and feelings of sadness, frustration, and lack of control over life.[83] Bartelink et al[84] confirmed that a breast conservation sample had a more intact body image, higher life satisfaction, and less fear of cancer recurrence.

We need to learn more about the partner's reaction[85] and whether conservation surgery helps preserve pleasure with breast caressing[86]; we also need detailed, before and after assessments of the frequency and variety of lovemaking. Our knowledge will increase as larger samples of women are studied, with clearer specification of the woman's role in actively choosing a therapy. The sense of having a choice may be as important as the treatment the women undergoes.

Women who seek breast reconstruction after mastectomy are no longer regarded as narcissistic. They have been characterized as healthy and assertive, with common motivations to feel whole again and dispense with a breast prosthesis.[87,88] For many women, breast reconstruction reduces the preoccupation with fear of recurrence that was elicited by the constant reminder of the mastectomy site.[88]

Research on the psychological and sexual benefits of reconstruction still lacks sophistication. Partners have not been included in the assessments, and measures of satisfaction with surgery often have been global and unfocused. Few researchers have specifically addressed the impact on sexuality. One issue studied has been the timing of reconstruction. Surgeons feared that woman undergoing immediate reconstruction at the time of mastectomy would be dissatisfied with less than perfect results, since they had not experienced the trauma of breast loss. Several studies comparing immediate versus delayed reconstruction have put this theory to rest, demonstrating that women are just as satisfied with surgical results after immediate reconstruction as after a delay.[89–91] Furthermore, immediate reconstruction seems to prevent psychological distress and facilitates a return to normal daily life.[91,92]

One study that assessed sexual function found that women were sexually dissatisfied before delayed reconstruction. After reconstruction, 75% reported increased sexual satisfaction. Immediate surgery was even more successful, however, in preventing sexual problems except in women undergoing chemotherapy.[90] Another study failed to find an advantage of immediate reconstruction in terms of sexual satisfaction at 1 year after mastectomy.[92]

Although "the sooner the better" is a reasonable recommendation for breast reconstruction,[91] some women are better off waiting. They may need time to weigh pros and cons or to finish adjuvant chemotherapy. Some worry about having a breast prosthesis inserted. For this last group, reconstructive surgery using the transverse rectus abdominis musculocutaneous flap can eliminate the need for an implant. One recent study reported fewer major complications and a higher patient satisfaction with this procedure than with implantation of a tissue expander.[93]

Recently, Wellisch et al[94] compared 26 women who did not have nipples added as part of breast reconstruction with 33 women who did. Women who chose to have nipples added were more satisfied with the size, softness, nude appearance, and sexual sensitivity of the reconstructed breast. These responses bear witness to the power of the woman's sense of restored bodily integrity in shaping her perception of herself and even her sexual pleasure.

The effectiveness of sexual counseling in enhancing sexual recovery after treatment for breast cancer has rarely been studied.[95] Another crucial issue is the impact of chemotherapy—not only the sexual impact of alopecia, weight gain, vaginal irritation and dryness, hot flashes, and general lack of well-being[96,97] but, for younger women, the threat to fertility. Despite fears that the hormonal elevations of pregnancy could trigger a cancer recurrence,[98] current evidence suggests that pregnancy at diagnosis or after successful cancer treatment does not affect disease-free survival in node-negative women.[99–101]

NERVE-SPARING RADICAL PELVIC SURGERY AND PRESERVATION OF ERECTILE FUNCTION

The introduction of nerve-sparing radical prostatectomy by Walsh and colleagues[5] has had an important impact on the treatment of localized carcinoma of the prostate. Surgery has gained in popularity over radiation therapy with the promise of effective treatment with low sexual and general morbidity.[102] Walsh and Mostwin[5] reported that 86% of a sample of previously potent men recovered erections 1 year after radical prostatectomy and at least 67% after nerve-sparing radical cystectomy. Catalona and Dresner[45] observed a 52% rate of recovery of erections sufficient for vaginal penetration in a comparable sample of 42 men followed up for at least 4 months. Their lower success rate may in part reflect the shorter duration of follow-up. According to Walsh's data,[5] the percentage of men recovering fully can be expected to increase at least through the first 12 months after surgery. Published data also suggest that nerve-sparing procedures do not compromise surgical margins when compared with standard radical retropubic prostatectomy.[45,103]

The issue of treatment of choice is not fully resolved, however. External beam radiation therapy has an excellent record in controlling for localized disease. Its morbidity includes rates of delayed proctitis of around 20%, with less than 2% of men requiring a bowel diversion. Urinary frequency, pain, or incontinence are delayed problems for about 20% of patients but resolve without a urinary diversion in all but 1% to 2%.[104,105] This compares with a 6% rate of urinary incontinence and 3% rate of bowel injury after radical prostatectomy in a recently published 5-year follow-up series.[106] Radiation therapy may offer an advantage in terms of local recurrence at 5- to 10-year follow-up, especially of Stage A2 and B2 disease,[104] and is the most effective treatment for Stage C tumors.[105]

The sexual morbidity of pelvic radiation therapy remains to be defined. The incidence of erectile dysfunction after external beam treatment for prostate cancer has ranged from 22% to 84% in various case series, but no large sample of men studied prospectively is available,[29] and in retrospective studies problems attributed by patients to cancer treatment often may have existed before the diagnosis.[14]

The recovery rates for erection after nerve-sparing surgery also need clarification. Although there is no question that nerve-sparing techniques increase the rate of sexual recovery, the magnitude of the improvement over standard procedures is an issue. With standard procedures, recovery of fully functional erections was reported after radical prostatectomy in 4 (11%) of 35 initially potent men[107] and 5 (7%) of 73 patients unselected for prior sexual capacity who underwent radical cystectomy.[44] Fully functional erections were defined in both case series as satisfactory in firmness with lasting rigidity until orgasm. Men who recovered partial erections comprised 43% of the prostatectomy[107] and 41% of the cystectomy[44] groups.

In the nerve-sparing series, Walsh and Mostwin[5] defined potency as "the ability to achieve successful vaginal penetration and orgasm." Catalona and Dresner[45] classified erections as "partial" or "sufficient for vaginal penetration." However, many men after radical surgery can achieve a semirigid erection sufficient for penetration with effort. These men describe penetration as "stuffing" the penis into the partner's vagina, using extra lubrication and support from a hand at the base of the penis. Such erections often decrease further in tumescence during the thrusting of intercourse. The man can reach orgasm with a flaccid penis. His partner's satisfaction is variable, depending on her ease in reaching orgasm without intense vaginal stimulation. In our experience, some men in this category are interested in further sexual rehabilitation but hesitate to ask for help if they know they have undergone a nerve-sparing procedure. We wonder whether some of these men are categorized as fully recovered in the case series reported thus far. More detailed studies are underway, and we await the results with interest.

We have observed clinically that men who recover fuller erections also report more intense orgasms after radical pelvic surgery. It would be interesting to look at this variable after nerve-sparing surgery.

LONG-TERM SEXUAL MORBIDITY OF TREATMENT FOR TESTICULAR CANCER

Although testicular cancer is a rare malignancy, it strikes men in their reproductive years. With the advent of radiation therapy for seminoma and combination chemotherapy for nonseminomatous tumors and advanced cases of seminoma, disease-free survival rates have climbed and the great majority of men can expect an excellent prognosis.[108]

Although early case series reported no excess of sexual problems in men after treatment for testicular cancer, more detailed surveys of long-term survivors revealed a significant amount of dysfunction in men treated either for seminoma or nonseminomatous disease.[20–22,31,109] Although divorce rates were similar to those of age-matched men in the general population, rates of low sexual desire ranged from 4% to 12%, erectile dysfunction from 10% to 15%, and difficulty reaching orgasm from 6% to 10%.[20–22] These percentages are slightly higher than one would expect in healthy young men. More saliently, about 20% of men were sexually inactive or had sex very infrequently.[20–22] Diminished pleasure with orgasm has also been a common complaint.[21,22,31] The subgroups of sexually dysfunctional men were also emotionally distressed[21] and reported more marital unhappiness.[20–22]

Some of the sexual impact of testicular cancer may reflect the emotional trauma of undergoing a life-threatening disease in young adulthood, the mourning of lost fertility, or the impact of surgical removal of a testicle.[109,110] Some sexual morbidity may be organically based as a result of radiation therapy[22] or retroperitoneal lymphadenectomy.[20,21]

Efforts at improving quality of life after treatment for testicular cancer have focused on limiting the dissection during retroperitoneal lymphadenectomy to reduce impairment of emission[60,111] or on avoiding node dissection altogether by careful surveillance programs for men with Stage I nonseminomatous tumors.[8,112,113] Surveillance alone has also been attempted as an alternative to prophylactic pelvic and para-aortic radiation therapy in men with Stage I seminoma.[112] Men who do undergo retroperitoneal lymphadenectomy and have impaired emission can be treated by sympathomimetic agents to try to induce antegrade ejaculation of semen.[31,60] We need prospective information on sexual function and psychological distress before and after limited node dissection or surveillance, however, to see if preserving fertility is also effective in reducing the emotional impact of testicular cancer.

ASSESSING SEXUAL FUNCTION IN CANCER PATIENTS

Every physician who treats cancer patients should ask briefly about sexuality during initial history-taking and at follow-up visits. This standard of care is rarely attained, however. For example, in one recent study only 2% of physicians asked about sexuality before or after mastectomy.[114] The most common reason clinicians give for not assessing sexuality is time pressure. Not only physicians but medical social workers and oncology nurses often feel overwhelmed by the demands of a busy clinic. Certainly it may take several moments to find out that a sexual problem exists and to refer the patient for more extensive services. Each clinician needs to decide on the priority to give to the sexual history. We hope this chapter will impress readers with the salience of these issues for patients.

Complaints about time pressure often mask clinicians' other common concerns—that discussing sexuality will be awkward or that they will not have remedies to offer for the patient's sexual problems. The section of this chapter on treatment should familiarize clinicians with the range of treatments for sexual dysfunction. We focus here on how to ease any discomfort about addressing sexuality.

We suggest that the health care professional who takes an initial history include one generic question about sex. The question should be prefaced by a normalizing statement: "I always ask patients about sexuality as part of a history," or, "One aspect of every person's health is sexual health." The actual assessment question should be open-ended, to elicit more than just a yes or no answer. For example, "What impact has your cancer diagnosis had on your sex life?" or "How important are any sexual side-effects of cancer treatment to you?" or "How well are you functioning now in your sex life?" When cancer treatment is likely to cause sexual problems, options for rehabilitation should be mentioned at least briefly at the time of treatment disposition. The same principles can be used to arrive at a sexuality question to ask at each routine follow-up visit. Some sexual dysfunctions, for example after radiation therapy, take time to become manifest.

Some clinicians may wish to refer all questions and problems regarding sex to one member of the health care team, for example a particular physician, psychologist, or social worker in the institution or community who assesses and treats sexual problems in cancer patients. If the primary physician is willing to invest a bit of extra time, however, we estimate that 80% to 90% of patients can benefit from brief sexual advice or counseling and do not need or desire a specialty consult. Providing sexual counseling requires a more thorough assessment of the sexual problem.

BRIEF SEXUAL ASSESSMENT INTERVIEW

Figure 61-3 provides a guide for the assessment interview. The clinician wants to know what specific sexual problems have occurred and what etiological factors are present in order to plan treatment. Often cancer patients have multiple sexual dysfunctions with a range of causes that interact to make the problems more severe. A good treatment plan will require more than one modality since more than one problem must be addressed.

We advocate including both partners in the interview whenever possible.[55] The benefit of a conjoint session is that both partners get across their point of view and have a chance to hear information given by the clinician. The partners' behavior with each other also provides valuable insights into their relationships. The risk is that the clinician will not find out about affairs, masturbation, or other "secrets." If time permits, a few minutes alone with each partner can be added to get a more complete picture in sensitive areas. The clinician must hold such information in confidence, however.

DEFINING THE DYSFUNCTION. The first section of this chapter gives the clinician a grasp of the types of problems cancer patients experience. Questions about sexual function should be detailed and specific. The clinician who is comfortable discussing sex helps the patient to be open. The clinician can begin with general questions about how often lovemaking occurs and who initiates sex. Does lovemaking include manual or oral genital caressing? Can each partner reach orgasm through noncoital caressing, or only during intercourse? We find that patients who have tried having orgasms with manual or oral stimulation are more likely to resume sex if cancer treatment impairs erections.[44] Can the patient and partner communicate their preferences for touch either verbally or nonverbally during sex? Cancer treatment can interfere with a long-term sexual routine, necessitating more sexual communication and negotiation than usual. How has sex changed since the cancer diagnosis? It is crucial to compare sexual frequency and function before and after cancer treatment.

Questions about specific sexual dysfunctions should include inquiries about whether the onset of the problems was sudden or gradual, and the timing of onset in relation to

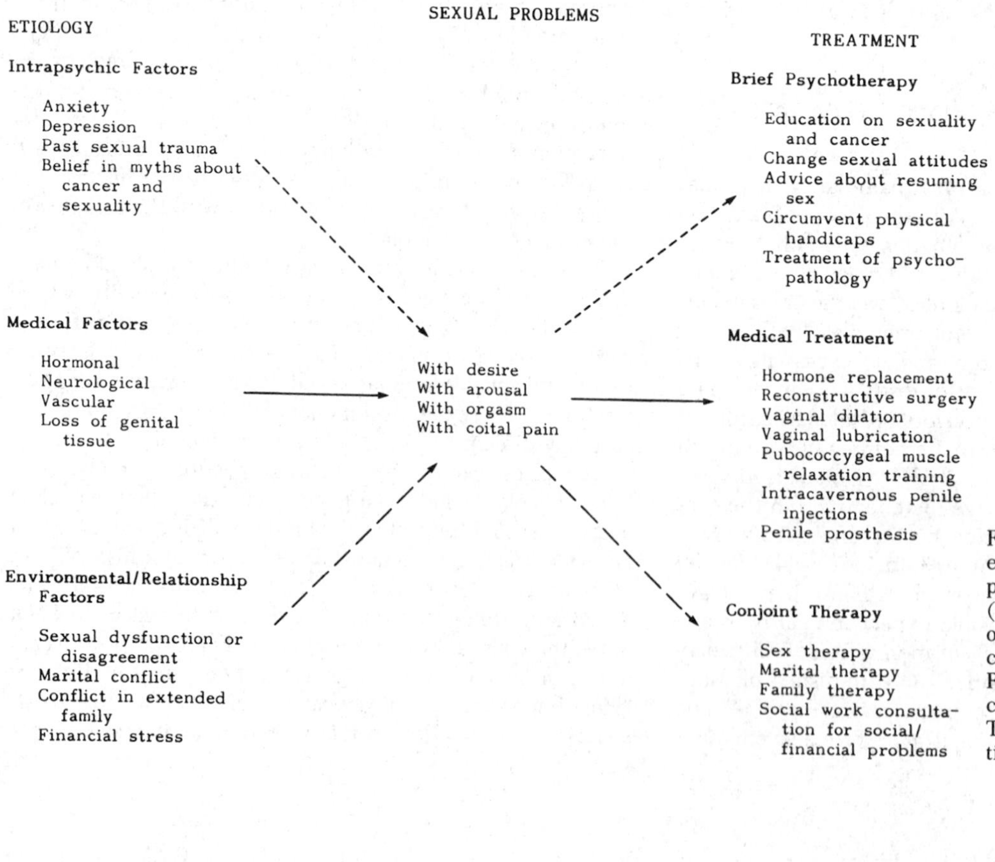

FIG. 61-3. An integrative model of etiology and treatment of sexual problems in cancer patients. (Schover LR: Sexual rehabilitation of the patient with gynecologic cancer. In Rutledge FN, Freedman RS, Gershenson DM [eds]: Gynecologic Cancer: Diagnosis and Treatment Strategies, p 462. Austin, TX, University of Texas Press)

cancer diagnosis and treatment. Other life stresses or medical problems that could have led to sexual dysfunction should not be overlooked.

The interviewer can ask about each phase of the sexual response cycle. How often does the patient feel a desire for sex? Can a man get and keep firm erections? If he loses erections, at what point in the lovemaking does the problem occur? Can a woman produce enough vaginal lubrication for comfort during genital caressing and intercourse? Is there pain during sex? What kinds of sexual acts help each partner to reach orgasm? Has the quality of orgasmic sensation changed? Does the male partner have premature ejaculation?

When a problem is pinpointed, the interviewer needs to ask if it occurs in all situations. How comfortable does the patient feel about masturbation? Does the sexual problem occur then too? Does the patient have more than one sexual partner? If so, is function different with different partners? What about response to erotic films, stories, or magazines? Does use of alcohol or drugs (including prescription medications) have a sexual impact?

Some cancer patients are seropositive for the human immunodeficiency virus (HIV) and are at risk for transmitting it to a partner. Others are seronegative or of unknown serologic status but are members of high-risk groups. Currently, any adult who is not in a monogamous relationship with a person known to be seronegative or at very low risk for HIV should be counseled about safe sex.[115]

ASSESSING INTRAPSYCHIC RISK FACTORS. The clinician should ask about emotional factors in the patient's history as well as current strategies for coping with cancer that could have an impact on sexuality.[11] Is the patient so overwhelmed by anxiety about the cancer that he or she is impaired in all aspects of daily living? Is the patient clinically depressed, so that loss of sexual desire is just one symptom of a more global affective disorder? The clinician should be familiar with diagnostic criteria for depression[9] and how it presents in cancer patients.[18,19]

ASSESSING ENVIRONMENTAL OR RELATIONSHIP RISK FACTORS. The patient's sexual function also depends on societal norms and relationship factors. The value a patient places on staying sexually active often is influenced by the mores of his or her ethnic group, religion, and immediate family. In the United States, black or Hispanic patients often believe that noncoital sex to orgasm is abnormal, but feel that continuing intercourse is important.[116] The result can be high distress if cancer treatment impairs the husband's erections or makes intercourse painful for the wife. The clinician needs to understand the patient's values to avoid suggesting strategies of sexual rehabilitation that will simply be rejected as distasteful or immoral.

The impact of illness on a relationship depends on the partners' capacities to communicate feelings, express caring and anger adaptively, meet each other's needs for intimacy, and reallocate the tasks of daily life when necessary. A detailed discussion of techniques of marital assessment in medical patients is beyond the scope of this chapter, but the interested reader can refer to a book by Schover and Jensen.[55] Some brief questions useful as an adjunct to the sexual assessment are the following:

- "How has the illness affected your private time with your partner?" Especially for young couples with children, cancer treatment disrupts the family schedule so much that spouses have little or no time just to sit together and talk, let alone have sex.
- "Have you noticed a change in the amount of physical affection you or your partner show to each other?" A decrease in sexual activity is often paralleled by declining expressions of love and caring, especially in couples with marital conflict or if the wife is the cancer patient.[11] Even when patients are terminally ill, touching and intimacy continue to be important to quality of life.[117]
- "Every couple has disagreements sometimes. If the two of you get angry with each other, how do you each express it?" The stress of cancer can accentuate marital conflict, sometimes even to the point of violence.[118]
- "Has the cancer diagnosis raised disagreements in the extended family?"
- "Are you under serious financial stress currently?" Financial stress related to the illness can contribute to marital and sexual conflict. In one study of men with erectile dysfunction, financial stress was the strongest predictor of a psychogenic etiology.[119]

USING QUESTIONNAIRES TO ASSESS SEXUAL FUNCTION

Asking patients to fill out questionnaires can sometimes save valuable clinician time. When large numbers of patients are being screened, giving questionnaires routinely allows the health care team to identify patients with high levels of sexual, marital, or psychological distress. Such patients can then be targeted for more detailed, interview assessment.

Patients receiving cancer treatment do not expect to fill out psychological testing. If a clinic or hospital uses screening questionnaires, the inventories should be presented to the patient by a member of the health care team with a rationale, a discussion of confidentiality, and an opportunity for the patient to ask questions or refuse to participate. In general, detailed information on sexuality, whether gathered by questionnaire or interview, should not become part of the patient's medical chart. Instead, we advocate that a sexual rehabilitation program keep private files.[55] Table 61-12 lists some questionnaires that we have found particularly useful.

TABLE 61-12. Questionnaires for Cancer Patients with Sexual Problems

Area of Assessment	*Questionnaire*
Sexual function	Sex History Form[55]
Marital satisfaction	Dyadic Adjustment Inventory[120]
Psychological distress	Brief Symptom Inventory[121]
Illness-related distress	Psychosocial Adjustment to Illness Scale[122]
Adjustment to cancer	Cancer Inventory of Problem Situations[123]

MEDICAL ASSESSMENT OF MALE SEXUAL DYSFUNCTION

Medical assessment of men's sexual problems has focused on ascertaining the causes of erectile dysfunction. A variety of specialized examinations are available, but some seem particularly relevant to the patient treated for cancer.

Although cancer treatment can damage hormonal, vascular, or neurologic aspects of erection, erectile dysfunction in a cancer patient often has a complex etiology, including psychological factors and medical conditions unrelated to cancer. Consider the case of a 62-year-old man with lymphoma, treated with combination chemotherapy and radiation therapy to the spine for leptomeningeal disease. He also has a history of alcohol abuse but has been sober for 5 years. His erections sporadically improve when he has a more arousing partner, suggesting a psychogenic component. Nevertheless, the erections are rarely fully rigid. An organic limitation on erections could result from hyperprolactinemia related to chronic antiemetic and opiate medication, a CNS effect from current use of opiates or chemotherapy agents, low levels of testosterone, spinal cord damage from tumor irradiation, or peripheral autonomic neuropathy. A proper evaluation should assess all these possibilities.

HISTORY. The evaluation begins with a clear definition of the sexual problem, as discussed above. The interviewer obtains a complete review of systems, a history of medication and illicit drug use, and a quantitative estimate of alcohol and tobacco consumption.

PHYSICAL EXAMINATION. The examiner observes the patient's affect and state of apparent general health, noting the presence or absence of secondary sex characteristics and gynecomastia. Following abdominal examination, the femoral pulses are palpated. The external genitalia are carefully examined. During a rectal examination, the anal sphincter tone, bulbocavernosus reflex, and prostate are checked. The patient's gait is observed. Motor strength, sensation, and deep tendon reflexes in the lower extremities are also assessed.

LABORATORY STUDIES. A complete blood count and SMA profile is a check for occult systemic disorders such as hepatic or renal disease. Serum testosterone and serum prolactin levels are also determined.[124] Hormonal levels are more often abnormal in some groups of cancer patients than in healthy men of similar age.[16,17] Because diabetes mellitus is a common cause of male erectile and ejaculatory disorders, a glucose tolerance test should be ordered unless the patient is already known to be diabetic.[125] Finally, thyroid function should be assessed by determining serum T_4 and TSH levels.

NOCTURNAL PENILE TUMESCENCE. From sleep studies we know that men have erections during rapid eye movement (REM) stages of sleep. Although abnormal sleep erections are often a sign of organic impotence,[126] they can also indicate depression[127] or a sleep disorder.[128] Nevertheless, full-scale nocturnal penile tumescence monitoring in a sleep laboratory, or screening with the Rigiscan device[129] or snap-gauges,[130] can help in planning appropriate treatment.

VASCULAR ASSESSMENT. Noninvasive vascular assessment consists primarily of systolic blood pressure determinations in the deep (cavernous) penile arteries using a 9 to 10 MHz Doppler stethoscope.[131] The ratio of penile systolic to brachial systolic pressure is known as the penile–brachial index (PBI). A PBI of less than 0.6 is considered highly suggestive of significant arterial disease.[132]

The nearly simultaneous discovery of Brindley and Virag[133,134] in the early 1980s that injection of vasoactive substances directly into the corpora cavernosa could produce erections led to the use of this technique both for diagnostic testing[135–137] and for treatment of erectile dysfunction.[138] For diagnostic purposes, papaverine hydrochloride (a potent smooth muscle relaxant) and phentolamine mesylate (an α-adrenergic blocking agent) are usually injected together directly into the corpora. A full, rigid erection implies that the penile circulation is normal. Thus, a full erectile response would be predicted in men with normal sexual function, psychogenically impotent men, and men with neurogenic impotence. A delayed or partial response suggests a circulatory abnormality: either arterial insufficiency or a corporeal-venous leak. If a patient has a poor response, normal saline is infused into the corpora. A good erection with saline infusion suggests that arterial insufficiency is the problem; a poor response suggests that a corporeal-venous leak exists.[27] These drug injection and corporeal infusion studies are commonly termed cavernosometry.

If cavernosometry suggests that arterial insufficiency exists and the patient wishes to consider the possibility of corporeal revascularization, penile (internal pudendal) arteriography is performed.[139] Likewise, if surgical treatment of a corporeal-venous leak is being considered, cavernosography is performed by injecting contrast material into the corpora and then obtaining radiographs of the corpora and their pelvic venous drainage.[28,140]

NEUROLOGIC ASSESSMENT. Vibratory perception threshold on the penis can be determined by applying a device known as a biothesiometer, which vibrates at a constant frequency while the amplitude is varied.[141] The bulbocavernosus reflex can be quantified by assessing the sacral evoked response.[142–144] When an electrical stimulus is applied to the penis, the evoked response is detected by an electromyographic needle placed in the bulbocavernosus muscle. If the evoked electroencephalographic wave form over the cerebral cortex is also recorded, this process is known as dorsal nerve somatosensory evoked potential testing.[145] Both the sacral evoked response and the dorsal nerve somatosensory evoked potential are tests of somatic nerve function. Unfortunately, no test can directly assess the autonomic innervation of the penis.

MEDICAL ASSESSMENT OF FEMALE SEXUAL DYSFUNCTION

We know less about the mechanisms of the female sexual response than we do about the male. The examinations available to the practitioner who wants to know the cause of a woman's sexual problems are thus far less sophisticated than the array available for erectile dysfunction.

The pelvic examination continues to be the mainstay of the evaluation for female sexual dysfunction. In women who may be experiencing ovarian failure, indices of vaginal atrophy such as skin elasticity, thickness of pubic hair, fullness of the labia, caliber of the vaginal introitus, color and rugation of the vaginal mucosa, and vaginal depth are important.[146] The physician can use a speculum or fingers to attempt to reproduce pelvic pain that a patient experiences during intercourse.[66] The cause of the pain then becomes more evident. Clinicians who examine women during systemic chemotherapy should look for an irritated vaginal mucosa. The effects of pelvic and vaginal irradiation can include reduced vascularization of the mucosa, vaginal ulcers or stenosis, or more diffuse fibrous changes in the vaginal walls or adnexae.[54]

Researchers continue to attempt to measure vaginal blood flow, analogous to noninvasive examinations of penile vascular integrity.[55] Unfortunately, such measurements in women must occur during sexual arousal and involve placing an instrument in the vagina.[147] Many women are not comfortable with erotic stimulation under laboratory conditions. The instruments used also have limited reliability, and thus far have not been very useful in measuring changes of menopause,[53] or in comparing healthy women to groups with some vaginal pathology.

Neurologic measures of genital reflex arcs in women have also proven unreliable and have no clear correlation with sexual symptoms.[148,149] Radioimmunoassays to measure serum levels of estradiol, prolactin, thyroid hormones, and follicle-stimulating hormone during amenorrhea or the first 5 days of a menstrual cycle can be helpful in deciding whether to prescribe replacement hormones for women showing signs of premature menopause after chemotherapy for cancers that are not hormone sensitive, for example leukemia or Hodgkin's disease.[48]

TREATING SEXUAL PROBLEMS IN CANCER PATIENTS

As Figure 61-3 illustrates, a treatment plan for a cancer patient's sexual problems often has multiple components. For example, even if a penile prosthesis would restore erections, brief sexual counseling might be needed to improve sexual communication or reduce marital conflict. The elements required depend on the causal factors that interacted to create the sexual dysfunction. We briefly describe current modalities of sexual rehabilitation in this section, citing resources for the clinician who wants to develop further skills in this area.

BRIEF SEXUAL COUNSELING

Brief sexual counseling is the backbone of sexual rehabilitation. Of patients referred for sexual consultation in a cancer center, 73% were seen only once or twice, and another 16% had only three to five sessions.[11] As we conceptualize it, brief sexual counseling includes five components: sex education, changing maladaptive sexual attitudes, advice on resuming sex comfortably, minimizing physical handicaps, and resolving marital conflict related to cancer treatment.[55]

SEX EDUCATION FOR CANCER PATIENTS. One of the most pressing needs of men and women with cancer is to understand how their bodies function and how cancer treatment changes that function. In the realm of sex, lifelike three-dimensional genital models that show internal and external anatomy are the clinician's most helpful educational tool.[55] Most men cannot identify their prostate gland or describe what it does. Few women have a clear picture of the location or appearance of the cervix. When cancer involves these areas of the body, patients usually have misconceptions about what to expect. Even when the tumor site is nongenital, the sexual impact of cancer treatment, for example on ovarian function, can best be understood in the context of a brief lesson on the sexual response cycle and pelvic anatomy. If a genital model is not available, a picture of the internal male organs or the female vulva can be valuable.

The American Cancer Society has also recently developed a guidebook for men and one for women on sexuality and cancer. These publications include diagrams, explanations of the sexual side-effects of cancer treatments, and advice on sexual rehabilitation.[150,151]

METHODS OF ATTITUDE CHANGE. Cancer patients sometimes believe myths about sexuality and cancer. Fear that sex could cause a recurrence or transmit cancer to the partner is a reason that many couples discontinue sex altogether. Rather than waiting for a patient to ask about such anxieties, the clinician who is familiar with common fears about sex and cancer[11,21–23] can bring up the topic routinely and debunk the myths.

A more stubborn area of maladaptive beliefs is the attitude that intercourse is the only "normal" type of sexual behavior, so that a noncoital orgasm or even body caressing without the goal of orgasm is considered off-limits. The clinician can discuss the wide range of normalcy in sexual practices and suggest that manual or oral genital caressing is a common and natural behavior. Many older patients or those with orthodox religious beliefs find oral sex frightening or disgusting. Strong preferences, or choices based on moral issues, should be respected. The clinician's role is to suggest alternatives, not to preach or proselytize. Self-help books about sex such as *Male Sexuality*[152] or *For Each Other*[153] can broaden a patient's perspective.

ADVICE ON RESUMING SEX. Cancer treatment often interrupts a couple's sex life completely for some period of time. Even when the patient recovers from surgery or chemotherapy and feels some return of sexual desire, initiating sex can be awkward. The partner also may fear hurting the patient or seeming to demand sex in a selfish way. Each perceives the other as uninterested in sex or fears rejection. The clinician's most important task is to help each partner discuss his or her desires to resume sex with the other. Fears about resuming sex, such as fear that the partner will be turned off by a surgical scar or ostomy, or that the patient will conceal pain during intercourse rather than disappoint the partner, should also be brought into the open.

Sensate focus exercises used in sex therapy provide an ideal framework for resuming sex.[55] Each partner takes turns giving and receiving a half-hour of all-over body caressing. At first the touching excludes the breasts and genitals to minimize any demand for sexual arousal, erections, or reaching orgasm. Over several sessions, more genital touching is allowed. Eventually the partners can help each other reach orgasm through manual or oral stimulation, and then proceed to intercourse. During the exercise, partners can practice communicating their desires for touch, either in words or by guiding each other's hands.

MINIMIZING PHYSICAL HANDICAPS. Cancer treatment can involve loss of a body part, as in limb amputation, vulvectomy, penectomy, or mastectomy. Other operative procedures create an ostomy. Chronic pain, fatigue, or limited range of motion are common sequelae of advanced disease or systemic treatments. Rather than expecting lovemaking to occur spontaneously, cancer patients may have to plan sexual activity for a time of day when they are not drowsy, nauseated, or in severe pain. Patients with ostomies can avoid foods that produce odor or gas and can empty their appliances before sex.[154]

No one coital position is right for every patient, but positioning for lovemaking is an important issue. Women with dyspareunia often have less pain when they sit or kneel over the male partner. That position allows the woman to control the angle of penetration and the speed and depth of thrusting. Women can reduce vaginal muscle tension by learning Kegel exercises.[66] Amputees or women with a mastectomy can use pillows to support tender areas of the body or to improve balance or stability during intercourse.

Some men and women are comfortable exposing an ostomy appliance, mastectomy site, or limb stump in the nude. Others feel more attractive and sensual when they create a "healthy illusion," using lingerie, a breast or limb prosthesis, makeup, or wigs to camouflage the physical changes wrought by cancer treatment.[155]

One group with special needs are head and neck cancer patients.[156] Many have facial deformities that affect self-esteem and perception by others. A laryngectomy interferes with sexual communication and presents problems of odor and mucous discharge if the patient is not meticulous. Clinicians need to devote more effort to developing sexual rehabilitation techniques to alleviate these problems.

RESOLVING COUPLE CONFLICT RELATED TO CANCER. The primary care team in a cancer treatment setting cannot do marital therapy, but they can often defuse minor conflicts between partners. The clinician can normalize disagreements, letting the couple know that a loss of private time, fear of losing one's role as wage-earner or nurturer in the family, and irritability are common during cancer treatments. Helping partners talk about areas of conflict with one another is often a big step in resolving the problems.

Common sense and an outsider's perspective aid the clinician in proposing solutions, such as suggesting a younger couple hire a babysitter and go out "on a date" once a week to have adult time together; encouraging an exhausted spouse to go home for the weekend instead of sleeping in the patient's hospital room; or rehearsing how a couple can jointly tell interfering in-laws to mind their own business.

INTENSIVE SEX THERAPY

Even the oncology clinician with interest and expertise in brief sexual counseling will find that perhaps 10% to 20% of patients have severe sexual dysfunctions that call for the specialty skills of a trained sex therapist.[55] Indications for referral to sex therapy include a sexual problem that preceded the cancer and is still a source of distress, sexual issues related to severe marital conflict, a dysfunction that has not responded to brief sexual counseling, or a sexual problem that appears to be just one feature of poor psychological coping. Some patients endure cancer treatments that are so mutilating, such as total pelvic exenteration, total penectomy, radical vulvectomy, or facial disfigurement, that consultation with a mental health professional trained in sex therapy should be routine during recovery, unless the patient objects.

Formal sex therapy is usually a short-term, symptom-focused treatment that ideally includes both partners.[154] The patients are given assigned tasks between sessions that include sensate focus exercises and learning other sexual techniques found effective in reversing specific dysfunctions. Work on marital communication and individual psychological well-being are often part of treatment. Sex therapy techniques have been useful in treating problems related to cancer and other chronic illnesses and may enhance the results of medical or surgical rehabilitation such as breast reconstruction or treatment of organic erectile dysfunction.[55]

TREATING ORGANIC ERECTILE DYSFUNCTION

Most cancer patients with organic erectile dysfunction will be candidates for either of two forms of treatment: therapeutic intracavernous injection or penile prosthesis implantation.

THERAPEUTIC INTRACAVERNOUS INJECTION. We have already discussed the usefulness of intracavernous injection in the evaluation of erectile function. Papaverine, alone or in combination with phentolamine, may also be used in many men for treatment of erectile dysfunction.[138] Men who do not develop any significant tumescence with the high doses of these agents used for testing are obviously poor candidates for therapeutic use, but those who achieve a partial erection in response to the test dose may still benefit, as sexual stimulation often increases the degree of response after injection.

Patients also need the cognitive ability to learn the self-injection program and the manual dexterity to perform the procedure. They should be compliant enough to come in for reversal if priapism occurs and committed to returning for regular follow-up examinations. Many cancer patients fit these criteria and see injection therapy as less drastic than a surgical intervention.

Complications of therapeutic intracavernous injections include prolonged erections (priapism), hematoma, infection, and fibrosis. The proper dosage for a patient produces an erection that will last 1 to 2 hours. If an erection persists beyond 3 to 4 hours, the patient must immediately return to his doctor for erection reversal. This is accomplished by aspirating blood from the corpora and then injecting a dilute solution of epinephrine (1 mg in 1000 ml of normal saline). Without reversal, the prolonged erection will result in corporeal hypoxia, which can produce severe intracavernous fibrosis.

Hematomas at the injection site can usually be avoided by directing the needle away from any visible blood vessels and by applying pressure to the injection site after the needle removal. Needles commonly used vary from 26 to 30 gauge and produce very little pain on injection. The patient is taught to avoid the dorsal midline neurovascular structures and the ventrally located urethra. Patients are also instructed to rotate the injection sites.

Infections are a theoretical complication of any injection procedure, and the patient must be appropriately cautioned to use proper sterile technique. Based on experience to date, infection is a very uncommon occurrence with these injections, but the risk of infection may be of special concern in an immunocompromised cancer patient.

At least one case of severe fibrosis has been reported following intracavernous injection therapy,[158] and there are increasing anecdotal and published reports of less severe cases.[159] Whether such fibrosis will necessitate stopping injection therapy or will complicate the subsequent implantation of a penile prosthesis remains to be seen.

PENILE PROSTHESIS IMPLANTATION. Although penile prosthesis implantation at the same time as pelvic cancer surgery has been advocated,[160] this practice has not gained widespread acceptance. Surgeons are reluctant to prolong the cancer operation or to incur the risk of periprosthetic infection. A certain percentage of patients also recover functional erections, especially with nerve-sparing techniques. This recovery process can take up to a year. The optimal time for prosthesis implantation appears to be at least 6 months following cancer surgery to give the patient time to recover and resume a normal life style.

Prosthesis implantation is often done through a single 2 to 4 cm incision. No tissue is removed and blood loss is minimal; blood transfusions are rarely if ever necessary. While penile prosthesis implantation has been done under local anesthesia on an outpatient basis,[161] most procedures are still performed under general or spinal anesthesia with a 1- to 2-day hospital stay.

Types of penile prostheses range from simple semirigid silicone rods to multiple component (cylinders, pump, fluid reservoir) hydraulic inflatable penile prostheses. A number of prostheses approach the simplicity of the semirigid rod devices but offer improved concealment. These include malleable penile prostheses, single-component hydraulic implants, and positionable, articulated rod prostheses (Figs. 61-4 and 61-5).[162]

Penile prosthesis surgery is successful in more than 95% of cases. Infection around the prosthesis occurs in approximately 2% to 5% of cases and invariably requires reoperation and removal of the prosthesis.[163] Later complications are usually mechanical device failures which, of course, require surgical revision. Device failures are least likely to occur with simple rod prostheses. The incidence of complications increases with increasing device complexity.

The fluid reservoir of a multiple-component inflatable prosthesis is usually implanted in the retropubic space. With special insertion tools the reservoir can be positioned through the same penoscrotal incision used to implant the other components of the prosthesis. In cancer patients who have had either pelvic irradiation or pelvic cancer surgery, a malleable or single-component hydraulic prosthesis without an abdominal reservoir is optimal. However, some patients desire the full penile girth and complete concealment of a multiple-component inflatable prosthesis. In those cases the surgeon can avoid the risk of injuring the bowel by placing the reservoir extraperitoneally behind a rectus muscle.[164] An inflatable prosthesis is best for the patient who needs repeated cystoscopic examinations. A multiple-component in-

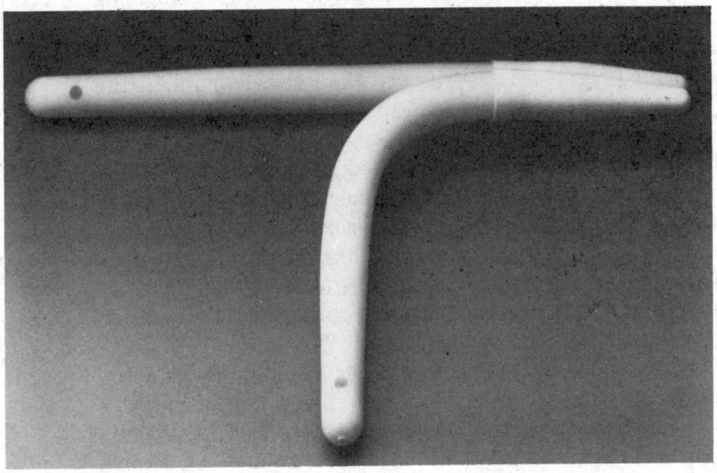

FIG. 61-4. A malleable penile prosthesis (AMS Malleable 600). (Courtesy of American Medical Systems, Inc, Minnetonka, MN)

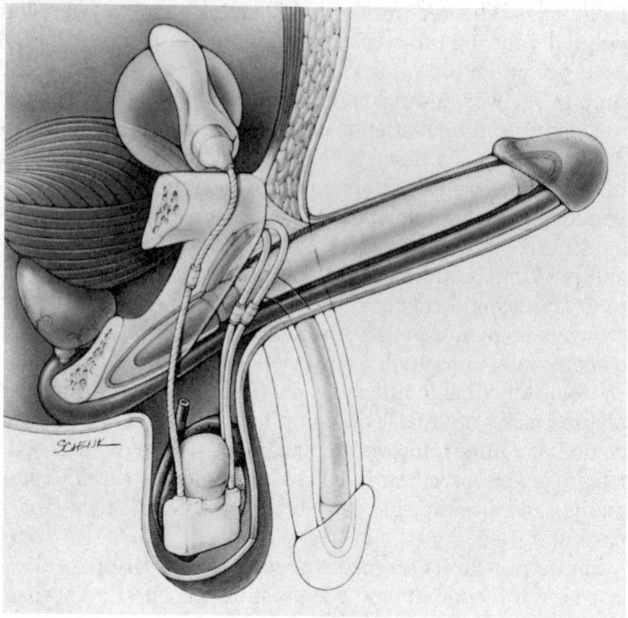

FIG. 61-5. A multiple component inflatable penile prosthesis (AMS Inflatable 700). (Courtesy of American Medical Systems, Inc, Minnetonka, MN)

flatable prosthesis can also compensate for some of the loss of penile girth after urethrectomy.

Surgeons debate about implanting a prosthesis in a man whose life expectancy is limited. We have seen patients benefit from a prosthesis, as long as their expected life span exceeds several months. For terminally ill patients, a simpler type of prosthesis minimizes the recovery time after surgery.

MEDICAL OR SURGICAL INTERVENTIONS FOR WOMEN

In contrast to the specific treatments for men's sexual problems, interventions for women are more closely linked to specific cancer therapies. Breast reconstruction can be considered a type of sexual rehabilitation, although enhancing sexual pleasure is not the primary motivation of most women who are candidates.

Vaginal reconstructive surgery more closely parallels the penile prosthesis in that it restores the functional capacity for intercourse. Split-thickness skin grafts have been helpful in enlarging the vagina after procedures such as vulvectomy or vaginectomy.[165] The disadvantages include the need to wear a vaginal stent for several weeks during healing, and then to practice regular vaginal dilation in order to keep vaginal size adequate. A positive feature is that the graft functions like a true vaginal mucosa, capable of expansion and lubrication with sexual arousal.[166]

For women undergoing total pelvic exenteration, simultaneous vaginal reconstruction with myocutaneous gracilis flaps has become the procedure of choice.[165,167] This technique creates a vagina with adequate size and cushioning. Although dilation is unnecessary, a woman does need to douche to minimize odor and must use extra lubrication for comfortable intercourse. Some women become coitally orgasmic after healing, but others find the neovagina has little erotic sensitivity. Recently, two clinicians suggested that vaginal reconstruction was often imposed on women by male surgeons who saw capacity for intercourse as the only criterion of sexual rehabilitation.[168] Their critique ignores the contribution of gracilis flaps to successful support of abdominal organs and postsurgical healing.[167] In our experience, even older women appreciate having a reconstructed vagina. The important point is to attend to psychological aspects of sexual rehabilitation as well as physical ones.[55]

Women who undergo premature menopause after cancer treatment need medical intervention. They should be considered for hormonal replacement unless an estrogen-sensitive tumor was involved.[4,50] With the use of topical and lower-dose regimes of estrogen and the addition of progestins to combination therapy, perhaps it is time to study the safety of hormonal therapy for women with node-negative breast cancer who have been free of disease for several years (Charles Vogel, personal communication). Nonhormonal medications such as clonidine are helpful for some women[169] but cannot relieve the vasomotor symptoms of many others. All women with vaginal dryness should be informed of the effective, water-based nonprescription lubricants now available. These include Transi-Lube foam (Carter-Wallace Co, New York), Lubrin suppositories (Upshur-Smith, Minneapolis, Minn), Astraglide (Astralube Co, North Hollywood, Fla), and Today Personal Lubricant (VLI Corporation, Irvine, Calif).

REFERENCES

1. Masters WH, Johnson VE: Human Sexual Inadequacy. Boston, Little, Brown & Co, 1970
2. Montague DK (ed): Disorders of Male Sexual Function. Chicago, Year Book Medical Publishers, 1987
3. Segraves RT, Schoenberg HW: Diagnosis and Treatment of Erectile Disturbances: A Guide for Clinicians. New York, Plenum Press, 1900
4. Ettinger B: Overview of the efficacy of hormonal replacement therapy. Am J Obstet Gynecol 156:1298–1303, 1987
5. Walsh PC, Mostwin JL: Radical prostatectomy and cystoprostatectomy with preservation of potency: Results using a new nerve-sparing technique. Br J Urol 56:694-697, 1984
6. Fischer MD, Bauer PH et al: Five-year results of a randomized clinical trial comparing total mastectomy and segmental mastectomy with or without irradiation in the treatment of breast cancer. N Engl J Med 312:665–673, 1985
7. Edwards CL, Stringer CA: Management of early carcinoma of the vulva, in Rutledge FN, Freedman RS, Gershenson DM (eds): Gynecologic Cancer: Diagnostic and Treatment Strategies, pp 285–290. Austin, Texas, University of Texas Press, 1986
8. Johnson DE, Lo RK, von Eschenback AC et al: Surveillance alone for patients with clinical stage I nonseminomatous germ cell tumors of the testis: Preliminary results. J Urol 131:491–493, 1984
9. American Psychiatric Association: Diagnostic and Statistical Manual of Mental Disorders, 3rd ed, rev. Washington, DC, American Psychiatric Association Press, 1987
10. Schover LR, Friedman J, Weiler S et al: The multiaxial problem-oriented diagnostic system for sexual dysfunctions. Arch Gen Psychiatry 39:614–619, 1982
11. Schover LR, Evans RB, von Eschenbach AC: Sexual rehabilitation in a cancer center: Diagnosis and outcome in 384 consultations. Arch Sex Behav 16:445–461, 1987
12. Miller BL, Cummings JL, McIntyre H et al: Hypersexuality or altered sexual preference following brain injury. J Neurol Neurosurg Psychiatry 49:867–873, 1986
13. Kaplan HS: Sexual Aversion, Sexual Phobias, and Panic Disorder. New York, Brunner/Mazel, 1987
14. Schover LR: Sexuality and fertility in urologic cancer patients. Cancer 60(suppl):553–558, 1987

15. Fossa SD, Klepp O, Molne K et al: Testicular function after unilateral orchiectomy for cancer and before further treatment. Int J Androl 5:179–184, 1982
16. Vigersky RA, Chapman RM, Berenberg J et al: Testicular dysfunction in untreated Hodgkin's disease. Am J Med 73:482–486, 1982
17. Bancroft J, Sanders D, Davidson D et al: Mood, sexuality, hormones, and the menstrual cycle: III. Sexuality and the role of androgens. Psychosom Med 45:509–516, 1983
18. Bukberg J, Penman D, Holland JC: Depression in hospitalized cancer patients. Psychosom Med 46:199–212, 1984
19. Derogatis LR, Morrow GR, Fetting J et al: The prevalence of psychiatric disorders among cancer patients. JAMA 249:751–757, 1983
20. Rieker PP, Edbril SD, Garnick MB: Curative testis cancer therapy: Psychosocial sequellae. J Clin Oncol 3:1117–1126, 1985
21. Schover LR, von Eschenbach AC: Sexual and marital relationships after treatment for nonseminomatous testicular cancer. Urology 25:251–255, 1985
22. Schover LR, Gonzales M, von Eschenbach AC: Sexual and marital relationships after radiotherapy for seminoma. Urology 27:117–123, 1986
23. Schover LR, Fife M, Gershenson DM: Sexual rehabilitation and treatment for early stage cervical cancer (unpublished manuscript)
24. Liss-Levinson WS: Clinical observations on the emotional responses of males to cancer. Psychother Theory Res Pract 19:325–330, 1982
25. O'Carroll R, Shapiro C, Bancroft J: Androgens, behaviour and nocturnal erection in hypogonadal men: The effects of varying the replacement dose. Clin Endocrinol 23:527–538, 1985
26. Michal V: Arterial disease as a cause of impotence. Clin Endocrinol Metab 11:725–748, 1982
27. Buvat J, Lemaire A, Dehaene JL et al: Venous incompetence: Critical study of the organic basis of high maintenance flow rates during artificial erection test. J Urol 135:926–928, 1986
28. Lue TF, Hricak H, Schmidt RA et al: Functional evaluation of penile veins by cavernosography in papaverine-induced erection. J Urol 135:479–482, 1986
29. Goldstein I, Feldman MI, Deckers PJ et al: Radiation-associated impotence: A clinical study of its mechanism. JAMA 251:903–910, 1984
30. Mittal B: A study of penile circulation before and after radiation in patients with prostate cancer and its effect on impotence. Int J Radiat Oncol Biol Phys 11:1121–1125, 1985
31. Nijman JM: Some Aspects of Sexual and Gonadal Function in Patients with Nonseminomatous Germ-Cell Tumor of the Testis (dissertation). Groningen, The Netherlands, Drukkerij Van Denderen BV, 1987
32. Lue TF, Hricak H, Marich KW et al: Evaluation of arteriogenic impotence with intracorporeal injection of papaverine and the duplex ultrasound scanner. Semin Urol 3:43–48, 1985
33. Bergman B, Sivertsson S, Suurkala M: Penile blood pressure in erectile impotence following cystectomy. Scand J Urol Nephrol 16:81–84, 1982
34. Tizzani A, Casetta G, Carone R et al: Defective erection in patients subjected to radical cystectomy: Diagnosis by Doppler test and stimulated sacral reflex. Minerva Urol Nefrol 37:335–339, 1985
35. Lepor H, Gregerman M, Crosby R et al: Precise localization of the autonomic nerves from the pelvic plexus to the corpora cavernosa: A detailed anatomical study of the adult male pelvis. J Urol 133:207–212, 1985
36. Lue TF, Zeineh SJ, Schmidt RA et al: Neuroanatomy of penile erection: Its relevance to iatrogenic impotence. J Urol 131:273–280, 1984
37. Balslev I, Harling H: Sexual dysfunction following operation of carcinoma of the rectum. Dis Colon Rectum 26:785–788, 1983
38. Danzi M, Ferulano GP, Abate S et al: Male sexual function after abdominoperineal resection for rectal cancer. Dis Colon Rectum 26:665–668, 1983
39. La Monica G, Audisio RA, Tamburini M et al: Incidence of sexual dysfunction in male patients treated surgically for rectal malignancy. Dis Colon Rectum 28:937–940, 1985
40. Neal D: The effects on pelvic visceral function of anal sphincter ablating and anal sphincter preserving operations for cancer of the lower part of the rectum and for benign colo-rectal disease. Ann R Coll Surg Engl 66:7–13, 1984
41. Kinn C, Ohman V: Bladder and sexual function after surgery for rectal cancer. Dis Colon Rectum 29:43–48, 1986
42. Williams NS, Johnston D: The quality of life after rectal excision for low rectal cancer. Br J Surg 70:460–462, 1983
43. Yeager ES, Van Heerden JA: Sexual dysfunction following proctocolectomy and abdominoperineal resection. Ann Surg 191:169–170, 1980
44. Schover LR, Evans RB, von Eschenbach AC: Sexual rehabilitation and male radical cystectomy. J Urol 136:1015–1017, 1986
45. Catalona WJ, Dresner SM: Nerve-sparing radical prostatectomy: Extraprostatic tumor extension and preservation of erectile function. J Urol 134:1149–1151, 1985
46. Hjortrup A, Kirkegaard P, Friis J et al: Sexual dysfunction after low anterior resection for midrectal cancer. Acta Chir Scand 150:687–688, 1984
47. Schilsky RL, Davidson HS, Magid D et al: Gonadal and sexual function in male patients with hairy cell leukemia: Lack of adverse effects of recombinant alpha-2-interferon. Cancer Treat Rep 71:179–181, 1987
48. Chapman RM: Effect of cytotoxic therapy on sexuality and gonadal function. Semin Oncol 9:84–94, 1982
49. Suttcliffe SB: Clinical problems and their management: Clinical problems in females with lymphoma. In: Proceedings of Workshop on Psychosexual and Reproductive Issues of Cancer Patients. Chicago, American Cancer Society, 1987
50. Chapman RM, Sutcliffe SB, Malpas JS: Cytotoxic-induced ovarian failure in Hodgkin's disease: II. Effects on sexual function. JAMA 242:1882–1884, 1979
51. Budel VM, Paridaens RJ, Spetschinsky A et al: Effects of aminoglutethimide plus hydrocortisone on the genital tract of postmenopausal women with advanced breast cancer: A clinical and cytologic survey. Anticancer Res 6:709–712, 1986
52. Semmens JP, Tsai CC, Semmens EC et al: Effects of estrogen therapy on vaginal physiology during menopause. Obstet Gynecol 66:15–18, 1985
53. Myers LS, Morokoff PJ: Physiological and subjective sexual arousal in pre- and postmenopausal women and postmenopausal women taking replacement therapy. Psychophysiology 23:283–292, 1986
54. Abitbol MM, Davenport JH: The irradiated vagina. Obstet Gynecol 44:249–256, 1974
55. Schover LR, Jensen SB: Sexuality and Chronic Illness: A Comprehensive Approach. New York, Guilford Press, 1988
56. Andersen BL, Hacker NF: Psychosexual adjustment after vulvar surgery. Obstet Gynecol 62:457–462, 1983
57. Moth I, Andreasson B, Jensen SB et al: Sexual function and somatopsychic reactions after vulvectomy. Dan Med Bull 30(suppl):27–30, 1983
58. Andersen BL, Hacker NF: Psychosexual adjustment following pelvic exenteration. Obstet Gynecol 61:331–338, 1983
59. Schover LR: Sexual function in female radical cystectomy: A case series. J Urol 134:465–468, 1985
60. Lange PH, Narayan P, Fraley EE: Fertility issues following therapy for testicular cancer. Semin Urol 11:264–274, 1984
61. Tomoda H, Furosawa M: Sexual and urinary dysfunction following surgery for sigmoid colon cancer. Jpn J Surg 15:355–360, 1985
62. Jamison KR, Wellisch DK, Pasnau RO: Psychosocial aspects of mastectomy: I. The woman's perspective. Am J Psychiatry 135:432–436, 1978
63. Alzate H, Hoch Z: The "G spot" and "female ejaculation": A current appraisal. J Sex Marital Ther 12:211–220, 1986
64. Edwards CL, Loeffler M, Rutledge FN: Vaginal reconstruction. In von Eschenbach AC, Rodriguez DB (eds): Sexual Rehabilitation of the Urologic Cancer Patient, pp 251–264. Boston, GK Hall, 1981
65. Morley GW, Lindenauer SM, Youngs D: Vaginal reconstruction following pelvic exenteration: Surgical and psychological considerations. Am J Obstet Gynecol 116:996–1002, 1973
66. Fordney DS: Dyspareunia and vaginismus. Clin Obstet Gynecol 21:205–221, 1978
67. Hansen MK: Surgical and combination therapy of the cervix uteri stages Ib and IIa. Gynecol Oncol 11:275–287, 1981
68. Andersen BL: Sexual difficulties for women following cancer treatment. In Andersen BL (ed): Women and Cancer: Psychological Perspectives, pp 257–288. New York, Springer-Verlag, 1986
69. Vincent CE, Vincent B, Griess FC et al: Some marital–sexual concomitants of carcinoma of the cervix. South Med J 68:552–558, 1975
70. Andersen BL: Longitudinal study of gynecologic oncology patients: Sexual and psychological outcomes. Presented at the American Cancer Society 28th Science Writers' Seminar, Daytona Beach, Fla, March 1986
71. Bard M, Sutherland AM: Psychological impact of cancer and its treatment: IV. Adaptation to radical mastectomy. Cancer 8:656–672, 1955
72. Renneker R, Cutler M: Psychological problems of adjustment to cancer of the breast. JAMA 148:833–838, 1952
73. Worden JW, Weisman AD: The fallacy in postmastectomy depression. Am J Med Sci 273:169–175, 1977
74. Andersen BL, Jochimsen PR: Sexual functioning among breast cancer, gynecologic cancer, and healthy women. J Consult Clin Psychol 53:25–32, 1985
75. Taylor SE, Lichtman RR, Wood JJ et al: Illness related and treatment related factors in psychological adjustment to breast cancer. Cancer 55:2506–2513, 1985
76. Jamison KR, Wellisch DK, Pasnau RO: Psychosocial aspects of mastectomy: I. The woman's perspective. Am J Psychiatry 135:432–436, 1978
77. Sanger CK, Reznikoff M: A comparison of the psychological effects of breast saving procedures with the modified radical mastectomy. Cancer 48:2341–2346, 1981
78. Cohen RS, Wellisch DK, Christensen A et al: Effect of mastectomy and lumpectomy on dimensions of mood, self-concept, impairment and marital satisfaction. Proc Am Soc Clin Oncol 3:72, 1984
79. Steinberg MD, Juliano MA, Wise L: Psychological outcome of lumpectomy versus mastectomy in the treatment of breast cancer. Am J Psychiatry 142:34–39, 1985
80. Baider L, Rizel S, Kaplan De-Nour A: Comparison of couples' adjustment to lumpectomy and mastectomy. Gen Hosp Psychiatry 8:251–257, 1986
81. Schain W, Edwards BK, Gorrell CR et al: Psychosocial and physical outcomes of primary breast cancer therapy: Mastectomy vs. excisional biopsy and irradiation. Breast Cancer Res Treat 3:377–382, 1983
82. Ashcroft JJ, Leinster SJ, Slade PD: Breast cancer-patient choice of treatment: Preliminary communication. J R Soc Med 78:43–46, 1985
83. Schain WS, Findley P, D'Angelo T et al: A prospective psychosocial assessment of breast cancer patients receiving mastectomy or radiation therapy in a randomized clinical trial. Proc Am Soc Chemother Oncol 4(No. C-968):248, 1985
84. Bartelink H, Van Dam F, Van Dongen J: Psychological effects of breast conservation therapy in comparison with radical mastectomy. Int J Radiat Oncol Biol Phys 2:381–388, 1985
85. Wellisch DK, Jamison KR, Pasnau RO: Psychological aspects of mastectomy: II. The man's perspective. Am J Psychiatry 135:543–546, 1978
86. Wabrek A, Wabrek CJ: Mastectomy: Sexual implications. Primary Care 3:803–810, 1976

87. Clifford E, Clifford M, Georgiade NG: Breast reconstruction following mastectomy: II. Marital characteristics of women seeking this procedure. Ann Plast Surg 5:343–346, 1980
88. Schain WS, Jacobs E, Wellisch DK: Psychosocial issues in breast reconstruction: Intrapsychic, interpersonal, and practical concerns. Clin Plast Surg 11:237–251, 1984
89. Noone RB, Frazier TG, Hayward CZ et al: Patient acceptance of immediate reconstruction following mastectomy. Plast Reconstr Surg 69:632–638, 1982
90. Stevens LA, McGrath MH, Druss RG et al: The psychological impact of immediate breast reconstruction for women with early breast cancer. Plast Reconstr Surg 73:619–626, 1984
91. Schain WS, Wellisch DK, Pasnau RO et al: The sooner the better: A study of psychological factors in women undergoing immediate versus delayed breast reconstruction. Am J Psychiatry 142:40–46, 1985
92. Dean C, Chetty V, Forrest AMP: Effects of immediate breast reconstruction on psychosocial morbidity after mastectomy. Lancet 2:459–462, 1983
93. McGraw J, Horton C, Grossman J et al: An early appraisal of the methods of tissue expansion and the transverse rectus abdominus musculocutaneous flap in reconstruction of the breast following mastectomy. Ann Plast Surg 18:93–113, 1987
94. Wellisch DM, Schain WS, Noone B et al: Psychological contribution of nipple addition in breast reconstruction. Plastic Reconstr Surg (in press)
95. Christensen D: Postmastectomy couple counseling: An outcome study of a structured treatment protocol. J Sex Marital Ther 9:267–270, 1982
96. Meyerowitz BE: Psychosocial correlates of breast cancer and its treatments. Psychol Bull 87:108–131, 1980
97. Knob P: Physical and psychological distress associated with adjuvant chemotherapy in women with breast cancer. J Clin Oncol 4:678–684, 1986
98. Nugent P, O'Connell TX: Breast cancer and pregnancy. Arch Surg 120:122–124, 1985
99. Bush H, McCredie JA: Carcinoma of the breast during pregnancy and lactation. In Allen HH, Nisker JA (eds): Cancer and Pregnancy: Therapeutic Guidelines, pp 91–101. Mount Kisco, New York, Futura, 1986
100. Querleu D, Laurent JC, Verhaeghe M: Pregnancy following surgery for cancer of the breast. J Gynecol Obstet Biol Reprod 15:633–639, 1986
101. Riberio G, Jones DA, Jones M: Carcinoma of the breast associated with pregnancy. Br J Surg 73:607–609, 1986
102. Lieber MM: Surgery vs. radiation for localized prostate cancer. Oncology 1:61–71, 1987
103. Eggleston JC, Walsh PC: Radical prostatectomy with preservation of sexual function: Pathological findings in the first 100 cases. J Urol 134:1146–1148, 1985
104. Zagars GK, von Eschenbach AC, Johnson DE et al: The role of radiation therapy in stages A2 and B adenocarcinoma of the prostate. Int J Radiat Ther Oncol Biol Phys (in press)
105. Zagars GK, von Eschenbach AC, Johnson DE et al: Stage C adenocarcinoma of the prostate: Analysis of 551 cases treated with external radiation therapy. Cancer (in press)
106. Middleton RG, Smith JA, Melzer RB et al: Patient survival and local recurrence rate following radical prostatectomy for prostatic carcinoma. J Urol 136:422–424, 1986
107. Pontes JE, Huben R, Wolf R: Sexual function after radical prostatectomy. Prostate 8:123–126, 1986
108. Li FP, Connelly RR, Myers M: Improved survival rates among testis cancer patients in the United States. JAMA 247:825–826, 1982
109. Gritz ER, Wellisch DK, Landsverk JA: Psychosocial sequelae in long-term survivors of testicular cancer. J Psychosoc Oncol (in press)
110. Schover LR, von Eschenbach AC: Sexual and marital counseling with men treated for testicular cancer. J Sex Marital Ther 10:29–40, 1984
111. Javadpour N, Moley J: Alternative to retroperitoneal lymphadenectomy with preservation of ejaculation and fertility in Stage I nonseminomatous testicular cancer. Cancer 55:1604–1606, 1985
112. Peckham MJ, Brada M: Surveillance following orchidectomy for stage I testicular cancer. Int J Androl 10:247–254, 1987
113. Donohue JP: Retroperitoneal lymphadenectomy (RPLND) in low stage disease: One point of view. Prog Clin Biol Res 203:287–311, 1985
114. Maguire P, Brooke M, Tact A et al: The effect of counseling on physical disability and social recovery after mastectomy. Clin Oncol 9:319–324, 1983
115. Goedert JJ: Sounding board: What is safe sex? Suggested standards linked to testing for human immunodeficiency virus. N Engl J Med 316:1339–1341, 1987
116. Wyatt GE, Strayer RG, Lobitz WC: Issues in the treatment of sexually dysfunctioning couples of Afro-American descent. In LoPiccolo J, LoPiccolo L (eds): Handbook of Sex Therapy, pp 441–450. New York, Plenum Press, 1978
117. Lieber L, Plumb MM, Gerstenzang ML et al: The communication of affection between cancer patients and their spouses. Psychosom Med 38:379–389, 1976
118. Chapman RM, Sutcliffe SB, Malpas JS: Male gonadal dysfunction in Hodgkin's disease: A prospective study. JAMA 245:1323–1328, 1981
119. Reid K, Surridge D, Harris C et al: The psychological correlates of psychogenic impotence: A retrospective comparison of psychogenically and organically impotent men. Sex Disabil (in press)
120. Spanier GB: Measuring dyadic adjustment: New scales for assessing the quality of marriage and similar dyads. J Marriage Fam 38:15–28, 1976
121. Derogatis LR, Melisaratos N: The Brief Symptom Inventory: An introductory report. Psychol Med 13:595–605, 1983
122. Derogatis LR: Psychosocial Adjustment to Illness Scale (PAIS and PAIS-SR): Scoring Procedures and Administration Manual—I. Baltimore, Md, Clinical Psychometric Research, 1983
123. Heinrich RL, Schag CC, Ganz P: Living with cancer: The Cancer Inventory of Problem Situations. J Clin Psychol 40:972–980, 1984
124. Maatman TJ, Montague DK, Martin LM: Cost-effective evaluation of impotence. Urology 27:132–135, 1986
125. Maatman TJ, Montague DK, Martin LM: Erectile dysfunction in men with diabetes mellitus. Urology 29:589–592, 1987
126. Karacan I: Clinical value of nocturnal erection in the prognosis and diagnosis of impotence. Med Aspects Hum Sex 4:27–34, 1970
127. Thase ME, Reynolds CE, Glanz LM et al: Nocturnal penile tumescence in depressed men. Am J Psychiatry 144:89–92, 1987
128. Pressman MR, DiPhillipo MA, Kendrick JI et al: Problems in the interpretation of nocturnal penile tumescence studies: Disruption of sleep by occult sleep disorders. J Urol 136:595–598, 1986
129. Kaneko S, Bradley WE: Evaluation of erectile dysfunction with continuous monitoring of rigidity. J Urol 136:1026–1029, 1986
130. Ek A, Bradley WE, Krane RJ: Nocturnal penile rigidity measured by the snap-gauge band. J Urol 129:964–966, 1983
131. Abelson D: Diagnostic value of the penile pulse and blood pressure: A Doppler study of impotence in diabetics. J Urol 130:636–639, 1975
132. deWolfe VG: Noninvasive evaluation of vasculogenic impotence. In Montague DK (ed): Disorders of Male Sexual Function. Chicago, Year Book Medical Publishers, 1988
133. Virag R: Intravenous injection of papaverine for erectile failure. Lancet 2:938, 1982
134. Brindley GS: Cavernosal alpha-blockade: A new technique for investigating and treating erectile impotence.
135. Virag R, Spencer PP, Frydman D: Artificial erection in diagnosis and treatment of impotence. Urology 24:157–161, 1984
136. Abber JC, Lue TF, Orvis BR et al: Diagnostic tests for impotence: A comparison of papaverine injection with the penile-brachial index and nocturnal penile tumescence monitoring. J Urol 135:923–925, 1986
137. Buvat J, Buvat-Herbaut M, Dehaene JL et al: Is intravascular injection of papaverine a reliable screening test for vascular impotence? J Urol 135:476–478, 1900
138. Zorgniotti AW, Lefleur RS: Auto-injection of the corpus cavernosum with a vasoactive drug combination for vasculogenic impotence. J Urol 133:39–41, 1985
139. Ginestie JF, Romieu A (eds): Radiologic Exploration of Impotency. The Hague, Martinus Nijhoff, 1978
140. Porst H, Altwein JE, Bach D et al: Venous outflow studies of cavernous bodies. J Urol 134:276–279, 1985
141. Newman HF: Vibratory sensitivity of the penis. Fertil Steril 21:791–793, 1970
142. Ertekin C, Reel F: Bulbocavernosus reflex in normal men and in patients with neurogenic bladder and/or impotence. J Neurol Sci 28:1–15, 1976
143. Siroky MB, Sax DS, Krane RJ: Sacral signal tracing: The electrophysiology of the bulbocavernosus reflex. J Urol 122:661–664, 1979
144. Krane RJ, Siroky MB: Studies on sacral-evoked potentials. J Urol 124:872–874, 1980
145. Goldstein I: Electromyography evoked-response evaluations. In Barrett DM, Wein AJ (eds): Controversies in Neuro-Urology. New York, Churchill-Livingstone, 1984
146. Leiblum SR, Bachmann G, Kemmann E et al: Vaginal atrophy in the postmenopausal woman: The importance of sexual activity and hormones. JAMA 249:2195–2198, 1983
147. Hoon PW: Physiologic assessment of sexual response in women: The unfulfilled promise. Clin Obstet Gynecol 27:767–780, 1984
148. Blaivas JG, Zayed AAH, Labib KB: The bulbocavernosus reflex in urology: A prospective study of 299 patients. J Urol 126:197–199, 1981
149. Haldeman S, Bradley WE, Bhatia WN et al: Pudendal evoked responses. Arch Neurol 39:280–283, 1982
150. Schover LR, Randers-Pehrson M: Sexuality and Cancer: For the Man Who Has Cancer, and His Partner. New York, American Cancer Society, 4658, 1988
151. Schover LR, Randers-Pehrson M: Sexuality and Cancer: For the Woman Who Has Cancer, and Her Partner. New York, American Cancer Society, 4657, 1988
152. Zilbergeld B: Male Sexuality. New York, Bantam Books, 1978
153. Barbach L: For Each Other: Sharing Sexual Intimacy. Garden City, New York, Anchor Press/Doubleday, 1982
154. Schover LR: Sexual rehabilitation of the ostomy patient. In Smith DB, Johnson DE (eds): Ostomy Care and the Cancer Patient: Surgical and Clinical Considerations, pp 103–120. Orlando, Fla, Grune & Stratton, 1986
155. Schain WS: Sexual and reproductive issues in breast cancer. In: Proceedings of the Workshop on Psychosexual and Reproductive Issues of Cancer Patients. New York, American Cancer Society, 1987
156. Petrucci RJ, Harwick RD: Role of the psychologist on a radical head and neck surgical service team. Professional Psychol Res Pract 15:538–543, 1984
157. Kaplan HS: The New Sex Therapy. New York, Brunner/Mazel, 1974
158. Larsen EH, Gasser TC, Bruskewitz RC: Fibrosis of corpus cavernosum after intracavernous injection of phentolamine/papaverine. J Urol 137:292–293, 1987
159. Althof SE, Turner LA, Levine SB et al: Intracavernosal injection in the treatment of impotence: A prospective study of sexual, psychological, and marital functioning. J Sex Marital Ther 13:155–167, 1987
160. Bennett AH: Placement of penile prosthesis during surgery for malignancies. Urology 20:276–277, 1982
161. Kaufman JJ: Penile prosthetic surgery under local anesthesia. J Urol 128:1190–1191, 1982

162. Montague DK: Penile prostheses. In Montague DK (ed): Disorders of Male Sexual Function. Chicago, Year Book Medical Publishers, 1988
163. Montague DK: Periprosthetic infections. J Urol 138:68–69, 1987
164. Scott FB, Light JK, Fishman IJ: Treatment of impotency caused by cancer therapy: The inflatable penile prosthesis. Cancer Bull 34:33–39, 1982
165. Edwards C, Loeffler M, Rutledge FN: Vaginal reconstruction. In von Eschenbach AC, Rodriguez DB (eds): Sexual Rehabilitation of the Urologic Cancer Patient, pp 250–265. Boston, GK Hall, 1981
166. Masters WH, Johnson VE: Human Sexual Response. Boston, Little, Brown & Co, 1966
167. Rutledge FN: Pelvic exenteration: An update of the U.T.M.D. Anderson Hospital experience and review of the literature. In Rutledge FN, Freedman R, Gershenson DM (eds): Gynecologic Cancer: Diagnosis and Treatment Strategies, pp 7–30. Austin, Texas, University of Texas Press, 1987
168. Cairns KV, Valentich M: Vaginal reconstruction in gynecologic cancer: A feminist perspective. J Sex Res 22:333–346, 1986
169. Laufer LR, Yohanan E, Meldrum DR et al: Effect of clonidine on hot flashes in postmenopausal women. Obstet Gynecol 60:583–586, 1982

GRACE CHRIST
LIBBY L. KLEIN
MATTHEW LOSCALZO
LOIS L. WEINSTEIN

SECTION 3

Community Resources for Cancer Patients

A patient diagnosed with cancer may require a range of assistive services. These resources have never been more essential to the patient's treatment and recovery than in the contemporary medical climate. An increasing number of cancer patients are being cured, and many other patients are living for a long time with cancer as a chronic illness. At the same time, with the introduction of prepayment systems in hospitals and greatly abbreviated hospital stays, more and more patients are being treated and cared for in outpatient settings. These changes, together with scientific advances in the treatment of cancer, have necessitated the development of different types of community services and more comprehensive systems of care to meet the broad range of patients' needs.

EMERGING PROBLEMS

Those for whom cancer is a prolonged chronic illness must deal with gradual debilitation, progression of disease, and fears of loss of control over the disease. The chronicity of the disease may interfere with fulfillment of normal developmental tasks and deplete financial, personal, and social resources. The stresses of chronic cancer often are heightened by the cost of medical care and surveillance, which can exhaust insurance and the family's resources. Finally, individuals with chronic cancer have few positive models to emulate. Social models tend to reflect cured patients who can continue in their roles in the community with no apparent impediments, or those who die heroically. There are few models of the courage it takes to live day by day in this society with a chronic, sometimes terminal illness.

Patients who are cured must reenter a culture that values individuals who emerge unscathed from a crisis, yet they must cope with their need for ongoing social and psychological rehabilitation. They may have lost hair, a breast, limb, or other organ; gained or lost weight; or suffered other effects of the disease or treatment, including infertility. They must live with the fear of recurrence of cancer or the development of a new cancer, possibly caused by the treatment for the original cancer. Finally, they may confront social discrimination in employment and in obtaining further health insurance. The notion that survivors can pick up where they left off is inconsistent with the experience of the majority of persons who have been successfully treated for cancer. Instead, the illness constitutes a major discontinuity in their lives that brings about lasting changes in the way they perceive themselves and their future.[1] Few support resources now exist in the community to help survivors deal with these obstacles to developing meaningful and productive lives.

Unfortunately, the health insurance system did not respond to the shift from hospital-based care to community care by providing greater coverage for outpatient treatment or home care. Thus, most outpatient costs—bills for care at clinics and travel costs—either are not covered or are inadequately reimbursed. In addition, home care services that traditionally have been covered by Medicare, Medicaid, and Blue Cross have been severely curtailed; in some cases, nursing care is reimbursed for only 2 hours a day. Moreover, health insurance policies rarely cover custodial care, focusing instead on skilled nursing care. The few resources that exist in some communities for these needs are often overwhelmed by the demand from many treatment institutions.

To deal with this problem, practitioners must be cognizant of a large network of agencies and community services that address patient needs. By so doing, they will be able to match individual patients quickly with the appropriate resources in the patients' locales.[2]

COMMUNITY RESOURCE NEEDS OF CANCER PATIENTS

Most of the literature on community resources available for cancer patients has focused on planning for the discharge of patients after an acute episode of illness[3–5] or on the care of cancer patients (at home or in a hospice) during the terminal phase of the illness.[6–10] Little has been written about the needs of patients in the chronic phase of cancer, when the progression of the disease and intensified treatment make the patient more and more debilitated but not yet in need of acute hospitalization or hospice care.[11–13]

In this chronic phase, patients may experience not only symptoms of the disease but the sequelae of chemotherapy and radiation therapy, such as nausea and vomiting, anorexia, weight loss, pancytopenia, and weakness.[12] Improved methods of medical management are increasing patients' tolerance of highly cytotoxic chemotherapeutic agents and have made it possible for any patient to be treated on an outpatient basis.[11] However, because of variations in the course of the disease and the unpredictability of the side-effects of chemotherapy and radiation, medical crises may arise suddenly and create concomitant changes in the types of home care the patients need.[11] Discharge plans that appear satisfactory immediately after hospitalization cannot always anticipate the patient's future needs as the disease progresses. Thus, when further deterioration occurs months later, the patient is an outpatient and is not as easily identified as requiring services,[14] since fewer screening mechanisms are in place for determining the resources that this population needs.

In recent years, the growing emphasis on discharge planning has heightened the awareness of oncology health professionals of the importance of the careful coordination of post-hospital care for cancer patients. Such coordination is crucial to ensure an uninterrupted flow of health services that will maximize the patient's chance of recovering his or her functional status and will minimize health expenditures.[15] Since the prospective payment system began to be phased into the health care system in 1983, the length of stay for inpatients has decreased and the demand for outpatient services has increased proportionately. Clearly, helping patients return home and remain at home have become national priorities. The identification of necessary supportive resources in the community and the development of new services are essential to this end.

The community resources that cancer patients need may be broken down into the following five categories:

1. *Financial assistance* for treatment and income maintenance.
2. *Home care*, including personal care and household assistance; *personal care*, including injections, the care of catheters, stoma management, nasogastric tube feeding, pain management, medical monitoring, grooming, bathing, dressing, and physical or occupational therapy[13,17]; and *household assistance*, including housecleaning, meal preparation, laundering, and shopping.[16]
3. *Equipment*, such as wheelchairs, walkers, bath benches, bed pans, urinals, commodes, hospital beds, alternating pressure mattresses, intravenous poles and pumps, and stoma bags.[16,17]
4. *Transportation*, including ambulances, ambulettes, taxis, car services, or volunteer drivers.[9]
5. *Emotional support and planning*, including psychological counseling, financial counseling, recreation, companionship, legal advice, and nutritional counseling.[16]

PREVALENCE OF PATIENTS' NEEDS

Many studies have estimated the extent to which cancer patients need community resources. Googe and Varricchio[17] noted that each of the 15 patients and family members they studied needed transportation, but that almost all the subjects thought that this need was being met satisfactorily. Two thirds or more of the patients acknowledged a need for help with activities of daily living; 25%, help with bathing; 30%, help with ambulation; and 80%, help with household chores, especially shopping. Financial help to pay for the additional expenses of care was also frequently mentioned.

The American Cancer Society's study of 810 patients found that daily home help was most often listed as a priority.[18] Twenty-two percent of the family members and 14% of the patients who responded cited home care as the most needed service, especially during the initial phase of treatment and on release from the hospital. More specifically, patients identified house cleaning, meal preparation, and assistance with shopping as their major concrete needs. In the same study, 27.4% of the patients reported difficulties with transportation.

In Siegel's study a clinical social worker conducted in-depth interviews with 200 patients receiving outpatient chemotherapy at Memorial Sloan–Kettering Cancer Center in New York City.[19] Of the 200 patients, 62%, or almost two out of three, reported at least one unmet need within the past month and 39% reported two or more; the mean number of unmet needs was about 1.7. Furthermore, these patients exhibited a marked lack of knowledge about the availability and accessibility of services in their community. The estimation of the prevalence of needs was based on a cross-sectional design and included patients who had been in treatment for various lengths of time. If the sample had been followed longitudinally, the proportion of patients with one or more unmet needs at any point in the course of treatment would have been significantly greater.

Putnam et al[9] found that patients had difficulty identifying the services they needed, and Rose[20] and Edstrom and Miller[12] stated that families were unaware of services available in the community. Grobe, Ahmann, and Alstrup[16] reported that the greatest barrier to the use of home care and other services was the lack of knowledge of their existence. The data from Siegel's study supported this contention.[19] In response to the question, "If the areas we have been talking about became a problem for you, would you know where to go to obtain help from an agency or a service?" 68% of the patients answered no. Parsons reported that many patients and their families have difficulty obtaining resources either because they are unaware of them or because they lack the mobility, strength, and knowledge to search them out.[13] Therefore, patients may not complete the arduous process of requesting help, establishing eligibility, and following through on an application.

Many authors have stressed the importance of informing patients and their families of the resources that are available and of providing guidance on how to utilize these resources to maximize comfort and functioning at home and to avoid unnecessary hospitalization. Dwyer and Held,[11] who emphasized the chronic phase of cancer and the possibility of periodic changes in needs, recommended that patients and families be told in advance of home care services so they will be able to request them when they need them. Lurie[22] suggested a case advocacy approach in this regard that would ensure that programs are made accessible for appropriate patients. Bennet[21] pointed out that the provision of information to physically ill patients is difficult and that professionals must take into account the patients' anxiety and capacity to comprehend and integrate the information. After distributing written materials on concrete resources to 80 patients, she found on follow-up interview that only 12 patients (15%) had read the materials and none was positive about its helpfulness. She concluded, therefore, that the distribution of written material must be done in conjunction with more individualized contact. Grobe et al[16] recommended that a glossary of available services be developed and used in an extensive educational program that would enhance patients' awareness of home health needs and available resources. Edstrom and Miller[12] used a three-session home care course to teach aspects of physical care and how to locate and use community services to meet concrete needs.

ATTITUDINAL AND PSYCHOLOGICAL BARRIERS TO THE USE OF RESOURCES

The study at Memorial Sloan-Kettering Cancer Center[19] and our clinical experience have revealed several attitudinal and psychological barriers to patients' learning about and using community resources. First, patients wish to hold onto their independence, and therefore would rather not ask for help. They generally do not spontaneously request assistance unless there is an emergency. If patients are asked about their needs, however, they are able to specify those that are not being met and often are interested in knowing about available services. In addition, asking patients if they could use certain kinds of assistance implies that these needs are commonplace among patients, which makes it easier for them to acknowledge these needs and legitimates the investigation of unmet needs. For these reasons, some system of universal outreach is essential.

Second, patients are so focused on their illness and its treatment that they find it difficult to assimilate information about services not relevant to their current needs, although the services may be related to future needs. Some patients find it threatening to receive information that forces them to acknowledge a probable deterioration in their functional status. Therefore, the timing of information given in this regard should be individualized and patient specific.

Third, since needs change over time with treatment and reactions to treatment, patients should be followed systematically so that such alterations can be dealt with. Because of the growing number of patients treated on an outpatient basis and the limited number of social work staff members available to serve them, social workers cannot regularly follow up all outpatients. Hence, patients frequently are left to recognize their own unmet needs and to make these needs known.

A range of new interventions are being developed to address the problems that typically arise in obtaining community resources and to monitor patients' care. The Social Work Department at Memorial Sloan-Kettering Cancer Center tested the feasibility and acceptability of utilizing a computer-automated telephone outreach system to assess the needs of chemotherapy outpatients for a range of practical services.[23] The fully automated system was programmed to place telephone calls to 97 patients; to conduct a 12-question survey in a high-quality, digitally stored voice; to interpret, confirm, and record the patients' answers; and to flag the names of patients who identified one or more unmet needs so that these patients could receive prompt, direct professional attention. The results of the pilot study indicated that computer-automated surveys are likely to have broad-based acceptance among cancer outpatients and that outpatients are able to comply with instructions for completing the interview. This method could provide a cost-effective, universal, and ongoing assessment of patients' needs that would facilitate timely intervention and the efficient use of professional staff.

FINANCIAL ASSISTANCE FOR TREATMENT AND INCOME MAINTENANCE

INSURANCE

Medical insurance coverage is usually obtained through one's place of employment or through the federally and state funded programs of Medicaid and Medicare. An employer may discontinue support of health insurance for someone on leave without pay for an extended period of time. Because individual policies are expensive and difficult to obtain, it is important that patients continue paying for their own work-related group policy and not allow it to lapse. Unfortunately, even people who have been free of disease for many years may find it difficult to obtain new or additional coverage. The state insurance representative and religious, fraternal, or advocacy organizations such as the American Association of Retired Persons may be of some help in locating individual policies for patients who have lost their insurance.

Medicaid is funded by both federal and state governments. It is designed to pay the medical expenses of individuals found to be disabled according to the Social Security definition as well as those who are supported by welfare. In most states, people who are considered disabled but whose income is greater than the Supplemental Security Income financial eligibility standards are still eligible for Medicaid benefits, especially if they owe large medical bills not covered by other insurance. In some hospitals certain applications for Medicaid can be made through the hospital billing department; otherwise the patient must apply at a local welfare or social services office.

Individuals over the age of 65 automatically receive Medicare coverage. In addition, Medicare is extended to individuals who have received Social Security disability benefits for a period of 2 years. Due to federal cost-saving efforts, Medicare benefits have been reduced in recent years, especially in their coverage of outpatient costs and home care.

The American Cancer Society, Inc (ACS), the Leukemia Society of America, Inc, and other local religious and philanthropic agencies may provide treatment assistance in specific areas such as equipment, home care, transportation, certain pharmacy costs, and prostheses. The Crippled Children's Fund, managed by state health departments and funded by the federal government, will also pay for some treatment costs such as hospitalization, surgeries, and appliances for individuals under 21 years of age. In most states, children who are diagnosed with cancer are eligible for these funds.

FINANCIAL ASSISTANCE FOR INCOME SUPPORT

Maintaining an ongoing source of income is a major concern for patients diagnosed with cancer once paid leave benefits from their place of employment are exhausted. Social Security disability benefits should be applied for early, as processing claims can be time-consuming. Individuals are eligible if they have accumulated sufficient quarters of Social Security coverage within the recent past. The availability of other assets is not considered in the determination of eligibility of this benefit. However, the disease must have been in existence for 6 months and be expected to last for at least 1 year, and the individual must be unable to work. The requirement that the disease exist for 6 months is often met while the application is being processed. Application forms and detailed information can be obtained from the individual's local Social Security office.

Supplemental Security Income (SSI) can be applied for at the same time as Social Security Disability. Under this program income is provided to the elderly and disabled who have very limited income and few assets—that is, it is means tested. The amount of income or assets allowable in order to be eligible for benefits varies from state to state. It may provide the individual with income while he or she is waiting for disability benefits, but then be terminated once disability benefits are obtained, as the individual's income is then over the limit. Children who have cancer may be eligible for this benefit if their parents' income meets the eligibility requirement.

Welfare provides financial assistance of various kinds, but this varies greatly from state to state and within different jurisdictions. In general, assets must be extremely limited in order to qualify for these programs, which include Aid to Dependent Children, food stamps, and general emergency relief funds.

Additional pension funds and income support may be available from the Veterans Administration and from religious and fraternal organizations with which the individual is affiliated.

HOME HEALTH CARE SERVICES

Home care for cancer patients consists of a wide range of health and assistance services and equipment provided in the home to support optimum recovery, restore functioning, and enhance the quality of life of patients and their families. The basic components of home care include home health services, medical care, skilled nursing, social work and therapies for specific problems, nutrition counseling, personal care, and homemaking services.

Because of the variety of personnel who may provide home care to an individual and the fact that titles used to denote these personnel vary according to geographic region, professionals and patients alike are often confused about the functions performed by home health staff. In general, home care personnel can be divided according to their level of skill and training into professional and nonprofessional categories. We will use the representative terms *companion, housekeeper, homemaker,* and *home health aide* to identify the nonprofessional staff in home care.

NONPROFESSIONAL STAFF. A companion may have little or no specific training and stays with patients either to supervise them or to ensure their safety because, for example, they are confused or demented despite good physical functioning. A housekeeper is responsible only for maintaining the household by performing such tasks as grocery shopping, cooking, and cleaning. (A homemaker usually takes care of children in addition to maintaining the household.) With some training in the essentials of caring for patients, a home health aide helps patients with bathing, dressing, toileting, and mobility, reminds them to take their medications, gets their prescriptions filled, accompanies them to medical appointments, and performs housekeeping tasks.

PROFESSIONAL STAFF. The professionally trained personnel who provide home care include registered nurses (RNs), licensed practical nurses (LPNs), social workers, physical therapists, and occupational therapists. An RN or LPN is responsible for monitoring the patient's medical status, communicating this information to the responsible physician, administering medication, supervising other home health care personnel, and teaching the patient and family how to manage special medical equipment or devices, such as oxygen tanks and Broviac catheters, and how to care for wounds or ostomas. The social worker makes home visits to the patient and the family and provides psychosocial counseling about issues of adjustment to cancer, the stress of caring for the patient, and the family's fears or anticipation of the patient's death. In addition, the social worker coordinates the provision of home care services by different organizations (a frequent occurrence) with the care rendered by the referring physician or hospital.

INDICATORS OF NEED

Medical Indicators

The kind and intensity of the home health care services needed by patients vary considerably and must be determined by evaluating several factors simultaneously. The indicators of need include the symptoms of the disease as defined by type, site, and stage of the cancer; the types of treatment that are required (surgery, radiation therapy, chemotherapy); and whether the treatment will be administered on an inpatient or outpatient basis. Differences in need can be seen most clearly at the time of the initial treatment, during treatment for recurrent or metastatic disease, and during palliative treatment for terminally ill patients.

Patients who have been recently diagnosed tend to be less symptomatic and more functional and hence usually require short-term (if any) home health care that is focused on their recovery from the initial treatment. Moreover, they frequently have surgical or radiation therapy procedures while they are inpatients. Unlike chemotherapy, surgery and radiation therapy are discrete and time-limited procedures. Such localized treatment means that the patients' functioning is either minimally compromised or affected significantly only for the immediate period of recuperation, and there is a realistic expectation of increased functioning as each day passes. Furthermore, any procedure that is done in the hospital lessens the need for home care because the patient receives complete care in the hospital and has the chance to recuperate somewhat before returning home. Thus, home care for such patients often includes teaching them to care for a surgical wound or ostomy or to manage a prosthesis; assisting with household maintenance while they regain their strength and stamina; and providing physical therapy, occupational therapy, or special equipment during the recuperation period.

Patients with recurrent or metastatic disease are often more symptomatic, and the treatment required frequently is long term rather than acute. Consequently, many of these patients require some form of home care, usually for an indefinite period. This type of care is particularly needed by patients who are receiving systematic chemotherapy, which in itself may be debilitating, aside from any disease-related symptoms that the patients may also be experiencing. In addition, chemotherapy is often administered on an outpatient basis, which taxes the patients' already limited energies by requiring frequent trips to the oncologist's office or hospital and increasing interactions with a complex medical system. Therefore, these patients (and those who receive the similarly fatiguing outpatient radiation therapy, especially if it requires many daily treatments) usually require home health care to help them manage not only the side-effects of treatment but the personal and household activities of daily living.

For patients with metastatic disease who enter the terminal stage of the disease and require palliative treatment, home health care is a primary issue. It is important to evaluate whether the patients can be managed at home rather than in an inpatient setting, given the nearly total care they require. Arranging appropriate home care for terminally ill patients is an emotionally stressful process, since it involves acknowledging and preparing for their death, both practically and psychologically. At this stage of the illness, most patients require home care from outside agencies because of their poor functional status and the exhaustion of their family members from caring for them during earlier stages of the disease.

The home health care team for terminally ill patients usually includes, in addition to traditional home health personnel, clergy, volunteers, and a physician who can make house calls. Hospice programs, which are frequently designed to help families to maintain their dying members safely and comfortably at home, attempt to provide such comprehensive services. For these reasons, the planning of appropriate home care for terminally ill patients is a complex process in which the medical, practical, and psychosocial needs of the patients and their families must be addressed. Because social workers have expertise in considering all these factors in relation to available home care resources, their involvement at this time is often helpful.

Social and Behavioral Indicators

A number of social and behavioral characteristics can be important indicators of the need for home health care. One such indicator is the commitment and ability of family members or friends to care for the patient. The home care needs of most patients are met by family members; patients who live alone are more likely to require help from outside agencies. However, even if patients live with their families or have relatives who live near them, the degree of the relatives' involvement in their care may vary greatly. The family members' availability and willingness to help usually can be demonstrated by their presence or absence at medical visits and the degree to which they take an active role in discussions about treatment, the symptoms and progress of the disease, medications, and the general care of their ill members.

A second behavioral indicator is the patient's Karnofsky status[24] and general appearance at medical appointments: Does the patient appear relatively well groomed? Does personal hygiene seem adequate? Are wounds or special medical devices being properly cared for? Is there any sign of decubitus or other symptoms that may indicate that the patient is not being well cared for? Is the patient's nutritional status adequate? Patients may hesitate to mention their need for home care until the situation has become serious. Therefore, the physician's observation of problems may provide an earlier indication of need for such services.

A third, often subtle, indicator is a noticeable change in the patient's or family's behavior and communication with the treatment team. For example, an increase in telephone calls about the patient's condition, especially if made outside standard office hours, from a patient or family member who has typically called infrequently and during office hours is often a sign that the patient is requiring more help at home than is available. Similarly, decreased contact with the medical system, as manifest in missed or canceled medical appointments, may also indicate that the patient is feeling too ill to make the visits without additional help done or that the family members can no longer assist as much as they had done. Finally, the patient who appears for an increased number of emergency visits, either at the hospital's emergency room or in unscheduled office visits, may well be signaling that he or she feels unsafe with the existing home care plan. In this situation, the family members may also be communicating that they feel overwhelmed by the responsibility of managing the patient's medical and emotional needs at home. Attention to these changes can alert the physician to patients or families who may be indirectly requesting additional help. In these cases, the social worker's skills in assessment and knowledge of resources may be necessary to identify the problem and design an appropriate home care plan.

LOCATING HOME CARE RESOURCES IN THE COMMUNITY

Patients who are receiving inpatient or outpatient care from a hospital may receive information and referral for home care services from a member of the hospital's social work department. The particular expertise of hospital-based social workers is to assess and enhance the problem-solving abilities of patients and families in relation to the medical plan and to link patients and families with the appropriate health resources in the community that will provide the needed services.

Patients who are not being treated by the hospital system can be helped with home care arrangements by social workers in community agencies or in private practice, or by a local unit of the American Cancer Society. Home care services in a specific region can be located by calling the department of social work or discharge planning of local hospitals, the American Cancer Society office, the local Visiting Nurse Association office, or the national clearing house organizations such as the National Home Caring Council (tel. 202–547–6586) or the National League for Nursing (212–582–1022). The type of care that patients require and their financial ability or insurance coverage for such care are two major factors in exploring home care resources. Three basic types of agencies provide home care services: (1) nonprofit (voluntary) home care agencies, (2) proprietary (for-profit) home care agencies, and (3) governmental tax-supported services.

Nonprofit home care agencies are community-based or hospital-based agencies that provide health services to people in their community. Reimbursement for services comes from Medicare, Medicaid, and insurance carriers. Often these agencies, which include Visiting Nurse Associations, have a sliding scale of fees, based on the individual's ability to pay. These agencies regulate criteria for eligibility and referral procedures. For example, the Visiting Nurse Association's referrals must demonstrate the need for some skilled nursing to activate other services, such as housekeeping. These agencies differ geographically in the number of hours of service per week they will provide to patients. Therefore, a patient who needs a great deal of care may require a plan that coordinates the services of a number of different agencies, including a visiting nurse for skilled nursing care, Meals on Wheels for nutrition, and a home health aide from another community agency for general care.

Proprietary home care agencies are privately owned businesses that often have a network of offices nationwide and are listed in the Yellow Pages of the telephone book under Home Health Agencies. These agencies recruit, train, and supervise a full range of home health care workers, whom they assign to clients under their supervision. The proprietary agencies provide comprehensive services and equipment at home 24 hours a day, 7 days a week. However, such services are costly and therefore accessible only to patients who are financially well off or who have excellent insurance coverage for home care. Only proprietary agencies that are certified by Medicare will be reimbursed (80%) by Medicare. A patient who is eligible for this type of home care under Medicare must meet the following criteria:

1. A physician must certify the need for home care services for a medical condition and then determine a specified plan of treatment.
2. The patient must require skilled care from a nurse or other therapist.
3. The patient must be homebound by this medical condition, that is, unable to leave the house without assistance from another person, special transportation, or the aid of equipment, such a crutch, cane, or wheelchair.

Referrals to proprietary agencies may be initiated directly by the patient or family. However, a social worker or other professional who is involved in discharge planning is more knowledgeable and therefore can coordinate a plan that will take into account the patient's financial situation.

Tax-supported home care services are a type of government-aided health care that can be found through county or state health departments or governmental offices on aging. Income and age requirements may have to be met to qualify for aid. A county home service is an example of this type of agency.

Medicaid is a state-administered health program of Title XIX of the Social Security Act for low-income or medically indigent people. It has stringent financial requirements for eligibility that vary among the states.

Medicaid coverage includes all the necessary services, although the number of hours of services may be limited in certain regions. Both voluntary and proprietary agencies have some Medicaid-certified programs or service. Social workers are familiar with the eligibility requirements for Medicaid in their state and can help patients apply for such aid. Cancer patients may be reluctant to apply for Medicaid because they regard it as a form of welfare or dependence on the state that they believe is intended for the poor or lower classes. However, the financial burden of cancer, especially as a chronic condition, can create financial problems for any family.

ALTERNATIVES TO HOME CARE

Cancer patients need care in an extended stay facility following acute care in the hospital primarily when their condition is preterminal or terminal. The most common social reason for long-term institutional care is that patients have no available family or need but cannot afford to pay for home services on a 24-hour basis. The usual *medical* indications for extended care are the progressive nature of the disease, coupled with a regimen of care that a family cannot manage at home. The decision to utilize this form of care must be made jointly by the patient, the family, and the treatment team to ensure that family relationships and the integrity of the family unit are maintained.

Many communities have institutions for the extended care of patients with chronic illnesses; in some instances, a floor or wing of a building may be designed for long-term care. Most extended-care institutions accept cancer patients, and a few are devoted exclusively to them. The institutions may be profit making or under voluntary or public auspices. Proprietary nursing homes accommodate the largest number of patients in extended-care institutions. Institutions that seek reimbursement from Medicare must meet the Social Security Administration's standards.

Terminal or preterminal cancer patients in particular tend to exceed Medicare's limit of 100 days for extended care. If their stay (which usually means, in effect, their life expectancy) is likely to exceed 100 days, their families must be prepared to assume the continuing financial responsibility. Many institutions, including some proprietary ones, make financial arrangements with families of limited means, such as helping them file an application for Medicaid, to avoid interrupting the patient's care.

TRANSPORTATION SERVICES FOR CANCER PATIENTS

In areas where services are accessible, transportation services are available to patients with certain levels of need and the financial resources to pay for them. However, since the first step in obtaining such services is an awareness of their existence and the ability to apply for them, it is best to have a social worker arrange for them. Although the level and quality of these services vary greatly in different parts of the country, the following are some general guidelines.

TYPES OF SERVICE

Ambulances

INDICATORS OF NEED. An ambulance is indicated when the patient's physical or mental condition is so severe that he or she cannot be transported by any other means. Thus, an ambulance is for patients who cannot sit, who experience intense pain when they move, who need to lie flat, or who have other conditions that require their rapid transportation to a hospital in optimal comfort and with advanced medical technology. Of all the forms of transportation to be discussed, only ambulances provide such medical equipment as intravenous poles and tubes, oxygen tanks, cardiac monitors, and suctioning devices.

COST. Transportation by ambulance is expensive and is seldom totally covered by insurance companies. Medicare usually pays up to 80% of the customary charges of a one-way trip. The costs of a transfer to the patient's home, to a nursing home, or to another hospital (if that hospital provides treatment that is not available at the present hospital) are also reimbursed. Under all these circumstances, however, reimbursement is made only when a hospital or a physician provides documentation of the need for the service.

Medicaid usually pays the entire cost of ambulance transportation for situations that are similar to those covered by Medicare. Because private or commercial insurance carriers vary greatly in their reimbursement policies for ambulance services, it is essential to review the specific policy. Social workers often are able to negotiate with the ambulance company and the insurance company to set up the best accommodations for all involved.

SERVICES. Social work departments in medical centers maintain lists of ambulance services and of the names of persons to be contacted in arranging for them. Although the Yellow Pages of the telephone book also list ambulance services, there is no way of determining the quality or reliability of these services from such listings. In an emergency, a local police emergency unit can be called; in New York City, patients are transported without cost to the emergency room of the nearest municipal hospital.

Ambulettes

INDICATORS OF NEED. An ambulette is the transportation of choice for patients who are unable to walk or climb stairs unassisted, who can sit in a wheelchair, and who do not require acute care while in transit. The most common medical and physical reasons for ambulette services include physical and or mental senility, functional orthopedic impairment, neuromuscular disorders that preclude unassisted movement, severe cardiac disease, and acute side-effects from treatments.

COST. An ambulette usually costs about 25% less than an ambulance. Although Medicare does not cover the cost of ambulette services, Medicaid in most states covers the entire cost. Under all circumstances, reimbursement requires the documentation of need by a hospital or a physician. Private or commercial carriers sometimes pay for this service. Although insurance carriers may initially refuse to pay for ambulette services, social workers are often able to negotiate with them to avoid the higher cost of an ambulance.

LOCATING SERVICES. Social work departments in medical centers maintain lists of ambulette services and the names of contact persons at these services, as they do for ambulance services. The Yellow Pages of the telephone book also list ambulette services, but again there is no way to know the quality and reliability of the services that are so listed.

Van Services, Car Services, and Taxis

INDICATORS OF NEED. Ambulatory patients who are sight impaired, feeble, physically disabled, cognitively compromised, weakened by illness or treatment, or otherwise unable to manage public transportation are best transported by a van or automobile.

COST. These services tend to be much less expensive than an ambulance or an ambulette and are more convenient than mass transportation in that they provide door-to-door service. Medicare and private or commercial insurance carriers do not pay for these services, although Medicaid usually does. Van services, however, generally pick up a number of patients at one time, so patients often are forced to wait and may become uncomfortable.

LOCATING SERVICES. Because of the competition among these services, it should be understood that the operators and drivers of these vehicles are not medically oriented and require monitoring by those who refer patients to them. More often than not, departments of social work in medical centers maintain lists and, at times, special relationships with vendors to ensure the quality of their services and to provide reduced rates to patients who require financial help.

Rail Services

INDICATORS OF NEED. For wheelchair-bound patients who are traveling long distance and prefer rail travel, 48-hour prior notice to the carrier is necessary for appropriate arrangements to be made. It is strongly suggested that reservations be made and confirmed before patients are actually transported. There are no facilities for stretcher patients on trains.

COSTS. There is no extra charge for wheelchair-bound patients who travel by train. Medicare and private and commercial insurance carriers generally do not pay for these services, although some Medicaid programs will if the circumstances warrant it.

LOCATING SERVICES. Under most circumstances, arrangements for travel for wheelchair-bound patients are easily made by calling the carrier's reservations desk. A slide board is useful for the easy transfer of a patient to a regular seat.

Airlines

INDICATORS OF NEED. The airlines are usually adept at transporting even acutely ill patients. Although each airline has different regulations, airlines generally require similar information—for example, a letter from a physician describing the patient's condition and stating that the patient is able to tolerate the trip. For a patient who needs to spend the entire trip on a stretcher, 48 hours is usually the minimum notice required.

COST. As with rail travel, Medicare and private and commercial insurance companies generally do not pay for these services. However, in many states Medicaid pays for air transportation under unusual circumstances. The cost of travel for a patient in a wheelchair who is moved to a regular seat is the same as for any other passenger. However, for a patient on a stretcher, the costs can be prohibitive. Generally, the patient will have to pay the price of a first-class seat (which must be physically removed) and perhaps also for a second or third first-class seat for an accompanying nurse or equipment, such as an intravenous pole and pump.

LOCATING SERVICES. Advance notice to the airline is essential. The necessary documentation should remain with the patient at all times. The airline should be called before the actual transfer occurs to ensure the timeliness of the flight and that all the necessary information is available. The patient should arrive at least 1 hour early. It is strongly suggested that a member of the health care team be available by telephone until the patient's plane has actually departed.

Volunteer Transportation

Volunteer services generally are underutilized because people do not know how to find them. In the case of cancer patients, one should first call the local chapter of the American Cancer Society, which often maintains lists of such resources. Other relevant sources of information about free or low-cost assistance include the Red Cross, volunteer police and fire departments, religious groups, local community men's and women's groups, visiting or public health nurses, and social work departments in hospitals.

Many of the vendors who serve hospitals provide free services for specific patients when asked. Often the free services are limited only by the imagination of those involved and the access to those who control them. When asking for help, always try to start at the top of the system. This often saves time and enables the person with the most control to consider your request.

Volunteer services for ground transportation are the most easily obtainable, but their availability, level of comfort, predictability, and reliability vary greatly, depending on the resources and commitment of the volunteers.

Limited free air travel is also available under certain circumstances. Corporate Angel Network (tel. 914–328–1313) offers free air travel by corporate jet planes primarily to cancer patients who can sit up and who do not require life-sustaining equipment. A physician's written clearance is required. This group also transports a member of the family and a bone-marrow donor (up to four people at a time, depending on the size of the aircraft).

In Toronto, Canada, and in Missouri, an air transportation network, in cooperation with the Canadian Cancer Society (tel. 416–924–9333), offers essentially the same services as does the Corporate Angel Network, although it also transports patients who do not have cancer.

Patients and their families can contact these services directly, or social workers can telephone them first to describe the specific situation involved. Advance notice and flexibility are essential for utilizing both these services.

ENSURING THE QUALITY OF TRANSPORTATION SERVICES

The transportation of most patients involves the use of services that are not directly provided by the institution. Therefore, the quality of the services must be constantly monitored in order to protect the patient and family and to ensure that medical treatments and protocols can be adhered to. Audits and surveys of or interviews with patients are a necessary part of the evaluation of transportation services. However, the most effective way to provide safe, reliable, and comfortable transportation is through ongoing communication with the vendors of these services. Such contact with vendors should include, in addition to standard evaluations, periodic education and orientation sessions to sensitize vendors to the specific needs and concerns of cancer patients. Establishing ongoing relationships with vendors and institutions ensures that the needs of all are presented and that changes are effectively made and maintained.

Despite the demand for such transportation services, financial support for them has not increased. Few insurance carriers reimburse patients for the most commonly utilized forms of transportation—automobiles, taxis, vans, and ambulettes. In the absence of this support it becomes increasingly important that local and community volunteer services communicate with medical centers to ensure that their efforts are mutually supportive and that patients' needs are articulated. The transportation needs of patients should be an integral part of any early psychosocial assessment of patients.

EMOTIONAL SUPPORT AND PLANNING SERVICES

Emotional support and planning include both self-help and professional, individual and group services that range in intensity from a single session to weekly traditional psychotherapy. Contacts with veteran patients are reported to be helpful to almost all patients in highlighting the normal and universal nature of their reactions and limiting their sense of isolation. Patients learn from other patients about different coping strategies used to deal with the myriad of stresses caused by the disease and treatment. While patients rarely report adverse reactions to meeting with other patients, they may feel these meetings are not sufficient to meet their emotional support needs. Professional help is recommended, therefore, when patients are emotionally overwhelmed by their disease and treatment, are in acute psychological crisis, have specific individual problems, or need to deal with preexisting personal and interpersonal problems that have been exacerbated by disease.

In hospitals, emotional support and planning services are typically provided by social workers, nurses, psychiatrists, psychologists, and chaplains. Patients may be referred directly to one of these professionals or may be automatically offered service after a routine psychosocial assessment. In the community, mental health professionals in private practice provide these therapies, or they may be offered by special agencies for cancer patients such as some local chapters of the American Cancer Society, by religious agencies or organizations, and by other mental health and family service agencies. Professionals who provide such counseling in the community include social workers, psychologists, psychiatrists, and oncology nurses; marriage, family, or child counselors; sex therapists; and religious counselors or pastoral care professionals. Most social work departments in medical centers maintain lists of competent professionals in the community.

SELF-HELP GROUPS

The number of self-help groups for people with a chronic illness such as cancer has grown astronomically. Gussow and Tracey[26] reported that there is a self-help group for every major disease listed by the World Health Organization. Locating self-help groups for cancer patients within a specific geographic area can be done through contacting the local office of the American Cancer Society or the National Self-Help Clearinghouse (1-800-422-6237).

All these groups share the philosophy that people who have experienced a crisis or a threatening situation have a unique contribution to make to others who are undergoing the same experience. Several mechanisms have been suggested to explain the appeal of self-help groups. First, because they have been through it themselves, "veterans" of a crisis can provide insight and understanding to those who are now coping with the crisis; that is, they have what Borkman called "experiential knowledge."[27] As Katz said, sharing a central problem is what defines members of a self-help group.[28]

A second mechanism through which group members experience benefits is the destigmatization and normalization of conditions and problems. A third mechanism is the helper-therapy principle, which suggests that "helpers" may benefit more than recipients of help because of their increased sense of interpersonal competence from their role as advisers, what they learn from those they help, the social approval they receive for helping others, and the reinforcement of their own success in coping.[29] Because members of self-help groups are both givers and receivers of care, all can benefit. Another way that self-help groups provide benefits is through the modeling of successful recovery—a role that veteran patients, such as Reach-to-Recovery volunteers, consciously adopt to encourage the successful adaptation to the illness.

Some groups are organized and run by mental health professionals, others are organized and controlled by patients. Some groups sponsor intense, short-term sessions that are held for several months and then are disbanded. Others have ongoing programs that involve the same members and are closed to newcomers. Still others are open to new members at all times. In all cases, the underlying mechanisms of the groups are the same: members help one another by sharing their problems, being role models of successful recovery, and destigmatizing the illness.

INDICATORS OF NEED FOR SERVICE

Although patients often experience emotional disequilibrium in response to a diagnosis of cancer, few request counseling, supportive interventions, psychiatric consultation, or even self-help. Despite their often overwhelming reactions, most are unable to request support for a variety of reasons. Some are psychologically immobilized and cannot exert the emotional energy needed to get help. Others view a request for support as reflecting inability to cope, a loss of autonomy, or a sign of mental illness. Furthermore, most patients are unaware that counseling may help assuage the existential terror that is evoked by a diagnosis of cancer or alleviate grief over the loss of body function or appearance. The dilemma is that these patients will later resent not receiving enough emotional help or support. Therefore, patients are most likely to use services to mitigate their normal distress if the services are universally prescribed and easily available.

Patients may be viewed as being on a continuum of need for psychosocial counseling services, from those who are seriously mentally ill, to those who are psychosocially vulnerable, to those who are normal and well supported. Although the majority of cancer patients can benefit from some counseling, others *must* receive it to maintain their functioning and prevent their social and emotional breakdown.

Cancer patients with a history of mental illness or psychiatric treatment generally have an ongoing relationship with a number of supportive services in the community that may need information about their medical condition. Such patients should be urged to communicate with their therapists or other mental health counselors about their medical condition or to have a social worker transmit this information and to arrange for their continued psychological treatment and care. The diagnosis of cancer may exacerbate their mental illness or seriously affect their day-to-day functioning. Early psychosocial intervention can prevent a breakdown in functioning that can have lasting negative effects on the quality of their lives, such as the loss of a job or the severance of important social relationships and the alienation of friends and relatives.

A much larger group of patients are not mentally ill but have a variety of social and psychological characteristics that place them at risk of an emotional and social breakdown when confronting a diagnosis of cancer. Such reactions may interfere with the individual's daily functioning and treatment compliance. These patients include, for example, those who are:

- Living alone, or who have few friends or relatives to help them.
- Over age 75.
- Children or young adults.
- Financially stressed (*e.g.*, have no or very limited insurance)
- Parents of dependent children.
- Multiply stressed—who have experienced a great deal of life stress or who are in the midst of other life crises, such as the recent loss of a job or a divorce.
- Members of highly conflicted family situations with, for example, a previous history of violence or abuse.
- Ill with other diseases or whose family members are ill and who therefore may have difficulty being realistic about their own diagnosis and prognosis.

These patients may be more difficult to identify. However, all such patients will benefit from recommendations that they obtain emotional support services.

Finally, some patients are resilient and psychologically strong and have numerous personal, social, practical, and financial resources. These patients often can be specific about their needs and are grateful when help is given. Therefore, their psychological and support needs are often overlooked by professionals. These individuals need to be informed of emotional support services because they can make rapid and highly effective use of them and they often resent not having access to them. As one patient said, "I knew I could cope well with a cancer diagnosis and I did, but I might have coped better with some help and would have liked to have known about counseling that could have been available to me."

APPENDIX: RESOURCES AND SERVICES

FINANCIAL ASSISTANCE FOR TREATMENT

Insurance/Individual or Group

Private insurance. State department of insurance can provide information.

Medicaid. Payment of expenses of disabled individuals. Eligibility requirements include very limited assets and income.

Medicare. Payment of medical expenses of individuals over 65 years of age or those who have received Social Security Disability for 2 years. Limited coverage for outpatient treatment and care.

Philanthropic Agencies and Government Entitlement Programs

American Cancer Society. Payment of some costs—transportation, treatment, home care, dressings.

Crippled Children's Program. Payment of approved hospitalizations, operations, and appliances.

Leukemia Society of America. Payment of some costs for leukemia patients—transportation, drugs, radiation in specific instances.

FINANCIAL ASSISTANCE FOR INCOME SUPPORT

Social Security Administration

Social Security/Disability. Monthly payments to those unable to work because of disease or treatment (not dependent on assets and income).

Supplemental Security Income. Monthly payment to disabled individuals with very limited income and assets.

Department of Social Services

Aid for Dependent Children. Monthly support to children of disabled parents.

General relief. Short-term emergency cash assistance.

Food Stamps. Coupons to purchase food items.

Veterans Administration

State Disability Benefits Office. Payments through employers.

HOME HEALTH CARE AND EQUIPMENT SERVICES

Hospital-based home care programs. Personnel and equipment to assist with home care.

Hospital departments of social work or discharge planning. Information about local home care resources.

Visiting Nurse Association or Public Health Nurses. Personnel to assist with home care and provide information about local proprietary agencies and other home care resources. Services covered by most insurances.

Meals on Wheels. Meals delivered to patients in their homes. Administered by a range of local social service and religious agencies.

Private home care agencies. Personnel to assist with home care; usually require private pay or major medical insurance cover for RN's only. Listed in the Yellow Pages of the phone directory or recommended by hospital departments of social work, discharge planning, or local Visiting Nurse Association.

Surgical supply companies. Durable medical equipment for the home.

Pharmacies. Specialized equipment for home.

Hospice. Coordinated home care for terminally ill patients utilizing VNS services and volunteers, insurance coverage for hospice varies.

American Cancer Society. Payment of some home health care fees and provision of dressings, prothesis, and equipment.

Leukemia Society of America. Selective provision of home care services.

ALTERNATIVES TO HOME CARE

Terminal care facilities or cancer-specific chronic care facilities. Provision of inpatient care for terminally ill patients.
Nursing homes. Chronic, terminal care of those who cannot be cared for in own home.
Veterans Administration Hospital. Residential placement of veterans.

TRANSPORTATION

Private transportation companies. Provide ambulance, ambulette, taxi, van, or car service transportation. Listed in Yellow Pages of phone directory.
American Cancer Society. Provides transportation or money for transportation to the treatment center.
Leukemia Society of America. Provides some money for transportation from home to the treatment center.
Hospital transportation service. Arranges transportation to and from the hospital and in some situations provides funding.
Corporate Angel Network. Provides free air transportation on corporate planes from home to treatment center when flights are available (for ambulatory patients only).
Local volunteer ambulance and fire departments. Often provide free transportation to and from treatment center when volunteers are available.
American Red Cross. Provides free transportation to and from treatment centers when volunteers are available.
Local religious organizations. Provide a range of vans and car services for members of their religious community.

EMOTIONAL SUPPORT AND PLANNING SERVICES

National Self-Help Clearing House. Provides information concerning self-help groups throughout the country.

American Cancer Society-sponsored self-help groups

Reach-to-Recovery. Emotional support, exercises, and temporary prosthesis for women undergoing mastectomy.
International Association of Laryngectomees. Provides emotional support and information to patients having larynx removed.
Cansurmount. Provides emotional support and information for patients with varying cancer diagnoses.
Candelighters. Provides emotional support and information to parents of children with cancer.
United Ostomy Association. Provides emotional support information, and advisory to ostomy patients.

Other Self-Help Groups

National Coalition of Cancer Survivors. A clearing house for publications and organizations of cancer survivors and a resource for political advocacy.
Make Today Count. Provides group and individual emotional support and problem-solving for cancer patients with all diagnoses.

Other Local Self-Help Groups

Professional Counseling

Hospital social work, psychiatric, nursing, or pastoral care staff. Provides information, emotional support, psychological and behavioral therapies.
Family service agencies. Provide information, practical help, emotional support, psychological and behavioral therapies.
Pastoral care or religious agencies. Provide emotional support and spiritual guidance.
Private practitioners. Provide emotional support and psychological and behavioral therapies.

EDUCATION AND INFORMATION

ACS. Source of information regarding prevention treatment, services, and rehabilitation.
Breast Cancer Advisory Center. Provides medical advice to people diagnosed as having breast cancer, makes referrals, disseminates information.
Cancer Information Service. A free, nationwide telephone information service, sponsored by the National Cancer Institute.
National Cancer Information Clearinghouse, NCI/NIH. Indexes, abstracts, and stores information and provides free searches of resources.

AGENCIES AND ORGANIZATIONS

American Cancer Society
National Headquarters
3340 Peachtree Road NE
Atlanta, GA 30326
(404-329-7625)

Voluntary organization offering programs of cancer research and education, and patient service and rehabilitation.

American Red Cross
National Headquarters
Washington, DC 20006
(202-737-8300)

Provides free transportation when volunteers are available.

Breast Cancer Advisory Center
11426 Rockville Pike
Suite 406
Rockville, MD 20859
(301-984-1020)

This organization, founded in 1985 by Rose Kushner, provides medical advice to people diagnosed as having breast cancer. The center makes referrals, disseminates information, and gives lectures. A library of breast cancer materials is maintained by the center.

Cancer Information Service
1-800-4-CANCER
New York business number for professionals: 212-794-7984

A free, nationwide telephone information service sponsored by the National Cancer Institute. It provides current, reliable information, including research about cancer and local sources of cancer care for the public. Answers are confidential. Free publications on a variety of subjects are available for mailing. The toll-free number will automatically connect caller to the CIS serving their area.

Candelighters
National Headquarters
2025 Eye Street, N.W.
Suite 1011
Washington, DC 20006
(202-659-5136)

Candelighters is an international organization devoted to providing emotional support to parents of children diagnosed with cancer. It offers family support, information services, and lobbying for legislation related to cancer programs and research. All services are provided free of charge. Candelighters publishes newsletters, pamphlets, and handbooks.

Compassionate Friends, Inc.
P.O. Box 1347
Oak Brook, IL 60521
(312-323-5010)

A self-help organization offering friendship and understanding to bereaved parents. Primary goals of organization chapters are to aid parents in the positive resolution of grief experienced after the death of a child, and to foster the physical and emotional health of bereaved parents and siblings.

Concern for Dying
250 West 57th Street
New York, NY 10019
(212-246-6962)

The nonprofit educational council dedicated to the belief in the individual's right to participate in treatment decisions made during terminal illness. It offers information on death, dying, burial information, and counseling and provides copies of The Living Will.

Corporate Angels Network
Westchester Company Airport Building
White Plains, New York 10604
(914-328-1313)

Provides free air transport on corporate planes *from home to treatment center when flights are available.*

Crippled Children's Program

Listed under Bureau of Handicapped Children in phone directory.

Hodgkin's Disease and Lymphoma Organization
518 Wingate Drive
East Meadow, NY 11154
(516-999-6813)

Provides information and emotional support for persons with Hodgkin's disease and their families.

International Association for Enterostomal Therapy
505 A Tustan Avenue
Suite 282
Santa Ana, CA 92705
(714-972-1725)

Organizes enterostomal therapy nurses for the promotion of education to patients, nurses, physicians, and other allied health professionals in the rehabilitation of persons with abnominal stomas, fistulas, draining wounds, incontinence, and pressure sores.

International Association of Laryngectomees
777 Third Avenue
New York, NY 10017
(212-371-2900)

A voluntary organization of 286 member clubs, it coordinates the activities of local laryngectomee clubs that provide mutual support and encourage total rehabilitation.

Leukemia Society of America, Inc.
National Headquarters
800 Second Avenue
New York, NY 10017
(212-573-8584)

A national voluntary health agency dedicated to seeking the control and eradication of leukemia, Hodgkin's disease, and the lymphomas. It supports a "three-pronged" program of research, patient aid, and public and professional education, supported primarily by donations from the community.

Make-a-Wish Foundation of America
Phoenix, Arizona
(602-234-0960)

Grants special wishes of a seriously or terminally ill child. Part of a network of 50 chapters.

National Cancer Information Clearinghouse, NCI/NIH
9000 Rockville Pike
Bethesda, MD 20205
(1-800-422-6237)

This organization, sponsored by NCI's Office of Cancer Communication, facilitates exchange of information on public and patient educational materials. It indexes, abstracts, and stores information received from individuals and organizations and provides free searches of resources.

National Home Caring Council
235 Park Avenue South
New York, NY 10003
(202-547-6586)

The service provides a quick reference to all homemaker/home health aide services across the country, including those it accredits.

National Hospice Organization
1901 North Fort Myer Drive
Suite 307
Arlington, VA 22209
(703-243-5900)

A nonprofit, privately funded association of health professionals dedicated to promoting better and more appropriate care for the terminally ill patient and ensuring that hospice care is kept at the highest level possible. NHO publishes a quarterly newsletter, locator directory, and several reports.

National League for Nursing
American Public Health Association
10 Columbus Circle
New York, NY 10019
(212-582-1022)

This organization provides a list of visiting nurse organizations in local areas.

National Self-Help Clearinghouse
Graduate School and University Center
City University of New York
33 West 42nd Street
New York, NY 10036

The organization provides information concerning self-help groups in a specific community. It will place an individual in contact with one of 27 regional clearinghouses. The regional clearinghouses may also be available to provide assistance in organizing a self-help group.

Starlight Foundation
9021 Melrose Avenue
Suite 204
Los Angeles, CA 90069
(213-205-0631)

Grants special wishes to terminally, chronically, and critically ill children.

United Ostomy Association, Inc.
2001 W. Beverly Blvd.
Los Angeles, CA 90057
(213-481-2811)

A nonprofit service agency organized and run by ostomates. Its purpose is to help ostomy patients return to normal living through mutual aid and moral support. At present, there are over 500 local chapters throughout the United States and Canada. The UOA educates patients and the public about ostomy and contributes to the improvement of ostomy equipment and supplies. It publishes the *Ostomy Quarterly* and educational literature for patients, the public and professionals.

REFERENCES

1. Siegel K, Christ GH: Psychosocial consequences of long-term survivorship. Hodgkin's Disease: Consequences of Survival. Philadelphia, Lea & Febiger, 1989
2. Polinsky ML, Ganz PA, Rofessart-O'Berry J et al: Developing a comprehensive network of rehabilitation resources for referral of cancer patients. J Psychosoc Oncol 5:1-10, 1987
3. Hunter G, Johnson SH: Physical support systems for the homebound oncology patient. Oncol Nurs Forum 7:21-23, 1980
4. Shragen J, Halman M, Myers D et al: Impediments to the cause and effectiveness of discharge planning. Soc Work Health Care 4:65-80, 1978
5. Wellisch DK, Fawzy FI, Landsverk J et al: Evaluation of psychosocial problems of the homebound cancer patient: The relationship of disease and the sociodemographical variables of patients to family problems. J Psychosoc Oncol 1:1-15, 1983
6. Amado A, Cronk BA, Mileo R: Cost of terminal care: Home hospice vs. hospital. Nurs Outlook 27:522-526, 1979
7. Cassileth BR, Donovan JA: History and implications of the new legislation. J Psychosoc Oncol 1:59-69, 1983
8. Market WM, Simon VB: The hospice concept. Cancer 28:225-237, 1978
9. Putnam ST, McDonald MM, Miller MM et al: Home as a place to die. Am J Nurs 80:1451-1453, 1980
10. Rosenbaum EH, Rosenbaum DR: Principles of home care for the patient with advanced cancer. JAMA 244:1484-1489, 1980
11. Dwyer JE, Held DM: Home management of the adult patient with leukemia. Nurs Clin North Am 17:665-675, 1982
12. Edstrom S, Miller MW: Preparing the family to care for the cancer patient at home: A home care course. Cancer Nurs 4:49-53, 1981
13. Parsons J: A descriptive study of intermediate stage terminally ill cancer patients at home. Nurs Dig 5:1-26, 1977
14. Lindenberg RE, Coulton C: Planning for post-hospital care: A follow-up study. Health Soc Work 5:45-50, 1980
15. Jessee WF, Doyle BJ: Discharge planning: Using audit to identify areas that need improvement. Quality Rev Bull 5:25-29, 1979
16. Grobe ME, Ahmann DL, Alstrup DM: Needs assessment for cancer patients and their families. Oncol Nurs Forum 9:26-30, 1982
17. Googe MC, Varricchio CG: A pilot investigation of home health care needs of cancer patients and their families. Oncol Nurs Forum 8:24-28, 1981
18. American Cancer Society: Social, Economic and Psychological Needs of Cancer Patients in California. San Francisco, American Cancer Society, 1979
19. Siegel K: Continuing care of cancer patients—concrete needs: Progress report. New York, Memorial Sloan-Kettering Cancer Center, 1987
20. Rose MA: Problems families face in home care. Am J Nurs 76:416-418, 1976
21. Bennet C: Testing the value of written information from patients and families in discharge planning. Soc Work Health Care 9:95-100, 1984
22. Lurie A: The social work advocacy role in discharge planning. Soc Work Health Care 8:75-85, 1982
23. Siegel K, Mesagno FP, Chen J et al: Computerized telephone assessment of the "concrete" needs of chemotherapy outpatients: a feasibility study. J Clin Oncol 6(11):1760-1767, 1988
24. Moer V, Laliberte L, Morris JN et al: The Karnofsky Performance Status Scale: An examination of its reliability and validity in a research setting. Cancer 53:2002-2007, 1984
25. 1986 National Hospice Organization Guide. Arlington, VA, National Hospice Organization
26. Gussow Z, Tracey GS: The role of self-help clubs in adaptation to chronic illness and disability. Soc Sci Med 10:407, 1976
27. Borkman T: A cross-national comparison of stutterers' self-help organizations. Speech Ther J 29:6, 1974
28. Katz S, Hedrick S, Henderson N: The measurement of long-term care needs and impact. Health Med Care Serv Rev 2:2-21, 1979
29. Riessman F: The helper therapy principle. Soc Work 10:27, 1965

SECTION 4 J. ANDREW BILLINGS

Specialized Care of the Terminally Ill Patient

> It is never true that "nothing more can be done" for a patient. It may be useless to continue treatment with curative drugs or surgery, but one can still give attention and friendship, relief and comfort.[1]

In the past quarter century medical understanding of the causes of cancer and ability to treat it have progressed enormously; at the same time, major advances have been made in the clinical care of the terminally ill. The "death and dying" movement is perhaps the most publicly evident manifestation of a revolution in attitudes toward persons facing death as both society at large and the medical profession in particular have expressed a new willingness to talk about fatal illness and to raise fresh notions of a "good" or "appropriate" death.[2-5] Death has been rediscovered.[6] Fine sociological and psychological investigations of dying and bereavement have provided a better appreciation of the plight of the terminally ill and their families while suggesting many areas in which treatment can be enhanced.[7-13]

For the practicing clinician, the modern hospice movement has been particularly important in asserting new standards for the medical and psychosocial management of dying persons and their families. This grassroots social reform emerged dramatically in the United States over the past 15 years.[14-16] Inspired by St. Christopher's Hospice in England and the pioneering efforts of Cicely Saunders and her colleagues,[1,17-20] clinicians and lay persons have come to recognize that terminally ill patients, too often relegated to profound isolation and suffering, could live well until death. Beginning with the British model, a variety of special programs have been developed in North America for both the inpatient and outpatient management of terminally ill patients and their families.

Physicians who work with cancer patients need to be familiar with modern standards of terminal care and the hospice approach, both to inform their daily clinical practice and to help their patients use special services. This chapter begins by outlining the hospice critique of contemporary terminal care and then describes general principles of modern care of dying persons and their families. It concludes with a description of formal hospice programs.

HOSPICE CRITIQUE OF CONTEMPORARY TERMINAL CARE

Although many people think of a hospice as a program or a place for the care of the dying, it is best appreciated first as a reform directed at the contemporary practice of terminal care. The hospice movement began and grew because of the dissatisfaction of lay persons and health care professionals with the care of dying patients. Several broad areas have been identified in which the special needs of dying persons and their families are often poorly met by existing medical practices and services; these are described below.

PAIN AND SYMPTOM CONTROL

Fear of pain and physical suffering is a foremost concern of cancer patients and their families. Too many patients suffer needlessly from uncontrolled pain. Despite the availability of straightforward and effective analgesic methods, over half of patients with far-advanced cancer have pain and a third are plagued by very severe or extreme pain.[21-24] Such distress has devastating physical and psychosocial effects on the patient and family. Additionally, many other common causes of physical discomfort in the dying—symptoms such as nausea, constipation, insomnia, or dry mouth—are not scrupulously managed.

PSYCHOSOCIAL SUPPORT

Communication among the patient, family members, and professional caretakers is often poor. Emotional support for the patient during the crises of terminal illness is deficient, and a full range of psychosocial services is not provided. Family members, who may play a major role in the patient's well-being and who likewise suffer from the terminal illness, tend to receive little attention while the patient is alive and during the period of bereavement.[25-28]

APPROPRIATE INTERVENTION

Finding a style of care that is appropriate to the dying patient can be difficult, but many diagnostic and therapeutic acts that are carried out almost reflexively by health care workers make little sense in the context of terminal illness. Dying patients may perceive diagnostic studies, surgery, and other procedures as an assault on their comfort, dignity, and desire to be allowed to die in peace. Clinicians who feel pressured to "do something" by the patient, the family, or their own personal standards may become preoccupied with aggressive interventions that add little to the patient's well-being and that detract attention from important comfort measures and the difficult emotional adjustment to facing oncoming death. Hence, increasing attention has been paid to such issues as "quality of life," "limiting treatment," and the "right to die."

A phase of zealous intervention may give way to neglect or abandonment—caretakers stop coming in to the patient's room, the doctor no longer sits down and touches the patient, or the dying person is sent home with little help or follow-up.[7,8] The physician may say, "We have nothing more to offer you," a terrible dismissal that is never true, since aggressive attention to comfort and support is appropriate for all patients until the moment of death.

SITE OF CARE

Institutions such as hospitals and nursing homes often seem poorly suited for meeting the personal needs of dying persons and their families. The hospital may be perceived as strange, cold, impersonal, and lacking in privacy. Family members who seek an active role in helping the dying person—by cooking a meal or providing other personal care—may feel useless.

Home care can offer great advantages to some terminally ill patients in terms of familiarity, comfort, security, a sense of autonomy, continuity with normal life, the closeness and involvement of family and friends, and cost. When well supported, many patients and families will choose to die at home.[29,30] However, patients must be appropriately advised about home care, a service that is often discouraged or poorly understood by hospital-based medical staff. Moreover, when patients are cared for at home, appropriate community services are not regularly available to ensure ongoing medical and nursing supervision and the other supports essential for good care.[31,32] Pain control has been particularly noted as deficient for many patients at home.[12,18,32]

A MODERN STANDARD OF TERMINAL CARE

Described below are some desirable elements of a modern system of care for cancer patients, as well as for patients with other chronic fatal diseases, particularly those in the terminal phase of illness. These elements are aspired to by hospices and other comprehensive or palliative care programs, while also setting a standard for the individual clinician and his or her referral network. Many of the topics addressed below—pain and symptom control, limiting treatment, communication about illness, emotional support for patient and family facing death, dying and bereavement, home care—are commonly neglected in general medical and oncology textbooks and in the training of physicians.

PAIN CONTROL

The hospice movement initially received wide attention because of its success in comforting patients who had intractable pain. Even among hospitalized cancer patients, roughly 20% suffer from severe and continuous pain. Reports from St. Christopher's Hospice in London indicate that over 98% of patients, many of whom are very near death and have been referred because their pain seemed unmanageable, can be made comfortable without being overly sedated.[19]

Techniques of pain control that were popularized partially by the hospice movement are now widely recognized, including the following[33-39]: careful attention to the sites and types of pain; prescription of doses of narcotics that are tailored to the individual patient and adequate to eradicate pain without causing drowsiness; the use of regular dosing intervals ("by the clock" rather than "as-needed" regimens) that are carefully adjusted to control pain at all times; education of staff, patients, and families on widespread but inappropriate concerns about narcotic tolerance and dependence; a favoring of oral medications, particularly elixirs of morphine, over parenteral treatment; awareness of the multidimensional contributions to pain (*e.g.*, depression, anxiety, social stress) and hence attention to control of other disagreeable symptoms and to the provision of good psychosocial support[40-42]; and use of a variety of additional methods for achieving excellent pain management, including such specific measures as nonsteroidal anti-inflammatory agents, steroids, antidepressants, radiation therapy, and simple nerve blocks. The avoidance of unnecessary, uncomfortable procedures or devices—intravenous lines, intramuscular injections, nasogastric tubes, venupunctures, and the like—also contributes to the patient's comfort.

CONTROL OF OTHER SYMPTOMS

Patients with advanced cancer experience a variety of disagreeable symptoms in addition to pain, including a high frequency of nausea, vomiting, anorexia, xerostomia, sore mouth, diarrhea, constipation, cough, dyspnea, bladder problems, pressure sores, edema and effusions, anorexia, fatigue, and a variety of neuropsychiatric disturbances.[1,17,39,43] Despite widespread attention to the nausea and vomiting associated with cancer treatment, 62% of terminal cancer patients experience these symptoms, mostly unrelated to chemotherapy or irradiation, yet only a third are prescribed antiemetics.[44]

Hospice clinicians have focused considerable attention on disagreeable symptoms and noted that careful attention to palliation can greatly improve the lot of the dying. Novel and generally simple methods of symptom control have been publicized. For instance, basic mouth care is considered preferable to the use of intravenous fluids for managing the discomfort of dehydration, while narcotics and other measures can be used safely to relieve the dyspnea that afflicts as many as 70% of dying cancer patients.[45] A discussion of the pathophysiology and clinical approach to common symptoms of advanced cancer is beyond the scope of this chapter, but a number of books are now available to guide the physician.[36,39,43,46-50]

COMMUNICATION ABOUT THE ILLNESS

Advanced cancer is a frightening condition for most patients. Patients anxiously monitor their bodies, interpreting new sensations as signs of progressing cancer. They worry about future suffering and often harbor fantasies of intractable pain, choking, deformity, and exsanguination. The clinician should be available to discuss the patient's condition in a leisurely manner, encouraging questions and the expression of concerns while allowing time for patient education. When worry is treated along with symptoms, well-being is greatly enhanced. Communication about the illness is a basic act for providing psychosocial support and reassurance, and lays the groundwork for the doctor and patient to develop an individualized approach to care.[51]

Contemporary standards of care dictate that patients be treated honestly and be allowed to participate fully in the decisions that bear on their well-being.[52-55] The great majority of patients appreciate being informed of the nature of their condition and having an opportunity to express their preferences about diagnostic and treatment options. The clinician should favor but not necessarily insist on full disclosure and participation in choosing management options; patients should be offered all the information they want, with the recognition that a few patients want limited information or prefer to delegate decision-making to family members or their doctor.

Similarly, family members, home health care workers, and other persons involved in the daily life of the dying person need information about the patient's illness and an opportunity to have their concerns addressed. Family members benefit from education that allows them to anticipate problems and rehearse appropriate actions (*e.g.*, how to handle worsening dyspnea, what to do when the patient dies at home).[51]

PSYCHOLOGICAL SUPPORT

A person who consciously faces death will inevitably undergo a psychological crisis. A healthy response to terminal illness for both the patient and family involves anticipatory grieving. No intervention will save the patient from some distress. However, loneliness, a sense of vulnerability, and other suffering can be alleviated, and coping can be enhanced.[13,56]

Methods for helping the dying person are generally quite simple. Indeed, most patients only need to be made physically comfortable, to be cared for in a supportive, personally satisfying environment, and to have the opportunity to talk openly about their feelings.[57] Many patients have their own support networks—family, friends, clergy, and others—but still benefit from talking with their physician, nurse, or social worker. Hospice programs have also trained volunteers to serve as "friendly listeners."

Similar emotional support should be available to family members. Terminal illness and the process of providing care for a dying relative regularly impose a severe psychological and social burden on relatives or close friends. New strains may develop among relatives or old wounds may be opened afresh, thus depriving family members of mutual support and causing further problems for themselves and the patient.

A subset of patients and family members want or need more specialized psychological services. Primary care providers (nurses and physicians) need to be trained to recognize problematic denial and other dysfunctional coping patterns, pathological anxiety, depression and dysfunctional grieving (as opposed to normal grief), sexual disorders, and evidence of other significant mental health disturbances. Counseling, psychopharmacologic treatment, or appropriate referral should then be provided. Mental health professionals and other clinicians with training and experience in working with the terminally ill and bereaved should be available for consultation to primary care providers and should provide individual and group therapy.[56,58–62]

SOCIAL SUPPORT

Illness and dying present a variety of social and economic problems to sick persons and their families. Home care particularly puts a burden on the family, who not only require professional supervision for their caretaking tasks, but also may need outside help in the form of homemakers, home health aides, and physical therapists. Assistance may be required for such matters as paying medical bills, obtaining equipment and services in the home, providing for minor children, settling financial affairs, and arranging for funeral services.[29,31,63] Good social supports facilitate bereavement and the family's eventual adjustment to loss.[56]

EXISTENTIAL AND SPIRITUAL CONCERNS

From a strictly biomedical viewpoint, sickness and death are facts of life. Humans, however, search for broader meaning in such events. In confronting death, patients and families turn to the physician for cure or palliation, but they simultaneously seek understanding and consolation from existential and spiritual viewpoints. Why did this happen to me? How can I bear up to this illness, withstand loss, and maintain a sense of worth? Where can I turn for hope? What sense can I make of my life? Existential and spiritual pain may be as troubling as physical or other psychological distress. Many patients and families find satisfactory ways of dealing with these issues on their own; others will benefit from rather simple counseling methods or referral to appropriately trained clergy or mental health workers.[64,65]

HELPING CHILDREN

The terminal illness and death of a parent is inevitably a psychological trauma for young children. Mental health consultation is regularly indicated. Few parents—either the sick person or the surviving spouse—are able to provide age-appropriate information for young children and optimal counseling and support, nor are many professional health care workers trained for this task. Special efforts should be made early in the course of the illness to work collaboratively with the parents and school personnel. When the parent is hospitalized, visits from the children should be carefully arranged. Additional attention is required in dealing with the death and funeral. Appropriate follow-up should be assured when the parent dies.[66]

BEREAVEMENT SERVICES

The morbidity and mortality of bereavement have been demonstrated in a number of studies.[67,68] Unresolved grief is a frequent source of psychological distress.[69] Clinical criteria have been developed for recognizing the differences between normal and dysfunctional grief, and a variety of interventions have been described for identifying and treating high-risk persons.[56,67,70–75] Bereavement counseling should be provided both to assist selected family members in the process of normal grief and to identify and treat persons with dysfunctional patterns.

INSTITUTIONAL CARE

The British hospices have suggested a new approach to inpatient care for the dying. The inpatient hospice is notable for a pleasant, light, homelike atmosphere. With a high nurse-to-patient ratio and conscientious selection and support of caregivers, the staff appear calm, unhurried, enthusiastic, and remarkably cheerful. The usual paraphernalia of institutional care are conspicuously absent. Patients are encouraged to wear their own clothes and to decorate their surroundings with personal items. They may be allowed to administer their own medication and to use alcohol. The staff fosters the involvement of the family in providing meals and personal care, and facilities may be offered for relatives to remain overnight. Access of guests, including children and pets, may be possible at any time. St. Christopher's Hospice has favored wards in which patients interact with each other and see each other die.[14–16]

The English model of free-standing hospice buildings has not been adopted in the United States, where only a handful of institutions dedicated solely to hospice care have been built. Inpatient wards, however, have been redesigned to emulate some of the features noted above, in a manner analogous to the development of home like birthing rooms. One testament to the value of such separate inpatient units comes from the report of a palliative care team: they were less successful in controlling pain while working on general medical wards than when they applied the same methods to patients in a special hospice unit.[76]

HOME CARE

In the United States, hospice has been primarily a home care program. Outpatient management is favored due to economic pressures to avoid institutional care and because many patients desire to be cared for in the home. Where adequate supervision and supports are available, most patients can remain at home, feeling comfortable and secure, throughout the course of a terminal illness. With proper support and training, rather intense or technical care, including intravenous therapy and parenteral administration of medicine, can often be managed by the family.

Terminally ill home care patients require regular visits from physicians or nurses trained to provide specialized palliative medical care and psychosocial support. Services must be available at all times of the day and night. Assistance with the burden of physical care may come from home health aides who, at times, may be required throughout the night.[31,77,78] Approaches to managing death in the home have been described.[79,80]

Brief admissions to an inpatient unit may be required to provide temporary relief for a family that is overburdened with around-the-clock patient care.

APPROPRIATE TREATMENT/LIMITING CARE

Steering between neglect and overzealous treatment is a constant tension in the care of the dying. There is always more that can be done, so limits to treatment inevitably must be set. The following basic principles are useful in thinking about decisions about appropriate treatment as death approaches.[81-86]

First, the physician's goal of restoring health becomes subservient to that of relieving suffering. Measures directed solely at prolonging life are rarely adopted. Aggressive palliation becomes a preoccupation for the clinician, including attention to both physical and psychosocial distress. Hospice care is sometimes contrasted to euthanasia, since vigorous measures that make life comfortable may obviate any desire to hasten death.

Second, the will of the patient is the supreme law in guiding action. Clinical management should reflect the patient's personal values, which may include a desire that "everything possible be done" or a desire for comfort measures only. Patients and family members need to be informed about the usefulness of various interventions and to develop realistic expectations for treatment. The physician should encourage the patient to express his or her own personal goals and to seek methods for achieving these goals. Competent patients are free to accept or reject any recommendations and to change their minds. Treatments need not be begun simply to prolong life, and treatments that are prolonging life may be discontinued if the patient so desires.

Third, when a patient is incompetent, treatment decisions should be based on that person's previously expressed values. Since many patients who are approaching death will lose their capacity to communicate their wishes, living wills and less formal measures for directing future decision-making are desirable.[87] In the absence of advance directives, family members may provide "substituted judgment," meaning that they try to convey what the patient would have wanted in the situation, not necessarily what they would want for themselves or the patient.

STAFF STRESS

Increased attention to the plight of the dying has led to greater awareness of the stress on caregivers. Caring for the dying presents both great rewards and great strains. On the one hand, clinicians note the unusual gratitude of terminally ill patients and their families, the pleasure of successfully providing physical and emotional support, the privilege and poignancy of sharing in the lives of people struggling with serious illness and facing death, and the personal value of reflecting on death. On the other hand, caregivers face the often desperate and time-consuming needs of the patient and family, high levels of anxiety, frequent crises, and daily encounters with deterioration, helplessness, loss, and death. Physicians and other staff regularly experience distress, manifested in such phenomena as "burnout," aversion toward or impersonal treatment of patients, false optimism, interpersonal problems at work or at home, demoralization, self-doubt, self-blame, and depression. Help for staff stress includes attending to the selection of personnel, to their personal and professional support network, and to many other aspects of the work milieu.[88-91]

HOSPICE PROGRAMS

In the past 15 years, diverse programs have emerged in North America under the hospice banner.[92,93] Hospice organizations, including inpatient-based units (special wards or palliative care teams that serve an entire hospital) and home health agency-based or free-standing programs, have offered a variety of services, delivered by mixtures of paid and volunteer, professional and nonprofessional workers. These programs may contract with other agencies for such functions as social work, volunteers, or bereavement follow-up and may develop alliances with inpatient and outpatient units in order to provide a full range of services. At the same time, many other organizations, some of which antedate the modern hospice movement, have provided similar services but under a different name.

In 1982, Congress added hospice coverage to the Medicare program. Hospice benefits have also been included in some insurance packages from Blue Cross and other third party payors. In practical terms, these hospice benefits tend to cover more community nursing and home health services than would be allowed under standard health insurance, and provide for short-term inpatient hospice care.

In order to be accredited and to receive third-party reimbursement for a full range of hospice services, a hospice program must meet standards set forth by the Joint Commission on the Accreditation of Hospitals, as well as by local and state regulations. With the emergence of hospice benefits, many health care organizations have sought to develop hospice programs, while existing hospice programs, many of which developed and flourished outside of mainstream health care, have been encouraged to join with established institutions and agencies in order to be accredited. Thus, hospice, which began as a reform movement, driven largely by volunteer efforts, has been transformed into a specially reimbursed program, and eventually is likely to develop into a hospice industry, analogous to the nursing home or home care industry.[94]

ELEMENTS OF AN ACCREDITED HOSPICE PROGRAM

Accredited hospice programs require an interdisciplinary team that is trained and supported in the provision of physical and psychosocial treatment for the dying patient and family. Care is directed to the patient and to the patient's family or other primary carepersons. At a minimum, personnel categories include physicians, nurses, psychologists or social workers, ministers, bereavement specialists, and volunteers. Emotional support for team members is offered. Services must be available in the home 24 hours a day, 7 days a week. Medicare also requires provision of medical supplies and equipment, drugs, home health aides, physical therapy, occupational therapy, and speech or language pathology services. Inpatient facilities are expected to attend to the privacy of patients and families and to their special nutritional and dietary needs, and must have access to emergency services, radiology, pathology, laboratory work, and pharmacy.

ADMISSION POLICY

In order to receive hospice reimbursement from Medicare, accredited hospices require the following criteria for admission: (1) a definite diagnosis of cancer; (2) certification by the hospice medical director or attending physician that the patient has a life expectancy of 6 months or less; (3) referral or consent of the primary physician; (4) informed consent of the patient and family, including acknowledgment of the prognosis and a desire for "noncurative" care and for remaining at home; and (5) a need for skilled services.

Three benefit periods, lasting 90, 90, and 30 days respectively, are allowed. Once patients have been accepted by a hospice, they may decide to leave the program (and are still eligible for standard Medicare benefits), but the hospice may not otherwise discharge or reduce services for patients, even for those who live beyond the 210-day period in which they are eligible for benefits. No more than 20% of the aggregate number of covered days for all of a program's patients may be spent in inpatient facilities, and a limit on average payments is now set at $7,391 per patient.

EVALUATION

A number of studies are available that convincingly validate specific components of specialized terminal care services. However, evaluation of entire hospice programs in the United States have been plagued with methodological problems: failure to randomize treatment or to identify satisfactory control groups; inadequate description of subjects and of the quality and types of services provided by the hospice and control groups; and questionable measurement instruments.[93,95]

Two major studies of accredited hospice programs in the United States have been published. Greer et al[96] and Mor et al[97] studied Medicare-approved hospice demonstration projects. They reported that the hospice programs, compared to conventional care providers, provided more social service support, less intravenous therapy, and cost less in the last weeks of life. No overall significant differences were noted in the measures of quality of life of patients or of family bereavement. Pain control was more efficient in hospital-based hospices than in home care hospices or conventional care settings. Hospital-based hospice programs, as compared to home care-based hospices, cost more per case ($6,148 *vs.* $5,492), had shorter lengths of stay (63 *vs.* 72 days), had fewer patient dying at home (27% *vs.* 62%), and used more inpatient days (29%–36% *vs.* 7%–16%).[93]

In a second study of a hospital-based unit at a Veterans Administration center,[98–100] hospice and nonhospice care were essentially indistinguishable in terms of survival, hospital days, control of pain and other symptoms, activities of daily living, patient affect, use of radiation, chemotherapy, and surgery, and costs. Hospice patients were more satisfied with their care, and their families were more involved in care, more satisfied, and less anxious.

These studies and others[17,101–103] indicate that hospice care is no more expensive than existing systems of terminal care, and that a favoring of home care may lead to cost savings. However, savings to the health care system may be offset by other societal costs of home care, particularly the financial burden assumed by the patient and family.[93,104]

One interpretation of the failure of some studies to show greater differences in outcomes has been that hospice methods have been widely adapted by clinicians who are not identified with a hospice program. A report from Great Britain has suggested that community standards of terminal care have greatly improved from 1967–69 to 1977–79, and that while hospice is associated with superior patient and family satisfaction, pain control is now well managed by generalists.[105]

In summary, hospice programs appear to do as well as or better than standard care. No study has shown inferior outcomes in a hospice. Clinicians working with an individual hospice, however, have no guarantee about the standards of training and care provided by a program and must judge it in the same manner as they might evaluate a hospital, nursing home, or home health care program.

THE EVOLUTION OF HOSPICE

Whereas reimbursement has provided financial viability for the hospice movement, certain features of the Medicare hospice program make little sense clinically. First, the limitation of services to patients in the last 6 months of life requires notoriously inaccurate prognostication, while erroneously implying that full palliative services would not be useful to patients in earlier phases of their illness. Second, an artificial and conceptually fuzzy distinction is promoted between "curative" treatment and services directed toward caring, support, or palliation. Rather than fostering inte-2cfgrated, comprehensive approaches to cancer management, an alternate system of care is established, potentially depriving patients in one system of the expertise and services available in the other. Why should a patient be asked to give up any interest in cure or life-prolonging measures in order to obtain important palliative services? Also, separate programs may force or encourage patients to leave a physician in whom they have developed confidence and trust. Third, the hospice concept is applicable to a wide variety of terminal illnesses, including progressive neurologic disease, end-stage heart and lung disease, and AIDS,[106] and should not be restricted to cancer patients. Fourth, meaningful standards for hospice staff training and quality of care have not been developed.

The hospice movement has developed and publicized many valuable approaches to caring for the dying and their families. No type of program, however, can claim a monopoly on fine terminal care, or necessarily offer all the quality services that patients deserve. The clinician's task is to provide fine biomedical and psychosocial care to his or her patients, either directly or by delegating key tasks to skilled colleagues. Declaring a patient's illness as irreversible, untreatable, or terminal and referring the patient to a program of specialized services will not solve the difficult problem of determining the best form of care for an individual. The popular rhetoric about the care of the dying—the antitechnology bias, the nostalgic and often unrealistic notions of "death with dignity" and "accepting death"—may obscure the difficult task for the patient, family, and clinician of finding skilled care that is appropriate for the individual, based on an appreciation of both medical expertise and the patient's personal values.

For further information about hospice programs, inquire at:

National Hospice Organization
1901 North Fort Myer Drive, Suite 307
Arlington, VA 22209
(703-243-5900)

REFERENCES

1. Lamerton R: Care of the Dying, rev ed. New York, Penguin, 1980
2. Feifel H (ed): The Meaning of Death. New York, McGraw-Hill, 1959
3. Kubler-Ross E: On Death and Dying. New York, Macmillan, 1969
4. Becker E: The Denial of Death. New York, Free Press, 1973
5. DeSpelder LA, Strickland AL: The Last Dance—Encountering Death and Dying. Palo Alto, Calif, Mayfield Publishing, 1983
6. Vovelle M: Rediscovery of death since 1960. Ann Am Acad Pol Soc Sci 447:89-99, 1980
7. Glaser BG, Strauss AL: Awareness of Dying. Chicago, Aldine, 1965
8. Glaser BG, Strauss AL: Time for Dying. Chicago, Aldine, 1968
9. Hinton J: Dying, 2nd ed. Baltimore, Penguin, 1972
10. Parkes CM: Bereavement: Studies of Grief in Adult Life. New York, International Universities Press, 1972
11. Weisman AD: On Dying and Denying: A Psychiatric Study of Terminality. New York, Behavioral Publications, 1972
12. Cartwright A, Hockey L, Anderson JL: Life Before Death. London, Routledge & Kegan Paul, 1973
13. Weisman AD: Coping with Cancer. New York, McGraw-Hill, 1979
14. Rossman P: Hospice: Creating New Models of Care for the Terminally Ill. New York, Fawcett Columbine, 1977
15. Stoddard S: The Hospice Movement: A Better Way of Caring for the Dying. Briarcliff Manor, New York, Stein and Day, 1978
16. DuBois PM: The Hospice Way of Death. New York, Human Science Press, 1980
17. Lack SA, Buckingham RW: First American Hospice. New Haven, Hospice, Inc, 1978
18. Parkes CM: Home or hospital? Terminal care as seen by surviving spouses. J R Coll Gen Pract 28:19-30, 1978
19. Saunders C: The Management of Terminal Disease. Chicago, Year Book Medical Publishers, 1978
20. Saunders C, Baines M: Living with Dying: The Management of Terminal Disease. New York, Oxford University Press, 1983
21. Angell M: Editorial: The quality of mercy. N Engl J Med 306:98-99, 1982
22. Daut RL, Cleeland CS: The prevalence and severity of pain in cancer. Cancer 50:1913-1918, 1982
23. Bonica JJ: Treatment of cancer pain: Current status and future need. In Fields HL et al (eds): Advances in Pain Research and Therapy, vol 9, pp 589-616. New York, Raven Press, 1985
24. Stjernsward J: Cancer pain relief: An important global public health issue. In Fields HL et al (eds): Advances in Pain Research and Therapy, vol 9, pp 555-558. New York, Raven Press, 1985
25. Krant MK: Family members' perceptions of communications in late stage cancer. Int J Psychiatry Med 8:203-216, 1977-1978
26. Cassileth BR, Lusk EJ, Strouse TB et al: A psychological analysis of cancer patients and their next-of-kin. Cancer 55:72-76, 1985
27. Lewis FM: The impact of cancer on the family: A critical analysis of the research literature. Patient Education Counseling pp 269-289, 1986
28. Tolle SW, Bascom PB, Hickam DH et al: Communication between physicians and surviving spouses following patient deaths. J Gen Intern Med 1:309-314, 1986
29. Martinson IM: Home Care for the Dying Child: Professional and Family Perspectives. New York, Appleton-Century-Crofts, 1976
30. Groth-Juncker A, McCusker J: Where do elderly patients prefer to die. J Am Geriatr Soc 31:457-461, 1983
31. Billings JA, Rubin F, Stoeckle JD: Home care. In Calkins E, Davis PJ, Ford AB (eds): The Practice of Geriatrics, pp 108-114. Philadelphia, WB Saunders, 1986
32. Parkes CM: Terminal care: Home, hospital, or hospice? Lancet 1:155-157, 1985
33. Marks RM, Sachar EJ: Undertreatment of medical inpatients with narcotic analgesics. Ann Intern Med 78:173-181, 1973
34. Mount BM, Ajemian I, Scott JF: Use of the Brompton Mixture in treating the chronic pain of malignant disease. Can Med Assoc J 113:122-124, 1976
35. Vere DW: Pharmacology of morphine drugs used in terminal care. In Vere DW (ed): Topics of Therapeutics 4, pp 75-83. Kent, England, Pitman Medical Publishing, 1978
36. Ajemian I, Mount MB (eds): The R.V.H. Manual on Palliative Hospice Care. New York, Arno, 1980
37. Twycross RG, Lack SA: Symptom Control in Far Advanced Cancer: Pain Relief. London, Pitman Publishing, 1983
38. Walsh TD: Common misunderstandings about the use of morphine for chronic pain in advanced cancer. CA 35:164-169, 1985
39. Billings JA: Outpatient Management of Advanced Cancer: Symptom Control, Support, and Hospice-in-the-Home. Philadelphia, JB Lippincott, 1985
40. Ahles TA, Blanchard EB, Ruckdeschel JC: The multidimensional nature of cancer-related pain. Pain 17:277-288, 1983
41. Spiegel D, Bloom JR: Pain in metastatic breast cancer. Cancer 52:341-345, 1983
42. Bond MR: Cancer pain: Psychological substrates and therapy. In Fields HL et al (eds): Advances in Pain Research and Therapy, vol 9, pp 559-567. New York, Raven Press, 1985
43. Baines MS: Control of other symptoms. In Saunders CM (ed): The Management of Terminal Disease. Chicago, Year Book Medical Publishers, 1978
44. Reuben DB, Mor V: Nausea and vomiting in terminal cancer patients. Arch Intern Med 146:2021-2023, 1986
45. Reuben DB, More V: Dyspnea in terminally ill cancer patients. Chest 89:234-236, 1986
46. Wilkes E: The Dying Patient: The Medical Management of Incurable and Terminal Illness. Ridgewood, New Jersey, George A. Bogden & Son, 1982
47. Corr CA, Corr DM (eds): Hospice Care: Principles and Practice. New York, Springer, 1983
48. Twycross RG, Lack SA: Therapeutics in terminal cancer. London, Pitman, 1984
49. Twycross RG, Lack SA: Control of alimentary symptoms in far advanced cancer. London, Churchill-Livingstone, 1986
50. Levy MH, Catalano RB: Control of common physical symptoms other than pain in patients with terminal disease. Semin Oncol 12:411-436, 1985
51. Billings JA: Feeling secure. In Billings JA (ed): Outpatient Management of Advanced Cancer: Symptom Control, Support, and Hospice-in-the-Home, pp 173-194. Philadelphia, JB Lippincott, 1985
52. Schoene-Seifer B, Childress JF: How much should the cancer patient know and decide? CA 36:85-94, 1986
53. President's Commission for the Study of Ethical Problems in Medicine and Biomedical and Behavioral Research: Making Health Care Decisions. Washington, DC, US Government Printing Office, 1982
54. Katz J: The Silent World of Doctor and Patient. New York, Free Press, 1984
55. Billings JA: Sharing bad news. In Billings JA (ed): Outpatient Management of Advanced Cancer: Symptom Control, Support and Hospice-in-the-Home, pp 236-259. Philadelphia, JB Lippincott, 1985
56. Block SD: Coping with loss. In Billings JA (ed): Outpatient Management of Advanced Cancer: Symptom Control, Support and Hospice-in-the-Home, pp 195-235. Philadelphia, JB Lippincott, 1985
57. Lack SA: Hospice—A concept of care in the final stage of life. Conn Med 43:367-372, 1979
58. Weisman AD: Early diagnosis of vulnerability in cancer patients. Am J Med Sci 271:187-196, 1976
59. Linn MW, Linn BS, Harris R: Effects of counseling for late stage cancer patients. Cancer 49:1048-1055, 1982
60. Weisman AD, Worden JW, Sobel HJ: Psychosocial Screening and Intervention with Cancer Patients. Boston, Project Omega, 1980
61. Spiegel D, Bloom JR, Yalom I: Group support for patients with metastatic cancer: A randomized prospective outcome study. Arch Gen Psychiatry 38:527-533, 1981
62. Cain EN, Kohorn EI, Quinlan DM et al: Psychosocial benefits of a cancer support group. Cancer 57:183-189, 1986
63. Billings JA: The tasks of physical care. In Billings JA (ed): Outpatient Management of Advanced Cancer: Symptom Control, Support and Hospice-in-the-Home, pp 155-171. Philadelphia, JB Lippincott, 1985
64. Frankl VE: Man's Search for Meaning: An Introduction to Logotherapy. New York, Simon and Schuster, 1959
65. Welch TA: Existential and spiritual concerns. In Billings JA (ed): Outpatient Management of Advanced Cancer: Symptom Control, Support and Hospice-in-the-Home, pp 260-268. Philadelphia, JB Lippincott, 1985
66. Adams-Greenly M, Moynihan R: Helping the children of fatally ill parents. Am J Orthopsychiatry 53:219-229, 1983 (See also Adams-Greenly M, Moynihan RT et al: Helping the children when a parent is dying. In Billings JA (ed): Outpatient Management of Advanced Cancer: Symptom Control, Support and Hospice-in-the-Home. Philadelphia, JB Lippincott, 1985)
67. Osterweis M, Solomon F, Green M (eds): Bereavement: Reactions, Consequences, and Care. Washington DC, National Academy Press, 1984
68. Bowling A: Mortality after bereavement: A review of the literature on survival periods and factors affecting survival. Soc Sci Med 24:117-124, 1987

69. Lazare A: Unresolved grief. In Lazare A (ed): Outpatient Psychiatry: Diagnosis and Treatment, pp 498–512. Baltimore, Williams & Wilkins, 1979
79. Raphael B: Preventive intervention with the recently bereaved. Arch Gen Psychiatry 34:1450–1454, 1977
71. Cameron J, Brings B: Bereavement outcome following preventive intervention: A controlled study. In Ajemian I, Mount B (eds): The R.V.H. Manual on Palliative/Hospice Care, pp 387–400. New York, Arno Press, 1980
72. Worden JW: Grief Counseling and Grief Therapy. New York, Springer, 1982
73. Cameron J, Parkes CM: Terminal care: Evaluation of effects on surviving family of care before and after bereavement. Postgrad Med J 59:73–78, 1983
74. Parkes CM, Weiss RS: Recovery from Bereavement. New York, Basic Books, 1983
75. Raphael B: The Anatomy of Bereavement. New York, Basic Books, 1983
76. Melzack R, Ofiesh JG, Mount BM: The Brompton mixture: Effects on pain in cancer patients. Can Med Assoc J 115:125–129, 1976
77. Rosenbaum EH, Rosenbaum IR: Principles of home care for the patient with advanced cancer. JAMA 244:1484–1487, 1980
78. Meyers AR, Master RJ, Kirk EM et al: Integrated care for the terminally ill: Variations in the utilization of formal services. Gerontologist 23:71–74, 1983
79. Billings JA: Death in the home. In Billings JA: Outpatient Management of Advanced Cancer: Symptom Control, Support and Hospice-in-the-Home. Philadelphia, JB Lippincott, 1985
80. Tolle SW, Elliot DL, Girard DE: How to manage patient death and care for the bereaved. Postgrad Med 78:87–95, 1985
81. Cassell ES: The nature of suffering and the goals of medicine. N Engl J Med 306:639–645, 1982
82. Micetich KC, Steinecker PH, Thomasma DC: Are intravenous fluids morally required for dying patients? Arch Intern Med 143:975–978, 1983
83. President's Commission for the Study of Ethical Problems in Medicine and Biomedical and Behavioral Research: Deciding to Forego Life-Sustaining Treatment: A Report on the Ethical, Medical, and Legal Issues in Treatment Decisions. Washington, DC, US Government Printing Office, 1983
84. Wanzer SH, Adelstein SJ, Cranford RE et al: The physician's responsibility toward hopelessly ill patients. N Engl J Med 301:955–959, 1984
85. Cassem EH: Appropriate treatment limits in advanced cancer. In Billings JA (ed): Outpatient Management of Advanced Cancer: Symptom Control, Support and Hospice-in-the-Home. Philadelphia, JB Lippincott, 1985
86. Hastings Center: Guidelines on the Termination of Life-Sustaining Treatment and the Care of the Dying. Briarcliff Manor, New York, Hastings Center, 1977
87. Bok S: Personal directions for care at the end of life. N Engl J Med 295:367–369, 1976
88. White LD: The self image of physicians and the care of dying patients. Ann NY Acad Sci 164:822–837, 1969
89. Weisman AD: Understanding the cancer patient: The syndrome of caregiver's plight. Psychiatry 44:161–168, 1981
90. Mount BM: Dealing with our losses. J Clin Oncol 4:1127–1134, 1986
91. Vachon MLS: Occupational Stress in the Care of the Critically Ill, the Dying, and the Bereaved. New York, Hemisphere Publishing, 1987
92. Torrens PR: Hospice Programs and Public Policy. Chicago, American Hospital Publishing, 1985
93. Mor V: Hospice Care Systems: Structure, Process, Costs, and Outcome. New York, Springer, 1987
94. Greer DS, Mor V: How Medicare is altering the hospice movement. Hastings Center Rep 15:5–13, 1985
95. Mount BM, Scott JF: Whither hospice evaluation? J Chronic Dis 36:73–76, 1983
96. Greer DS, Mor V, Morris JN et al: An alternative in terminal care: Results of the national hospice study. J Chronic Dis 39:9–26, 1986
97. Mor V, McHorney C, Sherwood S: Secondary morbidity among the recently bereaved. Am J Psychiatry 143:158–163, 1986
98. Kane RL, Bernstein L, Wales J et al: A randomised controlled trial of hospice care. Lancet 1:890–894, 1984
99. Kane RL, Klein SJ, Bernstein L et al: Hospice role in alleviating the emotional stress of terminal patients and their families. Med Care 23:189–197, 1985
100. Kane RL, Klein SJ, Bernstein L et al: The role of hospice in reducing the impact of bereavement. J Chronic Dis 39:735–742, 1986
101. Zimmer JG, Groth-Juncker A, McCusker J: Effects of a physician-led home care team on terminal care. J Am Geriatr Soc 32:288–292, 1984
102. Zimmer JG, Groth-Juncker A, McCusker J: A randomized controlled study of a home health care team. Am J Public Health 75:134–141,
103. McCusker J, Stoddard AM: Effects of an expanding home care program for the terminally ill. Med Care 25:373–385, 1987
104. Comptroller General of the United States: Home Health—The Need for a National Policy to Better Provide for the Elderly. Washington, DC, General Accounting Office, HRD-78-19, Dec 30, 1979
105. Parkes CM, Parkes J: 'Hospice' versus 'hospital' care: Reevaluation after 10 years as seen by surviving spouses. Postgrad Med J 60:120–124, 1984
106. Hughes AM, Martin JP, Franks P (eds): AIDS Home Care and Hospice Manual. San Francisco, Visiting Nurses Association of San Francisco (225 30th St, San Francisco, CA 94131), 1987

CHAPTER 62 *Treatment of Metastatic Cancer*

DONALD C. WRIGHT
THOMAS F. DELANEY

SECTION 1

Treatment of Metastatic Cancer to the Brain

Neurologic complications frequently arise in the patient with systemic cancer. The brain, which manifests an exquisite sensitivity to disturbances in the local environment, is unfortunately a favored site for metastatic spread. Brain metastases are common, life-threatening, and emotionally disabling; without successful management, patients frequently develop severe neurologic dysfunction and may ultimately die as a direct consequence of metastatic cerebral deposits despite adequate control of the primary cancer site.

Metastases to the brain occur in 25% to 35%[1] of all cancer patients, thus comprising a group representing the most common neoplasms of the brain.[2-4] This propensity for brain involvement by generalized cancers is aggravated by the fact that the more frequent primary cancer sites seen in the United States (*e.g.*, lung, breast) are associated with a high incidence of brain metastases. Table 62-1 is an epidemiologic estimate of the scope of metastatic brain tumors for the 1988 U.S. population. Symptomatic parenchymal metastases are forecast[1,5-7] to afflict 13.5% (133,000) of the total U.S. cancer population. This complication will also affect 13.5% (66,700) of the expected 1988 cancer deaths. Comparatively, primary brain tumors are forecast to account for 10,900 1988 deaths in the U.S. population.[2] Strict comparison of these two figures is not possible, as the cause of death in the two groups is not the same.

This chapter addresses the pathogenesis, clinical features, evaluation, therapy, and expected results of *parenchymal* metastases to the brain.

DEMOGRAPHIC PROFILE AND CLASSIFICATION OF BRAIN METASTASES

The reported incidence of metastatic involvement of the central nervous system (CNS) varies with the experience or material being analyzed.[1,6,8] Data for brain metastases may be derived from operative (clinical) series, necropsy material, and epidemiologic surveys compiled from death certificates, hospital records, and similar statistical sources. The exact incidence of metastatic brain tumors is unknown, but useful approximations suggest a figure of 25% as an accurate estimate for the overall prevalence of *intracranial* metastases in the cancer population.[6,9] The intradural (parenchymal and leptomeningeal) frequency approaches 20%; parenchymal involvement alone is present in 10% of patients.

There is an overall male preponderance (56%) in brain metastases reflecting the high incidence of lung cancer in males. Males are also preponderant in tumors involving the gastrointestinal tract, head and neck, and prostate as well as sarcomas.[6] Females are preponderant in breast and thyroid metastases. The average age of onset of a brain metastasis in

TABLE 62-1. Epidemiologic Estimates of Brain Metastases—*1988*

Site or Type	*Systemic Cancer 1988: New Cases*	*Frequency of Symptomatic Metastases**	*New Cases: Symptomatic Metastases†*	*1988 Deaths*	*Deaths with Symptomatic Metastases‡*
All sites	985,000	0.135	133,000	494,000	66,700
Lung	152,000	0.263	40,000	139,000	36,500
Breast	135,900	0.158	21,500	42,300	6,700
Colon and rectum	147,000	0.045	6,600	61,500	2,750
Urinary organs	68,900	0.128	8,800	20,000	2,550
Melanoma	27,300	0.37	10,100	5,800	2,150
Prostate	99,000	0.053	5,250	28,000	1,500
Pancreas	27,000	0.04	1,100	24,500	1,000
Leukemia	26,900	0.06	1,600	18,100	1,100
Lymphoma§	39,100	0.038	1,500	18,000	700
Liver	14,000	0.04	550	10,900	450
Female genital	70,700	0.015	1,050	23,100	350

Table developed from Silverberg E, Lubera JA: Cancer statistics, 1988. CA 38:5–22, 1988; Takakura K, Sano K, Hoho S et al: Metastatic Tumors of the Central Nervous System. Tokyo, Igaku-Shoin, 1982; Hildebrand J: Lesions of the Nervous System in Cancer Patients. Monograph series of the European Organization for Research on Treatment of Cancer, Volume 5, New York, Raven Press, 1978; and Galicich JH, Sundaresan N: Metastatic brain tumors. In Wilkins RH, Rengachary SS (eds): Neurosurgery, pp 597–610, New York, McGraw-Hill, 1985.

* Symptomatic parenchymal metastases only (does not include skull, dura, or leptomeninges).

† Estimated by (new 1988 cases) × (metastatic frequency).

‡ Estimated by (1988 cancer deaths) × (metastatic frequency of symptomatic parenchymal metastases).

§ Includes all lymphoma (Hodgkin's, and non-Hodgkin's types).

males is 56 years, whereas females have an average onset at 49 years.[6] There are two age peaks for metastatic deposits to the brain; the majority of patients develop tumors at 55 to 59 years,[6] and a childhood peak at 0 to 10 years is also noted. The childhood tumors (leukemia, lymphoma, neuroblastoma, and certain sarcomas) differ from those common to adults.

CLASSIFICATION

It is clinically useful to determine the specific anatomic site(s) or "compartments" involved in a metastatic process, as well as the primary histologic type, temporal patterns of involvement, and clinical status of the patient at the time of diagnosis.

ANATOMICAL DISTRIBUTION

The anatomical cerebral compartments commonly involved by metastasis are the skull, dura, leptomeninges (arachnoid and pia), and parenchymal substance of the brain (Fig. 62-1). Metastases to the pituitary and spinal canal complete the possible anatomical sites of central nervous system (CNS) involvement.

Parenchymal distribution patterns (Fig. 62-2) of cerebral metastases correlate with the relative brain weight and blood flow for a given region.[10–14] Approximately 80% of parenchymal metastases occur in the supratentorial compartment, whereas the cerebellum (representing about 13% of the brain by weight) "receives" approximately 15% of all metastases.[6,9]

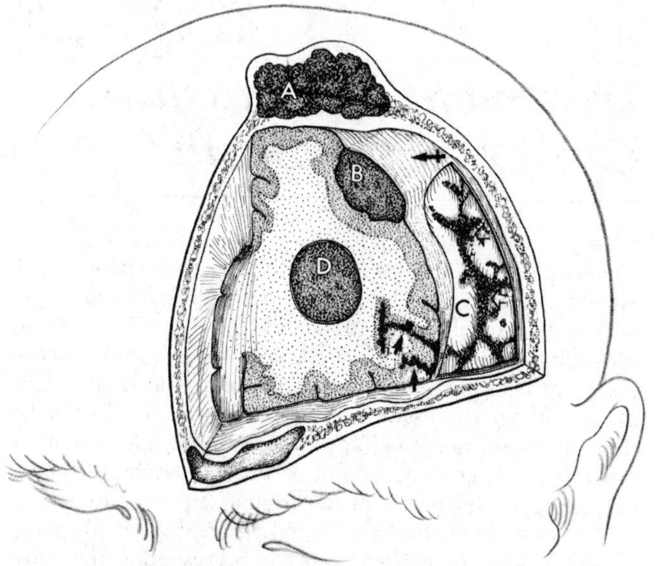

FIG. 62-1. Anatomical classification of brain metastases. Three-quarter view of left frontal cranium, showing **A** a large metastasis to the skull diploë; **B** a dural metastasis; **C** superficial leptomeningeal invasion; and **D** a parenchymal metastasis revealed by coronal cut made at posterior border of the frontal lobe. Open arrows indicate areas of leptomeningeal spread. Crossed arrow indicates convex surface of the brain with dura intact. Solid arrows indicate leptomeningeal spread into several sulci. (Courtesy of Pat Kenny, Medical Illustration Section, National Institutes of Health) (Wright DC: Surgical treatment of brain metastases. In Rosenberg SA [ed]: Surgical Treatment of Metastatic Cancer, pp 165–222. Philadelphia, JB Lippincott 1987)

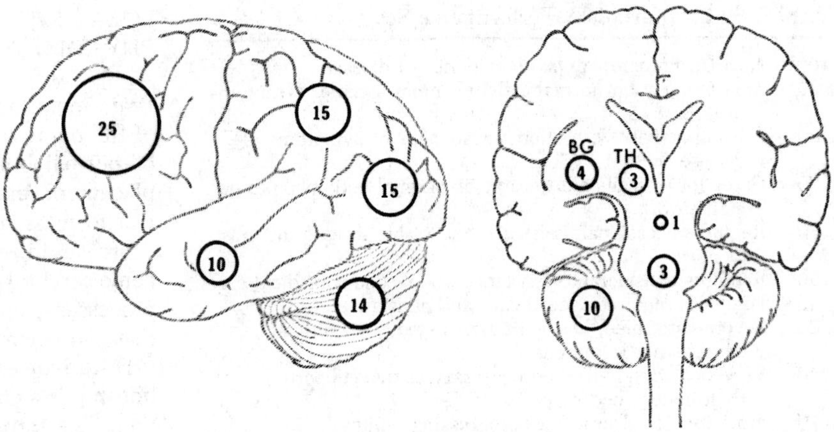

FIG. 62–2. Parenchymal distribution of brain metastases. The distribution and relative frequency (%) are diagrammed according to metastatic site. The subcortical gray structures (BG = basal ganglia, Th = thalamus) receive 7% of metastases, and cerebellar hemispheres receive 10% of metastases. (Adapted from Takakura K, Sano K, Hoho S et al: Metastatic Tumors of the Central Nervous System. Tokyo, Igaku-Shoin, 1982, and reproduced with permission from Wright DC: Surgical treatment of brain metastases. In Rosenberg SA [ed]: Surgical Treatment of Metastatic Cancer, pp 165–222. Philadelphia, JB Lippincott, 1987)

The detection of multiple metastatic deposits plays a critical role in the choice of therapy because most authors restrict surgery to single metastases. Multiple deposits are present in 53% of patients, although autopsy studies suggest that smaller (±3-mm) metastases are undetected, and the frequency of multiple tumors is higher.[5,6,9,15] Certain tumor types are associated with predominantly single (renal, ovarian, osteogenic sarcoma, breast) and multiple (lung, melanoma, seminoma) metastases.

HISTOLOGIC TYPE AND FREQUENCY OF METASTASES

Table 62-2 lists the parenchymal metastatic patterns for the more common cancers in a large autopsy series.[6] The overall parenchymal metastatic attack rate for this series was 17% (555/3359) of all cancer patients who were autopsied. Lung, gastrointestinal, and urinary tract primary tumors account for 80% of metastatic lesions in men, whereas breast, lung, gastrointestinal tract, and melanoma account for 80% of metastases in women. Lung carcinoma, by virtue of its relative frequency in the U.S. population, is the most common metastatic source, accounting for 40 to 60% of all parenchymal deposits.[6,7,16]

Melanoma has the highest likelihood of cerebral spread, with 65% of patients developing this complication; breast (51%), and lung (41%) contribute the greater number of overall patients by virtue of their prevalence.

TEMPORAL PATTERNS OF PRESENTATION

Brain metastases may present in three temporal patterns: precocious (occult primary), synchronous (simultaneous primary), and metachronous (antecedent primary).[8] Most patients (81%) present in a metachronous manner; the median interval from diagnosis of a primary tumor to the discovery of cerebral metastasis in a recent series was 17 months.[17] The mode of presentation is influenced by the primary tumor; lung, melanoma, and renal tumors tend to have brief intervals from the time of initial diagnosis to evolution of a brain metastasis, whereas breast, colon, and sarcomas have long intervals.

Classifying patients by their neurologic performance at

TABLE 62-2. Brain Metastases by Histologic Type*

Site of Primary Neoplasm	*No. of Patients*	*No. of Metastases**	*% Total†*	*Relative Frequency (%)‡*
Lung	774	266	7.9	48
Breast	526	111	3.3	20
Gastrointestinal	773	43	1.3	8
Urinary	199	34	1.0	6
Melanoma	69	34	1.0	6
Prostate	140	10	0.3	2
Liver and pancreas	293	14	0.4	3
Other	585	43	1.3	8
Total	3359	555	16.5	100

Modified from Takakura K, Sano K, Hoho S et al: Metastatic Tumors of the Central Nervous System. Tokyo, Igaku-Shoin, 1982.

* Parenchymal metastases only

† Expressed as $\frac{\text{Number (parenchymal) metastases}}{\text{Total number of cancer autopsies}} \times 100$

‡ Relative Frequency = $\frac{\text{Number (parenchymal) metastases by tumor type}}{\text{Total number of parenchymal metastases}} \times 100$

TABLE 62-3. Karnofsky Performance Scale

100	Normal; no complaints; no evidence of disease
90	Able to carry on normal activity; minor signs or symptoms of disease
80	Normal activity with effort; some signs or symptoms of disease
70	Cares for self; unable to carry on normal activity or to do active work
60	Requires occasional assistance but is able to care for most of needs
50	Requires considerable assistance and frequent medical care
40	Disabled; requires special care and assistance
30	Severely disabled; hospitalization is indicated although death is not imminent
20	Very sick; hospitalization necessary; active supportive treatment is necessary
10	Moribund; fatal processes progressing rapidly

the time when initial therapy is instituted has excellent prognostic value and a positive correlation with favorable outcome in patients selected for surgery. Several classification systems are employed,[8,18–21] most incorporating aspects of the performance scale originally developed by Karnofsky (Table 62-3).[22] The extent of nonneural disease associated with a cerebral metastasis also has prognostic value and is an important consideration in risk analysis for patients being considered for surgical therapy.

There are significant clinical, therapeutic, and pathophysiologic implications for patients with brain metastases when categorized in the manner as outlined. Choice of a therapeutic course for a given patient, and comparison of the efficacy of various treatment modalities in matched groups of patients are greatly facilitated by such classification.

PATHOGENESIS

The brain has a unique anatomic and physiologic organization that influences the localization, growth pattern, and spread of metastases. Brain metastases arise either from hematogenous dissemination of circulating tumor cells, or less commonly, by contiguous spread from adjacent tissues such as the skull, basal foramina (which transmit neural and vascular structures), and soft tissues of the head and neck. Hematogenous spread occurs by passive dissemination of tumor cells into the circulatory system.[6,8,23–25] Intrinsic tumor cell properties, characteristics of the target tissue, anatomic and hemodynamic influences are among the multiple factors affecting the patterns of tumor spread.[26] The typical generalizing secondary sites following penetration of the vascular system by a primary tumor are nonrandom, but most commonly involve the lung, liver, and lymph nodes. Tertiary deposits ("metastases of a metastasis") frequently develop from these secondary sites. Thus, brain metastases are generally a tertiary phenomenon, indicative of advanced disease.[27]

Certain primary tumors have "site-specific" target organs that are preferentially involved by metastatic disease.[28] The brain serves as a preferential site for melanoma and small-cell carcinoma of the lung, perhaps because of shared neuroendocrine features common to both tumor and host tissue.[29]

LOCAL EFFECTS OF METASTASES ON CEREBRAL PHYSIOLOGY

Brain metastases produce clinical symptoms by impairment of the homeostatic mechanisms necessary for maintenance of normal brain function. Mechanical distortion and displacement (herniations) by a progressively increasing neoplastic mass; increases in intracranial pressure (ICP) and decreases in cerebral blood flow (CBF); propagation of vasogenic cerebral edema; and derangement of metabolic energy processes, represent the major pathophysiologic changes that can occur.

Disturbances of the intracranial volume–pressure relationship is a common mechanism causing cerebral dysfunction. The intracranial volume is constant by virtue of the rigid confines of the skull and the incompressible nature of the cellular and fluid constituents of the brain (Monroe–Kellie doctrine).[30–32] The parenchymal compartment is fixed, but the brain can buffer changes in intracranial volume by reciprocal reductions of the cerebrospinal fluid (CSF) and vascular volumes or of the extracellular volume. These mechanisms of maintaining normal ICP can accommodate surprisingly large changes in intracranial volume, such as neoplasms, but only if the additional mass increases slowly in volume (months to years). Focal and rapid changes in volume tend to overwhelm the spatial (time) and volume compensatory mechanisms, and an increase in intracranial pressure occurs.

Intracranial masses that overwhelm the buffering capacity of the brain to accommodate increases in intracranial volume will result in various clinical herniation syndromes.[33] The midline falx, tentorium, and foramen magnum are anatomic sites at which herniation of cerebral tissue occurs when severe mechanical distortions arise. Even when recognized and quickly treated, herniations frequently result in permanent neurologic injury or death of the patient.

Brain swelling occurs as a result of mass lesions (*e.g.*, neoplasms, hematoma), obstruction of CSF pathways (hydrocephalus), increases in cerebrovascular blood volume (hyperemia), and brain edema. Brain edema is an increase in brain water and sodium,[34] occurring either by direct injury to cellular elements of the brain (cytotoxic edema) or arising from injury to the vascular endothelium (vasogenic edema). The former injury occurs by toxins, poisons, or hypoxic/ischemic insults,[34,35] whereas the latter is thought to be the primary form of edema associated with cerebral metastases. The *blood–brain* barrier (BBB) is a specialized membrane with a unique anatomic organization that normally restricts passage of large, water-soluble molecules from the vascular compartment to the brain extracellular space. Direct injury to endothelium by expanding mass lesions, dysplastic vascular structures present within neoplasms,[36] and biochemically mediated alterations of capillary permeability (phospholipid degradation products with vasoactive properties)[37–41] appear to play a role in the development of vasogenic edema, but the exact pathogenesis of this edema is unknown.

Injury to the vascular endothelium increases the permeability of the luminal plasma membrane and allows the passage of large molecules (*e.g.*, plasma proteins) normally restricted by the BBB. Edema develops as water and ions passively diffuse into the brain extracellular space to maintain isotonicity. The increase in extracellular water content primarily affects white matter, perhaps because of a less complex cytoarchitecture compared with that of gray matter. Edema fluid may travel along the longitudinally oriented white matter tracts and increase local extracellular water content at great distances from the focal "source" of increased capillary permeability.[42] Panhemispheric edema patterns occasionally arise by this mechanism from relatively small areas of BBB damage.

CLINICAL ASPECTS OF BRAIN METASTASES

The production of clinical symptoms and signs in the patient with brain metastasis does not differ substantially from development of other intracranial mass lesions. Thus, the definitive diagnosis of brain metastasis, particularly in the absence of a prior history of cancer, cannot be made solely on clinical examination.[7] Indeed, for the patient without an established diagnosis of cancer, a classic history suggestive of brain metastasis is elicitable in only a few patients.[43] Definitive diagnosis in such patients must rely on complementary diagnostic and pathologic examinations.

PRESENTATION: SYMPTOMS AND SIGNS

The presenting neurologic symptoms and signs (Table 62-4) from brain metastases are headache, weakness, cognitive or affective disturbance, and seizures.[5,16,43–48] Focal symptoms and signs (unilateral headache, weakness, seizures) are generally the result of direct parenchymal injury or destruction by neoplasm, whereas diffuse symptoms and signs (generalized headache, cognitive or behavioral changes, papilledema) reflect the more global effects of cerebral edema, metabolic dysfunction, or CSF obstruction.

Headache, the most common presenting symptom, is present in approximately half of patients and arises from traction of pain sensitive structures within the brain. The dura and dural sinuses, large blood vessels, and certain cranial nerves are subject to distortion by direct (tumor invasion) or indirect (edema, CSF obstruction) mechanisms. The headache is initially remitting, typically present in the morning, gradually increasing in duration and frequency, and it is soon associated with symptoms and signs of increased intracranial pressure (lethargy, confusion, papilledema). Unilateral headaches, when present, are of localizing value in most patients.[16]

Weakness, the most common focal sign, is symptomatic in 40% of patients and elicitable on examination in 65%.[43] Focal motor signs, particularly monoparesis, are also of localizing value when present. Ataxia may be present in patients with CSF obstruction and is a particular feature of cerebellar locations.

Disturbances in higher cerebral functions, including changes in behavior, memory, speech, and skilled integrative functions (reading, writing), form a large body of symptoms, generally reported in a third of patients as a presenting symptom. Careful testing will demonstrate such disturbances in 50% to 75% of patients.[43,49]

Seizures account for the most common acute onset of symptoms and, if focal, are of localizing value. Transient weakness (usually hemiparesis) may follow seizure activity (Todd's paralysis), or more permanent signs may occur in prolonged seizures (focal or generalized status epilepticus). Certain tumors (melanoma) and tumor patterns (leptomeningeal deposits) are associated with a high frequency of seizures because of their local proximity and irritative effects upon the cortex.[43,50] An abrupt evolution of symptoms occasionally arises as a result of tumoral hemorrhage and is usually manifested by seizure or focal weakness. Ten percent of patients with melanoma may present in this manner, whereas choriocarcinoma, lung, and renal metastases share a similar, although less common, tendency for tumoral hemorrhage.

DIFFERENTIAL DIAGNOSIS

Various disease processes mimic brain metastases by having a similar clinical profile or nonspecific appearance on diagnostic studies (Table 62-5). Benign, treatable conditions simulating a metastasis must be identified to avoid inappropriate or dangerous therapy. Presumptive diagnosis without pathologic verification has a high error rate,[15,51] even in patients with an established diagnosis of cancer. Other neoplasms (primary glial tumors, meningiomas) can often mimic metastatic disease, whereas infectious, cerebrovascular,[5,6,43,52] and toxic (iatrogenic) CNS complications frequently account for neurologic symptoms in patients with cancer and require specific evaluation and treatment. Those patients without a prior diagnosis of systemic cancer require an unequivocal pathologic diagnosis.

TABLE 62-4. Symptoms and Signs of Cerebral Metastases

Symptoms	*Frequency (%)*	*Signs*	*Frequency (%)*
Headache	53	Hemiparesis	66
Weakness, focal	40	Impaired cognition	77
Mental disturbance	31	Sensory loss, unilateral	27
Seizures	15	Papilledema	26
Gait disorder	20	Ataxia	24
Visual disturbance	12	Aphasia	19
Language disturbance	10		

Data from Refs. 6, 15, 17, 74, 99.

TABLE 62-5. Neurologic Dysfunction in the Cancer Patient: Differential Diagnosis*

Neoplastic	Primary brain tumors (glial series)
	Meningioma
Infectious	Abscess: pyogenic, tuberculous
	Fungal
	Toxoplasma
	Other
Cerebrovascular	Infarction
	Hemorrhage
	Sub- and epidural collections; acute and chronic
Toxic	Radiation necrosis

* Partial listing; not intended to serve as complete differential diagnostic list.

DIAGNOSTIC EVALUATION

There is no diagnostic test or procedure that substitutes for the clinical history and examination of a patient. The information gained from the clinician's interview and examination is the basis for localizing the neurologic lesion(s), developing a differential diagnosis, directing specific diagnostic studies, and assuring that the clinical diagnosis fully satisfies the extent of neurologic dysfunction in the patient.

GENERAL DIAGNOSTIC MEASURES

The diagnostic studies required for a given patient may vary considerably. The initial evaluation of a patient usually encompasses hematologic, coagulation, serum, urinary, and stool screening examinations. High quality chest x-ray examinations are an important screening test because of the disproportionate incidence of lung cancer in the U.S. population. Radionuclide studies (bone, liver), specialized contrast x-ray examinations (renal, gastrointestinal, breast), and endoscopic procedures may be indicated depending on the clinical presentation. Definitive therapy may occasionally be instituted on the basis of a single diagnostic study (usually a contrast CT scan).

SPECIALIZED NEURODIAGNOSTIC EVALUATION

Computed tomography (CT) scanning, magnetic resonance imaging (MRI), and arteriography are the primary studies currently employed in neurodiagnostic evaluation, whereas all other studies play a secondary or supplemental role. The principal use of these devices is for diagnosis and anatomic localization of a mass lesion. Accurate localization (Fig. 62-3D) is critical to the radiation therapist for treatment planning and to the surgeon in planning scalp flaps, bone openings, and cortical incisions.[7,53]

The initial diagnostic study in patients with suspected brain metastasis is the CT scan. Parenchymal metastases are typically spheroidal, surrounded by low-density edema formation, and located in the gray matter–white matter junction (see Fig. 62-3C,D). Most metastases are hypodense compared with the brain on noncontrast CT studies. Melanoma, choriocarcinoma, and colon metastases are exceptions and appear hyperdense on precontrast studies.[53] Greater than 90% of lesions will exhibit contrast enhancement by iodine conjugates. Enhancement occurs because of permeability changes in the blood–brain and blood–tumor barriers,[54,55] the large vascular volumes (neovascularity) characteristically found in tumors. This large neoplastic capillary surface area tends to increase the transit times for water-soluble molecules, such as the iodine conjugates used clinically to evaluate tumor contrast enhancement. The value of this diagnostic tool extends beyond the initial evaluation; serial CT scanning is a particularly effective means to monitor tumor development, progression, response to therapy, and detection of secondary complications.

Magnetic resonance imaging provides a spatial map of tissue ion density (*e.g.*, hydrogen protons associated with water molecules) without exposing patients to ionizing radiation. The resulting images derived from these data rival current CT scanners in anatomic resolution (see Fig. 62-3A,B). The MRI has superior clinical utility in certain disease processes (*e.g.*, multiple sclerosis) and CNS locations (posterior fossa, spinal cord), but it is currently limited by the inability to depict calcification or bone detail, nor can it readily differentiate tumor from surrounding edema. Enhancement of MRI contrast by paramagnetic conjugates (*e.g.*, gadolinium-DTPA) will likely solve the latter limitation, but the CT scanner currently has a higher specificity in typing various CNS lesions. Cerebral imaging technology, however, is a dynamic field, and MRI scanning has particular promise of further refinement in areas such as physiologic measurements (blood flow, phosphorous distribution), paramagnetic enhancement compounds, and specialized scanning techniques (T_1/T_2 weighting, time–scanning gated to physiologic events).

The respective diagnostic roles for CT and MRI scanning overlap because these devices have a high sensitivity for depicting metastatic involvement of the brain on an anatomic basis. Selection of appropriate therapy by localizing lesions to the specific anatomic compartment(s) involved, and identification of metastatic complications (hemorrhage, hydrocephalus, edema, infection) arising from treatment (surgical complications, radiation necrosis) has dramatically changed the short-term results of therapy by minimizing the morbidity of neoplastic and treatment-related complications.

Arteriography provides vascular detail such as the origin of arterial supply, routes of venous drainage and degree of neovascularity. It also provides some degree of local anatomic relationships not available by other imaging techniques. It is performed less frequently since the introduction of the CT scanner, and is generally reserved for the patient in whom tumor vascular characteristics play an important role in surgical planning.

Neurodiagnostic studies, such as radionuclide brain and CSF studies, skull films, and contrast ventricular and cisternal studies, have specific indications,[53] and are generally used to supplement CT, MRI, and angiographic studies.

A special note should be made on the use of lumbar puncture in the patient with suspected brain metastasis. This procedure has diagnostic value in situations in which infectious or neoplastic involvement of the CSF space is suspected; these represent the only entities for which a *specific* diagnosis can be inferred from examination of the cerebrospinal fluid. Lumbar puncture is a hazardous procedure in

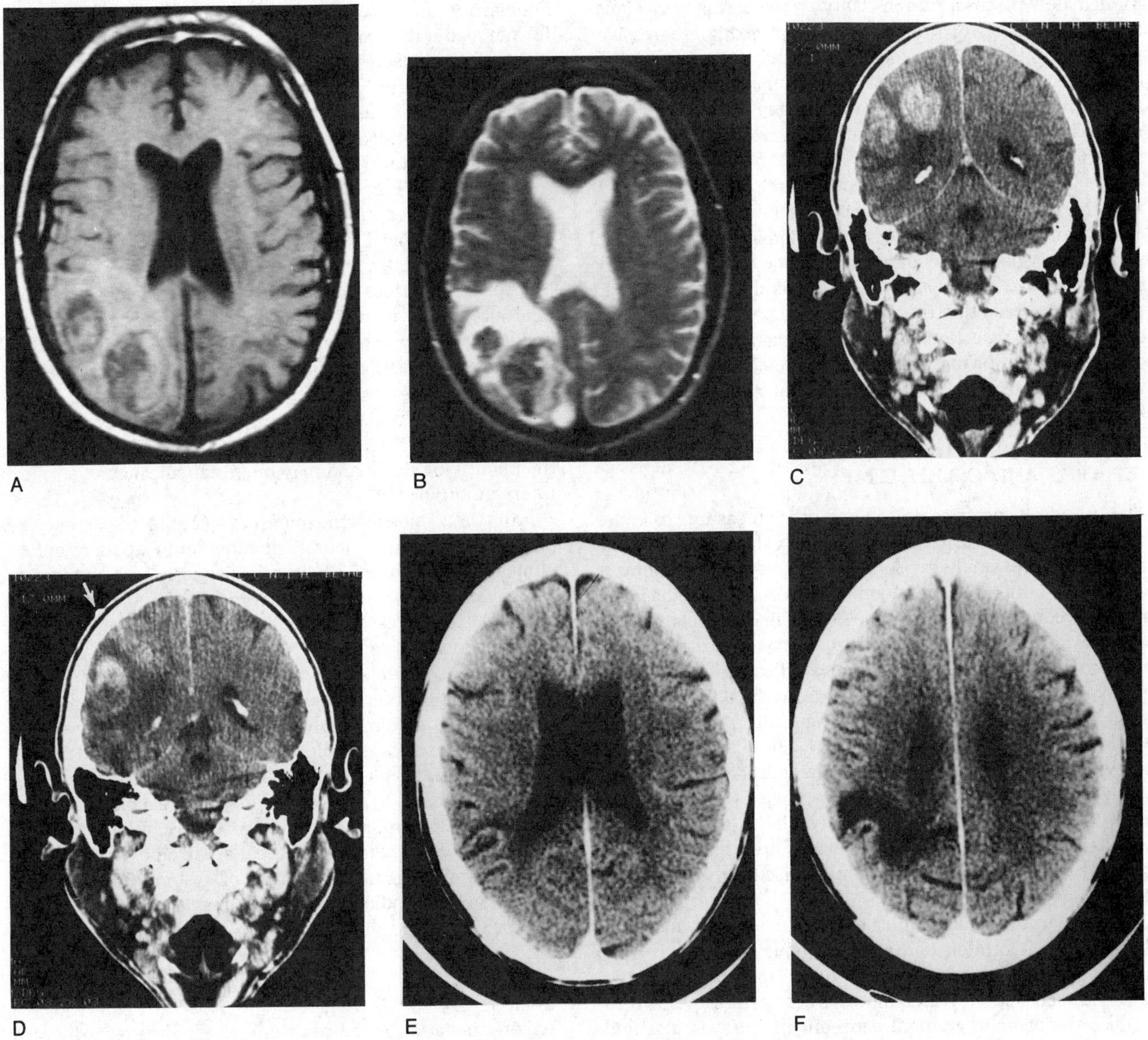

FIG. 62-3. Large, bilobed metastasis in the parieto-occipital lobe arising from a primary lung carcinoma. Magnetic resonance scanning (**A**, **B**) demonstrates heterogeneous nature of tumor on T_1-weighted image (**A**) and surrounding tumor-associated edema pattern evident on a T_2-weighted image (**B**). Coronal computed transmission (x-ray) scan (**C**, **D**) localizes tumor in an anterior-posterior plane and allows placement of external scalp landmarks (**D**, arrow) to assist placement of scalp, bone, and cortical incisions. Post-treatment contrast CT scans (**E**, **F**) show surgical site after gross total removal and adjuvant radiation 16 months after resection. The patient regained neurologic function (visual field deficit, parietal sensory loss) and has stable disease in both the primary and secondary (cerebral) sites.

any patient with increased intracranial pressure, particularly where focal masses produce regional transients of tissue pressure, commonly seen in brain metastases. Physical signs of increased intracranial pressure (papilledema), although reliable when present, require familiarity on the part of the observer and are not present in most patients. Before a lumbar puncture is done in a patient with known or suspected metastases, neurologic consultation and CT scanning should be performed, and a review of the indications and expected benefits of CSF examination should be carried out.

PRINCIPLES OF MANAGEMENT

GOALS OF THERAPY

The general goals of therapy are to maximize the quality and duration of neurologic function, which is generally achieved by successful eradication or control of intracranial deposits. The benefits of meaningful palliation or curative therapy of a secondary tumor deposit should not be underestimated. Recognition of the secondary spread of a cancer to the brain immediately places a responsibility on the caring physicians to institute means of preventing or minimizing progressive neurologic injury. Neurologic dysfunction, particularly of cognitive and motor skills, has a disproportionate affect on the quality of life in cancer patients, and aggressive treatment is warranted to sustain or restore neurologic performance.

The principal treatment regimens are radiation therapy alone, or surgery combined with postoperative radiation. Optimal therapy, or therapeutic combination for a given patient with a metastasis depends on the tumor type and clinical setting. All patients should receive general supportive care, steroids, and radiation therapy; selected patients should undergo surgical resection followed by radiation therapy. Surgery may play a primary or secondary role, depending upon whether it is used as a primary cytoreductive maneuver or for diagnostic biopsy.

STEROIDS AND OSMOTHERAPY

The use of glucocorticoids[56-58] and other measures to combat the effects of vasogenic edema secondary to metastasis represents the single most important adjunctive therapy available to this patient group. Steroids (dexamethasone, methylprednisolone, prednisone) exert their effects in several ways, none definitely understood, thus these drugs are used on an empiric basis. The clinical effects of steroids are rapid; noticeable within 6 to 24 hr[59,60] maximal within 3 to 7 days, and are successful in resolving clinical symptoms in 60% to 80% of patients.[15,56,61] The optimal dose is not known; starting dosages of 16 mg/day of dexamethasone (or equivalent dosage of other steroids) are used, and dosages as high as 100 mg/day have been successful in those patients refractory at lower dosages.[61] Steroids are able to relieve generalized symptoms (confusion, headache) more so than focal signs (hemiparesis).[15]

Osmotherapy reduces brain extracellular water and total body water. Mannitol, and similar agents (urea, glycerol), are normally excluded from the brain and remain in the intravascular space. Water moves freely across the BBB to reduce the osmotic gradient between the intravascular and brain extracellular fluid spaces. These agents require intact areas of the BBB to achieve this effect. The ICP is lowered by a reduction of brain extracellular volume, a situation that may promote movement of edema fluid out of the brain. Mannitol also has rheologic properties that act to increase cerebral blood flow to the brain.

The aim of these two pharmacologic maneuvers is to reduce intracranial pressure and bring about an increase in cerebral blood flow. Symptoms arising from metastases relapse within several weeks if no specific additional therapy is instituted.

EMERGENCY MANAGEMENT OF CEREBRAL METASTASES

On occasion, a patient will require emergent care when manifesting impairment of neurologic function.[62,63] A patient may rapidly evolve a neurologic deficit (*e.g.*, seizure, cerebral hemorrhage, CSF outflow obstruction) or develop subacute symptoms and signs (cerebral edema, expanding neoplastic mass, communicating hydrocelphalus). The former generally arises in patients in whom the cerebral lesion is unsuspected or occult, whereas the latter is more commonly a feature of relapsing symptoms in patients with known brain metastases for whom initial therapeutic efforts are ineffective. Regardless of the setting, this situation requires rapid clinical evaluation and treatment. Neurologic examination, CT or MRI scanning, and other specialized diagnostic studies are required to identify the underlying cause of the clinical syndrome. Focal neurologic symptoms and signs generally arise from intracranial pressure shifts that result in various herniation syndromes. Global, nonspecific alterations in neurologic function (headache, nausea and vomiting, impaired mental status, cognitive dysfunction, and the like) usually result from a generalized increase in intracranial pressure or an encephalopathic process (metabolic disturbances of electrolytes, hepatic/renal dysfunction, CNS infection). Treatment is directed toward correction of the underlying cause and may require medical care, surgical intervention, or both.

Immediate, nonspecific measures (Table 62-6) may be necessary to stabilize neurologic function in a patient before clinical evaluation until a specific diagnosis and appropriate therapy can be formulated. Such maneuvers include hyperventilation (decreases pCO_2), osmotherapy, steroids, and seizure control, if indicated. Occasionally, neurologic resuscitation for severely ill or rapidly deteriorating patients requires airway protection (intubation), ventilatory support, and induced motor paralysis. Neurosurgical intervention may be required for neurologic monitoring (ventricular catheter for drainage; placement of ICP monitoring devices) or, more commonly, to correct underlying treatable causes of increased ICP (tumoral hemorrhage, ventricular obstruction, etc.). Rational therapy requires a specific diagnosis as well as knowledge of the extent of systemic disease processes. Surgical indications and the results of emergent surgery are discussed in the following sections.

RADIATION THERAPY

Ionizing radiation is the most effective nonsurgical therapy available for the treatment of cerebral metastases. Radiation has been a component of therapy since the initial report of

TABLE 62-6. Emergency Measures for Cerebral Metastases

Maneuver	*Physiologic Effect*
Hyperventilation	Decreases pCO_2; cerebral vasoconstriction; decreases cerebral vascular volume; immediate effects
Head position ≥ 20°	Facilitates cerebral venous return; immediate effects
Osmotherapy (mannitol, glycerol)	Reduces cerebral extracellular volume; increases cerebral blood flow; maximal effects within 30–120 min
Steroids	Action poorly understood; reduces extracellular volume; blocks toxic vasoactive byproducts of tumor metabolism; 12–48 h for maximal effect to occur

palliative benefit in 1954[64] and today is used in nearly all patients with metastases, either as primary therapy or as adjuvant treatment after surgery. Subsequent studies[48,65-67] have further established efficacy; identified tumoral, host, and technical factors influencing the radiation response for a given patient; and developed guidelines for optimal time–dose treatment regimens.[65,67-77]

Radiation Technique: Time–Dose Schedules

Because of the high frequency of multiple brain metastases found at autopsy, there is assumed to be microscopic tumor present in the brain apart from clinically detectable lesions, even in patients with a single metastasis or a focal area of involvement. Thus, the radiation port generally encompasses the entire brain, despite the tendency that metastases have a distinct interface with the normal brain.

To investigate the optimal schedule for patients with brain metastases, several randomized prospective clinical trials have been conducted by the Radiation Therapy Oncology Group (RTOG).[78] In the first study (993 patients), four treatment schedules were employed: [1] 30 Gy/2 weeks, [2] 30 Gy/3 weeks, [3] 40 Gy/3 weeks, and [4] 40 Gy/4 weeks [1 Gy (Gray) = 100 rad]. Patients were stratified according to primary site (lung, breast, other) and the presence or absence of metastases to sites other than brain. None of the four schedules proved to be superior to the others when judged by treatment response or median survival. A second study was then undertaken evaluating even shorter treatment schedules.[78] This second study entered 1001 patients who were randomly assigned to receive: [1] 20 Gy/1 week, [2] 30 Gy/2 weeks, or [3] 40 Gy/3 weeks. No overall differences were seen among the three arms, although those patients with high initial functional performance scores receiving 40 Gy/3 weeks had a significantly longer median time to progression of disease (19 weeks) after a treatment response than did comparable patients treated at the lower doses (9 and 13, respectively). In both studies, patients were reported to improve faster if they received the shorter duration treatments. These results would suggest that the shorter time–dose fractionation schemes may be used preferentially over longer treatment programs with equal efficacy, less expense, and less patient inconvenience. A program of 30 Gy/2 weeks to the entire cranial cavity is generally well tolerated and can be followed by a boost of 9 Gy in three additional fractions to a defined area of gross disease as defined by CT or MRI scans.

The first two RTOG studies suggested significantly longer survivals in both ambulatory and nonambulatory patients when the brain was the only site of metastasis or when the primary lesion was controlled. An additional trial was conducted by the RTOG to investigate higher radiation doses. Patients with brain metastases and no evidence of other sites of disseminated disease were randomized to receive 50 Gy/ weeks or 30 Gy/2 weeks. This study group was predominated by patients with aggressive cancers (80% had lung cancer) and demonstrated no statistically significant advantage of one treatment over the other for symptom relief, median survival, or prevention of death by brain metastases.[79]

Very rapid fractionation programs have also been tested for palliation of brain metastases. The first two RTOG trials included an optional randomization arm into which patients could receive 10 Gy in one fraction or 12 Gy in two fractions. Response rates, promptness of neurologic improvement, treatment morbidity, and median survival were comparable with those of patients receiving 20 to 40 Gy. However, the duration of improvement, time to progression of neurologic status, and rate of complete disappearance of neurologic symptoms were generally less for those patients who received 1000 or 1200 rad, suggesting that ultrarapid, high-dose irradiation schedules might not be as effective as higher-dose schedules in the palliation of patients with brain metastases.[80] Harwood and Simpson reported the results of a randomized prospective clinical trial in which 100 patients received either 30 Gy/2 weeks or 10 Gy in a single dose.[73] No statistical difference between the two fractionation schemes was demonstrated in terms of survival, frequency or degree of response to treatment, complication rate, or local control rate. Forty percent of patients treated with the single-dose program had acute complications (increased headache, nausea and vomiting, increased neurologic deficit, or fall in level of consciousness) compared with 27% of patients treated with the fractionated radiation, although this difference was not significant.

Large-dose (10 Gy), single-fraction irradiation has also been reported to be effective palliation.[67,70] Hindo reported improvement in 65% of patients and a mean survival of 5.6 months, but both groups noted a high complication rate associated with this approach and suggested that moribund patients showing evidence of increased intracranial pressure were unsuitable candidates.

Specialized Radiation Approaches to Brain Metastases

Normal tissue (brain) radiation tolerance limits the dose (55–70 Gy) that can be safely delivered using conventional external radiation techniques. Brachytherapy (interstitial radiation) allows local application of continuous radiation exposure during the treatment interval (typically between 7–60 days) which is analogous to delivering a radiation dose in a large number of very small fractions. Radiation sources are surgically implanted within the tumor borders and configured to deliver higher doses (80–150 Gy) than those possible with conventional external radiation techniques.[81] The physical characteristic of the isotope used determines such factors as the dose rate and distance the emitted radiation travels in tissue, permitting relative control over the dose distribution. This strategy aims to achieve a high dose "local boost" to the tumor, creating a focal area of radiation necrosis within the borders of the neoplasm, while minimizing radiation exposure to normal tissues. Response is determined by such factors as tumor size and geometry, ability to accurately image the tumor–brain interface, and tumor radiosensitivity. A small number of patients with recurrent or resistant metastases have been treated using this approach,[81,82] and the preliminary results suggest brachytherapy may be useful in selected patients with radioresistant tumors (*e.g.*, lung, melanoma).

ADJUNCTIVE THERAPY

Clinical trials using conventional adjunctive chemotherapeutic agents and delivery methods have generally proved ineffective in the treatment of brain metastases.[83-86] Modest benefit is realized only when used in combination with other proven therapies such as radiation.[6,87] Recent chemotherapy trials have demonstrated greater efficacy for certain metastases (*e.g.*, lung carcinomas) when the agents are delivered using an intra-arterial route,[88,89] but widespread application of adjunctive chemotherapy to brain metastases cannot be justified with currently available agents and delivery methods.

Adoptive immunotherapy approaches may have potential efficacy against cerebral metastases because efficacy has been demonstrated against certain systemic cancers. Intravenously administered recombinant interleukin-2 and lymphokine-activated killer T cells penetrate the CSF levels that are sufficient to activate peripheral blood lymphocytes, but therapeutic efficacy with use of this promising approach has not yet been fully investigated.[90]

SURGICAL MANAGEMENT

General Aspects: Perioperative Care

One of the most important factors identified in the outcome in these patients treated by surgery is the preoperative condition.[7,17,19-21,44] Quality of postoperative neurologic function (a measure of morbidity), complications, and 30-day mortality are directly related to the preoperative classification of the patient subjected to surgery for brain metastasis.[7] Steps taken to optimize the general physical and neurologic status of a patient, although limited by the extent of the disease process, can only improve the potential for benefit from surgery. Cardiopulmonary function, immune status, and nutritional state are frequently disturbed by direct and indirect effects of systemic disease. Preoperative assessment and correction of underlying medical problems are a necessary prelude to successful surgery. Special emphasis is needed in this group of patients for the avoidance of coagulopathies (iatrogenic, malnutrition, thrombocytopenia, depressed clotting factors) and susceptibility to infections. Hemorrhagic and infectious hazards can be minimized by perioperative normalization of coagulation function, utilization of operative techniques to obtain complete hemostasis, obliteration or drainage of potential dead space in the wound, and intraoperative antibiotics. In a similar manner, measures to resist brain swelling in the perioperative period are employed. Favorable pressure–volume relationships and increases in cerebral blood flow generally result when steroids are administered (24–48 hr before surgery is preferable). Correction of underlying electrolyte disturbances (particularly hyponatremia) and hypo-osmolar states will minimize edema formation. Monitoring of ICP (with ventricular drainage capability) directs the management of brain swelling and protects patients from potential postoperative complications (edema, hemorrhage, CSF obstruction). Osmotherapy is generally reserved for the acutely deteriorating patient requiring neurologic resuscitation before instituting effective and more permanent means of lowering ICP. Stabilizing the decompensated patient with aggressive medical therapy (steroids, osmotherapy, respiratory support) is generally more successful than subjecting such patients to emergent surgical decompression.[18,44] Gross total removal of a metastasis is usually feasible, and when achieved, is effective in controlling ICP.

Surgical Indications, Goals, and Benefits

Surgery in this patient group is generally employed to obtain pathologic tissues for diagnosis, decompression of a mass lesion by subtotal or total removal, or to relieve CSF obstruction (Table 62-7). The indications for a particular surgical procedure are related to the therapeutic goals. Diagnostic uncertainties arising in patients with a history of systemic cancer require an unequivocal pathologic confirmation of the disease process. A diagnostic biopsy can identify a nonmalignant process and spare patients unnecessary or inappropriate therapy. The goals for a decompressive procedure for a resistant or relapsing metastasis are to rapidly reduce mass effect and remove the source of edema production. Gross total removal of a metastasis is possible in more than 80% of selected patients[6,7,19] and has superior benefit[6,7,19-21,91-93] over subtotal removal or biopsy. Figure 62-3E,F illustrates the posttreatment CT appearance of the brain following gross total removal and combined therapy for brain metastases.

Technical Aspects

Development of microneurosurgical technique in the late 1960s, instrumentation advances, superior preoperative localization, and effective medical means of managing ICP have led to advances in the surgical approach to metastatic disease. Judicious use of craniotomy for gross total removals in selected patients with solitary metastases has superseded the era when regional surgical procedures (wide tumor margins, lobectomy) sacrificing normal tissue were necessary to control perioperative swelling. Preservation of the normal brain and microcirculation adjacent to a metastatic lesion is now routinely possible using small cortical incisions that minimize normal tissue injury.[94]

Diagnostic biopsy has attained an impressive level of safety, precision, and utility since the introduction of stereotactic systems that use various imaging devices (CT, MRI).[95,96] Image-guided stereotactic biopsy is a widely available means of obtaining tissue for pathologic examination. Multiple sites can be sampled with safety and minimal stress

TABLE 62-7. Surgical Therapy of Brain Metastases: Selection Criteria*

Diagnostic uncertainty
Solitary metastasis
Life-threatening or critically located multiple metastatic lesions
Recurrent or persistent symptoms after nonsurgical therapy
Clinically resistant tumors
Treatment of metastatic complications: hemorrhagic, infectious, CSF obstruction
Placement of delivery devices for intrathecal access (Ommaya reservoir)

* Criteria are suggested guidelines rather than absolute indications; see text.

TABLE 62-8. Treatment: Selected Surgical* Series of Brain Metastases

Author	*Collection Interval*	*Cases*	*Mortality*† (%)	*Survival*	
				Median‡	*1-Year (%)*
Stortebecker[54]	1922–51	125	25	3.6	21
Richards[93]	1946–60	108	32	5.0	17
Lang[47]	1933–63	208	22	4.0	20
Vieth[101]	1938–62	155	15	6.0	13
Raskind[110]	1959–68	51	12	6.0	30
Haar[91]	1933–68	167	11	6.0	22
Ransohoff[21]	1970–73	100	10	6.0	28
Winston[19]	1967–77	79	10	6.0	22
Gamache[17]	1968–77	94	8.5	6.0	25
Galicich[94]	1977–80	75	9	9.0	45
Takakura[6]	1960–81	259	14§	9.1	26
Smalley[105]	1972–82	85	—	13.5‖	59‖

* Most patients in these surgical series were treated with adjuvant whole-brain radiation.
† Reported as 30-day mortality except Stortebecker (20 days), Vieth (14 days), Raskind (14 days).
‡ Median survival is given in months.
§ All mortality occurred before 1976 (before use of CT for patient selection).
‖ Overall results; results of surgery plus adjuvant radiation (34 patients) was superior to surgery alone (51 patients) (21 months versus 11.5 months median survival)

to the patients. The diagnostic procedure can also be combined with a formal craniotomy for resection, if indicated, or further surgical efforts undertaken as a separate procedure.

RESULTS

Despite a generous number of published studies (1960–present) employing a variety of treatment modalities for cerebral metastatic disease, relatively few definitive conclusions can be drawn about the effectiveness of a particular treatment approach. Random clinical studies lack comparably matched treatment groups and differ in defining such reported variables as response to therapy, relapse rates, morbidity, mortality, and cause of death. Selected clinical reports from the surgical and radiotherapy literature are presented in Tables 62-8 and 62-9. These reports span a period during which advances in diagnosis and treatment of brain metastases had a significant impact on the outcome of patients, thereby altering the interpretation of results from

TABLE 62-9. Treatment: Selected Radiation* Series of Brain Metastases

Author	*Collection Interval*	*Cases*	*Mortality (%)*	*Survival*		
				Median (mo.)	*Mean (mo.)*	*1-Year (%)*
Chu[66]	1954–58	218			6.5	
Order[99]	1958–66	108		3–6.0	6.3	9
Deeley[108]	Not given	88		<6.0		14
Hindo[67]	Not given	54			5.6	9
Nisce[48]	Not given	560		6.0		16
Montana[68]	1966–71	47		3.0		10
Young[70]	1967–72	162	4.3	3.0	3.4	
Deutsch[69]	1962–71	88	36†	3–6.0		10
Berry[74]	1964–73	124		4		9
Hendrickson[72]	1971–76	1001		5.8		15
Borgelt[78,80]	1971–73	993			4.5	
Cairncross[65]	1977–78	183	4.0	4.0		8
Kurtz[79]	1976–79	309		4.5		

* Most patients treated by radiation *only* except: Order, (26), Deeley (7), Nisce (376), Montana (15), Young (89), Deutsch (17), Berry (29), and Kurz (39); parentheses indicate number of patients undergoing surgery before radiation.
† Includes patients unable to complete therapy.

TABLE 62-10. Impact of Technical Advances in Treatment Results

Survival	*Winston*[19] *(1967–1977)* *(n = 79)*	*Galicich*[7] *(1977–1980)* *(n = 75)*
Median (mo.)	6.0	8.9
1 year (%)	22.0	44.0
2 year (%)	10.0	24.0
Mortality	10.0	9.0

preceding studies. An example of the impact modern imaging devices have had is possible by examining the reports of a representative series in the pre-CT era[19] with a comparably treated series[7] benefiting from this important diagnostic advance (Table 62-10). The improvement in 1- and 2-year survival rates in the latter study is probably a result of superior patient selection and preoperative localization of mass lesions.

There are some generalizations that can be safely drawn from these clinical reports. The natural history of untreated cerebral metastases is one of progressive neurologic deterioration, with a median survival of 1 to 2 months.[6,47,65,97] Steroids exert a salutary effect on neurologic performance, and extend medial survival to 2.5 months.[98] Radiation therapy (with or without steroids) further increases median survival to 3 to 6 months; and selected patients treated with surgery, radiation, and steroids[44] have a median survival exceeding 6 months.

RADIATION

Despite the high initial response rates (80% of patients benefit), radiation shows a surprisingly modest gain in survival compared with untreated and steroid groups. The associated morbidity and mortality further reduces the benefit because 10% to 20% of patients fail to complete the prescribed course of radiation, and approximately 5% of patients die during treatment because of neurologic deterioration.[80,99] Survival figures alone may not accurately reflect the efficacy of radiation therapy for cerebral metastases, because this treatment group tends to have unselected patients with poor prognostic factors and high mortality from uncontrolled systemic disease. Hence, it is also important to consider whether treatment improves functional status and the quality of survival. Order and co-workers noted palliation (defined as improvement in functional neurologic status) in 60% of patients treated with whole-brain irradiation for brain metastases.[99] Patients with mild pretreatment deficits had the highest rate of improvement. In the large RTOG studies, improvement in neurologic function was seen in approximately 50% of patients[80] and closely correlated with improvement in overall performance status. Ambulatory patients had a higher response rate than nonambulatory patients, as did patients whose only site of metastatic disease was in the brain. In reference to specific symptoms, headache was most predictably improved with a complete relief in 69% and partial or complete relief in 82%. Complete reversal of motor loss, on the other hand, occurred in only 37% of patients and partial restoration of motor function occurred in an additional 24%. However, only 57% of those patients with improvement in functional performance alive at 6 months remained improved.[99] A decreasing percentage of patients were able to maintain their improved state with the passage of time, illustrating a failure to permanently control intracranial disease in a substantial proportion of patients treated. Indeed, in patients who were irradiated for brain metastases in the two RTOG studies, persistent or uncontrolled disease in the brain was the cause of death in 31% and 49% of treated patients.[80] Although most irradiated patients will have unfavorable prognostic features, such as multiple metastases, it must be acknowledged that radiation alone in this setting fails to permanently control intracranial disease in a large proportion of treated patients.

Because of the high incidence of uncontrolled tumor in the brain (50% to 70%), the issue of retreatment with radiation will arise in many patients with brain metastases. Several reports[48,66,71] describe improvement in retreated patients with an average remission of 4 months with use of a rapid-fractionation scheme over 1 to 5 days.[71] Others are less sanguine about the prospects of retreatment,[73] noting transient benefit with a median survival following retreatment of only 8 weeks.[100] The benefits of radiation thus appear modest, but it may be appropriate for selected patients with limited extracranial disease and indolent tumor type.

SURGERY

The gradual introduction of modern surgical techniques and perioperative adjuncts has demonstrated declining mortality and morbidity, neurologic benefit, modest gains in median survival, and a small but consistent fraction of long-term survivors.[16,45,47,93,101–105] Although the gains in extending median survival are modest, the decline in mortality arising from surgery has been dramatic. The overall 30-day mortality associated with surgery has fallen from 32%[93] to less than 10%. If one excludes surgery performed under emergency situations for critically ill, postherniated, or moribund patients from the recent series, the 30-day mortality is approximately 3%.[6,7,17] One large study has achieved a zero mortality since the introduction of the CT scanner as an aid in patient selection.[6] These impressive gains have come about largely by improvements in selection criteria (*e.g.*, assuring solitary lesions), localization, neuroanesthesia, surgical microtechniques, and perioperative care. The mortality of surgery for metastatic brain disease is now largely determined by the extent of extra-CNS disease[7,44] and the preoperative condition of patients.

COMBINED THERAPY

The high rate of uncontrolled disease in the brain after radiation therapy alone, and the decline of morbidity associated with surgery suggests a combined treatment approach may offer the highest likelihood of a favorable and sustained treatment response in selected patients with cerebral metastases.[7] Two retrospective studies have examined the role of postoperative radiation after surgical resection of solitary brain metastatic lesions. Dosoretz[106] reviewed the treatment records of 33 patients (1962–1978) without evidence of systemic disease who were rendered clinically disease-free by the complete resection of a solitary brain metastatic lesion. Twelve of these patients received elective postoperative whole-brain irradiation. They saw no statistically significant difference in survival or local recurrence rate in the brain when comparing the patients who received adjuvant whole-brain irradiation compared with those patients who were observed after complete resection of tumor. Eleven of 21 patients had tumor recurrence in the brain after surgery alone, compared with 6 of 12 patients after treatment with both surgery and postoperative radiation. Twenty-seven percent of patients died with tumor limited to the brain. The majority of patients received either 30 Gy in 2 weeks or 40 Gy in 4 weeks.

A larger retrospective review (85 patients, 1972–1982) of a similar patient group rendered clinically disease-free by the resection of a solitary cerebral metastatic tumor did, however, demonstrate a significant reduction of subsequent brain relapse in the 34 patients who received adjuvant whole-brain radiotherapy compared with the surgery-only group (21% versus 85%, respectively).[105] The median survival was longer in the group receiving adjuvant radiotherapy (21 months versus 11.5 months). Those patients who received adjuvant irradiation to a dose ≥39 Gy manifested an 11% rate of subsequent brain failure as contrasted with a 31% rate seen in patients receiving ≤39 Gy, suggesting that higher doses may be appropriate for these prognostically favored patients with solitary brain metastatic lesions and no other clinical evidence of systemic disease.

In spite of the encouraging results with this combined surgical and radiotherapeutic approach, most (60% to 80%) patients are unsuited for a surgical approach and undergo irradiation (with or without steroids) as the primary treatment for intracranial metastatic disease. This direction in patient management is influenced by the clinical profile of the majority of patients with brain metastases (multiple metastatic intracranial lesions, widespread systemic disease, major neurologic dysfunction, or poor performance status). In addition, there is no effective chemotherapeutic, immunologic, or biologic treatment for brain metastases, and the lack of effective systemic therapy for many malignancies limits an aggressive surgical and radiotherapeutic approach for those patients with the combination of brain metastases and uncontrolled systemic disease.

PROGNOSTIC FACTORS: EXTENDED SURVIVAL IN BRAIN METASTASES

Overall survival for patients with brain metastases generally correlates with the intrinsic malignant behavior of a specific tumor type (Table 62-11) and the response of the systemic tumor burden to therapy. As previously discussed, the preoperative neurologic condition and extent of systemic disease constitutes the most important prognostic variables in predicting the short-term results for combined treatment (surgery, radiation, and steroids) and also correlates with the long-term survival pattern. Figures 62-4 and 62-5 reflect the influence of these two prognostic variables in the results for combined therapy.

The interval from the detection of a primary tumor to the development of a symptomatic metastatic lesion also has a strong correlation with survival (Fig. 62-6). The grouping of patients by temporal patterns of presentation (precocious, synchronous, metachronous) is essentially a classification by histologic type, because lung cancer (median interval 7.2–11 months),[6,20] melanoma, and renal cell carcinoma tend to have precocious or synchronous presentations, whereas breast carcinoma (median interval 42–51 months),[6,20] sarcoma, and colon cancer have longer intervals and a metachronous presentation.[7,44]

Extended survival (longer than 2 years) after treatment for highly malignant tumors[6,16,19,21,47,65,91,103,105,107–109] is an occasional feature of clinical reports. Most long-term survivors have been subjected to various forms of combined, multimodal therapy (surgery, radiation, steroids, chemotherapy.) Table 62-12 lists this intriguing category of patients from literature reports, who were predominantly treated by combined (surgery plus radiation) therapy methods. Surgical treatment is a consistent factor of nearly all reports of long-term survival, and a remarkable group of patients have received surgery as the only treatment,[19,47,101,105,106,110] indicating long survivals are possible without radiation. Patients with the more indolent tumors generally form the largest

TABLE 62-11. Brain Metastases: Survival by Primary Histologic Type*

Tumor	*Takakura*[6] (*n* = 259)		*Gamache*[17] (*n* = 80)		*Winston*† [19]	
	Survival					
	Median (mo.)	*1 Year (%)*	*Median (mo.)*	*1 Year (%)*	*Median (mo.)*	*1 Year (%)*
Lung	7.7	22.5	5.5	32.0	4.0	19.0
Breast	7.4	23.1	13.0	63.0	14.0	48.0
Gastrointestinal	3.8	14.3	5.5	0.0		27.0
Genitourinary	13.0	35.3	4.0	0.0	8.0	
Melanoma	20.2		3.5	31.0	2.0	32.0

* Data Compiled from surgical series.
† Compiled by Winston from literature sources.

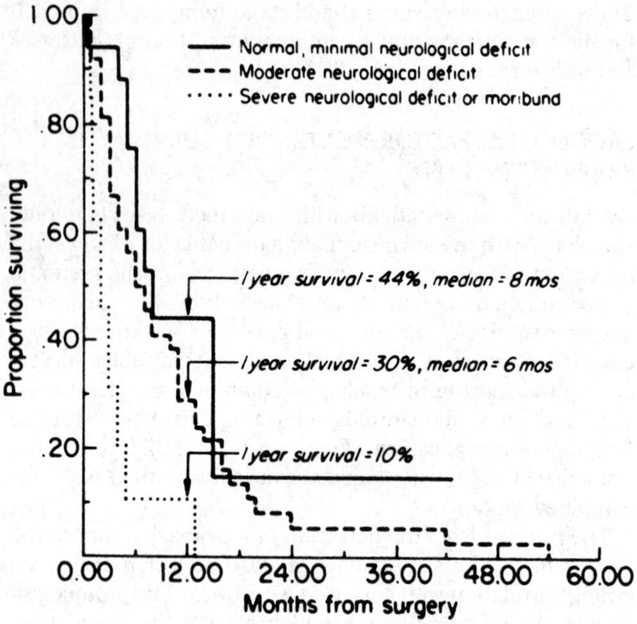

FIG. 62-4. Survival curve for patients treated with surgery and irradiation according to preoperative patient status. (Galicich JH, Sundaresan N, Arbit E et al: Surgical treatment of single brain metastasis: Factors associated with survival. Cancer 45:381–386, 1980)

group of long survivors; breast carcinoma, for example, has the highest (38%) patient 2-year survival rate, partly because of its inherent responsiveness to hormonal and chemotherapeutic manipulation. Long-term survival (3–5 years) is not exclusively restricted, however, to patients with less ma-

FIG. 62-5. Survival plot according to extent of disease. Group A represents patients without evidence of extra-CNS disease. Group B had evidence of disseminated disease outside the CNS. All patients were treated with surgery and irradiation. (Galicich JH, Sundaresan N: Metastatic brain tumors, pp 597–561. In Wilkins RH, Rengachary SS [eds]: Neurosurgery. New York, McGraw-Hill, 1985)

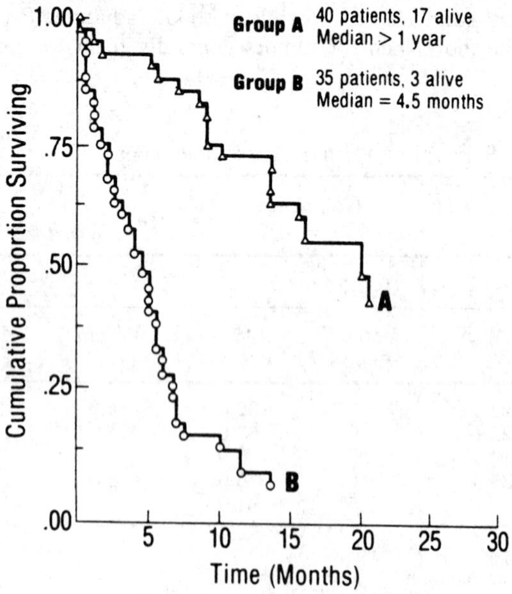

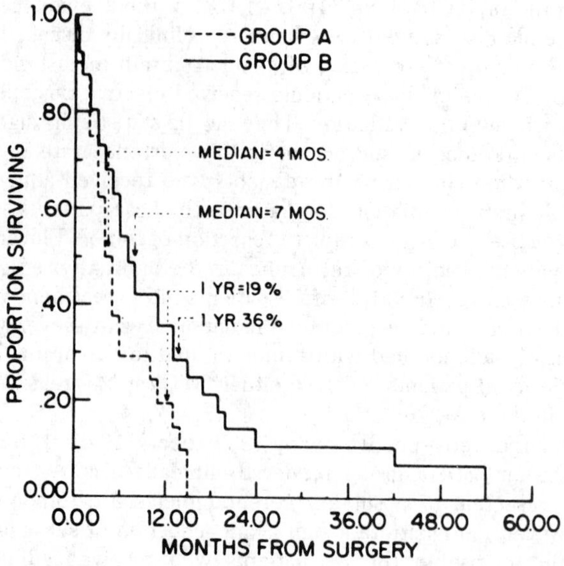

FIG. 62-6. Survival curve for patients treated with surgery and irradiation according to the metastatic interval. Group A had metastases detected within 12 months of diagnosis of primary site. Group B had an interval greater than 12 months. (Galicich JH, Sundaresan N, Arbit E et al: Surgical treatment of single brain metastasis: Factors associated with survival. Cancer 45:381, 1980)

lignant tumors. Extended survival correlates with neurologic status at the time of metastasis and does not strictly adhere to the usual outcome according to the histologic nature of the primary site.[6,19,21,111] The prognostic categories previously discussed (preoperative status, metastatic interval, extent of disease) apply in predicting survival. A precocious presentation with an occult systemic primary and no evidence of extraneural metastasis has favored long survivals in a few patients.[19,21] The specific identification of factors predicting survival beyond 3 to 5 years is not possible; by focusing upon the "ideal" candidates, benefit from maximal therapeutic efforts may yield a greater percentage of long-term survivors.

RELATIVE SURGICAL INDICATIONS

The surgical indications have been listed (see Table 62-7) and previously discussed; despite these guidelines, questions arise in some clinical settings about the role of surgery. Surgery for emergent situations, in which neurologic compromise has progressed rapidly, is occasionally rewarded with unexpected benefits,[7] but the practice of using surgical reduction of a metastatic lesion as a "last resort," or when "all else fails" for patients with "nothing to lose," is inappropriate. Emergent surgical intervention is advisable for situations in which obstructive hydrocephalus or hemorrhage has caused a rapid evolution of symptoms. Patients in poor neurologic condition before a sudden deterioration are best managed by intensive medical care and subjected to surgery only if their condition can be stabilized and neurologic state upgraded.

There are only occasional situations for which surgery is

TABLE 62-12. Brain Metastases: Long-Term Survival

Author	n	Survival (%) 1 Year	2 Year	5 Year	Comments
Veith[101]	155	13.5	12.2	2.5	Three patients > 10 yr
Lang[47]	208	20.0	13.0	4.8	
Haar[91]	167	13.5		4.0	
Ransohoff[21]	100	21.0	13.0		
Salerno (1978)	23	26.0	22.0	13.0	Three patients > 10 yr
Winston[19]	79	22.0	10.0		Surgery only for 4/8 long survivors
Galicich[7]	75	45.0	24.0	6.6	
Takakura[6]	259	26.5	12.6	2.7	Three patients > 8 yr
Smalley[105]	85	—	35.0	12.0	51 patients treated with surgery only

indicated for multiple metastatic deposits, because mortality is significantly increased.[98] There are anecdotal reports of benefit from excision of multiple metastatic lesions, but the risks associated with a surgical approach to multiple lesions usually exceed the potential benefit.

The situation in which patients are slowly deteriorating, despite the best available nonsurgical therapy or after completion of medical therapy, represents a therapeutic dilemma. The relapse rate for specific tumors is not known, except in the most general terms. Patients with limited treatment responses to radiation therapy do not necessarily realize significant benefit when subjected to surgery, typically showing high local recurrence rates and remaining steroid-dependent.[7] If such patients have favorable prognostic factors (*e.g.*, neurologic status, minimal extra-CNS disease), surgery may represent the only treatment option.

Metastatic complications such as hematoma formation, abscesses, and CSF obstruction should be treated much as if the metastasis were a secondary problem, unless severe risks attend surgical intervention. Patients can have dramatic responses to treatment of these associated complications.[7]

There is a logical tendency to assume a surgical approach for dominant hemispheric lesions in critical brain areas is associated with a higher frequency of morbidity. This has not proved to be true in recent (post-CT era) series.[6,7] The explanation for this is likely the excellent localization, careful patient selection, operative microtechnique, and the discrete nature of most metastatic neoplasms.

CONCLUSION

Rational selection of the appropriate therapy for maximal patient benefit requires accurate diagnosis and localization, and the determination of prognostic criteria. Technical advances in diagnostic imaging over the last 15 years have had a major impact in this area; parallel advances in surgical techniques have reduced the morbidity and mortality of surgical therapy, thus extending this modality to more patients, with reduced risk. The major prognostic variables identified for this group are the pretreatment neurologic state, metastatic interval, and extent of systemic disease. Therapeutic response is determined by the variable biologic behavior of the tumor, histology, radiosensitivity, tumor volume, location, hormonal responsiveness, and immune status of the host. The degree of response correlates with duration and quality of survival.

Cranial radiation, the primary treatment modality, is currently used in nearly all patients treated for brain metastases. Approximately 60% of patients will improve after radiation alone, with an anticipated median survival of 3 to 6 months. Nearly 50% of patients, however, will die from uncontrolled intracranial tumor after radiation alone. Hence, radiation should be combined with surgery in selected patients. For selected patients, surgery combined with adjuvant radiation is the best means of treating resistant malignancies of the lung, kidney, thyroid, colon, skin (melanoma), and many soft-tissue sarcomas. Superior benefit is realized if the dual goals of total resection and minimal neural tissue injury are achieved. The absolute and relative indications for surgery are now well established. The "ideal" patient will harbor a solitary lesion, with minimal neurologic impairment, limited extra-CNS disease, a long interval from the diagnosis of a primary cancer to dissemination to the brain, and precocious presentation or occult disease. The risks of surgery are a function of the preoperative state and extent of systemic disease.

Unfortunately, for most patients, this combination therapy is not possible because of unfavorable neurologic states, systemic tumor burden, and other factors that reduce the benefit and increase the risk of a surgical approach. Surgery of cerebral metastatic disease is applicable to 10% to 30% of patients for whom conservative selection criteria are used. Those patients who are not candidates for surgery should have radiation therapy delivered using one of the shorter treatment programs.

The potentially disastrous consequences of CNS involvement by cancer is a common problem confronting the oncologist. Symptomatic parenchymal lesions afflict approximately 133,000 patients in the United States annually, with lung, breast, gastrointestinal, renal, and melanoma composing the majority of tumors affecting the brain. Timely and effective therapy for cerebral metastases can restore function or prevent the neurologic complications of cancer for the duration of survival, but limiting neurologic disability is difficult, and available therapy is not fully effective. Future diagnostic and therapeutic advances will hopefully offer a greater fraction of these patients increasingly effective means of preventing the neurologic complications of metastatic disease.

REFERENCES

1. Posner JB: Brain metastases: A clinician's view. In Weiss L, Gilbert HA, Posner JB (eds): Brain Metastases, pp 2–29. Boston, GK Hall, 1980
2. Silverberg E, Lubera JA: Cancer statistics, 1988. CA 38:5–22, 1988
3. Walker AE, Robins M, Weinfeld FD: Epidemiology of brain tumors: The national survey of intracranial neoplasms. Neurology 35:219–226, 1985
4. Percy AK, Elveback LR, Okazaki H: Neoplasms of the central nervous system: Epidemiologic considerations. Neurology 22:40–48, 1972
5. Hildebrand J: Lesions of the Nervous System in Cancer Patients. Monograph Series of the European Organization for Research on Treatment of Cancer, Vol 5. New York, Raven Press, 1978
6. Takakura K, Sano K, Hoho S et al: Metastatic Tumors of the Central Nervous System. Tokyo, Igaku-Shoin, 1982
7. Galicich JH, Sundaresan N: Metastatic brain tumors. In Wilkins RH, Rengachary SS (eds): Neurosurgery, pp 597–610. New York, McGraw-Hill, 1985
8. Rubin R, Green J: Solitary Metastases. Springfield, CC Thomas, 1968
9. Posner JB, Chernik NL: Intracranial metastases from systemic cancer. Adv Neurol 19:575–587, 1978
10. Kindt GW: The pattern of location of cerebral metastatic tumors. J Neurosurg 21:54–57, 1964
11. Whisanant JP: Letter to the Editor. Stroke 13:720, 1982
12. Blacklock JB, Wright DC, Dedrick RL et al: Drug streaming during intra-arterial chemotherapy. J Neurosurg 64:284–291, 1986
13. McDonald DA, Potter JM: The distribution of blood to the brain. J Physiol (Lond) 114:356–371, 1951
14. Lutz RJ, Dedrick RL, Boretos JW et al: Mixing studies during intracarotid artery infusions as an in vitro model. J Neurosurg 64:277–283, 1986
15. Posner JB: Diagnosis and treatment of metastases to the brain. Clin Bull 4:47–57, 1974
16. Simionescu MD: Metastatic tumors of the brain. A follow-up study of 195 patients with neurosurgical considerations. J Neurosurg 17:361–373, 1960
17. Gamache FW Jr, Posner JB, Galicich JH: Treatment of brain metastases by surgical extirpation. In Weiss L, Gilbert HA, Posner JB (eds): Brain Metastases, pp 390–414. Boston, GK Hall, 1980
18. Posner JB: Management of central nervous system metastases. Semin Oncol 4:81–91, 1977
19. Winston KR, Walsh JW, Fischer EG: Results of operative treatment of intracranial metastatic tumors. Cancer 45:2639–2645, 1980
20. Galicich JH, Sundaresan N, Arbit E, Pase A: Surgical treatment of single brain metastasis: Factors associated with survival. Cancer 45:381–386, 1980
21. Ransohoff J: Surgical therapy of brain metastases. In Weiss L, Gilbert HA, Posner JB (eds): Brain Metastases, pp 380–389. Boston, GK Hall, 1980
22. Karnofsky DA, Burchenol JH: The clinical evaluation of chemotherapeutic agents in cancer. In MacLeod CN (ed): Evaluation of Chemotherapeutic Agents, pp 191–205. New York, Columbia University Press, 1949
23. Warren BA: Arrest and extravasation of cancer cells with special reference to brain metastases and the microinjury hypothesis. In Weiss L, Gilbert HA, Posner JB (eds): Brain Metastases, pp 81–99, Boston, GK Hall, 1980
24. Coman DR, DeLong RP: The role of the vertebral venous system in the metastasis of cancer to the spinal cord: Experiments with tumor-cell suspension in rats and rabbits. Cancer 4:610–618, 1951
25. Fidler IJ, Hart IR: Principles of cancer biology: Cancer metastasis. In DeVita VT, Hellman S, Rosenberg SA (eds): Cancer. Principles and Practice of Oncology. 2nd ed, pp 113–124. Philadelphia, JB Lippincott, 1985
26. Fisher B, Fisher ER: In 21st Symposium on Fundamental Cancer Research: Anderson Hospital and Tumor Institute: The Proliferation and Spread of Neoplastic Cells, pp 555–581. Baltimore, Williams & Wilkins, 1968
27. Weiss L: Metastatic brain tumors. Factors that govern the metastatic process. In Wilkins RH, Rengachary SS (eds): Neurosurgery, pp 591–596. New York, McGraw-Hill, 1985
28. Fidler IJ, Kripke ML: Metastasis results from pre-existing variant cells within a malignant tumor. Science 197:893–895, 1977
29. Katz DA, Liotta LA: Tumor invasion and metastasis in the central nervous system. In Zimmerman HM (eds): Progress in Neuropathology, Vol 6, pp 119–131, 1986
30. Lundberg N: Continuous recording and control of ventricular fluid pressure in neurosurgical practice. Acta Psychiatry Neurol Scand (suppl 149) 36:1–193, 1960
31. Langfitt TW: Increased intracranial pressure and the cerebral circulation. In Youmans JR (ed): Neurological Surgery, 2nd ed, pp 846–930. Philadelphia, WB Saunders, 1982
32. Miller JD: Volume and pressure in the craniospinal axis. Clin Neurosurg 22:76–105, 1975
33. Plum F, Posner JB: The Diagnosis of Stupor and Coma, 3rd ed. Philadelphia, FA Davis, 1980
34. Fishman RA: Brain edema. N Engl J Med 293:706–711, 1975
35. Fishman RA: Steroids in the treatment of brain edema (editorial). N Engl J Med 306:359–360, 1982
36. Hirano A, Zimmerman HM: Fenestrated blood vessels in a metastatic renal carcinoma in the brain. Lab Invest 26:465–468, 1972
37. Chan PH, Fishmam RA: Brain edema: Induction in cortical slices by polyunsaturated fatty acids. Science 201:358–360, 1978
38. Fishman RA, Chan PH: Metabolic basis of brain edema. Adv Neurol 28:207–215, 1980
39. Black KL, Hoff JT: Leukotrienes increase blood–brain barrier permeability following intraparenchymal injections in rats. Ann Neurol 18:349–351, 1985
40. Senger DR, Galli SJ, Dvorak AM et al: Tumor cells secrete a vascular permeability factor that promotes accumulation of ascites fluid. Science 219:983–985, 1983
41. Caronna JJ, Chan PH, Fishman RA: Protective effects of corticosteroids on fatty acid-induced cerebral edema. Trans Am Neurol Soc 105:200–202, 1980
42. Blasberg RG, Gazendam J, Patlak CS, Fenstermacher JD: Quantitative autoradiographic studies of brain edema and a comparison of multi-isotope autoradiographic techniques. Adv Neurol 28:255–270, 1980
43. Posner JB: Clinical manifestations of brain metastasis. In Weiss L, Gilbert HA, Posner JB (eds): Brain Metastasis, pp 189–207. Boston, GK Hall, 1980
44. Gamache FW, Posner JB, Patterson RH: Metastatic brain tumors. In Youmans JR (ed): Neurological Surgery, 2nd ed, Vol 4, pp 2872–2898. Philadelphia, WB Saunders, 1982
45. Stortebecker TP: Metastatic tumors of the brain from a neurosurgical point of view: A follow-up study of 158 cases. J Neurosurg 11:84–111, 1954
46. Paillas JE, Pellet W: Brain metastases. In Vinken PJ, Bruyn GW (eds): Handbook of Clinical Neurology, Vol 18, pp 201–232. Amsterdam, North-Holland Publishing, 1975
47. Lang EF Jr, Slater J: Metastatic brain tumors. Results of surgical and non-surgical treatment. Surg Clin North Am 44:865–872, 1964
48. Nisce IZ, Hilaris BS, Chu FCH: A review of experience with irradiation of brain metastasis. AJR 111:329–333, 1971
49. Strub RL, Black RW: The Mental Status Examination in Neurology. Philadelphia, FA Davis, 1977
50. Hayward RD: Secondary malignant melanoma of the brain. Clin Oncol 2:227–232, 1976
51. Raskind R, Weiss SR: Conditions simulating metastatic lesions of the brain. Report of eight cases. Int Surg 43:40–42, 1970
52. Mandybur TI: Intracranial hemorrhage caused by metastatic tumors. Neurology 27:650–655, 1977
53. Deck MDF: Computed tomography of metastatic disease of the brain. In Weiss L, Gilbert HA, Posner JB (eds): Brain Metastasis, pp 208–241. Boston, GK Hall, 1980
54. Gado MH, Phelps ME, Coleman RE: An extravascular component of contrast enhancement in cranial computed tomography (Parts I and II). Radiology 117:589–597, 1975
55. Takeda N, Tanaka R, Nakai O, Ueki K: Dynamics of contrast enhancement in delayed computed tomography of brain tumors: Tissue–blood ratio and differential diagnosis. Radiology 142:663–668, 1982
56. Galicich JH, French LA, Melby JC: Use of dexamethasone in the treatment of cerebral edema associated with brain tumors. J Lancet (Minneap) 81:46–53, 1961
57. French LA: The use of steroids in the treatment of cerebral edema. Bull NY Acad Med 42:301–311, 1966
58. Renaudin J, Fewer D, Wilson CB et al: Dose dependency of Decadron in patients with partially excised brain tumors. N Neurosurg 39:302–305, 1973
59. Gutin PH: Corticosteroid therapy in patients with cerebral tumor: Benefits, mechanisms, problems, practicalities. Semin Oncol 2:49–56, 1975
60. Ransohoff J: The effects of steroids on brain edema in man. In Reulen HJ, Schurmann K (eds): Steroids and Brain Edema, pp 211–217. Berling, Springer-Verlag, 1972
61. Ehrenkranz JRL, Posner JB: Adrenocorticosteroid hormones. In Weiss L, Gilbert HA, Posner JB (eds): Brain Metastasis, pp 340–363. Boston, GK Hall, 1980
62. Weiss HD: Neoplasms. In Samuels MA (ed): Manual of Neurologic Therapeutics, 2nd ed, pp 233–263. Boston, Little, Brown & Co, 1982
63. Quest DO: Increased intracranial pressure, brain herniation, and their control. In Wilkins RH, Rengachary SS (eds): Neurosurgery, pp 332–342. New York, McGraw-Hill, 1985
64. Chao J, Phillips R, Nickson JJ: Roentgen-ray therapy of cerebral metastases. Cancer 7:682–689, 1954
65. Cairncross JG, Kim J-H, Posner JB: Radiation therapy for brain metastases. Ann Neurol 7:529–541, 1980
66. Chu FCH, Hilaris BB: Value of radiation therapy in the management of intracranial metastasis. CA 14:577–581, 1961
67. Hindo WA, DeTrana FA, Lee MS et al: Large dose increment irradiation in treatment of cerebral metastases. Cancer 26:138–141, 1970
68. Montana GS, Meacham WF, Caldwell WL: Brain irradiation for metastatic disease of lung origin. Cancer 29:1477–1480, 1972
69. Deutsch M, Parsons JA, Mercado R Jr: Radiotherapy for intracranial metastases. Cancer 34:1607, 1974
70. Young DF, Posner JB, Chu FCH et al: Rapid-course radiation therapy of cerebral metastases: Results and complications. Cancer 34:1069–1076, 1974
71. Shehata WM, Hendrickson FR, Hindo WA: Rapid fractionation technique and retreatment of cerebral metastases by irradiation. Cancer 34:257–261, 1974
72. Hendrickson FR: The optimum schedule for palliative radiotherapy for metastatic brain cancer. Int J Radiat Oncol Biol Phys 2:165–168, 1977
73. Harwood AR, Simpson WF: Radiation therapy of cerebral metastases. A randomized prospective clinical trial. Int J Radiat Oncol Biol Phys 2:1091–1094, 1977
74. Berry HC, Parker RG, Gerdes AJ: Irradiation of brain metastases. Acta Radiol Ther 13:535–544, 1974
75. Fitzpatrick J, Keen CW: The Princess Margaret and Ontario Cancer Foundation

experience. In Weiss L, Gilbert HA, Posner JB (eds): Brain Metastases, pp 281–302. Boston, GK Hall, 1980
76. Brady LW, Bajpai D: The Hahnemann experience. In Weiss L, Gilbert HA, Posner JB (eds): Brain Metastases, pp 269–278. Boston, GK Hall, 1980
77. Gilbert H, Kagan AR, Wagner J et al: The Southern California Permanente Medical Group Experience: Functional results. In Weiss L, Gilbert HA, Posner JB (eds): Brain Metastases, pp 303–313. Boston, GK Hall, 1980
78. Borgelt B, Gelber R, Kramer S et al: The palliation of brain metastases: Final results of the first two studies by the Radiation Therapy Oncology Group. Int J Radiat Oncol Biol Phys 6:1–9, 1980
79. Kurtz JM, Gelber R, Brady LW et al: The palliation of brain metastases in a favorable patient population: A randomized clinical trial by the Radiation Therapy Oncology Group. Int J Radiat Oncol Biol Phys 7:891–895, 1981
80. Borgelt B, Gelber R, Larson M et al: Ultra-rapid high dose irradiation schedules for the palliation of brain metastases: Final results of the first two studies by the Radiation Therapy Oncology Group. Int J Radiat Oncol Biol Phys 7:1633–1638, 1981
81. Gutin PH, Phillips TL, Hosobuchi Y, et al: Permanent and removable implants for the brachytherapy of brain tumors. Int J Radiat Oncol Biol Phys 7:1371–1381, 1981
82. Prados M, Gutin P: Stereotaxic interstitial brachytherapy for metastatic brain tumors: Effective palliation after failure of external radiation (abstrt). American Society of Clinical Oncologists Annual Meeting, May 17, Atlanta, Georgia, 1987
83. Shapiro WR: Chemotherapy of metastatic central nervous system carcinoma. In Weiss L, Gilbert HA, Posner JB (eds): Brain Metastases, pp 328–339. Boston, GK Hall, 1980
84. Hildebrand J, Brihaye J, Wagenknecht L et al: Combination chemotherapy with CCNU, vincristine and methotrexate in primary and metastatic brain tumors. Eur J Cancer 11:585–587, 1975
85. Alexander M, Glatstein EJ, Gordon DS, Daniels JR: Combined modality treatment for oat cell carcinoma of the lung: A randomized trial. Cancer Treat Rep 61:1–6, 1977
86. Greig NH: Chemotherapy of brain metastases: Current status. Cancer Treat Rev 11:157–186, 1984
87. Chan PYM, Byfield JE, Campbell T et al: Combined chemotherapy and irradiation in the treatment of brain metastases from lung cancer. In Weiss L, Gilbert HA, Posner JB (eds): Brain Metastasis, pp 364–379. Boston, GK Hall, 1980
88. Cascino TL, Bryn TN, Deck MDF et al: Intra-arterial BCNU in the treatment of metastatic brain tumors. J Neurooncol 1:211–218, 1983
89. Madajewicz S, West CR, Park HC et al: Phase II study: Intra-arterial BCNU therapy for metastatic brain tumors. Cancer 47:653–657, 1981
90. Saris SC, Rosenberg SA, Friedman RB et al: Penetration of recombinant interleukin-2 across the blood-cerebrospinal fluid barrier. J Neurosurg 69:29–34, 1988
91. Haar F, Paterson RH JR: Surgery for metastatic intracranial neoplasm. Cancer 30:1241–1245, 1972
92. Galicich JH, Sundaresan N. Thaler HT: Surgical treatment of single brain metastasis: Evaluation of results by computerized tomography scanning. J Neurosurg 53:63–67, 1980
93. Richards P, MKcKissock W: Intracranial metastases. Br Med J 1:15–18, 1963
94. Galicich JH: Surgery of malignant brain tumors. In Vick NA (ed): Seminars in Neurology, Vol 1, pp 159–168. New York, Thieme–Stratton, 1981
95. Appuzo ML, Sabshin JK: Computed tomographic guidance stereotaxis in the management of intracranial mass lesions. Neurosurgery 12:227–284, 1983
96. Heilbrun MP, Roberts TS, Apuzzo ML et al: Preliminary experience with the Brown–Roberts–Wells (BRW) computerized tomography stereotaxic guidance system. J Neurosurg 59:217–222, 1983
97. Posner JB: Neurological complications of systemic cancer. Med Clin North Am 55:625–646, 1971
98. Horton J, Baxter DH, Olson DB et al: The management of metastases to the brain by irradiation and corticosteroids. AJR 111:334–336, 1971
99. Order SE, Hellman S, Von Essen CF et al: Improvement in quality of survival following whole-brain irradiation for whole brain metastasis. Radiology 91:149–153, 1968
100. Hazuka MB, Kinzie JJ: Brain metastases: Results and effects of re-irradiation (abstrt). Proceedings of the American Society for Therapeutic Radiology and Oncology 29th Annual Meeting, October 1987. Int J Radiat Oncol Biol Phys (Suppl 1) 13:89, 1987
101. Vieth RG, Odom GL: Intracranial metastases and their neurosurgical treatment. N Neurosurg 23:375–383, 1965
102. Bakay L: Results of surgical treatment of intracranial metastasis from pulmonary cancer. Report of a case with five-year survival. N Neurosurg 15:338–341, 1958
103. Lang EF Jr: Neurosurgical management of intracranial metastatic malignancy. Surg Clin North Am 47:737–742, 1967
104. Olivecrona H: The Metastatic Tumors. In Olivecrona H, Tonnis W (eds): Handbuch der Neurochirurgie, pp 292–298. Berlin, Springer-Verlag, 1967
105. Smalley SR, Schray MF, Laws ER, O'Fallon JR: Adjuvant radiation therapy after surgical resection of solitary brain metastasis: Association with pattern of failure and survival. Int J Radiat Oncol Biol Phys 13:1611–1616, 1987
106. Dosoretz DE, Blitzer PH, Russell AH et al: Management of solitary metastasis to the brain: The role of elective brain irradiation following complete surgical resection. Int J Radiat Oncol Biol Phys 6:1727–1730, 1980
107. Modesti LM, Feldman RA: Solitary cerebral metastasis from pulmonary cancer. Prolonged survival after surgery. JAMA 231:1064, 1975
108. Deeley TJ, Edwards JM: Radiotherapy in the management of cerebral secondaries from bronchial carcinoma. Lancet 1:1209–1213, 1968
109. Dayes LA, Rouhe SA, Barnes RW: Excision of multiple intracranial metastatic hypernephroma: Report of a case with a 7-year survival. J Neurosurg 46:533–535, 1977
110. Raskind R, Weiss RS, Manning JJ et al: Survival after surgical excision of single metastatic brain tumors. Am J Roentgenol Radium Ther Nucl Med 111:323–328, 1971
111. Weiss L, Gilbert HA, Posner JB: Introduction. In Weiss L, Gilbert HA, Posner JB (eds): Brain Metastases, pp xv–xxxi. Boston, GK Hall, 1980

SECTION 2

JACK A. ROTH

Treatment of Metastatic Cancer to Lung

The lungs represent the second most common site of metastasis in patients dying of malignancy, with 29% of patients having pulmonary metastases at autopsy.[1] However, patients dying of pulmonary metastases have no other detectable tumor foci at autopsy in up to 20% of cases, depending on the tumor histologic type.[2] For extremity soft-tissue sarcomas, the lungs represent the only site of early metastases in over 60% of patients.[3] The use of adjuvant combination therapy has reduced, but not eliminated, the frequency of pulmonary metastases in some tumors, including osteogenic sarcomas and carcinomas of the testes.

Pulmonary metastases are most often located subpleurally. Therefore, multiple metastatic lesions are easily resected, sparing normal pulmonary parenchyma, and complex operative procedures are not required.

Other approaches to the treatment of pulmonary metastases include chemotherapy or radiotherapy. Radiation therapy appears to be of marginal benefit, either as an adjuvant or as the primary treatment for established pulmonary metastatic lesions. Chemotherapy may offer some palliative benefits, but has not been curative for established pulmonary metastases. Thus, pulmonary resection remains the only potentially curative treatment for patients with metastatic lesions limited to the lung.

DIAGNOSIS

Because isolated pulmonary metastatic lesions are sometimes amenable to curative resection, patients at risk for developing these lesions should be closely followed with frequent chest roentgenograms. Conventional linear x-ray tomography (LT) is more sensitive in detecting new pulmonary modules than is the plain chest roentgenogram (Fig. 62-7). Additional pulmonary nodules are found in 30% to 35% of the patients by conventional tomography. However, this technique still underestimates by 50% the number of pulmonary metastases found at surgery. Computed tomogra-

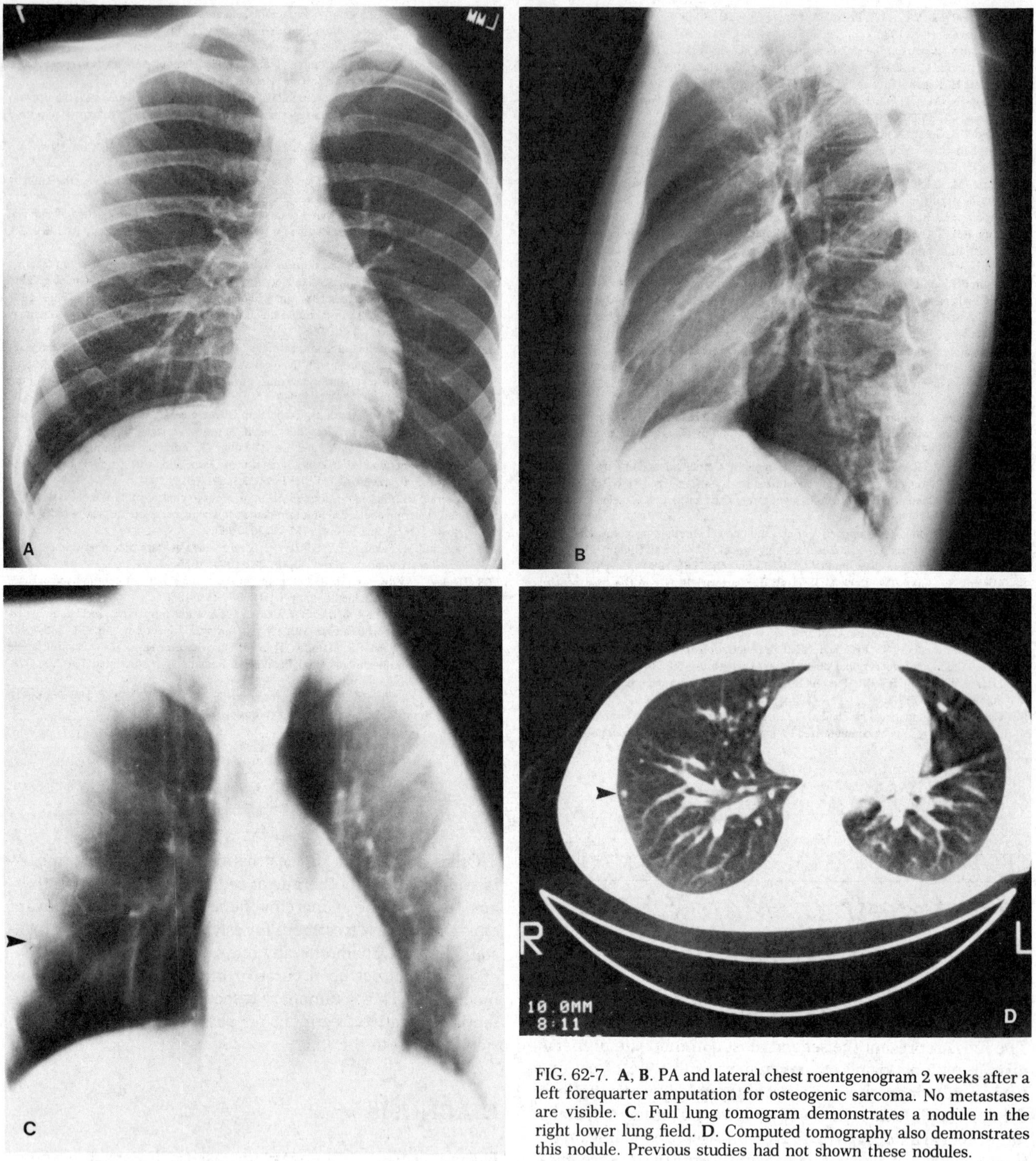

FIG. 62-7. **A**, **B**. PA and lateral chest roentgenogram 2 weeks after a left forequarter amputation for osteogenic sarcoma. No metastases are visible. **C**. Full lung tomogram demonstrates a nodule in the right lower lung field. **D**. Computed tomography also demonstrates this nodule. Previous studies had not shown these nodules.

phy (CT) is more sensitive than conventional tomography in detecting small pulmonary nodules. In a study by Chang and associates,[4] the CT detected 78% of all nodules larger than 3 mm in diameter subsequently removed at thoracotomy, compared with 59% for conventional linear tomography. However, 60% of the additional nodules detected were benign, thus reducing the specificity for identifying metastatic nodules. This study, however, compared CT and LT in a static time frame.

A subsequent study by Pass and associates from the Surgery Branch of the National Cancer Institute,[3] who used serial CT scans and dynamic criteria for defining pulmonary metastases, demonstrated superiority of CT over LT for detecting pulmonary metastases in sarcoma patients (Table

TABLE 62-13. Comparison of the Efficacy of Serial Computed Tomographic Scans (CT) and Conventional Linear Tomograms (LT) in Detecting Pulmonary Metastases from Sarcomas for 22 Preoperative Evaluations

	First Positive Study (No. of Patients)	*No. of Metastases Detected*	*Size (mm)*
CT	13	50	7.1 ± 1
LT	1	5	13.2 ± 3

62-13). In this study, simultaneous CT and LT were obtained, and the appearance of new nodules, as well as growth of existing nodules from baseline studies, was noted. For 8 of the 16 patients, CT was the first positive study, whereas LT was the first positive study for only one patient, with seven patients being CT- and LT-positive simultaneously. Significant by smaller metastases and greater numbers of metastases were detected by CT compared with LT (see Table 62-13). In this study, CT-detected nodules, which became apparent after a previously negative study, were histologically confirmed as metastases in 50 of 56 instances. Those nodules that increased in size also were metastatic (eight of eight). Caution must be used in extrapolating the findings of this study to all cancer patients. Patients with sarcomas are generally young and rarely have coexisting pulmonary abnormalities that may cause interpretative difficulties with the CT scan. The CT scan may not be as accurate in older patient populations with different tumor types.

Siegelman and associates have reported a technique for discriminating between benign and malignant pulmonary nodules that is based on the density, as determined by CT number.[5,6] Of those lesions with a CT number of 164H or higher, all were benign (20 of 33), and no malignant nodules had a CT number higher than 147H (45 primary lung malignancies and 13 metastases). The increased density of the benign nodules was attributed to calcification. This technique is dependent on the type of reconstructive algorithm, the design of the CT system, the true slice thickness, and the beam kilovoltage, and it has not been reproduced by all investigators.[6] Furthermore, some types of malignancy demonstrate calcification (primary lung carcinoma, metastases from osteogenic sarcoma) or may arise in juxtaposition to preexisting granulomas. A high percentage of pulmonary nodules are indeterminate with this technique, and occasional malignant lesions have benign-appearing characteristics.[7] Thus, it is unlikely that this technique will replace biopsy as the most accurate diagnostic modality for pulmonary nodules.

Because metastases are most often peripheral, symptoms are seldom present. Only 8 of 136 patients with metastases from osteogenic and soft-tissue sarcomas who were evaluated by the Surgery Branch of the National Cancer Institute (NCI) over the last 8 years presented with symptoms. Symptoms may include cough, hemoptysis, spontaneous pneumothorax, chest pain, and dyspnea. The paucity of early symptoms emphasizes the need for close roentgenographic follow-up. Diagnostic studies that are useful in other thoracic neoplasms are of limited value for the diagnosis of pulmonary metastases. In one series, sputum cytologic examination revealed malignant cells in only 5% of patients, and bronchoscopy provided notable findings in only 10% of the patients examined.[8] Percutaneous needle aspiration is also of limited usefulness for potentially resectable patients, because these patients will be explored with curative intent regardless of the diagnosis. However, in patients for whom resection is not an option, this technique can be useful in establishing the diagnosis of malignancy.[9]

For patients who have multiple lung nodules and a known extrapulmonary primary cancer, the lung lesions are most likely metastatic. The appearance of the solitary pulmonary lesion in patients with a known extrapulmonary primary lesion raises three possibilities: a carcinoma of the lung, which is a new and separate primary tumor; metastasis from the known primary; or a benign lesion. Although there is a less than 1% chance of a solitary nodule being a metastasis, if there is no history of cancer, this increases to 81% for patients with a history of malignancy.[2] However, the probability that the new solitary pulmonary nodule represents a metastasis varies with the type of the previous cancer. For example, Cahan and co-workers[10] found that in 72 breast cancer patients who developed solitary pulmonary nodules, only 23 (32%) of the nodules were metastases from the breast cancer. Forty-three of the patients had separate primary lung cancers. However, for 54 colon carcinoma patients with solitary lung shadows, 25 of the shadows were colon cancer metastases.[11] In our experience, for patients with sarcomas or melanomas, a new pulmonary nodule is almost always a metastasis.

SURGICAL TREATMENT OF PULMONARY METASTASES

The first removal of a pulmonary metastasis was accomplished by Weinlechner in 1882.[12] The metastasis was removed en bloc with the primary tumor during a chest wall resection for a sarcoma. In 1884 Krolein published a case history describing resection of a tumor nodule at the lung periphery after resection of a recurrent chest wall sarcoma. Divis, in Prague in 1926, performed metastastectomy as a separate procedure removing a metastasis from the right lower lobe. The report from Barney and Churchill, in 1939,[13] on resection of a solitary pulmonary metastasis from an adenosarcoma of the kidney and that patient's death 23 years later from coronary artery disease, was an impetus for further attempts at curative resection. In 1947, Alexander and Haight reported apparent cures in three of six patients after resection of metastases.[14]

Initially, surgical resection was offered to only highly selected patients with a solitary metastasis and a long tumor-free interval. However, in 1965 Thomford and co-workers found almost identical postthoracotomy survival rates for patients with solitary or multiple carcinoma and sarcoma lung metastases.[15] Martini and co-workers[16] and Morton and co-workers[17] later observed that survival rates after surgical resection of multiple metastatic lesions, even when bilateral, were similar to those after resection of solitary lung metastases.

Early diagnosis of pulmonary metastatic lesions is important because, if they are diagnosed at the symptomatic stage, the results are less favorable than resection when these lesions are asymptomatic. Thus, it is recommended that patients with primary tumors that have a propensity for pulmonary metastases undergo frequent radiographic examination. Serial CT scans at 3 to 6-month intervals are recommended for patients from high-risk groups (*e.g.*, testicular carcinoma, sarcoma) and when early resection of metastases offer a substantial probability for prolonged survival.

Preoperative evaluation differs according to the primary tumor type because the pattern of metastatic spread changes according to the histologic type. Sarcomas metastasize to the lung in preference to other sites. Generally, a thorough evaluation of the primary site and a radionuclide bone scan are all that are needed before exploration. Carcinomas, however, may metastasize to more than one distant site, including the liver; therefore, a careful evaluation of all potential metastatic sites is indicated. Malignant melanoma can spread simultaneously to any organ system, and the cause of death frequently is due to metastasis to the central nervous system. Because the chance of the disease being confined to the lungs is small, patients with metastatic lung lesions must fulfill the most stringent clinical criteria before resection of their pulmonary metastases.

Extensive pulmonary resections are rarely required for removal of pulmonary metastatic nodules. Nevertheless, an appropriate evaluation of the patient's pulmonary function must be made to assure adequate ventilatory reserve after the resection. If patients do not have symptomatic pulmonary disease and can climb two or more flights of stairs without shortness of breath, they can undergo thoracotomy and resection of a lobe with adequate function remaining. For the patient with compromised pulmonary function, spirometry can be useful in determining ventilatory reserve. If an extensive resection is planned, a quantitative ventilation–perfusion scan is a useful study for determining the residual 1-sec forced expiratory volume (FEV_1) after pulmonary resection.[18] In general, a patient must have a postoperative FEV_1 of 800 to 1000 cc to avoid being respirator-dependent.

CRITERIA FOR PATIENT SELECTION AND INFLUENCE OF PROGNOSTIC FACTORS ON SURVIVAL

Only a few patients undergoing resection of pulmonary metastases are cured, and another proportion have prolonged survival, compared with patients not amenable to resection. Various criteria have been proposed to select those patients who will benefit from resection. For most studies, there is agreement that patients must meet certain minimum criteria before undergoing resection. These include [1] local control of the primary tumor or the ability to gain local control if pulmonary exploration is performed first; [2] absence of metastatic lesions in nonpulmonary sites; [3] radiologic findings consistent with metastases on radiographic examination; and [4] potential for the operative resection to preserve adequate functioning lung tissue. A summary of the results of studies that have analyzed the correlation of the major prognostic criteria with survival following resection of pulmonary metastases is given in Table 62-14.

TABLE 62-14. Correlation of Prognostic Factors With Survival Following Resection of Pulmonary Metastases

Prognostic Factor	*Cancer*	*Author (Ref)*	*No. of Patients*	*Correlation*
Disease-free Interval	Osteogenic sarcoma	Burgers (20)	18	Positive
	Osteogenic sarcoma	Putnam (21)	18	None
	Osteogenic sarcoma	Meyer (23)	59	None
	Soft-tissue sarcoma	Creagen (24)	112	Positive <12 mo vs >12 mo
	Soft-tissue sarcoma	Putnam (22)	63	Positive <12 mo vs >12 mo
	Colon	Cahan (11)	25	None
	Breast	Cahan (10)	23	None
	Mixed histologies	Morrow (25)	167	Positive <5 yr vs >5 yr
	Mixed histologies	Takita (26)	234	Positive <8 mo vs >8 mo
	Mixed histologies	Turney (27)	68	Positive
Number of metastases	Colon	Cahan (28)	31	None-single vs multiple
	Colon	McCormack (29)	35	None-single vs multiple
	Osteogenic sarcoma	Telander (30)	28	None-single vs multiple
	Osteogenic sarcoma	Putnam (21)	38	Negative <4 vs >4 metastases
	Osteogenic sarcoma	Meyer (23)	59	Negative <4 vs >4 metastases
	Soft-tissue sarcoma	Putnam (22)	63	Negative <4 vs >4 metastases
	Mixed histologies	Takita (26)	234	Negative
	Mixed histologies	Morrow (25)	167	Negative-single vs multiple
	Mixed histologies	Ishihara (31)	77	None-single vs multiple
Tumor doubling-time	Mixed histologies	Joseph (32)	113	Positive <40 vs >40 days
	Mixed histologies	Takita (26)	234	Positive <45 vs >45 days
	Soft-tissue sarcoma	Putnam (22)	63	Positive <20 vs >20 days
	Osteogenic sarcoma	Putnam (21)	38	None

DISEASE-FREE INTERVAL FROM CONTROL OF THE PRIMARY TUMOR TO APPEARANCE OF A METASTASIS

There is good agreement in most reports of resection of pulmonary metastases from osteogenic and soft-tissue sarcomas that a longer disease-free interval (generally more than 1 year) indicates a more favorable prognosis. Huth and co-workers found, for a combined group of patients with osteogenic and soft-tissue sarcomas, a 70% 3-year survival if the disease-free interval is 1 year or longer, compared with a 28% 3-year survival for a disease-free interval of less than 1 year.[19] Burgers and co-workers observed a correlation between disease-free interval and prognosis following resection of metastases from osteogenic sarcoma.[20] Putnam and co-workers,[21,22] reviewing the National Cancer Institute experience, also found a significant correlation between disease-free interval and postresection survival for patients with soft-tissue sarcomas, although the correlation was of only borderline significance for osteogenic sarcoma patients (Fig. 62-8).

Cahan and co-workers, however, found no relationship between disease-free interval and survival following resection of solitary metastases from breast and colon carcinoma.[25-27] However, these series are heavily weighted with sarcomas, renal cell carcinomas, and testicular carcinomas. The possibility must be considered that the prognosis following metastasectomy for some tumor types may not be related to the disease-free interval. The importance of the disease-free interval is emphasized when patients with synchronous metastases are considered. Putnam and co-workers found that for 24 patients with soft-tissue sarcomas and synchronous pulmonary metastases only 46% were resectable,

FIG. 62-8. Actuarial survival for patients following resection of pulmonary metastases from soft tissue sarcomas. **A–C**. Patient survival is analyzed for tumor doubling time, disease-free interval (*DFI*), and nodules on conventional linear tomograms. **D**. Survival is analyzed for patients undergoing resection with favorable prognostic factors compared with unresectable metastases. (Putnam JB Jr, Roth JA, Wesley MN et al: J Thorac Cardiovasc Surg 87:260–268, 1984)

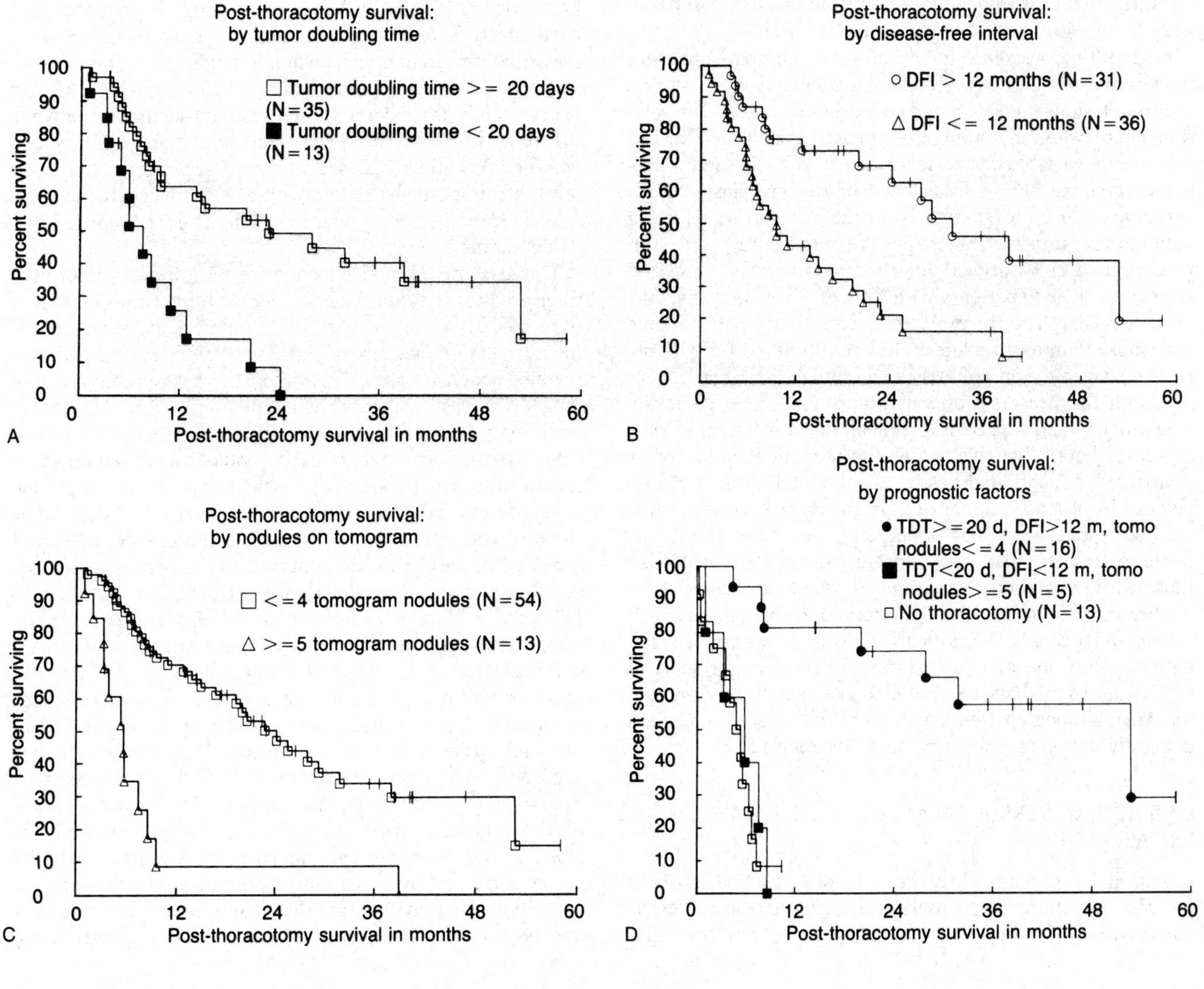

compared with an 80% resectability rate for patients with metachronous metastases.[22] However, postthoracotomy survival of patients with resectable metastases that were synchronous (22-months median survival) was similar to that of patients with metachronous metastases who underwent resection (23-months median survival).

NUMBER OF METASTASES

Early attempts at resection of pulmonary metastases were confined to patients with solitary lesions. Recently, it has become apparent that patients with multiple pulmonary metastases also will benefit from resection. Cahan and coworkers found no difference in survival for patients undergoing resection of solitary or multiple colon metastases to the lung.[28] Likewise, McCormack and Attiyeh noted similar survival for patients with solitary and multiple colon metastases.[29] In a series of 167 patients with various histologic types of pulmonary metastases, Morrow and co-workers observed a 27% 5-year survival for patients with multiple metastases that were resected, compared with 22% for patients with solitary metastases.[33] Telander and co-workers also found no difference for solitary compared to multiple metastases.[30] Ishihara and co-workers did not find improved survival in patients with a solitary metastatic lesion, compared with those with multiple metastases.[31]

In all of the foregoing studies, however, comparisons were made only between two groups of patients (solitary versus multiple lesions). Putnam and co-workers analyzed the relationship between the number of metastases and survival as a continuous variable for patients with soft-tissue and osteogenic sarcomas.[21,22] A knowledge of the prognosis before surgery would be of great help to the surgeon in selecting patients for surgery. The number of metastatic nodules on preoperative conventional lung tomograms was compared with survival. For patients with four or fewer nodules, survival was significantly prolonged, compared with patients with more than four nodules. This was observed for patients with osteogenic and soft tissue sarcomas (see Fig. 62-8). Although the presence of four metastases alone generally would not render a patient technically unresectable, it must be remembered that this is only the number seen on tomograms and, as such, underestimates the total number of metastases by at least a factor of 2. In the same series, patients with soft-tissue sarcomas undergoing resection with 15 or fewer metastases had a significantly longer survival than those with more than 15 metastases. Meyer and co-workers confirmed this with a similar observation for patients with osteogenic sarcoma.[23] Takita and co-workers also noted that patients with one or two metastases had a longer survival (13.5 months median) compared to five to eight (8.7 months median), although patients with more than eight lesions had a slightly better median survival (19.8 months).[26]

UNILATERAL VERSUS BILATERAL PULMONARY METASTASES

Takita and associates observed a median survival of 14.9 months in patients with unilateral multiple lesions, compared with 18.1 months for patients with bilateral multiple lesions.[26] Putnam and co-workers also found no difference in the survival of osteogenic or soft-tissue sarcoma patients with either unilateral or bilateral metastases when a correction for the total number of pulmonary nodules was made.[21,22]

TUMOR DOUBLING-TIME

A number of biologic systems grow exponentially at first, but, as the number of cells increases and there is competition for nutrients, the growth curve flattens. The growth of solid tumors is also characterized by retardation, which increases with time. This retardation may be caused by immunologic suppression, limitation of nutrition, or a decrease in blood supply, evident microscopically as tumor necrosis. These factors cause a longer generation time of cancer cells, with a resulting increase in the doubling-time. This tumor growth is best expressed by the gompertzian equation, which expresses exponential growth when the tumor is small and contains retarding factors; this increases exponentially with time to fit the decreasing growth rate when the tumor is large.

The growth of lung metastatic tumors in humans appears to be closer to an exponential rate than tumors in other locations. This may be because the lung tissue provides a particularly favorable environment. Actually, the interval between 10 mm in diameter, when a metastatic lesion is regularly visible on roentgenogram, and 100 mm, when the host is near death, is such a short and selected segment relative to the total life history of the neoplasm that arguments of whether the growth is logarithmic, gompertzian, linear, or other are impossible to resolve. Growth during this interval may be interspersed as a straight line when a lesion is measured at this time.

Tumor growth kinetics have been examined to determine their prognostic value.[34] The tumor doubling-times of pulmonary metastases or primary lung tumors have been studied most frequently because of the ease of precisely measuring a nodule, which is more dense than the surrounding aerated lung, on at least two chest roentgenograms taken under identical conditions and separated by a suitable time interval. The changing diameters of each nodule are plotted on semilogarithmic paper along the vertical axis, against time (in days), between determinations on the horizontal axis.[17] The slope of the line between the points represents the tumor growth rate, and the horizontal distance between any two doubling-points represents the tumor doubling-time in days (Fig.62-9). Most studies have found that the shorter the tumor doubling-time, the shorter the patient survival. This is demonstrated by the study of Joseph and co-workers of 113 patients with pulmonary metastases from sarcomas and carcinomas.[32] Eighty-nine patients who had no further treatment after the onset of metastatic lung lesions were grouped according to a tumor doubling-time of 20 days and fewer, 21 days to 40 days, and more than 40 days. The 1-year survivals of these groups were 11%, 45%, and 86%, respectively. None of the untreated patients survived 2 years. Of the 17 patients treated by resection of pulmonary metastases, all were dead within 18 months. There were no survivors beyond 30 months in the group of 17 patients with tumor

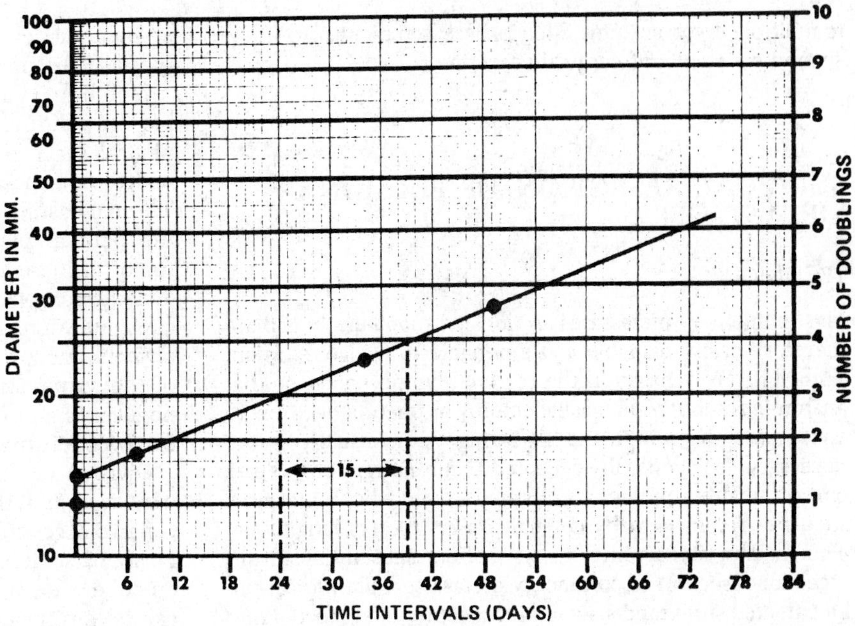

FIG. 62-9. Tumor doubling time is estimated by plotting the changing diameters of metastatic pulmonary nodules on semilogarithmic paper. (Joseph WL, Morton DL, Adkins PC: J Thorac Cardiovas Surg 61:23, 1971)

doubling-times of 20 days to 40 days who were treated surgically. Ninety-seven percent of patients with tumor doubling-times longer than 40 days undergoing surgical resection were alive at 2 years, and 63% were alive at 5 years. Of the 26 patients in this third group, 14 had undergone resection of bilateral pulmonary metastases.

Takita and colleagues reviewed 234 patients following resection of pulmonary metastases for a variety of histologically distinct primary tumors. Patients with a tumor doubling-time of 45 days or less had a significantly worse median survival (17.2 months) than patients with a tumor doubling-time of more than 45 days who had a median survival of 37.3 months.[26]

Putnam and associates found that soft tissue sarcoma patients with a tumor doubling-time of 20 days or more had a significantly longer postthoracotomy survival (22 months median) than patients with a tumor doubling-time of fewer than 20 days (6 month median).[21,22] Interestingly, Putnam and co-workers also found that the tumor doubling-time did not correlate with survival for patients with osteogenic sarcoma. Subsequent analysis showed that only the number of metastatic lesions on the preoperative tomograms predicted survival for both osteogenic and soft tissue sarcoma patients.[35] Tumor doubling-time and disease-free intervals were homogeneously distributed over a narrow range for osteogenic sarcoma patients and thus were not discriminating in terms of predicting prognosis. This raises the possibility that histologically distinct tumors may exhibit differences in biologic behavior and, consequently, patient selection must be made with differing criteria.

Therapeutic manipulation may alter the tumor doubling-time. In 12 patients with metastatic osteogenic sarcoma, Giritsky and co-workers reported that the tumor doubling-time averaged 22 days when patients received no chemotherapy or radiation, but during combination chemotherapy the tumor doubling-time was prolonged to 74 days.[36] Huth and associates also observed that chemotherapy would prolong the tumor doubling-time of patients with pulmonary metastases from sarcomas.[19] Those patients whose tumor growth slowed also had a prolonged survival compared with patients who did not respond, although the number of patients treated was small. This suggests that the preoperative response to chemotherapy may be used as a predictor of prognosis after surgical resection. It is also possible that the biologic character of the tumor might be modified such that improved results can be obtained by surgical resection.

The use of any of the foregoing prognostic criteria for patient selection remains controversial. No single factor is discriminating enough to select only those patients who will benefit, and some patients who may benefit will be excluded. Putnam and co-workers looked at combinations of prognostic factors and found that combining these significantly improved their predictive value.[22] Soft-tissue sarcoma patients with a tumor doubling-time of 20 days or more, four or fewer nodules on preoperative full-long tomograms, and a disease-free interval of more than 12 months, had a longer postthoracotomy survival (23 months median) than those patients with a tumor doubling-time of fewer than 20 days, five or more nodules on preoperative tomograms, and a disease-free interval of 12 months or less (5 months median). Postthoracotomy survival for patients in the latter group was no different from survival of patients with unresectable metastases (5 months median) who did not undergo thoracotomy (see Fig. 62-8).

HISTOLOGIC TYPE OF THE PRIMARY TUMOR

The histologic type of the primary tumor also influences its propensity for metastatic spread. The results of resection of pulmonary metastases vary greatly among differing tumor types. Resection of metastatic lesions from patients whose tumors have a propensity to spread initially only to the lungs generally have a more favorable outcome following resection than patients with metastases from tumors that disseminate to multiple organ systems. This is discussed more fully in the section on results of surgical resection.

SURGICAL RESECTION OF PULMONARY METASTASES

TECHNIQUE

Most pulmonary metastases are located subpleurally and are therefore easily palpable and amenable to wedge excision. Tumor is rarely found in the regional lymph nodes, so that anatomic resection such as lobectomy or pneumonectomy to encompass the lymph-node-bearing tissue usually is not necessary. It is generally accepted that a margin of 0.5 to 1 cm of healthy pulmonary tissue around the metastases should be removed with maximal conservation of lung tissue. The median sternotomy incision offers substantial advantages for resection of pulmonary metastases. Both lungs can be palpated simultaneously, and frequently unsuspected metastases in a radiographically uninvolved lung will be found. Roth and co-workers compared two groups of patients who underwent either median sternotomy or bilateral staged thoracotomies for resection of soft-tissue sarcoma pulmonary metastases.[37] No difference in survival was noted between the two groups (Fig. 62-10). However, 45% (9 of 20) of patients with unilateral metastases seen on CT scan had bilateral metastases at sternotomy. The median sternotomy incision is considerably less painful than the posterolateral incision and, in patients with known bilateral metastases, a second-staged operative procedure can be eliminated. A disadvantage of the median sternotomy approach is the increased difficulty in resecting posterior and medial lesions in the lower lobes. On occasion, combining a posterolateral thoracotomy with a sternotomy during a single operation has facilitated resection of lower lobe metastases requiring a lobectomy in patients with bilateral metastases. Patients must be carefully selected for such an approach and must have good preoperative pulmonary function. Intubation with a double-lumen endotracheal tube is essential during anesthesia if the median sternotomy incision is used.

Mobilization and adequate palpation of the lung are possible only during complete collapse of the lung. After the pleural space is opened, the mediastinal and hilar lymph nodes are inspected, and the parietal pleural space is opened. The mediastinal and hilar lymph nodes are inspected, and the parietal pleural surface is examined for seeding by tumor. If these areas are free of tumor, the lung is collapsed and carefully palpated sequentially by the surgeon and his assistant. All metastases are marked with a silk suture before any resection, because resection changes the configuration of the surrounding lung, making it difficult to identify the nodules. If an extensive resection is contemplated, it is useful to obtain frozen-section confirmation of malignancy.

Division of the inferior pulmonary ligaments facilitates mobilization of the lung and frequently makes posterior metastases accessible through the median sternotomy incision. For peripheral lesions a Duval lung clamp can be positioned on either side of the nodule or, for small nodules, the nodule can be positioned directly in the cutout area of the clamp. The TA automatic-stapling device is then placed across the base of the lesion. This instrument comes in 30-mm, 55-mm, and 90-mm sizes. For lesions deeper in the lung parenchyma, the GIA stapler, which staples and cuts simultaneously, may be used. This prevents the forceful traction sometimes needed when the TA stapler is used and minimizes the chance of an inadequate margin of resection. Resection of metastases with the lung inflated will avoid removal of excessive lung tissue and still provide an adequate margin. Other techniques for limited pulmonary resection are currently being evaluated including electrocautery and the neodymium : yttrium-aluminum-garnet (YAG) laser. The operative mortality and morbidity after resection of pulmonary metastases is very low (Table 62-15). There have been no deaths following 254 operative resections for pulmonary metastases at the National Cancer Institute over the past 8 years.[21,22] The complication rate has been 5.5%. Major complications are generally infectious or respiratory. Concomitant chemotherapy can contribute to increased

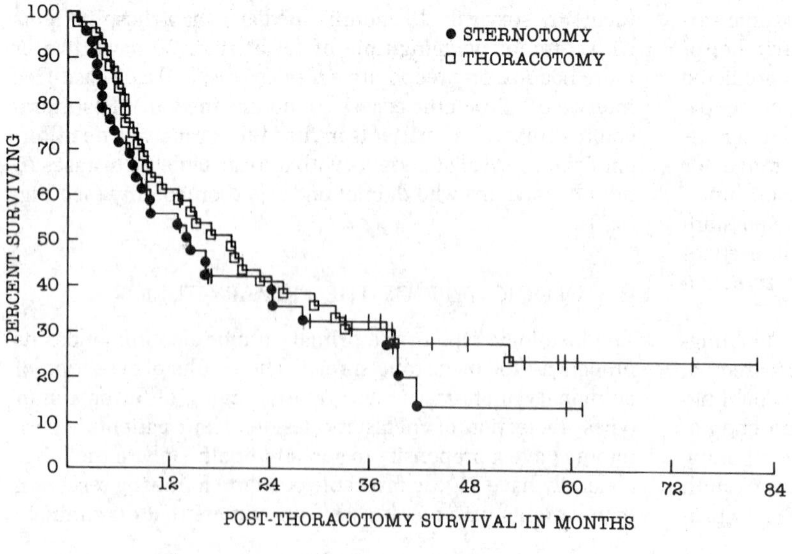

FIG. 62-10. Actuarial post-thoracotomy survival in adult soft-tissue sarcoma patients by type of incision. (P_2, 0.41; *, Median sternotomy; 0, Thoracotomy.) (Roth JA, Pass HI, Wesley MN et al: Ann Thorac Surg 42:134–138, 1986)

TABLE 62-15. Operative Mortality and Morbidity for Patients Undergoing Resection of Pulmonary Metastases

Author (Reference)		*Number of Patients*	*Operative Mortality (%)*	*Operative Morbidity (%)*
Giritsky	(36)	12	0	5
Telander	(30)	28	0	2
Putnam	(21)	39	0	5
Martini	(38)	102	1	NA*
Creagan	(24)	112	2	NA
Putnam	(22)	63	0	9
Wilkins	(39)	28	0	12
Cahan	(10)	31	0	0
Dahlback	(42)	8	0	0
Turney	(27)	68	1	NA

* NA = not available.

morbidity, especially if patients are granulocytopenic or immunosuppressed.

RESULTS OF SURGICAL RESECTION OF PULMONARY METASTASES

The metastases of many of the sarcomas and carcinomas are initially limited to the lungs. Except for trophoblastic choriocarcinomas and embryonal cell carcinoma of the testes, most physicians believe that there is currently no potentially curative treatment other than surgical removal. A summary of survival curves for various tumor types from the Memorial Hospital experience is shown in Figure 62-11.

The potential for prolonged survival after resection of pulmonary metastases depends, in part, on the pattern of spread of solid tumors to other organ systems. The most favorable pattern of spread for potential surgical resection is directly to the lungs, from which further metastases would have to disseminate. Tumors in this group include osteogenic and soft-tissue sarcomas, tumors of the head and neck, genitourinary carcinomas, and testicular tumors. A summary of survival rates following resection of pulmonary metastases for various tumor types is given in Table 62-16.

Osteogenic Sarcoma

Isolated pulmonary metastatic tumors are frequently the first site of metastases in patients with osteogenic sarcomas, although the percentage of initial extrapulmonary lesions has recently increased and may be associated with the use of adjuvant chemotherapy.[45]

Before the aggressive resection of pulmonary metastases in patients with osteogenic sarcoma, survival in patients treated by amputation alone was poor. Marcove and coworkers found only 17% of patients were tumor-free after 5 years.[46] Six months after amputation of the primary tumor, 50% of the 145 patients had developed pulmonary metastases and, by 12 months, this figure was approximately 80%. Of those who developed pulmonary metastases, 50% died within the first year, 88% within 2 years, 95% within 3 years, and none were alive at 5 years.

After institution of an aggressive resectional approach, survival of osteosarcoma patients has increased. Giritsky and associates, in a series of 12 patients, had a 57.8% survival at

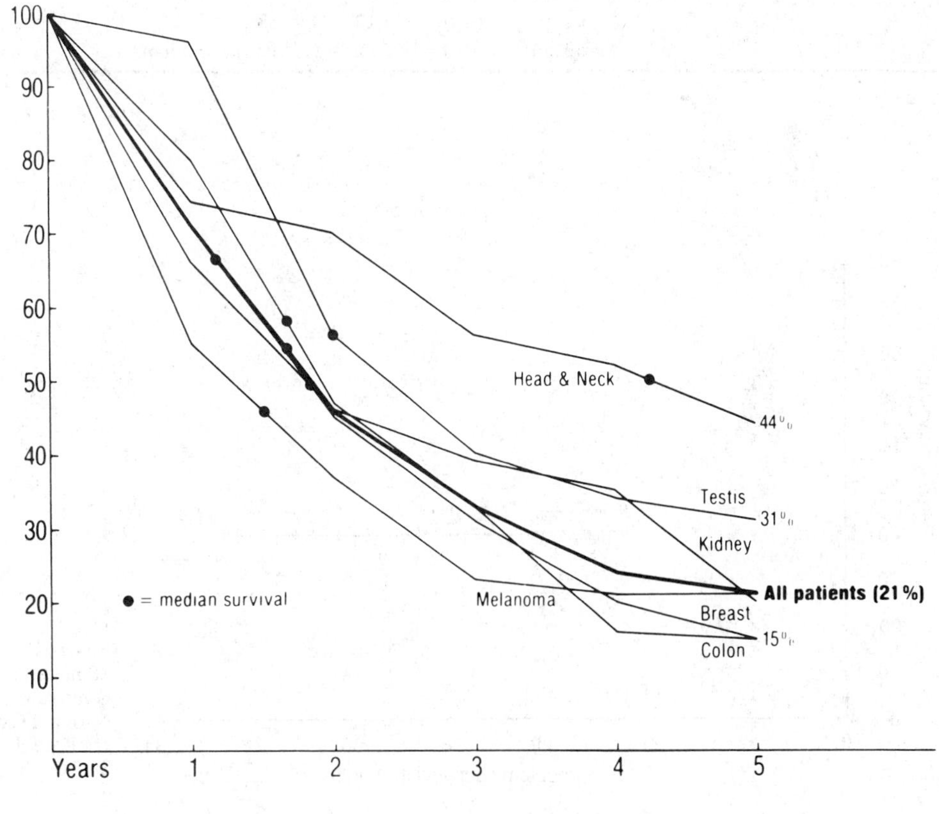

FIG. 62-11. Cumulative survival of patients (n = 215) after resection of pulmonary metastases from primary carcinomas. (McCormack P: Surgical treatment of pulmonary metastases: The Memorial Hospital experience. In Weiss L, Gilvert HA [eds]: Pulmonary Metastasis, pp 260–270. Boston, GK Hall, 1978)

TABLE 62-16. Survival Rates Following Resection of Pulmonary Metastases for Various Tumor Histologic Types

Cancer	*Author (Ref.)*		*No. of Patients*	*Survival (5-Year Actuarial Unless Otherwise Stated)*
Osteogenic Sarcoma	Girtisky	(36)	12	58 (3-yr)
	Terlander	(30)	28	57 (4 yr)
	Putnam	(21)	39	40
	Burgers	(20)	6	66
	Morrow	(33)	11	36
	Meyer	(23)	39	32
Soft-tissue sarcoma	Martini	(38)	102	26
	Creagen	(24)	112	29
	Putnam	(22)	63	30 (3 yr)
Urinary tract	Wilkins	(39)	28	37
	Mountain	(40)	16	50
	Morrow	(33)	6	30
Testicular	Morrow	(33)	30	24
	Mountain	(40)	11	30
Head and neck	McCormack	(29)	25	44
Colon–rectum	Cahan	(11)	31	30
	Morrow	(33)	16	13
	Mountain	(40)	28	28
	McCormack	(41)	40	15
	Mansel	(50)	66	38
Uterine–cervix	Morrow	(33)	22	8
	Mountain	(40)	31	19
Breast	Mountain	(40)	21	14
	McCormack	(41)	28	15
Melanoma	Morrow	(33)	12	12
	Dahlback	(42)	8	7 mo median
	Cahan	(43)	12	33
	Mathison	(44)	12	12 mo median

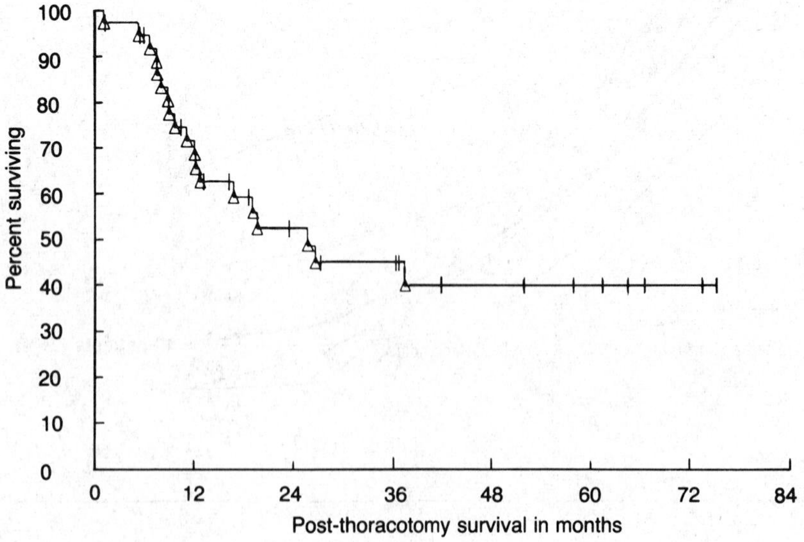

FIG. 62-12. Actuarial post-thoracotomy survival for 38 patients with pulmonary metastases from osteogenic sarcoma treated by the Surgery Branch of the National Cancer Institute over 8 years. (Putnam JB Jr, Roth JA, Wesley MN et al: Ann Thorac Surg 36:516–523, 1983)

3 years.[36] Telander and co-workers, in a series of 28 patients, had a 4-year actual survival of 57%.[30] In a series of 39 patients undergoing resection at the NCI, Putnam and co-workers noted a 5-year actual survival of 40% (Fig. 62-12).[21]

One difficulty with the interpretation of these studies is that intensive chemotherapy was also administered to many of these patients. Burgers and co-workers also reported resection of pulmonary metastases in six patients, and four were alive more than 5 years after resection without adjuvant treatment.[20] Thus, aggressive surgical resection of pulmonary metastases alone may prolong survival.

Soft-Tissue Sarcoma

Metastases from soft-tissue sarcomas, like osteogenic sarcomas, are confined to the lungs in most patients in the early stages of disease. Therefore, it is not surprising that the results of surgical resection of isolated pulmonary metastases are similar for both tumors. Of 102 patients operated on at Memorial Hospital, tumor was too extensive to permit complete resection in only 16 patients. In those patients for whom complete resection was possible, 26% were alive after 5 years and 17% of these patients were completely tumor-free.[38] At the Mayo Clinic the 5-year actuarial survival after the first thoracotomy for 112 patients was 29%, with a median survival of 18 months.[24] Putnam and co-workers, describing the NCI experience, reported that, of 63 patients undergoing exploration for resection of metastases, 51 patients had metastases that could be completely resected.[22] The median survival of patients undergoing resection was 18 months, and the actuarial disease-free survival at 3 years was 30% (Fig. 62-13). Survival correlated with tumor doubling-time, disease-free interval, and number of new nodules on preoperative full lung tomograms.

Patients undergoing two or more resections for isolated pulmonary metastases achieved similar survival rates irrespective of the number of operations.[47] Initial tumor doubling-time and the number of metastases before the first resection predicted survival (Fig. 62-14).

Urinary Tract

Favorable results have frequently been reported following resection of pulmonary metastases for carcinoma of the urinary tract. Wilkins and associates reported a cumulative 44.2% survival for 28 patients with the kidney as the primary site.[39]

Mountain and co-workers noted a 50% cumulative 5-year survival for 16 patients with tumors of the urinary tract.[40] Morrow and associates noted only a 24% cumulative 5-year survival in patients with metastases from primary renal tumors.[33]

Testicular

Nonseminomatous germ cell tumors of the testes are frequently widely disseminated when pulmonary metastases appear. Surgical excision of pulmonary metastases from other tumors is usually not indicated if the tumor has spread to other sites and, in general, there is no other effective therapy available. Germ cell tumors are extremely sensitive to chemotherapy, and this represents a primary treatment modality. Hence, surgery is recommended only when there is no response to chemotherapy, when there is a partial response followed by recurrence while receiving chemotherapy, or when it is necessary to determine if there is viable tumor present to decide on the advisability of continuing or changing chemotherapy. The histologic type of these tumors frequently will change during chemotherapy from embryonal carcinoma to benign teratoma. During surgical exploration all palpable tumor should also be resected with minimal sacrifice of lung tissue.

In a series from Memorial Sloan–Kettering, combination chemotherapy incorporating cyclophosphamide, dactinomycin, vinblastine, bleomycin, and high-dose cisplatin eliminated pulmonary metastases in 68% of patients with advanced disease and in 86% of patients with minimal disease.[48] All six patients with residual necrotic pulmonary lesions documented by resection were alive and tumor-free with a median follow-up of 26 months. Four of six patients

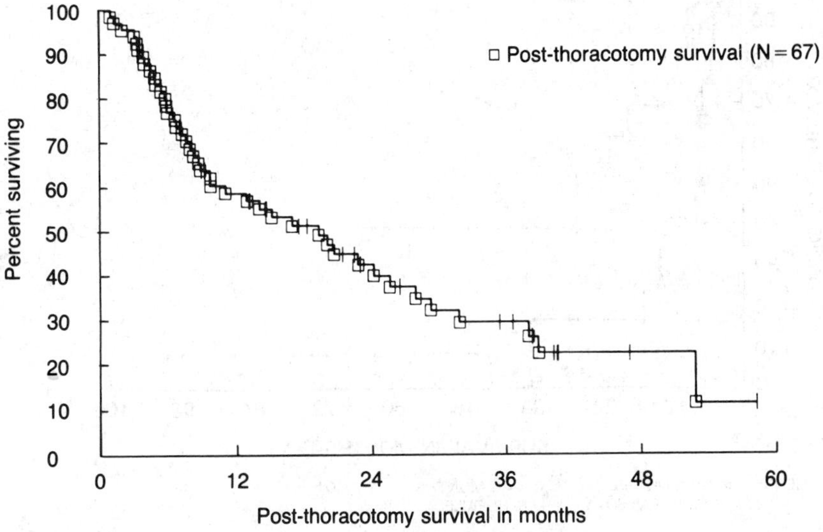

FIG. 62-13. Actuarial post-thoracotomy survival for 63 patients with pulmonary metastases from soft tissue sarcomas treated by the Surgery Branch of the National Cancer Institute over 8 years. (Putnam JB Jr, Roth JA, Wesley MN et al: J Thorac Cardiovasc Surg 87:260–268, 1984)

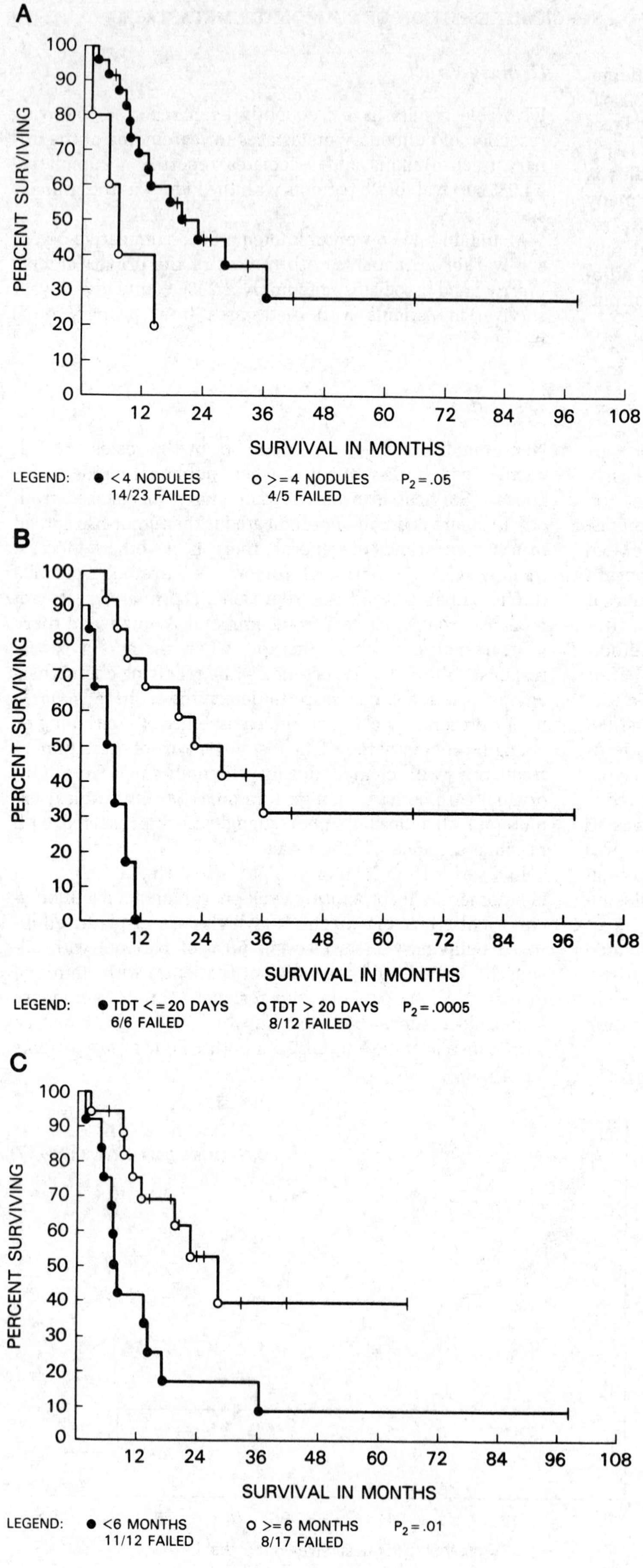

FIG. 62-14. Actuarial survival for patients following a second resection of pulmonary metastases from soft-tissue sarcomas. Patient survival is analyzed for number of metastases on tomography prior to the initial resection (**A**), tumor doubling time prior to the initial resection (**B**), and the interval between the first and second resections (**C**). (Rizzoni WE, Pass HI, Wesley MN et al: Arch Surg 121:1248–1252, 1986)

made tumor-free by pulmonary resection were disease-free with a median follow-up of 47 months. Morrow and associates achieved a cumulative survival of 60% for six patients with testicular carcinoma undergoing pulmonary metastasectomy.[33] Mountain and colleagues reported a 3% cumulative 5-year survival (median survival 10 months) for 11 resected patients.[40]

Head and Neck

Head and neck cancers, with the exception of cancers of the lip, tonsil, and adenoid, first spread to the lungs and from there to the liver, CNS, and endocrine system. Of 428 patients with primary cancers of the nose, nasopharynx, larynx, mouth, lip, tongue, salivary glands, oropharynx, tonsils, and combined head and neck, 105 patients had only lung metastases, and 16 patients had isolated liver metastases.[49] This emphasizes that the pattern of initial spread is primarily to the lungs. The 5-year, survival rate of 44% reported by McCormack and co-workers indicates that the results for these tumors are quite favorable (see Fig. 62-11). It should be remembered, however, that there is also a high prevalence of independently arising second primary lung tumors.

Colon-Rectum

The difference between the results of resection of pulmonary metastases from the rectum and colon is well illustrated by a 52% 5-year survival for solitary metastases from a rectal primary, but no 5-year survival when the colon is the primary site.[8] Other authors have not separated their results for rectal and colonic primaries and have reported combined survivals of 15% to 38%.[11,33,40,41,50] Mansel and co-workers found that patients with a solitary metastasis had a better survival than those with multiple pulmonary metastases.

Ovary

Although ovarian adenocarcinomas do not drain to the portal venous system, lymph-borne metastases originating in the pelvis and abdominal lymph nodes primarily spread to the liver. Very occasionally, metastatic disease will be isolated to the lungs, and long-term survivors have been reported following resection. Every effort should be made to detect other metastases before resecting pulmonary lesions.

Uterine–Cervix

The results of isolated metastases from uterine–cervix primary tumors are favorable. Five-year survival ranges from 8% to 40%.[25,40,51] Characteristically, these tumors grow slowly and are slow to metastasize. Favorable results have been achieved with both squamous and glandular carcinomas of uterine origin.

Breast

Adenocarcinoma of the breast may spread independently to the lungs, vertebrae, or liver. Metastases to the liver may arise by way of the lymphatics of the rectus abdominis muscle, or to the vertebrae by way of the intercostal veins and paravertebral plexuses (Batson's plexus), without lung involvement. However, the lung may be the first site of metastasis from the breast and may be the first site from which subsequent metastases can disseminate to the liver and bones without vertebral involvement.[49]

Despite the many women with breast cancer, there are relatively few reported cases of resection of metastatic breast pulmonary nodules. This reflects the difficulty of determining whether metastatic breast cancer is truly limited to the lungs. The 5-year survival results reported after resection are lower than for other tumors. Mountain and coworkers reported a cumulative 5-year survival of 14%.[40] McCormack and co-workers reported a 15% actuarial survival.[41]

The effects of chemotherapy may be particularly important in the treatment of micrometastases of breast carcinoma and, therefore, may affect resection results of pulmonary metastases.

Endocrine Tumors

The adverse effects of endocrine tumors initially result from inappropriate hormone production and not, until later, from the mass effect of the tumor. Therefore, when their hormonal effects cannot be controlled by other measures, occasionally resection of pulmonary metastases may make the disease easier to control. This has been temporarily effective for the hypercalcemia of metastatic parathyroid carcinoma.

Esophagus

Because of the difficulty of adequately resecting the primary tumor and because of the high local recurrence rate, any pulmonary metastases are generally considered part of the systemic disease, and no attempt is made at resection.

Melanoma

Although malignant melanoma initially spreads to the lungs after leaving its primary site or regional lymph nodes, it enjoys a reputation as an extraordinarily unpredictable disease. Mathisen and co-workers found that, for 22 patients who were operated on for isolated pulmonary metastases, no significant difference existed in mean survival between those rendered disease-free (12 months) and those deemed unresectable (10.5 months).[44] Other authors also report poor results, usually with no long-term survivors.[33,42] Cahan, on the other hand, reported a 33% 5-year survival for 12 patients undergoing pulmonary resection.[43] Thoracotomy is especially useful for staging purposes in patients with melanoma. Approximately one-third of the patients reported by Mathisen and co-workers had no metastases and, therefore, could be placed in a group with a much better prognosis.[44]

CHILDHOOD TUMORS

The lung is a principal site of metastatic spread for most childhood tumors (*e.g.*, nephroblastoma, or Wilms' tumor, hepatoma, hepatoblastoma, Ewing's sarcoma, and rhabdomyosarcoma), but it is rarely the only site of metastases. Patients with isolated pulmonary nodules from Ewing's sarcoma may benefit from exploration and resection.[52] Lanza and co-workers reported that 3 of 19 patients (16%) had benign disease, and the median survival of patients undergoing complete resection of metastases was 28 months compared with 12 months for patients with unresectable metastases.[52]

For nephroblastoma, the lungs are not only the most common metastatic site, but also the most frequent initial site of metastases. Romansky and Landing reported that of 26 patients with a nephroblastoma six had only pulmonary metastases.[53] Of these patients, five died of massive bilateral metastases, and one died of radiation pneumonitis. Rodgers and co-workers reported 12 patients with pulmonary metastases from nephroblastoma.[54] Of five patients who did not respond completely to chemotherapy, three died of progressive tumor growth, and two died of supervening infection. Three of seven were free of tumor 3 years to 7 years after detection of pulmonary metastases.[54]

The principal site of metastases for both hepatomas and hepatoblastomas is the lung. However, only 2 of 12 patients with hepatoblastoma, and four of seven patients with hepatoma, had metastases to the lung. The causes of death in those patients were often directly or indirectly associated with pulmonary metastases that were not isolated.[53] Rhabdomyosarcoma may metastasize to many different sites. Although the lung is the initial metastatic site for 20% of the entire group, no single anatomical primary site is peculiarly liable to produce only pulmonary metastases. Ballantine and co-workers reported three patients with localized pulmonary metastases, none of whom were cured by resection.[55] Rodgers and co-workers reported two of four patients disease-free at 24 months and 28 months following pulmonary resection.[54]

REFERENCES

1. Willis RA: Pathology of Tumors, p 175. London, Appleton–Century Crofts, 1967
2. Weiss L, Gilbert HA: Pulmonary Metastases, pp. 142–167. Boston, GK Hall, 1978
3. Pass HI, Dwyer A, Makuch R, Roth JA: Detection of pulmonary metastases in patients with osteogenic and soft-tissue sarcomas: The superiority of CT scans compared with conventional linear tomograms using dynamic analysis. J Clin Oncol 3:1261–1265, 1985
4. Chang AE, Schaner EG, Conkle DM et al: Evaluation of computed tomography in the detection of pulmonary metastases. Cancer 43:913, 1979
5. Siegelman SS, Zerhount EA, Leo FP et al: CT of the solitary pulmonary metastasis. Cancer 43:913, 1979
6. Zerhouni EA, Spivey JF, Morgan RH et al: Factors influencing quantitative CT measurements of solitary pulmonary nodules. J Comput Assist Tomogr 6:1075–1087, 1982
7. Zerhouni EA, Stitik FP, Siegelman SS et al: CT of the pulmonary nodule: A cooperative study in radiology. 160:319–327, 1986
8. Vincent RG, Choksi LB, Takita H et al: Surgical resection of the solitary pulmonary metastasis. In Weiss L, Gilbert HA (eds): Pulmonary Metastasis, p 224. Boston, GK Hall, 1978
9. Sagel SS, Ferguson TB, Forrest JV et al: Percutaneous transthoracic aspiration needle biopsy. Ann Thorac Surg 26:399–405, 1978
10. Cahan WG, Castro EG: Significance of a solitary lung shadow in patients with breast cancer. Ann Surg 181:137–143, 1975
11. Cahan WG, Castro EB, Hajdu SI: The significance of a solitary lung shadow in patients with colon carcinoma. Cancer 33:414–421, 1974
12. van Dongen JA, van Slooten EA: The surgical treatment of pulmonary metastases. Cancer Treat Rep 5:29–48, 1978
13. Barney JD, Churchill ED: Adeno-carcinoma of the kidney with metastasis to the lungs treated by pulmonary resection. J Urol 42:269–276, 1939
14. Alexander J, Haight C: Pulmonary resection for solitary metastatic sarcomas and carcinomas. Surgery 12:271–280, 1971
15. Thomford NR, Wodner LB, Clagett OT: The surgical treatment of metastatic tumors in the lungs. J Thorac Cardiovasc Surg 49:357–363, 1965
16. Martini N, Huvos AG, Mike V et al: Multiple pulmonary resections in the treatment of osteogenic sarcoma. Ann Thorac Surg 12:271–280, 1971
17. Morton DL, Joseph WL, Ketcham AS et al: Surgical resection and adjunctive immunotherapy for selected patients with multiple pulmonary metastases. Ann Surg 178:360–365, 1973
18. Boysen PG, Block AJ, Olsen GN et al: Prospective evaluation for pneumonectomy using the 99m technetium quantitative perfusion lung scan. Chest 72:422–425, 1977
19. Huth JF, Holmes EC, Vernon SE et al: Pulmonary resection for metastatic sarcoma. Am J Surg 140:9–16, 1980
20. Burgers JMV, Breur K, Van Dobbenburgh OA et al: Role of metastatectomy without chemotherapy in the management of osteosarcoma in children. Cancer 45:1664–1668, 1980
21. Putnam JB, Roth JA, Wesley MN et al: Survival following aggressive resection of pulmonary metastases from osteogenic sarcoma: Analysis of prognostic factors. Ann Thorac Surg 36:516–523, 1983
22. Putnam JB, Roth JA, Wesley MN et al: Survival following aggressive resection of pulmonary metastases from osteogenic sarcoma: Analysis of prognostic factors. Ann Thorac Surg 36:516–523, 1983
23. Meyer WH, Schell MJ, Kumar AP et al: Thoracotomy for pulmonary metastatic osteosarcoma: An analysis of prognostic indicators of survival. Cancer 59:374–379, 1987
24. Creagen ET, Fleming TR, Edmonson JH et al: Pulmonary resection for metastatic non-osteogenic sarcoma. Cancer 44:1908–1912, 1979
25. Morrow CE, Vassilopoulos P, Grage TB: Surgical resection for metastatic neoplasms of the lung. Cancer 45:2981–2985, 1980
26. Takita H, Edgerton F, Karakousis C et al: Surgical management of metastases to the lung. Surg Gynecol Obstet 152:191–194, 1981
27. Turney SZ, Haight C: Pulmonary resection for metastatic neoplasms. J Thorac Cardiovasc Surg 61:784–794, 1971
28. Cahan WG, Castro B, Hajdu SI: Therapeutic pulmonary resection of colonic carcinoma metastatic to the lung. Dis Colon Rectum 17:302–309, 1974
29. McCormack PM, Attiyeh FF: Resection of pulmonary metastases from colorectal cancer. Dis Colon Rectum 22:553–556, 1979
30. Telander RL, Pairolero PC, Pritchard DJ: Resection of pulmonary metastatic osteogenic sarcoma in children. Surgery 84:335–341, 1978
31. Ishihara T, Kikuchi K, Ikeda T: Metastatic diseases biologic factors and modes of treatment. Chest 63:227–232, 1973
32. Joseph WL, Morton DL, Adkins PC: Prognostic significance of tumor doubling time in evaluating operability in pulmonary metastatic disease. J Thorac Cardiovasc Surg 61:23–32, 1971
33. Morrow CE, Vassilopoulos P, Grage TB: Surgical resection for metastatic neoplasms of the lung. Cancer 45:2981–2985, 1981
34. Collins VP, Loeffler RK, Tivey H: Observations on growth rates of human tumors. AJR 76:988–1000, 1956
35. Roth JA, Putnam JB, Wesley MN, Rosenberg SA: Differing determinants of prognosis following resection of pulmonary metastases from osteogenic and soft tissue sarcoma patients with cancer. 55:1361–1366, 1985
36. Giritsky AS, Etcubanas E, Mark JBD: Pulmonary resection in children with metastatic osteogenic sarcoma. J Thorac Cardiovasc Surg 75:354–362, 1978
37. Roth JA, Pass HI, Wesley MN et al: A comparison of median sternotomy and thoracotomy for resection of pulmonary metastases in patients with adult soft tissue sarcomas. Ann Thorac Surg 42:134–138, 1986
38. Martini N, McCormack PM, Bains MS et al: Surgery for solitary and multiple pulmonary metastasis. NY State J Med 78:1711–1713, 1978
39. Wilkins, EW Jr: The status of pulmonary resection of metastases: Experience at Massachusetts General Hospital. In Weiss L, Gilbert HA (eds): Pulmonary Metastasis. Boston, GK Hall, 1978
40. Mountain CF, Khalil KG, Hermes KE et al: The contributions of surgery to the management of carcinomatous pulmonary metastases. Cancer 50:1057–1060, 1982
41. McCormack PM, Bains MS, Beattie JR et al: Pulmonary resection in metastatic carcinoma. Chest 73:163–166, 1978
42. Dahlback O, Hafstrom L, Johnsson PE et al: Lung resection for metastatic melanoma. Clin Oncol 6:15–20, 1980
43. Cahan WG: Excision of melanoma metastases to lung: Problems in diagnosis and management. Ann Surg 178:703–709, 1973
44. Mathisen DJ, Flye MW, Peabody J: The role of thoracotomy in the management of pulmonary metastases from malignant melanoma. Ann Thorac Surg 27:295–299, 1979
45. Giuliano AE, Fieg S, Eilber FR: Changing metastatic patterns of osteosarcoma. Cancer 54:2160–2164, 1984
46. Marcove RC, Mike V, Hajek JV et al: Osteogenic sarcoma under the age of 21: A review of 145 operative cases. J Bone Joint Surg 52:411–421, 1970
47. Rizzoni WE, Pass HI, Wesley MN et al: Reoperative pulmonary metastasectomies in patients with adult soft-tissue sarcomas. Ann Thorac Surg 121:1248–1252, 1986
48. Vugrin D, Whitmore WF, Bains M, Golbey RB: Role of chemotherapy and surgery in the treatment of thoracic metastases from nonseminomatous germ cell testis tumor. Cancer 50:1057–1060, 1982
49. Viadora E, Brass IDJ, Pickren JW: Cascade spread of blood-borne metastases in solid and non-solid cancers of humans. In Weiss L, Gilbert HA (eds): Pulmonary Metastases. Boston, GK Hall, 1978

50. Mansel JK, Zinsmeister AR, Pairolero PC, Jett JR: Pulmonary resection of metastatic colorectal adenocarcinoma: A ten year experience. Chest 89:109–112, 1986
51. Gallousis S: Isolated lung metastases from pelvic malignancies. Gyncecol Oncol 7:206–214, 1979
52. Lanza LA, Miser JS, Pass HI, Roth JA: Role of resection in the treatment of pulmonary metastases from Ewings sarcoma. J Thorac Cardiovasc Surg 94:181–187, 1987
53. Romansky SG, Landing BH: Metastatic patterns in childhood tumors. In Weiss L, Gilbert HA (eds): Pulmonary Metastatses. Boston, GK Hall, 1978
54. Rodgers BM, Talbert JL, Alexander JA: Pulmonary metatases in childhood sarcoma. Ann Thorac Surg 29:410–414, 1980
55. Ballantine TVN, Wiseman NE, Filler RM: Assessment of pulmonary wedge resection for the treatment of lung metastases. J Pediatr Surg 5:671–676, 1975

PAUL H. SUGARBAKER
NANCY KEMENY

SECTION 3

Treatment of Metastatic Cancer to Liver

Cooperative efforts at obtaining data confirm the single-institution reports of significant cure of metastatic cancer to the liver by surgical removal of the disease. Current use of serial carcinoembryonic antigen (CEA) assays to detect recurrence of cancer after large-bowel resection has led to a greater number of patients whose metastatic disease is at a stage compatible with resection. Radiology has made an important contribution to the clear definition of the surgical problem. Determination of the number of metastases, their location within the liver parenchyma, and their relationship to major vascular structures now provides the surgeon preoperatively with information available in the past only after considerable liver dissection. Liver anatomy has now been appreciated by the surgeon so that its segmental nature is utilized. Resections carried out through the relatively avascular intersegmental planes markedly decrease the blood loss during parenchymal transection. Finally, the surgical technology has been refined. Clean, bloodless, tumor-free margins of resection equate with low morbidity and mortality and optimal long-term survival.[1] The oncologist looks forward to the development of regional and systemic therapies that will augment hepatic resections for metastatic disease. Also, technologies aimed at the local or regional destruction of intrahepatic tumor promise to eliminate liver metastases as a cause of death from metastatic gastrointestinal malignancy.

LIVER ANATOMY

EXTERNAL ANATOMY OF THE LIVER

The liver is the largest internal organ of the human body excluding the skin. To perform its manifold metabolic tasks, the liver is richly supplied with arterial blood, portal venous blood, and hepatic venous drainage. It also has abundant lymphatic drainage.

Figure 62-15A and B shows the external anatomy of the liver. There are two external surfaces of the liver. Most evident to the surgeon upon opening the abdomen is the diaphragmatic surface of the liver. It is a large smooth surface, interrupted only by the falciform ligament. Unfortunately, little obvious help about the complex internal anatomy of the liver is revealed by its external anatomy. The visceral surface of the liver is adjacent to the right adrenal gland, upper pole of the right kidney, and the remainder of the abdominal viscera, including the hepatic flexure of the colon, the duodenum and pylorus, the gastric antrum, and the greater omentum.

For the surgeons, the right and left lobes of the liver present quite different technical problems. The left lobe is rather flat, very mobile after taking down the triangular ligament, and is covered by a tough fibrous capsule (Glisson's capsule).

In contrast, the right lobe of the liver is more spherical in its configuration, and it is attached to the vena cava by the hepatic veins and caudate veins. It is relatively immobile.

External Attachments of the Liver

The liver is suspended within the body from the falciform ligament and triangular ligaments. Both of these structures can be completely dissected off the liver without any noticeable compromise in its function. The falciform ligament is important in fetal life because it contains the venous drainage from placenta to fetus. What is referred to as the round ligament in adults is the umbilical vein in the fetus. Clinically, the umbilical vein has been used to deliver cytotoxic drugs into the portal system after it has been recannulated. It is seldom open in adult life, but it is accompanied by several sizable vessels. The falciform ligament marks the course of the left paramedian portal pedicle that separates liver segment 4 and 3. This is a unique anatomic feature of the falciform ligament, for all other liver segments are separated by hepatic veins.

Vascular Connections of the Liver

The portal vein receives blood from the small intestine and right colon through the superior mesenteric vein. Blood from the spleen drains through the splenic vein and connects beneath the head of the pancreas with the superior mesenteric vein. Entering the splenic vein at right angles is the inferior mesenteric vein which drains the left colon and upper rectum (Fig. 62-16).

The arterial blood supply to the liver is quite variable.[2] There is a consistent arterial blood supply to the right and the left lobes of the liver. Generally, there is a single left and a single right artery. It is the origin of these vessels that is so variable. Occasionally, however, three hepatic arteries will exist; generally, there are two arteries to the right lobe. There are three main sources for the hepatic arteries. These are the hepatic artery, the left gastric artery, and the superior mesenteric artery.

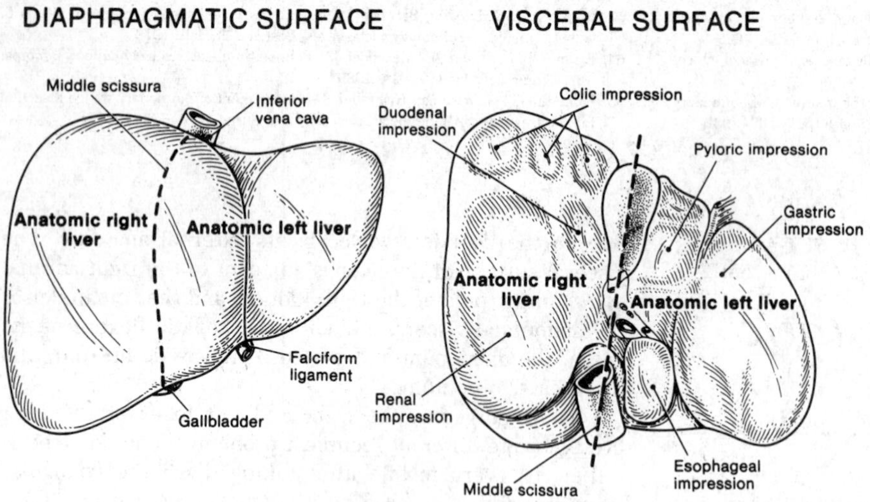

FIG. 62-15. **A**. Diaphragmatic surface of the liver. The dashed line separates anatomical right from anatomical left liver. **B**. Visceral surface of the liver. (Sugarbaker PH, Kemeny N: Management of metastatic liver metastases. Adv Surg [in press])

FIG. 62-16. Splanchnic veins. (Sugarbaker PH, Kemeny N: Management of liver metastases Adv Surg [in press])

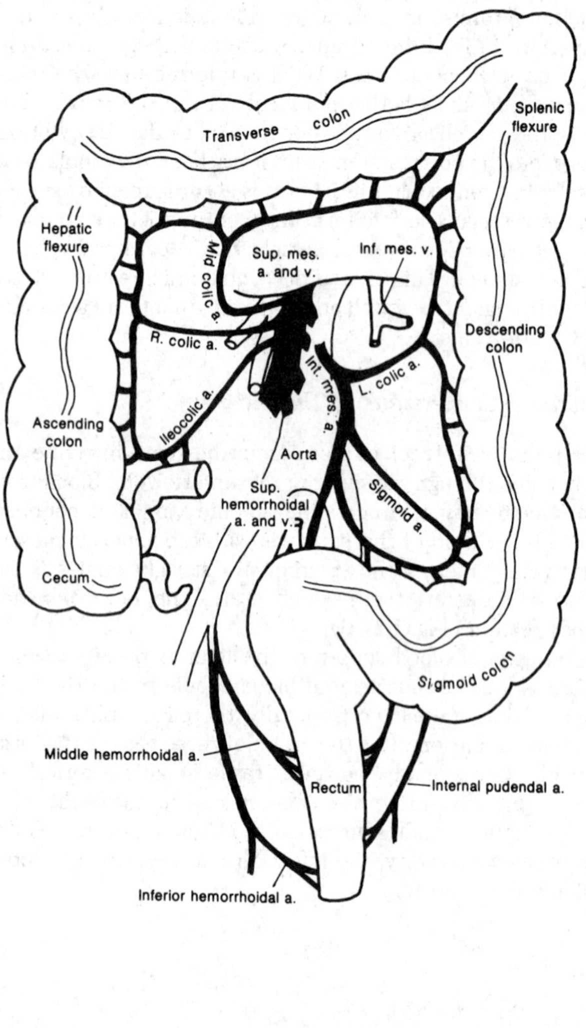

The three hepatic veins are barely visible externally between liver parenchyma and the vena cava. It is usually poor surgical practice to attempt to dissect these veins free from the suprahepatic space. The veins are completely accessible from within the hepatic parenchyma, and this is their proper surgical approach.

There are few or no lymphatic vessels going to the liver, but there is a rich lymphatic drainage from the liver. The lymphatic drainage is along the falciform ligament to the paraaortic and paraesophageal lymph nodes.[3] It may follow the phrenic lymphatics from the capsular surface of the liver. However, most of the lymphatic drainage from the liver parenchyma is retrograde along the porta hepatis into the hepatic and superior mesenteric lymph nodes. From here it courses upward into the thoracic duct.

Minor parabiliary veins and arteries exist. The parabiliary veins may become extremely important in providing venous drainage of the viscera if portal vein thrombosis or obstruction occurs. The arterial parabiliary arch may cause bothersome bleeding during dissection of the portal hepatis. Part of this plexus arises from the hepatic and cystic arteries. Other anastomoses are with the superior pancreaticoduodenal arteries. Hence, parabiliary arterial plexus liver dearterialization is only possible for a very brief time.

The nerve supply to the liver is poorly understood, and the function has not been well described. There apparently are sensory nerve fibers within Glisson's capsule, for pain is experienced upon penetration of the liver for liver biopsy. Also, the stretching of Glisson's capsule produces discomfort, as with acute vascular congestion of the liver or an expanding intrahepatic tumor mass. For the most part, liver pain is recognized as irritation of the adjacent sensory nerve supply to the parietal peritoneum or undersurface of the hemidiaphragm. Irritation of the diaphragm at its periphery is detected at that particular site, whereas irritation of nerve fibers over the major portion of the undersurface of the diaphragm is referred to the shoulder.

The common bile duct, extending from the porta hepatis toward the head of the pancreas, is fairly consistent in its anatomy. The common bile duct is the most superficial of the structures within the portal triad, and it is the first one to be damaged if errors occur in the dissection of this area.

INTERNAL ANATOMY OF THE LIVER

The anatomy of the liver within the parenchyma is considerably more complex than that of most other organs. There is a vasculature and duct system that is obscured by the large amount of hepatic parenchyma. The understanding of intrahepatic anatomy is further complicated because there is a dual segmentation. This dual division of intrahepatic structures is made up of two different vascular trees. There is a division of the liver parenchyma by portal venous segmentation and another division of the parenchyma by the hepatic venous segmentation.[4,5]

Division of the Liver through Portal Venous Segmentation

The hepatic ducts, hepatic arteries, and portal veins all run closely together within the liver parenchyma as part of the liver triad. The abundant lymphatic vessels are an additional structural complex that should be mentioned as a part of the triad.

The portal segmentation is vertically defined by scissurae that exist between the major branches of the portal vein. The middle portal scissura (Cantlie's line) is an imaginary line that runs from the middle of the vena cava to the middle of the gallbladder fossa. The middle hepatic vein exists within the plane beneath this line. The right scissura is defined by the right hepatic vein.

The left portal scissura follows the falciform ligament from hepatic veins midway across the dome of the left lobe of the liver. The left hepatic vein lies within the liver beneath this line. The left hepatic vein courses at an angle of 90° toward the left. The scissura continues as the falciform ligament, which contains the left paramedian portal triad. This is the only place in the liver where the portal triad separates the liver segments.

Segmentation of the Liver by the Hepatic Veins

There are three hepatic veins. The left vein drains the smaller anatomic left liver lobe and the large right hepatic vein drains the anatomic right liver lobe. The middle hepatic vein lies directly beneath the middle portal scissura and draws from both anatomic right and left liver lobes.

The left hepatic vein may join the middle hepatic vein to form a vessel that immediately enters the inferior vena cava. It may receive the left inferior phrenic vein. A frequent bothersome bleeding problem during dissection around the left hepatic veins is bleeding from a dissection injury to the left phrenic vein as it enters the left hepatic vein.

The right hepatic vein is the largest of the three vessels. It has three branches: the superior, middle, and inferior. The right hepatic vein follows the right portal scissura over most of its course.

The caudate veins drain directly from the caudate lobe into the anterior face of the retrohepatic vena cava. They number between one and five major veins. They present a particular hazard in performing a major liver resection unless they are ligated and then divided in continuity before any attempt at a major resection. If these veins are pulled out of the vena cava, severe hemorrhage can result.

DIAGNOSIS OF LIVER TUMORS

LIVER AS A COMMON SITE FOR TUMOR SPREAD

Because of its large size and protected position beneath the right rib cage, the liver is not readily accessible for examination by routine methods for physical diagnosis. Because of direct access of hematogenously disseminated tumor cells from the gastrointestinal tract, the liver is a common site for the spread of cancer. According to Pickren, Tsukada, and Lane, approximately 50% of patients with large-bowel cancer will eventually develop liver metastases.[6] The same is true for gastric cancer. Approximately 75% of patients with pancreatic cancer will show liver metastases at some time in their course. Also, endocrine tumors such as gastrinoma, insulinoma, or carcinoid frequently metastasize to the liver.

DIAGNOSIS FROM MEDICAL HISTORY

Even large tumors within the liver may cause no symptoms. The liver, itself, including the intrahepatic bile ducts, contains no sensory nerve supply. Glisson's capsule does contain somatic sensory fibers, and penetration of the capsule by a needle or its acute distention caused by liver swelling will result in pain or discomfort. A mass lesion in the liver may cause pain by irritation of the undersurface of the hemidiaphragm. Tumors that rub against the central portion of the diaphragm will result in pain in the shoulders. This is referred pain caused by irritation of phrenic nerve fibers. Irritation of the periphery of the diaphragm causes stimulation of the intercostal nerve, and that pain is detected at the site of irritation (Fig. 62-17).

PHYSICAL EXAMINATION

Physical examination of the liver is difficult, often impossible. For liver nodules to be detected by physical examination, they generally must be very large. Sometimes, a large tumor mass may displace the liver caudally and result in a large but normally textured organ.

LABORATORY TESTS

Approximately 90% of the patients who have had hepatic metastases from colorectal cancer will have an elevated carcinoembryonic antigen (CEA) assay.[9] Other tests such as the lactate dehydrogenase (LDH) and alkaline phosphatase may be used to screen patients preoperatively for liver abnormalities.[10] However, the truism, "negative" means nothing and must be used in interpreting these tests. Oftentimes, before the liver function tests become abnormal, metastases become evident by physical examination, and the clinical value of the diagnosis is minimal.

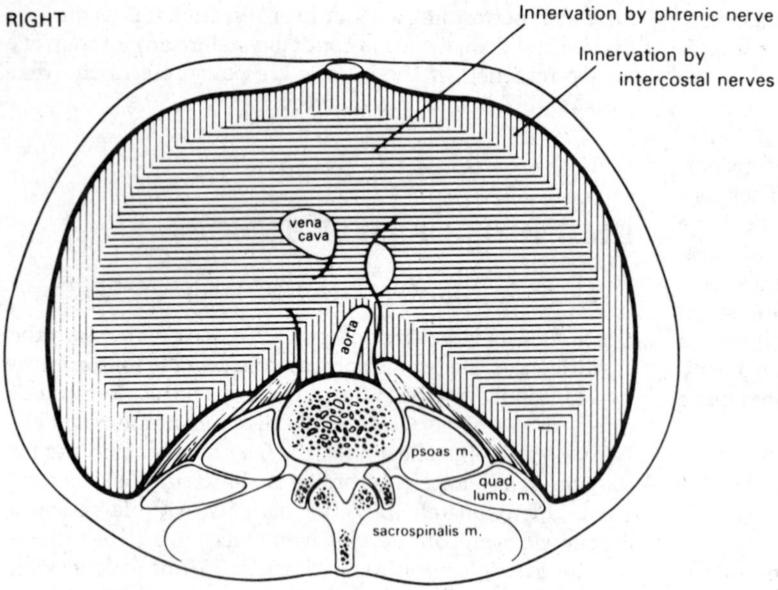

FIG. 62-17. Sites of pain reported from metastases on the diaphragmatic surface of the liver. Irritation of the periphery is detected by somatic sensory fibers and is felt at the tumor site. Irritation of the large central portion of the right or left hemidiaphragm is felt in the shoulders. (Sugarbaker PH, Reinig JW, Hughes KS: Diagnosis of hepatic metastases. In Rosenberg SA [ed]: Surgical Treatment of Metastatic Disease. Philadelphia, JB Lippincott, 1987)

RADIOLOGIC EXAMINATION OF THE LIVER

Determination of the presence or absence of hepatic metastases in patients with cancer is of great importance in making decisions about treatment. Many different radiologic tests have been developed and their usefulness tested in clinical studies. Smith and colleagues determined that the liver–spleen scan, the liver ultrasound, and the liver computed tomography (CT) scan (scans performed without contrast materials) were equally accurate in detecting hepatic mass lesions.[11] The size threshold for tumor identification was approximately 3 cm for all three tests, and they were considered equivalent for the radiologic study of hepatic metastases.

The CT scan has been used with several contrast agents to provide a large amount of information. In CT portography a bolus of soluble contrast medium is rapidly injected into the superior mesenteric artery while the CT scan is being performed.[12] Because the liver parenchyma is more richly vascularized by portal blood than are tumor nodules, the parenchyma is highlighted and the tumor nodules appear as filling defects. Tumor nodules as small as 0.5 cm in diameter are routinely detected. Also, the portal vein and its branches are distinctly seen, and the relationship of tumor masses to the portal structures can be readily determined. An example of CT portography in a patient with hepatic metastases is shown in Figure 62-18.

Bernardino and colleagues have explored the use of the delayed CT scan in patients with hepatic metastases.[13] If one waits 4 to 6 hr after the intravascular administration of soluble contrast material, approximately 10% of the dye is excreted in the bile. This makes the liver parenchyma denser

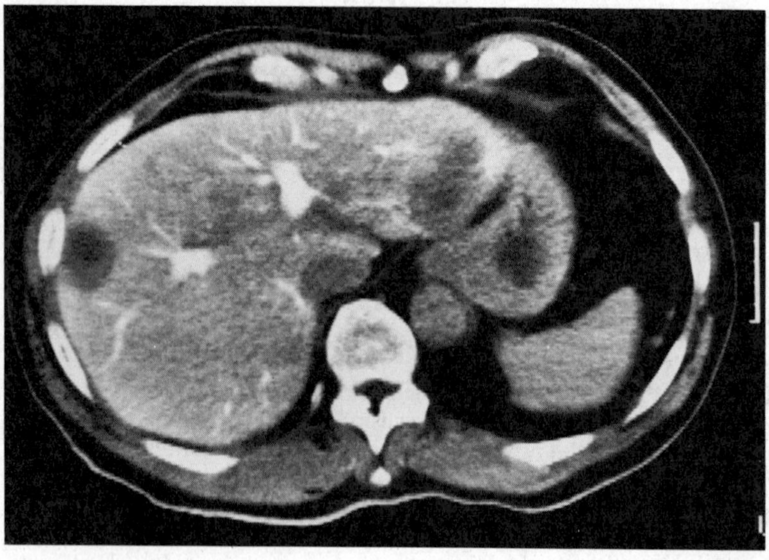

FIG. 62-18. Computed tomogram for the precise definition of liver metastases. A bolus of soluble contrast is infused through the superior mesenteric artery while the liver CT is performed. The portal structures and liver parenchyma are highlighted. Metastases show clearly as filling defects. The relationships of the tumor to portal vein and its branches are revealed. With this information the large right-side tumor was successfully resected.

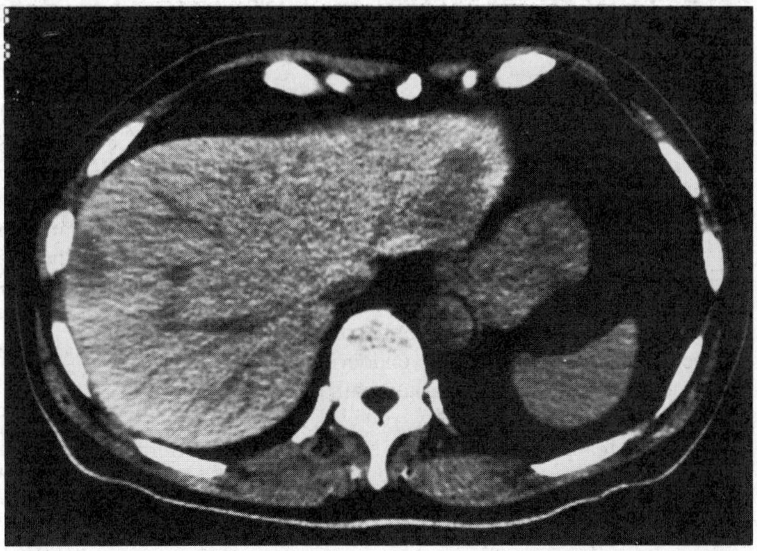

FIG. 62-19. Delayed computed tomogram for precise definition of liver metastases. If 50 g of iodine is infused intravascularly, sufficient contrast material will accumulate in the bile to increase the density of liver parenchyma 4 to 6 hours later. This will then function as a liver contrast agent.

than tumor tissue and denser than the portal and hepatic veins. An example of the delayed CT scan is shown in Figure 62-19. Cirrhotic livers will not image by delayed CT.

Magnetic resonance imaging (MRI) is emerging as a prominent new radiologic test to study the liver. Both the T1 and T2 effects have been studied. The experience of Reinig and colleagues suggests that MRI is as accurate as CT with contrast agents in the detection of hepatic lesions.[14] Unfortunately, MRI does not give as much information about the remainder of the abdominal cavity as does the CT scan. It does enable accurate detection of small lesions to 1 cm or less in diameter. These are lesions that may be missed by surgical palpations of the liver. As MRI increases in its availability and more is learned about its proper use, it may emerge as an important tool for the preoperative assessment of liver tumors.

Hypervascular liver metastases from endocrine tumors, hepatocellular carcinoma, and some metastases from gastrointestinal cancer can be visualized well with arteriography. A majority of metastatic lesions, however, are not well shown. Arteriography is often valuable in differentiating benign lesions, such as hemangioma, from metastases. Computed tomography scans after contrast infusion or the T2-weighted spin echo MRI can also help in this differentiation. The major role of arteriography in hepatic tumors is not in diagnosis but in therapy planning. Preoperative delineation of the hepatic arterial anatomy is helpful in defining the structures to be ligated within the portahepatis before performing a major liver resection.

Surgical palpation of the liver is still an accurate way to detect hepatic lesions. Minute surface lesions not currently detectable by any radiologic test are readily found, and their benign or malignant nature can be determined by biopsy. Lesions of 1 to 2 cm within the liver parenchyma can be detected accurately in the left liver. However, the thick right liver can hide lesions that cannot be palpable but they may be up to 2 cms in diameter. The sensitivity (true-positive percentage) of direct surgical examination is approximately 95%.[6,15–18] Therefore, meticulous hepatic imaging before surgical removal of hepatic metastases is essential.

Recently, intraoperative ultrasonography has become available for endocrine tumors and hepatomas.[19,20] Currently, studies are underway to determine the accuracy of intraoperative ultrasonography for hepatic metastases from colorectal or other gastrointestinal primary tumors.

At present, the major role of intraoperative ultrasonography comes from the ability to define the segmental anatomy of the liver. With this tool, the precise anatomic location of a metastasis within one or more of the eight anatomic segments can be determined.[21]

FIG. 62-20. Comparison of survival of resected and unresected hepatic metastases from colon cancer. The top survival curve shows the results over 5 years for 116 patients with solitary and multiple hepatic metastases that underwent potentially curative hepatic resections. The lower curves show solitary and multiple hepatic metastases without extrahepatic disease that were not resected. (Modified from Wagner JS, Adson MA, Van Heerden JA et al: The natural history of hepatic metastases from colorectal cancer. Ann Surg 147:502–508, 1984)

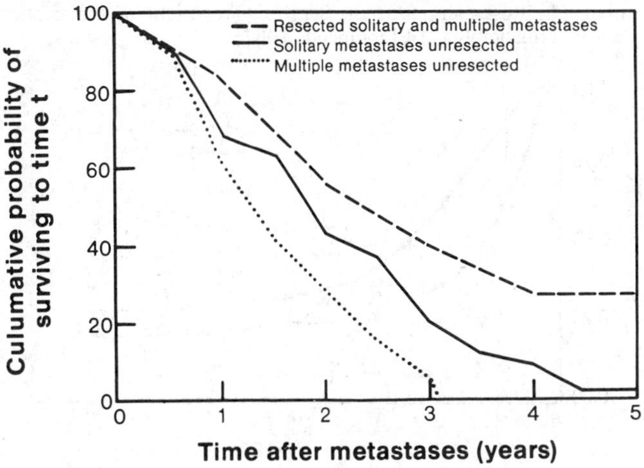

SELECTION OF PATIENTS FOR HEPATIC RESECTION

Studies by Wagner and colleagues show that the only curative treatment for metastatic solid tumors to the liver is hepatic resection (Fig. 62-20).[22-29] Resection of hepatic metastases has produced a 20% to 40% 5-year survival after removal of large-bowel cancer metastases isolated to the liver (Fig. 62-21).[30] Occasionally, long-term survivors have been reported after hepatic resection for metastatic Wilms' tumor, melanoma, leiomyosarcoma, pancreatic cancer, gastric cancer, renal cell cancer, and adrenal carcinoma. In addition, resection of metastatic endocrine tumors from the liver occasionally lead to a marked palliation and occasionally to a cure. This is particularly true with carcinoid tumors. The clinical features by which the surgeon selects patients for resection have been studied by many groups.[35-47] Our discussion will focus on the data provided by the Hepatic Metastases Registry (Table 62-17).[30]

NUMBERS OF HEPATIC METASTASES

In the past, surgeons recommended that resection be performed only in patients with solitary metastases. Others suggested that more than one metastasis might be resected in a good risk patient if it was confined to a single lobe of the liver. The data from the Hepatic Metastases Registry would expand these indications. Patients with one metastasis removed have essentially the same prognosis statistically as patients with two or three metastases. Those with over three metastases have only a slightly worse prognosis. From this data, it is impossible to exclude patients with a few metastases from a curative resection (Fig. 62-22). Current practice may be to recommend resection of four or fewer metastases in patients with metastatic colorectal cancer.

FIG. 62-21. Disease-free survival and survival of more than 800 patients who had a liver resection for colorectal metastases. About one-fourth of patients are cured of their metastatic disease by surgery. (Hughes KS, Sugarbaker PH: Treatment of metastatic liver tumors. In Rosenberg SA [ed]: Surgical Treatment of Metastatic Cancer. Philadelphia, JB Lippincott, 1987)

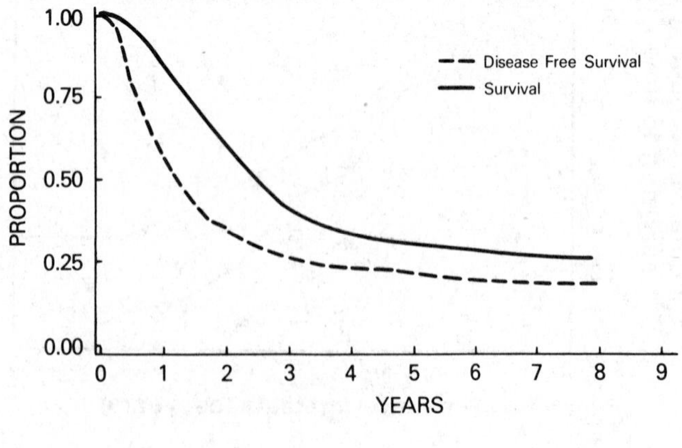

LOCATION OF TUMOR NODULES AS A PROGNOSTIC VARIABLE

If only patients with more than one metastases were examined, those with metastases on one side of the liver had the same 5-year survival and disease-free survival rates, as patients with metastases in both the right and left liver lobes. The distribution of metastases within the liver may have profound implications for the surgical techniques involved in liver resection, but it does not, in itself, have an effect on the prognosis (Fig. 62-23).

STAGE OF THE PRIMARY TUMOR

The strongest prognostic variable in patients with gastrointestinal malignancy is the status of the lymph nodes. Patients with positive lymph nodes have approximately a 30% 5-year survival, whereas those with negative lymph nodes have a 60% 5-year survival. Figure 62-24 shows that patients with potentially curative resections of Dukes' Stage B adenocarcinoma of the colon have a 40% 5-year survival, whereas those who had a Dukes' Stage C primary tumor have a 20% survival. Even in patients with hepatic metastases, lymph node invasion signifies a tumor biology more likely to result in distant disease spread.

It should be noted, however, that patients with Dukes' C adenocarcinoma of the large bowel with hepatic metastases have approximately 20% 5-year survival. A Dukes' Stage C primary lesion does indicate that hepatic resection should not be performed.

PATHOLOGIC MARGIN OF THE RESECTED SPECIMEN

Figure 62-25 shows that patients with less than 1-cm margin of resection or a positive margin of resection have a reduced 5-year survival. However, even in those patients with narrow or positive margins long-term survival was seen.

PREOPERATIVE CEA LEVEL

Patients with a preresection CEA level of less than 5 mg/ml do better than patients with an elevated CEA (40% survival versus 25%). Patients should not be denied a resection because the CEA is high.

DISEASE-FREE INTERVAL

The time interval between colon resection and hepatic resection does have an impact on prognosis. If patients had a disease-free interval of less than 1 month there was a 17% 5-year survival. A disease-free interval of 1 month to 1 year gave 22% 5-year survival, and if that interval was longer than 1 year there was a 26% disease-free survival. The absolute survival for the three groups was 27%, 31%, and 42%.

PRESENCE OF EXTRAHEPATIC METASTASES

Patients with extrahepatic metastases that were removed along with the disease in the liver had no significant difference in survival from patients with only hepatic metastasis,

TABLE 62-17. Prognostic Features as Defined by the Hepatic Metastases Registry for Patients Undergoing Resection of Hepatic Metastases in the Absence of Extrahepatic Disease

Prognostic Factor	*Survival (%)**	*Disease-Free Survival (%)†*
Number of Metastases		
1	37	25
2	37	25
3	7	0
≥4	23	7
Multiple (not specified)	18	15
Pathologic Margin on Liver Specimen (cm)		
0	19	13
>0 but <1	25	15
>1	47	33
Distribution of Multiple Metastases		
Unilobar	30	16
Bilobar	20	13
Stage of the Primary Tumor		
Dukes B (negative mesenteric nodes)	47	28
Dukes C (positive mesenteric nodes)	23	18
Disease-Free Interval		
<1 mo	27	17
1 mo to 1 yr	31	22
>1 yr	42	26
Age (yr)		
<40	37	27
40–70	33	21
>70	31	18
CEA Level Before Liver Resection (mg/ml)		
0–5	47	42
>5 and <30	30	19
>30	28	14
Size of Solitary Lesions (cm)		
<8	38	27
>8	27	21
Size of Largest Lesion in Multiple Metastases (cm)		
<2	27	18
2–4	17	10
4–8	27	18
>8	37	18
Type of Resection of Solitary Lesion		
Wedge	35	21
Anatomic	41	29
Type of Resection and Size of Solitary Lesions (cm)		
Anatomic, met <4	45	28
Wedge, met <4	37	25
Anatomic resection, met >4	35	25
Wedge, met >4	20	12.5

Data from Ref. 1.
* 5-yr actuarial survival.
† 5-yr actuarial disease-free survival.

but there was a trend toward reduced survival. Data reviewed by Wagner at the Mayo Clinic showed reduced survival when extrahepatic disease was resected.[22] It seems reasonable from these data to suggest that some good-risk patients who can be made clinically disease-free by hepatic surgery plus a resection of tumor at another site should undergo this potential curative surgery.

One site of cancer spread that did abrogate the beneficial effects of hepatic resection was disease in the hepatic lymph nodes. August and co-workers identified the hepatic lymph nodes as a site for metastatic spread of liver secondaries.[48] If the tumor biology is such that metastases from the liver to the local lymph nodes occurs, the chances for gaining control through liver resection must be extremely small.

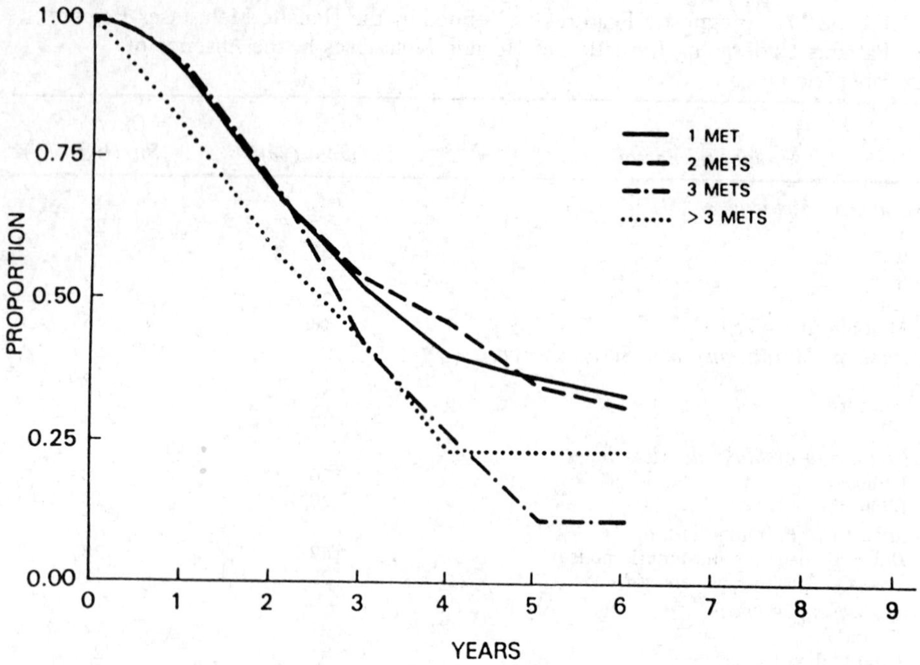

FIG. 62-22. Prognosis as determined by number of hepatic metastases resected. (Hughes KS, Sugarbaker PH: Treatment of metastatic liver tumors. In Rosenberg SA [ed]: Surgical Treatment of Metastatic Cancer. Philadelphia, JB Lippincott, 1987)

OTHER CLINICAL FEATURES

Age, size of solitary lesions, type of resection (metastasectomy versus major resection), and distribution of metastases are of little or no prognostic value. One prognostic feature related to size may be of some interest to surgeons. Large hepatic metastases, over 4 cm in diameter, seem to do less well with a local excision than with an anatomic right or left liver resection. Large lesions resected by metastasectomy may, of necessity, have a less adequate free margin.

CONTRAINDICATIONS TO HEPATIC RESECTION

The criteria by which patients are selected have become extremely generous. Few people who can be made clinically disease-free should be denied potential benefits for this surgical procedure. Only if one sees the mortality of the resection as 20% or more should the physical status of the patient be considered a contraindication. Another absolute contraindication to surgery is the presence of disease either within the liver or at another site that cannot be removed with curative intent. Multiple pulmonary metastases, peritoneal seeding, or retroperitoneal lymph node involvement should be considered absolute contraindications. Metastatic disease within the hepatic lymph nodes should be considered an absolute contraindication to hepatic resection, even though these nodes could be removed to make the patient clinically disease-free. Isolated foci of disease in the lungs or within the abdomen, especially at the anastomotic site, should not be considered contraindications to a curative approach (Table 62-18).

FIG. 62-23. Prognosis as determined by distribution of metastases within the liver: multiple metastases on one side of the liver as compared to lesions on both right and left sides of the liver. (Hughes KS, Sugarbaker PH: Treatment of metastatic liver tumors. In Rosenberg SA [ed]: Surgical Treatment of Metastatic Cancer. Philadelphia, JB Lippincott, 1987)

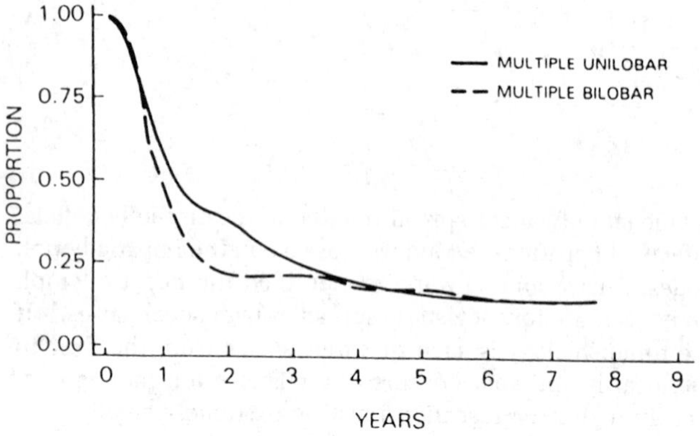

FIG. 62-24. Prognosis as determined by Dukes' classification. (Hughes KS, Sugarbaker PH: Treatment of metastatic liver tumors. In Rosenberg SA [ed]: Surgical Treatment of Metastatic Cancer. Philadelphia, JB Lippincott, 1987)

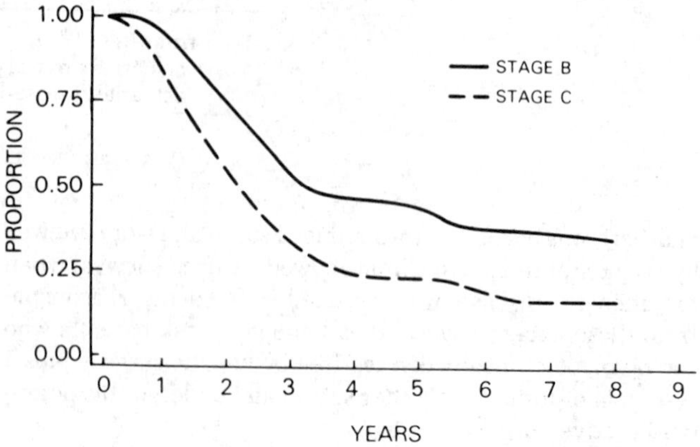

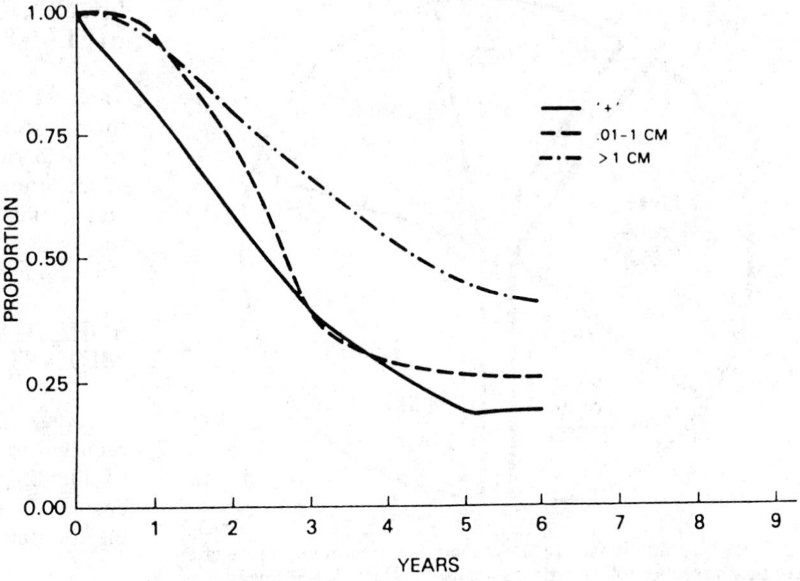

FIG. 62-25. Prognosis as determined by pathologic margin of resected specimen. (Hughes KS, Sugarbaker PH: Treatment of metastatic liver tumors. In Rosenberg SA [ed]: Surgical Treatment of Metastatic Cancer. Philadelphia, JB Lippincott, 1987)

RE-RESECTION OF HEPATIC METASTASES

Approximately one-third of the patients who fail hepatic resection will be found to have the cancer recurrence only in the liver.[49] In these patients, a careful workup for metastatic disease should be undertaken. If no other sites of disease recurrence are found and if the liver tumor is resectable, repeat resection should be considered. The experience with repeat-resection of hepatic metastases has been summarized.[50] In nine patients who had undergone a second hepatic resection with curative intent eight were free of disease with a median follow-up of 2 years. These patients seem to represent a select group who did very well with a second liver resection.

PATTERNS OF RECURRENCE

Steele and co-workers suggested that patients who fail the surgical treatment of hepatic metastases usually do so because of disease at other anatomic sites.[51] The liver usually remains free of metastatic disease through simple surgical removal of cancer.[52] Figure 62-26 shows the data from the Hepatic Metastases Registry regarding patterns of failure.[49] When one considers only the first site of recurrence, roughly, one-third of the patients recurred in the liver only, one-third recurred at other distant sites, including the lungs, and one-third remained disease free. Figure 62-27 shows the sites of recurrence seen initially and then with prolonged follow-up. The number of combined recurrences is markedly increased. Recurrences isolated to the liver only are infrequently observed. As suggested by Steele and co-workers, there is a need for effective systemic adjuvant therapy.[51]

TABLE 62-18. Contraindications for Hepatic Resection of Colorectal Metastases to the Liver

Operative mortality of 20% or greater
Moderate to severe cirrhosis
More than four hepatic metastatic lesions
Unresectable disease at another site
Involvement of hepatic lymph nodes

HEPATIC RESECTION FOR ENDOCRINE TUMORS

Resection of the liver for symptomatic metastases from endocrine tumors may be indicated even if patients are not made disease-free. Hughes collected literature reports on 54 patients. Alleviation of symptoms was reported in 33 of 36 patients to whom follow-up was available. Palliation lasted

FIG. 62-26. Initial sites of surgical treatment failure after surgical resection of hepatic metastases. (Hughes KS, Sugarbaker PH: Treatment of metastatic liver tumors. In Rosenberg SA [ed]: Surgical Treatment of Metastatic Cancer. Philadelphia, JB Lippincott, 1987)

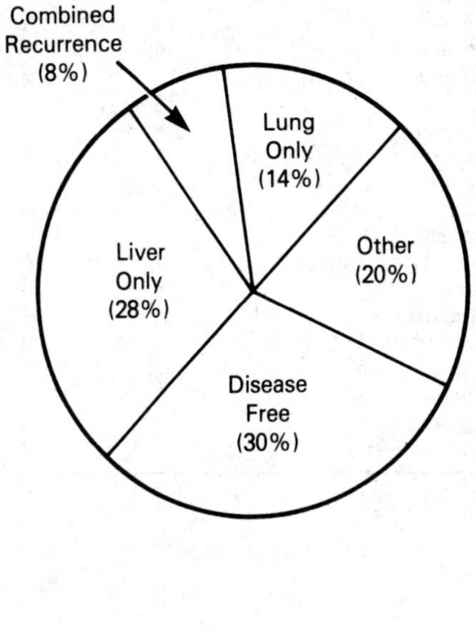

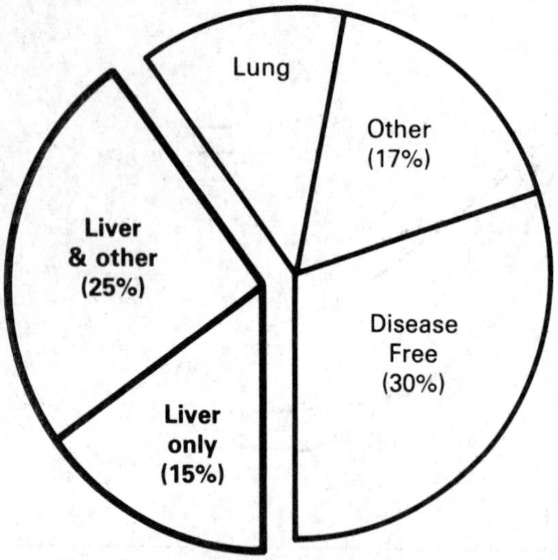

FIG. 62-27. Initial plus late sites of surgical treatment failure after surgical resection of hepatic metastases. (Hughes KS, Sugarbaker PH: Treatment of metastatic liver tumors. In Rosenberg SA [ed]: Surgical Treatment of Metastatic Cancer. Philadelphia, JB Lippincott, 1987)

up to 78 months in these patients.[53] Foster has suggested that hepatic resection to palliate the disabling symptoms of the carcinoid syndrome should be considered if 90% of the functioning tumor can be removed.[32]

Norton and co-workers have reported a curative approach to treatment of metastatic gastric tumors.[54] Resection of the primary tumor in the pancreas along with the hepatic spread of the disease may be considered a curative approach in some patients. In others, palliative efforts may be well worth the risks of surgery.[55]

NONCOLORECTAL, NONENDOCRINE METASTASES

Table 62-19 presents a summary of the literature concerning liver resection for metastatic cancer from noncolorectal, nonendocrine primary sites.[53] Long-term survivors with Wilms' tumor, renal cell cancer, adrenal cancer, leiomyosarcoma, melanoma, gastric and pancreatic cancer have been reported.

SURGICAL TREATMENT OF HEPATIC METASTASES

The year 1988 will make the 100th year since Garre was reported to have performed the removal of a liver tumor (Table 62-20). Certainly the modern era of liver surgery has begun. More and more surgeons will be methodically utilizing the new technology, oncology, and anatomy.[1,32,56–68]

PRE- AND POSTOPERATIVE CARE

Before surgery, the patient should be carefully evaluated for systemic spread of tumor. Also recurrent cancer or a new primary cancer within the colon should be ruled out. After surgery fresh-frozen plasma is frequently needed to maintain an adequate prothrombin time. Alblumin may be needed if edema from hypoalbuminemia is observed.

The incision is carefully planned to suite the expected procedure. For large tumors, a thoracoabdominal incision may be needed to keep blood loss at a minimum, deal with surgical misadventures should they occur, and keep tumor manipulation to a minimum. Not infrequently, tumors on the diaphragmatic surface of the right lobe of the liver are adherent to the right hemidiaphragm. If this is so, excision of

TABLE 62-19. Liver Resection for Metastatic Cancer from Noncolorectal, Nonendocrine Sites

Cancer Type	*Postoperative Survivors*	*5-Year Survivors*	*Died of Recurrence After 5 Years*
Wilms' tumor	20	6 (14, 17 yr)	?
Renal cell cancer	11	3 (5 yr, 7 yr, and 12 yr)	0
Adrenal carcinoma	4	2 (6 yr and 7 yr)	0
Leiomyosarcoma	16	2 (12 yr)	1
Melanoma	13	1	1
Pancreatic cancer	8	1	1
Stomach cancer	23	0	
Other adult sarcomas	9	0	
Breast cancer	7	0	
Ovarian cancer	5	0	
Uterine and cervical cancer	7	0	
Lung cancer	2	0	
Esophageal cancer	3	1 (13 yr)	
Rhabdomyosarcoma	1	0	
Neuroblastoma	1	0	
Thyroid cancer	1	0	
Choriocarcinoma	1	0	
Periampullary cancer	1	0	

Data from Ref. 53.

TABLE 62-20. One Hundred-Year Evolution of Techniques for Hepatic Surgery for Metastatic Colorectal Cancer

Date	*Author*	*Country*	*Comment*	*Reference*
1888	Garre	Germany	Metastasectomy	56
1889	Keen	USA	Left lateral segmentectomy	57
1908	Pringle	Great Britain	Inflow occlusion	58
1910	Wendel	Germany	Right lobectomy; partial hilar dissection	59
1952	Lortat-Jacob and Robert	France	Preliminary hilar ligation for anatomic lobectomy	60
1953	Healey	USA	Segmental anatomy	4
1958	Lin	Taiwan	Finger-fracture technique	62
1960	Couinaud	France	Segmental nomenclature and resections.	63
1971	Storm and Longmire	USA	Liver clamp	64
1975	Starzl	USA	Right trisegmentectomy	65
1976	Wilson and Adson	USA	Successful resection CRC metastasis	66
1977	Foster and Berman	USA	Liver tumor survey	32
1979	Hodgson	USA	Ultrasonic dissection	66
1981	Fortner	USA	Electrocautery	67
1982	Starzl	USA	Left trisegmentectomy	68
1986	Hughes	USA	Hepatic Metastases Registry	30

that portion of the diaphragm is indicated to prevent spillage of tumor cells.

Usually, a small incision is first made to explore the abdominal cavity. A complete examination should include node sampling of hepatic lymph nodes if these nodes are suspicious for malignant disease.[69] Another important site of disseminated disease is the peritoneal surfaces, especially in the pelvis. A third common site of disease spread is the large-bowel cancer resection site, and this should be carefully palpated. Finally the liver itself should be carefully inspected. Usually patients with four or fewer metastatic lesions remain candidates for hepatic resection.

The first step in the hepatic resection is complete mobilization of the portion of the liver that is to be removed. This is necessary so that tissue to be dissected can be placed on traction parenchymal dissection.

Preliminary occlusion of the right portal vein and right hepatic artery in an anatomic right liver resection will decrease blood loss and facilitate the accurate placement of the parenchymal incision. Preliminary occlusion of the right portal vein and right hepatic artery in an anatomic right liver resection lobe will facilitate the accurate placement of the parenchymal incision.

The preliminary occlusion of the hilar vessels clearly shows the portion of the liver supplied by these vessels. In patients with small tumors, preliminary ligation of the hilar vessels may not always be necessary. However, in patients with large tumor masses that distort the liver anatomy, demarcation of the division between anatomic right and anatomic left liver may be of great help. In patients who have had considerable liver hypertrophy, the same is true.

The entire portal pedicle is encircled by a Penrose drain before initiating parenchymal dissection. Vascular flow is interrupted (Pringle maneuver) whenever blood has become bothersome. This continues for 20 min and then blood flow is reestablished.[70]

With use of the ultrasonic dissector, a suction dissector, or a fracture technique, the parenchyma is divided, taking care not to traumatize major vascular or ductal structures before their ligation. Minor bleeding points on the parenchyma that exist between the major vessels are electrocoagulated or laser coagulated using the yttrium–aluminum–garnet (YAG) laser. Smaller ducts and vessels, up to 1 mm in size, are coagulated and divided using the electrocautery on coagulation current. Larger vessels and ducts are secured with silk ligatures.

A closed suction drain is placed in the bed of the excised liver; usually the end of the drain is placed through the foramen of Winslow. If the chest was opened, a large-bore chest tube is secured.

As the indications for hepatic resection have expanded and more liver surgery has been performed, surgeons have worked to improve their techniques for dissecting through hepatic parenchyma. The ideal instrument for hepatic resection will allow isolation of vascular and ductal structures, achieve small-vessel hemostasis, and leave minimal devitalized tissue behind.[71–76] Continued research in this field is needed to accumulate information about an important surgical technology. The surgical procedures used to remove liver tumors and a nomenclature to describe these techniques is shown in Figure 62-28.

SYSTEMIC CHEMOTHERAPY

The effect of systemic chemotherapy on hepatic metastases depends on the primary site of metastatic disease and the doses of agents used. Because certain tumors are responsive to chemotherapy, even when liver metastases develop, systemic chemotherapy may be the appropriate treatment. The response rates of liver metastases from breast carcinoma are well documented. In Carters' review of 5-fluorouracil (5-FU) or cyclophosphamide (CTX) used alone, the response rate for liver metastases was 20% versus a response rate in soft-tissue and osseous disease of 32% and 27%, respectively.[77] As work with combination chemotherapy regimens with or

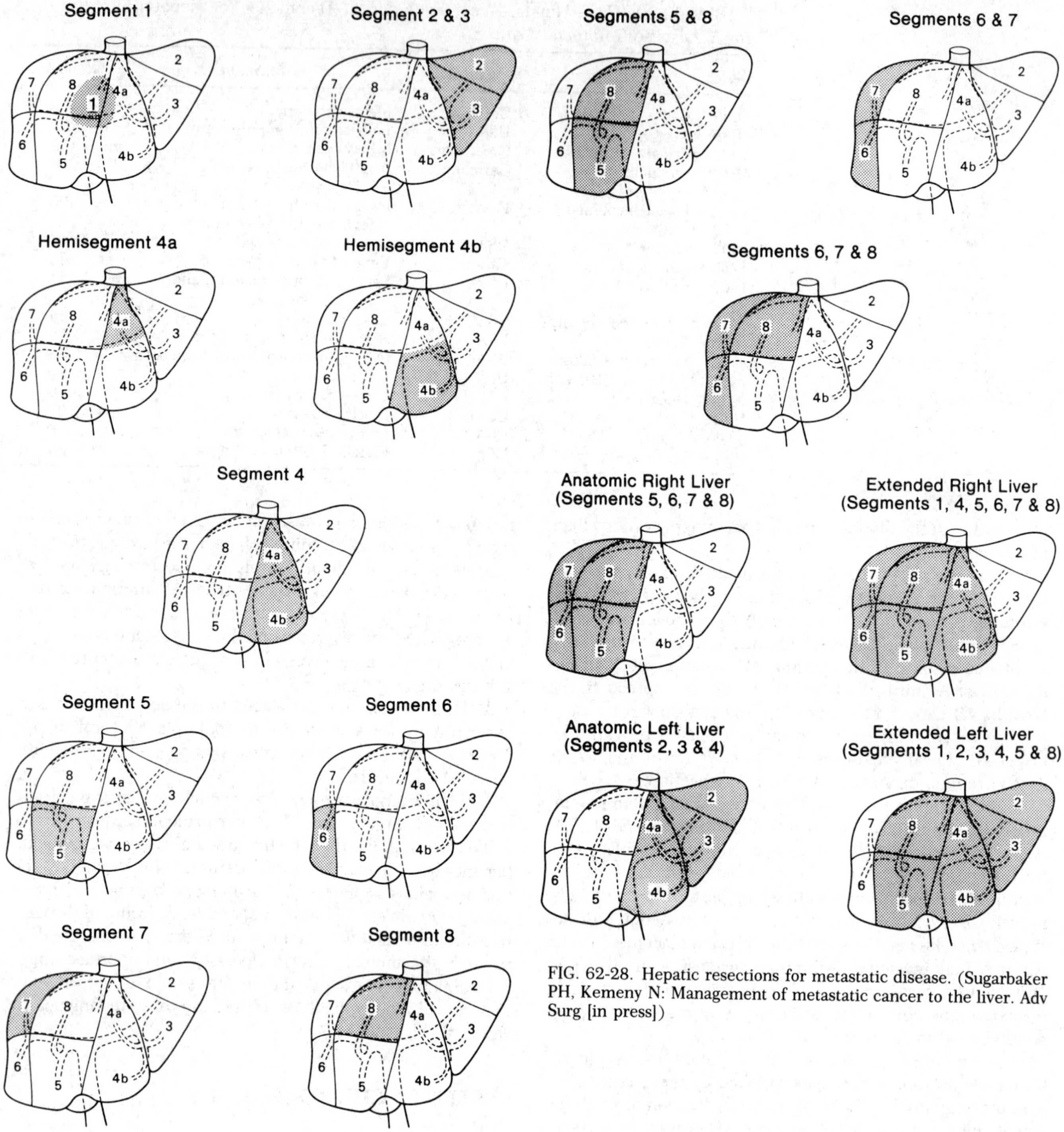

FIG. 62-28. Hepatic resections for metastatic disease. (Sugarbaker PH, Kemeny N: Management of metastatic cancer to the liver. Adv Surg [in press])

without hormones evolved, it became clear that the response rates for liver metastases could be higher.[78–86] The cumulative response rates for patients with or without liver metastases was 46% versus 53%, respectively ($p = 0.04$). In a Southwest Oncology Group (SWOG) study of 262 patients, 47% patients with liver metastases responded, versus 71% patients without liver involvement ($p = 0.001$).[87] The highest response rates for liver metastases from breast carcinoma are usually seen with doxorubicin, (Adriamycin)-containing regimens.

Colorectal carcinoma metastasizes to the liver in approximately 50% of the patients with advanced disease,[7,88,89] and in approximately half, the liver is the dominant or solitary metastatic site. The standard chemotherapeutic agent for advanced colorectal carcinoma has been 5-FU, with an average response rate of 20% and a median response duration of

TABLE 62-21. Response of Liver Metastases from Colorectal Carcinoma to Systemic Chemotherapy

Investigator (Ref.)	*No. of Patients*	*Response (%)*	*No. with Liver Metastases*	*Response (%)*
FU				
Moertel[91]	144	15	118	24
Baker[92]	42	10	11	0
Siefert[93]	36	17	5	20
Grage[94]	31	23	31	23
FU + MeCCNU ± VCR				
MacDonald[96]	25	40	14	43
Baker[92]	12	32	41	31
Buroker[97]	133	16	93	18
Kemeny[98]	69	11	41	11
FU + MeCCNU VCR + strep				
Kemeny[98]	35	34	29	30
Kemeny[99]	75	32	60	37
CF + FU				
Machover[101]	86	39	73	30
Meth + FU				
Kemeny[102]	43	32	33	31
Mit C + DDP VCR + FU				
Pandya[103]	23	48	15	30
DDP + FU				
Loehrer[104]	38	29	22	16
Kemeny[105]	105	28	77	20

FU, 5-fluorouracil; CF, leucovorin; DDP, cisplatin; MitC, mitomycin C; strep, streptozotocin; Meth, methotrexate.

6 months.[90] In a series in which response was clearly defined and in which response in liver metastases was indicated, the average response rate for all sites was 17%, and for patients with liver metastases the response was 22% (Table 62-21).

Combination therapy employing MOF [semustine (methyl-CCNU; MeCCNU), 5-FU, and vincristine (VCR)], originally yielded a response rate of 43%[95] in colorectal carcinoma, but subsequent trials employing a similar regimen failed to confirm this finding (see Table 62-21). Studies with 5-FU and MeCCNU with or without vincristine yielded a mean total response rate of 23% and a response rate in patients with liver metastases of 20%. When streptozotocin was added to methoxyflurane (MOF) (MOF-strep) the total response rate increased to 36%, and for those patients with liver metastases, the four-drug regimen achieved a partial rate of 30%.[100] Some of the newer combinations and the responses obtained in liver metastases are listed in Table 62-21. Generally, it is rare to obtain response rates higher than 30%, and this usually is only possible with considerable systemic toxicity.

Other common gastrointestinal malignancies in which patients develop hepatic metastases are gastric and pancreatic carcinoma. In a series of 307 patients at the Mayo Clinic, 22% eventually developed liver metastases.[106] Systemic treatment for gastric carcinoma produces an average response rate of 31%. The description of responses in patients with liver metastases is rarely mentioned, but in the studies that do, the mean response is 28%.[107–115] In the few studies documenting response in liver metastases from pancreatic carcinoma, the mean response rate is 22% and the mean survival is 3.1 months.[116]

In conclusion, for most malignancies the responses obtained in patients with liver metastases mirrors the overall response rate. For gastrointestinal malignancies, especially colorectal and pancreatic, this usually means a low response rate.

REGIONAL CHEMOTHERAPY

The rationale for the use of hepatic arterial infusion is to achieve higher drug levels in tumorous areas of the liver and lower systemic drug levels. This is possible because malignant lesions in the liver establish vasovascular connections with the arterial circulation and, therefore, most of their blood supply comes from the hepatic artery, whereas the normal hepatocytes derive most of their blood supply from the portal circulation. This observation was made on pathologic data from animal tumors,[117] and in a human study[118] using labeled floxuridine (fluorodeoxyuridine; FUDR). Ten patients were injected with [^{3}H]FUDR (1 μCi/kg) either into the hepatic artery or the portal vein. Liver biopsies obtained after injection demonstrated that the mean tumor FUDR levels after hepatic artery infusion were 12.4 nmol/g, whereas those after portal vein infusion were 0.8 nmol/g

TABLE 62-22. Drugs for Hepatic Arterial Infusion

Drug	*T½ (min)*	*Estimated Increased Exposure by Hepatic Arterial Infusion*
Fluorouracil (5-FU)	10	5- to 10-fold
Floxuridine (5-fluoro-2-deoxyuridine; 5-FUDR)	<10	100- to 400-fold
Carmustine (bischlorethylnitrosourea; BCNU)	<5	6- to 7-fold
Mitomycin	<10	6- to 8-fold
Cisplatin	20–30	4- to 7-fold
Doxorubicin hydrochloride (Adriamycin)	60	2-fold
Dichloromethotrexate (DCMTX)		6- to 8-fold

($p < 0.01$). This clearly demonstrated that regional chemotherapy for colorectal carcinoma should be administered through the hepatic artery.

Chemotherapeutic drugs that are most attractive for regional infusion are extracted by the liver during the first pass, thus producing lower systemic drug levels and toxicity.[119] Ensminger and colleagues[120] measured drug levels from hepatic venous catheters and showed that the hepatic extraction of FUDR was fourfold higher after hepatic arterial injection, compared with systemic injection. With hepatic arterial infusion, 94% to 99% of FUDR was extracted in the first pass. The ability to administer a higher dose locally exposes tumors to a higher drug concentration than can be achieved with systemic therapy. As most drugs have a steep dose–response curve, their antineoplastic efficacy should be increased by hepatic arterial infusion. On the basis of extraction data, the value of certain drugs for hepatic arterial infusion are listed in Table 62-22.

Collins reviewed the pharmacologic principles of regional delivery[122] and emphasized the need for drugs with a high total-body clearance and infusional sites with a low regional exchange. Because intra-arterial therapy has a high regional exchange rate (100 to 1500 ml/min), drugs with a high

TABLE 62-23. Regional Drug Delivery Advantage for Selected Anticancer Drugs when $Q_{HA} = 250$ ml/min

CL_{TB} (ml/min)	*Drug*	*R (ml/min)*
25,000	Floxuridine (5-FUDR)	101
4,000	5-FU	17
3,000	Cytarabine (Ara-C)	13
1,000	Carmustine (BCNU)	5
900	Doxorubicin (Adriamycin)	4.6
400	Diaziquinone (AZQ)	2.6
400	Cisplatin	2.6
200	Methotrexate	1.8
40	Etiposide (VP-16)	1.2

Adapted from Collins JM: Recent Results Cancer Res 100:143, 1987

CL_{TB}, Total body clearance of drug; R, regional drug delivery advantage given CL_{TB} and Q_{HA} and hepatic extraction of the drug; Q_{HA}, blood flow in hepatic artery.

TABLE 62-24. Hepatic Artery Infusional Therapy with External Pumps

Investigator	*No. of Patients*	*Tumor Type*	*Intrahepatic Dosage (mg/kg)*	*Prior Chemotherapy (%)*	*Response (%)*
Tandon[124]	122	Adeno	FU 25 × 9d, then FU 15 IV q wk	100	64
Ansfield[125]	419	Adeno GI	FU 25 × 4d then FU 15 × 17d	75	55
Buroker[126]	21	Colon	FUDR 0.3/d	100	35
Oberfield[127]	60	Colon	FU 20 × 10d, then FUDR 20/d		54
Watkins[128]	184	Adeno	FU 20 × 10d, then FUDR 20/d		71
Cady[129,130]	55	Colon	FUDR 20/d		61
Massey[131]	40	Adeno	FU 30 × 21 d		38
Petrak[132]	52	Adeno	FU 1 g × 21 d		43
Reed[133]	89	Colon	FUDR 0.3/d		73
Smiley[134]	166	Colon	FU 20 × 4 d	60	25

TABLE 62-25. Hepatic Arterial FUDR Infusion with Internal Pump: Responses

Investigator	*No. of Patients*	*Prior Chemotherapy (%)*	*PR*	*CEA Decrease (%)*	*Median Survival (mo.)*	*% > 50 Liver Metastasis*
Niederhuber[138]	70	45	83	91	25	
Balch[141]	50	40		83	26	
Kemeny[140]	41	43	42	51	12	53
Shepard[142]	53	42	32		17	
Cohen[143]	50	36	51			18
Weiss[144]	17	85	29	57	13	
Schwartz[145]	23		15	75	18	
Johnson[146]	40		47		12	34
Kemeny[147]	31	50	52		22	
Ramming[148]	55		8	88	11	

clearance rate are needed. Table 62-23 demonstrates that drugs, such as FUDR, 5-FU, and cytarabine (Ara-C) have high total-body clearance.[123]

In summary, intra-arterial infusion into the hepatic artery is effective because [1] a high concentration of the chemotherapeutic agent can be delivered to a localized area, [2] a significant amount of drug is extracted after the first pass, and [3] the blood flow of the artery receiving the infusion is small.

The first trials with hepatic artery infusion used external pumps and often required hospitalization and patient immobilization. The response rates and toxicity for this type of treatment are listed in Table 62-24. The average response rate from the studies was 51%, including previously treated patients. Arterial thrombosis (average incidence 9%; range 1%–22%) and catheter dislodgement were the main problems related to this type of treatment. The mean incidence of catheter dislodgement or punctures was 15% (range 1%–75%). Because of the hindrance to normal activity with external catheters, few oncologists advocated the use of hepatic arterial therapy, despite the apparently higher response rates.[133]

The development of a totally implantable infusion device provided a new stimulus for infusion.[135] Use of an implantable pump delivery system gave several potential advantages: [1] reduction in catheter-related sepsis, [2] ease of drug administration, and [3] greater patient acceptance because there are no bulky external devices.[136] Placement of the catheter at laparotomy eliminates the problem of catheter displacement and allows better determination of the presence of intra-abdominal extrahepatic disease. The surgical technique has been described by several groups.[137,138] In most patients, catheterization of the gastroduodenal artery is performed after ligation of the right gastric artery and dissection of the common hepatic, proper hepatic, and gastroduodenal arteries. It is important to take particular care to ligate all branches of the gastroduodenal artery, such as the supraduodenal artery which arises from the common hepatic artery. The beaded silastic catheter is inserted retrograde such that its tip lies at the junction of the common hepatic and gastroduodenal arteries.

In some patients, retrograde catheterization of the splenic artery is required and is performed after proximal ligation of the right gastric and gastroduodenal arteries (distal to the

Median Survival	*Thrombosis (%)*	*Catheters Displaced or Punctures (%)*	*Ulcer, GI Bleeding (%)*	*Diarrhea (%)*	*Stomatitis (%)*
8	1	1		2	32
7.3	2	16	3	15	6
8					
	18	75	0	23	
15*	14	12	2		
	22	8	9		
8	5	8	3	20	12
9*	4	17	6		
10	17	11	8		
7.5		24	6	23	23

* Median survival of patients with only colorectal carcinoma.

TABLE 62-26. Hepatic Arterial FUDR Infusion with Internal Pump: Toxicity

Investigator	*No. of Patients*	*Gastritis (%)*	*Ulcer (%)*	*SGOT (%)*	*Bilirubin (%)*	*Diarrhea (%)*	*Biliary Sclerosis (%)*
Niederhuber[138]	70	56	8	32	24		
Balch[141]	50		6	23	23	0	
Kemeny[140]	41	29	29	71	22	0	5
Shepard[142]	53		20	49	24		
Cohen[143]	50		40	10	25		
Weiss[144]	17	50	11	80	23	23	
Schwartz[145]	23	53		77	20	10	
Johnson[146]	40		8	50	13	0	5
Kemeny[147]	31	17	6	47		8	19
Ramming[148]	55		30	24	3		
Hohn[138]	61	35	2	0	78	11	29

take-off of the left hepatic artery) and ligation of the left gastric artery. The silastic catheter is inserted so that its tip lies within the celiac artery. In some patients the gastroduodenal artery is catheterized to allow infusion of the left hepatic artery while the replaced right hepatic artery is cannulated directly using a tapered Holter right arterial catheter to allow continued blood flow through the nonoccluded right hepatic artery.

After catheterization, 2.0 ml of a fluorescein solution is injected into the pump's side-port while the abdominal contents are exposed under Wood's ultraviolet light to establish a homogenous uptake in the liver and absence of infusion of the stomach and duodenum. The implantable pumps are then placed into left or right lower quadrant subcutaneous pockets below the belt line for patient comfort.

The first study with the implantable pump and continuous FUDR therapy suggested an 83% response rate.[139] Despite the fact that other investigators using this method could not reproduce these results (Table 62-25), the mean response rate of 44% in ten trials (in which 42% of the patients were previously treated) is higher than the mean response rate obtained with systemic chemotherapy.

TOXICITY OF INTRAHEPATIC THERAPY THROUGH AN IMPLANTABLE PUMP

Although the operative and technical complications with the implantable pump have been minimal, there have been chemotherapy complications.[140] In a pilot study at Memorial Sloan–Kettering Cancer Center (MSKCC), 29% of the patients developed endoscopically documented gastrointestinal ulcerations, and in a second study ulcers were seen in 19% of patients. The most likely mechanism for gastric toxicity from hepatic arterial infusion is inadvertent perfusion of the stomach and duodenum with drug through the small vessels from the hepatic artery. Hohn and colleagues found no ulcer disease in their patients and feel this is related to their surgical technique which involves very careful denuding of the vessels arising from the hepatic artery (distal to the cannulation) that supply the stomach and duodenum.[137] Other attempts to modify this toxicity include careful reduction of the dose with any gastrointestinal symptoms or serum glutamic oxaloacetic transaminase (SGOT) elevation. Drugs such as cimetidine, ranitidine, and antacids have been used, but have failed to prevent the development of ulcers in these patients. A summary of the gastrointestinal toxicities noted by investigators using the implantable pump are listed in Table 62-26. In some studies patients were not investigated with endoscopy when they experienced abdominal pain, and this may explain the lower rate of ulcer disease reported in some studies.

Another frequent side-effect of hepatic arterial infusion through an internal pump is hepatic toxicity. In a study at MSKCC, bilirubin elevations above 3 mg/ml were seen in 20% of the patients and transaminase elevations in 71%.[140] Hepatic toxicity was quite similar in the different pump studies. Approximately one-fourth of the patients developed bilirubin elevation. There is a disagreement about the nature of hepatic toxicity. Some feel it is like hepatic because of documented hepatocyte necrosis and cholestasis on liver biopsy.[151] Others believe the hepatic toxicity is due to pericholangitis and fibrosis of biliary radicals. In early stages of toxicity hepatic enzyme elevations will return to normal when the drug is withdrawn and the patient is given a rest period. In some patients, however, jaundice does not improve. These patients may develop biliary strictures, most commonly at the site of hepatic duct bifurcation, but also in the common bile duct or intrahepatic radicals. Radiographically, these lesions are similar to idiopathic sclerosing cholangitis. Because the ducts are sclerotic, sonograms are usually normal and the diagnosis must be made by endoscopic retrograde cholangiopancreatography (ERCP). Computed tomography of the liver should be done to exclude metastatic lesions as a curative cause of strictures. In some patients the strictures are more centralized and drainage procedures by ERCP or by transhepatic cholangiogram may be helpful.

Close monitoring is necessary to avoid biliary sclerosis. If bilirubin elevation is observed, no further treatment should be given until it returns to normal and then only with a small test dose (0.05 mg/kg per day). If there is no increase in the liver function tests after the pretest dose, the dose can be slowly escalated. In some patients who cannot tolerate a low dose for 2 weeks, it may be possible to continue treatment by giving the FUDR infusion for 1 week, rather than the usual 2 weeks. The rate of biliary sclerosis in the various trials is listed in Table 62-26. The studies with more extensive surgery[147,151] had a lower rate of ulcers, but a higher rate of biliary sclerosis, suggesting that efficient gastric devascularization (and greater hepatic arterial infusion) may increase the rate of biliary sclerosis.

At MSKCC it was found that a useful laboratory test to monitor hepatic toxicity was serum glutamic oxaloacetic transaminase (SGOT). A review of the liver function tests obtained over 2 weeks revealed a certain pattern of SGOT elevation in 23 of the original 45 patients: the SGOT increased at the end of FUDR infusion (2 weeks after treatment began) and then returned to the normal or almost normal levels before the next dose (4 weeks after treatment began). This pattern occurred in all of the patients who later developed severe hepatic toxicity (bilirubin valve > 3 mg/ml) and in 11 of 12 who developed ulcers. Alkaline phosphatase values should also be followed carefully. Bilirubin elevation is usually a late sign.

Another side-effect of hepatic arterial infusional chemotherapy is the development of cholecystitis which has been reported to occur in as many as 33% of patients.[152] In more recent series the gallbladder has been removed at the same time as catheter placement to prevent this complication and to avoid the confusion of these symptoms with other hepatic side-effects from pump treatment.

The usual side-effects of chemotherapy are almost never seen with intrahepatic therapy. Myelosuppression does not occur with FUDR. Although intrahepatic mitomycin or carmustine (BCNU) may depress platelet counts, this occurs to a lesser degree than with systemic administration. Nausea and vomiting are not usually seen from FUDR infusion, but if present, one should suspect that ulcer disease or gastritis has developed. Diarrhea, which is frequently a problem with systemic FUDR infusion, is rare with intrahepatic infusion. If it occurs, one should suspect high systemic drug levels caused by catheter disruption or shunting either to the lung or bowel.[150]

Randomized Studies

To understand the impact of hepatic infusional therapy on the natural history of patients with hepatic metastases, randomized studies were initiated in which patients were stratified for factors known to affect response and survival. The strong influence of the percentage of liver involvement on survival has been shown by many investigators.[152,154] At MSKCC the median survival for patients with less than 20% involvement (assessed medically or surgically) was longer than 29 months, whereas it was only 6 months for those with more than 60% involvement.[155] Certain laboratory parameters also influenced tumor response and patient survival. In one study patients whose initial LDH and CEA levels were normal had a median length survival of 32 months, versus only 8 months for those who originally had abnormal values.[156]

There now are a few completed, randomized studies in patients with metastatic colorectal carcinoma. The study at MSKCC compared intrahepatic infusion with systemic infusion, applying the same chemotherapeutic agent (FUDR), drug schedule, and method of administration.[157] The dosage of FUDR in the intrahepatic arm was 0.3 mg/kg a day for 14 days, and in the systemic arm the dosage was 0.125 mg/kg a day for 14 days. All patients underwent exploratory laparotomy to assess the percentage of liver involvement and to determine that there was no extrahepatic disease. At surgery, 33 of 162 patients were found to have disease outside the liver not detected on CT and were thus excluded from analysis.

Patients randomized to the systemic group had the hepatic artery connected to an Infus-A-Port, and the pump connected to an additional catheter placed in the cephalic vein. This allowed a crossover to intrahepatic therapy by a minor surgical procedure (ligation of the systemic catheter and Infus-A-Port, followed by a connection of the pump to the intrahepatic catheter) in the event of tumor progression during systemic therapy.

The study demonstrated a significantly higher response rate (>50% reduction in measurable disease) with hepatic therapy, 50% versus 20% for systemic infusion ($p = 0.001$). Thirty-one of the systemic patients crossed over to intrahepatic therapy after tumor progression. Twenty-five percent had a partial response, 22% stabilization of disease, and 50% of a drop in CEA with the intrahepatic therapy. The toxicity has been quite different between the two groups. The toxicity from intrahepatic treatment was similar to the other intrahepatic studies described earlier whereas the toxicity from systemic therapy was mostly diarrhea, occurring in 70% of patients and requiring admission for intravenous hydration in 9% of patients (Table 62-27).

Another potential problem with direct hepatic therapy is the development of extrahepatic disease. In the intrahepatic group, 27 patients developed extrahepatic disease, whereas in the systemic group, 19 patients developed extrahepatic disease ($p = 0.09$). The median survival for the intrahepatic and systemic groups was 17 and 12 months, respectively ($p = 0.424$). Survival information is difficult to interpret because 60% of the patients in the systemic group crossed over and received intrahepatic therapy. The patients who were unable to cross over (usually for mechanical reasons, such as clotting of the Infus-A-Port, had a median survival of 8 months, versus 18 months for those able to undergo the crossover.

A similar randomized study by the Northern California

TABLE 62-27. Intrahepatic Versus Systemic FUDR Infusion; Randomized Study, MSKCC

	Intrahepatic (n = 48)	*Systemic (n = 51)*	
Partial response	24 (50%)	10 (20%)	p = 0.001
>50% decrease in CEA	29	13	
Extrahepatic metastases	27	19	p = 0.09
Toxicity			
Ulcer	8	3	
Elevated enzymes	20 (42%)	12	
Bilirubin > 3	9	2	
Diarrhea	1	36 (70%)	
Survival (mo)			
Total	17	12	p = 0.424
Crossover		18	
No crossover		8	

Cooperative Cancer Group also used FUDR infusion in both the intrahepatic and systemic arms of the study and had similar response rates to the MSKCC study. They reported a 37% partial response rate in the intrahepatic infusion group and 12% in the systemic FUDR infusion group.[157] The dose of FUDR was lower in both arms: 0.2 mg/kg and 0.075 mg/kg for the intrahepatic and systemic groups, respectively. The median survival was 15 months for both the intrahepatic and systemic groups. Though a crossover design was not built into the study, many patients received intrahepatic therapy after failing systemic therapy, and again there was a difference in median survival: 22 months for those who went on to receive intrahepatic therapy versus 12 months for those who did not receive intrahepatic therapy after systemic failure.

A National Cancer Institute (NCI) study[158] also compared FUDR intrahepatic infusion versus systemic FUDR infusion. They reported a significant increase in response rate, 62% versus 17%, respectively. If patients with positive nodes are excluded, the 2-year survival was 47% versus 13%, respectively, ($p = 0.03$). Another randomized study done by a consortium of four institutions[159] was unable to enter enough patients and closed after 43 patients had entered. The response rates were 38%, 58%, and 56% for systemic 5-FU, intrahepatic FUDR infusion, and combined systemic and intrahepatic groups, respectively (Table 62-28).

It is still too early to form definite conclusions about the use of intrahepatic infusional therapy, but certain points appear valid. There are now randomized trials demonstrating a significantly higher response rate with intrahepatic infusion versus systemic infusion in the treatment of hepatic metastases from colorectal carcinoma. Because of the early successes with intrahepatic infusion, these studies allowed patients on the systemic arm to receive intrahepatic therapy after tumor failure of systemic therapy; therefore, the impact of intrahepatic treatment on survival is difficult to evaluate. The studies demonstrate survival differences between groups who never received intrahepatic treatment and those who did. A longer survival has been observed for those who received intrahepatic therapy, whether originally or after systemic failure. One might infer from this data that intrahepatic treatment is needed only after failure of systemic treatment. Two arguments against this viewpoint are the lack of systemic side-effects, and the ease of administration of continuous infusion through an implantable pump; and if one waits until a patient fails on systemic treatment, the patient may then be too sick to undergo surgery for hepatic artery cannulation. One could argue that a precutaneous catheterization of the hepatic artery could be performed before pump placement because this would allow one to see if there is a tumor response before laparotomy. However, this could lead to hepatic thrombosis and then destroy further chances for hepatic infusion.

Should this treatment be offered to all patients in the community? There is a definite "learning curve," so that in the hands of physicians who are not familiar with this type of treatment there may be more toxicity and a lower response rate. Before hepatic infusional therapy through the hepatic pump becomes a standard treatment, more work needs to be done on clearly defining whether or not there is a survival advantage; working on ways to decrease biliary sclerosis; and perhaps developing ways to increase response rate, particularly complete responses.

RADIATION THERAPY

The tolerance of the normal liver to radiation limits the total radiation dose and the use of this modality to treat hepatic metastases. Radiation toxicity of the liver consists of occlusion of small hepatic veins and centrilobular fibrosis.[160] Liver tolerance to radiation was obtained from studies using total abdominal irradiation in the treatment of ovarian carcinoma.[161] Of those treated with 3500 to 3950 rad, five of nine developed radiation hepatitis versus one of nine in those receiving ≤ 3000 rad. Radiation hepatitis can also be accompanied by ascites and Budd–Chiari-like syndrome.

The role of radiation in palliation of symptoms from liver metastases has been demonstrated. With an average dose of 2500 rad in 3 to 3.5 weeks, Prasad treated 27 patients (41% had failed to respond to chemotherapy) and reported symptomatic pain relief in 70%, with an average survival of 4 months.[162] Jaundice and ascites improved in 28% and 50% of patients, respectively; however, no follow-up radiologic studies were available. The Radiation Therapy Oncology Group[163] treated 109 patients (63% with gastrointestinal primaries) with 3000 rad in 15 fractions. Of the 51 patients with palpable liver masses, 49% had a reduction in size; improvement in abdominal pain without hepatic toxicity was accomplished in 55%. However, it was unclear how many patients received prior or concurrent therapy. Sherman and co-workers,[164] who used 2100 to 2400 rad in 300 rad/fractions, reported pain relief in 90% of patients with a median

TABLE 62-28. Randomized Studies of Intrahepatic Versus Systemic Chemotherapy for Hepatic Metastases

Group	No. of Patients	*Intrahepatic* Drug	*Intrahepatic* Response (%)	*Systemic* Drug	*Systemic* Response (%)	
MSKCC[156]	163	FUDR	50	FUDR	20	$p = 0.001$
NCOG[157]	143	FUDR	37	FUDR	10	$p = 0.002$
NCI[158]	64	FUDR	62	FUDR	17	
Consortium[159]	43	FUDR	56	5FU	38	
City of Hope[147]	41	FUDR	56	5FU	0	

survival of 4.5 months. Patients thought to have an excellent response had a median survival of 9 months. Sixty percent of the patients received concomitant chemotherapy and it is not clear if the better responses were seen in the combined treatment group.

Some investigators have combined chemotherapy with radiotherapy in an effort to increase response rates and survival. Experimental studies demonstrated that prolonged exposure of tumor cells to 5-FU following radiation produced enhanced cell killing.[165] In resectable colorectal carcinoma the addition of 5-FU to radiation, compared with radiation alone, increased the median survival.[166] Webber and associates[167] treated 48 patients with metastases in a nonrandomized sequential manner: 8 received FUDR hepatic infusion, 14 hepatic irradiation, and 25 combined treatment with intra-arterial chemotherapy and hepatic irradiation. The median survival times for the three groups were 190, 270, and 376 days, respectively. Raju and colleagues[168] used hyperfractionated whole-liver irradiation with FUDR or 5-FU infusion in 12 patients and obtained eight good responses, with a median survival of 20 weeks and no radiation hepatitis. Other studies that used combined radiation and chemotherapy are listed in Table 62-29. The average response rate obtained with combined treatment is no higher than that obtained with FUDR intrahepatic infusion alone. Few reports of combined treatment describe the patient population being treated, (*i.e.*, extent of liver involvement, liver function tests) or document the response (such as a 50% decrease in measurable liver metastases on scan). The possibility of increasing hepatic toxicity of FUDR by concurrent radiation was demonstrated in Yablonski's study[175] during which four of eight patients developed jaundice and a hepatitis-like syndrome after combined treatment. Because 5-FU is more of a radiosensitizer and has less hepatic toxicity than FUDR it may be more useful for future combined modality trials in the treatment of liver metastases.

Another method of radiation is interstitial radiation, which offers an opportunity for improved dose distribution by giving a higher dose to a smaller area and sparing of the normal liver. With a high-intensity iridium-192 source, doses of 5000 rad can be delivered in a single treatment. Dritschillo and colleagues[176] performed afterloading needle applicator placement by sonography in six patients with tumors ranging from 2.5 to 9.5 cm in size. One patient had a 25% regression, whereas the others remained stable, with little toxicity. The duration of response and survival were not mentioned.

OTHER THERAPEUTIC MODALITIES

HEPATIC ARTERIAL LIGATION

The concept for treating liver cancers by ligation of the hepatic artery has been in use since 1952.[177] It is based on the premise that tumors in the liver derive their blood supply from the hepatic artery, and that the normal liver is supplied by both the portal vein and hepatic artery. A summary of the reports using hepatic artery ligation is listed in Table 62-30. Very few studies use ligation alone; therefore, it is difficult to interpret the effect of ligation itself on survival. The studies that suggest most improvement used intrahepatic or portal infusion after the ligation. In Didoklar's study[182], although 14 of the 30 patients studied had greater than 50% involvement, 97% of the patients responded and had a median survival of 23 months. Laufman[189] described a 63% response rate in 19 patients (14 of whom had greater than 30% liver involvement with tumor) with portal vein infusion of 5-FU and mitomycin C and hepatic artery ligation. Because, theoretically, portal vein infusion should not be an effective treatment, the hepatic artery ligation must have played an important role in the response rate.

After ligation, tumor liquefaction and hepatic necrosis or abscesses may occur, and early studies reported a high mortality. Therefore, it is now felt that hepatic artery ligation should not be performed on patients with cirrhosis, severe liver impairment, ascites, jaundice, or occlusion of the portal vein.

HEPATIC ARTERY EMBOLIZATION

Although dramatic shrinkage has been reported after ligation, there is usually a rapid reestablishment of artery growth

TABLE 62-29. Hepatic Irradiation and Infusional Chemotherapy

Investigator	*Drug* (mg)*	*Radiation Dose*	*No. of Patients*	*Response (%)*	*Hepatic Toxicity (%)*	*Survival (mo)*
Barone (169)	FUDR 0.2 or FU 5–10	1000 R q4wk	18	56	22	8
Herbsman (170)	FUDR 0.25	2500–3000 R/15F	13	46	30	16
Rothman (171)	FU 25 × 5 d wk 1, 3, 5,	1000 R/wk wk 1, 3, 5	23	65	0	7
Webber (167)	FUDR 25	2500 rad/10F	25	33	1	12
Lokich (172)	FU 1 g	2500–3000 rad/12F	15	75		8
Raju (168)	FUDR 0.3 or FU 1000/m²	2100 R/14F 2F/day	12	83		17
Gansl (173)	FU 400/m² Meth 30/m²	3000 R in 4 wk	12	25		
Friedman (174)	FU 10–15 Ad 2.5–10/m²	1350–2100 300 R/F	22	55	0	

* Chemotherapy during RT in most studies.
R, rad; F, fraction(s); FU, 5-fluorouricil; FUDR, floxuridine; Meth, methotrexate; Ad, doxorubicin (Adriamycin).

TABLE 62-30. Hepatic Artery Ligation for Liver Metastases

Investigator	*No. of Patients*	*Hepa- toma*	*Colon*	*Drug*	*% with >50% Liver Involvement*	*Improve- ment (%)*	*Death from Procedure (%)*
Almersjo[178]	27	5	5	0			37
Balasegarem[179]	24		22	0		50	17
Larmi[180]	8	1	3	0		88	13
Petrelli[181]	97	97	0	FU*	100		2
Didolkar[182]	30	30		IA FU	47	97	3
Ramming[183]	9	9		IA FU		89	
Sparks[184]	19	13		FU		57	16
Kovdahl[185]	20	6	4	0			40
Zike[186]	38	25	5	IA FU			5
Fortner[187]	134	54	31	IA IP FU, Meth Act D			6
Cushieri[188]	17	8	9	IA FU Meth		50	
Zaufman[189]	19	19		IP FU Mit C	74	63	11

IA, intra-arterial; IP, intraportal.

through the development of collateral channels and, consequently, a regrowth of tumor. The rationale for arterial embolization is that a gradual and incomplete blockage of the hepatic artery may diminish the development of collateral circulation.

Most of the work with hepatic arterial embolization has been performed in patients with apudomas, and Gelfoam powder (The Upjohn Company, Kalamazoo, Michigan) or Ivalon (Unipoint Industries Inc., High Point, North Carolina) is used. Because the apudomas are slow-growing tumors, a reduction in the bulk of the tumor often gives significant palliation. In a series by Carrasco, 8 of 14 patients responded who underwent embolization after failure of systemic or hepatic chemotherapy.[190] Five of six patients experienced a dramatic improvement in the symptoms of carcinoid syndrome and reduction in 5-hydroxyindoleacetic acid (5-HIAA) levels. Nine of 13 patients with carcinoid syndrome treated by Maton[191] noted improvement in symptoms. He emphasized the necessity of blocking the actions of the substances produced by the tumor before embolization was attempted and also of assuring patency of the portal vein to avoid some of the complications of embolization. After embolization, almost all patients have fever, leukocytosis, and hepatic pain, and some develop hepatic abscesses, gas formation, or urate nephropathy. When using both hepatic artery occlusion and chemotherapy, Moertel noted systemic relief in nine of ten patients with carcinoid tumor.[192]

It is clear from these studies that embolization will decrease symptoms in patients with endocrine tumors and actually cause reduction in tumor size, but it is not clear whether or not these measures improve survival.

Another way to avoid revascularization after hepatic arterial ligation and to achieve temporary occlusion of the hepatic artery is by the use of microspheres. Degradable starch microspheres (DSM) are 40 μm in diameter and are degraded by amylase. When injected into the hepatic artery, they are entrapped in the arteriolar capillary bed and obstruct flow until they undergo degradation (approximately 30 min). If there is greater perfusion of the tumor compared with the normal liver, then microspheres should leads to a more prolonged tumor exposure to the chemotherapeutic agent.[194] Drugs with a short ½ or low extraction efficiency are the best to use with DSM.[195] Increase in local drug concentration depends on the flow rate of the infusing artery and the rate of drug elimination, that is, a low arterial blood flow will increase local drug levels.[119] Intrahepatic injection of labeled 5-FU and microspheres resulted in increased tumor labeling in the livers injected with the microspheres and a reduced peripheral blood [^{14}C]FU level compared with 5-FU alone.[196] With intrahepatic injections of doxorubicin (Adriamycin) or mitomycin and microspheres, there was a reduction in systemic levels of drugs (both peak values and area under the curve) when the drugs were injected with microspheres.[197,198]

In 16 patients with hepatic metastases (12 from colon), whose tumor failed to respond to systemic and intrahepatic chemotherapy, liver chemistry improvements were observed, but no objective responses were noted with microspheres and mitomycin. Toxicity of the combined treatment consisted of a transient increase in liver chemistries in 50% of the patients, myelosuppression in 20%, nausea in 40%, and right upper quadrant pain in 20%.[198]

There have been reported responses in breast cancer and cholangiocarcinoma with microspheres and doxorubicin or BCNU.[199,200] Myelosuppression has been limited. The usual side-effects are hepatic pain, hepatic enzyme elevations, and duodenitis. It is not clear yet whether or not the addition of microspheres to intrahepatic therapy adds to the response rate. Because microspheres cause transient obstruction to blood flow, a variable degree of extrahepatic shunting may occur, which may increase systemic drug levels.

Another type of microsphere is a resin particle in which

yttrium-90 has been entrapped, providing the opportunity for "internal radiotherapy." Grady and associates[201] reported six responses in 16 patients treated with intra-arterial yttrium-90 microspheres and hyperthermia. Toxicity included radiation hepatitis and peptic ulceration. Ariel and colleagues[202] treated 65 patients with hepatic metastases from colorectal carcinoma using infusion of 5-FU (1 g infused over 24 hr for 15 days) with yttrium-90 (estimated to deliver 10,000 rad to the liver). They obtained a 35% to 40% objective response rate and a median survival of 12 to 14 months. Abdominal pain and nausea and vomiting were present in half of the treated patients. It is not stated whether or not these patients had previous chemotherapy. Mantravadi[203] noted three responses in 15 previously treated patients when using yttrium microspheres alone and did not observe radiation hepatitis. It is not clear that these response rates are superior to hepatic infusional therapy alone.

MONOCLONAL ANTIBODY

With the development of technology to produce monoclonal or polyclonal antibodies to antigens on tumor surfaces or to tumor-associated proteins synthesized by tumors, new forms of treatment for liver metastases could be developed. The immunoglobulins can be applied alone or coupled with isotopes or chemotherapy.

LOCAL TUMOR DESTRUCTION PLUS REGIONAL CHEMOTHERAPY

Several groups have tried to combine the focal destruction of tumor nodules (to remove gross disease) with regional chemotherapy to maintain a disease-free status within the liver. Kemeny has reported using surgical removal of as many as 15 metastases combined with intra-arterial FUDR.[147] She found superior local control of tumor when patients had surgery plus intra-arterial FUDR, compared with intra-arterial FUDR alone. Steele and colleagues have used liver cryosurgery to destroy bulk disease in the liver. The extent of tumor destruction in the liver was monitored with intraoperative ultrasound.[204,205] Other groups have used the installation of absolute alcohol into a tumor mass to achieve a focal destruction of malignant disease.[206] Dritschillo used interstitial radiation therapy surgically positioned in the center of a tumor nodule to bring about its destruction.[176] The highly active radiation was left in place long enough to destroy tumor and a small margin of surrounding liver tissue. This modality promises to have few complications resulting from abscess formation or infection of metastases when patients with large metastases are excluded from treatment.

REFERENCES

1. Sugarbaker PA, Kemeny MM: Management of liver tumors. Adv Surg (in press)
2. Michaels NA: Blood Supply and Anatomy of Upper Abdominal Organs with Descriptive Atlas. Philadelphia, JB Lippincott, 1955
3. Hardy KJ, Wheatley IC, Anderson AIE, Bone RJ: The lymph nodes of the porta hepatis. Surg Gynecol Obstet 143:225–228, 1976
4. Healey JE: Vascular anatomy of the liver. Ann NY Acad Sci 170:8–17, 1970
5. Couinand C: Controlled hepatectomies and exposure of the intrahepatic bile ducts. Anatomical and technical study. Paris, France 1981
6. Pickren JW, Tsukada Y, Lane WW: Liver metastasis: Analysis of autopsy data. In Weiss L, Gilbert HA (eds): Liver Matastases, pp 2–18. Boston, GK Hall, 1982
7. Bismuth H: Surgical anatomy and anatomical surgery of the liver. World J Surg 6:3–9, 1982
8. Sugarbaker PH, Reinig JW, Hughes KS: Diagnosis of hepatic metastases. In Rosenberg SA (ed.): Surgical Treatment of Metastatic Disease. Philadelphia, JB Lippincott, 1987
9. Wanebo HG, Rao B, Pinsky C et al: Preoperative carcinoembryonic antigen level as a prognostic indicator in colorectal cancer. N Engl J Med 299:448–451
10. Kemeny MM, Sugarbaker PH, Smith TJ et al: A prospective analysis of laboratory tests and imaging studies to detect hepatic lesions. Ann Surg 195:163–167, 1982
11. Smith TJ, Kemeny MM, Sugarbaker PH et al: A prospective study of hepatic imaging in the detection of metastatic disease. Ann Surg 195:486–491, 1982
12. Matsui O, Kadoya M, Suzuki et al: Work in progress: Dynamic sequential computed tomography during arterial portography in the detection of hepatic neoplasms. Radiology 146:173–178, 1983
13. Bernardino ME, Erwin BC, Steinberg HV et al: Delayed hepatic scanning: Increased confidence and improved detection of hepatic metastase. Radiology 159:71–74, 1986
14. Reinig JW, Dwyer AJ, Miller DL, Sugarbaker PH: Liver metastases detection: Comparative sensitivities of MR imaging and CT scanning. Radiology 162:43–47, 1987
15. Hogg L Jr, Pack GT: Diagnostic accuracy of hepatic metastases at laparotomy. Arch Surg 72:251–252, 1966
16. Gray BN: Surgeon accuracy in the diagnosis of liver metastases at laparotomy. Aust NZ J Surg 50:524–526, 1980
17. Harbin WP, Wittenberg J, Ferrucci JT Jr et al: Fallibility of exploratory laparotomy in detection of hepatic and retroperitoneal masses. AJR 135:115–121, 1980
18. Finlay IG, Meek DR, Gray HW et al: Incidence and detection of occult hepatic metastases in colorectal carcinoma. Br Med J 284:803–805, 1982
19. Igawa SI, Sakai K, Kinoshita H, Kirohashi K: Intraoperative sonography: Clinical usefulness in liver surgery. Radiology 156:473–478, 1985
20. Gozzetti G, Mazziotti A, Bolondi L et al: Intraoperative ultrasonography in surgery for liver tumors. Surgery 99:523–529, 1986
21. Castaing D, Kunstlinger F, Habib N, Bismuth H: Intraoperative ultrasonographic study of the liver. Am J Surg 149:676–682, 1985
22. Wagner JS, Adson MA, van Heerden JA et al: The natural history of hepatic metastases from colorectal cancer. Ann Surg 197:502–508, 1984
23. Pestana C, Reitemeier RJ, Moertel CG et al: The natural history of carcinoma of colon and rectum. Am J Surg 108:826–829, 1964
24. Jaffe BM, Donegan WL, Watson F, Spratt JS Jr: Factors influencing survival in patients with untreated hepatic metastases. Surg Gynecol Obstet 127:1–11, 1968
25. Oxley EM, Ellis H: Prognosis of carcinoma of the large bowel in the presence of liver metastases. Br J Surg 56:149–152, 1969
26. Bengmark S, Hafstrom L: The natural history of primary and secondary malignant tumors of the liver. Cancer 23:198–202, 1969
27. Baden H, Anderson B: Survival of patients with untreated liver metastases from colorectal cancer. Scand J Gastroenterol 10:221–223, 1975
28. Wood C, Gillis CR, Blumgart LH: A retrospective study of the natural history of patients with liver metastases from colorectal cancer. Clin Oncol 2:285–288, 1976
29. Goslin R, Steele G, Zamcheck N et al: Factors influencing survival in patients with hepatic metastases from adenocarcinoma of the colon or rectum. Dis Colon Rectum 25:749–754, 1982
30. Hughes KS, Simon RM, Songhorabodi S, Sugarbaker PH: Hepatic Metastases Registry: Resection of the liver for colorectal carcinoma metastases: A multi-institutional study of indications for resection. Surgery (in press)
31. Wilson SM, Adson MA: Surgical treatment of hepatic metastases from colorectal cancers. Arch Surg 111:330–334, 1976
32. Foster JH, Berman MM: Solid Liver Tumors Philadelphia, WB Saunders, 1977
33. Morrow CE, Grage TB, Sutherland DER, Najarian JS: Hepatic resection for secondary neoplasms. Surgery 92:610–614, 1982
34. Aldrete JS, Agdemir D, Laws HL: Major hepatic resections: Analysis of 51 cases. Am Surg 48:118–122, 1982
35. Blumgart LH, Allison DJ: Resection and embolization in the management of secondary hepatic tumors. World J Surg 6:32–45, 1982
36. Thompson HH, Tompkins RK, Longmire WP Jr: Major hepatic resection: A 25 year experience. Ann Surg 197:375–388, 1983
37. Fortner JG, Silva JS, Golbey RB et al: Multivariate analysis of a personal series of 247 consecutive patients with liver metastases from colorectal cancer. Ann Surg 199:306–316, 1984
38. Cady B, McDermott WV: Major hepatic resection for metachronous metastases from colorectal cancer. Ann Surg 201:204–209, 1985
39. Adson MA, van Heerden JA, Adson MH et al: Resection of hepatic metastases from colorectal cancer. Arch Surg 119:647–651, 1984
40. Gennari L, Doci R, Bignami P: Surgical treatment of hepatic metastases from colorectal cancer. Ann Surg 203:49–54, 1985
41. August DA, Sugarbaker PH, Gianola FJ et al: Hepatic resection of colorectal metastases: Influence of clinical factors and adjuvant intraperitoneal 5-fluorouracil via Tenckhoff catheter on survival. Ann Surg 201:210–218, 1985
42. Petrelli NJ, Nambisan RN, Herrera L, Mittelman A: Hepatic resection for isolated metastases from colorectal carcinoma. Am J Surg 149:205–209, 1985

43. Coppa GF, Eng K, Ranson JHC et al: Hepatic resection for metastatic colon and rectal cancer: An elevation of preoperative factors. Ann Surg 202:203–208, 1985
44. Gall FP, Scheele J, Altendorf A: Typical and atypical resection techniques of hepatic metastases. In Recent Results in Cancer Research, pp 212–220. Berlin, Springer-Verlag
45. Iwatsuki S, Esquivel CO, Gordon RD, Starzl TE: Liver resection for metastatic colorectal cancer. Surgery 100:804–809, 1986
46. Ekberg H, Trangerg KG, Anderson R et al: Determinants of survival in liver resection for colorectal secondaries. Br J Surg 73:727–731, 1986
47. Butler J, Attiyeh F, Daly JM: Hepatic resection for metastases of the colon and rectum. Surg Gynecol Obstet 162:109–113, 1986
48. August DA, Sugarbaker PH, Schneider PD: Lymphatic dissemination of hepatic metastases. Cancer 55:1490–1494, 1985
49. Hughes KS: Hepatic Metastases Registry: Resection of the liver for colorectal metastases: A multi-institutional study of patterns of recurrence. Surgery 100:278–284, 1986
50. Griffith K, Chang AE, Sugarbaker PH: Beneficial effects of repeat resection of hepatic metastases.
51. Steel G Jr, Osteen RT, Wilson RE et al: Patterns of failure after surgical cure of large tumors. A change in the proximate cause of death and a need for effective systemic adjuvant therapy. Am J Surg 147:554–559, 1984
52. Hughes KS, August DA, Ottow RT, Gianola FJ: Hepatic resection for colorectal carcinoma metastasis: Present status and future prospects. In Mastromarino AJ (ed): Biology and Treatment of Colorectal Cancer Metastasis, pp 159–178. Boston, Martinus Nijhoff
53. Hughes KS, Sugarbaker PH: Treatment of metastatic liver tumors. In Rosenberg SA (ed): Surgical Cure of Metastatic Cancer. Philadelphia, JB Lippincott, 1987
54. Norton JA, Sugarbaker PH, Doppman JL et al: Aggressive resection of metastatic disease in selected patients with malignant gastrinoma. Ann Surg 203:352–359, 1986
55. Galland RB, Gart LH: Carconoid syndrome, surgical management. Br J Hosp Med 35:168–170, 1986
56. Garre C: Bietraege zur Leber-Chirurgie. Bruns Bietr Klin Chir 4:181, 1888
57. Keen WW: Report of case of resection of the liver for the removal of a neoplasm, with a table of seventy-six cases of resection of the liver for hepatic tumors. Ann Surg
58. Pringle JH. Notes on the arrest of hepatic hemorrhage due to trauma. Ann Surg 30:267, 1899
59. Wendel W. Beitraege zur Chirurgie der Leber. Arch Klin Chir 95:887, 1911
60. Lortat-Jacob JL, Robert HG: Hepatectomie droit reglee. Presse Med 60:549, 1952
61. Healey JE: Vascular anatomy of the liver. Ann NY Acad Sci 170:8–17, 1970
62. Lin TY, Hsu KY, Hsieh C, Chen CS. Study on lobectomy of ports on three cases of primary hepatoma treated with left lobectomy of the liver. J Formosan Med Assoc 57:742, 1958
63. Couinaud C: Principes directeurs des hepatectomies reglees. Chirurgie 106:8–10, 1980
64. Storm KF, Longmire WP JR: A simplified clamp for hepatic resection. Surg Gynecol Obstet 133:103, 1971
65. Starzl TE, Bell RH, Beart RW, Putnum CW: Hepatic trisegmentectomy and other liver resections. Surg Gynecol Obstet 141:429, 1975
66. Hodgson WJB, Afuses A Jr: Surgical ultrasonic dissection of the liver. Surg Rounds 2:68, 1979
67. Fortner JG, MacLean BJ, Kim DK et al: The seventies evolution in liver surgery for cancer. Cancer 47:2162, 1981
68. Starzl TE, Iwtsuki S, Shaw BW Jr et al: Left hepatic trisegmentectomy. Surg Gynecol Obstet 155:21, 1982
69. Lefor AT, Hughes KS, Shiloni E et al: Staging of patients with suspected isolated colorectal liver metastases. Curr Surg (in press)
70. Huget C, Nordlinger B, Galopin JJ et al: Normothermic hepatic vascular exclusion for extensive hepatectomy. Surg Gynecol Obstet 147:689–693, 1978
71. Hodgson WJB, DelGuercio LRM: Preliminary experience in liver surgery using the ultrasonic scalpel. Surgery 95:230–234, 1984
72. Ottow RT, Barbieri SA, Sugarbaker PH, Wesley RA: Liver transection: A controlled study of four different techniques in pigs. Surgery 97:596–601, 1985
73. Tranberg K, Rigotti P, Bracket KA et al: Liver resection: A comparison using the N-YAG laser, an ultrasonic surgical aspirator, or blunt dissection. Am J Surg 151:368–373, 1986
74. Tabuse K, Katsumi J, Kobyayashi Y et al: Microwave surgery: Hepatectomy using a microwave tissue coagulator. World J Surg 9:136–143, 1985
75. Joffe SN, Brackett KA, Sankar My, Daikuzono N: Resection of the liver with the ND laser. Surg Gynecol Obstet 163:437–442, 1986
76. Andrus CH, Kaminski DL: Segmental hepatic resection utilizing the ultrasonic dissector. Arch Surg 121:515–521, 1986
77. Carter SK: Single and combination nonhormonal chemotherapy in breast cancer. Cancer 30:1543–1555, 1972
78. Mattsson W, Arwidi A, von Eyben F et al: Phase II study of combined vincristine, Adriamycin, cyclophosphamide, and methotrexate with citrovorum factor rescue in metastatic breast cancer. Cancer Treat Rep 61:1527–1531, 1977
79. Muss HB, White DR, Richards F II et al: Adriamycin vs methotrexate in five-drug combination chemotherapy for advanced breast cancer. Cancer 42:2141–2148, 1978
80. Kennealey GT, Boston B, Mitchell MS et al: Combination chemotherapy for advanced breast cancer. Two regimens containing Adriamycin. Cancer 42:27–33, 1978
81. Tranum B, Hoogstraten B, Kennedy A et al: Adriamycin in combination for the treatment of breast cancer. Cancer 41:2078–2083, 1978
82. Jones SE, Durie BG, Salmon SE: Combination chemotherapy with Adriamycin and cyclophosphamide for advanced breast cancer. Cancer 36:90–97, 1975
83. Chauvergne J, Gary-Bobo J, Klein T et al: Polychimiotherapie des cancers mammaires en phase avancee. Association ternaire avec doxorubicine. Analyse de 209 observations. Bull Cancer 64:667–680, 1977
84. Russell JA, Baker JW, Dady PJ et al: Combination chemotherapy of metastatic breast cancer with vincristine, Adriamycin and prednisolone. Cancer 41:396–399, 1978
85. Smalley RV, Carpenter J, Bartolucci A et al: A comparison of cyclophosphamide, Adriamycin, 5-fluorouracil (CAF) and cyclophosphamide, methotrexate, 5-fluorouracil, vincristine, prednisone (CMFVP) in patients with metastatic breast cancer. A Southeastern Cancer Group study project. Cancer 40:625–632, 1977
86. Canellos GP, DeVita VT, Gold GL et al: Combination chemotherapy for advanced breast cancer: Response and effect on survival. Ann Intern Med 84:89–392, 1976
87. George SL, Hoogstraten B: Prognostic factors in the initial response to therapy by patients with advanced breast cancer. J Natl Cancer Inst 60:731–736, 1978
88. Abrams HL, Spiro R, Goldstein N: Metastases in carcinoma: Analysis of 1000 autopsied cases. Cancer 3:74–85, 1950
89. Bross IDJ, Viadana E, Pickren J: Do generalized metastases occur directly from the primary? J Chronic Dis 28:149–159, 1975
90. Wasserman T, Comis RL, Goldsmith M et al: Tabular analysis of the clinical chemotherapy of solid tumors. Cancer Chemother Rep 6:399, 1975
91. Moertal CG, Reitemeier RJ: Advanced Gastrointestinal Cancer—Clinical Management and Chemotherapy. New York, Harper & Row, 1969
92. Baker LH, Talley RW, Maiter R et al: Phase III comparison of the treatment of advanced gastrointestinal cancer with bolus weekly 5-FU vs methyl-CCNU plus bolus weekly 5-FU,. Cancer 38:1, 1976
93. Siefert P, Baker LH, Reed MD et al: Comparison of continuously infused 5-fluorouracil with bolus injection in treatment of patients with colorectal adenocarcinoma. Cancer 36:123, 1975
94. Grage TB, Vassilopoulos P, Shingleton WW et al: Results of a prospective randomized study of hepatic artery infusion with 5-fluorouracil vs intravenous 5-fluorouracil in patients with hepatic metastases from colorectal cancer: A Central Oncology Group Study. Surgery 86:550–555, 1979
95. Moertel CG, Schutt AJ, Hahn RG, Reifemeier RJ: Brief communications—therapy of advanced colorectal cancer with a combination of 5-fluorouracil, methyl-1,3-*cis*(2-chlorethyl)-1-nitrosourea and vincristine. J Natl Cancer Inst 54:69–71, 1975
96. MacDonald JS, Kisner DF, Smythe T et al: 5-Fluorouracil (5-FU), methyl-CCNU and vincristine in the treatment of advanced colorectal cancer. Phase II study utilizing weekly 5-FU. Cancer Treat Rep 60:1597, 1976
97. Buroker J, Kim PN, Groppe C et al: 5-FU infusion with methyl-CNU in the treatment of advanced colon cancer. Cancer 42:1228, 1978
98. Kemeny N, Yagoda A, Golbey RB: A randomized study of two different schedules of methyl-CCNU, 5-FU and vincristine for metastatic colorectal carcinoma. Cancer 43:78, 1979
99. Kemeny N, Yagoda A, Braun D: Metastatic colorectal carcinoma: A prospective randomized trial of methyl-CCNU, 5-fluorouracil (5-FU) and vincristine (MOF) versus MOF plus streptozotocin (MOF-strep). Cancer 51:20–25, 1983
100. Kemeny N, Yagoda A, Braun D et al: Therapy for metastatic colorectal carcinoma with a combination of methyl-CCNU, 5-fluorouracil, vincristine, and streptozotocin (MOF-strep). Cancer 45:876–881, 1980
101. Machover D, Goldschmidt E, Chollet P et al: Treatment of advanced colorectal and gastric adenocarcinomas with 5-fluorouracil and high-dose folinic acid. J Clin Oncol 4:685–696, 1986
102. Kemeny N, Ahmed T, Michaelson R et al: Activity of low dose methorexate and fluorouracil in advanced colorectal carcinoma: Attempted correlation with tissue and blood levels of phosphoribosylpyrophosphate. J Clin Oncol 2:311–315, 1984
103. Pandya KJ, Chans AYU, Qazi R et al: Combination chemotherapy for advanced colorectal cancer. A pilor study. Am J Clin Oncol 9:31–4, 1986
104. Loehrer PJ Sr, Einhorn LH, Williams SD et al: Cisplatin plus 5-FU for the treatment of adenocarcinoma of the colon. Cancer Treat Rep 69:1359–1363, 1985
105. Kemeny N, Reichman B, Botet J et al: Continuous infusion 5-fluorouracil (FU) and bolus cisplatin (DDP) for metastatic colorectal cancer. Proc ASCO 6:86, 1987
106. Moertel CG: The natural history of advanced gastric cancer. Surg Gynecol Obstet 126:1071–1074, 1968
107. Franks CR: Adriamycin and methotrexate in metastatic gastric cancer: A pilot study. Clin Oncol 6:309–315, 1980
108. Bitran JD, Desser RK, Kozloff MF et al: Treatment of metastatic pancreatic and gastric adenocarcinomas with 5-fluorouracil, Adriamycin, and mitomycin-C (FAM). Cancer Treat Rep 63:2049–2052, 1979
109. MacDonald JS, Schein PS, Wooley PV et al: 5-Fluorouracil, doxorubicin and mitomycin (FAM) combination chemotherapy for advanced gastric cancer. Ann Intern Med 93:533–536, 1980
110. Seligman M, Bukowski RM, Groppe CS et al: Chemotherapy of metastatic gastrointestinal neoplasms with 5-fluorouracil and streptozotocin. Cancer Treat Rep 61:1375–1377, 1977
111. Wooley PV III, MacDonald JS, Smythe TS et al: A Phase II trial of ftorafur, Adriamycin and mitomycin-C (FAM II) in advanced gastric cancer. Cancer 44:1211–1214, 1979
112. The Gastrointestinal Tumor Study Group: Phase II–III chemotherapy studies in advanced gastric cancer. Cancer Treat Rep 63:1871–1876, 1979
113. Bunn PA Jr, Nugent JL, Ihde DC et al: 5-Fluorouracil, methyl-CCNU, Adriamycin and mitomycin C in the treatment of advanced gastric cancer. Cancer Treat Rep 62:1287–1293, 1978

114. Cunningham D, Soukop M, McArdle CS et al: Advanced gastric cancer: Experience in Scotland using 5-fluorouracil, Adriamycin and mitomycin-C. Br J Surg 71:673–676, 1984
115. Moertel CG, Lavin PT: Phase II–III chemotherapy studies in advanced gastric cancer. Cancer Treat Rep 63:1863–1869, 1979
116. Kemeny N: The systemic chemotherapy of hepatic metastases. Semin Oncol 10:148–59, 1983
117. Breedis C, Young C: The blood supply of neoplasms in the liver. Am J Pathol 30:969, 1954
118. Sigurdson ER, Ridge JA, Kemeny N, Daly JM: Tumor and liver drug uptake following hepatic artery and portal vein infusion. J Clin Oncol (in press)
119. Chen HSG, Gross JF: Intra-arterial infusion of anti-cancer drugs: Theoretic aspects of drug delivery and review of responses. Cancer Treat Rep 64:31–40, 1980
120. Ensminger WD, Rosowsky A, Raso V: A clinical pharmacological evaluation of hepatic arterial infusions of 5-fluoro-2-deoxyuridine and 5-fluorouracil. Cancer Res 38:3784–3792, 1978
121. Ensminger WD, Gyves JW: Clinical pharmaology of hepatic arterial chemotherapy. Semin Oncol 10:176–183, 1983
122. Collins JM: Pharmacologic rationale for regional drug delivery. J Clin Oncol 2:498–504, 1984
123. Collins JM: Pharmacologic rationale for hepatic arterial therapy. Recent Results Cancer Res 100:140–148, 1986
124. Tandon RN, Bunnell IL, Copper RG: The treatment of metastatic carcinoma of the liver by percutaneous selective hepatic artery infusion of 5-fluorouracil. Surgery 73:118, 1973
125. Ansfield FJ, Ramirez G, Davis HL Jr et al: Further clinical studies with intrahepatic arterial infusion with 5-fluorouracil. Cancer 36:2413–2417, 1975
126. Buroker T, Samson M, Correa J et al: Hepatic artery infusion of 5-FUDR after prior systemic 5-fluorouracil. Cancer Treat Rep 60:1277–1279, 1976
127. Oberfield RA, McCaffrey JA, Polio J et al: Prolonged and continuous percutaneous intra-arterial hepatic infusion chemotherapy in advanced metastatic liver adenocarcinoma from colorectal primary. Cancer 44:414–423, 1979
128. Watkins E Jr, Khazei AM, Nahra KS: Surgical basis for arterial infusion chemotherapy of disseminated carcinoma of the liver. Surg Gynecol Obstet 130:581, 1970
129. Cady B, Oberfield RA: Regional infusion chemotherapy of hepatic metastases from carcinoma of the colon. Am J Surg 127:220–227, 1974
130. Cady B: Hepatic arterial patency and complications after catheterization for infusion chemotherapy. Ann Surg 178:156–61, 1973
131. Massey WH, Fletcher WS, Judkins MP: Hepatic artery infusion for metastatic malignancy using percutaneously placed catheters. Am J Surg 121:160–164, 1971
132. Petrek JA, Minton JP: Treatment of hepatic metastases by percutaneous hepatic arterial infusion. Cancer 43:2182–2188, 1979
133. Reed ML, Vaitkevicius VK, Al-Sarraf M et al: The practicality of chronic hepatic artery infusion therapy of primary and metastatic hepatic malignancies. Cancer 47:402, 1981
134. Smiley S, Schouten J, Chang A, Ramirez G: Intrahepatic arterial infusion with 5-FU for liver metastases of colorectal carcinoma. Proc Am Soc Clin Oncol 22:391, 1981
135. Buchwald H, Grage TB, Vassilopoulos PP et al: Intraarterial infusion chemotherapy for hepatic carcinoma using a totally implantable infusion pump. Cancer 45:866–869, 1980
136. Ensminger W, Niederhuber J, Dakhil S et al: Totally implanted drug delivery system for hepatic arterial chemotherapy. Cancer Treat Rep 65:393, 1981
137. Hohn DC, Stagg RJ, Price DC et al: Avoidance of gastroduodenal toxicity in patients receiving hepatic arterial 5-fluoro-2′-deoxyuridine. J Clin Oncol 3:1257–1260, 1985
138. Niederhuber JE, Ensminger W, Gyves et al: Regional chemotherapy of colorectal cancer metastatic to the liver. Cancer 53:1336, 1984
139. Ensminger W, Niederhuber J, Gyves J et al: Effective control of liver metastases from colon cancer with an implanted system for hepatic arterial chemotherapy. Proc Am Soc Clin Oncol 1:94, 1982
140. Kemeny N, Daly J, Oderman P et al: Hepatic artery pump infusion toxicity and results in patients with metastatic colorectal carcinoma. J Clin Oncol 2:595–600, 1984
141. Balch CM, Urist MM: Intraarterial chemotherapy for colorectal liver metastases and hepatomas using a totally implantable drug infusion pump. Recent Results Cancer Res 100:123–147, 1986
142. Shepard KV, Levin B, Karl RC et al: Therapy for metastatic colorectal cancer with hepatic artery infusion chemotherapy using a subcutaneous implanted pump. J Clin Oncol 3:161, 1985
143. Cohen AM, Kaufman SD, Wood WC, Greenfield AJ: Regional hepatic chemotherapy using an implantable drug infusion pump. Am J Surg 145:529–533, 1983
144. Weiss GR, Garnick MB, Osteen RT et al: Long-term hepatic arterial infusion of 5-fluorodeoxyuridine for liver metastases using an implantable infusion pump. J Clin Oncol 1:337–44, 1983
145. Schwartz SI, Jones LS, McCune CS: Assessment of treatment of intrahepatic malignancies using chemotherapy via an implantable pump. Anal Surg 201:560–567, 1985
146. Johnson LP, Wasserman PB, Rivkin SE: FUDR hepatic arterial infusion via an implantable pump for treatment of hepatic tumors. Proc Am Soc Clin Oncol 2:119, 1983
147. Kemeny MM, Goldberg D, Beatty JD et al: Results of a prospective randomized trial of continuous regional chemotherapy and hepatic resection as treatment of hepatic metastases from colorectal primaries. Cancer 57:492, 1986
148. Ramming KP, O'Toole K: The use of the implantable chemoinfusion pump in the treatment of hepatic metastases of colorectal cancer. Arch Surg 121:1440–1444, 1986
149. Hohn DC, Melnick J, Stagg R et al: Biliary sclerosis in patients receiving hepatic arterial infusions of floxuridine. J Clin Oncol 3:98–102, 1985
150. Gluck WI, Akwari OE, Kelvin FM et al: A reversible enteropathy complicating continuous hepatic artery infusion chemotherapy with 5-fluoro-2-deoxyuridine. Cancer 56:2424, 1985
151. Doria MI Jr, Shepard KV, Levin B et al: Liver pathology following hepatic arterial infusion chemotherapy. Cancer 58:855–861, 1986
152. Gennari L, Doci R, Bozzetti F, Veronesi U: Proposal for a clinical classification of liver metastases. Tumori 68:443–448, 1982
153. Wood CB, Gillis CR, Blumgart LH: A retrospective study on the natural history of patients with liver metastasis from colorectal cancer. Clin Oncol 2:285–288, 1976
154. Kemeny N, Daly J, Oderman P et al: Prognostic variables in patients with hepatic metastases from colorectal cancer: Importance of medical assessment of liver involvement. Proc Am Soc Clin Oncol 4:88, 1985
155. Kemeny N, Braun DW: Prognostic factors in advanced colorectal carcinoma: The importance of lactic dehydrogenase, performance status, and white blood cell count. Am J Med 74:786–794, 1983
156. Kemeny N, Daly J, Reichman B et al: Intrahepatic or systemic infusion of fluorodeoxyuridine in patients with liver metastases from colorectal carcinoma. Ann Intern Med 107:459–465, 1987
157. Hohn D, Stagg R, Friedman M et al: The NCOG randomized trial of intravenous (IV) vs hepatic arterial (IA) FUDR for colorectal cancer metastatic to the liver. Proc Am Soc Clin Oncol 6:85, 1987
158. Chang AE, Schneider PD, Sugarbaker PH: A prospective randomized trial of regional versus systemic continuous 5-fluorodeoxyuridine chemotherapy in the treatment of colorectal liver metastases. Ann Surg (in press)
159. Niederhuber JE: Arterial chemotherapy for metastatic colorectal cancer in the liver. Conference on Advances in Regional Cancer Therapy. Giessen, West Germany, 1985
160. Reed GB, Cox AJ: The human liver after radiation injury. Am J Pathol 46:597–611, 1966
161. Ingold JA, Reed GB, Kaplan HS, Bagsjaw MA: Radiation hepatitis. AJR 93:200–208, 1965
162. Prasad B, Lee M, Hendrickson FR: Irradiation of hepatic metastases. Int J Radiat Oncol Biol Phys 2:129–132, 1977
163. Borgelt BB, Gelber R, Brady LW et al: The palliation of hepatic metastases. Results of Radiation Therapy Oncology Group pilot study. Int J Radiat Oncol Biol Phys 7:587–591, 1981
164. Sherman DM et al: Palliation of hepatic metastases. Cancer 41:2013–2017, 1978
165. Barone RM, Calabro-Jones P, Thomas TN et al: Surgical adjuvant therapy in colon carcinoma: A human tumor spheroid model for evaluating radiation sensitizing agents. Cancer 47:2349–2357, 1981
166. Moertel DG, Childs PS, Reitmeier PJ et al: Combined 5-fluorouracil and supervoltage radiation therapy of locally unresectable gastrointestinal cancer. Lancet 2:865–867, 1969
167. Webber BM, Soderberg CH, Leone LA et al: A combined treatment approach to management of hepatic metastases. Cancer 42:1087–1095, 1978
168. Raju PI, Maruama Y, DeSimone P, MacDonald J: Treatment of liver metastases with a combination of chemotherapy and hyperfractionated external radiation therapy. Am J Clin Oncol 10:41–43, 1987
169. Barone RM, Byfield JE, Goldfarb PB et al: Intraarterial chemotherapy using an implantable infusion pump and liver irradiation for the treatment of hepatic metastases. Cancer 50:850–862, 1982
170. Herbsman H, Gardner B, Harshaw D et al: Treatment of hepatic metastases with a combination of hepatic artery infusion chemotherapy and external radiotherapy. Surg Gynecol Obstet 147:13–17, 1978
171. Rothman M, Kuruvilla AM, Choi K et al: Response of colorectal hepatic metastases to concomitant radiotherapy and intravenous infusion 5-fluorouracil. Int J Radiat Oncol Biol Phys 12:2179–2187, 1986
172. Lokich J, Kinsella T, Perri J et al: Concomitant hepatic radiation and intraarterial fluorinated pyrimidine therapy: Correlation of liver scan, liver function tests, and plasma CEA with tumor response. Cancer 48:2569–2574, 1982
173. Gansl RC, Hippolito J, Cutait R et al: Treatment of liver metastatic colorectal carcinoma with sequential methotrexate (MTX), fluorouracil (5-FU), and external hepatic radiation. Proc Am Soc Clin Oncol 5:94, 1986
174. Friedman MA, Cassidy MJ, Levine M et al: Combined modality therapy of hepatic metastases. Cancer 44:906–913, 1979
175. Yablonski-Peretz T, Freund H, Chisin R et al: Toxic hepatitis: A complication of intraarterial chemotherapy (IAC) and radiotherapy (XRT) for liver metastases. European Society for Therapeutic Radiology and Oncology, p. 307. Sept 9–15, 1984
176. Dritschilo A, Grant EG, Harter KW et al: Interstitial radiation therapy for hepatic metastases: Sonographic guidance for applicator placement. AJR 147:275–278, 1986
177. Markowitz J: The hepatic artery. Surg Gynecol Obstet 95:644–646, 1952
178. Almersjo O, Bengmark S, Rudenstam CM: Evaluation of hepatic dearterialization in primary and secondary cancer of the liver. Am J Surg 124:509, 1972
179. Balasegaram M: Complete hepatic dearterialization for primary carcinomas of the liver. Report of 24 patients. Am J Surg 124:340–345, 1972
180. Larmi TKI, Karkola P, Klintrup H et al: Treatment of patients with hepatic tumors and jaundice by ligation of the hepatic artery. Arch Surg 108:178–183, 1974
181. Petrelli NJ, Barcewicz PA, Evans JT et al: Hepatic artery ligation for liver metastasis in colorectal carcinoma. Cancer 53:1347–1353, 1984
182. Didolkar MS, Elias EG, Whitley NO et al: Unresectable hepatic metastases from carcinoma of the colon and rectum. Surg Gynecol Obstet 160:429–436, 1985

183. Ramming KP, Sparks FC, Eilber FR et al: Hepatic artery ligation and 5-fluorouracil infusion for metastatic colon carcinoma and primary hepatoma. Am J Surg 132:236-242, 1976
184. Sparks FC, Mosher MB, Hallauer WC et al: Hepatic artery ligation and postoperative chemotherapy for hepatic metastases: Clinical and pathophysiological results. Cancer 35:1074-1082, 1975
185. Koudahl G, Funding J: Hepatic artery ligation in primary and secondary hepatic cancer. Acta Chir Scan 138:289-292, 1972
186. Zike WL, Safaie-Shirazi S, Gulesserian HP et al: Hepatic artery ligation and cytotoxic infusion in treatment of liver neoplasms. Arch Surg 110:641-643, 1975
187. Fortner JG, Mulcare RJ, Solis A et al: Treatment of primary and secondary liver cancer by hepatic artery ligation and infusion chemotherapy. Ann Surg 178:162-172, 1973
188. Cuschieri A, Swain C: Hepatic artery ligation and prolonged cytotoxic therapy in advanced primary and secondary liver tumors. Proc Soc Med 68:678-80, 1975
189. Laufman LR, Nims TA, Guy JT: Hepatic artery ligation and portal vein infusion for liver metastases from colon cancer. J Clin Oncol 12:1382-1389, 1984
190. Carrasco H, Cuang VP, Wallace S: Apudomas metastatic to the liver: Treatment by hepatic artery embolization. Radiology 149:79-83, 1983
191. Maton PN, Camilleri M, Griffin G: Role of hepatic arterial embolisation in the carcinoid syndrome. Br J Med 287:932-935, 1983
192. Moertel CG, May GR, Martin JK et al: Sequential hepatic artery occlusion (HAO) and chemotherapy for metastatic carcinoid tumor and islet cell carcinoma (ICC). Proc Am Soc Clin Oncol 4:80, 1985
193. Allison DJ, Modlin IM, Jenkins WJ: Treatment of carcinoid liver metastases by hepatic artery embolization. Lancet 2:1323-1325, 1977
194. Aronsen KF, Hellenkant C, Holmberg J et al: Controlled blocking of hepatic artery flow with enzymatically degradable microspheres combined with oncolytic drugs. Eur Surg Res 11:99-106, 1979
195. Ziessman HA, Thrall JH, Ensminger WD et al: Quantitative hepatic arterial perfusion scintigraphy and starch microspheres in cancer chemotherapy. J Nucl Med 24:871-875, 1983
196. Lindell B, Aronsen KF, Nosslin B, Rothman U: Studies in pharmacokinetics and tolerance of substances temporarily retained in the liver by microsphere embolization. Ann Surg 187:95-99, 1978
197. Aronsen KF, Teder H, Lindberg B: Indications and therapeutic possibilities using degradable microspheres in liver malignancies. Recent Results Cancer Res 100:283-288, 1986
198. Gyves JW, Ensminger WD, VanHarken D et al: Improved regional selectivity of hepatic arterial BCNU with degradable microspheres. Clin Pharamacol Ther 34:259-265, 1983
199. Parker G, Regelson W: Treatment of primary and secondary liver cancers with intraarterial chemotherapy mixed with biodegradable starch microspheres. Proc ASCO 4:90, 1985
200. Dakhil S, Ensminger W, Cho K et al: Improved regional selectivity of hepatic arterial BCNU with degradable microspheres. Cancer 50:631-635, 1982
201. Grady ED, McLaren J, Auda SP et al: Combination of internal radiation therapy and hyperthermia to treat liver cancer. South Med J 76:1101-1105, 1983
202. Ariel IM, Padula G: Treatment of symptomatic metastatic cancer to the liver from primary colon and rectal cancer by the intraarterial administration of chemotherapy and radioactive isotopes. J Surg Oncol 10:327-335, 1978
203. Mantravadi RVP, Spigos DG, Tan WS et al: Intraarterial yttrium 90 in the treatment of hepatic malignancy. Radiology 142:783-786, 1982
204. Ravikumar TS, Kane R, Cady B et al: Hepatic cryosurgery with intraoperative ultrasound monitoring for metastatic colon carcinoma. Arch Surg 122:403-409, 1987
205. Onik G, Kane R, Steele G et al: Monitoring hepatic cryosurgery with sonography. AJR 147:655-669, 1986
206. Livragi T, Festi D, Monti F et al: Ultrasound guided alcohol injection of small hepatic and abdominal tumors. Radiology 161:309-312, 1986

SECTION 4

MARTIN M. MALAWER
THOMAS F. DELANEY

Treatment of Metastatic Cancer to Bone

Metastatic cancer is the most common neoplasm involving the skeletal system. Of approximately 965,000 new cancer patients each year in the United States, approximately 30 to 70% will develop skeletal involvement.[1-3] Like primary bone tumors, metastatic skeletal cancer is best treated with a multimodality approach that involves the combined expertise of the medical, surgical, and radiation oncologist. Major advances have been made in the early detection, diagnosis, and surgical/radiotherapeutic treatment of metastatic bone disease. The use of bone scintigraphy, computed tomography (CT), and magnetic resonance imaging (MRI) permits extremely early detection and localization of bone lesions and aids in treatment and preoperative planning.[4-9] During the early 1970s, paralleling the development of joint replacements and the use of a bone cement, polymethylmethacrylate (PMMA), orthopedic surgeons for the first time had a relatively simple and reliable method of treating patients with pathologic fractures.[10,11] The use of PMMA and prosthetic replacements enabled the reconstruction of large tumor defects without having to depend on bone healing. This permitted immediate and reliable stabilization of tumor defects and increased early function and ambulation. As these techniques have developed, so has an interest in identifying patients at high risk for pathologic fracture, and thus the development of the concept of prophylactic fixation. Similarly, improved techniques of spinal surgery have been applied to the treatment of metastatic cancer of the spine, resulting in marked improvement in the ability to decompress and stabilize the spine involved by tumor with resultant improvement of neurologic status.[12,13]

The large majority of patients do not require surgery; radiotherapy and medical management generally suffice. Megavoltage radiation, along with radioisotopes for specific tumor types, is permitting a substantial number of patients to be treated successfully.[14-20]

This chapter concentrates on the metastatic carcinomas. Sarcomas, melanomas, and the hematogenous malignancies are described briefly. Radiographic imaging techniques, mechanisms of bony metastases and biomechanical effects, biopsy/histologic techniques, and surgical/radiotherapeutic management are described. Specific emphasis is placed on the unique considerations of the different carcinomas and of the different anatomic sites.

INCIDENCE AND ANATOMICAL SITES OF SKELETAL METASTASES

Bone metastases occur primarily to the axial skeleton and lower extremities. Abrams and co-workers analyzed 1000 consecutive autopsies of patients who died of neoplasms of epithelial origin and reported bone metastasis in 272 cases.[2] The sites of the primary tumors associated with bony metastasis were breast (73.1%), lung (32.5%), kidney (24%), rectum (13%), pancreas (13%), stomach (10.9%), colon (9.3%), and ovary (9%). Clain analyzed 2000 patients who died of cancer with bone metastasis and reported involvement of the following sites: vertebra (69%), pelvis (41%), femur (especially the hip) (25%), and skull (14%).[20] The upper extremity is much less commonly involved; approximately 10% to 15% of bony metastases occur at this site.[2]

The pattern of involvement is similar for most carcinomas, although some tumors show a propensity for specific skeletal sites (*e.g.*, prostate tumors for the pelvic bones).

Pathologic fractures that require surgical intervention occur in approximately 9% of patients with metastatic bony disease.[21] Higinbotham and Marcove reported that 165 of 1800 patients with solitary or multiple metastatic cancers to the bone treated at the Bone Tumor Service at Memorial Hospital between 1931 and 1965 required surgery for fracture.[21] One hundred fifty had metastatic carcinoma, and 15 had metastatic sarcoma or myeloma. Most of these fractures were of the femur, humerus, or both. Four types of tumors accounted for nearly 80% of the fractures: breast (53%), kidney (11%), lung (8%), and thyroid (5%). Many studies have shown a similar distribution.[2,10,11,22,23]

GENERAL CONSIDERATIONS

CLINICAL CHARACTERISTICS

The hallmark of skeletal metastases, irrespective of histogenesis, is localized pain. The pain pattern is similar to that of primary bony tumors, that is, initially intermittent, unrelated to activity, and eventually becoming continuous and unrelenting. Many metastatic lesions, however, are not painful and are detected only by radiography or bone scintigraphy.[9,24] Additional characteristics are related to the specific sites involved. Shoulder girdle metastases often present as a "frozen" shoulder, whereas thoracic and vertebral body involvement may cause referred pain to the chest wall and the lower extremities, respectively. Lumbar vertebral disease often presents as "low-back pain," sciatica, or both. The most serious complication of vertebral metastases is secondary epidural compression of the spinal cord or cauda equina. Early cord compression is heralded by increasing back pain, followed by neurologic impairment. Patients who complain of increasing back pain must be immediately evaluated for this complication. Any cancer patient who develops skeletal pain should undergo plain radiography of the affected area and bone scintigraphy.

LABORATORY EVALUATION

Laboratory evaluation for the detection of skeletal disease includes assays of serum calcium and phosphorus, alkaline and acid phosphatase, and carcinoembryonic antigen (CEA) levels. None of these tests is specific for bony metastases. Hypercalcemia is not directly related to the extent of bony disease, although patients with bony metastases often have high serum calcium levels.[3,25,26]

DIAGNOSIS

The clinical presentation, plain radiography, and bone scintigraphy findings are usually typical of metastatic disease. A confirmatory pathologic evaluation is performed by simple needle or aspiration biopsy in most anatomic sites.[7,27] In the adult, entities that may be confused with metastatic cancer are the hematologic malignancies (myeloma, leukemia, lymphoma) and Paget's disease of bone. A primary sarcoma of bone may occasionally be mistaken for a metastatic cancer; therefore, a solitary metastasis must be appropriately staged and a biopsy taken. Radiation-induced sarcomas should also be considered if a bony lesion arises in a previous radiotherapy field after an appropriate latency period.

GOALS AND TYPES OF TREATMENT

Very few skeletal metastases require surgery. Radiotherapy, chemotherapy, hormonal manipulation, or all three, provide good symptomatic relief. A pending or actual pathologic fracture requires operative fixation because fractures through a tumor-bearing bone rarely heal without such intervention.

The goals of fixation are to relieve pain, to improve function and ambulation, to facilitate medical and nursing care, and to improve psychologic well-being.[28] This requires a different surgical approach from that used for nonneoplastic lesions. Immediate fixation must be provided. A variety of techniques are in use, including replacement by a prosthesis (especially about the hip) or a combination of internal fixation combined with PMMA.[10,22,23,28] Both provide immediate stability. In general, radiotherapy is used after wound healing to arrest local tumor growth, permit bony repair, and prevent regrowth of tumor around the fixation device.

MECHANISM AND PATHOGENESIS OF SKELETAL METASTASIS

The way in which tumor cells travel to the skeletal system and establish metastases, their relationship to the primary tumor, and the way in which they destroy normal bone are poorly understood. Attempts to explain the phenomenon have focused on the unique nature of the venous system, the bony microvascular structure and, more recently, the relationship of tumor cell to bone, termed the microenvironment.[29–31]

VASCULAR AND MICROVASCULAR CONSIDERATIONS

Normal bone does not contain lymphatic channels. Skeletal metastases occur hematogenously.[29,32] The pecularities of the venous system[33–40] are considered the main pathway of mechanical transport of cancer cells to the skeletal system.

Batson[31] initially emphasized the significant role of a complex network of vertebral, epidural, and perivertebral veins, a system heretofore not appreciated or named, in the transport of cancer cells to the skeleton (Fig. 62-29).[41,42] This system parallels, joins, and also *bypasses* the other three venous systems. External pressure, not valves, determines the flow within this system. Thus, blood within this system flows in different directions, depending upon the pressure exerted by physiologic activity. This network partially explains the frequency and distribution of metastases along the vertebral column, the pelvic and shoulder girdle, and apparent "aberrant" sites. In addition, the increased susceptibility of red marrow is related to the special hemodynamic and microanatomic aspects of its vasculature.[4,29] Its unique cellu-

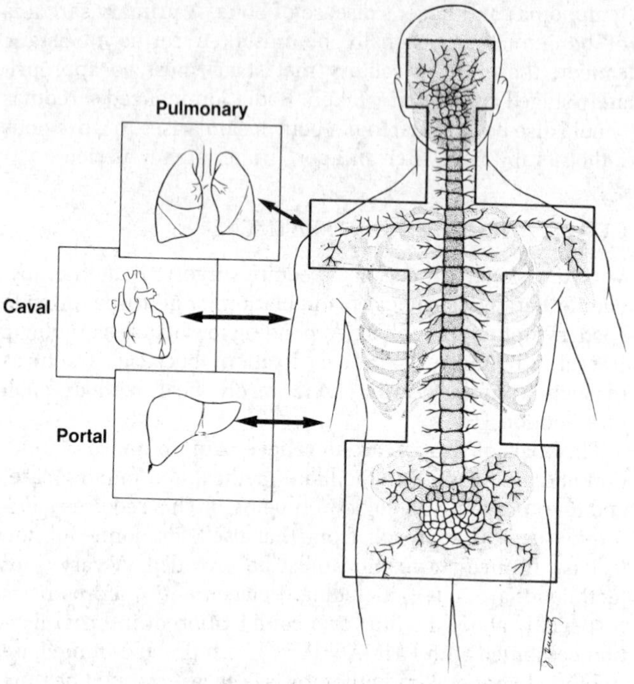

FIG. 62-29. Batson's plexus. (Modified from Batson OV: The function of the vertebral veins and their role in the spread of metastases. Ann Surg 112:138–149, 1940)

lar structure contributes to the propensity of tumor cell extravasation and to the formation of foci of tumor cells within the red marrow.[39]

TUMOR CELL–HOST BONE RELATIONSHIP

Tumor cells may destroy bone directly, produce mediators that stimulate resorption by osteoclasts, or produce other newly described mediators such as transforming growth factor (TGF) and prostaglandins (PGE_1 and PGE_2) (Fig. 62-30).[3,30,43] Much of this data comes from studies to patients with malignant hypercalcemia. Prostaglandins in bone act similarly to parathormone, that is, they stimulate cAMP, activate collagenase synthesis, and increase osteoclast number and activity.[32] Galasko demonstrated that osteoclastic proliferation and subsequent bony resorption occurred quite soon after tumor invasion.[3] An osteoclast-activating factor (OAF) has been identified (from lymphoma and myeloma cells) that might be dependent upon prostaglandins.[44] Interestingly, it has been suggested that tumor cells may have specific receptors for bone marrow.[45] Another possibility[46] is that resorbing bone itself can release chemoattractants that will cause tumor cell adherence and migration.

RADIOGRAPHIC DIAGNOSIS AND EVALUATION OF SKELETAL METASTASES

The diagnosis of metastatic cancer to the skeletal system is based upon one of several radiographic-imaging studies, followed by a definitive biopsy. The skeletal system can be easily and accurately imaged by several imaging modalities. The choice, indications, and advantages of each are summarized.

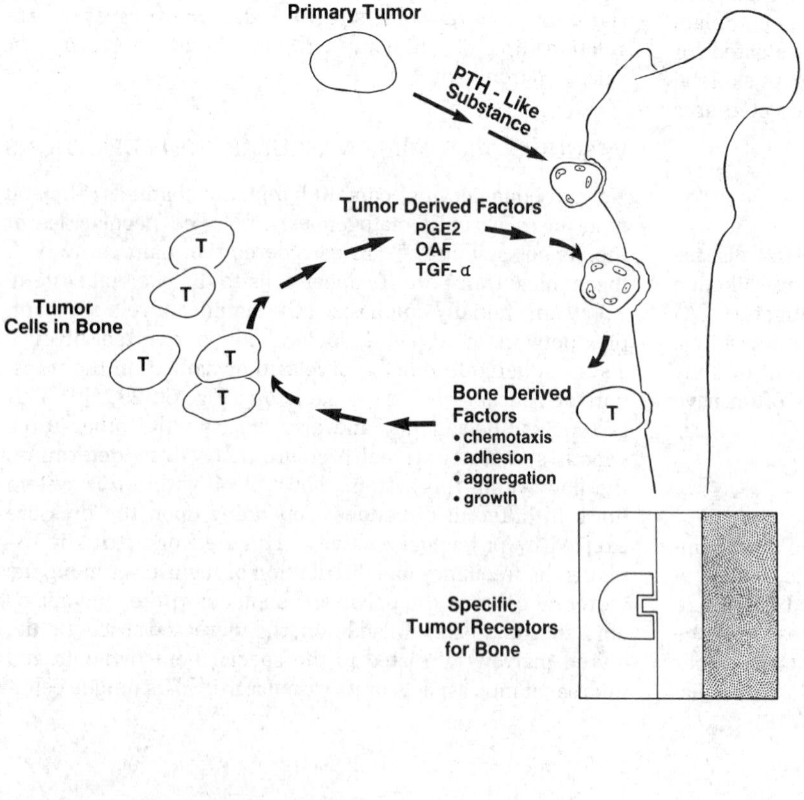

FIG. 62-30. Mechanisms of tumor cell growth and bone destruction. (Modified from Manishen WJ, Sivananthan K, Orr WF: Resorbing bone stimulates tumor cell growth. A role for the host microenvironment in bone metastasis. Am J Pathol 123:39–45, 1986)

TABLE 62-31. Radiographic Appearance of Skeletal Metastases

Primary Tumor	*Radiographic Appearance*
Common Primary Cancer	
Breast	Lytic; also mixed; frequently blastic
Lung	Lytic; also mixed; occasionally blastic
Kidney	Invariably lytic
Thyroid	Invariably lytic
Prostate	Usually blastic; occasionally lytic
Head and Neck	Usually lytic
Gastrointestinal Tract	
Esophagus	Lytic or mixed
Stomach	Lytic or mixed; occasionally blastic
Colon	Lytic or mixed; infrequently blastic
Rectum	Lytic or mixed; infrequently blastic
Pancreas	Lytic or mixed; occasionally blastic
Liver	Lytic or mixed
Gallbladder	Lytic or mixed
Genitourinary Tract	
Urinary bladder	Lytic; infrequently blastic
Adrenal	Lytic
Reproductive System	
Uterine cervix	Lytic or mixed; occasionally blastic
Uterine corpus	Lytic
Skin	
Squamous and basal cell carcinoma	Lytic
Malignant melanoma	Lytic
Carcinoid Tumors	
Bronchial and abdominal	Blastic; frequently mixed

Modified from Wilner D: Cancer metastasis to bone. In Wilner D (ed): Radiology of Bone Tumors and Allied Disorders, p 3646. Philadelphia, WB Saunders, 1982.

RADIOGRAPHY

Plain radiographs are highly accurate in differentiating metastatic carcinoma from other benign or malignant lesions of bone. Many times, no other tests may be required. Wilner acaceiisftese lesions.[47]

Location

The most common sites of metastasis are the spine, hip, and femur. When long bones are involved, the metaphyseal area and, less commonly, the mid-diaphyseal area are affected. Tumor generally reaches the medullary area before invading the cortex; primary cortical metastases are rare.

Size, Shape, and Number

Multiple bony lesions are the hallmark of metastatic disease. A solitary metastasis occurs occasionally and is difficult to differentiate from a primary bone tumor (see Chap. 42). In general, metastatic carcinomas are small (1–3 cm) and well defined. Lesions of the hip and pelvis may be larger. Appreciation of tumor size and shape, in conjunction with multiplicity, usually enables one to diagnose metastatic cancer with confidence. Extraosseous extension (*i.e.*, a soft-tissue component) rarely occurs with metastatic cancer; it is largely a characteristic of primary sarcomas of bone. Among the primary multiple tumors of bone that might be confused with metastatic carcinoma are histiocytosis, enchondromatosis, and fibrous dysplasia. Each of these tends to occur in the younger patient.

Radiographic Pattern

Bone that is invaded by metastatic cancer typically exhibits three patterns: osteolytic, osteoblastic and, less commonly, mixed (Table 62-31). A given patient may demonstrate a combination of patterns, often even within one bone. There are three types of osteolytic patterns: moth-eaten (multiple, small to medium-sized lesions that may coalesce to form large defects such as those often seen with breast cancer); diffuse infiltrative (often seen with round cell tumors such as lymphoma, neurobastoma, and Ewing's sarcoma); and large, expansile lesions (thyroid, hypernephroma); (Fig. 62-31).

Osteoblastic metastases, which are less common, are frequently seen in conjunction with cancers of the prostate and breast. They tend to be smaller than osteolytic lesions. There are three types of osteoblastic patterns: rounded, discrete (well-circumscribed, uniform density); mottled (irregular areas with varying sclerosis); and diffuse (large lesions). The osteoblastic component is *not* neoplastic osteoid tissue but, rather, represents the reaction of normal bone to the metastatic cancer. The amount and pattern of sclerosis indicate the growth rate of tumor: the denser the pattern, the slower the growth. If growth is fast, a mixed dense and lytic pattern is seen. Increasing sclerosis is a sign of repair.

Involvement of the cortex adjacent to metastatic cancer *rarely* causes periosteal elevation; when it does, one should consider cancer of the prostate or lung. In general, periosteal elevation is associated with primary bony neoplasms. In adults, primary tumors, such as Paget's sarcoma, malignant fibrous histiocytome (MFH) of bone, or primary fibrosarcoma, should be considered if periosteal elevation is present.

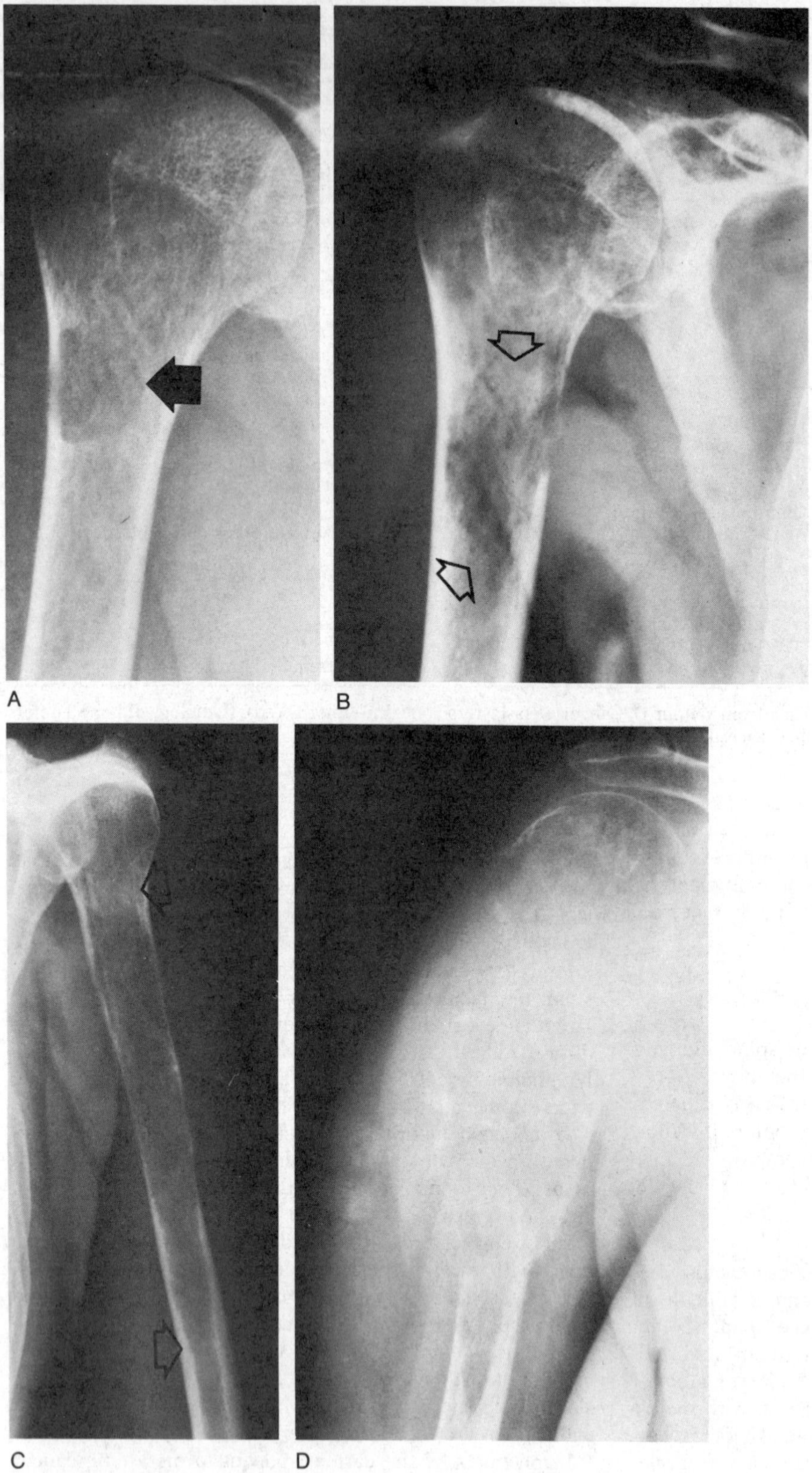

FIG. 62-31. Different radiographic patterns of osteolytic metastatic cancer. **A**. Sharply demarcated, punched-out defect (*solid arrow*) with well-delineated borders. **B**. Diffuse but well-localized lesion (*open arrows*). **C**. Large, diffuse, extensive osteolytic lesion. **D**. Large, expansile lesion, usually seen with thyroid or hypernephroma.

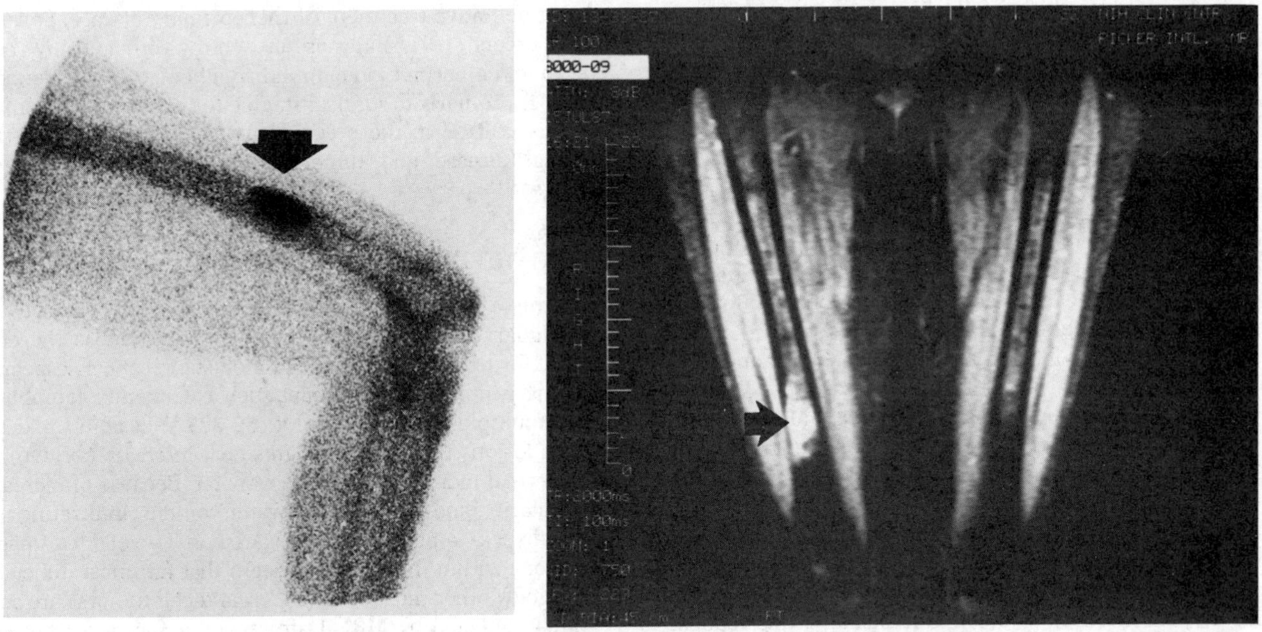

A B

FIG. 62-32. Radiographic imaging for metastatic cancer. Plain radiograph of the femur failed to demonstrate a metastatic lesion. **A**. Bone scintigraphy (lateral view) showing increased uptake in the anterior cortex of the distal femoral diaphysis. **B**. A T-2 weighted image that demonstrates an area of medullary tumor involvement seen as an area (*solid arrow*) of increased signal (*white*).

BONE SCINTIGRAPHY

Radionuclide imaging of the skeletal system is extremely useful in the diagnosis and management of the patient with skeletal metastasis.[2,8,9,24,48–50] With the development of whole-body imaging, the gamma camera, and a reliable bone imaging agent (^{99m}Tc-diphosphonate), bone scanning has become a routine method of evaluating the skeletal system for metastatic disease. It is utilized for detection and staging, for following the response of a bone lesion to treatment, and as a guide in performing needle biopsies for difficult lesions.[2,7–9,49,50]

In general, bone scans will detect metastatic lesions before they are evident on plain radiographs (Fig. 62-32). Wilner estimates that bone scans will detect lesions about 3 months earlier than plain radiographs.[47] Galasko reported a range of 2 months to 18 months, with 75% of breast cancer patients developing corresponding changes within 6 months.[32] Bone scans are most reliable for tumors of the breast, prostate, lung, and kidney. They are least accurate for the diagnosis of round cell tumors, myeloma, lymphoma, and the leukemias.[32] Areas of *decreased* uptake ("photopenic" areas) are often observed with myeloma and, occasionally, with breast and lung cancers.

The Solitary Lesion

A unique problem with bone scintigraphy in following patients with a known cancer is the appearance of a solitary lesion. This occurs in 6% and 8% of all patients.[9] McNeil reviewed 273 reports of such cases and reported that 55% represented metastatic disease.[9] Trauma (25%), infection (10%), and miscellaneous factors (10%) accounted for the nonmalignant causes. McNeil emphasized that anatomic site is important in this differentiation; 80% of the vertebral lesions, compared with 18% of the rib lesions, proved to be metastatic in patients with a known primary tumor. If scintigraphy reveals a solitary lesion, additional evaluation, including high-resolution plain radiographs. CT and possible biopsy, is recommended.

Bone Scan-Guided Needle Biopsy

Within the past few years, several reports have described the use of bone scintigraphy as an aid to biopsy.[7,8] The scan may be used to mark an area of abnormality before biopsy or may confirm that the correct area has been biopsied intraoperatively. These techniques have enhanced the accuracy of the biopsy in patients in whom other modalities have not demonstrated a lesion. Zegel and associates described a technique of localizing "hot" rib lesions with nuclear medicine guidance by the use of a lead ring.[7] Percutaneous biopsies reported in conjunction with positive scans revealed that 13 of 14 patients had metastatic tumor. Little and co-workers described a technique of marking the suspected rib under scintigraphic control with methylene blue and surgically excising the marked area.[8] None of their 15 patients had a grossly identifiable lesion, yet 10 patients had metastatic disease. Abnormal scans in the remainder had nonneoplastic causes. A portable gamma camera has been used in the operating room to localize a lesion following a preoperative injection of ^{99mm}Tc-diphosphonate for deeper structures (hip, femur, acetabulum). It avoids false-negative biopsies of these lesions.

Evaluation of Response to Treatment

Bone scan activity of a metastatic bony lesion generally decreases after chemotherapy/hormone therapy or radiotherapy, if a response is obtained.[9] Plain radiographs may demonstrate bone healing and reossification within a few months. The limitation of plain radiographs is that only a small percentage will show reossification, and changes in the osteoblastic lesions are difficult to determine. With bone scintigraphy, one can compare the activity. Most experience has been obtained with breast cancer patients. Healing is indicated as a decrease in activity. Approximately 10% to 15% of patients will demonstrate a "flare" phenomenon, that is, a period of increased uptake lasting 2 to 5 months as the lesions begins to reossify.[9] This increased uptake is presumably due to new, nonneoplastic reparative bone attempting to heal the tumor defect. Occasionally, this reponse is associated with pain. After this period, a repeat bone scan will show decreased uptake with no new lesions. In rare cases, previously unappreciated lesions will ossify, suggesting a new lesion; in retrospect, these can usually be identified as old lesions.

Quantitative Bone Scanning

Quantitative bone scanning (QBS) is a technique used to measure changes in bone scans to avoid the variations obtained in routine scintigraphy. The proportion of increased uptake in the diseased region is compared with the average uptake in the normal regions.[6] It gives an objective measurement of the change of activity in any region relative to the normal for a given patient. This technique has been used for comparing response to treatment in patients with metastatic as well as other diseases. Drelichman and colleagues described ten patients with prostate carcinoma in whom sequential QBS was performed.[6] Those patients with more than a 50% average decrease had a partial remission, as defined by their criteria. All patients had an increase within the first month (corresponding to the flare phenomenon), and no significant decrease occurred until 3 months. Similar results have been obtained with patients with breast carcinoma.

COMPUTED TOMOGRAPHY

Computed tomography (CT) has not been used in the evaluation of metastatic skeletal cancer as commonly as it has in other organ systems, although the literature of the usefulness of CT for malignant and benign primary bony neoplasms is extensive. Recently, CT has been shown to be useful in evaluating "hot" spots to confirm the presence of metastatic or other disease.[5] During and co-workers evaluated 44 breast cancer patients with positive bone scans and negative radiographs; 25 of these patients presented with solitary hot spots on bone scans, and 19 became positive after definitive treatment of their primary disease. Seventy-six percent (19/25) of those presenting with a positive bone scan and a normal radiograph had a benign cause identified by CT. Similarly to surgical staging for primary bony tumors, CT is utilized in the preoperative evaluation of metastatic spinal disease and tumors of the pelvis (see Surgical Stage).[51]

MAGNETIC RESONANCE IMAGING

Magnetic resonance imaging (MRI) accurately images the medullary (marrow) component of bone and is therefore ideal for the early detection of metastatic cancer, especially primary infiltrative neoplasms such as leukemia, lymphoma, and multiple myeloma (see Fig. 62-32).[4,5] Its ability to detect such lesions is due to the high signal intensity (brightness) of normal marrow, which is mostly fat. Because of increased cellularity, and thus a higher water content, infiltrating neoplasms will appear as a darker area on T_1-weighted images. Lesions within the skeletal system that are most difficult to image by other modalities (*e.g.*, round cell tumors) are accurately detected by MRI. Daffner and associates reported a prospective study of 80 patients with known malignancies; 50 had suspected metastases and 30 had multiple myeloma.[5] All patients were evaluated with plain radiographs, bone scintigraphy, and MRI. Of the 50 patients with suspected metastases based on bone scintigraphy,40 (80%) were shown to have disease. Ten (20%) had no evidence of metastasis, and the abnormalities on bone scintigraphy were shown to be due to other causes. Of the 30 patients with multiple myeloma, 6 (20%) had positive scans, 20 (67%) had abnormal radiographs, and 11 (37%) had abnormal CT scans. The MRI scan demonstrated abnormalities in all 30 patients; these were confirmed by needle aspiration. These authors emphasize the importance of correlating MRI with other studies, because infection, infarction, and other entities can also yield a decreased signal. In general, they recommend that MRI studies of the coronal sections of the pelvis and hips and the sagittal sections of the spine (*i.e.*, the hematopoietic-active sites) be performed when evaluating for metastatic cancer.

ANGIOGRAPHY

Angiography is rarely used for diagnosis of metastases to bone. Its main use is for preoperative assessment of large lesions and for embolization of vascular tumor (see Surgical Management).[52–55]

BIOMECHANICAL AND HEALING CONSIDERATIONS OF TUMOR DEFECTS AND PATHOLOGIC FRACTURES

BIOMECHANICAL CONSIDERATIONS

The strength of normal bone depends upon the continuity of the cortex and the underlying medullary/metaphyseal trabecular structure.[56,57] The torsional (rotational), compres-

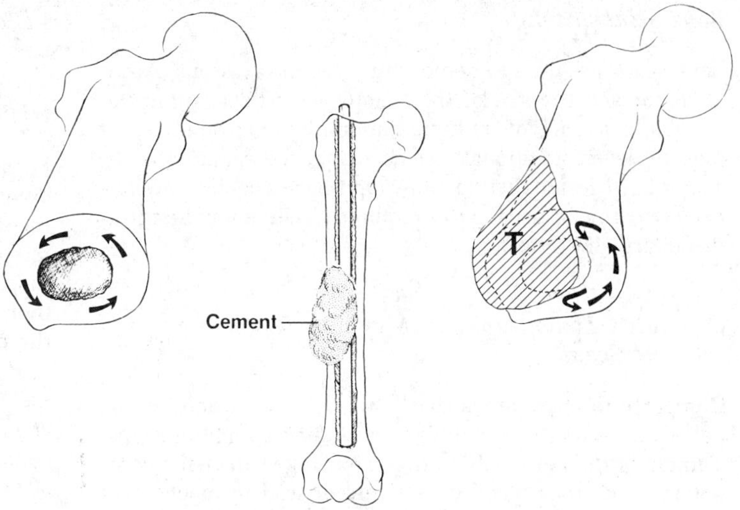

FIG. 62-33. Schematic demonstrating the biomechanical basis of intramedullary fixation of a bone with a large tumor defect. The normal rotational stress forces (*curved arrows*) are transmitted by the cortex in a uniform manner. A tumor defect (*T*) causes a stress riser that weakens the bone by 70% to 90% in torsion (rotation). The bone can be reconstructed by removing the tumor and reconstructing the defect with a combination of polymethylmethacrylate (PMMA) and intramedullary (IM) rod fixation.

sive, and bending forces are transmitted and absorbed by both components. A typical metastatic lesion of a long bone destroys a segment of the medullary structure and the corresponding cortical bone (Fig. 62-33). Cortical defects greatly weaken a bone, especially to torsional forces. A defect whose length is less than the diameter of the bone (termed a "stress riser") decreases torsional strength by 70%, whereas a defect larger than the diameter of the bone (termed an "open section" and the most common defect encountered clinically) effects a 90% reduction in strength.[56,57] The aim of an orthopedic procedure is to convert an open section to a closed section to allow substantial axial and torsional loads to be carried.

HEALING CONSIDERATIONS

The determinants of bony union following a pathologic fracture are quite different from those associated with nonneoplastic fracture. Bony union almost never occurs without surgical or radiotherapeutic treatment. Although pathologic fractures are quite common, few investigators have evaluated the rate and determinants of union. Gainor and Buchert reviewed 129 fractures of long bones in 123 patients treated between 1955 and 1979.[58] The overall healing rate was 36% (45 of 129 fractures). Individual healing rates were multiple myeloma (67%), hypernephroma (44%), and breast cancer (37%). None of the patients with lung cancer healed. The length of patient survival was the main determinant of fracture healing. Fracture healing was found to be multifactorial. Determinants of bony union of pathologic fractures are summarized in the following:[58]

1. *Type of Tumor:* Lung and colorectal tumors and melanomas tend not to heal. Multiple myelomas, tumors of the breast, and hypernephromas have the highest rate of healing.
2. *Type of Fixation:* Internal fixation combined with PMMA significantly increases the chance of osseous union.
3. *Duration of Survival:* Longer survival (more than six months) increases the rate of union.
4. *Amount of Postoperative Radiotherapy:* High-dose postoperative radiotherapy (greater than 3000–3500 rad) is associated with poorer healing.
5. *Effects of Chemotherapy:* There is little evidence on the impact of chemotherapy on bony repair.

PREOPERATIVE EVALUATION, LOCAL STAGING, AND BIOPSY CONSIDERATIONS

PREOPERATIVE CONSIDERATIONS

Special preoperative considerations are needed in cases of metastasis to bone because these patients often have extensive underlying metabolic, hematologic, and nutritional deficits. The risk of infection is increased because of multiple sources of possible sepsis (*e.g.,* colostomy, urinary tract infection), neutropenia from chemotherapy or other adjuvant modalities, and poor local skin condition from prior radiotherapy or other procedures. Perioperative antibiotics are recommended for all patients. All patients should have hematologic and clotting evaluation. Adequate blood replacement should be available because curettage of many carcinomas, especially myeloma, thyroid tumor, and renal cell carcinoma, often leads to substantial blood loss. Thrombocytopenia occasionally occurs intraoperatively and should be monitored. Disseminated intravascular coagulation (DIC) may occur.[59]

PREOPERATIVE-STAGING STUDIES

Evaluations of the extent of local disease, the amount of bone involved, and the presence of multiple lesions within the same bone are necessary to determine the optimal surgical approach, the amount of tumor to be removed, and the method of reconstruction. In general, the following studies are utilized; however, there is much variation, depending upon the unique considerations of the individual patient and tumor location and type.

Bone Scintigraphy

Bone scans are used to demonstrate the intraosseous extent of tumor and the site of the lesions and to determine the possible existence of multiple tumors. It is extremely common to detect additional lesions within the same bone. In general, all lesions within the same bone require simultaneous treatment; usually this requires placement of an intramedullary (IM) rod.

Computed Tomography or Magnetic Resonance Imaging Scans

Computed tomography is usually required for lesions of the pelvis and spine; it is rarely required for extremity lesions. Tumors of the bony pelvis often have large soft-tissue components that may bleed excessively or lead to mechanical failure of reconstruction if they are not recognized preoperatively. Vertebral body lesions are best evaluated by CT, MRI, or both. The amount of destruction and extent of epidural disease are best estimated on these studies (see Treatment of Vertebral Lesions).[13,51,60] Soft-tissue components rarely occur with carcinomas of the extremities; however, they are common with metastatic sarcoma (*e.g.*, primary sarcomas), some hypernephromas, and melanomas.

Angiography

Angiography is not routinely performed; specific indications are pelvic tumors with large extraosseous components and lesions in which preoperative embolization is considered. Patients with metastatic hypernephroma should undergo angiography with embolization.[52–54,61,62]

BIOPSY: TECHNIQUE AND CONSIDERATIONS

There are three situations in which a biopsy is warranted: to confirm metastatic disease in a patient with a known primary tumor; to evaluate a "suspicious" radiographic lesion; and to obtain tissue for hormonal/immunohistochemical evaluation. The technique of biopsy varies, depending upon the tumor location and specific answers sought.

In general, needle aspiration and cytologic evaluation can reliably confirm the diagnosis of cancer.[8,59,63,64] If the radiograph demonstrates a lesion, a biopsy should be performed under fluoroscopic guidance. Permanent x-ray films should be obtained to document that the correct area has been sampled. Several aspirations or cores should be obtained. The material should routinely be sent for culture, because indolent infections occasionally can present as metastatic lesions. Frozen sections or touch preparations should be obtained to determine the types of cells present. If the primary tumor is unknown, sufficient tissue should be obtained for special stains (see following section), especially immunohistochemical studies. This may require a large sample. If there is excessive bleeding, Gel-foam or PMMA should be packed into the defect. One must not assume that all "solitary" lesions in the adult are metastatic. A solitary lesion in the adult without a known primary tumor must be approached as if it were a primary sarcoma, despite the apparent "metastatic" appearance. The biopsy must be in line with the potential possible resection incision (see Chap. 42).

Histology

For most patients, the histologic diagnosis of metastatic carcinoma to bone is easily established. This depends on the recognition of squamous patterns of glandular structures, features of which are highly typical of the carcinomas that most frequently metastasize to bone. This diagnosis is further facilitated when representative microscopic slides from the primary neoplasm are available for comparison.

Metastatic, poorly differentiated carcinomas, and some melanomas, particularly those containing abundant spindled and pleomorphic cells, can closely mimic primary bone sarcomas such as fibrosarcoma or MFH. This pitfall is most often encountered with renal cell carcinoma. The application of selected histochemical studies to demonstrate cellular products has been helpful to confirm the presumption of metastatic carcinoma and to aid in determining the source of an unknown primary lesion. Alcian blue and mucicarmine stains will reveal the presence of epithelial mucins that are present in some adenocarcinomas of the breast, lung, and gastrointestinal tract. Abundant cytoplasmic glycogen typically occurs in renal cell carcinoma, as well as in some clear cell neoplasms from other organs. The demonstration of cytoplasmic melanin granules with the Fontana stain supports the diagnosis of melanoma.

The recent development of immunohistochemical techniques that can be applied to paraffin-embedded tissues has created a powerful diagnostic tool.[65,66] With this procedure, peroxidase-conjugated antibodies, directed against a variety of known antigenic markers, are detected at antibody–antigen reaction sites by the addition of peroxidase-sensitive chromogens. For example, an epithelial tumor (carcinoma) can contain a variety of cytokeratins, epithelial membrane antigen, or carcinoembryonic antigen. The application of an appropriately selected panel of antibodies will produce a recognizable pattern of positive staining of tumor cells that confirms the presence of carcinoma.[67] Similarly, there are antibodies available to identify specific markers of neuroendocrine tumors and melanoma (anti-S100 protein and anti–melanoma-specific antigens).[68] Both metastatic adenocarcinoma of the prostate and metastatic follicular carcinoma of the thyroid can appear quite similar. Immunohistochemical studies to detect either prostatic-specific acid phosphatase or thyroglobulin, respectively, will usually resolve this problem in differential diagnosis.[69] It must be noted, however, that immunohistochemical techniques require meticulous methodology and are fraught with numerous artifacts and interpretive pitfalls.[70]

PRINCIPLES OF SURGICAL TREATMENT FOR SKELETAL METASTASIS

Within the past 20 years, the surgical treatment of metastatic cancer involving the skeletal system has undergone dramatic change as a result of the development of techniques to replace and stabilize large segments of abnormal bone.[11,19a,21,22,28,33,60,71] These techniques have been paralleled by developments in total joint replacements as well as by procedures developed by the orthopedic oncologist in the treatment of primary bone tumors. Prosthetic replacements now permit the removal and immediate reconstruction of destroyed bone.[23] The use of PMMA, when combined with various metallic plates, rods, or prosthesis, or a combination, permits immediate filling and reconstruction of large defects and immediate stabilization.

The common local surgical procedures for metastatic tumors of the extremities are

1. *Composite osteosynthesis:* Curettage of tumor combined with internal fixation, either bone plates and screws (composite osteosynthesis) or intramedullary fixation with IM rods. This technique is most often used for the shafts (diaphysis) of long bones, most commonly, the humerus and femur.[22,28,71]
2. *Hemijoint replacement:* Resection of a joint with reconstruction by an endoprosthesis combined with PMMA. This technique is most often used for tumors of the hip.[23]
3. *Segmental resection:* Resection of a large segment of bone combined with custom segmental prosthetic replacement and PMMA. This technique is less common and involves substantially more surgical morbidity. It is most often used when no significant bone remains that can be reconstructed by the foregoing techniques.
4. *Cryosurgery:* Cryosurgery may be combined with any of the preceding procedures to increase local tumor control and control hemorrhage.[71,72]
5. *Amputations:* Amputations are occasionally necessary to control serious complications of extremity lesions, usually following inadequate tumor control.[73]

The general principles of management of pathologic or pending fractures are

1. Preoperative embolization for suspected vascular lesions
2. Perioperative antibiotics
3. Adequate hematologic evaluation and blood and component replacement
4. Modification of standard incisions, if necessary, to avoid prior radiation fields and to provide adequate soft-tissue coverage and closure to ensure healing
5. Curettage and removal of all gross disease, if possible
6. Composite reconstruction with internal fixation or prosthetic replacement and PMMA; assurance that PMMA fills the defect and extends proximal and distal to the abnormal area
7. Postoperative radiotherapy for local control

AMPUTATIONS

Amputations are rarely required today for metastatic cancer. Occasionally, radical amputation is indicated when advanced cancer of an extremity results in uncontrollable, intractable pain, a necrotic or functionless extremity, fungation and sepsis, or erosion and hemorrhage of a major vessel at the tumor site. These complications occur following inadequate tumor control. Elimination of pain and sepsis with restoration of function may be achieved by amputation.[73]

CRYOSURGERY

Cryosurgery is the use of liquid nitrogen as a surgical adjunct to tumor curettage to freeze (cryonecrosis) any residual tumor cells. The aim is to enhance local control.[71,72,74] Necrosis is obtained by a double or triple freeze-thaw cycle requiring temperatures between −20° and −40°C. Marcove at Memorial Hospital has treated several hundred patients with this technique since 1964.[71,72] It is useful for tumors that have recurred despite radiotherapy and those in difficult anatomic locations and in the treatment of hypernephromas.

GENERAL PRINCIPLES OF RADIATION THERAPY FOR SKELETAL METASTASIS

Radiation is an effective treatment for cancer that has metastasized to bone. Aims of treatment include pain relief, improved ambulation, and arrest of local tumor growth. With thoughtful treatment planning and megavoltage equipment, treatment can usually be delivered with minimal morbidity. The efforts of the radiation oncologist should be closely coordinated with those of other physicians and health care personnel. Careful consideration of the nature of the patient's disease is important in determining the most appropriate radiation therapy strategy and technique.

In the patient with symptoms of disease at multiple sites, a reasonable approach is to treat the most symptomatic areas with radiation.[25] If effective chemotherapy or hormonal therapy is available, they should be employed. The goal of treatment is to eliminate or greatly reduce the need for narcotics. If there is a single site of metastatic disease, appropriate radiation therapy may render the patient disease-free for an extended period.

TREATMENT PLANNING

The radiation fields should be planned using data from the history and physical examination, the bone scan, plain skeletal films and, where indicated, myelograms, CT scans and MRI (see Staging Studies). Soft-tissue masses, most often associated with bony metastases to the vertebral bodies or pelvis, must be included in the radiotherapy fields. The distribution of bone marrow is an important consideration, because irradiation for bony metastases will suppress hematopoiesis in the treatment field (see Table 62-32). Bone marrow suppression secondary to irradiation is more significant in patients who have received or are receiving myelosuppressive chemotherapy. Blood counts should be monitored closely during treatment. All previous radiation treatment portals must be reviewed. Damage to normal tissue can result from improperly matched or overlapping fields.

Lesions not responding to treatment should prompt another review of the diagnostic studies, particularly in a patient with multiple metastases in which a lesion not in the treatment field might, in fact, be causing persistent symptoms. Another possibility is that a soft-tissue mass adjacent to the bony lesion being radiated is not completely encompassed by the treatment field.

TABLE 62-32. Marrow Distribution in the Adult

Anatomical Site	*% of Total Red Marrow*
Head	13.1
Cranium	12.0
Mandible	1.1
Upper Limbs	8.3
2 humeri	2.0
2 scapulae	4.8
2 clavicles	1.5
Sternum	2.3
Ribs	7.9
Vertebrae	42.3
Cervical	3.4
Thoracic	14.1
Lumbar	10.9
Sacrum	13.9
Lower Limb Girdle	26.1
2 os coxae	22
	4

Extracted from Ellis RE: The distribution of active bone marrow in the adult. Phys Med Biol 5:255, 1961.

PAIN RELIEF

Approximately 80% to 90% of patients undergoing radiotherapy for pain from osseous metastases will have partial pain relief; 50% will have complete relief.[75-82] Most patients will begin to experience some response 10 to 14 days after the start of therapy. In one study, 70% of patients experienced pain relief by 2 weeks after the completion of treatment; 90% had relief within 1 to 3 months.[81] A sudden increase in pain during treatment should raise concern about a pathologic fracture, and appropriate films and orthopedic evaluation should be done. In a recent study, 70% of patients experiencing pain relief did not develop recurrent pain in the treatment field.[75] Another group noted sustained relief of pain in 55% to 65% of patients in the first year after treatment.[83]

In spite of the clinical impression that painful osseous metastases from the thyroid, lung, and kidney are more difficult to palliate with radiation, several small, nonrandomized studies failed to document any clear differences in overall response rates among different histologic types.[81,83,84] It was observed, however, that the time to achieve pain relief following treatment was longer with slowly proliferating tumors such as prostate cancer.[84] The final report from the large, randomized study by Radiation Therapy Oncology Group indicated that a significantly higher percentage of patients with metastases from breast and prostate primaries achieved complete pain relief when compared with patients with lung and other primaries. The sites of metastases have not been shown to correlate with the degree of pain relief.[18,75] Severe and frequent pain has been shown to be a poor prognostic feature.[75]

BONE HEALING

Radiation will necessarily affect both tumor and adjacent bone. The presence of tumor is a greater threat to the structural integrity of bone that the adverse effects of radiation on bone healing. Bone reossification will often occur after tumor eradication. Seventy-eight percent of osteolytic lesions treated in one study recalcified, and another 15% showed no further progression after radiation therapy.[80,85,86] In a study of bone reformation at the base of the skull after irradiation for carcinoma of the nasopharynx, 11 patients showed apparent bone reformation within 4 to 6 months of treatment.[87] These patients received treatment with doses of 5000 to 7000 rad, which are higher than those used in patients treated for metastatic lesions to the bone.

DOSE, FRACTIONATION, AND TYPES OF RADIATION

There is considerable debate among radiotherapists about the best approach for treating metastatic lesions to the bone. The radiation dose and the duration over which it should be delivered are major considerations. In patients with metastatic cancer in whom life expectancy is limited, one would like to deliver effective treatment with minimal morbidity over as short a time span as possible. One cooperative group studied pain relief in 759 patients randomized to a variety of dose-fractionation schedules: 270 cGy $\times$ 15 fractions, 300 $\times$ 10, 300 $\times$ 5, 400 $\times$ 5, and 500 $\times$ 5.[75] No significant difference in response was seen, although a subsequent independent reanalysis of the data suggested that the protracted fractionation schemes (270 $\times$ 15 or 300 $\times$ 10) were more effective.[87] Four retrospective studies of single (400–1500 rad) versus multiple (2000–4000 rad) treatment regimens have not shown any striking differences between the two.[16,17,80,88] A prospective randomized trial comparing single and multifractionation regimens is under way at the Royal Marsden Hospital in London.[79]

It might be considered expedient to give a single large fraction to a debilitated patient for whom resected, daily trips for treatment will be burdensome, yet single treatments with large fractions are poorly tolerated to such sites as the abdomen and brain. Hence, each radiotherapist must consider the site of disease, the patient's performance and social situation, and any normal tissue in the treatment field in deciding upon a treatment regimen. Patients with one or few sites of metastases and who have a good performance status and a primary disease that responds to systemic therapy may live for many years after irradiation for bony pain. Therefore, large fractions that are known to produce more late effects in normal tissue must be used with considerable caution, especially when radiation fields include the brain, spinal cord, kidneys, or significant portions of the liver or bowel. Such patients may survive long enough to have problems with recurrent tumor in bones that have not been radiated to high doses.

It has been difficult to demonstrate a clear dose–response relationship in treatment of bone metastases because the populations studied have been heterogeneous and have had different types of neoplasms and survival times after treatment. For patients whose expected survival after palliative radiotherapy is short, a high dose is less important because they do not survive long enough to manifest recurrent tumor.[89] Hence, in patients expected to live for a long time with metastatic disease, higher doses (4000–5000 rad) fractionated at 200 rad/day are recommended.

HEMIBODY IRRADIATION

Sequential hemibody irradiation has been proposed as an alternative to fractionated radiotherapy directed at specific sites of metastatic disease in patients with widely disseminated bony metastases.[15,18] It is designed to spare the patient with multiple sites of metastatic disease repeated trips to the hospital. One study reported complete relief of pain in 21% and partial relief in 77% of patients, most of whom had breast, prostate, or lung cancer.[15] Pain control was achieved rapidly, with half of these patients experiencing relief noting improvement within 2 days. Patients received 600 to 800 rad of irradiation to either the upper, middle, or lower portions of the body. Patients with metastases of the upper body were hospitalized for a day, hydrated, and premedicated with antiemetics and corticosteroids: those undergoing mid- and lower-body therapy were premedicated as outpatients to minimize nausea and vomiting. Treatment to the lower and midbody was tolerated relatively well, with severe or life-threatening nausea and vomiting, diarrhea, or hematologic toxicity occurring in 2%, 6%, and 8% of patients, respectively. Upper-body treatment induced severe or life-threatening nausea and vomiting, fever, or hematologic toxicity in 15%, 4%, and 32% of the patients, respectively. Hematologic complications were worse in patients who had received prior intensive courses of chemotherapy and had started treatment with low peripheral blood counts. There were no fatalities related to treatment, yet side-effects as just described were prominent, especially with the upper-body treatment. Such treatment should be undertaken only in centers prepared to support patients who encounter these treatment-induced complications.

SYSTEMIC RADIOISOTOPES

Systemically administered radioisotopes have been used to palliate pain caused by osseous metastases. Iodine-131 can provide pain relief in patients with well-differentiated thyroid carcinoma, whereas radioactive phosphorus (^{32}P) and subsequently strontium-89 (^{89}Sr), and iodine-131 (^{131}I) diphosphonates have been used for bone metastases from other primary sites. Phosphorus-32 has been administered to patients with metastatic prostate and breast cancers after priming with testosterone or parathyroid hormone to increase uptake into neoplastic tissue.[19a,91–94] Response rates and durations reported have been similar to those noted for sequential hemibody irradiation. Both methods induce significant bone marrow depression, but ^{32}P treatment does not have the concomitant risk of significant nausea, vomiting, pneumonitis, and alopecia seen with hemibody irradiation.[93] Phosphorus-32 therapy following testosterone administration, however, has been reported to cause transient exacerbation of pain, irreversible morbidity, such as spinal cord compression, or even death.[92,94] These complications are thought to be secondary to the administration of testosterone.

More recently, several groups have employed ^{89}Sr, a bone-seeking radionuclide with a lower energy β than ^{32}P. Two groups reported favorable response rates ranging from 72% to 91%, whereas a third institution noted improvement in 51% of patients so treated.[95–97] Much less toxicity has been reported in these patients, because testosterone administration is not required and marrow dose is lower with the lower energy β. Because toxicity was minimal, this isotope may prove to be a useful adjuvant therapy for palliation of pain from metastatic bone lesions. A recent Phase I study of ^{131}I-labeled diphosphonates, another radionuclide with a high affinity for bone, showed complete pain relief in 44% of patients, substantial pain relief in 6%, minimal improvement in 22%, and no change in 28%. Systemic and marrow toxicity was minimal.[19b]

SPECIFIC TUMORS: UNIQUE CLINICAL AND MANAGEMENT CONSIDERATIONS

In general, the medical management of bony metastases is similar to that of disseminated disease for each individual type.[97] The unique clinical characteristics and surgical and radiotherapeutic aspects of management of bony metastases are summarized for the most common tumors.

BREAST CANCER

Between 50% and 85% of all breast cancer patients will develop bony metastases.[2,9,32,49,50,98] In general, bony lesions respond well to radiotherapy, hormonal therapy, or chemotherapy.[75,97]

Radiation therapy is recommended for lesions not responding to endocrine or chemotherapy, for sites of pathologic fracture after fixation, and for areas such as the femoral neck and vertebral bodies, which are prone to complication in the event of tumor progression. The intent of radiation therapy should be to provide long-term control of symptomatic sites and to avoid late complications to normal tissue. This generally means fractionated, high-dose treatment to appropriately planned fields treated on megavoltage machines. To avoid any injury to normal tissue, one should be aware of any overlap with previous radiation fields involving the breast or draining nodal areas. Early (prophylactic) surgery is recommended for large lesions of their hip or femur to avoid fracture (see Prophylactic Fixation), especially, those that remain symptomatic despite radiotherapy. Pathologic fractures of the long bones are treated by a combination of intramedullary rod fixation combined with PMMA. A subgroup of breast cancer patients (with skeletal metastases only) has been recently described.[14,99,100] Because of their prolonged survival, it is recommended that these patients undergo aggressive management of skeletal metastases.[14]

RENAL CELL CARCINOMA (HYPERNEPHROMA)

Approximately one-fourth of patients with hypernephroma develop bony metastases.[101–103] One significant surgical consideration of metastatic hypernephromas is that they are extremely vascular; life-threatening hemorrhage can easily occur from a small incision. A second consideration is that unlike other metastatic carcinomas, hypernephromas are often associated with a large extraosseous component. Thus, before any surgical intervention, CT and angiography are recommended. Biopsy of a suspected hypernephroma should only be undertaken after careful planning; a needle biopsy is recommended. If an open biopsy is required, preoperative embolization should be performed. The need for surgery is indicated by large lesions, progressive bony destruction, instability, or pending fracture. Preoperative embolization and proximal vascular control is mandatory to avoid extensive hemorrhage.[45,62] Cryosurgery has been used as a surgical adjuvant in decreasing bleeding and in increasing local tumor control.[104–105] Palliative embolization alone (without surgery) for large tumors, especially those of the pelvis, has been reported to effect good pain relief.[62] Transient increases in pain and fever may occur as a postinfarction syndrome.

Many radiotherapists believe that the pain from renal cell carcinoma metastatic to bone is difficult to palliate. Experience at the National Cancer Institute indicates that adequate palliation has been achieved in most sites with moderate- to high-dose, fractionated radiation.[106] Extensive recurrences in the renal fossa with involvement of adjacent vertebral bodies, spinal cord, or nerve root may be difficult to palliate because doses administered to the adjacent spinal cord and bowel must be limited.

COLORECTAL CARCINOMA

Skeletal metastases (4%) occur infrequently from colorectal cancer; when they do, it is usually late in the course of the disease.[107] The most common sites of metastases are the lumbar spine and sacrum. Radiotherapy is the most effective mode of palliation in these anatomic sites.[108] Long bone fractures are rare.

LUNG CARCINOMA

Metastatic bony disease occurs in 20% to 40% of these patients.[102a,109] Palliative radiotherapy is usually successful: 3000 rad in 10 fractions is frequently employed. Fractures are less common in these patients than in others with osteolytic lesions, probably because the bony lesions do not have time to grow. When fractures do occur, treatment is similar to the other carcinomas.[22]

THYROID CANCER

McCormack reported bone metastases in 33 of 259 patients (12.7%) with thyroid cancer.[110] Most metastatic bony lesions can be treated with radioisotopes or external irradiation.

Well-differentiated thyroid tumors, follicular carcinomas, and some papillary tumors often retain their affinity for iodine. Thus, it is possible to deliver localized, radioactive ^{131}I to these lesions when they have metastasized to bone after appropriate ablation of normal thyroid by surgery. (see Fig. 62-37).[19a,20] Effective treatment with ^{131}I usually requires several doses given at 3-month intervals. Hence, sites of severe bone pain should be managed with local external beam radiation to achieve early pain relief.[33] For thyroid lesions that do not take up iodine, external beam irradiation usually provides relief. Pathologic fracture is rare. If surgery is required, bleeding may be excessive. Preoperative angiography and embolization may be useful. In the rare situation of a solitary bony metastasis, Niederle and co-workers have recommended surgical removal in lieu of radioiodine, especially for follicular or papillary carcinoma.[111]

MELANOMA

Stewart and associates reported an overall incidence of bony involvement of 6.9%.[112] The authors emphasized that these patients may not go through the sequential stage devised for the characterization of melanomas; approximately half of these patients were clinically Stage I before the detection of a bony lesion. Bone involvement is a grave prognosis; mean survival was only 3.6 months.[113] They strongly recommended nonoperative management unless the fracture was unstable, because radiotherapy provided good symptomatic relief and expected survival was short.

PROSTATE CANCER

Metastatic prostate cancer most often involves the axial skeleton and pelvis. Typically, bony metastases are osteoblastic (dense), multiple, and small. Occasionally, difficulty arises in distinguishing Paget's disease from metastatic lesions, and a solitary metastasis from a primary sarcoma. Acid phosphatase is almost always elevated in the presence of bony metastases and is helpful in these differentiations. Pathologic fractures tend not to occur because of the osteoblastic reaction. Despite the frequency of prostate cancer, only 4% of patients in most large series of pathologic fractures have prostate cancer.[9,10,22,23] Prophylactic surgery is rarely required.[19a,91,93,94]

LEUKEMIA, LYMPHOMA, AND MYELOMA

The leukemias and lymphomas, although exquisitely sensitive to radiation, are usually managed with systemic chemotherapy when metastases are present. Pathologic fractures are uncommon except with multiple myeloma. If surgery is required, the major problem is excessive bleeding because of thrombocytopenia, unexpected coagulopathy and, rarely, disseminated intravascular coagulopathy. Multiple myeloma tends to be notoriously vascular.

Should a metastasis involve a vertebral body with potential compromise of the spinal cord or nerve roots, localized radiation is recommended. Sites refractory to drug therapy can also be irradiated. For the indolent lymphomas and the leukemias, 2000 to 2500 rad should provide excellent palliation. For the aggressive lymphomas, doses in the 3000 to 4000 rad range should be used. Radiation treatment can provide excellent palliation for patients with symptomatic bony disease from multiple myeloma.[75–77]

SARCOMAS

Pathologic fractures through a primary sarcoma of bone is rare. In general, a pathologic fracture through a spindle cell sarcoma requires an amputation (see Bone Sarcomas). In general, radiotherapy offers good palliation for metastatic sarcomas to bone. If surgery is required, a primary prosthetic replacement is preferred to internal fixation to avoid progressive local disease.

SPECIFIC ANATOMIC SITES: CLINICAL, SURGICAL, AND RADIOTHERAPEUTIC CONSIDERATIONS

The surgical and radiotherapeutic considerations for metastatic tumors of the most common anatomic sites are discussed.

PROXIMAL FEMUR (HIP)

The hip is the most common site of pathologic fracture (Fig. 62-34).[10,22,23,32] The aim of treatment is to reduce pain and to keep the patient ambulatory. In general, all pathologic fractures of the hip require surgical reconstruction followed by postoperative radiotherapy. Even in the weakened, nonambulatory patient, surgery is often warranted to relieve pain, to permit simple nursing care, and to enable the patient to sit in a chair.

Indications for Prophylactic Fixation

Firm indications for pending fracture of the hip have not been established; criteria based on the experience at Memorial Hospital for operative repair are summarized here.[23] These authors noted that whenever one of the following three circumstances was present, significant loss of bone substance and continuity was found at surgery:

1. A painful intramedullary lytic lesion equal to, or greater than, 50% of the cross-sectional diameter of the bone
2. A painful lytic lesion involving a length of cortex equal to, or greater than, the cross-sectional diameter of the bone or larger than 2.5 cm in axial length
3. A lesion of bone in which pain was unrelieved after radiation therapy

Several investigators have described similar radiographic criteria for the high-risk fracture.[10,114,115] In the largest study to date, Keene and co-workers attempted to identify the clinical and radiographic risk factors for pathologic fracture of the femur.[115] The authors reviewed the skeletal surveys of 2673 patients with breast cancer. Eleven percent (293) of the patients had proximal femoral metastases, of which 203 patients could be evaluated. Overall, only 11% of these patients sustained pathologic fracture. There was no difference in the average age, height, weight, pain pattern, or response to radiotherapy of those sustaining fracture compared with those who did not. These authors were unable to identify either a specific percentage involvement of the bone or a critical diameter for metastases to fracture. The 12 measurable lesions that fractured had the same degree involvement as the 208 measurable lesions that did not fracture. There are no accurate criteria to select the patient at risk. Keene and colleagues concluded that radiographic measurements alone cannot identify the high-risk patient. Exact criteria for prophylactic fixation have not yet been determined.

Radiographs and bone scans of the entire femur and acetabulum must be obtained preoperatively. It is not uncommon to detect other lesions further down the shaft, a situation that indicates the need for simultaneous fixation. In general, a long-stem prosthesis will treat both the femoral neck and the diaphyseal lesion. The acetabulum must be evaluated. If there is substantial disease, surgery should include curettage of that lesion and total replacement of the hip and acetabulum. Harrington emphasizes the need for removal of all gross disease and replacement with PMMA and internal fixation (see next section).[11,61] Significant bleeding may occur, especially in patients with myelomas, thyroid tumors, and hypernephromas. Preoperative angiography and embolization of the profundus femoris artery should be considered.

Surgery Treatment

Metastatic fractures of the hip may be intracapsular, intertrochanteric, or subtrochantic. Surgical treatment of intracapsular fractures entails endoprosthetic replacement (usually long-stem) or total hip replacement. The treatment of intertrochanteric and subtrochanteric fractures varies; plate and screw fixation (with PMMA) and Zickoll rods, respectively, have been described with good success. More recently, Lane has recommended long-stem prostheses with PMMA for any of these three areas.[23] Endoprosthetic replacement has many advantages. It is reliable and simple, avoids late failure of fixation seen with other devices, simultaneously treats lesions more distal in the shaft, and permits early mobilization. Lane reported no instances of loosening or dislocation and only two infections in 167 patients (1.2%). A bicentric device is now preferred in lieu of a fixed head endoprosthesis.[23]

Technique

A standard posterolateral approach is used. The trochanter should not be osteotomized. The head and neck are removed and the canal is reamed with *flexible* reamers; solid reamers may perforate abnormally thin bone. The length of the stem of the prosthesis should be at least to the isthmus or distal to any shaft lesions. The incision may be extended to curette all gross tumor. Any absent bone can be reconstructed with PMMA. It is extremely important to obtain a good cement mantle around the stem of the prosthesis and distal to the tip. The PMMA should be cooled before injection to increase the time of polymerization. The patient is mobilized within 2 to 3 days. If there is extensive loss of proximal bone, a segmental prosthesis is utilized. This technique is associated with significant operative morbidity and is not routinely performed. When required, however, it can successfully reconstruct large proximal defects.

Radiotherapy

Radiation portals should encompass the involved area of the proximal femur and extend distally to any sites of involve-

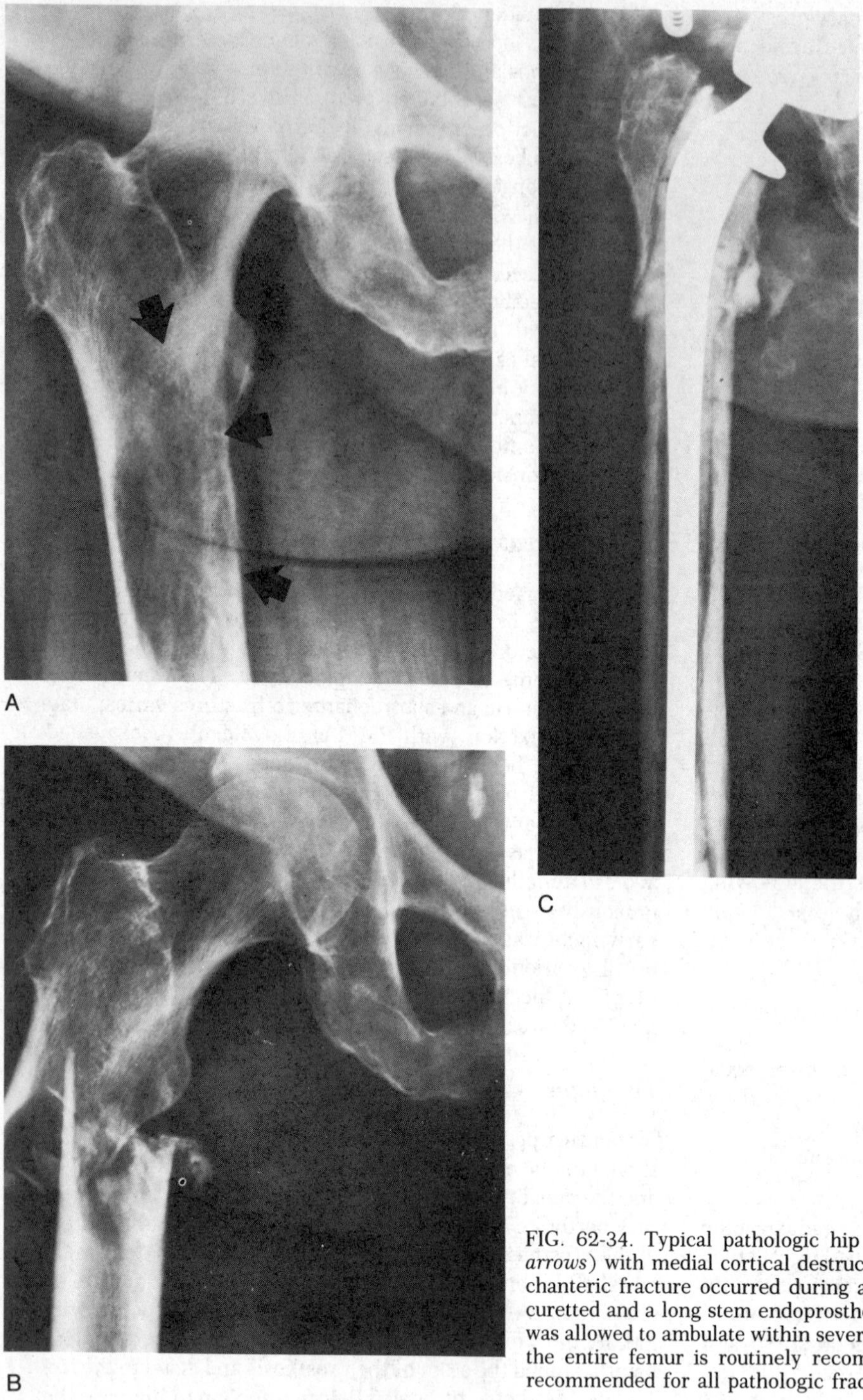

FIG. 62-34. Typical pathologic hip fracture. **A**. Large subtrochanteric lesion (*solid arrows*) with medial cortical destruction from a metastatic breast cancer. **B**. A subtrochanteric fracture occurred during administration of radiotherapy. **C**. The tumor was curetted and a long stem endoprosthesis was used with PMMA for fixation. The patient was allowed to ambulate within several days after surgery. Postoperative radiotherapy to the entire femur is routinely recommended. A long stem prosthesis with PMMA is recommended for all pathologic fractures of the hip.

ment of the femoral shaft. If surgery has been performed, radiotherapy should be started after the surgical wound has healed. Intramedullary or other fixation devices are generally included in the radiation field to encompass any microscopic tumor that might be dislodged by the surgery. Radiation fields should spare the knee joint unless there is frank tumor involvement of the adjacent distal femur. As is customary in other extremity sites, a strip of soft tissue should be left unirradiated to preserve lymphatic drainage.

FEMORAL SHAFT

Fractures of the femoral shaft should be treated by IM fixation and PMMA (Fig. 62-35). Combined osteosynthesis (*i.e.*, plate and screw fixation and PMMA) may be successful; however, it is not preferred because of the risk of fracture proximal and distal to the plate, increased operative time, and the need for a more extensive surgical exposure. In general, IM rod fixation is done by the "open" method: The

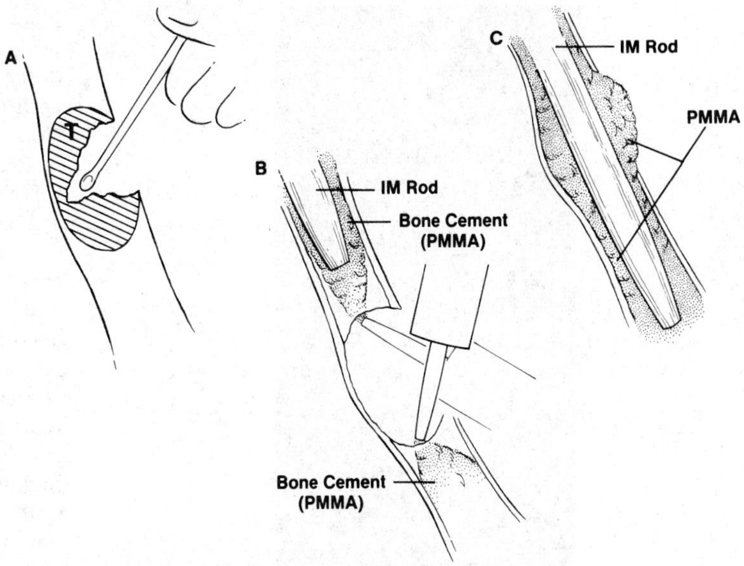

FIG. 62-35. Diaphyseal reconstruction for metastatic cancer. Metastatic tumors of the shafts (diaphysis) of long bones (femur and humerus) are reconstructed by a combination of intramedullary (IM) rod fixation combined with polymethylmethacrylate (PMMA). **A**. Curettage of the tumor. **B**. It is important to get the PMMA proximal and distal to the site of the tumor or fracture site, or both, in addition to filling the tumor defect. **C**. Stable fixation depends on this combined fixation. Small diaphyseal tumors may be treated prophylactically without opening the fracture site by using flouroscopic control.

tumor/fracture site is exposed, the tumor is curetted, PMMA is injected proximal and distal, and the IM rod is inserted. The proximal and distal fragments should be carefully reamed of all gross disease to permit easy insertion of the PMMA and rod. A uniform cement mantle should be obtained around the rod. Immediate ambulation with full weight-bearing is permitted within a few days after surgery.

Prophylactic Femoral Shaft Fixation

Small lesions of the femoral shaft may be treated prior to fracture by the "closed" method; that is, fluoroscopically inserting an IM rod from a small incision at the tip of the greater trochanter and anterograding it through the lesion to obtain good distal fixation. When utilizing this procedure, it is difficult to insert PMMA. This method is indicated only for small lesions of the femoral shaft with normal bone proximal. Careful preoperative evaluation of the hip is required, because progression and subsequent treatment of an undetected hip lesion would be extremely difficult with an IM rod in place.

PELVIS AND ACETABULUM

Metastatic tumors of the pelvis usually present with progressive pain; fractures are rare. The pelvis can be successfully treated nonoperatively with radiotherapy. Fortunately, marked bony destruction is uncommon; when it occurs, surgery can provide pain relief and enable the patient to walk again. Harrington classified and described the surgical management of 58 patients with severe acetabular insufficiency.[11,60] This classification is based upon the amount and location of bony destruction and the surgical procedure required for stabilization.

Extensive preoperative evaluation of the bony pelvis, extraosseous tumor extension, and tumor vascularity is required. The CT or MRI scan is more reliable than bone scintigraphy for evaluating pelvic tumor extent and is recommended for all patients. Angiography should be performed on all patients before surgery, with embolization of the vascular tumors. Significant blood loss must be anticipated; Harrington reported a mean blood loss of 1800 ml each for classes I and II and a loss of 2790 ml for class III (range 1125–8550 ml).[60] He emphasized that these procedures are indicated only in a *highly* select group of patients with a predictive long-term survival. For this select group, results are quite good. Sixty-seven percent of the patients reported excellent or good pain relief at 6 months, and 43% at 2 years. Eighty percent were ambulatory at 6 months.

Surgical Treatment

The surgical solution for overcoming the insufficiency of the roof or bony rim is to transmit the forces away from the local periacetabular bone into the superior part of the ilium and sacrum, which is still structurally intact. A standard anterior approach is used. It is unnecessary to enter the retroperitoneal space unless there is a large extraosseous component. All gross disease must be curetted. Hemostasis can be obtained by rapid tumor curettage and PMMA. Reconstruction is by a combination of Steinmann pins, protusio cups, and wire mesh. The trochanter should not be osteotomized. Close intraoperative monitoring of blood loss and hematologic values is required.

Pelvic Radiotherapy

Radiotherapy, following surgical procedures, is recommended for all symptomatic pelvic and acetabular lesions. Radiotherapy fields must encompass the area of bone involved by tumor and yet spare bone not grossly infiltrated by tumor to minimize radiation of the marrow. Consideration for the effect of radiation on bone marrow will be particularly important in patients receiving chemotherapy. If only a portion of the pelvis is treated, field edges should be designed to facilitate matching, should treatment elsewhere in

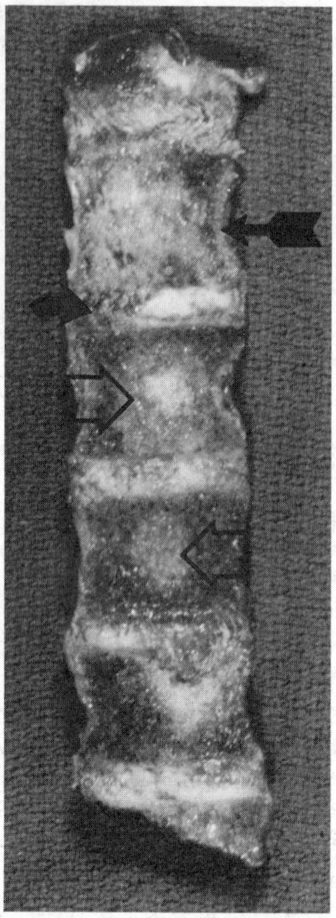

FIG. 62-36. Metastatic spinal disease. The spine is the most common site of metastatic disease. Metastatic cancer characteristically involves the anterior portion (vertebral body) of the spine. Shown is a gross specimen of the lumbar vertebra with characteristic metastatic tumor deposits within the vertebral bodies (*arrows*). The top vertebra (*straight solid arrow*) is almost completely replaced by tumor, and the adjacent disc space is being destroyed (*short curved arrow*). The lower two vertebrae show small, rounded central deposits of metastatic cancer (*open arrows*).

the pelvis be required at a later date. Pelvic fields will necessarily include some small bowel; the dose and fractionation must be within the limits of small-bowel tolerance.

SPINE

The vertebral bodies are most often affected by metastatic cancer (Fig. 62-36). Pain may be secondary to intraosseous disease, instability, collapse or pathologic fracture, or epidural compression, with or without nerve root involvement. Most vertebral pain can be treated with nonoperative modalities such as chemotherapy, radiotherapy, and external orthosis. The "radiosensitive" solid tumors, lymphomas, and myelomas, will respond with decreased pain and reossification. Indications for surgery are progressive neurologic symptoms, intractable pain, or progressive deformity. The traditional aim of such treatment has been decompression of the spinal canal by a posterior laminectomy and, occasionally, posterior stabilization with Harrington rods and PMMA. Recently, significant disagreement has arisen over the efficacy of posterior decompression.[12,13,116,117a] it is based on the fact that the site of metastatic disease to the spine is anterior, primarily involving the vertebral body. Several reports have described an anterior approach to the affected vertebrae, with removal of all gross disease, that permits decompression of the spinal cord and nerve roots and immediate stabilization by utilizing PMMA for vertebral body reconstruction.[12,13,116]

The use of CT, MRI, and myelography is required before surgery. The CT scan demonstrates the amount of bony destruction, whereas the MRI and myelogram localize the level and extent of epidural disease. The indications for anterior decompression are progressive neurologic deficit after surgery or radiotherapy and kyphosis with significant deformity (especially of the cervical spine).[12,13] All authors emphasize that this procedure is technically demanding, with significant morbidity and blood loss. It should be utilized only in highly select patients by skilled surgeons. Harrington initially reported 14 patients treated by vertebral body resection and PMMA replacement; 9 of 12 patients with major preoperative neurologic impairment recovered completely, 2 recovered partially, and 1 had no change.[12] Thirteen of the 14 patients had excellent pain relief. Average blood replacements for the cervical–thoracic and lumbar procedures were 200 and 1200 ml, respectively. More recently, Sundaresan and associates have performed 100 vertebral body resections and stabilizations for spinal metastases.[13] Eighty percent of these patients had notable pain relief immediately. Complications were related to previous treatment with intensive chemotherapy or radiotherapy. Minimal morbidity occurred in the de novo cases.

Surgical Technique

A thoracic or thoracoabdominal approach is used. The lumbar vertebrae are approached from the left side, and the aorta is mobilized and retracted. Care must be taken not to injure the segmental vessels, which must be carefully ligated. All gross disease is removed from the affected vertebral body and the adjacent disks are removed (Fig. 62-37). Gelfoam and continuous irrigation are used to protect the dura from the heat of polymerization before placing the PMMA. Steinmann pins or short distraction rods are placed as vertical supports between the vertebral bodies and then imbedded within the PMMA.[12,116] The adjacent bodies are undercut to permit snug PMMA fixation. Care must be taken not to put pressure on the cord.

Radiotherapy

Radiotherapy is recommended for symptomatic lesions and after surgical decompression. Radiation portals should include sites of symptomatic vertebral disease as well as other involved vertebrae that can be conveniently included without undue morbidity. Spinal cord tolerance must not be exceeded. Treatment of a portion of a vertebral body is not recommended because of the inherent danger of matching later treatment fields over the spinal cord should disease recur in the untreated portion of the vertebra. Paravertebral soft-tissue masses should be included in the treatment field.

FIG. 62-37. Technique of vertebral body reconstruction. The anterior aspect of the spine (vertebral bodies) can be approached successfully with reliable tumor removal, decompression of the spinal cord, and reconstruction in carefully selected patients. Significant morbidity and bleeding must be anticipated.

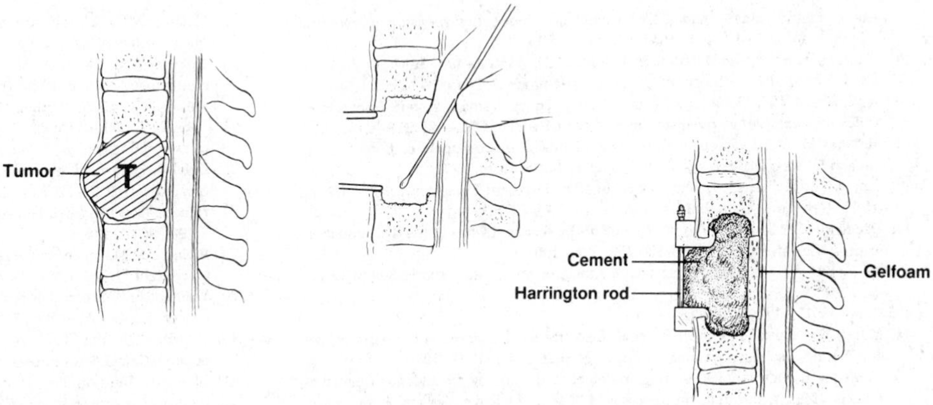

HUMERUS

Small lesions can be treated nonoperatively with radiotherapy and sling immobilization. Large lesions or those with a pathologic fracture are best treated by curettage, intramedullary fixation, and PMMA.[28] Proximal humeral lesions are approached through the standard deltopectoral interval. Tumors of the shaft require two incisions: one should be proximal, over the greater tuberosity, and the second over the tumor. Lesions of the supracondylar area are best treated by two rods inserted through the epicondyles. If the patient also has lower extremity lesions, early surgery for the humerus is recommended to permit crutch use and protect the lower extremities.

LESIONS DISTAL TO THE KNEE AND ELBOW

Leeson reported that 7% (57/827) of patients with metastatic cancer had distal extremity involvement.[117b] The most common primary cancers associated with distal metastases are the lung, breast, kidneys, and gastrointestinal tract. Tumors of the forearm or tibia are best treated by intramedullary fixation with PMMA. A recent poll of 163 hand surgeons recommended amputation of the digit in lieu of complicated surgical procedures and difficult radiation. Tumors of the hand often require amputation for local control and palliation.

REFERENCES

1. Silverberg E, Lubera J: Cancer statistics, 1987. CA 37:2–20, 1987
2. Abrams HL, Spiro R, Goldstein N: Metastases in carcinoma, Analysis of 1000 autopsied cases. Cancer 23:74–85, 1950
3. Galasko CSB: Mechanisms of lytic and blastic metastatic disease of bone. Clin Orthop 169:20–27, 1982
4. Porter BA, Shields AF, Olson DO: Magnetic resonance imaging of bone marrow disorders. Radiol Clin North Am 24:269–288, 1986
5. Daffner RH, Lupetin AR, Dash N, Sefczek RJ, Schapiro RL: MRI in the detection of malignant infiltration of bone marrow. AJR 146:353–358, 1986
6. Drelichman A, Decker DA, Al-Sarraf M et al: Computerized bone scan. A potential useful technique to measure response in prostatic carcinoma. Cancer 53:1061–1065, 1984
7. Zegel HG, Turner M, Velchik MG et al: Percutaneous osseous needle aspiration biopsy with nuclear medicine guidance. Clin Nucl Med 9:89–91, 1984
8. Little AG, DeMeester, Kirchner PT et al: Guided biopsies of abnormalities on nuclear bone scans. Technique and indications. J Thorac Cardiovasc Surg 85:396–403, 1983
9. McNeil BJ: Value of bone scanning in neoplastic disease. Semin Nucl Med 14:277–286, 1984
10. Harrington KD, Johnston JJ, Turner RH, Green DL: The use of methylmethacrylate as an adjunct in the internal fixation of malignant neoplastic fractures. J Bone Joint Surg 54A:1665–1676, 1972
11. Harrington KD: New trends in the management of lower extremity metastatis. Clin Orthop 169:53–61, 1982
12. Harrington KD: The use of methylmethacrylate for vertebral-body replacement and anterior stabilization of pathological fracture–dislocations of the spine due to metastatic malignant disease. J Bone Joint Surg 63A:36–46, 1981
13. Sundaresan N, Galicich JH, Lane JM et al: Treatment of neoplastic epidural cord compression by vertebral body resection and stabilization. J Neurosurg 63:676–684, 1985
14. Sherry MM, Greco FA, Johnson DH, Hainsworth JD: Metastatic breast cancer confined to the skeletal system, an indolent disease. AJR 81:381–386,
15. Salazar OM, Rubin P, Hendrickson et al: Single-dose half-body irradiation for palliation of multiple bone metastases from solid tumors: Final Radiation Therapy Oncology Group Report. Cancer 58:29–36, 1986
16. Vargha ZO, Glicksman AS, Boland J: Single-dose radiation therapy in the palliation of metastatic disease. Radiology 93:1180–1184, 1969
17. Penn CRH: Single dose and fractionated palliative irradiation for osseous metastases. Clin Radiol 27:405–408, 1976
18. Fitzpatrick PJ, Rider WD: Half-body radiotherapy. Int J Radiat Oncol Biol Phys 1:197–207, 1976
19a. Lawrence JH, Tobias CA: Radioactive isotopes and nuclear radiations in the treatment of cancer. Cancer Res 16:185–193, 1956
19b. Eisenhut M, Berberich R, Kimmig B, Oberhausen E: Iodine-131-labelled diphosphonates for palliative treatment of bone metastases: II. Preliminary clinical results with Iodine-131 BDP3. J Nucl Med 27:1255–1261, 1986
20. Clain A: Secondary malignant disease of bone. Br J Cancer 19:15–29, 1965
21. Higinbotham NL, Marcove RC: The management of pathological fractures. J Trauma 5:792–798, 1965
22. Haberman ET, Sachs R, Stern RE et al: The pathology and treatment of metastatic disease of the femur. Clin Orthop 169:70–82, 1982
23. Lane JM, Sculco TP, Zolan S: Treatment of pathological fractures of the hip by endoprosthetic replacement. J Bone Joint Surg 62A:954–959, 1980
24. Goris ML, Bretille J: Skeletal scintigraphy for the diagnosis of malignant metastatic diseases of bone. Radiother Oncol 4:319–329, 1985
25. Mundy GR, Ibbotson, D'Souza SM: Tumor products and hypercalcemia of malignancy. J Clin Invest 76:391–394, 1985
26. Beard DB, Haskell CM: Carcinoembryonic antigen in breast cancer. Clinical review. Am J Med 80:241–245, 1986
27. El-Khoury GY, Terepka RH, Mickelson MR et al: Fine-needle aspiration biopsy of bone. J Bone Joint Surg 65A:522–525, 1983
28. Sim F, Pritchard D: Metastatic disease of the upper extremity. Clin Orthop 169:83–94, 1982
29. Berrettoni BA, Carter JR: Mechanisms of cancer metastasis to bone. J Bone Joint Surg 68A:308–311, 1986
30. Manishen WJ, Sivananthan K, Orr FW: Resorbing bone stimulates tumor cell growth. A role for the host microenvironment in bone metastasis. Am J Pathol 123:39–45, 1986
31. Batson OV. The function of the vertebral veins and their role in the spread of metastases. Ann Surg 112:138–149, 1940
32. Galasko CSB. Skeletal metastases. Clin Orthop 210:18–30, 1986
33. Batson OV: Role of vertebral veins in metastatic processes. Ann Intern Med 16:38–45, 1942
34. Coman DR: Mechanisms responsible for origin and distribution of blood-borne tumor metastases. Review: Cancer Res 13:397–404, 1953
35. Coman DR, DeLong RP: The role of the vertebral venous system in the metastasis of

cancer to the spinal column. Experiment of tumor-cell suspension in rats and rabbits. Cancer 4:610–618, 1951
36. Turner JW, Jaffe HL: Metastatic neoplasms. AJR 43:479–492, 1940
37. Clark RL: Systemic cancer and the metastatic process. Cancer 43:790, 1979
38. Hollinshead WH, McFarlane JA: A collateral venous drainage system from kidney following occlusion of renal vein in dog. Surg Gynecol Obstet 97:213–219, 1953
39. Brookes M: Blood vessels in bone marrow. In The Blood Supply of Bone. An Approach to Bone Biology, pp 67–91. London, Butterworth, 1971
40. Enneking WF: Metastatic carcinoma. In *Musculoskeletal Tumor Surgery,* Vol 2, pp 1541. New York, Churchill-Livingstone. 1983
41. Dodds PR, Cardie VJ, Lytton B: The role of the vertebral veins in the dissemination of prostatic carcinoma. J Urol 126:753–755, 1981
42. del Regato JA: Pathways of metastatic spread of malignant tumors. Semin Oncol 4:33–38, 1977
43. Gephardt M: (Prostaglandins)
44. Mundy GR, Raisz LG, Cooper RA et al: Evidence for the secretion of an osteoclast-stimulating factor in myeloma. N Engl J Med 29:1041–1046, 1974
45. Kamenov B, Kiernan MW, Barrington-Leight et al: Homing receptors as functional markers for classification, prognosis, and therapy of leukemias and lymphomas. Proc Soc Exp Biol Med 177:211–219, 1984
46. Lam WC, Delikatny JE, Orr FW et al: The chemotactic response of tumor cells. A model of cancer metastasis. Am J Pathol 104:69–76, 1981
47. Wilner D: Cancer metastasis to bone. In Wilner D (ed): Radiology of Bone Tumors and Allied Disorders, pp. 3641–3908. Philadelphia, WB Saunders, 1982
48. Pollen JJ, Witztum, Ashburn WL: The flare phenomenon of radionuclide bone scan in metastatic prostate cancer. AJR 142:773–776, 1984
49. Hortobagyi GN, Lipshitz HI, Seabold JE: Osseous metastases of breast cancer. Clinical, biochemical, radiographic, and scintigraphic evaluation of response to therapy. Cancer 53:577–582, 1984
50. Hayward RB, Frazier TG: A re-evaluation of bone scans in breast cancer. J Surg Oncol 28:111, 1985
51. Weissman DE, Gilbert M, Wang H, Grossman SA: The use of computed tomography of the spine to identify patients at high risk for epidural metastases. J Clin Oncol 3:1541–1544, 1985
52. Wallace S, Granmayeh M, DeSantos LA et al: Arterial occlusion of pelvic bone tumors. Cancer 43:322–328, 1979
53. Wallace S, Charnsangavej C, Carrasco H, Bechtel W: Infusion-embolization. Cancer 54:2751–2765, 1984
54. Jonsson K, Johnell O: Preoperative angiography in patients with bone metastases. Acta Radiol Diag 23:485–489, 1982
55. Bowers TA, Murray JA, Charnsangavej C et al: Bone metastases from renal carcinoma, the preoperative use of transcatheter arterial occlusion. J Bone Joint Surg 64A:749–754, 1982
56. Pugh J, Sherry H, Futterman B et al: Biomechanics of pathologic fractures. Clin Orthop 169:109–114, 1982
57. Ryan JR, Begeman PC: The effects of filling experimental large cortical defects with methylmethacrylate. Clin Orthop 185:306–310, 1984
58. Gainor BJ, Buchert P: Fracture healing in metastatic bone disease. Clin Orthop 178:297–302, 1983
59. Unger AS, Boothe RE: Disseminated intravascular coagulopathy in a patient undergoing total hip arthroplasty. A case report. Clin Orthop 183:76–78, 1984
60. Harrington KD: The management of acetabular insufficiency secondary to metastatic malignant disease. J Bone Joint Surg 63A:653–663, 1981
61. Schobinger R: The arteriographic picture of metastatic bone disease. Cancer 11:1265–1268, 1958
62. Varma J, Huben RP, Wajsman Z, Pontes JE: Therapeutic embolization of pelvic metastases of renal cell carcinoma. J Urol 131:647–649, 1984
63. Mink J: Percutaneous bone biopsy in the patient with known or suspected osseous metastases. Radiology 161:191–194, 1986
64a. Michele AA, Krueger FJ: Surgical approach to the vertebral body. J Bone Joint Surg 31A:873–878, 1949
64b. Schajowicz F, Derqui JC: Puncture biopsy in lesions of the locomotor system. Review of results in 4050 cases, including 941 vertebral punctures. Cancer 21:531–548, 1968
65. Taylor CR, Kledzik G: Immunohistologic techniques in surgical pathology—a spectrum of "new" special stains. Hum Pathol 12:590–596, 1981
66. Pinkus GS: Diagnostic immunocytochemistry of paraffin-embedded tissues. Hum Pathol 13:411–415, 1982
67. Pinkus GS, Kurtin PJ: Epithelial membrane antigen—a diagnostic discriminant in surgical pathology. Hum Pathol 16:929–940, 1985
68. Kahn HJ, Marks A, Thom H, Baumal R: Role of antibody to S100 protein in diagnostic pathology. Am J Clin Pathol 79:341–347, 1983
69. Nadji M, Tabei SZ, Castro A et al: Prostatic origin of tumors. An immunohistochemical study. Am J Clin Pathol 73:735–739, 1980
70. Nadji M: Immunoperoxidase techniques I. Facts and artifacts. Am J Dermatopathol 8:32–36, 1986
71a. Sangeorzan BJ, Ryan JR, Salciccioli GG: Prophylactic femoral stabilization with the Zickel nail by closed technique. J Bone Joint Surg 68A:991–999, 1986
71b. Marcove RC, Miller TR: Treatment of primary and metastatic bone tumors by cryosurgery. JAMA 207:1890, 1969
72. Marcove RC: A 17-year review of cryosurgery in the treatement of bone tumors. Clin Orthop 163:231, 1982
73. Malawer MM, Baker A: Amputations for tumors. In Evarts CM (ed): Surgery of the Musculoskeletal System, 2nd ed. New York, Churchill-Livingstone, (In press)
74. Malawer MM, Marks A, McChecney D et al: The effect of cryosurgery and polymethylmethacrylate (PMMA) in dogs with experimental bone defects comparable to tumor defects. Clin Orthop (in press)
75. Tong D, Gillick L, Hendrickson FR: The palliation of symptomatic osseous metastases: Final results of the Radiation Therapy Oncology Group. Cancer 50:893, 1982
76. Delclos L: New and old concepts in radiotherapeutic treatment. Int J Radiat Oncol Biol Phys 1:1217–1220, 1976
77. Hendrickson FR, Sheinkop MB: Management of osseous metastases. Semin Oncol 2:399–404, 1975
78. Weber DA: The quantitative measurement of the response to treatment. Int J Radiat Oncol Biol Phys 1:1221–1222, 1976
79. Yarnold JR: Role of radiotherapy in the management of bone metastases from breast cancer. J R Soc Med Suppl 78:23–25, 1985
80. Garmatis CJ, Chu FCH: The effectiveness of radiation therapy in the treatment of bone metastases from breast cancer. Radiology 126:235–237, 1978
81. Allen KL, Johnson TW, Hibbs GG: Effective bone radiation as related to various treatment regimens. Cancer 37:984–987, 1976
82. Twycross RG: Analgesics and relief of pain. In Stoll BA, Parbhoo S (eds): Bone Metastasis: Monitoring and Treatment. New York, Raven Press, 1983
83. Gilbert HA, Kagan HR, Nussbaum et al: Evaluation of radiation therapy for bone metastases: Pain relief and quality of life. AJR 129:1095, 1977
84. Hendrickson FR, Shehata WM, Kirchner AR: Radiation therapy for osseous metastasis. Int J Radiat Oncol Biol Phys 1:275–278, 1976
85. Bhadrwaj S, Holland JF: Chemotherapy of metastatic cancer to bone. Clin Orthop 169:28–37, 1982
86. Greenburg EJ, Chu FCH, Dwyer AJ et al: Effects of radiation therapy on bone lesions as measured by 47-Ca and 85-Sr local kinetics. J Nucl Med 13:747–751, 1972
87. Blitzer PH: Reanalysis of the RTOG study of the palliation of symptomatic osseous metastasis. Cancer 55:1468–1472, 1985
88. Qasim MM: Single dose palliative irradiation for bony metastases. Strahlentherapie 153:531–532, 1977
89. McKenna WG, Barnes MM, Kinsella TJ et al: Combined modality treatment of adult soft tissue sarcomas of the head and neck. Int J Radiat Oncol Biol Phys 13:1127–1133, 1987
90. Ellis RE: The distribution of active bone marrow in the adult. Phys Med Biol 5:255–258, 1961
91. Maxfield JR, Maxfield JJG, Maxfield WS: The use of radioactive phosphorus and testosterone in metastatic bone lesions from breast and prostate. South Med J 51:320–327, 1958
92. Ariel IM, Hassouna H: Carcinoma of the prostate. The treatment of bone metastases by radioactive phosphorus (^{32}P). Int Surg 70:63–66, 1985
93. Aziz H, Choi K, Sohn C et al: Comparison of ^{32}P therapy and sequential hemibody irradiation (HBI) for bony metastases as methods of whole body irradiation. Am J Clin Oncol 9:264–268, 1986
94. Fowler JE Jr, Whitmore WF Jr: Considerations for the use of testosterone with systemic chemotherapy in prostatic cancer. Cancer 49:1373–1377, 1982
95. Firusian N, Mellin P, Schmidt CG: Results of ^{89} strontium therapy in patients with carcinoma of the prostate and incurable pain from bone metastases: A preliminary report. J Urol 116:764–768, 1976
96. Reddy EK, Robinson RG, Mansfield CM: Strontium-89 therapy for palliation of bone metastases. J Natl Med Assoc 78:27–32, 1986
97. Bhadrwaj S, Holland JF: Chemotherapy of metastatic cancer to bone. Clin Orthop 169:28–37, 1982
98. Miller F, Whitehill R: Carcinoma of the breast metastatic to the skeleton. Clin Orthop 184:121–127, 1984
99. Sherry MM, Greco A, Johnson DH, Hainsworth JD: Breast cancer with skeletal metastases at initial diagnosis. Cancer 58:178–182, 1986
100. Scheid V, Buzdar AU, Smith TL et al: Clinical course of breast cancer patients with osseous metastasis treated with combination chemotherapy. Cancer 58:2589–2593, 1986
101. Arkless R: Renal carcinoma: How it metastasizes. Cancer 84:496–501, 1965
102a. Garfield DH, Kennedy BJ: Regression of metastatic renal cell carcinoma following nephrectomy. Cancer 30:190–196, 1972
102b. Dorn W, Gladden MP, Rankin EA: Regression of a renal-cell metastatic osseous lesion following treatment. J Bone Joint Surg 57A:869–870, 1975
103. Chute R, Houghton JD: Solitary distant metastases from unsuspected renal carcinomas. J Urol 80:420–424, 1958
104. Marcove RC, Sadrieh J, Huvos AG et al: Cryosurgery in the treatment of solitary or multiple bone metastases from renal cell carcinomas. J Urol 108:540, 1972
105. Marcove RC, Searfoss RC, Whitmore WF et al: Cryosurgery in the treatment of bone metastases from renal cell carcinoma. Clin Orthop 127:220, 1972
106. Delaney TF: Personal experience
107. Bonnheim DC, Petrelli NJ, Herrera L et al: Osseous metastases from colorectal carcinoma. Am J Surg 151:457–459, 1986
108. Seife B: Osseous metastases from carcinoma of the large bowel. Cancer 119:414–418, 1973
109. Napoli LD, Hansen HH, Muggia FM et al: The incidence of osseous involvement in lung cancer, with special reference to the development of osteoblastic changes. Radiology 108:17–21, 1973

110. McCormack KR: Bone metastases from thyroid carcinoma. Cancer 19:181–184, 1966
111. Niederle B, Roka R, Schemper M et al: Surgical treatment of distant metastases in differentiated thyroid cancer: Indications and results. Surgery 100:1088–1097, 1986
112. Wilner D, Breckenridge RL: Bone metastasis in malignant melanoma. 62:388–394, 1949
113. Stewart WR, Gelerman RH, Harrelson JM et al: Skeletal metastases of melanoma, J Bone Joint Surg 60A:645–649, 1978
114. Beals RK, Lawton GD, Snell WE: Prophylactic internal fixation of the femur in metastatic breast cancer. Cancer 28:1350–1354, 1971
115. Keene JS, Sellinger DS, McBeath AA, Engber WD: Metastatic breast cancer in the femur. A search for the lesion at risk of fracture. Clin Orthop 203:282–288, 1986
116. Siegal T: Vertebral body resection of epidural compression by malignant tumors. Results of forty-seven consecutive operative procedures. J Bone Joint Surg 67A:375–382, 1985
117a. Harrison KM, Muss HB, Ball MR et al: Spinal cord compression in breast cancer. Cancer 55:2839–2844, 1985
117b. Leeson MC, Makley JT, Carter JR: Metastatic disease distal to the elbow and knee. Clin Orthop 206:94–99, 1986
118. Unger JD, Chiang LC, Unger GF: Apparent reformation of the base of the skull following radiotherapy for nasopharyngeal carcinoma. Radiology 126:779, 1978
119. Silberstein EB, Williams C: Strontium-89 therapy for the pain of osseous metastases. J Nucl Med 26:349, 1985

SECTION 5 HARVEY I. PASS

Treatment of Malignant Pleural and Pericardial Effusions

The occurrence of a new pleural or pericardial effusion in a cancer patient merits compulsive investigation by the oncologist. The degree of symptoms attending such effusions is variable and, indeed, the cause may not be due to malignancy. Appropriate therapy, however, must be dictated by objective documentation of a cause, especially when treatment may involve operative intervention or innovative therapy. This chapter will review the pathophysiology, incidence, diagnostic regimens, and modern treatment of pleural and pericardial effusions as they apply to the patient with a previous history of malignancy. Multiple options of treatment will be discussed for their efficacy, bearing in mind that most treatment regimens have been performed in a retrospective review of patient groups, as opposed to being under the auspices of prospective randomized trials.

PLEURAL EFFUSIONS

PATHOPHYSIOLOGY

Five to ten liters of fluid moves through the pleural space in 24 hr, of which 35% to 75% is turned over each hour, leaving 5 to 20 ml of fluid with a protein content of less than 2 g/dl.[1] Eighty to ninety percent of the fluid is reabsorbed, and abnormal fluid collections result from increased capillary permeability, increased hydrostatic pressure (congestive heart failure), increased negative intrapleural pressure (atelectasis), decreased oncotic pressure (hypoalbuminemia), or increased pleural fluid oncotic pressure (pleural tumor growth).[2] Processes that impair pleural lymphatic drainage also lead to effusion. There is a strong relationship between carcinomatous infiltration of mediastinal lymph nodes and pleural effusion; however, the extent of direct pleural involvement by metastases bears no relationship to the development of pleural effusion.[3] Therefore, the key elements in *malignant* pleural effusions include increased capillary permeability through inflammation or disruption of the capillary endothelium or impaired lymphatic drainage secondary to obstruction by tumor.[2] Although cancer patients may have transudative effusions on the basis of hypoalbuminemia, heart failure, or liver disease, malignant effusions are classically described as exudative with a protein content of >3 g/dl, specific gravity > 1.015, pleural protein/serum protein ratio >0.5, and pleural lactate dehydrogenase (LDH)/serum LDH ratio >0.6. As protein concentration in the pleura increases, pleural osmotic pressure increases, which impedes efflux of pleural fluid. Pleural tumor involvement leads to mesothelial shedding and subsequently pleural thickening. Capillary engorgement and lymphocyte infiltration of the pleura commonly leads to a lymphocyte-abundant, bloody pleural effusion from tumor directly invading the blood vessels, from occlusion of venules, or from capillary dilation by vasoactive substances. A bloody effusion is the single strongest positive predictive element toward malignancy.[4,5]

SYMPTOMS AND SIGNS

Twenty-three percent of patients are asymptomatic at the time of presentation and 50% to 90% of patients with primary or metastatic pleural malignancy will have pleural effusion as their initial presenting manifestation.[6] Most (90%) will have effusions of more than 500 ml, and approximately one-third will have bilateral effusions at the time of presentation.

Dyspnea, cough, and *chest pain* are the common presenting complaints. The degree of symptom severity is related to the rapidity with which the fluid develops rather than the amount of fluid present.[7] Dyspnea is related to pulmonary compression. Pleuritic chest wall pain occurs with parietal pleural inflammation, whereas dull continuous pain is usually associated with parietal pleural metastases.[1] Diaphragmatic pleural irritation may be referred to the ipsilateral shoulder. Cough is usually dry and nonproductive and is due to compression of bronchial walls by fluid.[7]

Objective findings include tachypnea, labored breathing, and restricted chest wall expansion. Dullness to percussion, decreased fremitus, increased intercostal fullness, and undetectable diaphragmatic excursion may be present. Massive effusions may cause contralateral tracheal deviation.

DIAGNOSTIC TECHNIQUES

Radiography

Blunting of the costophrenic angle seen in the upright posteroanterior (PA) x-ray film will be seen with as little as 175 to 525 ml, and a lateral decubitus film will detect as little as

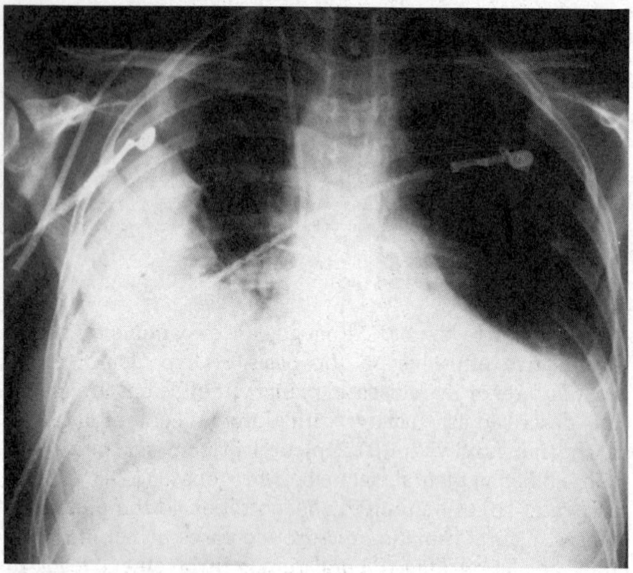

FIG. 62-38. Patient with right-side pseudotumor, pleural effusion, and large pericardial effusion from breast cancer.

100 ml.[8-11] Fluid can be loculated within pulmonary fissures (pseudotumors) or between the lung and the diaphragm (subpulmonic; Fig. 62-38).

An opacified hemithorax with mediastinal shift usually indicates massive effusion (>1500 ml): opacification without shift should alert one to the possibility of mainstem bronchial obstruction, mediastinal fixation with malignant lymph nodes, or malignant mesothelioma.[3]

Small pleural effusions can be detected on *computed tomography* (CT) and CT can sometimes delineate an underlying pleural malignancy. The use of CT attenuation numbers (Houndsfield units) is controversial for the differentiation of pleural fluid from pleural tumors.[12] The usual place for CT in the management of malignant pleural effusions is *after* pleural drainage, which then allows the radiologist to evaluate subtle changes in pleural structure, new parenchymal infiltrates or masses, or enlargement of mediastinal lymph nodes. This is especially useful if previous chest tomograms are available from before the development of the effusion. *Ultrasound* techniques using both A- and B-mode scans have been widely used to detect and sample pleural effusions.[13] Ultrasonography can identify pleural fluid as well as differentiate between pleural thickening and pleural fluid.[5] The use of ultrasonic guidance to determine the proper site for thoracentesis and establish the depth of the fluid decreases the risk of complications, especially in small effusions demonstrated by radiographic techniques.[5,14]

Cytology

Demonstration of malignant cells in pleural fluid is the sine qua non of a malignant pleural effusion. Samples prepared for examination of pleural fluid include wet mounts stained with toluidine blue; smears fixed in 95% alcohol or air-dried; membrane-filtered, cytocentrifuge preparations; and cell blocks for paraffin embedding and sectioning. Staining is by the modified Papanicolaou method, cytocentrifuge specimens by Wright-Giemsa, and paraffin sections by hematoxylin–eosin.

The rate of positivity for pleural cytologic specimens varies among large series. Sears,[15] Lopes,[16] and Johnson[17] have reported positive pleural cytologic appearances in 44%, 29%, and 9%, respectively, of all pleural specimens submitted. The results of the cytologic examination vary according to the site of the effusion, the type and site of the primary neoplasm, and the method of processing the specimen.[15,16,18-20] Cytologic specimens from patients *known to have neoplasms* have given positive results in 42% to 96% of patients, whereas the false-positive rates have ranged from zero to 3%.[16,18,19,21,22]

Recognition of cancer cells by cytopathologic techniques has become highly accurate when performed by an experienced clinical morphologist. Difficulties arise when trying to differentiate cancer cells from reactive mesothelial cells or when trying to classify the organ of origin. The use of immunocytochemical techniques as an adjunct to the diagnosis of malignant pleural effusions has, until recently, been limited by the availability, sensitivity, and specificity of the assays using polyclonal sera or monoclonal antibodies. Immunochemical techniques are now routinely performed in the diagnosis of malignancy. Anticarcinoembrionic antigen (anti-CEA) heteroantisera has demonstrated reactivity with approximately 50% of cancer cells, whereas no reactivity is noted with mesothelial cells or benign effusions.[23] Polyclonal antisera to epithelial membrane antigen has demonstrated reactivity with 54% of carcinomatous effusions and no reactivity with benign effusions.[24-26] B72.3, an IgG1 monoclonal antibody has recently been shown to recognize 100% of adenocarcinomas in patients with effusions from cancers of breast, ovary, and lung, and when additional metastatic adenocarcinomas from other sites are considered, overall recognition is 95%, including poorly differentiated squamous cell lung cancer.[27,28] Cytochemical staining with acid phosphatase, α-naphthylacetate esterase, periodicacid-Schiff, as well as sheep erythrocyte rosetting is useful in recognizing malignant lymphocytes.[29]

Cytogenetic analysis of pleural effusions combining cytologic and chromosome analyses of pleural effusions has correctly diagnosed 83% to 91% of malignant effusions, a result that was better than with either technique alone;[30] however, the false-positive rate is higher in chromosome analysis than in ordinary cytology.[5] Other studies[31,32] have yielded a close to 90% positive diagnosis of malignancy, with a 3% false-negative rate. Pleural cytogenetics, however, is limited by expense and time consumption.

Biochemical Analysis

The CEA levels in pleural fluid may be useful in detecting malignancy,[5] with a pleural fluid level of >20 ng/ml having a 91% sensitivity and 92% specificity in effusions caused by adenocarcinoma. In patients with metastatic bronchogenic adenocarcinoma in the pleura, the CEA level is higher than 10 ng/ml in 90% of the patients. Reported sensitivities in malignant effusion range from 25% to 57% using cutoff values between 10 and 20 ng/ml.[33-35] The CEA level assays are expensive, time-consuming, and lack sensitivity and specificity for malignancy in general. Hyaluronic acid levels have been noted to be elevated in patients with mesothelioma;[5] however, this assay lacks sensitivity and will not provide a definitive diagnosis.[36]

Thoracentesis

Thoracentesis of suspected malignant pleural effusions can be both diagnostic and therapeutic, although the symptomatic relief of fluid removal is usually short-lived without other adjuvant measures. The upright PA and lateral chest film helps to localize the effusion and, if available, should be correlated with CT findings to rule out loculations. Ideally, coagulation values should be close to normal.

After sufficient bactericidal preparation of the skin, the site of drainage is locally infiltrated with an anesthetic. Fluid can then be localized with a small-gauge needle to ensure correct placement of the drainage catheter. Disposable thoracentesis kits with specially designed catheters are available; otherwise, a simple 16- or 18-gauge needle attached to a syringe through a three-way stopcock can be used. It is important to differentiate a truly bloody effusion from a traumatic tap, and it only requires 1 ml of blood in 500 ml of effusion to give the appearance of a bloody effusion. Bleeding, pneumothorax with peripheral bronchopleural fistula, and "pleural shock," an exaggerated vagal response as the needle passes through the parietal pleura causing bradycardia, are possible complications. The latter is easily reversed with intravenous fluids, atropine, and Trendelenberg positioning. Oxygen therapy and narcotics may be necessary because of the pain of reexpansion. Thoracentesis of volumes larger than 1500 ml may cause reexpansion pulmonary edema.[37-39]

The fluid withdrawn is sent for cytologic and bacteriologic determinations, as well as for levels of protein, LDH, glucose, specific gravity, and cell count to determine the transudative or exudative nature of the fluid.

Pleural Biopsy

Closed pleural biopsy is a relatively easy technique that can be coordinated with CT guidance to try to decrease sampling error. The most commonly used needles are the Cope, Abrams, and Tru-cut. The pleural biopsy should be done before fluid aspiration to avoid pulmonary injury. Cytologic examination of pleural fluid alone has a higher sensitivity than needle biopsy,[40,41] and the yield of diagnosis of pleural neoplasm by needle biopsy alone ranges from 40% to 69%.[42-46] When pleural biopsy is combined with cytology, however, the diagnostic yield is increased from 81% to 90%.[47,48] Although several authors recommend that cytologic analysis and pleural biopsy be performed concurrently to increase the diagnostic rate for malignant effusions,[47-51] most investigators reserve pleural biopsy for patients suspected of malignant effusions but with negative cytologic evidence.[5,40,41,46] If an initial closed pleural biopsy is negative, the yield of a positive diagnosis increases slightly (2%–4%) with a second biopsy.[2,5,41]

The morbidity of pleural biopsy is 0.6%[52] with the most commonly reported complications being pneumothorax, pleural shock, hemothorax, subcutaneous emphysema, and inadequate biopsy. Cancer implantation, associated with the use of larger needles and hematoma formation, occurs in 4.1% of patients.[53]

Thoracoscopy

In undiagnosed suspected malignant pleural effusions with persistently negative cytologic results, thoracoscopy has been useful in establishing the diagnosis in 93% to 96% of the patients.[54-56] Boutin, in 215 cases of undiagnosed effusions, was able to correctly diagnose 131 of 150 malignant effusions.[54] Weissberg was able to diagnose the cause of effusion in 94% of 127 thoracoscopies performed.[56] The length of the procedure is 15 to 20 min, and complications include pain, subcutaneous emphysema, pneumothorax, hemorrhage, recurrence of tumor at the thoracoscopy site, and empyema (Fig. 62-39).[57] Thoracoscopic examination of patients with pleural effusion from lung cancer reveals that there is a higher percentage of metastatic disease in the visceral pleura in lung cancer as opposed to greater inferior mediastinal and diaphragmatic pleural involvement in cases of extrapulmonary origin of tumor.[58] Thoracoscopy has also been used, not only for documentation of disease in patients with malignant pleural effusions from breast cancer, but also to obtain sufficient tissue for hormone-receptor determination.[59] Synchronous sclerosis of malignant pleural effusions at the time of thoracoscopy has been reported with good success.[60,61]

Thoracotomy

The need for open thoracotomy in the management of malignant pleural effusion is reserved for the rare case of nondiagnostic studies and continued suspicion of malignant disease. Even after thoracotomy, a significant number of patients will be found not to have malignant disease.[2,5]

FIG. 62-39. Thoracoscopy with the Storz rigid thoracoscope permits visualization of pleural abnormalities and direct biopsy.

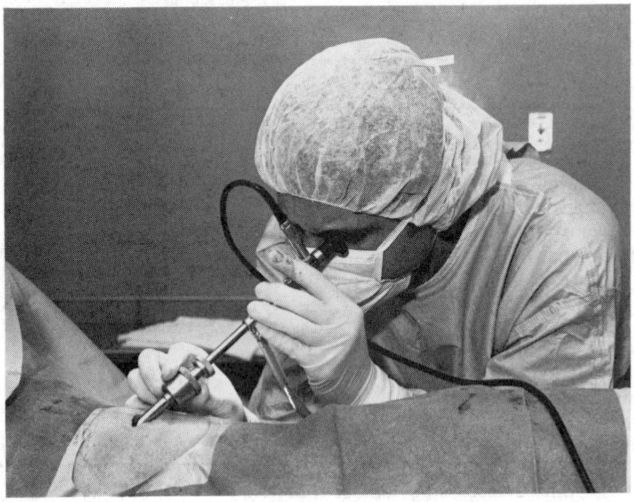

PROGNOSIS AND TREATMENT

The time for development of malignant effusion varies according to cell type, with breast cancer, lymphoma, and melanoma having an interval between primary diagnosis and effusion of 30 months,[15] whereas lung, gastric, esophageal, prostate, and thyroid cancers, have an interval of fewer than 10 months. The prognosis of patients who develop malignant pleural effusions varies with the histologic type of the primary tumor. When one considers all effusions regardless of the histologic type, 65% of the patients will be dead within 3 months and 80% within 6 months. Patients with breast cancer will have a mean survival of 7 to 15 months posteffusion[15,62] and a 3-year survival of 20%.[63] Mean survival time in patients with lung cancer has been reported to be as low as 2 months from the time of diagnosis of malignant pleural effusion,[62] and two-thirds of the patients will be dead by 3 months. One-third of patients with ovarian cancer will die within a mean time of 10 months after the diagnosis of malignant effusion, and the mean survival time is 3 months.[15]

Treatment should palliate symptoms in the most reliable, least complicated and, hopefully, most durable manner. In selected instances, local treatment can be combined with systemic regimens (i.e., testicular carcinoma, lymphoma, breast cancer), depending on the efficacy of the systemic agents for a given malignant histologic type. In the majority of cases of solid tumors with malignant effusions, only local therapy is considered, to control reaccumulation of pleural fluid and diminish or eliminate the need for repeated thoracenteses required by repeated bouts of respiratory compromise.

From the literature, it is difficult to objectively evaluate composites of large series for the success of treatment of malignant pleural effusions because of the differing criteria used to denote responsitivity. Moreover, time endpoints for evaluation differ among studies. The most useful criterion has been a failure of the effusion to recur at 4 to 6 weeks because patients treated by simple thoracentesis and followed for 1 month have a 97% recurrence rate. Some of the newer strategies (*e.g.*, the use of BCG and *Corynebacterium parvum*), which do not employ tube thoracostomy, define a complete response when there is no reaccumulation after one thoracentesis employing intrapleural treatment.

METHODS OF TREATMENT

Sclerotherapy

The management of malignant pleural effusions involves proper technique of sclerotherapy after space obliteration by placement of a large-bore thoracostomy tube. Initial removal of the effusion allows the visceral pleura to come into contact with the chest wall parietal pleura and thus obliterates, by continuous, underwater-seal suction drainage, the space occupied by the effusion. A sclerosing agent, either antibiotic, antineoplastic, or radioactive can then be delivered intrapleurally to produce mesothelial fibrosis and obliterate small pleural blood vessels, rather than produce specific antineoplastic activity.[64] Table 62-33 represents a recent updated survey of the available literature on the efficacy of intrapleural sclerotherapy.

TECHNIQUE OF PLEURAL SCLEROTHERAPY. The intrapleural installation of agents in patients with neoplastic pleural disease has been fairly standardized. The first order of business is a careful examination of the available roetgenographic studies including lateral decubitus films, upright PA and lateral chest films, as well as chest CT scans (if available). One must first determine whether or not this is a free-flowing pleural effusion without loculations, which may have developed because of initial multiple thoracenteses. The development of loculations in such a situation makes it difficult for a single chest tube placement to obtain adequate evacuation of the fluid. Fortunately, however, most patients have free-flowing pleural effusions without loculations.

Placement of the chest tube should be done by an experienced physician to minimize patient discomfort. The chest tube can usually be placed laterally in the sixth or seventh

TABLE 62-33. Management of Malignant Pleural Effusions*

	Histologic Type					
Treatment	*Lung*	*Breast*	*Lymphoma*	*Ovary*	*Other*	*Overall (%)*
Chest tube alone	1/6	18/38	—	—	1/10	20/54 (37%)
Tetracycline	17/28	24/44	0/1	0/1	20/40	61/114 (54)
Quinicrine	30/37	39/49	7/9	5/8	19/26	100/129 (78)
Bleomycin	7/11	33/38	4/6	5/6	32/55	81/116 (70)
Nitrogen mustard	35/53	109/225	7/19	8/11	24/50	183/358 (51)
5-FU						23/35 (66)
Thiotepa	0/1	11/21		2/2	0/2	14/26 (54)
Talc	54/59	71/75	4/4	8/9	71/90	208/237 (88)
Irradiation	8/10	2/3	9/10	—	11/15	30/38 (79)
Isotopes	102/190	234/413	22/44	32/54	85/177	475/878 (54)
BCG						5/9 (56)
C. parvum						57/70 (81)

* Number successful/number reported.

interspace, in a position lying in the anterior axillary line, such that the patient will not be lying on the chest tube when he is supine. Premedication with 75 to 100 mg of meperidine (Demerol) or 6 to 8 mg of morphine, subcutaneously, will relax the patient and decrease discomfort. The appropriate chest is sterilely prepared with an iodine-based cleansing solution and sterile towels are placed. The skin is infiltrated locally with 1% lidocaine (Xylocaine) at the appropriate site for chest tube placement. Usually 20 to 30 ml of 1% lidocaine, placed intra- and subdermally and down to the chest wall, will provide a satisfactory local block. Once the skin and chest wall is anesthetized, a quick thoracentesis is performed to document good flow of effusion in this designated area. If free flow of fluid is not obtained, another site that will guarantee good flow of fluid should be chosen for chest tube placement. A short 2- to 3-cm incision is then made in the skin and carried down to the subcutaneous tissues. A curved Mayo scissors is then used to create a tunnel through the chest wall musculature, directly down to the interspace of choice. The more care that is taken with the development of this subcutaneous tunnel down to the intercostal muscles over the appropriate rib, the less discomfort the patient will have when the chest tube is placed. Some physicians prefer the use of a trocar chest tube; however, the use of a surgical clamp to open into the pleural space under controlled conditions will allow the finger to be placed into the chest to assure that there are no adhesions that could be violated by chest tube placement. An appropriate-sized chest tube, either 28 or 32 French, is then placed through the subcutaneous tunnel into the pleural cavity and directed cephalad by having a clamp on the introducing end of the chest tube as well as a clamp at the end of the chest tube, closing it off to prevent open pneumothorax as well as a rush of fluid out of the chest tube. The chest tube is then connected to an underwater seal drainage system, using any of a variety of systems. A stitch of heavy silk is used to anchor the chest tube to the skin, and sterile dressings are applied. A chest x-ray film is then obtained and viewed for proper tube placement. We repeat chest x-rays daily after chest tube placement and subsequent sclerosis therapy.

For the first 24 hr the chest tube should be connected to underwater seal drainage with negative suction (approximately 15–20 cm H_2O) applied to the device. This will ensure maximum expansion of the compressed, underlying lung as well as total evacuation of the fluid. Because the use of a chest tube alone is associated with a low success rate (see Table 62-33), we always approach the patient who has a chest tube placed for neoplastic pleural disease as a candidate for intrapleural therapy. If the chest x-ray film, taken 24 hr after the placement of the chest tube, shows total evacuation of fluid with good lung expansion, the sclerotherapy can be started. Sclerotherapy should not be performed if the patient has a large volume of residual fluid left in the chest. Doing this will doom the treatment to failure because of dilution of the sclerosing medium as well as insufficient expansion of the underlying lung.

When the decision is made to give sclerotherapy, the patient is premedicated a half-hour before treatment with a narcotic agent. Tetracycline in a dose of 1 to 3 g in 100 ml of normal saline, or a 5% dextrose–water solution, is then instilled directly through the test tube with an irrigating catheter, followed by clamping of the chest tube and connecting the end of the chest tube back to the drainage system. Essentially, the tetracycline remains in the chest cavity because the chest tube is clamped, and the patient is instructed to change positions every 15 min for 4 hr (*i.e.*, lying flat, right-side-up, left-side-up, head-down, and head-up positions) to equally distribute this 100 ml throughout the pleural cavity. At the end of this 4 hr the chest tube clamp is them removed and the fluid allowed to drain, with suction for another 24 hr.

Twenty-four hours after the sclerotherapy, the patient is disconnected from suction and the chest allowed to drain by gravity. The patient is maintained connected to this underwater seal system, with daily monitoring of the amount of effluent. When the drainage is decreased substantially (*e.g.*, to 50–100 ml/24 hr), and the lung remains reexpanded, as seen on x-ray films, with the chest tube in, the tube is then removed and the site either closed with a stitch of 3-0 silk or with Vaseline gauze. We prefer suture closure of the chest tube site to ensure the absence of continued drainage onto the skin or a sucking chest wound. Twenty-four hours after chest tube removal the patient should have a chest x-ray that, it is hoped, reveals no further accumulation of fluid and total lung expansion, at which point the patient can be considered for discharge. A follow-up x-ray examination should be performed 1 month later.

Specific Sclerosing Agents

TETRACYCLINE. Intrapleural tetracycline (TCN) has gained popularity because of its overall efficiency, convenience, low cost, and minimal morbidity. Prospective trials comparing TCN to quinicrine,[65] to a comparable pH placebo,[66] or to tube thoracostomy alone,[67] show consistently better results with intrapleural TCN, with significantly less fever and pleuritic chest pain. Premedication of the patient with a narcotic, as well as addition of lidocaine (150 mg) to the sclerosis medium[68] may abate the pleurisy. Experimental models reveal that TCN increases pleural capillary permeability, allowing an accumulation of clotting factors into the pleural space and inactivation of the common fibrinolytic activity of pleural fluid. The fibrin matrix allows fibroblast attachment.[69] The effusion recurrence rate after TCN sclerosis is related to progression of the underlying malignancy and is independent of the dose of TCN given (500 mg to 3 g).[70] Patients may be successfully re-treated with TCN sclerosis.

QUINICRINE. The antimalarial, quinicrine, has been reported to be highly effective in pleural sclerotherapy, and compares favorably in efficacy with TCN[65] and with thiotepa in randomized studies.[71] Despite the high range of responses (64%–100%)[8,65,72–74] disadvantages include the necessity for repeated daily doses of 100 to 200 mg over a 2 to 5 day period, and greater morbidity than with other techniques that may not be quite as effective. These side-effects include persistent fever, pain, nausea, hypotension, hallucination, and seizures.[63,73,75]

TALC. The administration of intrapleural talc, either at the time of thoracoscopy under general anesthesia or by aerosolization through a chest tube, has been a popular means of controlling malignant pleural effusions in Great Britain and Europe, despite the absence of randomized trials.[56,76–80] When performed under general anesthesia at the time of thoracotomy or thoracoscopy, talc is 90% to 100% effective if there is complete expansion of the underlying lung. Unfortunately, even in highly selected patients, a mortality of 5% to 11%, which is related to the need for general anesthesia, exists.[64,80] Fever and pain complications are comparable with other forms of sclerotherapy; however, respiratory distress has been reported. Talc is less readily available than tetracycline, and despite optimistic reports of lower modern-day mortality from selected cancer centers,[1] it is generally agreed that the use of talc, either with general or local anesthesia, should be reserved for patients who have failed simpler forms of instillational therapy.[2,64]

ANTINEOPLASTIC AGENTS. The theoretical consideration that intracavitary cytotoxic agents would work, given their ability to kill tumor cells, does not take into account the mechanism of formation of effusions, and there does not appear to be a correlation between tumor cell count and response rate. Cytotoxic drugs most likely are effective by inducing inflammatory pleurodesis in the pleural space. Nitrogen mustard, thiotepa, bleomycin, doxorubicin and 5-fluorouracil have been used for intrapleural management of malignant effusions, with the major side-effects being bone marrow depression and leukopenia. Bleomycin seems to be the most successful, with the least side-effects at an instillation dose of 60 mg,[81] and with minimal myelosuppressive problems and minimal fever and pain. The only randomized study, however, comparing bleomycin with TCN revealed equal response rates.[82] Cost considerations also relegate this agent to a less-desirable therapy than TCN.

INTRAPLEURAL RADIOISOTOPES. Administration of radioactive isotopes has been associated with nausea and vomiting, high cost, special precautions, and response rates comparable with other forms of treatment. The use of ^{98}Au and ^{32}P are now of historical interest; however, conjugation of α- and β- emitters with selective monoclonal antibodies for intrapleural treatment is now under investigation.[83]

BIOLOGIC AGENTS. Intrapleural instillation of *C. parvum*, 5 to 10 mg, streptococcal preparation OK432, and BCG cell wall skeleton have demonstrated promising results in the management of malignant effusion. *Corynebacterium parvum* was noted to be superior in randomized trials compared with TCN,[84] bleomycin,[85] and nitrogen mustard,[86] with the advantage of the immunotherapy given by thoracentesis catheter. The *C. parvum* effect, however, is not associated with evidence of enhancement of local cell-mediated immunity.[87]

External Radiation

Only lymphomatous pleural effusions seem to respond favorably to external beam radiation. Close to 90%[1,88] of malignant lymphoma effusions could be controlled in a small series of patients using mediastinal and hemithorax irradiation (1.4–2.3 Gy). Systemic chemotherapy is also used.[89]

Surgical Interventions

PLEURECTOMY. Stripping of the parietal pleura from the rib cage and mediastinum, essentially removing 90% of the pleura, is infrequently used because of the modern-day success of sclerotherapy. Its limited reported applications[90–92] include highly selected patients who have failed all other approaches, usually because of the presence of trapped or nonexpansile lung. A 23% complication rate, consisting of air leak, bleeding, pneumonia, empyema, cardiac failure, pulmonary embolus, and respiratory insufficiency, is combined with a 9% mortality. Control of effusion is reported to be 87% to 100%. Candidates must be in a favorable functional class, and have slow-growing malignancies, such that the expected survival is 1 year or longer.

FIG. 62-40. *Top.* Placement of pleuroperitoneal shunt for drainage of intractable pleural effusions from chest to abdominal cavity. *Insert.* A small pursestring seals the entry site into the peritoneum. *Bottom.* View of the completed procedure. (Reprinted with permission of Denver Biomaterials, Inc)

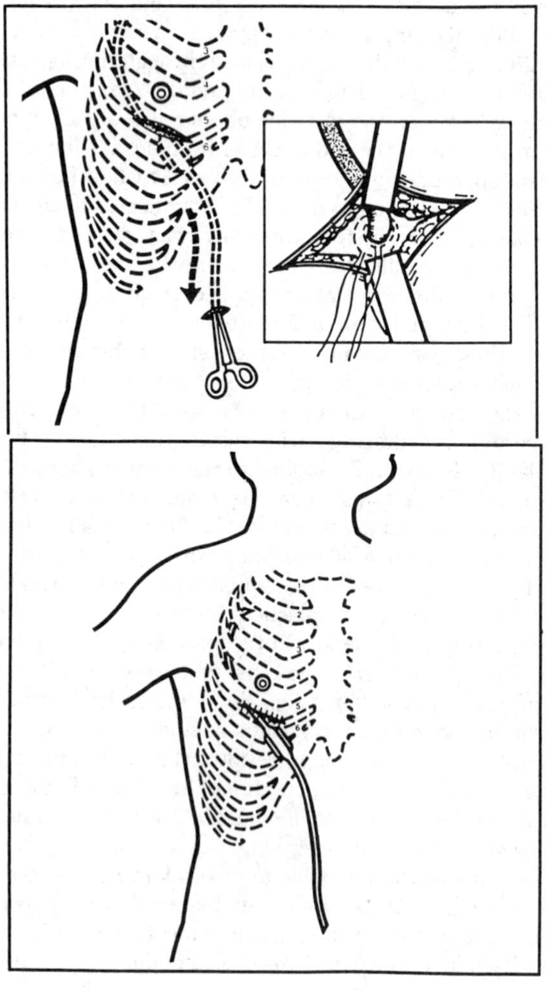

PLEUROPERITONEAL SHUNTING. Internal drainage of malignant pleural effusions to the abdomen was first described in 1984, in which the valved, pumping chamber of a Denver shunt was placed subcutaneously with a proximal limb in the pleural effusion and a distal limb in the abdomen (Fig. 62-40). Since that time, 23 patients have been described[93,94] of which 17 had relief of symptoms with or without significant (>50%) reduction of their pleural effusion. As of yet there has been no reported increased instance of malignant peritoneal seeding impinging on the patients' long-term course. The pleuroperitoneal shunt can be used in instances for which sclerotherapy has failed, particularly when this is due to inability of the lung to expand. The procedure can be performed under local anesthesia, and complications are minimal. Nuclear medicine studies confirm that the pleural fluid moves only with active pumping of the mechanism. Thus, patients must be sufficiently strong to pump the device, or the family taught to do this. Further controlled studies comparing TCN sclerosis with this technique for cost benefit, complications, and success of palliation are required before the endorsement of this device as a primary means of palliating malignant pleural effusions.

PERICARDIAL EFFUSIONS

INCIDENCE

Malignant involvement of the heart or pericardium is not uncommon in patients with advanced cancer, and its prevalence has been described in a number of autopsy studies. The prevalence of combined metastasis to the pericardium and heart has ranged from 0.1% to 21%.[95-98] In a series of 3327 autopsies, tumor lesions of the heart were detected in 5.1% of the cases.[99] When such data are available from autopsy series,[96,99-101] the pericardium is involved solely in 45% of the cases, the myocardium alone in 32%, and the myocardium and pericardium in 22%.

The most common malignancies involving the heart or pericardium include lung, breast, leukemia, Hodgkin's and non-Hodgkin's lymphoma, melanoma, gastrointestinal primaries, and sarcomas. Lung and breast predominate all autopsy series as the most likely neoplasms to cause myopericardial metastases, and it is estimated that 35% of patients with lung cancer will be found to have pericardial metastases at autopsy,[102] whereas as many as 25% of patients with breast cancer will have pericardial involvement at autopsy.[103-105]

PATHOPHYSIOLOGY

There is usually not in excess of 50 ml of pericardial fluid, which serves as a lubricant, normally in the pericardial sac. The increase in pericardial fluid seen in malignant pericardial effusions is due to obstruction of lymphatic and venous drainage of the heart, and this disturbs the level of intrapericardial pressure, depending on the rate of fluid accumulation, pericardial compliance, ventricular mass, and intravascular volume. Mediastinal nodal involvement, frequently seen with lung and breast cancer, disturbs lymphatic drainage through the cardiac nodes from the heart and pericardium.[106] Pathologically, pericardial metastases may extend and attach to a mediastinal mass and pericardium alone or to the heart. The pericardium may be diffusely studded with nodules, infiltrated with tumor, or be associated with solitary or multiple large nodular masses.[99]

SYMPTOMS

Malignant pericardial disease is unpredictable in its production of symptoms. The development of symptoms will depend on the rate of accumulation of pericardial fluid, the volume of fluid, and the underlying ventricular function. In a widely quoted study, Thurber reported that 71% of patients with cardiac metastases were asymptomatic; this figure, however, must be influenced by the degree of involvement, for in patients with large, nodular lesions, two-thirds of them are symptomatic, whereas only 27% of patients with small-nodular metastases were symptomatic.[99] Pericardial symptoms, usually tamponade, however, have been described as the initial feature of extracardiac malignancies in 36 patients, chiefly from lung cancer.[107]

Symptoms of neoplastic pericardial involvement include dyspnea, cough, chest pain, orthopnea, palpitations, weakness, fatigue, and dizziness. Cardiac tamponade is the most severe presenting symptom complex and is characterized by anxiety, chest pain, and dypsnea, with upright forward-leaning posturing to obtain maximal relief. Ashen faces with facial plethora, as well as vague gastrointestinal complaints from visceral congestion may be present.[101]

SIGNS

In the asymptomatic patient, signs of malignant pericardial/myocardial involvement may be absent. Physical examination, however, should be directed toward the presence of jugular venous distention, cardiac enlargement, distant heart sounds, pericardial friction rub, and arrhythmias. Hepatosplenomegaly and ascites may represent congestive phenomena. Tamponade is accompanied by the presence of pulsus paradoxus, hypotension, and significant tachycardia associated with weak heart sounds with or without a positive hepatojugular reflex.

DIAGNOSTIC TECHNIQUES

Radiography

A change in the contour of the heart shadow on an upright AP x-ray film of the chest, in association with the forementioned symptoms, in a patient with cancer should alert the clinician to the possibility of neoplastic pericarditis. A normal chest roentgenogram, however, does not exclude the possibility of effusion.[108] Classically, there is an enlargement of the cardiopericardial silhouette, described as a water-bottle heart, with bulging and loss of the normal contours of the pericardial reflection. Widening of the subcarinal angle[1] or associated pleural effusion may be present. The use of fluoroscopy for the diagnosis of pericardial effusion is now of historical interest, and cardiac catheterization is indicated only to delineate whether or not there is a constrictive component to the disease, as could be present after mediastinal irradiation. Fluoroscopy is useful, however, for guidance in the placement of catheters for diagnostic or therapeutic pericardiocentesis.

Computed tomography provides a more global view of the pericardium and its relation to the mediastinum as well as to the heart itself. The regular use of CT in diagnosing and staging lymphoma demonstrates periparacardial involvement earlier and with greater accuracy than conventional radiography.[109] Difficult-to-detect effusions, such as those distorted by pneumonectomy for lung cancer, are more readily detected by CT.[110] Malignant pericardial disease is suspected by CT criteria including [1] pericardial effusion with high CT density, [2] localized or diffuse pericardial thickening, [3] masses from or contiguous with the pericardium, and [4] obliteration of normal tissue planes between a paracardiac mass and the heart or pericardium.[111,112]

Echocardiography (ECHO) represents the least invasive, least time-consuming, and most precise method for rapid demonstration and quantitation of malignant pleural effusion. Portable ECHO can be performed at the bedside in less than 15 min and, with M-mode and two-dimensional techniques, describe and quantitate the distribution of pericardial fluid collections. Underlying myocardial function can be estimated as well as the presence of abnormal echoes within the pericardial sac that may point to the presence of pericardial metastases.[113] Precise bedside confirmation of placement of pericardial catheters can also be accomplished with ECHO.

Electrocardiographic Abnormalities

The ECG changes seen with neoplastic pericarditis include tachycardia, premature contractions, low QRS voltage, and nonspecific ST and T-wave changes.[1] Flattened or inverted T waves may be seen with constrictive pericarditis. Electrical alternans, alternating high- and low-voltage p waves, or ventricular complexes, correspond to superficial and deep positions of the heart relative to the anterior chest wall and is usually seen in tamponade. The alternans pattern will disappear with appropriate therapy for the effusion.[101]

Pericardiocentesis

TECHNIQUE AND USE IN DIAGNOSIS. The use of percutaneous pericardiocentesis guided by two-dimensional echocardiography is associated with a high diagnostic yield, a low frequency of complications, and rapid amelioration of symptoms of tamponade in patients with malignant pericardial effusions.[114] Risk-wise, pericardiocentis in patients with *malignant* pericardial effusion is very effective, both diagnostically and therapeutically, in comparison with other subgroups of patients requiring pericardial catheterization (*i.e.*, after open-heart surgery). The risk of pericardiocentesis is dependent on the amount and location of the fluid. Patients with loculated effusion in a posterior position usually cannot be drained by the usual approaches. The use of fluoroscopy or ECHO guidance decreases, to a minimum, the previously reported risk of cardiac chamber puncture, ventricular tachycardia, and tension pneumothorax.[115,116] In a recent series of 42 such catheterizations, there were no sudden deaths, and the complication rate (bradycardia–hypotension) was 5%.[115] A variety of self-contained kits are available for catheter drainage of the pericardium.

USE OF PERICARDIOCENTESIS FOR CYTOLOGIC DIAGNOSIS. The cause of the effusion in patients with cancer may be first surmised by the appearance of the fluid. Hemorrhagic fluid is usually associated with positive pericardial cytologic results, especially in lung cancer, and cytologic examination will demonstrate malignant cells in 80% to 90% of the patients with neoplastic pericarditis. There is, however, a significant percentage of false-negative cytologic results observed, and a negative report does not eliminate cancer from the differential diagnosis.[117,118] Moreover, the ability to make a cytologic diagnosis is more difficult in certain malignancies, including lymphoma and leukemia. There is a definite frequency of late effusive constrictive pericarditis that is seen very late in patients with lymphoma who have received mediastinal irradiation. A frequency of radiation-related pericardial effusion of 31% has been reported after upper mantle radiotherapy for Hodgkin's disease.[119] These patients will usually present with negative cytologic evaluations, yet will require management of the effusion and possible constrictive symptoms.

TREATMENT

The ultimate outcome for patients with malignant pericardial disease will depend on the performance status of the patients, the presence of metastatic disease, the availability of adjuvant systemic therapy, and the local management of the pericardial effusion for the long-term abolition of tamponade-like symptoms. Despite the prevalence of this manifestation of malignant disease, there are no prospective randomized trials comparing methods of local therapy to evaluate long-term effectiveness or survival.

Catheter Drainage Alone

The use of pericardial drainage alone has met with equivocal success in a small number of patients, as reported in the literature. Of six patients having a single pericardiocentesis or 24 to 48 hr of pericardial drainage, four had effusion control for 1 month or longer.[121] Of 16 patients with malignant effusions in another study,[115] only two required subsequent pericardiectomy for recurrence. Nine of the 16, however, had other nonsurgical therapy. In a more recent study of ten patients with histologically confirmed neoplastic (breast) pericarditis, all three patients treated by pericardiocentesis alone relapsed at 11, 40, or 1462 days after the tap. One of these patients died, upon relapse, of tamponade, and the other two required surgery.[103]

Instillational Local Therapy

Nitrogen mustard, thiotepa, and quinicrine were all used for intrapericardial instillation in the 1970s, but they were associated with severe pain and bone marrow toxicity. Treatment with TCN instillation usually requires multiple instillations for it to be effective. Of the 28 patients described, each treated with a mean TCN instillation of 500 mg/instillation, a success rate of longer than 1 month was seen in 75%, with a mean 120 days without recurrence.[121,122] Complications included mild fever, arrythmias, and pain. Bleomycin (four patients),[123] cisplatin (one patient),[124] and vinblastine (one patient)[125] have also been used for local instillation. These studies further verify that the pericardial catheter can be successfully left in place longer than 72 hr without infection and that catheter occlusion is more prevalent with continuous drainage as opposed to intermittent flushing.[115] The use of intrapericardial ^{98}AU has been largely relegated to historical interest.[1] Further trials of instillational therapy are required, to compare with catheter drainage alone or with surgical techniques, before this therapy can be adopted as a first-line option.

Radiotherapy

Although formerly used frequently for pericardial effusions related to various histolocic types of carcinoma, pericardial radiation is most suited for the management of pericardial effusions from lymphoma.[126] Recommended dosages are 2.0 to 3.0 Gy, fractionated over a 2 to 3 week period.

Surgery

Decisions about surgical intervention for the patient with neoplastic pericarditis must be influenced by the performance status of the patient, extent of disease, future therapeutic options, histologic type of the primary neoplasm, and the extent of surgical resection of the pericardium to provide the lowest surgical mortality with the least chance of the development of recurrent pericardial symptoms. Most of the patients will be able to have emergent placement of a pericardial catheter to relieve tamponade symptoms and thus be more favorable surgical–anesthetic candidates. It is generally agreed that surgical intervention should be considered in those medically fit patients whose effusive pericarditis is unresponsive to radiotherapy, or to intrapericardial therapy, or who have required repeated pericardiocentesis. Good-risk patients with effusions who have had repeated aspirations, in whom the cytologic results were inconclusive or negative, but in whom there is a high index of suspicion for neoplastic disease amenable to systemic or local therapy, should, for the most part, have surgical exploration. Finally, patients with constrictive pericarditis caused by radiation or neoplastic pericardial constriction, documented hemodynamically by catheterization, and who would be expected to have a reasonable long-term survival, should have pericardial resection.

Usually, patients will have effusive problems with tamponade symptoms. The subxiphoid approach has received many enthusiastic commendations in the literature, from a number of institutions, as being the procedure of choice in the management of malignant effusions. The use of local anesthesia; direct exposure of the pericardium; complete drainage of the pericardial space by chest tubes, allowing pericardial and epicardial symphysis; and the avoidance of a thoracotomy, have all been expounded as the advantages of this technique. When one examines the reports in the literature and defines the subset of patients with malignant effusions who had subxiphoid drainage (Table 62-34), it is difficult to label this procedure as the "cure all to end all" for neoplastic pericarditis. Ideally, the minimum mortality in cancer patients is 8%, and the ideal described recurrence rate is 7%. This procedure is probably superior to simple window formation by a left thoracotomy, relative to mortality and recurrence (Fig. 62-41). Moreover, the type of pericardiectomy does not seem to have any influence on the postoperative survival in patients with malignant disease. Survival in patients with malignant disease is affected by the tumor cell type, with lung cancer having a mean survival of 3.5 months; breast cancer, after surgical intervention having a survival of 9.3 to 18.5 months; and lymphoma survival is approximately 10 months. The amount of pericardium remaining after surgical drainage, however, does impinge directly on the development of late postoperative complications (*e.g.*, recurrence of effusion). Patients who have a complete pericardiectomy have significantly fewer late failures than those who have a window pericardiectomy. Therefore, in patients who have other salvage therapies, either radiation or chemotherapy, or those expected to have a

TABLE 62-34. Subxiphoid Approach for Malignant Pericardial Effusion

Author	*No. of Patients*	*Mortality*	*Recurrence*
Ghosh[127]	20	0	1
Hankins[128]	13	0	0
Raza[128]	49	0	3
Williams[128]	26	0	3
Osuch[129]	12	1	0
Berman[130]	3	0	0
Little[131]	19	6	0
Piehler[132]	10	1	3
Miller[132]	3	2	
Prager[133]	6	3	
TOTAL	161	13 (8%)	10 (7%)

FIG. 62-41. Pericardial "window" via left thoracotomy. Arrows denote edge of pericardium.

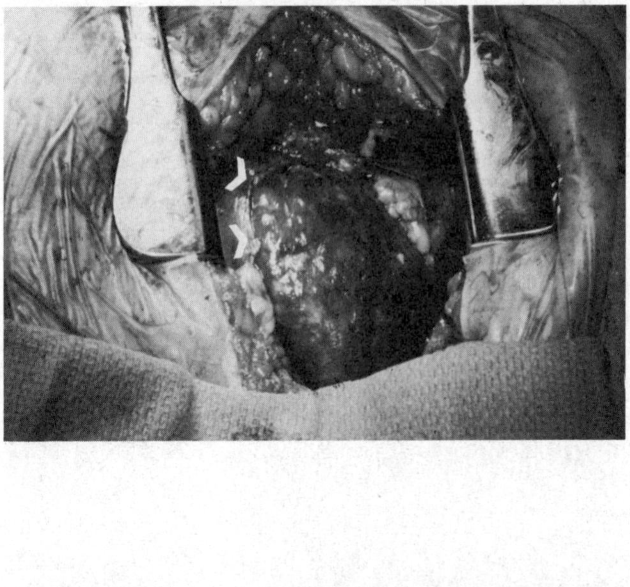

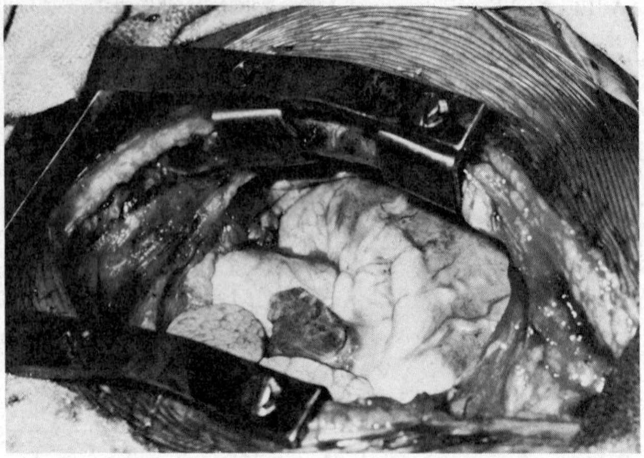

FIG. 62-42. Median sternotomy approach for complete pericardiectomy. View after completed resection.

longer survival (*e.g.*, lymphoma or breast cancer), the widest pericardial resection should be considered to prevent future recurrence (Fig. 62-42). Moreover, radiation-induced effusions should not be managed by a subxiphoid window because of a high late-failure rate.

REFERENCES

1. McKenna RJ, Ali MK, Ewer MS et al: Pleural and pericardial effusions in cancer patients. Curr Prob Cancer 9:1, 1985
2. Hausheer FH, Yarbro JW: Diagnosis and treatment of malignant pleural effusion. Semin Oncol 12:54, 1985
3. Sahn SA: Malignant pleural effusions. Clin Chest Med 6:113, 1985
4. Martensson G, Pettersson K, Thiringer G: Differentiation between malignant and non-malignant pleural effusion. Eur J Respir Dis 67:326, 1985
5. Dhillon DP, Spiro SG: Malignant pleural effusions. Br J Hosp Med 29:506, 1983
6. Chernow B, Sahn SA: Carcinomatous involvement of the pleura: An analysis of 96 patients. Am J Med 63:695, 1977
7. Zehner LC, Hoogstraten B: Malignant effusions and their management. Semin Oncol Nurs 1:259, 1985
8. Austin EH, Flye MW: The treatment of recurrent malignant pleural effusion. Ann Thorac Surg 28:190, 1979
9. Kaunitz J: Landmarks in simple pleural effusions. JAMA 113:1312, 1939
10. Peterson JA: Recognition of infrapulmonary pleural effusion. Radiology 74:34, 1960
11. Woodring JH: Recognition of pleural effusion on supine radiographs: How much fluid is required? AJR 142:59, 1984
12. Salonen O, Kivisaari L, Nordenstam G et al: Computed tomography of pleural lesions with special reference to the mediastinal pleura. Acta Radiol Diag 27:527, 1986
13. Doust BD, Baum JK, Maklad NF et al: Ultrasonic evaluation of pleural opacities. Radiology 114:135, 1975
14. Ravin CE: Thoracentesis of loculated pleural effusions using grey scale ultrasonic guidance. Chest 71:666, 1977
15. Sears D, Hajdu SI: The cytologic diagnosis of malignant neoplasm in pleural and peritoneal effusions. Acta Cytol 31:85, 1987
16. Lopes-Cardozo PL: A critical evaluation of 3000 cytologic analyses of pleural fluid, ascitic fluid, and peritoneal fluid. Acta Cytol 10:455, 1966
17. Johnston WW: The malignant pleural effusion: A review of cytopathologic diagnosis of 584 specimens from 472 consecutive patients. Cancer 56:905, 1985
18. Jarvi OH, Kunnas RJ, Laitio MT et al: The accuracy and significance of cytologic cancer diagnoses in pleural effusions. Acta Cytol 16:152, 1972
19. Johnson WD: The cytologic diagnosis of cancer in serous effusions. Acta Cytol 10:161, 1966
20. Melamed MR: The cytologic preparation of malignant lymphomas and related disease in effusions. Cancer 16:413, 1963
21. Ceelen GH: The cytologic diagnosis of ascitic fluid. Acta Cytol 8:175, 1964
22. Spriggs AI: Letter-to-the-Editor. Br Med J 282:1972, 1981
23. Sehested M, Ralfkiaer E, Rasmussen J: Immunoperoxidase demonstration of carcinoembryonic antigen in pleural and peritoneal effusions. Acta Cytol 27:124, 1983
24. To A, Coleman V, Dearnaley DP et al: Use of antisera to epithelial membrane antigen for the cytodiagnosis of malignancy in serous effusions. J Clin Pathol 24:1326, 1981
25. To A, Dearnaley DP, Ormerod G et al: Epithelial membrane antigen: Its use in the cytodiagnosis of malignancy in serous effusions. Am J Clin Pathol 77:214, 1982
26. Walts AE, Said JW, Banks-Schlegel S: Keratin and carcinoembryonic antigen in exfoliated mesothelial and malignant cells: An immunoperoxidase study. Am J Clin Pathol 80:671, 1983
27. Johnston WW, Szpak CA, Lottich SC et al: Use of a monoclonal antibody (B72.3) as an immunocytochemical adjunct to diagnosis of adenocarcinoma in human effusions. Cancer Res 45:1894, 1985
28. Martin SE, Moshiri S, Thor A et al: Identification of adenocarcinoma in cytospin preparations of effusions using monoclonal antibody B72.3. Am J Clin Pathol 86:10, 1986
29. Das DK, Gupta SK, Ayzagari S et al: Pleural effusions on non-Hodgkin's lymphoma: A cytomorphologic, cytochemical, and immunologic study. Acta Cytol 31:119, 1987
30. Musilova J, Michalova K: Cytogenetic study of cancer cells in effusions. Cancer Genet Cytogenet 19:271, 1986
31. Carlevaro C, Rossi GA, Cerri E et al: Cytogenetic study of pleural effusions. Tumori 64:335, 1978
32. Fraisse J, Brizard CP, Emonot A et al: Diagnosis of malignancy by cytogenetic means in effusions. Clin Genet 14:288, 1978
33. McKenna JM, Chandraesekhar AJ, Henkin RE: Diagnostic value of carcinoembryonic antigen in exudative pleural effusion. Chest 78:587, 1980
34. Rutgers RA, Loewenstein MS, Feinerman AE et al: Carcinoembryonic antigen levels in benign and malignant pleural effusions. Ann Intern Med 88:631, 1978
35. Vladutin AO, Brason FW, Adler RH: Differential diagnosis of pleural effusions: Clinical usefulness of cell marker quantitation. Chest 79:297, 1981
36. Rasmussen KN, Faher V: Hyaluronic acid in 247 pleural fluids. Scand J Respir Dis 48:366, 1967
37. Ratliff JL, Chavez CM, Jamchuk A et al: Reexpansion pulmonary edema. Chest 64:654, 1973
38. Trapnell DH, Thurston JGB: Unilateral pulmonary edema after pleural aspiration. Lancet 1:1367, 1970
39. Yamazaki S, Ogawa J, Shohyu A et al: Pulmonary blood flow to rapidly re-expanded lung on spontaneous pneumothorax. Chest 81:118, 1982
40. Prakash UBS: Malignant pleural effusions. Postgrad Med 80:201, 1986
41. Prakash UBS, Reiman HM: Comparison of needle biopsy with cytologic analysis for the evaluation of pleural effusion: Analysis of 414 cases. Mayo Clin Proc 60:158, 1985
42. Hanson G, Phillips T: Pleural biopsy in diagnosis of thoracic disease. Br Med J 2:300, 1962
43. Sisson BS, Weiss W: Needle biopsy of the parietal pleura in patients with pleural effusion. Br Med J 2:298, 1962
44. Scerbo J, Keltz H, Stone DJ: A prospective study of closed pleural biopsies. JAMA 218:377, 1971
45. Liss HP: Cope needle biopsy. South Med J 77:837, 1984
46. Bevelaqua FA, Aranda C, Leon W: The role of closed pleural biopsy in suspected malignant effusions. NY State J Med 84:229, 1984
47. Salyer WR, Eggleston JC, Eroyan YS: Efficacy of pleural needle biopsy and pleural fluid cytopathology in the diagnosis of malignant neoplasm involving the pleura. Chest 67:536, 1975
48. Winkelman M, Pfitzer P: Blind pleural biopsy in combination with cytology of pleural effusions. Acta Cytol 25:373, 1981
49. Levine H, Cugell DW: Blunt-end needle biopsy of pleura and rib. Arch Intern Med 109:516, 1962
50. Mayer HR: Closed pleural biopsy. NY State J Med 70:1763, 1970
51. Poe RH, Israel RH, Utell MJ et al: Sensitivity, specificity, and predictive values of closed pleural biopsy. Arch Intern Med 144:325, 1984
52. Schools GS: Needle biopsy of parietal pleura: Current status. Tex State J Med 59:1056, 1963
53. Jones FL: Subcutaneous implantation of cancer: A rare complication of pleural biopsy. Chest 57:189, 1970
54. Boutin C, Cargrino P, Viallat JR: Thoracoscopy in the early diagnosis of malignant pleural effusions. Endoscopy 12:155, 1980
55. Weissburg D, Kaufman M, Zurkowski Z: Pleuroscopy in patients with pleural effusions and pleural masses. Ann Thorac Surg 29:205, 1980
56. Weissburg D, Kaufman M: Diagnostic and therapeutic pleuroscopy: Experience with 127 patients. Chest 78:732, 1980
57. Thoracoscopy. In Vladutin AO (ed): Pleural Effusion, p. 160. Mount Kisco, Futura, 1986
58. Canto A, Fener G, Romagosa V et al: Lung cancer and pleural effusion: Clinical significance and study of pleural metastatic locations. Chest 87:649, 1985
59. Levine MN, Young JE, Ryan E et al: Pleural effusion in breast cancer. Cancer 57:324, 1986
60. Oakes DD, Sherck JP, Brodsky JB et al: Therapeutic thoracoscopy. J Thorac Cardiovasc Surg 87:269, 1984
61. Weissberg D: Talc pleurodesis: A controversial issue. Poumon-Coeur 37:291, 1981
62. Chernow B, Sahn SA: Carcinomatous involvement of the pleura. Am J Med 63:695, 1977
63. Roy RH, Can DT, Payne WS: The problem of chylothorax. Mayo Clin Proc 42:457, 1967
64. Leff A, Honeywell PC, Costello J: Pleural effusion from malignancy. Ann Intern Med 88:532, 1978

65. Bayly TC, Kisner DL, Sybert A et al: Tetracycline and quinacrine in the control of malignant pleural effusions: A randomized trial. Cancer 41:1188, 1978
66. Zaloznek AJ, Oswald SG, Langin M: Intrapleural tetracycline in malignant pleural effusions: A randomized study. Cancer 51:752, 1983
67. O'Neill W, Spurr C, Muss H et al: A prospective study of chest tube drainage and tetracycline sclerosis versus chest tube drainage in the treatment of malignant pleural effusion. Proc Am Soc Clin Oncol 21:349, 1980
68. Wallach H: Letter-to-the-Editor. Chest 73:246, 1978
69. Sahn SA, Good JT: The effect of common sclerosing agents on the rabbit pleural space. Am Rev Respir Dis 124:65, 1981
70. Dunkel TB: Intrapleural tetracycline in the treatment of malignant pleural effusions. Minn Med 69:717, 1986
71. Mejer J, Martensen KM, Hansen HH: Mepacrine hydrochloride in the treatment of malignant pleural effusion: A randomized trial. Scand J Resp Dis 58:319, 1977
72. Taylor SA, Hooton NS, MacArthur AM: Quinacrine in the management of malignant pleural effusions. Br J Surg 64:52, 1977
73. Hickman JA, Jones MC: Treatment of neoplastic pleural effusions with local instillation of quinacrine (mepacrine) hydrochloride. Thorax 25:226, 1970
74. Arvastson B, Boe J, Stiksu J et al: Mepacrine in malignant pleural effusion. Scand J Respir Dis 54:132, 1973
75. Boya ET, Pugh RP: Single-dose quinacrine (Atabrine) and thoracostomy in the control of pleural effusion in patients with neoplastic disease. Cancer 31:899, 1973
76. Sorensen PG, Svendsen TL, Enk B: Treatment of malignant pleural effusion with drainage, with and without instillation of talc. Eur J Respir Dis 65:131, 1984
77. Adler RH, Sayek I: Treatment of malignant pleural effusion: A method using tube thoracostomy and talc. Ann Thorac Surg 22:8, 1976
78. Starkey GW: Recurrent malignant pleural effusions: N Engl J Med 270:436, 1964
79. Jones GR: Treatment of malignant pleural effusion by iodized talc pleurodesis. Thorax 24:69, 1969
80. Shedbalkar AR, Head JM, Head LR et al: Evaluation of talc pleural symphysis in management of malignant pleural effusion. J Thorac Cardiovasc Surg 61:492, 1971
81. Ostrowski M: An assessment of the long term results of controlling the reaccumulation of malignant effusions using intracavitary bleomycin. Cancer 57:721, 1986
82. Gupta N, Opfell RW, Padova C et al: Intrapleural bleomycin vs tetracycline for control of malignant pleural effusions. A randomized study. Am Soc Clin Oncol Abstr C-189:366, 1980
83. Pectasides P, Stewart S, Courtenay-Luch N et al: Antibody-guided irradiation of malignant pleural and pericardial effusions. Br J Cancer 53:727, 1986
84. Leahy BC, Honeybourne D, Brear SG et al: Treatment of malignant pleural effusions with intrapleural *Corynebacterium parvum* or tetracycline. Eur J Respir Dis 66:50, 1985
85. Hillerdal G, Kiviloog J, Nou E et al: *Corynebacterium parvum* in malignant pleural effusion. A randomized prospective study. Eur J Respir Dis 69:204, 1986
86. Millar JW, Hunter AM, Horne NW: Intrapleural immunotherapy with *Corynebacterium parvum* in recurrent malignant pleural effusions. Thorax 35:856, 1979
87. Rossi GA, Felletti R, Balbi R et al: Symptomatic treatment of recurrent malignant pleural effusions with intrapleurally administered *Corynebacterium parvum*. Am Rev Respir Dis 135:885, 1987
88. Weick JK, Killy JM, Harrison EG et al: Pleural effusion in lymphoma. Cancer 31:848, 1973
89. Xaubet A, Duimenjo MC, Maren A et al: Characteristics and prognostic value of pleural effusion in non-Hodgkin's lymphoma. Eur J Respir Dis 66:135, 1985
90. Martini N, Bains M, Beattie EJ: Indications for pleurectomy in malignant effusion. Cancer 35:734, 1975
91. Jensik R, Cagle JE, Melloy F et al: Pleurectomy in the treatment of pleural effusion due to metastatic malignancy. J Thorac Cardiovasc Surg 46:322, 1963
92. Anderson CB, Philpott GW, Ferguson TB: The treatment of malignant pleural effusions. Cancer 33:916, 1974
93. Cemochowski GE, Joyner LR, Farden R et al: Pleuroperitoneal shunting for recalcitrant pleural effusions. J Thorac Cardiovasc Surg 92:866, 1986
94. Little AG, Ferguson MK, Golomb HM et al: Pleuroperitoneal shunting for malignant pleural effusions. Cancer 58:2740, 1986
95. Yates WM: Tumors of the heart and pericardium. Arch Intern Med 48:627, 1931
96. Scott RW, Garvin CF: Tumors of the heart and pericardium. Am Heart J 17:431, 1939
97. Bisel HF, Wroblewski F, LaDue JS: Incidence and clinical manifestations of cardiac metastases. JAMA 153:712, 1953
98. Thurber DL, Edwards JE, Achor RWP: Secondary malignant tumors of the pericardium. Circulation 26:228, 1962
99. Skhvatsabaju LV: Secondary malignant lesions of the heart and pericardium in neoplastic disease. Oncology 43:103, 1986
100. Goudie RB: Secondary tumors of the heart and pericardium. Br Heart J 17:183, 1955
101. Theologides A: Neoplastic cardiac tamponade. Semin Oncol 5:181, 1978
102. Shenkai T, Tomenagu K, Saijo N et al: The incidence of cardiac metastases in primary lung cancer and the management of malignant pericardial effusion. Jpn J Clin Oncol 12:23, 1982
103. Buck M, Ingle JN, Guilani ER et al: Pericardial effusion in women with breast cancer. Cancer 60:263, 1987
104. Hagemeister FB, Buydan AU, Luna MA et al: Causes of death in breast cancer. Cancer 46:162, 1980
105. Nakayama R, Yoneyama T, Takatani O et al: A study of metastatic tumors to the heart, pericardium and great vessels. Jpn Heart J 7:227, 1966
106. Oruigbo WIB: The spread of lung cancer to the heart, pericardium, and great vessels. Jpn Heart J 15:234, 1974
107. Shende SR, Shana PB, Shetty PA: Cardiac tamponade as the only initial feature of malignancy: A case report and review of the literature. J Surg Oncol 32:96, 1956
108. Pories WJ, Gaudiani VA: Cardiac tamponade. Surg Clin North Am 55:573, 1975
109. Jochelson MS, Balikian JP, Mauch P et al: Peri- and paracardial involvement in lymphoma: A radiographic study of 11 cases. AJR 140:483, 1983
110. Dighton DH, Golding R, de Feytes PJ: Post-pneumonectomy pericardial effusion. Chest 82:389, 1982
111. Golding RD, Zanten TEG: Computed tomography in malignant conditions affecting the pericardium. J Belge Radiol 67:371, 1984
112. Johnson FE, Wolverson MIL, Sundaram M et al: Unsuspected malignant pericardial effusion causing cardiac tamponade. Chest 82:501, 1982
113. Chandraratna DAN, Aronow WS: Detection of pericardial metastases by cross sectional echocardiography. Circulation 63:197, 1981
114. Callahan JA, Seward JB, Nishimura RA et al: Two-dimensional echocardiographically guided pericardiocentesis: Experience in 117 consecutive patients. Am J Cardiol 55:476, 1985
115. Kopecky SL, Callahan JA, Tajek AJ et al: Percutaneous pericardial catheter drainage: Report of 42 consecutive cases. Am J Cardiol 58:633, 1986
116. Wong B, Murphy J, Chang CJ et al: The risk of pericardiocentesis. Am J Cardiol 44:1110, 1979
117. Zepf RE, Johnston WW: The role of cytology in the evaluation of pericardial effusions. Chest 62:593, 1972
118. Reyes CV, Strinden C, Banerji M: The role of cytology in neoplastic tamponade. Acta Cytol 26:299, 1982
119. Applefeld MM, Cole JF, Pollock SH et al: The late appearance of chronic pericardial disease in patients treated by radiotherapy for Hodgkin's disease. Ann Intern Med 94:338, 1981
120. Flannery EP, Gregoratos G, Corder MP: Pericardial effusions in patients with malignant diseases. Arch Intern Med 135:976, 1975
121. Pavis S, Sharma SM, Blumberg ED et al: Intrapericardial tetracycline for the management of cardiac tamponade secondary to malignant pericardial effusion. N Engl J Med 299:1113, 1978
122. Shepherd FA, Ginsberg JS, Evans WR et al: Tetracycline sclerosis in the management of malignant pericardial effusion. J Clin Oncol 3:1678, 1985
123. Maher FR, Buckman R: Intrapericardial installation of bleomycin in malignant pericardial effusion. Am Heart J 111:613, 1986
124. Markman M, Howell SB: Intrapericardial instillation of cisplatin in a patient with a large malignant effusion. Cancer Drug Deliv 2:49, 1985
125. Primrose WR, Clee MD, Johnston RN: Malignant pericardial effusion managed with vinblastine. Clin Oncol 9:67, 1983
126. Terry LN, Klegerman MM: Pericardial and myocardial involvement by lymphomas and leukemias: The role of radiotherapy. Cancer 25:1003, 1970
127. Ghosh SC, Larrieu A, Ablaza S et al: Clinical experience with subxyphoid pericardial decompression. Int Surg 70:5, 1985
128. Hankins JR, Sattersfield JR, Aisner J et al: Pericardial window for malignant pericardial effusion. Ann Thorac Surg 30:465, 1980
129. Osuch JR, Khandehar JN, Fry WA. Emergency subxyphoid pericardial decompression for malignant pericardial effusion. Am Surg 51:298, 1985
130. Berman K, Fielding MB, Richi AA: Diagnosis and treatment of malignant pericardial effusion: The subxyphoid approach. Conn Med 48:701, 1984
131. Little AG, Krimser PC, Wade JL et al: Operation for diagnosis and treatment of pericardial effusions. Surgery 96:738, 1984
132. Piehler JM, Pluth JR, Schaff HV et al: Surgical management of effusive pericardial disease. J Thorac Cardiovasc Surg 90:506, 1985
133. Prager PL, Wilson CH, Bender AW: The subxyphoid approach to pericardial disease. Ann Thorac Surg 34:6, 1982

SECTION 6

ALAN R. BAKER

Treatment of Malignant Ascites

The development of a malignant peritoneal effusion during a tumor patient's clinical course is a not infrequent, prognostically adverse, and often symptomatically troublesome event. Loss of a sense of well-being, anorexia, and early satiety; difficulty with ambulation; and respiratory compromise can all impose significant quality-of-life debits. With a median life expectancy on the order of months (see Table 62-36), therapy measures, if successful, can provide very meaningful palliation. That numerous treatment alternatives have been explored—diuresis, paracentesis, systemic chemotherapy, intraperitoneal chemotherapy, external beam x-ray and intracavitary radiocolloid instillation, immunotherapy, and internal ascitic fluid shunting—attest as much to the lack of singular success with any one approach, as to the conceptual and technical bias and expertise of the variety of physician subspecialists who have tried to alter this problem. Lacy and co-workers[1] have provided a recent extensive and thoughtful review of this subject.

The pathogenesis of malignant ascites can be multifactorial. Compromised drainage of the peritoneal cavity by tumor-caused obstruction of subdiaphragmatic lymphatic channels and plexuses as demonstrated by Feldman[2,3] and others[4,5] is doubtless a factor of major importance. Although excess fluid production is probably a more important factor in the genesis of cirrhotic ascites, Hirayashi[6] has demonstrated that it occurs in the setting of ovarian cancer, and Garrison and colleagues[7] have suggested that tumor can elaborate humoral factors that cause increased capillary leakage, even across normal peritoneal surfaces and omentum. Hydrodynamic disequilibria caused by hypoalbuminemia or portal venous or hepatic venous obstruction, noted when the liver is extensively replaced by metastatic tumor, probably favor the production of ascitic fluid as well.

DIAGNOSIS AND WORKUP

Ascites may be the presenting problem, as is often the case for patients with ovarian cancer, or it may develop later during the patient's clinical course. Even for the patient with cancer, nonneoplastic causes, such as congestive heart failure, cirrhosis, nephrosis and, on less frequent occasions, complications of radiotherapy or chemotherapy directed at the underlying malignancy, can be responsible and should be ruled out.

Abdominal paracentesis, with complete removal of the ascitic collection, permits quantitation of its volume, diagnostic assessment of its profile, usually temporary resolution of any symptomatic sequellae, and an opportunity to assess the time for significant reaccumulation. To prevent the infrequently seen orthostatic changes or electrolyte abberations that may follow removal of a large volume of ascitic fluid, the patient should be encouraged to take fluids liberally or be supported parenterally and cautioned about dizziness and lightheadedness.

The character of the aspirated fluid should be noted and can offer immediate clues to its etiology. Bloody (malignant or traumatic), serous (cirrhotic, nephrotic, pancreatic, or cardiopathic), cloudy (infectious peritonitis), or chylous (lymphoma or gut lymphatic or thoracic duct injury) collections suggest alternative etiologic explanations that are, unfortunately, not mutually exclusive.

Although no single feature in the chemical profile of ascitic fluid is pathognomonic for a malignant cause, the presence of an elevated total protein ($>$40% of the serum protein,[7] elevated lactic acid dehydrogenase (LDH; ratio of ascitic fluid LDH/serum LDH $>$1.0),[8] or a significant concentration of carcinoembryonic antigen (CEA $>$10 ng/ml)[9,10] or another tumor marker are factors that favor a neoplastic explanation. The presence of red blood cells ($>$10,000 RBC/mm^3) and various morphologic types of white blood cells ($>$1000 WBC/mm^3), as well as the absence of bacteria on Gram stain and sterility on microbiologic culture, further characterize a malignant effusion. Malignant cells seen on cytologic examination by Papanicolaou staining of the spun pellet or cell block confirm the clinical suspicion of a malignant cause. Unfortunately, even in the setting of cancer, only about 50% of such specimens will prove positive.[7]

The information in Table 62-35 summarizes important features in the evaluation of a patient with a peritoneal effusion.

TREATMENT

No critically controlled trials comparing the several alternative modes of management for patients with recalcitrant malignant ascites have been reported. The problem of evaluating a treatment modality is further compounded by nonuniform, or often nonexistent, definition of patient selection, as well as objective response criteria to the varied published regimens. Limited longevity (average survival about 2 months; see Table 62-36) seems to be a common denominator for cancer patients with this distressing problem managed by any of a variety of measures. Because none of these

TABLE 62-35. Assessment of the Patient with a Peritoneal Effusion

- Diagnosis/Workup
  - History
    - Increasing abdominal girth "clothes don't fit"
    - Indigestion and early satiety
    - Ankle swelling
    - Easy fatigability
    - Shortness of breath
  - Physical examination
    - Fluid wave
    - Shifting dullness
  - x-ray studies
    - Abdominal flat plate: generalized ground-glass appearance, air-filled small-bowel loops occupy central position and are separated by fluid between loops, psoas shadows obscured
    - Ultrasound, Abdominal CT: Both are sensitive tests that definitively diagnose small amounts of ascites
  - Paracentesis
    - Gross character on inspection: bloody, serious, milky, turbid
    - Cell count and differential
    - Chemistries: total protein, LDH, CEA, OC .25 amylase levels
    - Cytology
    - Microbiology: Gram stain and culture

TABLE 62-36. Reported Experience with Peritoneovenous Shunt Management of Malignant Ascites

	Underlying Malignancy						*Patient Survival*	
Series (year)	*Ovary*	*GI**	*Breast*	*Unknown Adenocarcinoma*	*Other*	*Author's Comments*	*Median (wk)*	*% Alive at 1 Year*
Straus (1979)[39]	13	10	3	2	9	27/37 (73%), Good shunt function and palliation	8	
Oosterlee (1980)[40]	6	7	2	1	4	13/20 (65%), Good shunt function and palliation	7	5
Raaf (1980)[41]		2	1	1	1	5/5 (100%), Ascites controlled	5	0
Lokich (1980)[42]	3		3	1	1	6/8 (75%), Ascites controlled and meaningful palliation	8	12
Downing (1982)[43]		2	3	1	1	4/7 (57%), Good shunt function and palliation	13	0
Lund (1982)[44]	14	9	5		7	Excellent initial and long-term therapy for ascites	16	11
Qazi (1982)[45]	28	4	8			28/40 (70%), Effective palliation		
Cheung (1982)[46]	2	7	4		9		5	10
Reinhold (1983)[47]	6	3	6		4	6/19 (32%), Excellent symptomatic relief	6	
Souter	9	4	4	4	5	23/26 (88%), Satisfactory palliation	16	12
Gough (1984)[49]	4	4	2		7	13/17 (76%), Ascites controlled, worthwhile palliation	13	6
Kostroff (1985)[50]	11	8	5		7		8	0
Campioni (1986)[51]	8	14	7	7	6	Safe and effective way to improve quality of life	7	7
Sonnenfeld (1986)[52]		16		5	6	19/27 (70%), Good palliation	8	0
Roussel (1986)[53]	12	10	11		3	Effective palliation for most patients	13	0
Total	116	100	64	22	70		5–16	0–12

*GI, gastrointestinal (colon, stomach, pancreas, hepatobiliary).

measures consistently or meaningfully prolongs survival and each can provide some degree of palliation, physician bias, tempered by common sense considerations, often dictates the treatment choice. Efforts should be directed at maximizing out-of-hospital time and minimizing treatment-imposed morbidity, complications, and quality-of-life debits. With these considerations in mind, and proceeding from the less invasive to the more invasive alternatives, a brief discussion of the therapy options follows.

DIET AND DIURESIS

Although often a useful adjunct in the management of cirrhotic ascites, dietary salt restriction and aldosterone-inhibiting and loop diuretics have little impact on malignant ascites. Sodium retention, as a pathogenetic factor in this setting, is probably less important than excess fluid elaboration from the tumor-involved expanded peritoneal surface area and the lymphatic obstruction that inhibits resorption. Pathogenetic considerations notwithstanding, Greenway and co-workers[11] have reported success in 13 of 15 patients treated with larger doses of spironolactone (150 mg/day in one patient, 300 mg/day in eight patients, and 450 mg/day in four patients) than customarily used. The only treatment toxicity observed was nausea in 2 of 15 patients. Baseline elevated plasma renin levels were measured in five of five patients, whereas above-normal aldosterone levels were noted in three of five patients.

REPEATED PARACENTESIS

Although advocated by some[12,13] as an approach to chronic management, repeated frequent abdominal taps should probably be discouraged. They contribute, under catabolic circumstances, to further protein depletion and electrolyte aberration, can cause injury to intra-abdominal viscera, and can lead to bacterial inoculation with resultant infection of the peritoneal fluid.

INTRACAVITARY THERAPY

Intracavitary therapy has consisted of intraperitoneal instillation with either a radioactive colloidal suspension or a chemotherapeutic drug.

Judging from the paucity of recent reports involving intraperitoneal instillation of radioactive agents to manage malignant ascites, enthusiasm for this treatment approach has clearly waned. Initially described over 40 years ago by Muller[14] the use of radioactive ^{63}Zn was soon supplanted by ^{198}Au,[15] which for reasons of safety, simplicity, and practicality has been essentially replaced by colloidal suspensions of ^{32}P-containing $CrPO_4$. Two substantial series[16,17] suggest that about 50% of patients derive some palliative benefit from this approach while suffering minimal treatment-related toxicity.

The topical application of chemotherapeutic agents by intracavitary instillation is designed to provoke an inflammatory response on the exposed surface, with the irritative reaction leading to sclerosis and space obliteration. Although this strategy is quite useful in the management of malignant pleural effusions, it appears less successful in the treatment of ascites. By intraperitoneal instillation, direct delivery to the tumor of a high drug concentration (2.5–8.0 times higher than with systemic administration) for prolonged periods with no increase in systemic toxicity lends added conceptual appeal.[18]

A resurgence of general interest in locoregional drug treatment for certain patterns of tumor dissemination has, nevertheless, led to several publications describing the response of patients with malignant ascites to intraperitoneal drug instillation. Paladine and associates[19] reported using bleomycin (60–120 mg diluted in 100 ml of normal saline) to manage 11 patients with ascites resulting from ovarian, gastrointestinal, lymphoma, lung, or renal cancers. With the exception of the patient with hypernephroma, all patients received concurrent systemic chemotherapy. Four of the 11 patients were categorized as complete or partial responders to intraperitoneal bleomycin instillation (no fluid reaccumulation, or minimal fluid reaccumulation, without symptoms or need for paracentesis). Median survival for the whole group was 2.5 months. Bitran and co-workers[20] treated ten patients with malignant ascites with a similar bleomycin regimen instilled through a Tenkoff catheter and noted complete resolution in six. Ostrowski,[21] again using intraperitoneal bleomycin, reported on 22 patients whose malignant peritoneal effusions were similarly treated. Of the 16 who survived for more than 1 month, 63% had complete or partial response that lasted at least 2 months. None of the authors reported serious side-effects. Other intraperitoneal drug regimens have been tried as well. Ozols and colleagues[22] in a Phase I study, reported on ten patients with advanced, drug-refractory ovarian cancer, treated with intraperitoneal doxorubicin (Adriamycin), instilled through a Tenkoff catheter. The two patients with severe malignant ascites both escaped need for continuing paracentesis. Kefford and co-workers[23] in a randomized study, sought to compare the efficacy of intraperitoneal instillation of doxorubicin, nitrogen mustard, and tetracycline. Complete or partial responses were noted for doxorubicin (four of four) and nitrogen mustard (two of eight), whereas none (zero of 3) was observed for tetracycline. And finally, Lopez and associates,[24] in a Phase I study of intraperitoneal instillation with cisplatin, noted "therapeutic benefit" in two of seven patients treated for malignant ascites.

Additional experience with the efficacy of this approach is accumulating and will need to be reported before its proper role can be determined. Catheter-related complications, such as malfunction and sepsis occur[25,26] and represent a caveat that must somewhat temper enthusiasm for this approach.

PERITONEOVENOUS SHUNTING

Although the concept of returning an ascitic fluid collection to the intravascular space is over 75 years old,[27,28] the technology to accomplish the objective in a minimally cumbersome fashion, with continuous reinfusion has evolved significantly over only the past 25 years.[29–32] The availability of several relatively simple, reasonably effective peritoneovenous (PV) shunt devices (LeVeen and Denver) has led to their fairly widespread use.

The devices consist of [1] a length of multiply perforated tubing to be implanted in the free peritoneal cavity, [2] a length of tubing to be inserted into the superior vena cava or right atrium, and [3] a unidirectional flow valve connecting the two limbs.

The principal difference between the LeVeen and Denver shunts is that the one-way valve in the Denver shunt can be manually pumped by physician or patient to flush it clear of possibly accumulating debris at periodic intervals. Despite this potentially theoretic advantage, the literature fails to demonstrate functional superiority for one or the other of these devices, thus, either may be chosen on the basis of personal preference.

This approach, with substantial pathophysiologic rationale,[33] was initially applied to the management of intractable ascites from cirrhosis.[34–38] Numerous series[39–53] have been more recently published that address its applicability in the management of malignant ascites.

In principle, the PV shunt takes advantage of the fact that a 5- to 15-cmH_2O pressure head exists between the ascites-laden peritoneal cavity and the central venous circulation. On inspiration, when intrathoracic pressure becomes more negative, the pressure differential further increases. Whenever the pressure gradient exceeds about 3 to 5 cmH_2O the unidirectional flow valve opens, and ascitic fluid moves through the tubing from peritoneal cavity to central circulation. Several excellent reports that describe details of shunt placement are available[31,32,35,54–56] and might profitably be perused by the uninitiated in an effort to avoid any one of the numerous technical pitfalls responsible for early shunt malfunction.

Figure 62-43 represents a schematic illustration of the shunt in place. In brief summary, the operation may be performed under either general anesthesia or local, supplemented with sedation. Prophylactic antibiotics are used. The peritoneal limb of the shunt is placed first through a roughly 3-in. long, muscle-splitting, subcostal incision. A nonabsorbable pursestring suture, which includes some transversus abdominus muscle, secures this limb in a watertight fashion. If the Denver shunt is used, a subcutaneous pocket overlying the lower rib cage is made for the pump device, and it is secured in position. Free flow of ascitic fluid is demonstrated by holding the open end of the venous limb several inches below heart level. Most surgeons remove about one-half the patient's ascitic fluid burden at this point, submitting some for culture and perhaps the rest for cytologic analysis. A cervical incision is then made exposing the internal jugular vein and a fine Prolene pursestring suture placed in its anterior wall. A uterine sound can then be used to make a graceful subcutaneous tunnel linking the abdominal and neck incisions such that all tubing will lie in a kink-free manner. The venous limb is then passed through the tunnel exiting into the cervical incision. After again demonstrating free flow of ascitic fluid and cutting the venous limb to permit its tip to lie in the superior vena cava or right atrium, it is placed through a stab wound in the vein and advanced centrally. It is useful to confirm the position of the PV shunt at this point, either fluoroscopically or with portable chest and abdominal x-ray films. Wounds are then irrigated with antibiotic solution, inspected and perfect hemostasis assured, and closed.

Although able to afford palliation, PV shunting is no panacea. Before proceeding to a PV shunt procedure, the patient's ascites, at the very least, should have proved refractory to first-line treatment for the underlying malignant condition. This is particularly true in the setting of ovarian cancer, for which ascites can be a component of relatively early stage (Ic or IIc) disease and come under control with hysterectomy–salpingo-oophorectomy alone. Further, mul-

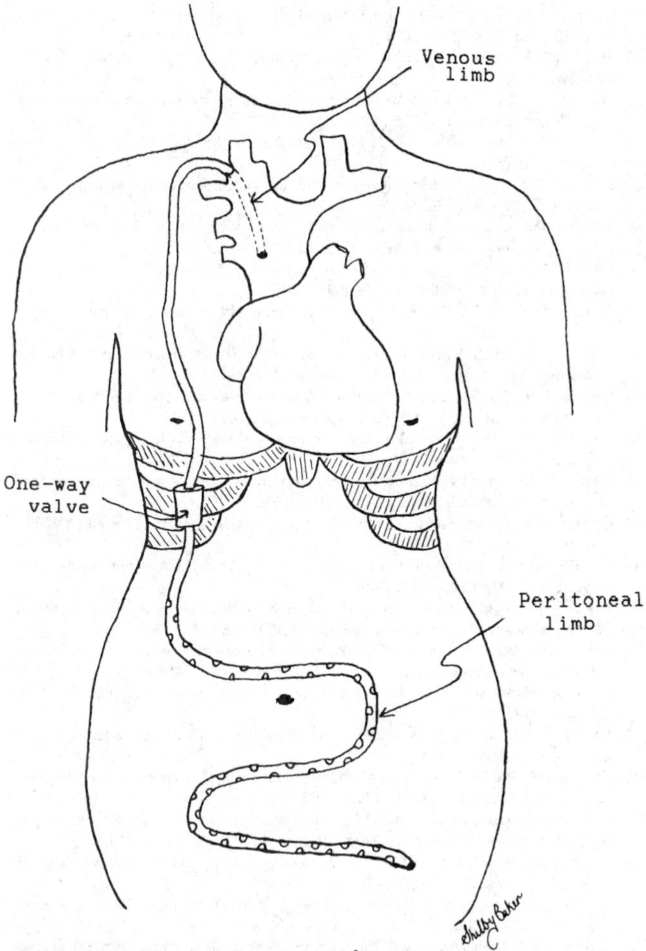

FIG. 62-43. The peritoneovenous shunt in situ.

tidrug regimens have proved quite successful, at least initially, in controlling the manifestations of much more extensive intra-abdominal dissemination and may significantly impinge on the ascitic fluid component of the tumor-imposed burden.

The data in Table 62-36 summarize the results of 15 reported studies of patients managed by placement of a PV shunt to control malignant ascites. Although each includes only a modest number of patients, 372 patients in all are reported, with the majority suffering cancer of the ovary (31%), gastrointestinal tract (27%), and breast (17%). That endstage illness is an apt characterization of the patient populations clinical condition is attested to by median survivals of about 2 to 4 months, and 1 year survivals of about 10%. Although, for the most part, the authors emphasize that patient's derive significant symptomatic relief and improvement in qualitative existence, this regrettably translates into substantial quantitative postshunt survival only anecdotally.

COMPLICATIONS

Although the litany of potential and reported complications is long, with the exception of shunt malfunction, they tend to occur infrequently and, on occasion, are preventable.

Shunt occlusion, with flow cessation can occur at any time after insertion. Between 10% and 42% of shunts placed, cease to function before the patient's death.[39-44,49,50,52,53,56,57] Immediate malfunction often is due to technical factors, such as tube kinking or tip malposition. Later failures may be secondary to fibrin clot formation and debris accumulation at the valve. Heavily blood-tinged ascites, particularly rich in protein with a somewhat viscous character, portend this complication. Valve chamber pumping (Denver) and shunt flushing with thrombolytic agents,[44] on occasion, can restore flow, but revision or replacement, if clinically indicated, is usually required. Late occlusion may also reflect thrombosis of the venous system about that limb of the PV shunt.

Ascitic fluid leakage at the peritoneal insertion site is reported, predisposes to infection, and it is perhaps best prevented by using a double-pursestring suture buttressed by transversalis muscle and fascia at this location.[35,52]

Acute postinsertion problems with fluid overload, pulmonary congestion, and respiratory insufficiency occur infrequently.[44,50] To help avoid this problem, most authors recommend removing about one-half of the ascitic fluid accumulation at the time of shunt placement. Careful postoperative monitoring is required and includes central venous pressure assessment, input–output determination, daily weight and abdominal girth measurement. A Foley catheter facilitates management of the often brisk post-PV shunt insertion diuretic-abetted diuresis and can help to more accurately monitor fluid fluxes. Judicious intravenous fluid support and the liberal use of diuretics and potassium replacement are often necessary to prevent intravascular volume overload and hypokalemia. Because shunt flow volume is hydrostatically determined, simply raising or lowering the head of the patient's bed will alter significantly the flow pressure gradient. Need for this maneuver can be monitored by central venous pressure determination and made accordingly.

Although disseminated intravascular coagulation (DIC) and bleeding diatheses occur often[58-60] after PV shunt management of cirrhotic ascites, they are rarely a clinical problem when shunts are placed in the neoplastic ascites context.[39,45,57] Laboratory evidence for the ongoing process at a subclinical level is readily demonstrable. Mild decreases in platelet count, slight prolongation in prothrombin time and partial thromboplastin time, and measurable increases in fibrin degradation products, all have been reported.[45,60] Significant preshunt hepatic dysfunction, particularly as evidenced by a serum bilirubin level higher than 3 mg/dl, may well presage clinical coagulopathy and probably contraindicate the procedure.[59,61]

Although shunt-induced tumor dissemination is a potentially adverse complication, it appears more of a theoretical consideration than a clinical contraindication. Although several reports, particularly in the setting of ovarian malignancy, suggest this both can occur and can produce serious consequences,[40,42,57,62,63] in the vast majority of instances this problem has not been incurred. Tarin and coworkers[64,65] prospectively studied a series of 29 PV shunt recipients, 15 of whom came to autopsy. All had large numbers of viable malignant cells ($8-600 \times 10^6$/100 ml ascites —95+% viable) in their ascitic fluid. Most formed colonies when grown in soft agar. Postshunt peripheral blood samples often revealed bizarre multinucleated cells, morphologically suggestive of tumor. Eight of the 15 patients had no evidence of hemotologic dissemination at postmortem examination, the longest survivor, a patient with an ovarian primary lesion, lived 27 months after initial shunt placement. The seven patients with evidence of hematogenous spread survived 1 to 9 months after shunt placement; six of seven had evidence of multiple, uniform-sized, small pulmonary nodules, possibly of iatrogenic origin but clinically not felt to have caused the patient's death. It may well be that the otherwise limited longevity of the PV shunt recipient precludes this theoretic difficulty from becoming a problematic clinical reality. Not unexpectedly, tumor growth along the subcutaneous shunt tunnel[41,66] and at the venotomy site of the venous limb[34,45] has been reported.

Although fever in the immediate postoperative period has been noted by most authors,[49,50] it usually remits spontaneously and is only rarely the harbinger of serious sepsis.[36,46]

REFERENCES

1. Lacy JH, Wieman TJ, Shively EH: Management of malignant ascites. Surg Gynecol Obstet 159:397–412, 1984
2. Feldman GB, Knapp RC, Order SE, Hellman S: The role of lymphatic obstruction in the formation of ascites in a murine ovarian carcinoma. Cancer Res 32:1663–1666, 1972
3. Feldman GB, Knapp RC: Lymphatic drainage of the peritoneal cavity and its significance in ovarian cancer. Am J Obstet Gynecol 119:991–994, 1974
4. Coates G, Bush RS, Aspin N: A study of ascites using lymphoscintigraphy with ^{99}Tc-sulfur colloid. Radiology 107:577–583, 1973
5. Bronskill MJ, Bush RS, Ege GN: A quantitative measurement of peritoneal drainage in malignant ascites. Cancer 40:2375–2380, 1977
6. Hirabayashi K, Graham J: Genesis of ascites in ovarian cancer. Am J Obstet Gynecol 106:492–497, 1970
7. Garrison RN, Kaelin LD, Heusser LS, Galloway RH: Malignant ascites. Ann Surg 203:644–651, 1986
8. Greene LS, Levine R, Gross MJ, Gordon S: Distinguishing between malignant and cirrhotic ascites by computerized step-wise discriminant functional analysis of its biochemistry. Am J Gastroenterol 70:448–454, 1978
9. Nystrom JS, Dyce B, Wada J et al: Carcinoembryonic antigen titers on effusion fluid. Arch Intern Med 137:875–879, 1977
10. Lowenstein MS, Rittgers RA, Kupchik HZ et al: Improved detection of malignant ascites and pleural effusions by combined assay of fluid CEA and cytology. Clin Res 23:596A, 1975
11. Greenway B, Johnson PJ, Williams R: Control of malignant ascites with spironolactone. Br J Surg 69:441–442, 1982
12. Appelqvist P, Silvo J, Salmela L, Kostiainen S: J Surg Oncol 20:238–242, 1982
13. Lifshitz S: Ascites, pathophysiology and control measures. Int J Radiat Oncol Biol Phys 8:1423–1426, 1982
14. Muller JH: Zur medizinisch-therapeutischen verwendung der kunstlichen radioaktivitat. Bull Schweiz Akad Med Wiss 5:584, 1949
15. Rose RG: Intracavitary radioactive colloidal gold: Results in 257 cancer patients. J Nucl Med 3:323–331, 1962
16. Ariel IM, Oropeza R, Pack GT: Intracavitary administration of radioactive isotopes in the control of effusions due to cancer. Cancer 19:1096–1102, 1966
17. Jackson GL, Blosser NM: Intracavitary chromic phosphate (32-P) colloidal suspension therapy. Cancer 48:2596–2598, 1981
18. Pretorius RG, Petrelli ES, Kean C et al: Comparison of the IV and IP routes of administration of cisplatin in dogs. Cancer Treat Rep 65:1055–1062, 1981
19. Paladine W, Cunningham TJ, Sponzo R et al: Intracavitary bleomycin in the management of malignant effusions. Cancer 38:1903–1908, 1976
20. Bitran JD: Intraperitoneal bleomycin—pharmacokinetics and results of a Phase II trial. Cancer 56:2420–2423, 1985
21. Ostrowski MJ: An assessment of the long term results of controlling the reaccumulation of malignant effusions using intracavitary bleomycin. Cancer 57:721–727, 1986
22. Ozols RF, Young RC, Speyer JL et al: Phase I and pharmacological studies of Adriamycin administered intraperitoneally to patients with ovarian cancer. Cancer Res 42:4265–4269, 1982
23. Kefford RF, Woods RL, Fox RM, Tattersall MHN: Intracavitary Adriamycin, nitrogen mustard and tetracycline in the control of malignant effusions. Med J Aust 2:447–448, 1980
24. Lopez JA, Krikorian JG, Reich SD et al: Clinical pharmacology of intraperitoneal cisplatin. Gynecol Oncol 20:1–9, 1985
25. Kaplan RA, Markman M, Lucas WE et al: Infectious peritonitis in patients receiving intraperitoneal chemotherapy. Am J Med 78:49–53, 1985
26. Piccart MJ, Speyer JL, Markman M et al: Intraperitoneal chemotherapy: Technical experience at five institutions. Semin Oncol 12:90–96, 1985
27. Routte M: De l'abouchement des veines saphenes internes au peritoine abdominal dans certains cas d'ascite a reproduction. Lyon Med 114:911–921, 1910
28. Evler T: Autoserotherepie bei bauchfelltuberkulose durch dauerdrainage des Aszites unter die haut. Med Klin 16:627–628, 1910
29. Hyde GL, Eisman B: Peritoneal atrial shunt for intractable ascites. Arch Surg 95:369–373, 1967
30. Pollock AV: The treatment of resistant malignant ascites by insertion of a peritoneo-atrial Holter valve. Br J Surg 62:104–107, 1975
31. LeVeen HH, Christoudias G, Ip M et al: Peritoneo-venous shunting for ascites. Ann Surg 180:580–591, 1974
32. Lund RH, Newkirk JB: Peritoneo-venous shunting system for surgical management of ascites. Contemp Surg 14:31–45, 1979
33. Stanley MM: Treatment of intractable ascites in patients with alcoholic cirrhosis by peritoneovenous shunting (LeVeen). Med Clin North Am 63:523–536, 1979
34. LeVeen HH, Wapnick S, Grosberg S et al: Further experiences with peritoneo-venous shunt for ascites. Ann Surg 184:574–581, 1976
35. Reinhardt GF, Stanley MM: Peritoneovenous shunting for ascites. Surg Gynecol Obstet 145:419–424, 1977
36. Greig PD, Langer B, Blendis LM et al: Complications after peritoneovenous shunting for ascites. Am J Surg 139:125–131, 1980
37. Greenlee HB, Stanley MM, Reinhardt GF: Intractable ascites treated with peritoneovenous shunts (LeVeen). Arch Surg 116:518–524, 1981
38. Bernhoft RA, Pellegrini CA, Way LW: Peritoneovenous shunts for refractory ascites. Arch Surg 117:631–635, 1982
39. Straus AK, Roseman DL, Shapiro TM: Peritoneovenous shunting in the management of malignant ascites. Arch Surg 114:489–491, 1979
40. Osterlee J: Peritoneovenous shunting for ascites in cancer patients. Br J Surg 67:663–666, 1980
41. Raaf JH, Stroehlein JR: Palliation of malignant ascites by the LeVeen peritoneo-venous shunt. Cancer 45:1019–1024, 1980
42. Lokich J, Reinhold R, Silverman M et al: Complications of peritoneovenous shunt for malignant ascites. Cancer Treat Rep 64:305–309, 1980
43. Downing R, Black J, Windsor CW: Palliation of malignant ascites by the Denver peritoneovenous shunt. Ann R Coll Surg Engl 66:340–343, 1984
44. Lund RH, Moritz MW: Complications of Denver peritoneovenous shunting. Arch Surg 117:924–928, 1982
45. Qazi R, Savlov ED: Peritoneovenous shunt for palliation of malignant ascites. Cancer 49:600–602, 1982
46. Cheung DK, Raaf JH: Selection of patients with malignant ascites for a peritoneovenous shunt. Cancer 50:1204–1209, 1982
47. Reinhold RB, Lokich JJ, Tomashefski J et al: Management of malignant ascites with peritoneovenous shunting. Am J Surg 145:455–457, 1983
48. Souter RG, Tarin D, Kettlewell MGW: Peritoneovenous shunts in the management of malignant ascites. Br J Surg 70:478–481, 1983
49. Gough IR: Control of malignant ascites by peritoneovenous shunting. Cancer 54:2226–2230, 1984
50. Kostroff KM, Ross DW, Davis JM: Peritoneovenous shunting for cirrhotic versus malignant ascites. Surg Gynecol Obstet 161:204–208, 1985
51. Campioni N, Pasquali Lasagni R et al: Peritoneovenous shunt and neoplastic ascites: A 5 year experience report. J Surg Oncol 33:31–35, 1986
52. Sonnenfeld T, Tyden G: Peritoneovenous shunts for malignant ascites. Acta Chir Scand 152:117–121, 1986
53. Roussel JGJ, Kroon BBR, Hart GAM: The Denver type for peritoneovenous shunting of malignant ascites. Surg Gynecol Obstet 162:235–240, 1986
54. Hyde GL, Dillon M, Bivins BA: Peritoneal venous shunting for ascites: A 15 year perspective. Am Surg 48:123–127, 1982
55. Holman JM, Albo D Jr: Peritoneovenous shunting in patients with malignant ascites. Am J Surg 142:774–776, 1981
56. LeVeen HH, Vujic I, D'Ovidio NG, Hutto RB: Peritoneovenous shunt occlusion—etiology, diagnosis and therapy. Ann Surg 200:212–223, 1984
57. Souter RG, Wells C, Tarin D et al: Surgical and pathologic complications associated with peritoneovenous shunts in the management of malignant ascites. Cancer 55:1973–1978, 1985
58. Ragni MV, Lewis JH, Spero JA: Ascites-induced LeVeen shunt coagulopathy. Ann Surg 198:91–95, 1983
59. Schwartz ML, Swaim WR, Vogel SB: Coagulopathy following peritoneovenous shunting. Surgery 85:671–676, 1979
60. Harmon DC, Demirjian Z, Ellman L, Fischer JE: Disseminated intravascular coagulation with the peritoneovenous shunt. Ann Intern Med 90:774–776, 1979
61. Tempero MA, Davis RB, Reed E et al: Thrombocytopenia and laboratory evidence of disseminated intravascular coagulation after shunts for ascites in malignant disease. Cancer 55:2718–2721, 1985
62. Maat B, Oosterlee J, Spaas JAJ et al: Dissemination of tumor cells via LaVeen shunt. Lancet 1:988, 1979
63. Smith RRL, Sternberg SS, Paglia MA et al: Fatal pulmonary tumor embolization following peritoneovenous shunting for malignant ascites. J Surg Oncol 16:27–35 1981
64. Tarin D, Price JE, Kettlewell MGW et al: Mechanisms of human tumor metastasis studied in patients with peritoneovenous shunts. Cancer Res 44:3584–3592, 1984
65. Tarin D, Vass ACR, Kettlewell MGW et al: Absence of metastatic sequellae during long term treatment of malignant ascites by peritoneo-venous shunting. Invasion Metastasis 4:1–12, 1984
66. Berger A, Goldberg MI: Subcutaneous cancer growth complicating the peritoneovenous shunting of malignant ascites. Surgery 93:374–376, 1983

JOEL A. DeLISA
ROBERT M. MILLER
ROSALIE RAPS MELNICK
LYNN H. GERBER
ALLEN D. HILLEL

CHAPTER 63 *Rehabilitation of the Cancer Patient*

Of the approximately 965,000 newly diagnosed cases of cancer in the United States each year and the approximately 1.5 million Americans who are considered to be cured, a significant number will experience functional limitations because of their disease or its treatment.[1] In a random sample of 805 cancer patients, Lehmann demonstrated that a significant number of these patients had functional disabilities that could be treated by rehabilitation techniques.[2] The primary barriers to optimal rehabilitation in the cancer patients were the physician's failure to identify functional problems, unfamiliarity with the concepts of rehabilitation and its value for cancer patients, and the resulting lack of appropriate referrals. Table 63-1 identifies a number of functional problems of cancer patients and the results of rehabilitation techniques.

Whereas physicians failed to identify the functional problems when queried, the cancer patients, even outpatients with controlled disease, were able to identify their functional problems.[3] With a clear understanding of the principles and effects of rehabilitation, the primary care physician should be able to identify patients with functional problems and make appropriate rehabilitation referrals. Rehabilitation should start as soon as diagnosis is made and continue through all phases of care and recovery.

Rehabilitation is best defined as the development of the disabled patient to his fullest physical, psychological, social, vocational, avocational, and educational potential. Goals must be realistic and consistent with physiologic and environmental limitations. The patient and rehabilitation professionals share responsibility in setting goals that allow them to work together toward maximum independence, while remaining flexible to respond to illness, symptom management, and difficulties in medical treatment that might be encountered. Throughout the process, rehabilitation considers the affected anatomic site, histologic type and stage of cancer, treatments used, possible metastases, patient age, and prognosis in establishing goals. While addressing physical rehabilitation factors, psychological and social issues must also be considered because they can be very important for patient motivation to obtain and sustain increased independence.

INTERDISCIPLINARY TEAM APPROACH

Comprehensive rehabilitation requires the expertise of professionals from multiple disciplines using a team approach to care. Although the appropriate team members and the specifics offered will vary with each patient or diagnosis, the principles are consistent. When patients are referred to rehabilitation professionals, the first emphasis is on a functional assessment, which includes evaluating physical performance within the mobility spectrum, basic and advanced activities of daily living (ADL), psychological status, and social situations. Throughout the rehabilitation assessment, areas of ability, as well as disability, are noted for future consideration.

This chapter is dedicated to Mary Ann Mikulic, R.N., M.N.

TABLE 57-1. Percentage of People in Sample With One or More Rehabilitation Problems

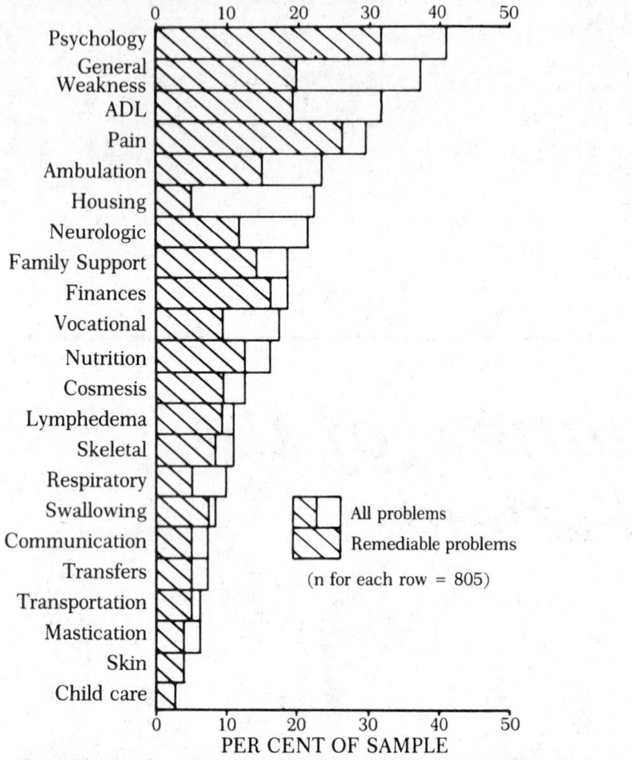

(Lehmann JF, DeLisa JA, Warren CG et al: Cancer rehabilitation: Assessment of need, development, and evaluation of a model of care. Arch Phys Med Rehabil 59:410–419, 1978)

After assessment, therapeutic interventions are directed toward maximizing functional capabilities and prevention of secondary complications. To attain the desired goals, principles such as energy conservation, work simplification, and the use of adaptive equipment may be employed: for example, reorganization of the kitchen to improve work flow or the use of a utility cart to move heavy objects when strength and energy are reduced. By using the specific physical treatment regimens and environmental changes, improved function can be achieved. Patients may also be assisted in making behavioral changes to attain their psychological and social goals.

Rehabilitation services exist in most medical facilities, although the variety offered and their degree of sophistication will vary. As the survival rates for cancer patients increase, it becomes increasingly important that patients be offered as many of these services as may be necessary. Therefore, where the services are available, access routes must be established. To aid in the process, Lehmann devised a successful model. All cancer patients are automatically screened by a trained cancer rehabilitation coordinator, and those with functional problems are seen by a physiatrist, who makes referrals to appropriate specialists on the rehabilitation team. Thereafter, as leader of the rehabilitation team, the physiatrist provides the link between the clinical oncology team (radiation oncologist, general surgeon, medical oncologist, gynecologist, otolaryngologist, and other medical and surgical specialists) and the comprehensive rehabilitation team.

Because rehabilitation uses a holistic and comprehensive approach, the combined expertise of a multidisciplinary team is necessary. In a study of 36 cancer rehabilitation programs in cancer centers, university hospitals, and community hospitals, Harvey and colleagues[4] found the most common team members to be the physician (oncologist or physiatrist), social worker, psychologist, physical therapist, oncology nurse, and occupational therapist. Others frequently included were the speech pathologist, dietitian, vocational rehabilitation counselor, chaplain, and rehabilitation nurse.

Team members evaluate patients according to their clinical specialty and then join in a team conference to develop a comprehensive functional problem list. Usually the conference is led by the physician in charge. An individual therapeutic rehabilitation plan is defined and implemented such that the patient may function within the limitations imposed by the disease. The multidisciplinary team uses an approach that accentuates the patient's remaining abilities.

The team must be prepared to deal with death and dying and to adjust to radical fluctuations in the patient's medical, physical, and psychological states. Pain has to be taken into account, as well as treatment-induced problems such as nausea and fatigue, and alternative goals must be available to accommodate declines in physical status or advancing disease. The team must also recognize that some patients will choose less-than-independent function. These factors may cause difficulties in determining clear and realistic performance expectations. The successful team will allow for this and strive to promote coordination, cooperation, and open communication among all involved parties to optimize the chances for success, whatever the goals. Table 63-2 identifies common members of a comprehensive rehabilitation team and indicates ways in which each member may contribute to the team approach for the rehabilitation of cancer patients.

PSYCHOLOGICAL, SOCIAL, VOCATIONAL, AND DISCHARGE PLANNING ISSUES

There are many psychological and social issues related to cancer rehabilitation that can have a sizable effect on rehabilitation, quality of life, and life-styles. Their effects are likely to begin with the first suspicion or diagnosis of cancer and may remain throughout the patient's lifetime. The type and magnitude of the concerns, fears, and problems will vary with the type and site of cancer and will fluctuate in intensity and focus throughout the course of the disease.

The effect of cancer and its treatment on the quality of life has been described by Devlin, Plant, and Griffin in an article on the aftermath of anorectal surgery.[5] They concluded that there is an "immense price paid in physical discomfort and in psychological and social trauma" and, additionally, that "society has determined life must be saved at all costs, and the skill of the surgeon is directed to this end. We have shown that it is now time to look more closely at the costs and at those who bear them; more emphasis must now be

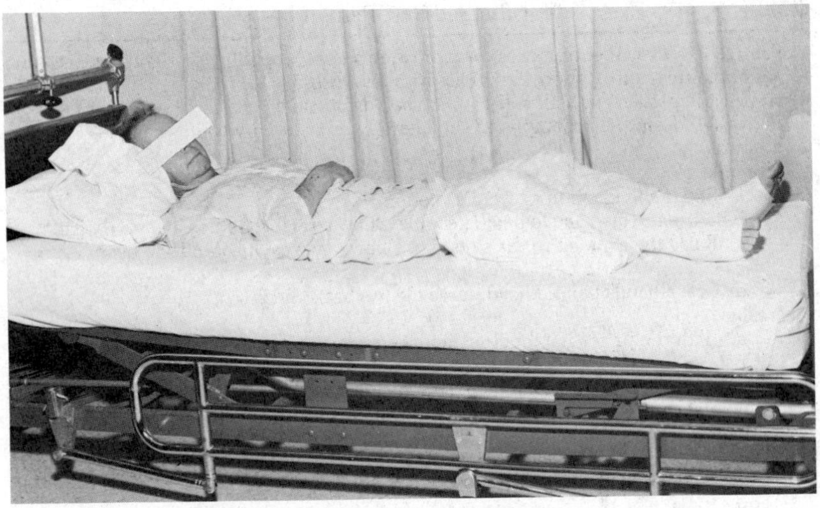

FIG. 63-1. Improper bed positioning (pillows under neck and knees) contributes to development of flexion contractures.

using ultrasound and static stretch because it is hard to stabilize the pelvis adequately to establish three-point pressure. Knee contractures of more than 15° can also be difficult to stretch manually, even with the use of heat. This is especially true in elderly patients.

A patient confined to bed will lose muscle strength and endurance and develop muscle atrophy. In normal subjects, a muscle at complete rest (no muscle tension exerted) will lose 10% to 15% of its physical strength weekly—approximately 3% to 5% daily.[7,9] Persons at bed rest and who are immobilized for 3 to 5 weeks will lose half of their muscle strength. Additional disease processes, preexisting weaknesses, or age may further reduce strength. Conversely, it takes about 60 days to increase muscle strength 10%; hence, it is much easier to lose than to gain. Fortunately, muscle strength can be maintained if the normal muscle undergoes an isometric contraction at a tension that is 20% to 30% of maximum for several seconds daily.[9] If the tension generated by the contraction is less than 20% of maximum, strength continues to decrease. Isolated muscle group atrophy and weakness may be prevented by using electrical stimulation. Motor strength is measured clinically by the manual muscle-testing and grading scheme described in Table 63-3.

TABLE 63-3. Quantifying Manual Motor Strength

Grade	*Test Performance*
5/5	Normal power. The muscle can move the joint through the full ROM, against gravity and against maximum resistance applied by the examiner.
4/5	The muscle can move the joint through the full ROM, against gravity and against some, but not full, examiner resistance.
3/5	The muscle can move the joint through the full ROM, against gravity, but with no examiner resistance.
2/5	The muscle can move the joint through full ROM, but only with gravity eliminated and no examiner resistance.
1/5	Contraction of the muscle can be seen or felt but is of insufficient strength to produce movement even with gravity eliminated.
0/5	Complete paralysis. No visible or palpable contraction of the muscle even with gravity removed.

Examples of exercises to maintain strength while the patient is bedridden are noted in Table 63-4 and in Figures 63-2, 63-3, and 63-4.

Endurance decreases from disuse. In fact, disuse affects muscle endurance more than instantaneous strength because it affects blood supply and metabolic demand of the muscle adversely.[7] Reduced endurance may cause CNS fatigue, reduce patient motivation, and decrease the beneficial effects of rehabilitation.

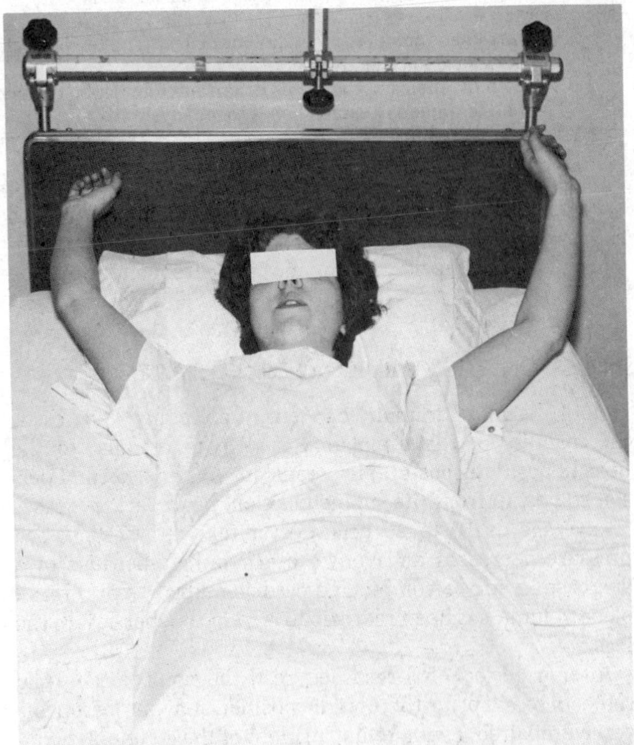

FIG. 63-2. To maintain active shoulder ROM in the supine position, the patient raises both arms out to the side, bends the elbow, and reaches behind the head. The sequence is completed by having the patient return the arms to the sides.

TABLE 63-4. Exercise for the Bed Rest Patient

1. Passive ROM to all extremities once or twice a day, depending on tightness and tone abnormalities, until patient can assist with exercises.
2. Have patient assist with all self-care as soon as possible.
3. Active ROM may be accomplished unilaterally or bilaterally while the patient is in the supine position.

   Shoulder
   a. Shrug shoulders in a circular motion.
   b. Raise the arm above head, keeping elbow straight. Return arm to the side.
   c. Raise the arm out to the side, flex elbow, and reach behind the head. Return arm to the side.
   d. Grasp hands behind head, force elbows back and down.

   Elbow
   a. With the palms up, touch hand to shoulder, return with palm down.

   Wrist
   a. Make circular motions with the wrist.
   b. Make an "O" with the thumb and each fingertip.

   Finger
   a. Squeeze a ball.
   b. Make an "O" with the thumb and each fingertip.

   Hip
   a. Raise one leg up at hip, keeping the knee straight, then relax. Repeat with the opposite leg.
   b. Flex knee and hip up toward chest, relax. Repeat with opposite leg.
   c. Flex knees up and place feet flat on the bed. Tighten buttock muscles, lifting buttocks up. Relax.
   d. Perform isometric quadriceps sets.
   e. With the leg straight, move the leg out to side. Return. Repeat with opposite leg.
   f. With the leg straight, roll the knee in and out.

   Foot
   a. Dorsiflex and plantarflex the ankles.
   b. Make a circular motion with the feet.

   Trunk
   a. With the hip and knees flexed and the feet flat on the bed, flex the chin and slowly curl up reaching for the knees. Hold 3 to 5 sec. Relax.

   Hip and Trunk
   a. Flex knees and place feet flat on the bed. Tighten buttock muscles, lifting buttocks up. Hold for 3 to 5 sec. Relax.
   b. With the hips and the knees flexed and feet flat on the bed, rotate both legs to the right, then to the left, keeping knees together.

Prescriptions for bedside exercises to maintain strength can prevent these complications. Prescriptions should include type, intensity, duration, and frequency of the exercise.[8]

EFFECT ON THE CARDIOVASCULAR SYSTEM

One of the most dramatic dangers of prolonged bed rest is the inability of the circulatory system to readjust to the upright position (postural hypotension). When a normal person stands up from the supine position, heart rate increases an average of 10 to 20 beats per minute.[10] Systolic blood pressure decreases an average of 14 mmHg because of a decrease in stroke volume and cardiac output, as 500 ml of blood volume has been redistributed from the thorax into the legs.[11]

After a period of forced bed rest, the ability of normal subjects to adapt to the upright position may be lost or severely impaired, owing to impairment of the autonomic control of the heart and the peripheral circulation. This may occur faster in a patient who is receiving chemotherapy. Deitrick, studying the effects of 3 weeks of forced bed rest on normal subjects, found a significantly increased heart rate and a 40% to 70% blood pressure drop with frequent fainting episodes when subjects resumed the upright position.[12] Subjects were unable to maintain stable pressure, despite a strong sympathetic response that was manifested by sweating, pallor, and restlessness. Reestablishment of the normal orthostatic reflexes and return of pre-bed rest pulse and blood pressure took 3 to 4 weeks after the subject became ambulatory. Older people are slower to reestablish normal blood pressure and heart rate levels during remobilization.

The specific therapies used to reestablish the orthostatic reflexes are [1] early mobilization of body parts not affected by the pathology, [2] active and passive ROM exercises, [3] utilization of the tilt table with the goal of tolerating 20 min at 75° of tilt, and [4] use of an electrical hospital bed. Supportive garments such as abdominal binders, elastic stockings, and Ace wraps are often used. Ephedrine or phenylephrine may be helpful.

With bed rest, a decrease in plasma volume and an increase in blood viscosity result in an increased risk of thrombophlebitis. Greenleaf found that the reduction in plasma volume can be limited by exercises, isotonic being more effective than isometric.[13] Low-dose anticoagulants have been used in some patients to prevent the risk of thrombophlebitis and pulmonary embolus. However, patients receiv-

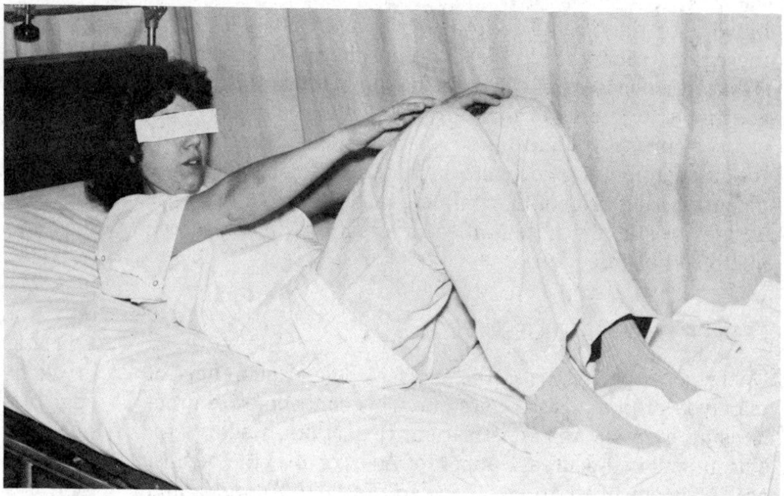

FIG. 63-3. Active ROM exercises for the trunk are performed while supine with the hips and knees flexed with the feet flat on the bed. The patient then flexes the chin and slowly curls up reaching for the knees. The patient holds for 3 to 5 seconds and then relaxes.

ing chemotherapy carry a higher risk for bleeding when using anticoagulants.

EFFECT ON THE RESPIRATORY SYSTEM

Because of the splinting effect of the bed, breathing tends to be shallower and less frequent, with reduced aeration of the posterior lungs. Decreased clearance of secretions from the bronchial tree may result in atelectasis and an increased incidence of respiratory infection. Pulmonary embolus is another frequent complication. Early mobilization and turning, deep breathing, coughing, and coughing exercises may help prevent some of these problems. Percussion and postural drainage may be indicated in some patients.

EFFECT ON THE ENDOCRINE SYSTEM

During bed rest, tissue anabolism is slowed, whereas the catabolic process that breaks down tissues is increased. An increase in protein catabolism, which leads to a negative nitrogen balance, contributes to decubitus formation and slow wound healing.[12] Significant carbohydrate intolerance has been noted after 8 weeks of immobilization.

A negative calcium balance also exists after prolonged recumbency.[12] Despite a normal calcium level, these patients have marked hypercalciuria. This, in part, is due to calcium being absorbed from bones that are not stressed by body weight or muscle contraction and may result in disuse osteoporosis from increased resorption. In osteoporotic bone, strength and density are decreased, with potentially resultant fractures. Exercises, activity, and diet can reverse this negative calcium balance.

EFFECT ON THE URINARY SYSTEM

Inactivity may lead to the development of urinary retention, renal stones, and urinary tract infections. Difficulty in urination is directly related to position. Incomplete emptying is a function both of the stasis in the entire urinary tract and decreased muscle functioning that interferes with normal voiding.

Excessive calcium loss and its excretion in the urine, com-

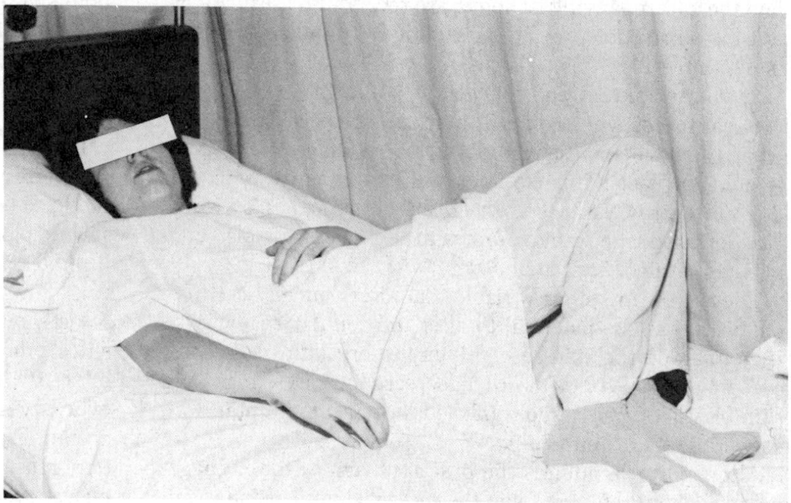

FIG. 63-4. Another hips and trunk active ROM exercise in the supine position is to have the hips and knees flexed with the feet flat on the bed, keeping the knees together. The legs are then rotated from the right to the left.

bined with the altered ratio of citric acid/calcium and the increased urinary excretion of phosphorus, plus urinary stasis, predisposes to stone formation. Other factors that contribute to stone formation are alkaline urine and decreased urine volume. Intervention should be directed toward maintaining adequate hydration, keeping the urine pH acidic, and promoting complete bladder-emptying in the upright position. These same interventions decrease the likelihood of infection.

EFFECT ON THE DIGESTIVE SYSTEM

Decrease in peristalsis is the primary deleterious effect of inactivity on the digestive system. This contributes to problems of anorexia and constipation. Reduction in energy requirements will decrease appetite. Additionally, the bedfast patient is not likely to take in adequate fluid. Anorexia and dehydration also have an impact on the decrease in intestinal peristalsis and contribute to constipation.

Intervention should include exercises to increase activity, surveillance of fluid and dietary intake, and establishment of a bowel program. Bowel programs can be enhanced by taking advantage of the gastrocolic reflex, which is strongest after intake of a meal, abdominal massage, digital stimulation, and suppositories.[14]

Constipation, as a side-effect of pain medication, may be a notable problem in cancer patients. It is not uncommon for these persons to require laxatives in conjunction with their bowel program. Lactulose shows some promise in the treatment of chronic constipation and establishment of normal defecation patterns.[15]

EFFECT ON THE SKIN

Reduced bed mobility owing to general debilitation, painful movements, lethargy from pain medications, or a depressed psychological response frequently leads to skin breakdown over bony prominences. Comprehensive skin care programs should include both preventive techniques and specific treatments of pressure ulcers (decubitus).

Pressure ulcer is the preferred diagnostic term because it addresses the primary cause. Obstruction of capillary flow and the accompanying ischemia are recognized as the mechanisms responsible for ulcer formation.[16] Capillary pressure is 32 mmHg.[16–18] Tissue damage can be avoided if the pressure is intermittent and relieved at 5-min intervals.[19]

Shear forces will also result in tissue necrosis. These exist when the bone and the underlying tissues move and the skin is held in place. This commonly occurs when a person is pulled up in bed or when the head of the bed is elevated. Friction from mechanical forces to the epidermis also contributes to ulcer formation.[20]

Edema, or any other variable that alters normal cell metabolism, has the potential to alter the cellular response to ischemia and the skin susceptibility to breakdown. Greater susceptibility also exists with a decrease in muscle mass and skin elasticity and with diminished food and fluid intake, all concomitants of immobility.

Although prevention is the best approach to the management of skin problems, even the most vigilant care may fail when the effects of the disease or its treatment render tissue incapable of withstanding pressures equal to normal capillary pressure. Available body-resting surface may be so limited that adequate turning and changes of position cannot be effected.

Prevention requires recognition of the multiple risk factors, including paralysis, pain (especially aggravated by movement), spasticity, edema, contractures, sedation, altered mental status, and psychological stress. Nutritional deficiencies reflected by hematocrit, hemoglobin, serum protein, iron, zinc, and vitamin C levels should be corrected.[21,22] Education of staff, patient, and family to the causes of skin breakdown, the identification of patients at risk, and knowledge of body sites most frequently involved are prerequisites of preventive care. Patients at risk should be protected by pressure-dispersing padding on operating tables during prolonged surgery, because vulnerability is further increased under these conditions.

Observation is the key to prevention. Skin inspection techniques should be taught to patients or to significant others. Exposed areas should also be palpated for temperature increases and induration. The area exposed to excessive pressure will become erythematous after pressure release. If erythema and induration persist for more than 20 min, the exposure interval has been too long and the areas should be kept free of pressure until these conditions disappear. Graphs depicting duration of pressure and fade time permit analysis of individual response and the development of safe position-change schedules.

In addition to specific turning schedules, small shifts of weight or "pushups" will also contribute to the prevention of breakdown. This is especially important when patients cannot be turned because of the nature of their illness or injury or for patients in chairs who are too weak to lift themselves off the chair frequently. Frequency of pushup varies from 5-min to 15-min intervals, depending on tissue tolerance. Electronic buzzers are available to assist in conditioning the patient to perform this necessary protective behavior. Massage to high pressure areas, exercise, and antiembolic stockings may be used to improve circulation.

Numerous mechanical devices are used in preventive skin management. Generally, these devices are intended to alter points of pressure at regular intervals or to provide a molding effect to disperse pressure over a wider area. None of these devices has proved totally effective in the prevention of pressure ulcers, and their use will not reduce the need for continued intensive surveillance.

Electric rotating beds are available but are cumbersome and confining. Turning frames, circle electric beds, and air-fluidized beds may be considered for people who experience severe pain on movement. Alternating air mattresses are limited in that they only partially reduce pressure at intervals. For maximum effect the patient should be positioned directly over the air cells with only a sheet over the mattress, since pillows, sheepskin, and the like will only negate its effect. Other mattresses are designed to disperse pressure over larger surfaces. Water mattresses are more efficient in accomplishing this than any of the foam varieties, but caution must be exerted to establish and maintain adequate buoyancy.

Bed-positioning techniques include elevation of heels and malleoli off the bed with pillows or foam. Pillows or split foam mattresses can provide a bridging effect to remove pressure over the sacrum and trochanters. Pillows to support the patient in the desired position also add to general comfort, and sheepskin adds to comfort and reduces shear. Use of a lifting and turning sheet can reduce shear and friction. A light dusting of cornstarch or use of satin sheets and pillowcases further reduce friction and improve bed mobility.

Wheelchair cushions reduce pressures exerted over the ischial tuberosities.[23] In a comparison of several types, Souther found that a 2-in. latex foam pad can substantially reduce ischial pressure; however, a water-filled cushion (Jobst Hydro-Float) was the most effective.[24] The height of the wheelchair footrest should be adjusted to allow pressure to be dispersed along the undersurface of the leg. Steps to prevent pressure ulcers are listed in Table 63-5.

Treatment of pressure ulcers, when they do occur, should address the intrinsic factors just discussed, relative to prevention as well as local and surgical interventions. Forty-six agents have been identified in an analysis of local treatment, yet well-designed clinical and laboratory studies to evaluate proposed therapies are lacking.[25]

The basic tenets of treatment are the following:

1. Remove all pressure
2. Treat infection if present
3. Debride and keep the ulcer clean
4. Protect from further injury

Topical antibiotics are not indicated because of the bacterial resistance factor. Debridement can be mechanical—by means of wet to dry dressings—surgical or biochemical. A variety of debriding enzymes are useful. A combination of sutlains and collagenase appears to effect faster debridement. Dextranomer beads (Debrisan) can assist in cleaning wounds and promoting healing.[26] Pace reports clinical evidence of faster healing with local application of benzoyl peroxide.[27] Surgical closure should be considered when lesions involve muscle, bone, or joints.

TABLE 63-5. Steps to Prevent the Development of Pressure Ulcers

1. Staff and patient/family education as to cause
2. Identification of patients at risk
   a. Decreased mobility—pain, paralysis, sedation
   b. Mental status—unconscious, anesthetized, confused
   c. Incontinence
   d. Malnutrition—nausea, hematocrit, serum protein, and so forth
   e. Dehydration—vomiting, diarrhea, fever, poor intake
   f. Edema—circulatory impairments
3. Intensive surveillance for those at risk
   a. Monitoring of above risk factors
   b. Daily skin inspection (especially over bony prominences)
4. Institution of specific protective regimens
   a. Positioning and turning schedules
   b. Determine tissue tolerance to pressure (observe and record fade times)
   c. Pressure dispersion equipment (special mattresses and wheelchair pads)
   d. Reduce shear and friction (sheepskin, cornstarch)
   e. Pressure relief maneuvers: bridging over body prominences, "pushups"
   f. Remove *all pressure* from reddened areas that do not fade in 20 min GET OFF THAT SPOT

PSYCHOLOGICAL AND SOCIAL EFFECTS

Inactivity resulting from bed rest can lead to psychological and social problems that may require professional intervention, although awareness of potential problems may allow prevention. The patient on bed rest will need a degree of assistance with routine self-care and treatment-related activities. For brief periods, dependence may be satisfactory; however, if it is long-term, psychological problems may develop.

For patients at home, bed rest can also cause problems for family members who take on added responsibilities. For patients without family assistance, the recruitment of aides can be frustrating and expensive. The possible psychological and social impact of these frustrations and expenses on rehabilitation is evident and must be addressed early in treatment if preventive measures for the disuse syndrome are to be successful.

Another complication of total bed rest is social and intellectual isolation, which may lead to depression, withdrawal, and anxiety. It also allows the patient to dwell on his situation, which may exacerbate existing psychological problems. Isolation must be minimized and its effects treated to allow participation in rehabilitation.

SPECIFIC REHABILITATION PROBLEMS

BREAST CANCER

In the adult woman, breast cancer accounts for more new cases and more deaths than cancer of any other organ. This disease is rare in men, with about one case to every 100 to 120 in females.[1] Treatment may involve removal of the breast with some or all of the axillary nodes. The pectoralis major and pectoralis minor muscles are removed during a standard radical mastectomy, which will affect shoulder strength. The pectoralis major is left intact in modified radical mastectomy, and there is usually little functional shoulder deficit. Adjuvant therapy, including radiotherapy or chemotherapy, may lead to substantial disability.

Resulting disability may be minimized by initiating rehabilitation as soon as the diagnosis is made. The goals for rehabilitation of the postmastectomy patient include the following:[28]

1. Physical restoration: obtain functional pain-free use of the affected arm with full ROM
2. Psychosocial rehabilitation: to help the patient accept the loss of her breast and to help both the patient and significant others to cope with their fears and anxieties concerning death and dying, physical attractiveness, and sexuality
3. Cosmetic rehabilitation: restoration of the external physical appearance by use of a temporary breast form, external breast prosthesis, or breast reconstruction

4. Occupational or vocational rehabilitation: includes patient education to prevent excessive edema and infection of the affected arm, as well as returning the patient to employment

Physical Restoration

HISTORY AND PHYSICAL EXAMINATION. Rehabilitation of the patient with breast cancer focuses on preventive measures. It is important to know preoperatively whether the patient has shoulder trauma, tendonitis, bursitis, arthritis, adhesive capsulitis, C5-C6 radiculopathy, or a rotator cuff tear on the same side as the proposed mastectomy. These conditions and any functional shoulder limitations will affect the rehabilitation outcome relative to shoulder ROM and strength. It is essential to perform and record an exact musculoskeletal examination of the shoulder and upper extremity (UE), recording the shoulder ROM for external rotation, internal rotation, abduction, extension, and forward flexion. Motor strength of the UE and scapulohumeral muscles must be recorded, and any atrophy noted. The UE baseline circumference measurements should be taken before surgery and at regular intervals after surgery to note the onset of lymphedema. The brachium is measured above the lateral epicondyle of the humerus and the antibrachium 3 in. below the lateral epicondyle. Measurements are also taken at the wrist and across the metacarpal phalangeal joints. Some centers use volumetric measurement instead of circumferential measurement.

The UE deep tendon reflexes should be recorded and a careful sensory examination performed. Because both the long thoracic (serratus anterior) and the thoracodorsal (latissimus dorsi) nerves may be injured with axillary nerve dissection, it is essential to check these muscles both before and after surgery.

The thoracodorsal nerve is often surrounded by metastatic nodes; consequently, it may be necessary to sacrifice the nerve.[29] However, the long thoracic nerve that innervates the serratus anterior usually does not have nodes running with it and should be spared, because its injury will result in medial winging of the scapula with weakness in forward flexion against resistance. Upward rotation of the scapula is almost completely abolished, thus limiting shoulder abduction and forward flexion. In one series evaluating 37 patients with 41 axillary dissections, 30% had transient serratus anterior palsy, probably secondary to a traction injury. These completely recovered at 3 to 6 months after the operation.[30]

TREATMENT. Patients first seen with far-advanced disease may receive palliative radiation followed by chemotherapy. Radiation fibrosis may cause marked periarticular fibrosis of the shoulder, with limitation of shoulder ROM, arm lymphedema, and ulcerations of the skin, as well as brachial plexus injury with corresponding pain and motor and sensory loss. These patients require individualized, closely monitored rehabilitation plans to maximize function.[31]

The rehabilitation plan used for patients who have a normal shoulder (ROM and strength) and who will be receiving preoperative radiation therapy should include baseline goniometric shoulder ROM measurements, which should be reviewed periodically during the course of the radiation. The patient should also be instructed in a home program to maintain ROM. These exercises are to be performed two to three times daily for 6 months, then at least daily for 1 or 2 years after radiation therapy.[31] Patients who have restricted shoulder ROM and are receiving radiation should be placed on a daily supervised active assistive ROM to obtain maximum function, and then shifted to a daily home program, possibly with heat and static stretch, that is closely supervised.[31]

Immediately after surgery, the arm should be compressed with an elastic wrap to minimize the development of edema. To reduce the risk of developing a frozen shoulder, the arm should not, in our opinion, be pinned to the chest wall after the surgery. Degenshein suggests a postoperative position technique in which the arm is placed at right angles to the chest with the shoulder in external rotation and a towel placed around the arm and attached to the bed sheet. This keeps the elbow free.[32] Even if the arm is kept in this position for 24 to 48 hr, the patient will have a 90° painless abduction ROM at the shoulder and all internal and external rotation.

When the axilla has been dissected or the shoulder musculature disrupted, a suggested treatment plan would be referral to physical therapy on the third to fifth postoperative day, when wound healing has been well established. Before the physical therapy prescription is written, it is essential to consider the following:

1. Stage of wound healing and placement of suture lines
2. Adherence or lack of adherence of the skin grafts
3. Presence or absence of drainage tubes, and the amount of drainage
4. Local instability of the chest wall
5. Laboratory or radiographic evidence of metastasis

In the supine position, the amount of tension on the suture line is assessed as the patient is carefully progressed toward full passive ROM, especially in abduction, external rotation, and flexion. This will allow evaluation of shoulder mobility without applying undue tension to the surgical wound or mobilizing the skin flaps.

As mentioned earlier, one must consider the presurgical complications involving the musculoskeletal system of the affected extremity, such as the brachial plexus injury and long thoracic or thoracodorsal nerve injury.[33] Electrodiagnostic studies may prove helpful in documenting the injury and predicting the prognosis for neurologic recovery.[34] Obviously, these complications will cause a modification in the postmastectomy rehabilitation prescription noted in Table 63-6.

At the first therapy visit, the patient should be instructed in active ROM exercises for the elbow, wrist, and fingers of the involved extremity. One-handed ADLs, using the noninvolved arm, are also taught at this time.

By the fifth postoperative day, the suction catheters usually have been removed, and the therapy program can be accelerated, for there is less risk of separation of the skin flaps and the formation of seromas. Active ROM exercises in the supine position to the affected shoulder should be initiated, avoiding stretch of the suture line. If needed, muscle relaxation exercises (*e.g.*, deep-breathing exercises) can be

TABLE 63-6. Exercise Program for the Postmastectomy Patient

1. Three to 5 days postoperative: Patient is supine with the operative side elevated and the arm wrapped.
   a. Active ROM to fingers, wrist, and elbow on the operative side. Some examples of these exercises follow.
      1. With palm up, touch hands to shoulder on operated side. Return with palm down.
      2. Make circular motions with wrist on operative side.
      3. Make a fist, then straighten fingers on operated side (squeeze a ball).
   b. Active ROM of nonoperated UE.
2. Five days postoperative: Patient is supine with operated UE Ace wrapped.
   a. Isometric exercises to operated UE for strengthening, using opposite arm for assistance.
   b. Gentle, straight active shoulder ROM of operated side, that is, abduction—raise arm sideways and upward, keeping elbow straight.
   c. Continue with active elbow and hand exercises.
   d. Relaxation breathing exercises.
3. Nine to 12 days postoperative: Or when sutures are removed.
   a. Active assistive shoulder ROM to the operated side, that is, sitting, overhead pulleys, clasp hands in front midline, raise arms forward and up as far as tolerated.
   b. Upper back isometrics in sitting position.
   c. Active shoulder ROM of operated side in sitting position.

taught to the patient to aid in the decreasing of muscle tension and the improving of pain tolerance. Isometric exercises to the biceps, triceps, forearm musculature, and the hand intrinsics should be initiated to improve the pumping efficiency of the affected extremity. These exercises should be performed with the affected arm wrapped and elevated. Daily ROM and circumference measurement must be obtained and recorded to document the patient's progress and to look for evidence of postmastectomy lymphedema. Isometric exercises to the rotator cuff musculature on the affected side should be taught to maintain strength. Positioning is utilized to increase gradually the shoulder flexion, abduction, and external rotation. Simultaneously, maintenance active assistance ROM exercises should be performed on the unaffected extremity to avoid the complications of immobilization.

When the sutures have been removed, usually 10 to 14 days after surgery, exercises can then be prescribed for the erect position. Progressive active and active assistive exercises are used to increase the ROM to 180° of forward flexion and abduction at the affected shoulder and to obtain full range of external rotation. Wand exercises, use of the overhead pulley, and wall-climbing exercises are designed to increase elevation (Fig. 63-5A–C). If the pectoralis group has been removed, progressive resistive exercises to the shoulder abductors and adductors are used to prevent possible shoulder dislocation. Wall weights or sandbags can be used to perform these exercises. Skin mobilization, friction massage, and stretching of the subcutaneous fibrosis of the glenohumeral joint are prescribed for chest wall adhesions.

To prevent swelling of the affected extremity, the arm should be elevated when sitting for an extended period. For elevation to be effective, it must be maintained for at least 30 min.

In persons who have developed chronic capsulitis from prolonged immobilization, diathermy modalities (short-wave diathermy and ultrasound) can be particularly helpful when combined with active stretching at the shoulder.[35] Diathermy is contraindicated in the presence of infection or carcinoma.[36]

Before discharge, the patient must be able to demonstrate the various exercises that have been prescribed to facilitate rehabilitation. With proper physical therapy, full ROM of the affected shoulder can be obtained. However, full muscular strength will not be obtained if the pectoralis major and minor have been removed, and weakness will be noted in horizontal adduction.

Cosmetic Rehabilitation

Temporary breast forms are used by the patient until a permanent prosthesis is obtained. Permanent prostheses usually are not ordered until 6 to 12 weeks after surgery or after radiation therapy has been completed. Temporary breast forms can be made from such materials as fluff, cotton, lamb's wool, nylon stockings, or facial tissues.

The fitting of the permanent breast prosthesis must consider size, weight, symmetry, feel, comfort, and cost. There is a wide range of prostheses available: foam-filled, custom-made sculptured models, and a liquid silicone-filled type.[37] Consultation with the American Cancer Society will be helpful in identifying local resources. It may be necessary to assist some patients in locating sources of modified clothing.

Breast reconstruction can technically be performed for any of these patients, even those who have received radiation therapy. Patient selection is based on the patient's general health and perception of the deformity.[38] Reconstruction may contribute to better psychological adjustment. Some surgeons believe that breast reconstruction should be performed even in patients who have a poor prognosis. The percentage of patients with mastectomy who undergo breast reconstruction probably will increase because many patients are dissatisfied with the available external prostheses. Most surgeons prefer to delay the reconstructive procedures for 2 to 6 months after mastectomy and until the patient has completed radiation and chemotherapy (see Chap. 38 for further discussion of breast reconstruction).[39]

Reach to Recovery Program of the American Cancer Society

The American Cancer Society has a voluntary program in which all of the volunteers have undergone mastectomy and have become successfully rehabilitated. This group aids the patient in physiologic, psychological, and cosmetic rehabilitation. The volunteers will not see the patient unless it is requested by the physician, who may request all or a portion of the program.[40] When they visit the patient, they bring with them a kit containing a booklet of exercises for the affected shoulder, a temporary breast prosthesis, and information about clothing. They also provide exercise equipment. Not every patient is a candidate for this type of visit, and some patients may even resent this approach.

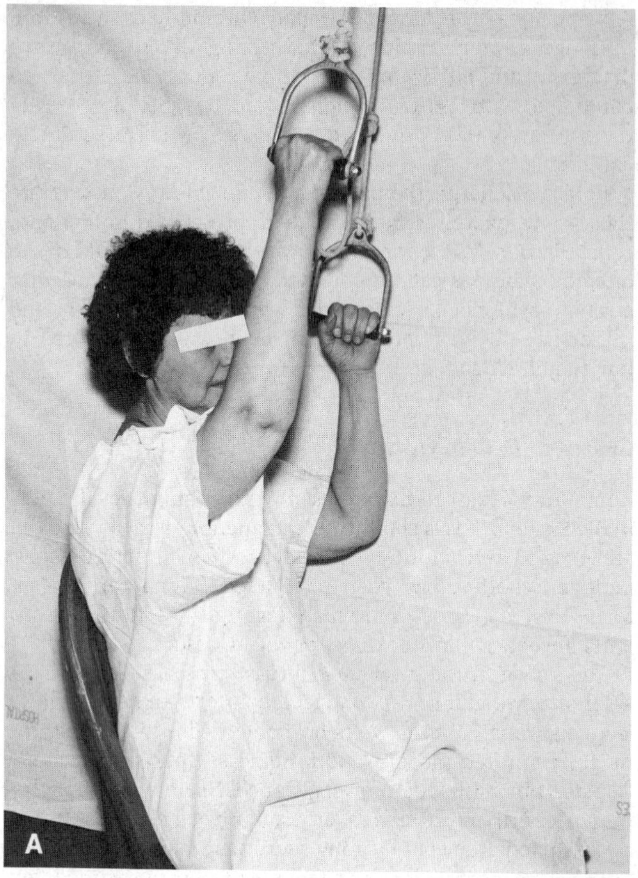

FIG. 63-5. Overhead pulley, wand exercises, and wall-climbing exercises are used to obtain full shoulder ROM. **A**. Pulley. **B**. Wand. (*Figure continues.*)

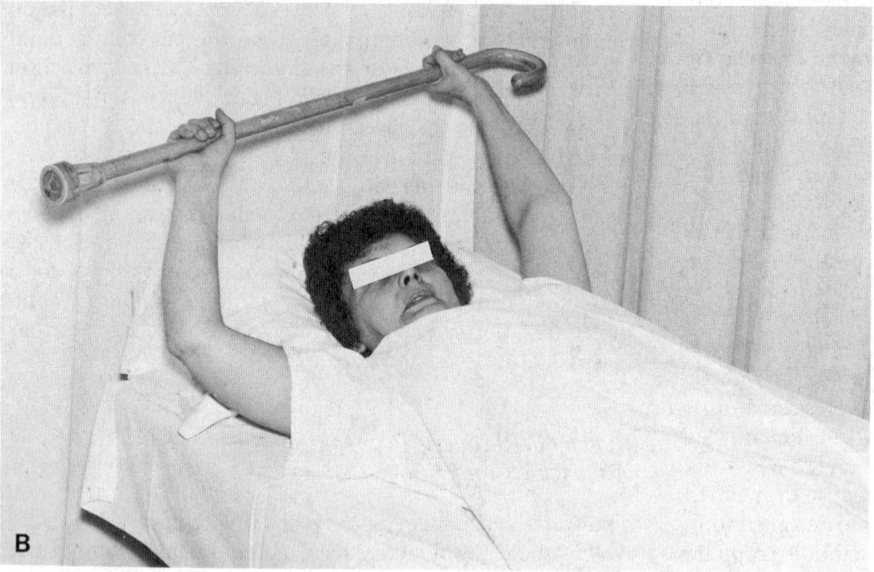

Postmastectomy Lymphedema

Reports on the incidence of postmastectomy lymphedema vary from 6.7% to 62.5%.[41] Severe edema, defined as an increase of 35% in volume, occurs in approximately 10% of these patients.[42] The disability from lymphedema is proportional to its amount and disfigurement. It has never been explained why some mastectomy patients develop lymphedema and others do not. Some may go several years with no lymphedema, only to develop massive lymphedema later, for no known reason. An onset 6 months after mastectomy should arouse suspicion of occult infection or recurrent tumor.

Multiple factors such as radiation therapy, infections, delayed wound healing, surgical ablation of lymphatic nodes and vessels, fibrosis from radiation or chronic edema,

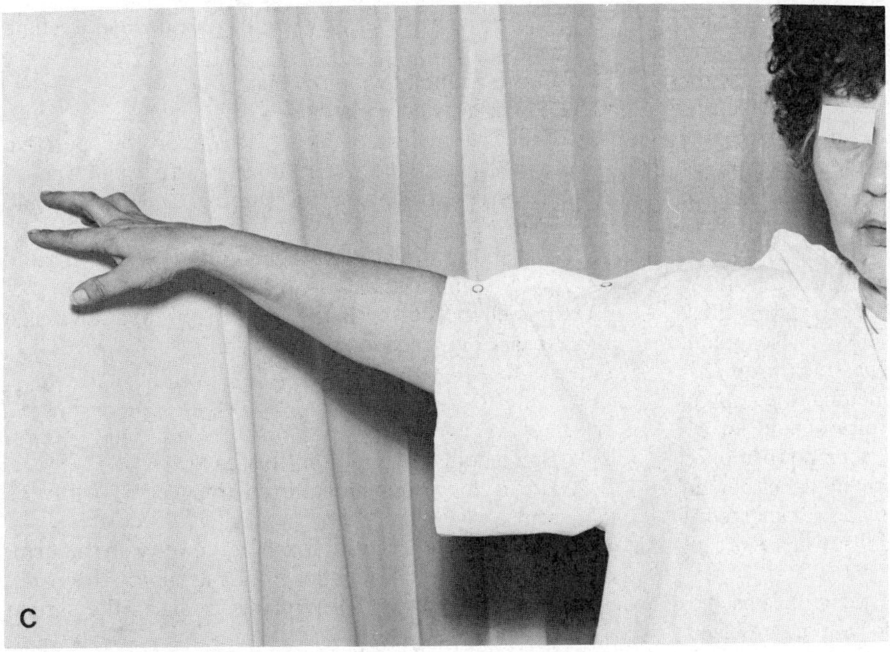

thrombophlebitis, inadequate regeneration of lymphatic vessels, or recurrent tumor have been suggested as possible etiologic factors. However, it is generally believed that a combination of multiple factors is operating.[43,44] To help determine the functional abnormality and to aid with treatment, it is important to know whether the cause of the lymphedema is disease of the lymphatics or venous system. Venograms and lymphangiography may aid in making this differential diagnosis.

Prevention of lymphedema is much better than any surgical or medical treatment designed to remedy the situation once it has occurred.[29] The axillary vein should not be damaged, and prevention of infection is a necessity. Postoperatively, the arm should be elevated, and a supervised exercise program to obtain full ROM should be initiated. Elastic compression bandage or sleeves are also helpful in preventing lymphedema.[43]

Multiple surgical procedures have been devised for treatment of lymphedema.[45,46] The aim of these surgical procedures has been to reestablish the lymphatic flow. The procedures include the following:

1. Lymphangioplasty, which creates new lymphatic pathways
2. Bridging procedures, which form a bypass of normal tissue with intact lymphatics over a disease or blocked area
3. Lymphaticovenous shunts, which develop an anastomosis between the lymph and venous systems[47]
4. Superficial-to-deep lymphatic anastomosis, which connects lymphatics by converting shaved pedical strips of deep fascia into bone or muscle[48]
5. Lysis of axillary vein adhesions[49]
6. Amputation, when the edema is severe and disabling and the hand is nonfunctional

None of these procedures has proved to be universally successful or accepted. Goldsmith's intact omentum-bridging transposition, in which the omentum, with its rich lymphatic and vascular supply, is pulled through the subcutaneous tunnel in the chest wall and laid on the underlying muscle of the lymphedematous arm, may possibly be the most successful.[50]

Medical treatment of postmastectomy lymphedema includes elevation of the hand higher than the elbow, which in turn is higher than the shoulder.[51] To be effective, the elevation must persist for at least 30 min each session, and the frequency of elevation is determined by the clinical status. During all or part of the night, the arm should be elevated while the patient is supine.

The patient should be instructed in isometric exercises of the affected arm and hand to increase the active muscle pump. To take advantage of gravity, these exercises should be done with the distal part of the extremity elevated higher than the proximal. The exercises are isometric, rather than isotonic, to reduce joint motion and cause less constriction.[45] The frequency of these isometric contractions needs to be determined by the patient's response during the therapy. An example would be isometric contractions for 1 sec then a 2- to 3-sec rest period, for a total of 20 contractions.[45] When established, this should be repeated frequently throughout the day. These isometric exercises need to be supplemented with isotonic exercises to obtain full shoulder ROM.

Pneumatic intermittent compression (pneumomassage) can be helpful in increasing the flow of fluid out of the limb. The most common one is produced by a Jobst unit and is composed of a number of cuffs that inflate, then deflate sequentially. This pumping results in milking the limb from the distal to the proximal points. The common adjustment settings for intervals of pressure are 45 sec on and 15 sec off.[52] The pressure setting usually is slightly lower than the diastolic blood pressure of the patient. In persistent cases, the circulation unit, if available, works better than the Jobst unit because it inflates from distal to proximal, whereas the Jobst unit fills all at once. Both units empty simultaneously. The pressure phase forces the edema fluid up the lymphatic channels, and the exhaust phase allows them to refill assisted by gravity in the slightly elevated limb. The treatment may vary from 2 hr twice daily, up to a maximum of 12 hr/day.[45] The duration of treatment depends on the amount of lymphedema and its response to pneumomassage.[6] Pitting edema seems to respond better than the brawny variety. Rest periods may be necessary if problems such as nausea, pain, or finger tingling occur. Circumference measurements should be taken before and after each pneumatic compression session to document progress. Jewelry should be removed and a wrinkle-free, full-cuff, hand stockinette applied to absorb perspiration. It can be performed on either an inpatient or an outpatient basis, but it is contraindicated if there is evidence of acute phlebitis, cellulitis, or recurrent carcinoma.

After each treatment, a figure-eight elastic wrap is used to provide compression and keep the fluid volume reduced. Instruction in proper figure-eight wrapping technique must be provided. The elastic wrap is applied upon arising.

When the volume of the affected arm and hand has been reduced and stabilized, a custom-fitted, pressure-gradiated elastic sleeve should be provided. The patient should wear it throughout waking hours. To remain effective, it must be replaced every 2 to 3 months.[44] Before replacement, it may be necessary, once again, to treat the patient with intermittent pneumatic compression before measuring for a new elastic sleeve. Some people find the elastic sleeve uncomfortable, and others find it cosmetically unacceptable. For patients who, for social or occupational reasons, choose not to have an elastic sleeve, a Jobst pneumomassage home unit can be prescribed for daily use.

Diuretic therapy and salt restriction are used as adjuvant therapy to the pneumatic compression, particularly for patients who live in hot humid areas and for those with cardiovascular problems. A higher prevalence of postmastectomy lymphedema has been noted with obese patients, and weight loss should be encouraged.[53]

Lymphedema provides an excellent culture medium, and low-grade cellulitis (usually streptococcal) may occur. Erythromycin, 250 mg q.i.d. for 7 days, should be initiated at the first sign of infection.[33] Some physicians prescribe prophylactic erythromycin 48 hr before pneumomassage.

The programs just discussed are not rigid and will need to be modified for each patient. Upon discharge, the patient should have regular measurements, circumferential or volumetric, of the affected arm.

The patient must be educated on the performance and avoidance of specific behaviors to protect the arm. These are designed to avoid excessive use of the arm, constrictive clothing, local or generalized heating, and trauma.[33,54,55]

Some "DOs"

1. Wear canvas gloves when gardening, wear rubber gloves when cleaning utensils with steel wool.
2. Wear a loose rubber glove on this hand when washing dishes.
3. Wear a thimble when sewing.
4. Keep dress sleeves loose.
5. Wash the smallest break in the skin on the operative side with soap and water, cover it with a bandage.
6. Use an electric razor for shaving, avoid nicks and scrapes.
7. Keep the arm elevated when sitting.
8. Apply a lanolin hand cream several times daily.
9. Contact the doctor if the arm on the operative side appears hot, reddened, or swollen.

Some "DON'Ts"

1. Don't hold a cigarette in this hand.
2. Don't carry your purse or anything heavy with this arm.
3. Don't wear a wristwatch or other jewelry on this arm.
4. Don't cut or pick at cuticles or hangnails on this hand.
5. Don't work near thorny plants or dig in the garden barehanded.
6. Don't reach into a hot oven with this arm.
7. Don't permit injections or vaccinations in this arm.
8. Don't allow blood to be drawn from this arm (an obvious exception would be if you were receiving chemotherapy and have no other veins remaining).
9. Don't allow your blood pressure to be taken in this arm.
10. Don't get sunburned; tan gradually.

Results of rehabilitation programs for postmastectomy lymphedema are widely reported in the literature. Zeissler has shown that 67% of 123 patients benefitted from this type of treatment program.[44]

HEAD AND NECK CANCER

Areas of major functional concern in head and neck cancer patients include nutrition and deglutition problems, shoulder dysfunction, self-care considerations, altered speech communication, and disfigurement.

In planning for the rehabilitation needs of patients with head and neck cancer, some pretreatment data must be gathered. This data base should include medical and social history, including life-style, nutritional habits, and intellectual learning ability. Head and neck cancer patients frequently have a long history of alcohol abuse and heavy smoking, the combination of which contributes to the development of squamous cell carcinoma in the head and neck.[56,57] These habits may also contribute to deterioration of intellectual functioning, noncompliant behavior, and possibly recurrent disease.[58] To improve the chance of cure and to enhance compliance, the patient may need assistance in altering smoking and drinking habits.

Nutrition and Deglutition

Maintenance of optimal nutrition is a prime concern because of the frequent impairment to the deglutitory mechanism.

Alterations in dentition; jaw musculature; tongue mobility; palatal function; taste appreciation; saliva, laryngeal and pharyngeal musculature; or esophageal function each contribute to potential deglutitory impairment.

An optimal nutritional state before and during treatment may enhance the patient's chances for recovery.[59] Many patients have had symptoms of their illness for weeks and months before diagnosis. Often, during that time, they have failed to have an adequate intake and progressed to a negative nitrogen balance. It is important that the patient reverse this trend by increasing nutritional intake and creating a protein-synthesizing (positive nitrogen balance) state before treatment begins.

Generally, the patient's nutritional state is monitored by weight. High protein dietary supplements may be encouraged in an attempt to effect weight gain. If weight declines in excess of 4.5 kg (10 lb), a nasogastric tube is often inserted to provide primary nutritional needs or supplement what the patient can take by mouth (see Chap. 59, Sect. 1 for discussion of nutritional management).[60]

Swallowing impairments often are anticipated during the course of treatment or in advancing disease. If it is anticipated that the patient will be unable to take adequate oral alimentation for a significant time, minor surgical procedures can provide a tube placement more comfortable than the nasogastric route. Feeding esophagostomies[61] place the feeding tube through the skin of the lower part of the neck. On occasion, feeding esophagostomies are performed during the surgical treatment of the cancer. Gastrostomies or jejunostomies may be performed if the abdomen is the preferred location for the feeding tube. Recently, gastrostomies have been performed percutaneously,[62] a procedure that can be done under local anesthesia. Feeding through a tube can easily provide a nutritionally complete diet.[63] Because canned formulas are expensive, some patients are instructed in blenderized diets. The instructions should address nutritional education and procedural techniques relative to food preparation, cleaning, and storage to avoid spoilage.[64]

Radiation and chemotherapy in these patients present special problems in nutritional management and deglutition. Alteration in taste, noxious sensations, or loss of taste is common.[65] A decrease in salivary flow may lead to xerostomia. Saliva may be altered to a thick sticky consistency, interfering with swallowing and speech. Mucositis, loss of appetite, nausea, and esophagitis are common sequelae of these treatment modes.[66] Therefore, it is important that patients receiving radiation and chemotherapy as outpatients are closely followed with weekly weighing and counseling.

To counteract the foregoing effects and to reduce the likelihood of anorexia, careful dietary planning is necessary. Because red meat may taste rancid, fish, poultry, eggs, and dairy products can be substituted to provide the required protein.[65] Menus that emphasize gravy, sauces, and butter will help compensate for dry oral mucosa. An increase in total fluid intake will aid the patient who has decreased saliva, and dryness can be relieved by providing artificial saliva, sugarless gum, or sugarless lemon drops. Papain, a proteolytic enzyme from papaya fruit, will dissolve thick secretions. Its effect can be obtained by dissolving a papase tablet in the mouth or coating a cotton swab with meat tenderizer and swabbing the mouth 10 min before the meal.[67,68] Episodes of nausea can be minimized by providing the patient with frequent small meals, avoiding cooking fragrances, and using antiemetic drugs.[60] Pain from mucositis may contribute to an anorexic state. Viscous lidocaine (Xylocaine) 10 min before a meal, or diphenhydramine (Benadryl) mixed with nondairy whipped cream and placed in the mouth, acts as a soothing topical analgesic.[67]

The teeth are particularly susceptible to damage from radiation. Caries may result from the direct effect of irradiation on teeth or supporting structures. Alterations in salivary flow change bacterial flora and raise the oral pH, thus creating a medium for bacterial growth.[66] Dental consultation before radiation therapy, with prophylactic treatment often can prevent rampant caries. Evidence suggests that fluoride treatment can aid in the prevention of decay and also reduce postradiation hypersensitivity to hot, cold, and sweet foods.[69]

Before radiation, all necessary extractions in the field should be performed, and the gums allowed to heal. When extractions are required in an already radiated field, the risk of osteoradionecrosis is increased. Hence, all nonrestorable teeth and those in the direct path of radiation often are removed.[66,69]

The risk of osteoradionecrosis is reduced when bone is covered by normal mucosa and contains healthy teeth. Therefore, a program of oral hygiene should be established before radiation therapy. Dentures should not be worn during therapy because of the risk of developing mucosal sores, and complete recovery of radiated mucosa should be allowed before dentures are refitted.[70]

Excision of structures important to swallowing during surgery has a greater influence on deglutition than does impaired mobility of residual structures.[71] Patients who have undergone either partial or total glossectomy will experience some disruption in ability to move a bolus from the anterior to the posterior oral cavity.[68] All partial and total glossectomy patients must be evaluated on an individual basis. It has been reported that patients with partial glossectomies have remarkable adaptation to swallowing, and in one series more than 50% of patients with total glossectomy were able to take adequate oral nutrition.[72,73] Some may be able to take adequate liquid diets by adjusting body and head posture to allow swallowing.[74] Others may need to adapt a large syringe by attaching a length of tubing that reaches to the uvula to place fluids in the oropharynx for swallowing (Fig. 63-6).[64] Soft foods that do not require mastication can be inserted in the mouth on a long-handled spoon or plunger and placed near the uvula to be swallowed.[68,74,75] It is important, however, to be sure that the hypopharynx is capable of handling a food bolus dropped in the posterior oropharynx without the usual oral phase of swallowing. Finger foods can be placed in the posterior mouth and manipulated by remaining muscles for swallowing. These patients should avoid food that falls apart in the mouth (corn, applesauce, dry ground meat) and include food that holds together (custards, puddings, ground meat combined with gravy).

Orogastric tube feedings can be used as either an intermediate mode of nutritional intake or as a permanent solution for nutritional management. A lubricated feeding tube intermittently passed orally allows the patient to take canned or

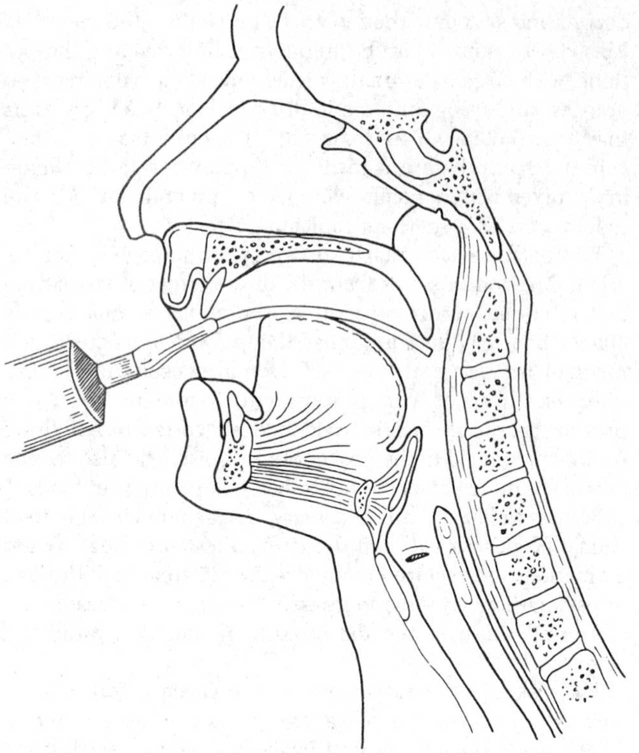

FIG. 63-6. Use of modified syringe to introduce fluids into oropharynx of patients with dysphagia mechanica.

blenderized diets, all fluids, and medications. It is surprising how easily many patients learn to swallow an orogastric tube without difficulty. These patients avoid the need for a surgically placed feeding tube and avoid the constant interference of a nasogastric tube.[67,74]

Other surgery patients with mechanical dysphagia have had resections of the soft or bony palate. The major problem here is leakage of food and liquid through the defect into the nose and sinuses. Prosthetic obturators designed to separate the cavities are often successful in solving these mechanical swallowing problems;[76] however, soft palate defects are difficult to correct with an obturator and some of these patients cannot manage nutritionally without tube feedings.

Patients who have undergone partial laryngectomies, especially those having had supraglottic laryngectomies, are susceptible to aspiration because of interruption of the pharyngeal phase of swallowing. The incidence of persistent dysphagia in these patients has varied greatly among reports[77–82] and may be related to the exact structures resected during the procedure. Although some patients do eventually swallow with minimal aspiration, resections that impair the mobility of the arytenoids and include the pyriform sinuses and base of the tongue result in persistent and significant aspiration. Conversely, an unresected base of tongue, laryngeal elevation that meets the tongue base, and mobile arytenoids that provide for glottal closure are positive indicators for swallowing. For those with supraglottic laryngectomies who can learn and intellectualize the swallowing act, a technique can be taught to protect the airway and minimize aspiration. The patient learns to [1] flex the neck, [2] inhale before swallowing, [3] consciously hold a breath while swallowing, and [4] gently cough or clear the throat immediately after swallowing is complete.[67]

Shoulder Dysfunction

The trapezius is the muscle most responsible for normal shoulder alignment, function, and cosmesis. It can be divided functionally into upper, middle, and lower fibers. Its motor innervation is by the spinal accessory nerve. Some authors feel that there are also motor contributions from C3, C4, and C5,[83] but most evidence points to their contribution being for proprioception (Table 63-7).[84]

Neck dissections are performed for removal of the regional nodes for a malignancy in the head and neck area. In many cases, the 11th nerve can be spared during the surgery. However, occasionally, when it is felt that there is disease near the course of the 11th nerve, the nerve is sacrificed during the surgery. Almost all patients who have their nerve removed suffer from 11th nerve syndrome: weakness and limitation of abduction in the coronal plane, drooping of the shoulder, and pain in the shoulder. Many patients who have their 11th nerve preserved also suffer the 11th nerve syndrome.[85] Many of these patients have recovery of function at 6 to 12 months, although some never regain function.

The trapezius is the primary upward rotator during shoulder abduction and forward flexion, and the main stabilizer of the scapula. With the loss of the trapezius function after neck dissection, the remaining scapular musculature is inadequate to maintain normal shoulder alignment and function. The deeper posterior scapular muscles lack the size and direction of pull to adequately oppose the action of the pectoral group (pectoralis major and minor), to stabilize the scapula during glenohumeral motion, or to support the weight of the affected arm when it hangs at the side. Muscles that are synergistic with the trapezius for one motion are, unfortunately, antagonistic during another. Hence, substitution is not completely adequate because the substituted muscles cannot perform shoulder abduction and forward flexion in a coordinated functional manner.[86]

Injury to the accessory nerve will affect shoulder function after surgery. This is true whether the injury is partial owing to neurapraxia, or complete, with or without nerve continuity. Electrodiagnosis can be helpful in documenting and differentiating partial from complete nerve injury and in predicting prognosis.[34] Preoperative shoulder pathology such as bursitis or adhesive capsulitis will affect postoperative shoulder function.

TABLE 63-7. Function of Various Positions of the Trapezius

Parts of the Trapezius	*Function*
Upper fibers	Elevates scapula
Middle fibers	Retracts (adducts) scapula
Lower fibers	Depresses scapula
Upper and lower fibers	Upward rotator of scapula
All fibers	Hold scapula tightly to the thoracic cage during movement of the arm

To test the trapezius, the patient must be examined with the clothes removed above the waist. One way to test the upper trapezius is to ask the patient to elevate the shoulder (shrug) against resistance. This test can give inaccurate results, however, because muscular patients may have a well-developed levator scapula that can provide this function. To avoid misjudgment, it is better to view the patient from behind, with the arms relaxed at the side of the body and the shoulder at rest. With a weak or paralyzed trapezius, the scapula is displaced downward (drooped) and laterally (lateral winging) owing to the unopposed pull of the serratus anterior, and the superior angle is rotated further from the spine than the inferior angle.[31]

Following sacrifice or injury of the accessory nerve, active ROM of the involved shoulder will have limited abduction in the horizontal position of only 60° to 70° owing to the scapula's upward rotation (Fig. 63-7).[87] A few very strong patients can abduct to 160°, providing that they move the arm forward 20° to 25° while abducting.[86] A functional test is to have the patient stand with his chest against a wall, head turned opposite to the side tested, and perform abduction of the arm in the coronal plane with the hand externally rotated. This position isolates the trapezius and deltoid muscles. It is important that the examiner does not allow the patient's shoulder to rotate away from the wall which lets the arm leave the coronal plane and allows substitution to occur. The deltoid alone can achieve abduction of about 70°. The trapezius and deltoid together achieve abduction of 170° to 180° in normal persons.[88]

The main antagonist of the trapezius is the pectoralis group. The resulting shoulder alignment is mainly due to the pull of the unopposed pectoralis when the trapezius is weakened or paralyzed, resulting in a contracture in the protracted (abducted) position.

A dropped shoulder is not only painful and cosmetically unacceptable to many patients, but also has marked functional limitations, such as the inability to push, lift, or carry heavy objects. Although uncommon, some patients with severe 11th nerve syndromes and marked shoulder droop suffer brachial plexus traction injuries.

Patients with the 11th nerve syndrome cannot actively reach shoulder level or above, and loading them at their maximum shoulder ROM produces or increases pain. These patients often find the shoulder problems to be the major long-term functional disability. For a laborer, it can mean the end of employment. This can be a devastating, painful problem to a patient who has had a bilateral radical neck dissection. Whenever possible, the accessory nerve should be preserved.

After surgery, shoulder external and internal ROM are usually preserved, but because of scapular instability, strength is decreased. Excessive shoulder internal rotation must be avoided because this further protracts and depresses the shoulder, aggravating the disability. Proper body mechanics and shoulder posture (shoulders back) are essential to maximize function and reduce pain. The role of physical therapy in rehabilitating patients with the 11th nerve syndrome has not yet been proved. It is certainly advisable for such patients to undergo an individualized program to maintain passive ROM and to preserve active ROM.

Rehabilitation can be started during the second week after surgery in a patient who has had no postoperative complications. Early therapy should consist mostly of passive ROM exercises and care should be taken not to stress suture lines or put tension on flaps used for reconstruction.

By the fourth postoperative week, most patients can undergo thorough active ROM exercises. By 2 months after surgery, the patient can participate in fully active strengthening exercises.

For those patients with severe 11th nerve syndrome, phys-

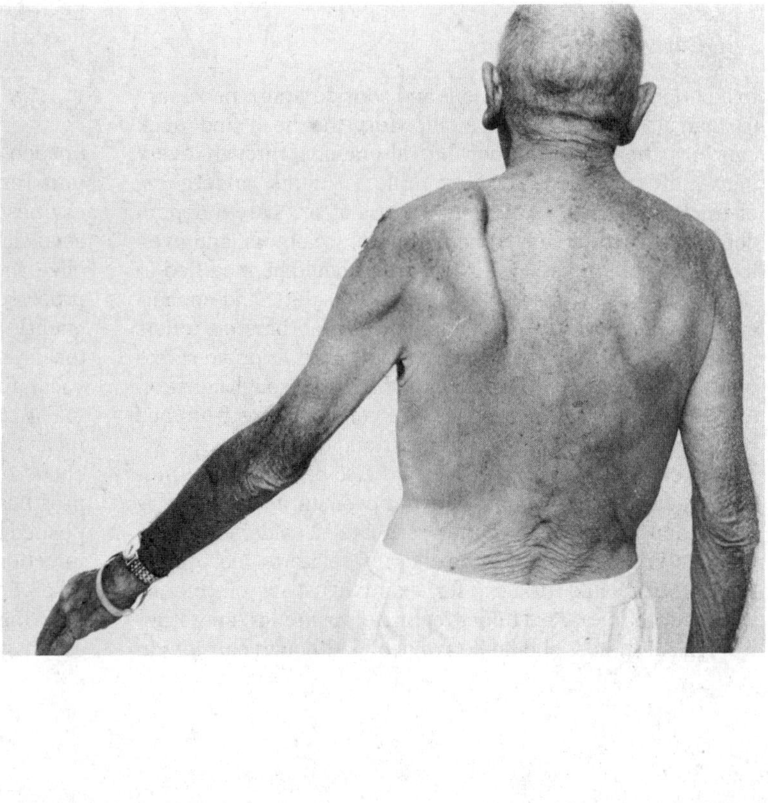

FIG. 63-7. Maximum active abduction in this patient following severance of accessory nerve.

ical therapy can perhaps maintain ROM and encourage active use of the shoulder. However, many patients persist with their symptoms, in spite of the most thorough and long-term physical therapy. These patients can be considered for use of a sling.[86] Some authors report that 11th nerve grafting during the original operative procedure can preserve shoulder function.[89] Animal studies have shown reinnervation to occur[90] and, recently, human studies have electromyographically demonstrated reinnervation.[91] There are also reported cases of static procedures to sling the shoulder, but these techniques are not widely practiced.[92]

Recent reconstructive techniques have utilized myocutaneous flaps employing the pectoralis muscle[93] and the trapezius muscle.[94] These reconstructive techniques transfer a muscle–skin paddle based upon a specific arterial and venous supply from the chest wall or upper back to a site in the head and neck area when a large defect has been created after a surgical extirpation of a tumor. The resulting defects in the donor muscles might add to further shoulder dysfunction. Studies evaluating these considerations have not yet been completed.

Neck Dysfunction

During most neck dissections, the sternocleidomastoid muscle is removed. In a unilateral neck dissection, most patients do not notice major morbidity in terms of neck motion. Postoperatively, very few patients need a physical therapy program for rehabilitation because of removal of the sternocleidomastoid muscle. Patients who have had bilateral neck dissections with removal of both sternocleidomastoid muscles have difficulty coming up to a sitting position from a supine position. Usually this is managed by the use of the hands to stabilize the neck during that movement. Turning of the head to the right and left is usually not a major problem, even in bilateral neck dissections.

Self-Care Considerations

In addition to the modifications and considerations necessary to manage nutrition and swallowing, the head and neck cancer patient faces other life alterations through every phase of treatment. For example, patients undergoing chemotherapy often experience a loss of self-care independence owing to fatigue, general muscle weakness, and even loss of muscle mass.[95] Daily activities should be modified in such a way as to conserve energy, stress safety, and encourage hygiene. Assistive devices such as grab bars on toilets and tubs will aid in energy conservation and improve safety on transfers. The ROM must be maintained through conservative exercise, and the avoidance of complications from bed rest becomes a principal consideration.

Range of motion exercises should also be performed prophylactically to reduce restrictive movement brought on by irradiation of tissues.[95] Other self-care considerations for patients undergoing radiation therapy relate to the protection of irradiated tissues; for example, soap, ointments, salves, deodorants, perfumes, cologne, cosmetics, and other foreign substances should be avoided.[64] Although hair loss in irradiated fields is common, shaving, when necessary, with an electric razor is safer than with a blade. When bathing, lukewarm water is recommended and the skin should be blotted dry. Clothing should be loose fitting around irradiated areas.[64]

Patients undergoing radiation therapy that involves the posterior aspect of the jaw also can develop trismus resulting from fibrosis of the fibromuscular tissues involved in mastication. It is important that patients are counseled during their radiation to maintain ROM of their temporomandibular joints. If necessary, tongue blades can be used to "prop" the jaw open as a stretching exercise.

Head and neck surgery often involves either temporary or permanent creation of a tracheostoma. Patient education on stoma care is vital. Swimming must be avoided and bathing done with care to avoid aspiration. Showers should be taken while wearing a special protective bib. Because the air entering the tracheal stoma has not been humidified by the nose, mouth, and pharynx, most neck breathers require humidified air to prevent dryness and crusting that can block the airway. Patients must be weaned gradually from the continuous mist they received during the first days after surgery. Patients with permanent tracheostomas may eventually adjust to the dry air and may only need room humidifiers for sleeping.

With a tracheostoma, patients are unable to occlude the glottis to perform the Valsalva maneuver. Because this maneuver is important in functional activities (defecation, lifting, and pushing), patients must learn to compensate. For example, during defecation, patients should occlude the stoma with a thumb to hold a breath and develop abdominal push.

Neck breathers should be instructed to wear medical alert bracelets and to carry medical data on their persons. The American Cancer Society provides emergency cards for neck breathers that describe pulmonary resuscitation procedures, such as keeping the neck opening clear, giving mouth-to-neck breathing only, and giving oxygen to the neck when needed.

Speech Communication

Speech is accomplished through the processes of cerebration, respiration, phonation, and articulation. The resonating cavities of the nose, mouth, and pharynx influence the acoustic product. Head and neck cancers and their treatment have the potential to interfere with one or more of these processes; for example, cancer of the larynx is treated frequently with total laryngectomy, thus diverting the respiratory system from the oral articulators and eliminating the vocal apparatus.

For patients with laryngectomies, the most common means of speech rehabilitation are esophageal speech, tracheoesophageal puncture (TEP) with placement of a voice prosthesis, and electrolarnyx. Esophageal voice is accomplished by training patients to force air into the esophagus by injection or suction methods, to trap the air in an esophageal reservoir, and to release the air in a controlled manner, allowing it to pass up through the remnants of the pharyngoesophageal sphincter. The esophagus, therefore, acts as a false lung, using trapped air under pressure to produce vibration of tissues at its uppermost end.[96] The resulting voice is then articulated in the usual manner of speech.

With good esophageal speech, the product is remarkably similar to normal laryngeal speech;[97] however, up to 75% of laryngectomy patients are unable to learn this method.[98,99] Failure may be due to problems of pharyngoesophageal sphincter relaxation, scarring, or nerve damage. Pharyngectomy, along with laryngectomy, usually precludes esophageal speech.[97] Impaired intellectual ability and hearing loss interfere with the learning process. Abdominal distension, excessive flatulence, and even peptic ulcers are sequelae related to aerophagia, a potential complication of esophageal speech.

In 1980, Singer and Blom[100] described a relatively simple procedure for voice restoration using the TEP technique and a one-way valved silicone voice prosthesis. The prosthesis is inserted through the TEP to prevent fistula closure and aspiration. By occluding the tracheostoma with a finger, or in some cases a lightweight tracheostoma valve, pulmonary air is shunted through the prosthesis into the esophagus allowing for the production of esophageal voice (Fig. 63-8). Success in attaining fluent speech with the Singer and Blom method has been reported in almost 90% of the patients,[101,102] although it has been emphasized that careful patient selection is mandatory. Factors to consider in patient selection include motivation; intellect; dexterity; hygiene; eyesight; stoma size, configuration and sensitivity; surgical risk; and cost. Voice restoration using the TEP can be performed either primarily at laryngectomy[103] or as a secondary procedure months or years after laryngectomy, with either general or local anesthesia.[104]

Preoperative studies should be performed to rule out pharyngoesophageal spasm and esophageal structure abnormalities. An esophageal air insufflation test[105] and radiographic studies of the esophagus should be obtained. Pharyngoesophageal spasm is cited as a major factor contributing to failure in attaining both esophageal speech and TEP speech. When spasm is identified as a problem, selective myotomy of the pharyngeal constrictor muscles frequently helps in voice acquisition.[101]

Prosthetic devices such as the electrolarynx or pneumatic external reed are also available for speech rehabilitation. The electrolarynx, either intraoral or neck type, is the most commonly used speech aid (Fig. 63-9). A neck type electrolarynx is a battery-powered tone generator that conveys sound through neck tissue to resonate within the oral cavity, where it can be articulated as speech. When the neck is not suitable for transmitting the sounds because of edema or pain, an intraoral electrolarynx can be used to transmit the generated tone directly into the mouth through a small catheter. In general, the speech produced by the neck-type electrolarynx is more intelligible, but training with an intraoral electrolarynx can begin almost immediately after surgery without stressing neck wounds.

The pneumatic external reed larynx diverts pulmonary air from the tracheostoma past a vibrating membrane, reed, or rubber band (Fig. 63-10). The sound produced by the vibrator is directed into the mouth by way of a length of tubing and then articulated as speech. Although some patients use this method of speech quite satisfactorily, many lack the respiratory support to drive the vibrator.[96]

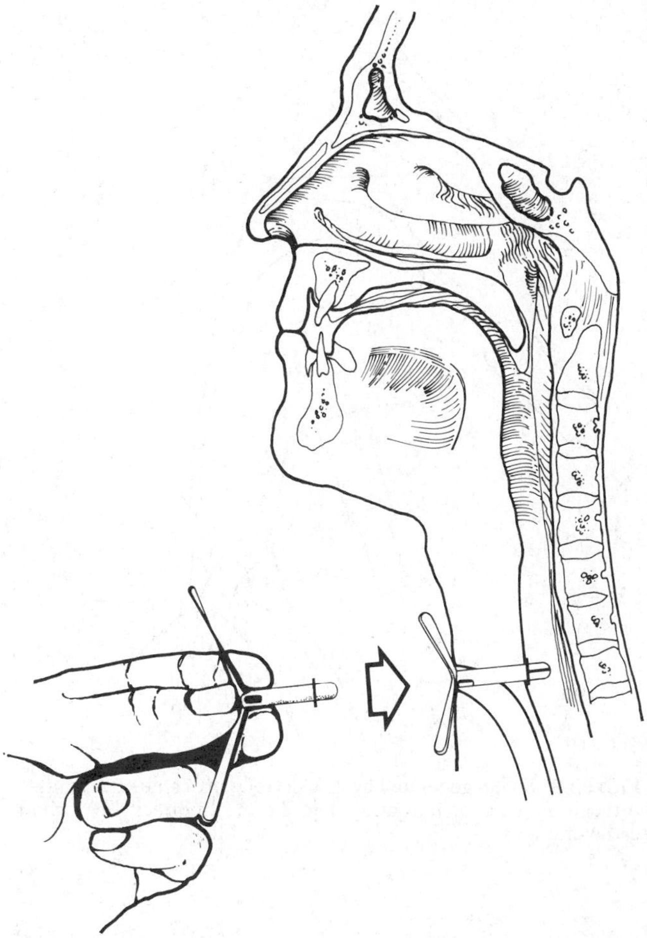

FIG. 63-8. A one-way valved voice prosthesis can be placed in a surgically created tracheal-esophageal puncture to allow the shunting of pulmonary air into the esophagus for esophageal voice production.

Rehabilitation of patients with laryngectomies should begin with preoperative counseling. Some will benefit from a preoperative visit by a person with a laryngectomy who has functional speech, whereas others will be discouraged by such a visit.[106] The American Cancer Society and International Association of Laryngectomees (IAL) have booklets available that explain anatomic changes and first-aid for a laryngectomee and list resources available to patients after treatment. Many communities have laryngectomee clubs or "lost chord clubs" that can serve as a useful resource for information and support as well as a social outlet for interested patients and their families.

Glossectomy patients may also require speech rehabilitation. Skelly and her co-workers have shown that many patients with partial and total glossectomies can achieve intelligible speech with therapy.[73,107–110] Patients with partial glossectomies tend to use the remaining tongue stump for articulation and need to be taught modifications of normal articulatory patterns to improve speech intelligibility.[107]

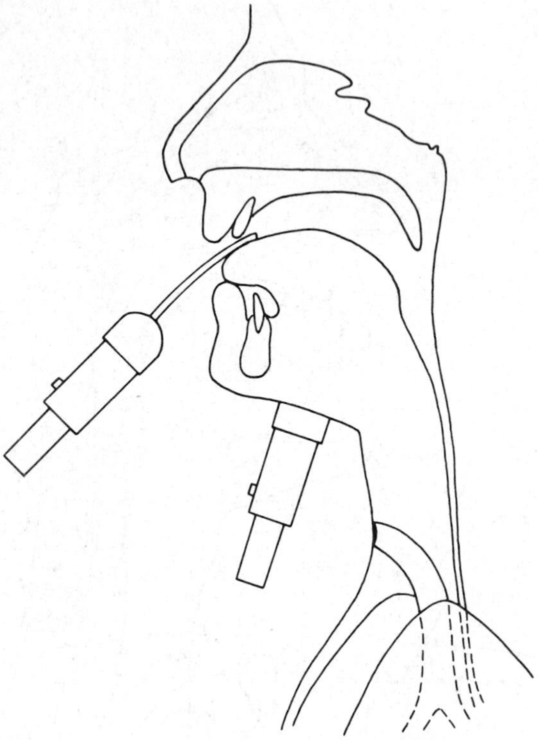

FIG. 63-9. Sound generated by an electrolarynx can be transmitted through the neck or introduced into the mouth directly by a short catheter.

Those with a total glossectomy must master the use of lips, cheeks, soft palate, mandible, and floor of the mouth to substitute for the missing tongue in producing approximations of phonemes.[73,107]

Intelligible speech has been achieved in up to 50% of patients with total glossectomies, with 57% of these same patients able to swallow adequately.[73] In general, patients who learn to swallow without difficulty also develop intelligible speech.[73,107] Speech therapy may begin as soon as wounds are healed. Early training consists of practice occluding the stoma and producing vocal tones.[73] The therapy generally is long and intense, with 6 to 8 months of elapsed time before usable gains in intelligibility occur.[109]

The total glossectomy patient learns to produce vowels by varying the degree of mandibular thrust.[110] Consonants approximated by substituting sounds produced by the compensating articulators, for example, the phoneme /z/ can be approximated by creating bilabial tension and obstructing the airstream, and the phoneme /d/ can be produced by lower lip contact with the upper teeth or alveolar ridge.[107] Once these compensations are mastered, the therapist emphasizes consistency of substitution to improve intelligibility.[109]

Prosthetic management of partial and total glossectomy patients has reportedly assisted with oral rehabilitation.[111,112] A maxillary augmentation prosthesis may assist patients who have partial tongue resection to improve the functions of speech, mastication, and swallowing by enhancing palate-tongue interaction.[113] For the total glossectomy patient, a mandibularly based tongue replacement prosthesis may improve vocal resonance characteristics by reducing the size of the oral cavity, providing an additional contact point for articulation, and serving as a guide for a food bolus to enter the esophagus.

Disfigurement

As more patients survive longer with head and neck cancers and as surgical procedures become necessarily more sophisticated and extensive, the need for restoring acceptable appearance and function presents an enormous challenge. The disfigurement of head and neck surgery can be managed by facial reconstructive surgery, implantable devices, and prosthetic devices.

Reconstructive surgery has advanced tremendously in recent years. Pectoralis major and trapezius flaps are able to provide large amounts of healthy tissue outside the field of radiation to repair large defects. Some surgeons have had success with leaving bone attached to myocutaneous flaps,[114] although the success rate of these procedures remains variable. Calvarial bone can be harvested in large quantity and has the advantages of undergoing minimal resorption, having the ability to be contoured, and having minimal morbidity at the donor site.[115] Numerous other standard techniques of facial cosmetic surgery can also be employed in recon-

FIG. 63-10. A pneumatic external voice prosthesis diverts air from the lungs to vibrate a membrane, reed, or rubber band and transmits the sound to the mouth.

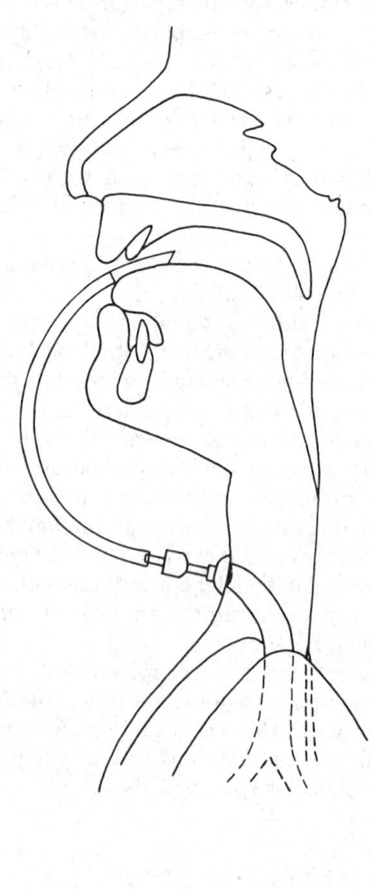

structive procedures. It is important to counsel the patient that reconstructive surgery usually involves a number of small procedures at intervals to achieve the best result.

Alloplastic implantation with synthetic plastics or metal can be useful in some patients, although most surgeons try to avoid their use in an irradiated field for many months after treatment has been completed. Reconstruction in the zygomatic, nasal, and mental area are often helped significantly by the availability of permanently implanted devices. On occasion mandibular reconstruction is performed with the use of metal or plastic trays that provide a contour and create a pocket for an autograft of cancellous bone.

Prosthetic devices are also most useful to handle the disfigurement of surgery for large cancers. Defects resulting from orbital exenteration, auriculectomy, and rhinectomy are often managed best by custom-made prosthetic devices.[31]

Presurgical consultation with a maxillofacial prosthodontist is necessary for the preparation or modification of the surgical site to facilitate retention of the prosthesis. This also allows the prosthodontist to obtain impressions and diagnostic casts of teeth and jaw arches and to collect necessary data on the mold, shade, and alignment of existing dentition.[76]

Surgical splints, stents, and obturators fabricated for use in the primary surgical procedure may be helpful in promoting healing and reducing the period of hospitalization.[31,76] In the case of maxillectomy, an obturator inserted at wound closure may permit early intelligible speech, limited chewing, and swallowing.[76]

Interim prostheses are also devised to promote functional return following extensive surgery; for example, an interim obturator to fill palatal defects is fabricated once major healing has occurred. This interim palatal obturator generally extends into the defect to improve voice and stability of the prosthesis, and artificial teeth are added to aid in mastication.[31] Another example of interim prosthesis is one used to correct mandibular discontinuity after unilateral mandibular resection. The remaining mandible tends to drift toward the defect and rotate back, resulting in malocclusion. This may be corrected by using simple hand pressure to guide the mandible to proper occlusion.[76] More severe occlusions require a maxillomandibular guiding prosthesis to reinforce movement of the mandible away from the defect toward functional occlusion.[31,76]

Some clinicians believe that because aged and debilitated patients often cannot tolerate staged extended surgical restoration, especially in the face, they are best treated by prosthetic rehabilitation.[116] The maxillofacial prosthodontist attempts to develop a facial prosthesis that is comfortable, natural in appearance, and durable. Acrylics, silicones, polyvinyl chlorides, and urethans are most commonly used in the fabrication of these prostheses.[76,117] Regardless of the material used, the prosthesis has to be altered frequently as the tissues change. Because the material wears out, the prosthesis should be replaced about once a year and a new facial moulage obtained as needed. Temporary removable facial prostheses are frequently used when delayed surgery is elected. These can also be used in cases of the uncontrolled primary, allowing the surgeon to remove the prosthesis and view the defect during follow-up.[116]

The most noticeable part of the facial prosthesis is the margin, and the maxillofacial prosthodontist tries to conceal this beneath hair, glasses, or natural facial line.[76] These prostheses usually are held in place with skin adhesives, although glasses and intraoral prostheses can provide mechanical reinforcement for added stability. When a facial prosthesis approaches the oral cavity, retention problems are greater because of saliva leakage and movement of support structures.[76]

The psychological and social effects of head and neck cancer can be particularly severe owing to the visibility of the cancer and the effect of radiation and surgery. The psychological and social intervention must begin with diagnosis, and supporting relationships should be developed. When more is known about the extent of the disease, the treatments for it, and the prognosis, individualized psychological and social intervention programs can be developed. Because of the poor prognosis for many of these patients, counseling services about death and dying should be available for the patients and significant others.

Staff members who work with these patients must be sensitive to the psychological needs of the patient and should convey attitudes of acceptance and support. Careful staff selection is appropriate, and consideration should be given to providing staff members with psychological support.

BONE AND SOFT-TISSUE MALIGNANCY: AMPUTATIONS, PATHOLOGIC FRACTURES, AND RECONSTRUCTIVE (LIMB-SPARING) SURGERY

Amputation

Amputation of a limb poses a major loss and often precipitates a substantial change in functional status. The role of the rehabilitation team is to restore near-normal function as quickly as possible. Evaluation and treatment should be given before surgery because there is evidence that surgical technique is important for good prosthetic fit and good rehabilitation outcome.[118] Excess stump tissue may result in poor socket fit, and tissue pulled too tightly may result in continual skin breakdown. Preserving as much stump length as possible often results in a more functional extremity.[119] Consultation with the surgeon before surgery concerning these issues may improve the outcome of rehabilitation.

Before surgery, the patients should be instructed in crutch walking when balance is better and pain is less, and the patient should be oriented to the rehabilitation program and the postoperative time schedule of mobility and self-care. For patients with scheduled forequarter amputations, if a shoulder cosmesis is to be made (Fig. 63-11), it must be molded from the affected side before surgery.

There is ample evidence to suggest that rigid dressings for the amputated stump reduce pain and control edema, thus decreasing the time required to develop a mature stump and allow fitting with a definitive limb.[120,121] The use of a rigid dressing may also decrease the likelihood of developing phantom limb pain by allowing early ambulation or upper extremity use, thereby providing early sensory and proprioceptive feedback. Phantom limb sensation is common after surgery, but persistent phantom limb pain is uncommon, occurring in less than 15%. When it occurs, the use of a

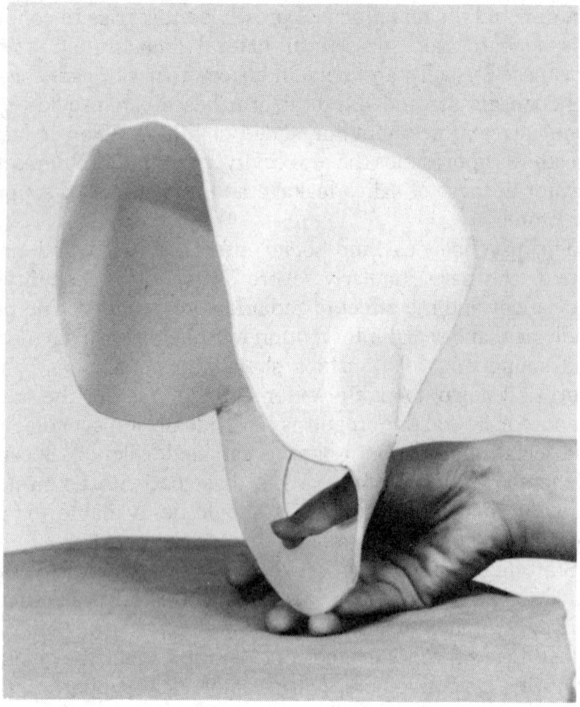

FIG. 63-11. Cosmetic shoulder cap for the interscapulothoracic level amputation.

transcutaneous nerve stimulator has been associated with pain relief. A rigid dressing is also used in some settings for hip disarticulation or hemipelvectomy patients in an attempt to encourage ambulation.[122] However, most use an Ace wrap or a girdle within 24 hr for support and limb-shaping.

The average time interval between amputation and cessation of stump shrinkage necessary for prosthetic prescription is 34 days for below-knee (BK) and 55 days for above-knee (AK) amputations.[123] In our experience, the interval between surgery and prosthetic fit for hip disarticulation (HD) and hemipelvectomy (HP) is 90 days, and a below- or above-elbow amputation matures in approximately 60 to 75 days. During this time, therapy should be prescribed to prevent contractures and to strengthen appropriate muscles.

Below- and above-elbow level amputations are treated with rigid dressings and temporary prosthesis with good results. A prosthesis is usually not used by a forequarter amputee, but the shoulder mold made before amputation is used to fashion a cosmetic shoulder cap, which is given at the time of suture removal. All upper extremity (UE) amputees are trained in one-handed activities and should be provided with self-care aids as needed. If the dominant hand has been lost, training should be extended to include handwriting and dexterity.

A prosthesis should be prescribed for any patient with a cancer-related LE amputation who desires one, provided the surgical wound has healed and ambulation is a reasonably safe goal. Residual malignant disease is not a contraindication to prosthetic prescription, and the key consideration should be the patient's need, both functionally and psychologically. Each case has to be judged individually.

Although a prosthesis of functional value can be provided for any LE amputation, the type of prosthesis socket and its suspension may be of concern in patients with healing problems resulting from radiation or chemotherapy. Patients undergoing chemotherapy often experience weight fluctuations, resulting in rapid changes in stump size.[124] It is important to remember that prosthesis fitting must be determined individually, with clinical circumstances and the experience of the physician and prosthetist modifying the prescriptions.

Prosthetics are exoskeletal or endoskeletal. The former is a wood laminate that is recommended for particularly active children or adults. The latter is foam covered, more cosmetic, and lighter; however, because the cover snags easily, it is harder to maintain. Endoskeletal units are modular and offer easier assembly with interchangeable parts.

Major advances in lower extremity prosthetic design and manufacture have occurred during the last several years. Flexible sockets have been gaining widespread use in AK prosthetics and their use in BK prostheses is increasing. Surlyn seems to be well tolerated, with no appreciable increase in skin problems.[125] Natural alignment sockets with narrow AP dimensions and wider ML with high lateral wall and slightly adducted socket have been reported to be well tolerated and associated with relatively rapid gait retraining.[126]

Sports and recreational activity occupy much of leisure time in our population. Amputee athletes and sports persons are increasing in number with over 5000 participating in organized competition.[127] Their interests have stimulated new developments in prosthetic design, manufacture, and rehabilitation techniques, as well as the establishment of sports organizations for amputees.

Limb care has been improved with the use of materials that reduce friction between skin and prosthesis. One of these materials, 2nd Skin, is a polyethylene oxide and water compound; another is Skin Care Pad, which is a closed cell elastomer. These materials should be used as preventive measures in decreasing skin breakdown caused by overactivity, but they also may be used for dysvascular patients with partial insensitivity that leads to skin breakdown.

Upper extremity prostheses have been adapted to meet the myriad of needs of sports participants. Proper conditioning is the first step, and using weight harnesses for barbell and other weight-lifting activity is the recommended approach. Major advances in the design of terminal devices have been made to permit specialized grasps for rods, reels, guns, clubs, gymnastics, and so forth.[128]

Advances in LE prosthetic design include the development of energy-storing feet that could assist in push off. The Seattle Foot and Flex Foot offer reduced weight, compared with conventional articulated ankle/foot assemblies. They provide a more propulsive gait. The Flex Foot offers multiaxial movement. A good review of the currently available feet is available.[129]

Finally, an improvement in socket design for below-knee

amputees is available through a suction socket. Total surface-bearing and anatomic accuracy of fit are essential for proper suspension and minimal skin breakdown.[130] Similar improvements have been noted for above-knee amputees using flexible sockets as well.[125]

HIP DISARTICULATION AND HEMIPELVECTOMY. Hip disarticulation and hemipelvectomy prosthetic limbs are usually Canadian style (Figs. 63-12, 63-13) and weigh approximately 11 lb for exoskeletal and 8 lb for the endoskeletal units. The knee component most frequently used is a single-axis knee. Occasionally, an extension aid is added for stability or, rarely, a hydraulic unit is used if the patient is a strong ambulator. The foot unit prescribed is usually a single-axis ankle when there is a need for walking on rough terrain or sports interest. Sometimes a solid ankle cushion heel (SACH) can be prescribed. The gait pattern is usually hip hiking, or an exaggerated pelvic tilt and trunkal bend. A cane or crutch may be used to decrease the amount of Trendelenburg gait. The HD and HP patient expends a substantial amount of energy to ambulate and ambulates at a slower speed than any other level amputee.[131] Younger patients are more likely to be prosthesis users than those over 50. Those who do not use prostheses usually are crutch walkers and do not use wheelchairs.[132] Back pain and scoliosis are commonly seen[133] and should be monitored, especially in the

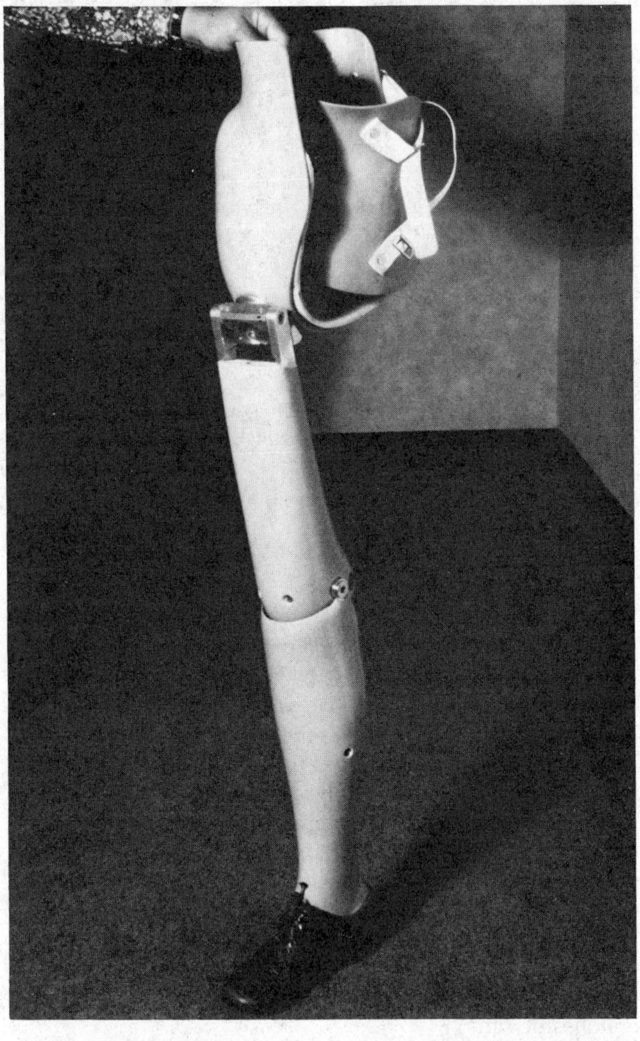

FIG. 63-12. Canadian hemipelvectomy prosthesis. The sitting surface is unstable, and patient must vault for the leg to clear the floor during the swing phase of gait. The patient will use a cane or crutch, and many patients tend to use these prostheses only for special occasions.

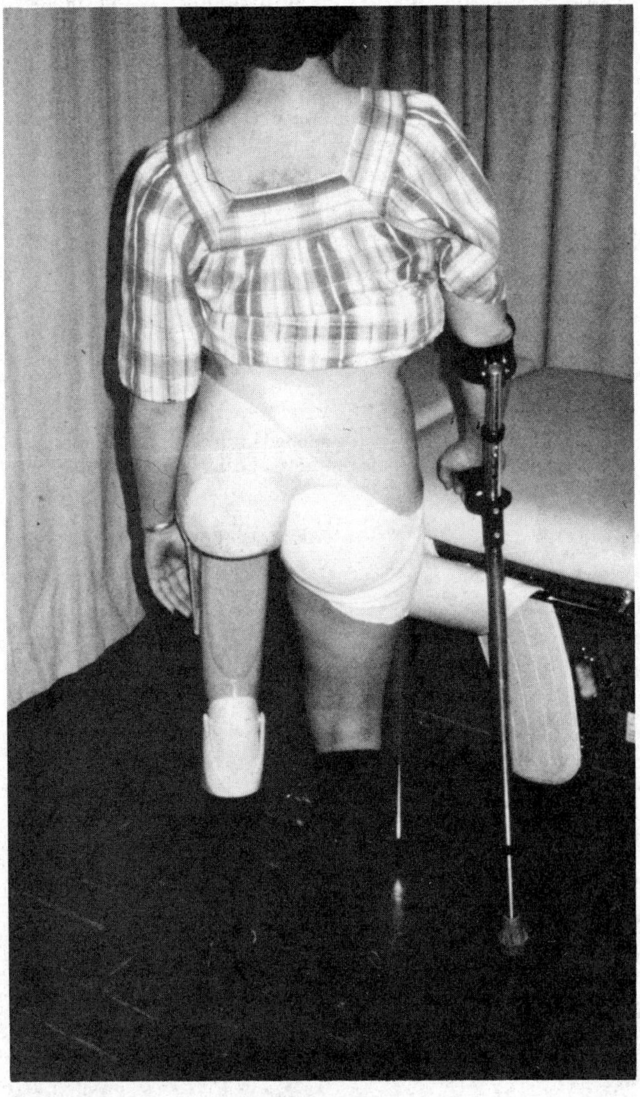

FIG. 63-13. Canadian hip disarticulation prosthesis. The patient clears the swing prosthesis leg by hip hiking and uses a cane when walking on uneven ground and thick carpets.

growing child. If a limb is impractical or not wanted, a sitting jacket may be useful in providing support.

The patient usually begins ambulation on the fifth day after surgery. The process is begun with tilt-table standing, and then advances to parallel bars, walker, and crutches. When the medical condition permits and flap integrity is assured, the patient may sit in a chair—usually 14 days following surgery. The HP patient should be given a wedge-shaped cushion under the operative side for comfortable sitting. Bathroom safety, with encouragement to use a tub seat, grab bars, and other adaptive equipment, should be reviewed before hospital discharge.

ABOVE-KNEE LEVEL. The midthigh is the most frequent site of amputation for femoral lesions. This anatomic location is associated with the greatest flexion and extension power.[134] The short AK stump (less than 15 cm) is usually associated with more phantom limb sensation and marked flexion, abduction, and external rotation.[134] Nonetheless, short AK amputees can be successful prosthetic users.[135]

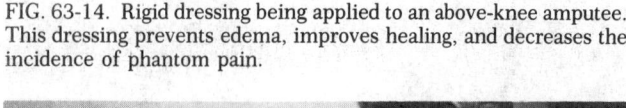

The AK socket usually is quadrilateral, ischial weight-bearing, and total contact. Most amputees will suspend this socket with suction. (A vacuum is created by the intimate fit of total contact). When stump length is too short for this type of socket, a silesian or pelvic band is added to suspend the prosthesis. Extremely short stumps (less than 8 cm) are fit into a gluteal weight-bearing, free-formed socket that is suspended using a pelvic band. A constant friction knee component or the more expensive hydraulic, hydrocadence, or Henschke-Mauch units can be prescribed. The most frequently used foot component is the SACH foot, but an articulated ankle should be prescribed for those walking on uneven terrain or those actively involved in sports.

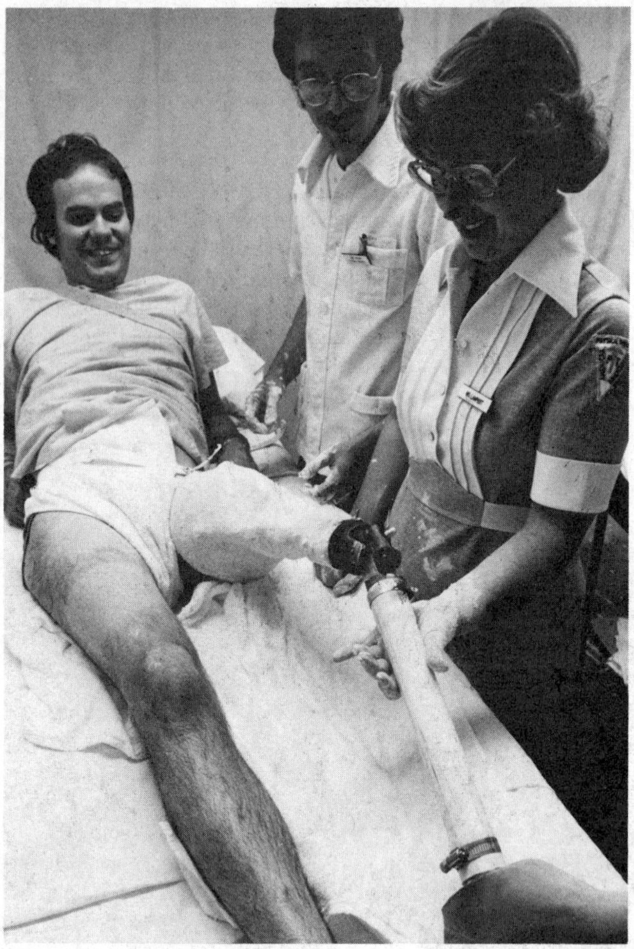

FIG. 63-15. Incorporated into the rigid plaster of Paris dressing is a coupling device with the pylon and artificial foot attached.

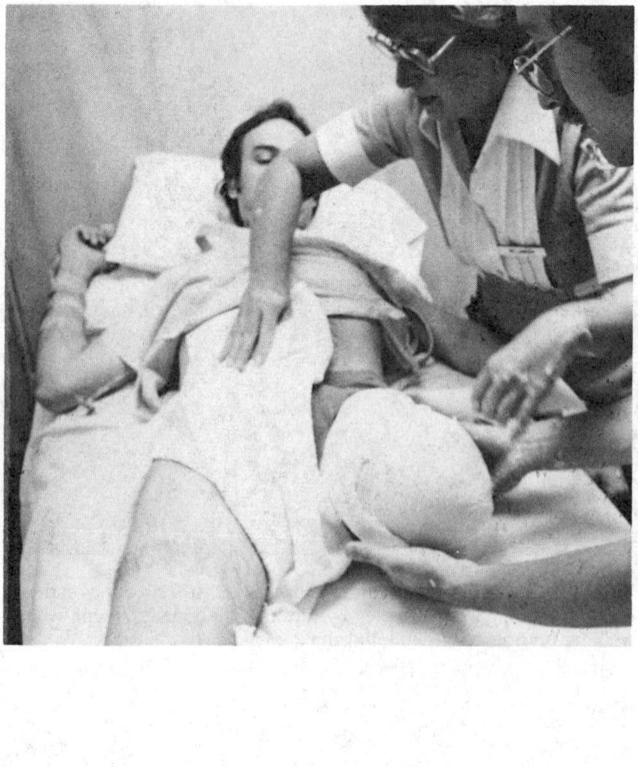

FIG. 63-14. Rigid dressing being applied to an above-knee amputee. This dressing prevents edema, improves healing, and decreases the incidence of phantom pain.

Patients undergoing AK amputations are fit with rigid dressings (Fig. 63-14) and are ambulated 24 hr after surgery using parallel bars and advanced to crutches when able. A temporary pylon (Fig. 63-15) is added after suture removal, and the socket is replaced as changes in stump size dictate. Gait training for younger patients with the definitive limb usually takes 3 days. Many AK amputees walk without crutches or cane.

BELOW-KNEE LEVEL. The BK prosthesis most frequently prescribed is patella tendon-bearing (PTB) with a SACH foot. Often one prescribes this unit with a soft liner, which permits some additional cushioning as the stump matures and the tissues become firmer. The unit is usually suspended by a supracondylar strap or occasionally a wedge. Gait training for younger patients usually takes 2 days, and gait patterns and energy requirements are near normal.[119] A cane or crutch is rarely used by BK amputees.

HEMICORPORECTOMY LEVEL. Hemicorporectomy, or translumbar amputation, has been performed for advanced cancer in a final life-saving effort.[136,137] The amputation is usually between the L4 and L5 levels. The procedure requires the fecal stream to be diverted by a colostomy or an ileostomy. With the latter, continuous liquid drainage causes special prosthetic concerns. The urine is diverted by an ilioloop procedure, emptying into a collection bag.

A sitting bucket prosthesis, mounted on a platform so that the socket can rotate, allows the patient to sit and perform wheelchair ambulation.[136,137] These patients should be evaluated by a rehabilitation team before prosthetic prescription.

UPPER EXTREMITY LEVEL. *Shoulder Disarticulation Level.* The UE amputee undergoing forequarter (interscapulothoracic) amputation should have a shoulder cap to provide symmetry and feedback for head and neck position, as well as to provide a shelf for clothing. A forequarter prosthesis unit has very limited function and tends to be used as a stabilizer. Prescription of such a unit should be delayed until chemotherapy or radiation is complete and a thorough assessment of a patient's functional needs can be met. Hence, we recommend a cosmetic soft-shoulder-without-arm unit, or an endoskeletal non-cable-driven unit. Fabrication and training time are prolonged for functional forequarter prostheses. Functional units are available with cables, manual locks to position the elbow, or electrically driven elbows with myoelectric terminal devices.

Above-Elbow Level. Above-elbow (AE) prostheses are easier to don and use than forequarter prostheses. The AE prosthesis is a functional unit that can be body-powered using a shoulder harness or externally powered using an electric motor and battery or myoelectric control.[138] This latter unit depends upon a surface electrode to pick up EMG signals when a muscle or muscle groups contract. The signal is amplified and sent to a signal processor and then the direct current motor of a mechanical hand or elbow. The most frequent prescription is for a microswitch-controlled elbow (Utah or Boston elbow) and a myoelectric hand. These units allow flexion-extension as well as humeral rotation. Formal training requires a week. The AE prosthesis is usually suspended by a figure-eight harness and an elbow unit with an internal locking unit. The forearm piece can be endoskeletal or exoskeletal.

Below-Elbow Level. By far the greatest number of UE amputees are those of below-elbow (BE) level. Many of these patients are fitted with a body-powered system of hook and harness. For short BE a triceps cuff may be added. Terminal devices may be voluntary closure hooks, which are open during the relaxed state, or voluntary opening hooks, which are closed during the relaxed state. The voluntary closure relies on patient effort to maintain grasp. Many patients prefer this to passive closure. Myoelectric BE prostheses are widely accepted (Fig. 63-16). The unit is worn without a harness, has superior pinch force (15-25 lb versus 7-8 lb for the hook) and, because the terminal device is a hand, is more cosmetic. The unit is powered by the flexors and extensors of the wrist, which are usually intact and not used in lifting or reaching. Hence, they are ideal for myoelectric use. Training requires 2 to 3 days. Stump length can be as short as 3.5 in. from the olecranon. The patient must be able to elicit control over the myoelectric signal and hold different levels of muscle tension reliably (*e.g.*, relaxation, moderate, and strong contractions).

Proper fit, alignment, and function must be assured before releasing any amputee patient with a prosthetic unit. Patients are educated about prosthetic maintenance, skin care, and the need for routine rehabilitation follow-up. For the growing child, regular return appointments must be scheduled to correct prosthetic lengths during growth and to guard against the development of significant scoliosis.

Sports activities are encouraged. Some persons with particularly good balance play football, soccer, and cycle without prosthetics. Return to work or school is a critical part of the rehabilitation process.

Limb-Sparing Procedures

Advances in early detection of tumors, using magnetic resonance imaging and computerized tomography have permitted early and more definitive surgical planning in the management of extremity neoplasms.[139,140] There are three parts to the surgical procedure itself: resection, reconstruction,

FIG. 63-16. Myoelectric prosthesis with a hand terminal device in a below-elbow amputee.

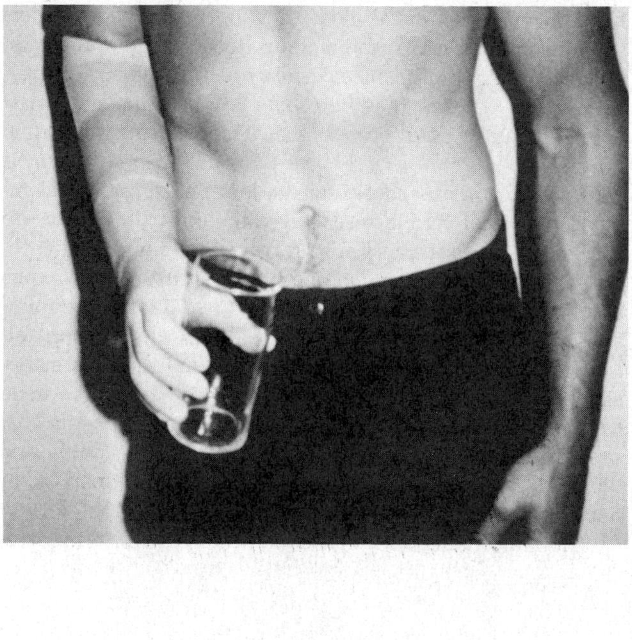

and skin coverage. The decision about what type of reconstruction to be used should include information about the patient's life-style, as well as vocational and avocational goals.

The surgical decision about how much soft tissue to resect and whether to use arthrodesis or arthroplasty will, in part, determine the functional outcome, but the main determinant of function is the soft tissue that is resected and the reconstruction required. The UE treatment options include scapulectomy, Tikhoff-Lindberg procedure, and forearm bone excisions. Scapulectomy patients have a reasonably good functional outcome with preservation of the use of the elbow and hand, with some flexion and minimal abduction of the shoulder. Pain is often a problem, and patients report a sense of drag on the arm. Edema of the forearm and hand can occur when the arm is always dependent. Normal arm use is encouraged, and passive ROM to the shoulder is prescribed.

The Tikhoff-Lindberg procedure (see Chap. 42) offers the patient with a high UE lesion an opportunity for excellent functional outcome and is clearly superior to a forequarter amputation. In this procedure, there is en bloc removal of the scapula, clavicle, and proximal humerus.[141] If some scapula can be preserved, a proximal humeral spacer or autograft can be placed to help stabilize the elbow.[142] The surgery produces minimal disfigurement and only mild pain and edema. Shoulder function is lost, and motion is only passive, but elbow and hand function are retained. A cosmetic shoulder should be molded before surgery, and an arm sling provided to support the arm after surgery. The sling should be worn until sutures are removed at 14 days, and shoulder motion should be restricted for this period. Hand and forearm muscle pumping, plus the use of an elastic sleeve should control edema. The sling may be maintained for longer periods. It is important to begin passive ROM of the shoulder by 2 weeks to avoid the development of joint contracture. Once the arm is out of the sling, full ROM of elbow and shoulder should be done for several minutes daily. Normal daily activities are encouraged, but lifting more than 20 lb with the operative side should be avoided.

When the distal radius is removed, the wrist is usually fused and a small distal ulna resection performed to allow some pronation/supination motion. Reconstruction using an allograft or autograft can be performed. If the ulna is centralized, wrist function may be retained.[143] A functional wrist splint should be used for tasks that require lifting more than 10 lb.

Limb-sparing procedures for the lower extremity (LE) include proximal femur resection with hip arthroplasty, en bloc excisions for tumors arising around the knee joint (provided posterior tibial nerve and popliteal artery are intact) can be treated with arthrodesis or arthroplasty. Femoral shaft resection or fibulectomy can also be done when followed by an allograft. A new expandable/adjustable prosthesis has been used in the treatment of childhood bone tumors.[144] Generally, the rehabilitation team has as its goal preservation of ROM, strength, and control of edema and pain. Patients with LE sarcoma are at significant risk of developing mobility problems when they receive wide local excision and radiation.[145] These patients may need an orthosis to help control knee extension if the quadriceps has been excised or to maintain dorsiflexion of the foot if the peroneal nerve has been sacrificed. Long after surgery has been completed, ROM exercises and edema control must still be practiced.

Fibulectomy, either partial or total, is usually associated with footdrop because the peroneal nerve is sacrificed.[146] Usually the knee is stable because the capsule has not been violated. These patients are usually in a cast that immobilizes the extremity at 30° flexion for 2 weeks, and then they are allowed partial weight-bearing on crutches for 2 weeks.[147] At the same time of cast removal, an ankle–foot orthosis is provided to control footdrop. Knee and ankle ROM and quadriceps strengthening are prescribed. Often a cane is temporarily recommended. Delayed wound healing and numbness of the foot are frequently observed. Distal femur lesions, when removed en bloc, are treated with arthrodesis or joint replacement.[147] Arthrodesis creates a slow, energy-inefficient gait. To ambulate with knee arthrodesis, good ankle ROM is mandatory; without this, it is impossible to walk. Postoperatively, patients are in a long leg brace and non–weight-bearing for 6 weeks. They are advanced to partial weight-bearing with a posterior splint for at least 3 months.

When these lesions are treated with knee joint arthroplasty, knee motion is preserved. The functional outcome depends on the amount of soft tissue excised, but a limp of the gluteus maximus type is observed.[148] Following surgery, ROM exercises and quadriceps strengthening are begun, then walking with a walker until the patient is ready for crutches or a cane. Ischial weight-bearing long leg braces[149] are sometimes recommended; control of the knee motion is critical; however, we have not used these and have had no biomechanical failures. The patient is kept non–weight-bearing for 2 to 3 weeks followed by partial weight-bearing for at least 3 weeks.

Clearly, limb-sparing procedures have greater potential than do amputations for functional outcome. Successful outcome, however, depends on selection of appropriate patients.

Psychological Considerations

Because patients with amputations owing to cancer are usually young, the impact of the cancer and amputation on their education process and return to school may be significant and require professional intervention. The patient and family should be offered counseling about body image change, cancer-related fears, full participation in rehabilitation, and how to deal with others around these issues. The teacher and classmates should also be provided with information on changes to expect and how to be supportive, while allowing the patient to be as independent as possible.

Vocational considerations must be addressed from the beginning. If the amputation will necessitate adaptive changes in the work environment, they should be initiated. If a new job or retraining is needed, this should also be addressed early to provide a tangible goal and to increase motivation for the overall rehabilitation process.

LUNG CANCER

Rehabilitation goals in patients with lung cancer are to prevent pulmonary disability after radiation or surgery by facilitating bronchial drainage, improving ventilation, augmenting coughing, helping to maintain mobilization of the thorax, and preventing postural deformity such as scoliosis.[150]

Surgery to remove cancerous lung tissue (thoracotomy, lobectomy, and pneumonectomy) may be associated with a postoperative limitation of pulmonary function and impairment of the mechanics of breathing. The decrease in respiratory reserve depends on the amount of lung tissue resected. Breathing is impaired because of chest wall resection with transected muscles, pain, and restrictive bandaging in the postoperative period.[151]

Treatment before surgery is helpful, because many of these patients already have restricted pulmonary function that will only be aggravated by the thoracotomy and lung tissue resection. It is best before surgery to have the patient quit smoking and to try inhaled or oral bronchodilators. If the sputum is purulent, antibiotics should be prescribed.

The preoperative rehabilitation program should emphasize breathing retraining to increase diaphragmatic excursion with a resultant reduction in the work of breathing, increased tidal volume, and improvement in the distribution of inspired gas.[152] Diaphragmatic abdominal breathing is usually combined with pursed-lips breathing, which is an effective method of altering the respiratory pattern, slowing down the respiratory rate, and decreasing airway collapse during expiration.[153] It is best to teach these exercises before surgery, when there is no incision pain; however, some patients quickly revert to their old breathing patterns when not being supervised. Segmental breathing can be taught to allow certain areas to expand, and the lateral basal, posterior basal, and diaphragmatic areas should receive special attention.[154] These techniques are much more difficult for patients with pulmonary disease than for normal persons.

Postural drainage is used to help clear bronchial secretions from a particular segment or lobe of the lung and is most effective in patients who have bronchiectasis or an infiltrate. The frequency and the duration of drainage depend on the patient's individual needs and tolerance.[155]

Preoperatively, effective coughing is taught using correct respiratory control, rather than by simply increasing force or volume of expelled air.[156] It is best to have the patient fully inspire and cough two or three times in one breath,[155] which will allow evacuation throughout the tracheobronchial tree segments. Postoperatively, therapy begins as soon as the patient awakens. The intensity of the program will depend on the patient's overall medical condition, tolerance to exercise, and specific respiratory problems.[150]

Manual hand splinting of the chest by the patient or staff helps to reduce the patient's discomfort and apprehension, because incision pain plays a major role in cooperation with therapy. Initially, respiratory accessory muscle activity of the thorax and neck should be eliminated to further reduce discomfort. It is sensible to treat these patients 20 to 30 min after the administration of analgesics so that they can comply with the therapeutic plan. The postoperative treatment program should include breathing exercises, positional drainage, and proper coughing. The intensity of the program depends on the patient's needs, physical condition, and response to exercise.

Chest percussion and vibration may be added to the program when they can be tolerated. These methods are used to loosen secretions that may adhere to the inner lumen of the small bronchi. Direct pressure to the wound site should be avoided, and percussion should not be used in cases of suspected pneumothorax, chest trauma, rib fracture, or pathologic fracture.[155] As the patient improves and the incisional pain decreases, a more active exercise program is initiated to restore ROM and muscle strength. The program will focus on correction and prevention of scoliosis and any ipsilateral shoulder restriction. Contracture of this shoulder could impede such ADLs as dressing, bathing, and grooming. In some patients, dyspnea may be so severe that it interferes with self-care and day-to-day activities, and they need to be instructed in energy conservation techniques.

Some of the extrapulmonary effects of lung cancer are peripheral neuropathies, myositis, cortical cerebellar degeneration, and the myasthenic syndrome. All of these will potentially affect the patient's ability to function with respect to ADLs and mobility. Problems that stem from the remote effects should be addressed in the comprehensive rehabilitation plan.

OSTOMIES FOR BOWEL AND BLADDER CANCER

Surgical treatment of bowel and bladder cancer may result in ostomies to divert feces and urine. For patients with ostomies, rehabilitation must address the individual's adjustments to a drastically altered self-concept, the ability to control elimination, and the need to learn ostomy management in a manner that facilitates optimum psychosocial function. A nurse specialist or enterostomal specialist, who is skillful in utilizing knowledge relative to a body image, learning theories, and the effects of the disease and its treatment, and who is competent in all aspects of stoma management, can provide continuity.

The concept of trained enterostomal therapists is credited to Dr. Rupert Turnbull of the Cleveland Clinic. Certification has been administered by their official organization, the International Association for Enterostomal Therapy, and currently includes persons of diverse backgrounds, some with ostomies themselves.[157]

Acceptance of an altered body image and learning self-care programs are faster if rehabilitation is initiated at the time of the diagnosis. Clear explanations of the physical and functional outcome expectations of surgery should be given. Although this is primarily the surgeon's role, the enterostomal therapist should help clarify and amplify the physiologic and psychological consequences. Initially, the psychological impact of this information may interfere with the patient's ability to assimilate it, but it sets the state for future interventions aimed at self-care independence. Persons who are ill-prepared before surgery will require more time, support, and assistance in their rehabilitation.[158]

It has been demonstrated that patients provided with the continuous services of an enterostomal therapist have shorter hospital stays and require fewer home visits to attain successful management.[157]

To help the patient resolve conflicts and eventually accept an altered body image, the following rehabilitation steps have been proposed:

1. Accepts the importance of viewing the operative site
2. Touches and explores the operative site
3. Accepts the necessity of learning to care for the stoma
4. Develops independence and competence in daily care
5. Reintegrates the new body image and adjusts to a possibly altered life-style[159]

This process may be modified by cultural attitudes and values and the patient's actual ability to perform the procedures.

Participation of the enterostomal therapist in the selection of the stoma site can also contribute to problem prevention. The stoma should be on a flat surface without creases or wrinkles and away from scars, bony protuberances, the waistline, umbilicus, and other stomas. To best assess the site, the patient should be checked in the supine, sitting, and forward-bending positions. The stoma should protrude about a half-inch above the skin level to allow for more effective collection and liquid drainage.[160]

The procedural steps for teaching the behaviors to accomplish control of urine and feces should reflect the competence of the enterostomal therapist and the familiarity with the specific equipment and appliances to be used. The prescribed appliance system should be consistently available during hospitalization, at discharge, and in the community. The patient should be made aware of the various component parts and help select them. The care and use of each component should be explained to the patient.

About 50% of patients with a descending or sigmoid colostomy develop a natural evacuation at regular intervals, thus avoiding a collecting device. Other patients with colostomies may require irrigation to control elimination. This should be encouraged in those who have regular bowel movements before surgery and who desire to try this method to avoid using a collecting device. Patients whose bowel movements were irregular and unpredictable before surgery will most likely have to wear a collecting device, even if they use irrigation to stimulate bowel evacuation. Perforation from colostomy irrigations may occur, although the risk can be reduced by using an irrigation cone or inserting the catheter tip less than 5 cm.[160]

A typical colostomy irrigation program would involve training the bowel on a fixed daily, or every-other-day, schedule. The time chosen would be convenient and without distraction, taking usually an hour to start. The gastrocolic reflex is stimulated by using food or hot or cold liquids to increase peristalsis. The irrigation is used to stimulate the colon from below. A bag or can containing 500 to 1000 ml of lukewarm water is hung 60 cm above the stoma. The patient should sit on the toilet with the soiled appliance bag or dressing removed. An irrigation bag is attached with the long end in the toilet bowl, and the water is then allowed to run through the tubing to remove all air. The lubricated cone or catheter is inserted into the stoma, and the water is released to enter at a rate that is determined by the patient's comfort. Rapid distension of the bowel may produce cramps. It usually takes 5 to 10 min for the water to run into the bowel. The return from the irrigation occurs in two stages. The first occurs with the removal of the cone or the catheter and drainage through the irrigation bag into the toilet bowl; 30 min later the rest of the drainage occurs. Most persons will then remove the appliance, clean it, dry it, and cover the colostomy with a gauze pad.[160]

Bromley presented this rehabilitation process covering preoperative counseling to posthospital follow-up using Orem's self-care theory.[161] Her interventions are designed to bring about a transition from dependence to independence, relative to ostomy management. Although limited to physical abilities immediately after operation, the patient is able to learn through the modeling of the enterostomal therapist. Explaining and giving information also prepare the patient for participation. Other learning concepts to be used in developing self-care include building in a measure of success for each session, positively reinforcing appropriate behaviors, and shaping these through stages of successive approximations from dependence to independence.[162]

A resource for patient information and psychological support is a member of the Ostomy Association, who will visit patients upon request. These volunteers all have ostomies and can be located through the American Cancer Society. Another "normalizing" approach used in physical rehabilitation is to have patients wear their own clothing while still in the hospital. This practice can also resolve the patient's fears about visibility of appliances.

For the patient with an ostomy, skin care will always be important. During the operation, and immediately afterward, it is essential to avoid skin damage. Sutures must not be placed through the epidermis of the periostomal skin, and accumulation of blood and serum in the subcutaneous tissue adjacent to the stoma must be avoided. To avoid leakage, the appliance must fit exactly to the skin around the stoma, leaving only an ⅛-in. to 1/16-in. margin between the stoma and the appliance edge, to allow for contraction and relaxation of the stoma. Any complaint of stomal itching or burning should be interpreted as leakage, and the appliance must be changed immediately.[160]

The most common postoperative skin problems are maceration or candidal infection. Skin maceration should be treated with nonadherent bandage and topical steroid cream or spray. Candidal infection will respond to nystatin powder.[160] Contact dermatitis may develop and should be treated by removing the irritant (adhesive tape or material comprising the appliance or the barrier) and by using local steroids. Folliculitis is best treated by trimming the hairs around the stoma, not by pulling them out or shaving them with a razor.[160] The continent ileostomy procedure offers the advantage of freedom from the external appliance and a decrease in skin problems.[163]

Diet information for the colostomy and ileostomy patient should not consist of long lists of restrictive prohibitions but rather a more positive approach of experimenting to determine individual tolerance.[164] Foods that cause gas or diarrhea before surgery are likely to continue to be a problem. Patients with a colostomy should be advised to chew foods well to avoid constipation, especially nuts, seeds, popcorn, and celery. New foods should be tried one at a time to discover their effect on the ostomy. Patients with diabetic or antihypertensive diets should continue them after surgery.[160]

Gas is produced in an empty intestine and is a consequence of abdominal surgery. The gas, although harmless, is uncomfortable and embarrassing. Patients should avoid skipping meals to prevent an empty intestine. They should be informed that anxiety, gum chewing, candy sucking, and cigarette smoking will increase gas.[160]

Ileostomy patients may experience problems with fluids and electrolytes. When the terminal ileum is removed, vitamin B_{12} supplements are required. Diarrhea, caused by infection (influenza), medications, impacted sigmoid colostomy, or bowel irradiation, may lead to rapid dehydration in ileostomy patients. Urine output of less than 400 ml in 12 hr indicates impending dehydration and requires intravenous electrolytes.[160]

Discharge planning and follow-up are the real tests of hospital-initiated rehabilitation programs. A smooth transition back to community living depends on early communication among the patient, family, hospital team, and community resource people. Written information for home reference should include instructions to reinforce teaching and sources of equipment, appropriate medication, and dietary information. Patients need printed material on the resumption of activities, including sexual intercourse; Ostomy Association information; follow-up appointments; and names of people to call for assistance. In some states, the American Cancer Society will contribute to the cost of equipment. Referrals to a home nursing service may enhance the transition. The community nurse, using technical knowledge and sensitivity, can further stimulate the resumption of normal activities. This nurse also brings a knowledge of community resources and how to coordinate them on behalf of the patient's optimal functioning in the community.

Unless there are complicating mechanical problems, most patients with ostomies should be able to return to their previous employment. This will not be true for many laborers, because heavy, prolonged lifting should be avoided.[160]

Although rapid changes in atmospheric pressure may produce more intestinal gas, there should be no travel restrictions as far as the ostomy is concerned. Patients should take along any equipment required for routine ostomy care. Seat belts should be fastened below or well above the stoma.[162] No special clothing is required, but too tight or too rigid clothing tends to put too much pressure on the stoma. The patient should be able to participate in all exercise and sports and can even enjoy swimming, provided he uses a non–water-soluble appliance seal.[162]

CANCER OF THE BRAIN

Cancer of the central nervous system (CNS) represents only about 2% of all cancers, but up to 15% of patients with systemic cancer develop neurologic symptoms.[165] The nervous system is susceptible to anatomic lesions and to toxic or destructive effects of surgery, chemotherapy, and radiation. Cancer of the vital organs also may have a remote effect on the nervous system.[166]

Primary brain tumors, metastatic lesion, remote cancers, and brain damage from a treatment modality may cause functional deficits in areas of cognition, mobility, ADL, and bowel and bladder continence that should be addressed by a rehabilitation team. Rehabilitation should be a concomitant of diagnosis to prevent unnecessary loss of function and to minimize the effect of the deficit on the patient's quality of life.

The degree of deficit and ability to respond to rehabilitation measures may fluctuate during and after treatment. During radiation and chemotherapy, there may be a decline in the patient's neurologic or hematologic condition, but completion of these therapies may result in a cure or rapid improvement.

Changes in cognitive functions are common in patients with cancer of the brain and may resemble those of stroke patients.[167] Because many rehabilitation techniques depend on learning and cooperation, cognitive functioning should be evaluated. The deficits themselves may not be subject to change, but the rehabilitation plan should develop with full knowledge of the patient's learning capabilities and weaknesses. For those who cannot learn, the team should work with care providers to develop a management plan. Early intellectual assessment is important for establishing a baseline of activities that can be used to follow disease progression.

Patients with lesions in the left cerebral hemisphere may develop communication and intellectual deficits of aphasia. A speech pathologist should assess all language modalities (speaking, writing, gesturing, listening, and reading) to develop a communication management plan. Assessment of other learning modalities, including visual–spatial skills, memory, and problem solving, is also essential. Benefits may be realized by educating and organizing the patient's family and care providers about the degree of impairment and prevention of patient frustration. Some severely aphasic patients learn self-care activities when the clinician demonstrates the performance in a stepwise fashion and either eliminates or simplifies the verbal input. It is important not to isolate the patient by assuming more intellectual deficit than is present; therefore, each patient deserves careful assessment and an individualized plan.

Because fluent speech is often retained in cancer patients with right brain lesions, problems related to visual–motor–perceptual and spatial difficulties that impair performance are frequently missed. These problems include judging form, distance, rate of movement, and position of body parts. Patients may have problems performing simple actions such as putting on a shirt, brushing teeth, or propelling a wheelchair through a doorway. The lack of initiation of action or performance becomes a major problem, and patients are often incorrectly described as obstinate, uncooperative, unmotivated, or depressed. Because of these patients' good verbal skills, their rehabilitation potential can be overestimated and, with their impulsiveness and perceptual problems, they are at high risk for an accident. It is particularly important that their care providers are cognizant of the patient's limitations and understand the discrepancy between their language and performance. Furthermore, care providers should be instructed to talk the patient through activities that are otherwise performed incompletely, inaccurately, or with poor judgment.[168,169]

Memory processes need a totally functioning brain for maximum efficiency. Patients with recent memory deficits may recall details of past events, names of old acquaintances, and occasions long past, yet be unable to retain new information, which drastically affects their rehabilitation. Patients with memory deficits may use written aids such as a printed daily schedule and step-by-step instruction cards. As with other brain-damaged patients, they need a fixed routine and predictable environment to reduce frustrations and ease management.

Mobility

As mentioned earlier, proper bed-positioning techniques and passive or active ROM are essential to avoid contractures. Specific strengthening exercises must be initiated if there is any return.

Extremely weak patients need to work on bed mobility and practice coming to a sitting position. Sitting balance is essential for safe transfers. The most common transfers are the standing pivot and the sliding transfer described by Stolov.[170] It is much easier to transfer to an equal height; hence, environmental modifications such as hospital beds, raised toilet seats, and grab bars are essential. Ambulation may be by wheelchair on bipedal, with or without aids, and the degree of independence may vary with the environment. The patient may be independent in a level home but need assistance for stairs, ramps, and uneven ground.

The best mode of ambulation for the patient may be the wheelchair. The prescription must consider the patient's needs, cost, size, and special adaptive components, such as removable armrests to facilitate side transfers, desk arms to allow the chair to fit under a table or desk, and detachable elevating foot rests for patients with LE edema.[171] Thin, solid tires move easier on level smooth surfaces, whereas balloon tires are better for thick carpeting, grass, or gravel. A manual one-arm drive or electric wheelchair may be indicated.[172] All wheelchairs must have brakes.

Free-standing balance is a prerequisite for independent bipedal ambulation. Most patients want to walk, but some, such as those with severe cerebellar ataxia, are not safe. Most patients with hemiparesis, and many with hemiplegia, can be taught to walk using an ankle–foot orthosis (AFO) provided they do not have significant hip or knee flexion contractures. The hemiplegic patient neurologically recovers in a proximal to distal distribution with an extensor synergy pattern present in the LE. To maximize this recovery and to minimize the effects of bed rest, the hip and knee extensors and hip abductor muscles, should receive strengthening exercises. The dorsiflexors frequently do not return, and the AFO compensates for this function. This orthosis works best with the ankle in neutral position or with passive ROM to 5° dorsiflexion. It is important to actively range the ankle joint and prevent muscle imbalance, extensor synergy, and spasticity from developing static contractures.[173]

Many assistive devices are available for walking, with the four-legged (quad) cane being the most common for the patient with hemiplegia or hemiparesis.[174] This allows a slow, wide-based gait in which much of the body weight is supported through the hand. Before discharge, the patient should be trained on stairs, ramps, uneven ground, and getting up from a fall. The patient and significant others must know safety limits and when assistance is needed.

Problems with Activities of Daily Living

The ADL retraining and management should be guided by the patient's prognosis, needs, desires, degree of intellectual impairment, presence of other diseases and complications, and the care provider's requirements and skills. In patients with a poor prognosis, the aim should be to restore basic self-care functions to ease care and to improve the quality of life.

For patients who have lost the use of one UE, training in one-handed techniques may be indicated. Assistive aids such as Velcro straps instead of buttons, shoes modified for one-handed closure, and silverware for one-handed self-feeding are available.[175] Some patients with rotator cuff paresis need slings to support the affected arm to prevent glenohumeral subluxation and shoulder pain.[149] Bathing can be facilitated by using tub benches for stability, a grab-bar on the wall for transfers, long-handled sponges, and hand-held shower heads.

Some patients with brain cancer will experience dysphagia, which is often related to intellectual deficits, particularly impaired judgment (pseudobulbar dysphagia). In this case, meals should be supervised in a simplified, distraction-free setting. If productive cough and gag reflex are present, the patient can usually be fed safely by being positioned upright with the neck flexed, chin toward the chest. The patient is more likely to choke on liquids and foods that fall apart in the mouth and will do better on textures that hold together as a single bolus. A patient with paralysis of swallowing reflex (paralytic dysphagia) may be unable to eat safely and must receive nutrition by an alternate route.

Bowel and Bladder Incontinence

Brain cancer that alters a patient's sensorium, mobility, communication, or performance can lead to bowel and bladder incontinence. Incontinence can interfere with ambulation and ADL training, prolong hospitalization, make nursing home placement difficult, or preclude home care. The neurogenic bowel is trained by instituting a regular consistent program that utilizes the gastrocolic reflex by positioning on a stable commode, by digital stimulation, bisacodyl (Dulcolax) or glycerine rectal suppositories, consistent high-fiber diet, and adequate fluids.[14] For patients who cannot be transferred easily from bed, disposable pads can be used. Medications to provide bulk or soften the stool, such as docusate sodium (Colace), may also be indicated. The goal is to enable the individual to defecate at a predictable time and place and to prevent accidents and social embarrassment.

A program to control urinary incontinence should establish a consistent daily schedule in which the patient is taken to the toilet or provided with a urinal or bedpan at regular time intervals. The male can often be managed by external condom drainage, although the confused patient does not allow it to remain in place.[176] The patient with a neurogenic bladder can be managed by establishing bladder-training programs that address the findings of the complete bladder workup including urodynamic flow studies.[177] Intermittent in-and-out straight catheterization is preferred to an indwelling retention catheter because this is more likely to keep the urine sterile.

For a hyperreflexic upper motor neuron bladder, propantheline bromide (Pro-Banthine), an anticholinergic drug, can be prescribed to block the detrusor activity and enlarge bladder capacity. Bethanencol, a cholinergic drug, can be used to stimulate the detrusor bladder musculature to contract in an areflexic lower motor neuron neurogenic bladder. When the bladder neck fails to relax during voiding, an α-receptor blocker, such as phenoxbenzamine hydrochloride (Dibenzyline), will reduce the internal sphincter resistance. To reduce external-sphincter dyssynergia, diazepam (Valium), baclofen (Lioresal), or dantrolene sodium (Dantrium) may be helpful.

SPINAL CORD TUMORS

Cancer of the spinal cord, whether primary or metastatic, can produce various forms of paralysis (paraparesis, paraplegia, quadriparesis, quadriplegia), with paraplegia or paraparesis the most common. Spinal metastasis is usually epidural and affects about 5% of patients with systemic cancer.[165] The common primary sites are lung, breast, lymphomas, and prostate.

The anatomic patterns of cord involvement result from either direct cord compression or ischemic compromise of the arterial blood supply to the spinal cord. The most common sites of spinal cord ischemia are the T3 to T9 segments, where a marginal arterial blood supply is present.[178] Arterial compromise can give rise to sudden permanent paraplegia within hours, whereas direct cord compressions are usually characterized by a slow, steady neurologic progression over days to weeks. Early diagnosis, when there are soft neurologic signs (*i.e.*, radicular pain), is the key, because these patients may show reversibility of neurologic deficits with irradiation and steroids. In many patients, pain will precede the neurologic symptoms by many months. Myelography is the method of choice to establish the diagnosis.

Rehabilitation treatment strategies and techniques are basically the same whether the cause is trauma or cancer. The functional limitations of patients with spinal cord cancer vary greatly depending on the level of the lesion and whether it is complete or incomplete. Motivation problems, depression, contracture, decubitus, spasticity, deconditioning, or other medical problems may prevent the patient from obtaining an optimal functional level.[179,180]

With a complete spinal cord lesion, impairment of function to varying degrees is present in dressing, feeding, ambulation, transfers, and personal hygiene. Higher level lesions and more complete lesions result in more extensive disabilities. Patients with high lesions are best treated in specialized centers that use skilled treatment techniques and adaptive equipment to maximize function.

C2 Through C4 Lesions

Patients with C2 through C4 lesions are completely dependent for all of their self-care activities and transfers. They can propel an electric wheelchair with a mouth wand, chin attachment, or by breath control. The C2 through C3 patients usually require tracheostomy and assisted ventilation. A battery-powered portable respirator can be fitted to the wheelchair. An environmental control system, which allows the patient to control a telephone, television, light switch, call button, and so forth, can be purchased. These patients require a full-time attendant. Male patients usually have undergone a urethral sphincterotomy and wear an external collecting device consisting of a condom, a tube, and a collecting bag. Female patients use a continuous indwelling urinary catheter, because no satisfactory external collecting device exists for women.

C5 Lesion

With training, these patients can propel their electric wheelchairs using a "joy stick." With their food cut and mobile arm supports, they can feed themselves, using a plate guard and universal cuff with a spoon or an electric or carbon dioxide-powered splint. They are usually dependent on an attendant for personal hygiene, dressing, transfers, and writing. They can be taught to type with a head wand. A few can be taught to drive with special adaptive vans. Bladder management does not change until lumbar innervation.

C6 Through C7 Lesions

The C6 root allows the patient to have wrist extension (dorsiflexion), and with the wrist-driven flexor hinge splint, patients can feed themselves, write, and drive, using hand controls and special vans. The wrist-driven flexor hinge orthosis uses dorsiflexion to create opposition of the thumb and the second and third fingers. Some patients may choose to eat using a universal cuff, which has a slot for a spoon or fork. The patient can also dress and bathe with partial assistance after training. The clothes usually have loops and Velcro closures to replace buttons and snaps. Transfers require standby assistance and a sliding board. Ambulation is independent using manual wheelchair with "quad" knobs, although some may require an electric wheelchair. These patients require an attendant.

T1 Through T2 Lesions

Patients with T1 through T2 lesions, with proper training, can live alone because they are independent in dressing, eating, personal hygiene, and can drive an automobile with hand controls and trunk support. Ambulation is independent with a manual wheelchair. Transfers may require standby assistance and a sliding board.

T2 Through T6 Lesions

Patients with T2 through T6 lesions have additional trunk stability. They can become independent in all self-care activities with training, and they ambulate independently in a manual wheelchair. Bipedal ambulation is not practical. They can drive with hand controls but may require additional external trunk support. An attendant usually is not required.

T7 Through T12 Lesions

Patients with T7 through T12 lesions have greater trunk stability and are independent in self-care activities. They ambulate independently, using a manual wheelchair, and drive with hand controls. Bilateral knee–ankle–foot orthosis (KAFO) can be prescribed for exercise and to allow the patient to obtain the upright posture. Excessive energy consumption makes bipedal ambulation impractical. An attendant is not required.

L1 Through L2 Lesions

Patients with L1 through L2 lesions, with training, are independent in all self-care activities, including bowel and bladder functions. Because of some dribbling, males may choose to wear an external collecting device and females may use absorbent pads. The patient can drive, using hand controls, and can ambulate, usually with a manual wheelchair. Bipedal ambulation with bilateral KAFOs and crutches for a walkerette can be functional for short distances using a four-point swing-through or swing-to-gait pattern.

L4 Through S1 Lesions

Wheelchair use is limited to long distances. Independent bipedal ambulation is achieved using bilateral AFOs and two canes. After training, patients will be independent in self-care activities, transfers, driving with hand controls, and bowel and bladder functions. They do not usually require urinary catheters. Male patients may use an external collecting system, and female patients might wear an absorbent pad.

CRANIAL AND PERIPHERAL NERVES

Cranial and peripheral nerves can also be injured by the cancer or its treatment. The functional deficit will depend on the function of the specific muscles innervated by that nerve whether the lesion is complete or incomplete, the training of other musculature, and the use of adaptive equipment that may substitute for the impaired function. Remote or secondary cancer effects on the nervous system such as encephalomyelitis, cerebellar dysfunction, subacute cerebellar degeneration, Eaton–Lambert syndrome, neuropathy, myopathy, polymyositis, dermatomyositis, and peripheral neuropathy may also result in significant disability.[165,166] The incidence of the various syndromes varies, but the overall incidence is reported to be about 70%.[181] The occurrence may precede the cancer diagnosis, and control of the cancer usually causes a disappearance of the syndromes. The avoidance of the complications of inactivity and the use of therapeutic exercise, self-care training, adaptive equipment, and environmental modification can improve the patient's functional levels and quality of life.

It is important to recognize that a deficit in a specific cranial nerve function can have some significant effect on an entire functional mechanism. For example, an isolated injury to the superior laryngeal nerve can cause anesthesia in one side of the throat above the vocal cords. The deficit can precipitate tremendous problems with swallowing and can lead the patient to chronic aspiration. An injury to the distal vagus nerve or recurrent laryngeal nerve can cause a temporary or permanent paralysis of one vocal cord. Not only will this deficit affect the patient's ability to phonate, it could cause an ineffectual cough, difficulty with Valsalva maneuvers, and occasionally, airway compromise.

In many cases of isolated facial nerve dysfunction, rehabilitative techniques can be very effective in ameliorating the resultant deficit. An injured facial nerve can often be grafted directly to the proximal stump. If this is not possible, anastomoses from the hypoglossal nerve to the distal facial nerve can restore facial tone.[182] Injuries to the recurrent laryngeal nerve can occasionally be compensated by vocal cord injections of Teflon[183] of collagen.[184]

Overall, the multiple cranial and peripheral nerve injuries that can result from cancer and cancer therapy can be addressed by a myriad of rehabilitative techniques. It is important to consider each patient individually and to pursue the specialty evaluation necessary to thoroughly consider rehabilitative techniques.

PEDIATRIC CONSIDERATIONS

Many of the problems seen in the patient with cancer in the pediatric age group are similar to those seen in adults, for example, the weakness commonly seen in leukemia can be due to either the disease process or the peripheral neuropathy associated with chemotherapy. Contractures could further impair mobility and self-care skills; thus they need to be prevented by ROM exercises and proper bed positioning. Fixed contractures that interfere with function should be treated with heat and static stretch. Adaptive equipment and environmental modification, as well as work simplification techniques, are all used to conserve energy and improve function.

For children with cancer, many of their possible psychological and social problems related to the cancer, or the residual effects of surgery, chemotherapy, or radiation, are similar to those previously discussed. Additional areas of psychological and social concern in pediatric patients include the reactions of parents and peers and the school situation.

For parents, the fact that their child has cancer is very traumatic. Many issues may come to the surface, including feelings of guilt – "Could we have prevented this?" – fear for the child's survival, and anxiety over the treatment and its effects. It is remarkable that the child's attitude is usually extremely positive and that the parents are helped by this.[185]

The parents' plans for their healthy child's future, and the impact of the cancer and its treatment on that future, is also a factor in the patient's ability to cope. Cancer-related stress can put a strain on the parents' relationship and can alter the parent–child relationship, particularly in the direction of overprotectiveness. Health care providers must be cognizant of these issues and keep track of how the parents are coping, as well as following the child's own progress.

Children can be very cruel to each other, as well as very understanding and accepting, depending on the circumstances. For children who are already experiencing anxiety and stress because of cancer and the residuals of treatment, looking or acting different can be very difficult, particularly if this fact is noted by peers. For children undergoing cancer treatment that will result in a change in their physical appearance, it is important that health care providers help young patients to be assimilated back into their peer group. Understanding and knowledgeable adults, such as the physician, parent, or other health care provider, should spend some time trying to explain the obvious changes to patients and their friends. The intent is not to foster sympathy, but rather to develop understanding among the peer group about the body and functional changes observed, and enlisting their assistance to help rather than to hinder the rehabilitation process. One way to do this is by working with the schoolmates, perhaps the entire classroom, explaining briefly what has happened to the child, what changes to expect, areas in which help may be needed, and areas in which the child should be expected to function independently. The teacher may be recruited to help put the issue into perspective, but the parent or health care provider must explain the needed information to the teacher if this course of action is selected.

If the cancer or the effect of its treatment will interfere with the child's normal classroom performance, then adaptations must be made so that education can continue. This may include environmental changes or a tutor.

Children can be remarkably resilient after physical trauma, surgery, or illness. The adults in their environment frequently have a more difficult time in adjusting and responding to the cancer-induced changes that can interfere with the child's rehabilitation. It is imperative that when cancer rehabilitation is in progress, professional counseling be available for the child as well as for the adults in the environment.

It would be extremely unfortunate if, 10 or 20 years from now, we were to find cases in which the cancer had been successfully treated, and physical rehabilitation provided, only to find that parents' attitudes and peer treatment had caused long-term psychological and social problems. A little treatment, and a little understanding at the right time, will go a long way toward helping the child with cancer develop along "normal" lines.

CONCLUSION

A limited number of forms of cancer and the rehabilitation aspects of treatment have been discussed herein. For almost all forms of cancer, rehabilitation is a vital component of the treatment and care plan and should be addressed in a multidisciplinary manner. The first step in selecting appropriate rehabilitation techniques is to identify what physical and functional limitations or deficits will result from the cancer or the treatment procedures. These areas then become the focal point for rehabilitation procedures. Keeping in mind the special precautions needed because of the natures of radiation, surgery, chemotherapy, and cancer cells, rehabilitation procedures are similar to those used for other functional losses and deficits from noncancer reasons.

The rehabilitation process, whether for adults or for children, should start as soon as the diagnosis is made. With an understanding of the rehabilitation techniques described in this chapter, physicians should be able to identify the patient in need of rehabilitation. They should be able to address the cancer patient's needs relative to prevention, specific therapy, and restoration. With a knowledge of rehabilitation concepts and expertise of team members, appropriate referrals can be made to ensure adequate rehabilitation of cancer patients. Rehabilitation programs should be individualized for each patient and designed to improve the quality of each life.

REFERENCES

1. Silverberg E, Lubera J: Cancer statistics, 1983, CA 37:2–19, 1987
2. Lehmann JF, DeLisa JA, Warren CG et al: Cancer rehabilitation: Assessment of need, development and evaluation of a model of care. Arch Phys Med Rehabil 59:410–419, 1978
3. Habeck RV, Blandford KK, Sacks R, Malec J: WCCC cancer rehabilitation and continuing care needs assessment study report. University of Wisconsin Cancer Control Program, 1981
4. Harvey RF, Jellinek HM, Habeck RV: Cancer rehabilitation: An analysis of 36 program approaches. JAMA 247:2127–2131, 1982
5. Devlin HB, Plant JA, Griffin M: Aftermath of surgery for anorectal cancer. Br Med J 3:413–418, 1971
6. Healy JE Jr, Villanueva R, Donovan ES: Principles of rehabilitation. In Holland JF, Frei E III (eds): Cancer Medicine, pp 1917–1929, Philadelphia, Lea & Febiger, 1973 1973
7. Kottke FJ: The effects of limitation of activity upon the human body. JAMA 196:825–830, 1966
8. DeLisa JA, de Lateur BJ: Therapeutic exercise: Types and indications. Am Fam Physician 28:227–233, 1983
9. Muller EA: Influence of training and of inactivity on muscle strength. Arch Phys Med 51:449–462, 1970
10. Bevegard S, Holmgren A, Jonsson B: The effect of body position on the circulation at rest and during exercise, with special reference to the influence on the stroke volume. Acta Physiol Scand 49:279–298, 1960
11. Waterfield RL: The effect of posture on the volume of the leg. J Physiol 72:121–131, 1931

12. Deitrick JE, Whedon GD, Shorr E: Effects of immobilization upon various metabolic and physiologic functions of normal men. Am J Med 4:3–36, 1948
13. Greenleaf JE, Bernauer EM, Young HL et al: Fluid and electrolyte shifts during bed rest with isometric and isotonic exercise. J Appl Physiol 42:59–66, 1977
14. Taylor N, Berni R, Horning MR: Neurogenic bowel management. Am Fam Physician 7:126–128, 1973
15. Med Lett 22:2–3, January 11, 1980
16. Kosiak M: Etiology and pathology of decubitus ulcer. Arch Phys Med 40:62–69, 1959
17. Landis EM: Micro injection studies of capillary blood pressures in human skin. Heart 15:209–228, 1930
18. Lindan O, Greenway RM, Piazza JM: Pressure distribution of the surface of the human body: I. Evaluation in lying and sitting positions using a "bed of springs and nails." Arch Phys Med 46:378–385, 1965
19. Kosiak M: A mechanical resting surface: Its effect on the prevention of ischemic ulcers. Arch Phys Med Rehabil 56:547, 1975
20. Dinsdale SM: Decubitus ulcers: Role of pressure and friction in causation. Arch Phys Med Rehabil 55:147–152, 1974
21. Agate J: Pressure sores mechanical and medical factors. Nurs Mirror (suppl) V:144, March 17, 1977
22. Kavchak-Keyes MA: Four proven steps for preventing decubitus ulcers. Nursing 7(9):58–61, 1977
23. deLateur BJ, Berni R, Hongladarom T et al: Wheelchair cushions designed to prevent pressure sores: An evaluation. Arch Phys Med Rehabil 57:129–135, 1976
24. Souther SG, Carr SD, Vistnes LM: Wheelchair cushions to reduce pressure under bony prominences. Arch Phys Med Rehabil 55:460–464, 1974
25. Mikulic MA: Decubitus: An analysis of current methods of prevention and treatment. Am J Nurs 80:1125–1128, 1980
26. McClemont EJ, Shand IG, Ramsay B: Pressure sores: A new method of treatment. Br J Clin Pract 33:21–25, 1979
27. Pace WE: Treatment of cutaneous ulcers with benzoyl peroxide. Can Med Assoc J 115:1101–1106, 1976
28. Burdick D: Rehabilitation of the breast cancer patient. Cancer 36:645–648, 1975
29. Maier WP: The technique of modified radical mastectomy. Surg Gynecol Obstet 145:68–74, 1977
30. Lotze MT, Duncan MA, Gerber LH et al: Early versus delayed shoulder motion following axillary dissection; a randomized prospective study. Ann Surg 193:288–295, 1981
31. Villaneuva R, Drane JB, Gunn AE et al: Rehabilitation of the cancer patient. In Clark RL, Howe CD (eds): Cancer Patient Care at M.D. Anderson Hospital and Tumor Institute, pp 671–691. Chicago, Year Book Medical Publishers, 1976
32. Degenshein GA: Mobility of the arm following radical mastectomy. Surg Gynecol Obstet 145:77, 1977
33. Nelson PA: Recent advances in treatment of lymphedema of the extremities. Geriatrics 21:162–173, 1966
34. DeLisa JA, Kraft GH, Gans BM: Clinical electromyography and nerve conduction studies. Orthop Rev 7:75–84, 1978
35. DeLisa JA: Practical use of the therapeutic physical modalities. Am Fam Physician 27(5):129–138, 1983
36. Lehmann JH: Diathermy. In Krusen FH, Kottke FJ, Elwood PM (eds): Handbook of Physical Medicine and Rehabilitation, 2nd ed. pp 273–345. Philadelphia, WB Saunders, 1971
37. Winkler WA: Breast cancer. Confronting one's changed image. Choosing the prosthesis and clothing. Am J Nurs 77:1433–1436, 1977
38. Bostwick J III: Breast reconstruction: A comprehensive approach. Clin Plast Surg 6:143–162, 1979
39. Thomas SE, Yates MM: Breast cancer: Confronting one's changed image. Breast reconstruction after mastectomy. Am J Nurs 77:1438–1442, 1977
40. Markel WM: Rehabilitation after mastectomy. Proc Natl Cancer Conf 7:851, 1973
41. Britton RC, Nelson PA: Causes and treatment of postmastectomy lymphedema of the arm: Report of 114 cases. JAMA 180:95–102, 1962
42. Farrow JH: Rehabilitation following radical breast surgery. Cancer 16:222–223, 1966
43. Leis HP Jr, Bowers WF, Dursi J: Post mastectomy edema of arm. NY J Med 66:618–624, 1966
44. Zeissler RH, Rose GB, Nelson PA: Postmastectomy lymphedema: Late results of treatment in 385 patients. Arch Phys Med Rehabil 53:159–166, 1972
45. Grabois M: Rehabilitation of the postmastectomy patient with lymphedema. Cancer 26:75–79, 1976
46. Stone EG, Hugo NE: Lymphedema. Surg Gynecol Obstet 135:625–631, 1972
47. Neilubowicz J, Olszewski W, Sokolowski J: Surgical lymphovenous shunts. J Cardiovasc Surg 6:262–267, 1968
48. Thompson N: The surgical treatment of chronic lymphedema of the extremities. Surg Clin North Am 47:445–503, 1967
49. Larson NE, Crampton AR: A surgical procedure for postmastectomy edema. Arch Surg 106:475–481, 1973
50. Goldsmith HS, Santos R de Ros, Beatie EJ Jr: Omental transportation in the control of chronic lymphedema. JAMA 203:1119–1121, 1968
51. Stillwell GK: Treatment of postmastectomy lymphedema. Mod Treat 6:396–412, 1969
52. Sanderson RG, Fletcher WS: Conservative management of primary lymphedema. Northwest Med 64:584–588, 1965
53. Treves N: An evaluation of the etiological factors of lymphedema following radical mastectomy: An analysis of 1007 cases. Cancer 10:444–459, 1957
54. Robbins GJ, Markel WM: The postmastectomy lymphedematous arm. Med Ann DC 42:495–497, 1973
55. Robbins GF, Markel WM: The postmastectomy lymphedematous arm. J Med Assoc Ga 62:319–321, 1973
56. Rothman KJ: The effect of alcohol consumption on risk of cancer of the head and neck. Laryngoscope (suppl) 88:51–55, 1978
57. Lowry WS: Alcoholism in cancer of the head and neck. Laryngoscope 85:1275–1280, 1975
58. Dropkin MJ: Compliance in postoperative head and neck patients. Cancer Nurs 379–384, 1979
59. Van Pellon M: Feeding the cancer patient. Nursing 78(10):87–88, 1978
60. Bradford K: A practical application of nutrition for the patient with head and neck cancer. Cancer Bull 29:35–36, March/April, 1977
61. Acquarelli MJ, Fenno G, Ward PH: Cervical esophagostomy. Arch Otolaryngol 96:453–456, 1972
62. Russell TR, Brotman M, Norris F: Percutaneous gastrostomy. Am J Surg 148:132–137, July, 1984
63. Aker S, Tilmont G, Harrison V: A guide to good nutrition during and after chemotherapy and radiation. Health Sciences Learning Research Center, Fred Hutchinson Cancer Research Center, 1976
64. Dudgeon B, DeLisa J, Miller R: Head and neck cancer, a rehabilitation approach. Am J Occup Ther 34:243–251, 1980
65. DeWys WD, Walters K: Abnormalities of taste sensation in cancer patients. Cancer 36:1888–1896, 1975
66. Donaldson SS: Nutritional consequences of radiotherapy. Cancer Res 37:2407–2413, 1977
67. Larsen GL: Guidelines for head and neck rehabilitation. Fred Hutchinson Cancer Research Center, 1979
68. Larsen GL: Rehabilitating dysphagia mechanica, paralytica, pseudobulbar. J Neurosurg Nurs 8(1):14–17, 1976
69. Keyes HM, McCasland JP: Techniques and results of a comprehensive dental care program in head and neck cancer patients. Int J Radiat Oncol Biol Phys 1:859–865, 1976
70. Mossman KL, Sheer AC: Complications of radiotherapy of head and neck cancer. Ear Nose Throat J 56:145–149, 1977
71. Doberneck RC, Antoine JE: Deglutition after resection of oral, laryngeal, and pharyngeal cancers. Surgery 75:87–90, 1974
72. Trible WM: The rehabilitation of deglutition following head and neck surgery. Laryngoscope 77:518–523, 1967
73. Donaldson RC, Skelly M, Paletta FX: Total glossectomy for cancer. Am J Surg 116:585–590, 1968
74. Agullar NV, Olson ML, Shedd DP: Rehabilitation of deglutition in patients with head and neck cancer. Am J Surg 138:501–507, 1979
75. Dobie RA: Rehabilitation of swallowing disorders. Am Fam Physician 17(5):84–95, 1978
76. Desjardins RP, Laney WR: Prosthetic rehabilitation after cancer resection in the head and neck. Surg Clin North Am 57:809–822, 1977
77. Staple TW, Ogura JH: Cineradiography of the swallowing mechanism following supraglottic subtotal laryngectomy. Radiology 87:226–230, 1966
78. Litton WB, Leonard JR: Aspiration after partial laryngectomy: Cineradiographic studies. Laryngoscope 79:887–908, 1969
79. Weaver AW, Fleming SM: Partial laryngectomy. Analysis of associated swallowing disorders. Am J Surg 136:486–489, 1978
80. Schoenrock LD, King AY, Everts EC et al: Hemilaryngectomy: Deglutition evaluation and rehabilitation. Trans Am Acad Ophthalmol Otolaryngol 76:752–757, 1972
81. Bocca E, Pignataro O, Mosciaro O: Supraglottic surgery of the larynx. Ann Otol 77:1105–1026, 1968
82. Flores TC, Wood BG, Koegel L et al: Factors in successful deglutition following supraglottic laryngeal surgery. Ann Otol Rhinol Laryngol 91:579–583, 1982
83. Hoaglund FT, Duthie RB: Surgical reconstruction for shoulder pain after radical neck dissection. Am J Surg 118:796–799, 1969
84. Corbin KB, Harrison F: The sensory innervation of the spinal accessory and tongue musculature in the rhesus monkey. Brain 62:191–197, 1939
85. Carenfelt C, Eliason K: Occurrence, duration and prognosis of unexpected accessory nerve paresis in radical neck dissection. Acta Otolaryngol 90:470–473, 1980
86. Villaneuva R: Orthosis to correct shoulder pain and deformity after trapezius palsy. Arch Phys Med Rehabil 58:30–34, 1977
87. Saunders WH, Johnson EW: Rehabilitation of the shoulder after radical neck dissection. Ann Otol Rhinol Laryngol 84:812–816, 1975
88. Daniels L, Worthingham C: Muscle Testing Techniques of Manual Examination. Philadelphia, WB Saunders, 1980
89. Ballantyne AJ, Guinn GA: Reduction of shoulder disability after neck dissection. Am J Surg 112:661–665, 1966
Anderson R, Flowers RS: Free grafts of the spinal accessory nerve during radical neck dissection. Am J Surg 118:796–799, 1969
90. Eisele DW, Trachy RE, Little JW et al: Reinnervation of the trapezius muscle. Otolaryngol Head Neck Surg 98:34–44, 1988
91. Weisberger EC, Lingeman R: Cable grafting of the spinal accessory nerve for rehabil-

itation of shoulder function after radical neck dissection. Laryngoscope 97:(8 Pt1):915–918, 1987
92. Dewar FP, Harris RI: Restoration of function of the shoulder following paralysis of the trapezius by fascial sling fixation and transplantation of the levator scapulae. Ann Surg 132:1111–1115, 1950
93. Ariyan S: The pectoralis major myocutaneous flap: A versatile flap for reconstruction in the head and neck. Plast Reconstr Surgery 63:73–81, 1979
94. Netterville JL, Panje WR, Naves MD: The trapezius myocutaneous flap. Dependability and limitations. Arch Otolaryngol Head Neck Surg 113:271–281, 1987
95. Villaneuva R, Chandra A: The role of rehabilitation medicine in physical restoration of patients with head and neck cancer. Cancer Bull 29:46–54, 1977
96. Kelly D: Speech rehabilitation of the laryngectomized patient. Cancer Bull 29:39–41, 1977
97. Calcaterra TC, Zwitman DH: Vocal rehabilitation after partial or total laryngectomy. Calif Med 117:12–15, 1972
98. Schaefer SD, Johns DF: Attaining functional esophageal speech. Arch Otolaryngol 108:647–649, 1982
99. Gates GA, Ryan W, Cooper JC et al: Current status of laryngectomy rehabilitation: I. Results of therapy. Am J Otolaryngol 3:1–7, 1982
100. Singer MI, Blom ED: An endoscopic technique for restoration of voice after laryngectomy. Ann Otol Rhinol Laryngol 89:529–533, 1980
101. Singer MI, Blom ED, Hamaker RC: Further experience with voice restoration after total laryngectomy. Ann Otol Rhinol Laryngol 90:498–502, 1981
102. Wetmore SJ, Johns ME, Baker SR: The Singer-Blom voice restoration procedure. Arch Otolaryngol 107:674–676, 1981
103. Hamaker RC, Singer MI, Blom ED et al: Primary voice restoration of laryngectomy. Arch Otolaryngol 111:182–186, 1985
104. Singer MI: Tracheoesophageal speech: Vocal rehabilitation after total laryngectomy. Laryngoscope 93:1454–1465, 1983
105. Blom ED, Singer MI, Hamaker RC: An improved esophageal insufflation test. Arch Otolaryngol 111:211–212, 1985
106. Gilchrist AG: Rehabilitation after laryngectomy. Acta Otolaryngol 75:511–518, 1973
107. Skelly M, Spector DJ, Donaldson RC et al: Compensatory physiologic phonetics for the glossectomee. J Speech Hear Disord 36:101–114, 1971
108. Skelly M, Donaldson RC, Fust RS et al: Changes in phonatory aspects of glossectomee intelligibility through vocal parameter manipulation. J Speech Hear Disord 37:379–389, 1972
109. Skelly M, Donaldson R, Schinsky I: Substitution consistency as a factor in glossectomy intelligibility. J Missouri Heart Assoc 5(3):21–23, 1972
110. Skelly M, Donaldson R: Rehabilitation of speech after total glossectomy. Presented to Twelfth World Congress of Rehabilitation International, Sydney, Australia, 1972
111. Lanciello FR, Vergo T, Schaaf NG, Zimmerman R: Prosthodontic and speech rehabilitation after partial and complete glossectomy. J Prosthet Dent 43:204–211, 1980
112. Aramy MA, Down JA, Berry QC et al: Prosthodontic rehabilitation for glossectomy patients. J Prosthet Dent 48:78–81, 1982
113. Davis JW, Lazarus C, Logemann J, Hurst PS: Effect of a maxillary glossectomy prosthesis on articulation and swallowing. J Prosthet Dent 57:715–719, 1987
114. Panje WR: Mandibular reconstruction with the trapezius osteomusculocutaneous flap. Arch Otolaryngol 111:223–229, 1985
115. Powell NB, Riley RW: Cranial bone grafting in facial aesthetic and reconstructive contouring. Arch Otolaryngol Head Neck Surg 113:713–719, 1987
116. Drane J: Role of maxillofacial prosthetics. Cancer Bull 29:41–45, 1977
117. Gonzalez JB: Recently developed elastomers for facial prostheses. Mayo Clin Proc 53:423–431, 1978
118. Burgess EM: Surgery as related to prosthetics and orthotics. Bull Prosthet Res pp 15–21, Fall 1974
119. Gonzalez EG, Corcoran PJ, Reyes RL: Energy expenditure in below-knee length amputees: Correlation with stump length. Arch Phys Med Rehabil 55:111–119, 1974
120. Burgess E, Romano R: The management of amputees using immediate post-surgical prosthesis. Clin Orthop 57:137–146, 1968
121. Thorpe W, Gerber LH, Lampert M et al: A prospective study of rehabilitation of the above-knee amputee with rigid dressings. Clin Orthop Related Res 133:137, 1979
122. Nora PF: The extremities. In Operative Surgery, pp 1036, 1074. Philadelphia, Lea & Febiger, 1980
123. Kegel B, Carpenter ML, Burgess EM: A survey of lower limb amputees: Prostheses, phantom sensations, and psychosocial aspects. Bull Prosthet Res pp 43–60, Spring 1977
124. Muilenberg AL: Prosthetic considerations for the cancer amputee. In Rehabilitation of the Cancer Patient, pp 654–673. Chicago, Year Book Medical Publishers, 1972
125. Davies RM: The rapid form process for automated thermoplastic socket production. Prosthet Orthotics Int 9:27–30, 1985
126. Foort J: Innovation in prosthetics and orthotics. Prosthet Orthotics Int 10:61–71, 1986
127. Riley R: The amputee athlete. Sports Med 4:31–32, 1984
128. Radocy B: Upper extremity prosthetics: Considerations and designs for sports and recreation. Clin Prosthet Orthot 11:131–153, 1987
129. Michael J: Energy storing feet: A clinical comparison. Clin Prosthet Orthot 11:154–168, 1987
130. Sabolich J, Guth T: Below knee prosthesis with total flexible socket: Preliminary report. Clin Prosthet Orthot 10:93–99, 1986
131. Nowroozi F, Salvanelli M, Gerber LH: Energy expenditure in hip disarticulation and hemipelvectomy amputees. Arch Phys Med Rehabil 64:300–303, 1983
132. Sneppen O, Johansen T, Heerfordt J et al: Hemipelvectomy. Postoperative rehabilitation assessed on the basis of 41 cases. Acta Orthop Scand 49:175–179, 1978
133. Burke MJ, Roman V, Wright V: Bone and joint changes in lower limb amputees. Ann Rheum Dis 37:252–254, 1978
134. Chodera JD: Relation between the anatomical properties and output of the thigh stump. In Murdoch G (ed): Conference on Priorities in Prosthetic and Orthotic Practice, 1969, Dundee, Scotland. Sect 5, pp 181–189. London, Edward Arnold Publishing, 1970
135. Gerber LH, Mathai MM, Rosenberg SA: Above-knee prosthesis for very short femur length (abstr). Arch Phys Med Rehabil 61:465, 1980
136. deLateur BJ, Lehmann JF, Winterscheid LC et al: Rehabilitation of the patient after hemicorporectomy. Arch Phys Med Rehabil 50:11–16, 1969
137. Simons BC, Lehmann JF, Taylor N et al: Prosthetic management of hemicorporectomy. Orthop Prosthet 22:63–68, 1968
138. Schmidl H: The INAIL experience fitting upper limb dysmelia patients with myoelectric control. Bull Prosthet Res pp 17–42, 1977
139. Simon M: Current Concepts Review: Causes of increased survival of patients with osteosarcoma: Current controversies. J Bone Joint Surg 66A:306–310, 1984
140. Sundaram J, McGuire MH et al: Magnetic resonance imaging in planning limb salvage surgery for primary malignant tumors of bone. J Bone Joint Surg 68A:809–819, 1986
141. Marcove RC, Lewis MM, Huvos AG: En bloc upper humeral interscapulothoracic resection. Clin Orthop Related Res 124:219–228, 1977
142. Mankin HJ, Doppelt SH et al: Osteoarticular and intercalary allograft transplantation in the management of malignant tumors of bone. Cancer 50:613–630, 1982
143. Mnaymneeh W, Malinin TI et al: Massive osteoarticular allografts in the reconstruction of extremities following resection of tumors not requiring chemotherapy and radiation. Clin Orthop 197:76–87, 1985
144. Lewis M: The use of an expandable and adjustable prosthesis in the treatment of childhood malignant bone tumors of the extremity. Cancer 57:499–502, 1986
145. Lampert MH, Gerber LH, Glatstein E et al: Functional outcome of patients undergoing wide local excision and radiation therapy for soft tissue sarcoma. Arch Phys Med Rehabil 65:477–480, 1984
146. Marcove RC, Jensen MJ: Radical resection for osteogenic sarcoma of the fibula with preservation of the limb. Clin Orthop 125:173, 1977
147. Malawer MM: Distal femoral osteogenic sarcoma. In Chao E, Irvins J (eds): Tumor Prostheses, Chap 37. New York, Grune & Stratton, 1983
148. Marcove RC: En bloc resections for osteogenic sarcoma: Cancer Treat Rep 62:225–231, 1978
149. Dietz JH Jr: The cancer patient after amputation of an extremity of neurologic disability. In Schottenfield D (ed): Cancer Epidemiology and Prevention: Current Concepts, pp 511–521. Springfield, Charles C Thomas, 1975
150. Hinterbuchner C: Rehabilitation of physical disability in cancer. NY State J Med 78:1066–1069, 1978
151. Dietz JH Jr: Rehabilitation of the cancer patient. Med Clin North Am 53:607–624, 1969
152. Lertzman MM, Cherniack RM: Rehabilitation of patients with chronic obstructive pulmonary disease. Am Rev Respir Dis 114:1145–1165, 1976
153. Petty TL: Pulmonary rehabilitation. Basis of respiratory disease. Am Thorac Soc 4:1–6, 1975
154. Zislis JM: Rehabilitation of the cancer patient. Geriatrics 25:150–158, 1970
155. Cassara EL: Chest physical therapy. Int Anesthesiol Clin 9:159–171, 1971
156. Rusk MA: Rehabilitation Medicine, 4th ed. pp 623–627. St Louis, CV Mosby, 1977
157. Frey GS: The effect of special preparation of the therapist on the rehabilitation of the ostomate. Int Assoc Enterostomal Ther 6:26–28, 1979
158. Watson PG, Wood RY, Wechsler NL et al: Comprehensive care of the iliostomy patient. Nurs Clin North Am 11:427–444, 1976
159. Costello AM: Supporting the patient with problems relating to body image, pp 36–40. Proc Natl Conf Cancer Nursing, Chicago, Am Cancer Soc, 1974
160. Guidelines for ostomy rehabilitation. In Guidelines for Managing Cancer, developed by Fred Hutchison Cancer Research Center, Sect 5, 6, 1979
161. Bromley B: Applying Orem's self-care theory in enterostomal therapy. Am J Nurs 80:245–249, 1980
162. Fordyce WE: Psychological assessment and management. In Krusen FH, Kottke FJ, Ellwood PM (eds): Handbook of Physical Medicine and Rehabilitation, 2nd ed. pp 168–195. Philadelphia, WB Saunders, 1971
163. Hartter C, Berghtol MJ, Abdelkader S: What's a continent ileostomy? Nursing 11(11):84–89, 1981
164. Gazzard BG, Saunders B, Dawson AM: Diets and stoma function. Br J Surg 65:642–644, 1978
165. Posner JB: Neurological complications of systemic cancer. Med Clin North Am 63:783–800, 1979
166. Horstein S: Distal effects of neoplasm on the nervous system. Postgrad Med 50:85–90, 1971
167. DeLisa JA, Miller RM, Melnick RR et al: Guidelines for the family practitioner: Comprehensive stroke rehabilitation, part 1. Am Fam Physician 26:207–214, 1982
168. Fowler RS Jr, Fordyce W: Adapting care for the brain damaged patient. Am J Nurs 72:1832–1835, 2056–2059, 1972

169. Stanton KM, Flowers CR, Kuhl PK et al: Language-oriented training program to teach compensation of left side neglect. Arch Phys Med Rehabil 60:540, 1979
170. Stolov WC: Progressive ambulation (mobility). Postgrad Med 47:229–235, 1970
171. DeLisa JA, Greenberg S: Wheelchair prescription guidelines. Am Fam Physician 25:145–150, 1982
172. Spiegler JH, Goldberg MJ: The wheelchair as a permanent mode of mobility. A detailed guide to prescription: I. Frame, armrest, and brakes. Am J Phys Med 47:315–316, 1968; II. Upholstery, leg supports, wheels and accessories. Am J Phys Med 48:25–37, 1969
173. DeLisa JA, Little JW: A comprehensive approach to the management of spasticity. Am Fam Physician 26:117–122, 1982
174. Jebsen RH: Use and abuse of ambulation aids. JAMA 199:5–10, 1967
175. Hale G (ed): The Source Book for the disabled. New York, Paddington Press, 1979
176. Kester NC, Block JM: Rehabilitation of patients after surgery for brain tumor. In Vinkin PJ, Bruyn GW (eds): Handbook of Clinical Neurology, Vol 18, Part II: Tumors of the Brain and Skull, pp 523–529. Amsterdam, North-Holland Publishing, 1975
177. Koff SA, Diokno AC, Lapides J: Neurogenic bladder dysfunction. Am Fam Physician 19:100–109, 1979
178. Gilbert H, Apuzzo M, Marshall L et al: Neoplastic epidural spinal cord compression: A current perspective. JAMA 240:2771–2773, 1978
179. Long C II, Lawton EB: Functional significance of spinal cord lesion level. Arch Phys Med 36:249–255, 1955
180. Symington DC, McKay DW: A study of functional independence in the quadriplegia patient. Arch Phys Med 47:378–392, 1966
181. Dietz JH: Adaptive rehabilitation of the cancer patient. Curr Prob Cancer 5(5):3–56, 1980
182. Colemer CC: Results of facio-hypoglossal anastomosis in the treatment of facial paralysis. Ann Surg 3:958–970, 1940
183. Dedo HH, Uckea RD, Lawson L: Intracordal injection of Teflon in the treatment of 135 patients with dysphonia. Ann Otol Rhinol Laryngol 82:661–667, 1973
184. Ford CN, Bless DM: Clinical experience with injectable collagen for vocal cord augmentation. Laryngoscope 96:863–869, 1986
185. Voute PA, Burgers JMV, Van Putten WJ et al: Amputations in children: Clinical indications and psychological complications. Arch Chir Neerlandicum 25:427–433, 1973

SUSAN MOLLOY HUBBARD
CLAUDIA A. SEIPP
PATRICIA L. DUFFEY

CHAPTER 64 *Administration of Cancer Treatments: Practical Guide for Physicians and Oncology Nurses*

EVOLUTION OF ROLES FOR ONCOLOGY NURSES

Nurses have always cared for patients with cancer, but it was not until the early 1970s when oncology began to emerge as a medical specialty, that it began to evolve as a specialized area of clinical nursing practice.[1-9] The rapid expansion in the National Cancer Institute's (NCI) drug development program that occurred during this period created a need for skilled nurses to share major responsibilities for the safe administration of drug regimens under evaluation to cancer patients. Initially, guidance and supervision by experienced oncologists was necessary for such a nurse to acquire the requisite knowledge and clinical expertise, but nurses soon became skilled in the safe administration of cancer therapy. Integration of a single nurse into a research team at NCI permitted a 25% increase in outpatient visits for chemotherapy within 1 year and a significant reduction in errors related to the intravenous administration of drugs.[1] As the chemotherapy research nurses became knowledgeable about research methodology, they began to actively participate in clinical trials through the collection, analysis, and publication of research data.[6-10]

With increasing experience, the chemotherapy research nurse became a primary source of practical information for patients about their disease and the management and reduction of side-effects of therapy. Patient care and clinical research both benefited from their contribution in this area.[7-9] Further role expansion and growth in the specialty have occurred in response to advances in cancer treatment, a revolution in biotechnology, and changes within the nursing profession. Greater integration of surgery, chemotherapy, radiotherapy, and biologic agents into multimodal approaches to primary cancer treatment has created opportunities for independent investigation as well as participation in collaborative research and treatment.[6-12] As a result, oncology nursing has become one of the most challenging and diverse areas of clinical practice, with ongoing opportunities for role expansion in cancer treatment, detection and prevention, and supportive care.[14-27]

The membership of the Oncology Nursing Society (ONS) has increased from 20 nurses in 1976 to over 14,000 members in 1988. Overall, 60% of the members are directly involved in patient care, with 65% providing care to cancer patients in a hospital setting and 24% providing care in ambulatory settings; 8% now classify research as their principal function.[28] The Association of Pediatric Oncology Nurses has over 600 members.[29] The development of widely circulated peer-reviewed professional journals with increasing numbers of subscribers further attests to the growth of this nursing subspecialty.

As the demand for sophisticated clinical services has grown, nurses have collaborated with oncologists to design and run well-organized inpatient and outpatient units in which clinical research and highly specialized cancer care can be successfully performed in a diversity of clinical settings.[30-37] This type of multidisciplinary collaboration has helped to establish a collegial relationship between the nurse and physician as a standard of cancer nursing practice. It is now commonly expected that, as members of research teams, oncology nurses will develop and implement sophisticated programs of nursing care for patients as new treatments and treatment modalities are being developed. In addition, nurses are expected to design and implement structured education programs for patients that are designed to reduce disease and treatment-related morbidity and to facilitate self-care, home care, and rehabilitation of the cancer patients in their care. Given the current emphasis on research for new therapies against the acquired immunodeficiency syndrome (AIDS) and the relatively high incidence of neoplasms in this patient population, oncology nurses must be knowledgeable about AIDS and its complications.[38-40]

To ensure that the quality of care delivered to cancer patients is consistently high, the ONS has developed practice and educational standards that have been implemented, and evaluated in a variety of clinical settings. The ONS has also formulated guidelines for the development and evaluation of continuing education programs to foster continued professional growth among its members and has established a program of professional certification in the specialty of oncology nursing.[41-52]

Graduate programs that provide advanced education and clinical training in oncology and permit nurses to assume greater clinical responsibilities for the management of adult and pediatric patients have flourished over the last decade. At the end of 1988, there were 43 university-based programs with graduate educational curricula leading to a master's degree in oncology nursing; 14 of these universities provide advanced education in pediatric oncology.[53-55] These programs prepare nurses to function as clinical specialists or nurse practitioners who can assume accountability for the total nursing care required by their patients.[56-58] Their advanced knowledge and clinical skills have prepared these nurses to assume their own case loads and to manage complex patient needs, taking on major responsibilities for the care of cancer patients who have major chronic and continuing care needs. Under guidelines established in collaboration with oncologists, they perform diagnostic and therapeutic procedures, interpret study results, as well as order and administer a variety of therapeutic regimens, and coordinate patient and family teaching, counseling, rehabilitation, home care, and hospice or terminal care at home.

Changes in the financing of health care have exerted a significant influence on the delivery of health care and will continue to do so in the foreseeable future. Traditional concepts about hospital- and office-based medical practice, professional roles, and role relationships have come under scrutiny and are undergoing change.[53-65] This process offers nurses real opportunities for role expansion and increased professional collaboration in a variety of clinical settings. Integration of clinical specialists and nurse practitioner roles in oncology have stimulated the development of collaborative practice models in hospital and office practice settings in which physicians and nurses share clinical and administrative responsibilities for all aspects of patient care.[66-72] Data on joint practice models suggest that patient and physician satisfaction is high, and there is an increase in the efficiency and cost-effectiveness of health care delivery.

Cancer prevention and early detection guidelines have been incorporated into the ONS' outcome standards for cancer nursing practice and public education.[41-44] Oncology nurses are also making substantial contributions to cancer screening and detection programs.[20,73-88] Numerous projects have demonstrated that trained nurses can conduct screening programs effectively.[73-88] For example, data on colorectal screening by nurses with flexible fiberoptic sigmoidoscopy indicate that positive findings are comparable with those expected when the procedure is performed by physicians.[86] Health care programs developed by nurses for individuals with a hereditary predisposition to cancer or with premalignant lesions, such as dysplastic nevi, educate patients and their families about the importance of regular self-examination, close observation of suspicious lesions, regular medical follow-up, and the need for preventive health care to decrease their cancer risk.[80-82] Programs that emphasize incorporating cancer prevention (*e.g.*, smoking cessation) and early detection into the life-style have been developed by nurses utilizing creative techniques, such as mobile vans, closed-circuit TV, videotapes, and "hot lines" to reach and provide follow-up to target populations more effectively.[89] In addition, the ONS actively supports community-based programs that address social aspects of motivation and behavior change.[77]

PRACTICAL ISSUES AFFECTING PATIENT CARE

INTRAVENOUS CHEMOTHERAPY

Because nurses have assumed major responsibilities for the administration of parenteral chemotherapy, it is essential that they know the potential effects of each agent and any precautions that should be taken to maximize patient safety and comfort during administration.[23,45,90] Tables 64-1 and 64-2 list the major chemotherapeutic and hormonal agents used in cancer treatment. Although basic dose and schedule information is provided, readers are referred to Chapter 18, "Clinical Pharmacology of Cancer Chemotherapy," for a more detailed discussion of structure, mechanism of action, dose and schedule, clinical pharmacology and pharmacokinetics, and acute and chronic toxicity, in as much as these data will not be discussed here. Data in these tables are designed to assist nurses in establishing guidelines for safe drug administration and in developing patient care plans that

(*Text continues on page* 2375)

TABLE 64-1. Major Chemotherapeutic Agents Used in Cancer Treatment

Drug (Synonyms)	*Patient Management Considerations*
Alkylating Agents	
Mechlorethamine hydrochloride (Nitrogen mustard, Mustargen, HN_2) 0.4 mg/kg IV q4wk 6 mg/m² d1 and 8 q4wk 0.2–0.4 mg/kg (intracavitary) 10 mg in 50ml aqueous solution tiw then qwk	Bone marrow depression (BMD). Severe nausea and vomiting (N/V) in ½ to 2 h lasting 2–12 h. Anorexia. Potent tissue vesicant; give only in established IV line. Sodium thiosulfate may decrease tissue damage if extravasated. Chemical thrombophlebitis and venous discoloration common. Allergic and anaphylactic reactions rare. Maculopapular rash, alopecia, and tinnitus also occur. Avoid direct eye contact. Metallic taste. Fever, diarrhea, chills in 1 h. Pain common, due to intense inflammatory reaction. Turn patient immediately to maximize drug distribution. Fever, chills, malaise, milder N/V Gloves should be worn during application. Topical and intralesional application of aqueous solution is applied in mycosis fungoides. Hypersensitivity reactions occur frequently with topical use. Desensitization is generally effective.
10 mg% ointment in Aquaphor base qd	Hyperpigmentation, urticaria, and pruritus occur. Ointment has simplified application and appears to increase absorption into the skin. Lower incidence of hypersensitivity reactions. Decrease in dry skin compared with aqueous preparation.
Cyclophosphamide (CYT, Cytoxan, Endoxan) 500–1500 mg/m² IV q3–4wk	BMD. Dose-related N/V starting 3–12 h, may last 8–10 h. Anorexia. Dizziness, sinus congestion can occur with rapid infusion of high doses. Vigorous hydration with oral or IV fluids (>3 liter/d) to maintain adequate urine output and encourage frequent voiding to minimize drug contact with bladder to decrease risk of hemorrhagic cystitis which can be severe, even fatal. Discontinue if dysuria or hematuria develop. Barbiturates and phenytoin may increase toxic effects. Gonadal suppression resulting in amenorrhea or azoospermia has been reported and appears dose-related. May be temporary.
60–120 mg/m² po qd based on WBC	Interstitial pulmonary fibrosis after prolonged administration. Potentiation of anthracycline cardiotoxicity. Daily oral CYT may be taken in divided doses with meals.
Ifosfamide (Ifex, Holoxan) 1200 mg/m² IV 5d q3wk 4 mg/m² IV q3wk	Mild BMD; Dose-related N/V in 2–10 h, often persisting several days. Chemical thrombophlebitis. Alopecia. Hemorrhagic cystitis. Hydration of >2 liter/d to maintain urine output and frequent voiding. Administration of *N*-acetylcysteine protects bladder. Ascorbic acid may also reduce bladder toxicity. Nephrotoxicity, lethargy, and confusion at high doses. Hepatic microsomal enzyme activation affected by phenytoin and barbiturates.
Mesna (Uromitexan, sodium 2-mercaptoethanesulfonate) [NSC 20581] 1500 mg/m² × 5 d IV then po	Not an antineoplastic agent. Prevents lesions of the urinary bladder mucosa by binding to reactive metabolites of cyclophosphamide or ifosphamide without interfering with antitumor activity. No adverse effects <60 mg/kg. Above >60 mg/kg may result in N/V and diarrhea. May be given po at end of CYT and ifosphamide infusions. Report of CNS toxicity with mesna/ifosfamide therapy have been reported including confusion, somnolence, generalized clonic seizures; one case of irreversible encephalopathy after multiple courses possibly related to progressive renal failure.[274]
L-Phenylalanine mustard (L-PAM, melphalan, Alkeran) 0.2 mg/kg po qd × 5 d q3wk 0.05–0.1 mg/kg po qd	Well tolerated. Delayed and cumulative BMD can occur. Chronic nausea/anorexia can occur. Little alopecia. Occasional dermatitis and stomatitis. Serious hypersensitivity reactions reported with IV use (investigational). Amenorrhea. Leukemogenic and chromosomal damage in humans.
Chlorambucil 0.5–0.2 mg/kg po qd continuous based on WBC	BMD. Severe bone marrow suppression. Occasional dermatitis. Well tolerated at standard doses. GI distress only at high doses. Oral absorption reliable. Carcinogenic in humans and probably teratogenic. Gonadal dysfunction. May be irreversible. Potential benefit must be weighed against risk of secondary malignancy. Pulmonary infiltrates and fibrosis. Hepatic toxicity.
Busulfan (Myleran) 0.05–2.0 mg/kg po qd continuous based on WBC	Well tolerated. Reliable absorption. Cumulative and prolonged BMD. Recovery can take from 1 mo to 2 yr. BM function should be monitored closely. Prolonged use associated with pulmonary fibrosis. Hyperpigmentation; gynecomastia; adrenal insufficiency; ovarian failure and azoospermia; pregnancy has occurred during therapy; effective contraception is required. Leukemogenic, chromosomal aberrations; cataracts.
Triethylenethiophosphoramide (thio-TEPA, TSPA) 0.2 mg/kg iv or im qd × 5 q 3–4 wk 0.5 mg/kg q1–4wk 10–60 mg q3–4wk for intracavitary use	BMD. Dose reductions required for patients with existing hepatic, renal, or bone marrow dysfunction. Myelosuppression potentiated by prior radiation and other alkylating agents. Can be given im or sc. Poor oral absorption; well tolerated. Allergic reactions and dermatitis. Paresthesias reported after IT administration (1–10 mg/m²). Amenorrhea and interference with spermatogenesis. Local irritation can occur. Pain, N/V, dizziness, headaches can occur with intracavitary and instillation. Leukopenia can occur after intravesicular bladder instillation.
Prednimustine [NSC 134087] 8–25 mg/m² qd po	BMD. Mild N/V usually transient. Emotional lability. Rash and urticaria can occur. Mild diarrhea; edema.

TABLE 64-1. Major Chemotherapeutic Agents Used in Cancer Treatment (*Continued*)

Drug (Synonyms)	*Patient Management Considerations*
Estramustine (Estracyte, Emcyt) [NSC 89199] 280–600 mg/qd po (1 mo) 150 mg qd iv	Severe N/V. Administer with food or antacids or both to decrease GI toxic effects; delayed and intractable N/V can occur in 6–8 wk requiring cessation of therapy. Nipple tenderness and gynecomastia. Exacerbation of CHF. Mild paresthesia with IV use. Transient perineal itching and pain after IV administration. IV preparation is a potent tissue vesicant. Thrombocytopenia may occur rarely.
Cisplatin (Platinol, DDP) 60–120 mg/m² iv q3–4wk	Nephrotoxicity. Administration of DDP with 250 ml hypertonic (3%) saline and vigorous hydration with NS and KCl can protect against renal damage. IV hydration and furosemide or mannitol diuresis can reduce or eliminate renal toxicity. Check RFTs, creatinine clearance and electrolytes before each dose. Anaphylactic reaction with tachycardia, hypotension, erythema, wheezing, and facial edema.[272,273] Treat with epinephrine, steroids, and antihistamines, and pretreat with same for future doses. Peripheral neuropathy may be dose-limiting in high doses (40 mg/m²).
15–20 mg/m² iv qd × 5 q3–4wk	Ophthalmic and ototoxicity. Magnesium-wasting requiring replacement for neuromuscular irritability. Mild–moderate BMD depending on dose and schedule. Severe N/V in 1 h lasting 6–24 h.
Intraperitoneal use 90 mg/m² in 2-L dialysate q3wk	N/V. Dwell time/4 hr. Abdominal discomfort; sterile ascites. Catheter care is critical. Nephrotoxicity dose-limiting at 90 mg/m². Use of mannitol and sodium thiosulfate (7.5 g/m² loading dose and 2.13 g/m² q12h) permits ip DDP at 270 mg/m² without nephrotoxicity.
CBDCA (carboplatin, JM8) 200–400 mg/m² iv q4wk	BMD. No renal toxicity. Mild neurologic toxicity in patients previously treated with cisplatin. Minimal N/V. No ototoxicity.
Aziridinylbenzoquinone (AZQ) 6–8 mg/m² × 5 d q4wk	Cumulative BMD, especially thrombocytopenia. Mild N/V. Stomatitis, diarrhea, anorexia. Penetration of CSF. Do not give unless solution is clear. Dissolution of particles in IV preparation is extremely slow.
Nitrosoureas	
Carmustine (BCNU, BiCNU) 150–200 mg/m² po q4–6wk	Delayed and cumulative BMD. Severe N/V in 2–4 hr. Enters CNS. Venous discoloration. Local pain. Tissue vesicant. Chemical thrombophlebitis often occurs in several days. Marked facial flushing and venous spasm 2% alcohol diluent. Avoid direct contact with eyes. Increase volume and slow infusion to decrease venous pain. Hepatotoxicity in 20%. Pulmonary fibrosis and renal damage seen with prolonged use. Refrigerate and protect from light.
Lomustine (CCNU, CeeNU) 100–130 mg/m² po q4–6wk	Delayed and cumulative BMD; stomatitis; alopecia. Renal toxicity with prolonged use. Moderate–severe N/V in 2–6 h. May be reduced if taken at bedtime with antiemetics. Enters CNS. Diarrhea. Anorexia often lasts several days.
Semustine (Me-CCNU, methyl CCNU, MCCNU) 150–200mg/m² po q4–6wk	Delayed and cumulative BMD. Stomatitis. Take on empty stomach at bedtime. GI absorption in 30–60min. Moderate–severe N/V in 1–4h. Anorexia may be persistent. Renal failure and pulmonary fibrosis after prolonged administration.
Chlorozotocin (DCNU) 150mg/m²iv 40mg/m² qd × q6wk	Mild BMD with prominent thrombocytopenia. Diabetes with ketoacidosis. Mild N/V. Chemical thrombophlebitis. Transient hepatotoxicity. Interstitial pulmonary fibrosis. Renal toxicity can occur as with other nitrosoureas.
Streptozotocin (STZ, Zanosar) 500mg/m² iv qd × 5d q3–4wks	Mild BMD. Tissue vesicant. Reactive hypoglycemia due to insulin release. Hydrate to prevent nephrotoxicity. Check for proteinuria, glycosuria, and hypophosphatemia before each dose. Management of insulin shock. Diarrhea and abdominal cramps can occur. Educate patients about hypoglycemia and insulin shock. Mild anemia and hepatotoxicity. Slow infusion to decrease local venous pain and burning.
Antimetabolites	
Cytosine arabinoside (Ara-C, Cytosar, cytarabine, arabinosyl cytosine) 100mg/m² q 12 h sc or iv 7–21d 100mg/m² continuous infusion	Marked BMD. N/V dose- and schedule-dependent. Less N/V with slow infusions. Anorexia and mild mouth ulcers common. Flu-like syndrome with fever and headache. Diarrhea. Arthralgias. Rashes and sensitivity to sunlight; use of sunscreens recommended. Systemic effects from IT use (20–30mg/m²) uncommon. Neurotoxicity is common. Reconstitute with Elliott's B solution. Experimental doses: high-dose Ara-C at 3g/m² q12h × 5–7d used to induced BM aplasia causes CNS, GI, pulmonary toxicity not seen at standard doses. Cerebral and cerebellar dysfunction occur. Early identification is essential to prevent irreversible toxicity. Photophobia. Conjunctivitis can be minimized by steroid eye drops. Low-dose (20mg/m² q12h sc or continuous infusion under investigation as potential differentiating agent). May cause BMD.[275]
5-Fluorouracil [5-FU, Adrucil, Efudex (topical)] 7.5–12mg/kg iv × 5 d then 12–15mg/kg q wk	Dose-related BMD. Promote oral hygiene. Stomatitis often preceded by sore mouth and tongue. Pharyngitis, diarrhea, and proctitis may be severe. Interrupt therapy when GI toxicity appears.

(*continued*)

TABLE 64-1. Major Chemotherapeutic Agents Used in Cancer Treatment (*Continued*)

Drug (Synonyms)	*Patient Management Considerations*
Intraperitoneal use up to 4mM in 2L dialysate × 8 q 2 wk	GI toxicity often immediately precedes serious myelotoxicity. Oral absorption erratic.
	Increased toxicity postadrenalectomy. Decreased myelotoxicity with intra-arterial use.
	N/V is dose- and schedule-dependent. Anaphylaxis has been reported. Cerebellar ataxia, visual disturbances. Diffuse hair thinning, nail cracking and loss occur. Conjunctival irritation.
	Topical 5-FU (Efudex) in malignant keratosis. Sensitivity to sunlight. Use of sunscreen is recommended. Hyperpigmentation; dermatitis.
	Abdominal discomfort with ip administration. Dwell time 4hr/exchange. Catheter care is critical.
	Chemical peritonitis at 5mM dose. Addition of 50mEq $NaHCO_3$ increases solubility.
	Minimal systemic toxcity.
Methotrexate (MTX, Folex, Mexate, amethopterin) 20–80mg/m^2 iv/im/po	BMD. Renal impairment delays excretion and increases systemic toxicity. Renal function must be checked before each dose. Diarrhea and ulcerative stomatitis frequent. GI tract ulcers can require drug discontinuation. Serious pulmonary and hepatotoxicity can occur at high doses or with prolonged use. Acute reversible pneumonitis occurs with prolonged administration. Stop MTX and treat with steroids. Protein-bound. Avoid sulfonamides, aspirin, tetracycline, phenytoin, and chloral hydrate which displace MTX from plasma proteins. Mild–moderate N/V.
10–15 mg/m^2 it q wk or 15mg	Dilute preservative-free MTX in Elliott's solution for IT use. May cause systemic toxicity.
	Reduce systemic dose appropriately. Chemical arachnoiditis, vomiting, fever, and headache.
High-dose MTX 1–10g/m^2 iv with iv CF then po	Mild–moderate N/V, diarrhea. Maintain urinary pH >6.5–7.0 and high output to prevent precipitation in renal tubules. Check pH q3–6h during therapy. Adjust urinary pH with $NaHCO_3$ to maintain alkalinity. Check RFTs and LFTs before each dose. Use only preservative-free MTX. Continue CF until plasma MTX <10–8 molar (0.45g/100ml) when high-dose MTX regimens are used.
Folinic acid (citrovorum factor, CF, calcium leucovorin)	Allergic sensitization occurs but unusual; no other toxicity. Dose, schedule and duration of CF depends on dose and schedule of MTX and plasma MTX levels drawn at 48h.
Hydroxyurea (Hydrea) 25mg/kg po continuous 100mg/kg iv qd × 3d	BMD. Minimal N/V, anorexia. GI toxicity at high doses >70mg/kg. Pretreat with allopurinol as rapid fall in leukemic cells occurs. Monitor blood counts frequently. Renal toxicity.
	Neurologic toxicity. May be potential mutagenic agent. Rash.
6-Mercaptopurine (6-MP, Purinethol) 1–2.5 mg/kg po qd (based on toxicity)	BMD. Nausea, anorexia, fever. Reduce 6-MP to 25%–33% if concurrent allopurinol is given. Allopurinol inhibits 6-MP degradation. Hepatic/renal dysfunction requires dose reduction.
	Stomatitis and cholestatic jaundice occur at high doses. When used with doxorubicin, liver toxicity may be increased. Oral bioavailability is variable; iv preparation is investigational.
6-Thioguanine (6TG, Thioguanine, Tabloid) 1–3 mg/kg po qd 100 mg/m^2 iv × 5d	BMD. Well tolerated. Reduce dose if stomatitis/diarrhea develop. Dose reduction not required for concurrent allopurinol. Monitor for hepatotoxicity. Administer oral dose on an empty stomach to facilitate complete absorption. Myelosuppression is more severe after iv administration.
5-Azacytidine [NSC 102816] 150–300 mg/m^2 iv × 5d	BMD. Dose- and schedule-dependent N/V and profound diarrhea, fever, and hypotension with rapid infusions. Give in four 6-h infusions. Reconstituted drug stable only 6 h. Use Ringer's lactate for optimal pH and stability. Stomatitis; hypophosphatemia; pruritic rash.
	Neurologic toxicity (weakness, lethargy) reported but rare. Hepatotoxicity rare but serious.
	Care be given sc but causes pain and brown skin discoloration.
2-Deoxycoformycin (DCF, pentostatin) [NSC 218321] 2–4 mg/m^2 iv q2wk	BMD. N/V, anorexia, fatigue. Nephrotoxicity. Acute renal failure at high doses. Check RFTs before each dose. Hepatotoxicity; ocular pain, conjunctivitis; fever; skin rash.
	CNS depression, drowsiness, lethargy, rarely, seizures and coma.
Antitumor Antibiotics	
Dactinomycin (actinomycin-D ACT-D, Cosmegen) 15 μg/kg iv × 5 q3–4wk	Marked BMD. Moderate–severe N/V in 2–5 h, lasts 12–24h. N/V tends to decrease with daily use.
	Prolonged anorexia common. Use preservative-free diluent to prevent precipitation. Calculated in micrograms. Tissue vesicant. Severe radiation recall reactions can occur with necrosis.
	Acneiform rash, alopecia, hyperpigmentation, stomatitis, glossitis, diarrhea, proctitis.
	Dose modification may be required for severe hepatic dysfunction.
Bleomycin (Bleo, Blenoxane) 5–15 units/m^2 iv/im/sc intralesional q wk	Little BMD. Mild N/V; anorexia. Chills and fevers to 103–105°F. Acetaminophen and antihistamines can decrease febrile reactions. Dehydration; stomatitis; alopecia; hyperpigmentation.
	Cutaneous toxicity may be dose-limiting. Anaphylaxis and hypotension (immediate or delayed or several hours). Test doses of 1–2 units are recommended, then observe 2–4h. Pulmonary toxicity (fibrosis) is dose-limiting. Total cumulative dose

(*continued*)

TABLE 64-1. Major Chemotherapeutic Agents Used in Cancer Treatment (*Continued*)

Drug (Synonyms)	*Patient Management Considerations*
	should not exceed 400 units to decrease risk of pulmonary fibrosis, which often presents as an interstitial pneumonitis.
Doxorubicin hydrochloride (Adriamycin)	BMD. Dose-related N/V. Tissue vesicant. Treat extravasation with cooling. Hypersensitivity reactions with local venous spasm, erythema, urticaria, pain, and pruritus along vein.
	Radiation recall reactions. Stomatitis; proctitis: alopecia totalis; red urine.
30–75 mg/m² iv q3–4wk 30–60 mg/m² (intravesicular)	Cardiotoxicity is dose-limiting and cumulative. Limit total dose to 550 mg/m². Monitor with serial radionuclide angiocardiography to predict CHF.[276] Dose modification for severe hepatic dysfunction. Bladder instillation can cause urgency and chemical cystitis.
Intraperitoneal use 40 mg in 2 L dialysate	Incompatible with heparin and 5-FU. Mild leukopenia with ip administration of 40 mg/m².
	Sterile ascites and adhesions can occur.
Daunomycin hydrochloride (daunorubicin, DNR rubidomycin, Cerubidine) 30–60 mg/m² iv q3–4wk	BMD. Moderate–severe N/V. Tissue vesicant. Stomatitis and diarrhea unusual; red urine; allergic reactions; alopecia. Reduce dose with severe hepatic dysfunction. Cardiotoxicity. Limit total dose to 550 mg/m². Monitor with serial radionuclide angiocardiography to predict CHF. Local pain in veins. Dose modifications may be required for severe hepatic dysfunction.
Mithramycin 0.025–0.05mg/kg iv qod to toxicity 0.025mg iv × 1–3 d	BMD, particularly thrombocytopenia. Moderate–severe N/V in 6h lasting 12–14h. Fever; tissue vesicant; hemorrhagic diathesis; coagulation abnormalities and hemorrhage often preceded by flushing and epistaxis. CNS toxicity, neuromuscular excitability, severe headache. Dermatitis.
	Proteinuria, azotemia, and electrolyte abnormalities (decreased PO, K, Mg, Ca). Unstable in acid solutions. Dilute with sterile water. Cumulative renal toxicity can occur. D/C for abnormal RFTs/LFTs. Effects on calcium metabolism valuable for control of malignant hypercalcemia.
Mitomycin C (Mutamycin) 2 mg/m² iv qd × 5 d 15–20 mg/m² iv q6–8wk 20–60mg (1 mg/ml) intravesicular	Delayed and cumulative BMD. Mild-moderate N/V in 1–2 h lasting 2–3 days. Fever; alopecia.
	Tissue vesicant. Chemical phlebitis and skin reactions. Stomatitis, diarrhea, anorexia, malaise.
	Weight loss common, even in responders. Hepatic activation and metabolism.
	Pulmonary toxicity infrequent but may be severe. Palmar rash that resolves with antihistamines or topical steroids. Hemolytic uremic syndrome with serious, often fatal hemolytic anemia, thrombocytopenia, renal failure, and hypertension reported.
	Bladder instillation causes dysuria, urgency. No BMD noted.
Plant Alkaloids	
Vincristine (Oncovin, VCR) 0.5–2 mg/m² iv q wk	Mild BMD. N/V unusual. Tissue vesicant. Treat extravasation with local hyaluronidase and heat.
	Biliary excretion. Decrease dose for hepatic dysfunction. Hyponatremia and syndrome of inappropriate ADH secretion. Peripheral neuropathy is dose-limiting. Paresthesias, loss of DTRs, jaw and abdominal pain, hoarseness, and constipation are common. Use of stool softener or mild laxatives is recommended. Bladder atony, vocal cord paresis, increased hepatic and neurotoxicity in elderly and immobile.
Vinblastine (VLB, Velban) 6 mg/m² iv q wk 0.1–0.4 mg/kg iv q wk 1.5–2 mg/m³/d × 5 q4wk	Dose-related BMD. N/V unusual. Tissue vesicant. Treat extravasation with local hyaluronidase and heat. Reduce dose for hepatic dysfunction. Stomatitis. Corneal ulceration if splashed into eyes. Neurotoxicity only at high doses (>20mg). Alopecia.
Etoposide (VP-16-213 EPEG, Vepesid, epipodophyllotoxin) 50–100 mg/m²/d iv × 5 d 200–250 mg/m² iv q wk 125–140 mg/m² iv TIW q4w	BMD. Mild N/V. Phlebitis; headache, fever/chills; anaphylactoid reactions.
	Hypotension may occur following rapid infusion. Give over 30–60 min. Peripheral neuropathy.
	D/C if hypersensitivity reactions develop. Continue saline infusion; treat with antihistamines and epinephrine. Alopecia. May precipitate. Stability of reconstituted drug is concentration-dependent. Examine solution; give only clear solution. Oral formulations (liquid and capsules) cause GI toxicity, N/V, and diarrhea and are investigational.
Teniposide (VM-26, PTG, thenylidene, Vumon) [NSC 14150] 60–80 mg/m² iv q wk 60 mg/m² qd × 5q4w	BMD. Tissue vesicant. Chemical phlebitis common. Infuse slowly over 15–30min.
	Fever, hypotension, bronchospasm, anaphylaxis with cardiovascular collapse. If hypersensitivity reaction develops, stop drug and treat with epinephrine and antihistamines. Continue infusion of normal saline or D5W. Alopecia.
Vindesine (Eldisine, vinblastine amide desacytyl) [NSC 132819] 3–4 mg/m² iv q1–2 wk 1.5–2 mg/m² iv BIw	BMD. Occasional N/V/diarrhea. Tissue vesicant. Do not administer with other vinca alkaloids because of potential for cumulative neurotoxicity. Neurotoxicity is dose-limiting.
	Loss of DTRs and paresthesias common. Proximal muscle weakness. Severe jaw pain. Abdominal cramping; diarrhea. Paralytic ileus rare; hoarseness; mild stomatitis.

(*continued*)

TABLE 64-1. Major Chemotherapeutic Agents Used in Cancer Treatment (*Continued*)

Drug (Synonyms)	*Patient Management Considerations*
Miscellaneous Agents	
L-Asparaginase (Elspar Crasnitin, L-ASP, L-asnase, colaspase) 1,000–20,000 IU/m^2 q10–14d 1000 IU/kg/d iv × 10d	Anaphylaxis precautions.[272,273] Give over 30 min. Desensitization and skin testing may help prevent anaphylaxis. Prophylactic antihistamines and slowing the infusion may decrease risk of reactions. Risks increase with use; significantly less common with im than iv use. If hypersensitivity reactions develop, *Erwinia* preparation may be substituted for *Escherichia coli* preparation. Moderate–severe N/V, fever, chills, urticaria, malaise. Hepatotoxicity common within 2 wk. Hyperglycemia. Coagulation abnormalities. Pancreatitis; azotemia; CNS toxicity, lethargy. Use only clear solutions.
Acridinylaniside (AMSA, m-AMSA) [NSC 249992] 90–120 mg/m^2 iv q4wk 25–40 mg/m^2 iv × 3d q3wk	BMD. Moderate–severe N/V. Tissue vesicant; chemical phlebitis. Increase diluent to 500 ml and slow rate to decrease venous spasm and pain. Do not infuse in less than 1 h. Unstable in chloride solutions. Reduce dose for hepatic dysfunction. Renal toxicity. Diarrhea; orange urine; stomatitis; paresthesias; yellow skin discoloration.
Hexamethylmelamine (HXM, HMM) [NSC 13875] 6–12 mg/kg po qd × 14–21 d or continuous	Mild BMD. Moderate–severe N/V. GI toxicity may be dose-limiting at high doses, with diarrhea and abdominal cramping. Take after meals to minimize GI symptoms. Rash. Neurotoxicity with peripheral neuropathy, agitation, confusion, hallucinations, petit mal seizures. May exacerbate vincristine-related neuropathy.
Dacarbazine (DTIC, Imidazole carboxamide DTIC-Dome) 250 mg/m^2 × 5d iv q3–4wk 800–1200 mg/m^2 iv q3–4wk	Mild BMD. Severe N/V in 1–3 h. Tissue vesicant. Flu-like syndrome with fever, myalgia, and malaise lasting 7–10 d. Facial flushing and paresthesias; alopecia. Slow rate of infusion to decrease pain from venous spasm. Protect from light. Change in color from yellow to pink denotes drug decomposition. Metabolic activation by liver. Precipitates hydrocortisone sodium succinate (Solu-Cortef).
Mitotane *o,p′*-DDD Lysodren) 2–10 g po qd continuous	Severe N/V. Anorexia; CNS toxicity with lethargy, vertigo, visual disturbance. Acute adrenal insufficiency; allergic rash; sensitivity to sunlight.
Procarbazine methylhydrazine (Matulane) 100–200 mg/m^2 po × 14 d	BMD. Moderate–severe N/V subsiding with daily use. Flu-like syndrome that decreases over time. Dose reductions for renal dysfunction. Hypersensitivity reactions with fever, rash, urticaria angioedema. Sympathomimetics, tricyclic antidepressants, other MAO inhibitors, and foods rich in tyramine can cause acute hypertensive crisis. Alcohol can cause Antabuse-like reaction. Azoospermia and amenorrhea at high doses. Often not reversible. CNS abnormalities, depression, nightmares, mania, psychosis. Barbiturates, phenothiazines, antihistamines may increase CNS-depressive effects. Postural hypotension. Interstitial pneumonitis/pulmonary fibrosis.
Mitoxantrone hydrochloride (DHAD, Novantrone) [NSC 301739]	BMD with platelet sparing. Mild N/V. Little GI toxicity. Cardiac arrhythmias in some doxorubicin-treated patients. No renal, hepatic, or cardiac toxicity reported to date. Bluish discoloration in vein used for infusion. Greenish urine.
Methyl-GAG (MGBG, mitoguazone) [NSC 32946] 10–14 mg/m^2 iv q3wk 3–4 mg/m^2 × 3–5d iv q4wk 260–600 mg/m^2 iv q wk 3–4mg/kg deep im q wk	Hypotension, N/V, dizziness, weakness, and malaise, persistent anorexia. Toxicity is dose- and schedule-dependent. Little BMD. Severe mucositis with 5-day infusions. Anorexia and weight loss common. Hypotension with rapid infusions; give over 30min. Deep im injections can be given if venous access is difficult. However, im injections are associated with severe dizziness and a transient burning feeling that spreads from the face to the entire body. Neuropathy; chemical thrombophlebitis; delayed hypoglycemia; vasculitis; skin ulcers.
13-*cis*-retinoic acid (13-CRA) 20 mg/d po 2.5 mg/kg/d po continuous	Well tolerated. Under investigation in myelodysplastic syndromes as a potential differentiating agent. No serious toxicity at low doses. Mild to moderate dermatologic toxicity including cheilosis, skin dryness, conjunctival irritation, drying of mucous membranes. Hepatotoxicity with chronic or high doses.[275,276]

adequately address the potential adverse effects of treatment. Nurses have played a pivotal role in the development of structured educational programs that teach patients and their families about the beneficial as well as the adverse effects of treatment and the interventions that can be used to prevent or ameliorate toxicity. By doing so, they have enabled the administration of complex treatment regimens to move safely from inpatient units to ambulatory settings that maximize the patient's potential for maintaining normal activities and reduce the costs of cancer care.[91–94]

The text of this section is focused on the technical aspects of parenteral drug administration. Special emphasis is placed on guidelines for the education and training of nurses in parenteral therapy; vein selection and venipuncture technique; the selection and maintenance of the various cannulae, catheters, and infusion ports/pumps that are used for vascular access; the educational needs of patients and families for the care of vascular access devices; the complications of parenteral therapy; the safe administration of parenteral antitumor agents; and guidelines for the management of extravasation.

Knowledge and Skills

Recommendations for the education and training of nurses and policies for the administration of parenteral therapy have been developed and widely implemented.[95–99] Nurses

TABLE 64-2. Major Hormonal Agents Used in Cancer Treatment

Drug (Synonyms)	*Patient Care Considerations*
Androgens	
Fluoxymesterone (Halotestin) 10–30 mg/d po	Cholestatic jaundice. Dosage reductions required for hepatic dysfunction. Increased appetite and weight gain; anorexia and N/V at high doses. Hypercalcemia in immobilized patients, especially those with bone metastases. Masculinization, hirsutism, acne, patchy alopecia, voice change. Decreased libido. Sodium and fluid retention—monitor weight; low salt diet. Injectable products are poorly soluble oil-based esters, which result in slow release and prolonged biologic activity. Patients may become sensitized to oil carriers.
Calusterone (Methosarb) 40 mg qid po, or 0.3 mg/kg/d po	
Testolactone (Teslac) 250 mg qid po or 100 mg im 3 times/wk	
Testosterone propionate (Oreton) 50–100 mg im 3 times/wk	
Testosterone enanthate (Delatestryl) 600–1200 mg im q wk	
Dromostanolone propionate (Drolban) 100 mg im 3 times/wk	
Estrogens	
Diethylstilbestrol (DES, stilbesteron) 1–15 mg po qd (prostate cancer 1–3 mg po qd)	Rapid rise in serum calcium in patients with bone metastases. Sodium and fluid retention with hypertension → CHF and thromboembolic complications. Monitor weight; low-salt diet. Feminization, gynecomastia, endometrial hypertrophy, uterine bleeding, areolar hyperpigmentation. Urinary frequency. Sensitization to oil carrier. Natural and synthetic compounds vary with regard to onset of activity, bioavailability, and duration of action. Chlorotrianisene is extremely fat-soluble and considerable fat storage occurs, accounting for delayed onset and prolonged duration. Individual products should be chosen selectively based on such properties. N/V at high doses resembling morning sickness. N/V often subsides with continued administration.
Diethylstilbestrol diphosphate (Honvan, Stilphostrol) 500–1000 mg iv × 5 day then 250–100 mg iv q wk	
Chlorotrianisene (TACE) 12–25 mg po tid	
Conjugated equine estrogenic compound (Premarin) 1–10 mg po tid	
Ethinyl estradiol (Estinyl) 0.5–1 mg po tid	
Antiestrogenic Compounds	
Tamoxifen citrate (Nolvadex) 10–80 mg po qd	Induction of ovulation and lactation: hot flashes. Transient "flare" in skin, soft tissue, and bone metastases. Hypercalcemia. Mild leukopenia and thrombocytopenia. Mild estrogenic activity seen; vaginal discharge, bleeding, and pruritus. Corneal opacity and retinopathies with prolonged high doses >240 mg/d >1 yr.
Progestins	
Hydroxyprogesterone caproate (Delalutin) 1.0–2.5 g im 2 times/wk	Generally well tolerated. Minimal fluid retention; alopecia. Occasional hypercalcemia in patients with bone metastases. Cholestatic jaundice. Use with care in patients with hepatic dysfunction. Thromboembolic phenomena. Patients may become sensitized to oil carrier. Natural progestins are rapidly inactivated. Slow release formulations administered intramuscularly.
Medroxyprogesterone acetate (Provera; po) 20–200 mg po qd (Depo-Provera; im) 200–800 mg im 2 times/wk	
Megestrol acetate (Megace) 40–300 mg po qd	
Adrenocortical steroids	
Prednisone (Deltasone) 40–60 mg/m^2 po qd	Agents vary with respect to mineralocorticoid potency (sodium and fluid retention); intermittent administration can increase the risk of serious toxicity. Adrenalectomized patients must increase steroids in stress, infection, trauma. Oral preparations irritate GI mucosa; administer with antacids or take with meals.
Prednisolone (Delta-Cortef) 40–60 mg/m^2 im qd	
Methylprednisolone (Medrol) Sodium succinate (Solu-Medrol)	Prolonged use may produce immunosuppression. GI ulceration and hemorrhage; hyperglycemia, diabetes, hyperlipidemia, weight gain; sodium and fluid retention, hypertension, edema, potassium wasting; emotional lability, euphoria, psychosis; muscle wasting, osteoporosis; aseptic necrosis of bones; glaucoma, cataracts;

TABLE 64-2. Major Hormonal Agents Used in Cancer Treatment (*Continued*)

Drug (Synonyms)	*Patient Care Considerations*
M. acetate (Depo-Medrol) 10–25 mg iv or im Hydrocortisone (Cortef) H. sodium succinate (Solu-Cortef) 100–500 mg iv or im qd Dexamethasone (Decadron) 0.5–16 mg po, iv, im qd	cushingoid appearance, acne; secondary amenorrhea, growth failure. Suppression of pituitary–adrenal axis requires slow withdrawal.
Chemical adrenalectomy	
Aminoglutethemide (Cytadren, Elipten) 750–2000 mg po qd (Cytadren, Elipten) 40–60 mg/m² po qd	Skin rash with 5–7 days lasting 8 days. Lethargy; somnolence. Addisonian characteristics; secretion of aldosterone with postural hypotension and hyponatremia; hypothyroidism; virilization; mild nausea, vertigo, nystagmus; BMD rare.

have also established standards of practice and a program for professional certification in parenteral therapy.[100–102] Technical proficiency in the aseptic insertion of vascular access devices must be acquired under the supervision of an experienced preceptor. At a minimum, most institutions require a nurse to demonstrate knowledge about the anatomy and physiology of veins and arteries, clinical pharmacology, and safe and effective drug administration in written and practical examinations before assuming responsibilities for drug administration. In addition, nurses are expected to develop and implement care plans that facilitate the anticipatory management of disease and treatment-related morbidity and to assess the physical and psychological needs of patients in their care.

Technique

Preparation of the patient is an important step in intravenous (IV) technique. Before venipuncture, ambulatory patients should be comfortably positioned for the infusion in bed or in chairs with arm rests. The purpose and duration of the infusion should always be reiterated just before the venipuncture is performed, even if the nature and purpose of the therapy has already been explained by the physician.

Vein selection should be based on the type of cannula to be used, the purpose of the infusion, its duration, and the patient's age, general condition, and activity level.[103–106] Ideally, the vein that is selected should follow a straight course for a distance that is long enough to permit full insertion of the needle or catheter. The choice of needle gauge should be based on the size of the vein. Large, easily accessible veins found along the forearm, such as the cephalic, median, and basilic veins, provide safe, convenient venipuncture sites. The bones of the forearm provide a natural split that eliminates the need for immobilizing the arm. The use of large veins reduces the risk of chemical thrombophlebitis when caustic agents are to be infused, especially when the drug is injected into the vein as a bolus (IV push). Extreme care must always be exercised when administering irritating solutions/drugs into veins that lie in the antecubital fossa or over the wrist joint. If the patient has undergone an axillary node dissection, the venous circulation can be greatly compromised so the affected arm should be avoided whenever possible. If the affected arm must be used for an intravenous infusion, the use of strict aseptic technique during venipuncture is absolutely critical. Infusions in the veins of lower extremities should be avoided because the risk of thrombophlebitis and embolism is significantly increased, especially in adults.

Before cleansing the skin, the vein should be palpated for resilience. Thrombosed veins feel hard and cord-like. When a prolonged course of parenteral therapy is anticipated, the distal portion of veins should be used for venipuncture so that inadvertent thrombosis will not preclude future use of the proximal portion. Veins located over areas of joint flexion, such as the antecubital fossa, should be avoided when prolonged infusions are planned, to decrease the risk of infiltration and the need for limb immobilization. Aseptic technique is essential.

The selection of a specific intravenous cannula depends on the purpose and length of the infusion, as well as the size and condition of the patient's veins. Stainless steel scalp vein ("butterfly") needles, centered and held by plastic wings, are employed for most short-term infusions (Fig. 64-1). Scalp vein needles range from 25 to 16 gauge in diameter. They are manufactured with a short length of plastic tubing and a female Luer-Lok adaptor that connects the winged needle to the tubing of commercially available administration sets. The plastic wings of scalp vein needles provide stability and maximal control of the needle during insertion and reduce mechanical irritation from traction after insertion. A short strip of tape should be placed over the plastic wings to anchor the needle. The tubing should be looped and taped independently to prevent a pull on the tubing from dislodging the needle. Arm boards are useful for immobilizing the extremity when a long infusion is planned or sudden movements, such as vomiting, are anticipated. Tape placed over the needle and tubing should not be secured to the arm board, nor should it tightly constrict any part of the hand or arm. If an agent that is a tissue vesicant is to be administered

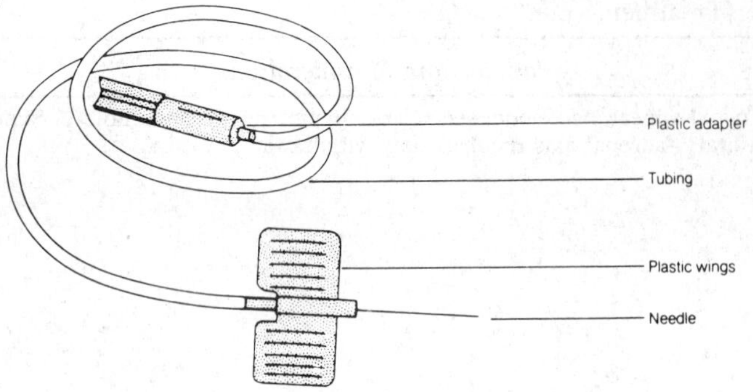

FIG. 64-1. Steel infusion cannula often referred to as the "scalp vein" or "butterfly" needle.

as an IV bolus following venipuncture, the area above the venipuncture site should not be completely obscured by tape or a dressing until after the drug has been completely infused, permitting the puncture site to be observed carefully for subtle evidence of extravasation. If the cannula is to remain in place after the drug is administered, a topical polyantibiotic ointment and sterile dressing should be applied.

For patients with impaired venous access or fragile veins, flexible small-bore, polyethylene, Teflon, or Silastic catheters offer an alternative to a steel scalp vein needle.[106] The two types of cannulas are shown in Figures 64-2A and B. When the catheter is introduced over the needle, it is slipped off the steel needle into the vein; then the needle is removed. Local anesthesia (ethyl alcohol spray or intradermal lidocaine/procaine) can be used to decrease the discomfort patients experience during catheter insertion. When the catheter is inside the needle, it is pushed through the needle until the desired length is within the lumen of the vein. Because the tip can be inadvertently severed during insertion, placement of a peripheral intravenous catheter should be limited to experienced individuals. Radiopaque catheters are recommended so that a severed tip can be visualized radiographically. Once the catheter is inserted, the cutting edge of the needle is then protected by a shield to prevent the catheter from being severed.

Although the scalp vein needle is unquestionably the easiest cannula to insert and the least expensive, steel needles tend to infiltrate easily. The tendency of steel needles to infiltrate is a source of added cost in terms of time, effort, and materials, and must be kept in mind when vascular irritants are to be administered. Given their relatively low rate of infiltration, short (1–1.5 in.), small-bore plastic, Teflon, or Silastic catheters offer an alternative to steel needles when vesicants are to be infused. However, the risk of infusion-related infection and phlebitis is substantially greater with synthetic catheters if the devices remain in place for more than 48 hr.[107–109]

Steel scalp vein needles are also available with a self-sealing cap at the end of the tubing that can be used when IV therapy can be administered intermittently.[110–112] These devices, which are known as heparin locks, are available as short 19- and 21-gauge needles that are manufactured with foreshortened bevels to reduce the risk of puncturing the posterior wall of the vein during insertion and maintenance. In addition, capped Teflon catheters are available for intermittent IV therapy.[110] Injection caps and plugs can also be attached to an open-ended needle or catheter to create an intermittent device. Factors influencing the decision to employ a heparin lock include the frequency of drug administration or of blood sampling, the volume and length of the infusion, properties of the infusate, and the general condition of the patient's veins. Nonirritating chemotherapeutic and antibiotic agents that are administered on an intermittent basis in IV boluses or short infusions are well suited for delivery through heparin locks. A dilute solution of heparin (10 units/ml) equal to the volume of the cannula (0.2–0.4 ml) is generally instilled into the self-sealing diaphragm of the heparin lock after insertion and at 6-hr intervals to flush the tubing and prevent the development of a blood clot at the needle tip.[112] Once they are taught how to flush the device using aseptic technique, patients who might otherwise have remained hospitalized for IV chemotherapy can be discharged and treated as outpatients. Sterile saline has been successfully used to maintain the patency of intermittent devices and should be considered for patients in whom heparin is contraindicated.[113,114]

Central Venous Catheters

Percutaneously placed single- or multiple-lumen right atrial catheters, such as the Centrasil and Quinton central venous catheters, are often used in acute care settings for short-term vascular access when multiple solutions need to be infused simultaneously, and frequent blood samples must be withdrawn. Catheters are generally placed into the subclavian, internal jugular and, rarely, the femoral vein by percutaneous puncture at the bedside under local anesthesia. The size (2.2–3.9 mm external diameter) and inflexibility of percutaneously placed central venous catheters, especially those made of stiff polymers such as Teflon, make sterility of the skin exit site somewhat difficult to maintain. Because the risk of infection is increased with a central line catheter, strict attention must be paid to aseptic technique during all dressing changes. When a lumen is not in use, a dilute (100 unit/ml) solution of heparin (2–3 ml) should be instilled to prevent backflow of blood into the catheter and then clamped and sealed with Luer-Lok plugs.

The Intrasil catheter is a 20-in. 16- to 18-gauge central venous line that is inserted into a peripheral vein. This catheter has been utilized for the administration of vesicants in patients with impaired venous access. Catheter maintenance

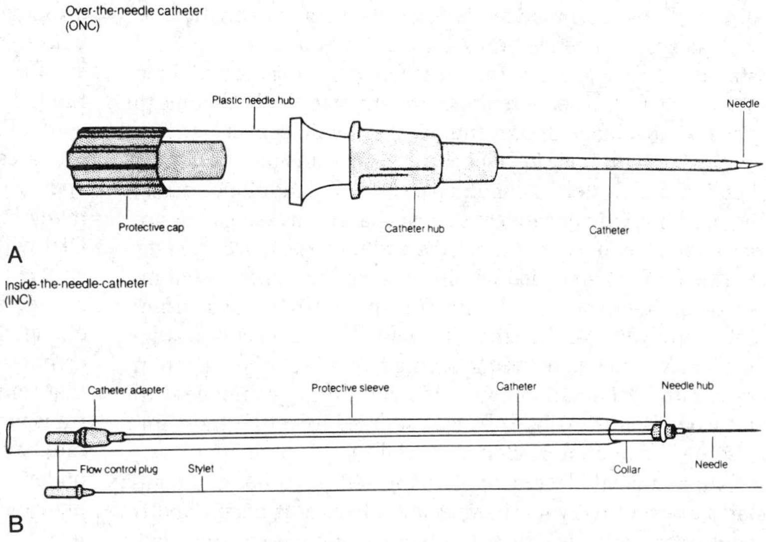

FIG. 64-2. **A.** ONC (over-the-needle) infusion catheter. **B.** INC (inside-the-needle) infusion catheter.

requires strict adherence to sterile technique; blood sampling through peripherally placed central lines is not recommended.

INDWELLING CENTRAL VENOUS CATHETERS. When frequent access to the circulation is anticipated for prolonged periods or when peripheral access has deteriorated to the point at which venipuncture is traumatic, patients are often considered candidates for placement of an indwelling central venous line that is composed of a flexible, durable, and nonirritating Silastic elastomer, such as the Hickman, Broviac, Raaf, or Groshong catheters.[115-121] These catheters can maximize comfort in patients receiving intensive remission induction regimens or bone marrow transplantation and have been used successfully as all-purpose intravascular lifelines for the prolonged administration of hyperalimentation and antineoplastic, biologic, antiviral, antibiotic, and antifungicidal agents, in both inpatients and outpatients.

Implantation of indwelling catheters can be performed in the operating room either utilizing "peel away" introducers into the subclavian, internal jugular, or femoral vein or by surgical cutdown into the external jugular or saphenous vein in the groin. The catheter is positioned at the entrance to the right atrium by advancing it into the superior vena cava through the subclavian, cephalic, or external jugular vein.[121-125] Correct placement is confirmed by fluoroscopy or a chest x-ray film. The extravascular portion of the catheter is threaded through a subcutaneous tunnel that extends from the point of insertion to a skin exit site on the chest or abdominal wall approximately 10 cm away. Ideally, the catheter should exit the subcutaneous tunnel in an area that is accessible and cosmetically acceptable to the patient so that the potential for self-care can be maximized. A Dacron cuff fused to the surface of the catheter is positioned about 2 cm from the exit site, firmly securing the catheter in the subcutaneous tissue. The Dacron elicits a fibroblastic reaction in the subcutaneous tissue that provides a mechanical barrier to microbial contamination. Patients with open chest wounds, tumor involvement of the chest wall, radiation fibrosis, a tracheostomy, or an enterocutaneous fistula, have special catheter placement needs that may require peripheral placement of a central venous catheter as just described.

Double- and triple-lumen catheters that allow one lumen to be used for hyperalimentation, and the other(s) to be used for parenteral fluids, drug administration, blood product support, blood sampling, or plasmapheresis, are widely available.[126-128] The increase in the external diameter of multilumen catheters may represent a consideration in patient selection. After each line entry, it is recommended that the lumen be flushed with a dilute solution of heparin. When a lumen is not in use for therapy, it should be capped with a Luer-Lok injection cap. A dilute solution of heparin (100 units/ml), equal to the volume of the lumen, should be instilled daily into the catheter to prevent backflow.[127] Nurses should avail themselves of information about the benefits and disadvantages of the various catheters that are available so that they can evaluate which can best meet the individual needs of their patients.

Catheter Care

Although indwelling central venous catheters can theoretically remain in place indefinitely in the absence of complications, successful maintenance is highly dependent on compliance with maintenance procedures for care of the catheter and the exit site.[129-146] Preoperatively, patients should be educated about the catheter, the technique for its placement, its uses, and care in the postoperative period. Special emphasis should be placed on catheter maintenance, especially if home care and treatment are planned. Patients should be taught sterile dressing changes and procedures for flushing the catheter with heparin as soon as they are willing and able to assume these responsibilities. Catheter maintenance can be assumed by the patient and family over time with careful instruction. Most nursing services have developed written manuals that help patients and families develop confidence in catheter care.[139] Mastery of catheter self-care is essential before discharge from the hospital. Adherence to dressing change procedures, exit site skin sensitivities, as well as cost and convenience have been evaluated in several studies. Transparent semipermeable dressings have some advantage for inspection of the site and stability but seems to have no advantage in preventing infection in cancer patients compared with traditional occlusive gauze and tape materials applied under sterile conditions.[150,152,155] Traditional dressings are initially cheaper than transparent dressings but are less stable and cost more, in time and materials, over a 72-hr period.[150] Povidone–iodine ointment did not affect local infection rates when used with transparent dressings in another study.[155] Neither the ointment nor the weekly changing of IV extension tubing seemed to affect the infection rate; rather, the maintenance of strict sterile technique with insertion and dressings changes seemed to be the most important factor in a randomized trial of 435 patients.[155]

After surgical placement of an indwelling catheter, a regular pattern of daily sterile dressing changes is begun and is continued until the exit site is healed, sutures are removed, the Dacron cuff is firmly anchored, and the patient is without signs of infection. Although dressing change procedures may vary from one institution to another, some basic principles seem universal. Strict adherence to sterile technique is required for all procedures to reduce the risk of infection. Masks should be worn during periods of high risk (*e.g.*, severe neutropenia). The catheter exit site should be thoroughly cleansed with alcohol swabs followed by povidone–iodine swabs. Then povidone–iodine ointment is applied, and a dry sterile dressing is put in place. Once the Dacron cuff is secure and the sutures are removed, patients are generally allowed to bathe normally. When patients with Hickman catheters bathe, the exit site should not be submerged in the bath water.

Sterile, transparent waterproof polyurethane adhesive dressings that permit moisture to evaporate from the skin while repelling fluid and preventing bacterial contamination, such as Op-site, Uniflex, and Tegaderm, have been introduced as alternatives to occlusive gauze dressings for central venous catheters.[148–157] When these dressings are used, ointment should not be applied to the skin surface after the exit site is cleansed. A dry skin surface under these dressings is important. Transparent dressings permit direct visualization of the catheter insertion site, in addition to stabilizing the catheter. In addition, their semipermeable characteristics preclude the need for daily dressing changes. Use of these dressings increases patient comfort because the dressings stretch to accommodate body movements. The comfort and convenience that transparent dressings offer has made them a popular alternative to occlusive dressings in patients with catheters that do not require daily dressing changes.[156] Waterproof dressings are recommended when there is a tracheostomy, an open wound, or a fistula near a catheter exit site. Swimming is often permitted if the catheter exit site is covered with an occlusive dressing and protected by a transparent dressing, with the understanding that the exit site will be cleansed and redressed afterward.

A prospectively randomized trial evaluating the safety and efficacy of a transparent polyurethane dressing versus a traditional occlusive dressing composed of gauze and tape applied under sterile conditions reported that polyurethane dressings protected the catheter (short percutaneously placed catheters) exit site from bacterial contamination and significantly reduced the incidence of phlebitis.[153] Several randomized trials performed subsequently have provided conflicting data on the risks of phlebitis and infection, but the rates of catheter-related infection were low in all studies, and the statistical power of the conclusions was weak in many.[154–159] Recent data from a prospectively randomized trial with 2088 small Teflon catheters indicate that complication rates (infection, local inflammation, and phlebitis) are equivalent among sterile gauze and tape dressings, changed every 48 hr; sterile gauze left in place until the catheter was removed; transparent polyurethane dressing that remained in place until the catheter was removed; and a transparent dressing with an iodophor antiseptic incorporated into the adhesive.[160] Moisture or blood accumulated under the two transparent dressings more frequently than under gauze dressings but did not significantly increase infectious complications among the four groups. At least half of the catheters had been in place for over 48 hr. Given these data, the use of a transparent dressing in afebrile patients for the duration that a catheter remains in place must be considered safe and cost-effective. In diaphoretic patients, transparent dressings adhere poorly and should be replaced at least every 48 hr.

Self-sealing Luer-Lok catheter injection plugs have eliminated the need for repetitious opening of the catheter system. Some caps are manufactured with an inner needle stabilizing center that reduces the risk of inadvertent needle puncture of the catheter sidewall.[110] The cap should be carefully cleansed before all line entries. For security, the plug should be taped in place. The catheter is generally coiled loosely and taped to the chest wall or tucked into a bra. When not in use, it is generally recommended that the catheter be clamped over an adhesive tag. Patients must be taught how to close the system with a catheter clamp to prevent air embolus in the event there is an accidental break in the line. A catheter clamp, worn around the neck or carried by the patient, should be readily available at all times. A smooth-surfaced catheter clamp should always be used; rubber-shod hemostats should not be used. Catheters should never be allowed to dangle freely. Patients should be cautioned that pets and small children can inadvertently dislodge catheters when picked up or held near the chest and that great care should also be exercised when using scissors or any other sharp objects near the catheter to avoid severing the lines.

Although generally safe, the use of indwelling catheters can be associated with serious morbidity.[109,161–169] Expert nursing care is critical if the risk of complications is to be minimized, especially in neutropenic and immunosuppressed patients, who must be closely monitored for subtle signs of local and systemic infection. A new fever in a patient who has no other obvious source of infection warrants a prompt evaluation for a catheter-related bacteremia. In the great majority of centers, including the National Cancer Institute, bacteremias from Hickman catheters are successfully treated with antibiotics without catheter removal. Catheter removal is required only in the face of refractory infection, ongoing sepsis, or fungal infections. Local (exit site) infections can also be treated successfully with antibiotics without catheter removal. However, established tunnel infections are rarely cured by antibiotics and are an indication for catheter removal. Extrusion of the Dacron cuff is an indication that the catheter has migrated. Because the physical barrier to infection is lost and the tip is often malpositioned, catheter removal is generally warranted.

Difficulty with blood withdrawal may indicate an occlusion of the catheter. Blood withdrawal should be gentle to prevent catheter collapse and suction adherence to the vessel wall. Often a change in the patient's position will move the catheter away from the vessel wall. Occasionally, a small clot at the tip will act as a ball valve, preventing blood withdrawal without affecting fluid flow. Catheter occlusion from thrombus formation, once the major cause of premature catheter removal, can frequently be handled by lysing the clot with fibrinolytic enzymes that act on plasminogen or plasmin within the clot.[170-176] Before instituting therapy, correct catheter placement should be verified by an x-ray film. Then, the following procedure may be utilized to lyse the occlusion. A dilute solution containing a fibrinolytic enzyme (250 IU/ml of streptokinase or 5000 IU/ml of urokinase) should be instilled into the catheter, preferably after clot retraction starts to occur, in a volume equal to the internal volume of the central venous catheter (0.2–0.6 ml). The solution should be allowed to interact with the clot for 5 to 10 min. Then, an attempt should be made to aspirate the clot at 5-min intervals. Catheter patency can often be restored with one injection of enzyme after 20 to 25 min. In some instances, several enzyme injections may be required. In a study conducted at the M. D. Anderson Cancer Center, 1624 (98.6%) of 1647 occluded catheters were cleared with urokinase; 81% were cleared with a single enzyme instillation.[174] Although urokinase is much more expensive than streptokinase, many prefer it because it is nonantigenic and rapidly cleared by the liver.

Catheter occlusion from drug precipitates are not easy to dissolve. Great care must always be exercised to avoid mixing incompatible drugs or solutions in the line. Occlusions from drug precipitates generally mandate catheter removal.

If swelling, pain, or tenderness at the catheter entrance site or in the neck, shoulder, or arm are noted, a subclavian or axillary thrombosis should be suspected and a venogram performed through a peripheral vein (as opposed to the catheter) to confirm the diagnosis. Although catheters have traditionally been removed if the venogram is positive, recent reports indicate that low-dose infusions of thrombolytic enzymes are effective in lysing axillary–subclavian vein thromboses as well as peripheral arterial occlusions.[175-176] Because the use of thrombolytic enzymes increases the risk of bleeding, urokinase therapy is contraindicated in patients with active or recent internal bleeding, recent intraspinal or intracranial surgery, an intracranial neoplasm, or a recent cerebrovascular accident.

Mechanical damage (tear, puncture, rupture) to indwelling catheters is an infrequent problem.[134-138] However, it is essential that patients know that they should immediately clamp the line proximal to the damaged area to prevent air embolism. If the damage is at least 4 cm away from the skin exit site, the catheter can usually be temporarily repaired with a repair kit available from the manufacturer.

Portable Infusion Pumps

Infusions that must be administered with a precision that exceeds the accuracy of simple flow clamps, which use the force of gravity, require the use of a controller or an infusion pump. Controllers, such as the IVAC, utilize a photoelectric sensor and an electronic feedback mechanism to eliminate the need to count drops and manually regulate flow rates. Most models have an alarm that is set off if the bottle of solution empties, the tubing becomes occluded, or sufficient backpressure builds because of a positional or infiltrated infusion.[178] Infusion pumps that minimize flow rate changes caused by viscosity, tubing characteristics, and positional changes, are useful for medications that can do harm if they infuse too quickly. Volumetric and nonvolumetric pumps are available. Volumetric models provide precise flow rates and are particularly well adapted to handle slow infusions.

Light-weight reusable microvolume infusion pumps such as the one shown in Figure 64-3 are well suited for use by ambulatory patients and have facilitated the evaluation of chemotherapy administered in continuous infusions.[179-183] Three types of portable volumetric infusion pumps are currently in use: battery-powered piston-valve (syringe-cassette) pumps [Autosyringe, Graseby]; battery-powered peristaltic (roller drum and linear devices) pumps [Cormed, Infumed, Deltec-Pharmacia CADD, Pancretec 2000]; and balloon pumps [Travenol Infusor]. Advantages and disadvantages of each product relate to the overall cost of purchase or rental, accuracy, ease of operation, fluid capacity, sensor alarm features, as well as weight and bulk. However, most

FIG. 64-3. Example of a microvolume ambulatory infusion pump. These self-powered infusion systems can deliver continuous parenteral infusions of solutions in microvolumes. (Courtesy of Travenol Inc)

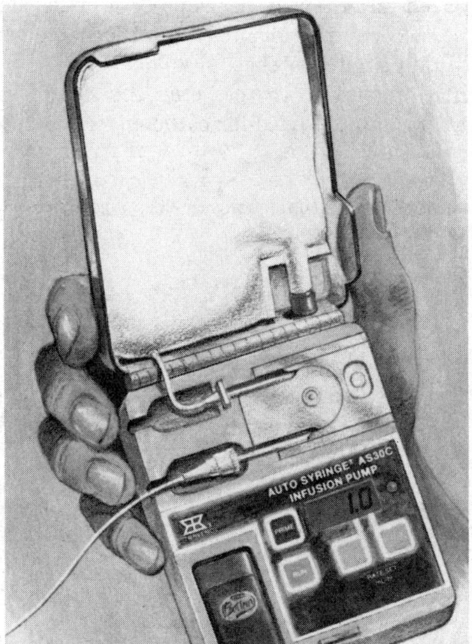

models are manufactured with the capacity to deliver an intermittent bolus of drug, in addition to a fixed rate of drug delivery. Additional considerations include the availability of instructional materials and services from the supplier. Because patients can be taught to change the cartridge, bag, or syringe that holds the infusate without risk of contamination, parenteral chemotherapy can even be administered at home under the guidance and supervision of an oncology nurse. Although the use of an ambulatory infusion pump can minimize life-style disruption when continuous infusions are administered over protracted periods, they do require patient participation. Good vision, manual dexterity, the ability to learn and follow instructions reliably are important considerations.

Use of ambulatory infusion pumps can circumvent many of the problems associated with long-term parenteral analgesic administration. Continuous analgesic infusions achieve relief at lower doses without the peak-and-trough effects associated with intermittent drug administration. Pump design now permits patients to titrate their dose of analgesic based on the intensity of the pain by delivering a predefined dose of the analgesic on demand at measured intervals. A prescriber-defined lockout period during which the infusor cannot be activated prevents overmedication.[183]

Implantable Vascular Access Devices: Infusion Ports and Pumps

When a patient is unable or unwilling to assume responsibility for the care of the catheter and the exit site, a totally implantable injection port (Infusaport, Port-A-Cath, Norport, Mediport) or infusion pump (Infusaid, Medtronic) provides an alternative that is safe and convenient.[184–195] An infusion port is a small plastic or metal drug reservoir with a self-sealing silicone rubber septum that is attached to a Silastic central venous outlet catheter (Fig. 64-4). After the catheter is placed into the superior vena cava under local anesthesia, the reservoir is implanted into a subcutaneous pocket, generally on the anterior chest (Fig. 64-5). Because there is no external opening to the catheter, the risk of infectious complications and the need for catheter maintenance is reduced. Subcutaneous implantation of the port frees patients from external dressing changes and provides obvious cosmetic advantages, making these devices particularly acceptable to children.[195]

FIG. 64-4. Mediport infusion access device and deflected tip Huber needle. (Courtesy of Cormed Inc)

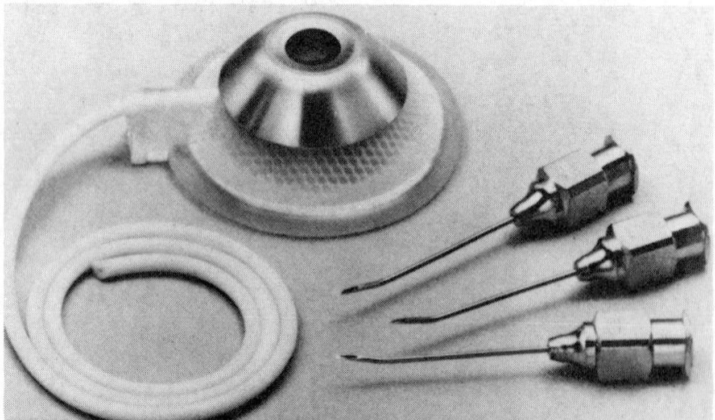

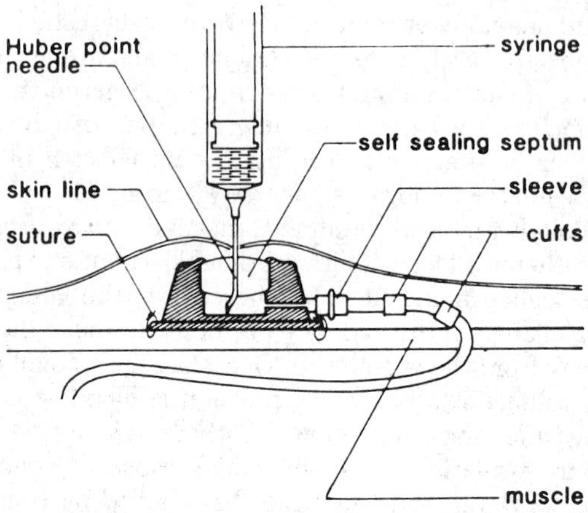

FIG. 64-5. A subcutaneously implanted port with Huber point needle penetrating the skin and the injection septum.

Implantable infusion ports are heparinized after each port entry. When not in use, the system is generally heparinized every 28 days with 3 to 5 ml of heparin (100 units/ml). Whenever blood is aspirated through an implanted vascular access device, the system must be flushed with 20 ml of sterile saline before heparinization to ensure that the catheter is completely cleared of blood. Subcutaneous ports require no other maintenance.

Because a regular hypodermic needle will core the Silastic rubber septum, permanently damaging the port, a special 19 to 22-gauge, 90° deflected point, Huber needle is used to gain vascular access. Because the skin must be punctured each time the port is entered, skin cleansing and attention to aseptic technique is required. The needle should be secured with tape and covered with a sterile dressing to decrease traction at the insertion site. Ports attached to small-bore (0.5-mm) catheters will infuse at rates up to 200 to 250 ml/hr without a positive pressure pump; larger-bore (1.0-mm) catheters accommodate infusions of 450 to 500 ml/hr. A recent, prospectively randomized trial comparing externalized venous access with Hickman catheters with a subcutaneously implanted Port-A-Cath in cancer patients suggests that infectious complications with implanted infusion ports are lower than with indwelling central venous catheters.[196]

The septum of most implantable infusion ports is designed to withstand 2000 injections for drug administration, blood product support, and blood sampling, permitting these devices to remain in place for a year or more. The cost of most implantable ports ranges from 300 to 450 dollars. Recently, manufacturers have begun to market double-port/double-lumen devices and ports with catheters suitable for intraperitoneal drug delivery.

The Infusaid is a miniaturized (8-oz), totally implantable, drug delivery system that is FDA approved for commercial use for continuous infusions of 5-fluorouracil, methotrexate, intra-arterial floxuridine (FUDR), heparin, morphine, insulin, and certain aminoglycosides. It provides another attrac-

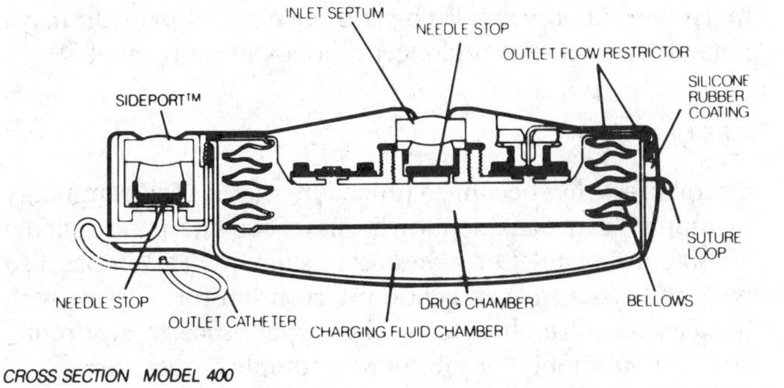

FIG. 64-6. The inside of an Infusaid pump. (Courtesy of the Infusaid Corp)

tive alternative to external pumps for the delivery of timed infusions. The drug delivery system is composed of a shallow (8.7 × 2.8-cm) titanium disk that houses a pump and a radiopaque Silastic outlet catheter. The disk has three chambers: a 50-ml drug reservoir; a chamber that holds a volatile fluorocarbon that serves as the power source; and a side port that permits bolus administration of drugs (Fig. 64-6). The pump is permanently powered by the vapor pressure of the fluorocarbon and is virtually maintenance free. The flow rate is calibrated by the manufacturer and can be set to infuse as slowly as 1 ml/day, permitting pumps to be refilled as infrequently as every 30 days. The disk is implanted in a subcutaneous pouch during catheter placement. [194–204] Similarly to implantable ports, the pump requires no maintenance other than heparinization when the device is not in use. Because the vapor pressure of the fluorocarbon that powers the Infusaid pump is influenced by changes in body temperature, atmospheric pressure, and viscosity, patients must become quite familiar with how the pump functions because fever and changes in altitude can significantly change flow rates. For each 1°C rise in body temperature, flow rate increases approximately 10%.[198] Educational materials for professionals and patients are available from the manufacturer. Infusaid pumps range in cost from 2750 to 4750 dollars.

The treatment of patients with hepatic artery infusions using external pumps and angiographically placed catheters is demanding and has restricted the clinical evaluation of intra-arterial chemotherapy. The development of a totally implanted drug delivery system that is safe and reliable, such as the Infusaid pump, has simplified the administration of intra-arterial infusions and stimulated clinical trials of hepatic artery infusions in patients with tumor limited to the liver.[197–199,205–213] Surgical placement of the catheter to ensure complete perfusion of the liver without extrahepatic infusion is crucial to maximize response and minimize biliary and gastrointestinal toxicity. Catheter displacement with implanted pumps occurs less frequently than with transcutaneous intra-arterial catheters attached to external pumps, and patient mobility is greatly increased. The use of these devices may offer major improvements in quality of life during treatment. In one study, over 70% of the employed patients with implanted pumps returned to work.[209] Aside from infection, thrombosis is the major complication of arterial infusions. Therefore, patients should be taught to report pain, fever, and changes in temperature, color, and sensation.[197]

The Medtronic pump, an investigational implantable drug delivery system, is a 7.0 × 2.8-cm titanium disk with a peristaltic roller pump powered by a lithium battery with an expected lifetime of 2 years.[198,214–217] It contains a microprocessor that can be reprogrammed after implantation to deliver drug by infusion (2–200 ml/day), bolus, or bolus delay by electromagnetic signals emitted from a hand-held telemetry wand. This device is being used to explore dose schedule interventions that explore the use of circadian shaping of infusion times.[214] The initial cost of this device is high (17,140 dollars plus monthly maintenance of 349 dollars). However, a cost analysis performed by a group evaluating the pump for low-dose continuous doxorubicin infusions indicates that the pump becomes less costly than inpatient 96-hr infusions after the fifth month of therapy.[217]

Infusaid and Medtronic pumps have also been used successfully to manage intractable cancer pain.[215–218] Intrathecal and subcutaneous infusions of low-dose narcotics has been shown to achieve pain relief at lower doses, circumvent adverse effects, decrease the need for supplemental opiates, in addition to enhancing patient mobility.

Complications associated with the use of implanted infusion ports have begun to appear in the literature. Problems have included flow rate changes, inversion of the device in the subcutaneous pocket, occlusion from thrombi, tissue necrosis from drug extravasation in the subcutaneous pocket because of needle displacement from the inlet septum or catheter occlusion with retrograde drug pooling, and occlusion from metastatic tumor.[219–224] The incidence of these complications has yet to be determined.

Intraperitoneal Drug Administration

A technique for intraperitoneal drug administration that uses a semipermanent Tenckhoff catheter has been developed to bathe the entire peritoneal surface with the antitumor agents. Steep concentration gradients between intraperitoneal and plasma drug levels can be achieved with a number of chemotherapeutic agents (5-fluorouracil, methotrexate, cisplatin, melphalan, cytosine arabinoside, and doxorubicin).[225–233] A Tenckhoff indwelling catheter is placed in the peritoneal cavity through an incision in the anterior abdominal wall. The tip is positioned in the peritoneal cavity and the catheter is implanted in the subcutaneous tissue. The intraperitoneal portion of the catheter has many small holes that facilitate the instillation and drainage of peritoneal fluids. Like indwelling central venous lines, the intraperitoneal catheter is secured by a Dacron cuff that is positioned near the exit skin site. The Tenckhoff catheter may also be connected to a subcutaneous infusion port to create a closed system. When an infusion port is used, the reservoir is anchored by suturing it to the fascia over a bony area, usually the rib cage in the anterior abdominal wall.[232]

Catheter patency is preserved while the incision is healing by daily instillation of warmed solutions of heparinized dialysis fluid (Inpersol 1.5%). To prevent bacterial peritonitis, sterile technique is used to place the catheter and to care for it during the first 10 to 14 days.[234-239] Once the exit site has healed, chemotherapy is administered into the cavity in a warmed 2-liter solution of dialysis fluid through the catheter (or infusion port) using a Y-tube administration set. Instilling the drug in a large volume of dialysate increases the area of peritoneal surface exposed to the drug. The dialysate remains in the cavity for a specific dwell time (20 min to 5 hr) before it is drained, to maximize exposure of tumor cells to the drug, based on the properties of the drug. Therapy is generally administered continuously for a 48-hr period or given once daily for 5 days. Clinical trials with intraperitoneal chemotherapy have shown that the objective tumor regression can be achieved and that therapy can be safely administered on an outpatient basis. A comparison of IV and intraperitoneal 5-fluorouracil suggests that patients experience less hematologic and hepatic toxicity after the intraperitoneal therapy.[231]

Nurses play a major role in fluid exchange, catheter maintenance, and the education of patients about the therapy and catheter care.[234-241] Most problems that are encountered during intraperitoneal therapy relate to catheter function (inflow and drainage of dialysate) or discomfort related to abdominal distention and poor drainage of the dialysate. These problems are managed symptomatically. As with central venous catheters, the most significant threat to catheter longevity is infection.[240] Educational programs, developed by nurses, allow patients to gradually assume total responsibility for dressing changes and enable them to care for their catheters safely at home. Until recently, catheter maintenance generally involved daily or every-other-day sterile dressing changes. Data from a prospectively randomized trial evaluating the incidence of infection in patients with healed catheter exit sites have shown that peritonitis and exit site infections are not increased in patients who perform catheter care using "clean" procedures, when compared with those who perform sterile dressing changes.[241] Catheters with infusion ports require no special care between treatments.

Intrathecal Therapy

Tumor involvement of the central nervous system caused by infiltration of the leptomeninges can be managed without repeated lumbar punctures by instilling chemotherapy directly into a lateral ventricle utilizing implantable access devices, such as the Ommaya reservoir.[242-246] Nurses are generally responsible for the maintenance of these devices and for intraventricular drug administration. A procedure has been established for safe and effective drug administration through this device. First, the reservoir is pumped several times to fill the device with spinal fluid. Then, the skin is prepared and the reservoir is obliquely punctured, using sterile technique, with a 25- to 27-gauge scalp vein needle. Enough spinal fluid is removed for laboratory studies and to keep exchanges isovolumetric. A chemotherapeutic agent is then slowly injected into the reservoir through the scalp vein needle which is then flushed with Elliott's B solution. After the needle is removed, the reservoir is pumped to distribute the drug into the intraventricular space. Preservative-free morphine sulfate can also be administered into an Ommaya reservoir to achieve prolonged periods of pain relief.[244]

Cytapheresis

Cytapheresis has become a procedure that is used commonly to support cancer patients who have become pancytopenic and require platelet or granulocyte support.[247-249] It has also been utilized as a therapeutic intervention for patients with leukostasis, thrombocytosis, the hyperviscosity syndrome, and autoimmune or immune complex disorders.[250,251] Nurses have played a major role in the development of collection procedures to maintain maximal viability and function of cells and in the establishment and the operation of cytapheresis units in which specific blood components can be collected safely from many individuals on a daily basis. Cytapheresis using continuous flow centrifugation collection techniques or intermittent nylon filtration is safe and effective when administered properly by trained nurses. Strict aseptic techniques are essential to prevent nosocomial infection as well as hepatitis transmission. Throughout the collection procedures, cytapheresis nurses must be prepared to manage side-effects such as hypotension, hypothermia, hypovolemia, and other untoward reactions. If substances such as etiocholanolone, hydroxyethyl starch, or dextran are used to enhance the separation of red blood cells from leukocytes to increase the yield of granulocytes, hypersensitivity and anaphylactic reactions can occur. Therefore, these nurses must be skilled in the management of anaphylactic reactions and the provision of emergency care. In centers at which trials of immunomodulators are in progress, the role of cytapheresis as a mechanism for obtaining lymphocytes for therapeutic purposes is expanding.[252]

Complications of Parenteral Therapy

Infection is the most serious complication of parenteral therapy. Almost all infections are preventable if insertion and maintenance techniques preserve sterility.[100-109,160,253-259] Effective disinfection of the insertion site and meticulous attention to aseptic technique is particularly important in neutropenic and immunosuppressed patients. To minimize the risk of infusion-related bacteremia, strict aseptic technique must be observed during cannula insertion; the device should be carefully anchored to minimize traction; a topical polyantibiotic and sterile dressing should be applied; and the venipuncture site should be labeled with the date, time, and type of device. Special attention must also be paid to aseptic technique during all line entries to preserve the sterility of the stopcocks, tubing, solutions, and inline filters. Although the lowest rates of sepsis have been reported from organizations with established IV teams, the cost-effectiveness of using such teams has not been established by controlled trial.

Most septicemias originate as local infections of the transcutaneous cannula tract. Inevitably, the organisms involved are normal skin flora that have entered the body through the intravenous needle or an infected catheter hub.[109,160,253] Medical personnel commonly carry gram-negative pathogens on their hands. Vigorous hand-washing should always precede venipuncture. Given concerns about the transmission of the human immunodeficiency virus (HIV) in the health care setting, the CDC now recommends the routine use of "appropriate barrier precautions" when contact with the blood body fluids of *any patient* is anticipated. These recommendations specify the routine use of gloves in addition to vigorous hand-washing before each patient contact.[254]

Although every parenteral cannula carries some risk of infection, the relative risk is greater with plastic catheters than with small steel needles; with long catheters than with short ones; and with central rather than with peripheral lines. Synthetic catheters induce the formation of a fibrin sheath around the intravascular portion of the device within 24 to 48 hr of placement. Microorganisms migrating down the transcutaneous cannula tract multiply within the sheath protected from antibiotics and host defenses.[109] Fibrin sheath formation does not occur with steel needles.

The duration that the device remains in place has a direct influence on the risk of bacteremia. Few devices produce sepsis until they have been left in place for at least 48 hr. However, in most studies, the rate of sepsis sharply increases when a peripheral cannula remains in place for over 48 hr. Peripherally placed plastic catheters are probably more hazardous because they are left in place for longer periods. In neutropenic and immunocompromised cancer patients, even steel needles are associated with significant risk of sepsis when the needle remains in place for more than 72 hr. A large, prospectively randomized study that evaluated infusion-related sepsis with steel needles and small Teflon catheters in 954 cannula insertions, found that catheters posed no greater risk of infection if inserted under aseptic conditions and removed within 72 hr.[107] Therefore, unless extenuating circumstances exist, it is widely advocated that all peripheral intravenous catheters should be replaced at least every 72 hr.[109,160] Data from a randomized trial performed in 487 patients have demonstrated that the risk of extrinsic contamination of IV fluids from the administration sets is low ($<3\%$) and that it is unnecessary to replace the administration set more frequently than every 72 hr.[255]

Catheter-related infections can be divided into two types. The first includes infections that present with local tenderness or erythema at the exit site or the subcutaneous tunnel without evidence of sepsis. These infections generally resolve with antibiotic therapy without catheter removal. The second type of catheter-related infection is associated with clinical evidence of bacteremia and requires catheter removal. Clinical features of catheter-related sepsis are indistinguishable from bacteremias arising from other sites. In granulocytopenic patients, classic signs and symptoms of overwhelming sepsis are often masked until the precipitous onset of shock. If a patient with a central venous line develops a fever without an obvious source of infection, blood cultures should be drawn peripherally and from the line; then empiric treatment with broad-spectrum IV antibiotics should be instituted immediately. The persistence of a fever or the appearance of clinical signs of sepsis, despite antibiotic therapy, warrants additional blood cultures, catheter removal, and culture of the catheter tip.[109,259] In those clinical situations in which the catheter is not judged to be the primary source of infection, the existing catheter may be exchanged for a new one over a guide wire.[260] If the culture of the old catheter is positive, the new catheter, in the old, presumably infected tract is immediately removed. Conversely, if the cultures are negative, it is possible to exclude the device as the cause of infection without subjecting the patient to the risks of another subclavian catheter insertion. When in doubt, take it out.

As previously noted, synthetic catheters are associated with the development of a fibrin sheath that forms within 24 to 48 hr of insertion.[109] Microorganisms can multiply within the sheath, protected from host defenses and antibiotics. Septic or suppurative phlebitis, the most serious form of infusion-related infection, occurs most often after prolonged venous catheterization and can involve central veins in patients receiving parenteral hyperalimentation. The infected vein literally becomes an intravascular abscess that continually seeds the bloodstream with microorganisms, producing overwhelming and refractory sepsis that cannot be controlled without surgical excision of the affected vessel. The incidence of infectious complications with intra-arterial catheters also increases with time. Traumatic cannulation and the need to reposition the catheter increase the risk.[109] Local pain or inflammation, or clinical evidence of bacteremia in the absence of an obvious source warrant the removal and culture of an intra-arterial line.

Infusion phlebitis is an extremely common complication of intravenous infusions that is manifest by pain, erythema, tenderness, or a palpable inflamed and thrombosed vessel. Major factors contributing to the development of infusion phlebitis include cannula-catheter size and composition, the site of insertion, traumatic cannula insertion, trauma during insertion, vessel size and blood flow, mechanical irritation, irritating diluents and drug additives, particulate matter in the solution, the duration of infusion (most occur between 24 and 48 hr), hypertonicity, higher acidic or alkaline pH, concentration, and microbial contamination.[265-271] However, in about 20% of patients, infusion phlebitis is directly related to infection.[109] Given that it is associated with an increased risk of infusion-related septicemia, phlebitis should always be considered a potential sign and symptom of infection. Studies on the routine use of inline final filters provide conflicting data on the clinical efficacy and cost-effectiveness of these devices in reducing phlebitis related to contaminated and particulate matter introduced during admixture procedures.[266-271]

In patients receiving frequent infusions of IV chemotherapy, antibiotics, or other vascular irritants, infusion phlebitis is often a major care problem. Whenever patients complain of pain during an infusion, the site should be carefully inspected for obvious signs of infiltration or phlebitis (warmth, redness, and tenderness). If none are present, the infusion should be slowed and heat applied. If the discomfort is caused by venous spasm rather than phlebitis, local application of heat can relieve pain by dilating the vessel and increasing the blood flow.

Mechlorethamine frequently produces a severe chemical phlebitis and venous discoloration 1 to 3 days after administration, even when the agent is diluted by administering it as a slow bolus in a large vein which is rapidly being infused with an isotonic solution. Amsacrine (acridinylaniside;

AMSA), dacarbazine (DTIC), and carmustine (BCNU) also cause irritation of the vascular endothelium, and often produce venous spasm, severe pain, and evidence of thrombophlebitis during and after infusion. An attempt should be made to alleviate the pain by increasing the volume of fluid in which the agent is diluted and slowing the rate of infusion, because venous spasm can restrict blood flow and increase the likelihood of extravasation. Application of heat may also reduce discomfort.

Local hypersensitivity ("flare") reactions, manifested by urticaria, erythematous streaking, with or without localized pruritus, or pain, have been reported with at least four agents: mechlorethamine, doxorubicin, aclarubicin, and daunorubicin. Pain associated with this type of reaction is often a dull ache over the course of the vein as opposed to localized burning or stinging. Resolution of symptoms associated with local hypersensitivity reactions generally occur spontaneously within 30 min, and the agent can generally be administered in a new vein without the reaction recurring.

Although relatively infrequent, type I hypersensitivity reactions (anaphylaxis) can occur after the administration of an antineoplastic agent. Acute systemic reactions usually occur within minutes of exposure, and are characterized by dysphoria, agitation, dizziness, nausea, generalized pruritus, substernal chest discomfort or inability to speak, and dyspnea. These symptoms may be accompanied by local or generalized urticaria, angioedema, stridor, cyanosis, bronchospasm, or life-threatening hypotension and shock. L-Asparaginase and cisplatin are the two agents most commonly associated with hypersensitivity reactions. However, bleomycin, cyclophosphamide, doxorubicin, daunorubicin, etoposide (VP-16), methotrexate, topical mechlorethamine, IV melphalan, teniposide (VM-26), and zinostatin can cause hypersensitivity reactions.[272,273] If any of the foregoing symptoms are noted by the patient or nurse, the drug infusion should be terminated and the IV line should be maintained with saline in case drug therapy is required to manage the anaphylactic reaction. Emergency equipment should always be readily available to patients receiving parenteral chemotherapy.

Extravasation

Many antineoplastic agents have the potential for causing serious toxicity to local tissues if extravasated during parenteral administration.[45,278–288] Those that are listed in Table 64-3 are known to be tissue vesicants or have been reported to cause local irritation. Whenever venipuncture is traumatic or the position of the needle bevel is in doubt, it is always wise to infuse a sterile solution of normal saline or 5% dextrose and water (D5W) before the administration of chemotherapy, to ensure that the infusate is not extravasating into subcutaneous tissues. When there is doubt about the needle's placement in the vein, a rubber tourniquet should be tied around the extremity proximal to the venipuncture site. If the entire bevel of needle is in the vein, the rate of infusion will slow rapidly from the pressure exerted by the tourniquet. If the needle has penetrated the vessel wall and the infusion is extravasating, the flow rate will be unaffected by the tourniquet.

TABLE 64-3. Antineoplastics Agents That Are Vesicants or Local Irritants

Aclarubicin
Actinomycin-D
Amsacrine
BCNU
Bisantrene
Cisplatin
Dacarbazine
Daunorubicin
Doxorubicin
Estramustine phosphate
Etoposide
Mechlorethamine
Mithramycin
Mitoguazone
Mitomycin-C
Mitoxantrone
Streptozotocin
Teniposide
Vinblastine
Vincristine
Vindesine
Zinostatin
Zorubicin

If the needle is dislodged or the vein bursts during an infusion, infiltration and extravasation of the infusate into tissues can occur. Many chemotherapeutic agents, as well as other solutions that are hypertonic, or highly acidic or alkaline, can cause serious tissue damage if extravasated. While pain and burning are often early indicators of an infiltration, even the most potent tissue vesicants can extravasate without producing immediate symptoms. Any evidence of infiltration, (blanching, edema, unexplained slowing of the infusion rate, or loss of blood return) should be considered sufficient cause to interrupt an infusion when a solution containing chemotherapy is administered. Even if the agent is not a tissue vesicant, extravasation of the drug into tissues adversely affects drug absorption, reducing the potential therapeutic effect, and predisposes the area to infection. Factors that alter normal vascular anatomy and restrict or obstruct normal blood flow increase the risk of extravasation. Risk factors should be considered when selecting a site for venipuncture when vesicants are to be administered.

Estimates on the overall incidence of extravasation of antineoplastic agents range between 0.1% and 6%.[278–288] However, the true incidence of drug extravasation and the local tissue damage that is produced are difficult to ascertain from the literature because many of the data are gleaned from small series and anecdotal case reports. As the use of indwelling Hickman catheters and subcutaneously implanted ports and pumps has increased, reports of extravasations have begun to appear in the literature. Although it is not possible to assess the risk of extravasation with infusion devices, recent reports emphasize the need for staff, patients, and families to carefully monitor implanted devices for malfunctions during infusions and to pay special attention to securing the position of the Huber needle in the rubber septum, particularly in sleeping patients.[222–224,289] Drug extravasations complicated five of ten continuous infusions in outpatients with implanted ports in one case report.[289] Despite that none of the agents was a known vesicant, all five extravasations caused substantial local tissue damage; three were severe enough to require port removal. A 6% rate of extravasation complicated the use of infusion devices in 211 port placements.[222] Six were caused by displacement of the Huber needle from the septum; one was a pocket extravasation caused by the separation of the port from the catheter; the others were due to retrograde extravasation following the development of a catheter tip thrombus.

Extravasation injuries are divided into two categories: those that are caused by agents that do not bind to nucleic acids and those caused by agents that do.[287,290] Agents, such as doxorubicin, that bind to tissue nucleic acids, cause immediate tissue damage similar to a burn injury. Because the agent remains in the infiltrated tissues, it continues to cause injury. Progressive tissue damage, manifested by enlarging ulcers, presumably occurs as drug complexes are released locally by necrotic cells and are taken up by healthy cells.[281] High doxorubicin concentrations have been identified in tissues surrounding an extravasation for as long as 5 months.[291–293] Agents such as vinca alkaloids, that do not bind to nucleic acids, also cause immediate tissue damage. However, metabolism, inactivation, or drug egress permit repair mechanisms to operate normally.

The degree of local tissue injury after the extravasation of doxorubicin varies from mild erythema, with induration and pain, to severe necrosis of the skin and subcutaneous tissues, with progressive involvement of underlying vessels and tendons that requires surgical excision and skin grafting and, in extreme cases, amputation.[278–288] Nerve compression syndromes, contractures, and infectious complications are also common. One series has reported a 59% incidence (20/34) of sepsis from microorganisms cultured from the extravasation site.[283] Early and complete surgical excision of all doxorubicin-containing tissues can relieve pain, reduce morbidity, preserve function, and is widely advocated in patients who develop anthracycline-induced ulcerations.[282–287]

A variety of compounds have been proposed as pharmacologic antidotes based on their chemical structure or a hypothetical interaction that would neutralize the toxic interaction. Although tissue damage appears to be dose-dependent, relatively little is known about the biochemical mechanisms that actually produce local tissue damage or could counteract a specific vesicant's toxic effects. In addition, it is often difficult to firmly establish when the extravasation began or to quantify the amount of drug that has actually infiltrated. These uncertainties complicate the interpretation of clinical data on extravasation.

Most experimental data on the management of extravasation come from studies of doxorubicin in the mouse, the rat, and the pig. Anatomic similarities between pig and human skin lend particular credence to the pig as a model. However, extensive testing in these animals has been precluded by their size and expense. Differences between rodent and human skin make extrapolation of data on the efficacy of antidotes tested in these animals to the human situation difficult. Rodents have a thin muscle layer adherent to the skin that provides a blood supply to the skin, the panniculus carnosus. Although necrosis is produced consistently when doxorubicin is injected into rodent skin above the panniculus carnosus, tissue toxicity often does not progress as it does in human tissues.[294] In addition, large lesions that eventually heal in rodents do not heal in humans.

Compounds that have been evaluated as pharmacologic antidotes in animal models include sodium bicarbonate, corticosteroids, propranolol, isoproterenol, *N*-acetylcysteine, glutathione, lidocaine, bupivacaine, hyaluronidase, diphenhydramine, cimetidine, α-tocopherol, dimethyl sulfoxide (DMSO), and butylated hydroxytoluene (BHT); hyperbaric oxygen and topical heat and cold have been tested as well.[294–317] Potential antidotes are generally evaluated for reduced ulcer formation and the speed with which lesions heal after an intradermal injection of a specified doxorubicin dose and concentration.

Local injections and topical application of corticosteroids have been reported to reduce doxorubicin-induced tissue toxicity in patients.[280,318–322] However, doxorubicin-damaged tissues reveal ischemic necrosis rather than inflammatory changes on histologic examination, data that do not lend support for the use of anti-inflammatory agents.[283,323] Although one study in the mouse model showed a decrease in ulcer size with low doses of intradermal hydrocortisone, large doses did not prevent local toxicity and were inherently toxic to the skin.[296] Subsequent studies in rats, mice, and pigs have failed to demonstrate significant benefit from hydrocortisone, and some have suggested that intradermal injections can increase toxicity.[287,290,297,301,311,316,324] It is possible that the benign course that has been reported in patients treated with steroids reflect the relatively indolent natural history of extravasation with small doses of doxorubicin.

Data on the protective effects of sodium bicarbonate are anecdotal.[318,325,326] The rationale for its use was based on data that suggested that DNA and tissue binding was pH-dependent and required an acidic environment. Although dermal necrosis was reduced in one study with rats, subsequent studies in mice and rats have been inconclusive, negative, or associated with necrosis.[287,298,301,316] Recent data suggest that increasing the pH from 5 to 8 with sodium bicarbonate may actually increase the cellular uptake of anthracyclines and enhance cytotoxicity.[327] Extravasation of sodium bicarbonate (4.2% and 8.4%) has been reported to cause tissue necrosis in patients.[287,328]

Protective effects have also been reported for the topical use of the free-radical scavenger, dimethyl disulfoxide (DMSO), with and without α-tocopherol, in pigs and rats. The rationale for the use of these agents presumes that drug-induced damage is related to hydroxyl radical formation that can be decreased by free-radical scavengers. Interest in DMSO stems from its rapid absorption into skin after topical application. Topical application of DMSO for 7 days significantly reduced or prevented doxorubicin tissue toxicity in rats and pigs.[290,303,304,310,317] Topical DMSO was well tolerated in mice but did not reduce ulcers when used with or without α-tocopherol.[309] However, another study suggests that topical DMSO does reduce local tissue toxicity caused by daunorubicin extravasation in mice.[290]

Clinical reports on 12 patients have also suggested that topical DMSO (70%–100%) for 2 to 14 days alone or in combination with topical α-tocopherol (eight patients) or 2 to 5 ml of 8.4% sodium bicarbonate (four patients) exerted a protective effect in these 12 patients, none of whom developed ulcers, after the extravasation of ulcerogenic amounts of doxorubicin, daunomycin, or mitomycin.[325,326] The only toxic effect of DMSO was transient skin irritation. Further clinical investigation appears warranted. Butylated hydroxytoluene (BHT), another free-radical scavenger, has also significantly reduced doxorubicin-induced ulcerations in mice and rats.[312,315,316]

Experimental data in the mouse suggest that the topical application of cold significantly reduces doxorubicin-induced local tissue damage, and that heat enhances toxicity.[313] These results are consistent with experimental data that demonstrate that heat increases the effect of doxorubicin in experimental tumor systems, and that cytotoxicity is reduced in cell lines that are cooled before doxorubicin exposure.[330,331] Local cooling for 60 min produced statistically significant reductions in induration, erythema, and ulceration. The degree of benefit was duration-dependent. Local toxicity was reduced, even if cooling was delayed, as long as the cooling was maintained for at least 45 min. Equivocal results have been reported by others.[312,315] However, a controlled study in pigs has suggested that local cooling reduced ulcer size and speeded the healing of doxorubicin-induced lesions more effectively than did topical DMSO.[317] This study confirmed that the degree of protection could be correlated to the duration that cold was applied. The application of ice packs for 10 hr on the first day and then four times daily for 20 min on days 2 through 7 was more effective than a single 10-hr application of cold. A clinical report has confirmed the effectiveness of topical cooling in 119 patients conservatively managed with immediate application of cold and elevation of the extremity.[286] Only 13 patients (11%) required surgical intervention. In 56 patients treated with a variety of other topical interventions by the same surgeon, 26 (46%) required surgery.[282,286] Experimental mouse data suggest that local cooling may reduce local toxicity from dactinomycin as well.[334]

Recently, a novel radical dimer [bi(3,5-dimethyl-5-hydromethyl-2-oxomorpholin-3-yl); DHM3], that reacts with doxorubicin in vitro to produce an insoluble and pharmacologically inactive compound (7-deoxydoxorubicin aglycone) has been shown to reduce ulcer size by 80% and healing time from 7 to 5 weeks after doxorubicin extravasation in weanling swine.[324,332] DHM3 also reduces local tissue toxicity from mitomycin-C. No clinical trial has been conducted.

MANAGEMENT OF EXTRAVASATION. Chemotherapeutic agents should be administered only by skilled individuals. A high index of suspicion, early detection with immediate drug discontinuation, and aspiration of residual drug from the tissues are all required to minimize local injury. When an antidote is to be administered intravenously after a drug extravasation, every attempt should be made to aspirate any residual drug remaining in the needle, tubing, and tissues before administration of the antidote. If no antidote will be given, the needle should be removed, the incident carefully documented, and the area closely observed for progressive tissue damage. As new data become available, recommendations may change. Therefore, it is essential for those administering vesicants to remain current with the literature on the management of extravasation. Current guidelines include:

Anthracyclines. The recommended treatment for anthracycline extravasation is the topical application of cold to the area for 20 min every 6 hr for 3 days, elevation, and close observation. Evidence of ulceration warrants prompt surgical intervention. The duration of local cooling and benefit is currently being addressed by an ECOG clinical trial that is randomizing patients with doxorubicin extravasations to local cooling for 24 hr with or without intermittent cooling every 6 hr for 7 days.[333] The use of DMSO should be considered investigational given current data.

Mitomycin. Experimental and clinical data suggest that topical application of DMSO reduces local tissue toxicity from extravasated mitomycin.[324,329,335] Like the anthracyclines, mitomycin extravasation often produces progressive local tissue toxicity that requires surgical intervention.[336–339] Use of DMSO should be considered investigational.

Mechlorethamine. Although mechlorethamine rapidly alkylates protein and DNA, it is not recycled locally because of metabolic degradation. Isotonic sodium thiosulfate (0.17 molar), an alkaline solution that is well tolerated locally, provides an alternative substrate to tissue alkylation. Its use is recommended by the manufacturer based on experimental data and one case report of an accidental intramuscular injection of mechlorethamine (Mustargen) successfully treated with sodium thiosulfate.[340,341] The antidote is prepared by mixing 4 ml of 10% sodium thiosulfate with 6 ml of sterile water. Experimental data in mice suggest that sodium thiosulfate may also reduce dacarbazine-induced local toxicity.[342]

Vinca Alkaloids. Experimental data support the administration of hyaluronidase as an effective antidote in the management of vinca alkaloid (vincristine, vinblastine, and vindesine) and epipodophyllotoxin (VP16 and VM26) extravasations.[305,308,314] Hyaluronidase (500–1000 units), injected directly into the extravasation site, dilutes the vesicant drug, promotes the absorption of these drugs from local tissues, and significantly decreases local tissue toxicity.

RISK ASSESSMENT ASSOCIATED WITH HANDLING ANTINEOPLASTIC AGENTS

Many antineoplastic agents are known to be mutagenic, teratogenic, and carcinogenic. Although mutagenic activity does not directly correlate with carcinogenicity, 83% to 89% of known carcinogens are mutagenic when tested in short-term assays using bacterial strains in the salmonella/mammalian microsomal mutagenic assay developed by Ames.[343,344] A letter published in the *Lancet* in 1979 reported that significant levels of mutagenic activity could be detected in the urine of nurses preparing chemotherapeutic agents and in the urine of patients receiving the drugs, although mutagenic activity could not be detected in the urine of unexposed control subjects working in the same general environment.[345] These data and subsequent reports of increased urinary excretion of mutagenic substances by health care workers involved in admixture procedures and unusual symptoms attributed to antineoplastic drug exposure have led to increased concern about health risks associated with drug handling during admixture procedures.[346-359] Symptomatic complaints that include lightheadedness, dizziness, facial flushing, nausea, headaches, hair loss, nasal sores, rash, vomiting, and malaise are, for the most part, derived from case reports or uncontrolled studies. In addition, two studies have reported an increased risk of fetal loss in personnel handling antineoplastic agents during the first trimester of pregnancy.[355,360]

Evidence that systemic drug absorption has occurred has been inferred from the presence of increased levels of urinary mutagens in exposed workers, compared with unexposed controls, as shown by the Ames test or a similar assay or by detecting intact drug in blood or urine.[343-355] However, not all investigators have detected evidence of systemic exposure with these assays.[361-366] Assays from nonsmoking nurses who administer but do not prepare antineoplastic agents have generally been negative, although one study has reported positive urine mutagenicity studies in nurses who only administered parenteral antineoplastic agents.[355,365] The interpretation of conflicting data is complicated by the small sample numbers; uncertainties about the sensitivity of the assays; concerns about differences in assay procedures and the collection, processing, and storage of samples; and significant differences in the admixture procedures used at each site. Attempts to measure exposure through chromosomal aberrations and sister chromatid exchanges induced in peripheral lymphocytes have been performed in health care workers handling antineoplastic agents. Several studies have reported a slight increase in the induction of sister chromatid exchanges in personnel handling antineoplastic agents.[367-369] However, negative findings have been reported by others.[349,353,370]

A critical problem in data interpretation is the failure of many studies to rule out the effects of cigarette smoking. A striking association between cigarette smoking and increased urinary excretion of mutagenic substances, as well as an increase in sister chromatid exchanges, has been documented in a number of studies.[371-377] Dietary factors and certain medications can also increase the urinary excretion of mutagenic substances. Of the studies that have evaluated smoking among study subjects, two have found significant increases in the urinary excretion of mutagens in exposed personnel after adjustment for smoking habits, although in one study the increase in urinary mutagens was statistically significant only for nurses who had handled alkylating agents, nitrosoureas, mitomycin, or cisplatin on the day of the collection.[354,355] Other reports indicate that, although exposed workers who smoke had increased urinary mutagens, urine mutagenicity or chromosomal abnormalities in nonsmoking exposed workers were not statistically different from unexposed nonsmoking controls.[348,353,354,366]

Exposure during preparation or administration may occur by direct contact, through transdermal absorption or ingestion (through unwashed hands), or by inhalation of aerosols. Cyclophosphamide has been detected in the urine of individuals who have permitted small amounts to be applied to their skin.[351] Assays of air samples taken from inside a laminar airflow hood and from the ambient air of a drug preparation area not equipped with laminar airflow hoods have detected appreciable drug levels that are eliminated when a vertical-flow air hood is utilized.[378-380] Data on the permeability of gloves and protective apparel indicate that latex and polyvinyl chloride gloves and disposable protective garments made of nonporous polymers offer limited protection against contact exposure, as determined by mutagenicity and chemical assays.[381,382] Cloth laboratory coats and disposable isolation gowns are completely absorbent. These data have led many institutions, and more recently, the U.S. Occupational Safety and Health Administration (OSHA) to recommend the use of class II vertical-flow safety cabinets and gloves as precautionary measures to minimize the risk of exposure.[383]

A number of studies that have not detected increased levels of mutagenic substances or intact drug in exposed health care workers, report the use of protective measures (masks, gloves, vertical-flow safety cabinets) by personnel during admixture and administration procedures.[361-366] The literature suggests, however, that although protective apparel and procedures have been adopted in pharmacies, they are not consistently employed by nurses.[355,359,365,384-391] This is not surprising because these measures are not easily implemented in office settings, and the cost of protective measures are not insignificant.[392,393] The cost of a class II vertical-flow safety cabinet is approximately 6700 dollars. The overall cost of protective measures (including the purchase of a safety cabinet) for a 704-bed VA facility with a comprehensive cancer treatment program was estimated at 57,115 dollars for 1 year.[393] Despite the reports that there is an increased risk of systemic drug absorption, especially in unprotected personnel, many nurses do not perceive themselves at risk. An evaluation of work practices by one investigator indicated that less than 20% of the 59 nurses interviewed had *ever* worn protective apparel for anything other than the preparation of mechlorethamine for parenteral use.[359]

Because the precise risk resulting from low-level exposure to these agents over a prolonged period is unknown, available data dictate prudence. To reduce systemic exposure during drug preparation and administration and during contact with patients who have been treated with antineoplastic agents, the following guidelines were issued by OSHA in January 1986 for the handling of antineoplastic drugs:[383]

1. Whenever possible, a special area should be set aside for the preparation of injectable agents. A class II vertical-flow biologic safety cabinet (BSC) should be used. Open-faced horizontal-flow laminar air hoods are not recommended because contaminated air is blown out at the operator.[346,394] If a vertical-flow BSC is not currently available, a respirator with a high-efficiency filter provides the best protection until one can be installed. Surgical masks do not protect against the breathing of aerosol. Therefore, if a BSC is not available, a plastic face shield or splash goggles should be worn. Eating, drinking, smoking, applying

cosmetics, and storing food in or near the area should be forbidden.

2. A disposable plastic-backed sheet of absorbent paper should be used to cover the work surface inside the cabinet to allow complete cleanup of inadvertent spills. The paper should be changed after any overt spills.
3. Surgical latex gloves should be used. Latex gloves have been found to be less permeable to most chemotherapy drugs than polyvinyl chloride. Powdered gloves should never be used. A double layer of gloves is less permeable. Double-gloving is advised if it does not interfere with proper technique.[381] Because permeability of gloves increases with time, hourly glove changes are recommended. Gloves should be discarded whenever torn or punctured. A long-sleeved disposable gown should be worn to protect the skin from drug contact.
4. Drug ampules should be opened away from the face. The ampules should be wrapped with sterile gauze at the anticipated breakpoint to minimize the risk of inhaling powders or aerosols and to protect against broken glass.
5. When reconstituting a drug, the diluent should be injected slowly down the side of the vial. The needle should be kept from coming in contact with the solution.
6. A sterile alcohol swab should be placed over the needle as it is withdrawn from a vial to prevent aerosolization.
7. The needle should be covered by a vacuum vial or sealed waste bottle when air bubbles are ejected from a filled syringe to prevent aerosolization. If done at the bedside, gauze in a plastic bag should be used as a receptacle.
8. After reconstitution, the old needle should be replaced by a new one. A volume of air that is less than the volume of solution to be withdrawn should be introduced into the vial. Excess solution should be injected into a waste bottle.
9. The external surface of syringes and IV bottles should be wiped clean after reconstitution or admixture procedures, labeled, and dated.
10. All syringes and needles used in the course of preparation should be placed in the puncture-proof container for disposal. The container should be placed in a cytotoxic drug container bag and disposed of in accordance with the hospital's toxic-waste disposal procedures.
11. For administration of antineoplastic agents, a gown and latex gloves should be worn. Although a mask may also be used, it provides minimal protection against aerosols compared with a vertical-flow BSC. Proper technique should be used for optimal protection.
12. Personnel caring for patients who have received chemotherapy within the last 48 hr should wear surgical latex gloves and disposable gloves when handling blood, vomitus, or excreta from that patient. Gloves and gowns should be discarded after use.
13. Hands should be washed carefully after gloves have been removed.

The creation of satellite pharmacies for ambulatory care clinics where drugs are mixed by pharmacists in laminar airflow cabinets has reduced the need for nurses to mix IV medications, ensures the sterility of solutions, minimizes delays, and enables nurses to spend more time educating patients about their therapy and the measures that should be taken to prevent or manage potential side-effects. The presence of a pharmacist in the clinic enables nurses to verify drug doses and dilutions directly and to resolve any questions about drug administration (*e.g.*, potential drug interactions).

The disposal of antineoplastic drugs and contaminated materials is a potential source of drug exposure to support and housekeeping staff as well as other health-care personnel. To ensure that all materials are handled properly, each syringe and IV bottle sent to a clinic or an inpatient unit should be labeled with instructions indicating that the item should not be discarded on the unit but returned to the pharmacy for proper disposal. The Clinical Center of the NIH has adopted a policy of disposing of all such materials under the guidelines used for the disposal of hazardous wastes.[395] Needles, syringes, empty drug vials and ampules, gloves, used alcohol swabs, are carefully packaged in leak proof puncture-resistant containers and incinerated in an on-site incinerator. Bottles of unused IV solutions and partially filled drug vials and syringes are disposed of in land internment facilities approved by the Environmental Protection Agency. Because the ultimate fate and the effect of introducing these drugs into the environment by disposing of them with incineration and the use of landfills are not known, the NIH is committed to further investigation into disposal options.

INFORMED CONSENT

Although primary responsibility for obtaining informed consents rests with the physician, it is a legal and ethical responsibility shared by nurses, who therefore must be knowledgeable about its components.[397–401] These elements are outlined in Chapter 19, *"Design and Conduct of Clinical Trials."* The exact role that the nurse plays in this process varies depending on the practice setting, the level of responsibility of nurses in that practice, whether the treatment is standard or investigational, and institutional policies. To ensure that a consent is truly informed and voluntary, nurses should assess the patient's understanding about the proposed treatment plan, the potential benefits and risks, and the therapeutic alternatives, especially if the therapy is investigational. Protecting the patients' rights of self-determination is a fundamental component of the nurse's role as a patient advocate, a responsibility that involves concern for the patients' rights, insight into their concerns, and a willingness to act independently on their behalf to resolve problems.[399–404] Although most physicians encourage patients to ask questions about the proposed procedure or treatment, it is often difficult for the physician to determine if the patient understood the explanation or to identify areas of conflict. The anxiety that is experienced by a patient during this process can compromise comprehension. A trial to evaluate patient comprehension of information provided during the consent process, found that patients given several days to digest information understood the information significantly better than those who gave consent immediately, suggesting that in situations for which treatment does not have to begin immediately, patient comprehension appears to improve when written consent is postponed until that patient has time to absorb the information provided about the proposed therapy.[404] A nurse who can explore the patient's feelings about the therapy that has been proposed can serve as an information liaison and communicate misunderstanding and concerns to the physician.

Because informed consent must be maintained to be valid, it is an ongoing process. Therefore, it is essential to consider the nurse's ethical responsibilities relative to consent within the framework of patient education. At the outset of any educational program, the nurse should assess the nature of the patient's previous health care experiences, identify exactly what the patient knows, what the patient thinks that he needs to know or learn, and his level of anxiety. Only by identifying the patient's perceived needs can a teaching/learning program be designed that will actively involve the patient. Explanations should be simple, concise, provided in a language and manner that the patient can comprehend, and supplemented by written information that can be shared with family members and saved for future reference. Written information should also contain the names and telephone numbers of persons who can be contacted for supplemental information or assistance during the course of treatment. Patients should be encouraged to write down any questions as they occur for later discussion. Education about the proposed therapy should also provide specific information about exactly how the treatment will be administered. This information should be reiterated and supplemented on a regular basis. The educational process should encourage the development of a continuing dialogue between the patient, the family, and all of the care-givers to foster the development of realistic goals and expectations.[401-407]

By developing educational materials that help patients understand why certain procedures and treatments are being used, the nurse can assist patients to become actively involved in their care and treatment. When primary physicians change frequently, the knowledge and experience of nurses assume even greater importance because they ensure that the quality and continuity of care are maintained during transitions. This is especially important for patients who are managed as outpatients and must assume major self-care responsibilities.[402,403]

SURGERY

Changes in the philosophy of the surgical management of cancer patients have produced noticeable changes in traditional surgical nursing care. Because many cancer patients admitted to a hospital for surgical procedures will ultimately receive multimodal treatment, surgical nurses must be knowledgeable about the fundamentals of medical oncology, radiotherapy, and immunology, as well as about surgical and critical care nursing.[408,409]

Preoperative Preparation

Preparing patients for their operations is a responsibility shared by the surgeon, anesthesiologist, and the surgical nursing staff. Because patients and families often need clarification about the ramifications of surgical procedures, lines of effective communication must be established by team members. Preoperative teaching, coordinated by the patient's primary nurse, should evaluate the patient's perceptions about what the operation involves, supplementing and reinforcing information as required. Nursing care during the preoperative period focuses on the reduction of surgical morbidity and the education of patients about the postoperative period. This requires a thorough understanding of the patient's diagnosis and stage, of the proposed treatment plan, and a knowledge of the patient's physical and laboratory examinations.

Risk assessment for surgical morbidity should include the identification of potential problems that may complicate wound healing, and physical, psychological, and sexual rehabilitation. Information about preoperative radiotherapy or chemotherapy, as well as nutritional status and medications that the patient is taking, can provide predictive data and should be obtained through a nursing history. Aspirin, anticoagulants, antihypertensives, hormones, antibiotics, chemotherapy, and steroids can contribute to surgical risk, as can a history of alcohol, tobacco, or drug dependence.[410] Meticulous oral care, taught preoperatively, can significantly reduce infectious complications in the oral mucosa of the patient having head and neck surgery.

To prepare patients for physiologic changes after the surgical procedure, the nurse should encourage patients to express fears about deformity and loss of control, because these represent serious threats to the patients' self-images and their self-esteem. Patients should also be encouraged to express their fears concerning what the surgical procedure will reveal in terms of prognosis and treatment. By allowing patients and families to express these fears, the nurse can identify needs that should be addressed by the care and treatment plan. Temporary and permanent alterations in body functions should be reviewed before surgery, and the purpose of Foley catheters, tracheotomy tubes, and colostomy or other wound drainage systems should be discussed.[410-415] When a stoma will be required, an enterostomal therapist can provide valuable input on site selection. For postoperative management, the site should be visible to the patient.

If monitoring devices will be required in the postoperative period, the patient should be taught, before the surgery, how they function so that anxiety in the surgical intensive care unit is minimized. Because the risk of cardiac and pulmonary complications are increased in patients with preexisting cardiovascular disease, they should be taught respiratory exercises and how to breathe with the ventilation devices before surgery. Time spent teaching deep-breathing and effective coughing can assist patients to perform respiratory exercises despite incisional pain. The availability of pain medications after surgery should be emphasized. Details concerning where the family can wait, when they can see the patient, and when they can talk to the surgeon should also be provided routinely.

Care After Surgery

In the immediate postoperative period, the prevention of complications in the surgical wound should be given priority. If skin flaps have been raised, tissue transferred, or free skin applied to the site, tissue viability must be maintained by assuring that drainage tubes sutured into the wound effectively remove blood, plasma, and air, and all suction tubes operate properly. Intact skin coverage is necessary to prevent infection, fistula formation, wound breakdown, and flap necrosis. Ensuring the viability of skin flaps requires regular assessments by skilled nurses. Tension and pressure on flaps should be avoided, and careful attention to positioning can improve circulation at graft sites.[411] The potential for hematoma or frank bleeding in the surgical wound must be recognized. The formation of a hematoma in the surgical wound, or frank brisk bleeding in the drainage tubing, demands surgical exploration and ligation of bleeding sites. Pressure dressings over amputation sites require frequent inspection for drainage and circulation. If the amputated stump is placed in an occlusive plaster dressing, the patient's signs and subjective symptoms must be monitored carefully.

The potential for development of postoperative complications in patients who have had radical head and neck explorations must be assessed.[412] Chyle leak, wound breakdown, and carotid artery rupture may necessitate emergency nursing interventions. Emergency equipment near the patient's bedside should include a tracheotomy tray, pressure dressings, and bull-dog clamps for hemorrhage control.[416,417] Visible chart flow sheets that provide critical physiologic, biochemical, and pharmacologic data for a 24 hr period must be readily available to the surgeon. Intake and output records must be designed to reflect the status of each separate drainage site.

If patients develop a wound complication, such as incision breakdown, infection, fistula, or frank necrosis of skin edges, the incision may be opened and allowed to heal by secondary intention. Debridement of grossly infected sites, followed by a systematic program of irrigation, has been identified as an effective technique for wound management. Hydrotherapy, using a showerhead, water pick, or whirlpool agitation, can aid in granulation of the wound.[418]

Normal hematologic defense mechanisms may be diminished or absent in the cancer surgical candidate. Temperature elevation, drainage, or erythema must be reported promptly. Compromise of host defense mechanisms in the cancer patients increase the likelihood of a nosocomial infection in the postoperative period. Length of hospitalization, disease status, and the number of invasive procedures performed preoperatively correlate directly with the frequency of infection.[414–419] Because the most frequent source of sepsis from nosocomial infection is the urinary tract, it is important to prevent postoperative bladder catheterization whenever possible. If indwelling catheters are necessary, sterile, closed catheter drainage systems minimize infectious complications. Because poor ventilation is a significant cause of infectious complications, deep breathing exercises and early ambulatory activity are considered essential.

Ostomy Care

The drainage from enterocutaneous fistulas must be isolated from the skin so that the highly alkaline or acid fluids will not excoriate the surrounding tissues. A skin barrier and adhesive bond are chosen to provide a leak-proof seal between the appliance and the skin. Techniques for skin care and pouching can be applied to feeding stomas such as esophagostomy and gastrostomy as well as colostomies, urinary diversions, and fistulas. Skin sealants such as Bard's Protective Barrier Film and United's Skin Prep around the drainage site may provide protection from maceration. Solid skin barriers (*e.g.*, Stomahesive or Premium Barrier) may be used around a fistula site alone or in conjunction with a pouch or dressing, depending on the volume of the drainage. In high-volume output fistulas, dressings may be contraindicated. For containment of drainage (to observe and measure the drainage), volume, odor control, and skin protection, pouching is the technique of choice.[420–424] Basic guidelines have been proposed by enterostomal therapists for managing these complicated surgical wounds, regardless of dimensions.[424]

- Cleaning and drying skin with a mild soap
- Use of a hypoallergenic adhesive: an adhesive collodion spray or cement, Stomahesive face plate, karaya ring
- Use of a skin barrier: Karayapaste, Stomahesive, silicone spray, gelatin-based pastes
- Use of a collecting pouch: many designs of odor-proof materials; most open at the bottom for emptying wastes and are disposable
- Securing pouch with hypoallergenic tape or use of a belt

Skin integrity should be maximized by excellent hygiene, protection from irritants, a well-fitted appliance, and testing all adhesives for skin sensitivity. Descriptions of pouching procedures are thoroughly detailed in most general surgical nursing and cancer nursing texts. The choice of an ostomy appliance is influenced by the nature of the drainage, anatomic considerations, and the patient's preferences and capacity for self-care. A variety of temporary and permanent appliances and supplies are available. Specific brands of materials may be selected by central supply departments in hospitals or the preference of enterostomal therapists in each institution.[420,422–425] Diet, irrigation, and medications can often be synchronized to achieve maximum bowel control. The level of control will vary with the type of surgical intervention. Nursing care goals include protection of the skin from urine or fecal contaminants and odor control. Not all colostomates can or should irrigate.

When a bowel enterostomy is made for primary control of a pelvic tumor, patients must adjust to permanent changes in bowel or bladder function.[420,422–425] A positive attitude and an effective teaching program can lead to confident self-care whether support is provided by a trained primary nurse or by consultation with an enterostomal therapist. Rehabilitation must be carefully planned and should involve an interdisciplinary team. Education must include detailed information and opportunities for practice sessions before discharge from the hospital to reduce the frustration of dealing with changes in elimination patterns. Sharing this information with a spouse or family member is often the most important contribution that a nurse can make to the patient's physical and emotional adjustments. When family members know what to expect, they can often modify home life to facilitate long-term rehabilitation. Visual teaching aids are often the best approach to conveying this information. Nurses should be prepared to discuss sexual concerns with patients and options for reconstructive surgery (*e.g.,* long bone replacement, penile implant, mammoplasty, vaginoplasty) to counsel patients about their options.[425–431] A detailed discussion of sexual issues is provided in Chapter 61, Section 2.

Before discharge, patients should be made aware of the ostomy association in their locality. Emotional support, education, and practical knowledge can be provided by members of the United Ostomy Association (UAO) who visit patients in hospitals and at home to share experiences, assist adaptation, and encourage patients and families to resume an active life after the surgery. Most patients can benefit from the continuity of care that community nursing services provide after hospitalization.

RADIATION THERAPY

Radiation plays a major role in the cure and palliation of many human cancers. It is the definitive treatment for many types of cancer and is commonly integrated into a multimodal approach to the primary treatment with surgery or chemotherapy. Because the major focus of the nursing care of cancer patients undergoing radiotherapy is education and symptom management, it is crucial for the nurse to be cognizant of the therapeutic intent. To anticipate the supportive care that the patient may need during and after radiation therapy, nurses must be knowledgeable about the principles of radiotherapy, the relationship between radiosensitivity and tissue tolerance, methods of administration, the onset and character of commonly encountered side-effects, the measures that can be taken to prevent or reduce morbidity, and the management of local and systemic toxicity.[432–444] In addition, the nurse should know whether the radiation will be administered alone or in combination with other treatment modalities.

Knowledge about normal tissue tolerance in the radiation field enables the nurse to anticipate the onset and severity of complications and to provide practical information about dealing with the adverse effects of the treatment to patients and their families.[442–451] Facts about the actual treatment techniques should be reiterated after the radiotherapist has discussed the treatment with the patient.[452–455] Information about the procedures that are employed to establish treatment portals, shield normal tissues, and maintain a correct position should be reviewed and supplemented as required. Because the administration of radiation generally requires isolation of patients during treatment, the nurse should orient the patient to the equipment that will be used before treatment is initiated whenever possible.[456]

Nurses also need to teach patients how to deal with the adverse effects of radiotherapy. Common symptoms include anorexia, dysphagia, esophagitis, xerostomia, nausea, vomiting, mucositis, diarrhea, and skin reactions.[457–466] To provide the patient with useful information, the nurse needs to be familiar with the onset, frequency, duration, and severity of side-effects that can be anticipated. Guidelines for symptom management are generally established by the radiotherapy department on the basis of institutional policies. Self-care measures taught by the nurse should be simple, easily carried out, and logical in relation to anticipated toxicities. They should be shared with family members when the patient will be managed as an outpatient. Education of patients in self-care can decrease avoidable morbidity and also assist patients to play an active role in their treatment.

The care of irradiated skin may vary from one institution to another and is usually outlined by a radiotherapy nurse. Generally, these instructions are written so the materials can be taken home, reread, shared with family members, and reinforced. A detailed discussion of the acute and chronic effects of radiotherapy on normal tissues can be found in Chapter 15 and throughout the book in the discussion of radiotherapy for specific tumors. Specific guidelines for dietary support are provided in Chapter 59, Section 1, and those for the amelioration of other adverse effects can be found in Chapter 60.

BIOTHERAPY

Scientific developments in immunotherapy and the expansion of clinical trials with biological agents have implications for changes in oncology nursing practice.[13,27,467–473] Nurses need to become better educated in basic immunology to plan nursing strategies to assist patients receiving these agents. In addition, they will need to be conversant in the biologic basis of these treatment regimens to educate patients and their families as well as their own peers. With understanding about the rationale for this investigative approach to cancer treatment, practical methods for dealing with the potential side-effects of these agents can be devised. There is a role for nurses administering the biologic agents to establish safe and efficient patient care procedures, patient assessment tools, and data collection methods in a standardized manner, so that accurate patient observations can be made and reported.[474–477] Because several of these therapies can be self-administered or given in outpatient facilities, patients need to be able to recognize and report toxicities. Careful preparation of the patient and his family can avoid complications and provide reassurance.

A variety of biologic agents are now being evaluated in Phase I and II clinical trials. Only one agent, interferon-α has been approved by the FDA for treatment of hairy cell leukemia and is commercially available to oncologists. Responses have been reported for a variety of tumors in studies with other biologic response modifiers, but their future place in cancer therapy is uncertain. These clinical trials have received much publicity, and it is important for nurses to remain abreast of the status of the trials so that they can respond to patient queries with a realistic perspective on the meaning of the results of the agent's therapeutic efficacy.

The application and evaluation of several nonspecific intradermal skin test antigens is frequently a responsibility assumed by nurses. Cell-mediated immune function can be evaluated in both the immunosuppressed cancer patient or the patient with AIDS. Nurses should be aware of the intention and expected results of their intervention and should be certain that authority for this practice has been specifically delegated to them through the institutions in which they are employed. Although the risks to the patient from anaphylaxis are small, precautions should be taken.

Intradermal injections of five common agents are given in the volar area of the forearms in adults and the paravertebral area in children. Ethyl chloride spray, a local anesthetic, can be applied immediately before the procedure. The skin tests are always performed in a consistent predetermined order, 3 to 4 cm apart. The skin surface is cleansed with alcohol. Each antigen is prepared in a separate tuberculin syringe and a small-gauge (25- to 27-gauge) needle is used. Common recall antigens usually include all or some of the following:

Trichophyton	1:30 dilution	Use 0.1 ml
Purified protein derivatives (PPD)	5 TU (intermediate)	Use 0.1 ml
Candida	1:100 dilution	Use 0.1 ml
Streptokinase–Streptodornase (SKSD)	75U	Use 0.05 ml
Mumps		Use 0.1 ml

Although some institutions measure the reactions more frequently, a reading at 48 hr is usually chosen for convenience.[478] An accurate recording of the area of induration is made in two dimensions. Reactions to recall antigens can be considered positive when the diameter measures more than 5 mm. When patients are provided instructions and appropriate measuring tools, it is feasible to have them read and report their own skin test results.[479] The nurse must then document these results so the physician will have these readings available for retrieval and interpretation.

In addition to assessing the immune response and evaluating skin tests, nurses who are administering new biologic agents frequently schedule blood specimen procurement and distribution of tissue samples for laboratory analysis. Immunocompetence and treatment must be assessed before initial therapy, during treatment, and after completion of the immunotherapy regimen. As program coordinator, the nurse can assure that the number of samples and the amount of blood drawn are not excessive and that the venipunctures required to evaluate the patient's immune system are coordinated, so that the patient suffers minimal discomfort.[474–476] Frequent x-ray studies and scans are ordered to monitor the patient's response to therapy and often require creative planning so that the patient is at the proper place, prepared to undergo the test.

Education of the patients and their families about the practical methods of dealing with the side-effects of these agents is as important a new role for the nurse as the responsibility of data collection for the evaluation of treatment efficacy.

Nurses must recognize that, unlike traditional medications, biologic agents can have very limited and unstable storage requirements. Patients who self-medicate with interferons or colony-stimulating factor, for example, must have refrigeration available for the proper storage of prefilled syringes or continuous infusion pump cartridges.

It is important that patients and their families receive instruction that some products are not standardized in their measurements and that variations exist between manufacturers, batches, and dosage units. As a rule, the side-effects of biologicals are dose-related and may be acute or chronic, but are usually limited to the time period during which the agent is being administered.[468]

Subjective side-effects can be severe and dose-limiting. Patient management is supportive with the liberal use of antiemetics and antidiarrheal agents. Acetaminophen (Tylenol) is used to control fever, but when chills begin, intravenous narcotic administration prevents the progression to full shaking rigors. Nurses have a major influence on improving patient comfort by anticipating patient needs, by encouraging small, frequent, nonirritating foods and beverages, and providing oils and cream lotions for relief of pruritus.[470–472]

Some unique neurologic and cardiovascular reactions have been seen, particularly with the use of interleukin-2. Sometimes patients need the care and skills of nurses in critical care areas for cardiac or hemodynamic monitoring. The problems of profound malaise and acute and chronic skin reactions seem universal for many biologicals for which supportive nursing measures have been explored, but for which there is also an obvious need for nursing research to identify effective strategies for nursing management.[468]

Apprehension and anxiety about treatment failure and their individual prognosis and suffering can become major problems for the patients in these treatment programs. Compliance with an extended course of adjuvant chemotherapy or immunotherapy when there may be no personal benefit can be difficult for patients. If nurses recognize these conflicts as potential problems, they can better assist patients to deal with their ambivalence with realistic expectations. In these situations, patient education must be reinforced with reassurance, encouragement, and support that will assist patients to reestablish a sense of control over their lives, and the door of hope can be kept open (absolutely essential for some patients) by the possibility of their participation in new and promising immunotherapeutic trials.[468–474]

CONTINUING CARE

Thorough discharge planning can facilitate adjustment and continued recovery, and is an important facet of patient rehabilitation.[480] Services that are coordinated by a knowledgeable oncology nurse can provide assistance to patients and their families and direct them to the appropriate community resources that are available to help defray the costs of continuing health-care services and rehabilitation.[480–486] Ideally, discharge planning should begin shortly after admission.[142] Realistically, it is often begun as the patients begin to recover and demonstrate that they no longer require hospitalization. Often a nurse is the discharge-planning coordinator who identifies community resources for home care. With strong support from a community-based visiting health care team, many patients can be cared for in the home, even when their physical needs are great. If discharge to the home is not feasible, the discharge coordinator must identify appropriate extended care facilities. When a patient's condition is deteriorating, a hospice or home-care program approach provide sensitive terminal care for patients. The types of resources available in any community and the roles played by nurses in placing patients into continuing home care programs vary widely.[482-502] Communication is essential to avoid gaps in the provision of services and duplication of efforts.

The financial cost of cancer to a family is, by no means, limited to medical expense. Nonmedical, out-of-pocket expenses are major sources of anxiety because these expenses, unlike medical bills, are not reimbursable. Loss of income, or productivity because of absence from work for clinic or hospital visits, and the cost of transportation, food, or housing for lengthy outpatient treatment, child care expenses, and miscellaneous expenses, all make significant contributions to the financial cost associated with cancer treatment. Several studies reporting on the cost of cancer care have indicated that "out-of-pocket" expenses add 50% to the cost of disease-related care and consumed anywhere from 38% to 50% of gross family income.[503-505]

A major research interest of oncology nurses is the development of programs to optimize the care and treatment of homebound cancer patients. Most studies emphasize the importance of family members as the primary care providers and the role of nurses as care coordinators and consultants who assist families to identify and avail themselves of the community resources that are available to the homebound.[482-491] There is a continued need for nurses to conduct research on community-based home care programs to define care needs, the relationship between patient symptoms and family coping patterns, and to establish systems for monitoring the quality and cost-effectiveness of the care provided.[486-500] Although there is a growing sentiment that nursing care for the homebound should be covered on a fee-for-service basis, there is a need for research data that will demonstrate that skilled nursing services decrease the cost of care and significantly improve the quality of care that can be provided.

Insurance coverage for home health care services has been greatly expanded over the past several years by private insurers.[61-63,146,506-512] Although there are differences in reimbursement policies of private carriers and Medicare, most private carriers follow Medicare requirements to some degree. Although prior hospitalization is not always a prerequisite for home care coverage, patients must be homebound and in need of skilled nursing services. Nursing care must be ordered by a physician, be intermittent, reasonable and necessary, and follow an established treatment plan. In 1983, the Health Care Financing Administration (HCVA) approved coverage for medical supplies to include infusion pumps and any sterile supplies required for the maintenance of indwelling catheters if a vascular access/infusion device is required to administer chemotherapy.

Nurses delivering home chemotherapy must employ the same standards of practice for drug administration (*i.e.*, hydration, premedication, postadministration monitoring) that are utilized in more traditional settings, and they must be especially well prepared to manage acute drug reactions. The nurse must ensure that patients and their families are informed about the status of the disease, the nature and goal of therapy, technical aspects of home care that are associated with treatment (*e.g.*, catheter care, pump operations), the potential adverse effects of disease and the treatment, and how disease or treatment-related complications should be handled in the home setting.[23,45,130-137,142-146]

Oncology nurses have begun to utilize the expertise they have developed by collaborating with oncologists in clinical research to design and perform clinical trials to investigate new ways to reduce disease and treatment-related morbidity. Although close approximation between basic and clinical researchers may well simplify treatment in the future, the rapid evolution of new therapeutic concepts is likely to make the administration of cancer therapy increasingly complex in the short term, demanding an ever expanding base of knowledge and skills from nurses. The introduction of new techniques and devices as therapeutic tools, and the likelihood that some of the current crop of biologics will be incorporated into multimodal treatment regimens that may well include conventional antineoplastic agents, will most certainly require nurses who share responsibilities for the care and support of patients receiving these agents to continually augment their knowledge base and refine their clinical skills. Research performed by nurses and referenced in this chapter provides substantive evidence that they are continuing to break new ground and are playing key roles in the development, evaluation, and delivery of improved cancer care. Interventions developed by nurses involved in chemotherapy administration have done much to minimize morbidity and to improve the quality of life that patients achieve during therapy by ameliorating treatment-induced toxicities. Numerous creative approaches, such as relaxation, guided imagery, and play therapy, are undergoing evaluation as techniques to assist patients cope with the rigors of therapy without the use of drugs.[513-519] When effective, these interventions can increase feelings of control and psychological well-being, a benefit of no small significance that deserves clinical investigation by nurses.

The creation of the National Center for Nursing Research (NCNR) in 1985, under auspices of the Health Research Extension Act of 1985 (Public Law 99-158), offers the potential for developing a national resource to support nurses who wish to perform clinical research. Established as an integral component of the NIH, this Center was established to advance nursing knowledge and focus on studies of nursing intervention, procedures, delivery methods, and ethics of patient care.[520] This center will establish a program of grants and awards that will assist nurses to acquire the support to perform research designed to answer questions of concern to nurses and to complement biomedical research concerned with the cause and treatment of disease. Research innovation in nursing practice have been, and must continue to be, developed with systematic evaluation in improved outcome of patient care, enhanced patient satisfaction, and demonstrated cost-effectiveness.

REFERENCES

1. Hubbard SM: The role of the chemotherapy nurse in medical oncology. Proc ASCO 16:256, 1974
2. Hubbard SP, DeVita V: Chemotherapy research nurse. Am J Nurs 76:560–565, 1976
3. Hubbard SM: The practice of cancer nursing. Proc 2nd Natl Conf Cancer Nurs, pp 23–29. New York, American Cancer Society, 1977
4. Hubbard SM, Donehower M: The nurse in a cancer research setting. Semin Oncol 7:9–18, 1980
5. Hubbard SM: Clinical research and cancer nursing. Oncol Nurs Forum 8:17–23, 1981
6. Hubbard SM: Principles of clinical research. In Johnson BL, Gross J (eds): *Handbook of Oncology Nursing,* pp 67–92. New York, John Wiley & Sons, 1985
7. Hilkemeyer, R: A historical perspective in cancer nursing. Oncol Nurs Forum 9:47–56, 1982. (Reprinted in ONF (suppl) 12:6–15, 1985)
8. Gross J: Clinical research in cancer chemotherapy. Oncol Nurs Forum 11:59–64, 1986
9. Hubbard SM: Reflections on the oncology nurse's role in cancer therapy: Future challenges. Semin Oncol Nurs 3:154–158, 1987
10. Benoliel JQ: The historical development of cancer nursing research in the United States. Cancer Nurs 6:261–268, 1983
11. Grant MM, Padilla GV: An overview of cancer nursing research. Oncol Nurs Forum 10:58–69, 1983
12. Fernsler J, Holcombe J, Pulliam L: A survey of cancer research: January 1975–June 1982. Oncol Nurs Forum 11:46–52, 1984
13. Suppers VJ, McClamrock EA: Biologicals in cancer treatment: Future effects on nursing practice. Oncol Nurs Forum 12:27–32, 1985
14. Sexuality and Cancer. Semin Oncol Nurs 1(1):1–75, 1985
15. Cancer Pain. Semin Oncol Nurs 1(2):81–154, 1985
16. Nursing Management of Breast Cancer. Semin Oncol Nurs 1(3):155–227, 1985
17. Acute Complications of Cancer. Semin Oncol Nurs 1(4):230–306, 1985
18. Nutrition and Cancer. Semin Oncol Nurs 2(1):1–69, 1986
19. The Adolescent with Cancer. Semin Oncol Nurs 2(2):73–141, 1986
20. Cancer Prevention and Early Detection. Semin Oncol Nurs 2(3):145–224, 1986
21. The Ostomy: Colorectal, Urinary, and Gynecologic Cancer. Semin Oncol Nurs 2(4):227–292, 1986
22. Brachytherapy: Nursing Challenges. Semin Oncol Nurs 3(1):1–81, 1987
23. Current Concepts in Chemotherapy Administration. Semin Oncol Nurs 3(2):83–158, 1987
24. Nursing Care of the Patient with Lung Cancer. Semin Oncol Nurs 3(3):163–236, 1987
25. Symptom Distress Semin. Oncol Nurs 3(4):241–315, 1987
26. Biotherapy: Nursing Challenges. Semin Oncol Nurs 4(2):83–150, 1988
27. Abernathy E, Hood LE, Jassak PF: The new immunology: Helping the body heal itself. Am J Nurs 87:455–473, 1987
28. Personal communication. Oncol Nurs Soc 1988
29. Personal communication. Assoc Pediatr Oncol Nurs 1987
30. Torosian LC, De Stephano M, Dietrick-Gallagher M: Day gynecologic chemotherapy unit: An innovative approach to changing health care systems. Cancer Nurs 4:221–227, 1985
31. Clark M: A day hospital for cancer patients: Clinical and economic feasibility. Oncol Nurs Forum 13:41–45, 1986
32. Brown JK: Ambulatory services: Mainstay of cancer nursing care. Oncol Nurs Forum 12:57–59, 1985
33. Moseley JR, Brown JS: The organization and operation of oncology units. Oncol Nurs Forum 12:17–24, 1985
34. Tighe MG, Fisher SG, Hastings C: A study of the oncology nurse role in ambulatory care. Oncol Nurse Forum 12:23–27, 1985
35. Moldawer NP, Murray JL: The clinical uses of monoclonal antibodies in cancer research. Cancer Nurs 8:207–213, 1985
36. Wiley FM, DeCuir-Whalley S: Allogenic bone marrow transplantation for children with acute leukemia. Oncol Nurs Forum 10:49–53, 1983
37. Schryber S, LaCasse CR, Barton-Burke M: Autologous bone marrow transplantation. Oncol Nurs Forum 14:74–80, 1987
38. Viele CS, Dodd MJ, Morrison C: Caring for acquired immunodeficiency syndrome patients. Oncol Nurs Forum 11:56–60, 1984
39. Donehower MG: Malignant complications of AIDS. Oncol Nurs Forum 14:57–64, 1987
40. Brown ML: AIDS and ethics: Concerns and considerations. Oncol Nurs Forum 14:69–73, 1987
41. Outcome Standards for Cancer Nursing Practice. Pittsburgh, Oncol Nurs Soc 1979
42. Outcome Standards for Cancer Nursing Education: Fundamental Level. Pittsburgh, Oncol Nurs Soc 1982
43. Outcome Standards for Cancer Patient Education. Pittsburgh, Oncol Nurs Soc 1982
44. Outcome Standards for Public Cancer Education. Pittsburgh, Oncol Nurs Soc 1982
45. Cancer Chemotherapy: Guidelines and Recommendations for Nursing Education and Practice. Pittsburgh, Oncol Nurs Soc, 1984
46. Nevidjon B, Detrich J (eds): Implementing the ONS education standards. Oncol Nurs Forum 12:57–67, 1985
47. Kinney MR: Certification for specialty nursing practice. NITA 5:246–248, 1982
48. Steel JE: Getting our "C's" in order. Oncol Nurs Forum 12:88–89, 1985
49. Ziegfield CR (ed): Core Curriculum for Oncology Nursing. Philadelphia, WB Saunders, 1987
50. Guidelines for Assessing Continuing Education Programs. Oncol Nurs Forum 10:94–95, 1983
51. Moskowitz RZ: Long term continuing education programs in cancer nursing. Oncol Nurs Forum 13:89–95, 1986
52. Fernsler J (ed): Developing continuing education programs in cancer nursing. Oncol Nurs Forum 14:59–70, 1987
53. Piemme J: Oncology clinical nurse specialist education. Oncol Nurs Forum 12:45–48, 1985
54. McMillan S: Survey of graduate programs in cancer nursing. Oncol Nurs Forum 15:825–831, 1986
55. Chiaviello JM: Graduate education in pediatric oncology nursing. J Assoc Pediatr Oncol Nurse 4:47–49, 1987
56. Spross J: An overview of the oncology clinical nurse specialist role. Oncol Nurs Forum 10:54–58, 1983
57. Hamric A, Spross J (eds): The Clinical Nurse Specialist in Theory and in Practice New York, Grune & Stratton, 1983
58. Welch-McCaffrey D: Role performance issues for oncology clinical nurse specialists. Cancer Nurs 9:287–294, 1986
59. Arenth LM: The development and validation of an oncology patient classification system. Oncol Nurs Forum 12:17–22, 1985
60. Bednash GP: Federal funding for nursing education: Competition for federal dollars. Nurse Pract 12:15–18, 1987
61. Yasko JM, Fleck A: Prospective payment (DRGs): What will be the impact on cancer care? Oncol Nurs Forum 11:63–72, 1984
62. Bonorris JS, Kapuy-Carlos IE: Health care trends, DRGs and community hospital oncology units. Prog Clin Biol Res 216:183–190, 1986
63. Obtaining Third-Party Reimbursement: A Nurse's Guide to Methods and Strategies. Kansas City, American Nurses Association, 1984
64. Stanfill PH, McDonnell JW: Determining nursing costs: A strategy for professional survival. Oncol Nurs Forum 12:79–82, 1985
65. Yasko JM: The predicted effect of recent health care trends on the role of the oncology clinical nursing specialist. Oncol Nurs Forum 12:58–61, 1985
66. Makadon HJ, Gibbons MP: Nurses and physicians: Prospects for collaboration. Ann Intern Med 103:134–136, 1985
67. Prescott PA, Bowen SA: Physician–nurse relationships. Ann Intern Med 103:127–133, 1985
68. Ryan L, Edwards RL, Rickles FR: A joint practice approach to cancer care. Oncol Nurs Forum. 7:8–12, 1980
69. Koerner B, Armstrong D: Collaborative practice cuts costs of patient care: Study. Hospitals 58(10):52–54, 1984
70. Diers D, Hamman A, Molde S: Complexity of ambulatory care: Nurse practitioner and physician caseloads. Nursing Res 35:310–314, 1986
71. Crowley SA, Wollner IS: Collaborative practice: A tool for change. Oncol Nurs Forum. 14:59–63, 1987
72. Goldberg HI, Cohen DI, Hershey CO et al: A randomized controlled trial of academic group practice. JAMA 257:2051–2055, 1987
73. Yancik R: Frame of reference: Old age as the context for the prevention and treatment of cancer. In Yancik R (ed): Perspectives on Prevention and Treatment of Cancer in the Elderly. New York, Raven Press, 1983
74. Waskerwitz MJ, Leonard M: Early detection of malignancy: From birth to twenty years. Oncol Nurs Forum 13:50–57, 1986
75. White L: Cancer prevention and detection: From twenty to sixty-five years of age. Oncol Nurs Forum 13:59–64, 1986
76. Frank-Stromberg M: The role of the nurse in early detection of cancer: Population sixty-six years of age and older. Oncol Nurs Forum 13:66–74, 1986
77. Nevidjon B: Cancer prevention and early detection: Reported activities of nurses. 13:76–80, 1986
78. Lindberg SC: Adult preventive health screening. Nurse Pract 12:19–41, 1987
79. Burdman GDM, Benoliel JQ, Dohner CW et al: A focus on cancer: Development of a course on prevention and detection. J Cont Educ Nurs 18:93–96, 1987
80. Fraser MC: The role of the nurse in the prevention and early detection of malignant melanoma. Cancer Nurs 5:351–360, 1982
81. McGuire DB: Preventive health practices and educational needs in families with hereditary melanoma. Cancer Nurs 8:29–36, 1985
82. Jamison DS: Hereditary predisposition to cancer: Opportunities for early detection and prevention. Oncol Nurs 2:176–183, 1986
83. White LN, Faulkenberry JE: Screening by nurse clinicians in cancer prevention and detection. Curr Probl Cancer 9:1–42, 1984
84. du Toit JP: The role of the nurse in the early detection of cervical carcinoma in a developing country. Cancer Nurs 8:121–127, 1985
85. Roosevelt J, Frankl H: Colorectal cancer screening by nurse practitioner using 60-cm flexible fiberoptic sigmoidoscope. Dig Dis Sci 29:161–163, 1984
86. Schapiro M, Gillman L, Kerlin J et al: Flexible sigmoidoscopy by the GI assistant in the community. Gastrointest Endosc 27:138, 1981
87. Melillo KD: Who needs health maintenance? Teaching aged women to care about health prevention exams. J Gerontol Nurs:11–21, 1985
88. Love RR, Olsen SJ: An agenda for cancer prevention in nursing practice. Cancer Nurs 8:329–338, 1985
89. Love RR: Research in cancer prevention and screening: A community challenge. Health Care Financing Res 216:13–22, 1986
90. Hubbard SM: Cancer Treatment. In, Johnson BL, Gross J (eds): Handbook of Oncology Nursing, pp 21–65. New York, John Wiley & Sons, 1985

91. Garvey E, Kramer R: Improving cancer patients' adjustment to infusion chemotherapy: Evaluation of a patient education program. Cancer Nurs 6:373–378, 1983
92. Teich CJ, Raia K: Teaching strategies for an ambulatory chemotherapy program. Oncol Nurs Forum 11:24–28, 1984
93. Stromborg MF: Developing patient education materials. Oncol Nurs Forum 11:70–72, 1984
94. Battista EM: Educational needs of the adolescent with cancer and his family. Semin Oncol Nurs 2:123–125, 1986
95. Pagliaro AM: Preparation, administration, and monitoring of Medications. In Pharmacologic Aspects of Nursing, pp 30–67. St Louis, CV Mosby, 1986
96. Knobf, MK: IV therapy guidelines for oncology practice. Oncol Nurs Forum 9:30–34, 1982
97. Plumer AL: Principles and Practice of IV Therapy, 4th ed. Boston, Little, Brown & Company, 1987
98. Millam DA: A study of IV therapy education. NITA 8:393–407, 1985
99. Welsh-McCaffrey D: Rationale, development, and evaluation on a chemotherapy certification course for nurses. Cancer Nurs 8:255–262, 1985
100. The national IV therapy association standards of practice (IV and parenteral nutrition therapy). NITA 5:19–34, 1982
101. Spartanburg, General Hospital Policy Book on IV Therapy Administration. NITA 9:267–288; 9:252–384, 1986
102. Crudi C (ed.): Core Curriculum for IV Nursing, pp 1–186. Philadelphia, JB Lippincott, 1987
103. Blust JE, Commerton RN: Consideration for venipuncture: Selection, utilization and maintenance. NITA 3:238–241, 1980
104. Huff NL: Practical considerations in pediatric IV therapy. NITA 4:436–438, 1981
105. Streckfuss BL: Pediatric IV care. NITA 8:75–82, 1985
106. Pauley SY: A new generation of catheter: The third option. NITA 3:203–206, 1980
107. Tully JL, Friedland GH, Baldini LM et al: Complications of IV therapy with steel needles and Teflon catheters. Am J Med 70:702–706, 1981
108. Williams DN, Gibson J, Vos J, Kind AE: Infusion thrombophlebitis and infiltration associated with IV cannula types. NITA 5:379–382, 1982
109. Maki DG: Infections due to infusion therapy. Bennett JV, Brachman PS (eds): Hospital Acquired Infections, pp 561–580. Boston, Little, Brown & Co 1986
110. Millam D: Intermittent devices. NITA 4:142–145, 1981
111. Levitt DZ: Use of heparin lock on an outpatient basis. Cancer Nurs 4:115–119, 1981
112. Turco S: Heparin locks. Am J IV Ther Clin Nutr 1:78–79, 1983
113. Harrigan CA: Intermittent therapy without heparin: A study. NITA 8:519–520, 1985
114. Shearer J: Normal saline flush versus dilute heparin flush: A study of peripheral intermittent IV devices. NITA 10:425–427, 1987
115. Broviac JW, Cole JJ, Scribner BH: A silicone rubber atrial catheter for prolonged parenteral alimentation. Surg Gynecol Obstet 136:602–606, 1973
116. Hickman RO, Buckner CE, Cliff RA et al: A modified right atrial catheter for access to the venous system in marrow transplant recipients. Surg Gynecol Obstet 148:871–875, 1979
117. Meguid MM, Eldar S, Wahga A: The delivery of nutritional support. A potpourri of new devices and methods. Cancer 55:279–289, 1985
118. Reed WP, Newman KA, deJongh C et al: Prolonged venous access for chemotherapy by means of Hickman catheter. Cancer 52:185–192, 1983
119. Raaf JH: Two Broviac catheters for intensive long-term support of patients with cancer. Surg Gynecol Obstet 158:173–176, 1984
120. Legha SS, Haq M, Rabinowitz M et al: Evaluation of silicone elastomer catheters for long-term IV chemotherapy. Arch Intern Med 145:1208–1211, 1985
121. Raaf JH: Results from use of 826 vascular access devices in cancer patients. Cancer 55:1312–1321, 1985
122. Slater H, Goldfarb IW, Jacob HE et al: Experience with long-term outpatient venous access utilizing percutaneously placed silicone elastomer catheters. Cancer 56:2074–2077, 1985
123. O'Donnell JJ, Clague MB, Dudrick SJ: Percutaneous insertion of a cuffed catheter with a long subcutaneous tunnel for IV hyperalimentation: South Med J 76:1344–1348, 1983
124. Nidus BD, Speyer JL, Bottino J et al: Repeated femoral vein cannulation for administration of chemotherapeutic agents. Cancer Treat Rep 67:185–186, 1983
125. Troxel M, Mansour R: A new technique for placement of tunnelled subclavian right atrial catheters: Experience with 130 cases. J Clin Oncol 5:131–136, 1987
126. Warren J: The multi-lumen subclavian catheter. NITA 8:151–156, 1986
127. Pituk TL, DeYoung JS, Levin HJ: Volumes of selected central venous catheters: Implications for heparin flush use. NITA 6:98–100, 1983
128. Kaufman JL, Nissenblatt MJ: New options for central venous access in cancer chemotherapy: Multiple lumen catheters. Am Surg 52:105–107, 1986
129. Bjeletich J, Hickman RO: The Hickman indwelling catheter. Am J Nurs 80:62–65, 1980
130. Daeffler RJ, Lewinski J: Home care of the Hickman/Broviac catheter. Oncol Nurs Forum 9:59–63, 1982
131. Duval A, Hennessey K: Care of the Broviac catheter. NITA 6:40–42, 1983
132. Terry J: Home care utilizing Silastic catheters. NITA 6:348–350, 1983
133. Wilson JM: Right arterial catheters (Broviac and Hickman): Indications, maintenance and protocol for home care. NITA 6:23–27, 1983
134. Wilson JM, Schaeffer N, Nolan KR et al: Silicone catheters: Patient teaching pamphlet. NITA 7:169–172, 1984
135. Ford R: History and organization of the Seattle-area Hickman catheter committee. NITA 8:123–135, 1985 [Detailed care procedures provided]
136. Simon RC: Small gauge central venous catheters and right atrial catheters. Semin Oncol Nurs 3:87–95, 1987
137. Jenkins J: Parenteral chemotherapy. In Johnson BL, Gross J (eds): Handbook of Oncology Nursing, pp 535–566. New York, John Wiley & Sons, 1985
138. Howser DM, Meade CD: Hickman catheter care: Developing organized teaching strategies. Cancer Nurs 10:70–76, 1987
139. Patient Teaching Guide: Hickman or Broviac Catheter. Nursing Department, Clinical Center, NIH
140. Wainstock JM: Making a choice: The vein access method you prefer. [A patient education booklet] Oncol Nurs Forum 14:79–82, 1987
141. Standards of practice: Home IV therapy. NITA 7:93–95, 1984
142. Bledsoe L: Discharge planning for the home care IV therapy patient. NITA 8:486–487, 1985
143. Konstantinides NN: Home parenteral nutrition: A viable alternative for patients with cancer. Oncol Nurs Forum 12:23–29, 1985
144. Miller P: Home blood component therapy: An alternative. NITA 9:213–217, 1986
145. Pluth NM: A home care transfusion program. Oncol Nurs Forum 14:43–46, 1987
146. Garvey E: Current and future nursing issues in the home administration of chemotherapy. Semin Oncol Nurs 3:142–147, 1987
147. Fulton JS, Tischenko MM: Hickman catheter exit site skin sensitivities in an oncology patient population. NITA 8:63–68, 1985
148. Cook DA: Op-Site An alternative in IV dressings: A survey report. NITA 4:218–219, 1981
149. Curtas S, Grant JP: Evaluation of Op-Site as a total parenteral nutrition dressing. NITA 4:414–415, 1981
150. Haessler RM: Transparent IV dressing versus traditional dressings: An in service evaluation. NITA 4:169–171, 1981
151. Peterson PJ, Freeman M: Use of a transparent polyurethane dressing for peripheral IV catheter care. NITA 5:387–390, 1982
152. Gantz NM, Presswood GM, Goldberg R et al: Effects of dressing type and change interval on IV therapy complication rates. Diag Microbiol Infect Dis 2:325–332, 1984
153. Nicola M, De Chairo R: A transparent polyurethane membrane used as an IV dressing. NITA 7:139–142, 1984
154. Kelsey MC, Gosling M: A comparison of the morbidity associated with occlusive and non occlusive dressings applied to peripheral IV devices. J Hosp Infect 5:313–321, 1984
155. Powell CR, Traetow MJ, Fabri PJ et al: Op-Site dressing study: A prospectively randomized study evaluating povidone iodine ointment and extension set changes with 7-day Op-Site dressings applied to parenteral nutrition subclavian sites. J Parenter Enter Nutr 9:443–446, 1985
156. Popovsky MA, Ilstrup DM: Randomized clinical trial of transparent polyurethane dressings. NITA 9:107–110, 1986
157. Craven DE, Lichtenberg A, Kunches LM: A comparative evaluation of transparent polyurethane dressing to a dry gauze dressing for peripheral IV catheter sites. Infect Control 6:361–366, 1985
158. Ricard P, Martin R, Marcoux JA: Protection of indwelling vascular catheters: Incidence of bacterial contamination and catheter-related sepsis 13:541–543, 1985
159. Lawson M, Kavanagh T, McCredie K et al: Comparison of transparent dressing to paper tape dressing over central venous catheter sites. NITA 9:40–43, 1986
160. Maki DG, Ringer M: Evaluation of dressing regimens for prevention of infection with peripheral IV catheters JAMA 258:2396–2403, 1987
161. Lazarus HM, Lowder JN, Herzig RH: Occlusion and infection in Broviac catheters during intensive cancer therapy. Cancer 52:2342–2348, 1983
162. Lokich JJ, Bothe A, Benotti P, Moore C: Complications and management of implanted venous access catheters. J Clin Oncol 3:710–717, 1985
163. Schuman ES, Winters V, Gross GF, Hayes JF: Management of Hickman catheter sepsis. Am J Surg 149:627–628, 1985
164. Jacobs MB, Yeager M: Thrombotic and infectious complications of Hickman–Broviac catheters. Arch Intern Med 44:1597–1599, 1984
165. Jones PM: Indwelling central venous catheter-related infections and two different procedures of catheter care. Cancer Nurs 10:123–130, 1987
166. Wistbacka J, Nuutinen LS: Catheter-related complications of total parenteral nutrition (TPN). Acta Anaesthesiol Scand 29:84–88, 1985
167. Brismar B, Nystrom B: Thrombophlebitis and septicemia: Complications related to intravascular devices and their prophylaxis. A review. Acta Chir Scand (suppl) 530:73–77, 1986
168. Pessa ME, Howard RJ: Complications of Hickman–Broviac catheters. Surg Gynecol Obstet 161:257–260, 1985
169. Lawson M, McCredie KB, Bottino J: Use of silicone elastomer central venous catheters for IV therapy in cancer patients. NITA 4:245–249, 1980
170. Hurtubise MR, Bottino JC, Lawson M et al: Restoring patency of occluded central venous catheters. Arch Surg 115:212–213, 1980
171. Glynn MFX, Langer B, Jeejeebhoy KN: Therapy for thrombotic occlusion of long term IV alimentation catheters. J Parenter Enter Nutr 4:387–390, 1980
172. Hess H, Ingrisch H, Mietaschk A et al: Local low-dose thrombolytic therapy of peripheral arterial occlusions. N Engl J Med 307:1627–1630, 1982
173. Faubion WC: Ventral venous catheter occlusion treated by thrombolytic agents. Nutr Support Serv 3:24–26, 1983
174. Weinstein SM: Thrombolytic therapy. NITA 9:31–35, 1986
175. Rubin RN: Local instillation of small doses of streptokinase for treatment of thrombotic occlusions of long-term access catheters. J Clin Oncol 9:572–573, 1983
176. Fraschini G, Jadeja J, Lawson M: Local infusion of urokinase for the lysis of thrombo-

sis associated with permanent central venous catheters in cancer patients. J Clin Oncol 5:672–678, 1987

177. Carlson RW, Sikic BI: Continuous infusion or bolus injection in cancer chemotherapy. Ann Intern Med 99:823–833, 1983
178. Storc R: Current concepts in flow control. NITA 7:517–520, 1984
179. Ensminger WD, Gyves J: Regional cancer chemotherapy. Cancer Treat Rep 68:101–115, 1984
180. Mioduszewski J, Zarbo AG: Ambulatory infusion pumps: A practical view at an alternative approach. Semin Oncol Nurs 3:106–111, 1987
181. Jenkins J, Culnane M: The autosyringe infusion pump: A patient guide. Oncol Nurs Forum 11:87–91, 1984
182. Bender CM, Bast JF, Drapac D et al: Patient teaching in hepatic artery infusion. Oncol Nurs Forum 11:61–65, 1984
183. Bruera E, Brenneis C, MacDonald RN: Continuous SC infusion of narcotics for the treatment of cancer pain. Cancer Treat Rep 71:953–958, 1987
184. Gyves J, Ensminger W, Neiderhuber JE: A totally implanted system for IV chemotherapy for blood sampling and chemotherapy administration. JAMA 251:2538–2541, 1984
185. Brincker H, Saeter G: Fifty-five patient years' experience with a totally implanted system for IV chemotherapy. Cancer 57:1124–1129, 1986
186. Strum S, McDermed J, Korn A et al: Improved methods for venous access: The Port-A-Cath, a totally implanted catheter system. J Clin Oncol 4:596–603, 1986
187. Goodman M, Wickham R: Venous access devices: An overview. Oncol Nurs Forum 11:16–23, 1984
188. Winters V: Implantable vascular access devices. Oncol Nurs Forum 11:25–30, 1984
189. Hughes CB: A totally implantable central venous system for chemotherapy administration. NITA 8:523–527, 1985
190. Speciale JL: Infuse-A-Port: New path for IV chemotherapy. Nursing 15:40–43, 1985
191. Newton R, DeYoung JL, Levin HJ: Volumes of implantable vascular access devices and heparin flush requirements. NITA 8:137–140, 1985
192. Kilbride SS: A patient's guide to the implanted port. Oncol Nurs Forum 13:83–85, 1986
193. Moore C, Erickson KA, Yanes CB et al: Nursing care and management of venous access ports. Oncol Nurs Forum 13:35–39, 1986
194. Nieweg R, Greidanus J, de Vries EGE: A patient education program for a continuous infusion regimen on an outpatient basis. Cancer Nurs 10:177–182, 1987
195. Bagnall H, Ruccione K: Experience with a totally implanted venous access device in children with malignant disease. Oncol Nurs Forum 14:51–56, 1987
196. Skelton J, Leong S, Hathorn J et al: A prospectively randomized trial comparing externalized venous access Hickman catheter (HC) to a subcutaneously implanted Port-A-Cath (PAC) in cancer patients. Proc ICAAC, 1986
197. Perri J, Erikson KA: Nursing issues for hepatic arterial infusion therapy. Semin Oncol Nurs 10:191–198, 1983
198. Hagle ME: Implantable devices for chemotherapy access and delivery. Semin Oncol Nurs 3:96–105, 1987
199. Niederhuber JE, Ensminger W, Gyves JW et al: Totally implanted venous and arterial access system to replace external catheters in cancer treatment. Surgery 92:706–712, 1982
200. Lokich JJ, Perry J, Bothe A et al: Cancer chemotherapy via ambulatory infusion pump. Am J Clin Oncol 6:355–363, 1983
201. Keizer HJ, Pinedo HM: Cancer chemotherapy: Alternative routes of drug administration. Cancer Drug Deliv 2:147–169, 1985
202. McGovern B, Solenberger R, Reed K: A totally implantable venous access system for long-term chemotherapy. J Pediatr Surg 20:725–727, 1985
203. Khoury MD, Lloyd LR, Burrows J: A totally implanted venous access system for the delivery of chemotherapy. Cancer 56:1231–1234, 1985
204. Cozzi E, Hagle M, McGregor ML et al: Nursing management of patients receiving hepatic arterial chemotherapy through an implanted infusion pump. Cancer Nurs 7:229–234, 1984
205. Ensminger W, Niederhuber J, Dakhill S et al: Totally implanted drug delivery system for hepatic arterial chemotherapy. Cancer Treat Rep 65:393–400, 1981
206. Lokich J, Ensminger W: Ambulatory pump infusion devices for hepatic artery infusion. Semin Oncol 10:183–190, 1983
207. Niederhuber JE, Ensminger W, Gyves J et al: Regional chemotherapy of colorectal cancer metastatic to the liver. Cancer 53:1336–1343, 1984
208. Ensminger WD: Management, complications, and evaluation of intra-arterial infusion. Dev Oncol 26:33–40, 1984
209. Balch CM, Urist MM, Soong SJ et al: A prospective Phase II clinical trial of continuous FUDR chemotherapy for colorectal metastases to the liver using a totally implantable infusion pump. Ann Surg 198:567–573, 1983
210. Daly JM, Kemeny N, Oderman P, Botet J: Long-term hepatic arterial infusion chemotherapy. Arch Surg 119:936–941, 1984
211. Hohn DC, Rayner AA, Economou JS et al: Toxicities and complications of implanted pump hepatic arterial and IV floxuridine infusion. Cancer 57:465–470, 1985
212. Schwartz SI, Jones LS, McCune CS: Assessment of treatment of intrahepatic malignancies using chemotherapy via an implantable pump. Ann Surg 201:560–567, 1985
213. Kemeny N, Daly JM, Reichman B et al: Intrahepatic or systemic infusion of fluorodeoxyuridine in patients with liver metastases from colorectal carcinoma: A randomized trial. Ann Intern Med 107:459–465, 1987
214. Roemeling R, MacDonald M, Langevin T et al: Chemotherapy via implanted infusion pump: New perspectives for delivery of long-term continuous treatment. Oncol Nurs Forum 13:17–24, 1986
215. Paice JA: Intrathecal morphine infusion for intractable cancer pain: A new use for implanted pumps. Oncol Nurs Forum 13:41–47, 1986
216. Vogelzang NJ, Ruane M, DeMeester TR et al: Phase I trial of an implanted battery-powered, programmable drug delivery system for continuous doxorubicin administration. J Clin Oncol 3:407–414, 1985
217. Vogelzang NJ, Ruane M, Ratain MJ et al: A programmable and implantable pumping system for systemic chemotherapy: A performance analysis in 52 patients. J Clin Oncol 5:1968–1976, 1985
218. Coyle N, Mauskop A, Maggard J, Foley KM: Continuous subcutaneous infusions of opiates in cancer patients with pain. Oncol Nurs Forum 13:53–57, 1986
219. Seeger J, Woodcock TM, Richardson JD: Complications of implantable chemotherapy pump. Cancer 56:2428–2429, 1985
220. Schulmeister L, Herfarth L: Port occlusion by tumor growth. Oncol Nurs Forum 12:8, 1985
221. Stellato TA, Gauderer MW, Kazura J: Tumor metastasis from multiple myeloma and Burkitt's lymphoma in Broviac catheter tracts. Cancer 55:2715–2717, 1985
222. Reed WP, Newman KA, Applefield MM et al: Drug extravasation as a complication of venous access ports. Ann Intern Med 102:788–789, 1985
223. Lokich JJ, Moore C: Drug extravasation in cancer chemotherapy. Ann Intern Med 104:124, 1986
224. Steele CA: A complication of hepatic chemotherapy via implantable pump: A case report. Oncol Nurs Forum 13:25–27, 1986
225. Myers CE, Collins JM: Pharmacology of intraperitoneal chemotherapy. Cancer Invest 1:395–407, 1983
226. Jenkins J, Hubbard S, Howser D: The use of intraperitoneal chemotherapy in the management of ovarian cancer. Nursing'82 12:76–83, 1982
227. Howell SB, Pfeifle CL, Wung WE et al: Intraperitoneal cisplatin with systemic thiosulfate protection. Ann Intern Med 97:845–851, 1982
228. Markman M, Howell SB, Lucas WE et al: Combination intraperitoneal chemotherapy with cisplatin, cytarabine and doxorubicin for refractory ovarian carcinoma and other malignancies principally confined to the peritoneal cavity. J Clin Oncol 2:1321–1326, 1984
229. Markman M, Clearly S, Lucas WE et al: Intraperitoneal chemotherapy with high-dose cisplatin and cytosine arabinoside for refractory ovarian carcinoma and other malignancies principally involving the peritoneal cavity. J Clin Oncol 3:925–931, 1985
230. Howell SB, Pfeifle CE, Olshen RA: Intraperitoneal chemotherapy with melphalan. Ann Intern Med 101:14–18, 1984
231. Sugarbaker PH, Gianda FJ, Speyer JL: Prospective randomized trial of IV versus intraperitoneal 5-FU in patients with advanced primary colon or rectal cancer. Semin Oncol 12:101–111, 1985
232. Pfeifle CE, Howell SB, Markman M et al: Totally implantable system of peritoneal access. J Clin Oncol 2:1277–1280, 1984
233. Piccart MJ, Speyer JL, Markman M et al: Intraperitoneal chemotherapy: Technical experience at five institutions. Semin Oncol 12:90–96, 1985
234. Jenkins J, Sugarbaker PH, Gianola FJ, Myers CE: Technical considerations in the use of intraperitoneal chemotherapy administered by Tenckhoff catheter. Surg Gynecol Obstet 154:858–864, 1982
235. Caring for your Tenckhoff Catheter During Intraperitoneal Chemotherapy. Nursing Dept, Clinical Center, NIH, 1983
236. Swenson KK, Eriksson JH: Nursing management of intraperitoneal chemotherapy. Oncol Nurs Forum 13:77–81, 1986
237. Eriksson JH, Swenson KK: Guide to intraperitoneal chemotherapy. Oncol Nurs Forum 13:77–81, 1986
238. Hoff ST: Concepts in intraperitoneal chemotherapy. Semin Oncol Nurs 3:112–117, 1987
239. Jenkins J: Managing intraperitoneal chemotherapy: A medical, nursing and personal challenge. Semin Oncol 12:97–100, 1985
240. Kaplan RA, Markman M, Lucas WE: Infectious peritonitis in patients receiving intraperitoneal chemotherapy. Am J Med 78:49–53, 1985
241. Ostchega Y, Gianola FJ, Jenkins J et al: Prospective assessment of two methods of exit-site home care for the patient with a Tenckhoff catheter. Cancer Nurs (in press)
242. Ommaya AK: Implantable devices for chronic access and drug delivery to the central nervous system. Cancer Drug Deliv 1:169–179, 1984
243. Daklil S, Ensminger W, Kindt G et al: Implanted system for intraventricular drug infusion in central nervous system tumors. Cancer Treat Rep 65:401–411, 1981
244. Esparza DM, Weyland J: Nursing care for the patient with an Ommaya reservoir. Oncol Nurs Forum 9:17–20, 1982
245. Wujcik D: Meningeal carcinomatosis: Diagnosis, treatment and nursing care. Oncol Nurs Forum 10:35–40, 1983
246. Dyck P: Lumbar reservoirs for intrathecal chemotherapy. Cancer 55: 2771–2773, 1985
247. Patterson P: Granulocyte transfusion: Nursing considerations. Cancer Nurs 3:101–104, 1980
248. Graham V, Rubal BJ: Recipient and donor response to granulocyte transfusion and leukopheresis. Cancer Nurs 4:97–100, 1980
249. Button G: Pheresis. NITA 4:224–226, 1981
250. Baer MR, Steun RS, Dessypris EN: Chronic lymphocytes leukemia with hyperleukocytosis: Hyperviscosity syndrome. Cancer 56:2865–2869, 1985
251. Liebert A, Quietzsch D, Zimmerman S: Immunomodulation with apheresis techniques. Allergy Immunol 32:5–18, 1986
252. Yannelli JR, Thurman GB, Dickerson SG: An improved method for the generation of human lymphokine activated killer cells. J Immunol Methods 100:137–145, 1987

253. Sitges-Serra A, Linares J, Garau J: Catheter sepsis: The clue is the hub. Surgery 97:355–367, 1985
254. Centers for Disease Control: Recommendations for prevention of HIV transmission in health care settings. MMWR 36:1–18S, 1987
255. Maki DG, Botticelli JY, LeRoy ML, Thielke TS: Prospective study of replacing administration sets for IV therapy at 48 vs 72 hour intervals. JAMA 258:1777–1781, 1987
256. Henderson DK, Myers RF, Laniak, JM: Catheter-acquired infection in total parenteral nutrition. NITA 5:62–68, 1982
257. Fulton JS, Valanis B: Sepsis related to IV and hyperalimentation catheters: A summary of research findings. NITA 4:248–255, 1981
258. The CDC's Guidelines for Prevention of Intravascular Infection. NITA 5:39–50, 1982
259. Heimenz J, Skelton J, Pizzo PA: Perspective on the management of catheter-related infection. Pediatr Infect Dis 5:6–11, 1986
260. Maher MM, Henderson DK, Brennan MF: Central venous catheter exchange in cancer patients during total parenteral nutrition. NITA 5:54–60, 1982
261. Faulkner LA, Miller D: An analysis of phlebitis in a 240 bed hospital. NITA 4:274–277, 1981
262. Jones ER: Relationship between pH of IV medications and phlebitis: An experimental study. NITA 5:273–276, 1982
263. Jemison-Smith P, Thrupp LD: Phlebitis, infections and filtration. NITA 5:328–335, 1982
264. Larson E, Lunche S, Tran JT: Correlates of IV phlebitis. NITA 7:203–205, 1984
265. Gill S: Is filtration cost-effective in routine IV therapy? NITA 7:227–229, 1984
266. Falchuk KH, Peterson L, McNeil BJ: Microparticulate induced phlebitis: Its prevention by in-line filtration. N Engl J Med 312:78–82, 1985
267. Hessof I: Prevention of infusion thrombophlebitis. Acta Anaesthesiol Scand 29:33–37, 1985
268. Adams SD, Killen M, Larson E: Inline filtration and infusion phlebitis. Heart Lung 15:134–140, 1986
269. Lewis GBH, Heckler JF: Infusion thrombophlebitis. Br J Anaesthesiol 57:22–223, 1985
270. Harrigan CA: Care and cost-justification of final filtration. NITA 8:426–430, 1985
271. Ervin SM: The association of potassium chloride and particulate matter with the development of phlebitis. NITA 10:145–149, 1987
272. Weiss RB, Bruno S: Hypersensitivity reactions to cancer chemotherapy agents. Ann Intern Med 94:66–72, 1981
273. Kreamer KM: Anaphylaxis resulting from chemotherapy. Oncol Nurs Forum 8:13–16, 1981
274. Salloum E, Flamant F, Ghosm M: Irreversible encephalopathy with ifosphamide/mesna (letter). J Clin Oncol 5:1303–1304, 1987
275. Picozzi VJ, Swanson GF, Morgan R et al: 13-*cis*-Retinoic acid treatment for myelodysplastic syndromes. J Clin Oncol 4:589–595, 1986
276. Clark RE, Ismail SAD, Jacobs A et al: A randomized trial of *cis*-retinoic acid with or without cytosine arabinoside in patients with myelodysplastic syndrome. Br J Haematol 66:77–83, 1987
277. Schwartz RG, McKenzie WB, Alexander J et al: Congestive heart failure and left ventricular dysfunction complicating doxorubicin therapy. Am J Med 82:1109–1118, 1987
278. Wang JJ, Cortes E, Sinks L: Therapeutic effect and toxicity of Adriamycin in patients with neoplastic disease. Cancer 28:837–843, 1971
279. Rudolph R, Stein R, Patillo RA: Skin ulcers due to Adriamycin. Cancer 38:1087–1094, 1976
280. Reilly JJ, Neifield JP, Rosenberg SA: Clinical course and management of accidental Adriamycin extravasation. Cancer 40:2053–2056, 1977
281. Ignoffo RJ, Friedman MA: Therapy of local toxicities caused by extravasation of cancer chemotherapeutic drugs. Cancer Ther Rev 7:17–27, 1980
282. Larson DL: Treatment of tissue extravasation by antitumor agents. Cancer 49:1796–1799, 1982
283. Linder PM, Upton J, Osteen R: Management of extensive doxorubicin hydrochloride extravasation injuries. J Hand Surg 8:32–38, 1983
284. Harwood KV, Aisner J: Treatment of chemotherapy extravasation: Current status. Cancer Treat Rep 68:939–944, 1984
285. Hankin FM, Louis DS: Extravasation of chemotherapeutic agents. Am Fam Physician 3:147–150, 1985
286. Larson DL: What is the appropriate management of tissue extravasation by antitumor agents? Plast Reconstr Surg 75:397–402, 1985
287. Rudolph R, Larson DL: Etiology and treatment of chemotherapeutic agent extravasation injuries: A review. J Clin Oncol 5:1116–1126, 1987
288. Montrose PA: Extravasation management. Semin Oncol Nurs 3:128–132, 1987
289. Diekmann J, Ransom J: Extravasation of doxorubicin from a Hickman catheter: A case presentation. Oncol Nurs Forum 12:50–52, 1985
290. Soble MJ, Dorr RT, Breckenridge S: Dose dependent skin ulcers in mice treated with DNA binding antitumor antibiotics. Cancer Chemother Pharmacol 20:33–36, 1987
291. Garnick M, Israel M, Ketarpal V: Persistence of anthracycline levels following dermal and subcutaneous Adriamycin extravasation. Proc Am Soc Clin Oncol 22:173, 1981
292. Cohen FJ, Manganaro J, Bezozo RC: Identification of involved tissue during surgical treatment of doxorubicin-induced extravasation necrosis. J Hand Surg 8:43–45, 1983
293. Sonnevald P, Wassenaar HA, Nooter K: Long persistence of doxorubicin in human skin after extravasation. Cancer Treat Rep 68:895–896, 1984
294. Rudolph R, Suzuki M, Luce JK: Experimental skin necrosis produced by Adriamycin. Cancer Treat Rep 63:529–537, 1979
295. Cohen MH: Amelioration of Adriamycin skin necrosis: An experimental study. Cancer Treat Rep 63:1003–1004, 1979
296. Dorr RT, Alberts DS, Chen G: The limited role of corticosteroids in ameliorating experimental doxorubicin skin toxicity in the mouse. Cancer Chemother Pharmocol 5:17–20, 1980
297. Seigel DM, Giri SN, Scheinholtz RM et al: Characteristics and effect of anti-inflammatory drugs on Adriamycin-induced inflammation in the mouse paw. Inflammation 4:233–248, 1980
298. Bartkowski-Dodds L, Daniels J: Use of sodium bicarbonate as a means of ameliorating doxorubicin-induced dermal necrosis in rats. Cancer Chemother Pharmacol 4:179–181, 1980
299. Dorr RT, Alberts DS, Chen G: Experimental model of doxorubicin extravasation in the mouse. J Pharmacol Methods 4:237–250, 1980
300. Dorr RT, Alberts DS: Pharmacologic antidotes to experimental doxorubicin skin toxicity: A suggested role for beta-adrenergic compounds. Cancer Treat Rep 65:1001–1006, 1981
301. Ropka M: Comparison of effectiveness of immediate treatment of doxorubicin extravasation with sodium bicarbonate and hydrocortisone in a rat model Second Conf Cancer Nurs Res, A25, 1981
302. Barr RD, Sertic J: Soft tissue necrosis induced by extravasated cancer chemotherapeutic agents. Br J Cancer 44:267–269, 1981
303. Svingen BA, Powis G, Appel PL, Scott M: Protection against Adriamycin-induced skin necrosis in the rat by dimethyl sulfoxide- and alpha-tocopherol. Cancer Res 41:3395–3399, 1981
304. Desai MH, Teres D: Prevention of doxorubicin-induced skin ulcers in the rat and pig with dimethylsulfoxide (DMSO). Cancer Treat Rep 66:1371–1374, 1982
305. Dorr RT, Alberts DS, Woods MW: Vinca alkaloid ulceration: Experimental mouse model and effects of local antidotes. Proc Am Assoc Cancer Res 23:109, 1982
306. Wolgenmuth RL, Myers CA, Luce JK et al: Doxorubicin extravasation ulceration; animal model; development and testing of potential antidotes. Proc Am Assoc Cancer Res 23:673, 1982
307. Van Sloten, Harwood K, Gill M et al: Treatment of doxorubicin extravasation in a rat model. Proc 7th ONS Cong 7:70, 1982
308. Dorr RT, Alberts DS: Skin ulceration potential without therapeutic anticancer activity for epipodophyllotoxin commercial diluents. Invest New Drugs 1:151–159, 1983
309. Dorr RT, Alberts DS: Failure of DMSO and vitamin E to prevent doxorubicin skin ulceration in the mouse. Cancer Treat Rep 67:499–501, 1983
310. Okano T, Ohnuma T, Efremidis A et al: Doxorubicin-induced skin ulcer in the piglet. Cancer Treat Rep 67:1075–1078, 1983
311. Coleman JJ, Walker AP, Didolkar MS: Treatment of Adriamycin-induced skin ulcers: A prospective controlled study. J Surg Oncol 22:129–135, 1983
312. Daugherty JP, Khurana A, Simpson TA: Protective effect of butylated hydroxytoluene on Adriamycin-induced skin necrosis in the rat. Res Commun Chem Pathol Pharmacol 45:289–292, 1984
313. Dorr RT, Alberts DS: Cold protection and heat enhancement of doxorubicin skin toxicity on the mouse. Cancer Treat Rep 69:431–437, 1985
314. Dorr RT, Alberts DS: Vinca alkaloid skin toxicity: Antidote and drug disposition studies in the mouse. J Natl Cancer Inst 74:113–120, 1985
315. Daugherty JP, Khurana A: Amelioration of doxorubicin-induced skin necrosis in mice by butylated hydroxytoluene. Cancer Chemother Pharmacol 14:243–246, 1985
316. Upton PG, Yamaguch KT, Myers S et al: Effects of antioxidants and hyperbaric oxygen in ameliorating experimental doxorubicin skin toxicity in the rat. Cancer Treat Rep 70:503–507, 1986
317. Harwood KV, Bachur N: Evaluation of DMSO and local cooling as antidotes for doxorubicin extravasation in a pig model. Oncol Nurs Forum 14:39–44, 1987
318. Zweig J, Kabakow B: An apparently effective countermeasure for doxorubicin extravasation. JAMA 239:2116–2117, 1978
319. Barlock A, Howser D, Hubbard SM: Nursing management in Adriamycin extravasation. Am J Nurs 79:94–98, 1979
320. Swartz AJ: Chemotherapy extravasation. Cancer Nurs 2:405, 1979
321. Satterwhite B: What to do when Adriamycin extravasates. Nursing 80 10:37, 1980
322. Hirsh JD, Conlon PF: Implementing guidelines for managing extravasation of antineoplastics. Am J Hosp Pharm 40:1516–1519, 1983
323. Luedke DW, Kennedy PS, Rietchel RL: Histopathogenesis of skin and subcutaneous injury induced by Adriamycin. Plast Reconstruc Surg 63:463–465, 1979
324. Averbuch SD, Boldt M, Gaudiano G et al: Experimental chemotherapy-induced skin necrosis in swine. J Clin Invest 81:142–148, 1988
325. Olver IA, Schwarz MA: Use of dimethyl sulfoxide in limiting tissue damage caused by extravasation of doxorubicin. Cancer Treat Rep 67:407–408, 1983
326. Lawrence HJ, Goodnight SH: Dimethyl sulfoxide in extravasation of anthracyline agents. Ann Intern Med 98:1026, 1983
327. Kappel B, Hindenburg AA, Taub RN: Treatment of anthracycline extravasation: A warning against the use of sodium bicarbonate (letter). J Clin Oncol 5:825–826, 1987
328. Gaze NR: Tissue necrosis caused by commonly used IV infusions. Lancet 2:417–419, 1978
329. Ludwig CU, Stoll HR, Obrist R et al: Prevention of cytotoxic drug-induced skin ulcers with dimethyl sulfoxide (DMSO) and alpha-tocopherol. Eur J Cancer Clin Oncol 23:327–329, 1986
330. Hahn GM, Shavde DP: Cytotoxic effects of hyperthermia and Adriamycin on Chinese hamster cells. J Natl Cancer Inst 57:1063–1067, 1976
331. Herman TS, Baustian AM, Kundrat MA: Enhancement of hyperthermia-induced le-

thality and modulation of Adriamycin cytotoxicity by cooling. Proc Am Assoc Cancer Res 21:221, 1981

332. Averbuch SD, Gaudiano G, Koch TH et al: Doxorubicin-induced skin necrosis in the swine model: Protection with a novel radical dimer. J Clin Oncol 4:88–94, 1986
333. Harwood KV: Treatment of anthracycline extravasation: Recommendations for practice (letter). J Clin Oncol 5:1705, 1987
334. Buchanan GR, Buchsbaum HJ, Gojer B et al: Extravasation of dactinomycin, vincristine, and cisplatin: Studies in an animal model. Med Pediatr Oncol 13:375–380, 1985
335. Dorr RT, Soble MJ, Liddil JD et al: Mitomycin-C skin toxicity studies in mice: Reduced ulceration and altered pharmacokinetics with topical dimethyl sulfoxide. J Clin Oncol 4:1399–1404, 1986
336. Duvall E, Baumann B: An unusual accident during the administration of chemotherapy. (letter). Cancer Nurs 3:305–306, 1980
337. Johnson-Early A, Cohen MH: Mitocycin C-induced skin ulceration remote from infusion site (letter). Cancer Treat Rep 65:529, 1981
338. Wood HA, Ellenhorst-Ryan JA: Delayed adverse skin reaction associated with mitomycin-C administration. Oncol Nurs Forum 11:14–18, 1984
339. Bartkowski-Dodds L: Extensive tissue ulceration due to apparent sensitivity reactions to mitomycin. Cancer Treat Rep 69:925–927, 1985
340. Whitehouse MW, Beck FW: Question of cyclophosphamide derived aldehydes and their effect on lymphocyte distribution in vivo: Protective effect of thiols and bisulphate ions. Agents Actions 5:541–548, 1975
341. Owen OE, Dellatore DL: Accidental intramuscular injection of mechlorethamine. Cancer 45:2225–2226, 1980
342. Dorr RT, Alberts DS, Einspar J et al: Experimental dacarbazine antitumor activity and skin toxicity in relation to light exposure and pharmacologic antidotes. Cancer Treat Rep 71:267–272, 1987
343. Ames BN, Mc Cann J, Yamasaki E: Methods for detecting carcinogens and mutagens with the *Salmonella*/mammalian microsomal mutagenic test. Mutat Res 31:347–364, 1975
344. Benedict WF, Baker MS, Haroun L et al: Mutagenicity of cancer chemotherapeutic agents in the *Salmonella*/microsome test. Cancer Res 37:2209–2213, 1977
345. Falck K, Grohn P, Sorsa M et al: Mutagenicity in urine of nurses handling cytostatic drugs. Lancet 1:1250–1251, 1979
346. Anderson RW, Puckatt WH, Dana WJ et al: Risk of handling injectable antineoplastic agents. Am J Hosp Pharm 39:881–887, 1982
347. Jagun O, Ryan M, Waldron H: Urinary thioether excretion in nurses handling cytotoxic drugs. Lancet 1:443–444, 1982
348. Bos R, Leenaars A, Theuws J et al: Mutagenicity of urine from nurses handling cytostatic drugs, influence of smoking. Int Arch Occup Environ Health 50:359–369, 1982
349. Kolmodin-Hedman B, Hartvig P, Sorsa M et al: Occupational handling of cytostatic drugs. Arch Toxicol 54:25–33, 1983
350. Venitt S, Crofton-Sleigh C, Hunt J et al: Monitoring exposure of nursing and pharmacy personnel to cytotoxic drugs: Urinary mutation assays and urinary platinum as markers of absorption. Lancet 1:74–76, 1984
351. Hirst M, Tse S, Mills DG: Occupational hazard to cyclophosphamide. Lancet 1:186–188, 1984
352. Sorsa M, Hemminki K, Vainio H et al: Occupational exposure to anticancer drug—potential and real hazards. Mutat Res 154:135–149, 1985
353. Stucker I, Hirsh A, Doloy T et al: Urine mutagenicity, chromosomal abnormalities and sister chromatid exchanges in lymphocytes of nurses handling cytostatic drugs. Int Arch Occup Environ Health 57:195–205, 1986
354. Benhamou S, Callais F, Sancho-Garnier H et al: Mutagenicity in urine from nurses handling cytostatic agents. Eur J Cancer Clin Oncol 22:1489–1493, 1986
355. Rogers B, Emmett EA: Handling antineoplastic agents: Urine mutagenicity in nurses: Image. J Nurs Scholarship 19:108–113, 1987
356. Ladik CF, Stoehr GP, Mawrer MA: Precautionary measures in the preparation of antineoplastics. Am J Hosp Pharm 37:1184–1186, 1980
357. Crudi CB: I've kept the drug sterile but have I contaminated myself? NITA 3:77–78, 1980
358. Reynolds R, Ignoffo R, Lawrence J et al: Adverse reactions to AMSA in medical personnel. Cancer Treat Rep 66:410, 1983
359. Rogers B: Work practices of nurses who handle antineoplastic agents. AAOHN J 35:24–31, 1987
360. Seleven SG, Lindbohm ML, Hornung RW et al: A study of occupational exposure to antineoplastic drugs and fetal loss in nurses. N Engl J Med 313:1173–1178, 1985
361. Hoffman D: The handling of antineoplastic drugs in a major cancer center. Hosp Phar 15:301–303, 1980
362. Staiano N, Galleli JF, Adamson RH et al: Lack of mutagenic activity in hospital pharmacists admixing antitumor drugs. Lancet 1:615–616, 1981
363. Johnson BH, Gross J: Handling methotrexate: A safety program. Am J Nurs 82:1531, 1982
364. Gibson JF, Gomperts D, Hedworth-Whitty RB: Mutagenicity of urine from nurses handling cytotoxic drugs. Lancet 1:100–101, 1984
365. Cloak M, Connor T, Stevens KR et al: Occupational exposure of nursing personnel to antineoplastic agents. Oncol Nurs Forum 12:33–39, 1985
366. Everson RB, Ratcliffe JM, Flack PM et al: Detection of low levels of urinary mutagen excretion by chemotherapy workers which was not related to occupational drug exposures. Cancer Res 45:6487–6497, 1985
367. Waksvik H, Klepp O, Brogger A: Chromosome analyses of nurses handling cytostatic agents. Cancer Treat Rep 63:607–611, 1981
368. Norppa H, Sorsa M, Vainio H et al: Increased sister chromatid exchange frequencies in lymphocytes of nurses handling cytostatic drugs. Scand J Work Environ Health 6:299–301, 1980
369. Nikula E, Kivinitty K, Leisti J et al: Chromosome aberrations in lymphocytes of nurses handling cytostatic agents. Scand J Work Environ Health 10:71–74, 1984
370. Stiller A, Obe G, Boll I et al: No elevation of the frequencies of chromosomal alteration as a consequence of handling cytostatic drugs. Mutat Res. 121:253–259, 1983
371. Yamasaki E, Ames BL: Concentration of mutagens from urine by adsorption with the nonpolar resin XAD-2: Cigarette smokers have mutagenic urine. Proc Natl Acad Sci 7:3555–3559, 1977
372. Dolara P, Mazzoli S, Rosi D et al: Exposure to carcinogenic chemicals and smoking increases urinary excretion of mutagens in humans. J Toxicol Environ Health. 8:95–103, 1981
373. Hannan MA, Recio L, Duluca PP et al: Co-mutagenic effects of 2-aminoanthracene and cigarette smoke condensate on smoker's urine in the Ames salmonella assay system. Cancer Lett 13:203–212, 1981
374. Trell E, Janzon L, Pero RW et al: Mutagen sensitivity, smoking habits and enzyme induction in healthy middle-aged men. Environ Res 35:421–429, 1984
375. Hopkin JM: Sister chromatid exchange induction by cigarette smoke. Basic Life Sci 29:927–937, 1984
376. Watanabe T, Endo A: The SCE test as a tool for cytogenetic monitoring of human exposure to occupational and environmental mutagens. Basic Life Sci Part B 29:939–955, 1984
377. Sasson IM, Coleman DT, LaVoie EJ et al: Mutagens in human urine: Effects of cigarette smoking and diet. Mutat Res 158:149–157, 1985
378. Kleinberg M, Quinn M: Airborne drug levels in a laminar flow hood. Am J Hosp Pharm 38:1301–1303, 1981
379. deWerk NA, Wadden RA, Chiou WL: Exposure of hospital workers to airborne antineoplastic agents. Am H Hosp Pharm 40:597–601, 1983
380. McDiarmid MA, Egan T, Furio M et al: Sampling for airborne fluorouracil in a hospital drug preparation area. Am J Hosp Pharm 43:1942–1945, 1986
381. Connor TH, Laidlaw JL, Theiss JC et al: Permeability of latex and polyvinyl chloride gloves to carmustine. Am H Hosp Pharm. 41:676–679, 1984
382. Laidlaw JL, Connor TH, Theiss JC et al: Permeability of four disposable protective clothing materials to seven antineoplastic drugs. Am J Hosp Pharm. 42:2449–2454, 1985
383. Yodaiken RE, Bennett D: OSHA work-practice guidelines for personnel dealing with cytotoxic (antineoplastic) drugs, occupational safety and health administration. Am J Hosp Pharm 43:1193–1204, 1986 (Exerpted from OSHA Instruction Publ. #8-1-1, Washington DC, 1/29/86)
384. Knowles RS, Virden JE: Handling of injectable antineoplastic agents. Br Med J 281:589–591, 1981
385. Crudi CB, Stephens BL, Maier P: Possible occupational hazards associated with the preparation of antineoplastic agents. NITA 5:264–266, 1982
386. Stolar MH, Power LA, Viele CS: Recommendations for handling cytotoxic drugs in hospitals. Am J Hosp Pharm 40:1163–1171, 1983
387. Valanis B, Browne M: Use of protection by nurses during occupational handling of antineoplastic drugs. NITA 8:218–222, 1985
388. Barry LK, Booher RB: Promoting the responsible handling of antineoplastic agents in the community. Oncol Nurs Forum 12:41–46, 1985
389. Stajich GV, Barnett CW, Turner SV et al: Protective measures used by oncologic office nurses handling parenteral antineoplastic agents. Oncol Nurs Forum 13:47–49, 1986
390. Barhamand BA: Difficulties encountered in implementing guidelines for handling antineoplastics in the physician's office. Cancer Nurs 9:138–143, 1986
391. Valanis R, Shortridge L: Self protective practices of nurses handling antineoplastic drugs. Oncol Nurs Forum 14:23–27, 1987
392. Cohen IA, Newland SJ, Kirking DM: Injectable-antineoplastic-drug practices in Michigan hospitals. Am H Hosp Pharm 44:1096–1105, 1987
393. Murphy CP, Goldspiel BR, Koeller J: Cost of implementing veterans administration directives for handling antineoplastic agents. Am J Hosp Pharm. 44:788–791, 1987
394. Avis KE, Levchuk JW: Special considerations in the use of vertical laminar flow workbenches. Am J Hosp Pharm 41:81–88, 1984
395. Vaccari PL, Tonat K, DeChristoforo R, et al: Disposal of antineoplastic wastes at the NIH. Am J Hosp Pharm 41:87–93, 1984
396. Provost GJ: Legal issues associated with the handling of cytotoxic drugs. Am J Hosp Pharm. 41:1115–1121, 1984
397. Curtin L: Ethical issues in informed consent. Proc 3rd Natl Conf Cancer Nurs, pp 71–73. New York, American Cancer Society, 1981
398. Benoliel JQ, McCorkle R: Ethical considerations in treatment. Proc 2nd Natl Conf Cancer Nurs, pp 63–68, New York, Am Cancer Soc, 1978
399. Whitman H, Donovan CT, Spross J, Gadow S: Ethical issues in cancer nursing. Oncol Nurs Forum. 7:37–47, 1980
400. Federal Register 46:8389–8952 January 27, 1981
401. Rimer B, Jones WL, Keintz MK: Informed consent: A crucial step in cancer patient education. Health Educ Q (Suppl) 10:30–42, 1984
402. Frei E III: Ethical considerations in patient care. Proc 4th Natl Conf Human Values and Cancer, p 28. New York, Am Cancer Soc, 1984
403. Mayer DK: Information. In Johnson BL, Gross J (eds): Handbook of Oncology Nursing, pp 115–127. New York, John Wiley & Sons, 1985
404. Rostad M: Simplifying the process (letter). Oncol Nurs Forum 14:92, 1987
405. Brody D: The patient's role in clinical decision-making. Ann Intern Med. 95:718–722, 1980

406. Cassileth BR, Zupkis RV, Sutton-Smith K et al: Informed consent; why are its goals imperfectly realized? N Engl J Med 302:896–900, 1980
407. Schain W: Patients rights in decision-making: The case for personalism versus paternalism in health care. Cancer 46:1035–1041, 1980
408. Hubbard SM: Neoplasia. In Jones DA, Girovec MM, Dunbar CF (eds): Medical-Surgical Nursing. A Conceptual Approach, 2nd ed, pp 141–186. New York, McGraw-Hill, 1982
409. Rickel LH, Davis A, Sigler G: Solid neoplasms. In Jones DA, Girovec MM, Dunbar CF (eds): Medical-Surgical Nursing, A Conceptual Approach, 2nd ed, pp 187–274. New York, McGraw-Hill, 1982
410. Schumann D: Preoperative measures to promote wound healing. Nurs Clin North Am 14:695, 1979
411. Mahon SM: Nursing interventions for the patient with a myocutaneous flap. Cancer Nurs 10:21–31, 1987
412. O'Dell AJ: Objectives and standards in the care of the patient with a radical neck dissection. Nurs Clin North Am 8:159–164, 1973
413. Byrne N: Critical care of the thoracic surgical patient. Cancer Nurs 1:135–144, 1978
414. Robichaud KJ, Hubbard SM: Infection and cancer. In Groenwald S (ed): Cancer Nursing: Principles and Practice. pp 221–244. Boston, Jones & Bartlett Publ. 1986
415. Harris RB: National survey of aseptic tracheostomy care techniques in hospitals with head and neck surgical departments. Cancer Nurs 7:23–32, 1984
416. Kane K: Carotid artery rupture in advanced head and neck patients. Oncol Nurs Forum 10:14–18, 1983
417. Lesage C: Carotid artery rupture: Prediction, prevention and preparation. Cancer Nurs 9:1–7, 1986
418. Starck P: Hydrotherapy for open wounds. Oncol Nurs Forum 8:42, 1981
419. Gorrell CR: Frequency of infection in hospitalized patients with colon cancer. Proc 5th ONS Congr, San Diego, 1980
420. Jackson BS: The growing role of nurses in enterostomal therapy. Semin Oncol 7:48–55, 1980
421. Jackson BS, Broadwell DC: Ostomy surgery: An overview of historical current and future perspectives. Semin Oncol Nurs 2:227–234, 1986
422. Dobkin KA, Broadwell DC: Nursing considerations for the patient undergoing colostomy surgery. Semin Oncol Nurs 2:249–255, 1986
423. Watt RL: Nursing management of a patient with a urinary diversion. Semin Oncol Nurs 2:265–269, 1986
424. Boarini JH, Bryant RA, Irrgang SJ: Fistula management. Semin Oncol Nurs 2:287–292, 1986
425. Hampton B: Nursing management of a patient following pelvic exenteration Semin Oncol Nurs 2:281–286, 1986
426. Fisher SG: Psychosexual adjustment following total pelvic exenteration. Cancer Nurs 2:219–225, 1979
427. Burkhalter P: Sexuality in the cancer patient. In Burkhalter P, Donley D (eds): Dynamics of Oncology Nursing. New York, McGraw–Hill, 1978
428. Jusenius K: Sexuality and gynecologic cancer. Cancer Nurs 4:479–484, 1981
429. Springer M: Radical vulvectomy: Physical, psychological, social, and sexual implications. Oncol Nurs Forum 9:19–21, 1982
430. Shipes E, Lehr S: Sexuality and the male cancer patient. Cancer Nurs 5:375–381, 1982
431. Fisher SG: The psychosexual effects of cancer and cancer treatment. Oncol Nurs Forum 10:63–68, 1983
432. Hilderley L: Radiation therapy. In Groenwald S (ed): Cancer Nursing: Principles and Practice, pp 320–347. Boston, Jones & Bartlett, 1987
433. Glicksman AS: Radiobiologic basis of brachytherapy. Semin Oncol Nurs 3:3–6, 1987
434. Maddock PG: Brachytherapy sources and applicators. Semin Oncol Nurs 3:15–22, 1987
435. Hassey KM: Principles of radiation safety and protection. Semin Oncol Nurs 3:23–29, 1987
436. Strohl RA: Head and neck implants. Semin Oncol Nurs 3:30–46, 1987
437. Phillips TL, Wasserman TH: Promise of radiosensitizers and radioprotectors in the treatment of human cancer. Cancer Treat Rep 68:291–302, 1984
438. Richter MP, Coia LR: Palliative radiation therapy. Semin Oncol 12:375–383, 1985
439. Bucholtz JD: Radiolabeled antibody therapy. Semin Oncol Nurs 3:67–73, 1987
440. Held J, McLaughlin P: Antiferritin immunoglobulin therapy for treatment of hepatoma. Oncol Nurs Forum 14:27–31, 1987
441. Dudjak LA: Future directions of brachytherapy. Semin Oncol Nurs 3:74–77, 1987
442. Smith DS, Chamorrow TP: Nursing care of patients undergoing combination chemotherapy and radiotherapy. Cancer Nurs 1:129–134, 1978
443. Strohl RA, Salazar O: Management of the patient receiving hemibody irradiation. Oncol Nurs Forum 9:13–16, 1982
444. Yasko JM: Care of the patient receiving radiation therapy. Nurs Clin North Am 17:631–648, 1982
445. Wilson CA, Strohl RA: Radiation therapy as primary treatment for breast cancer. Oncol Nurs Forum 9:12–18, 1982
446. Hassey K: Demystifying care of patients with radioactive implants. Am J Nurs 85:788–792, 1985
447. Hassey K: Radiation therapy for breast cancer: A historic review. Semin Oncol Nurs 1:181–188, 1985
448. McCarthy CP: The role of interstitial implantation in the treatment of primary breast cancer. Semin Oncol Nurs 3:47–53, 1987
449. McNaull FW: Radiation therapy for lung cancer: Nursing considerations. Semin Oncol Nurs 3:194–201, 1987
450. Shell JA, Carter J: The gynecological implant patient. Semin Oncol Nurs 3:54–56, 1987
451. Witt ME, McDonald-Lynch A, Grimmer D: Adjuvant radiotherapy to the colorectum: Nursing implications. Oncol Nurs Forum 14:17–21, 1987
452. Cassileth BR, Volckmar D, Goodman RL: The effect of experience on radiation therapy patients' desire for information. Int J Radiat Oncol Biol Phys 6:493–496, 1980
453. Israel MJ, Mood DW: Three media presentations for patients receiving radiation therapy. Cancer Nurs 5:57–63, 1982
454. Kreamer K, Aquila K, Haller M et al: Information about radiation therapy. Oncol Nurs Forum 11:67–71, 1984
455. Dodd MJ: Patterns of self care in cancer patients receiving radiation therapy. Oncol Nurs Forum 11:23–27, 1984
456. King K, Nail W, Kreamer K et al: Patients' descriptions of the experience of receiving radiotherapy. Oncol Nurs Forum 12:55–61, 1985
457. Schoot JAM, Hanewald GJ, Van Dam FS et al: Assessment of malaise in cancer patients treated with radiotherapy. Cancer Nurs 8:306–313, 1985
458. Haylock PJ, Hart LK: Fatigue in patients receiving localized radiation. Cancer Nurs 6:461–467, 1979
459. Welch D: Radiation-related nausea and vomiting. A review of the literature. Oncol Nurs Forum 6:8–11, 1979
460. Beck S: Impact of a systematic oral care protocol on stomatitis after chemotherapy. Cancer Nurs 2:185–199, 1979
461. Welch D: Assessment of nausea and vomiting in cancer patients receiving external beam radiotherapy. Cancer Nurs 3:365–371, 1980
462. Hassey KM, Rose CM: Altered skin integrity in patients receiving radiation therapy. Oncol Nurs Forum 9:44–50, 1982
463. Hilderly L: Skin care in radiation therapy: A review of the literature. Oncol Nurs Forum 10:51–56, 1983
464. Strohl R: Management of moist desquamation due to radiotherapy (letter). Oncol Nurs Forum 11:68,1984
465. O'Rourke M: Enhanced cutaneous effects in combined modality therapy. Oncol Nurs Forum 14:31–35, 1987
466. Dudjak LA: Mouth care for mucositis due to radiation therapy. Cancer Nurs 10:131–140, 1987
467. Abernathy E: Biotherapy: An introductory overview. Oncol Nurs Forum (suppl) 14:13–15, 1987
468. Irwin MM: Patients receiving biological response modifiers: Overview of nursing care. Oncol Nurs Forum (Suppl) 14:(6) 32–37, 1987
469. Galluci B: The immune system and cancer. Oncol Nurs Forum 14:3–12, 1987
470. Jassak PF, Sticklin LA: Interleukin 2: An overview. Oncol Nurs Forum 13:17–22, 1986
471. Corey BF, Collins JL: Implementation of an rIL-2/LAK cell clinical trial: A nursing perspective. Oncol Nurs Forum 13:31–36, 1987
472. Garvey E, Matuat RJ, Bolten D: Care of the patient undergoing interferon therapy. Cancer Nurs 6:303–306, 1983
473. Moldawar NP, Murray JL: The clinical use of monoclonal antibodies in cancer research. Cancer Nurs 8:207–213, 1985
474. Seipp CA, Simpson C, Rosenberg SA: Clinical trials with IL-2. Oncol Nurs Forum 13:25–29, 1986
475. Scogna DM, Schoenburger CS: Biological response modifiers: An overview and nursing implications. Oncol Nurs Forum 9:45–49, 1982
476. Jeffs C, Laszlo J: A coordinating role for the nurse clinician in a Phase I interferon study. Cancer Nurs 6:379–386, 1983
477. Jassak PF: Future trends in biotherapy. Oncol Nurs Forum 14:38–40, 1987
478. Morris DL, Hersh EM, Gutterman JU et al: Recall antigen delayed-type hypersensitivity skin testing: Standardization of self reading by patients. Cancer Immunol Immunother 6:5–8, 1979
479. Dean JC: Application and reading of skin tests. In Dorr DT, Fritz WL (eds): Cancer Chemotherapy Handbook, pp 194–200. New York, Elsevier, 1980
480. Stromborg MF, Wright P: Ambulatory patients perceptions of the physical and psychosocial changes in their lives since the diagnosis of cancer. Oncol Nurs Forum 7:117–130, 1984
481. Dietz JH: Adaptive rehabilitation in cancer. Cancer Rehabil 68:145–153, 1980
482. McCorkle R, Germina B: What nurses need to know about home care. Oncol Nurs Forum 11:63–64, 1984
483. Googe MC, Varricchio CG: A pilot investigation of home health care needs of cancer patients and their families. Oncol Nurs Forum 8:24–28, 1981
484. May DM, Oleske D, Justo-Ober PK et al: The role of the area wide oncology nurse coordinator in the home care of cancer patients. Oncol Nurs Forum 9:39–43, 1982
485. Monaco GP: Resources available to the family of the child with cancer. Cancer 58:516–521, 1986
486. Wood CA, Baily LR, Yates JW: Advanced cancer pain management in a community setting. Oncol Nurs Forum 9:32–36, 1982
487. Oleske D, Hauk W, Heide E: Characteristics of cancer patient referrals to home care: A regional perspective. Am J Publ Health 73:768–682, 1983
488. Ballard S, McNamara R: Quantifying nursing needs in home health care. Nurs Res 32:236–241, 1983
489. Garvey EC: Guidelines for caring for the AIDS patient in the home setting. NITA 8:481–483, 1985
490. White EJ: Home care of the patient with advanced lung cancer. Semin Oncol Nurs 3:216–221, 1987
491. Oleske DM, Otte DM, Heinze S: Development and evaluation of a system for moni-

toring the quality of oncology nursing care in the home setting. Cancer Nurs 10:190–198, 1987
492. Benoliel J, McCorkle R: A holistic approach to terminal illness. Cancer Nurs 1:143–149, 1978
493. Ferszt G, Houck J: Integration of the community health nurse in a hospital based hospice program. Oncol Nurs Forum 10:36–39, 1983
494. Vinguerra V, Degnan TJ, Sciortino A et al: A comparative assessment of home versus hospital comprehensive treatment for advanced cancer patients. J Clin Oncol 4:1521–1528, 1986
495. Hays JC: Patient symptoms and family coping. Predictors of hospice utilization patterns. Cancer Nurs 9:317–325, 1986
496. Hadlock DC: The hospice: Intensive care of a different kind. Semin Oncol 12:357–367, 1985
497. Swinehart PS: Hospice home care: How to get patients home and help them stay there. Semin Oncol 12:461–465, 1985
498. Stephany TM: Quality assurance for hospice programs. Oncol Nurs Forum 12:33–40, 1985
499. Lauer ME, Mulhern RK, Hoffmann RG et al: Utilization of hospice/home care in pediatric oncology. Cancer Nurs 9:102–107, 1986
500. Greer DS, Mor V, Morris JN et al: An alternative in terminal care: Results of the national hospice study. J Chronic Dis 39:9–26, 1986
501. Caring for the Terminally Ill Patient at Home: A Guide for Family Caregivers. U of Penn Cancer Center Hospice Home Care Programs, 1986
502. Otte DM, Allen KS: Ethical principles in the nursing care of the terminally ill adult. Oncol Nurs Forum 14:87–91, 1987
503. Lansky SB, Cairns N, Clark G et al: Childhood cancer and non-medical costs of the illness. Cancer 43:403–408, 1979
504. Houts PS, Lipton A, Harvey HA et al: Non medical costs to patients and their families associated with outpatient chemotherapy. Cancer 52:2388–2392, 1984
505. Bloom BS, Knorr RS, Evans AE: The epidemiology of disease expenses; the cost of caring for children with cancer. JAMA 253:2393–2397, 1985
506. Davis CK: Health care economic issues: Projections for oncology nurses. Oncol Nurs Forum 12:17–22, 1985
507. Curtiss FR: Third party reimbursement for home parenteral nutrition and IV therapy. NITA 6:193–197, 1983
508. Jencks SF, Dobson A: Strategies for reforming Medicare's physician payments. N Engl J Med 312:1492–1499, 1985
509. Studebaker E: Home health agencies, functions and reimbursement, NITA 8:43–46, 1985.
510. Weinstein SM: Regulatory concerns: Home care. NITA 10:175–184, 1987
511. Joel LA: DRGs: The state of the art of reimbursement for nursing services. Nurs Health Care 4:560–563, 1983
512. Joel LA: DRGs and RIMs: Implications for nursing. Nurs Outlook 32:42–49, 1984
513. Klopovich P: Research on problems of chronicity in childhood cancer. Oncol Nurs Forum 10:72–75, 1983
514. Hubbard SM: Chemotherapy-induced alopecia. In Mead GM, Whitehouse JMA (eds): Early and Late Effects of Cancer Treatment: Clinics in Oncology, Vol 4. East Sussex, England, WB Saunders, 1985
515. Lindsey AM: Building the knowledge base for practice: Nausea and vomiting. Oncol Nurs Forum. 12:49–56, 1986
516. Lindsey AM: Building the knowledge base for practice: Alopecia, breast self-exam and other human responses. Oncol Nurs Forum. 12:27–34, 1986
517. Cotanch P, Hockenberry M, Herman S: Self-hypnosis as antiemetic therapy in children receiving chemotherapy. Oncol Nurs Forum. 12:41–46, 1985
518. Frank JM: The effects of music therapy and guided visual imagery on chemotherapy induced nausea and vomiting. Oncol Nurs Forum 12:47–52, 1985
519. Scott DW, Donahue DC, Mastrovito RC: Comparative trial of clinical relaxation and an antiemetic drug regimen in reducing chemotherapy-related nausea and vomiting. Cancer Nurs 9:178–187, 1986
520. Merritt DH: National center for nursing research. Image 13:84–85, 1986

EDWARD H. SHORTLIFFE

SUSAN MOLLOY HUBBARD

CHAPTER 65 *Information Systems in Oncology*

The rapid growth of knowledge about carcinogenesis, prognoses, and treatment options has made the practice of oncology particularly complex. As in other fields of medicine, investigators are developing computer programs to help oncologists effectively deal with the clinical information they need to provide optimal care.

This chapter summarizes the available tools for information management and describes current research indicative of the evolving information systems for oncology. The emphasis is on computer-based tools to help physicians and other health workers deliver improved care to cancer patients through rapid access to general information and to data and advice about specific patients.

Imagine the day when physicians and other health-care providers will manage all patient data through a simple and familiar computer workstation.[1] Data will be gathered automatically from clinical laboratories, radiology departments, hospitals, and other sources, and the user's interaction with the machine will be based on voice input, perhaps coupled with pointing devices, such as a mouse, a light pen, or even a finger tip, used with a portable display screen the size of a clipboard. This single workstation will be a transparent window into myriad information sources, many running on other computers and connected through electronic pathways as invisible to the user as are today's telephone connections. Physicians will be able to review their patients' data, to seek relevant references from the recent literature, to request information about available treatment options or about nearby providers for possible referrals, and even to seek patient-specific advice regarding proper management. Although this scenario is futuristic, many of the technologies necessary to achieve it are already available. The challenge is to build on the results of current systems, integrating individual tools into coherent environments that simplify the physician's tasks. In the meantime, many available computational tools are already of value to oncologists.

HISTORICAL PERSPECTIVE

ORGANIZING THE MEDICAL LITERATURE

Index Medicus, inaugurated in 1879, was the first systematic classification of current medical literature. The first year's volume contained 17,000 citations from 700 periodicals. In 1988, a single month of the *Index* averages 21,000 citations; annual coverage exceeds 250,000 articles.[2,3] Rapid growth in medical knowledge made manual preparation of the *Index* a logistical nightmare by the early 1950s, prompting the National Library of Medicine (NLM) to develop MEDLARS. This computer-based MEDical Literature Analysis and Retrieval System automated the process of organizing, indexing, and publishing the *Index*. The pioneering use of early computer technology to facilitate citation retrieval led to interactive computer searching and to the introduction in 1971 of MEDLINE, an online version of *Cumulated Index Medicus.* The medical and scientific community rapidly accepted MEDLINE, stimulating the evolution of a nationwide access system via telecommunication networks and the development of a variety of related databases for distribution over the MEDLARS system.

ONCOLOGY RESOURCES

In 1971, the National Cancer Act mandated the creation of an international databank to foster rapid and effective exchange of cancer data throughout the world.[4] Faced with responsibility for organizing, updating, and disseminating a rapidly growing collection of knowledge, the National Cancer Institute (NCI) decided to establish a computer-based information program to complement its scientific journals. This led to the development of the CANCERLINE databases for distribution on MEDLARS and of a series of database-derived publications for those who did not have direct access to online systems.[5-7] These products continue to provide data required for cancer research and patient care.

The NCI has developed a comprehensive database on the subject of cancer treatment.[8] Physician Data Query (PDQ), compiled especially for distribution to physicians by a computer network, is described later in this chapter.

CLINICAL INFORMATION SYSTEMS

The need for automated collection, retrieval, and analysis of information in clinical settings led to the development of computer-based hospital information systems (HIS).[9,10] One example of large hospital-based programs is the HELP system developed at Latter Day Saints Hospital in Salt Lake City.[11] HELP processes comprehensive, time-oriented clinical, laboratory, and administrative data to support inpatient care, clinical research, and hospital operations. Unlike most HIS programs, HELP also uses computer-based logic to support clinical decision making. Integration of the decision logic with programs that store and retrieve information from a comprehensive patient database enables HELP to assist physicians and other health workers without additional data-entry requirements. For over 2000 clinical topics, the logic incorporated in the HELP system generates medical alerts for interpreting physiologic data and medical advice about topics like drug interactions, diagnostic suggestions, or clinical test recommendations.[12]

New decision-support systems for ambulatory care, such as RMIS, also use computer-based medical logic to alert physicians to clinical circumstances that warrant their attention (*e.g.*, the need for testing serum potassium levels in patients receiving diuretics and digitalis preparations).[13] Other outpatient information systems such as COSTAR generate time-oriented, patient-specific encounter forms from a comprehensive patient database for each clinic or office visit.[14] These guide the physician in the efficient management of patients based on their past medical histories and current problem lists.

Information systems have been designed to deal specifically with diagnostic or therapy-selection problems. For example, DXplain suggests possible diagnoses to explain the spectrum of findings that a physician may encounter in a patient with a complex disorder.[15] DXplain was released in 1987 by the American Medical Association for access by a national computer network.[16]

Researchers in medical computer science have developed experimental decision-support systems that formulate advice by following lines of reasoning similar to those used by human experts.[17] Drawing on symbolic reasoning techniques from the field of artificial intelligence, these programs, called expert systems, often use rules of the form "if A and B are true, then it is likely that C is true" to represent the inference steps used by experts. Experimental prototypes deal with medical diagnosis (*e.g.*, the INTERNIST-1/QMR program for general internal medicine diagnosis) and with therapy advice (*e.g.*, the MYCIN system for antimicrobial therapy selection).[18-20] These systems capture and analyze patient data, apply medical knowledge to the management of individual patients, and interact with the physician to provide recommendations for treating a specific patient.

USE OF COMPUTERS IN CLINICAL ONCOLOGY

In the field of oncology, computer-based information systems have provided assistance with clinical decisions such as the administration of complex treatment regimens. Protocol-derived clinical algorithms have been developed to specify requirements for data collection (*e.g.*, the frequency of radiologic studies or laboratory tests), to flag abnormal values, and to help physicians administer therapy according to the protocol. Many of the oncology systems developed during the last decade have provided clinical databanks for statistical analysis, often with special displays or prompts to remind physicians about protocol details.[21-23] Johns Hopkins Hospital has implemented a particularly comprehensive Oncology Clinical Information System (OCIS).[24] The OCIS provides an online medical record system coupled to scheduling programs, other clinical databases at Johns Hopkins Hospital, and limited advisory functions to ensure adherence to protocols for patients who are enrolled in clinical studies.

Advice provided through computer algorithms was shown by workers at the University of Alabama to improve oncology protocol compliance significantly for the cooperative group with which they worked.[23,25] However, the Alabama system was unable to analyze complex, ambiguous, or unusual clinical situations; required data entry and program management at the university, rather than at the cooperating oncologist's office; and required considerable effort to prepare the appropriate algorithm for each clinic visit. These limitations precluded the system's use in routine practice settings.

An experimental chemotherapy advice system known as ONCOCIN has been developed at Stanford University.[26,27] A clinical data management program is integrated with an underlying expert system that provides tailored therapy advice for patients enrolled in chemotherapy protocols. Although ONCOCIN is currently available only for limited use in the outpatient oncology clinic at Stanford Hospital, it serves as a model for the kind of active advisory tools that will become available to all health workers in the field of clinical oncology.

In the remainder of this chapter, we will discuss two of the current computer systems for clinical oncology. PDQ has been selected for inclusion because it is widely available and makes extensive use of current database and computer-networking techniques. ONCOCIN is presented as an example of the integration of computer-aided decision making with patient database systems and advanced computer graphics. PDQ and ONCOCIN provide a glimpse of the spectrum of computational resources that will affect the efficiency and quality of care delivery in clinical oncology.

THE PDQ SYSTEM

Current epidemiologic data indicate that aggressive and widespread use of existing cancer therapies could reduce national cancer mortality by 10% to 20% within the next decade.[28] To speed diffusion of information about new cancer treatments and to facilitate integration of research advances into clinical practice, the NCI developed PDQ. The PDQ system provides therapeutic information that is peer reviewed and updated by cancer experts, summaries of cancer trials that are open to patient accrual, and a directory of physicians and organizations providing cancer treatment (Fig. 65-1). The system is simple to use and provides a retrieval mechanism that internally links diverse types of clinical information about cancer and treatment protocols. Users can search for and display information easily, without learning a specialized query language. The PDQ data enable users to determine the full range of treatment alternatives for all major cancers. Users can identify clinical trials for appropriate patients and can locate physicians and treatment facilities for consultation or referral.[29]

PDQ treatment overviews summarize therapies for all major cancers and help clinicians decide whether or not standard therapy is appropriate for their patients. Each statement provides information on prognosis, relevant staging and histologic classifications, standard therapies, and references to key literature. An editorial board of cancer specialists develops the information contained in these overviews. This board actively solicits input from specialists throughout the country to determine treatment options that should be listed in PDQ as the standard of care for each cancer. These recommendations are written using specific guidelines:

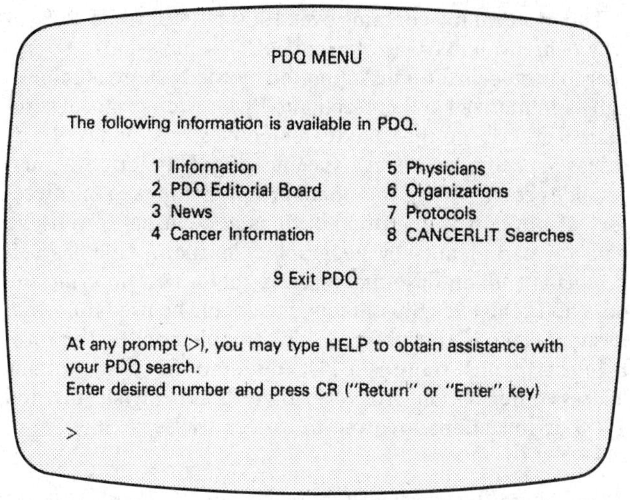
PDQ MENU
The following information is available in PDQ.
1 Information
2 PDQ Editorial Board
3 News
4 Cancer Information
5 Physicians
6 Organizations
7 Protocols
8 CANCERLIT Searches
9 Exit PDQ
At any prompt (>), you may type HELP to obtain assistance with your PDQ search.
Enter desired number and press CR ("Return" or "Enter" key)
>

FIG. 65-1. The files in PDQ. The main PDQ menu lists the files that are in the system. By selecting the desired number at the prompt, users can retrieve the following: 1) *Information*—a description of the data files and searching hints; 2) *PDQ editorial board*—the names, addresses, and affiliations of the medical board responsible for maintaining the accuracy and currency of the treatment recommendations in the PDQ system; 3) *News*—announcements about new developments in cancer treatment and new features; 4) *Cancer information*—summaries of the most current thinking on the prognosis, staging, and treatment of all major cancers; 5) *Physicians*—a directory of more than 12,000 physicians who specialize in cancer treatment and who are either clinical investigators participating in a clinical trial described in the PDQ protocol file or belong to one of 17 medical specialty organizations; 6) *Organizations*—a directory of more than 1500 organizations that are affiliated with an NCI research program, participate in one or more clinical trials listed in the PDQ protocol file, or have programs of cancer care certified by the American College of Surgeons Commission on Cancer; 7) *Protocols*—a directory of treatment protocols with outlines of 1000+ active investigational studies that describe study objectives, eligibility criteria, the treatment plan, and the location of all study participants as well as standard therapy protocols for established regimens that have gained acceptance as standard treatment options; 8) *CANCERLIT searches*—preformulated literature searches that allow users to rapidly and easily retrieve current citations on highly focused aspects of treatment from CANCERLIT, NCI's bibliographic database.

1. Open with a prognostic statement that clearly describes the success of treatment in terms of curability (or treatability) with current modalities and discloses whether prognostic variables influence treatment outcome.
2. Provide clinically relevant information on the histopathologic classification of the malignant cells.
3. Describe the most clinically useful and widely accepted staging classification.
4. Provide current survival data for each stage and histologic type.
5. Provide information about standard and investigational treatment options according to stage of dissemination or other prognostic factors such as histologic type (*e.g.*, rhabdomyosarcoma), sites of involvement (*e.g.*, metastatic to lung), or location of the primary tumor (*e.g.*, brain neoplasm).
6. Indicate if the therapeutic alternatives produce equivalent results and if there are reasons for selecting one treatment over another in a particular clinical setting.
7. List only those therapies with superior and documented efficacy with references that document treatment efficacy whenever cure or prolonged disease-free survival is achievable.
8. Clearly state that patients should be considered candidates for investigational therapies currently under evaluation if no effective treatment exists.

Treatment recommendations are reviewed by panels selected from a group of over 400 consultants.[8] Abstracts for all citations referenced in PDQ can be retrieved by users. Because a goal of PDQ is to inform users about ongoing therapeutic research, the treatment guidelines direct users to another part of the database that contains active protocols if effective therapies do not exist or if investigational protocols represent important therapeutic alternatives.

The protocol file contains over 1000 clinical trials, 20% of which are voluntary (not from NCI) submissions. All research protocols directly supported by the NCI are automatically summarized and entered into PDQ. Each protocol summary describes the study objectives, is indexed by disease-specific and stage-specific eligibility criteria, and provides details of the treatment program. Links to the directory of physicians and organizations allow users to retrieve data on participants by geographic location. All Phase III protocols contain dose-modification tables that describe the dose and schedule adjustments that should be used if normal tissue toxicity is encountered.[30] To complement these protocol descriptions, there is a PDQ directory file that contains address information on more than 12,000 physicians and 1400 organizations involved in cancer trials.

SYSTEM IMPLEMENTATION

As implemented on the NLM computers, PDQ is a menu-driven system that guides users through the data displays and allows information retrieval from files stored in the machine. A main menu prompts users to select a description of the database, a news file, instructions, a list of the editorial board members, cancer information, the directory, or the protocol file. The options of prognostic and treatment information contained in the cancer information file are provided when the user selects the cancer diagnosis of interest. This information is provided in state-of-the-art or patient-specific formats (Fig. 65-2).

Users can examine protocols for a particular cancer diagnosis and stage by selecting them from the main menu or by typing a brief command at most prompts. PDQ can retrieve protocols by diagnosis, stage, ID number, phase of clinical investigation, treatment, key words, the state in which investigators practice, or by any combination of these parameters (Fig. 65-3). Summaries of currently accepted chemotherapeutic regimens are provided as standard therapy protocols. After the relevant protocols are defined, PDQ informs the user how many of the protocols meet the search criteria. The user can either redefine the criteria or decide to display or print the information.

Users can examine protocols directly from the related place in the information file (see Fig. 65-2). A menu option automatically retrieves from the PDQ protocol file all trials that are open to a patient with the stage or type of cancer of interest (see Fig. 65-3).

Users can retrieve information about physicians by entering a name or a medical specialty, by specifying a particular geographic location, or by using a combination of these. PDQ offers a variety of print and display options for reviewing physician and organizational profiles in varying degrees of detail. Linkages between files allow a user to view protocols that are being conducted at a specific institution or for which a particular physician is a principal investigator.

FIG. 65-2. The cancer information file. Users can seek information about a particular cancer through a series of screens that allow them to select a specific body site. This figure shows the series of displays, starting with the main menu, through which the physician would pass in seeking state-of-the-art information about prostate cancer.

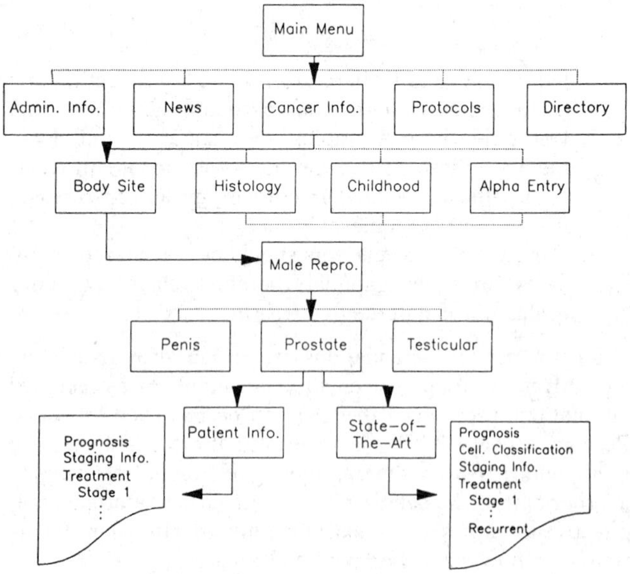

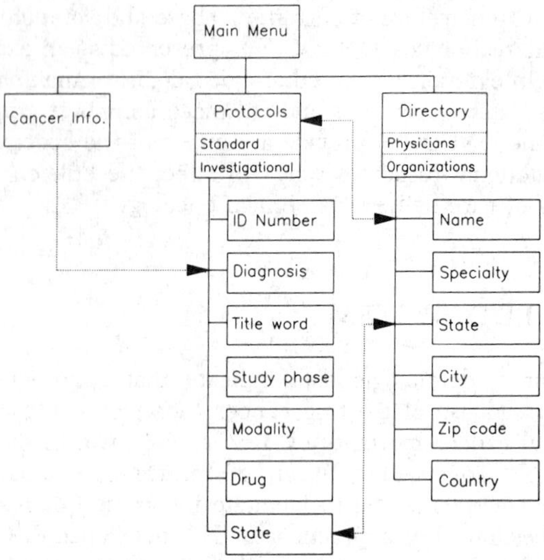

FIG. 65-3. The protocol information file. A user can access protocol descriptions while examining information on a specific cancer (through the cancer information file) or by directly selecting the protocol information file from the main menu. There are extensive cross-linkages between the protocol descriptions and other data files such as the directory of physicians and organizations. This allows protocol information to be sought using a variety of search strategies.

MAINTENANCE OF THE DATABASE

State-of-the-art treatment recommendations in the cancer information file are continually updated by a two-tiered editorial board of experts. A core board meets monthly to discuss new treatment data, and the associate editors provide data and peer review by mail. Board members review current statements and submit articles with new data. Modifications to the database are made after discussing these data. Articles that provide data suggesting improved outcome with investigational regimens are reviewed and highlighted or referenced in the text. On average, 20% to 25% of the statements are modified each month. Because the system provides a current and critically analyzed body of knowledge that encompasses an entire specialty, online use has been certified for Category I continuing medical education credits.

The accuracy and currency of the PDQ protocol file are maintained every month by local coordinators who review and edit the summaries and the lists of the protocol participants. In an average month, 60 new protocols are abstracted, indexed, and entered in PDQ; about 50 protocols close and are deleted from the file. About 35% of the protocol file is modified every month. The entire directory is updated by mail, with one-twelfth of the file revalidated each month.

CURRENT STATUS

PDQ is accessible on the NLM's MEDLARS computer system at 6800 medical libraries and health-care organizations in the United States and through 16 online MEDLARS centers located abroad. Current use of PDQ averages 570 hours each month, making it one of the top five databases at the NLM, and use of the system has been increasing 20% annually. PDQ also is licensed to commercial vendors and to health-care organizations. The system is available by subscription on optical disk (CD-ROM) as part of a comprehensive cancer library.[31]

Since PDQ's inception, the NCI has solicited recommendations from users, and improvements increasing clinical and educational value and its ease of use are frequently incorporated into the system. A telecommunications program (PDQ Access) has been developed to automate the sign-on procedures, to transfer information from search sessions to the user's disk, and to allow PDQ users to search the CANCERLIT database during a PDQ search session.[32] Future enhancements will include an information file on investigational drugs, an interface that will permit CANCERLIT search specifications using natural language, and smooth interconnections between the PDQ protocol file and supplemental systems, such as ONCOCIN, that are designed to provide advice for specific patients.

THE ONCOCIN SYSTEM

ONCOCIN is an experimental system developed at Stanford University to assist oncologists with the management of chemotherapy for patients participating in formal clinical trials. As with other oncologic advice systems, ONCOCIN was developed to meet the need for a comprehensive computer system that could provide protocol guidance and manage clinical trial data in both university and community settings.[21–24] Unlike the other systems, the Stanford system is designed for direct access by the physician caring for the patient with cancer. It incorporates heuristic methods that supplement the straightforward rules of a protocol, assuring that therapy is tailored to the subtle variations among patients. Unlike PDQ, ONCOCIN is not yet widely available. However, we have included a description of the program here so that readers will understand the capabilities and interactive style of similar advisory programs for oncology that may become available in the future.

CLINICAL DATA MANAGEMENT

ONCOCIN runs on powerful, relatively small, dedicated computers that are fully integrated into a cancer treatment program for outpatients. Because its developers believed that advisory tools would appeal to physicians only if the programs were in routine use, the program is designed to replace the traditional paper flowsheet filled out by oncologists as they track a patient's progress during a course of chemotherapy. ONCOCIN presents, on a picture-quality display screen, a flowsheet that duplicates the familiar paper version (Fig. 65-4). After the physician has seen the patient in the examining room, he leaves to sit at an ONCOCIN workstation in the office or clinic. The patient's flowsheet is displayed so that old data may be reviewed and current data entered. Data entry uses a mouse pointing device, eliminating the need for the physician to type. The graphic flowsheet is divided into sections, similar to those that separate classes of data on the paper flowsheet, and the physician can open sections for review or data entry by selecting them with the mouse. In Figure 65-4, the sections labeled "Mass/x-ray" and "Hematology" have been opened; the other data sections remain closed. The "Time" section opens automatically to show the dates corresponding to the columns of data in the opened sections.

Figure 65-4 demonstrates three additional features of ONCOCIN:

1. *Registers and menus for data entry:* When the physician enters data, such as the current white blood cell (WBC) count, he or she selects the corresponding box on the flowsheet. An appropriate register appears on the screen. The mouse is used to select the proper value (in this case, 1.4 thousand or 1400/ml^3) and the word "done," after which the register disappears and the entered value appears in the appropriate box on the flowsheet.
2. *Graphic data entry:* The paper flowsheet traditionally has included drawings of the human torso and chest x-ray views on which the physician is able to draw the areas of disease involvement. ONCOCIN also permits data to be entered and retrieved in this way. The "Mass/x-ray" section shown in Figure 65-4 permits the physician to select anatomic regions or organs (in this case, a left axillary lymph node and the spleen).
3. *Guidance during data entry:* Because ONCOCIN uses current and past patient data to assess appropriate protocol-directed treatment for each visit, it knows what information it needs to make a recommendation. Although the physician may enter data on the flowsheet in any order and need not fill in all items, ONCOCIN asks unobtrusively for information by displaying question marks in areas of particular interest. In Figure 65-4, for example, question marks indicate that ONCOCIN needs the WBC count and asks the physician to complete the "Toxicity" and "Chemistry" sections.

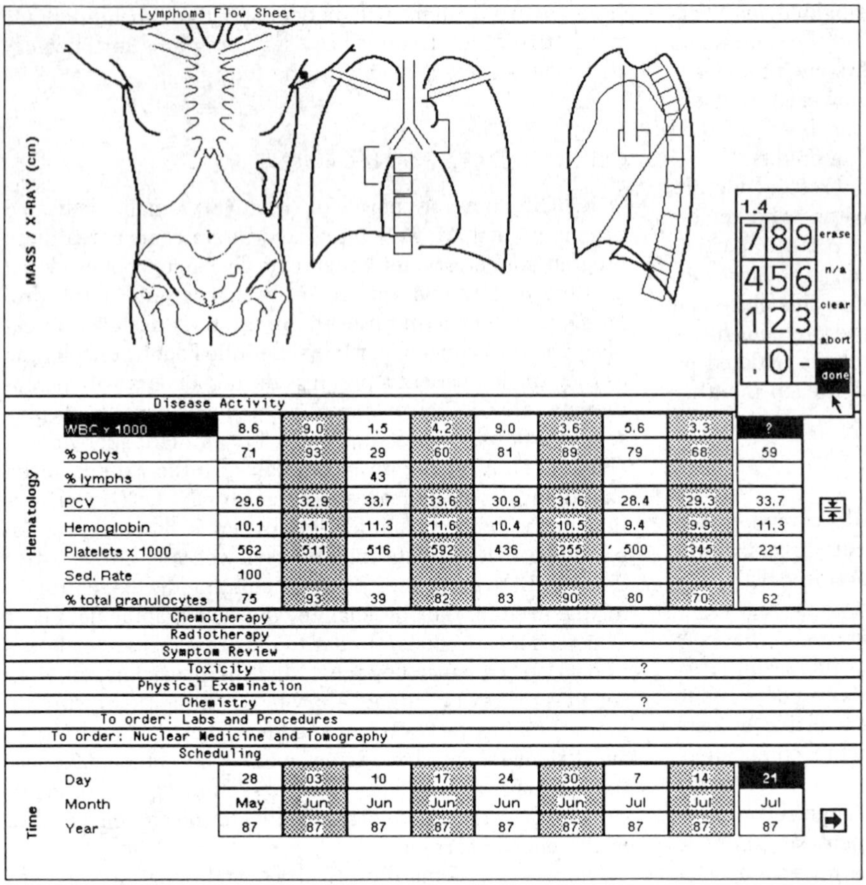

FIG. 65-4. The ONCOCIN flowsheet for data entry. The appearance of the display screen during the entry of the current white blood cell count for a patient with lymphoma. The user can select with the mouse the double-arrow element at the right side of an opened flowsheet section to close that portion of the form. The single-arrow element in the bottom "Time" section may be selected to shift the columns of data to the right, thereby displaying information on outpatient visits before May 28.

THERAPY ADVICE

Although the program can be used for the routine management of oncologic data for outpatients, a principal goal of ONCOCIN is determining the proper therapy for patients receiving complex chemotherapeutic treatment in trials. As clinical data are entered on the graphic flowsheet, they are passed to a program that uses them and knowledge about the protocol or treatment program to consider the dosage and type of chemotherapy administered for each visit. This support program, known as the Reasoner, then displays its recommendations in the appropriate column on the flowsheet when the physician opens the "Chemotherapy" section (Fig. 65-5). ONCOCIN provides recommendations by assisting with the portion of the flowsheet on which the physician usually would enter the therapy plan.

Consider the flowsheet in Figure 65-5, which shows ONCOCIN's advice for a patient with lymphoma who is receiving MACOP-B (methotrexate, doxorubicin, cyclophosphamide, vincristine, prednisone, and bleomycin). Patients normally receive weekly therapy for 12 weeks, with methotrexate administered at weeks 2, 6, and 10 and bleomycin at weeks 4, 8, and 12. On week 9, ONCOCIN recommended treatment by suggesting doses for doxorubicin, cyclophosphamide, and prednisone. In accordance with protocol rules, because the patient had neutropenia (WBC count is 1400), the program suggested appropriate dosage attenuation for the two myelosuppressive agents. If the physician wishes to administer different dosages or to delay therapy until the patient's WBC count has partially recovered, he or she selects the appropriate box and enters the new dose on a register, such as the one shown in Figure 65-4. ONCOCIN is designed to permit overrides of this sort, emphasizing its role as an assistant to the oncologist, rather than as a source of protocol dogma.

Figure 65-5 also demonstrates ONCOCIN's ability to adjust to unusual circumstances. On week 2, when methotrexate normally would have been required by the protocol, it happened that the patient had a significant pleural effusion. The MACOP-B documentation made no mention of what action should be taken in this situation, but the oncologist was aware of the potential toxicity from methotrexate sequestration in the effusion and chose to administer bleomycin instead of methotrexate. The effusion resolved by week 4, and ONCOCIN recognized that an adjustment to the protocol was required because the patient had received bleomycin rather than methotrexate at week 2. ONCOCIN switched the schedule for the two drugs, recommending methotrexate at weeks 4, 8, and 12, alternating with bleomycin at weeks 6 and 10. This example demonstrates that it is crucial for an advisory program to have access to data from previous treatment cycles; it would be inappropriate for ONCOCIN to recommend therapy based on current data without first reviewing recent trends and therapy adjustments.

Lymphoma Flow Sheet										
Mass / X-ray										
Disease Activity										
Hematology	WBC x 1000	8.6	9.0	1.5	4.2	9.0	3.6	5.6	3.3	1.4
	% polys	71	93	29	60	81	89	79	68	59
	% lymphs			43						
	PCV	29.6	32.9	33.7	33.6	30.9	31.6	28.4	29.3	33.7
	Hemoglobin	10.1	11.1	11.3	11.6	10.4	10.5	9.4	9.9	11.3
	Platelets x 1000	562	511	516	592	436	255	500	345	221
	Sed. Rate	100								
	% total granulocytes	75	93	39	82	83	90	80	70	62
CHEMOTHERAPY (includes non-cytoxic drugs)	BSA (m2)	1.71								
	Arm assignment									
	Combination Name	MACOP-B	MACOP-B	MACOP-B	MACOP-B	MACOP-B	MACOP-B	MACOP-B	MACOP-B	MACOP-B
	Subcycle	week 1	week 2	week 3	week 4	week 5	week 6	week 7	week 8	week 9
	Visit type	TREAT	TREAT	TREAT	TREAT	TREAT	TREAT	TREAT	TREAT	TREAT
	Methotrexate 400 MG/M2				700				700	
	Doxorubicin 50 MG/M2	85		55		85		85		55
	Cytoxan 350 MG/M2	600		390		600		600		390
	Vincristine 1,4 MG/M2		2.0		2.0		2.0		2.0	
	Prednisone 75 MG	75	75	75	75	75	75	75	75	75
	Bleomycin 10 U/M2		17				17			
	Folinic Acid 15 MG				15				15	
	Septra DS 2 TABLETS	2	2	2	2	2	2	2	2	2
	Ketoconazole 200 MG	200	200	200	200	200	200	200	200	200
	Sodium Bicarbonate 3000 MG				3000				3000	
	Cum, Bleomycin (mg/m2)		10				20			
	Cum, Doxorubicin (mg/m2)	50		82		132		181		213
Radiotherapy										
Symptom Review										
Toxicity										
Physical Examination										
Chemistry										
To order: Labs and Procedures										
To order: Nuclear Medicine and Tomography										
Scheduling										
Time	Day	28	03	10	17	24	30	7	14	21
	Month	May	Jun	Jun	Jun	Jun	Jun	Jul	Jul	Jul
	Year	87	87	87	87	87	87	87	87	87

FIG. 65-5. ONCOCIN displays its recommendation on the flowsheet. The appearance of the display screen after ONCOCIN has indicated (in the rightmost column) its suggested dosing of agents to be administered for a patient with lymphoma. The "Chemotherapy" section of the flowsheet, unlike the sections used by the physician when entering data, is filled out by ONCOCIN based on patient-specific data and on a knowledge base of information regarding the treatment protocol in which the patient is enrolled.

In addition to knowing the rules for chemotherapy administration in specific clinical trials, ONCOCIN keeps track of the data required by the protocol and provides reminders to the physician if laboratory studies or radiologic examinations are indicated. Two sections of the graphic flowsheet deal with test ordering (labeled "To order" in Fig. 65-5). Selected items are used to generate order forms, which are printed and used by the scheduling desk when the patient is arranging for subsequent appointments. When the clinic visit ends, ONCOCIN also prints a flowsheet, similar to the traditional paper document, which is placed in the patient's chart for back-up and review. The entire interaction between ONCOCIN and the physician usually requires less than 5 minutes.

MAINTENANCE OF THE DATABASE: OPAL

ONCOCIN must maintain a description of a protocol to advise physicians managing patients enrolled in that protocol. It would be impractical if ONCOCIN had to be reprogrammed every time a new protocol was developed. The developers therefore devised a second system that can be used by clinical researchers to describe for ONCOCIN the details of a new protocol. This knowledge-entry system, known as OPAL, takes advantage of the graphic capabilities of the computer workstation. After a cancer specialist has described or edited a protocol using OPAL, special programs create a corresponding knowledge base that ONCOCIN can use when it helps physicians manage patients enrolled in that protocol.

OPAL provides two graphic environments for use by the cancer specialist.[33] In the first, the expert describes the overall organization and temporal sequence of the steps in the protocol, using the mouse to create and manipulate on the screen objects that correspond to individual therapies or decisions. For example, Figure 65-6 shows the high-level schema for a protocol (#2091), a treatment plan for small cell carcinoma of the lung. In Figure 65-6A, the expert has created a diagram indicating that all patients initially are managed using a standard treatment. The details of this initial treatment, represented in a subschema using the same conventions, are shown in Figure 65-6B. Patients first receive a cycle of POCC (procarbazine, vincristine, cyclophosphamide, and CCNU) chemotherapy. Those having a complete response then receive VAM (VP-16, doxorubicin, and methotrexate) chemotherapy with concurrent brain irradiation; those without a complete response to POCC receive as many as three cycles of alternating POCC and VAM, stopping earlier if they demonstrate a complete response.

When the initial treatment is complete (Fig. 65-6A), sub-

A

B

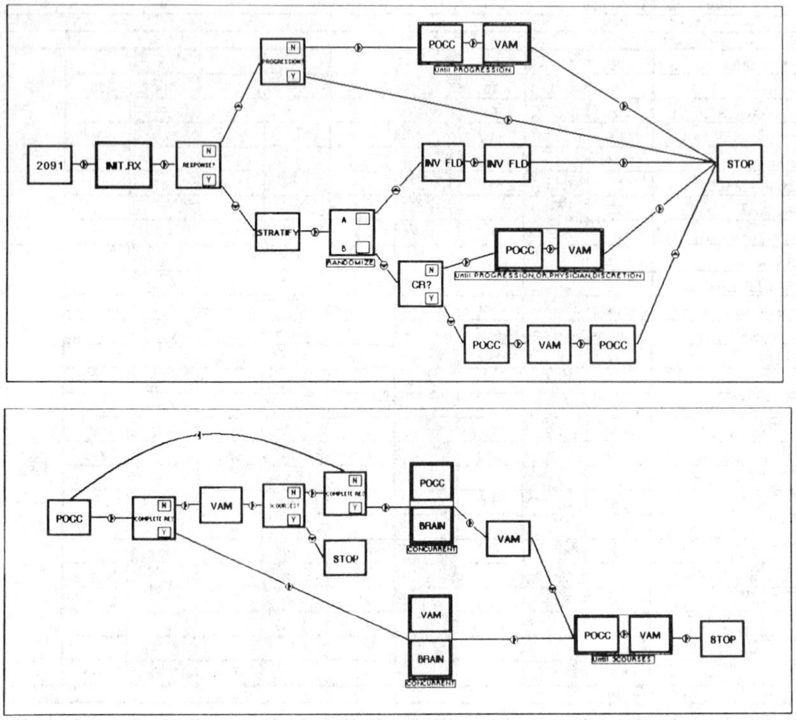

FIG. 65-6. Entry of a protocol schema using OPAL. The clinical researcher describes the overall schema for a protocol using the graphical environment shown here. He creates the individual boxes using mouse selections and then positions and joins them as desired. **A**. The top-level schema for protocol #2091, used in the treatment of small-cell lung carcinoma. The experimental question (note the randomization between arms A and B) is whether involved field irradiation is an adequate alternative to further (perhaps indefinite) treatment with POCC and VAM chemotherapies in patients who have had a complete or partial response to the drugs. **B**. The subschema corresponding to the box labeled INIT.RX (initial treatment) in **A**.

sequent management depends on whether the patient has achieved a complete or partial remission. Those who have responded are stratified and randomly assigned to receive involved-field irradiation or additional therapy with POCC and VAM.

The expert using OPAL does not need to understand either computer programming or the internal organization of ONCOCIN's knowledge. The physician describes the protocol's overall organization using a flow diagram that is intuitive. It is based on the kinds of diagrams that appear in many printed protocol documents. OPAL interprets the diagram and translates that knowledge to a form that is useful to ONCOCIN. This is an example of "visual programming."

Many of the protocol details are not captured in diagrams such as the ones shown in Figure 65-6. In particular, there is no information about dosage, dose attenuation, timing of drug administration, or criteria for aborting cycles or deleting specific agents. These kinds of details are entered using the second part of OPAL, a system of fill-in-the-blank forms (Fig. 65-7). These forms, displayed by OPAL in a logical sequence that guides the expert through protocol definition, permit the specific treatment rules to be entered and used by ONCOCIN. In Figure 65-7, for example, the physician has entered a table that indicates the attenuation schedule for procarbazine in POCC therapy as a function of the patient's platelet count and WBC count. In many circumstances, the

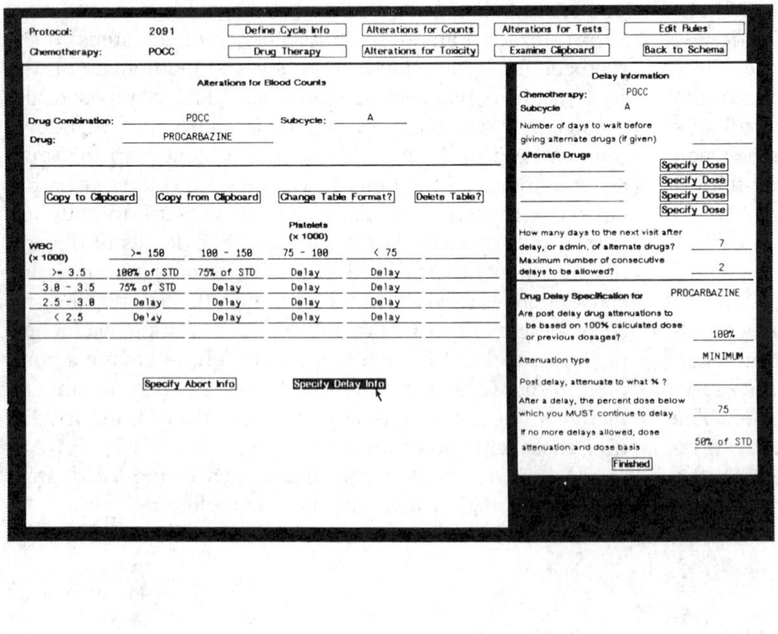

FIG. 65-7. OPAL forms for entering dose attenuation criteria. The expert has used the mouse and a series of menus to indicate the appropriate response to combined reductions in white blood cell and platelet counts when treating with procarbazine in POCC chemotherapy. For example, a platelet count less than 75,000/ml^3 requires a delay in therapy even if the WBC count is normal. The subform at the right defines the proper management of such delays. The top of the form provides access to other forms used for protocol definition.

protocol calls for a delay in therapy if there is evidence of significant marrow suppression; the subform displayed to the right in Figure 65-7 permits the expert to enter information about what to do when therapy is delayed. There are many similar graphic forms that deal with appropriate responses to nonhematologic toxicities, with test ordering criteria, and with similar issues routinely defined in protocol documents.

OPAL is a graphic environment designed for use by clinical researchers who wish to define the details of protocols so that ONCOCIN can, in turn, assist physicians who are managing patients enrolled in those protocols. OPAL permits experts to enter new protocols, but it may also be used to refine extant protocols. The knowledge structures created with OPAL are translated directly for use by ONCOCIN. If a physician notices toxicity or other complicating factors in a patient enrolled in a protocol, ONCOCIN is able to help determine the proper course of action.

CURRENT STATUS

The ONCOCIN program described here is being tested and refined in the Stanford University Oncology Day Care Center. Clinical researchers have used OPAL to enter over 35 protocols for use by ONCOCIN. Although ONCOCIN has favorably affected data collection for patients enrolled in protocols and provided excellent management advice based on protocol guidelines, it runs only on advanced computer workstations, which are impractical for widespread dissemination.[26,27] ONCOCIN and OPAL are best viewed as experimental prototypes. The Stanford team that developed these programs is exploring mechanisms for implementing the system on common and less expensive computing hardware.

CHALLENGES FOR ONCOLOGY INFORMATION SYSTEMS

Although it has been documented that data management and clinical consultation systems can exert a significant influence on physician behavior, the overall impact of computer information systems on medical practice has been limited to selected settings. Nonetheless, there is increasing interest in computational tools as a practical mechanism for meeting the practicing physician's need for current medical information and expert medical advice.[9,33–36] The interest is stimulated by the availability of powerful, sophisticated microcomputers and affordable, easily used software, coupled with growing concern about the increase in medical knowledge, legal accountability, and cost-effective practice.

The barriers to widespread implementation of these systems are only partially scientific. Currently available technologies could be of great value to clinical oncologists and other health personnel if logistic, psychologic, and financial constraints could be overcome.[9] For example, many observers believe that physician acceptance of information systems depends on smooth integration of programs into the routine of patient care. Narrowly defined systems that serve a single purpose and that require their users to make a special effort to access them have met with limited success, even though the information they provide has been valuable for patient care. The ONCOCIN system provides its advice about chemotherapy management as a byproduct of the physician's routine use of a graphic flowsheet. ONCOCIN automatically offers advice for managing clinical data. Integration of data management with laboratory, financial, and office-management systems and with information resources such as PDQ will further enhance the appeal of advisory programs.

The problems are not simply logistic. We also need new approaches to representing the oncologic literature in computers. A future MEDLINE-style system should help physicians find pertinent articles and determine how those articles apply to a specific clinical question.[37] Other research subjects include the development of improved models of chemotherapeutic kinetics and mechanisms of drug action, so that advisory systems can creatively propose therapeutic approaches based on first-principle considerations of pathophysiology and pharmacology. An improved understanding of the nature of medical knowledge and of the way it should be used for optimal decision making is a goal for basic researchers in medical computer science.

As investigators have improved our understanding of the complex nature of medical knowledge, it has become clear that the role of computer-based decision tools always will be to assist trained practitioners. There is no evidence that a machine's abilities will ever equal those of the human mind in dealing with unexpected situations, in integrating visual and auditory data that reveal subtleties of a patient's problem, or in weighing the social and ethical issues that often determine proper medical decisions.

A simple example illustrating the inadvisability of computer-based dogma arose in the experimental testing of ONCOCIN.[9] When a young woman with lymphoma was seen in the clinic one Friday afternoon, ONCOCIN recommended 100% dosing with all drugs in her regimen, but her physician overrode this advice and chose to give no treatment. The clinic data manager later sought an explanation for this disagreement, and the physician explained that the patient was to be a bridesmaid the next day and had asked to delay her treatment, which routinely caused 1 or 2 days of nausea, until after the weekend. Her request was eminently reasonable, but formulating a proper response required both medical expertise and world knowledge. Such commonsense insights, used routinely in patient care, are totally foreign to decision-support systems. This observation argues cogently for the discretion of the physician in the proper use of decision-support tools.

REFERENCES

1. Rennels GD, Shortliffe EH: Advanced computing for medicine. Sci Am 255:154–161, 1987
2. Association of American Medical Colleges: Medical Education in the Information Age. Washington DC, 1986
3. Lindberg DAB, Schoolman HM: The National Library of Medicine and medical informatics. West J Med 145:786–790, 1986
4. 92nd Congress: National Cancer Act of 1971. Public Law 92–218, Sec 1828 December 23, 1971
5. Holt RL, Buzzerd PM, Schneider JH: International Cancer Research Data Bank: A system for selecting, processing, organizing, and disseminating cancer research information. NCI Monogr 40:25–29, 1974

6. Tancredi SA, Amacher RA, Schneider JH et al: CANCERLINE: A new NLM/NCI database. J Chem Inf Comput Sci 16:128–130, 1976
7. Masys DR, Hubbard SM: Technical information progress of the National Cancer Institute. J Am Soc Inf Sci 38:60–64, 1987
8. Hubbard SM, Henney JE, DeVita VT: A computer database for information on cancer treatment. N Engl J Med 316:315–318, 1987
9. Shortliffe EH: Computer programs to support clinical decision making. JAMA 258:67–74, 1987
10. Blum BI: Clinical information systems: A review. West J Med 145:791–797, 1986
11. Pryor TA, Gardner RM, Clayton PD et al: The HELP system. J Med Syst 7:87–102, 1983
12. Warner HR: Computer-Assisted Medical Decision-Making. New York, Academic Press, 1979
13. McDonald CJ, Hui SL, Smith DM et al: Reminders to physicians from an introspective computer medical record. Ann Intern Med 100:130–138, 1984
14. Barnett GO: The application of computer-based medical-record systems in ambulatory practice. N Engl J Med 310:1643–1650, 1984
15. Barnett GO, Cimino JJ, Hupp JA et al: DXplain: An evolving diagnostic decision-support system. JAMA 258:67–74, 1987
16. Harris DK: Editorial: Computer-assisted decision support: A new available reality. JAMA 258:86, 1987
17. Shortliffe EH: Medical expert systems: Knowledge tools for physicians. West J Med 145:830–839, 1986
18. Miller RA, Pople HE, Myers JD: Internist-1: An experimental computer-based diagnostic consultant for general internal medicine. N Engl J Med 307:468–476, 1982
19. Miller RA, McNeil MA, Challinor SM et al: The Internist-1/Quick Medical Reference project: Status report. West J Med 45:816–822, 1986
20. Buchanan BG, Shortliffe EH (eds): Rule-Based Expert Systems: The MYCIN Experiments of the Stanford Heuristic Programming Project. Reading, MA, Addison-Wesley, 1984
21. Friedman RH, Frank AD: Use of a conditional rule structure to automate clinical decision support: A comparison of artificial intelligence and deterministic programming techniques. Comput Biomed Res 16:378–394, 1983
22. Friedman RB, Entine SM, Carbone PP: Experience with an automated cancer protocol surveillance system. Am J Clin Oncol 6:583–592, 1983
23. Wirtschafter DD, Scalise M, Henke C et al: Do information systems improve the quality of clinical research? Results of a randomized trial in a cooperative multi-institutional cancer group. Comput Biomed Res 14:78–90, 1981
24. Lenhard RE, Blum BI, Sunderland JM: The Johns Hopkins' oncology clinical information system. J Med Syst 7:147–174, 1983
25. Wirtschafter DD, Carpenter JT, Mesel E: A consultant-extender system for breast cancer adjuvant chemotherapy. Ann Intern Med 90:396–401, 1979
26. Hickam DH, Shortliffe EH, Bischoff MB et al: The treatment advice of a computer-based chemotherapy protocol advisor. Ann Intern Med 103:928–936, 1985
27. Kent DL, Shortliffe EH, Carlson RW et al: Improvements in data collection through physician use of a computer-based chemotherapy treatment consultant. J Clin Oncol 3:409–417, 1985
28. Greenwald P, Sondik E (eds): Division of Cancer Prevention and Control: Cancer control objectives for the nation: 1985–2000. NCI Monogr 2:1–105, 1986
29. Hubbard SM, DeVita VT: PDQ: An innovation in information dissemination linking cancer research and clinical practice. In DeVita VT, Hellman S, Rosenberg SA (eds): Important Advances in Oncology: 1987, pp 263–277. Philadelphia, JB Lippincott, 1987
30. Perry DJ, Hubbard SM, Masys DR et al: Dose modification for PDQ. Proceedings of the 11th Symposium on Computer Applications in Medical Care, Los Angeles, CA, 1987, pp 739–742.
31. Schipma PB, Cichocki EM, Ziemer SM: Medical information on optical disc. Proceedings of the 11th Symposium on Computer Applications in Medical Care, Los Angeles, CA, 1987, pp 732–738
32. Perry DJ, Sloan EM, Hubbard SM et al: Keeping up with the cancer literature: PDQ and CANCERLIT. (submitted)
33. Walton JD, Musen MA, Combs DM et al: Graphical access to medical expert systems: III. Design of a knowledge acquisition environment. Methods Inf Med 26:78–88, 1987
34. Schwartz WB, Patil RS, Szolovits P: Artificial intelligence in medicine: Where do we stand? N Engl J Med 316:685–688, 1987
35. Haynes RB, McKibbon A, Fitzgerald D et al: How to keep up with the medical literature: V. Access by personal computer to the medical literature. Ann Intern Med 105:810–824, 1986
36. Juckett M, Spratt JS: What is the value of the computer for the physician? J Surg Oncol 34:1–5, 1987
37. Rennels GD, Shortliffe EH, Miller PM et al: A computational model of reasoning from the clinical literature. Comput Methods Programs Biomed 24:139–149, 1987

CHAPTER 66 *Newer Methods of Cancer Treatment*

SECTION 1

ALBERT B. DEISSEROTH

Molecular and Genetic Approaches to Cancer Diagnosis and Treatment

The advent of genetic engineering has spawned a revolution in medicine and biology that provides the oncologist with a new level of understanding of neoplastic diseases, as well as novel approaches to its treatment. These developments will help us define, with precision, the defects that lead to cancer or hematopoietic neoplasms and to tailor-make therapy for each patient. This chapter will summarize the recent discoveries that have occurred in the understanding of the biology of malignancy and then will describe the new directions of therapy that this knowledge will create.

USE OF POLYMERASE CHAIN REACTION TO DETECT MINIMAL RESIDUAL DISEASE

Since the morphology of neoplastic cells in the bone marrow was first described at the light microscopic level, clinicians and pathologists have tried to devise means of increasing the sensitivity for detection of neoplastic cells in aspirates of hematopoietic cells from marrow. Several chemotherapeutic programs have resulted in reduction of the total body tumor or leukemia cell burden by 2 to 3 logs below the level of detection by clinical means. It has not been possible to detect residual abnormal cells in marrow during clinical remission when they are present at dilutions higher than 1 : 1000 normal cells. It has not been possible to exclude the presence of tumor or leukemia cells in populations of marrow used for exogenous hematopoietic reconstitution after intensive therapy for refractory neoplasms. No techniques are available to define the number of therapy cycles that are required to completely remove all tumor cells from the marrow after the induction of a clinical remission in leukemia or lymphoma.

Two developments have combined to make the detection of residual tumor cells possible at a dilution of 1 : 10^6 normal cells. First, the molecular locations of chromosomal translocations, which are specific for a number of leukemias and lymphomas,[1–24] have been established as shown in Table 66-1. Second, an in vitro method has recently been developed for amplifying by 1 million times the amount of rearranged DNA associated with a chromosomal translocation junction point that is a specific marker for the neoplastic cell.[25] This reaction is called the polymerase chain reaction (PCR). As shown in Figure 66-1, cloned pieces from each of the strands of the DNA double helix on each side of the chromosomal translocation junction, called primers, are added to the clinical DNA sample. These primers are necessary to start a synthetic reaction catalyzed by *Escherichia coli* polymerase I. This enzyme uses the primers that anneal to the two strands of the DNA double helix on either side of the translocation junction as starting points to replicate the DNA

TABLE 66-1. Chromosomal Translocations in Hematopoietic Neoplasms

Disease	Chromosomes Involved	Oncogene Close to Translocation	Significance
CML chronic phase[1]	(9;22)	*abl/bcr*	Present in 95%, absence conveys poor prognosis
CML blast crisis	Monosomy 7, isochromosome 17, trisomy 8,18	?	Poor prognosis
M1 ANLL	(9;22)	*abl/bcr*	Present in 5%; poor prognosis
M2 ANLL[2,3]	(8;21)	*ets*	Good prognosis
M3 ANLL[4,5]	(15;17)		Good prognosis
M4, ANLL[6,7] with eosinophilia[8]	Inversion 16		Good prognosis, but associated with CNS involvement
M5, ANLL[8]	Translocations of 11q23	*ets*-1	Poor prognosis
M1, M2, M4, M5 ANLL[8]	Trisomy 8		Poor prognosis
M1, M2, M4 ANLL[8]	Monosomy 7, 5		Poor prognosis
M2 ANLL with basophilia[23]	(6;9q)		Less than 1% of ANLL
ANLL + thrombocytopenia (megakaryoblastic)[24]	3 Deletion or inversion		
M6 ANLL	Monosomy 3,5,7, Trisomy 8		
ALL[9]	(9;22)	*abl/bcr*	20% of adult cases; poor prognosis
ALL (Hyperdiploidy)[8]			Good prognosis
Burkitt's lymphoma, leukemia[10]	(8;14) (also (2;8), (8;22))	*myc*	Poor prognosis
Nodular non-Hodgkins, lymphoma*[11-13]	(14;18)	*bcl*-2, immunoglobulin	
T-cell lymphomas	Inversion 14	*tcl*-1, alpha chain of T-cell antigen receptor	
T-cell leukemias and lymphomas[15]	(11;14)	*tcl*-2, alpha chain of T-cell antigen receptor	
T-cell neoplasms[15]	7q 34	Beta chain of T-cell receptor[1]	
CLL[17]; B-cell leukemias and other B-cell neoplasms[8] (small-cell lymphocyte lymphoma, diffuse large cell lymphoma)	(11;14) (p13; q13)	*bcl*-1	
CLL[18]	Trisomy 12	?	Poor prognosis
Myelodysplasia[19]	Monosomy 7	*met* ?	Poor prognosis
	5q-monosomy 5		Poor prognosis
Secondary ANLL following chemoradiotherapy[20]	Monosomy 7	*met* ?	Poor prognosis
	5q-trisomy 8		Poor prognosis
	Monosomy 5		
Myeloma[21]	Trisomies 3,5,9,15, Monosomies 13,16 t(11;14) (p13;q13)	?	Poor prognosis
Biphenotypic leukemia (lymphoid/monocyloid)[22]	(4;17) (11q;4)	?	Poor prognosis

*Follicular small cleaved cell.
Follicular mixed cell.
Follicular large cell.

on both sides of the translocation junction, as shown in Figure 66-1. Because there is no location in the normal cell to which both primers bind in proximity to both strands of the DNA double helix, no complete double-stranded gene sequence in the normal DNA is replicated. As shown in Figure 66-1, by repeating this cycle of denaturation and replication 20 times, the relative ratio of the abnormal junctional DNA/normal DNA (cancer cell/normal cell) can be increased 1 million-fold. The DNA must be denatured between each synthetic reaction to reestablish a double-stranded helix with primers on each side of the translocation junction for the polymerization reaction to work.

This technique will enable one to measure residual tumor cells in the marrow cells of patients in complete remission, even when they are present at a ratio of 1 abnormal cell/10^6 normal cells instead of at a ratio of only 1 abnormal cell/1000 normal cells, as is currently the case. In addition, this technique will permit us to screen for contaminating abnormal cells in marrow collections that are used to support patients being treated with intensive therapy. It will be possible to test if there is a threshold of cytoreduction beyond which the immune system of the body can permanently control a neoplasm. It will be possible to define more precisely the therapeutic endpoints of our experimental protocols. Thus, more objective means are now available to define the optimal duration of therapy required to rid each patient's body of all tumor cells. Primers for the polymerase chain reactions are available for the *bcr–abl* translocation of chronic myelocytic leukemia (CML), the 14/18 translocation of follicular lymphoma, and for diseases that carry clonal rearrangements of the T-cell receptor gene or the immunoglobulin gene. Further application of this technique will depend on the cloning of junction fragments to be used as primers from translocations that are specific for additional solid tumors and hematopoietic neoplasms.

USE OF LOSS OF HETEROZYGOSITY TO LOCALIZE CANCER SUPPRESSOR GENES (ANTIONCOGENES)

The existence of stable variations in the population at the nucleotide sequence level (termed *genetic polymorphisms*) and the presence in each normal cell of two chromosomal analogues, one maternal and one paternal, result in the ability to detect two separate copies (*alleles*) of each gene in every normal cell (as shown in Figs. 66-2A–C). It has been estimated that there are, on the average, differences in the nucleotide composition of DNA in at least 1 in every 200 nucleotides throughout the genome in corresponding positions of any two individuals randomly selected from the population at large. This variation in DNA composition has made possible the isolation of probes for polymorphisms in regions of every chromosome. Another variation in DNA, the insertion of repeat sequences called *minisatellite DNA*, has permitted the development of a diagnostic technique called *DNA fingerprinting*.[26] The use of DNA fingerprinting can distinguish between the DNA of different siblings in a family and, therefore, is useful, as is restriction fragment length polymorphism analysis, in determining the origin of cells (donor or recipient) after bone marrow transplantation.

As shown in Table 66-2, allelic alterations around biologically important genes, as well as in anonymous areas of the genome, have been used to define variations (termed *heterozygosity*), which are used as markers for genes, in the DNA of normal cells.[27–43] Because of the clonal nature of many leukemias, lymphomas, and some solid tumors, it has been possible to use the existence of these DNA polymorphisms to determine that specific pieces of DNA have been lost in many solid tumors and hematopoietic malignancies such as carcinomas of the breast, colon, and lung, as well as retinoblastoma, Wilms' tumor, and osteogenic sarcoma (see Table 66-2). The DNA that is lost during the evolution of cancer may involve coding regions of cancer suppressor genes or

TABLE 66-2. Deletion of Cancer Suppressor Genes (Antioncogenes) by Loss of Heterozygosity

Disease	*Chromosomal Location of Loss of Heterozygosity*	*Reference*	*Genes in the Region*
Rhabdomyosarcoma	11p 15.5 → 11pTer	(27)	Unknown
Myelodysplastic syndrome	5q	(28)	*GMCSF*, *IL-3* PDGF receptor, *CSF-1*, c-*FMS*
	7q21–22	(29)	*met*
Renal cell carcinoma	3p (also 3,11) or (3,8) translocation	(30)	
Wilms' tumor	11p13	(31)	*ras*
Retinoblastoma	13q14	(32)	Retinoblastoma antioncogene
Osteogenic sarcoma	13q14		
Ewing's sarcoma/neuroepithelioma	t(11;22)	(33)	
Bladder cancer	11p	(34)	*ras*
Embryonal Tumors	11p13	(35)	
Beckwith–Wiedeman syndrome (rhabdomysarcoma and hepatoblastomas)			
Small-cell	3p(14–23)	(36)	?
Colorectal cancer	5q	(37)	?
Acoustic neuroma	1p	(38)	?
Neuroblastoma	1p(31–36)	(39)	?
Prostate	10q(23–24)	(40)	?
Testicular	Isochromosome 12q	(41)	?
Melanoma	1p22	(42)	?
Meningioma	Monosomy 22	(43)	?

Note: The examples of loss of heterozygosity in each chromosome listed may not be specific for each neoplasm (the data are very early in their analysis) and, in some cases cited, it is found in only a small percentage of patients (*e.g.*, 5q in colon cancer). In addition, "benign" or the malignant conditions (benign polyps of the colon, midline granuloma) have been found to exhibit loss of heterozygosity.

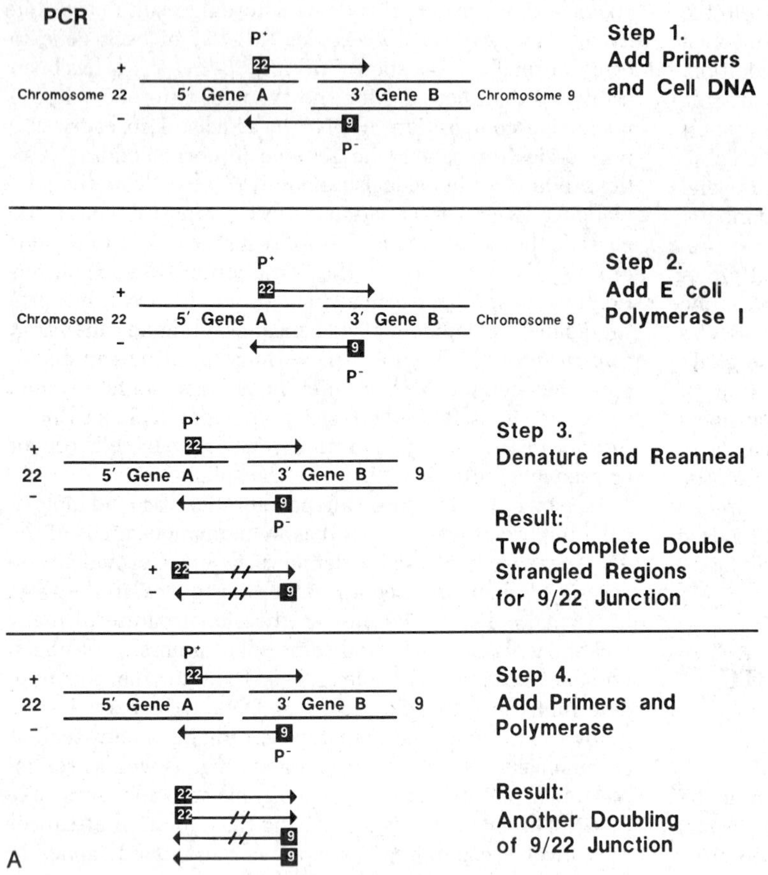

FIG. 66-1. Polymerase chain reaction of normal (**A**) and translocated (**B**) material. Pr^+ = primer for the plus strand of DNA; Pr^- = primer for the minus strand of DNA. Because the two primers are cloned from each side of the translocation junction, they bind on both strands of DNA on either side of the translocation junction. This results in the complete duplication of the abnormal chromosomal junctional DNA each time the PCR reaction is run. In normal DNA, there is no region to which the two primers can bind in proximity to each other on the positive and negative strands of DNA. Therefore, no normal DNA is doubled by the PCR reaction. This leads to selective enrichment of the chromosomal junctional DNA 1 million-fold during 22 cycles of the PCR.

antioncogenes, the products of which are involved in the normal regulation of cellular proliferation and differentiation. Antioncogene regions, corresponding to the areas lost from chromosome 13 in retinoblastoma and from chromosome 11 in Wilms' tumor, have been recently cloned and isolated. Probes for these regions are being studied for their diagnostic value as well as for establishing prognosis in several solid tumors. Once the gene products responsible for the putative antioncogenes action are established, they may become useful for therapy based on reprogramming the neoplastic cell to more regulated patterns of growth and differentiation.

It is possible that persons who develop cancer carry a congenital cryptic mutation in one of their two antioncogene alleles and subsequently lose the remaining normal antioncogene allele, as detected by restriction fragment length polymorphism analysis, minisatellite probes, or cytogenetic detectable deletions. This results in a marked increase in their susceptibility to developing cancer in a given organ site. This characterization of the biologic role of each genetic locus modified in each organ site may help in developing new therapeutic interventions based on gene replacement therapy for tumors of each organ site in the future.

CHARACTERIZATION OF THE ANTIONCOGENE LOST IN RETINOBLASTOMA: AN EXAMPLE OF THE USE OF REVERSE GENETICS TO CHARACTERIZE THE MOLECULAR BASIS OF CANCER

Before 1980, to identify the genetic locus responsible for any disease, it was necessary to know the protein involved and often its biologic function. Investigation then proceeded to the isolation of RNA and, after this, the DNA associated with a given molecular disease. Because of the ability to localize abnormalities in genes by the restriction fragment length polymorphism analysis just summarized and to clone these genes from DNA, it has now become possible to identify the

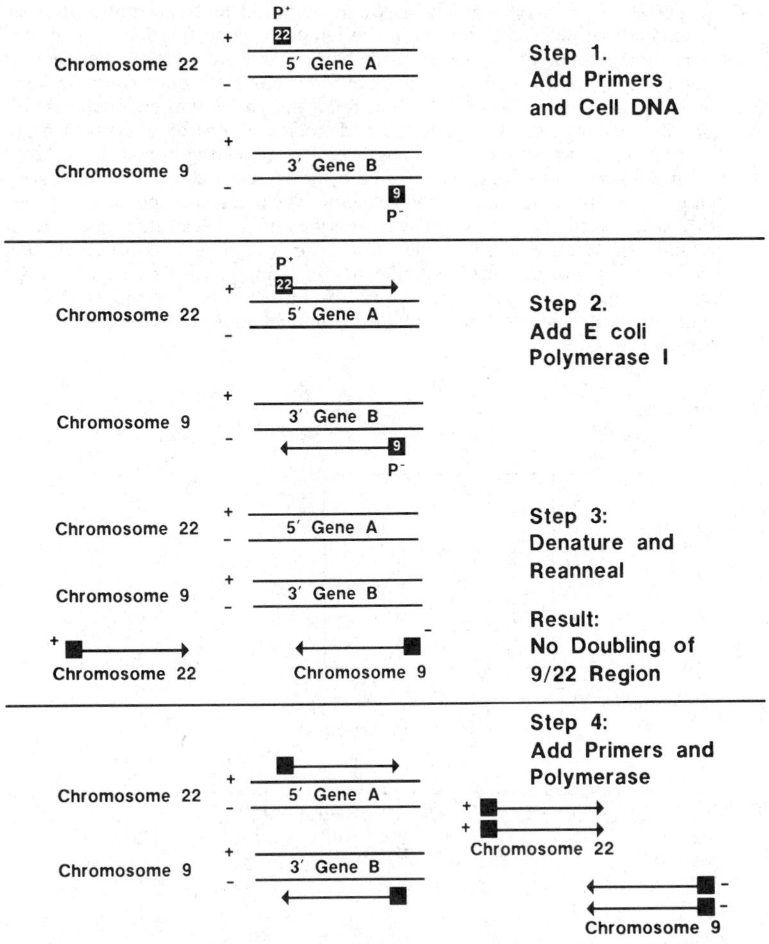

B Result: No Accumulation of Doublestanding DNA from 9/22 Region

existence of a genetic locus, the abnormality of which is responsible for a given disease, without knowing the protein product of the gene or its role in the disease. One can often then clone the gene that causes a disease before the protein product of the gene is known or even before biologic function of the gene product is known. The characterization of the biologic nature of the protein product of the gene may then become clear through structural analysis of the gene itself. This is called reverse genetics (discovering an unknown gene, the product of which is missing in a disease and then discovering its protein product). An example of this is provided by the discovery of the cancer suppressor gene in retinoblastoma (see previous section and Table 66-2). For many years, statistical and family studies of retinoblastoma had suggested the existence of a genetic locus, the loss of which was a necessary prerequisite for the development of retinoblastoma.[44] Subsequent use of enzyme phenotyping and cytogenetic analysis suggested that this locus was on chromosome 13. The discovery that loss of restriction fragment length polymorphisms in this region accompanied the evolution of retinoblastoma was critical to the discovery of the retinoblastoma "susceptibility gene" or the retinoblastoma "cancer suppressor gene" termed *RB*, the loss of which is a step in the development of retinoblastoma.

It has now been determined that the protein product of this gene is probably a transcriptional regulatory protein that governs the expression of genes through binding to their regulatory regions.[45] Several other DNA-binding proteins involved in the evolution of cancer have been discovered (*e.g.*, *myb*, *myc*, *fos*). Clearly the means of discovering genetic changes at the DNA level, which are operative in neoplastic diseases, has led to the discovery of new mechanisms of oncogenesis. These advances undoubtedly will provide new targets for novel therapeutic interventions in the future.

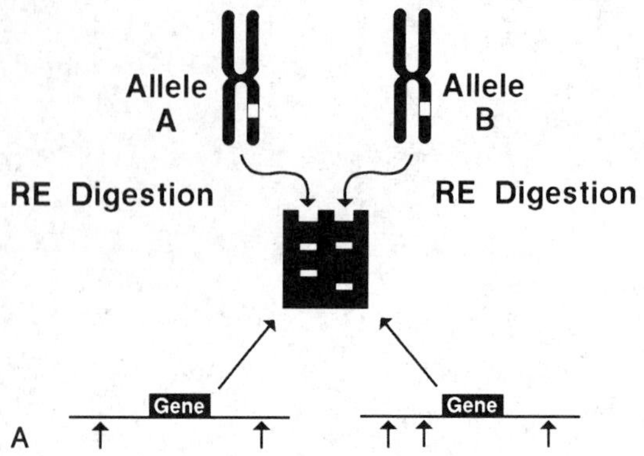

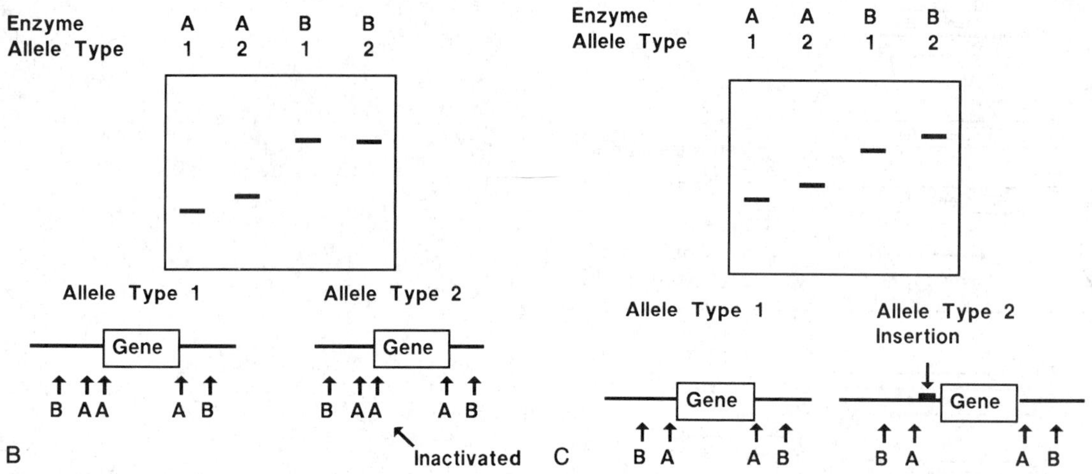

FIG. 66-2. **A**. Variations in the DNA in maternal and paternal chromosomal homologues result in differences in the length of gene fragments generated by restriction endonuclease. Arrows at the bottom indicate restriction endonuclease sites; the symbols by allele A and B are chromosomes; the curved arrows from the chromosomes lead to a Southern blot following restriction endonuclease digestion. **B**. Loss of a single restriction endonuclease site for enzyme A by point mutation leads to an increased length of the gene fragment released by that enzyme. Fragments of genes generated by other restrictions endonucleases (enzyme B) will still be normal, as shown below. The box shows the molecular weight of the gene fragments generated by restriction endonuclease digestion in a Southern blot. **C**. Mechanisms by which restriction fragment length polymorphisms lead to changes of diagnostic significance in humans. In the case of restriction fragment length polymorphisms caused by insertion or deletion of DNA, fragments generated by several restriction endonucleases will all exhibit a variant fragment length.

ROLE OF EXTRACELLULAR MATRIX IN CANCER AND LEUKEMIA

From the past 10 years, it has become clear that the growth of solid tumor cells depends not only on the presence of internal growth stimulatory signals and altered interactions between extracellular growth regulatory signals (growth factors), but also on the type of surface upon which the tumor cells grow. Epithelial neoplasms of specific organ sites exhibit growth dependencies on extracellular matrix proteins (proteins on which the normal and neoplastic epithelial cells grow) such as fibronectin and laminin.[46] Highly metastatic fibrosarcoma cells exhibit an independence of laminin for their growth, whereas fibrosarcoma cells of low metastatic potential required the presence of laminin to grow well.[47] The surface of the "laminin-independent" highly metastatic cells contained a molecule immunologically similar to laminin, suggesting that the development of the metastatic phenotype (the ability to grow in many different tissue environments) evolved from the ability of the tumor cells to synthesize its own extracellular matrix protein and to deploy it on its surface.

Breast cancer cells have been found to contain an autocrine growth regulatory molecule, *tumor autocrine mobility factor*, that stimulates extension of pseudopodia on which a 20-fold increase of laminin and fibronectin receptors reside.[48] Thus, the tumor-angiogenesis factor (TAF) autocrine factor stimulates tumor locomotion and metastasis by improving the ability of the tumor cell to interact with extracellular matrix and develop pseudopodia.[48] Fibrosarcoma tumors have been reported to secrete factors (transforming growth factor-β; TGF-β) that stimulate the production of the extracellular matrix.

Extracellular matrix proteins specific for hematopoietic cells (*e.g.*, hemonectin) have also recently been discovered.[49] Differences in the binding of normal and CML hematopoietic stem cells to extracellular matrix are now being exploited in many laboratories in an attempt to separate CML cells from residual normal hematopoietic stem cells for use in intensive therapeutic options in CML that require autologous stem cell support.[50]

The characterization of the extracellular matrix proteins and their cellular receptors on the hematopoietic neoplasms and solid tumors may provide new molecular approaches to the therapy of these diseases. Attempts to develop monoclonal antibodies to the extracellular matrix receptors on cells or molecules that can mask these receptors on tumor cells may provide additional approaches to the prevention of metastases and result in the eventual control of epithelial malignancies as well as hematopoietic neoplasms.

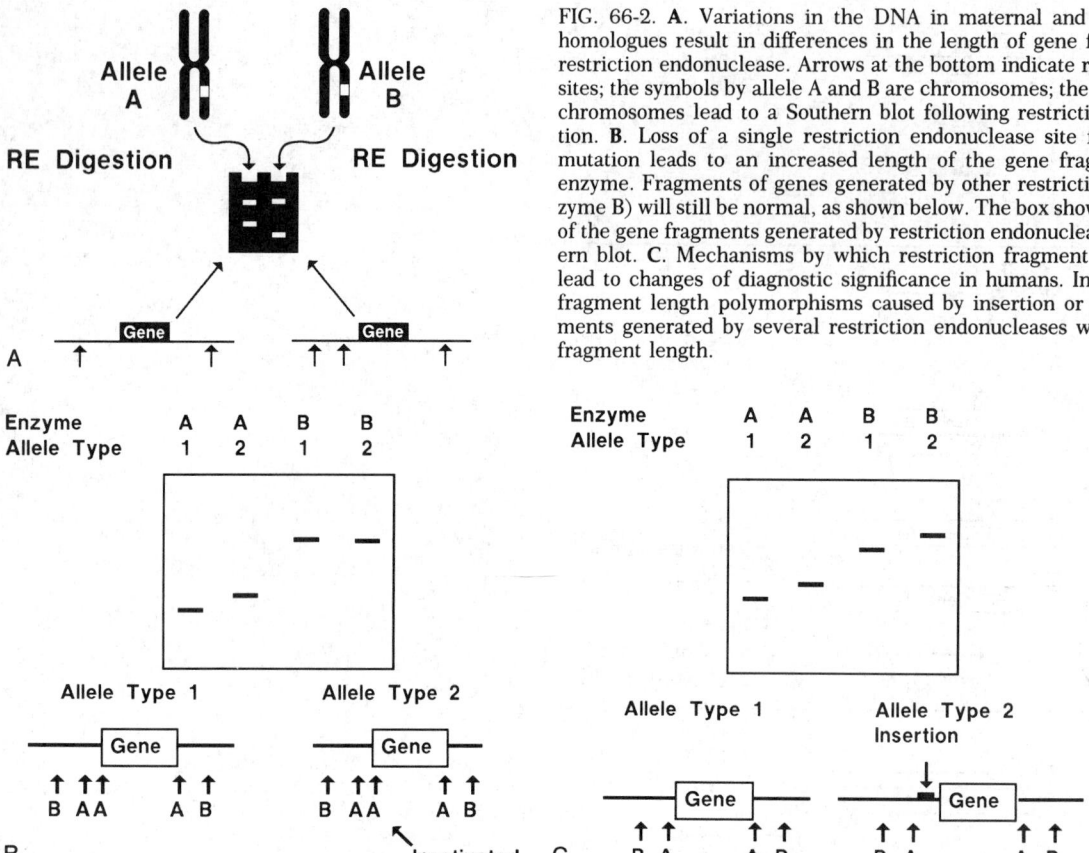

ONCOGENES: TARGETS OF MOLECULAR APPROACHES TO DIAGNOSIS AND TREATMENT OF CANCER

The discovery of genes in RNA tumor and leukemia viruses, termed *oncogenes*, that are responsible for the rapid transformation by viruses of rodent and avian tissue, led to the recognition that cellular homologues of these transforming genes, called *proto-oncogenes*, exist in normal cells, and that alteration of the structure and expression of these genes occur in tumors. Oncogenes have been found to code for growth factor receptors (*Erb*-b), growth factors (*sis, TGF-β*), protein kinases (*abl, src*), and DNA-binding proteins (*myb, fos, myc*). Mutational change, induced by environmental carcinogens or by errors in normal cellular processes, alters the protein products of the proto-oncogenes so that they are similar in biologic effect to the protein products of the transforming genes of retroviral oncogenes. Altered expression of several proto-oncogenes in human tumors has been documented (Table 66-3A). Such abnormal states of proto-oncogene expression produces useful markers for a wide variety of tumors, as shown in Table 66-3A. Altered expression of these genes takes place through at least three mechanisms as shown in Figure 66-3.

1. Point mutations (Fig. 66-3A) alter the biologic activity of the gene. Mutations in the *ras* genes at amino acid positions 12 and 61 have been documented in leukemia,[51] myelodysplastic syndrome,[52] colon cancer,[53] breast cancer,[54] bladder cancer,[55] and papillomas. This mutation decreases the GTPase activity of the *ras* gene.
2. Amplification of a gene (Fig. 66-3B) leads to elevation of the level of the protein product of the N-*myc* oncogene in neuroblastoma and retinoblastoma,[56,57] c-*Erb*-b in breast cancer,[58,59] c-*myb* in colon cancer,[60] c-*myc* and N-*myc* in small cell carcinoma of the lung,[61,62] and epidermal growth factor (*EGF*) receptor gene in glial tumors,[63] as shown in Table 66-3.
3. Translocation (see Fig. 66-3 and Table 66-1) of the oncogene into a transcriptionally active domain, such as occurs with c-*myc* into immunoglobulin in Burkitt's lymphoma,[10] and c-*abl* into *bcr* in CML,[1] leads to unregulated expression or to a protein of altered biologic activity, respectively.

TABLE 66-3A. Activation of Cellular Oncogenes in Human Cancer

Disease	Oncogene
Colon	*ras, myb*
Prostate	*ras*
Breast	*ras, Her, Erb*-b-2
Myelodysplastic disease	*ras*
Burkitt's lymphoma	c-*myc, bcl*-1
Small-cell carcinoma of the lung	N-*myc*, c-*myc*
Non–small-cell carcinoma of the lung	*Erb*-b
Neuroblastoma	N-*myc, ets*-1
Wilms' tumor	N-*myc*
Ewing's sarcoma	c-*myc*
Neuroepithelioma	c-*myc*
Squamous cell head and neck	*Erb*-b
CML	*abl*
T-cell ALL	*tcl*-2
Follicular non-Hodgkin's lymphoma	*bcl*-2
Myeloma	*myc, ras*
Glioblastoma	*sis*

TABLE 66-3B. Mutational Change in Oncogenes

	Oncogene	Disease
Point Mutation	*ras*[52–56]	AML[51], myelodysplastic disease[52]
		Colon cancer[53]
		Breast cancer[54]
		Bladder cancer[55]
		Papillomas[56]
Amplification	N-*myc*[57]	Neuroblastoma, retinoblastoma
	c-*Erb*-b[58,59]	Breast cancer
	c-*myb*[60]	Colon cancer
	c-*myc*, N-*myc*[61,62]	Small-cell carcinoma—lung
	c-*Erb*-b[63]	Glial tumors
Translocation	c-*myc*[10]	Burkitt's lymphoma
	c-*abl*[1]	CML

Patterns of oncogene expression have recently been used to identify specific types of tumors that are hard to define on the histopathologic level alone (*e.g.*, neuroepithelioma, in which expression of c-*ets*-1 is variable, N-*myc* is low, and c-*myc* is high; and neuroblastoma, in which expression of c-*ets*-1 is positive, N-*myc* is high, and c-*myc* is low).[64] There are undoubtedly many more mechanisms through which alteration of proto-oncogenes may lead to cancer. Whether any of these constitute the initial transforming event or are acquired late in the evolution of the disease is not known.

As discussed previously, several of the oncogenes are DNA-binding proteins and may exert a pleotropic effect on gene expression in the cell. At least one of the so-called antioncogenes (the deleted sequence on chromosome 13 that is associated with neuroblastoma) has been found to be a DNA-binding protein.[45] Because structural analysis of some of the transcriptional regulatory factors has shown them to consist of a DNA-binding domain and a phosphoprotein domain, the hypothesis outlined in Figure 66-3D has been proposed to explain the mechanism by which gene expression is altered in cancer. In this formulation, altered expression of kinase genes by translocation or point mutation could lead to loss of specificity of the protein kinase. The inappropriate phosphorylation of transcriptional regulatory proteins alters the effect of these proteins at the regulatory regions of growth-stimulatory genes, which leads to their activation. This hypothesis could conceivably explain the manner in which the *bcr–abl* kinase alters gene expression in CML.

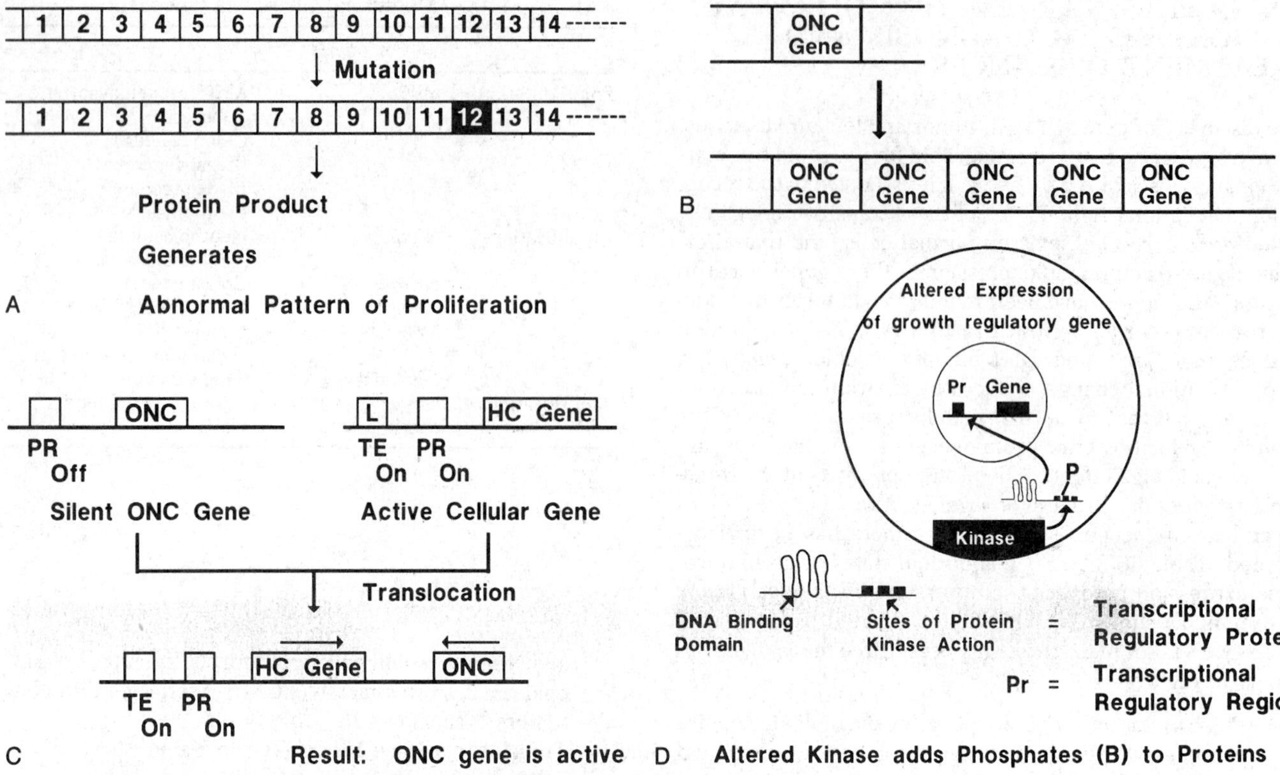

FIG. 66-3. Alteration of oncogene expression by point mutation, amplification, and translocation. **A.** A point mutation in the codon for the 12th amino acid changes the biologic properties of the protein so as to lead to unregulated growth (*e.g.*, *ras* in bladder cancer cell line T24). **B.** Amplification of an oncogene leads to the acquisition of multiple copies of the gene, resulting in abnormally high levels of the protein product of the gene, which leads to abnormal growth (*e.g.*, n-*myc* in neuroblastoma). **C.** Translocation of a silent proto-oncogene (*ONC*) that splits the gene from its 5′ regulatory region into the domain of a very active transcriptional enhancer (*TE*), and transcriptional promoter (*PR*) linked to a highly active cellular gene (*HC*) leads to unregulated expression of the cellular proto-oncogene (*e.g.*, c-*myc* in the [8; 14] translocation of Burkitt's lymphoma) or to a change in the biologic nature of the protein product of the proto-oncogene (*e.g.*, *abl* in CML). **D.** Relationship of abnormal kinase function and altered behavior of DNA binding protein oncogenes. Chromosomal translocation (such as [9; 22] in CML) alters a protein kinase. The activity of this enzyme results in modification of transcriptional regulatory protein (DNA binding protein) by adding phosphates to the kinase domain. This alters the affinity or biologic activity of the DNA binding domain in the regulatory regions (*Pr*) of the genes that govern proliferation or differentiation resulting in the disease state (such as CML).

ALTERED GROWTH FACTOR AND GROWTH FACTOR RECEPTORS IN NEOPLASTIC DISEASE

Alterations in the expression and function of growth factors and growth factor receptor genes have been identified in many solid tumors and hematopoietic neoplasms. Examples of such genes include *fms*, *Erb*-b, *Erb*-a, *sis*, *TGF-α*, *TGF-β*, *PDGF*-1, and *PDGF*-2. These and other cellular homologues of retroviral oncogenes are being studied for their use as predictors of prognosis in both solid tumors and hematopoietic neoplasms. Amplification or increased expression of c-*myc* in small-cell carcinoma of the lung,[65] of N-*myc* in neuroblastoma,[56,57] or of the *Neu* oncogene in carcinoma of the breast,[58] have been associated with differences in responsiveness to chemotherapy or with survival.

Other growth regulatory peptides, such as bombesin, have been shown to be secreted by the tumor tissues themselves, as in small-cell carcinoma of the lung. These molecules have become the targets for therapy. Monoclonal antibodies to the bombesin receptor are being used to inhibit the stimulatory effect of bombesin on small-cell carcinoma cells. Similar experiments are underway with EGF receptors in squamous cell malignancies. As more examples of altered states of expression of the growth regulatory molecules are discovered in solid tumors and hematopoietic malignancies, they will become the targets of therapeutic interventions. Table 66-4 summarizes the growth factors or their receptors that are associated with tumors of specific organ sites. The ultimate goal of current biologic research in cancer and leukemia is to understand the mechanisms by which regulation of expression of these growth regulatory genes is mediated and

TABLE 66-4. Growth Factors as Markers of Cancer

Organ Site of Cancer	*Growth Regulatory Molecule That Is Marker of Cancer*
Pancreas	Cholecystokinin
Breast, lung	EGF receptor (ERB-b)
Small-cell carcinoma of the lung	Bombesin
Glioblastoma	PDGF
Acute T-cell leukemia	IL-2 receptor
Acute myeloid leukemia	IL-3, GM-CSF
Melanoma	MSH
Thyroid cancer	TSH

how this affects the natural history of cancer and their response to therapy. Once we are able to modulate the activity of growth regulatory proteins, we may be able to use this knowledge on a therapeutic level.

USE OF TARGETING AGENTS FOR THERAPY IN CANCER

For many years, cancer biologists and clinicians have been studying how to use monoclonal antibodies that recognize differentiation antigens in hematopoietic neoplasms and solid tumors. These efforts have been limited by the toxicity of these reagents to normal cells, as well as to tumor cells. The escape of the neoplastic cell by clonal evolution or antigenic modulation, and the heterogeneity of the tumor cells for the expression of such antigens, have also limited the usefulness of this approach.

The first phase of research in this field focused on the use of monoclonal antibodies directly for therapy. A number of monoclonal antibodies have been identified for radionuclide-imaging studies of tumors as well as for targeting radioisotopes, chemotherapeutic agents, and biologic toxins for therapy of hematologic malignancies and solid tumors, as shown in Table 66-5. Although these reagents have almost uniformly been of value in imagining studies, the value of unconjugated monoclonal antibody infusions as therapeutic tools for lymphomas, leukemias, and solid tumors currently remain unproved. This has largely been due to heterogeneity of the expression of the antigens to which the monoclonal antibodies are directed on the tumor cells and their tendency to undergo mutational change. Current attempts to improve the results achievable with antibodies have focused on the development of anti-idiotype antibodies and vaccines.

The second phase of research with monoclonal antibodies as therapeutic tools has involved the conjugation of monoclonal antibodies to radioisotopes, chemotherapeutic agents, and biologic toxins (see Table 66-5). Once such reagent composed of a conjugate between anti–T-cell antibodies and the ricin toxin has been shown to be of value in the treatment of steroid-resistant graft-versus-host disease. Several major problems have now been identified with such therapy: [1] nonspecific uptake of the monoclonal conjugates into the liver or kidney; [2] myelosuppression with radionucleotide conjugates; [3] the evolution of neutralizing antibodies; [4] limited equilibration with extravascular space and tumor penetration, often because of the high molecular weight of these conjugates.

To attempt to solve many of these problems, the so-called third-generation targeting reagents have been created at the DNA level through genetic engineering (see Table 66-5). In this work, a family of biologic toxins (diphtheria toxin or pseudomonas exotoxin) has been modified at the gene level to remove binding domains that mediate attachment of the toxins to most cells of the body, as shown in Figure 66-4. The remaining parts of the molecule, the cellular uptake domain and the toxin domain (usually an inhibitor of protein synthesis), are then attached at the DNA level to a targeting molecule, such as the interleukin-2 (IL-2) growth factor, which mediates the attachment of the toxin to a specific abnormal

TABLE 66-5. Monoclonal Antibodies Used in Diagnosis and Treatment of Cancer

Monoclonal Reagents for Diagnosis and Imaging
Melanoma
Pancreatic cancer
Prostate cancer
Colonic cancer
Ovarian cancer
Head and neck cancer
Small-cell cancer of the lung
Neuroblastoma
T-cell and myeloid antigens
Ferritin
Carcinoembryonic antigen
Hybrid Toxins for Therapy
Diphtheria toxin
Pseudomonas exotoxin
Ricin toxin

FIG. 66-4. Construction of hybrid toxin genes for therapy. The nonselective binding domain of a bacterial toxin is replaced by a ligand for a receptor specific for a target neoplastic cell having the cellular uptake and toxic domain intact. This results in a molecule that is specifically lethal for tumor cells (*e.g.,* work of Jack Murphy in Boston, Ira Pastan at the NIH, or Ellen Vitteta in Dallas). T, toxin domain (often an inhibitor of elongation in protein synthesis); CU, cellular uptake domain; B, binding domain.

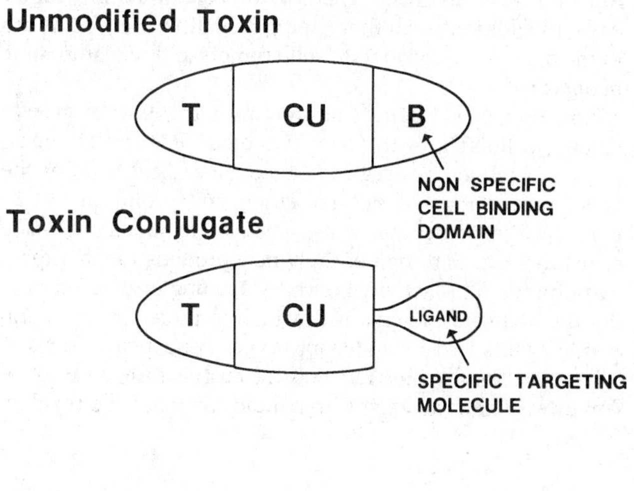

cell (HTLV-1 leukemia) or activated T cells that express the IL-2 growth factor receptor and are participants in pathogenetic disease-related processes such as graft-versus-host disease.

A recent example of implementation of this strategy is the construction of a hybrid toxin gene composed of the cellular uptake and binding domain of pseudomonas exotoxin and a monoclonal antibody, developed by Ira Pastan's group of NIH, which is directed against the drug-resistance genes that become amplified in tumor cells in the presence of chemotherapy. If one were to give a patient the drug-resistance monoclonal–toxin conjugate alone, the tumor cells that are resistent to chemotherapy would die but those sensitive to chemotherapy would survive. Application of both chemotherapy and the immunoconjugate would prevent escape of the neoplastic population by clonal evolution. In the next few years, the synchronous delivery of therapy directed to several such targets may help improve results in both solid tumors and hematopoietic neoplasms.

Drs. J. Murphy and T. Strom of Boston have taken the diphtheria toxin gene and removed the cellular-binding domain and replaced it with the IL-2 gene that binds to the antigen recognition receptor of the T-cell lymphocyte. This fusion gene has been placed into expression vectors in bacterial cells in which quantities of the fusion protein are produced that are sufficient for therapy. In contrast to immunoconjugates made at the protein level, which are very large, this reagent is of low molecular weight thus permitting it to equilibrate with the extravascular space. Because it lacks the variable and constant regions of mouse monoclonal antibodies, which are often used for targeting, it is less immunogenic, thus reducing the problem with neutralizing antibodies. It is not covered with carbohydrates and, therefore, is not taken up by the liver. It is totally specific in its binding because the Tac antigen-binding domain has replaced the nonspecific diphtheria toxin-binding domain and thus will not cause myelosuppression or mucositis. Finally, its destructive action is dose-dependent and, therefore, one can titrate the dose to kill those cells with the highest levels of receptors. This property of the reagent makes it ideal for the modulation of graft-versus-host disease because the attacking populations of T cells in graft-versus-host disease have the highest number of Tac antigen receptors. Such immunoconjugates may also be of value in cleansing normal marrow, that is to be used to reconstitute normal hematopoietic function after intensive therapy, of contaminating tumor cells. In addition, such therapeutic modalities may be of use in the systemic treatment of solid tumors and hematopoietic neoplasms.

Now that the sequences of proteins and genes for growth factors, cellular growth factor receptors, ion and chemical pumps which act as drug-resistance genes, and most of the cellular mediators of differentiation and proliferation are being worked out, it becomes possible to modify existing structures and to design entirely new proteins for therapeutic purposes. This activity is already ongoing in an attempt to develop delivery systems with which to target chemotherapeutic agents and recombinant toxins to neoplastic cells.

These examples illustrate how the custom design of a gene can provide the therapist with a molecule that is better than those Mother Nature has produced. The ability to analyze structure–function relationships by computer virtually provides one unlimited opportunity to create new therapeutic reagents. The cancer researcher can accomplish in a few months of computer modeling and automated synthesis what required millions of years to be produced by evolution. Clearly we are entering an exciting era in which the oncologist–hematologist may be a genetic engineer who will be in a position to design new therapeutic reagents that are based on the understanding of neoplastic disease at the molecular level.

REPROGRAMMING THERAPY FOR CANCER

Strategies designed to destroy or remove neoplastic tissue are currently the cornerstone of cancer and leukemia treatment. The current accumulation of knowledge about the mechanisms that govern cellular proliferation and differentiation may make possible *reprogramming therapy* as a new approach to the management of these diseases. Not only are growth regulatory factors being cloned and produced in quantities sufficient for therapy, but the intranuclear signals that mediate the activation and inhibition of gene expression are being purified and characterized. The set of proteins in the nucleus that regulates gene expression represent a final common pathway through which all signals affecting gene expression must pass. In addition, it is possible that each intranuclear regulatory protein regulates many genes. If we are able to characterize the mechanisms by which factors involved in the regulation of proliferation and differentiated gene expression, we may be able to forge therapeutic approaches to many neoplastic diseases with one or two reagents.

Such an approach has many advantages. It might not be as toxic or functionally disabling as current treatment programs. Once the mechanisms by which these regulatory proteins act is known, it is possible that drugs could be designed that would amplify or inhibit the interaction of each regulatory protein with DNA. Finally, because these treatments are affecting the final common pathway of signal transduction in the cell, the modulation of a single regulatory protein might be appropriate for hundreds of different types of mutations in evolving leukemic or solid tumor populations from different patients. Thus, the problem posed by tumor cell heterogeneity and genetic instability of neoplastic populations for therapy could potentially be solved.

GENE REPLACEMENT THERAPY FOR CANCER

Constitutional or acquired abnormalities in the function of structural genes can result in "molecular diseases" that involve virtually every organ of the body and every physiologic system in the body. Those diseases that affect the hematopoietic system and result in uncontrolled proliferation of abnormal differentiation result in diseases that have been the area of interest of the hematologist–oncologist. Culture systems permit the short-term growth in vitro of cells from the skin, muscle, liver, breast, as well as the mucosal cells of the gastrointestinal, respiratory, and urothelial tracts, as well as the hematopoietic cells. Methods of stably introducing functional genes into mammalian cells are available. Thus, it is time to develop systems for the replacement of genes, the malfunction of which result in neoplastic diseases in humans. Examples of diseases that arise from the malfunction of single genes include: phenylketonuria; Gaucher's disease; accelerated atherosclerosis (congenital deficiency of the lipoprotein carriers of cholesterol and triglycerides or the cellular receptors for their disposition); α_1-antitrypsin deficiency; adenosine deaminase deficiency, which leads to severe combined immunodeficiency disease; factor VIII deficiency, which leads to hemophilia; deficiency of α- or β-globin gene expression, which leads to thalassemia; and deficiency of antithrombin III, protein S, and protein C, all of which lead to hypercoagulable states (Table 66-6). One can either attempt to introduce functional genes into hematopoietic cells or into autologous fibroblasts that one can then engraft either into the marrow or onto the skin of recipients. Although the technology of engraftment has been worked out for several years, the gene delivery systems required for the introduction of single-copy genes in a form that permits expression of genes at the level required for physiologic amounts of the missing gene product are not yet available. Most workers in the field are experimenting with viral or plasmid gene delivery systems.

Introduction of the plasmid gene delivery systems that are currently available into mammalian cells results in cell lines that express physiologically significant and appropriate levels of the missing gene product in only a very tiny fraction of the starting cells. This weakness imposes the necessity for genetic selection systems and in vitro or in vivo selection to maintain the modified cells in the population. Despite these constraints, experiments with retroviral vectors that contain the hematopoietic growth factors GM-CSF and IL-3 have led to model systems for CML.[66] Retroviral systems, as shown in Figures 66-5 and 66-6 are attracting a lot of attention by workers who are attempting to design vectors that do not spread horizontally in the population; that provide adequate levels of expression of the missing gene; that do not recombine in the host cell to produce unwanted gene products; and that persist in the setting of bone marrow transplant, if hematopoietic cells are modified, or in the setting of organ or skin transplant.

These systems have the potential not only to replace missing genes but also to modify important cellular processes such as graft rejection in organ (heart, lung, liver, and kidney) transplant and graft-versus-host disease in bone marrow transplantation. We may be in a position to modify gene expression in organs by in vitro perfusion of virus or plasmid gene transfer systems into these organs, or into hematopoietic cells in vitro. The challenge that remains before such strategies can be implemented include working out the technology to modify or replace genes on a molecular level in 100% of the cells in a population.

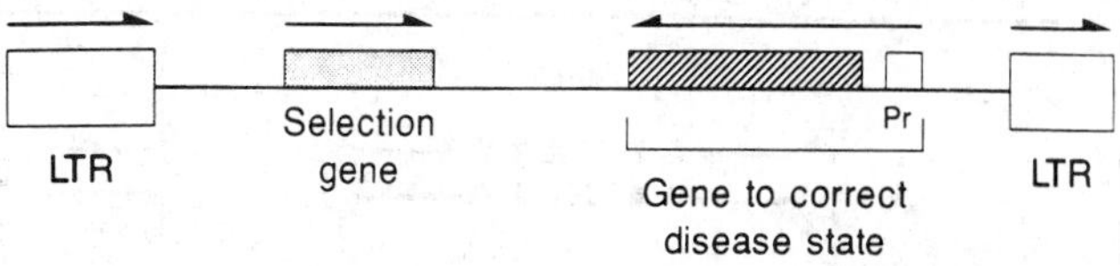

FIG. 66-5. Components of retroviral vectors used for introducing genes into mammalian cells. LTR, long terminal repeat, which contains sequences for transcriptional activation of genes as well as the polyadenylation of mRNA; Pr, transcriptional promoter. Arrows indicate the direction of transcription.

TABLE 66-6. Examples of Genes and Growth Regulatory Molecules That Have Been Cloned

Cloned Genes That Are Known to be Missing in Diseases
Tissue plasminogen activator (hypercoaguable stages)
Factor VIII (antihemophilic factor; hemophilia)
Von Willebrand factor (Von Willebrand disease)
α_1-Antitrypsin (chronic obstructive pulmonary disease)
Insulin (diabetes)
Growth hormone (dwarfism)
Adenosine deaminase (severe combine immunodeficiency disease)
Globin (thalassemia)
Hypoxanthire-guanine phosphoribosy transferases (Lesch–Nyhan disease)
Glucosylceramidase (Gancher's disease)
Pyruvate kinase (mental retardation)
Low-density lipoprotein (atherosclerosis)
Growth Regulatory Molecules That Have Been Cloned
Erythropoietin (EPO)
Granulocyte colony-stimulating factor (GCSF)
Granulocyte macrophage colony-stimulating factor (GM-CSF)
Colony-stimulating factor (CSF)
Platelet-derived growth factor (PDGF)
Platelet-derived growth factor receptor
Interleukins (IL-) (1, 2, 3, 4, 6)
Colony-stimulating factor-1 receptor (c-FMS)
Oncogenes (*myc, myb, Erb*-a, *Erb*-b, *src, abl, mos, fos, fms, met,* etc).
Lymphotoxin
T-Cell receptor genes α and β
Epidermal growth factor and its receptor
Tumor-derived growth factors α and β
Tumor necrosis factor
Interferons (IFN-) α, β, and γ

FIG. 66-6. Infection of a hematopoietic cell by a retrovirus leads to the production by the cell of a protein that is designed to correct a molecular defect disease state.

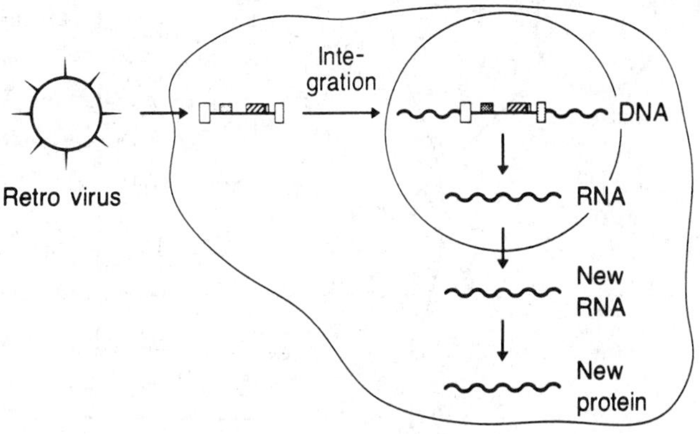

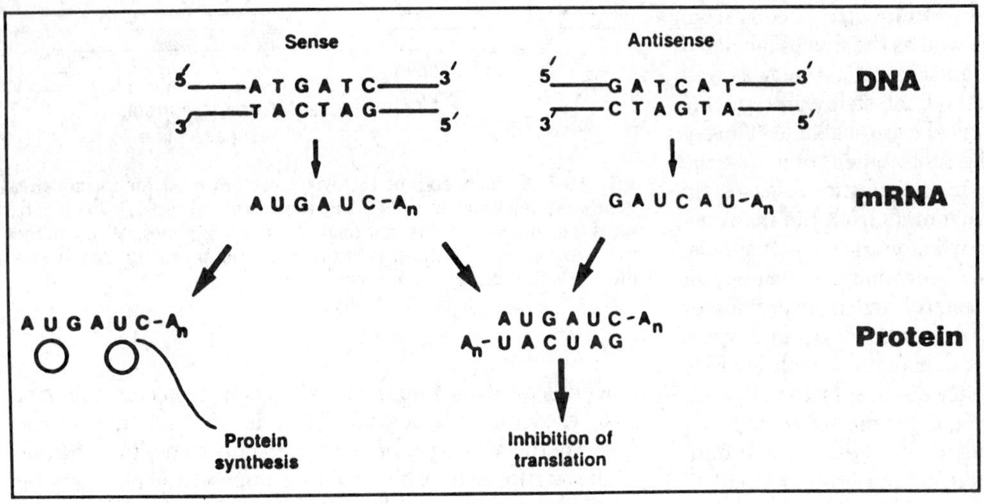

FIG. 66-7. Antisense mRNA.

ANTISENSE RNA INHIBITION OF ONCOGENE EXPRESSION FOR CANCER TREATMENT

Molecular strategies to downregulate unwanted genes are also now being experimented with. One such approach involves the generation of an RNA, called antisense RNA, which is homologous to the normal mRNA product of a gene to be inhibited.[67] Antisense RNA, the nature of which is outlined conceptually in Figure 66-7, is being used in an attempt to downregulate unwanted oncogene expression in malignant cells and to identify the biologic nature of genes, the protein product of which is unknown. Sense mRNA is usually read off one of the two strands of double-stranded DNA, called the coding strand. If one reverses the orientation of a gene to a transcriptional promoter, (see Fig. 66-7), an RNA, called antisense RNA, is produced which is homologous in sequence to the normal mRNA product of the gene. The formation of such duplexes of RNA in the nucleus inhibits mRNA processing and egress of mRNA from the nucleus (see Figs. 66-7 and 66-8). Alternatively, the antisense RNA can also inhibit translation by formation of duplexes if it is introduced with the cytoplasm of cells (Fig. 66-8). Thus, one can inhibit the production of the protein product of any unwanted gene (such as one that is stimulating proliferation of a cell in an uncontrolled manner).

There are three criteria to be met if such an antisense system is to work: [1] the amount of antisense mRNA must be equal to or greater than the level of the sense mRNA, the processing of which is to be inhibited; [2] the level of sense mRNA must be reduced to a level at which the protein product of the mRNA is thereby reduced such as to produce the desired change in cell behavior; and [3] the target cell must not contain enzymes that antagonize the effect of antisense mRNA. As an example, high levels of an enzyme "unwindase" have been identified that dissociate RNA duplexes between sense and antisense mRNA, thereby inhibiting the effect of the antisense mRNA.[68]

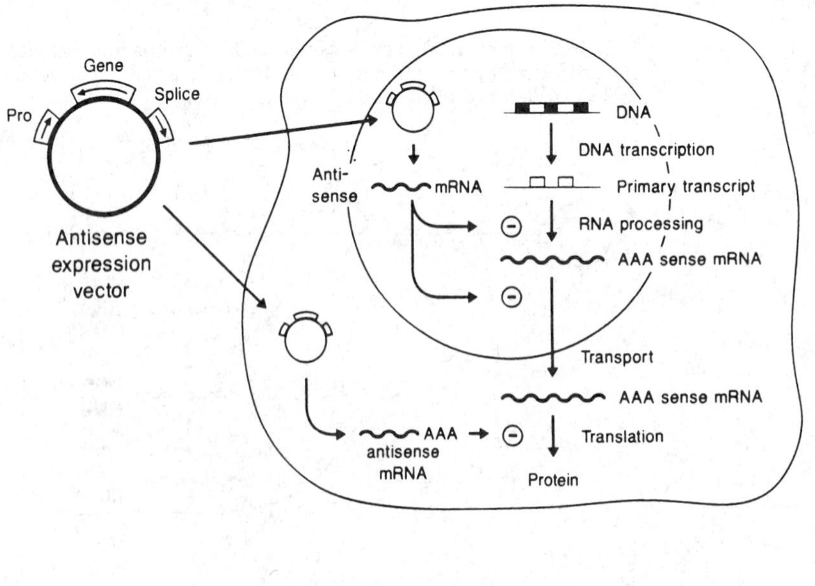

FIG. 66-8. Inhibition of gene expression by plasmid vector that produces antisense mRNA. As noted in the diagram, if the plasmid containing the gene in a transcription unit in the antisense orientation is introduced into the nuclease, the formation of RNA duplexes inhibits the egress of mRNA to the cytoplasm. If the antisense plasmid is introduced into the cytoplasm, the formation of RNA duplexes inhibits translation of mRNA into protein.

Despite all of these constraints, considerable progress has been made in the use of antisense RNA to inhibit oncogene expression. Holt and Nienhuis,[69] as well as Nisbikury and Murray,[70] have shown that introduction of anti-*fos* mRNA antisense vectors inhibits the proliferation of 3T3 cells. Workers have also found that addition of large quantities of synthetic DNA oligonucleotides that contained antisense *myc* sequence could induce differentiation of HL60 acute promyelocytic leukemia cells in which the c-*myc* gene is expressed at high levels.[70,71]

Antisense oligonucleotides have successfully been used to interrupt in vitro the replicative cycle of the Rous sarcoma virus,[72] the human immunodeficiency virus,[73,74] and the herpes simplex virus type 1.[75] The oligonucleotides are also being studied as targeting agents for chemotherapeutic agents to cells that contain specific and unique mRNAs.[76] Finally, it may be possible to attach molecules to the antisense RNA that will inactivate the mRNA of an unwanted protein.[76] Obviously, if one is to use direct addition of synthetic oligonucleotides to completely inhibit the expression of an unwanted gene, a vast excess of the antisense oligonucleotide must be produced. Several chemical modifications of the oligonucleotides have been devised to make them more stable and resistant to nuclease attack.[76] The ultimate utility of this approach remains to be established.

SUMMARY

Once we can use molecular biology to identify the precise defect present in the tumor of each patient, it is conceivable that we will have the means to tailor-make therapy to each patient's specific molecular defect and to use molecular replacement or modification strategies to correct these defects. Thus, a new kind of medicine is coming of age that will provide the oncologist–hematologist with a battery of new weapons with which to conquer neoplastic disease. Although these new technologies present their own problems, the potential rewards will be decisive therapeutic interventions and the reduction of human suffering.

The author acknowledges helpful discussion with Gary Spitzer, Michael Keating, Alan Oliff, Mark Israel, Frank Dunfy, Jack Cohen, and Bart Barlogie.

REFERENCES

1. Heisterkamp N, Stephenson J, Groffen JR et al: Localization of the c-*abl* oncogene adjacent to a translocation breakpoint in chronic myelocytic leukemia. Nature 306:239–242, 1983
2. Rowley JD, Alimena G, Garson O et al: A collaborative study of the relationship of the morphological type of ANLL with patient age and karyotype. Blood 59:1013–1022, 1982
3. LeBean MM, Rowley JD, Sacchi N et al: Hu-*ets*-2 is translocated to chromosome 8 in the t(8;21) in acute myelogenous leukemia. Cancer Genet Cytogenet 23:269–274, 1986
4. De Braekeleer M: The occurrence of translocation (15;17) in acute promyelocytic leukemia: An update. Cancer Genet Cytogenet 23:275–277, 1986
5. Rowley JD, Golomb H, Daugherty C: 15/17 Translocation, a consistent chromosomal change in acute promyelocytic leukemia. Lancet 1:549–550, 1977
6. LeBeau M, Larson R, Bitter M et al: Association of an inversion of chrosomome 16 with abnormal eosinophils in acute myelomonocytic leukemia. N Engl J Med 309:630–636, 1983
7. Yunis J, Brunning R, Howe R, Labell M: High-resolution chromosomes as an independent prognostic indicator in adult acute nonlymphocytic leukemia. N Engl J Med 311:812–818, 1984
8. Keating MJ: Leukemia cell characterization: Clinical and therapeutic implications in adult acute leukemia. In Stass SA (ed): The Acute Leukemias, pp 435–468. New York, Marcel Dekker, 1987
9. Hermans A, Heisterkamp N, Von Lindern M et al: Unique fusion of *bcr* and c-*abl* genes in Philadelphia chromosome positive ALL. Cell 51:33–40, 1987
10. Dalla-Favera R, Martinotti S, Gallo RC et al: Translocation and rearrangements of the c-*myc* oncogene locus in human undifferentiated lymphoma. Science 219:963–967, 1983
11. Cleary ML, Smith SD, Sklar J: Cloning and structural analysis of cDNAs for *bcl*-2 and a hybrid *bcl*-2/immunoglobulin transcript resulting from the t(14;18) translocation. Cell 47:19–28, 1986
12. Tsujimoto Y, Finger LR, Yunis J et al: Cloning of the chromosome breakpoint of neoplastic B cells with the t(14;18) chromosome translocation. Science 226:1097–1099, 1984
13. Bakhshi A, Jensen JP, Goldman P et al: Cloning the chromosomal breakpoint of t(14;18) human lymphomas: Clustering around *tH* on chromosomal 14 and near a transcriptional unit on 18. Cell 41:899–906, 1985
14. Zesh L, Gahrton G, Hammarston L et al: Inversion of chromosome 14 marks the human T-cell CLL. Nature 308:858–860, 1984
15. Erikson J, Williams D, Finan J et al: Locus of the alpha chain of the T cell receptor is split by chromosome translocation in T cell leukemias. Science 229:784–786, 1985
16. Smith S, Morgan R, Gernmell R et al: Clinical and biological characterization of T-cell neoplasias with rearrangements of chromosome 7 band of 34. Blood 71:395–402, 1988
17. Erikson J, Finan J, Tsujimoto Y et al: The chromosome 14 breakpoint in neoplastic B cells with the (11;14) translocation involves the immunoglobulin heavy chain locus. Proc Natl Acad Sci USA 81:4144–4148, 1984
18. Juliasson G, Robert KH, Ost A et al: Prognostic information from cytogenetic analysis in chronic B-lymphocytic leukemia. Blood 65:134–141, 1985
19. Kere J, RuuTu T, Lak Tinen R, dela Chapelle: Molecular characterization of chromosome 7 long arm deletions. Blood 70:1349–1353, 1987
20. Whang-Peng J, Young R, Lee E et al: Cytogenetic studies in patients with secondary leukemia/dysmyelopoietic syndrome after different treatment modalities. Blood 71:403–414, 1988
21. Gould J, Alexanian R, Goodacre A et al: Plasma cell karyotype in multiple myeloma. Blood 71:453–456, 1988
22. Strong RC, Karsemeyer S, Parkin J et al: Human acute leukemia cell line with the t(4;11) chromosomal rearrangement exhibits B cell lineage and monocytic characteristics. Blood 65:21–31, 1985
23. Pearson M, Vardiman J, LeBean M: Increased numbers of marrow basophils may be associated with t(6;9) in ANLL. Am J Hematol 18:393–403, 1985
24. Bernstein R, Pinto M, Behr A, Mendelow B: Chromosome 3 abnormalities in ANLL with abnormal thrombopoiesis. Blood 60:613–617, 1982
25. Saiki RK, Scharf S, Faloona F et al: Enzymatic amplification of beta-globin genomic sequences and restriction site analysis for diagnosis of sickle cell anemia. Science 230:1350–1354, 1985
26. Jeffreys AJ, Wilson V, Thein SL: Hypervariable "minisatellite" regions in human DNA. Nature 314:67–73, 1985
27. Scrable H, Witlee DP, Lampkin BC, Lavenee WX: Chromosomal localization of the human rhabomyosarcoma locus by mitotic recombination mapping. Nature 329:645–647, 1987
28. LeBeau MM, Westbrook CA, Diaz MO: Evidence for the involvement of GMCSF and FMS in the deletion (5q) in myeloid disorders. Science 231:984–987, 1986
29. Hutter J, Hecht F, Kaiser et al: Bone marrow monosomy 7. Hematol Oncol 2:5–12, 1984
30. Zbar B, Brauch H, Talmadge C, Linehan M: Loss of alleles in loci in the short arm of chromosome 3 in renal cell carcinoma. Nature 327:721–724, 1987
31. Schroeder W, Chao LY, Dao D et al: Nonrandom loss of material chromosome 11 alleles in Wilms tumors. Am J Human Genet 40:413–420, 1987
32. Cavanee W, Hansen M, Nordenskjold M et al: Genetic origin of mutations predisposing to retinoblastoma. Science 228:501–503, 1985
33. Turc-Carel C, Philip I, Bager M et al: Chromosomal translocation in Ewing's sarcoma. N Engl J Med 309:497–498, 1983
34. Fearon ER, Feinberg AB, Hamilton S, Vogelstein B: Loss of genes on the short arm of chromosome 11 in bladder cancer. Nature 318:377; 380, 1985
35. Koufos A, Hansen M, Copeland N et al: Loss of heterozygosity in three embryonal tumors suggest a common pathogenetic mechanism. Nature 316:330–334, 1985
36. Naylor S, Johnson B, Minna J, Sakaguchi A: Loss of heterozygosity in small cell lung cancer. nature 329:451–453, 1987
37. Solomon E, Vass R, Hall V et al: Chromosome 5 allele loss in human colorectal carcinomas. Nature 328:616–619, 1987
38. Slezinger BR, Martuza R, Gusella JF: Loss of genes on chromosome 22 in tumorigenesis of human acoustic neuroma. Nature 322:644–647, 1986
39. Gilbert F, Feder M, Balaban G et al: Human neuroblastomas and abnormalities of chromosomes 1 and 17. Cancer Res 44:5444–5447, 1984
40. Atkin NB: Chromosome 10 deletion in carcinoma of the prostate. N Engl J Med 312:315, 1985
41. Delozier-Blanchet CD, Engel E, Wolt H: Isochromosome 12p in malignant testicular tumors. Cancer Genet Cytogenet 15:375–376, 1985

42. Semple TV, Moore GE, Morgan RT et al: Multiple cell lines from patients with malignant melanoma. J Natl Cancer Inst 68:365–380, 1982
43. Zanel H, Zang KD: Correlations between clinical and cytogenetical data in 180 human meningiomas. Cancer Genet Cytogenet 1:351–356, 1980
44. Knudson AG: Mutation and cancer statistical study of retinoblastoma. Proc Natl Acad Sci USA 68:820–823, 1971
45. Lee WH, Shen JY, Hong FD et al: The retinoblastoma susceptibility gene encodes a nuclear phosphoprotein associated with DNA binding activity. Nature 329:642–645, 1987
46. Hand PH, Thor A, Siblom J et al: Expression of a laminim receptor in normal and carcinomatous human tissues as defined by a monoclonal antibody. Cancer Res 45:2713–2714, 1985
47. Verini J, Lovett EJ, McCoy JP et al: Differential expression of a laminin like substance by high and low metastatic tumor cells. Am J Pathol 111:27–34, 1983
48. Guirguis R, Margulies I, Taraboletti G et al: Cytokine induced pseudopodial protrusion is coupled to tumor cell progression. Nature 329:261–263, 1987
49. Campbell A, Long M, Wicha M: Haemonectin, a bone marrow adhesion protein specific for cells of granulocyte lineage. Nature 329:744–745, 1987
50. Takobashi M, Keating A, Singer J: A functional defect in initiated adherent layers from chronic myelogenous leukemia long term cultures. Exp Hematol 13:926–931, 1985
51. Bos JL, de Vries MV, van der Eb AJ et al: Mutations in N-*ras* predominate in acute myeloid leukemia. Blood 69:1237–1241, 1987
52. Liu E, Hjelle B, Morgan R et al: Mutations of the Kirsten-*ras* protooncogene in human preleukemia. Nature 330:186–188, 1987
53. Bos JL, Fearon ER, Hamilton SR et al: Prevalence of *ras* gene mutations in human colorectal cancers. Nature 327:293–297, 1987
54. Kozina S, Bogaard M, Buser K et al: The human c-Kirsten *ras* gene is activated by a novel mutation in codon 13 in the breast carcinoma cell line MDA-MB231. Nucleic Acid Res 15:5963–5971, 1987
55. Reddy EP, Reynolds RK, Santos E, Barbacid M: A point mutation is responsible for the acquisition of transforming properties by the T24 human bladder carcinoma oncogene. Nature 300:149–152, 1982
56. Seager R, Brodeur G, Sather H et al: Association of multiple copies of the N-*myc* oncogene with rapid progression of neuroblastomas. N Engl J Med 313:1111–1116, 1985
57. Nakagawara A, Iheda K, Tsuda T, Higashi: N-*myc* oncogene amplification and prognostic factors of neuroblastoma in children. J Pediatr Surg 22:895–898, 1987
58. Slamon DJ, Clark GM, Wong SG et al: Human breast cancer correlation of relapse and survival with amplification of the *Her-2/neu* oncogene. Science 235:177–182, 1987
59. Zhou D, Battiford H, Yokota J, et al: Association of multiple copies of the c-*erb*-2 oncogene with spread of breast cancer. Cancer Res 47:6123–6125, 1987
60. Rosen N, Israel M: Genetic abnormalities as biological tumor markers. Semin Oncol 14:213–221, 1987
61. Little CD, Nau MM, Carney DN et al: Amplification and expression of the c-*myc* oncogene in human lung cancer cell lines. Nature 306:194–196, 1983
62. Wong AJ, Ruppert J, Eggleston J et al: Gene amplification in small cell carcinoma of the lung. Science 233:461–464, 1986
63. Libermann TA, Nusbaum HR, Razon N et al: Amplification, enhanced expression and possible rearrangement of EGF receptor gene in primary human brain tumors of glial origin. Nature 313:144–147, 1985
64. Thiele CJ, McKeon C, Triche TJ et al: Differential protooncogene expression characterizes histopathologically indistinguishable tumors of the peripheral nervous system. J Clin Invest 80:804–811, 1987
65. Funa K, Steinholtz L, Nou E, Bergh J: Increased expression of N-*myc* in human small cell lung cancer biopsies predicts lack of response to chemotherapy and poor prognosis. Am J Clin Pathol 88:216–220, 1987
66. Wong PC, Chung SW, Nienhuis AW: Retroviral transfer and expression of the interleukin-3 gene in hematopoietic cells. Genes Dev 1:358–365, 1987
67. Izant JG, Weintraub H: Constitutive and conditional suppression of exogenous and endogenous genes by antisense RNA. Science 229:345–352, 1985
68. Wagner R, Nishikura K: Cycle expression of RNA duplex unwindase activity in mammalian cells. Mol Cell Biol 8:770–777, 1988
69. Holt JT, Gopal TV, Moulton AD, Nienhuis A: Inducible production of c-*fos* antisense RNA inhibits 3T3 cell proliferation. Proc Natl Acad Sci USA 83:4794–4798, 1986
70. Nishikura K, Murray JM: Antisense RNA of proto-oncogene c-*fos* blocks renewed growth of NIH 3T3 cells. Mol Cell Biol 7:639–649, 1987
71. Holt JT, Redner RL, Nienhuis A: An oligoma complementary to c-*myc* RNA inhibits proliferation of HL60 promyelocytic cells and induces differentiation. Mol Cell Biol 8:963–973, 1988
72. Stephenson M, Zamecnik P: Inhibition of Rous sarcoma viral RNA translation by a specific oligodeoxyribonucleotide. Proc Natl Acad Sci USA 75:285–288, 1978
73. Zamecnik PC, Goodchild J, Yoguchi Y, Sarin P: Inhibition of replication and expression of human T-cell lymphotrophic virus type III in cultured cells by exogenous synthetic oligonucleotides complementary to viral RNA. Proc Natl Acad Sci USA 83:4143–4146, 1986
74. Malsukura M, Shinuzuka K, Zon G et al: Phosphorotheonate analogs of oligonucleotides inhibitors of replication and cytopathic effects of human immunodeficiency virus. Proc Natl Acad Sci USA 84:7706–7710, 1987
75. Smith C, Aurelian L, Reddy M et al: Antiviral effect of an oligo(nucleotide methylphosphonate) complementary to the splice junction of herpes simplex virus type I immediate pre-mRNAs 4 and 5. Proc Natl Acad Sci USA 83:2787–2791, 1988
76. Stein CA, Cohen JS: Oligonucleotides as inhibitors of gene expression: A review. Cancer Res (in press), 1989

SECTION 2

JAMES R. OLESON

Hyperthermia

Temperature elevation to 42° to 45°C for 10 to 60 min can lethally damage bacterial and mammalian cells. This fact, first observed in ancient times, was rediscovered in the nineteenth century when patients with malignant tumors that had fevers related to bacterial infections occasionally had regressions in tumor size. Coley deliberately induced fevers in cancer patients by using pyrogenic bacterial toxins and noted some partial responses.[1] The development of radiofrequency generators in the early 1900s allowed the testing of effects caused by temperature rise localized to a tumor, rather than whole-body hyperthermia.[2,3] Although investigation of combined hyperthermia and radiation soon followed,[4–5] a series of reports by Crile in the 1960s probably stimulated the modern quantitative study of effects of hyperthermia on cancer.[6] With water bath heating, Crile demonstrated thermal enhancement of radiation effect and cure of melanomas implanted on the feet of mice: no normal tissue damage was observed from exposures to 44°C for 30 min. Since the early 1960s, systematic laboratory investigation of hyperthermia has expanded, and these investigations continue to support use of hyperthermia in cancer therapy. Several recent reviews provide further information.[7–10]

BIOLOGICAL BACKGROUND

EFFECTS OF HYPERTHERMIA ALONE

When the logarithm of the surviving fraction of cells is plotted as a function of time of exposure to given temperatures above 41°C, the resulting cell survival curve is similar to that resulting from radiation exposure (Fig. 66-9). An initial shoulder region for short-exposure times is followed by a linear portion representing cell killing that is an exponential function of time.[11] At temperatures below 42.5°C, the rate of cell killing diminishes with exposure times longer than about 200 min, providing evidence of the development of thermotolerance, a fundamentally important and universal phenomenon.[12] For a given effect such as percentage of cell kill, the exposure time must be reduced by one-half for each 1°C increase in temperature. For temperatures below 42.5°C in thermotolerant cells, the heating time must be doubled for

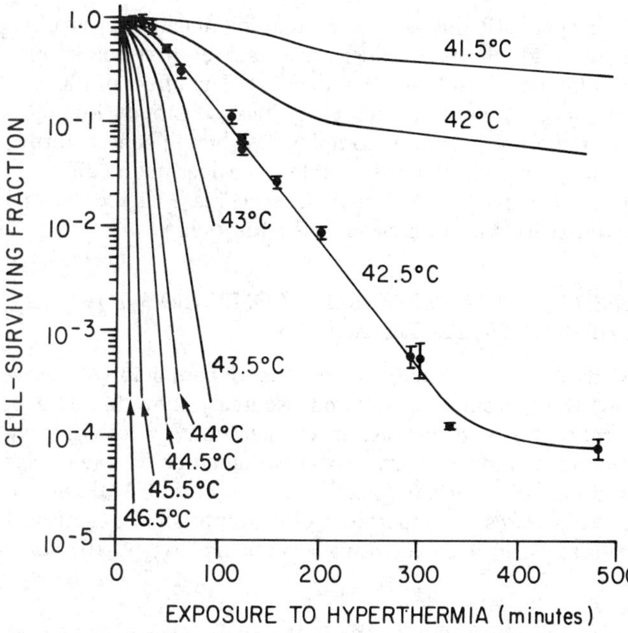

FIG. 66-9. Survival curves for Chinese hamster ovary cells in vitro exposed to varying temperatures for varying lengths of time. Similarly to radiation survival curves, there is a shoulder and an exponential portion. Prolonged exposure to 42.5 °C and below leads to flattening of the curves with minimal further cell kill, corresponding to thermotolerance induction. (Modified from Dewey W, Hopwood L, Sapareto S et al: Cellular responses to combinations of hyperthermia and radiation. Radiology 123:463–474, 1977)

each 0.5°C increase in temperature for an isoeffect. Thermal sensitivity varies during the cell cycle: Chinese hamster ovary (CHO) cells exhibit the greatest thermal sensitivity during the M and S phases,[13] and mild thermal exposure of CHO causes a cell cycle delay in G_2 of about 6 hr.[14] Relative thermal sensitivity varies with different cell lines and is not correlated with the radiation sensitivity.[15] Earlier reports suggested, erroneously, that malignant cells were *intrinsically* more thermally sensitive than normal cells;[16] however, the altered physiologic milieu of malignant cells in vivo may lead to thermal sensitization relative to normal cells.[17] The shoulder of the survival curve of preheated cells is reproduced with a second exposure, thereby implying recovery from sublethal damage produced with the first exposure; part of this recovery is separate from thermotolerance induction.[18]

The ratio of slopes of survival curves for preheated and single-heated cells, respectively, gives a thermotolerance ratio (TTR) that varies as a function of the fractionation interval. Exposure to temperatures above 42.5°C for more than 30 min induces a maximum TTR at 6 to 16 hr of 4 to 6, respectively, after the first or priming exposure; this effect requires at least 24 hr for complete decay in L1A2 cells.[19] The magnitude and kinetics of thermotolerance vary with cell lines[20] and may even vary within subclonogenic lines.[21] Acidic pH inhibits the magnitude and rate of expression of thermotolerance,[22,23] although the pH effects in cells adapted to low pH are less marked.[24] Induction of thermotolerance is associated temporally with synthesis of proteins with a molecular mass in the range of 20 to 100 kD, called heat-shock proteins (HSP).[25–27] If these proteins are induced by agents other than heat, cells become thermotolerant. Whether the HSP are enzymes or structural proteins is unknown, and the causal link between thermal stress and HSP is not completely established. A possible link is that HSP may participate in "rescuing" denatured proteins.[28]

Other agents and conditions, in addition to pH, can modify the cellular effects of hyperthermia from those illustrated in Figure 66-9. Incubation of cells at temperatures from 40° to 43°C after an initial exposure at 45°C for 20 min ("step-down heating") leads to cell survival curves lacking a shoulder region and having significantly increased slopes.[29] Presumably, the initial exposure at 45°C blocks the development of the thermotolerance observed during subsequent lower-temperature exposure. Under conditions controlled for pH and nutrient levels, no variation in thermal sensitivity with Po_2 level exists in CHO cells,[30] and the Po_2 level does not affect the magnitude or kinetics of thermotolerance development.[31] Nutrients in the culture medium do affect the level of cellular recovery from potentially lethal damage.[32] Other classes of substances that can modify the exposure of cells to hyperthermia, perhaps through alteration of membrane structure or biosynthetic pathways, include alcohols, anesthetics, polyamines, thiols, and hypoxic cell sensitizers.[7,33] The use of such agents to increase thermal sensitivity of malignant cells could have clinical importance by lowering the temperatures required for direct thermal cytotoxicity. The exposure of Chinese hamster ovary cells to α-difluoromethylornithine (DFMO), for example, can increase cell kill at 43°C by two orders of magnitude relative to cells not exposed to DFMO.[34]

Mechanisms for thermal damage are not clear, although effects on the cell membrane[35,36] and nucleus[37] occur in association with heat exposure. An Arrhenius plot analysis gives the energy of activation of the assumed chemical reaction that is rate-limiting for thermal cell killing to be about 140 to 150 kcal/mol,[14] similar to that required for protein denaturation. An event such as protein denaturation could initiate a multistep cascade of events leading to induction of thermotolerance or cell killing. A calcium ion-mediated cascade, perhaps linked to a triggering event on the cell membrane, may explain the separate pieces of evidence documenting thermal effects on so many cellular structures and processes.[38–40] Ionic permeabilities, in general, are little affected by heat, but at 45°C a marked increase in calcium ion uptake by HA-1 CHO cells occurs.[39] The time required for maximum increase in calcium ion permeability corresponds to the shoulder region of the survival curve. The blocking of calcium ion uptake induces heat-shock proteins and partial thermotolerance. These data support the concept that changes in the calcium cation are fundamental to cell killing and thermotolerance.

EFFECTS OF COMBINED HYPERTHERMIA AND RADIATION

In 1963, Belli and Bonti[41] demonstrated temperature dependence of the radiation response of mammalian cells in tissue culture, suggesting thermal lability of enzymes involved in repair of radiation damage. Ben Hur and associates[42] showed that temperature elevation above 41 °C increases the slope of the exponential portion of the radiation survival curve of CHO cells, thus confirming enhancement of lethal damage expression. The effects of incubation at temperatures below 40.5 °C after irradiation are principally on the shoulder of the survival curve, indicating a reduced capacity for sublethal damage repair. At 41 °C the shoulder of the survival curve is absent. Survival of CHO cells depends on the sequence of hyperthermia and radiation, sixfold lower survival resulting from simultaneous exposure to 42.5 °C and radiation compared with heat preceding or following the irradiation by more than 5 min.[43] Thermal radiosensitization is greater for S-phase cells than G_1 cells,[13] complementary to the cell cycle dependence of survival after irradiation alone. Survival also is lower for very low dose rates typical of brachytherapy than for those used in teletherapy.[44] Cell survival with hyperthermia and radiation is markedly dependent upon pH; this is of particular significance in vivo because acid pH also reduces the rate of thermotolerance development at 42° to 42.5 °C.[24,45–47] The effect of thermotolerance on thermal cytotoxicity, radiosensitivity, and thermal radiosensitization is complex,[48–51] but, in general terms, we may conclude that thermotolerance does not modify radiation sensitivity of cells but does decrease direct thermal cytotoxicity and thermal radiosensitization.

EFFECTS OF HYPERTHERMIA COMBINED WITH CHEMOTHERAPEUTIC AGENTS

Many chemotherapeutic agents [*e.g.* doxorubicin (Adriamycin), bleomycin, cisplatin, nitrosoureas] show increase in cytotoxicity with increase in temperature.[7] When thermotolerance is induced, an associated tolerance for the effects of drugs sometimes occurs.[52,53] Recent work of Wallner and Li[54] illustrates the importance of the duration of exposure of cells to a drug and heat–drug sequencing (Fig. 66-10). Max-

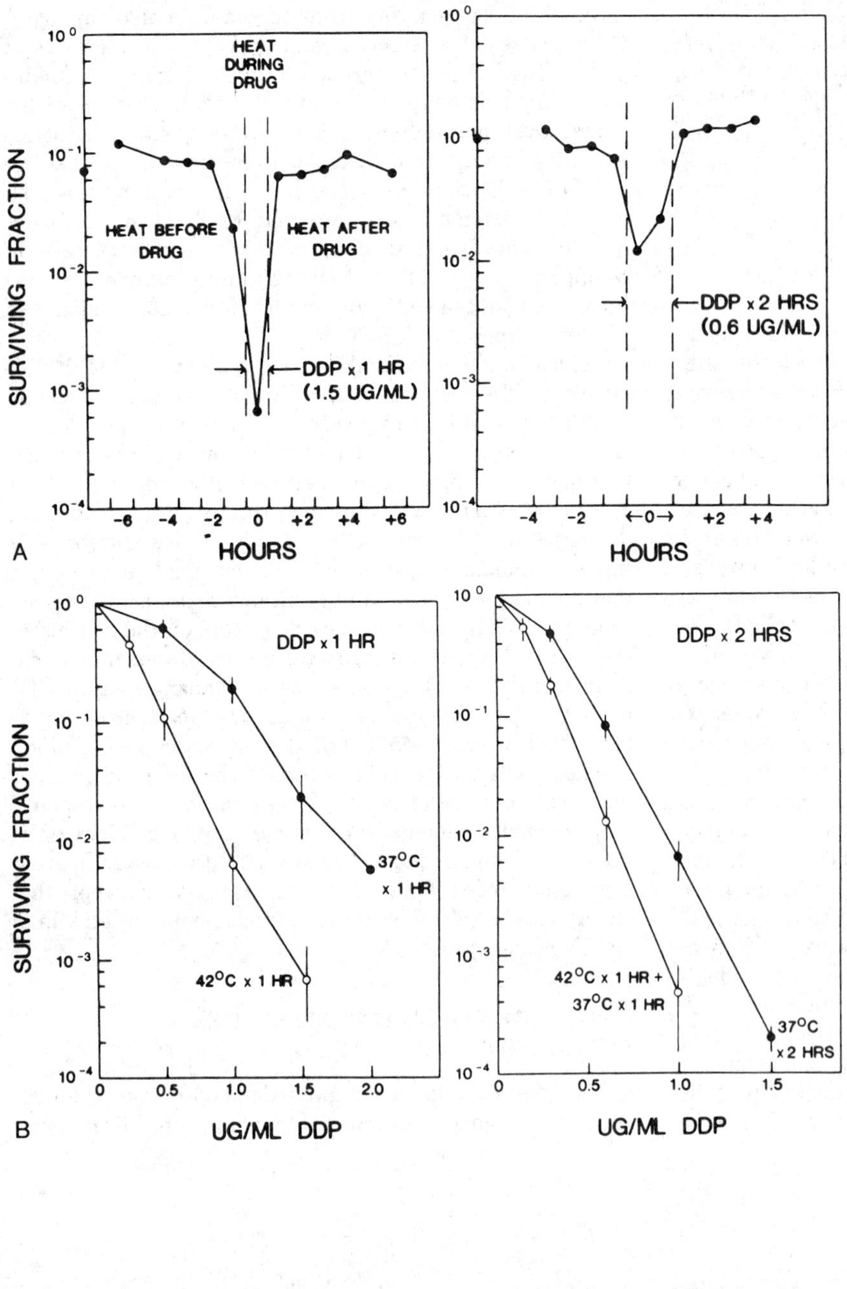

FIG. 66-10. **A.** The effect of increasing time of exposure to cisplatin (*DDP*) and sequencing of hyperthermia (42 °C × 60 min) and cisplatin on Chinese hamster cells in vitro. **B.** Increasing cytotoxicity with increasing duration and concentration of cisplatin exposure at 37 °C versus 42 °C. (Wallner K, Li G: Effect of drug exposure duration and sequencing on hyperthermia potentiation of mitomycin-C and cisplatin. Cancer Res 47:493–495, 1987)

imum potentiation with simultaneous exposure also occurs with cyclophosphamide and mitomycin. Although an increased number of DNA crosslinks in CHO cells exposed to cisplatin at 43°C, compared with 37°C, exists,[55] the precise mechanisms of thermal potentiation of drug effects are not known.

IN VIVO EFFECTS OF HYPERTHERMIA

The effects of hyperthermia alone or in combination with other agents in vivo have been studied in rodents, large animals, and humans. Many variables can influence the effects of hyperthermia in vivo.[56] Most importantly, blood circulation is a mechanism for transporting heat, thereby affecting the temperatures produced in tissues with heating by any means.[57,58] The amount of blood flow and the temperature dependence of the flow itself influence the delivery of nutrients to the cells and, hence, the metabolic status and pH.[59] Tumor vessels resemble leaky capillaries and venous sinusoids without the vascular smooth muscle that allows normal vasoactivity, such as thermally induced vasodilation.[58] Stasis of blood flow and vascular destruction can occur in tumor microcirculation under conditions that produce only reversible reactive change in normal tissues, creating one of the most important rationales for advantageous differential effects of hyperthermia between tumors and normal tissues (Fig. 66-11). Areas of low blood perfusion in tumors can reach preferentially higher temperatures than normal tissue, further enhancing the differential effects of heat. Recent measurements of extracellular pH in animal and human tumors[47] confirm that acidic pH occurs in some tumors, presumably from low Po_2 and nutrient levels, producing anaerobic glycolysis and high lactic acid levels. The pH shift does not correlate consistently with tumor size, histologic type, or other characteristics. Glucose infusions to lower tumor pH during hyperthermia may take advantage of increased thermal cytotoxicity, reduced thermotolerance, and reduced recovery from sublethal hyperthermic damage.[60,61] Thermotolerance clearly occurs in vivo:[62] a priming treatment of 43.5°C for 30 min in C3H mammary carcinoma tumors, for example, leads to maximum thermotolerance 16-hr later and a complete decay time of 120 hr.[63] The implications of thermotolerance development for fractionation of hyperthermia and radiation in treatment regimens are complex and of considerable potential significance. The kinetics of repair of sublethal damage and thermotolerance induction and decay in vivo also may vary between tumor and normal tissue. Simultaneous application of irradiation and heat results in equal sensitization of tumor and normal tissue and, hence, no therapeutic gain.[64,65] When a time interval of at least 2 hr separates irradiation and heat, especially in this order, there is consistently a ratio of enhancement of radiation effect in tumor versus normal tissue (therapeutic gain) between 1.2 and 1.5. The expression of direct thermal injury in normal tissues follows that expected from interphase death of cells, rather than postmitotic death, as with radiation injury. Studies involving scoring of development of rodent leg contracture, for instance, show peak damage between 2 and 15 days after hyperthermia, whereas radiation damage peaks at 20 to 25 days, then progresses for

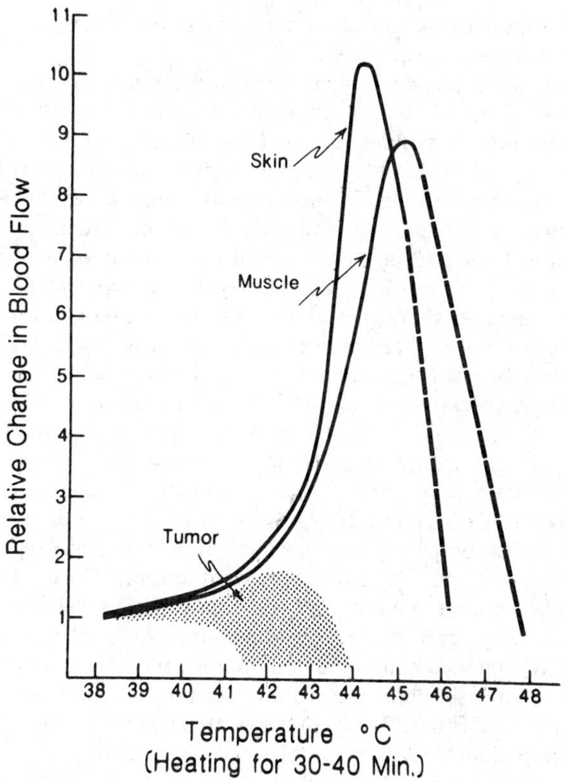

FIG. 66-11. Relative change in tumor versus normal tissue blood flow during heating at various temperatures for 30 to 40 minutes in laboratory animals based on data in various reports. Note thermally induced vasodilation followed by stasis. (Song C, Lokshina A, Rhee J et al: Implication of blood flow in hyperthermic treatment of tumors. IEEE-Trans BME 31:9–16, 1984)

as long as 365 days.[66] This pattern of difference is found in intestinal crypts, testis, and kidney. In the normal feline brain, the histologic appearance and time course of repair of thermal injury are similar to the acute necrosis produced by vascular infarction.[67] In murine jejunal tissue[68] hyperthermia accelerates the expression and increases the magnitude of late radiation fibrosis. The threshold for normal tissue injury is sharply marked as a function of time and temperature of exposure. A 20% increase in time of exposure or a 0.5°C increase in temperature, in the range of 42.0° to 45.5°C, increases the likelihood of necrosis from zero to 100% in rodent tissue.[69] Few clinical studies report severe normal tissue thermal injury or potentiation of radiation effect in superficial tissues when there has been careful monitoring of temperatures achieved and patient perceptions. Normal tissue temperatures rarely exceed safe limits of 42°C to 43°C and usually reach the highest levels corresponding to locations that predictably receive the greatest power deposition. Hyperthermia techniques causing temperature elevation in deep visceral sites also infrequently cause serious injury; on the other hand, the potential location and magnitude of temperature elevation is more difficult to predict and is less well perceived by the patient. There is little information in the literature on toxic or therapeutic in vivo effects of combined hyperthermia and chemotherapeutic agents, although significant alteration of drug pharmacology by hyperthermia can exist.[70-72]

Relating the tissue effects of hyperthermia to a thermal dose is a desirable but, thus far, elusive goal. From Arrhenius relationships, formulas for combinations of time and temperature can be derived that give isoeffects in cultured cells and in animal tissues.[73] Such formulas may be useful for comparing clinical treatments, but they do not predict absolute levels of effects, they are difficult to apply to nonuniform temperature distributions, they do not express effects of fractionated therapy, and they may not express correctly the variation of thermal radiosensitization with pH.[74] The use of thermal isoeffective dose is still investigational.

The prospective randomized Phase III study of Dewhirst and collaborators[75] is one of the most important therapeutic trials in animals. Treatment with combined hyperthermia and radiotherapy produced a statistically significant improvement in freedom from disease progression, compared with radiotherapy or hyperthermia alone. The complete response (CR) rate and duration were inversely correlated with the tumor volume, but the relative improvement in response was greater for large tumors than for small tumors. The average site-nonspecific minimum temperature was the thermal measure best correlating with response: the equivalent of 41.3°C for 30 min, plus radiation, nearly doubled the CR rate from 35% to 65% relative to RT alone.

TECHNICAL ASPECTS

THERMOMETRY

Typical temperature distributions in tumors are very nonuniform. Methods for measuring temperatures are limited in practice to invasive placement of probes at only a few sites,[76] introducing the problem of inferring the overall temperature distribution from spatially limited samples.[77] Corry and coworkers[78] have shown that estimates of minimum and maximum temperatures depend on the number of sites monitored (Fig. 66-12). Methods of calculating temperature distributions are being developed but cannot now be applied routinely, because the principal determinants of temperature rise—absorbed power density and blood perfusion rate—are not accurately known.[79] Proper choice, use, and calibration of thermometers to limit errors of measurement require many different considerations for each hyperthermia technique.[80] Standard practice includes use of single sensors, multiple sensors, or periodically translated sensors[81] within catheters placed into tumor sites. The selection of the number of sensors and sites of measurement bears directly upon the likelihood of sampling prognostically important temperatures or, conversely, of defining prospectively what temperature distributions are required for efficacious treatment.

METHODS OF HEATING

Available heating methods include ultrasound (US) or electromagnetic (EM) applicators. The principle of heat production is that energy is absorbed in tissue in doing work against the molecular viscosity or electrical resistance of tissue constituents.[82,83] These dissipative processes that cause heat production do not involve ionization, in contrast with absorption mechanisms for diagnostic and therapeutic radiation. Local heat production results in a temperature rise that depends upon the specific heat of the tissue and the heat transport processes of conduction and convection (blood flow); chemical or metabolic heat production levels are themselves temperature-dependent and may contribute to the local temperature rise.[57] The heating methods consist of noninvasive and invasive techniques of depositing power in localized volumes, regional vascular perfusion techniques, and whole-body hyperthermia techniques. Heating superficial tumors in a water bath is common for laboratory study of small rodent tumors, but this technique is inappropriate for bulky human tumors. Special techniques are required for achieving temperature uniformity, even in small rodent tumors.[84] The *International Journal of Hyperthermia* is publishing results of a 5-year National Cancer Institute (NCI)-funded multi-institu-

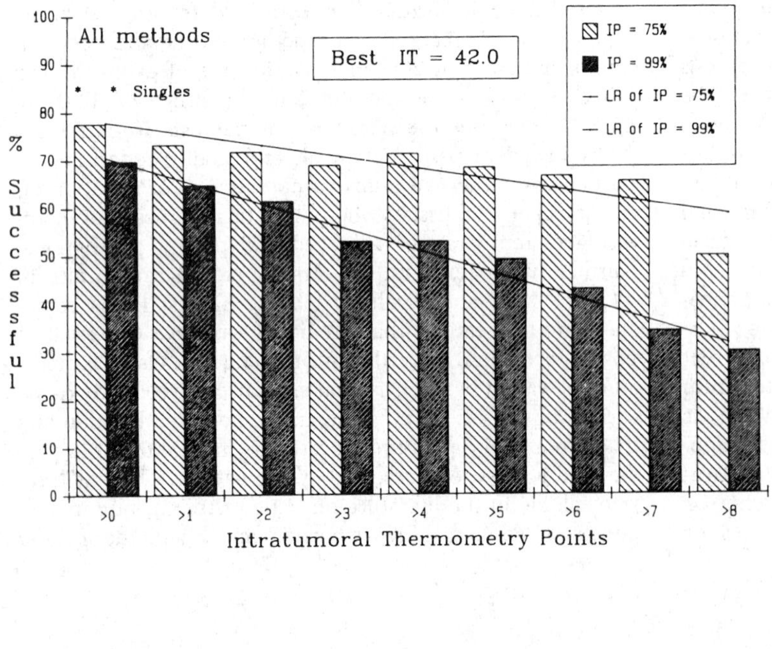

FIG. 66-12. Percentage of successful hyperthermia treatments, based on temperatures achieved, versus the number of sites of temperature measurement for a series of patients treated with ultrasound or magnetic induction heating methods. The criterion for success was that the best observed intratumoral average temperature exceeded an index temperature (*IT*) of 42 °C at a specified index percentage (IP = 75% or 99%) of monitored sites. As the number of monitored sites increased, the average of the observed temperatures decreased, leading to a lower score of successful treatments. These data demonstrate the nonuniformity of temperature distributions and the inaccuracy of basing estimates of the temperature distribution on a small number of monitored sites. The linear regression (*LR*) lines are shown for IP = 75% and 99%. (Corry PM et al: Clinical experience with plane-wave ultrasound systems. In Steeves RA, Paliwal BR [eds]: Syllabus: A Categorical Course in Hyperthermia, p 151. Oak Brook, IL, Radiological Society of North America, 1987)

tional evaluation of a wide variety of hyperthermia and thermometry devices that will be an excellent reference on this topic.

LOCAL HYPERTHERMIA TECHNIQUES. Ultrasonic applicators with focused or unfocused stationary beams and with focused scanning beams, are available for the frequency range of 0.5 to 10 MHz, for which the penetration depth in tissue varies from about 10 to 0.5 cm, respectively. Lack of US propagation across air spaces, marked absorption in bone, and reflections from tissue interfaces constitute fundamental problems with US. The depths of penetration and ability to focus, however, are advantages relative to EM techniques, especially for deep-seated tumors.[85] Electric currents, in the frequency range of 0.2 to 13 MHz, can be capacitively coupled into tissue to result in resistive heating by using two or more surface electrodes or plates.[82] The currents flow in divergent paths between the plates, and large plates must be used for substantial power absorption in deep sites relative to superficial sites near the plates. The power absorption is not focused or localized in tumor, and excessive superficial fat heating is a problem for fat layers thicker than about 1.5 cm. At frequencies of 10 to 30 MHz, current-carrying coils external to the body can create an intense magnetic field that, in turn, induces eddy current flow within the body.[86] The resulting power deposition generally diminishes with increasing depth, so these techniques are best suited for tumors at superficial and intermediate depths. Radiated EM fields in the frequency range of 60 to 2450 MHz penetrate to depths of about 15 to 1.5 cm, respectively. Single microwave applicators commonly are limited to heating superficial lesions, whereas multiapplicator arrays can achieve heating at depth in the body without excessive heating of superficial normal tissue.[87] Sharp focusing of the power is not generally possible with these techniques, thus, as with the other EM approaches, one must rely upon a lower blood perfusion in the tumor than in normal tissue for preferential temperature elevation in the tumor.

Greater localization and control of power deposition with a tumor volume is possible when one uses interstitial techniques[88] that can be combined with conventional interstitial radiation treatments. Electric current at 0.5 MHz, flowing between implanted metallic needles, results in resistive heating of an intervening tumor.[89] Alternatively, nonmetallic catheters can accommodate miniature microwave antennae operating at 433 to 2450 MHz that radiate power into a surrounding tumor.[90] Soon to be tested in the human clinic are implants using ferromagnetic seeds that can be heated by an externally applied magnetic field that induces eddy current flow preferentially in the seeds.[91] Proper selection of magnetic properties can result in seeds that self-regulate the temperature rise.

REGIONAL VASCULAR PERFUSION. Isolation of the major artery and vein of an extremity from the systemic circulation and connection of these vessels to an extracorporeal heated perfusion circuit results in temperature elevation of an entire limb.[92] This approach has been used for treating extremity melanoma and sarcoma with chemotherapy-containing heated perfusates.

WHOLE-BODY HYPERTHERMIA TECHNIQUES. Methods of inducing systemic temperature rise depend upon limiting the heat loss from the body while introducing heat absorption through conduction across the skin surface from heated wax[93] or water;[94] through direct superficial electromagnetic[95] or infrared power absorption[96] with systemic redistribution; or through blood circulation through an extracorporeal heat exchanger.[97]

CLINICAL RESULTS

EVIDENCE FOR EFFICACY OF COMBINED HYPERTHERMIA AND RADIOTHERAPY

Several studies report treatment to small superficial metastatic nodules by hyperthermia alone, radiotherapy alone, or combined radiotherapy and hyperthermia. A variety of heating techniques and radiation fractionation schemes was used, and temperature distributions were not always characterized. Despite these problems, there is surprising consistency in results as summarized recently by Overgaard[98] and as updated in Table 66-7. Complete response rates with hyperthermia alone are about 15%, with radiotherapy about 35%, and with combined radiotherapy and hyperthermia about 70%. Toxicity, principally thermal burns and blisters, is usually about 10% to 15%. No evidence exists of enhanced late effects of radiotherapy in these studies. These trials have established safety and efficacy for combined treatment in superficial lesions, particularly when prior radiotherapy limits additional doses to suboptimal levels. Other recent trials, summarized in Table 66-8, confirm that tumor volume, radiation dose, and measures of minimum tumor temperature are prognostic factors for response to hyperthermia and radiotherapy. Arcangeli and co-workers[99] found a highly significant correlation of complete response rate with minimum thermal isoeffective dose. With increase in tumor volume, an increasing isoeffective dose was needed to achieve a given response rate, radiation dose being fixed. Dunlop and associates[100] found improvement in response rates from 35% to 86% with at least two hyperthermia treatments in which a tumor minimum isoeffective dose of 20 min Eq43 was achieved.[100] Kapp and colleagues[101] randomized prospectively treatment to small superficial lesions to radiotherapy plus two versus six weekly fractions of hyperthermia and observed no difference in complete response rate or duration of response. Leopold and associates[102] prospectively randomized preoperative treatment to patients with bulky high-grade sarcomas to 50 Gy/5 wk, plus one versus two hyperthermia treatments per week. Histologic scoring of resected specimens showed a highly significant increase in complete or nearly complete necrosis in the two hyperthermia per week group, compared with the one hyperthermia per week group. Average minimum and mean temperatures achieved

TABLE 66-7. Complete Response (CR) of Superficial Tumors to RT Versus RT plus HT

Authors	*Lesions*	*Total No. of Tumors*	*RT-alone*	*RT + HT*	*p*
Valdagni *et al*[117]*	Neck nodes	43	CR = 36.8%	CR = 82.3%	0.015
Arcangeli *et al*[99,118]	Neck nodes;	81	CR = 42%	CR = 79%	<0.05
	Melanoma metastases		CR at 24 mo = 14%	CR at 24 mo = 58%	<0.05
Steeves *et al*[119]	Superficial tumors	90	CR = 31%	CR = 65%	
Lindholm *et al*[120]	Superficial tumors	85	CR = 25%	CR = 46%	0.0027
	Superficial matched pairs only	56	CR = 25%	CR = 57%	
van der Zee *et al*[121]	Breast cancer recurrences	113	CR = 55%	CR = 90%	<0.001
Kim *et al*[122]	Melanoma recurrences	97	CR = 45%	CR = 66%	
Li *et al*[123]	Superficial tumors	124	CR = 29%	CR = 53.8%	
	Superficial matched pairs only	62	CR = 29%	CR = 68%	
Scott *et al*[124]	Superficial tumors matched pairs only	62	CR = 39%	CR = 87%	<0.01
Corry *et al*[125]	Superficial tumors	21	CR = 30%	CR = 62%	

* Prospective, randomized trial; p values shown when reported.

(38.1°C versus 40.5°C, respectively) imply that direct thermal cytotoxicity was unlikely in most of the tumor volume and that hyperthermia probably contributed only to thermal radiosensitization. All of these results lead to the tentative conclusion that the minimum number of hyperthermia fractions required for a high probability of response depends upon the temperatures achieved (*i.e.*, relative amount of direct thermal cytotoxicity versus thermal radiosensitization), the tumor volume, and the radiation dose.[99]

Evaluation of Hyperthermia for Deep Tumors

The reported trials on superficial tumors define important biologic aspects of treatment with hyperthermia and radiotherapy. Control of bulky deep locoregional disease, however, limits curability of many common human tumors.[103] Development and Phase I equipment evaluation for inducing hyperthermia in deep sites, especially interstitial techniques, magnetic induction coils, capacitively coupled plates, annular microwave phased arrays, and focused ultrasound, is the subject of extensive current investigation.[104] When deep sites can be implanted, interstitial hyperthermia techniques can provide higher average temperatures than noninvasive techniques.[105] Toxicity is similar to radiation alone except that in pelvic sites, tumor necrosis and slough can occur suddenly, precipitating development of fistulas. The potential for thermal toxicity is high with this technique, especially in sites such as the brain.[90] Trials using a commercially available magnetic induction coil (Magnetrode) include a multi-institutional Phase I/II study of 1170 patients with hyperthermia alone or in combinations with radiotherapy and chemotherapy.[106] Reported toxicity was <0.3%, but the paucity of measured temperatures leads to difficulty in identifying the contribution of hyperthermia to subjective and objective responses. Other studies that include extensive temperature measurements reveal that most intratumoral sites do not exceed 42°–43°C with this device,[107,108] although marked temperature elevation in core regions of bulky tumors is possible, presumably because of low blood perfusion. Japanese investigators have reported clinical testing of capacitively coupled radiofrequency devices (13.6 and 8 MHz). Most of the reports describe temperature measurements only in the center of tumors,[109] but a recent report[110] of multipoint measurements in 60 deep-seated tumors revealed a maximum tumor center temperature >43°C in 38% of tumors, a lowest intratumoral temperature >42°C in 11%, and temperature variation >2°C in 81%. Localized pain was the major power-limiting factor.[111] The capacitively coupled radiofrequency device thus can produce significant temperature rise in deep tumors at a variety of anatomic locations with limited toxicity, and with significant nonuniformity of the temperature distribution. Investigators at the University of Utah have extensively evaluated an annular microwave array (AA) for heating intra-abdominal and pelvic malignancies.[108,112] Measurement of temperature distributions across at least one tumor diameter was typical. In pelvic tumors, pain during the hyperthermia treatments occurred in most of 43 patients, and there were eight instances of serious late complications. In 73% of 175 treatments in 43 patients, temperatures over 42°C were achieved. The minimum intratumoral isoeffective dose was 6.3 min Eq43, on average, and an average of 18% of monitored sites exceeded

TABLE 66-8. Prognostic Variables for Complete Response to HT plus RT

Author	*Prognostic Variables*
Kim *et al*[126]	Volume, RT dose/fx, T_{min}
Dewhirst and Sim[75]	Volume, T_{min} (non–site-specific)
Oleson *et al*[105]	Volume, RT dose, T_{min} averaged over all treatments, HT technique
Sims *et al*[127]	Volume, rad dose, HT technique, number of intratumoral sites ≥42.5°C
Arcangeli *et al*[99,118]	Volume, minimum equivalent time at 42.5°C
Luk *et al*[128]	Total rad dose, recurrence status, minimum daily average temperature, volume
Kapp *et al*[129]	T_{min} and T_{ave} averaged over all treatments
van der Zee *et al*[130]	Min HT dose
Dunlop *et al*[100]	Number of HT treatments for which T_{min} ≥20 min Eq43
Scott *et al*[131]	T_{ave} ≥43°C, greatest tumor diameter, site/histology

the desired goal of the equivalent of 30 min at 43°C. In a comparison in the same patients of temperatures achieved with the Magnetrode and the AA in deep abdominal and pelvic sites,[108] these investigators reported 59% of intratumoral sites in 12 patients exceeded 30 Eq43 with the AA compared with 18% of sites with the Magnetrode: a similar frequency of treatment-limiting conditions and toxicity was found with the Magnetrode and the AA. Applied EM power levels are limited by patient discomfort and safety considerations, and power cannot be focused sharply within the tumor target volume. Serious toxicity with these techniques has, however, been infrequent. In most of the tumor volume, temperature elevation may be insufficient to result in direct thermal cytotoxicity and enhancement of radiation effect by hyperthermia may be more limited than is evident in superficial tumors. Determining the extent and distribution of temperature elevation and number of treatments needed for significant improvement in local control will require prospective studies.

Study of focused US for treatments of deep tumors has been limited. Lele has used scanned focused US transducers to treat tumors at depths ≤12 cm with volumes up to about $10 \times 10 \times 10$ cm³.[85] The frequency of pain from bone or periosteum heating and other toxicity was negligible and desired temperatures of 43°C were achieved in 43 of 44 tumors in 30 patients. Further development and clinical testing of scanned focused US techniques is in progress.[113]

Most reports of whole-body hyperthermia have been Phase I trials, which showed considerable toxicity. However, a radiant-heating device has allowed routine heating of mildly sedated patients to 41.8°C for 2 hr with minimal toxicity:[96] this device promises to facilitate more systematic study of whole-body hyperthermia with chemotherapy and localized radiotherapy. Although no clear evidence of therapeutic gain with whole-body hyperthermia and chemotherapeutic agents exists, altered pharmacokinetics of systemic agents[114] and acid pH in tumors[115] are factors one might exploit for therapeutic gain.

FUTURE DIRECTIONS

Early phenomenologic observations on anticancer effects of hyperthermia have led to recent advances in understanding mechanisms of cellular effects of hyperthermia and confirmation of marked enhancement of drug and radiation effects at elevated temperature. Trials in superficial tumors show clinical efficacy of hyperthermia and radiotherapy. Application of hyperthermia in deep body sites for locoregionally advanced disease in which there is a possibility of cure remains a high priority that has required extensive development of thermometry systems and techniques as well as sophisticated energy delivery systems. Although these approaches are feasible and have limited toxicity, efficacy will require improved localization, control, and extent of temperature rise. Hyperthermia, thus, is a therapy based upon a solid rationale that is now accepted as an adjunct to radiotherapy in treatment of superficial tumors but is still investigational in all other situations. The laboratory evidence for enhancement of drug effects at elevated temperature continues to stimulate interest in this combination, but selection of suitable patients, the underlying limited efficacy of many current drugs as sole agents, and limitations in current hyperthermia technology impede clinical testing. Directions for future research in hyperthermia have been detailed in reports sponsored jointly by the American College of Radiology, the Intersociety Council for Radiation Oncology, and the National Cancer Institute.[10,116] In addition to improvement in power delivery and temperature measurement systems, approaches are needed for hyperthermia treatment planning, prediction of temperature distributions, and expression of thermal dose. Basic biologic research must continue on mechanisms of cellular effects and interactions among hyperthermia, radiotherapy, and drugs. In many respects, hyperthermia is proving to be a probe for cellular processes that are common to all mammalian cells. Clinical research must optimize the therapeutic gain for the number and frequency of hyperthermia fractions, length of treatment, and range of temperatures. This requires Phase II testing with appropriate selection of sites and disease for which current hyperthermia techniques may be likely to produce safe heating to temperatures 42° to 43°C. Increasing availability of commercial hyperthermia equipment is facilitating the conduct of standardized multi-institutional protocols.

In summary, hyperthermia continues to show promise in improving results of treatment in cancer patients for whom conventional therapy has low efficacy. Current research emphasizes an increasing understanding of the basic mechanisms of action of hyperthermia alone and in combination with other modalities, improving the techniques for heating tumors in a variety of sites, and conducting clinical trials ranging from Phase I through Phase III.

REFERENCES

1. Coley-Nauts H, Swife W, Coley B: The treatment of malignant tumors by bacterial toxins as developed by the late William B. Coley, M.D. reviewed in light of modern research. Cancer Res 6:205–216, 1946
2. Susskind C: The "story" of nonionizing radiation research. Bull NY Acad Med 55:1152–1163, 1979
3. Westermark N: The effect of heat upon rat-tumors. Skand Arch Physiol 52:257–322, 1927
4. Rohdenburg GL, Prime F: The effect of combined radiation and heat on neoplasms. Arch Surg 2:116–129, 1921
5. Selawry OS, Carlson JC, Moore GE: Tumor response to ionizing rays at elevated temperatures. AJR 80:833–839, 1958
6. Crile G Jr: The effects of heat and radiation on cancers implanted on the feet of mice. Cancer Res 23:372–380, 1963
7. Hahn GM: Hyperthermia in Cancer. New York, Plenum Press, 1982
8. Storm FK (ed): Hyperthermia in Cancer Therapy. Boston, GK Hall Medical Publ, 1983
9. Hand JW, James JR (eds): Physical Techniques in Clinical Hyperthermia. Letchworth, England, Research Studies Press, 1986
10. Oleson JR, Calderwood SR, Coughlin CT et al: Biological and clinical aspects of hyperthermia in cancer therapy. Am J Clin Oncol 11:368–380, 1988
11. Dewey WC, Hopwood LE, Sapareto SA et al: Cellular responses to combinations of hyperthermia and radiation. Radiology 123:463–474, 1977
12. Gerner E, Schneider M: Induced thermal resistance in HeLa cells. Nature 256:500–502, 1976
13. Westra A, Dewey WC: Variation in sensitivity to heat shock during the cell-cycle of Chinese hamster cells in vitro. Int J Radiat Biol 19:467–477, 1971
14. Sapareto SA, Hopwood LE, Dewey WC et al: Effects of hyperthermia on survival and progression of Chinese hamster ovary cells. Cancer Res 38:393–400, 1978
15. Gerweck LE, Burlett P: The lack of correlation between heat and radiation sensitivity in mammalian cells. Int J Radiat Oncol Biol Phys 4:283–285, 1978
16. Giovanella BC, Stehlin JS Jr, Morgan AC: Selective lethal effect of supranormal temperatures on human neoplastic cells. Cancer Res 36:3944–3950, 1976

17. Overgaard J, Nielsen OS: The role of tissue environmental factors on the kinetics and morphology of tumor cells exposed to hyperthermia. Ann NY Acad Sci 335:254–278, 1980
18. Nielsen OS, Overgaard J: Effect of extracellular pH on thermotolerance and recovery of hyperthermic damage in vitro. Cancer Res 39:2772–2778, 1979
19. Nielsen OS, Overgaard J: Influence of time and temperature on the kinetics of thermotolerance in L1A2 cells in vitro. Cancer Res 42:4190–4196, 1982
20. Rofstad EK, Midthjell H, Brustad T: Heat sensitivity and thermotolerance in cells from five human melanoma xenografts. Cancer Res 44:4347–4354, 1984
21. Leith JT, Bliven SF, Glicksman AS: Similarity of thermotolerance characteristics in heterogeneous human colon tumor subpopulations after exposure to fractionated heat doses (44°C). Radiat Res 104:128–139, 1985
22. Gerweck LE: Modification of cell lethality at elevated temperatures: The pH effect. Radiat Res 70:224–235, 1977
23. Holahan PK, Dewey WC: Effect of pH and cell cycle progression on development and decay of thermotolerance. Radiat Res 106:111–121, 1986
24. Hahn GM, Shiu EC: Adaptation to low pH modifies thermal and thermochemical responses of mammalian cells. Int J Hyperthermia 2:379–387, 1986
25. Hahn GM, Li GC: Thermotolerance and heat shock proteins in mammalian cells. Radiat Res 92:452–457, 1982
26. Li GC: Elevated levels of 70,000 Dalton heat shock protein in transiently thermotolerant Chinese hamster fibroblasts and in their stable heat resistant variants. Int J Radiat Oncol Biol Phys 11:165–177, 1985
27. Lindquist SL: The heat shock response. Annu Rev Biochem 55:535–572, 1986
28. Pelham HRB: Speculations on the function of the major heat shock proteins. Cell 46:959–961, 1986
29. Henle KJ: Sensitization to hyperthermia below 43°C induced in Chinese hamster ovary cells by step-down heating. J Natl Cancer Inst 64:1479–1483, 1980
30. Gerweck LE, Richards B, Jennings M: The influence of variable oxygen concentration on the response of cells to heat or x-irradiation. Radiat Res 85:314–320, 1981
31. Gerweck LE, Bascomb F: Influence of hypoxia on the development of thermotolerance. Radiat Res 90:356–361, 1982
32. Li GC, Shiu EC, Hahn GM: Recovery of cells from heat-induced potentially lethal damage: Effects of pH and nutrient environment. Int J Radiat Oncol Biol Phys 6:577–582, 1980
33. Stone HB, Dewey WC: Biologic basis and clinical potential of local–regional hyperthermia. In Phillips T, Wara W (eds): Radiation Oncology Vol 2, pp 1–41. New York, Raven Press, 1987
34. Fuller DJM, Gerner EW: Sensitization of Chinese hamster ovary cells to heat shock by alpha-difluoromethylornithine. Cancer Res 47:816–820, 1987
35. Lepcock JR: Involvement of membranes in cellular responses to hyperthermia. Radiat Res 92:433–438, 1982
36. Konings AWT, Ruifrok ACC: Role of membrane lipids and membrane fluidity in thermosensitivity and thermotolerance of mammalian cells. Radiat Res 102:86–98, 1985
37. Roti Roti JL, Uygur N, Higashikubo R: Nuclear protein following heat shock: Protein removal kinetics and cell cycle rearrangements. Radiat Res 107:250–261, 1986
38. Campbell AC: Intracellular Calcium: Its Role as a Universal Regulator. Chichester, John Wiley & Sons, 1983
39. Stevenson MA, Calderwood SK, Hahn GM: Effect of hyperthermia (45°C) on calcium flux in Chinese hamster ovary HA-1 fibroblasts and its potential role in cytotoxicity and heat resistance. Cancer Res 47:3712–3717, 1987
40. Li GC, Fisher GA, Hahn GM: Induction of thermotolerance and evidence for a well-defined thermotropic cooperative process. Radiat Res 89:361–368, 1982
41. Belli JA, Bonte FJ: Influence of temperature on the radiation response of mammalian cells in tissue culture. Radiat Res 18:272–276, 1963
42. Ben-Hur E, Elkind MM, Bronk BV: Thermally enhanced radioresponse of cultured Chinese hamster cells: Inhibition of repair of sublethal damage and enhancement of lethal damage. Radiat Res 58:38–51, 1974
43. Sapareto S, Raaphorst G, Dewey WC: Cell killing and the sequencing of hyperthermia and radiation. Int J Radiat Oncol Biol Phys 5:343–347, 1979
44. Gerner EW, Oval JH, Manning MR et al: Dose-rate dependence of heat radiosensitization. Int J Radiat Oncol Biol Phys 9:1401–1404, 1983
45. Gillette EL, Ensley BS: Effect of heat, radiation, and pH on mouse mammary tumor cells. Int J Radiat Oncol Biol Phys 9:1521–1525, 1983
46. Wike-Hooley JL, Haveman J, Reinhold HS: The relevance of tumour pH to the treatment of malignant disease. Radiother Oncol 2:343–366, 1984
47. Thistlethwaite AJ, Leeper DB, Moylan DJ III et al: pH distribution in human tumors. Int J Radiat Oncol Biol Phys 11:1647–1652, 1985
48. Haveman J: Influence of pH and thermotolerance on the enhancement of x-ray induced inactivation of cultured mammalian cells by hyperthermia. Int J Radiat Biol 43:281–289, 1983
49. Holahan EV, Highfield DP, Holahan PK et al: Hyperthermic killing and hyperthermic radiosensitization in Chinese hamster ovary cells: Effects of pH and thermal tolerance. Radiat Res 97:108–131, 1984
50. Holahan PK, Dewey WC: Effect of pH and cell cycle progression on development and decay of thermotolerance. Radiat Res 106:111–121, 1986
51. Haveman J, Luinenburg M, Wondergem J et al: Effects of hyperthermia on the linear and quadratic parameters of the radiation survival curve of mammalian cells: Influence of thermotolerance. Int J Radiat Biol 51:561–565, 1987
52. Morgan JE, Honess DJ, Bleehen NM: The interaction of thermal tolerance with drug cytotoxicity in vitro. Br J Cancer 39:422–428, 1979
53. Herman TS, Sweets CC, White DM et al: Effect of heating on lethality due to hyperthermia and selected chemotherapeutic drugs. J Natl Cancer Inst 68:487–491, 1982
54. Wallner KE, Li GC: Effect of drug exposure duration and sequencing on hyperthermic potentiation of mitomycin-C and cisplatin. Cancer Res 47:493–495, 1987
55. Meyn RE, Corry PM, Fletcher SE et al: Thermal enhancement of DNA damage in mammalian cells treated with *cis*-diaminadichloroplatinum(II). Cancer Res 40:1136–1139, 1980
56. Urano M, Gerweck LE, Epstein R et al: Response of a spontaneous murine tumor to hyperthermia: Factors which modify the thermal response in vivo. Radiat Res 83:312–322, 1980
57. Jain RK, Ward-Hartley K: Tumor blood flow—characterization, modifications, and role in hyperthermia. IEEE Trans Sonics Ultrasonics 31:504–526, 1984
58. Reinhold HS, Endrich B: Tumor microcirculation as a target for hyperthermia. Int J Hyperthermia 2:111–137, 1986
59. Streffer C: Metabolic changes during and after hyperthermia. Int J Hyperthermia 1:305–319, 1985
60. Ward-Hartley KA, Jain RK: Effect of glucose and galactose on microcirculatory flow in normal and neoplastic tissues in rabbits. Cancer Res 47:371–377, 1987
61. Thistlethwaite AJ, Alexander GA, Moylan DJ III et al: Modification of human tumor pH by elevation of blood glucose. Int J Radiat Oncol Biol Phys 13:603–610, 1987
62. Urano M: Kinetics of thermotolerance in normal and tumor tissues: A review. Cancer Res 46:474–482, 1986
63. Nielsen OS, Overgaard J, Kamura T: Influence of thermotolerance on the interaction between hyperthermia and radiation in a solid tumor in vivo. Br J Radiol 56:267–273, 1983
64. Dewey WC, Freeman ML, Raaphorst GP et al: Cell biology of hyperthermia and radiation. In Meyn RE, Withers HR (eds): Radiation Biology in Cancer Research, pp 589–621. New York, Raven Press, 1980
65. Overgaard J: Simultaneous and sequential hyperthermia and radiation treatment of an experimental tumor and its surrounding normal tissue in vivo. Int J Radiat Oncol Biol Phys 6:1507–1517, 1980
66. Stone HB, Harding RP: Reversible injury after mild hyperthermia. Int J Radiat Oncol Biol Phys 12:823–827, 1986
67. Lyons BE, Obona WG, Borcich JK et al: Chronic histological effects of ultrasonic hyperthermia on normal feline brain tissue. Radiat Res 106:234–251, 1986
68. Peck JW, Gibbs FA Jr: Assay of premorbid murine jejunal fibrosis based on mechanical changes after x-irradiation and hyperthermia. Radiat Res 112:525–543, 1987
69. Morris CC, Meyers R, Field SB: The response of the rat tail to hyperthermia. Br J Radiol 50:576–580, 1977
70. Marmor JB: Interactions of hyperthermia and chemotherapy in animals. Cancer Res 39:2269–2276, 1979
71. Zakris EL, Dewhirst MW, Riviere JE et al: Pharmacokinetics and toxicity of intraperitoneal cisplatin combined with regional hyperthermia. J Clin Oncol 5:1613–1620, 1987
72. Page RL, Price GS, Heidner GL et al: Phase I study of cisplatin combined with whole body hyperthermia in tumor-bearing dogs. Int J Hyperthermia (in press)
73. Field SB: Studies relevant to a means of quantifying the effects of hyperthermia. Int J Hyperthermia 3:291–296, 1987
74. Overgaard J: Some problems related to the clinical use of thermal isoeffect doses. Int J Hyperthermia 3:329–336, 1987
75. Dewhirst MW, Sim DA: The utility of thermal dose as a predictor of tumor and normal tissue responses to combined radiation and hyperthermia. Cancer Res 44:4772s–4780s, 1984
76. Fessenden P, Lee ER, Samulski TV: Direct temperature measurement. Cancer Res 44:4799s–4804s, 1984
77. Divrik AM, Roemer RB, Cetas TC: Inference of complete temperature fields from a few measured temperatures: An uncontstrained optimization method. IEEE-Trans BME 31:150–160, 1984
78. Corry PM et al: Clinical experience with plane-wave ultrasound systems. In Steeves RA, Paliwal BR (eds): Syllabus: A Categorical Course in Hyperthermia, p 151. Oak Brook, Il, Radiological Society of North America, 1987
79. Strohbehen JW, Roemer RB: A survey of computer simulations of hyperthermia treatments. IEEE-Trans BME 31:136–149, 1984
80. Cetas TC: Thermometry. In Lehmann JR (ed): Therapeutic Heat and Cold, 3rd ed, pp 35–69. Baltimore, Williams & Wilkins, 1982
81. Gibbs FA Jr: "Thermal mapping" in experimental cancer treatment with hyperthermia: Description and use of a semiautomatic system. Int J Radiat Oncol Biol Phys 9:1057–1063, 1983
82. Guy AW: Biophysics of high frequency currents and electromagnetic radiation. In Lehmann JF (ed): Therapeutic Heat and Cold, 3rd ed, pp 199–277, Baltimore, Williams & Wilkins, 1982
83. Frizzell LA, Dunn F: Biophysics of ultrasound. In Lehmann JF (ed): Therapeutic Heat and Cold, 3rd ed, pp 353–385. Baltimore, Williams & Wilkins, 1982
84. Gibbs FA Jr, Peck JW, Dethlefsen LA: The importance of temperature uniformity in the study of radiosensitizing effects of hyperthermia in vivo. Radiat Res 87:187–197, 1981
85. Lele PP: Physical aspects and clinical studies with ultrasonic hyperthermia. In Storm FK (ed): Hyperthermia in Cancer Therapy, pp 333–365. Boston, GK Hall Medical Publ, 1983
86. Oleson JR: A review of magnetic induction methods for hyperthermia treatment of cancer. IEEE-Trans BME 31:91–97, 1984

87. Bach Andersen J: Regional electromagnetic heating. In Hand JW, James JR (eds): Physical Techniques in Clinical Hyperthermia, pp 65–97. Letchworth, England, Research Studies Press, 1986
88. Oleson JR: Interstitial hyperthermia. In Withers HR, Peters LJ (eds): Innovations in Radiation Oncology Research, pp 303–312. Berlin, Springer-Verlag, 1987
89. Joseph C, Astrahan M, Lipsett J et al: Interstitial hyperthermia and interstitial iridium-192 implantation: A technique and preliminary results. Int J Radiat Oncol Biol Phys 7:827–833, 1981
90. Lyons BE, Britt RH, Strohbehn JW: Localized hyperthermia in the treatment of malignant brain tumors using an interstitial microwave antenna array. IEEE-Trans BME 31:53–62, 1984
91. Stauffer PR, Cetas TC, Fletcher AM et al: Observations on the use of ferromagnetic implants for inducing hyperthermia. IEEE-Trans BME 31:76–90, 1984
92. Cavaliere R, Mondovi B, Moricca G et al: Regional perfusion hyperthermia. In Storm FK (ed): Hyperthermia in Cancer Therapy, pp 369–399. Boston, GK Hall Medical Publ, 1983
93. Pettigrew R, Galt J, Ludgate C et al: Clinical effect of whole body hyperthermia in advanced malignancies. Br Med J 4:679–682, 1974
94. Bull J, Lees D, Schuette W et al: Whole body hyperthermia: A phase I trial of a potential adjuvant to chemotherapy. Ann Intern Med 90:317–323, 1979
95. Reinhold H, van der Zee J, Faithful N et al: Use of the Pomp–Siemens hyperthermia cabin. Natl Cancer Inst Monogr 61:371–375, 1982
96. Robins HI, Dennis WH, Neville AJ et al: A nontoxic system for 41.8°C whole body hyperthermia. Results of a Phase I study using a radiant heat device. Cancer Res 45:3937–3944, 1985
97. Parks L, Minaberry C, Smith D et al: Treatment of far advanced bronchogenic carcinoma by extracorporeally induced systemic hyperthermia. J Thorac Cardiovasc Surg 78:883–892, 1979
98. Overgaard J: Rationale and problems in the design of clinical studies. In Overgaard J (ed): Hyperthermic Oncology 1984, Vol 2, pp 325–338. London, Taylor & Francis, 1985
99. Arcangeli G, Benassi M, Cividalli A et al: Radiotherapy and hyperthermia. Analysis of clinical results and identification of prognostic variables. Cancer 60:950–956, 1987
100. Dunlop PRC, Hand JW, Dickinson RJ et al: An assessment of local hyperthermia in clinical practice. Int J Hyperthermia 2:39–50, 1986
101. Kapp DS, Bagshaw MA, Meyer JL et al: Optimization of hyperthermia and low dose irradiation in the treatment of superficial tumors: A prospective randomized trial of 2 vs 6 heat treatments (abstr). Radiat Res Soc, 33rd Annual Meeting, 1985
102. Leopold KA, Harrelson J, Prosnitz L et al: Preoperative hyperthermia and radiation for soft tissue sarcomas: Advantage of two vs one hyperthermia treatments per week. Int J Radiat Oncol Biol Phys 16:107–115, 1989
103. Kapp DS: Site and disease selection for hyperthermia clinical trials. Int J Hyperthermia 2:139–156, 1986
104. Gibbs FA Jr: Regional hyperthermia: A clinical appraisal of noninvasive deep-heating methods. Cancer Res (suppl) 44:4765s–4770s, 1984
105. Oleson JR, Sim DA, Manning MR: Analysis of prognostic variables in hyperthermia treatment of 161 patients. Int J Radiat Oncol Biol Phys 10:2231–2239, 1984
106. Storm FK, Baker HW, Scanlon EF et al: Magnetic-induction hyperthermia. Results of a 5-year multi-institutional national cooperative trial in advanced cancer patients. Cancer 55:2677–2687, 1985
107. Oleson JR, Manning MR, Heusinkveld RS: Hyperthermia by magnetic induction: II. Clinical experience with concentric electrodes. Int J Radiat Oncol Biol Phys 10:2231–2239, 1984
108. Sapozink MD, Gibbs FA Jr, Thomson JW et al: A comparison of deep regional hyperthermia from an annular phased array and a concentric coil in the same patients. Int J Radiat Oncol Biol Phys 11:179–190, 1985
109. Abe M, Hiraoka M, Takahashi M et al: Multi-institutional studies on hyperthermia using an 8-MHz radiofrequency capacitive heating device (Thermotron RF-8) in combination with radiation for cancer therapy. Cancer 58:1589–1595, 1986
110. Hiraoka M, Shiken J, Alzuta K et al: Radiofrequency capacitive hyperthermia for deep-seated tumors. I. Studies on thermometry. Cancer 60:121–127, 1987
111. Hiraoka M, Shiken J, Akuta K et al: Radiofrequency capacitive hyperthermia for deep-seated tumors. II. Effects of thermoradiotherapy. Cancer 60:128–135, 1987
112. Sapozink MD, Gibbs FA Jr, Egger MJ et al: Regional hyperthermia for clinically advanced deep-seated pelvic malignancy. J Clin Oncol 9:162–169, 1986
113. Hynynen K, Roemer R, Anhalt D et al: A scanned, focussed, multiple transducer ultrasonic system for localized hyperthermia treatments. Int J Hyperthermia 3:21–35, 1987
114. Riviere JE, Page RL, Dewhirst MW et al: Effect of hyperthermia on cisplatin pharmacokinetics in normal dogs. Int J Hyperthermia 2:351–358, 1986
115. Tobari C, Kersen TV, Hahn GM: Modification of pH of normal and malignant tissue by hydralazine and glucose, with and without breathing of 5% CO_2 and 95% air. Radiat Res (in press)
116. Stewart J, Bagshaw M, Corry P et al: Hyperthermia as a treatment of cancer. Cancer Treat Symp 1:135–145, 1984
117. Valdagni R, Armichetti M, Pani G: Radical radiation alone versus radical radiation plus microwave hyperthermia for N_3 (TNM-UICC) neck nodes: A prospective randomized clinical trial. Int J Radiat Oncol Biol Phys 15:13–24, 1988
118. Arcangeli G, Arcangeli GC, Guerra A et al: Tumor response to heat and radiation: Prognostic variables in the treatment of neck node metastases from head and neck cancer. Int J Hyperthermia 1:207–217, 1985
119. Steeves RA, Severson SB, Paliwal BR et al: Matched-pair analysis of response to local hyperthermia and megavoltage electron therapy for superficial human tumors. Endocurietherapy/Hyperthermia Oncol 2:163–170, 1986
120. Lindholm CE, Kjellen E, Nilsson P et al: Microwave-induced hyperthermia and radiotherapy in human superficial tumors: Clinical results with a comparative study of combined treatment versus radiotherapy alone. Int J Hyperthermia 3:393–411, 1987
121. van der Zee J, van Rhoon GC, Wike-Hooley et al: Thermal enhancement of radiotherapy in breast carcinoma. In Overgaard J (ed): Hyperthermic Oncology 1984, Vol 1, pp 345–348. London, Taylor & Francis, 1985
122. Kim JH, Hahn EW, Ahmed SA et al: Clinical study of the sequence of combined hyperthermia and radiation therapy of malignant melanoma. In Overgaard J (ed): Hyperthermic Oncology 1984, Vol 1, pp 387–390. London, Taylor & Francis, 1985
123. Li R-Y, Zhang T-Z, Lin S-Y et al: Effects of hyperthermia combined with radiation in the treatment of superficial malignant lesions in 90 patients. In Overgaard J (ed): Hyperthermic Oncology 1984, Vol 1, pp 395–397. London, Taylor & Francis, 1985
124. Scott RS, Johnson RJR, Story KV et al: Local hyperthermia in combination with definitive radiotherapy: Increased tumor clearance, reduced recurrence rate in extended follow-up. Int J Radiat Oncol Biol Phys 10:2119–2123, 1984
125. Corry PM, Spanos WJ, Tilchen EJ et al: Combined ultrasound and radiation therapy treatment of human superficial tumors. Radiology 145:165–169, 1982
126. Kim JH, Hahn EW, Antich P: Radiofrequency hyperthermia for clinical cancer therapy. Natl Cancer Inst Monogr 61:339–342, 1982
127. Sim DA, Oleson JR, Grochowski KJ: An update of the University of Arizona human clinical hyperthermia experience including estimates of therapeutic advantage. In Overgaard J (ed): Hyperthermic Oncology 1984, Vol 1, pp 367–370. London, Taylor & Francis, 1985
128. Luk KH, Pajak TF, Perez CA et al: Prognostic factors for tumor response after hyperthermia and radiation. In Overgaard J (ed): Hyperthermic Oncology 1984, Vol 1, pp 353–358. London, Taylor & Francis, 1985
129. Kapp DS, Samulski TV, Meyer JL et al: Metastatic breast cancer with chest wall recurrences in previously irradiated areas: Management with low–moderate dose irradiation therapy and hyperthermia (abstr). Radiat Res Soc 33rd Annual Meeting, 1985
130. van der Zee J, van Putten WLJ, van den Berg AP et al: Retrospective analysis of the response of tumors in patients treated with a combination of radiotherapy and hyperthermia. Int J Hyperthermia 2:337–349, 1986
131. Scott R, Gillespie B, Perez CA et al: Hyperthermia in combination with definitive radiation therapy: Results of a Phase I/II RTOG study. Int J Radiat Oncol Biol Phys 15:711–716, 1988

SECTION 3

C. NORMAN COLEMAN

Chemical Modification of Radiation and Chemotherapy

The field of chemical modification of cancer therapy, initially developed in relation to radiation therapy, has expanded rapidly in the last few years. Included under the heading of chemical modifiers are agents that interact by chemical or physical means with known cytotoxic treatments—radiation and chemotherapy. In general, the chemical modifiers were not designed to be cytotoxic by themselves, rather they modify the tumor or the host tissue in such a way that the standard cytotoxic therapy becomes either more (sensitization) or less (protection) toxic. Chemical modification includes maneuvers used in biochemical modification (*e.g.*, depletion or augmentation of intracellular thiols), and it potentially overlaps with combined modality therapy in which two or more cytotoxic modalities are given together. Indeed, cytotoxic agents such as cisplatin and 5-fluorouracil can be administered in schedules that minimize the cytotoxic effects and enhance the radiation-sensitizing properties of the drug. The hypoxic cell sensitizers may be cytotoxic, as well, in addition to enhancing the efficacy of irradiation.

This chapter will focus on the general approaches toward hypoxia, as this has the potential to influence the clinical use of radiation and chemotherapy. It will include hypoxic cell sensitizers, radioprotectors, chemosensitizers, and chemoprotectors, all of which are currently being tested in clinical trials. Combined modality therapy that uses standard chemotherapeutic agents and radiation therapy will not be discussed. The use of chemical modifiers that are based on mechanisms other than hypoxia will be mentioned briefly. A more detailed and extensively referenced overview of this subject has recently been published.[1]

HYPOXIA

THE POTENTIAL IMPORTANCE OF HYPOXIC CELLS

It has been known for many years that hypoxic cells are relatively resistant to cell killing by radiation. To achieve the same proportion of cell kill, about three times the radiation dose is required for hypoxic cells compared with that for well-oxygenated cells. The ratio of dose required for a given level of cell killing under hypoxia compared with the dose needed in air is called the oxygen enhancement ratio (OER; Fig. 66-13).[2] At relatively large single doses of radiation the OER is in the range of 3, whereas for clinically relevant doses of 200 cGy/fraction the OER is approximately 2.[3,4] Thus, oxygen has the ability to sensitize cells to ionizing radiation at clinically relevant radiation doses.

Given that hypoxic cells are relatively radioresistant, how important is hypoxia in clinical radiotherapy? Although the answer to this question is not yet known, a good deal of information suggests that hypoxia may be important in certain situations. It should be emphasized that hypoxia is certainly not the sole cause for the failure of radiation to achieve local control of tumors,[5] therefore, an effective hypoxic cell sensitizer will not be a panacea for local tumor persistence. Conceptual knowledge of the physiology of hypoxia, the mechanism of radiation cell killing, and the competition model is necessary to understand the current therapeutic approaches.

TYPES OF HYPOXIA

The classic model of hypoxia is that of chronic hypoxia.[2] In tissue, oxygen can diffuse approximately 150 μm from a vessel as it is metabolized and consumed by the cells closest to the vessel. Cells beyond the diffusion limit will be anoxic and necrotic. Surrounding the necrotic zone are cells that are hypoxic and relatively radioresistant, yet they remain viable and clonogenic (Fig. 66-14, left-hand side). In this model it is assumed that the nutrient vessel remains patent and that the hypoxic cells are confined to the area surrounding the necrosis. These chronically hypoxic cells have diffusion-limited hypoxia.

A second type of hypoxia, acute hypoxia, has been postulated to be important.[6] Recently, such acute, intermittent hypoxia has been demonstrated in animal tumors [7-9] as illus-

FIG. 66-13. Oxygen enhancement and sensitizer enhancement ratios at clinically relevant radiation doses. OER/SER curves at a low radiation dose are less than that seen at the higher single doses often used in the laboratory (approximately 1500 cGy). Both oxygen and the 2-nitroimidazole sensitizers are effective at clinically relevant radiation doses. (Brown JM, Yu NY: Radiosensitization of hypoxic cells *in vivo* by SR 2508 at low radiation doses. Int J Radiat Oncol Biol Phys 10:1207–1212, 1984)

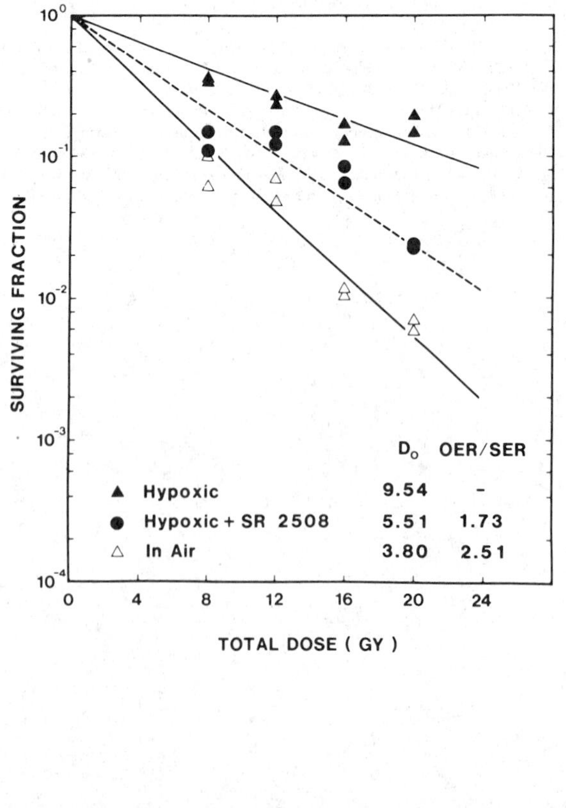

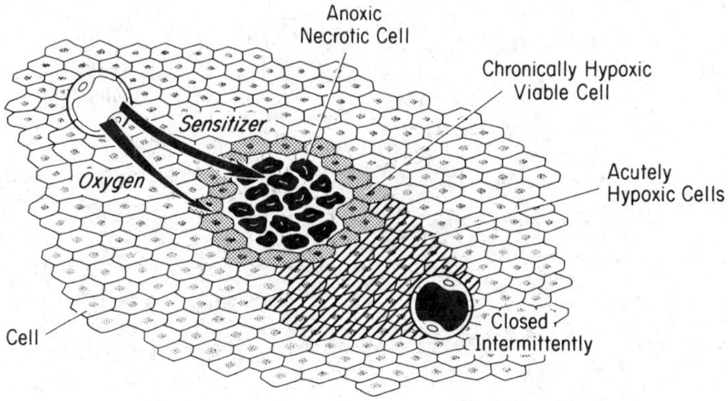

FIG. 66-14. Chronic and acute hypoxia. Chronically hypoxic cells are "diffusion-limited." Acutely hypoxic cells are "perfusion-limited," that is, they are hypoxic only when blood flow transiently stops in their nutrient vessel.

trated in Fig. 66-14 (right-hand side). In the acute hypoxia model, a small blood vessel within a tumor has intermittent blood flow. Cells irradiated when blood flow is present will behave radiobiologically as oxygenated cells. However, when blood flow transiently stops, the existing oxygen and other nutrients are rapidly exhausted, thereby leaving the cells that are perfused by that vessel in a temporarily hypoxic state. If radiation is given when the cells are not perfused, these cells will behave radiobiologically as hypoxic cells. These acutely hypoxic cells can be conceived as having "perfusion-limited" hypoxia. Many tumors undergo a process called reoxygenation, whereby the proportion of hypoxic cells remains relatively constant during a course of treatment.[2,10] Although the extent of reoxygenation that occurs clinically is unknown, the acute hypoxia model could account for the rapidity of reoxygenation observed in the laboratory. Because oxygen is the best hypoxic cell sensitizer, and because the reoxygenation process goes on between each fraction of radiation, regimens that use few fractions of radiation will not optimize this important reoxygenation process. Such few-fraction regimens were used in the early trials of hyperbaric oxygen and hypoxic cell sensitizers.

Although the presence and extent of acute and chronic hypoxia in human tumors are unknown, the existence of two types of hypoxia has implications for attempts to overcome hypoxic radioresistance. Because chronically hypoxic cells are diffusion-limited, an increase in the diffusion distance of oxygen would make more cells oxygenated. Similarly, a sensitizer that is diffusible without being rapidly metabolized would reach these cells. The acutely hypoxic cells present a different problem. While blood is flowing through the nutrient vessel the cells are well perfused with oxygen, or hypoxic sensitizer. However, when the blood flow ceases, the oxygen content will be quickly depleted, whereas the concentration of other slowly metabolized substances will remain at their preexisting level. Maneuvers that increase oxygen diffusion would not be expected to sensitize these cells, unless they were fortuitously within the diffusion distance of oxygen from a neighboring vessel. A slowly metabolized hypoxic cell sensitizer would be effective for these cells. Other processes to be described, such as hypoxic cell cytoxicity and chemosensitization, depend on the extent and duration of hypoxia and are likely to be affected differently by acute and chronic hypoxia. Fig. 66-15 illustrates some potential mechanisms for overcoming the two types of hypoxia.

MECHANISM OF RADIATION CELL KILLING AND COMPETITION MODEL

Cell killing by ionizing is caused by damage to the DNA. The target radical in the DNA, designated DNA· in Fig. 66-16, is produced by either direct ionization or by reaction with hydroxyl radicals produced from radiolysis of neighboring water molecules (termed the *indirect effect*).[2] Reaction with oxygen will produce a peroxyl radical, DNA-0_2·, which will next form products that are different from the original target molecules (irreversible damage). Reducing species, such as the thiols (-SH), can react with the target radical by hydrogen donation, resulting in restoration of the original target molecule. The oxygen-mimetic hypoxic cell radiosensitizers are designed to replace oxygen by producing irreversible damage, DNA-sensitizer· (Fig. 66-16). In each instance, the reaction of DNA with thiol (termed *protection*), or with oxygen or sensitizer (termed *sensitization*), depends on the reaction rate constant, *k*, and the concentration of the particular constituents.

The ability of oxygen or sensitizer to enhance cell killing is described by the enhancement ratio—OER for oxygen—and sensitizer enhancement ratio (SER) for sensitizer (see Fig. 66-13). The OER is dependent on the concentration of oxygen present at the target at the time of irradiation. Similarly, the oxygen-mimetic effect of hypoxic cell sensitizers depends on the concentration of sensitizer at the target at the time of irradiation. As will be discussed later, prolonged contact with the radiosensitizer can have effects beyond the oxygen-mimetic effects. It must be remembered that the oxygen-mimetic sensitizers will only affect the hypoxic cells, which usually compose about 20% of the tumor.[11] Therefore, in estimating the degree of enhancement in cell killing, the SER would apply to only the hypoxic cells, not to the entire tumor. To apply it to the entire tumor would over-estimate the potential impact of the hypoxic cell sensitizer.

Although the exact role of hypoxic cells in the failure of radiation to cure tumors is unknown, there is evidence to suggest that these cells are important in clinical radiother-

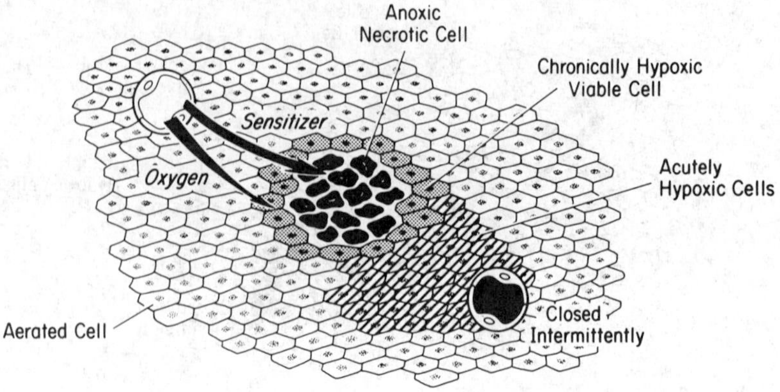

Approaches to Chronic Hypoxia

- Increase Oxygen Delivery
  - Transfusion
  - Hyperbaric Oxygen
  - Perfluorochemical
  - Altered Hgb Affinity for O_2
- Hypoxic Cell Sensitizers
  - ± Thiol modification
- Bioreductive Agents
  - Mitomycin-C
  - Nitroimidazoles
- ? Hyperthermia

Approaches to Acute Hypoxia

- Altered Oxygen Delivery
  - Likely to have minimal impact
- Hypoxic Cell Sensitizers
  - ± Thiol modification
- Bioreductive Agents
  - Would need rapid action under hypoxia
- ? Hyperthermia
- ? Chemotherapy

FIG. 66-15. Theoretical means of overcoming treatment resistance due to hypoxia. Possible methods of overcoming acute and chronic hypoxia are listed. The efficacy of the specific approaches against the different hypoxic cell populations remains to be established.

apy. Trials using hyperbaric oxygen have yielded variable and, at times, conflicting results.[5] In these trials, hyperbaric oxygen was administered to patients who were in compression chambers at 3 atm of oxygen. Because of the difficulty in oxygen administration, the radiation therapy was often administered in few-fraction regimens that did not take full advantage of reoxygenation. Many of the tumors treated were quite large, and the incurability of the tumor may have been due to the well-oxygenated cells rather than to hypoxia. Despite the limitations of the trials, the use of hyperbaric oxygen produced positive results in moderate-sized lesions of the cervix and head and neck.[20] In addition, a number of authors have suggested that patients with certain cancers, including cervix, head and neck, and bladder, who had higher hemoglobin levels, had better local tumor control than those with lower levels.[13-15] Such data were sufficiently encouraging to lead to the effort to develop other methods of overcoming hypoxia.

HYPOXIC CELL, OXYGEN-MIMETIC RADIOSENSITIZERS

The major class of drugs of clinical interest has been the nitroimidazole compounds. The first such compound tested was the 5-nitroimidazole, metronidazole. In the classic randomized trial by Urtasun and co-workers[16] patients with glioblastoma were treated with 330 cGy, three times a week for 3 weeks with either metronidazole plus radiation or radiation alone. The median survival of the sensitizer group was

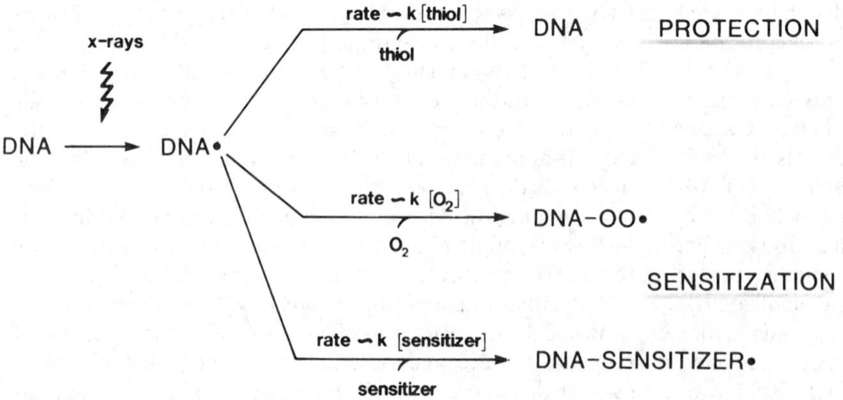

FIG. 66-16. Competition model. The DNA radical formed by ionizing irradiation can undergo chemical restitution (protection) or can be made into a permanent lesion in the presence of oxygen or a sensitizer (sensitization). (Coleman CN, Bump EA, Kramer RA: Chemical modifiers of cancer therapy. J Clin Oncol 6:709–733, 1988)

approximately 7 months, which was statistically superior to the 3-month median survival of the control ($p = 0.02$). However, almost all patients died by 1 year. Therefore, the result with sensitizer was no better than that of historical controls. The few-fraction regimen did not optimize reoxygenation, and the total radiation dose was somewhat lower than that used in conventional treatment. This study illustrated that an oxygen-mimetic sensitizer could demonstrate clinical activity, but that such a sensitizer should be added to the best possible radiation scheme.

MISONIDAZOLE

Misonidazole was the first in the class of 2-nitroimidazole drugs to be evaluated in the clinic. The 2-nitroimidazoles are more electron affinic and, therefore, more potent as sensitizers than metronidazole. In the laboratory, these compounds are definitely effective sensitizers. As with the OER, the SER is somewhat lower at the standard radiation fraction size (180–200 cGy)[3,4] than it is at a higher dose per fraction (approximately 1500 cGy) often used in the laboratory. Nevertheless, sensitization can occur at clinically relevant radiation doses. The amount of oxygen-mimetic sensitization obtained depends on the concentration of sensitizer in the tumor at the time of irradiation. Therefore, in planning a clinical trial it is desirable to use the sensitizer in a dose that would provide good drug levels in the tumor. However, regimens that use few high-dose fractions should be avoided so that reoxygenation can be maximized. One should be able to give the ideal sensitizer at an adequate dose with every radiation treatment, and it should not be toxic to the well-oxygenated normal tissues. Because none of the sensitizers can be given in unlimited amounts, it has not been possible to meet all of these ideal criteria. However, as will be discussed, optimizing the timing of sensitizer based on the "natural history" of hypoxia during a course of treatment or by using a combination of approaches against hypoxia is in the future plans for the clinical use of hypoxic sensitizers.

The development of clinical trials with the hypoxic cell sensitizers has recently been reviewed.[5] In the Phase I trials, misonidazole was observed to have a dose-limiting neurotoxicity.[17,18] At a cumulative dose of 10 to 12 g/m^2, approximately 30% to 50% of patients developed a peripheral sensory neuropathy. Approximately 10% had central nervous system toxicity. If the neuropathy was mild, it resolved relatively promptly; however, the more severe neuropathies could be very persistent and debilitating. To achieve an adequate level of sensitizer in the tumor, a single dose of approximately 2 g/m^2 was needed. Therefore, because of its dose-limiting neurotoxicity, only five or six doses of misonidazole could be administered. Alternatively, more doses could be given but at a dose size that was not likely to produce clinically detectable hypoxic cell sensitization. In retrospect, it would have been very surprising had misonidazole produced much therapeutic advantage given its dose-limiting neurotoxicity, as only a small proportion of the total number of radiation treatments could be sensitized. Dische[19] reviewed the results of 33 trials with misonidazole, five of which showed some possible benefit to the use of this drug. Four of the five positive trials were from 12 head and neck cancer studies. A large randomized trial in Denmark (1979–1985) suggested that misonidazole was of benefit for male patients with pharnygeal cancer, with an overall disease-free survival of 46% for the misonidazole group versus 26% for controls ($p < 0.02$). The misonidazole group has a superior 3-year survival rate, 59% versus 39% (p value not stated).[20]

Desmethylmisonidazole is an endogenously formed metabolite of misonidazole that, because of its pharmacokinetic properties to be described later, was predicted to be better tolerated than misonidazole. Although this drug was less neurotoxic and produced no central neurotoxicity, it was not sufficiently better than misonidazole so that the trials did not proceed beyond the Phase I studies.[21]

DEVELOPMENT OF LESS TOXIC SENSITIZERS

The further development of hypoxic cell sensitizers included [1] 2-nitroimidazoles that are less toxic so that more can be administered, [2] 2-nitroimidazoles that concentrate in tumors, [3] nonnitro compounds that might not be expected to have the same dose-limiting toxicity, [4] agents that are cytotoxic to hypoxic cells, and [5] dual-function molecules that are activated in the presence of hypoxia to bifunctional alkylating agents.

Brown and co-workers developed a series of misonidazole analogues that had the same electron affinity (a measure of ability to react in place of oxygen in the free-radical reaction illustrated in Fig. 66-13). The drugs of interest were less lipid-soluble than misonidazole, thus they would be excluded from the central nervous system by the lipid blood–brain barrier. Moreover, these compounds would be expected to be cleared more rapidly, resulting in reduced drug exposure.[22,23] The drug judged to be best was SR 2508, a nonpolar 2-nitroimidazole with an amide side chain.[24] This drug has completed Phase I testing[25,26] with the maximum tolerated dose of approximately 34 to 36 g/m^2. Like misonidazole, it has a dose-limiting peripheral neuropathy, however a dose of SR 2508 that is three to four times that of misonidazole can be administered. The central nervous system and ototoxicity seen with misonidazole[17] have not been encountered.

A retrospective analysis of the patients in the Phase I trial suggested that the risk of developing neuropathy in a given patient can be estimated by the pharmacokinetic parameters obtained at the time of initial drug administration. The drug exposure, as described by the area-under-the-curve of plasma concentration versus time (AUC), is the parameter used to predict toxicity.[27] Because the single-dose AUC remains constant throughout a course of treatment, multiplying the AUC by the number of doses gives the total AUC, a measure of drug exposure. The correlation between total AUC and the risk of developing neurotoxicity in the Phase I trial is shown in Fig. 66-17. If this observation is corroborated in the Phase II and III trials, it will be possible to use SR 2508 with only a small risk of producing a neuropathy, and if a neuropathy was to occur, it would likely be mild with prompt resolution. Thus, SR 2508 is much superior to misonidazole [1] by producing a better SER for a single dose of 2 g/m^2 dose (approximately 1.6 for the hypoxic tumor cells for SR 2508 versus 1.4 for misonidazole),[28] [2] by being able

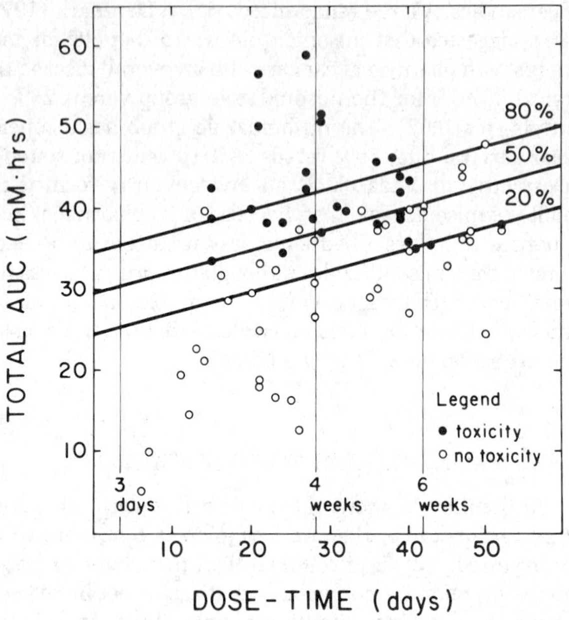

FIG. 66-17. Correlation between drug exposure and the risk of developing peripheral neuropathy. In the Phase I trial of SR 2508, drug exposure as assessed by the total-AUC correlated with the risk of developing neurotoxicity. Although this model requires confirmation and possible refinement in Phases II and III trials, it can be used to reduce the risk of development of severe neurotoxicity in individual patients. (Coleman CN, Halsey J, Cox RS, et al: Prediction of the neurotoxicity of the hypoxic cell radiosensitizer SR 2508 from the pharmacokinetic profile. Cancer Res 47:319–322, 1987)

to be utilized for three to four times the number of doses, and [3] by possibly having predictable toxicity. However, efficacy remains to be established.

Phase II and III trials with SR 2508 are in progress or planned for sites including head and neck cancer, inoperable bladder and prostate cancer, and esophageal tumors. Sites were carefully selected: for head and neck cancer, results from the hyperbaric oxygen trials or misonidazole trials suggested that hypoxia might be important; prostate and bladder cancers were selected because SR 2508, being in high concentration in the urine, could theoretically reach high concentrations in these tumor sites.[25] The starting dose in the Phase II and III trials is 34 g/m^2 given in 17 fractions of 2 g/m^2 over 5 to 6 weeks with dose escalation planned, depending on drug tolerance. All patients are monitored pharmacologically to direct drug usage. In addition, a Phase I trial is in progress utilizing SR 2508 in a continuous infusion during interstitial radiotherapy in an attempt to exploit both oxygen-mimetic sensitization and the prolonged exposure effect (to be described later).[29]

Another 2-nitroimidazole currently under clinical development in England is Ro-03-8799. Because this compound has a basic side chain, it accumulates in the acidic environment of tumors, producing a tumor/plasma ratio of approximately 3:1. Of interest, Ro-03-8799 has a different dose-limiting toxicity than SR 2508. It does not produce the cumulative peripheral neurotoxicity seen with SR 2508, but rather it causes an acute central nervous system toxicity of dizziness, nausea, and affective mental changes that last for 30 to 60 min. after injection. A single dose of 750 mg/m^2 is tolerable and is predicted to produce an SER for the hypoxic cells of approximately 1.6, similar to that obtained with SR 2508 at a dose of 2 g/m^2.[30–32] There does not appear to be a cumulative toxicity. Because it is desirable to give as much sensitizer as possible and to give drug with each treatment, there is interest in administering SR 2508 and Ro-03-8799 in combination. Limited clinical data available at present suggest that there is no pharmacokinetic interaction between the sensitizers[32] and that both drugs can be given in doses close to their individual maximal tolerated dose.[33] However, it remains to be seen whether this multisensitizer approach will be employed, or whether drugs will be used singly, possibly with thiol modifiers.

A series of 2-nitroimidazole compounds are under development that have a dual action—the oxygen-mimetic sensitization as seen with SR 2508 plus a biochemical process that leads to cytotoxicity because of the presence of an aziridine ring in the side chain.[34–36] In addition to the dual function there is preferential uptake in tumors, possibly caused by the low pH of tumors or to the alkylating function of the molecule.[36] Clinical trials with the prototype compound RSU-1069 were limited by gastrointestinal toxicity;[35] however, newer analogues are under development (RSU-1164 and RB-7040), which may be less toxic and which appear to concentrate in tumors. In the immediate future, the efforts in the development of the 2-nitroimidazoles will likely be limited to the aforementioned groups of compounds. A program is in progress developing nonnitro sensitizers.

Although SR 2508 is far superior to misonidazole, its usefulness is limited by a dose-related neuropathy. Because of this limitation, there has been an interest in studying the mechanism of neurotoxicity of misonidazole and its analogues with the goal of somehow ameliorating this toxicity. Under certain conditions in the laboratory, misonidazole can be toxic to oxygenated cells with inhibition of key enzymes, which might be an important aspect in the development of the neuropathy.[37,38] However, the mechanism of the neurotoxicity remains to be determined. The pathologic finding is axonal degeneration.[39,40] Empiric clinical and laboratory efforts to lessen the toxicity of misonidazole and DMM, including the use of dexamethasone,[41] pyridoxine,[42] and antioxidants, have been largely unsuccessful. Further laboratory studies are in progress using in vitro nerve culture techniques.

PROLONGED EXPOSURE OF HYPOXIC CELLS TO SENSITIZERS

After prolonged exposure of hypoxic cells to the 2-nitroimidazole compounds, the drug can reduce the size of the shoulder of the radiation survival curve and, with further exposure, produce direct cytotoxicity. In addition the 2-nitroimidazoles can act as chemosensitizers, as will be described in the following discussion. These processes require hypoxic conditions. The effect of continuous exposure of hypoxic cells to misonidazole was first noted when the hypoxic cells were given a prolonged exposure to misonidazole before they

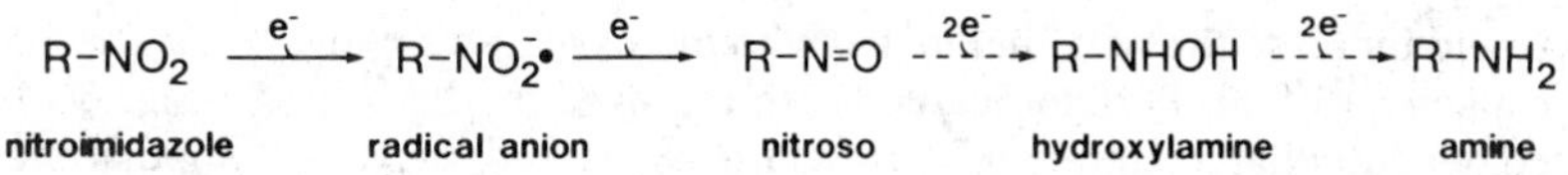

FIG. 66-18. Nitroreduction of the 2-nitroimidazole compounds under anoxic conditions. Without oxygen, the nitro (NO_2) group undergoes reduction to the amine (NH_2). The metabolites, some of which are not yet known, can be cytotoxic or can act as chemomodifiers. (Coleman CN, Bump EA, Kramer RA: Chemical modifiers of cancer therapy. J Clin Oncol 6:709–733, 1988)

were irradiated. Therefore, this continuous exposure effect is often referred to as the "preincubation" effect.[43]

The mechanism by which the prolonged hypoxic exposure to misonidazole produces shoulder reduction, cytotoxicity, or chemosensitization remains to be fully elucidated.[44] Under hypoxia the nitro ($-NO_2$) group is completely reduced to the amine ($-NH_2$) including the intermediates shown in Fig. 66-18.

In addition to these reduction products, a number of other metabolic products have been identified. These various reduction and metabolic products are believed to contribute to the cytotoxicity, chemopotentiation, and macromolecular binding seen under hypoxic conditions. The presence of oxygen will inhibit the formation of these products, some of which are capable of limited diffusion to neighboring cells.[45] Thus, a product formed in hypoxic cells could diffuse into neighboring cells and cause DNA damage or could become cytotoxic with reoxygenation.

Is there any application for this "continuous hypoxic exposure" effect? Efforts to detect hypoxia in situ have made use of this effect. Chemosensitization, to be discussed later, depends on hypoxic metabolism of misonidazole or its analogues. Of interest, Taylor and associates have recent data indicating that continuous, prolonged exposure may enhance the therapeutic efficacy of the sensitizer over that seen from the oxygen-mimetic mechanisms alone[46] (*i.e.*, the SER can be greater than the OER). This is in contradistinction to the pure oxygen-mimetic effect for which the OER is larger than the SER (*i.e.*, oxygen is the best sensitizer). Thus, it is conceivable that having the ability to utilize a sensitizer with many fractions of radiation will produce a therapeutic benefit at least as great as that predicted by the OER or SER.[28]

It is possible to utilize the continuous-exposure effect by administering a continuous infusion of SR 2508 with interstitial radiotherapy. Animal data from Fu and colleagues indicate that this might be an effective approach.[29] The continuous exposure of tumor to drug and radiation over a 2- to 3-day period will enable more of the acutely hypoxic cells to experience both the metabolic effects of the sensitizer and the oxygen-mimetic effects. The chronically hypoxic cells will also be sensitized by both effects but, perhaps, with a greater amount of the continuous exposure effect compared with that achieved with daily fractionated therapy accompanied by only a short infusion of sensitizer. Furthermore, the total amount of drug necessary to achieve an effective plasma concentration of sensitizer during the infusion (approximately 50–70 μg/ml) may permit the safe administration of sensitizer with both the daily fractionated, and the interstitial irradiation. Preliminary data from a Phase I continuous infusion trial indicate that this approach is, indeed, feasible.

ALTERATION IN OXYGEN DELIVERY TO TISSUES

The development of new sensitizers has been paralleled by the development of methods of altering oxygen delivery to tissues. Methods include altering the affinity of hemoglobin for oxygen; increasing the oxygen-carrying capacity of blood by the use of transfusion; or administrating perfluorochemicals and hyperbaric oxygen.[47–49] The major problem with alteration in oxygen delivery is that the tumor will undergo rapid adaptation to the new oxygen level. For example, in animal tumors alteration of radiosensitivity by either the production of anemia or by the administration of a blood transfusion lasts only about 24 hr.[47] Transfusion will transiently increase radiosensitivity; however, the tumor will soon adapt to the new oxygenation state and have sensitivity identical with that in the anemic state.

Despite this problem of adaptation, some clinical trials have shown a benefit from increasing hemoglobin concentration.[13–15,47] Even with an initial hemoglobin level within the normal range, the alteration of hemoglobin from 12 to 15 g/dl, theoretically, can rapidly increase tumor oxygenation by 30%.[50] Hirst postulated that the growth inhibitory effect of radiation on the tumor might partly account for the benefit to the transfusion seen in the clinical trials, that is, the theoretical compensatory growth of the cells surrounding the vessel might be prevented by the irradiation. Because of the presence of possible confounding variables it is not possible to conclude from the data that transfusion is appropriate therapy, nevertheless, as reviewed by Bush,[13] a number of clinical studies indicate that maintaining a hemoglobin level in the range of 12 g/dl might be of clinical benefit.

An alternative to blood transfusion is intravenous administration of a perfluorochemical emulsion (which dissolves oxygen) plus oxygen-breathing at the time of irradiation.[48,51] The amount of extra oxygen available depends on the amount of blood volume replaced by the perfluorocarbon (*i.e.*, the fluorocrit). One attractive aspect of the use of perfluorocarbons with oxygen-breathing is that the tumor is exposed to the increased oxygenation only transiently, during the actual period of oxygen-breathing. This may lessen the adaptation of the tumor to the increased oxygen delivery, thereby making the daily exposure more effective.[47]

A 5% fluorocrit will increase the non–hemoglobin-bound oxygen-carrying capacity of the blood twofold.[48] With a fluorocrit of 5%, breathing oxygen at 3 atm of pressure would increase the non–hemoglobin-bound oxygen-carrying capacity 13-fold. Perfluorocarbons are removed by the reticuloendothelial system and can cause a marked hepatosplenomegaly.[52,53] Preliminary results from a Phase I/II trial using Fluosol-DA (8–9 ml/kg IV once weekly), with the patients breathing 100% oxygen during irradiation, showed that 8 of 15 patients exhibited mild liver function abnormalities that returned to normal after the completion of therapy. The authors felt that both the acute normal tissue reactions and rate of tumor clearance were somewhat enhanced.[54]

As noted earlier, efforts to increase oxygen delivery will affect the diffusion-limited, chronically hypoxic cells. Acutely hypoxic cells should not be affected because even an augmented supply of oxygen would be quickly utilized once the blood supply stops. Oxygen-mimetic compounds would be expected to reach both types of hypoxic cells. Conceivably, both strategies could be used together, an approach that is being investigated in the laboratory (see Fig. 66-15).

AGENTS THAT ARE TOXIC TO HYPOXIC CELLS

Given the existence of hypoxia in tumors, it is sensible to develop strategies to take advantage of its presence. One such approach is the use of agents that are toxic to hypoxic cells. The 2-nitroimidazole compounds can be toxic to hypoxic cells after prolonged incubation under hypoxia.[55,56] Zeman and co-workers recently developed on a nonnitro compound, SR-4233, which is substantially more toxic to hypoxic human tumor cells in vitro.[57] Hypoxic cell killing occurred at concentrations 15- to 50-fold less than that needed for the same degree of cell killing of oxygenated cells. A much less pronounced effect was seen in vivo. Although these new approaches are interesting, their usefulness may be limited because the degree of hypoxic cytotoxicity depends on the duration of contact between the sensitizer and the hypoxic cells. This approach would be less effective for acutely hypoxic cells unless the time required for hypoxic cytotoxicity to occur is short, or the damage done during the time under hypoxia is only slowly repaired, thereby allowing the damage from multiple short exposures to acute hypoxia to be added together.

In summary, a number of approaches have been undertaken toward overcoming the radioresistance caused by hypoxic cells (see Fig. 66-15). From a slightly different perspective, Adams and co-workers[58] have investigated the use of a drug, BW12C, that increases the oxygen affinity of hemoglobin, thereby producing increased hypoxia. By decreasing the availability of oxygen, this drug acted as a radioprotector to normal tissues. Furthermore, the increase in tumor hypoxia produced tumor necrosis. Our having the ability to both increase and decrease the extent of hypoxia is of great benefit in understanding the tumor biology of oxygen and in the development of effective clinical strategies.

THIOL MODIFICATION

The next general approach to be considered is thiol modification. This can be approached in two general ways—thiol depletion to enhance cell killing and thiol augmentation as a means of radioprotection.

The competition model of radiation injury, illustrated in Fig. 66-16, suggests that it might be possible to direct the radiation-induced target radical, DNA·, toward an irreversible lesion using oxygen or an oxygen-mimetic sensitizer, or toward chemical restitution by providing a reducing agent such as a thiol (-SH) compound. In addition, one could direct the DNA· toward a permanent lesion by the depletion of the thiol species, thereby driving the reaction toward DNA-O_2· or, if sensitizer were used, toward DNA-sensitizer·.

THIOL DEPLETION TO ENHANCE CELL KILLING BY RADIATION

The nonprotein thiol present in the largest quantity in the cell is the tripeptide, glutathione (GSH). With the recent development of agents that can deplete GSH relatively selectively, there has been an intense interest in GSH depletion as a means of enhancing the effects of radiation and of certain chemotherapeutic agents in the clinic.[59,60] Although the biochemistry of GSH can be perturbed in many ways, the initial approach to depletion of GSH in clinical medicine will be with a compound, L-buthionine sulfoximine (L-BSO), that inhibits the synthesis of GSH.

Although agents such as L-BSO and diethylmaleate (DEM) have their major effect on GSH, other cellular processes may be affected.[61–63] Glutathione is important in many biochemical processes. Severe depletion of GSH can alter activity of enzymes that utilize GSH as a cofactor or substrate[37] and, through subsequent impairment of the ability to maintain protein thiols, alter the structure and function of proteins.[64] Within a tumor, there is likely to be heterogeneity in GSH concentration among cells. Thus, depleting a tumor to a certain level may leave some cells with a relatively high residual concentration.[65]

The difference in endogenous concentrations of GSH may alter the response of the cell lines to radiation therapy and might alter the ability of an oxygen-mimetic sensitizer to sensitize a hypoxic cell.[66,67] Cells with a high endogenous concentration of GSH require higher concentrations of SR 2508 to produce radiosensitization similar to that of cells with lower GSH concentrations.

Glutathione depletion, by itself, has been shown to sensitize hypoxic cells to cell killing by radiation to only a small extent.[1] A better potential use of GSH depletion would be to enhance the hypoxic cell sensitization of the electron affinic sensitizers.[1,61,68] This enhancement of radiosensitization will be particularly important in cells that have a high endogenous concentration of GSH.[66] L-Buthionine sulfoximine has enhanced the sensitization of SR 2508 in such cell lines after only a modest depletion of GSH to approximately 30% of control.[66,67] Thus, L-BSO could be effective clinically without causing severe GSH depletion that would produce a wide variety of biochemical perturbations.[37]

L-Buthionine sulfoximine is currently completing preclinical evaluation. The agent will likely be tested in clinical trials as both a radiation modifier and a chemomodifier (see later discussion). The problem in using L-BSO is knowing the proper dosage. It is not the L-BSO level per se that is important but, rather, it is the concentration of GSH in the critical cell population. The level of depletion and rate of replenishment in a given tissue will vary with the pharmacokinetics of the L-BSO, the endogenous concentration of GSH, and the rate of GSH resynthesis after removal of the L-BSO. The complexity of the GSH effect is exemplified by recent data looking at the addition of exogenous GSH after depletion of intracellular GSH to very low levels.[69–71] Very small concentrations of extracellular GSH are able to reverse the radiosensitization seen by the depletion of intracellular GSH. This suggests that part of the protection afforded by GSH may be a membrane-associated process. Thus, the interaction of GSH with radiation and radiation modifiers is highly complex and is far from being well understood. Nevertheless, with empiric data suggesting that thiol depletion will be of therapeutic benefit, Phase I clinical trials will soon be started.

THIOL AUGMENTATION AND RADIOPROTECTORS

The competition model in Fig. 66-16 suggests that an increase in the thiol content of the cell would direct the target free radical. DNA,· toward chemical restitution, thereby leaving no permanent damage. Extensive work has been done in this area by Yuhas and colleagues.[72] Elevating thiol levels cannot be accomplished by simply administering thiol compounds such as cysteamine or GSH, as these can be toxic and will not necessarily be transported into the cell of interest. As with thiol depletion, an increment in thiol concentration can have numerous complex effects beyond the simple competition theory.[1] Strategies have been developed to increase the thiol content of cells and to develop clinical radioprotectors such as the drug WR-2721.[72]

Russo and associates produced a twofold increase in intracellular GSH concentration using a compound 2-oxothiazolidine-4-carboxylate (OTZ), which is cleaved intracellularly providing cysteine which stimulates GSH synthesis.[73] This degree of elevation of GSH did not protect fully aerated cells, whereas modest protection was observed at intermediate oxygen tensions. The oxygen tension at the target normal tissues is unknown. It is possible that some normal tissues may be at intermediate oxygen tension and, thus, can be protected by a modest increase in GSH concentration. It can be inferred from the data of Russo and co-workers that a protection factor of up to 1.3 could be achieved by a doubling of GSH in cells exposed to 4% oxygen.[73] Additional strategies are being developed that might lead to a greater increase in GSH than that produced by OTZ. These include agents such as glutathione esters that bypass the regulatory enzyme in GSH biosynthesis (γ-glutamylcysteine synthetase).[74]

After an extensive preclinical evaluation that demonstrated that a wide range of normal tissues are protected from radiation injury by WR-2721,[72] this drug has been used in Phase I and II clinical trials. WR-2721 is an aminothiol in which the thiol group is "covered" by a phosphate and requires dephosphorylation by alkaline phosphatase[75] to become active. It is cleared from the blood of patients in minutes, and only small amounts of the dephosphorylated compound (WR-1065) or the disulfide of WR-1065 (WR-33278) are excreted in the urine.[75] In mice, the maximal tissue level of the thiol, WR-1065, is seen 5 to 15 min after intravenous administration of WR-2721.[76] Furthermore, intracellular GSH levels did not appear to be altered by WR-2721, but it should be noted that there is a relatively wide range of normal GSH levels dependent on diurnal variation and diet.[76] Therefore, the mechanism of protection by WR-2721 remains to be elucidated.

The effectiveness of the protector is assessed by the *protection factor* (PF), defined as the radiation dose needed to produce a certain endpoint in the presence of WR-2721 divided by the radiation dose to produce the same endpoint without WR-2721. In concept it is analogous to the oxygen or sensitizer enhancement ratio. In assessing the efficacy of protectors, it is important to evaluate the therapeutic ratio to assess whether the effect will be greater on the normal tissues than on the tumor. An interesting aspect of WR-2721 was that, in mice, relatively low levels of drug reached the tumor compared with normal tissues.[77]

A number of recent animal studies have been done looking at PFs for tumors[78–80] and normal tissues at radiation doses and fractions similar to those used clinically.[80] These data are somewhat discouraging in that low PFs are seen with relatively small single doses of radiation ($PF = 1.1-1.3$),[80] and that a small degree of protection is seen in some tumors depending, in part, on the endpoint chosen.[78] These data indicate the complexities of protectors that are not yet resolved.

1. What is the mechanism of protection?
2. Is there a pharmacologic differential for protector uptake between normal tissues and tumors, and can certain normal tissues be targeted with specific compounds?
3. Is there a time after administration at which treatment should be given to achieve the greatest therapeutic gain?
4. Is there preferential normal tissue protection?

These issues remain to be clarified in both the laboratory and the clinic and should lead to advances in the area of protectors. However, despite these potential pitfalls, early clinical trials have suggested that WR-2721 does protect normal tissues from the adverse effects of radio- and chemotherapy, without obvious tumor protection.

In the Phase I clinical trials, WR-2721 was found to produce hypotension and vomiting, which limited the tolerable dose to 740 mg/m^2 in single doses and 340 mg/m^2 four times a week in multidose regimens.[81] When comparing hematologic toxicity following hemibody irradiation plus WR-2721 with that seen in a historical control group, Constine and associates[82] observed protection with WR-2721 as assessed by the patients experiencing less of a white blood cell and platelet count nadir and a more rapid return to baseline after treatment. At this point, multi-institution trials are planned through the RTOG to test the efficacy of WR-2721 with fractionated radiation therapy.

RADIOSENSITIZATION BY NONHYPOXIC CELL SENSITIZERS

A wide variety of approaches are being studied that are beyond the scope of this chapter. These have been included in the recent review and include efforts to develop inhibitors of potentially lethal damage repair, inhibitors of the enzyme poly(ADP-ribose) polymerase, the use of differentiating agents, and the use of agents that alter the redox state of the cell.[1] The halogenated pyrimidines will be discussed because they are currently in clinical trials.

HALOGENATED PYRIMIDINES

The halogenated pyrimidines, broxuridine (bromodeoxyuridine; BRDU) and idoxuridine (iododeoxyuridine; IDU) were designed as thymidine analogues that would be incorporated into the DNA of cycling cells and make them more sensitive to irradiation. The rationale, current status, and future prospects for these compounds were recently reviewed by Kinsella and colleagues[83] and by Mitchell and associates.[84]

Early clinical trials showed little efficacy and excessive normal tissue toxicity, the latter, in part, because of the disease site selected. Patients treated for head and neck cancer had increased normal tissue toxicity, because of the rapid cell cycling of the mucosa which rapidly incorporated BRDU. After a number of years of inactivity in this area, clinical trials have been undertaken by the National Cancer Institute. Broxuridine was initially tested but produced photosensitivity, a phenomenon not encountered with IDU.[85] Idoxuridine is now in clinical trials as a radiosensitizer. The results of the Phase I trial have been published,[86] and Phase II trials are in progress for sarcomas and gliomas, with some encouraging results.[87] As yet, there are insufficient data to assess the clinical efficacy of the halogenated pyrimidines.

Russo and colleagues[88] have preliminary data suggesting that the halogenated pyrimidines might be effective as chemosensitizers for melphalan, doxorubicin (Adriamycin), cisplatin, and zinostatin (neocarzinostatin).[88] In general, the therapeutic gain for these compounds used as radio- or chemosensitizers depends on greater incorporation into tumors than normal tissues. Therefore, the cellular kinetics of the tumor and dose-limiting normal tissues should be understood so that the proper clinical setting will be selected for use of these agents.

CHEMICAL MODIFICATION OF CHEMOTHERAPY

Drug resistance to chemotherapeutic agents, a major clinical problem,[89] is discussed elsewhere in this book. An empiric observation by Rose and co-workers[90] led to the investigation of the use of misonidazole and its analogues as a clinical chemosensitizer. Although the mechanism of chemosensitization by misonidazole remains to be elucidated, some empiric and mechanistic data are available and will be presented in brief. Additional information can be found in recent reviews.[1,91,92]

The agents whose activity has been shown to be modifiable by misonidazole and its analogues are the alkylating agents, such as melphalan and cyclophosphamide, and the nitrosoureas.[91,92] Because chemomodification emerged from observations with misonidazole, most of the sensitizers studied have been in the 2-nitroimidazole class. Virtually all of the 2-nitroimidazole radiosensitizers described in the foregoing have been shown to have chemosensitization properties.[1] However, the sensitizers are not necessarily "interchangeable," because in the laboratory, a particular sensitizer–chemotherapeutic drug combination may be superior to a different sensitizer with the same chemotherapeutic drug. From the data available, there is no one superior sensitizer for use with all agents. Misonidazole appears to be a very good chemosensitizer and, because chemosensitization is given on an intermittent schedule (misonidazole dose 4 g/m^2 every 3–4 weeks), the dose-limiting neuropathy should be much less of a problem with misonidazole used as a chemosensitizer rather than as a radiosensitizer.

The early experiments testing the efficacy of sensitizers used a large single dose of sensitizer. This turned out to produce a number of effects that led to the conclusion that the mechanism of action of the sensitizer is that of altering the pharmacokinetics of the chemotherapeutic agent. A large single dose of misonidazole causes a significant drop in body temperature of the mouse, which could alter pharmacokinetics and drug activation, distribution, and metabolism. Brown and Hirst and others helped clarify the situation by using a multiple-dose misonidazole schedule that closely mimicked the human pharmacokinetics.[93,94] With this approach, sensitization was still seen, indicating that the large single dose of sensitizer was not necessary. By using such scheduling, the pharmacokinetics of melphalan or cyclophosphamide were unaltered by misonidazole.[95–97] It is generally accepted that when used in a clinically relevant schedule the sensitizers do not produce a major perturbation of the pharmacokinetics of the alkylating agents.

What is not clear is the relationship between plasma concentration of sensitizer and chemosensitization for the alkylating agents. Randhawa and co-workers felt that to obtain chemosensitization of melphalan by misonidazole in mice a sensitizer concentration above 70 μg/ml is needed.[97] Although not investigating a threshold effect, other authors have observed sensitization with concentrations of approximately 100 μg/ml.[96] Increasing the concentration of sensitizer produced only a small increase in chemosensitization.[98] These observations suggest that to obtain chemosensitization in the clinic it might not be necessary to give the maximally tolerated sensitizer dose with each treatment but, rather, enough drug should be given to obtain a certain sensitizer concentration.

For chemosensitization to occur, there is a critical need for a low oxygen tension, as will be described next. A lower sensitizer concentration in the presence of hypoxia would produce sensitization, whereas any sensitizer concentration without hypoxia would likely be ineffective.[99] Thus, the effect will likely be dependent to an unknown degree on sensitizer concentration,[99,100] duration of exposure,[101,102] and extent of exposure to hypoxia. Consideration must again be given to the two types of hypoxia. For the chronically hypoxic cells the sensitizer could undergo reductive metabolism throughout its duration of contact with the cell. However, for intermittently hypoxic cells, reductive metabolism would take place only during the time of hypoxia. Therefore, some prolongation of drug exposure may be best for the acutely hypoxic cells. Some of the hypoxia-related metabolites of misonidazole can diffuse to other cells; therefore, it is possible that some cells will benefit from the hypoxic reductive metabolism of misonidazole but not be hypoxic themselves. In short, the optimal pharmacokinetic approach to the use of misonidazole has not been defined and may vary with the clinical setting.

In vitro data indicate that the presence of low oxygen concentration is required for chemosensitization to occur.[92,99,101] It should be recalled that under low oxygen conditions the sensitizer itself can become cytotoxic.[103] Comparison of the shape of the curves relating oxygen tension to cytotoxicity of the sensitizer, and oxygen tension to chemosensitization suggests that a similar process is ongoing. As indicated from Fig. 66-18, a number of misonidazole reduction products are obtained and a variety of them could be involved in chemosensitization and cytotoxicity. As noted, the degree of cytotoxicity or chemosensitization seen is dependent on the oxygen concentration, the duration of exposure,[101,102] and the sensitizer concentration.[99,100] The need for hypoxia for tumor sensitization in vivo can be inferred from data of Spooner and associates demonstrating no sensitization of micrometastases, a situation in which hypoxia is not expected to be present, whereas gross tumors of the same cell type were sensitized.[104] Therefore, based on these data it would not be expected that misonidazole or its analogues would enhance the efficacy of adjuvant chemotherapy of micrometastatic disease.

Metabolism of misonidazole or its analogues under hypoxic conditions can produce an array of products that can lead to a number of cellular changes. These include macromolecular binding, GSH depletion, altered levels of intracellular calcium, lower threshold to oxidative stress, enhancement of DNA crosslinking, and possibly alteration in DNA repair.[1] The GSH depletion per se is not a major factor in chemosensitization, because matching the extent of GSH depletion seen with misonidazole using the reagent diethylmaleate (DEM) resulted in only slight chemosensitization, even though it was accompanied by an equal extent of enhancement of melphalan binding to macromolecules.[105] Alkylating agents first form a monoadduct before forming a crosslink; the crosslinking will not be maximal for a number of hours.[105–107] Data from both Taylor and co-workers[105,107] and Mulcahy[106] indicate that there is no interference with monoadduct formation. The chemoenhancement occurs after monoadduct formation and may involve inhibition of the repair of the monoadduct or alteration of the repair of the DNA–DNA crosslink. The precise mechanism of chemoenhancement and the misonidazole metabolite necessary for enhancement to occur remain to be elucidated.

CLINICAL CHEMOSENSITIZER TRIALS

There have been few trials studying the efficacy of chemosensitization. A Phase I trial using melphalan plus misonidazole indicated that both drugs could be given at their known maximum tolerated single dose.[108] In a nonrandomized Phase II trial using lomustine (CCNU) with benznidazole for patients with metastatic melanoma, Bleehan and associates observed four partial responses in 16 patients, interpreted as showing equivocal evidence for chemosensitization.[109] Glover and co-workers saw only one response in 30 patients treated with cyclophosphamide plus misonidazole for metastatic renal cell cancer.[110]

The results of random Phase II trial studying melphalan, with and without misonidazole for non–small-cell lung cancer will soon be reported.[111] Of 43 patients given melphalan alone none responded. Of 42 patients given the sensitizer there were two complete and four partial remissions ($p = 0.024$). There was a small effect of misonidiazole on the melphalan plasma pharmacokinetics. The total melphalan concentration was about 25% higher in six patients in the chemosensitizer group, compared with a similar number of patients in the melphalan group. Additionally, the plasma concentration of misonidazole was >100 μg/ml for five of the six patients studied. This concentration is above the threshold for chemosensitization suggested by Randawa and co-workers.[97] There was no difference in bone marrow toxicity between the groups, suggesting that the small increase in melphalan concentration did not affect normal tissue toxicity. Therefore, an increase in therapeutic index was obtained.

GLUTATHIONE MODIFICATION WITH CHEMOTHERAPY: CHEMOPROTECTORS

Alterations in GSH metabolism can have an important impact on the cytotoxicity of various chemotherapeutic agents. Recent reviews on the role of GSH as a determinant of therapeutic efficacy have been published by Arrick and Nathan[60] and by Russo and colleagues.[112] Figure 66-19 shows some of the GSH reactions that potentially interact with chemotherapeutic agents.

The GSH depletion with L-BSO has been reported to increase the in vitro cytotoxicity of a number of chemotherapeutic agents including cisplatin, mitomycin, melphalan, cyclophosphamide, nitrogen mustard, chlorambucil, and doxorubicin. Similar sensitization has been observed in vivo for cyclophosphamide, mitomycin, cisplatin, bleomycin, and melphalan.[1] In a fibroblast cell line, elevation of intracellular GSH by OTZ can lead to some degree of resistance to melphalan, cisplatin, and bleomycin.[113] Similarly, cell lines[114] and normal tissues have been reported to become resistant to alkylating agent damage following the development of an increase in intracellular GSH.[115–117] For the alkylating agents, the likely interaction is between GSH and the electrophilic alkylating moiety, with the drug being more cytotoxic when a smaller quantity of GSH is present. This reaction can occur directly with GSH or can be catalyzed by the enzyme glutathione-*S*-transferase.[118]

Exposure of tumor[119] and bone marrow[120] to alkylating agents has produced an increase in GSH[120] and an increase in glutathione-*S*-transferase activity.[119,120] This overshoot in GSH concentration and transferase activity after treatment with cyclophosphamide resulted in a protective effect to subsequent treatments with cyclophosphamide.[116] Carmichael and co-workers have demonstrated that this overshoot in GSH is prevented with L-BSO. Although severe GSH depletion can affect glutathione-*S*-transferase activity,[1] in the study by Carmichael and associates,[116] L-BSO treatment did not affect this enzyme's activity, which suggests that it was the elevation of GSH rather than that of transferase activity that conferred resistance. The use of L-BSO before the administration of melphalan[117] did not increase marrow

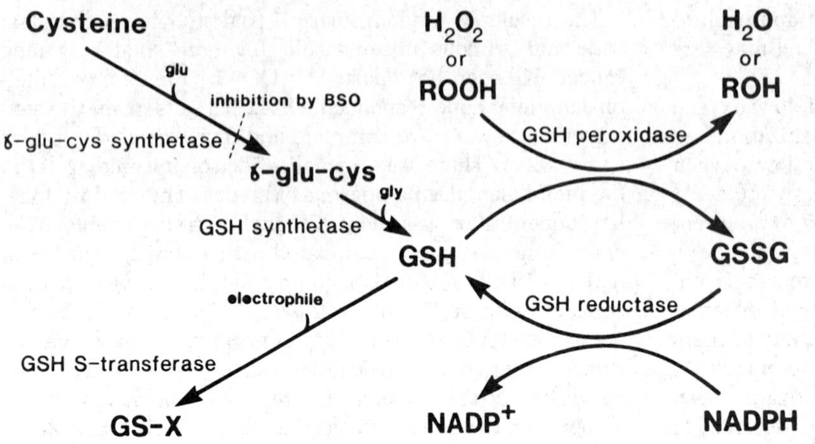

FIG. 66-19. GSH metabolism. GSH is a critical molecule in cellular detoxification processes. In addition to acting in the competition model, GSH reacts with electrophiles such as alkylating agents to detoxify these agents with an enzyme glutathione-S-transferase. By inhibiting the rate-limiting enzyme gamma-glutamyl synthetase, L-BSO can prevent the synthesis of GSH, leading to GSH depletion. (Coleman CN, Bump EA, Kramer RA: Chemical modifiers of cancer therapy. J Clin Oncol 6:709–733, 1988)

toxicity. Therefore, it appears that L-BSO may, in certain instances, produce a therapeutic gain with alkylating agents.[121] However, thiol depletion by L-BSO was shown to increase the renal and hepatic toxicity of the nitrosourea, semustine-(methyl-CCNU).[122] Additional studies on the organ toxicity of specific agents that may be used in combination with L-BSO are necessary.

The use of L-BSO as a chemomodifier is of great interest, and the drug will soon be tested clinically. The ubiquitous role of GSH in intermediary metabolism is complex; therefore, clinical studies of GSH depletion will require extreme care.

In parallel with the investigation of WR-2721 as a radioprotector, Yuhas and co-workers[36,123,124] demonstrated that this drug can protect against the bone marrow toxicity of alkylating agents and the nephrotoxicity of cisplatin. The mechanism of this protection is unknown. Glover and colleagues have conducted a number of Phase I/II trials with WR-2721 as a chemoprotector. Compared with retrospective series, WR-2721 appeared to offer protection against cisplatin-induced nephrotoxicity and neurotoxicity.[125] In a controlled Phase II study with a crossover design using cyclophosphamide by itself and then with WR-2721, the protector reduced the hematologic toxicity of the cyclophosphamide.[126] In neither study was there a suggestion of protection of tumor response. Results of a phase II trial for patients with melanoma, including patients who had received prior chemotherapy, suggested that WR-2721 increased the therapeutic efficacy of cisplatin in this disease.[127] Further disease-specific randomized studies are to be conducted to confirm these observations.

In summary, there is a clinical observation of chemoprotection of normal tissues for cyclophosphamide and cisplatin with an increase in therapeutic index produced by WR-2721 by an, as yet, unknown mechanism. The understanding of this clinical observation in the laboratory would be of enormous benefit in the further development of chemoprotecting agents.

POTENTIAL CROSS-RESISTANCE BETWEEN CHEMOTHERAPY AND RADIOTHERAPY CAUSED BY CHEMOTHERAPY-INDUCED INCREASE IN INTRACELLULAR GLUTATHIONE

Recently, Louie and co-workers[128] studied the development of radioresistance in an ovarian cancer cell line made resistant to doxorubicin, melphalan, and cisplatin by stepwise incubation with drugs. Compared with the parent cell line and to the doxorubicin-resistant line, the melphalan- and cisplatin-resistant lines were more radioresistant and had a higher concentration of intracellular GSH. Treatment of the melphalan and cisplatin-resistant lines with L-BSO led to a reduction in the intracellular GSH and to restored radiosensitivity. This implies that the development of drug resistance can lead to radioresistance by causing an increase in GSH, and that this resistance can be abrogated by the use of L-BSO. In contrast with this are the findings with ovarian cancer cell lines that were resistant to melphalan at the time of their establishment, (*i.e.*, they were not made resistant in the laboratory). Two such cell lines had high concentrations of GSH that could be reduced by L-BSO. However, in neither of these lines was the radiation sensitivity changed by L-BSO. The findings from these inherently chemoresistant lines contradict the finding from the lines made chemoresistant in the laboratory in that, for the inherently resistant cell lines, GSH depletion by L-BSO did not alter radiosensitivity. The area of cross-resistance between modalities caused by GSH elevation, hypoxia-related gene amplification,[129] or other mechanism might have a major impact on the therapeutic strategies of combined modality therapy.

IDENTIFICATION OF HYPOXIC CELLS IN TUMORS

Given that hypoxic cells are probably important in clinical outcome, it would be advantageous to be able not only to identify such cells at diagnosis, but to follow these populations during treatment. Using radiolabeled misonidazole, Urtasun and associates[130] have detected hypoxia in some tumors; however, the degree of hypoxia seen was less than that expected from the laboratory. Although this technique is of interest, it might well underestimate the extent of hypoxia, because detection of hypoxia with this method requires the presence of relatively prolonged hypoxia so that enough drug is bound; nitroreductase activity (for reactions in Fig. 66-18); sufficient glucose to provide reducing equivalents (glucose could be consumed in poor-nutrition zones).[1] Therefore, such techniques could miss both acutely and chronically hypoxic cells. Work is in progress to develop radiolabeled and nuclear magnetic resonance techniques.[1]

CONCLUSION

The field of chemical and biochemical modifiers of cancer treatment is a rapidly evolving one in both the laboratory and the clinic. The agents used are, in general, not cytotoxic, but rather, they modify the effects of radiation or drugs on tumors and normal tissues. Hypoxic tumor cells were an early target approached by the use of drugs and physiologic maneuvers designed to eliminate the hypoxic fraction of tumors. Techniques are becoming available to image both chronically and acutely hypoxic cells. The use of such techniques in the laboratory should assist in the development of superior clinical strategies.

Endogenous thiols play a role in the efficacy of radiation and certain drugs. Glutathione concentration can be decreased or increased to alter cellular sensitivity. The radioprotector WR-2721 also has activity as a chemoprotector, with the mechanism of protection to either modality still to be elucidated. The observation that hypoxic cell sensitizers are also chemosensitizers by mechanisms different than those of radiosensitization has opened up a new avenue of investigation.

Although a great deal of additional information on the mechanisms of action of these various approaches is needed, a substantial amount of information has been accumulated that has permitted the development of agents for clinical trials. Despite the fact that the drugs used in the initial clinical trials were early prototypes, there have been some trials that suggest therapeutic efficacy of hypoxic cell radiosensitization, chemosensitization, radiation protection, and chemoprotection. Although there is, as yet, no definitive proof of efficacy, the positive preliminary results and the rapid expansion in the understanding of the basic mechanisms of action, are encouraging.

REFERENCES

1. Coleman CN, Bump EA, Kramer RA: Chemical modifiers of cancer therapy. J Clin Oncol 6:709–733, 1988
2. Hall EH; Radiobiology for the Radiologist, pp 79–110. New York, Harper & Row, 1978
3. Brown JM, Yu NY: Radiosensitization of hypoxic cells in vivo by SR 2508 at low radiation doses. Int J Radiat Oncol Biol Phys 10:1207–1212, 1984
4. Skarsgard LD, Harrison I, Durand RE et al: Radiosensitization of hypoxic cells at low doses. Int J Radiat Oncol Biol Phys 12:1075–1078, 1986
5. Coleman CN: Hypoxic cell radiosensitizers: Expectations and progress in drug development. Int J Radiat Oncol Biol Phys 11:323–329, 1985
6. Brown JM: Evidence for acutely hypoxic cells in mouse tumors, and a possible mechanism for reoxygenation. Br J Radiol 52:650–656, 1979
7. Chaplin DJ, Olive PL, Durand RE: Intermittent blood flow in a murine tumor: Radiobiological effects. Cancer Res 47:597–601, 1987
8. Chaplin DJ, Durand RE, Olive PL: Acute hypoxia in tumors: Implications for modifiers of radiation effects. Int J Radiat Oncol Biol Phys 12:1279–1282, 1986
9. Olive PL, Chaplin DJ, Durand RE: Pharmacokinetics, binding and distribution of Hoechst 33342 in spheroids and murine tumors. Br J Cancer 52:739–746, 1985
10. Howes AE: An estimation of the changes in the proportions and absolute numbers of hypoxic cells after irradiation of transplanted C3H mouse mammary tumors. Br J Radiol 42:441–447, 1969
11. Moulder JE, Rockwell S: Hypoxic fractions of solid tumors: Experimental techniques, methods of analysis, and a survey of existing data. Int J Radiat Oncol Biol Phys 10:695–712, 1984
12. Henk JM: Does hyperbaric oxygen have a future in radiation therapy? Int J Radiat Oncol Biol Phys 7:1125–1128, 1981
13. Bush RS: The significance of anemia in clinical radiation therapy (editorial). Int J Radiat Oncol Biol Phys 12:2047–2050, 1986
14. Overgaard J, Sand Hansen H, Jorgensen K et al: Primary radiotherapy of larynx and pharynx carcinoma—an analysis of some factors influencing local control and survival. Int J Radiat Oncol Biol Phys 12:515–521, 1986
15. Quilty PM, Duncan W: The influence of hemoglobin level on the regression and long term local control of transitional cell carcinoma of the bladder following photon irradiation. Int J Radiat Oncol Biol Phys 12:1735–1742, 1986
16. Urtasun RC, Band P, Chapman JD et al: Radiation and high-dose metronidazole in supratentorial glioblastomas. N Engl J Med 294:1364–1367, 1976
17. Wasserman TH, Phillips TL, Johnson RJ et al: Initial United States clinical and pharmacologic evaluation of misonidazole (RO-07-0582), and hypoxic cell radiosensitizer. Int J Radiat Oncol Biol Phys 5:775–786, 1979
18. Dische S, Saunders MI, Flockhart IR et al: Misonidazole—a drug for trial in radiotherapy and oncology. Int J Radiat Oncol Biol Phys 5:851–860, 1979
19. Dische S: Chemical sensitizers for hypoxic cells. A decade of experience in clinical radiotherapy. Radiother Oncol 3:97–115, 1985
20. Overgaard J, Sand Hansen H, Anderson AP et al: Misonidazole as an adjuvant to radiotherapy in the treatment of invasive carcinoma of the larynx and the pharynx (abstr). 2nd interim analysis of the Danish Head and Neck Cancer study (personal communication and Proceedings of the conference on Chemical Modifiers of Cancer Treatment, Clearwater, FL 1–23), 1985
21. Coleman CN, Wasserman TH, Phillips TL et al: Initial pharmacology and toxicology of intravenous desmethylmisonidazole. Int J Radiat Oncol Biol Phys 8:371–375, 1982
22. Brown JM, Lee, WW: Pharmacokinetic considerations in radiosensitizer development. In Brady L (ed): Radiation Sensitizers, Their Use in the Clinical Management of Cancer, pp 2–13. New York, Masson, 1980
23. Brown JM: Clinical perspectives for the use of new hypoxic cell sensitizers. Int J Radiat Oncol Biol Phys 8:1491–1497, 1982
24. Brown JM, Yu NY, Brown DM et al: SR-2508: A 2-nitroimidazole amide which should be superior to misonidazole as a radiosensitizer for clinical use. Int J Radiat Oncol Biol Phys 7:695–701, 1981
25. Coleman CN, Urtasun RC, Wasserman TH et al: Initial report of the Phase I trial of the hypoxic cell radiosensitizer SR 2508. Int J Radiat Oncol Biol Phys 10:1749–1753, 1984
26. Coleman CN, Wasserman TH, Urtasun RC et al: Phase I trial of the hypoxic cell radiosensitizer SR 2508: The results of the five to six week schedule. Int J Radiat Oncol Biol Phys 12:1105–1108, 1986
27. Coleman CN, Halsey J, Cox RS et al: Prediction of the neurotoxicity of the hypoxic cell radiosensitizer SR 2508 from the pharmacokinetic profile. Cancer Res 47:319–322, 1987
28. Brown JM: Clinical trials of radiosensitizers: What should we expect? Int J Radiat Oncol Biol Phys 10:425–429, 1984
29. Fu K, Hurst S, Begg AC, Brown, JM: The effects of misonidazole during continuous low dose rate irradiation. In Brady L (ed): Radiation Sensitizers, Their Use in the Clinical Management of Cancer, pp 267–275. New York, Masson, 1980
30. Saunders MI, Anderson PJ, Bennett MH et al: The clinical testing of Ro 03-8799-pharmcokinetics, toxicology, tissue and tumor concentrations. Int J Radiat Oncol Biol Phys 10:1759–1763, 1984
31. Roberts JT, Bleehan NM, Walton JI et al: A clinical phase I toxicity study of Ro 03-8799: Plasma, urine, tumour and normal brain pharmacokinetics. Br J Radiol 59:107–116, 1986
32. Minchinton AL, Stratford MRL: A comparison of tumor and normal tissue levels of acidic, basic and neutral 2-nitroimidazole radiosensitizers in mice. Int J Radiat Oncol Biol Phys 12:1117–1120, 1986
33. Newman H, Bleehan NM, Workman P: A Phase I study of the combination of two hypoxic cell radiosensitizers, Ro-03-8799 and SR 2508: Toxicity and pharmacokinetics. Int J Radiat Oncol Biol Phys 12:1113–1116, 1986
34. Stratford IJ, O'Neill P, Sheldon PW et al: RSU 1069, a nitroimidazole containing an aziridine group. Biochem Pharmacol 35:105–109, 1986
35. Ahmed I, Jenkins TC, Walling JM et al: Analogues of RSU-1069: Radiosensitization and toxicity in vitro and in vivo, Int J Radiat Oncol Biol Phys 12:1079–1081, 1986

36. Deacon JM, Holliday SB, Ahmed I et al: Experimental pharmacokinetics of RSU-1069 and its analogues: High tumor/plasma ratios. Int J Radiat Oncol Biol Phys 12:1087–1090, 1986
37. Biaglow JE, Varnes ME, Roizen-Towle J et al: Biochemistry of reduction of nitroheterocycles. Biochem Pharmacol 35:77–90, 1986
38. Varnes ME, Biaglow JE: Misonidazole-induced biochemical alterations of mammalian cells: Effects on glycolysis. Int J Radiat Oncol Biol Phys 8:683–686, 1982
39. Melgaard B, Hansen HS, Kamieniecka Z et al: Misonidazole neurotoxicity: A clinical, eletrophysiological, and histological study. Ann Neurol 12:10–17, 1982
40. Wasserman TH, Nelson JS, VonGerichton D: Neuropathy of nitroimidazole radiosensitizers: Clinical and pathological description. Int J Radiat Oncol Biol Phys 10:1725–1730, 1984
41. Tanasichuk H, Urtasun RC, Fulton DS et al: Misonidazole with dexamethasone rescue: An escalating dose toxicity study. Int J Radiat Oncol Biol Phys 10:1735–1737, 1984
42. Coleman CN, Hirst VK, Brown DM et al: The effect of vitamin B_6 on the neurotoxicity and pharmacology of desmethylmisonidazole and misonidazole: Clinical and laboratory studies. Int J Radiat Oncol Biol Phys 10:1381–1386, 1984
43. Hall EJ, Astor MA, Biaglow J et al: The enhanced sensitivity of mammalian cells to killing by x-rays after prolonged exposure to several nitroimidazoles. Int J Radiat Oncol Biol Phys 8:447–451, 1982
44. Panicucci R, McClelland RA, Rauth AM: Stable reduction products of misonidazole. Int J Radiat Oncol Biol Phys 12:1227–1230, 1986
45. Laderoute KR, Eryavec E, McClelland RA et al: The production of strand breaks in DNA in the presence of the hydoxylamine of SR-2508 (1-[N(2-hydroxylethyl)acetamido]-2-nitroimidazole) at neutral pH. Int J Radiat Oncol Biol Phys 12:1215–1218, 1986
46. Taylor YC, Brown JM: Radiosensitization in multifraction schedules: II. Greater sensitization by 2-nitroimidazoles than by oxygen. Radiat Res 112:134–145, 1987
47. Hirst DG: Anemia: A problem or an opportunity in radiotherapy? Int J Radiat Oncol Biol Phys 12:2009–2017, 1986
48. Fischer JJ, Rockwell S, Martin DF: Perfluorochemicals and hyperbaric oxygen in radiation therapy. Int J Radiat Oncol Biol Phys 12:95–102, 1986
49. Siemann DW, Macler LM: Tumor radiosensitization through reductions in hemoglobin affinity. Int J Radiat Oncol Biol Phys 12:1295–1297, 1986
50. Degner FL, Sutherland RM: Theoretical evaluation of expected changes in oxygenation of tumors associated with different hemoglobin levels. Int J Radiat Oncol Biol Phys 12:1291–1294, 1986
51. Teicher BA, Rose CM: Effects of dose and scheduling on growth delay of the Lewis lung carcinoma produced by the perfluorochemical emulsion, Fluosol-DA. Int J Radiat Oncol Biol Phys 12:1311–1313, 1986
52. Goodman RL, Moore RE, Davis ME et al: Perfluorcarbon emulsions in cancer therapy: Preliminary observations on presently available formulations. Int J Radiat Oncol Biol Phys 10:1421–1424, 1984
53. West L, McIntosh N, Gendler S et al: Effects of intravenously infused Fluosol-DA 20% in rats. Int J Radiat Oncol Biol Phys 12:1319–1323, 1986
54. Rose C, Lustig R, McIntosh N et al: A clinical trial of Fluosol-DA 20% in advanced squamous cell carcinoma of the head and neck. Int J Radiat Oncol Biol Phys 12:1325–1327, 1986
55. Stratford IJ, Adams GE, Horsman MR et al: The interaction of misonidazole with radiation, chemotherapeutic agents, or heat. Cancer Clin Trials 3:231–236, 1980
56. Chaplin DJ, Durand RE, Stratford IJ: The radiosensitizing and toxic effects of RSU-1069 on hypoxic cells in a murine tumor. Int J Radiat Oncol Biol Phys 12:1091–1095, 1986
57. Zeman EM, Brown JM, Lemmon MJ et al: SR-4233: A new bioreductive agent with high selective toxicity for hypoxic mammalian cells. Int J Radiat Oncol Biol Phys 12:1239–1242, 1986
58. Adams GE, Barnes DWH, du Boulay C et al: Induction of hypoxia in normal and malignant tissues by changing the oxygen affinity of hemoglobin—implications for therapy. Int J Radiat Oncol Biol Phys 12:1299–1302, 1986
59. Meister A: Selective modification of glutathione metabolism. Science 220:472–477, 1983
60. Arrick BA, Nathan CF: Glutathione metabolism as a determinant of therapeutic efficacy: A review. Cancer Res 44:4224–4232, 1984
61. Bump EA, Yu NY, Taylor YC et al: Radiosensitization and chemosensitization by diethylmaleate. In Nygaard O, Simic M (eds): Radioprotectors and Anticarcinogens, pp 297–323, New York, Academic Press, 1983
62. Dethlefsen LA, Biaglow JE, Peck VM et al: Toxic effects of extended glutathione depletion by buthionine sulfoximine on murine mammary carcinoma cells. Int J Radiat Oncol Biol Phys 12:1157–1160, 1986
63. Reed DJ: Defense mechanisms of normal and tumor cells. Int J Radiat Oncol Biol Phys 12:1457–1461, 1986
64. Brigelius R: Mixed disulfides: Biological functions and increase in oxidative stress. In Sies H (ed): Oxidative Stress, pp 243–272, London, Academic Press, 1985
65. Clark EP: Thiol-induced biochemical modification of chemo- and radioresponses. Int J Radiat Oncol Biol Phys 12:1121–1126, 1986
66. Mitchell JB, Phillips TL, DeGraff W et al: The relationship of SR-2058 sensitizer enhancement ratio to cellular glutathione in human tumor cell lines. Int J Radiat Oncol Biol Phys 12:1143–1146, 1986
67. Phillips TL, Mitchell JB, DeGraff W et al: Variation in sensitizing efficiency for SR 2508 in human cells dependent on glutathione content. Int J Radiat Oncol Biol Phys 12:1627–1635, 1986
68. Yu NY, Brown JM: Depletion of glutathione in vivo as a method of improving the therapeutic ratio of misonidazole and SR 2508. Int J Radiat Oncol Biol Phys 10:1265–1269, 1984
69. Koch CJ, Stobbe CC, Baer KA: Combined radiation-protective and radiation-sensitizing agents III: Radiosensitization by misonidazole as a function of concentrations of endogenous glutathione or exogenous thiols. Int J Radiat Oncol Biol Phys 12:1151–1155, 1986
70. Rice GC, Bump EA, Shrieve DC et al: Quantitative analysis of cellular glutathione by flow cytometry utilizing monochlorobimane: Some applications to radiation and drug resistance in vitro and in vivo. Cancer Res 46:6105–6110, 1986
71. Clark EP, Epp ER, Morse-Gaudio M et al: The role of glutathione in the aerobic radioresponse: I. Sensitization and recovery in the absence of intracellular glutathione. Radiat Res 108:238–250, 1986
72. Yuhas JM, Spellman JM, Culo F: The role of WR-2721 in radiotherapy and/or chemotherapy. Cancer Clin Trials 3:211–216, 1980
73. Russo A, Mitchell JB, Finkelstein E et al: The effects of cellular glutathione elevation on the oxygen enhancement ratio. Radiat Res 103:232–239, 1985
74. Wellner VP, Anderson ME, Puri RN et al: Radioprotection by glutathione ester: Transport of glutathione ester in human lymphoid cells and fibroblasts. Proc Natl Acad Sci USA 81:4732–4735, 1984
75. Shaw LM, Turrisi AT, Glover DJ et al: Human pharmacokinetics of WR-2721. Int J Radiat Oncol Biol Phys 12:1501–1504, 1986
76. Utley JF, Seaver N, Newton GL et al: Pharmacokinetics of WR-1065 in mouse tissue following treatment with WR-2721. Int J Radiat Oncol Biol Phys 10:1525–1528, 1984
77. Yuhas JM: On the potential application of radioprotective drugs in solid tumor radiotherapy. In Sokol GH, Maickel RP (eds): Radiation-Drug Interactions in the Treatment of Cancer, pp 113–135 New York, John Wiley & Sons, 1981
78. Milas L, Hunter N, Ito H et al: Effect of tumor type, size, and endpoint on tumor radioprotection by WR-2721. Int J Radiat Oncol Biol Phys 10:41–48, 1984
79. Rojas A, Denekamp J: The influence of x-ray dose levels on normal tissue radioprotection by WR-2721. Int J Radiat Oncol Biol Phys 10:2351–2356, 1984
80. Rojas A, Stewart FA, Soranson JA et al: Fractionation studies with WR-2721: Normal tissues and tumour. Radiother Oncol 6:51–60, 1986
81. Kligerman MM, Glover DJ, Turrisi AT et al: Toxicity of WR-2721 administered in single and multiple doses. Int J Radiat Oncol Biol Phys 10:1773–1776, 1984
82. Constine LS, Zagars G, Rubin P et al: Protection by WR-2721 of human bone marrow function following irradiation. Int J Radiat Oncol Biol Phys 12:1505–1508, 1986
83. Kinsella TJ, Mitchell JB, Russo A et al: The use of halogenated thymidine analogues as clinical radiosensitizers: Rationale, current status, and future prospects: Non-hypoxic cell sensitizers. Int J Radiat Oncol Biol Phys 10:1399–1406, 1984
84. Mitchell JB, Russo A, Kinsella et al: The use of non-hypoxic cell sensitizers in radiobiology and radiotherapy. Int J Radiat Oncol Biol Phys 12:1513–1518, 1986
85. Mitchell JB, Morstyn G, Russo A et al: Differing sensitivity to fluorescent light in Chinese hamster cells containing equally incorporated quantities of BUdR and IUdR. Int J Radiat Oncol Biol Phys 10:1447–1451, 1984
86. Kinsella TJ, Russo A, Mitchell JB et al: A Phase I study of intravenous iododeoxyuridine as a clinical radiosensitizer. Int J Radiat Oncol Biol Phys 11:1941–1946, 1985
87. Kinsella TJ, Glatstein E: Clinical experience with intravenous radiosensitizers in unresectable sarcomas. Cancer 59:908–915, 1987
88. Russo A, DeGraff W, Kinsella TJ et al: Potentiation of chemotherapy cytotoxicity following iododeoxyuridine incorporation in Chinese hamster cells. Int J Radiat Oncol Biol Phys 12:1371–1374, 1986
89. Chabner BA: The oncologic end game. J Clin Oncol 4:625–638, 1986
90. Rose CM, Millar JL, Peacock JH et al: Differential enhancement of melphalan cytotoxicity in tumor and normal tissue by misonidazole. In Brady LW (ed): Radiation Sensitizers. Their Use in the Clinical Management of Cancer, pp 250–257 New York, Masson, 1980
91. McNally NJ: Enhancement of chemotherapy agents. Int J Radiat Oncol Biol Phys 8:593–598, 1982
92. Siemann DW: Modification of chemotherapy by nitroimidazoles. Int J Radiat Oncol Biol Phys 10:1585–1594, 1984
93. Brown JM, Hirst DG: Effect of clinical levels of misonidazole on the response of tumour and normal tissues in the mouse to alkylating agents. Br J Cancer 45:700–708, 1982
94. McNally NJ, Hinchliffe M, de Ronde J: Enhancement of the action of alkylating agents by single high, or chronic low doses of misonidazole. Br J Cancer 48:271–278, 1983
95. Hinchliffe M, McNally NJ, Stratford MRL: The effect of radiosensitizers on the pharmacokinetics of melphalan and cyclophosphamide in the mouse. Br J Cancer 48:375–383, 1983
96. Horsman MR, Evans JW, Brown JM: Enhancement of melphalan-induced tumour cell killing by misonidazole: An interaction of competing mechanisms. Br J Cancer 50:305–316, 1984
97. Randhawa VS, Stewart FA, Denekamp J et al: Factors influencing the chemosensitization of melphalan by misonidazole. Br J Cancer 51:219–228, 1985
98. Hirst DG, Horsman MR, Brown JM et al: The effect of timing on chemosensitization by clinical levels of SR-2508. Int J Radiat Oncol Biol Phys 10:1641–1645, 1984
99. Durand RE, Olive PL: Potentiation of CCNU toxicity by AF-2 in V79 spheroids: Implications for mechanisms of chemosensitization. Int J Radiat Oncol Biol Phys 12:1375–1378, 1986
100. Koch CJ, Stobbe CC, Baer KA: Metabolism induced binding of ^{14}C-misonidazole to

hypoxic cells: Kinetic dependence on oxygen concentration and misonidazole concentration. Int J Radiat Oncol Biol Phys 10:1327–1331, 1984
101. Spooner D, Peacock JH, Stephens TC: Enhancement of cytotoxic drugs by misonidazole in Lewis lung tumors of different sizes, and in mouse bone marrow. Int J Radiat Oncol Biol Phys 8:643–646, 1982
102. Mulcahy RT: Effect of oxygen on misonidazole chemosensitization and cytotoxicity in vitro. Cancer Res 44:4409–4413, 1984
103. Franko AJ: Misonidazole and other hypoxia markers: Metabolism and applications. Int J Radiat Oncol Biol Phys 12:1195–1202, 1986
104. Roizen-Towle L, Hall EJ, Pirro JP: Oxygen dependence for chemosensitization by misonidazole. Br J Cancer 54:919–924, 1986
105. Taylor YC, Evans JW, Brown JM: Mechanism of sensitization of Chinese hamster ovary cells to melphalan by hypoxic treatment with misonidazole. Cancer Res 43:3175–3181, 1983
106. Mulcahy RT: Cross-link formation and chemopotentiation of EMT-6/Ro cells exposed to miso after CCNU treatment in vitro. Int J Radiat Oncol Biol Phys 12:1389–1392, 1986
107. Taylor YC, Sawyer JM, Hsu B et al: Mechanism of melphalan crosslink enhancement by misonidazole pretreatment. Int J Radiat Oncol Biol Phys 10:1603–1607, 1984
108. Coleman CN, Friedman MK, Jacobs C et al: Phase I trial of intravenous L-phenylalanine mustard plus the sensitizer misonidazole. Cancer Res 43:5022–5025, 1983
109. Bleehan NM, Roberts JT, Newman HFV: A Phase II study of CCNU with benznidazole for metastatic malignant melanoma. Int J Radiat Oncol Biol Phys 12:1401–1403, 1986
110. Glover D, Trump D, Kvols L et al: Phase II trial of misonidazole and cyclophosphamide in metastatic renal cell carcinoma. Int J Radiat Oncol Biol Phys 12:1405–1408, 1986
111. Coleman CN, Carlson RC, Halsey J et al: Enhancement of the clinical activity of melphalan by the sensitizer misonidazole. Cancer Res 48:3528–3532, 1988
112. Russo A, Carmichael J, Friedman N et al: The role of intracellular glutathione in antineoplastic chemotherapy. Int J Radiat Oncol Biol Phys 12:1347–1354, 1986
113. Russo A, DeGraff W, Friedman N et al: Selective modulation of glutathione levels in human normal versus tumor cells and subsequent differential response to chemotherapy drugs. Cancer Res 46:2845–2848, 1986
114. Green JA, Vistica DT, Young RC et al: Potentiation of melphalan cytotoxicity in human ovarian cancer cell lines by glutathione depletion. Cancer Res 44:5427–5431, 1984
115. Adams DJ, Carmichael J, Wolf CR: Altered mouse bone marrow glutathione and glutathione transferase levels in response to cytotoxins. Cancer Res 45:1669–1673, 1985
116. Carmichael J, Friedman N, Tochner Z et al: Inhibition of the protective effect of cyclophosphamide by pre-treatment with buthionine sulfoximine. Int J Radiat Oncol Biol Phys 12:1191–1193, 1986
117. Russo A, Tochner Z, Phillips T et al: In vivo modulation of glutathione by buthionine sulfoximine: Effect on marrow response to melphalan. Int J Radiat Oncol Biol Phys 12:1187–1189, 1986
118. Chasseaud LF: The role of glutathione and glutathione S-transferases in the metabolism of chemical carcinogens and other electrophilic agents. Adv Cancer Res 29:175–273, 1979
119. Wang AL, Tew KD: Increased glutathione-S-transferase activity in a cell line with acquired resistance to nitrogen mustards. Cancer Treat Rep 69:677–682, 1985
120. Carmichael J, Adams DJ, Ansell J et al: Glutathione and glutathione transferase levels in mouse granulocytes following cyclophosphamide administration. Cancer Res 46:735–739, 1986
121. Russo A, DeGraff W, Friedman N et al: Selective modulation of glutathione levels in human normal versus tumor cells and subsequent differential response to chemotherapy drugs. Cancer Res 46:2845–2848, 1986
122. Kramer RA, Greene K, Ahmad S et al: Chemosensitization of L-phenylalanine mustard (L-PAM) by the thiol modulation agent buthionine sulfoximine (BSO). Cancer Res 47:1593–1597, 1987
123. Yuhas JM: Differential protection of normal and malignant tissues against the cytotoxic effects of mechlorethamine. Cancer Treat Rep 63:971–976, 1979
124. Yuhas JM, Culo F: Selective inhibition of the nephrotoxicity of *cis*-dichlorodiamineplatinum (II) by WR-2721 without altering its antitumor properties. Cancer Treat Rep 64:57–64, 1980
125. Glover D, Glick JH, Weiler C et al: Phase I/II trials of WR-2721 and cis-platinum. Int J Radiat Oncol Biol Phys 12:1509–1512, 1986
126. Glover D, Glick JH, Weiler C et al: WR-2721 protects against the hematologic toxicity of cyclophosphamide: A controlled phase II trial. J Clin Oncol 4:584–588, 1986
127. Glover D, Glick JH, Weiler C et al: WR-2721 and high-dose cisplatin: An active combination in the treatment of metastatic melanoma. J Clin Oncol 5:574–578, 1987
128. Louie KG, Behrens BC, Kinsella TJ et al: Radiation survival parameters of antineoplastic drug-sensitive and -resistant human ovarian cancer cell lines and their modification by buthionine sulfoximine. Cancer Res 45:2110–2115, 1985
129. Rice GC, Hoy CA, Schimke RT: Transient hypoxia enhances the frequency of dihydrofolate reductase gene amplification in Chinese hamster ovary cells. Proc Natl Acad Sci USA 83:5978–5982, 1986
130. Urtasun RC, Chapman JD, Raleigh JA et al: Binding of ^{3}H-misonidazole to solid human tumors as a measure of tumor hypoxia. Int J Radiat Oncol Biol Phys 12:1263–1267, 1986

ANGELO RUSSO
JAMES B. MITCHELL
HARVEY I. PASS
ELI J. GLATSTEIN

SECTION 4

Photodynamic Therapy

Photodynamic therapy (PDT) was first used in 1900 when acridine and light were combined to kill paramecia,[1] and the first oncologic use of PDT was in 1903 when eosin and light were employed in the treatment of skin cancer.[2] In the following years, many chemicals have been used to promote photochemically induced cytotoxicity.[3] However, since Hauseman's initial experiments in 1911 with hematoporphyrin (HP) there has been a continued interest in porphyrin-based photosensitizers.[4] During the 1940s a key development was made. HP (probably a fairly impure preparation) was found to selectively concentrate or to be preferentially retained in malignant tissues.[5,6] Lipson improved the tumor-localizing properties of HP by synthesizing a complex porphyrin mixture named hematoporphyrin derivative (HPD)[7-10] Gregorie extended Lipson's observations by demonstrating that HPD is retained in a large percentage of squamous and adenocarcinomas.[11] Lipson's work on tumor detection also resulted in a single attempt to manage a large, recurrent breast cancer by multiple injections of HPD and light treatments. The tumorous lesion was not cured, but there was objective evidence of a photodynamically induced cytotoxic effect.[12] Several years later, Kelly reported results with intravenous HPD followed by light delivered through a fiber-optic device to treat a patient with recurrent bladder cancer. Shortly afterward, Dougherty described his first of a sustained series of studies throughout the 1970s and 1980s exploring the mechanism and applications of HPD-based PDT for the treatment of diverse human malignancies.[13-18] It was through Dougherty's continued efforts that PDT evolved to the level it is practiced today.

What is distinctly unique about PDT is that some time after sensitizer injection, greater retention of the sensitizer can be found in malignant tissue than in most normal tissue. Thereafter, the tumor is exposed to the appropriate light wavelength that corresponds to an absorbance peak of the sensitizer. Photodynamic therapy, as practiced today, is a relatively new cancer treatment modality that depends on the concerted action of a three-component system: sensitizer, light, and oxygen. Over the past few years PDT has undergone several name changes, being previously known as photochemotherapy and photoradiation therapy. The evolution in terminology led from the specific term *photodynamic effect*, which refers to an oxygen-dependent photochemical oxidative process.[19] Photodynamic therapy should not be confused with psoralen-based light therapy or laser techniques that employ either the carbon dioxide (10,600 nm) or the neodymium–yttrium–aluminum–garnet (YAG, 1064 nm) lasers. What differentiates PDT from psoralen light therapy, as well as from carbon dioxide or YAG lasers, is that PDT utilizes light to activate a photosensitizing agent that, once excited, inverts spin to become an excited triplet species. Thereafter, in a spin-conserving reaction, the excited triplet-state photosensitizer transfers energy to ground-state triplet oxygen to produce an excited-state species (singlet oxygen). Singlet oxygen subsequently reacts with cellular components and results in cytotoxicity. As is seen in Fig. 66-20, the light excites the sensitizer, the sensitizer transfers energy to oxygen, and singlet oxygen causes subsequent tumoricidal effects. This manner of photo-oxidation is described as being a type II process. Had the process proceeded through a path in which the excited-state sensitizer initiated a free-radical reaction, and oxygen subsequently reacted with one of the free-radical intermediates, the mechanism would be described as a type I photooxidative process.[20] The products from either process are frequently indistinguishable, and because the internal reductive milieu of the cell usually eliminates peroxides and endoperoxides in short order, the exact mechanism by which the cytotoxicity is initiated remains obscure.[20] Certain benzofuran derivatives are thought to react specifically with singlet oxygen; whereas others, such as cholesterol when reacted with singlet oxygen, result in a specific stereoisomer. The cytotoxicity of PDT has been shown to be markedly reduced when HPD-treated cells are exposed to light in the presence of 1,3-diphenylisobenzofuran (DPBF).[21] Although the reduction in cytotoxicity is suggestive of a singlet–oxygen-mediated cytotoxicity, unfortunately, DPBF is not entirely specific, and other activated oxygen species (hydroxyl radical, hydroperoxyl radical) could also be trapped.[20] Deuterated water increases the lifetime of singlet oxygen and, in so doing, is expected to influence in vitro survival studies; however, experimental conditions are exquisitely sensitive to deuterium oxide concentration. An example of such was found for PDT with the phthalocyanine photosensitizers. Unless the deuterium oxide concentration was higher than 98%, little isotopic effect could be found.[22,23] Direct spectrophotometric detection of the short-lived singlet oxygen species (lifetimes, in aqueous environments, span several microseconds) in an in vitro cell system or in an in vivo system, and correlation of the presence and quantity of singlet oxygen with survival, would be definitive proof of the pivotal role of singlet oxygen cytotoxicity. Because of the potential multiple active photosensitizer components in HPD, there is no concrete knowledge of the active component within the cell, and calculations based on the quantum yields (defined as the number of molecules of product formed per 100 photons absorbed) from any one active species are subject to great uncertainties. Yet, with so many apparent ambiguities, singlet oxygen has been reported to have been measured in an animal model. By use of a liquid nitrogen-cooled germanium diode and temporal resolution techniques, singlet oxygen phosphorescent emission at 1270 nm has been detected from the surface of a murine tumor previously treated with dihematoporphyrin ether.[24] It is not clear whether the 1270-nm phosphorescence represents singlet oxygen being generated within the tumor or, rather, purely from the surface of the tumor as oxygen from the environment penetrates the tumor's outermost surface layer.

FIG. 66-20. Photodynamic oxidation process.

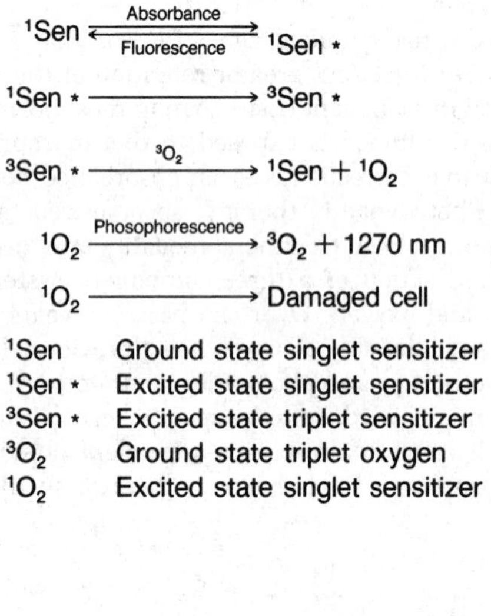

What is clear is that PDT does require oxygen. Several laboratories have shown that at oxygen concentration less than 10% cell survival decreases and that below 2% cells are resistant to PDT.[25–27] Moreover, induced tissue hypoxia in an animal model has been shown to definitely lessen the photodynamic effect.[28] The implications of a hypoxic effect in the use of PDT for human tumors remain undefined. There is evidence that murine tumors have a cellular fraction that is hypoxic[29] and likewise, tumor hypoxia probably also exists in human tumors.[30]

Although, currently, there is an intense search for new photosensitizers that will broaden the scope of PDT, the agent that has been most widely used in clinical studies has been either HPD (Photofrin I) or a further purified mixture of HPD named dihematoporphyrin ether/ester, DHE (Photofrin II).[18,31] HPD or DHE localizes in tumors and has a large therapeutic index in clinically meaningful dosages. Additionally, HPD absorbs light at a wavelength (630 nm) that allows greater tissue penetration (the longer the wavelength, the greater tissue penetration) and obviates the problem associated with light absorbance by naturally present biologic chromophores such as hemoglobin. These two features permit more light to reach tumors that have preferentially retained the photosensitizer. Why HPD is retained to a greater extent in tumors, as opposed to normal tissues, is not known. In aqueous environments HPD and DHE are known to aggregate into structures with a molecular weight greater than 25 kD.[31] In vitro studies to determine if tumor cells are more photosensitive or selectively retain HPD, for the most part, indicate that there is no difference between normal and cancerous cells. However, Andreoni and associates did find that transformed thyroid cells are more sensitive than control cells.[32] What the study did not address is the possible differences in cell volume and the effects that cell volume might have on drug uptake. Moan and co-workers demonstrated that, once cell volume normalization by flow cytometry had been accounted for, there is little difference in HPD and subsequent PDT sensitivity between a mouse fibroblast cell line and three of its transformants.[33] The difference in in vivo tumor versus normal cell sensitizer uptake and retention probably resides in a multitude of environmental factors, and perhaps cell volume differences account for some of the preferential drug uptake. However, heterogeneity of the HPD or DHE mixture and aggregates tend to obfuscate the issues of in vivo HPD tumor retention. But leaky tumor neovascular effects; retention within tumor vasculature endothelial cells, with subsequent disruption of tumor oxygen and nutrient delivery; poorly developed tumor lymphatics; lower tumor pH; and binding to lipoproteins and subsequent receptor mediated endocytosis, all may contribute to in vivo tumor retention and cytotoxicity.[34–40] Studies addressing these issues are indecisive because distribution studies with tritiated radiolabeled sensitizers may suffer from isotope exchange, and fluorescence-based methods may be inaccurate because porphyrin aggregates, which are apparently important in the localization and retentive properties of the actual most important component of the drug, may contribute little fluorescence, and, lastly, tissue scattering and quenching may decrease measurable fluorescence.[40–44]

Figure 66-21 diagrams a mammalian cell and the subcellular components that have been reported to be damaged by PDT. The most striking and immediate cellular response observed following PDT is damage to membranes, particularly the plasma membrane.[45,46] Shortly after light treatment, cells are noted to withstand trypsin removal from plastic surfaces.[47,48] Such early changes imply that membrane proteins have cross-linked with residual double bonds of the plastic. Within hours after treatment, visible damage is seen by cessation of normal cellular movement (time-lapse photography) and the formation of multiple membrane blebs.[49] The blebs, which are often as large as the cell itself, develop as balloon-like structures protruding from the cell membrane and indicate severe membrane damage.[50,51] After cell blebbing, there is no longer cell division, and cell lysis follows (personal observation by time-lapse photography). Other experimental indications of membrane distortion after PDT are constituent leakage from intact cells[52] or isotope from red blood cell ghosts.[23] As shown in Fig. 66-21, other cellular membranes, in addition to the plasma membrane, may be at risk, including the nucleus, mitochondria, lysosome, Golgi apparatus, and endoplasmic reticulum. Membranes, therefore, by virtue of the HPD or DHE water–lipid partition coefficient, are good targets for PDT damage. Mitochondrial damage after PDT has been shown by noting specific inhibition of oxidative phosphorylation and electron transport enzymes[53] and reduction in cellular ATP levels.[54] Although production of DNA strand breaks has been observed after PDT, such lesions may not be responsible for cellular death.[55,56] Incorporation of bromodeoxyuridine into cellular DNA has been shown to sensitize cells to ionizing radiation and chemotherapy drugs.[57,58] but not to PDT (per-

FIG. 66-21. Diagrammatic representation of a mammalian cell and the subcellular components that have been reported to be damaged by PDT. Mitochondrial insert shows the location of three mitochondrial enzymes that have been found to be inhibited by PDT with hematoporphyrin derivative. (Mitochondrial insert courtesy of R. Hilf)

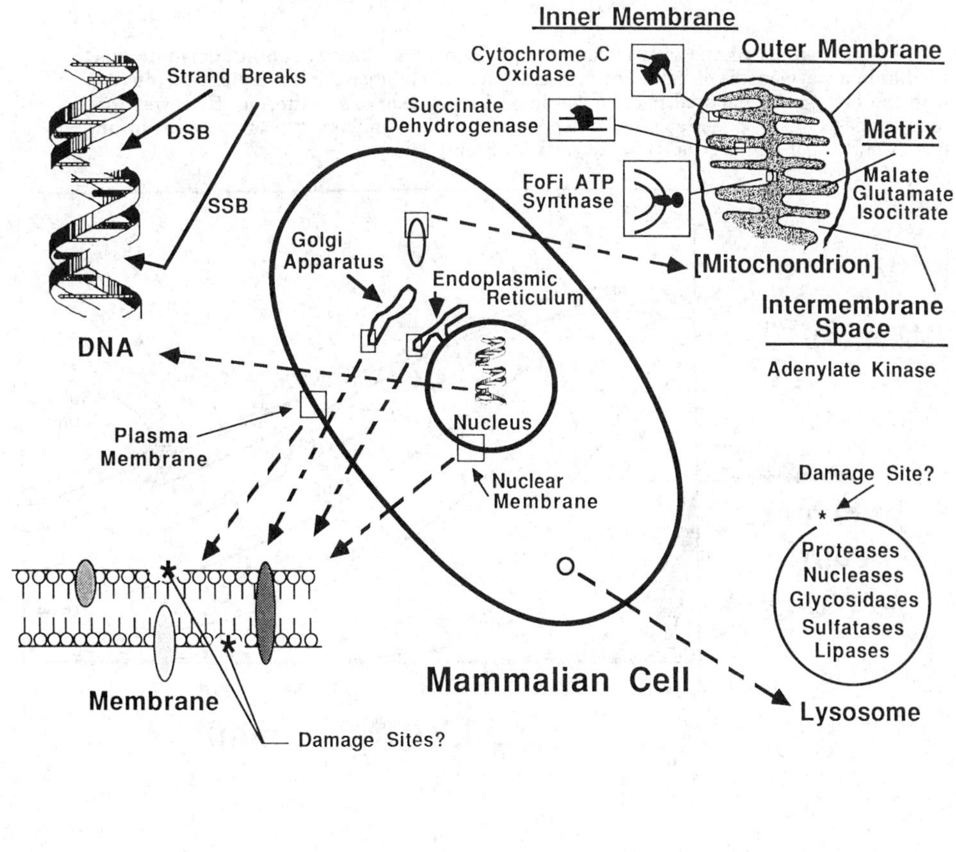

sonal observation). Additionally, PDT has been shown not to be mutagenic in in vitro systems.[59,60] Together the last two facts indicate that DNA is not a primary target for PDT-induced cytotoxicity. The HPD or DHE uptake studies clearly define initial binding within the plasma membrane, followed, in time, by migration to internal cellular regions.[61] Figure 66-21 is not meant to be inclusive of all the possible sites damaged by PDT. Particularly because highly reactive oxygen species may react relatively indiscriminately with cellular constituents and, therefore, yet to be determined sites may be at risk. If with time the biologically active photosensitizer partitions into multiple sites, there may not be one site or a specific singular biochemical disruption but, rather, multiple concurrent damage sites resulting in cytotoxicity.

Dihematoporphyrin ether/ester is purported to be at least twice as active as HPD.[31,62] Both sensitizers are usually administered 48 to 72 hr before light treatment to allow tumor retention and clearance from most normal tissues. The HPD LD_{50} in mice is 275 mg/kg, death is from hepatic toxicity; whereas, if whole-body irradiation is used after HPD injection, the LD_{50} is 7.5 mg/kg, death is from a shock-like syndrome. The doses used in humans in various published studies vary slightly, 2 to 5 mg/kg for HPD and 1 to 2.5 mg/kg for DHE.[18,31] Clear data showing quantifiable advantages of HPD or DHE retention in tumors versus normal tissue are sparse, but fluorescent measurements from tissue as a function of time after HPD administration show that, with time, there is greater retention in tumors than in normal tissues, the ratio of which varies widely.[38,45,62-65] In general, 24 to 48 hr after administration of HPD, the tumor/normal tissue ratio is greater than 1. Kaye and co-workers showed, in a rodent brain model, that the tumor/normal brain ratio was approximately 12 to 16.[65] In addition to malignant tumors, tissues that attain high levels of HPD or DHE are liver and spleen reticuloendothelial cells, kidney parenchymal cells, vascular stroma, skin, endometrium, and ovary.[18,36,38,66] The HPD serum T½ in humans is approximately 20 hr. Slow skin clearance (4–8 weeks) accounts for the primary untoward effect of PDT: dermal photosensitivity. The dermal photosensitivity, although entirely preventable by restricting light exposure, is usually only of minimal concern, yet toxicity may range from minimal erythema to severe sunburn.[18,31] Because PDT is an experimental modality, it has been used primarily after patients have failed previous treatment with surgery, radiation or chemotherapy. It may be used in areas previously treated with surgery, radiation, or chemotherapy. However, concurrent or recent ionizing radiation, as well a history of previous treatment with doxorubicin (Adriamycin), may increase dermal photosensitivity.[18,31]

What dictates the choice of the wavelength of light to be used to initiate PDT is the absorbance characteristics of the photosensitizing agent. As is seen in Fig. 66-22, light penetration attenuates rapidly because of absorbance and scattering. Any source of light with appropriate spectral characteristics can be used for PDT. Initial work with HPD employed wavelength-filtered lamps as an energy source, but lasers offer a more effective means of light delivery through emission of a monochromatic form of intense collimated light energy.[42,66-70] Currently, 18 to 24 W CW argon lasers are frequently used to excite (pump) dyes, commonly Kiton red or rhodamine B, in an optical cavity to produce up to 5 W red laser light—630 nm corresponds to one of the minor peaks of DHE. In the event that a photosensitizer with a different

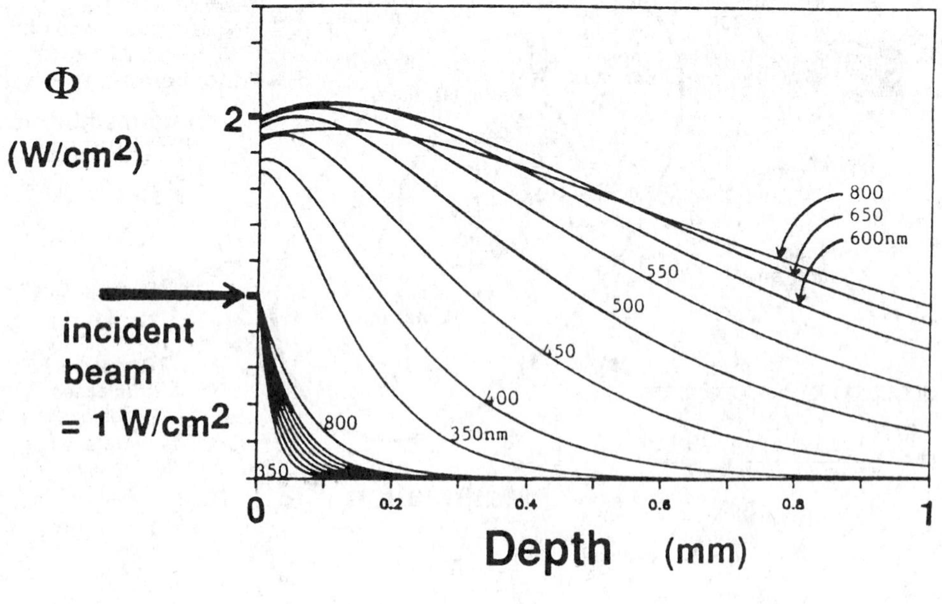

FIG. 66-22. Collimated and total radiant energy fluence rate distribution in human dermis for different wavelengths of light. The incident 1 W/cm^2 collimated beam rapidly attentuates with the first couple hundred microns because of absorption and scattering. However, the total fluence rate, Φ, penetrates much deeper into tissue. Numbers indicate wavelength in nm. (Courtesy of SL Jacques, D Zrakit, and SA Prahl)

absorbance spectrum is used for PDT, it is relatively easy to change the dye to attain the appropriate light emission. Pulsed gold vapor lasers that emit at 628 nm are also used for PDT.[69] Preliminary reports comparing pulsed gold vapor with argon-pumped dye lasers suggest equal tumoricidal efficacy.[69] The laser can be coupled to one or multiple durable optical fibers which virtually lose no light during propagation and provide energy, depending on configuration, according to fiber tip design (Fig. 66-23). In addition to surface illumination, the fibers can be placed through endoscopic instruments, allowing treatment of previously inaccessible sites. Likewise, the optical fiber may be implanted into larger tumors, thereby providing treatment of larger and deeper-seated tumors. Modification of optical fibers or multiple fibers allows various geometric distributions of light.[42,69–71] Cleaved-tipped fibers project light forward along the optical axis, with the numerical aperture of the fiber determining the divergence; bulbed-tipped fibers yield isotropic spherical distribution, and cylindrical scattering material applied to the fiber tip yields peak light 90° from the midpoint of the fiber axis.

FIG. 66-23. Different types of illumination possible to a surface, interstitium, or cavity by the use of direct illumination or specially designed optical fibers.

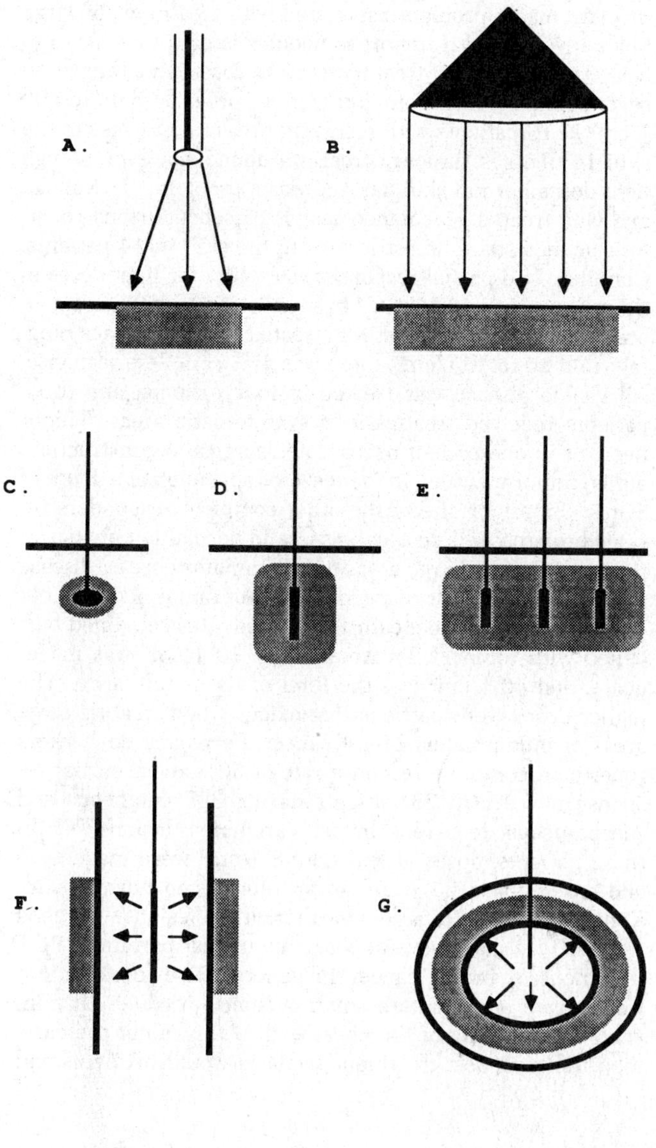

CLINICAL STUDIES

Except for the early work on fluorescence detection and two separate case reports, HPD-based PDT began in 1976. It is now estimated that more than 3000 patients have been treated with PDT. Since 1984 most patients within the United States have been treated with DHE. Most of these patients had advanced-stage malignancies or else were refractory to conventional therapy. Debulking of large tumors with subsequent PDT has largely been unsuccessful and interstitial therapy, although promising, has limited success because of limited light penetration at 630 nm. In general, the tendency in most institutions is to treat earlier-stage primary cancers. Most of the published results have been accrued from studies that vary in the dose of photosensitizer used, the total energy and rate of administration of light, the time after photosensitizer injection, the number of treatments, and the light delivery techniques. No study has yet been published from randomized trials. The degree and duration of tumor response is not always easily gleaned from the literature. Most studies report follow-up times of less than 1 year. But even with all of the apparent pitfalls of different treatments and reporting, PDT does cause tumor necrosis in patients refractory to other treatment modalities.

CUTANEOUS AND SUBCUTANEOUS TUMORS

The treatment of either cutaneous or subcutaneous malignancies exemplifies both the advantages and disadvantages of PDT. Epidermal malignancies are readily accessible and suitable to treatment. Patient selection, particularly for extensive treatment areas, is necessary to avoid disfigurement or acute medical problems. Yet an adequate cosmetic result normally follows successful tumor treatment. Treatment includes basal cell and squamous cell carcinoma, malignant melanoma, Bowen's disease, Kaposi's sarcoma, mycosis fungoides, and metastatic epidermoid and recurrent or metastatic breast cancer (Table 66-9).

Dougherty reported excellent treatment results of basal cell carcinoma. Of the 50 sites treated in 15 patients there was a 70% to 80% complete response and a 20% to 30% partial response, with the longest patient follow-up without recurrence being 4 years.[17,18] Kennedy[72] reported results from treatment of 38 basal cell carcinoma lesions.[72] Complete response was achieved in all lesions, the longest time of follow-up without recurrence was 35 months. Tokuda[73] showed an 82% complete response in 40 lesions from three patients with nevoid basal cell carcinoma syndrome. The recurrence rate was 11% at 14 months. Tomio and coworkers[74] reported three cases of basal cell carcinoma responding completely to PDT with hematoporphyrin. Bowden's disease has been treated in two patients with ten lesions, with a complete response of all lesions, with the longest follow-up being 1.5 years.[75] Results of the treatment

TABLE 66-9. Summary of Clinical Results of PDT Use in Cutaneous Malignancies

Cutaneous Malignancies	*Lesions Treated*	*CR (%)*	*PR (%)*	*NR (%)*	*Reference*
Basal Cell	50	75	25		18
Basal Cell	38	100			72
Bowen Disease	10	100			18
Squamous Cell	10	20	80		18
Squamous Cell*	114	21	37	42	78
Melanoma	1000	50	30	20	17
Melanoma	16	0	0	100	79
Mycosis Fungoides	5	20	60	20	
Kaposi's Sarcoma†	100	80	20		18,80
Breast‡	1000	60–70	20–30		18
Breast	395	56	19	25	77,78

*Metastatic head and neck.
†Endemic Kaposi's.
‡Metastatic to skin.

of squamous cell carcinoma are not nearly as good as that seen for basal cell carcinoma. Of the ten lesions in five patients treated, there was a 20% complete and a 70% to 80% partial response; the longest follow-up was 1 year.[18] Similar complete responses were reported from Bern's group, wherein metastatic squamous cell carcinoma of the head and neck in 39 patients, who had 114 sites treated, showed a complete response of 21% and partial response of 37%.[76,77] Kennedy, likewise, reported poor results for complete response in squamous cell carcinoma.[72] In one patient who had metastatic squamous cell carcinoma of head and neck origin, 13 cutaneous and subcutaneous lesions were treated with doses ranging from 10 to 20 J/cm^2; there was an initial complete response of 61% and partial response of 23%. Persisting lesions were retreated 25 days later with complete response in all lesions. The duration of response was 9 months, at which time the patient died of metastatic lesions.[78] This one case illustrates that retreatment is effective, and apparently antineoplastic drug resistance does not translate into resistance to PDT.

The composite results from several studies for treatment of 50 patients with more than 1000 malignant melonoma lesions indicate approximately 50% had a complete response and 30% had a partial response.[18] However, response may be highly dependent on size and degree of pigmentation of the tumor.[72,79] Light penetrates highly melanotic tissue sparingly, and significant heat is generated if high-power densities are used. Of 16 deeply pigmented bluish-black lesions that were treated with 500 mW/cm^2, varying the field sizes from 0.5 to 1.0 cm and the dose from 80 to 160 J/cm^2 none responded.[78] Yet, even though Kaposi's sarcoma is pigmented, there appears to be excellent response to PDT, with complete responses seen in 80% of more than 100 lesions treated in five patients.[18,72,80] With the increasing incidence of epidemic Kaposi's sarcoma and the limited second-line drug regimens available, PDT may find increased use in the treatment of the disfiguring and potential life-threatening disease.

Probably the greatest experience with treatment of superficially located tumors is in recurrent and metastatic breast cancer. Dougherty reported a complete response rate of 60% to 70%, and a partial response of 20% to 30%, in results form 120 patients compositely having more than 1000 lesions treated in various centers.[18] Original reports of recurrent breast nodules showed an 88% complete response rate.[81] With further experience, the response rates are in the range 60% to 70%. Usually, the response begins to be seen with 2 hr. The major problem associated with treatment of large fields involved with tumorous nodules is pain that may necessitate cessation of treatment. Light doses have ranged, in several studies, from 5 to 250 J/cm^2. Forbes used 40 to 250 J/cm^2 in 16 patients with recurrent breast metastases to the skin. In all cases, tumor necrosis was found; however, at high light doses normal skin damage was a problem.[82,83] Konoka and Ono treated 71 cutaneous and 16 subcutaneous recurrent or metastatic breast lesions to the skin in 14 patients. Complete and partial responses were 40% for light doses in the range of 5 to 43 J/cm^2.[84] In seven patients with recurrent breast cancer on the chest wall treated with light doses ranging from 20 to 40 J/cm^2, there was 42% complete response. All visible disease was treated in four patients, and three patients received treatment to symptomatic areas. Tumor necrosis in one patient necessitated surgical reconstruction, but no tumor was seen in the resected specimen at a depth of 5 mm. Biopsy of one of the other complete responders revealed microscopic residual disease in dermal lymphatics of the treated area. Large areas of inflammatory breast disease in two of the patients resulted in areas of tumor necrosis, but dermal lymphatics beneath the treated sites remained burdened with tumor.[78] Treatment with 10 J/cm^2 was inadequate, and 40 J/cm^2 was the limit of tissue tolerance. The higher doses were particularly noxious when treating large areas of inflammatory breast cancer. Berns and co-workers reported a complete response rate of 56% and a partial response of 19% in 33 patients having 395 cutaneous and subcutaneous recurrent breast carcinoma lesions.[76,77] In these patients, doses of less than 8 J/cm^2 were inadequate and doses above 25 J/cm^2 were injurious to normal skin. Kennedy treated 16 patients with multiple lesions with good results.[72] He made several observations that pertain to PDT treatment of breast cancer in general. The ideal patient would have one or more small cutaneous nodules that involve a small area of the chest wall. If this is not the case, then the next best treatment scenario would involve small subcutaneous nodules restricted to a small area of the chest wall. Treatment of large areas should be attempted in two fractionated doses; the first treatment reduces the tumor burden to a more manageable size. When treating inflammatory breast cancer during phototherapy there can be a strong reaction with itching and erythema commencing during treatment. He advises pretreatment with antihistamines, not just for comfort, but also to reduce or prevent the severe skin reaction that may be anticipated. Lastly, Kennedy noted that in one patient there was one nodule among many that was exquisitely resistant to PDT. The experience with breast cancer certainly appears to indicate that there is a distinct place for PDT in the treatment of recurrent breast cancer unresponsive to other modalities, yet the experience in the use of PDT for breast cancer does provide insight into the limitations of the use of PDT for both this cancer and other tumors. Large treatment areas result in pain that may require narcotic analgesics. Smaller nodules respond better than do larger ones. The major shortcoming now appears limited only by lack of light penetration into subdermal lymphatics and uptake of photosensitizer by inflamed skin. As new photosensitizing agents with absorbance bands at longer wavelengths become available, both of these limitations will undoubtedly be circumvented.

HEAD AND NECK CANCERS

Nearly all patients who were treated with PDT for cancers of the head and neck had recurrent squamous cell carcinoma refractory to, or not suited for, traditional treatment. Several tumors were accessible only by endoscopic procedures. Bern and Wile[77] reported a 29% complete response and a 62% partial response rate for patients with recurrent head and neck cancers (tongue 9, nasopharynx 3, floor of mouth 2, soft palate 2, miscellaneous 5) recurrent in the primary site. Retreatment with a second or third course was used in eight patients. Three nasopharyngeal tumors and one vocal cord tumor were treated endoscopically; all other sites were treated with external light irradiation. Two large exophytic tumors were treated interstitially with no response noted. Two of the nine tongue cancers treated resulted in durable complete responses, and six of the nine had partial responses. Kennedy[73] treated four patients with head and neck cancers originating in the mucous membrane of the mouth and nose with disappointing results. No differential cytotoxicity was noted between tumor and normal skin. Taketa and Imakiire treated two laryngeal, two tongue, and two oropharyngeal cancers with surface irradiation through a endoscope.[85] Although partial tumor necrosis was seen in all patients, treatment effect was limited by virtue of poor tissue penetration through surface illumination. Also in the area of larynx, treatment precision is necessary to limit induction of obstruction secondary to edema. Treatment of nasopharyngeal carcinoma has given mixed responses.[86] Most of the treated tumors were large. After treatment, nearly all tumors were reduced in size and contained central necrosis, but subsequent biopsies showed residual malignancy. Shuller and associates reported complete response in one patient treated with tongue cancer.[87] In the same study five complications in 24 treated patients occurred. Complications included orocutaneous fistula, necrosis of a previous skin graft, exsanguination secondary to treatment of a tumor infiltrating the carotid, and chronic ulceration. These complications emphasize the need for careful patient selection when using PDT to eradicate tumor in areas involving vital structures. In general, the experience of PDT for head and neck involved treatment of patients with recurrence of primary tumors who, despite successful local tumor eradication, tended to fail outside of the treatment field. Such results beg for studies that use PDT in an earlier setting as an adjunct in combination with surgery or radiation therapy.

BLADDER CANCER

More than 100 patients with bladder cancer have now been treated with PDT. The responses are encouraging (Table 66-10) and indicate that the modality will have a place in the care of patients with diffuse carcinoma in situ, Ta, T1, and in a select group of T2 lesions. With bladder lesions, there is strong evidence that there is selective retention of HPD by bladder cancer, as was shown by fluorescence mapping of the bladder cancer in 16 patients who underwent subsequent radical cystectomy for invasive or widespread carcinoma in situ.[88] One hundred percent correlation was found between presurgical localization of tumors and subsequent histopathologic bladder mapping. In a similar study Tsuchiya and co-workers used an image intensifier to detect fluorescence of HPD at all tumor sites in eight patients.[89] Such data appear to hold when PDT is used because the treatment is well tolerated with little trauma to normal bladder mucosa. Furthermore, the fact that there has been highly successful therapy after injection of varying amounts of HPD, varying intervals before treatment after HPD injection, and varying energy levels supports the overall efficacy of the modality for treatment of bladder cancer. Treatment either of individual lesions or the entire bladder surface is achieved by inflating the bladder with gas, saline, or a diffusing medium and subsequently cystoscopically inserting the appropriate geometrically tipped optical fiber.[90–94] After treatment of tumors, surface edema is noted within 20 min, and tumor necrosis with edema and hyperemia of the surrounding normal mucosa is evident within 3 to 7 days, which is most pronounced after 2 weeks. Normal mucosa returns in 4 to 9 weeks after PDT. Superficial lesions were treated by Tsuchiya and associates[89] and Hisazumi and co-workers,[91] who respectively reported 75% and 83% complete response with 6 to 18 month disease-free follow-up. Benson and coworkers reported complete responses in four patients with eventual recurrence in two patients, both of whom were successfully retreated.[90] Misaki *et al* treated 32 superficial

TABLE 66-10. Results of PDT for Bladder Cancer

Patients	*CR (%)*	*PR (%)*	*NR (%)*	*Reference*
10	60	40		92
6	33	50	17	94
16	69	18	13	95
9	67	33		96
19	47	47	6	97

papillary lesions with complete responses in 67% and partial responses in the remainder.[95] Shumaker *et al* treated 16 patients who had received previous treatments; all had superficial, noninvasive bladder carcinoma.[96] Of the 16 patients, 11 (69%) complete responses and three partial responses were achieved. Prout and associates reported their results from a clinical trial wherein dosing of photosensitizer (2.0 mg/kg DHE), light energy (100–200 J/cm²), treatment time after DHE (48 hr), and techniques were standardized.[97] Patient selection was well described and treatment results were meticulously recorded. In the study, 37 patients with bladder carcinoma were evaluated for treatment, 20 patients were selected. Of these 20 patients all were considered evaluable except one in whom the diagnosis was revised to cystitis cystica with moderate atypia and urothelial hyperplasia. All tumors, except two, were less than 2.5 cm. Two patients received whole-bladder light irradiation; one patient received a total light dose of 5.5 J/cm², and the other, because of decrease of bladder volume during the course of treatment, received between 5.5 J/cm² and 10 J/cm². At the time of each cystoscopy, at least three urologists were present to verify findings. Assessment of the effect of treatment was carried out 3 months after treatment. Nine of 19 patients (47%) had complete responses. Treatment results within the remaining 10 patients showed that 13 of 50 tumors could not be eradicated, but nine of the ten patients had reduction in tumor size, number, or both, of more than 50%. The overall eradication in the ten patients that did not achieve a complete response was 37 of 50 (74%) tumors. Of the patients treated 18 experienced adverse effects, 11 had irritable bladder symptoms. In most patients, there were only mild symptoms of frequency, hematuria, dysuria, and spasm persisting for less than a week. Two patients who had total bladder treatment and one patient who had 13 lesions treated had moderate symptoms. Of all the patients, only one had severe irritative symptoms and at the 3-month follow-up was found to have extensive granulation tissue present. In no patient was there a decrease in vesicle volume. In the United States there are now ongoing controlled randomized trials addressing the efficacy of PDT versus intravesical chemotherapy in early-stage bladder carcinoma. With the development of new photosensitizers, the encouraging results with early-stage bladder may be extended to more invasive lesions.

ENDOBRONCHIAL CANCER

Photodynamic therapy has been effectively employed for the diagnosis of early lung cancer, for curative or palliative treatment of primary lung cancer, or for malignancies metastatic to the tracheobronchial tree. One of the major issues in oncology is the early detection of lung cancer. Radiologically occult lung cancer is usually squamous and primarily involves males in their fifth through eighth decade. The tumors evolve from in situ lesions, may be multicentric, may grow slowly, and usually metastasize relatively late. The heavy smoker who develops lung cancer is oftentimes less than an ideal pulmonary or cardiac risk for major thoracic surgery that may involve pulmonary resection. Likewise, the patient with lung or with cancer metastatic to the bronchus causing pulmonary obstructive symptoms is usually a poor operative risk and, not infrequently, the obstructive lesion obscures the distal lung, thereby making presurgical evaluation difficult. It is in these settings that PDT may have a role in the management of endobronchial lesions. As mentioned previously, one of the first uses of HPD was to determine by fluorescent examination the possibility of detecting squamous cell cancer of the lung.[9] Use of PDT in early lung cancer may be indicated for patients with sputum-positive cytologies and negative chest x-ray films, or in patients with a peripheral nodule and squamous cells in the sputum in which simultaneous occult squamous cancer may be present.[98] Use of PDT in larger obstructive lesions is usually palliative for those accessible lesions in which the obstruction does not extend extrinsically; however, PDT may extend indications for surgery or may reduce the extent of lung resection. The advantage of PDT over carbon dioxide laser therapy is that flexible optical fibers for transmission of 10.6-μm laser light are not available and, therefore, rigid bronchoscopy must be used; the advantage over 1.06 μm neodynium-YAG laser therapy is that control of the fiber optical output is critical, requiring considerable expertise. However, a good argument can be made for the use of neodynium-YAG laser therapy in the treatment of large, obstructing, endobronchial lesions.[98] PDT offers tumor-selective therapy with no, or only limited, damage to surrounding normal tissue.

Because of the location of tumors within the tracheobronchial tree fiber-optic transmission of laser light is usually delivered through flexible bronchoscopes. Superficial lesions can be treated directly to the surface by a flat-ended fiber; obstructive lesions can be treated either interstitially or circumferentially with a cylindrical emitting fiber. The HPD or DHE is usually injected 2 to 6 days before light treatment. The light doses used are in the range of 50 to 675 J/cm², with a power density of 90 to 600 mW. In 1984 Hayata and associates presented their work using PDT for the treatment of 73 patients with endobronchial lesions.[99] Eight of the 13 patients with early-stage squamous cell carcinoma were considered inoperable and, therefore, were candidates for PDT, either because of poor pulmonary function or refusal of surgery. In all eight patients complete responses were obtained. They reported that follow-up times ranged from 8 to 36 months. In the five patients who were resected after PDT, two complete responses were verified histologically, and three patients had significant reduction of tumor but were not considered to have had adequate light treatment because of the location of the tumor or laser mechanical problems. The overall complete response within the 13-patient group was 77%. In advanced cases intraluminal opening was accomplished in 48%.[100,101] There were several adverse effects reported other than dermal photosensitivity. A viscuous proteinaceous material with potential for obstruction had to be removed daily for several days by cleanup bronchoscopy, and two cases of bronchial pulmonary fistulas developed. Caution was advised in cases that required treatment of advanced tumor with invasion to the pulmonary artery. Kato and associates have extended their series of patients and have reported the first case of 5-year disease-free survival with only PDT treatment.[102,103] They have now reported their work on preoperative PDT for early-stage central-type lung cancer in 30 patients.[104] Of the 30 patients, 17 were not candidates for surgery, all had complete responses. Eight of these patients are disease-free from 23 to 70 months. Six died without lung disease from 16 to 46 months after PDT and three developed recurrent lung cancer 12, 16, and 20 months after treatment. Thirteen of the 30 patients were resected after PDT. Complete responses were found in four and only tumor nests were observed in nine. All patients remain disease-free from 12 to 70 months after therapy.

Edsell and Cortese reported their results of PDT in 38 patients with cancer involving the tracheobronchial tree.[105] The HPD doses used varied between 2 and 5 mg/kg and the light dose varied from 90 to 675 J/cm^2, for tumors treated with surface illumination, and 54 to 600 J/cm^2 for tumors treated intralesionally. Five cancers required a second HPD/PDT course. A complete response occurred in 13 patients, and 11 did not recur during follow-up from 3 to 53 months.

After having developed the technique of endobronchial tumor localization and having acquired experience in earlier trials treating 38 patients with varying concentrations of sensitizer and light doses, Dorion and co-workers reported their experience with a standardized approach to PDT for palliation of 22 patients with extensive obstructing endobronchial lesions.[106,107] All of the patients were treated with 3 mg/kg HPD 72 hr before PDT. Tumors were treated with a flat-surface fiber or cylindrical fiber either directly (100 J/cm^2) or interstitially (200 J/cm^2). The energies used were less than those used in Hayata's studies. Nineteen of the patients had partial obstruction (40 to 90%), 15 patients required one treatment, 7 required two treatments. Of the 22 patients treated, 20 had complete responses. There were no deaths nor complications during the procedure; two patients developed a pneumothorax (1 and 5 days) after the procedure. All patients received cleanup bronchoscopy 2 to 3 days after PDT for removal of tumor debris and mucous plugs. Their work was extended to include patients with metastatic tumor to the bronchus, and they achieved a 97% complete response, defined as complete opening of the bronchus to its full extent, or a wall with no visible residual endobronchial tumor remaining.[108] They have now treated 236 patients with endobronchial tumors obstructing up to 90% of the trachea and up to 100% of the main lobar or segmental airways. Their last report is complete response (airway open to the bronchial wall) in all patients.[109]

Other smaller series treating endobronchial lesions include 21 patients treated by Lin and co-workers,[110] with obstructing lesions reported by Vincent and associates,[111] and 7 patients treated by Forbes and associates.[112] In the Lin study there were only 12.5% complete responses, and 83% had some response; however, the tumors were treated only on their surfaces, and only 120 J/cm^2 was used. In the Vincent study 7 of 17 patients had greater than 50% shrinkage of tumor, and of those seven patients, two achieved biopsy-proven complete responses. The Forbes' study showed no benefit in six of seven patients and was attributed to technically inadequate treatment. There is one preliminary report of a randomized trial comparing the safety and efficiency of palliative radiation therapy alone versus radiation and phototherapy for inoperable obstructive non-small bronchogenic carcinoma.[113] Preliminary results for the very small group of patients (five in one arm and four in the other) suggest that the addition of PDT before radiation therapy provides significantly longer-lasting benefits. Results of the various studies are summarized in Table 66-11.

TABLE 66-11. Results of PDT for Endobronchial Tumors

Patients	*CR (%)*	*PR (%)*	*NR (%)*	*Reference*
13*	77	23		100
60†		48‡	52	101, 102
30	70	30§		105
38	34	66		106
22	91	9		107, 108
236#	100‖			109
21	12	83**	5	111
17	22	30	48	112
7	0	14	86	113

* Early-stage bronchogenic.
† Advanced-stage bronchogenic.
§ Tumor nest residual.
‖ Defined as airway open to bronchial wall.
Including metastatic tumor to bronchus.
** Response but not complete.

ESOPHAGEAL AND GASTROINTESTINAL CANCER

Phototherapy has been used for cure and palliation of esophageal carcinoma (Table 66-12). Early stage esophageal carcinoma usually requires routine screening practices and, therefore, the vast majority of patients that would come to PDT would be expected to have advanced disease. Hayata and colleagues reported the use of PDT for treatment of four patients, with squamous cell carcinoma of the esophagus, using flexible endoscopy.[99] Light energies of 120 to 240 J/cm^2 were used. Complete remissions were achieved in three patients and a significant response in the fourth. Two of the three patients with complete remission were not resected and were disease-free at 15 and 25 months. Okuda and co-workers treated two patients with squamous cell carcinoma of the esophagus.[114] The size of the lesion in the first patient was 3 cm^2, whereas the size in second patient was 14 cm^2. The first patient was treated with 204 J/cm^2, which resulted in complete remission for 14 months. The second patient was treated with 45 J/cm^2 and achieved a partial

TABLE 66-12. Results of PDT for Esophageal Cancer

Patients	*CR (%)*	*PR (%)*	*NR (%)*	*Reference*
4	75	25		100
2	50	50		115
2	50	50		116
7		100*		117
14	28	72		118
15	47	33	20	119

* Tumor responded/swallowing improved.

remission. Corti *et al* treated two patients with squamous cell carcinoma of the esophagus.[115] The first patient achieved a complete response documented by endoscopy, cytology, and histology at 6 months. The patient follow-up at the time was 10 months. Although the second patient was incompletely treated, a partial response was achieved.

McCaughan and co-workers reported the use of interstitial PDT with cylindrical fibers for seven patients who had complete, or nearly complete, esophageal obstruction.[116] Patients received 3 mg/kg HPD 3 to 6 days before treatment. Patients received one to four treatments with PDT and, in one patient, a neodynium-YAG laser was also used. The tumor types included three squamous cell carcinomas, three adenocarcinomas, and one melanoma. All tumors responded, and swallowing was improved. Thomas and associates treated 14 patients with inoperable advanced esophageal cancer.[117] Patients received between 2.5 and 5.0 mg/kg (the first seven patients received 2.5 mg/kg, the second seven patients received 5.0 mg/kg) 3 days before receiving light doses ranging from 60 to 337 J/cm^2. To control the dose of light delivered to the tumor, a polyethylene cannula with a thin-walled balloon was bronchoscopically inserted into the tumor. Once in the tumor, the balloon was inflated with a dispersing medium 0.5% lipid emulsion, after which the optical fiber was moved within the balloon. A total of 24 PDT treatments were given to 14 patients. All patients responded to therapy. Two patients had pathologically confirmed complete responses. Tomio and colleagues reported their results of treatment of 15 patients with esophageal carcinoma with doses of light ranging from 35 to 200 J/cm^2 and power densities of 100 to 250 mW/cm^2.[118] Among the seven superficial lesions, five complete responses were achieved and one partial response; whereas, in the advanced esophageal cancers two complete responses and two partial responses were achieved.

Treatment of stomach carcinoma (Table 66-13) has been attempted, but gastric folds and the tumor site presented significant technical difficulties. Nevertheless, Hayata and associates treated 14 cases of early-stage gastric cancer.[101] Three patients were not resected because of refusal or poor surgical risks. All three patients were complete responders and disease-free 16 to 29 months after PDT. Eleven patients underwent resection after PDT. Of these 11 patients, 4 were complete responses (total complete responses, 50%), 1 was a partial response, and 6 were considered to have had significant remission of tumor. The reasons given for not having achieved complete responses were: difficult illumination angles because of the location of the tumor (three cases), overlooking an accessory lesion (one case), technical failure (one case), submucosal growth (one case), and light obstruction by gastric folds (one case). Okuda and co-workers, using a dose range from 54 to 117 J/cm^2, treated five patients with early- and one with advanced-stage gastric carcinoma.[114] Complete response was achieved in four of five early-stage lesions, the remaining patient was considered a partial response. The advanced-stage lesion was treated twice (40 and 52 J/cm^2), only a minimal response was noted. Spinelli *et al* treated and recorded a complete response in one patient with early-stage gastric carcinoma.[119] The results from China were much less impressive. Zhonghe and co-workers treated ten patients with gastric carcinoma and saw only one complete response.[120] Eight patients achieved a partial response, and one patient had no response. In this study, power densities of 80 to 250 mW/cm^2, 48 to 72 hr after HPD injection, were used. The extent of tumor was not described. Douglass and associates described tumor responses of gastric carcinoma treated with PDT in four patients.[121]

GYNECOLOGIC TUMORS

Treatment of unifocal, small, low-grade intraepithelial neoplasia of gynecologic origin may be approached by using a diversity of techniques—CO_2 laser vaporization, local excision, cryotherapy, electrocautery, or topical chemotherapy. However, large, multifocal, and higher-grade lesions frequently require extensive surgery because of the invasive potential and recurrence outside of the treated areas. Exenterative surgical treatment of recurrences is unacceptable for many candidates because of perioperative risk. Kyriazis and co-workers, in 1973, used HPD as a diagnostic test to study 20 patients for atypical metaplasia, dysplasia, and carcinoma in situ of the cervix.[122] Seventeen showed positive HPD fluorescence. There were no false-negative results. Of the three patients with negative fluorescence, one had squamous metaplasia, and two had chronic cervicitis. Ten years later Soma and Nutahara used PDT to treat 12 cases of gynecologic malignancies (Table 66-14): five carcinomas in situ of the cervix, four vaginal carcinomas, and three cancers of the vulva.[123] Optical fibers delivered 90 to 346 J/cm^2 at a power density of 100 to 400 mW/cm^2. A 58% complete response was recorded. Rettenmaier and colleagues treated six cases of recurrent gynecologic cancers.[124] Two complete and three partial responses were recorded. In addition to these recurrences, three premalignant lesions (one vaginal and two vulvar intraepithelial neoplasia) refractory to conventional therapy were treated with laser light after having had topical HPD applied. Of these premalignant lesions one responded partially, one did not, and in one case no treatment response was recorded.

TABLE 66-13. Use of PDT for Stomach Carcinomas

Patients	*CR (%)*	*PR (%)*	*NR (%)*	*Reference*
14	50	7	43	100
6	66	17	17	115
10	10	80	10	121

TABLE 66-14. Use of PDT for Gynecologic Malignancies

Patients	*CR (%)*	*PR (%)*	*NR (%)*	*Reference*
12	58	?	?	123
6	33	50	17	124

BRAIN

Wise and Taxdall first illustrated that HPD is retained in cerebral lesions and excluded in normal brain,[125] and Diamond and associates in 1972, first used PDT to treat a transplanted glioma.[126] Since 1978, 64 patients with cerebral tumors have been treated with PDT.[127] In 1980, Perria and co-workers reported their results in nine patients treated (three glioblastoma, five astrocytoma, one sarcoma) with PDT.[128] Patients received 2.5 to 10.0 mg/kg HPD 24 to 96 hr before surgical resection of the tumor. After bulk tumor resection, the bed was treated with 9 J/cm^2. Tumor necrosis was apparent, yet there was no improvement in survival. Laws *et al* treated five patients with recurrent glioblastoma with 5 mg/kg HPD and light doses of 500 to 1260 J/cm^2, administered after stereotaxic-controlled fiber-optic placement.[129] The interstitial treatment resulted in tumor response but no complete responses, the limitation being lack of light diffusion. McCulloch and associates reported their results in the treatment of four metastatic tumors to the brain (kidney, breast, lung, malignant melanoma), nine glioblastomas, 2 oligodendrogliomas, and one astrocytoma.[130] Forty-eight hours before surgery patients received 5 mg/kg HPD. After having completed conventional neurosurgical resection, visible or microscopic tumors were treated with light doses ranging from 1260 to 2520 J/cm^2. Two of the four patients with metastatic cancer were alive with no CT evidence of tumor at 10 and 16 months. Three of the glioblastoma patients were alive with no evidence of disease at 42, 35, and 2 months. One patient with oligodendroglioma and the other with astrocytoma were alive with no evidence of disease at 10 and 13 months. Although the study is encouraging, the results are clouded by patients receiving postoperative radiotherapy. Furthermore, light sources were changed throughout the study, and in several patients temperature changes from 37° to 45°C were recorded.

CONCLUSION

At this time, PDT appears to provide a therapeutic option for patients requiring treatment of early bladder cancer, early esophageal and gastric cancers, basal cell carcinoma, Kaposi's sarcoma, and early central non–small-cell carcinoma of the lung, as well as obstructing lung and metastatic lesions to the tracheobronchial tree. There also appears to be a role for treatment of certain recurrent breast cancers to the chest, as well as early accessible primary gynecologic cancers. The modality may have a use in clearing macro- and microscopic cancer from the borders of surgical fields. The use of PDT in the treatment of other sites, such as the abdominal and thoracic cavities, may extend PDT to the treatment of pleural and abdominal carcinomatosis. There is the promise that alternative sensitizers will extend the use of PDT to more deeply seated tumors, and the use of chemiluminescent materials as light delivery systems may allow access to the central nervous system, as well as provide more uniform light distribution to cavitary spaces. The major impact of this modality may well await a further understanding of the tumor retentive properties of photosensitizers. Efforts by the NIH Drug Development Branch are underway to standardize and allow access to promising new photosensitizers to be used with PDT. Such efforts should allow better interstudy comparisons. As the field of PDT progresses, more stringent standardized documentation of patient selection criteria, treatment variables, results, and follow-up will be forthcoming. Trials, such as the controlled randomized study currently underway in the United States for endobronchial and bladder carcinoma, will lead PDT into the mainstream of cancer treatment. And lastly, as with radiation therapy, the requirements of lasers and optical dosimetry may well restrict PDT to larger institutions at which optics, electronics, and bioengineering support is available.

REFERENCES

1. Raab O: Uber die Wirkung Fluoreszierenden Stoffen. Infusoria Z Biol 39:524, 1900
2. Jesionek A, Tappeiner VH: Zur Behandlung der Hautcarcinomit mit Fluorescierenden Stoffen. Muench Med Wochenshr 47:2042, 1903
3. Spikes JD, Straight R: Sensitized photochemical processes in biological systems. Annu Rev Phys Chem 18:409, 1967
4. Hausmann W: Die sensibilisierende Wirkung des Hematoporphyrins. Biochem Z 30:276, 1911
5. Auber H, Banger G: Unter Suchungen uber die Rolle der Porphyrine bei geschwulstkranken Menschen und Tieren. Z Krebsforsch 53:65, 1942
6. Figge FHJ, Weiland GS, Manganiello LOJ: Cancer detection and therapy. Affinity of neoplastic embryonic and traumatized tissue for porphyrins and metalloporphyrins. Proc Soc Exp Biol Med 68:640, 1948
7. Lipson RL, Baldes EJ: The photodynamic properties of a particular hematoporphyrin derivative. Arch Dermatol 82:508, 1960
8. Lipson RL, Blades EJ: The use of a derivative of hematoporphyrin in tumor detection. J Natl Cancer Inst 26:1, 1961
9. Lipson RL, Baldes EJ: Hematoporphyrin derivative: A new aid for endoscopic detection of malignant disease. J Thorac Cardiovasc Surg 42:623, 1961
10. Grey M, Lipson RL, Mack JVS et al: Use of hematoporphyrin derivative in detection and management of cervical cancer. Am J Obstrt Gynecol 9:766, 1967
11. Gregorie HG, Horger EO, Ward JL et al: Hematoporphyrin-derivative fluorescence in malignant neoplasm. Ann Surg 167:820, 1968
12. Lipson RL, Gray MJ, Baldes EJ: Hematoporphyrin derivative for detection and management of cancer. Proc 9th Int Cancer Cong, Tokyo, Japan p 393, 1966
13. Kelly JF, Snell NE, Berenbaum MC: Photodynamic destruction of human bladder carcinoma. J Urol 115:150, 176
14. Dougherty RJ: Activated dyes vs anti-tumor agents. J Natl Cancer Inst 51:1333, 1974
15. Dougherty TJ, Grindley GE, Fiel R et al: Photoradiation therapy II. Cure of animal tumors with hematoporphyrin and light. J Natl Cancer Inst 55;115, 1975
16. Dougherty TJ, Kaufman JE, Goldfarb A et al: Photoradiation therapy for the treatment of malignant tumors. Cancer Res 38:2628, 1978
17. Dougherty TJ: Photoradiation therapy. Urol Suppl 23:61, 1984
18. Dougherty TJ: Photosensitizers: Therapy and detection of malignant tumors. Photochem Photobiol 45:874, 1987
19. Fowlks WL: The mechanism of the photodynamic effect. J Invest Dermatol 32;233, 1959
20. Foote CS: Mechanisms of photooxygenation. In Doiron DR, Gomer CJ (eds): Porphyrin Localization and Treatment of Tumors, p 3. New York, Alan R Liss, 1984
21. Weishaupt KR, Gomer CJ, Dougherty TJ: Identification of singlet oxygen as the cytotoxic agent in photoinactivation of 2 murine tumors. Cancer Res 36:2326, 1976
22. Ben-Hur E, Rosenthal I: The phthalocyanines: A new class of mammalian cell photosensitizers with a potential for cancer phototherapy. Int J Radiat Biol 47:145, 1985
23. Sonoda M, Murali-Krishna C, Riesz P: The role of singlet oxygen in the photohemolysis of red blood cells sensitized by phthalocyanine sulfonates. Photochem Photobiol 46:635, 1987
24. Parker JG: Optical detection of the photodynamic production of singlet oxygen in vivo. Laser Surg Med 6:258, 1986
25. Lee See K, Forbes IJ, Betts WH: Oxygen dependency of phototoxicity with haematoporphyrin derivative. Photochem Photobiol 39:631, 1984
26. Mitchell JB, McPherson S, DeGraff W et al: Oxygen dependence of hematoporphyrin derivative-induced photoinactivation of Chinese hamster cells. Cancer Res 45:2008, 1985
27. Moan J, Sommer S: Oxygen dependence of the photosensitizing effect of hematoporphyrin derivative in NHIK 3025 cells. Cancer Res 45:1608, 1985
28. Gomer CJ, Razum NJ: Acute skin response in albino mice following porphyrin photosensitization under oxic and anoxic conditions. Photochem Photobiol 40:435, 1984
29. Powers WE, Tolmach LJ: A multicomponent x-ray survival curve for mouse lymphosarcoma cells irradiated in vivo. Nature 197:710, 1963

30. Thomlinson RH, Gray LH: The histological structure of some human lung cancers and the possible implications for radiotherapy. Br J Cancer 9:539, 1977
31. Dougherty TJ, Potter WR, Weishaupt KR: The structure of the active component of hematoporphyrin derivative. In Doiron DR, Gomer CJ (eds): Porphyrin Localization and Treatment of Tumors, p 301. New York, Alan R Liss, 1984
32. Andreoni A, Cubeddu R, DeSilvestri S et al: Effects of laser irradiation on hematoporphyrin-treated normal transformed thyroid cells in culture. Cancer Res 43:2076, 1983
33. Moan J, Steen HB, Feren K, Christensen T: Uptake of hematoporphyrin derivative and sensitized photoinactivation of C3H cells with different oncogenic potential. Cancer Lett 14;291, 1981
35. Jori GM, Battrammi E, Reddi B et al: Evidence for a major role plasma proteins as hematoporphyrin carriers in vivo. Cancer Lett 33:183, 1984
36. Musser DA, Wagner JM, Datta-Gupta N: The interaction of tumor localizing porphyrins with collagen and elastin. Res Commun Chem Pathol Pharmacol 36:251, 1982
37. Henderson BW, Dougherty TJ, Malone PB: Studies on the mechanism of tumor destruction by photoradiation therapy. In Dorion DR, Gomer CJ (eds): Porphyrin Localization and Treatment, p 601. New York, Alan R Liss, 1984
38. Bugelski PJ, Porter CW, Dougherty TJ: Autoradiographic distribution of hematoporphyrin derivative in normal and tumor tissue. Cancer Res 41:4606, 1981
39. Henderson BW, Waldow SM, Mang TS et al: Tumor destruction and kinetics of tumor cell death in two experimental mouse tumors following photodynamic therapy. Cancer Res 45:572, 1985
40. Moan J: The photochemical yield of singlet oxygen from porphyrins in different states of aggregation. Photochem Photobiol 39:445, 1984
41. Wilson BC, Adam G: A Monte Carlo model for the absorption and flux distribution of light in tissues. Med Phys 10:824, 1983
42. Wilson BC, Patterson MS: The physics of photodynamic therapy. Phys Med Biol 31:327, 1986
43. Kessel D, Chou TH: Tumor-localizing components of the porphyrin preparation hematoporphyrin derivative. Cancer Res 43:1994, 1983
44. Kessel D: Hematoporphyrin and HPD: Photophysics, photochemistry and phototherapy. Photochem Photobiol 39:851, 1984
45. Kessel D: Effects of photoactivated porphyrins at the cell surface of leukemia L1210 cells. Biochemistry 16:3443, 1977
46. Belliner DA, Dougherty TJ: Membrane lysis in Chinese hamster ovary cells treated with hematoporphyrin derivative plus light. Photochem Photobiol 36:43, 1982
47. Christensen T, Moan J, Smedshammer L et al: Influence of hematoporphyrin derivative (HPD) and light on the attachment of cells to the substratum. Photochem Photobiophys 10:53, 1985
48. Denstaman SC, Dillehay LE, Williams JR: Enhanced susceptibility to HPD-sensitized phototoxicity and correlated resistance to trypsin detachment in SV40 transformed IMR-90 cell. Photobiochem Photobiol 43:145, 1986
49. Volden G, Christensen T, Moan J: Photodynamic membrane damage of hematoporphyrin derivative-treated NHIK 3025 cells in vitro. Photobiochem Photobiophys 3:105, 1981
50. Jewell SA, Bellomo G, Thor H et al: Bleb formation in hepatocytes during drug metabolism is caused by disturbances in thiol and calcium ion homeostasis. Science 217:1257, 1982
51. Borrelli MJ, Wong RSL, Dewey WC: A direct correlation between hyperthermia-induced blebbing and survival in synchronous G_1 CHO cells. J Cell Physiol 126:181, 1986
52. Dubbelman TMAR, Smeets M, Boegheim JPJ: Cell models. In Moreno G, Potter RH, Truscott TG (eds): Photosensitization: Molecular and Medical Aspects NATO AST series (in press).
53. Hilf R, Murant RS, Narayanan U, Gibson SL: Hematoporphyrin derivative-induced photosensitivity of mitochondrial succinate dehydrogenase and selected cytosolic enzymes of R3230AC mammary adenocarcinomas of rats. Cancer Res 44:1483, 1984
54. Hilf R, Murant RS, Narayanan U, Gibson SL: Relationship of mitochondrial function and cellular adenosine triphosphate levels to hematoporphyrin derivative-induced photosensitization in R3230AC mammary tumors. Cancer Res 46:211, 1986
55. Gomer CJ: DNA damage and repair in CHO cells following hematoporphyrin photoradiation. Cancer Lett 11:161, 1980
56. Moan J, Waksvik H, Christensen T: DNA single-stand breaks and sister chromatid exchanges induced by treatment with hematoporphyrin and light or by x-rays in human NHIK 3025 cells. Cancer Res 40:2915, 1980
57. Mitchell JB, Russo A, Kinsella TJ, Glatstein E: The use of non-hypoxic cell sensitizers in radiobiology and radiotherapy. Int J Radiat Oncol Biol Phys 12:1513, 1986
58. Russo A, DeGraff W, Kinsella TJ et al: Potentiation of chemotherapy cytotoxicity following iododeoxyuridine incorporation in Chinese hamster cells. Int J Radiat Oncol Biol Phys 12:1417, 1986
59. Gomer CJ, Rucker N, Banerjee A, Benedict WF: Comparison of mutagenicity and induction of sister chromatid exchange in Chinese hamster cells exposed to hematoporphyrin derivative, ionizing radiation, or ultraviolet radiation. Cancer Res 43:2662, 1983
60. Ben-Hur E, Fujihara T, Suzuki F, Elkind MM: Genetic toxicology of the photosensitization of Chinese hamster cells by phthalocyanines. Photochem Photobiol 45:227, 1987
61. Kessel D: Sites of photosensitization by derivatives of hematoporphyrin. Photochem Photobiol 44:489, 1986
62. Gomer CJ, Dougherty TJ: Determination of [^{3}H]- and [^{14}C]hematoporphyrin derivative distribution in malignant and normal tissue. Cancer Res 39:146, 1979
63. Wharen REJ, Anderson RE, Laws ERJ: Quantization of hematoporphyrin derivative in human gliomas, experimental central nervous system tumors and normal tissues. Neurosurgery 12:446, 1983
64. Tochner Z, Mitchell JB, Smith P et al: Photodynamic therapy of ascites tumours within the peritoneal cavity. Br J Cancer 53:733, 1986
65. Kaye AH, Morstyn G, Ashcroft RG: Uptake and retention of hematoporphyrin derivative in an in vivo/in vitro model of cerebral glioma. Neurosurgery 17:883, 1985
66. Manyak MJ, Nelson LM, Stillman RJ et al: Fluorescent detection of endometriosis with HPD and light. Soc Gyncol Invest, Baltimore, 1988
67. Fuller TA: Fundamentals of lasers in surgery and medicine. In Dixon (ed): Surgical Application of Lasers, p 11. Chicago, Year Book Medical Publisher, 1983
68. Cowled PA, Grace JR, Forbes IJ: Comparison of the efficacy of pulsed and continuous wave red laser light in induction of phototoxicity by hematoporphyrin derivative. Photochem Photobiol 39:115, 1984
69. Pottier R, Truscott TG: The photochemistry of hematoporphyrin and related systems. Int J Radiat Biol 50:421, 1986
70. Russo V, Righini G, Trigari S: Side radiation fibers for medical applications. In Andreoni A, Cubedda R (eds): Porphyrin in Tumor Phototherapy, p 309. New York, Plenum Press, 1983
71. Russo V, Tighini G, Scottini S et al: Lens-ended fibers for medical applications: A new fabrication technique. Appl Optics 23:3277, 1984
72. Kennedy J: HPD photoradiation therapy for cancer at Kingston and Hamilton. In Kessel D, Dougherty TJ (eds): Porphyrin Photosensitization, p 53. New York, Plenum Press, 1983
73. Tokuda Y: Primary skin cancer. In Hayata Y and Dougherty TJ (eds): Lasers and Hematoporphyrin Derivative in Cancer, p 88. Tokyo, Igaku-Shoin, 1983
74. Tomio L, Calzavara F, Zorat PL et al: Photoradiation therapy for cutaneous and subcutaneous malignant tumors using hematoporphyrins. In Dorion DR, Gomer CJ (eds): Porphyrin Localization and Treatment of Tumors, p 829. New York, Alan R Liss, 1984
75. Dougherty TJ: Photosensitization of malignant tumors. Semin Surg Oncol 2:24, 1986
76. Wile AG, Coffey J, Nahabedian MY et al: Laser photoradiation therapy of cancer: An update of the experience at the University of California, Irvine. Lasers Surg Med 4:5, 1984
77. Bern MW, Wile AG: Hematoporphyrin phototherapy of cancer. Radiother Oncol 7:233, 1986
78. Delaney T, Bonner R, Smith P: Photodynamic therapy for surface malignancies: Clinical results with blood flow effects secondary to photoirradiation. Int J Radiat Oncol, Biol, Phys 13:186, 1987
79. Kennedy JC, Oswald K: Hematoporphyrin derivative photoradiation therapy in theory and practice. In Andrioni A, Cubedda R (eds): Porphyrin in Tumor Phototherapy, p. 365. New York, Plenum Press, 1983
80. Zorat PL, Romio L, Corti L et al: Hematoporphyrin phototherapy of malignant tumors. In Andreoni A, Cubedda R (eds): Porphyrins in Tumor Phototherapy, p. 381. New York, Plenum Press, 1983
81. Dougherty TJ, Lawrence G, Kaufman JH et al: Photoradiation in the treatment of recurrent breast carcinoma. J Natl Cancer Inst 62:231, 1979
82. Forbes IJ, Cowled PA, Leong AS-Y et al: Phototherapy of human tumors using hematoporphyrin derivative. Med J Aust 2:489, 1980
83. Forbes IJ, Ward AD, Jacka FJ et al: Multidisciplinary approach to phototherapy of human tumors. In Doiron DR, Gomer CJ (eds): Porphyrin Localization and Treatment of Tumors, p 693. New York, Alan R Liss, 1984
84. Konaka C, Ono J: Skin metastases from breast cancer. In Hayata Y, Dougherty TJ (eds): Lasers and Hematoporphyrin Derivative in Cancer, p 11. Tokyo, Igaka-Shion, 1983
85. Taketa C, Imakiira M: Cancer of the ear, nose, and throat. In Hayata Y, Dougherty TJ (eds): Lasers and Hematoporphyrin Derivatives in Cancer, p 70. Tokyo, Igaka-Shion, 1983
86. Dougherty TJ: Excerpts from photodynamic therapy workshop, Western Institute for Laser Treatment, Santa Barbara, Calif. Oct, 1984
87. Schuller DE, McCaughan JS Jr, Rock RP: Photodynamic therapy in head and neck cancer. Arch Otolaryngol 111:351, 1984
88. Benson RC Jr, Farrow GM, Kinsey JH et al: Detection and localization of in site carcinoma of the bladder with hematoporphyrin derivative. Mayo Clin Proc 57:548, 1982
89. Tsuchiya A, Obara N, Miwa M: Hematoporphyrin derivative and photoradiation in the diagnosis and treatment of bladder cancer. J Urol 130:79, 1983
90. Benson RC, Kinsey JH, Cortese DA et al: Treatment of transitional cell carcinoma of the bladder with hematoporphyrin derivative phototherapy. J Urol 130:1090, 1983
91. Hisazumi H, Miyoshi N, Naito K et al: Whole bladder wall photoradiation therapy for carcinoma in the site of the bladder: A preliminary report. J Urol 131:884, 1984
92. Benson RC Jr: Treatment of diffuse transitional cell carcinoma in situ by whole bladder hematoporphyrin derivative photodynamic therapy. J Urol 134:675, 1985
93. Jocham D, Unsold E, Staehler G: Use of light dispersion medium for an integrated dye laser therapy of bladder tumors after photosensitization with hematoporphyrin derivative. In Doiron D, Gomer CJ (eds): Porphyrin Localization and Treatment of Tumors, p 249. New York, Alan R Liss, 1984
94. Nseyo UO, Wolf R, Dougherty TJ: Whole bladder photodynamic therapy for transitional carcinoma of bladder. Urology 26:274, 1985
95. Misaki T, Hisazumi H, Miyoshi N: Photoradiation therapy of bladder tumors. In Dorion DR, Gomer CJ (eds): Porphyrin Localization and Treatment of Tumors, p 785. New York, Alan R Liss, 1984
96. Shumaker BP, Hetzel FW: The practical use of laser photodynamic therapy in the

treatment of bladder carcinoma. Presented at the Clayton Foundation Conference on Photodynamic Therapy, Los Angeles, Calif, Feb 18, 1987
97. Prout GR Jr, Lin C-I, Benson R Jr et al: Photodynamic therapy with hematoporphyrin derivative in the treatment of superficial transitional-cell carcinoma of the bladder. N Engl J Med 317:1251, 1987
98. Cortese D: Endobronchial management of lung cancer. Chest 89:234S, 1986
99. Hayata Y, Kato H, Konaka C et al: Photoradiation therapy in early stage cancer of the lung, esophagus, and stomach. In Andreoni A, Cubedda R (eds): Porphyrin in Tumor Phototherapy, p 405. New York, Plenum Press, 1983
100. Kato H, Konaka C, Ono J et al: Effectiveness of HPD and radiation therapy in lung cancer. In Kessel D, Dougherty TJ (eds): Porphyrin Photosensitization, p 23. New York, Plenum Press, 1983
101. Kato H: Lung cancer. In Hayata Y, Dougherty TJ (eds): Lasers and Hematoporphyrin Derivative in Cancer, p 39. Tokyo, Igaka-Shion, 1983
102. Kato H, Konaka C, Ono J et al: Preoperative laser photodynamic therapy in combination with operative lung cancer. J Thorac Cardiovas Surg 90:420, 1985
103. Kato H, Konaka C, Kawate N et al: Five-year disease-free survival of a lung cancer patient only by photodynamic therapy. Chest 90:768, 1986
104. Hayata Y, Kato H, Konaka C et al: Photodynamic therapy in early stage lung cancer. Presented at Clayton Foundation Conference on Photodynamic Therapy, Los Angeles, Calif, Feb 15, 1987
105. Edsell ES, Cortese DA: Bronchoscopic phototherapy with hematoporphyrin derivative for treatment of localized bronchogenic carcinoma: A 5-year experience. Mayo Clin Proc 62:8, 1987
106. Dorion DR, Balchum OJ: Hematoporphyrin derivative photoradiation therapy of endobronchial lung cancer. In Andreoni A, Cubedda R (eds): Porphyrin in Tumor Phototherapy, p 195. New York, Plenum Press, 1983
107. Balchum OJ, Dorion DR, Huth GC: Photodynamic therapy obstructing lung cancer. In Dorion D, Gomer CJ (eds): Porphyrin Localization and Treatment of Tumors, p 721. Alan R Liss, 1984
108. Balchum OJ, Dorion DR, Huth GC: Photoradiation therapy of endobronchial lung cancers employing the photodynamic action of hematoporphrin derivative. Laser Surg Med 4:13, 1984
109. Balchum OJ: Photodynamic therapy (PDT) of endobronchial lung tumors. Presented at Clayton Foundation Conference on Photodynamic Therapy, Los Angeles, Calif, Feb 15, 1987
110. Lin JH, Chen Y-P, Zhao SD et al: Application of hematoporphyrin and laser induced photodynamic reaction in the treatment of lung cancer: A preliminary report on 21 cases. Lasers Surg Med 4:31, 1984
111. Vincent RG, Dougherty TJ, Rao U et al: Photoradiation therapy in the treatment of advanced carcinoma of the trachea and bronchus. In Dorion DR, Gomer CJ (eds): Porphyrin Localization and Treatment of Tumors, p 759. New York, Alan R Liss, 1984
112. Forbes IJ, Ward AD, Jacka FJ et al: Multidisciplinary approach to phototherapy in tumors. In Doiron DR, Gomer CJ (eds): Porphyrin Localization and Treatment of Tumors, p 759. New York, Alan R Liss, 1984
113. Lam S, Kostashuk EC, Coy P et al: A randomized comparative study of the safety and efficacy of photodynamic therapy using Photofrin II combined with palliative radiotherapy versus palliative radiotherapy alone in patients with inoperable non-small bronchogenic carcinoma: A preliminary report. Presented at Clayton Foundation Conference on Photodynamic Therapy, Los Angeles, Calif, Feb 15, 1987
114. Okuda S, Mimura S, Otani T et al: Experimental and clinical studies on HPD-photoradiation therapy for upper gastrointestinal cancers. In Andreoni A, Cubedda R (eds): Porphyrin in Tumor Phototherapy, p 413. New York, Plenum Press, 1983
115. Corti L, Tomio F, Calzavara F et al: Evaluation of hematoporphyrin photodynamic therapy to treat malignant tumors. In Jori G, Perria C (eds): Photodynamic Therapy of Tumors and Diseases, p 317. Podova, Italy, Libreria, 1985
116. McCaughan JS, Hicks W, Laufman L et al: Palliation of esophageal malignancies with photoradiation therapy. Cancer 54:2905, 1984
117. Thomas RJ, Abbott M, Bhathal PS et al: High dose radiation of esophageal cancer. Ann Surg 206:193, 1987
118. Tomio L, Calzavara F, Corti L et al: Photodynamic therapy in the treatment of malignant tumors of the upper aerodigestive tract. Presented at Clayton Foundation Conference on Photodynamic Therapy, Los Angeles, Calif, Feb 15, 1987
119. Spinelli P, Andreola S, Marchesini R et al: Endoscopic HPD-laser photoradiation (PRT) of cancer. In Andreoni A, Cubedda R (eds): Porphyrin in Tumor Phototherapy, p 423. New York, Plenum Press, 1983
120. Zhonge G, Yingcai H, Zangmin W: Evaluation of photoirradiation therapy (PRT) in 20 cases of cancers. In Andreoni A, Cubedda R (eds): Porphyrin in Tumor Phototherapy, p 375. New York, Plenum Press, 1983
121. Douglass HO, Nava HR, Weishaupt KR et al: Intra-abdominal applications of hematoporphyrin photoradiation therapy. In Kessel D, Dougherty TJ (eds): Porphyrin Photosensitization, p 15. New York, Plenum Press, 1983
122. Kyriazis GA, Balin H, Lipson RL: Hematoporphyrin-derivative-fluorescence test colposcopy and colpophotography in the diagnosis of atypical metaplasia, dysplasia, and carcinoma in situ of the cervic uteri. Am J Obstret Gynecol 117:375, 1973
123. Soma H, Nutahara S: Cancer of the female genitalia. In Hayata Y, Dougherty TJ (eds): Lasers and Hematoporphyrin Derivatives in Cancer, p 97. Tokyo, Igaka-Shion, 1983
124. Rettenmaier MA, Berman ML, Disaia PJ et al: Gynecologic uses of photoradiation therapy. In Doiron DR, Gomer CJ (eds): Porphyrin Localization and Treatment of Tumors, p 767. New York, Alan R Liss, 1984
125. Wise BL, Taxdal DR: Studies of the blood brain barrier utilizing hematoporphyrin. Brain Res 4:387, 1967
126. Diamond I, Granelli S, McDonagu AF et al: Photodynamic therapy of malignant tumors. Lancet 2:1175, 1972
127. Kaye AH, Morstyn G, Apuzzo M: Photoradiation therapy and its potential in the management of neurological tumors. J Neurosurg 69:1, 1988
128. Perria C, Capuzzo T, Cavagnaro G et al: First attempts at the photodynamic treatment of human gliomas. J Neurosurg Sci 24:119, 1980
129. Laws ER, Cortese DA, Kinsey JH et al: Photoradiation in the treatment of malignant brain tumors: A Phase I (feasibility) study. Neurosurgery 9:672, 1981
130. McCulloch GAJ, Forbes IJ, Lee See K et al: Phototherapy in malignant brain tumors. In Dorion DR, Gomer CJ (eds): Porphyrin Localization and Treatment of Tumors, p 709. New York, Alan R Liss, 1984

SECTION 5

THOMAS W. GRIFFIN

Particle Beam Radiation Therapy

Over the last two decades, advances in the field of radiation oncology have resulted in a substantial improvement in the outlook for patients with various malignancies. This improvement has been largely due to an increased understanding of the biology of the disease process and to the development of machines capable of optimizing radiation dose distributions. Nevertheless, there are still many patients in whom failure to control local disease contributes materially to death. For the reasons outlined in the following pages, heavy particle beam radiation therapy might be expected to offer a therapeutic gain, compared with conventional photon and electron beam therapy, in the management of these patients.

Currently, the following heavy particle beams are being clinically tested: fast neutrons, protons, helium ions, heavy ions [carbon (C), neon (Ne), argon (Ar)], and negative pions. Fast neutrons are being investigated because they have radiobiologic properties that potentially are superior to those of conventional x-rays and gamma rays. Protons and helium ions are being studied because the dose distributions that may be achieved with these particles are superior in many clinical situations to those obtainable with photons or electrons. Heavy ions and pions have both a potential biologic advantage and a dose distribution advantage.

BIOLOGIC EFFECTS OF PARTICLE BEAMS

The biologic effects of a radiation beam depend on the spatial distribution of the ionizing events produced in tissue. The rate at which charged particles deposit energy per unit distance is known as the *linear energy transfer* (LET), expressed in keV/μm. Protons, helium ions, electrons, and photons are sparsely ionizing, characterized by a low LET. Conversely, fast neutrons, heavy ions, and pions are densely ionizing and are referred to as high LET radiations.

Review of the possible causes of treatment failure in various cancers with conventional radiation therapy suggests that there are major areas in which neutrons and other high LET radiations may offer a biologic advantage.

TUMOR CELL HYPOXIA

Numerous studies in many biologic systems have shown that hypoxic cells are significantly more resistant to the effects of x-irradiation and gamma irradiation than are well-oxygenated cells. Whereas cells in most normal tissues are well oxygenated, most solid tumors are thought to have hypoxic regions, that have outgrown their vascular supply. It has been postulated that these cells, nevertheless, remain viable and provide a focus for local tumor recurrence.[1]

The *oxygen enhancement ratio* (OER) is defined as the ratio of the dose of radiation required to produce a specified biologic effect under anoxic conditions to the dose required to produce the same effect under well-oxygenated conditions. With photons, the OER for most mammalian cells is 2.5 to 3.0. With neutrons, heavy charged particles, or pions, the OER is significantly smaller (1.4 to 1.7) and, therefore, the protection conferred on tumor cells by hypoxia is diminished. Figure 66-24 illustrates survival curves for Chinese hamster ovary cells irradiated with ^{60}Co gamma rays or 50-MeV neutrons (from deuteron-on-beryllium reactions). The OER for neutrons is 1.4, appreciably improved over the value of 2.4 for ^{60}Co gamma rays.

In practice, the clinical advantage of high LET radiation may be less than that suggested by this difference in OER. Not all tumor cells are severely hypoxic, and reoxygenation may occur during intervals between dose fractions, diminishing the influence of hypoxic cells on tumor recurrence.

RELATIVE BIOLOGIC EFFECTIVENESS

The *relative biologic effectiveness* (RBE) of an ionizing radiation is the ratio of the dose of that radiation compared with the dose of a reference radiation required to produce a specific endpoint in a specific tissue.

A potential area of therapeutic gain from high LET radiation exists when tumor cells are relatively radioresistant because of increased capacity to accumulate sublethal radiation injury. This situation is reflected in a wide shoulder for the tumor cell survival curve. With neutrons and other high LET radiation, most cell killing results from single lethal events, leading to survival curves that are almost exponential in the range of clinical relevance (Fig. 66-25). Tumors characterized by a large capacity to accumulate and repair sublethal radiation injury should have a higher RBE for neutrons than for normal tissue.[2] It should be noted, however, that Howlett and others have shown that RBEs of neutrons for different experimental tumors vary considerably, and no general statement about which types of tumors are best treated with high LET radiation can be made at present.[3]

FIG. 66-24. Survival curves for Chinese hamster ovary (CHO) cells irradiated with ^{60}Co gamma rays or 50 MeV d⇒Be fast neutrons under aerated and anoxic conditions. At the survival level illustrated, the OER for neutrons is 1.4 compared with 2.4 for ^{60}Co gamma rays.

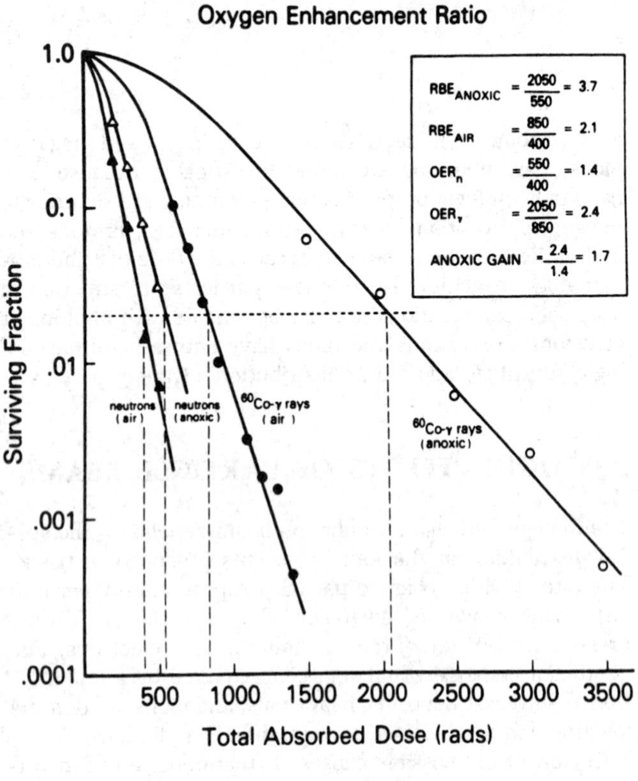

FIG. 66-25. Survival curves for CHO cells exposed to ^{60}Co gamma rays or 50 MeV d⇒Be fast neutrons, illustrating the increase in RBE with decreasing dose per fraction. With fast neutron irradiation, most cell killing results from single-hit lethal events, leading to survival curves with little or no shoulder.

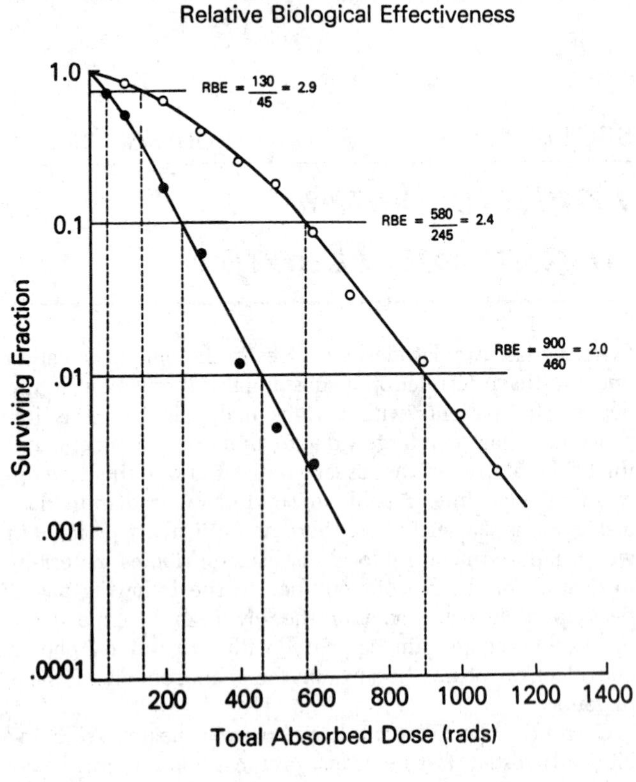

TUMOR CELL KINETICS

Because of the variation in radiosensitivity between cells in different stages of the cell cycle, redistribution between dose fractions results in an effective sensitization of proliferating cells that is not shared by nonproliferating normal cells. The latter are probably responsible for late radiation sequelae, which are the usual dose-limiting factors in radiation therapy. The cell cycle-dependent variation of radiosensitivity is similar for neutrons and gamma rays, but the magnitude of the difference is smaller for neutrons (Fig. 66-26).[4] Whether or not this property constitutes a therapeutic advantage for high LET radiation cannot be predicted. Tumors whose cells redistribute poorly or whose spectrum is demonstrated by cells in resistant phases would be more effectively treated with high LET radiation.

REPAIR OF POTENTIALLY LETHAL DAMAGE

The recovery from potentially lethal damage occurs over a period of hours in cells irradiated in vitro when the postirradiation conditions are suboptimal for growth. Repair of potentially lethal damage occurs after x-irradiation and gamma irradiation but is observed less frequently after neutron irradiation (Fig. 66-27).[5] If, as has been suggested by Hall and Kraljevic, potentially lethal damage repair after x-irradiation and gamma irradiation occurs in nutritionally deprived tumor cells but not in normal tissue cells, then the use of high LET beams would be therapeutically advantageous.[6]

FIG. 66-26. Survival curves for synchronized CHO cells irradiated with ^{60}Co gamma rays or 50 MeV d⇒Be fast neutrons illustrating the variation in radiosensitivity with the position in the cell cycle. The cells were irradiated in three different positions in the cell cycle: mitosis, late G1/early S, and mid-to-late S phase. The cell cycle-dependent variation in radiation sensitivity is qualitatively similar for neutrons and gamma rays, but the magnitude of the variation is reduced by a factor of four for neutrons.

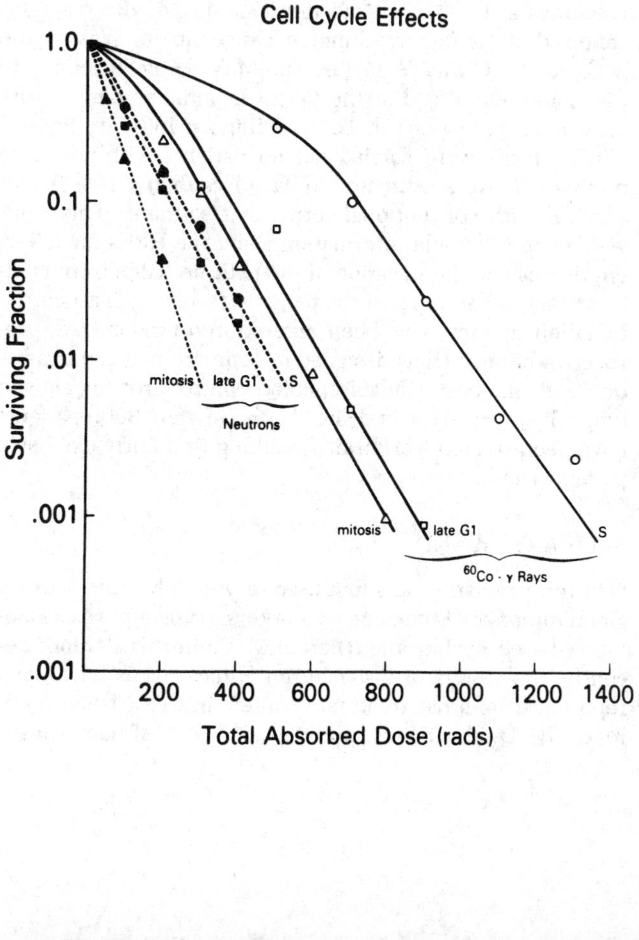

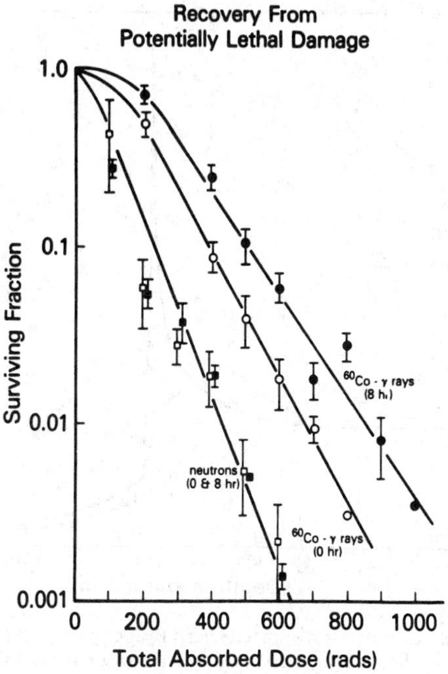

FIG. 66-27. Potentially lethal damage: survival curves for plateau-phase CHO cells irradiated with ^{60}Co gamma rays (*circles*) or 50 MeV d⇒Be fast neutrons (*squares*) and plated either immediately (*open symbols*) or 8 hours after irradiation (*closed symbols*). Repair of potentially lethal damage occurs after irradiation with gamma rays but is not observed after neutron irradiation.

PHYSICAL EFFECTS OF PARTICLE BEAMS

Fast neutron beams can be generated for radiation therapy either by bombarding a target containing tritium (T) with accelerated deuterium (D) ions in a D–T generator or by bombarding a suitable target such as beryllium (Be) with protons (p) or deuterons (d) accelerated in a cyclotron or linear accelerator. The D–T generator produces a monoenergetic 14-MeV neutron beam, whereas the proton-on-beryllium (p→be) reactions produce neutron beams with a spectrum of energies. High-energy particle accelerators are required to produce medically useful heavy charged particle treatment beams.

Neutrons have no dose distribution advantages over photons, whereas protons, helium ions, heavy ions, and negative pions all have significant dose distribution advantages over conventional photons and electrons. These charged particles have a preferential deposition of energy and a more effective destruction of tumor cells near the end of their path. By appropriate determination of range (or path length) in tissue and by spreading of the peak area, the high-effect region

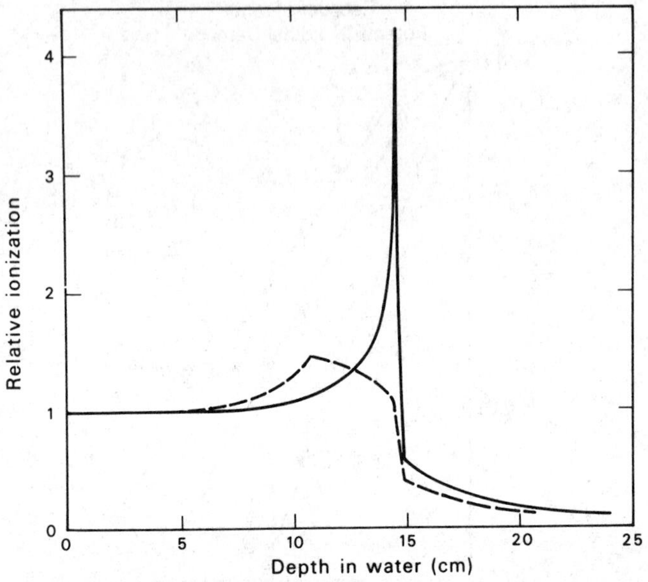

FIG. 66-28. Comparison of usual sharp Bragg peak (*solid curve*) and spread (modified) Bragg peak (*dashed curve*) used for radiation therapy. The dimensions and depth in tissue of the spread Bragg peak can be modified as appropriate for the clinical target volume.

(called the *spread Bragg peak*) can be made to correspond to the target volume (Fig. 66-28).

The effects of heavy particles in tissues and tumors are complex and are a function of the energy, weight, velocity, and track structure of the accelerated particle and the technique of beam delivery. Figure 66-29 shows a comparison of the physical parameters of the clinically useful heavy particles. Figure 66-30 illustrates both the biologic and physical characteristics of these particles.

FIG. 66-29. Comparison of depth dose (spread peak curves) for various charged particles of clinical interest.

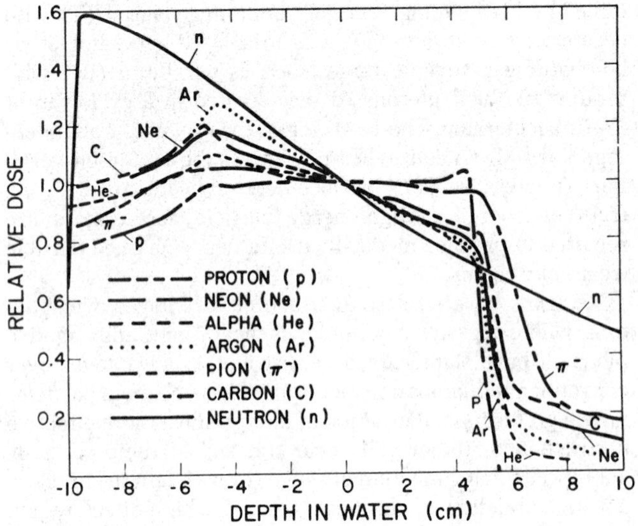

FAST NEUTRON CLINICAL STUDIES

Fast neutron radiation therapy dates back to the 1940s, when Stone used a neutron beam to treat patients with various advanced malignancies.[7] Almost all of the long-term survivors from that clinical trial had severe radiation sequelae in the normal tissue surrounding the tumor sites. This effect was initially interpreted as being due to an increased RBE for late effects as compared with acute effects, and it deterred further clinical investigation of high LET radiation for approximately 20 years. In the 1950s, mammalian cell culture techniques were developed, and it became apparent that the shapes of postirradiation cell survival curves were very different for high-energy photons and fast neutrons. This difference demonstrated that the clinically used neutron fraction sizes corresponded to much higher RBEs than were extrapolated from the large-dose increment animal model studies before Stone's clinical work. Hence, nearly all of Stone's patients with serious radiation sequelae had inadvertently received extremely high radiation doses.

Clinical trials were first resumed at Hammersmith Hospital in London in the 1960s. After several hundred patients with extensive cancer were treated, it was concluded that fast neutron radiation therapy was well tolerated and that many advanced malignancies responded amazingly well to fast neutron irradiation.[8,9] On the basis of these very encouraging results, various centers throughout the world again began clinical trials with fast neutrons.[10] In the United States, patient treatments were started in 1972 at the M. D. Anderson Hospital, using the Texas A&M University variable energy cyclotron (50-MeV d→Be reaction). Clinical trials were next instituted at the University of Washington, using a fixed energy cyclotron (22-MeV d→Be reaction), in 1973. Additional patients were treated on physics laboratory-based machines at the MANTA facility (35-MeV d→Be reaction) centered at George Washington University in Washington D.C., at the GLANTA facility (25-MeV d→Be reaction) in Cleveland, Ohio, and at the Fermi Laboratory facility (66-MeV p→Be reaction) in Batavia, Illinois. Initially, Phase I clinical trials were carried out on patients with advanced tumors who were estimated to have less than a 10% 5-year survival with conventional forms of treatment. This work yielded considerable information about the RBEs for different tissues and the variation of the neutron RBEs from facility to facility. More recently, patients receiving fast neutron radiation therapy have been entered into randomized, prospective clinical trials designed to compare neutron irradiation with the best available photon control arm for a given tumor histologic type and site. Approximately 8000 patients have been treated worldwide, resulting in a fairly extensive patient data base.

SALIVARY GLAND

Neutron irradiation was first used to treat advanced salivary gland tumors by Stone and co-workers, using a physics laboratory-based cyclotron in Berkeley, California.[11] More recently, the results of fast neutron clinical trials have been reported from other treatment centers in Great Britain, Europe, the United States, and Japan.[8,9,12–19] Although insti-

HIGH LET ADVANTAGE ??	Protons	Helium	Pions	Neutrons	Heavy Ions C	Heavy Ions Ne	Heavy Ions Si	Heavy Ions Ar
PHYSICAL DEPTH-DOSE	+++	+++	+++	no	+++	+++	++	+
RBE	no	+	+	++	++	++	+++	+++
OER	no	+	+	+++	+	++	+++	+++

FIG. 66-30. Comparison of relative physical and biologic parameters of particles in clinical use.

tuted on a more-or-less empirical basis, these results have been consistently encouraging, and it has been suggested that salivary gland tumors are much more responsive to neutrons than to photons.[13] The radiobiology results strongly support this conclusion.

The first radiobiologic evidence that neutrons should be particularly effective in the treatment of salivary gland tumors came from Batterman and associates.[20] Batterman and co-workers measured the RBE of neutrons produced by a d→T reaction relative to ^{60}Co radiation using human tumors metastatic to the lung. They determined the RBE for growth delay in terms of the time required for tumor mass to return to its preirradiation volume as evaluated on serial radiographs. Patients having two or more metastases had lesions simultaneously treated with the two types of radiation. The RBE for adenoidcystic carcinoma was 5.7 for a single radiation dose and 8.0 for fractionated radiation, such as would correspond to clinical treatment schemes. The RBEs for most other tumors were in the range of 2.5 to 4.0.

On the basis of the encouraging results from earlier nonrandom clinical trials, and the strong supporting evidence from Dr. Batterman's radiobiology studies, the Radiation Therapy Oncology Group (RTOG) in the United States and the Medical Research Council (MRC) of Great Britain sponsored a prospective, randomized study comparing fast neutron irradiation with low LET photon or electron treatment of inoperable malignant salivary gland tumors.

A total of 32 patients were entered into this study. Twenty-five were entered from the United States and seven were entered from Scotland. Seventeen patients were randomized to receive neutrons and 15 were randomized to receive standard photon or electron radiation therapy, or both. Sixty-one percent of the neutron-treated patients and 75% of the photon-treated patients presented with inoperable or unresectable primary tumors, whereas 39% of the neutron-treated and 25% of the photon-treated patients presented with unresectable recurrent disease. The minimum follow-up period at the time of this analysis is 2 years.

The complete tumor clearance rates at the primary site were 85% for neutrons and 33% for photons following protocol treatment ($p = 0.01$). The complete tumor clearance rates in the cervical lymph nodes were 86% for neutrons and 25% for photons. The overall locoregional complete tumor response rates were 85% and 33% for neutrons and photons, respectively (Fig. 66-31). The locoregional control rates at 2

FIG. 66-31. Complete response rates for neutron-treated and photon-treated patients. The difference is statistically significant at the $p = 0.01$ level.

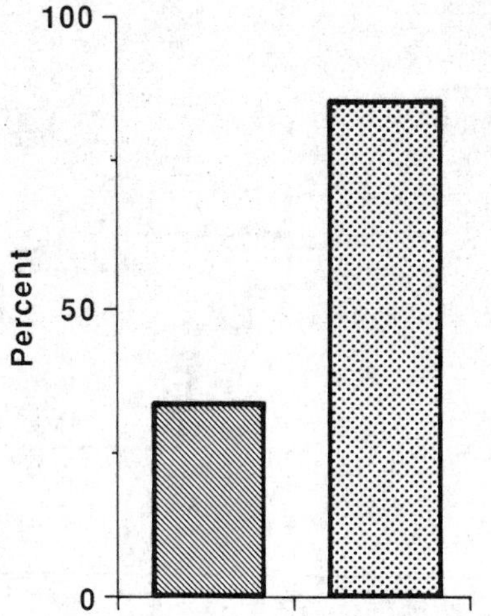

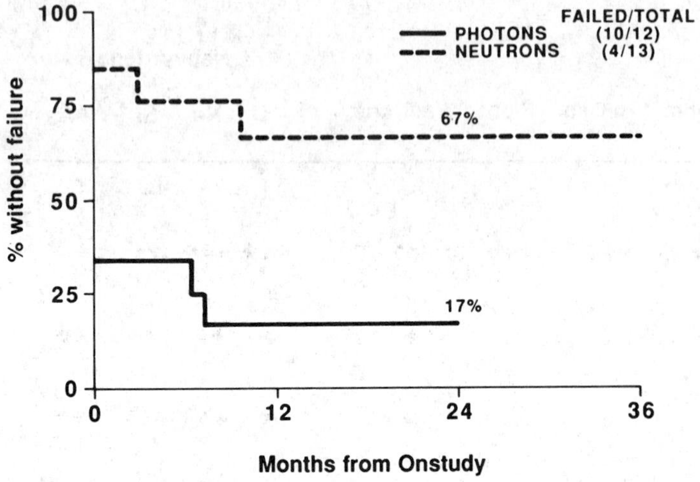

FIG. 66-32. Locoregional tumor control rates for neutron-treated and photon-treated patients. The difference is statistically significant at the $p < 0.005$ level.

years as illustrated in Figure 66-32 for the two groups are 67% for neutrons and 17% for photons ($p < 0.005$). The 2-year survival rates as illustrated in Figure 66-33 are 62% and 25% for neutrons and photons, respectively ($p = 0.10$). There was no significant difference between the normal tissue complication rates of the two groups.

Before this study, the results of neutron treatment of 289 patients with inoperable salivary gland tumors had been reported in the literature. This number excludes patients who were treated for presumed residual disease after surgery. Some of these patients were treated with "mixed beam" treatment (⅖ neutrons, ⅗ photons); others were treated with neutrons alone. Treatment was delivered in 12 to 38 fractions over 4 to 7 weeks. In spite of this variability, the results are remarkably consistent. Table 66-15 lists the reported neutron experience in this tumor system. The composite local control rate is 67% (194/289).[8,9,12-19]

Local tumor control rates following low LET photon and/or electron irradiation for inoperable salivary gland carcinomas are less satisfactory. Table 66-16 lists the photon treatment results in this clinical situation. The composite local control rate following photons in these series is 24% (61/254).[10,16,21-29]

Table 66-17 compares the randomized study results with the historical results. Taken as a whole, the data from the radiobiologic studies, the nonrandom clinical studies, and the prospective randomized clinical trial overwhelmingly support the contention that fast neutron radiotherapy offers a significant advance in the treatment of inoperable and unresectable primary and recurrent malignant salivary gland tumors. There was no observable difference in tumor response to neutron therapy according to histologic type.

PROSTATE

Ninety-five patients with Stages C and D carcinomas of the prostate were entered in a Phase III randomized study comparing mixed beam radiation (⅖ neutrons and ⅗ photons) against standard photon radiation therapy.[30] Patients were randomized to receive either 50 Gy whole pelvis photon irradiation with a prostate boost to 70 Gy, or its equivalent with mixed beam treatment.

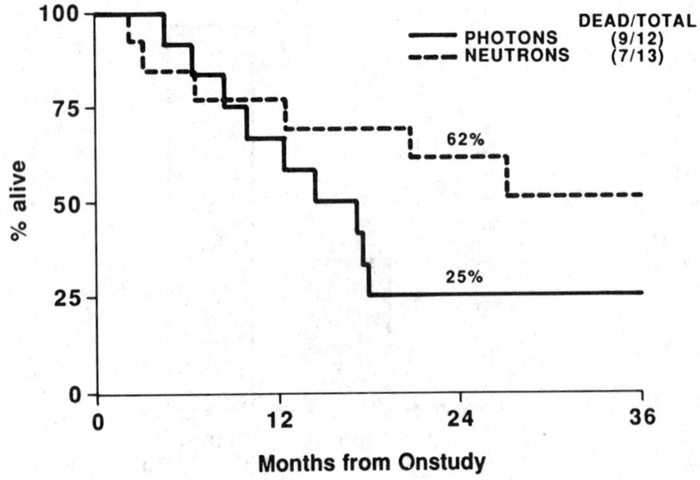

FIG. 66-33. Survival rates for neutron-treated and photon-treated patients. The difference is significant at the $p = 0.10$ level.

TABLE 66-15. Neutron Locoregional Tumor Control Rates for Malignant Salivary Gland Tumors

	No. of Patients	*Locoregional Tumor Control (%)*
Saroja[a*]	113	63 (71/113)
Catterall[24]	65	77 (50/65)
Batterman[12]	32	66 (21/32)
Griffin[35,60]	32	81 (26/32)
Duncan[28]	22	55 (12/22)
Maor[32]	9	67 (6/9)
Ornitz[61]	8	38 (3/8)
Eichhorn[10]	5	60 (3/5)
Skolyszewski[b*]	3	67 (2/3)
Total	289	67 (194/289)

*See Supplementary References at the end of Chap. 66.

TABLE 66-16. Low LET (Photon/Electron) Locoregional Tumor Control Rates for Malignant Salivary Gland Tumors

	No. of Patients	*Locoregional Tumor Control (%)*
Fitzpatrick[c*]	50	12 (6/50)
Vikram[d*]	49	4 (2/49)
Borthne[e*]	35	23 (8/35)
Rafla[62]	25	36 (9/25)
Fu[59]	19	32 (6/19)
Stewart[64]	19	47 (9/19)
Dobrowsky	17	41 (7/17)
Shidnia[63]	16	38 (6/16)
Elkon[f*]	13	15 (2/13)
Rossman[g*]	11	54 (6/11)
Total	254	24 (61/254)

*See Supplementary References at the end of Chap. 66.

The decision to make the experimental arm a neutron/photon mix rather than neutrons alone arose from the poor depth–dose characteristics of the neutron beams available at the time this study was conducted. All of these neutron beams were produced by accelerators located in nuclear physics laboratories. The poor penetration of many of these beams would have resulted in unacceptably high radiation doses to pelvic subcutaneous tissues and bowel in the process of treating the deep-seated primary tumors and lymph nodes to tumoricidal doses with neutrons alone. The resulting complications would have been unacceptable. To avoid this problem, it was decided to dilute the neutrons with better-penetrating photons, resulting in the "mixed beam" treatment delivered in this study.

At the time of the analysis, with a median follow-up time of 6.7 years, 81% of the neutron-treated patients remained clinically free of local tumor recurrence compared with 61% of the patients treated with photons alone (Fig. 66-34). This difference is statistically significant ($p < 0.01$). Although no standard approach to routine posttreatment biopsy was mandated in this study, 11 patients had their prostates rebiopsied a minimum of 2 years after treatment while in clinical remission. Combining the pathologic criterion of a positive biopsy with the clinical criteria, 77% of the neutron-treated patients versus 31% of the photon-treated patients remained free of local disease. These differences remain statistically significant ($p < 0.01$), and the positive biopsy rate for photon-treated patients is consistent with other reports in the literature.

TABLE 66-17. Comparison of the RTOG–MRC Study Results with Historical Results

	No. of Patients	*Locoregional Tumor Control (%)*
Low LET		
Low LET historical experience	254	24
ROTG–MRC photon controls	12	17
Neutron		
Historical neutron experience	289	67
ROTG–MRC neutron results	13	67

Survival data are graphically displayed in Figure 66-35. Sixty-three percent of the neutron-treated group are alive at 8 years as opposed to 13% of the photon-only treated cohort ($p = 0.01$). There were a large number of intercurrent deaths on this study, presumably because of the advanced average age of the patients entered.

When one excludes intercurrent deaths from causes other than prostate cancer, the corresponding disease-specific survival data are summarized in Figure 66-36. The disease-specific survival rate for the neutron-treated group of patients at 8 years is 82%, compared with 54% for the photon-only treated group. The difference remains statistically significant ($p = 0.02$).

A stepwise Cox analysis has been used to identify the important patient parameters relating to overall survival in this study. The most significant factor associated with patient survival was type of treatment (mixed beam versus photons, $p < 0.01$). The second most significant factor was patient age ($p < 0.05$). No significant differences were noted for either acute or late-normal tissue toxicity.

The results of this trial suggest that a local modality (neutrons + photons) can have a favorable survival impact on locally advanced prostate cancer. Because these are the only data available using this treatment modality in this disease, these results need to be confirmed.

Since the completion of this study, three high-energy, hospital-based cyclotrons have been installed in the United States. Additional machines are under construction. These new machines are capable of isocentric beam delivery with doses at depth comparable with the dose distributions of megavoltage linear accelerators. They present the opportunity to study the efficacy of neutrons used alone (undiluted with photons) in the treatment of prostate cancer. Currently, the efficacy of neutrons used alone is being tested in a national cooperative study in an attempt to confirm and, it is hoped, improve upon the results obtained with mixed beam treatment.

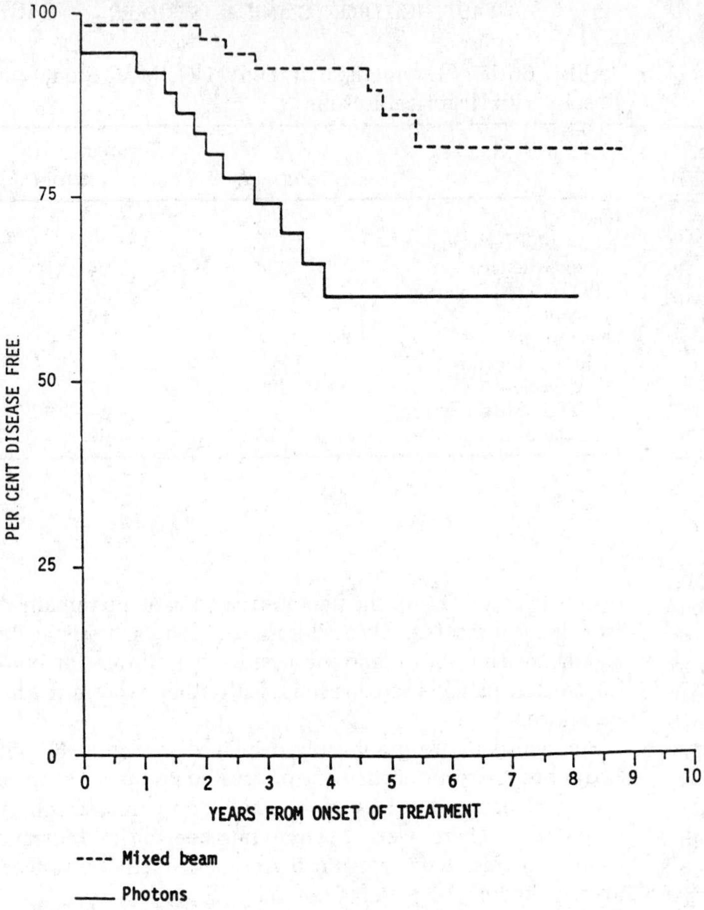

FIG. 66-34. Freedom from locoregional tumor recurrence. The two curves are different at the $p < 0.01$ level.

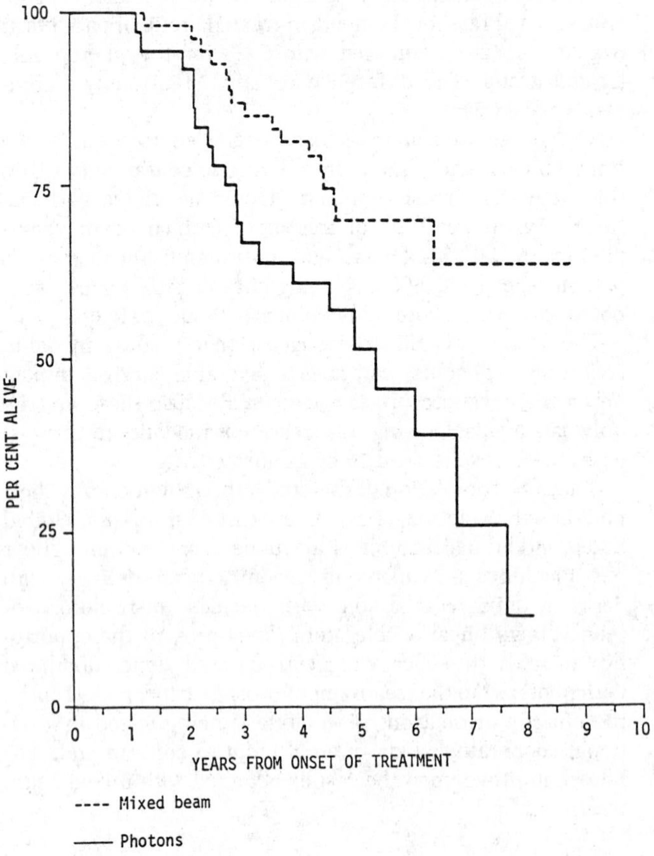

FIG. 66-35. Patient survival as a function of treatment. The two curves are different at the $p = 0.01$ level.

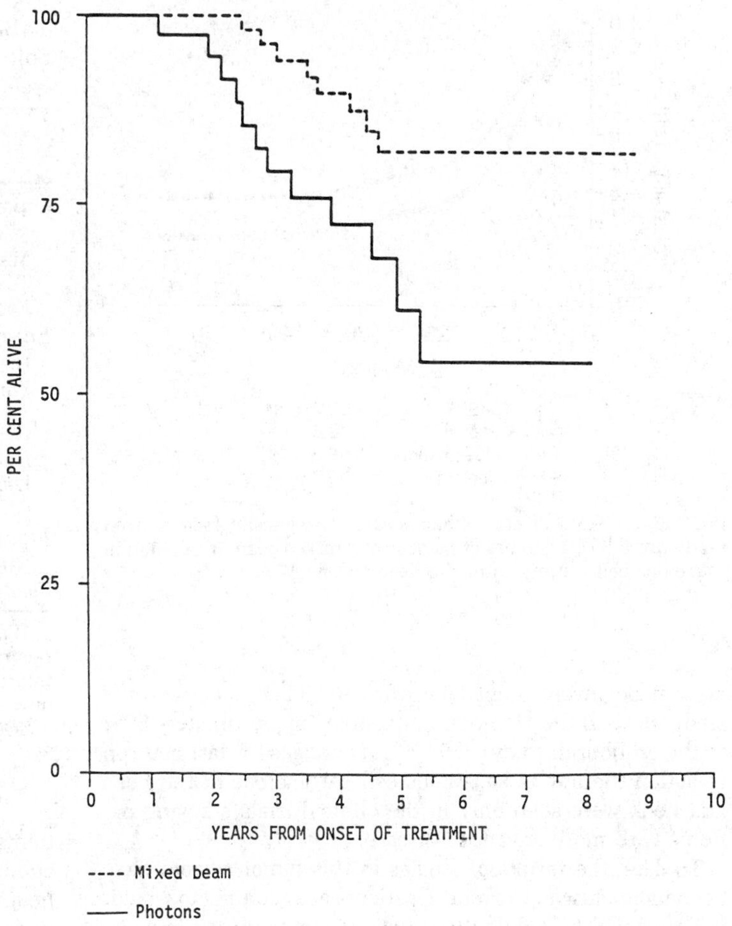

FIG. 66-36. Patient survival as a function of treatment using active cancer (local or distant) at the time of death as the endpoint. Deaths due to intercurrent disease with no evidence of cancer present are treated as censored observations. The two curves are different at the $p = 0.02$ level.

HEAD AND NECK

The use of fast neutron radiation therapy for the treatment of patients with squamous cell head and neck cancer has been studied intermittently for four decades. Following Stone's early work, Catterall and co-workers conducted a randomized study in the 1960s at Hammersmith Hospital in London, reporting a significant advantage for neutrons over conventional photon treatment for this group of tumors. With use of the low-energy MRC cyclotron, they observed a 76% (53/70) local control rate for neutrons, compared with a 19% (12/63) local control rate for photons in a group of patients with advanced disease.[17] The survival rates were poor in both treatment groups. Their early work led to many follow-up studies in Europe, Japan, and the United States.[31-33]

A second randomized study of fast neutrons in head and neck cancer has recently been reported by Duncan and colleagues on a group of patients with earlier stage disease.[18] They reported the results of a randomized, cooperative study conducted at the Antoni van Leeuwenhoek Ziekenhuis in Amsterdam, the Department of Clinical Oncology in Edinburgh, and Universitatsklinikun in Essen. No significant advantage for neutrons over photons could be demonstrated in this study. The complete response rate for neutrons was 70% (70/100), and the complete response rate for photons was 66% (63/95). The ultimate local control rates were 44% (44/100) for neutrons and 40% (38/95) for photons. There was no significant difference in the overall survival rates between the two groups. These results stand in contrast with the results obtained at Hammersmith Hospital.

A third major randomized study of neutrons in head and neck cancer was carried out in the United States by the RTOG.[34,35] More than 300 patients were entered in this study, which compared both neutrons used alone and neutrons used in a mixed beam treatment schedule (⅖ neutrons and ⅗ photons) against photons for inoperable squamous cell carcinomas. There were no significant differences between the mixed beam and photon control treatments in terms of either primary tumor control or survival; however, significant advantages were seen for neutrons given alone. The complete response rates were 52% for neutrons compared with 17% for photons ($p = 0.035$), with a major complication rate of 18% for neutrons and 33% for photons. Figure 66-37 illustrates the survival rates adjusted for prognostic factors for the three randomizations. This study demonstrated a 37% improvement in 5-year survival for neutron-treated patients over photon-treated patients, which is significant at the $p = 0.04$ level.

The patient populations in these three randomized studies were distinctly different as evidenced by differences in photon local control rates and the percentage of patients with

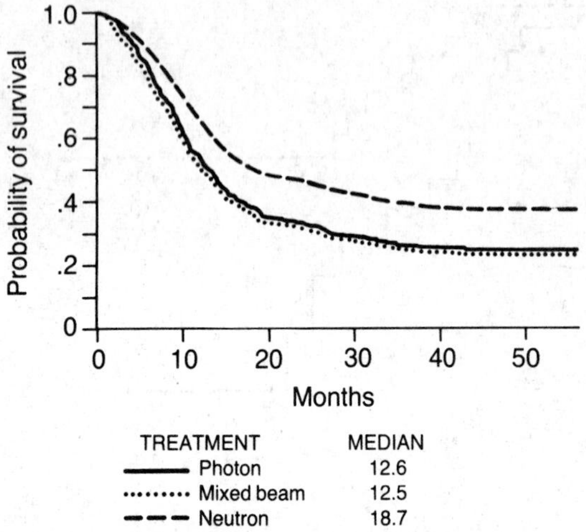

FIG. 66-37. Survival curves balanced for prognostic factors from randomized RTOG studies of neutron and mixed beam irradiation in squamous cell carcinoma of the head and neck.

neck node involvement (83% for the RTOG neutron-only study; 66% in the Hammersmith study; approximately 50% in the Edinburgh study).[17,28,34,35] Advantages for fast neutron radiation therapy in squamous cell carcinomas of the head and neck were seen only in the clinical trials studying patients with more advanced disease.

To date, the results of studies in this tumor system have been inconclusive. Currently, patients are accruing to what it is hoped will be a definitive study of fast neutrons in squamous cell carcinomas of the head and neck using the newer hospital-based, high-energy, isocentric neutron beams.

SOFT-TISSUE SARCOMAS

Soft-tissue sarcomas have been considered radioresistant because of poor results achieved with conventional photon irradiation. More recently it has been shown that a "complete" local excision coupled with either postoperative[36,37] or preoperative[38] radiation therapy yielded excellent local control rates of approximately 90%, with good preservation of function and cosmetic appearance. These excellent results require excision of all gross tumor, however, and frequently this is not possible. Soft-tissue sarcomas often present as deep-seated masses that can grow to large dimensions before being detected. This is especially true of lesions of the trunk, retroperitoneum, and proximal thigh. It is for such lesions that fast neutron radiation therapy may be significant.

At present, no definitive randomized studies have compared fast neutrons with megavoltage photons or electrons in the treatment of inoperable soft-tissue sarcomas; however, review of the world literature is quite encouraging. A total of 286 patients with large, inoperable tumors have been treated with fast neutrons and followed long enough to establish local control rates. (This number excludes patients treated for microscopic or limited macroscopic residual disease after a surgical excision.) The results[12,26,39–41] are summarized in Table 66-18. This clearly represents a diverse group of patients treated in many different ways (*e.g.*, neutrons alone, combined neutrons and photons in mixed beam schemes, or neutron boosts after photon irradiation), but the results are generally consistent, with the overall local control rate being 50% (144/286). The incidence of severe complications from the treatment was about 39%. This generally consisted of severe subcutaneous fibrosis with several instances of skin necrosis. In many patients, the fibrosis was sufficient to compromise limb function, but one must remember that the alternative was amputation. It is hoped that the higher energy beams and more sophisticated treatment abilities of the newer neutron facilities will allow improvement of this local control rate and at the same time, reduce treatment-related morbidity. A cooperative Phase III randomized trial is currently directly comparing neutron and photon irradiation for this tumor system.

TABLE 66-18. Summary of Local Control Rates for Soft Tissue Sarcomas Treated Definitively with Neutron Irradiation*

Facility	*Patients Achieving Local Control/Patients Treated (%)*
United States	
Seattle[57]	5/10 (50)
MANTA[39]	4/10 (40)
Texas A&M[40]	18/29 (62)
Fermi Lab[26]	13/26 (50)
Europe	
Hammersmith[9]	17/22 (77)
Edinburgh[28]	6/18 (33)
Amsterdam[12]	11/19 (58)
Hamburg/Eppendorf[29]	28/52 (54)
Heidelberg/Essen[58]	31/60 (52)
Louvain[41]	4/28 (14)
CICR[11]	42/62 (68) CR only
Japan	
NIRS[45]	7/12 (58)
Total	144/286 (50)†

*Patients treated de novo and for gross disease after a postsurgical recurrence are included, but not patients treated postoperatively for microscopic residual disease or very limited macroscopic residual disease.

†CR only data from CICR.

SARCOMA OF BONE

Sarcoma of bone refers to osteosarcomas and chondrosarcomas that arise in the bony or cartilaginous skeleton. Conventional radiation therapy for these lesions requires very high doses, with substantial subsequent morbidity in the treated areas. DeMoor describes 43 osteosarcoma cases treated radically with 6600 to 7700 cGy in 6 to 8 weeks.[27] All patients with lower extremity lesions who were followed for more than 1 year had significant subcutaneous fibrosis and partial flexion ankylosis of the knee joint. Eleven patients required postirradiation amputation—in three patients there was no viable tumor, in another three patients there was significant radiation change with tumor cells of questionable viability being present, and in five patients necrosis without active tumor was found. Twenty-seven patients were followed until their death or a minimum of 5 years; 9 of the 27 (33%) exhibited local control. Beck and co-workers reported a series of 21 patients with osteogenic sarcomas treated definitively with low LET radiation therapy, and they had only one long-term survivor with local control.[13] This patient had a mandibular lesion and received 5200 cGy with external beam and an additional 5600 cGy by means of an implant.

The situation is similar for chondrosarcomas. Harwood and others described a series of 31 cases treated by radiation therapy with an overall control rate of 23%.[42] However, only 20 of these cases were treated "radically" with curative intent and of these, 7 out of 20 (35%) were reported as having achieved local control for minimum follow-up times of approximately 3 years. It was noted that clinical regression was quite slow and, in many cases, a residual, calcified mass remained. McNaney and colleagues reported on seven patients treated with curative intent using megavoltage photons, and only one in seven (14%) exhibited long-term local control.[43]

International experience with fast neutron irradiation for these lesions is summarized in Tables 66-19 and 66-20 for osteosarcomas and chondrosarcomas, respectively.[26,39-41] A total of 64 patients with osteosarcomas have been treated definitively at the various facilities, with the overall local control rate being 43 in 64 (67%). The largest series is from the NIRS facility in Japan.[44,45] Their patients received chemotherapy [doxorubicin (Adriamycin), vincristine, and high-dose methotrexate] along with fast neutron irradiation as part of a combined method of treatment. After this combined treatment, 17 of their patients underwent either amputation or a "second-look" incisional biopsy, and 15 of 17 (88%) were histologically free of viable tumor. The three patients treated at the Amsterdam facility all had persistent residual calcification at the tumor site but no further growth.[41] The attending physicians reported these lesions as being "uncontrolled," and we have followed this in tabulating the data.

TABLE 66-19. Summary of Local Control Rates for Osteosarcomas Treated Definitively with Neutron Irradiation

Facility	*Patients Achieving Local Control/Patients Treated (%)*
United States	
Seattle[57]	7/9 (78)
MANTA[39]	1/1 (100)
Texas A&M[40]	0/1 (0)
Fermi Lab[26]	2/9 (22)
Europe	
Amsterdam[12]	0/3 (0)*
Japan	
NIRS[44]	33/41 (80)†
Total	43/64 (67)

*Persistent calcification but no growth.
†15 of 17 histologically negative on posttreatment surgical procedure.

TABLE 66-20. Summary of Local Control Rates for Inoperable Chondrosarcomas Treated Definitively with Neutron Irradiation

Facility	*Patients Achieving Local Control/Patients Treated (%)*
United States	
Seattle[57]	2/4 (50)*
MANTA[39]	7/9 (78)
Texas A&M[40]	4/4 (100)
Fermi Lab[26]	9/16 (56)
Europe	
Amsterdam[12]	0/6 (0)
Japan	
NIRS[44]	1/2 (50)
Total	23/41 (56)†

*Preliminary analysis.
†Persistent calcification but no local growth in three patients.

Because most of the tumors treated were quite large, with radiographically defined volume in excess of 1000 cm^3, the overall results appear considerably better than expected for photon irradiation for both types of bone sarcomas. Again, neutrons are currently being tested with a Phase III randomized study in this tumor system.

OTHER TUMOR SITES

Neutron studies have been carried out in the central nervous system, esophagus, lung, breast, pancreas, bladder, and cervix. Although some of the early results from these studies look promising, no definitive advantages have been demonstrated for neutrons in these sites, as yet.

HEAVY CHARGED PARTICLE CLINICAL STUDIES

As with neutrons (uncharged particles), which were introduced into clinical therapy at the Radiation Laboratory of the University of California shortly after the development of the cyclotron by Ernest Lawrence, charged particle radiation therapy was first suggested by physicists.[11,46-53] However, despite two decades of small-volume treatment of pituitary diseases, study of large field charged particle cancer therapy did not begin until the mid 1970s.

American clinical trials began in 1975 with helium ions (α particles) at the University of California Lawrence Berkeley Laboratory and at the Harvard cyclotron using protons (hydrogen nuclei).[54] Introduced later were pi mesons (subatomic particles) at the Los Alamos Scientific Laboratory (1976) and heavier nuclei such as carbon, neon, and silicon at the Lawrence Berkeley Laboratory (1977 to 1981).[25,55]

The experience with protons and helium ions in the United States has now reached over 1000 patients, and pions[56] and heavier ions have been used in about 250 patients each.[14-16,22,23] Because of limitations on beam availability and the need to develop new pioneering treatment techniques, accumulation of clinical data has been slow.

TABLE 66-21. Proton and Helium Ion Therapy of Choroidal Melanoma*

Tumor Size	Total No. of Patients	Status: Local Control	Status: Distant Metastasis
Small (>5 mm)			
Protons	24	23	0
Helium Ions	2	2	1
Medium (10–15 × 2–5 mm)			
Protons	198	195	4
Helium Ions	65	61	1
Large (>15 × >5 mm)			
Protons	244	242	22
Helium Ions	123	116	16
Total	656	639	44

*Minimum 1-yr follow-up.

PRECISION HIGH-DOSE CHARGED PARTICLE THERAPY

The results of precision high-dose proton and helium treatment of selected malignant tumors, such as melanoma of the uveal tract of the eye and tumors lying close to the spinal cord or base of brain (chordoma, chondrosarcoma, or meningioma), are shown in Tables 66-21 and 66-22.

These patients had tumors such as chordoma, low-grade chondrosarcoma, or meningioma lying at the base of the brain or near the spinal cord, which could not have complete surgical extirpation, and conventional radiotherapy could not deliver a sufficiently high tumor dose without serious risk of severe complication. With charged particle therapy, tumor doses of 6000 to 7500 ^{60}Co-equivalent cGy (particle cGy equivalent to low LET cobalt or x-ray treatment) have been given in 25 to 35 fractions over 6 to 8 weeks (Fig. 66-38).

Local control rates have been high; however, many patients have had low-grade malignancies with slow-growth patterns, and many years of follow-up are needed to fully evaluate tumor control and complications.

A large number of patients have been treated with protons and helium ions for arteriovenous malformations (AVMs) in Phase II studies. Although more follow-up is needed, the early results of these studies have been highly encouraging. Other studies are ongoing for carcinomas of the brain, head and neck, lung, retroperitoneum, prostate, and sarcomas in selected anatomic sites.

HIGH LET CHARGED PARTICLES

Phase I–II studies have been carried out with negative pions and carbon, neon, and silicon ions. At the present time, studies are centered on neon ions in the United States and negative pions in Canada and Switzerland. Carcinomas of the brain, head and neck, esophagus, lung, pancreas, stomach, biliary tract, and sarcomas of various sites have been studied. The impression is that promising results have been observed in patients with sarcoma of soft tissue and bone, tumors of the head and neck, unresectable carcinoma of the

TABLE 66-22. Proton and Helium Ion Therapy for Tumors of Base of Skull or Cervical Spine Abutting CNS*

Histologic Type	Total No. of Patients	Mean Follow-up (mo)	Status: Local Control	Status: Marginal Failure	Status: Distant Metastasis
Protons					
Chordoma, chondrosarcoma	88	26	78	4	2
Meningioma, craniopharyngioma	19	23	18		
Total	107	25	96	4	2
Helium Ions					
Chordoma, chondrosarcoma	28	24	16		3
Meningioma, craniopharyngioma	10	27	9		
Total	38	25	25		3

*Follow-up of 6–98 mo.

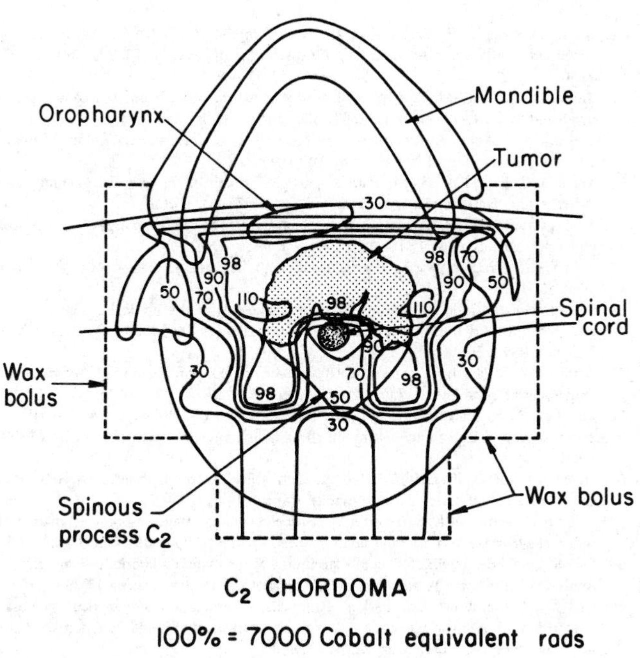

FIG. 66-38. Composite treatment plan for precision high-dose helium irradiation of chordoma of upper cervical spine.

lung, and locally advanced carcinoma of the prostate. However, these impressions are based, at this date, on small numbers of patients. Phase III trials are planned for the near future.

SUMMARY AND FUTURE DIRECTIONS

The biologic advantages of high LET radiations when compared with low LET radiations can be summarized in terms of a decreased oxygen enhancement ratio, a diminished capacity for cellular sublethal damage repair, a diminished capacity for potentially lethal damage repair, and diminished variability of radiosensitivity of cells in different stages of the cell cycle. These potential biologic advantages led to the neutron and high LET charged particle trials outlined in the preceding pages. Dose distribution advantages led to the low LET charged particle trials. Until recently, heavy particle radiation research has been limited by equipment availability and versatility. Laboratory-based fixed horizontal beam machines have placed a severe handicap on the development of these treatment modalities. The installation of hospital-based high-energy cyclotrons capable of isocentric beam delivery for neutrons and the development of a hospital-based synchrotron capable of isocentric proton therapy have greatly improved the situation; however, cost and size considerations still make these machines impractical for most hospital settings. New developments in superconducting technology hold a promise for the future of small, relatively inexpensive (at least compared with today's technology) particle accelerators suitable for heavy particle radiation therapy. If this promise is realized, proton, neutron, and heavy ion therapy may indeed become practical for a large number of treatment centers.

REFERENCES

1. Gray LH, Conger AE, Ebert M et al: Concentration of oxygen dissolved in tissues at time of irradiation as factor in radiotherapy. Br J Radiol 26:638, 1953
2. Withers HR, Thames HD, Peters LJ: Biological bases for high RBE values for late effects of neutron irradiation. Int J Radiat Oncol Biol Phys 8:2071, 1982
3. Howlett JF, Thomlinson RH, Alper T: A marked dependence of the conformative effective causes of neutrons on tumor line and its implications for clinical trials. Br J Radiol 48:40, 1975
4. Gragg RL, Humphrey RM, Thomas HT et al: The response of Chinese hamster ovary cells to fast neutron radiotherapy beams. I. Variations in RBE with position in the cell cycle. Radiat Res 76:283, 1978
5. Gragg RL, Humphrey RM, Meyn RE: The response of Chinese hamster ovary cells to fast neutron radiotherapy beams. II. Sublethal potentially lethal damage recovery capabilities. Radiat Res 71:461, 1977
6. Hall EJ, Kraljevic J: Repair of potentially lethal radiation damage: Comparison of neutron and x-ray RBE and implications for radiation therapy. Radiology 121:731, 1976
7. Stone RS: Neutron therapy and specific ionization. AJR 59:771, 1940
8. Catterall M, Bewley DK: Fast Neutrons in the Treatment of Cancer, pp 14–27. London, Academic Press, 1973
9. Catterall M: The treatment of advanced cancer by fast neutrons from the Medical Research Council's cyclotron at Hammersmith Hospital, London. Eur J Cancer 10:343, 1974
10. Eichhorn HJ: Results of a pilot study on neutron therapy with 600 patients. Int J Radiat Oncol Biol Phys 8:1561, 1982
11. Fowler PH, Perkins DH: The possibility of therapeutic applications of beams of negative pi mesons. Nature 189:524, 1981
12. Batterman JJ, Breur K: Fast neutron therapy for locally advanced sarcomas. Int J Radiat Oncol Biol Phys 7:1051, 1981
13. Beck JC, Wara WM, Bovill Jr EG et al: The role of radiation therapy in the treatment of osteosarcoma. Radiology 120:163, 1976
14. Castro JR: Heavy charged particle irradiation of human cancers. In Radiation Medicine, Vol 1-1, pp 70–75. Tokyo, Radiation Medicine Association, University of Tokyo, Faculty of Medicine, 1983
15. Castro JR, Quivey JM, Lyman JT et al: Current status of clinical particle radiotherapy at Lawrence Berkeley Laboratory. Cancer 46:633, 1980
16. Castro JR, Saunders WM, Tobias CA et al: Treatment of cancer with heavy charged particles. Int J Radiat Oncol Biol Phys 8:2191, 1982
17. Catterall M, Bewley DK, Sutherland I: Second report on a randomized clinical trial of fast neutrons with x or gamma rays in the treatment of advanced cancers of the head and neck. Br Med J 1:1942, 1977
18. Duncan W, Arnott SJ, Batterman JJ et al: Fast neutrons in the treatment of advanced head and neck cancers: The results of a multi-centre randomly controlled trial. Radiother Oncol 2:293, 1984
19. Duttenhaver JR, Shipley WU, Perrone T et al: Protons or megavoltage x-rays as boost therapy for patients irradiated for localized prostatic carcinoma. Cancer 51:1599, 1983
20. Batterman JJ, Breur K: Results of fast neutron teletherapy for locally advanced head and neck tumors. Int J Radiat Oncol Biol Phys 7:1045, 1981
21. Batterman JJ, Breur K, Hart BAM et al: Observations on pulmonary metastases in patients after single doses and multiple fractions of fast neutrons and cobalt-60 gamma rays. Eur J Cancer 17:539, 1981
22. Castro JR, Saunders WM, Quivey JM et al: Clinical problems in radiotherapy of carcinoma of the pancreas. Am J Clin Oncol 5:579, 1982
23. Castro JR, Chen GTY, Pitluck S et al: Helium charged particle radiotherapy of locally advanced carcinoma of the esophagus, stomach and biliary tract. Am J Clin Oncol 6:629, 1983
24. Catterall M: The treatment of salivary gland tumors with fast neutrons. Int J Radiat Oncol Biol Phys 7:1737, 1981
25. Chen GTY, Castro JR, Quivey JM: Heavy charged particle radiotherapy. Annu Rev Biophys Bioeng 10:419, 1981
26. Cohen L, Hendrickson F, Mansell J et al: Response of sarcomas of bone and soft tissue to neutron beam therapy. Int J Radiat Oncol Biol Phys 10:821, 1984
27. DeMoor NG: Osteosarcoma: A review of 72 cases treated by megavoltage radiation therapy with or without surgery. S Afr J Surg 13:137, 1975
28. Duncan W, Arnott SJ, Orr JA et al: The Edinburgh experience of fast neutron therapy. Int J Radiat Oncol Biol Phys 8:2155, 1982
29. Franke HD, Hess A, Brassow F et al: Clinical results after irradiation of intracranial tumors, soft tissue sarcomas, and thyroid cancers with fast neutrons at Hamburg-Eppendorf. In Karcher KH (ed): Progress in Radio-Oncology II, pp 123–137. New York, Raven Press, 1982
30. Laramore GE, Griffin TW, Maor MH: Mixed beam radiation therapy for carcinoma of the prostate: The results of a randomized RTOG study. Int J Radiat Oncol Biol Phys 112:1621, 1985

31. Laramore GE, Griffin TW, Tesh DW et al: Phase I pilot study on fast neutron teletherapy for advanced carcinoma of the head and neck region: Final report on local control rate and survival. Cancer 51:192, 1983
32. Maor MH, Hussey DH, Fletcher GH et al: Fast neutron therapy for locally advanced head and neck tumors. Int J Radiat Oncol Biol Phys 7:155, 1981 (private communication also)
33. Morita S, Tsunemoto H, Kurisu A et al: Results of fast neutron therapy at NIRS. Presented at Fourth High LET Radiotherapy Seminar. Sponsored by the United States–Japan Cooperative Cancer Research Program, Philadelphia, Pa, June 19, 1978
34. Griffin TW, Davis R, Laramore GE et al: Fast neutron irradiation of metastatic cervical adenopathy: The results of a randomized RTOG study. Int J Radiat Oncol Biol Phys 9:1267, 1983
35. Griffin TW, Davis R, Hendrickson FR: Fast neutron radiation therapy for unresectable squamous cell carcinomas of the head and neck: The results of a randomized RTOG study. Int J Radiat Oncol Biol Phys 10:2217, 1984
36. Lindberg RD: The role of radiation therapy in the treatment of soft tissue sarcomas in adults. Semin Oncol 16:883, 1976
37. Lindberg RD, Martin RG, Romsdahl MD et al: Conservative surgery and postoperative radiotherapy in 300 adults with soft tissue sarcoma. Cancer 47:2391, 1981
38. Suit H, Proppe K, Mankin H et al: Preoperative radiation therapy for sarcoma of soft tissue. Cancer 47:2269, 1981
39. Ornitz R, Herskovic A, Schell M: Treatment experience: locally advanced sarcomas with 15 MeV fast neutrons. Cancer 45:2712, 1980
40. Salinas R, Hussey DH, Fletcher GH: Experience with fast neutron therapy for locally advanced sarcomas. Int J Radiat Oncol Biol Phys 6:267, 1980
41. Wambersie A: The European experience in neutron therapy at the end of 1981. Int J Radiat Oncol Biol Phys 8:2145, 1982
42. Harwood AR, Krajbich JI, Fornasier VL: Radiotherapy of chondrosarcoma of bone. Cancer 45:2769, 1980
43. McNaney D, Lindberg RD, Ayala AG et al: Fifteen-year radiotherapy experience with chondrosarcoma of bone. Int J Radiat Oncol Biol Phys 8:187, 1982
44. Hodaka E, Maruyama K, Takada N et al: Multimodality treatment, including fast neutron radiotherapy, for osteosarcoma. Cancer Bull 31:216, 1979
45. Tsunemoto H, Morita S, Arai T et al: Results of clinical trials with 30 MeV d-Be neutrons at NIRS. In Sakamoto MAK, Phillips TL (eds): Treatment of Radioresistant Cancers. Amsterdam, Elsevier-North Holland, 1979
46. Goldstein LS, Phillips TL, Fu KK: Biological effects of accelerated heavy ions. I. Single doses in normal tissues, tumors and cells in vitro. Radiat Res 86:529, 1981
47. Ngo FQH, Blakely EA, Tobias CA: Sequential exposures of mammalian cells to low and high LET radiation. I. Lethal effects following x-ray and neon ion irradiation. Radiat Res 87:59, 1981
48. Roots RJ, Yang TCH, Craise L et al: Rate of rejoining of DNA breaks induced by accelerated carbon and neon ions in the spread Bragg peak. Int J Radiat Res 38:203, 1980
49. Tenforde TJ, Azal SM, Parr SS et al: Cell survival in rat rhabdomyosarcoma tumors irradiated in vivo with extended peak silicon ions. Radiat Res 92:208, 1982
50. Tobias CA, Blakely EA, Alpen EL et al: Molecular and cellular radiobiology of heavy ions. Int J Radiat Oncol Biol Phys 8:2109, 1982
51. Tobias CA, Todd PW: Heavy charged particles in cancer therapy: Radiobiology and radiotherapy. Natl Cancer Inst Monogr 24:1, 1967
52. Tobias CA, Anger HO, Lawrence JH: Radiobiological use of high energy deuterons and alpha particles. AJR 67:1, 1952
53. Tobias CA: Pretherapeutic investigations with accelerated heavy ions. Radiology 108:145, 1973
54. Suit H, Munzenrider GJ, Verhey L et al: Evaluation of the clinical applicability of proton beams in definitive fractionated radiation therapy. Int J Radiat Oncol Biol Phys 8:2199, 1982
55. Griffin TW, Blasko J, Laramore GE: Results of fast neutron beam pilot studies at the University of Washington. Eur J Cancer (suppl):23, 1979
56. Von Essen CF, Blattman H, Crawford JF et al: The PIOTRON: Initial experience, preparation and experience with pion therapy. Int J Radiat Oncol Biol Phys 8:1499, 1982
57. Henry LW, Blasko JC, Griffin TW: Evaluation of fast neutron teletherapy for advanced carcinomas of the major salivary glands. Cancer 44:814, 1979
58. Schmitt G, Schnabel K, Sauerwein W et al: Neutron and neutron-boost irradiation of soft tissue sarcomas: A 4.5 year analysis of 139 patients. Radiother Oncol 1:23, 1983
59. Fu KK, Leibel SA, Levine MG et al: Carcinoma of the major and minor salivary glands: Analysis of treatment results and sites and causes of failure. Cancer 40:2882, 1977
60. Griffin TW, Laramore GE, Parker RG et al: An evaluation of fast neutron beam teletherapy of metastatic cervical adenopathy from squamous cell carcinomas of the head and neck region. Cancer 42:2517, 1978
61. Ornitz R, Herskovic A, Bradley E: Clinical observations of early and late normal tissue injury and tumor control in patients receiving fast neutron irradiation. In Barendsen GW, Broerse J, Breur K (eds): High LET Radiations in Clinical Radiotherapy, pp 44–50. New York, Pergamon Press, 1979
62. Rafla S: Malignant parotid tumors: Natural history and treatment. Cancer 40:136, 1977
63. Shidnia H, Hornback NB, Hamaker R et al: Carcinoma of major salivary glands. Cancer 45:693, 1980
64. Stewart JG, Jackson AW, Chew MK: The role of radiation therapy in the management of malignant tumor of salivary glands. AJR 102:100, 1968

SECTION 6

RAINER STORB

Bone Marrow Transplantation

Toxicity to the marrow is a serious limitation of cancer therapy. Higher—and potentially curative—doses of chemoradiotherapy may be given if the patient is treated by marrow transplantation. Under these circumstances therapy would be limited only by nonhematopoietic toxicity. It follows then that the most efficacious application of marrow transplantation would be for the treatment of cancer originating in hematopoietic tissues, whereas benefit might be less impressive in the therapy of nonhematopoietic tumors.

Because the donor marrow must be free of all clonogenic tumor cells, the graft usually comes from a separate, healthy individual—raising all the problems of immunologic incompatibility and restricting treatment to those with suitable donors, either a monozygous twin (syngeneic graft) or a human leukocyte antigen (HLA)-identical sibling (allogeneic graft). A way around this restriction is possible if marrow is taken from the affected individual before chemoradiotherapy, cleared of tumor cells without destroying the hematopoietic stem cells and then used for autologous transplantation.

Initially, marrow transplantation was considered experimental and used only as a last, desperate procedure. The early results highlighted both the potential benefits and limitations of this new procedure.[1] The conditioning programs, involving cyclophosphamide (Cy) and total-body irradiation (TBI), permanently eradicated leukemia in 30% of chemotherapy-resistant patients but failed to do so in the remaining 70%. Results were improved when marrow grafting was used at earlier disease stages, and the technique has now progressed to a therapeutically effective modality for selected patients with malignant disease (reviewed in detail in Refs. 1–5). This chapter will review the clinical results, contrast autologous and allogeneic transplantation, and highlight the principal problems that must still be overcome.

GENERAL PRINCIPLES

THE SOURCE OF MARROW

Presently, most marrow donors are genetically different allogeneic individuals, usually HLA-A, -B, -DR, and -D-identical siblings. The genes coding for HLA antigens are located on the short arm of chromosome 6. Every individual inherits one HLA haplotype from each parent. Thus, within any given family there can be only four haplotypes, and every patient has a 25% chance of having a genotypically HLA-identical sibling. Syngeneic grafts are from twins, completely identical at all genetic loci, providing an ideal source of marrow. Recent interest has focused on identifying acceptable HLA nonidentical donors within families. These may include siblings, parents, children, aunts, uncles, cousins, and grandparents genotypically identical for one HLA haplotype and phenotypically matched for one or more of the HLA loci on the nonshared haplotype. Acceptable donors are found in approximately 10% of the cases. Successful transplants have also been reported with marrow from phenotypically HLA-identical unrelated donors. Finally, an ever-increasing number of autologous marrow grafts are being carried out.

MARROW HARVEST AND INFUSION

Between 400 ml and 1000 ml of marrow is obtained by multiple aspirations from the iliac crests of the donor under anesthesia.[6] The marrow is placed into heparinized tissue culture medium, screened through wire mesh to remove bone and tissue particles, and infused intravenously into the recipient within 1 to 24 hr of TBI, usually in an amount of 1×10^8 to 8×10^8 nucleated marrow cells per kilogram. The hematopoietic stem cells needed for engraftment circulate through the lungs, "home" into the marrow cavity, and divide. There is no permanent loss to the donor. Apart from varying degrees of temporary local soreness, donor complications are unusual, although isolated potentially life-threatening complications have been described, including cardiac arrest, ventricular tachycardia, aspiration pneumonitis, and septicemia.

MARROW CRYOPRESERVATION

Autologous transplantation requires cryopreservation of viable marrow cells which are harvested while the patient is in chemotherapy-induced remission (reviewed in Refs. 7, 8). Often, the marrow is treated before cryopreservation either with certain monoclonal antibodies plus complement, immunotoxins, or certain chemicals (*e.g.*, 4-hydroxyperoxycyclophosphamide) in attempts at removing clonogenic leukemia cells. Preservation of marrow for more than 24 hr usually involves freezing in the presence of a cryoprotective agent, most often dimethylsulfoxide (DMSO). The cryoprotective agent serves to prevent ice crystal formation inside the cell during freezing. The freezing process is done under careful control of the rate of cooling. Frozen cells are stored at ultralow temperatures in liquid nitrogen at −196°C. Studies in animals, and the experience to date in humans, have indicated that pluripotent hematopoietic stem cells can survive under these conditions for periods measured in months or even years.

At some future date, after completion of the conditioning program for the patient, the plastic bag containing the marrow is removed from the freezer, placed in a 40°C waterbath, and the marrow is rapidly thawed. After thawing, marrow cells are infused intravenously, often without any further manipulations, but occasionally, slow dilution with Hanks balanced salt solution is used to reduce problems with cellular osmotic stress.

GRAFTS OF PERIPHERAL BLOOD STEM CELLS AND OF MARROW DERIVED FROM LONG-TERM CULTURE

On the basis of studies in experimental animals, stem cells derived from peripheral blood have recently been used for autologous transplantation.[9] This may be a useful alternative for those patients in whom marrow is difficult to harvest because of marrow damage by preceding radiotherapy. Although allogeneic grafts with peripheral blood stem cells are feasible, the contamination of peripheral blood with T cells would carry a high risk for graft-versus-host disease (GVHD).

Another development has been the successful transplantation of marrow maintained in long-term culture.[10] It appears that long-term culture conditions favor survival of normal pluripotent stem cells over that of their leukemic counterparts, thereby permitting "purging" of malignant cells. As our understanding of culture conditions and the use of recombinant hematopoietic growth factors increase, this technique may become increasingly attractive because it may permit propagation of desirable, and elimination of undesirable, cells.

CONDITIONING PROGRAMS USED BEFORE TRANSPLANTATION

The conditioning programs are critical for the success of marrow grafting. Their aim is to both eradicate the malignant cells and suppress host immunity sufficiently to prevent rejection of allogeneic grafts. A common regimen consists of Cy (60 mg/kg on each of 2 days) followed by TBI.[1] Radiation dose rates range from 2.5 to 85 cGy/min, delivered by either opposing ^{60}Co sources or, more commonly, linear accelerators. More recently, fractionated TBI has been used in attempts to reduce toxicity and perhaps increase leukemic cell kill. Doses per fraction range from 1.25 to 3.3 Gy, fractionation intervals from 3 to 24 hr, and total doses from 5.0 to 15.75 Gy. Fractionation of TBI has reduced the long-term toxicity of irradiation.

The possible schedules of TBI dose fractionation are infinite. Examples of commonly used regimens are shown in Table 66-23. Total-body irradiation is attractive because it has an antitumor effect, it penetrates privileged sites for tumor (*e.g.*, central nervous system and testicles) for which chemotherapy is ineffective, and it provides sufficient immunosuppression. A number of institutions have begun sub-

TABLE 66-23. Commonly Used Conditioning Programs

		Total Body Irradiation			
Institution	*Chemotherapy**	*Total Dose (cGy)*	*Dose Rate (cGy/min)*	*Regimen (cGy/d)*	*Compensation/Bolus*
Case Western Reserve[76]	Ara-C, 6 g/m^2/d × 6 d	1200	22	2 × 200/d × 3 d	Reduction of dose to head and legs
City of Hope[75]	Etoposide, 60 mg/kg	1320	20	3 × 120/d × 3.6 d	Electron boost chest and testes
Fred Hutchinson Cancer Research Center[1,11,12]	Cy, 60 mg/kg/d × 2 d	1200	5–8	200/d × 6 d	
	Cy, 60 mg/kg/d × 2 d	1575	5–8	225/d × 7 d	
Johns Hopkins Univ[16,80]	Cy, 60 mg/kg/d × 2 d	1200	7–8	300/d × 4 d	Lungs blocked 25%
	Cy, 50 mg/kg/d × 4 d and busulfan, 4 mg/kg/d × 4 d	<----- None ----->			
M. D. Anderson Hosp[97]	Piperazinedione, 25 mg/m^2/d × 2 d	1020	26	2 × 170/d × 3 d	Bolus to head and legs
	Cy, 4.5–6.0 g/m^2 and BCNU, 300 mg/m^2 and etoposide, 600 mg/m^2	<----- None ----->			
Memorial Sloan–Kettering[79,98]	Cy, 60 mg/kg/d × 2 d	1320	9–18	3 × 120/d × 3.6 d	Lungs by 1 HLV, electron boost
Princess Margaret Hosp[99]	Ara-C, 100 mg/m^2/d × 5 d and Cy, 60 mg/kg/d × 2 d	500	50–85	Single dose	Extensive bolus
Royal Marsden Hosp[19]	Cy, 60 mg/kg/d × 2 d	950	2.5	Single dose	
UCLA[18]	Cy, 60 mg/kg/d × 2 d	1125	6–7	2 × 225/d × 2.5 d	
Univ of British Columbia[100]	Cy, 60 mg/kg/d × 2 d	1260	20	2 × 180/d × 3.5 d	Compensation for head and lower leg
Univ of Minnesota[102,103]	Ara-C, 2 × 3 g/m^2/d × 6 d	850	26	Single dose	Compensation for head and lower leg
	Cy, 60 mg/kg/d × 2 d	1320	10	2 × 165/d × 4 d	
Univ of Pennsylvania[104]	Cy, 60 mg/kg/d × 2 d	1320	8	2 × 165/d × 4 d	
Washington Univ[96]	Cy, 60 mg/kg/d × 2 d	999	8	333/d × 3 d	
	Cy, 60 mg/kg/d × 2 d	1200	45	2 × 200/d × 3 d	Body compensation
Royal Free Hosp[101]	Cy, 60 mg/kg/d × 2 d	750	26	Single dose	

*Ara-C, cytosine arabinoside; Cy, cyclophosphamide; BCNU, bischloroethylnitrosourea.

stituting other chemotherapeutic agents for cyclophosphamide (see Table 66-23). The Johns Hopkins team has replaced TBI by busulfan in patients with myeloid leukemias (see Table 66-23).

CLINICAL RESULTS OF MARROW GRAFTING

ACUTE NONLYMPHOBLASTIC LEUKEMIA

Allogeneic Marrow Grafts

RELAPSE ACUTE NONLYMPHOBLASTIC LEUKEMIA. Until the mid-1970s, marrow grafting was employed only after failure of all other therapy. Between 1970 and 1975, 54 patients with acute nonlymphoblastic leukemia (ANL) in relapse were given HLA-identical marrow grafts in Seattle, and six are living and well 12 to 16 years later in unmaintained remission (Fig. 66-39).[11] The actuarial relapse rate was 65%. An improvement in these statistics was seen in 132

FIG. 66-39. Kaplan-Meier product limit estimates for disease-free survival after marrow transplantation in 110 patients with advanced acute lymphoblastic leukemia (*ALL*) and acute nonlymphoblastic leukemia (*ANL*). Patients were given CY and 10 Gy single-dose TBI followed by HLA-identical sibling marrow and intermittent methotrexate for the first 100 days postgrafting. Circles indicate disease-free survivors as of September 1987.

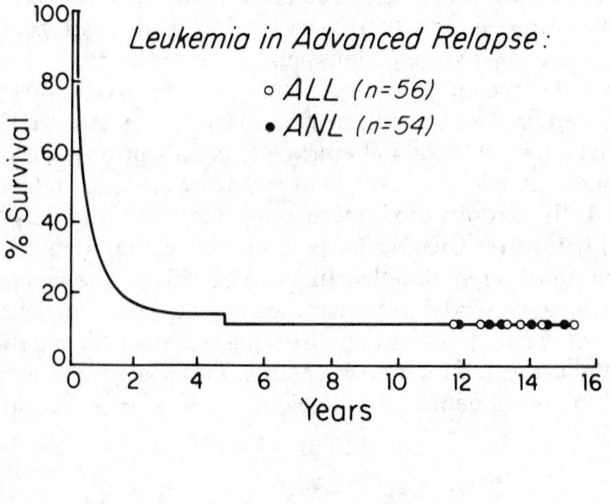

more-recent patients.[12] Survival at 3 years was comparable (34%) for those grafted in untreated first relapse or second remission but only 24% for those grafted in resistant first relapse. This suggests that patients should receive marrow transplants in early first relapse, rather than after an attempt has been made to induce another remission, in particular because some patients may die during remission induction.

ACUTE NONLYMPHOBLASTIC LEUKEMIA IN FIRST REMISSION. In 1976, the Seattle team began to transplant marrow into patients with ANL in first remission. This approach promised improved disease-free survival because the body burden of leukemic cells is smaller, cells probably are less resistant to therapy, and patients are clinically well and, therefore, better able to tolerate a transplant. Results have borne out the expectations.[12] Twelve of the first 22 patients are surviving between 9 and 11 years after grafting (Fig. 66-40). By 1986, 231 patients had received transplants in Seattle, and 49% are alive at 3 years. The relapse rate has been 25%. Best results were seen in patients under 20 years of age, with 70% survival as opposed to 40% to 50% for those over that age. Results are similar in other transplant centers, as summarized by the European and International Marrow Transplant Registry reports.[13,14]

Allogeneic Versus Autologous Marrow Grafts

Recent reports have shown up to 45% survival at 2 years after autologous marrow transplantation in first remission, and 30% with transplants in second remission, regardless of whether the marrow was treated to remove clonogenic leukemic cells.[15,16] Survival seemed comparable with that seen after allogeneic grafts. Results reconfirm that conditioning programs are more effective in eradicating leukemic cells than conventional chemotherapy and, surprisingly, suggest that many times the infused marrow lacks sufficient clonogenic leukemic cells to lead to relapse. Although autologous grafts have been carried out in a small and perhaps highly select group of patients with a still short follow-up, results are sufficiently encouraging to question whether an allogeneic or autologous graft should be preferred in a given patient in whom there is a choice. Allogeneic transplants avoid the infusion of potentially clonogenic leukemic cells and have the advantage of a potential graft-versus-leukemia effect, which could lead to lower relapse rates. Autologous grafts, in turn, have the advantage of avoiding GVHD, its complications, and the toxicity incurred from its treatment. The question of what the best approach is for any given patient will be answered by prospective trials comparing allogeneic and autologous transplants. Another unanswered question in autologous transplantation concerns the effectiveness and potential toxicity of methods of purging the marrow from leukemic cells.

FIG. 66-40. Kaplan-Meier product limit estimates for survival of the first patients given HLA-identical marrow grafts for acute nonlymphoblastic leukemia (*ANL*) in first remission and acute lymphoblastic leukemia (*ALL*) in second or subsequent remission. Tick marks indicate disease-free survivors as of September 1987. Reversed mark shows a patient with ALL who died in a car accident without evidence of leukemia.

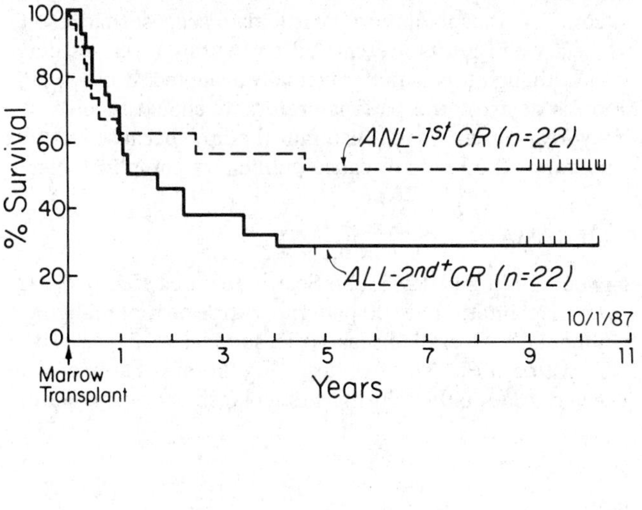

When to Carry out Marrow Grafts in Patients with Acute Nonlymphoblastic Leukemia

The question of when to give a transplant to a patient with ANL is unresolved. Prospective studies comparing the outcome of allogeneic transplantation in first remission with conventional chemotherapy showed either statistically significant or suggestive advantages of transplantation.[17-19] The dilemma arises from the variable proportion of transplantation patients (20%–35%) who would have been cured by chemotherapy alone.[17-20] After transplantation, 25% of these otherwise cured patients may die from complications. On the other hand, 65% to 75% of the patients will not be cured by chemotherapy, and of these, approximately 40% can be cured by transplantation in first remission. In the absence of appropriate markers predicting which patient will relapse and who will remain in remission on a chemotherapy regimen, the dilemma will persist. An argument could be made for transplantation at early first relapse, when transplantation will cure approximately 30% of patients. Adding this figure to the 25% to 35% cure rate expected with chemotherapy alone would be close to the 50% achieved with transplantation early in first remission. However, the recent improvements in cure rates with chemotherapy have yet to be substantiated with longer follow-up. Previous cure rates have been only in the range of 20% to 25%, and survival curves have clearly not yet reached plateaus. Therefore, to determine whether or not transplantation in first remission is superior to transplantation after first relapse, prospective comparative trials are required.

ACUTE LYMPHOBLASTIC LEUKEMIA

Allogeneic Marrow Grafts

RELAPSE ACUTE LYMPHOBLASTIC LEUKEMIA. Similarly to ANL, marrow transplantation was first employed to treat patients with advanced disease.[11] Of 56 patients receiving transplants between 1970 and 1975 in Seattle, six are currently alive between 11.5 and 15.5 years after transplantation (see Fig. 66-41). The actuarial relapse rate was 75%.

ACUTE LYMPHOBLASTIC LEUKEMIA IN REMISSION. Results are better when marrow transplantation is carried out in remission.[13,14,21,22] Figure 66-40 shows the survival curve of the first 22 Seattle patients with ALL who were grafted in second or subsequent remission, showing a plateau at 27%, 9 to 10.5 years after grafting. Leukemic relapse in cells of host type continues to be the major problem, with an incidence of 60%. Survival for patients who received a transplant during first remission is about 30% to 45%, with a relapse rate of 35%.

Autologous Versus Allogeneic Marrow Grafts

Long-term disease-free survival has been reported in a proportion of patients with ALL given autologous transplants in second or subsequent remission.[23] In many cases, marrow has been purged from clonogenic leukemic cells with the help of antibodies and complement or immunotoxins. As with transplantation for ANL, autologous transplants are safer, but allogeneic grafts will result in fewer relapses. Head-to-head comparisons of autologous versus allogeneic transplants, as yet, have not been made.

When to Carry out Marrow Transplants in Patients with ALL

Given the grim prognosis of patients with ALL resistant to chemotherapy, there is little doubt that these patients should receive marrow transplants. A prospective study in children showed transplantation to be superior to chemotherapy in patients who had relapsed at least once.[24] Children who relapse long after chemotherapy has been discontinued, however, may do as well with renewed chemotherapy as with transplantation.[25] Adults who have relapsed are unlikely to be cured by chemotherapy and should receive transplants. Transplantation for ALL in first remission is controversial in view of the good results with current chemotherapy for normal-risk children and also adults.[26,27] However, children with a high risk for relapse on conventional therapy (*e.g.*, those with Philadelphia chromosome-positive ALL, Burkitt-type leukemia, mediastinal mass, with an extremely high white blood cell count at diagnosis, and those under 2 years of age) may benefit from transplantation in first remission. Adults with null-ALL, those older than 35 years, those with more than 30,000 leukocytes/mm^3 at diagnosis, and those who need more than 4 weeks of induction chemotherapy to achieve remission are at high risk for relapse and should also be considered candidates for marrow transplantation during first remission.[28]

CHRONIC MYELOCYTIC LEUKEMIA

Allogeneic Marrow Grafts

BLAST CRISIS AND ACCELERATED PHASE. The experience with marrow transplantation for the treatment of patients with chronic myelocytic leukemia (CML) in blast crisis parallels that in patients with acute leukemia in advanced relapse.[29–31] Long-term disease-free survival is approximately 15%, with actuarial probabilities of relapse of between 50% to 75%. Marrow cells in surviving patients do not show the Philadelphia chromosome, suggesting cure of the disease, a unique and impressive result. Attempts to improve results by transplanting in the accelerated phase have been only marginally successful, with 15% to 28% disease-free survival, and relapse rates of 40% to 56%.

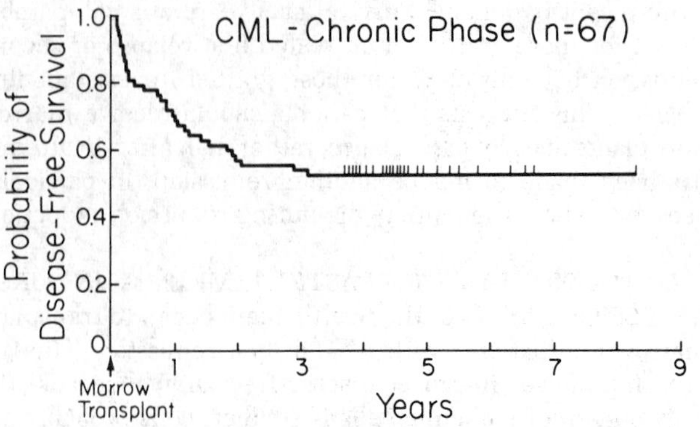

FIG. 66-41. Kaplan-Meier product limit estimates for survival of the first 67 patients with chronic myelocytic leukemia (*CML*) transplanted in the chronic phase. Vertical marks indicate disease-free survivors as of September 1987.

CHRONIC PHASE. In 1976, the Seattle team began a clinical trial in 19 patients who had cytogenetically normal identical twins to serve as marrow donors. Twelve of these patients are alive and in apparent remission, without the Philadelphia chromosome, 1 to 11.5 (median 8) years later. These results have encouraged studies of allogeneic transplantation with marrow from HLA-identical siblings.[29–31] Long-term disease-free survival has been 49% to 56% (Fig. 66-41). The actuarial probability of relapse is 12% to 20%.

When to Transplant Patients with Chronic Myelocytic Leukemia

Currently, transplantation is the only form of cure for CML. Any patient under the age of 50 years who has a suitable donor should receive a transplant. Results are best with transplantation during the chronic phase. However, because of associated complications, the lives of some patients may be shortened by early transplantation. Delaying the transplant may result in disease progression, and with it a poor outcome of transplantation. Seattle data suggest that results are best when grafts are carried out within 1 year of diagnosis, although this is not universally accepted. If transplantation is delayed, the patient preferably should receive hydroxyurea rather than busulfan therapy because of the potential of the latter to cause pulmonary complications.

LYMPHOMA

Between 1970 and 1985, the Seattle team carried out marrow transplantation in 100 patients with recurrent malignant lymphoma.[32] Overall disease-free survival at 5 years was 22%, with a 60% risk of relapse (Fig. 66-42). Patients who received grafts either during first relapse or second remis-

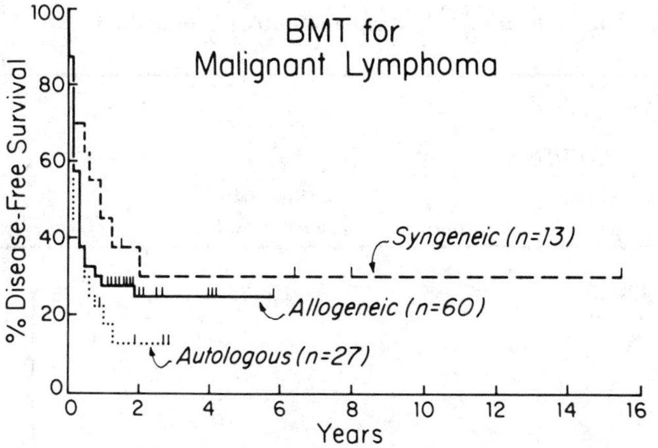

FIG. 66-42. Kaplan-Meier product limit estimates for survival of patients with malignant lymphoma. Shown are results of patients given syngeneic, allogeneic, and autologous marrow transplants. Vertical marks indicate disease-free survivors as of September 1987.

sion did significantly better than those with more advanced disease, with a 2-year disease-free survival of 42%, and a relapse rate of 41%. Neither the source of marrow (autologous versus allogeneic versus syngeneic) nor the histologic type of the disease (high-grade versus intermediate-grade non-Hodgkin's lymphoma versus Hodgkin's disease) were predictive of outcome. These results[32] and those obtained by other centers[33] indicate that marrow transplantation for recurrent malignant lymphoma yields better results than those with any salvage chemotherapy.[34]

OTHER HEMATOLOGIC MALIGNANCIES

Marrow grafting has also been successful in a few patients with myelofibrosis, multiple myeloma, hairy cell leukemia, and histiocytic medullary reticulosis. Of interest are patients with preleukemic syndromes who, although occasionally responding to chemotherapy, suffer from an incurable disease. Recent reports suggest approximately 50% disease-free survival in patients who receive transplants for de novo preleukemia, whereas results in patients with secondary preleukemia are not as encouraging, although occasional long-term survivors have been observed.[35]

SOLID TUMORS

Pilot studies have been reported with autologous marrow grafts for radiosensitive solid tumors, such as ovarian, testicular, and small-cell lung cancers, and neuroblastoma, usually after failure of other therapy (reviewed in Ref. 36). Results have been poor, with the exception of metastatic neuroblastoma, in which long-term disease-free survival and probable cures have been seen.

HLA-NONIDENTICAL MARROW GRAFTS

Considerable data from experimental animals support the general concept that best results can be expected with marrow from genotypically HLA-identical siblings and that HLA-nonidentity can affect several outcomes, including engraftment, graft rejection, GVHD, and immune reconstitution. However, only 35% to 40% of patients have an HLA-identical sibling, a fact that limits the applicability of allogeneic grafts unless other donors can be identified.

HLA-NONIDENTICAL FAMILY MEMBER DONORS

Results with marrow from less well-matched family members have shown that transplant-related complications will increase commensurate with the degree of HLA-disparity.[37,38] Engraftment can be delayed, granulocyte and platelet counts remain low, and the risk of graft rejection is clearly increased. Furthermore, among those patients who have sustained engraftment, the rate of onset, severity, and overall incidence of acute GVHD are increased, as shown in Figure 66-43. Surprisingly, despite the somewhat higher frequency of graft failure and of GVHD, survival of phenotypically HLA-identical or one HLA-locus mismatched patients is not

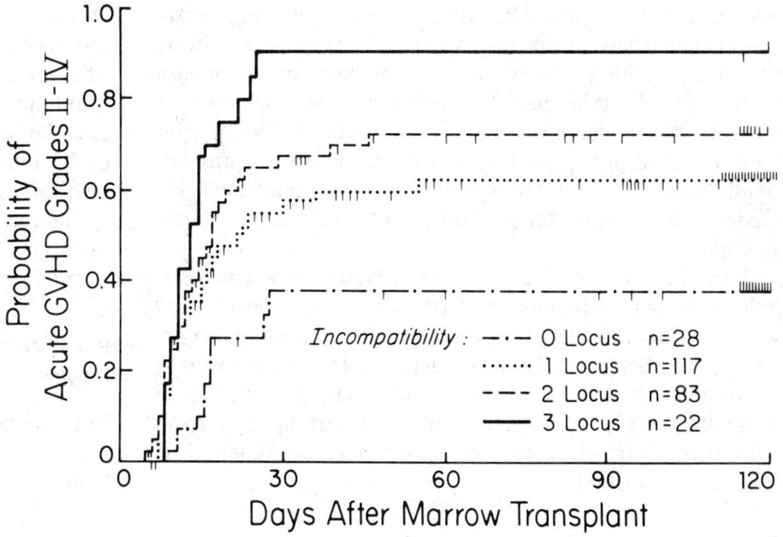

FIG. 66-43. Probability of Grades II–IV acute graft-versus-host disease in patients given HLA-haploidentical marrow grafts for hematologic malignancy. Shown are data in patients phenotypically HLA-identical on the nonshared haplotype and those in patients with a one-locus, two-locus, and three-locus difference.

TABLE 66-24. Incidence and Types of Complications and Long-term Survival After Transplantation of Unmodified Marrow from HLA-Identical Siblings for Patients with Leukemia

Disease	*Disease Phase*	*Disease-free Long-term Survival (%)*	*Relapse (%)*	*GVHD (%) Acute, Grade 2–4*	*GVHD (%) Chronic*	*Interstitial Pneumonia (%)**	*VOD (%)*
ANL	1st CR	50	22				
	2nd + CR	25	45	40–45	25–35	15–35	28
	1st REL	34	31				
ALL	1st CR	54	35				
	2nd CR	35	45	35	25	15	7
	3rd CR	30	58				
	2nd + REL	18	75				
CML	1st CP	58	17				
	AP	30	45	45	35	22	25
	BC	20	70				

Data from Refs. 11–14, 23, 29, 30, 42–48, 66, 71, 105–107.

ANL, acute nonlymphoblastic leukemia; ALL, acute lymphoblastic leukemia; CML, chronic myelocytic leukemia; CR, complete remission; REL, relapse; CP, chronic phase; AP, accelerated phase; BC, blast crisis; GVHD, graft-versus-host disease; VOD, veno-occlusive disease of the liver; VZV, varicella–zoster virus.

*Includes both idiopathic and cytomegalovirus interstitial pneumonias.

†Includes cardiorenal failure, bleeding, encephalitis, leukoencephalopathy, adult respiratory distress syndrome.

‡% applies to patients given fractionated total body irradiation; % usually considerably higher with single dose irradiation.

significantly different from that of patients given genotypically HLA-identical grafts. However, patients mismatched for two or more of the HLA loci on the nonshared haplotype clearly fare worse, and actuarial survival is only 10% to 20%. In these patients, autologous transplantation should be considered first.

UNRELATED DONORS

Studies in a canine model suggest that marrow grafts from phenotypically DLA-identical unrelated donors, although better than those from DLA haplo-identical littermates, do worse than those from genotypically DLA-identical littermates. The clinical experience accumulated so far concurs with those observations.[38,39] There are now a number of patients given marrow grafts from unrelated donors who have achieved prolonged disease-free survival, but many patients have died from transplant-related complications, including slow engraftment, GVHD, and interstitial pneumonitis.

With the computerization of HLA-typing data and with federal support, a national registry is now being developed, which will include data on 50,000 to 80,000 potential marrow donors. Some centers have suggested storage of marrow from cadaveric donors. It is conceivable that, as conditioning programs and GVHD prevention improve, unrelated marrow will be more widely used, and its ultimate usefulness will become established.

CURRENT PROBLEMS AND FUTURE APPROACHES

The principal complications after transplantation of unmodified marrow for patients with leukemia are listed in Table 66-24. Complications vary somewhat with the underlying disease for which the transplant has been carried out and include [1] toxicities from the conditioning programs and postgrafting immunosuppression (*e.g.*, mucositis, cardiorenal failure, leukencephalopathy, nephrotoxicity, veno-occlusive disease of the liver, idiopathic interstitial pneumonia, and late secondary malignancies); [2] infections related to the early granulocytopenia and the only slowly recovering immunologic reactivity of the graft; [3] transplant-related immunologic problems (*e.g.*, acute and chronic GVHD and graft failure); and [4] relapse of the original leukemia. Table 66-25 illustrates the impact of these complications on survival in a group of patients grafted for ANL.

The following paragraphs will attempt to place these complications into perspective and outline future approaches at overcoming them.

RECOVERY OF HEMATOPOIESIS AND THE IMMUNE SYSTEM

In an uneventful marrow transplant, normal granulocyte and platelet levels may be recovered by day 40 to 50, and normal hematocrit values by day 60 to 90. In most cases, hemato-

Bacterial and Fungal Infections During First 3 Mo (%)									
Before Engraftment	*After Engraftment*	*After 3 Months*	*Nephrotoxicity (%)*	*Moderate to Severe Mucositis (%)*	*Other† (%)*	*Graft Failure (%)*	*VZV Infections (%)*	*Cataracts (%)*	*Late Secondary Malignancies (%)*
20	12	20	13	38	5	<1	40	18‡	1–2

poiesis is entirely of donor origin, although some patients may show a persistent mixture of donor and host cells. Hematopoiesis is stable, as shown by observations in patients for up to 16 years. Recovery of monocytes and return of bronchoalveolar and hepatic macrophages are equally prompt. Nevertheless, certain prolonged functional impairments exist, including deficient granulocyte chemotaxis, reduction in the number of clonogenic precursors in the marrow, and decreased immune function (reviewed in Refs. 40, 41).

Three components contribute to the recipient's immunologic status after transplantation, all of which may provide some protection against infections. First, there may still be vestiges of the host's original immune system, as documented by transient production of host-type isohemagglutinin titers in ABO-incompatible recipients for as long as 12 months. Second, immunologically active donor cells may be grafted along with the marrow, thereby conveying "instant" immune function. Transfer of immunity to keyhole-limpet hemocyanin, tetanus toxoid, measles, and diphtheria has been documented in 85% of patients without GVHD and 45% of those with chronic GVHD. Finally, the most important component is the "rebirth" of the recipient's immune system originating from the infused stem cells. All recipients, regardless of the kind of graft, underlying disease, conditioning program, acute GVHD, and postgrafting immunosuppression, have profound impairment of most immune functions during the first 4 to 5 months. Exceptions include rapidly restored activity of monocyte–macrophages and of cytotoxic effector cells mediating natural killing, antibody-

TABLE 66-25. Causes of Death Among 363 Patients Given HLA-Identical Sibling Marrow Grafts for Acute Nonlymphoblastic Leukemia in First or Second Remission or in First Relapse

		Bacterial and Fungal Infections				
Time After Marrow Graft	*Interstitial Pneumonia (%)*	*With GVHD (%)*	*Without GVHD (%)*	*VOD (%)*	*Relapse (%)*	*Other* (%)*
First 100 days	13.5	5	3	3	1	4
After 100 days	5	5	5	0	20	6
Total	17	8	7	3	16	9

Data from Ref. 12.

GVHD, graft-versus-host disease; VOD, veno-occlusive disease of the liver.

*Includes hepatorenal failure, cardio-renal failure, bleeding, encephalitis, adult respiratory distress syndrome, graft failure, and late secondary malignancy.

dependent and lectin-dependent killing, all of which are normal after 30 days. Beyond the first 4 to 5 months, recipients of autologous and syngeneic grafts, and those with allogeneic grafts and no GVHD, show a return to normal of many immunologic values. Nevertheless, even among healthy, long-term survivors, there are a few who fail to produce appropriate humoral antibody to neo- and recall antigens, and 30% to 40% of these show persistent in vitro B-cell defects and decreased T-cell help. Long-term survivors with chronic GVHD more often fail to produce normal antibody and do not convert from IgM to IgG antibody after antigenic challenge; in vitro studies show B-cell dysfunction, lack of T-cell help, and in many, T-cell suppression.

It would be important to accelerate the rate of return of immunity and restore it in those patients who have persistent immunologic deficits. Attempts to do so by grafts of thymic tissue and thymic epithelial monolayers, and injection of thymosin fraction V and thymopoietin, however, have as yet been unsuccessful. Perhaps infusion of cloned donor B cells or the use of recombinant B-cell growth factors and other immune response modifiers will prove to be effective for correcting immunologic deficits and reducing the risk of infection.

OPPORTUNISTIC INFECTIONS

Bacterial and Fungal Infections

Despite supportive care, including transfusions, antibiotics, antifungal agents, and sometimes, the use of protective environments, 5% of HLA-identical marrow graft recipients may die from bacterial or fungal infections during the early granulocytopenic period.[42,43] This figure is increased in patients with HLA-nonidentical grafts. Furthermore, certain antibiotics and antifungal agents may increase the organ toxicity of the conditioning programs. Shortening the period of pancytopenia would help to reduce both the frequency of infections and the use of potentially toxic drugs needed to treat them. Perhaps recombinant human hematopoietic growth factors, such as interleukin-3 (IL-3), granulocyte–macrophage colony-stimulating factor (GM-CSF), IL-1-α, and the like, will prove useful for this. Results in murine models have been promising, and first trials in patients with autologous transplants are underway. A potential problem is that growth factors may also enhance the growth of leukemic cells, thereby increasing the risk of relapse.

Viral and Protozoan Infections

The most serious infections during the first 3 to 4 months are viral.[42–46] Activation of herpes simplex virus immediately postgrafting is common, but it can now be controlled with acyclovir. Varicella–zoster infections, seen in approximately 40% of all patients, are also treatable with acyclovir, and prevention studies with low-dose acyclovir are underway. *Pneumocystis carinii* formerly caused about 10% of interstitial pneumonias, but this has now been prevented with prophylactic trimethoprim–sulfamethoxazole. By far the most important infection is due to cytomegalovirus (CMV). Evidence of CMV activation is seen in about 75% of patients who have antibody to CMV before transplantation. Although often asymptomatic and manifested only by viral excretion in the urine or by rises in antibody titers, activation can become a serious complication in the form of CMV pneumonia. This pneumonia is seen in about 15% of patients who have received transplants for malignancy, and it has a case fatality rate of about 85%. Patients who are CMV seronegative before transplantation can be protected from infection by the exclusive use of CMV seronegative blood products. Perhaps CMV-negative blood products should be considered for any CMV-negative leukemic patient who is a transplant candidate. Immunoprophylaxis using CMV immunoglobulin has been controversial. Currently, there is no effective proven therapy for established CMV infection.[46] A trial of an acyclovir derivative, dihydroxymethylethoxymethylguanine, although ineffective in treating CMV pneumonia, resulted in a significant reduction in the amount of virus in the lung tissues. Thus, it is reasonable to contemplate using this drug in prophylactic trials.

TOXICITIES RELATED TO CONDITIONING PROGRAMS

Conditioning programs have been intensified to a point at which serious nonhematopoietic toxicity has been observed. Mucositis of varying degrees of severity is common, but it generally subsides sometime after day 14.[47] Similarly, diarrhea is frequent, but reversible. More serious has been veno-occlusive disease of the liver, a problem that has been particularly frequent in patients with underlying liver damage.[47] It is clearly caused by the conditioning programs, but it can be magnified by postgrafting immunosuppression, in particular cyclosporine. Veno-occlusive disease may be seen in 15% to 28% of patients, and may have a morbidity as high as 30%. Acute myocarditis can be a problem in patients with extensive previous exposure to anthracyclines. The incidence of idiopathic interstitial pneumonia has been 8% to 10% in patients conditioned with single-dose TBI, but this has dropped to 3% with the use of fractionated TBI.[44] Leukoencephalopathy can be a problem in children with ALL who have had previous cranial radiation therapy. Other long-term side-effects may include impairment of growth and sexual development in children.[48] It is rare for irradiated patients to have offspring. Cataracts have been seen in 80% of patients given single-dose TBI but only in 18% of those given fractionated TBI.[48] Late secondary malignancies can be expected, as suggested by studies in long-term canine radiation chimeras showing a sixfold increase in cancer compared with healthy dogs.[48]

It is clear that current conditioning programs involving systemic exposure of patients to toxic agents have been pushed to their limit, and new regimens causing more specific destruction of malignant cells while sparing normal tissues need to be developed.

GRAFT FAILURE, GRAFT-VERSUS-HOST DISEASE, RECURRENCE OF MALIGNANT DISEASE

The long-term success of marrow grafts for the treatment of hematologic cancer depends on avoiding all of three mutually related problems: graft failure, GVHD, and recurrence of underlying malignancy. Hallmarks of success are stable hematopoietic engraftment, immunologic graft–host tolerance, and eradication of malignant disease. Graft failure and recurrence of leukemia both reflect on the relative ineffectiveness of current conditioning programs to eradicate host immune and cancer cells. For complete eradication to occur, an allogeneic graft-versus-leukemia effect may be needed.

Graft Failure

Graft failure is rare in recipients of unmodified HLA-identical sibling marrow (<1% incidence). Occasionally poor graft function is seen, which may be due to drug toxicity, (*e.g.*, methotrexate, trimethoprim–sulfamethoxazole, interferon) or related to certain infections (*e.g.*, CMV). When incriminating drugs are discontinued or recovery from viral infection occurs, graft function frequently recovers.

Failure of engraftment and graft rejection have been recognized to occur in two settings. The first is with marrow from donors who are HLA-nonidentical.[38] Failure of sustained engraftment is seen in 5% of phenotypically HLA-matched pairs, 7% to 10% of one HLA locus-mismatched pairs, and 15% to 25% of two and three HLA locus-mismatched pairs. The second setting occurs with HLA-identical or HLA-nonidentical T-cell–depleted marrow.[5,49–51] Presumably, donor T cells are needed to destroy those host cells that cause rejection of the marrow graft. Graft failure has an extremely high case fatality rate.

Understanding the mechanisms of graft failure in humans is important in designing ways to overcome the problem. Animal studies have suggested that the mechanisms depend upon the particular donor–recipient combination. Studies in a canine model have implicated radioresistant Ia-positive non-T cells in destruction of DLA-nonidentical marrow grafts, whereas host T cells may be responsible for rejection of DLA-identical grafts.[52] Canine studies also suggest that an increase in the dose of TBI from 9.2 to 18.0 Gy or recipient pretreatment with anti-Ia antibody are capable of overcoming resistance to mismatched grafts, whereas treatment with antithymocyte globulin is effective in overcoming the problem of failure of histocompatible grafts.

Clinically, more intensive conditioning programs, including the addition of total lymphoid irradiation, decreased the incidence of graft rejection, but the concomitant increase in regimen-related toxicities may negate any survival advantage. The addition to the conditioning regimen of antibodies directed at immune cells is being explored. Antithymocyte globulin and anti-Ia antibodies have been prime candidates for this approach. The animal studies have already shown that antibodies are not uniformly successful in overcoming the problem of graft failure.[52–53] Current efforts are therefore directed toward coupling certain monoclonal antibodies to short-lived radioactive isotopes to further abrogate resistance to marrow grafts without too much added toxicity (see upcoming section, Radiolabeled Monoclonal Antibodies).

It is also conceivable that the T cells in the marrow inoculum that cause GVHD may be different from those needed to overcome graft rejection. Animal studies, as yet, have not provided unequivocal answers to this question. However, clinical trials are in progress that use antibodies, with the specific aim of removing cells causing GVHD from the marrow, while leaving other immune cells that may be needed for successful engraftment. The role of hematopoietic growth factors in establishing marrow grafts is also being explored.

Acute GVHD

PATHOPHYSIOLOGY. The clinical and histologic criteria for acute GVHD have been described in detailed reviews.[54–58] The disease is presumably caused by T cells in the donor marrow that attack targets in skin, liver, and gastrointestinal tract. It manifests itself by skin rash, abdominal pain, diarrhea, and liver function abnormalities. Between 20% and 50% of patients given marrow grafts from HLA-identical siblings develop significant acute GVHD. GVHD signifies the advent of life-threatening complications. For example, patients with aplastic anemia with no or only very mild acute GVHD have a survival of 90% compared with 45% survival in those with significant GVHD.[55] Similarly, among 231 Seattle patients with ANL who received transplants during their first remission, clinically significant GVHD was associated with a 2.5 times higher risk of fatality.[12] Death is often due to infections, for which GVHD may set the stage by creating portals of entry through lesions in skin and intestinal tract and through enhancement of the postgrafting immunodeficiency. Prevention of infection by decontamination and laminar airflow room isolation can decrease the incidence and delay the onset of acute GVHD and increase survival.[55] The mechanism by which this is achieved remains conjectural. Perhaps decontamination prevents a process in which infections cause lymphocytes to secrete lymphokines which, in turn, may increase the expression of the class II histocompatibility antigens on certain target cells (*e.g.*, gut epithelium), thereby making them targets for GVHD.

RELATIONSHIP BETWEEN GVHD AND LEUKEMIC RECURRENCE: "GRAFT-VERSUS-LEUKEMIA EFFECT." Some of the apparent cures seen after marrow transplantation may have been due to a graft-versus-leukemia effect directed at normal and perhaps also leukemia-associated antigens present on the patient's leukemic cells. This hypothesis is based on animal studies and retrospective analyses of clinical results. Among patients who have lived at least 150 days after grafting, the likelihood of being in remission 2 years later is significantly higher in allogeneic recipients with acute or chronic GVHD than in those without GVHD or than in syngeneic recipients.[59] Also, recipients of T-cell–depleted marrow have less GVHD, but a higher incidence of leukemic recurrence than those given unmanipulated marrow.[49–51,60] The increase in the incidence of relapse may outweigh any survival advantage gained from the reduction in GVHD. Figure 66-44 illustrates this point and shows that the disease-free survival at 2 years is 62% for patients with CML in chronic phase who were given transplants of unmodified marrow compared with only 42% for those given T-depleted marrow.[60] These data suggest that certain T cells in the donor marrow are capable of eliminating residual leukemic cells in the host. Attempts at inducing GVHD,

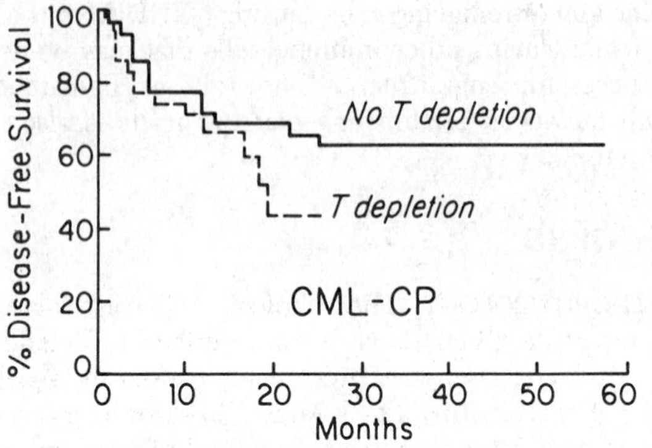

FIG. 66-44. Probability of disease-free survival for two groups of patients transplanted for chronic myelocytic leukemia in chronic phase following conditioning with high-dose cyclophosphamide and total body irradiation.[60] All patients were given marrow grafts from HLA-identical siblings. One group of patients (n = 35) was given unmodified marrow and the other (n = 28) was given marrow that was T-cell depleted by the Campath 1 antibody.

thereby decreasing the incidence of leukemic relapse and improving survival, have as yet not met with success because the lessened incidence of relapse is offset by a greater risk of other fatal complications.[61]

Certain murine studies suggest that a graft-versus-leukemia effect can be distinguished from GVHD.[62] Results of these studies imply that some cells in the graft specifically react with surface antigens expressed on leukemic cells, whereas others react more broadly with minor histocompatibility antigens expressed on host tissue cells. It remains to be seen whether or not these findings in the mouse can be verified in humans. In one marrow transplant recipient, it was possible to isolate clones of donor-derived lymphoid cells that showed spontaneous cytotoxicity against cryopreserved host leukemic cells but no activity against activated T-lymphocytes from the host.[63] It was suggested that cells of this type might have an antileukemic effect without causing GVHD. Thus, measures taken to prevent GVHD may not always be accompanied by an increased risk of leukemic relapse. A preliminary suggestion that this might be so has come from the observation that the decrease in incidence and severity of acute GVHD associated with the use of postgrafting methotrexate/cyclosporine, discussed later, has not yet had an adverse effect on the risk of leukemic relapse (Fig. 66-45). Finally, parallel to findings in murine models, it might be possible to expand in vitro T cells sensitized to tumor antigens with the help of IL-2, before infusion into the tumor-bearing host, along with in vivo infusion of IL-2.[64,65]

FIG. 66-45. Probability of disease-free survival and of relapse for two groups of patients with chronic myelocytic leukemia in chronic phase (*CML-CP*) given HLA-identical sibling marrow transplants after conditioning with high-dose cyclophosphamide and total body irradiation.[69] One group of patients received a methotrexate/cyclosporine combination for prevention of graft-versus-host disease (n = 26), and the other was given cyclosporine alone (n = 29).

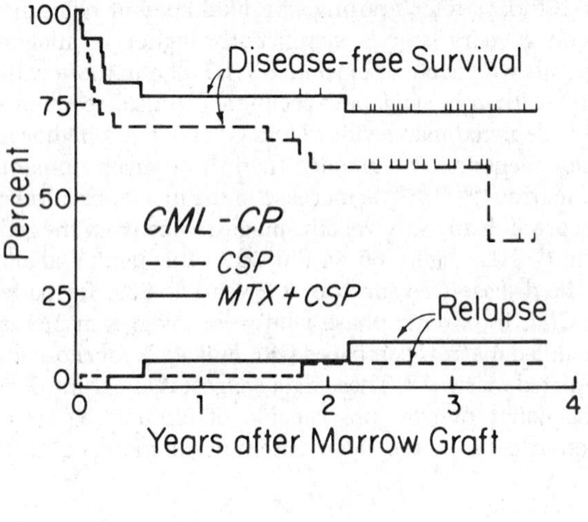

PREVENTION OF ACUTE GVHD. Prevention of GVHD has customarily involved the use of immunosupressive drugs postgrafting.[5,54,55,58,66] In contrast with patients with solid organ transplants, marrow graft recipients do not need to be given immunosuppression for an indefinite period of time. In many patients, immunosuppression can be discontinued by 3 to 6 months after grafting when a stable state of graft–host tolerance has been reached. It is not entirely clear what maintains transplantation tolerance in these patients, although earlier data suggest that specific suppressor cells of donor origin are involved.[67] Omission of these drugs in patients given unmanipulated marrow has caused an unacceptably high incidence of acute GVHD, with resultant poor survival.[68] Prospective randomized trials have shown methotrexate and cyclosporine to be equally effective in preventing GVHD, whereas Cy is less effective. The addition of prednisone to methotrexate or cyclosporine may further improve the results, although this remains to be proved in prospective trials. A combination of methotrexate along with cyclosporine is significantly better than either drug alone and leads to improved survival.[69] For example, among 29 patients with CML in chronic phase randomized to receive cyclosporine alone, seven developed grade 2, four grade 3, and four developed grade 4 acute GVHD. This compares with five patients with grade 2, two with grade 3, and none with grade 4 GVHD among 26 patients given methotrexate combined with cyclosporine. Figure 64-45 illustrates disease-free survival and relapse rates in the two groups of patients. Although these results are encouraging, both methotrexate and cyclosporine have associated toxicities often necessitating dose reductions, thereby impairing their efficacy in GVHD prevention. Also, although acute GVHD is lessened, chronic GVHD continues to be seen.

Another way to prevent GVHD has been the removal of T cells from the marrow through monoclonal antibodies used either to target lytic activities of complement or toxins or for immunoadsorption. T cells have also been depleted by their selective agglutination to soybean lectin or through E-rosetting and elutriation. With any of these techniques, there is a reduction in the number of infused T cells by 1 to 3 logs.[3,5,49–51,60] This way, virtually all differentiated cells involved in generating GVH reactions would be removed, and the immune system returned to an early prenatal state. Any new stem cell-derived immune cell would accept the host antigenic environment as "self" and become tolerant. The strategy of T-cell depletion has worked well in preventing GVHD in rodent models, whereas results in a large random-bred animal, the dog, have been less encouraging. The canine studies already pointed at the problem of graft failure. Graft failure is almost certainly the result of rejection of the graft through host immune cells that have survived the conditioning program and whose continued survival is assured through the absence of a GVH reaction. For patients given HLA-identical marrow, results in nearly all studies have demonstrated a significant reduction in acute GVHD if at least a 1.5 log T-cell depletion is achieved, regardless of the technique used. Significant GVHD was seen in 11% of HLA-identical marrow graft recipients and only 28% of HLA-nonidentical recipients. These data provide convincing evidence for a favorable effect of T-cell depletion on GVHD. However, the beneficial effect of T-cell depletion on acute, and possibly also chronic GVHD, was achieved at the price of substantial increases in graft rejection and leukemic relapse. The overall incidence of graft rejection in HLA-identical marrow transplant recipients increased from less than 1% to 10% to 20% and in HLA-nonidentical recipients from 5% to 35%. Additionally, most studies showed an increase in the risk of leukemic relapse after T-cell depletion. An example of this is given in Figure 66-44.

Given that rejection and leukemic relapse almost uniformly result in death, an improvement in survival in patients given T-cell–depleted marrow has not been realized. Nevertheless, the significant decrease in the incidence of GVHD seen with T-cell depletion suggests that the technique is promising if the risk of graft rejection and leukemic relapse can be lessened. To achieve this aim two different approaches can be envisioned. One is improved pretransplant conditioning programs leading to significantly better eradication of both malignant and immune cells of the host type. As will be discussed, this aim may be achievable through innovative approaches using antibody isotope conjugates. The other approach is based on the hope that T cells causing GVHD are distinct from those involved in enhancing allogeneic engraftment and causing graft-versus-leukemia effects. A better understanding of the precise role lymphocytes play in mediating these diverse immune functions is needed. Better knowledge might result in the development of strategies to specifically eliminate GVHD without affecting engraftment and the graft-versus-leukemia effect.

TREATMENT OF ESTABLISHED ACUTE GVHD. Based in part on animal studies, treatment of acute GVHD has been tried in humans with prednisone, antithymocyte globulin, cyclosporine, and various monoclonal antibodies directed against T cells with variable responses (reviewed in Refs. 55, 66). As the repertoire of monoclonal anti–T-cell antibodies increases, reagents may be found that specifically interact with those cells that are actively involved in acute GVHD. Perhaps antibodies will have to be coupled to immunotoxins for optimum effect.

Chronic GVHD

Chronic GVHD can be diagnosed in 30% to 50% of patients some time between 3 and 15 months after transplantation (reviewed in Refs. 55, 57, 58, and 66). The clinical manifestations, ranging from mild to extreme, resemble those seen in systemic collagen vascular diseases and include skin lesions, keratoconjunctivitis, buccal mucositis, esophageal and vaginal strictures, intestinal involvement, chronic liver disease, generalized wasting, and pulmonary insufficiency. Acute GVHD predicts a high incidence of chronic GVHD, as does increasing patient age. When untreated, the disease has a poor prognosis, and most patients die or become disabled. The most effective drug to treat chronic GVHD is prednisone given alone or combined with cyclosporine.[70] Azathioprine is less effective. With therapy, approximately one-half of the patients with extensive chronic GVHD are living with Karnofsky Performance scores of 100%, and an additional 25% with scores of between 80% and 90%. In about half of the patients, therapy can be discontinued after 9 to 12 months. Despite this apparent success, however, the management of patients with chronic GVHD remains unsatisfactory. Of the affected patients, 25% die with infections, mainly from encapsulated gram-positive bacteria, resulting from their poor immunologic status.[71]

Recurrence of Malignant Disease

INCIDENCE AND ORIGIN OF RECURRENT DISEASE. Recurrent disease remains a major cause of failure of marrow transplantation. Recurrence rates range from 20% to 80%. In more than 95% of the patients, this means reappearance of the original malignant cell population as determined by blood genetic markers. This demonstrates the inability of current conditioning programs to eradicate all clonogenic leukemic cells and emphasizes the need for improvement. Occasional leukemia recurrences (less than 5% of patients) have involved donor type cells[72] (reviewed in Refs. 1, 48, 73). Whether this is due to transfection of donor cells with DNA derived from host cells, or the result of influences of the marrow stroma, is presently unclear. A small number of malignant disease recurrences have been in the form of immunoblastic lymphosarcoma in cells of donor origin, usually in patients given T-depleted marrow or in patients treated with monoclonal antibodies for steroid-resistant GVHD (reviewed in Refs. 48, 73). These lymphosarcomas have detectable Epstein-Barr virus. The proliferation of Epstein-Barr virus-transformed cells suggests that normal immune surveillance mechanisms must be compromised in these patients.

MODIFICATIONS OF CHEMOTHERAPY OR TBI (SEE TABLE 66-23). The most commonly used conditioning program for marrow transplantation has been Cy and TBI. To improve results with transplantation, numerous chemotherapeutic agents have been administered in addition to, or in lieu of, Cy, including etoposide, high-dose cytosine arabinoside, piperazine dione, carmustine (bischloroethylnitrosourea, BCNU), and others[74–77] (see also Refs. 94–104). Results of uncontrolled studies have suggested advantages with these newer programs. Since 1977, fractionated TBI has begun replacing single-dose TBI. A prospective comparison of these two radiation modalities showed that fractionated TBI was better tolerated, resulted in fewer long-term complications, and caused no alteration in the rate of postgrafting relapse.[78] Hyperfractionated TBI followed by Cy has been used by the Sloan–Kettering transplant team in patients with ALL in second or subsequent remission, with apparently superior results.[79] The Johns-Hopkins transplant team has used busulfan and Cy without TBI.[80] They reported very low leukemic recurrence rates in patients with ANL in first remission, whereas relapse rates in patients with ANL in second remission or ALL appeared to be no different from those seen after TBI regimens. The teams at the M. D. Anderson Hospital and the University of British Columbia have used a combination of Cy, BCNU, and etoposide (see Refs. 97, 100). For all approaches involving systemic chemotherapy and TBI, the limits of nonhematopoietic toxicity have been reached and, barring unexpected developments, no quantum improvements can be anticipated from these approaches.

RADIOLABELED MONOCLONAL ANTIBODIES. The most effective way to eradicate cancer would be through agents that specifically interact with the malignant cells. The approach that comes closest to this ideal is the use of monoclonal antibodies directed against tumor-associated antigens. Monoclonal antibodies injected in vivo can concentrate on tumor cells;[81–84] however, the antitumor effect is limited. In part, this is because some tumor cells lack target antigens, whereas others, although coated by antibody, are not killed by it.[85] Investigations are in progress with antibodies linked to toxins (*e.g.*, the ricin A chain) for more effective tumor cell kill. An additional promising way to use monoclonal antibodies is to attach them to a short-lived radioactive isotope. In this way cells expressing the target antigen will be killed, as well as neighboring cells, which may be antigen-negative. Of course, if this approach is applied to hematologic malignancies, normal marrow cells will also be ablated. Thus, subsequent marrow "rescue" would still be an obligatory requirement.

Initial experiments in a canine model have shown appropriate antibody–isotope conjugates to localize preferentially in marrow and spleen and, to some extent, also in lymph nodes.[86,87] The amount of isotope in the marrow, compared with other organs, achieves a ratio of 5:1 or better. Such radiolabeled antibodies are capable of producing fatal marrow aplasia, which can be reversed by infusion of cryopreserved autologous marrow 8 days later, at a time when very little radioactivity is left. These studies, done initially with radioactive iodine, are continuing, and combinations of chemotherapy, TBI, and radiolabeled antibody are being explored for their efficacy in preparing dogs for grafts of T-cell–depleted marrow. These experiments will set the stage for the clinical application of this technique. It is likely that refinements of this approach, particularly the use of high-energy β-emitting isotopes with short linear energy transfer, will ultimately result in less toxic, but more efficient, programs, not only providing better eradication of malignant disease, but also ameliorating the problem of graft failure.

BONE-SEEKING RADIOISOTOPES. An approach similar to that of radiolabeled antibodies involves bone-seeking substances such as those used for scanning purposes. It is possible to link β-emitting isotopes to such bone-seeking substances (*e.g.*, ^{153}Sm complexed to ethylenediaminetetramethylene phosphoric acid) which, upon intravenous infusion, localizes within minutes to bone. Samarium-153 deposits most of its energy within a 1- to 2-mm radius. It also emits very low-intensity gamma radiation, permitting external camera scanning. This approach is of interest because marrow cells are rarely ever more than 1 to 2 mm away from bony trabeculae and are thus within reach of the radiation emitted by the ^{153}Sm. Initial results in the dog have shown that marrow ablation can be accomplished without toxicity to other organs, and marrow/other organ ratios of 20:1 have been achieved.

GENE TRANSFER IN HEMATOPOIETIC STEM CELLS

The marrow is composed of a mixture of cells including large numbers of differentiated and mature cells, many committed progenitors with defined function and limited proliferation potential, and rare pluripotent stem cells that have broad developmental and proliferative potential. The ability of pluripotent stem cells not only to self-renew but also to differentiate into the various committed hematopoietic precursors has made them potential targets for attempts at somatic gene therapy. Recent years have seen advances in gene cloning and transfer. It is now reasonable to contemplate the replacement of missing or defective genes in hematopoietic tissues to cure potentially lethal hereditary disorders. It is also conceivable that the therapeutic index of chemotherapy could be substantially improved if a patient's bone marrow could be made resistant to one or more of the antineoplastic agents. The cloning of genes that confer resistance to chemotherapeutic drugs may make this feasible. Gene transfer also may provide a new approach to addressing questions on stem cell commitment and proliferation. It may be possible to introduce lineage-specific genes or oncogenes into stem cells and their progeny, thereby modulating the system in a defined way. Finally, site-specific insertion of new genetic material will make it possible to mark the progeny of individual stem cell clones as they move along their differentiation pathways.

Retroviral vectors have many advantages for gene transfer into hematopoietic cells.[88–95] These include the high efficiency of gene transfer that is required for successful introduction of genes into the very rare pluripotent stem cells, the stable integration of the provirus into the genome of the target cell so that the transduced genes will be passed on to the differentiated progenitors and mature cells, the wide spectrum of tissue and species specificity, and finally the precise single-copy colinear structure of the transduced provirus. In vitro studies have shown successful use of retroviral vectors to transfer genes into murine, canine, and human hematopoietic cells. Additionally, these vectors have been used to infect pluripotent stem cells capable of reconstituting the hematopoietic systems in mice, dogs, and nonhuman primates. Best results have generally been observed in mice. Nevertheless, even in this animal model, expression of the transferred genes is generally poor and the frequency of cells expressing the gene of interest can decrease over time. Attempts to improve results in large animals by selectively enriching for stem cells that carry the gene of interest by concurrently infecting cells with a methotrexate-resistance gene and using methotrexate for in vivo selection have, as yet, met with limited success.

It is clear that much work still needs to be done to increase the relatively low levels of gene expression in vivo through improvements in the development both of retroviral vectors and of packaging cell lines so that the highest possible virus titers can be generated in the absence of any detectable helper virus. Perhaps results can be improved through the use of various hematopoietic growth factors. Perhaps improved infection can be achieved in stem cells that have been maintained in long-term culture. As our understanding of gene transfer techniques increases and our knowledge of gene regulation in the course of differentiation improves, gene transfer for the treatment of hematopoietic disorders may one day become clinical reality.

OUTLOOK

Seventeen years ago marrow transplantation was restricted to patients with advanced acute leukemia. Since then, the technique has proved to be beneficial and even curative for patients with many different hematologic conditions. In younger patients, transplantation is the treatment of choice for any acute leukemia that has recurred at least once, for ANL in first remission and for CML. For patients with CML in the chronic phase and ANL in first remission, the risk of early death due to complications of marrow grafting must be weighed against the benefit of long-term survival and cure.

Despite impressive improvements in the results of marrow grafting, major problems still need to be solved. These include recurrence of malignant disease, graft failure in patients given T-cell–depleted or HLA-nonidentical marrow grafts, acute and chronic GVHD, infections associated with the prolonged immunodeficiency, and late complications resulting from the conditioning programs. Crucial developments must come in the area of more effective and less toxic conditioning programs. Approaches such as the use of monoclonal antibodies linked to short-lived radioisotopes, or the use of bone-seeking isotopes, hold much promise in this regard. More effective conditioning programs are likely to reduce drastically the problems of recurrence of malignant disease and of graft failure. They will also permit a broader application of T-cell depletion to prevent GVHD, thus extending transplantation to include more HLA-nonidentical and unrelated patients. Efficient conditioning programs will also enlarge the scope of autologous marrow grafting, in particular if they are combined with better purging methods. As combinations of immunosuppressive agents have already decreased the incidence of GVHD, the use of recombinant hematopoietic growth factors might reduce the risk of infections. In the distant future, gene transfer into stem cells might find clinical application to confer drug resistance and to inhibit or alter the function of genes involved in the generation of disease.

REFERENCES

1. Thomas ED, Storb R, Clift RA et al: Bone-marrow transplantation. N Engl J Med 292:832–843; 895–902, 1975
2. Santos GW: History of bone marrow transplantation. Clin Haematol 12:611–639, 1983
3. O'Reilly RJ: Allogeneic bone marrow transplantation: Current status and future directions. Blood 62:941–964, 1983
4. Storb R, Thomas ED: Allogeneic bone-marrow transplantation. Immunol Rev 71:77–102, 1983
5. Storb R: Critical issues in bone marrow transplantation. Transplantation Proc 19:2774–2781, 1987
6. Thomas ED, Storb R: Technique for human marrow grafting. Blood 36:507–515, 1970
7. Buckner CD, Appelbaum FR, Thomas ED: Bone marrow and fetal liver. In Karow AM, Pegg DE (eds): Organ Preservation for Transplantation, pp 355–375. New York, Marcel Dekker, 1981
8. Schaefer UW: Preservation of bone marrow for transplantation. In van Bekkum DW, Lowenberg B (eds): Bone Marrow Transplantation, pp 513–538. New York, Marcel Dekker, 1985
9. Korbling M, Martin H, Fliedner TM et al: Autologous blood stem cell transplantation. In Gale RP, Champlin R (eds): Progress in Bone Marrow Transplantation, pp 877–888. New York, Alan R Liss, 1987
10. Chang J, Morgenstern G, Deakin D et al: Reconstitution of haematopoietic system with autologous marrow taken during relapse of acute myeloblastic leukaemia and grown in long-term culture. Lancet 1:294–295, 1986
11. Thomas ED, Buckner CD, Banaji M et al: One hundred patients with acute leukemia treated by chemotherapy, total body irradiation, and allogeneic marrow transplantation. Blood 49:511–533, 1977
12. Clift RA, Buckner CD, Thomas ED et al: The treatment of acute nonylmphoblastic leukemia by allogeneic marrow transplantation. Bone Marrow Transplantation 2:243–258, 1987
13. Champlin R, for the Advisory Committee of the International Bone Marrow Transplant Registry: Bone marrow transplantation for acute leukemia: A preliminary report from the International Bone Marrow Transplant Registry. Transplantation Proc 19:2626–2628, 1987
14. Gratwohl A, Hermans J, Lyklema A, Zwaan FE: Bone marrow transplantation for leukaemia in Europe: Report from the Leukaemia Working Party 1987. Bone Marrow Transplantation (Suppl 1) 2:15–18, 1987
15. Linch DC, Burnett AK: Clinical studies of ABMT in acute myeloid leukemia. Clin Haematol 15:167–186, 1986
16. Yeager AM, Kaizer H, Santos GW et al: Autologous bone marrow transplantation in patients with acute nonlymphocytic leukemia, using ex vivo marrow treatment with 4-hydroperoxycyclophosphamide. N Engl J Med 315:141–147, 1986
17. Appelbaum FR, Dahlberg S, Thomas ED et al: Bone marrow transplantation or chemotherapy after remission induction for adults with acute nonlymphoblastic leukemia: a prospective comparison. Ann Intern Med 101:581–588, 1984
18. Champlin RE, Ho WG, Gale RP et al: Treatment of acute myelogenous leukemia: A prospective controlled trial of bone marrow transplantation versus consolidation chemotherapy. Ann Intern Med 102:285–291, 1985
19. Powles RL, Clink HM, Bandini G et al: The place of bone-marrow transplantation in acute myelogenous leukaemia. Lancet 1:1047–1050, 1980
20. Tallman MS, Appelbaum FR, Amos D et al: Evaluation of intensive post-remission chemotherapy for adults with acute nonlymphocytic leukemia using high-dose cytosine arabinoside with L-asparaginase and amsacrine with etoposide. J Clin Oncol 5:918–926, 1987
21. Thomas ED, Sanders JE, Flournoy N et al: Marrow transplantation for patients with acute lymphoblastic leukemia: A long-term follow-up. Blood 62:1139–1141, 1983
22. Sanders JE, Flournoy N, Thomas ED et al: Marrow transplant experience in children with acute lymphoblastic leukemia: An analysis of factors associated with survival, relapse and graft-versus-host disease. Med Pediatr Oncol 13:165–172, 1985
23. Gorin NC, Aegerter P: Autologous bone marrow transplantation for acute leukaemia in remission: 4th EBMTG survey. Bone Marrow Transplantation (Suppl 1) 2:320–323, 1987
24. Johnson FL, Thomas ED, Clark BS et al: A comparison of marrow transplantation with chemotherapy for children with acute lymphoblastic leukemia in second or subsequent remission. N Engl J Med 305:846–851, 1981
25. Rivera GK, Buchanan G, Boyett JM et al: Intensive retreatment of childhood acute lymphoblastic leukemia in first bone marrow relapse. N Engl J Med 315:273–278, 1986
26. Hoelzer D, Thiel E, Loffler H et al: Intensified therapy in acute lymphoblastic and acute undifferentiated leukemia in adults. Blood 64:38–47, 1984
27. Schauer P, Arlin ZA, Mertelsmann R et al: Treatment of acute lymphoblastic leukemia in adults: Results of the L-10 and L-10M protocols. J Clin Oncol 1:462–470, 1983
28. Hoelzer D, Thiel E, Buchner T et al: Prognostic factors in a multicenter study for treatment of acute lymphoblastic leukemia in adults. Blood 71:123–131, 1988
29. Thomas ED, Clift RA, Fefer A et al: Marrow transplantation for the treatment of chronic myelogenous leukemia. Ann Intern Med 104:155–163, 1986
30. Goldman JM, Apperley JF, Jones L et al: Bone marrow transplantation for patients with chronic myeloid leukemia. N Engl J Med 314:202–207, 1986

31. Speck B, Bortin MM, Champlin R et al: Allogeneic bone-marrow transplantation for chronic myelogenous leukaemia. Lancet 1:665–668, 1984
32. Appelbaum FR, Sullivan KM, Buckner CD et al: Treatment of malignant lymphoma in one hundred patients with chemotherapy, total body irradiation and marrow transplantation. J Clin Oncol 5:1340–1347, 1987
33. Goldstone AH, for the European Bone Marrow Transplant Group: EBMT experience of autologous bone marrow transplantation in non-Hodgkin's lymphoma and Hodgkin's disease. Bone Marrow Transplantation (Suppl 1) 1:289–292, 1986
34. Cabanillas F, Hagemeister FB, Bodey GP et al: IMVP-16: An effective regimen for patients with lymphoma who have relapsed after initial combination chemotherapy. Blood 60:693–697, 1982
35. Appelbaum FR, Storb R, Ramberg RE et al: Treatment of preleukemic syndromes with marrow transplantation. Blood 69:92–96, 1987
36. Spitzer G, Ventura G, Hortobagyi G et al: High dose chemotherapy studies with autologous marrow support in human solid tumors: What have we done and where should we be going. In Gale RP, Champlin R (eds): Progress in Bone Marrow Transplantation, pp 827–845. New York, Alan R Liss, 1987
37. Beatty PG, Clift RA, Mickelson EM et al: Marrow transplantation from related donors other than HLA-identical siblings. N Engl J Med 313:765–771, 1985
38. Hansen JA, Beatty PG, Anasetti C et al: Treatment of leukemia by marrow transplantation from donors other than HLA genotypically identical siblings. In Gale RP, Champlin R (eds): Progress in Bone Marrow Transplantation, pp 667–675. New York, Alan R Liss, 1987
39. Ash RC, Casper J, Serwint MS et al: Extending the application of allogeneic marrow transplantation for leukemic patients who lack matched sibling donors, utilizing partially matched donors in concert with T-cell depletion for GVHD prophylaxis. In Gale RP, Champlin R (eds): Progress in Bone Marrow Transplantation, pp 365–379. New York, Alan R Liss, 1987
40. Witherspoon RP, Lum LG, Storb R: Immunologic reconstitution after human marrow grafting. Semin Hematol 21:2–10, 1984
41. Lum LG: A review: The kinetics of immune reconstitution after human marrow transplantation. Blood 69:369–380, 1987
42. Bowden RA, Meyers JD: Infectious complications following marrow transplantation. Plasma Ther Transfusion Technol 6:285–302, 1985
43. Winston DJ, Ho WG, Champlin RE et al: Infectious complications of bone marrow transplantation. Exp Hematol 12:205–215, 1984
44. Meyers JD, Flournoy N, Thomas ED: Nonbacterial pneumonia after allogeneic marrow transplantation: A review of ten years' experience. Rev Infect Dis 4:1119–1132, 1982
45. Weiner RS, Bortin MM, Gale RP et al: Interstitial pneumonitis after bone marrow transplantation. Assessment of risk factors. Ann Intern Med 104:168–175, 1986
46. Meyers JD, Thomas ED: Infection complicating bone marrow transplantation. In Rubin RH, Young LS (eds): Clinical Approach to Infection in the Immunocompromised Host, Chap. 20, pp 525–556. New York, Plenum Press, 1988
47. McDonald GB, Shulman HM, Sullivan KM et al: Intestinal and hepatic complications of human bone marrow transplantation. Gastroenterology 90:460–477; 770–784, 1986
48. Deeg HJ, Storb R, Thomas ED: Bone marrow transplantation: A review of delayed complications. Br J Haematol 57:185–208, 1984
49. Martin PJ, Hansen JA, Storb R et al: Applications of monoclonal antibodies for prevention of graft-versus-host disease. In Grignani F, Mantelli MF, Mason DY (eds): Monoclonal Antibodies in Haematopathology, pp 139–148. New York, Raven Press, 1986
50. Butturini A, Gale RP: T-cell depletion in bone marrow transplantation for leukemia: Current results and future directions. Bone Marrow Transplantation 3:185–192, 1988
51. Hale G, Waldmann H: Depletion of T-cells with Campath-1 and human complement: Analysis of GVHD and graft failure in a multi-centre study. Bone Marrow Transplantation (Suppl 1) 1:93–94, 1986
52. Storb R, Deeg HJ: Failure of allogeneic canine marrow grafts after total body irradiation: Allogeneic "resistance" vs transfusion induced sensitization. Transplantation 42:571–580, 1986
53. Deeg HJ, Sale GE, Storb R et al: Engraftment of DLA-nonidentical bone marrow facilitated by recipient treatment with anti-class II monoclonal antibody and methotrexate. Transplantation 44:340–345, 1987
54. van Bekkum DW, Lowenberg B (eds): Bone Marrow Transplantation: Biological Mechanisms and Clinical Practice. New York, Marcel Dekker, 1985
55. Storb R, Thomas ED: Graft-versus-host disease in dog and man: The Seattle experience. Immunol Rev 88:215–238, 1985
56. Sale GE, Shulman HM (eds): The Pathology of Bone Marrow Transplantation. New York, Masson, 1984
57. Sullivan KM, Witherspoon R, Deeg HJ et al: Chronic graft-versus-host disease in man. In Gale RP, Champlin R (eds): Progress in Bone Marrow Transplantation, pp 473–487. New York, Alan R Liss, 1987
58. Santos GW, Hess AD, Vogelsang B: Graft-versus-host reactions and disease. Immunol Rev 88:169–192, 1985
59. Weiden PL, Sullivan KM, Flournoy N et al: Antileukemic effect of chronic graft-versus-host disease. Contribution to improved survival after allogeneic marrow transplantation. N Engl J Med 304:1529–1533, 1981
60. Apperley JF, Jones L, Hale G et al: Bone marrow transplantation for patients with chronic myeloid leukaemia: T-cell depletion with Campath-1 reduces the incidence of graft-versus-host disease but may increase the risk of leukaemic relapse. Bone Marrow Transplantation 1:53–66, 1986
61. Sullivan KM, Buckner CD, Weiden P et al: Antileukemic effect of high dose fractionated total body irradiation (TBI) and manipulation of graft-versus-host disease (GVHD) immunosuppression following bone marrow transplantation (BMT) (abstr). Blood (Suppl 1) 64:221A, 1984
62. Truitt RL, LeFever AV, Shih CC-Y: Graft-versus-leukemia reactions: Experimental models and clinical trials. In Gale RP, Champlin R (eds): Progress in Bone Marrow Transplantation, pp 219–232. New York, Alan R Liss, 1987
63. Hercend T, Takvorian T, Nowill A et al: Characterization of natural killer cells with antileukemia activity following allogeneic bone marrow transplantation. Blood 67:722–728, 1986
64. Cheever MA, Greenberg PD, Fefer A: Specific adoptive therapy of established leukemia with syngeneic lymphocytes sequentially immunized in vivo and in vitro and nonspecifically expanded by culture with interleukin 2. J Immunol 126:1318–1322, 1981
65. Greenberg PD, Cheever MA, Fefer A: Eradication of disseminated murine leukemia by chemoimmunotherapy with cyclophosphamide and adoptively transferred immune syngeneic Lyt 1^+2^- T lymphocytes. J Exp Med 154:952–963, 1981
66. Storb R: Graft-versus-host disease after marrow transplantation. In Meryman HT (ed): Transplantation: Approaches to Graft Rejection, pp 139–157. New York, Alan R Liss, 1986
67. Tsoi M-S, Storb R, Dobbs S, Thomas ED: Specific suppressor cells in graft-host tolerance of HLA-identical marrow transplantation. Nature 292:355–357, 1981
68. Sullivan KM, Deeg HJ, Sanders J et al: Hyperacute GVHD in patients not given immunosuppression after allogeneic marrow transplantation. Blood 67:1172–1175, 1986
69. Storb R, Deeg HJ, Whitehead J et al: Marrow transplantation for leukemia and aplastic anemia: Two controlled trials of a combination of methotrexate and cyclosporine versus cyclosporine alone or methotrexate alone for prophylaxis of acute graft-versus-host disease. Transplantation Proc 19:2608–2613, 1987
70. Sullivan KM, Witherspoon RP, Storb R et al: Alternating-day cyclosporine and prednisone for treatment of high-risk chronic graft-versus-host disease. Blood 72:555–561, 1988
71. Atkinson K, Farewell V, Storb R et al: Analysis of late infections after human bone marrow transplantation: Role of genotypic nonidentity between marrow donor and recipient and of nonspecific suppressor cells in patients with chronic graft-versus-host disease. Blood 60:714–720, 1982
72. Thomas ED, Bryant JI, Buckner CD et al: Leukaemic transformation of engrafted human marrow cells in vivo. Lancet 1:1310–1313, 1972
73. Martin PJ, Hansen JA, Storb R et al: Human marrow transplantation: An immunological perspective. Adv Immunol 40:379–438, 1987
74. Badger C, Buckner CD, Thomas ED et al: Allogeneic marrow transplantation for acute leukemia in relapse. Leukemia Res 6:383–387, 1982
75. Blume KG, Forman SJ, O'Donnell MR et al: Total body irradiation and high-dose etoposide: A new preparatory regimen for bone marrow transplantation in patients with advanced hematologic malignancies. Blood 69:1015–1020, 1987
76. Herzig RH, Coccia PF, Lazarus HM et al: Bone marrow transplantation for acute leukemia and lymphoma with high-dose cytosine arabinoside and total body irradiation. Semin Oncol 12:184–186, 1985
77. Champlin R, Jacobs A, Gale RP et al: High-dose cytarabine in consolidation chemotherapy or with bone marrow transplantation for patients with acute leukemia: Preliminary results. Semin Oncol 12:190–195, 1985
78. Thomas ED, Clift RA, Hersman J et al: Marrow transplantation for acute nonlymphoblastic leukemia in first remission. Int J Radiat Oncol Biol Phys 8:817–821, 1982
79. Brochstein JA, Kernan NA, Groshen S et al: Allogeneic bone marrow transplantation after hyperfractionated total-body irradiation and cyclophosphamide in children with acute leukemia. N Engl J Med 317:1618–1624, 1987
80. Santos GW, Tutschka PJ, Brookmeyer R et al: Marrow transplantation for acute nonlymphocytic leukemia after treatment with busulfan and cyclophosphamide. N Engl J Med 309:1347–1353, 1983
81. Bernstein ID, Nowinski RC: Monoclonal antibody treatment of transplanted and spontaneous murine leukemia. In Mitchell MS, Oettgen HF (eds): Hybridomas in Cancer Diagnosis and Treatment, pp 97–112. New York, Raven Press, 1982
82. Badger CC, Shulman H, Peterson AV et al: Monoclonal antibody therapy of spontaneous AKR T-cell leukemia. Cancer Res 46:4058–4063, 1986
83. Meeker TC, Lowder J, Maloney DG et al: A clinical trial of anti-idiotype therapy for B cell malignancy. Blood 65:1349–1363, 1985
84. Press OW, Appelbaum F, Ledbetter JA et al: Monoclonal antibody 1F5 (anti-CD20) serotherapy of human B cell lymphomas. Blood 69:584–591, 1987
85. Badger CC, Bernstein ID: Therapy of murine leukemia with monoclonal antibody against a normal differentiation antigen. J Exp Med 157:828–842, 1983
86. Appelbaum FR, Badger C, Deeg HJ et al: Use of iodine-131-labeled anti-immune response-associated monoclonal antibody as a preparative regimen prior to bone marrow transplantation: Initial dosimetry. Natl Cancer Inst Monogr 3:67–71, 1987
87. Appelbaum FR, Brown PA, Graham TC et al: Characterization of malignant lymphoma in dogs and use as a model for the development of treatment strategies. In Baum SJ, Santos GW, Takaku F (eds): Recent Advances and Future Directions in Bone Marrow Transplantation (Experimental Hematology Today 1987), pp 31–35. New York, Springer-Verlag, 1988
88. Dick JE, Magli MC, Estrov Z et al: Retrovirus-mediated gene transfer and expression in murine and human hematopoietic stem cells. In Gale RP, Champlin R (eds): Progress in Bone Marrow Transplantation, pp 951–962. New York, Alan R Liss, 1987
89. Belmont JW, Henkel-Tigges J, Wager-Smith K et al: Transfer and expression of human adenosine deaminse gene in murine bone marrow cells. In Gale RP, Champlin

R (eds): Progress in Bone Marrow Transplantation, pp 963–972. New York, Alan R Liss, 1987

90. Anderson WF, Kantoff P, Eglitis M et al: An autologous bone marrow transplantation/gene transfer protocol in non-human primates using retroviral vectors. In Gale RP, Champlin R (eds): Progress in Bone Marrow Transplantation, pp 973–981. New York, Alan R Liss, 1987
91. Williams DA, Orkin SH, Mulligan RC. Retrovirus-mediated transfer of human adenosine deaminase gene sequences into cells in culture and into murine hematopoietic cells in vivo. Proc Natl Acad Sci USA 83:2566–2570, 1986
92. Lemischka IR, Raulet DH, Mulligan RC: Developmental potential and dynamic behavior of hematopoietic stem cells. Cell 45:917–927, 1986
93. Hock RA, Miller AD: Retrovirus-mediated transfer and expression of drug resistance genes in human haematopoietic progenitor cells. Nature 320:275–277, 1986
94. Kwok WW, Schuening F, Stead RB, Miller AD: Retroviral transfer of genes into canine hematopoietic progenitor cells in culture: A model for human gene therapy. Proc Natl Acad Sci USA 83:4552–4555, 1986
95. Stead RB, Kwok WW, Storb R et al: Canine model for gene therapy: Inefficient gene expression in dogs reconstituted with autologous marrow infected with retroviral vectors. Blood 71:742–747, 1988
96. Herzig RH, Coccia PF, Lazarus HM et al: Bone marrow transplantation for acute leukemia and lymphoma with high-dose cytosine arabinoside and total body irradiation. Semin Oncol 12:184–186, 1985
97. Dicke KA, Jagannath S, Spitzer G et al: The role of autologous bone marrow transplantation in various malignancies. Semin Hematol 21:109–122, 1984
98. Dinsmore R, Kirkpatrick D, Flomenberg N et al: Allogeneic bone marrow transplantation for patients with acute lymphoblastic leukemia. Blood 62:381–388, 1983
99. Messner HA, Curtis JE, Minden MM: The combined use of cytosine arabinoside, cyclophosphamide, and total body irradiation as preparative regimen for bone marrow transplantation in patients with AML and CML. Semin Oncol 12:187–189, 1985
100. Phillips GL, Connors JM: Bone marrow transplantation for malignant lymphoma. In Gale RP, Champlin R (eds): Progress in Bone Marrow Transplantation, pp 799–825. New York, Alan R Liss, 1987
101. Prentice HG, Brenner MK, Grob J-P et al: Bone marrow transplantation in the treatment of acute leukaemia in first remission using T-lymphocyte depleted marrow from HLA identical sibling donors. In Gale RP, Champlin R (eds): Progress in Bone Marrow Transplantation, pp 337–341. New York, Alan R Liss, 1987
102. Kim TH, Khan FM, Galvin JM: A report of the work party: Comparison of total body irradiation techniques for bone marrow transplantation. Int J Radiat Oncol Biol Phys 6:779–784, 1980
103. Kersey J, Weisdorf D, Nesbit M et al: Allogeneic and autologous bone marrow transplantation for acute lymphoblastic leukemia (ALL). In Gale RP, Champlin R (eds): Progress in Bone Marrow Transplantation, pp 77–90. New York, Alan R Liss, 1987
104. Serota FT, Burkey ED, August CS et al: Total body irradiation as preparation for bone marrow transplantation in treatment of acute leukemia and aplastic anemia. Int J Radiat Oncol Biol Phys 9:1941–1949, 1983
105. Ringden O, Zwann F, Hermans J: European experience of bone marrow transplantation for leukemia. Transplantation Proc 19:2600–2604, 1987
106. Meyers JD, Petersen FB, Counts GW et al: Bacterial, fungal and protozoan infection after marrow transplantation. In Baum SJ, Santos GW, Takaku F (eds): Recent Advances and Future Directions in Bone Marrow Transplantation (Experimental Hematology Today 1987), pp 171–176. New York, Springer-Verlag, 1988
107. Atkinson K, Storb R, Prentice RL et al: Analysis of late infections in 89 long-term survivors of bone marrow transplantation. Blood 53:720–731, 1979

SUPPLEMENTARY REFERENCES, SECTION 5 (TABLES 66-15, 66-16)

a. Saroja KR, Mansell J, Hendrickson RR, Cohen L, Lennox A: An update on malignant salivary gland tumors treated with neutrons at Fermilab. Int J Radiat Oncol Biol Phys 13:1319–1325, 1987
b. Skolyszewski J, Byrski E, Chrzanowska A et al: A preliminary report on the clinical application of fast neutrons in Krakow. Int J Radiat Oncol Biol Phys 8:1781–1786, 1982
c. Fitzpatrick PJ, Theriault C: Malignant salivary gland tumors. Int J Radiat Oncol Biol Phys 12:1743–1747, 1986
d. Vikram B, Strong EW, Shah JP, Spiro RH: Radiation therapy in adenoid-cystic carcinoma. Int J Radiat Oncol Biol Phys 10:221–223, 1984
e. Borthne A, Kjellevold K, Kaalhus O, Vermund H: Salivary gland malignant neoplasms: Treatment and prognosis. Int J Radiat Oncol Biol Phys 12:747–754, 1986
f. Elkon D, Colman H, Hendrickson FR: Radiation therapy in the treatment of malignant salivary gland tumors. Cancer 41:502–506, 1978
g. Rossman KJ: The role of radiation therapy in the treatment of parotid carcinomas. Am J Radiol 123:492–499, 1975

Index

Index

Page numbers in *italics* indicate figures; page numbers followed by *t* indicate tabular material.